TEXTBOOK OF
SURGERY
The Biological Basis of
Modern Surgical Practice

TEXTBOOK OF
SURGERY

The Biological Basis of Modern Surgical Practice

FIFTEENTH EDITION

DAVID C. SABISTON, JR., M.D.

James B. Duke Professor of Surgery
Director of International Programs
Duke University Medical Center
Durham, North Carolina

Associate Editor for Basic Surgical Science

H. KIM LYERLY, M.D.

Associate Professor of Surgery
Assistant Professor of Pathology and Immunology
Clinical Director, Molecular Therapeutics Program
Duke University Medical Center
Durham, North Carolina

W.B. SAUNDERS COMPANY

A Division of Harcourt Brace & Company
Philadelphia   London   Toronto   Montreal   Sydney   Tokyo

1997

W.B. SAUNDERS COMPANY
A Division of Harcourt Brace & Company

The Curtis Center
Independence Square West
Philadelphia, Pennsylvania 19106

Library of Congress Cataloging-in-Publication Data

Textbook of surgery: the biological basis of modern surgical practice.—15th ed. /
[edited by] David C. Sabiston, Jr.; editor for basic surgical science, H. Kim Lyerly.

p.   cm.

Includes bibliographical references and index.

ISBN 0–7216–5887–3

1. Surgery.   I. Sabiston, David C.   II. Lyerly, H. Kim.
 [DNLM: 1. Surgery.   WO 100 T3552 1997]
 RD31.T49 1997

617—dc20

DNLM/DLC   95-46939

TEXTBOOK OF SURGERY: The Biological Basis of Modern Surgical Practice   ISBN 0–7216–5887–3

Printed in the United States of America.

Last digit is the print number: 9   8   7   6   5   4   3   2   1

CONTRIBUTORS

JOHN G. ADAMS, JR., M.D.
Clinical Assistant Professor of Surgery, University of Missouri–Columbia School of Medicine, Columbia, Missouri.
Thoracic Outlet Syndrome

N. SCOTT ADZICK, M.D.
C. Everett Koop Professor of Pediatric Surgery, University of Pennsylvania School of Medicine. Surgeon-in-Chief, Children's Hospital of Philadelphia, Philadelphia, Pennsylvania.
Wound Healing: Biologic and Clinical Features

ROBERT W. ANDERSON, M.D.
The David C. Sabiston, Jr., Professor and Chairman, Department of Surgery, and Professor, Biomedical Engineering, Duke University Medical Center. Chief of Staff and Senior Attending Surgeon, Duke University Medical Center; Consultant, Durham Veterans Administration Medical Center, Durham, and Oteen Veterans Administration Hospital, Asheville, North Carolina.
Shock: Causes and Management of Circulatory Collapse; The Use of Cardiovascular Pharmacologic Agents in Surgical Patients

PAUL S. AUERBACH, M.D., M.S.
Chief Operating Officer, Sterling Healthcare Group, Coral Gables, Florida.
Bites and Stings

ERLE H. AUSTIN III, M.D.
Professor of Surgery, University of Louisville Medical School. Chief, Pediatric Cardiac Surgery, Kosair Children's Hospital, Louisville, Kentucky.
Disorders of Pulmonary Venous Return; Tricuspid Atresia; Hypoplastic Left Heart Syndrome; Congenital Aortic Stenosis

WILLIAM H. BAKER, M.D.
Professor of Surgery, Loyola University Chicago Stritch School of Medicine. Attending Surgeon and Chief, Division of Peripheral Vascular Surgery, Loyola University Medical Center, Maywood, Illinois.
Arterial Injuries

CLYDE F. BARKER, M.D.
Professor of Surgery, University of Pennsylvania School of Medicine. Chairman, Department of Surgery, University of Pennsylvania Medical Center, Philadelphia, Pennsylvania.
Renal Transplantation

ROBERT H. BARTLETT, M.D.
Professor of Surgery, University of Michigan School of Medicine. Professor of Surgery, University of Michigan Medical Center, Ann Arbor, Michigan.
Extracorporeal Membrane Oxygenation

JAMES M. BECKER, M.D.
James Utley Professor and Chairman, Department of Surgery, Boston University School of Medicine. Surgeon-in-Chief, Boston University Medical Center Hospital, Boston, Massachusetts.
Ulcerative Colitis

FOLKERT O. BELZER, M.D. (deceased)
Late Professor of Surgery and Chairman, Department of Surgery, University of Wisconsin Medical School, Madison, Wisconsin.
Organ Preservation

MICHAEL E. BEREND, M.D.
Senior Resident in Orthopaedic Surgery, Duke University Medical Center, Durham, North Carolina.
Fractures and Dislocations: General Principles

JOHN J. BERGAN, M.D.
Professor of Surgery, Loma Linda University Medical School, Loma Linda. Clinical Professor of Surgery, University of California, San Diego, California. Clinical Professor of Surgery, Uniformed Services University of the Health Sciences, Bethesda, Maryland. Attending Staff Surgeon, Scripps Memorial Hospital, La Jolla, California.
Visceral Ischemic Syndromes: Obstruction of the Superior Mesenteric Artery, Celiac Axis, and Inferior Mesenteric Artery

AMITAVA BISWAS, M.D.
Clinical Fellow, Harvard Medical School, Boston, Massachusetts.
Acute Arterial Occlusion

R. RANDAL BOLLINGER, M.D., PH.D.
Professor of Surgery and Chief of General Surgery, Duke University Medical Center, Durham, North Carolina.
Acute Renal Failure in Surgical Patients: Prevention and Treatment; Transplantation: Historical Aspects; Autotransplantation

R. MORTON BOLMAN III, M.D.
C. Walton and Richard C. Lillehei Professor and Chief of Division of Cardiovascular and Thoracic Surgery, University of Minnesota, Minneapolis, Minnesota.
Cardiac and Cardiopulmonary Homotransplants

WILLIAM Z. BORER, M.D.
Associate Professor, Department of Pathology, Anatomy, and Cell Biology, Thomas Jefferson University. Director, Clinical Chemistry Section, Thomas Jefferson University Hospital, Philadelphia, Pennsylvania.
Appendix: Laboratory Reference Values of Clinical Importance

JOHN BOSTWICK III, M.D.
Professor of Surgery and Chairman of Plastic and Reconstructive Surgery, Emory University School of Medicine, Atlanta, Georgia.
Plastic and Maxillofacial Surgery

GENE D. BRANUM, M.D.
Assistant Professor of Surgery and Assistant Director, Gastrointestinal Surgery, Emory University School of Medicine, Atlanta. Chief, General Surgery, Atlanta Veterans Administration Medical Center, Decatur, Georgia.
Adenocarcinoma of the Stomach; Pyogenic and Amebic Liver Abscess

KENNETH L. BRAYMAN, M.D., PH.D.
Assistant Professor of Surgery, University of Pennsylvania School of Medicine, Philadelphia, Pennsylvania.
Renal Transplantation

ALYSON J. BREISCH, R.N., M.S.
Clinical Associate, Duke University School of Nursing. Cardiovascular Clinical Nurse Specialist, Duke University Medical Center, Durham, North Carolina.
Percutaneous Transluminal Angioplasty

MURRAY F. BRENNAN, M.D.
Professor of Surgery, Cornell University Medical College. Alfred P. Sloan Chair in Surgery, Memorial Sloan-Kettering Cancer Center, New York, New York.
Soft Tissue Sarcomas

GERT H. BRIEGER, M.D., Ph.D.
Chairman, Department of the History of Science, Medicine, and Technology, The Johns Hopkins University School of Medicine, Baltimore, Maryland.
The Development of Surgery: Historical Aspects Important in the Origin and Development of Modern Surgical Science

JOHN H. CALHOON, M.D.
Associate Professor and Head, Division of Cardiothoracic Surgery, University of Texas Health Science Center at San Antonio. Active Staff, University Hospital and Audie L. Murphy Veterans Administration Hospital, San Antonio. Consultant, Brooke Army Medical Center, Fort Sam Houston, and Wilford Hall Medical Center, Lackland Air Force Base, Texas.
Aneurysms of the Sinus of Valsalva

JOHN L. CAMERON, M.D.
Professor and Director, Department of Surgery, The Johns Hopkins University School of Medicine. Surgeon-in-Chief, The Johns Hopkins Hospital, Baltimore, Maryland.
The Pancreas

DAVID N. CAMPBELL, M.D.
Professor of Surgery, University of Colorado Health Sciences Center, Denver, Colorado.
Aneurysms of the Sinus of Valsalva

GRANT W. CARLSON, M.D.
Assistant Professor of Surgery and Plastic Surgery and Associate Chief of Surgical Oncology, Emory University School of Medicine, Atlanta, Georgia.
Plastic and Maxillofacial Surgery

C. JAMES CARRICO, M.D.
Professor and Chairman, Department of Surgery, University of Texas Southwestern Medical Center. Chief of Surgery, Parkland Memorial Hospital, Dallas, Texas.
Trauma: Management of the Acutely Injured Patient

JAMES CERILLI, M.D.
Former Professor of Surgery, University of Rochester Medical Center, Rochester, New York.
Vascular Access Procedures for Renal Dialysis (Including Peritoneal Dialysis)

RAVI S. CHARI, M.D.
Fellow in Transplant Surgery, University of Toronto, Toronto, Canada.
The Liver: Anatomy and Physiology; Hemobilia

WILLIAM G. CHEADLE, M.D.
Associate Professor of Surgery, University of Louisville School of Medicine. Associate Chief of Staff for Research and Development and Director of Surgical Intensive Care Unit, Veterans Administration Medical Center, Louisville, Kentucky.
Principles of Preoperative Preparation of the Surgical Patient.

LAURENCE Y. CHEUNG, M.D.
Professor and Chairman, Department of Surgery, University of Kansas School of Medicine. Chief of Surgery, University of Kansas Hospital, Kansas City, Kansas.
The Pathogenesis, Prophylaxis, and Treatment of Stress Gastritis

W. RANDOLPH CHITWOOD, Jr., M.D.
Professor and Chairman, Department of Surgery, East Carolina University School of Medicine. Chairman, Department of Surgery; Chief, Division of Cardiothoracic Surgery; Director, Heart Center, Pitt County Memorial Hospital, Greenville, North Carolina.
Intra-Aortic Balloon Counterpulsation: Physiology, Indications, and Techniques

BRYAN M. CLARY, M.D.
Senior Assistant Resident, Department of Surgery, Duke University Medical Center, Durham, North Carolina.
Meckel's Diverticulum

PIERRE A. CLAVIEN, M.D., Ph.D.
Associate Professor of Surgery and Chief, Hepatobiliary Surgery; Director, Liver Transplant Program, Duke University Medical Center, Durham, North Carolina.
Liver Transplantation

JOEL D. COOPER, M.D.
Joseph C. Bancroft Professor of Surgery, Washington University School of Medicine. Head, Section of General Thoracic Surgery, Barnes Hospital, St. Louis, Missouri.
Lung Transplantation; Surgical Management of Myasthenia Gravis

JAMES L. COX, M.D.
Evarts A. Graham Professor of Surgery, Washington University School of Medicine. Cardiothoracic Surgeon-in-Chief, Barnes–Jewish Hospital, St. Louis, Missouri.
Surgical Treatment of Cardiac Arrhythmias

FRED A. CRAWFORD, Jr., M.D.
Professor and Chairman, Department of Surgery; Head, Division of Cardiothoracic Surgery, Medical University of South Carolina, Charleston, South Carolina.
Penetrating Cardiac Injuries

ROBERT D. CROOM III, M.D.
Professor Emeritus of Surgery, University of North Carolina School of Medicine and University of North Carolina Hospitals, Chapel Hill, North Carolina.
The Spleen

THOMAS A. D'AMICO, M.D.
Assistant Professor of Surgery, Duke University Medical Center, Durham, North Carolina.
Carcinoma of the Lung; Kawasaki's Disease

MARK G. DAVIES, M.D., Ph.D.
Chief Resident in General Surgery, Duke University Medical Center, Durham, North Carolina.
Physiology of the Arterial System, Including the Effects of Nitric Oxide

R. DUANE DAVIS, Jr., M.D.
Assistant Professor of Surgery and Director of Cardiopulmonary Transplantation, Duke University Medical Center, Durham, North Carolina.
Percutaneous Transluminal Angioplasty; The Mediastinum; The Coronary Circulation

RICHARD H. DEAN, M.D.
Professor of Surgery and Chairman, Department of General Surgery, Bowman Gray School of Medicine. Chief of Surgery, North Carolina Baptist Hospital, Winston-Salem, North Carolina.
Aneurysms of the Carotid Artery; Carotid Body Tumors; Carotid Artery Occlusive Disease

HAILE T. DEBAS, M.D.
Maurice Galante Distinguished Professor of Surgery and Dean, School of Medicine, University of California, San Francisco, California.
Carcinoid Tumors and the Carcinoid Syndrome

JEROME J. DeCOSSE, M.D., Ph.D.
Lewis Thomas University Professor, Cornell University Medical College. Attending Surgeon, New York Hospital, New York, New York.
Radiation Injury to the Intestine

E. PATCHEN DELLINGER, M.D.
Professor of Surgery, Vice-Chairman, Chief of General Surgery, University of Washington School of Medicine. Attending Surgeon and Associate Medical Director, University of Washington Medical Center, Seattle, Washington.
Surgical Infections and Choice of Antibiotics

MARK E. DENTZ, M.D.
Assistant Professor of Anesthesiology, Duke University Medical Center, Durham, North Carolina.
Anesthesia and Postoperative Analgesia

ARNOLD G. DIETHELM, M.D.
Professor and Chairman, Department of Surgery, University of Alabama School of Medicine, Birmingham, Alabama.
The Acute Abdomen

GERARD M. DOHERTY, M.D.
Assistant Professor of Surgery, Section of Endocrine and Oncologic Surgery, Washington University. Attending Surgeon, Barnes–Jewish Hospital, St. Louis, Missouri.
The Parathyroid Glands

ROGER R. DOZOIS, M.D.
Professor of Surgery, Mayo Medical School. Chair, Division of Colon and Rectal Surgery, Mayo Clinic, Rochester, Minnesota.
Disorders of the Anal Canal

ANDRÉ DURANCEAU, M.D.
Professor of Surgery, Department of Surgery and Division of Thoracic Surgery, Université de Montréal. Staff, Division of Thoracic Surgery, Hotel-Dieu de Montreal, Montreal, Quebec.
Perforation of the Esophagus; Hiatal Hernia and Gastroesophageal Reflux

DAVID W. EASTER, M.D.
Associate Professor of Surgery and Program Director, General Surgery, University of California, San Diego, San Diego, California.
Surgical Complications

JAMES M. EDWARDS, M.D.
Assistant Professor, Division of Vascular Surgery, Oregon Health Sciences University. Staff Surgeon, Division of Vascular Surgery, Portland Veterans Affairs Medical Center, Portland, Oregon.
Raynaud's Syndrome

JOSEPH R. ELBEERY, M.D.
Assistant Professor of Surgery, East Carolina University School of Medicine, Greenville, North Carolina.
Intra-Aortic Balloon Counterpulsation: Physiology, Indications, and Techniques

STEVE EUBANKS, M.D.
Assistant Professor of Surgery, Director of Surgical Endoscopy, and Director of the Duke/U.S. Surgical Endosurgery Center, Duke University Medical Center, Durham, North Carolina.
Laparoscopic Surgery; Hernias

SAMIR M. FAKHRY, M.D.
Associate Professor of Surgery, University of North Carolina. Chief, Surgical Critical Care, University of North Carolina School of Medicine. Director, Surgical Intensive Care Unit, University of North Carolina Hospitals, Chapel Hill, North Carolina.
Blood Transfusions and Disorders of Surgical Bleeding

JOHN A. FEAGIN, M.D.
Associate Professor of Surgery, Division of Orthopaedic Surgery and the Duke Sports Medicine Center, and Associate Professor of Biomedical Engineering, Duke University Medical Center, Durham, North Carolina.
Fractures and Dislocations: General Principles

AARON S. FINK, M.D.
Professor of Surgery, Emory University School of Medicine, Atlanta. Chief, Surgical Service, Atlanta Veterans Administration Medical Center, Decatur, Georgia.
Adenocarcinoma of the Stomach

JOSEF E. FISCHER, M.D.
Christian R. Holmes Professor and Chairman of Surgery, University of Cincinnati College of Medicine. Surgeon-in-Chief, University Hospital, Cincinnati, Ohio.
Metabolism in Surgical Patients: Protein, Carbohydrate, and Fat Utilization by Oral and Parenteral Routes

ROBERT D. FITCH, M.D.
Associate Professor of Surgery, Division of Orthopaedic Surgery, Duke University Medical Center, Durham, North Carolina.
Fractures and Dislocations of the Shoulder, Arm, and Forearm

WILLIAM R. FLINN, M.D.
Professor of Surgery and Chief, Division of Vascular Surgery, University of Maryland Medical School and Hospital. Staff, Baltimore Veterans Administration Medical Center and Mercy Hospital, Baltimore, Maryland.
Visceral Ischemic Syndromes: Obstruction of the Superior Mesenteric Artery, Celiac Axis, and Inferior Mesenteric Artery

M. WAYNE FLYE, M.D., Ph.D.
Professor of Surgery, Molecular Microbiology, and Immunology, Washington University School of Medicine. Senior At-

tending Staff, Barnes–Jewish Hospital and St. Louis Children's Hospital, St. Louis, Missouri.
Venous Disorders

THOMAS J. FOGARTY, M.D.
Professor of Surgery, Stanford University School of Medicine and The Vascular Center, Stanford University Medical Center, Stanford, California.
Acute Arterial Occlusion

DOUGLAS L. FRAKER, M.D.
Associate Professor of Surgery, University of Pennsylvania School of Medicine. Chief of Oncology Surgery, Hospital of the University of Pennsylvania, Philadelphia, Pennsylvania.
Tumor Markers

ALLAN H. FRIEDMAN, M.D.
Professor of Surgery, Division of Neurosurgery, Duke University Medical Center, Durham, North Carolina.
Spontaneous Intracranial and Intraspinal Hemorrhage; Craniocerebral Injuries; Neurosurgical Relief of Epilepsy

DAVID FROMM, M.D.
Penberthy Professor and Chairman, Department of Surgery, Wayne State University. Surgeon-in-Chief, Detroit Medical Center; Chief of Surgery, Harper Hospital, Detroit, Michigan.
Carcinoma of the Gallbladder

HERBERT E. FUCHS, M.D., Ph.D.
Assistant Professor of Surgery, Division of Neurosurgery, and Assistant Professor of Pediatrics, Duke University Medical Center, Durham, North Carolina.
Congenital Abnormalities

DAVID A. FULLERTON, M.D.
Professor of Surgery and Chief, Cardiothoracic Surgery, Northwestern University, Chicago, Illinois.
Acquired Disorders of the Aortic Valve and Subaortic Valve

STANLEY A. GALL, Jr., M.D.
Department of Surgery, St. John's Hospital, Springfield, Illinois.
Reoperative Coronary Surgery

WILLIAM E. GARRETT, Jr., M.D., Ph.D.
Professor of Orthopaedic Surgery and Director of the Duke Sports Medicine Center, Duke University Medical Center, Durham, North Carolina.
Fractures of the Tibia, Fibula, Ankle, and Foot

WILLIAM A. GAY, Jr., M.D.
Professor of Surgery, Division of Cardiothoracic Surgery, Washington University School of Medicine. Attending Surgeon in Cardiothoracic Surgery, Barnes–Jewish Hospital and St. Louis Children's Hospital, St. Louis, Missouri.
Ventricular Aneurysm

J. WILLIAM GAYNOR, M.D.
Assistant Professor of Surgery, Children's Hospital of Philadelphia, Philadelphia, Pennsylvania.
Patent Ductus Arteriosus, Coarctation of the Aorta, Aortopulmonary Window, and Anomalies of the Aortic Arch

COHAVA GELBER, Ph.D.
Assistant Research Professor, Department of Surgery, Duke University Medical Center, Durham, North Carolina.
Immunobiology and Immunotherapy of Neoplastic Disease

ANNETINE C. GELIJNS, Ph.D.
Associate Professor of Public Health and Surgery, Columbia University School of Public Health, College of Physicians and Surgeons. Director, International Center for Health Outcomes and Innovation Research (InCHOIR), Columbia University, New York, New York.
Clinical Outcomes in Surgery

GREGORY S. GEORGIADE, M.D.
Associate Professor, Divisions of General and Thoracic Surgery and of Plastic, Reconstructive, Maxillofacial, and Oral Surgery, Duke University Medical Center, Durham, North Carolina.
Reconstructive and Aesthetic Breast Surgery

FARID GHARAGOZLOO, M.D.
Associate Professor, Cardiothoracic Surgery, Anatomy, and Cell Biology, Georgetown University School of Medicine, Washington, D.C. Consultant Cardiothoracic Surgeon, National Cancer Institute, Bethesda, Maryland. Chief of Thoracic Surgery, Harbor Hospital Center, Baltimore, Maryland.
Clinical and Physiologic Evaluation of Respiratory Function

DONALD D. GLOWER, M.D.
Associate Professor of Surgery, Duke University Medical Center, Durham, North Carolina.
Bronchiectasis; Cardiopulmonary Resuscitation; Mitral and Tricuspid Valve Disease

J. LEONARD GOLDNER, M.D.
James B. Duke Professor Emeritus of Orthopaedic Surgery, Duke University Medical Center, Durham, North Carolina.
Fracture of the Carpal Scaphoid; Fractures and Dislocations of the Hand; The Hand: Tendon Injury and Repair; Compression Neuropathies of the Hand and Forearm

RICHARD D. GOLDNER, M.D.
Associate Professor of Orthopaedic Surgery, Duke University Medical Center, Durham, North Carolina.
Fracture of the Carpal Scaphoid; Fractures and Dislocations of the Hand; Compression Neuropathies of the Hand and Forearm

CLEON W. GOODWIN, Jr., M.D.
Commander and Director, U.S. Army Institute of Surgical Research, Fort Sam Houston, Texas.
Burns: Including Cold, Chemical, and Electric Injuries

JOHN GORECKI, M.D.
Assistant Professor of Surgery, Division of Neurosurgery, Duke University Medical Center, Durham, North Carolina.
Neurosurgical Relief of Pain

LAWRENCE J. GOTTLIEB, M.D.
Professor of Clinical Surgery, University of Chicago School of Medicine, Chicago, Illinois.
Acute Suppurative Mediastinitis

JOHN P. GRANT, M.D.
Professor of Surgery and Director of Nutritional Support Service, Duke University Medical Center, Durham, North Carolina.
Malabsorption Syndromes

PAUL D. GREIG, M.D.
Associate Professor, Department of Surgery, University of Toronto. Director, Gastrointestinal Transplantation, The Toronto Hospital and The University of Toronto, Toronto, Ontario, Canada.
Peritoneovenous Shunts for Intractable Ascites

KATHERINE P. GRICHNIK, M.D.
Assistant Professor of Anesthesiology, Duke University Medical Center, Durham, North Carolina.
Anesthesia and Postoperative Analgesia

HERMES C. GRILLO, M.D.
Professor of Surgery, Harvard Medical School. Emeritus Chief of General Thoracic Surgery, Massachusetts General Hospital, Boston, Massachusetts.
Tracheostomy and Its Complications

JAY L. GROSFELD, M.D.
Professor and Chairman, Department of Surgery, Indiana University School of Medicine. Surgeon-in-Chief, James Whitcomb Riley Hospital for Children, Indianapolis, Indiana.
Pediatric Surgery

FREDERICK L. GROVER, M.D.
Professor and Head, Division of Cardiothoracic Surgery, University of Colorado Health Sciences Center. Chief, Surgical Service, Denver Department of Veterans Affairs Medical Center, Denver, Colorado.
Aneurysms of the Sinus of Valsalva

J. CAULIE GUNNELLS, Jr., M.D.
Professor Emeritus of Medicine, Duke University Medical Center, Durham, North Carolina.
Renovascular Disease

JEFFREY A. HAGEN, M.D.
Assistant Professor of Surgery, University of Southern California and LAC/USC Medical Center, Los Angeles, California.
Surgical Management of Myasthenia Gravis

PER-OTTO HAGEN, M.D.
Research Professor of Surgery, Duke University Medical Center, Durham, North Carolina.
Physiology of the Arterial System, Including the Effects of Nitric Oxide

CARL E. HAISCH, M.D.
Professor of Surgery, East Carolina University. Director of Surgical Immunology and Transplantation; Attending Surgeon in Transplant, Trauma, and General Surgery, University Medical Center of Eastern North Carolina, Greenville, North Carolina.
Vascular Access Procedures for Renal Dialysis (Including Peritoneal Dialysis)

JOHN D. HAMILTON, M.D.
Professor of Medicine, and Chief, Infectious Diseases and International Health, Duke University Medical Center. Staff Physician and Research Director of Center for AIDS and HIV Infection, Durham Veterans Administration Medical Center, Durham, North Carolina.
Viral Hepatitis and the Surgeon

CHARLES B. HAMMOND, M.D.
E. C. Hamblen Professor and Chairman, Department of Obstetrics and Gynecology, Duke University Medical Center, Durham, North Carolina.
Gynecology: The Female Reproductive Organs

WILLIAM T. HARDAKER, Jr., M.D.
Associate Professor, Division of Orthopaedic Surgery, Duke University Medical Center. Staff, Veterans Administration Medical Center and Lenox Baker Children's Hospital, Durham, North Carolina.
Fractures of the Spine

ALDEN H. HARKEN, M.D.
Professor of Surgery and Chairman, Department of Surgery, University of Colorado, Denver, Colorado.
Acquired Disorders of the Aortic Valve and Subaortic Valve

DAVID H. HARPOLE, Jr., M.D.
Associate Professor of Surgery, Division of Thoracic Surgery, and Director, Thoracic Oncology Program, Duke University Medical Center. Chief of Cardiothoracic Surgery, Durham Veterans Administration Medical Center, Durham, North Carolina.
Benign Tumors of the Trachea and Bronchi; Bronchial Adenomas

JOHN M. HARRELSON, M.D.
Associate Professor, Division of Orthopaedic Surgery, Duke University Medical Center, Durham, North Carolina.
Fractures and Dislocations: General Principles; Amputation and Limb Substitution; Infections and Neoplasms of Bone

MARQUIS E. HART, M.D.
Assistant Professor, Department of Surgery, University of California, San Diego. Attending Surgeon, University of California, San Diego Medical Center, San Diego, California.
Surgical Complications

JEFFREY S. HEINLE, M.D.
Boston Children's Hospital and Brigham and Women's Hospital, Boston, Massachusetts.
Congenital Deformities of the Chest Wall

JULIO HOCHBERG, M.D.
Associate Professor and Chief, Section of Plastic and Reconstructive Surgery, Department of Surgery, West Virginia University Health Sciences Center and Ruby Memorial Hospital of West Virginia University, Morgantown, West Virginia.
Principles of Operative Surgery: Antisepsis, Technique, Sutures, and Drains

WILLIAM L. HOLMAN, M.D.
Associate Professor of Surgery, Division of Cardiothoracic Surgery, University of Alabama at Birmingham. Staff Surgeon, University of Alabama Hospital and Veterans Administration Hospital, Birmingham, Alabama.
Cardiopulmonary Bypass for Cardiac Surgery

RICHARD A. HOPKINS, M.D.
Professor of Surgery, Pediatrics, and Physiology and Chief, Division of Cardiothoracic Surgery, Brown University School of Medicine. Chief of Cardiothoracic Surgery, The Miriam Hospital, Rhode Island Hospital, and Hasbro Children's Hospital, Providence, Rhode Island.
Clinical and Physiologic Evaluation of Respiratory Function; Truncus Arteriosus

J. DIRK IGLEHART, M.D.
Professor of Surgery, Associate Professor of Pathology, and Assistant Professor of Cell Biology, Duke University Medical Center, Durham, North Carolina.
The Breast

SUZANNE T. ILDSTAD, M.D.
Professor and Chief, Department of Surgery, Division of Cellular Therapeutics, University of Pittsburgh School of Medicine, Pittsburgh, Pennsylvania.
Principles of Therapeutic Immunosuppression

ANTHONY L. IMBEMBO, M.D.
Professor and Chairman, Department of Surgery, University of Maryland School of Medicine. Surgeon-in-Chief, University of Maryland Hospital, Baltimore, Maryland.
Diverticular Disease of the Colon; Benign Neoplasms of the Colon, Including Vascular Malformations; Volvulus of the Colon

GLYN G. JAMIESON, M.D.
Dorothy Mortlock Professor of Surgery, Department of Surgery, University of Adelaide. Chairman, Department of Surgery, Royal Adelaide Hospital, Adelaide, South Australia, Australia.
Hiatal Hernia and Gastroesophageal Reflux

MICHAEL E. JESSEN, M.D.
Associate Professor of Surgery, University of Texas Southwestern Medical Center at Dallas. Chief, Cardiothoracic Surgery, Veterans Affairs Medical Center, Dallas, Texas.
Surgical Disorders of the Pericardium

OLGA JONASSON, M.D.
Professor, University of Illinois at Chicago; Adjunct Professor, Northwestern University. Director, Education and Surgical Services, American College of Surgeons, Chicago, Illinois.
Surgical Aspects of Diabetes Mellitus

R. SCOTT JONES, M.D.
S. Hurt Watts Professor and Chairman, Department of Surgery, University of Virginia School of Medicine, Charlottesville, Virginia.
The Small Intestine: Anatomy; Physiology; Intestinal Obstruction

ROBERT H. JONES, M.D.
Mary and Deryl Hart Professor of Surgery, Duke University Medical Center. Chief Medical Officer, Duke University Hospital, Durham, North Carolina.
Radionuclide Evaluation of Coronary Artery Disease

GREGORY J. JURKOVICH, M.D.
Professor of Surgery, University of Washington. Chief of Trauma and Director, Emergency Department Surgical Services, Harborview Medical Center, Seattle, Washington.
Trauma: Management of the Acutely Injured Patient

LARRY R. KAISER, M.D.
Professor of Surgery, University of Pennsylvania School of Medicine. Director, General Thoracic Surgery, University of Pennsylvania Medical Center, Philadelphia, Pennsylvania.
Thoracoscopy

STEVEN S. KANG, M.D.
Assistant Professor of Surgery, Loyola University Chicago Stritch School of Medicine. Attending Surgeon, Loyola University Medical Center, Maywood, Illinois.
Arterial Injuries

KEITH A. KELLY, M.D.
Professor of Surgery, Mayo Medical School, Rochester. Chair, Department of Surgery, Mayo Clinic, Scottsdale, Minnesota.
Crohn's Disease (Regional Enteritis)

ALLAN D. KIRK, M.D., PH.D.
Assistant Professor of Surgery, University of Wisconsin Health Center, Madison, Wisconsin.
Liver Transplantation

JAMES K. KIRKLIN, M.D.
Professor of Surgery, Division of Cardiothoracic Surgery, University of Alabama at Birmingham School of Medicine. Professor and Surgeon, Director of Cardiothoracic Transplantation, University Hospital, University of Alabama at Birmingham Medical Center, Birmingham, Alabama.
Ventricular Septal Defects; Cardiopulmonary Bypass for Cardiac Surgery

STUART J. KNECHTLE, M.D.
Assistant Professor of Surgery, University of Wisconsin School of Medicine. Staff Surgeon, University of Wisconsin Hospital and Clinics, Madison, Wisconsin.
Pancreas Transplantation

THEODORE C. KOUTLAS, M.D.
Assistant Professor of Surgery, East Carolina University School of Medicine, Greenville, North Carolina.
Ebstein's Anomaly

THOMAS J. KRIZEK, M.D.
Professor of Surgery and Vice-Chairman, Department of Surgery, University of South Florida. Chief, Division of Plastic Surgery, Tampa General Hospital, Tampa, Florida.
Acute Suppurative Mediastinitis

TERRY C. LAIRMORE, M.D.
Assistant Professor of Surgery, Surgical Oncology, and Endocrinology, Washington University School of Medicine, St. Louis, Missouri.
Multiple Endocrine Neoplasia Syndromes

GREGORY J. LANDRY, M.D.
Research Resident, Division of Vascular Surgery, and Surgical Resident, Department of Surgery, Oregon Health Sciences University, Portland, Oregon.
Raynaud's Syndrome

BERNARD LANGER, M.D.
Professor of Surgery, University of Toronto. Head, Surgical Oncology Program, The Toronto Hospital, Toronto, Ontario, Canada.
Peritoneovenous Shunts for Intractable Ascites

JEFFREY H. LAWSON, M.D., PH.D.
Research Fellow in General and Thoracic Surgery, Duke University Medical Center, Durham, North Carolina.
The Use of Cardiovascular Pharmacologic Agents in Surgical Patients

ALAN T. LEFOR, M.D.
Associate Professor of Clinical Surgery, University of California, San Diego. Program Director in General Surgery, Kern Medical Center, Bakersfield, California.
Benign Neoplasms of the Colon, Including Vascular Malformations

GEORGE S. LEIGHT, JR., M.D.
Professor of Surgery, Duke University Medical Center, Durham, North Carolina.
Nodular Goiter and Benign and Malignant Neoplasms of the Thyroid

L. SCOTT LEVIN, M.D.
Assistant Professor of Surgery, Division of Orthopaedic Surgery and Chief, Division of Plastic, Reconstructive, Maxillofacial, and Oral Surgery, Duke University Medical Center, Durham, North Carolina.
Fractures of the Tibia, Fibula, Ankle, and Foot

JONATHAN J. LEWIS, M.D., PH.D.
Assistant Professor of Surgery, Cornell University Medical College. Assistant Attending Physician, Memorial Sloan-Kettering Cancer Center, New York, New York.
Soft Tissue Sarcomas

R. ERIC LILLY, M.D.
Senior Resident, Duke University Medical Center, Durham, North Carolina.
Disorders of the Lungs, Pleura, and Chest Wall: Anatomy

JAMES E. LOWE, M.D.
Professor of Surgery, Division of Thoracic Surgery, and Associate Professor of Pathology, Duke University Medical Center, Durham, North Carolina.
Congenital Lesions of the Coronary Circulation; Cardiac Pacemakers

H. KIM LYERLY, M.D.
Associate Professor of Surgery, Assistant Professor of Pathology and of Immunology. Clinical Director, Molecular Therapeutics Program, Duke University Medical Center, Durham, North Carolina.
Molecular Biology in Surgery; Surgical Aspects of Acquired Immunodeficiency Syndrome; Immunobiology and Immunotherapy of Neoplastic Disease; The Thyroid Gland: Physiology; Hyperthyroidism; Thyroiditis; Meckel's Diverticulum; Carcinoma of the Colon, Rectum, and Anus; Arteriovenous Fistulas

GREG J. MACKAY, M.D.
Director of Aesthetic and Reconstructive Craniofacial Surgery, The Nalle Clinic, Charlotte, North Carolina.
Plastic and Maxillofacial Surgery

RAYMOND G. MAKHOUL, M.D.
Assistant Professor of Surgery and Director, Noninvasive Vascular Laboratory, Medical College of Virginia, Richmond, Virginia.
Femoral Artery Aneurysms; Popliteal Artery Aneurysms

JOHN A. MANNICK, M.D.
Mosely Distinguished Professor of Surgery, Harvard Medical School. Surgeon-in-Chief Emeritus, Brigham and Women's Hospital, Boston, Massachusetts.
Subclavian Steal Syndrome

JAMES F. MARKMANN, M.D., PH.D.
Instructor in Surgery, University of Pennsylvania School of Medicine, Philadelphia, Pennsylvania.
Renal Transplantation

G. ROBERT MASON, M.D., PH.D.
Professor of Surgery and Professor of Thoracic and Cardiovascular Surgery, Loyola University Chicago Stritch School of Medicine. Chairman, Department of Thoracic and Cardiovascular Surgery, Loyola University Medical Center, Maywood, Illinois
Tumors of the Duodenum and Small Intestine

DOUGLAS J. MATHISEN, M.D.
Associate Professor of Surgery, Harvard Medical School. Chief of General Thoracic Surgery, Massachusetts General Hospital, Boston, Massachusetts.
Tracheostomy and Its Complications

JAMES R. MAULT, M.D.
Teaching Scholar, Division of Cardiothoracic Surgery, Duke University Medical Center, Durham, North Carolina.
Surgical Management of Pulmonary Emphysema; Extracorporeal Membrane Oxygenation

RICHARD L. McCANN, M.D.
Professor of Surgery and Chief, Section of Vascular Surgery, Duke University Medical Center, Durham, North Carolina.
Disorders of the Lymphatic System; Femoropopliteal and Femoro-infrapopliteal Bypass; Renovascular Disease

DONALD E. McCOLLUM, M.D.
Professor of Surgery, Division of Orthopaedic Surgery, Duke University Medical Center, Durham, North Carolina.
Fractures of the Pelvis, Femur, and Knee

JOHN C. McDONALD, M.D.
Professor and Chairman, Louisiana State University School of Medicine, Shreveport, Louisiana. Chief of Surgery, LSU Hospital, Shreveport, Louisiana.
Abdominal Wall, Umbilicus, Peritoneum, Mesenteries, Omentum, and Retroperitoneum

DAVID C. McGIFFIN, M.D.
Associate Professor of Surgery and Staff Surgeon, University of Alabama at Birmingham, Birmingham, Alabama.
Cardiopulmonary Bypass for Cardiac Surgery

ANTHONY A. MEYER, M.D., PH.D.
Professor of Surgery, University of North Carolina School of Medicine and University of North Carolina Hospitals, Chapel Hill, North Carolina.
The Spleen

WILLIAM C. MEYERS, M.D.
Professor and Chairman, Department of Surgery, University of Massachusetts Medical Center, Worcester, Massachusetts.
The Liver: Anatomy and Physiology; Pyogenic and Amebic Liver Abscess; Neoplasms of the Liver; Hemobilia

GREGORY L. MONETA, M.D.
Associate Professor of Surgery, Oregon Health Sciences University. Staff Surgeon, Portland Veterans Affairs Hospital, Portland, Oregon.
Arterial Substitutes

FRANK G. MOODY, M.D.
Denton A. Cooley Professor, Department of Surgery, The University of Texas Medical School, Houston, Texas.
Ulcerative Colitis

A. R. MOOSA, M.D.
Professor and Chairman, Department of Surgery, University of California, San Diego. Surgeon-in-Chief, Department of Surgery, UCSD Medical Center, San Diego, California.
Surgical Complications

JON F. MORAN, M.D.
Professor of Surgery, Division of Cardiac Surgery, East Carolina University School of Medicine, Greenville, North Carolina.
Surgical Treatment of Pulmonary Tuberculosis

ALAN J. MOSKOWITZ, M.D.
Assistant Professor of Clinical Medicine in Surgery and Public Health, Columbia University, College of Physicians and Surgeons, School of Public Health. Associate Director, International Center for Health Outcomes and Innovation Research (InCHOIR), Columbia University, New York, New York.
Clinical Outcomes in Surgery

JOSEPH A. MOYLAN, M.D.
Professor of Surgery and Chairman, Department of Surgery, University of Miami School of Medicine. Chief, Surgical Hospital Center at Jackson Memorial Hospital, Miami, Florida.
Fat Emboli Syndrome

GORDON F. MURRAY, M.D.
Professor and Chairman, Department of Surgery, West Virginia University Health Sciences Center. Chairman of Surgery, Ruby Memorial Hospital of West Virginia University, Morgantown, West Virginia.
Principles of Operative Surgery: Antisepsis, Technique, Sutures, and Drains

DAVID L. NAHRWOLD, M.D.
Loyal and Edith Davis Professor and Chairman, Department of Surgery, Northwestern University Medical School. Surgeon-in-Chief, Northwestern Memorial Hospital, Chicago, Illinois.
The Biliary System: Acute Cholecystitis; Chronic Cholecystitis and Cholelithiasis; Cholangitis

ALI NAJI, M.D., PH.D.
Professor of Surgery, University of Pennsylvania School of Medicine, Philadelphia, Pennsylvania.
Renal Transplantation

ELAINE E. NELSON, M.D.
Chief Resident, Emergency Medicine, Stanford Medical Center/Kaiser Permanente, Stanford, California.
Bites and Stings

JEFFREY A. NORTON, M.D.
Professor of Surgery, Washington University School of Medicine. Chief of Endocrine and Oncologic Surgery and Attending Surgeon, Barnes–Jewish Hospital, St. Louis, Missouri.
Tumor Markers

JAMES A. NUNLEY, M.D.
Professor of Surgery, Division of Orthopaedic Surgery, Duke University Medical Center, Durham, North Carolina.
The Hand: Tendon Injury and Repair

JOHN A. OLSON, JR., M.D., PH.D.
Research Fellow in Surgery, Washington University School of Medicine and Barnes–Jewish Hospital, St. Louis, Missouri.
The Pituitary and Adrenal Glands

SUSAN L. ORLOFF, M.D.
Transplant Fellow and Clinical Instructor, Department of Surgery, University of California, San Francisco, California.
Carcinoid Tumors and the Carcinoid Syndrome

MARK B. ORRINGER, M.D.
Professor and Head, Section of Thoracic Surgery, University of Michigan Medical School, Ann Arbor, Michigan.
The Esophagus: Historical Aspects and Anatomy; Physiology; Disorders of Esophageal Motility; Diverticula and Miscellaneous Conditions of the Esophagus; Esophagoscopy; Tumors of the Esophagus

ALBERT D. PACIFICO, M.D.
John W. Kirklin Professor of Surgery, University of Alabama at Birmingham School of Medicine. Director, Division of Cardiothoracic Surgery, and Vice-Chairman, Department of Surgery, University of Alabama at Birmingham Hospital, Birmingham, Alabama.
Ventricular Septal Defects; Double Outlet Right Ventricle

THEODORE N. PAPPAS, M.D.
Professor of Surgery, Division of General Surgery, Duke University Medical Center, Durham, North Carolina.
The Stomach and Duodenum: Historical Aspects, Anatomy, Pathology, Physiology, and Peptic Ulcer Disease; Lymphoma of the Stomach

DAVID F. PAULSON, M.D.
Professor of Surgery and Chief, Division of Urologic Surgery, Duke University Medical Center, Durham, North Carolina.
The Urinary System

JOSE A. PEREZ, M.D.
Assistant Professor of Medicine, Division of Cardiology, Duke University Medical Center, Durham, North Carolina.
Percutaneous Transluminal Angioplasty

WILLIAM S. PIERCE, M.D.
Professor of Surgery and Associate Chairman, Department of Surgery, College of Medicine, The Pennsylvania State University. Staff Surgeon, The Milton S. Hershey Medical Center, The Pennsylvania State University, Hershey, Pennsylvania.
The Artificial Heart

JEFFREY L. PLATT, M.D.
Joseph W. and Dorothy W. Beard Professor, Departments of Surgery, Pediatrics, and Immunology, Duke University Medical Center, Durham, North Carolina.
The Immunology of Transplant Antigens; Mechanisms and Characteristics of Allograft Rejection

HIRAM C. POLK, JR., M.D.
Ben A. Reid, Sr., Professor and Chairman, Department of Surgery, University of Louisville School of Medicine, Louisville, Kentucky.
Principles of Preoperative Preparation of the Surgical Patient

WALTER J. PORIES, M.D.
Professor and Chairman, Department of Surgery, East Carolina University School of Medicine. Chief of Surgery, University Medical Center of Eastern North Carolina and Pitt County Memorial Hospital, Greenville, North Carolina.
The Surgical Approach to Morbid Obesity

JOHN M. PORTER, M.D.
Professor of Surgery and Chief, Division of Vascular Surgery, Oregon Health Sciences University, Portland, Oregon.
Arterial Substitutes; Raynaud's Syndrome

BASIL A. PRUITT, JR., M.D.
Clinical Professor of Surgery, University of Texas Health Science Center at San Antonio. Consultant, U.S. Army Institute of Surgical Research, Fort Sam Houston, Texas.
Burns: Including Cold, Chemical, and Electric Injuries

SCOTT K. PRUITT, M.D., PH.D.
Chief Resident, Department of Surgery, Duke University Medical Center, Durham, North Carolina.
Burns: Including Cold, Chemical, and Electric Injuries

CEMIL M. PURUT, M.D.
Resident in Cardiothoracic Surgery, Duke University Medical Center, Durham, North Carolina.
Lesions of the Chest Wall

MICHAEL F. REED, M.D.
Research Fellow in Surgery, Harvard Medical School. Senior Resident in Surgery, Brigham and Women's Hospital, Boston, Massachusetts.
Mesothelioma

KEITH REEMTSMA, M.D., MED. SC.D.
Professor of Surgery, Columbia University College of Physicians and Surgeons. Founder and Chairman, International Center for Health Outcomes and Innovation Research (InCHOIR), Columbia University, New York, New York.
Clinical Outcomes in Surgery

J. G. REVES, M.D.
Professor and Chairman, Department of Anesthesiology, Duke University Medical Center, Durham, North Carolina.
Anesthesia and Postoperative Analgesia

NORMAN M. RICH, M.D.
Professor and Chairman, Department of Surgery, and Chief, Division of Vascular Surgery, F. Edward Hebert School of Medicine, Uniformed Services University of the Health Sciences, Bethesda, Maryland.
Venous Injuries

WILLIAM J. RICHARDSON, M.D.
Associate Professor of Orthopaedic Surgery and Assistant Professor of Neurosurgery, Duke University Medical Center, Durham, North Carolina.
Fractures of the Spine

LAYTON F. RIKKERS, M.D.
Anthony Curreri Professor and Chairman, Department of Surgery, University of Wisconsin Clinical Science Center, Madison, Wisconsin.
Surgical Complications of Cirrhosis and Portal Hypertension

MICHELLE L. ROBBIN, M.D.
Assistant Professor and Chief of Ultrasound, Department of Radiology, University of Alabama at Birmingham School of Medicine. Radiologist, University of Alabama Hospital, Birmingham, Alabama.
The Acute Abdomen

CARY N. ROBERTSON, M.D.
Associate Professor of Surgery, Division of Urology, Duke University Medical Center, Durham, North Carolina.
The Male Genital System

MICHAEL S. ROHR, M.D., PH.D.
Professor of Surgery and Director of Transplantation Services, Bowman Gray School of Medicine. Medical Director, Carolina LifeCare, The Organ Procurement Agency of the North Carolina Baptist Hospital, North Carolina Baptist Hospital, Winston-Salem, North Carolina.
Abdominal Wall, Umbilicus, Peritoneum, Mesenteries, Omentum, and Retroperitoneum

ROLANDO ROLANDELLI, M.D.
Associate Professor of Surgery, Medical College of Pennsylvania and Hahnemann University, Philadelphia, Pennsylvania.
The Colon and Rectum: Surgical Anatomy and Operative Procedures; Physiology; Diagnostic Studies; Intestinal Antisepsis

FRANCIS E. ROSATO, M.D.
Samuel D. Gross Professor of Surgery and Chairman of the Department of Surgery, Jefferson Medical College of Thomas Jefferson University. Attending Surgeon and Chief of Surgery, Thomas Jefferson University Hospital, Philadelphia, Pennsylvania.
Gallstone Ileus and Fistula

ERIC A. ROSE, M.D.
Chairman, Department of Surgery, and Valentine Mott/Johnson & Johnson Professor of Surgery, Columbia University, College of Physicians and Surgeons. Surgeon-in-Chief and Director, Surgical Service, Columbia-Presbyterian Medical Center, New York, New York.
Clinical Outcomes in Surgery

JOEL J. ROSLYN, M.D.
Alma Dea Morani Professor and Chairman, Department of Surgery, Medical College of Pennsylvania and Hahnemann University, Philadelphia, Pennsylvania.
The Colon and Rectum: Surgical Anatomy and Operative Procedures; Physiology; Diagnostic Studies; Intestinal Antisepsis

PABLO RUBINSTEIN, M.D.
Director, Fred H. Allen Laboratory of Immunogenetics, New York Blood Center, New York, New York.
The Immunology of Transplant Antigens; Mechanisms and Characteristics of Allograft Rejection

DAVID C. SABISTON, JR., M.D.
James B. Duke Professor of Surgery and Director of International Programs, Duke University Medical Center, Durham, North Carolina.
Appendicitis; Pulmonary Embolism; Chronic Pulmonary Embolism; Disorders of the Arterial System: Introduction; Anatomy; Aneurysms; Subclavian Artery Aneurysms; Visceral Arterial Aneurysms; Aortic Abdominal Aneurysms; Thrombo-Obliterative Disease of the Aorta and Its Branches; Takayasu's Arteritis; Thrombotic Obliteration of the Abdominal Aorta and Iliac Arteries (Leriche's Syndrome); Iliac Arterial Occlusion; Arteriovenous Fistulas; Carcinoma of the Lung; Congenital Deformities of the Chest Wall; The Mediastinum; Patent Ductus Arteriosus, Coarctation of the Aorta, Aortopulmonary Window, and Anomalies of the Aortic Arch; The Coronary Circulation; Congenital Lesions of the Coronary Circulation; Cardiac Neoplasms

JAMES D. ST. LOUIS, M.D.
Resident in Surgery, Duke University Medical Center, Durham, North Carolina.
Congenital Lesions of the Coronary Circulation

PHILIP R. SCHAUER, M.D.
Assistant Professor of Surgery, University of Pittsburgh School of Medicine and Medical Center, Pittsburgh, Pennsylvania.
Laparoscopic Surgery

BRUCE D. SCHIRMER, M.D.
Professor of Surgery, University of Virginia School of Medicine and Health Sciences Center, Charlottesville, Virginia.
Vascular Compression of the Duodenum

STEVE J. SCHWAB, M.D.
Professor of Medicine and Clinical Director, Renal Division, Duke University Medical Center, Durham, North Carolina.
Acute Renal Failure in Surgical Patients: Prevention and Treatment

STEWART M. SCOTT, M.D. (deceased)
Late Clinical Professor of Surgery, Duke University Medical Center, Durham. Late Chief, Surgical Service, Oteen Veterans Administration Hospital, Asheville, North Carolina.
Pulmonary Infections; The Pleura and Empyema

SEAN P. SCULLY, M.D., Ph.D.
Assistant Professor of Surgery, Division of Orthopaedic Surgery, Duke University Medical Center, Durham, North Carolina.
Amputation and Limb Substitution; Infections and Neoplasms of Bone

MARK W. SEBASTIAN, M.D.
Assistant Professor of Surgery, Duke University Medical Center, Durham, North Carolina.
Benign Tumors of the Stomach; Pilonidal Cysts and Sinuses; Pulmonary Embolism; Chronic Pulmonary Embolism

H. F. SEIGLER, M.D.
Professor of Surgery and of Microbiology and Immunology, Duke University Medical Center, Durham, North Carolina.
Melanoma

GEORGE F. SHELDON, M.D.
Zack D. Owens Professor and Chair, Department of Surgery, University of North Carolina School of Medicine. Professor and Chairman, Department of Surgery, University of North Carolina Hospitals, Chapel Hill, North Carolina.
Blood Transfusions and Disorders of Surgical Bleeding; The Spleen

G. TOM SHIRES, M.D.
Peter C. Canizaro, M.D., Distinguished Professor of Surgery, Texas Tech University School of Medicine. Attending Staff, Texas Tech University Health Sciences Center at Lubbock, Lubbock, Texas.
Fluid and Electrolyte Management of the Surgical Patient

G. TOM SHIRES III, M.D.
Associate Professor of Surgery, University of Texas Southwestern Medical Center at Dallas. Attending Staff, Parkland Memorial Hospital of Dallas and Zale Lipshy University Hospital at Dallas, Texas.
Fluid and Electrolyte Management of the Surgical Patient

JOSEPH B. SHRAGER, M.D.
Resident, Cardiothoracic Surgery, Massachusetts General Hospital, Boston, Massachusetts.
Thoracoscopy

KAREN S. SIBERT, M.D.
Assistant Professor of Anesthesiology and Director of Perioperative Services, Duke University Medical Center, Durham, North Carolina.
Anesthesia and Postoperative Analgesia

DONALD SILVER, M.D.
W. Alton Jones Distinguished Professor, Department of Surgery, University of Missouri–Columbia School of Medicine. Chairman, Department of Surgery, University of Missouri Hospital and Clinics, Columbia, Missouri.
Circulatory Problems of the Upper Extremity; Thoracic Outlet Syndrome

NORMAN A. SILVERMAN, M.D.
Professor of Surgery, Case Western Reserve School of Medicine, Cleveland, Ohio. Division Head, Cardiac and Thoracic Surgery, Henry Ford Hospital, Detroit, Michigan.
Cardiac Neoplasms

RICHARD L. SIMMONS, M.D.
Distinguished Service Professor of Surgery; George V. Foster Professor of Surgery and Chair; and Professor of Molecular Genetics and Biochemistry, University of Pittsburgh School of Medicine. Chair, Department of Surgery, University of Pittsburgh Medical Center, Pittsburgh, Pennsylvania.
Principles of Therapeutic Immunosuppression

KEVIN M. SITTIG, M.D.
Associate Professor of Surgery, Louisiana State University School of Medicine. Director, LSU Burn Center, Louisiana State University Medical Center, Shreveport, Louisiana.
Abdominal Wall, Umbilicus, Peritoneum, Mesenteries, Omentum, and Retroperitoneum

CRAIG L. SLINGLUFF, Jr., M.D.
Associate Professor of Surgery and Chief, Division of Surgical Oncology, University of Virginia School of Medicine, Charlottesville, Virginia.
Melanoma

MILTON M. SLOCUM, M.D.
Clinical Instructor of Surgery and Resident Physician in Vascular Surgery, University of Missouri–Columbia School of Medicine, Columbia, Missouri.
Circulatory Problems of the Upper Extremity

JAMES B. SNOW, Jr., M.D.
Director, National Institute on Deafness and Other Communication Disorders, National Institutes of Health, Bethesda, Maryland.
Surgical Disorders of the Ears, Nose, Paranasal Sinuses, Pharynx, and Larynx

HANS W. SOLLINGER, M.D., Ph.D.
Professor of Surgery and Pathology and Chairman, Division of Organ Transplantation, University of Wisconsin School of Medicine. Staff Surgeon, University of Wisconsin Hospital and Clinics, Madison, Wisconsin.
Pancreas Transplantation

JAMES H. SOUTHARD, Ph.D.
Professor, Department of Surgery, University of Wisconsin Medical School, Madison, Wisconsin.
Organ Preservation

KEVIN P. SPEER, M.D.
Assistant Professor, Division of Orthopaedic Surgery, Duke University Medical Center, Durham, North Carolina.
Fractures and Dislocations of the Shoulder, Arm, and Forearm

THOMAS L. SPRAY, M.D.
Professor of Surgery, University of Pennsylvania School of Medicine. Chief, Cardiothoracic Surgery, The Children's Hospital of Philadelphia, Philadelphia, Pennsylvania.
Transposition of the Great Arteries

ROBERT J. STANLEY, M.D.
Professor and Chairman, Department of Radiology, University of Alabama School of Medicine. Radiologist-in-Chief, University of Alabama Hospital, Birmingham, Alabama.
The Acute Abdomen

DELFORD L. STICKEL, M.D.
Professor of Surgery, Duke University Medical Center, Durham, North Carolina.
Transplantation: Historical Aspects

DAVID J. SUGARBAKER, M.D.
Associate Professor of Surgery, Harvard Medical School. Chief, Division of Thoracic Surgery, Brigham and Women's Hospital, Boston, Massachusetts.
Mesothelioma

BRUCE A. SULLENGER, PH.D.
Assistant Professor, Departments of Surgery and Genetics, Duke University Medical Center, Durham, North Carolina.
Molecular Biology in Surgery

R. SUDHIR SUNDARESAN, M.D.
Assistant Professor of Surgery, Washington University School of Medicine and Barnes–Jewish Hospital, St. Louis, Missouri.
Lung Transplantation

SCOTT J. SWANSON, M.D.
Instructor in Surgery, Harvard Medical School. Associate Thoracic Surgeon, Brigham and Women's Hospital, Boston, Massachusetts.
Mesothelioma

TIMOTHY TAKARO, M.D.
Former Clinical Professor of Surgery, Duke University Medical Center, Durham. Former Chief of Staff, Oteen Veterans Administration Hospital, Asheville, North Carolina.
Pulmonary Infections; The Pleura and Empyema

JAMES L. TALBERT, M.D.
Professor of Surgery and Pediatrics and Chief of Children's Surgery, University of Florida College of Medicine. Staff, Shands Hospital at the University of Florida and Veterans Administration Medical Center, Gainesville, Florida.
Corrosive Strictures of the Esophagus

MARK TEDDER, M.D.
Senior Cardiothoracic Surgery Fellow, Duke University Medical Center, Durham, North Carolina.
Bronchoscopy

ANGUS W. THOMSON, PH.D., D.SC.
Research Professor of Surgery and Molecular Genetics and Biochemistry, University of Pittsburgh School of Medicine.

Director of Transplant Immunology, Thomas E. Starzl Transplantation Institute, University of Pittsburgh, Pittsburgh, Pennsylvania.
Principles of Therapeutic Immunosuppression

ROBERT D. TIEN, M.D., M.P.H.
Associate Professor of Radiology, Section Head of Neuroradiology, Director of Neuro-MR, and Co-Director of MR, Duke University Medical Center, Durham, North Carolina.
Neuroradiology

DENNIS A. TURNER, M.D., M.A.
Associate Professor of Neurosurgery and Neurobiology, Duke University Medical Center. Chief, Neurosurgery, Durham Veterans Administration Medical Center, Durham, North Carolina.
Stereotactic Neurosurgery

DOUGLAS TYLER, M.D.
Assistant Professor of Surgery, Duke University Medical Center. Chief, General Surgery Service, Durham Veterans Administration Medical Center, Durham, North Carolina.
Surgical Aspects of Acquired Immunodeficiency Syndrome

ROSS M. UNGERLEIDER, M.D.
Professor of General and Thoracic Surgery and Chief, Pediatric Cardiac Surgery, Duke University Medical Center, Durham, North Carolina.
Bronchoscopy; Atrial Septal Defects, Ostium Primum Defects, and Atrioventricular Canals; Tetralogy of Fallot

JAMES R. URBANIAK, M.D.
Virginia Flowers Baker Professor and Chief of Orthopaedic Surgery and Vice Chairman, Department of Surgery, Duke University Medical Center, Durham, North Carolina.
Replantation of Amputated Limbs and Digits

THOMAS PARKER VAIL, M.D.
Assistant Professor of Orthopaedic Surgery, Duke University Medical Center, Durham, North Carolina.
Fractures of the Pelvis, Femur, and Knee

PETER VAN TRIGT III, M.D.
Cardiovascular and Thoracic Surgeons of Greensboro, Greensboro, North Carolina.
Surgical Management of Failed Angioplasty

STEVEN N. VASLEF, M.D., PH.D.
Assistant Professor of Surgery and of Biomedical Engineering, Duke University Medical Center. Consultant, Durham Veterans Administration Medical Center, Durham, North Carolina.
Shock: Causes and Management of Circulatory Collapse

ROBERT B. WALLACE, M.D.
Professor of Surgery and Chief, Thoracic and Cardiovascular Surgery, Georgetown University Medical Center, Washington, D.C.
Truncus Arteriosus

HENRY L. WALTERS III, M.D.
Assistant Professor of Surgery, Wayne State University School of Medicine. Co-Chief, Department of Cardiovascular Surgery, Children's Hospital of Michigan, Detroit, Michigan.
Ventricular Septal Defects; Double Outlet Right Ventricle

JOHN L. WEINERTH, M.D.
Professor of Surgery, Divisions of General Surgery and of Urology, Duke University Medical Center. Director and Associate Dean, Graduate Medical Education, Duke University School of Medicine, Durham, North Carolina.
The Male Genital System

SAMUEL A. WELLS, JR., M.D.
Bixby Professor and Chairman, Department of Surgery, Washington University School of Medicine. Surgeon-in-Chief, Barnes–Jewish Hospital, St. Louis, Missouri.
Multiple Endocrine Neoplasia Syndromes; The Parathyroid Glands; The Pituitary and Adrenal Glands

H. BROWNELL WHEELER, M.D.
Harry M. Haidak Distinguished Professor of Surgery, University of Massachusetts Medical School, Worcester, Massachusetts.
Thromboangiitis Obliterans (Buerger's Disease)

ANTHONY D. WHITTEMORE, M.D.
Professor of Surgery, Harvard Medical School. Chief, Vascular Surgery, Brigham and Women's Hospital, Boston, Massachusetts.
Subclavian Steal Syndrome

ROBERT H. WILKINS, M.D.
Professor of Surgery and Chief, Division of Neurosurgery, Duke University Medical Center, Durham, North Carolina.
Neurosurgery: Historical Aspects; Intracranial Tumors; Intracranial Infections; Intraspinal Tumors; Ruptured Lumbar Intervertebral Disc; Cervical Disc Lesions; Peripheral Nerve Injuries

DOUGLAS W. WILMORE, M.D.
Frank Sawyer Professor of Surgery, Harvard Medical School. Staff Surgeon and Director, Nutritional Support Service, Brigham and Women's Hospital, Boston, Massachusetts.
Homeostasis: Bodily Changes in Trauma and Surgery

WALTER G. WOLFE, M.D.
Professor of Surgery, Division of Thoracic Surgery, Duke University Medical Center, Durham, North Carolina.
Traumatic Aneurysms of the Aorta; Dissecting Diseases of the Aorta; Aneurysms of the Thoracic Aorta; Disorders of the Lungs, Pleura, and Chest Wall: Anatomy; Clinical and Physiologic Evaluation of Respiratory Function

BRUCE G. WOLFF, M.D.
Professor of Surgery, Mayo Medical School. Consultant, General and Colon and Rectal Surgery, Mayo Medical Center, Rochester, Minnesota.
Crohn's Disease (Regional Enteritis)

ROBERT J. WOOD, M.D.
Assistant Professor of Surgery and Director of the Center for Cleft and Craniofacial Anomalies, Emory University School of Medicine, Atlanta, Georgia.
Plastic and Maxillofacial Surgery

CHARLES J. YEO, M.D.
Professor of Surgery and Oncology, The Johns Hopkins University School of Medicine. Attending Surgeon, The Johns Hopkins Hospital, Baltimore, Maryland.
The Pancreas

KARL A. ZUCKER, M.D.
Professor of Surgery, University of New Mexico School of Medicine, Albuquerque, New Mexico.
Volvulus of the Colon

PREFACE

It is astonishing how much new information has appeared in the field of surgery since the Fourteenth Edition of the *Textbook of Surgery* was last published five years ago. As in previous editions of this text, the prime criterion in the selection of contributors is their recognition as authorities in their fields. A thorough update of each chapter, including the basic science contributions, clinical features, illustrations, and bibliography, have again been emphasized.

Increasingly, the role of basic science in the understanding, diagnosis, and treatment of disease is expanding, and additional emphasis is placed on this feature in the current edition. The importance of basic science is increasingly stressed in medical school, on licensure examinations by the American Board of Surgery, and by the specialty surgical boards. The contributors to the current edition have each updated their section with emphasis on an improved understanding of the pathogenesis of surgical disorders.

Six *new* and quite important chapters have been added and include

"Molecular Biology in Surgery" by Drs. H. Kim Lyerly and Bruce A. Sullenger
"Clinical Outcomes in Surgery" by Drs. Alan J. Moskowitz, Keith Reemtsma, Eric A. Rose, and Annetine C. Gelijns
"Laparoscopic Surgery" by Drs. Steve Eubanks and Philip R. Schauer

"Plastic and Maxillofacial Surgery" by Drs. Greg J. Mackay, Grant W. Carlson, Robert J. Wood, and John Bostwick III
"Surgical Management of Pulmonary Emphysema" by Dr. James R. Mault
"Mesothelioma" by Drs. David J. Sugarbaker, Michael F. Reed, and Scott J. Swanson.

In addition, *all* chapters have been thoroughly revised and updated.

The reader will find that each chapter is organized with a consistent format, including the pertinent anatomic, pathologic, physiologic, bacteriologic, biochemical, pharmacologic, immunologic, and genetic features of each surgical disorder. Emphasis is placed on the findings on physical examination, a review of the modern diagnostic procedures necessary in each instance, and the therapeutic aspects of each disorder.

It is fortunate that the *Textbook of Surgery* has had far-reaching impact in many nations, with translations into Spanish, Japanese, Portuguese, Italian, and Indonesian. For the past 60 years, the goal of this *Textbook of Surgery* has been to present as effectively as possible the entire field of surgery to medical students, surgical residents, practicing surgeons, and teachers of surgery throughout the world.

DAVID C. SABISTON, JR.

ACKNOWLEDGMENTS

It is the view of the Editor that this edition of the *Textbook of Surgery: The Biological Basis of Modern Surgical Practice,* 15th edition, is the most complete yet to be published, with appropriate emphasis on *basic* and *clinical* surgical science. The contributors are due great credit for updating each chapter with diligence and adding the latest contributions in each field.

Six additional texts authored by the Editor and published by W.B. Saunders Company are closely associated with the *Textbook of Surgery* and are additional resources. These include the *Textbook of Surgery Pocket Companion,* the *Sabiston Review of Surgery,* the *Atlas of General Surgery,* the *Atlas of Cardiothoracic Surgery,* the *Sabiston Essentials of Surgery* with Dr. H. Kim Lyerly, and the *Surgery of the Chest* with Dr. Frank C. Spencer. To the contributors to these texts, sincere appreciation is also due.

Special appreciation is due to Mr. Lewis Reines, President of the W.B. Saunders Company, and his staff for their unflagging interest and commitment in publishing these texts and their attention to every detail. It has been a genuine pleasure to work with the entire staff during preparation and publication of these texts. Their dedication to excellence is gratefully acknowledged.

To those at W.B. Saunders who have been closely associated with the editing and publication of this edition, I am especially grateful. These include Ms. Janice Gaillard, associate developmental editor; Ms. Lori Irvine, production manager; and Ms. Sue Reilly, supervising copy editor for the *Textbook of Surgery.* As in previous editions, Ms. Carolyn Naylor, assistant director, book production, has provided valued support and continuing interest. My appreciation is also expressed to Ms. Lisette Bralow, vice-president and editor-in-chief.

To my editorial assistant, Dr. Catherine Macek, I am especially grateful, as she has been both thorough and accurate in her reviews of the manuscripts. Her efforts have been of monumental proportions, requiring many hours of tedious work. Her participation and enthusiasm merit my grateful thanks in making this edition a reality.

DAVID C. SABISTON, JR.

CONTENTS

CHAPTER **51**

DISORDERS OF THE LUNGS, PLEURA, AND CHEST WALL **1775**

CHAPTER 1

THE DEVELOPMENT OF SURGERY

Historical Aspects Important in the Origin and Development of Modern Surgical Science

Gert H. Brieger, M.D., Ph.D.

The history of surgery in the major surgical textbooks has a long and honorable tradition. Every field has its great contributors and each has its heroes. A history of surgery without Paré, Vesalius, Hunter, Lister, and Halsted would be a strange history indeed; the magnitude of the achievements of these men warrants discussion of their lives and work. Nevertheless, many justly famous names will be missing. The emphasis will be placed on the *recent* past, especially the last 100 years, although the reader should keep in mind always that surgery's history is as old as that of humans on earth.

The history of disease is at least as old as the history of mankind. One can assume that the surgical response to disease is of similar antiquity. The basic forms of disease—tumors, infections, trauma, and congenital abnormalities—have existed unchanged. Today's surgeons obviously manage them in different ways than did their prehistoric colleagues, yet some aspects of the surgeon's work are timeless. Ackerknecht, who wrote extensively on primitive medicine, emphasized that surgery was not defined as a special field by the primitives,[1] yet much of their medical treatment would be termed *surgical*. They treated wounds and tried to stop hemorrhage, and they trephined for injury to the head as well as for ritual reasons, such as the release of demons.

In Greek and Roman antiquity the surgeon existed as a specialist, but only when diet and drugs were of no avail did doctors resort to surgery. In cases of injury, of course, the surgeon might be called upon immediately. Among the great Greek medical works that are ascribed to Hippocrates (but certainly not all written by him) are books on fractures, dislocations, and other surgical disorders. One of the most interesting is simply entitled *On the Surgery*. Here the author described what surgeons should know, how they should proceed with the treatment, and what general qualifications they should possess. Much of the work relates to bandaging of various types of injuries. "The things related to surgery," the Hippocratic author wrote around 400 B.C., "are the patient; the operator; the assistants; the instruments; the light; where and how; how many things, and how; where the body, and the instruments; the time; the manner; the place."

Besides the 70 books of the Hippocratic works, one of our best authorities for Greek medicine is the Roman encyclopedist of the early first century A.D., Aulus Cornelius Celsus. His *De re medicina* reflects much learning, although its author was himself probably not a medical practitioner. This book was one of the earliest medical books to be printed (1478) after the invention of movable type. Of interest to surgeons is the classic description Celsus left us of inflammation: "Now the characteristics of inflammation are four: redness

and swelling, with heat and pain" (Book III). Of more direct interest, though, is what he had to say about surgery. He went into great detail regarding some surgical remedies, but his general comments found in the *Prooemium* of Book VII are timeless and bear repeating:

The third part of the Art of Medicine is that which cures by the hand.... It does not omit medicaments and regulated diets [the other two parts of medicine], but does most by hand. The effects of this treatment are more obvious than any other kind; in as much as in diseases since luck helps much, and the same things are often salutary, often of no use at all, it may be doubted whether recovery has been due to medicine or a sound body or good luck.... But in that part of medicine which cures by hand, it is obvious that all improvement comes chiefly from this, even if it be assisted somewhat in other ways....

Now a surgeon should be youthful or at any rate nearer youth than age; with a strong and steady hand which never trembles, and ready to use the left hand as well as the right; with vision sharp and clear, and spirit undaunted; filled with pity, so that he wishes to cure his patient, yet is not moved by his cries, to go too fast, or cut less than is necessary; but he does everything just as if the cries of pain cause him no emotion.

In the later Middle Ages, when medicine was in a stagnant state except for the contributions of the Arabs, surgery was the branch that began again to show progress. Surgery was separated from medicine during the time of Galen (ca. 200 A.D.) or before, and the two branches of medicine took quite different paths in the following 1500 years. There were probably many reasons why the surgeons were accorded less prestige and became a much less learned group than their medical colleagues, but the separation of surgery from medicine was not decreed by the Church, as history books said for years. What misled historians of surgery was the phrase *Ecclesia abhorret a sanguine* (the Church abhors blood). This is not to be found in the text of the Council of Tours (1163), as was commonly claimed, or in any papal decree, although certainly the idea that the Church wished its monks to spend more time on matters of religion and less on such secular things as medicine and surgery seems reasonable enough. It was Quesnay, the eighteenth century French historian of surgery, who disseminated the mistaken notion that the Church actually forbade surgery, and the phrase and his interpretation were repeated over and over again.[37]

By the thirteenth and fourteenth centuries, surgery was denigrated and avoided by physicians, who had received their education in the universities that were now arising all over Europe. Along with theology and law, medicine was usually one of the basic faculties. Surgeons, on the other hand, were often unlettered, lower-class men scorned in clerical circles. The surgeons were taught the ways of their craft by apprenticeship. However, as Sir Clifford Allbutt has written, "by the expulsion of surgery from the liberal arts medicine herself was eviscerated."[3]

That surgery had also declined there is no doubt. The Salernitan surgeons of the twelfth century, when a rebirth of medicine and surgery occurred, believed that surgery's decadence could be ascribed to two causes: its division from medicine and the neglect of anatomy. It was not long thereafter, however, that two major developments greatly affected the future course of surgery: the invention of gunpowder and its use in human warfare beginning in the fourteenth century, and the beginning of a renewed interest in the study of anatomy at about the same time. Thus, with greater call for their services and with the beginnings of greater fundamental knowledge from which advances could be made, the surgeons can be credited with taking medicine forward from the time of the fourteenth century. The texts of Guy de Chauliac, who unfortunately favored suppuration in healing, and the works of Theodoric and Henri de Mondeville, whom we like to honor because they stressed clean wounds, reflected great credit upon the whole of medicine.

From the year 1200 on, there is little doubt that surgeons existed as separate practitioners. They were especially to be found in the newly rising cities, where they joined guilds. Earlier, they had sometimes been admitted to the universities, where they could even lecture. As time passed, however, they were excluded and thus formed their own colleges, such as the Collège de St. Côme in Paris. Along with these surgeons of the long robe, who were often clerics, arose the barbers, the even less learned surgeons. The physicians usually favored the barbers because, being simpler men, they were more likely to be at the beck and call of the learned doctors.

The barbers and surgeons of England had belonged to separate guilds since the fourteenth century. In 1540 a compromise over the rights and duties of each was achieved, and a single company of Barbers and Surgeons was formed. Surgeons agreed to do no barbering, and the barbers restricted their surgery to dentistry. The union lasted 200 years. In 1745 it was dissolved and the surgeons' company again existed independently, jealously guarding its prerogatives and protecting its interests. In 1800 George III chartered the Royal College of Surgeons of London, which by charter from Queen Victoria in 1843 became the Royal College of Surgeons of England.

The surgeons of four centuries ago had many of the same aims as their counterparts today. Witness, for instance, what the British surgeon Peter Lowe (1550–1613) had to say in his *A Discourse of the Whole Art of Chirurgerie* (1597), the first real textbook of surgery written in English. Lowe asks: "What is chirurgerie?" "It is a science or Arte that sheweth the manner howe to work on man's body, exercising all manuall operations necessary to heal man, or as much as is possible by using of most expedient medicines." Lowe's textbook, incidentally, is arranged under five headings, also used by Paré: to take away, to help and add, to put in place that which is out, to separate, and to join what is separated. These early surgeons also had a clear conception of what the surgeon should be. Who can improve upon the qualifications set forth by Thomas Vicary, mid–sixteenth century surgeon and author?:

Now then to know what properties and conditions this man must have before he be a perfect chirurgien. I doe note foure things most specially that every chirurgien ought so to have: the first, that he be learned; the second, that he be expert; the third, that he be ingenious; the fourth, that he be well mannered.[40]

Some physicians in the Renaissance saw clearly that medicine and surgery, united in ancient times, must be brought together again. During the Renaissance, surgery did slowly begin to attain a higher social position once again. No longer primarily in the hands of barbers, surgery was taught and practiced by some of the most illustrious physicians and anatomists. Vesalius and Fabricius of Aquapendente, the teacher of William Harvey, were but two of many.

Few men in the history of medicine have been more popular than Ambroise Paré (1510–1590). There are many reasons for his high standing. His superb work, his pleasing personality, his humility, and, not least, the loving study made of his life and work by the nineteenth century surgeon Joseph Malgaigne all help to account for Paré's place in the history of surgery.

Born of humble parents in the province of Maine in 1510, Paré received his medical training as an apprentice barber-surgeon and then went to Paris, where he was appointed a house surgeon at the Hôtel-Dieu, already a famous charity hospital. Here he learned anatomy and surgery and began to develop the superb manual dexterity and sound general knowledge of the medicine of his time that led to his success. He served four successive kings of France as a military surgeon and wrote books in his own tongue instead of Latin, in which he and his fellow barber-surgeons were not schooled. Thus, in his writing as well as in his surgical treatment, Paré achieved a victory of experience over tradition.

The use of a digestive solution of egg yolk, rose oil, and turpentine to dress gunshot wounds was a discovery Paré made when the hot oil normally used to cauterize wounds ran out during the war between Francis I and Charles V. Those men treated by Paré's improvised methods, he tells us, did much better, and he resolved to treat all gunshot wounds without boiling oil in the future. Remarkable as were his results, it is of equal note that Paré here knowingly challenged authority.

One can readily see in Paré's approach a great similarity to our own—doubtless still another reason why he should be so attractive to us today. He stressed, for instance, the importance of anatomy, which in his time was beginning to come out of its doldrums.

ANATOMY

The origins of the study of anatomy are veiled in obscurity, but early wound surgeons and those who butchered animals must have had some notions of structure. The Greeks pursued animal anatomy, and it must be kept in mind that ancient anatomy, except in the school of Alexandria in the time of Herophilus and Erasistratus in the third century B.C., was largely animal anatomy. It was one of the great accomplishments of the Renaissance to rediscover the fine structure of the body and to impress upon the medical world the essential knowledge of anatomy that underlies all medical knowledge.

Anatomic dissection began to be more common again at the end of the thirteenth century. With the first manual for dissection written by Mondino de Luzzi in 1316, students had some guidelines. The early dissections were still often confined to the bodies of animals and sometimes were really autopsies performed to ascertain the cause of death, especially if foul play was suspected. These dissections were usually the responsibility of the surgeon. Only by the middle of the fifteenth century did anatomic dissection become so common that a special theater for it was built in Padua.

A basic requirement of any descriptive science is the ability to make pictures that can be readily duplicated so that they can be used for instruction and learning. Woodcuts with pictures began to be made in Europe probably late in the fourteenth century, mainly as a labor-saving device for turning out sacred images. It was some time before biologists

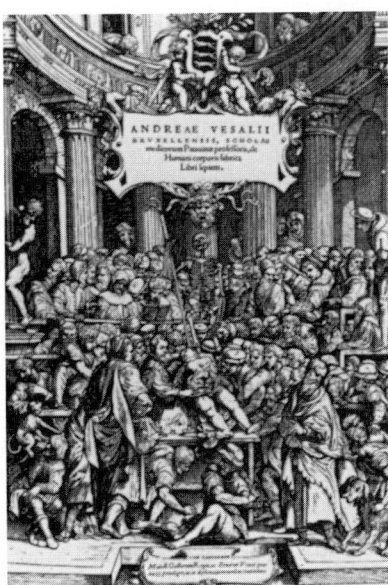

Figure 1–1. Frontispiece from Vesalius' *Fabrica*, published in 1543.

took up the idea, but by the end of the fifteenth century and early in the sixteenth, occasional illustrated medical works began to appear. One of the best and most lasting proved to be the *De humani corporis fabrica* of Andreas Vesalius. The publication of the *Fabrica* of 1543 coincided with the publication of another great book in the history of science, the *De revolutionibus orbium coelestium* of Nicolaus Copernicus. Thus, in a single year the modern understanding of both microcosm and macrocosm was under way.

The importance of Vesalius is that by his work and example he set forth a program. The famous frontispiece depicting him at the dissecting table, knife in hand, is itself programmatic (Fig. 1–1). This young man, born in Louvain in 1514 and educated in Brussels and Paris, went to Padua to finish his medical studies. At the age of 23, upon receiving his degree, he was appointed professor of anatomy and surgery, an important academic combination for centuries to come. Vesalius was certainly not alone in his attack upon the ancients, particularly the anatomic physiologic system of Galen, yet his great achievements set a tone. One must also remember that in the same year as the *Fabrica* Vesalius also published the *Epitome*, a shorter book intended to serve as a guide for students. The great rarity of original editions of the *Epitome* probably attests to its heavy use.[30]

The surgeon-anatomists, Vesalius being one of their number, played an increasingly important role as time went on and knowledge of anatomy advanced. Thomas Vicary in his anatomy text quoted Galen's remark that it is as possible for a surgeon not knowing anatomy to work in man's body without error as it is for a blind man to carve an image and make it perfect. The tradition of teaching both surgery and anatomy was carried on by the professors of surgery in medical schools until the early twentieth century.

Henry Gray, a surgeon who in 1859—the year of Darwin's *Origin of Species*—introduced the first edition of his *Anatomy*, gave his book the title *Anatomy, Descriptive and Surgical.*

PATHOLOGY AND EXPERIMENTAL SURGERY

One of the great medical events of the eighteenth century was the publication of *On the Seats and Causes of Disease Investigated by Anatomy (De sedibus et causus morborum . . .)*

by Giovanni Battista Morgagni, Padua's gifted professor of anatomy for nearly 60 years, in 1761 when the author was 79 years old. It represented a lifetime of work and stands as one of the great classics of medicine. Morgagni insisted that clinical observations be correlated with postmortem findings. He intended his book to be a useful one; he dealt with common diseases faced by physicians, not the rare and unusual ones usually written about by previous authors. Morgagni wrote his book as a series of 70 letters, composed in elegant Latin. Not until 1793 did Matthew Baillie, a nephew of the Hunters, write a book on morbid anatomy in English. In the tradition of Morgagni, then, John Hunter was to bring pathologic study to surgery.

John Hunter (Fig. 1–2), born in Scotland in 1728, was the youngest son in a large family.[24] He was a poor student and was little interested in his studies except for those having to do with natural history. At age 20 he was apprenticed to his brother William, 10 years his senior, who earlier that year had begun giving private anatomy lessons for surgeons in London.

Although John Hunter had been a poor student, he took to dissection immediately, and his brother quickly recognized his talents. This was the beginning of John Hunter's long illustrious career as a naturalist who collected a large museum of specimens, as an anatomist and experimental surgeon, and as a teacher of great influence (Fig. 1–3). That he should have been the preceptor of so many pupils who later became famous in their own right is the more remarkable when one considers that he was a poor lecturer and an obtuse writer. Nevertheless, his precepts were stimulating and his writings widely read. His work on venereal disease confused syphilis and gonorrhea but was a major study of the subject. In 1794, a year after Hunter's death, his *Treatise on the Blood, Inflammation and Gun-Shot Wounds* appeared. Inflammation thus became "the first principle of surgery."

Equally well known was Hunter's study of ligation of arterial vessels in cases of aneurysm. By supposed experimental study on the antlers of deer, he realized that collateral circulation would probably suffice if the vessel involved by aneurysm were ligated in its healthy part. By this means, amputation, if the aneurysm was in the femoral or popliteal

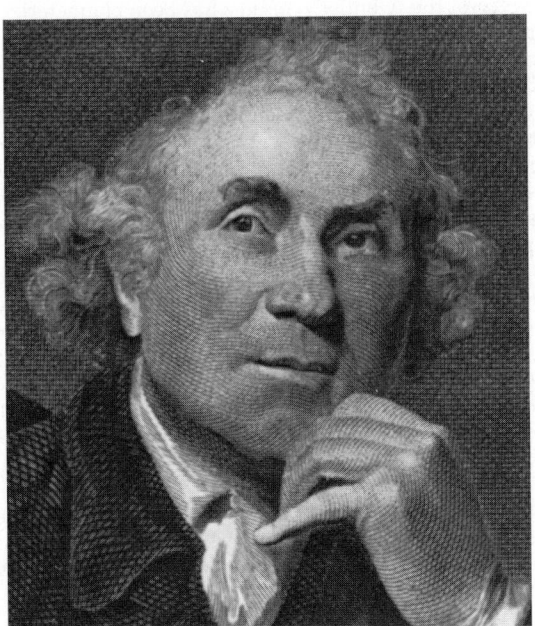

Figure 1–2. John Hunter (1728–1793), the father of experimental surgery and a superb anatomist and teacher.

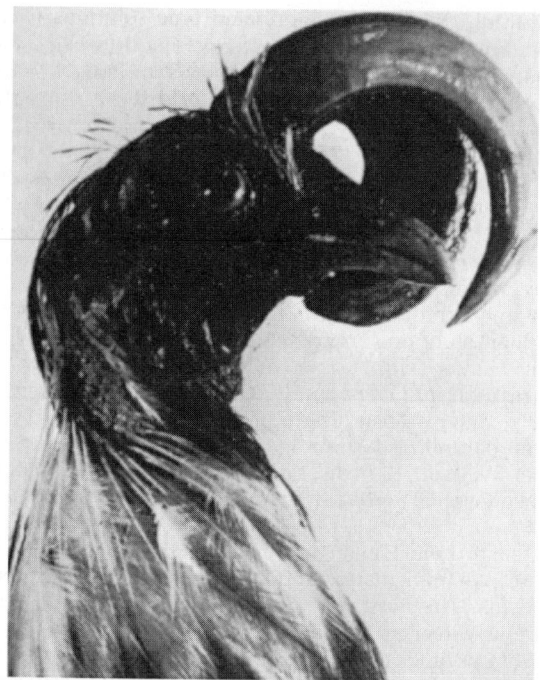

Figure 1–3. Photograph of a specimen from the Royal College of Surgeons of England of a spur that grew after being transplanted to the cock's comb by John Hunter (example of tissue transplantation).

arteries, for instance, could be avoided. This was a major advance in surgical therapy and was the real beginning of what came to prominence in the nineteenth century as conservative surgery. Thus, Hunter amply earned the epitaph given him by the medical historian Fielding H. Garrison, who said: "With the advent of John Hunter, surgery ceased to be regarded as a mere technical mode of treatment, and began to take its place as a branch of scientific medicine, firmly grounded in physiology and pathology."[16]

ANESTHESIA AND ANTISEPSIS

Surgery of the twentieth century has been characterized by "a lifting of the eyes from the local lesion and the operation designed to deal with it to regard the more general aspects of surgical disorders," according to Churchill.[9] While this approach is certainly a hallmark of our time, we did not invent it. The institutes of surgery, as they were called in previous times, "are its settled principles," Henry J. Bigelow told his students in 1849.[4] Although the principles were still excessively general, discussion of constitution and disease was not entirely neglected by the surgeons. However, in the field of operative surgery, Bigelow confessed, "we occupy more directly what is popularly considered to be the province of the surgeon. The surgeon, with the public, is associated with surgical operations, and his notoriety is in measure with the belief which the world may entertain of the number of or magnitude of the operations he may perform."[4] The public may be impressed, warned Bigelow, and the surgeon should guard against much of the exaggerated sense of worth and of drama.

Both Bigelow and his Boston colleague J. Mason Warren wrote about the all too frequent sepsis that appeared after the drama in the amphitheater had run its course. Primary healing was seldom attained in city practice. Union by first intention had been rare for 20 years, Warren claimed. Part of the blame, he believed, could be laid at the doors of the city fathers who were responsible for the unhygienic conditions

then prevalent. Thus, some surgeons looked well beyond the local lesion, but they were usually powerless to make changes.

The surgeons of the nineteenth century, incidentally, played an honorable part in the movement for sanitary reform. For instance, Edmund Parke and John Simon in England, and Stephen Smith and Willard Parker in New York, were both surgeons and sanitarians. The French surgeon E. Doyen, in his *Surgical Therapeutics and Operative Technique* of the early twentieth century, entitled one chapter "Parallelism of the Evolution of Surgical Asepsis and the Progress of Public Hygiene."

In the early nineteenth century, surgical operations were still infrequent. Many hospitals in England and America had their weekly operating days, on which one or two procedures might be performed. In many major hospitals there were fewer operations in 1 year than are performed in 2 days in one of our modern busy surgical services. The surgery for tuberculosis, especially its bony complications, accounted for a significant proportion of operations; accidents, strangulated hernias, abscesses, and aneurysms made up most of the rest. Mortality rates varied from hospital to hospital and differed in different countries.[36] They were generally highest on the Continent of Europe, amounting to 40% to 60%, depending on the operative procedure.

Pain, infection, hemorrhage, and shock were four of the most difficult obstacles to the progress of surgery. As each was dealt with, the bounds of surgery enlarged. As the limits of surgery were extended, the field of the individual surgeons seems to have become more and more restricted.

Since the fundamental aim of all medical art and science has always been to alleviate human pain and suffering, the development of anesthesia for use during surgical operations ranks as one of the most dramatic discoveries in the annals of medicine. The use of alcohol, mandrake root, opium, and even bleeding or reduction of blood flow to the brain to reduce sensibility was known to the ancients in a crude sense, but the really effective use of general anesthesia can be very precisely dated to the 1840s. In 1842 a rural Georgia practitioner, Crawford W. Long, used ether to remove small skin tumors, but he did not report his results until 3 years after William Morton (Fig. 1–4) successfully etherized a patient for John Collins Warren on October 16, 1846, at the Massachusetts General Hospital. James Young Simpson of

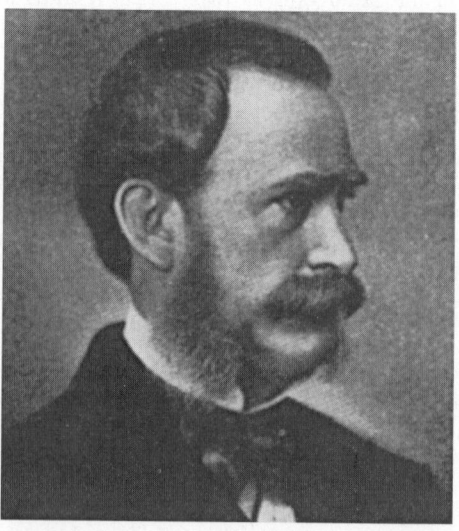

Figure 1–4. William T. G. Morton (1819–1868), a Boston dentist whose successful demonstration of ether anesthesia on October 16, 1846, at the Massachusetts General Hospital was a landmark in the history of surgery.

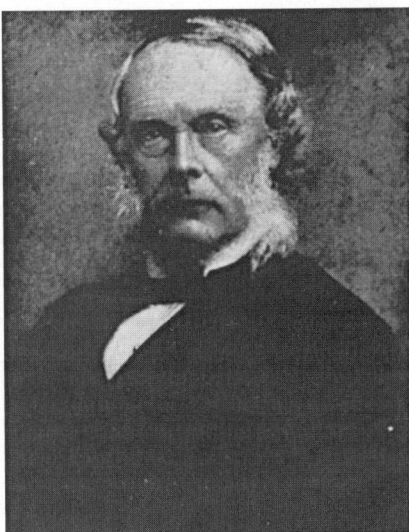

Figure 1–5. Joseph Lister (1827–1912), the originator of antiseptic surgery.

Edinburgh introduced chloroform in the next year, and a new age in surgery was born. Speed of operation would now no longer be the hallmark of the great surgeons.

Although the mid–nineteenth century English physician John Snow, famous for his writing about cholera and the Broad Street pump, was one of the first to call himself an anesthesiologist, the specialty of anesthesiology did not really begin to develop until the years just before World War II. No longer was it sufficient for a surgical house officer or even a medical student to be delegated the task of administering the anesthetic and monitoring the patient, who was often neglected as the student eagerly watched the surgeon operate.

Anesthesia found speedy acceptance. The same, unfortunately, cannot be said for the attempts to control infection. Wound healing in the days before Lister was a confused and depressing aspect of surgery. Wounding, either accidental or caused by the surgeon, was often followed by what was called irritative fever, usually lasting a few days and resulting in accumulation of pus in the wound. Sometimes the pus was creamy white; this thick exudate was often called "laudable pus." If the patient was fortunate, there was a slow healing process to recovery. This was the state of surgery seen from the patient's view, and it had existed for centuries.

Even with the most ingenious technique, the most agile and skilled operators all too often found that their work went for naught because the patient succumbed to postoperative infection. The term *hospitalism* was used by surgeons to describe the postsurgical infections so commonly found in surgical wards: erysipelas, pyemia, septicemia, and hospital gangrene.[25] The causes of these infections may have been guessed by some shrewd surgeons of the prebacteriologic era, but by and large most surgeons felt helpless in their wake. Simpson, the Scottish surgeon who introduced chloroform, strongly urged his colleagues to do their operating on kitchen tables or in small cottage hospitals, for here the patients stood much less chance of becoming infected.

Joseph Lister (Fig. 1–5), faced with these problems, watched the wretched patients in his surgical wards with increasing frustration and concern. Although he was not alone, he was the first to combat this major surgical obstacle successfully. The Hungarian obstetrician Ignaz Semmelweis and the American anatomist and writer Oliver Wendell Holmes had clearly shown in the 1840s that puerperal fever was carried to parturient women on the hands of their doctors. Simple washing in chlorinated lime solutions was extremely successful in Semmelweis' wards, but his Viennese colleagues and the world paid scant heed. Thus, it was left to Lister doggedly to convince the world that wound infection was evil, not laudable, and that it could be effectively prevented.

Lister was born in Essex in 1827[18] and attended University College, London, the common school for dissenters such as the Quaker Listers. He was graduated in 1847 and received his medical degree in 1852. In the following year he journeyed to Edinburgh to work and study with James Syme, one of the outstanding surgeons and surgical teachers of the midcentury. Syme was a leader in the movement toward a conservative surgery, one that tried to conserve limbs by excision of parts of bone, with preservation of the limb as a whole. Lister remained in Edinburgh, became a member of the surgical staff of the Royal Infirmary, and married Syme's eldest daughter Agnes. In 1861 Lister moved to the chair of surgery at the Royal Infirmary in Glasgow, and it was during 8 fruitful years there that he began to develop his principles and practice of antisepsis. In 1869 he was called back to Edinburgh to fill Syme's chair, and in 1877 he moved to King's College Hospital in London. In 1897 he became the first physician to be elevated to the peerage.

In his earlier Edinburgh and Glasgow years, Lister investigated a number of problems closely related to surgery, such as inflammation, wound healing, and the role of blood coagulation in both. His approach to the problems of surgery was distinctly modern, in the sense that it was scientific and physiologic. Despite Lister's attempts to clean up his wards and to perform surgery as cleanly as possible, there was still an appalling rate of the common surgical complications of hospital gangrene, pyemia, and erysipelas among his patients.

In the years just before 1865, the French scientist Louis Pasteur (Fig. 1–6) slowly developed what came to be a germ theory of disease. He clearly showed that fermentation and putrefaction, observed since ancient days, were caused by living, multiplying matter. He reasoned that pus formation, wound infection, and some fevers must also be caused by minute organisms from the environment.[12]

Lister's first papers describing his method and its success appeared in 1867. In the following years he changed the technical details of his method, added the steam-powered spray for the operating environment, and continued to fight for his idea in many publications. As years went by, he was able to perform operations safely that previously no capable surgeon would have dared attempt. The successful wiring of a fractured patella in 1877, which converted a closed fracture

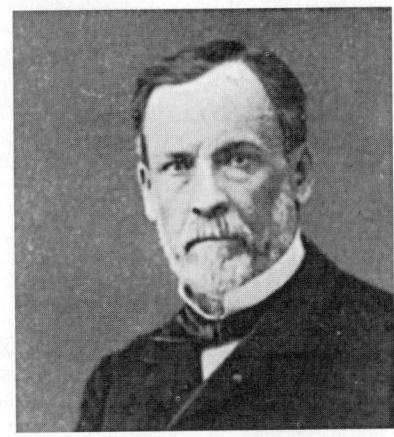

Figure 1–6. Louis Pasteur (1822–1895), the originator of the germ theory of disease.

to an open one, brought much scorn upon him, but patience, doggedness, and scrupulous attention to detail led eventually to complete success. Lister admitted in the 1880s that the spray was not necessary and indeed may have been harmful to operators and patients alike. He gracefully accepted the development of aseptic surgery by the Germans, acknowledging that it was but a step beyond his own work and a logical extension of it.

The acceptance of listerism, as I have already indicated, was uneven and, in our eyes, with the advantage of retrospective view, quite slow. There were many reasons for this, most of them not tied to simple conservatism or resistance to change. Lister's method was complicated; the carbolic acid was an unpleasant nuisance that could actually be harmful; the method was time-consuming and expensive, and required assistance. Some surgeons and physicians believed the germ theory to be mere speculation; hence, the underlying theory or the rationale for Lister's technique was also slow to be accepted. Also, one must remember that many leading surgeons simply could not duplicate Lister's good results, hard as they might try. Theodor Billroth was one who tried the method, wanting to accept it, but found it somewhat frustrating. By the late 1870s he had adopted listerism fully but not without much discouragement.

Other surgeons reported that they used Lister's techniques but that their results were not much improved. In reading case reports in medical journals of the period, one must evaluate carefully such phrases as "listerism used" or "Lister's technique followed throughout." In the case of President James Garfield in 1881, for instance, the extensive medical bulletins issued during his 2-month lingering battle with an abdominal gunshot wound inflicted through the back often reported, "Lister's dressings used." Yet we know, too, that fingers and instruments probed the wound from the first day on. Little real understanding of the germ theory can be ascribed to surgeons who carefully soaked their instruments in carbolic acid but then reused them without resoaking after they had been dropped on the floor, or, even more commonly, used them after they had been wiped on the operator's nonsterile apron or held between his teeth. Thus, the full realization by Lister of the meaning of Pasteur's work is perhaps his greatest achievement.

Rudolph Matas (Fig. 1–7) recalled that in the 1880s the head, chest, and abdomen were still sanctuaries not to be opened, unless by accident.[27] It has frequently been stressed

that the development of anesthesia and antisepsis greatly increased the numbers of operations performed, but a look at the statistics reveals that the increase was very slow. Halsted in 1904 showed that in the decade following the fairly wide acceptance of antisepsis in the United States (1878 to 1888), the number of operations performed increased only slightly.[20] This decade, we must remember, was the second after Lister's first enunciation of his principles in 1867. Matas gave the figures for the Charity Hospital in New Orleans, where in 1881 only 172 operations were performed among 5300 admissions, or about 3.2%. In 1890, the Charity Hospital admitted 6083 patients, but only 291, or 4.7%, had major surgical procedures. By 1939, about 40% of admissions were surgical.[27] As Charles Rosenberg has so clearly shown in his history of hospitals, *The Care of Strangers,* it was the increasing use of hospitals by surgeons that helped to shift the locus of medical care in the early decades of this century to the hospital.[35]

In the decade after Lister's momentous papers on the efficacy of antisepsis, there was still much reticence about accepting the method as well as its theoretical foundation, the germ theory of disease. There was also some reluctance to hope for much more improvement in the art of surgery. After the Napoleonic wars at the beginning of the century, the French surgeon and author of surgical texts, Alexis Boyer, is supposed to have said: "Surgery seems to have attained the highest degree of perfection of which it is capable."[32] Despite anesthesia and the development of many new techniques and despite the promise of antisepsis, John Eric Erichsen, one of the most perceptive and influential surgeons of late nineteenth century Britain, came to similar conclusions in 1873:

That there must be a final limit to development in this department of our profession there can be no doubt. . . . Like every other art, be it manipulative, plastic, or imitative, it can only be carried to a certain definite point of excellence. An art may be modified, it may be varied, but it cannot be perfected beyond certain attainable limits. . . . There cannot always be fresh fields for conquest by the knife; there must be portions of the human frame that will ever remain sacred from intrusion, at least in the surgeon's hands. That we have nearly, if not quite, reached these final limits there can be little question.[32]

The story of the years since 1873 has proved Erichsen a poor prophet, yet most of those engaged in medicine have at one time or another shared his feelings.

ABDOMINAL SURGERY

Among the many difficult technical problems faced by nineteenth century surgeons was that of reconnecting the divided ends of hollow tubes, especially blood vessels and intestine. Just as cardiovascular surgery has captured both public and professional attention in the past two or three decades, it was abdominal surgery that played the same role about 100 years ago. The successful removal of an inflamed appendix before rupture, the Billroth operations for esophageal and gastric cancer causing obstruction, the improved hernia operations of Bassini and Halsted, and abdominal operations for such other reasons as diseases of the ovary all caused great excitement in the medical world of the late nineteenth century.

The problem of intestinal obstruction faced surgeons long before the 1880s. Strangulated hernia, for instance, was not uncommon. Before antisepsis was introduced, laparotomy was not usually performed. Ephraim McDowell, the Kentucky physician who successfully removed a huge ovarian tumor from Mrs. Jane Todd Crawford in 1809, was skilled, to be sure, but also very lucky. An indication of how his townsmen felt is that they gathered in large numbers around

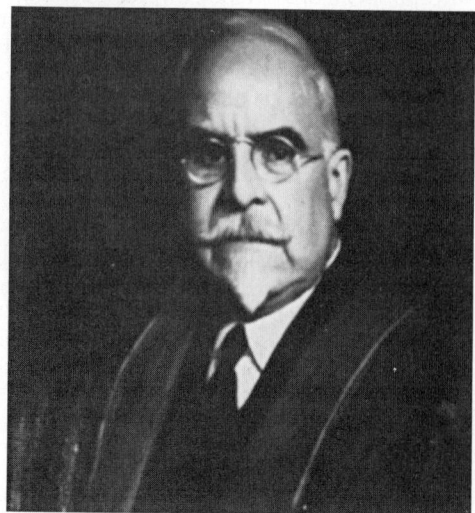

Figure 1–7. Rudolph Matas (1860–1957), professor of surgery at Tulane University in Louisiana and a pioneer in vascular surgery. He introduced the technique of endoaneurysmorrhaphy in the treatment of arterial aneurysm.

his house on that Christmas Day in Danville, Kentucky, with a rope slung over a tree, ready for use if the doctor should fail in the butchery they were convinced he was committing. They might well have hanged him had his patient died.

The basic principle of intestinal suture—that the serous coats must be brought into contact—was not discovered until early in the nineteenth century and not put into use until some decades later. The British surgeon Benjamin Travers in 1812 published *An Inquiry Into the Process of Nature in Preparing Injuries of Intestines.* About the same time, Guillaume Dupuytren, one of the best trained and ablest surgeons of France, whose approach to surgery was much like John Hunter's in the use of experimental physiology and pathology, also concerned himself with intestinal suture. Although apparently quite a mean and unscrupulous man, he was a great teacher and surgical innovator. Unfortunately, his name is associated today mainly with an uncommon malady of the hand caused by contraction of the palmar fascia. Dupuytren's student, Antoine Lembert, is known for his suture, which resulted from the observation that careful approximation of the peritoneal coats of divided intestine would produce good healing. Not until the German and German-trained surgeons (including Swiss and Austrians) began putting antiseptic and aseptic principles to work did the techniques of abdominal surgery find their way into common practice.

In America, one of the important contributions to the advance of surgery stemmed from the work of a pathologist, Reginald Heber Fitz of Boston, and the surgeons Charles McBurney and Henry B. Sands of New York and John B. Murphy of Chicago. Fitz in 1886 published his classic paper on appendicitis, a term he coined.[14] Known for centuries under a variety of names such as perityphlitis and iliac passion, acute inflammation of the vermiform appendix was a surgical disease, according to Fitz.

Charles McBurney, professor of surgery at the College of Physicians and Surgeons, working mainly at Roosevelt Hospital in New York, in 1889 described the point of maximal tenderness now bearing his name, and 5 years later proposed a new incision for appendectomy. J. B. Murphy in the United States, Lord Moynihan of Leeds in England, and others at the turn of the century led the vigorous campaign for withholding purgatives and for resorting to prompt surgery. It should be noted that the understanding of this common disease and the operative concept for it were worked out by the cooperative efforts of physicians of several specialties.

This use of surgery, self-evident to us today, took some years to become assimilated into standard medical practice. In 1900 abdominal surgery was not yet something undertaken lightly by most doctors and patients. The successful drainage of an appendiceal abscess in King Edward VII of England, forcing the delay of his coronation in 1902, helped make appendicitis a fashionable disease and also helped break down further the resistance to surgery.

TRAINING OF THE SURGEON

Much has been written about the training of the surgeon, the proper qualifications, and what it means to be a surgeon. Between the simple apprenticeship or even the transfer of knowledge from father to son that held sway until the nineteenth century and the thorough grounding in pathology, research, and operative and postoperative management required of today's surgeon, much surgical history has passed.[7]

The subject of surgical training in America invariably brings to mind the name of William S. Halsted (Fig. 1–8), no doubt partly because of his famous address entitled "The Training of the Surgeon" delivered at Yale in 1904.[20] Halsted, who was born in New York City in 1852 and died in Baltimore 70 years later, made numerous important contributions

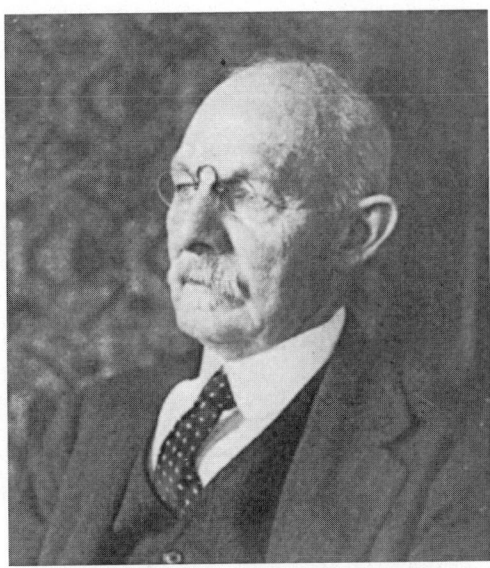

Figure 1–8. William S. Halsted (1852–1922), prominent American surgeon who introduced the German system of residency training to the United States. He also made fundamental contributions to the surgery of the thyroid, breast, and blood vessels and to the surgical treatment of hernia.

to surgical technique and teaching.[21] After graduation from the College of Physicians and Surgeons and a trip to Europe, he quickly established himself as an energetic researcher, a gifted operator, and a popular young teacher in New York. While working with cocaine for nerve block anesthesia, he and some of his associates became addicted. Only after hospitalization and prolonged convalescence, and with the faithful help of his friend William H. Welch, who invited him to Baltimore in 1886, did Halsted recover. Historians are still working at unraveling the circumstances of further addiction during his later and very productive years.

When the Johns Hopkins Hospital opened in 1889, Halsted was appointed acting surgeon and head of the outpatient clinic. He became professor of surgery in 1892, the year before admission of the first medical school class. Halsted developed improved methods for operating on hernias and cancer of the breast, he introduced the use of rubber gloves in surgery, and he constantly stressed the relationship of surgery to physiology. Careful handling of tissues and the minimization of blood loss were concepts he passed on to the many fine surgeons he trained over 30 years. Justifiable as has been his fame, Halsted was not solely responsible for establishing the surgical residency system as we know it. He himself would have been the first to note that the great German teachers of surgery, especially von Langenbeck (Fig. 1–9) and his pupils, including Billroth (Fig. 1–10), were his models. Furthermore, Halsted's colleague William Osler deserves equal credit for instituting the residency system at Johns Hopkins.

Why was it in Germany that the surgeons first adopted antisepsis, Halsted asked in his Yale lecture. The answer lay, he believed, "in the character of the scientific and practical training of surgeons in Germany." The assistants or "residents" in these programs enjoyed good research facilities, ample clinical material, and excellent instruction, and this is what Halsted successfully duplicated in Baltimore. "We need a system," he said at Yale in 1904, "and we shall surely have it, which will produce not only surgeons but surgeons of the highest type, men who will stimulate the first youths of our country to study surgery and to devote their energies and their lives to raising the standard of surgical science."[20] Reforms, Halsted stressed, had to come from

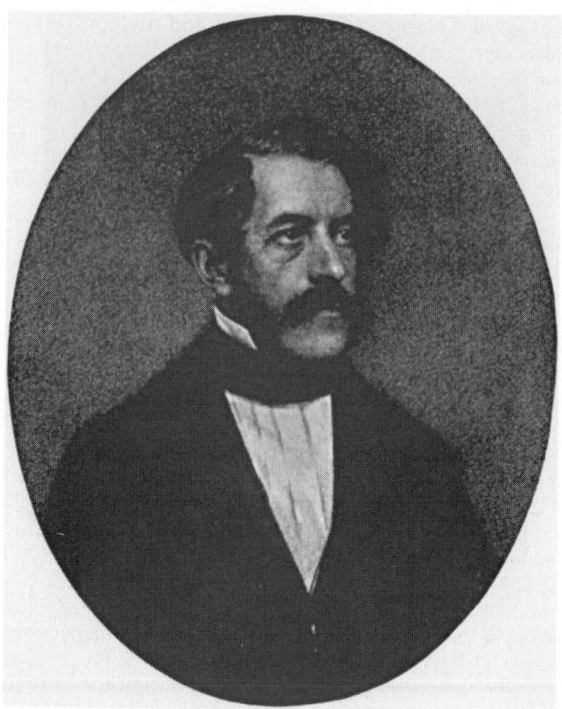

Figure 1–9. Bernhard von Langenbeck (1810–1887), master German surgeon who is acknowledged by many to be the father of the modern residency system in surgery. His students included Billroth and Kocher.

both hospital and university, and the medical school should control a hospital of its own.

Halsted spent 2 years studying surgery, histology, and pathology in various German centers. He watched the work of Bergmann, Volkmann, Billroth, Esmarch, and Mikulicz in their surgical clinics. He was thus favorably inclined to the use of antisepsis, and the German thoroughness and insistence on knowledge of the basic sciences as a foundation for surgery were to be the hallmarks of his own career as well. Halsted's 17 residents and more than 50 assistant residents

carried this "German method" to many teaching centers in the United States. The second and third generations from this "Johns Hopkins school" are still to be seen in American academic centers.

Halsted was a keen judge of surgical talent among both his peers and his students. That he considered Theodor Kocher of Berne (Fig. 1–11) perhaps the greatest surgeon of his time was one reason why Kocher was very popular with American students. Kocher was known for his work on the brain and spinal cord and especially for his careful techniques and study of the thyroid gland. His surgical treatment of goiter, a particularly severe disease in his native Switzerland, earned Kocher the Nobel Prize in 1909, the first time it was awarded to a surgeon.

In his work on the surgical relief of goiter, Kocher not only developed the surgical technique necessary for removal of the thyroid but also added immeasurably to the understanding of its role in the body's metabolism. In his early thyroidectomy patients, if removal was complete, myxedema developed, accompanied by all its unpleasant and stunting side effects. When his colleagues pointed out this tragic aftereffect, Kocher took positive steps to learn from his mistake instead of engaging in the scientific polemics so common in his era.

NEUROSURGERY AND THORACIC SURGERY

It should be clear that the latter decades of the nineteenth century gave rise to numerous developments in surgery and that these developments clearly set the stage for advances in our own century. Changing concepts in pathology during the nineteenth century greatly influenced surgery. Especially important was the idea that disease was localized and hence remediable by surgical attack. In addition to his many other talents, the pathologist Rudolf Virchow, who in 1858 published his *Cellular Pathology*, was also a superb historian. He spoke in his essays about the "anatomical idea," the progressive localization of life and disease in the body. The "anatomical idea" originated in the mid–eighteenth century with Morgagni, who believed that disease had its seat within the organs of the body. At the beginning of the nineteenth

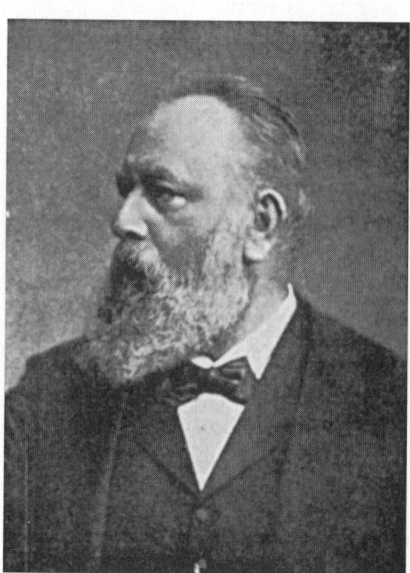

Figure 1–10. Theodor Billroth (1829–1894), professor of surgery at the University of Vienna and pioneer abdominal surgeon. Billroth was one of the most influential teachers of his time.

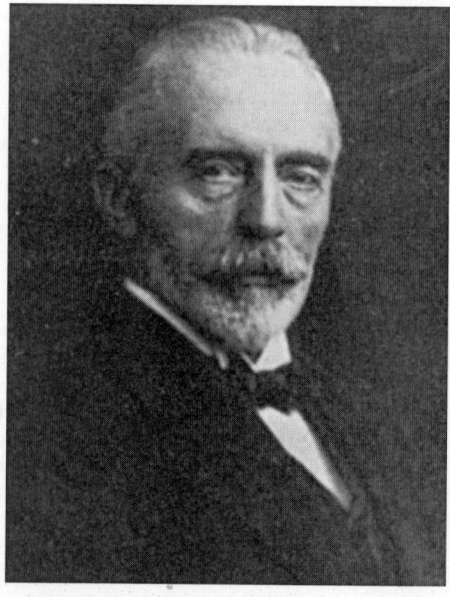

Figure 1–11. Theodor Kocher (1841–1917), professor of surgery at the University of Berne and pioneer in the development of surgery of the thyroid. He received the Nobel Prize in 1909.

century, the French surgeon Xavier Bichat claimed that it was to the tissues that one must look.[2] He identified 21 kinds, such as muscle, bone, and nerve, and pointed out that when epithelium becomes inflamed, the reaction is similar no matter where in the body it may occur. Virchow took the last step and localized disease processes within the cell. This view has held sway since, although today we also discuss disease on the molecular or even the submolecular level.[38]

Some aspects of the surgical approach to disease that the student of the 1990s may take for granted have actually quite a short history. The twentieth century is the century especially of neurosurgery, thoracic surgery, and the whole field of transplantation.

The field of neurosurgery, so much of it brought to its modern state by the work of Harvey Cushing, Walter Dandy, and others, is similar in its historical development to general surgery in a variety of ways. Trephination of the skull is one of the oldest operations in the annals of surgery, but since it was done only to release evil spirits, to relieve pressure from injuries, or to treat epilepsy, it hardly qualifies for pride of place as neurosurgery. Not until the work on cerebral localization in the latter nineteenth century could the surgeon really begin to attack lesions within the cranium effectively. As in other branches of surgery, diagnostic means had to be developed along with safe and efficient operative measures.

Harvey Cushing, like all neurosurgeons until fairly recent times (after World War II), was trained in general surgery.[15] He was Halsted's resident, although emotionally and personally he felt much closer to the professor of medicine at Johns Hopkins, William Osler. While still a medical student at Harvard, Cushing devised a chart for continuous recording of respiration and blood pressure by the anesthetist, and some years later brought to American operating rooms the practice of sphygmomanometry. While at Johns Hopkins, he helped found the "hunterian" surgical laboratory, where the modern practice of experimental surgery in dogs began for medical students.[7]

In thoracic surgery, the story is much the same. Basic cardiac and pulmonary physiology had to be understood before surgical therapy could be contemplated. The problems of operating on a beating heart were as hard to overcome as the difficulty of maintaining pressure relationships within the chest. Not until the 1890s were direct wounds of the heart successfully sutured. Before this time, chest surgery primarily involved evacuation of empyema or drainage of a pericardial sac filled with fluid or blood. The story of the surgical treatment of cardiac lesions (traumatic, congenital, degenerative, or postinfective) has been told in some detail in books by Meade,[28] Richardson,[34] and Johnson.[22]

The history of valvular surgery has been one of steady progress since the operations were reintroduced in the late 1940s. The progress relates not only to direct improvements in operative approach and technique, but also, as is the case in most thoracic surgery, to technical developments by which physiologic conditions can be made suitable for surgery. There is an interesting connection between surgeons and internists in the story of the surgical alleviation of valvular disease. As has been true throughout the history of medicine, the underlying theory regarding causation of disease has been closely intertwined with the therapy made available. In the case of mitral valve disease, for instance, a great English clinician, the London cardiologist Sir Lauder Brunton, suggested in 1902 that animal experiments showed the feasibility of a surgical approach to the disease. This suggestion was not well received, and no surgeon seems to have acted upon it until a London colleague, Henry Souttar, operated on a woman in 1925. Souttar, instead of inserting an instrument into the ventricle to reach the valve, used his finger to push through the valve from the atrium. The patient, a 19-year-old girl, lived in fair health for 5 years and died of a cerebral embolus.

New theories and innovations should not be accepted uncritically. The medical profession has been accused of being too conservative, but for the sake of our patients this is a necessary trait. Other aspects of the resistance to change are not so defensible, as the story of listerism has shown. Once again, in the story of mitral valve surgery, a major theoretical hurdle had to be overcome before real progress could be made. James MacKenzie, who was Britain's leading cardiologist and a respected teacher, hastened to condemn Souttar's attempted treatment, basing his objections on the belief that the abnormality of mitral stenosis was in the myocardium, not in the valve. With this theory, as with that of a basically humoral pathology, surgical therapy made little sense. Theory must affect practice; one cannot be divorced from the other, as this example clearly illustrates.

By 1928 Elliot Cutler and Claude Beck could summarize only 12 known cases of valvular surgery, and the results were discouraging. Mortality was 83%. The truly remarkable changes that have occurred in the years since 1955 are now known to all students of surgery.

Experimental cardiac surgery began in the early 1880s. M. H. Block, a German surgeon, published a report on wounds of the heart in 1882 in which he described successful suture of rabbit hearts, and strongly urged that the procedure be used in humans. In the best surgical circles of the time, however, resistance to his innovation was strong. Billroth is reported to have said a year later: "A surgeon who would attempt such an operation should lose the respect of his colleagues." The technical problems of pressure relationships in the chest, stilling the heart, and maintaining the circulation during surgery had to be mastered before practical application was possible.

One of the very basic physiologic obstacles that had already been overcome was the problem of negative pressure within the pleural cavity. Ferdinand Sauerbruch, working in the clinic of his teacher Mikulicz in Breslau, devised an apparatus in which negative pressure for the open thorax could be maintained. These experiments in 1903 and 1904 led to the construction of a large chamber in the following years, and the technical difficulties involved were soon alleviated by the introduction of endotracheal or insufflation anesthesia around 1910. Not until the late 1930s was a reliable apparatus available that would give good control of respiration.

Hypothermia and the heart-lung machine are even more recent developments. Hypothermia had been used in the treatment of cancer and other medical problems when it was adapted for surgery by groups in Philadelphia, Minneapolis, and Denver in the 1950s. Many of the same surgeons also did much to develop a safe and efficient means of extracorporeal circulation. John H. Gibbon (Fig. 1–12) began to work on this problem before World War II.[17] He and others, especially C. Walton Lillehei and Clarence Dennis and their co-workers, made the possibility of extensive cardiac surgery an everyday reality in large hospital surgical services.

The problem of shock is important for all surgery, especially in times of war. Major surgical texts of the late nineteenth century rarely devoted more than a page to the subject. Loss of blood was known to be a cause, but beyond that not much more was known, nor could much have been done to counteract the effects. The list of credit for unraveling the story is a long one, but certainly two American surgeons, George Crile and Alfred Blalock, deserve special mention.

Blalock (Fig. 1–13), while at Vanderbilt University in the late 1920s and the 1930s, published significant papers on the cause and treatment of shock. The prevailing theory of the time was that the most likely cause of shock was release of

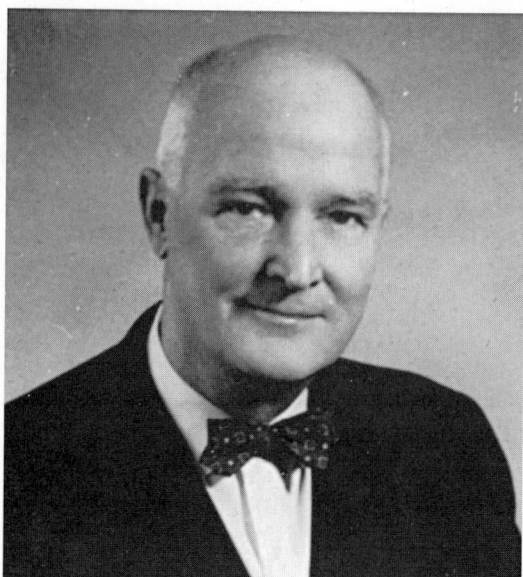

Figure 1–12. John H. Gibbon (1903–1973), pioneer cardiothoracic surgeon who developed extracorporeal circulation.

to Vanderbilt, a new medical center with many young men ambitious to do research. His former Johns Hopkins roommate, Tinsley Harrison, was a resident in medicine at Vanderbilt when Blalock was a resident in surgery, and Harrison's influence, though hard to measure exactly, was doubtless important. After returning to Johns Hopkins in the early 1940s, Blalock worked in one of the finest medical research centers in any academic institution. His cooperation with the pediatrics department, particularly with Edwards A. Park and Helen Taussig, and with help from his gifted technician Vivien Thomas, produced the discovery of a successful method of surgical treatment of tetralogy of Fallot.[39] This in no way detracts from what Blalock or any other single individual may have contributed. It merely illustrates that an important change in scientific medicine has come about since the time when Claude Bernard or Louis Pasteur worked in inadequate quarters with a handful of students and assistants. Science today is, more than ever before, a great cooperative venture. To conduct such a venture successfully, academic and scientific leadership of high quality is required. Perhaps it is for this kind of leadership, for the stimulus provided to a whole school of research rather than for individual surgical feats, that the more recent great teachers such as Blalock and Owen Wangensteen (Fig. 1–14) will be best remembered.

a toxin, very possibly histamine. In studies of shock produced by muscle injury, Blalock and his colleagues found a large accumulation of blood at the site of trauma, whether in an extremity or the intestinal tract.

The contributions of surgical teachers and investigators such as Blalock, to single out just one among many, also illustrate the importance and influence of the scientific and academic environment. Blalock was fortunate in having gone

ELECTROLYTE AND FLUID BALANCE, NUTRITION, CHEMOTHERAPY, SURGICAL ENDOCRINOLOGY, AND RADIOLOGY

Not until the 1850s and the work of Claude Bernard was a definition of the role of the blood and the body fluids clearly enunciated. In his *Liquids of the Organism,* a series of lectures published in 1859, Bernard first used the word *milieu* to express the internal environment. In the following years he elaborated his concept of the *milieu intérieur,* the physiologic state that allows the organism to exist independently. In our own century these earlier ideas of Bernard were taken over by many, including Walter Cannon of Harvard, who coined the term *homeostasis,* and Lawrence J. Henderson, also of Harvard, who wrote much on the mechanism of acid-base balance, and whose name is familiar to all medical students

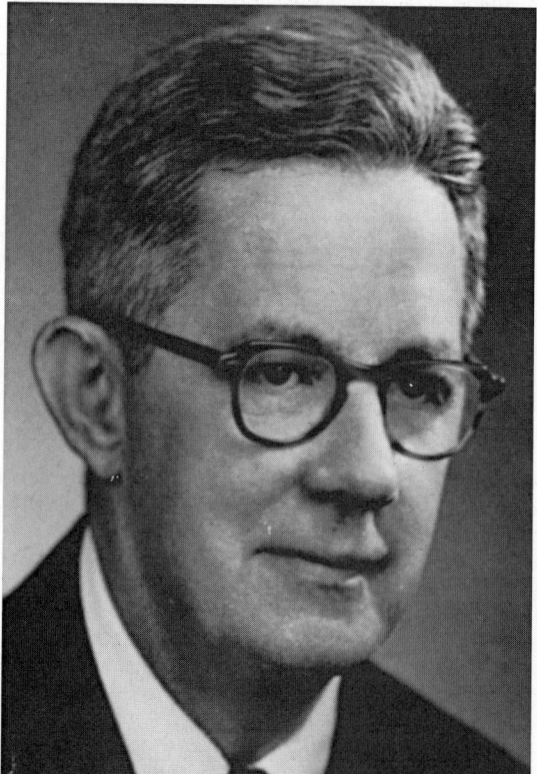

Figure 1–13. Alfred Blalock (1889–1964), noted investigator and clinical surgeon who made basic contributions to the understanding of the pathogenesis of shock. He also was a pioneer and innovator in the field of cardiac surgery.

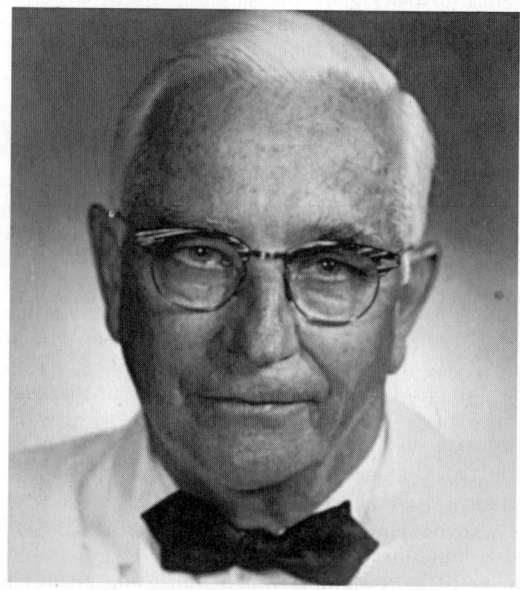

Figure 1–14. Owen H. Wangensteen, who for more than half a century was a leading teacher of surgeons at the University of Minnesota.

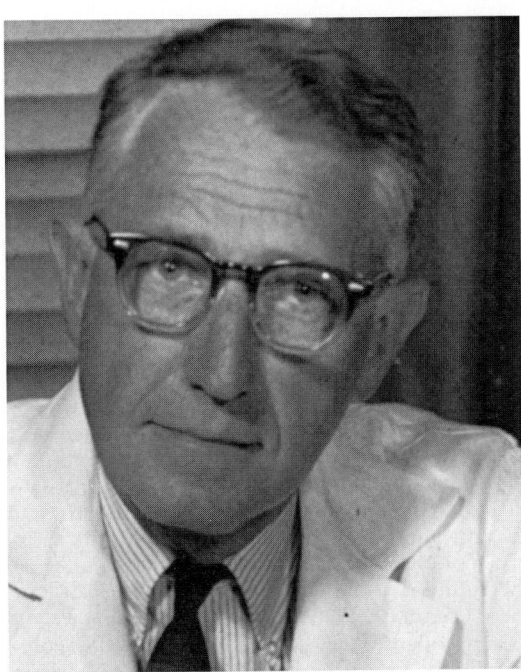

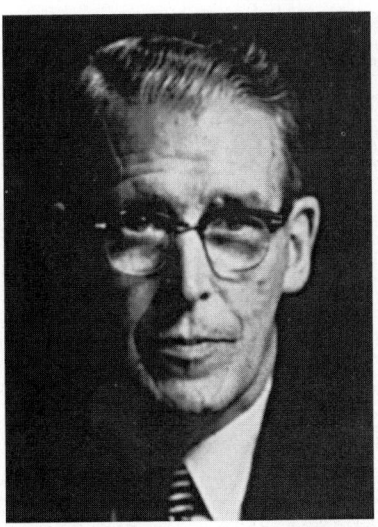

Figure 1–16. Jonathan Rhoads, distinguished professor of surgery at the University of Pennsylvania, editor, author, and investigative surgeon, who has made many contributions to surgery and teaching. His work in the field of surgical nutrition is outstanding, especially the introduction of total parenteral hyperalimentation. He is also known for his contributions to the field of surgical oncology.

Figure 1–15. Francis D. Moore, leading investigative surgeon who defined objective aspects of metabolism in surgical patients.

who have mastered the Henderson-Hasselbalch equation, at least for biochemistry examinations.

Neither Cannon nor Henderson was a surgeon, and although both were medically trained, neither practiced. Another Harvard physician, the Moseley Professor of Surgery Francis D. Moore (Fig. 1–15), early in his career became interested in the metabolic problems of surgical patients. The Coconut Grove fire in 1942 was a sad stimulus to learning for many. Moore continued to learn and write and in 1952 published *Metabolic Response to Surgery*, a surgical landmark. He greatly expanded his ideas in *Metabolic Care of the Surgical Patient*, which has been a standard work since it was published in 1959.

The nutritive needs of surgical patients have been the subject of much attention and investigation. In this field, Jonathan Rhoads (Fig. 1–16) has been a pioneer and distinctive leader. Together with his colleague Stanley Dudrick, he introduced total parenteral hyperalimentation in the 1960s. This has become a very important aspect of preoperative and postoperative care, particularly in severely ill patients.

The role of the endocrine glands in the pathogenesis and control of neoplastic disease has long been a subject of much interest. A major contribution in this area was made in 1940 when Charles Huggins (Fig. 1–17) showed that antiandrogenic treatment consisting of orchiectomy or the administration of estrogens could produce long-term regression in patients with advanced disseminated prostatic carcinoma. His further studies of serum enzymes and protein chemistry, including the role of the renal glands in the control of metastatic neoplastic disease, have been monumental, and for these landmark observations he was awarded the Nobel Prize in 1966.

In 1921 Sir Alexander Fleming described and isolated an inhibiting agent and called it lysozyme. Unfortunately, the bacteria inhibited by this natural enzyme are not those harmful to humans. However, the lysozyme work alerted him to be on the lookout for other suitable antagonistic candidates. In the fall of 1928 Fleming noted that some of his plates of staphylococcal cultures contaminated by laboratory air grew a mold that inhibited growth of the bacteria.

Fleming's observation, so often ascribed to chance, was actually made in the course of careful laboratory investigation. Part of Fleming's goal was to find just such a substance. What did prove to be extremely fortuitous was that the product of the contaminating mold—penicillin—was a powerful antibacterial substance, effective against some of the common human pathogens, yet remarkably free of toxicity for humans. Why Fleming's important discovery was not commercially produced until the war years is not entirely clear. Fleming himself claimed that physicians became interested in the possibility of antibiotics only after the demonstrated usefulness of the sulfonamide drugs introduced by

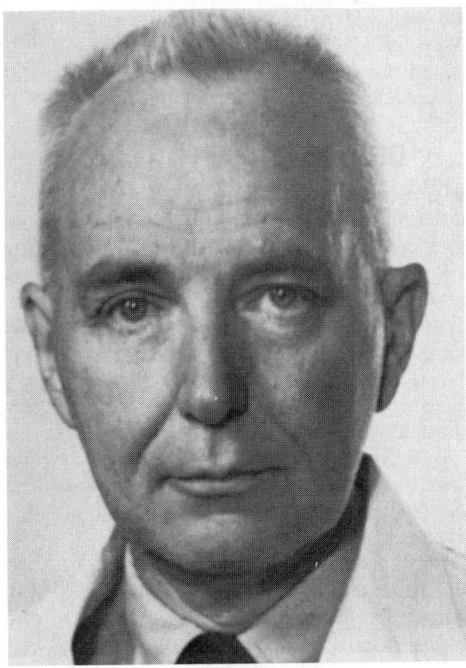

Figure 1–17. Charles B. Huggins, distinguished cancer researcher at the University of Chicago, who received the Nobel Prize in 1966 for his studies of the effects of hormones on tumor growth.

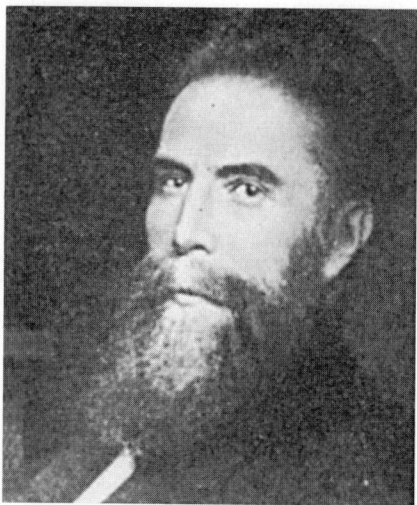

Figure 1–18. Wilhelm K. Röntgen (1845–1923), who discovered x-rays in 1895.

Gerhard Domagk in 1935. Not until several American manufacturing plants entered the picture in the early 1940s was there enough penicillin for a clinical trial.

If Fleming fully recognized the momentous nature of his discovery, and every indication points to the fact that he did, the question still remains why he and others did not push harder for earlier synthesis or isolation of penicillin.

Another development that deserves emphasis is the discovery of x-rays by Röntgen (Fig. 1–18) in 1895, which, although part of a general physical investigation, was accidental. Moreover, it was the first modern scientific discovery to receive banner headlines in the newspapers. The public was fascinated and frightened. "Old ladies," Derek Price tells us, "went into their baths fully clothed, being convinced that the scientists now had mystery rays that could look through brick walls and round corners."[33] It was only a matter of months following the discovery that Frau Röntgen's hand and wrist bones could be clearly visualized that clinical application of the finding was made. Within a few years the use of rays was expanded to include physiologic studies, such as those of swallowing and intestinal motion. Walter B. Cannon used fluoroscopy for this purpose while still a medical student in 1901.

ORGAN TRANSPLANTATION

Probably no recent development in surgery has so captured the public interest as has organ transplantation. Like some other contemporary aspects of medicine, transplantation has a long history. An integral part of the story of transplantation is to be found in the annals of plastic surgery. The ancient Hindus were adept at transplanting skin from the buttocks area to refashion noses and ears. Even more common was the forehead flap method given wide publicity with a picture in *The Gentleman's Magazine* in 1794. This can be traced back to much earlier times.

In the sixteenth century the Italian surgeon Gasparo Tagliacozzi gained fame for his method of rhinoplasty. One sees in the history of plastic surgery a close connection between social customs and civilization as a whole and the surgeon's responses to the resultant needs. During the Renaissance and beyond, frequent street brawls, the cutting off of nose or ears as punishment for thievery and adultery, and the devastating effects of leprosy, syphilis, and mercury treatment all made the need for a method to rebuild the face very evident. The history of plastic surgery can be seen in terms of an increasing facility in transplanting skin.

Another aspect of transplantation that has direct bearing on surgery is tissue and cell culture, more properly called *explantation*. Here, medicine and biology met and joined forces in the early twentieth century. What happened in this field is thus a typical case study for the development of twentieth century medicine and surgery generally. To understand the story of tissue culture and cell culture, one must go back into the history of botany, especially that of plant grafting, and also into the history of experimental embryology, because it was the embryologists at the end of the last century who made extensive use of explantation of embryos to observe their subsequent growth and development.

The history of tissue culture is really one of the more recent episodes in the history of medicine. It began with the work of Ross G. Harrison in the first decade of this century. Born in Germantown near Philadelphia in 1870, Harrison was among many illustrious students in the early years of the Johns Hopkins University, where he received his undergraduate degree in biology in 1889. After further study, including medical education, Harrison went to Yale in 1907, and in the same year published the paper generally considered to contain the rudiments of the method of modern tissue culture so widely used today.

Harrison hoped to settle the controversy then being aired in the scientific journals over the growth of the nerve cell. Was its long process an outgrowth of the cell or was it an independent unit, growing toward the cell body? By means of a hanging-drop preparation, Harrison was able to observe under direct vision the growth of frog embryo nervous tissue in clotted lymph. Soon after Harrison moved to New Haven, Montrose Burrows came from the newly established Rockefeller Institute in New York to learn about the method of independent cell growth.[10] Burrows suggested improvements in the medium, and incidentally probably also deserves credit for suggesting the term *tissue culture*. He returned to New York to report his findings to the man who had sent him to New Haven, the French-born surgeon Alexis Carrel (Fig. 1–19).

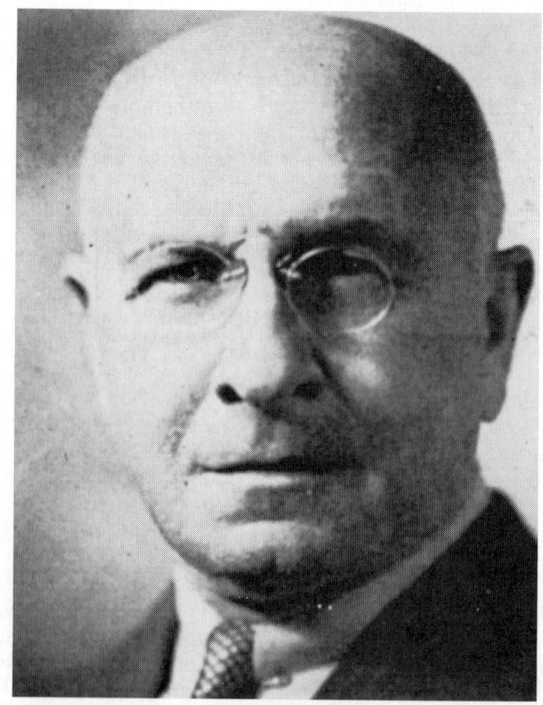

Figure 1–19. Alexis Carrel (1873–1944), an experimental surgeon interested in wound healing, tissue culture, organ transplantation, and blood vessel anastomosis. He was awarded the Nobel Prize in 1912.

Carrel, born in Lyon in 1873, was one of the most colorful and interesting figures in medicine in the first half of this century. He was trained in France and became a skilled and imaginative experimental surgeon who developed the finest of techniques. Carrel was much interested in Harrison's work because he saw its potential for his own work on wound healing and tissue proliferation. The problems could be much better studied if they were isolated from the body as a whole. Carrel and Burrows did indeed manage to grow tissues in flasks. The next step was to grow entire organs. Carrel had already been involved in extensive transplantation of organs in the decade from 1902 to 1912.

Here, in the work of this one man, there is a close connection between surgery and transplantation of organs and the growth of cells and tissues. What Carrel accomplished with the delicate instruments he devised was to suture blood vessels, end to end, without leaving tissue hanging into the lumen that could then act as a focus for clot formation (Fig. 1–20). Previous attempts to transplant organs and re-establish their blood supply had met with failure because of infection and thrombosis. Carrel first reported his technique in 1902, when he was not yet 30 and only 2 years after he had obtained his M.D. degree. His method was to use three retaining sutures, thereby converting a round hole to a triangular one, which could then be easily sutured—a simple but lasting technique for which he was awarded the Nobel Prize in 1912.

Carrel came to the United States in 1905 and that summer worked with Charles Claude Guthrie at the Hull Physiological Laboratory at the University of Chicago. Guthrie, medically trained but a physiologist for most of his career, is the unsung hero in the story of vascular suture and hence organ transplantation. Guthrie suggested improvements in Carrel's technique, and the two men collaborated in numerous experiments and papers. Guthrie urged Carrel to include all layers of the vessel wall, even the endothelium, in the suture to prevent wrinkling.

In 1990 Joseph E. Murray of the Brigham and Women's Hospital and Harvard received the Nobel Prize for his contributions to renal transplantation (Fig. 1–21). He successfully transplanted the kidney from an identical twin to another twin with severe kidney disease. He had done much experimental work before the clinical procedure and recognized that the immunologic barrier is lacking between identical

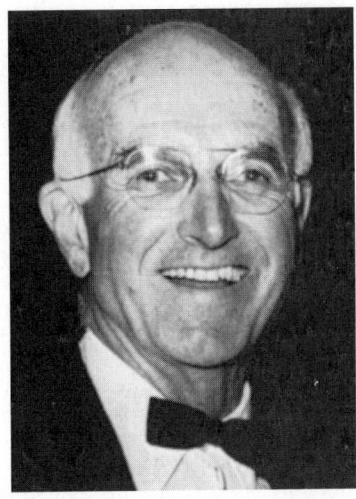

Figure 1–21. Joseph E. Murray received the Nobel Prize in 1990 for his contributions to kidney transplantation.

twins. Later, it was found that immunosuppressants could reduce the effects of the immunologic barrier, and this greatly expanded the applicability of renal transplantation.

One of the prime contributors to the field of cardiovascular surgery has been Michael E. DeBakey (Fig. 1–22) of Houston. In 1934 he first described the occlusive roller pump, which has been widely used throughout the world in extracorporeal circulation. After this basic contribution, he became a leader in the field of direct surgery for the treatment of thoracic and abdominal aneurysms, including complicated resections of lesions of the aortic arch. Moreover, he and his associates dedicated much time and effort to the development of plastic prosthetic arterial substitutes, which have been widely adopted and highly successful. He was the first to perform a successful carotid endarterectomy in 1953, and he and his colleagues were also the first to report the successful use of a saphenous vein bypass graft for coronary arterial occlusion, a procedure they accomplished in 1964.

Besides his important surgical contributions, DeBakey has

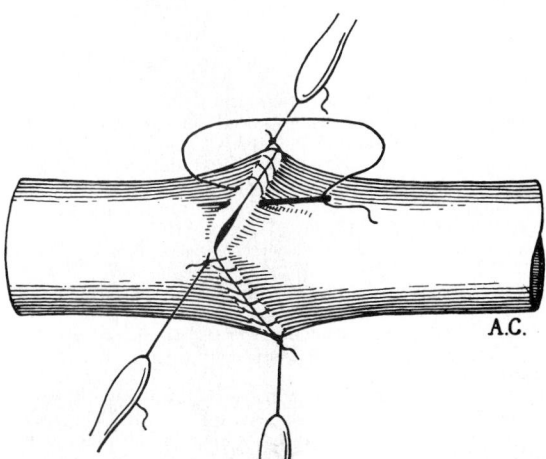

Figure 1–20. Joining blood vessels by suture anastomosis. This representation is adapted from the line drawing by Alexis Carrel published in *Lyon Medical* in 1902. The walls of the two blood vessels (here drawn as about 5 mm. in diameter) are held together by three holding sutures. Another is then used to sew over and over, with very fine needles ("aiguilles extrêmement fines"). This method of suture anastomosis, demonstrated initially by Carrel, is still used throughout surgery, and particularly in the transplantation of organs.

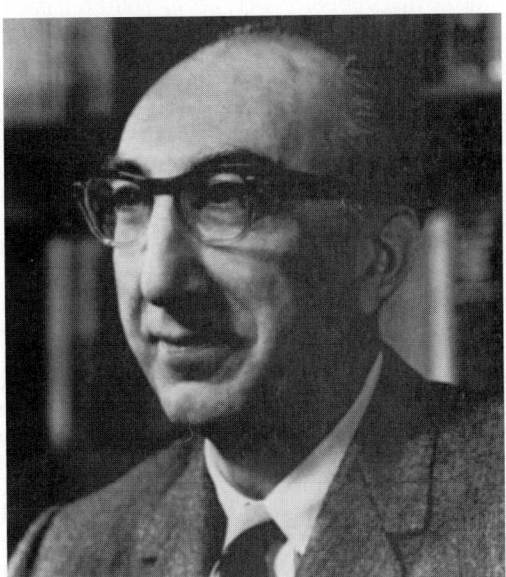

Figure 1–22. Michael E. DeBakey, an American pioneer in cardiovascular surgery who has been a leading spokesman for medicine and medical research.

for many decades been an influential member of an advisory group that has been important in shaping biomedical research. His influence on Mary and Albert Lasker and on members of Congress was instrumental in the evolution of support for research and health care.

As surgery has progressed, it has also become increasingly specialized. Surgery as a specialty began with the wound surgeons of early antiquity. From later antiquity to the early twentieth century, surgeons for the most part did not confine themselves to operative therapy; they were also charged with care for a variety of dermatologic disorders, especially syphilis. It is no accident that Sir Jonathan Hutchinson (1828–1913), a surgeon, described the triad of congenital syphilis: deformed incisor teeth, interstitial keratitis, and deafness. It was not until the great advances made by surgery in the nineteenth century that surgeons as a group began to regain prestige, which they did for themselves as well as for the medical profession as a whole.

In the United States, most historians have pointed out, no definite separation of medicine and surgery ever existed, despite the early attempts of John Morgan to have university-educated physicians desist from the work of the apothecary and the surgeon. The most widely known statement regarding the lack of separation comes from a long review article by Samuel D. Gross on the achievements of surgery in the first 100 years of the country:

Although this paper is designed to record the achievements of American surgeons, there are, strange to say, as a separate and distinct class, no such persons among us. It is safe to affirm that there is not a medical man on this continent who devotes himself exclusively to the practice of surgery. On the other hand, there are few physicians, even in our larger cities, who do not treat the more common surgical diseases and injuries. . . . In short, American medical men are general practitioners, ready for the most part, if well-educated, to meet any and every emergency, whether in medicine, surgery or midwifery.[19]

A few years later, Gross welcomed the newly founded American Surgical Association to its inaugural meeting in 1882. He justified the existence of the new society by pointing out that there were in the United States about 60,000 medical men, many being surgeons.

In a general sense, surgeons doubtless practiced family medicine or the like, but there is evidence that they did exist as a distinct specialty even at the time of Gross and before. According to the *Seventh Census of the United States* (1850), the State of New York, for instance, is credited with 5060 physicians for a population of 3,097,394. In addition, listed separately among the occupations are 54 surgeons. Five years later, in a census of New York State, the City of New York claimed 1252 physicians and 19 surgeons. More and more, as the nineteenth century progressed, surgery was performed by those who called themselves surgeons. This became true especially in the urban areas and for the increasingly complex operations within the abdomen after the introduction of antisepsis. In rural areas there was less reluctance among those not specifically trained to do so to perform surgery. This is still true for some family practitioners today. The founding of the American Surgical Association in 1880, the American College of Surgeons in 1913, and the American Board of Surgery in 1937 played an important part in setting and maintaining high professional standards and providing a forum for communication among men with similar scientific interests. Like their European predecessors, these surgical organizations have thus aided the process of professionalization by insisting on standards for both surgeons and hospitals.[11]

All the people, events, and institutions discussed in this chapter have contributed to the science and practice of surgery today. Perhaps nothing is more indicative of the great changes that have occurred than the fact that surgery has moved from the theatricality and drama of the operating theater to the privacy and relative sterility of the operating room. No longer is the drama of the operation or the technical skill or virtuosity of the surgeon on center stage. In the old surgery it was the art that predominated. In the new surgery it is science. The focus has thus shifted increasingly from the operation itself to the results that now provide the drama.[8]

SELECTED REFERENCES

Gelfand, T.: Professionalizing Modern Medicine: Paris Surgeons and Medical Science and Institutions in the Eighteenth Century. Westport, CT, Greenwood Press, 1980.
A superior book that uses surgeons to illustrate the formation of modern medicine.

Johnson, S. L.: The History of Cardiac Surgery 1896–1955. Baltimore, Johns Hopkins University Press, 1970.
This short but superior book describes the advances in physiology and technology that necessarily preceded or accompanied the development of cardiac surgery. The illustrations help make the story more readily understandable for those who are not specialists in thoracic surgery.

Lawrence, C.W. (Ed.): Medical Theory, Surgical Practice, Studies in the History of Surgery. London, Routledge, 1992.
Rather than putting the emphases on the main names and principal ideas in the history of surgery, this collection of essays examines medical and surgical concepts of disease and their relation to the practice of surgery. Thus, medical and surgical theories are related to the social contexts in which they developed.

Majno, G.: The Healing Hand, Man and Wound in the Ancient World. Boston, Harvard University Press, 1975.
A superbly illustrated book describing wound care and the treatment of inflammation in the ancient cultures of Mesopotamia, Egypt, Arabia, China, India, and Greece.

Pernick, M.S.: A Calculus of Suffering: Pain, Professionalism and Anesthesia in Nineteenth Century America. New York, Columbia University Press, 1985.
This book explores how the use of anesthesia changed medicine in the nineteenth century.

REFERENCES

1. Ackerknecht, E. H.: Primitive surgery. Am. Anthropol., 49:25, 1947.
2. Ackerknecht, E. H.: Medicine at the Paris Hospital 1794–1848. Baltimore, Johns Hopkins University Press, 1967.
3. Allbutt, T. C.: The Historical Relations of Medicine and Surgery to the End of the Sixteenth Century. London, Macmillan, 1905.
4. Bigelow, H. J.: Introductory Lecture. Boston, Mussey, 1850.
5. Billings, J. S.: The history and literature of surgery. In Dennis, F. (Ed.): System of Surgery. Vol. 1. Philadelphia, Lea, 1895, pp. 17–144.
6. Billroth, T.: The Medical Sciences in the German Universities. New York, Macmillan, 1924.
7. Brieger, G. H.: In Numbers, R. L. (Ed.): The Education of American Physicians: Historical Essays. Berkeley, University of California Press, 1980, pp. 175–204.
8. Brieger, G. H.: A Portrait of Surgery, Surgery in America, 1875–1889. Surg. Clin. North Am., 67:1181, 1987.
9. Churchill, E. D.: Surgery in the twentieth century. In Nardi, G. L., and Zuidema, G. D. (Eds.): Surgery, A Concise Guide to Clinical Practice, 2nd ed. Boston, Little, Brown, 1965, pp. 1–8.
10. Corner, G. W.: A History of the Rockefeller Institute 1901–1953. New York, Rockefeller Institute Press, 1964.
11. Davis, L.: Fellowship of Surgeons, A History of the American College of Surgeons. Springfield, IL, Charles C Thomas, 1960.
12. Dubos, R.: Louis Pasteur: Free Lance of Science. Boston, Little, Brown, 1950, 1976.
13. Faber, K.: Nosography in Modern Internal Medicine. New York, Paul B. Hoeber, 1923.
14. Fitz, R. H.: Perforating inflammation of the vermiform appendix; with special reference to its early diagnosis and treatment. Trans. Assoc. Am. Physicians, 1:107, 1886.
15. Fulton, J. F.: Harvey Cushing: A Biography. Springfield, IL, Charles C Thomas, 1946.
16. Garrison, F. H.: History of Medicine, 4th ed. Philadelphia, W. B. Saunders, 1960.
17. Gibbon, J. H.: Development of the artificial heart and lung extracorporeal blood circuit. JAMA, 206:1983, 1968.
18. Godlee, R. J.: Lord Lister. London, Macmillan, 1917.
19. Gross, S. D.: A century of American medicine, 1776–1876. II. Surgery. Am. J. Med. Sci., 71:431, 1876.
20. Halsted, W. S.: The training of the surgeon. Bull. Johns Hopkins Hosp., 15:267, 1904.

21. Heuer, G. W.: Dr. Halsted. Bull. Johns Hopkins Hosp. (Suppl.), *90*:1, 1952.
22. Johnson, S. L.: The History of Cardiac Surgery 1896–1955. Baltimore, Johns Hopkins University Press, 1970.
23. Keys, T. E.: The History of Surgical Anesthesia. New York, Dover Publications, 1963.
24. Kobler, J.: The Reluctant Surgeon. A Biography of John Hunter. New York, Doubleday, 1960.
25. Koch, R.: Investigations into the Etiology of Traumatic Infective Diseases, trans. W. W. Cheyne. London, New Sydenham Society, 1880.
26. Malgaigne, J. F.: Surgery and Ambroise Paré, trans. W. B. Hamby. Norman, University of Oklahoma Press, 1965.
27. Matas, R.: Surgical operations fifty years ago. Am. J. Surg., *82*:111, 1951.
28. Meade, R. H.: A History of Thoracic Surgery. Springfield, IL, Charles C Thomas, 1960.
29. Moore, F. D.: Metabolic Care of the Surgical Patient. Philadelphia, W. B. Saunders, 1959.
30. O'Malley, C. D.: Andreas Vesalius of Brussels 1514–1564. Berkeley, University of California Press, 1965.
31. Paré, A.: The Apologie and Treatise of Ambroise Paré. G. Keynes (Ed.). New York, Dover Publications, 1968.
32. Poland, J.: A Retrospect of Surgery During the Past Century. London, Smith, Elder, 1901.
33. Price, D. J. D.: Science Since Babylon. New Haven, Yale University Press, 1961.
34. Richardson, R. G.: The Scalpel and the Heart. New York, Charles Scribner's Sons, 1970.
35. Rosenberg, C. E.: The Care of Strangers, The Rise of America's Hospital System. New York, Basic Books, 1987.
36. Smith, S.: The comparative results of operations in Bellevue Hospital. Med. Rec., *28*:427, 1885.
37. Talbot, C. H.: Medicine in Medieval England. New York, American Elsevier, 1967.
38. Temkin, O.: The role of surgery in the rise of modern medical thought. Bull. Hist. Med., *25*:248, 1951.
39. Thomas, V.: Pioneering Research in Surgical Shock and Cardiovascular Surgery: Vivien Thomas and His Work with Alfred Blalock. Philadelphia, University of Pennsylvania Press, 1985.
40. Vicary, T.: The English-Man's Treasure. With the True Anatomie of Man's Body. London, 1633.
41. Warren, J. M.: Recent Progress in Surgery. Boston, Clapp, 1864.
42. Zimmerman, L. M., and Veith, I.: Great Ideas in the History of Surgery. Baltimore, Williams & Wilkins, 1961.

CHAPTER 2

MOLECULAR BIOLOGY IN SURGERY

H. Kim Lyerly, M.D., and Bruce A. Sullenger, Ph.D.

Deoxyribonucleic acid (DNA) is the hereditary material of the cell.[2] A remarkable series of events (Table 2–1) has occurred over the past 50 years to elucidate the critical role of inherited and acquired genetic abnormalities in human disorders. As of 1995, approximately 3000 of the more than 100,000 genes in the human genome have been mapped, and advancements in molecular biology have led not only to new diagnostic tests and treatments but also to a greater appreciation of the fundamental pathways underlying human biology. This core of knowledge in cell and molecular biology is becoming increasingly important in the clinical practice of surgery. Therefore, a brief overview of the field in relation to the practice of surgery is presented. For more extensive discussion, several recent monographs and reviews are cited in the Selected References at the end of this chapter.

STRUCTURE AND FUNCTION OF HUMAN GENES

More than a century ago, Mendel defined genes as inheritable factors that pass from parent to offspring. In the 1940s, two discoveries revolutionized the concept of genes. In 1941, Beadle and Tatum demonstrated that genes can encode proteins, and in 1944, Avery proved that DNA was the material of which genes are made. Subsequent studies illustrated that the genetic information encoded in a given gene determines the order in which amino acids are added to a corresponding peptide chain. This conversion of the genetic instructions embedded in DNA into the necessary proteins depends on many large biologic molecules and is a multistage process detailed in the following sections.

TABLE 2–1. Major Events in Molecular Biology

Year	Event
1941	Genes are found to encode proteins
1944	DNA is determined to be the hereditary material
1953	Structure of DNA is determined
1961–1967	Genetic code is deciphered
1968	Restriction endonucleases are discovered
1973	Technique for recombining genes in living cells is established
1976	First oncogene is discovered
1977	Human growth hormone is produced in bacteria
1978	Gene for human insulin is cloned; Humulin is marketed in 1982
1983–1985	Polymerase chain reaction is developed and published in 1985
1985	First tumor suppressor gene is discovered
1990	Human genome project is created
1995	*BRCA-1* gene is discovered

DNA, deoxyribonucleic acid.

Structure of DNA and Genes

DNA consists of two strands of nucleotides wrapped around each other to form a complex double helix (Fig. 2–1). The building blocks of each strand are deoxyribonucleotides, which consist of one of four bases—adenine (A), guanine (G), cytosine (C), and thymine (T)—a sugar-deoxyribose, and a covalently joined phosphate group.[36] The deoxyribose molecules are linked by phosphates to form the backbone of DNA. Thus, the only variable part of a DNA molecule lies within its sequence of bases. The double helix is held together by the hydrogen bonds that form between the bases on the two complementary strands oriented in antiparallel directions. The sequence of a DNA strand can be predicted if the sequence of its complementary strand is known because a given deoxyribonucleotide pairs with a specific partner: A always pairs with T, and C always pairs with G. Therefore, a DNA strand of AAGCCT (written in the 5′-to-3′ direction) has a complementary strand of TTCGGA (written in the 3′-to-5′ direction).

The double-helical structure of DNA allows for the direct copying or replication of genetic instructions. During replication, the intertwined strands of DNA are unwound, separated, and then copied by an enzyme known as *DNA polymerase,* which uses one strand as a template for the synthesis of its complementary partner. This copying always occurs in a 5′-to-3′ direction by the stepwise addition of the prescribed deoxyribonucleotide triphosphates. Each of the new double-stranded DNAs consists of one old and one new strand, and completed replication results in the production of two identical copies of the original molecule.[23]

As mentioned, the only variable part of a DNA strand is the arrangement of the four bases along the deoxyribose-phosphate backbone. This sequence of bases in a gene encodes the genetic instructions for the building of a specific peptide chain. In the process of translation, each amino acid is coded for by a specific set of three nonoverlapping nucleotide triplets known as *codons.* Specific codons are employed to denote which regions of genes are to be translated; the DNA codon ATG corresponds to the translation initiation signal, whereas the codons TAA, TAG, and TGA are used to signal the termination of translation of messenger ribonucleic acid (mRNA) into protein. A gene must include the instructions about the amino acid chain to be made (the coding region), and it must also contain sequences that regulate the transcription of the gene to ensure that the protein product is made in its appropriate amounts, in the correct tissues, and at particular times during cellular development and differentiation. A schematic of a single gene is shown in Figure 2–2. Almost all mammalian genes analyzed to date have important flanking regulatory regions as well as sequences known as *introns* that interrupt their coding segments at varying positions along their length. These introns vary in size and number from gene to gene and can often be considerably longer than the coding regions, called *exons.*

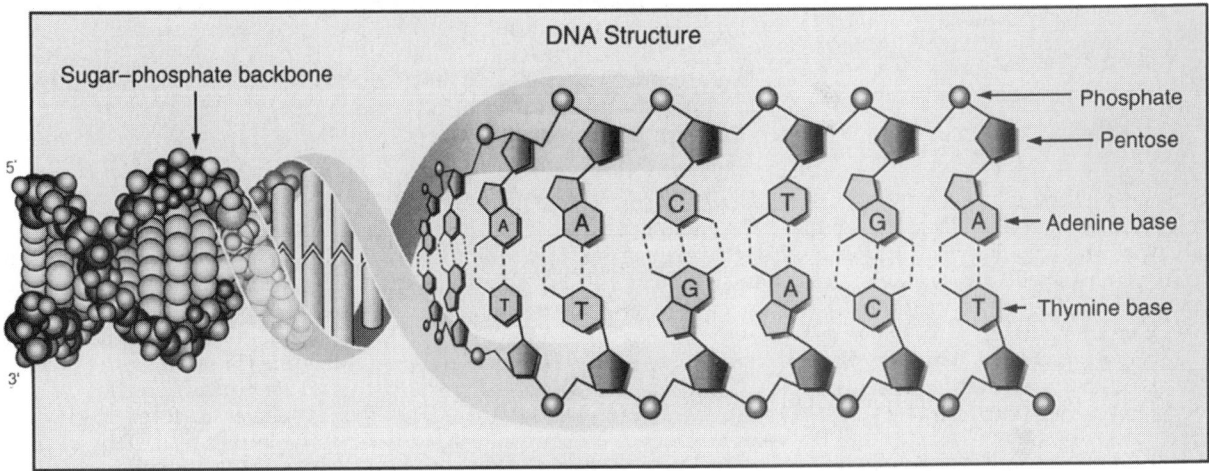

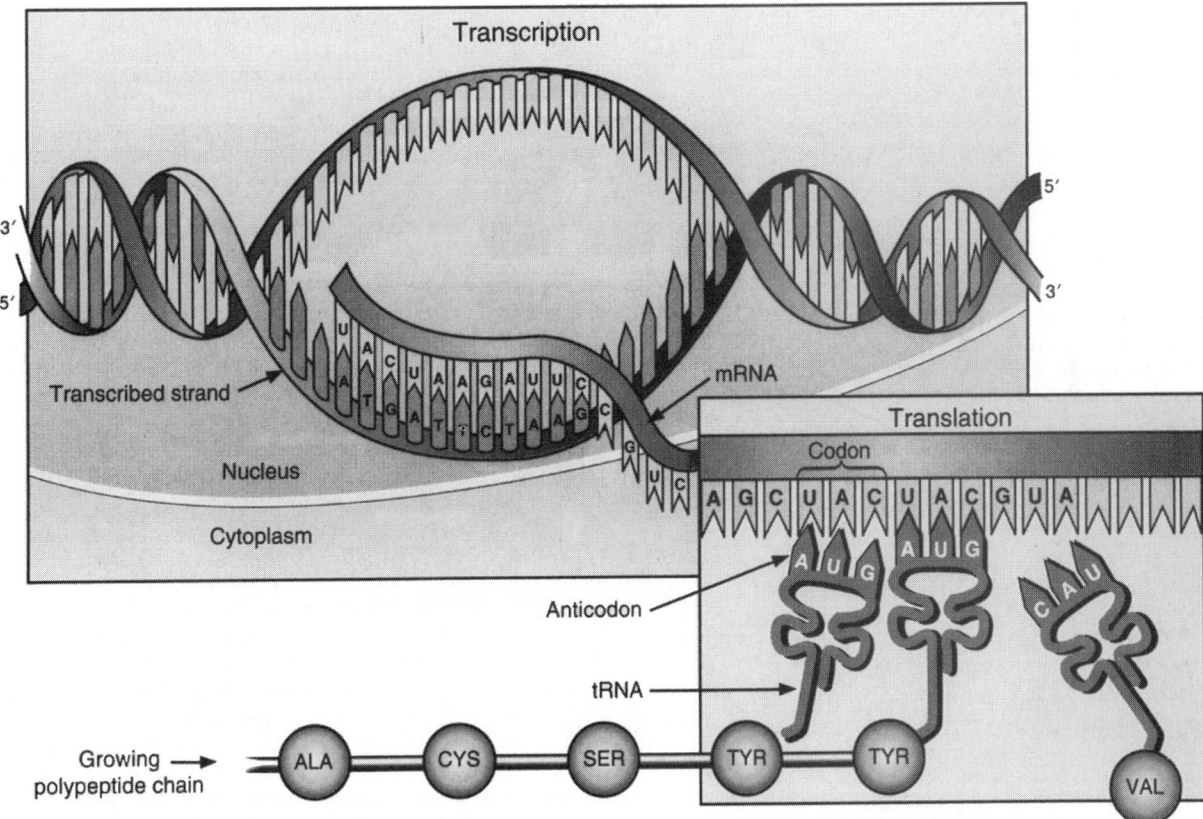

Figure 2–1. The DNA double helix and the flow of genetic information. The top panel shows the sequence of four bases (guanine [G], adenine [A], thymine [T], and cytosine [C]), which determines the specificity of genetic information. The bases face inward from the sugar-phosphate backbone and form pairs (dashed lines) with complementary bases on the opposing strand. In the larger bottom panel, transcription in the nucleus creates a complementary nucleic acid copy (messenger RNA [mRNA]) from one of the DNA strands in the double helix. The mRNA leaves the nucleus and associates with ribosomes in the cytoplasm, where it is translated into protein (smaller bottom panel). Special transfer RNAs (tRNAs) align the corresponding amino acids along the mRNA using the three-base genetic code to transform the nucleic acid sequence into a protein sequence. (Reprinted by permission of *The New England Journal of Medicine* from Rosenthal, N.: DNA and the genetic code. N. Engl. J. Med., *331*[1]:39–41, Copyright 1994, Massachusetts Medical Society.)

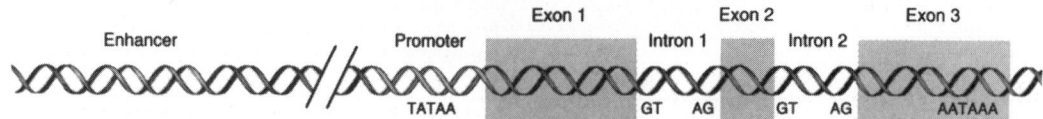

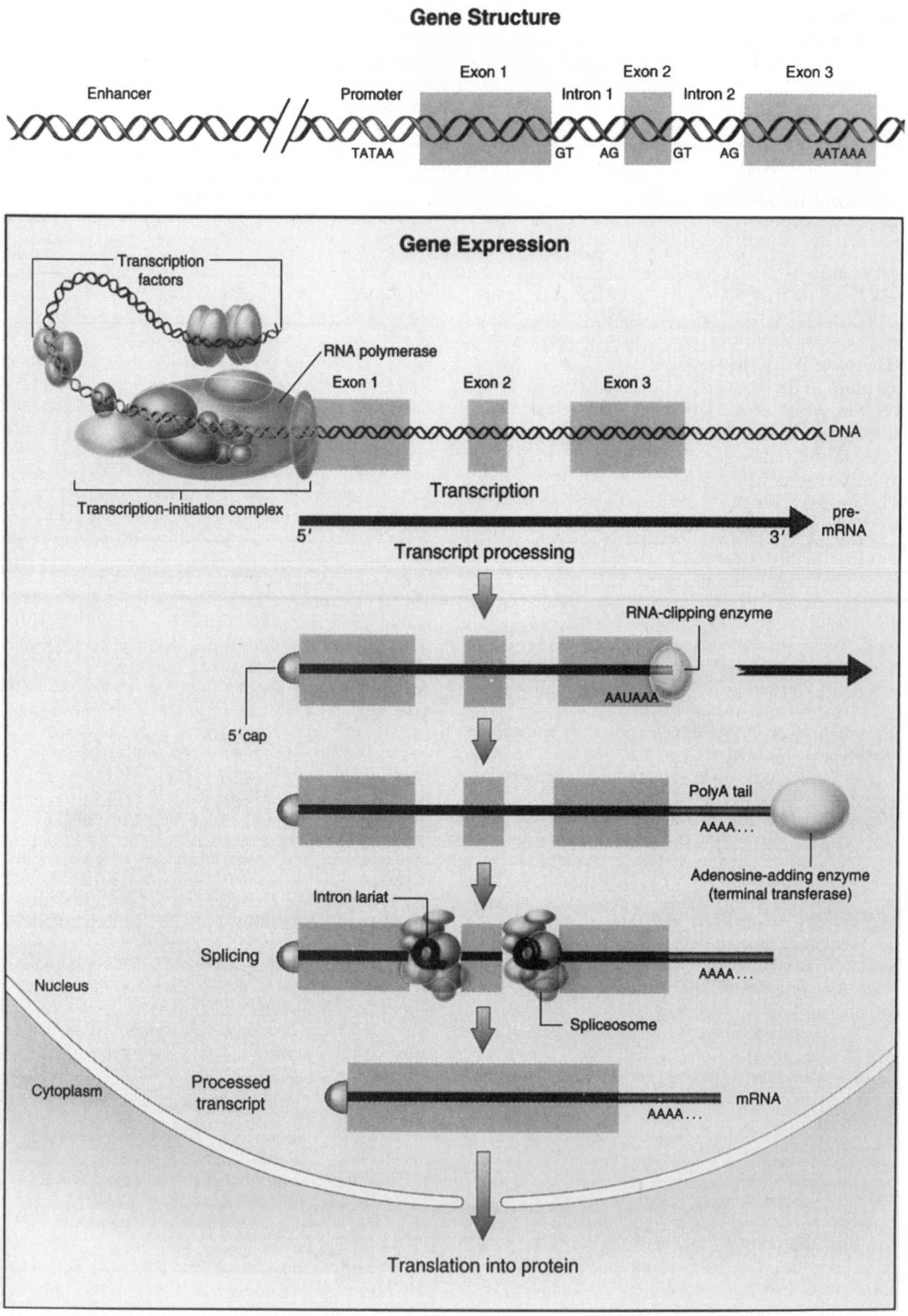

Gene Structure

Figure 2–2. Gene structure and expression in higher organisms. The DNA sequences that are transcribed as RNA are collectively called the *gene* and include exons (expressed sequences) and introns (intervening sequences). Introns invariably begin with the nucleotide sequence GT and end with AG. An AT-rich sequence in the last exon forms a signal for processing the end of the RNA transcript. Regulatory sequences that make up the promoter and include the TATA box occur close to the site where transcription starts. Enhancer sequences are located at variable distances from the gene.

Gene expression begins with the binding of multiple protein factors to enhancer sequences and promoter sequences. These factors help form the transcription-initiation complex, which includes the enzyme RNA polymerase and multiple polymerase-associated proteins. The primary transcript (pre-messenger RNA [mRNA]) includes both exon and intron sequences. Posttranscriptional processing begins with changes at both ends of the RNA transcript. At the 5' end, enzymes add a special nucleotide cap; at the 3' end, an enzyme clips the pre-mRNA about 30 base pairs after the AAUAAA sequence in the last exon. Another enzyme adds a polyA tail, which consists of as many as 200 adenine nucleotides. Next, spliceosomes remove the introns by cutting the RNA at the boundaries between exons and introns. The process of excision forms lariats of the intron sequences. The spliced mRNA is now mature and can leave the nucleus for protein translation in the cytoplasm. (G, guanine; A, adenine; U, uracil.) (Reprinted by permission of *The New England Journal of Medicine* from Rosenthal, N.: Regulation of gene expression. N. Engl. J. Med., *331*[14]:931–933, Copyright 1994, Massachusetts Medical Society.)

Other genetic instructions are required to properly control the expression of genes. Gene expression can be regulated at a number of points, including transcription, translation, and protein modification, as seen in Figure 2–2 and discussed in the following section.

Transcription and Processing of Messenger RNA

mRNA is synthesized from a DNA template in the 5'-to-3' direction by the action of RNA polymerases.[37] RNA is similar to DNA except that the deoxyribose sugar of DNA is replaced by a ribose moiety in RNA, and instead of T, RNA contains the closely related pyrimidine, uracil (U). The synthesis of RNA on the DNA template is similar in principle to the process of DNA replication and involves the formation of complementary base pairs. In this instance, G is complementary to and pairs with C, but A is complementary to and pairs with U, in place of T. Thus, an mRNA carries a complementary replica of the sequences of bases present on the DNA template from which it is transcribed. This transcription initially results in the production of a precursor messenger RNA (pre-mRNA) that contains both intron and exon sequences. This molecule undergoes a series of processing steps before it is ready for delivery to the cell cytoplasm for translation. The introns are excised and the exons are ligated together in a two-stage splicing process that results in a mature mRNA that can be exported from the nucleus and translated to produce the desired protein. While still in the nucleus, the spliced mRNA undergoes further processing. The 5' end of the RNA is capped by a guanosine derivative, and a string of adenylic acid residues (polyA) is added to its 3' end to stabilize the transcript for transit within the cellular environment.

Once in the cytoplasm, the spliced and processed mRNA acts as a template for protein synthesis. In a separate series of events, amino acids are attached to transfer RNAs (tRNAs) by cellular enzymes. These charged tRNAs are then brought to the mRNA template, where they recognize the different codons that specify which particular amino acid is to be incorporated into the growing peptide chain (see Fig. 2–1). Protein synthesis occurs on ribosomes, each of which consists of a large and a small subunit composed of several proteins and ribosomal RNAs. The initiation of translation occurs when a ribosome encounters the initiation codon, AUG, and the corresponding initiator tRNA pairs with this codon. A second charged tRNA, specified by the next codon, is then brought into place, and the ribosome catalyzes the formation of a peptide bond between the two attached amino acids. The peptide chain is then extended as the ribosome moves along the mRNA, adding the prescribed amino acids to the growing protein. The ribosome moves over the mRNA in a 5'-to-3' direction from codon to codon until a specific termination codon is reached. The completed protein is then released from the translation complex. However, many proteins have to undergo a considerable amount of posttranslational modification before they are fully functional. These modifications include phosphorylation, glycosylation, and cleavage.

Regulation of Gene Expression

The expression of a gene can be under the guidance of a number of regulatory elements that either flank the coding sequence or lie within the sequence itself. Although a mammalian cell possesses the genetic instructions to make thousands of different proteins, only a subset of those proteins, perhaps 10% to 20%, is found in any single cell. This fact suggests that in each type of cell, some genes are expressed while others remain silent. Moreover, different sets of genes are expressed in different types of cells, and among those that are expressed, the actual amount of protein finally generated can vary as much as a millionfold. This means that in addition to the presence of the coding sequences, genes must also contain instructions that regulate the production of the proteins in the correct amounts, at the correct times, for each cell type.

As discussed, the most obvious and common area of regulation resides in the control of transcription, which directly affects the amount of mRNA produced from a single gene. Transcription can vary by many orders of magnitude. For example, the synthesis of mRNAs encoding the protein components of hemoglobin occurs at an extremely high rate in red blood cell precursors but at negligible levels in most other cells, even though all cells carry the genes for making hemoglobin proteins. Some knowledge does exist about the specific DNA sequences involved in gene activation. At the 5' and 3' ends of genes, there are sequences of varying lengths that determine the structure and length of the untranslated regions of mRNA. For example, the highly conserved AATAAA sequence in the 3' noncoding region of all mammalian genes is essential for the normal processing and polyadenylation of mRNA (see Fig. 2–2).

Most mammalian genes have blocks of sequences in their 5' flanking regions—the upstream regions—that are similar to those found in many other species, indicating their importance in the general phenomenon of gene regulation. These regions are involved in the regulation of transcription of mRNA. For this reason they are called *promoters,* or *upstream promoter elements,* and are believed to represent regions of DNA to which RNA polymerases or transcription factors bind and initiate RNA synthesis (see Fig. 2–2). It is apparent that other major regulatory elements are involved in determining whether genes are transcribed in particular tissues. These so-called enhancer elements may be located at some distance along the DNA chain from the structural genes whose expression they help regulate. However, they may be brought into close proximity to other promoter elements during control of gene expression via DNA bending. Many DNA-binding proteins interact with these enhancer and promoter elements, and several have been purified from nuclear extracts and biochemically characterized. These proteins fall into several different classes, distinguishable by particular structural motifs. They bind to specific regulatory regions close to, or at a distance from, particular genes and may help activate or suppress gene expression by altering the DNA-chromatin structure or by recruiting RNA polymerase or other transcription proteins to specific genes.

In addition to the regulatory elements of transcription detailed earlier, other factors can influence the general state of transcription. DNA exists in a highly compressed form in nuclei, complexed with histones and other proteins to constitute chromatin; major alterations in this chromatin structure can lead to changes in transcriptional activity in an individual cell. Another useful indicator of the state of gene activation lies in its degree of methylation; that is, actively transcribed genes are hypomethylated, and vice versa.

In addition to transcription, later steps in the overall process of gene expression also afford points of control. Beyond nuclear transcriptional activity, the concentration of mRNA can be regulated by its rate of transport from the nucleus to the ribosomes, where translation occurs, and by the relative stability of the transcript in the cytoplasm. If the mRNA is stable, it can be used repeatedly to make new protein chains; if quickly degraded, its capacity to direct protein synthesis is correspondingly limited.

Still other constraints operate on translation, influencing, for example, the likelihood that a ribosome would use a given mRNA molecule as the template for protein synthesis.

In addition, the long- or short-term stability of a newly synthesized protein can determine whether it accumulates in a cell. Finally, posttranslational modifications of a protein can influence its biologic activity. Some proteins, for example, must have certain chemical groups—sugars or phosphates—attached to them to perform their normal functions; others must be cleaved at defined positions. Thus, the ability or inability to modify certain proteins can result in functional differences in various cell types. In summary, gene expression is regulated by a complex series of molecular events that often occur in response to external signals. Such regulation ensures that genes are expressed at their proper levels in the appropriate tissues during the various stages of development and differentiation.

CELL GROWTH AND REGULATION: SIGNAL TRANSDUCTION AND CELL DIVISION

Although understanding the mechanisms of gene regulation is important, determining the function of normal and abnormal genes has led to important insights into how cell division is turned on and off in the healthy organism.[4, 32] Many cellular genes associated with abnormal growth are involved in signal transduction and cell division pathways. Therefore, a review of signal transduction and the cell cycle provides some needed insight into the function of many genes and their effects on cellular growth and metabolism.[5, 6, 32]

Signal transduction is defined as the conversion of an extracellular signal (e.g., binding of a soluble growth factor ligand to its membrane-bound cellular receptor) into the series of intracellular events that results in a cellular function, as depicted in Figure 2–3.

After the ligand binds to a specific cell surface receptor, the consequent conformational change, usually receptor dimerization, results in its activation. The receptor then associates with a coupler protein, usually a G protein, which, in turn, binds to an effector. Effectors catalyze the production of small molecules that act as second messengers in the cell. These molecules bind to intracellular proteins that directly affect processes such as the opening of a channel that, for example, results in the flow of ions. The net effect is a physiologic process, such as muscle contraction, secretion, and cell growth. Some processes are promptly evoked. Others, such as cell division, require new protein synthesis, and the transcription factors involved in that process are also considered part of the signal transduction pathway.

For most receptor systems involved in oncogenic transformation, the ligands are growth factors that bind to transmembrane enzyme/receptors containing a *tyrosine kinase* domain. These membrane receptors are generally involved in the promotion of cellular growth and division, and they share a common structure: a single transmembrane glycoprotein consisting of an extracellular ligand-binding domain, a transmembrane region, and a cytoplasmic or intracellular kinase domain. On binding of its cognate ligand, receptor dimerization occurs. This is believed to allow molecular interactions between the adjacent cytoplasmic domains, and it results in the activation of kinase activity. Once activated, each of these receptors becomes autophosphorylated and phosphorylates other cellular substrates. Because signal transduction plays such a central and unifying role in the understanding of cell growth and regulation, a brief discussion of each class of signal transduction proteins follows.

Growth Factors

Growth factors and their receptors are believed to work via autocrine or paracrine mechanisms; that is, the growth factors produced and secreted by cells act directly on themselves or on neighboring cells. Normal cells commonly produce a number of factors, including transforming growth factor-α (TGF-α), related to epidermal growth factor (EGF); TGF-β, a family of factors structurally unrelated to the EGF family; platelet-derived growth factor (PDGF); fibroblast growth factor; and insulin-like growth factor. In addition, under normal physiologic circumstances, certain growth factors, such as EGF and PDGF, are produced at a few major sites, from which they enter the systemic circulation to act on distant targets.

Growth Factor Receptors

Structurally, nearly all the receptors involved in human cancers share a distinct pattern: a typically glycosylated extracytoplasmic domain that binds the growth factor and a single transmembrane domain that connects the external and intracytoplasmic regions together.[47] The internal domain may be responsible for interacting with G proteins (discussed later). When receptors bind growth factors, they undergo a conformational change leading to their dimerization, which, in turn, activates the kinase portion. The first substrate to be phosphorylated is the receptor itself. Phospholipase C (PLC, discussed later), one of the effector molecules of signal transduction, then couples directly with the receptor.

Several proteins possess tyrosine kinase activity yet have neither an extracellular domain nor a ligand-binding region. (The *src* oncogene exemplifies this class of proteins.) They are tethered to the membrane by a modified lipid, but until recently, it was unclear how they were otherwise coupled to a classic signal transduction cascade. It had been known for some time that the members of the *src* family have in common two domains, called SH2 and SH3 (for *src* homology). A recent discovery is that many non-*src* proteins also possess SH2 domains that can bind to tyrosine-phosphorylated proteins.[33] This provides a novel interaction between signal transduction proteins and either receptors or substrates. In addition, it has been shown that SH3 domains can bind to proteins that regulate G proteins. Thus, the *src*-like proteins may interact with all the standard components of a signal transduction system via the SH2 and SH3 interactions.

Transducers of Growth Factor Responses

G Proteins. The typical G protein involved in receptor signaling is made up of three subunits: α, β, and γ. The α subunit binds the nucleotide guanosine diphosphate (GDP) and, when activated via receptor interaction, exchanges GDP for guanosine triphosphate (GTP), which renders the G protein active and able to stimulate an effector molecule. An endogenous guanosine triphosphatase (GTPase) activity then hydrolyzes GTP to GDP, deactivating the G protein. In addition to heterotrimeric G proteins, single polypeptide proteins similar to the α subunit of the heterotrimeric G protein, called the *small-G proteins*, bind GTP. The prototypes of these small-G proteins are the *ras* oncogenes: Ha-*ras*, Ki-*ras*, and N-*ras*.

Although originally discovered through both retroviral oncogenic and chemical carcinogenetic studies in animals, the *ras* oncogene has had a major influence on the field of oncogenes and signal transduction because it was one of the first oncogenes to be linked directly to human tumors. In 1979, researchers had shown that cells transformed by a chemical carcinogen carried an active oncogene, suggesting that oncogenes were a target for the chemical. Later work showed that *ras* was activated in both the chemically transformed cells and human bladder cancer cells, thus establishing the link to a specific human tumor.

The three *ras* genes have a remarkably similar mechanism

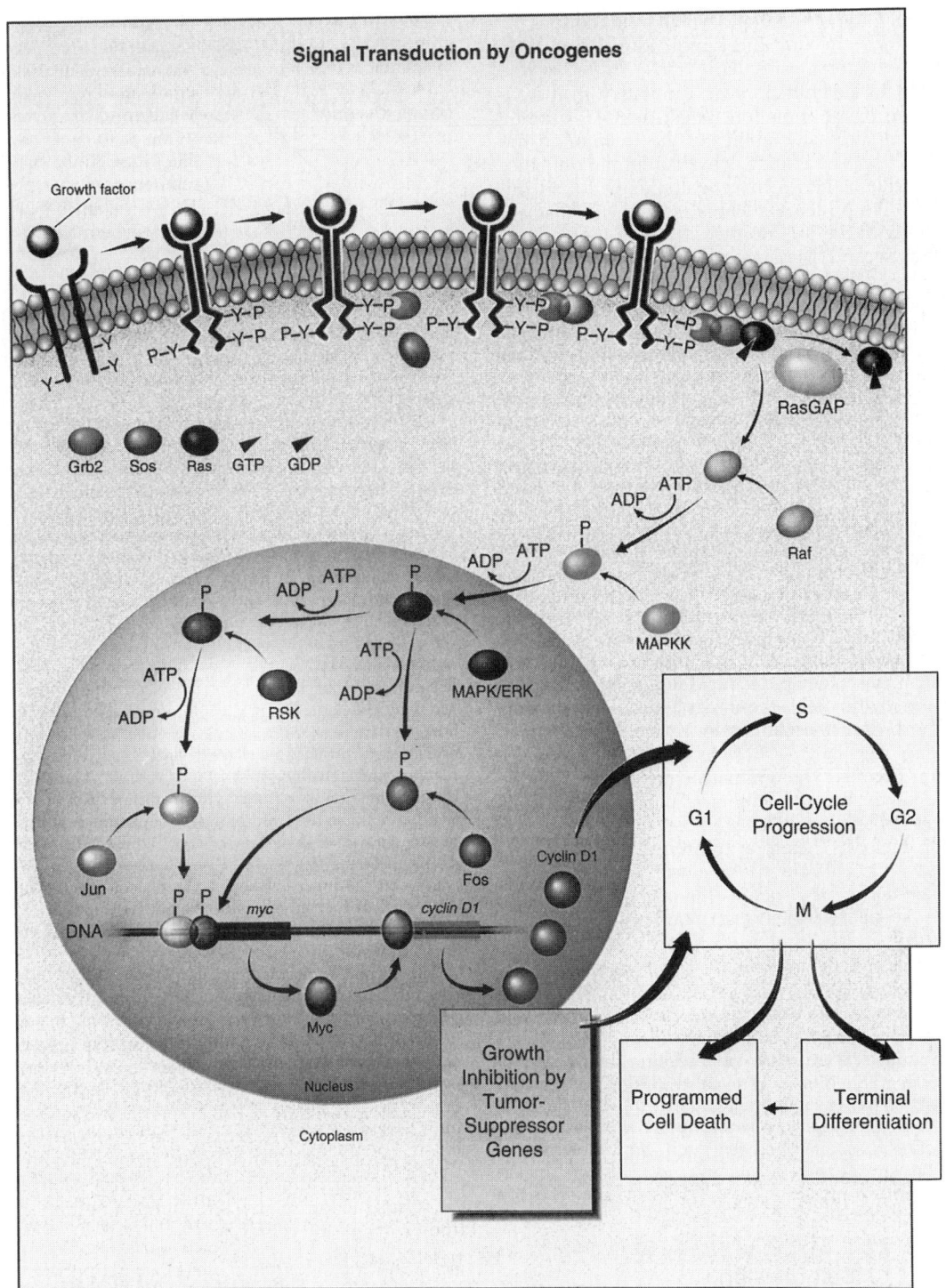

Figure 2–3. Mitogenic signal transduction through a series of proteins encoded by oncogenes. In the cell cycle, the progression from DNA synthesis (S) to mitosis (M) includes phases before (G$_1$) and after (G$_2$) the replication of DNA. On receiving signals to differentiate, cells leave the cycle and enter the pathway of terminal differentiation. Under certain circumstances, cells may enter the pathway to programmed cell death, or apoptosis.

Signal transduction begins with the binding of a growth factor to its transmembrane receptor (upper left-hand corner). Usually, the next step is the dimerization of the receptor. The receptor subunits then phosphorylate one another on tyrosine residues (Y). The phosphotyrosines (P) create docking sites on the receptor for many proteins, some of which undergo phosphorylation, whereas others recruit multicomponent complexes to the plasma membrane. One such interaction, shown here, is the activation of the Ras guanosine triphosphatase (GTPase).

In the cascade of phosphorylation initiated by the activation of Ras, the Raf kinase phosphorylates another kinase (mitogen-activated protein kinase kinase [MAPKK]), which in turn phosphorylates a third kinase, the mitogen-activated protein kinase (MAPK). (MAPK is also known as extracellular signal-regulated kinase [ERK].) MAPK directly activates transcription factors and ribosomal S6 protein kinase (RSK), which also phosphorylates transcription factors. MAPK probably represents at lease two related proteins.

For clarity, only two transcription proteins, Fos and Jun, are shown. They join to form a fully active transcription factor. The phosphorylation of Fos by MAPK, and of Jun by RSK, causes them to bind to specific DNA sequences near the *myc* gene, thereby initiating transcription of the gene. The Myc protein itself is a transcription factor with several binding partners (not shown). The binding of Myc to its specific recognition sites on DNA activates another set of genes. An important member of this set, *cyclin D1*, initiates the progression of cells through G$_1$ to the S-phase. (Reprinted by permission of *The New England Journal of Medicine* from Krontiris, T. G.: Oncogenes. N. Engl. J. Med., *333*[5]:303–306, Copyright 1995, Massachusetts Medical Society.)

of activation involving point mutations that affect codons 12, 13, or 61. Mutations affecting the same codons have been found in human tumors, particularly those of the colon, where more than 40% of tumors bear a mutation in the Ki-*ras* or Ha-*ras* gene. These mutations affect the GTP binding region, thereby impairing the ability of the receptor to hydrolyze GTP and trapping it in an active conformation. Since the discovery of the *ras* genes, investigators have found numerous other *ras*-like proteins, such as *rac* and *rho*, that apparently interact with the SH3 domains of other proteins.

Effectors and Second Messengers. The effector protein most definitively linked to an oncogenic receptor is PLC. This family has at least seven members, but only the γ form interacts with tyrosine kinase receptors. PLC-γ contains SH2 domains that mediate direct binding to some but not all tyrosine kinase receptors. Phosphorylation by the growth factor receptor activates PLC-γ so that it cleaves phosphatidylinositol into inositol triphosphate (IP_3) and diacylglycerol (DAG), both potent second messengers.[3] Because PLC-γ does not interact with all receptors, other effector molecules such as phosphatidylinositol-3 kinase must play important roles as well.

As stated earlier, the signal transduction pathway of PLC has two arms, IP_3 and DAG. IP_3 binds to specific intracellular receptors—in particular, ion channels that allow the efflux of Ca^{2+}. These ions then activate a wide variety of proteins, such as proteases and calmodulin. The second activation sequence, initiated by DAG, activates protein kinase C, a serine-threonine kinase that phosphorylates a wide variety of other proteins. Ultimately, these signals are sent to the nucleus, but the precise mechanism by which they are sent is unclear.

Transcription Factors. The ultimate consequence of the activation of growth factor receptors is cell division. This process involves protein synthesis and, hence, the activation of transcription factors. Therefore, transcription factors are believed to play a critical role in the control of cell growth. It is clear that certain genes, such as the oncogenes *fos*, *jun*, and *myc*, are responsible for the transcription of new genes in response to growth factors, and, in fact, each was originally identified in an oncogenic retrovirus. The *myc* family has three members (c-*myc*, L-*myc*, and N-*myc*), and each has a strong association with human cancer. The c-*myc* gene is activated by the chromosome 8;14 translocation of endemic Burkitt's lymphoma and is frequently amplified in lung tumors, as is L-*myc*. The N-*myc* gene is amplified in neuroblastoma and has a strong correlation with poor prognosis. In addition to *fos*, *jun*, and *myc*, many other putative transcription factors have been identified, including some that fall under the classification of tumor-suppressor genes, such as p53, and the Wilms' tumor genes WT-1 and WT-2.

Cell Division

In addition to the fundamental understanding of cell growth and regulation that has been elucidated from the study of signal transduction pathways, a second line of basic studies involving oncogenes and their proteins has led to a new understanding of the regulation of the cell cycle. Studies have identified a set of genes and their products that are essential for progression of cells through the division cycle, as depicted in Figure 2–4.

The cyclins, proteins that increase or decrease at different stages of the cell cycle, regulate cyclin-dependent kinases, which in turn phosphorylate critical targets at specific points in the cell cycle. In addition to the cyclin control of cell division, another set of genes appears to regulate the cell cycle at a series of points that may serve to stop progression

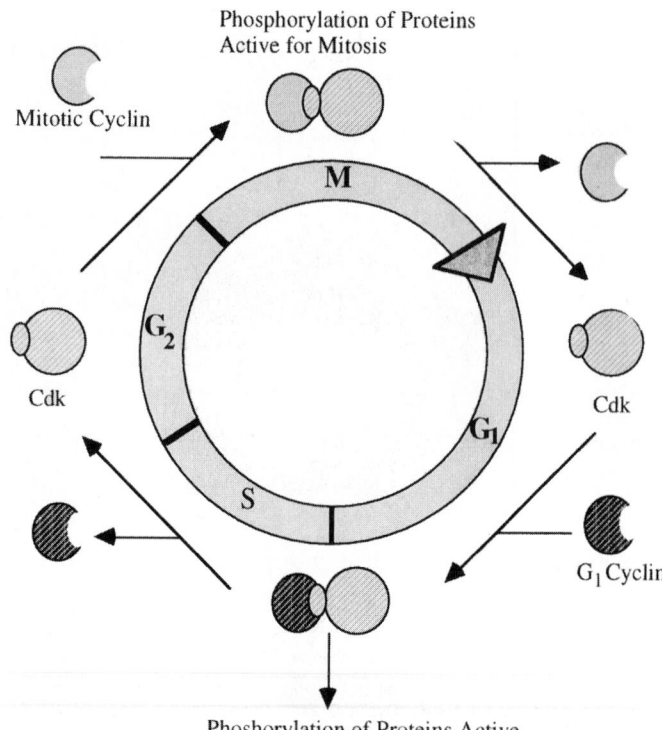

Figure 2–4. Through their association with the cyclin proteins, the cyclin-dependent kinases (Cdks) regulate cell cycle events by phosphorylating selected proteins critical to the different phases.

of the cell cycle if something has gone wrong, as shown in Figure 2–5.

For example, the proto-oncogene cyclin D1 regulates another proto-oncogene, cyclin-dependent kinase 4, which phosphorylates the tumor-suppressor gene product *Rb* in the late G_1 phase of the cell cycle. This releases the transcription factor E2F-1 and promotes entry into S-phase. When the DNA in a cell is damaged, a checkpoint control mechanism is activated and causes the p53 tumor-suppressor gene product to rise. This leads to the enhanced synthesis of a protein that blocks the activity of cyclin-dependent kinase 4; the *Rb* protein is no longer phosphorylated by this kinase, and the cell is blocked in late G_1. This then permits time in G_1 for the cell to repair its DNA damage before faulty genetic information is propagated. This series of events emphasizes how oncogenes and tumor-suppressor genes, along with the signal transduction pathways, interact within the complete framework of the cell cycle.

THE HUMAN GENOME

Current estimates of the human genome put it between 3 and 3.5×10^9 base pairs. However, it is apparent that more than half the human genome consists of noncoding DNA of no known function, so-called junk DNA. It has been estimated that there may be somewhere between 50,000 and 200,000 important genes to be found and mapped.[16, 31a]

A number of critical tools are required to analyze these genes. Restriction endonucleases are enzymes that occur naturally, mainly in bacteria and that cleave foreign DNA. For example, if DNA from one strain of *Escherichia coli* is introduced into another strain, it is fragmented by the host restriction endonucleases; the bacterium's own DNA is not attached because its vulnerable sites are protected by methylation. The restriction enzymes used most commonly in genetic engi-

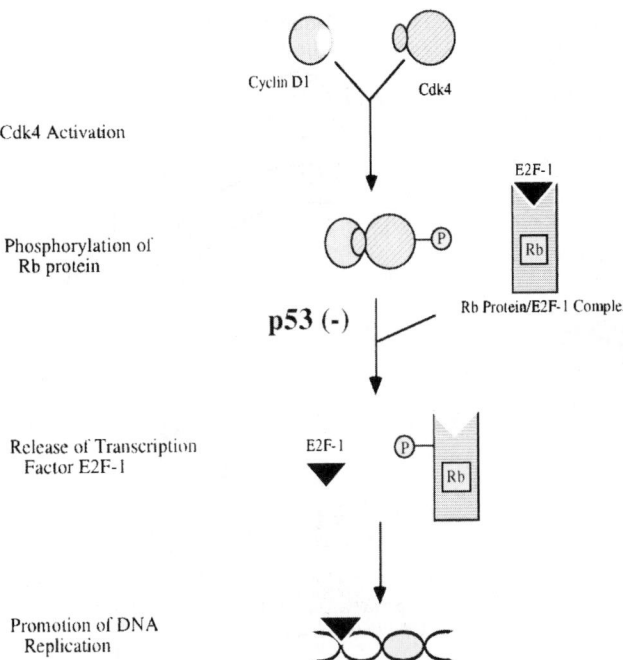

Cyclin D1   Cdk4

Cdk4 Activation

E2F-1

Phosphorylation of
Rb protein

Rb

p53 (-)

Rb Protein/E2F-1 Complex

Release of Transcription
Factor E2F-1

E2F-1   P

Rb

Promotion of DNA
Replication

Figure 2–5. Regulation of the cell cycle involves the action of proto-oncogenes and tumor-suppressor genes. Cyclin D association with cyclin-dependent kinase 4 (Cdk4) results in kinase activation and subsequent phosphorylation of the retinoblastoma (Rb) protein/E2F-1 transcription factor complex. This causes release of E2F-1, which promotes entry into the S-phase. The tumor-suppressor gene *p53* inhibits the association of Cdk4 with cyclin D1 by increasing the production of an inhibitory protein.

neering recognize signals consisting of a specific sequence of bases, often palindromes such as GAATTC, which is recognized by the restriction enzyme *Eco* RI. More than 400 restriction enzymes with 100 different specificities have now been isolated, many of which are in regular use for recombinant DNA technology.

The insertion of human DNA into bacterial plasmids or bacteriophage is the keystone of recombinant DNA technology (Fig. 2–6). Plasmids are closed, circular DNA molecules that replicate autonomously in bacteria. A plasmid has an origin of replication, which means that it can be replicated in a bacterium by exploiting the latter's DNA-synthesizing machinery. It usually contains one or two genes for antibiotic resistance and sites where restriction enzymes can cleave the DNA circle, thereby opening it to produce a linear molecule. The DNA to be inserted into the plasmid is fragmented by the same restriction enzyme. Plasmid and DNA fragments are then mixed and associate with each other by virtue of the *sticky* ends of the DNA. A permanent union is achieved by adding an enzyme called *DNA ligase*. Some plasmids rejoin and form the original circular DNA, but others, recombinants, incorporate the foreign DNA. Suitable bacteria are then transformed by the plasmids (i.e., plasmids and bacteria are mixed, and a small number of plasmids enter the bacteria). The frequency of transformation is such that each bacterium usually contains only one plasmid. The latter are selected by a variety of microbiologic tricks, usually by allowing the recombinant plasmids to confer antibiotic resistance on their bacterial hosts and growing the latter on selected media. Bacterial colonies can be screened by hybridization with appropriate gene probes for the presence of foreign DNA inserts, and when such a colony is identified, it can be grown in large quantities to provide the required DNA fragment.[38]

Southern Blotting

It is often desirable to identify an individual DNA fragment in a complex mixture that has been resolved by gel electrophoresis. This is accomplished by a technique termed *Southern blotting* (Fig. 2–7), used to transfer DNA from its position in an agarose gel to a nitrocellulose or nylon filter placed directly above the gel. The DNA is denatured, neutralized, and transferred in a high-salt buffer by capillary action. The denatured, single-stranded DNA binds to the filter, is permanently bonded by baking the filter (or by ultraviolet cross-linking), and is later hybridized to a radiolabeled probe to detect hybridizing DNA species. This approach is widely used to identify specific fragments in a digest of total genomic DNA.

Polymerase Chain Reaction

Recently, some ingenious techniques have been developed for increasing the speed of analysis of human DNA. The polymerase chain reaction (PCR) is a rapid procedure for *in vitro* enzymatic amplification of a specific segment of DNA (see Fig. 2–6). The theoretic basis of PCR is amplification of a specific DNA molecule. There are three nucleic acid segments: the segment of double-stranded DNA to be amplified and two single-stranded oligonucleotide primers flanking this segment. Additionally, there are a protein component (a DNA polymerase), appropriate deoxynucleotide triphosphates to be used to generate new fragments of DNA, a buffer, and salts.

The primers are added in vast excess compared with the DNA to be amplified. They hybridize to opposite strands of the DNA and are oriented with their 3′ ends facing each other, so that synthesis by DNA polymerase (which catalyzes growth of new strands in a 5′-to-3′ direction) extends across the segment of DNA between them. One round of synthesis results in new strands of indeterminate length that, like the parental strands, can hybridize to the primers on denaturation and annealing. These products accumulate only arithmetically with each subsequent cycle of denaturation, annealing to the primers, and synthesis. However, the second cycle of denaturation, annealing, and synthesis produces two single-stranded products that together compose a discrete double-stranded product that is exactly the length between the primer ends. Each strand of this discrete product is complementary to one of the two primers and can therefore participate as a template in subsequent cycles. The amount of this product doubles with every subsequent cycle of synthesis, denaturation, and annealing, accumulating exponentially so that 30 cycles should result in a great amplification of the discrete product.[44]

Genetic Mapping

A genetic map consists of a collection of polymorphic markers ordered not by physical means but by linkage studies—the more often two markers are inherited together in a family, the closer they are presumed to be in the genome.[18] Because these markers are followed through families, it is necessary for them to be polymorphic so that individual chromosomes within the family can be distinguished (Fig. 2–8). The unit of measurement is that of recombination; markers 1 centimorgan (cM.) apart are said to be separated by a recombination event approximately once every 100 meioses. The physical distance corresponding to 1 cM. varies within the genome, because some regions are more prone to recombination than others; on the average, however, 1 cM. is equivalent to approximately 1 million bases.

The polymorphic marker traditionally used to generate genetic maps is the restriction fragment length polymor-

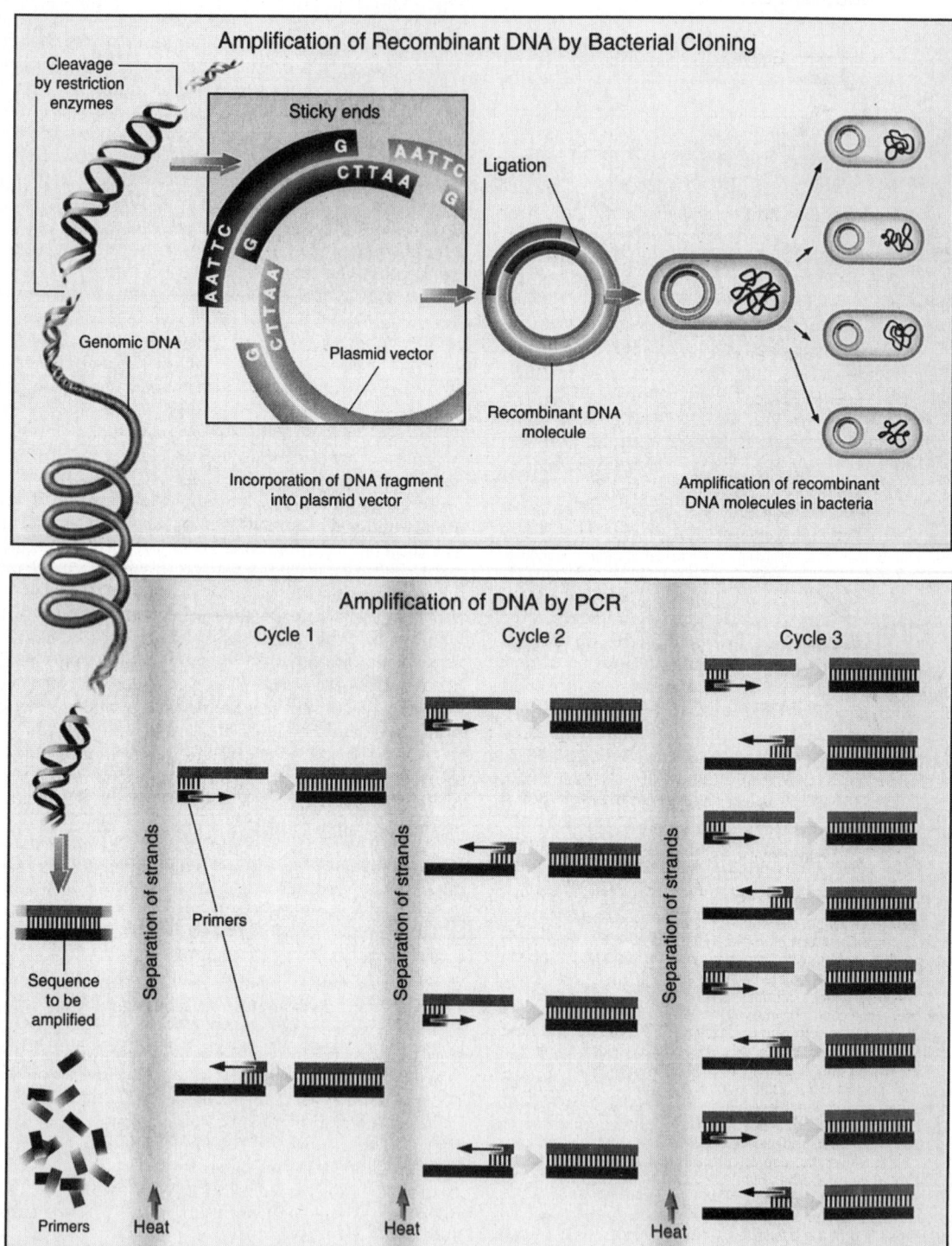

Figure 2–6. Amplification of recombinant DNA and amplification by polymerase chain reaction (PCR). In the amplification of recombinant DNA (top panel), the DNA segment to be amplified is separated from surrounding genomic DNA by cleavage with a restriction enzyme. The enzymatic cuts often produce staggered or *sticky* ends. In the example shown here, the restriction enzyme *Eco*RI recognizes the sequence GAATTC and cuts each strand between guanine (G) and adenine (A); the two strands of the genomic DNA are shown as black (C denotes cytosine and T, thymine). The same restriction enzyme cuts the circular plasmid DNA (gray) at a single site, generating sticky ends that are complementary to the sticky ends of the genomic DNA fragment. The cut genomic DNA and the remainder of the plasmid, when mixed together in the presence of a ligase enzyme, form smooth joints on each side of the plasmid-genomic DNA junction. This new molecule—recombinant DNA—is carried into bacteria, which replicate the plasmid as they grow in culture.

In the amplification of DNA by PCR (bottom panel), the DNA sequence to be amplified is selected by primers, which are short, synthetic oligonucleotides that correspond to sequences flanking the DNA to be amplified. After an excess of primers is added to the DNA, together with a heat-stable DNA polymerase, the strands of both the genomic DNA and the primers are separated by heating and allowed to cool. A heat-stable polymerase elongates the primers on either strand, thus generating two new, identical double-stranded DNA molecules and doubling the number of DNA fragments. Each cycle takes just a few minutes and doubles the number of copies of the original DNA fragment. (Reprinted by permission of *The New England Journal of Medicine* from Rosenthal, N.: Tools of the trade: Recombinant DNA. N. Engl. J. Med., *331*[5]:315–317, Copyright 1994, Massachusetts Medical Society.)

Southern Blotting

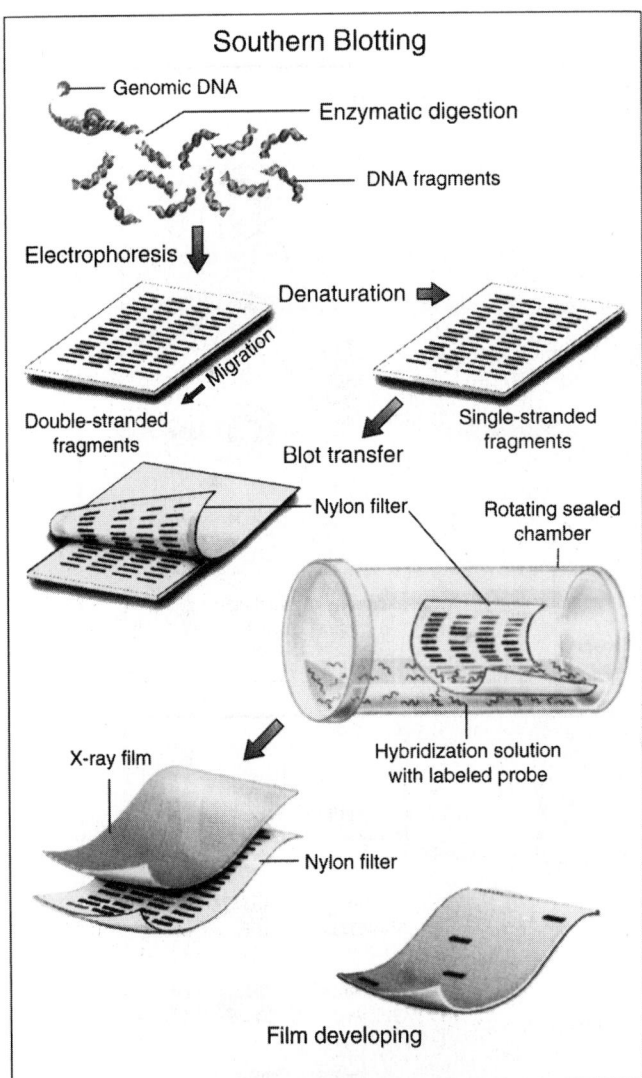

Genomic DNA — Enzymatic digestion

DNA fragments

Electrophoresis

Denaturation

Migration

Double-stranded fragments

Single-stranded fragments

Blot transfer

Nylon filter

Rotating sealed chamber

X-ray film

Hybridization solution with labeled probe

Nylon filter

Film developing

Figure 2–7. Analysis of DNA by gel electrophoresis and Southern blotting. The procedure is termed *Southern blotting* when DNA is analyzed and *Northern blotting* when RNA is analyzed. In Southern blotting, genomic DNA is cut with restriction enzymes into fragments before being separated according to size by gel electrophoresis. The four lanes on the gel represent the digestion of the DNA with four different restriction enzymes. In Northern blotting, total cellular RNA, including messenger RNA, can also be separated according to size. After electrophoresis, the nucleic acids in the gel are transferred directly onto a charged nylon filter to which they are tightly bound. Thus, the filter contains a precise replica of the nucleic acid distribution in the gel. The filter is then hybridized in a rotating sealed chamber with a DNA or RNA probe specific for the target of interest (in this instance, sequences in a microbial pathogen). Probes have traditionally been radioactively labeled with nucleotides containing phosphorus-32; however, the use of nonradiolabeled probes is becoming more common. After the probe has hybridized to its target sequence, the nonhybridized probe is washed away and the filter is exposed to x-ray film. A DNA sequence complementary to the probe is seen as a dark band on the developed film. The position of the hybridized target sequence in each lane is unique to the restriction enzyme used to digest the DNA. (Reprinted by permission of *The New England Journal of Medicine* from Naber, S. P.: Molecular pathology: Diagnosis of infectious disease. N. Engl. J. Med., *331*[18]:1212–1215, Copyright 1994, Massachusetts Medical Society.)

phism (RFLP). As soon as restriction enzymes were discovered and human DNA was digested, it became clear that humans show a remarkable variability in the structure of DNA. Single-base changes in the genetic code may result in the production of the identical protein and may in themselves be harmless. Single-base polymorphisms occur on average every few hundred kilobases and can be detected by means of several techniques. For example, these single-base changes

can be identified by the fact that they alter the cutting sites for restriction enzymes, as depicted in Figure 2–8. Thus, the size of the DNA fragments generated by those enzymes varies. By using a series of different enzymes that cleave the DNA either within or outside the gene or genes being studied, and by orienting some of the fragments in the appropriate direction, it is possible to build up restriction enzyme maps to certain areas of the genome. Almost all these markers have only two alleles at each locus (presence or absence of a restriction site) and are therefore limited in their informativeness (i.e., the ability to differentiate between individuals). However, RFLPs can be extremely valuable genetic markers if their chromosomal location can be identified, because they are then excellent markers for linkage analyses.

In addition to RFLPs, there are some regions of DNA scattered about the genome that are highly polymorphic and often represent blocks of repeated segments of DNA, varying in length from person to person. Such minisatellite or microsatellite DNA has turned out to be a particularly valuable source of linkage markers.[31]

Physical Mapping

Physical mapping has also moved forward quickly. At low resolution, one of the most useful approaches has been a technique called *somatic cell hybridization*. If human cells and rodent tumor cells are cultured together with Sendai virus, they tend to fuse together. After fusion, the chromosomes of each cell become mixed together, and many of them are subsequently lost from the now-hybrid cell; human chromosomes are preferentially lost in a random fashion. Thus, it is possible to propagate cells in culture that contain only a limited number of human chromosomes, allowing for the creation of a panel of such somatic cell hybrids. These can then be used to assign human genes to particular chromosomes by looking for the products of those genes in hybrid lines that contain only a select number of human chromosomes.

Genes can also be assigned to chromosomes by a technique known as in situ *hybridization,* in which a radioactive probe for the particular gene is used to hybridize directly to complementary sequences on a particular chromosome (Fig. 2–9). Recently, the development of highly sophisticated microscopic techniques has revolutionized the field of chromosomal analysis. For example, the development of multichannel confocal fluorescent microscopy has made it possible to label entire chromosomes with chromosome-specific libraries, a procedure referred to as *chromosome painting.* Furthermore, equally sophisticated techniques have been developed for sorting human chromosomes and isolating them.

At higher resolution, physical mapping involves the isolation of chromosomal DNA, the fragmentation of the DNA by restriction enzymes, the generation of a library of cloned fragments, and the ordering of the clones to reflect the original order of the particular fragments along the chromosome. This approach can be used to link the physical and genetic mapping techniques. For example, starting with an RFLP marker, it is possible to build up a series of overlapping phage or cosmid clones and, in essence, walk along the chromosome until the gene of interest is encountered. All these techniques have been facilitated by the increasing ability to handle larger pieces of DNA by cloning into yeast. Finally, it is often possible to obtain clues to where specific genes may be by studying patients with a particular phenotype associated with a chromosomal abnormality, such as a deletion. In these instances, it is reasonable to assume that the patients' clinical picture may be related to loss of genetic material in the deleted region of DNA. Thus, the deletion can serve as a reference point for locating a specific gene.

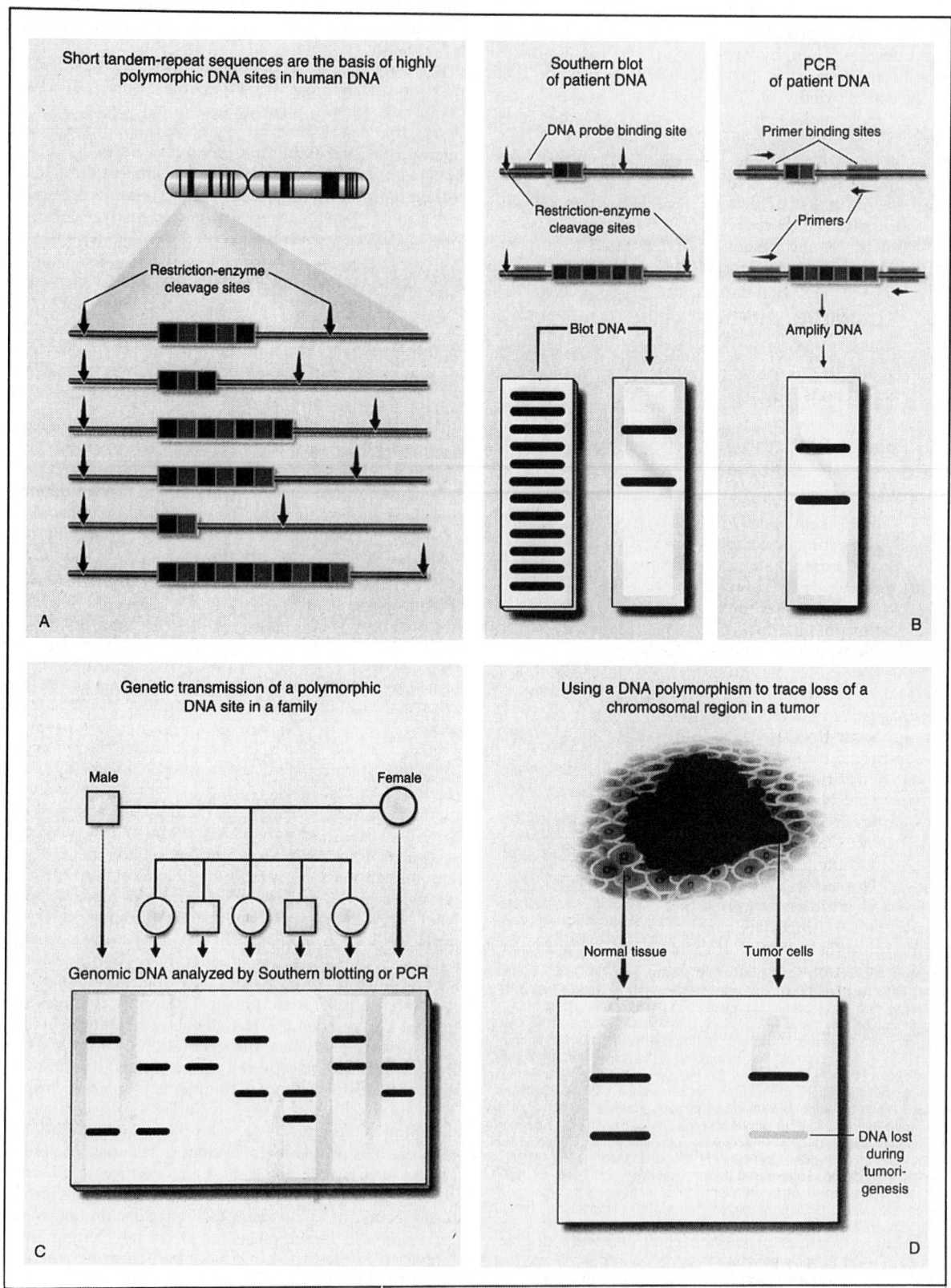

Figure 2–8 *See legend on opposite page*

Mapping techniques of this type have led to some remarkable success stories in clinical genetics. In particular, it has been possible to discover the underlying cause of some important genetic diseases. The first step is to define an RFLP linkage, which may approach within a few million bases of the gene in question. Then, by various chromosomal walking or jumping techniques, it is possible to move toward the gene and eventually define it. The next step is to sequence the gene and then make educated guesses regarding the likely protein structure and physiologic function encoded by such a sequence. Finally, the mutations in the gene are determined, and insights are gained into how these changes might affect the normal structural and functional integrity of the protein product. The discoveries of the genetic effects in Duchenne's dystrophy and cystic fibrosis are prime examples of the power of this approach.

CLINICAL APPLICATIONS

It is beyond the scope of this chapter to outline all the possible clinical applications of molecular biology to surgery. In the following sections, specific examples are considered.

Molecular Pathology of Single-Gene Disorders

Although it has only been a few years since the first human gene was cloned and sequenced, a great deal of progress has been made in dissecting the molecular basis of disease in disorders resulting from a disorder of a single gene. One of the most informative diseases includes the inherited hemoglobin disorders, of which examples exist that represent the broad spectrum of possible mutations, including single-base changes or deletions, and deletions of entire genes. Furthermore, mutations include insertions of new genetic material and inversions of stretches of DNA. Finally, in addition to mutations that directly affect the encoded protein product, mutations can occur that affect the regulatory regions of the gene that control the transcription and ultimately expression, as well as base substitutions that interfere with the processing or translation of mRNAs.

These examples provide evidence for two broad classifications of mutations. Obviously, there are those mutations that result in altered protein products. Most of these mutations involve single-base substitutions, which may continue to encode for the same amino acid (a so-called polymorphism), or a single-base substitution may cause a single amino acid substitution within the encoded protein, a so-called missense mutation. A single amino acid mutation, especially at a noncritical location within the protein, may cause no ill effects in many cases. However, a single amino acid substitution in a critical location within the protein may change the function

or stability of the protein and may result in a clinical disorder. The best known example of this type of mutation is in sickle cell disease, in which a single-base substitution results in a single amino acid substitution (a valine for an aspartic acid in position 6 of the β-globin chain), which leads to sickle cell disease.

The other class of mutations concerns those that cause the defective synthesis of proteins without changing their structure. For example, mutations that affect the promotor region of a gene may lead to a decrease in the ability of RNA polymerase to bind and actively transcribe the gene, resulting in a decrease in expression of the normal protein; that is, it would be present, but in smaller quantities. In addition, the stability of mRNA is critical for translation, and mutations that would have an effect on the rate at which the RNA of a gene was transported or degraded would have a similar effect on the expression of the normal protein.

There are a number of other examples of mutations that can profoundly influence the expression of a mammalian gene. For example, a base substitution that results not in a substituted amino acid but rather an instruction for RNA processing has a profound influence on gene expression. A base substitution may produce a premature stop codon, so that when the mRNA is translated, rather than producing a full-length polypeptide molecule, translation will be terminated prematurely, resulting in only shortened and functionally useless peptide chains being produced. Such lesions are called *nonsense mutations,* and they result in truncated protein. Many of the mutations found in the gene associated with hereditary breast cancer, *BRCA-1,* have been found to be nonsense mutations, resulting in truncated protein production.

Another major result from an apparently minor base loss or insertion can result because amino acids are encoded by a triplet code; that is, they are read as a set of three base pairs. For example, the triplets AAA-GAA-AAT-ATC would encode a protein with an amino acid sequence of lysine-glutamine-asparagine-isoleucine. A loss of the first adenosine would result in a series of triplets AAG-AAA-ATA-TC that would encode a protein with an amino acid sequence arginine-lysine-isoleucine. The loss of reading frame that results from the loss or insertion of one, two, or four bases in a gene results in an mRNA that cannot be translated beyond the frame shift.

Finally, even more subtle changes can result in massive aberrations in the types of protein product being encoded. As mentioned earlier, most genes have their coding regions (exons) divided into several pieces of introns. Because the introns have to be cut out and the exons precisely spliced together before the mRNA moves into the cell cytoplasm, several types of single-gene disorders can result from mutations that interfere with this splicing mechanism. Single-base

---

Figure 2–8. Visualization of highly variable DNA sequences in human DNA. Variable-length sequences in human DNA can be created by variations in the number of copies of a tandem-repeat DNA sequences *(A)*. Each line in the figure represents a copy of a human DNA sequence. The copies are identical in sequence except for the tandemly repeated DNA sequence indicated by the boxes. The number of copies of the tandemly repeated DNA sequence is indicated by the number of boxes. The size of the DNA fragment that includes the tandem-repeat sequence is measured between two fixed points. In Southern blotting, the sites of restriction-enzyme digestion are the fixed points that determine the ends of the DNA fragment.

In *B*, the number of copies of the tandem-repeat sequence determines the total length of the fragment that can be visualized by Southern blotting. In the polymerase chain reaction (PCR), the binding sites of oligonucleotide primers are the fixed points that determine the ends of the DNA fragment. The number of copies of the tandem-repeat sequence determines the total length of the fragment that can be visualized by separating the products of the PCR reaction on a polyacrylamide gel.

In *C*, a family in which a highly polymorphic marker is used for genetic analysis is illustrated. Note that the two copies of the DNA fragment from the offspring can be distinguished from the two copies of the fragment from the father, making the inheritance pattern from each parent clear for this chromosomal site. Detection may be carried out by Southern blotting or PCR, depending on the size of the tandem-repeat sequence.

In *D*, a highly polymorphic site distinguishes the two copies of a chromosomal region in a person's normal cells. During tumorigenesis, one copy of the chromosomal region is lost. Only one of the variable DNA fragments (the one marking the chromosome that is not lost during tumorigenesis) remains in the tumor. A light band is evident in the tumor DNA sample at the position characteristic of the chromosomal region that has been lost during tumorigenesis, perhaps indicating contamination of the tumor sample by normal tissue. Detection may be carried out by Southern blotting or PCR, depending on the size of the tandem-repeat sequence. (Reprinted by permission of *The New England Journal of Medicine* from Housman, D.: Human DNA polymorphism. N. Engl. J. Med., *332*[5]:318–320, Copyright 1995, Massachusetts Medical Society.)

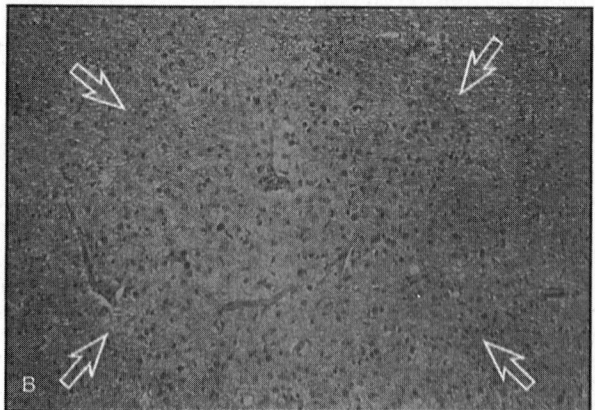

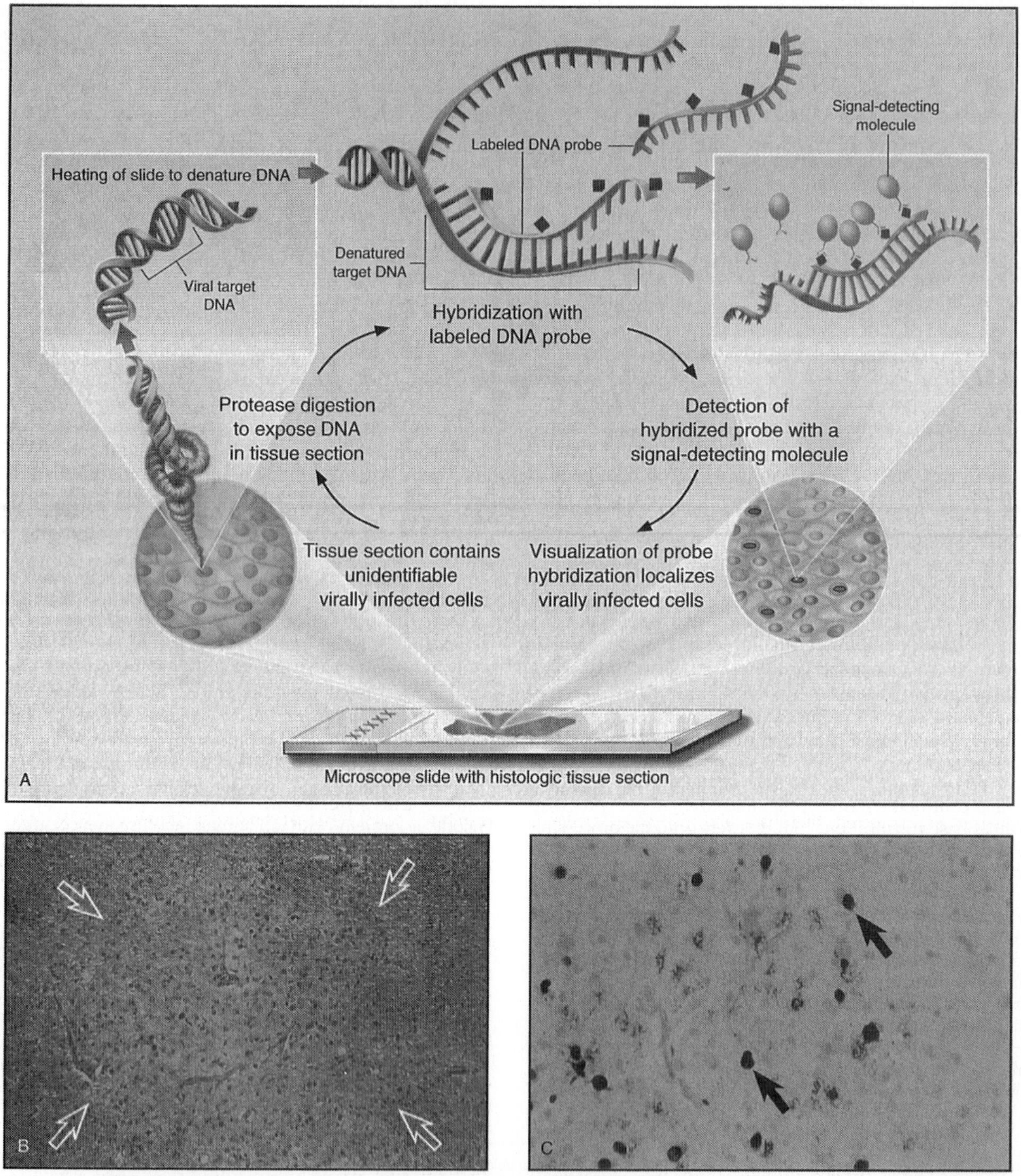

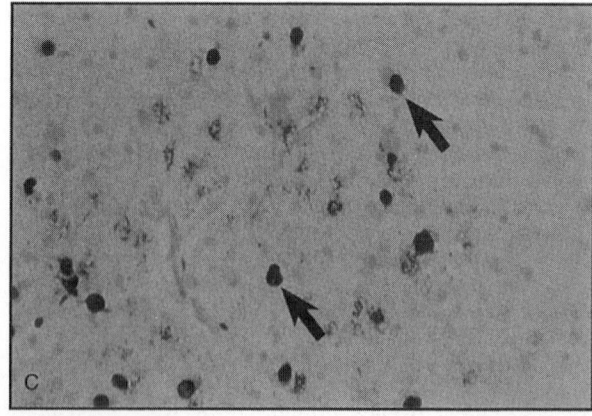

Figure 2–9. Detection of cells infected with a double-stranded DNA virus in a formalin-fixed, paraffin-embedded tissue section by *in situ* hybridization. In *A*, tissue fixation with formalin cross-links proteins and partially entraps the target DNA. Therefore, the tissue sections must be specially prepared to expose the target DNA for hybridization while preserving cellular morphology. The steps include digestion of the tissue section by a mild protease and heat denaturation of double-stranded DNA to single-stranded DNA to hybridize with the probe. The temperature is then lowered during an incubation of several hours, allowing the probe to hybridize to its complementary target DNA sequence. After the nonhybridized probe is washed away, the specifically bound probe can be detected by means of its label. In this example, the label incorporated into the probe is not radioactive; it can be detected by an antibody against the label or, in the case of a biotin-tagged probe, by means of avidin linked to a chromogenic substrate. The tissue section is then counterstained to reveal histologic details. The hybridization signal localizes the virally infected cells in the tissue section. This procedure can be completed in 1 day. *B* shows a section of cerebral white matter from a brain biopsy in a patient with progressive multifocal leukoencephalopathy. The Luxol fast blue stain reveals a pale area of demyelination (arrows) with numerous glial cells, which are predominantly oligonucleotides (×75). *C* shows the results of in situ hybridization of the lesion shown in *B* with a biotinylated DNA probe for JC virus. There is strong hybridization of the JC virus probe to oligodendrocytes in the demyelinated area (arrows) (×200). (Reprinted by permission of *The New England Journal of Medicine* from Naber, S. P.: Molecular pathology: Diagnosis of infectious disease. N. Engl. J. Med., *331*[18]:1212–1215, Copyright 1994, Massachusetts Medical Society.)

changes at the junctions between introns and exons may prevent correct splicing, resulting in the production of no normal mRNA. In addition, base changes within introns or exons can produce alternative splice sites, resulting in the production of normal and abnormally spliced mRNA. As expected, the presence of an exon within the protein reading frame results in a massive aberration within the mRNA, and this cannot be used as a template for peptide chain synthesis.

Thus, there may already exist a reasonable idea of the repertoire of molecular abnormalities underlying single-gene disorders. Recent studies of the appropriate genes of patients with Christmas disease, hemophilia, Duchenne's dystrophy, cystic fibrosis, growth hormone deficiency, antithrombin III deficiency, and low-density lipoprotein receptor deficiency support this prediction; the molecular pathology of these disorders is turning out to be similar to the thalassemias.

Common Polygenic Diseases

Although the single-gene disorders have provided information regarding the nature of abnormalities that can occur and disrupt the expression of specific protein, when common disorders are considered, the potential for even more subtle changes within the context of complementary or confounding aberrations to have a profound influence on the cell function is enormous. For this reason, the complexities of more common disorders have not lent themselves to the molecular dissection portrayed in the less common single-gene disorders. In addition to the complexities involved in multiple-gene disorders evoked by the interaction of each of the genes involved, many of them have environmental factors that play a major role in their etiology.

Studies that have analyzed the occurrence of common diseases in identical twins have suggested that the genetic contribution and the clinical expression of the disease vary considerably between disorders. For example, the common form of maturity-onset diabetes, type II diabetes, can be considered a complex genetic disease, because if one of a pair of identical twins is affected, there is a high likelihood that the other twin will also become diabetic. Similar findings have been obtained in many common diseases, although often the genetic component is not as clear. However, for many common diseases little is known about the basic pathologic defect involved, except that in some instances environmental factors, such as smoking, control of blood glucose level, and diet in vascular disease, may play an important role. One of the principal reasons to identify a gene or genes that confer susceptibility to complex disorders is that an understanding of these genes and their function may lead to considerable insights into the underlying causes of these diseases.

There are several different approaches to defining the major genes in these complex polygenic systems. One is to find large families in which more than one member is affected. By using random RFLP linkage markers and carrying out extensive family studies, it might be possible to obtain a linkage to a susceptibility gene that could then be identified by reverse genetics. This approach has been used to identify a number of genes involved in inherited susceptibility to breast, ovarian, colon, and pancreatic cancer.

Another more elegant approach is to deduce which genes might be involved by postulating that the aberration of a particular function of a gene would lead to disease. For example, it would be reasonable to suppose that genes involved in cholesterol metabolism might be important in the pathogenesis of atherosclerosis. Thus, having isolated these so-called candidate genes and obtained appropriate RFLP

markers, family studies can be carried out to see if any polymorphisms segregate with a particular disease.

With these different approaches, considerable progress has already been made in defining some of the genes that are likely to be involved in susceptibility or resistance to common diseases. Useful progress has also been made in defining some of the major genes involved in susceptibility to coronary artery disease. For example, certain polymorphisms of the apolipoprotein genes involved in cholesterol and lipid metabolism seem to be strongly related to the development of premature vascular disease and obesity. It also seems likely that genetic variability in the coagulation system, particularly fibrinogen production, may be an important factor in the generation of coronary artery disease and myocardial infarction.

Cancer

The development of cancer is a complex, multistep process, originating in a phenotypically normal cell and culminating in the development of cells with deregulated growth characteristics and the ability to invade and metastasize. Cancer, even the nonhereditary forms, is considered a collection of polygenic disorders, because alterations in a number of genes have been shown to contribute to its origin and progression.[46] Generally, the genes that are altered in the development of cancer fall into three broad categories: (1) oncogenes, the presence of which may cause cellular transformation; (2) tumor-suppressor genes, the absence of which may cause cellular transformation; and (3) mutator genes. The genetic changes that are found in otherwise normal cells that lead to their transformation can be caused by inherited defects, in which case a hereditary predisposition to cancer is found.[1] In addition, genetic changes leading to cancer may be caused by DNA rearrangements during the cell cycle, viral infection, exposure to mutagenic agents, or inherited defects in DNA replication or repair.[43] These latter defects do not in themselves lead to transformation, but, as discussed later, may lead to an increase in the mutation rate in other genes directly responsible for the development of cancer.

Proto-oncogenes are genes present in normal cells that, when activated (to become oncogenes), may lead to the transformation of the cell.[42] The alterations that convert the normal cellular gene to its oncogenic counterpart include gene amplifications, translocations, and point mutations. Amplifications result from an increase in the copy number of the gene; translocations refer to the exchange of DNA segments between two chromosomes; and point mutations are single nucleotide changes or deletions that can result in an alteration of the gene product (discussed later).[9] When activated, oncogenes such as *ras, neu/erb B2,* and *myc* acquire or gain function and begin to act in a more dominant fashion. Therefore, mutations in a single allele may contribute to cancer development. About 70 oncogenes have been identified since the first oncogene (*src*) was discovered in 1975, and some of the more well-known ones are shown in Table 2–2.

In contrast with the proto-oncogenes and oncogenes, researchers have also identified about 12 tumor-suppressor genes. Tumor-suppressor genes are different from oncogenes in that it is their loss of function rather than gain of function that may contribute to cancer development. Unlike the oncogenes, mutations must occur in both alleles of a tumor-suppressor gene before it can contribute to a malignant phenotype. Although the first known tumor-suppressor gene (*Rb*) was not cloned until 1986, they have been found in recent years to be common defects in many cancers. For example, the tumor-suppressor gene p53 is mutated in as

TABLE 2–2. Normal Cellular Function of Commonly Encountered Oncogenes

Oncogene	Location in Cell	Function
sis	Secreted	Growth factor (PDGF)
erb B	Cell membrane	Part of EGF receptor
Her-2/neu (c-erb B2)	Cell membrane	Protein tyrosine kinase
src	Cell membrane	Protein tyrosine kinase
RET	Cell membrane	Protein tyrosine kinase
raf/mil	Cytoplasm	Protein serine kinase
ras	Cell membrane	GTP binding/ GTPase
myc	Nucleus	Transcription factor
fos	Nucleus	Transcription factor
jun	Nucleus	Transcription factor
bcl-1 (cyclin D1)	Nucleus	Activates cell cycle kinases
bcl-2	Internal membranes	Antagonizes programmed cell death

PDGF, platelet-derived growth factor; EGF, epidermal growth factor; GTP, guanosine triphosphate; GTPase, guanosine triphosphatase.

many as 50% of human cancers. In addition, a series of inherited cancer-susceptibility genes have been found to encode tumor-suppressor genes.

The third class of genes that contribute to cancer development, the mutator gene, is responsible for enhancing the fidelity of the DNA replication process. When mutator gene products fail to function, the mutation rate in the cell increases and an inherent predisposition to cancer is observed. Presumably, the tumor-suppressor genes and oncogenes may become mutated by this faulty DNA editing process. Other mutatable genes may be responsible for the repair of DNA damage that, when lost in a cell, also results in an inherent predisposition to a variety of cancers. The inability to repair DNA and the subsequent duplication of damaged genetic information result in a high DNA mutation rate, leading to an increase in activated oncogenes and inactivated tumor-suppressor genes.

Mechanisms of Proto-Oncogene Activation

Efforts to find out what causes the src gene of respiratory syncytial virus (RSV) to make cells cancerous led to an understanding of the mechanisms that convert a proto-oncogene to an oncogene. One early clue to the difference between the normal gene and its transforming counterpart was the finding that the RSV src gene is much more active than the normal cellular gene at producing its src protein. In addition, a comparison of the RSV src and cellular src revealed that the RSV src gene had undergone mutations making the encoded protein function more effectively, that is, a gain-of-function mutation. Together, these changes in the RSV src gene, leading to quantitative and qualitative changes in the RSV src gene product, provide a powerful growth stimulus to cells infected with RSV. Currently, a more complete understanding of the changes that can activate proto-oncogenes to oncogenes exists at the molecular level. The three molecular changes that can occur in a proto-oncogene that may convert it into an oncogene include gene amplification, translocation, and point mutation.

True gene amplification is caused by increased replication of the discrete locus where the gene is found, leading to production of many extra copies of the gene. Although the proto-oncogene is not altered itself, the extra copies of the proto-oncogene lead to an increase in the amount of protein encoded by the gene. The increase in the amount of protein leads to an increase in activity and therefore a gain of function. For example, gene amplification can produce as many as 50 extra copies of the EGF receptor gene in breast, skin, and glial tumors, leading to production of large amounts of the EGF receptor protein. Another example of amplification occurs in a related growth factor receptor called neu in the rat and its human homologue erb B2, also called HER-2. Increased production of the HER-2/neu gene product occurring partly as a consequence of gene amplification is found in approximately 30% of breast and ovarian cancers.

Another mechanism of oncogene activation involves the chromosomal abnormality called translocation, in which two chromosomes exchange segments.[9, 15, 17, 35, 41] The consequence of this exchange may be that genes are placed under regulatory elements that would not normally control them. For example, a gene placed downstream from a promoter element after translocation would be much more actively transcribed, resulting in an increase in mRNA and protein production. The increase in the amount of protein leads to an increase in activity and therefore a gain of function. In 1982, several researchers found that the myc oncogene is located at or near the translocation breakpoints in cells of the cancer called Burkitt's lymphoma; this shift in the proto-oncogene's position may place it adjacent to powerful promoter and/or enhancer elements, which may lead to its activation. Although translocation is one mechanism of proto-oncogene activation, it is by no means the exclusive mechanism by which myc is activated. In addition to activation by translocation, the myc proto-oncogene can also become activated by gene amplification, as seen in neuroblastoma and lung carcinoma.

A proto-oncogene may also be activated through a point mutation, a good example of which occurs in the oncogene ras. The ras gene has been found to have a mechanism of activation involving point mutations specifically affecting codons 12, 13, or 61. Mutations affecting the same codons of this highly conserved family of genes have been found in human tumors, particularly those of the colon and pancreas, where more than 40% and 80% of tumors, respectively, bear a mutation in the ras gene, leading to its activation. In addition, mutations that generate a stop codon result in the premature halting of protein translation and the truncation of the gene product. This mutated product and its function may be altered from the wild-type protein and may reflect a change to either an active or inactive state. In the case of oncogenes, the truncation that activates the proto-oncogene leads to the loss of a regulatory element, locking the protein in a constitutively active state, whereas the normal protein fluctuates between both inactive and active states. The increase in the amount of activated protein relative to the inactive protein leads to an increase in activity and therefore a gain of function.

Although understanding the mechanisms of proto-oncogene activation is important in understanding carcinogenesis, determining the normal function of proto-oncogenes has led to important insights into how cell division is turned on and off in the healthy organism. Some of the normal functions that have been widely found for the products of cellular proto-oncogenes involve signal transduction and cell division.

Molecular Oncogenesis

Although the presence of an oncogene can cause a cell to become transformed, the development of a cancer is a complex, multistep process in which a series of progressive changes culminates in deregulation of cell proliferation.[20] Therefore, a review of the understanding of the multiple steps required for the development of cancer, and the contributions of oncogenes, is presented. The best characterized model of stepwise carcinogenesis is the colon, which has been extensively studied by Fearon and Vogelstein.[11a] Carcinogenesis in the colon is appreciated to evolve through a series of pathologically recognizable steps, from hyperplastic epithelium to adenomatous polyps to invasive carcinoma. The first histologically recognized step in neoplasia is a shift in the normal epithelium to continuous proliferation, leading to the formation of an adenomatous polyp. With time, certain adenomas grow and undergo pathologic changes in their morphology (see Chapter 32).

As mentioned, several genetic abnormalities commonly occur during the genesis of colorectal carcinoma, and the cumulative total of genetic abnormalities appears to be more important than the order of their appearance. Most of the early genetic studies of colon cancer involved analysis of karyotype and large fragments of DNA; not surprisingly, the early abnormalities found in colon cancer were caused by deleted fragments of chromosomes. Consequently, a number of tumor-suppressor genes were implicated as loss-of-function mutations. Among the tumor-suppressor genes, deletion of the APC (*a*denomatous *p*olyposis *c*oli locus, on the long arm of chromosome 5) appears to be an early event. In addition to its association with familial colon cancer, the APC gene is deleted frequently in sporadic tumors, suggesting that it plays an important and early role in every type of colon carcinogenesis. In addition to deletion of APC, DNA methylation throughout the genome is an early event, detectable even in small adenomas. The deleted colorectal carcinoma (DCC) gene, on the long arm of chromosome 12, is also frequently detected in sporadic tumors. Deletion of this gene is much more frequent in carcinomas than in the adenomas from which they arose, suggesting that, rather than being important in the genesis of adenomas, DCC may play a role in the progression from adenoma to carcinoma. The gene most strikingly associated with the transition from adenoma to carcinoma is the p53 gene on the short arm of chromosome 17. Deletions and mutations of p53 are far more frequent in carcinomas than in adenomas, suggesting that it too may also play a role in the progression from adenoma to carcinoma.[12]

As more sophisticated methods of detecting genetic abnormalities became available, minor changes in the genome, including the presence of point mutations, could be detected. This led to an increase in the detection of acquired, single-allele events such as the activation of proto-oncogenes. Among the oncogenes, activating mutations in *ras*, on the short arm of chromosome 12, appear to be relatively early events in the adenoma-carcinoma sequence. These mutations commonly involve codon 12 of the Ki-*ras* gene. Similarly, activation of *src* also occurs in adenomas.

Recently, four genes that may be responsible for hereditary non-polyposis colorectal carcinoma in most kindreds have been isolated.[8] These genes are human homologues of the bacterial mut-HLS complex, involved in genetic proofreading (the repair of mismatched base pairs in DNA). Loss of this function is believed to allow base pair mismatches to accumulate, resulting in a replication-error phenotype that is seen in a high percentage of patients with hereditary non-polyposis colorectal cancer and approximately 15% of the cases of sporadic colon cancer.

Development, Differentiation, Repair, and Congenital Malformation

A major question in human biology is how a single fertilized egg with its 10^9 base pairs of DNA turns into a human being. This field of study has enormous implications for all aspects of clinical practice. It is becoming clear that developmental work in such an apparently unpromising organism as the fruit fly, *Drosophila*, has important implications for understanding major developmental abnormalities in humans. As in much of modern biologic research, the ideas are not new, but the availability of the tools of recombinant DNA technology allows them to be explored in a novel fashion. In 1894 Bateson suggested that the study of chance deviation in normal developmental patterns might provide clues about the rules that govern the regulation of development. This is turning out to be the case. For example, it has been found that the homeotic genes of *Drosophila*, which regulate the development of body segments, have DNA sequences in common with many other species, including humans. Furthermore, the products of these genes are expressed in different tissues during mammalian development. Homeotic mutations in insects result in major developmental abnormalities, including substitutions of one or more segments normally found elsewhere along the body axis. Thus, the discovery of the human equivalent of the homeotic genes represents a particularly promising new area of research into human development and its abnormalities.

Another major area of advance in developmental genetics is the isolation of genes for proteins that are involved in the regulation of growth and differentiation and, of particular interest for surgery, repair. In addition to the more general regulatory molecules, such as the insulin-like growth factors, there are many proteins that are involved in the differentiation of specific tissues. For example, a battery of regulatory proteins has been isolated that plays a role in the complex program in which hematopoietic stem cells divide and give rise to progeny that mature into red blood cells, white blood cells, and platelets. Similarly, many other important tissue-specific growth factors have been isolated and are available for the study of the regulation of growth and differentiation of particular cell populations. Further studies along these lines have important implications for intractable problems such as nerve repair and the control of regenerative and healing processes in general.

It has been known for a long time that many congenital abnormalities result from chromosomal defects. Hitherto, it has been possible to identify only gross abnormalities of this type, using light microscopy. Recently, however, it has become apparent that much more subtle structural changes of chromosomes (e.g., submicroscopic deletions or insertions) can be identified with the use of restriction enzymes.

DIAGNOSIS AND TREATMENT OF DISEASE

It seems likely that the applications of recombinant DNA technology and cell biology have practical implications for all aspects of clinical practice.[21] Major efforts into developing and producing diagnostic and therapeutic agents are in progress.[39]

Diagnosis

Recombinant DNA and monoclonal antibody technology promise to revolutionize diagnostic medicine. The earliest diagnostic uses of gene probes were for prenatal screening of fetal DNA and the detection of carrier states for genetic diseases. This new technology promises to revolutionize preventive genetics and offers the possibility of controlling many inherited diseases.

Gene probes, together with the use of PCR technology, will have wide application in diagnostic pathology.[30] Probes will become increasingly valuable for the rapid identification of malignant transformation (Fig. 2–10). As demonstrated ear-

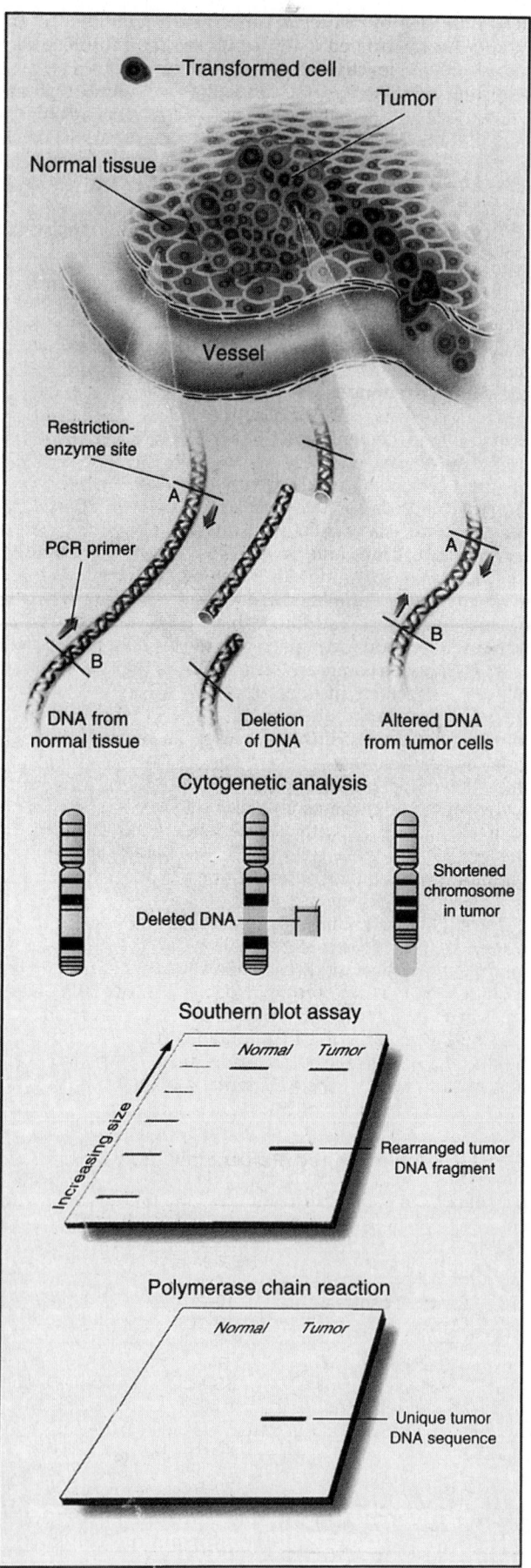

Figure 2–10. Cytogenetic and molecular analysis of tumor cells. Three methods of detecting the specific genetic alterations shared by all the neoplastic cells in a tumor are shown: (1) If the genetic alteration is large enough, as in the deletion of a region of DNA between loci A and B, cytogenetic analysis can detect grossly visible karyotypic changes; (2) Southern blot analysis can detect small changes in gene structure that routine karyotyping studies cannot find. In this example, a probe to locus A normally detects a large DNA restriction fragment, as shown by the band for the normal DNA sample. Because of the deleted DNA segment in the tumor cells, the probe for the region between loci A and B hybridizes to a smaller, rearranged, tumor-specific restriction fragment. The normal, larger band shown on the blot is from DNA contributed by nonneoplastic stromal and reactive cells; (3) In many applications, the polymerase chain reaction (PCR) can detect alterations in DNA structure with the highest degree of sensitivity. Here, the primers that anneal to loci A and B in normal DNA are too far apart to yield an amplified PCR product. The deletion shown in the tumor DNA brings the two annealing sites close to one another, allowing the generation of a novel amplified PCR product. (Reprinted by permission of *The New England Journal of Medicine* from Naber, S. P.: Molecular pathology: Detection of neoplasia. N. Engl. J. Med., *331*[22]:1508–1510, Copyright 1995, Massachusetts Medical Society.)

lier in the case of colorectal cancer, the common adult solid tumors are associated with a number of activated proto-oncogenes and inactivated tumor-suppressor genes. The relative frequency of these abnormalities for the most widely studied oncogenes and tumor-suppressor genes in the common adult solid tumors is shown in Table 2–3.

The practical applications of this knowledge are currently limited to a select number of cancers discussed in the following paragraphs.

Medullary Thyroid Cancer and the RET Proto-oncogene. Twenty per cent of medullary thyroid cancers (MTCs) are associated with familial patterns of occurrence. These include those cancers occurring in the setting of multiple endocrine neoplasia (MEN) Types 2A and 2B and, less commonly, non-MEN familial MTC (FMTC). Each syndrome is inherited in a mendelian dominant fashion and is characterized by near-complete penetrance. MTC is the most common cause of death in patients with MEN 2 and occurs early in life. The primary management goal in MEN 2 is to provide early treatment of affected presymptomatic people. Until recently, the most commonly used method of screening people within afflicted kindreds for the presence of MTC or premalignant C-cell hyperplasia was the measurement of plasma calcitonin levels after calcium and pentogastrin stimulation. Although this method of screening can be effective in diagnosing MTC, as many as 10% of patients have metastatic disease at the time of diagnosis. In addition, this method of testing is associated with discomforting symptoms that reduce compliance with annual screening and also requires lifelong testing for all family members of affected people. In 1987, the gene for MEN 2A (and subsequently for MEN 2B and FMTC) was localized by genetic linkage analysis to the centromeric region of chromosome 10. Recent studies have identified mutations in the RET proto-oncogene, which resides in the centromeric region of chromosome 10, in afflicted people in more than 90% of kindred with MEN 2A and MEN 2B and approximately 70% of those with FMTC. RET is a tyrosine kinase receptor expressed in normal human thyroid tissue, MTC, and pheochromocytoma.[10, 11, 28, 45]

These genetic findings have dramatically altered the approach to presymptomatic people with MEN 2 and FMTC kindred. People related to patients with MTC in whom a mutation in the RET proto-oncogene has been detected all are screened for the RET mutation. Asymptomatic family members who carry the RET mutation are then offered prophylactic thyroidectomy. Thyroidectomy in children identified to be carriers of the RET mutation is recommended at 5 years of age or any time thereafter, once the diagnosis is established. People who by mutational analysis are negative for the RET mutation are considered to have essentially the same risk as the general population for MTC and thus warrant no further evaluation.

Neuroblastoma and the N-*myc* Proto-oncogene. Neuroblastoma is a tumor of the autonomous nervous system and is the fourth most common pediatric malignancy. The clinical course of neuroblastoma can be unpredictable, with intra-stage variability in response to similar treatments being especially common in advanced stages. N-*myc*, a proto-oncogene encoding a gene regulatory protein, has been demonstrated to be amplified within neuroblastoma cells. The number of copies of the N-*myc* gene in tissue present at different sites is similar to the number present in primary versus metastatic lesions. The copy number is related to the clinical aggressiveness of the tumor and is a prognostic indicator independent of stage and age. N-*myc* amplification associated with any clinical stage or age places the patient at high risk for recurrence. Patients with stage III or IV disease with high amplification of N-*myc* benefit from complete versus subtotal resection, whereas aggressive resection of all tumors does not seem to affect survival intervals for those with low amplification of N-*myc*. Patients with stage I, II, or IV disease with high amplification of N-*myc* should be selected to undergo more aggressive therapy.

Breast Cancer and Overexpression of p53 and HER-2/*neu*. Mutations of p53 and overexpression of HER-2/*neu* are present in 25% to 50% and 25% to 40% of breast cancer patients, respectively.[12, 25] Recent retrospective reviews have demonstrated that in node-negative groups of patients at low risk for recurrence after operation, mutant p53 and HER-2/*neu* overexpression are independent prognostic indicators associated with an increased risk of recurrence and poorer survival. Although not reported in prior retrospective analyses, Marks and colleagues[25] found an additive effect in risk with overexpression of both. It is unclear how best to proceed with this information, and it remains to be seen whether changes in treatment strategies based on these parameters will improve outcome.

Treatment

There is already enough information to suggest that therapeutics will be changed dramatically by the use of recombinant DNA and monoclonal antibody technology. The ability to clone and express genes for human proteins in micro-

TABLE 2–3. Frequency (Percentage) of Proto-oncogene Activation/Tumor-Suppressor Gene Inactivation for Selected Common Adult Tumors

Tumor	Oncogenes			Tumor Suppressor Genes			
	HER-2/*neu*	*ras*	*myc*	p53	Rb	APC	DCC
Exocrine: pancreas	10–20	75–90		40	20	30	50
Colon	10–20	65	5–65	70–75	35	70–80	70–80
Lung							
Small cell	Rare	0	25	99–100	95–100	—	—
NSCLC	55–60	40 (adeno)	48	50	10–20	30	15
Ovarian: epithelial	30	20–25	10–40	50	10	Rare	35 (LOH)
Breast	25–40	Rare	20–30	25–50	20	5–10	30 (LOH)
Prostate	70–80	0–5	50	10–20	25	20	25
Esophageal	20	Rare	5–10	33–50	35–55	5–15	5–10
Gastric	20	20	5–20	20–50	Rare	20	50

LOH, loss of heterozygosity, insufficient data to comment on mutation rate; APC, adenomatous polyposis cell; DCC, deleted colorectal carcinoma; NSCLC, non–small cell lung carcinoma.

organisms provides a remarkable effective way of producing large quantities of absolutely pure products for therapeutic purposes.[13]

Because the gene products of proto-oncogenes are required for normal cellular function, drugs that seek to inhibit oncogene expression or function are likely to be associated with some levels of toxicity.[22] Despite this concern, strategies that embrace this approach are currently being tested and/or developed. The use of retinoic acid to treat patients with acute promyelocytic leukemia (PML), who harbor a translocation of the retinoic acid receptor to form the *PML/RARa* oncogene, is one example. Leukemia cells possessing this genetic abnormality are induced to undergo terminal differentiation when exposed to retinoic acid, resulting in a temporary clinical remission in as many as 90% of patients.[7]

Ras proteins, which require the posttranslational addition of farnesyl for their membrane association and biologic activity, offer another potential target for oncogene-directed drug therapy. Agents that inhibit farnesyl-protein transferase have been shown to reverse the transformed phenotype of *ras*-transformed cells without appearing to inhibit normal cell growth, a phenomenon not clearly understood.[19]

The immune system presents a unique opportunity to achieve selective killing of tumor cells expressing proto-oncogenes activated by mutations. Cytotoxic T-lymphocytes (CTL), through recognition of peptide fragments in association with the major histocompatibility complex, can discriminate between normal cells and those expressing mutant genes, even when the mutation involves a single amino acid change. Recent studies have demonstrated that cells transformed by mutated K-*ras* can be lysed by CTLs generated by immunization with mutated *ras* peptide.[34] These studies suggest that with the use of an appropriate immunization regimen, the immune systems of patients with tumors possessing mutated oncogenes can be manipulated to selectively kill oncogene-transformed cells (see Chapter 21).

An alternative approach is to prevent the translation of oncogene mRNA transcripts by the use of antisense oligonucleotides. These nucleotides bind mRNA transcripts to form double-stranded RNA molecules that are more susceptible to the action of cellular ribonucleases. Selectivity is achieved by using oligonucleotides precisely complementary to the unique nucleotide sequence of the mRNA transcribed from the mutated proto-oncogene. To achieve continuous exposure of cells to the oligonucleotides, Roth and colleagues have used gene transfer vehicles to introduce a gene encoding the antisense oligonucleotide sequence complementary to a mutated K-*ras* species into *ras*-transformed lung cancer cells.[40] Following gene transfer, the transformed phenotype of the cells *in vitro* is significantly inhibited. *In vivo* transfection of *ras*-transformed human lung cancer cells inoculated into the lungs of immunodeficient mice, with retroviral vectors encoding antisense to K-*ras,* is effective in preventing tumor growth. These studies have prompted phase I clinical trials using this approach in patients with non–small cell lung cancer.

Gene Therapy

As mentioned earlier, the advent of recombinant DNA technology has allowed researchers to elucidate the genetic basis for an increasing number of inherited diseases. Gene therapy has been championed as a new and exciting approach for the treatment or prevention of such diseases.[14, 26, 29] In its conception, gene therapy seemed quite simple: to treat a genetic deficiency, a functional copy of the defective gene was introduced into the cells of the deficient patient. The potential applications of gene therapy have expanded to include the treatment of acquired diseases. Thus, gene therapy

can best be defined as the transfer of therapeutically useful genetic material to the cells of a patient.

Because transfer of DNA into human cells is the first critical step in gene therapy, much effort has focused on developing a variety of gene transfer modalities.[24] Both physicochemical- and viral-based approaches have been evaluated. However, viral-based gene transfer methods have become the method of choice because they can more efficiently deliver genes to target cells. These viral delivery strategies capitalize on the natural ability of viruses to enter cells and bring their genetic contents with them. Several viruses have now been modified to serve as vectors for the transfer of therapeutic genes to human cells. Certain viral vectors, such as retroviral vectors and adeno-associated virus vectors, stably integrate the transferred DNA into the chromosomal DNA of the infected cell. Thus, transduced cells and their progeny permanently contain a copy of the delivered gene. Most physical methods and other viral vectors, such as those derived from adenovirus, deliver genes to the nucleus but do not stably integrate them into the genome of the transduced cell. These transfer modalities can result in high but transient levels of gene transfer. Although there are a number of options for gene transfer, potential problems still exist for each gene transfer method. For example, murine retroviral vectors require mitotic cell division for stable vector integration. Unfortunately, mitotic stimulation of primary cells may be deleterious to cell function or impair the subsequent development and differentiation of the cells. Thus, much effort in the gene therapy field is still focused on developing improved gene transfer methods for therapeutic applications.

After gene transfer, the next critical step in gene therapy is to ensure that a therapeutic gene is expressed at proper times and at proper levels during the development and differentiation of the patient's transduced cells. Much less attention has been focused on this task, because researchers had to initially concentrate their efforts on how to get genes into human cells. Now that such gene transfer is becoming feasible, the problem of controlling gene expression after gene transfer is getting more consideration. Regulated gene expression may be difficult to obtain from the gene transfer vectors currently being employed, because only small pieces of DNA can be incorporated into such viral vectors. These vectors cannot accommodate the large pieces of genomic DNA that encompass all the elements known to constitute an endogenous gene. Therefore, most gene therapy procedures attempt to transfer a cDNA version of a gene (a copy of the gene that lacks the intron sequences) under the control of a heterologous promoter to a patient's cells harboring a mutant version of the gene for therapeutic applications.

If the human genome were a simple warehouse of genetic information, this approach would probably be quite successful. Unfortunately for the gene therapist, the human genome appears to be extremely complicated, and expression of the information contained within it is apparently highly regulated. This complexity may severely limit the usefulness of the simple *add-back* approach to gene therapy.[40] Regrettably, cDNA versions of genes that are integrated in incorrect locations in the genome and that are expressed from heterologous promoters almost assuredly will not recapitulate the normal expression pattern of their endogenous counterparts. Therefore, significant technical advances must be made if the simple gene add-back approach is to become useful for the treatment of genetic disorders associated with genes that require regulated expression to function properly for therapeutic applications.

Such regulated expression may be especially critical when attempting to replace genes associated with tumorigenesis. Because such genes normally control cell growth and differentiation, their expression most likely has to be tightly regulated to coordinate cell cycle progression and development. Several observations support this theory. For example, deregulated expression of the transcription factor E2F-1, which normally turns on the genes that are required for S-phase, has been shown to engender premature entry into S-phase and lead to p53-dependent apoptosis. In addition, it has been demonstrated that modest overexpression of the wild-type *p53* gene aberrantly alters growth and differentiation of normal human keratinocytes, even though these cells normally express some natural level of the p53 protein from their wild-type, endogenous genes. In these experiments, the extra *p53* gene was introduced into primary keratinocytes using a retroviral vector, and this *p53* cDNA version of the gene was expressed from the Moloney murine leukemia virus long terminal repeat promoter. The cells transduced with the *p53* gene were shown to express only a twofold to fourfold increase in the wild-type p53 protein as compared with cells transduced with control vectors. Nevertheless, this modest additional *p53* expression resulted in extremely reduced growth rate, altered morphologic differentiation, and aberrant expression of genes normally associated with correct differentiation of keratinocytes. Thus, coordinated expression of the *p53* gene is apparently important for proper growth, development, and differentiation of primary human cells, and incorrect expression can lead to dramatic phenotypic aberrations.

SELECTED REFERENCES

Leder, P., Clayton, D. A., and Rubenstein, E.: Introduction to Molecular Medicine. New York, Scientific American, 1994.

Lewin, B.: Genes V. New York, Oxford University Press, 1994.

Lyerly, H. K., and DiMaio, J. M.: Gene delivery systems in surgery. Arch. Surg., *128*:1197, 1993.

REFERENCES

1. Aaltonen, L. A., Peltomäki, P., Leach, F. S., et al.: Clues to the pathogenesis of familial colorectal cancer. Science, *260*:812, 1993.
2. Berg, P., and Singer, M.: Dealing with Genes: The Language of Heredity. Mill Valley, CA, University Science Books, 1992.
3. Berridge, M. J.: Inositol trisphosphate and calcium signaling. Nature, *361*:315, 1992.
4. Bishop, J. M.: Oncogenes and retroviruses 11. *In* Les Prix Nobel: The Nobel Prizes—1989. Stockholm, Almqvist & Wiksell International, 1989, pp. 220–238.
5. Bishop, J. M.: Molecular themes in oncogenesis. Cell, *64*:235, 1991.
6. Cantley, L. C., et al.: Oncogenes and signal transduction. Cell, *64*:281, 1991.
7. Castaigne, S., Chomienne, C., Daniel, M. T., Ballerini, P., Berger, R., Fenauw, P., Castaigne, S., and Degos, L.: All-*trans* retinoic acid as a differentiation therapy for acute promyelocytic leukemia: I. Clinical results. Blood, *76*:1704, 1990.
8. Chapelle, A., and Peltomaki, P.: Genetics of hereditary colon cancer. Annu. Rev. Genet., *29*:329, 1995.
9. Croce, C. M.: Role of chromosome translocations in human neoplasia. Cell, *49*:155, 1987.
10. Donis-Keller, H., Dou, S., Chi, D., Carlson, K. M., Toshima, K., Lairmore, T. C., et al.: Mutations in the RET proto-oncogene are associated with MEN 2A and FMTC. Hum. Mol. Genet., *2*:851, 1993.
11. Eng, C., Smith, D. P., Mulligan, L. M., Nagai, M. A., Healey, C. S., Ponder, M. A., et al.: Point mutation within the tyrosine kinase domain of the RET proto-oncogene in multiple endocrine neoplasia type 2B and related sporadic tumours. Hum. Mol. Genet., *3*:237, 1994.
11a. Fearon, E. R., and Vogelstein, B.: A genetic model for colorectal tumorigenesis. Cell, *61*:759, 1990.
12. Fraumeni, J. F., Jr., Devesa, S. S., Hoover, R. N., and Kinlen, L. J.: Epidemiology of cancer. *In* DeVita, V. T., Hellman, S., and Rosenberg, S. A. (Eds.): Cancer: Principles and Practice of Oncology, 4th ed. Philadelphia, J. B. Lippincott, 1993.
13. Gibbs, J. B., and Oliff, A.: Pharmaceutical research in molecular oncology. Cell, *79*:193, 1994.
14. Gilboa, E., and Lyerly, H. K.: Specific active immunotherapy with cytokine gene–modified tumor. *In* Biologic Therapy of Cancer Updates. Philadelphia, J. B. Lippincott, 1994.
15. Gu, Y., et al.: The t(4;11) chromosome translocation of human acute leukemias involves fusion between the ALL-1 gene encoding a protein with homology to *Drosophila trithorax* gene and a gene AF-4 on chromosome 4. Cell, *71*:701, 1992.
16. Gyapay, G., Morissette, J., Vignal, A., et al.: The 1993–94 Généthon human genetic linkage map. Nat. Genet., *7*:246, 1994.
17. Haluska, F. G., Tsuimoto, Y., and Croce, C. M.: Oncogene activation by chromosome translocation in human malignancy. Annu. Rev. Genet., *21*:321, 1987.
18. Housman, D.: Human DNA polymorphism. N. Engl. J. Med., 332:318, 1995.
19. Kohl, N. E., Mosser, S. D., deSolms, S. J., Giuliani, E. A., Pompliano, D. L., Graham, S. L., Smith, R. L., Scolnick, E. M., Oliff, A., and Gibbs, J.: Selective inhibition of *ras*-dependent transformation by a farnesyltransferase inhibitor. Science, *260*:1934, 1993.
20. Krontiris, T.: Oncogenes. N. Engl. J. Med., 333:303, 1995.
21. Leder, P., Clayton, D. A., and Rubenstein, E.: Introduction to Molecular Medicine. New York, Scientific American, 1994.
22. Levitzki, A., and Gazit, A.: Tyrosine kinase inhibition: An approach to drug development. Science, *267*:1782, 1995.
23. Lewin, B.: Genes V. New York, Oxford University Press, 1994.
24. Lyerly, H. K., and DiMaio, J. M.: Gene delivery systems in surgery. Arch. Surg., *128*:1197, 1993.
25. Marks, J. R., Humphrey, P. A., Wu, K., Berry, D., Bandarenko, N., Kerns, B. M., and Iglehart, J. D.: Overexpression of p53 and HER-2/*neu* proteins as prognostic markers in early-stage breast cancer. Ann. Surg., *219*(4):332, 1994.
26. Morgan, R. A., and Anderson, W. F.: Human gene therapy. Annu. Rev. Biochem., *62*:191, 1993.
27. Mukhopadhyay, T., Cavender, A., Tainsky, M., and Roth, J. A.: Expression of antisense K-*ras* message in a human lung cancer cell line with a spontaneous activated K-*ras* oncogene alters the transformed phenotype. Proc. Am. Assoc. Cancer Res., *31*:304, 1990.
28. Mulligan, L. M., Kwok, J. B., Healey, C. S., Elsdon, M. J., Eng, C., Gardner, E., et al.: Germ-line mutations of the RET proto-oncogene in multiple endocrine neoplasia, type 2A. Nature, *363*:458, 1993.
29. Mulligan, R. C.: The basic science of gene therapy. Science, *260*:926, 1993.
30. Naber, S. P.: Molecular pathology: Detection of neoplasia. N. Engl. J. Med., *331*:1508, 1994.
31. Nakamura, Y., Leppert, M., O'Connell, P., et al.: Variable number of tandem repeat (VNTR) markers for human gene mapping. Science, *235*:1616, 1987.
31a. Olson, M. V.: The human genome project. Proc. Natl. Acad. Sci. USA, *90*:4338, 1993.
32. Pawson, T.: Protein modules and signaling networks. Nature, *373*:573, 1995.
33. Pawson, T., and Gish, G. D.: SH2 and SH3 domains: From structure to function. Cell, *71*:359, 1992.
34. Peace, D. J., Smith, J. W., Chen, W., You, S., Cosand, W. L., Blake, J., and Cheever, M. A.: Lysis of *ras* oncogene-transformed cells by specific cytotoxic t lymphocytes elicited by primary *in vitro* immunization with mutated *ras* peptide. J. Exp. Med., *179*:473, 1994.
35. Rabbitts, T. H.: Chromosomal translocations in human cancer. Nature, *372*:143, 1994.
36. Rosenthal, N.: DNA and the genetic code. N. Engl. J. Med., *331*:39, 1994.
37. Rosenthal, N.: Regulation of gene expression. N. Engl. J. Med., *331*:931, 1994.
38. Rosenthal, N.: Stalking the gene—DNA libraries. N. Engl. J. Med., *331*:599, 1994.
39. Rosenthal, N.: Tools of the trade recombinant DNA. N. Engl. J. Med., *331*:315, 1994.
40. Roth, J. A.: Modulation of oncogene and tumor-suppressor gene expression: A novel strategy for cancer prevention and treatment. Ann. Surg. Oncol., *81*:79, 1994.
41. Sklar, J., and Longtine, J.: The clinical significance of antigen receptor gene rearrangements in lymphoid neoplasia. Cancer, 70(Suppl):1710, 1992.
42. Varmus, H. E.: Oncogenes and retroviruses 1. *In* Les Prix Nobel: The Nobel Prizes—1989. Stockholm, Almqvist & Wiksell International, 1989, pp. 194–211.
43. Wainscoat, J. S., and Fey, M. F.: Assessment of clonality in human tumors: A review. Cancer Res., *50*:1355, 1990.
44. Weber, J. L., and May, P. E.: Abundant class of human DNA polymorphisms which can be typed using the polymerase chain reaction. Am. J. Hum. Genet., *44*:388, 1989.
45. Wells, S. A., and Donis-Keller, H.: Current perspectives on the diagnosis and management of patients with multiple endocrine neoplasia type 2 syndromes. Endocrinol. Metab. Clin. North Am., *23*:215, 1994.
46. Witkowski, J. A.: The inherited character of cancer—an historical survey. Cancer Cells, *2*:229, 1990.
47. Wong, A. J., et al.: Structural alterations of the EGFR gene in human gliomas. Proc. Natl. Acad. Sci. U S A, *89*:2965, 1992.

CHAPTER 3

CLINICAL OUTCOMES IN SURGERY

Alan J. Moskowitz, M.D., Keith Reemtsma, M.D., Med. ScD., Eric A. Rose, M.D., and Annetine C. Gelijns, Ph.D.

Over time, a wide variety of methods (clinical trials, quasi-experimental techniques, decision analysis, economic analysis, and meta-analysis) have evolved to assess patient outcomes. This chapter reviews the strengths and weaknesses of these various methods in the context of a range of surgical examples. It then closes by discussing the promise, as well as the problems, of applying the results of outcomes research in surgical practice.

A BRIEF HISTORY OF OUTCOMES RESEARCH

In a broad sense, the assessment of patient outcomes is as old as medicine itself. During the twentieth century, however, the assessment of such outcomes has undergone a complex conceptual and institutional evolution.[39] In the early part of this century, the rapidly developing laboratory sciences stimulated those in clinical practice to attempt to remain current with these developments and to make clinical medicine more scientific. This desire led to the introduction of increasingly rigorous methods of clinical investigation. In the 1930s, for example, the British Medical Research Council (MRC) institutionalized the testing of drugs under controlled conditions, which produced the famous streptomycin trial in 1946.[48] Subsequent decades saw the clinical trial concept make further inroads into clinical medicine. This process was stimulated in 1962 by the expansion of drug regulation in the United States to include efficacy as well as safety. The Food and Drug Administration (FDA), the agency charged with implementing the Food, Drug, and Cosmetic Act, determined that randomized controlled clinical trials (RCTs) were the gold standard for determining the efficacy of new drugs, boosting their widespread application.

This surge of activity in the clinical evaluative sciences went hand in hand with the rapid expansion of medicine's technological armamentarium, which, in turn, was stimulated by powerful supply- and demand-side forces that were embedded in the postwar U.S. health care system. On the supply side, an impressive growth occurred in federal funding for biomedical research and education. In fact, the research budget of the National Institutes of Health (NIH) grew from roughly $26 million in 1945 to nearly $7 billion in 1990 (both in 1988 inflation-adjusted dollars). The increase in federal funds for biomedical research strengthened the role of the university as the primary performer of medical research and development (R&D). It also contributed to tilting the medical educational system toward specialization and subspecialization, a movement that has been crucial in terms of accelerating technological change in medicine. At the same time, on the demand side, health insurance of the American population underwent a major expansion with the introduction of Medicare and Medicaid legislation in 1966. This expansion was coupled with a retrospective reimbursement system for hospitals and fee-for-service payment for physicians. Such reimbursement systems incorporated strong incentives for the rapid development and diffusion of new medical and surgical interventions, often regardless of their cost.

In the mid-1970s, concerns began to emerge about the rapidly expanding costs of health care, and new medical technologies were identified as being the culprit behind these rising expenditures. Two major medical technologies were pivotal in creating these concerns.[39] The first was renal dialysis. The introduction of dialysis, and particularly the enactment of the end-stage renal disease (ESRD) program that provided universal coverage, far exceeded initial cost projections. The second technology was computed tomography (CT), a so-called big-ticket technology that underwent rapid adoption and diffusion. These technologies stimulated further interest in assessment activities as a way to identify the cost-effectiveness of medical practices. This interest was reflected in a flurry of institutional activity: the Medical Device Amendments to the Food, Drug, and Cosmetic Act were introduced in 1976; the NIH created its consensus development conferences in 1977 to assess the significance of emerging medical interventions; and the National Center for Health Care Technology was established in 1978 to coordinate the federal government's assessment activities.[39]

During the 1980s, two important factors further reshaped the contours of outcomes research. The first was the far-reaching transformation, under ongoing pressure to contain escalating costs, of the financing and delivery of U.S. health care. In the early 1980s, for example, the prospective payment system (PPS), based on diagnosis-related groups (DRGs), was introduced for Medicare recipients. PPS led to great changes in hospitals' financial incentives. Cost-plus reimbursement, which had a built-in reward for maximizing resource use, was rapidly replaced by a reimbursement method that encouraged less diagnostic testing, shorter hospital stays, and outpatient care. Financial incentives to reduce technology expenditures have subsequently been reinforced by the rapid growth in managed care initiatives such as health maintenance organizations (HMOs) and preferred provider organizations (PPOs), which actively employ utilization controls. In fact, cost-conscious managed care organizations more than quadrupled their membership during the 1980s. In the current medical marketplace, hospitals and individual practitioners have to compete with other providers for managed care contracts. This competition undoubtedly takes place on the basis of price, but also increasingly on the basis of quality. As a result, these changes have increased the demand for better information about both the effectiveness and the cost of current health care practices. In addition, they have stimulated new efforts to monitor, and especially preserve, the quality of care in an environment of stringent cost control.

The second major factor that reshaped outcomes research was the emergence of strong evidence that significant geographic variations exist in the utilization of medical and surgical interventions. Researchers found more than 3-fold differences in the rates of prostatectomy, 5-fold differences for lower back surgery, and almost 20-fold differences for endarterectomies among four regions in the United States.[40, 51] Surprisingly, these variations could not be explained by differences in disease prevalence. Rather, they appeared to be largely a result of insufficient evidence about the ultimate health effects of alternative medical practices, leading to major variations in use based on physician discretion.[9]

These developments underscored the need to improve our understanding of what does and does not work in medicine and introduced what is commonly referred to as the current era of assessment and accountability.[38] To get at these issues, not only has the level of activity increased but also the questions being asked have become broader than, and in some cases quite different from, those asked in traditional clinical research. What are these differences? In the past, outcomes studies emphasized determining the benefits and risks of interventions under carefully controlled, often idealized conditions of use (i.e., *efficacy*; see Table 3–1). It became increasingly clear, however, that the full range of information about the benefits and risks of a procedure may not emerge under such carefully controlled conditions of use. Efficacy studies have traditionally excluded all but the most experienced providers and included only a narrow spectrum of patients (the elderly, pregnant or lactating women, or patients with comorbidities were often ineligible). For example, Hlatky and colleagues[21] compared the patient population in their cardiovascular disease data bank with patients involved in some large RCTs of coronary artery surgery. They found that only 8% of their patients met the eligibility criteria for the European Coronary Surgery Study, 13% met the criteria for the large Veterans Administration study, and 4% met those for the Coronary Artery Surgery Study. As a result, current outcome studies have begun to emphasize determining the benefits and risks of interventions under general or routine conditions of use (i.e., *effectiveness*; see Table 3–1).

The second major change in perspective concerns the end-points considered in outcomes research. A spectrum of relevant end-points, ranging from physiologic or anatomic parameters to mortality, morbidity, functional status, and quality of life, can be evaluated. Traditionally, clinical research has often focused on short-term biologic end-points or mortality. Undoubtedly, death is still the oldest and simplest and often a highly relevant clinical end-point. However, because many new therapeutic interventions for chronic degenerative diseases treat only symptoms and functional limitations, improvements in quality of life and functional status have become increasingly important end-points in clinical evaluation. Indeed, the primary outcomes in many of today's studies are functional status and quality of life. With the shift of emphasis toward less dramatic and often nonlifesaving interventions came the question of whether society could afford the sometimes marginal improvements in health status. This led to the inclusion of cost data and cost-effectiveness analysis in clinical practice evaluations, which was often done after the fact. More recently, an increasing number of clinical studies have begun to include costs as a relevant end-point during primary data collection and analysis.

The third change concerns the methods employed. There has been an increasing recognition that both experimental and observational methods play a role in outcomes research. Whereas RCTs are the gold standard for measuring efficacy and can also capture effectiveness, the cost of doing so is often prohibitive. The stronger emphasis on measuring what works in daily practice has refocused some attention from experimental to nonexperimental methods. This is being facilitated by the recent proliferation of large-scale automated observational databases, such as those maintained by HMOs or Medicare, which are opening up a wealth of new possibilities for monitoring hospital use and surgical outcomes in everyday practice. At the same time, advances in psychometrics have established a range of reliable and valid instruments for measuring quality of life. Furthermore, the methodology for capturing health care costs has expanded. In addition to these improvements in methods of primary data analysis, methods for synthesizing existing data (such as meta-analysis) have been considerably strengthened. In the following section, the strengths and weaknesses of these various methods are discussed.

BASIC NOTIONS OF CLINICAL EVIDENCE AND THE METHODOLOGIC FOUNDATIONS OF CLINICAL RESEARCH

Ideas or hypotheses about causes of disease and usefulness of treatment arise from a variety of activities within medical science, at both the microscopic and the macroscopic levels. Once generated, these ideas need to be substantiated or tested to derive clinical evidence of validity and usefulness for patient care. Clinical evidence is based on observations of patients. Observations are differentiated by whether or not reliable techniques were utilized at the data acquisition stage to control for variables that can impose ambiguity in the interpretation of results. The prospective, randomized, double-blind, controlled clinical trial is the consummate clinical *experiment*, which averts such ambiguity by ensuring equity of comparison groups at the time of their assembly and by controlling for bias that could be imposed during treatment and observation. It is widely regarded as the most powerful and sensitive tool for comparing therapies and regimens of care. Despite the strengths of the method, the time and expense required to implement such trials make it impossible to use them to investigate every medical intervention or diagnostic test for clinical use. Furthermore, not all clinical questions can be addressed through this experimental format. Much of what is known and what will be known in medicine has and will be learned from patient experiences that were either unplanned or deliberately not controlled for bias at the data acquisition stage. Consequently, such quasi-experimental methods (commonly referred to as *epidemiologic methods*), which include cohort studies, case-control studies, and case series, are regarded as less powerful techniques for testing therapeutic hypotheses than RCTs. To make up for the absence of control for bias at the data acquisition stage, these quasi-experimental methods employ techniques that control for bias at the analysis stage. Although they do not offer the same level of confirmation as controlled clinical trials, these techniques have special value in generating and supporting hypotheses. These techniques can be applied to the evaluation of clinical data deliberately collected for research, as well as data routinely collected in the care of patients (hospital charts), in the processing of health care services (administrative databases), or in the regulation of professional activities (statewide quality assurance programs). Over the years, both clinical trials and quasi-experimental methods have been used to compare the broader array of outcomes that are germane to patient care, including mortality, morbidity, quality of life, and cost. These outcome measures each have their own theories of measurement and calculus, which have developed considerably in the last 30 to 40 years.

With the advancement and proliferation of these methods,

TABLE 3–1. Definitions

Efficacy—The effect of a health care intervention on the outcome of care under ideal or experimental conditions.

Effectiveness—The effect of a health care intervention on the outcome of care under usual conditions of use.

clinical investigators have generated a wealth of clinical studies to address important clinical issues. Unfortunately, not all these studies are conclusive, often because not enough patients were evaluated. Occasionally, the results of clinical investigations conflict with existing pieces of evidence, and this may lead to even more studies to attempt to resolve the conflicts. All too often, this process contributes more evidence to the chain rather than resolving the conflict. Statistical techniques that quantitatively combine the results of different experiments (meta-analysis) have been under development since the turn of the century and have entered the medical mainstream in the last 10 years. These techniques have been useful for summarizing current states of medical knowledge and providing pooled estimates of effect with sufficient statistical power to support conclusions that can resolve conflicts in the existing data or at least explain why they exist.

As noted earlier, not all clinical questions can be answered by traditional forms of clinical research. More often than not, clinicians are forced to select among therapeutic interventions for patients for whom definitive studies addressing a particular dilemma are not available, may never be available, or at least will not be available in time to influence the decision at hand. The patient in question may have a unique constellation of comorbidities that can affect the outcome of the therapy, making it unlikely that a group of similar patients will ever be collected to evaluate the circumstance systematically. Or the decision at hand may involve a new and risky prophylactic intervention for a rare but dreaded disease for which the patient is at risk. Here the rarity of the outcome and the unknown effectiveness of the therapy may demand thousands of similar exposures to conduct a clinical trial that will lead to a definitive conclusion, and such a trial may not be feasible. To address such questions, medicine has increasingly turned to probabilistic modeling techniques, such as decision analysis, to provide a way to simulate the future and play out scenarios related to the known and potential risks and benefits of therapy. Such reasoning techniques often identify the therapeutic strategy that will do the most good and the least harm.

The following is a synopsis of the aforementioned methods. Each section gives a brief description of the method, followed by typical uses, capabilities, and limitations. Where appropriate, examples are given from real clinical situations that address common surgical problems.

RANDOMIZED, CONTROLLED CLINICAL TRIALS

Generally, clinical trials are any form of planned experiment that involves patients and is designed to elucidate the most appropriate treatment, management strategy, diagnostic test, or preventive measure for the future care of patients with a given medical condition or a population at risk of developing a particular condition.[35] At the core of such an experiment is the notion of using the results from the study of a limited sample of representative patients to draw inferences about how treatment should be conducted in a broader patient population who will require such care in the future. Similar inferences cannot be drawn from clinical experience with only one patient, because individuals vary biologically and their response to treatment varies accordingly. Thus, to evaluate the results of treatment, researchers must be able to examine the variation in the outcome of treatment, which requires examination of the effects of treatment on a group of patients. The results can then be interpreted probabilistically, describing the level of confidence in the observed outcome and the likelihood that the results could have been achieved by random variation or chance alone.

Although the specifics of design of RCTs vary, in general, they employ techniques that help avoid biases that can distort the results of a study. Key features that function to avert bias in the data collection and analysis stages of these studies are shown in Table 3–2.

Comparative Control Groups. RCTs are comparative: the experience of a control group of patients receiving standard therapy (or no therapy when standard therapy does not exist) is compared with the experience of the experimental treatment group, also referred to as the intervention group. The control group gives the *expected rate* of the study outcome under the null hypothesis of no effect of the investigational intervention, and the intervention group gives the *observed rate* of this outcome under the investigational treatment.

For a controlled clinical trial to be a valid test of whether the intervention effect differs from the effect under the null hypothesis, both groups must have an equal probability of achieving the study outcome prior to administering the intervention, i.e., they must be equally constituted in terms of their pretreatment likelihood of developing the outcome for study. To accomplish this, patients are randomly assigned to a treatment group. It is easy to see how the selective assignment of patients to the various treatment groups could alter the groups' prior likelihood of experiencing the outcome of interest by considering the following flawed scheme for assigning treatment in a study of coronary bypass surgery: If, because of differences in operative mortality risk, investigators selectively assigned the more stable angina patients to coronary artery bypass surgery and the less stable angina patients to medical therapy, there would immediately be an inequity between the groups. The more symptomatic medical therapy patients would be at higher risk of developing myocardial infarction (MI) or coronary mortality than the surgery group, even if they were treated the same. Thus, the *expected rate* of MI and coronary death, which would be the outcomes of interest in such a study, may be higher than anticipated in the control group, and the relative advantages and disadvantages of coronary bypass surgery may be overestimated and underestimated, respectively.

Intention-to-Treat Principle. Even though patients are assigned to a particular therapy at randomization, they do not always receive it. For a variety of reasons, patients may actually *cross over* from the experimental to the control treatment group, or vice versa. Factors that predict failure to receive therapy and crossovers almost invariably also predict the study outcome. Consequently, an analysis based on the treatment that the patient actually received (*as-treated analysis*) no longer compares randomly chosen groups that are equally likely to develop the outcome of interest. To appreciate how the factors that predict failure to receive assigned therapy and crossover are also predictive of the outcome event, the hypothetical trial that compared coronary bypass surgery and medical management for severe angina pectoris can be used. If surgical therapy is delayed several weeks after randomization, (1) some patients who were assigned to operation may expire before they are operated on (patients at higher risk of the outcome event); (2) others who were assigned to operation may stabilize preoperatively, refuse a bypass operation, and select continued medical therapy

---

TABLE 3–2. Design Features for Averting Bias in Randomized, Controlled Clinical Trials

Concurrently assessed comparative control group
Random assignment of patients to treatment groups
Blinding or masking of investigators and patients
Equivalent follow-up care for comparison groups
Analysis of primary outcome by intention-to-treat principle

(crossover patients would be at lower risk of the outcome event); and (3) some patients who were assigned to medical management may deteriorate and require emergency bypass operation (crossover patients with a higher risk of the outcome event). Thus, an *as-treated analysis* in this experiment would not compare comparable groups of patients. To ensure comparability between the study groups, the analysis should compare the groups that were composed at randomization, regardless of whether all patients received the assigned treatment. This analytic technique, which is referred to as analysis by the *intention-to-treat principle*, is the only valid method for testing the main hypothesis in a clinical trial. However, it may be supplemented by an *as-treated analysis* to support other points, such as the analysis of complication rates.

Chronologic Bias. The concurrent comparison of control and experimentally treated patients is essential for avoiding chronologic bias. Chronologic bias can occur because diagnostic and therapeutic abilities change over time, and comparisons between control and intervention groups who are treated at different times, perhaps years apart, may reflect differences in an aspect of care other than the effect of the intervention itself. For example, such a bias would arise if we were to compare early and delayed repair of Ebstein's anomaly and assigned infants with such anomalies to either early childhood or adult repairs. By the time delayed-treatment patients reached adulthood, the differences in outcome of repair might have as much to do with the differences in the diagnostic and surgical techniques of the two time periods as it would with the timing of the operation in the life of the patient.

Observational Bias. Observational bias can occur whenever there are differences in how outcome observations are made in the control and experimental treatment groups. An obvious form of this bias would occur, for example, in a clinical trial evaluating a new treatment modality for peptic ulcer disease, in which fiberoptic endoscopy was used to detect healing and recurrence in one group and upper gastrointestinal radiographic series was used in the other. Differences in discrimination capabilities between these two imaging modalities could easily affect the outcome tally for the various treatment groups in the study. However, even if the same diagnostic modality were used in these two study groups (e.g., endoscopy in both groups), observational bias could still be imposed if, for example, endoscopy follow-up time were different in the study groups or if different endoscopists with unequal observational skills were used in the two groups. A more subtle form of observational bias can ensue if the observer is aware of the treatment group to which the patient belongs. In the peptic ulcer disease example, if the endoscopist is aware of which treatment group the patient belongs to and has personal leanings toward one therapy, it might affect how he or she designates borderline endoscopic findings. Furthermore, if patients are aware of the treatment group they belong to, it might affect how they interpret symptoms they experience, which could conceivably affect whether they seek medical attention and, therefore, receive further diagnostic evaluation. Observational biases such as these can be prevented by (1) denying both the investigator and the patient knowledge of which treatment was received (i.e., *double blinding*), (2) ensuring identical follow-up care for both groups of patients, and (3) documenting all outcome observations so that they can be verified by an independent, blinded observer.

Being able to establish these controls for bias in a thoughtfully conceived and rigorously specified research plan has established the double-blind, randomized, controlled clinical trial as the strongest form of clinical evidence available today. Over the years, the questions addressed by clinical trials have broadened to include issues concerning the quality of life produced by treatments as well as the feasibility and efficiency of the delivery of the health care. Accordingly, the outcome measures included in clinical trials have broadened from the traditional mortality and frequency of morbid events to include patient preferences, health status indices, resource utilization, and dollar cost.

Clinical Trials in Surgery

The methodology of clinical trials has advanced considerably in the last 40 years, largely through the process of pharmaceutical development, for which FDA regulation has provided a framework requiring RCTs. However, there is no analogous regulatory structure for clinical procedures, including surgical procedures. As discussed in greater detail below, there are some real practical and conceptual difficulties regarding the use of RCTs in evaluating surgical procedures. Consequently, there are fewer clinical trials in the surgical literature. The delay in engaging in randomized surgical trials can also be attributed to the fact that early investigations in surgical treatment, in the form of case series, often demonstrated such dramatic patient responses that formal trials were unnecessary. However, as our efforts increasingly focus on the treatment of diseases that are not immediately life threatening, dramatic and unequivocal patient responses are not seen as often, and the need to engage in rigorous studies to demonstrate efficacy has become important. Significantly, the failure to engage in clinical trials early in the evaluation of a new surgical procedure often causes the loss of the opportunity to perform such a trial; once a new procedure is in widespread use, even when this use is based on inadequate evidence of efficacy, it is nearly impossible to motivate investigators and patients to engage in a randomized trial. Examples of treatments that have become standard practice in the absence of controlled clinical trials include radical mastectomy, laparoscopic cholecystectomy, and cesarean section for fetal distress.

The ethical dilemma in randomly assigning patients to treatment, for surgical procedures as well as for other forms of therapy, has contributed to the slow embrace of this methodology. This is especially true for the treatment of life-threatening illnesses. For random allocation of treatment to be ethically justifiable, it must be unknown whether the experimental treatment is more or less effective than the control treatment. If a clinician has a strong opinion as to whether an experimental treatment is more or less effective than the control treatment, he or she has an ethical responsibility to give the patient the treatment believed to be superior. However, one must be objective in analyzing the strength of the evidence on which such opinions are based. Case series, quasi-experimental studies, and animal studies rarely offer irrefutable evidence concerning effectiveness. When the evidence concerning the effectiveness of an important procedure is promising but less than unequivocal, confirmative evidence should be sought. Unlike supportive evidence, which merely adds weight to a hypothesis, confirmative evidence requires maximal control for bias and, hence, involves random assignment of patients to therapy. There is another important ethical consideration concerning clinical trials: not performing them when an important difference between treatments may exist could mean that an inferior treatment continues in use, resulting in suboptimal care for many patients for generations to come.

Patients' difficulty with accepting random assignment of treatment has also contributed to the slow development of clinical trials in surgery.[1a, 2] This is especially true when the experimental and control treatments are radically different, such as the comparison of amputation and limb-sparing therapy for osteogenic sarcoma of an extremity.[16] In a conventional randomization scheme, patients would need to be willing to consent, in advance, to either losing or saving a limb. They would then learn their fate after what amounts to a roll of the dice. Alternatives, such as the randomized consent design, allow the patient a choice after randomization, and yet establish equally constituted groups with respect to the risk of the outcome event.[52] In this scheme, patients are randomized to a *consent group* or a *no-consent* group. The no-consent group receives standard therapy, as if they were not in the trial. However, they actually serve as the control group for the trial. Those patients assigned to the consent group are given a choice between the experimental and the standard therapy. The consent group and the no-consent group have equal probabilities of the study outcome, and it is the outcomes of these two groups that are compared. With this design, not all the patients in the consent group receive the experimental treatment, and the degree to which this happens determines the statistical efficiency of the design. However, this may be compensated for by the fact that the randomized consent design may attract more patients into the trial than would be the case with conventional consent procedures.

Although many of the logistic problems of conducting a clinical trial have been solved for pharmacologic interventions, analogous solutions for surgical interventions are not always feasible. For instance, as discussed above, one important technique for controlling observational bias in a clinical trial is to keep both the investigator and the patient ignorant of what therapy was given to the patient. Unfortunately, in clinical trials of surgical procedures, it is impossible for the treating surgeon to be blinded from this fact. A partial solution to this dilemma is to have outcome events judged by independent, blinded observers who did not participate in the care of the study patients. Patient blinding is more problematic. If the two interventions being compared are both surgical procedures, it may be possible for the patient to be kept in the dark about which procedure was administered. However, patient blinding is not possible if one of the comparative therapies is nonsurgical. Furthermore, it is generally accepted that a sham surgical procedure as a means of accomplishing patient blinding is unethical.

Also, unlike clinical trials of pharmaceutical agents, in which each and every dose of medication that is dispensed in treatment is presumably the same or at least varies insignificantly, the skills of the surgeons in a multisurgeon trial can vary considerably, and this can dramatically affect the outcome of the trial. The results of a comparative surgical trial in which there is selective assignment of surgeons or clinical centers to one procedure versus another may have more to do with differences in the skills of the surgeons or the resources of the clinical centers than with the inherent differences between the two surgical approaches. Along this same line, the skill of the surgeon and the clinical center involved in a clinical trial also affect the generalizability of the results. Routine clinical practice often does not demonstrate the same measures of outcome achieved by the most skilled surgeons participating in a study at an academic institution. Consequently, widespread use of a particular procedure may not always be appropriate. To make results more generalizable, trials now include a variety of venues of care, both university and community based.

Another important difference between surgical and pharmaceutical trials is that surgical procedures often undergo extensive refinement, and later achievements usually far surpass those of the first experimental operations. Consequently, the results of a comparative clinical trial of a new surgical intervention depend on when the comparison was made. This poses a problem in selecting the optimal time to bring a surgical procedure to trial: waiting too long often results in

widespread use of the procedure and a loss of the opportunity to perform a trial, and proceeding too early can mean that a procedure is not fully developed and does not reflect the procedure that may eventually go into widespread use.[35]

UNCONTROLLED CLINICAL TRIALS

Trials are called *uncontrolled* if they do not contain a comparative control group and therefore describe the course of disease in only a single group of patients who have been exposed to a particular intervention. Such trials are problematic because the clinical courses of many diseases are fairly unpredictable: spontaneous remissions in disease activity can occur, which can be misinterpreted as a treatment effect. Moreover, patients in clinical trials may show greater improvement than would be expected with standard care by virtue of the special attention they receive and not because of the treatment itself. Such effects cannot be sorted out without a comparative control group. Regression to the mean is a phenomenon that can make using patients as their own controls problematic. This phenomenon is most apparent when patients are selected for entry into a clinical trial because of an extreme measure on first presentation (e.g., blood pressure elevation). Subsequent blood pressure determinations are likely to show lower readings, purely for statistical reasons; thus, such improvements in blood pressure may be misinterpreted as a treatment effect.

When the outcome of interest is irrefutable (e.g., death) and the natural history is well defined (e.g., uniformly fatal without treatment), uncontrolled trials can produce valid and highly informative results. Such is the case for congenital heart surgery, such as transposition of the great vessels, in which longitudinal studies of all patients treated at one center using a particular procedure have yielded important results.[36]

CASE REPORTS AND CASE SERIES

Case reports, which are detailed presentations of a single patient or several patients, have a long tradition in medicine and have contributed greatly to its advancement.[13] These reports are an important format for presenting the medical community with a description of an unusual disease, an unusual presentation of a disease, a new or novel procedure or treatment approach, or an unusual consequence of treatment. They are often the source of new hypotheses about disease frequency, risk, prognosis, and treatment. Moreover, they can illuminate the mechanisms of disease and treatment by reporting detailed and methodologically sophisticated clinical and laboratory studies of a patient or group of patients. A detailed report of an unusual case drew the link between the anesthetic halothane and postexposure hepatitis.[24] The case concerned an anesthetist who developed recurrent hepatitis and subsequently cirrhosis. His hepatitis recurred regularly within hours of returning to work. Exposure to small doses of halothane under experimental conditions produced hepatitis that was well-documented clinically, biochemically, and pathologically. Prior to this case report, a cause-and-effect relationship between halothane and hepatitis was only suspected, as it is a relatively rare consequence of exposure.

What cannot be discerned from case reports is the frequency of occurrence of the reported events. This limitation may unduly affect clinical behavior, because the high visibility of the report may make the event seem more common than it really is. Furthermore, using this form of publication in a literature search to establish therapeutic efficacy is fraught with problems, due to the proclivity of authors and journal editors to publish only successful cases. Because of the inherent biases in this form of reporting and the inability of this technique to estimate the frequency of the described events, case reports should not be the basis for altering clinical practice.

In contrast to case reports, *case series* are prevalence surveys. They are used to delineate the picture of a rare disease or rare treatment complication by describing the prevalence of specific characteristics in the affected population. Because these studies do not report on the outcomes of patients followed over time, they do not provide prognostic information and, therefore, do not address issues of cause and effect. Also, without a comparison group, the within-group associations that are observed cannot be put into context.

CASE-CONTROL STUDIES

Case-control studies are a method for analyzing nonexperimental or observational data to discern the association between the exposure to a suspected risk factor and the development of disease.[13, 25, 44] Patients who have a disease (cases) and a group of otherwise similar people who do not have the disease (controls) are selected, and investigators then look backward in time to determine the frequency of exposure to the suspected risk factor in the two groups. An estimate of the relative risk for developing disease related to the suspected risk factor can be calculated. Neither case reports nor case series are suited to delineate this association, because neither contains a nondiseased comparison population. Cohort studies (see below) may have a nondiseased comparison group, but because large numbers of people may need to be followed for long periods of time to gather enough cases, they are often impractical for this purpose. Case-control studies are more efficient (i.e., quicker) and less expensive than other methodologies for evaluating uncommon clinical associations, but they are highly susceptible to bias, which requires caution in their interpretation.

One clinical question that has been addressed by this approach is whether cholecystectomy increases the risk of colon cancer. The reasoning behind this controversial hypothesis is that a high intake of animal fat, animal protein, and bile acids increases the risk for developing colon cancer. Cholecystectomized patients have been reported to have an increased output of total bile acids and an increased concentration of fat in the stool, possibly predisposing them to a higher risk of colon cancer. One group of researchers compared the frequency of prior cholecystectomy in patients undergoing laparotomy for colorectal carcinoma *(cases)* to patients hospitalized concurrently with other forms of cancer that were not associated with cholelithiasis *(controls)*, during a period of 8 years.[22] To reduce the direct contribution of the gallstones themselves to the development of colon cancer in those who underwent cholecystecomy, the investigators excluded patients with colon cancer that developed within 2 years of the gallbladder surgery. The exposure to the purported risk factor, which in this case was cholecystectomy, was ascertained retrospectively, after the disease (colon cancer) developed. Consequently, such studies are occasionally referred to as retrospective studies. The selection of the control population for case-control studies is critical in determining the magnitude of the odds ratio. Control patients must be similar to the case patients with respect to all factors that might determine the risk of developing colon cancer, other than the history of cholecystectomy.

The *odds ratio* is the measure used in the study to determine whether cholecystectomy increases the risk of developing colon cancer. With respect to the current example, the odds ratio is defined as the odds that a case patient with colon cancer had previously undergone cholecystectomy divided by the odds that a colon cancer–free control patient had previously undergone cholecystectomy. Odds and probabilities are related concepts that express likelihood. Probabilities range from zero to one, and odds range from zero to infinity. The odds that a case patient has undergone cholecystectomy is the probability that a case patient has undergone cholecystectomy divided by the probability that a case patient has not undergone cholecystectomy. An analogous odds calculation is done for control patients, and the ratio of the two odds is the metric of interest, the odds ratio. Although the odds ratio compares the frequency of exposure (e.g., cholecystectomy) among case and control patients, it actually provides a measure of risk that is conceptually and mathematically similar to *relative risk*. With respect to our cholecystectomy example, relative risk describes how much more likely the development of colon cancer is among patients who received cholecystectomy than among those who did not. A measurement of true relative risk can come only from cohort studies, which are described later in this chapter. Values of the odds ratio less than one suggest that the exposure was in some way protective against the development of disease, and values greater than one suggest that the exposure in some way induced the disease. As with all population-based measures, the odds ratio should be accompanied by some measures of certainty, such as the 95% confidence interval and p value. In the cholecystectomy example, the investigators found that the odds ratio for men was greater than one. This finding, however, was statistically insignificant; i.e., the p value was greater than conventional criteria for significance (0.05), and the 95% confidence interval crossed one. The odds ratio they found was 3.04, with a 95% confidence interval of 0.95 to 9.69 and a corresponding p value of 0.2573. However, for women, the odds ratio was 1.88, with a 95% confidence interval of 1.01 to 3.51 and a p value of 0.0458. This result suggests that cholecystectomy increased the risk of colon cancer by 88% over what was experienced by the control patients.

Susceptibility to bias in case-control studies is related to two features of study design: (1) the groups to be compared are selected by the researcher and are not constituted naturally, as in a cohort study (see below); and (2) the exposure to the suspected risk factor is measured after the disease has already occurred. An important decision in selecting cases is whether to select *incident* (newly developed while the study is in progress) or *prevalent* (existing) cases. This is an important consideration if the form of the disease caused by the risk factor is different from, perhaps more lethal than, the disease that is not associated with the risk factor. In the above example, if colon cancer that is associated with cholecystectomy were more lethal than colon cancer that is not, such patients would die sooner and lower the proportion of prevalent cases that were exposed to cholecystectomy. This would inappropriately lower the calculated odds ratio compared with what would be calculated in an *incident* case-control study.

Any systematic differences between cases and controls that might be related to exposure could distort the odds ratio and therefore the estimate of relative risk. One can minimize this bias by selecting both the cases and the controls from an unbiased sample of the same population (e.g., from a particular city or county). When this is not feasible, one can match controls so that for each case, one or more control patients are selected who possess characteristics in common with the cases (e.g., age, race, gender, and other factors other than the suspected risk factor), which can minimize differences in determinants of disease. This process carries the risk of overmatching, whereby the investigator unknowingly matches on a factor that itself is related to the suspected risk factor, giving the cases and controls the same frequency of risk factor exposure, which would move the estimate of relative risk toward one. Rather than matching to restrict entry into the study, the results can be stratified by the presence or absence of other factors that might be related to the outcome or adjusted for their effects on the overall results (see the section on cohort studies).

Beyond these issues of selection bias, case-control studies face measurement biases because the exposure is measured after the disease or outcome has occurred. This is especially important when the investigator has to rely on patient recollection to establish exposure, which is not the case in the cholecystectomy example. It is well known that people with a disease are likely to recall an exposure to a risk factor differently than someone without it (recall bias) and that knowledge of the purpose of the investigation may *lead* the patient. Furthermore, the interviewers themselves can impose bias if they alter their vigor in questioning based on whether the patient is a case or a control. To avoid such biases, exposure histories should be obtained from alternative sources of the same information (e.g., medical records, patients, and physicians), and both the study subjects and the interviewers should be blinded to the specific purposes of the study.

It is this vulnerability to bias that relegates such studies to hypothesis generation and hypothesis support rather than hypothesis confirmation. However, the efficiency of conducting case-control studies cannot be surpassed. Such studies are often the first piece of important evidence of disease association, which was the case with identifying maternal DES use as a risk factor for developing clear cell carcinoma of the vagina.[20] With rigorous attention to possible sources of bias, such studies can provide valid estimates of risk for rare clinical associations.

COHORT STUDIES

The epidemiologic concept of a *cohort* refers to a group of individuals who, at the time of their assembly, have characteristics in common, including not having yet experienced the outcome for study.[13, 25, 41] Cohorts must be followed over time to study whether the outcome event of interest develops. Such studies are suitable for studying the risk of developing disease, prognosis following the development of disease, or response to treatment. In a study of risk factors, patients in a cohort are classified at the time of assembly according to whether they possess particular characteristics that might be related to outcome. It is then possible to see how these characteristics relate to the development of the outcome of interest. Such was the case with the most famous of all cohort studies, the Framingham Study, which was started in 1949 to identify risk factors for developing coronary artery disease.[15] A representative sample of 30- to 60-year-old people from the town of Framingham, Massachusetts, who were without a history of cardiovascular disease (over 5000 in number) was monitored for manifestations of that disease for over 30 years. This study established the association between hypertension, smoking, hypercholesterolemia, and diabetes mellitus and the development of symptomatic cardiovascular disease. Cohort studies are alternatively referred to as longitudinal studies, prospective studies, and incidence studies. These designations relate to the fact that the patients being studied are followed prospectively, over time, and that the evaluation process looks at the diseases or outcome states that develop during the period of observation (incident diseases or outcome states).

In true cohort studies, the entire group is assembled at a synchronous point in their illness or before the development of illness, and their course is described as it evolves from that point. Such studies can be classified into two types: *concurrent cohort studies*, in which the group is assembled in the present and followed into the future, and *historic cohort studies*, in which people are identified from past records and followed from that time to the present. Historic cohort studies are suitable for studying pre-existent data, possibly data that were collected for nonresearch purposes (e.g., patient care records from hospital charts and administrative databases used for billing or regulatory purposes). A concern of using such incidentally collected data is that they will not be of adequate quality for precise research purposes.

A true cohort study must be distinguished from a *survival cohort* or *available cohort* study. In the latter, patients are assembled after they develop the outcome of interest rather than before they develop it. Their clinical course is then constructed retrospectively, from a point before the outcome developed. The selection bias that occurs here is caused by selecting cohort members from surviving or available patients. For lethal outcomes, all the nonsurvivors will have been excluded from the cohort. For remitting diseases, all patients in remission will have been excluded from the cohort. Such studies look only at the past history of prevalent disease and not at the full experience of what evolves in a cohort of patients at risk for developing the outcome of interest.

Two constructs to measure risk in cohort studies are relevant to individuals: *attributable risk* and *relative risk*. Both are based on incidence. The epidemiologic definition of incidence is as follows: the number of new cases of disease that develop in a designated population during a circumscribed period of time. This is just the number of new cases of a disease or outcome that develops during the course of a cohort study. It is expressed as the number of new cases of disease (or outcome event) per person at risk for developing the disease (or outcome event). Attributable risk and relative risk compare the incidence of disease in two or more cohorts that have had different exposures to some possible risk factor. Attributable risk (risk difference) is defined as the incidence of disease that is attributable to the risk factor exposure and is calculated by subtracting the incidence of disease in the unexposed cohort from the incidence of disease in the exposed cohort. This measure gives an absolute increase in the incidence of disease among those exposed to the risk factor. Relative risk (risk ratio) designates how many times more likely it is that an exposed person will become diseased than a nonexposed person. The relative risk can be deceiving, in that even if the absolute increase in risk is insignificant, the relative risk increase may appear to be impressively large. A population-based cohort study was conducted to study the relative risk of colon cancer among cholecystectomy patients.[10] The investigators followed the course of 62,515 cholecystectomy patients for up to 23 years and compared their frequency of colorectal cancer with that found in the general public. They discovered 633 (incidence 0.0101) colorectal cancers, compared with the 637.9 (incidence 0.0102) that would have been expected in a similar-sized sample of the general population. This difference was not statistically significant. However, looking at women only, they demonstrated an increased risk of proximal colon cancer (relative risk 1.24, with 95% confidence interval of 1.03 to 1.48). Thus, in this subgroup, right colon cancer was 24% more likely, or 1.24 times more frequent, in women who underwent cholecystectomy than in those who did not.

Cohort studies are inefficient for studying rare associations and for studying diseases that have a long latency between risk factor exposure and manifestation of disease. Great time and expense are often needed to collect such data prospectively.

Although cohort studies are the next best thing to RCTs for evaluating prognosis and the effects of treatment, they are more susceptible to bias. Without the use of randomization, caution must be taken to avoid selection bias in the assembly of comparative cohorts. Comparative cohorts must be equivalent in all characteristics that are related to developing the outcome of interest, with the exception of the risk factor or exposure under study. If characteristics that differ are themselves predictive of the study outcome, then any observed difference in incidence of disease or outcome of treatment may simply reflect differences in the cohorts that existed before the study started and not differences in the exposure or treatment being evaluated. As with clinical trials, cohort studies are susceptible to patient dropout and crossover between cohorts, which can alter the composition of the two groups and, consequently, the risk of the outcome event in the two groups. Measurement bias is also possible if patients in one cohort are more likely to have their developed disease or outcome detected than are those in the comparative cohort.

Controlling for selection bias (Table 3–3) can be accomplished by (1) restriction—limiting the range of characteristics of patients entered into the study, producing relatively homogeneous cohorts but risking the loss of generalizability; (2) matching—for each patient in one cohort, selecting one or more patients with similar characteristics for the comparative cohort, which can be difficult to accomplish for more than a few characteristics; (3) stratification—comparing rates within subgroups with clinical characteristics that put them at the same risk of the outcome event, which can be done for only a few characteristics before statistical power is lost; and (4) adjustment for differences in clinical characteristics between the cohorts. When differences between the cohorts are few, adjustment can be accomplished by standardizing the crude outcome rates between the cohorts so that equal weight is given to subgroups of similar risk. When differences are multiple, adjustment can be accomplished by using multivariable analysis. This method requires that the investigator construct a mathematical model (an equation) that relates the pertinent clinical characteristics of the patients to a prediction of the outcome event. This equation can be employed to adjust for the predictive effects of many of the clinical characteristics that differ between the two cohorts, thereby allowing the calculation of the relative risk that has controlled for the differences between the cohorts. This is actually the only realistic way of dealing with multiple clinical characteristic differences at one time.

STRENGTH OF VARIOUS RESEARCH DESIGNS

Each of the research designs used to establish clinical evidence has a slightly different susceptibility to systematic error or bias (selection, measurement, and confounding), and the strength of evidence provided by each is judged by its susceptibility. The strongest design, with respect to control for bias, is the randomized controlled clinical trial (Table 3–4). This design uses randomization to guard against differences in the comparison groups (both known and unknown factors), sufficient sample size to avoid errors of chance, and both blinding (of patients and researchers) and standardization (of measurement procedures and analysis methods) to

TABLE 3–3. Methods to Control for Selection Bias in Epidemiologic Studies

Restriction
Matching
Stratification
Adjustment (standardization or multivariable analysis)

TABLE 3–4. Strength of Clinical Research Designs (in Order of Decreasing Ability to Control for Bias)

Randomized controlled trial
Cohort study
Case-control study
Case series
Case reports

avoid bias. Next on the list is the clinical cohort study, which can be designed and analyzed to minimize the effects of known confounding factors, selection bias, and measurement bias. Next is the case-control study. Such studies offer less design control to avoid selection and measurement bias, as well as confounding. But, like with cohort studies, some of these effects can be minimized at the point of analysis. Next is the case series, a cross-sectional prevalence survey of a defined population, e.g., by disease group. Such studies can minimize the effects of selection bias, but they do not have a comparison group, and therefore cannot put the findings into context; they do not have a time dimension, and therefore cannot provide direct evidence of the sequence of events that led to the disease; and they do not guard against biases in measurement or confounding. Case series or individual case reports offer the weakest form of evidence. Neither has a defined population or comparison group, and neither guards against selection bias, measurement bias, or confounding. Regardless of the study design employed, the quality of the research conducted can mitigate the strength of the evidence.

In recent years, the proliferation of large-scale automated data systems and improved methods of database linkage make it possible to monitor utilization patterns and outcomes. These databases have been useful for identifying regional practice variations that point to unsubstantiated physician discretion as an important cause of treatment differences. Moreover, Wennberg and others have used claims data to evaluate health outcomes following surgical procedures such as prostatectomy, hysterectomy, and cholecystectomy.[51] Given the increased availability of computerized data banks, the possibilities of inexpensive monitoring are appealing. Their relevance for individual patient care decisions, however, requires a more extensive examination not only of the advantages (such as lowered costs and ease of patient follow-up over long periods) but also of the disadvantages (such as adequacy of the data for case severity adjustment and lack of outcome information on quality of life and functional status) of these databases.

QUANTITATIVE SYNTHESIS: META-ANALYSIS

Meta-analysis is a formal process for critically reviewing and statistically combining the results of previous research.[6, 42] Alternative designations include data pooling, literature synthesis, data synthesis, quantitative synthesis, and quantitative review. Although meta-analysis has been applied to clinical research only in the last 15 years, some of the statistical methods used in the process actually date back to the turn of the century.[33] When the definitive study of the effectiveness of a therapy is impractical or impossible to perform or is currently in progress, and the decision to use this therapy must be made on the basis of existing studies, which may be multiple in number, small in sample size, and inconclusive, meta-analysis can help the decision-making process by giving quantitative estimates of the weight of available evidence. This methodology can be used to analyze both randomized trials and epidemiologic data. The process of pooling existing studies can increase statistical power for measuring primary and secondary study end-points, as well as increase the statistical power for subgroup analyses. It can help resolve uncertainty when studies disagree and can answer questions that were not posed at the start of the individual studies. Moreover, it can improve estimates of therapeutic effect size or diagnostic accuracy.

Statistical Techniques for Combining Studies

There is a variety of statistical techniques for combining the results from different clinical studies. In general, they all calculate a weighted average of study-specific results. This keeps the comparison of treatment (or exposure) groups within the original study and is distinct from the process of simply pooling the data from all studies and calculating an average treatment outcome, which is an invalid method of combining the results of different studies. The weighting process allows one to give more weight to studies with large sample sizes and less weight to those with small sample sizes. All the techniques for combining studies make one of two assumptions: a fixed-effects assumption or a random-effects assumption.

Fixed-effects methods assume that each of the studies to be combined is drawn from the same population and, therefore, that each provides an estimate of the single, underlying, true treatment (or exposure) effect. According to the fixed-effects assumption, the reason that the individual study estimates might differ is experimental error, i.e., within-study variation. Random-effects methods assume that each of the studies to be combined is drawn from a different population. This reflected the fact that patients from different studies may have met different entry criteria or been given slightly different care or had different comorbidities and, therefore, that each individual study is an estimate of a slightly different treatment (or exposure) effect. Thus, according to the random-effects assumption, the individual study estimates may differ because the study populations differ (between-study variability) and because of experimental error (within-study variability).

Methods based on either assumption can combine effects measured in odds ratios, risk ratios, and risk differences. Fixed-effects techniques have been developed for combining means or mean differences in outcome. Both fixed- and random-effects techniques generate similar point estimates of pooled effect. However, confidence intervals around that point estimate differ: random-effects methods produce broader (more conservative) 95% confidence intervals than fixed-effect methods. There are a variety of methods for deciding which of the two model types is more appropriate. These are based on the degree of effect differences (heterogeneity) of the studies to be combined. Techniques that employ the random-effects assumption can accommodate a greater degree of heterogeneity than the fixed-effects assumption methods can. However, when the degree of heterogeneity is significantly larger than expected from random variation, as measured by a statistical test—especially when the individual studies disagree on the direction of treatment or exposure effects—it may not be reasonable or meaningful to pool results.

Graphic Presentation

Meta-analyses are often presented graphically. Usually, point estimates of effect and associated confidence intervals (e.g., odds ratio) of the individual studies are presented in a list, and a summary or pooled effect measure is given at the end of this list. The schemes for ordering the list vary and can be done chronologically, by study size, by quality of study, or by a variety of other criteria. The presentation is

valuable because it gives an overall impression of the variability of patient responses and the degree of overlap in effect sizes. Figures 3–1 and 3–2 are graphic presentations from a meta-analysis that compiled the epidemiologic investigations of the association of colon cancer and cholecystectomy.[14] This analysis categorized individual studies by whether they were of a cohort type or a case-control type and, for the latter study type, by whether the control group was selected from the catchment population from which the cases arose (population based) or from hospitalized patients at the institution where the cases were diagnosed. Overall, the five cohort studies did not demonstrate an increased risk of colon cancer associated with cholecystectomy (relative risk 0.97, 95% confidence interval [CI] 0.82 to 1.14). However, the pooled results from 38 case-control studies did demonstrate a significantly increased risk of colorectal cancer associated with cholecystectomy (odds ratio 1.21, 95% CI 1.04 to 1.4). Figure 3–1 addresses the risk of proximal colon cancer. Restricting the analysis to population-based case-control studies, there were seven studies that distinguished proximal (up to the distal end of the transverse colon) from other tumor locations. The meta-analysis was conducted using a random-effects method.[5] For each study, the individual odds ratio (point) and 95% CI (line) are plotted. The individual point estimates vary (odds ratios from 0.79 to 2.15), but the CIs around these estimates overlap, indicating that it is unlikely that they are truly different. On the bottom of the chart is the overall pooled estimate of 1.41, which was significantly different from 1 (95% CI from 1.16 to 1.7, p = 0.000435), based on observations among 32,774 patients. Figure 3–2 is the analogous graphic plot for left-sided colorectal tumors. The individual odds ratios have about the same range of variation as was seen in Figure 3–1, and the 95% CIs of the individual studies overlap as well. The overall pooled odds ratio was 1.03, based on observations in 35,149 patients, which was not significantly different from 1 (95% CI 0.88 to 1.2, p = 0.375). Together, these epidemiologic studies suggest (but do not confirm) that cholecystectomy increases the risk of proximal colorectal cancer by 40%, but that such operations do not increase the risk of distal colorectal cancer.

INDIVIDUAL STUDY QUALITY

As discussed in the above sections on study design, bias can significantly alter the degree and direction of treatment or exposure effect. Thus, study quality, as defined by adherence to scientific standards that avoid bias in the collection and analysis of primary data, is an important consideration in the data synthesis process. A measure of study quality can be useful for determining which studies to include in a meta-analysis and for examining the relationship between study quality and outcome. Several scoring systems have been proposed for judging quality. In general, they generate numeric scores for each study by assigning points for adherence to a list of techniques that avoid bias and offer documentation. One such score was proposed by Thomas Chalmers, which utilizes 25 separate quality criteria for clinical trials.[2b] Another simplified system has been proposed and is based on an evaluation of the method of randomization, the method of handling withdrawals in the analysis, and the blinding of those assessing outcome.[2a]

Bias

Just as with primary data collection and analysis, one must guard against the introduction of bias into the meta-analysis process. *Selection bias* can be imposed into a meta-analysis if strict criteria for including or excluding studies from the analysis are not adhered to; the decision to include a paper

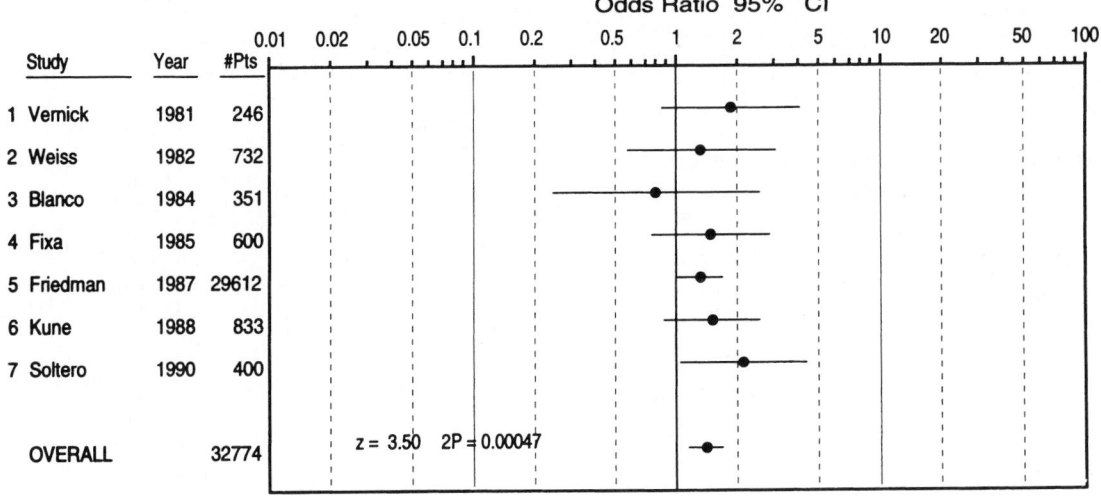

Figure 3–1. Meta-analysis of studies addressing the association of cholecystectomy with proximal colon cancer. This figure depicts the odds ratios (plotted as points) and associated 95% confidence intervals (plotted as horizontal lines) for each of seven case-control studies that investigated the relationship between proximal colon cancer and prior cholecystectomy. It also contains the *overall* estimated odds ratio and 95% confidence interval calculated by pooling these seven studies (bottom of figure). For each of the seven studies, the name of the first author, year of publication, and number of patients investigated are included. The complete citations are located at the end of the reference list. For the overall estimate, the total number of patients in the pool, the value of the z statistic used in performing the analysis, and the corresponding p value multiplied by 2 are included. Odds-ratio values greater than one (on the right side of the diagram) portend an increased risk of developing proximal colon cancer. Odds-ratio values less than one (on the left side of the diagram) suggest a reduced risk of colon cancer associated with cholecystectomy. When the confidence interval crosses one, the associated effect is not statistically significant.

should be made by looking only at its methods and not at its results, or possibly by looking at both, but under separate and blinded conditions. The authors must outline how they searched for the articles they included; different search strategies are certain to turn up different sets of references. The presentation of the results of a meta-analysis should always include the list of articles excluded from the analysis and the reasons for exclusion.

Data extraction bias can be introduced in the meta-analytic process if there is not uniformity in the techniques used to

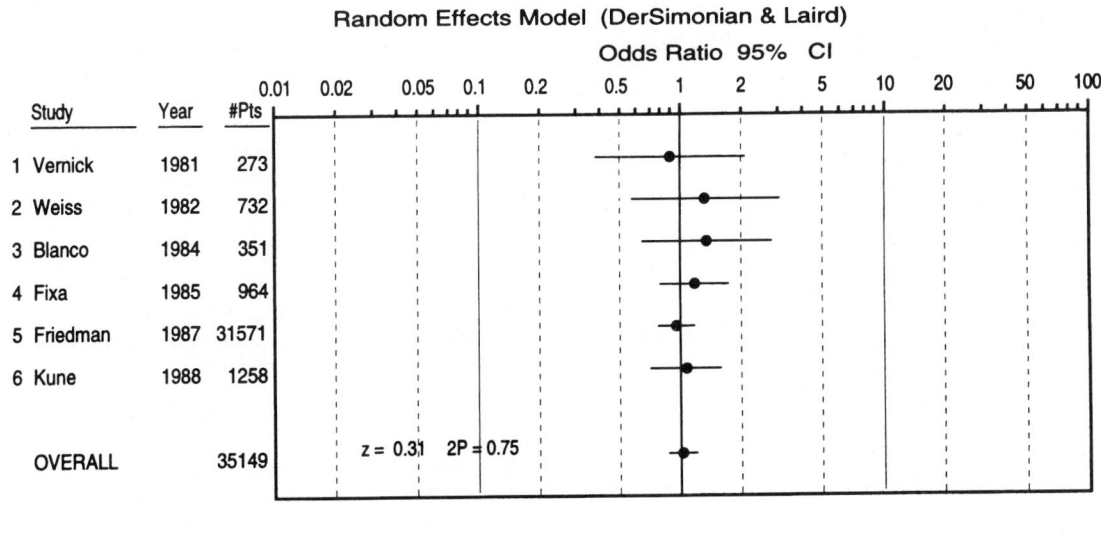

Figure 3–2. Meta-analysis of studies addressing the association of cholecystectomy with distal colon cancer. This figure depicts the odds ratios (plotted as points) and associated 95% confidence intervals (plotted as horizontal lines) for each of six case-control studies that investigated the relationship between distal colon cancer and prior cholecystectomy. It also contains the *overall* estimated odds ratio and 95% confidence interval calculated by pooling these six studies (bottom of figure). For each of the six studies, the name of the first author, year of publication, and number of patients investigated are included. For the overall estimate, the total number of patients in the pool, the value of the z statistic used in performing the analysis, and the corresponding p value multiplied by 2 are included. Odds-ratio values greater than one (on the right side of the diagram) portend an increased risk of developing proximal colon cancer. Odds-ratio values less than one (on the left side of the diagram) suggest a reduced risk of colon cancer associated with cholecystectomy. When the confidence interval crosses one, the associated effect is not statistically significant.

extract the data from the individual studies. Studies report on a variety of subgroups, end-points, and exclusion criteria, which may be interpreted differently by different individuals. To control for bias at this stage, data should be extracted by more than one observer, and each should be blinded to the treatment groups. The agreement between observers can be measured and conflicting observations rectified.

Publication bias is another concern that is particularly germane to the meta-analytic process. It occurs when study results are differentially reported, depending on the direction and strength of their findings. Publication bias is not an uncommon phenomenon, and it appears that the failure to publish the results of a particular study actually lies more with the investigator than with the editor. Investigators acknowledge that they are less likely to pursue publication when they have obtained uninteresting results. Moreover, authors can also impose publication bias if they selectively exclude data from a publication based on the nature of the findings. Methods have been devised to estimate the size of the problem in a given analysis. A *funnel plot* (Fig. 3–3) has been proposed to ascertain the presence of publication bias in a set of individual articles for meta-analysis.[26] When estimates of effect size from the individual studies are plotted against a measure of sample size (usually inverse variance), the plotted points should take on the shape of a funnel, scattered around the true value of the point estimate of effect. The larger the sample size, the smaller the spread of points from the true effect size—hence, the funnel plot. Should a portion of this funnel formation be absent, publication bias should be suspected. Clearly, the limitation of this method is that numerous studies are required to visualize the funnel.

The need to make the most of existing information in making clinical decisions rather than waiting for definitive studies to be completed and the unfortunate decrease in funding for new studies have been major stimuli to the development of the meta-analytic process in medical research.

MEASURING QUALITY OF LIFE AND PATIENT PREFERENCES

An essential aspect of clinical care is assessing the impact of disease on the lives of patients. Whereas the effects of disease can be characterized by changes in physiologic parameters, the impact on the patient is ultimately measured in its effects on survival and quality of life. This section reviews some of the concepts related to the quantitative measurement of quality of life. Overall quality of life is an all-inclusive concept that incorporates the ability of an individual to function physically, emotionally, and socially.[17] For measuring the impact of medical interventions, however, a more limited definition is appropriate: health-related quality of life (HRQOL) includes those factors that immediately affect the health of the individual. Thus, factors such as socioeconomic status, which does not affect the health of the individual in the short term but may do so in the long term, are excluded from the definition.

Instruments for measuring HRQOL fall into two broad categories: *generic* and *specific*. Generic measures assess general aspects of HRQOL that are applicable to a variety of populations and, thus, allow broad comparisons of the relative impact of disparate health care interventions. An example of this type of measure is the MOS 36-Item Short-Form Health Survey (SF-36).[49] Specific instruments are geared to particular diseases or populations and focus on the functional limitations or disabilities produced by the disease of interest or experienced by the population of interest. An example of this type of measure is the Minnesota Living with Heart Failure Questionnaire.[37] By focusing on only important aspects of HRQOL that are relevant to the patients being studied, the measurement is more likely to be responsive to subtle changes in the function of those individuals over time. The choice of instrument category depends on the task at hand. When discriminating or differentiating the quality of life of people with different illnesses, a generic instrument would be more suitable. When evaluating changes in quality of life over a period of time for a particular group of patients, a specific instrument may be more suitable.

Within these two broad categories of measurement there are two types of instruments: *health profiles* and *utility instruments*. Health profiles capture health status through questionnaires that ask about patients' functional capabilities and symptomatology. These questionnaires are multidimensional constructs; that is, they are composed of questions that address each of the different concepts (dimensions or domains)

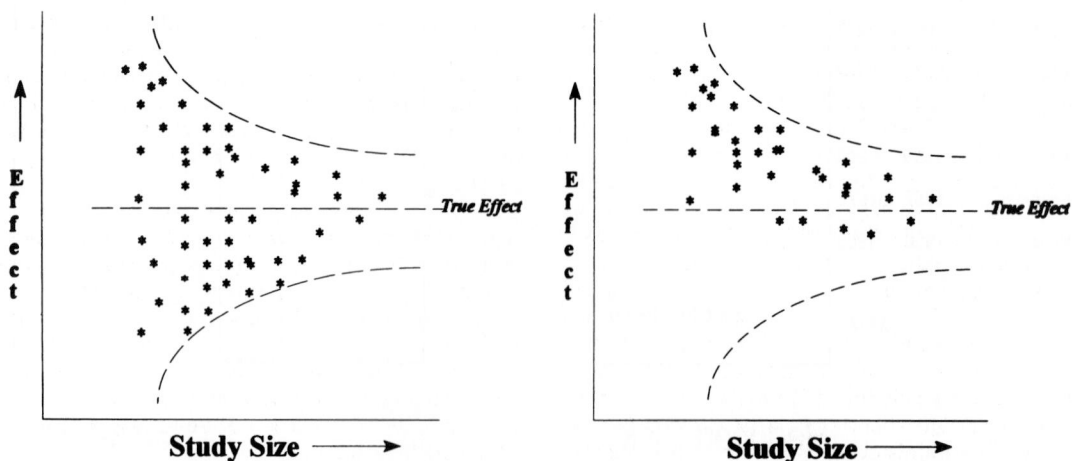

Figure 3–3. Hypothetic funnel plot addressing publication bias. This figure contains two examples of a graphic technique to ascertain the presence of publication bias in a set of articles for meta-analysis. In each of the two graphs, the effect size is on the vertical axis and the sample size is on the horizontal axis. Each point (asterisk) represents a different study. In the absence of publication bias (graph on the left), the points take on the shape of a funnel, scattered around the true value of the point estimate of effect: the larger the sample size, the smaller the spread of points (estimates) from the true effect size. When a portion of this funnel formation is absent (graph on the right), publication bias should be suspected. The graph on the left depicts what would be seen if there were no smaller studies with negative effects found in the literature, as would be expected from the theoretical relationship.

that, together, are thought to define HRQOL. In general, such concepts include physical function, mobility, cognitive function, self-care, emotional status, sensory function, and pain. The questionnaires can be interviewer-administered or self-administered. Ideally, the questionnaire respondent is the patient. However, surrogate respondents (e.g., close family members or caregivers) are resorted to when patients are incapable of responding. Numeric scoring is accomplished by assigning points to the responses to each question and summing the scores for each concept or domain covered in the questionnaire. For some profiles, the domain scores can then be compiled to generate a single overall score. These scores have ordinal measurement properties with arbitrary magnitude. More extreme values are better or worse than less extreme values (depending on the profile being used).

An example of the type of information obtainable from such profiles is a comparison of the quality of life of cardiac transplantation candidates and recipients, measured by the SF-36 health profile.[37] The results of *recipients* versus *candidates* are as follows: general health perception (70 versus 33), vitality (62 versus 39), physical function (71 versus 36), ability to perform roles without physical limits (62 versus 27), and social function (85 versus 63). All these differences were statistically significant. Interestingly, for questions relating to mental function and ability to perform roles without emotional problems, both groups scored relatively high, and the differences did not reach statistical significance. Such profiles are useful to see which areas of quality of life have improved or worsened over time, as well as for performing a cross-sectional analysis of different groups of patients at the same time. Because the measurements generated by these profiles have ordinal scale properties, reasoning about magnitude of differences is limited.

Utility measurements, which are also referred to as *preference-based measurements,* capture both the quality of life experienced by the patient and the strength of the patient's preference for the health state relative to full health (assigned a score of one) and death (assigned a score of zero). Scores less than zero, representing states worse than death, are possible. These scores are cardinal measures with interval scale properties and, accordingly, offer a greater ability to reason about the magnitude of scoring differences. This form of measurement was derived from economic and decision theory and is classically elicited from the patient by structured, face-to-face interviews.[47] One technique, the standard gamble, relates value for quality of life to the amount of risk that a patient would be willing to take to improve it.[47] Presumably, the better the quality of life that the patient was experiencing, the less the risk that he or she would be willing to incur to improve it. A related technique, referred to as the *time trade-off,* relates value for quality of life to the number of years of future life that a patient would be willing to give up to improve it.[46] Table 3–5 lists the utility values of patients with several chronic medical problems derived by utility interviews using the standard gamble and time trade-off techniques.

Based on the more recently derived multiattribute utility theory, utility measures can now be derived through a questionnaire format, which facilitates assessing utilities in large-scale research efforts. Questionnaires, such as the Health Utility Index, can be administered to patients and scored in the same fashion as other health profile instruments.[12] The domain scores are then converted to a utility score by using a preference-based scoring function, derived previously, through classic utility interviews of other groups of patients or community groups. Thus, utility scores derived by multi-

TABLE 3–5. Utility Values of Patients with Chronic Medical Problems

Health State	Utility
Full health (reference state)	1.00
Cardiac transplant recipients	0.91[29a]
Kidney transplant recipients	0.84[3a]
LVAD implant recipients	0.81[29a]
Severe rheumatoid arthritis patients	0.70[1]
Hospital dialysis patients	0.57[3a]
Dead (reference state)	0.00

LVAD, left ventricular assist device.

attribute techniques reflect a reference population's values for the health profile descriptions given by patients.

Quality-adjusted survival, measured in quality-adjusted life years (QALYs), is a complex outcome measure that captures features of both the survival and the quality of life of the individuals under study.[34] Its calculation entails using quality-adjustment factors to modify the measured survival for the quality of life experienced. Utility scores are commonly used as the quality-adjustment factors for calculating this product. If, for example, an individual lives 70 years at full quality of life, he or she would have accumulated 70 QALYs (70 years $\times$ 1.0 quality units). If, however, this patient's entire 70-year survival was at half of full quality, he or she would have accumulated only 35 QALYs (70 years $\times$ 0.5 quality units). Actual calculations must take into consideration the multiple fluctuations of quality of life that occur throughout the life of an individual. Calculating the quality-adjusted survival of a cohort of patients requires several steps: (1) utility scores need to be assessed for each member of the cohort at periodic intervals, and an average utility for the time period needs to be calculated; (2) the survival for the cohort must be calculated for the analogous time periods; and (3) the products of the average survival and average utility for each time period are summed to yield average QALYs. Figure 3–4 is a hypothetical survival curve for patients undergoing treatment for a malignancy. The area under the curve would be the 5-year survival for the cohort. The sum of the shaded areas beneath the curve is the 5-year quality-adjusted survival for the cohort, measured in QALYs. As would be expected, the shaded area is less than the full area beneath the curve, because life with a malignancy is not always at full quality. In particular, quality of life is often significantly impaired during the primary therapy (operative therapy and/or chemotherapy), which can last months or years. Also, quality usually drops after tumor recurrence.

Having a single, unified outcome measure, such as QALYs, that reflects the multiple attributes of health believed to be germane to making therapeutic choices facilitates the decision-making process considerably. Consider the choice between limb-sparing therapy and amputation for soft tissue and osteogenic sarcoma of the extremity. Limb-sparing therapy saves a functional extremity and therefore provides a better quality of life than amputation, but the survival with this modality of care is not quite as long as with amputation. Choosing between these two therapeutic options is extremely difficult to do, because it requires that the patient trade off life (survival) for limb. Unifying these two outcome features into a single measurement facilitates decision making, allowing patients to choose the treatment option that offers the best overall quality-adjusted survival.[29]

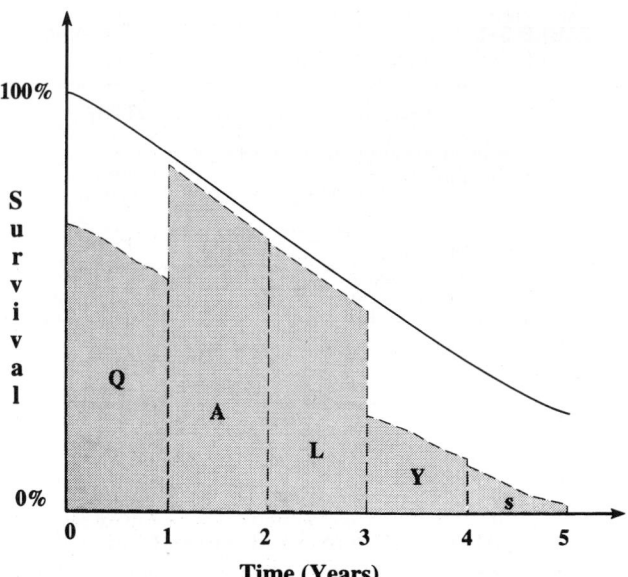

Figure 3–4. Hypothetic 5-year survival curve for cancer patients, depicting the concept of quality-adjusted life years (QALYs). This figure plots a hypothetical 5-year survival curve for a population with cancer. Survival is on the vertical axis, and time, in years, is on the horizontal axis. The smooth curve, which depicts the percentage of the cohort that is alive at a given time during the 5 years after diagnosis, naturally decreases with time. The area under this curve is the 5-year survival of the cohort. The shaded area represents the quality-adjusted 5-year survival, measured in QALYs. To measure quality-adjusted survival, the quality of life for each member of the cohort was measured annually, using a utility scale. The average utility value for each time period is used as the quality adjustment factor for the period and multiplied by the interval survival. The entire area beneath the curve would have been shaded if the patients had experienced full quality of life throughout the 5 years. It is more typical, however, to see decrements in quality of life during periods of morbidity, especially during the course of a cancer patient's life. Thus, during year 1, the reduction in accumulated QALYs may have been from primary treatment of the tumor. During years 2 and 3, QALY accumulation is near maximal, which is what may be seen during the disease-free remission period. Accordingly, years 4 and 5 may represent the years following recurrence, in which there is usually a dramatic falloff in quality of life.

DECISION MAKING UNDER UNCERTAINTY

Not uncommonly, physicians must contemplate administering a risky therapy to patients when only animal studies or clinical logic suggests that the therapy will eliminate the suffering or potential mortality of the patient's condition. Ideally, such decisions should be based on the results of well-planned, controlled clinical trials. Unfortunately, it often takes years from study initiation for the results of clinical trials to become available. This may be because the disease under consideration may take years to evolve before the relevant outcome events occur. For some clinical problems, clinical trials may not even be feasible, because the outcome events of interest are so uncommon that it would be impossible to enroll a large enough population to ensure a sufficient number of events to be confident about the results of the study. One difficulty of basing clinical decisions on the results of clinical trials is that existing studies may not adequately address the patient at hand. Sometimes the patient under consideration is so unique in terms of comorbidities that it is unlikely that the patient would ever be adequately represented in a clinical trial. Thus, when such trials are not feasible, unavailable, or unrepresentative of the patient at hand, clinicians are forced to make decisions based on their perception about the likely effect of a therapeutic option on the natural course of the patient's disease. Fortunately, decision analysis, a formal analytic approach to making decisions under conditions of uncertainty, provides techniques to ana-

lyze such questions and project whether the benefits of the proposed intervention outweigh the risks, based on the various facts at hand.[23] The *facts* in such instances are derived from a variety of sources, including published reports and expert opinion.

The general process of decision analysis involves five steps.[45] First, the problem is structured explicitly, separating choices (decisions) from chance events (prognoses) and assigning a relative value to each possible outcome. A decision tree (Fig. 3–5) or another representational structure is used for this purpose. Second, each possible result of each chance event is assigned a relative likelihood on a probability scale. Third, each potential outcome is assigned an appropriate outcome measure on a single consistent scale. Percent survival, years of survival, and quality-adjusted survival, measured in QALYs, are commonly used outcome scales. Fourth, the average or expected outcome of each treatment or diagnostic strategy is calculated, using a weighted averaging process. The strategy offering the higher expected outcome is the preferred one. Finally, and most importantly, the decision model is explored by sensitivity analysis, in which the analysis is repeated, using a range of plausible probability and outcome values in the decision model to see whether these variations in the assumptions made in constructing the base-case decision model affect the identification of the preferred strategy. When the identification of the preferred strategy is invariant to changes in the assumptions in the model, the decision is said to be insensitive to these assumptions, and the case for choosing the identified preferred option is strengthened. The process has been applied to decisions affecting the care of individual patients and groups as well as to questions of health policy.

The decision to take zidovudine prophylactically after an accidental needle-stick exposure to an HIV-contaminated needle is an example of a problem in which the risk of developing a devastating disease is perceptible, the efficacy of treatment is entirely unknown, but the risks of treatment are tangible. Although recent experience in using this treatment to prevent vertical transmission from mother to fetus supports the notion of zidovudine prophylaxis, for years the decision to use this treatment for needle-stick exposures had no supporting evidence other than animal data. The manufacturer's efforts to conduct a clinical trial for needle-stick exposures came to no avail, as fewer than 100 patients were recruited during the first year of enrollment. Estimates of the sample size needed to achieve statistical certainty for a 20% efficacy in preventing HIV seroconversion are on the order of 60,000 needle-stick exposures. Thus, it is unlikely that such a clinical trial would ever be completed. A decision analysis was undertaken that used existing information about rates of needle-stick transmission of the virus and worst-case estimates for the risk of fatal toxicity from a short course of zidovudine to determine what the threshold of efficacy would need to be for the benefits of prophylactic treatment to outweigh the risks.[43] Figure 3–6 depicts the results of this analysis, which was done from the perspective of a 30-year-old—the age group of many staff members who face this decision. On the vertical axis is life expectancy, in years of survival. On the horizontal axis is the efficacy of zidovudine in preventing HIV conversion. The average expected outcome of the strategy of not taking zidovudine prophylactically is plotted as a horizontal line. The line is horizontal because the outcome of this strategy is unaffected by the efficacy of zidovudine. The average expected outcome of taking zidovudine is plotted as three diagonal lines, each at a different assumed rate of fatal toxicity of this therapy. As would be expected, the higher the effectiveness in preventing seroconversion, the higher the life expectancy from taking zidovudine prophylactically. The point where the plotted

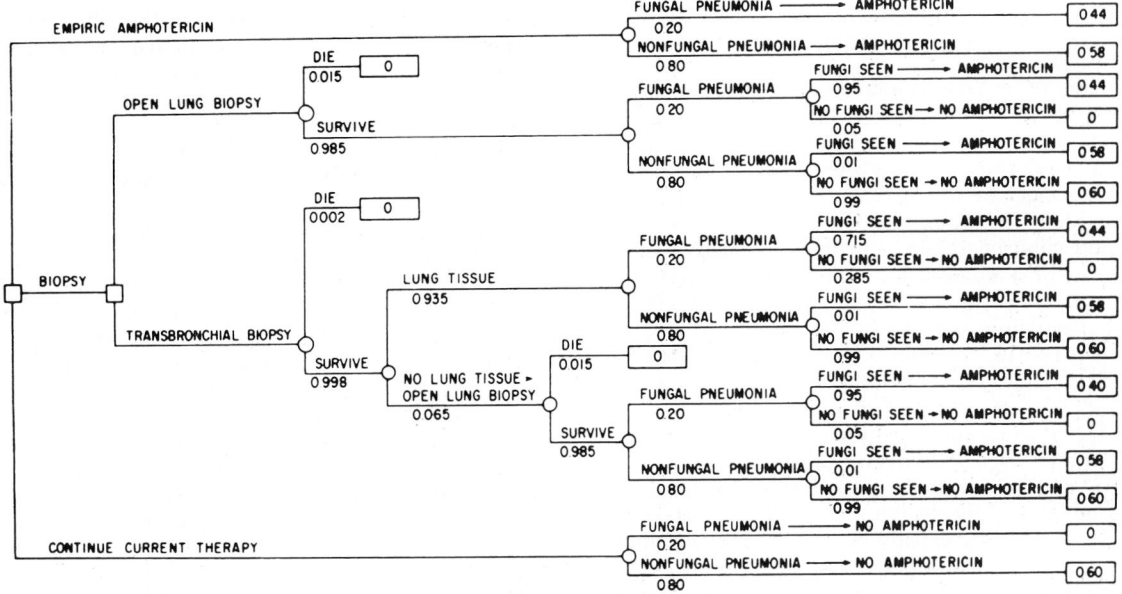

Figure 3–5. This decision tree is the problem representation used to determine the best treatment for a specific patient with preleukemia and granulocytopenia who failed to respond to a course of broad-spectrum intravenous antimicrobial therapy. Decision points are depicted by square nodes, chance points by circular nodes, and outcome points by rectangular nodes. Starting on the left, the decision maker must select among three options: (1) empiric amphotericin to treat the suspected fungal pneumonia, (2) biopsy (either open or transbronchoscopic) to look for the presence of fungi before treatment, or (3) continuation of the current antimicrobial therapy. The events (branches) following each circular chance node are associated with a probability that they will occur, which is represented by the number beneath the line. The outcome of interest here is expected survival, and a value for expected survival following each path of events in the decision tree is placed in the terminal or outcome nodes on the right-hand side of the tree. Thus, for the top strategy in the tree (empiric therapy), there is a 0.2 chance that the patient has fungal pneumonia, and a 0.8 chance that he does not. In either case, the patient will receive amphotericin, because no diagnostic test will be performed to guide therapy. If the patient has fungal pneumonia, the probability of survival is 0.44. If the patient does not have fungal pneumonia (nonfungal pneumonia), the survival is better, 0.58. The expected survival, if the patient takes amphotericin empirically, is equal to the sum of the products of path probabilities and outcome values (0.2 × 0.44) + (0.8 × 0.58), or 0.552. A similar calculation scheme is used for the other strategies and yields survivals of 0.555 for open lung biopsy, 0.542 for transbronchoscopic biopsy, and 0.48 for continuation of the current therapy. For this particular patient, open lung biopsy provides a slightly better survival than empiric therapy, followed closely by transbronchoscopic biopsy and more distantly by continuing current therapy. (From Moskowitz, A. J., Kuipers, B. J., and Kassirer, J.: Dealing with uncertainty, risks, and tradeoffs in clinical decisions: A cognitive science approach. Ann. Intern. Med., *108*:435, 1988.)

lines for the strategies of prophylactic zidovudine and no prophylactic zidovudine cross is the point where they offer equivalent life expectancy. This is known as the threshold point. The location of this point depends on the assumed fatal toxicity rate associated with zidovudine. The literature demonstrates this risk to be 1 in 15,000. The upper limit of a 95% CI for this estimate is 3 in 15,000. Using the worst-case assumption of 3 in 15,000, zidovudine must prevent only more than 8% of seroconversions to outweigh the risks of that therapy and become the therapeutic option of choice. Although a good estimate of effectiveness in prophylaxis

is still not available, the threshold value needed to make prophylactic zidovudine the optimal choice is within the realm of possibility. The efficacy of zidovudine observed in preventing vertical transmission was several times this threshold value (67.5%).[4]

There are a variety of applications for decision analysis in clinical practice. However, it is the methodology's ability to collate cost in the decision-making process for health policy that has brought it to the forefront during the last 10 years. The economic issues of medical care are addressed in the section that follows.

Figure 3–6. Two-way sensitivity analysis in the decision to take zidovudine (Retrovir, AZT) empirically following a stick from a needle that was contaminated with blood from an HIV-positive patient. This analysis examines the effects of varying the assumed fatal toxicity of AZT and effectiveness of AZT in preventing seroconversion on the decision to take prophylactic AZT. The vertical axis is life expectancy, in years, and the horizontal axis is AZT effectiveness, on a scale of 0 to 100%. Each solid upsloping diagonal line represents the expected outcome of the strategy of taking AZT, each with a different underlying assumption about drug toxicity (from 0 to 3 in 15,000). The expected outcome of the decision not to take AZT prophylactically is represented by the horizontal broken line. For all values of effectiveness greater than 8%, regardless of the assumed value of toxicity, the expected outcome of taking AZT, measured in years of life expected, exceeds that of not taking AZT. (From Sacks, H. S., and Rose, D. N.: Zidovudine prophylaxis for needlestick exposure to human immunodeficiency virus: A decision analysis. J. Gen. Intern. Med., *5*:132–137, 1990. Reprinted by permission of Blackwell Science, Inc.)

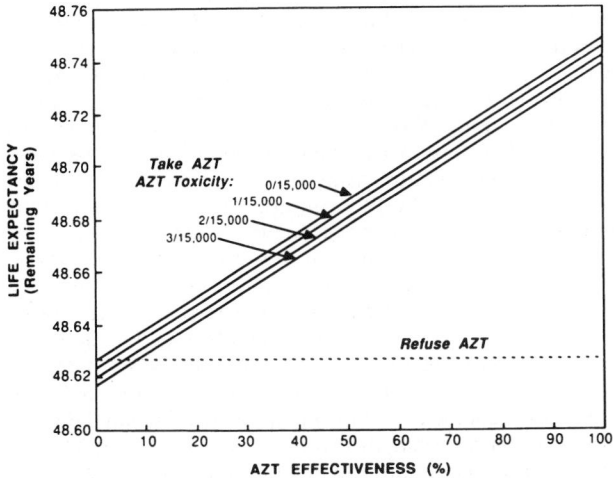

ASSESSING THE ECONOMIC IMPACT OF CLINICAL CARE

The objective of an economic evaluation of a medical or surgical intervention is to measure the resources consumed (i.e., costs) in relation to the health benefits provided. An economic analysis can be undertaken from four different perspectives: society or the health care system, third-party payers, providers (including managed care organizations, hospitals, and clinicians), and patients. Obviously, the perspective from which an analysis is undertaken matters: what may be cost-effective for one party (e.g., a hospital) may not be cost-effective for another (e.g., a third-party payer).[27] Generally, economists favor the societal viewpoint. From this broad point of view, the constrained resource is the total economic output of society, and the analytic objective is to maximize the health benefit achieved by society through optimal allocation of the limited resources available for health care.[49] By contrast, if the perspective was limited to medical providers or the health care system, costs could spuriously be affected by expanding or contracting patients' responsibility for certain services, such as home care.

The rational allocation of scarce resources presupposes information about the value of a particular intervention in comparison to alternative modes of intervention or, in some cases, to no intervention or watchful waiting. Most economic studies compare a new or modified clinical procedure or practice (e.g., laparoscopic cholecystectomy) with an existing one (e.g., open cholecystectomy). In addition to therapeutic modalities, economic studies may examine alternative diagnostic procedures (e.g., transhepatic cholangiograms versus endoscopic retrograde cholangiopancreatography for diagnosing common bile duct stones), preventive versus curative services, or different settings of care (e.g., ambulatory versus inpatient operations).

Cost-Minimization Analysis, Cost-Benefit Analysis, and Cost-Effectiveness Analysis

There are different methods of economic evaluation. Cost-minimization analyses are the least commonly used. These analyses are appropriate if the health effects of alternative clinical practices are identical and the focus of the analysis is on finding the least costly alternative.[7] A case in point is ambulatory surgical procedures. If clinical studies find no differences in efficacy or complication rates following a particular surgical procedure performed on an outpatient as opposed to an inpatient basis, the analysis can focus solely on the relative costs of treatment under inpatient and outpatient conditions. Cost-benefit and cost-effective analyses both examine the costs as well as the benefits of alternative technologies. In a cost-benefit analysis, however, all costs and benefits are expressed in monetary terms. Expressing certain benefits, such as reduction in pain or increase in life expectancy, in dollar values is complex and requires a number of gross assumptions. Various techniques, such as the *human capital* approach or the *willingness-to-pay* method, have been employed, but they still have important limitations, and the results tend to be controversial. As a result, the field has increasingly moved away from cost-benefit analyses and toward cost-effectiveness analyses.[8]

In a cost-effectiveness analysis, the health benefits are expressed in the most appropriate natural units, such as *cases successfully detected* or *years of life gained*.[8] Most of today's interventions, however, affect not one but multiple clinical outcomes. For example, treatment modalities for end-stage heart failure, such as mechanical assist devices, may extend life but decrease quality of life. At the same time, certain pharmacologic agents for this condition, such as flosequinan,

have been found to increase quality of life but decrease survival. In such cases, it is desirable to use QALYs as a common metric for integrating mortality and morbidity data. As described earlier, the quality adjustment is based on a set of values or weights, called *utilities* or *preferences*, that reflect the relative desirability of a particular health state. In a so-called cost-utility analysis, which is a special form of cost-effectiveness analysis, the results are expressed as the cost per QALY gained.

Cost-effectiveness and cost-utility ratios are calculated by dividing the net costs of an intervention by the net health effects of an intervention. Thus, the lower the value of the ratio, the higher the priority, in terms of maximizing benefits derived from a given health expenditure. Table 3–6 compares several cardiovascular interventions in terms of their cost-effectiveness ratios. This table underscores that certain interventions may be highly cost-effective for one indication but very cost-ineffective for another (e.g., coronary artery bypass surgery for left main stenosis is $6900 per QALY, whereas for one-vessel stenosis with mild angina it is $899,300).[32]

The following cost-effectiveness analysis demonstrates that even seemingly inexpensive and routine practices may turn out to be extravagant when subjected to a rigorous economic analysis: The AIDS epidemic has increased the concern about transmitting infectious diseases through blood transfusions. Although efforts to screen the blood supply for HIV and hepatitis C have improved, there has been a dramatic increase in preoperative autologous blood donations. Autologous blood donation entails greater administrative expense and a longer, more labor-intensive process of collection than allogeneic blood donation. More importantly, the frequency of positive test results for infectious diseases in autologous blood has caused most centers to destroy unused units of such blood rather than using them for other patients. Needless to say, this raises the cost of autologous transfusions. A recent cost-effectiveness analysis conducted at the University of California–Los Angeles made the case for abandoning autologous blood donations on economic grounds.[11] The results of this analysis were that the substitution of autologous for allogeneic blood would result in little expected health benefit (between 0.0002 and 0.00044 QALY saved per unit of blood), at considerable additional cost (between $68 and

TABLE 3–6. Cost-Effectiveness Ratios of Selected Cardiovascular Treatments

Treatment	Cost per Life Year or QALY Gained (1991 Dollars)
Coronary artery bypass surgery	
Left main coronary artery disease	$6900
3-vessel coronary artery disease	
Severe angina	$14,400
Very mild angina, poor LV function	$9500
Very mild angina, good LV function	$143,800
2-vessel coronary artery disease	
Severe angina	$33,500
Very mild angina	$89,900
1-vessel coronary artery disease	
Severe angina	$57,400
Very mild angina	$899,300
Percutaneous transluminal coronary angioplasty	
Severe angina	$6900–12,700
Mild angina	$47,200–102,400
Cardiac transplantation	$32,000

LV, left ventricular.
Reprinted with permission from THE ARTIFICIAL HEART: PROTOTYPES, POLICIES, AND PATIENTS. Copyright 1991 by the National Academy of Sciences. Courtesy of the National Academy Press, Washington, D.C.

$4783 per unit of blood) for four surgical procedures (total hip replacement, coronary artery bypass grafting, abdominal hysterectomy, and transurethral prostatectomy). The cost-effectiveness values ranged from $235,000 to over $23 million per QALY saved.

Measuring Costs

Measuring health care costs is fraught with practical and conceptual difficulties. Although analyses have historically used the charges that providers bill as proxies for the cost of resources, charges may differ substantially from the resource costs of delivering care. This divergence may stem from cross-subsidization of less lucrative products and services by more profitable ones, and cost-shifting to some patients and third-party payers from those that cannot pay all or part of their medical bills.[27] A less-than-perfect proxy for measuring costs is the *ratio-of-costs-to-charges* (RCC) method. With this method, charges billed are converted to actual hospital expenditures using a ratio of the actual costs to the charges billed; however, hospitals calculate RCCs only down to the department level. This means that the RCC loses accuracy when applied to individual patients who have undergone specific procedures, such as a lung transplantation. Furthermore, overhead allocation rules that are factored into the ratios do not have a strong relationship with per-patient resource use, which creates further inaccuracies. Payments relate to actual financial transactions but reflect differences in resource use only for services that are paid separately. Diagnosis-related group (DRG) payments for hospitalizations, for example, might not capture differences in resources used for particular diagnostic or therapeutic procedures because they are not paid for separately. *Resource costs*, the monetary value of actual resources used to deliver care, are the most desirable conceptually but usually require extensive data collection to obtain.

Different types of costs can be examined within an economic evaluation. Direct costs include those resource categories directly related to the technology being studied, such as personnel, medication, diagnostic testing, outpatient visits, cost of treatment required to manage side effects, or cost of treatment averted as a result of the health effects of a program. Direct costs can also include nonmedical costs, such as transportation of patients to and from the hospital, home health care services, or nursing home care.[49] Indirect costs include earnings gained or lost by patients and the economic value of intangible costs, such as pain, suffering, or quality of life; as mentioned, current methodology is limited in capturing such costs. An important analytic distinction concerns the difference between average and marginal costs. Generally, the interesting question in health care is, What are the additional, or marginal, benefits of additional, or marginal, increases in resource expenditures? Neuhauser and Lewicki conducted one of the more telling analyses in this respect.[31] They examined the marginal costs of a recommendation by the American Cancer Society to conduct six sequential stool tests for detecting cancer of the large bowel and found that conducting the sixth test would cost society $47 million per case detected!

Interpretation and Extrapolation of Economic Results

Historically, economic analyses were often conducted separately from clinical trials, and they used the evidence from existing clinical and epidemiologic studies to determine the health effects of a particular practice or treatment modality. One of the arguments for not integrating economic studies into clinical trials was that the care provided in these trials is so atypical of normal practice that it would be unwise to extrapolate from the data on resource use.[8] Furthermore, if a new clinical practice was just emerging, it was likely that the manner of use, clinical results, and costs associated with its use were undergoing continuous change. In recent years, however, pressures have been mounting to understand both the clinical and the cost implications of new technologies before they are widely diffused into clinical practice. As a result, more economic studies are incorporated into clinical trials of new and emerging interventions. This raises a number of methodologic issues about the generalizability of results from the clinical experiment to the real world. For instance, it is important to identify whether the frequency of consumption of particular resources, such as diagnostic tests, is determined by the trial and may differ from routine practice. Also, clinical trials of new procedures are often conducted in academic health centers that differ from other practice settings. Sensitivity analysis is the tool for assessing the external validity of the results of economic analysis, and it can be used to extend the analysis to different clinical and economic circumstances. Thus, to increase the value of economic evaluations for health care decision making, it is important that these evaluations not restrict themselves to data from a particular trial, modeling exercises must be conducted in which trial data are combined with data obtained from a mixture of sources.

IMPACT OF THE OUTCOMES MOVEMENT ON THE PRACTICE OF SURGERY

In recent years, rigorous methods of clinical evaluation have increasingly supplanted subjective clinical experience in the assessment of new and existing surgical procedures. The dramatic restructuring of the U.S. health care system is reinforcing this trend. This chapter reviews a diverse set of methods that may be employed to measure the outcomes of clinical practices. These methods can be used to evaluate an increasingly broad range of end-points, including clinical effectiveness, quality of life, patient preferences, and costs. As such, the results of evaluative studies can be used by the different players in the U.S. health care system to improve the quality of medical care.

In what ways can this type of research contribute to surgical practice? Obviously, these studies provide critical information to surgeons, as well as other physicians, about the effectiveness and cost-effectiveness of alternative surgical treatments. Presumably this information should lead to more evidence-based use of existing surgical treatments and, more generally, the use of health care resources. In addition, outcomes studies may identify the elements of care that account for the outcomes achieved, thereby facilitating efforts by clinicians and hospitals to improve the outcomes of care in their institutions. In New York State, for example, cardiovascular surgeons and cardiologists created the cardiac advisory committee, which has provided important risk-adjusted outcomes information on open-heart surgery in the state. These profiles are available on specific institutions and practitioners and are commonly referred to as *practice profiling*.

These profiles, and outcomes research in general, have use beyond self-assessment. First, they provide information on the risks and benefits of clinical interventions to prospective patients and the general public. This allows patients, in consultation with their physicians, to have a realistic look at the outcomes facing them, which facilitates making more informed choices based on willingness to accept risk. As such, outcomes research may contribute to a clinical decision-making process that better reflects patient preferences. Finally, outcomes research may provide important information to federal and state authorities, as well as to health care payers. In particular, it may assist in guiding licensure decisions, identifying centers of excellence for advanced tertiary care, and determining appropriate benefit packages—all of these, in turn, affect the quality and cost of care.

Realizing the potential of outcomes research, however, requires certain conditions to be fulfilled. First, in a dramatically changing health care environment, managed care organizations, with their large patient populations and vast databases, need to be encouraged to participate more fully in evaluative research. In fact, several managed care organizations are beginning to do so. For instance, in response to pressures from patients who want access to new procedures, a number of managed care providers have agreed to offer coverage for certain costly experimental interventions (such as autologous bone marrow transplants to treat advanced breast cancer), but only on the condition that the patient enrolls in a research protocol designed to assess that technology. Such efforts need to be expanded to include the evaluation of new medications, devices, and procedures, as well as the assessment of older but inadequately evaluated ones.

Second, investigators need to find more effective ways to disseminate the product of outcomes research. The evidence, so far, indicates that merely publishing outcomes information is insufficient to change clinical practice significantly. Other factors, such as the opinion of clinical colleagues, economic incentives, and administrative mechanisms (such as utilization review), are quite influential in determining practice patterns. As such, health care policymakers should untangle the complex of influences for given clinical practices and use that information to influence physician behavior.

Third, there is a clear need for more appropriate levels of funding for research to assess outcomes. In 1990, the federal government established the Agency for Health Care Policy and Research (AHCPR), whose mission includes outcomes research and technology assessment. Its goal is to encourage studies that will permit science-based consensus on the numerous clinical conditions for which there are wide and inexplicable variations in practice patterns. It should be noted, however, that this is still a very tentative step. Although the AHCPR is at the same administrative level as the NIH, its budget is minuscule compared with that of the NIH. The fundamental biomedical research supported by the NIH has provided a rich science base from which much of tomorrow's medical technology will be developed. At a time of severe budget constraints, however, it will not be easy to balance the competing claims of fundamental biology and the clinical evaluative sciences. In making those hard choices, government policy makers should keep in mind that clinical evaluation is an essential, albeit costly, part of medical innovation. Moreover, it provides important information for the reallocation of resources within the current system of expenditures.

ACKNOWLEDGMENT

One of the authors (A. C. G.) acknowledges the generous support of the Robert Wood Johnson Foundation's Investigator Awards in Health Policy Research.

REFERENCES

1. Chalmers, T. C.: Randomized clinical trials in surgery. *In* Varco, R.L.,and Delaney, J. P. (Eds.): Controversy in Surgery. Philadelphia, W. B. Saunders, 1976.
1a. Bombardier, C., Ware, J., Russell, I. J., et al.: Auranofin therapy and quality of life in patients with rheumatoid arthritis: Results of a multicenter trial. Am. J. Med., 81:565, 1986.
2. Chalmers, T. C., Block, J. B., and Lee, S.: Controlled studies in clinical cancer research. N. Engl. J. Med., 287:75, 1972.
2a. Chalmers, I., Hetherington, J., Elbourne, D., et al.: Methods used in synthesizing evidence to evaluate the effects of care during pregnancy and childbirth. *In* Chalmers, I., Enkin, M., and Keirse, M. J. (Eds.): Effective Care in Pregnancy and Childbirth. Oxford, Oxford University Press, 1989.
2b. Chalmers, T. C., Smith, H., Jr., Blackburn, B., et al.: A method for assessing the quality of a randomized control trial. Control. Clin. Trials, 2:31, 1981.
3. Churchill, D. N., Morgan, J., and Torrance, G. W.: Quality of life in end-stage renal disease. Peritoneal Dialysis Bulletin, January–March 1994, p. 20.
3a. Churchill, D. N., Torrance, G. W., Taylor, D. W., et al.: Measurement of quality of life in end-stage renal disease: The time trade-off approach. Clin. Invest. Med., 10:14, 1987.
4. Connors, E. M., Sperling, R. S., Gelber, R., et al.: Reduction of maternal-infant transmission of human immunodeficiency virus type 1 with zidovudine treatment: Pediatric AIDS clinical trials group protocol 076 study group. N. Engl. J. Med., 331:1173, 1994.
5. DerSimonian, R., and Laird, N.: Meta-analysis in clinical trials. Control Clin. Trials, 7:177, 1986.
6. Dickersin, K., and Berlin, J. A.: Meta-analysis: State of the science. Epidemiol. Rev., 14:154, 1992.
7. Drummond, M. F., Stoddart, G. L., and Torrance, G. W.: Methods for the Economic Evaluation of Health Care Programmes. Oxford, Oxford University Press, 1987.
8. Drummond, M. F., and Davies, L.: Economic analysis alongside clinical trials: Revisiting the methodological issues. Int. J. Technol. Assess. Health Care, 7:561, 1991.
9. Eddy, D. M.: Variations in physician practice: The role of uncertainty. Health Aff., 3:74, 1984.
10. Ekbom, A., Yuen, J., Adami, H. O., et al.: Cholecystectomy and colorectal cancer. Gastroenterology, 101:286, 1993.
11. Etchason, J., Petz, L., Keeler, E., Caloun, L., Kleinman, S., Snider, C., Fink, A., and Brook, R.: The cost effectiveness of preoperative autologous blood donations. N. Engl. J. Med., 332:719, 1995.
12. Feeney, D. H., Torrance, G. W., Goldsmith, G. H., Fulong, W., and Boyle, M. H. A multi-attribute approach to population health status. Proceedings of 153rd annual meeting of the American Statistical Association, session 180, Measuring Health Status: Survey-Based Approaches, San Francisco, August 10, 1993.
13. Fletcher, R. H., Fletcher, S. W., and Wagner, E. H.: Clinical Epidemiology: The Essentials. Baltimore, Williams & Wilkins, 1988.
14. Giovannucci, E., Codlitz, G. A., and Stampfer, M. J.: A meta-analysis of cholecystectomy and risk of colorectal cancer. Gastroenterology, 105:130, 1993.
15. Gordon, T., and Kannel, W. B.: Predisposition to atherosclerosis in the head, heart and legs: The Framingham study. JAMA, 221:661, 1972.
16. Grage, T. B., and Zelen, M.: The controlled randomized trial in the evaluation of cancer treatment—the dilemma and alternative designs. UICC Tech. Rep. Ser., 70:23, 1980.
17. Guyatt, G. H., Feeney, D. H., and Patrick, D. L.: Measuring health-related quality of life. Ann. Intern. Med., 118:622, 1993.
18. Herbst, A. L., Green, T. H., Jr., and Ulfelder, H.: Primary carcinoma of the vagina: An analysis of 68 cases. Am. J. Obstet. Gynecol., 106:210, 1970.
19. Herbst, A. L., and Scully, R. E.: Adenocarcinoma of the vagina in adolescence: A report of 7 cases including 6 clear-cell carcinomas (so-called mesonephromas). Cancer, 25:745, 1970.
20. Herbst, A. L., Ulfelder, H., and Poskanzer, D. C.: Adenocarcinoma of the vagina: Association of maternal stilbestrol therapy with tumor appearance in young women. N. Engl. J. Med., 284:8778, 1971.
21. Hlatky, M. A., Leek, L., Harrell, F. E., Califf, R. M., Pryor, P. B., March, D. B., and Rosatti, R. A.: Tying clinical research to patient care by use of an observational database. Stat. Med., 3:375, 1984.
22. Janowitz, P., Gessner, F., Wechsler, J. G., et al.: Increased incidence of gallstones and prior cholecystectomy in patients with large bowel cancer. Am. J. Gastroenterol., 97:1120, 1992.
23. Kassirer, K. P., Moskowitz, A. J., Lau, J., and Pauker, S. G.: Decision analysis: A progress report. Ann. Intern. Med., 106:275, 1987.
24. Klatskin, G., and Kimberg, D. V.: Recurrent hepatitis attributable to halothane sensitization in an anesthetist. N. Engl. J. Med., 280:515, 1969.
25. Klieinbaum, D., Kuupper, L. L., and Morgenstern, H.: Epidemiologic Research: Principles and Quantitative Methods. New York, Van Nostrand Reinhold, 1982.
26. Light, R. J., and Ploymer, D. B.: Summing Up: The Science of Reviewing Research. Cambridge, Harvard University Press, 1984.
27. Luce, B. R., and Alixhauser, A.: Estimating costs in the economic evaluation of medical technologies. Int. J. Technol. Assess. Health Care, 6:57, 1990.
28. Moskowitz, A. J., Kuipers, B. J., and Kassirer, J.: Dealing with uncertainty, risks and tradeoffs in clinical decisions: A cognitive science approach. Ann. Intern. Med., 108:435, 1988.
29. Moskowitz, A. J., and Pauker, S. G.: A decision analytic approach to limb-sparing treatment for adult soft tissue and osteogenic sarcoma. Cancer Treat. Symp., 3:11, 1985.
29a. Moskowitz A. J., Weinberg, A. D., Oz, M. C., and Williams, D. L.: Quality of life with a ventricular assist device: The potential for destination therapy. J. Heart Lung Transplant., 15:S75, 1996.
30. Neuhauser, D.: Ernest Amory Codman, M.D., and end results of medical care. Int. J. Technol. Assess. Health Care, 6:307, 1990.
31. Neuhauser, D., and Lewicki, A. M.: What do we gain from the sixth stool guaiac? N. Engl. J. Med., 293:226, 1975.
32. Neumann, P. J., and Weinsteind, M. C.: The diffusion of new technology:

Costs and benefits to health care. *In* Gelijns, A. C., and Halm, E. A. (Eds.): The Changing Economic of Health Care: Medical Innovation at the Crossroads. Vol. 2. Washington, D.C., National Academy Press, 1991.

33. Pearson, K.: Report on certain enteric fever inoculation statistics. Br. Med. J., 3:1243, 1904.
34. Pliskin, J. S., Shepard, D. S., and Weinstein, M. C.: Utility functions for life years and health status. Operations Res., 28:206, 1980.
35. Pocock, S. J.: Clinical Trials: A Practical Approach. New York, John Wiley and Sons, 1983.
36. Quaegebeur, J. M., Rohmer, J., Ottenkamp, J., Buis, T., Kirklin, J. W., Blackstone, E. H., and Brom, A. G.: The arterial switch operation—an eight year experience. J. Thorac. Cardiovasc. Surg., 92:361, 1986.
37. Rector, T. S., Kubo, S. P., and Cohn, J. N.: Validity of the Minnesota living with heart failure questionnaire as a measure of therapeutic response to enalapril or placebo. Am. J. Cardiol., 71:1106, 1993.
38. Relman, A. S.: Assessment and accountability: The third revolution in medical care. N. Engl. J. Med., 319:1220, 1988.
39. Rettig, R. A.: Health policy in radiology: Technology assessment—an update. Invest. Radiol., 26:165, 1991.
40. Roos, L. L.: Nonexperimental data systems in surgery. Int. J. Technol. Assess. Health Care, 5:341, 1989.
41. Sackett, D. L., Haynes, R. B., and Tugwell, P.: Clinical Epidemiology: A Basic Science for Clinical Medicine. Boston, Little, Brown, 1985.
42. Sacks, H. S., Berrier, J., Reitman, D., Ancona-Berk, V. A., and Chalmers, T. C.: Meta-analyses of randomized controlled trials. N. Engl. J. Med., 316:450, 1987.
43. Sacks, H. S., and Rose, D. N.: Zidovudine prophylaxis for needlestick exposure to human immunodeficiency virus: A decision analysis. J. Gen. Intern. Med., 5:132, 1990.
44. Schlesselman, J. J.: Case-Control Studies: Design, Conduct, Analysis. New York, Oxford University Press, 1982.
45. Sox, H. C., Blatt, M. A., Higgins, M. C., and Marton, K. I.: Medical Decision Making. Stoneham, Mass., Butterworth, 1988.
46. Torrance, G. W.: Utility approach to measuring health-related quality of life. J. Chron. Dis., 40:6, 1987.
47. von Neumann, J., and Morgenstern, O.: Theory of Games and Economic Behavior, 2nd ed. Princeton, N.J., Princeton University Press, 1947.
48. Vos, R.: Drugs Looking for Disease [Dissertation]. Groningen, C. Regenboog, 1989.
49. Ware, J. E., and Sherbourne, C. D.: The MOS 36-item short-form health survey (SF-36). 1. Conceptual framework and item selection. Med. Care, 30:473, 1992.
50. Weinstein, M. C.: Principles of cost-effective resource allocation in health care organizations. Int. J. Technol. Assess. Health Care, 6:93, 1990.
51. Wennberg, J. E., Roos, N. P., Sola, L., Schori, A., and Jaffe, R.: Use of claims data system to evaluate health care outcomes: Mortality and reoperation following prostatectomy. JAMA, 257:933, 1987.
52. Zelen, M.: A new design for randomized clinical trials. N. Engl. J. Med., 300:1242, 1980.

Figure 3–1 Citations

1. Vernick, L. J., and Kuller, L. H.: Cholecystectomy and right-sided colon cancer: An epidemiological study. Lancet, 2:381, 1981.
2. Weiss, N. S., Daling, J. R., and Chow, W. H.: Cholecystectomy and the incidence of cancer of the large bowel. Cancer, 49:1713, 1982.
3. Blanco, D., Ross, R. K., Paganini-Hill, A., and Henderson, B.E.: Cholecystectomy and colonic cancer. Dis. Colon Rectum, 27:290, 1984.
4. Fixa, B., Komarkova, O., Zaydlar, K., Bures, J., and Erben J.: Is there an increased risk of colorectal cancer after cholecystectomy? Neoplasma, 32:513, 1985.
5. Friedman, G. D., Goldhaber, M. K., and Quesenberry, C. P., Jr.: Cholecystectomy and alare bowel cancer. Lancet, 1:906, 1987.
6. Kune, G. A, Kune, S., and Watson, L. F.: Large bowel cancer after cholecystectomy. Am. J. Surg., 156:359, 1988.
7. Soltero, E., Cruz, N. I., Nazario, C. M., Lopez, R. E., Alonso, A., and Carols, F. R.: Cholecystectomy and right colon cancer in Puerto Rico. Cancer, 66:2249, 1990.

CHAPTER 4

HOMEOSTASIS

Bodily Changes in Trauma and Surgery

Douglas W. Wilmore, M.D.

Surgeons care for patients who experience sudden, rapid, and intense changes in normal physiologic function and metabolism. Such alterations occur after an elective operative procedure, an event that causes pain, interrupts normal food and fluid intake, and usually involves tissue removal and/ or disruption, often of a vital organ. A more dramatic perturbation occurs after major accidental injury, which involves rapid blood loss, tissue underperfusion, massive cellular damage, and disturbance of vital organ function.

The human body responds to these stresses with dramatic resilience. For example, after injury, clotting mechanisms are immediately activated to reduce blood loss; body fluids shift from the extravascular compartment to restore blood volumes; blood flow is redistributed to ensure perfusion of vital organs; and respiratory and renal functions compensate to maintain acid-base neutrality and body fluid tonicity. After these acute adaptations, other changes occur; these responses are more gradual and prolonged but are apparently necessary for recovery of the injured organism. Numerous immunologic alterations are initiated; leukocytes are mobilized, macrophages and specialized T cells are produced, and "acute-phase" plasma proteins are synthesized by the liver. Inflammatory cells invade the injured area, set up a perimeter defense, and engulf the dead and dying cells and other wound contaminants. These initial steps are followed rapidly by ingrowth of blood vessels, appearance of fibroblasts that build collagen scaffolding, and a host of other local changes that aid wound repair.

Local changes that occur at the injury site are accompanied by systemic alterations in body physiologic processes and metabolism. Cardiac output is elevated, minute ventilation is increased, and the patient becomes febrile. Lipolysis and skeletal muscle proteolysis are accelerated, providing an ongoing fuel supply and an immediate source of amino acids that are used for wound healing and synthesis of "acute-phase" proteins and new glucose. The glucose provides essential energy for the brain and other vital organs and for healing of the wound.

These biologic functions following injury and other stresses reflect a unique and indelible program that is encoded in higher species, particularly *Homo sapiens.* In strict Darwinian terms, these responses follow an evolutionary process that favors survival of the fittest in the struggle for existence. In teleologic terms, these responses have a purpose: to benefit the organism and aid recovery. Although a direct cause-and-effect relationship has not been established between many of these posttraumatic events and recovery, these adaptive responses occur during the same period when the wound heals and the patient returns to health. Elective operative procedures without complications, accompanied by appropriate anesthesia and adequate postoperative pain control, cause minimal changes in bodily functions in the low-risk patient. Thus, intervention on the part of the surgeon is rarely necessary and can even be meddlesome. However, critical illnesses secondary to major injury or infection require significant therapy to aid eventual recovery. Knowledge of homeostatic adjustments that occur in critically ill patients is essential for optimal patient care and reflects the physician's insight into blood volume regulation, nutritional requirements, cardiovascular resuscitation, wound healing, and physical and psychological rehabilitation and recovery from a life-threatening illness.

Whereas constancy of biologic systems was appreciated as early as the time of Hippocrates, it was not until the 1800s, when Claude Bernard established physiology as a new discipline, that regulation of body systems to maintain internal constancy was actually proposed. Bernard suggested that all living processes were attributable to biochemical and physiologic reactions and that a detailed analysis of these functions would allow a more complete understanding of the process of life. In his *Introduction to the Study of Experimental Medicine,* Bernard detailed a number of studies that described the digestion of food, the maintenance of blood glucose, and the vasomotor control of circulation. He proposed that living organs did not exist "in the *milieu extérieur"* (the atmosphere, or salt or fresh water), but in a liquid *milieu intérieur* formed by circulating organic liquid that surrounds and bathes all of the tissue elements; this is the lymphoplasma, the liquid part of the blood, which in the higher animals is perfused through the tissue and is the basis of all local nutrition and the common factor of all elementary changes. The stability of the *milieu intérieur* is the primary condition for freedom and independence of existence.[2] Thus, Bernard's description of the constancy of the chemical composition of the body formed the basis for understanding the uniqueness of animal life.

The next major contributor to the field of body homeostasis was Walter B. Cannon, an American who served as a physiologist at the Harvard Medical School for most of his professional career. Much like Bernard, Cannon worked in a number of different areas, including digestion, metabolism, control of hunger and thirst, maintenance of blood glucose, tissue energetics, thermoregulation, and maintenance of oxygen supply. However, Cannon is best known for his detailed studies of the autonomic nervous system; he described the sympathetic and parasympathetic nervous system and proved that autonomic nervous system control maintained constancy and autoregulatory adjustments after stress. Cannon coined the word *homeostasis* and defined it as "the coordinated physiological process which maintains most of the steady states in the organisms."[6] He noted that homeostatic responses were extremely complex, involving brain, nerves, heart, lungs, kidneys, and spleen; these organs worked cooperatively to maintain body constancy.

While these physiologic mechanisms were being observed, the description and categorization of responses that occurred in patients after injury and other critical illnesses were also being recorded. John Hunter, an English surgeon and biologist in the eighteenth century, commented on the response that occurred after tissue injury and noted: "There is a circumstance attending accidental injury which does not belong to disease, namely that the injury done, has in all cases a tendency to produce, both the deposition and means of cure."[14] This was the first suggestion that the responses to injury were beneficial to the host.

In the latter part of the nineteenth century, an extremely imaginative group of German scientists focused their energies on the study of protein metabolism and the thermogenesis of food. These individuals, led by Carl Voit, performed nitrogen balance studies and built large calorimeters for the study of food oxidation and heat production. Both energy and nitrogen balance studies were performed under a variety of experimental conditions in animals and humans. With these techniques, the impact of infection on protein metabolism was studied and a view contrary to that suggested by Hunter was proposed.[25] The German scientists described the accelerated proteolysis that accompanies infection as the "toxic destruction of protein," implying that this process was maladaptive rather than an appropriate response to illness.

The "modern era" of understanding injury responses was initiated by the careful and thorough studies of David Patton Cuthbertson, a young Scottish clinical chemist working in Glasgow in the early 1930s. Cuthbertson studied the urinary excretion of calcium and phosphorus in patients who sustained long bone fractures. He hoped to relate abnormal mineral excretion to delayed fracture healing. Extensive balance studies were performed in normal individuals confined to bed and in patients with long bone fractures. Cuthbertson noted that the injured patients had increased urinary excretion of phosphorus and exaggerated urinary losses of nitrogen and potassium.[8] He also determined energy requirement, using indirect calorimetry in the injured patients, and found that increased oxygen consumption accompanied the protein catabolic response. Cuthbertson described a constant rise in body temperature in uninfected, injured patients and characterized this response as "posttraumatic fever." In subsequent studies he attempted to modify the injury response by altering food intake but noted that the increased nitrogen excretion could not be diminished by nutrient intake. Because of the large quantity of nitrogen lost, he suggested that the nitrogen excreted in the urine was due to a generalized proteolytic response throughout the skeletal muscle mass and did not follow protein breakdown at the site of injury.

Some years later, Francis D. Moore, Moseley Professor of Surgery at the Harvard Medical School, collected, tabulated, categorized, and applied much of the knowledge concerning homeostatic responses following trauma and surgery to patient care. He brought sophisticated scientific techniques to the bedside, used isotopic dilution methodology to measure body composition in patients, and developed an intensive care unit where careful balance studies could be performed in critically ill patients. He evaluated the impact of specific components of the injury response such as bed rest, anesthesia, volume loss, and starvation on metabolic responses and described various stages of convalescence after injury. This information is summarized in his classic volume *The Metabolic Care of the Surgical Patient*.[20] More important, however, this information was translated into knowledge that could be applied by the practicing surgeon to improve the care of the critically ill surgical patient.

Many others have contributed to the field of homeostatic alterations following injury. Other authorities have directed their attention to specific areas, and much of this knowledge serves as the basis for chapters in this textbook. In addition to focusing on specific areas, a body of knowledge has evolved that addresses responses to stress and the control of biologic systems.

Proposed models for the regulation of homeostasis define a signal detector, a processor, and an effector organ, all elements necessary for maintaining the internal milieu. In classic physiologic terms, such systems are controlled by negative feedback servomechanisms (Fig. 4–1). In addition, open loop controllers may function in the trauma patient. One example is the constant demand for glucose by the healing wound; provision of dietary glucose fails to suppress the accelerated gluconeogenesis and marked insulin resistance that occur after injury, suggesting that the usual feedback signal is absent. Only wound closure and/or healing returns these alterations to normal, indicating that an open loop stimulus-response system may be operative. Much of the knowledge of biochemical controls is incorporated in the field of endocrinology, but more specific areas of study have evolved, such as cybernetics and control theory. These areas of knowledge have improved understanding of biologic processes and, with computer application, may lead to the development of artificial intelligence.

ANATOMY

Body Composition and Its Response to Surgical Stress. The body is composed of two major components: a *nonaqueous* and an *aqueous* phase.[20] Body fat and extracellular solids such as bone matrix, tendon, fascia, and collagen make up the nonhydrous portion. The aqueous phase is, in general, the sum of three compartments: extracellular water, blood volume, and intracellular fluid. Cells of the body are supported within the aqueous phase, and the heterogeneous mass of body cells and the supporting aqueous environment is called the *lean body mass*. The *body cell mass* is the metabolically active portion of the body and is composed of the lean body mass minus the extracellular fluid. This is the portion of the body that consists of all hydrated cells and represents the functioning, actively exchanging component of the body. The body cell mass consists of skeletal muscle, visceral organs, and a smaller portion of cells that lies on the periphery and includes connective tissue, skin, and areolar cells and the red cell mass. The measure of total body nitrogen by neutron activation analysis allows quantitation of the body cell mass. The determination of total exchangeable potassium has also been used to measure this compartment but appears to be more imprecise. In contrast, extracellular fluid is relatively depleted of potassium but is rich in sodium. Extracellular fluid is determined by one of a variety of isotope dilutional techniques or other body compositional measurements that quantitate the size of the extracellular fluid compartments. Body composition of normal individuals varies with age and sex.[7, 20] Normal composition is shown in Figure 4–2.

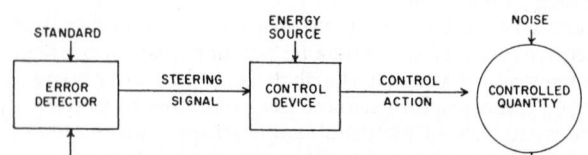

Figure 4–1. An early model of a biologic control system. The error detector serves as a monitor and elicits signals (usually hormonal or nervous), which affect the control device that imparts a change. This perturbation is generally larger than the background *noise* level, and the correction is perceived by the detector. A biologic example would be the response to hypoglycemia (glucose being the "controlled quantity"). This would be detected in the hypothalamus, which would *signal* via hormones and the sympathetic nervous system to the liver ("control device") to liberate more glucose. When the blood glucose level is corrected, the *error detector* diminishes its signal. (From Brookhaven Symposia in Biology, 10, Homeostatic Mechanisms. Office of Technical Services, Washington, D.C., 1958.)

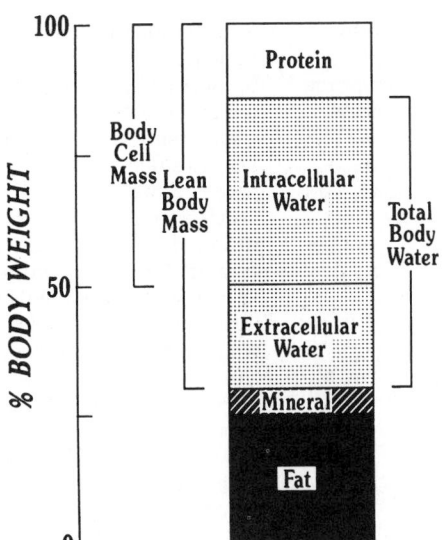

Figure 4–2. Normal body composition. The body weight is the sum of body fat, mineral content, water, and protein. The *lean mass* is defined as the nonfat and nonmineral-containing tissue, whereas the body cell mass is the lean without the extracellular fluid compartment. The total body water is subdivided into the extracellular water and the intracellular water.

NORMAL REFERENCE VALUES

	Male	Female
Body Weight (kg)	70.0	60.0
Lean Body Mass (kg)	54.0	40.4
Body Cell Mass (kg)	36.7	26.7
Extracellular Water (L)	17.3	14.0
Intracellular Water (L)	22.1	15.5
Total Body Water (L)	39.4	29.5
Protein (kg)	14.6	10.9
Minerals (kg)	2.9	2.5
Fat (kg)	13.1	17.1

Alteration in Body Composition with Disease. The components of the body change with disease. For example, obesity increases the absolute (or relative) quantity of adipose tissue, whereas starvation decreases both fat and lean body mass. Patients with disorders of fluid homeostasis have alterations in the size of the aqueous compartments. For example, an individual with congestive heart failure has an expanded extracellular fluid volume associated with an increase in total exchangeable body sodium. A common response also occurs after loss of body protoplasm. This is characterized by loss of body cell mass as measured by a decrease in total exchangeable potassium and an observable diminution of skeletal muscle mass associated with loss of body fat, expansion of the extracellular fluid compartment, and increase in total exchangeable sodium. Thus, the extracellular fluid compartment enlarges and salt is retained, while the body mass (functional tissue) is reduced (Fig. 4–3). These changes may be greatly exaggerated by specific organ dysfunction (such as heart or renal failure) and/or accelerated weight loss, which occurs in unfed patients after severe injury or infection. Because of the avidity of the body to retain water and sodium, critically ill patients become extremely sensitive to volume and sodium loads; sodium-containing solutions should be administered judiciously in such patients.

Body Energy Stores. The components of the body cell mass represent active, functioning tissue. These cells and the adipose tissue also represent a form of stored energy. The greatest energy component is fat, which is a nonhydrous portion of the body that yields approximately 9 calories per gm. (Table 4–1). Thus, this calorically dense storage form of energy provides a source of lightweight and transportable fuel to be used by highly mobile species. The protein component of the body is the next largest substrate mass but yields considerably fewer calories than body fat because of its caloric content of only 4 calories per gm. Moreover, because the body cell mass is hydrated, body protein, when expressed as caloric potential, is quite different from fat on a weight basis. This is because hydrated muscle tissue contains three parts water and one part protein, which yield only 1 calorie per gm. of hydrated protein. These differences between nonhydrous fat and hydrated protein highlight the relative inefficiency of body protein as a transportable caloric source. Body protein is thus not a primary storage fuel but rather serves as structural and functional components of the body; *loss of body protein is associated with loss of body function.* Reduction of body protein is not without consequence. During catabolic

states, protein is broken down and used primarily to synthesize new glucose, which does not exist in storage form to a great extent and is rapidly oxidized after stress (see Table 4–1). Because several vital organs, including the brain, peripheral nerves, renal medulla, red cells, white cells, and inflammatory tissue, all use glucose as a primary fuel, the need for an ongoing glucose supply is imperative if the organism is to survive. An ongoing glucose supply is provided via proteolysis (primarily skeletal muscle) and accelerated hepatic gluconeogenesis. The conversion of amino acids

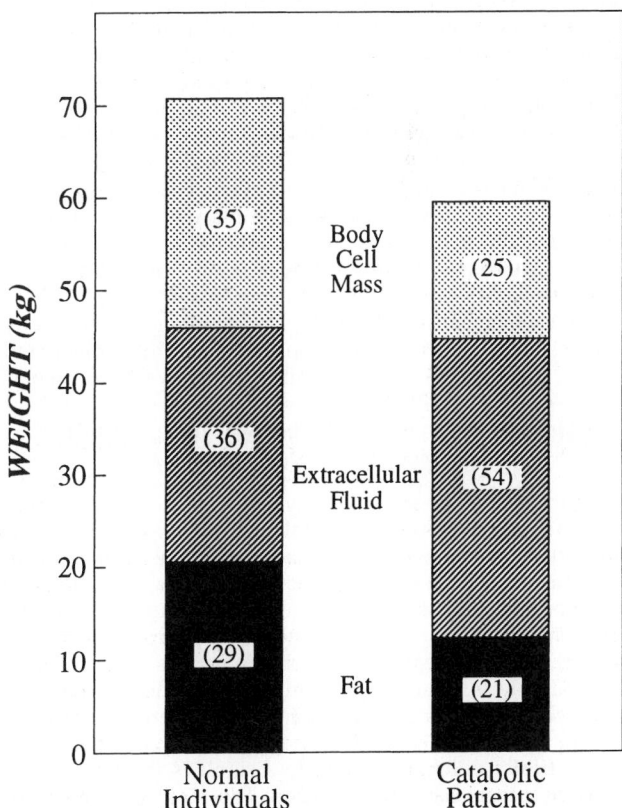

Figure 4–3. Changes in body composition with catabolic illness. Numbers in parentheses denote percentage of the total. (Data from Shizgal, H. M.: Body composition. *In* Fischer, J. E. [Ed.]: Surgical Nutrition. Boston, Little, Brown, 1983, pp. 1–17.)

TABLE 4–1. Estimated Fuel Consumption of Normal Individuals

	kg.	kcal.
Tissues		
Fat	15.0	141,000
Protein	6.0	24,000
Glycogen (muscle)	0.150	600
Glycogen (liver)	0.075	300
Total		165,900
Circulating		
Glucose (extracellular water)	0.020	80
Free fatty acids (plasma)	0.0003	3
Triglyceride (plasma)	0.003	30
Total		113

Adapted from Cahill, G. F., Jr.: Starvation in man. N. Engl. J. Med., *282*:668, 1970. Copyright 1970. Massachusetts Medical Society.

to glucose is a necessary step because the enzymatic machinery is not present in humans to convert long-chain fatty acids to glucose.

The alterations in body compartments following critical illness have been quantitated using compositional studies and balance techniques. Most normal individuals can lose up to 10% of body weight with minimal changes in physiologic function, but weight loss greater than this compromises normal responses and may limit survival. Approximately one half of the weight loss after a catabolic illness reflects a decrease in body fat; the remaining portion reflects loss of protein and its associated water (body cell mass).[20] Limitations in body function are reflected primarily by loss of body protein, excreted in the urine as nitrogen, and large losses may be extensive in a critically ill patient. If a normal individual undergoes 5 days of starvation, total protein loss may average approximately 1600 gm. of muscle tissue. If this same individual sustains injury and cannot eat, total protein loss is accelerated to 550 to 600 gm. over the same period, representing loss of more than 2 kg. of muscle tissue. Whereas these quantities are relatively small in terms of overall body protein, associated complications that may occur in the traumatized patient, coupled with adequate food intake, further accelerate proteolysis. Since death, secondary to starvation, is associated with losses of body protein of approximately 30% to 40%, such a tremendous drain on body nitrogen stores exerts an additional stress on the patient, and may be associated with the inability to survive major injury.

HOMEOSTATIC RESPONSES TO SPECIFIC COMPONENTS OF INJURY

Critical illness creates a variety of complex interacting homeostatic responses. The clinical features observed are the sum of changes known to occur after single perturbations. In the following section, events frequently observed in surgical patients are discussed as responses to one single change. These adjustments include volume loss, underperfusion, starvation, tissue damage, and invasive infection.

Volume Loss. Acute volume reduction associated with accidental injury or an elective surgical procedure is a nonlethal stimulus for the mechanisms that maintain circulation and restore blood volume. Volume loss signifies the decrease of effective circulating blood volume. The most frequent form of volume reduction in the surgical patient is simple hemorrhage. With blood loss there is no initial change in plasma osmolality or tonicity, and serum sodium and/or osmolality remains normal (this is referred to as *isotonic volume reduc-*

tion). Various responses are initiated after simple volume reduction, including the stimulation of pressor receptors in the arterial tree and volume receptors in the heart. These and other signals lead to the elaboration of aldosterone and vasopressin, which augment fluid retention.

In addition to the hormonal responses to a volume loss, there is a marked shift of fluid across capillary beds into the bloodstream.[20] This "refill" phenomenon decreases concentration of red cells (as measured by the hematocrit) and may slightly dilute the serum protein concentration. Transcapillary refill is stimulated by as little as a 15% to 20% loss in blood volume and, with other mechanisms, requires about 24 hours to restore blood volume.

In addition to hemorrhage, volume reduction occurs by other mechanisms. There may be acute *desalting water loss* associated with vomiting, diarrhea, pancreatic fistula, uncontrolled ileostomy loss, or intestinal obstruction. In these cases, there is minimal loss of red cell mass but often a decrease in tonicity after mobilization of cell water, which is relatively free of sodium. If osmotic changes in the plasma are marked because of loss of sodium, the plasma electrolyte alterations become quite distinct from those of isotonic volume reduction, as seen with mild to moderate hemorrhage.

Fluid losses may also cause the *desiccation-dehydration syndrome*, and excessive water is lost from the skin or lungs without accompanying salt loss. Such marked dehydration is characteristic of exposure to heat but can also occur with acute renal dysfunction, diarrhea associated with tube feedings, diabetic ketoacidosis, and simple dehydration. A rise in serum sodium, and thus in plasma tonicity, is characteristic of these states.

Underperfusion. Volume reduction is characterized by a set of compensatory responses that attempt to maintain circulating volume and plasma tonicity. However, blood volume reduction of any type, if severe enough, causes a prolonged low-flow state. During a low-flow state, oxygen delivery is inadequate for oxygen demands of the tissues despite compensatory mechanisms, and cell deterioration occurs. Inadequate perfusion causes accumulation of acid products, particularly lactic acid, within the body, and this is associated with profound acidosis of both the intracellular and extracellular fluid compartments. Compensatory adjustments are stimulated by the kidney and respiratory tract. However, with underperfusion, minimal quantities of urine are excreted, and this, accompanied by the presence of abnormal pigments in the plasma such as hemoglobin or myoglobin, may cause acute renal failure. If a low-flow state persists, cellular damage increases, disturbing membrane function. This effect is manifested by the need for large volumes of fluid to resuscitate the patient, referred to in animal shock models as the "reuptake phenomenon." In addition, reperfusion may be associated with the generation of free oxygen radicals, which cause tissue oxidative injury and cellular disruption. Thus, recovery from low-flow states depends on the extent and duration of the insult. Brief periods of underperfusion cause little sustained cellular damage, whereas more prolonged episodes cause marked acidosis, renal failure, central nervous system (CNS) hypoxia, and generalized disruption of cell function. Often, the patient does not recover if these alterations are irreversible.

Starvation. In many surgical patients, fluid and nutrient intake is interrupted and inadequate, or insufficient energy and protein are provided. When this occurs during simple starvation, fat mobilization proceeds and ketosis results. Concentration of plasma substrate generally reflects the decrease in glucose as a primary oxidizable fuel and the increase in fatty acids as the body's major energy source.[5] Insulin appears to have a central role in adaptation to fasting. As glucose and insulin levels fall, mobilization and utilization of fatty acids are favored at high rates of oxidation. Increased concentrations of fatty acids compete with glucose for entry into muscle cells and therefore are potent peripheral glucose antagonists. After several days of starvation, fatty acids are primarily oxidized in the liver to form acetoacetate, acetone, or beta-hydroxybutyrate, all referred to as *ketone bodies*. During total starvation, concentrations of blood ketone rise markedly and serve as signals to a variety of tissues to decrease glucose utilization or minimize protein breakdown. In addition, ketone bodies serve as oxidizable fuel, since these compounds are a water-soluble form of fat and can be used by the CNS during prolonged starvation. However, surgical patients frequently receive some glucose in their intravenous solutions, which stimulates insulin elaboration and limits ketosis.

Because carbohydrate stores are limited and because these glycogen stores are used rapidly after stress, an ongoing supply of glucose must be provided. Skeletal muscle proteolysis provides amino acids that serve as glucose precursors, although glycerol from triglyceride breakdown may also be used as a carbon source for new glucose.[5] Gluconeogenesis results and is generally proportional to the proteolysis and increased loss of urea in the urine.

Tissue Damage. Unlike the responses to simple starvation, which are characterized by a generalized decrease in metabolism, injured patients demonstrate heightened metabolic responses. These stem from the increased elaboration of catabolic hormones that stimulate respiration, cardiac output, and mobilization and utilization of fuel. All the processes contribute to the accelerated loss of body tissue. This response is characterized by increased oxidation of fat and marked proteolysis, primarily in skeletal muscle. Volume loss, underperfusion, and simple starvation may be additional components of this response, but the specific presence of damaged tissue appears to be the initiator of this hypercatabolic response. Tissue injury causes afferent nerve signals that increase elaboration of adrenocorticotropic hormone

(ACTH) and other pituitary hormones. However, other substances, such as cell breakdown products or mediators released during inflammation, may have additional metabolic effects. Many new inflammatory cells appear in the wound soon after injury. Initially, leukocytes predominate, but later macrophages and fibroblasts are the major cell types present. These cells release a variety of mediator substances, including cytokines, soluble biochemical signals that influence the proliferation, development, and function of surrounding cells to aid host resistance and wound repair. Many of these substances have been identified and include the interleukins, tumor necrosis factor (TNF)-alpha, the interferons, and various other growth factors (Table 4–2). These factors predominantly modify local cellular proliferation and regulate wound repair, through their paracrine action, but they may also reach the bloodstream to exert systemic effects, such as mediating fever, stimulating the elaboration of acute-phase proteins, and causing redistribution of trace elements. These responses to inflammation are collectively referred to as the acute-phase response. In addition, cytokines may stimulate the elaboration of pituitary hormones and activate the cyclooxygenase pathway, causing prostaglandin synthesis. Elaboration of prostaglandins, particularly PGE_2, may also contribute to some of the systemic responses observed after tissue injury.

Invasive Infection. One major complication observed in surgical patients is infection. The infective organisms are generally opportunistic bacteria that, under normal circumstances, are ubiquitous, noninvasive, and therefore benign. However, the multiple sites of entry via wounds and tubes that are present in the critically ill patient, coupled with alterations in host defense mechanisms, cause increased susceptibility of injured patients to infection. Infection alone initiates catabolic responses that are similar to (but not the same as) those described after injury in noninfected patients. Both processes cause fever, hyperventilation, tachycardia, accelerated gluconeogenesis, increased proteolysis, and lipoly-

TABLE 4–2. Sources and Targets of Some Cytokines and Other Peptide Regulatory Factors

Regulatory Factor*	Sources	Target Tissues/Cells
Interleukins (ILs)		
IL-1α, IL-1β (endogenous pyrogen, lymphocyte-activating factor, leukocyte endogenous mediator, hemopoietin-1)	Monocytes/macrophages; many endothelial, epithelial, and hematopoietic cells	Thymocytes, T and B cells, hematopoietic cells, fibroblasts, chondrocytes, receptors in brain and liver
IL-2 (T cell growth factor)	T cells	T and B cells, thymocytes, natural killer cells
IL-6 (B cell–stimulating factor 2, interferon-beta₂, hepatocyte-stimulating factor, hybridoma growth factor, B cell differentiation factor, 26-kd. protein)	Monocytes/macrophages, T cells, fibroblasts, epithelial cell types	T and B cells, fibroblasts, hepatocytes, hematopoietic stem cells
Tumor Necrosis Factors (TNFs)		
TNF (TNF-α, cachectin)	Monocytes/macrophages, lymphocytes, natural killer cells, glial cells, Kupffer cells	Endothelial cells, monocytes/macrophages, neutrophils, fibroblasts, receptors in liver, muscle, lung, gut, kidney
Interferons		
Gamma interferon (immune interferon, macrophage-activating factor)	Multiple cell types (antigen-antibody reaction)	T and B cells, phagocytic cells
Other Growth and Regulatory Factors		
Epidermal growth factor	Salivary gland, kidney, ? mammary tissue	Epidermal/epithelial cells, angiogenesis factor
Platelet-derived growth factor	Platelets, macrophages, vascular endothelium, astrocytes	Fibroblasts, skeletal muscle
Transforming growth factors (TGFs) TGF-α	Embryonic cells, placenta, keratinocytes	Epidermal/epithelial cells, angiogenesis factor
TGF-β	Macrophages, neural cells, platelets, bone, connective tissue	Many cell types (stimulates extracellular matrix components)

*The terms in parentheses are terms that have been, and in some cases are, used for the same substance or group of substances.

sis, with fat utilized as the principal fuel.[10] If the infection is sudden and severe (such as would occur with dehiscence of a colonic anastomosis), hypotension and *septic shock* may result. It is now realized that the mediators for all these events are cytokines, products of the host's own cells. In some cases the signal that initiates these alterations is bacterial endotoxin, a lipopolysaccharide elaborated by gram-negative organisms. However, antigen-antibody reactions may also trigger these events, and this mechanism is thought to be responsible for the responses observed after gram-positive infections and antigenic stimulation, such as blood transfusion reactions and responses following organ rejection.

After endotoxin, monocytes, macrophages, and lymphocytes are stimulated to produce TNF, which mediates many of the systemic responses associated with infection (Fig. 4–4). Many of the cellular events are mediated via the cyclooxygenase reaction and can be markedly attenuated by administration of nonsteroidal anti-inflammatory agents, which block the generation of prostaglandins. The systemic responses observed after infection are related to the amount of cytokine elaborated; this has been demonstrated by studies examining the response characteristics after infusion of increasing doses of TNF into patients (Table 4–3). In addition, other cytokines have been shown to stimulate similar responses, and cytokines may interact and amplify the responses. Because various cytokines serve as inflammatory signals, the response probably depends on the specific disease process, the size of the initial inflammatory focus, and the type and extent of bacterial colonization or infection.[17]

RESPONSES TO ELECTIVE OPERATIVE PROCEDURES

Endocrine Changes and Their Metabolic Consequences. Most patients requiring elective operative procedures are adequately nourished. They fast overnight and receive intravenous solution containing 5% glucose. They then receive a general anesthetic; the skin is prepared and the operative site draped. An incision is made.

One of the earliest consequences of the surgical incision is the rise in levels of circulating cortisol that occurs when afferent nervous signals from the operative site reach the hypothalamus to initiate the stress response, which then stimulates the elaboration of cortisol. This hormone remains at two to five times normal levels for approximately 24 hours after a major operation. Cortisol has generalized effects on tissue catabolism and mobilizes amino acids from skeletal muscle that provide substrates for wound healing and serve as precursors for the hepatic synthesis of acute-phase proteins or new glucose.[26] Associated with the activation of the adrenal cortex is stimulation of the adrenal medulla through the sympathetic nervous system, with elaboration of epinephrine. Urinary catecholamines may be elevated for 24 to 48 hours after operation and may then return to normal. This circulating neurotransmitter has an important role in circulatory adjustment, but it may also stimulate hepatic glycogenolysis and gluconeogenesis in concert with glucagon and glucocorticoids.

The neuroendocrine responses to operation also modify the various mechanisms in salt and water excretion. Alterations in serum osmolarity and tonicity of body fluids secondary to anesthesia and the operative stress stimulate the secretion of aldosterone and antidiuretic hormone (ADH). The ability to excrete a water load after elective surgical procedures is reduced. The usual postoperative patient concentrates urine to 1 to 2 ml. water per mOsm. solute excreted, corresponding to a urine osmolarity of 500 to 1000 mOsm. per liter, even in the presence of adequate hydration. Hence, weight gain secondary to salt and water retention is usual

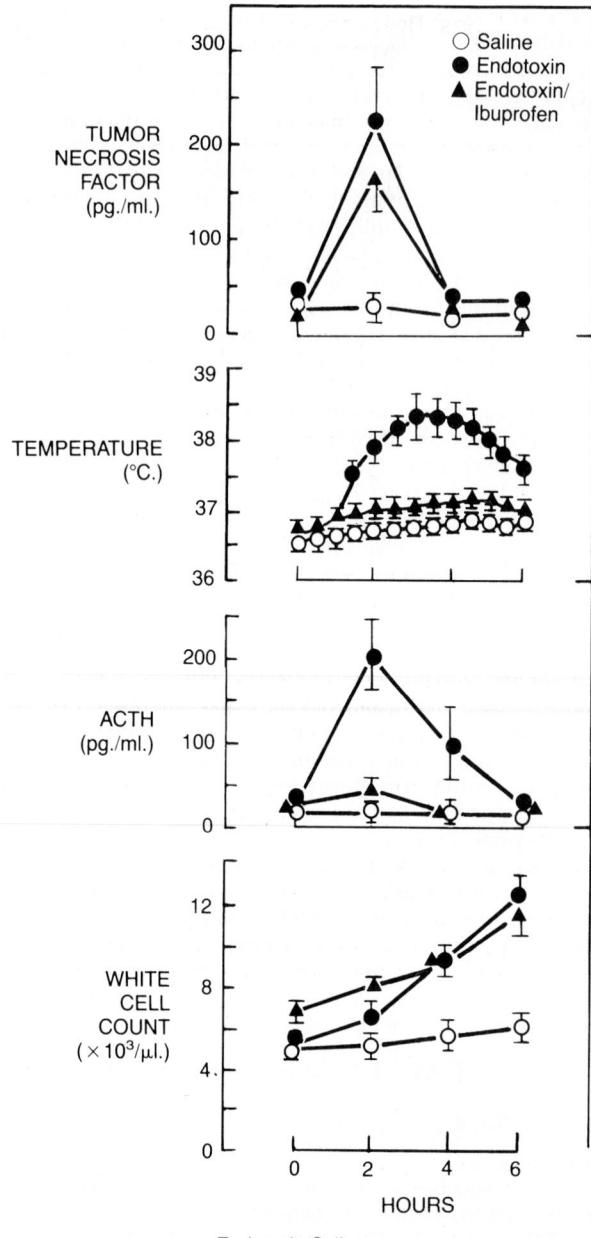

Figure 4–4. Changes in plasma concentrations of tumor necrosis factor and metabolic responses after endotoxin administration in 13 subjects without ibuprofen pretreatment and in 8 subjects with ibuprofen pretreatment. The data obtained in the group pretreated with ibuprofen were similar to those obtained during saline studies in the group that was not pretreated, and the data from both groups have been pooled. (Adapted from Michie, H. R., Manogue, K. R., Spriggs, D. R., Revhaug, A., O'Dwyer, S. T., Dinarello, C. A., Cerami, A., Wolff, S. M., and Wilmore, D. W.: N Engl J Med, 1988, *318*, 1481. Copyright 1988. Massachusetts Medical Society. All rights reserved.)

after operation (Fig. 4–5). Edema occurs to a varying extent in all surgical wounds, and this accumulation is proportional to the extent of tissue dissection and local trauma. Administration of sodium-containing solutions during operation replaces this functional volume loss as extracellular fluid redistributes in the body. This *third-space* fluid eventually returns to the circulation as the wound edema subsides, and diuresis begins 2 to 4 days after the operation.

Alterations occur in the response of the endocrine pancreas after elective operation. In general, insulin elaboration is

TABLE 4–3. Host Responses to Various Doses of Tumor Necrosis Factor

Dose of TNF Infused (μg./m.²/24 hr.)	Response	Clinical Correlate
1	Hypoferremia	Subclinical infection
20	Myalgia and headache, anorexia, fever, tachycardia, elevated acute-phase proteins	Influenza, acute appendicitis
>500	Rigors, elevated stress hormones, fluid retention, lymphopenia, hypotension	Intra-abdominal abscess, major thermal injury
>620	Decreased consciousness, profound hypotension, pulmonary edema, oliguria	Septicemia, severe acute pancreatitis, infected massive burns

diminished and glucagon concentrations rise. This response may be related to increased sympathetic activity or to the rise in levels of circulating epinephrine, which is known to suppress insulin release. The increased elaboration of glucagon may be related to increased stimulation of the sympathetic nervous system or to alterations in circulating mediators. The rise in glucagon and the corresponding fall in insulin are a potent signal to accelerate hepatic glucose production, and, with other hormones (epinephrine and glucocorticoids), gluconeogenesis is maintained.

The postoperative hormonal responses are thought to orchestrate physiologic and biochemical changes that benefit the host. Salt and water conservation support the circulating blood volume. Augmented hepatic glucose production provides adequate essential fuel for the nervous system, the red and white blood cells, and the healing wound. Skeletal muscle proteolysis provides amino acid precursors for gluconeogenesis and hepatic protein synthesis, although negative nitrogen balance occurs. Postoperative lipolysis provides abundant quantities of free fatty acid, as an additional energy source. Current techniques of postoperative care minimize, but do not reverse, these responses.

States of Surgical Recovery. The period of catabolism initiated by operation, a combination of inadequate nutrition and alteration of the hormonal environment, has been termed the adrenergic-corticoid phase.[20] This period is followed by the onset of anabolism, which occurs at a variable time in the patient's convalescence. In general, in the absence of postoperative complications, this phase starts 3 to 6 days after open laparotomy of the magnitude of a colectomy or gastrectomy, often concomitant with the start of oral feedings. This turning point from catabolism to anabolism is referred to as the corticoid-withdrawal phase because it is characterized by a spontaneous sodium and free-water diuresis, a positive potassium balance, and a reduction in nitrogen excretion. This transitional phase usually lasts only 1 to 2 days.

The patient then enters a prolonged period of early anabolism characterized by positive nitrogen balance and weight gain. Protein synthesis is increased after sustained enteral feedings, and this change is related to the return of lean body mass and muscular strength.

The fourth and final phase of surgical convalescence is late anabolism, the hallmark of which is much slower weight gain. During this period, the patient is in nitrogen equilib-

rium but in positive carbon balance, which follows deposition of body fat.

Modifying Postoperative Responses. Early investigators who studied the catabolic responses after operation concluded that these responses were obligatory and irreversible. However, Riegel and associates supplied adequate energy and nitrogen to postoperative patients by feeding tube and greatly diminished the catabolic response to operation.[22] Holden and associates supported gastrectomy patients with intravenous nutrients and noted that weight was maintained and near nitrogen balance achieved.[12] Thus, the catabolic response to an elective operation is due in large part to

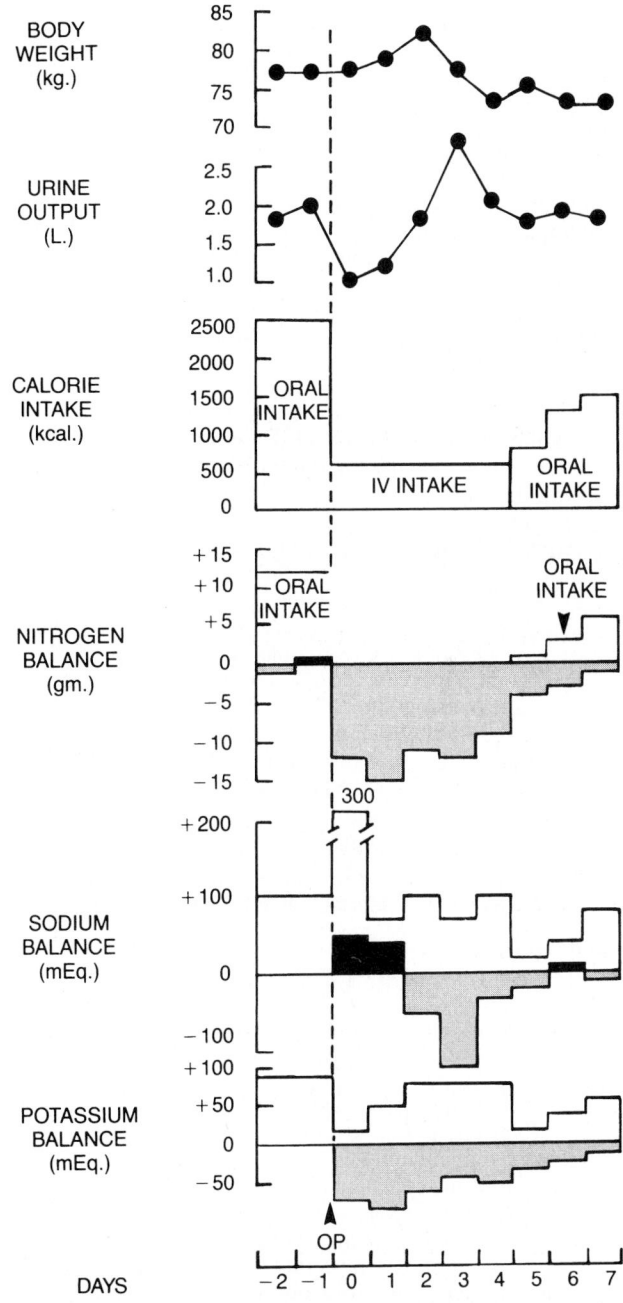

Figure 4–5. The metabolic response of a previously healthy subject to an elective operative procedure. Intake is plotted upward from zero, output downward from the top of the intake line. Negative balance is represented by the shaded, with positive balance solid black. (Redrawn from Wilmore, D. W., and Souba, W. W.: Diet and nutrition in the care of the patient with surgery, trauma and sepsis. *In* Shils, M. E., and Young, V. R. [Eds.]: Modern Nutrition in Health and Disease. Philadelphia, Lea & Febiger, 1988, p. 1309.)

inadequate food intake and is not an obligatory consequence of operative stress.

Laparoscopic or thoracoscopic procedures have greatly reduced the postoperative impulses. Such operations obviate the need for an open wound into the abdominal or thoracic cavities. As a result, there is decreased postoperative pain, reduced postoperative respiratory complications, decreased hospital stay, and an early return to normal activity, such as food intake and exercise. Studies of patients undergoing open versus laparoscopic cholecystectomy have shown that the minimally invasive approach is associated with a reduced or comparable endocrine response[19] but a more normal immunologic response.[21] Such minimal access approaches will be more useful in the future and will be particularly helpful in decreasing patient debility.

Various human studies have shown that many postoperative responses can be ablated after denervation of the wound. Kehlet used epidural or spinal anesthesia in women undergoing elective abdominal hysterectomy.[16] With epidural anesthesia extending from S5 to T4, plasma concentrations of cortisol, aldosterone, glucose, and free fatty acids remained normal, in contrast to increased concentrations in patients receiving general anesthesia alone. Other workers have extended these observations and reported that low spinal anesthesia blocks the elevation of catecholamines, hyperglycemia, and inhibition of insulin release observed in patients undergoing surgical procedures on the lower half of the body. These observations suggest that regional anesthetic techniques block afferent signals from the wound and interrupt sympathetic nervous efferent signals to the adrenal gland and possibly the liver. The effect of sympathetic blockade is a reduction in the apparent magnitude of the stress response.

Growth hormone is an anabolic hormone that may improve the response to injury. Small doses of growth hormone (approximately 3 to 4 mg. per day) and a hypocaloric diet were administered to patients after elective gastrectomy or colectomy.[15] The subjects received parenteral nutrition containing 20 calories per kg. per day and 1 gm. protein per kg. per day. The nine control subjects lost 3.3 kg. (5.9% of preoperative weight) and had a cumulative nitrogen loss of 32.6 ± 4.2 gm. per 8 days. The patients receiving growth hormone lost significantly less weight (1.3 kg.) and nitrogen loss was 7.1 ± 3.1 gm. per 8 days (p <.001) (Fig. 4–6). Body compositional analysis of other patients receiving growth hormone demonstrated significant gain in lean body mass compared with controls (Fig. 4–7).[4]

RESPONSES TO ACCIDENTAL INJURY

General Features and Time Course. Events that occur after injury are generally graded responses: the more severe the injury, the greater is the response (Fig. 4–8). The response generally increases until a maximal level is reached; severity of injury over and above this level simply causes a maximal response.

Responses to injury change with time, and events occurring at various points in time were initially described as periods of *ebb* and *flow*. The early phase (ebb or low-flow phase) occurred immediately after injury and was characterized by a fall in metabolic functions and a decrease in core temperature but increased levels of stress hormones.[27] Blood glucose might fall to hypoglycemic levels if the patient could not be resuscitated, and measurements were made in the terminal state. With restoration of blood flow and with time, the patient's responses changed (Table 4–4). The metabolic rate rose, body temperature became elevated, and blood insulin levels were normal or even increased, as were catecholamines, glucose, and blood lactate. Levels of free fatty acids were generally normal or decreased. These changes occurred

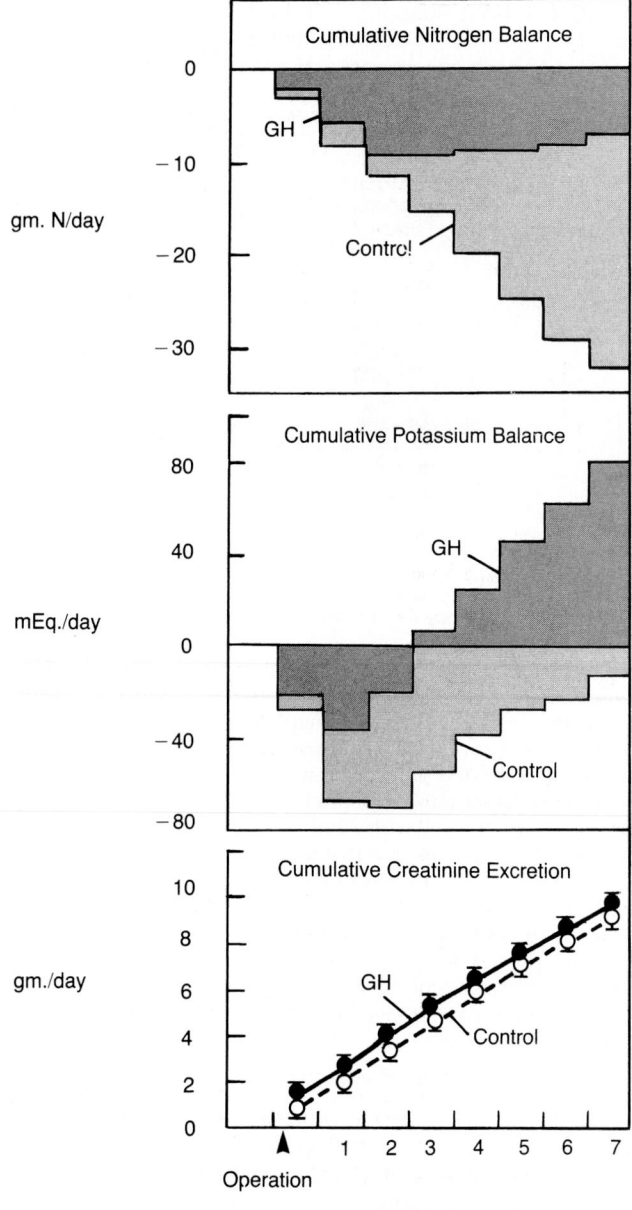

Figure 4–6. The cumulative nitrogen balance was significantly different between groups from postoperative days 3 to 7. Potassium balance tended to follow nitrogen balance. Creatinine excretion was similar in both groups of patients, confirming the adequacy of urinary collection. (Redrawn from Jiang, Z. M., He, G. Z., Zhang, S. Y., Wang, X. R., Yang, N. F., Zhu, Y., and Wilmore, D. W.: Low-dose growth hormone and hypocaloric nutrition attenuate the protein-catabolic response after major operation. Ann. Surg., *210*:514, 1989.)

during the flow phase, which is also referred to as the chronic or hyperdynamic phase of injury. It was later realized that many of the early changes were related to hypovolemia and organ perfusion; with resuscitation of the patient and restoration of circulating blood volume, flow-phase responses occurred rapidly. Aside from research directed toward improved shock resuscitation, most investigative work has now been focused on the later or hyperdynamic phase of injury when wound closure, nutritional support, prevention of infection, and respiratory support are central to patient care.

Several other characteristics of the metabolic responses to injury may confound interpretation of the patient's response. *Complications* occur in injured patients, particularly the com-

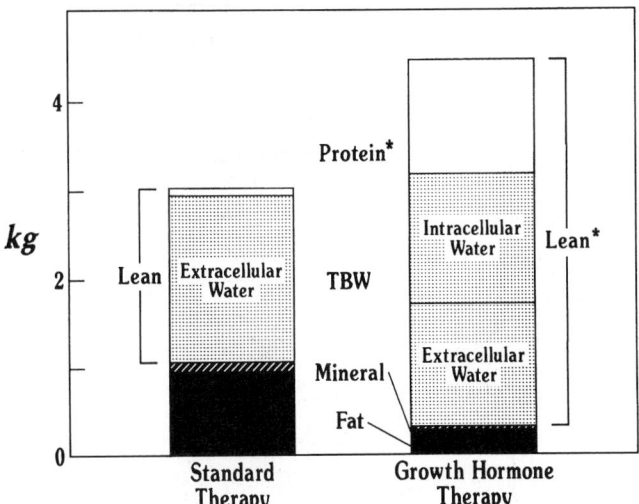

Figure 4–7. Weight gain during 3 weeks of therapy. Growth hormone–treated patients gained significantly more lean mass and protein-containing mass than did patients receiving standard therapy (* p <.05). This was accomplished without a significant increase in fat or an inappropriate expansion of extracellular water. Standard therapy was associated with fat deposition and a disproportionate gain in extracellular water. (Data from Byrne, T. A., et al.: Anabolic therapy with growth hormone accelerates protein gain in surgical patients requiring nutritional rehabilitation. Ann. Surg. *218*:400, 1993.)

TABLE 4–4. Alterations That Occur Following Injury

"Ebb" Phase	"Flow" Phase
Blood glucose elevated	Glucose normal or slightly elevated
Normal glucose production	Increased glucose production
Free fatty acids elevated	Free fatty acids normal or slightly elevated—flux increased
Insulin concentration low	Insulin concentration normal or elevated
Catecholamines and glucagon elevated	Catecholamines high-normal or elevated; glucagon elevated
Blood lactate elevated	Blood lactate normal
Oxygen consumption depressed	Oxygen consumption elevated
Cardiac output below normal	Cardiac output increased
Core temperature below normal	Core temperature elevated

plication of infection, and these effects appear additive to injury responses. *Treatment variables* alter injury responses, and repeated operative procedures, use of glucocorticoids, patient paralysis during mechanical ventilation, use of positive end-expiratory pressure ventilation, and administration of pressor drugs are therapies that alter hemodynamics and metabolism and thus may influence usual responses.

Other factors unique to each individual patient influence the metabolic responses to injury. These include nutritional state, body composition, and other disease processes.

Signals That Initiate the Injury Responses

1. *Afferent sensory nerve fibers* provide the most direct and the quickest route for signals to arrive at the CNS after stress. It has frequently been suggested that pain may serve as the

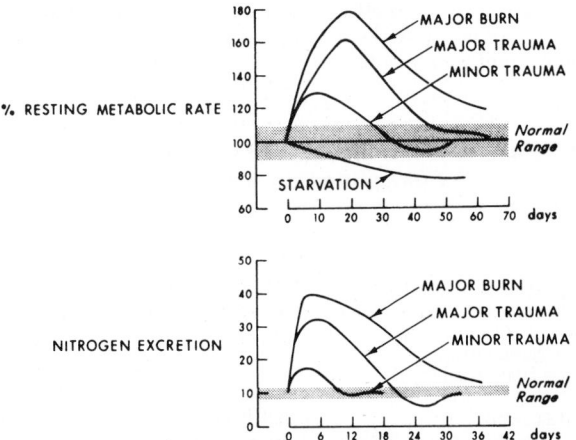

Figure 4–8. Hypermetabolism and increased nitrogen excretion are closely related following minor or major trauma or major burn injury. Patients received 12 gm. of nitrogen intake per day. (Adapted from Kinney, J. M.: Energy deficits in acute illness and injury. *In* Morgan, A. P. [Ed.]: Proceedings of a Conference on Energy Metabolism and Body Fuel Utilization. Cambridge, Harvard University Press, 1966, p. 174.)

initial afferent signal after injury, and many studies suggest that the afferent nerve signals from the injured area are essential to stimulate the pituitary-adrenal axis.[13] The adrenocortical response to injury was not observed in animals after section of the peripheral nerves to the area of injury, transection of the spinal cord above the injury, or section through the medulla oblongata. A similar pattern of response to denervation before injury has been described in humans. Both growth hormone and ACTH levels in the serum rise within 1 hour after incision in patients receiving general anesthesia and undergoing cholecystectomy or inguinal herniorrhaphy. However, this hormonal response did not occur in patients undergoing abdominal procedures when epidural blockade was employed in conjunction with the general anesthetic.[16] Nerve afferents also appear to stimulate the elaboration of ADH after trauma. In addition, several factors that accompany the stress of critical illness—restraint, immobilization, environmental disturbances—most likely alter afferent nerve impulses and affect the response to injury.

2. *Fluid loss from the vascular compartment* stimulates volume and pressure receptors, initiating a series of CNS-mediated cardiovascular adjustments. Cardiac output falls, peripheral resistance increases, and blood is redistributed to vital organs to maintain function. With progressive volume loss into the area of injury, the resulting hypoperfusion reduces tissue oxygenation and disturbs the acid-base equilibrium. Chemoreceptor stimulation thus serves as additional afferent input to both vasomotor and respiratory centers during hypovolemia. Because loss of fluid volume after injury is closely related to the extent of tissue damage, these specific mechanisms allow a quantitative response to occur after trauma (i.e., the response is directly proportional to the size of the injury).

3. *Circulating substances* may directly or indirectly stimulate the CNS and set in motion the injury response. Alterations in serum electrolytes, release of cell breakdown products, changes in the amino acid pattern, and elaboration of endotoxin and the release of cytokines, all originating from or a direct result of the wound, may initiate homeostatic adjustments that develop after injury.

Signal Integration and Effector Mechanisms: Role of the CNS. The brain receives a variety of signals that stress has occurred and integrates this afferent input. Although the sympathetic nervous system is not essential to the adaptation to simple starvation, the CNS is essential to the hypermetabolic response to injury; patients with *brain death* and associated soft tissue injury failed to mount a flow-phase response. Similarly, in severely burned patients, morphine anesthesia, which markedly reduced hypothalamic function, caused a prompt decrease in hypermetabolism, rectal temperature, and cardiac output.[27] In patients with an intact CNS, various adjustments are observed within the hypothalamus and pituitary gland; these alterations in neurohormonal control appear to be specific compensatory adjustments to stress. These alterations in CNS control have an impact on thermoregulation, substrate mobilization, and intraorgan energy transfer.

Cytokines produced in the wound may signal the brain to initiate these changes. Conversely, it has been demonstrated that cytokines are produced within the brain and have been found in the cerebrospinal fluid of patients after head injury and meningitis.[18] There is an extensive network of interleukin-1 (IL-1) nerve fibers innervating the hypothalamus, and this cytokine may be central in initiating and directing the metabolic response to stress. For example, chronic CNS exposure to IL-1 produced catabolism in the rat.[11] Significant loss of weight, negative nitrogen balance, and hyperpyrexia were demonstrated in the animals infused with IL-1 into the cerebral ventricle compared with saline-infused controls. This stress response was also associated with activation of the hypothalamic-pituitary axis.

Hormonal Environment. Hypothalamic stimulation creates a variety of hormonal alterations in patients after injury: in all phases of injury there is a marked rise in the counterregulatory hormones glucagon, glucocorticoids, and catecholamines. In contrast, plasma concentrations of the patient's anabolic hormone insulin may be low, normal, or elevated (Fig. 4–9). During the *flow* or hypermetabolic phase of injury, insulin concentrations are normal or increased. However, the effects of these elevated insulin concentrations on peripheral tissues (skeletal muscle and fat) are blunted. The cause of the marked insulin resistance is related to diminished food intake and an altered hormonal environment that exerts anti-insulin activity.[3] The counterregulatory hormones glucagon, cortisol, and catecholamines oppose the storage or anabolic functions of insulin. In the short term, they maintain blood glucose levels and prevent hypoglycemia. More chronic hormonal elaboration accelerates body catabolism.

Glucocorticoids are also released after stress, and steroids have potent effects on substrate and mineral metabolism. Cortisol is elaborated in response to increasing concentrations of ACTH released from the anterior pituitary gland. Cortisol mobilizes amino acids from skeletal muscle and increases hepatic gluconeogenesis; it also causes marked insulin resistance, and these effects cause the marked hyperglycemia associated with acute illness.[3]

Catecholamines. Elaboration of catecholamines—epinephrine and norepinephrine—may be the most basic of the hormonal responses to stress.[27] These hormones exert regulatory effects on cardiac output, regional circulation, blood glucose, and oxidative metabolism. Epinephrine stimulates glycogenolysis, which, in skeletal muscle, promotes lactate production. In addition, epinephrine at higher concentrations markedly inhibits insulin elaboration, thus facilitating amino acid and fat mobilization.

The infusion of any one of these catabolic hormones alone in normal individuals causes minimal alterations in metabolism and circulation. However, when the three hormones are infused together, the effects are synergistic and sustained. Negative nitrogen balance, gluconeogenesis, and hypermetabolism are observed, associated with salt and water retention, all major components of the injury response (Table 4–5). Thus, it appears that the simultaneous elaboration of the counterregulatory hormones glucagon, cortisol, and epinephrine is responsible in part for the posttraumatic changes.

Role of Cytokines. Another regulatory component appears to mediate other changes that occur after injury. Inflammation associated with wound repair generates a variety of

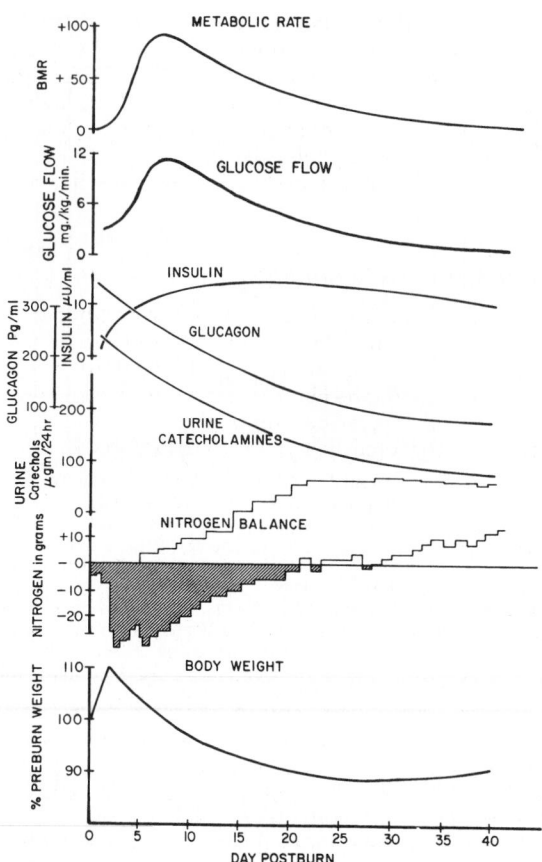

Figure 4–9. The increased rate of hepatic glucose production (glucose flow) parallels the hypermetabolic response after thermal injury. Increased gluconeogenesis is associated in time with negative nitrogen balance and high levels of glucagon and catecholamines relative to insulin. Cortisol concentrations (not shown) parallel glucagon and catecholamine alterations. As these hormonal mediators return to normal, oxygen consumption and hepatic glucose production fall and nitrogen balance becomes positive.

signals such as substance P, bradykinin, and prostaglandins. Whereas most of these signals direct local inflammatory events, some may reach the bloodstream and alter systemic metabolism. Such a molecule is IL-1, which stimulates a variety of responses commonly observed in the critically ill host, including the mobilization of leukocytes, the stimulation of fever, the redistribution of circulating iron and other trace minerals, and the hepatic stimulation of acute-phase protein synthesis. Other substances that participate in the

TABLE 4–5. Effect of Infusion of Cortisol, Glucagon, and Epinephrine on Metabolism

	Saline	Hormones*
Metabolic rate (kcal./m.²/hr.)	32.24 ± 1.05	38.42 ± 1.31
Nitrogen balance (gm./day)	−0.2 ± 0.4	−3.2 ± 0.4
Protein catabolic rate (gm. N/day)	38.4 ± 1.9	46.5 ± 2.5
Plasma glucose (mg./100 ml.)	94 ± 2	133 ± 4
Serum insulin (μ.unit/ml.)	8 ± 1	22 ± 3
Glucose production rate (mg./kg./min.)	2.08 ± 0.06	2.55 ± 0.06
Insulin-mediated glucose disposal (mg./kg./min.)	8.62 ± 0.51	3.22 ± 0.51
Insulin-mediated forearm glucose uptake (mg./100 ml. forearm/min.)	1.03 ± 0.09	0.48 ± 0.12

*All significantly different from control values.

Adapted from Bessey, P. Q., Watters, J. M., Aoki, T. T., and Wilmore, D. W.: Combined hormone infusion simulates the metabolic response to injury. Ann. Surg., 200:264, 1984.

nous mediators of inflammation. Further support of the role of hypovolemia in the pathogenesis of shock was provided by a number of investigators, including Parsons and Phemister and Cournand and co-workers.[25, 73] Cournand and co-workers, in 1943, applied cardiac catheterization techniques to document the relationship between blood volume loss and the fall in cardiac output. The rise of blood banking in the 1940s only seemed to confirm the importance of hypovolemia in shock and its treatment with correction of blood volume.

The extensive physiologic research of Wiggers in the early 1940s defined for the first time the concept of irreversible shock, a state Wiggers characterized as progressive systemic circulatory decompensation.[88] In addition, he antedated the era of critical care medicine by integrating the concepts of impaired oxygen delivery, oxygen debt, and tissue injury or death.

The study of shock during the Korean and Vietnam conflicts, and thereafter, became more focused on resuscitation, individual organ dysfunction, and cellular derangements. More prompt and aggressive resuscitative efforts caused a declining incidence of renal failure among those who survived, but the reasons for massive volume requirements and interstitial fluid depletion were not clarified until the work of Shires,[81] who demonstrated shock-induced defects in cell membrane function and vascular permeability. Such changes at the cellular level were thought to be responsible for the development of the *shock lung* syndrome that became evident with increasing frequency after successful initial resuscitations in the Vietnam conflict. With the introduction of the flow-directed pulmonary artery catheter in 1970, it became clear that the pulmonary edema of the shock lung syndrome, which later became more widely known as the adult respiratory distress syndrome (ARDS), was of a noncardiogenic nature and therefore not due to volume overload.

Much of the recent work in the field of shock, spurred on by rapid advances in molecular biology, has dealt with the identification and possible manipulation of numerous inflammatory mediators, such as cytokines, leukotrienes, and prostaglandins, that are thought to be activated after severe injury, ischemia, or sepsis. Other areas of active research have concentrated on metabolic support, oxygen delivery, and the prevention of organ ischemia.

DEFINITION

Shock, regardless of the cause, may be defined as a syndrome that results from inadequate perfusion of tissues. Tissue perfusion in shock is insufficient to meet the metabolic demands of those tissues. Consequently, alterations in cellular metabolism occur that lead to cellular dysfunction, elaboration of inflammatory mediators, and cellular injury. If tissue perfusion can be restored in an expeditious fashion, cellular injury may be limited, but shock may become irreversible if cellular injury and metabolic dysfunction become widespread. Thus, current interpretations of shock view the syndrome as a continuum, ranging from subclinical deficits in perfusion to multiple organ dysfunction syndrome (MODS) or frank organ failure. Recognition that shock can manifest as progressive degrees of severity and metabolic dysfunction is a central concept that is important when considering the initiation of measures to prevent or treat shock.

The corollary of tissue hypoperfusion is tissue hypoxia. Oxygen, as an essential nutrient to maintain normal cellular metabolism and function, becomes less available in shock, relative to tissue oxygen demands. An oxygen debt is established in shock whereby the oxygen demand exceeds the oxygen supply. Therefore, even in hyperdynamic states such as sepsis, in which the oxygen delivery may be *normal*, the hypermetabolism that ensues from the systemic inflammatory response leads to increased oxygen demands that may not be met by the existing level of oxygen delivery.

CLASSIFICATION OF SHOCK

Although there is a growing tendency to avoid traditional classification schemes of shock and to concentrate, instead, on the common defect in all shock states (i.e., tissue hypoperfusion), a useful classification system, as shown in Table 5–1, serves to delineate the various causes of shock and to provide a framework for establishing the diagnosis and instituting treatment. There are limitations to such a classification system, however. Not infrequently, a combination of one or more etiologic processes may contribute to the clinical syndrome of shock. For example, traumatic injuries may cause shock from hemorrhage alone, but a vasogenic component may be present owing to the elaboration of inflammatory mediators or tissue toxins. Sepsis may also complicate the clinical picture, particularly after trauma, causing difficulty assigning the patient to one etiologic category.

Hypovolemic Shock. Hypovolemic shock occurs from hemorrhagic losses, such as with trauma, gastrointestinal bleeding, or ruptured aneurysms, or from plasma volume losses. Shock arising from plasma volume losses may be due to extravascular fluid sequestration, as might occur in pancreatitis, burns, and bowel obstruction, or it may arise from excessive gastrointestinal, renal, or insensible fluid losses.

Cardiogenic Shock. Cardiogenic shock occurs when the heart is unable to generate an adequate cardiac output to maintain tissue perfusion. Both intrinsic cardiac dysfunction and extrinsic causes of diminished cardiac output are incorporated in the category of cardiogenic shock. Intrinsic causes of cardiac dysfunction include myocardial infarction, cardiomyopathy, valvular heart disease, cardiac rhythm disturbances, and myocardial depression from drug toxicity or trauma. Extrinsic mechanisms of cardiogenic shock produce cardiac dysfunction by compressive or obstructive means. Thus, tension pneumothorax, pericardial tamponade, and high levels of positive-pressure ventilation may all cause external compression of the heart, which impedes diastolic filling and decreases cardiac output. Pulmonary embolism is an example of an obstructive cause that precipitates right-sided heart failure by causing an increased vascular resistance, thereby limiting systolic ejection.

Neurogenic Shock. Neurogenic shock may occur after spinal cord injury, severe head injury, or spinal anesthesia as the result of failure of the sympathetic nervous system to maintain normal vascular tone. Arteriolar and venous vasodilation, with a reduction of peripheral vascular resistance

TABLE 5–1. Classification of Shock

Hypovolemic
   Hemorrhage
   Plasma volume loss

Cardiogenic
   Intrinsic
   Extrinsic

Neurogenic

Vasogenic
   Systemic inflammatory response syndrome
      Infectious (septic)
      Noninfectious
   Anaphylactic
   Hypoadrenal
   Traumatic

and an increase in venous capacitance, are characteristic of neurogenic shock.

Vasogenic Shock. Vasogenic shock is similar to neurogenic shock in that arteriolar and venous vasomotor tone are decreased; however, the mechanisms responsible for the development of these two entities are quite different. Whereas sympathetic denervation is implicated in the clinical syndrome of neurogenic shock, this mechanism is absent in vasogenic shock. Endogenous or exogenous vasoactive mediators are believed to play a major role in the development of vasogenic shock. Included in this category are shock associated with the systemic inflammatory response syndrome (SIRS), sepsis, anaphylaxis, adrenocortical insufficiency, and traumatic injuries.

Many previous classifications of shock have included septic shock as a separate category, but the present scheme denoting SIRS as a subclassification of vasogenic shock emphasizes the importance of inflammatory mediators in the pathogenesis of shock due to SIRS, irrespective of the presence *or* absence of microbial evidence of infection.

Anaphylaxis, hypoadrenal shock, and traumatic shock are also included under the category of vasogenic shock because these forms of shock, which are particularly virulent, have in common the mechanism of vasomotor collapse. Traumatic shock is not always easily differentiated from hypovolemic shock that occurs after injury and hemorrhage. However, the pathogenesis of traumatic shock appears to involve a more intense elaboration of vasoactive inflammatory mediators or tissue toxins, and this form of shock is more refractory to treatment.

PATIENT MONITORING

Expeditious restoration of perfusion and correction of the underlying pathology are the goals of resuscitation of patients in shock.[36] Any delays in restoring adequate perfusion may lead to irreversible tissue injury. Ongoing assessment of the patient's response to resuscitative efforts is essential to determine the efficacy of therapy. Because therapy is aimed at restoring perfusion, the ideal monitoring technique is one that provides an accurate measure of tissue and cellular perfusion yet is noninvasive and has a high safety profile.

Unfortunately, such an ideal monitor does not exist, and the physician has to rely on other monitoring techniques to assess the patient's response to therapy. In general, selection of appropriate monitoring techniques is dependent on a number of variables, including the patient's individual characteristics, the severity and duration of the physiologic insult, and the patient's initial response to resuscitative measures. A previously healthy patient who experiences a brief episode of hypovolemic shock but responds quickly to resuscitation and treatment measures may not require intensive care monitoring. However, most patients in moderate or severe shock, patients at high risk for developing postshock sequelae, or those patients suspected of being incompletely resuscitated are optimally managed in a critical care setting, where frequent, and often continuous, monitoring of a patient's clinical status may be undertaken by highly trained personnel.

Conventional Monitoring Techniques. Conventional monitoring techniques used to assess the adequacy of resuscitation in patients in shock have employed a number of modalities based on physical examination or laboratory data. Some measures, such as blood pressure, heart rate, central venous pressure, hematocrit, arterial blood gases, and urine output are more objective than assessments of capillary refill or of skin temperature and turgor. All of these measures, however, are somewhat insensitive in diagnosing or evaluating the treatment of shock because *abnormal* values reflect secondary effects of shock or tissue hypoxia.[82] Abnormal values, therefore, are late manifestations of shock. Furthermore, *normal* values may not accurately reflect reversal of the shock state because these measurements do not assess oxygen debt or overall tissue perfusion. Thus, end-points such as adequate urine output or mean arterial pressure greater than 80 mm. Hg may not be appropriate or sensitive indicators of occult tissue hypoxia. Shippy and associates have provided some evidence that several of these commonly monitored parameters, including heart rate, mean arterial pressure, hematocrit, central venous pressure, and even pulmonary capillary wedge pressure, are unreliable indicators of blood volume because of the complex interactions of compensatory mechanisms and resuscitative interventions (Fig. 5–1).[80] Nevertheless, such measures are useful in guiding the initial resuscitation from shock.

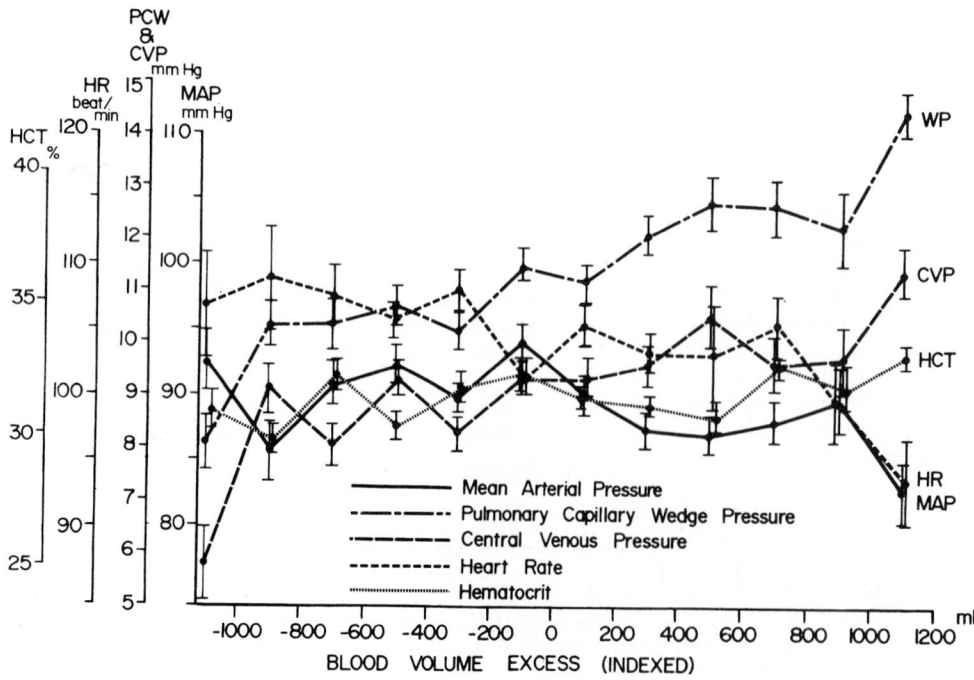

Figure 5–1. Relationship of blood volume to commonly measured hemodynamic parameters. Mean ± S.E. for hematocrit, central venous pressure, pulmonary capillary wedge pressure, heart rate, and mean arterial pressure on the y-axis plotted against the corresponding blood volume excess (+) or deficit (−) induced. Overall, these are poor relationships between measured blood volumes and commonly measured variables. (From Shippy, C. R., Appel, P. L., and Shoemaker, W. C.: Reliability of clinical monitoring to assess blood volume in critically ill patients. Crit. Care Med., *12*:107, 1984. Copyright © Williams & Wilkins.)

Adjunctive Monitoring Techniques. In addition to the conventional parameters just described, there are some monitoring techniques, such as pulse oximetry, that are employed fairly routinely in the intensive care unit. The decision to use further measures, some of which are invasive, costly, and potentially hazardous, must be made on an individual basis.

Pulmonary Artery Catheterization. The use of the flow-directed pulmonary artery catheter has revolutionized the practice of critical care medicine since its introduction by Swan and associates in 1970. When used in conjunction with an indwelling arterial cannula and blood gas analysis, the Swan-Ganz catheter can provide considerable hemodynamic and oxygen transport data that are extremely useful in directing therapy aimed at optimizing cardiac function and oxygen delivery. The catheter is introduced percutaneously, preferably through the internal jugular or subclavian vein, and advanced sequentially through the right atrium and right ventricle into the pulmonary artery. Proper placement of the catheter in the pulmonary artery is recognized by the characteristic transformation of transduced pressure waveforms (Fig. 5–2),[34] as well as by the rise in diastolic pressure and the appearance of a dicrotic notch in the pulmonary artery tracing. A chest radiograph confirms proper placement of the catheter.

Inflation of the balloon at the tip of the catheter yields the pulmonary capillary wedge (occlusion) pressure (PCWP). For PCWP to accurately reflect left ventricular preload (i.e., left ventricular end-diastolic volume), several conditions must be met. First, PCWP must approximate left atrial pressure. This condition may not be met if PCWP is measured incorrectly, if the catheter is not in correct position, or if a pulmonary venous or left atrial pathologic process exists. Correct measurement of PCWP should take place during end-expiration, when ventilatory artifacts are minimized (Fig. 5–3).[1] The tip of the catheter should lie in West's zone III of the lung (mean pulmonary artery pressure > pulmonary venous pressure > alveolar pressure) during end-expiration so that PCWP reflects pulmonary venous pressure and not alveolar pressure (Fig. 5–4).[70] Second, left atrial pressure must reflect left ventricular end-diastolic pressure. This condition may be violated in the presence of mitral valve disease or aortic valve

insufficiency. Third, left ventricular end-diastolic pressure must accurately represent left ventricular end-diastolic volume. This third condition may not be met in the presence of altered ventricular compliance. These factors that influence the accuracy of PCWP to measure left ventricular preload are summarized in Figure 5–5.

Cardiac output may be measured by the Swan-Ganz catheter using the thermodilution technique. In this method, a known amount of fluid at a known temperature is injected into the proximal (right atrial) lumen, where it mixes with and is warmed up by blood. The temperature change, dependent on cardiac output, is detected by a thermistor at the tip of the catheter in the pulmonary artery. A bedside computer calculates the cardiac output based on the change in blood temperature over time. For this technique to be reliable, injectate volumes and temperatures must be accurate, several injections should be made and averaged at the same time in the respiratory cycle, and appropriate computational constants must be entered into the computer. Furthermore, the presence of cardiac arrhythmias, tricuspid regurgitation, or intracardiac shunts will affect the measurement of cardiac output by this method. Despite these limitations of this technique, which has a precision no better than 4% to 9% in the best hands, cardiac output determination by the bolus thermodilution method is considered the clinical standard. In addition to measuring left- and right-sided filling pressures and cardiac output, the pulmonary artery catheter may also provide some measures of oxygen balance for adequacy of tissue perfusion. From the cardiac output, hemoglobin concentration, and arterial and mixed venous blood gas analysis, one can calculate arteriovenous oxygen content difference, oxygen delivery ($\dot{D}O_2$), oxygen consumption ($\dot{V}O_2$), and oxygen extraction ratio (O_2ER). Intermittent monitoring of these oxygen transport parameters can detect imbalances between oxygen delivery and consumption; therefore, it provides a nondynamic means of globally assessing tissue perfusion and adequacy of resuscitation from shock. Evidence of ongoing shock by proper interpretation of these oxygen transport parameters may appear well before the late, clinical manifestations of shock and end organ dysfunction become obvious. Table 5–2 summarizes the normal hemodynamic

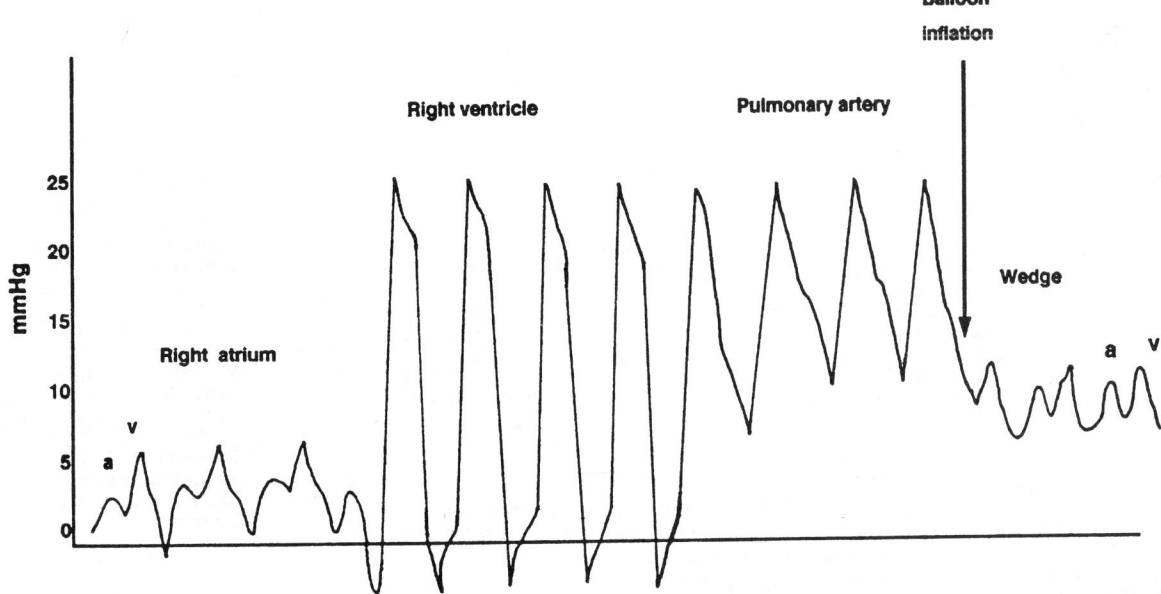

Figure 5–2. Pulmonary artery catheter tracing as catheter is advanced from atrium to pulmonary artery position. Balloon inflation yields the pulmonary capillary wedge pressure waveform as shown. (From Fakhry, S. M., and Rutledge, R.: Monitoring. *In* Moylan, J. A. [Ed.]: Surgical Critical Care, St. Louis, C. V. Mosby, 1994, p. 88.)

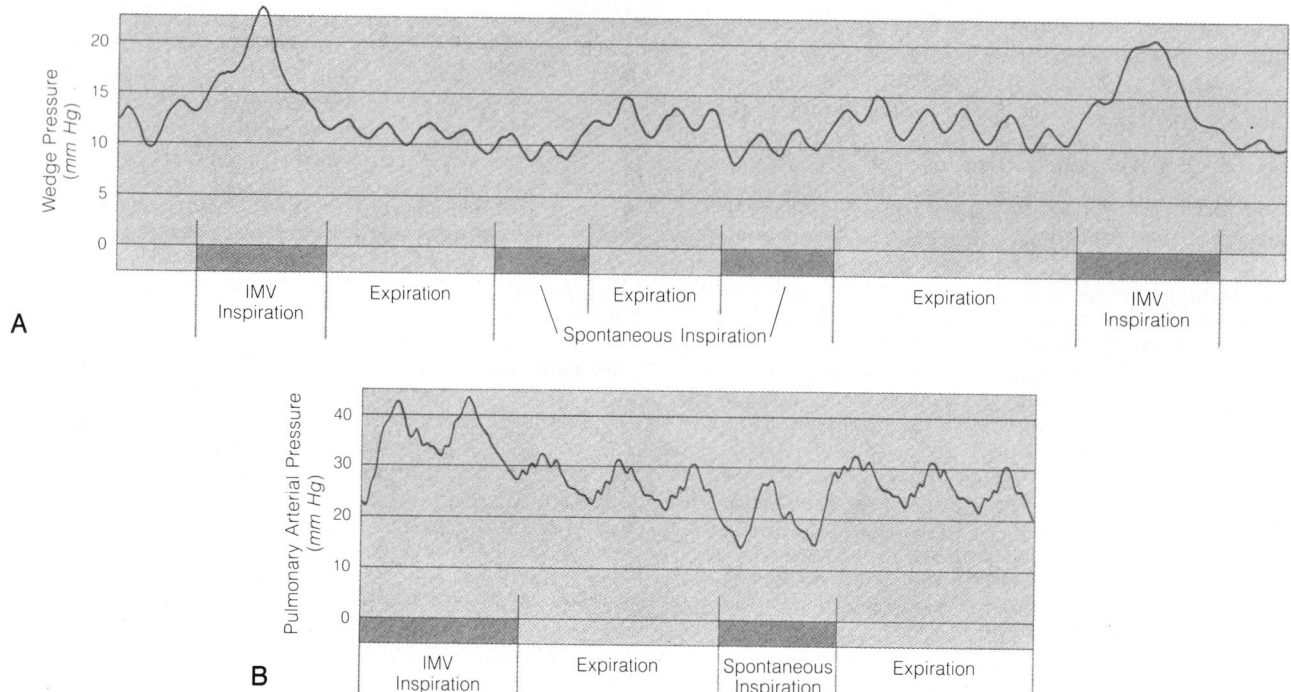

Figure 5–3. Influence of spontaneous and positive-pressure mechanical ventilation on wedge pressure and pulmonary artery pressures. Intermittent mandatory ventilation (IMV) causes *(A)* an increase in wedge pressure during inspiration due to the positive pressure and an increase in intrathoracic and intravascular pressures. Spontaneous inspirations cause a decrease in wedge pressure. The correct reading is the end-expiratory pressure, which is the plateau pressure between the two extremes, or approximately 12 mm. Hg in this patient. Pulmonary artery pressures *(B)* may vary widely between systole and diastole, as well as during respirations. Mean pulmonary artery pressure may be measured between the extremes at end-expiration, or approximately 26 mm. Hg in this patient. (From Abrams, J. H., Cerra, F., and Holcroft, S. W.: Cardiopulmonary monitoring. *In* Wilmore, D. W., Brennan, M. F., Harken, A. H., Holcroft, J. W., and Meakins, J. L. [Eds.]: Care of the Surgical Patient. Vol. 1, Critical Care. A Publication of the Committee on Pre- and Postoperative Care, American College of Surgeons. New York, Scientific American, 1989.)

and oxygen transport parameters that are commonly evaluated in conjunction with use of the pulmonary artery catheter.

Complications from use of the pulmonary artery catheter

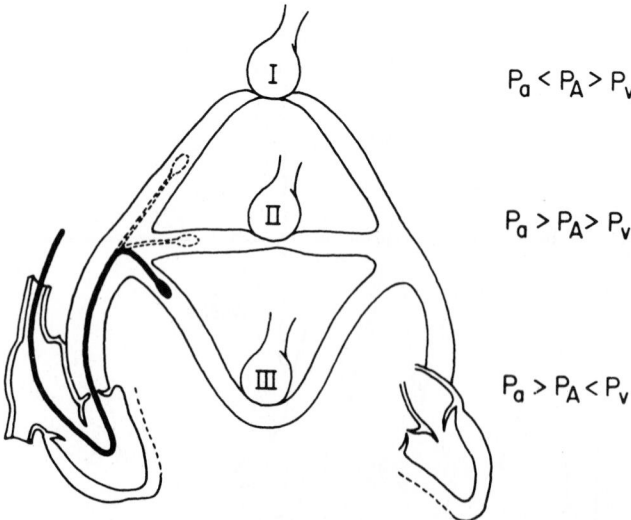

Figure 5–4. Effect of pulmonary artery catheter tip location on estimation of wedge pressure in the various physiologic lung zones. Only in zone III does the wedge pressure accurately estimate pulmonary venous pressure. In zones I and II, alveolar pressure (P_A) is greater than P_v; hence the wedge pressure would reflect P_a, rather than P_v. P_a, pulmonary artery pressure. (From O'Quin, R., and Marini, J. J.: Pulmonary artery occlusion pressure: Clinical physiology, measurement, and interpretation. Am. Rev. Respir. Dis., *128*:319, 1983.)

are not infrequent and include pneumothorax, hemothorax, arterial injury, air embolism, venous thrombosis, pulmonary artery rupture, knotting of the catheter, valvular injury, line sepsis, and dysrhythmias. The incidence of major complications appears to be 3% to 5%.

Mixed Venous Oximetry. Continuous measurement of mixed venous oxygen saturation ($S\bar{v}O_2$) is possible by use of a modified pulmonary artery catheter that incorporates a fiberoptic bundle and the technology of reflectance spectrophotometry. A normal $S\bar{v}O_2$ of 75% indicates a balance between oxygen delivery and consumption, while a decrease in $S\bar{v}O_2$ suggests a reduction in oxygen delivery (owing to low cardiac output, decreased hemoglobin concentration, or decreased arterial oxygen saturation) or an increase in oxygen consumption. $S\bar{v}O_2$ monitoring is thus a dynamic way to provide early warning signs of inadequate oxygen delivery or hemodynamic compromise. Cardiac output may be inferred from continuous $S\bar{v}O_2$ monitoring if one assumes constant oxygen consumption and arterial oxygen content. However, such an inference may lead to misinterpretation in a dynamic critical care environment where oxygen consumption and arterial oxygen content may frequently change. A sudden change in $S\bar{v}O_2$, therefore, may alert the clinician to measure the cardiac output, such as by the thermodilution method, to grasp a more complete picture of the hemodynamic profile. Continuous mixed venous oximetry has been shown to be accurate and reliable, but criteria for its optimal use have not been clearly defined.

Continuous Cardiac Output Monitoring. Recent trends in critical care technology have emphasized the development of data acquisition systems that permit continuous on-line measurements. Automated, continuous patient monitoring, when compared with intermittent monitoring, permits more

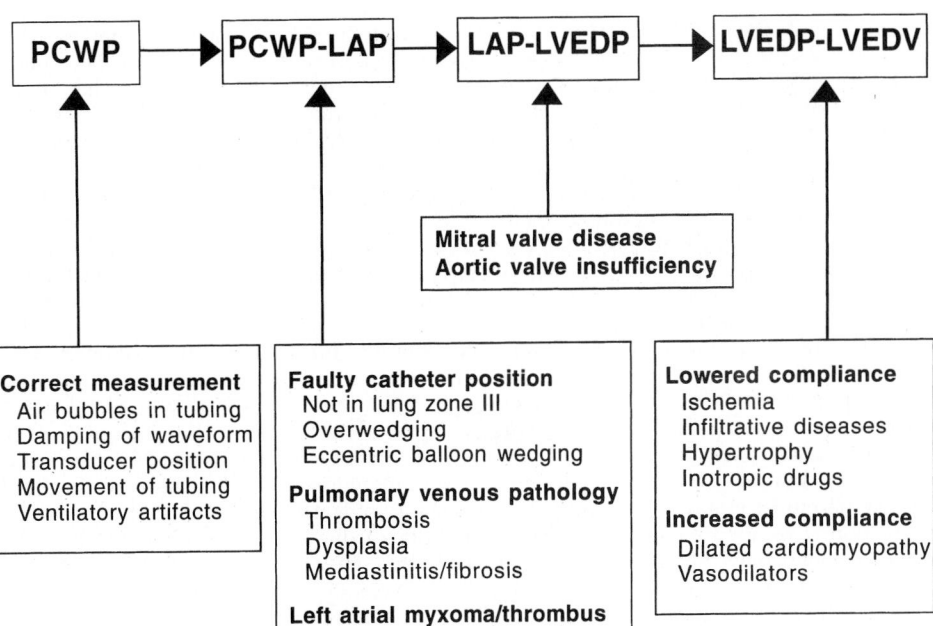

Figure 5–5. Influences on the PCWP–LVEDV relationship. PCWP, pulmonary capillary wedge pressure; LAP, left trial pressure; LVEDP, left ventricular end-diastolic pressure; LVEDV, left ventricular end-diastolic volume. (Adapted from Bossaert, L. L., Demey, H. E., De Jongh, R., and Heytens, L.: Haemodynamic monitoring: Problems, pitfalls, and practical solutions. Drugs, *41*:857, 1991.)

information to be obtained in a more efficient manner. The implications of continuous monitoring are well known. Previously undetected events may become unmasked, more prompt recognition of adverse events may be achieved, earlier therapeutic intervention may be accomplished, and the physiologic response to various interventions may be quickly assessed.

A number of methods have been developed that allow the continuous measurement of cardiac output. Thoracic electrical bioimpedance is a method by which impedance (resistance to alternating current) changes in the thoracic cavity are used to determine cardiac output. The impedance change induced by each cardiac ejection is a function of the stroke volume. The most widely used configuration is noninvasive, utilizing skin electrodes to transmit and sense a small-amplitude alternating current. The correlation between thoracic electrical bioimpedance and thermodilution methods to measure cardiac output has been variable, and further refinements are required before widespread clinical use of thoracic electrical bioimpedance becomes feasible. A semi-invasive

TABLE 5–2. Normal Hemodynamic and Oxygen Transport Parameters

Abbreviation	Parameter	Normal Range	Units	Derivation
CVP	Central venous pressure	1–8	mm. Hg.	Measured
MAP	Mean arterial pressure	75–100	mm. Hg.	Measured
MPAP	Mean pulmonary arterial pressure	10–16	mm. Hg.	Measured
PCWP	Pulmonary capillary wedge pressure	5–12	mm. Hg.	Measured
CO	Cardiac output	4–6	L./min.	Measured
CI	Cardiac index	2.5–3.5	L./min./m.^{2}	CO/BSA
SVR	Systemic vascular resistance	800–1400	dynes • sec./cm.^{5}	$(MAP - CVP) \times 80/CO$
SVRI	Systemic vascular resistance index	1500–2400	dynes • sec./(cm.^{5} • m.^{2})	$SVR \times BSA$
PVR	Pulmonary vascular resistance	100–200	dynes • sec./cm.^{5}	$(MPAP - PCWP) \times 80/CO$
PVRI	Pulmonary vascular resistance index	150–300	dynes • sec./(cm.^{5} • m.^{2})	$PVR \times BSA$
CaO$_2$	Arterial oxygen content	16–22	ml.O$_2$/100 ml. (vol.%)	$(SaO_2 \times Hgb. \times 1.39) + (PaO_2 \times 0.0031)$
CvO$_2$	Venous oxygen content	12–17	ml.O$_2$/100 ml. (vol. %)	$(S\bar{v}O_2 \times Hgb. \times 1.39) + (P\bar{v}O_2 \times 0.0031)$
C(a − v)O$_2$	Arteriovenous oxygen difference	3.5–5.5	ml. O$_2$/100 ml. (vol. %)	$CaO_2 - CvO_2$
ḊO$_2$	Oxygen delivery	700–1400	ml./min.	$CaO_2 \times CO \times 10$
ḊO$_2$I	Oxygen delivery index	400–600	ml./(min. • m.^{2})	$CaO_2 \times CI \times 10$
V̇O$_2$	Oxygen consumption	150–300	ml./min.	$C(a - v)O_2 \times CO \times 10$
V̇O$_2$I	Oxygen consumption index	100–150	ml./(min. • m.^{2})	$C(a - v)O_2 \times CI \times 10$
O$_2$ER	Oxygen extraction ratio	0.23–0.32	Dimensionless	$\dot{V}O_2/\dot{D}O_2$

BSA, body surface area; SaO$_2$, arterial oxygen saturation; S$\bar{v}$O$_2$, mixed venous oxygen saturation; PaO$_2$, arterial oxygen partial pressure; P$\bar{v}$O$_2$, mixed venous oxygen partial pressure.

modification of thoracic electrical bioimpedance that reportedly increases the reliability of the technique uses esophageal electrodes mounted on an esophageal probe. Standardized placement of the esophageal probe is thought to reduce the variability associated with placement of the skin electrodes. This modality also awaits further study.

A promising, though invasive, method of continuous cardiac output monitoring is an automated modification of the intermittent thermodilution technique that is currently widely used. In this method, a pulmonary artery catheter is modified by incorporating a thermal filament on the catheter that transfers a safe level of heat to the bloodstream at pulsed intervals. The temperature change is detected downstream by a distal thermistor. Thus, no fluid injectate is required. There is presently a 3- to 6-minute averaging time before the cardiac output reading is updated; therefore, the applicability of this method in situations of rapidly changing hemodynamics may be limited. Furthermore, thermodilution methods may be inaccurate in low cardiac output states owing to heat dissipation.[4] Despite these limitations, the continuous cardiac output catheter, which is commercially available, has been generally validated against standard cardiac output measurement techniques (Fig. 5–6).[90] An even more recent modification has electronically linked the continuous thermodilution cardiac output measurement system with standard critical care patient monitoring systems to provide a continuous measurement of systemic vascular resistance.

Another method to continuously monitor cardiac output is arterial pulse contour analysis, in which arterial pressure waveforms are used to estimate stroke volume. Both invasive and noninvasive techniques have been described. The noninvasive method uses a finger cuff to yield an arterial pressure waveform, from which the cardiac output is derived. Although the technique is conceptually attractive, inconsistencies remain with respect to accuracy and reproducibility.[35] Cardiac output estimates derived from arterial pulse contour analysis cannot be relied on at the present time to base intervention decisions in critically ill patients.

The Fick method is a standard, accurate technique for intermittently determining cardiac output from measurements of oxygen consumption (as measured by respiratory gas analysis) and of arteriovenous oxygen content difference. Attempts have been made to use the Fick principle to provide continuous cardiac output estimates using a combination of invasive oximetry and on-line metabolic gas analysis.[10] This method may become applicable in cases in which the continuous thermodilution method may be inaccurate, such as in low cardiac output states.

Invasive and noninvasive Doppler methods have been used to provide continuous measurements of cardiac output.[79] In these techniques, blood flow velocity is measured using ultrasonic transducers mounted on pulmonary artery catheters, endotracheal tubes, esophageal probes, or suprasternally positioned devices. A limitation of these methods is that they generally make assumptions about great vessel geometry or blood flow velocity profiles. Such assumptions may lead to considerable error in estimating cardiac output. Ultrasound probe positioning is also critical but subject to high degrees of variability. Doppler methods have not proven to be consistently reliable or accurate in determining continuous cardiac output.

Transcutaneous Oxygen Monitoring. Transcutaneous oxygen monitoring is a noninvasive technique of continuously measuring skin PO_2 ($PtcO_2$). $PtcO_2$, which is dependent on PaO_2, cardiac output, and skin perfusion, appears to correlate well with PaO_2 measurements in hemodynamically stable patients but not in patients in shock.[84] On the other hand, $PtcO_2$ seems to correlate with cardiac output in severe shock. Although more work needs to be done in this area, the major use of transcutaneous oxygen monitoring may be to identify trends or sudden drops in perfusion or PaO_2. This technique, which presently is not widely used, may prove to be more valuable than pulse oximetry, which is relatively insensitive to small changes in PaO_2 when hemoglobin is nearly saturated with oxygen, that is, when PaO_2 is greater than about 80 mm. Hg.

Serum Lactate Concentration. Measurements of the serum lactate concentration have been used with varying success as a metabolic monitor of shock. Mild to moderate hyperlactatemia (2 to 5 mmol. per liter) may be seen in hypermetabolic states but is not necessarily associated with tissue hypoxia. Similarly, lactic acidosis, which is a metabolic acidosis associated with hyperlactatemia (usually >5 mmol. per liter), may be seen in a number of clinical conditions unassociated with shock or tissue hypoxia, such as liver disease or toxin ingestion. Thus, the absolute level of the serum lactate may be difficult to interpret. Moreover, normal serum lactate levels have been observed in the presence of shock. Probably a more useful interpretation of serum lactate levels in shock involves monitoring trends of a rising or falling lactate level (Fig. 5–7).[85] The lactate to pyruvate ratio, normally about 10:1, is increased in the presence of anaerobic metabolism and appears to be a good indicator of the adequacy of cellular oxygenation.

Gastrointestinal Tonometry. Gastrointestinal tonometry is a minimally invasive technique that can be used to assess the adequacy of tissue oxygenation in a particular organ system. This method of assessment of regional tissue oxygenation is in sharp contrast to methods previously discussed that attempt to provide information about tissue oxygenation from global indices. Global measures do not take into account regional variations in oxygen consumption and delivery, whereas gastrointestinal tonometry focuses on an organ system that is thought to be particularly susceptible at an early stage to the consequences of hypoperfusion and ischemia. Therefore, gastrointestinal tonometry may provide early warning signs of inadequate tissue perfusion in critically ill patients.[36] This method is based on the principle that intraluminal PCO_2 of the gut reflects intramucosal, or tissue, PCO_2. In the most common configuration, gastric tonometry,

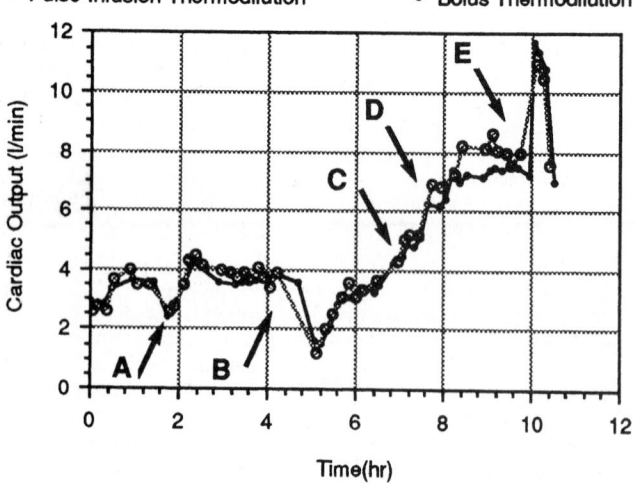

Figure 5–6. Comparison of intermittent and continuous thermodilation cardiac output measurements in a sheep model. At A, mechanical ventilation is initiated. At B, approximately 20% of blood volume is exsanguinated. Blood is reinfused at time C. At D, 1 liter of lactated Ringer's solution is infused, and at E, an isoproterenol infusion is started. Over a wide range of cardiac outputs there is good agreement between the two methods of measurement. (From Yelderman, M. L., Quinn, M. D., McKown, R. C., et al.: Continuous thermodilution cardiac output measurement in sheep. J. Thorac. Cardiovasc. Surg., *104*:315, 1992.)

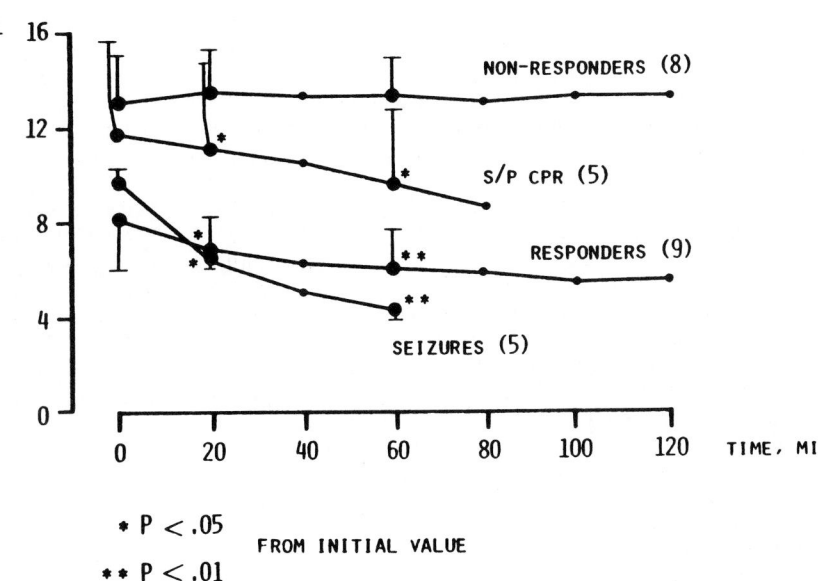

Figure 5–7. Time course of serum arterial lactate concentrations in patients in shock who respond to treatment shows slower resolution than in patients with hyperlactatemia after grand mal seizures or after successful cardiopulmonary resuscitation. Nonresponders (fatal outcome) showed no change in the lactate level. Serial lactate level determinations may be useful in monitoring response to therapy in shock. (From Vincent, J–L., Dufaye, P., Berré, J., et al.: Serial lactate determinations during circulatory shock. Crit. Care Med., *11*:449, 1983.)

a silicone balloon permeable to carbon dioxide is attached to the end of a nasogastric tube. Equilibration of the PCO_2 between the gastric lumen and saline in the balloon occurs in approximately 30 minutes, after which time the saline is anaerobically collected and measured for PCO_2 using a conventional blood gas analyzer. Simultaneously, the arterial bicarbonate concentration is measured. Intramucosal pH can then be calculated using the bicarbonate concentration and the intraluminal PCO_2 in the Henderson-Hasselbalch equation.

Intramucosal pH of the gastrointestinal tract appears to be a reliable index of regional anaerobic activity, and thus of local tissue hypoxia. Gastric intramucosal pH (pH_i) was found in one study to be the most reliable indicator of tissue oxygenation in a group of 83 critically ill patients with acute circulatory failure.[61] In that study, survivors had a significantly higher gastric pH_i than nonsurvivors. A low gastric pH_i (<7.35) in the first 24 hours after admission was highly sensitive in predicting death, and an abnormal value at 24 hours was even more predictive of outcome. Thus, the gastric pH_i may be useful in distinguishing those patients who respond well to resuscitation from those who do not. Another study by Gutierrez and associates[47] used the gastric pH_i as a therapeutic index to guide therapy in 260 patients in an intensive care unit. Patient outcome was significantly better in the group of patients admitted with a normal pH_i whose therapy was guided by gastric tonometry measurements. However, there was no difference in survival between protocol and control groups if the admission pH_i was below 7.35 (Fig. 5–8).[47] Further studies are needed to validate these outcomes, but the technique of gastrointestinal tonometry appears to be an effective, simple, relatively inexpensive way to monitor the adequacy of splanchnic tissue oxygenation.

PATHOPHYSIOLOGY OF SHOCK

Shock, by definition, is the result of impaired tissue perfusion. Hypoperfusion is the common feature of all shock syndromes, regardless of the inciting cause. Shock syndromes, however, vary in degrees of severity, ranging from occult tissue hypoxia to full-blown cardiovascular collapse or multiple organ dysfunction. Appreciation of this wide spectrum of shock presentations may lead to earlier awareness, thus earlier treatment, of the milder forms of shock. Consequences of tissue hypoperfusion may include tissue hypoxia, anaerobic metabolism, acidosis, elaboration of inflammatory mediators, circulatory redistribution with early involvement of the splanchnic circulation, cellular injury, septic complications, and MODS (Fig. 5–9).

Role of Hypoxia

Impaired tissue hypoperfusion, the primary pathophysiologic mechanism in shock, leads to decreased oxygen delivery relative to oxygen needs. In the resting state, oxygen delivery ($\dot{D}O_2$) and oxygen consumption ($\dot{V}O_2$) are well matched, resulting in a $\dot{D}O_2$ that normally exceeds $\dot{V}O_2$ by threefold to fourfold. This corresponds to an oxygen extraction ratio (O_2ER) of 0.25 to 0.33. Under conditions of either increased energy expenditure or decreased $\dot{D}O_2$, the normal $\dot{D}O_2$–$\dot{V}O_2$ relationship is disrupted. The physiologic response to restore homeostasis under such conditions is to increase the O_2ER to supply the basal oxygen requirements and preserve aerobic metabolism. The increased O_2ER may become clinically apparent by a fall in $S\bar{v}O_2$, although this global measure may be relatively insensitive to regional tissue hypoxia. As long as the tissues are able to extract enough oxygen to maintain aerobic metabolism, $\dot{V}O_2$ remains constant and independent of $\dot{D}O_2$. If, on the other hand, further increases in O_2ER are inadequate to maintain tissue oxygenation, a critical O_2ER ($O_2ERcrit$) is reached, above which $\dot{V}O_2$ becomes dependent on $\dot{D}O_2$ and anaerobic metabolism supervenes. This critical O_2ER threshold may also be regarded as the critical $\dot{D}O_2crit$, below which $\dot{V}O_2$ is dependent on $\dot{D}O_2$.

Figure 5–10 is a schematic illustration of the relationship between $\dot{V}O_2$ and $\dot{D}O_2$. The biphasic relationship between $\dot{V}O_2$ and $\dot{D}O_2$, as depicted, was first described in animal models.[20] A similar relationship has been observed in some studies in humans, but other investigations have not corroborated the biphasic nature of the $\dot{V}O_2$–$\dot{D}O_2$ relationship, particularly in sepsis,[6, 76] although the existence of a critical oxygen delivery

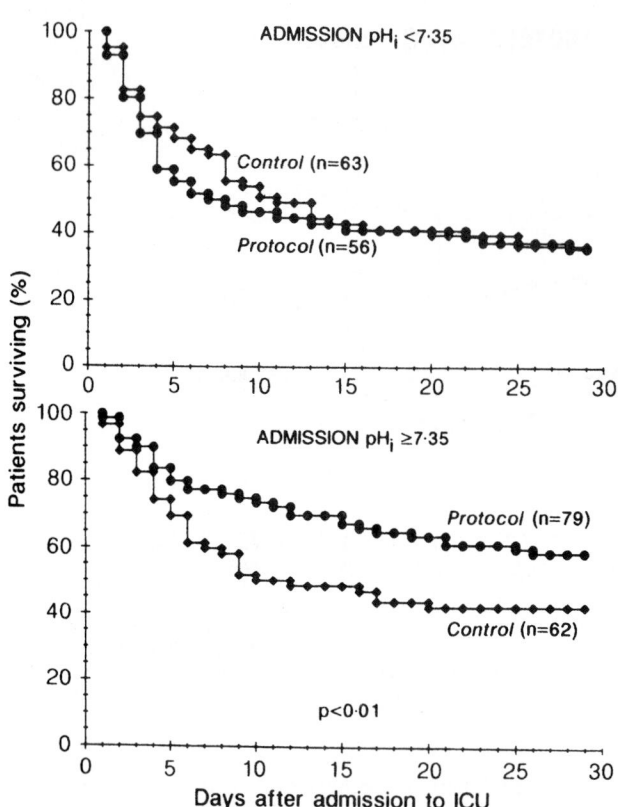

Figure 5–8. Kaplan-Meier Hospital survival curves according to admission gastric intramucosal pH (pH$_i$) as determined by gastric tonometery. Control patients were treated according to standard intensive care unit practices, and protocol patients were given therapy guided by pH$_i$ for pH$_i$ less than 7.35. There were more interventions in the protocol group for both pH$_i$ categories. Interventions were aimed at increasing perfusion and normalizing pH$_i$. Survival was significantly improved in the protocol patients whose admission pH$_i$ was greater than or equal to 7.35. (From Gutierrez, G., Palizas, F., Doglio, G., et al.: Gastric intramucosal pH as a therapeutic index of tissue oxygenation in critically ill patients. Lancet, *339*:195–199. © by The Lancet Ltd, 1992.)

threshold below which anaerobic metabolism occurs is not disputed. The value of O$_2$ERcrit (or D̊o$_2$crit) has not been definitively established in humans and may vary substantially from patient to patient.[28]

The issue of whether D̊o$_2$crit is increased in patients with ARDS or sepsis is debated, as are the implications for treatment. In these patients, a continued dependence of V̊o$_2$ on

D̊o$_2$ has been identified in some instances, prompting some investigators to recommend treatment aimed at providing *supranormal* levels of oxygen delivery in critically ill patients.[39, 92] Such treatment strategies are based on the premises that (1) delivery-dependent oxygen uptake reflects cellular hypoxia; (2) cellular hypoxia plays a key role in the pathogenesis of MODS; and (3) provision of supranormal levels

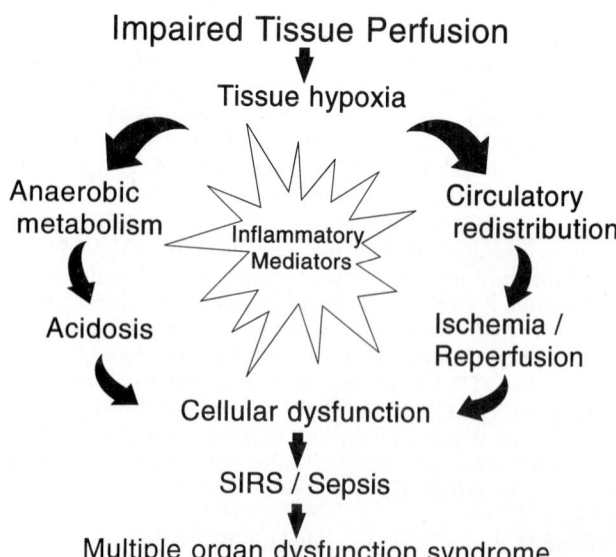

Figure 5–9. Simplified schematic diagram of shock. The fundamental abnormality of impaired tissue perfusion leads to tissue hypoxia, anaerobic metabolism, acidosis, end organ ischemia, and cellular dysfunction. The role of inflammatory mediators appears to be central to the progression of shock, which ultimately may lead to the systemic inflammatory response syndrome (SIRS), sepsis, and the multiple organ dysfunction syndrome.

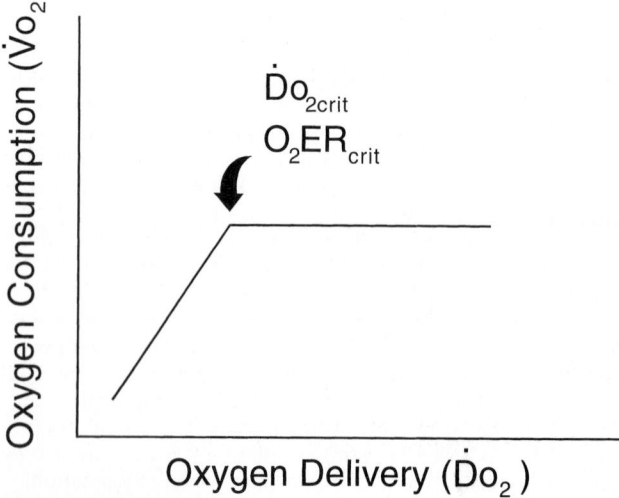

Figure 5–10. Relationship of oxygen consumption to oxygen delivery, showing that as oxygen delivery decreases, oxygen consumption remains constant (delivery independent), until a critical threshold is reached below which oxygen consumption becomes dependent on oxygen delivery. This threshold has been termed the critical oxygen delivery (D̊o$_2$crit) or the critical oxygen extraction ratio (O$_2$ERcrit). Below this threshold, oxygen consumption falls dramatically and the oxygen extraction ratio rises, signaling inadequate oxygen delivery to match cellular oxygen needs. Anaerobic metabolism supervenes, therefore, when oxygen delivery falls below the critical threshold.

of oxygen may reverse cellular hypoxia and prevent the progression of MODS. The premise that delivery-dependent oxygen uptake signifies cellular hypoxia may not be correct in all instances. Studies on critically ill patients have shown, for example, that the lactate/pyruvate ratio is not increased, as would be expected if cellular hypoxia were present.[42] Furthermore, delivery-dependent oxygen uptake has been observed in groups of patients, other than those with sepsis, without any evidence of oxygen starvation. At the present time, the validity of treating critically ill patients by increasing oxygen delivery to supranormal has not been verified by some recent studies,[50] and further evaluation of this approach needs to be carried out to resolve the ongoing debate.

Another metabolic abnormality that has been observed in septic patients is a decreased O_2ER, corresponding to an increase in $S\bar{v}O_2$ and a decrease in the arteriovenous oxygen content difference. Explanations that have been proposed to account for this finding include the presence of microcirculatory derangements such as arteriovenous shunting, defective oxygen utilization at the cellular level (bioenergetic failure), and down-regulation of the process of oxidative metabolism, at least in some organs. True anatomic shunting at the capillary level has not been documented in septic patients, but microcirculatory maldistribution leading to physiologic shunting has been postulated. However, the failure to observe an increase in the lactate/pyruvate ratio is evidence against the theory of inadequate microvascular perfusion in many cases of sepsis. Defective oxygen utilization at the cellular level has also been proposed to explain the frequently observed decrease in O_2ER in sepsis.[6] Proponents of this theory would argue that defects in the pathways of oxidative metabolism lead to decreased production of high-energy phosphates (adenosine triphosphate, phosphocreatine, inorganic phosphate), hence, bioenergetic failure. Results of experimental studies using phosphorus-31 nuclear magnetic resonance spectroscopy to measure high-energy phosphates, however, are not consistent with bioenergetic failure in skeletal muscle, brain, or myocardium.[51] Thus, it appears unlikely that this theory can satisfactorily explain the alterations in oxygen utilization observed in early sepsis in all instances. On the other hand, bioenergetic failure may play a significant role in late sepsis, in hemorrhagic or traumatic shock, or in cases of early sepsis with inadequate volume resuscitation. All of these uncompensated conditions will cause cellular hypoperfusion, inadequate oxygen delivery, and the onset of anaerobic metabolism. Finally, the hypothesis that metabolic down-regulation may occur in some organs in patients with sepsis might explain the inappropriately low oxygen consumption and low O_2ER observed in sepsis.[51] Evidence to support this hypothesis includes the observation that endotoxin may cause a decrease in oxidative metabolism in skeletal muscle.[77] Moreover, interleukin-1, an inflammatory mediator thought to play an important role in the systemic inflammatory response syndrome and sepsis, has been shown to induce slow-wave sleep and neurologic depression.[32]

Clearly, the role of hypoxia in the pathogenesis and perpetuation of the shock state is complex and incompletely defined, particularly in shock associated with SIRS or sepsis. As techniques improve to assess organ-specific oxygen metabolism, this role should become better elucidated.

Anaerobic Metabolism and Acidosis

When oxygen delivery is insufficient to meet cellular oxygen demands, anaerobic glycolysis occurs (Fig. 5–11). In the absence of oxygen, pyruvate is converted to lactate in the cytosol, yielding only two molecules of adenosine triphosphate per molecule of glucose. In contrast, under aerobic

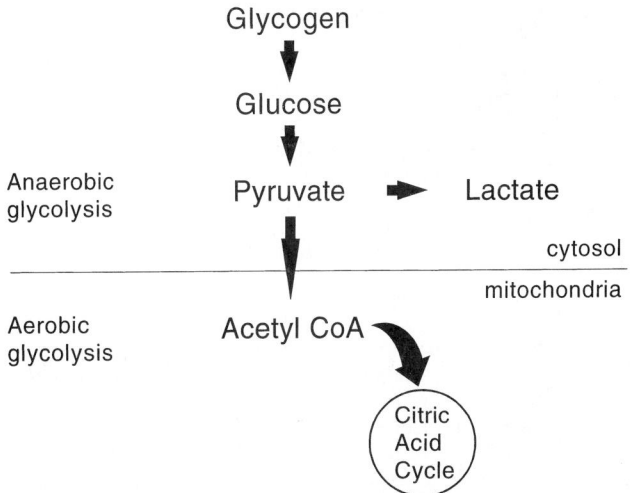

Figure 5–11. Schematic of glucose metabolism under aerobic and anaerobic conditions. If adequate oxygen is available, pyruvate, the end-product of the Embden-Meyerhof pathway, enters the mitochondria where it is metabolized to acetyl coenzyme A, which enters the citric acid cycle. Under anaerobic conditions, pyruvate is converted to lactate in the cytosol, resulting in an accumulation of lactate and an increased lactate–pyruvate ratio. This latter process is much less efficient in generating adenosine triphosphate (ATP) than aerobic glycolysis (2 ATP versus 38 ATP per molecule of glucose metabolized).

conditions, pyruvate enters the mitochondria and is metabolized to acetyl coenzyme A, which, through the citric acid cycle and electron transport chain, results in the net production of 38 molecules of adenosine triphosphate per molecule of glucose oxidized.

As cellular oxygen supply diminishes, lactate production increases and pyruvate concentration diminishes. Thus, increases in the blood lactate concentration and the blood lactate/pyruvate (L/P) ratio have been observed under conditions of anaerobic metabolism. The degree of hyperlactatemia has been correlated with patient outcome in studies that indicate that the probability of survival decreases markedly as blood lactate concentration increases beyond the normal range of 0 to 2 mmol. per liter.[19] It is noteworthy, however, that cellular hypoxia may not account for elevated blood lactate concentrations in all cases. Delayed clearance of lactate due to hepatic dysfunction, for instance, may cause persistent elevations of blood lactate in the absence of hypoxia.[89] Also, overproduction of lactate under aerobic, but hypermetabolic conditions, has been observed. Accelerated glycolysis and hyperlactatemia may occur during sepsis, despite the lack of other evidence, such as bioenergetic studies of high-energy phosphate balance, to indicate cellular hypoxia. The L/P ratio, on the other hand, has been considered an excellent indicator of cellular hypoxia and may be used to differentiate hyperlactatemia due to ischemia from that due to enhanced aerobic glycolysis in hypermetabolic states. The L/P ratio has been observed to increase dramatically once the anaerobic threshold is reached, and L/P ratios exceeding 15 to 20 (normal <10) are indicative of ongoing cellular hypoxia.

The pathophysiologic effects of metabolic acidosis depend, to some extent, on the degree of acidosis. In mild acidemia (pH >7.2), catechol stimulation may cause tachycardia, increased cardiac output, and vasoconstriction. In more severe acidemia (pH <7.2), direct effects of acidosis predominate, causing decreased responsiveness to the effects of circulating catechols, bradycardia, vasodilation, and decreased cardiac output. A direct, negative inotropic effect is also observed, probably owing to alteration of the slow calcium ion flux into the cell. The net cardiovascular response to metabolic acidosis, therefore, is determined by the relative influences of the direct effects of acidosis and the effects due to catechol stimulation. Other effects of metabolic acidosis include a decreased threshold for ventricular fibrillation and a rightward shift of the oxyhemoglobin dissociation curve. This latter effect, which causes a decreased affinity of hemoglobin for oxygen, is partially opposed by a decrease in concentration of 2,3-diphosphoglycerate in red blood cells.

Circulatory Redistribution

The homeostatic response to hypoperfusion and hypoxia is to preserve oxygen delivery to the heart and brain by selectively diverting blood flow from other tissues, particularly the skin, subcutaneous tissues, and the gastrointestinal tract. The splanchnic circulation is especially vulnerable to this redistribution of blood flow, which occurs in response to local, as well as humoral, influences. Hypodynamic forms of shock such as cardiogenic or hypovolemic shock are usually associated with a predominantly vasoconstrictive effect. In such cases, the observed increase in systemic vascular resistance is due largely to the disproportionate increase in splanchnic vascular resistance. A number of vasoconstrictive factors have been identified that may contribute to splanchnic hypoperfusion, including catechols, angiotensin II, vasopressin, endothelin, and thromboxane A_2. Although redistribution of blood flow to *vital* organs protects those organs from the deleterious effects of ischemia, impairment of gut perfusion may perpetuate the shock state and lead to irreversibility, a heightened systemic inflammatory response, and MODS.

In some forms of shock, such as vasogenic shock due to sepsis, a hyperdynamic cardiovascular profile is frequently observed, along with a reduction in systemic vascular resistance. However, the reduction in vascular resistance is not uniform across all vascular beds, and significant maldistribution of blood flow may result. A functional shunt may occur, whereby relatively well-perfused tissues *steal* oxygenated blood from more ischemic regions. Thus, despite an overall reduction in systemic vascular resistance and a *normal blood pressure*, ongoing hypoperfusion and ischemia may occur in some organs or in some regions of particular organs. Some of the vasodilatory mediators that may play a role in this process include nitric oxide, prostaglandin E_2, prostacyclin, interleukin-2, bradykinin, and others.

On the microcirculatory level, redistribution of blood flow may occur in some capillary beds due to intrinsic or extrinsic obstruction. Low-flow states, hypothermia, and increased viscosity may predispose to capillary sludging. Intravascular coagulation, platelet aggregation, and other intraluminal debris may occlude capillary channels, preventing red blood cells from reaching tissues nourished by those capillaries. Extrinsic compression of capillaries from local tissue inflammation, edema, or hemorrhage may also lead to microcirculatory obstruction. Damage to the endothelial cells themselves from the effects of direct tissue injury, ischemia, or reperfusion injury may contribute to cellular and organ dysfunction.[63]

Role of the Gut in Shock

The gut has emerged as a central organ in the pathophysiology of shock. Gut dysfunction may be a manifestation of the *effect* of shock, but it may also be an important *cause* of the perpetuation of various shock syndromes. As a result of circulatory redistribution in shock, splanchnic blood flow, which normally comprises 15% to 20% of cardiac output, is reduced. Mucosal ischemia and cellular hypoxia ensue, leading to further injury and deleterious systemic effects. For these reasons, the gut has been termed the *motor* of irreversible shock and MODS.[22]

Lillehei, as early as 1957, concluded that an intestinal factor existed and contributed to the high mortality in irreversible shock.[58] His studies in dogs demonstrated that perfusion of the gut with blood from normovolemic, healthy dogs reduced mortality. Other investigators have shown that intraluminal instillation of oxygen reduces mucosal ischemia.

The pathogenesis of gut injury involves at least two different mechanisms: (1) those related to hypoxia and (2) those related to reperfusion injury once blood flow is reestablished. Hypoxic injury causes mucosal ischemia, which leads to the disruption of the normal epithelial cell barrier. Reperfusion causes the accumulation of toxic oxidants,[43] such as superoxide anion ($O_2 \bullet$), hydroxyl radical ($OH \bullet$), and hydrogen peroxide (H_2O_2), which may lead to cellular injury by the process of lipid peroxidation and the disruption of cell membrane integrity (Fig. 5–12).[30] In addition to causing tissue injury directly, these oxidants may have a chemotactic role, leading to granulocyte infiltration of the injured tissue, granulocyte activation and release of cytotoxic proteases, and further injury mediated by the elaboration of proinflammatory mediators such as tumor necrosis factor-alpha (TNF-α), platelet activating factor (PAF), interleukin (IL)-1 and IL-6, and others.

As a consequence of intestinal mucosal injury, gut permeability may increase, allowing enteric flora or bacterial toxins to *translocate* across the gut wall and invade the host through lymphatic or portal venous routes.[29] This breakdown of the normal intestinal epithelial barrier with subsequent bacterial or toxin translocation may amplify the systemic inflammatory response and contribute to the development of MODS.[5]

MEDIATORS OF SHOCK AND SEPSIS

Shock, like sepsis, induces a complicated cascade of physiologic events that is brought about through the action of a number of inflammatory and neuroendocrine mediators. The mediators of the inflammatory response, which may have either local or systemic effects, include a large and growing cadre of molecules with important, but incompletely defined roles in the development, progression, and perpetuation of the various shock syndromes. Depending on the severity of the injury or insult, the systemic inflammatory response may be self-limited or it may escalate to the point of multiple organ dysfunction. Not all of the mediators discussed in this section are involved in each shock syndrome, and some are likely to predominate in certain forms of shock, for example, in shock due to sepsis. The precise roles of specific mediators, as well as the interactions between mediators, are still being elucidated.

Endotoxin. Endotoxin is a cell wall component of gram-negative bacteria and a potent mediator in the development of septic shock. Other bacterial cell wall components and various exotoxins from gram-negative or gram-positive organisms may also induce a septic response in the host, but the actions of endotoxin are the most thoroughly studied. Endotoxin is a lipopolysaccharide molecule consisting of three major regions: (1) O-antigen or side chain that is responsible for the O serotype of gram-negative bacteria, (2) the core, and (3) lipid A, which is the region responsible for most of the toxicity of endotoxin. The host responses to endotoxin are multiple and include the activation of macrophages, activation of the complement and coagulation systems, and the release of numerous mediators, including TNF-α, IL-1, IL-6, PAF, nitric oxide, and various oxidants. The activation of macrophages by endotoxin with subsequent release of proinflammatory cytokines appears to be a key

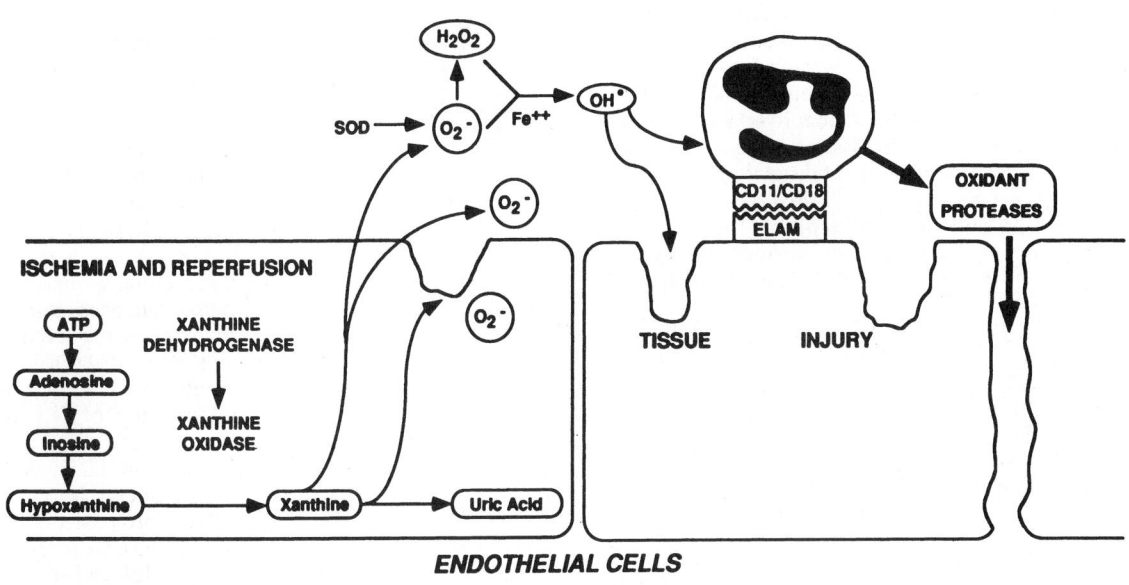

Figure 5–12. Pathophysiology of ischemia–reperfusion injury. Under ischemic conditions, xanthine oxidase accumulates. When oxygen becomes available again during the reperfusion stage, superoxide anion ($O_2\cdot$), hydrogen peroxide (H_2O_2), and hydroxyl radical ($OH\cdot$) are produced. These toxic oxidants cause tissue damage directly and by promoting neutrophil activation, which leads to further release of toxic oxidants and proteases. (From Demling, R., La Londe, C., Saldinger, P., and Knox, J.: Multiple-organ dysfunction in the surgical patient: Pathophysiology, prevention, and treatment. Curr. Probl. Surg., *30*:345, 1994.)

factor in the development of the physiologic derangements associated with sepsis.

Complement Fragments. The complement cascade is activated in response to infection, shock, and tissue injury. The anaphylatoxins C3a and C5a are the components of the complement system that exert the most apparent physiologic effects. Both C3a and C5a cause histamine to be released from basophils and mast cells. Systemic effects include vasodilatation and increase in vascular permeability. C5a is also a potent chemoattractant for neutrophils and mononuclear phagocytes, which then become activated and can amplify the inflammatory response through the actions of other mediators, such as oxygen radicals and thromboxane.

Eicosanoids. Eicosanoids form a group of compounds that arise from the metabolism of arachidonic acid. Arachidonic acid is produced when cell membrane phospholipids react with the enzyme phospholipase in response to injury or sepsis. The metabolism of arachidonic acid through the lipoxygenase and cyclooxygenase pathways results in the formation of the biologically active leukotrienes and prostanoids, respectively (Fig. 5–13).

The cyclic endoperoxides prostaglandin G_2 (PGG$_2$) and PGH$_2$ are the precursors of the prostaglandins and the thromboxanes, collectively known as prostanoids. Prostaglandins and thromboxanes are cyclic fatty acid derivatives containing either a five-member ring, in the case of the former, or a six-member ring, in the case of the latter. The principal prostaglandins, PGI$_2$ (prostacyclin), PGD$_2$, PGE$_2$, and PGF$_{2\alpha}$, are metabolized quickly and exert most of their physiologic effects locally. Prostacyclin, produced largely by vascular endothelium, causes vasodilatation, bronchodilation, and inhibits platelet aggregation. Its effects are balanced by those of thromboxane A$_2$, which is a potent vasoconstrictor, bronchoconstrictor, and platelet aggregating agent produced mainly by platelets. Prostacyclin and thromboxane thus act to achieve an appropriate balance of vascular tone and blood flow in the region of injury, but excessive thromboxane production may also potentiate tissue ischemia by limiting blood

flow to the area of injury and causing maldistribution of blood flow. PGE$_2$ acts as a vasodilator and a bronchodilator, causes fever, and has immunodepressant activity by inhibiting TNF-α and IL-1 synthesis.

Leukotrienes are produced by a number of cells, including mast cells, macrophages, neutrophils, and vascular smooth muscle. Leukotriene B$_4$ is a chemoattractant for neutrophils and promotes neutrophil adhesion. Leukotrienes C$_4$ and D$_4$, which produce bronchoconstriction, vasoconstriction, and in-

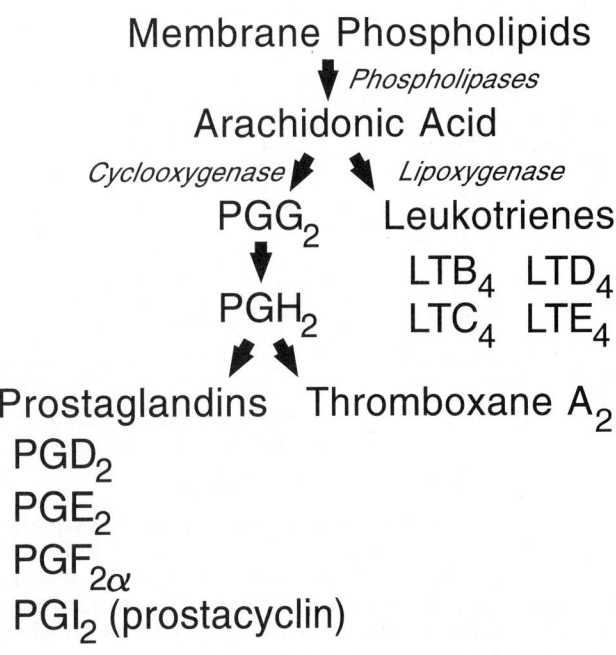

Figure 5–13. Arachidonic acid metabolism. Prostaglandins and thromboxane are synthesized by means of the cyclooxygenase pathway, whereas leukotrienes are synthesized by means of the lipoxygenase pathway.

creased vascular permeability, may be involved in the early pulmonary changes of ARDS in addition to the hemodynamic changes associated with anaphylaxis and sepsis.

Kinins. Bradykinin and kallidin (lysyl bradykinin) are low-molecular-weight peptides that are thought to play a role in the development of inflammation, anaphylaxis, and septic shock. The principal effects of the kinins include vasodilatation, an increase in capillary permeability, and local edema formation. They have also been implicated as causative factors of pain at local wound sites. In addition, the kinins may activate phospholipase, leading to the formation of eicosanoids and further amplification of the inflammatory response.

Nitric Oxide. Nitric oxide, formerly called endothelium-derived relaxing factor, is a potent vasodilator and inhibitor of platelet aggregation. Produced from the metabolism of L-arginine, nitric oxide activates guanylate cyclase in vascular smooth muscle cells to cause cyclic guanosine monophosphate–dependent vasodilatation. Through a similar mechanism in platelets, endothelium-derived nitric oxide also inhibits platelet aggregation and adherence to help maintain vascular patency. Nitric oxide appears to be involved in the regulation of basal vascular tone, as well as the pathophysiologic decreases in blood pressure and systemic vascular resistance seen in sepsis and other shock syndromes associated with refractory hypotension.

Cytokines. Cytokines are small peptide molecules that are synthesized and secreted by a number of cell types in response to injury, inflammation, and infection. These compounds are now recognized as key mediators in SIRS, shock, sepsis, and MODS. In addition to acting directly on target cells, cytokines also exert their effects by potentiating one another to produce an amplified host response that may lead to a state of persistent shock, progressive cellular and physiologic dysfunction, and irreversibility.

Cytokines comprise a number of different categories of compounds, including interleukins, tumor necrosis factors, colony stimulating factors, and interferons (Table 5–3). Of the interleukins, IL-1, IL-2, and IL-6 have been the most widely studied in the settings of injury, infection, and inflammatory response. IL-1 is a major proinflammatory cytokine produced primarily by monocytes and tissue macrophages but also by endothelial cells, neutrophils, B lymphocytes, and keratinocytes. IL-1, secreted in response to endotoxin and tumor necrosis factor release, has numerous effects, including induction of fever, acute-phase protein production and release, stimulation of T and B cells, potentiation of other inflammatory mediator release, and promotion of endothelial cell procoagulant activity. In addition, IL-1 appears to regulate skeletal muscle proteolysis in patients with sepsis or after significant injury.

IL-2, produced by T lymphocytes, stimulates T-cell proliferation and cell-mediated cytotoxic T-cell function and may induce hypotension. IL-6, produced by numerous cell types, including monocytes, macrophages, fibroblasts, and neutrophils, is a major stimulant of hepatic acute-phase protein synthesis. Other actions of IL-6 include the promotion of T- and B-cell activation and the induction of fever. Serum IL-6 levels increase markedly after trauma or sepsis and may correlate with the severity of illness.

TNF-α has a central role in the stress response, particularly in the inflammatory response to endotoxemia.[65] Although it has a plasma half-life of about 15 minutes, TNF-α, or cachectin, is thought to be the principal mediator of sepsis and MODS because of the secondary cascades that it stimulates.[11] Evidence to support this claim includes the following[30]: (1) rapid increases in circulating TNF-α levels are seen after the onset of invasive systemic infection; (2) the physiologic response to TNF-α administration in healthy persons is

TABLE 5–3. Major Effects of Principal Cytokines in Shock and Sepsis

Cytokine	Effects
Interleukins	
IL-1	Stimulates release of TNF-α, IL-6, IL-8, platelet activating factor, prostaglandins
	Stimulates T and B cells
	Induces skeletal muscle proteolysis
	Causes fever
	Promotes acute-phase protein production and release
	Increases expression of adhesion molecules
	Increases endothelial procoagulant activity
IL-2	Stimulates release of TNF-α and IFN-γ
	Causes hypotension
	Enhances T-cell proliferation and cytotoxic T-cell function
IL-6	Stimulates acute-phase protein production and release
	Promotes T- and B-cell activation
	Causes fever
	Enhances neutrophil activation and accumulation
Tumor Necrosis Factors	
TNF-α	Stimulates release of IL-1, IL-6, platelet activating factor, prostaglandins
	Promotes activation of neutrophils, eosinophils, monocytes
	Increases expression of adhesion molecules
	Activates complement and coagulation cascades
	Increases vascular permeability
	Causes hypotension
	Causes fever
Colony Stimulating Factors	
GCSF	Stimulates growth of granulocytes
GM-CSF	Stimulates growth of granulocytes, eosinophils, and macrophages
Interferons	
IFN-γ	Stimulates release of TNF-α, IL-1, IL-6
	Promotes macrophage activation and function

virtually identical to that seen in sepsis; (3) detectable levels of TNF-α are observed before those of other inflammatory mediators; and (4) pretreatment with TNF antibodies prevents the systemic inflammatory response. Like IL-1, TNF-α is secreted primarily by monocytes and macrophages, but also by lymphocytes, Kupffer cells, and other cell types. Some of the physiologic responses seen after the administration of TNF-α include hypotension, fever, lactic acidosis, disseminated intravascular coagulation, increased systemic and pulmonary vascular permeability, and the release of stress hormones such as catecholamines, glucagon, and cortisol. Many of the effects of TNF-α at the tissue level are mediated through oxidant release and eicosanoid production.

Colony stimulating factors promote the bone marrow production and maturation of various cell lines. Granulocyte colony stimulating factor (GCSF) has a more limited influence than granulocyte-macrophage colony stimulating factor (GM-CSF), which stimulates the growth and activity of macrophages and eosinophils, as well as of granulocytes.

Interferon gamma, derived from T cells and some macrophage populations, potentiates the actions of other cytokines, particularly TNF-α, and promotes macrophage activation and function. Unlike other interferons, interferon gamma possesses no antiviral activity.

Platelet Activating Factor. Platelet activating factor is a lipid mediator that amplifies the actions of TNF-α and IL-1, resulting in the exacerbation of shock and ischemia through its multiple physiologic effects. PAF release causes platelet aggregation, leukocyte activation, bronchoconstriction, increased vascular permeability, cardiodepression, and hypotension. PAF also stimulates the synthesis of leukotrienes and may mediate bowel necrosis in endotoxemia.[52]

Endogenous Opioids. Endogenous opioids, such as the enkephalins and beta-endorphins, are peptides produced by the pituitary gland and other neurologic tissues. The plasma levels of these substances are elevated in various stress and toxic states, leading some investigators to believe that opiate receptor blockade with naloxone can ameliorate the hemodynamic depression associated with opioids.[45] The ultimate role of the endogenous opioids in shock and sepsis in humans is still uncertain.

Oxidants. Oxidants are reactive oxygen metabolites that may be more appropriately classified under effectors of cellular injury rather than as inflammatory mediators. Oxidants have a physiologic role, such as in cytochrome P-450–mediated oxidations, but most of the attention given to these potent oxidizing agents is directed at their pathophysiologic roles in inflammation, injury, and infection.[9, 49] The production of oxidants in ischemia-reperfusion injury has been alluded to (see Fig. 5–12), whereby the enzyme xanthine oxidase catalyzes the production of superoxide anion ($O_2 \cdot$).[30, 40] Other mechanisms may be involved, as well, in the generation of $O_2 \cdot$. Another oxidant, hydrogen peroxide (H_2O_2), is formed from the dismutation of $O_2 \cdot$. The extremely reactive hydroxyl radical ($OH \cdot$) is produced by means of the Fenton reaction, in which the transformation of H_2O_2 occurs in the presence of transition ions such as iron (Fe^{2+}). Activated neutrophils are another source of oxidants, specifically of hypochlorous acid ($HOCl$), which is generated from H_2O_2 and chloride by a reaction catalyzed by myeloperoxidase.

The deleterious effects of oxidants are multiple and include (1) lipid peroxidation and cell membrane disruption, leading to cell death; (2) inhibition of adenosine triphosphate synthesis in both glycolytic and mitochondrial pathways; (3) oxidative damage to deoxyribonucleic acid; (4) reduction in the levels of cellular nicotinamide-adenine dinucleotide; (5) interference of intracellular calcium regulation; and (6) oxidative damage to amino acids and proteins.

Neuroendocrine Mediators. In response to injury, stress, or infection there is an increase in the circulating levels of catabolic, or stress, hormones. Thus, the metabolic responses observed in such states are largely due to the outpouring of catechols, cortisol, and glucagon. Stimulation of the sympathetic nervous system causes the release of both epinephrine and norepinephrine, which produce the cardiovascular effects of tachycardia, increased inotropy, and peripheral vasoconstriction, as well as increased metabolic rate, increased glycogenolysis, increased gluconeogenesis, and inhibition of insulin secretion by the pancreas. Release of adrenocorticotropic hormone (ACTH) by the anterior pituitary stimulates cortisol output by the adrenal cortex. The catabolic effects of cortisol include proteolysis, lipolysis, and gluconeogenesis.

Glucagon release also contributes to gluconeogenesis and glucose intolerance.

The renin-angiotensin system may be activated due to adrenergic vasoconstriction in the kidneys. The resultant release of angiotensin II leads to further vasoconstriction, which may exacerbate ischemia and shock. Aldosterone and vasopressin are also released, leading to salt and water retention.

DIAGNOSIS AND MANAGEMENT OF SHOCK: GENERAL APPROACH

The ultimate goals in the management of shock are to restore perfusion and adequate oxygen delivery to tissue. No matter what the cause of shock, the basic algorithm to restore hemodynamic stability and tissue perfusion is the same in the initial evaluation (Fig. 5–14). To improve oxygen delivery, three parameters may be manipulated: arterial oxyhemoglobin saturation (SaO_2), hemoglobin concentration, and cardiac output. The SaO_2 should be kept above 90%. Beyond that level there is little change in the arterial oxygen content. Transfusions of packed red blood cells should be considered in patients who do not quickly respond to initial volume expansion measures. Indiscriminate transfusions should be condemned, but patients with persisting perfusion deficits may benefit from a hemoglobin concentration of 11 to 13 gm. per 100 ml., although the optimal hemoglobin concentration has not been well defined.

Cardiac output is the parameter most effectively manipulated to increase oxygen delivery. Assessment of volume status (preload) is done early in the evaluation of a patient in shock. Patients who have mild forms of shock may respond to volume administration alone, without the need for invasive hemodynamic monitoring. Many patients, however, will likely need a pulmonary artery catheter placed to optimize cardiac output and oxygen delivery.

Volume expansion to a PCWP of between 15 and 18 mm. Hg is a reasonable goal. Patients with a PCWP greater than 18 mm. Hg should be suspected of having cardiogenic causes of shock and should be treated for their underlying disease with diuretics and cardiac-directed therapy. Frequent reassessment of the patient's hemodynamic and physiologic status should be carried out after each significant intervention. Reasonable initial resuscitation goals include (1) maintaining PCWP between 15 and 18 mm. Hg; (2) achieving a mean arterial pressure between 60 and 80 mm. Hg; (3) maintaining $S\bar{v}O_2$ greater than 65% to 70%; and (4) achieving delivery-independent oxygen consumption. To reach these goals, patients may require the use of pharmacologic agents to improve cardiac inotropy (dobutamine, dopamine, epinephrine), decrease afterload (nitroglycerin, nitroprusside), or increase perfusion pressure (agents with alpha-adrenergic effects, such as norepinephrine, moderate doses of epinephrine, and phenylephrine).

Once the initial resuscitation goals are met, therapy should continue to provide optimal oxygen delivery. In addition, measures should be instituted to treat the inciting cause of shock, eliminate infectious or inflammatory foci with appropriate surgical intervention and antibiotics, and provide early nutritional support.

SPECIFIC SHOCK SYNDROMES

Hypovolemic Shock. Hypovolemia accounts for the most commonly encountered shock syndrome in surgical patients. Hypovolemic shock occurs when a loss of body fluids is sufficient to cause intravascular volume depletion and when compensatory mechanisms fail to restore normal tissue perfusion. Fluid losses may vary, depending on the cause of hypo-

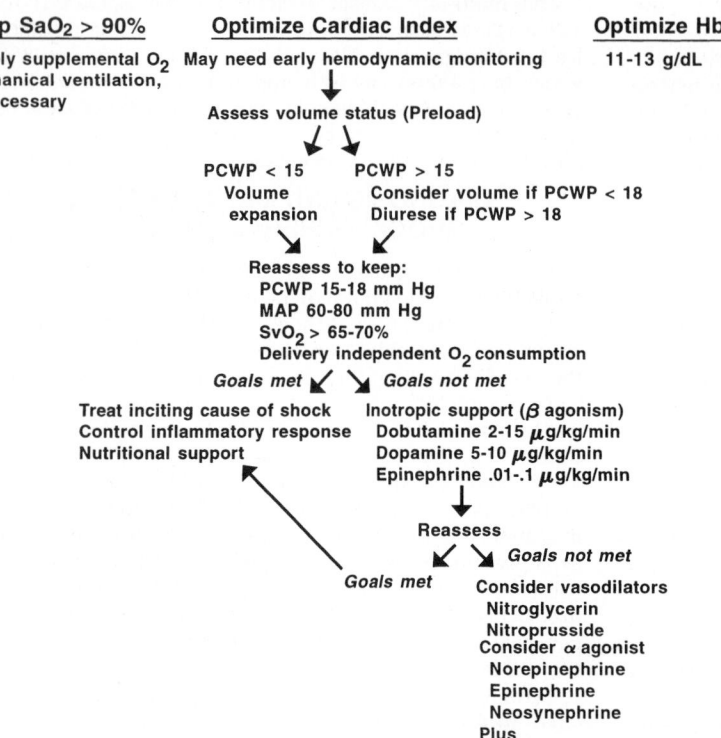

Optimize Oxygen Delivery

Keep SaO₂ > 90%

Supply supplemental O₂
Mechanical ventilation,
if necessary

Optimize Cardiac Index

May need early hemodynamic monitoring

Assess volume status (Preload)

PCWP < 15
Volume
expansion

PCWP > 15
Consider volume if PCWP < 18
Diurese if PCWP > 18

Reassess to keep:
PCWP 15-18 mm Hg
MAP 60-80 mm Hg
SvO₂ > 65-70%
Delivery independent O₂ consumption

Goals met   *Goals not met*

Treat inciting cause of shock
Control inflammatory response
Nutritional support

Inotropic support (β agonism)
Dobutamine 2-15 μg/kg/min
Dopamine 5-10 μg/kg/min
Epinephrine .01-.1 μg/kg/min

Reassess

Goals not met

Goals met
Consider vasodilators
Nitroglycerin
Nitroprusside
Consider α agonist
Norepinephrine
Epinephrine
Neosynephrine
Plus
Dopamine 2-3 μg/kg/min

Optimize Hb

11-13 g/dL

Figure 5–14. Simplified algorithm for the initial resuscitation of patients in shock. The ultimate goal is to restore perfusion and adequate oxygen delivery to tissue.

volemia. Whole blood loss, for example, is seen in hemorrhagic shock after trauma, whereas plasma or free water losses may be seen with extracellular fluid sequestration, unreplaced gastrointestinal fluid loss, or excessive insensible fluid loss. Hemorrhagic losses are normally recognized readily, but occult fluid losses may not be so easily diagnosed. Irrespective of whether the hypovolemia is secondary to hemorrhage, pancreatitis, or intestinal obstruction, the systemic response, as well as the initial treatment, is essentially the same.

Although the clinical signs and symptoms of hypovolemic shock depend on the severity of the intravascular volume deficit, it is imperative to realize that minimal findings on physical examination may still be associated with significant volume losses (Table 5–4). A loss of 15% or less of the circulating blood volume is generally well tolerated by most patients without any hemodynamic signs of shock. The first

sign of hypovolemic shock may be a decrease in the pulse pressure (difference between systolic and diastolic pressures) due to an increase in catecholamine levels. As the circulating blood volume is reduced even further, exceeding 30%, a graded increase in both tachycardia and hypotension becomes evident. Concomitantly, urine output falls, normal skin turgor is lost, and mental status changes occur in a progressive fashion, ranging from apprehension and anxiety to complete obtundation.

A number of compensatory mechanisms are evoked that aim to restore homeostasis and preserve blood flow to the heart and brain. *Baroreceptors* in the aortic arch and carotid sinus respond to a fall in blood pressure by transmitting less afferent stimuli to the vasomotor center in the medulla, which, in turn, enhances sympathetic neural output. The increase in sympathetic tone results in arteriolar and venous constriction, which leads to increased systemic vascular resis-

TABLE 5–4. Clinical Signs and Symptoms of Hemorrhagic Shock Based on Severity of Blood Loss

Percent Loss of Circulating Blood Volume (Volume Loss for 70-kg. Male)	Pulse Rate	Systolic Pressure	Pulse Pressure	Capillary Refill	Respirations	Central Nervous System	Urine Output
<15% (<750 ml.)	Normal	Normal	Normal	Normal	Normal	Normal	Normal
15%–30% (750–1500 ml.)	>100	Normal	Decreased	Delayed	Mild tachypnea	Anxious	20–30 ml./hr.
30%–40% (1500–2000 ml.)	>120 Weak	Decreased	Decreased	Delayed	Marked tachypnea	Confused	20 ml./hr.
>40% (>2000 ml.)	>140 Nonpalpable	Marked decrease	Marked decrease	Absent	Marked tachypnea	Lethargic	Negligible

tance and increased venous return to the heart. Arteriolar vasoconstriction is most evident in cutaneous tissue, skeletal muscle, and renal and splanchnic vascular beds, whereas this effect is negligible in the coronary and cerebral circulations. Adrenal medullary output of norepinephrine and epinephrine causes tachycardia and enhanced myocardial contractility. Sympathetic discharge is enhanced with excitation of peripheral chemoreceptors and in response to cerebral ischemia. Cerebral ischemia, which occurs when mean arterial blood pressure falls below 50 mm. Hg, is a potent stimulus for sympathetic output, leading to intense vasoconstriction and augmentation of cardiac contractility and heart rate.

Antidiuretic hormone is released by the posterior pituitary in response to hypovolemia. It produces vasoconstriction, particularly in the splanchnic circulation, and increases water reabsorption in the distal tubule of the kidney. Renin secretion is stimulated in hypovolemic shock because of hypoperfusion of the juxtaglomerular apparatus in the kidney. The secretion of renin leads to the formation of angiotensin I in the liver and subsequently to the formation of angiotensin II in the lungs. Angiotensin II is a powerful vasoconstrictor that also causes aldosterone release from the adrenal cortex. Aldosterone acts to restore circulating blood volume by promoting the reabsorption of sodium in the renal tubules. Intravascular fluid reabsorption is also enhanced by microcirculatory autoregulation, whereby precapillary vasoconstriction effectively causes a reduction in capillary hydrostatic pressure. The lower capillary hydrostatic pressure, in conjunction with the increased intravascular osmolarity associated with the hyperglycemic response to hypovolemic shock, results in the net reabsorption of interstitial fluid into the vascular compartment.

Diagnosis of Hypovolemic Shock. The diagnosis of hypovolemic shock may be straightforward in certain clinical settings, such as acute hemorrhage, in which the history and physical findings, as described earlier, are consistent with intravascular volume losses and adrenergic compensatory responses. Blood tests are infrequently helpful in situations of acute volume losses because of the fluid shifts that occur, but they may be helpful in detecting less acute, occult fluid losses. Thus, in bowel obstruction, for instance, hemoconcentration may occur, as evidenced by an increase in hemoglobin concentration, hematocrit, and the blood urea nitrogen–creatinine ratio. Hypernatremia may be observed after excessive free water losses, as with insensible losses due to a large burn wound.

If the clinical picture of hypovolemic shock is unclear, it is helpful to place a central venous line or, preferably, a pulmonary artery catheter for hemodynamic monitoring. The characteristic hemodynamic profile of hypovolemic shock reflects low right- and left-sided filling pressures (low central venous pressure and low PCWP), decreased cardiac output, decreased $S\bar{v}O_2$, and increased systemic vascular resistance.

Treatment. Initial management of hypovolemic shock includes an assessment of the patient's airway and a determination of the adequacy of ventilation and oxygenation. Essentially all patients with severe shock and circulatory collapse will require tracheal intubation and mechanical ventilation. Patients with less severe symptoms and signs of shock may frequently be managed without the need for mechanical ventilation, as long as a patent airway is present that allows for adequate ventilation and oxygenation.

Once the airway and breathing have been addressed, an assessment of the patient's circulatory status must be performed. Direct pressure on bleeding external wounds may be applied to control obvious hemorrhage. Two large-bore intravenous lines should be established, and an initial fluid bolus should be administered. A decision must be made at this point regarding the rate and volume of fluid replacement, as well as the choice of fluid. Ordinarily, isotonic electrolyte solutions, such as Ringer's lactate solution, are infused in the initial stages of resuscitation. In severe shock with hypotension, an initial 1- to 2-liter bolus of fluid is rapidly infused. If hypotension persists after a 2-liter fluid challenge, ongoing volume losses are likely. If the clinical situation is compatible with hemorrhagic shock, and there is no response or a transient response to initial crystalloid administration, blood transfusion must be considered. Fully crossmatched blood is preferred, but type-specific or type O packed red blood cells may be necessary in life-threatening, exsanguinating hemorrhage. Immediate volume resuscitation may be detrimental in the face of uncontrolled, ongoing hemorrhage.[12] This seeming paradox to conventional surgical wisdom is based on the concerns that aggressive fluid resuscitation before surgical control of hemorrhage may lead to disruption of thrombus, increased bleeding, and decreased survival.

The placement of a central venous line to monitor the central venous pressure or a pulmonary artery catheter for more extensive hemodynamic monitoring may be necessary, as previously discussed, to guide fluid replacement, optimize oxygen delivery, and ensure the adequacy of resuscitation. In the absence of central venous pressure or pulmonary artery catheter monitoring, initial end-points for volume resuscitation include the reestablishment of urinary output to a rate of 0.5 to 1.0 ml. per kg. per hour, a normal heart rate and blood pressure, adequate capillary refill, and normal sensorium.

Continuing fluid replenishment should extend beyond the initial resuscitative phase. After hemorrhagic shock there is an initial extracellular fluid volume contraction that lasts about 1 day. The importance of restoring extracellular fluid volume during this period was demonstrated by Shires and others,[62] who showed that a reduction in mortality could be achieved in hemorrhagic shock by adding crystalloid or nonblood colloid solutions to blood replacement. The volume of sequestered fluid is related to the severity of trauma and the degree of tissue damage. Failure to accommodate this obligatory extravascular fluid sequestration by restricting fluids or administering diuretics results in an exacerbation of the shock state, metabolic acidosis, multiple organ dysfunction, and death. After the sequestration phase, the diuretic phase begins, in which the sequestered extravascular fluid is mobilized and diuresed to restore the body fluid compartments to their normal, preinjury levels.

Adjunctive Measures. The pneumatic antishock garment (PASG) is an inflatable suit composed of an abdominal and two lower extremity compartments. The three compartments, which may be inflated independently, compress blood vessels, thereby increasing systemic vascular resistance. Initially it was thought that the PASG provided an autotransfusion effect by increasing venous blood return to the heart, but it is now recognized that it acts primarily to increase the resistance in both arterial and venous channels. Application of this device, therefore, increases the possibility of further decreasing peripheral perfusion and potentiating ischemia and the shock syndrome. Contraindications to the use of the PASG include cardiogenic shock, diaphragmatic rupture, significant chest injury, and pregnancy. Enhanced survival has not been demonstrated with use of the PASG in hypovolemic shock, and the potential detrimental effects of its use and misuse generally preclude its use in the hospital care of the shock victim. Nevertheless, the PASG may be useful in the prehospital setting, particularly to stabilize pelvic fractures and to tamponade bleeding arising from such injuries.

Controversy exists regarding the use of colloid solutions, hypertonic saline solutions, or a combination of colloid and hypertonic saline solutions in the treatment of hypovolemic shock.[53] Theoretical advantages of colloid solutions, such as albumin, fresh frozen plasma, dextran, and hetastarch, or of hypertonic saline solutions, such as 3% NaCl or 7.5% NaCl, are that they restore plasma volume quicker and with less volume requirement than isotonic crystalloid solutions. Whereas the administration of isotonic crystalloids causes a large increase in interstitial fluid volume, as well as the restoration of intravascular volume, the infusion of colloid or hypertonic saline solutions causes a quick expansion of the intravascular compartment. Thus, less volume of colloid or hypertonic saline is required to restore baseline hemodynamic parameters. The use of these solutions may therefore be especially beneficial in the prehospital care and resuscitation of the injured patient. A prospective, multicenter trial demonstrated that the prehospital use of a hypertonic saline/dextran solution is as effective as standard isotonic resuscitation fluids for posttraumatic hypotension.[91] Another purported advantage of using colloid solutions is that there might be a reduction in interstitial pulmonary edema. Unfortunately, this perceived benefit has not been observed in laboratory or clinical studies. Because of the lack of definitive evidence showing that colloid resuscitation is better than crystalloid resuscitation in terms of patient benefit or outcome, and because of the greatly increased cost of colloid solutions, the use of colloid solutions in the resuscitation of patients with hypovolemic shock cannot be recommended for routine use at this time. The use of hypertonic saline or of hypertonic saline/colloid solutions requires further study to resolve this controversy.[44]

The use of blood substitutes in the treatment of acute blood loss is being investigated. Both the perfluorocarbon-based solutions and various stroma-free hemoglobin solutions are undergoing clinical trials and are currently restricted to investigative protocols.

Traumatic Shock. Traumatic shock is a type of vasogenic shock that begins as hypovolemic shock. In contrast to simple hypovolemic shock, traumatic shock is associated with larger volume losses, greater fluid sequestration in the extravascular compartments, more intense activation of inflammatory mediators, and development of SIRS. This form of shock, which may develop, for example, with large burns or devastating soft tissue injuries, is particularly refractory to fluid replacement therapy. Microcirculatory derangements are common, leading to increased microvascular permeability and excessive fluid requirements. Patients with this type of shock frequently require mechanical ventilation, pulmonary artery catheter monitoring, and cardiovascular support with inotropic agents such as dobutamine or dopamine. Despite aggressive resuscitation efforts, multiple organ dysfunction is frequently observed.

Cardiogenic Shock. Cardiogenic shock occurs when the heart fails to generate an adequate cardiac output to maintain tissue perfusion. This type of shock, whether due to intrinsic or extrinsic causes (Table 5–5), may be regarded as pump failure. Intrinsic causes of cardiogenic shock include myocardial dysfunction secondary to ischemic heart disease, arrhythmias, myocarditis, cardiomyopathy, metabolic abnormalities, cardiodepressant drugs or toxins, or valvular dysfunction. Extrinsic causes of cardiogenic shock may be either obstructive or compressive. Obstructive causes produce mechanical or functional obstruction that results in increased left ventricular or right ventricular afterload. Coarctation of the aorta and malignant hypertension are examples of obstructive causes of increased left ventricular afterload, whereas pulmonary embolism and various other causes of pulmonary hypertension lead to increased right ventricular afterload and right ventricular failure. Compressive cardiogenic shock encompasses those disease processes that cause an increase in external pressure on the heart. Pericardial

TABLE 5–5. Causes of Cardiogenic Shock

Intrinsic Causes

Myocardial infarction
Myocardial ischemia
Myocardial contusion
Myocardial depression—due to drugs, toxins, etc.
Metabolic abnormalities—acidosis, hypocalcemia, hypophosphatemia
Cardiomyopathy—hypertrophic, restrictive
Myocarditis
Aortic valve dysfunction—stenosis, insufficiency
Mitral valve dysfunction—stenosis, insufficiency, papillary muscle dysfunction
Arrhythmias

Extrinsic Causes

Obstructive—increased left or right ventricular afterload
  Coarctation of aorta
  Malignant hypertension
  Pulmonary embolism
  Pulmonary hypertension—primary, or due to hypoxic vasoconstriction, pulmonary fibrosis, adult respiratory distress syndrome, chronic obstructive pulmonary disease, thromboembolic disease, hypoventilation syndromes, restrictive lung diseases
Compressive
  Pericardial tamponade
  Constrictive pericarditis
  Tension pneumothorax
  Massive hydrothorax
  Positive-pressure ventilation
  Large mediastinal hematoma
  Diaphragmatic hernia

tamponade, restrictive pericarditis, tension pneumothorax or massive hydrothorax, positive-pressure ventilation, and diaphragmatic hernia are all included in this category. The physiologic effects of increased compressive forces on the heart are to impair diastolic filling, reduce cardiac compliance, and reduce cardiac output.

Diagnosis of Cardiogenic Shock. The appearance of the patient in cardiogenic shock is similar to that of the patient in hypovolemic shock, in that signs of adrenergic stimulation and of peripheral and end-organ hypoperfusion are present. Thus, the patient may appear anxious, tachycardic, and tachypneic, with cool, clammy, mottled skin and oliguria. In addition, there may be signs of increased preload, such as distended neck veins, the presence of an S_3 heart sound, pulmonary rales, and peripheral edema. Prior history of cardiovascular disease may be useful in establishing the diagnosis.

Laboratory data, particularly arterial blood gases, serum electrolytes, and cardiac enzymes may be useful in the diagnosis and management of cardiogenic shock. A chest radiograph and electrocardiogram should be obtained in all cases of suspected cardiogenic shock to identify acute, as well as chronic, disease. An echocardiogram can provide valuable information about cardiac function, as well as about any structural abnormalities of the heart. If pulmonary embolism is considered, a ventilation-perfusion scan or pulmonary angiogram should be obtained.

Invasive monitoring using a pulmonary artery catheter is frequently required to optimize cardiac function and oxygen delivery in cases of cardiogenic shock. Typical hemodynamic findings in cardiogenic shock include a low cardiac output (< 2.2 liters per minute per square meter), an elevated systemic vascular resistance, and elevated filling pressures.

The diagnosis of compressive cardiogenic shock must be entertained in any patient with a history of trauma who presents with hypotension. The diagnosis may be difficult, but the distinction between cardiogenic and hypovolemic shock is critical, because the management of the two shock states is different. Patients with *tension pneumothorax* may present with profound hypotension, absence of breath sounds on the affected side, hyperresonance to percussion on the affected side, distended neck veins, and a trachea deviated to the opposite side. The development of tension pneumothorax may be rapid and dramatic, especially in patients who have sustained chest trauma or who are on positive-pressure ventilation. In such instances, with cardiovascular collapse, immediate treatment by decompression of the pleural space may be lifesaving and should be carried out without obtaining a confirmatory chest radiograph. *Pericardial tamponade* may be seen after trauma, particularly after penetrating wounds to the heart, but it may also be seen with pericardial effusions due to renal failure or malignant processes. The findings of Beck's triad, consisting of hypotension, distended neck veins, and muffled heart sounds, and of pulsus paradoxus, in which the systolic pressure falls by more than 10 mm. Hg with inspiration, may be helpful in diagnosing pericardial tamponade, but the absence of these findings does not exclude the diagnosis. Echocardiography is very sensitive in detecting pericardial effusions, and this modality is frequently employed in the evaluation of parasternal or mediastinal penetrating trauma.

Treatment of Compressive Cardiogenic Shock. Tension pneumothorax should be treated as soon as the condition is diagnosed or suspected. Immediate treatment consists of inserting a 14- or 16-gauge needle into the chest on the affected side at the level of the second or third intercostal space in the midclavicular line. This maneuver effectively releases the pressure in the chest and restores hemodynamic stability. Definitive therapy requires the placement of a thoracostomy tube, usually under less urgent circumstances, to treat the simple pneumothorax.

Patients in shock due to pericardial tamponade may initially respond to the administration of intravenous fluids to increase preload. Pericardiocentesis should be performed in patients suspected of having a pericardial effusion who fail to respond or transiently respond to initial measures. Patients with pericardial effusion and chest trauma require either pericardiocentesis or subxiphoid pericardiotomy to diagnose the presence of blood in the pericardial sac. The finding of a bloody effusion, with an appropriate history of chest trauma, mandates cardiac exploration to identify and repair a myocardial injury.

Treatment of Noncompressive Cardiogenic Shock. Principles of management of cardiogenic shock, like other forms of shock, are to optimize cardiovascular function, improve oxygen delivery, and restore tissue perfusion. To achieve these goals, manipulation of preload, afterload, and cardiac contractility is necessary, as is the optimization of the myocardial oxygen supply-to-demand ratio. Supplemental oxygen should be administered and mechanical ventilation instituted, if indicated. Initial hemodynamic interventions should be aimed at correcting arrhythmias and optimizing preload. Most patients in cardiogenic shock have higher than normal filling pressures, with the PCWP greater than 15 mm. Hg. Patients with a noncompliant left ventricle, however, may require high filling pressures with the PCWP in the range of 18 to 20 mm. Hg. Ordinarily, if the plasma colloid oncotic pressure is normal, pulmonary edema will not develop until the PCWP exceeds 20 mm. Hg. Therefore, a reasonable initial goal is to manipulate the preload until PCWP is between 15 and 18 mm. Hg. This may be accomplished with fluid administration to increase preload or with pharmacologic intervention to decrease preload. Both morphine and furosemide have venodilating effects that serve to reduce preload, in addition to their respective analgesic and diuretic effects. The use of these agents, and of other venodilator drugs such as the nitrates, must be used cautiously, if at all, in the presence of hypotension, which may be exacerbated. In such instances, an inotropic agent may be the first drug of choice.

The sympathomimetic inotropic agents commonly used include dopamine, dobutamine, and epinephrine. The choice of which agent to use depends on the patient's hemodynamic parameters. In moderate doses of 5 to 10 µg. per kg. per minute, dopamine acts primarily to stimulate beta$_1$-adrenergic receptors, resulting in positive inotropic and chronotropic effects. Left ventricular wall stress may also be increased with the use of dopamine; therefore, myocardial oxygen consumption and myocardial ischemia may be exacerbated with its use. Dobutamine, in addition to its inotropic properties, produces arterial vasodilation, which may limit its use in hypotensive states and decreases ventricular filling pressures. Dobutamine generally produces less tachycardia than other adrenergic agents. When both afterload reduction and inotropic support are desirable, dobutamine is frequently the drug of choice. Epinephrine stimulates beta$_1$-, beta$_2$-, and alpha-adrenergic receptors, although the alpha effects predominate at higher doses. Like dopamine, epinephrine may induce myocardial ischemia because of the increased cardiac work that occurs from its use.

Amrinone and milrinone are inotropic and vasodilating agents that inhibit phosphodiesterase, thereby increasing the cellular availability of cyclic adenosine monophosphate. The net hemodynamic results observed with the use of these agents are similar to those of dobutamine, in that there is an increase in cardiac output, a decrease in filling pressures, and a decrease in systemic vascular resistance.

Vasodilators to reduce afterload in patients with cardiogenic shock may be useful in patients with evidence of elevated filling pressures, low cardiac output, elevated systemic vascular resistance, and normal or raised blood pressure. By reducing myocardial wall tension and improving the myocardial oxygen supply-to-demand ratio, afterload-reducing agents may cause improvement in cardiac output. Nitroprusside and nitroglycerin are the two vasodilating drugs most commonly used in this scenario and require careful monitoring of the patient's hemodynamic response.

If pharmacologic manipulations of preload, afterload, and contractility fail to improve cardiac function, the use of the intra-aortic balloon pump (IABP) may be considered. This device, positioned in the descending thoracic aorta, inflates during diastole and deflates before systole. The effects of the IABP (Fig. 5–15) are (1) to provide diastolic augmentation, hence increased coronary artery perfusion; (2) to reduce left ventricular afterload; and (3) to reduce myocardial oxygen consumption. The IABP is particularly useful in postcardiotomy patients with low cardiac output, in patients with acute myocardial infarction complicated by mitral insufficiency or ventricular septal defect, and in patients who are considered candidates for surgical revascularization or angioplasty procedures. Other mechanical cardiac assist devices are being evaluated or developed for temporary support, as a bridge to transplantation, or for permanent implantation.

Thrombolytic therapy with tissue plasminogen activating factor or streptokinase has shown to be beneficial in acute myocardial infarction if therapy is instituted within 6 hours of onset of symptoms.[48] Emergency coronary angioplasty, however, has had a greater impact on survival rate in myocardial infarction complicated by cardiogenic shock. Gacioch and colleagues showed that the 30-day survival rates in patients with failed angioplasty, no attempt at angioplasty, and successful angioplasty were 7%, 14%, and 61%, respectively.[41] This difference was maintained over a 12-month fol-

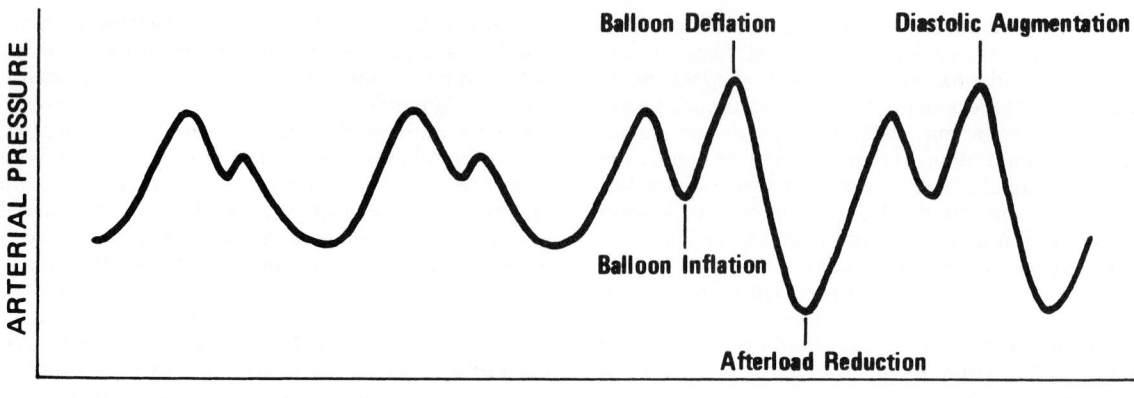

Figure 5–15. Arterial pressure tracing showing the effect of an intra-aortic balloon pump. Diastolic inflation of the balloon results in diastolic augmentation of pressure, and balloon deflation just before the onset of systole leads to afterload reduction. (Reprinted with permission from Mouchawar, A., and Rosenthal, M.: A pathophysiological approach to the patient in shock. Int. Anesthesiol. Clin., *31*:1, 1993.)

low-up period. Thus, early restoration of coronary blood flow is critical for successful outcomes.

Neurogenic Shock. Neurogenic shock occurs when sympathetic denervation produces an impairment in vasomotor tone. Severe head injury, spinal cord injury, or pharmacologic sympathetic blockade, as with high spinal anesthesia, all may cause neurogenic shock. Loss of vasomotor tone in both the arteriolar and venous systems leads to a decrease in systemic vascular resistance, a large increase in venous capacitance, a decrease in venous return to the heart, and a decrease in cardiac output. Hypotension and bradycardia are included in the classic description of neurogenic shock, but tachycardia is frequently observed. In contrast to cardiogenic or hypovolemic shock, the patient's extremities are warm and dry. In traumatic injuries to the spinal cord, an initial systemic sympathetic response may be seen, followed in several minutes by the findings of neurogenic shock. However, even with complete cord injuries, the classic presentation of neurogenic shock is not commonly observed. Hypovolemia from associated injuries must always be considered when hypotension is present after trauma.

The mainstay of treatment of neurogenic shock is to improve cardiac filling by intravenous volume administration. Several liters of fluid may be required to achieve adequate venous return because of the greatly expanded intravascular volume. Placement of the patient in the Trendelenburg position may assist in increasing venous return to the heart. The use of alpha-adrenergic agonist agents such as phenylephrine is rarely indicated if restoration of an effective intravascular volume has been carried out.

Anaphylactic and Anaphylactoid Shock. Anaphylaxis is an allergic response mediated by IgE antibody. Antigens associated with anaphylaxis include insect venom, drugs, and certain foods. Anaphylactoid reactions are not immunologically mediated. Examples of substances producing anaphylactoid responses include intravenous radiographic contrast dyes, narcotics in high doses, and various colloids, such as the dextrans and hydroxyethyl starch. The symptoms of both anaphylactic and anaphylactoid reactions are similar and are due to the activation and release of inflammatory mediators, such as the anaphylatoxins C3a and C5a, histamine, kinins, prostaglandins, and others. The profound release of these mediators leads to vasodilatation, increased capillary permeability, bronchospasm, airway edema, and circulatory collapse secondary to a sudden decrease in systemic vascular resistance and a fall in cardiac output. Initial management consists of ensuring an adequate airway, providing supplemental oxygen, and administering epinephrine. For mild to moderate reactions, 0.3 to 0.5 ml. of epinephrine in a 1:1000 dilution is administered subcutaneously. This dose may be repeated in 10 to 20 minutes. For more severe reactions resulting in hypotension, intravenous fluids, as well as intravenous epinephrine, should be given. Epinephrine may be administered as a continuous infusion at a rate of 0.5 to 5 μg. per minute or as a bolus of 0.1 to 0.2 ml. of a 1:1000 solution in 10 ml. of saline. Bronchospasm may further be treated initially by inhaled nebulized solutions of metaproterenol or albuterol. Secondary therapy may include the use of aminophylline (5–6 mg. per kg. load, followed by 0.3–0.9 mg. per kg. per hour maintenance intravenous), corticosteroids (250 mg. hydrocortisone intravenous every 6 hours), and antihistamines (25–50 mg. hydroxyzine or diphenhydramine intramuscular, and 300 mg. cimetidine intravenous). Persistent hypotension may be more responsive to a continuous infusion of norepinephrine because of its increased alpha-adrenergic activity.

Hypoadrenal Shock. Shock due to adrenocortical insufficiency is a relatively uncommon form of shock but should be considered in patients who have a history of glucocorticoid therapy or in patients with no previous history of adrenocortical insufficiency who develop severe shock refractory to volume and pressor resuscitation. Especially in this latter group, a high index of suspicion must be maintained to make the diagnosis. Patients with high metabolic stress due to trauma, operation, or serious medical illness may not exhibit symptoms of adrenocortical insufficiency in the unstressed state; thus, a relative glucocorticoid deficiency may manifest itself only under conditions of severe stress. Clinical features of acute adrenocortical insufficiency may be similar, but more severe, than those of Addison's disease; however, the absence of such features, such as hyperpigmentation, weight loss, and gastrointestinal symptoms does not exclude the diagnosis. Hypoglycemia in a hypotensive patient may suggest the diagnosis, which may be supported by the findings of hyponatremia and hyperkalemia.

The diagnosis should be established by performance of the rapid ACTH stimulation test, but institution of corticosteroid therapy should not be delayed in unstable patients while waiting for the laboratory results. Baseline serum cortisol levels should be drawn before and 30 and 60 minutes after the intravenous administration of 250 μg. of synthetic ACTH (cosyntropin). The test may be performed at any time of day. Interpretation of a positive test is somewhat controversial, but the demonstration of a peak cortisol level greater than 20 μg. per 100 ml. has been proposed as a sufficient single criterion for normal adrenal function.[60] A peak cortisol level less than 20 μg. per 100 ml. suggests abnormal adrenal function.

Treatment of acute adrenocortical insufficiency includes the administration of *stress* doses of corticosteroids and hydration with glucose-containing saline solutions. Dexamethasone, 4 mg. given intravenously will not interfere with the cortisol assay and should be given to hemodynamically unstable patients in whom the diagnosis is suspected. Because dexamethasone does not have mineralocorticoid activity, hydrocortisone, 100 mg. intravenously every 6 hours, should be substituted once the rapid ACTH stimulation test is concluded.

Shock Associated with SIRS, Sepsis, and Multiple Organ Dysfunction. Multiple organ failure is the most common cause of death in intensive care units. In the 1970s and early 1980s, it was generally believed that progressive organ failure was causally related to the presence of uncontrolled infection, usually in the abdomen or chest. More recently, it has become increasingly clear that noninfectious insults, such as trauma, pancreatitis, burns, and massive transfusions, may produce a syndrome of multiple organ dysfunction that is clinically indistinguishable from that due to culture-proven infectious causes.[16] Recognition that numerous distinct entities, both infectious and noninfectious, may lead to the same clinical syndrome suggests that common mediators may be involved in the systemic inflammatory response. This syndrome has been termed the *sepsis syndrome* or *septic syndrome*, but confounding definitions of this entity, as well as of *sepsis, septicemia, septic shock,* and so on led to a reappraisal of this issue in 1992 by members of the American College of Chest Physicians/Society of Critical Care Medicine Consensus Conference Committee. Their proposal to standardize the terminology in a precise manner included the following definitions, which are adhered to here[2]:

Systemic inflammatory response syndrome (SIRS): The systemic inflammatory response to a variety of severe clinical insults. SIRS is characterized by two or more of the following: (1) temperature greater than 38° C. (100.4° F.) or less than 36° C. (96.8° F.); (2) heart rate greater than 90 beats per minute; (3) respiratory rate greater than 20 breaths per minute or $PaCO_2$ less than 32 mm. Hg; and (4) white blood cell count greater than 12,000 per cu. mm., less than 4000 per cu. mm., or greater than 10% band forms.

Sepsis: The presence of SIRS in association with culture-proven infection

Septic shock: Sepsis with hypotension despite adequate fluid resuscitation, along with the presence of manifestations of hypoperfusion, including, but not limited to, lactic acidosis, oliguria, or an acute alteration in mental status

Multiple organ dysfunction syndrome (MODS): The presence of altered organ function in an acutely ill patient such that homeostasis cannot be maintained without intervention

Whereas these definitions admittedly have their limitations, they are nonetheless very useful in providing a framework of standardized terminology that can be expanded as our understanding of these disorders becomes elucidated through advances in clinical and basic research. Moreover, these definitions conceptually imply that there is a clinically recognizable pathophysiologic progression from SIRS to sepsis to shock and, ultimately, to MODS. A prospective epidemiologic study of the natural history of SIRS and related conditions provides evidence to strengthen the theory that there exists a potential continuum of increasing clinical severity in patients who have manifestations of a systemic inflammatory response to infectious or noninfectious insults.[74] In that study, 26% of patients with SIRS developed sepsis and 4% developed septic shock. The mortality rates were found to increase from 7% for SIRS to 16% for sepsis and to 46% for septic shock. A similar progression from SIRS to shock, as well as a corresponding increase in mortality, was observed in a group of patients who did not have culture-proven microbiologic infection.

Appreciation of the clinical continuum that ranges from SIRS to MODS serves several purposes. First, earlier recognition of organ *dysfunction* may allow earlier therapeutic interventions to be instituted before frank organ *failure* becomes evident. Despite improvements in critical care and in the understanding of the pathogenesis of multiple organ failure, the mortality rate, once organs have failed, has not significantly improved over the past two decades. Depending on the number of organs that have failed, the mortality ranges from 20% to 100%.[56] It is likely that only with earlier intervention to attempt to halt the progression of MODS will a significant impact on outcome be possible. To recognize organ dysfunction at an earlier stage, however, it becomes necessary to modify existing arbitrary criteria of individual organ failure to reflect the dynamic continuum of organ dysfunction. Thus, various organ scoring systems have appeared in the literature that enable one to grade the severity of individual organ dysfunction based on clinical parameters.[30, 68] Second, a widespread understanding that a multitude of noninfectious, as well as infectious, insults may predispose a host to the development of SIRS, sepsis, and eventually MODS may provide an incentive to stimulate further advances in prehospital care, initial hospital care aimed at expeditious resuscitation, and critical care medicine. Perhaps because of recent advances in these areas, the syndrome of progressive organ dysfunction has become increasingly recognized[22] in intensive care units since its first description in 1973 by Tilney,[83] and its incidence will probably continue to rise. Third, the ability to classify patients in a standardized fashion facilitates the identification of patients for inclusion in clinical research protocols and, in conjunction with various *severity of illness* scoring systems, may aid in risk stratification for predicting the development of MODS and for predicting clinical outcome.

MODS may be either primary or secondary.[2] Primary MODS arises early as the direct result of a distinct insult to the host. Pulmonary contusion due to thoracic trauma and renal insufficiency due to rhabdomyolysis are examples of primary organ dysfunction. Primary MODS may also develop from the sequelae of hypovolemic shock, which leads to organ dysfunction by the mechanisms of ischemic injury and reperfusion injury previously described. Even though these mechanisms involve activation of the host stress response, the response is *normal,* not exaggerated, and the organ dysfunction that occurs can be attributed to the initial inciting event. Once the host inflammatory response has been primed, even a relatively minor second insult can reactivate the process in a more amplified form. This has been termed a *two-hit* model to produce secondary MODS (Fig. 5–16).[64] Secondary MODS, then, occurs from a persistently exaggerated and uncontrolled systemic inflammatory response that involves organs remote from the initial insult. It thus represents a late stage in the evolution of SIRS characterized by a self-perpetuating, autodestructive inflammatory response. Unless the accentuated inflammatory response *and* the cause of the persistent activation of inflammatory mediators can be tempered, the vicious cycle cannot be broken.

Clinical Features. Patients in shock associated with sepsis or SIRS frequently have a characteristic clinical picture consisting of fever, tachycardia, hypotension, oliguria, and altered mental status. The hemodynamic profile may vary, depending where on the continuum of illness severity a particular patient fits. In the early stages, a hyperdynamic profile exists, manifested by elevated cardiac index and a decreased systemic vascular resistance. The intravascular vol-

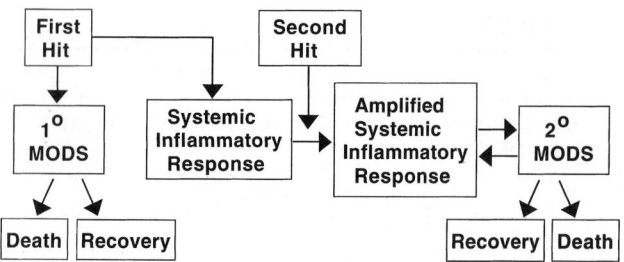

Figure 5–16. The *two-hit* theory of the development of the multiple organ dysfunction syndrome (MODS). An initial insult may directly lead to the development of primary MODS, as well as the priming of inflammatory cells and mediators. A second hit, or insult, then leads to an exaggerated inflammatory response and the subsequent development of secondary MODS.

ume is expanded, and vasodilatation occurs in peripheral arterial and venous capacitance vessels, while the splanchnic circulation may remain underperfused. As with neurogenic shock, the patient's extremities feel warm to touch. Along with the hyperdynamic cardiovascular profile, hypermetabolism is typically seen,[23] reflected by increases in resting energy expenditure, gluconeogenesis, catabolism, and oxygen consumption. In contrast, during the late, or preterminal, stage of shock associated with sepsis or SIRS, a hypodynamic response is sometimes seen. The hypodynamic response, which is associated with a high morbidity and mortality, is indicative of a decompensated circulatory state, characterized by an inappropriately low cardiac index, tachycardia, fever or hypothermia, hypotension, oliguria, leukocytosis or leukopenia, increased or decreased systemic vascular resistance, and deterioration of mental status to obtundation or coma. Patients with preexisting cardiovascular dysfunction are more prone to developing a hypodynamic response.

Patients in septic shock, by definition, have positive microbial cultures. Most commonly, gram-negative bacteria, such as *Escherichia coli, Klebsiella, Pseudomonas,* and *Bacteroides,* are isolated from patients with this clinical syndrome, but *Staphylococcus* and *Streptococcus* species may also be found. Less commonly, fungal, viral, and protozoal infections may cause septic shock, although the clinical presentation may be indistinguishable from that due to bacterial causes of septic shock. In adults, septic shock is most frequently associated with pneumonia, gastrointestinal perforation, biliary tract infection, urinary tract infection, burn wounds, and line sepsis from indwelling intravascular catheters.

MODS—The Clinical Syndrome. The continuum of illness severity that encompasses MODS spans a wide range of clinical presentations. Organ dysfunction, as opposed to organ failure, is not an *all-or-none* phenomenon. Gradations of organ dysfunction, therefore, are sometimes used to identify MODS and to provide a relative severity score (Table 5–6). Unfortunately, such scoring systems based on commonly measured laboratory or physiologic parameters are not sensitive enough to detect organ hypoperfusion and organ dysfunction at the very earliest stages when there is probably the greatest chance to make potentially beneficial therapeutic interventions. As our understanding of MODS improves, so will our ability to describe organ dysfunction at an earlier point on the continuum. The development of MODS, and its subsequent clinical course in a given patient, depends on a number of factors, including the presence of pre-existing disease or advanced age, the nature and intensity of the inciting event and of the *second hit,* and the presence of sepsis. The number of organs involved continues to be a prognostic indicator of mortality,[8] as is the existence of particular combinations of dysfunctional organs (e.g., liver and lung). Sequential organ failure is the classic description that

characterizes this syndrome. Pulmonary failure, followed by hepatic, gastrointestinal, and renal failure predictably occurs in that order, unless preexisting organ dysfunction is present. With the current emphasis on organ dysfunction, rather than failure, this sequence may no longer be applicable when describing the evolution of MODS.[8] Pulmonary dysfunction, however, still appears at an early stage of MODS. The acute lung injury in MODS reflects the pathophysiologic pulmonary manifestations of a systemic inflammatory process. Recruitment of leukocytes into the pulmonary vascular bed occurs early. A complex interaction of activated neutrophils, macrophages, platelets, endothelial cells, and inflammatory mediators ensues, resulting in pulmonary capillary endothelial injury.[87] The increase in microvascular permeability leads to interstitial edema. Alveolar injury occurs secondary to ischemia and the activation of inflammatory mediators, causing progressive alveolar edema, loss of surfactant, and alveolar collapse. The clinical consequence of these changes is the development of ARDS. ARDS is characterized by ventilation–perfusion abnormalities, noncardiogenic pulmonary edema, decreased functional residual capacity, refractory hypoxemia, diffuse infiltrates on chest x-rays, and decreased lung compliance. Treatment is largely supportive, including the use of mechanical ventilation. The mortality for ARDS exceeds 50%, but progression of MODS, rather than hypoxemia, accounts for the majority of fatalities.[66]

Gastrointestinal dysfunction in MODS may include gastritis or ulcerations, ileus, pancreatitis, acalculous cholecystitis, malabsorption, and mucosal atrophy. Breakdown of the gut mucosal barrier predisposes to the translocation of bacteria or toxins that can perpetuate the inflammatory process. In addition, endogenous enteric flora may be the source of microbial infections complicating SIRS or MODS.[59]

The liver appears to play a pivotal role in the progression and outcome of MODS. The vital metabolic functions of the liver, as well as the host defense functions of the Kupffer cells, are key processes, that, when perturbed, contribute to the high morbidity and mortality associated with MODS when severe hepatic dysfunction exists. In the early stages of MODS, gluconeogenesis is stimulated, as is acute-phase protein synthesis. Protein catabolism and increased amino acid load to the liver contribute to the hypermetabolic state. With progressive hepatic dysfunction, the synthetic and metabolic roles of the liver deteriorate, causing substantial increases in the plasma levels of glucose, triglycerides, amino acids, bilirubin, urea, and lactate. The importance of the macrophage in the elaboration of inflammatory mediators and in the development of MODS should be underscored.[17] The Kupffer cells residing in the liver constitute about 70% of the total body macrophage population. As part of the hepatic reticuloendothelial system, the Kupffer cells are responsible for detoxifying the blood of circulating bacteria and toxins that may be present in larger amounts in MODS due to gut dysfunction or other sources of infection. Prolonged stimulation or activation of the Kupffer cells is thought to be a critical factor in the continued and uncontrolled release of inflammatory mediators that contribute to the pathogenesis of MODS. Activated Kupffer cells are also believed to have an integral interactive role with hepatocytes, as demonstrated by their ability to modulate hepatic protein synthesis.[55]

Renal dysfunction in MODS may arise due to tissue hypoperfusion or direct tissue damage by activated inflammatory cells and their mediators.[78] Vasoconstrictive mechanisms, including increased levels of circulating catecholamines, activation of the renin-angiotensin system, and reduced synthesis of vasodilating prostaglandins, lead to a reduction in renal blood flow and in glomerular filtration rate. Additionally, redistribution of blood flow preferentially affects the outer cortex, causing cortical ischemia at an early stage. In hyper-

TABLE 5–6. Organ Dysfunction Score

Organ	Grade 1	Grade 2	Grade 3
A. Kidneys	Creatinine >1.8 mg./100 ml.	Creatinine >2.5 mg./100 ml.	Creatinine >5.0 mg./100 ml.
B. Liver*	Bilirubin >2.0 mg./100 ml.	Bilirubin >4.0 mg./100 ml.	Bilirubin >8.0 mg./100 ml.
C. Heart†	Minimal inotropes	Moderate inotropes	High inotropes
D. Lungs‡	ARDS score >5	ARDS score >9	ARDS score >13

Organ dysfunction score = A + B + C + D not due to chronic diseases.
*Not due to biliary obstruction or resolving hematoma.
†Cardiac index <2.2 L./min./M.^{2} requiring inotropic support:
   Minimal dose = dopamine or dobutamine <5 μg./kg./min.
   Moderate dose = dopamine or dobutamine 5–15 μg./kg./min.
   High dose = dopamine or dobutamine >15 μg./kg./min.
‡Adult respiratory distress syndrome (ARDS) score = a + b + c + d + e when pulmonary capillary wedge pressure ≤18 cm. H_2O or when there is no clinical reason to suspect hydrostatic pulmonary edema:

Variable	Grade 1	Grade 2	Grade 3	Grade 4
a. Pulmonary/radiographic	Diffuse, mild interstitial marking/opacities	Diffuse, marked interstitial/mild air-space opacities	Diffuse, moderate air-space consolidation	Diffuse, severe air-space consolidation
b. Pao_2/Fio_2 (mm. Hg.)	175–250	125–174	80–124	<80
c. Minute ventilation (L./min.)	11–13	14–16	17–20	>20
d. Positive end-expiratory pressure (cm. H_2O)	6–9	10–13	14–17	>17
e. Static compliance (ml./cm. H_2O)	40–50	30–39	20–29	<20

Adapted from Moore, F. A., and Moore, E. E.: Evolving concepts in the pathogenesis of postinjury multiple organ failure. Surg. Clin. North Am., 75: 257, 1995.

dynamic states, as occurs with shock associated with sepsis or SIRS, redistribution of blood flow or inadequate perfusion pressure may contribute to renal dysfunction. Aggressive resuscitative measures, avoidance of nephrotoxic drugs, and control of inflammatory foci at other sites may help prevent the progression of renal dysfunction, but the development of renal failure with its associated problems of uremia and electrolyte disturbances may require dialysis.

The etiology of cardiac dysfunction remains controversial in the setting of MODS. Preexisting cardiovascular disease predisposes the patient to more severe cardiac dysfunction during the course of MODS. In other cases, however, the cause of the observed increases in ventricular volumes and decreased ejection fractions is not as clear. Depressed coronary blood flow, direct endotoxin toxicity, and the presence of a circulating myocardial depressant factor have all been proposed as possible mechanisms. Coronary blood flow during septic shock was found by Cunnion and colleagues to be normal or increased, and the level of lactate extraction by the myocardium from the coronary circulation was similar in septic patients with or without myocardial depression.[27] Thus, global myocardial ischemia seems unlikely to account for the myocardial depression in septic shock. There is no evidence that endotoxin directly affects myocardial function; however, studies indicate that a circulating myocardial depressant factor may exist.[72] Although the exact identity of this substance has not been confirmed, tumor necrosis factor may be the elusive agent responsible for myocardial depression in sepsis or SIRS.[71]

Central nervous system manifestations of MODS may appear at variable times in the course of the syndrome. Because compensatory mechanisms in shock are aimed at preserving blood flow to the brain and heart, as previously discussed, central nervous system manifestations may appear late, unless a prolonged period of hypoxemia can be identified during the patient's clinical course. Mental status is frequently measured objectively using the Glasgow Coma Scale, which takes into account, on a graded scale, the patient's best eye opening, verbal, and motor responses.

Treatment. The best treatment for shock associated with sepsis or SIRS is preventing the progression to MODS. As with other forms of shock, aggressive resuscitation to establish optimal levels of oxygen delivery and oxygen consumption should be the goal. Evidence exists proving that increased survival may be seen in patients who can generate a hyperdynamic response early in the course of sepsis or SIRS.[39] Thus, attempts to improve oxygen delivery and oxygen consumption to achieve delivery-independent oxygen consumption seem warranted, at least in the early stages of SIRS or sepsis. Such therapy has not proven to be of benefit when MODS is fully developed.

As discussed and illustrated (see Fig. 5–14) previously, oxygen delivery can be optimized by using a rational combination of volume expansion, provision of red blood cell mass, and appropriate use of pharmacologic agents. Beta-agonists, vasodilators, and, occasionally, alpha-agonists may improve cardiac contractility, decrease afterload, and increase mean arterial or perfusion pressure, respectively. Appropriate monitoring must be employed that allows frequent evaluation of the patient's hemodynamic and other physiologic parameters. Invasive pulmonary artery catheters or other less invasive techniques should be routinely used, as outlined earlier, in patients with shock due to sepsis or SIRS because of the high (>50%) mortality seen with this syndrome as it progresses to MODS.

Patients with sepsis or presumed sepsis should be started on broad-spectrum antibiotics, which should be changed to narrower-spectrum agents once culture results are confirmed. Indiscriminate use of antibiotics should be avoided. Careful, thorough examination of the patient should be performed routinely to identify possible sources of infection. Examination may be supplemented by radiographic or laboratory studies, as indicated, to detect the presence of possible sources of infection. Surgical débridement and drainage may be required to remove devitalized tissue and eliminate foci of infection. Reduction of nosocomial infections, or second hits, through meticulous and attentive care to lines and catheters should be achieved. Selective decontamination of the gut using oral antibiotics is controversial but has been shown in some studies to reduce nosocomial pneumonia.[24] Improvement in mortality, however, has not been demonstrated with this technique. Similarly, the use of sucralfate, instead of H$_2$ blockers, as a prophylaxis against stress gastritis has been shown to decrease nosocomial pneumonia, particularly in mechanically ventilated patients, without an effect on mortality.[33]

Nutritional support should be addressed early in the care of the critically ill patient. Positive protein balance without the administration of excessive calories is the goal. Overfeeding of carbohydrate and fatty acid calories can lead to hyperglycemia, hepatic steatosis, and carbon dioxide retention, in the case of the former, and hypoxemia, bacteremia, and immune deficiencies in the case of the latter. The administration of 25 to 35 kcal. per kg. per day, including 1.5 to 2.0 gm. per kg. per day of protein, accomplishes most of the nutritional goals.

Enteral nutrition is the preferred route of alimentation for a number of reasons. Compared with total parenteral nutrition, enteral nutrition (1) is much more cost effective; (2) maintains the integrity of the gut and the villus architecture; (3) stimulates gallbladder contraction, reducing the likelihood of biliary complications; (4) reduces septic morbidity[67]; and (5) promotes less bacterial translocation from the gut.[3] In addition, newer enteral feeding formulas, including one that incorporates arginine, nucleotides, and omega-3 polyunsaturated fatty acids, may enhance immune function, reduce septic complications, and contribute to decreased length of hospital stay.[18]

Therapies for shock due to sepsis or SIRS and for MODS have been primarily directed at supporting organ function. With recent advances in the molecular understanding of the systemic inflammatory response, new approaches are being evaluated that aim to modulate the stress response by blocking the activation or action of key mediators or by enhancing immune function. Numerous agents have been tried, including corticosteroids,[15] nonsteroidal anti-inflammatory drugs,[75] various antioxidants, antiendotoxin antibodies,[86] IL-1 receptor antagonists,[37] monoclonal antibodies against tumor necrosis factor,[38] platelet activating factor receptor antagonists,[31] macrophage-specific immunomodulators,[7] and many others. Despite promising effects of many of these agents in experimental animal studies, the results of human clinical trials have not been as encouraging thus far. No clear-cut benefits have been unequivocally demonstrated from the use of antimediator therapy. Indeed, because of the complex interactions that occur between inflammatory cells and their mediators, single-agent therapy may not halt the uncontrolled inflammatory response seen in shock associated with sepsis, SIRS, and MODS. Further studies need to be carried out in carefully controlled, well-conducted, clinical protocols, as well as in research laboratories, before such therapies become available in the routine treatment—or prevention—of this shock syndrome.

REFERENCES

1. Abrams, J. H., Cerra, F., and Holcroft, S. W.: Cardiopulmonary monitoring. In Wilmore, D. W., Brennan, M. F., Harken, A. H., Holcroft, J. W., and Meakins, J. L. (Eds.): Care of the Surgical Patient. Vol. 1, Critical Care. A Publication of the Committee on Pre and Postoperative Care of the American College of Surgeons. New York, Scientific American, 1989.
2. ACCP/SCCM: American College of Chest Physicians/Society of Critical Care Medicine Consensus Conference: Definitions for sepsis and organ failure and guidelines for the use of innovative therapies in sepsis. Crit. Care Med., 20:864, 1992.
3. Alverdy, J. C., Aoys, E., and Moss, G. S.: Total parenteral nutrition promotes bacterial translocation from the gut. Surgery, 104:185, 1988.
4. Anstadt, M. P., Tedder, M., Stonnington, M. J., et al.: Thermodilution techniques erroneously predict flow alterations during cardiac failure. J. Am. Coll. Cardiol., 19:135A, 1992.
5. Antonsson, J. B., and Fiddian-Green, R. G.: The role of the gut in shock and multiple system organ failure. Eur. J. Surg., 157:3, 1991.

6. Astiz, M. E., Rackow, R. C., Falk, J. L., Kaufman, B. S., and Weil, M. H.: Oxygen delivery and consumption in patients with hyperdynamic septic shock. Crit. Care Med., 15:26, 1987.
7. Babineau, T. J., Marcello, P., Swails, W., et al.: Randomized phase I/II trial of a macrophage-specific immunomodulator (PGG-Glucan) in high-risk surgical patients. Ann. Surg., 220:601, 1994.
8. Barie, P. S., Hydo, L. J., and Fischer, E.: A prospective comparison of two multiple organ dysfunction/failure scoring systems for prediction of mortality in critical surgical illness. J. Trauma, 37:660, 1994.
9. Bast, A., Haenen, G. R. M. M., and Doelman, C. J. A.: Oxidants and antioxidants: State of the art. Am. J. Med., 91:S3C, 1991.
10. Baxley, W. A., Cavender, J. B., and Knoblock, B.: Continuous cardiac output monitoring by the Fick method. Cathet. Cardiovasc. Diagn., 28:89, 1993.
11. Beutler, B., and Cerami, A.: Cachectin: More than a tumor necrosis factor. N. Engl. J. Med., 316:379, 1987.
12. Bickell, W. H., Wall, M. J., Pepe, P. E., et al.: Immediate versus delayed fluid resuscitation for hypotensive patients with penetrating torso injuries. N. Engl. J. Med., 331:1105, 1994.
13. Blalock, A.: Experimental shock, the cause of the low blood pressure produced by muscle injury. Arch. Surg., 22:959, 1930.
14. Blalock, A.: Principles of Surgical Care, Shock, and Other Problems. St. Louis, C. V. Mosby, 1940.
15. Bone, R. C., Fisher, C. J., Jr., Clemmer, T. P., et al.: A controlled clinical trial of high-dose methylprednisolone in the treatment of severe sepsis and septic shock. N. Engl. J. Med., 317:653, 1987.
16. Bone, R. C., Fisher, C. J., Jr., Clemmer, T. P., et al.: Sepsis syndrome: A valid clinical entity. Crit. Care Med., 17:389, 1989.
17. Border, J. R.: Hypothesis: Sepsis, multiple systems organ failure, and the macrophage. Arch. Surg., 123:285, 1988.
18. Bower, R. H., Cerra, F. B., Bershadsky, B., et al.: Early enteral administration of a formula (Impact) supplemented with arginine, nucleotides, and fish oil in intensive care unit patients: Results of a multicenter, prospective, randomized, clinical trial. Crit. Care Med., 23:436, 1995.
19. Broder, G., and Weil, M. H.: Excess lactate: An index of reversibility of shock in human patients. Science, 143:1457, 1964.
20. Cain, S.M.: Oxygen delivery and uptake in dogs during anemic and hypoxic hypoxia. J. Appl. Physiol., 42:228, 1977.
21. Cannon, W. B., and Bayliss, W. M.: Notes on muscle injury in relation to shock: Special report of the Medical Research Commission, 26:19, 1919.
22. Carrico, C. J., Meakins, J. L., Marshall, J. C., Fry, B., and Maier, R. V.: Multiple-organ-failure syndrome. Arch. Surg., 121:196, 1986.
23. Cerra, F. B.: Hypermetabolism, organ failure, and metabolic support. Surgery, 101:1, 1987.
24. Cerra, F. B., Maddaus, M. A., Dunn, D. L., et al.: Selective gut decontamination reduces nosocomial infections and length of stay but not mortality or organ failure in surgical intensive care unit patients. Arch. Surg., 127:163, 1992.
25. Cournand, A., Riley, R. L., Bradley, S. E., et al.: Studies of the circulation in clinical shock. Surgery, 13:964, 1943.
26. Crile, G. W.: An Experimental Research into Surgical Shock. Philadelphia, J. B. Lippincott, 1899.
27. Cunnion, R. E., Schaer, G. L., Parker, M. M., et al.: The coronary circulation in human septic shock. Circulation, 73:637, 1986.
28. Dantzker, D. R., Foresman, B., and Gutierrez, G.: Oxygen supply and utilization relationships. Am. Rev. Respir. Dis., 143:675, 1991.
29. Deitch, E., Winterton, J., Li, M., and Berg, R.: The gut as a portal of entry for bacteremia. Ann. Surg., 205:681, 1987.
30. Demling, R., LaLonde, C., Saldinger, P., and Knox, J.: Multiple-organ dysfunction in the surgical patient: Pathophysiology, prevention, and treatment. Curr. Probl. Surg., 30:345, 1993.
31. Dhainaut, J. F. A., Tenaillon, A., Le Tulzo, Y., et al.: Platelet-activating factor receptor antagonist BN 52021 in the treatment of severe sepsis: A randomized, double-blind, placebo-controlled, multicenter clinical trial. Crit. Care Med., 22:1720, 1994.
32. Dinarello, C. A.: Interleukin-1 and the pathogenesis of the acute-phase response. N. Engl. J. Med., 311:1413, 1984.
33. Driks, M. R., Craven, D. E., Celli, B. R., et al.: Nosocomial pneumonia in intubated patients given sucralfate as compared with antacids or histamine type 2 blocker: The role of gastric colonization. N. Engl. J. Med., 317:1376, 1987.
34. Fakhry, S. M., and Rutledge, R.: Monitoring. In Moylan, J. A. (Ed.): Surgical Critical Care. St. Louis, C. V. Mosby, 1994, p. 88.
35. Farquhar, I. K.: Continuous direct and indirect blood pressure measurement (Finapres) in the critically ill. Anaesthesia, 46:1050, 1991.
36. Fiddian-Green, R. G., Haglund, U., Gutierrez, G., and Shoemaker, W. C.: Goals for the resuscitation of shock. Crit. Care Med., 21:S25, 1993.
37. Fisher, C. J., Jr., Dhainaut, J. F. A., Opal, S. M., et al.: Recombinant human interleukin-1 receptor antagonist in the treatment of patients with sepsis syndrome: Results from a randomized, double-blind, placebo-controlled trial. JAMA, 271:1836, 1994.
38. Fisher, C. J., Jr., Opal, S. M., Dhainaut, J. F., et al.: Influence of an anti-tumor necrosis factor monoclonal antibody on cytokine levels in patients with sepsis. Crit. Care Med., 21:318, 1993.
39. Fleming, A., Bishop, M., Shoemaker, W., et al.: Prospective trial of supranormal values as goals of resuscitation in severe trauma. Arch. Surg., 127:1175, 1992.

40. Friedl, H. P., Smith, D. J., Till, G. O., Thomson, P. D., Louis, D. S., and Ward, P. A.: Ischemia-reperfusion in humans: Appearance of xanthine oxidase activity. Am. J. Pathol., 136:491, 1990.
41. Gacioch, G. M., Ellis, S. G., Lee, L., et al.: Cardiogenic shock complicating acute myocardial infarction: The use of coronary angioplasty and the integration of the new support devices into patient management. J. Am. Coll. Cardiol., 19:647, 1992.
42. Gammaitoni, C., and Nasraway, S. A.: Normal lactate/pyruvate ratio during overwhelming polymicrobial bacteremia and multiple organ failure. Anesthesiology, 80:213, 1994.
43. Granger, D. N.: Role of xanthine oxidase and granulocytes in ischemia-reperfusion injury. Am. J. Physiol., 255:H1269, 1988.
44. Gross, D., Landau, E. H., Klin, B., and Krausz, M. M.: Treatment of uncontrolled hemorrhagic shock with hypertonic saline solution. Surg. Gynecol. Obstet., 170:106, 1990.
45. Gurll, N. G., Vargish, T., Reynolds, D. G., and Lechner, R. D.: Opiate receptors and endorphins in the pathophysiology of hemorrhagic shock. Surgery, 80:364, 1981.
46. Guthrie, G. J.: On Gunshot Wounds of the Extremities. London, Longman, 1815.
47. Gutierrez, G., Palizas, F., Doglio, G., et al.: Gastric intramucosal pH as a therapeutic index of tissue oxygenation in critically ill patients. Lancet, 339:195, 1992.
48. GISSI: Effectiveness of intravenous thrombolytic treatment in acute myocardial infarction. Lancet, 1:871, 1987.
49. Halliwell, B.: Reactive oxygen species in living systems: Source, biochemistry, and role in human disease. Am. J. Med., 91:145, 1991.
50. Hayes, M. A., Timmins, A. C., Yau, E. H. S., Palazzo, M., Hinds, C. J., and Watson, D.: Elevation of systemic oxygen delivery in the treatment of critically ill patients. N. Engl. J. Med., 330:1717, 1994.
51. Hotchkiss, R. S., and Karl, I. E.: Reevaluation of the role of cellular hypoxia and bioenergetic failure in sepsis. JAMA, 267:1503, 1992.
52. Hsueh, W., Gonzalez-Grussi, F., and Arroyave, J. L.: Platelet-activating factor: An endogenous mediator for bowel necrosis in endotoxemia. FASEB J., 1:403, 1987.
53. Imm, A., and Carlson, R. W.: Fluid resuscitation in circulatory shock. Circ. Shock, 9:313, 1993.
54. Keith, N. M.: Blood Volume Changes in Wound Shock and Primary Hemorrhage: Reports of the Special Investigations Committee on Surgical Shock and Allied Conditions, Vol. 9, London, 1919.
55. Keller, G. A., West, M. A., Cerra, F. B., and Simmons, R. L.: Multiple system organ failure: Modulation of hepatocyte protein synthesis by endotoxin-activated Kupffer cells. Ann. Surg., 201:87, 1985.
56. Knaus, W. A., Draper, E. A., Wagner, D. P., and Zimmerman, J. E.: Prognosis in acute organ-system failure. Ann. Surg., 202:685, 1985.
57. Latta, T.: Treatment of malignant cholera. Lancet, 2:1831, 1832.
58. Lillehei, R. C.: The intestinal factor in irreversible hemorrhagic shock. Surgery, 42:1043, 1957.
59. Marshall, J. C., Christou, N. V., Horn, R., and Meakins, J. L.: The microbiology of multiple organ failure. Arch. Surg., 123:309, 1988.
60. May, M. E., and Carey, R. M.: Rapid adrenocorticotropic hormone test in practice. Am. J. Med., 79:679, 1985.
61. Maynard, N., Bihari, D., Beale, R., et al.: Assessment of splanchnic oxygenation by gastric tonometry in patients with acute circulatory failure. JAMA, 270:1203, 1993.
62. McClelland, R. N., Shires, T., Baxter, C. R., Coln, C. D., and Carrico, J.: Balanced salt solution in the treatment of hemorrhagic shock. JAMA, 199:166, 1967.
63. McMillen, M. A., Huribal, M., and Sumpio, B.: Common pathway of endothelial-leukocyte interaction in shock, ischemia, and reperfusion. Am. J. Surg., 166:557, 1993.
64. Meakins, J. L.: Etiology of multiple organ failure. J. Trauma, 30(12 Suppl):S165, 1990.
65. Michie, H. R., Manogue, K. R., and Spriggs, et al.: Detection of circulating tumor necrosis factor after endotoxin administration. N. Engl. J. Med., 318:1481, 1988.
66. Montgomery, A., Stager, M., Carrico, J., et al.: Causes of mortality in patients with the adult respiratory distress syndrome. Am. Rev. Respir. Dis., 132:485, 1985.
67. Moore, F. A., Feliciano, D. V., Andrassy, R. J., et al.: Early enteral feeding,

68. compared with parenteral, reduces postoperative septic complications. Ann. Surg., 216:172, 1992.
68. Moore, F. A., and Moore, E. E.: Evolving concepts in the pathogenesis of postinjury multiple organ failure. Surg. Clin. North Am., 75:257, 1995.
69. Moore, F. A., Moore, E. E., Poggetti, R., et al.: Gut bacterial translocation via the portal vein: A clinical perspective with major torso trauma. J. Trauma, 31:629, 1991.
70. O'Quin, R., and Marini, J. J.: Pulmonary artery occlusion pressure: Clinical physiology, measurement, and interpretation. Am. Rev. Respir. Dis., 128:319, 1983.
71. Parrillo, J. E.: Pathogenetic mechanisms of septic shock. N. Engl. J. Med., 328:1471, 1993.
72. Parrillo, J. E., Burch, C., Shelhamer, J. H., et al.: A circulating myocardial depressant substance in humans with septic shock: Septic shock patients with a reduced ejection fraction have a circulating factor that depresses in vitro myocardial cell performance. J. Clin. Invest., 76:1539, 1985.
73. Parsons, E., and Phemister, D. B.: Hemorrhage and shock in traumatized limbs: Experimental study. Surg. Gynecol. Obstet., 50:196, 1930.
74. Rangel-Frausto, M. S., Pittet, D., Costigan, M., et al.: The natural history of the systemic inflammatory response syndrome (SIRS). JAMA, 273:117, 1995.
75. Revhaug, A., Michie, H. R., Manson, J. M., et al.: Inhibition of cyclo-oxygenase attenuates the metabolic response to endotoxin in humans. Arch. Surg., 123:162, 1988.
76. Ronco, J. J., Fenwick, J. C., Tweeddale, M. G., et al.: Identification of the critical oxygen delivery for anaerobic metabolism in critically ill septic and nonseptic humans. JAMA, 270:1724, 1993.
77. Samsel, R. W., Nelson, D. P., Sanders, W. M., Wood, L. D. H., and Schumacker, P. T.: The effect of endotoxin on systemic and skeletal muscle oxygen extraction. J. Appl. Physiol., 65:1377, 1988.
78. Sandin, R.: Kidney function in shock. Acta. Anaesth. Scand., Supp 98:14, 1993.
79. Segal, J., Gaudiani, V., and Nishimura, T.: Continuous determination of cardiac output using a flow-directed Doppler pulmonary artery catheter. J. Cardiothorac. Vasc. Anesth., 5:309, 1991.
80. Shippy, C. R., Appel, P. L., and Shoemaker, W. C.: Reliability of clinical monitoring to assess blood volume in critically ill patients. Crit. Care Med., 12:107, 1984.
81. Shires, G. T., Cunningham, J. N., Baker, C. R. F., et al.: Alterations in cellular membrane function during hemorrhagic shock in primates. Ann. Surg., 176:288, 1972.
82. Shoemaker, W. C., Kram, H. B., and Appel, P. L.: Therapy of shock based on pathophysiology, monitoring, and outcome prediction. Crit. Care Med., 18:S19, 1990.
83. Tilney, N. L., Bailey, G. L., and Morgan, A. P.: Sequential system failure after rupture of abdominal aortic aneurysms: An unsolved problem in postoperative care. Ann. Surg., 178:117, 1973.
84. Tremper, K. K., and Shoemaker, W. C.: Transcutaneous oxygen monitoring of critically ill adults with and without low flow shock. Crit. Care Med., 9:706, 1981.
85. Vincent, J. L., Dufaye, P., Berré, J., et al.: Serial lactate determinations during circulatory shock. Crit. Care Med., 11:449, 1983.
86. Warren, H. S., Danner, R. L., and Munford, R. S.: Anti-endotoxin monoclonal antibodies. N. Engl. J. Med., 326:1153, 1992.
87. Welbourn, C. R. B., and Young, Y.: Endotoxin, septic shock and acute lung injury: Neutrophils, macrophages and inflammatory mediators. Br. J. Surg., 79:998, 1992.
88. Wiggers, C. J.: Myocardial depression and shock: Survey of cardiodynamic studies. Am. Heart J., 33:633, 1947.
89. Woll, P. J., and Record, C. O.: Lactate elimination in man: Effects of lactate concentration and hepatic dysfunction. Eur. J. Clin. Invest., 9:397, 1979.
90. Yelderman, M. L., Ramsay, M. A., Quinn, M. D., et al.: Continuous thermodilution cardiac output measurement in intensive care unit patients. J. Cardiothorac. Vasc. Anesthesiol., 6:270, 1992.
91. Younes, R. N., Aun, F., Accioly, C. Q., et al.: Hypertonic solutions in the treatment of hypovolemic shock: A prospective, randomized study in patients admitted to the emergency room. Surgery, 111:380, 1992.
92. Yu, M., Levy, M. M., Smith, P., et al.: Effect of maximizing oxygen delivery on morbidity and mortality rates in critically ill patients: A prospective, controlled study. Crit. Care Med., 21:830, 1993.

CHAPTER 6

FLUID AND ELECTROLYTE MANAGEMENT OF THE SURGICAL PATIENT

G. Tom Shires III, M.D., and G. Tom Shires, M.D.

Management of fluids and electrolytes is an integral part of the care of surgical patients, and it may be a critical factor in certain patients. Many diseases, injuries, and operative trauma have a great effect on the physiology of body fluids and electrolytes, far greater than the changes associated with a simple lack of alimentation. Therefore, a thorough understanding of the metabolism of salt, water, and other electrolytes and of certain metabolic responses is essential to the care of surgical patients.

This chapter defines the anatomy of body fluid compartments and the physiologic principles relating to fluids and electrolytes. In addition to normal functions, a classification of derangements will be developed so that therapy may be described.

ANATOMY OF BODY FLUID COMPARTMENTS

A prerequisite to the understanding of fluid and electrolyte management is knowledge of the extent and composition of the various body fluid compartments. Early attempts to define these compartments were relatively accurate, but a more precise definition has been obtained by many investigators through the use of isotopic tracer techniques. The wide range of normal values is a function of body size, weight, and sex, but these compartments are relatively constant in size for the individual patient in the normal steady state. The figures used in this section are approximate and reported as percentages of body weight.

Total Body Water

Water constitutes between 50% and 70% of total body weight. With deuterium oxide or tritiated water used to measure total body water, the average normal value is 60% of body weight for young adult males and 50% for young adult females. A normal variation of ±15% applies to both groups. The actual figure for a healthy individual is remarkably constant and is a function of several variables, including lean body mass and age. Because fat contains little water, the lean individual has a greater proportion of water to total body weight than the obese person. Thus, an extremely obese individual may have 25% to 30% less body water than a lean individual of the same weight. The lower percentage of total body water in females correlates with a larger amount of subcutaneous adipose tissue and smaller muscle mass. Moore and colleagues have shown that total body water, as a percentage of total body weight, decreases steadily and significantly with age to a low of 52% and 47% in males and females, respectively.[17] Conversely, the highest proportion of total body water is found in newborn infants, with a maxi-

mum of 75% to 80%. During the first several months after birth there is a gradual *physiologic* loss of body water as the infant adjusts to the environment. At 1 year of age, the total body water averages approximately 65% of body weight and remains relatively constant throughout the remainder of infancy and childhood.

The water of the body is divided into three functional compartments (Fig. 6–1). The fluid within the body's diverse cell population, intracellular water, represents between 30% and 40% of body weight. The extracellular water represents approximately 20% of body weight and is divided between intravascular fluid, or plasma (5% of body weight), and interstitial, or extravascular, extracellular fluid (15% of body weight).

Intracellular Fluid. Measurement of intracellular fluid (ICF) is determined indirectly by subtraction of the measured extracellular fluid (ECF) from the measured total body water. The intracellular water is between 30% and 40% of body weight, with the largest proportion in the skeletal muscle mass. Because of the smaller muscle mass in the female, the percentage of intracellular water is lower than in the male.

The chemical composition of ICF is shown in Figure 6–2, with potassium and magnesium the principal cations, and phosphates and proteins the principal anions. This is an approximation, because few data concerning ICF are available.

Extracellular Fluid. The total ECF volume represents approximately 20% of body weight. The ECF compartment has two major subdivisions. The plasma volume is approximately 5% of body weight in the normal adult. The interstitial, or extravascular, ECF volume, obtained by subtracting the plasma volume from the measured total ECF volume, accounts for approximately 15% of body weight.

The interstitial fluid is further complicated by having a rapidly equilibrating or functional component as well as

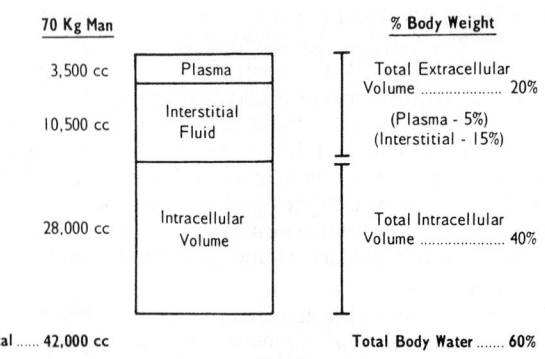

Figure 6–1. Functional compartments of body fluids.

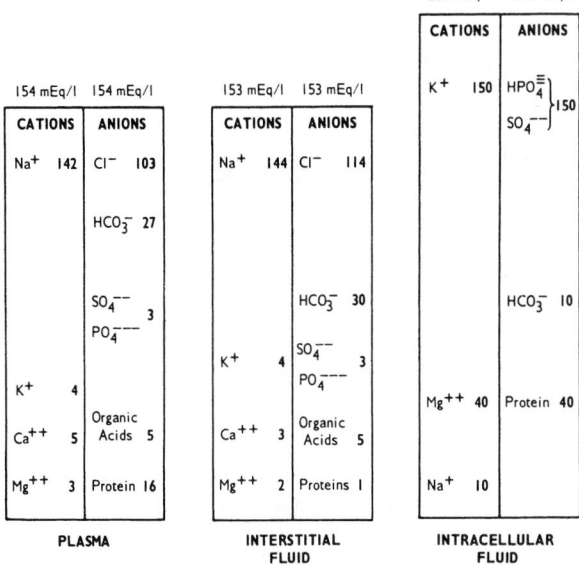

Figure 6–2. Chemical composition of body fluid compartments.

several more slowly equilibrating, or relatively nonfunctioning, components. The nonfunctioning components include connective tissue water as well as transcellular water, which includes cerebrospinal and joint fluids. This nonfunctional component normally represents only 10% of interstitial fluid volume (1% to 2% of body weight) and is not to be confused with the relatively nonfunctional ECF, often called a *third space,* found in burns and soft tissue injuries.

The normal constituents of ECF are shown in Figure 6–2, with sodium the principal cation and chloride and bicarbonate the principal anions. Minor differences in ionic composition between the plasma and the interstitial fluid are occasioned by the difference in protein concentration. Because of the higher protein content (organic anions) of the plasma, the total concentration of cations is higher and the concentration of inorganic anions somewhat lower than in the interstitial fluid, as explained by the Gibbs-Donnan equilibrium equation.* For practical considerations, however, they may be considered equal. The total concentration of intracellular ions exceeds that of the extracellular compartment and would seem to violate the concept of osmolar equilibrium between the two compartments. This apparent discrepancy occurs because the concentration of ions is expressed in milliequivalents (mEq.) without regard to osmotic activity. In addition, some of the intracellular cations probably exist in undissociated form.

Osmotic Pressure. Relevant to a discussion of the complicated interactions between the various body fluid compartments is the definition of commonly used terms. The physiologic and chemical activity of electrolytes depends on the number of particles present per unit volume (moles or millimoles [mM.] per liter), the number of electrical charges per unit volume (equivalents or milliequivalents [mEq.] per liter), and the number of osmotically active particles, or ions per unit volume (osmoles or milliosmoles [mOsm.] per liter). The use of the term *grams* or *milligrams per 100 milliliters* expresses the weight of the electrolytes per unit volume but does not allow a physiologic comparison of the solutes in a solution.

A mole of a substance is the molecular weight of that

---

*The product of the concentrations of any pair of diffusible cations and anions on one side of a semipermeable membrane will equal the product of the same pair of ions on the other side.

substance in grams, and a millimole is that figure expressed in milligrams. For example, a mole of sodium chloride is 58 grams (Na, 23; Cl, 35), and a millimole is 58 milligrams. This expression, however, gives no direct information as to the number of osmotically active ions in solution or the electrical charges that they carry.

The electrolytes of the body fluids, then, may be expressed in terms of chemical combining activity, or *equivalents.* An equivalent of an ion is its atomic weight expressed in grams divided by the valence, whereas a milliequivalent of an ion is that figure expressed in milligrams. In the case of univalent ions, a milliequivalent is the same as a millimole. However, in the case of divalent ions, such as calcium or magnesium, 1 millimole equals 2 milliequivalents. The importance of this expression is that a milliequivalent of any substance will combine chemically with a milliequivalent of any other substance; in any given solution, the number of milliequivalents of cations present is balanced precisely by the same number of milliequivalents of anions.

When the osmotic pressure of a solution is considered, it is more descriptive to employ the terms *osmole* and *milliosmole.* These terms refer to the actual number of osmotically active particles present in solution, but do not depend on the chemical combining capacities of the substances. Thus, 1 millimole of sodium chloride, which dissociates nearly completely into sodium and chloride, contributes 2 milliosmoles, and 1 millimole of sodium sulfate (Na_2SO_4), which dissociates into three particles, contributes 3 milliosmoles. One millimole of an un-ionized substance such as glucose is equal to 1 milliosmole of the substance.

The differences in ionic composition between ICF and ECF are maintained by the cell wall, which functions as a semipermeable membrane. The total number of osmotically active particles is 290 to 310 mOsm. in each compartment. Although the osmotic pressure of a fluid is the sum of the partial pressures contributed by each of the solutes in that fluid, the effective osmotic pressure depends on those substances that fail to pass through the pores of the semipermeable membrane. The dissolved proteins in the plasma, therefore, are primarily responsible for effective osmotic pressure between the plasma and the interstitial fluid compartments; this is frequently referred to as the colloid osmotic pressure. The effective osmotic pressure between the ECF and ICF compartments is contributed to by any substance that does not traverse the cell membranes freely. Thus, sodium, which is the principal cation of ECF, contributes a major portion of the osmotic pressure, but any substance that fails to penetrate the cell membrane freely, such as glucose, also increases the effective osmotic pressure.

Since the cell membranes are completely permeable to water, the effective osmotic pressures in the two compartments are considered equal. Any condition that alters the effective osmotic pressure in either compartment causes redistribution of water between the compartments. Thus, an increase in effective osmotic pressure in ECF, which would occur most frequently through increased sodium concentration, causes a net transfer of water from the ICF to the ECF compartment. This transfer of water continues until the effective osmotic pressures in the two compartments are equal. Conversely, a decrease in the sodium concentration in ECF causes a transfer of water from the ECF to the ICF compartment. Depletion of ECF volume without a change in the concentration of ions, however, will not transfer free water from the intracellular space.

Thus, ICF shares in losses that involve a change in concentration or composition of ECF, but shares slowly in changes involving loss of isotonic volume alone. For practical considerations, most losses and gains of body fluid occur directly from the extracellular compartment.

CLASSIFICATION OF BODY FLUID CHANGES

The disorders in fluid balance may be classified into three general categories: disturbance of volume, concentration, and composition. Of primary importance is the concept that although these disturbances are interrelated, each is a separate entity.

If an isotonic salt solution is added to or lost from the body fluids, only the volume of the ECF is changed. The acute loss of an isotonic extracellular solution, such as intestinal juice, is followed by a significant decrease in ECF volume and little, if any, change in ICF volume. Fluid is not transferred from the intracellular space to refill the depleted extracellular space as long as the osmolality remains the same in the two compartments.

If water alone is added to or lost from the ECF, the concentration of osmotically active particles changes. Sodium ions account for most of the osmotically active particles in ECF and generally reflect the tonicity of other body fluid compartments. If ECF is depleted of sodium, water passes into the intracellular space until osmolality is again equal in the two compartments.

The concentration of most other ions within the ECF compartment can be altered without significant change in the total number of osmotically active particles, thus producing only a compositional change. For instance, a rise of the serum potassium concentration from 4 to 8 mEq. per liter would have a significant effect on the myocardium, but it would not significantly change the effective osmotic pressure of the ECF compartment. Normally functioning kidneys minimize these changes considerably, particularly if the addition or loss of solute or water is gradual.

An internal loss of ECF into a nonfunctional space, such as the sequestration of isotonic fluid in a burn, peritonitis, ascites, or muscle trauma, is termed a distributional change. This transfer or functional loss of ECF internally may be extracellular (e.g., as in peritonitis) or intracellular (e.g., as in hemorrhagic shock).[20] In any event, all distributional shifts or losses cause a contraction of the functional ECF space.

Volume Changes

An excess or deficit of ECF volume must be diagnosed by clinical examination of the patient. Direct measurement of ECF volume using sodium bromide or radioactive sodium sulfate is feasible in a research setting but is of limited use clinically because of the complexity of the tests. However, several laboratory tests indirectly reflect changes in ECF volume. The blood urea nitrogen (BUN) rises with an ECF deficit of sufficient magnitude to reduce the glomerular filtration rate (GFR). The serum creatinine level may not increase proportionally in young people with healthy kidneys, and this discrepancy is often used as one test to differentiate prerenal and renal azotemia. (Importantly, the rise in serum creatinine often parallels the increase of BUN in elderly patients and in those with chronic renal disease.)

The concentration of formed elements in the blood (red blood cells [RBCs], white blood cells [WBCs], platelets, plasma proteins) increases with an ECF deficit and decreases with an ECF excess. The concentration of serum sodium, however, is not related to the volume status of extracellular fluid: a severe ECF volume deficit may exist with a normal, low, or high serum sodium level.

Volume Deficit. ECF volume deficit is by far the most common fluid disorder in the surgical patient. The loss of fluid is not water alone but water and electrolytes in approximately the same proportion as that in which they exist in normal ECF. The most common disorders leading to an ECF

volume deficit include losses of gastrointestinal fluids due to vomiting, nasogastric suction, diarrhea, and fistula drainage. Other common causes include sequestration of fluid in soft tissue injuries and infections, intra-abdominal and retroperitoneal inflammatory processes, peritonitis, intestinal obstruction, and burns. The signs and symptoms of this state are easily recognized and are listed in Table 6–1. The central nervous system (CNS) and cardiovascular signs occur early with acute rapid losses, whereas tissue signs may be absent until the deficit has existed for at least 24 hours. The CNS signs are similar to those of barbiturate intoxication and may be missed by the casual observer if the volume deficit is mild. The cardiovascular signs are secondary to a decrease in plasma volume and may be associated with varying degrees of hypotension in a patient with severe ECF volume deficit. Skin turgor may be difficult to assess in an elderly patient or in a patient with recent weight loss and is not diagnostic in the absence of other confirmatory signs. Body temperature tends to vary with the environmental temperature. In a cool room a patient may be slightly hypothermic, and the febrile response and increased WBC count expected with infection may be suppressed. This occurs frequently and can be misleading during clinical evaluation of a septic patient. After partial correction of the volume deficit, the temperature and WBC usually rise to appropriate levels.

Severe volume depletion depresses all body systems (including the CNS) and interferes with the clinical evaluation of a patient. For example, a volume-depleted patient with severe sepsis from peritonitis may have a normal temperature and WBC count, complain of little pain, and have unimpressive findings on abdominal examination. The clinical picture will change dramatically, however, as the ECF volume is restored.

The oliguria is secondary to renal hypoperfusion (prerenal azotemia) and occasionally may be difficult to distinguish from oliguria caused by intrinsic renal disease (renal azotemia). In addition to the clinical setting and examination of urinary sediment, the tests of urinary function listed in Table 6–2 may be beneficial.[16] Some of these tests are of limited value in the differential diagnosis of oliguria in elderly patients because of the diminished ability to concentrate urine generally associated with aging. Many patients, however, retain the ability to conserve sodium. Of the listed tests, the renal failure index and the fractional excretion of filtered sodium are the most accurate.

Volume Excess. ECF volume excess is generally iatrogenic or secondary to renal insufficiency. Both the plasma and the interstitial fluid volumes are increased. In a healthy young adult the signs are generally those of circulatory overload, manifested primarily in the pulmonary circulation, and of excessive fluid in other tissues (see Table 6–1). In an elderly patient, congestive heart failure with pulmonary edema may develop rather quickly with a moderate volume excess.

Concentration Changes

The serum sodium level is used to estimate total body fluid osmolality. Since the ECF and ICF compartments are separated by a membrane that is freely permeable only to water, osmolality is approximately the same in the two spaces. Any change in the number of particles (osmolality) in one compartment initiates an appropriate transfer of water between the two spaces. Therefore, even though the sodium ion is largely confined to the extracellular compartment, its level reflects total body fluid osmolality. Hyponatremia and hypernatremia can be diagnosed by clinical manifestations (Table 6–3), but discernible signs and symptoms are not generally present until the changes are severe. Changes in concentration should be noted early by appropriate laboratory

TABLE 6–1. Extracellular Fluid Volume

	Deficit		Excess	
	Moderate	*Severe*	*Moderate*	*Severe*
Central nervous system	Sleepiness Apathy Slow responses Anorexia Cessation of usual activity	Decreased tendon reflexes Anesthesia of distal extremities Stupor Coma	None	None
Gastrointestinal	Progressive decrease in food consumption	Nausea, vomiting Refusal to eat Silent ileus and distention	*At Operation:* Edema of stomach, colon, lesser and greater omenta, and small bowel mesentery	
Cardiovascular	Orthostatic hypotension Tachycardia Collapsed veins Collapsing pulse	Cutaneous lividity Hypotension Distant heart sounds Cold extremities Absent peripheral pulses	Elevated venous pressure Distention of peripheral veins Increased cardiac output Loud heart sounds Functional murmurs Bounding pulse High pulse pressure Increased pulmonary second sound Gallop	Pulmonary edema
Tissue signs	Soft, small tongue with longitudinal wrinkling Decreased skin turgor	Atonic muscles Sunken eyes	Subcutaneous pitting edema Basilar rales	Anasarca Moist rales Vomiting Diarrhea
Metabolism	Mild decrease of temperature, 97°–99° F.	Marked decrease of temperature, 95°–98° F.	None	None

tests and corrected promptly. Clinical signs of hyponatremia or hypernatremia tend to occur early and with greater severity if the rate of change is rapid.

Hyponatremia. Acute symptomatic hyponatremia clinically is characterized by CNS signs of increased intracranial pressure and tissue signs of excessive intracellular water. There are no cardiovascular signs *per se*. The hypertension is induced by the rise in intracranial pressure, since the blood pressure generally returns to normal after correction of the sodium level. Of importance with severe hyponatremia is the relatively rapid development of oliguric renal failure, which may not be reversible if therapy is delayed.

Many hyponatremic states are asymptomatic until the serum sodium level falls well below 120 mEq. per liter. One important exception is the patient with increased cerebrospinal fluid pressure, as after closed head injury, in which mild hyponatremia may be extremely deleterious, even fatal. This is due to the progressive increase in intracellular water (further increasing intracranial pressure) as the ECF osmolality falls.

Hypernatremia. CNS and tissue signs (listed in Table 6–3) characterize acute symptomatic hypernatremia. This is the only state in which dry, sticky mucous membranes are characteristic. This sign does not occur with ECF volume deficit alone and usually is only an indication that the patient is breathing through the mouth. Body temperature is generally elevated and may approach a lethal level, as in the patient with heat stroke. Although volume changes occur frequently without a change in serum sodium concentration (osmolality), the reverse is not true. Disease states that cause acute alterations in serum sodium levels frequently produce concomitant changes in ECF volume.

Mixed Volume and Concentration Abnormalities

Mixed abnormalities in volume and concentration may develop as a consequence of the disease state or occasionally from inappropriate parenteral fluid therapy. Moyer noted that the clinical picture associated with a combination of fluid abnormalities tends to be an algebraic composite of the signs and symptoms of each state.[30] Equal signs produced by both abnormalities are additive, and opposing signs tend to nullify one another.

One of the more common mixed abnormalities is an ECF deficit and hyponatremia. This state is readily produced in a patient who continues to drink water while losing large

TABLE 6–2. Oliguria

	Prerenal	Renal
Urine osmolality (mOsm./kg. H_2O)	>500	<350
Urine sodium (mEq./L.)	<20	>40
BUN/serum creatinine	>15	<10
Urine/plasma urea	>8	<3
Urine/plasma creatinine	>40	<20
Renal failure index	<1	>1.5
$RFI = \dfrac{Urine\ Na}{U/P\ creatinine}$		
Fractional excretion sodium	<1	>1.5
$FE_{Na} = \dfrac{U/P\ Na}{U/P\ Cr} \times 100$		

Patients with early acute glomerulonephritis may have indices similar to prerenal patients. Indices are not reliable in patients with obstructive uropathy.

Adapted from Miller, T. R., et al.: Urinary diagnostic indices in acute renal failure. Ann. Intern. Med., *89*:47, 1978.

TABLE 6–3. Acute Changes in Osmolar Concentration

	Hyponatremia (Water Intoxication)		Hypernatremia (Water Deficit)	
Central nervous system	*Moderate* Muscle twitching Hyperactive tendon reflexes Increased intracranial pressure (compensated phase)	*Severe* Convulsions Loss of reflexes Increased intracranial pressure (decompensated phase)	*Moderate* Restlessness Weakness	*Severe* Delirium Maniacal behavior
Cardiovascular	Changes in blood pressure and pulse secondary to increased intracranial pressure		Tachycardia Hypotension (if severe)	
Tissue signs	Increased salivation, lacrimation Watery diarrhea "Fingerprinting" of skin (sign of intracellular volume excess)		Decreased saliva and tears Dry and sticky mucous membranes Red, swollen tongue Flushed skin	
Renal	Oliguria progressing to anuria		Oliguria	
Metabolic		None	Fever	

volumes of gastrointestinal fluids. It may also occur postoperatively when gastrointestinal losses are replaced with only 5% dextrose in water or a hypotonic sodium solution. An ECF volume deficit accompanied by hypernatremia may be produced by the loss of a large amount of hypotonic salt solution, such as an osmotic diuresis due to glucosuria in a hyperglycemic patient.

The prolonged administration of excessive quantities of sodium salts may eventually cause an ECF volume excess and hypernatremia. This may also occur when pure water losses (such as insensible loss of water from the skin and lungs) are replaced with sodium-containing solutions only. Similarly, excessive administration of water or hypotonic salt solutions to a patient with oliguric renal failure may rapidly produce an ECF volume excess and hyponatremia.

Normally functioning kidneys minimize these changes to some extent and compensate for many of the errors associated with parenteral fluid administration. In contrast, the patient in anuric or oliguric renal failure is particularly prone to develop these mixed volume and osmolar concentration abnormalities. Management of fluids and electrolytes in these patients must therefore be precise. Unfortunately, the fact that a patient with normal kidneys who develops a significant volume deficit may be in a state of *functional* renal failure is often not appreciated. As the volume deficit progresses, the GFR falls precipitously, and the kidneys' unique mechanisms for maintaining fluid and electrolyte homeostasis are compromised. Such changes may occur with only mild volume deficits in elderly patients with borderline renal function. In these patients, the BUN level may rise higher than 100 mg. per 100 ml. in response to the fluid deficit, with a concomitant rise in the serum creatinine level. Fortunately, the changes are usually reversible with early and adequate correction of the ECF volume deficit.

Composition Changes

Compositional abnormalities of importance include changes in acid-base balance and concentration changes of potassium, calcium, and magnesium.

Acid-base Balance. The pH (the negative logarithm of the hydrogen ion concentration) of the body fluids is normally maintained within narrow limits despite the rather large load of acid produced endogenously as a by-product of body metabolism. The acids are neutralized efficiently by several buffer systems and subsequently excreted by the lungs and kidneys. The important buffers include proteins and phosphates, which play a primary role in maintaining intracellular pH, and the bicarbonate–carbonic acid system, which operates principally in the ECF space. Proteins have only minor influence in the ECF space, but hemoglobin is of prime significance as a buffer in the red cell.

A buffer system consists of a weak acid or base and the salt of that acid or base. The buffering effect is produced by the formation of an amount of weak acid or base equivalent to the amount of strong acid or base added to the system. The resultant change in pH is considerably less than if the substance were added to water alone. Thus, inorganic acids (e.g., hydrochloric, sulfuric, phosphoric) and organic acids (e.g., lactic, pyruvic, keto) combine with base bicarbonate, producing the sodium salt of the acid and carbonic acid:

$$(HCl + NaHCO_3 \rightarrow NaCl + H_2CO_3)$$

The carbonic acid formed is then excreted via the lungs as carbon dioxide (CO_2). The inorganic acid anions are excreted by the kidneys with hydrogen or as ammonium salts. The organic acid anions are generally metabolized as the underlying disorder is corrected, although some renal excretion may occur with high levels.

The functions of the buffer systems are expressed in the Henderson-Hasselbalch equation, which defines the pH in terms of the ratio of the salt and acid. The pH of the ECF is defined primarily by the ratio of the amount of base bicarbonate (majority as sodium bicarbonate) to the amount of carbonic acid (related to the CO_2 content of alveolar air) present in the blood:

$$pH = pK + \log \frac{BHCO_3}{H_2CO_3} = [6.1] +$$

$$[\log \frac{27\,mEq./L.}{1.35\,mEq./L.} = \frac{20}{1} = 1.3] = 7.4$$

pK represents the dissociation constant of carbonic acid in the presence of base bicarbonate and by measurement is 6.1. At a body pH of 7.4, the ratio must be 20:1, as depicted. From a chemical standpoint this is an inefficient buffer system, but the unusual ability of CO_2 to behave as an acid or to change to a neutral gas subsequently excreted by the lungs makes it quite efficient biologically.

As long as the 20:1 ratio is maintained, regardless of the absolute values, the pH remains at 7.4. When an acid is added to the system, the concentration of bicarbonate (the numerator in the Henderson-Hasselbalch equation) decreases. Ventilation immediately increases to eliminate larger quantities of CO_2 with a subsequent decrease in the carbonic acid (the denominator in the Henderson-Hasselbalch equa-

TABLE 6–4. Acidosis-Alkalosis

	Defect	Common Causes	$\dfrac{BHCO_3}{H_2CO_3} = \dfrac{20}{1}$	Compensation
Respiratory acidosis	Retention of CO_2 (decreased alveolar ventilation)	Depression of respiratory center by morphine Central nervous system injury Pulmonary disease—emphysema, pneumonia	↑ Denominator Ratio less than 20:1	Renal Retention of bicarbonate, excretion of acid salts, increased ammonia formation Chloride shift into red cells
Respiratory alkalosis	Excessive loss of CO_2 (increased alveolar ventilation)	Hyperventilation: emotional disturbances, severe pain, assisted ventilation, encephalitis	↓ Denominator Ratio greater than 20:1	Renal Excretion of bicarbonate, retention of acid salts, decreased ammonia formation
Metabolic acidosis	Retention of fixed acids or loss of base bicarbonate	Diabetes, azotemia, lactic acid accumulation, starvation Diarrhea, small bowel fistulas	↓ Numerator Ratio less than 20:1	Pulmonary (rapid): increased rate and depth of breathing Renal (slow): as in respiratory acidosis
Metabolic alkalosis	Loss of fixed acids Gain of base bicarbonate Potassium depletion	Vomiting or gastric suction with pyloric obstruction Excessive intake of bicarbonate Diuretics	↑ Numerator Ratio greater than 20:1	Pulmonary (rapid): decreased rate and depth of breathing Renal (slow): as in respiratory alkalosis

tion) until the 20:1 ratio is re-established. Slower, more complete compensation is effected by the kidneys with increased excretion of acid salts and retention of bicarbonate. The reverse occurs if an alkali is added to the system. Respiratory acidosis and alkalosis are produced by disturbances of ventilation, with an increase or decrease in the denominator and a resultant change in the 20:1 ratio. Compensation is primarily renal, with a retention of bicarbonate and increased excretion of acid salts in respiratory acidosis and the reverse process in respiratory alkalosis.

The four types of acid-base disturbances are listed in Table 6–4. Use of the CO_2 combining power (approximates the plasma bicarbonate) or CO_2 content (includes bicarbonate, carbonic acid, and dissolved CO_2) and knowledge of the patient's disease may allow an accurate diagnosis in the uncomplicated case. However, use of the CO_2 content or CO_2 combining power alone is generally inadequate as an index of acid-base balance. Both these tests principally reflect the level of plasma bicarbonate, since dissolved CO_2 and carbonic acid contribute no more than a few millimoles under most circumstances. In the acute phase, therefore, respiratory acidosis or alkalosis may exist without any change in the CO_2 content; determinations of the pH and P_{CO_2} from a freshly drawn arterial blood sample are necessary for diagnosis. Thus, measurements of pH, bicarbonate concentration,

and P_{CO_2} are required for a more complete understanding of the acid-base status in most patients (Table 6–5).

Unfortunately, more complex acid-base disturbances are frequently encountered. Combinations of respiratory and metabolic changes occur and may represent compensation for the initial acid-base disturbance, or may indicate two or more coexisting primary disorders (e.g., a primary respiratory acidosis complicated by a primary metabolic acidosis or alkalosis).

Usually, primary acid-base disturbances are compensated to some extent. A primary metabolic disturbance is initially compensated by changes in pulmonary ventilation, while respiratory disturbances are compensated by renal mechanisms. For example, the initial compensation for an acute metabolic acidosis is an increase in the rate and depth of breathing to lower the arterial P_{CO_2}. As pointed out by Astrup and associates, the actual state of the acid-base disorder may be characterized by the degree of compensation—not compensated (early or compensatory mechanisms not functioning), partially compensated (pH has not returned to a normal value), compensated, or overcompensated.[1] Physiologically, complete compensation or overcompensation cannot occur; when tempted to believe that it can, one should consider the presence of a mixed acid-base disturbance as the explanation.[19]

TABLE 6–5. Respiratory and Metabolic Components of Acid-Base Disorders

	Acute (Uncompensated)			Chronic (Partially Compensated)		
	pH	*P$_{CO_2}$ (respiratory component)*	*Plasma HCO$_3^-$ * (metabolic component)*	pH	*P$_{CO_2}$ (respiratory component)*	*Plasma HCO$_3^-$ * (metabolic component)*
Respiratory acidosis	↓↓	↑↑	N	↓	↑↑	↑
Respiratory alkalosis	↑↑	↓↓	N	↑	↓↓	↓
Metabolic acidosis	↓↓	N	↓↓	↓	↓	↓
Metabolic alkalosis	↑↑	N	↑↑	↑	↑?	↑

*Measured as standard bicarbonate, whole-blood buffer base, CO_2 content or CO_2-combining power. The *base excess value* is positive when the standard bicarbonate is above normal (N), and negative when the standard bicarbonate is below normal.

As previously noted, a knowledge of the pH, bicarbonate concentration, and P_{CO_2} allows an accurate diagnosis of most acid-base disturbances. However, the clinical interpretation of these measurements is associated with some inherent problems. Although the arterial P_{CO_2} is considered an accurate index of primary respiratory disturbances, changes in the level may represent compensation for a primary metabolic alteration. Thus, a depressed P_{CO_2} (below 40 mm. Hg) characterizes respiratory alkalosis but also represents the normal compensatory response to a metabolic acidosis. Similarly, the level of plasma bicarbonate cannot be regarded exclusively as an index of metabolic disturbances. An elevated plasma bicarbonate level may indicate a primary metabolic alkalosis or a compensatory response to chronic respiratory acidosis.

In an effort to separate the respiratory and metabolic components of acid-base disorders, two other approaches have been introduced. In 1948 Singer and Hastings introduced the concept of whole blood buffer base,[28] and later Astrup and colleagues proposed the use of the standard bicarbonate and base excess values.[1] The approach advocated by Astrup has been the more popular of the two, although both are attempts to quantify the metabolic, or nonrespiratory, component in an acid-base disturbance and separate it from the respiratory component.

The standard bicarbonate value is defined as the concentration of bicarbonate in plasma, when whole blood with fully oxygenated hemoglobin has been equilibrated with CO_2 at a P_{CO_2} of 40 mm. Hg at a temperature of 38° C. This value may be rapidly determined using the Astrup technique by measuring pH values at two known levels of P_{CO_2} and reading the standard bicarbonate directly from a nomogram. The normal mean value for standard bicarbonate is 24.5 mEq. per liter of plasma. Base excess (or deficit) directly expresses the amount, in milliequivalents, of fixed base (or fixed acid) added to each liter of blood. This value is obtained by multiplying the deviation of standard bicarbonate from the normal mean by a factor of 1.2. This factor corrects for the buffering capacity of the red cells and varies slightly with changes in hemoglobin concentration.[1] To avoid calculations, the base excess may be read directly from a nomogram. When the term *base excess* is used exclusively, the *positive* values represent the excess of base, and the *negative* values reflect the deficit of base (or excess of acid).*

In an excellent review of the Singer-Hastings and Astrup systems, Schwartz and Relman stated that neither system offers any advantage over the classic approach for the diagnosis of acid-base disorders.[22] They questioned the validity of using an *in vitro* CO_2 titration curve as a measure of *in vivo* acid-base changes. They also noted that the use of either of the two systems may be misleading in the analysis of chronic disorders. For example, a low pH with an elevated P_{CO_2}, a normal standard bicarbonate value, and a base excess value of zero are compatible with a diagnosis of primary uncompensated respiratory acidosis. After several hours or days, compensatory renal mechanisms would cause elevation of the standard bicarbonate level above normal, creating a positive base excess value. This partially compensated respiratory acidosis, then, could be erroneously interpreted as a respiratory acidosis *plus* a metabolic alkalosis as indicated by a significant base excess.

Despite these shortcomings, either approach may be useful when properly interpreted as a single laboratory test. Other systems have been recommended, some with ingeniously devised nomograms, but all are subject to misinterpretation.

---

*The deficit or excess of base in the extracellular compartment can be estimated in milliequivalents by multiplying the negative or positive value for base excess, in milliequivalents per liter of blood, by 0.5 times the body weight in kilograms.[19]

Unfortunately, there are no shortcuts. Regardless of the methods used, proper analysis of complex acid-base disorders requires a thorough knowledge of the clinical situation, good judgment, and a sound understanding of acid-base physiology.

Respiratory Acidosis. In most instances the underlying cause of a respiratory-induced disorder is readily apparent by history and physical examination (Table 6–6), and special tests are generally not required. Respiratory acidosis is caused by retention of CO_2 secondary to decreased alveolar ventilation. Initially, P_{CO_2} is elevated and plasma bicarbonate concentration is normal. In the chronic form, P_{CO_2} remains elevated and bicarbonate concentration rises as renal compensation occurs.

Numerous conditions causing inadequate ventilation (airway obstruction, pneumonia, atelectasis, pleural effusion, and hypoventilation due to the pain of abdominal incisions or to abdominal distention limiting diaphragmatic excursion) may exist singly or in combination to produce respiratory acidosis. The problem is particularly serious in patients with chronic pulmonary disease, in whom preexisting respiratory acidosis may be accentuated by another illness or injury. With surgical patients a not infrequent problem in the postoperative period is restlessness, hypertension, and tachycardia. These may be caused by pain, although similar signs are associated with inadequate ventilation and hypercapnia compounded by the use of narcotics.

Management of respiratory acidosis involves prompt correction of the pulmonary defect, when feasible, and measures to ensure adequate ventilation. This is particularly important in trauma patients with closed head injury or hypoxic brain damage. Acute hypercapnia aggravates existing cerebral edema because it causes cerebral vasodilation and increased cerebral blood flow. Maintenance of mild hypocapnia may be useful for temporarily reducing cerebral edema in such patients. In contrast, correction of chronic, well-compensated respiratory acidosis should be accomplished slowly.[7] Sudden lowering of P_{CO_2} in such patients may produce severe alkalosis because bicarbonate concentration is already greatly elevated (as compensation for the original disorder) and will not return to normal for many hours. Additionally, oxygen administration may depress or arrest ventilation if the P_{CO_2} is above 65 mm. Hg. Normally, increased P_{CO_2} stimulates the

TABLE 6–6. Causes of Respiratory Disturbances

Acidosis (Hypoventilation)	Alkalosis (Hyperventilation)
Airway obstruction Foreign body, pneumonia, emphysema, laryngospasm	Central nervous system disorders Injury, tumor, stroke, anxiety
Central nervous system depression	Hypoxia
Narcotics, anesthetics, injury, tumor	Adult respiratory distress syndrome, pulmonary embolus, atelectasis, anemia
Thoracic injury Pneumothorax, flail chest, tracheal tear	Mechanical ventilation Excess tidal volume and/or rate
Mechanical ventilation Inadequate rate and/or tidal volume, increased dead space	Hypermetabolism Fever, injury, sepsis
Miscellaneous Congestive heart failure, myopathy, severe obesity	Miscellaneous Congestive heart failure, salicylate intoxication, cirrhosis

respiratory center; above 65 mm. Hg, however, the respiratory center is depressed and hypoxia is the principal stimulus for respiration.

Respiratory Alkalosis. Hyperventilation due to apprehension, pain, hypoxia, CNS injury, and assisted ventilation are common causes of respiratory alkalosis. Any of these conditions may cause rapid depression of arterial P_{CO_2} and elevation of pH. Concentration of plasma bicarbonate is normal in the acute phase but falls with renal compensation if the condition persists.

Most patients who require ventilatory support develop varying degrees of respiratory alkalosis. This may be inadvertent, due to improper use of a mechanical respirator, or it may occur during attempts to raise the P_{O_2} in a hypoxic patient. Proper management requires frequent measurements of blood gases and appropriate corrections of the ventilatory pattern when indicated. Generally, P_{CO_2} can be maintained at an acceptable level by adjustments of ventilatory rate and volume. Increasing the pulmonary dead space to raise P_{CO_2} is of doubtful benefit, while adding 5% CO_2 to inspired air is potentially dangerous and poorly tolerated by many patients.

Severe respiratory alkalosis may cause serious impairment of both cardiovascular and cerebral functions. The predisposition for development of cardiac arrhythmias and cardiac arrest is particularly acute in patients who are digitalized or have preexisting hypokalemia. Hypokalemia may develop suddenly and is related to entry of potassium ions into cells in exchange for hydrogen and excessive urinary potassium loss in exchange for sodium. Additionally, an abrupt fall in the level of ionized calcium (caused by acute alkalosis) alone may produce serious arrhythmias. Cerebral ischemia and acidosis due to cerebral vasoconstriction may also occur with the sudden onset of severe respiratory alkalosis.[13] This is of little consequence in some patients but may cause irreparable damage in patients with impaired cerebral blood flow from obstructive arterial disease or during performance of a carotid endarterectomy. Another effect of alkalosis that is often not appreciated is a shift of the oxygen dissociation curve to the left, which may limit the ability of hemoglobin to unload oxygen to tissues.[5]

Severe and persistent respiratory alkalosis is often difficult to correct and may be associated with a poor prognosis because of the underlying cause of hyperventilation (e.g., intracranial injury). Treatment is directed primarily toward the cause of the disorder. Moreover, it is important to prevent the condition by proper use of mechanical ventilators and correction of any existing potassium deficit.

Metabolic Acidosis. Metabolic acidosis results from the retention or production of acids (diabetic ketoacidosis, lactic acidosis, azotemia) or loss of bicarbonate (diarrhea, pancreatic or small bowel fistula). The excess hydrogen ion lowers pH and causes plasma bicarbonate concentration to decrease. Initial compensation is pulmonary, with an increase in the rate and depth of breathing and depression of arterial P_{CO_2}; more definitive control is effected by the kidneys. Coexisting renal insufficiency, however, compounds the problem. A decreased GFR causes retention of acid metabolites, and renal tubular dysfunction interferes with the excretion of hydrogen in exchange for sodium and the production of ammonia. The acidosis may be greatly accentuated and difficult to control.

The causes of metabolic acidosis can be divided into two manageable groups by determining the anion gap.[19] This value should be determined routinely when evaluating a set of serum electrolytes; one simply subtracts the sum of serum chloride and bicarbonate from the serum sodium concentration. The normal value is 10 to 15 mEq. per liter. The anion gap is a laboratory anomaly, since routine clinical laboratory tests measure the cations sodium and potassium and the anions chloride and bicarbonate. The unmeasured anions

Figure 6–3. The anion gap.

that account for the gap are sulfate and phosphate plus lactate and other organic anions (Fig. 6–3). If the acidosis is due to loss of bicarbonate (e.g., diarrhea) or gain of a chloride acid (e.g., administration of ammonium chloride), the anion gap will be normal. Conversely, if the acidosis is due to increased production of an organic acid (e.g., lactic acid in circulatory shock) or the retention of sulfuric or phosphoric acid (e.g., renal failure), the concentration of unmeasured anions (anion gap) will be increased.

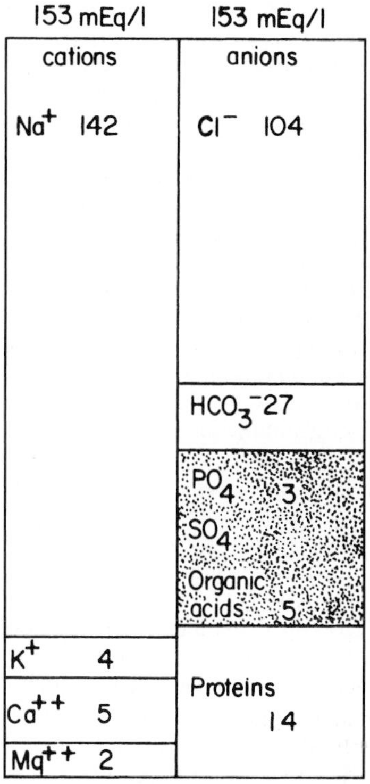

Conditions associated with an elevated anion gap are listed in Table 6–7. By far the most common is shock or inadequate tissue perfusion from any number of causes, accumulating large quantities of lactic acid. Diabetic ketoacidosis, starvation, and ethanol intoxication elevate the anion gap by the formation of keto acids; renal failure and uremia cause such

TABLE 6–7. Causes of Metabolic Acidosis

Causes	Mechanisms
Normal Anion Gap	
Diarrhea, small bowel fistula, ureterosigmoidostomy	Loss of HCO_3
Proximal renal tubular acidosis	Decreased tubular reabsorption of HCO_3
Distal renal tubular acidosis	Decreased acid excretion
Acid administration (NH_4Cl, HCl)	Increased acid load
"Dilutional" acidosis	Volume expansion with HCO_3^- free fluids
Elevated Anion Gap	
Shock (inadequate perfusion)	Increased lactic acid
Diabetes, starvation, alcohol intoxication	Increased ketoacids
Uremia	Retention of sulfuric and phosphoric acids
Ingestion of methanol, ethylene glycol, aspirin	Conversion to formic, oxalic, and salicylic acids

elevation by the retention of sulfuric and phosphoric acids. Poisoning by methanol, ethylene glycol, and aspirin produces increased anion gaps by elevation of their organic acid counterparts (formic, oxalic, and salicylic acids). In a patient with an elevated anion gap, therefore, one or more of these causes should be considered.

Metabolic acidosis associated with a loss of bicarbonate or retention of chloride acids is characterized by a normal anion gap. Diarrhea, small bowel fistula, and ureterosigmoidostomy all cause significant losses of bicarbonate, while the resorption of bicarbonate is decreased in patients with proximal renal tubular acidosis. The anion gap is also normal in patients with distal renal tubular acidosis, in whom the excretion of fixed acids (containing chloride) is decreased. Metabolic acidosis may also develop in patients who have large losses of gastrointestinal fluids containing bicarbonate (biliary, pancreatic, and small bowel secretions) replaced with normal saline. Use of a balanced salt solution containing sodium lactate or bicarbonate is more appropriate. Additionally, massive replacement of ECF volume with bicarbonate-free solutions may cause dilutional acidosis associated with a normal anion gap.[24]

The most common cause of severe metabolic acidosis in surgical patients is acute circulatory failure with accumulation of lactic acid. Acute hemorrhagic shock causes a rapid and profound drop in pH, and attempts to raise the blood pressure with vasopressors simply compound the problem. Attempts to correct the acidosis by infusion of large quantities of sodium bicarbonate without restoration of flow are futile. After restoration of adequate tissue perfusion by volume replacement, lactic acid is cleared rapidly and the pH returns toward normal. Concomitant with administration of blood, use of lactated Ringer's solution to replace the ECF deficit caused by severe, prolonged hemorrhagic shock and associated injuries does not accentuate the lactic acidosis. Instead, the lactic acid level rapidly decreases and the pH returns to normal, unlike the results of using blood alone.[6]

Routine use of sodium bicarbonate during the resuscitation of patients in hypovolemic shock is discouraged. Mild metabolic alkalosis is a common finding after resuscitation, which is in part due to the alkalinizing effects of blood transfusions and administration of lactated Ringer's solution. After infusion (and partial restoration of hepatic blood flow), the citrate contained in the transfused blood and the lactate in lactated Ringer's solution are metabolized, producing bicarbonate. Production of lactic acid ceases, excess hydrogen ion is buffered and excreted, and the organic anion lactate is metabolized by the liver. If excessive quantities of sodium bicarbonate are administered during resuscitation, severe metabolic alkalosis can occur. A highly alkaline pH is undesirable, particularly in patients with hypoxia or low fixed cardiac outputs, since the oxygen dissociation curve is shifted to the left. Other factors shifting the curve to the left that may be operative in such patients include hypothermia and depressed levels of erythrocyte 2,3-diphosphoglycerate in stored transfused blood. If the curve shifts far enough to the left, interference with oxygen unloading at the cellular level may occur.

The treatment of metabolic acidosis is directed toward correcting the underlying disorder when possible. Bicarbonate therapy is appropriately reserved for the treatment of severe metabolic acidosis, particularly after cardiac arrest, when partial correction of pH may be essential to restore myocardial function. Previous studies[4] have indicated that the acidosis accompanying cardiac arrest is compensated for a time if the patient is well ventilated and not previously acidotic (although cardiac arrest after prolonged hypovolemic shock is invariably associated with severe metabolic acidosis). Furthermore, administration of bicarbonate in the usually recommended doses may induce acute, severe hypernatremia and a hyperosmolar state. Thus, bicarbonate should be used judiciously during cardiac arrest.

Correction of pH in more protracted states of metabolic acidosis may be indicated and should be accomplished slowly. Frequent measurements of bicarbonate and blood pH are the best guides to therapy, since a satisfactory formula to estimate the amount of alkali needed has not been devised.

Metabolic Alkalosis. Metabolic alkalosis results from the loss of fixed acids or gain of bicarbonate and is aggravated by any existing potassium deficit. Both the pH and the plasma bicarbonate concentration are elevated. Compensation occurs primarily through renal mechanisms, because respiratory compensation is generally small and cannot be detected in many patients. The expected respiratory response would be a decrease in ventilation to retain CO_2; PO_2 would also fall, however, so that hypoxia imposes a limit on the amount of respiratory compensation that can occur. In the rare situation in which hypercapnia is thought to represent a compensatory response to metabolic alkalosis, rapid reduction of PCO_2 by mechanical ventilation should be avoided. Rather, the PCO_2 falls as the metabolic alkalosis is corrected.

The causes of metabolic alkalosis can be divided into two major groups, chloride responsive (urine chloride less than 10 to 20 mEq. per liter) and chloride resistant (urine chloride more than 10 to 20 mEq. per liter), depending on the amounts of chloride in the urine of untreated patients (Table 6–8).[3] States of chloride-resistant metabolic alkalosis are usually associated with a normal or slightly increased ECF volume. Most are secondary to adrenal disorders, in which the high levels of steroid secretion cause maximal tubular resorption of sodium and bicarbonate and an excessive loss of chloride in the urine. The result is metabolic alkalosis and (because of increased sodium reabsorption) expansion of the ECF compartment. Therapy is directed toward the underlying cause.

Chloride-responsive types of metabolic alkalosis are considerably more common and are often associated with ECF volume deficits. In addition to volume replacement, the provision of an adequate quantity of chloride is a prerequisite to restoration of normal acid-base and potassium equilibrium, for the following reasons. First, sodium reabsorption occurs along the entire renal tubule, although the responsible mechanisms vary in the proximal and distal portions of the tubule. Most sodium filtered by the glomerulus is removed in the proximal tubule; electroneutrality is maintained by simultaneous reabsorption of an anion, principally chloride. If there is a deficit of chloride ion, more sodium must be reabsorbed in the *distal* tubule in exchange for hydrogen or potassium. Second, in the distal tubule, sodium is reabsorbed in exchange for hydrogen or potassium, depending on their relative availability. This process also involves the generation

---

TABLE 6–8. Metabolic Alkalosis

Chloride Responsive
(Urine Chloride <10–20 mEq./L.)
Vomiting, gastric suction with obstructed pylorus
Diuretics
Villous adenoma of colon

Chloride Resistant
(Urine Chloride >10–20 mEq./L.)
Primary hyperaldosteronism
Cushing's disease
Exogenous corticosteroids
Chronic hypokalemia

Unclassified
Alkali ingestion or infusion

of one bicarbonate ion for each sodium ion that is reabsorbed, which perpetuates the alkalosis. Giving the patient an adequate quantity of chloride is critical to reverse this imbalance and allow more sodium to be reabsorbed with chloride in the proximal tubule.[9]

The prototype for chloride-responsive, hypochloremic, hypokalemic metabolic alkalosis is that which occurs from persistent vomiting or prolonged nasogastric suction in the presence of an obstructed pylorus. Unlike vomiting with an open pylorus (involving a loss of gastric, pancreatic, biliary, and intestinal secretions), this entity produces loss of fluid with high chloride and hydrogen ion concentrations in relation to sodium. In addition to a chloride deficit, the accompanying depletion of ECF volume (often marked) stimulates maximal reabsorption of sodium in the distal renal tubule to maintain volume. Since there is less chloride in the glomerular filtrate for reabsorption of sodium in the proximal tubule, more sodium must be reabsorbed in the distal tubule in exchange for hydrogen and potassium. The developing hypokalemia from continued vomiting causes even greater excretion of hydrogen, since less potassium is available for exchange. If hypokalemia is severe enough, the initially alkaline urine becomes acidic (paradoxical aciduria). Treatment involves replacing the ECF volume deficit with isotonic sodium chloride solution and potassium. The provision of chloride allows increased reabsorption of sodium in the proximal tubule, and less sodium is presented to the distal tubule. As the amount of sodium reabsorbed in the distal tubule decreases, the alkalosis begins to resolve as less hydrogen ion is secreted and less bicarbonate is generated. Also, hydrogen secretion is decreased further as hypokalemia is corrected, because more potassium is now available for exchange with sodium. Although severe potassium depletion invariably occurs, volume repletion should be started and satisfactory urinary output obtained before potassium is administered.

Rarely, severe metabolic alkalosis in a patient with pyloric outlet obstruction may be refractory to standard therapy. This is seen most often in patients who also have severe hypochloremia and several liters of nasogastric drainage daily. The infusion of ammonium chloride or arginine hydrochloride has been the usual method of increasing the level of nonvolatile acids in this situation. However, use of the first may produce ammonia toxicity, and the latter solution is no longer available commercially. The use of 0.1 N to 0.2 N hydrochloric acid has proven to be safe and effective therapy for the correction of severe, resistant metabolic alkalosis.[19] A 0.15 N hydrochloric acid solution is prepared by addition of 150 ml. of 1 N hydrochloric acid to 1 liter of isotonic saline or 5% dextrose solution. This is infused into a large vein at a rate of 25 to 50 ml. per hour, and measurements of pH, P_{CO_2}, and serum electrolytes are obtained every 4 to 6 hours. Generally, 1 or 2 liters of solution over a period of 24 hours is sufficient, although one should not hesitate to give additional hydrochloric acid when the need is based on appropriate clinical and laboratory evidence. Temporary control of alkalosis is usually successful, but the pyloric outlet obstruction should be corrected as soon as possible.

Alkalotic patients are invariably hypokalemic, and potassium depletion itself may induce metabolic alkalosis. In the latter instance, potassium lost from body cells is replaced in part by hydrogen, causing ECF alkalosis. The same process occurs in the distal renal tubular cells, so there is less potassium to exchange for sodium; therefore, more hydrogen must be excreted in the urine in exchange for sodium. Conversely, alkalosis affecting both the ICF and ECF compartments increases the urinary loss of potassium. As hydrogen leaves the cell, it is replaced in part by potassium. In the renal tubular cell more potassium than hydrogen is available for exchange with sodium, raising urinary potassium.

Potassium Abnormalities. The normal dietary intake of potassium is approximately 50 to 100 mEq. daily, and in the absence of hypokalemia, most of this is excreted in the urine. Ninety-eight per cent of the potassium in the body is located in the intracellular compartment at a concentration of approximately 150 mEq. per liter, and it is the major cation of intracellular water. Although the total extracellular potassium in a 70-kg. male would approximate only 63 mEq. (4.5 mEq. per liter $\times$ 14 liters), this small amount is critical to cardiac and neuromuscular function. In addition, the turnover rate in the ECF compartment may be extremely rapid.

The intracellular and extracellular distribution of potassium is influenced by many factors. Significant quantities of intracellular potassium are released into the extracellular space in response to severe injury or surgical stress, acidosis, and the catabolic state. A significant rise in serum potassium may occur in these states in the presence of oliguric or anuric renal failure, but dangerous hyperkalemia (greater than 6 mEq. per liter) is rarely encountered if renal function is normal. After severe trauma, however, normal or excessive urinary volumes may not reflect the kidneys' ability to clear solutes or to excrete potassium. (See the later section on high-output renal failure.)

Hyperkalemia. The signs of significant hyperkalemia are limited to the cardiovascular and gastrointestinal systems. The gastrointestinal symptoms include nausea, vomiting, intermittent intestinal colic, and diarrhea. The cardiovascular signs are apparent on the electrocardiogram (ECG) initially, with high peaked T waves, widened QRS complex, and depressed S-T segments. Disappearance of T waves, heart block, and diastolic cardiac arrest may develop with increasing levels of potassium.

Treatment of hyperkalemia consists of immediate measures to reduce the serum potassium level, withholding of exogenously administered potassium, and correction of the underlying cause when possible.[31] Temporary suppression of the myocardial effects of a sudden rapid rise of potassium can be accomplished by intravenous administration of 1 gm. of 10% calcium gluconate under ECG monitoring. Infusion of calcium ions does not affect serum potassium concentration but does counteract the effects of hyperkalemia on cardiac cells by restoring a more normal differential between threshold and resting cellular transmembrane potential. Serum potassium levels may be transiently decreased by administration of bicarbonate and glucose with insulin (45 mEq. $NaHCO_3$ in 1000 ml. of $D_{10}W$ with 20 units regular insulin). The administration of dextrose stimulates insulin release, which augments cellular potassium uptake. Rapid alkalinization of the ECF with either sodium lactate or bicarbonate promotes transfer of potassium into cells; it is particularly valuable when hyperkalemia is partially due to a metabolic acidosis. These maneuvers are temporary and allow time for definitive removal of excess potassium by cation-exchange resins, peritoneal dialysis, or hemodialysis.

Hypokalemia. A more common problem in the surgical patient is hypokalemia, which may occur as a result of excessive renal excretion, movement of potassium into cells, prolonged administration of potassium-free parenteral fluids with continued obligatory renal loss of potassium (more than 20 mEq. per day), parenteral nutrition with inadequate potassium replacement, and loss of gastrointestinal secretions.

Potassium plays an important role in the regulation of acid-base balance. Increased renal excretion occurs with both respiratory and metabolic alkalosis. Potassium competes with hydrogen ion for renal tubular excretion in exchange for sodium ion. Thus, in alkalosis, the increased potassium ion excretion in exchange for sodium ion permits hydrogen ion conservation. Hypokalemia itself may produce a metabolic alkalosis, since an increase in excretion of hydrogen ions occurs when the concentration of potassium in the tubular cells is low. In addition, movement of hydrogen ions into the cells as a consequence of potassium loss is partly responsible for the alkalosis. In metabolic acidosis the reverse process occurs, and the excess hydrogen ion exchanges for sodium with retention of greater amounts of potassium.

Renal tubular excretion of potassium ion is increased when large quantities of sodium are available for excretion. The more sodium ion available for resorption, the more potassium is exchanged for it in the lumen. Potassium requirements for prolonged or massive isotonic fluid volume replacement are increased, probably on this basis. The same mechanism may also explain the increased potassium ion excretion with steroid administration.

The renal excretion of potassium may be small compared with the amount of potassium that can be lost in gastrointestinal secretions. The amount per liter in various types of gastrointestinal fluids is shown in Table 6–9. Although the average potassium concentration of some of these fluids is relatively low, significant hypokalemia results if potassium-free fluids are used for replacement.

Hypokalemia may also be a problem in the patient maintained on intravenous nutrition. Large quantities of supplemental potassium are generally necessary to restore depleted intracellular stores and meet the requirements for tissue synthesis during the anabolic phase.

In summary, most of the factors that influence potassium metabolism produce excess excretion, and a tendency toward hypokalemia occurs frequently in the surgical patient, except when shock or acidosis interferes with the normal renal handling of potassium.

The signs of potassium deficit are related to failure of normal contractility of skeletal, smooth, and cardiac muscle and include weakness that may progress to flaccid paralysis, diminished to absent tendon reflexes, and paralytic ileus. Sensitivity to digitalis with cardiac arrhythmias and ECG signs of low voltage, flattening of T waves, and depression of S-T segments are characteristic. However, signs of potassium deficit may be masked by those of a severe ECF volume deficit. Repletion of the volume deficit may further aggravate the situation by lowering the serum potassium level secondary to dilution.

The treatment of hypokalemia involves, first, prevention of this state. In the replacement of gastrointestinal fluids, it is safe to replace the upper limits of loss, since an excess is readily handled by the patient with normal renal function. No more than 40 mEq. should be added to 1 liter of intravenous fluid, and the rate of administration should not exceed 20 mEq. per hour unless the ECG is being monitored.[10] In the absence of specific indications, potassium should not be

given to an oliguric patient or during the first 24 hours after severe surgical stress or trauma.

Calcium Abnormalities. Most of the 1000 to 1200 gm. of body calcium in the average-sized adult is found in the bone in the form of phosphate and carbonate. Normal daily intake of calcium is between 1 and 3 gm. Most of this is excreted via the gastrointestinal tract, and 200 mg. or less is excreted in the urine daily. The normal serum level is between 8.5 and 10.5 mg. per 100 ml., depending on the individual laboratory's normal range, and approximately half of this is not ionized and is bound to plasma protein. An additional nonionized fraction (5%) is bound to other substances in the plasma and interstitial fluid; the remaining 45% is the ionized portion that is responsible for neuromuscular stability. Determination of the plasma protein level is therefore essential for proper analysis of the serum calcium level. The ratio of ionized to nonionized calcium is also related to the pH: acidosis increases the ionized fraction, whereas alkalosis decreases it.

Disturbances of calcium metabolism are generally not a problem in the uncomplicated postoperative patient, except for skeletal loss during prolonged immobilization. Routine administration of calcium to the surgical patient is therefore not needed in the absence of specific indications.

Hypocalcemia. The symptoms of hypocalcemia (serum level less than 8 mg. per 100 ml.) are numbness and tingling of the circumoral region and the tips of the fingers and toes. The signs are of neuromuscular origin and include hyperactive tendon reflexes, a positive Chvostek sign, muscle and abdominal cramps, tetany with carpopedal spasm, convulsions (with severe deficit), and prolongation of the Q-T interval on the ECG.

The common causes include acute pancreatitis, massive soft tissue infections (necrotizing fasciitis), acute and chronic renal failure, pancreatic and small intestinal fistulas, and hypoparathyroidism. Transient hypocalcemia is a frequent occurrence in the hyperparathyroid patient after removal of a parathyroid adenoma until the remaining parathyroid tissue resumes normal hormone secretion. Severe postoperative hypocalcemia is likely if marked bone resorption was present preoperatively or if the normal parathyroid glands were injured during surgery. Asymptomatic hypocalcemia may occur with hypoproteinemia (normal ionized fraction), whereas symptoms may appear with a normal serum calcium level in a patient with severe alkalosis. The latter is due to a decrease in the physiologically active or ionized fraction of total serum calcium. Calcium levels may also fall with a severe depletion of magnesium.

Treatment is aimed at correction of the underlying cause with concomitant repletion of the deficit. Acute symptoms may be relieved by intravenous administration of calcium gluconate or calcium chloride. Calcium lactate may be given orally, with or without supplemental vitamin D, in a patient requiring prolonged replacement.

Routine administration of calcium during massive transfusions of blood remains controversial. Most patients receiving blood transfusions do not require calcium supplementation.[8] The binding of ionized calcium by citrate is generally compensated for by the mobilization of calcium from body stores. However, for patients receiving massive transfusion, calcium administration may be indicated. Intravenous bolus therapy of 300 to 1000 mg. may be given in patients who have rapidly received more than 10 units of blood.[29] During massive transfusions, some attempt should be made to monitor the calcium level. A rough approximation of calcium ion concentration can be obtained by monitoring the Q-T interval on the ECG, although techniques for rapid measurement of the ionized calcium concentration are now available.

Hypercalcemia. The symptoms of hypercalcemia are rather

TABLE 6–9. Composition of Gastrointestinal Secretions

	Volume (ml./24 hr.)	Na (mEq./L.)	K (mEq./L.)	Cl (mEq./L.)	HCO₃ (mEq./L.)
Salivary	1500 (500–2000)	10 (2–10)	26 (20–30)	10 (8–18)	30
Stomach	1500 (100–4000)	60 (9–116)	10 (0–32)	130 (8–154)	—
Duodenum	(100–2000)	140	5	80	—
Ileum	3000 (100–9000)	140 (80–150)	5 (2–8)	104 (43–137)	30
Colon	—	60	30	40	—
Pancreas	(100–800)	140 (113–185)	5 (3–7)	75 (54–95)	115
Bile	(50–800)	145 (131–164)	5 (3–12)	100 (89–180)	35

vague and of gastrointestinal, renal, musculoskeletal, and CNS origin. The early manifestations of hypercalcemia include easy fatigue, lassitude, weakness of varying degree, anorexia, nausea, vomiting, and weight loss. With higher serum calcium levels, lassitude gives way to somnambulism, stupor, and finally coma. Other symptoms include severe headaches, pains in the back and extremities, thirst, polydipsia, and polyuria. The critical level for serum calcium is between 16 and 20 mg. per 100 ml., and unless treatment is instituted promptly, the symptoms may rapidly progress to death. The two major causes of hypercalcemia are hyperparathyroidism and cancer with bony metastasis. The latter is most frequently seen in a patient with metastatic breast cancer.

A serum calcium concentration of 15 mg. per 100 ml. or higher requires emergency treatment. Most patients have an ECF volume deficit due to the effects of hypercalcemia (vomiting, polyuria), and vigorous volume repletion with salt solutions lowers the calcium level by dilution and increased urinary calcium excretion. Concomitant use of large doses of intravenous furosemide has been recommended to increase urinary calcium excretion, but careful monitoring and replacement of resultant losses of fluids and electrolytes are necessary.

Oral or intravenous inorganic phosphates effectively lower serum calcium levels by inhibiting bone resorption and forming calcium-phosphate complexes that are deposited in soft tissues and bone. However, intravenous use may cause an abrupt fall in calcium, and tetany, hypotension, and acute renal failure have been reported with this form of therapy. If used, intravenous phosphorus should be given slowly over a period of approximately 12 hours once daily for no more than 2 or 3 days. Inorganic phosphates are contraindicated in patients with hyperphosphatemia or renal failure. Intravenous sodium sulfate also lowers serum calcium by increasing urinary excretion of this ion. It is less effective than phosphate salts, however, and is probably no more effective than normal saline.

Corticosteroids decrease resorption of calcium from bone and reduce the intestinal absorption of vitamin D. They have been found useful for treating hypercalcemic patients with sarcoidosis, myelomas, lymphomas, and leukemias, although the reduction in serum calcium may not be apparent for 1 or 2 weeks. Plicamycin, a cytotoxic drug, effectively lowers serum calcium in 24 to 48 hours by direct action on the bones. The drug is relatively safe in the small doses used, and the calcium level may remain normal for several days to weeks after a single dose. Calcitonin induces a moderate decrease in serum calcium, but the effect is diminished with repeated administration. Prompt surgery remains the definitive treatment of acute hypercalcemic crisis in patients with hyperparathyroidism.

Treatment of hypercalcemia in a patient with metastatic cancer is primarily that of prevention. The serum calcium level is checked frequently; if it is elevated, the patient is placed on a low-calcium diet, and measures to ensure adequate hydration are instituted.

Magnesium Abnormalities. The total body content of magnesium in the average adult is approximately 2000 mEq., about half of which is incorporated in bone and only slowly exchangeable. The distribution of magnesium is similar to that of potassium, the major portion being intracellular. Serum magnesium concentration normally ranges between 1.5 and 2.5 mEq. per liter. The normal dietary intake of magnesium is approximately 20 mEq. (240 mg.) daily. The larger part is excreted in the feces and the remainder in the urine. The kidneys have a remarkable ability to conserve magnesium; on a magnesium-free diet, renal excretion of this ion may be less than 1 mEq. per day.

Magnesium Deficiency. Magnesium deficiency is known to occur with starvation, malabsorption syndromes, protracted losses of gastrointestinal fluid, prolonged parenteral fluid therapy with magnesium-free solutions, and parenteral nutrition when inadequate quantities of magnesium have been added to the solution. Other causes include acute pancreatitis, diabetic acidosis during treatment, primary aldosteronism, and chronic alcoholism.

The magnesium ion is essential for proper function of most enzyme systems, and depletion is characterized by neuromuscular and CNS hyperactivity. The signs and symptoms are quite similar to those of calcium deficiency, including hyperactive tendon reflexes, muscle tremors, and tetany with a positive Chvostek sign. Progression to delirium and convulsions may occur with a severe deficit. A concomitant calcium deficiency is occasionally noted and is refractory to treatment in the absence of magnesium repletion.

The diagnosis of magnesium deficiency depends on an awareness of the syndrome and clinical recognition of the symptoms. Laboratory confirmation is available but not reliable, because the syndrome may exist in the presence of a normal serum magnesium level. The possibility of magnesium deficiency should always be considered in a surgical patient who exhibits disturbed neuromuscular or cerebral activity in the postoperative period. This is particularly important in patients who have had protracted dysfunction of the gastrointestinal tract with long-term maintenance on parenteral fluids, and in patients on total parenteral nutrition. Routine administration of magnesium is always indicated in the management of these patients.

Treatment of magnesium deficiency is usually by parenteral administration of magnesium sulfate or magnesium chloride solution. In asymptomatic patients, oral replacement is an option. If renal function is normal, as much as 2 mEq. of magnesium per kg. of body weight can be administered in a day in the face of severe depletion. Magnesium sulfate (50% solution contains approximately 4 mEq. of magnesium ion per ml.) may be given intravenously or intramuscularly. The intravenous route is preferable for the initial treatment of a severe symptomatic deficit. This can be accomplished by infusion of 600 mg. of elemental magnesium administered over a 3-hour period.[21] The possibility of acute magnesium toxicity should be kept in mind when giving this ion intravenously. When large doses are given, the heart rate, blood pressure, respiration, and ECG should be monitored closely for signs of magnesium toxicity, which could lead to cardiac arrest. It is advisable to have calcium chloride or calcium gluconate available to counteract any adverse effects of a rapidly rising serum magnesium level.

Partial or complete relief of symptoms may follow this infusion as a result of increased concentration of magnesium ion in the ECF compartment, although continued replacement over a 1- to 3-week period is necessary to replenish the ICF compartment. For this purpose and for an asymptomatic patient who is likely to have significant magnesium depletion, 10 to 20 mEq. of 50% magnesium sulfate solution is given daily by the intramuscular route or in infusion fluids. When magnesium sulfate is used, it should be given in divided doses or at multiple sites, since the intramuscular injection of this salt is painful. After complete repletion of intracellular magnesium and in the absence of abnormal loss, balance may be maintained by administration of as little as 300 mg. of magnesium daily.[23]

Magnesium should not be given to an oliguric patient or in the presence of severe volume deficit unless there is actual magnesium depletion. If magnesium is given to a patient with renal insufficiency, considerably smaller doses are used, and the patient is carefully observed for signs or symptoms of toxicity.

Magnesium Excess. Symptomatic hypermagnesemia, although rare, is most commonly seen with severe renal insufficiency. Retention and accumulation of magnesium may occur in any patient with impaired glomerular or renal tubular function, and the presence of acidosis may rapidly compound the situation. Serum magnesium levels tend to parallel changes in potassium concentration in these cases. Therefore, magnesium levels should be carefully monitored in patients with acute and chronic renal failure and in selected patients with borderline renal function. Magnesium-containing antacids and laxatives may be administered in quantities sufficient to produce toxic serum levels of magnesium in patients with impaired renal function. Other conditions that may be associated with symptomatic hypermagnesemia include early-stage burns, massive trauma or surgical stress, severe ECF volume deficit, and severe acidosis.

The early signs and symptoms include lethargy and weakness with progressive loss of deep tendon reflexes. Interference with cardiac conduction occurs with increasing levels of magnesium, and ECG changes (increased P-R interval, widened QRS complex, and elevated T waves) resemble those seen with hyperkalemia. Somnolence leading to coma and muscular paralysis occurs in the later stages, and death is usually caused by respiratory or cardiac arrest.

Treatment consists of immediate measures to lower the serum magnesium level by correcting any acidosis, replenishing any preexisting ECF volume deficit, and withholding exogenously administered magnesium. Acute symptoms may be temporarily controlled by slow intravenous administration of 5 to 10 mEq. of calcium chloride or calcium gluconate. If elevated levels or symptoms persist, peritoneal dialysis or hemodialysis is indicated.

NORMAL EXCHANGE OF FLUID AND ELECTROLYTES

Knowledge of the basic principles governing both the internal and the external exchanges of water and salt is mandatory for care of the patient undergoing major operative surgery. The stable internal fluid environment, which is maintained by the kidneys, brain, lungs, skin, and gastrointestinal tract, may be compromised by severe surgical stress or direct damage to any of these organs.

Water Exchange

The normal individual consumes an average of 2000 to 2500 ml. of water per day; approximately 1500 ml. of water is taken by mouth, and the rest is extracted from solid food, either from the contents of food or as the product of oxidation (Table 6–10). The daily water losses include 250 ml. in stools, 800 to 1500 ml. as urine, and approximately 600 to 900 ml. as insensible loss. A patient deprived of all external access to water must still excrete a minimum of 500 to 800 ml. of urine per day in order to excrete the products of catabolism, in addition to the mandatory insensible loss through the skin and lungs.

Insensible loss of water occurs through the skin (75%) and the lungs (25%) and is increased by hypermetabolism, hyperventilation, and fever. The insensible water loss through the skin occurs not from evaporation of water from sweat glands but from water vapor formed within the body and lost through the skin. With excessive heat production (or excessive environmental heat), the capacity for insensible loss through the skin is exceeded, and sweating occurs. These losses may, but seldom do, exceed 250 ml. per day per degree of fever. An unhumidified tracheostomy with hyperventilation increases the loss through the lungs and produces a total insensible loss up to 1.5 liters per day.

TABLE 6–10. Water Exchange (60- to 80-kg. Man)

	Average Daily Volume (ml.)	Minimal (ml.)	Maximal (ml.)
H_2O Gain—Routes			
Sensible			
Oral fluids	800–1500	0	1500/hr.
Solid foods	500–700	0	1500
Insensible			
Water of oxidation	250	125	800
Water of solution	0	0	500
H_2O Loss—Routes			
Sensible			
Urine	800–1500	300	1400/hr. (diabetes insipidus)
Intestinal	0–250	0	2500/hr.
Sweat	0	0	4000/hr.
Insensible			
Lungs and skin	600–900	600–900	1500

A frequently overlooked source of gain is the *water of solution*, which is another name for cell water. Normally, gain of water from this source is zero, but after 4 to 5 days without food intake a patient may begin to gain significant quantities of water (maximum 500 ml. daily) from excessive cell catabolism and release of its water. The amount depends on the degree of trauma and the complications occurring postoperatively.

Salt Gain and Losses

In a normal individual the daily salt intake varies between 50 and 90 mEq. (3 to 5 gm.) as sodium chloride (Table 6–11). Balance is maintained primarily by the kidneys, which excrete the excess salt. Under conditions of reduced intake or extrarenal losses, normal kidneys can reduce sodium excretion to less than 1 mEq. per day within 24 hours after restriction. In a patient with salt-wasting kidneys, however, the loss may exceed 100 mEq. per liter of urine. Sweat represents a hypotonic loss of fluids with an average sodium concentration of 15 mEq. per liter in an acclimatized patient. In an unacclimatized individual the sodium concentration in sweat may be 60 mEq. per liter or more. Insensible fluid lost from the skin and lungs, by definition, is pure water. For practical considerations, then, normal losses may be relatively free of salt in the healthy individual with normal renal function.

The volume and composition of various types of gastrointestinal secretions are shown in Table 6–9. Gastrointestinal losses are usually isotonic, although there is considerable variation in their compositions. These should be replaced by isotonic salt solutions. It is also important to reiterate that

TABLE 6–11. Sodium (Salt) Exchange (60- to 80-kg. Man)

Sodium Exchange	Average	Minimal	Maximal
Sodium Gain			
Diet	50–90 mEq./day	0	75–100 mEq./hr. (oral)
Sodium Loss			
Skin (sweat)	10–60 mEq./day*	0	300 mEq./hr.
Urine	10–80 mEq./day	<1 mEq./day†	110–200 mEq./L.‡
Intestine	0–20 mEq./day	0	300 mEq./hr.

*Depending on the degree of acclimatization of the individual.
†With normal renal function.
‡With renal salt wasting.

distributional or sequestration losses of ECF at any point in the operative or postoperative course also represent isotonic losses of salt and water.

FLUID AND ELECTROLYTE THERAPY

Parenteral Solutions

The composition of various parenteral fluids is shown in Table 6–12. There is sufficient variety to satisfy most fluid requirements in the surgical patient. The proper choice of parenteral fluid in a given situation corrects the abnormalities but imposes minimal demands on the kidneys.

A good available isotonic salt solution for replacing gastrointestinal losses and ECF volume deficits, in the absence of gross abnormalities of concentration and composition, is lactated Ringer's solution. This solution is *physiologic* and contains 130 mEq. of sodium balanced by 109 mEq. of chloride and 28 mEq. of lactate. Lactate is used instead of bicarbonate, since the former is more stable in intravenous fluids during storage. The lactate is readily converted to bicarbonate by the liver after infusion. Concern about the liver's ability to metabolize lactate is unwarranted even when large quantities of lactated Ringer's solution are infused into patients in hemorrhagic shock.[6] This fluid has minimal effects on normal body fluid composition and pH even when infused in large quantities. Other balanced salt solutions are available, some with sodium acetate or bicarbonate instead of lactate; all are considered interchangeable.

The other solutions listed in Table 6–12 are used to correct specific deficits. Choice of a particular fluid depends on the volume status of the patient and the type of concentration or compositional abnormality present.

Isotonic sodium chloride contains 154 mEq. of sodium and 154 mEq. of chloride per liter. The high concentration of chloride above the normal serum concentration of 103 mEq. per liter imposes on the kidneys an appreciable load of excess chloride that cannot be rapidly excreted. Thus, a dilutional acidosis may develop.* This solution is ideal, however, for the initial correction of an ECF volume deficit in the presence of hyponatremia, hypochloremia, and metabolic alkalosis.

A frequent choice for maintenance fluid in the postoperative period, 0.45% sodium chloride in 5% dextrose solution provides free water for insensible losses and some sodium for renal adjustment of serum concentration. With added potassium, this is a reasonable solution to use for maintenance requirements in an uncomplicated patient requiring only a short period of parenteral fluids.

A 5% sodium chloride solution may be used to correct symptomatic hyponatremic states. After correction of concentration and compositional abnormalities by use of specific

---

*Infusion of a large volume of isotonic sodium chloride solution may induce or aggravate an existing acidosis by reducing the amount of base bicarbonate in the body relative to the carbonic acid content.[24]

electrolyte solutions, a balanced salt solution is given to replenish the remaining volume deficit.

Preoperative Fluid Therapy

Preoperative evaluation and correction of existing fluid disorders are integral parts of surgical care. An orderly approach to these problems requires both an understanding of the common fluid disturbances associated with surgical illness and adherence to a few simple guidelines. There are no shortcuts; close observation of the patient and frequent reevaluation of the clinical situation are the most rewarding approaches.

The analysis of a fluid disorder may be facilitated by categorizing the abnormalities into volume, concentration, and compositional changes. Although some disease states produce characteristic changes in fluid balance, much confusion may be avoided by regarding each disturbance as a separate entity. For example, volume changes cannot be accurately predicted from a knowledge of the level of serum sodium, since an ECF volume deficit or excess may exist with a normal, low, or high sodium concentration. Similarly, any of the four primary acid-base disturbances may be associated with any combination of volume and concentration abnormalities.

Correction of Volume Changes. Changes in the volume of ECF are the most frequent and important abnormalities encountered in the surgical patient. Depletion of the ECF compartment without changes in concentration or composition is a common problem. The diagnosis of volume changes is made almost entirely on clinical grounds. The signs present in an individual patient depend not only on the relative or absolute quantity of ECF that has been lost but also on the rapidity with which it is lost and the presence or absence of signs of associated disease.

Volume deficit in the surgical patient may result from external loss of fluids or from an internal redistribution of ECF into nonfunctional compartments. Often, it involves a combination of the two, but the internal redistribution is frequently overlooked.

The phenomenon of internal redistribution or translocation of ECF is peculiar to many surgical diseases; in the individual patient, the loss may be quite large. Although the concept of a third space is not new, it is generally considered only in relation to patients with massive ascites, burns, or crush injuries. Of more importance, however, is the third-space loss into the peritoneum, the bowel wall, and other tissues associated with inflammatory lesions of the intra-abdominal organs. The magnitude of these losses may not be fully appreciated without realizing that the peritoneum alone has approximately 1 sq. meter of surface area. A slight increase in thickness from sequestration of fluid, which would not be appreciated on casual observation, may cause a functional loss of several liters of fluid. Swelling of the bowel wall and mesentery and secretion of fluid into the lumen of the bowel will cause even larger losses. Similar deficits may occur with massive infection of the subcutaneous tissues (necrotizing fasciitis) or with severe crush injury.

These *parasitic* losses remain a part of the ECF space and may be measured as a slowly equilibrating volume. The term *nonfunctional* is used because the fluid is no longer able to participate in the normal functions of the ECF compartment and may just as well have been lost externally. Any transfer of ICF to the ECF compartment for replenishment of the loss is insignificant. The patient with ascites may have an enormous total ECF volume even though the functional component is severely depleted. The same is true of extensive inflammatory or obstructive lesions of the gastrointestinal tract, although the loss is not as obvious. These losses evoke

---

TABLE 6–12. Composition of Parenteral Fluids: Electrolyte Content (mEq./L.)

Solution	Cations				Anions	
	Na	K	Ca	Mg	Cl	HCO$_3^-$
Extracellular fluid	142	4	5	3	103	27
Lactated Ringer's	130	4	2.7		109	28*
0.9% sodium chloride (saline)	154				154	
D$_5$/0.45% sodium chloride	77				77	

*Present in solution as lactate, which is converted to bicarbonate.

the signs and symptoms of an ECF volume deficit with or without concomitant external loss of fluids.

Exact quantification of these deficits is impossible. The defect can be estimated on the basis of the severity of the clinical signs. A mild deficit represents a loss of approximately 4% of body weight (e.g., 70 kg. × 0.04 = 2.8 liter deficit); a moderate deficit, a loss of 6% to 8% of body weight; and a severe deficit, a loss of approximately 10% of body weight. It is important to emphasize that cardiovascular signs predominate when there is acute rapid loss of fluid from the ECF compartment with few or no tissue signs. In addition to the estimated deficit, fluids lost during the period of treatment must be replaced.

Fluid replacement should be started and changed according to the response of the patient as noted on frequent clinical observation. Reliance on a formula or single clinical sign to determine the adequacy of resuscitation is unwise. Rather, reversal of the signs of the volume deficit, stabilization of the blood pressure and pulse, and an hourly urinary volume of 30 to 50 ml. are used as general guidelines. However, an adequate hourly urinary output, although usually a reliable monitor for volume replacement, may be totally misleading. For example, excessive administration of glucose (over 50 gm. in a 2- to 3-hour period) may cause osmotic diuresis, while an osmotic agent such as mannitol will produce urine at the expense of the vascular volume. Patients with chronic renal disease or incipient acute renal damage from shock and injury may also have inappropriately high urinary volumes. Also, rapid administration of salt solutions may transiently expand the intravascular volume, increase the GFR, and produce an immediate outpouring of urine, although the total ECF space remains quite depleted.

The choice of a proper fluid for replacement depends on the existence of concomitant concentration or compositional abnormalities. With pure ECF volume loss or when only minimal concentrations or compositional abnormalities are present, the use of a balanced salt solution is desirable.

Rate of Fluid Administration. This rate varies considerably, depending on the severity and type of fluid disturbance, the presence of continuing losses, and the cardiac status. In general, the most severe volume deficits may be safely replaced initially with isotonic solutions at a rate of 1000 ml. per hour, reducing the rate as the fluid status improves. Constant observation by a physician is mandatory when administration exceeds 1000 ml. per hour. At these rates, however, a significant portion may be lost as urinary output owing to a transient overexpansion of the plasma volume.

In elderly patients, associated cardiovascular disorders do not preclude correction of existing volume deficits, but they do require slower, more careful correction with appropriate monitoring, including the central venous or pulmonary artery and wedge pressures.

Correction of Concentration Changes. If severe *symptomatic* hyponatremia or hypernatremia complicates the volume loss, prompt correction of the concentration abnormality to the extent that symptoms are relieved is the first step. Volume replenishment should then be accomplished, with slower correction of the remaining concentration abnormality. For immediate correction of severe symptomatic hyponatremia, a 5% sodium chloride solution is used. The sodium deficit can be estimated by multiplying the decrease in serum sodium concentration below normal (in milliequivalents per liter) times the liters of total body water. Total body water averages 60% of body weight in young adult males and 50% in young adult females.

Example: A 24-year-old woman with symptomatic hyponatremia, weight = 60 kg., serum sodium = 120 mEq. per liter:

Total body water = 60 kg. × 0.50 = 30 liters
Sodium deficit = (140 − 120 mEq. per liter) × 30 liters = 600 mEq.

Note that this estimate is based on total body water, since the effective osmotic pressure in the ECF compartment cannot be increased without increasing this fraction proportionally in the ICF compartment. Although absolute reliance on any formula is undesirable, proper use of this estimate will allow a safe quantitative approximation of the sodium deficit. Generally, only a portion of the total deficit is replaced initially to relieve acute symptoms. Further correction is facilitated when renal function is restored by correction of the volume deficit. If the total calculated deficit is given rapidly, symptomatic hypervolemia may occur, particularly in patients with limited cardiac reserve. Of more importance, central pontine and extrapontine myelinolysis may occur during *rapid* correction of hyponatremia and cause irreversible CNS damage or death.[14] It is recommended, therefore, that the serum sodium level not be increased more than 12 mEq. per liter during the first 24 hours and even less during each subsequent 24-hour period. In practice, the infusion of small, successive increments of hypertonic saline solution with frequent evaluation of the clinical response and serum sodium concentration is recommended.

In the treatment of moderate hyponatremia with an associated volume deficit, volume replacement can be started immediately with concomitant correction of the serum sodium deficit. Isotonic sodium chloride solution (normal saline) is used initially in the presence of metabolic alkalosis, whereas M/6 sodium lactate is used to correct an associated acidosis. Only a few liters of these solutions may be necessary to correct the serum sodium concentration; the remainder of the volume deficit can be repaired with a balanced salt solution.

Treatment of hyponatremia associated with volume excess is by restriction of water. In the presence of severe symptomatic hyponatremia, a small amount of hypertonic salt solution may be infused cautiously to alleviate symptoms. Because this will cause additional volume expansion, it is contraindicated in patients with limited cardiac reserve; peritoneal dialysis or hemodialysis is preferred in this situation.

For the correction of severe, symptomatic hypernatremia with an associated volume deficit, 5% dextrose in water may be infused slowly until symptoms are relieved. If the extracellular osmolarity is reduced too rapidly, however, convulsions and coma may result. For this reason, initial correction of hypernatremia concomitant with repletion of the volume deficit by balanced salt solution is safer in most cases.[18] In the absence of a significant volume deficit, water should be administered cautiously, since hypervolemia may result; constant observation and frequent determinations of the serum sodium concentration are indicated. The problem is somewhat simplified once a sufficient quantity of fluid has been given to permit renal excretion of the solute load.

Composition and Miscellaneous Considerations. Correction of potassium deficits should be started *after* an adequate urinary output is obtained. The concentration of potassium chloride should not exceed 40 mEq. per liter of intravenous fluids, with rare exceptions, such as the treatment of digitalis intoxication, during which the ECG must be monitored. Calcium and magnesium are rarely needed during preoperative resuscitation but should be given if indicated, particularly to patients with massive subcutaneous infections, those with acute pancreatitis, and those who have been chronically starved.

Fluid abnormalities also must be suspected in the patient for whom an elective procedure is planned. Chronic illnesses are frequently associated with ECF volume deficits, and concentration and compositional changes are not uncommon. Correction of anemia and recognition of the fact that a contracted blood volume may exist in the chronically debilitated patient are of obvious importance.

Of equal importance is the prevention of volume depletion

during the preoperative period. Prolonged periods of fluid restriction in preparation for various diagnostic procedures, the use of cathartics and enemas to prepare the bowel, and osmotic diuresis from contrast agents may cause a significant acute loss of ECF. Prompt recognition and treatment of these losses are necessary to prevent complications during the operative procedure.

Intraoperative Management of Fluids

If preoperative replacement of ECF volume has been incomplete, hypotension may develop promptly with the induction of anesthesia. This can be insidious, because the ability of the awake patient to compensate for a mild volume deficit is revealed only when compensatory mechanisms are abolished with anesthesia. This problem is prevented by maintaining baseline requirements and replacing abnormal losses of fluids and electrolytes by intravenous infusions in the preoperative period.

Blood lost during the operative procedure should be replaced steadily. It is usually unnecessary to replace blood loss of less than 500 ml. (even more in young, healthy patients), but after the loss has exceeded this amount, replacement may be required. The warnings against the use of a single transfusion during operation have been somewhat confusing. There may be a definite need for a single-unit transfusion in the patient who loses between 500 and 1000 ml. of blood during operation.

In addition to blood losses during operation, there are ECF losses during major operative procedures. Some of these, including edema from extensive dissection, fluid collections within the lumen and the wall of the small bowel, and accumulations of fluid in the peritoneal cavity, are clinically discernible and well recognized. They are generally thought to represent distributional shifts, in that the functional volume of ECF is reduced but not externally lost from the body. These functional losses are often referred to as *a parasitic loss of extracellular fluid, third-space edema,* or *sequestration* of ECF. Another source of ECF loss during major operative trauma is the wound itself. This is a relatively small loss that is difficult to quantify except in extensive operative procedures.

At the beginning of this century, surgeons became aware that many changes occurred in urinary output, blood volume, and fluid and electrolyte composition during and after surgery. Assessment of these changes, however, awaited the development of analytic techniques and their application to patient studies. In the following 25 years, saline solutions in varying combinations were given to patients undergoing operation, often in excessive amounts. Work in the late 1930s and early 1940s by Moyer and others indicated that during and after operative procedures, saline and water solutions should be withheld entirely because most of the fluid administered is retained.[15]

The possibility existed, however, that the operative and postoperative retention of salt and water might simply be physiologic retention to replace a deficit of salt and water incurred by the operative procedure.[32] Subsequent studies revealed that functional ECF decreases with major abdominal operations, largely as a sequestered loss into the operative site.[20, 25, 26] Intraoperative correction of this volume deficit with a balanced salt solution eliminates *postoperative salt intolerance.* Salt solution is not intended to be a substitute for blood replacement; rather, it is to replace the ECF volume deficit.

Thus, the pendulum swung from indiscriminate use of salt solutions in the first quarter of this century to almost total withholding of fluids and electrolytes from surgical patients in the second quarter of the century; proper management lies somewhere between these two extremes. Some guidelines are necessary, since exact quantification of the deficit is not possible. The amount of lost or sequestered ECF directly correlates with the amount of operative trauma: e.g., only a few hundred milliliters during a 1-hour cholecystectomy in a thin patient compared with several liters during a prolonged and difficult low anterior colon resection in an obese person. The loss is also directly related to the amount of surface area of the traumatized tissues. Characteristically, the largest losses occur during intra-abdominal surgical procedures because of the extensive surface area of the peritoneum, bowel, mesentery, and so on. Smaller losses are incurred during thoracic and orthopedic procedures, because fluid is sequestered primarily into retracted muscle and subcutaneous tissues. Losses during head and neck surgery are negligible.

Some arbitrary but clinically useful guidelines follow: (1) blood should be replaced as lost, regardless of any additional fluid and electrolyte therapy; (2) the replacement of ECF should begin during the operative procedure; and (3) balanced salt solution needed during operation is approximately 0.5 to 1 liter per hour, but only to a maximum of 2 to 3 liters during a 4-hour major abdominal procedure, unless there are other measurable losses.

The use of albumin solutions, in addition to balanced salt solutions, to replace ECF deficits incurred during surgery, is not only unnecessary but potentially harmful. Measurements of cardiac function and extravascular lung water indicate optimal function after replacement of blood loss and the administration of balanced salt solution without the addition of albumin.[27]

In summary, the replacement of ECF deficits during surgery with an appropriate volume of balanced salt solution, in addition to blood replacement, has markedly improved the ability to maintain intraoperative homeostasis and avoid organ injury associated with inadequate volume replacement.

Postoperative Management of Fluids

Immediate Postoperative Period. Orders for postoperative fluids are not written until the patient is in the recovery room and the fluid status has been assessed. Evaluation at this point should include a review of preoperative fluid status, the amount of fluid loss and gain during operation, and clinical examination of the patient with assessment of vital signs and urinary output. Initial fluid orders are written to correct any existing deficit, followed with maintenance fluids for the remainder of the day. For a patient with complications who has received or lost large amounts of fluid, it is frequently difficult to estimate the fluid requirements for the ensuing 24 hours. In this situation, intravenous fluids are ordered 1 liter at a time, and the patient is checked frequently until the situation is clarified. Proper replacement of fluids during this relatively short period facilitates subsequent fluid management.

After operation, sequestration of ECF into the sites of injury or operative trauma may continue for 12 hours or more. Unrecognized deficits of ECF volume during the early postoperative period are not uncommon and are manifested primarily as circulatory instability. Evaluation of the level of consciousness, pupillary size, airway patency, breathing patterns, pulse rate and volume, skin warmth, color, body temperature, and a 30- to 50-ml. hourly urinary output, combined with critical review of the operative procedure and the operative fluid management, is usually rewarding. In addition, several liters of extravascular ECF can be sequestered in areas of injury and manifested only by oliguria and mild depression of the blood pressure with a rapid pulse. For a patient with circulatory instability, further volume replacement of an additional 1000 ml. of balanced salt solution, while it is determined whether continuing losses or other causes are present, often resolves the problem.

It is unnecessary and probably unwise to administer potassium during the first 24 hours postoperatively, unless a definite potassium deficit exists. This is particularly important for a patient subjected to prolonged operative trauma involving one or more episodes of hypotension and for a posttraumatic patient with hemorrhagic hypotension. Oliguric renal failure or the more insidious high-output renal failure may develop, and administration of even a small quantity of potassium may be detrimental.

Late Postoperative Period. The problem of volume management during the postoperative convalescent phase is one of accurate measurement and replacement of all losses. In an otherwise healthy individual, this involves replacement of measured sensible losses, which are generally of gastrointestinal origin, and estimation and replacement of insensible losses.

The insensible loss is usually relatively constant and averages 600 to 900 ml. daily. This may be increased by hypermetabolism, hyperventilation, and fever to a maximum of approximately 1500 ml. daily. The estimated insensible loss is replaced with 5% dextrose in water. This loss may be partially offset by an insensible gain of water from excessive tissue catabolism in the postoperative patient with complications, particularly if these are associated with oliguric renal failure.

Approximately 1 liter of fluid should be given to replace that volume of urine required to excrete the catabolic end products of metabolism (800 to 1000 ml. per day). In an individual with normal renal function, this may be given as 5% dextrose in water, since the kidneys are able to conserve sodium, with excretion of less than 1 mEq. daily. It is probably unnecessary to stress the kidneys to this degree, however, and a small amount of salt solution may be given in addition to water to cover urinary loss. In an elderly patient with salt-losing kidneys or in patients with head injuries, an insidious hyponatremia may develop if urinary losses are replaced with water. Urinary sodium in these circumstances may exceed 100 mEq. per liter and create a daily loss of significant amounts of sodium. Measurement of urinary sodium facilitates accurate replacement. Urinary volume is not replaced on a milliliter-for-milliliter basis. A urinary output of 2000 to 3000 ml. on a given day may simply represent diuresis of fluids given during operation or may result from excessive fluid administration. If these large losses are completely replaced, the urinary output will progressively increase.

Sensible losses, by definition, can be measured or, as in the case of sweating, estimated. Gastrointestinal losses are usually isotonic or slightly hypotonic, and are replaced with an essentially isotonic salt solution. When the estimated loss is slightly above or below isotonicity, appropriate corrections can be made in the daily water administration, while isotonic salt solutions are used to replace these losses volume for volume. Sweating is not usually a problem except in the febrile patient in whom losses may, but seldom do, exceed 250 ml. per day per degree of fever. Excessive sweating may also represent a considerable loss of sodium in an unacclimatized individual.

Determination of serum electrolyte levels is generally unnecessary in a patient with an uncomplicated postoperative course maintained on parenteral fluids for 2 to 3 days. A more prolonged period of parenteral replacement or one complicated by excessive fluid losses requires frequent determinations of serum sodium, potassium, and chloride levels and CO_2 combining power. Adjustments can then be made with intravenous fluids of appropriate composition. For example, gastrointestinal losses should be replaced with isotonic sodium chloride solution in a patient with hypona-

tremia, hypochloremia, and mild metabolic alkalosis, and this should be continued until these abnormalities are corrected. In a hyponatremic patient with obvious volume overload, the amount of free water given is restricted. In the presence of hyponatremia and mild metabolic acidosis, lactated Ringer's solution with added sodium bicarbonate may be used. In this way, severe concentration and compositional changes can be avoided while an adequate ECF volume is maintained by appropriate maintenance fluids.

Maintenance fluids are administered at a steady rate over an 18- to 24-hour period as the losses are incurred. If given over a shorter period, renal excretion of the excess salt and water may occur while the normal losses continue over the full 24-hour period. For the same reason, fluids of different composition are alternated, and additives to intravenous fluids are evenly distributed in the total volume of fluid given.

In summary, daily fluid orders should begin with an assessment of the patient's volume status and a check for possible concentration or compositional disorders as reflected by proper laboratory determinations. All measured and insensible losses are replaced with fluids of appropriate composition, allowing for any preexisting deficit or excess. The amount of potassium replacement is 40 mEq. daily for baseline renal excretion of potassium, in addition to approximately 20 mEq. per liter for replacement of gastrointestinal losses. Inadequate replacement may prolong the usual postoperative ileus and contribute to the insidious development of a resistant metabolic alkalosis. Calcium and magnesium are replaced when needed, as previously discussed.

Special Considerations in the Postoperative Patient

Volume Excess. Administration of isotonic salt solutions in excess of volume losses (external or internal) may cause overexpansion of the ECF space. An otherwise normal person in a postoperative state tolerates an acute overexpansion extremely well. Excesses administered over a period of several days, however, will soon exceed the kidney's ability to excrete sodium; since water losses continue, hypernatremia may ensue. Therefore, it is important to determine as accurately as possible from intake and output records and serum sodium concentrations the actual needs of the patient managed over several postoperative days. Attention to the signs and symptoms of overload usually prevents this fluid abnormality. It arises most frequently with attempts to meet excessive volume losses that are not measurable, such as those occurring from incompletely controlled fistula drainage.

The earliest sign is a weight gain (when measurable) during the catabolic period, when the patient should be losing ¼ to ½ pound per day. Heavy eyelids, hoarseness, or dyspnea on exertion may rapidly appear. Circulatory and pulmonary signs of overload appear late and represent a rather massive overload. Peripheral edema may be a sign, but it does not necessarily indicate an excess of *functional* ECF volume. Without additional evidence of volume overload, other causes of peripheral edema should be considered. Of particular importance is the fact that overexpansion of the *total* ECF may coexist with *depletion* of the functional ECF compartment (e.g., in a patient with ascites). Central venous pressure measurements may be helpful during volume replacement but may be misleading: a rapid rise may indicate an excessive rate of fluid administration or primary pump failure, but it may not accurately establish volume status. Measurement of pulmonary wedge pressure is a more sensitive indicator of volume status.

Hyponatremia. Significant postoperative alterations in serum sodium concentration are not frequently observed if the fluid resuscitation during operation has included adequate volumes of isotonic salt solutions. The kidneys retain the ability to excrete moderate excesses of salt water administered in the early postoperative period if functional ECF has been adequately replaced during the operative or immediate postoperative period. Previous studies of sodium balance have revealed that patients do excrete sodium after the functional deficit incurred by the shift of ECF has been replaced. Thus, the commonly described hyponatremia associated with surgical procedures and traumatic injury is prevented by the replacement of ECF deficits. Thereafter, the daily maintenance of normal osmolarity is simplified by the replacement of observable losses of known sodium content.

Hyponatremia may easily occur when water is given to replace losses of sodium-containing fluids or when water administration consistently exceeds water losses. The latter may occur with oliguria or in association with decreased water loss through the skin and lungs, intracellular shifts of sodium, or cellular release of excessive amounts of endogenous water. Severe or refractory hyponatremia, however, is difficult to produce if renal function remains normal.

In the presence of hyperglycemia, knowledge of the glucose concentration is necessary to evaluate the significance of a depressed serum sodium level. Since glucose does not enter cells by passive diffusion, it exerts an osmotic force in the ECF compartment. This contribution to osmotic pressure is normally small, but with an elevated glucose concentration, the increased osmotic pressure causes the transfer of cellular water into the ECF compartment, producing a dilutional hyponatremia. Hyponatremia may therefore be observed when the total effective osmotic pressure in the ECF compartment is normal or even above normal. In terms of tonicity, each 100 mg. per 100 ml. rise in blood glucose above normal will cause a fall in serum sodium concentration variously estimated to be between 1.6 and 2.8 mEq. per liter. The figure 2.8 is based on the assumption that the shift of water from the cells will continue until osmolality is restored to normal in the ECF compartment. This does not occur because the flow of water will stop before normal osmolality is obtained (i.e., the addition of solute to the ECF compartment will increase osmolality in both compartments after equilibration). Katz therefore suggested use of the lower figure 1.6.[12] This is also inaccurate since renal and thirst mechanisms usually have already been activated in attempts to normalize ECF osmolality. To resolve the dilemma, the authors have arbitrarily chosen a whole number between the two extremes for use in clinical practice; that is, serum sodium will fall approximately 2 mEq. per liter for each 100 mg. per 100 ml. rise of serum glucose above normal. Consider a patient with a serum sodium concentration of 128 mEq. per liter and a blood glucose level of 500 mg. per 100 ml. The glucose is approximately 400 mg. per 100 ml. above normal, which should cause an 8 mEq. per liter fall in serum sodium; the low sodium level is therefore primarily due to high glucose concentration. In this instance, therapy is directed toward lowering the glucose concentration; once that is accomplished, the serum sodium will rise to approximately 136 mEq. per liter as the excess water leaves the ECF compartment. In a similar manner, urea elevation will cause a fall in extracellular sodium concentration. For clinical purposes, each 30 mg. per 100 ml. rise in BUN concentration above normal is expected to reduce the serum sodium concentration 2 mEq. per liter.

Replacement of Sodium Losses with Water. A common error is replacement of gastrointestinal and other isotonic salt losses with D_5W or a hypotonic salt solution. Also, patients with head injury or renal disease (loss of concentrating ability) may elaborate urine with a high salt concentration (50 to 200 mEq. per liter) that must be replaced. The former is usually secondary to excessive secretion of antidiuretic hor-

mone with consequent water retention, whereas the latter (*salt-wasting kidneys*) may be a problem in elderly patients. This source of sodium loss is frequently not anticipated, since the BUN and creatinine levels may be normal. Continued replacement of these urinary losses with D_5W may eventually cause marked hyponatremia. The urine sodium concentration should be determined if the diagnosis is in doubt; with hyponatremia and normal renal function, the urine should be virtually free of sodium.

Decreased Urinary Volume. Oliguria, from whatever cause (prerenal or renal), reduces the daily water requirements if not corrected. Cellular catabolism and the metabolic acidosis produced by the retention of nitrogenous waste products increase the cellular release of water. Therefore, the gain of endogenous water decreases the total water requirement beyond that expected when the urinary volume is low.

Endogenous Water Release. Between the fifth and tenth postoperative days, a patient maintained on intravenous fluids without adequate caloric intake gains significant quantities of water (maximum 500 ml. daily) from excessive cellular catabolism, thus decreasing the quantity of exogenous water required per day.

Intracellular Shifts. Systemic bacterial sepsis is often accompanied by a precipitous drop in serum sodium concentration. This sudden change is poorly understood, but usually accompanies loss of ECF as either interstitial or intracellular sequestrations. This can be treated by withholding free water, restoring ECF volume, and initiating treatment of the sepsis.

Hypernatremia. Hypernatremia (serum sodium concentration above 150 mEq. per liter), although uncommon, is a dangerous abnormality. Unlike decreased serum sodium concentration, hypernatremia is easily produced when renal function is normal. The ECF hyperosmolarity causes a shift of intracellular water to the ECF compartment; in this situation, a high serum sodium level may indicate a significant deficit of total body water. In surgical patients, hypernatremia arises most often from excessive or unexpected water losses, although it may result from use of salt-containing solutions to replace water losses. The following classification of water losses may be helpful in preventing and treating this abnormality.

Excessive Extrarenal Water Losses. With increased metabolism from any cause, but particularly associated with fever, the water loss through evaporation of sweat may reach several liters daily. Patients with tracheostomies in dry environments can (with excessive minute volume air exchange) lose as much as 1 to 1.5 liters of water per day by this route. Increased water evaporation from a burn wound is often of significance in the thermally injured patient.

Increased Renal Water Losses. Extremely large volumes of solute-poor urine may result from hypoxic damage to the distal tubules and collecting ducts or loss of antidiuretic hormone stimulation from damage to the CNS. In both instances, facultative water resorption is impaired. The former occurs in high-output renal failure; in the authors' experience, this is the most common type of renal failure after severe injury or operative trauma. The latter occurs with extensive head injuries accompanied by temporary diabetes insipidus.

Solute Loading. High protein intake may produce an increased osmotic load of urea, which necessitates the excretion of large volumes of water. Hypernatremia, azotemia, and ECF volume deficits follow. In general, these can be prevented by an intake of 7 ml. of water per gm. of dietary protein.

Osmotic diuretics such as mannitol, urea, and glucose cause the obligatory excretion of large volumes of urine, with free water losses greatly exceeding those of sodium. Uncontrolled hyperglycemia during intravenous nutrition is a most common cause of serious hypernatremia. The associated glucosuria causes an osmotic diuresis of large volumes of salt-poor urine, creating hypernatremia and an ECF volume deficit. If these are not corrected for several days, nonketotic, hyperosmolar coma may ensue. Treatment involves measures to lower serum glucose and replacement of the severe volume deficit with 0.45% sodium chloride solution.

High-output Renal Failure. Acute renal insufficiency after trauma or surgical stress may be a lethal complication. The diagnosis is classically based on persistent oliguria and chemical evidence of uremia after stabilization of the circulation. The clinical course is characterized by oliguria lasting from several days to several weeks, followed by a progressive rise in daily urinary volume until both the excretory and the concentrating functions of the kidneys are gradually restored.

Uremia, occurring without a period of oliguria and accompanied by a daily urinary volume greater than 1000 to 1500 ml., is a more frequent but less well recognized entity.[2] Clinical experience and laboratory experiments suggest that high-output renal failure represents the renal response to a less severe or modified episode of renal injury than that required to produce classic oliguric renal failure. Its importance lies in the fact that it is a milder form of renal insufficiency, and realization of its presence by serial measurements of BUN and serum electrolytes permits intelligent fluid volume management with a much greater latitude because of the daily urinary volume excretion. Normal ECF volume and serum sodium concentration are therefore quite easily maintained when accurate daily outputs of each are obtained and replaced accordingly. The sodium-containing fluids may be administered as lactate to control the mild metabolic acidosis that occurs. More severe acidosis may develop if isotonic losses from the gastrointestinal tract or from renal excretion of sodium are replaced with sodium chloride.

The chief dangers of high-output renal failure are failure to recognize its existence because of normal urinary output, and the intravenous administration of potassium salts. Initially, the patient may be very sensitive to exogenously administered potassium, not unlike an individual in oliguric renal failure. Later in the course of the disease, normal amounts of maintenance potassium are usually required.

The typical course of high-output renal failure begins without a period of oliguria. The daily urinary volumes are normal or greater than normal, often reaching levels of 3 to 5 liters per day, while BUN increases. An attempt to decrease urinary output by water restriction rapidly causes hypernatremia without a change in urinary volume. On average, BUN continues to increase for 8 to 12 days before a downward trend occurs. The blood/urine urea ratio is about 1:10 until a decrease occurs in the BUN concentration.

Functionally, the lesion is characterized by a GFR less than 20% of normal and complete resistance to vasopressin for 1 to 3 weeks after the BUN has declined. During the next 6 to 8 weeks the GFR gradually rises and the response to vasopressin becomes normal. Early recognition of high-output renal failure by serial blood determinations of BUN is important. Failure to recognize its presence may result in death from hyperkalemia, hypernatremia, or acidosis.

SELECTED REFERENCES

Maxwell, M. H., Kleeman, C. R., and Narins, R. G. (Eds.): Clinical Disorders of Fluid and Electrolyte Metabolism, 4th ed. New York, McGraw-Hill, 1987.
Encyclopedic coverage of fluid and electrolyte metabolism.

Mengoli, L. R.: Excerpts from the history of postoperative fluid therapy. Am. J. Surg., 121:311, 1971.
An interesting historical review, beginning in 1831 with W. B. O'Shaughnessy's suggestion that saline solution be given intravenously for the treatment of cholera and ending with a discussion of the work of Shires and associates advocating the replacement of extracellular fluid volume deficits incurred during surgery. The seesaw pattern of recommendations made between 1913 and 1967 for the administration or withholding of salt solutions during operative procedures is particularly illuminating.

Roberts, J. P., Roberts, J. B., Skinner, C., Shires, G. T., III, Illner, H., Canizaro, P. C., and Shires, G. T.: Extracellular fluid deficit following operation and its correction with Ringers lactate: A reassessment. Ann. Surg., 202:1, 1985.
An update of the original report by the senior author of this chapter quantitating the loss of functional extracellular fluid during abdominal surgical procedures.

Schwartz, W. B., and Relman, A. S.: A critique of the parameters used in the evaluation of acid-base disorders. N. Engl. J. Med., 268:1382, 1963.
This classic work critiques the systems for analysis of acid-base problems advocated by Singer and Hastings (buffer base) and Astrup (standard bicarbonate and base excess). Specifically, the authors discuss the limitations of these techniques and conclude that traditional measurements of pH, Pco₂, and plasma bicarbonate, combined with appropriate clinical information, allow proper evaluation of even the most complicated acid-base disorders.

Valeri, C. R.: Physiology of blood transfusion. In Barie, P. S., Shires, G. T. (Eds.): Surgical Intensive Care. Boston, Little, Brown, 1993.
Authoritative review by a noted surgical research professor whose career has focused on blood physiology.

REFERENCES

1. Astrup, P., Jorgensen, K., Anderson, O. S., and Engel, K.: The acid-base metabolism: A new approach. Lancet, 1:1035, 1960.
2. Baxter, C. R., Zedlitz, W. H., and Shires, G. T.: High output acute renal failure complicating traumatic injury. J. Trauma, 4:467, 1964.
3. Bear, R. A., and Dyck, R. F.: Clinical approach to the diagnosis of acid-base disorders. Can. Med. Assoc. J., 120:172, 1979.
4. Bishop, R. L., and Weisfeldt, M. L.: Sodium bicarbonate administration during cardiac arrest: Effect of arterial pH, Pco₂, and osmolality. JAMA, 235:506, 1976.
5. Canizaro, P. C.: Oxygen transport in shock. In Shires, G. T. (Ed.): Shock and Related Problems. Edinburgh, Churchill Livingstone, 1984, p. 95.
6. Canizaro, P. C., Prager, M. D., and Shires, G. T.: The infusion of Ringer's lactate solution during shock. Am. J. Surg., 122:494, 1971.
7. Christensen, M. S., Brodersen, P., Olesen, J., et al.: Cerebral apoplexy (stroke) treated with or without prolonged artificial hyperventilation. II. Cerebrospinal fluid acid-base balance and intracranial pressure. Stroke, 4:620, 1973.
8. Collins, J. A.: Problems associated with the massive transfusion of stored blood. Surgery, 75:274, 1974.
9. Emmett, M., and Seldin, D. W.: Clinical syndromes of metabolic acidosis and metabolic alkalosis. In Seldin, D. W., and Giebisch, G. (Eds.): The Kidney: Physiology and Pathophysiology. New York, Raven Press, 1985, pp. 1611–1639.
10. Freedman, B. I., and Burkart, J. M.: Hypokalemia. Crit. Care Clin., 7:143, 1991.
11. Kassirer, J., Berkman, P., Lawrenz, D., et al.: The critical role of chloride in the correction of hypokalemic alkalosis in man. Am. J. Med., 38:172, 1965.
12. Katz, M. A.: Hyperglycemia-induced hyponatremia: Calculations of expected serum sodium depression. N. Engl. J. Med., 289:843, 1973.
13. Lassen, N. A.: Control of cerebral circulation in health and disease. Circ. Res., 34:749, 1974.
14. Laurens, R., and Karp, B. I.: Pontine and extrapontine myelinolysis following rapid correction of hyponatremia. Lancet, 1:1439, 1988.
15. Mengoli, L. R.: Excerpts from the history of postoperative fluid therapy. Am. J. Surg., 121:311, 1971.
16. Miller, T. R., Anderson, R. J., Linas, S. L., Henrich, W. L., Berns, A. S., Gabow, P. A., and Schrier, R. W.: Urinary diagnostic indices in acute renal failure. Ann. Intern. Med., 89:47, 1978.
17. Moore, F. D., Olesen, K. H., McMurrey, J. D., Parker, H. V., Ball, M. R., and Boyden, C. M.: The Body Cell Mass and Its Supporting Environment. Philadelphia, W.B. Saunders, 1963.
18. Oh, M. S., and Carroll, H. J.: Disorders of sodium metabolism: Hypernatremia and hyponatremia. Crit. Care Med., 20:94, 1992.
19. Riley, L. J., Ilson, B. E., and Narins, R. G.: Acute metabolic acid-base disorders. Crit. Care Clin., 5:699, 1987.
20. Roberts, J. P., Roberts, J. B., Skinner, C., Shires, G. T., III, Illner, H., Canizaro, P. C., and Shires, G. T.: Extracellular fluid deficit following operation and its correction with Ringer's lactate: A reassessment. Ann. Surg., 202:1, 1985.
21. Salem, M., Munoz, R., and Chernow, B.: Hypomagnesemia in critical illness: A common and clinically important problem. Crit. Care Clin., 7:225, 1991.
22. Schwartz, W. B., and Relman, A. S.: A critique of the parameters used in the evaluation of acid-base disorders. N. Engl. J. Med., 268:1382, 1963.
23. Seelig, M. S.: Mg requirements in human nutrition. J. Med. Soc. N.J., 79:849, 1982.
24. Shires, G. T., and Holman, V: Dilutional acidosis. Ann. Intern. Med., 28:551, 1948.
25. Shires, G. T., and Jackson, D. E.: Postoperative salt tolerance. Arch. Surg., 84:703, 1962.

26. Shires, G. T., Williams, J., and Brown, F.: Acute changes in extracellular fluids associated with major surgical procedures. Ann. Surg., *154*:803, 1961.

27. Shires, G. T., III, Peitzman, A. B., Albert, S. A., et al.: Response of intraoperative lung water to intraoperative fluids. Ann. Surg., *197*:515, 1983.

28. Singer, R. B., and Hastings, A. B.: An improved clinical method for the estimation of disturbances of the acid-base balance of human blood. Medicine, *27*:223, 1948.

29. Valeri, C. R.: Physiology of blood transfusion. *In* Barie, P. S., Shires, G. T. (Eds.): Surgical Intensive Care. Boston, Little, Brown, 1993.

30. Vanatta, J. D., and Fogelman, M. J.: Moyer's Fluid Balance, 3rd ed. Chicago, Year Book, 1982.

31. Williams, M. E.: Hyperkalemia. Crit. Care Clin., *7*:155, 1991.

32. Wright, H. K., and Gann, D. S.: Correction of defect in free water excretion in postoperative patients by extracellular fluid volume expansion. Ann. Surg., *158*:70, 1963.

CHAPTER 7

PRINCIPLES OF PREOPERATIVE PREPARATION OF THE SURGICAL PATIENT

Hiram C. Polk, Jr., M.D., and William G. Cheadle, M.D.

The modern preparation of a patient for operation characterizes the emergence of the surgical disciplines from an art to a science. The development of anesthesia, followed by the introduction of the antiseptic concepts of Semmelweis and Lister, was a monumental achievement, but it can be viewed best as providing the basis for the healthy growth and development of modern surgery. Preparation for most elective operations is now made in the outpatient setting. This has made teaching such preparation to surgeons in training challenging, because exposure to the patient is limited.

ASSESSMENT OF OPERATIVE RISK

Inherent in a discussion of operative risk is the determination each physician must make regarding the relative rewards and risks in treating a specific illness. Surgeons are perhaps fortunate that the dramatic nature of their methods magnifies the significance of adverse results and permits clear understanding of this expression in the therapeutic ratio. In its simplest terms, such a ratio defines the relative harm (risk) and the relative good (benefit) that are likely to follow a specific operation for a specific illness in a specific patient. There are few more valuable parameters than the natural history of the disease process—that is, the course of the disease and its ultimate outcome if untreated. Especially good examples concern the natural history of abdominal aortic aneurysms and the course of untreated mammary carcinoma. One must further ascertain that the stages of disease being considered are clinically comparable. More often than not, alleged differences among treatments are attributable to differences in clinical staging of the patient populations under comparison[18] and not to different results of the putative therapies.[12]

The urgency of a specific procedure is in part a function of the relative risks and rewards. In suspected appendicitis, the rewards of treatment entail prompt control of an inflamed focus or management of a systemic complication that is likely to be fatal if untreated. The benefits of surgery compared with nonoperative treatment or diagnostic delay point strongly toward prompt operation. The potential for an adverse effect recently has been redefined in an analysis of the gatekeeper and managed care trends in American practice today.[3] Whereas the urgency of an operation may determine the amount of time available and indirectly limit measures taken to prepare the patient, it is important that these preparations be accomplished promptly.

Elderly patients often require concurrent management of multiple organ degenerative disease. When one disease produces a complication that can be controlled only by operation, particular attention should be given to the often subtle but physiologically important alterations of the other organs essential for life support, as well as to nutritional status.[5] The influence of age on operative risk is important. Elderly patients often tolerate operations well but complications poorly. Age *per se* should not contraindicate operative intervention but should be taken into account in the overall therapeutic ratio.

The capacity for sound clinical judgment is the ultimate characteristic of the mature physician. The parameters involved in clinical decisions are difficult to define, but quantification of these factors is desirable to affirm the physician's initial professional judgment and to provide the younger physician with a means to learn this attribute of professional excellence. Linn and associates[15] found that the presence of systemic and local disease is generally additive in determining the probability of death during hospitalization, profoundly influencing some decisions for operation. Despite general agreement about principles of intraoperative decisions in a common major operation, practicing board-certified surgeons often deviate from accepted standards; these deviations are associated with significant increases in death after operation and in decreased cure of some colorectal cancers.[14] Algorithms may help delineate more of these crucial but often overlooked concepts (Table 7–1).

For the determination of operative risk and factors requiring specific preoperative correction, a simple list should be part of each physical examination, including personal and familial history of any bleeding tendency, with laboratory definition of its significance; allergic responses to medication or prior treatment; and current medications, with awareness that patients often forget to list some drugs or to recognize that nonprescription products may contain active medicinal agents.

PERSONAL RELATIONSHIPS

When a surgical procedure is being considered, a genuine bond of communication and personal responsibility must be established between the surgeon and the patient. The patient's confidence is based on true understanding, allowing

TABLE 7–1. Basic Factors Affecting Operative Risk

Age >70 yr.
Overall physical status
Elective vs. emergency operation
Physiologic extent of procedure
Number of associated illnesses

him or her to participate, when appropriate, in judgments affecting risks, future lifestyle, and the process of postoperative recovery. The rarity of legal action taken by a patient when a careful effort has been made by the physician to achieve such understanding before operation is noteworthy and depends on a carefully informed and accurate statement of the relative risks and rewards of the operation. Many patients today have growing insight regarding such matters and should be allowed to participate actively in the decisions. The physician must not convey a sense of hurry or allow an inadequate time for explanations, no matter how small or seemingly minor the operation might be. Finally, on some occasions, a definite answer may not be possible, in which case honesty is the best approach. If there is reasonable question on the part of a patient that an operation is indicated, the surgeon should seek confirmation by obtaining the independent view of another surgeon.

For young surgeons, few concepts are as poorly understood as the importance of effective relationships with referring physicians. In most situations, patients are referred to surgeons by physicians in other disciplines; it is important to have an understanding of the wishes and views of the referring physician at the outset. On some occasions the referring physician will have made certain judgments that differ from those of the surgeon—differences that must be discussed with the surgeon and, occasionally, with the patient. This may become a more frequent problem in tightly managed care scenarios. Further, it is helpful to have a clear understanding of the projected course of treatment and the relative participation of the referring physician in the postoperative care so that duplicative or, more important, contradictory efforts and orders are avoided.

The specific permission for conduct of an operation is a focal point of medical, legal, and sociologic discussion. Local custom and recent legal practice often determine which of these is most appropriate. The surest perception of true informed consent can be attained in a setting in which there is a full and frank discussion with the patient in the presence of a close relative and an appropriate professional witness. The surgeon should concisely record a summary of this encounter in the hospital chart. Moreover, when writing such a note, the surgeon should enumerate those patient characteristics that determine the need for operation; the special risk factors recognized, with further notation as to their amelioration; and the special intraoperative and postoperative problems anticipated. This also serves as a checklist for possible errors of omission.

Some procedures have such major measurable risk that the real possibility of death or disability must be discussed as part of the mutual decision making. It is usually sufficient to inform the patient that there are risks of both complication and death, no matter how well or carefully the operation is conducted. One must truly respect the patient's options, but it is also important to avoid undue arousal of fear.

GENERAL PREPARATION OF THE PATIENT

The basic principles of patient preparation for a major operative procedure can be readily enumerated, but it is much more difficult to determine the rapidity with which such preparation must be accomplished. The disease process usually dictates the timing of operation, so there is a measurable spectrum of urgency that substantively determines the rapidity and completeness of preoperative preparation.

Psychologic Preparation

A frank, but optimistic, discussion of the possibilities ahead is of great value for the patient who is to undergo a

major surgical procedure. The preoperative steps should be enumerated, justified, and explained in detail. The use of drainage devices and various forms of intubation is better tolerated, both physiologically and psychologically, if their need has been previously explained. The patient then anticipates and understands the benefits and realizes that the discomfort serves an identifiable purpose. The surgeon must not equivocate in discussing possible disfiguring operations, such as those involving the head and neck, the breasts, or the genital organs, and especially with respect to methods of urinary or fecal elimination.

When an illness is apt to have a clinically significant course beyond the duration of the early posthospital follow-up, it is usually reassuring for the surgeon to explain the continuing commitment to the patient. This is particularly helpful for a patient with neoplastic disease. Both the reassurance of anticipated longevity for the patient and the assurance that the surgeon will be a partner in the long-term management of the disease or any complication that may arise from the treatment are most helpful. Well-intentioned friends or family members often wish to shield the patient from unpleasant facts. This is generally unwise, and the surgeon's contract ordinarily is with the patient. When the medical facts are unpleasant, it is important to allow the patient an opportunity to recover from the immediate effects of the operation and to ascertain that he or she is alert before such information is provided. Within a period of several days, the surgeon should take the initiative and review with the patient the operative finding and the probable prognosis. At the point of first information, the prognosis, if poor, should *not* be presented as hopeless. This is unjustified biologically and also denies the patient the small degree of justifiable optimism that supports an individual with a grim prognosis surprisingly well.

Physiologic Preparation

Blood Volume Considerations. Various chronic disease processes are associated with anemia; however, such patients have a normal total blood volume. They have compensated for a significantly decreased red blood cell volume by expansion of the plasma volume to supernormal levels.[17] Although acute intravascular volume deficiencies are manifested by an increased pulse rate or decreased blood pressure, on a chronic basis, volume is restored by expanding the plasma volume, often at the expense of the extracellular fluid, to compensate for the loss or nonproduction of red blood cell mass.

Correction of these concentration deficits before an elective operation requires recognition that even large deficits in red blood cell mass occurring over a long period are well tolerated. Although 10 gm. per 100 ml. of hemoglobin is regarded by many as minimal for general anesthesia, what must be determined are the physiologically safe limits for tissue oxygen delivery. Enhanced oxygen delivery can be achieved by increased cardiac output, hemoglobin concentration, and/or oxygen extraction. The last may be least amenable to improvement, and an increased stroke volume or pulse rate places a definite physiologic stress on the heart, which is often diseased itself in the elderly patients who acquire such chronic illnesses. Indeed, if one could ascertain that no unforeseen blood losses or inadvertent hypoxia would occur, a patient could expect to safely undergo an elective operation with a very low hemoglobin concentration. However, the risk of one of these untoward events is greater than the hazard of transfusion. Thus, patients being prepared for operation who have an anemia commonly associated with chronic disease should have replacement of the red blood cell mass up to 10 gm. per 100 ml. A useful rule when attempting physiologic correction of chronic anemia is to administer no more than 1 unit of blood per day, thereby allowing time for excretion of excess plasma.

Other Fluid Deficits. Whereas blood deficits are primarily concentrational, plasma and extracellular fluid deficits are significant in both volume and concentration in terms of the preoperative preparation of most patients. Special problems are presented when the volume deficiencies are preexisting or concealed. For example, preexisting losses may represent vomitus and/or diarrhea occurring for 3 to 4 days before hospitalization. Although some losses occur visibly, as in a fracture of the femur or in a major third-degree burn of an extremity, and are manifested by visible swelling, more often such fluid losses are concealed and thus inadequately estimated.

The problem of concealed loss is particularly difficult. These third-space losses in which blood, plasma, and/or extracellular fluid are extravasated are often associated with major burns, fractures, and generalized peritonitis. Objective estimation of preexisting and continuing fluid deficits should be made, and one of the most ubiquitously useful measurements is hourly urinary output through a urinary catheter to determine the efficacy of replenishment. Serial central venous pressures or measurement of end-diastolic filling pressures and cardiac output via pulmonary artery catheter is helpful in complicated cases with underlying cardiopulmonary disease. Standard losses in these circumstances total approximately 3 liters a day, or 125 ml. per hour in adults. Therefore, the rate of fluid resuscitation in a deficit situation should begin at twice that rate. The hourly urinary output should be assessed over 3 to 4 hours to determine volume deficiency and the rate at which replenishment should continue. A common error in quantitating concentrational deficits is to assume that the normal serum concentration of a specific electrolyte ensures that there has been no loss. Isotonic losses of water, sodium, chloride, and potassium may produce profound volume deficiencies with maintenance of normal concentrations of the commonly measured serum electrolytes. Reasonably normal kidneys conserve all sodium and chloride administered, and infusion of solutions proportionate to total losses (i.e., isotonic) is usually appropriate.

Timing and Parameters. Not all volume and concentrational deficits need be corrected before operation is undertaken, but a significant fraction of the total deficit should be replaced to enhance the safety of anesthesia and operation. Resuscitation may be initiated with lactated Ringer's solution with added potassium at a rate of 500 ml. in the first hour. If the urinary response to such administration is only 10 ml., another 500 ml. should be infused during the next hour. Should urinary output increase to 20 ml. per hour, one might reasonably anticipate proceeding with the operation. In general, the longer a patient has been ill, the more time one can take to correct the deficiencies. The overly rapid correction of fluid deficits could induce pulmonary edema, particularly in elderly patients with marginal cardiovascular compensation. This risk, however, might be tolerated in a young patient with a normal cardiovascular system and an acutely encountered disease.

Nutrition

Although nutritional replenishment and supplementation have become a common (and expensive) worldwide surgical practice, their specific role in improved survival from certain illnesses or after certain operations continues to defy documentation and certainly defies cost-benefit analysis. Such preoperative support applies only to a patient who awaits an elective operation. Skin test anergy is associated with subsequent infection and appears to have shown that non-specific nutritional repletion reverses both anergy and the tendency to infection.[23] A recent Veterans Affairs cooperative study demonstrated that 2 weeks of preoperative parenteral nutrition was helpful only to those patients who were severely depleted, as measured by serum albumin levels less than 2 gm. per 100 ml. or by a greater than 10% loss of body weight.[2] Often the disease process itself defines the ability to correct malnutrition, as is the case with malignancy. However, patients with chronic gastric outlet obstruction, pancreatitis, and alcoholism may benefit from preoperative nutritional support.

Prevention of Infection

Infection continues to be a major source of morbidity and a disconcerting source of mortality in surgical patients. A patient who is badly injured or who undergoes a major operation and survives despite the development of secondary shock and electrolyte disturbances is at very high risk for serious infection. During preoperative evaluation, the patient should be protected from any patient with extramural or hospital-acquired infections. The proposed operative site should be washed with an appropriate antiseptic agent several times before operation, and shaving should be done either as close to the time of operation as is feasible or not at all, substituting either clipping or depilatory agents when removal of hair is desired.

A primary factor that should be considered in preparing the patient is antibiotic prophylaxis. Evidence supports the commonly accepted practice of preoperative intestinal preparation with poorly absorbed oral antimicrobial agents for colon operations.[24] Explicit laboratory studies[16] were confirmed by multiple clinical trials that showed systemic antibiotics to be highly effective when used just before, during, and immediately after an operation.[1, 19] However, one must always balance the risk of an antibiotic's adverse effect with its potential benefit. To date, most studies showing a clearcut benefit from such antibiotics have involved operations that bore an appreciable risk of infection; the other characteristics varied considerably (Table 7–2). The agent selected should manifest sustained antibiotic activity in the surgical wound.[20] Declining wound antibiotic activity is an indication to readminister the agent or to seek a drug that produces more sustained activity levels. Another major factor is unanticipated delays in elective operations.[7] With regard to delivery of antimicrobial protection to the wound itself, one may administer systemic antibiotics or apply topical antibiotics to the wound.

SPECIFIC ORGANS AND SYSTEMS

Cardiovascular. The efforts of Goldman[10] did much to advance the whole line of inquiry toward precise determina-

TABLE 7–2. Operations in Which Systemic Antibiotic Prophylaxis Is of Benefit

Head and neck, which require opening the upper aerodigestive tract
Esophageal, excluding hiatal hernia repair
Gastroduodenal, except for complications of uncorrected hyperacidity
Biliary tract for patients aged >70 yr., with acute cholecystitis, and/or requiring choledochostomy
Small and large bowel resections
Appendectomy for gangrenous or perforated appendix
Hysterectomy
Abdominal and lower extremity revascularizations, including prosthetic grafts
Other clean operations implanting high-risk prostheses, e.g., hip, knee, aortic valve

TABLE 7–3. Weighting of Cardiac Risk Factors

Criteria	Points
Historical	
Age >70 yr.	5
Myocardial infarction previous 6 months	10
Examination	
S_3 gallop or jugular venous distention	11
Significant aortic valvular stenosis	3
Electrocardiogram	
Premature atrial contractions or rhythm other than sinus	7
>5 premature ventricular contractions/min.	7
General status	3
Abnormal blood gases	
K^+/HCO_3 abnormalities	
Abnormal renal function	
Liver disease or bedridden	
Operation	
Emergency	4
Intraperitoneal, intrathoracic, aortic	3
Total possible	53

tion of operative risk, and those efforts have recently been updated.[21] The patient's capacity to increase cardiac output in response to intraoperative and postoperative challenges is perhaps the most fundamental determinant of survival after complex operations.[4]

Several risk factors were found by Goldman and associates[11] to be useful predictors of fatal or life-threatening complications of cardiac origin after noncardiac operations. Such factors allowed them to develop a weighting scheme for these factors (Table 7–3), which then correlated accurately with the likelihood of significant cardiac risk. Although the statistical soundness of a negative observation depends on limited numbers fulfilling such negative criteria, their work did not confirm the significance of diabetes mellitus, smoking, hypertension, hyperlipidemia, stable angina pectoris, remote myocardial infarctions, ST-segment or T-wave changes on the electrocardiogram, bundle branch blocks, mitral valvular disease, or cardiomegaly. These conditions must not be ignored but are apparently less pertinent determinants of cardiac risk than had been thought. Note further that 28 of the 53 points in the cardiac risk weighting scheme are potentially treatable. The operation could be deferred until there is improvement in the overall cardiac status and the prognosis is more favorable.

Also significant in detecting unsuspected high-risk patients is preoperative pulmonary wedge pressure monitoring with and without volume challenge.[9] More important, this method has unmasked some patients with prohibitive cardiac risk and allowed others to be improved before operation. Not suprisingly, successful myocardial revascularization ameliorates much of the excess risk of coronary ischemia.[6]

Thromboembolism is generally an infrequent but potentially lethal clinical event. Patients at increased risk include those with a clear history of prior thrombosis or embolism; those likely to have prolonged operations, with special emphasis on procedures that temporarily interfere with lower extremity blood flow; and those with certain reconstructive operations on the hip. Given these and other parameters, the clinician may employ a variety of methods to reduce the risk of thromboembolism, including pneumatic compression stockings, exercises, and early ambulation. Anticoagulation with low-dose heparin should be reserved for those patients with morbid obesity or a history of prior pulmonary embolism or deep venous thrombosis.

Respiratory. Respiratory complications occur in two major patient groups: those with grossly normal lungs who develop respiratory abnormalities secondary to anesthetic agents and operation, and those with overt chronic lung disease in whom the problems of anesthesia and operation are superimposed on intrinsically diseased pulmonary tissue. Some risk factors are outlined in Table 7–4.

Preoperative pulmonary insufficiency requires the surgeon to determine whether operation can be tolerated at all and the optimal preparation if operation is to be undertaken. The distinction between nonobstructive and obstructive pulmonary emphysema can be made with the standard tests of pulmonary function. These tests are particularly important when pulmonary resection is being contemplated. Estimation of the capacity of the remaining lung tissue is critical to ensure tolerance of the procedure without ventilatory dependence. Although several specific tests delineate minimal function, careful evaluation by the surgeon, in consultation with pulmonary medicine specialists, is often indicated.[22] A simple, useful test is having the patient take a brisk walk up a flight of stairs and observing his or her tolerance. Arterial blood gases should be obtained as a baseline in symptomatic patients and in those who will undergo major procedures, especially in the chest.

Preoperative preparatory maneuvers aimed at preventing postoperative respiratory complications include cessation of smoking, use of bronchodilators, chest physiotherapy, education, and occasionally antibiotics, if sputum is purulent. Such maneuvers are especially important for those with chronic obstructive pulmonary disease.[13]

Renal. With appropriate perioperative hydration, renal complications of major surgical endeavors have become relatively uncommon. With the screening procedures of blood urea nitrogen and creatinine determinations and urinalysis, one may proceed with an operation and subsequent fluid therapy and be reasonably confident that the patient will tolerate judiciously managed fluid loads. Patients requiring dialysis are chronically anemic and have acquired platelet dysfunction but tolerate most procedures under general anesthesia quite well. Timing of dialysis and appropriate transfusion are important preparations, as is the decision to use heparin. A special type of renal disease is associated with obstruction in the lower urinary tract, exemplified by prostatic hypertrophy in elderly men. If time permits, catheter drainage of the obstructed urinary tract and elimination of infection should be done before an elective procedure to allow return of adequate function.

TABLE 7–4. Risk Factors for Postoperative Pulmonary Complications

Thoracic and upper abdominal surgery
Preoperative history of chronic obstructive pulmonary disease
Preoperative purulent productive cough
Anesthesia time >3 hr.
History of cigarette smoking
Age >60 yr.
Obesity
Poor preoperative state of nutrition
Symptoms of respiratory disease
Abnormal findings on physical examination
Abnormal chest film findings

TABLE 7–5. Sample Preoperative Checklist

Operative permit—appropriately signed and witnessed
Dietary considerations
  For abdominal operation, liquid diet and laxatives to ensure clean, collapsed bowel
  Nothing by mouth at least 6 hr. before operation
Review of life-support systems
  Vital signs recorded often enough to establish normal
  Pulmonary system—chest films; other studies as indicated
  Cardiac function—electrocardiogram; other studies as indicated
  Renal function—urinalysis; blood urea nitrogen and possibly creatinine determinations
Adequate hydration up to time of operation—especially to compensate for laxatives and fasting
Area of operation washed with appropriate germicidal detergent and shaved, clipped, or cleansed with depilatory agent
Blood transfusions prepared as anticipated
Order that patient should void on call to operating room
Preoperative medications—vagolytic and sedative drugs
Special medications—digitalis, insulin, and so forth

Modified from Houston, M. C., Ratcliff, D. G., Hays, J. T., and Gluck, F. W.: Preoperative medical consultation and evaluation of surgical risk. South. Med. J., *80*:1385, 1987.

Hepatic. The signs and symptoms of significant liver impairment are detectable on a number of standard clinical and laboratory examinations. With cirrhotic patients, a substantial preoperative period, concentrating on nutrition and avoidance of hepatotoxins in any form, must be allowed if any recovery of function is to be achieved. Risk of operation is directly correlated with the Child's classification of the patient, which can be improved by nutritional support and the reduction or elimination of ascites and encephalopathy. The overwhelming risk of cirrhosis in nonshunting operations has been a subject of great importance, and ascites prevention in the postoperative period is especially prudent.[8] Some factors are particularly important and preclude all but absolutely life-saving operations; they include Child's Class C, bacterial contamination, bilirubinemia higher than 3 mg. per 100 ml., albumin levels lower than 3 mg. per 100 ml., and malnutrition.

Neurologic. Maintaining cerebral function via appropriate oxygenation and circulation is vitally important to the anesthesiologist and the surgeon. Of special concern is the prevalence of occult cerebrovascular disease in elderly people, who constitute a large proportion of patients requiring surgical attention. Several lines of evidence now suggest that significant occult asymptomatic carotid lesions are rare and that corrective procedures undertaken before the primary operation are seldom justified. Asymptomatic carotid stenoses rarely produce problems without prior development of symptoms, and these patients are not as susceptible to stroke as are patients with transient ischemic attacks. All in all, a careful history remains the best determinant of whether cerebrovascular disease poses a real or imagined risk to a patient requiring another operation.

SPECIAL PROBLEMS

Several special problems demand preoperative correction. Foremost among these is incomplete evacuation and cleansing of the alimentary tract. Pulmonary aspiration is a dreaded surgical complication whose treatment remains inadequate; prevention, however, is simple. In almost no circumstances should general anesthesia be induced without specific attention to evacuation of the patient's stomach. Aspiration remains a common cause of surgical mortality. A useful checklist of considerations that should be reviewed when writing preoperative hospital orders is provided in Table 7–5.

SELECTED REFERENCES

Bolt, R. J.: Medical Evaluation of the Surgical Patient. Mount Kisco, N.Y., Futura, 1987.
  Although organized as a medical consultant's handbook, this monograph brings the current, largely medical, literature to bear on risk factors, the correction thereof, and the "tuning up" of the surgical patient.

Kinney, J. M., Egdahl, R. H., and Zuidema, G. D.: Manual of Preoperative and Postoperative Care. Philadelphia, W. B. Saunders, 1971.
  This work, produced under the auspices of the American College of Surgeons, is a standard text that covers issues of preoperative and postoperative care of the surgical patient, including critical care.

Norton, L. W., Steele, G., Jr., and Eiseman, B.: Surgical Decision Making, 3rd ed. Philadelphia, W. B. Saunders, 1993.
  The use of algorithms is especially helpful in determining options in the surgical patient with multiple associated or underlying illnesses.

REFERENCES

1. Bernard, H. R., and Cole, W. R.: The prophylaxis of surgical infection: The effect of prophylactic antimicrobial drugs on the incidence of infection following potentially contaminated operations. Surgery, 56:151, 1964.
2. Buzby, G. P.: Overview of randomized clinical trials of total parenteral nutrition for malnourished surgical patients. World J. Surg., *17*:173, 1993.
3. Cacioppo, J. C., Diettrich, N. A., Kaplan, G., and Nora, P. F.: The consequences of current constraints on surgical treatment of appendicitis. Am. J. Surg., *157*:276, 1989.
4. Clowes, G. H. A., Jr., DelGuercio, L. R., and Barwinsky, J.: The cardiac output in response to surgical trauma: A comparison between patients who survived and those who died. Arch. Surg., *81*:212, 1960.
5. Corti, M. C., Guralnik, J. M., Salive, M. E., and Sorkin, J. D.: Serum albumin level and physical disability as predictors of mortality in older persons. JAMA, *272*:1036, 1994.
6. Fudge, T. L., McKinnon, W. M. P., Schoettle, G. P., et al.: Improved operative risk after myocardial revascularization. South. Med. J., *74*:799, 1981.
7. Galandiuk, S., Polk, H. C., Jr., Jagelman, D. G., and Fazio, V. W.: Reemphasis of priorities in surgical antibiotic prophylaxis. Surg. Gynecol. Obstet., *169*:219, 1989.
8. Garrison, R. N., Cryer, H. M., Howard, D. A., and Polk, H. C., Jr.: Clarification of risk factors for abdominal operations in patients with hepatic cirrhosis. Ann. Surg., *199*:648, 1984.
9. Garrison, R. N., Wilson, M. A., Matheson, P. J., and Spain, D. A.: Preoperative saline loading improves outcome after elective, noncardiac surgical procedures. Am. Surg., *62*:223, 1996.
10. Goldman, L.: Cardiac risks and complications of noncardiac surgery. Ann. Surg., *198*:780, 1983.
11. Goldman, L., Caldera, D. L., Nussbaum, S. R., et al.: Multifactorial index of cardiac risk in noncardiac surgical procedures. N. Engl. J. Med., *297*:845, 1977.
12. Greenfield, S., Aronow, H. U., Elashoff, R. M., and Watanabe, D.: Flaws in mortality data: The hazards of ignoring comorbid disease. JAMA, *260*:2253, 1988.
13. Houston, M. C., Ratcliff, D. G., Hays, J. T., and Gluck, F. W.: Preoperative medical consultation and evaluation of surgical risk. South. Med. J., *80*:1385, 1987.
14. Knutson, C. O., Fry, D. E., Barbie, R. D., et al.: Reassessment of intraoperative decisions—why operations for cancer of the large bowel fail. Ann. Surg., *187*:549, 1978.
15. Linn, B. S., Linn, M. W., and Wallen, N.: Evaluation of results from studies of surgery in the elderly. Ann. Surg., *195*:90, 1982.
16. Miles, A. A., Miles, E. M., and Burke, J.: The value and duration of defense reactions of the skin to primary lodgement of bacteria. Br. J. Exp. Pathol., *38*:79, 1957.
17. Peden, J. E., Jr., Maxwell, M., Ohin, A., et al.: A consideration of indications for preoperative transfusion based on analysis of blood volumes and circulating proteins in normal and malnourished patients with or without cancer. Ann. Surg., *151*:303, 1960.
18. Polk, H. C., Jr.: The mathematics of clinical judgment, including an evaluation of operative risk. In Polk, H. C., Jr., Gardner, B., and Stone, H. H. (Eds.): Basic Surgery, 5th ed. St. Louis, Quality Medical Publishing, 1995, p. 10.
19. Polk, H. C., Jr., and Lopez-Mayor, J. F.: Postoperative wound infection: A prospective study of determinant factors and prevention. Surgery, *66*:97, 1969.
20. Polk, H. C., Jr., Trachtenberg, L., and Finn, M. P.: Human incisional antibiotic activity. JAMA, *244*:1353, 1980.
21. Rose, S. D.: Cardiac risk factors in patients undergoing non-cardiac surgery.

In Bolt, R. J. (Ed.): Medical Evaluation of the Surgical Patient. Mount Kisco, N. Y., Futura, 1987, p. 253.

22. Siefkin, A. D., and Lillington, G. A.: Pulmonary complications of surgery. *In* Bolt, R. J. (Ed.): Medical Evaluation of the Surgical Patient. Mount Kisco, N. Y., Futura, 1987, p. 307.

23. Tchervenkov, J. I., Diano, E., Meakins, J. L., and Christou, N. V.: Susceptibil-ity to bacterial sepsis: Accurate measurement by the delayed-type hyper-sensitivity skin test score. Arch. Surg., *121*:37, 1986.

24. Washington, J. A., II, Dearing, W. H., Judd, E. S., et al.: Effect of preopera-tive antibiotic regimen on development of infection after intestinal surgery: Prospective, randomized, double-blind study. Ann. Surg., *180*:567, 1974.

CHAPTER 8

BLOOD TRANSFUSIONS AND DISORDERS OF SURGICAL BLEEDING

Samir M. Fakhry, M.D., and George F. Sheldon, M.D.

The administration of blood products and the management of bleeding disorders are important therapeutic modalities employed by surgeons caring for patients with a wide variety of acute and chronic problems. When used with a thorough understanding of appropriate indications, risks, and benefits, blood transfusion is safe and effective. Congenital and acquired bleeding disorders are encountered by surgeons in a variety of clinical settings. Congenital conditions such as hemophilia present challenges for elective as well as emergent operations. Acquired bleeding disorders are associated with conditions such as infection, systemic inflammatory states, massive transfusion, hypothermia, severe malnutrition, liver dysfunction, and drugs (e.g., heparin and warfarin). A knowledge of the fundamentals of normal and deranged hemostasis is critical to the successful conduct of operative procedures and the complete care of surgical patients.

In this chapter the preparation and clinical use of blood components, the potential risks of hemotherapy, and the available substitutes and alternatives to blood transfusion is reviewed. Normal hemostatic mechanisms are discussed, and appropriate diagnostic and therapeutic measures for disorders of surgical bleeding are reviewed. Because blood transfusion is lifesaving in many patients, a knowledge of appropriate indications, potential risks, and available alternatives should allow clinicians to exercise judgment in using this important resource.

BLOOD TRANSFUSIONS

Although it is now routine, the ability to successfully transfuse blood is relatively recent. Accounts of blood letting and phlebotomy, but not blood transfusion, appear in many early historical references and were recommended for many ailments, including insanity. Transfusions were reportedly performed several hundred years ago to change the *nature* of individuals and were attempted in those accused of being witches to infuse them with the *proper spirits*. The first known successful transfusion recorded was by Jean-Baptiste Denis in France. In 1667, he gave three pints of sheep blood to a person with no apparent ill effects. Subsequent attempts to give blood to a young man "to mollify his fiery nature" failed, with the patient dying shortly after the transfusion. A lawsuit resulted, and Denis went to trial but was ultimately exonerated. However, the Paris medical faculty subsequently forbade blood transfusions, which led to bans on transfusion throughout France and Italy that lasted until modern times. An 1825 medical journal noted a transfusion administered by Dr. Philip Syng Physick of Philadelphia, perhaps the first recorded successful transfusion of human blood.[45] In 1828, Blundell administered human blood to a patient with post-partum hemorrhage, and the patient reportedly felt better.[4] The routine, safe administration of blood products, however, required several important scientific advances. The discovery of the A, B, and O blood types by Landsteiner in 1900 and the AB blood type by Von Decastello and Sturli in 1902 began the era of modern blood transfusion. By the 1940s, techniques of crossmatching, anticoagulation, and storage of blood and the establishment of blood banks made routine blood transfusion possible. The first blood bank was established in the United States in 1937, and the introduction of plastic storage containers and apheresis instruments made component therapy possible.

The ability to replace blood lost intraoperatively is an important prerequisite in modern surgical practice. Approximately 60% of all blood products given to patients are transfused at or near the time of operation. Blood component therapy has made successful operation possible in patients with symptomatic anemia, thrombocytopenia, or coagulopathy. In 1992, the American Red Cross reported that 15.5 million units of blood products were produced for transfusion in the United States.[1] Of this total, 5.8 million were units of packed red blood cells (RBCs), 3.1 million were units of platelets, and 5.2 million units were plasma. The use of packed RBCs doubled from 1970 to 1980, but the increase appears to have stabilized since the mid 1980s.[47] However, the use of other components, especially platelets, has increased.[47] Because only 4% to 5% of eligible donors ever donate blood, future increases may cause shortages.

PREPARATION OF BLOOD COMPONENTS

Component therapy is the accepted standard for the optimal management of the blood supply. Blood is collected and separated into its individual components (packed red blood cells, plasma, platelets) to optimize therapeutic potency. This strategy maximizes the benefit derived from each individual unit collected while minimizing the risk to each recipient. Blood is withdrawn from the donor and mixed with a solution containing citrate to prevent coagulation by binding calcium. The solutions used most commonly today are citrate phosphate dextrose (CPD) and citrate phosphate dextrose adenine (CPDA-1). Solutions containing extra nutrients (AS-1, AS-2) extend the storage life of cells. The unit is gently centrifuged (Fig. 8–1) to pack the RBCs and leave about 70% of the platelets suspended in plasma. The platelet-rich plasma is removed and centrifuged again at a faster speed to "pellet" the platelets. All but 50 ml. of supernatant plasma is removed and rapidly frozen at less than −30° C. The platelets are resuspended to yield platelet concentrate. Frozen plasma that is stored at less than −18° C. is termed fresh frozen plasma (FFP). If the frozen plasma is allowed to thaw

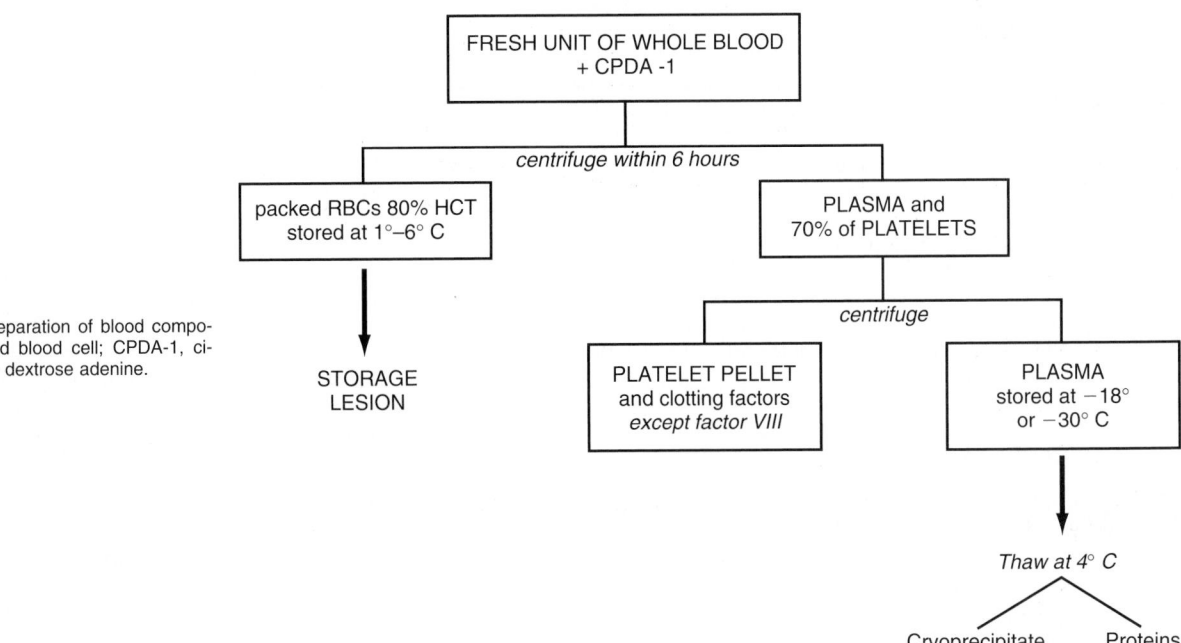

Figure 8–1. Preparation of blood components. RBC, red blood cell; CPDA-1, citrate phosphate dextrose adenine.

at 4° C., the precipitate that remains can be collected to yield cryoprecipitate. Proteins, such as albumin, can be isolated from the remaining supernatant plasma by ethanol fractionation. A summary of available blood components is presented in Table 8–1.

Manual or mechanical apheresis can be employed to collect leukocytes, platelets, or plasma. In manual apheresis, a unit of whole blood is drawn from the donor and centrifuged; plasma or platelets or both are removed, and the blood is returned to the donor. In mechanical apheresis, blood is withdrawn continuously from the donor using an automated device. The blood is separated by centrifuge, and the desired component is removed. Blood is then returned to the donor in a continuous loop. Large numbers of units of leukocytes

TABLE 8–1. Summary of Blood Components

Component	Composition	Shelf Life
Whole blood	RBCs; nonfunctional WBCs and platelets; plasma (450 ml. total volume contains 200 ml. of RBCs)	CPDA-1: 35 days (1° to 6° C.)
Packed RBCs	RBCs; some plasma; nonfunctional WBCs and platelets (250 to 350 ml. total volume contains 200 ml. of RBCs)	AS-1: 42 days CPDA-1: 35 days (1° to 6° C.)
Washed RBCs	RBCs; minimum plasma and nonfunctional WBCs and platelets (200 ml. total volume contains 170 to 190 ml. of RBCs)	24 hours (1° to 6° C.)
Deglycerolized RBCs	RBCs; no plasma, minimum WBC and platelet debris (200 ml. total volume contains 170 to 190 ml. of RBCs)	24 hours after deglycerolization (1° to 6° C.); 3 years ($<-65°$ C.)
Platelets (single unit from whole blood donation)	Platelets; some nonfunctional WBCs; few RBCs; plasma (50 to 70 ml. total volume contains 5.5×10^{10} platelets); levels of labile clotting factors depend on storage time	5 days (20° to 24° C.)
Platelets (apheresis from random donor)	As above; usually contains as many platelets as 6 to 10 single units ($>30 \times 10^{10}$)	Usually 24 hours; up to 5 days (20° to 24° C.)
Leukocyte concentrate	WBCs; may contain large numbers of platelets, some RBCs (600 ml. total volume contains 5 to 30×10^9 granulocytes)	24 hours (20° to 24° C.)
Fresh frozen plasma	Plasma, all coagulation factors (180–250 ml. contain 0.7 to 1 U./ml. of factor II, factor V, factor VII, factor VIII, factor IX, factor XII, factor XIII, and 500 mg. of fibrinogen)	Frozen: 1 year ($<-30°$ C.) Thawed: 24 hours (1° to 6° C.)
Cryoprecipitate	Fibrinogen, factor VIII, factor XIII, von Willebrand's factor, fibronectin (10–20 ml. contains 80 U./ml. factor VIII, 200 mg. fibrinogen)	Frozen: 1 year ($<-30°$ C.) Thawed: 4 hours if pooled (20° to 24° C.)
Albumin	Albumin (12.5 gm. albumin in 50 or 250 ml.)	3 years (room temperature)

RBCs, red blood cells; WBCs, white blood cells; CPDA-1, citrate phosphate dextrose adenine; AS-1, Adsol.

or platelets can thus be removed in a relatively short period.

The storage and refrigeration of packed RBCs creates progressive changes, known as *storage lesions*[42] (Table 8–2), which include altered affinity of hemoglobin for oxygen; decrease in pH; changes in RBC deformability; hemolysis; an increase in the concentration of potassium, phosphate, and ammonia; development of microaggregates; release of vasoactive substances; and denaturation of proteins. The survival of RBCs is shortened the longer cells are stored, and this is associated with a decrease in intracellular 2,3-diphosphoglycerate (2,3-DPG). The transfusion of cold blood may also contribute to the development of hypothermia, especially in patients receiving large volumes of banked blood rapidly. Many of the changes described can be reversed within a short time after transfusion or may cause different metabolic patterns than predicted based on the content of the unit.

CLINICAL USE OF BLOOD COMPONENTS

Transfusion based on sound physiologic principles and an understanding of relative risks and benefits should give maximal benefit to the patient with efficient use of a valuable and finite resource. The following guidelines for transfusion from our hospital provide a general basis for sound transfusion practice but should not be considered a mandate. Such guidelines cannot substitute for the clinical judgment of an experienced clinician and are designed to allow flexibility in practice. The specific needs of some patients may require consultation with specialists in transfusion medicine.

Whole Blood

Whole blood may be used for patients with acute blood loss who have lost over 15% of the blood volume. Giving whole blood instead of packed RBCs and plasma is less expensive and carries half the infectious risk of packed RBCs plus FFP each from different donors. However, storage of whole blood precludes the production of components and is highly inefficient. Whole blood is thus unavailable in most blood banks in the United States, because oxygen-carrying capacity and replacement of volume can be achieved with packed RBCs and crystalloid solutions. There are currently few indications for whole blood besides acute blood loss, and many blood banks in the United States do not routinely store this product.

Red Blood Cells

Packed RBCs can be stored in CPDA-1 for 35 days at 1° to 6° C. With longer storage, fewer than 70% of the RBCs remain viable in circulation 24 hours after transfusion, which is the current Food and Drug Administration definition of an outdated unit. Storage in AS-1 solution prolongs the shelf life to 42 days. Platelets degenerate at refrigerator temperatures, so banked packed RBCs contain essentially no functioning platelets. The levels of factors V and VIII decrease significantly over 24 hours at 1° to 6° C., although the levels of other factors remain essentially unchanged.

Packed RBCs. Packed RBCs provide oxygen-carrying capacity and maintain oxygen delivery provided intravascular volume and cardiac function are adequate. Packed RBC transfusion should be used only when time or the clinical situation precludes other therapy. The decision to transfuse and the amount to transfuse depend on the clinical situation. The use of a hematocrit of 30% (or a hemoglobin of 10 gm. per 100 ml.) as a *transfusion trigger* is no longer acceptable without considering the clinical situation.[51] Oxygen delivery is maintained by a series of complex interactions and compensatory mechanisms when the red cell mass (as measured by hemoglobin or less precisely by hematocrit) falls. This includes increased cardiac output, increased extraction ratio, rightward shift of the oxyhemoglobin curve, and expansion of volume.[51] Many chronically anemic patients tolerate hemoglobin levels of 7 to 8 gm. per 100 ml. or less, as has been demonstrated in patients with chronic renal failure and in Jehovah's Witnesses. Such patients compensate for a lowered red cell mass by an increase in concentrations of 2,3-DPG in the RBC with shift of the oxyhemoglobin curve to the right and greater release of oxygen to the tissues. The cardiac output in such patients does not increase until the hemoglobin falls below approximately 7 gm. per 100 ml. Young healthy patients tolerate acute anemia to hemoglobin levels of 7 gm. per 100 ml. or less provided they have a normal intravascular volume and high arterial oxygen saturation. The primary compensation in this setting is an increased cardiac output (heart rate and stroke volume). The response to the lowered RBC mass and the need for RBC transfusion can be assessed by clinical criteria such as ongoing blood loss, increased heart rate, dizziness, and oxygen delivery and weighed against potential untoward effects. In patients with significant cardiopulmonary disease, especially advanced coronary artery disease, increases in cardiac output can cause myocardial ischemia. Such patients should receive RBC transfusion whenever clinically indicated to prevent cardiac ischemia. A stable, asymptomatic patient should not generally receive packed RBCs solely for a hematocrit below 30%.

Each unit of packed RBCs usually raises the hematocrit 2% to 3% in a 70-kg. adult, although this varies depending on the donor, the recipient's fluid status, the method of storage, and its duration. Suggested guidelines for packed RBC transfusion are shown in Table 8–3.

Washed RBCs. Washed RBCs are given to patients who require packed RBCs but cannot tolerate the plasma and leukocyte or platelet debris normally found in units prepared in standard fashion. This includes patients who have febrile reactions caused by leukoagglutinins and patients with renal dysfunction who cannot tolerate the potassium present in the

TABLE 8–2. Metabolic and Related Changes During Storage; Value for Third Week of Storage of Whole Blood in CPD

Metabolic acid load	25–40 mEq./L.
Citrate	5 mEq./L.
Phosphate	6–10 mg./L. plasma
Ammonia	Up to 1 mg./100 ml.
Plasma hemoglobin	20 mg./100 ml.
Particulate matter	Up to 2–4 gm./unit
Negative thermal load	14.4 kcal./unit at 4° C.
Plasticizer	20–25 mg./unit
Red blood cells	
Posttransfusion early loss	20–25%
2,3-Diphosphoglycerate	0
Adenosine triphosphate	Very low
Membrane lipids	Depleted
Osmotic fragility	Increased
Coagulation	
Factor V	Probably 10% or less
Factor VIII	Probably 30% or less
Platelets	0
Antigenic debris	Considerable (HLA, platelet, red blood cell, leukocyte, plasma protein antigens)
Transmissible diseases	See text
Denatured proteins	Likely but undefined
Vasoactive substances	Serotonin, bradykinin, histamine, ?others

TABLE 8–3. Suggested Transfusion Guidelines for Red Blood Cells

Hemoglobin ≤8 gm./100 ml. or acute blood loss in an otherwise healthy patient with signs and symptoms of decreased oxygen delivery with two or more of the following:
  Estimated or anticipated acute blood loss of ≥15% of total blood volume (750 ml. in 70-kg. male)
  Diastolic blood pressure ≤60 mm. Hg
  Systolic blood pressure drop ≥30 mm. Hg from baseline
  Tachycardia (>100 beats per minute)
  Oliguria/anuria
  Mental status changes

Hemoglobin ≤10 gm./100 ml. in patients with known increased risk of coronary artery disease or pulmonary insufficiency who have sustained or are expected to sustain significant blood loss

Symptomatic anemia with any of the following:
  Tachycardia (>100 beats per minute)
  Mental status changes
  Evidence of myocardial ischemia including angina
  Shortness of breath or dizziness with mild exertion
  Orthostatic hypotension
Unfounded/questionable indications:
  To increase wound healing
  To improve the patient's sense of well-being
  7 ≤hemoglobin ≤10 (or 21≤hematocrit ≤30) in otherwise stable, asymptomatic patient
  Mere availability of pre-donated autologous blood without medical indication

plasma of banked blood. Such cases should generally be discussed with a transfusion specialist.

Deglycerolized RBCs. RBCs may be stored for up to 3 years at lower than −65° C. in special glycerol-containing media. This technique permits the stockpiling of rare blood units. When such a unit is needed, the RBCs are thawed and washed before transfusion. These units may also be used for patients requiring washed RBCs, as described earlier.

Platelets

Platelet transfusions are indicated for patients suffering from or at significant risk of bleeding due to thrombocytopenia and/or platelet dysfunction. Three types of platelet concentrate are available. A single, random-donor unit of platelets is prepared from a single donation of whole blood from one donor (see Fig. 8–1). Patients receive 6 to 10 units of this product (a *six-pack* or a *ten-pack* of platelets). Multiple-unit, single-donor platelets are harvested from one donor by apheresis.[44] This yields as many platelets as 6 to 10 single random-donor units. Multiple-unit, single-donor platelets can be obtained by apheresis from donors who are selected by human leukocyte antigen (HLA) type to yield HLA-matched platelets. Beside monitoring the patient for evidence of improved hemostasis, follow-up platelet counts at 1 hour and at 12 or 24 hours can provide an estimate of platelet survival. After platelet transfusion in the adult, the platelet count obtained at 1 hour should rise at least 5000 platelets per cu. mm. for each unit of platelets transfused. Patients may experience a lesser response especially after repeated transfusion and the development of alloimmunization or because of fever, sepsis, splenomegaly, drug effects, or uremia. When alloimmunization causes the poor response, single-donor units may provide an adequate response. Platelets from a donor of HLA type similar to that of the patient may also be needed.[19]

Basic guidelines for platelet transfusion are outlined in Table 8–4. In general, platelets should not be transfused prophylactically in the absence of microvascular bleeding, a low platelet count in a patient undergoing a surgical procedure, or a platelet count that has recently fallen below 10,000 per microliter. Previous guidelines used a guideline of 20,000 per microliter for prophylaxis in stable patients without oozing or in those not undergoing surgical or invasive procedures. More recent data, however, suggest that a threshold of 10,000 per microliter causes no added bleeding while significantly reducing use of the resource. Patients receiving massive transfusion should not automatically receive prophylactic platelets in the absence of microvascular bleeding.[18, 40] In such patients, hypothermia effects depressed platelet function, and platelet transfusion is generally ineffective.[34, 49] Restoration of a normal temperature returns platelet function to normal and ameliorates microvascular bleeding. Ideally, platelets should be transfused after the temperature has been corrected.

TABLE 8–4. Suggested Transfusion Guidelines for Platelets

Recent (within 24 hours) platelet count ≤10,000/cu. mm. (for prophylaxis)
Recent (within 24 hours) platelet count ≤50,000/cu. mm. with demonstrated microvascular bleeding ("oozing") or a planned surgical/invasive procedure
Demonstrated microvascular bleeding and a precipitous fall in platelet count
Adult patients in the operating room who have had complicated procedures or have required more than 10 units of blood *and* have microvascular bleeding. Giving platelets assumes adequate surgical hemostasis has been achieved.
Documented platelet dysfunction (e.g., prolonged bleeding time greater than 15 minutes, abnormal platelet function tests) with petechiae, purpura, microvascular bleeding ("oozing"), or surgical/invasive procedure
Unfounded/questionable indications:
  Empiric use with massive transfusion when patient is not having clinically evident microvascular bleeding ("oozing")
  Prophylaxis in thrombotic thrombocytopenic purpura/hemolytic-uremic syndrome or idiopathic thrombocytopenic purpura
  Extrinsic platelet dysfunction (e.g., renal failure, von Willebrand's disease)

Leukocyte Concentrate

Leukocyte transfusions are indicated in profoundly granulocytopenic (less than 500/cu. mm.) patients with evidence of infection (e.g., positive blood culture, persistent temperature above 38.5° C.) unresponsive to antibiotic therapy. Daily transfusions are given until the infection is under control or the granulocyte count is greater than 1000 per cu. mm. Because leukocyte concentrate is usually prepared by mechanical apheresis from donors typically premedicated with corticosteroids to increase the number of circulating granulocytes, using hydroxyethyl starch to enhance the separation of cells, there is more risk to the donor than with a routine blood donation. Consultation with specialists in infectious disease is recommended before leukocyte concentrate is given.

Fresh Frozen Plasma

Fresh frozen plasma is used to replace labile clotting factors in patients with coagulopathy and documented deficiency of clotting factors. This condition may derive from liver dysfunction, congenital absence of clotting factor, or transfusion of factor-deficient blood products. A unit of FFP contains near-normal levels of all clotting factors, including about 400 mg of fibrinogen. A unit of FFP increases clotting factor levels by about 3%. Adequate clotting is usually achieved with factor levels above 30%, although higher levels are advisable in patients undergoing operative or invasive procedures. The prothrombin time (PT) and the activated partial thromboplastin time (aPTT) can be used to assess patients for FFP transfusion and to follow the efficacy of administered FFP.

Guidelines for administration of FFP are listed in Table 8–5. Documentation of factor deficiency or abnormal PT or aPTT in a patient with clinical bleeding minimizes unnecessary use of FFP. FFP should not be used routinely by preset formula after RBC transfusion (e.g., 2 units of FFP for every 5 units of packed RBCs) or *prophylactically* after cardiac bypass or other procedures. With the availability of equally effective but safer (albumin, hetastarch) and less expensive (crystalloids) solutions, FFP should not be used as a volume expander.[38]

Cryoprecipitate

Cryoprecipitate is useful in treating factor deficiency (hemophilia A), von Willebrand's disease, and hypofibrinogenemia and may help treat uremic bleeding.[20] Each 5- to 15-ml. unit contains 80 units of factor VIII and about 200 mg. of fibrinogen. Fibronectin is also present. Because the proteins mentioned previously are in relatively high concentration, a smaller volume may be given than would be required if FFP were used. Cryoprecipitate is usually administered as a transfusion of 10 single units.

PERIOPERATIVE TRANSFUSION

The decision to transfuse a patient before operation should address several factors. No specific hematocrit is an indication for preoperative transfusion in a stable patient. However, a symptomatic patient with anemia who is about to undergo a procedure that involves significant blood loss is best transfused before the operation. Preoperative transfusion allows an *in vivo* test of compatibility between donor blood and recipient, thus avoiding a potential intraoperative transfusion reaction. If the patient is anemic with a low (or normal) reticulocyte count, transfusion may be the only way to raise the hemoglobin level before operation. As discussed earlier, patients with chronic anemia whose condition is otherwise stable should not be routinely transfused based on a criterion such as a hematocrit of 30%.[50] The goal of transfusion of a symptomatic patient is the relief of symptoms. The single-unit transfusion has been justifiably condemned; but if one unit is sufficient to alleviate symptoms, no additional transfusion should be given because each unit adds to the risk of transmission disease.

The maximal surgical blood order schedule was designed to minimize the use of RBC-containing products perioperatively[16] and is usually based on the institution's or physician's record of transfusion for certain operative procedures. When a surgeon requests blood preoperatively, a *type and screen* procedure is performed to determine the patient's ABO and D types and to detect preformed antibodies to RBC antigens. If the antibody screen is negative and the probability that the patient will require blood in the operating room is less than 10%, RBCs are not crossmatched unless the patient needs blood during the procedure. An abbreviated crossmatch is then performed within a few minutes and blood is released. If the probability of transfusion is greater than 10%, blood is crossmatched preoperatively. The number of units prepared is a function of the number of units transfused during the procedure in the past. In operations in which blood is frequently used, such as open heart or vascular procedures, the minimal number of units are crossmatched, and additional units are made available if they are needed. When a procedure is completed, blood is held for 24 to 48 hours and then automatically released for other patients. This process allows the most efficient use of blood products and avoids the full, three-phase crossmatch, which is not necessary.

TRANSFUSION OF THE PATIENT IN SHOCK

During World War I, it was believed that vascular collapse in injured patients was caused by toxins.[28] Experiments in the 1930s by Phemister and Blalock showed that fluid was lost from the circulation into damaged tissues. This was in keeping with the concept of a *third space*. In World War II, plasma was the resuscitation solution of choice. Although

---

TABLE 8–5. Suggested Transfusion Guidelines for Fresh Frozen Plasma

Treatment of multiple or specific coagulation factor deficiency with abnormal prothrombin time and/or activated partial thromboplastin time
Abnormal specific factor deficiency in the presence of one of the following:
   Congenital deficiency of antithrombin III; factors II, V, VII, IX, X, and XI; protein C or S; plasminogen or antiplasmin
   Acquired deficiency related to warfarin therapy, vitamin K deficiency, liver disease, massive transfusion, or disseminated intravascular coagulation
Also indicated as prophylaxis for the above if a surgical/invasive procedure is planned
Unfounded/questionable indications:
   Empiric use during massive transfusion if patient does not exhibit clinical coagulopathy
   Volume replacement
   Nutritional supplement
   Hypoalbuminemia

solutions containing electrolytes were used for children with diarrhea and advances had increased the understanding of metabolic and endocrine changes seen with injury, the use of plasma solutions prevailed until the Korean conflict. Subsequent experimental work indicated that extracellular fluids shifted into the intracellular space after significant hemorrhage with shock.[12] Providing volume resuscitation in excess of shed blood then became an acceptable practice to maintain adequate circulation.

During World War II, acute tubular necrosis was a common consequence of hypovolemic shock. Because fluid resuscitation became more prevalent during the Korean and Vietnam conflicts, the incidence of acute tubular necrosis dramatically decreased. Although acute tubular necrosis after hypovolemic shock became less of a problem with better fluid resuscitation, the *shock lung* syndrome (i.e., adult respiratory distress syndrome) became increasingly common. The lung injury in adult respiratory distress syndrome is a function of the shock state rather than the resuscitation solution used.

The goal of resuscitation from shock is prompt restoration of adequate perfusion and transport of oxygen. Restoration of circulation allows the cell to clear products of anaerobic metabolism and restore aerobic metabolism. The American College of Surgeons Committee on Trauma developed a classification of shock that permits useful guidelines for resuscitation. Crystalloid is infused at a 3:1 ratio for every unit of RBCs administered, and therapy is monitored by hemodynamic response. Because crystalloid solutions are universally available and some delay is required to prepare blood products, crystalloid is the proper initial resuscitation fluid. Resuscitation then proceeds with the use of blood products depending on the patient's response. The choice of a colloid solution (e.g., albumin, plasma) or a crystalloid solution (e.g., lactated Ringer's solution) has been controversial. Both can expand the extracellular space and provide effective resuscitation. However, crystalloid solutions are favored because they are less expensive, need not be crossmatched with the patient, do not transmit disease, and probably create less fluid accumulation in the lung. No experimental data indicate that using colloid rather than crystalloid solutions can prevent pulmonary edema.[24, 39]

Several crystalloid solutions are available for resuscitation, but isotonic solutions should be used to avoid overload of free water. Lactated Ringer's solution is recommended as initial therapy. Metabolic alkalosis is common after successful resuscitation with lactated Ringer's solution and blood products, because the lactate in Ringer's solution and the citrate in banked blood are both converted to bicarbonate if the patient has a functioning, perfused liver. Lactated Ringer's solution contains calcium; and if it is mixed with a unit of blood product, the blood may clot in the bag. Normal saline solution is an acceptable alternative to lactated Ringer's solution, but large volumes can produce a hyperchloremic metabolic acidosis, which may complicate the care of the patient in shock.

MASSIVE TRANSFUSION

Massive transfusion has been defined as replacement of the patient's blood volume with stored RBCs in 24 hours or as transfusion of more than 10 units of blood over a few hours. As many as 186 units of blood have been transfused intraoperatively over a 12-hour period.[32] Massive transfusion can create significant changes in the patient's metabolic status because of the infusion of large volumes of cold citrate-containing blood that has undergone changes during storage.[42] When blood is stored at 1° to 6° C., changes occur over time, including leakage of intracellular potassium, decrease in pH, reduced levels of intracellular adenosine triphosphate

and 2,3-DPG in the RBCs with increased affinity of hemoglobin for oxygen, degeneration of functional granulocytes and platelets, and deterioration of clotting factors V and VIII (see Table 8–2). Thus, if a large volume of stored blood is infused rapidly, significant effects may be seen in the recipient, depending on his or her metabolic state. Many of the expected changes can be reversed after transfusion or may produce different metabolic patterns than predicted.[42] Consequently, the use of standard formulas for the infusion of FFP, platelets, calcium, bicarbonate, and other substances for a specific number of units of packed RBCs transfused is contraindicated and may add risk for the patient.

Thermal Load. Significant degrees of hypothermia occur with rapid transfusion of large volumes of cold blood products. This is exacerbated in patients who have an open thoracic or abdominal cavity, which accelerates heat loss. Hypothermia increases the affinity of hemoglobin for oxygen, as do alkalosis and reduced 2,3-DPG in the transfused RBCs. Hypothermia impairs function of platelets.[34, 40, 49] Patients who have a core temperature below 34° C. do not clot normally, even if the levels of clotting factors and platelets are normal. Low temperature also increases the potential for hypocalcemia because the cold liver does not metabolize citrate as well, an effect exacerbated by shock. If the blood is being rapidly infused through a central line with its tip near the sinoatrial node, fatal arrhythmias can result. Hypothermia can be ameliorated by warming intravenous fluids before they are given. However, care must be taken to not heat RBCs above 40° C. because shortened survival or acute hemolysis can result.

Acid-Base Changes. Even though stored RBCs and whole blood have an acid pH (about 6.3), alkalosis is the usual result of massive transfusion. Sodium citrate, the anticoagulant in blood products, is converted to sodium bicarbonate in the liver. The alkalosis initially increases the oxygen affinity of hemoglobin. However, because it stimulates enzymes in the Embden-Meyerhof pathway of glycolysis, the net effects of alkalosis are to increase intracellular 2,3-DPG and restore RBC transport of oxygen. The posttransfusion pH may range from 7.48 to 7.50 and is associated with an increased excretion of potassium. The routine administration of bicarbonate with large transfusion volumes causes more severe alkalosis in the patient with undesirable effects on myocardial contractility and greater affinity of hemoglobin for oxygen, so that less oxygen is released to tissues.

Changes due to Citrate. Massive transfusion of citrated blood products can lead to transiently decreased levels of ionized calcium. The effects of hypocalcemia include hypotension, narrowed pulse pressure, and elevated left ventricular, end-diastolic, pulmonary artery, and central venous pressures. Electrocardiographic abnormalities (e.g., prolonged QT intervals) also occur. Commercially available electrodes can determine ionized calcium. Most normothermic adults who are not in shock can withstand the infusion of 1 unit of RBCs every 5 minutes without requiring calcium supplementation. Indiscriminate administration of calcium can produce transient hypercalcemia and should be avoided.

Changes in Potassium. Hyperkalemia is theoretically possible with massive blood transfusion because stored blood commonly has elevated potassium concentrations, as high as 30 to 40 mEq. per liter by 3 weeks of storage. However, unless the transfusion rate exceeds 100 to 150 ml. per minute, clinical problems associated with potassium are rare. Most patients requiring rapid transfusion are in shock and have an increase in aldosterone, antidiuretic hormone, and the permissive steroid hormones. Therefore, most massively transfused patients are hypokalemic unless renal function ceases. Hyperkalemia may cause peaked T waves on the electrocardiogram. Hyperkalemia, especially if associated with hypocalcemia, may significantly alter cardiac function.

Changes in 2,3-Diphosphoglycerate. Because 2,3-DPG is greatly reduced in RBCs after about 3 weeks of storage, massive transfusion of a patient with blood near the end of its storage life may decrease oxygen off-loading. Rapid correction occurs in most cases after the RBCs are transfused and rewarmed. If the patient's hematocrit is low with depressed cardiac function, as in the case of elderly persons with atherosclerosis, the reduced level of 2,3-DPG may be detrimental.

Hemostasis. Dilutional thrombocytopenia may occur in a patient who is massively transfused because the number of viable platelets is almost nil in blood stored for 24 hours at 1° to 6° C. The decrease is often less than one would expect on the basis of simple dilution, and this effect is not completely understood. Release of platelets from the spleen and the bone marrow may account for part of this difference. Despite the fact that platelet counts may fall with massive transfusion, dilutional thrombocytopenia alone usually does not account for microvascular bleeding.[18] As previously noted, prophylactic use of platelet concentrate in the massively transfused patient is not justified without evidence of microvascular bleeding.[18] Platelet concentrate contains significant amounts of all clotting factors except factor VIII, a factor often increased in shock victims. Patients receiving large-volume blood transfusion who experience microvascular bleeding unrelated to hypothermia are best treated with platelet concentrate, which provides clotting factors in addition to platelets. The PT and aPTT provide a reliable indicator for the need for FFP and factor replacement. The prophylactic use of FFP along with transfusion of RBCs is no longer acceptable in light of convincing data from several studies and the added risk of transfusion.[13, 42] In patients who develop disseminated intravascular coagulation (DIC), large doses of platelet concentrate, FFP, and cryoprecipitate may be required.

In summary, the major changes in the massively transfused patient are opposite to what one might expect based on the changes that occur during the storage of RBCs. In patients requiring massive transfusion, packed RBCs should be transfused to provide oxygen-carrying capacity, platelets given for microvascular bleeding in a normothermic patient, and crystalloid solution infused to restore intravascular volume. In most instances, addition of bicarbonate or calcium and prophylactic transfusion of FFP are contraindicated.

RISKS OF BLOOD TRANSFUSION

The transfusion of blood products can cause numerous serious complications, even death,[25, 43] and blood products should be considered potentially dangerous *drugs*. Physicians should exercise judgment when prescribing a blood transfusion; a transfusion that is not clearly indicated is contraindicated. A transfusion of incompatible RBCs is potentially fatal, but other significant concerns exist when a patient receives blood products, including infectious hazards and immunologic effects. The acquired immune deficiency syndrome and viral hepatitis remain the major infectious risks of transfusion. Data from the 1980s indicated that as many as 1 in 10 patients transfused would show evidence of hepatitis infection. With the introduction of donor screening for surrogate markers for non-A, non-B hepatitis and for antibodies to hepatitis C virus, the risk of posttransfusion hepatitis should fall to less than 1% per patient.[15] Other risks include hemolytic disease of the newborn in females of child-bearing age who become pregnant after Rh-incompatible transfusion. Because a transfusion exposes the recipient to a complex mixture of donor cells and proteins it is in many ways a *trans-*

plant. Blood components contain viable lymphocytes that can provoke a graft-versus-host response in the severely immunocompromised recipient.[50] Transfusion can modify the recipient's immune response, as has been demonstrated in patients undergoing renal transplantation.

Transfusion Reactions

The most severe transfusion reactions involve complement-mediated RBC destruction. As the RBCs are rapidly destroyed intravascularly, peptides derived from complement are released and produce hypotension, compromise renal blood flow, activate the clotting cascade, and lead to DIC. The conscious patient may become aware that almost immediately something is wrong. Signs and symptoms include pain and redness along the infused vein, chest tightness and pain, a feeling of *doom*, hypotension, oozing from intravenous sites, hematuria, oliguria, chills, and fever. In the unconscious patient, hypotension, hemoglobinuria, and diffuse oozing may be the only clues.

Most reported fatalities from transfusion reactions result from ABO incompatible transfusions.[25, 43] Most have occurred when a type O person received type A RBCs because of a clerical error in identification either at the time the blood sample was drawn, during laboratory processing, or when the unit was administered.[11] Such deaths are preventable, and extreme care should be employed throughout the process of drawing blood and labeling samples, during laboratory processing, and during identification of the proper recipient before transfusion.

When a transfusion reaction is suspected, the infusion should be stopped immediately and the label on the unit checked against the recipient's wristband. The unit, with all attached intravenous solutions and tubing, should be sent to the blood bank with blood samples drawn from a site remote from the infusion line. Urine should be tested for free hemoglobin. The blood bank should immediately check all samples and records, note whether the posttransfusion plasma is pink, and perform a direct antiglobulin test. The patient should receive aggressive fluid resuscitation to correct hypotension and maintain renal blood flow. Mannitol may be useful for diuresis. Patients who develop hypotension and DIC early are at greatest risk of death.

A hemolytic reaction can occur hours to days after transfusion. The degree of hemolysis may be particularly significant in the patient whose total RBC mass has been replaced by massive transfusion. A transfused patient who develops an unexplained fall in hematocrit, fever, or jaundice should be evaluated for the possibility of a hemolytic reaction. Nonhemolytic transfusion reactions are caused by antibodies against white blood cells (WBCs) or plasma proteins. The former usually cause chills and fever, whereas the latter lead to allergic symptoms such as urticaria or anaphylaxis. Febrile reactions can be prevented by transfusing leukocyte-poor RBCs or by premedicating the patient with acetaminophen before giving non–RBC-containing components such as platelet concentrate. Allergic reactions are usually prevented by premedication with diphenhydramine.

Transmission of Infection

Viral and bacterial diseases may be transmitted by blood transfusion. Viruses include Epstein-Barr virus, cytomegalovirus, hepatitis viruses, the human immunodeficiency virus (HIV), and human T-cell leukemia virus (HTLV) type I and II. Bacterial diseases include syphilis, malaria, and infection with *Yersinia enterocolitica, Babesia microti,* or *Trypanosoma cruzi.* The risk of transmission of bacterial infection is probably less than one in 1 million with current methods of testing.

Advances in the ability to detect the hepatitis C virus and more efficient screening of blood products have made the blood supply currently available in the United States from volunteer donors extremely safe and the risk of posttransfusion infection significantly reduced (Table 8–6). Blood transfusion represents a relatively safe therapeutic modality in comparison with other therapies employed in the care of patients.

Cytomegalovirus. Cytomegalovirus is the most common viral agent transmitted by means of blood transfusion.[8] Routine screening for cytomegalovirus is not performed in the United States because the infection is endemic. About 20% of blood donors are infected with cytomegalovirus by 20 years of age, and approximately 70% are infected by 70 years of age. The infection is carried in WBCs. Most patients who encounter problems related to cytomegalovirus are immunocompromised, especially transplant recipients on immunosuppressive drugs. Such patients require transfusion with cytomegalovirus-negative blood products to avoid the transmission of this viral infection.

Human Immunodeficiency Virus. Estimates of the risk of HIV transmission from blood transfusion range widely. Data suggest that the infectious window for HIV infection is approximately 45 days and that the overall risk of transmitting infection by transfusion is about 1 in 220,000 per unit.[14, 52] Previous estimates had ranged from 1 in 40,000 to 1 in 60,000 based on studies conducted in areas with high HIV prevalence.

Because infection with HIV causes active disease and ultimately death, transmission of this infectious agent must be viewed with great concern. It is encouraging that the number of cases of HIV infection related to transfusion have declined with the institution of effective methods to exclude infected donors. The latency period for development of antibody to the virus continues to pose a problem with the ability to detect all seropositive donors. Efforts to improve the safety of the blood supply have resulted in a reduction of the overall prevalence of HIV antibody–positive blood donors from 0.04% in 1985 to 0.015% in 1987.[51]

Hepatitis. Transmission of the infectious agents for hepatitis is among the most serious risks of blood transfusion. Past estimates of posttransfusion hepatitis were approximately 10%. Current data suggest that the infectious risk of hepatitis is closer to 1% or less per unit transfused.[14, 15] All blood is screened for the hepatitis B surface antigen, which should effectively eliminate transmission of the hepatitis B virus. In addition, blood is screened for surrogate markers for non-A, non-B hepatitis and for the hepatitis C virus. These screening techniques should produce high rates of detection for units with the potential for transmitting infection. The risk of transfusion-associated hepatitis B virus infection is approximately 1 in 200,000 per unit.[15] With the development of screening tests for the hepatitis C virus, studies suggest that the infectious risk for hepatitis C is about 1 in 3300 per unit.[14, 15]

TABLE 8–6. Estimated Risk (per Unit) of Transmission of Infection by Transfusion

Human immunodeficiency virus infection	1:225,000
Hepatitis B	1:200,000
Hepatitis C	1:3300
Human T-cell lymphotrophic virus type I and II infection	1:50,000
Malaria and *Yersinia enterocolitica*, *Babesia microti*, and *Trypanosome cruzi* infections	<1:1 million

Approximately half of the blood recipients who contract hepatitis B viral infection develop symptoms. A much smaller percentage require hospitalization. Approximately half of patients who contract posttransfusion hepatitis C infection develop a chronic form of the disease. Many of those patients eventually develop significant liver dysfunction, including cirrhosis.

Human T-Cell Leukemia Virus. In addition to the transmission of cytomegalovirus, hepatitis infection, and HIV, blood transfusion carries the risk of transmission of HTLV I and II infection. The prevalence of HTLV I seropositivity in the United States is quite low—approximately 0.025% of the donors tested.[7] Transmission of the virus especially to immunocompromised patients may cause a variety of illnesses, such as T-cell leukemia, spastic paraparesis, and myelopathy, and has prompted routine screening of donors in the United States since 1989.

Graft-Versus-Host Reaction

Blood transfusion exposes the recipient to a variety of cells and proteins from the donor. These include viable lymphocytes, which in an immunocompromised patient can produce a graft-versus-host reaction,[50] with fever, rash, nausea, vomiting and diarrhea, as well as abnormalities in liver function tests and depressed cell counts. A large proportion of these reactions have been fatal (as many as 90%). The prevalence of this complication in the United States is not known. Gamma irradiation of blood products can decrease the risk of this reaction.

Immunosuppression

The transfusion of packed RBCs depresses the immune response in patients undergoing renal transplantation. Studies on the effect of perioperative blood transfusion on the survival of patients with a variety of tumors have been noted.[3, 10] Controversy exists regarding the exact relationship of blood transfusions to increased recurrence of tumor and poor prognosis. The possibility that blood transfusion may represent a co-variable exists, because very ill patients and those undergoing more difficult procedures for more extensive disease are the ones most likely to receive blood transfusion. A comparison of autologous blood to allogeneic blood for perioperative transfusion produced no difference in outcome.[10] The impact of blood transfusions on the prognosis of colorectal cancer was thought to be that of a co-variable rather than a cause. Other studies have implicated blood transfusion as an independent prognostic factor for patients with colorectal cancer. Tarrter showed that patients whose tumor recurred had received approximately twice as many blood transfusions as patients without recurrence, an effect that was independent of other variables such as the patient's age, sex, tumor characteristics, extent of involvement of nodes, blood loss, duration of operation, and other variables.[48] Other studies using retrospective analysis and meta-analysis suggested a causative relationship between blood transfusion and recurrence of tumor and recommended a policy of blood conservation to minimize any negative impact of blood transfusion.

In view of the data on immunosuppression from blood transfusion, it would seem reasonable to adopt a policy of blood conservation in the perioperative period in the absence of clear indications and acute symptoms. Further studies may clarify the exact relationship between perioperative blood transfusion and the recurrence of solid tumors.

BLOOD SUBSTITUTES AND ALTERNATIVES TO TRANSFUSION

Red Blood Cell Substitutes. Red blood cell transfusion is the only acceptable clinical method for increasing oxygen-carrying capacity. Development of RBC substitutes would eliminate the infectious risk of blood transfusion and provide a ready source of universally compatible product. Several substances have been considered as RBC substitutes and can be divided into two general groups: (1) synthetic molecules, such as the porphyrins and the perfluoro compounds, and (2) molecules that incorporate hemoglobin in their structure, such as the conjugated and polymerized stroma-free hemoglobin solutions. Acceptable RBC substitutes must be able to carry at least as much oxygen as hemoglobin normally carries (1.34 ml. of oxygen per gram of hemoglobin). In addition, these molecules should be stable and have an acceptable half-life. The RBC substitute should have properties that allow it to become completely saturated with oxygen at standard fraction of inspired oxygen, while unloading substantial portions of its transported oxygen at tissue partial pressure of oxygen levels. The solutions prepared must be highly purified and free of contaminants and endotoxin.

Perfluorocarbons efficiently transport significant quantities of oxygen and carbon dioxide and thus have the potential to be an effective RBC substitute. Perfluorocarbons can transport 40 to 50 ml. of oxygen per 100 ml. of solution, which is greater than twice the quantity of oxygen that completely saturated hemoglobin carries in the normal adult. Several perfluorocarbon molecules have been tested in humans with limited success.[46] At present they have no clinical application as RBC substitutes.

Early attempts to prepare hemoglobin solutions consisted of pooling outdated blood, breaking the RBCs open, and extracting the hemoglobin molecules. Because the antigenic properties of RBCs are associated with the membrane, hemoglobin solution so prepared can be infused into patients of all blood types. This solution is termed *stroma-free hemoglobin*. Limitations to the use of stroma-free hemoglobin include its very short half-life in the circulation, its relatively low oxygen-carrying capacity, and its clearance through the kidneys, causing significant side effects. To circumvent these problems, the hemoglobin solutions were polymerized and pyridoxylated. The resultant solution has the same oxygen-carrying capacity as normal blood and stays in circulation 4 to 5 days without being cleared through the kidneys. Such solutions can keep experimental animals alive for several hours in the complete absence of any native RBCs.[46] Subsequent trials in healthy volunteers demonstrated the safety of the solution in humans. Clinical trials are underway to determine the efficacy of the solution for acute blood loss and perioperative applications.

Intraoperative Hemodilution. Intraoperative hemodilution was introduced by Messmer.[18] The procedure removes 1 to 3 units of the patient's blood and replaces it with crystalloid or in some cases a combination of crystalloid and colloid to restore the intravascular volume. This is done before an operative procedure and is tolerated well in all patient populations. The blood that is withdrawn is anticoagulated and maintained at room temperature for up to 4 hours. It is reinfused into the patient as needed during the surgical procedure. If this procedure is combined with autologous predonation, 6 or more units of blood can be available for a procedure in which significant blood loss is expected. Data suggest that the actual benefits of this procedure are minimal, especially when used in isolation to minimize blood transfusion.[17] There is no role for this technique in acute hemorrhage.

Intraoperative Cell Salvage. The salvage of intraoperative blood loss effectively minimizes the need for blood transfusion. This technique has had successful applications in various operative procedures, including cardiac surgery, spine surgery, liver transplantation, trauma procedures, and vascular surgery. Reports of intraoperative cell salvage in trauma patients with enteric contamination have demonstrated that the procedure can be used safely in such situations, provided the cells are washed before reinfusion.[6] The use of devices for collecting blood lost from the thoracic cavity through a chest tube can also decrease the amount needed for transfusion.

Autologous Blood. Patients scheduled for elective procedures in which significant blood loss requiring transfusion is expected should be considered for autologous predisposition. Autologous blood transfusion has many advantages, including compatibility and the lack of infectious transfusion risk. If the patient is free of infection and has a hematocrit of at least 30%, he or she should be able to predonate. Many patients can have blood withdrawn every 3 to 4 days until 3 days before operation. Predonation can begin up to 1 month before the procedure. Autologous donors must receive iron supplementation and should maintain good nutrition. Patients ordinarily thought to be at high risk, such as those with cardiac disease, have successfully predonated blood,[29] and patients of all ages can predonate safely. The success of an autologous blood transfusion program requires the collaboration of surgeons and blood bank personnel.

SURGICAL BLEEDING DISORDERS

Hemostasis is the physiologic cessation of bleeding. The ability to achieve adequate hemostasis is critical to the success of surgical operations and the recovery from injury. Under normal circumstances, blood maintains its fluidity because of the balance of various procoagulant and anticoagulant influences, including interactions at the blood-endothelial interface and a variety of circulating factors.[36] Hemostatic and coagulation mechanisms allow the prompt repair of a local injury in the microcirculation without progression to a systemic reaction. Injured blood vessels can therefore be repaired and hemorrhage can be controlled locally, while blood continues to flow normally in other uninjured areas. Once the injury to the blood vessel has been repaired, lysis of clots formed in the area begins and the vessel may ultimately regain patency. Localized injury to the vascular system thus activates hemostatic mechanisms at the injury site and circulating coagulation mechanisms. Once healing has occurred, a system of fibrinolysis reestablishes patency of the blood vessel and degrades the products of coagulation.

A series of highly interrelated events is responsible for hemostasis[22, 27] (Table 8–7). Advances in the understanding of the molecular processes involved in hemostasis and coagulation have led to a fundamental reappraisal of the coagulation cascade, especially its initiation and regulation. When injury to a vessel occurs, subendothelial tissue factor (TF) and collagen are exposed. Platelets adhere to the site of injury and undergo a release phenomenon with further platelet aggregation. A platelet *plug* forms. Vasoconstriction occurs in response to the release of vasoactive substances from platelets (e.g., thromboxane A_2 and serotonin) and endothelin from endothelial cells. The interaction of coagulation factor VII with TF, its high-affinity receptor and cofactor, initiates the coagulation cascade. Thrombin is produced, as are fibrin monomers from fibrinogen. A thrombus is formed from fibrin and entrapped platelets and other blood elements and is stabilized by cross-linking of the fibrin monomers. Ultimately, clot retraction follows the interaction of platelets and the fibrin strands. Under normal circumstances, local blood flow, vasodilatory substances, and regulatory feedback mech-

TABLE 8–7. Key Events in Hemostasis

Blood vessel injury with exposure of tissue factor and collagen

Platelet aggregation and adherence with formation of platelet "plug"

Vasoconstriction

Initiation of coagulation cascade by interaction of tissue factor with factor VII, with conversion of prothrombin to thrombin and activation of the coagulation cascade

Thrombin converts fibrinogen to fibrin

Fibrin monomers and entrapped platelets form a hemostatic thrombus

Stabilization of the fibrin clot by cross-linking of fibrin monomers

Organized clot formation and arrest of bleeding

Local blood flow, vasodilatory influences, and regulatory feedback mechanisms limit extension of thrombus

Fibrinolysis with dissolution of the fibrin thrombus. Thrombus protects itself from unimpeded fibrinolysis by incorporating inhibitors in the clot

anisms limit the clotting process to the area of injury. The thrombus is ultimately dissolved by fibrinolysis, which involves the formation of plasmin from plasminogen. These processes are highly interrelated and interdependent *in vivo* and are involved in regulatory feedback loops that maintain a fine balance between procoagulant hemostatic mechanisms and normal anticoagulant functions.

Local Hemostatic Mechanisms

Blood Vessels and Endothelial Cells. Vasoconstriction is an important early response to vessel injury. Thromboxane A_2 is produced locally at the site of injury and is a very potent constrictor of smooth muscle, especially in smaller and medium-sized vessels. Larger vessels constrict in response to innervation and to circulating constrictive factors such as norepinephrine. Completely transected vessels are more likely to seal effectively than are partially transected vessels. Arteries are more muscular than veins and thus undergo vasoconstriction more readily. Veins experience a lower perfusion pressure than arteries and are therefore more likely to cease bleeding with local tamponade.

Although endothelial cells were considered relatively quiescent, they are highly active cells with many important products and effects, including both antithrombotic and procoagulant effects[36] (Table 8–8). Under normal conditions, endothelial cells are crucial in the maintenance of a nonthrombogenic interface between vessels and the circulating blood. Among the contributory mechanisms identified thus far are the elaboration of prostacyclin (a potent inhibitor of platelet aggregation), nitric oxide, thrombomodulin, tissue plasminogen activator (tPA), and binding of the anticoagulant antithrombin III to heparan sulfate on the endothelial cell surface. Thrombomodulin is a membrane-bound glycoprotein that binds thrombin. The thrombomodulin-thrombin complex activates protein C, which, along with its cofactor protein S, degrades activated factors Va and VIIIa, thus decreasing thrombin generation. Endothelial cell injury exposes subendothelial TF and collagen, reduces thrombomodulin availability, increases phospholipid sites for coagulation protein binding, and expresses TF on the cell surface. These changes promote the procoagulant effect of injury. In addition, inflammatory agents such as endotoxin, interleukin-1, and tumor necrosis factor promote the procoagulant effects described.[33]

Platelets. Platelets participate in hemostasis through a sequence of adherence to the site of injury, release of the contents of their alpha and dense granules, aggregation to form a platelet plug, and promotion of coagulation by providing a procoagulant surface on their phospholipid membranes.[22] Platelets rapidly adhere to exposed subendothelial collagen and other basement membrane proteins. The presence of fibrinogen and von Willebrand's factor (vWF) is important for the successful adherence of platelets. It is known that vWF binds to collagen and undergoes a conformational change. The vWF then binds the platelet surface receptor glycoprotein Ib/IX. After adhering to the subendothelium, platelets develop pseudopods. Platelets are then activated with release of the contents of their alpha granules (platelet factor 4, beta-thromboglobulin, thrombospondin, platelet-derived growth factor, fibrinogen, vWF) and dense granules (adenosine diphosphate, serotonin). With the release of platelet granule contents, particularly adenosine diphosphate, further platelet aggregation at the site of injury occurs. The glycoprotein IIb/IIIa receptors on adjacent platelets are joined by a molecule of fibrinogen. Platelet activation also produces platelet procoagulant activity through surface coagulation factors. These events lead to the formation of a platelet plug within 1 to 3 minutes of vessel injury. Ionized calcium and thromboxane A_2, a potent platelet aggregator, are important in many steps of this process. The expression of coagulation factor Va on the platelet phospholipid surface promotes interaction of coagulation factors and ultimately the formation of thrombin on the platelet surface. This causes further platelet degranulation and aggregation with incorporation of more platelets into the clot. As fibrin is deposited, the clot is stabilized. Retraction of the clot occurs with a reduction in clot size within 10 minutes of the initial injury.

The production of prostacyclin by the endothelial cell serves to counterbalance the local hemostatic process. In particular, prostacyclin elevates levels of adenyl cyclase with an increase in cyclic adenosine monophosphate levels within platelets, decreasing available ionized calcium and limiting further aggregation of platelets. Because of its potent vasodilatory effects, prostacyclin also limits the progress of localized coagulation.

TABLE 8–8. Endothelial Cell Products That Regulate Hemostasis

Product	Properties
Prostacyclin	Labile secreted inhibitor of platelet aggregation; vasodilator
Nitric oxide	Labile secreted inhibitor of platelet aggregation and adhesion; vasodilator
Platelet activating factor	Secreted and cell surface–associated platelet and leukocyte stimulant
Ectonucleotidases	Surface enzymes that regulate breakdown of platelet: active and vasoactive nucleotides
von Willebrand's factor	Stored and secreted cofactor for platelet adhesion and clotting factor VIII
Thrombomodulin	Surface-expressed anticoagulant
Tissue factor (thromboplastin)	Procoagulant only expressed on activated endothelium
Tissue plasminogen activator	Stored and secreted regulator of fibrinolysis
Plasminogen activator inhibitor	Secreted, circulating and matrix-bound inhibitor of tissue plasminogen activator

From Pearson, J. D.: Endothelial cell function and thrombosis. Baillieres Clin. Haematol., 7:441–452, 1994.

Circulating Coagulation Mechanisms

Hemostasis is initiated by interactions between the vessel wall and circulating platelets. Ultimately, however, the formation of a stable fibrin clot is necessary for adequate hemostasis to occur. The process leading to clot formation is highly regulated. The interactions of this system occur on the phospholipid surfaces and involve core factors, enzymes, and substrates (see Table 8–7). Several inactive precursors (zymogens) are sequentially converted to serine proteases that interact in an amplification reaction to generate the enzyme thrombin that converts insoluble fibrinogen to a soluble fibrin clot (Table 8–9). Fibrin monomers are then cross-linked to form the stable fibrin clot under the effect of factor XIII. Regulatory proteins and inhibitory substances are produced concurrently that limit the propagation of the clot and ensure that the thrombosis is limited to the site of injury.

Previous concepts of coagulation held that two pathways exist by which coagulation could occur: the intrinsic pathway and the extrinsic pathway (Fig. 8–2). In the intrinsic pathway, interaction of circulating factors already within the blood initiates coagulation. This begins with the binding of factor XII to negatively charged surfaces, whereby it undergoes a conformational change. Partial activation thus results, and factor XII then interacts with prekallikrein and high-molecular-weight kininogen. More complete activation of factor XII to factor XIIa thus occurs. In the process, factor XIIa activates prekallikrein to kallikrein, which itself becomes a potent activator of factor XII. Activated factor XIIa then activates factor XI. Activated factor XI converts factor IX to factor IXa in the presence of calcium. Activated factor IXa then forms a complex with activated factor VIIIa, calcium ion, and phospholipids to activate factor X. Activated factor Xa is then able to convert prothrombin to thrombin, thus changing fibrinogen into fibrin. Factor XIII converts the fibrin monomers into a cross-linked fibrin clot in the presence of calcium. The clinical relevance of the intrinsic pathway is not clear. Deficiency of some components of the intrinsic pathway is not associated with clinically significant bleeding, although it does produce aberrations in tests of coagulation. In particular, deficiencies of factor XII or of prekallikrein are not associated with a bleeding tendency in humans, whereas patients with defi-

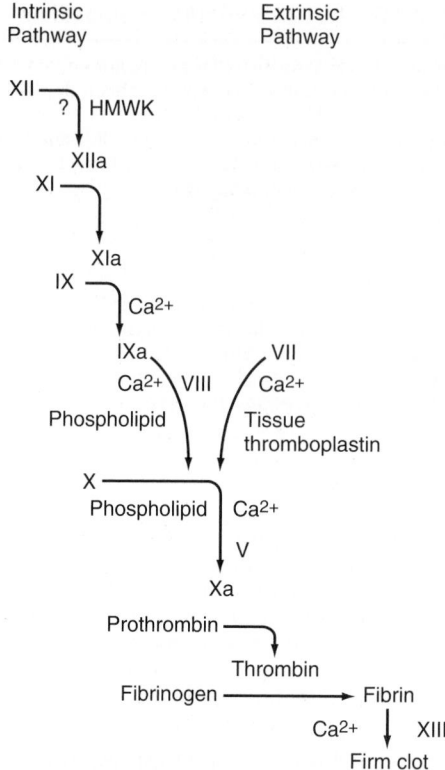

Figure 8–2. Traditional schematic version of the coagulation system. HMWK, high-molecular-weight kininogen.

ciencies of factor VIII or factor IX exhibit pronounced bleeding disorders (hemophilia A and B, respectively). The role of the intrinsic pathway in *in vivo* coagulation has not been established. The extrinsic pathway involves the interaction of factor VII with TF. In the presence of calcium, the factor VII–TF complex is formed and activates factor X to factor Xa. Activated factor Xa then converts prothrombin to thrombin, and the reaction proceeds as described previously.

TABLE 8–9. Hemostatic and Coagulation Factors

Factor	Synonym	*In Vivo* Half-Life (hr.)	Source for Therapy
I	Fibrinogen	100–150	FFP, cryoprecipitate, platelets
II	Prothrombin	50–80	FFP, platelets
III	Tissue factor		
IV	Calcium ion		
V	Proaccelerin, labile factor	24	FFP, minimal in platelets
vWF	von Willebrand's factor	24	FFP, cryoprecipitate, full concentrate
VII	Serum prothrombin conversion accelerator, stable factor	6	FFP, platelets
VIII	Antihemophilic factor	12	FFP, cryoprecipitate, factor VIII concentrate (plasma derived or recombinant)
IX*	Christmas factor	24	FFP, prothrombin complex concentrate, factor IX concentrate, platelets
X*	Stuart-Prower factor	25–60	FFP, platelets
XI	Plasma thromboplastin antecedent	40–80	FFP, minimal in platelets
XII	Hageman factor	50–70	FFP, platelets
XIII	Fibrin stabilizing factor	150	
Platelets		Variable	Platelets

*Vitamin K–dependent factors.
FFP, fresh frozen plasma; platelets, platelet packs.

Recent discoveries have increased emphasis on the TF pathway (Fig. 8–3).[22, 27] When the integrity of the blood vessel wall is disrupted, subendothelial substances are exposed, including TF, collagen, and plasminogen activator (which initiates fibrinolysis). The exposure of cells expressing TF to plasma activates the coagulation system. The distribution of TF is highly cell specific and includes adventitial cells, outer layers of the epidermis, other squamous epithelial cells, and myoepithelial cells. This corresponds to a *hemostatic envelope* surrounding blood vessels and organs.[27] Factor VII binds to TF and is rapidly activated to factor VIIa. The TF–factor VIIa complex catalyzes the activation of factor IX to IXa. In addition, the TF–factor VIIa complex can directly convert factor X to factor Xa, converting prothrombin to thrombin. The amounts of thrombin formed by the direct activation of factor X to factor Xa are relatively small, however, and cannot account for observed hemostatic effects. This is in part due to the rapid inactivation of the TF–factor VIIa–factor Xa complex by TF pathway inhibitor (TFPI).[9] The small amounts of thrombin formed, however, are sufficient to induce the activation of factors VIII and IX, thereby perpetuating the cascade. Factor IXa creates a complex with factor VIIIa, calcium, and phospholipid. This complex activates factor X to factor Xa with the production of significant amounts of thrombin. Deficiencies of either factor VIII or IX are associated with significant bleeding disorders in humans (hemophilia A and B, respectively). These observations suggest that the activation of factor X to factor Xa by the factor VIII–factor IX–phospholipid complex is the predominant mechanism for the generation of thrombin *in vivo*. Factor V is a cofactor for the activation of factor X to factor Xa. The activity of TF–factor VIIa complex is inhibited by the action of antithrombin III, a member of the serine protease inhibitor superfamily, in the presence of heparin. This revised scheme of blood coagulation explains the observed clinical syndromes of deficiency of the various factors and clarifies the relatively limited role that factor XII plays in coagulation *in vivo*.

Thrombin is a potent enzyme transforming fibrinogen into fibrin. Thrombin also converts factor VIII to activated factor VIIIa and factor XI to activated factor XIa. It also has a role in the activation of factor V, an important cofactor for factor X activation. Factor XI deficiencies are associated with a mild bleeding disorder in humans. Factor XI can also be activated by activated factor XIIa, as previously described. The interaction of activated factor XIa with factor IX explains the relatively limited role that factor XI has in coagulation. It may have a significant role in cases of severe bleeding. The activation of factor XI by thrombin requires the presence of a number of cofactors, including high-molecular-weight dextran sulfate. The importance of these observations for coagulation *in vivo* is still incompletely determined.

In addition to its other effects, thrombin activates anticoagulant pathways. Thrombin binds thrombomodulin on the cell surface of endothelial cells. The thrombin-thrombomodulin complex activates protein C in the presence of its cofactor protein S, rapidly inactivating factors Va and VIIIa. This is a clinically important anticoagulant pathway in humans, because either protein C or protein S deficiency is known to cause a significant tendency toward thrombosis. Thrombin is inactivated by antithrombin III in the presence of heparin. Deficiency of antithrombin III is also associated with a tendency to venous thrombosis. Antithrombin III also inactivates factors VIIa, IXa, Xa, XIa, kallikrein, and plasmin. Heparin accelerates all these reactions by causing a conformational change in antithrombin III. Heparin cofactor 2 is similar to antithrombin III in that it is a naturally occurring anticoagulant. However, heparin cofactor 2 inhibits only thrombin. Its activity is enhanced by both heparin and dermatan sulfate.

Fibrinogen is a large plasma protein composed of two pairs of polypeptide chains. Cleavage of portions of these chains by thrombin produces fibrin monomers. The fibrin monomers are then cross-linked in the presence of factor XIII to form a stable clot.

Von Willebrand's factor (vWF) is a large protein that produces several important effects in hemostasis and coagulation. In addition to its role in the adhesion of platelets to injured vessel walls, it is a carrier for factor VIII in plasma, thus protecting it from degradation.

Fibrinolysis. Numerous advances have been made in understanding the biochemical mechanisms of the fibrinolytic system.[5] Several activators of plasminogen have been characterized and the mechanism of the activation reaction studied. The fibrinolytic system is important in opposing the tendency toward blood coagulation and maintaining the fluid charac-

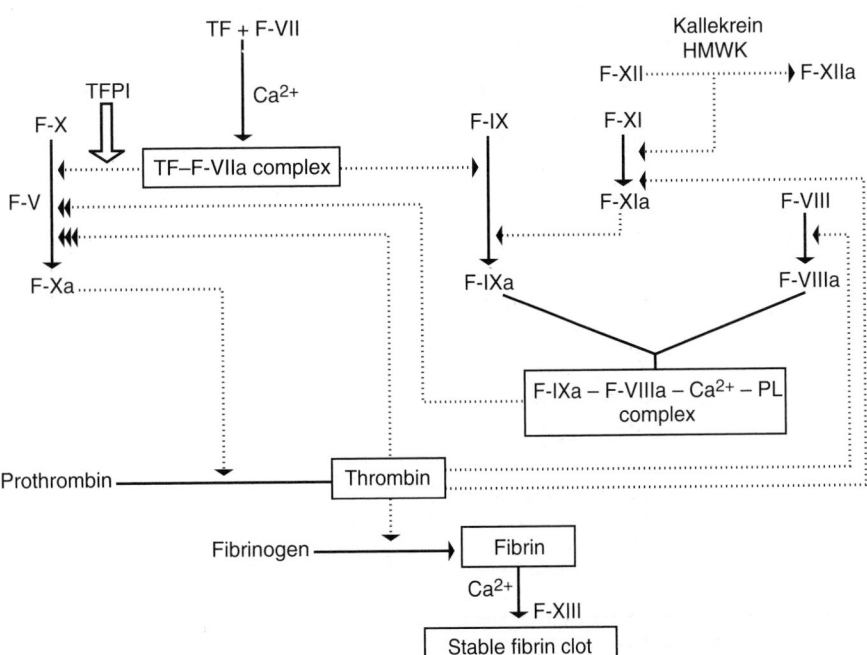

Figure 8–3. Updated coagulation scheme emphasizing the tissue factor pathway. TF, tissue factor; TFPI, tissue factor pathway inhibitor; F, factor; HMWK, high-molecular-weight kininogen.

teristics of blood in the intravascular space. The main reaction of the fibrinolytic pathway is the activation of plasminogen to plasmin by the plasminogen activators, tissue plasminogen activator (tPA) and urokinase (Fig. 8–4). The reactions of the fibrinolytic cascade are catalyzed by serine proteases in a manner analogous to the coagulation cascade. These reactions are believed to occur on the surface of endothelial cells. The serine proteases are regulated by inhibitors from the serine protease inhibitors superfamily, which act as pseudosubstrates for the proteases. The major inhibitors of plasminogen are plasminogen activator inhibitor 1 (PAI-1) and plasminogen activator inhibitor 2 (PAI-2). The major inhibitor of plasmin is alpha$_2$-antiplasmin (also called alpha$_2$ plasmin inhibitor). Fibrin helps regulate fibrinolysis in addition to serving as its major substrate. Physiologic fibrinolysis is a reparative process that occurs in response to hemostatic plug or formation of thrombus. The final enzymatic step, fibrin proteolysis, results from a coordinated interaction of enzymes and inhibitors, which produces effective action at the site of the disease and spares the proteins of the blood or uninvolved parts of the vascular system.

Plasmin is a serine protease and its main *in vivo* target is fibrin. Plasmin is a powerful proteolytic enzyme that breaks down fibrin into soluble fragments. Like other coagulation factors, plasmin is formed from plasminogen, a circulating precursor. Plasmin acts not only on fibrin but also on fibrinogen and factors II, V, and VIII and, some data suggest, on factors IX and XI. It effectively metabolizes a number of other proteins, including adrenocorticotropic hormone, growth hormone, and insulin. It also activates factor XII and thus activates the coagulation, complement, and kinin systems. The interactions among these multiple, complex systems are incompletely understood.

Plasminogen circulates in plasma at relatively high concentrations, whereas tPA is found in low concentration. Plasma tPA concentrations are markedly increased by release from endothelial cells in response to stress and injury. The activation of plasminogen by tPA is inefficient in the absence of fibrin. In the presence of fibrin, activation proceeds rapidly, providing an important regulatory role for fibrin in the process of its degradation. Urokinase efficiently activates plasminogen in the absence of fibrin, but its plasma levels are low and its role in hemostasis is poorly defined. Epithelial cells lining excretory ducts of the body (e.g., renal tubules, mammary ducts) secrete urokinase, which is the physiologic activator initiating lysis of fibrin that may be formed in these areas. Streptokinase, a bacterial product not normally found in the body, is a potent activator of plasminogen and has been used to induce fibrinolysis therapeutically.

The major inhibitor of plasminogen activation is PAI-1, which is found in low concentration in plasma but at higher concentration within platelets. Plasma PAI-1 is probably synthesized in endothelial cells and/or hepatocytes. This inhibitor of the fibrinolytic system increases after trauma and operation. The synthesis of PAI-1 is affected by a variety of compounds, including endotoxin, thrombin, transforming growth factor-beta, interleukin-l, and tumor necrosis factor-alpha. The major inhibitor of plasmin, alpha$_2$-antiplasmin, circulates in plasma at relatively high concentrations and can neutralize large amounts of plasmin. It can also bind plasminogen. Alpha$_2$-antiplasmin binds to fibrin during the process of fibrin cross-linking by factor XIII and protects the thrombus from fibrinolysis. Both plasminogen activator inhibitors and plasmin inhibitors are important regulators. The plasminogen activators, predominantly tPA, and their main inhibitor, PAI-1, circulate at low concentrations and are readily cleared from the circulation. Small changes in their production or elimination significantly change the balance of their activities in plasma. Because PAI-1 levels are higher than tPA levels, tPA is generally highly bound in plasma. Under stress conditions, significant amounts of tPA are released from the endothelium and unbound tPA is available to promote activation of plasminogen. The ability of alpha$_2$-antiplasmin to neutralize free (nonfibrin-bound) plasmin prevents inappropriate systemic activation of fibrinolysis. This control is superseded in certain conditions, such as with the therapeutic administration of plasminogen activators to lyse pathologic thrombi or when plasmin degrades plasma fibrinogen into degradation fragments (X, Y, D, and E). Degradation of cross-linked fibrin creates distinctive products characterized by cross-linked (factor XIIIa–induced) derivatives such as D-dimer. Disease states occurring after abnormalities in the fibrinolytic system include both hemorrhagic disorders, resulting from excessive fibrinolysis, and thrombotic disorders, from deficient fibrinolysis. Hyperfibrinolysis can result from pharmacologic administration of activators such as streptokinase, urokinase, and tPA or from defective inhibition produced by alpha$_2$-antiplasmin deficiency. Hyperfibrinolytic thrombosis can result from hereditary defects of plasminogen or from pharmacologic inhibition of fibrinolysis, such as with epsilon-aminocaproic acid. Laboratory evaluation of fibrinolysis can aid assessment of thrombotic disorders and bleeding. It includes the specific measurements of plasminogen activators, plasminogen, plasmin inhibitors, and circulating fibrinogen and products of cross-linked fibrin degradation.

EVALUATION OF PATIENTS WITH DISORDERS OF HEMOSTASIS OR COAGULATION

The surgeon may encounter disorders of hemostasis and coagulation either in the preoperative evaluation of the patients for elective surgery or in the perioperative care of patients with acute bleeding disorders. Diagnosis of the specific disorder involved requires an evaluation of the patient's history, a review of available medical records, especially as they relate to risk factors for bleeding or previously obtained laboratory data, a physical examination, and appropriate laboratory tests.[31]

An accurate history and physical examination of a patient scheduled to undergo elective operation offers the most valuable source of information regarding the risk of bleeding during operation. A patient with a history of bleeding, easy bruisability (either spontaneous or traumatic), frequent or unusual mucosal bleeding, exceptionally high menstrual flow in females, prior history of significant or life-threatening hemorrhage associated with invasive procedures, or a family

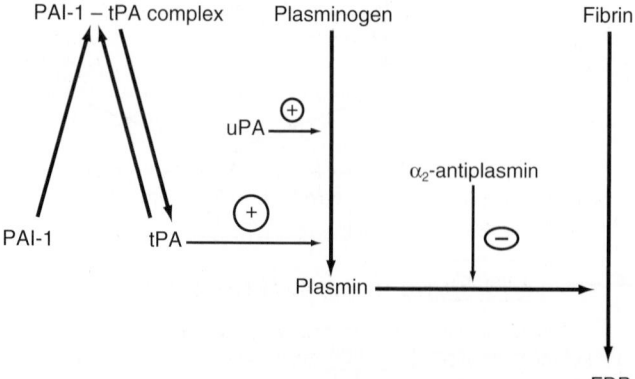

Figure 8–4. Schematic representation of fibrinolysis. PAI-1, plasminogen activator inhibitor 1; tPA, tissue plasminogen activator; uPA, urokinase plasminogen activator; FDP, fibrin degradation products.

history of such problems may be at risk. A history of repeated severe epistaxis or abnormal laboratory tests may also be significant. The intake of medications should always be elicited. Especially important are drugs such as aspirin and nonsteroidal anti-inflammatory drugs (NSAIDs); and because these preparations are widely available "over the counter," it is important to inquire specifically about them. Patients may not consider the intake of aspirin or NSAIDs as being important enough to mention when interviewed unless a specific question is asked. In addition, a history of liver dysfunction, renal dysfunction, or major metabolic or endocrine disorder is useful in directing preoperative screening. Physical examination also provides valuable information. Evidence of excessive bruising, joint deformities, petechiae or ecchymosis, hepatosplenomegaly, excessive mobility of joints, or increased elasticity of the skin are symptoms of disorders associated with excessive perioperative bleeding. Evidence of amyloidosis (such as thickening of the skin or tongue), multiple myeloma, or other hematologic malignancies is also revealing.

Screening Tests for Bleeding Disorders

The extent of laboratory testing needed for patients with a normal history and physical examination has been debated. For most patients undergoing either minor operations or procedures that do not involve extensive dissection, laboratory testing is unlikely to provide additional information over a properly performed history and physical examination. Routine preoperative laboratory screening is useful for patients undergoing major procedures, especially involving body cavities or operations with significant dissection and the creation of raw surfaces, or patients with an abnormal history or physical examination. Patients with infection, sepsis syndrome (or the systemic inflammatory response syndrome), malnutrition, organ failure, and other major systemic disorders also warrant preoperative screening before surgical intervention. In general, the commonly recommended tests include the prothrombin time (PT), the activated partial thromboplastin time (aPTT), a complete blood cell count with platelet count, and, in some patients, a bleeding time. The PT measures the function of factor VII as well as the *common pathway* factors (factor X, prothrombin/thrombin, fibrinogen, fibrin). The aPTT measures the *intrinsic pathway* factors as well as those of the common pathway. The platelet count identifies numbers of platelets, whereas the bleeding time estimates qualitative platelet function. None of the commonly recommended screening tests measures fibrinolytic function. Additional screening tests that may be used for specific patients include a fibrinogen level, the thrombin time (TT), and screens for factor XIII levels. The TT detects abnormalities of globulin, fibrinogen, excess fibrinolysis, and heparin-like substances. In patients suspected of having platelet dysfunction, additional assessments include platelet function tests (aggregation with epinephrine, adenosine diphosphate, collagen, and ristocetin). If a deficiency or specific factor is suspected, as in patients with a family history of hemophilia, then specific factor assays should be obtained.

Patients with familial thrombocytopenia (May-Hegglin anomaly) have a relatively common autosomal dominant disorder associated with petechiae and hyperpigmentation of the distal lower extremities. These patients may have abnormal bleeding due to decreased platelet numbers. Patients with Marfan's syndrome, the Ehlers-Danlos syndrome, or osteogenesis imperfecta may have abnormal bleeding and poor wound healing despite normal screening tests. Other bleeding disorders often missed by routine coagulation testing include mild von Willebrand's disease, platelet function

defect, factor XIII deficiency, hyperglobulinemic states, alpha$_2$-antiplasmin deficiency, and amyloidosis.

If a patient scheduled for an elective procedure has a history of significant risk factor for bleeding, or if abnormal findings on physical examination suggest a bleeding disorder or deranged screening laboratory tests, the procedure should be postponed pending a more complete evaluation and any necessary treatment. Patients about to undergo emergency operative procedures may require urgent correction of their hemostatic abnormalities before and during operation (using the guidelines previously presented).

The PT is identified by adding a thromboplastin (TF + phospholipid and calcium) to citrated platelet-poor plasma. The time until a fibrin clot is formed is measured in seconds and reported as the PT. A control specimen provides the baseline normal value. The PT detects deficiencies of factor VII and the common pathway protein factors (fibrinogen, factor II, factor V, factor X). Warfarin therapy and vitamin K deficiency deplete the vitamin K–dependent proteins (factor II, factor VII, factor IX, factor X, protein C, protein S) and prolong the PT.

The aPTT is performed by adding a partial thromboplastin (a mixture of phospholipids), an activating substance, and calcium chloride to citrated plasma. The aPTT detects decreased levels of the intrinsic pathway factors (high-molecular-weight kininogen, prekallikrein, factor XII, factor XI, factor IX, and factor VIII) and the "common pathway" factors (fibrinogen, factor II, factor V, and factor X). The anticoagulant heparin is a commonly employed drug that causes prolongation of the aPTT without significantly prolonging the PT by depleting the intrinsic pathway factors. The aPTT is therefore useful for monitoring heparin therapy.

The PT and aPTT can be used together in an attempt to localize coagulation defects. A normal PT with an abnormal aPTT suggests deficiency of the proximal intrinsic pathway factors. A prolonged PT with a normal aPTT suggests abnormalities of the vitamin K–dependent factors such as factor VII. In addition, an abnormal PT or aPTT may indicate the presence of an inhibitor (e.g., lupus anticoagulant, heparin, or an inhibitor of a specific factor). To differentiate an inhibitor from a factor deficiency, a mixing study is performed by mixing the patient's plasma in a 1:1 ratio with normal plasma and repeating the abnormal PT or aPTT. If the abnormal value corrects to the normal range, this indicates the presence of a coagulation factor deficiency in the patient's plasma. However, if the abnormality does not correct, an inhibitor is presumed to exist.

The bleeding time is a somewhat crude screening test for platelet function that also reflects, to some degree, endothelial cell function. This test is performed by placing a standardized cut in the skin of either the forearm (Ivy method) or the earlobe (Duke method). Because the bleeding time is affected by many variables, including the manner in which the cut is placed, the location of the cut, endothelial cell function, platelet counts, and overall platelet function, it is a somewhat difficult test to standardize. Data suggest that although the bleeding time may be useful in evaluating patients with bleeding disorders, it has limited value as a screening test in predicting whether an otherwise normal patient will develop bleeding during an operation.[41]

ACQUIRED BLEEDING DISORDERS

A variety of coagulation abnormalities may be present in the surgical patient. Acquired defects are more common than congenital defects.

Vitamin K Deficiency. Several proenzymes of the coagulation system contain carboxyglutamic acid, which has two carboxy groups attached to the carbon of glutamic acid. The extra carboxy group acts as a binding site for calcium. Vitamin K is necessary for the reaction that attaches the additional carboxy group to glutamic acid, and the proteins containing carboxyglutamic acid residues are therefore called vitamin K–dependent clotting factors (including factors II, VII, IX, and X and protein C and protein S). When synthesized in the absence of vitamin K, these proteins, lacking carboxyglutamic acid residues, cannot bind calcium normally. Vitamin K is a cofactor of hepatic microsomal carboxylase. This is also the site of action of the coumarin oral anticoagulants. The causes of vitamin K deficiency may be inadequate dietary intake, malabsorption, lack of bile salts, obstructive jaundice, biliary fistula, oral administration of antibiotics, or parenteral alimentation. A number of broad-spectrum antibiotics can cause a vitamin-dependent coagulopathy, including cefoperazone, moxalactam, cefamandole, and ceftizoxime.

Vitamin K may be administered parenterally and produces a measurable correction in clotting times within 6 to 12 hours. Up to 5 mg. intravenously is given slowly as an initial dose. Older preparations of vitamin K were less purified than those used at present, and anaphylaxis and death were reported with intravenous administration of these older agents. The more purified forms are less likely to cause complications, but intravenous vitamin K should be given cautiously. Intramuscular or subcutaneous vitamin K may be given in doses of 10 to 25 mg. per day. Repeated doses of intramuscular or subcutaneous vitamin K allow total body repletion (10–25 mg. daily for 3 days). Administration of FFP rapidly corrects the coagulation deficit and should be given with vitamin K to patients with ongoing bleeding.

Anticoagulant Drugs. Derivatives of warfarin (Coumadin) act by blocking the synthesis of vitamin K–dependent coagulation factors. Warfarin prolongs the prothrombin time and causes a slight elevation of the aPTT by reducing the levels of prothrombin (factor II) and factors VII, IX, and X. Warfarin has a half-life of 40 hours, and treatment of major bleeding caused by warfarin consists of either administration of vitamin K or infusion of FFP for life-threatening bleeding.

Heparin blocks the activation of factor X by binding with antithrombin III to the thrombin molecule, inactivating it. All coagulation tests can be affected by heparin, including the PT, but the aPTT is most sensitive. A dose of heparin is cleared from the blood in approximately 6 hours, but this varies depending on other factors such as hepatic function, body temperature, and shock. Because heparin is strongly negatively charged, it can be neutralized on a milligram-for-milligram basis with intravenous protamine sulfate, which is strongly positively charged (100 units of heparin is equal to 1 mg. of protamine). The dose of protamine given should be approximately equal to the dose of heparin given, considering the half-life. Heparin can cause thrombocytopenia in up to 5% of patients; rarely, it causes a profound thrombocytopenia with secondary arterial thrombosis.[21] In these patients, all heparin should be withdrawn immediately, and another anticoagulant such as citrate initiated if necessary.

Hepatic Failure. Liver diseases including major hepatic trauma, cirrhosis, and biliary obstruction regularly impair coagulation. The liver is the major site of synthesis of all the coagulation factors except factor VIII. Hemostasis may be further impaired by an associated thrombocytopenia or platelet dysfunction, which also occur frequently with liver disease. Studies have shown that the prolonged bleeding times frequently seen in cirrhotic patients can be improved by administration of desmopressin.[23] The compound is often ineffective in patients with thrombocytopenia or congenital platelet dysfunction. The liver is important in clearing blood of the activated metabolites of both fibrinolysis and coagulation, and the coagulation system may be pushed either toward coagulation or bleeding in patients with liver dysfunction.

Liver disease is commonly associated with a low level of serum fibrinogen, a prolonged PT, and a normal to slightly increased aPTT. An elevated TT usually indicates abnormal or decreased fibrinogen. In patients with severe liver dysfunction, whether caused by cirrhosis, shock, or hepatic trauma, extremely large volumes of FFP may be required to maintain normal factor levels. Up to 2 units of FFP may be needed every 2 hours in patients with complete liver failure to maintain adequate coagulation factor levels, normalize clotting tests, and control bleeding.

Renal Failure. Renal disease and uremia cause a reversible bleeding disorder largely related to platelet dysfunction. There is a decrease in aggregation and adhesiveness of platelets, in the levels of platelet factor II, and in a prolonged bleeding time. The nature of the lesion caused by renal insufficiency is not known. The administration of desmopressin helps decrease bleeding problems after a variety of procedures in these patients.[23] The intravenous administration of desmopressin, 0.3 µg. per kg., in uremic patients decreases bleeding time, increases platelet retention on glass beads, and increases activity of factor VIII. Cryoprecipitate also helps normalize the prolonged bleeding times. The administration of conjugated estrogens effectively shortens the bleeding time in patients with renal failure.

Thrombocytopenia. Normal platelet counts range from 150,000 to 400,000 per cu. mm. A platelet count of less than 100,000 per cu. mm. generally constitutes thrombocytopenia. With platelet counts between 40,000 and 100,000 per cu. mm., bleeding may occur after injury or operation, but spontaneous bleeding is uncommon. Spontaneous bleeding may occur with platelet counts between 10,000 and 20,000 per cu. mm.; with counts below 10,000 per cu. mm., spontaneous bleeding is frequent and often severe.

Thrombocytopenia may be secondary to failure of production of platelets, splenic sequestration, increased destruction of platelets, increased use of platelets, or dilution. Defects in platelets often cause spontaneous bleeding into the skin, manifested by petechiae, purpura, or confluent ecchymoses. Thrombocytopenia also causes mucosal bleeding and excessive bleeding after operation. Heavy gastrointestinal bleeding and bleeding into the central nervous system may be life-threatening manifestations of thrombocytopenic bleeding. Thrombocytopenia does not generally cause massive bleeding into tissues or hemarthroses.

Drugs (e.g., quinidine, sulfa preparations, oral antidiabetic agents, gold salts, rifampin, and heparin) can cause thrombocytopenia. Contributing factors include a recent blood transfusion with posttransfusion purpura, heavy consumption of alcohol (alcohol-induced thrombocytopenia), and underlying immunologic disease (e.g., arthralgia, Raynaud's phenomenon, unexplained fever). The presence or absence of fever is an important point of differential diagnosis. It is usually present in thrombocytopenia secondary to infection or active systemic lupus erythematosus and in thrombotic thrombocytopenic purpura but absent in idiopathic thrombocytopenic purpura and in drug-related thrombocytopenias. Size of the spleen on physical examination is a second important diagnostic point. The spleen is not palpably enlarged in most thrombocytopenias caused by increased destruction of platelets (e.g., idiopathic thrombocytopenic purpura, drug-related immune thrombocytopenias), whereas it is usually palpably enlarged in thrombocytopenia secondary to splenic sequestration of platelets and often in patients with thrombocytopenia secondary to a lymphoma or a myeloproliferative disorder.

The peripheral blood cell count provides clues to the diagnosis and severity of thrombocytopenia. An increased proportion of large platelets (determined by scanning the blood smear or by measuring mean platelet volume with an electronic blood counter) suggests compensatory increased production of platelets and is often found in thrombocytopenias secondary to increased destruction or utilization of platelets. The bleeding time is routinely prolonged in severe thrombocytopenia of any cause. Bone marrow aspiration is useful.

Management of thrombocytopenia secondary to decreased production is directed toward correcting its cause (e.g., to induce a remission in a patient with acute leukemia). Platelet concentrates can be given to raise the platelet count temporarily; however, repeated use reduces their effectiveness due to development of platelet alloantibodies. If rapid correction of bone marrow failure is not expected, transfusions of platelets are often saved to treat an active bleeding episode. Corticosteroids have not proved beneficial in the management of patients with thrombocytopenia secondary to bone marrow failure.

Thrombocytopathy. Drugs to consider with important effects on platelets include chemotherapeutic agents, thiazide diuretics, alcohol, estrogen, antibiotics such as the sulfa agents, quinidine and quinine, methyldopa, and gold salts. The most common drugs that block platelet function are probably prostaglandin inhibitors, particularly aspirin, indomethacin, and other NSAIDs. Aspirin and other NSAIDs act to block prostaglandin metabolism in the platelet. Aspirin permanently acetylates cyclooxygenase, and affected platelets remain dysfunctional throughout their 7-day life span after exposure to aspirin. NSAIDs cause a reversible defect that lasts 3 to 4 days. Desmopressin may be effective in normalizing the prolonged bleeding time caused by aspirin.[23]

Hypothermia. Hypothermia is one of the most common and least well recognized causes of altered coagulation in surgical patients, especially those receiving massive transfusion. The coagulation system is a series of proteolytic enzymes, and all enzyme activity decreases with decreasing temperature. Hypothermia is characterized by a marked increase in fibrinolytic activity, thrombocytopenia, and a decrease in collagen-induced platelet aggregation. These abnormalities can cause severe bleeding complications.

Hypothermia and bleeding usually occur in a patient who receives large volume resuscitation during an extensive surgical procedure or in the perioperative period. Temperatures as low as 30° C. to 34° C. can occur in this setting. In these patients, nonmechanical bleeding frequently occurs and can be uncontrollable and lethal. The best course is to complete the surgical procedure as expeditiously as possible, pack bleeding areas as needed, close the surgical incision, and attempt to rewarm the patient as rapidly as possible in the intensive care unit. Continued administration of FFP, platelets, and other blood products often worsens hypothermia and continues bleeding. Hypothermia clearly creates abnormalities in coagulation and excessive bleeding. Cold has been associated with hepatic dysfunction and increased levels of blood citrate with transfusion. Hemorrhage accounts for 90% of deaths after abdominal injury, and half of these deaths are secondary to a recalcitrant coagulopathy.[35]

CONGENITAL BLEEDING DISORDERS

Congenital disorders of coagulation usually involve a single coagulation protein. Diagnosis depends on the history, physical examination, PT and aPTT determinations, and assay of levels of plasma factor. Surgical procedures can be performed on patients with congenital disorders of coagulation with a high degree of confidence and an acceptable, but somewhat increased, incidence of complications. Ideally, the coagulation defect should be diagnosed preoperatively, which may not be possible in the emergency or trauma patient. If available, a history of bleeding problems before presentation usually suggests the presence of this disease. Careful management should include specific factor replacement, meticulous intraoperative hemostasis, and careful monitoring of blood coagulation in the perioperative period. Early consultation with a coagulation specialist is important.

Hemophilia

Hemophilia A (classic hemophilia) is a congenital coagulation disorder that results from a deficiency or an abnormality of factor VIII. It is transmitted as an X-linked recessive disorder, with males being affected almost exclusively. A large number of different mutations accounting for the genetic abnormality have been identified. Up to 30% of cases of hemophilia A represent spontaneous mutations. In patients with hemophilia who have normal platelet function, the onset of bleeding is often delayed by several hours or days after injury, because the platelet plug is the first line of defense against bleeding, followed later by formation of thrombus. Bleeding may then persist for several days or weeks. The severity of the disease can be categorized based on the functional levels of factor VIII. This is termed *factor VIII:C* in contradistinction to *factor VIII:Ag*, which refers to the antigenic level. Patients with factor levels less than 2% generally have very severe bleeding, whereas those with levels between 2% and 5% have moderate bleeding and those in the range of 5% to 30% have mild disease. The patient with hemophilia A generally presents with bleeding into the deep tissues and joints. Large hematomas and hemarthroses are more common than the mucosal bleeding commonly seen with platelet disorders. The long-term complications of the repeated hematomas and hemarthroses can be crippling.

The laboratory work-up of patients with hemophilia A reveals a prolonged aPTT with decreased factor VIII:C in a male with normal PT, bleeding time, and vWF:Ag (antigenic level of von Willebrand's factor). The determination of vWF:Ag excludes the diagnosis of von Willebrand's disease, which may occur with a normal bleeding time (although that is generally not the case). A female patient with laboratory abnormalities consistent with hemophilia A is unusual but may represent a carrier state, an unusual chromosomal aberration, or other rare disorder. A small proportion of patients with hemophilia A (10–20%) develops inhibitors to factor VIII:C. These are usually IgG antibodies, and they complicate therapy. The detection of inhibitors requires a mixing study. The actual level of the inhibitor can be quantified using a Bethesda assay.

Hemophilia B is also known as Christmas disease. It is an inherited X-linked bleeding disorder similar to hemophilia A. The symptoms are identical to those of hemophilia A. Deep bleeding and hemarthroses occur in males and ultimately cause crippling dysfunction in those with severe disease. The disorder reflects a deficiency or defect in factor IX levels. The severity of symptoms correlates directly with the level of circulating factor IX in a manner analogous to hemophilia A.

The laboratory diagnosis of hemophilia B consists of the detection of an abnormal aPTT with decreased factor IX levels in a male patient with a normal PT, bleeding time, and platelet count. In the work-up of a familial bleeding disorder, the determination of factor VIII, factor IX, and vWF:Ag is helpful in differentiating the three major congenital disorders: hemophilia A, hemophilia B, and von Willebrand's disease. Because factor IX is a vitamin K–dependent factor, vitamin K deficiency may produce depressed levels. In cases of vitamin K deficiency, however, the PT is prolonged and levels subsequently correct with the administration of exogenous vitamin K. As is the case with hemophilia A, inhibitors can develop to factor IX. Mixing studies will demonstrate the presence of an inhibitor, and a Bethesda study quantitates their levels.

Therapy. The use of desmopressin may temporarily raise factor VIII levels in the patient with mild hemophilia A (basal factor VIII levels of 5% to 10%). Its administration to such patients after minor trauma or before elective dental surgery may obviate or reduce the need for replacement therapy. An intravenous dose of 0.3 μg. per kg. raises factor VIII levels 2-fold to 10-fold. Intranasal desmopressin is also effective and raises factor VIII levels 2-fold to 3-fold. Desmopressin is uniformly ineffective in severe hemophilia A.[26]

FFP contains both factors VIII and IX. However, unless plasma exchange is done, sufficient whole plasma cannot be given to patients with severe hemophilia to raise factor VIII or IX concentrations to levels that effectively prevent or control bleeding episodes. Cryoprecipitate is a good source of factor VIII but is rarely used when specific factor VIII concentrates are available. Plasma concentrates have therefore been developed. Prior serious problems with transmission of HIV and hepatitis have been addressed previously, and viral transmission is now unlikely with preparations available in the United States. Two types of concentrates are available for treatment of hemophilia A: (1) plasma-based factor VIII preparations, and (2) recombinant preparations. Plasma-based preparations are available in intermediate- and high-purity strengths and are significantly less costly than recombinant preparations. Factor VIII activity is expressed in units, with 1 unit being defined as the amount of factor VIII in 1 ml. of normal plasma. In general, 1 U. per kg. of factor VIII raises levels by 2%. Although the concentration of factor VIII in individual bags of cryoprecipitate varies, a bag may be assumed to contain 80 U. of factor VIII in calculating the number of bags needed for replacement therapy. In the event of a major surgical procedure or an injury, factor VIII levels should be maintained well above 50% of normal initially, and above 30% of normal at all times until complete healing has occurred. In general, these levels can be achieved by administering 50 U. per kg. and then about 30 U. per kg. every 8 hours for the first 2 days after operation or injury. Subsequent infusions given every 12 hours are suitably adjusted, depending on serum factor VIII assays.

For treatment of hemophilia B, the traditional therapy is prothrombin complex concentrate, which contains not only factor IX but all of the vitamin K–dependent clotting factors. High-purity factor IX concentrate is now available. For unknown reasons, only about half the number of factor IX units listed on a bottle of prothrombin complex concentrate can be recovered after infusion into patients. Therefore, when prothrombin complex concentrate is given for factor IX replacement therapy, an amount double that calculated as necessary is given. Because prothrombin complex concentrate may contain variable amounts of activated clotting factors, patients receiving repeated doses of factor IX concentrate are, paradoxically, at increased risk for thrombosis. For this reason, heparin (5 to 10 U.) is often added to each milliliter of reconstituted prothrombin complex concentrate.

The level of factor VIII or IX should be raised transiently to about 30% to protect against bleeding after dental extraction or to abort a beginning joint hemorrhage; to 50% if major joint or intramuscular bleeding is already evident; and to 100% in life-threatening bleeding or before major operation. In hemophiliacs with a factor VIII inhibitor who are bleeding, treatment is difficult and should be undertaken in consultation with a coagulation specialist experienced in such care. If possible, musculoskeletal bleeding is managed without giving factor VIII, because it will stimulate further production of antibodies and a rise in plasma titer of antibody within 3 to 4 days. In patients with serious bleeding and a low initial

antibody titer, a large dose of factor VIII, calculated to overcome the inhibitor and temporarily raise the concentration of plasma factor VIII, may be given. If this does not control the bleeding, further infusion of factor VIII is useless because of the rapid rise in antibody induced. Prothrombin complex concentrate contains variable amounts of a poorly characterized activity that bypasses the role of factor VIII in coagulation; therefore, these concentrates are used to manage serious bleeding in patients with a high titer inhibitor. Special preparations of prothrombin complex concentrate with increased amounts of this activity are available but expensive. Recombinant factor VIII preparations are often effective in patients with inhibitors.

Von Willebrand's Disease

Von Willebrand's disease is the most common of the congenital bleeding disorders, and its frequency has been estimated as high as 1%. Most patients have a mild bleeding disorder. The symptoms of von Willebrand's disease are related to its role as an important stimulus to platelet aggregation at the site of tissue injury and as the major carrier protein for circulating factor VIII. A large number of subtypes have been described, most of which are rare. The three major groups are type I, inherited as an autosomal dominant trait and characterized by a quantitative decrease of an otherwise normally functioning vWF; type II, which is variably inherited and characterized by qualitative defects in vWF; and type III, an autosomal recessive severe bleeding disorder with essentially absent levels of vWF. Bleeding encountered in patients with von Willebrand's disease is similar to that of patients with bleeding from platelet dysfunction. Unlike patients with hemophilia who develop deep hematomas and hemarthroses, patients with von Willebrand's disease develop mucosal bleeding, petechiae, epistaxis, and menorrhagia similar to patients with platelet disorders.

The laboratory diagnosis of von Willebrand's disease varies by subtype. Type I von Willebrand's disease is characterized by a normal PT, a mildly prolonged aPTT, an abnormal bleeding time, a normal platelet count, and a mild reduction in both factor VIII:C and vWF:Ag. The reduction in factor VIII:C occurs because vWF is the serum carrier for factor VIII. Patients with blood type O have lower normal levels of factor VIII:C and vWG:Ag and may occasionally be erroneously thought to have mild type I von Willebrand's disease. The diagnosis of type II von Willebrand's disease is complicated by the many described subgroups. In general, decreased functional activity of vWF produces a depressed ristocetin cofactor assay (vWF R:Cof), which measures the effectiveness of vWF in agglutinating platelets when stimulated with the antibiotic ristocetin. A further subtype of type II von Willebrand's disease, called pseudo–von Willebrand's disease, is a platelet disorder characterized by the presence of very large platelets that aggregate in the presence of cryoprecipitate. Type III von Willebrand's disease is characterized by near-complete absence of factor VIII:C, vWF:Ag, and R:Cof. These patients have prolonged aPTT levels, abnormal bleeding times, and low platelet counts. The help of a specialist in coagulation is important in determining the exact subtype and ultimate treatment of such patients.

The administration of desmopressin, 0.3 μg. per kg., causes significant shortening in the bleeding time and normalization of factor VIII and vWF activities. It is effective in reducing blood loss in the perioperative setting.[23] About 48 hours must elapse for new endothelial stores of vWF to accumulate and so permit a second injection of desmopressin to be as effective as an initial dose. Replacement of vWF by infusing cryoprecipitate is effective in the control or prevention of bleeding in von Willebrand's disease. Dosage is often selected empirically (e.g., 1 bag per 10 kg. every 8 to 12 hours for several days to prevent excessive bleeding after major operation).

Other Congenital Deficiencies

A variety of other congenital deficiencies may be encountered rarely. These include deficiencies of factor XI, factor XII, prekallikrein, and high-molecular-weight kininogen, also called the contact factors. In addition, deficiencies of factor VII, factor V, and factor II have been described but are extremely rare. Disorders of fibrinogen, including afibrinogenemia, hypofibrinogenemia, and dysfibrinogenemia may occur. Bleeding disorders in these patients range from severe to very mild depending on the level and function of factor in circulation. Factor XIII deficiency creates abnormalities of the cross-linking of fibrin monomers. This is a rare disorder inherited through an autosomal recessive route and characterized by poor wound healing and delayed postsurgical bleeding. Standard laboratory testing is not diagnostic in this disorder, and determination of factor XIII levels is necessary for the diagnosis.

DISSEMINATED INTRAVASCULAR COAGULATION

Disseminated intravascular coagulation (DIC) is a syndrome rather than a specific disease. Much confusion and controversy surrounds the diagnosis and treatment. Although DIC is generally considered a hemorrhagic disorder because of the obvious bleeding problems encountered, it is important to recognize the very serious sequelae resulting from microvascular (and sometimes large vessel) thrombosis that always accompanies true DIC and leads to end-organ failure and death. DIC is a systemic thrombohemorrhagic disorder seen in association with well-defined clinical situations with laboratory evidence of procoagulant activation, fibrinolytic activation, inhibitor consumption, and biochemical evidence of end-organ damage or failure.[2] The disorder may have a spectrum of presentations, from *low grade* DIC, with minimal symptoms and minor laboratory abnormalities, to *fulminant* DIC presenting with life-threatening bleeding and protean coagulation abnormalities producing end-organ dysfunction and death. Various disorders ranging from sepsis to malignancy have been described in association with DIC (Table 8–10). Although the diagnosis of DIC is often attached to patients who are receiving massive transfusion, in those patients the diagnosis of platelet dysfunction due to hypothermia or a specific factor deficiency should be excluded before making a diagnosis of DIC. In most cases, such patients will respond to rewarming and replenishment of coagulation factors and platelets (see discussion on massive transfusion).

With the activation of the coagulation and fibrinolytic systems, both thrombin and plasmin are in circulation. Thrombin cleaves fibrinopeptides A and B from fibrinogen, converting it to fibrin monomers. These monomers form soluble fibrin clots, causing microvascular thrombosis with entrapment and depletion of platelets. A simultaneous degradation of these factors by plasmin occurs. Depressed levels of fibrinogen and elevated levels of fibrinogen degradation products (also called fibrin split products) result. These degradation products inhibit the normal coagulation of blood by delaying polymerization of fibrin. Fibrin degradation products may also interpose themselves between fibrin and polymers, forming a weak fibrin clot. The fibrin degradation products include X, Y, D, and E fragments, and platelet dysfunction is attributable to the latter two fragments. Plasmin also degrades factors V, VIII, IX, and XI and activates the complement system. These changes produce the clinically observed changes characteristic of DIC.

Laboratory abnormalities in DIC are variable and related to the many diseases that are associated with this condition. Common abnormalities include abnormal PT and aPTT levels with depressed fibrinogen levels and abnormal platelet counts. Levels of fibrin degradation products and D-dimer are commonly elevated. The peripheral smear reveals fragmented RBCs, but this finding is not specific. Because of the continued activation of coagulation, thrombin-antithrombin complexes will be formed and can be measured. Levels of thrombin-antithrombin and antithrombin III are depressed. In addition, various fragments of coagulation factor degradation are elevated, including F1.2 and FpA. Because of the activation of the fibrinolytic system, plasminogen and alpha$_2$-antiplasmin inhibitor levels are decreased.

Low-grade DIC generally responds to management of the underlying disorder, with some patients requiring heparin therapy. The appropriate therapy for fulminant DIC remains somewhat controversial, and this is compounded by the lack of objective studies and the many underlying causes. The help of a physician experienced in managing DIC is valuable. The treatment of the underlying condition is critical to the successful management of DIC. Also important is the treatment of the thrombotic intravascular process that causes end-organ failure. Therapy with heparin is begun if treatment of the underlying pathology does not ameliorate DIC after 6 to 8 hours. Either subcutaneous or intravenous heparin is administered in doses of 80 to 100 U. per kg. every 4 to 6 hours.[2] Higher doses of heparin may be needed if the patient does not respond. Antithrombin concentrates administered to attain a serum level of 125% of normal have been useful in some patients. Continued bleeding may be related to depletion of components, but random administration of blood products may exacerbate the syndrome, especially those containing fibrinogen. Washed packed RBCs, platelets, antithrombin III concentrate, and crystalloid and colloid volume expanders may be used as needed in DIC. If other therapeutic measures are unsuccessful, inhibition of fibrinolysis may be employed. Epsilon-aminocaproic acid may be given along with heparin and can resolve hemorrhage. Despite improved diagnostic and therapeutic modalities, mortality from DIC remains high and closely related to the underlying disorder.

TABLE 8–10. Conditions Associated with the Syndrome of Disseminated Intravascular Coagulation

Hemolysis
Massive transfusion
Amniotic fluid embolism
Placental abruption
Retained fetus
Gram-negative and gram-positive sepsis
Viremia
Burns
Crush injury and tissue destruction
Leukemia
Malignancy, especially metastatic
Liver disease
Miscellaneous inflammatory and autoimmune conditions including vasculitis

SELECTED REFERENCES

Bick, R. L.: Disseminated intravascular coagulation: Objective criteria for diagnosis and management. Med. Clin. North Am., 78:511, 1994.
This review of a difficult and sometimes confusing clinical entity provides a

comprehensive assessment of the various conditions leading to the diagnosis of DIC and explores the available therapeutic options. Many of the recently described findings in patients with DIC are addressed, including molecular markers of the disorder and useful diagnostic approaches.

Dodd, R. Y.: Transfusion-transmitted hepatitis virus infection. Hematol. Oncol. Clin. North Am., 9:137, 1995.
The status of transfusion-transmitted hepatitis virus infection is reviewed by one of the leading experts in this area. The overall analysis is extremely reassuring in terms of the rather high success rate in detecting and avoiding viral transmission, especially with hepatitis virus.

Kottke-Marchant, K.: Laboratory diagnosis of hemorrhagic and thrombotic disorders. Hematol. Oncol. Clin. North Am., 8:809, 1994.
The diagnosis and management of a variety of bleeding disorders, as well as disorders of thrombosis and fibrinolysis, are presented in an excellent review. In addition to a thorough discussion of fundamental principles and recent discoveries, various disorders of bleeding and coagulopathy and available treatment modes are considered.

MacLean, L. D.: Shock: A century of progress. Ann. Surg., 201:407, 1985.
The author presents a very interesting and informative historical review of progress in the management of shock throughout this century. The discoveries and advances that have radically altered management of this condition are discussed.

Rutledge, R., Sheldon, G. F., and Collins, M. L.: Massive transfusion. Crit. Care Clin. 2:791, 1986.
This is a comprehensive review of massive blood transfusion and the changes that accompany it in patients with a variety of conditions. The authors provide available data in regard to appropriate therapeutic interventions that should accompany blood transfusion.

Welch, H. G., Meehan, K. R., and Goodnough, L. T.: Prudent strategies for elective red cell transfusion. Ann. Intern. Med., 116:393, 1992.
A number of reasonable approaches to the use of red blood cell transfusion in the elective setting are addressed, and various approaches to red blood cell transfusion are discussed. The compository mechanisms in anemia and the value of volume infusion are also discussed.

REFERENCES

1. American Red Cross: Annual Statistics. Washington, DC, American Red Cross, 1992.
2. Bick, R. L.: Disseminated intravascular coagulation: Objective criteria for diagnosis and management. Med. Clin. North Am., 78:511, 1994.
3. Blumberg, N., and Heal, J. M.: Transfusion in host defenses against cancer recurrence and infection. Transfusion, 29:236, 1989.
4. Blundell, J.: Successful case of transfusion. Lancet, 1:431, 1828.
5. Booth, N. A., and Bennet, B.: Fibrinolysis and thrombosis. Bailliéres Clin. Haematol., 7:559, 1994.
6. Boudreaux, J. P., Bornside, G. H., and Cohn, I.: Emergency autotransfusion: Partial cleansing of bacteria-laden blood by cell washing. J. Trauma, 23:31, 1983.
7. Bove, J. R., and Sandler, S. G.: HTLV I and blood transfusion. Transfusion, 28:93, 1988.
8. Bowden, R. A.: Transfusion-transmitted cytomegalovirus infection. Hematol. Oncol. Clin. North Am., 9:155, 1995.
9. Broze, G. J.: The role of tissue factor pathway inhibitor in a revised coagulation cascade. Semin. Hematol., 29:159, 1992.
10. Busch, O. R. C., Hop, W. C. J., et al.: Blood transfusions and prognosis in colorectal cancer. N. Engl. J. Med., 328:1372, 1993.
11. Camp, F. R., and Monsghan, W. P.: Fatal blood transfusion reactions. Am. J. Forensic Med. Pathol., 2:143, 1981.
12. Canizaro, P. C., and Shires, G. T.: Fluid resuscitation in injured patients. Surg. Clin. North Am., 53:1341, 1973.
13. Ciavarella, D., Reed, R. L., Counts, R. B., et al.: Clotting factor levels and the risk of diffuse microvascular bleeding in the massively transfused patient. Br. J. Haematol., 67:365, 1987.
14. Dodd, R. Y.: The risk of transfusion transmitted infection (Editorial). N. Engl. J. Med., 327:419, 1992.
15. Dodd, R. Y.: Transfusion-transmitted hepatitis virus infection. Hematol. Oncol Clin. North Am., 9:137, 1995.
16. Friedman, B. A., Oberman, H. A., Chadwick, R., and Kingdon, I.: The maximum surgical blood order schedule and surgical blood use in the United States. Transfusion, 16:380, 1976.
17. Goodnough, L. T., Grishaber, J. E., Monk, T. G., and Catalona, W. J.: Acute preoperative hemodilution in patients undergoing radical prostatectomy: A case study analysis of efficacy. Anesth. Analg., 78:932, 1994.
18. Harrigan, C., Lucas, C. E., Ledgerwood, A. N., et al.: Serial changes in primary hemostasis after massive transfusion. Surgery, 98:836, 1985.
19. Hecht, T., Wolf, J. L., Niraz, L., Scott, E. P., and Petz, L. D.: Platelet transfusion therapy in an alloimmunized patient: The value of crossmatch procedures for donor selection. JAMA, 248:2301, 1982.
20. Janson, P. A., Jubelirer, S. J., Weinstein, M. J., and Deykin, D.: Treatment of the bleeding tendency in uremia with cryoprecipitate. N. Engl. J. Med., 303:1319, 1980.
21. King, D. J., and Kelton, J. G.: Heparin-associated thrombocytopenia. Ann. Intern. Med., 100:535, 1984.
22. Kottke-Marchant, K.: Laboratory diagnosis of hemorrhagic and thrombotic disorders. Hematol. Oncol. Clin. North Am., 8:809, 1994.
23. Lethagen, S.: Desmopressin (DDAVP) and hemostasis. Ann. Hematol., 69:173, 1994.
24. Lewis, F. R., Elings, V. B., and Sturm, J. A.: Bedside measurement of lung water. J. Surg. Res., 27:250, 1979.
25. Linden, J. V., Paul, B., Dressler, K. P.: A report of 104 transfusion errors in New York State. Transfusion, 32:601, 1992.
26. Lusher, J. M.: Transfusion therapy in congenital coagulopathies. Hematol. Oncol. Clin. North Am., 8:1167, 1994.
27. McVey, J. H.: Tissue factor pathway. Bailliéres Clin. Haematol., 7:469, 1994.
28. MacLean, L. D.: Shock: A century of progress. Ann. Surg., 201:407, 1985.
29. Mann, M., Sacks, H. J., and Goldfinger, D.: Safety of autologous blood donation prior to elective surgery for a variety of potentially "high-risk" patients. Transfusion, 23:229, 1983.
30. Messmer, K.: Hemodilution. Surg. Clin. North Am., 55:659, 1975.
31. Messmore, H. L., and Godwin, J.: Medical assessment of bleeding in the surgical patient. Med. Clin. North Am., 78:625, 1994.
32. Michelsen, T., Salmela, L., Tigerstedt, I., Makelainen, A., and Linko, K.: Massive blood transfusion: Is there a limit? Crit. Care Med., 17:699, 1989.
33. Nawroth, P. P., and Stern, D. M.: Modulation of endothelial hemostasis properties by tumor necrosis factor. J. Exp. Med., 163:740, 1986.
34. Oung, C. M., Li, M. S., Shum-Tim, D., et al.: In vivo study of bleeding time and arterial hemorrhage in hypothermic versus normothermic animals. J. Trauma, 35:251, 1993.
35. Patt, A., McCroskey, B. L., and Moore, E. E.: Hypothermia induced coagulopathy in trauma. Surg. Clin. North Am., 68:775, 1988.
36. Pearson, J. D.: Endothelial cell function and thrombosis. Bailliéres Clin. Haematol., 7:441, 1994.
37. Perking, H. A., Cordell, R., Bueno, C., et al.: The progressive decrease in the proportion of blood donors with antibody to the human immunodeficiency virus. Transfusion, 27:502, 1982.
38. Plasma Consensus Panel: Fresh frozen plasma: Indications and risks. JAMA, 253:551, 1985.
39. Poole, G. V., Meredith, J. W., and Pennell, T.: Comparison of colloids and crystalloids in resuscitation from hemorrhagic shock. Surg. Gynecol. Obstet., 154:577, 1982
40. Reed, R. L., Ciavarella, D., Heimbach, D. M., et al.: Prophylactic platelet transfusion during massive transfusion: A prospective double-blind clinical study. Ann. Surg., 203:40, 1986.
41. Channing-Rodgers, R. P., and Levin, J.: A critical reappraisal of the bleeding time. Semin. Thromb. Hemost., 16:1, 1990.
42. Rutledge, R., Sheldon, G. F., and Collins, M. L.: Massive transfusion. Crit. Care Clin., 2:791, 1986.
43. Sazama, K.: Reports of 355 transfusion associated deaths: 1976 through 1985. Transfusion, 30:583, 1990.
44. Schiffer, C. A., and Slichter, S. J.: Platelet transfusions from single donors. N. Engl. J. Med., 307:245, 1982.
45. Schmidt, P. J.: Transfusion in America in the eighteenth and nineteenth centuries. N. Engl. J. Med., 279:1319, 1968.
46. Seaghell, L. R., Rosen, A. L., Gould, S. A., et al.: Artificial blood: Current status of fluorocarbon and hemoglobin solution. Anesthesiol. Rev., 17(suppl. 3):38, 1990.
47. Surgenor, D. M., Wallace, E. L., Hoe, S. H., and Chapman, R. H.: Collection and transfusion of blood in the United States, 1982–1988. N. Engl. J. Med., 322:1646, 1990.
48. Tarrter, P. I.: The association of peri-operative blood transfusion with colorectal cancer recurrence. Ann. Surg., 216:633, 1992.
49. Valeri, C. R., Cassidy, G., Khuri, S., et al.: Hypothermia induced reversible platelet dysfunction. Ann. Surg., 205:175, 1987.
50. Von Fliedner, V., Higby, D. J., and Kim, U.: Graft-versus-host reaction following blood product transfusion. Am. J. Med., 72:951, 1982.
51. Welch, H. G., Meehan, K. R., and Goodnough, L. T.: Prudent strategies for elective red cell transfusion. Ann. Intern. Med., 116:393, 1992.
52. Williams, A. E., and Sullivan, M. T.: Transfusion-transmitted retrovirus infection. Hematol. Oncol. Clin. North Am., 9:115, 1995.

CHAPTER 9

METABOLISM IN SURGICAL PATIENTS

Protein, Carbohydrate, and Fat Utilization by Oral and Parenteral Routes

Josef E. Fischer, M.D.

When the history of medicine in the twentieth century is written, nutritional support, along with antibiotics, blood transfusions, critical care monitoring and support, advances in anesthesia, modification of the immune system, and cardiopulmonary bypass, will rank high among advances in surgery. Priorities are clearly established in this case. In Europe, safe parenteral fat emulsions and protein hydrolysates were first used with small amounts of glucose but were inappropriate for the critically ill. Dudrick, working in Rhoads' laboratory at the University of Pennsylvania, first demonstrated total nutritional support in puppies. Infusion of hypertonic dextrose with a calorie-nitrogen ratio that would support nitrogen equilibrium was made possible by application of Aubiniac's subclavian venipuncture. Nutritional support began to be widely applied in the United States.

Parenteral nutrition has evolved from initial enthusiastic acceptance (1968–1975) to more critical review, with demands for efficacy (1975–1985). More recently, nutritional needs in specific disease states have been proposed. Nutritional pharmacology has proposed the use of specific nutrient components as drugs, which is only possible when pathophysiologic mechanisms are defined. Currently, utilization of the gut for nutritional support has relegated total parenteral nutrition (TPN) to instances when enteral support cannot be achieved, either because the gut cannot be used or because caloric requirements cannot be met by the gut alone and must be supplemented parenterally.

SURGICAL ANATOMY: INTERORGAN RELATIONSHIPS

The anatomic arrangements of the various metabolic organs have not been stressed. The liver, the central metabolic powerhouse, drains the portal vein—receiving, processing, and storing ingested nutrients for release in response to neural and hormonal signals. It is not clear that the liver, which may extract between 75% and 100% of all portal vein nutrients in one pass, requires this input to maintain functional integrity. Is the enormous postprandial urea production (56%) from absorbed amino acids wasteful or required for hepatic functional integrity? Only one fourth of ingested protein ever becomes available to the free amino acid pool. If required for hepatic functional integrity, this may explain in part the superior results reported with posttraumatic gut feeding.

The anatomic relationship between the gut, liver, and lung is important with respect to glutamine as the major fuel source of the gut and the ability to transpose glutamine to alanine with the release of ammonia under the cover of the liver's detoxification. When hepatic function fails, the lung may detoxify as well. This may be deleterious; for example, in the carcinoid syndrome, substances normally cleared by the liver adversely affect the heart and lung.

Insulin and glucagon are trophic for hepatic function, as are other gut-produced hepatotrophic substances. The relationships between Kupffer cells and hepatocytes make this a fruitful research area.

Liver and kidney play a role in the disposition of nitrogen excess to urea. In the metabolic cycle between skeletal muscle and viscera (e.g., heart), the liver metabolizes proteolytically released amino acids to form glucose.

PROTEIN

Protein is the most important nutrient, as the effector of all organic functions, whether enzymatic, contractile, or immunologic. Protein is unique, because it alone is specific for genus and species. Protein synthesis and degradation both require energy. Breakdown yields only one fourth of the energy as synthesis requires. Thus, utilization of protein for energy is wasteful.

AMINO ACIDS

Basic Structure. Amino acids have a core configuration of an amino and a carboxyl group adjacent to a carbon atom from which a side chain extends. In glycine, this side chain is a hydrogen atom; in all other amino acids, it is composed of one or more carbon atoms. Amino acids also exist as optically active isomers that rotate a plane of polarized light to the left (the more biologically important levorotatory, or L-form) or to the right (dextrorotatory, or D-form). Amino acids are grouped based on electrical charge and the side chain.

The neutral amino acid group comprises 12 amino acids, including glycine and alanine; the hydroxy amino acids serine and threonine; the branched-chain amino acids valine, leucine, and isoleucine; and the aromatic amino acids phenylalanine, tyrosine, and tryptophan (more properly, a heterocyclic amino acid); as well as the sulfur-containing amino acids methionine and cysteine. Aspartic and glutamic acid are diacidic; arginine, lysine, and histidine are dibasic. These features also determine transport across membranes.

Essential Versus Nonessential Amino Acids. The essential or indispensable amino acids are those whose carbon skeleton cannot be synthesized. These include the classic eight (determined by Rose and colleagues): valine, leucine, isoleucine, lysine, methionine, phenylalanine, threonine, and tryptophan. Cysteine and tyrosine are conditionally indispensable and are synthesized from the essential amino acids methionine and phenylalanine, respectively. Histidine, proline, hydroxyproline, glutamine, and arginine are also conditionally indispensable, certainly in infants and when needs are increased, as the low synthetic rates fall short of increased requirements. The remaining seven amino acids—alanine, aspartic acid, asparagine, glutamic acid, glycine, proline, and serine—are not essential.

Basic Principles. Three major fates of amino acids are (1) protein synthesis; (2) catabolic reactions leading to the production of urea from nitrogen and carbon dioxide from carbon-energy and/or storage of the carbon as carbohydrate and/or fat; and (3) synthesis of nonessential amino acids and other small molecules, such as purines and pyrimidines.

Transport. Transport of free amino acids across cell membranes has been studied in only a few types of cells; it is probably universal. Christensen has proposed several transport systems:

1. The A-system is an energy- and sodium-dependent system with a high affinity for alanine and other neutral amino acids, including the synthetic amino acids alpha-aminoisobutyric acid and, more specifically, alpha-methylaminoisobutyric acid. It is concentrative against a gradient and is stimulated by insulin.

2. The L-system is sodium independent and transports the branched-chain amino acids—leucine, isoleucine, and valine—and the aromatic amino acids—phenylalanine, tyrosine, and tryptophan—and probably methionine and histidine. It operates by exchange for intracellular amino acids and is competitive.

3. Two transport systems are available for the basic amino acids. The carriers for transport of dibasic amino acids and the L-system may be linked in some as yet unknown way.

4. Dicarboxylic amino acids have their own transport system.

Changes in muscle amino acid transport in sepsis may prove important in understanding the metabolic changes. Current knowledge about amino acid transport in muscle is summarized in Table 9–1.

Turnover: Synthesis and Degradation. Synthesis of protein requires energy and begins with DNA transmitting messages

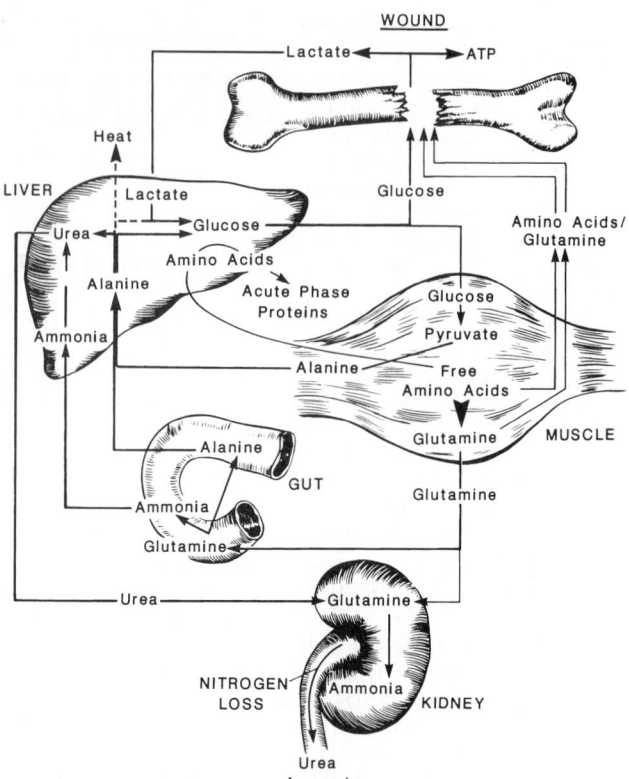

Figure 9–1. Overall scheme of the metabolic response to illness. This scheme includes the metabolic relationship between organs. This feature has heretofore not been very prominently addressed but is now receiving increased attention. One of the articles of faith is that such responses occur in response to injury and are teleologically correct and beneficial. Thus, the wound requires glucose, probably glutamine, and certainly arginine with respect to certain cellular elements. The movement of amino acids from the periphery (muscle) to the liver presumably results in the secretion of acute-phase protein, the purpose of which in turn is to fight infection. The muscle-gut-liver-alanine-glutamine-glucose cycle is prominently displayed. (Adapted from Bessey, P. Q.: Metabolic response to critical illness. Scientific American Surgery, Wilmore, D. W., Cheung, L. Y., Harken, A. H., et al. [Eds.]. Section II, Subsection 11, © 1996 Scientific American, Inc. All rights reserved.)

TABLE 9–1. Amino Acid Transporters in Muscle

Transporter	Na+ Coupling	Typical Substrates	Comments
X⁻A,G	Yes	Glutamate, aspartate	Insulin insensitive
y⁺	No	Lysine, cystine, arginine, ornithine	Insulin insensitive
L	No	Neutral amino acids	Insulin insensitive
A	Yes	Short-chain neutral amino acids	Insulin sensitive, reduced by starvation
ASC	Yes	Alanine, cysteine, serine, threonine	Insulin insensitive
Nᵐ	Yes	Glutamine, histidine, asparagine	Insulin sensitive

through messenger RNA to charge tRNA, to polysomes where amino acids are aligned on a template and split off as protein is synthesized.

Degradation of protein is a mechanism by which worn-out, three-dimensionally damaged protein is recycled to free amino acids for reutilization. Amino acids are catabolized to ammonia and urea, carbon dioxide, energy, and glucose. Of the indispensable amino acids, 7 of the 10 are degraded by the liver, the exceptions (in the conventional wisdom) being the branched-chain amino acids—valine, leucine, and isoleucine—a view that has been challenged. Skeletal muscle plays a major role in the catabolism of the branched-chain amino acids.

Twelve of the 20 amino acids are initially transaminated to an alpha-ketoacid, which then has two fates: (1) conversion to glucose and (2) oxidation to carbon dioxide (and high-energy phosphate) by means of the tricarboxylic acid cycle.

Two amino acids—alanine and glutamine—are carriers for organ exchanges of nitrogen. The branched-chain amino acids are initially transaminated with pyruvate to alanine and with glutamate to glutamine (Fig. 9–1). Oxidative deamination is a less important pathway. A third protein degradative pathway involves urea synthesis, in which both the liver and the kidney participate.

Regulation of Amino Acid Levels. The liver is most important in regulation of plasma amino acid levels. The Kms of enzymes involved in degradation are high, and those of synthesis are low, favoring synthesis, but excessive accumulation of plasma amino acids is prevented. This is understandable in view of the sudden postprandial peaks of amino acids, which could result in rapid increases in amino acid brain neurotransmitter precursors. Only 25% of ingested protein reaches the general (nonportal) circulation as free amino acids. Most (almost 60%) is converted to urea, a small amount (6%) is synthesized to plasma protein, and 14% becomes liver protein. Because protein turnover is much higher than exogenous protein intake, most of the free amino acid pool is derived from breakdown of endogenous protein.

In parenteral nutrition, nutrients are first supplied to the systemic, rather than the portal, circulation, thus overriding the liver, normally the principal controlling factor. Thus, at least amino acid and probably most nutrient regulation is bypassed by parenteral nutrition.

Other Regulation. The plasma amino acid pool is also influenced by exchange of amino acids between skeletal muscle, gut, and viscera. In muscle, the branched-chain amino acids are transaminated to alanine and glutamine. Alanine is processed by the liver to glucose and glutamine is transaminated to alanine by the gut, with alanine going to the liver. The kidney also participates in gluconeogenesis and has a major role in the metabolism of glutamine, particularly as concerns acid-base balance.

The lung may have a greater role in regulation of amino acid levels (glutamine in particular) than has heretofore been hypothesized, especially when the liver is bypassed or diseased (and thus incapable of modifying portal flow).

Regulation of Amino Acid Levels Within Organs, Including Muscle. The study of transport systems into skeletal muscle, which contains the bulk of amino acids, has been comparatively neglected. Glutamine comprises between 50% and 60% of white, fast-twitch, and mixed muscle. Within 24 hours of operation or trauma (even after laparoscopic cholecystectomy), much of this glutamine store has disappeared and is roughly equivalent to the urinary excretion of urea. It is not fully replaced until as long as 8 weeks later. The significance of the glutamine export is not clear, nor is it clear why refilling this store takes so long. It is also not clear whether return of stamina, as some have claimed, requires reconstitution of skeletal muscle glutamine.

Attempts to prevent depletion of muscle-free glutamine by glutamine supplementation in parenteral nutrition solutions have shown some muscle glutamine sparing. However, the marginal improvements in nitrogen balance are unlikely to improve clinical outcome.

Control of muscle protein synthesis and degradation appears different in the white fast-twitch muscle as opposed to the red slow-twitch muscle in response to various stimuli, particularly sepsis. Protein synthesis is stimulated by insulin, amino acid administration, increased concentration of branched-chain amino acids, and likely by human growth hormone and somatomedin and/or insulin-like growth factor-1. Release of insulin and human growth hormone is stimulated by individual amino acids, such as arginine, which is also a preferred fuel for macrophages, especially within the healing wound. The branched-chain amino acids play a special role. In health, in nitrogen equilibrium, the postprandial uptake of branched-chain amino acids into skeletal muscle accounts for 60% to 100% of daily nitrogen retention. Plasma levels of the branched-chain amino acids are a tertiary but real controlling factor in the efflux of amino acids from muscle.

In sepsis, protein synthesis continues, but at a decreased rate; the response to stimuli that normally promotes increased protein synthesis, such as the branched-chain amino acids, is diminished. The slope of the response to insulin is

normal, but the baseline is depressed, so that the actual response to insulin is about half that of the normal muscle.

With the recent ability to study breakdown of muscle, a more accurate picture emerges. Proteolysis in sepsis is principally in the white, fast-twitch (and mixed) muscle, of which the principal indicator is 3-methylhistidine. Although a good indicator of proteolysis in isolated muscle, 3-methylhistidine is not a good indicator of whole-body protein turnover, because it measures other organs such as small intestine. Catabolic stimuli include the classic counterregulatory hormones—glucagon, steroids, and epinephrine (Fig. 9–2). In addition, cytokines, such as interleukin (IL)-1, tumor necrosis factor (TNF)/cachectin, IL-6, and perhaps proteolysis-inducing factor, a 4200-dalton protein described by Clowes and coworkers, and a host of other cytokines also contribute. Studies suggest that, in rats, at least 50% of muscle breakdown in sepsis is due to corticosterone; other studies indicate that at least some of the actions previously attributed to TNF/cachectin are mediated by corticosteroids. A novel apparent cytokine of approximate molecular weight of 1500 daltons prevents the muscle transport of amino acids so they cannot be incorporated into muscle protein synthesis.[38] This cytokine thus diverts plasma amino acids derived from proteolysis for hepatic protein synthesis. The current list of cytokines is shown in Table 9–2.

Muscle proteolysis includes lysosomal and nonlysosomal, calcium-dependent and calcium-independent, and energy-requiring and non–energy-requiring pathways. Of the energy-requiring pathways, the ubiquitin pathway is one of the most prominent.[16, 20] Proteolysis in white, fast-twitch muscle in sepsis appears primarily due to the ubiquitin energy-requiring pathway, controlled at the transcriptional level (Fig. 9–3).[12, 34]

Using both glucose and amino acid clamps, Abumrad has demonstrated that the non–glucose-responsive portion of muscle protein breakdown is responsive to leucine. However, in sepsis, proteolysis is responsive neither to glucose nor to pharmacologic doses of leucine, emphasizing the altered control systems in sepsis. However, nonconventional fuels, such as short-chain fatty acids, may decrease muscle proteolysis in sepsis when conventional fuels fail, but whether this is clinically applicable is not yet clear.

Hypocaloric feeding and *safe amounts* of amino acids administered with recombinant growth hormone to patients with ample fat stores result in significant retention of nitrogen, phosphorus, and potassium, suggesting accretion of small (but likely not clinically significant) amounts of lean body mass. These effects of growth hormone may be mediated by insulin-like growth factor-1.

ROLES OF THE KIDNEY

The roles of the kidney in protein metabolism include (1) the production of urea (with the liver) from ammonia by means of the argininosuccinate cycle; (2) the production of ammonia (from glutamine) for urinary acid-base balance; and (3) to a lesser degree, metabolism of other amino acids, such as the branched-chain amino acids. The role of the kidney in amino acid metabolism has not been as well studied as that of muscle or liver but is probably more important than heretofore supposed. The kidney is a source of glucose as well.

TOTAL INTEGRATION OF BODY PROTEIN

In a 70-kg. man there are between 10 and 11 kg. of protein. Daily protein turnover is 250 to 300 gm., or 3%; the gut is the largest component of this turnover, which is composed mostly of shed enterocytes and secreted digestive enzymes.

INTEGRATED CONCEPT OF SEPSIS

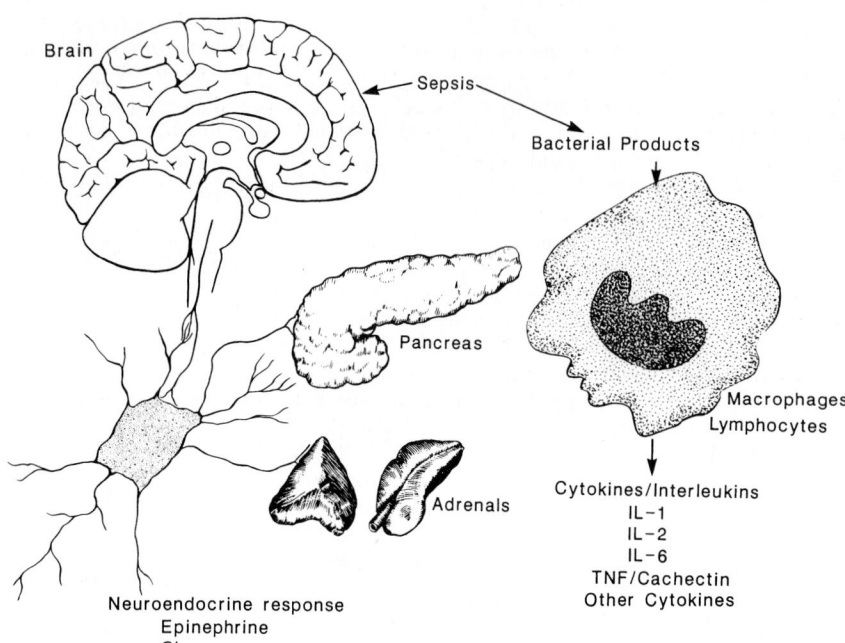

Figure 9–2. An emerging concept of the response to stress and sepsis. In previous years, the neurosympathetic response to sepsis was emphasized, with the secretion of epinephrine, glucagon, and corticosteroids—the so-called counterregulatory hormones. It is now clear that this is but one half of the efferent limb and that cytokines, including those listed here and in Table 9–2, are extremely important.

After digestion, all amino acids are absorbed, save 1 gm. of nitrogen excreted in the stool. Proteolysis accounts for another 50 to 70 gm. of amino acids. In total, ingested amino acids contribute only 25 gm. to the free amino acid pool (Fig. 9–4), whereas 250 gm. of amino acids is provided by endogenous breakdown. If adequate energy is present, most of these amino acids are resynthesized. Whether protein synthesis proceeds if only a source of energy and a small amount of essential amino acids are supplied is still controversial. It is proposed that the other nonessential amino acids are synthesized from carbon skeletons and sources of nitrogen such as glutamine through transamination. Twenty grams of plasma protein, 8 gm. of hemoglobin, 20 gm. of white blood cells, and a few grams of skin constitute the remainder of total body protein synthesis (see Fig. 9–4).

Protein turnover decreases with age. Turnover in a neonate approximates 25 gm. of protein per kg. per 24 hours, which decreases to 7 gm. per kg. per 24 hours at 1 year. In adults, turnover falls to 3 gm. per kg. per 24 hours and is slightly greater in males. Thus, with age, turnover rate decreases, but as lean body mass increases, total body turnover remains approximately the same.

Caloric supply is important. Carbohydrate increases muscle protein synthesis under the influence of insulin; fat increases hepatic and other visceral protein synthesis as well as muscle protein synthesis, the latter to a lesser extent as compared with carbohydrate. Carbohydrate depresses albumin synthesis as compared with optimal calories as fat.

PROTEIN REQUIREMENTS

After several days on a calorically adequate protein-free diet, 37 mg. per kg. of nitrogen is excreted into the urine, whereas 12 mg. per kg. of nitrogen is lost in the feces. Integumentary losses account for another 5 mg. per kg., with another 2 to 3 mg. of nitrogen per kg. by evaporation, making a total of 56 to 57 mg. of nitrogen per kg. or, in terms of whole protein, 0.34 gm. of protein per kg. per day. With various corrections, the average normal requirement is 0.8 gm. of protein per kg. or between 56 to 60 gm. of protein per

day. Trauma increases the requirement. Normal protein intake is twice that amount (100 to 120 gm.) in affluent American society.

Most amino acids can be recycled provided there is adequate energy. Thus, small amounts of essential amino acids with adequate energy are sufficient for nitrogen equilibrium. In infants, 40% to 50% of the protein intake should be essential amino acids, whereas in an adult in nitrogen equilibrium without stress, sepsis, or trauma, 19% to 20% is sufficient. The percentage of essential amino acids should increase with injury or depletion. A *safe* intake figure for patients on parenteral nutrition is 200 to 250 mg. of nitrogen per kg. of body weight or 1.7 gm. of protein equivalent per kg. per day, although some have advocated higher levels, especially in sepsis.

CALORIES

Caloric Sources. There are three major sources of energy—protein, carbohydrate, and fat. Amino acids contribute 15% of normal energy expenditure, with branched-chain amino acids, oxidized directly to high-energy phosphate without going through glucose, contributing 6% to 7% of energy requirements. The remaining 8% to 9% is derived from gluconeogenesis. The remaining 85% of energy expenditure is derived from carbohydrate or fat, with 70% to 75% from fat, either oxidized directly or metabolized by the liver to ketone bodies.

In TPN, most calories are administered as glucose; it is not clear that fat is used in all states, particularly in sepsis. Utilization of caloric sources is estimated from the respiratory quotient (RQ), the relationship between carbon dioxide produced and oxygen consumed, as follows.*

---

*Metabolic rate $= 4.83 \times V_{O_2}$ (resting subject, average American diet—4.83 kcal. generated for every liter of oxygen consumed). Heat per unit time (energy equivalent—kcal. per min.) $= 3.941\ V_{O_2} + 1.106\ V_{CO_2}$. Heat per unit time (energy equivalent—kcal. per min.) $= V_{O_2}\ (3.941 + 1.106$ respiratory quotient). If urinary nitrogen measurements are included, the formula described by Weir can be used: heat production per unit time (energy equivalent—kcal. per min.) $= 3.94\ V_{O_2} + 1.11\ V_{CO_2} - 2.17$ urinary nitrogen.

TABLE 9–2. Sources and Targets of Cytokines and Other Peptide Regulatory Factors

Regulatory Factor*	Sources	Target Tissues/Cells
Interleukins (ILs)		
IL-1α, IL-1β (endogenous pyrogen, lymphocyte-activating factor, leukocyte endogenous mediator, hemopoietin-1)	Monocytes/macrophages; many endothelial, epithelial, and hematopoietic cells	Thymocytes, T and B cells, hematopoietic cells, fibroblasts, chondrocytes, receptors in brain and liver, hepatocytes
IL-2 (T-cell growth factor)	T cells	T and B cells, thymocytes, natural killer cells
IL-3 (multipotential colony-stimulating factor, hematopoietic growth factor)	T cells, myelomonocytic cells	Hematopoietic cells, pre–B cells
IL-4 (B-cell stimulating factor 1, B-cell growth factor I)	T cells, mast cells	T and B cells, mast cells, other hematopoietic cells
IL-5 (T-cell replacing factor, eosinophil differentiation factor, B-cell growth factor II, eosinophil colony-stimulating factor, IgA-enhancing factor)	T cells	B cells, eosinophils, thymocytes
IL-6 (B-cell stimulating factor 2, interferon beta₂, hepatocyte-stimulating factor, hybridoma growth factor, B-cell differentiation factor, 26-kd protein)	Monocytes/macrophages, T cells, fibroblasts, epithelial cell types	T and B cells, fibroblasts, hepatocytes, hematopoietic stem cells
IL-7 (lymphoprotein-1, pre–B-cell growth factor)	Stomal cells, thymus	Pre–B cells, thymocytes
IL-8	Macrophages, neurotrophils, endothelial cells, hepatocytes, fibroblasts	Neutrophils, fibroblasts
IL-9	T cells	Lymphoid cells, myeloid cells
IL-10	Monocytes/macrophages, B cells, T-helper cells	Macrophages, cytokines, antigens, IL-1 receptors
IL-11	Lung stromal cells, bone marrow stromal cells	Progenitor cells, B cells
IL-12	Monocytes/macrophages, B cells, skin Langerhans cells	T-cell growth factor, cytokines
IL-13	T-helper cells	Monocytes, endothelial cells, B cells
IL-14	B cells	B cells (B-cell growth factor)
IL-15	Mononuclear cells, muscle	T cells, B cells
Tumor Necrosis Factors (TNFs)		
TNF (TNF-α, cachectin)	Monocytes/macrophages, lymphocytes, natural killer cells, glial cells, Kupffer cells	Endothelial cells, monocytes/macrophages, neutrophils, fibroblasts, receptors in liver, muscle, lung, gut, kidney
Lymphotoxin (TNF-β)	Monocytes/macrophages	?Same receptors as TNF
Interferons		
Interferon alpha (leukocyte interferon)	Monocytes/macrophages	Multiple immune cells
Interferon beta (fibroblast interferon)	Fibroblasts, epithelial cells	Multiple immune cells
Interferon beta₂ [see IL-6]		
Interferon gamma (immune interferon, macrophage-activating factor)	Multiple cell types (antigen–antibody reaction)	T and B cells, phagocytic cells
Insulin-like Growth Factors (IGFs)		
IGF-1 (somatomedin C)	Fibroblasts, astrocytes, other neuronal and nonneuronal cells	Most cell types (necessary for cell survival), muscle and cartilage, precursor cells
IGF-2 (somatomedin A)	Astrocytes	Most cell types

*The terms in parentheses are alternative terms that have been, and in some cases still are, used for the same substance or group of substances.
Note: This is but a partial and likely outdated list, because new cytokines are being discovered constantly.
Adapted from Bessey, P. Q.: Metabolic response to critical illness. Scientific American Surgery, Wilmore, D. W., Cheung, L. Y., Harken, A. H., et al. (Eds.). Section II, Subsection 11. © 1996 Scientific American, Inc. All rights reserved.

$$RQ = \frac{V_{CO_2}}{V_{O_2}}$$

Metabolic charts determine which fuel is being consumed in a clinical setting. An RQ of 1 indicates pure carbohydrate utilization. Theoretically the RQ with lipogenesis can be as high as 9; an RQ of greater than 1 is rarely seen. An RQ of 0.7 indicates fat utilization; one of less than 0.7 indicates ketogenesis.

Without such measurements, when fat is administered intravenously, indirect measures of fat utilization, such as absence of plasma lipemia and presence of ketone bodies, are necessary to confirm fat utilization.

Calorie-Nitrogen Ratio. A calorie-nitrogen ratio of 100 to 150 to 1 (i.e., 100 to 150 nonprotein calories per gram of nitrogen) is required for protein synthesis in normal patients. The calorie-nitrogen ratio changes in different disease states; in sepsis, increased nitrogen and decreased nonprotein calories are appropriate (100 to 1), whereas in uremia, between 300 and 400 to 1 (calorie per gram of nitrogen) has been advocated. The manner of investigation is critical; that is, keeping nitrogen adequate and varying the calorie-nitrogen ratio is the preferred method. When inadequate amounts of protein are given and caloric intake varied, erroneous data and conclusions may result.

Energy Requirements. Metabolic cart measurements help determine caloric requirements. With such measurements, it is clear that in the past, oversupplementation was the rule, resulting in excessive lipid deposition. Whereas 15 years ago it was common for patients to receive 3500 to 4000 calories per day, at present, 1800 to 2000 calories is usual, increased to 2500 calories in stress states. The Harris-Benedict equation with an activity correction may also be used (BEE = basal energy expenditure):

$$BEE = 66.5 + 13.7 \times weight\ (kg.) + 5.0 \times height\ (cm.) - 6.8 \times age\ (yr.)\ [male]$$

$$BEE = 655.1 + 9.56 \times weight\ (kg.) + 1.85 \times height\ (cm.) - 4.68 \times age\ (yr.)\ [female]$$

The estimate shown in Figure 9–5 may be used; it may overestimate caloric requirements. When metabolic cart measurements are used, patients are in a basal state: thus, a 15% activity correction is necessary. Studies in the Cincinnati unit suggest that reasonable accuracy can be achieved by either method.

Carbohydrates. Glucose is the preferred carbohydrate source in traditional TPN. Other carbohydrates include fruc-

141

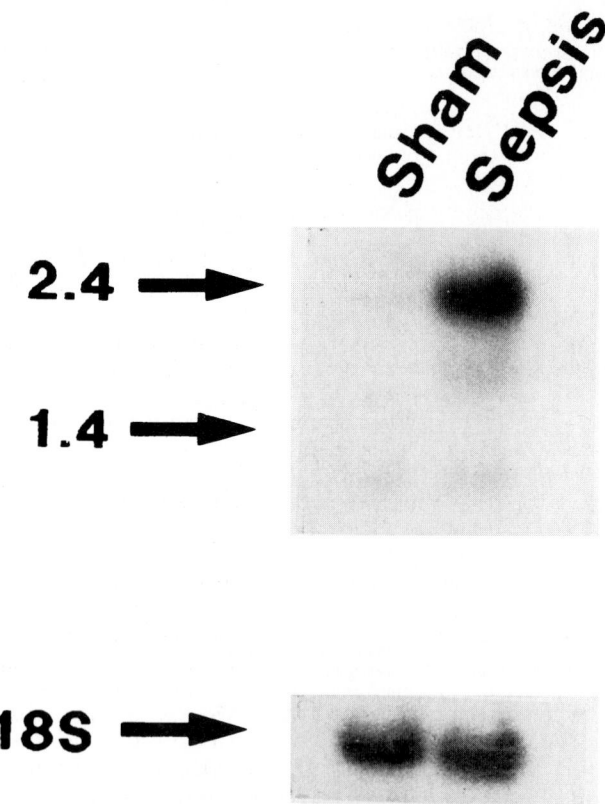

Figure 9–3. Northern blots of RNA extracted from extensor digitorum longus muscles of sham-operated control rats and septic rats 16 hours after cecal ligation and puncture. The blots were hybridized with a rat ubiquitin cDNA probe, stripped, and rehybridized with an 18-S rat ribosomal oligonucleotide probe to control for equal loading of RNA in the two lanes. The numbers to the left indicate the location of standard markers in kilobases run concurrently with the samples. (From Tiao, G., Fagan, J. M., Samuels, N., James, J. H., Hudson, K., Lieberman, M., Fischer, J. E., and Hasselgren, P. O.: Sepsis stimulates nonlysosomal, energy-dependent proteolysis and increases ubiquitin mRNA levels in rat skeletal muscle. J. Clin. Invest., *94*:2255, 1994. Reproduced from The Journal of Clinical Investigation, 1994, by copyright permission of The American Society for Clinical Investigation.)

BODY PROTEIN

Protein Intake — 100 gm

Protein Losses:
  Fecal Nitrogen – 10 gm
  Urinary Nitrogen – 80 gm
  Skin – 2 gm

Secreted Gut Protein [70 gm]

BODY PROTEIN SYNTHESIS [250 gm]

Muscle [50 gm]

Plasma [20 gm]:
  Albumin [12 gm]
  Fibrinogen [2 gm]
  γ-Globulin [3 gm]

Absorbed Gut Protein [160 gm]

Free Amino Acids [70 gm]
(NEAA: 60 gm;
EAA: 10 gm)

White Blood Cells [20 gm]

Hemoglobin [8 gm]

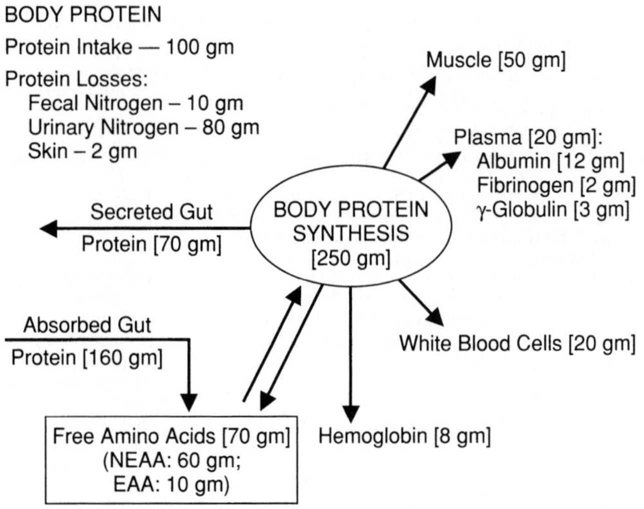

Figure 9–4. Diagram to show the daily flux of amino acids in the body of a 70-kg. man. Note that total body protein synthesis is 250 gm. per 24 hours, of which 50 gm. is muscle; proteolysis contributes approximately the same. Thus, with adequate amounts of energy, nitrogen equilibrium is the result. (Data from Munro, H. N.: Parenteral nutrition: Metabolic consequences of bypassing the gut and liver. *In* Clinical Nutrition Update: Amino Acids. Chicago, American Medical Association, 1977, p. 141.)

Deleterious effects of excessive glucose include hepatic steatosis (see under Metabolic Complications). Blood glucose levels in excess of 300 mg. per 100 ml. adversely affect neutrophil function.

Other carbohydrate sources have not achieved popularity in the United States. Fructose, which some have proposed for use in glucose resistance, may cause fatal lactic acidosis. Fructose requires expenditure of high-energy phosphate through the pentose-monophosphate shunt for conversion to

tose, sorbitol, xylitol, and glycerol. There are little carbohydrate stores beyond a 24-hour fast. Liver glycogen is exhausted; small amounts of muscle glycogen may remain. Glucose oxidized completely through the Krebs tricarboxylic acid cycle produces a larger yield of high-energy phosphate (aerobic glycolysis) than incomplete oxidation to lactate (anaerobic glycolysis). The exact circumstances of aerobic and anaerobic glycolysis are vague; in sepsis, low-flow states, and neoplasia, gluconeogenesis is increased, yet the maximal energy value from the produced glucose is not obtained because of anaerobic (incomplete) glycolysis, for reasons poorly understood. Recent studies in the author's laboratory suggest that the conventional views concerning the reasons for anaerobic glycolysis are incorrect.

Glucose is the gold standard for protein sparing, with a minimum of 400 calories per 24 hours (based on Gamble's classic work); and up to 1800 calories in the resting fasting state minimizes proteolysis, particularly after adaptation to starvation. Glucose will not decrease proteolysis beyond 50%; the remainder is apparently amino acid sensitive. Red blood cells, white blood cells, and the central nervous system prefer glucose—the red and white blood cells because of limited metabolic apparatus; the central nervous system can adapt to other energy sources. Wound repair requires glucose, although some cellular elements utilize amino acids, such as arginine, extensively.

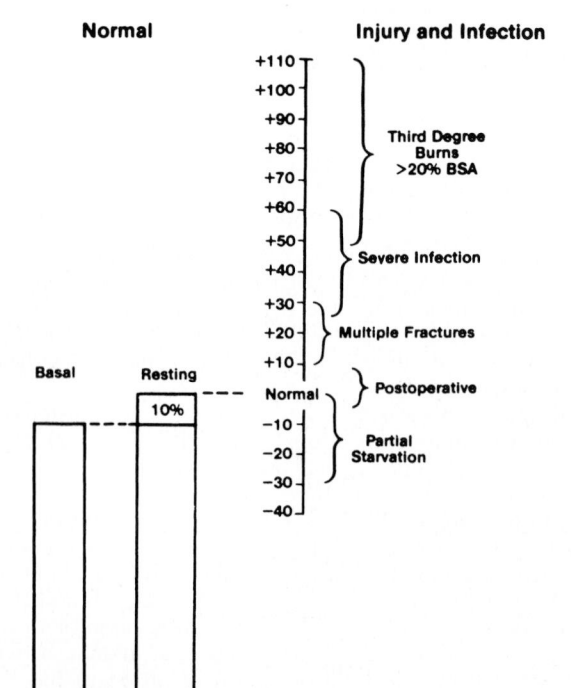

Figure 9–5. The increases in resting energy expenditure that have been shown to occur during the acute catabolic phase of injury or infection, when compared with the decreases that develop during partial starvation. (From Kinney, J. M.: The application of indirect calorimetry to clinical studies. *In* Kinney, J. M. [Ed.]: Assessment of Energy Metabolism in Health and Disease. Columbus, OH, Ross Laboratories, 1980.)

glucose, with 80% of fructose metabolized as glucose; use of fructose thus appears illogical.

The polyalcohols xylitol and sorbitol also undergo transformation to glucose. Xylitol is hepatotoxic and has caused several deaths in the Australian experience. Despite this, xylitol and sorbitol are again being examined for specialized circumstances.

Glycerol, another potential source of glucose, is advantageous in that it may be sterilized in solution with amino acids, without the caramelization reaction. In addition, its osmolality is low. These properties of glycerol are utilized in a new solution, ProcalAmine (McGaw, Inc., Irvine, CA), that does not require mixing and thus saves pharmacy costs. This solution, administered peripherally, is intended as an intermediate solution for temporary support in patients who are not critically ill and in whom it is not clear TPN will be needed. Its place in the armamentarium remains to be determined. Glycerol in large doses may cause renal failure in experimental animals. The doses of glycerol administered clinically are not those in experimental renal failure; deleterious effects may result in patients with already compromised organ function, and caution is appropriate.

The safety and efficacy of glycerol in patients who were recovering from major trauma or surgery was studied in 34 patients receiving either 10% (Group I) or 20% (Group II) lipid emulsion as their caloric source. The groups were not comparable; blood loss in Group II was three times that of Group I. Nitrogen equilibrium was achieved in Group I and was significantly negative in Group II, which may reflect decreased fat utilization with suboptimal glucose supply, or the more severely traumatized group receiving the 20% lipid.[39]

Controlling Mechanisms. Normally, insulin, released by glucose administration, inhibits lipolysis. In sepsis, and possibly stress, these *shut-off* valves do not function, and gluconeogenesis continues, despite the administration of either fat or carbohydrate. The trauma patient becomes desensitized to insulin and becomes hyperglycemic. The basis for this insulin resistance is unknown. There are many signals released in response to injury, and the various mediators may either impair insulin release or render insulin less effective. Insulin resistance results in elevated hepatic gluconeogenesis, even when extraneous glucose is provided. Additionally, in burn patients, glucose is preferentially metabolized through anaerobic glycolysis,[35] resulting in production of excess lactate that is converted by the liver to glucose, thus exacerbating the problem. Thus, appropriate nutritional support is difficult, as it is difficult to supplement calories without elevating glucose concentrations. A number of strategies have been proposed.

One approach is by lipid supplementation. As lipid cannot be converted into glucose, such supplementation will not prevent continuing gluconeogenesis (the brain still requires a continual supply of glucose). However, lipid reduces circulating glucose because lipid is replacing glucose as an energy source. Thus, lipid may reduce hyperglycemia despite continuing gluconeogenesis. Paradoxically, fat metabolism is continuously active in these patients, despite hyperglycemia. Whether lipid metabolism continues normally or in accelerated fashion in sepsis is still a matter of controversy. It may be that in moderate sepsis, fat continues to be utilized, while in severe sepsis, fat is not efficiently utilized (but perhaps no energy source is). Because the patient has become insulin resistant, the adipose tissue is responding to released glucagon, which activates fat metabolism. To truly understand why these metabolic profiles are altered requires a better understanding at the molecular level of the effect of the various mediators released after trauma on the pancreatic beta cell and insulin release. It is believed that pancreatic beta cell glucokinase is involved in the *switching mechanism*

regulating glucose sensing and insulin secretion.[33, 36] Once that process is better understood, it may be possible to more rationally design a proper diet for the trauma or septic patient.

Fat as a Caloric Source. In resting starvation, fat provides the bulk of calories as ketone bodies manufactured by the liver from long-chain fatty acids. Lipolysis is promoted by steroids, catechols, glucagon, and some cytokines and is extremely sensitive to inhibition by insulin. In stress, generous lipolysis occurs. In the American diet, 25% to 45% of calories are supplied by fat. Fat was omitted in early parenteral nutrition because of absence of a safe fat emulsion. When it became clear that the practice of administering plasma twice weekly was an insufficient source of trace metals and essential fatty acids, fat was given to supply 4% of the calories to prevent essential fatty acid deficiency. Currently, fat is a calorie source as well as a source of essential fatty acids. Because fatty acids are precursors of the prostaglandins, alternative fats are being investigated to modify the inflammatory and immunologic response.

The use of fat in severe stress and sepsis has been previously discussed. Under normal circumstances or in moderate stress, fat and carbohydrate are indistinguishable with respect to nitrogen balance, with 25% of nonprotein calories as fat seemingly optimal for hepatic protein synthesis. What is not clear is at which point in stress and/or sepsis, fat oxidation and/or utilization becomes impaired. Most agree that while hepatic manufacture of ketone bodies is impaired early in sepsis, fat clearance remains relatively normal until comparatively late, but fat oxidation is impaired earlier.

The specific dynamic action of carbohydrate when given with amino acids appears trivial at physiologic concentrations. In patients with severe sepsis, one must either measure RQ and/or monitor lipemia to ensure fat clearance. A limit of 2 gm. of fat emulsion per kg. per day in adults prevents fat overload syndrome, manifested by fever, back pain, chills, pulmonary insufficiency, and blocking of the reticuloendothelial system. In infants, who are anatomically mainly viscera with little skeletal muscle, up to 4 gm. per kg. per day is tolerated. Whether in severe sepsis normal fat intake blocks the reticuloendothelial system is not clear.

Alternative or Nonconventional Fuels. Glutamine as a fuel for enterocytes has received much attention, with several clinical trials. Small, clinically insignificant changes in nitrogen balance result from the administration of a dipeptide glutamine ester. However, in severe stress, such as bone marrow transplant, a beneficial effect of glutamine in decreasing hospital stay, improving nitrogen balance, and decreasing infection has been demonstrated.[40] These effects have been attributed to improved gut barrier function, but improved gut protein and hepatic protein synthesis are equally possible.

The ketone bodies—acetoacetate, propionate, and butyrate—are the subjects of considerable investigation, again with respect to their beneficial effect on the gut and especially the effect of butyrate on the ileum and colon.

No clinical studies of ketone bodies are available, but experimental studies are. Monoacetoacetin, a water-soluble neutral monoacylglycerol ester of acetoacetate, is nontoxic when given intravenously. It is hydrolyzed to glycerol, which in turn may be used as a fuel, and to acetoacetate, of which only 10% is consumed locally and 90% exported to the portal system. Yet animals receiving monoacetin show greater preservation of jejunal mucosal weight, protein, RNA, and DNA. An effect on colonic DNA was lacking. No differences in nitrogen balance or weight gain were noted, despite a predominance of calories furnished by monoacetin. In burned rats, monoacetin and a dextrose-based TPN solution were equally efficacious. From the literature, butyrate might be more efficacious and beneficial to both colonocytes and ileal enterocytes. When produced from soluble pectin by gut bacteria, 80% of the butyrate is utilized locally by colonocytes and only 20% is released into the portal vein, suggesting that butyrate may be a more effective trophic agent. Short-chain fatty acids derived from soluble pectin prevent and heal chemotherapy-related gut mucosal damage. The protective effects of enteral diets on radiation enteritis may be due to the glutamine content.

CATABOLISM

Causes of Inadequate Nutrition. Lack of food is a cause of malnutrition in poor urban populations, especially in alcoholics. In the usual United States hospital setting, however, starvation is usually the result of either anorexia, such as occurs with cancer, sepsis, or liver disease, or poor intake due to obstruction. Obstruction may, in turn, be due to neoplasia or stricture of the esophagus secondary to reflux or lye or may be distal in the gastrointestinal tract, such as carcinoma of the colon. Less common intra-abdominal illness, such as scleroderma, motility disorders, pseudo-obstruction, major gastric resection, or a short-bowel syndrome, also result in inadequate absorption. Inadequate nutrition may also be due to excessive losses, as with gastrointestinal fistulas, or from malabsorption, as with inflammatory bowel disease or protein-losing enteropathies. However, the most common causes of in-hospital malnutrition are poor food unappetizingly served, with timing for the benefit of personnel rather than patients. Patients are given nothing by mouth for the most trivial reasons (chest or abdominal films). Diets are not advanced rapidly after trivial operations. The hospital administration regards food as an area in which to save money.

Reasons for Protein Loss. Whereas not all muscles are under similar controls, most understanding of muscle metabolism has been derived from *in vitro* preparations such as rat hemidiaphragm, an atypical muscle that is highly catabolic and probably dying *in vitro*. Work in other preparations such as epitrochlearis and soleus has revealed different results. The major controls of nitrogen accrual in muscle include (1) tension-exercise, the most potent controlling mechanism; (2) presence of insulin, the principal storage hormone; (3) presence of glucose; and (4) presence of branched-chain amino acids. The *in vitro* and *in vivo* beneficial effects of the branched-chain amino acids on nitrogen accrual and decreasing amino acid efflux have been seen in very hypercatabolic and/or metabolically rapid turnover situations and have been much more difficult to establish in normal patients or in less catabolic preparations.

Hormonal Changes. The hormonal milieu provides for either a storage or a breakdown state. Insulin is *the* storage factor, inhibiting lipolysis and increasing nitrogen accrual in muscle. Insulin probably also increases protein synthesis and fat storage in the liver, especially portally supplied insulin. Growth hormone is also an anabolic hormone and has been tested primarily in hypocaloric supplementation. Insulin growth factor-1 may be the active mediator. Glucagon, catecholamines, and steroids promote proteolysis and gluconeogenesis but also increase hepatic protein synthesis.

Cytokines. In the past 5 years, cytokines, materials produced by macrophages and at least T lymphocytes, have been extensively studied (see Table 9–2; Fig. 9–2). Although there are probably more than 100 products of macrophages, attention has focused largely on only a few—IL-1, IL-2, IL-6, TNF/cachectin, and interferon gamma. Investigators have studied etiocholanolone (as a cause of fever) with IL-1 and TNF/cachectin to elucidate some of the metabolic responses to sepsis. To summarize both *in vivo* and *in vitro* studies:

(1) prostaglandins probably have little role in the control of skeletal muscle proteolysis; (2) TNF has little role *in vitro* in muscle proteolysis. TNF *in vivo* requires steroids, either as a permissive or cofactor in proteolysis. The author's *in vitro* studies suggest that at least 50% of the proteolytic activity in sepsis is due to steroids. TNF, promoted as an early cytokine, may trigger, with other stimuli, the *cytokine cascade*.

IL-1 and IL-6 are promoters of the catabolic response, acting in concert with the classic neuroendocrine response. Enterocytes, in addition to perhaps serving as targets for cytokines, may serve as sources of IL-6, TNF, and IL-1.[21–23, 26]

The effects of cytokines on the liver are complex. IL-1 is associated with increased hepatic protein synthesis of some of the complement intermediates, whereas synthesis of transferrin is steroid dependent. IL-6 (hepatocyte-stimulating factor) increases synthesis of some of the alpha-glycoproteins. Undoubtedly, other cytokines are involved as well.

A complete discussion of cytokines is beyond the scope of this chapter; the reader is referred to recent reviews. However, cytokines may not act directly but may in turn be regulated by systems such as nitric oxide. A basic question is whether cytokines are endocrine mediators or act solely as paracrine or autocrine mediators. If paracrine, the high level of cytokines in the plasma is overflow, and the view that circulating cytokines contribute to such deleterious effects as the multiple organ failure syndrome becomes much more plausible.

Many of the effects of sepsis can be mimicked by the *in vivo* injection of endotoxin, while incubating endotoxin *in vitro* is without effect, suggesting that a release of, or synergism with, other substances is necessary. It is of interest that Fine's endotoxin hypothesis is now being revisited 50 years after it was discredited.

Clowes proposed that proteolysis-inducing factor (PIF), of molecular weight 4200 daltons and perhaps a split product of IL-1, was responsible for both proteolysis and increased hepatic protein synthesis, which stimulated recent interest in the cytokines. Consequently, it is ironic that efforts to confirm PIF have proved very difficult.[15] It appears that the very peculiar experimental conditions used by Clowes may produce the effects attributed to PIF.[15] Unfortunately, controls were not done in the initial study. Nonetheless, the contribution of Clowes is enormous.

Nitric Oxide. More than 1000 papers on nitric oxide appeared in 1993, just 8 years after the first description of synthesis of nitric oxide by mammalian cells by Stuehr and Marletta. Nearly every cell type thus far studied has the capacity to synthesize nitric oxide by one of three nitric oxide synthetase isoforms. Depending on the location, the targets, and the local environment, nitric oxide performs a variety of very different functions. A small amount of nitric oxide released at nerve termini may act as a neurotransmitter and may regulate relaxation of various muscular sphincters within the gastrointestinal tract. In very small amounts, nitric oxide may serve as a neurotransmitter in the central nervous system. Nitric oxide released by the vascular endothelium, again in small amounts, probably regulates the relaxation state of adjacent smooth muscle. Much larger amounts released in the response to stimuli, such as cytokines, can kill pathogens and protect or, in excessive amounts, destroy host tissues. Such different effects, depending on the amounts released, appear entirely dependent on the isoform of nitric oxide synthetase at a specific site.

Nitric oxide is a normal atmospheric component. A single atom of nitrogen and a single oxygen atom form, creating the smallest synthetic product of mammalian cells. The configuration of a single oxygen atom is also a molecule with an unpaired electron, and thus highly unstable. Target molecules that accept electrons include oxygen, other free radicals, thiol groups, and various metals. Nitric oxide has a very short half-life (a few seconds or less). If the nitric oxide free radical interacts with oxygen, the resultant oxidation to nitrite and nitrate inactivates the molecule; it also enables measurement of nitric oxide indirectly by the measurement of nitrite or nitrate. Nitric oxide exerts some of its effect by interaction with prosthetic iron groups or thiol groups and proteins, as it forms complexes that activate or inactivate target enzymes. For example, a combination with iron results in activation of soluble guanate cyclase, which increases cellular cyclic guanosine monophosphate concentrations and results in vasorelaxation.

L-Arginine is the sole substrate for nitric oxide synthesis. The relevant synthetic pathway is a five-electron oxidation, with the reduced form of nicotinamide-adenine dinucleotide phosphate acting as a nitric oxide donor; oxygen is derived from molecular oxygen. It is thought N^G-hydroxy-L-arginine may be a short-lived intermediate. Citrulline is formed as a coproduct.

Of the three isoforms of nitric oxide synthetase, the inducible nitric oxide synthetase (INOS) is most important because, once induced, large and sustained amounts of nitric oxide may be produced. In addition to its role in vasodilatation and neurotransmission, a major role of nitric oxide is in the area of infection and inflammation. The capacity to express the INOS protein is widespread and, in animals, includes macrophages, chondrocytes, neutrophils, hepatocytes, vascular smooth muscle cells, and pancreatic islets. The highest expression of the inducible enzyme is in response to a combination of multiple simultaneous agents that may vary from cell to cell and include lipopolysaccharide, interferon gamma, IL-1, and TNF. In the relationship between the Kupffer cells and the hepatocytes, both respond to nitric oxide, which may increase hepatic protein synthesis. The interested reader is referred to several recent reviews.[3, 25]

Causes of Increased Protein Loss. The normal turnover of protein is 2.5% to 3% of lean body mass per day (see Fig. 9–4). With normal protein and calorie intake, and without strenuous exercise, only minuscule daily accrual of nitrogen occurs. Proteolysis occurs in response to starvation, stress, and sepsis and is mediated by glucagon, catechols, and steroids, with a considerably smaller increase in insulin and (in trauma or sepsis) cytokines. Proteolysis supplies the necessary amino acids to increase hepatic protein synthesis for host defense and for glucose production by gluconeogenesis (alanine-glucose cycle). The alanine-glucose cycle is not a true cycle, because nitrogen is lost during each turn of the cycle, with ammonia going to urea. Thus, although glucose, which originates from pyruvate, is returned to the periphery, there is net destruction of muscle and loss of nitrogen.

In starvation, as much as 300 gm. of protein per day may be lost initially. There is rapid adaptation to resting starvation, and proteolysis is minimal after as little as 4 days. The metabolic tragedy of sepsis is that this adaptation to starva-

tion does not occur, and breakdown of protein, to supply amino acids either for hepatic protein synthesis for host defense or for gluconeogenesis for the energy needs of the organism, continues.

The calorie stores of the body are given in Table 9–3, with fat constituting the bulk of calories available. The additional metabolic tragedy of stress and sepsis is that fat is not utilized to its maximal potential and protein is continually broken down for glucose. The controls are inoperative; administration of either fat or glucose does not abolish proteolysis.

Recent work suggests that in the muscle from a septic animal or patient, the branched-chain amino acids, which normally decrease the efflux of amino acids from muscle, do not decrease muscle breakdown even in pharmacologic quantities (5 mM.). Leupeptin, an inhibitor of lysosomal breakdown, diminishes proteolysis.

METHODS OF ASSESSMENT

Accumulation of lean body mass is the principal objective of nutritional support; thus, determination of lean body mass is the most appropriate means of nutritional assessment. Such determinations are usually available only on a research basis.

Displacement. Probably the most sensitive determination of lean body mass is displacement. Various body components are estimated by displacement of water volume. This is beyond the capacity of most institutions.

Exchange of Labeled Ions. This procedure is available only in research centers. Total body water may be determined by administration of tritiated water. Lean body mass is estimated by exchangeable potassium (^{42}K) and extracellular water by total exchangeable sodium (^{22}Na). Shizgal has suggested that a ratio of exchangeable sodium to exchangeable potassium of greater than 1.22 indicates the increased extracellular water and decreased body mass accompanying malnutrition. Shizgal also proposed derivative ratios to estimate total body fat, but because of compounded error in the ratios, these are probably inaccurate.

Neutron Activation Analysis. This technique is accurate but requires sophisticated apparatus in which the body is bombarded with activated neutrons. Nitrogen, indicative of lean body mass, is then measured. Other ions may also be determined.

Total Body Counters. There are approximately 13 body counters in the United States. These large installations measure spontaneous decay of naturally occurring isotopes, such as potassium-40, which reflect lean body mass. However, these measurements are not suitable for patients who are ill, because one must remain stationary within the counter for prolonged periods of time.

Magnetic Resonance Imaging. Magnetic resonance imaging may accurately measure lean body mass. Most of the current work has focused on energy stores and the relation-

---

TABLE 9–3. Normal Stores of Available Energy and Rates of Utilization in a Man Weighing 65 kg.

	Total Body Content (gm.)	Available Store			Daily Utilization* (gm.)	Exhaustion Time (days)
		(gm.)	(mJ.)	(kcal.)		
Carbohydrate	500	150	2.5	600	All used in first 24 hr.	<1
Protein	11,000	2400	40	9600	60	About 40†
Fat	9000	6500	235	58,500	150	About 40†

*Assuming an energy expenditure of about 6.7 mJ. (1600 kcal.)/day.

†Experience in voluntary starvation suggests that the limit of resting starvation in young men in excellent physical condition may be as much as 60 to 70 days (Maize Prison).

From Passmore, R., and Robson, J. S.: A Companion to Medical Studies. Vol. 3. Oxford, Blackwell Scientific Publications, 1974.

ships between phosphocreatine, adenosine triphosphate, adenosine diphosphate, creatine, and adenosine monophosphate in starvation and refeeding. In rats, changes are detected after 6 to 8 days of starvation, with decreased phosphocreatine. This is interpreted as being utilized to maintain adenosine triphosphate. Other studies suggest that there may be some decrease in efficiency in the starved muscle.

History and Physical Examination. Weight loss, anorexia, or a disease process that interferes with intake, such as esophageal carcinoma, should alert the examiner to the possibility of malnutrition. On physical examination, muscle wasting, loss of thenar muscles, loose flabby skin, the edema of hypoproteinemia, weakness, loss of body fat, and pallor confirm. In several studies, a careful history and physical examination by a seasoned clinician is as accurate as multiple complex tests, particularly when functionality is assessed. Loss of ability to carry out normal function is especially significant.

Clinical Methodologies. Simple tests available in most hospitals are most useful.

Nitrogen Balance. For research purposes, nitrogen balance is a tedious technique that requires the measurement of expired nitrogen and the collection of all integumentary, wound, and excretory losses. In the clinical setting, nitrogen balance is determined by measuring urinary and gastrointestinal losses. Because most patients on parenteral nutrition do not eat, stool nitrogen can be assumed to be 1 gm. per day when present or disregarded if absent. One can measure nitrogen balance in two ways, depending on instrumentation available. Any hospital laboratory can measure urinary urea nitrogen, but urinary collection must be accurate; this can be monitored by measuring urinary creatinine. Two to 3 gm. of nitrogen should be added to urinary urea nitrogen for insensible and nonurea losses. An alternative is to measure total urinary nitrogen by chemiluminescence, in which case a small amount of nitrogen, less than 1 gm., should be added for insensible losses. This is compared with nitrogen intake, and nitrogen balance is obtained.

Nitrogen Breakdown. Nitrogen turnover, particularly that of lean body mass, is estimated by urinary excretion of 3-methylhistidine (3-MH), a methylated derivative of histidine. 3-MH, a product of actin and myosin, once methylated is not reutilized for nitrogen synthesis. Its urinary excretion does not merely measure breakdown, but probably turnover as well. It is likely that 3-MH measures not only muscle lean body mass but also a relatively small, rapidly turning-over protein pool derived from the gut. This does not invalidate 3-MH as a measurement of breakdown or turnover of lean body mass; it merely invalidates it as a measurement of turnover of skeletal muscle. Most investigators now believe that 3-MH reflects lean body mass but not skeletal muscle alone.

Indirect Calorimetry. Indirect calorimetry, now available as bedside metabolic carts, is used increasingly to measure energy balance, which may be as important as nitrogen balance. Metabolic carts are also used to estimate caloric requirements. The measurement is carried out in the resting state; 15% should be added for activity. In one study from the author's institution, the Harris-Benedict equation, with some correction for the clinical state, compared favorably with metabolic cart measurements as an estimation of patient requirements. The caloric requirement is considerably lower than it was originally thought to be 10 or 15 years ago, more in the range of between 1800 and 2200 kcal. per 24 hours than the 3500 or 4000 kcal. per 24 hours as was common practice at that time.

Delayed Cutaneous Hypersensitivity or Anergy. Delayed cutaneous hypersensitivity was widely used early in studies of nutritional assessment. Although in most studies there was a statistical relationship between anergy and mortality, investigators have concluded that delayed cutaneous hypersensitivity was without value for measuring specific operative risk. More recent data, using different antigens and injection techniques, suggest that when carefully performed by trained personnel, and done at defined times—on admission rather than at random throughout the hospital course—skin reactivity may have value. In patients admitted after trauma or with infection, anergy to cutaneous recall antigens is associated with a high mortality and morbidity. These patients are likely those with severe malnutrition. However, not all malnourished patients are at risk; the defect is immunologic, not nutritional. In subsequent studies, anergy and malnutrition were related in another logit function, using albumin (ALB) and reactivity to recall antigens as a specific function equation:

$$P \mid death \mid = 1/\{1 + e^{(-3-45 + 1.75^* [ALB]) + 0.3^* (In[DTH\ score])}\}$$

Delayed cutaneous hypersensitivity is complicated by extraneous factors such as operation, which is followed by immediate anergy in many patients. Patients with cancer are anergic; this is reversed after resection. Thus, delayed cutaneous hypersensitivity must be assessed in concert with other tests.

Functional Studies of Muscle Function. Because many of the tests described earlier are not readily available, muscle strength, either as evaluated by hand-grip dynamometry or as force frequency characteristics, and rate of recovery from fatigue after electrical stimulation of the ulnar nerve have been evaluated. Although not perfect, these studies when properly conducted provide a functional counterpart of severe protein-calorie malnutrition. In most studies, however, patients with deficits in hand dynamometry are easily identifiable by other means such as a simple functional history, physical examination, or *global nutritional assessment.*

NUTRITIONAL ASSESSMENT

Nutritional assessment, a clinical term, estimates changes in body nutritional composition to predict risk for surgery. Although the ability to predict risk in large, severely malnourished populations is well established, risk for an *individual patient* cannot be predicted accurately.

The confusion in this area is due to inaccuracies of concept. Theoretically, one should measure lean body mass functionally, including muscular, respiratory, cardiac, hepatic, renal, immunologic, and host defense functions. How is this done?

In the light of the aforementioned goals, current practices are disappointing. Midarm muscle circumference and height-weight ratio indicate stores but do not reflect function. Triceps skinfold thickness measures fat stores, which have little to do with function. Neutrophil function is at least one order of magnitude removed from cell-mediated immunity, most commonly tested by delayed hypersensitivity to skin recall antigens.

Acceptable studies should be randomized, prospective, and *consecutive* and have blinded observers. When these criteria are used, few studies qualify. Most published studies are retrospective for selected patients, usually those judged severely at risk. Studies that emphasize hepatic synthesis of short-turnover proteins and immunologically related proteins and neutrophil function may be more successful in identifying patients at risk for infection. The University of Pennsylvania group suggested a *prognostic nutritional index,* but the patients were nonconsecutive and studied retrospectively.[5] Consecutive patients studied prospectively failed to reveal a group at risk. Accurate observation by experienced observers provides the same accuracy as extensive tests. A careful functional history may be equally accurate at identifying the patient at risk. Once this subset of patients can be identified, one can concentrate on repairing the defect. In a Veterans Administration Hospital cooperative study, a group of severely malnourished patients at risk was treated with perioperative TPN, with resulting decreased operative morbidity.[5]

When all studies are evaluated, the patient at risk can be recognized as follows:

1. Recent weight loss of greater than 10% body weight and/or body weight of 80% to 85% ideal body weight
2. Serum albumin in a stable, hydrated patient of less than 3.0 gm. per 100 ml.

These two simple parameters will probably define the population at risk. Corroborative information includes the following:

3. Anergy to injected skin recall antigens
4. True transferrin of less than 200 mg. per 100 ml.
5. A history of functional impairment
6. Significant deficits in hand dynamometry or muscle response to nerve stimulation

The critical importance of albumin is shown by juxtaposing two logit functions that attempt to identify the patient at risk:
From Mullen and co-workers:

$$PNI = 158 - 16.6 \text{ ALB} - 0.78 \text{ triceps skinfold} - 0.20 \text{ TFN} - 5.8 \text{ DTH}$$

where PNI is prognostic nutritional index, DTH is delayed-type hypersensitivity, and TFN is transferrin.
From Christou's work:

$$P\,|\,death\,| = 1/\{1 + e^{(-3-45 + 1.75*[\text{ALB}]) + 0.3*(\ln[\text{DTH score}])}\}$$

What is it about albumin? In subsequent studies in Montreal, the anergic group is the same group that has an exchangeable sodium-potassium ratio of greater than 1.22, thus making them malnourished. With an increased exchangeable sodium-potassium ratio of greater than 1.22, one can expect an increase in extravascular volume. With greater extravascular volume, there is likely to be a greater amount of albumin in the extravascular space; because the serum concentration of albumin is directly proportional to its degradation, increasing the amount of albumin in the extravascular space will increase the degradation rate, thus decreasing serum concentration.

There has always been controversy over the meaning of the lowered serum albumin in patients malnourished and at risk. Some have attributed the low serum albumin to decreased synthesis, others to increased degradation. Still others have suggested that perhaps low-grade sepsis results in down-regulation of albumin synthesis. This latter point is probably not tenable because in a long-term sepsis model, von Allmen and associates found that whereas albumin synthesis was decreased for the first 24 hours, after 4 days albumin synthesis was increased.[37]

Thus, decreased albumin synthesis because of down-regulation is not tenable in long-term malnutrition. That there is increased albumin in the extravascular space with an increased rate of degradation may very well explain the lowered serum albumin in patients who are at risk. It is of interest that two different bodies of work have come together on this conclusion.

INDICATIONS FOR NUTRITIONAL SUPPORT

Indications for nutritional support should consider the following: (1) the premorbid state (healthy or otherwise); (2) nutritional status; (3) age of the patient; (4) duration of starvation; (5) degree of the anticipated insult; (6) the likelihood of resuming normal intake soon; (7) weight loss of 15%; and

(8) a serum albumin value less than 3.0 gm. per 100 ml. Confirmatory values indicating a possible problem with sepsis include a true transferrin of less than 200 mg. per 100 ml. and anergy to injected antigens. In patients meeting these criteria, a 60% rate of sepsis may occur.

Each practitioner must choose the criteria in a given patient. However, patients in the seventh and eighth decades lose lean body mass, although their percentage of lean body mass as a percentage of total body composition is greater with fewer fat reserves. Patients up to 60 years of age can tolerate a 12- to 14-day period of fast, beyond which continued starvation is deleterious. In septuagenarians, 7 to 8 days is the limit, and probably 5 to 6 days is the limit in patients of 80 years or more. Obviously, in critically ill patients, nutritional supplementation should be undertaken more readily than in those less severely stressed.

ROUTES OF ADMINISTRATION

Two routes are possible: the enteral route, using stomach or preferably small intestine, and the parenteral route. The enteral route is more physiologic—the liver is not bypassed and hepatic ability to take up, process, and store the various nutrients for later release on nervous or hormonal command is maintained. Furthermore, there is some evidence that increased cardiac output is required when the gut is bypassed. With parenteral nutrition, gut blood flow increases about 15% to 20%, presumably to allow the gut to perform its usual metabolic functions, such as transamination.

It is often said that enteral nutrition is safer and more efficacious than the parenteral route. Although earlier studies in experimental animals and man did not demonstrate improved outcome using enteral nutrition, more recent studies in the trauma and burn settings have suggested improved outcome. The initial study indicating that there might be an advantage to survival with enteral feeding came from a study of burned children.[1] The study found that increasing the percentage of calories with whey protein from the standard 15% to 25% in severely burned children statistically improved survival. The children who survived with the increased amount of protein received a greater percentage of their feeding by gut as opposed to vein. Alexander and co-workers, in a classic series of investigations, subsequently provided evidence that gut feedings early in burns in guinea pigs and subsequently in man prevented, in part, the burn hypercatabolism.[17] The working hypothesis was that early gut feeding in guinea pigs and in man, but not in rats, prevented bacteria and/or their products from translocating the gut mucosa, releasing catecholamines and other counterregulatory stimuli, and thus prevented the hypercatabolism.

In posttraumatic situations, two prospective and randomized studies showed that early gut feedings result in lower mortality and septic complication rates. That much is clear—enteral nutrition is superior to parenteral nutrition with respect to outcome. What is not clear is the mechanism. There is an unfortunate tendency to equate a better result through enteral feeding with decreased translocation of bacteria and their products and improved mucosal barrier integrity. Although this might be *the* mechanism, or at least *a* mechanism, there is no evidence to this point. On the other hand, increased substrate supply to the liver and improved hepatic acute phase protein synthesis might be another mechanism by which outcome is improved. In any event, there is finally evidence demonstrating that the use of the gut may be superior to parenteral nutrition in severely traumatized or burned individuals.

In comparing enteral and parenteral nutrition in postoperative experimental animals, enteral nutrition is not more efficacious than parenteral nutrition when animals in which the catheters are septic (as judged either by mediastinal culture or section) are eliminated. Similar results are obtained in *normal* postoperative patients in whom enteral and parenteral feeding are compared. It is also not true that enteral nutrition is safer. Deaths in persons receiving enteral nutrition are generally due to aspiration; gastric motility suddenly changes with the onset of sepsis. One death from aspiration is equivalent to the mortality over 2 to 3 years of a well-operated parenteral nutrition program, despite the danger of catheter sepsis (which in well-operated units is now less than 3%).

Despite this, the gut should be used preferentially. There are several reasons for this: (1) enteral nutrition costs less; (2) it likely protects and improves hepatic function; (3) it mimics the normal ingress of nutrients so that the liver can store, process, and release nutrients as it normally does; and (4) gut mucosal integrity is maintained, particularly in burns and hemorrhagic shock. When mucosal integrity is not protected, increased translocation of bacteria or their products may occur, or at least decreased bacterial clearance occurs.[14]

The Translocation Hypothesis. A possible deleterious role of the gut and/or its contents in the pathophysiology of severe injury, particularly burns, was first proposed by Alexander and co-workers, who prevented hypercatabolism by immediate enteral feeding in burned guinea pigs. When feedings were delayed by 24 hours, even increases in the caloric intake from 175 to 200 calories per kg. did not prevent hypercatabolism and weight loss as well as early feeding. Similar results have been obtained in patients.[17]

Translocation is a normal process that teleologically may be important in releasing small amounts of endotoxin to prime the immune systems. Translocation is increased in burns and in hemorrhagic shock but not by pure starvation. Whereas the bacteria are normally cleared by the lymph nodes, it is the bacterial products in the portal circulation, presumably interacting with the Kupffer cells and hepatocytes, that may contribute to the hepatic dysfunction and multiple organ system failure.[11] One study comparing enteral with parenteral nutrition in critically ill patients showed no improvement in outcome or decrease in frequency of multiple organ system failure. There are two studies of early gut feeding in traumatized patients that seem to indicate that early posttraumatic jejunal feeding results in a lower rate of mortality and sepsis in patients receiving the jejunal feeding than those receiving parenteral nutrition.[18]

One problem with the translocation hypothesis as a whole is that a number of results have been ascribed to it that cloud, rather than clarify, the issue. Any beneficial result of enteral feeding is automatically attributed to improvement in gut mucosal barrier integrity. As stated earlier, there are other possible explanations for beneficial results obtained from gut feeding. Although it is true that in pre-agonal patients, total breakdown of gut mucosal integrity results in random bacteremias without a focal area of infection, clinically significant loss of gut mucosal integrity has been demonstrated only in burns, trauma, and perhaps hemorrhagic shock. In the latter study, although the bacteria were labeled, it is not clear that the label that was recovered was still on the bacteria, and no identification procedure was carried out. The final common pathway is lack of perfusion of the gut. Finally, one should focus on clearance, that is, the number of viable bacteria rather than translocation *per se.*[14]

Enterocyte-Specific Nutritional Substrates. The inclusion of enterocyte-specific nutrients, such as glutamine and the short-chain fatty acid products of bacterial action on soluble pectin, will, it is hoped, prevent gut atrophy and maintain gut mucosal integrity.

Glutamine. Glutamine was first described as a gut fuel by Spaeth and Windmueller. Forty percent of the available glutamine is taken up by the gut from the general circulation. It had been assumed that glutamine was taken up by the liver, but the liver's role normally is secondary. In sepsis, however, the liver takes up a great deal of glutamine.

It is likely that the enterocytes take most of the glutamine, although lymphocytes and macrophages may contribute to this uptake. Glutamine is taken up both by the basolateral membrane and from the lumen (Fig. 9–6). Most of the uptake across the basolateral membrane is from the plasma rather than the red blood cells. Luminal transport of glutamine is conducted by system B, a brush-border mucosal transporter. The gut is a very efficient utilizer of glutamine, seeking to maintain its own internal concentration. When the internal concentration decreases, glutamine synthetase increases, with ammonia and glutamate serving as the principal precursors under the influence of steroids. Other fuels may substitute for glutamine. Acetoacetate may replace glutamine on a mole-for-mole basis with equivalent protein synthesis.

The lung has a high capacity for synthesizing glutamine. Normally, the lung is active in the exchange of glutamine, but in sepsis the lung produces large amounts of glutamine, participating in the wholesale changes in the sources and the fates of glutamine.

The role of glutamine in interorgan nitrogen transfer, both normally as well as in sepsis, has not been as well studied, but there are different fates of glutamine and interorgan glutamine flow in sepsis. After induction of a sepsis-like state with lipopolysaccharide in the experimental animal and based on studies with pulmonary artery catheters measuring lung flux in man, in sepsis, lung release of glutamine at least doubles, presumably as the result of glutamine synthetase in the type II pneumocytes. Glutamine uptake by the small intestine decreases, and glutamine uptake by the liver in-

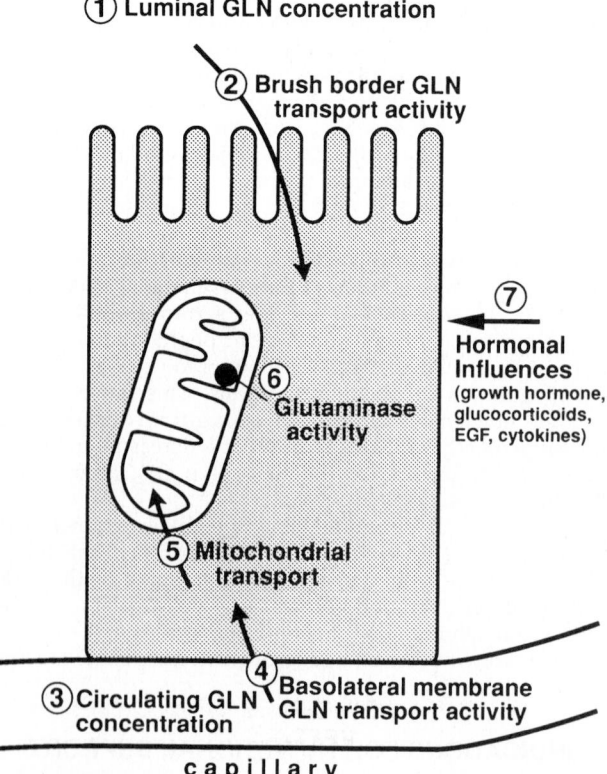

Figure 9–6. Several factors can influence the uptake and release of glutamine by the small intestinal epithelial cell. These include substrate delivery, membrane transport, and intracellular metabolism. (Reprinted by permission of the publisher from Souba, W. W.: Intestinal glutamine metabolism and nutrition. J. Nutr. Biochem., 4:2. Copyright 1993 by Elsevier Science, Inc.)

creases dramatically. The benefit of these changes is not clear. A detailed review of the interorgan relationships of glutamine and their flux is available.[32]

It has been proposed that the addition of glutamine to parenteral nutrition solutions may prevent the gut atrophy that normally accompanies parenteral nutrition. In experimental studies, addition of 2% glutamine to parenteral nutrition solution has shown maintenance of jejunal or ileal mucosal thickness, protein content, and DNA. Not all agree, however. It is difficult to obtain reproducible technical studies. The beneficial results occur after 2 weeks, a biologically long time for a rat, and likely longer in humans. In one study, gut DNA was slightly increased at 1 week, but gut protein, RNA, and wall thickness were unchanged.[19] Epidermal growth factor is much more efficacious in preventing gut wall atrophy than is glutamine. Glutamine's effects in either preventing or healing chemotherapeutic or radiation toxicity, and the regrowth after massive small bowel resection, are more impressive. However, in neoplastic disease, one should remember that glutamine is a principal nitrogen source for many tumors, thus raising a cautionary flag. Early studies in postoperative patients whose TPN was supplemented with a glutamine dipeptide show a small, clinically insignificant positive difference in nitrogen balance in the group supplemented with glutamine.

Short-Chain Fatty Acids. Acetoacetate, propionate, and butyrate are produced by the fermentation of soluble pectin by colonic bacteria. Only 10% of acetoacetate is utilized locally, with 90% exported into the portal vein. With propionate, 50% is exported, and of beta-hydroxybutyrate 80% is consumed locally by the colonocytes and only 20% enters the portal vein. Intravenous beta-hydroxybutyrate results in wall thickening and increased protein content of both the colon and ileum. Use of ketone bodies in preventing diversion colitis has been promising.

As compared with the other common fuels, butyrate is the principal metabolic fuel for colonocytes, with acetoacetate, L-glutamine, and D-glucose following in sequential order of importance. The short-chain fatty acids, principally butyrate, provide approximately 70% of the energy supply of the colonic mucosa. Butyrate may stimulate ketogenesis by the hydroxymethylglutaryl–acetyl coenzyme A pathway. Adenosine triphosphate generation, lipolysis, and absorption of sodium and potassium are enhanced by short-chain fatty acid and principally butyrate oxidation. Diminished short-chain fatty acid oxidation may disrupt the colonic mucosal barrier and presumably, although certainly not proven in man, its immune function. Some investigators have proposed a deficiency of short-chain fatty acids to colonocytes as a cause or precursor to ulcerative colitis,[29] but evidence has been difficult to obtain.

Butyrate and propionate are primarily metabolized by the colonic mucosa, and the remnants are exported in the portal vein by the liver. Acetate passes into the peripheral circulation, where it nourishes the colon by absorption through the basolateral membrane. Because the short-chain fatty acids are not synthesized endogenously, the colonic mucosa can only obtain these respiratory fuels from bacterial fermentation. Further information on the role of short-chain fatty acids is provided elsewhere.[30]

GENERAL PRINCIPLES OF ENTERAL FEEDING

The stomach is the principal defense against an enteral osmotic load. After bolus administration of hyperosmotic fluid, gastric motility stops and gastric secretion proceeds until gastric contents are iso-osmotic, at which point transfer across the pylorus begins. The small bowel is less able to

dilute osmotic loads when they are administered directly. Moreover, gastric acid secretion, which normally prevents bacterial contamination of the gastrointestinal tract, may be neutralized by constant infusion into the stomach; thus, bacterial overgrowth in the gastrointestinal tract may occur. If nutritional solutions are not properly refrigerated, bacterial overgrowth may occur in the container.

The small bowel is the principal area for nutrient absorption. Dipeptides and oligopeptides are preferred for protein absorption, not single amino acids, although this has been challenged recently. With normal gut function, this is unimportant, because protein is completely absorbed in the first 120 cm. of jejunum. With short or diseased bowel, there may be an advantage to dipeptides. Carbohydrate is also absorbed high in the jejunum, with simple sugars preferred. Complex sugars, such as disaccharides, require enzymatic cleavage. A common difficulty with patients who are ill is acquired lactase deficiency, which often corrects itself in time, but in the early recovery phase, lactose-containing foods may cause diarrhea. Fat is most difficult to absorb, depending on proper release and mixing of bile and pancreatic enzymes. After gastrectomy, pancreatic resection, or complex upper abdominal operations, such relationships are disturbed, and proper mixing of bile and pancreatic enzymes does not occur. Fat absorption after gastrectomy is diminished after Billroth II, less so with Billroth I, procedures. Calcium, iron, and other metals are absorbed in the duodenum. Consequently, duodenal bypass (as after Billroth II gastrectomy) results in long-term deficiencies of these ions.

Other Functions of the Gut. At least 22 putative gut hormones have been described, and immunohistochemical examinations have revealed an equally complex series of endocrine-like cells. These functions are covered elsewhere in this volume.

Immunologic Functions of the Gut. The gut is the largest immunologic organ in the body and contains large numbers of lymphocytes, plasma cells, and macrophages, often in large accumulations, such as Peyer's patches. A variety of immunoglobulins are produced by the gut, including IgM and perhaps IgA. Secretion of IgA by the liver is stimulated by gut feeding. It has been suggested that TPN not only does not promote IgA secretion but also may suppress IgA secretion. The evidence for this is scant.

The immunologic functions of the gut are important because of the improvements in survival and outcome in post-traumatic patients receiving enteral as opposed to parenteral nutrition. Whereas some have focused on gut mucosal barrier integrity as the principal cause of this improvement, an equally likely alternative might be improvement in overall immunologic function.

Another important and poorly understood function of the gut is the secretion of mucin, presumably as a protective feature. Production of mucin is dramatically increased in sepsis. Its purpose is not yet clear.

PRACTICALITIES OF ENTERAL FEEDING

A major recent change in nutritional support is the realization that the gut may be more efficacious, at least in burns and trauma, as compared with parenteral nutrition. Enteral nutrition has not been emphasized as much as parenteral nutrition, because it has been assumed that in many disease states, the gut will not work. With effort, it turns out that the gut works and can be used but that perhaps it cannot provide total nutritional support. Still, there is probably significant benefit from utilizing the gut for partial nutritional support. It is not clear to what extent gut feeding must be utilized to obtain the immunologic, hepatic protein synthesis, and bacteriologic advantages to gut feeding. It may be that the percentage of nutrients that should be administered to the gut is not large, perhaps as little as 20%.

Therefore, one should approach nutritional support with two goals in mind: (1) to use the gut if possible and (2) if total nutritional supplementation cannot be provided by gut, to administer at least 20% of the caloric and protein requirements by gut.

Because hyperosmolar solutions are better tolerated by the stomach than by the intestine, enteral feeding is best given by the smallest possible nasogastric tube; to prevent aspiration the tube should end in duodenum or intestine. Mortality from enteral feeding is largely due to aspiration, and gastric motility may be suddenly altered in sepsis. A 10-French Silastic catheter is adequate for most enteral diets; an 8-French tube will not accept some of the thicker hydrolysates because it plugs easily. Long-term indwelling tubes probably render the cardia incompetent, and the resultant prolonged reflux may (rarely) yield an esophageal stricture. Patients should be infused constantly, with the bolus technique reserved for special situations. To prevent reflux and aspiration, patients should be kept at a 30-degree angle, and gastric tube feedings should be stopped at 11 P.M., when only skeletal nursing shifts are present. From the standpoint of safety but not physiology, it is safer to give diets into the small intestine, by passing a tube through a nostril by gastrostomy into the duodenum or by needle catheter jejunostomy or 12- or 14-French catheter jejunostomy.

Administration. For gastric feeding, first osmolality and then volume is increased, usually beginning with solutions that are slightly hyposmolar. With iso-osmolar formulations, additional water is essential. If administration is into the small bowel, volume is increased first, then osmolality. Most patients do not tolerate small bowel administration of greater than 500 to 600 mOsm.

Diets Available. There are a wide variety of enteral products. For patients with normal gut function, a less expensive commercial version of blenderized meal, a *hydrolysate,* is well tolerated. Patients in this category include those who cannot eat, such as the elderly, those with carcinoma of the head and neck, and those with neurologic disease. Additionally, there are products with various degrees of complexity, ranging from oligopeptides to individual amino acids. The caloric supply varies from dextrose to complex starches (Table 9–4). Complex starches have solved a major problem in gut feeding—hyperosmolality. Modular diets are those in which the protein, fat, and carbohydrate components can be individually supplied. A partial listing of available products is given in Table 9–4.

With reasonably normal gut function, there appears to be no advantage of elemental diets over hydrolysates, except that elemental diets are more easily administered through needle catheter jejunostomies or 8-French catheters.

Complications of Enteral Administration. In addition to malpositioning of the catheter (i.e., within the pharynx or trachea) and/or aspiration due to sudden changes in gastric motility or overloading, the most common complications of enteral feedings result from solute overload. Inappropriately rapid administration of hyperosmolar solutions results in diarrhea, dehydration, electrolyte imbalance, and hyperglycemia (with glucose-containing solutions) as well as loss of potassium, magnesium, and other ions lost in diarrhea. If aggressive administration of hyperosmolar solute continues despite diarrhea, pneumatosis intestinalis with perforation, which may cause death, occurs. Hyperosmolar, nonketotic coma can occur with enteral feedings as well as with parenteral nutrition. Perforation may occur with the new catheters with rigid styluses to aid in their passage. Malposition in the bronchus with perforation into the pleural cavity seems associated with the more rigid EntriFlex tube.

All these complications are avoidable with care. Aspiration is prevented by the head-up position, placing the catheter into the duodenum, and monitoring of gastric residual, particularly in febrile patients. Dehydration is prevented by carefully increasing osmolality and using Kaopectate and opiates to slow diarrhea, as well as by the addition of free water.

Enteral feeding is much less expensive, costing as little as $25 to $50 per day, compared with up to $200 per day for parenteral nutrition. In the author's studies, comparable nitrogen retention is achieved at 30% to 50% of the cost. However, enteral nutrition is often not possible in patients who are very ill and whose situation is complicated by intra-abdominal sepsis; the parenteral approach is then necessary.

THE PARENTERAL ROUTE

In discussing the parenteral route, several assumptions will be made:

1. Protein is a mixture of single amino acids of synthetic origin, produced from *intelligent bacteria* cultures. At present, Japan is the sole source. Although hydrolysates are available, there is much protein wastage in the hydrolysates, because hydrolysis is incomplete. Legally, 55% of the protein is hydrolyzed to amino acids to qualify as a hydrolysate. The residual dipeptides and tripeptides are not efficiently utilized when infused intravenously. A further advantage of synthetic amino acid solutions is different solutions for different disease states (hepatic and renal disease).

2. Caloric supply is hypertonic dextrose. A few solutions, intended for peripheral administration, use fructose and/or glycerol.

3. Fat consists of 10% or 20% emulsions of soy or safflower oil, usually stabilized with egg phosphatide and lecithin. Newer fat sources using omega-3 sources are not yet available for intravenous use. *Structured lipids*—mixtures of different side chains on a single glycerol molecule—are not yet available for commercial use.

THE PERIPHERAL ROUTE

Parenteral Administration. The peripheral route is used largely in hospitals without formal nutritional support programs. It is useful only under very limited circumstances, when the duration of parenteral nutrition will be limited or one is not certain that parenteral nutrition will be required. When the risk of catheter sepsis is significant because of the lack of a protocol and a nutritional support team to enforce that protocol, *peripheral hyperalimentation* may be safer, but the needs of sick patients are rarely satisfied by this approach.

In the *lipid system,* caloric need is satisfied by 10% or 20% fat emulsions given with amino acids and 5% dextrose. In the author's experience, veins are quickly exhausted, and fat, even with heparin, does not protect against phlebitis. Amino acids given in water without dextrose have no advantage. The hypothesis of Flatt and Blackburn, which proposed the administration of dextrose-free amino acids by allowing the utilization of endogenous fat secondary to lower plasma levels of insulin, has been thoroughly discredited by at least 12 laboratories. The rationale for (hypocaloric) amino acids and 5% dextrose, or glycerol, is an attempt to minimize nitrogen breakdown for limited periods of time. In one European trial, a limited 14-hour infusion of amino acids and 5% dextrose after operations of modest severity did not show improved nitrogen balance.[8]

It is not clear what role the new mixture of amino acids and glycerol (ProcalAmine; McGaw, Inc., Irvine, CA) will play. Theoretically, glycerol is an acceptable carbohydrate, and the avoidance of expense of pharmacy mixing is an advantage.

Text continued on page 159

TABLE 9–4. Enteral Nutritional Products

	Blenderized Formulas		Defined Formula Diets
	Compleat-Modified (Sandoz)	*Compleat-Regular (Sandoz)*	*Criticare HN (Mead-Johnson)*
kcal./ml.	1.07	1.07	1.06
Protein, gm./L. (source)	43 (beef, Ca caseinate)	43 (beef, nonfat milk)	38 (casein hydrolysate, amino acids)
Fat, gm./L. (source)	37 (canola oil, beef)	43 (corn oil, beef)	5.3 (safflower oil, polyglycerol esters of fatty acids)
Carbohydrate, gm./L. (source)	140 (maltodextrin, vegetables, fruits)	130 (maltodextrin, vegetables, fruits, nonfat milk)	220 (maltodextrin, modified corn starch)
Lactose, gm./L.	0	24	0
Minerals/L.			
Calcium, mg.	670	670	530
Phosphorus, mg.	870	1200	530
Magnesium, mg.	270	270	210
Iron, mg.	12	12	9.5
Sodium, mEq.	43	55	27
Potassium, mEq.	36	36	34
Chloride, mEq.	32	32	30
Iodine, μg.	100	100	79
Zinc, mg.	15	15	10.6
Copper, mg.	1.3	1.3	1.1
Manganese, mg.	2.7	2.7	2.6
Volume required to meet 100% RDA, ml.	1500	1500	1890
Nonprotein kcal./gm. N_2	131/1	131/1	149/1
mOsm./kg. H_2O	300	450	650
Preparation	Ready to use	Ready to use	Ready to use
Comments	Commercially prepared blenderized tube feeding	Complete, commercially prepared blenderized formula	Increased nitrogen, elemental tube feeding, uses peptide carrier system + free amino acids, absorbed in upper gut

	Defined Formula Diets (continued)		
	Reabilan (Clintec)	*Reabilan HN (Clintec)*	*Tolerex (Sandoz)*
kcal./ml.	1	1.33	1
Protein, gm./L. (source)	31.5 (hydrolyzed whey protein, casein and whey peptides)	58.2 (hydrolyzed whey protein, casein and whey peptides)	21 (free amino acids)
Fat, gm./L. (source)	39 (MCT, primrose oil, soy oil)	52 (MCT, primrose oil, soy oil)	1.5 (safflower oil)
Carbohydrate, gm./L. (source)	131.5 (maltodextrin, tapioca)	158 (maltodextrin, tapioca)	230 (glucose oligosaccharides)
Lactose, gm./L.	0	0	0
Minerals/L.			
Calcium, mg.	499	451	560
Phosphorus, mg.	499	499	560
Magnesium, mg.	251	331	220
Iron, mg.	10	13.3	10
Sodium, mEq.	30.4	43.5	20
Potassium, mEq.	32	42.4	31
Chloride, mEq.	56.3	70.4	27
Iodine, μg.	74.7	101.3	83
Zinc, mg.	10	13.3	8.3
Copper, mg.	1.6	1.3	1.1
Manganese, mg.	2	2.7	1.6
Volume required to meet 100% RDA, ml.	3000	2857	3160
Nonprotein kcal./gm. N_2	175/1	117/1	282/1
mOsm./kg. H_2O	350	490	550
Preparation	Ready to use—liquid	Ready to use—liquid	Powder—mix with water
Comments	Contains small peptides, enteral only	Contains small peptides, enteral only	Complete, tube feeding, absorbed in upper gut, supplemental

Table continued on following page

TABLE 9–4. Enteral Nutritional Products *Continued*

	Defined Formula Diets (continued)		Lactose-Free Formulas
	Travasorb STD *(Clintec)*	*Vital HN* *(Ross)*	*Attain* *(Sherwood)*
kcal./ml.	1	1	1
Protein, gm./L. (source)	30 (enzymatically hydrolyzed lactalbumin)	41.7 (partially hydrolyzed whey, meat, soy)	40 (Na + Ca caseinates)
Fat, gm./L. (source)	14 (MCT, sunflower oil)	10.8 (safflower oil, MCT)	35 (MCT, corn oil)
Carbohydrate, gm./L. (source)	190 (glucose, oligosaccharides)	185 (hydrolyzed corn starch, sucrose)	135
Lactose, gm./L.	0	0	0
Minerals/L.			
Calcium, mg.	501	667	NA
Phosphorus, mg.	501	667	NA
Magnesium, mg.	201	267	NA
Iron, mg.	9	12	NA
Sodium, mEq.	40	25	35
Potassium, mEq.	30	36	41
Chloride, mEq.	42	29	NA
Iodine, μg.	75	100	NA
Zinc, mg.	7.5	15	NA
Copper, mg.	0.99	1.4	NA
Manganese, mg.	1.26	3.4	NA
Volume required to meet 100% RDA, ml.	2000	1500	1250
Nonprotein kcal./gm. N_2	184/1	125/1	134/1
mOsm./kg. H_2O	560	500	300
Preparation	Powder	Powder—mix with water	Ready to use—liquid
Comments	Complete, gluten- and lactose-free, balanced oral or tube feeding, readily digested and rapidly absorbed	Complete, partially hydrolyzed, oral or tube feeding, HN for patients with impaired gastrointestinal function	Complete, isotonic tube feeding, lactose free

	Lactose-Free Formulas (continued)		
	Ensure *(Ross)*	*Ensure HN* *(Ross)*	*Ensure Plus* *(Ross)*
kcal./ml.	1.06	1.06	1.5
Protein, gm./L. (source)	37 (Na + Ca caseinates, soy protein isolate)	44 (Na + Ca caseinates, soy protein isolate)	55 (Na + Ca caseinates, soy protein isolate)
Fat, gm./L. (source)	37 (corn oil)	36 (corn oil)	53 (corn oil)
Carbohydrate, gm./L. (source)	145 (corn syrup, sucrose)	141 (corn syrup, sucrose)	200 (corn syrup, sucrose)
Lactose, gm./L.	0	0	0
Minerals/L.			
Calcium, mg.	530	758	705
Phosphorus, mg.	530	758	705
Magnesium, mg.	212	303	282
Iron, mg.	9.6	14	12.7
Sodium, mEq.	37	35	46
Potassium, mEq.	40	40	50
Chloride, mEq.	37	38	54
Iodine, μg.	80	114	106
Zinc, mg.	12	17	16
Copper, mg.	1.1	1.6	1.41
Manganese, mg.	2.7	3.8	3.53
Volume required to meet 100% RDA, ml.	1887	1321	1420
Nonprotein kcal./gm. N_2	153/1	125/1	146/1
mOsm./kg. H_2O	470	470	690
Preparation	Ready to use	Ready to use	Ready to use—liquid
Comments	Balanced supplement or total feeding, oral or tube feeding	High-quality protein, supplemental tube feeding, low residue, lactose and gluten free	Complete, HC, supplemental oral or tube feeding

TABLE 9–4. Enteral Nutritional Products *Continued*

	Lactose-Free Formulas (continued)		
	Ensure Plus HN *(Ross)*	*Isocal* *(Mead-Johnson)*	*Isocal HN* *(Mead-Johnson)*
kcal./ml.	1.5	1.06	1.06
Protein, gm./L. (source)	63 (Na + Ca caseinates, soy protein isolate)	34 (Ca + Na caseinates, soy protein isolate)	44 (Ca + Na caseinates, soy protein isolate)
Fat, gm./L. (source)	50 (corn oil)	44 (soy oil, MCT)	45 (soy oil, MCT)
Carbohydrate, gm./L. (source)	200 (hydrolyzed cornstarch, sucrose)	135 (maltodextrin)	123 (maltodextrin)
Lactose, gm./L.	0	0	0
Minerals/L.			
Calcium, mg.	1056	630	850
Phosphorus, mg.	1056	530	850
Magnesium, mg.	423	210	340
Iron, mg.	19	9.5	15
Sodium, mEq.	51	23	40
Potassium, mEq.	47	34	41
Chloride, mEq.	46	30	41
Iodine, μg.	159	79	127
Zinc, mg.	24	11	17
Copper, mg.	2.12	1.06	1.69
Manganese, mg.	5.28	1.6	2.5
Volume required to meet 100% RDA, ml.	947	1890	1180
Nonprotein kcal./gm. N_2	125/1	167/1	125/1
mOsm./kg. H_2O	650	270	270
Preparation	Ready to use	Ready to use	Ready to use
Comments	Supplemental tube feeding, HC, ultra-trace minerals	Complete, moderate level of high-quality protein, low residue	Complete, isotonic tube feeding, high protein, ultra-trace elements

	Lactose-Free Formulas (continued)		
	Isosource *(Sandoz)*	*Magnacal* *(Sherwood)*	*Osmolite* *(Ross)*
kcal./ml.	1.2	2	1.06
Protein, gm./L. (source)	43 (Na + Ca caseinates, soy protein isolate)	70 (Na + Ca caseinates)	37.2 (Na + Ca caseinates, soy protein isolate)
Fat, gm./L. (source)	41 (MCT, canola oil)	80 (partially hydrogenated soybean oil)	37.6 (high-oleic safflower oil, canola oil, MCT)
Carbohydrate, gm./L. (source)	170 (hydrolyzed cornstarch)	250 (maltodextrin, surcrose)	145 (hydrolyzed cornstarch)
Lactose, gm./L.	0	0	0
Minerals/L.			
Calcium, mg.	670	1000	530
Phosphorus, mg.	670	1000	530
Magnesium, mg.	270	400	212
Iron, mg.	12	28	9.54
Sodium, mEq.	52	43.5	27.8
Potassium, mEq.	43	32	26
Chloride, mEq.	31	26.8	24
Iodine, μg.	100	150	79.5
Zinc, mg.	17	30	12
Copper, mg.	1.3	2	1.06
Manganese, mg.	3.3	5	2.65
Volume required to meet 100% RDA, ml.	1500	1000	1887
Nonprotein kcal./gm. N_2	148/1	157/1	153/1
mOsm./kg. H_2O	360	590	300
Preparation	Ready to use	Ready to use—liquid	Ready to use
Comments	Complete, supplemental oral or tube feeding	Complete, oral or tube feeding	Isotonic, low residue, tube or oral feeding, ultra-trace minerals, lactose and gluten free, low cholesterol

Table continued on following page

TABLE 9–4. Enteral Nutritional Products *Continued*

	Lactose-Free Formulas (continued)		
	Osmolite HN *(Ross)*	*Sustacal Basic* *(Mead-Johnson)*	*Sustacal Liquid* *(Mead-Johnson)*
kcal./ml.	1.06	1.06	1.01
Protein, gm./L. (source)	44.4 (Na + Ca caseinates, soy protein isolate)	37 (casein, soy protein isolate)	61 (Na + Ca caseinates, soy protein isolate)
Fat, gm./L. (source)	36 (high-oleic safflower oil, canola oil, MCT)	35 (soy oil)	23 (partially hydrogenated soy oil)
Carbohydrate, gm./L. (source)	141 (glucose polymers)	148 (corn syrup, sugar)	139 (sugar, corn syrup)
Lactose, gm./L.	0	0	0
Minerals/L.			
Calcium, mg.	758	530	1010
Phosphorus, mg.	758	530	930
Magnesium, mg.	304	210	380
Iron, mg.	13.7	9.7	17
Sodium, mEq.	40.4	37	40
Potassium, mEq.	40.25	41	54
Chloride, mEq.	40.6	41	42
Iodine, μg.	114	79	139
Zinc, mg.	17.1	10.6	14
Copper, mg.	1.52	1.06	2
Manganese, mg.	3.79	1.6	2.8
Volume required to meet 100% RDA, ml.	1321	1890	1060
Nonprotein kcal./gm. N_2	125/1	153/1	78/1
mOsm./kg. H_2O	300	500	650
Preparation	Ready to use	Ready to use	Ready to use
Comments	Supplemental tube or oral feeding, HN, lactose and gluten free, low residue	Complete, oral or tube feeding, low residue	Complete, high-protein, low-fat, oral or tube feeding, lactose and fiber free, low residue

	Lactose-Free Formulas (continued)		Lactose-Free Formulas with Fiber
	Sustacal Plus *(Mead-Johnson)*	*Ultralan* *(Élan)*	*Ensure with Fiber* *(Ross)*
kcal./ml.	1.52	1.5	1.1
Protein, gm./L. (source)	61 (Na + Ca caseinates)	60 (Na + Ca caseinates)	39.7 (Na + Ca caseinates, soy protein isolate)
Fat, gm./L. (source)	57 (corn oil)	50 (MCT, corn oil)	37.2 (corn oil)
Carbohydrate, gm./L. (source)	190 (corn syrup solids, sugar)	202 (maltodextrin)	162 (hydrolyzed cornstarch, sucrose, soy fiber)
Lactose, gm./L.	0	0	0
Minerals/L.			
Calcium, mg.	850	1000	719
Phosphorus, mg.	850	1000	719
Magnesium, mg.	340	400	288
Iron, mg.	15.2	18	13
Sodium, mEq.	37	51	36.8
Potassium, mEq.	38	49	43.4
Chloride, mEq.	36	48	38
Iodine, μg.	127	150	108
Zinc, mg.	17	15	16.2
Copper, mg.	1.69	2	1.5
Manganese, mg.	2.5	2.5	3.6
Volume required to meet 100% RDA, ml.	1180	1000	1391
Nonprotein kcal./gm. N_2	134/1	131/1	148/1
mOsm./kg. H_2O	630	540	480
Preparation	Ready to use	Ready to use	Ready to use
Comments	Complete, oral or tube feeding, HC, lactose-free, ultra-trace elements	Lactose and gluten free, kosher, increased calorie intake	Oral supplement or tube feeding

TABLE 9–4. Enteral Nutritional Products *Continued*

Lactose-Free Formulas with Fiber (continued)

	Fibersource (Sandoz)	Fibersource HN (Sandoz)	Jevity (Ross)
kcal./ml.	1.2	1.2	1.06
Protein, gm./L. (source)	43 (Na + Ca caseinates)	53 (Na + Ca caseinates)	44.4 (Na + Ca caseinates)
Fat, gm./L. (source)	41 (MCT, canola oil)	41 (MCT, canola oil)	35.9 (oleic safflower oil, canola oil, MCT)
Carbohydrate, gm./L. (source)	170 (hydrolyzed cornstarch, soy fiber)	160 (hydrolyzed cornstarch, soy fiber)	151.7 (hydrolyzed cornstarch, soy fiber)
Lactose, gm./L.	0	0	0
Minerals/L.			
Calcium, mg.	670	670	909
Phosphorus, mg.	670	670	758
Magnesium, mg.	270	270	304
Iron, mg.	12	12	13.7
Sodium, mEq.	48	48	40.4
Potassium, mEq.	46	46	40.3
Chloride, mEq.	31	31	37
Iodine, μg.	100	100	114
Zinc, mg.	17	17	17.1
Copper, mg.	1.3	1.3	1.52
Manganese, mg.	3.3	3.3	3.79
Volume required to meet 100% RDA, ml.	1500	1500	1321
Nonprotein kcal./gm. N_2	151/1	118/1	125/1
mOsm./kg. H_2O	390	390	300
Preparation	Ready to use	Ready to use	Ready to use
Comments	Complete for maintenance, oral or tube feeding	HN with fiber, oral or tube feeding	Complete, tube feeding

Lactose-Free Formulas with Fiber (continued)

	Nutren 1.0 with Fiber (Clintec)	Sustacal with Fiber (Mead-Johnson)	Ultracal (Mead-Johnson)
kcal./ml.	1	1.06	1.06
Protein, gm./L. (source)	40 (Ca + K caseinates)	46 (Na + Ca caseinates, soy protein isolate)	44 (Na + Ca caseinates)
Fat, gm./L. (source)	38 (canola oil, MCT, corn oil)	35 (corn oil)	45 (corn oil, MCT)
Carbohydrate, gm./L. (source)	127 (maltodextrin, corn syrup solids, polysaccharides)	139 (maltodextrin, sugar, soy fiber)	123 (maltodextrin, oat fiber, soy fiber)
Lactose, gm./L.	0	0	0
Minerals/L.			
Calcium, mg.	700	840	850
Phosphorus, mg.	700	700	850
Magnesium, mg.	340	280	340
Iron, mg.	12	12.7	15.2
Sodium, mEq.	21.7	31	40
Potassium, mEq.	32	36	41
Chloride, mEq.	28.2	39	41
Iodine, μg.	100	105	127
Zinc, mg.	14	14	17
Copper, mg.	1.4	1.39	1.69
Manganese, mg.	2.7	1.78	2.5
Volume required to meet 100% RDA, ml.	1500	1420	1180
Nonprotein kcal./gm. N_2	133/1	120/1	128/1
mOsm./kg. H_2O	303–412	480	310
Preparation	Ready to use—liquid	Ready to use	Ready to use
Comments	Lactose and gluten free, oral or tube feeding, complete, high fiber	Complete supplement, oral	HN, complete, isotonic tube feeding with fiber

Table continued on following page

TABLE 9–4. Enteral Nutritional Products *Continued*

	Milk-Based Formulas		
	Sustacal Powder *(Mead Johnson)*	*Sustacal Pudding* *(Mead Johnson)*	*Sustagen* *(Mead Johnson)*
kcal./ml.	1.09	1.7	1.6
Protein, gm./L. (source)	79 (nonfat milk, whole milk)	6.8/5-oz. can (nonfat milk)	100 (nonfat milk, powdered milk, Ca caseinate)
Fat, gm./L. (source)	5.6 (butter fat)	9.5/can (partially hydrogenated soybean oil)	14.6 (milk fat)
Carbohydrate, gm./L. (source)	180 (sugar, corn syrup solids, lactose)	32/can (sucrose, modified starch, lactose)	275 (corn syrup solids, lactose, dextrose)
Lactose, gm./L.	NA	646	105
Minerals/L.			
Calcium, mg.	2200	220/can	2958
Phosphorus, mg.	1880	220/can	2208
Magnesium, mg.	500	60/can	366.6
Iron, mg.	23	2.7/can	16.6
Sodium, mEq.	52	5.2/can	40
Potassium, mEq.	92.3	8.2/can	75.8
Chloride, mEq.	50.8	5.6/can	62
Iodine, μg.	188	23/can	137.5
Zinc, mg.	18.8	2.3/can	18.3
Copper, mg.	2.6	0.3/can	1.8
Manganese, mg.	3.8	0.67/can	4.58
Volume required to meet 100% RDA, ml.	NA	Provides 15–20% per can	NA
Nonprotein kcal./gm. N_2	61/1	196/1	78/1
mOsm./kg. H_2O			1130
Preparation	Powder	Ready to use	Powder
Comments	High protein and fat, palatable	Supplemental	Supplemental, high calorie, high protein

	Modular Formulas		
	Microlipid *(Sherwood)*	*Propac* *(Sherwood)*	*Sumacal* *(Sherwood)*
kcal./ml.	4.5	3.95	3.8/100 gm. powder
Protein, gm./L. (source)	0	75/100 gm. powder (whey)	0
Fat, gm./L. (source)	500 (safflower oil emulsion)	8/100 gm. powder	0
Carbohydrate, gm./L. (source)	0	NA	95/100 gm. powder (maltodextrin)
Lactose, gm./L.	0	6	NA
Minerals/L.			
Calcium, mg.	0	350/100 gm. powder	<1 mEq./100 gm.
Phosphorus, mg.	0	300/100 gm. powder	<1 mEq./100 gm.
Magnesium, mg.	0	50/100 gm. powder	0
Iron, mg.	0	NA	0
Sodium, mEq.	0	9.8/100 gm. powder	4.3/100 gm. powder
Potassium, mEq.	0	12.8/100 gm. powder	<1/100 gm. powder
Chloride, mEq.	0	1.4/100 gm. powder	5.9/100 gm. powder
Iodine, μg.	0	0	0
Zinc, mg.	0	0	0
Copper, mg.	0	0	0
Manganese, mg.	0	0	0
Volume required to meet 100% RDA, ml.	NA	3 packets = 100% RDA for protein	NA
Nonprotein kcal./gm. N_2	NA	NA	NA
mOsm./kg. H_2O	60	490	NA
Preparation	Liquid—mix with formula, food, or beverages	Powder	Powder
Comments	Oral or tube feeding, fat supplement	Oral or tube feeding, protein supplement	Oral or tube feeding, carbohydrate supplement

TABLE 9–4. Enteral Nutritional Products *Continued*

	Special Formulations		
	Amin-Aid **(McGaw)**	*Hepatic-Aid II* **(McGaw)**	*Immun-Aid* **(McGaw)**
kcal./ml.	2	1.2	1
Protein, gm./L. (source)	19.4 (amino acids)	44 (amino acids, high in branched chain amino acids, low in aromatic amino acids)	37 (lactalbumin, free amino acids)
Fat, gm./L. (source)	46.2 (partially hydrogenated soybean oil, lecithin, mono- and diglycerides)	36.2 (soy oil, mono- and diglycerides)	22 (canola oil, MCT)
Carbohydrate, gm./L. (source)	365.6 (maltodextrin, sucrose)	168.5 (maltodextrin, sucrose)	120 (maltodextrin)
Lactose, gm./L.	0	0	0
Minerals/L.			
Calcium, mg.	0	0	500
Phosphorus, mg.	Trace	0	500
Magnesium, mg.	0	Negligible	200
Iron, mg.	0	Negligible	9
Sodium, mEq.	<15	<15	25
Potassium, mEq.	Negligible	<15	27
Chloride, mEq.	Negligible	Negligible	25
Iodine, μg.	0	Negligible	75
Zinc, mg.	0	Negligible	25
Copper, mg.	0	Negligible	2
Manganese, mg.	0	Negligible	2.5
Volume required to meet 100% RDA, ml.	0	No vitamins or minerals	2000
Nonprotein kcal./gm. N_2	800/1	148/1	113/1
mOsm./kg. H_2O	700	560	460
Preparation	Powder	Powder	Powder
Comments	Comes in orange, lemon-lime, strawberry, supplement for patients with acute or chronic hepatic failure	Supplement, tube feeding with low electrolytes, high branched chain amino acids and low aromatic amino acids, for patients with liver failure, contains aspartame for liver disease	Complete, low residue, HN enteral diet for immunocompromised patients

	Special Formulations (continued)		
	Impact **(Sandoz)**	*Impact (with Fiber)* **(Sandoz)**	*Introlite* **(Ross)**
kcal./ml.	1	1	0.5
Protein, gm./L. (source)	56 (Na + Ca caseinate, L-arginine)	56 (Na + Ca caseinates, L-arginine)	22 (Na + Ca caseinate, soy protein isolate)
Fat, gm./L. (source)	28 (structured lipid from palm kernel oil + sunflower oil, refined menhaden oil)	28 (structured lipid from palm kernel oil + sunflower oil, refined menhaden oil)	18.4 (MCT, corn oil)
Carbohydrate, gm./L. (source)	130 (hydrolyzed cornstarch)	140 (hydrolyzed cornstarch, soy polysaccharide + enzymatically modified guar)	70.5 (hydrolyzed cornstarch)
Lactose, gm./L.	0	0	0
Minerals/L.			
Calcium, mg.	800	800	758
Phosphorus, mg.	800	800	758
Magnesium, mg.	270	270	304
Iron, mg.	12	12	13.7
Sodium, mEq.	48	48	40.4
Potassium, mEq.	33	33	40.3
Chloride, mEq.	37	37	40.7
Iodine, μg.	100	100	114
Zinc, mg.	15	15	17.1
Copper, mg.	1.7	1.7	1.52
Manganese, mg.	2	2	3.79
Volume required to meet 100% RDA, ml.	1500	1500	1321
Nonprotein kcal./gm. N_2	71/1	71/1	127/1
mOsm./kg. H_2O	375	375	220
Preparation	Ready to use	Ready to use	Ready to use
Comments	Meets metabolic and nutritional needs of critically ill patients with or at risk of infection, increased protein, complete	Tube feeding for critically ill, hypermetabolic patients at risk of immune dysfunction, with fiber	Introductory to tube feeding

Table continued on following page

TABLE 9–4. Enteral Nutritional Products *Continued*

	Special Formulations (continued)		
	Nepro *(Ross)*	*Perative* *(Ross)*	*Suplena* *(Ross)*
kcal./ml.	2	1.3	2
Protein, gm./L. (source)	70 (Ca + Na caseinate)	66.6 (partially hydrolyzed Na caseinate, lactalbumin hydrolysate, L-arginine)	30 (Na + Ca caseinates)
Fat, gm./L. (source)	95.6 (oleic safflower oil, soy oil)	37.4 (canola oil, MCT, corn oil)	95.6 (high oleic safflower oil, soy oil)
Carbohydrate, gm./L. (source)	215 (hydrolyzed corn starch, sucrose)	177 (hydrolyzed cornstarch)	255 (hydrolyzed cornstarch, sucrose)
Lactose, gm./L.	0	0	0
Minerals/L.			
Calcium, mg.	1373	867	1385
Phosphorus, mg.	686	867	728
Magnesium, mg.	211	347	211
Iron, mg.	19	16	19
Sodium, mEq.	36	45	34
Potassium, mEq.	27	44.4	28.6
Chloride, mEq.	28.5	46.6	26
Iodine, μg.	158	130	158
Zinc, mg.	23.6	19.5	23.6
Copper, mg.	2.1	1.74	2.1
Manganese, mg.	5.26	4.34	5.26
Volume required to meet 100% RDA, ml.	947	1155	947
Nonprotein kcal./gm. N_2	154/1	97/1	393/1
mOsm./kg. H_2O	635	385	600
Preparation	Ready to use	Ready to use	Ready to use
Comments	Oral or tube feeding, balanced for patients requiring dialysis	Complete for metabolically stressed, unflavored tube feeding	HC, low protein, low electrolytes, low fluid, balanced for nondialyzed renal patients, oral or tube feeding

	Special Formulations (continued)	
	TwoCal HN *(Ross)*	*Vivonex T.E.N.* *(Sandoz)*
kcal./ml.	2	1
Protein gm./L. (source)	83.7 (Na + Ca caseinates)	38 (free amino acids)
Fat, gm./L. (source)	91 (corn oil, MCT)	2.8 (safflower oil)
Carbohydrate, gm./L. (source)	217 (hydrolyzed cornstarch, sucrose)	210 (maltodextrin)
Minerals/L.		
Calcium, mg.	1052	500
Phosphorus, mg.	1052	500
Magnesium, mg.	421	200
Iron, mg.	19	9
Sodium, mEq.	60	20
Potassium, mEq.	63	20
Chloride, mEq.	46.6	23
Iodine, μg.	158	75
Zinc, mg.	23.7	10
Copper, mg.	2.2	1
Manganese, mg.	5.3	0.9
Volume required to meet 100% RDA, ml.	947	2000
Nonprotein kcal./gm. N_2	124/1	149/1
mOsm./kg. H_2O	690	630
Preparation	Ready to use	Powder—mix with water
Comments	HC, HN, for stressed patients with increased caloric and protein needs, tube feeding	HN for patients with gastrointestinal impairment, supplement, tube feeding, enriched with branched chain amino acids, absorbed in upper gut

MCT, medium-chain triglycerides; NA, not available.

This table was originally prepared by Carol Lang, R.D., revised 11/17/89 by Joseph Lacy, M.S., R.D., and updated 2/10/95 by Kimberly Ann Fahrmeier, R.D., University Hospital Nutrition Services, University of Cincinnati Medical Center.

Central Approach. In central hyperalimentation (TPN), the catheter terminates in the superior vena cava, although the inferior vena cava may be used. Silastic or Teflon-coated catheters have replaced polyvinyl chloride–coated catheters; they are less reactive and probably associated with a lower incidence of subclavian and vena caval thrombosis. Percutaneous (or open through the axilla) placement of indwelling *permanent* (Broviac or Hickman) catheters is being done early in patients in whom the need of a central indwelling line for weeks is obvious, because it is likely that the incidence of thrombosis and/or sepsis is lower with these catheters. Infuse-A-Ports are being used with increasing frequency, although the incidence of sepsis is higher.

Safe TPN requires an organization composed of nurses, physicians, and pharmacists and an enforced protocol. In this institution, such organization decreased the catheter sepsis rate from 27% to 0.64%.

Requirements for Nutrition. *Safe* protein requirements are 250 mg. of nitrogen per kg. per day or 1.7 gm. of protein equivalent per kg. per day. Normally, 35 kcal. per kg. per day is adequate. Twenty to 25% of nonprotein calories as fat is probably optimal for hepatic protein synthesis. Adequate vitamins and trace minerals should be given, but knowledge is incomplete as to what amounts. Most authorities advocate two to five times the requirement for water-soluble vitamins and minimal daily requirements for the fat-soluble vitamins that are toxic in excess. Thiamine deficiency in patients receiving normal amounts of thiamine has occasionally been seen, usually in a very depleted patient given a sudden carbohydrate load. The clinical syndrome consists of disturbed mentation, diabetes insipidus, hyperbilirubinemia, thrombocytopenia, and lactic acidosis mimicking sepsis. The plasma amino acid pattern is very distorted, with high levels of proline and hydroxyproline. Once recognized, thiamine deficiency is easily treated with 100 mg. of thiamine per day. Trace metals are given to prevent deficiency states and meet increased needs (Table 9–5).

TABLE 9–5. Suggested Dosage of Vitamins and Trace Metals During Severe Illness

Vitamin	Suggested Dosage (mg./day)
Water soluble	
Thiamine	25
Riboflavin	25
Niacin	200
Pantothenic acid	50
Pyridoxine	50
Folic acid*	2.5
B_{12}†	5
Fat soluble	
A†	5000 µg.
D†	400 µg.
E†	100 µg.
K*	10
Trace Metal	
Zinc	10–20
Copper	0.5–2.0
Chromium	20 µg.
Selenium	70–150 µg.
Manganese	2–2.5
Iron	25

*Inactivated (oxidized) by addition to hypertonic glucose amino acid solutions.
†Sufficient stores of these vitamins exist so that deficiency states are unlikely during short-term (2 to 4 weeks) parenteral nutrition. In practice, however, it is wise to provide them.

TABLE 9–6. Indications for Parenteral Nutrition

Primary Therapy
Efficacy shown*
  Gastrointestinal cutaneous fistulas
  Renal failure (acute tubular necrosis)
  Short bowel syndrome
  Acute burns
  Hepatic failure (acute decompensation superimposed on cirrhosis)
Efficacy not shown
  Crohn's disease
  Anorexia nervosa

Supportive Therapy
Efficacy shown*
  Acute radiation enteritis
  Acute chemotherapy toxicity
  Prolonged ileus
  Weight loss preliminary to major surgery
Efficacy not shown
  Before cardiac surgery
  Prolonged respiratory support
  Large wound losses

Areas Under Intensive Study
  Patients with cancer
  Patients with sepsis

*This indicates that randomized prospective trials or similar investigations have suggested that such nutritional intervention results in changed (improved) outcome.

INDICATIONS FOR PARENTERAL NUTRITION

Indications for parenteral nutrition may be organized into three categories, depending on desired outcome: (1) primary therapy: parenteral nutrition is thought to influence disease process; (2) supportive therapy: nutritional support is achieved and does not alter disease processes; and (3) controversial or under intensive study. These indications are listed in Table 9–6.

Primary Therapy: Efficacy Shown

Gastrointestinal-Cutaneous Fistulas. Patients with gastrointestinal-cutaneous fistulas represent the classic indication for TPN. Increased oral intake increases fistula output. Two longitudinal reviews of fistulas concluded the following:

1. TPN increases spontaneous closure of fistulas.
2. TPN has not resulted in decreased mortality in centers experienced in the treatment of fistulas. The major decrease in mortality in the series at Massachusetts General Hospital and the University of California at San Francisco occurred in the 1960s, probably the result of improved parasurgical intensive care, including monitoring, respiratory care, and better fluid and electrolyte balance.
3. TPN probably has contributed to decreased mortality in patients with fistulas in most other institutions.
4. The treatment of patients with fistulas has been altered by nutritional support. If spontaneous closure does not occur because of fistula anatomy, patients are in better condition for operation.

Respectable rates of fistula closure are also achieved with enteral nutrition, although slightly lower than with TPN. Initially, fistula drainage increases and then decreases toward closure. A useful compromise, if total caloric replacement is not possible enterally, is to give 20% to 30% of calories enterally, which is likely to give all of the benefits of enteral feeding, the remainder given parenterally.

Renal Failure. TPN results in decreased mortality in patients with acute renal failure, but controversy persists concerning the amino acid solution to use. Abel and co-workers, using a mixture of essential amino acids with hypertonic dextrose largely in patients with surgically related renal failure, described decreased urea appearance, earlier diuresis, and a statistically significant improvement in survival in treated patients as opposed to those receiving dextrose alone. Others have argued for a more complete amino acid formula, dealing with the rise in blood urea nitrogen by dialysis. Whereas a few studies have attempted to compare the two formulas, no study with adequate patients concurrently studied is available. The author's practice is as follows.

If it is not clear whether dialysis will be necessary or if dialysis should be delayed, essential amino acids and hypertonic dextrose are used. An additional advantage is that early after operations, such as for ruptured abdominal aortic aneurysm, patients may not tolerate the cardiovascular stress of hemodialysis, and the retroperitoneum may not be sufficiently sealed for peritoneal dialysis. Dialysis will thus be delayed until better tolerated, because accumulation of blood urea nitrogen and hyperkalemia is decreased by the use of the essential amino acid solution. After regular dialysis is established, a conventional mixture of essential and nonessential amino acids is used.

It has been proposed that protein excess may be injurious to patients with renal failure. Patients with chronic renal failure on a low-protein diet deteriorated more slowly, while the use of alpha-ketoanalogs maintained renal function over a period of several years. This does, however, suggest that the use of essential amino acids may have other advantages.

The Short Bowel Syndrome. Repeated small bowel resections for Crohn's disease or major enterectomy after mesenteric thrombosis or volvulus are the three major causes of short bowel syndrome. No randomized prospective trials have been undertaken, but patients with short bowel syndrome have no alternative to long-term home TPN. It is now common for patients on home TPN who would otherwise almost certainly have died to survive for 10 years.[13] Some undergo sufficient hypertrophy of remaining small bowel to ultimately decrease or obviate the need for home TPN. If a patient is left with 1½ feet of small bowel anastomosed to the left colon, hypertrophy in 1 or 2 years will in most cases enable survival without daily parenteral nutritional support, although twice-weekly supplementation may be necessary. Efforts to promote more rapid hypertrophy of small bowel using gut-specific hormones, fuels, and isotonic solutions have been reported.

Burns. The sharp decrease in mortality in patients with burns from 1965 to 1970 is likely the result of aggressive nutritional support. A prospective trial by Alexander and colleagues[1] randomized children with major burns for either normal protein (15% of calories as protein) versus a high-protein (25% of calories as protein) diet, with all other treatment identical. The high-protein diet group showed improved survival as well as improved immunologic parameters and improved neutrophil function. The group receiving the high-protein diet received more of their nutrition enterally. Early aggressive nutritional support in patients with major burns is associated with improved survival.[17]

With the striking finding that early enteral feeding in a guinea pig burn model prevented hypercatabolism, and verification of this work by Warden, Alexander, and co-workers in burned patients,[17] aggressive enteral feeding within 3 hours of burn injury is being increasingly practiced. Parenteral nutritional support is reserved for those few patients in whom enteral nutrition cannot meet the patient's caloric needs. Moreover, *nutritional pharmacology* is increasingly utilized in enteral diets specifically designed for burned patients. Thus, increasing the concentration of arginine as well

as changing the composition of the fatty acid source to omega-3 fats in fish oil, with the resultant production of the prostaglandin E_3 series of prostaglandins and thromboxanes rather than prostaglandin E_2, and thus using eicosapentaenoic acid rather than the arachidonic acid metabolites, have drastically altered nutritional support of burned patients. A product pioneered by Alexander and co-workers (Impact; Sandoz Pharmaceuticals, Minneapolis, MN) was tested in a multicenter trial after upper gastrointestinal surgical procedures. Patients receiving this diet have a lower sepsis rate, fewer days of bacteremia, lower mortality, and shorter hospital stay.[4]

Hepatic Failure. Improved survival is also seen in patients with hepatic failure given aggressive parenteral nutritional support. Patients with liver disease are often malnourished secondary to excessive alcohol and decreased food intake and have decreased tolerance to stress. Protein is the important nutritional component they require, but they are specifically protein intolerant with hepatic encephalopathy. The amino acid–neurotransmitter hypothesis proposed by Fischer and Baldessarini and as elaborated in the *unified hypothesis* proposes that under circumstances of decreased hepatic function and functional or anatomic shunting of portal blood around the liver, amino acid imbalance in the plasma, specifically of the amino acid precursors of central monoamine neurotransmitters, leads to deranged neurotransmitters within the central nervous system. Correcting the plasma amino acid imbalance by the administration of solutions enriched with branched chain amino acids and deficient in aromatic amino acids results in increased tolerance to administered protein and arousal from hepatic encephalopathy. Of the seven randomized prospective trials thus far, in the five in which hypertonic dextrose was used as the caloric source, branched chain–enriched amino acid solutions were at least as effective as lactulose or neomycin in the treatment of hepatic encephalopathy. In two studies, improved survival was seen. In studies in which the major caloric source was fat, efficacy for the branched chain–enriched amino acid solutions was not seen.[27]

The mechanism of this apparently improved survival may be improved regeneration of the liver, better cooperation of the patient with therapy, and decreased infection.

Fan and associates randomized 124 patients undergoing hepatic resection for hepatocellular carcinoma.[11] Half of the patients received only oral nutrition; the other half received perioperative intravenous nutritional support using a branched chain–enriched solution. Dextrose and lipid were the caloric sources, with medium chain triglycerides comprising 50% of the lipids. There was a statistically significant reduction in the overall postoperative morbidity rate in the perioperative nutrition group as compared with the control group (34% vs. 55%, p<.05), predominantly because of fewer septic complications (17% vs. 37%, p<.05). In addition, there was a lower incidence of diuretic agents to control ascites (25% vs. 50%, p<.05), less weight loss (0 kg. vs. 1.4 kg., p=.01), and less deterioration of liver function as measured by change in the rate of indocyanine green clearance (−2.8% vs. 4.8%, p<.05). However, the difference in mortality (5/64 in the perioperative nutrition group and 9/60 in the control group) did not reach statistical significance.[11] Thus, in hepatectomy in cirrhotic patients, outcome can be considerably improved by perioperative parenteral nutrition.

Parenteral Nutrition as Primary Therapy: Efficacy Not Shown

Inflammatory Bowel Disease. In patients with inflammatory bowel disease, oral intake often provokes diarrhea, protein-losing enteropathy, bleeding, and so on. Although TPN and bowel rest are useful in the treatment of Crohn's disease (particularly limited to the small bowel, in which a remission rate of 75% can be expected), such therapy has never been subjected to a randomized prospective trial. The mean duration of remission is approximately 11 months. Patients with colonic involvement do less well; their rates of initial remission and duration are considerably less than those of patients with small-bowel disease alone. Such recurrences can be prevented by maintaining such patients who go into remission on low doses of prednisone, 5 or 10 mg. per day, but this has not been generally accepted. In one long-term study of parenteral nutrition for acute exacerbations of Crohn's disease, after 15 months only 26% of patients had avoided operation.[31]

Patients with extensive, severe, and chronically recurrent Crohn's disease are suitable for home hyperalimentation, particularly when surgical therapy would leave the patient almost anenteric. Chemically defined diets are utilized not only to promote but also to maintain remission achieved by other means.

Ulcerative colitis does not respond to short-term parenteral nutrition, nor is long-term TPN indicated to induce remission, because sphincter-saving operation produces long-term cure. TPN may be useful in preparation for the Soave procedure. In-hospital TPN for usually less than 2 weeks, but occasionally longer, in conjunction with intravenous antibiotics (chloramphenicol or metronidazole) allows rectal mucosa to heal, thereby facilitating rectal mucosal stripping. Home parenteral nutrition in ulcerative colitis is a misuse of an expensive technique.

Anorexia Nervosa. Patients with anorexia nervosa starve to a moribund state, with enormous losses of lean body mass, tissue and protein. For psychotherapy to be successful, some repletion of brain protein is essential. Anorectic patients are difficult to treat; they are self-destructive by disconnecting their intravenous lines, inviting air embolism. A prospective trial has never been carried out in patients with anorexia nervosa.

SUPPORTIVE THERAPY

Supportive Therapy: Efficacy Shown

Acute Radiation Enteritis or Chemotherapy Toxicity. Acute radiation enteritis and/or gastrointestinal complications of chemotherapy may prevent oral intake. Elemental diets are not of value except in preventing radiation damage (probably glutamine content). Rombeau and co-workers have proposed, with good evidence, that the use of soluble pectin in rats receiving 5-fluorouracil chemotherapy prevents toxicity and promotes earlier healing. No clinical trials in patients have been carried out. TPN until the gut mucosa heals will enable the patient to survive. Chronic radiation enteritis with multiple strictures may render the patient a candidate for home parenteral nutrition or, rarely, enteral feeding with minimal residue diets, provided the original neoplasm has been cured.

Prolonged Ileus. Prolonged ileus after an abdominal procedure may necessitate a course of TPN until the ileus subsides. Obviously, this is only supportive.

Supportive Therapy: Efficacy Probably Present

Weight Loss Preliminary to Major Surgery (Perioperative Parenteral Nutrition). There are four major questions concerning the use of parenteral nutrition in patients who have lost weight before major surgery: (1) Are operative complications of major surgical procedures increased in patients who have lost weight? (2) If so, can these patients be identified?

(3) If they are identified, does short-term parenteral nutrition *change the outcome*? (4) If all of these conditions are met, what mode of nutritional repletion should be used and/or for how long?

1. *Are surgical complications of major operative procedures increased in patients who have lost weight?* In a review analyzing 18 randomized and pseudo-randomized studies, Detsky and colleagues concluded that the case had not yet been made for the use of TPN before major operation.[10] Yet the Veterans Administration study appears to identify a group at risk: patients who lost greater than 15% of body weight.[5] The operant defect is not malnutrition, *per se*, but immunologic dysfunction. The two are different: there are patients who are malnourished and have lost 15% of their body weight who remain immunologically capable; other patients with similar weight loss are immunologically dysfunctional. In Graham Hill's work, the group that lost greater than 15% of their body weight and manifested functional impairment was most likely at risk.

2. *Can this group be identified?* Studley suggested that patients with profound (20%) weight loss and low serum albumin experienced increased complications and mortality after gastrectomy. The group at risk can probably be identified statistically, but the individual patient at risk cannot yet be identified. Thus, identifying the group at risk would include careful history and global assessment. A history of greater than 10% or certainly 15% weight loss and an albumin value of less than 3 gm. per 100 ml. would place these patients into a high-risk group. Delayed cutaneous hypersensitivity testing by injected antigens, hand dynamometry, and serum transferrin are confirmatory and optional.

3. *Does short-term nutritional intervention change the outcome?* Yes, provided that nutritional intervention is limited to the group with severe malnutrition and immunologic dysfunction. In the Veterans Administration multicenter trial,[5] in patients judged severely malnourished who had lost greater than 15% of their body weight, preoperative nutritional intervention for 7 to 10 days decreased operative septic complications. In the group stratified as having mild to moderate malnutrition, the decrease in surgical complications was more than offset by the increase in non–catheter-related infectious complications. Thus, TPN, even in the absence of hyperglycemia of greater than 300 mg. per 100 ml. (which interferes with neutrophil function, not the case in these studies), increased the risk of non–catheter-related infection. These presumably nosocomial infections may be due to the lengthy hospital stay or the relative overfeeding (the study being designed in the late 1970s). Whether fewer calories or a shorter hospital repletion would have resulted in greater benefit to the minimally or moderately malnourished group is not clear.

4. *How long should preoperative repletion be?* The period of preoperative parenteral nutrition is likely 5 to 7 days. In previous studies, with 3 days of parenteral nutritional support before operation, there was a trend toward decreased sepsis, but statistical significance was not achieved because of a small number of patients. With preoperative repletion, patients begin to feel better at approximately 5 days, which generally coincides with an increase in the shortest turnover proteins, retinol-binding protein and thyroxin-binding prealbumin. In the Veterans Administration cooperative study,[5] the duration of preoperative parenteral nutrition was between 7 and 10 days, and efficacy was seen. Thus, 5 to 7 days should be used for preoperative nutritional repletion.

Malignant Disease. It is likely that the current form of TPN, especially with overfeeding, may increase growth of tumors (see later); preoperative TPN should be limited to 5 days.

Cardiac Surgery. Patients with cardiac cachexia are at increased risk for complications and mortality after cardiac surgery. The conventional wisdom is based on Starling's pronouncement in 1912 that the heart is spared the ravages of starvation. This is not true. Protein depletion in experimental animals results in decreased myocardial contractility, with distortion of cardiac histology, edema, disruption, and necrosis of myofibrils, which are not totally reversed even after prolonged nutritional repletion. In the single prospective randomized trial in which nutritional supplementation was begun on the day of operation (and thus unlikely to show efficacy), no improvement in outcome was seen. A study in which patients with cardiac cachexia about to undergo surgery are subjected to prolonged nutritional repletion has yet to be done. Anecdotal clinical evidence suggests that patients with cardiac cachexia require nutritional supplementation for 2 to 3 weeks before operation, a finding supported by experimental evidence. Fluid limitations in such patients require more concentrated solutions.

Respiratory Failure and Requirements for Prolonged Respiratory Support. It is barely conceivable that while severely ill patients are receiving the best in intensive care support, nutritional support is neglected; yet it is common. There is no evidence that pulmonary function itself, rather than muscles of respiration, is improved by nutritional support. Although there is some information concerning the metabolic needs of the alveolar cells responsible for surfactant production and gas exchange, a proposed solution has not appeared. Because these cells represent such a small proportion of the structure of the lung, such attempts are complicated.

Whereas weaning from ventilators may improve with nutritional support, a potential deleterious effect of hypertonic dextrose is overproduction of carbon dioxide, especially in patients who are septic, very depleted, and given a sudden glucose load. Although this has been given extensive publicity, it is not common; occasionally in patients with marginal pulmonary function, carbon dioxide overproduction may require replacing glucose calories with fat calories to promote weaning. Carbon dioxide production can be measured in most intensive care units.

Large Wounds and Other Sources of Nitrogen Loss. Many patients with large wounds such as decubiti are unable to eat. Provision of nutritional support to improve wound healing is logical, but no randomized studies exist.

AREAS UNDER INTENSE STUDY

Patients with Cancer. Patients with neoplastic disease may suffer profound weight loss. Anorexia is common, even when the tumor is small, suggesting deranged central nervous system satiety mechanisms.[7] Obstruction of the gastrointestinal tract and mechanical interference with digestion and absorption also contribute to cachexia. During the past decade, the initial enthusiasm for adjunctive nutritional support in patients with cancer has waned, because evidence suggests that tumor growth is stimulated at least in direct proportion to supply of protein and calories. Some clinical evidence suggests that nutritional supplementation of patients undergoing chemotherapy and/or radiation therapy may decrease survival and/or remission-free interval and thus alter cell kinetics.

This important area is plagued by a lack of uniformity in studies, by differences in patient populations, in that both malnourished and normally nourished patients have been included in studies, and by the fact that response to adjunctive nutritional support may differ depending on whether the treatment modality is to be radiation therapy or chemotherapy and/or resection (Table 9–7). The types of calories currently supplied may be inappropriate in the patient with cancer. Although different tumors require different growth factors, glucose, not fat, may be utilized preferentially by tumors. Studies from this laboratory in specific tumor models indicate that by employing specific metabolic blocking agents, it may be possible to treat animals with TPN, adding nitrogen to the carcass without increasing tumor growth. For example, TPN given with acivicin, a glutamine blocker (glutamine is a preferred fuel for tumors), and insulin, which diverts glucose from the tumor to the normal body mass, added lean body mass to the host rat, while averting tumor growth. Unfortunately, this combination is too toxic for use in patients.

The beta-agonists enable better accrual of nitrogen to lean body mass and muscle in experimental animals with experimental tumors.[6] However, clenbuterol, the index drug, is likely too toxic for patients, but subsequent drugs may not be.

In the future, patients may receive TPN with a combination of medications that prevent tumor growth. Such studies also suggest that the *magical* primacy of the tumor is not correct and that metabolic analysis of tumor needs may be important therapeutically.

Randomized prospective trials in patients with cancer have been efficacious in providing preoperative nutritional support only with upper gastrointestinal tumors. Patients with carcinoma of the esophagus or gastric cardia benefit from perioperative nutritional support, with decreased mortality and morbidity without apparent stimulation of the tumor. Caution is justified; adjunctive nutritional therapy is indicated only for patients who are severely malnourished and unable to survive a contemplated course of therapy or operative procedure.[5] In the pediatric age group, the needs of growth are additive to the requirements of stress of operative or other therapy, and adjunctive nutritional support results in decreased concurrent infection.

Sepsis. Sepsis is the major cause of surgical mortality. The metabolic response to sepsis includes proteolysis, with a flow of amino acids from muscle to the liver. Hepatic protein synthesis is increased. The metabolic stimuli for proteolysis include hyperglucagonemia in excess of the corresponding hyperinsulinemia, increased steroids and catecholamines, and cytokines such as IL-1 and IL-6, TNF/cachectin, interferon gamma, and additional cytokines such as those that block amino acid transport into the muscle (see Table 9–2). Many of the amino acids supplied to the liver are metabolized to urea. Is this excess required for a specific purpose? Is the excessive glucose generated by gluconeogenesis appropriate, in view of the glucose resistance? Several years ago, it was suggested that modified nutritional substrate might be more appropriate for patients with sepsis. In overwhelming sepsis, glucose resistance, the failure of ketone body manufacture, and inefficiencies in lipid utilization suggested that a fuel that did not require metabolism through glucose might be more efficient. In addition, because the amount of amino acids supplied to the liver may be excessive, provision of the branched chain amino acids, which supply energy and decrease the breakdown of lean body mass, might be more appropriate.

The branched chain amino acids—valine, leucine, and isoleucine—are utilized as energy without going through glucose, stimulate protein synthesis, and decrease proteolysis in muscle. High branched chain amino acid solutions decreased proteolysis in experimental animals with sepsis. In patients, prospective randomized trials using a high branched chain solution that is either balanced with respect to all three—leucine, isoleucine, and valine—or containing more leucine showed marginal efficacy in preventing breakdown of lean body mass and perhaps increasing hepatic protein synthesis in septic patients. No difference in outcome

TABLE 9–7. Studies of the Effects of Parenteral Nutrition on Patients with Cancer Undergoing Surgery, Radiation, or Chemotherapy

	No. of Patients	Type of Tumor	Type of Therapy	Nutritional Effects (PN vs. Control)	Response to Therapy (%) PN	Response to Therapy (%) Control	Complications of Therapy (%) PN	Complications of Therapy (%) Control	Survival (%) PN	Survival (%) Control	Comments
Holter & Fischer (1977)	56	Gastrointestinal cancer	Surgery	Decreased weight loss and increased albumin level with PN	Same		13	19	93.4	92.4	Lower major complication rate with PN
Moghissi et al. (1977)	15	Esophageal cancer	Surgery	Better nitrogen balance with PN	Same		0	20	NA		Lower rate of wound infection with PN
Issell et al. (1978)	26	Squamous cell lung cancer	Chemotherapy	Improved weight gain and arm circumference with PN	31	7	15	77	NA		Less myelosuppression, less toxic effects of chemotherapy with PN
Heatley et al. (1979)	74	Esophageal/gastric cancer	Surgery	Same	Same		35	83	15	22	Significant reduction in postoperative wound infection
Simms et al. (1980)	30	Esophageal/gastric cancer	Surgery	Improved nitrogen balance and albumin level with PN	Same			NA	10	10	
Lanzotti et al. (1980)	56	Non-oat cell lung cancer	Chemotherapy	NA	10	23		NA	Median 11 wk	Median 12 wk	Significantly better long-term survival curve for PN
Sako et al. (1981)	69	Head and neck cancer	Surgery	Weight gain and better nitrogen balance with PN	Same		50	56	NA		
Valdivieso et al. (1981)	49	Small cell bronchogenic cancer	Chemotherapy	Weight gain with PN	85	59		NA	Survival advantage for PN		PN did not ameliorate hematologic, gastrointestinal, or infectious morbidity
Thompson et al. (1981)	41	Gastrointestinal cancer	Surgery	Improved weight gain with PN; no other differences	Same		17	11	100	100	
Popp et al. (1981)	36, 42	Diffuse lymphoma	Chemotherapy	Marked weight gain with PN; lean body mass, anthropometry albumin, transferrin, and total lymphocytes similar for both groups			11% subclavian vein thrombosis		69	66	No difference in drug tolerance or total drug dose between control and TPN
Nixon et al. (1981)	45	Metastatic colon cancer	Chemotherapy	Weight gain with PN; no other differences	15	12			79 days	308 days	
Serrou et al. (1981)	19	Anaplastic lung cancer	Chemotherapy	Same	83	80	Same; Increased incidence of noncatheter infections with PN		84	80	
Samuels et al. (1981)	30	Metastatic testicular cancer	Chemotherapy	Less weight loss with PN	63	79			75	79	
Linn et al. (1981)	24	Esophageal cancer	Surgery	Better weight gain and nitrogen balance with PN			6 complications	12 complications	90	80	Preoperative TPN and gastrostomy feeding compared
Muller et al. (1982)	125	Gastrointestinal cancer	Surgery	Improved weight gain, visceral proteins, and immunologic status with PN			17	32	96	81	
Shamberger et al. (1983)	27	Sarcomas	Chemotherapy				42	33	Long-term survival rate similar		Similar granulocyte and platelet recovery after chemotherapy-induced myelosupression
Shamberger et al. (1984)	32	Sarcomas	Chemotherapy	Improved nitrogen, balance with PN, but similar visceral proteins	71	86					Shorter remissions for PN
Clamon et al. (1985)	119	Small cell lung cancer	Chemotherapy	Higher colonic and protein intake with PN	48	43		NA	Same		Significantly more febrile episodes with TPN
Muller et al. (1986)	110	Gastroesophageal	Surgery	Improved visceral proteins and immunocompetence with PN	NA		8	17	4	11	Improvement in surgical technique limited value of TPN

PN, parenteral nutrition; NA, not available.

163

was seen, although the number of patients studied was small. The sicker the patient, the more likely improvement in amino acid flux, nitrogen balance, short-turnover proteins, and decreased requirement for insulin after administration of high (45%) branched chain amino acid solutions.

Future solutions for septic patients should stimulate hepatic protein synthesis and improve neutrophil function. Given the apparently specific cytokine blocking amino acid transport into muscle, it may be difficult to maintain lean body mass.

COMPLICATIONS OF PARENTERAL NUTRITION

Complications of parenteral nutrition may be grouped as technical, metabolic, and septic.

Technical Complications

Technical Complications of Catheter Placement. These complications of TPN are related to catheter placement through a crowded thoracic inlet. They decrease with experience, but even the most experienced physician may occasionally experience one of the following:

1. Pneumothorax is more common in elderly and/or cachectic patients. In these patients, an internal jugular line is safer, although dressing is more difficult.
2. Arterial lacerations, although rare, can be avoided by keeping the needle no deeper than 10 degrees to the horizontal.
3. Hemothorax is the result of leakage of blood from the subclavian vein.
4. Mediastinal hematoma occurs especially in patients with deficient clotting factors.
5. Nerve injury may occur to the brachial plexus.
6. Hydrothorax results from catheter malposition and fluid administration into the thoracic cavity.
7. Sympathetic effusions (usually bilateral transudates in response to mediastinal hematoma), substernal pain, and fever may occur.
8. Injury is possible to the thoracic duct after left-sided cannulation.
9. Air embolism is usually the result of improper technique, with the patient not in proper Trendelenburg position or sufficiently hydrated.
10. Catheter embolism may result from shearing of the catheter by the needle when removing a catheter without removing the needle.

Late Technical Complications
1. Erosion of the catheter may occur into bronchus, right atrium, or other structures.
2. Subclavian thrombosis occurs in 5% to 10% of patients. Signs include upper arm swelling and/or pain at the base of the neck. When thrombosis is suspected, the catheter should be removed and, after confirmation, thrombolytic therapy begun. After completion of streptokinase therapy, heparin should be continued for 1 or 2 weeks, followed by warfarin therapy for 6 months.
3. Septic thrombosis is a life-threatening complication. If antibiotics and anticoagulation are not successful, excision of the subclavian vein or Fogarty catheter embolectomy may occasionally be successful.

Metabolic Complications

Metabolic complications are categorized as (1) deficiency states due to inadequate administration of needed nutrients;
(2) disorders of glucose metabolism; and (3) metabolic complications specific for parenteral nutrition.

Plasma Electrolyte Abnormalities

Abnormalities in plasma electrolytes are relatively common and are minimized by careful monitoring. At least 50 mEq. of sodium, 40 mEq. of potassium, 90 to 100 mEq. of phosphorus, and 28 to 32 mEq. of magnesium and calcium should be administered daily to all patients receiving parenteral nutrition. Patients who are rapidly anabolic may require additional potassium, phosphorus, and/or magnesium. Acid-base imbalance is prevented by adding acetate to patients with acidosis and potassium chloride to patients with large gastric output. If potassium chloride is insufficient to prevent metabolic alkalosis, administration of hydrochloric acid or arginine hydrochloride may be necessary.

Trace Metal Deficiencies

Zinc Deficiency. Patients who are very catabolic or have excessive diarrhea may develop zinc deficiency. Neither plasma nor hair zinc is an accurate reflection of total body stores. Three to 6 mg. of elemental zinc per day is required in patients with normal stool losses and between 12 and 20 mg. in patients with short bowel syndrome or excessive diarrhea. Zinc deficiency is characterized by a perioral pustular rash, darkening of the skin creases, and neuritis and is similar to the zinc deficiency seen in sheep (acrodermatitis enteropathica).
Copper Deficiency. This deficiency has been observed in a few patients receiving home parenteral nutrition as a microcytic anemia, which may be mistaken for pyridoxine deficiency. Up to 2 mg. of copper per day is given as the sulfate.
Chromium Deficency. This deficiency is likely to occur only in patients on long-term TPN with minimal or no oral intake. Chromium is necessary for the adequate utilization of glucose. Chromium deficiency is manifest as a sudden diabetic state in which blood sugar is difficult to control, along with peripheral neuropathy and encephalopathy. Fifteen to 20 μg. per day of chromium is adequate to meet daily requirements. To treat chromium deficiency, 150 μg. of chromium per day is given for several days.
Selenium Deficiency. Selenium deficiency has not been clearly established. Abnormalities in basement and plasma membranes have been seen in skeletal muscle biopsies. It is rare.

Biotin Deficiency

Biotin deficiency has been reported by Dudrick (personal communication). Because biotin is ubiquitous, deficiency almost never occurs in patients taking anything by mouth.

Essential Fatty Acid Deficiency

The deficiency of essential fatty acids may be prevented by administration of between 4% to 6% of the daily calories as either soybean or safflower oil fat emulsion. Plasma alterations, which occur within 1 week of fat-free parenteral nutrition, include decreases in linoleic and arachidonic acid and increases in 5,8,11-eicosatrienoic acid and the triene/tetraine ratio; the latter is not uniform. The principal lesion is dry, flaky skin with small reddish papules and alopecia. Prostaglandin deficiency results in decreased intraocular pressure (a convenient noninvasive method of testing for essential fatty acid deficiency). Essential fatty acid deficiency can also be prevented by oral ingestion of 25 to 50 ml. of corn, sunflower, or safflower oil or margarine per day, made palatable with toast. Patients with essential fatty acid deficiency will absorb essential fatty acids through the skin, but this is not practical except in infants.

Disorders of Glucose Metabolism

Hypoglycemia. Other than excessive insulin administration, the most common cause of hypoglycemia is a sudden slowing of the glucose infusion. A curious form of hypoglycemia may be caused by oversecretion of endogenous insulin at high infusion rates. Slowing of the infusion will decrease the hyperinsulinism.

Hyperglycemia. The most dangerous metabolic complication, hyperglycemia is most commonly caused by too rapid initiation of the infusion. This is best prevented by initiation of the infusion at 40 to 60 ml. per hour (25% glucose base) and an increase of 20 ml. per hour every 24 or 48 hours, depending on the age of the patient, the presence of sepsis, and tolerance to infused glucose. Patients with normal glucose tolerance may manifest glycosuria for the first 48 hours of parenteral nutrition, but before initiating insulin one must verify that the blood sugar level is high and that glycosuria is not secondary to a reduced renal threshold for glucose; the blood sugar level is often normal, and the glycosuria disappears with continued parenteral nutrition. The most common cause of sudden hyperglycemia is sepsis, and hyperglycemia may antedate sepsis by 24 hours. Sudden appearance of hyperglycemia should initiate a thorough search for the source of infection.

The Diabetic Patient. Patients with adult-onset diabetes are not difficult to control. Although secretion of insulin in response to glucose is deranged in these patients, adequate insulin release is elicited by amino acid administration. Hyperosmolar nonketotic coma is a potentially fatal complication, with blood sugars in excess of 700 mg. per 100 ml. that result in osmotic diuresis and dehydration, fever, obtundation, and coma. Death occurs unless treatment is begun by administration of up to 200 units of insulin per day and of large volumes of dextrose-free hypo-osmotic solution, generally 0.45% saline with added potassium.

Liver Function Derangements. Patients receiving any hyperalimentation solution, regardless of composition, may manifest increased aspartate aminotransferase, alanine aminotransferase, gamma-glutamyl transferase, and alkaline phosphatase. Hyperbilirubinemia is rare, and when it occurs in a patient on TPN the cause is generally sepsis. All components of parenteral nutrition have been accused of causing the hepatic steatosis that occurs with parenteral nutrition, including metabolic products of tryptophan and preservatives. Consider the following: Hepatic steatosis is most common secondary to excessive glucose administration. Although it has been proposed that translocation of gut bacteria or their products (such as endotoxin) are responsible for increased hepatic fat, using a very specific chromogenic assay, in the laboratory at the author's institution endotoxin has not been identified in the portal circulation.

There is an excellent correlation between the portal vein insulin and glucagon molar ratio and hepatic fat content. This appears logical, because the portal concentrations of insulin and glucagon are what the liver *sees*. Insulin results in hepatic lipogenesis and glucagon in fat mobilization. Incubation of mice hepatoma cells with insulin and glucagon will decrease the number of insulin receptors, thus decreasing the fat storage function of insulin by the presence of glucagon. Once established, hepatic steatosis is cleared by the addition of small amounts (15 μg.) of glucagon to TPN in experimental animals despite continuing glucose overload. Similarly, when fat is added to parenteral nutrition or enteral feedings, or, as recently suggested, glutamine, the decrease in the portal vein insulin-glucagon molar ratio to normal is associated with clearance of hepatic steatosis. Peripheral venous concentrations of insulin and glucagon do not correlate with hepatic steatosis.

In infants, hepatic dysfunction is a more serious and different disease. It is frequently associated with cholestasis. Even when enteral feeding is begun and TPN is discontinued, hepatic dysfunction may persist and progress to cirrhosis and death. Whether translocation of gut bacteria or their products across the immature gut, immaturity of other enzyme systems, or other factors play a role is not clear, but the disease in infants clearly is different from that seen in adults.

Septic Complications

Catheter Infection

Catheter sepsis is potentially the most lethal complication in patients receiving TPN. Bacterial catheter sepsis is directly related to catheter care and can be reduced to the current minimum of less than 1% (in a well-run program) by careful attention to detail and the avoidance of multi-use catheters. Fungemia, a far more serious complication, has accounted for more than 50% of the septicemias in one study, but the rate of disseminated candidiasis was low. The entry site of *Candida*, the most common fungal pathogen, is probably the gastrointestinal tract. Large oral doses of nystatin will not prevent candidemia in the susceptible patient. It is probably more important to treat colonization with *Candida* (defined as two positive site cultures, e.g., urine and skin) with either fluconazole or amphotericin in patients with normal white blood cell counts, because the two drugs appear equally efficacious.[28]

Most hyperalimentation patients are malnourished and thus more prone to infection. Corticosteroid administration apparently also predisposes patients to infection, as do multiple antibiotics and chemotherapy. The following factors contribute to the development of catheter sepsis:

1. The absence of a protocol. At the University of Cincinnati Medical Center, the sepsis rate decreased from 27%, before the establishment of a hyperalimentation team and a rigid protocol, to 0.6%.

2. Catheter sepsis is correlated with the degree of colonization of the pericatheter skin. When the skin around catheters was quantitatively cultured, those catheters whose surrounding skin showed colonization of 10^3 organisms or greater had associated sepsis. There was a gradient of colonization from the skin to the intravascular portion of the catheter.

3. Gram-positive organisms originating from other sites may seed the fibrin sleeve along the catheter. Consequently, in a patient with established gram-positive bacteremia, the catheter should be removed. Gram-negative organisms do not implant as readily, and antibiotic treatment may be sufficient to sterilize the catheter.

4. *Candida* seeds the bloodstream through the gut. Once *Candida* infection is established, all intravenous nutritional regimens must be stopped, because they all support *Candida* sepsis. Nutrition must be given enterally.

Management of the Patient with Suspected Catheter Sepsis. If one is carrying out serial quantitative cultures, a catheter with surrounding skin showing colonization of greater than 10^3 organisms per sq. cm. is removed. If quantitative cultures are less than 10^3, removal of a catheter rarely (<5% of the time) confirms catheter sepsis. In situations in which rigid protocols are not followed and quantitative cultures are not obtained, the following protocol is proposed: If a patient who was previously afebrile suddenly spikes a fever, the bottle should be taken down, the tubing and filter changed, and a new bottle suspended; the bottle and tubing should then be cultured. Blood cultures should be drawn, and a thorough search should be made of other possible sources of fever, such as pneumonia, intra-abdominal abscess, or urinary tract and wound infection. If the fever persists after an 8-hour period, the catheter should be removed and the tip cultured. Four of five catheters removed under these circumstances will be innocent and sources of sepsis ultimately found elsewhere. When a septic catheter is removed, it is not necessary to treat the patient with antibiotics unless the fever persists for longer than 24 hours. Catheters are not changed over guidewires when catheter infection is suspected, because the causative infected skin tract is still present. However, when another source is suspected, it is reasonable to change catheters over guidewires. When triple-lumen catheters are used, they should be changed every 72 hours over a guidewire to reduce infection, because the incidence of infection is higher.

Prevention of Catheter Complications

Catheter Placement. Catheter placement is never an emergency procedure and should be done only under proper conditions, with the patient well hydrated and lightly sedated and with adequate assistance. A subclavian approach is preferred: The patient is positioned with a roll between the shoulder blades, arms at the sides, head relaxed, and bed tilted at 15 degrees in the Trendelenburg position. The subclavian vein is the most anterior structure in the thorax (Fig. 9–7). On the left side, the subclavian catheter takes a more transverse arch as compared with the right (Fig. 9–8). Right-handed persons will find it easier to pass a left subclavian catheter. The patient is carefully prepped and draped, and the vein is located with a No. 22 needle through which lidocaine (Xylocaine) is infiltrated along the anticipated track, infiltrating the periosteum as well. The point of insertion is 1 cm. medial and 1 cm. caudad to the midpoint of the clavicle (Fig. 9–9). The needle is no more than 10 to 15 degrees to the horizontal and is aimed toward a point one fingerbreadth above the suprasternal notch. After the vein is located with the small needle, the larger needle is inserted; a pop will be felt. After blood is aspirated freely with a syringe, the patient

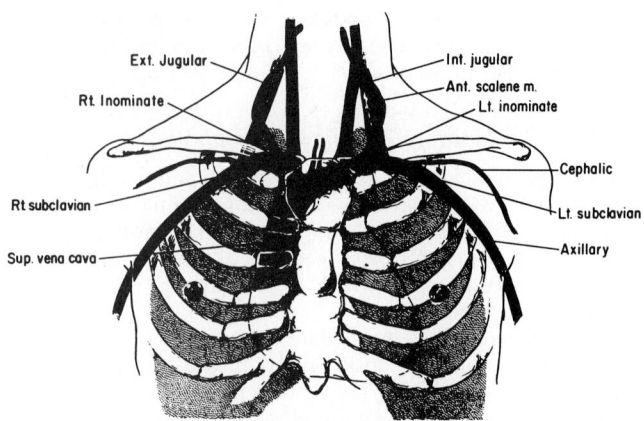

Figure 9–8. The venous anatomy of the thoracic inlet. Note the transverse position of the subclavian veins. The horizontal course of the subclavian vein is longer on the left than on the right. It is also easier for a right-handed person to cannulate the left subclavian vein. (From Fischer, J. E., and Freund, H. R.: Central hyperalimentation. *In* Fischer, J. E. [Ed.]: Surgical Nutrition. Boston, Little, Brown & Co, 1983, p. 696.)

is asked to do a Valsalva maneuver, the hub of the needle is tipped cephalad, and the guidewire is inserted with the patient still holding his or her breath. If the wire does not thread and is not easily withdrawn, both the needle and the wire should be withdrawn together to prevent the wire from shearing off. The catheter is inserted over the wire after the needle has been withdrawn and the tract dilated. The catheter is secured with a single 3-0 or 4-0 suture. After the dressing, tubing, and intravenous line have been hung, the bottle should be depressed to confirm backflow of blood through the catheter and a confirmatory chest x-ray is taken. For an internal jugular catheter, the operator uses a point 2 cm. above the clavicle at the posterior edge of the posterior belly of the sternocleidomastoid. The internal jugular vein may be approached by aiming the needle toward the suprasternal notch with a lifting motion immediately under and in the plane of the fissure of the sternocleidomastoid (Fig. 9–10). In the anterior approach, the internal jugular vein may

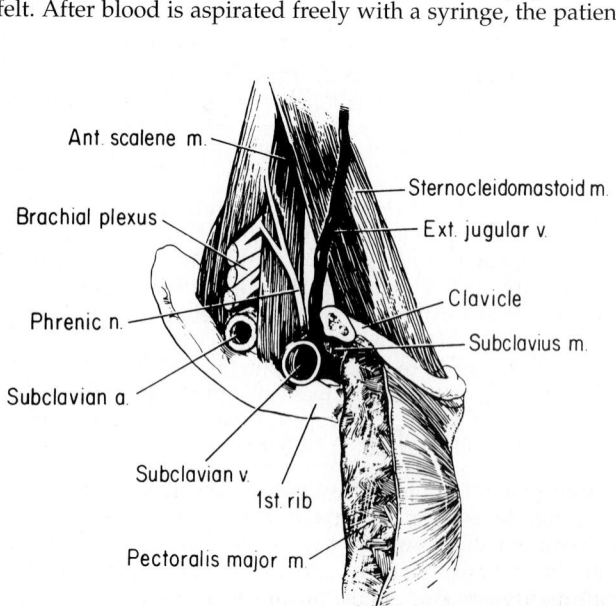

Figure 9–7. A section of the thoracic inlet through the area of the subclavian vein. Note that the subclavian vein is the most anterior structure in a thoracic inlet. (From Fischer, J. E., and Freund, H. R.: Central hyperalimentation. *In* Fischer, J. E. [Ed.]: Surgical Nutrition. Boston, Little, Brown & Co, 1983, p. 695.)

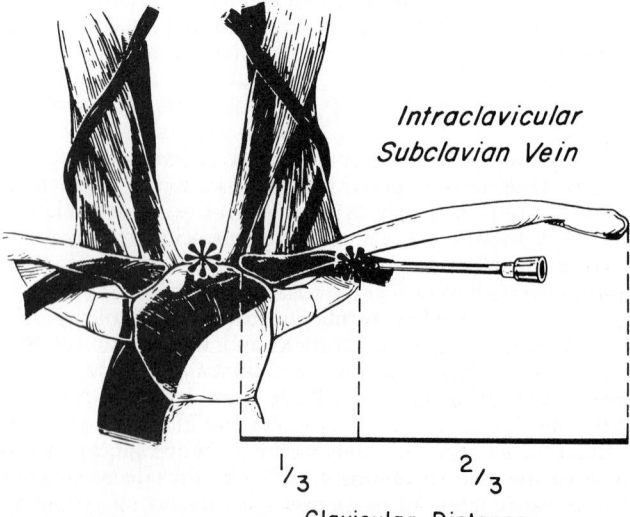

Figure 9–9. The position of the needle in cannulating the subclavian vein. Note that one approaches the subclavian vein through the medial third of the thoracic inlet, aiming for that portion of the subclavian vein behind the clavicle. (From Fischer, J. E., and Freund, H. R.: Central hyperalimentation. *In* Fischer, J. E. [Ed.]: Surgical Nutrition. Boston, Little, Brown & Co, 1983, p. 697.)

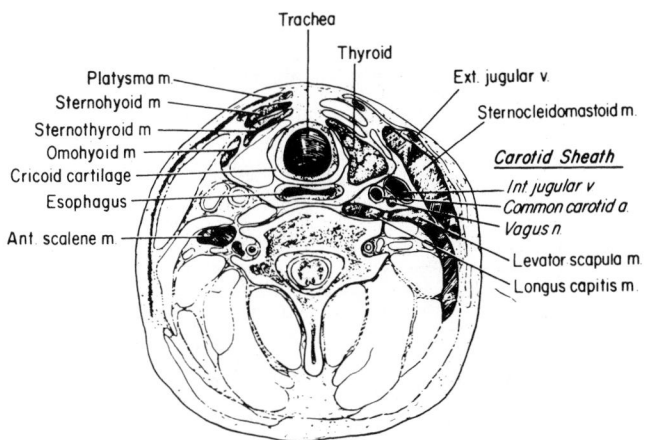

Figure 9–10. A cross-section of the neck at the level of insertion of an internal jugular catheter. Note that the internal jugular vein lies in relationship to the sternocleidomastoid muscles and is lateral to the common carotid artery. (From Fischer, J. E.: Nutritional support in the seriously ill patient. In Ravitch, M. M., and Steichen, F. M. [Eds.]: Current Problems in Surgery, Vol. XVII, No. 9, Sept. 1980, p. 515. Copyright © 1980 by Year Book Medical Publishers, Inc., Chicago.)

be entered at a point directly posterior where the external jugular vein crosses the sternoclavicular head.

Nutritional Support Teams and Protocols. Because of current budget constrictions, hospital administrators are resistant to a nutritional support team, which should include physicians, pharmacists, dietitians, and nurse clinicians for the supervision of parenteral nutritional support throughout the hospital. Rigid protocols must be established in catheter care, because clinical catheter sepsis may require from 2 to 6 weeks in the hospital and expensive intravenous antibiotics. If the infection rate is decreased from 10% to 2%, the nutritional support team is more than cost effective.

The pharmacy is responsible for the manufacture and quality control of solutions. This process is carried out in a clean room, using a laminar-flow hood. A variety of mechanisms may be utilized for safe ordering of parenteral nutrition. At the University of Cincinnati Medical Center, a multiple-copy order form (Figs. 9–11 and 9–12) is used—orders before 9:30 A.M. are promptly hung at 2 P.M. when staffing is most plentiful. A list of maximum allowable additives is given in Table 9–8. The protocol is placed in the patient's orders (Figs. 9–13 and 9–14).

Other Considerations

The Pediatric Patient Population. Requirements for pediatric patients differ from those for adults. Growth is more rapid. The distribution of viscera versus lean body mass is considerably different in an infant—an infant is all viscera in a skin envelope, with little fat or muscle. Enzyme systems are incompletely developed and excessive administration of certain amino acids may result in abnormally high concentrations of potentially toxic amino acids in the brain and perhaps other viscera. Surface area in the infant is proportionally greater, with little fat insulation, and heat loss is more of a problem.

Requirements for nutritional support in infants are given in Table 9–9. The requirement for protein is far in excess of that for adults and decreases progressively with age. Energy requirements are also greater than for adults but may be decreased by providing a thermoneutral environment. The amount of lipid that can safely be administered is approximately 4 gm. per kg. in the infant, whereas the upper normal limit in the adult is thought to be 2 gm. per kg. Whether this is due to proportionally larger amounts of viscera, the caloric requirements of which are largely met by fat, is unclear.

Vitamins and trace metals must be carefully administered because stores are limited; yet the opportunity for toxicity is greater. Access is a problem; the use of the umbilical artery or vein is mentioned only to be condemned, because catheter sepsis here is a disaster.

In certain catastrophes, such as meconium ileus, gastroschisis, and neonatal enterocolitis, the increased survival now seen is almost certainly the result of aggressive nutritional support as well as monitoring and perioperative care. The contribution of nutritional support to the survival of low-birth-weight babies is suggestive but unproven.

Home Hyperalimentation. Patients have been maintained in a functional state on parenteral nutrition for decades with minimal oral intake. Home hyperalimentation has now been standardized, using Silastic catheters with long subcutaneous tunnels or ports; these may be used only intermittently, provided they are regularly filled with heparin. Mean catheter life of a properly cared for catheter is now approaching 7 years. The Cincinnati experience with ports has not been as good, with sepsis more frequent, which is unfortunate because patients can swim with the ports. Home hyperalimentation is performed overnight, using sophisticated pumps with an impressive array of protective alarms.

Most patients requiring home parenteral nutrition have lost a large portion of the gastrointestinal tract, either by repeated resections for Crohn's disease or by massive small bowel resection after midgut volvulus and/or mesenteric thrombosis. Rare indications include sprue, pseudo-obstruction, chronic radiation enteritis, and scleroderma. Home hyperalimentation for patients with cancer is rarely indicated except for patients in whom leukemia has been successfully treated and who are on continued suppressive therapy or in patients on aggressive therapy in whom there is a reasonable chance for survival.

A Silastic catheter is placed either in open manner or percutaneously through an introducer. Whereas percutaneous placement is most popular, an axillary approach is favored, using a small branch of the axillary vein and a long tunnel onto the abdominal wall (Fig. 9–15). Although many patients no longer require parenteral nutrition after gut hypertrophy in the first 1 or 2 years, there will be a number of patients in whom several catheter sites will be required. It is logical to sacrifice as few of the large veins as necessary, because one may have to rotate catheters using the axilla and branches of the internal jugular vein over the years.

Patients with home hyperalimentation manifest a special series of complications. Deficiency states that are almost never seen in human nutrition, such as biotin deficiency (because of biotin's ubiquitous nature), may be seen in patients in whom the only nutrient supply is from the intravenous fluid administered. Catheter complications are largely those of sepsis. Thrombosis of the superior vena cava and subclavian vein is less often seen because of the inert nature of the Silastic catheter inserted. Infection of the catheter exit site is treated with antibiotics if the catheter tunnel is not severely infected.

The cost of home hyperalimentation is a source of consternation to most working in that field. Depending on the area of the country and the technique used, such costs may run anywhere from $30,000 to $60,000 per year. Clearly, patient function, rehabilitation, quality of life, and other considerations enter the cost-benefit ratio. Such patients are extremely well motivated, and almost all of them work and/or have returned to their premorbid situation.

Acquired Immunodeficiency Syndrome (AIDS). The place of home TPN in the treatment of patients with AIDS is controversial and probably dependent on the current debate

UNIVERSITY OF CINCINNATI HOSPITAL

PARENTERAL NUTRITION
<u>ORDER FORM</u>

Deadline for orders at 9:30 A.M.

Date: _____   Time: _____

UMC-375, 8/92

STEP 1:   SELECT BASE FORMULA:

Total Nutrient Admixture (TNA) contains: Fat emulsion, Dextrose, & Amino acids.
Non-TNA contains: Dextrose & Amino acids.

Standard Formula:		
	❏ TNA	❏ NON-TNA
Each Liter contains:		
Non-Protein Calorie: N	119	67
Total kcal/ml	1.1	0.71
Dextrose (15%)	150 gm	
Amino Acids (5%)	50 gm	
Fat Emulsion (4%)	40 gm (as TNA)	

MVI-12 (10 ml) & Trace elements-5 (3 ml) daily
Vit K   5 mg weekly

Standard Electrolytes (mEq/L)

Na	K	Ca	Mg	P(mM)	Cl	Acetate
30	18	4.5	5	10	37	55

High Dextrose Formula:		
	❏ TNA	❏ NON-TNA
Each Liter contains:		
Non-Protein Calorie: N	141	89
Total kcal/ml	1.3	0.88
Dextrose (20%)	200 gm	
Amino Acids (5%)	50 gm	
Fat Emulsion (4%)	40 gm (as TNA)	

MVI-12 (10 ml) & Trace elements-5 (3 ml) daily
Vit K   5 mg weekly

Standard Electrolytes (mEq/L)

Na	K	Ca	Mg	P(mM)	Cl	Acetate
30	18	4.5	5	10	37	55

STEP 2:   ORDER <u>TOTAL</u> ADDITIVES IF DIFFERENT FROM ABOVE:

Total Na _____ mEq/L   Other per Liter:

Total K _____ mEq/L   _____

Total Ca _____ mEq/L   _____

Total Mg_____ mEq/L   _____

Total Phos _____ mM/L   _____

Reg. Insulin _____ units/L   _____

MAXIMUM TOTAL CONC/LITER	
K+	80 mEq
Ca	9.4 mEq
Mg	12 mEq
Phos	15 mM
Ac	80 mEq

DAILY TRACE ELEMENTS	
Zn	3.0 mg
Cu	1.2 mg
Cr	12 mcg
Mn	0.3 mg
Se	60 mcg

STEP 3:   SELECT INFUSION RATE:

INFUSE AT _____ ml/hr or Cycle: _____ ml Total Volume

PHYSICIAN SIGNATURE _____   PAGER #: _____

WHITE—CHART   YELLOW—PHARMACY

Figure 9–11. Physician's order form for parenteral formulation used at the University of Cincinnati Medical Center. Carbon copies are collected by the pharmacy each morning and the orders are manufactured and delivered by 2 P.M. The variety of solutions minimizes the chance of error and enables one to handle almost any metabolic situation. Note that the various possible contents of each solution are given.

UNIVERSITY OF CINCINNATI HOSPITAL

SPECIALTY PARENTERAL
NUTRITION ORDER FORM

Deadline for orders at 9:30 A.M.

Date: _____ Time: _____

UMC-376, 7/92

STEP 1: SELECT BASE FORMULA:

Total Nutrient Admixture (TNA) contains: Fat emulsion, Dextrose, & Amino acids.
Non-TNA contains: Dextrose & Amino acids.

Hepatic Formula:

❑ TNA ❑ NON-TNA

Each Liter contains:

Non-Protein Calorie: N	208	142
Total kcal/ml	1.3	1.0
Dextrose (25%)	250 gm	
Amino Acids (4%)	40 gm	
Fat Emulsion (4%)	40 gm (as TNA)	

MVI-12 (10 ml) & Trace elements-5 (3 ml) daily
Vit K 5 mg weekly

Standard Electrolytes (mEq/L)

Na	K	Ca	Mg	P(mM)	Cl	Acetate
5	12	4.7	8	5	13.5	31

Renal Formula:

❑ NON-TNA (see step 4) *

Each Liter contains:

Non-Protein Calorie: N	794
Total kcal/ml	1.65
Dextrose (46.7%)	467 gm
Amino Acids (1.7%)	17 gm

MVI-12 (10 ml) & Trace elements-5 (3 ml) daily
Vit K 5 mg weekly

Standard Electrolytes (mEq/L)

Na	K	Ca	Mg	P(mM)	Cl	Acetate
2	0	0	0	0	1	14

Cardiac Formula:

❑ NON-TNA (see step 4) *

Each Liter contains:

Non-Protein Calorie: N	156
Total kcal/ml	1.4
Dextrose (35%)	350 gm
Amino Acid (5%)	50 gm

MVI-12 (10 ml) & Trace elements-5 (3 ml) daily
Vit K 5 mg weekly

Standard Electrolytes (mEq/L)

Na	K	Ca	Mg	P(mM)	Cl	Acetate
5	0	0	8	5	2	45

Peripheral Formula:

❑ TNA

Each Liter contains:

Non-Protein Calorie: N	104
Total kcal/ml	0.71
Dextrose (5%)	50 gm
Amino Acids (3.5%)	35 gm
Fat emulsion (4%)	40 gm

MVI-12 (10 ml) & Trace elements-5 (3 ml) daily
Vit K 5 mg weekly

Standard Electrolytes (mEq/L)

Na	K	Ca	Mg	P(mM)	Cl	Acetate
40	10	4.7	8	5	40	52

STEP 2: ORDER TOTAL ADDITIVES IF DIFFERENT FROM ABOVE:

Total Na _____ mEq/L   Other per Liter:

Total K _____ mEq/L   _____

Total Ca _____ mEq/L   _____

Total Mg _____ mEq/L   _____

Total Phos _____ mM/L   _____

Reg. Insulin _____ units/L   _____

MAXIMUM TOTAL CONC/LITER

K+	80 mEq
Ca	9.4 mEq
Mg	12 mEq
Phos	15 mM
Ac	80 mEq

DAILY TRACE ELEMENTS

Zn	3.0 mg
Cu	1.2 mg
Cr	12 mcg
Mn	0.3 mg
Se	60 mcg

STEP 3: SELECT INFUSION RATE:

Infuse Base Formula at _____ ml/hr

* STEP 4: SELECT IF NON-TNA FAT EMULSION DESIRED:

❑ 20% FAT EMULSION (250 ML) INFUSE OVER 10 HOURS.

PHYSICIAN SIGNATURE _____ PAGER #: _____

WHITE—CHART   YELLOW—PHARMACY

Figure 9–12. Physician's order form for specialty parenteral formulations used at the University of Cincinnati Medical Center.

TABLE 9–8. Allowable Additive Supplementation (at University of Cincinnati Hospital)

Additives	Available Products (Injection)	Maximum Allowable Total Per Liter
Calcium	Calcium gluconate Calcium chloride	9 mEq.
Magnesium	Magnesium sulfate	12 mEq.
Phosphate	Sodium phosphate Potassium phosphate	15 mmol.
Potassium	Potassium chloride Potassium acetate	80 mEq.
Sodium	Sodium chloride Sodium acetate	Patient tolerance and/or need
Chloride	Sodium chloride Calcium chloride Potassium chloride	Limited by amount of cation
Acetate	Sodium acetate Potassium acetate	Limited by amount of cation
Insulin	Regular insulin	100 units (in conjunction with fingerstick blood sugars)

Some Points to Remember:
1. Bicarbonate salts must not be added to parenteral nutrition formulations since they create a number of incompatibilities and are ineffective given in this manner.
2. Medicinal agents not mentioned must not be admixed or administered with parenteral nutrition formulations unless compatibility data are available.
3. Phosphate supplementation must be ordered in terms of millimoles (mmol.) of phosphate. Please note that phosphate is available only as the sodium or potassium salt and that when the potassium salt is used for "added" phosphate it must not exceed the maximum allowable concentration of potassium (i.e., 80 mEq.).

on the proper locale for treatment. The author is not an expert in this area but understands from infectious disease authorities that it is appropriate to treat AIDS patients in an acute hospital setting for the first infection; thereafter, the issue becomes uncertain.

Advances in Nutritional Pharmacology. Nutritional pharmacology is a term that emphasizes the use of nutritional support to change either the milieu or the pathophysiology of a disease process to affect outcome. Early examples include the application of essential amino acids to patients in acute renal failure, and the modified amino acid mixtures for the treatment of patients with acute hepatic failure superimposed on cirrhosis. Areas of nutritional pharmacology under investigation include the use of specific nutrients to enhance host defenses.

Glutamine and Ketone Bodies. These have been discussed previously.

Arginine. A deficiency of arginine and the dibasic amino acids in the plasma of patients with overwhelming sepsis was observed as early as 1978.[13] Although arginine was thought to be a nonessential amino acid, it is now recognized that the ability to synthesize arginine in the presence of increased requirements may be exceeded; and it probably is semiessential. Arginine is used not only by the host but apparently by macrophages, lymphocytes, and perhaps other cells in healing wounds. Arginine-supplemented diets are utilized in patients with burns as a new enteral formula and may also be useful in trauma. Arginine enhances the responsiveness of T lymphocytes to mitogenic stimulation. There has also been interest in the use of the response of the T lymphocytes to arginine in patients with cancer. In a controlled study, arginine in an enteral diet was administered to 30 cancer patients; the controls received an L-glycine–supplemented, isonitrogenous enteral diet.[9] Whereas nitrogen accumulation was no different between the two groups, the beneficial effect of arginine on T-lymphocyte response to

TABLE 9–9. Nutritional Requirements in Infants

Protein (gm./kg./day)	Newborn to 6 months 2.5–3	6–12 months 2.0–2.5	School age 1.75	Adolescent 1.2	kcal./Nitrogen 150:1
Calories (kcal./kg./day)	Newborn or premature 120	Infant (to 10 kg.) 100	10–20 kg. 100 + 50	Over 20 kg. 100 + 50 + 20	
Fat	? 35% of calories (up to 3.5 gm./kg./day)				

Electrolytes (mEq./kg./day)		Trace Elements (per day)		Vitamins (per day)	
Na$^+$	24	Term Infants		A	700 mg.
K$^+$	1–2	(assuming 1200 kg./day fluid intake)		C	80 mg.
Urine Na$^+$:K$^+$	>1.0 adequate	Ca^{2+}	500–600 mg./L.	D	400 IU
		Mg^{2+}	50–70 mg./L.	B$_1$	1.2 mg.
		P	400–450 mg./L.	B$_2$	1.4 mg.
		Zn	800 gm./L.	B$_6$	1.0 mg.
		Cu	100 gm./L.	E	7 IU
		Children >1 year		Niacin	17 mg
		Ca^{2+}	200–400 mg./L.	Dexpanthenol	5 mg.
		Mg^{2+}	20–40 mg./L.	Folic acid	140 μg.
		P	150–300 mg./L.	B$_{12}$	1 μg.
				K	200 μg.

UNIVERSITY OF CINCINNATI HOSPITAL

PHYSICIAN'S CHECKLIST/ORDER SHEET

All applicable orders have been checked. A line has been placed through orders that have been voided. ORDERS NOT CHECKED ARE NOT TO BE FOLLOWED. Orders have been modified according to the medical condition of the patient. These orders have been dated, timed and signed by a physician. As an order is filled, the individual doing so must date/time and initial in the space provided. Further orders will be added as needed.

UMC-396, Rev. 6/94

❑ None Known

ALLERGIES: ❑ Yes, Drug/Reaction:_____

PAGE ___1___ OF ___1___

ORDER NUMBER	✔	ENTERAL NUTRITION (EN) STANDING ORDERS	ORDER NOTED (DATE/TIME)	(INITIAL)
1.	√	Obtain confirmation of appropriate position of feeding tube prior to initiating EN.		
2.	√	Elevate head of bed at least 30° during feeding.		
3.	√	Check residuals q4h for continuous feeding and prior to each intermittent feeding. If residuals are ≥ twice the infusion rate or ≥ 1/2 the volume of intermittent feedings, stop the feeding and notify the physician.		
4.	√	Irrigate tube with 60 ml tap H_2O q4h and prn.		
5.	√	Administer continuous feeding with an enteral pump.		
6.	√	Hang time = 24h for closed system and 8h for all others.		
7.	√	Change administration sets q24h.		
8.	√	Vital signs q8h. I & O q8h.		
9.	√	Finger stick or serum glucose b.i.d. x 3 days unless patient is diabetic, then FSBS q _____. Call MD for >250 mg/dl.		
10.	√	Measure initial height and weight. Record weight q Monday, Wednesday, Friday.		
11.	√	Avoid use of small bore feeding tube (<10Fr) for any medications; however, if medication must be given, use only liquid form.		
12.	√	Irrigate tube before and after medications with 20ml tap H_2O.		
13.	√	Laboratory studies (Use low volume tubes when possible). Prior to starting EN		
		Renal (4203) Retinol Binding Protein (4707)		
		Bone (4041) Magnesium (4229)		
		Hepatic (4162) Magnesium (4229)		
		Transferrin (4706) (See, also, Nursing Procedures)		

White–Chart Yellow–UD Copy
Pink–IV Copy Goldenrod–Floor Copy

Physician signature _____

Date _____ Time _____

Developed by __Robert H. Bower, M.D.__ Date ___5/94___ Review Date ___6/95___

Figure 9–13. Standard enteral nutrition orders at the University of Cincinnati Medical Center.

UNIVERSITY OF CINCINNATI HOSPITAL

PHYSICIAN'S CHECKLIST/ORDER SHEET

All applicable orders have been checked. A line has been placed through orders that have been voided. ORDERS NOT CHECKED ARE NOT TO BE FOLLOWED. Orders have been modified according to the medical condition of the patient. These orders have been dated, timed and signed by a physician. As an order is filled, the individual doing so must date/time and initial in the space provided. Further orders will be added as needed.

UMC-374, Rev. 6/94

❑ None Known

ALLERGIES: ❑ Yes, Drug/Reaction:_____

PAGE ___1___ OF ___1___

ORDER NUMBER	✔	PARENTERAL NUTRITION (PN) STANDING ORDERS	ORDER NOTED (DATE/TIME)	(INITIAL)
1.	√	Obtain confirmation of appropriate position of central venous access device prior to initiating PN.		
2.	√	Initial and subsequent dressings per nursing procedure.		
3.	√	Phlebotomy by peripheral venipuncture unless peripheral access is exhausted.		
4.	√	Vital signs q8h.		
5.	√	I & O q8h.		
6.	√	Measure initial height and weight. Record weight q Monday, Wednesday, Friday.		
7.	√	If PN is temporarily interrupted, infuse $D_{10}W$ at PN infusion rate.		
8.	√	Do not infuse IVPB into PN.		
9.	√	Finger stick or serum glucose b.i.d. x 3 days unless patient is diabetic, then FSBS q _____. Call MD for >250 mg/dl.		
10.	√	Laboratory studies (use low volume tubes when possible).		
		PRIOR TO STARTING PN EVERY MONDAY EVERY THURSDAY		
		Renal (4203) Renal (4203) Renal (4203)		
		Bone (4041) Bone (4041) Bone (4041)		
		Hepatic (4162) Hepatic (4162)		
		Transferrin (4706) Transferrin (4706)		
		Retinol Binding Retinol Binding		
		Protein (4707) Protein (4707)		
		Magnesium (4229) Magnesium (4229)		
		CBC (4032) CBC (4032)		
		Triglyceride (4726)		
		Prothrombin Time (4204)		
		(See, also, Nursing Procedures)		

White–Chart Yellow–UD Copy
Pink–IV Copy Goldenrod–Floor Copy

Physician signature _____

Date _____ Time _____

Developed by ___Robert H. Bower, M.D.___   Date _____5/94_____   Review Date _____6/95_____

Figure 9–14. Standard parenteral nutrition orders at the University of Cincinnati Medical Center.

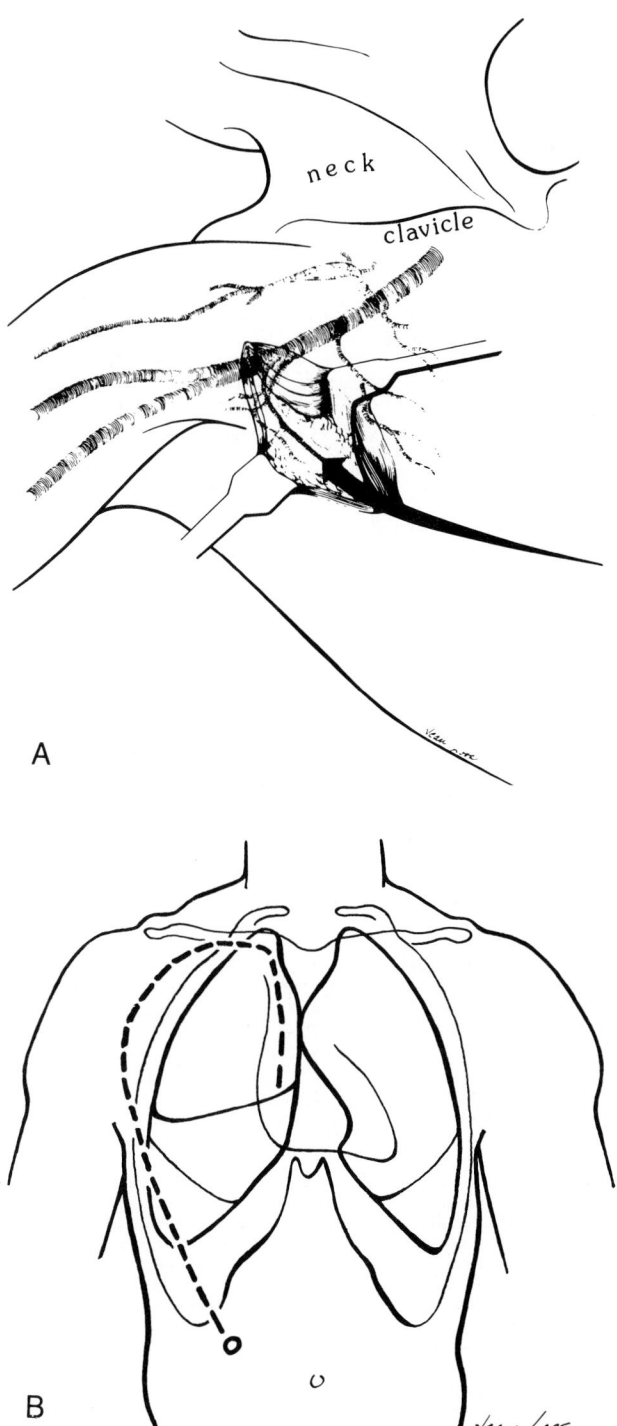

Figure 9–15. *A,* Open axillary approach to placement of long-term indwelling catheter. The incision is posterior and parallel to the pectoralis major and is hidden (an important consideration in females). A branch of the axillary vein is cannulated under direct vision. This approach is especially useful in patients with bleeding tendencies. *B,* Hickman catheter in place, with tip in right atrium and exit site over right upper quadrant of the abdomen. (From Freund, H. R., Benson, D. W., Bower, R. H., and Fischer, J. E.: Enteral and parenteral nutrition. *In* Moody, F. G., Carey, L. C., Jones, R. S., Kelly, K. A., Nahrwold, D. L., and Skinner, D. B. [Eds.]: Surgical Treatment of Digestive Disease, 2nd ed. Chicago, Year Book Medical Publishers, 1990, p. 864.)

concanavalin A was verified, but it was also associated with increased helper T-cell activity. There was an increased T-cell proliferation to both concanavalin A and phytohemagglutinin in the arginine-supplemented patients. Although the

dietary supplements in the study published by Daly and colleagues[9] was not isonitrogenous, the nationwide trial published by Bower and co-workers[4] addressed this issue. Patients fed with the alternate diet had a shorter postoperative stay and fewer infectious complications; and if complications did develop, the patients survived them more easily.

Alterations in Lipid Profile and Their Possible Effects on the Inflammatory Response. Arachidonic acid is the substrate for the synthesis of prostaglandins, thromboxanes, and leukotrienes through lipoxygenase-mediated pathways. Although the evidence that prostaglandins contribute to proteolysis and catabolism in sepsis has been challenged, the prostaglandins may have a role in transplantation rejection. Studies in patients with burns using a fish oil derivative as a lipid source, instead of arachidonic acid, suggest that the inflammatory response is modified. In transplantation immunology, substitution of a fish oil lipid source together with cyclosporine and pretransplantation transfusion results in indefinite survival of transplanted rat hearts. These exciting developments suggest that in patients with inflammatory disease and in patients about to undergo transplantation, dietary manipulation by substitution of the lipid source may result in improvement in outcome. One word of caution: When one modifies essential responses, timing may be very important; it is conceivable that with improper timing, as with all immunomodulation, harm may result as well.

As surgeons become more facile biochemically and continue to investigate the basis for some of the pathophysiologic responses in sepsis and injury, the ability to modify the milieu will yield enormous dividends to patients in various disease states.

SUMMARY

Nutritional support has been available for approximately two decades. It has proved its value as one of the most important therapeutic modalities in this century and perhaps in the history of medicine. It is still in its infancy. A new phase of nutritional support is emerging. As investigators who are equally familiar with the operating room and biochemistry, physiology, and immunology laboratories have been trained, the basic mechanisms and pathophysiology of disease at even molecular levels are being elucidated. Advances in nutritional pharmacology are due to various investigators, but largely surgeons, elucidating disease states. Only the surface of the ability to modify the internal milieu of patients, the response to cytokines, or the pathophysiologic and biochemical mechanisms in diseases has been scratched. The next several decades should prove very exciting, and nutritional support and especially advances in nutritional pharmacology will contribute to improvements in outcome in disease states that are today the cause of significant mortality in patients. As the knowledge of nutrition, biochemistry and pathophysiology becomes more sophisticated, it is only natural that the route of physiologic entry for nutrients—the gut—becomes more of a focus for administration of nutrients. The gut has been a major focus of nutritional support over the past decade, and this is likely to continue.

SELECTED REFERENCES

Articles

Abel, R. M., Beck C. H., Jr., Abbott, W. M., Ryan, J. A., Barnett, G. O., and Fischer, J. E.: Improved survival from acute renal failure after treatment with intravenous essential L-amino acids and glucose: Results of a prospective, double-blind study. N. Engl. J. Med., 288:695, 1973.
An early, randomized, double-blinded trial showed improved survival after the application of techniques of parenteral nutrition and a specialized solution to patients with renal failure. The eight essential L-amino acids in hypertonic dextrose were administered to patients with renal failure and compared with a group

receiving isocaloric hypertonic dextrose alone. Improved survival and perhaps early healing of the renal lesion were seen. At present, because dialysis techniques are more widely used, there is controversy as to what solution should be used in patients with renal failure: essential amino acids alone or a low dose of a standard solution. This article, however, represents an excellent early effort in defining needs of patients with specialized disease states.

Askanazi, J., Rosenbaum, S. H., Hyman, A. I., Silverberg, P. A., Milic-Emili, J., and Kinney, J. M.: Respiratory changes induced by the large glucose loads of total parenteral nutrition. JAMA, 243:1444, 1980.
In this paper, the effects of glucose in generating excess CO_2, particularly in patients with sepsis, is described. Although one should be aware of this phenomenon, which has been given wide publicity, it occurs largely in patients who are septic and whose glucose loads are increased suddenly and dramatically, as in this study. Nonetheless, in patients with marginal pulmonary reserve who have difficulty weaning from the ventilator because of carbon dioxide retention, decreasing the glucose load and substitution of fat calories will sometimes enable successful weaning. If possible, CO_2 production should be measured.

Clowes, G. H. A., George, B. C., Villee, C. A., and Saravis, C. A.: Muscle proteolysis induced by a circulating peptide in patients with sepsis or trauma. N. Engl. J. Med., 308:545, 1983.
Few papers have inspired as much interest and excitement as this description of a 4200-dalton protein isolated in the plasma of patients with sepsis. This hypothetical cytokine, PIF, increased hepatic protein synthesis and muscle breakdown. Subsequent experiments have revealed that the particular conditions used in these experiments may have contributed to these findings. Nonetheless, this paper probably contributed more to the research in surgery of cytokines than any other paper, exciting a great deal of work over the subsequent years.

Cuthbertson, D. P.: Observations on the disturbance of metabolism produced by injury to the limbs. Q. J. Med., 1:233, 1932.
This study may well have begun contemporary nutritional support. This classic description of loss of nitrogen and breakdown of lean body mass after injury is a careful study in a classic tradition.

Dominioni, L., Trocki, O., Mochizuki, H., Fang, C. H., and Alexander, J. W.: Prevention of severe postburn hypermetabolism and catabolism by immediate intragastric feeding. J. Burn Care Rehabil., 5:106, 1984.
The first demonstration that changes in gut flora and the translocation of bacteria or absorption of bacterial products after thinning of mucosa in burns contributes to the hypermetabolism is presented. With the confirmation of similar results in patients with burns, it is clear that this hypothesis with respect to gut products is operant in patients as well.

Dudrick, S. J., Wilmore, D. W., Vars, H. M., and Rhoads, J. E.: Long-term total parenteral nutrition with growth, development, and positive nitrogen balance. Surgery, 64:134, 1968.
This is one of the classic papers originally describing high-glucose central total parenteral nutrition from which stems the current popularity of parenteral nutrition in the United States. In this ambitious project, the biochemical requirements for growth in puppies were investigated with astounding results: normal growth comparable to puppies eating ad lib. could be achieved without any oral intake, provided that one infused the necessary nutrients by vein.

Fischer, J. E., Rosen, H. M., Ebeid, A. M., James, J. H., Keane, J. M., and Soeters, P. B.: The effect of normalization of plasma amino acids on hepatic encephalopathy in man. Surgery, 80:77, 1976.
An approach to liver disease and the intolerance to protein in patients with hepatic encephalopathy is described. This study represents the culmination of a hypothesis of hepatic encephalopathy, depending on altered plasma amino acid patterns, changes subsequently discovered to be amplified by changes in the blood-brain barrier secondary to disturbed metabolism in liver disease. It represents an early anecdotal attempt to enable patients with severe hepatic deficiency to receive adequate nutrition at the same time as awakening from hepatic encephalopathy while receiving increased protein equivalent in the form of a branched chain–enriched (to 36%) amino acid solution now commercially available as HepatAmine.

Ryan, J. A., Jr., Abel, R. M., Abbott, W. M., Hopkins, C. C., Chesney, T., Colley, R., Phillips, K., and Fischer, J. E.: Catheter complications in total parenteral nutrition: A prospective study of 200 consecutive patients. N. Engl. J. Med., 290:757, 1974.
A study of the complications of parenteral nutrition was done in a large hospital with one of the first centralized nutritional support teams. This study confirmed that rigid asepsis in the care of catheters and minimizing catheter manipulation were the most important factors in preventing line catheter sepsis.

Wilmore, D. W., and Dudrick, S. J.: Treatment of acute renal failure with intravenous essential L-amino acids. Arch. Surg., 99:669, 1969.
This study represents the earliest approach to disease-specific parenteral nutrition. The principle of attempting to define the metabolic abnormalities in a given patient and infusing an appropriate nutritional substrate was first proposed in this study. The intravenous equivalent of a Giordano-Giovanetti diet, containing only the eight L-essential amino acids—a high biologic value oral diet—was used.

Books

Fischer, J. E. (Ed.): Total Parenteral Nutrition, 2nd ed. Boston, Little, Brown & Co., 1991.

This book represents an attempt to standardize the practical approach to total parenteral nutrition. It is still current.

Fischer, J. E. (Ed.): Nutrition and Metabolism in Surgical Patients. Boston, Little, Brown & Co., 1996.
An attempt to collate basic science knowledge and practical knowledge is presented in one volume. The various chapters also address efficacy of parenteral nutrition.

Grant, J. P. (Ed.): Handbook of Total Parenteral Nutrition. Philadelphia, W. B. Saunders, 1980.
This short version is an attempt to detail knowledge in the area of parenteral nutrition. The bibliography is particularly exhaustive and very useful. A second edition is being prepared.

Greep, J. M., Soeters, P. B., Wesdorp, R. I. C., Phaf, C. W. R., and Fischer, J. E. (Eds.): Current Concepts in Parenteral Nutrition. The Hague, Martinus Nihjoff Medical Division, 1977.
Of historic interest, the meeting was held at a time when there were many controversies in parenteral nutrition, and many authorities were present. The discussion, which is published in its entirety, is of particular interest.

Rombeau, J. L., and Caldwell, M. D. (Eds.): Clinical Nutrition, 2nd ed. Vol. 1 (1990), Enteral and Tube Nutrition and Vol. 2 (1993), Parenteral Nutrition. Philadelphia, W. B. Saunders, 1993.
This is the most recent large textbook on enteral and parenteral nutrition. It is well done and has been updated. There are a large number of specialized chapters.

Wilmore, W. W. (Ed.): The Metabolic Management of the Critically Ill. New York, Plenum Press, 1977.
This excellent summary goes into great detail in certain metabolic areas, particularly in critically ill patients. Although much of the basic science components have subsequently been enlarged upon, it is still of benefit.

REFERENCES

1. Alexander, J. W., MacMillan, B. G., Stinnett, J. D., Ogle, C. K., Bozian, R. C., Fischer, J. E., Oakes, J. B., Morris, M. J., and Krummel, R.: Beneficial effects of aggressive protein feeding in severely burned children. Ann. Surg., 192:505, 1980.
2. Baue, A. E.: Nutrition and metabolism in sepsis and multisystem organ failure. Surg. Clin. North Am., 71:549, 1991.
3. Billiar, T. R., and Simmons, R. L.: Arginine and nitric oxide. In Fischer, J.E. (Ed.): Surgical Nutrition, 2nd ed. Boston, Little, Brown & Co., 1996.
4. Bower, R. H., Cerra, F. B., Bershadsky, B., Licari, J. J., Hoyt, D. B., Jensen, G. L., van Buren, C. T., Rothkopf, M. M., Daly, J. M., and Adelsberg, B. R.: Early enteral administration of a formula (Impact®) supplemented with arginine, nucleotides and fish oil in intensive care unit patients: Results of a randomized prospective clinical trial. Crit. Care Med., 23:436, 1995.
5. Buzby, G. P. (Veterans Affairs Total Parenteral Nutrition Cooperative Study Group): Perioperative total parenteral nutrition in surgical patients. N. Engl. J. Med., 325:525, 1991.
6. Chance, W. T., Cao, L., Zhang, F. S., Foley-Nelson, T., and Fischer, J. E.: Clenbuterol treatment increases muscle mass and protein content of tumor-bearing rats maintained on total parenteral nutrition. J. Parenter. Enter. Nutr., 15:530, 1991.
7. Chance, W. T., Balasubramaniam, A., and Fischer, J. E.: Neuropeptide Y and the development of cancer anorexia. Ann. Surg., 221:579, 1995.
8. Culebras, J. M. (EUROPAN: Concerted Action on the Effect of Hypocaloric Peripheral Parenteral Nutrition in Surgical Patients): The effect of hypocaloric peripheral parenteral nutrition in surgical patients. In Baya, C. (Ed.): Advances in Medical Biology. Leon, Spain, Commission of the European Communities, 1994, pp. 216–232.
9. Daly, J. M., Reynolds, J., Thom, A., Kinsley, L., Dietrick-Gallagher, M., Shou, J., and Ruggieri, B.: Immune and metabolic effects of arginine in the surgical patient. Ann. Surg., 208:512, 1988.
10. Detsky, A. S., Baker, J. P., O'Rourke, K., and Goel, V.: Perioperative parenteral nutrition: A meta-analysis. Ann. Intern. Med., 107:195, 1987.
11. Fan, S. T., Lo, C. M., Lai, E. C. S., Chu, K. M., Liu, C. L., and Wong, J.: Perioperative nutritional support in patients undergoing hepatectomy for hepatocellular carcinoma. N. Engl. J. Med., 331:547, 1994.
12. Fang, C. H., Tiao, G., James, J. H., Ogle, C., Fischer, J. E., and Hasselgren, P. O.: Burn injury stimulates multiple proteolytic pathways in skeletal muscle, including the ubiquitin-energy-dependent pathway. J. Am. Coll. Surg., 180:161, 1995.
13. Galandiuk, S., O'Neill, M., McDonald, P., Fazio, V., and Steiger, E.: A century of home parenteral nutrition for Crohn's disease. Am. J. Surg., 159:540, 1990.
14. Gennari, R., Alexander, J. W., Gianotti, L., Eaves-Pyles, T., and Hartmann, S.: Granulocyte macrophage colony-stimulating factor improves survival in two models of gut-derived sepsis by improving gut barrier function and modulating bacterial clearance. Ann. Surg., 56:530, 1994.
15. Hasselgren, P. O., James, J. H., Benson, D. W., Li, S., and Fischer, J. E.: Is there a circulating proteolysis inducing factor (PIF) during sepsis? Arch. Surg., 125:510, 1990.
16. Hershko, A., and Ciechanover, A.: The ubiquitin system for protein degradation. Ann. Rev. Biochem., 61:761, 1992.
17. Jenkins, M., Gottschlich, M., Alexander, J. W., and Warden, G. D.: Effect of

immediate enteral feeding on the hypermetabolic response following severe burn injury. J. Parenter. Enter. Nutr., *13*(Suppl. l):12s, 1989.

18. Kudsk, K. A., Croce, M. A., Fabian, T. C., Minard, G., Tolley, E. A., Poret, H. A., Kuhl, M. R., and Brown, R. O.: Enteral versus parenteral feeding: Effects on septic morbidity after blunt and penetrating abdominal trauma. Ann. Surg., *215*:503, 1992.

19. Li, S., Nussbaum, M. S., McFadden, D. W., Zhang, F. S., LaFrance, R. J., Dayal, R., and Fischer, J. E.: Addition of L-glutamine to total parenteral nutrition (TPN) and its effects on portal insulin and glucagon and the development of hepatic steatosis in rats. J. Surg. Res., *48*:421, 1990.

20. Mayer, R. J., Arnold, J., Laszlo, L., Landon, M., and Lowe, J.: Ubiquitin in health and disease. Biochim. Biophys. Acta, *1089*:141, 1991.

21. Mester, M., Tompkins, R. G., Gelfand, J. A., Dinarello, C. A., Burke, J. F., and Clark, B. D.: Intestinal production of interleukin-1α during endotoxemia in the mouse. J. Surg. Res., *54*:584, 1993.

22. Meyer, T. A., Noguchi, Y., Ogle, C. K., Tiao, G., Wang, J. J., Fischer, J. E., and Hasselgren, P.O.: Endotoxin stimulates IL-6 production in intestinal epithelial cells: A synergistic effect with PGE$_2$. Arch. Surg., *129*:1290, 1994.

23. Meyer, T. A., Tiao, G. M., James, J. H., Noguchi, Y., Ogle, C. K., Fischer, J. E., and Hasselgren, P.O.: Nitric oxide inhibits LPS-induced IL-6 production in enterocytes. J. Surg. Res., *58*:570, 1995.

24. Moore, F. A., Feliciano, D. V., Andrassy, R. J., McArdle, A. H., Booth, F. V., Morgenstein-Wagner, T. B., Kellum, J. M., Jr., Welling, R. E., and Moore, E. E.: Early enteral feeding, compared with parenteral, reduces postoperative septic complications: The results of a meta-analysis. Ann. Surg., *216*:172, 1992.

25. Morris, S. M., Jr., and Billiar, T. R.: New insights into the regulation of inducible nitric oxide synthesis. Am. J. Physiol., *266*:E829, 1994.

26. Nathens, A. B., Ding, J. W., Marshall, J. C., Ribeiro, M., and Rotstein, O. D.: The gut as a cytokine generating organ: Small bowel TNF-α production during systemic endotoxemia (Abstract). Presented at the Surgical Infection Society, 14th Annual Meeting, Toronto, April 1994.

27. Naylor, C. D., O'Rourke, K., Detsky, A. S., and Baker, J. P.: Parenteral nutrition with branched-chain amino acids in hepatic encephalopathy: A meta-analysis. Gastroenterology, *97*:1033, 1989.

28. Rex, J. H., Bennett, J. E., Sugar, A. M., Pappas, P. G., van der Horst, C. M., Edwards, J. E., Washburn, R. G., Schield, W. M., Karchmer, A. W., Dine, A. P., Levenstein, M. J., and Webb, C. D.: A randomized trial comparing fluconazole with amphotericin B for the treatment of candidemia in patients without neutropenia. N. Engl. J. Med., *331*:1325, 1994.

29. Roediger, W. E. W.: The place of SCFAs in colonocyte metabolism in health

and ulcerative colitis: The impaired colonocyte barrier. *In* Cummings, J. H., Sakata, T., and Rombeau, J. L. (Eds.): Physiologic and Clinical Aspects of Short-Chain Fatty Acids. Cambridge, England, Cambridge University Press, 1993.

30. Rombeau, J. L., and Lew, J. I.: Intestinal fuels: Implications for improvement of intestinal growth and function. *In* Fischer, J.E. (Ed.): Surgical Nutrition, 2nd ed. Boston, Little, Brown & Co., 1996.

31. Shiloni, E., Coronado, E., and Freund, H. R.: The role of total parenteral nutrition in the treatment of Crohn's disease. Am. J. Surg., *157*:180, 1989.

32. Souba, W. W: Glutamine: Physiology, Biochemistry and Nutrition in Critical Illness. Austin, R. G. Landes Co., 1992.

33. Stoffel, M., Froguel, P., Takeda, J., Zouali, H., Vionnet, N., Nishi, S., Weber, I. T., Harrison, R. W., Pilkis, S. J., Lesage, S., Vaxillaire, M., Velho, G., Sun, F., Iris, F., Passa, P., Cohen, D., and Bell, G. I.: Human glucokinase gene: Isolation, characterization, and identification of two missense mutations linked to early-onset non-insulin-dependent (type 2) diabetes mellitus. Proc. Natl. Acad. Sci. USA, *89*:7698, 1992.

34. Tiao, G. M., Fagan, J. M., Samuels, N., James, J. H., Hudson, K., Lieberman, M., Fischer, J. E., and Hasselgren, P. O.: Sepsis stimulates non-lysosomal, energy-dependent proteolysis and increases ubiquitin mRNA levels in rat skeletal muscle. J. Clin. Invest., *94*:2255, 1994.

35. Tredgett, E. E., and Yu, Y. M.: The metabolic effects of thermal injury. World J. Surg., *16*:68, 1992.

36. Vionnet, N., Stoffel, M., Takeda, J., Yasuda, K., Bell, G. I., Zouali, H., Lesage, S., Velho, G., Iris, F., Passa, P., Froguel, P., and Cohen, D.: Nonsense mutation in the glucokinase gene causes early-onset non-insulin-dependent diabetes mellitus. Nature *356*:721, 1992.

37. von Allmen, D., Hasselgren, P. O., and Fischer, J. E.: Hepatic protein synthesis in a modified septic rat model. J. Surg. Res., *48*:476, 1990.

38. Warner, B. W., Hasselgren, P. O., James, J. H., Hummel, R. P. III, Rigel, D. F., and Fischer, J. E.: Reduced amino acid transport in skeletal muscle caused by a circulating factor during endotoxemia. Ann. Surg., *211*:323, 1990.

39. Waxman, K., Day, A. T., Stellin, G. P., Tominaga, G. T., Gazzaniga, A. B., and Bradford, R. R.: Safety and efficacy of glycerol and amino acids in combination with lipid emulsion for peripheral parenteral nutrition support. J. Parenter. Enter. Nutr., *16*:374, 1992.

40. Ziegler, T. R., Young, L. S., Benfall, K., Scheltinga, M., Hortos, K., Bye, R., Morrow, F. D., Jacobs, D. O., Smith, R. J., Antin, J. H., and Wilmore, D. W.: Clinical and metabolic efficacy of glutamine-supplemented parenteral nutrition after bone marrow transplantation: A randomized, double-blind, controlled study. Ann. Intern. Med., *116*:821, 1992.

CHAPTER 10

SURGICAL ASPECTS OF DIABETES MELLITUS

Olga Jonasson, M.D.

Diabetes mellitus is a disorder of carbohydrate metabolism that causes hyperglycemia. The consequences of diabetes derive from elevated levels of blood glucose and a deficiency in insulin. More than 10% of the population of the United States has intolerance to glucose, with abnormally elevated blood glucose levels after ingestion of a meal or of a glucose challenge, and progression to clinical diabetes occurs in more than 7% of the general population. The direct costs for care of diabetic patients in 1992 exceeded $45 billion.[20]

PATHOPHYSIOLOGY

Insulin is normally produced in the beta cells of pancreatic islets. A single-chain peptide, proinsulin, is packaged into granules (together with other peptides) where it is cleaved into equimolar amounts of insulin and a connecting peptide (C peptide). When it is necessary to measure insulin production in patients receiving exogenous insulin, it is advisable to measure the C peptide molecule because both endogenous and exogenous insulin will be measured in an insulin assay.

On sensing an increase in blood glucose, insulin stored in beta cell granules is released in a burst, followed by a second phase of synthesis and secretion. Insulin secretion is pulsatile, even when islets are isolated from excised pancreatic tissue; the periodicity of secretions, about every 10 minutes, is regulated by a pacemaker within the beta cell.[24] Oral glucose stimulates insulin production to a greater degree than intravenous glucose, probably by release of enteric hormones. Amino acids and free fatty acids also stimulate secretion of insulin, as does glucagon. Somatostatin inhibits insulin secretion. Cholinergic alpha fibers inhibit insulin secretion whereas beta fibers stimulate insulin secretion; after transplantation of the pancreas with the customary systemic venous drainage, the denervated response is changed such that peripheral hyperinsulinism, if found, is possibly due to systemic venous drainage of the transplant as well as the denervated state.[10]

Insulin lowers blood glucose levels by inhibiting hepatic glucose production (glycogenolysis and gluconeogenesis) as well as stimulating glucose use in skeletal muscle and other tissues by increasing blood flow and glucose extraction and by promoting glucose transport into cells. Insulin binds to receptors on cells, and then internalization and intracellular processes lead to utilization of glucose, synthesis of protein, and inhibition of glycogenolysis and fatty acid breakdown. Conversely, insulin deficiency promotes release from fat tissue of free fatty acids, which are metabolized by hepatic mitochondria to acetyl coenzyme A and then to ketoacids, and also creates hyperglycemia by increasing the production of hepatic glucose and reducing use of peripheral glucose. Defects in insulin receptors on cells or in intracellular processing may cause insulin resistance, an important factor in the etiology of the most common form of diabetes.

In islets, beta cells are centrally located and are supplied by arterial blood flow from the center to the periphery of the islet where the other types of islet cells are found. Paracrine control of islet hormone secretion is an important phenomenon, with insulin from the beta cells probably acting to control the output of other cells, such as glucagon from alpha cells. In the absence of insulin, for instance, hyperglucagonemia is usually found.

DIAGNOSIS

Diabetes mellitus is diagnosed by measurement of the blood glucose level. Fasting levels greater than 140 mg. per 100 ml. on at least two occasions indicate the presence of diabetes. Measurement of glycosylated hemoglobin assesses mean blood glucose levels over time and is more valuable in long-term follow-up than sporadic blood glucose levels or self-reported home blood glucose monitoring. Some individuals have fasting blood glucose levels less than 140 mg. per 100 ml. but have abnormal glucose tolerance tests and elevated glycosylated hemoglobin levels; these patients do not maintain consistent blood glucose control and should be treated as diabetics during an acute illness or a perioperative period. Many factors—starvation, infection, pregnancy, medical illnesses and inactivity, drugs such as corticosteroids, thiazide diuretics, and oral contraceptives, and age—influence the glucose tolerance test and may make interpretation difficult. Patients with hyperglycemia from any cause must be treated appropriately with insulin to normalize their blood glucose levels during any acute illness, stress, or operation.

CLASSIFICATION

Diabetes is classified into two major categories: primary diabetes—both Type I, or insulin-dependent diabetes mellitus (IDDM), and Type II, or non–insulin-dependent diabetes mellitus (NIDDM); and secondary diabetes—pancreatic disease, drug- or chemical-induced, hormonal excess, genetic syndromes, and abnormalities in the insulin receptor. Most diabetics have primary diabetes, the vast majority being Type II (NIDDM) (Table 10–1).

IDDM and NIDDM differ in a number of respects. IDDM (Type I) usually develops in childhood or adolescence. Insulin-producing beta cells of the pancreatic islets are destroyed by a chronic autoimmune process directed specifically at beta cells and sparing other islet cells (alpha, delta, PP cells). Susceptibility to IDDM is influenced by genetic factors, particularly HLA-DR3 and HLA-DR4 and certain HLA-DQ phenotypes and the genotypes containing HLA-A1, B8, and DR3 or DR4. These genes may act by presenting a beta cell autoantigen in a manner inducing autoimmunity or may direct the immune responsiveness to the autoantigen. The particular antigen(s) responsible for the autoimmune destruction of beta cells is not known, but candidate antigens are the enzyme glutamic acid decarboxylase or heat shock protein 60, which is coexpressed with insulin in the beta cell secretory

TABLE 10–1. Diagnosis and Classification of Diabetes Mellitus

Type I	Insulin-dependent diabetes mellitus (IDDM) ~20% of all diabetes mellitus Onset in childhood or adolescence; patients not obese Autoimmune disease, genetic risk factors Entirely dependent on exogenous insulin Prone to develop ketosis and acidosis Visual impairment, nephropathy, and neuropathy major chronic complications
Type II	Non–insulin-dependent diabetes mellitus (NIDDM) ~80% of all diabetes mellitus Onset after age 30 years; patients usually obese Risk factors are obesity and family history of NIDDM Insulin resistance, insulin levels may be normal or high Treated with diet, exercise, oral hypoglycemics Atherosclerosis, coronary artery disease, and stroke major chronic complications but may have visual impairment, nephropathy, and neuropathy

Secondary Diabetes	Pancreatic disease or resection
	    Occurs with pancreatic insufficiency such as chronic pancreatitis, cystic fibrosis, and hemochromatosis
	    Insulin dependent
	    May be "brittle"; prone to hypoglycemia due to no glucagon, exocrine insufficiency, and poor food absorption
	Hormonal excess diabetes; Cushing's disease, acromegaly, pheochromocytoma, stress
	Drug-induced diabetes; corticosteroids, thiazide diuretics

granules.[12] Immune tolerance to glutamic acid decarboxylase or injection of a component of heat shock protein 60 prevents diabetes from occurring in diabetes-susceptible strains of mice and may abort the autoimmune insulitis in progress. Similarly, immunosuppression with cyclosporine acts to control the T-cell–mediated destructive inflammatory insulitis (at the expense of the toxicity of cyclosporine).[5] The insulitis is a chronic process that usually takes years to destroy most (at least 90%) of the beta cells; when this threshold is reached, the classic manifestations of hyperglycemia and ketoacidosis herald the onset of IDDM. During the development of the disease, administration of prophylactic insulin with strict normalization of blood glucose may reduce the damage to residual beta cells and preserve some endogenous insulin secretory capacity; this is desirable because endogenous insulin, even in small amounts, serves to protect the patient from ketoacidosis. Because intervention early in the disease process is rarely possible, most patients with IDDM have no endogenous insulin production and depend entirely on exogenous insulin administration. They are prone to develop severe hyperglycemia, ketosis, and dehydration. About 20% of diabetic patients have IDDM.

In NIDDM, the predominant form of the disease, two defects are present: (1) the action of insulin on peripheral tissues to stimulate glucose metabolism and to inhibit production of glucose by the liver is impaired (insulin resistance); and (2) beta cells of the pancreas are unable to compensate for insulin resistance, causing a relative insulin deficiency (actual levels of insulin may be normal or high as an attempt to compensate for insulin resistance). In the past few years before clinical diabetes occurs, insulin secretion falls and diabetes becomes evident. Insulin resistance is strongly associated with obesity and inactivity and is influenced by genetic factors. Individuals who are obese and inactive and have a family history of NIDDM are at high risk for developing NIDDM. These patients also have lipid disturbances and hypertension as atherogenic risk factors and have a high rate of morbidity and premature death from coronary artery disease and stroke.[35] In high-risk patients (obese, positive family history, middle-aged and older) insulin resistance can be detected by testing glucose tolerance (through such simple tests as a postprandial blood glucose measurement). NIDDM can be delayed or prevented in these patients through diet and lifestyle changes, emphasizing exercise and cessation of smoking. These measures reverse insulin resistance and preserve beta cell function. If weight loss cannot be accomplished, sulfonylureas or biguanides may be used to stimulate insulin secretion, but strict normalization of blood glucose is rarely achieved. Exogenous insulin is given if oral drugs fail to normalize blood glucose levels and during any time of stress, such as infection or a surgical procedure. Patients with NIDDM are not ketosis prone but are subject to all of the other consequences of chronic hyperglycemia, detailed later. Treatment of NIDDM is difficult because compliance with diet and lifestyle changes, the cornerstone of successful management, is rarely achieved. Prevention, through early intervention in high-risk patients, is more effective and should become a high health care priority, given the human and economic burdens imposed by NIDDM.

Secondary diabetes is most often due to pancreatic insufficiency or disease, such as chronic pancreatitis with islet fibrosis, hemochromatosis, cystic fibrosis, or after extensive pancreatic resection. These patients have lost all islet cell function and are *brittle*, in that the important counterregulatory hormones such as glucagon are also absent. They depend entirely on exogenous insulin; and because of the absence of glucagon, concomitant pancreatic exocrine deficiency, and poor food absorption, they are especially prone to the development of hypoglycemia. With better treatment and longer survival for patients with cystic fibrosis, pancreatic diabetes has appeared in as many as 15% of long-term survivors and 50% to 75% of patients have impaired insulin secretion and glucose intolerance.[27] Because some insulin production is preserved, these patients tend not to be ketosis prone. Hormonal excess states, such as Cushing's disease, functional adrenal cortical neoplasms or exogenous administration of corticosteroids, acromegaly, and pheochromocytoma are associated with hyperglycemia and relative insulin insufficiency. Whatever the cause of the hyperglycemia, patients must be treated with insulin if simple dietary measures are insufficient and during stress, sepsis, or a surgical procedure.

ACUTE COMPLICATIONS

Metabolic Disorders

Hyperglycemia and insulin deficiency cause metabolic complications, and each of these complications must be managed with the liberal use of exogenous insulin to strictly control (normalize) blood glucose levels. The risks of these complications are especially important to the surgical patient who is undergoing stress or is injured, and in these patients great care must be taken to precisely manage their insulin needs and control blood glucose levels (Table 10–2).

The immediate effect of hyperglycemia is glucosuria and osmotic diuresis. Patients note polyuria and polydipsia and may become dehydrated to the point of shock owing to depletion of extracellular volume. Absence of insulin causes breakdown of fatty acids into ketoacids as fuel for the brain,

TABLE 10–2. Complications of Diabetes Mellitus

Acute	Chronic
Susceptibility to infections	Retinopathy, cataracts
Metabolic derangements	Nephropathy
Hyperglycemic	Proteinuria
Hyperosmolar state	Renal failure
Acidosis	Neuropathy
Hypertriglyceridemia	Peripheral
Iatrogenic hypoglycemia	Autonomic
Impaired wound healing	Hypercoagulable state
	Hypertension
	Macrovascular disease
	Peripheral arterial insufficiency
	Coronary artery disease
	Mesenteric vascular insufficiency
	Cerebral arterial insufficiency
	Chronic diabetic encephalopathy

and the excess ketone bodies appear in the plasma and urine. Severe electrolyte losses occur in the urine as a result of the osmotic glucose diuresis to buffer the ketoacids. The excess sodium presented to the distal tubule promotes the secretion of aldosterone with resultant potassium losses; although serum potassium levels might be elevated in these severely dehydrated patients, total body potassium is depleted. If uncorrected, the condition of diabetic ketoacidosis occurs, with extreme hyperglycemia, ketosis, and acidosis (Table 10–3). The acidosis produced by ketoacids is worsened when volume depletion and shock cause peripheral underperfusion and lactic acidemia. Patients become obtunded and display deep and prolonged Kussmaul respirations, and the odor of the ketones is detected on their breath. Leukocytosis and abdominal pain due to delayed gastric emptying are often present. The inciting cause for this catastrophic metabolic cascade is often sepsis or stress, which must be corrected to treat the patient successfully. During their lifetime most patients with IDDM experience diabetic ketoacidosis, and the mortality of the condition may be as high as 50%, reflecting the severity of the inciting disease as well as the metabolic derangement.

Patients with NIDDM may develop even more serious hyperglycemia associated with coma. Because these patients produce enough endogenous insulin to prevent lipolysis and ketogenesis but insufficient to utilize glucose, the syndrome is that of nonketotic hyperosmolar hyperglycemia. It is associated with such serious medical complications as bacterial or viral sepsis or myocardial infarction and usually occurs in elderly patients. The syndrome is characterized by extreme hyperglycemia (blood glucose levels may exceed 1000 mg. per 100 ml.). Osmolarity may exceed 350 mOsm. per liter. There is only mild acidosis, and ketonemia is absent. Dehydration is severe, and prerenal azotemia is common. Changes in mental status, obtundation, or coma is present. Because these patients are elderly and usually have a serious underlying condition, the mortality rate for the nonketotic hyperosmolar syndrome is at least 50%.

Infection

Hyperglycemia is directly related to the well-known heightened susceptibility of diabetics to infections. Polymorphonuclear cell phagocytic and intracellular bactericidal killing activities are depressed, as is chemotaxis of leukocytes to the site of inflammation. There is no measurable effect of diabetes on the immune system.

The most common site of infection in diabetics is the urinary tract. Pyelonephritis, papillary necrosis, emphysematous pyelonephritis, and perinephric abscesses are all more common in diabetics. Pulmonary infections with common bacterial organisms such as *Streptococcus pneumoniae*, *Escherichia coli*, and *Staphylococcus aureus* also occur frequently and are associated with high mortality rates. Unusual infections are also seen, including rhinocerebral mucormycosis, an invasive fungal infection of the nose and sinuses, and malignant external otitis, an invasive bacterial infection of the auditory canal usually caused by *Pseudomonas aeruginosa*. Necrotizing cellulitis and fasciitis can occur, especially in the perineal region of male diabetics who have recently had urethral catheterization. Known as Fournier's gangrene, this polymicrobial infection with aerobic and anaerobic organisms must be treated with prompt aggressive surgical débridement, colostomy, and systemic antibiotics. A troublesome infectious complication of hyperglycemia is gingivitis and pyorrhea, with periodontal infections, abscesses, and loss of teeth. Dental sepsis may often cause systemic symptoms and precipitate hyperglycemia and even diabetic ketoacidosis, and it often complicates major surgical procedures especially in immunosuppressed diabetic recipients of organ transplant. Great care must be taken with oral hygiene, including professional control of plaque and hypertrophic gingivitis.

Impaired Wound Healing

Impaired wound healing in poorly controlled diabetic patients is a multifactorial problem. Wound infection, with de-

TABLE 10–3. Hyperglycemic Crises in the Surgical Patient

Symptoms	Signs	Laboratory Values
Diabetic Ketoacidosis		
Type I (IDDM) diabetic	Hypotension	Blood glucose >300 mg./100 ml.
Missed insulin doses	Dehydration	Arterial pH <7.3
Polyuria, polydipsia	Hypothermia	Elevated plasma ketones
Vomiting, abdominal pain	Abdominal rigidity	Leukocytosis
Weakness	Kussmaul breathing	NaHCO$_3$ <15 mEq./L.
Blurred vision	Fruity odor	Osmols >300
Nonketotic Hyperosmolar Syndrome		
Type II (NIDDM) diabetic	Severe dehydration	Blood glucose >600 mg./100 ml.
	Oliguria	Elevated blood urea nitrogen, creatinine
Mental status changes	Obtundation or coma	Arterial pH >7.3
Complicating medical illness	Urosepsis, pneumonia, congestive heart failure, myocardial infarction	Osmols >330

fective phagocytosis and migration of inflammatory cells during hyperglycemia, is a prominent factor. When glucose fuel is unavailable to cells for normal aerobic metabolism, fibroblasts and leukocytes in the wound become dysfunctional, and impaired fibroblast and endothelial cell proliferation and epithelialization, decreased collagen deposition, and decreased wound strength ensue. Well-controlled diabetics with adequate insulin availability and normal blood glucose levels show no defects in wound healing or in ultimate wound strength.

Cholelithiasis

Cholelithiasis is more prevalent in diabetic than in nondiabetic patients of comparable age. The mortality and morbidity of gallstone-related complications, including gangrene of the gallbladder, is high in diabetic patients, but studies containing controls for coexisting medical conditions such as ischemic heart disease have found that increased risk is related to the medical conditions rather than the diabetic state.[3] Consequently, there is no justification for prophylactic cholecystectomy for asymptomatic cholelithiasis in diabetic patients. However, given the strong propensity for diabetic patients, especially those with NIDDM, to have established ischemic heart disease or other atherosclerotic complications, cholelithiasis should be dealt with electively as soon as symptoms appear, when perioperative preparation and management can be optimal. Waiting for complications of acute cholecystitis or choledocholithiasis to appear before surgical intervention is chosen converts a controlled elective procedure into an emergency with substantial increased mortality. Nonoperative methods for dissolution or fragmentation with dissolution of gallstones have little or no role, especially in diabetic patients in whom symptoms should prompt early cholecystectomy.

CHRONIC COMPLICATIONS

Diabetes mellitus is associated with long-term microvascular, neurologic, and macrovascular complications that are caused, almost entirely, by hyperglycemia. These long-term complications shorten life expectancy and severely compromise the quality of life for the diabetic patient. Premature disability and mortality affect patients with all types of diabetes. Blindness, renal failure, peripheral neuropathy, and accelerated advanced atherosclerosis are the major disorders of concern in the diabetic patient.

Vision Impairment and Blindness

After 15 years, essentially all patients with diabetes have some visual impairment due to diabetic retinopathy or cataracts or both. Many of these patients are blind. Diabetes is the leading cause of new blindness in adults.[11] Retinopathy stems from chronic hyperglycemia, and its development and severity depend on the duration of diabetes and the degree of glycemic control. Retinopathy begins as *background* lesions; these are microaneurysms, dot and blot hemorrhages, and hard exudates formed from plasma leakage into the retina. Later, occlusion of vessels occurs with ischemia and infarction, and cotton-wool exudates indicate neovascularization with proliferation of new vessels into the vitreous in association with the appearance of endothelial growth factors in ocular fluids.[1] Because of the prevalence of hypertension in these patients and the fragility of the neovessels, anticoagulation of the patient with diabetic retinopathy may not be safe. Patients with any type of diabetes may develop retinopathy if blood glucose levels are not controlled. Cataracts form as a consequence of high blood glucose levels,

probably through the polyol pathway. When blood glucose is elevated it enters the cells of the lens where, in the presence of aldose reductase, it is converted to sorbitol, creating intracellular hyperosmolarity, water influx, cell swelling, and injury.

Neuropathy and the Diabetic Foot

A peripheral, symmetric sensorimotor neuropathy with paresthesias is common in diabetic patients and is found in most patients after 5 to 10 years of diabetes. The development of neuropathy has also been attributed to the polyol pathway, with sorbitol accumulation in Schwann cells during periods of hyperglycemia damaging to the nerve fibers.[13] Severe pain may be present but is uncommon. The most common manifestation is peripheral neuropathy of the feet and distal lower extremity, with loss of protective sensation in the foot. Minor trauma may develop into a serious necrotizing infection with tissue loss. Normal adjustments of the foot in weight bearing do not occur, and heavy calluses form over pressure points, adding to the pressure and causing necrosis under the callus. Foot problems are the most common indication for hospital admission in diabetics.[33] Necrobiosis lipoidica diabeticorum is a skin lesion occurring over the shins of patients with peripheral neuropathy. When abraded by the patient because of dysesthesias and itching, the lesion may become ulcerated and infected.

Autonomic neuropathy, usually involving the gastrointestinal and cardiac systems, is a late complication that can occur in patients with established peripheral neuropathy. Gastroparesis with delayed gastric emptying and gastric dilatation may cause hypoglycemia in patients receiving insulin. Bethanecol, metoclopramide, and erythromycin have been somewhat effective in increasing gastric motility, but surgical procedures such as gastric resection or pyloroplasty have been ineffective. Intractable diarrhea and steatorrhea are advanced manifestations of gastrointestinal autonomic neuropathy.[36] Diarrhea is often nocturnal, profuse, and watery and is related not only to disordered neurologic control of intestinal motility but also to bacterial overgrowth occurring in poorly draining segments, including the stomach. Oral antibiotics and cholestyramine to bind bile acids may be of some benefit, but there is no effective surgical treatment. Dysmotility may also occur in the esophagus in patients with advanced autonomic neuropathy. Esophagoscopy should be performed in diabetic patients with dysphagia because *Candida* infection of the esophagus is commonly found in patients with oral candidiasis (thrush) and will also cause dysphagia. The diagnosis of esophageal candidiasis is made by mucosal brushings and biopsies and can be further differentiated from diabetic esophageal dysmotility by manometry. *Candida* infection should be treated with fluconazole because the infection is invasive and may cause deep ulceration and bleeding. Esophageal candidiasis may be prevented by nystatin mouthwashes to swish and swallow; this therapy should be administered to all diabetic patients during periods of surgical stress or antibiotic administration.

Similar hypotonicity and failure to empty occur in the urinary bladder and contribute to the high rate of urinary tract infections in diabetics. This problem may be treated successfully initially, by educating the patients in double-voiding techniques and in clean, intermittent self-catheterization.

Cardiac autonomic neuropathy is also a late complication. The symptoms are principally those of postural hypotension or hemodynamic instability with tachycardia, especially seen during hemodialysis. Diabetic patients should be evaluated preoperatively for the presence of cardiac neuropathy by measuring the electrocardiographic RR interval during a Valsalva maneuver or measuring orthostatic changes in pulse rate and blood pressure.

Nephropathy

In contrast to retinopathy, which occurs in nearly all patients with diabetes, diabetic nephropathy occurs in less than 40% of patients, and its incidence is declining as tight control of blood glucose levels becomes standard practice.[4] Nonetheless, diabetic nephropathy strongly correlates with poor glucose control and hypertension. Sodium retention is characteristic of diabetes, and some genetic correlates with hypertension and renal sodium handling have been proposed but not proven.

In early diabetes, hyperglycemia and hyperosmolarity cause afferent renal vasodilatation and glomerular hyperfiltration. The kidneys and the individual glomeruli become visibly enlarged, and measurements of renal plasma flow and glomerular filtration rate are markedly elevated. Albumin, a small molecule, is present in the urine in amounts detectable only with sensitive assays and in insufficient amounts (less than 0.5 gm. per 24 hours) to give a positive *dipstick* test (microalbuminuria). The amount of albumin excreted in the urine is related to the degree of hyperfiltration and increases with exercise and with the degree of hypertension present in the capillary loops of the glomerulus. The basement membrane of the capillary loops widens irregularly and becomes more permeable; with glomerular hypertension and hyperfiltration, protein leaks into the mesangium of the glomerulus, and mesangial cell expansion occurs with gradual encroachment on the filtration surface of capillary loops. Glomerular sclerosis is the end point of this process. At this point, usually more than 15 years after the onset of diabetes, overt dipstick-positive proteinuria appears and the composition of the proteinuria changes to include many larger plasma proteins (global proteinuria). Renal function then fails at a rapid and accelerating rate as additional nephrons are lost and the remaining glomeruli are exposed to even more severe hyperfiltration. The survival of patients with proteinuria for 5 years is 55%.[7]

The pre-existing hyperfiltration in poorly controlled diabetic patients and their chronic osmotic diuresis and dehydration make such patients highly susceptible to the nephrotoxic effects of iodinated radiologic contrast agents, especially (but not exclusively) if these are given intravenously. Diabetic patients who are scheduled for angiography, computed tomography, or even oral cholecystography must be prepared by correction of pre-existing dehydration with infusion of 0.45% saline for 12 hours before and 12 hours after administration of the contrast agent.[32]

Angiotensin-converting enzyme (ACE) inhibitors effectively reduce intraglomerular hypertension by reducing glomerular afterload and systemic hypertension, and they have been shown to delay or halt progression of early diabetic nephropathy in normotensive patients.[23, 37] Although control of hyperglycemia and protein restriction decreases afferent vasodilatation and glomerular hyperfiltration, ACE inhibitors increase efferent vasodilatation and are the first choice of antihypertensive drugs for use in diabetic patients.

Pathogenesis and Prevention of Microvascular Complications

Hyperglycemia has long been implicated as the cause of microvascular and neurologic complications, and strong and convincing clinical evidence that strict glycemic control would prevent their development has only recently been obtained. A multicenter trial (Diabetes Control and Complications Trial [DCCT]), beginning in 1983, enrolled 1441 patients with IDDM, ages 13 to 39, who had no evidence of severe diabetic complications or medical conditions. A group of patients with IDDM for 1 to 5 years and no evidence of diabetic retinopathy or microalbuminuria was randomized into an intensive therapy group treated with at least three insulin injections a day or with an external insulin delivery pump and closely monitored by blood glucose measurements at least four times a day, to maintain normoglycemia both preprandial and postprandial. The control group received conventional insulin therapy with one or two insulin injections a day and blood or urine glucose measurements once daily. All received education regarding diet and exercise. A second group of patients had IDDM for 1 to 15 years and had mild-to-moderate retinopathy and moderate microalbuminuria. They were similarly randomized. After a mean follow-up time of 6.5 years, intensive therapy reduced the risk of first development of retinopathy by 76% and substantially impeded the progression of retinopathy once present, the occurrence of microalbuminuria by 39%, the development of proteinuria by 54%, and the development of neuropathy by 60%. Aside from some weight gain in most patients, the major side effect of intensive insulin therapy was a twofold to threefold increase in hypoglycemic episodes.

On the basis of these dramatic results, intensive insulin therapy with close glucose monitoring is now recommended as standard treatment for most patients with IDDM.[2, 11, 28, 29, 38] Patients with complicating medical illnesses, especially cardiac ischemia, may best be treated with conventional treatment regimens if the risk/benefit ratio of intensive therapy is unfavorable. Two important clinical questions remain unresolved by the DCCT: (1) whether the benefits of more strict glycemic control also apply to patients with NIDDM and (2) whether strict glycemic control can ameliorate macrovascular disease. Many indications show that poor blood glucose control predicts the development and progression of long-term microvascular complications in NIDDM, and the rate and severity of complications directly correlate with mean blood glucose and glycosylated hemoglobin levels. NIDDM is associated with atherogenic changes of serum lipids and lipoproteins, and improvement is seen with better glycemic control; obesity adversely affects lipoprotein concentrations, especially in the presence of insulin resistance (the typical NIDDM state), and weight loss also improves the lipoprotein profile. There is no evidence that intensive insulin therapy worsens macrovascular disease, as might have occurred if hyperinsulinism contributes to the development of atherosclerosis, but the weight gain and worsened insulin resistance with even higher requirements for insulin may not be worth the risks to patients with NIDDM. Simpler measures, such as diet with exercise, may be sufficient.

The major impediment to intensive insulin therapy for patients with IDDM is hypoglycemia.[8] Some patients with long-standing diabetes fail to develop the symptoms of hypoglycemia (tremor, palpitations, diaphoresis) and are unaware of the precarious low level of their blood glucose. Although the condition of *hypoglycemia unawareness* is found most commonly in patients with severe autonomic neuropathy, this is not always the case. Intensive insulin therapy and recent previous episodes of hypoglycemia predispose to more episodes—a vicious cycle. These patients have lost their ability to secrete the major counterregulatory hormones, epinephrine and glucagon, perhaps because the brain fails to recognize the hypoglycemia or a selective autonomic neuropathy affects the peripheral mechanisms responsible for the secretion of epinephrine.[18] Beta blockade appears to worsen the unawareness. Much care must be taken by patients to monitor their blood glucose levels often and take preemptive measures to treat incipient hypoglycemia before they become unable to assist themselves.

Macrovascular Disease

The greatest risk to survival and to quality of life of diabetic patients is the development of macrovascular atherosclerotic disease. Atherosclerosis and coronary artery disease have a considerably higher prevalence in diabetic than in nondiabetic patients of a similar age.[14] Vascular insufficiency of the lower extremities together with the propensity of diabetic patients for foot infections and ulcers accounts for the observation that nearly half of all amputations of the leg are carried out in diabetic patients. Large-vessel atherosclerotic lesions appear at an earlier age than in a normal population, and tibial artery occlusion is often the first lesion to appear. Small vessel disease, at one time believed to be uniformly present and to constitute a contraindication to surgical revascularization, is no longer believed to be a factor in lower leg ischemia.[33] In contrast to findings in nondiabetic patients with occlusive vascular disease in the leg, the foot vessels of the diabetic patient are usually spared. Medial calcification of arterial walls makes Doppler evaluation unreliable because the vessels are poorly compressible. When dealing with lower leg ischemia in the diabetic patient, septic foci must be dealt with by aggressive débridement and local amputations. Only when the infection is controlled should surgical reconstruction be considered. Appropriate bypass procedures, often infrainguinal, have good rates of patency and limb salvage. Sepsis, not ischemia, is the greatest cause of major amputation.

Diabetes is associated with a hypercoagulable state. Platelet aggregation is enhanced, fibrinogen levels are increased, natural anticoagulants in the blood such as protein C are decreased, and there is decreased plasminogen activator and fibrinolysis. Combined with hypertension and endothelial cell dysfunction and damage, the hypercoagulable state contributes to the high incidence of thrombotic complications in diabetic patients.[21]

The principal threat to life of the diabetic patient is coronary artery disease.[19, 31] The incidence is high, and the mortality from an acute myocardial infarction is twice that of a nondiabetic; this combination makes coronary artery disease the major cause of premature mortality in diabetic patients. Women are also at high risk; compared with a nondiabetic group of a similar age range, diabetic women who were age 40 to 54 at the time of diagnosis had a 39% death rate from heart disease by age 70, whereas nondiabetic women had a 10% rate for the same period.[15] In a prospective angiographic study of IDDM patients awaiting renal transplantation, a 40% incidence of significant coronary artery occlusion or left ventricular dysfunction was detected.[6]

The strong likelihood of significant coronary artery occlusive disease must be taken into account when undertaking surgical treatment of any diabetic patient (Table 10–4). A careful history must be taken to detect angina or previous myocardial infarction, postural hypotension, or treatment with antihypertensive drugs, beta-blockade (see previous section on hypoglycemia unawareness), coronary vasodilators, calcium channel blocking agents, and diuretics, because all of these drugs influence perioperative management and may cause drug-related complications. Electrocardiography with attention to signs of cardiac neuropathy and ischemia, echocardiography, stress myocardial function tests, and coronary angiography may be indicated should any evidence of heart disease be uncovered or in any event if the patient is older than age 30 years. Perioperative management in a facility in which heart rate, rhythm, and blood pressure can be continuously monitored is required. Invasive monitoring of hemody-

TABLE 10–4. Preoperative Workup of the Diabetic Patient

History
Duration of diabetes; episodes of diabetic ketoacidosis or hypoglycemia
Insulin, diet, or oral hypoglycemic therapy
Complications: visual impairment, neuropathy, symptoms of renal or peripheral vascular disease, neurogenic bladder
History of heart disease: angina, congestive heart failure, myocardial infarction, arrhythmias
Drug history: ACE inhibitors, beta-blockade, calcium channel blockers, diuretics, coronary vasodilators
Symptoms of infection at any site: urinary tract, lungs, skin and subcutaneous tissues, gums, feet, intra-abdominal sites

Physical Examination
Body habitus: NIDDM patients obese
Ophthalmoscopy: background or proliferative retinopathy
Blood pressure: often elevated, predicts renal and visual impairment
Circulation: evidence of congestive heart failure or peripheral vascular insufficiency
Neurologic examination: sensory neuropathy especially in feet, mental status changes
Status of feet: ischemia, ulcers, infection, loss of sensation

Laboratory Examination
Blood glucose, serum sodium, potassium, and sodium bicarbonate levels
Renal function: proteinuria, blood urea nitrogen, and creatinine
Cardiac evaluation: electrocardiogram, stress test, echocardiogram, possible coronary angiogram

namic status with a pulmonary artery catheter may be indicated in a patient with existing heart disease who has had a major surgical procedure. It is unwise to perform any but the most simple procedures on a diabetic patient in an outpatient setting.

Central Nervous System Disorders

Diabetes increases stroke risk as much as sixfold, especially in elderly patients with NIDDM, through the combined effects of chronic hypertension, macrovascular disease, and a hypercoagulable state. Attacks of hypoglycemia, if not treated immediately, may cause seizure disorders and permanent damage to the brain. Hyperglycemia impairs consciousness and acutely raises the risk of stroke, perhaps from increased viscosity of the blood and other factors contributing to a hypercoagulable state. Hyperglycemia also changes brain electrolyte transport as well as brain blood flow and metabolism and may cause a chronic encephalopathy.[25]

Diabetes and Pancreatic Cancer

Diabetes occurs more frequently in patients with pancreatic cancer than in the general population and is a risk factor for the development of pancreatic cancer. In a large multicenter study of patients in Italy who were hospitalized for a variety of conditions including pancreatic cancer, age-matched subjects were compared; 23% of patients with pancreatic cancer and 8% of nondiabetic patients matched for age and other characteristics had NIDDM. Most patients with pancreatic cancer had diabetes of recent onset, and there was no statistically significant association of pancreatic cancer in patients with long-standing diabetes. The tumor had apparently caused the diabetes in most cases.[17]

MANAGEMENT OF THE DIABETIC PATIENT

The basic goal of management of diabetes is the consistent maintenance of a normal blood glucose. Diet is the corner-

TABLE 10–5. Targets for Management of Diabetic Patients

	Good	Acceptable	Poor
Blood glucose:			
Fasting (mg./100 ml.)	80–134	≤150	≥150
	90–180	<200	>200
Glycosylated hemoglobin (% of upper limit of normal)	<110%	≤140%	>150%
Serum cholesterol:			
Total (mg./100 ml.)	<200	<250	>250
HDL (mg./100 ml.)	>42	>35	<35
Fasting serum triglycerides (mg./100 ml.)	<170	<220	>220
Body-mass index:			
Men	<25	<27	>27
Women	<24	<26	>26
Blood pressure (mm. Hg)	<140/90	<160/95	>160/95

Adapted from Williams, G.: Management of non–insulin-dependent diabetes mellitus. Lancet, *343*:95, 1994. © by The Lancet Ltd, 1994.

stone of long-term therapy for patients with any type of diabetes.[39] Dietary fat should not exceed 30% of calories and saturated fat should not make up more than 10% of fat. Daily protein intake should not exceed 0.8 gm. per kg. of ideal body weight. Patients should eat at least three meals a day, and those receiving insulin should also take a bedtime snack, with meals spaced to achieve best glycemic control. Weight reduction and exercise reverses much of the characteristic insulin resistance of patients with NIDDM, and the objective for these patients is to achieve ideal body weight. All diabetic patients should be strongly encouraged to become active participants in their own care. Targets are set for blood glucose, glycosylated hemoglobin, lipid profile, weight (body mass index), and blood pressure; and patients must participate in reaching these goals (Table 10–5). They must learn, practice, and record home glucose monitoring and learn to recognize signs and symptoms of impending hypoglycemia. All diabetic patients should examine their feet daily and strictly avoid walking barefoot or in constricting shoes (Table 10–6).

Patients with NIDDM respond well to diet and exercise if they are cooperative.[39] If hyperglycemia persists or occurs later in the disease as beta cell compensation fails, sulfonylurea or biguanide drugs (oral hypoglycemic agents) are begun to stimulate higher levels of insulin secretion. Even later in the disease, insulin may be required. At this point, NIDDM patients are managed similarly to IDDM patients with intensive insulin therapy and frequent blood glucose monitoring, unless the risks of hypoglycemia outweigh the benefits of blood glucose control, such as in patients with ischemic heart disease. Treatment of hypertension should be initiated and maintained with ACE inhibitors; single drug treatment with diuretics is not appropriate because these patients are often chronically dehydrated. Beta-blockade may complicate the management of the diabetes because hypoglycemic awareness may be blocked.

TABLE 10–6. Rules for Care of Diabetic Patient's Feet

1. Always wear roomy and comfortable well-padded shoes.
2. Keep feet warm, dry, and clean.
3. Inspect feet daily; place cotton between toes. (If vision is poor, have someone else do this.)
4. Avoid hot soaks or baths.
5. Trim toenails and calluses expertly.
6. Never walk barefoot.
7. Get prompt medical attention for any injury or blister.

Patients with IDDM and many patients with secondary diabetes require insulin. Insulin administration is coordinated with meals to mimic a normal physiologic beta cell response. Insulin is available as human recombinant, beef, pork, or semisynthetic. Human insulin is the preferred form. Various preparations have different times of peak activity and duration so that an individualized regimen can be developed for each patient, related to diet and activity habits (Table 10–7). The normal daily insulin production in a nondiabetic is approximately 25 units; this number can be used as a baseline for planning an initial schedule, with two thirds of the dose planned for morning and one third before dinner. Some patients prefer a continuous subcutaneous insulin infusion administered by an externally worn pump. Intraperitoneal insulin delivery through an implanted catheter and external pump device is superior to peripheral delivery because absorption into the portal bloodstream is accomplished with first pass extraction by the liver, thus lowering peripheral insulin levels.[9]

Hypoglycemia occurs frequently, especially in intensively treated patients. Patients with gastroparesis are especially at risk, as are those with pancreatic insufficiency who absorb food poorly and have an inability to secrete glucagon as a counterregulatory hormone. Patients with frequent recent hypoglycemic events are often unaware of impending hypoglycemia. Severe hypoglycemia should be treated by oral carbohydrates, but an unconscious patient requires an intra-

TABLE 10–7. Insulin Preparations and Regimens

Preparations of Human Insulin	Onset	Peak	Duration
Regular human insulin	30 min.	2–5 hr.	6–8 hr.
Intermediate acting:			
Lente	2.5 hr.	7–15 hr.	22 hr.
NPH	1.5 hr.	4–12 hr.	24 hr.
Long acting: Ultralente	Slow		28 hr.

(Many other preparations—beef, pork, combinations of beef and pork, combinations of regular and intermediate- or long-acting concentrations, delivery systems, etc.—are available.)

Regimens
Maintenance:
　Intermediate + regular (two thirds + one third) in A.M., supplemental regular for meals, additional intermediate- or long-acting insulin in afternoon based on blood glucose monitoring records. Usual total dose: 25 units/day or 0.5 unit/kg./day
Intensive insulin therapy:
　Intermediate + regular in A.M., supplemental regular for meals based on blood glucose checks four to six times a day, or continuous subcutaneous insulin infusion with an external pump.
(Regular insulin should not be given at bedtime without close monitoring of blood glucose.)
Perioperative:
　Discontinue oral hypoglycemics 24 hours before operation.
　Discontinue intermediate- and long-acting insulin preparations on morning of operation.
　Give nothing by mouth after midnight.
　Start IV infusion of D_5W or D_5NS with 20 mEq./L. KCl at 6 A.M.; run at 100–200 ml./hr.
　Start second IV infusion of insulin, 25 units/250 ml. NS. Run 75 ml. through the IV tubing (to occupy protein-binding sites on tubing); then discard.
　Administer at 1–2 units/hr. via infusion pump.
　Monitor blood glucose at 30-min. intervals until stable at 150–200 mg./100 ml.; then monitor hourly until patient is awake, every 4 hours until diet is resumed.
　Convert to maintenance regimen when diet is begun by giving 80% of previous day's total insulin, two thirds as intermediate and one third as regular. Adjust using blood glucose levels.

venous bolus of 20 ml. of 50% glucose, repeated as necessary, and an intravenous infusion of 5% or 10% dextrose until the blood glucose value is above 100 mg. per 100 ml. and the patient is conscious.

Perioperative Management

Approximately half of the 12 million diabetics in the United States will undergo at least one operation in their lifetime. Many operations are for infections, and a substantial number are for emergency conditions. Many patients presenting for elective or emergency operations have previously undiagnosed NIDDM and are hyperglycemic or have hyperglycemia secondary to sepsis or stress. The acute management of the hyperglycemic patient depends on achieving and maintaining a normal blood glucose level. Except for the patient with NIDDM who is easily managed by diet alone and is normoglycemic, diabetic patients require insulin infusions during illness and operative stress to maintain euglycemia. Fluid and electrolyte imbalance, blood pressure abnormalities, infection, and diminished wound healing are the risks of hyperglycemia in the surgical patient, and they are more serious than the risks of hypoglycemia during insulin treatment in a well-monitored surgical patient.

For elective procedures, patients who will miss a meal should have oral hypoglycemic agents discontinued for at least 24 hours before operation. Insulin-dependent patients should not receive their full dose of either intermediate- or long-acting insulin on the day of operation; the most effective management is to omit intermediate- and long-acting insulin entirely and manage the blood glucose levels with intravenous insulin infusion. An infusion of glucose is begun at a rate of 5 to 10 gm. per hour (5% dextrose in water at 100 to 200 ml./hr. with potassium chloride, 20 mEq./L.), and a separate infusion of insulin is added (25 units of regular human insulin in 250 ml. of normal saline, discarding the first 75 ml. by flushing through the tubing) at a rate of 1 to 2 units per hour. The blood glucose is measured by venous or capillary blood samples 1 hour after beginning this infusion and at intervals thereafter, and the rate of insulin infusion is adjusted to maintain the blood glucose between 150 and 200 mg. per 100 ml. Postoperatively the patient is maintained with glucose, potassium, and insulin until a normal diet is resumed and then is converted back to an intermediate- or long-acting subcutaneous insulin regimen. This is done by taking 80% of the total previous day's insulin and giving two thirds as long-acting and one third as regular; then fasting and late-afternoon blood glucose values are measured to adjust and tailor the regimen. Particular care must be taken when performing gastric bypass procedures for morbid obesity, because patients with NIDDM who have been taking insulin for blood glucose control have an abrupt decrease in insulin requirements immediately after the procedure, perhaps related to increased release of gastric inhibitory polypeptide from proximal small bowel. It is incorrect to use urine glucose levels to determine insulin doses because factors relating to renal threshold for glucose, urine flow rates, and concentration of the urine influence the results.

Hyperglycemic Crises

Diabetic patients who have infections or other acute illnesses and stress and some who are noncompliant with their medical management may develop severe hyperglycemia. Diabetics with IDDM who have not had sufficient insulin or are undergoing sepsis or stress may present with diabetic ketoacidosis, and patients with NIDDM may have nonketotic hyperosmolar syndrome. Although patients with severe hyperglycemia may have abdominal pain and rigidity mimicking an acute abdomen, it is important to remember that the precipitating cause for the development of diabetic ketoacidosis or the nonketotic hyperosmolar syndrome might be an acute abdominal condition. Urosepsis, pneumonia, and myocardial infarction are common inciting conditions, especially in patients with NIDDM.

The treatment of severe hyperglycemia must precede any operative intervention and should be accomplished as expeditiously as possible because the root cause may require surgical treatment (Table 10–8). The basic principles of treatment, even in patients with NIDDM, include intravenous insulin, resuscitation with intravenous fluids and electrolytes, and treatment of the underlying medical condition. It is most important to treat the acidosis and dehydration; correction of the blood glucose follows. Resuscitation should take place in a monitored setting, such as the intensive care unit. Invasive monitoring with a pulmonary artery catheter is advisable because many patients with IDDM may have coronary artery disease and all patients with NIDDM can be assumed to have established organic heart disease. Patients with mental status changes likely require endotracheal intubations and a nasogastric tube must be placed because all severely hyperglycemic patients have gastric stasis.

Fluid resuscitation is begun with normal saline supplemented with potassium chloride (lactated solutions are avoided). As much as 10 to 12 liters of electrolyte solution may eventually be required. Replacement is based on hemodynamic parameters, not on urine flow rate, because renal dysfunction and osmotic diuresis are usually present. When the serum sodium approaches 150 mEq. per liter, the solution is changed to 0.45% saline. A separate intravenous infusion of regular insulin in normal saline is begun, with an intravenous loading dose of 0.1 to 0.2 units per kg. (10–15 units). Insulin is then infused at a rate of 5 to 10 units per hour until the blood glucose level is about 300 mg. per 100 ml.; the rate is then reduced to 1 to 2 units per hour, and the

---

TABLE 10–8. Treatment of Hyperglycemic Crises in the Surgical Patient

1. Admit to intensive care unit.
   Insert nasogastric tube.
   Consider endotracheal intubation.
   Institute cardiac monitoring, including central venous pressure measurement or placement of a Swan-Ganz pulmonary artery catheter for hemodynamic monitoring.

2. Begin IV infusion of normal saline solution through large-bore catheter. Avoid lactated solutions.
   Base fluid requirements on hemodynamic and biochemical parameters, not urine flow rate.
   Plan on 5–10 L. of fluid for resuscitation.

3. Through a separate IV line, begin insulin infusion, using solution of 1 unit insulin/10 ml. normal saline.
   Discard first 75 ml. after running through the tubing. Give loading dose of 1–2 units/kg. and then infuse at 0.1 unit/kg./hr. Rate can be doubled if necessary.

4. Monitor blood glucose hourly. Goal is to reduce hyperglycemia by 100 mg./100 ml./hr. More rapid reduction may cause cerebral edema.
   When serum sodium ≥ 150 mEq./L., change IV fluids to 0.45% saline with 20 mEq./L. potassium chloride.
   Monitor serum potassium levels closely.

5. When blood glucose is ≤ 250 mg./100 ml., reduce insulin infusion to 1–2 units/hr. and change IV fluids to D₅W with 20 mEq. potassium chloride at 50–100 ml./hr.
   Monitor serial 1:2 dilutions of patient's plasma for ketones and continue to resuscitate with glucose-potassium-insulin solutions until ketones have disappeared. (Use Acetest tablets.)

intravenous fluids are changed to 5% dextrose in 0.45% saline with potassium chloride, 20 mEq. per liter. Blood glucose may respond sooner than the ketonemia, but intravenous fluid resuscitation must continue until plasma ketones become undetectable. A simple bedside method for assessing ketonemia is to serially dilute the patient's serum from 1:1 to 1:32 and place a drop onto an Acetest tablet. This will estimate acetoacetate levels; beta-hydroxybutyrate is converted to acetoacetate during treatment. The presence of a purple color is a positive test for acetoacetate. Sodium bicarbonate is not used routinely, owing to its effect on oxygen delivery.

Potassium should always be given cautiously in patients with renal insufficiency. Magnesium may also be necessary, although replacement of phosphorus is not advisable. Throughout resuscitation, capillary or venous blood glucose is monitored every 30 to 60 minutes until it is near normal, and the insulin rate is adjusted accordingly. The goal is to reduce the blood glucose by approximately 100 mg. per 100 ml. per hour. A more rapid decrease in the blood glucose level may cause cerebral edema. The response of ketoacidosis and hyperglycemia to insulin is usually prompt and reliable.

Transplantation of the Pancreas and Other New Developments in Treatment

Transplantation of the pancreas has been attempted since 1966, but in recent years the transplantation of vascularized whole pancreas has become a relatively safe procedure and has achieved normoglycemia and near-normal insulin production in selected patients with IDDM. By mid-1993, nearly 5000 procedures had been performed.[34] Arterial blood supply is established by an end-to-side anastomosis to the iliac artery and venous drainage is to the iliac vein; a small portion of duodenum surrounding the pancreatic duct opening is anastomosed to the urinary bladder. Recent graft survival rates reach 75% in most centers, and patient survival rates exceed 90%. Patients with a successful pancreas transplant report improvement in quality of life and feeling of well-being. Pancreas transplantation is performed in patients with established end-stage renal disease and is usually done in conjunction with a renal transplant from the same cadaver donor. In some patients, a well-matched related kidney donor is available; a pancreas transplant may then be performed at a later date. Although it would be preferable to provide beta cell replacement before complications of diabetes have occurred, and thus prevent their development, the consequences of immunosuppressive therapy have precluded isolated pancreas transplantation in nonuremic patients. With advances in surgical technique leading to improved safety of the procedure and with improved management of immunosuppression, a small number of pre-uremic patients whose diabetes is extremely difficult to control and associated with numerous episodes of diabetic ketoacidosis or severe hypoglycemia unawareness have been treated successfully with a pancreas transplant.

Transplantation of isolated pancreatic islets would seem to be a preferred technique. Isolation of sufficient islets to achieve normoglycemia from human adult donors has proven difficult, as has the establishment of survival of islets implanted into the portal bloodstream. Attempts at islet xenotransplantation using porcine islets have been unsuccessful; although they are morphologically intact when transplanted under the kidney capsule of a renal allograft, insulin production is insignificant.[16] Other investigators have developed immunoisolation techniques, placing islets into chambers, capsules, or intravascular devices with a selectively permeable membrane to allow insulin to diffuse out but prevent immune cells or antibodies from permeating into the islets. These biohybrid techniques, though promising, have yet to become clinically applicable.[22]

Molecular strategies are also being developed. Attempts have been made to engineer cell lines to serve as surrogates for islets, implanted in chambers or other devices. Gene therapy directed at repair of the beta cell dysfunction of NIDDM is being investigated.[26] Immune tolerance to certain products of the beta cell granules may avert the development of autoimmune destructive insulitis,[12] and Bacille Calmette-Guérin may redirect the immune response in insulitis away from beta cell lysis.[30]

SUMMARY

Diabetes mellitus is a serious disease affecting millions of people worldwide. Nearly one fourth of patients needing an emergency surgical procedure have undiagnosed diabetes. Diabetes accounts for a large proportion of major amputations. Premature death from coronary artery disease and stroke is common. Acute metabolic complications, foot infections, urinary tract infections, and pneumonia produce many hospitalizations and large medical costs. Long-term microvascular complications lead to blindness and renal failure in many patients with diabetes of long standing. Peripheral and autonomic neuropathy adversely affect the quality of life.

Most of these conditions can be prevented by achievement of normal blood glucose levels. Early recognition and treatment of patients at high risk for developing NIDDM prevent the development of hyperglycemia. Intensive insulin therapy of patients with IDDM has been clearly demonstrated to prevent most microvascular complications. Treatment of diabetic patients, even if normotensive, with ACE inhibitors prevents progression of renal insufficiency. The perioperative patient with diabetes must be managed with great attention to consistent maintenance of blood glucose levels within the normal range. Frequent monitoring of the blood glucose level is required for proper management, and the active participation of the patient in achievement of treatment goals is essential. Strict control of blood glucose level through intensive therapy is not possible in patients unable or unwilling to participate actively in the management of their disease.[2]

SELECTED REFERENCES

Atkinson, M. A., and Maclaren, N. D.: The pathogenesis of insulin-dependent diabetes mellitus. N. Engl. J. Med., 331:1428, 1994.
This is a comprehensive review, with nearly 100 references, of the various genetic and environmental factors leading to the autoimmune beta cell destruction of type I diabetes. Especially interesting are the prevention strategies that have been successful in delaying, or perhaps even averting, the insulitis and the diabetes.

Caputo, G. M., Cavanagh, P. R., Ulbrecht, J. S., Gibbons, G. W., and Karchmer, A. W.: Assessment and management of foot disease in patients with diabetes. N. Engl. J. Med., 331:854, 1994.
The manifestation of neuropathy that causes most morbidity (and most of the lower leg amputations in diabetic patients) is the "diabetic foot." Caputo recommends use of a simple monofilament thread to detect loss of protective sensation; however, because most long-term diabetics have already lost this protection, management and healing of ulcers on the feet with the use of a total-contact boot cast is recommended. The United States Department of Health has set a goal for the year 2000 of a 40% reduction in amputations in diabetics; reading and practicing the methods in this paper will advance this goal.

The Diabetes Control and Complications Trial Research Group: The effect of intensive treatment of diabetes on the development and progression of long-term complications in insulin-dependent diabetes mellitus. N. Engl. J. Med., 329:977, 1993.
The report from this large, extensive multicenter trial of intensive insulin therapy, long awaited, has put to rest any lingering doubts that normalization of blood glucose levels was worth the effort, cost, and risks. Over a mean follow-up time of more than 6 years, the improvement in glycemic control successfully prevented much of the microvascular disease progression. The major complication of the therapy was iatrogenic hypoglycemia; this risk is the major deciding factor in the decision to also intensively treat NIDDM patients because many of these patients are older and have established heart disease. The days of loose management of blood glucose levels have come to an end.

Nathan, D. M.: Long-term complications of diabetes mellitus. N. Engl. J. Med., *328*:1676, 1993.

This comprehensive review (126 references) presents the microvascular complications of diabetes. Of special note are the excellent color fundus photographs of the various stages of diabetic retinopathy and a complete table of neuropathy manifestations and recommended treatment modalities.

Yki-Järvinen, H.: Pathogenesis of non-insulin-dependent diabetes mellitus. Lancet, *343*:91, 1994.

The complex disorders of insulin production and utilization that characterize the development of NIDDM are clearly presented in this comprehensive review of the state of knowledge in this disease. Immediately after this article in Lancet is an article by Williams (reference 39), who presents a very sensible approach to the management of NIDDM.

REFERENCES

1. Aiello, L. P., Avery, R. L., Arrigg, P. G., Keyt, B. A., et al.: Vascular endothelial growth factor in ocular fluid of patients with diabetic retinopathy and other retinal disorders. N. Engl. J. Med., *331*:1480, 1994.
2. American Diabetes Association: Implications of the diabetes control and complications trial. Diabetes, *42*:1555, 1993.
3. Aucott, J. N., Cooper, G. S., Bloom, A. D., and Aron, D. C.: Management of gallstones in diabetic patients. Arch. Intern. Med., *153*:1053, 1993.
4. Bojestig, M., Arnqvist, H. J., Hermansson, G., Karlberg, B. E., et al.: Declining incidence of nephropathy in insulin-dependent diabetes mellitus. N. Engl. J. Med., *330*:15, 1994.
5. Bougneres, P. F., Carel, J. C., Castano, L., Boitard, C., et al.: Factors associated with early remission of type I diabetes in children treated with cyclosporine. N. Engl. J. Med., *318*:663, 1988.
6. Braun, W. E., Phillips, D., Vidt, D. G., Novick, A. C., et al.: The course of coronary artery disease in diabetics with and without renal allografts. Transplant. Proc., *15*:1114, 1983.
7. Carella, M. J., Gossain, V. V., and Rovner, D. R.: Early diabetic nephropathy: Emerging treatment options. Arch. Intern. Med., *154*:624, 1994.
8. Cryer, P. E.: Hypoglycemia: The limiting factor in the management of IDDM. Diabetes, *43*:1378, 1994.
9. Duckworth, W. C., Saudek, C. D., and Henry, R. R.: Why intraperitoneal delivery of insulin with implantable pumps in NIDDM? Diabetes, *41*:657, 1992.
10. Earnhardt, R. C., Kindler, D. D., Weaver, A. M., Cornett, G., et al.: Hyperinsulinemia after pancreatic transplantation: Prediction by a novel computer model and in vivo verification. Ann. Surg., *218*:428, 1993.
11. Eastman, R. C., Siebert, C. W., Harris, M., and Gorden, P.: Clinical Review 51: Implications of the diabetes control and complications trial. J. Clin. Endocrinol. Metab., *77*:1105, 1993.
12. Elias, D., and Cohen, I. R.: Peptide therapy for diabetes in NOD mice. Lancet, *343*:704, 1994.
13. Frank, R. N.: The aldose reductase controversy. Diabetes, *43*:169, 1994.
14. Garg, A.: Lipid-lowering therapy and macrovascular disease in diabetes mellitus. Diabetes, *41*(Suppl. 2):111, 1992.
15. Gordon, T., Castelli, W. P., Hjortland, M. C., Kannel, W. B., et al.: Diabetes, blood lipids, and the role of obesity in coronary heart disease risk for women: The Framingham study. Am. J. Cardiol., *87*:393, 1977.
16. Groth, C. G., Korsgren, O., Tibell, A., Tolleman, J., et al.: Transplantation of porcine fetal pancreas to diabetic patients. Lancet, *344*:1402, 1994.
17. Gullo, L., Pezzilli, R., Morselli-Labate, A. M., and the Italian Pancreatic Cancer Study Group: Diabetes and the risk of pancreatic cancer. N. Engl. J. Med., *331*:81, 1994.
18. Hoeldtke, R. D., and Boden, G.: Epinephrine secretion, hypoglycemia unawareness, and diabetic autonomic neuropathy. Ann. Intern. Med., *120*:512, 1994.
19. Jarrett, R. J.: Risk factors for coronary heart disease in diabetes mellitus. Diabetes, *41*(Suppl. 2):1, 1992.
20. Keen, H.: Insulin resistance and the prevention of diabetes mellitus (Editorial). N. Engl. J. Med., *331*:1226, 1994.
21. Kwaan, H. C.: Changes in blood coagulation, platelet function, and plasminogen-plasmin system in diabetes. Diabetes, *41*(Suppl. 2):32, 1992.
22. Lanza, R. P., Sullivan, S. J., and Chick, W. L.: Islet transplantation with immunoisolation. Diabetes, *41*:1503, 1992.
23. Lewis, E. J., Hunsicker, L. G., Bain, R. P., Rohde, R. D., et al.: The effect of angiotensin-converting-enzyme inhibition on diabetic nephropathy. N. Engl. J. Med., *329*:1456, 1993.
24. Marchetti, P., Scharp, D. W., McLear, M., Gingerich, R., et al.: Pulsatile insulin secretion from isolated human pancreatic islets. Diabetes, *43*:827, 1994.
25. McCall, A.: The impact of diabetes on the CNS. Diabetes, *41*:557, 1992.
26. Newgard, C.: Cellular engineering and gene therapy strategies for insulin replacement in diabetes. Diabetes, *43*:341, 1994.
27. Pfeifer, T.: Diabetes in cystic fibrosis. Clin. Pediatr., *31*:682, 1992.
28. Reichard, P., Nilsson, B-Y., and Rosenqvist, U.: The effect of long-term intensified insulin treatment on the development of microvascular complications of diabetes mellitus. N. Engl. J. Med., *329*:304, 1993.
29. Santiago, J. V.: Lessons from the diabetes control and complications trial. Diabetes, *42*:1549, 1993.
30. Shehadeh, N., Calcinaro, F., Bradley, B. J., Bruchlim, I., et al.: Effect of adjuvant therapy on development of diabetes in mouse and man. Lancet, *343*:706, 1994.
31. Singer, D. E., Moulton, A. W., and Nathan, D. M.: Diabetic myocardial infarction: Interaction of diabetes with other preinfarction risk factors. Diabetes, *38*:350, 1989.
32. Solomon, R., Werner, C., Mann, D., D'Elia, J., et al.: Effects of saline, mannitol, and furosemide on acute decreases in renal function induced by radiocontrast agents. N. Engl. J. Med., *331*:1416, 1994.
33. Stonebridge, P. A., and Murie, J. A.: Infrainguinal revascularization in the diabetic patient. Br. J. Surg., *80*:1237, 1993.
34. Sutherland, D. E. R.: Pancreas transplants. Br. J. Surg., *81*:2, 1994.
35. Taskinen, M-R.: Quantitative and qualitative lipoprotein abnormalities in diabetes mellitus. Diabetes, *41*(Suppl. 2):12, 1992.
36. Valdovinos, M. A., Camilleri, M., and Zimmerman, B. R.: Chronic diarrhea in diabetes mellitus: Mechanisms and an approach to diagnosis and treatment. Mayo Clin. Proc., *68*:691, 1993.
37. Viberti, G., Mogensen, C. E., Groop, L. C., Pauls, J. F., et al.: Effect of captopril on progression to clinical proteinuria in patients with insulin-dependent diabetes mellitus and microalbuminuria. JAMA, *271*:275, 1994.
38. Wang, P. H., Lau, J., and Chalmers, T. C.: Meta-analysis of effects of intensive blood-glucose control on late complications of type I diabetes. Lancet, *341*:1306, 1993.
39. Williams, G.: Management of non-insulin-dependent diabetes mellitus. Lancet, *343*:95, 1994.

CHAPTER 11

ANESTHESIA AND POSTOPERATIVE ANALGESIA

Mark E. Dentz, M.D., Katherine P. Grichnik, M.D., Karen S. Sibert, M.D., and J. G. Reves, M.D.

THE ROLE OF THE ANESTHESIOLOGIST IN THE CARE OF THE SURGICAL PATIENT

The anesthesiologist, like the surgeon, has a critical role in caring for the patient undergoing a surgical procedure. This care covers the preoperative, the operative, and the postoperative periods. Comprehensive preoperative evaluation is vital to the safe delivery of anesthetic care. The patient's history and physical examination, a review of medication use, laboratory values, electrocardiograms, radiographs, and consultative notes must all be carefully scrutinized. Considerations unique to the anesthesiologist include the history of prior anesthetics with any associated complications, review of anatomy for the placement of vascular catheters or regional anesthetics, and examination of the head and airway to predict difficulty with intubation. The anesthesiologist must then integrate the considerations unique to a particular surgical procedure with the patient's preoperative status to formulate an anesthetic care plan. It is the responsibility of the anesthesiologist, with the surgeon, to ensure that the patient is ready for a surgical procedure.

Once the preoperative evaluation is complete, the anesthesiologist's role is then to provide the anesthesia and analgesia suitable for a particular patient and a particular surgical procedure. This may be as simple as providing sedation for a procedure done under local anesthesia or as complex as providing anesthesia for a critically ill patient, with management of invasive monitoring. This intraoperative period starts with assumption of the patient's care immediately before operation. Intraoperative care includes placement of vascular catheters and invasive monitors, placement of catheters for postoperative analgesia, induction and maintenance of anesthesia, determination of the postoperative disposition of the patient, and, if indicated, management of emergence from anesthesia. The intraoperative responsibility for the care of the surgical patient continues until the patient's care is turned over to another physician after the surgical procedure. This may occur in a postoperative care unit, an ambulatory care unit, an intensive care unit, or a postsurgical ward.

Postoperatively, anesthesiologists remain vital to the care of the surgical patient. Many anesthesiologists assume postoperative care for surgical patients in the intensive care setting, including pediatric, neonatal, surgical, neurosurgical, and cardiothoracic intensive care units. Furthermore, anesthesiologists care for the average surgical patient through postoperative pain management and respiratory care services.

Adjunctive care of hospitalized patients, an important part of an anesthesiologist's job, includes care of patients during procedures outside of the operating suite, care of patients for radiologic procedures or hyperbaric medicine, and care of the patient with chronic pain. Additionally, the skills of the anesthesiologist are often required to manage patients who suffer cardiopulmonary arrests.[3]

An anesthesiologist's job is comprehensive, sharing the responsibility for patient outcome. Preoperative, intraoperative, and postoperative skills are needed as part of the medical team providing care for the surgical patient.

PREOPERATIVE ASSESSMENT AND ANESTHETIC RISK

Thanks to advances in anesthetic pharmacology and in physiologic monitoring, most patients safely undergo anesthesia and operations today who would never have been subjected to operation in decades past because of severe underlying medical disease. The challenge for the anesthesiologist is to function as the patient's internist in the perioperative period as well as to provide anesthesia safely during the operation. During the preoperative assessment, the anesthesiologist's goal is to determine whether the patient's underlying medical problems are under the best possible control and management. If not, optimal management should be implemented before anesthesia and the operation. At the point where the patient's condition cannot be improved further, the anesthesiologist devises the best possible plan of care, taking into account the needed surgical procedure, the patient's medical problems, and the multiple possible interactions between the patient's current medications and the drugs needed during the anesthetic. Although consultants may be highly beneficial, ensuring that cardiac, pulmonary, and other underlying medical problems are managed to best effect, the final responsibility for determining the patient's readiness for anesthesia belongs to the anesthesiologist.

During the preoperative interview with the patient, the anesthesiologist obtains all pertinent information that will give him or her a complete portrait of the patient's physical health status, level of anxiety, and specific risk factors for complications from anesthesia. The anesthesiologist asks about symptoms of underlying cardiopulmonary disease or other major organ system problems and seeks information about previous anesthetic complications the patient or a direct relative may have sustained. Physical examination focuses on the airway, heart, and lungs, looking for evidence of respiratory infection, congestive failure, or any previously unrecognized disease, and on any factors that could render airway management and intubation difficult, such as morbid obesity, restricted jaw mobility, a recessed chin, or cervical spine disease. Instructions are given to the patient about whether to take or abstain from routine medications and about the amount of time during which oral intake should be avoided before the operation. At its best, the preanesthetic interview allows the patient and anesthesiologist to establish a personal rapport that facilitates the discussion of the risks and benefits of different types of anesthesia and provides the patient with the education necessary to give a truly informed consent.

The planned surgical procedure is the major determinant in assessing an individual patient's risk for perioperative complications and in deciding which anesthetic technique—local anesthesia alone or with sedation, regional anesthesia, or general anesthesia—is most appropriate. Good communication between the surgeon and the anesthesiologist is vital; the surgeon knows better than anyone else the extent of the planned operation, the time required, and whether the patient has any fears or preferences that might alter the anesthetic plan. For example, an inguinal herniorrhaphy may be performed under general, spinal, epidural, or even local anesthesia, and each technique has advantages and disadvantages. If the surgeon contends that the hernia is recurrent and may take a long time and be difficult to repair, the anesthesiologist considers these problems in suggesting options for anesthesia and in selecting drugs with a longer duration of action for use during the case. A history of previous nausea and vomiting under general anesthesia may make the choice of a spinal or epidural anesthetic more attractive, but the presence of a cardiac condition such as aortic stenosis could favor local anesthesia with sedation, which would confer greater hemodynamic stability. Consultants in other fields usually are not fully aware of the anesthetic implications of medical illnesses; numerous cases have occurred in which a medical consultant has *cleared* a patient and has recommended, for example, a spinal anesthetic that in fact would be contraindicated in the case of active infection or coagulopathy. The role of the medical consultant, then, is to assess the patient from a medical perspective, not to prescribe an anesthetic. Regardless of underlying health risk, there is no alternative to general anesthesia with endotracheal intubation for many procedures involving the airway, the thorax, or the head and neck. Some adult patients and virtually all small children will be unable to cooperate for a surgical procedure under any condition other than general anesthesia. The anesthesiologist's specialized training enables him or her to take all these factors into account during preoperative assessment to plan safe anesthetic care for the patient and optimal operating conditions for the surgeon.

The American Society of Anesthesiologists (ASA) has adopted a five-point evaluation scale for preoperative physical status, which helps provide an overall stratification of the patient's risk for anesthetic morbidity and mortality.[32] Each patient's ASA classification summarizes the patient's degree of illness before anesthesia and also assesses the increased risk inherent in unplanned, emergency procedures. The following is a description of the ASA scale:

ASA Class 1. The patient is healthy with no systemic disease, and the pathologic process for which operation is to be performed is localized. *Example:* a fit patient to undergo knee arthroscopy.

ASA Class 2. There is mild to moderate systemic disturbance caused either by the condition to be treated surgically or by pathophysiologic processes. *Examples:* mild diabetes, smoking, essential hypertension, or anemia. Extremes of youth or age are often included in this category, as is pregnancy.

ASA Class 3. The patient either has multiple-system disease or well-controlled major system disease. *Examples:* chronic obstructive lung disease, chronic stable angina; or a combination of related problems, such as obesity, diabetes, and hypertension.

ASA Class 4. The patient has a severe systemic disorder that is already life threatening and may not be correctable by operation. *Examples:* congestive heart failure, unstable angina, advanced degrees of pulmonary or hepatic insufficiency, major trauma.

ASA Class 5. The patient is already moribund, with little chance of survival, but is submitted to operation in desperation. *Examples:* ruptured abdominal aneurysm, major cerebral trauma, massive pulmonary embolism. In some cases, the patient may have been relatively healthy before the catastrophic event that led to the current medical condition.

Emergency Operation (E). Any patient in one of the classes just listed who undergoes operation in an emergency situation is considered to be in poorer physical condition, and the operation confers an additional degree of risk. *Examples:* an inguinal hernia that is incarcerated with symptoms of bowel obstruction, or an acute appendix, in an otherwise healthy patient, who would then be classified 1E.

Questions are often raised, by both surgeons and patients, concerning the chance of survival or the risk involved in undergoing anesthesia. Although it is difficult to separate the risks of anesthesia from those of the operation, most studies have suggested that approximately one death per 10,000 anesthetics is totally attributable to anesthesia, and approximately two deaths per 10,000 anesthetics are either totally or in major part due to anesthesia management. The major risks of anesthesia include allergic drug reactions, failure to intubate or otherwise provide adequate oxygenation and ventilation, nerve damage, and malignant hyperthermia (a potentially fatal hypermetabolic syndrome induced by certain anesthetic drugs). The morbidity and mortality from major regional anesthetics (spinal and epidural) do not differ substantially from those of general anesthesia. Morbid events that occur after operation and anesthesia include myocardial infarction, stroke, and pulmonary embolism. The mortality rates for patients in ASA Class 4 and 5 are much higher, ranging in different studies from 7% to 50%. However, because far fewer anesthetics are administered to patients in ASA Class 4 and 5, the overall mortality statistics (1–2 deaths per 10,000 anesthetics) reflect the real risk to relatively healthy patients. This risk should be considered in the context of the overall mortality after surgery, which is 0.6%, or 60 deaths per 10,000 surgical patients, within the first 6 postoperative days.[12, 24]

Preoperative Evaluation and Testing

A dramatic change has occurred in the practice of medicine in the United States over the past 10 years, as the volume of ambulatory surgery has increased steadily and the custom of admitting healthy elective patients to the hospital the night before surgical procedures has been nearly abandoned. At Duke University Medical Center, patients now are admitted on the day of their operation even for complex procedures such as lung resection, total joint replacement, and cardiac surgery. The need for an organized approach to preoperative assessment becomes critical when the entire work-up must be managed on an outpatient basis, and insurance carriers are increasingly reluctant to pay for batteries of tests without documented benefit. To balance patient safety against the need to control health care costs, anesthesiologists and surgeons must work in tandem to evaluate preoperative patients in the most cost-effective manner. The former standard of practice, in which the intern or resident ordered a complete blood cell count, chemistry panel, coagulation profile, electrocardiogram, and chest radiograph on every patient, is no longer acceptable. Instead, only those tests should be ordered that contribute directly to evaluation of the surgical problem or of any underlying medical condition that may affect the patient's risk for anesthetic complications.[46]

Is any laboratory test mandatory before anesthesia and the operation? At Duke University, the answer is an unequivocal *no.* The history and physical examination, together with knowledge of the planned surgical procedure, should guide the ordering of preoperative tests. Unnecessary testing may harm the patient, because invasive studies (with the risk of serious complications) may be ordered to investigate false-positive results from the original tests.[36] The ordering of unnecessary tests also carries a liability risk for the responsible physician, who has a duty to follow up on any abnormal result no matter how insignificant it may seem. Thus, no preoperative testing would be indicated for the healthy young male patient who presents for elective repair of an inguinal hernia, and many female patients of menstruating age require only a preoperative hematocrit. In the authors' hospital, a hematocrit is checked routinely on infants younger than the age of 6 months to rule out anemia, but there is no minimal requirement for preoperative testing in healthy older infants and children. Electrolytes are obtained only with an indication, such as the use of diuretic medications or a history of renal insufficiency, and coagulation profiles are ordered only if there is a history of abnormal bleeding or if the surgical procedure may involve major blood loss or intraoperative anticoagulation. A preoperative electrocardiogram and chest radiograph is required only in the patient who is 60 years of age or older, unless there is a positive indication from the patient's history or physical examination (Table 11–1).

The Anesthesiologist as Consultant

Patient care is served best when the anesthesiologist and surgeon collaborate in their efforts preoperatively as well as during operation. A collegial relationship between the anesthesiology and surgery teams prevents miscommunication, ill feelings, and potentially disastrous clinical errors. Anesthesiologists are pleased to serve as a resource at any time, whether a quick telephone call can help settle a clinical question, or full consultant expertise is required to plan the preoperative evaluation and management of a patient with complex medical problems. The anesthesiologist should be viewed by the surgeon as a partner in patient care as well as an operating room medical consultant.

MONITORING

Monitoring of a patient's physiologic functions during surgical procedures is one of the primary responsibilities of the anesthesiologist. Historically, this has been accomplished by qualitative measurements. Inspection of the surgical field, palpation of the pulse, percussion of the lungs, and auscultation of the heart and breath sounds all provide subjective data on the condition of the patient. Today, electronic monitors objectively measure various organ systems. The purpose of physiologic monitoring is twofold: (1) it provides a record of intraoperative events for comparison before future surgery and (2) it enables the surgeon and anesthesiologist to optimize the patient's current care to allow appropriate therapeutic intervention.[49]

Routine Monitors. The standards for basic intraoperative monitoring, as stated by the ASA, require that the patient's ventilation, circulation, oxygenation, and temperature be evaluated continually during all anesthetics. Precordial and esophageal stethoscopes record the level and effectiveness of ventilation, heart sounds, and early signs of cardiac rhythm changes. The circulation is assessed by intermittent blood pressure measurements and a continuous electrocardiogram. Although blood pressure can be determined by sphygmomanometry, it is usually measured by an oscillotomometric device (automatic noninvasive blood pressure cuff). The electrocardiogram assesses cardiac dysrhythmias (lead II) and/or myocardial ischemia (lead V_5). The pulse oximeter pro-

TABLE 11–1. Department of Anesthesiology Guidelines for Preoperative Testing

Preoperative Conditions	HGB M	HGB F	WBC	PT/ PTT	PLT, BT	Elect	Creat/ BUN	Blood-Glucose	AST/Alk Phos	X-ray	ECG	Pregnancy	T/S
Surgical procedure													
With blood loss	X	X											X
Without blood loss													
Neonates	X	X											
Age 6 mo–13 yr.													
13–40 yr.	X												
40–59 yr.	X										±		
≥60 yr.	X	X									X		
Cardiovascular disease							X			X	X		
Pulmonary disease										X	X		
Malignancy	X	X	*	*						X			
Radiation therapy			X										
Hepatic disease	X	X		X		X	X		X				
Exposure to hepatitis									X				
Renal disease	X	X				X	X				X		
Bleeding disorder	X	X		X	X								
Diabetes						X	X	X			X		
Smoking ≥20 pk.-yr. history	X	X								X	±		
Possible pregnancy												X	
Diuretic use						X	X						
Digoxin use						X	X				X		
Steroid use						X		X					
Anticoagulant use	X	X		X									

Note: Not all diseases are included in this table. Please use your own judgment on patients with diseases not included.

Symbols: ±, maybe; *, leukemias only; X, obtain.

Abbreviations: HGB, hemoglobin; PT, prothrombin time; PTT, partial thromboplastin time; PLT, platelet count; BT, bleeding time; Elect, Na$^+$, K$^+$, Cl$^-$, CO$_2$; Creat/BUN, creatinine or blood urea nitrogen, plasma/serum; AST, aspartate aminotransferase; Alk Phos, alkaline phosphatase, serum; T/S, blood typing and screen for unexpected antibodies. The test results are acceptable for 6 months, unless the patient's underlying disease would dictate that testing be repeated closer to the scheduled procedure; chest radiographs and electrocardiograms taken within the past 1 year are acceptable if they were normal and the patient has no cardiorespiratory abnormality.

vides beat-to-beat information on systemic oxygenation and heart rate. Skin, rectal, nasal, or esophageal temperature probes permit intervention to maintain normothermia for optimal physiologic performance.

Special Monitors. Depending on the surgical procedure and the physical status of the patient, specialized monitors may be required to assess specific organ systems.

Cardiovascular. Continuous intra-arterial pressure monitoring allows constant measurement of the blood pressure as well as access for blood gas sampling. The potential for myocardial ischemia is often monitored by ST-segment analysis. A central venous catheter or a pulmonary artery catheter is indicated for patients whose cardiovascular system requires accurate assessment. Also, the incorporation of mixed venous oxygen saturation ($S\bar{v}O_2$) to pulmonary artery catheters may help predict physiologic problems. Decreases in $S\bar{v}O_2$ may reveal early detection of cardiac decompensation, acidosis, cellular injury, light anesthesia, or reduced oxygen-carrying capacity. Increases in $S\bar{v}O_2$ can warn of sepsis, physiologic or anatomic shunting, hypothermia, or catheter malfunction. Finally, transesophageal echocardiography may be useful in patients who might benefit from intraoperative evaluation of myocardial performance, valvular status, ventricular filling, and regional wall myocardial function.[18]

Pulmonary. End-tidal carbon dioxide measurement (capnography) gives valuable information on the effectiveness of ventilation as well as certain disease states, such as chronic obstructive pulmonary disease and pulmonary embolism. For general anesthesia, the use of capnography and pulse oximetry has become so prevalent that they can be considered routine monitors. Inspired gases are often monitored with an oxygen analyzer to prevent delivery of hypoxic gas mixtures. Changes in peak airway pressure, tidal volume, expiratory time, and minute ventilation may indicate abnormal pulmonary physiology. These variables, which are usually connected to pressure and/or volume alarm systems, may warn of ventilation disconnection, endotracheal tube kinking, and partial or total obstruction.

Neurologic. Monitoring of the electroencephalogram may allow the early diagnosis of potentially reversible brain ischemia or injury, while motor- and sensory-evoked potential monitoring permits on-line analysis of spinal cord integrity. Loss of electroencephalographic or evoked potential activity should alert the physician that an intervention is necessary to prevent permanent neurologic damage. Intracranial pressure monitoring may also serve this purpose. Assessment of such variables as cerebral blood flow, cerebral perfusion pressure, and cerebral blood oxygenation may have a role in monitoring the central nervous system (CNS) as rapidly evolving technology improves.

Other Organ Systems. Bladder catheterization (urine output) is the most practical method to monitor the renal system during the operation. The coagulation system can be assessed through a variety of laboratory tests as well as intraoperative use of thromboelastography. Finally, metabolic and electrolyte abnormalities can be followed by arterial blood gas and chemistry analysis.

Complications. Specialized monitoring provides useful physiologic data to aid the physician in minute-to-minute management of the patient. Nevertheless, these monitors have risks. Arterial cannulation may cause blood vessel perforation, infection, and thrombogenesis, although it occurs rarely. The most frequent complications from central venous and pulmonary artery catheters occur with placement and include cardiac arrhythmias, pneumothorax, hemothorax, nerve injury, and hematoma and, after placement, vessel injury. Because of complications, the use of specialized monitors should be based on the patient's condition, in an attempt to optimize the risk-benefit ratio.

ANESTHETIC DRUG PHARMACOLOGY

A variety of drugs may be used to provide anesthesia. Anesthesia groups include intravenous (including neuromuscular blockade), inhalational, and local. The surgeon should be familiar with some aspects of the pharmacology of these drug groups. Anesthesiologists use knowledge of pharmacokinetics (the absorption, distribution, biotransformation, and excretion of drugs) and pharmacodynamics (effects and mechanism of action of drugs) as the basis for selecting a drug for a particular patient.

Intravenous Drugs

Intravenous anesthetic drugs are used to induce and maintain general anesthesia, and some are employed perioperatively for sedation and analgesia (Table 11–2). With general anesthesia the objective is to provide unconsciousness, amnesia, analgesia, and usually muscle relaxation.

Pharmacodynamics. The pharmacodynamic properties of intravenous drugs are established by relating the possibility of response to drug level. This approach is used to calculate the effective dose (ED). The ED_{50}, or concentration producing the desired response in 50% of patients, is used to compare potency of intravenous anesthetics. The time to reach effect is also computed and is important in deciding which drug to use for induction.

Hypnosis (Unconsciousness) and Amnesia. Drugs that produce sleep are hypnotics. Among the most commonly used hypnotics in anesthesia are thiopental, midazolam, etomidate, propofol, and ketamine. Except for ketamine, none of these drugs produces analgesia, so they must be given with analgesic drugs to produce satisfactory anesthesia. They are also devoid of muscle paralysis properties and therefore must be supplemented with neuromuscular blocking drugs if muscle relaxation is required. In general, hypnotics produce a dose-related effect on the CNS that reflects the plasma/brain equilibrium; however, the dose-response relationship varies widely among individuals. Benzodiazepines (diazepam, lorazepam, and midazolam) are very specific amnestic drugs. They produce dose-related amnesia that can persist for hours after administration. Benzodiazepines can be antagonized with a specific antagonist, flumazenil.[19]

Analgesia. Analgesic drugs block pain stimuli and thereby protect against the physiologic responses to noxious stimuli and other stresses. Opioids such as morphine, meperidine, fentanyl, sufentanil, alfentanil, and remifentanil maintain analgesia during surgical procedures and in the postoperative period. As anesthetic drugs, the opioids are not reliable hypnotics or amnestics, and thus require supplemental hypnotics or inhalation anesthetics. Like the hypnotics, opioids have a wide interindividual dose-response as well as a ceiling effect in some patients (giving more drug does not produce greater analgesia).

Muscle Relaxants. Muscle relaxants facilitate endotracheal intubation, provide the surgeon with optimal working conditions during anesthesia, and optimize mechanical ventilator support in some patients. Because the neuromuscular block-

TABLE 11–2. Doses of Commonly Used Sedatives

Drug	Loading Dose (μg./kg.)	Maintenance Infusion (μg./kg./min.)
Midazolam	10–50	0.10–0.50
Ketamine	500–750	10–15
Propofol	200–500	10–50
Methohexital	200–500	10–50

ers do not produce analgesia, sedation, or amnesia, they cannot substitute for other supportive care in the potentially conscious patient. Therefore, muscle paralysis should not be induced without sedation or general anesthesia.

Mechanism of Action and Classification. The drugs are classified as either *depolarizing* or *nondepolarizing,* depending on their mechanism of block. A depolarizing neuromuscular blocker mimics the neural transmitter acetylcholine and produces changes in sustained membrane permeability that prevent further depolarization of the postsynaptic membrane until the drug dissipates. Onset of muscle paralysis is very rapid. The nondepolarizing blockers are competitive antagonists that prevent acetylcholine binding and subsequent depolarization. Because of the relative excess of receptors, more than 70% of them must be blocked before there is clinically significant muscle weakness. The onset of nondepolarizers is slow compared with depolarizers, often requiring several minutes for the full paralyzing effect. These relaxants also exhibit characteristic responses to electrical nerve stimulation: diminished twitch response, fade during tetany, posttetanic potentiation, and reversibility with anticholinesterases.

Administration Guidelines. Succinylcholine, the prototypic depolarizing neuromuscular blocker, is metabolized principally by plasma cholinesterase. Succinylcholine's rate of metabolism is rapid but may be reduced by a loss of effective hydrolysis enzyme in severe liver disease or by genetically atypical plasma cholinesterase. This may create unexpected prolongation in neuromuscular blockade. Because of this and other potential side effects (bradycardia, hypotension, dysrhythmias, hyperkalemia, postoperative myalgia, increased intracranial pressure, malignant hyperthermia), succinylcholine is not recommended for routine use except during anesthetic induction and for specific clinical situations.

The nondepolarizing blockers undergo hepatic and/or renal degradation leading to their elimination and return of muscle function. Many factors can alter drug distribution, metabolism, and elimination, creating potentially wide variability in dosing requirements and cautions. These factors include renal disease, hepatic disease, protein binding, age, temperature, and concomitant drugs. Table 11–3 lists commonly used relaxants and their frequently recommended doses.

The specific drugs, when compared, may have advantages and/or disadvantages as relaxants. The major differences between the nondepolarizers involve duration of block (intermediate versus long-acting), mechanism(s) of metabolism and clearance, and autonomic side effects. Pancuronium provides an excellent long-acting state of muscle relaxation but may increase heart rate, especially if administered rapidly or in large doses. Atracurium has a unique mechanism of metabolism, Hoffman degradation, which occurs at a predictable *in vivo* rate so that clearance of the drug is unaltered even in the presence of severe hepatic or renal disease.[54] Vecuronium has the lowest autonomic side effect profile and produces little hemodynamic alteration.

Muscle Relaxant Reversal. The depolarizing relaxants cannot be pharmacologically reversed. Patients with a prolonged effect may improve with intravenous enzyme administration through a plasma transfusion. However, sedation and ventilatory support until the drug is metabolized is generally sufficient.

The nondepolarizing relaxants can be reversed once the patient has recovered partial neuromuscular function. Anticholinesterase drugs (e.g., neostigmine, physostigmine, pyridostigmine, edrophonium) inhibit the acetylcholinesterase enzyme and permit accumulation of the acetylcholine at the postsynaptic junction. Acetylcholine competitively displaces residual nondepolarizing muscle relaxants. Potential problems in routine reversal of nondepolarizing drugs may complicate the clinical situation. Anticholinesterases increase ganglionic neural transmission, thus necessitating the usual concomitant administration of an anticholinergic drug. If the duration of action of the competitive reversal agent is shorter than the duration of the muscle relaxant, unexpected postreversal weakness and potential muscle paralysis can occur. Properly administered and monitored, however, nondepolarizing relaxants and reversal agents can provide periods of optimal relaxation.[51]

Pharmacokinetics. A drug is eliminated from the blood by redistribution, biotransformation, and excretion. Major factors that are important in determining the pharmacokinetic fate of drugs are tissue solubility of the drug and hepatic and renal metabolism (clearance) of the drug. To maintain therapeutic levels of intravenous drugs, continuous infusion of the drugs is the most appropriate method of delivery.[26] The termination of an intravenous anesthetic action after a single-bolus administration is due to the distribution of the drug from the blood and well-perfused tissues, such as the brain, to other less well-perfused tissues, such as muscle and fat. Drugs with high tissue solubility disappear from the blood rapidly and have a short context-sensitive half-time (time for drug level to decrease 50%)[31] (Fig. 11–1). The context-sensitive half-time increases for each drug with the duration of infusion. This information is necessary in considering the choice of drug as well as anticipating the need for redosing and estimating awakening. Drugs with short half-times are used for short operations and those with long half-times are more appropriate for longer surgical procedures or for prolonged sedation postoperatively.

Inhalation Drugs

Specific Inhalation Anesthetics. Contemporary inhalation anesthesia includes the use of four drugs: the volatile liquids halothane, enflurane, and isoflurane, and the inert gas nitrous oxide (N_2O). Sevoflurane and desflurane are new volatile anesthetics, and their place in anesthesia is not yet established. The physical properties of these anesthetic gases determine how they are supplied, influence the systems involved in their administration, and, most important, influence uptake and distribution in the body. The laws of physics governing diffusion, solubility, differential partial pressures, and temperature underline the differences in pharmacologic effects and clinical use of these anesthetics. Nevertheless, all inhalational anesthetics produce varying degrees of unconsciousness, amnesia, analgesia, and muscle relaxation.

TABLE 11–3. Neuromuscular Blocking Drug Pharmacology and Dosing

Drug	Initial Dose (mg./kg.)	Expected Duration (min.)
Depolarizer		
Succinylcholine	1–1.5	3–5
Nondepolarizer		
D-Tubocurarine	0.5	60–90
Pancuronium	0.07–0.1	45–90
Atracurium	0.2–0.4	30–45
Vecuronium	0.1–0.2	30–45
Mivacurium	0.1–0.13	8–10
Pipecuronium	0.05–0.15	80+*
Doxacurium	0.04–0.06	80+*

*Follow neuromuscular blockade depth with twitch monitor.

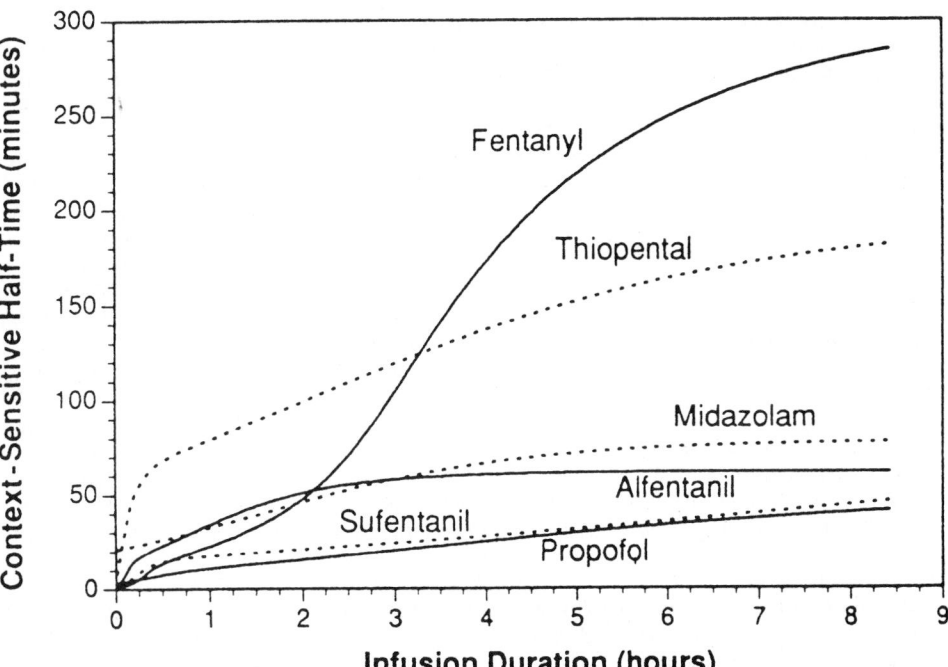

Figure 11–1. Context-sensitive half-times (time for drug blood level to decrease 50% with cessation of infusion) as a function of infusion duration for each of the pharmacokinetic models simulated. Solid and dashed line patterns are used only to permit overlapping lines to be distinguished. Note that each drug tends to accumulate with duration of infusion but that each drug has a different pattern. (From Hughes, M., Jacobs, J., and Glass, P.: Context-sensitive half-times in multi-compartment pharmacokinetic models for intravenous anesthetic drugs. Anesthesiology, 76:334, 1992.)

Uptake and Distribution. The inhalation anesthetics rely on the respiratory tract for entry and elimination from the body. Although the precise mechanism for the action of inhalation agents is not completely understood, it is clear that the primary site of action is within the CNS.[21] Thus, an adequate partial pressure of drug in the brain is required for anesthesia. The brain and other tissues in the body equilibrate with the partial pressure of the anesthetic drug delivered to them by arterial blood. The partial pressure of the inhalation drug in blood, in turn, is determined by the alveolar partial pressure. Because the alveolar partial pressure governs the partial pressure of anesthetic in all body tissues, including the brain, the relationship between inspired and alveolar anesthetic partial pressures is an important first step in producing an anesthetic state.[21]

Three factors determine the rate at which alveolar anesthetic tension rises toward the concentration of the anesthetic being inspired: (1) increasing the inspired tension of the anesthetic directly increases delivery of the drug and increases alveolar anesthetic tension; (2) increasing the minute ventilation promotes increased alveolar anesthetic tension; and (3) changing the physical characteristics of the breathing system (e.g., the volume of the breathing circuit) may alter the alveolar anesthetic tension. Additional factors that influence the level of alveolar anesthetic tension and ultimately general anesthesia can be observed in the relationship between alveolar and blood anesthetic partial pressure. Decreased removal of anesthetic by the blood promotes an increase in alveolar anesthetic tension and a greater anesthetic effect. Decreased removal may occur through a decrease in cardiac output, a decrease in alveolar-venous anesthetic gradient, or a decrease in solubility of the specific anesthetic agent. Conversely, increased cardiac output, use of a very soluble drug, or a large alveolar-venous anesthetic gradient promotes increased removal of the drug into the bloodstream, limiting the alveolar anesthetic tension build-up. Under the latter conditions this delays the anesthetic effect.

The factors that govern the rate at which alveolar anesthetic concentration rises during the induction of anesthesia also apply to the emergence from anesthesia. Recovery from anesthesia is triggered by the elimination of the anesthetic from the brain by reversing the pressure gradient process. The anesthetic is removed through the differential gradient from brain to blood to alveoli that is created when the inspired concentration is reduced to zero. As ventilation reduces the concentration of anesthetic from alveoli, an anesthetic partial pressure gradient develops from the returning venous blood to the alveoli. This gradient drives the anesthetic into the alveoli, where it can be removed. Ultimately this reversal of gradient decreases the partial pressure of anesthetic in the brain and permits recovery.[21] Therefore, induction, maintenance, and recovery from inhalation anesthesia are controlled by alterations in the inspired concentration of the specific gas.

Pharmacodynamics. As with intravenous anesthetic drugs, it is important to assess the anesthetic potency of inhalation agents. The concept of minimum alveolar concentration (MAC) was developed as an index of anesthetic potency that facilitated the comparison of pharmacodynamic properties of all the inhalation anesthetic agents.[21] MAC is the anesthetic concentration at 1 atmosphere of pressure that produces immobility to a noxious stimulus in 50% of subjects. Because MAC is measured at equilibrium between inspired and alveolar concentrations, the alveolar concentration and brain partial pressures are assumed to be equal. Therefore, MAC represents the anesthetic concentration at the anesthetic site of action. Measurements of MAC indicate that patient susceptibility to inhalation anesthetics is not altered significantly by gender, duration of anesthesia, metabolic alkalosis or acidosis, respiratory acidosis, anemia, or hypertension. However, increased susceptibility to anesthetic effects occurs with hypercarbia, hypoxemia, increasing age, decreasing body temperature, and exposure to other CNS depressants. Specifically, opioids, benzodiazepines, and the barbiturates decrease the amount of inhalation anesthetic required because they depress the CNS. The ultimate clinical criterion for appropriate anesthetic depth is the patient's unique response to the balance between anesthetic-induced CNS depression and surgical stimulation.

Pharmacokinetics. All the potent inhalation anesthetic agents undergo some biotransformation in the liver.[10] Under normal circumstances, the biotransformation of these agents is minimal and safe because an oxidative reaction forms nontoxic, inert metabolites. However, hepatic necrosis may develop after the administration of halothane, enflurane, or isoflurane through a chance combination of events, which include genetic background, exposure to other drugs, reduced hepatic blood flow or hypoxia, the dose or molecular structure of the agent, and certain properties promoting retention of anesthetic in tissues.

Local Anesthetics

The local anesthetics are widely used to provide anesthesia for localized surgical procedures as well as to produce regional anesthesia (spinal, epidural, caudal, nerve block, intravenous or Bier block). Their specific membrane-altering properties also explain the use of many drugs with local anesthetic properties to treat cardiac dysrhythmias.

Like the neuromuscular blocking drugs, local anesthetics interfere with neural transmission to produce their effects, although by different mechanisms. Local anesthetics act within the nerve membrane, where they inhibit transmission of nerve impulses by reducing sodium membrane permeability and the displacement of ionized calcium. Thus the threshold potential for depolarization activation is not reached, and an action potential is not conducted. The duration of action is proportional to the time the anesthetic is in direct contact with the nerve fiber. Subsequent recovery of conduction occurs spontaneously. These drugs produce no permanent structural damage to neural tissue and can produce both sensory and motor block.

All local anesthetics consist of a hydrophobic region (usually an aromatic ring) and a hydrophilic region (usually a tertiary amine) separated by an intermediate alkyl chain. The bond of the alkyl chain with the aromatic ring is either an ester (—CO—) or an amide bond (—NHC—). Thus, these drugs are classified as esters or amides depending on their linkage. Local anesthetics are weak bases and poorly water soluble and are therefore marketed as their water-soluble, hydrochloride salts. All local anesthetics except cocaine produce peripheral vasodilation by direct relaxation of vascular smooth muscle. Epinephrine is often added to local anesthetics to produce local vasoconstriction, reduce systemic drug absorption, and, thus, maintain a high drug concentration at the injection site. The properties of local anesthetics are determined by their lipid solubility (potency), pKa (onset time), and protein binding (duration).

There are important differences in the pathways of drug metabolism for the two classes of local anesthetics, as well as differences in their potentials for producing allergic reactions and other side effects. Ester local anesthetics are metabolized by plasma cholinesterase with p-aminobenzoic acid as a metabolite. This metabolite makes esters more likely to produce allergic reactions than are amide local anesthetics, which are metabolized in the liver to multiple metabolites, none of which are particularly allergenic. Although preservative agents (e.g., methylparaben) added to ester or amide local anesthetics may cause allergic reactions, allergy from local anesthetics remains a rare event.

Administration Guidelines. The onset of anesthesia after injection of a local anesthetic depends on the site of injection, dose, concentration, characteristics of the drug, protein binding, and blood supply of the area.[16] Acidosis at the site of injection causes a greater portion of the drug to become ionized and less diffusible across cell membranes. This is consistent with poor conduction analgesia produced in an area of infection and tissue acidosis.

Local anesthetic toxicity arises from a relative or absolute overdose of the drug through inadvertent intravascular injection or excessive intravascular absorption of local anesthetic from its injection site. Local anesthetic toxicity produces toxicity of both the CNS and the cardiovascular system.[17] Fortunately, the toxicity of local anesthetics is progressive, with CNS toxicity occurring well before cardiac toxicity. CNS toxicity is manifested by lightheadedness, tinnitus, and circumoral numbness, leading to seizures. Concurrently, there may be signs of sympathetic nervous system activation as the result of increased cerebral activity. With further increases in plasma local anesthetic concentration, signs of cardiovascular toxicity can occur in the cardiac electrical system, the myocardium, and the peripheral vascular smooth muscle. Cardiac electrical effects include increases in the ratio of the effective refractory period to the action potential duration, prolonged PR and QRS intervals, AV nodal dysrhythmias, and, ultimately, sinus bradycardia and arrest. The mechanical effect of local anesthetics on cardiac muscle is one of negative inotropy, which is directly related to potency. Dosages should be adjusted based on site of injection, use of vasoconstrictors, patient comorbid disease, and volume of drug necessary (Table 11–4). Local anesthetic toxicity is prevented by having a relatively alert patient who can report onset of symptoms, by dividing doses, by aspiration for heme, and by careful needle placement. Treatment of local anesthetic toxicity involves securing an airway and establishing ventilation. Seizures may be treated with benzodiazepines or barbiturates. Cardiovascular toxicity can be treated with catecholamines, atropine, and bretylium as necessary.

ANESTHESIA TECHNIQUES

Numerous anesthesia techniques are used in the care of the surgical patient. These techniques range from the type of anesthesia chosen to specialized techniques such as acute normovolemic hemodilution. The unique considerations for different types of operations are discussed.

Types of Anesthesia

The induction of anesthesia, in general, falls into two categories: general and regional anesthesia. General anesthesia involves inducing a state of unconsciousness with analgesia, amnesia, and immobility. This goal can be accomplished with a combination of intravenous and inhalational medications. Furthermore, some degree of control of a patient's airway is usually part of the induction of a general anesthetic. Preoperatively, the anesthesiologist may choose to allay anxiety with a premedicant, usually a benzodiazepine and/or an opioid. Induction of unconsciousness is usually accomplished with a short-acting intravenous agent. Because each induction drug has a unique profile of effects, the anesthesiologist can choose a drug best suited to an individual patient. After the induction of unconsciousness, the patient is often unable to main-

TABLE 11–4. Doses and Toxic Levels of Commonly Used Local Anesthetics

	Dose (mg./kg.)	Toxic Blood Levels (μg./ml.)
Esters		
Procaine	10–12	20
Chloroprocaine	7–10	20
Tetracaine	2	1.5–4
Amides		
Lidocaine	5–7	5–10
Mepivacaine	5–7	5–10
Bupivacaine	2–4	1.5–4
Prilocaine	6–8	5–10
Etidocaine	3–5	1.5–4

tain a patent airway due to relaxation of the pharyngeal muscles. Mask ventilation is usually accomplished with positive-pressure ventilation as necessary. Depending on the surgical procedure and the patient's comorbid disease, the anesthesiologist may choose to continue mask ventilation (spontaneous or controlled), place a laryngeal mask airway,[42] or intubate the patient with cuffed or uncuffed endotracheal tube. Placement of an endotracheal tube is facilitated by the use of a neuromuscular blocking agent as well. Adequacy of ventilation and oxygenation is then established in part through assessment of breath sounds, production of end-tidal CO_2, and adequacy of pulse oximetry. Some complications of induction of general anesthesia include laryngospasm, breath holding, airway obstruction, aspiration, esophageal intubation, damage to the teeth or airway, undesirable physiologic reflexes, and cardiac ischemia.[57]

Anesthesia is maintained with intravenous drug delivery (bolus or infusion) and/or inhalational drug delivery through the ventilating circuit. Most often a combined approach is taken, with both intravenous and inhalational drugs given. Such an approach may allow the anesthesiologist to give smaller doses of individual drugs and thereby avoid their side effects. Some commonly used drugs are opioids, benzodiazepines, neuromuscular blocking agents, and inhalational agents. The drugs and combinations chosen are tailored to the patient's disease processes and the needs of the surgical procedure. The maintenance period of anesthesia involves adjusting the level of anesthesia to the surgical stimulus, monitoring vital body functions, treating abnormalities of hemodynamics or other organ function, and ensuring a quiet surgical field.

At the end of the operation the disposition of the patient is determined by the anesthesiologist in conjunction with the surgeon. If the patient is to be transferred to an intensive care unit (ICU), the anesthesiologist may elect not to allow the patient to emerge from anesthesia and may take the patient to the ICU anesthetized and with ventilation controlled. However, if the patient is to be transferred to the postanesthesia care unit (PACU) in anticipation of going home or to a ward bed, the anesthesiologist usually allows the patient to emerge from anesthesia. This involves decreasing and eliminating the anesthetic agents delivered, reversing neuromuscular blockade, and ensuring that the patient has control of vital body functions such as spontaneous ventilation, has protective airway reflexes, and can maintain stable hemodynamics. After a general anesthetic, the patient must be observed in a monitored care setting before being transferred to an ambulatory care unit or a ward bed.

Regional anesthesia is often divided into major conduction anesthesia and major nerve block. Major conduction anesthesia includes epidural and spinal anesthesia. Epidural and spinal anesthesia interrupt afferent neural impulses by depositing drugs close to the spinal cord. Epidural anesthesia is most often accomplished by epidural space cannulation and subsequent infusion of local anesthetic agents and/or opioids. The epidural space is a potential space above the dura and is identified through a loss of resistance technique with a large-bore (17- or 18-gauge) hollow needle. Anesthetic drugs may be delivered directly through the needle (a one-shot technique), or a catheter may be threaded through the needle into the epidural space. This allows incremental dosing of anesthetic agents, which can be adjusted to the length and intensity of the surgical procedure. Epidural space may be cannulated at lumbar, thoracic, or cervical levels depending on the site of the surgical procedure. The major risks of an epidural anesthetic are a spinal headache from dural puncture with a large needle, adverse hemodynamic alterations, bleeding, total spinal anesthesia, intravenous injection of local anesthetic, and minor back pain postoperatively.[15]

Spinal anesthesia involves the placement of anesthetic drugs into the subarachnoid space through puncture of the dura mater with a small-bore needle (24- to 28-gauge). Usually this allows the use of smaller (tenfold) doses of drugs than those used epidurally, a quicker onset of analgesia, and perhaps a denser block in the sacral fibers. Usually spinal anesthesia is given as a one-time bolus through a needle placed in the subarachnoid space, but catheters can be passed into this space for repetitive dosing. The major risks of a spinal anesthetic are similar to those for an epidural anesthetic but may also include cauda equina syndrome or dysrhythmias.[35, 60]

The benefits of major conduction anesthesia are multifold. Patients can control their own respiratory function, they receive less medication to achieve anesthesia, and postoperative analgesia is enhanced. Furthermore, there may be beneficial effects on respiratory function, cardiac function, release of stress hormones, coagulation, and blood loss.[56, 63]

Major nerve blockade is also a form of regional anesthesia. Many surgical procedures can be performed under nerve block. Blocks used most often are the brachial plexus blocks (interscalene, supraclavicular, and axillary) for arm and shoulder procedures, cervical plexus block for neck and carotid procedures, femoral-sciatic nerve blocks for upper and lower leg procedures, 3-in-1 nerve (femoral, obturator, and lateral femoral cutaneous nerves) blocks for upper leg procedures, popliteal fossa nerve blocks for lower leg procedures, and ankle blocks for foot procedures. In addition, paravertebral blocks may be used to perform certain upper abdominal and thoracic procedures, and retrobulbar blocks are used for eye procedures. Major nerve block has the advantage of providing profound analgesia and muscle relaxation to a limited portion of the body, allowing the patient to maintain respiratory, cardiac, and neurologic functions. Further major nerve blockade often provides prolonged postoperative analgesia (up to 24 hours of pain relief).

Anesthetic techniques may also be combined to achieve the benefits of each single technique while possibly using less of each agent. For example, epidural anesthesia may be obtained with a general anesthetic for a repeat hip replacement, and the patient will reap the benefits of the anesthesia intraoperatively and postoperatively. The general anesthetic is used because the patient may not be able to lie in the lateral position for the time necessary to perform a repeat hip replacement. This dual anesthesia keeps the patient comfortable and anesthetized for the duration of the procedure with less of the general anesthetic agents than one would have to use without concurrent epidural anesthesia.

Anesthesiologists also use techniques designed to minimize blood loss, including acute normovolemic hemodilution and hypotensive anesthesia. For acute normovolemic hemodilution an anesthesiologist phlebotomizes a portion of the patient's blood, stores it, and replaces it with a crystalloid or colloid fluid to maintain normovolemia.[53] When a patient undergoes a procedure associated with heavy blood loss, such as an operation to correct scoliosis, he or she loses less red blood cell mass during the operation because the blood lost has a lower hematocrit. Furthermore, the patient can be given his or her own blood at the end of the period of blood loss and thereby avoid homologous transfusion of blood. Similarly, hypotensive anesthesia can be induced to control mean arterial blood pressure at a level that allows the surgical team to complete difficult dissections and lose less blood. This technique is useful for clipping of cerebral artery aneurysms.[34]

ANESTHESIA FOR SPECIALIZED OPERATIONS

Anesthetic management for all specialized operations includes common concerns for patient welfare, optimal anesthesia, appropriate monitoring, and close communication with the surgeon. Below are listed certain concerns unique to various subspecialties.

Cardiac Operations

The preanesthetic evaluation focuses on the individual patient and his or her hemodynamic status. Special investigations that must be reviewed include comparison of rest and exercise electrocardiograms, echocardiography, radioisotope scanning, and cardiac catheterization with angiography. The information from these tests is both informative and prognostic and allows one to plan the type of monitors and anesthetic needed, including a postoperative plan for the patient.

Monitoring must be individualized to the preoperative condition of the patient and the anticipated surgical procedure. Minimally, a precordial stethoscope, blood pressure cuff, temperature probe urinary bladder catheter, continuous electrocardiograph with recorder and V_5 lead, continuous arterial blood pressure, and a method to determine anticoagulant activity are needed. Some patients may also require central venous pressure, pulmonary artery pressure, cardiac output, mixed venous saturation, and transesophageal echocardiographic monitoring.

No absolute indications or contraindications exist for a specific anesthetic technique for cardiac operations. Intravenous and inhalational anesthetics are used in most cases, although inhalation drugs are used less than in other types of general anesthesia because of myocardial depression.

A knowledge of cardiopulmonary bypass (CPB) is essential for the safe and effective management of extracorporeal circulation. Although a CPB pump technician actually operates the pump, the anesthesiologist must understand the CPB circuit, the oxygenators, the priming solutions used, and the various malfunctions that can occur. Before the great vessels are cannulated, intravenous anticoagulation is achieved with heparin. Serial measurements of the activated clotting time are performed before, during, and after CPB to ensure adequate anticoagulation during CPB and the reversal of anticoagulation at the end of the operation. CPB introduces a significant physiologic stress for the patient with hemodynamic alterations that may require pharmacologic intervention. The pump flow must be ensured to be adequate with no obstruction to venous return or arterial flow. Mean arterial blood pressure is usually adjusted to a range of 40 to 70 mm. Hg with the aid of various vasoactive agents. The hematocrit is generally kept at 20% or greater. Normal blood gas values are derived and maintained. An understanding of myocardial preservation and the role of temperature and cardioplegia (antegrade and retrograde) is essential.[39] The monitoring used during CPB may include serial arterial blood gas analysis (using alpha-stat),[43] in-line venous and arterial saturation, activated clotting time determinations, and various line pressure monitors.

During the rewarming phase of CPB, the anesthesiologist must evaluate the depth of anesthesia and administer additional drugs as needed, assess the hematocrit, serum potassium, and arterial blood gases, monitor the hemodynamics, and evaluate the adequacy of anticoagulation. Before CPB is discontinued, the core temperature should be greater than 36° C., the cardiac rhythm should be able to generate an adequate cardiac output, ventilation of the lungs should be adequate, and venting of arterial air should have been done. Preload, afterload, rate, rhythm, and ventricular contractility should be optimized with vasoactive agents as indicated. After decannulation of the major blood vessels, anticoagulation is reversed with protamine titrated to effect. Serial cardiac output, arterial blood pressure, pulmonary arterial pressure, and systemic venous saturation measurements may guide vasoactive drug therapy and transfusion requirements.

Safe transport of the patient after a cardiac operation is similar to the transport of any critically ill patient: it requires assurance of adequate ventilation and oxygenation, continuous monitoring of electrocardiogram and arterial blood pressure, and the availability of drugs and tools needed to treat an emergency during transport. Most patients are transferred to an ICU that can provide advanced circulatory and ventilatory support. The anesthesiologist must carefully relay pertinent information about the patient, including history, medications given, intraoperative course, and laboratory data, to the care team in the ICU. Most cardiac patients require a period of ventilatory support, and the decision to extubate the patient depends on mental status, hemodynamic stability, temperature, and ability to oxygenate and ventilate independently. Normal convalescence includes extubation 3 to 6 hours after operation, at which time anesthetic drug effects should be minimal.

Thoracic Operations

Patients undergoing pulmonary resection and thoracic procedures require the safe, careful preoperative evaluation that all patients coming for surgery require. Pulmonary function must be assessed especially with consideration for the amount of pulmonary tissue to be resected. The effect of the intrathoracic disease process on other physiologic systems must also be evaluated. History and physical examination should include an assessment of exercise tolerance, smoking history, symptoms of respiratory distress, determination of clubbing and cyanosis, and determination of the depth and quality of the breath sounds. Laboratory and diagnostic tests may include chest x-rays, arterial blood gas analysis, routine blood analysis, electrocardiography, sputum analysis, and flow-volume loops. Preoperatively, patients for thoracic operations must be in the best condition possible because they are at high risk for postoperative complications.[23] The process may include discontinuation of smoking, vigorous pulmonary toilet, antibiotic therapy, and bronchodilator therapy.

The anesthetic technique may be determined by the degree of respiratory dysfunction, the need to share an airway and respiratory tract, and the functional status of other organ systems, such as the cardiovascular system. Special monitoring should include arterial blood pressure and arterial blood gas analysis in addition to routine intraoperative monitors. The need for other invasive monitoring should be determined by the pathophysiology of the patient and the expected course of the operation. A variety of anesthetic techniques and agents may be used, most of which involve intubation with general anesthesia. The particular anesthetic technique may be individualized to obtain stable hemodynamics, adequate oxygenation, and ventilation and to minimize ischemia and achieve control of blood or secretions from the airway.

The need to place a double-lumen endotracheal tube (bronchial intubation) with individual lung isolation may be dictated by the underlying pathology and the type of procedure planned. The absolute indications for a double-lumen tube are to protect one lung from the other, and include ventilation with a bronchopleural fistula, massive hemorrhage from one lung, pulmonary air cyst resection, unilateral infection, and unilateral bronchopulmonary lavage. Relative indications include facilitation of surgical exposure such as for pneumonectomy,[5] upper lobectomy, and thoracic aneurysm repair. The patient's ability to tolerate one-lung ventilation is dictated by preoperative pulmonary function, the distribution of ventilation and blood flow to each lung, and the ability of an individual lung to achieve hypoxic pulmonary vasoconstriction. Methods to improve oxygenation during one-lung ventilation include the addition of continuous positive airway pressure to the deflated lung, the addition of positive end-expiratory pressure to the ventilated lung, adjustment of tidal volume and respiratory rate, control of pulmonary artery pressures, and, ultimately, clamping of the ipsilateral pulmonary artery as needed to control the absolute shunt created by one-lung ventilation. Intraoperatively, the anesthesiologist should anticipate the need to optimize oxygenation and ventilation, be wary of dysrhythmias caused by direct mechanical stimulation, watch for acid-base disturbances or ischemia, and be alert to changes in endotracheal tube position.

Postoperatively, the timing of extubation is based on the degree of preoperative pulmonary disease, the type of operation, the intraoperative course of events, and the postoperative status of the patient. Some surgical procedures may benefit from extubation shortly after the operation; for example, it is best to extubate a patient soon after a pneumonectomy to decrease the stress on the bronchial suture line caused by positive-pressure ventilation. Pain must be effectively controlled to allow patients to maintain adequate lung mechanics, to cough, and to cooperate with physical and respiratory therapy. Pain may be controlled most effectively with thoracic epidural analgesia, intercostal nerve blocks, or patient-controlled analgesia.

Vascular Operations

Patients who present for vascular operations often have a multitude of underlying medical problems that must be addressed in conjunction with the assessment for the operation. Most patients have cardiopulmonary disease, peripheral vascular disease, extensive smoking histories, and perhaps renal disease. Patients present for procedures in any of three main categories: carotid operations (cerebrovascular), peripheral arterial operations (usually bypass procedures in the extremities or arterial-venous fistula placement for dialysis), and major arterial operations (abdominal aortic repairs). To care for these patients adequately, one must understand the underlying vascular disease process, the extent of the vascular disease process, and the comorbid diseases that may influence surgical and anesthetic outcome.[22, 37]

Patients presenting for carotid surgical procedures usually have had a cerebrovascular insufficiency event that led to the diagnosis.[55] Thus, a patient may present for carotid endarterectomy who has recently had a stroke or a reversible neurologic defect. However, as indications for this procedure broaden, some patients present with a high-grade stenosis or ulcerated plaque of the carotid artery in the absence of a prior neurologic event.

Common coexisting problems in this population of patients include hypertension, coronary artery disease, and smoking. It is not prudent to try to lower pre-existing hypertension before operation in a patient with a recent neurologic event because the patient may need a high blood pressure for cerebral perfusion. However, other disease processes should be controlled before operation. Preanesthetic evaluation rests on assessment of the neurologic dysfunction, examination of the surgical work-up, the extent of plaque or ulceration within the carotid artery, documentation of coexisting diseases, and examination for arterial line placement.

Monitoring is critical to the success of this operation. Most anesthesiologists place routine monitors as well as a continuous arterial line for beat-to-beat blood pressure monitoring. Neurologic monitoring may also be warranted. Communication with the surgeon is crucial to formulate an intraoperative care plan. For example, surgical plans to electively shunt across the carotid lesion may obviate the need for intraoperative neurologic monitoring, because the treatment for a

change in the electroencephalogram under anesthesia with carotid cross-clamping is to shunt and maintain adequate arterial pressure. Contrarily, if no shunting is planned unless needed, one may choose to monitor the patient with an electroencephalogram to ensure adequate cerebral blood flow during the period of carotid cross-clamping.[29] Other monitors of neurologic function include somatosensory evoked potentials, cerebral blood flow measurement, and transcranial Doppler study. It should be decided ahead of time in which arm to place the arterial line to ensure adequate vascular flow. Ideally, the arterial line should be placed in an accessible extremity in the event of a mechanical problem intraoperatively (usually the contralateral arm). The need for vasopressors and vasodilators to control blood pressure intraoperatively should be evaluated and intravenous access planned accordingly. A range of normal blood pressures for the particular patient should be sought, with plans to control blood pressure within 10% to 20% of these values.

No single anesthetic technique has proven to be superior to another. This surgical procedure can be done under local anesthesia, under regional anesthesia (cervical plexus block), or under general anesthesia. Advantages to the local and regional anesthetic techniques are that the patient can serve as his or her own cerebral function monitor and that the need for intubation, with the stress and hemodynamic changes associated with induction and emergence, is avoided. Disadvantages include difficult airway control should a seizure or loss of consciousness occur with cross-clamping, possible patient movement, and possibly more labile hemodynamics. General anesthesia obviates these problems. Intraoperatively, blood pressure must be controlled carefully with higher mean arterial pressures for the times when the carotid is cross-clamped without a shunt in place. This goal must be balanced with the needs of the patient's heart so as not to induce myocardial ischemia. The goal for any anesthetic technique is an awake, alert patient soon after the end of the procedure so that neurologic evaluation can be done quickly. At the end of the operation blood pressure is often very labile and may require multiple vasoactive interventions.

Anesthesia for peripheral vascular procedures involves many of the same considerations as for cerebrovascular operations. Preoperative considerations must include investigation of coexisting diseases, evaluation of the peripheral vascular insufficiency, and communication with the surgeon about the procedure planned and which blood vessels are to be clamped and bypassed. A thorough history and physical examination are directed toward the cardiopulmonary functions and the planned site of operation. Furthermore, should the anesthetic technique planned be a regional technique, the site for needle insertion must be examined and coagulation status determined.

Monitoring of the patient for peripheral vascular operations is guided by the extent of the underlying cardiovascular and pulmonary disease. This surgical procedure usually does not involve major artery cross-clamping nor large volume shifts. Thus, central venous catheterization should be considered in the patient with severe cardiac or pulmonary disease, but not done routinely. An arterial line is useful to monitor blood pressure carefully and allow blood to be drawn. Also in place are the standard monitors used for any surgical procedure.

The anesthetic technique may be regional or general. Regional anesthesia may confer some benefit in that the patient does not suffer the stress of intubation and emergence, postoperative pain can be relieved regionally, and some studies have shown a decrease in graft clotting with a regional technique intraoperatively and postoperatively.[9, 25, 48] These factors should be weighed against the risk of bleeding within the epidural space, because most patients are heparinized intraoperatively and perhaps postoperatively. General anesthesia confers a secure airway, a quiet surgical field, and no problems with heparinization.

Usually, clamping of peripheral arteries has no major hemodynamic consequence and does not require vasoactive drug infusion. Unclamping does require care because ischemic metabolites can transiently lower arterial blood pressure by vasodilation and perhaps myocardial depression. Postoperatively, patients must be monitored closely for graft function and cardiopulmonary status. Clotting of the grafts and myocardial ischemia are not uncommon complications.

Anesthesia for major aortic reconstructive procedures can be a challenging task for the anesthesiologist. Not only do most patients have underlying cardiac, pulmonary, cerebrovascular, and renal disease, but the operation itself may also induce adverse physiologic effects in each of these major organ systems. Preoperative evaluation must focus on improving the patient's underlying disorders in preparation for the stress of aortic cross-clamping.

Specialized monitors include continuous arterial blood pressure, central venous pressure (with pulmonary artery catheterization as necessary), and urinary catheters. Other monitors are those used for any surgical procedure. Adequate intravenous access must be ensured before the operation.

Most anesthetic techniques involve a general anesthetic with or without a regional anesthetic. Any agent or combination of agents that confers myocardial stability and optimal hemodynamics is suitable. An intimate knowledge of the physiologic consequences of aortic cross-clamping and unclamping is needed to manage intraoperative events. In brief, with aortic cross-clamping, an acute rise in afterload with increased heart work should be anticipated; the result may be myocardial ischemia or failure. With unclamping, acute hypotension can occur with an acute decrease in afterload and reperfusion of ischemic tissue. Again, myocardial ischemia can ensue. As the aorta is opened, the surgical team must also be prepared for hemorrhage, with good intravenous access and availability of blood products and/or a cell saver. Hypothermia can also become a problem with a large incision and an open abdomen; steps must be taken to prevent or manage this occurrence.

Patients are usually monitored in an intensive care setting for the first postoperative night to watch for potential complications of this procedure, including myocardial dysfunction with ischemia, renal failure, bleeding, clotting and embolization, neurologic dysfunction, pulmonary failure, and cerebrovascular accidents. If not extubated in the operating room, patients are usually extubated after they are warm and hemodynamically stable.

Neurosurgery

One must have a thorough knowledge of neurophysiology to care optimally for the patient undergoing a neurosurgical procedure. This includes knowledge of cerebral blood flow, intracranial pressure control, the dynamics of CNS injury, and specialized airway management. Of particular importance is awareness of the effects of various disease states and drugs on cerebral circulation and intracranial pressure.

The intracranial contents include brain tissue, cerebral blood volume, and cerebrospinal fluid (CSF). These contents together are incompressible, so an increase in pressure or volume of one of the contents affects the other two. The translocation of CSF to extracranial areas serves as a major mechanism for volume equilibration with brain expansion. After this mechanism is exhausted, intracranial pressure rises rapidly, with small changes in volume causing large changes in pressure. To limit rises in intracranial pressure, it is neces-

sary to reduce cerebral blood flow and thus cerebral blood volume. Determinants of cerebral blood flow include arterial carbon dioxide (PCO_2) and oxygen (PO_2) tensions, systemic arterial pressure, and temperature.[41] Increasing PCO_2 increases cerebral blood flow, and decreasing PCO_2 decreases cerebral blood flow. At physiologic PO_2 tensions, there is little effect on cerebral blood flow; however, when PO_2 drops below 50 mm. Hg, cerebral blood flow increases. Cerebral autoregulation maintains cerebral blood flow between mean arterial blood pressures of 60 to 160 mm. Hg, with cerebral blood flow becoming linearly related to mean arterial pressure outside these limits. Other factors that may affect cerebral blood flow and intracranial pressure are head position, jugular venous obstruction, positive end-expiratory pressure, and temperature.

Management of anesthesia for neurosurgical procedures includes special attention to maneuvers that could increase or decrease intracranial pressure. Before anesthesia is activated, a plan must be formulated to control intracranial pressure. Important considerations are the absence of coughing or straining, maintenance of an adequate airway and ventilation, hyperventilation when indicated, use of agents that minimally affect cerebral blood flow, and a rapid return to consciousness at the end of the procedure. Other considerations include assessing the need for fiberoptic intubation (for patients who present in halos or with unstable cervical spines).

Induction should be rapid and smooth, possibly after voluntary hyperventilation. One must anticipate known stimulations such as endotracheal intubation, head clamping, dural opening and closing, and skin closure with adjustments in anesthetic depth. All volatile anesthetics may increase cerebral blood flow and intracranial pressure, although the effect is dose related and, in the case of isoflurane, may be prevented with hyperventilation before its use. Hyperventilation is continued when N_2O is used. Osmotherapy is used when a negative fluid balance is desirable. Isotonic solutions without glucose are preferred so that rebound cerebral edema is avoided and hyperglycemia is avoided in the event of cerebral ischemia.

During emergence, *bucking* on the endotracheal tube must be avoided. Thus, neuromuscular blockade is not reversed until the head bandage is applied and small intermittent doses of thiopental or lidocaine may be used to titrate anesthesia. In the recovery area, the patient must be observed carefully for changes in neurologic function, consciousness, hemodynamics, and urine output. When the technology is available, intracranial pressure may also be monitored. Patients recovering from anesthesia may be placed in the semisitting position, and sedatives and narcotics are avoided because most neurosurgical procedures cause minimal pain. Furthermore, these drugs may depress ventilation and thus may interfere with appropriate assessment of the patient. Postoperative problems include cerebral edema, cerebral vasospasm, intracranial hemorrhage, seizures, fluid and electrolyte disturbances, inadequate ventilation, hypertension, and fever. Rapid recognition of these problems and appropriate therapy are the cornerstones of management of the postoperative neurosurgical patient.

Anesthesia for Organ Transplantation

Commonly transplanted organs include the heart, lung, kidneys, liver, and pancreas. For each of these transplants, the anesthesia for the donor must preserve organ function, oxygenation, and perfusion. To successfully manage the anesthesia for a transplant surgical procedure, one must have a complete knowledge of the anatomy, physiology, pharmacology, and pathology of the organ being transplanted. Furthermore, the effects of that organ's dysfunction on the rest of the patient's physiology must be considered. Specialized techniques and their management, unique to each type of transplant, are also important. For example, cardiopulmonary bypass is needed with heart transplants; double-lumen tubes and strategies to manage right-sided heart failure are necessary for lung transplants; and venovenous bypass with severe metabolic, electrolyte, coagulation, and hemodynamic abnormalities must be managed in liver transplants. Anesthetics for these procedures are among the most challenging for the anesthesiologist.

Pediatric Operations

The risks of a specific anesthetic for a surgical procedure are greater for patients who are younger than age 1 year compared with the risks for older pediatric patients and adults.[11] However, in the past two decades there has been a significant reduction in perioperative morbidity and mortality among children, even those critically ill. This trend is partly due to major advances in pediatric anesthesiology with increased understanding of the physiology of the neonate, advances in clinical pharmacology of intravenous and inhalational drugs, improved hemodynamic monitoring, and significant improvements in postoperative care, including intensive care.

Management rests on the understanding that the pediatric patient differs from the adult and that the principles of adult anesthesiologic care may not apply to pediatric anesthesiology. A child's anatomy, physiology, and disease states are all different from an adult's.

The preoperative visit allows the physician not only to evaluate the child but also to prepare the child and the parent psychologically for anesthesia and operation. A standard review of systems should be done, with attention to the child's present illness and any comorbid disease that may have an effect on the anesthesia and operation. Further review of prior anesthetics, intrauterine development (if a neonate), history of prematurity, and familial diseases should be done. The physical examination should include an assessment of the patient's general health and exercise tolerance, the cardiopulmonary system, and the state of hydration. Laboratory work should be dictated by the patient's underlying disease processes and use of medication. A hemoglobin determination should be ordered for all children 6 months and younger as well as for girls of menstruating age. Preoperative feeding orders should be individualized for age with attention to the hydration status of the patient, the time of operation, and the procedure to be done.[14] Most anesthesiologists allow patients older than 6 months no solid food after midnight, but allow clear liquids up to 3 hours before the operation. Children younger than 6 months old may be fed up to 4 hours before the procedure and allowed clear liquids up to 2 hours beforehand. Similarly, preoperative medications for the pediatric patient should be individualized according to the patient's needs and institutional practices. Preoperative sedation may be provided by intramuscular, intravenous, rectal, or oral agents. These premedications should be individualized, but a skillful anesthetic preoperative interview may obviate the need for a premedicant.

Airway management requires an appreciation of both quantitative and qualitative differences in anatomy and physiology. Specialized circuits to administer anesthesia are designed to minimize dead space and flow resistance as well as to provide adequate humidification. Endotracheal tubes must be sized to the individual patient, with uncuffed endotracheal tubes used in children younger than 8 years of age because the narrowest portion of their larynx is subglottic (Fig. 11–2). A small leak should be present around the endotracheal tube with positive-pressure ventilation to avoid subglottic injury in children with uncuffed endotracheal tubes.

All of the common inhalational and intravenous agents and techniques have been used in children. Mask inductions with inhalational agents are performed much more frequently in children than in adults owing to children's fear of needles and their relatively easy inductability. Furthermore, parents are often allowed to accompany a child to the operating room for induction of anesthesia, thus decreasing the apprehension of the child. Halothane is often chosen because it has a relatively pleasant smell and may induce less breathholding than some of the other inhalational agents. When the child loses consciousness, an intravenous cannula may be placed and appropriate drugs given to facilitate intubation and surgical procedures. For older children, a routine intravenous induction is normally used. Tracheal intubation and controlled ventilation are indicated in operations of the head and neck, intrathoracic and intraperitoneal procedures, operations in the prone position, most procedures in infants younger than 1 year of age, and all emergency procedures.

Fluid therapy in children must be meticulous to avoid excessive or deficient amounts of intravenous fluid. Calculations for such therapy are based on preoperative weight, the

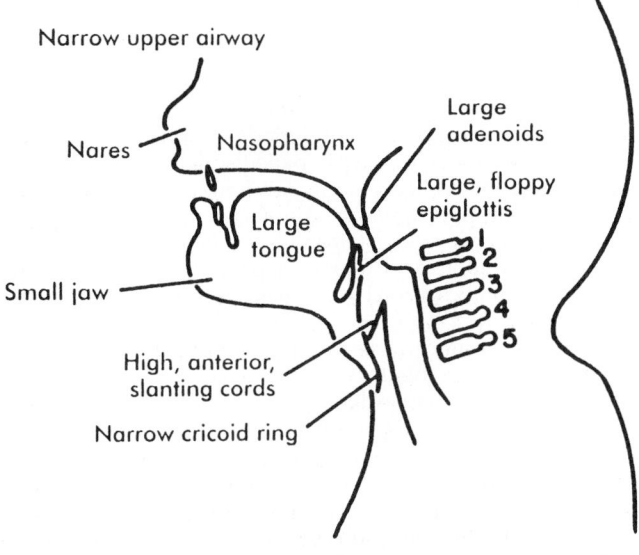

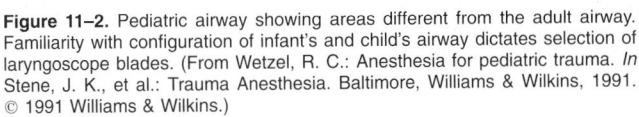

Figure 11–2. Pediatric airway showing areas different from the adult airway. Familiarity with configuration of infant's and child's airway dictates selection of laryngoscope blades. (From Wetzel, R. C.: Anesthesia for pediatric trauma. *In* Stene, J. K., et al.: Trauma Anesthesia. Baltimore, Williams & Wilkins, 1991. © 1991 Williams & Wilkins.)

time of last oral intake, intraoperative maintenance fluid requirements, and replacement of blood losses. Careful administration and monitoring of fluid therapy are very important and are instituted through a calibrated infusion pump or a calibrated gravity-dependent infusion system. When the procedure is concluded, the decision to extubate must be made with respect to the intraoperative course and the anticipated postoperative problems. Under most circumstances, neuromuscular blockade will be reversed and the patient extubated after return of muscle strength and ability to protect the airway. Children should be transported to the recovery room along with a precordial stethoscope and may be placed on their side in case of postoperative vomiting. As with adults, oxygen is usually administered until full awakening. Problems in the recovery room may include delirium, pain, anxiety, nausea and vomiting, airway obstruction, and loss of intravenous cannulation.

Geriatric Anesthesia

Anesthesia and surgical procedures for older adults may carry more risk than procedures in younger adults. This depends partly on the physiologic state of the patient (as opposed to the chronologic age) and the number of coexisting diseases. However, even for healthy adults, age-related declines occur in almost all physiologic parameters, including cardiovascular and autonomic nervous systems; respiratory, hepatic, and renal systems; and the CNS. These deteriorations may significantly affect the anesthetic and the perioperative course of the patient. Additionally, most operations performed in this population are major or emergent or involve major organ systems. Finally, the pharmacokinetics and pharmacodynamics of anesthetic drugs are altered by age; most drugs last longer and are relatively more potent in geriatric patients.[28]

The cardiovascular system of the elderly patient is characterized by changes in myocardial function, vascular tone, autonomic nervous system function, and responses to stress. Myocardial pump function declines with decreases in cardiac output and cardiac index and changes in responsiveness to catecholamines.[33] Furthermore, with progressive atherosclerosis, the myocardium may be pumping against an increased afterload. Many patients may have had further myocardial dysfunction in the form of a myocardial infarction or congestive heart failure. Hypertension is exceedingly common and may contribute to these problems. Baroreceptor responses to changes in volume or tone may not be as brisk as in younger patients.[13] The result is a limited response to cardiac depression, which may decrease the margin of safety for anesthetic agents and surgical stress. Elderly patients experience functional differences in respiratory control as well.[52] These changes are manifested by an altered CO_2 response curve, low resting closing volumes, diminished gag reflexes, and natural sleep characterized by periods of apnea or periodic breathing. Additionally, elderly patients may have anatomic changes such as scoliosis, decreased lung elasticity, and decreased chest wall compliance. All of these factors may cause resting hypoxemia and an inability to increase respiratory function in response to stress. Hepatic and renal system changes are characterized by declines in synthesizing, metabolizing, clearance, and elimination functions.[62] Thus, one must be exceedingly careful with the drugs given to the elderly patient and should anticipate altered volumes of distribution and elimination half-times. CNS function also declines, primarily characterized by a lower requirement for anesthetic agents and perhaps for pain medication.[30] The clinician should also be aware of all of the comorbid diseases that the patient may have in each of these organ systems in addition to normal physiologic declines in function (e.g.,

smoking and chronic obstructive pulmonary disease). The clinical consequence of all of these changes is a fragile patient; care must be taken to titrate all anesthetics and help the patient meet the stresses of anesthesia and operation.

No anesthetic technique is of greater benefit than others to the elderly patient; attention to detail and titrating of agents used is more important. Other considerations during anesthetic management should include avoidance of hypothermia during the surgical procedure, careful fluid and electrolyte management in the perioperative period, optimization of myocardial oxygen balance, and preservation of adequate cerebral blood flow. Should such problems arise, these patients experience the usual postoperative problems related to the particular operation and their comorbid diseases. They may need a longer period of observation in a monitored care setting.

Outpatient Anesthesia

Outpatient operations are performed in patients who are not expected to be admitted to the hospital and may be discharged to home from an ambulatory surgery unit. Increasingly, many surgical procedures that had required lengthy hospitalizations in the past are being done on an outpatient basis. Improved surgical technique, improved anesthetic agents, recognition that many people rehabilitate more quickly at home, and pressure to enhance use of medical resources have made outpatient procedures increasingly viable. Such patients generally require a limited procedure with minimal systemic hemodynamic or fluid balance impact. Usually they have few or well-controlled systemic disease processes. Advantages of outpatient operations include decreased medical costs, optimal use of hospital beds, operating room time, decreased risk of a hospital-acquired infection, and decreased hospital stay, obviating the need for extended separation from one's family or job. Disadvantages include the need for outpatient preoperative evaluation, the need for patients to do preoperative procedures at home, such as bowel preparation, and occasionally patient anxiety. Provisions must be made for unexpected hospital admissions for a variety of reasons. A preoperative screening visit is vital to complete the surgical preoperative evaluation, complete the anesthetic preoperative evaluation, and order appropriate tests and consults. It is also important to educate the patient about how to get to the hospital, be admitted, what to expect surgically, and what to expect postoperatively.

Rapid recovery with minimal procedure and drug-related side effects is the cornerstone of anesthetic management for the outpatient. Various anesthetic agents and techniques have been chosen for outpatient anesthesia; none has proven to be superior to the others. As with any patient, the anesthetic should be tailored to the individual's physiology and the surgical need, with consideration for a quick recovery. Pain control, as well as ability to ambulate, ability to urinate, and oral intake should be addressed; each of these factors may delay a patient's discharge after an otherwise uncomplicated anesthetic and operation. After the procedure, a more extended period of observation may be indicated for patients who received general anesthesia or sedatives or those who required treatment for nausea and vomiting.[59]

Discharge criteria must include the patient's being fully awake and oriented, the ability to have protective airway reflexes, stable vital signs, adequate hydration with the ability to hold down oral intake, ability to ambulate, and adequate pain control. All patients must have a competent person with them to transport them and ideally to stay with them on the first postoperative night. A physician must discharge each patient. Written and verbal instructions must be given for the treatment of anticipated postoperative problems and complications.

The most frequent complications after outpatient anesthesia and operation are sore throat, croup, headache, vomiting, pain, bleeding, and slow emergence. Rarely, complications such as poor pain control, nausea and vomiting, or inability to care for oneself may necessitate admission to the hospital.[58] Of course, serious complications related to the operation or anesthesia require admission. In most cases, outpatient operation and anesthesia can be performed safely in a time- and cost-efficient manner to the benefit of all parties. Maintenance of high standards for patient care in this setting is the cornerstone for its continued existence.

POSTANESTHESIA CARE UNIT

The postoperative period is one of multiple physiologic and pharmacologic changes. Complex pharmacology surrounds emergence and reversal of anesthesia and physiologic changes derive from surgical trauma. Intensive care for a period of time in the PACU is therefore critical to successful surgical outcomes. Patients are transported immediately to the PACU after the conclusion of the surgical procedure, usually after emergence from anesthesia. The PACU is an intensively monitored setting that allows observation, therapeutic intervention, and observation of patients as they more fully recover from the effects of the surgical procedure and anesthetic.

A detailed report about the patient (including preoperative history, intraoperative events, drug delivery, and fluid management) is given to the PACU team. Subsequently the patient's vital signs, hemodynamics, and recovery are closely monitored, usually in a low patient-to-nursing care ratio. Initial postoperative orders from the primary care team are fulfilled as the patient is prepared for eventual transfer to a ward bed. If patients come to the PACU intubated, they require further monitoring and ventilatory management. During this period, the patient should stabilize with respect to vital signs and hemodynamics, be extubated, become awake and alert, and have pain due to the surgical procedure treated. Furthermore, any complications from the surgical procedure and/or the anesthetic should be treated. Airway management is exceedingly important as patients are being readied for transfer to a ward bed with fewer monitoring capabilities.

Common problems in the PACU include hypertension, hypotension, alterations in heart rate, hypothermia, hypoventilation, low urine output, bleeding, pain, and nausea and vomiting. Both the source and the symptoms of the problem should be sought and corrected. Most PACUs have close physician supervision for management of these problems.

The PACU can function as a critical care unit should a critically ill patient be transferred to the PACU or should a patient become critically ill in the PACU. Additionally, procedures such as cardioversions and epidural blood patches may be done in the PACU.

ACUTE PAIN MANAGEMENT

The alleviation of acute pain has made major progress since the mid 1980s. Much attention has been focused on the concept of preemptive analgesia through opioids, nonsteroidal anti-inflammatory drugs (NSAIDs), and regional analgesia. Preventing and alleviating pain may be associated with reduced morbidity and mortality.

Historically, pain after operative procedures has been managed with intramuscular opioids. Because the frequency of the intramuscular dosing is restricted, larger doses than necessary are usually given, producing blood levels that exceed the analgesic threshold. Patients may thus experience side effects from the large dose, fall to the analgesic range for a period of time, and then become subtherapeutic for a period of time. This form of analgesia leads to recurring cycles of pain, a wait for the next dose of medication, and relief from pain (possibly with side effects).[38]

Because the intramuscular route for giving pain medication has been determined to be inadequate, many other modes of analgesia have been developed. They include intravenous medication by means of patient-controlled analgesia (PCA), epidural analgesia, intrapleural analgesia, peripheral nerve block, transdermal and transmucosal analgesia, and adjuvant medications.

Intravenous Patient-Controlled Analgesia

PCA provides individualized opioid dosing without extensive nursing intervention.[4] However, the pharmacodynamics and pharmacokinetics of the drugs administered and the variables of the PCA delivery system must be understood for its safe and effective use.

PCA allows patients to give themselves pain medication in a highly controlled manner. After analgesia has been established with a loading dose of opioid, patients give themselves small doses of opioids to maintain their level of analgesia. Thus, patients do not have to wait for a third party to assess their pain, nor must they wait for an intramuscular opioid to work. Lockout intervals and safe maximum doses are built into the program so the patients will not overdose.

Reduced contact with the nursing staff and the patient's fear of inadvertently administering an overdose or of addiction to the opioid are potential disadvantages of PCA. These fears can be allayed by adequate education of the patients and personnel. Advantages of PCA are immediate delivery of medication, rapid onset of analgesia, and patient control over pain medication. In some studies comparing PCA with conventional intramuscular medication, patients on PCA used less analgesia medication, suffered less sedation, ambulated earlier, suffered less ileus, and had a reduced incidence of postoperative fever.[2, 6, 20]

Clinical Use. When PCA is initiated, the factors that need to be considered are loading dose, the maintenance dose, the lockout interval, the continuous infusion, opioid selection, monitoring protocols, complications of PCA, and weaning from PCA.

Loading Dose. An adequate loading dose given under the supervision of a physician will enable patients to rapidly achieve a pain-free state. If the maintenance dose is used without the benefit of a loading dose, an analgesic state will not be reached for a prolonged period. The loading dose is best titrated to effect. Most PCA units have a loading mode that will limit the need for any separate analgesics. This facility also limits the amount of paperwork required to control opioids.

Maintenance Dose. PCA units use an intermittent bolus dose that is self-administered by the patient. The maintenance dose can be administered by pressing and releasing a button either on a hand-held pendant or on the PCA unit itself. The aim of the small, frequently injected dose in PCA is to safely maintain an analgesic blood level without producing sedation. The dose required to produce this effect is highly individualized, because pain tolerance and response to analgesics are extremely variable. Poor analgesia can result from maintenance doses that are set either too small or large. The patient's weight is a useful guide in initiating PCA dosing even though the ultimate correlation between analgesic requirements and weight is poor. The effectiveness of the dose selected must be appraised intermittently to optimize the level of analgesia and thus patient satisfaction. The pa-

TABLE 11–5. Doses of Opioids and Settings for Patient-Controlled Analgesia

Drug	Dose (μg./kg.)	Lockout Interval (min.)	Loading Dose (μg./kg.)
Morphine	20–30	8–12	50–100
Meperidine	200–250	8–12	500–750
Fentanyl	20–40	5–8	0.5–1
Hydromorphone	2–4	6–10	20–40
Sufentanil	0.01–0.02	5–8	0.1–0.2

tient should not have to make too many repeated demands over too long a period. Doses that are commonly used are summarized in Table 11–5. If the patients demonstrate inadequate analgesia despite making sufficient demands, the dose is increased by 20% to 50%. This must not be an automatic increase because the patient must be evaluated before the dose is increased to exclude an alteration in the patient's condition, such as a tight limb cast. Similarly, if the patient manifests signs of an overdose, such as excessive sedation, the dose is also reduced by 20% to 50%.

Lockout Interval. This is the period during which the PCA unit is refractory to further demands by the patient. The lockout interval is a needed safeguard to prevent patients from taking a further dose before they appreciate the full effect of the preceding dose. The lockout interval should therefore take into account the speed of onset of the agent and the time during which adequate concentrations of the opioid are available. It is also influenced by the size of the maintenance dose; with a larger maintenance dose the lockout interval can be widened. The average lockout intervals are depicted in Table 11–5.

Continuous Infusion. Constant-rate infusion alone and constant-rate infusion plus PCA can be administered through the PCA machine. A constant-rate infusion of opioids provides pain relief to patients after operation. When an infusion is started, the plasma level of the opioid gradually increases until the rate of infusion matches the rate of elimination. The time taken for the analgesic to reach the plateau level is dictated by the elimination half-life of the drug selected. With the use of a simple constant-rate infusion, the final level is reached after 20 to 24 hours. With a constant-rate infusion, the rate of infusion must be continuously tailored to the patient's analgesic requirements and needs constant adjustments in the infusion rate in both directions. Constant-rate infusion adjusted by the nursing staff to the patient's pain level required more morphine than a continuous infusion of morphine supplemented with PCA.[64]

In the *continuous plus PCA mode,* a continuous or *background* infusion is used in addition to intermittent bolus doses. Although the addition of a low-dose constant infusion was expected to minimize the fluctuation in the plasma concentration of the analgesic and provide better analgesia, in fact, the addition of a continuous infusion to a normal PCA dose and lockout intervals has not been shown to improve analgesia and has been shown to increase overall narcotic use. Furthermore, the potential for side effects such as respiratory depression may be increased. Therefore, a continuous infusion should not be used routinely to manage acute pain, even when combined with PCA. A continuous infusion would have to have specific indications for use in the management of acute pain states.

Opioid Selection. The ideal PCA agent would have a rapid onset of action with a medium duration of action. There should not be a ceiling to the analgesic effect, and the agent should not cause nausea, vomiting, or respiratory depression or impair bowel motility. Because no opioid is available with

these properties, the agents selected for use in PCA represent a compromise.

Morphine is one of the most commonly used analgesics for PCA. It has been used extensively with safety, is inexpensive, and is familiar to most medical personnel. The onset of action of morphine is slow when compared with the more lipid-soluble opioids, but its duration of action is longer.

Meperidine is the only opioid other than morphine that has been approved by the Food and Drug Administration for PCA use. Comparisons of meperidine and morphine found no differences between these two agents in the level of analgesia (at rest) and side-effect profile. Although meperidine is an effective analgesic, its use is complicated by the possible accumulation of normeperidine, a renally excreted metabolite of meperidine. Normeperidine causes dose-related CNS excitement, manifesting as agitation, insomnia, and tremors that can culminate in seizures.

Fentanyl has been used extensively to provide postoperative analgesia. It has a more rapid onset than less lipid-soluble drugs but has extremely variable interpatient requirements. It does not release histamine, has no active metabolites, and has a paucity of other side effects. Other opioids that have been used successfully for PCA include alfentanil, sufentanil, and hydromorphone.

Monitoring Protocols. Before a PCA service is initiated, protocols must be established for effective and safe use of this form of analgesia. These include detailed instruction to the staff on the use of the PCA device, opioid control, and patient monitoring and care. The patient monitoring should include at least four hourly assessments of the patient's level of pain and sedation and respiratory rate (Table 11–6). A simple verbal pain scale will track the patient's pain level and alert the staff if alterations in PCA settings are necessary. Patient education helps ensure optimal pain relief. The patient is educated preoperatively with instructions about pushing the PCA button often enough to keep pain at a minimum rather than waiting until it is severe; use of the PCA before such painful activities as movement or breathing exercises; reassurance regarding the unlikelihood of overdosage or addiction; reporting of side effects to the nursing staff; and when to expect a change to oral medication. In addition, relatives and/or friends may be instructed to encourage the patient to use the PCA device to treat pain. *However, relatives and/or friends may not be allowed to press the button for the patient.* The authors' institution uses a label attached to PCA pumps warning the patient's relatives that the PCA pump is only safe if used by the patient.

Complications. The most-feared complication of opioid use is respiratory depression. Respiratory rate and sedation scale checks are both used to detect the onset of respiratory depression. A decrease in respiratory rate or depth reflects the classic signs of respiratory depression induced by opioids. CO_2 may accumulate and produce CO_2-induced narcosis. This can be detected by observation of the patient's level of sedation on at least a 4-hour basis (see Table 11–6). A sedation scale of 3 or more indicates respiratory depression and warrants immediate therapy, which includes oxygen and naloxone and discontinuation of the opioid.

Anesthesia and surgical procedures are associated with a

TABLE 11–6. Sedation Scale Used to Monitor Patients Receiving Analgesic Therapy

1	None	Awake, alert, oriented
2	Mild	Sleepy but aroused by soft voice
3	Moderate	Required physical stimulus to arouse, then oriented
4	Severe	Required physical stimulus to arouse, not oriented

high incidence of nausea and vomiting. Opioids contribute to the nausea and vomiting by directly stimulating the chemoreceptor trigger zone and sensitizing the vestibular apparatus to movement. Nausea and vomiting with PCA can be managed by adjustment of the PCA dose, change of analgesic, the use of an antiemetic, or a scopolamine patch. Opioids may depress the peristaltic activity of the large and small intestine and increase the tone of the ileocecal and anal sphincters. Pruritus is a common complaint with the use of opiates through the PCA, although it is less than that associated with epidural morphine. Mild itching can be treated with an antihistamine and more severe itching with an alteration of analgesic or a low-dose infusion of naloxone. Urinary retention can be treated similarly.

Weaning. The aim of PCA is to continue with this modality until the postoperative patient is able to take oral analgesics. After bowel function has returned it is easily possible to replace the opioid requirements of the patient with oral analgesics. This dictates a knowledge of oral equivalence of the parenteral opioid (Table 11–7).

Epidural Analgesia

Epidural analgesia using opioids and local anesthetics has been used extensively to manage acute postoperative pain. Epidurally administered opioids diffuse to the spinal cord through multiple routes to act presynaptically and postsynaptically at specific receptors ($\mu\delta\kappa$). Opioids also bind in the substantia gelatinosa of the dorsal horn. Epidural opioid analgesia does not affect other sensory modalities or motor functions.[7]

Local anesthetics inhibit nerve impulses (including pain impulses) by inhibiting sodium channels along nerve fibers. Local anesthetics may act on the nerves in the intervertebral foramina or on the spinal roots in dural sleeves. In addition, local anesthetics may act on the periphery of the spinal cord after penetrating the subarachnoid space. Local anesthetics affect multiple sensory modalities, including pain, sensation, and motor function. The degree of loss of sensory or motor function depends on the local anesthetic and the concentration of local anesthetic used.

Epidural analgesia can relieve pain in a segmental manner, producing localized analgesia with fewer systemic effects than intravenous analgesia. Epidural analgesia may be effected with opioids, local anesthetics, or a combination of the two.

Advantages of epidural analgesia include excellent pain relief, decreased sedation with more rapid recovery to presurgical levels of consciousness, earlier mobilization after the operation, and increased ability to cooperate with respiratory therapy and physical therapy. This may decrease the incidence of pulmonary complications and venous thrombosis. Furthermore, epidural analgesia may also improve graft flow in patients after vascular surgery through mild sympathetic blockade. Earlier return of bowel function, decreased stress response, shorter hospitalizations, and decreased morbidity have all been associated with epidural analgesia.[9, 40, 50, 56, 63]

Epidural analgesia effectively treats pain emanating from sites in the body below the upper thoracic level. Orthopedic, urologic, gynecologic, upper abdominal, and thoracic procedures particularly benefit from epidural anesthesia and analgesia. In addition, trauma victims can be aided by epidural analgesia after a flail chest.

Local anesthetic agents—most commonly lidocaine and bupivacaine—often provide analgesia and anesthesia for patients undergoing operation. In general, lidocaine is limited to use in a bolus form to establish or rescue a block, whereas bupivacaine is used as an infusion or in bolus form, because systemic accumulation is more marked with the shorter-acting local anesthetics (lidocaine), with greater potential for toxicity over time. Bupivacaine has a long duration of action and has a differential between its sensory and motor blockade. Analgesia can be provided with minimal muscle weakness when bupivacaine is used in appropriate concentrations.

Bolus techniques for the administration of local anesthetic are short-lived, and the doses required to re-establish the desired level of analgesia may precipitate physiologic alterations, a drop in blood pressure, or the potential for systemic toxicity from a rapidly rising level of absorbed local anesthetic. Continuous infusions of local anesthetics may circumvent these difficulties. Potential problems in the use of local anesthetic agents alone are tachyphylaxis and systemic accumu-

TABLE 11–7. Equianalgesic Opioid Conversions

Drug	Equianalgesic Dose (mg.)		Comments	Precautions
	Oral	Intramuscular		
Morphine	30–60	10	Gold standard	Oral MSO$_4$ q8–12hr.
Fentanyl		0.1	Transdermal form available 25 μg./hr. minimum dose	12-hr. delay in onset and offset of transdermal patch, local heat and fever including rate of absorption
Meperidine	300	75	Oral form not recommended	Toxic metabolite (normeperidine) causes seizures, especially dose >600 mg./day. Do not use with renal failure or in patients on monoamine oxidase inhibitors; use with caution in patients with sickle cell anemia
Methadone	20	10	Long half-life of 24–36 hours	Accumulates, sedation after 2–3 days
Hydromorphone	7.5	1.5	Duration slightly shorter than MSO$_4$	
Oxycodone	15–30		Usually prepared with acetaminophen 325–500 mg./tablet	Acetaminophen dose not more than 4000 mg./day

Note: For all opioids, exercise caution in patients with sedation, marginal ventilation, asthma, increased intracranial pressure, liver failure, and renal failure.
Adapted from Principles of Analgesic Use in the Treatment of Acute and Cancer Pain, 3rd ed. Skokie, IL, American Pain Society, 1992.

TABLE 11–8. Local Anesthetic Concentrations for Use in Epidural Analgesia

Percentage	Percentage	mg./ml.
1/16	0.0625	0.625
1/8	0.125	1.25
1/4	0.25	2.5

TABLE 11–10. Ideal Analgesic Pump Criteria

1. Accurate dose delivery over a wide range of doses
   a. Ability to dose in mg./μg./ml.
   b. Simple to use and program
2. Alarms
   a. High pressure
   b. Prevention of free flow
   c. Device malfunction (low batteries)
   d. Low drug reservoir
3. Physical characteristics
   a. Small, portable, and lightweight
   b. Clear display of drug and doses
   c. Locks to prevent drug tampering
   d. Printer capability
   e. No infusion ports on connecting tubing
   f. Both battery and AC power
4. Adaptable
   a. Has many modes of delivery

lation of the local anesthetic agent. Systemic accumulation may cause CNS depression, convulsions, or cardiac arrest. The concentration of local anesthetic that is used will influence the analgesia and the profile of side effects. A constant rate infusion of 0.5% bupivacaine may induce hypotension, muscle weakness, sensory block, and the possible accumulation of toxic systemic levels of bupivacaine. Side effects may be attenuated by using lower concentrations of bupivacaine, such as 0.1%. If a low concentration of bupivacaine is ineffective, it may be combined with epidural opioids to increase efficacy.

Multiple opioids can be used in the epidural space. Once introduced into the epidural space, opioids can diffuse in a number of directions. The quantity of the opioid that is absorbed into the systemic circulation depends on the dose of the opioid used and the lipid solubility of the opioid. Opioids that are more lipid soluble (fentanyl) have a faster onset and more systemic absorption. Less-soluble opioids have a slow onset but less systemic absorption with more sustained CSF levels of opioid. If the systemic level of the opioid exceeds the minimal effective analgesic concentration, this will contribute to the analgesia following epidural administration as may occur with fentanyl. However, the analgesia that occurs from epidurally administered morphine (a less lipid-soluble opioid) does not depend on the systemic levels. In addition, the duration of analgesia after epidural administration of morphine exceeds the time during which morphine can be detected in significant amounts in the plasma.

An alternative method of providing pain relief is to infuse a combination of local anesthetics and opioids into the epidural space. Local anesthetics and opioids are thought to act synergistically and thus may allow decreased concentrations and dosages of each agent to be used, limiting the potential for side effects. Bupivacaine has been used most often in concentrations ranging from 0.1% to 0.25% with morphine, fentanyl, or meperidine. Tables 11–8 and 11–9 review commonly used bupivacaine concentrations and epidural opioid concentrations.

Epidural analgesia may be administered in multiple forms. Bolus analgesia is used with both opioids and local anesthetics. The duration of effect of the opioids or local anesthesia determines the interval dosing time. In general, morphine, meperidine, and hydromorphone (Dilaudid) are used in bolus form because these opioids last 6 to 12 hours. Fentanyl is rarely used repeatedly in bolus form because its duration of action is 2 to 4 hours. Local anesthetics may be used for analgesia in bolus form, but this mode of analgesia may be limited by side effects such as hypotension. Epidural analgesia may also be administered as a continuous infusion. The continuous infusion may consist of opioids, local anesthetics, or combinations of the two. A third form of epidural analgesia is patient-controlled epidural analgesia, which is similar to patient-controlled analgesia using intravenous opioids. Small boluses of opioids and/or local anesthetics are available at defined intervals with defined maximum allowable dosages. A continuous background infusion of opioids and/or local anesthetics may be added to the patient-controlled intermittent mode. Multiple pumps have been designed and marketed for epidural analgesia. Table 11–10 lists several criteria that are important considerations when choosing a pump to deliver drugs through the epidural catheter.

Common side effects of epidural opioids include nausea, pruritus, and urinary retention. These can usually be treated with low-dose naloxone infusion (while retaining pain relief) or by altering the local anesthetic/opioid concentration (Table 11–11). More serious complications include sedation and delayed respiratory depression. Delayed respiratory depression (6–12 hours) is thought to be due to the rostral spread of epidural opioid to the brain stem with effects on the respiratory control centers in the floor of the fourth ventricle. The incidence of respiratory depression ranges from 0.09% to 0.25% to 0.4%, being highest in the elderly, those with excessive concomitant sedatives or thoracic epidurals, and debilitated patients. Epidural local anesthetics may cause hypotension, motor block, or sensory loss in the dermatomal distribution of the catheter. Subarachnoid migration of the catheter is an extremely rare complication whose symptoms are increasing sensory and motor function loss. Agitation and seizures may also result from migration of the catheter to a blood vessel or from systemic absorption of local anesthetics. Appropriate monitoring of the patient allows for

TABLE 11–9. Commonly Used Epidural Opioids

Drug	Bolus Dose (mg./kg.)	Infusion Concentration (mg./ml.)	Infusion Rates (ml./hr.)
Fentanyl	0.001–0.002	0.0025–0.01	4–10
Morphine	0.03–0.10	0.1–0.2	1–5
Meperidine	0.35–0.7	1–2.5	4–10
Hydromorphone	0.01–0.02	0.05–0.1	1–5

TABLE 11–11. Treatment of Side Effects from Epidural Opioids

Side Effect	Treatment	Dosage/70 kg.
Respiratory depression	Naloxone IV	0.04–0.4 mg. or an infusion
Urinary retention	Urinary catheter Naloxone IV	0.1–0.4 mg. or infusion*
Pruritus	Antihistamine (less effective) Naloxone IV	0.1–0.4 mg. or infusion*
Nausea and vomiting	Metoclopramide IV/IM	10 mg.
	Naloxone IV	0.1–0.4 mg. or infusion*
	Droperidol IV	1.25–2.5 mg.
Constipation	Laxatives	

*Infusion = 0.4–0.8 mg./hr., titrate to effect.
IV, Intravenous; IM, intramuscular.
Data from Decastro et al., 1991, Bromage et al., 1982, and Rawal and Wattwill, 1984.

prevention, early recognition, and treatment of these complications. These side effects can be managed further by changes in the local anesthetic concentration or by intravenous fluid infusion.

Monitoring regimens are set up to detect and treat side effects if they occur. Guidelines for monitoring epidural analgesia have been established by many hospitals. Sensible protocols include the following: For every patient following or during epidural anesthesia, analgesia monitoring equipment and emergency drugs and equipment must be readily available. The patient's room should be equipped with at least oxygen, an ambu mask, and a blood pressure cuff. Naloxone, 0.4 mg. per ml., with a syringe should be present in a prominent position in each room, such as taped to the epidural pump or above the patient's bed. Patients with epidural analgesia should have their respiratory rate and depth assessed with a sedation scale once every 1 to 2 hours. Epidural opioids may depress the depth of ventilation without affecting the rate. Treatment is based on the amount of sedation and respiratory depression. It may range from simple stimulation to the administration of naloxone. Absolutely no additional opioids or CNS depressant medication should be given without the approval of the pain treatment service.

Patients receiving a continuous infusion with local anesthetics should be assessed every 4 hours for vital signs, sensory levels, and the degree of motor block. Patients with lumbar or low thoracic epidural analgesia should not be allowed to ambulate. Patients with higher thoracic catheters may ambulate with assistance.

The most important monitor, however, is good nursing personnel with good communication between the nursing staff and the members of the pain treatment service or primary care physician. A member of the pain treatment service who is familiar with the patients with epidural analgesia should be available immediately to cope with problems and should be easily reachable to answer questions. Whether these monitoring guidelines are applied in an intensive care setting or on routine postoperative floors may be determined by the level of expertise and training of the team (anesthesiologist, surgeon, and nursing staff) caring for the patient, by the resources available in the hospital, and at the discretion of the individuals responsible for the epidural analgesia.[45]

Patients receiving epidural medications on a long-term basis (more than 1 to 2 weeks) usually have catheters implanted. Implanted catheters are sutured in place and are much less likely to be removed accidentally. These catheters are designed to prevent infection via the exit site by using a Dacron cuff to help prevent infection from tracking by means of the exit wound. The implanted catheters are also tunneled to the lower chest, and the exit site is made easily accessible to the patient and/or caretaker. The catheter can then be externalized, like venous access devices, or it can be made into a MediPort access (in which a needle is required to puncture the skin and access the catheter).

Intrapleural Analgesia

Intrapleural analgesia provides effective pain relief for many procedures, including upper abdominal and thoracic procedures.[47] Intrapleural analgesia involves placement of analgesic agents (usually a local anesthetic) in the intrapleural space, usually through a single shot or catheter. The action of intrapleural local anesthetic agents is believed to occur principally by diffusion through the parietal pleura to anesthetize the intercostal nerves. The intercostal nerves are separated from the parietal pleura by only a layer of fat in the paravertebral region. Lateral to this fascial layer, the posterior intercostal membrane separates the nerves from the pleura. At the level of the angle of the ribs the membrane is replaced by the fibers of the internal intercostal membrane. Local anesthetic deposited in the pleural space must diffuse through one of these layers to be effective. The close proximity of the thoracic sympathetic chain indicates that the sympathetic nervous system could be involved after an intrapleural blockade. However, little alteration of hemodynamic parameters has been noted, probably due to the unilateral nature of these blocks.

The easiest and safest technique for inserting an intrapleural catheter is under direct vision by the surgeon at the time of a thoracotomy. A catheter is laid between the parietal and visceral pleura and then tunneled through the chest wall to exit laterally at the side of the chest. Many techniques have been used to identify the intrapleural space in closed chest patients. Most use a well-lubricated glass syringe attached to a Tuohy needle that is advanced immediately above the rib. In a spontaneously breathing patient the intrapleural space is identified by the inward suction of the entire needle-syringe combination from negative pressure in the pleural space. Alternatively, a loss of resistance to pressure as the syringe is advanced through the pleural space may be an indication. The hanging drop technique can also indicate the negative pressure in the pleural space in a spontaneously breathing patient.

Controversy exists regarding the optimal concentration and volume of local anesthetic agent to use with the intrapleural technique. Both bupivacaine and lidocaine have been used successfully to provide analgesia. Bupivacaine concentrations have ranged from 0.25% to 0.75%, with volumes ranging from 8 to 30 ml. Most studies have used 0.5% bupivacaine in volumes ranging from 20 to 30 ml. The mean duration of analgesia ranged from 285 minutes in the low concentration to 500 minutes with 0.5% bupivacaine.

Systemic absorption of the local anesthetic may limit the use of a continuous infusion of local anesthetics into the pleural space. A contraindication to the use of local anesthetic intrapleural analgesia is inflammation or fibrosis of the pleura due to increased absorption and the technical difficulty of isolating the pleural space. The presence of blood or fluid in the pleural space is also a contraindication, owing to the dilution of the local anesthetic and increased absorption of the local anesthetic. Test doses of local anesthetic with epinephrine may decrease the risk of injecting a larger amount of local anesthetic into the pleural space.

Transdermal Opioids

Transdermal fentanyl has been approved for use in patients with cancer-induced pain. Many studies have already been performed exploring the role of transdermal fentanyl in the management of postoperative pain.[8] Transdermal fentanyl may obviate the need for a functioning gastrointestinal tract or an intravenous or epidural catheter.

Fentanyl meets the criteria for use in a transdermal delivery system in that it is both highly lipid soluble and potent enough for transdermal use. A system, TTS fentanyl (Transdermal Therapeutic System, Alzo Corporation, Palo Alto, CA), has been developed. The TTS is self-adhesive with a selectively permeable membrane, which comes in various sizes to vary the rate of delivery. These patches provide the predicted amount of medication in the range of 25 to 100 μg. per hour. Because the skin is not uniform, the rate of transfer varies with the site on which the patch is placed as well as the patient's gender, age, skin, blood flow, sweat gland activity, temperature, and pH of the skin.

There is a significant lag time before a therapeutic level of fentanyl is detected in the plasma (up to 2 hours before any detectable plasma fentanyl levels). Therefore, several rescue treatments are necessary at the beginning of therapy. Full effectiveness of the fentanyl patch may take up to 24 hours. Likewise, there is a long elimination half-life (up to 22 to 24 hours) after the removal of the patch. Thus the skin acts as a reservoir as well as a barrier for fentanyl. Fentanyl patches have been used for up to 5 months and have provided excellent pain control with good correlation between the plasma fentanyl level and the predicted rate of delivery.

Fever or local heating, such as the use of a heating pad, increases the release of fentanyl, which may precipitate respiratory depression. Respiratory depression, nausea, and vomiting all are reported side effects. When initiating fentanyl, patch analgesia one must monitor for these complications. Furthermore, the adhesive can cause a transient period of redness when the patches have been removed. Transdermal fentanyl provides an effective form of analgesia but is difficult to titrate, with a slow onset and prolonged elimination half-life limiting its usefulness.

Transmucosal Opioids

With recent advances in technology, opioid administration has become available in a transmucosal delivery system.[1] The mucosa of the mouth and nose has long been used for drug delivery (e.g., desmopressin, nifedipine). To be effective transmucosally, a drug must be potent and nonirritating and have a high solubility. Such potent drugs with high solubility include buprenorphine, fentanyl, and methadone.

Transmucosal administration can occur in a number of sites, including the mouth (sublingual, buccal, and gingival), the nose, and the rectum. Each site presents advantages and disadvantages. The nose and mouth can yield a swift absorption and onset of action with little first-pass metabolism. However, transmucosal medications given through the mouth (as compared with oral administration) may be diluted by saliva and those given nasally may be irritating. Rectal delivery may have advantages in uncooperative patients. However, absorption may be limited by bowel movements, mucosal irritation, and variable absorption because the rectum has venous plexi that drain to the systemic and portal systems.

Advantages of a transmucosal drug delivery system are clear in the hospital and in outpatient settings: for patients without intravenous access who present in the emergency department, for premedication before operation, and for patients whose intravenous access has been discontinued or is difficult to obtain. For an outpatient, transmucosal opioids may be used as maintenance pain management therapy or as rescue therapy for the treatment of breakthrough pain.

Transmucosal opioids are not currently marketed but are in the investigative stage of development.

Nonsteroidal Anti-inflammatory Drugs

NSAIDs may be used to manage postsurgical pain both as a sole agent or in combination with other analgesics.[45] The use of NSAIDs may reduce the requirements for opioids. NSAIDs all have the ability to produce antipyretic, analgesic, and anti-inflammatory effects, but the relative proportions vary with the different agents.

Multiple forms of NSAIDs have been used, including oral, rectal, intramuscular, and intravenous. One of the most commonly used agents is ketorolac tromethamine, an NSAID that is approved by the Food and Drug Administration for intravenous, intramuscular, and oral administration. This agent is an effective analgesic with a paucity of side effects. Ketorolac is absorbed rapidly and completely after oral and intramuscular administration. The dose that is usually effective in young healthy individuals is 30 mg. given intravenously or intramuscularly every 6 to 8 hours. It is routinely recommended that the dose should be reduced by 50% in patients younger than 65 years of age or those with severe systemic disease. In addition, ketorolac should not be used for more than 5 consecutive days.

Multiple studies have demonstrated effective analgesia with ketorolac both as a sole agent and when used in combination with opioids.[27] Some studies have demonstrated increased blood loss with ketorolac used preoperatively or intraoperatively, but other studies have failed to demonstrate this phenomenon. As with all NSAIDs, there is potential for enhanced surgical or gastrointestinal bleeding, renal dysfunction, and platelet dysfunction. Further anaphylaxis to ketorolac has been reported in patients with a history of nasal polyps, allergy to aspirin, and/or asthma.

Acute Pain Management—A Team Approach

The management of chronic pain has long been recognized to be superior if a team approach is applied. The purpose of an acute pain service is to coordinate the skills and knowledge of all the personnel into a uniform plan to manage postoperative pain relief.[44]

A physician is essential on the team to provide medical knowledge and to direct the team. The primary physician can be from any discipline but is typically an anesthesiologist. Other physicians include the patient's primary care service and significant consulting services, such as oncology or radiology. A full-time nurse can help provide continuity throughout the institution and be responsible for nursing in-services pertaining to pain management throughout the hospital. A pharmacist may be a member of the acute pain service to coordinate decisions about products to be used, to establish stability and sterility data about products to be used, and even to evaluate monitoring of side effects of the treatment being used. Consultative membership of the acute pain service will be dictated by the evolution of the patient's postoperative course.

SUMMARY

The art and science of anesthetic practice has existed as a unique medical specialty for a relatively short time. The focus of the anesthesiologist has changed from merely providing amnesia, analgesia, and muscle relaxation for surgical procedures to aggressive management of surgical stress, prior co-existing diseases, and hemodynamic parameters as part of an anesthetic. This requires an extensive knowledge of pharmacology, physiology, anatomy, and pathology integrated with knowledge about the actions and effects of anesthetic agents and techniques. Furthermore, the anesthesiologist's role in care of the patient has extended beyond the borders of the operating room to the critical care unit, to pain management teams, to respiratory care teams, and to emergency response teams. Advances in pharmacology and molecular biology continue to expand the knowledge of anesthetic mechanisms and to provide improved agents. As more powerful agents and techniques become available, the need for increasingly sophisticated physicians to practice anesthesia will increase. The mutually dependent relationship of surgeons and anesthesiologists is unique to medicine: Two specialists work side by side at the same time, each with respective duties but both ensuring optimal patient care through communication, cooperation, and competence.

SELECTED REFERENCES

Bromage, P. R.: Epidural Anesthesia. Philadelphia, W. B. Saunders, 1978.
This text gives a detailed account of epidural analgesia and anesthesia, bringing together clinical and laboratory information. Included is a section on the pharmacology of local anesthetics, which serves as a basis for logical use of these drugs in practice. Several clinical illustrations and actual case descriptions make this a complete resource.

Cottrell, J. E., and Smith, D. S.: Anesthesia and Neurosurgery. St. Louis, C. V. Mosby, 1994.
This multiauthored text presents the application of basic information concerning CNS disease in a context of understanding the intracranial effects of anesthetic drugs and techniques. Neuroanesthesia practice is presented as an amalgam of neurology, neurosurgery, and anesthesia.

Cousins, M. J., and Bridenbaugh, P. O. (Eds.): Neural Blockade in Clinical Anesthesia and Management of Pain, 2nd ed. Philadelphia, J. B. Lippincott, 1987.
This is one of the most comprehensive texts covering the pharmacology, principles, and practice of neural blockade in anesthetic practice.

Estafanous, F., Barash, P. G., and Reves, J. G. (Eds.): Cardiac Anesthesia: Principles and Clinical Practice. Philadelphia, J. B. Lippincott, 1994.
This is a comprehensive text on the practice of cardiac anesthesia. In this excellent text known principles of the care of the acutely unstable cardiovascular patient are collated and a scientific basis is presented for their medical management. Considerable effort has been expended to ensure that each major topic is covered thoroughly by experienced investigative anesthesiologists, cardiologists, and surgeons.

Ferrante, F. M., and Vadeboncoeur, T. R. (Eds.): Postoperative Pain Management. New York, Churchill Livingstone, 1993.
This informative and interesting text has much practical advice regarding the management of acute pain.

Gregory, G. A. (Ed.): Pediatric Anesthesia. New York, Churchill Livingstone, 1981.
This is the most comprehensive text for anesthetic care of the infant and child. It provides a physiologic and pharmacologic approach to anesthesia for the pediatric patient.

Jacobs, J. R., Reves, J. G., and Glass, P. S. A.: Continuous infusions for maintaining anesthesia. Int. Anesthesiol. Clin., 29(4), 1991.
This monograph is a succinct guide to the theory and practice of the administration of intravenous anesthetics. It is a classic in clarity, because it is not multiauthored.

Miller, R. D. (Ed.): Anesthesia, 4th ed. New York, Churchill Livingstone, 1994.
Anesthesia is the most current, comprehensive textbook of anesthesia available. Its two volumes were written by 31 contributors, all recognized experts in their particular subspecialty of anesthesia. This book is invaluable as a resource for both theoretical and practical knowledge.

Scurr, C., and Feldman, S. (Eds.): Scientific Foundations in Anaesthesia. London, Heineman Medical Books, 1974.
This is an excellent review of the scientific principles that are the basis of the clinical practice of anesthesia, resuscitation, and intensive care. It details the physics, mathematics, and measurement techniques of practice with emphasis on practical knowledge.

Shoemaker, W. C., Thompson, W. L., and Holbrook, P. R. (Eds.): Textbook of Critical Care. Philadelphia, W. B. Saunders, 1984.
This multiauthored text offers comprehensive information regarding the practice of critical care medicine.

Sinatra, R. S., Hord, A. H., Ginsberg, B., and Preble, L. M. (Eds.): Acute Pain: Mechanisms and Management. St. Louis, Mosby–Year Book, 1992.
This detailed text has much theory as well as much information about the management of pain in general and in specific situations.

Critical Care Medicine References

Blitt, C. D. (Ed.): Monitoring in Anesthesia and Critical Care Medicine. New York, Churchill Livingstone, 1985.

Chernow, B. (Ed.): The Pharmacologic Approach to the Critically Ill Patient, 2nd ed. Baltimore, Williams & Wilkins, 1988.

Civetta, J. M., Taylor, R. W., and Kirby, R. R. (Eds.): Critical Care. Philadelphia, J. B. Lippincott, 1988.

Lyerly, H. K. (Ed.): The Handbook of Surgical Intensive Care, 2nd ed. Chicago, Year Book Medical Publishers, 1989.

Shoemaker, W. C., Thompson, W. L., and Holbrook, P. D. (Eds.): Textbook of Critical Care, 2nd ed. Philadelphia, W. B. Saunders, 1988.

Snyder, J. V., and Pinsky, M. P. (Eds.): Oxygen Transport in the Critically Ill. Chicago, Year Book Medical Publishers, 1987.

REFERENCES

1. Ashburn, M. A., Lind, G. H., Gillie, M. H., et al.: Oral transmucosal fentanyl citrate (OTFC) for the treatment of postoperative pain. Anesth. Analg., 76:377, 1993.
2. Atwell, J. R., Flanigan, R. C., Bennet, R. L., et al.: The efficacy of patient controlled analgesia in patients recovering from flank incisions. J. Urol., 132:701, 1984.
3. Bagdonoff, D. L., and Stone, D. J.: Emergency management of the airway outside of the operating room. Can. J. Anaesth., 39:1069, 1993.
4. Bennett, R. L., Batenhorst, R. L., and Bivens, B. A.: Patient-controlled analgesia: A new concept of postoperative pain relief. Ann. Surg., 195:700, 1982.
5. Benumof, J. L., and Alfrey, D. D.: Anesthesia for thoracic surgery. In Miller, R. D. (Ed.): Anesthesia, 4th ed. New York, Churchill Livingstone, 1994.
6. Bollish, S. J., Collins, C. L., Kirking, D. M., et al.: Efficacy of patient controlled versus conventional analgesia for postoperative pain. Clin. Pharm., 4:48, 1985.
7. Bromage, P. R., Camporesi, E., and Chestnut, D.: Epidural narcotics for postoperative pain relief. Anesth. Analg., 59:473, 1980.
8. Caplan, D. M., Ready, B. L., Oden, R. V., et al.: Transdermal fentanyl for postoperative pain management. JAMA, 26:1036, 1989.
9. Christopherson, R., Beattie, C., Frank, S. M., et al.: Perioperative morbidity in patients randomized to epidural or general anesthesia for lower extremity vascular surgery. Anesthesiology, 79:422, 1993.
10. Cohen, E. N., Trudell, J. R., and Edmunds, H. N.: Urinary metabolites of halothane in man. Anesthesiology, 43:392, 1970.
11. Cohen, M. M., Cameron, C. B., and Duncan, P. G.: Pediatric anesthesia morbidity and mortality in the perioperative period. Anesth. Analg., 70:160, 1990.
12. Cohen, M. M., and Duncan, P. G.: Physical status score and trends in anesthetic complications. J. Clin. Epidemiol., 41:83, 1988.
13. Collins, K. J., Exton-Smith, A. N., James, M. H., and Oliver, D. J.: Functional changes in autonomic nervous system responses with aging. Age Aging, 9:17, 1980.
14. Cote, C. J.: NPO after midnight for children—A reappraisal. Anesthesiology, 72:589, 1990.
15. Cousins, M. J., and Bromage, P. R.: Epidural neural blockade. In Cousins, M. J., and Bridenbaugh, P. O. (Eds.): Neural Blockade in Clinical Anesthesia and Management of Pain, 2nd ed. Philadelphia, J. B. Lippincott, 1987.
16. Covino, B. G., and Vassallo, H. L.: Local Anesthetics: Mechanisms of Action and Clinical Use. New York, Grune & Stratton, 1976.
17. Covino, B. G.: Clinical pharmacology of local anesthetic agents. In Cousins, M., and Bridenbaugh, P. O. (Eds.): Neural Blockade, 2nd ed. Philadelphia, J. B. Lippincott, 1992, p. 111.
18. deBruijn, N. P., and Clements, F. M.: Transesophageal Echocardiography. Boston, Martinus Nijhoff, 1987.
19. Dunton A, Schwam, E., and Pitman, V.: Flumazenil: U. S. clinical pharmacology studies. Eur. J. Anaesthesiol., 2:81, 1988.
20. Egberts, K. M., Parks, L. H., Short, L. M., and Burnett, M. L.: Randomized trial of postoperative patient controlled analgesia versus intramuscular narcotics in elderly men. Arch. Intern. Med., 150:1897, 1990.
21. Eger, E. I.: Anesthetic Uptake and Action. Baltimore, Williams & Wilkins, 1974.
22. Fleisher, L. A., and Barash, P. G.: Preoperative cardiac evaluation for noncardiac surgery: A functional approach. Anesth. Analg., 74:586, 1992.
23. Ford, G. T., and Guenta, C. A.: Toward prevention of postoperative pulmonary complications. Am. Rev. Respir. Dis., 130:4, 1984.
24. Fowkes, F. G. R., Lunn, J. N., Farrow, S. C., et al.: Epidemiology in anaesthesia: III. Mortality risk in patients with coexisting physical disease. Br. J. Anaesth., 54:819, 1982.
25. Gelman, S.: General versus regional anesthesia for peripheral vascular surgery: Is the problem solved? Anesthesiology, 79:415, 1993.
26. Glass, P. S. A., Shafer, S. L., Jacobs, J. R., and Reves, J. R.: Intravenous drug delivery systems. In Miller, R. (Ed.): Anesthesia, 4th ed. New York, Churchill Livingstone, 1994, p. 389.
27. Grass, J. A., Sakima, N. T., Valley, M., et al.: Assessment of ketorolac as an adjuvant to fentanyl patient controlled analgesia after radical retropubic prostatectomy. Anesthesiology, 78:642, 1993.
28. Greenblatt, D. J., Sellers, E. M., Shader, R. I.: Drug disposition in old age. N. Engl. J. Med., 306:1081, 1982.
29. Halsey, J. H.: Risks and benefits of shunting in carotid endarterectomy: The international Doppler collaborators. Stroke, 23:1583, 1992.
30. Harkins, S. W., and Chapman, C. R.: Detection and decision factors in pain perception in young and elderly men. Pain, 2:253, 1976.

31. Hughes M., Jacobs, J., and Glass, P.: Context sensitive half-time in multi-compartment pharmacokinetic models for intravenous anesthetic drugs. Anesthesiology, 76:334, 1992.

32. Keats, A. S.: The ASA classification of physical status—A recapitulation. Anesthesiology, 49:233, 1978.

33. Kennedy, R. D., and Claird, F. L.: Physiology of aging of the heart. Cardiovasc. Clin., 12:1, 1981.

34. Lagerkranser, M.: Controlled hypotension in neurosurgery. J. Arch. Neurosurg. Anesth., 3:150, 1991.

35. Lambert, D. H.: Continuous spinal anesthesia. Anesthesiol. Clin. North Am., 10:87, 1992.

36. Macario, A., Roizen, M. F., Thisted, R. A., et al.: Reassessment of preoperative laboratory testing has changed the test-ordering patterns of physicians. Surg. Gynecol. Obstet., 75:539, 1992.

37. Mangano, D. T., Bronner, W. S., Hollenberg M., et al.: Association of perioperative myocardial ischaemia with cardiac morbidity and mortality in men undergoing noncardiac surgery. N. Engl. J. Med., 323:1781, 1990.

38. Marks, R. M., and Sachar, E. J.: Undertreatment of medical inpatients with narcotic analgesics. Ann. Intern. Med., 78:173, 1973.

39. Menache, P., and Piwnica, A.: Cardioplegia by way of the coronary sinus for valvular and coronary surgery. J. Am. Coll. Cardiol., 28:628, 1991.

40. Modig, J., Borg, T., Karlstrom, G., et al.: Thromboembolism after total hip replacement: Role of epidural and general anesthesia. Anesth. Analg., 62:174, 1983.

41. Paulson, O. B., Strandgaard, S., and Edvinsson, L.: Cerebral autoregulation. Cerebrovasc. Brain Metab. Rev., 2:161, 1990.

42. Pennant, J. H., and White, P. F.: The laryngeal mask airway: Its uses in anesthesiology. Anesthesiology, 79:144, 1993.

43. Prough, D. S., Stump, D. A., and Troost, B. T.: PaCO$_2$ management during cardiopulmonary bypass: Intriguing physiological rationale, convincing clinical data, evolving hypothesis? Anesthesiology, 73:3, 1990.

44. Ready, L. B., Oden R., Chadwick, H. S., et al.: Development of an anesthesiology based postoperative pain management service. Anesthesiology, 68:100, 1988

45. Rhodes, M., Conacher, I., Morritt, G., et al.: Nonsteroidal antiinflammatory drugs for post-thoracotomy pain: A prospective controlled trial after lateral thoracotomy. J. Thorac. Cardiovasc. Surg., 103:17, 1992.

46. Roizen, M. F., Kaplan, E. B., Schreider, B. D., et al.: The relative roles of the history and physical examination, and laboratory testing in preoperative evaluation for outpatient surgery: The "Starling" curve in preoperative laboratory testing. Anesthesiol. Clin. North Am., 5:15, 1987.

47. Rosenberg, P. H., Scheinin, B. M., Lepantalo, M. J., and Lindfors, O. L.: Continuous intrapleural infusion of bupivacaine for analgesia after thoracotomy. Anesthesiology, 67:311, 1987.

48. Rosenfeld, B. A., Beattie C., Christopherson, R., et al.: The effects of different anesthetic regimens on fibrinolysis and the development of postoperative arterial thrombosis. Anesthesiology, 79:435, 1993.

49. Saidman, L. J., and Smith, N. T.: Monitoring in Anesthesia. Stoneham, MA, Butterworth Publishers, 1984.

50. Scott, N. B., Mogenson, T., Big, D., et al.: Continuous thoracic extradural 0.5% bupivacaine with or without morphine: Effect on quality of blockade, lung function and the surgical stress response. Br. J. Anaesth., 62:253, 1989.

51. Shanks, C. A.: Pharmacokinetics of the nondepolarizing neuromuscular relaxants applied to calculation of bolus and infusion dosage regimens. Anesthesiology, 64:72, 1986.

52. Smith, T. C.: Respiratory effects of aging. Semin. Anesth., 5:14, 1986.

53. Stehling, L., Zauder, H. L.: Acute limited normovolemic hemodilution. Transfusion, 31:857, 1991.

54. Stenlake, J. B., Waigh, R. D., Urwin, J., et al.: Atracurium: Conception and inception. Br. J. Anaesth., 55:3s, 1983.

55. Taylor, D. W.: Beneficial effect of carotid endarterectomy in symptomatic patients with high-grade stenosis. N. Engl. J. Med., 325:445, 1991.

56. Tuman, K. J., McCarty, R. J., March, R. J., et al.: Effects of epidural anesthesia and analgesia on coagulation and outcome after major vascular surgery. Anesth. Analg., 73:696, 1991.

57. Utting, J. E., Gray, T. C., and Shelley, F. C.: Human misadventure in anesthesia. Can. Anaesth. Soc. J., 26:472, 1979.

58. Warner, M. A., Shields, B. E., and Chute, C. G.: Major morbidity and mortality within one month of ambulatory surgery and anesthesia. JAMA, 270:1437, 1993.

59. Watcha, M. F., and White, P. F.: Postoperative nausea and vomiting: Its etiology, treatment and prevention. Anesthesiology, 77:162, 1992.

60. Wetstone, D. L., and Wong, K. C.: Sinus bradycardia and asystole during spinal anesthesia. Anesthesiology, 41:87, 1974.

61. Wetzel, R. C.: Anesthesia for pediatric trauma. In Stene, J. K. (Ed.): Trauma Anesthesia. Baltimore, Williams & Wilkins, 1991.

62. Woodhouse, K. W., Mutch, E., Williams, F. M., et al.: The effect of age on pathways of drug metabolism in human liver. Age Aging, 13:328, 1984.

63. Yeager, M. P., Glass, D. D., Neff, R. K., and Brinck-Johnsen, T.: Epidural anesthesia and analgesia in high risk surgical patients. Anesthesiology, 66:729, 1987.

64. Zacharias, M., Pfeifer, M. V., and Herbison, P.: Comparison of two methods of intravenous administration of morphine for postoperative pain. Anaesth. Intensive Care, 18:205, 1990.

CHAPTER 12

WOUND HEALING
Biologic and Clinical Features

N. Scott Adzick, M.D.

Surgeons depend on wound repair, and understanding the mechanisms that control wound healing is fundamental to the practice of surgery. Although surgeons can now anticipate and often prevent problems of infection and inadequate or excessive tissue repair, this was not always the case. For most of human history, incomplete or complicated healing after injury or surgery was the rule, not the exception. The basic principles of wound care and antisepsis introduced during the past century improved surgery dramatically. The past decade has seen an explosive growth of wound healing research that promises to facilitate clinical wound repair. The impending translation of recent basic science discoveries into clinical reality reflects the application of a new cellular and molecular biologic approach to the study of wound healing.

TISSUE INJURY AND TYPES OF HEALING

Tissue loss or damage causes either regeneration or repair by scar tissue, or a combination of both. Some amphibians can regenerate amputated appendages, but mammals have almost no organ regeneration capability except for bone and liver. Repair by scar, the postnatal mammalian response to injury, occurs with a sequential cascade of overlapping processes that restore tissue integrity.

The amount of tissue injury and degree of contamination influence the speed and quality of healing. Injury may follow surgery or accidental trauma, burns or cold exposure, or contact with chemical agents or foreign bodies. A superficial skin injury may remove only the epithelial cell layer, leaving the epithelial-dermal basement membrane intact. Healing then occurs rapidly by simple re-epithelialization, with no scar. Small, clean, closed wounds heal quickly with little scar formation, whereas large, open, dirty wounds heal slowly with significant scarring.

The types of healing are customarily divided into repair by first, second, or third *intention* (Fig. 12–1). Primary or *first intention* healing occurs in closed wounds in which the edges are approximated, such as a clean skin incision closed with sutures. The incisional defect re-epithelializes rapidly, and matrix deposition seals the defect. *Second intention* healing occurs when the wound edges are not apposed, such as an open punch skin biopsy wound, a deep burn, and an infected wound left open to granulate. Granulation tissue fills the wound, and the wound contracts and re-epithelializes. Delayed primary or *third intention* healing occurs when an open wound is secondarily closed several days after injury. Such a wound is initially left open because of gross contamination. A classic example is wound management after removal of a ruptured appendix. After the peritoneum and fascia are closed to prevent evisceration, the skin and subcutaneous tissue are left open and the wound is packed loosely with sterile moist gauze. The wound is closed several days later after wound contamination has markedly diminished. Par-

tial-thickness wounds are defects in which only the epithelium and superficial portion of the dermis have been removed. A good example is the donor site for a split-thickness skin graft. These wounds heal almost entirely by re-epithelialization, with little need for the matrix synthesis and remodeling that are characteristic of other wounds.

Both open and closed wounds heal with the same basic repair mechanisms: Epithelialization seals the wound, and matrix synthesis provides structural strength. When tissue has been lost, contraction enhances wound closure by pulling normal tissue over the defect. Contraction is distinct from contracture, which is the loss of tissue mobility due to a shrinking scar. Dermal appendages such as sweat glands and hair follicles can repair themselves in a partial-thickness injury but cannot regenerate in full-thickness wounds.

Understanding these concepts allows therapeutic modulation of the healing process. For instance, the level of bacterial contamination governs the subsequent risk of wound infection. The conversion of a heavily injured or grossly contaminated wound into a clean incisional wound with coapted edges can help achieve acceptable tissue repair with less morbidity and improved function.

Most research on wound repair has been done on skin (cutaneous) healing, and the principles described for cutaneous repair can be applied to most tissues. Although certain tissues, such as nerve, bladder, intestine, trachea, artery, and peritoneum, have distinctive healing characteristics, they all share common features: the formation of granulation tissue to fill the wound space, and resurfacing with epithelium, serosa, mucosa, endothelium, or mesothelium.

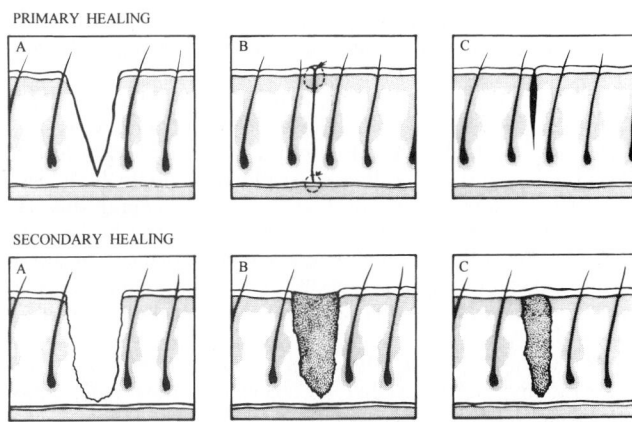

Figure 12–1. Wound healing classification. Top, Primary or first intention healing: a clean incision is made *(A)* and the wound margins are brought together *(B)* with sutures, staples, or adhesive strips. *C*, There is minimal scarring. Bottom, Secondary intention healing: the wound is left open to heal *(A and B)* by a combination of contraction, granulation, and epithelialization. *C*, A large scar results.

REPAIR PROCESSES

For ease of description, wound repair events are conceptually defined as inflammation, epithelialization, granulation, fibroplasia, and contraction. However, wound healing is really a concert of simultaneously occurring processes rather than a series of discrete steps. Of note, there are striking parallels between the cellular and molecular events of wound healing, regeneration, embryogenesis, and neoplasia.[8] There are many similarities in the stroma generated in both wounds and tumors, but a major difference is the factor of control: The wound repair process is self-limited, whereas tumor growth is not. Understanding the regulation of these phenomena should provide substantial potential clinical benefit.

Inflammation

Inflammation is the first stage of wound healing. After tissue injury, vessels immediately constrict, thromboplastic tissue products are exposed, and the coagulation and complement cascades are initiated. Platelets trapped in the wound degranulate, releasing a cadre of biologically active substances that are important for wound repair. At least three types of storage organelles are involved in platelet degranulation: (1) *alpha granules* contain growth factors such as platelet-derived growth factor (PDGF), transforming growth factor-beta (TGF-β), and insulin-like growth factor-1 (IGF-1), as well as adhesive glycoproteins such as fibronectin, fibrinogen, thrombospondin, and von Willebrand's factor; (2) *dense bodies* store vasoactive amines such as serotonin, which increase microvascular permeability; and (3) *lysosomes* contain hydrolases and proteases. Coagulation and platelet activation limit loss of blood and generate biologically active products that convert fibroblasts and endothelial cells into a reparative mode. The coagulation mechanisms activate prothrombin to thrombin, which converts fibrinogen to fibrin. Fibrin is then polymerized into stable clot. If the clot is exposed to air it will desiccate, forming a scab as a temporary wound cover. Fibrin and fibronectin within the clot provide the provisional matrix for early cell migration into the wound.

Products of the coagulation cascade regulate the cells in the injury area. Intact thrombin functions as a potent growth factor for fibroblasts and endothelial cells. Degraded thrombin fragments stimulate monocytes and platelets. Fibrinogen contains growth-promoting peptide sequences, and some fibrinopeptides are chemoattractant to monocytes. The clot also induces angiogenesis with directed capillary endothelial cell ingrowth. This complex pattern of interactions is easier to understand when one realizes that many growth factor peptides involved in wound healing are contributed by several sources.

As thrombus is formed, hemostasis in the wound is achieved. After the transient vasoconstriction, local small vessels dilate in response to kinin, complement components, and prostaglandins. White blood cells (first neutrophils, later monocytes) and plasma proteins enter the wound site. The early neutrophil infiltrate scavenges cellular debris, dirt, and bacteria. Activated complement fragments such as C5a attract neutrophils and aid in bacterial killing. Of note, healing may progress normally in the absence of neutrophils in a clean wound.[33]

Monocytes infiltrate later at the wound site and differentiate into macrophages that are crucial in the orchestration of tissue repair. Most wound macrophages are converted monocytes that are recruited from the circulation, but some are tissue macrophages that can proliferate locally. Macrophages continue to consume tissue and bacterial debris but, more important, secrete a plethora of growth factors.[29] These peptide growth factors attract and activate local endothelial cells, fibroblasts, and epithelial cells to begin their respective repair functions and initiate the next phase of wound repair—granulation tissue formation. Depletion of monocytes and macrophages causes a severe alteration in wound healing, with poor débridement, delayed fibroblast proliferation, and inadequate angiogenesis.[21] If wound conditions warrant, macrophages continue to recruit additional inflammatory cells. Lymphocytes enter the wound much later, and their role in wound repair is unclear. Interleukin-1 is a lymphocyte product that regulates collagenase activity, so the lymphocyte may be involved in collagen remodeling.

A unique environment is created in the wound space by the combination of the initial lack of microcirculation and the influx of white blood cells. As measured by microelectrodes, the wound space is hypoxic, hypoglycemic, acidotic, hyperkalemic, hyperlactic, and hypercarbic.[18]

Granulation

Granulation tissue is characterized by its beefy-red appearance, a consequence of endothelial cell division and migration to form a rich bed of new capillary networks (angiogenesis) at the wound site. Wound fibroblasts are derived from cells surrounding the wound that change their differentiated phenotypes and become mobile during the process of replication. Fibroblasts migrate into the wound, using the newly deposited fibrin and fibronectin matrix as a scaffold. Fibroblasts proliferate (fibroplasia) and synthesize new extracellular matrix. The directed growth of vascular endothelial cells occurs simultaneously with fibroplasia during granulation tissue formation, stimulated by platelet and activated macrophage products. Thus, granulation tissue is a loose matrix that appears in open wounds and is composed of collagen, fibronectin, and hyaluronic acid, with dense infiltration by macrophages, fibroblasts, and capillary endothelial cells. Granulation is most prominent in wounds healing by second intention. The new tissue that unites simple coapted wounds is not quite the same as granulation tissue, although it is composed of the same tissue elements.

The initial provisional wound matrix is composed of fibrin, fibronectin, and the glycosaminoglycan (GAG) hyaluronic acid. Because of its large water or hydration shell, hyaluronic acid provides a matrix that enhances cell migration. Adhesion glycoproteins, including fibronectin, laminin, and tenascin, are present throughout the early matrix and facilitate cell attachment and migration. Integrin receptors on cell surfaces bind to the matrix GAGs and glycoproteins. As fibroblasts enter and populate the wound, they use hyaluronidase to digest the provisional hyaluronic acid–rich matrix and then deposit larger, sulfated GAGs. Concomitantly, fibroblasts deposit collagen onto a fibronectin and GAG scaffold in a disorganized array. Collagen Types I and III are the major fibrillar collagens composing skin extracellular matrix. Type III collagen is initially more predominant in wounds compared with normal skin, but as the wound matures, Type I collagen is deposited in increasing amounts. Most collagen in both wounds and normal skin is Type I.

Epithelialization

Within minutes after injury, morphologic changes in keratinocytes at the wound margin are evident. In skin wounds, the epidermis thickens, and marginal basal cells enlarge and migrate over the wound defect. Once a cell begins migrating, it does not divide until epidermal continuity is restored. Fixed basal cells in a zone near the cut edge of the wound continue to divide, and their daughter cells flatten and migrate over the wound matrix as a sheet. Cell adhesion glycoproteins such as fibronectin, vitronectin, and tenascin provide a *railroad track* to facilitate epithelial cell migration over the wound matrix. Keratinocytes lay down laminin and Type IV collagen as part of their basement membrane. The keratinocytes then become columnar and divide as the layering of the epidermis is established. Necrotic tissue or foreign bodies are gradually separated from the wound as the epithelial cells migrate under them. Once epithelial integrity is completed, the cells reform hemidesmosomes and attach to the new basement membrane, thus completing a barrier to further contamination and moisture loss. Keratin forms as the cells mature.

Keratinocytes can respond to foreign body stimulation with migration as well. Sutures in skin wounds provide tracts along which these cells can migrate. Subsequent epithelial thickening and keratinization produce fibrotic reactions, cysts, and/or sterile abscesses centered on the suture.

Fibroplasia

Ultimately, the outcome of mammalian wound healing is scar formation. Scar is defined morphologically as the lack of tissue organization compared with surrounding normal tissue architecture. Disorganized collagen deposition plays a prominent role in scar formation. New collagen fibers secreted by fibroblasts are present as early as 3 days after wounding. As the collagenous matrix forms, densely packed fibers fill the wound site. The balance of collagen synthesis and degradation favors collagen deposition.

The wound remodels slowly over months to form a mature scar. The initially dense capillary network and fibroblast infiltrate regress until relatively few capillaries and fibroblasts remain. Wounds become stronger with time. The tensile strength of a skin wound increases rapidly from 1 to 6 weeks after wounding (Fig. 12–2). Thereafter, tensile strength increases at a slower pace and has been documented to increase up to 1 year after wounding in animal studies. The overall tensile strength of various wounded tissue varies; for exam-

ple, by 3 weeks after wounding, skin obtains 30% of normal tensile strength, fascia about 20%, intestine 65%, and urinary bladder about 95%. At best, the tensile strength of wounded skin reaches only about 80% that of unwounded skin. The final result of repair is scar, which is brittle and less elastic than normal skin, lacks skin appendages such as hair follicles or sweat glands, and is therefore less functional than the surrounding uninjured tissue. The major benefit of repair by scar is the relatively rapid reformation of tissue integrity.

Contraction

The destruction of soft tissue and its eventual repair involve the migration of a number of different cell types into the wound site, forming a new connective tissue matrix. In an open wound, surrounding uninjured skin is pulled over the defect by the process of wound contraction. The appearance of normal skin in the repair site is not due to skin regeneration but rather to the centripetal movement of skin. The newly deposited tissue that occupies the area between skin edges is scar, lacking normal dermal architecture and skin appendages. The skin that has been pulled over the defect has normal dermal fiber structure and skin appendages. In general, wound contraction is beneficial because a reduced area of scar tissue covers the defect.

In contrast to wound *contraction* is scar *contracture*, in which the contractile process follows completed wound closure. Scar contracture can be detrimental because established fibrotic tissue undergoes a reduction in surface area that can disrupt the mechanical function of neighboring tissue or structures. Examples include scar contracture occurring over a joint, restricting joint movement; esophageal stricture after caustic ingestion; and common bile duct stricture after injury. Although the mechanisms of wound contraction are still being defined, the process involves interaction between cellular forces and connective tissue organization.[9]

Compelling evidence shows that the cell responsible for wound contraction is the *myofibroblast* (Fig. 12–3), although wound matrix components undoubtedly play a role as well.[31] The myofibroblast is a mesenchymal cell with functional and structural characteristics in common with fibroblasts and smooth muscle cells. It is the cellular component of granulation tissue or scar connective tissue that generates contractile forces involving cytoplasmic actin-myosin muscular contractile activity. The dynamic contraction of these cytoplasmic structures produces the force that reorients surrounding connective tissue. This specialized cell is a classic feature of contracting wounds and is also observed in abundance in fibrocontractive diseases such as fibromatoses, hepatic cirrhosis, renal and pulmonary fibrosis, Dupuytren's contracture, and neoplasia-induced desmoplastic reactions. Consequently, the appearance of myofibroblasts indicates wound contraction, and persistence of myofibroblasts at the wound site correlates with scar contracture.

The myofibroblast is derived from the wound fibroblast, and the hallmark of the myofibroblastic phenotype is expression of alpha-smooth muscle actin, the actin isoform prevalent in vascular smooth muscle cells.[5] The actin microfilaments are arranged along the long axis of the fibroblasts and are associated with dense bodies for attachment to the surrounding extracellular matrix. Myofibroblasts show other characteristics of smooth muscle cells. Gap junctions connect granulation tissue myofibroblasts but are not found in normal tissue fibroblasts. Myofibroblasts also possess a unique attachment entity connecting the cytoskeleton to the extracellular matrix called the *fibronexus*. The fibronexus is essentially a connection that spans the cell membrane between intracellular microfilaments and extracellular fibronectin. Granulation tissue responds to the same drugs as does smooth mus-

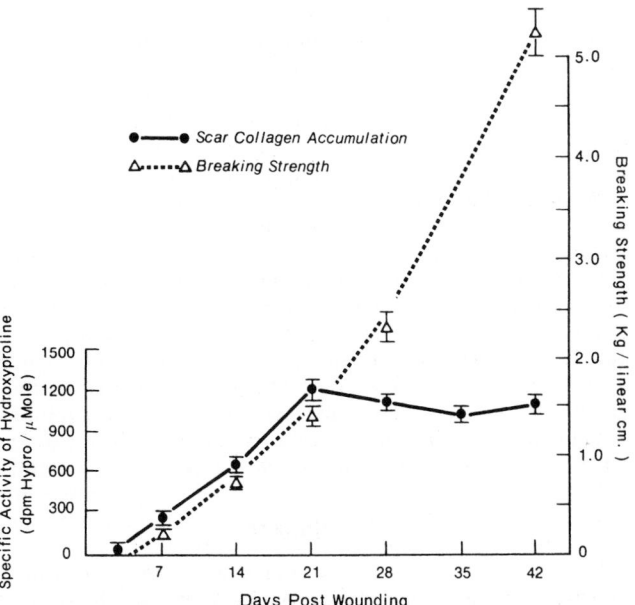

Figure 12–2. Comparison of scar collagen accumulation and breaking strength of rat skin wounds. Note that over the first 3 weeks, strength and collagen content correlate. After 21 days, strength increases with no change in wound collagen, reflecting scar remodeling. There is no correlation between collagen content and strength after 3 weeks. (From Madden, J. W., and Peacock, E. E., Jr.: Studies on the biology of collagen during wound healing: III. Dynamic metabolism of scar collagen and remodeling in dermal wounds. Ann. Surg., *174*:511, 1971.)

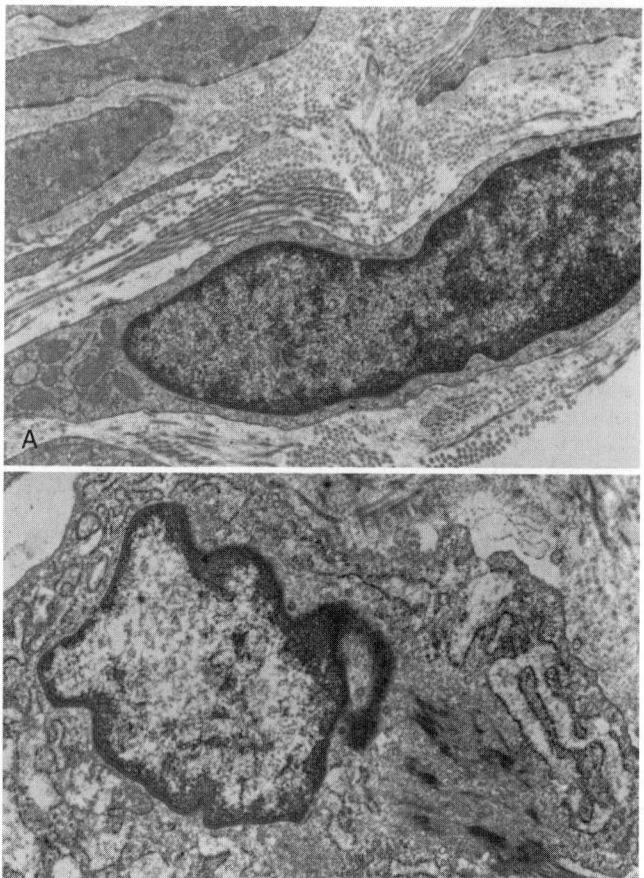

Figure 12–3. *A*, Normal resting fibroblast from human connective tissue. Note the large, smooth, oval nucleus; normal mitochondria; and a small amount of rough endoplasmic reticulum. The cell is surrounded by collagen fibrils cut in longitudinal and cross section. The cell fragments seen in the upper left are typical smooth muscle cells. Electron micrograph, ×22,000. *B*, Myofibroblast from a patient with plantar fasciitis. Compared with the fibroblast, note the highly irregular nucleus, the large amount of rough endoplasmic reticulum, and the dense collection of myofilaments. There are numerous dense bodies adjacent to and intermingled with the myofilaments. No basal lamina is seen, and the cell is surrounded by numerous collagen fibrils. This cell has ultrastructural features typical of both a fibroblast and a smooth muscle cell. Electron micrograph, ×25,000. (Courtesy of Edward C. Carlson, Ph.D.)

cle, by either contracting or relaxing. Thus, the force of wound contraction is probably generated by actin bundles in the myofibroblasts, and it is transmitted to the sides of the wound by cell-cell and cell-matrix links.

GROWTH FACTORS: REGULATORS OF REPAIR

Growth factors play a prominent role in the regulation of wound healing. These polypeptides are released by a variety of activated cells at the wound site, and they can stimulate or inhibit cell proliferation, movement, and biosynthetic activity (Fig. 12–4). They can act as autocrine (produced by the cell to act on itself) or paracrine (produced by one cell type to act on another in the local area) factors. Growth factors also chemoattract new cells to the wound. Myriad growth factors can be present in wounds. Many growth factors have overlapping functions, and their various biologic effects are only beginning to be understood.

Of the many cytokines that have been implicated in wound healing, TGF-β affects all phases of healing, including the inflammatory response and matrix accumulation. The topical

application of TGF-β accelerates normal healing. The name TGF-β is derived from the observation that normal cells exposed to TGF-β while grown in soft agar proliferate as though they had been virally transformed. The mammalian TGF-β family consists of three known isoforms—β1, β2, and β3—that are closely related both structurally and functionally. TGF-β is released from platelets and macrophages in the wound. In addition, TGF-β is released from fibroblasts and acts in an autocrine manner to further stimulate its own synthesis and secretion. Many cells secrete TGF-β in a latent form associated with a binding protein that makes the TGF-β biologically inactive. This inactive, or latent, complex may be a storage form of the cytokine until it is activated by macrophages or local conditions. Through autocrine and paracrine mechanisms, TGF-β stimulates the deposition of collagen and other matrix components by fibroblasts, inhibits collagenase, blocks plasminogen inhibitor, enhances angiogenesis, and is chemotactic for fibroblasts, monocytes, and macrophages.[34] Through these mechanisms, TGF-β can augment fibrosis at the wound site (Fig. 12–5).

PDGF is released from platelet alpha granules immediately after injury. PDGF attracts neutrophils, macrophages, and fibroblasts to the wound and serves as a powerful mitogen. Macrophages, endothelial cells, and fibroblasts also synthesize and secrete PDGF. PDGF stimulates fibroblasts to synthesize new extracellular matrix, predominantly noncollagenous components such as GAGs and adhesion proteins. PDGF also increases the amount of fibroblast-secreted collagenase, indicating a role for this cytokine in tissue remodeling.[28]

Angiogenesis is the formation of new blood vessels by directed endothelial cell migration and growth. This widespread process occurs in development, cancer, and wound healing.[14] Angiogenesis is stimulated by acidic and basic fibroblast growth factors (aFGF and bFGF, respectively). Both endothelial cells and macrophages produce aFGF and bFGF. Although bFGF is about 10 times as potent as aFGF, it has identical effects because it binds to the same FGF receptor. These growth factors are bound by heparin and the GAG heparan sulfate in the extracellular matrix. Basement membrane serves as a storage depot for bFGF, which is released when the basement membrane is degraded by collagenases and other hydrolytic enzymes after injury. Other stores of FGF include the intracellular spaces of endothelial cells, smooth muscle cells, and fibroblasts, which may be released on cell damage or ischemia. The FGFs stimulate endothelial cells to divide and form new capillaries. They also chemoattract endothelial cells and fibroblasts.

Epithelialization is directly stimulated by at least two growth factors: epidermal growth factor (EGF) and keratinocyte growth factor (KGF). EGF is released by keratinocytes to act in an autocrine manner, whereas KGF is released by fibroblasts to act in a paracrine manner to stimulate keratinocyte division and differentiation.[37] EGF is the same protein as urogastrone, a peptide found in human urine that inhibits gastric acid secretion. The major effect of EGF is to encourage cells to continue through the cell cycle. In wounds, it has this effect on epithelial cells, fibroblasts, and endothelial cells. EGF is also chemotactic for epithelial cells and increases the secretion of collagenases by fibroblasts, which is an important step in tissue remodeling.

Many other growth factors affect wound repair. For example, IGF-1 stimulates collagen synthesis by fibroblasts and functions synergistically with PDGF and bFGF to facilitate fibroblast proliferation. Interferon-gamma has been shown to downregulate collagen synthesis. The various interleukins mediate inflammatory cell functions at the wound site.

Surgeons may soon be able to enhance repair by adding or deleting growth factors from healing wounds. The use of recombinant deoxyribonucleic acid (DNA) technology has

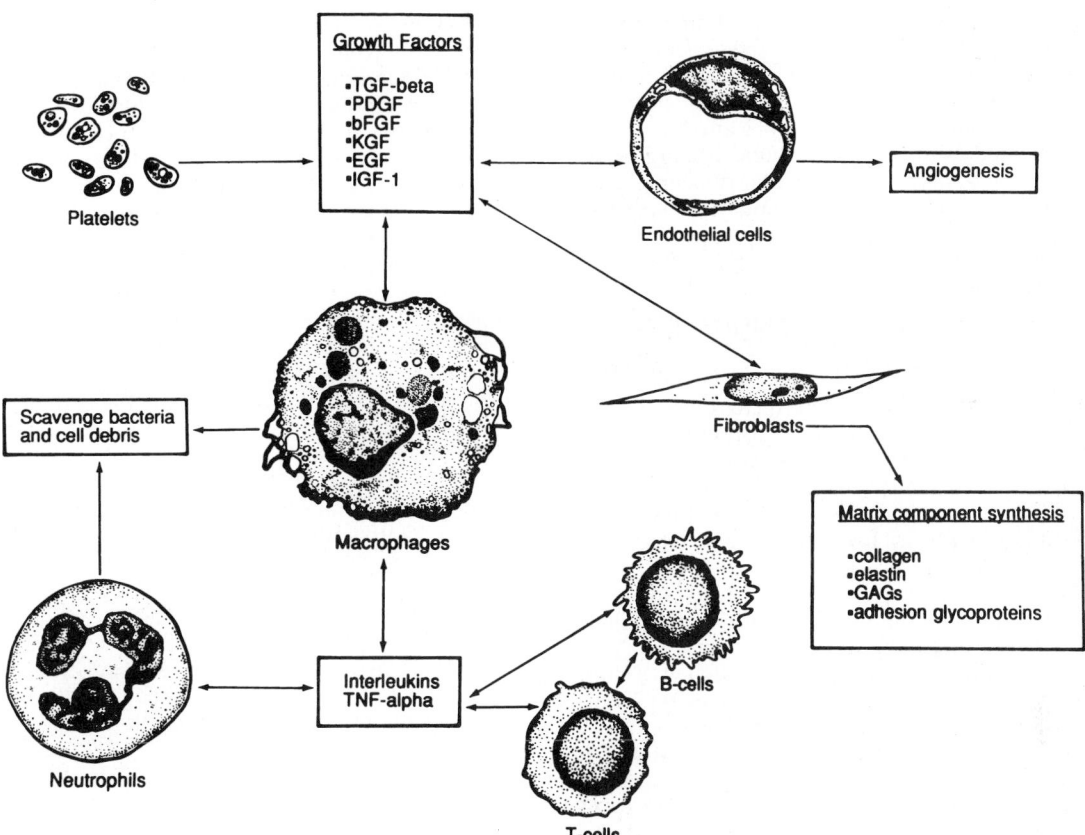

Figure 12–4. Schematic of the complex interrelationships between cells and growth factors involved in wound repair. Growth factors regulate each cell type involved in wound healing. For abbreviations, see text.

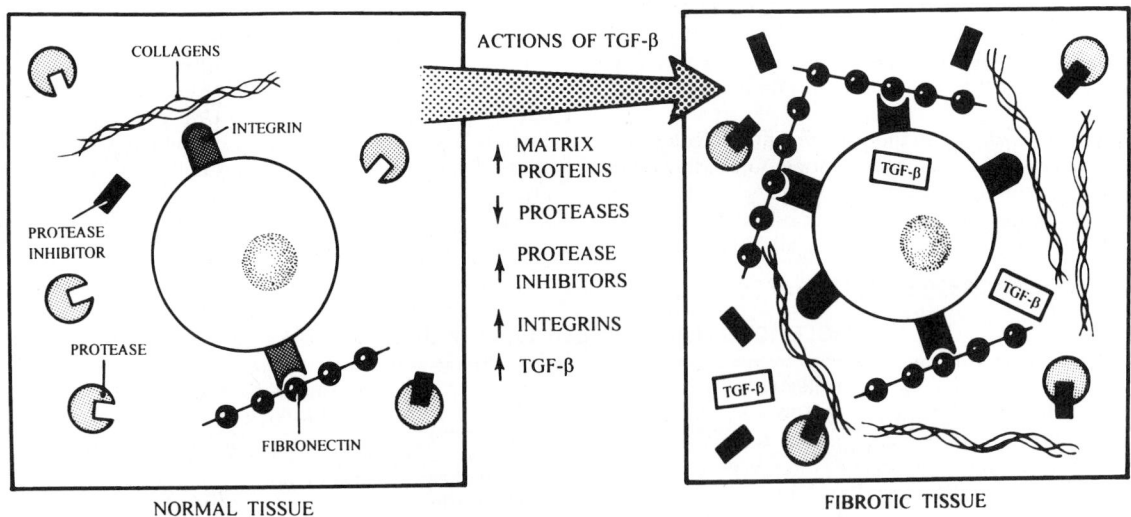

ACTIONS OF TGF-β IN THE FIBROTIC RESPONSE TO INJURY

Figure 12–5. The sustained production of transforming growth factor-beta (TGF-β) at the wound site leads to tissue fibrosis. Platelets and macrophages release TGF-β at the site of injury. To repair the damage, TGF-β induces the deposition of extracellular matrix by simultaneously stimulating the production of new matrix proteins (fibronectin, collagens, and proteoglycans), blocking matrix degradation by decreasing the synthesis of proteases and increasing the synthesis of protease inhibitors, and modulating the expression of cell-surface integrins in a manner that enhances cell-matrix interaction and matrix assembly. TGF-β also induces its own production by cells, thus amplifying its biologic effects. (Adapted from Border, W. A., and Noble, N. A.: Transforming growth factor beta in tissue fibrosis. N. Engl. J. Med., *331*:1286, 1994. Copyright 1994. Massachusetts Medical Society. All rights reserved.)

permitted the development of an increasing number of endogenous growth regulatory peptides for therapeutic biologics. Investigators have accelerated healing rates in normal wounds by adding exogenous EGF, TGF-β, PDGF, or bFGF.[4, 30] Addition of these same growth factors has also augmented repair in animal models of impaired wound healing conditions such as diabetes, chronic steroid use, duodenal ulcer, and chemotherapy.[36] Clinical trials are under way. Further studies are needed to determine the precise growth factor combination that is optimal for specific wound types.

MATRIX FORMATION AND REMODELING
Collagen

The extracellular matrix is the complex, cross-linked structure of proteins and polysaccharides that surrounds cells and organizes the geometry of tissues. Collagen is the principal component of the extracellular matrix (25% of total body protein), and a scar is loosely defined as an abnormal, disorganized collection of collagen following wound repair. The collagens are a large group of triple-helix structural matrix proteins (Table 12–1). Type I collagen is the major structural component of bones, skin, and tendons. Type II is found predominantly in cartilage. Type III is found in association with Type I, although the ratio varies in different tissues. Type IV collagen is found in basement membranes in association with mucopolysaccharides and laminin, whereas Type V is found in the cornea in association with Type III and is important in maintaining transparency. Other types of collagen (up to Type XII) are found in small amounts in many tissues and serve unknown functions.

Collagen is a key component of all phases of wound repair. Immediately after injury, the exposure of fibrillar collagen to blood promotes aggregation and activation of platelets and the release of chemotactic factors that initiate healing. Collagen fragments released by leukocytic collagenases attract fibroblasts to the injured area. Later, collagen becomes the foundation of the new extracellular matrix. Normal dermis contains about 80% Type I collagen and 20% Type III collagen. The amount of Type III collagen in healing wounds is elevated for 3 to 4 days before the levels of Type I collagen increase. As early as 24 hours after injury, invading fibroblasts synthesize and secrete Type I and III collagen to form the neomatrix. Granulation tissue has higher levels of Type III collagen than most normal tissues, although Type I is still the major component.

The fibroblast manufactures the procollagen molecule (tropocollagen) intracellularly on membrane-bound ribosomes, packages procollagen into secretory vesicles in the Golgi apparatus, and then exports it across the cell membrane into the extracellular space. Once outside the fibroblast, procollagen undergoes enzymatic cleavage of the nonhelical portion to release the collagen molecule, which then forms intramolecular and intermolecular cross-links, leading to alignment in collagen fibrils followed by aggregation into cable-like collagen fibers. Overall, some important structural features of collagen include three alpha-peptide chains in a right-handed helix, the presence of glycine in every third position, and the presence of two unique amino acids—hydroxylysine and hydroxyproline.

Several steps of collagen synthesis are unusual compared with standard protein synthesis. For instance, although extracellular collagen contains significant amounts of hydroxyproline—the only major protein to do so—its genes code only for proline. As the growing alpha-peptide chain leaves the ribosomal network, it is inserted into the endoplasmic reticulum, where it is glycosylated, and 14% of its prolines are hydroxylated by two dioxygenases called *lysyl hydroxylase* and *prolyl hydroxylase*. Prolyl hydroxylase is one of the rate-limiting enzymes in collagen synthesis. Substrates and cofactors such as iron, alpha-ketoglutarate, ascorbate, and oxygen are important participants in this process. If insufficient prolines are hydroxylated, the alpha-peptide chains cannot assume a stable triple helix, the collagen cannot be exported, and the incomplete unassociated alpha chains are broken down. Thus, ascorbate deficiency (scurvy) and hypoxia have similar effects on collagen synthesis. Once the triple-helical procollagen molecule is exported, the telopeptide ends of the molecule that prevent polymerization are cleaved. The collagen molecule is polymerized by several types of chemical bonds, among which lysines are oxidized and condensed to lysyl-lysine bonds by lysyl oxidase. This step is fundamental to collagen cross-linking. Without these bonds, collagen fails to gain structural stability. Formation of cross-links can be inhibited by two pharmacologic agents: beta-aminopropionitrile inhibits lysyl oxidase, and D-penicillamine binds to collagen substrate directly to prevent collagen cross-link formation.

What starts and stops collagen synthesis is being actively investigated. Many signals influence collagen synthesis, including growth factors, nutritional elements, the partial pressure of oxygen, and lactate concentration. For example, a gradient of oxygen tension extends from the perfused wound periphery to the hypoxic microenvironment at the center of the wound, which in turn can affect proline hydroxylation.[16] Fibroblasts exposed to hypoxia or high lactate concentrations, conditions found in the wound microenvironment, increase their rate of collagen synthesis when oxygen levels are increased. Hypoxia causes accumulation of lactate in the cell, and lactate stimulates collagen synthesis by at least two mechanisms: increased collagen gene transcription and increased prolyl hydroxylase activity.

TABLE 12–1. Major Collagen Types and Distribution

Type*	Molecular Formula	Tissue Distribution
I	$[\alpha1(I)]_2\alpha2(I)$	All connective tissues except cartilage and basement membranes; accounts for 90% of body collagen
II	$[\alpha1(II)]_3$	Cartilage, vitreous humor, intervertebral disc
III	$[\alpha1(III)]_3$	Skin, blood vessel, internal organs
IV	$[\alpha1(IV)]_2\alpha2(IV)$	Basement membrane
V	$[\alpha1(V)]_2\alpha2(V)$	Essentially all tissues
VI	$[\alpha1(VI),\alpha2(VI),\alpha3(VI)]$	Essentially all tissues

*Collagen Type VI is composed of three types of alpha chain, Types I and IV are composed of two types of alpha chain, and Types II and III are composed of only one type of alpha chain. Most collagens contain three alpha chains interacting in a helical structure. Only 6 types of collagen are shown, but more than 12 types have been described to date.

Modified from Alberts, B., Bray, D., Lewis, J., Raff, M., Roberts, K., and Watson, J.D.: The Molecular Biology of the Cell. New York, Garland, 1989, p. 810.

The control mechanisms for collagen synthesis appear to involve several steps (Fig. 12–6). Lactate (and hypoxia) reduces the nicotinamide adenine dinucleotide (NAD^+) pool by converting NAD^+ to NADH. This reduces the amount of the metabolite of NAD^+, adenosine diphosphoribose (ADPR), which is merely NAD^+ with its nicotinamide removed. The polymerized form of ADPR (PADPR) may normally downregulate collagen gene transcription in the resting state. Prolyl hydroxylase is also inhibited by ADPR; ADPR removal activates the enzyme by decreasing levels of NAD^+. Thus, lactate alters both the genetic expression of unhydroxylated procollagen gene transcripts in the cell nucleus and the cytoplasmic hydroxylation of these peptides. This system is then limited only by the prolyl hydroxylase substrates ascorbate and oxygen.[17]

Accumulation of collagen in the wound area depends on the ratio of collagen synthesis to collagen degradation by local enzymes. Early in the wound healing phase, the amount of collagen degradation is low, but it increases as the wound matures. Interstitial collagenases are the principal degradative enzymes. They are secreted by granulocytes, macrophages, fibroblasts, and epithelial cells as inactive zymogens that are activated by proteases. Interstitial collagenases cleave all three chains of the collagen Type I and III triple helix at a specific bond, creating two characteristic fragments that represent three fourths and one fourth of the original molecule. This allows the collagen to denature and become susceptible to other nonspecific proteases. The synthesis and activity of collagenases are modulated by growth factors and local protease inhibitors.

Control of collagen synthesis, secretion, cross-linking, and degradation is incompletely understood but is the subject of much wound healing research. Collagen is obviously important in all phases of wound healing and is critical for return of tissue integrity and strength.

Proteoglycans

Alterations in the synthesis of proteoglycans (PGs) and their constituent GAGs correlate with the cell proliferation, migration, and collagen synthesis that accompany adult wound healing.[2] PGs are a heterogeneous group of polyanionic macromolecules consisting of a protein core to which a variable number of linear, sulfated GAG chains are covalently bound (Table 12–2). These PGs include versican, a large chondroitin sulfate proteoglycan (CSPG); decorin, a small dermatan sulfate proteoglycan (DSPG); and heparan sulfate proteoglycan (HSPG). Hyaluronic acid (HA), often a massive GAG molecule without either sulfated groups or a core protein, consists of variable lengths of repeating disaccharide, leading to a broad range of molecular weights. The sulfated GAGs temporally follow HA in the healing process, and the decline of HA and the appearance of sulfated GAGs have been shown in several embryologic systems to correlate with the onset of cytodifferentiation.

The variations in protein cores and types of sugar moieties create tremendous variability in PG structure, but all share a polyanionic charge that influences their interactions with other macromolecules and cells. They appear to create a charged, hydrated environment that facilitates cell mobility. In addition, PGs and GAGs affect wound collagen organization and fibrillogenesis and, by binding to specific sites on collagen, control its rate of degradation.

Adhesion Glycoproteins and Integrins

As cells become mobile during wound repair, specific interactions occur between them and the extracellular matrix that allow cells to detach and migrate. The matrix provides the scaffolding for cell attachment and migration through various glycoprotein components, such as fibronectin, tenascin, laminin, fibrinogen, thrombospondin, and vitronectin. Cells bind to these adhesion glycoproteins with cell-surface adhesion receptors called *integrins,* which are a family of membrane glycoproteins consisting of two types of subunits, alpha and beta. Integrins provide a bond among a cell's cytoskeleton, its surrounding extracellular matrix, and adjacent cells. Cell motility direction may be determined by the relative integrin-ligand binding affinities of the various adhesion glycoproteins bound to a particular cell.

Fibronectins are prominent matrix molecules involved in wound contraction, cell migration, collagen matrix deposi-

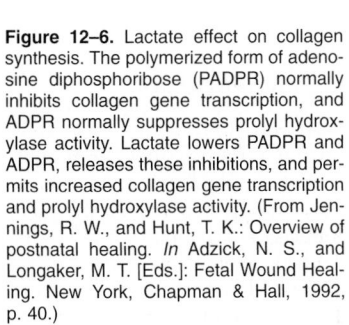

Figure 12–6. Lactate effect on collagen synthesis. The polymerized form of adenosine diphosphoribose (PADPR) normally inhibits collagen gene transcription, and ADPR normally suppresses prolyl hydroxylase activity. Lactate lowers PADPR and ADPR, releases these inhibitions, and permits increased collagen gene transcription and prolyl hydroxylase activity. (From Jennings, R. W., and Hunt, T. K.: Overview of postnatal healing. *In* Adzick, N. S., and Longaker, M. T. [Eds.]: Fetal Wound Healing. New York, Chapman & Hall, 1992, p. 40.)

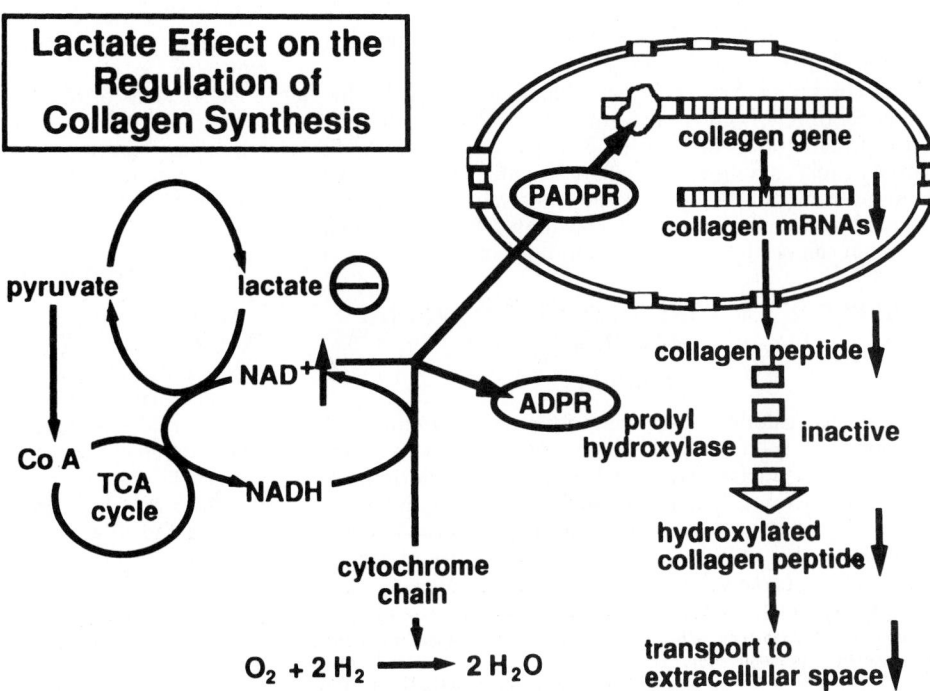

Lactate Effect on the Regulation of Collagen Synthesis

TABLE 12–2. The Glycosaminoglycans

Glycosaminoglycan	Molecular Weight	Repeating Disaccharide (A-B)		Linked to Protein	Other Sugar Components	Tissue Distribution
		Monosaccharide A	Monosaccharide B			
Hyaluronic acid	4000–8 × 10⁶	D-glucuronic acid	N-acetyl-D-glucosamine	–	None	Most connective tissues, skin, cartilage, synovial fluid, vitreous humor
Chondroitin sulfate	5000–50,000	D-glucuronic acid	N-acetyl-D-galactosamine	+	D-galactose D-xylose	Skin, cartilage, bone, cornea
Dermatan sulfate	15,000–40,000	D-glucuronic acid or L-iduronic acid*	N-acetyl-D-galactosamine	+	D-galactose D-xylose	Skin, blood vessels, heart
Heparan sulfate	5000–12,000	D-glucuronic acid or L-iduronic acid*	N-acetyl-D-glucosamine	+	D-galactose D-xylose	Lungs, arteries, cell surfaces
Heparin	6000–25,000	D-glucuronic acid or L-iduronic acid*	N-acetyl-D-glucosamine	+	D-galactose D-xylose	Skin, lungs, liver, mast cells
Keratan sulfate	4000–19,000	D-galactose	N-acetyl-D-glucosamine	+	D-galactosamine D-mannose L-fucose Sialic acid	Cartilage, cornea, intervertebral disc

*L-iduronic acid is produced by the epimerization of D-glucuronic acid at the position where the carboxyl group is located. Thus, dermatan sulfate is a modified form of chondroitin sulfate, and the two types of repeating disaccharide sequences usually occur as alternating segments in the same glycosaminoglycan chain.

From Alberts, B., Bray, D., Lewis, J., Raff, M., Roberts, K., and Watson, J.D.: The Molecular Biology of the Cell. New York, Garland, 1989, p. 805.

tion, and re-epithelialization. Fibronectin is one of the first proteins to be laid down in a wound and forms part of the preliminary matrix. Fibronectin acts as the scaffold for cell migration and collagen deposition. The molecule is a complex glycoprotein made up of two subunits, each of which has specific collagen binding sites. The differences between soluble plasma fibronectin and stromal fibronectin, as well as the differences between its two subunits, result from post-translational modification of a single fibronectin gene product.[12] Fibronectin is produced by fibroblasts, epithelial cells, and macrophages, and it can bind a wide variety of molecules involved in wound healing, including collagens, actin, fibrin, HA, heparin, fibronectin itself, and cell-surface receptors on fibroblasts. Granulation tissue fibroblasts are coated with a layer of fibronectin matrix, and myofibroblasts are covered with fibronectin, which forms part of the fibronexus attachment that effects wound contraction.

Tenascin is a matrix glycoprotein that inhibits the cell adhesion effect of fibronectin and permits cells to detach from the matrix and migrate. The appearance of tenascin in the wound matrix correlates with the initiation of epithelial and mesenchymal cell migration. Laminin, an important component of basement membrane, must be reconstituted before epithelial migration can occur across the wound defect.

CLINICAL FACTORS THAT AFFECT WOUND HEALING

Nutrition

The precise caloric requirements for optimal wound healing have not been defined. Large injuries such as burns greatly increase metabolic rate, whereas smaller injuries such as isolated fractures do not increase nutritional requirements. Protein depletion impairs wound healing if recent weight loss exceeds 15% to 25% of body weight. The risk of wound dehiscence is increased in hypoalbuminemic patients, signifying the detrimental effect of chronic malnutrition on repair.

Vitamin C (ascorbic acid) deficiency causes scurvy. In patients with this deficiency, wound healing is arrested during fibroplasia. Normal amounts of fibroblasts are present in the wound, but they produce an inadequate amount of collagen. Vitamin C is necessary for hydroxylation of proline and lysine residues. Without hydroxyproline, newly synthesized collagen is not transported out of cells. Without hydroxylysine, collagen fibrils are not cross-linked. In severe scurvy, not only do new wounds fail to heal but old healed scars open, because ongoing collagen lysis greatly outstrips new collagen production.

Vitamin A (retinoic acid) requirements increase during injury. Severely injured patients require supplemental vitamin A to maintain normal serum levels. Vitamin A also partially reverses the impaired healing in chronically steroid-treated patients.

Vitamin B₆ (pyridoxine) deficiency impairs collagen cross-linking. Vitamin B₁ (thiamine) and vitamin B₂ (riboflavin) deficiencies cause syndromes associated with poor wound repair.

Deficiencies of trace metals such as zinc and copper have been implicated in poor wound repair, since these divalent cations are cofactors in many important enzymatic reactions. Zinc deficiency is associated with poor epithelialization and chronic, nonhealing wounds.

Oxygen, Anemia, and Perfusion

Wounds require adequate oxygen delivery to heal well. Oxygen is required for successful inflammation, angiogenesis, epithelialization, and matrix deposition. Ischemic wounds heal poorly and have a much greater risk of infection. Wound infection is influenced by a variety of factors, such as occlusive vascular disease, vasoconstriction, and hypovolemia. The increased oxygen demand resulting from infection, and the concomitant neutrophil response further increase the total oxygen and nutrient demand. Excessive suture tension causes local wound ischemia and complications in wound healing. Conversely, increased oxygen delivery at the wound improves healing. Experimentally, collagen synthesis by fibroblasts is increased with supplemental oxygen.

Anemia in a normovolemic patient is not detrimental to

wound repair as long as the hematocrit is greater than 15%, because oxygen content in blood does not affect wound collagen synthesis. However, increasing the P_{O_2} in blood levels high above 100% hemoglobin saturation allows more oxygen to diffuse to the relatively poorly vascularized wound edge, which upregulates collagen synthesis.

Tissue perfusion is the ultimate determinant of wound oxygenation and nutrition.[18] To optimize wound repair, those factors leading to wound ischemia should be prevented. Sutures should not be placed too tightly. The patient should be kept warm, pain should be well controlled to prevent catecholamine-mediated vasoconstriction, and hypovolemia should be treated.

Diabetes Mellitus and Obesity

Wound healing is impaired in diabetic patients by unknown mechanisms. Healing is enhanced if glucose levels are well controlled. The high incidence of chronic cutaneous wounds in these patients often relates to the combination of neuropathy, vasculopathy, impaired host defense against infection, and metabolic disorders. Obesity interferes with repair independently of diabetes. Obese patients with diabetes have impaired wound healing regardless of the degree of glucose control and insulin therapy. Poor wound perfusion and necrotic adipose debris probably impair healing in both diabetic and nondiabetic obese patients.

Corticosteroids, Chemotherapy, and Radiation Therapy

Use of pharmacologic steroids impairs healing, especially when given in the first 3 days after wounding. Steroids reduce wound inflammation, epithelialization, and collagen synthesis.

Both radiation and chemotherapeutic agents have their greatest effects on dividing cells. The division of endothelial cells, fibroblasts, and keratinocytes is impaired in irradiated tissue, which slows wound healing. Irradiated tissue usually has some degree of residual endothelial cell injury and endarteritis, which causes atrophy, fibrosis, and poor tissue repair. Chemotherapeutic agents are not administered until at least 5 to 7 days postoperatively to prevent impairment of the initial healing events.

Infection

Wound contamination by bacteria causes clinical wound infection and delays healing if more than 10^5 organisms per mg. tissue are present. In antiquity, the host response to local infection was described as rubor, dolor, calor, and tumor (erythema, pain, heat, and swelling). Thus, infected wounds are erythematous and tender and commonly have drainage. The patient may be febrile. Immediate wound opening with suture removal and débridement is essential. Administration of antibiotics treats surrounding cellulitis.

FETAL WOUND HEALING

Fetal skin wounds heal rapidly and without the scarring and inflammation that accompany adult skin wounds. In all species examined (mice, rats, rabbits, pigs, sheep, and monkeys), the prenatal wound healing process is faster and more efficient than adult repair and produces new tissue rather than scar. Similarly, human fetal surgery has shown that the younger the fetus is at the time of surgery, the less likely it is that he or she will be born with surgical scars. How does this happen? A summary of some of the phenomenologic differences between adult and fetal repair is shown in Table 12–3.

Fetal wound healing may represent a paradigm for ideal tissue repair.[1] The therapeutic goal is to apply the lessons of fetal wound healing to control the quality of healing. This model may provide the tools for surgeons to regulate each step of the adult wound healing process.

Problem of Scar Formation

Scarring and fibrosis dominate some diseases in virtually every branch of medicine and surgery (Table 12–4). Surgeons confront the consequences of excessive scar formation daily. Skin incisions heal with scar, and sometimes pathologic processes such as keloids and hypertrophic scars are the unanticipated sequelae. Abdominal surgery invariably leads to intraperitoneal fibrous adhesions, and repeated bouts of mechanical intestinal obstruction can result. Strictures occur at anastomotic sites, whether of the bowel, blood vessel, trachea, ureter, or bile duct. Pediatric surgeons are frustrated by the tragic problem of biliary atresia in infants—a progressive, fibrotic obliteration of the hepatobiliary tree. Other examples include esophageal stricture after caustic ingestion, posttraumatic urethral stricture, tendon adhesions after hand surgery, and transmission loss after peripheral nerve injury.

Pathologic scarring and fibrosis also frequently occur in nonsurgical specialties. Ophthalmologists observe retrolental fibroplasia in premature infants as well as a similar fibrotic retinopathy in diabetics. Gastroenterologists attempt to mollify the bleeding, liver failure, and encephalopathic complications of hepatic cirrhosis. Pulmonologists detect bronchopulmonary dysplasia in tiny premature infants and diagnose

TABLE 12–3. Comparison of Adult and Fetal Skin Wound Healing Characteristics

Wound Healing Characteristic	Adult	Fetus
Scar	Present	Absent
Cell proliferation	Slower	Faster
Speed to closure	Slower	Faster
Scab	Present	Absent
Oxygen tension	Greater	Lesser
Fluid environment	Absent	Present
Sterile environment	Absent	Present
Skin temperature	Cooler	Warmer
Acute inflammation	Greater	Lesser
Matrix deposition	Slower, disorganized	Faster, organized
TGF-β and bFGF	Greater	Lesser
Angiogenesis	Greater	Lesser
Keratinization	Present	Immature

TABLE 12–4. Consequences of Scar Formation

Organ/System	Effect
Skin	Keloid
	Hypertrophic scar
	Burn contracture
	Scleroderma
Gastrointestinal tract	Stricture
	Adhesions
	Chronic pancreatitis
Liver	Cirrhosis
	Biliary atresia
Lung	Interstitial fibrosis
	Bronchopulmonary dysplasia
Heart	Rheumatic heart disease
	Ventricular aneurysm
Eye	Retrolental fibroplasia
	Diabetic retinopathy
Nerve	Transmission loss
Bone	Ankylosis
	Osteoarthritis
Kidney	Glomerulonephritis

pulmonary fibrosis in aging cigarette smokers. Radiotherapists worry about radiation-induced fibrosis. Cardiologists wish to ameliorate the fibrotic end-points of rheumatic heart disease—shortened, distorted chordae and scarred valve leaflets. Dermatologists deal with scleroderma. And this is only a partial list.

All these problems are notoriously difficult to prevent or treat. Clinicians' therapeutic role is largely to hope for the best, much as physicians did in the past when confronted with what were then unsolved problems: appendicitis until 100 years ago, bacterial infections until 50 years ago, and organ replacement until recently. An understanding of fetal wound healing may lead to therapeutic strategies to help avert scarring and fibrosis. Healing without scar would have a tremendous impact on both medical and surgical practice.

Fetal Skin

The less-developed state of fetal skin at the time of wounding may be important for scar-free tissue repair. The human fetal epidermis begins with two cell layers, the basal layer and the periderm, at about 4 weeks' gestation. The periderm is the outermost single-cell layer of the fetal skin. Peridermal cells have microvilli and blebs projecting off the surface of the skin into the amniotic fluid. Although the function of the periderm has not been determined, a secretive or absorptive process has been hypothesized. As development continues, an intermediate epidermal cell layer develops. Keratinization begins at 9 to 16 weeks' gestation. During this period, primordial hair follicles and sebaceous glands become apparent. By 24 weeks' gestation, the epidermis has completely keratinized and stratified into adult morphologic layers.[20]

The dermis, which is the location of scar in adult wounds, is similarly undergoing morphologic and biochemical changes. Early in gestation, the fetal dermis is thin and cellular, owing to the paucity of extracellular matrix. As development progresses, dermal collagen is deposited, and sulfated GAGs replace nonsulfated GAGs, among which HA is predominant. The rapid growth and the relatively undifferentiated state of fetal skin set the stage for the unique response of fetal skin to injury.

Fetal Environment

Differences between the fetal and adult environments may affect wound repair. The fetal wound environment is quite different from the wound environment after adult tissue injury. The fetus is profoundly hypoxemic, with an arterial Po_2 of 20 mm. Hg, which is lower than the arterial Po_2 of a maskless mountaineer on top of Mount Everest. In addition, fetal skin wounds are continually bathed in warm, sterile amniotic fluid, which is rich in growth factors that are crucial for development.

The lower fetal oxygen tension and the amniotic fluid environment might each dramatically influence wound healing. However, the contribution of these differences to tissue repair may be partially discounted by recent results from fetal animal studies. Fetal tissue oxygenation remains consistently low throughout gestation, yet fetal wound healing is affected by gestational age: Skin wound healing in the rat, lamb, or rhesus monkey fetus becomes adultlike, with scar formation, late in gestation.[10, 26] Thus, despite a relatively constant intrauterine environment, fetuses heal without scar formation early in gestation and begin to scar late in gestation. Several other lines of evidence suggest that amniotic fluid exposure is not crucial for scarless tissue repair. At birth, the opossum is physiologically and anatomically a fetus and remains attached to the mother's nipple for 4 to 5 weeks before weaning. Although the *fetal* development of the marsupial continues in the nonsterile environment of the pouch and in the absence of an amniotic fluid milieu, scarless skin healing still occurs in 2-day-old pouch young, whereas 28-day-old opossums heal with scar (Fig. 12–7).[15] Similarly, isolated fetal rat or mouse tissue grown in organ culture media can heal wounds without scar formation, demonstrating that amniotic fluid and fetal blood components such as platelets are not required for scarless repair.[27] Finally, fetal lamb studies have shown that exclusion of wounds from amniotic fluid by a Silastic patch does not obviate repair, and that adult skin transplanted to the fetus heals with scar formation despite exposure to the fluid intrauterine environment.[24] This research suggests that scarless fetal skin healing properties are intrinsic to fetal skin and are not due to the fetal environment.

These experiments led to the hypothesis that fetal healing must involve different cellular and connective tissue events than adult repair and that this process is independent of the unique fetal environment. In addition, we have learned that the type of healing that occurs in fetal animals also depends on the extent of tissue damage—large excisional fetal skin wounds scar earlier in gestation than incisional wounds; the type of tissue that is injured—internal fetal tissues such as the diaphragm muscle, stomach, and peritoneum heal with scar formation; and the species of animal—fetal rabbits do not heal excisional skin wounds.

Fetal Fibroblast

Several recent studies suggest that the fetal fibroblast plays a central role in coordinating scarless healing. An exciting new technique to study human fetal skin wound healing in the postnatal environment has been developed, and this model has helped delineate the relative importance of fetal tissue properties and the absence of certain inflammatory cytokines in scarless repair.[25] Grafts of human fetal skin placed onto adult athymic mice retain the morphologic features of normal fetal skin development. Human fetal skin that is transplanted to a subcutaneous location on an adult athymic mouse and subsequently wounded heals without scar formation, whereas the same skin heals with scar formation when transplanted to a cutaneous location. *In situ* hy-

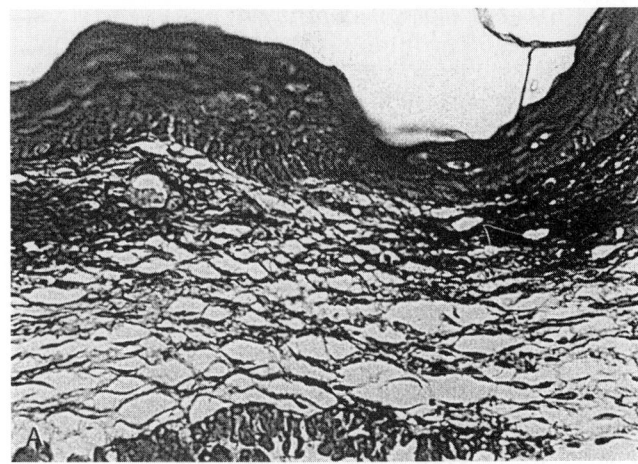

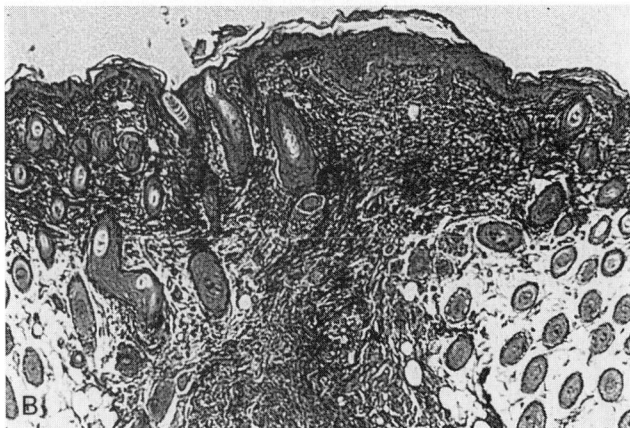

Figure 12–7. Comparison of scar-free repair and healing with scar using Mallory's trichrome staining. *A,* Healed skin wound in a 2-day-old opossum pouch young, 2 days after wounding, illustrating the absence of scar formation in the dermis and the very rapid repair process. There is epithelial thickening at the wound site and a fine reticular collagen pattern in the healed dermis. *B,* Day 28 pouch young wound, 7 days postoperatively, demonstrating extensive scarring in the dermis as well as abnormal orientation of the collagen fibers perpendicular to the dermis.

bridization and immunohistochemical studies have shown that cutaneous human fetal grafts heal with an influx of adult mouse fibroblasts and macrophages as well as mouse collagen in a scar pattern. Subcutaneous human fetal grafts demonstrate exclusively human fetal fibroblasts and human collagen in the wound environment, an absence of inflammatory cells, and scar-free repair. Thus, scarless fetal repair appears to be a consequence of a unique extracellular matrix produced by the fetal fibroblast in the absence of an adultlike inflammatory response to injury.[22]

The identification of cytoskeletal differentiation markers in fibroblasts has led to the recognition of their phenotypic heterogeneity. During wound healing and fibrocontractive diseases in adults, some fibroblasts acquire morphologic and biochemical features of smooth muscle cells (myofibroblasts), including the expression of alpha-smooth muscle actin. In turn, alpha-smooth muscle actin expression and myofibroblast function can be modulated by the wound matrix and growth factors, and these interactions change during development. Wound fibroblasts later in gestation acquire more smooth muscle–like elements, suggesting a relationship to the development of scar seen at that time.[11] Within late-gestation fetal wounds or adult wounds, the forces of wound contraction generated by myofibroblasts and the surrounding *stiffer* matrix may alter the alignment of collagen fibrils, establishing an early, abnormal, scarlike orientation.

Fetal Wound Extracellular Matrix

Recent studies have focused on the principal components of the fetal dermal matrix: collagen and PGs produced by the fetal fibroblast. Fetal wounds synthesize most of the matrix molecules present in adult wounds, but differences occur in the timing and pattern of these molecules in fetal wounds. For example, the cell adhesion molecule called tenascin is deposited much more rapidly and persists longer in fetal wounds, perhaps accounting for the rapid epithelialization and cellular ingrowth that occurs in fetal wound healing.[40]

Because a scar is defined as abnormal collagen organization after wound repair compared with normal surrounding tissue, the pattern of collagen deposition in fetal and adult wounds is of particular interest. The orderly deposition of collagen in fetal animal models has been demonstrated using histologic, immunohistochemical, biochemical, and biophysical techniques. The collagen pattern in fetal wounds is reticular and indistinguishable from adjacent normal tissue, whereas adult wounds contain large, parallel collagen bundles that are oriented perpendicular to the wound surface. Thus, scarless fetal wound healing must reflect the *organization* of collagen rather than the absence of collagen in the fetal wound matrix.

Although collagen Types I, III, V, and VI are present in both fetal and adult wounds, there are a few known differences in fetal and adult dermal collagen. The presence of aminopropeptides of Type I collagen in heterogeneous collagen fibrils is more common in the fetus than in the adult. The fetal dermis also contains a preponderance of Type III collagen, and as the fetus develops, the ratio of Type III to Type I collagen decreases, perhaps influencing collagen fibril size.[13] Small-diameter collagen I fibrils with a high turnover and a similar configuration to fetal collagen occur adjacent to the epidermal-dermal junction in adult skin, which is the region that shows minimal scarring in adult wounds. These minor differences between collagen in fetal and adult dermis may be important in modulating the nature of the wounding response.

The fetal wound matrix is rich in GAGs—in fetal rabbit wounds, the GAG content is approximately three times that of adult wounds during the same period, and approximately 10 times that found in unwounded fetal skin.[6] HA is the principal GAG present in fetal wounds, and it is a large molecule composed of alternating units of glucuronic acid and *N*-acetylglucosamine. An HA-rich matrix permits cell motility and proliferation, and a prolonged presence of HA in fetal wounds may provide the matrix signal that orchestrates healing by regeneration. Mammalian HA also has associated binding proteins, which have been implicated in the biologic activity of HA. Fetal wound fluid, fetal urine, and amniotic fluid can stimulate and sustain HA synthesis through a unique hyaluronic acid–stimulating activity (HASA). Recent support for the important role of HA in the fetal wound healing process is that levels of both HA and HASA in fetal lamb wound fluid decrease significantly during the transitional period from fetal-like to adult healing at 120 days' gestation in fetal sheep.[10, 23] Finally, CSPG is present within fetal mouse wounds at the time of collagen fibril formation but is absent at that time in adult mouse wounds. Thus, HA and chondroitin sulfate are likely to be important for scar-free repair, whereas other sulfated GAGs may play a role in scar formation.[39]

The primary wound scaffolding into which fibroblasts migrate has an important influence on collagen fibrillogenesis. In fetal wounds, fibroblasts can migrate rapidly into a loose honeycomb matrix containing high levels of HA. In contrast, adult wounds exhibit slow fibroblast migration into a denser, more resistant wound matrix, where fibroblast migration occurs more easily along the wound margins. These initial differences in the migration and orientation of fibroblasts may establish the pattern of collagen fibrils deposited in the respective wounds, with a loose reticular structure in the fetus and a closely packed, disorganized arrangement in the adult.

Role of Inflammation and Cytokines

Major differences appear in the degree of inflammation in fetal and adult wounds. Until midgestation, the fetus is significantly neutropenic and has not developed self–non-self immunologic identity. Histologically, there are few, if any, polymorphonuclear leukocytes in fetal wounds, and there may be a defect in immature polymorphonuclear leukocyte chemotactic ability. Recent studies have correlated the absence of scarring in fetal wounds with the sparse inflammatory response, as evidenced by markedly reduced macrophage and monocyte infiltrates, absence of endogenous immunoglobulins at the wound site, reduced angiogenesis, and altered levels of peptide growth factors.[40] The transition of the fetal healing phenotype to a scarring, adult phenotype in the marsupial correlates directly with the amount of inflammatory reaction at the wound site. These studies suggest that immature fetal immune cells do not respond to the wounding stimulus in the same way as adult cells do.

Peptide growth factors are released by inflammatory cells, and they help provide a cell-to-cell and cell-to-matrix communication system. These cytokines can affect matrix synthesis, matrix degradation, cell proliferation, and cell recruitment to the wound site. Because inflammation plays a prominent role in adult tissue repair, the characteristic inflammatory mediators of adult wound healing may be absent or modified in fetal wounds. A different cytokine profile of fetal wounds, occasioned by the relative lack of inflammatory cells, may cause matrix molecule differences that lead to scar-free healing.

Overproduction of TGF-β in Fibrosis

Of the many cytokines that have been implicated in wound healing, TGF-β affects all phases of the healing process, including the inflammatory response and matrix accumulation. In adult wounds, the macrophage is a crucial inflammatory cell that releases TGF-β as well as other cytokines. Through autocrine and paracrine mechanisms, TGF-β stimulates the deposition of collagen and other matrix components by fibroblasts, inhibits collagenase, blocks plasminogen inhibitor, enhances angiogenesis, and is chemotactic for fibroblasts, monocytes, and macrophages. Thus, TGF-β is capable of stimulating fibrogenesis by the fibroblast.[3]

TGF-β may provide the links among injury, inflammation, and fibrosis (see Fig. 12–5). After tissue injury, activated macrophage-derived TGF-β disturbs the balance of synthesis and degradation of collagens and causes accumulation of extracellular matrix. TGF-β induces alpha-smooth muscle actin expression in fibroblasts, and this finding correlates with scar formation and pathologic wound contraction.[7] The ability of TGF-β to induce its own production may be crucial for the development of progressive scarring in chronic diseases that leads to eventual obliteration of normal tissue architecture. The correlation between TGF-β levels and scar formation holds true for a variety of fibrotic diseases.

When TGF-β is administered intraperitoneally, adhesions form. There is enhanced expression of TGF-β$_1$ at the site of scar in the rat brain after localized cerebral injury. In proliferative vitreoretinopathy, total TGF-β levels in intraocular fluid increase as the retinal scarring progresses from mild to moderate to severe. Markedly increased amounts of TGF-β are present in fibrogenic diseases such as cirrhosis, interstitial pulmonary fibrosis, glomerulonephritis, and scleroderma.[3]

Exogenously applied TGF-β promotes scar formation in both adult and fetal wounds. Specifically, the addition of TGF-β to polyvinyl alcohol sponges implanted in fetal rabbits produces fibrosis.[19] It has been demonstrated that when TGF-β is added to human fetal skin wounds via a slow-release disc, scar formation results. In vitro studies have shown that exposure of fetal dermal fibroblasts to TGF-β produces marked upregulation of collagen gene expression. Thus, the cellular and matrix machinery that is necessary for scar formation exists in fetal wounds.[35]

This series of studies led to the hypothesis that scarless fetal wounds may be relatively TGF-β deficient. Indeed, Whitby and Ferguson performed TGF-β immunostaining studies in fetal mouse wounds and found that TGF-β was absent, whereas TGF-β staining was abundant in neonatal and adult mouse wounds.[38] The author has shown an absence of immunostaining for either TGF-β$_1$ or TGF-β$_2$ from 1 hour to 28 days after wounding of human fetal skin. In contrast, wounds in adult human skin grafts demonstrated TGF-β$_1$ at the wound edge at 6 hours through 21 days and TGF-β$_2$ at 12 hours through 7 days after wounding. It is possible that TGF-β levels in fetal wounds are below the threshold for detection by immunohistochemical techniques, but compared with adult wounds, fetal wounds are at least relatively TGF-β deficient.

Macrophages are the principal source of TGF-β in adult wounds, and the reduced TGF-β level in fetal wounds may reflect the absent or minimal macrophage infiltrate in these wounds. In adult wounds, TGF-β is also released from the alpha granules of activated platelets, so it is possible that fetal platelets may not synthesize or release TGF-β at the fetal wound site. The relative lack of TGF-β, a cytokine known to induce fibrosis, may be an important reason that the fetus heals by regeneration rather than by scarring. TGF-β may be important in adult tissue repair, but excessive action of this cytokine may be responsible for the tissue damage caused by scarring in many serious diseases. These findings suggest that anti-TGF-β therapeutic strategies may ameliorate scar formation in adult fibrotic diseases.

Cytokine Excess in Adult Wounds

Shah and colleagues[32] mimicked the fetal wound situation within healing adult rat wounds by using an anti-TGF-β polyclonal neutralizing antibody to experimentally reduce TGF-β levels. This manipulation markedly diminished scarring in adult wounds. The wounds treated with neutralizing antibody had normal tensile strength and a nearly normal dermal architecture compared with untreated wounds, and this salutary effect was accompanied by deposition of less collagen and fibronectin and infiltration by fewer macrophages and blood vessels. Injection of TGF-β alone had the opposite effects. Application of TGF-β neutralizing antibody at the time of wounding (and not later) was essential to reduce active TGF-β levels, prevent autoinduction of TGF-β messenger ribonucleic acid, and limit macrophage infiltration and further TGF-β release. The effectiveness of this approach has been demonstrated in another fibrotic process, since administration of either TGF-β$_1$ antiserum or decorin to neutralize TGF-β biologic activity suppresses the pathologic increase in matrix synthesis that occurs in an animal model of glomerulonephritis. Although injection of cytokine antibodies into wounds has limited clinical potential because of antigenicity problems, there are other promising ways to reduce wound levels of TGF-β. Various other theoretical anti-TGF-β therapeutic strategies, such as flooding the wound with soluble

TGF-β receptors to compete effectively with cellular TGF-β binding sites, preventing TGF-β activation, and adding antisense oligonucleotides to inhibit TGF-β gene expression, may also make adult wounds heal in a fetal-like manner. Inhibitors of TGF-β may be important future drugs for the control of fibrosis. Thus the relationship of TGF-β to scar formation fulfills Koch's postulates: TGF-β is absent in scarless fetal wounds, adding TGF-β to fetal wounds results in scarring, the presence of TGF-β after adult injury correlates with the degree of fibrosis observed, and blocking TGF-β in adult wounds has a potent antiscarring effect.

The repair of injured tissue in adults is a complex event that culminates in the return of tissue integrity and exclusion of the external environment. In contrast to fetal wound healing, it does so at the not-trivial expense of scar tissue formation with some loss of function. In evolutionary terms, it appears that adult wounds may be optimized for speed of healing under adverse conditions (dirt, foreign bodies), and the result is an excessive inflammatory infiltrate and cytokine profile. The potential *fetal* regenerative response in adult wounds may be overrun by an inflammation-induced cytokine surplus, leading to scar. This phenomenon is an example of *cytokine poisoning*, in which the inappropriate reparative response of the patient may prove detrimental to outcome.

FUTURE DIRECTIONS

Surgeons should all be students of wound repair and its sequelae. Fetal wound healing studies may help surgeons understand what accounts for scarring and, perhaps more important, how scar formation can be prevented. Unraveling the biology of fetal repair has led to novel strategies for the prevention and treatment of scarring and fibrosis. The matrix and cellular response of healing adult wounds might be manipulated in numerous ways to reduce scarring: inhibit the wound inflammatory response by blocking inflammatory cytokines such as TGF-β, bFGF, and PDGF; add exogenous tenascin to facilitate keratinocyte and fibroblast migration into the wound; transplant fibroblasts with fetal characteristics to the adult wound site; or provide a more porous wound scaffold by adding HA or HASA to enhance fibroblast migration and promote regeneration of a normal reticular collagen organization in the wounded dermis. Although all these potential therapeutic strategies require rigorous scientific testing, it may be possible to alter adult wound healing toward a scar-free fetal-like phenotype by modifying one or more of the components that are different in fetal and adult repair.

SELECTED REFERENCES

Adzick, N. S., and Longaker, M. T. (Eds.): Fetal Wound Healing. New York, Chapman and Hall, 1992.
This monograph reviews the morphologic, cellular, and molecular aspects of scarless fetal tissue repair. Several interesting in vivo and in vitro repair models are described.

Border, W. A., and Noble, N. A.: Transforming growth factor beta in tissue fibrosis. N. Engl. J. Med. 331:1286, 1994.
This review article depicts the "dark side" of repair characterized by tissue fibrosis associated with excess production of transforming growth factor beta. Potential therapeutic strategies to avert scar formation are discussed based on recent experimental and clinical studies.

Clark, R. A. F., and Henson, P. M. (Eds.): The Molecular and Cellular Biology of Wound Healing. New York, Plenum Press, 1988.
This is the first systematic review of the application of modern cellular and molecular biologic methods to the study of wound healing.

Cohen, I. K., Diegelmann, R. F., and Lindblad, W. J. (Eds.): Wound Healing: Biochemical and Clinical Aspects. Philadelphia, W. B. Saunders, 1992.
The editors have assembled an impressive array of contributors from diverse areas, including molecular biology, biochemistry, immunology, pharmacology, and surgery, to share their unique perspectives on tissue repair. After a broad overview of the principles of wound healing with an emphasis on basic biology, the book

approaches specific wound healing responses by organ systems. This textbook is the most comprehensive work on wound healing available.

Peacock, E. E., Jr., and Van Winkle, W., Jr.: Surgery and Biology of Wound Repair. Philadelphia, W. B. Saunders, 1976.
This classic volume was written by a surgeon and a biologist. It reviews many of the important experiments on the biology of repair. The practical considerations given to difficult wound healing problems are still clinically relevant.

REFERENCES

1. Adzick, N. S., and Longaker, M. T.: Scarless fetal healing: Therapeutic implications. Ann. Surg., 215:3, 1991.
2. Alexander, S. A., and Donoff, R. B.: The glycosaminoglycans of open fetal wounds. J. Surg. Res., 29:422, 1980.
3. Border, W. A., and Noble, N. A.: Transforming growth factor beta in tissue fibrosis. N. Engl. J. Med., 331:1286, 1994.
4. Brown, G. L., Naney, L. B., Griffen, J., Cramer, A. B., Yancey, J. M., Curtsinger, L. J., Holtzin, L., Schultze, G. S., Jurkiewicz, M. J., and Lynch, J. B.: Enhancement of wound healing by topical treatment with epidermal growth factor. N. Engl. J. Med., 321:76, 1989.
5. Darby, I., Skalli, O., and Gabbiani, G.: Alpha-smooth muscle actin is transiently expressed by myofibroblasts during experimental wound healing. Lab. Invest., 63:21, 1990.
6. DePalma, R. L., Krummel, T. M., Durham, L. A., Michna, B. A., Thomas, B. L., Nelson, J. M., and Diegelmann, R. F.: Characterization and quantification of wound matrix in the fetal rabbit. Matrix, 9:224, 1990.
7. Desmouliere, A., Geinoz, A., Gabbiani, F., and Gabbiani, G.: Transforming growth factor-β1 induces alpha-smooth muscle actin expression in granulation tissue myofibroblasts and in quiescent and growing fibroblasts. J. Cell Biol., 122:103, 1993.
8. Dvorak, H. F.: Tumors: Wounds that do not heal. N. Engl. J. Med., 315:1650, 1986.
9. Ehrlich, H. P.: The role of connective tissue matrix in wound healing. Prog. Clin. Biol. Res., 266:243, 1988.
10. Estes, J. M., Adzick, N. S., Longaker, M. T., Harrison, M. R., and Adzick, N. S.: Hyaluronate metabolism undergoes ontogenetic transition during fetal development: Implications for scarless wound healing. J. Pediatr. Surg., 28:1227, 1993.
11. Estes, J. M., Vande Berg, J. S., Adzick, N. S., MacGillivray, T. M., Desmouliere, A., and Gabbiani, G.: Phenotypic and functional features of myofibroblasts in fetal wounds. Differentiation, 56:173, 1994.
12. Ffrench-Constant, C., Vanderwater, L., Dvorak, H. F., and Hynes, R. O.: Reappearance of an embryonic pattern of fibronectin splicing during wound healing in the adult rat. J. Cell Biol., 10:903, 1989.
13. Fleischmajer, R., Perlish, J. S., Burgeson, R. E., Shaikh-Bahai, F., and Timpl, R.: Type I and type III collagen interactions during embryogenesis. Ann. N. Y. Acad. Sci., 580:161, 1990.
14. Folkman, J., and Shing, Y.: Angiogenesis. J. Biol. Chem., 267:10931, 1992.
15. Howarth, G., and Ferguson, M. W. J.: Marsupial models of fetal wound healing. In Adzick, N. S., and Longaker, M. T. (Eds.): Fetal Wound Healing. New York, Chapman and Hall, 1992, p. 95.
16. Hunt, T. K., Connolly, W. B., Aronson, S. B., and Goldstein, P.: Anaerobic metabolism and wound healing: A hypothesis for the initiation and cessation of collagen synthesis in wounds. Am. J. Surg., 135:328, 1978.
17. Hussain, M. Z., Ghani, Q. P., and Hunt, T. K.: Inhibition of prolyl hydroxylase by poly(ADP-ribose) and phosphoribosyl-AMP. J. Biol. Chem., 264:7850, 1989.
18. Jonsson, K., Jensen, J. A., Goodson, W. H., Scheuenstuhl, H., West, J., Hopf, H. W., and Hunt, T. K.: Tissue oxygenation, anemia, and perfusion in relation to wound healing in surgical patients. Ann. Surg., 214:605, 1991.
19. Krummel, T. M., Michna, B. A., Thomas, B. L., Diegelmann, R. F., and Cohen, I. K.: TGF-β induces fibrosis in a fetal wound model. J. Pediatr. Surg., 23:647, 1988.
20. Lane, A. L.: Human fetal skin development. Pediatr. Dermatol., 3:487, 1986.
21. Leibovich, S. J., and Ross, R.: The role of the macrophage in wound repair: A study with hydrocortisone and antimacrophage serum. Am. J. Pathol., 78:71, 1975.
22. Lin, R. Y., Sullivan, K. M., Argenta, P. A., Lorenz, H. P., and Adzick, N. S.: Scarless human fetal skin repair is intrinsic to the fetal fibroblast and occurs in the absence of an inflammatory response: In situ hybridization and immunohistochemical studies. Wound Repair Regeneration, 2:297, 1994.
23. Longaker, M. T., Chiu, E. S., Adzick, N. S., Stern, M., Harrison, M. R., and Stern, R.: Studies in fetal wound healing: V. A prolonged presence of hyaluronic acid characterizes fetal wound fluid. Ann. Surg., 213:292, 1991.
24. Longaker, M. T., Whitby, D. J., Ferguson, M. W. J., Lorenz, H. P., Harrison, M. R., and Adzick, N. S.: Adult skin wounds in the fetal environment heal with scar formation. Ann. Surg., 219:692, 1994.
25. Lorenz, H. P., Longaker, M. T., Perkocha, L. A., Jennings, R. W., Harrison, M. R., and Adzick, N. S.: Scarless wound repair: A human fetal skin model. Development, 114:253, 1992.
26. Lorenz, H. P., Whitby, D. J., Longaker, M. T., and Adzick, N. S.: The ontogeny of scar formation in the non-human primate. Ann. Surg., 217:391, 1993.

27. Martin, P., and Lewis, J.: Actin cables and epidermal movement in embryonic wound healing. Nature, *360*:179, 1992.

28. Pierce, G. F., Vande Berg, J., Rudolph, R., Tarpley, J., and Mustoe, T. A.: Platelet-derived growth factor-BB and transforming growth factor beta$_1$ selectively modulate glycosaminoglycans, collagen, and myofibroblasts in excisional wounds. Am. J. Pathol., *138*:629, 1991.

29. Rappolee, D. A., Mark, D., Banda, M. J., and Werb, Z.: Wound macrophages express TGF-alpha and other growth factors *in vivo*: Analysis by mRNA phenotyping. Science, *241*:708, 1989.

30. Robson, M. C., Phillips, L. G., Thomason, A., Robson, L. E., and Pierce, G. F.: Recombinant human platelet-derived growth factor-BB for the treatment of chronic pressure ulcers. Lancet, *339*:23, 1992.

31. Sappino, A. P., Schurch, W., and Gabbiani, G.: Differentiation repertoire of fibroblastic cells: Expression of cytoskeletal proteins as markers of phenotypic modulations. Lab. Invest., *63*:144, 1990.

32. Shah, M., Foreman, D. M., and Ferguson, M. W. J.: Control of scarring in adult wounds by neutralizing antibody to transforming growth factor beta. Lancet, *339*:213, 1992.

33. Simpson, D. M., and Ross, R.: The neutrophilic leukocyte in wound repair: A study with antineutrophil serum. J. Clin. Invest., *51*:2009, 1972.

34. Sporn, M. B., and Roberts, A. B.: Transforming growth factor-β: Recent progress and new challenges. J. Cell Biol., *119*:1017, 1992.

35. Sullivan, K. M., Lorenz, H. P., Meuli, M., Lin, R. Y., and Adzick, N. S.: A model of human fetal skin repair is deficient in transforming growth factor beta. J. Pediatr. Surg., *30*:198, 1995.

36. Szabo, S., Folkman, J., Vattay, P., Morales, R. E., Pinkus, G. S., and Kato, K.: Accelerated healing of duodenal ulcers by oral administration of a mutein of basic fibroblast growth factor in rats. Gastroenterology, *106*:1106, 1994.

37. Werner, S., Peters, K. G., Longaker, M. T., Fuller-Pace, F., Banda, M. J., and Williams, L. T.: Large induction of keratinocyte growth factor expression in the dermis during wound healing. Proc. Natl. Acad. Sci., *89*:6896, 1992.

38. Whitby, D. J., and Ferguson, M. W. J.: Immunohistochemical localization of growth factors in fetal wound healing. Dev. Biol., *147*:207, 1991.

39. Whitby, D. J., and Ferguson, M. W. J.: The extracellular matrix of lip wounds in fetal, neonatal, and adult mice. Development, *112*:651, 1991.

40. Whitby, D. J., Longaker, M. T., Harrison, M. R., Adzick, N. S., and Ferguson, M. W. J.: Rapid epithelization of fetal wounds is associated with early deposition of tenascin. J. Cell Sci., *99*:583, 1991.

CHAPTER 13

BURNS

Including Cold, Chemical, and Electric Injuries

Basil A. Pruitt, Jr., M.D., Cleon W. Goodwin, Jr., M.D., and Scott K. Pruitt, M.D., Ph.D.

BURN INJURY

It is estimated that between 1.4 million and 2 million persons are burned in the United States each year. In 1991, there were 5053 fire- and burn-related deaths.[26] The cause and risk of burn injury as well as the risk of burn death are influenced by age, economic circumstances, geographic location, season of the year, and occupation. The risks of burn injury and fire death are greatest in the very young, the elderly, the economically disadvantaged, those who reside in the southeastern states, and in the winter months. Seventy-three per cent of all burn-related deaths result from house fires, and the death rates are highest among young children and the elderly, who have difficulty escaping from the fire. Flame injury, most often caused by a house fire or ignition of clothing, is the predominant type of injury in patients admitted to burn centers. Scald burns are the most frequent form of burn injury overall and lead to over 100,000 visits to hospital emergency departments each year but are responsible for slightly less than one third of all burns requiring hospital treatment.[68]

The majority of burn injuries are of limited severity and extent (more than 80% of all burns involve less than 20% of the total body surface area) and can be cared for in an outpatient setting. The remainder, approximately 270 patients per million population per year, require hospital care because of the extent of the burn or a complicating factor such as associated injury, pre-existing disease, or either extreme of age. Three fourths of these patients have burn injuries that involve less than 20% of the total body surface, and most of those are adequately cared for in a general hospital by personnel experienced in burn care.

Among the burn patients requiring in-hospital care is a smaller group (82 per million population per year) who are classified, on the basis of burn size and complicating comorbid factors, as having major burn injury. As outlined by the American Burn Association, all patients with the burn injuries listed in Table 13–1 are best cared for in a burn center where specialized staff, equipment, and facilities ensure optimal treatment. There are 138 self-designated burn centers in the United States and 21 in Canada, with a total of 1951 beds. The geographic distribution of those burn centers necessitates the use of rotary or fixed-wing aircraft to transport burn patients from distant and remote areas.

Prehospital and Emergency Department Care of Burn Patients

At the scene of the injury the first responder should remove the patient from the source of heat, extinguish burning clothing, remove the patient from electric contact without making contact with the current, dilute with copious lavage any chemical agent causing tissue injury, and remove all clothing, including footwear and gloves, contaminated by a chemical agent. The need for cardiopulmonary resuscitation is uncommon in burn patients, except for those who have sustained high-voltage electric injury. If transportation to a treatment facility will take less than 45 minutes, the first responder should not attempt to place an intravenous line unless the patient has evidence of cardiac irregularity or hypotension due to blood loss from other injuries.

The application of ice or cold water soaks is effective in decreasing pain in areas of second-degree burn and should be used for analgesic effect if the burns involve less than 25% of the total body surface. However, systemic hypothermia must be avoided. Cold applications may help reduce tissue heat content and thus thermal injury from severe burns if applied within 10 minutes of the time of burning but exert little effect beyond that time. Following cooling procedures, the burns should be covered with a clean sheet, over which a blanket can be placed to conserve the patient's body heat. If feasible, the burned parts should be elevated to minimize edema formation both before and during transport.

Carbon monoxide poisoning, which is most likely to be present in patients who were burned in a closed space, impairs tissue oxygenation by reducing the oxygen-carrying capacity of the blood, shifting the oxygen-hemoglobin dissociation curve to the left, binding to myoglobin, and binding to the terminal cytochrome oxidase. Because symptoms of carbon monoxide poisoning correlate poorly with measured

---

TABLE 13–1. American Burn Association Burn Center Referral Criteria

I. Second- and third-degree burns involving more than 10% of the body surface area in patients younger than 10 or older than 50 years of age

II. Second- and third-degree burns involving more than 20% of the body surface area in other age groups

III. Significant burns of the face, hands, feet, genitalia, perineum, or the skin overlying major joints

IV. Full-thickness burns that involve more than 5% of the total body surface area in patients of any age

V. Significant electric injury, including lightning injury

VI. Significant chemical injury

VII. Lesser burn injuries with associated inhalation injury, concomitant mechanical trauma, or significant pre-existing medical disorders

VIII. Burn injury in patients who will require special social, emotional, or long-term rehabilitative support, including cases of suspected or actual child abuse and neglect

TABLE 13–2. Characteristics of First-, Second-, and Third-Degree Burns

	First-Degree Burns	Second-Degree Burns	Third-Degree Burns
Cause	Exposure to sunlight	Limited exposure to hot liquid, flash, flame or chemical agent	Prolonged exposure to flame, hot object, or chemical agent Contact with high-voltage electricity
Color	Red	Pink or mottled red	Pearly white, charred, translucent, or parchment-like Deeply tanned—strong acid burns Dark red—in young children
Surface	Dry or small to moderate sized blisters	Bullae or moist weeping surface	Dry, with thrombosis of superficial vessels Focal tissue loss—high-voltage electric injury Soapy tissue necrosis—strong alkali
Sensations	Painful	Painful Deep second-degree burns may be anesthetic to pinprick with intact pressure sensation	Insensate surface
Healing	3–6 days	10–21 days—superficial second-degree > 21 days—deep second-degree	Requires grafting

carboxyhemoglobin levels, little purpose is served by attempting to estimate carboxyhemoglobin levels in the field. The first responder should administer 100% oxygen by nonrebreathing mask to accelerate the dissociation of carboxyhemoglobin in any patient suspected of having inhaled significant amounts of carbon monoxide. An endotracheal tube should be inserted to maintain airway patency in patients with severe inhalation injury, in whom edema of the upper airway may develop rapidly. Hyperbaric oxygen therapy has been advocated for those patients with carbon monoxide poisoning who are comatose. Although treatment unquestionably accelerates the dissociation of carbon monoxide from hemoglobin, improvement in neurologic outcome remains undocumented.

Hydrogen cyanide, present in the smoke from nitrogen-containing polymers, inhibits cellular respiration and impairs adenosine triphosphate generation. Cyanide poisoning in patients without carbon monoxide poisoning is rare. Consequently, treatment of cyanide poisoning need be considered only for unconscious burn patients with signs of hypoxia. Hydroxycobalamin, the antidote of choice, has few toxic effects. Sodium thiosulfate, an agent that enhances enzymatic detoxification of cyanide to thiocyanate and has no significant side effects, can be administered intravenously but acts slowly. The beneficial effects of both agents are realized if 80 ml. of a solution containing 4 gm. of hydroxycobalamin and 8 gm. of sodium thiosulfate is given intravenously over 3 to 5 minutes.

In the emergency department, patency of the airway and ventilatory status should be assessed to determine the need for oxygen administration, endotracheal intubation, and ventilatory support. Fluid resuscitation should be initiated by infusing a balanced salt solution through a large-caliber intravenous cannula placed, in order of preference, in a peripheral vein underlying unburned skin, a peripheral vein underlying the burn wound, or a central vein. Insofar as is possible, a history should be obtained to determine the circumstances of the injury, the presence of pre-existing diseases and allergies, and any medications taken before injury. A swift but thorough physical examination should be performed to identify any associated injuries. An arterial blood sample for determination of pH, blood gases, carboxyhemoglobin level, electrolytes, urea nitrogen, glucose, and hematocrit should be obtained for any patient with a major burn injury.

The patient should be weighed, the depth of the burns assessed (Table 13–2 and Fig. 13–1), and the extent of burn estimated using the Rule of Nines* or any of several burn diagrams (Fig. 13–2). Fluid needs are then estimated on the basis of the total extent of second- and third-degree burns and body weight, and the fluid infusion rate is adjusted accordingly. The volume and type of all fluids administered must be recorded on a flow sheet. A urethral catheter should be placed in all burn patients requiring intravenous fluid therapy, and the hourly urinary output should be measured and recorded. In patients who have sustained high-voltage electric injury, electrocardiographic (ECG) monitoring should be initiated.

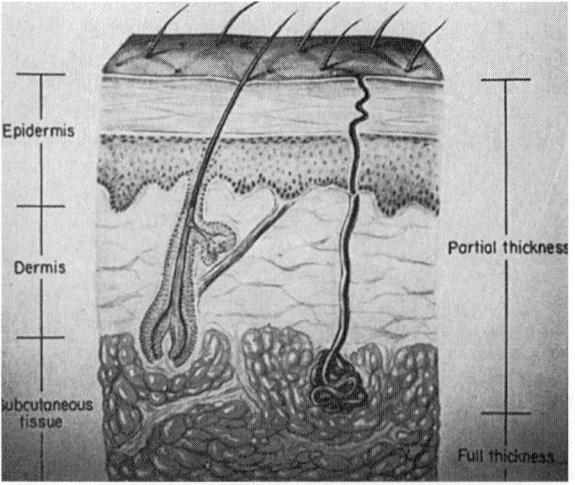

Figure 13–1. Diagram of skin and subcutaneous tissue showing relationship of depth of burn to location of adnexal structures. A partial-thickness or second-degree burn, if protected from infection, desiccation, and subsequent ischemia, will heal spontaneously as epithelial cells migrate from residual viable hair follicles and sweat glands. Since all adnexa are destroyed in full-thickness or third-degree burns, such wounds will not re-epithelialize and must be closed by skin grafting.

*The Rule of Nines describes the percentage of the body surface represented by various anatomic areas (i.e., each upper limb, 9%; each lower limb, 18%; anterior and posterior trunk, each 18%; head and neck, 9%; and perineum and genitalia, 1%).

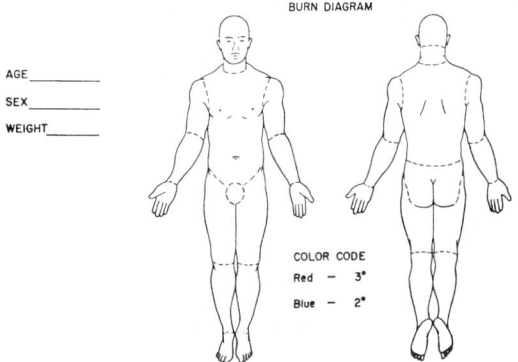

BURN ESTIMATE AND DIAGRAM

AGE vs. AREA

Area	Birth 1 yr.	1–4 yr.	5–9 yr.	10–14 yr.	15 yr.	Adult	2°	3°	Total	Donor Areas
Head	19	17	13	11	9	7				
Neck	2	2	2	2	2	2				
Ant. Trunk	13	13	13	13	13	13				
Post. Trunk	13	13	13	13	13	13				
R. Buttock	2½	2½	2½	2½	2½	2½				
L. Buttock	2½	2½	2½	2½	2½	2½				
Genitalia	1	1	1	1	1	1				
R.U. Arm	4	4	4	4	4	4				
L.U. Arm	4	4	4	4	4	4				
R.L. Arm	3	3	3	3	3	3				
L.L. Arm	3	3	3	3	3	3				
R. Hand	2½	2½	2½	2½	2½	2½				
L. Hand	2½	2½	2½	2½	2½	2½				
R. Thigh	5½	6½	8	8½	9	9½				
L. Thigh	5½	6½	8	8½	9	9½				
R. Leg	5	5	5½	6	6½	7				
L. Leg	5	5	5½	6	6½	7				
R. Foot	3½	3½	3½	3½	3½	3½				
L. Foot	3½	3½	3½	3½	3½	3½				
						TOTAL				

BURN DIAGRAM

AGE_____
SEX_____
WEIGHT_____

COLOR CODE
Red — 3°
Blue — 2°

Figure 13–2. Burn diagram and table used to estimate extent of burn. Note that the fractions of total body surface represented by head and lower limbs change with age and assume constant proportions after age 15.

Initial burn wound care should be carried out in the emergency department for those patients whose burns are of such limited extent that they do not require in-hospital care. The burned areas should be gently cleansed using a surgical detergent disinfectant, after which loose, nonviable skin should be débrided. Bullae larger than 2 cm. should be excised since they commonly rupture and are thereafter easily infected. Burns of limited extent are not at significant risk of infection, and topical antimicrobial agents need not be used. Such small burns can be dressed with any of several nonadherent, pliable synthetic dressings. The patient should be seen in follow-up at least every 3 days. If healing is proceeding uneventfully and the wound is free of infection, the dressing is reapplied, and that sequence is repeated as many times as necessary until healing has occurred. If infection is evident, the dressing should be removed, the patient admitted to the hospital, and topical antimicrobial therapy initiated.

In the case of patients requiring in-hospital care, transfer to the appropriate treatment facility is made after completion of emergency department procedures. The wound should be covered by a clean, dry sheet (and a blanket if necessary) during transfer.

Pathophysiology of Thermal Injury

Thermal injury causes coagulation necrosis of the skin and underlying tissues to variable depth. Burn injury also exerts deleterious effects on all other organ systems, with the extent and duration of organ dysfunction proportional to the extent of burn.[67] The biphasic changes in organ function (typically

TABLE 13–3. Extent of Burn Associated with a 50% Mortality (LA$_{50}$), 1987–1991, United States Army Institute of Surgical Research

Age	LA$_{50}$
5	72.154
21	81.905
40	71.881
60	46.391

early hypofunction and later hyperfunction, except for the central nervous and immunologic systems in which that sequence is reversed) are readily identified in patients with extensive burns. Mortality is similarly related to extent of burn in a sigmoid dose-response fashion and is further influenced by age (Table 13–3).

Hemodynamic Changes. Immediately following thermal injury the changes that occur in the cardiovascular system predominate and assume treatment priority to limit volume deficits and prevent the development of burn shock (Fig. 13–3). The direct effect of heat as well as the liberation of vasoactive materials from the area of injury alter transvascular pressure relationships and capillary permeability as well as the microvascular endothelial surface area exposed to those forces, all of which promote loss of fluid and protein from the intravascular into the extravascular compartment. The magnitude of these volume shifts is proportional to the extent of the burn and clinically evident in the edema that occurs in areas of thermal injury and may also develop in unburned tissues as resuscitation proceeds in patients with extensive burns (i.e., those involving more than 25% of the total body surface).

Within minutes after burning, cardiac output decreases in proportion to burn size in association with an increase in peripheral vascular resistance. Later (but still early post burn) the depression of cardiac output is maintained or even accentuated by the combined effect of a decreasing blood volume and increasing blood viscosity, as indexed by a rising hematocrit. Animal studies have largely discounted the presence of a circulating myocardial depressant factor. In burn patients with depressed cardiac output in the first 24 hours post burn, the heart is typically hyperdynamic, as indexed by elevation

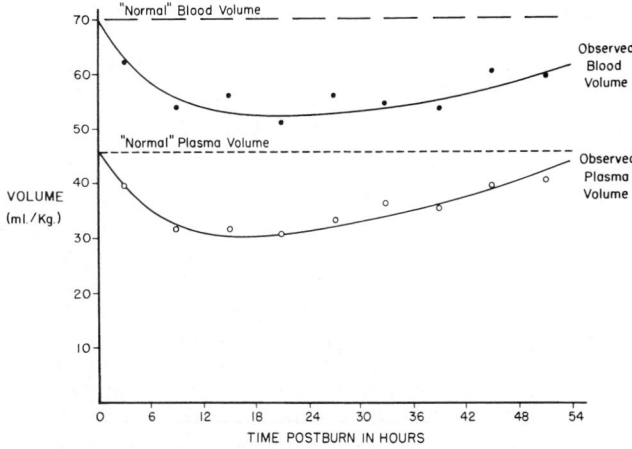

Figure 13–3. Mean blood and plasma volume changes during the first 54 hours after injury in 10 patients with burns involving an average of 65% of the total body surface. Fluid resuscitation guided by the Brooke formula permitted an early modest volume loss (the velocity of which decreased with time), defended against further loss, and restored plasma volume to near predicted levels by 54 hours.

of ejection fraction and velocity of myocardial fiber shortening. Hypovolemia, manifested by a depressed left ventricular end diastolic volume, is an obvious cause of the depressed cardiac output in those patients.

The loss of fluid from the vascular tree has been generally attributed to an increase in microvascular permeability due to the direct effects of heat and the effects of a variety of humoral factors liberated from damaged tissue as well as cytokines produced by activated leukocytes. The most frequently incriminated cell product is histamine, the plasma concentration of which rises in proportion to burn size within 1 minute of thermal injury. Additionally, arachidonic acid metabolites (principally, thromboxane A_2 and the leukotrienes), substance P (apparently originating in sensory nerve endings and causing a receptor-mediated increase in nitric oxide production and formation of water-filled interendothelial cell convective pathways), fibrin degradation product D, activated proteases, and platelet activating factor (PAF) have all been reported to increase vascular permeability. Antagonists of each of those agents (when administered before burn injury) have been reported to reduce but not eliminate the increase in transcapillary filtration that occurs following burning.

Activation of the immune system also results in the production of factors that can increase microvascular permeability, including products of complement activation, lysosomal enzymes, increased xanthine oxidase activity, oxygen radicals, activated killer lymphocytes, lymphokines (interleukin [IL]-1, IL-6, and IL-8), as well as neutrophil cathepsin G.[16, 64, 88] Till and associates have reported that neutrophil depletion protects against post-burn lung injury but has no effect on burn wound edema formation.[82] Oxygen-derived free radicals appear to be of little importance in local vascular changes.[50]

Changes in capillary and interstitial fluid hydrostatic pressures may be important in the formation of post-burn edema. Capillary filtration during the first 3 hours following a scald burn is increased, owing to increased capillary pressure.[65] A strongly negative interstitial fluid hydrostatic pressure and an abnormal tissue osmotic gradient have also been noted within 15 to 30 minutes following burning in an animal model.[42, 43]

The rate of edema formation is greatest immediately post burn, and edema volume reaches peak values from 3 to 24 hours post burn. The subsequent time-related decrease in edema formation has been related to restoration of capillary integrity. Studies in a murine burn injury model have revealed a progressive rise in burn wound edema for the first 6 hours and a subsequent slow rise over the next 18 hours to reach a peak of burn wound water and protein content at 24 hours post injury. At that time capillary permeability, as measured by albumin flux rates, was still elevated, but edema formation ceased because a new equilibrium of fluid and protein flow through the wound had been established.

The diminished blood volume and cardiac output cause a post-burn decrease in renal blood flow and glomerular filtration rate. The resulting oliguria, if untreated, may progress to acute renal failure. Post-burn hypovolemia may also impair flow to other organs as well, and restlessness (a reflection of impaired cerebral blood flow) is a frequent early sign of blood volume depletion. Following resuscitation, renal blood flow and glomerular filtration rate increase to supranormal levels in concert with the increase in cardiac output characteristic of post-burn hypermetabolism. The hyperdynamic renal circulation often necessitates adjustment of the dosage of antibiotics and other drugs that are renally excreted.

Pulmonary Changes. Alterations of pulmonary function following burn injury are variable. In those patients with circumferential burns of the thorax, the constricting eschar and underlying edema may produce a restrictive ventilatory defect requiring relief by placement of escharotomy incisions, as described below. In patients without burns of the thorax or inhalation injury, the initial hypovolemia may result in rapid shallow respirations. Following resuscitation, hyperventilation (two to two and one-half times normal minute ventilation) with modest, if any, evidence of parenchymal dysfunction is customarily observed. This response, considered to be a reflection of post-injury hypermetabolism, may be associated with modest hypoxemia, especially during the period of edema resorption. As a consequence of this hyperventilation, a mild respiratory alkalosis is the most frequent acid-base disturbance in burn patients following resuscitation. If secondary pulmonary complications supervene, the hyperventilation may be accentuated. If pulmonary reserve is exceeded, the acid-base status may quickly change from alkalosis to acidosis, hypoxemia may develop, and mechanical ventilatory support may be necessary. Burn-related hyperventilation typically recedes as the burn wound heals.

Pulmonary vascular resistance increases in the immediate post-burn period. The rarity of pulmonary edema during the resuscitation phase, even when large volumes of fluid are infused, is consistent with the site of increased resistance being in a precapillary location and being protective in nature. Studies using an ovine model have identified differential changes in the lymph/plasma protein ratios in the lymph draining from burned tissue, unburned subcutaneous tissue, and the lung, indicating that burn injury has no apparent effect on pulmonary capillary permeability.[18, 35]

Burn injury and initial fluid therapy appear to evoke other immediate and delayed changes in the pulmonary vasculature and alter pulmonary function. Post-burn generation of the chemotactic peptide C5a, as a result of complement activation, is temporally related to neutropenia, aggregation of leukocytes in pulmonary capillaries, and intra-alveolar hemorrhage. The eicosanoids appear to be involved in the lung injury induced by complement activation but to play no role in the associated pulmonary hypertension, since both cyclooxygenase and lipoxygenase inhibitors attenuate the former and exert little, if any, effect on the latter.[20, 53] During the period of lung dysfunction, thromboxane levels in the lymph from the burned areas and in venous plasma are increased, and the preburn administration of ibuprofen reduces post-injury lung dysfunction.[20]

The burn wound may also serve as the source of cell metabolites that are produced by infection and exert deleterious effects on the lungs. In laboratory studies, the injection of endotoxin into the subcutaneous tissue beneath a burn increased the thromboxane B_2 content in lymph draining from the burned area and in venous plasma and was associated with a coincident increase in pulmonary artery pressure and a decrease in mean arterial oxygen tension.

Hematologic Changes. In addition to the loss of plasma from the circulation in the early post-burn period, there is immediate red blood cell destruction in direct proportion to the extent of the burn, particularly third-degree burn. In patients with extensive burns there is a continuing red blood cell loss of variable extent (8% to 12% of red cell mass per day) from the aggregate effect of lysis of cells damaged by heat, microvascular thrombosis in areas of damaged tissue that subsequently undergo necrosis, and the blood sampling required for patient care.

A biphasic alteration of the coagulation system also characterizes the response to thermal injury. Animal studies have identified vascular occlusion by platelet microthrombi, not leukocyte adherence, as the major factor causing progressive postburn dermal ischemia. That process is reflected in the early marked depression of platelet and fibrinogen levels accompanied by a parallel increase in fibrin split product levels observed in patients with extensive burns. These changes are followed by a prompt post-resuscitation return to normal and subsequent elevation of those coagulation factors in association with an increase in factors V and VIII. As early as 3 days post burn, marked depression of antithrombin III and protein C levels has been identified. Although thromboembolic disease is surprisingly rare in patients with extensive burns, when such does occur and anticoagulation is necessary, the antithrombin III deficit may markedly elevate the dose of heparin required for effective anticoagulation.

Gastrointestinal Changes. The gastrointestinal tract also responds in a stereotypic burn size–related manner to thermal injury. Ileus is virtually universal in patients with burns of more than 25% of the total body surface. Following resuscitation, gastrointestinal motility returns by the third to fifth post-burn day. Animal studies have identified an early diminution of gastric mucosal blood flow following injury, which is corrected by fluid resuscitation. Gastric and duodenal mucosal damage, secondary to focal ischemia, can be observed as early as 3 to 5 hours post burn. If the mucosa is unprotected, the early erosions may progress to frank ulceration. Later in the post-burn period, sepsis and/or hypovolemia can produce similar ischemic mucosal, even transmural, changes throughout the gastrointestinal tract to produce focal mucosal ulcerations, mural scarring, and perforation.

Gastrointestinal permeability, as reflected by the lactulose-mannitol excretion ratio, was increased on post-burn day 2 in a group of burn patients who developed clinically significant infections within the first 2 weeks of injury. Studies in a murine model with a 30% full-thickness burn have identified the presence of radiolabeled *Escherichia coli* and *E. coli* endotoxin in the mesenteric lymph nodes as early as 1 hour after burn injury.[2] The relationship between translocation and subsequent infection remains uncertain.

Endocrine Changes. In the early post-burn period a catabolic endocrine pattern develops characterized by elevated glucagon, cortisol, and catecholamine levels and depressed insulin and triiodothyronine levels. These changes are associated with a burn size–related increase in metabolic rate, glucose flow, and negative nitrogen balance.

Neurologic Changes. Specific neurologic changes are most commonly seen in patients with high-voltage electric injury or in association with mechanical trauma. Nonspecific neurologic changes are similar to those that can occur in other injured patients.

Immunologic Effects

The global effects of burn injury on host defense mechanisms are reflected by the fact that infection remains the major cause of death in burn patients. While destruction of the mechanical barrier of the skin contributes to the increased susceptibility to infection, post-burn alterations in immune function may also be of critical importance.

Numerous examples of suppressed cellular immune responsiveness have been noted, including prolonged skin allograft survival, inhibited delayed-type hypersensitivity, and reduced peripheral blood lymphocyte proliferation in the mixed lymphocyte reaction.[8, 48, 71] In patients with burns of 20% or more of the body surface area, impairment of cell-mediated immunity is proportional to burn size.

After thermal injury, alterations in lymphocyte number and phenotype occur, with reduction in peripheral blood lymphocyte counts and inversion of the normal CD8/CD4 ratio.[8, 44, 48, 71, 72] All of these indices normalize during the second post-burn week in normally recovering patients. A late (>14 days post burn) increase in the CD8/CD4 ratio may correspond to patient death from sepsis,[48] but experimental studies suggest that this alteration may be an effect, rather than a cause, of sepsis.[7]

While the absolute number of lymphocytes is reduced 48 hours post burn, Maldonado and associates[44] noted that the expression of cell surface markers of lymphocyte activation (CD25, CD69, and CD71) was increased, as was the expression of integrin adhesion molecules (CD11c, CD49a, CD54). Similarly, Schluter and colleagues[72] noted increased CD25 expression by peripheral blood lymphocytes following thermal injury, an increase not seen in studies performed by Zapata-Sirvent and Hansbrough.[94] Elevated serum levels of IL-2 and soluble IL-2 receptor, also indicative of T-cell activation, have also been observed in burn patients.[81] These studies and others [17] seem to suggest that early, possibly nonspecific, activation of the cellular immune system by burn injury may preclude further specific T-cell responses, leading to functional cellular immunosuppression.

The expression of surface receptors on lymphocytes is differentially affected by injury and infection. The surface expression of a variety of receptors was measured serially for 6 weeks following injury in 19 burn patients. The percentage of CD4+ and CD8+ lymphocytes that expressed various receptors changed with time post burn and was influenced by the occurrence of infection. In those patients who developed infection, the proportion of CD4+ and CD8+ cells was greater than in uninfected patients. Natural killer cells were decreased by 50% in the infected patients. The percentage of cells expressing the alpha integrin CD11b was markedly decreased in the infected patients. The percentage of memory cells (CD45RO+) was slightly decreased in the infected patients while the percentage of lymphocytes expressing the IL-2 receptor and the early activation antigen receptor (CD69) was significantly increased. Discriminant function analysis has identified patient variables that can be used to predict the likelihood that infection will develop in a burn patient. A classification function involving age, burn size, and the percentage of CD4+ cells expressing CD69 and HLA-DR antigens and the total percentage of cells expressing CD69 identified infected patient samples with 87% accuracy.[6] This classification system may be useful in identifying those patients who require intensive monitoring and those who may benefit from prophylaxis.

A variety of studies suggest that altered cytokine production and regulation may contribute to the immune defects associated with burn injury. The decreased *in vitro* IL-1 production by circulating monocytes in those burn patients who developed evidence of multiple organ failure has been interpreted as indicative of hyperstimulation.[41] Plasma levels of IL-1-beta are highest during the first week after injury, and the elevation correlates with extent of burn. There does not appear to be a correlation between IL-1 levels and infection. Elevated plasma levels of a naturally occurring inhibitor of IL-1, IL-1 receptor antagonist (IL-1Ra), have been detected in patients experiencing thermal injury.[46] Because IL-1Ra, which like IL-1 itself is produced by macrophages, blocks the action of the inflammatory cytokine IL-1, it is possible that IL-1Ra secretion may contribute to burn-induced immunosuppression. However, IL-1Ra may simply be a marker of stress or nonspecific inflammation, since levels rose following burn excision and grafting and levels did not normalize in patients with fatal burns.

A well-documented alteration in cellular immune function is the impaired mitogenic responses of lymphocytes harvested from patients following burn injury.[72] One factor thought to contribute to this reduced T-cell responsiveness is decreased IL-2 production.[30, 39] IL-2 gene transcription appears to be downregulated, in part due to reduced expression of the c-*fos* proto-oncogene, the product of which forms part of a transcriptional factor that interacts with the IL-2 promoter,[39] and to defective transmembrane signaling. In thermally injured patients, Wood and associates found a direct correlation between burn size and the reduction of IL-2 production by peripheral blood lymphocytes.[89] Soluble IL-2Ra, levels of which are elevated in serum from burn patients in proportion to burn size,[80, 90] may bind IL-2 and competitively inhibit IL-2–dependent immune responses, producing some of the immune dysfunction in burn patients. Lymphocytes from burn patients also demonstrate reduced surface expression of IL-2R.[27, 79]

In vivo administration of IL-2 to thermally injured mice before septic challenge produces significantly improved survival following cecal ligation and puncture, suggesting a potential for therapeutic applications of IL-2 administration to enhance host immune competence in the burned patient.[30] Conflicting results have been obtained in an animal model of burn wound sepsis, in which the administration of IL-2 had no effect on mortality.

In contrast to these studies suggesting intrinsic T-cell immune suppression following burn injury, several investigators have found that the diminished responsiveness in these *in vitro* assays may be due to the presence of nonlymphoid cells contaminating the lymphocyte preparations and altering normal cytokine regulation.[7, 91] When these contaminated cells are removed, burn patient peripheral blood lymphocytes have been found to respond normally to mitogens and alloantigens,[91] a response also observed in a murine model of burn injury.[92] Mediators implicated in this inhibition of responsiveness include prostaglandin E$_2$, which is produced by burn- and infection-activated monocytes and macrophages and inhibits lymphocyte IL-2 production by T cells,[31] and IL-6, which when added to cultured murine splenocytes has been shown to suppress mitogen responsiveness.[96]

Macrophage and monocyte secretion of IL-6 is enhanced after burn injury,[62] and an elevation in serum IL-6 levels occurs in burn patients within hours of injury and persists for several weeks.[60] This cytokine, induced by both IL-1 and tumor necrosis factor (TNF), is released by activated monocytes and macrophages and is known to cause fever, enhance the production of acute-phase proteins such as C-reactive protein and fibrinogen, stimulate hepatocytes to produce alpha$_1$-antitrypsin, and induce immunoglobulin production, all of which to a variable degree occur post burn. Bacterial infection may further stimulate IL-6 production, since in response to lipopolysaccharide, secretion of this cytokine from adherent splenocytes harvested from burned mice was significantly enhanced over that observed from unburned control mice.[62] Studies by He and associates[36] in a murine burn injury model suggest that TNF as well as IL-6 may exert deleterious effects following a burn. However, neither IL-1 nor TNF levels appear to change in relation to the extent of burn.[23]

Stimulated Kupffer cells may be an additional source of enhanced TNF-alpha production following burn injury.[21] Alveolar macrophages from thermally injured rats also demonstrate increased TNF-alpha secretion,[51] and TNF release may also be important in the pathogenesis of inhalation injury. The administration of pentoxifylline has been shown to attenuate smoke inhalation injury in a sheep model. This effect may have been due to the ability of this agent to block TNF mRNA transcription by macrophages, to reduce leukocyte expression of CD11b/CD18, and to inhibit the stimulatory effects of IL-1, platelet activating factor, and granulocyte-macrophage colony stimulating factor (GM-CSF) on polymorphonuclear leukocytes. These activities may have been responsible for the reduced numbers of polymorphonuclear leukocytes within bronchoalveolar lavage fluid as well as the reduced lung injury observed with pentoxifylline therapy.

Studies by Napolitano and Campbell[58] of murine spleno-cytes harvested 4 days following a 20% body surface area burn demonstrated reduced production of both interferon-gamma and IL-10, a cytokine that downregulates macrophage cytokine production and inhibits NO production by activated macrophages. Pharmacologic inhibition of NO synthesis in culture normalized the IL-10 response and improved mitogen-induced proliferation.

Granulocytosis and B-lymphocytosis also occur early in the post-burn course (beginning on post-burn day 1),[8] but serum immunoglobulin G (IgG) levels are decreased after burn injury and gradually return to normal over the next 2 to 4 weeks. The reduced expression of the B-cell activation marker CD23 by unstimulated cells as well as by cells stimulated with IL-4 observed by Teodorczyk-Injejan and coworkers[81] in patients during weeks 2 through 5 post burn suggests that B cells in thermally injured patients may be downregulated and unable to respond normally to cytokine stimulation. Studies in a murine model suggest that a defect in the ability of B cells to propagate a normal IgG response may occur following burn injury.[45] Similarly, Tabata and Meyer[77] observed increased numbers of IgM+ cells in murine mesenteric lymph nodes and spleens following burn injury but reduced IgM production by these cells in culture. Again, this is consistent with a B-cell defect in immunoglobulin secretion following burn injury. Exogenous administration of IgG to burned patients promptly restores IgG to normal levels but exerts no demonstrable effect on morbidity or mortality.

In addition to lymphocytes, other populations of immune cells are known to be adversely affected by burn injury. Natural killer cell activity of peripheral blood lymphocytes is reduced in thermally injured patients, possibly because of circulating endotoxin, but the number of circulating natural killer cells (CD16+) in the peripheral blood of thermally injured patients does not seem to be significantly altered.[72]

In burn patients, polymorphonuclear leukocyte dysfunction has been thought to contribute to immunosuppression and increased susceptibility to infection. Polymorphonuclear leukocytes from burn patients exhibit a reduction in chemotactic activity, which is proportional to burn size and can be restored by incubation with normal serum, and also demonstrate defects in phagocytosis.[1] Increased neutrophil expression of CR1 and CR3 receptors and an elevation of neutrophil resting cytosolic oxidative activity are consistent with early activation being the cause of such neutrophil hyporesponsiveness. Other investigators have documented downregulation of neutrophil C5a receptors and a decreased chemotactic response to an f-Met-Leu-Phe gradient. The observed chemotactic dysfunction of neutrophils appears to be multifactorial, as indicated by studies incriminating oxidation of cell components, abnormalities in actin polymerization and depolymerization, and increased synthesis of prostaglandin E$_1$.

Studies of neutrophil function have demonstrated a variable immediate response to burn injury with a generally greater depression of granulocyte oxidative activity in patients with burns of over 40% of the body surface.[4] After resuscitation, neutrophil oxidative activity is influenced by the patient's clinical condition. In burn patients with infection, granulocyte peroxidase activity is typically elevated in association with toxic granulation. Granulocyte membrane–associated oxidase is depressed and progressively decreases in patients who die. A preterminal decrease in peroxidase activity appears to reflect bone marrow exhaustion.

Peripheral blood monocyte HLA-DR expression is reduced by day 1 following burn injury, is maximally suppressed on day 4, and remains below normal through day 21.[72] This reduced class II MHC expression may prevent monocytes from effectively presenting antigens to CD4+ T cells and thus contribute to decreased immune responsiveness in burn patients.

Because of these apparent defects in polymorphonuclear leukocyte and monocyte activity, therapy with granulocyte-macrophage colony-stimulating factor (GM-CSF) is being evaluated as a means of augmenting host defense in burn patients. GM-CSF has a variety of immunostimulatory effects, including prolongation of neutrophil and macrophage life span, enhancement of killing and phagocytosis by neutrophils, enhancement of the response of these cells to chemotactic agents, and induction of increased cell-surface expression of HLA class II, CD11b, and complement receptors CR1 and CR3. After a 5-day course of pretreatment of mice with GM-CSF, their survival in response to a combined transfusion/bacterial gavage/burn injury insult was significantly improved as compared with that of untreated controls.[28] This GM-CSF pretreatment also significantly reduced bacterial translocation to the mesenteric lymph nodes, spleen, and liver. These findings are consistent with a defect in nonspecific inflammatory cell function being detrimental to the burn patient but could also suggest that enhancement of neutrophil and macrophage function with GM-CSF can compensate for other host defense defects. As a note of caution, since sustained polymorphonuclear leukocyte activation appears to be present after burn injury and could be responsible for detrimental effects on tissues, especially the pulmonary vasculature, the clinical administration of agents to enhance polymorphonuclear leukocyte function might not be warranted.

Numerous investigators, utilizing a number of experimental methods, have demonstrated immunosuppressive factors in serum from burn patients. Both Hakim and Constantian have described an immunosuppressive polypeptide of approximately 10,000 daltons molecular weight obtained from burn patient serum that inhibits mitogen-stimulated lymphocyte proliferation.[14] Similar but elevated immunosuppressive activity has also been detected in subeschar fluid and may be a contributing factor to burn wound invasion.[25] Burn serum has also been noted to inhibit neutrophil chemotaxis and to impair neutrophil chemiluminescence.[4]

In addition to a suppressive peptide, other proposed immunosuppressive factors in burn serum include complement degradation products that inhibit phagocyte function,[1] immunoglobulin fragments, breakdown products of the coagulation and fibrinolytic systems,[63] prostaglandins, and endotoxin.[85] Although serum suppressive activity appears to be present in all severely burned patients, levels of activity do not correlate with patient survival.

Burn injury and other pathologic changes that induce tissue ischemia lead to increased expression of heat shock proteins by hypoperfused cells. Autoantibodies, which bind to a 68-kd. protein closely related to the 70-kd. heat shock protein (HSP70), have been identified in the sera of burn patients. Topical application of epidermal growth factor in an ointment containing the protease inhibitor nafamostat has been reported to increase messenger RNA for superoxide dismutase and significantly reduce the content of heat shock protein (HSP70) in the burned tissue. Another heat shock protein (HSP90) must bind to the hormone-binding domain of the glucocorticoid receptor for that receptor to assume a high-affinity steroid binding conformation. HSP70 is required for assembly of that glucocorticoid receptor-HSP90 complex, which functions as a *foldosome* to effect proper receptor folding necessary for the activation of steroid binding activity. Manipulation of heat shock proteins may thus influence both the local and systemic responses to burn injury.

It is difficult to define the specific cause-and-effect relationship between changes in various components of the immune system and infection in human burn patients. Even so, Moss and colleagues,[54] using an animal model of thermal injury, have convincingly demonstrated a correlation between defects in cellular immune function and susceptibility to sepsis. Thus, to reduce the susceptibility to infection in the burn patient, methods to correct depressed immune function are being developed. Among the therapies investigated, early burn wound excision with grafting has been shown to restore defective neutrophil migration in an animal model.[78] Administration of polymyxin B to severely burned patients has been shown to enhance depressed natural killer cell activity; and, as previously mentioned, administration of recombinant IL-2 has been shown to improve resistance to a secondary septic challenge in a murine model of thermal injury.[8] The limited or total lack of effectiveness of various vaccines, immunomodulators and serologic agents, such as IgG, IL-2, and interleukin receptor antagonists in preventing invasive burn wound infection and improving survival of burn patients may simply represent the inability of any single agent to correct the multiple immune deficits induced by an extensive burn. Newly developed immunomodulatory drugs (soluble complement receptor Type 1 and anti-L-selectin [CD62L] preparations are being evaluated) and recombinant lymphokines (IL-4 and IL-10 are attractive candidates), used individually or in combination therapy, may have a future clinical role in reducing the burn patient's susceptibility to infection.

Fluid Resuscitation

Fluid resuscitation should be started in all patients with burns of 15% or more of the total body surface. Because of ileus (see earlier), oral resuscitation is precluded, and the fluid should be infused intravenously. Several formulas, most of which are based on the weight of the patient and the extent of the burn, have been proposed for estimating a burn patient's fluid needs. The fluid estimates of each of the commonly used formulas are shown in Table 13–4.

Several studies have indicated that during the first 24 hours post burn, colloid-containing fluids are not essential for resuscitation. During that time period, these fluids appear to be retained within the circulation to no greater extent than an equal volume of colloid-free electrolyte containing fluid, such as lactated Ringer's solution. In a randomized prospective clinical trial, resuscitation using only crystalloid fluids during the first 24 hours was compared with resuscitation using a combination of crystalloid- and colloid-containing fluids (2.5% albumin and Ringer's lactate). When resuscitation was guided by hourly urinary output as an index of adequate organ perfusion, the colloid-containing regimen restored cardiac output more rapidly than did crystalloid solution alone. However, by the end of the first 48 post-burn hours, the two resuscitation regimens had been equally effective in restoring cardiac output and intravascular volume.

Those patients who received colloid continued to gain weight throughout the first 3 post-injury days, and they retained more sodium and had a lesser urinary output as compared with those patients who received crystalloid fluid only. The potential hemodynamic advantages of the colloid-containing resuscitation regimen appeared to be offset by deleterious effects of colloid-containing fluids on the lungs. Extravascular lung water remained essentially unchanged during the first post-burn week in those patients who initially received only crystalloid-containing fluids but increased significantly above normal in those patients who received colloid-containing fluids as a component of initial resuscitation. Late pulmonary complications and mortality were also higher in the colloid-treated patients.

Although the formulas in Table 13–4 vary considerably, each formula has been found to be clinically effective. It is evident that the physiologic tolerance of the majority of burn patients allows them to adapt to the variations in formula-based fluids. There are, however, subsets of patients who

TABLE 13–4. Commonly Used Burn Resuscitation Formulae for Adult Patients

Formula	First 24 Hours Post Burn			Second 24 Hours Post Burn		
	Electrolyte-Containing Solution	Colloid-Containing Fluid Equivalent to Plasma	Glucose in Water (D_5W)	Electrolyte-Containing Solution	Colloid-Containing Fluid Equivalent to Plasma	Glucose in Water (D_5W)
Burn Budget of F.D. Moore	Lactated Ringer's 1000–4000 ml. 0.5 Normal saline 1200 ml.	7.5% of body weight	1500–5000 ml.	Lactated Ringer's 1000–4000 ml. 0.5 Normal saline 1200 ml.	2.5% of body weight	1500–5000 ml.
Evans	Normal saline 1.0 ml./kg./% burn	1.0 ml./kg./% burn	2000 ml.	One half of first 24-hour requirement	One half of first 24-hour requirement	2000 ml.
Brooke	Lactated Ringer's 1.5 ml./kg./% burn	0.5 ml./kg./% burn	2000 ml.	One half to three fourths of first 24-hour requirement	One half to three fourths of first 24-hour requirement	2000 ml.
Parkland	Lactated Ringer's 4.0 ml./kg./% burn				20% to 60% of calculated plasma volume	As necessary to maintain urinary output
Hypertonic Sodium Solution	Volume of hypertonic lactated saline (HLS) containing 250 mEq. of sodium per liter to maintain hourly urinary output of 30 ml.			0.6% ml. of HLS/kg./% burn plus oral Haldan's Solution to replace insensible water loss *or* One third isotonic salt solution orally up to 3500 ml. limit		
Modified Brooke	Lactated Ringer's 2.0 ml./kg./% burn				0.3–0.5 ml./kg./% burn	As necessary to maintain urinary output

predictably require modifications of the resuscitation regimen and individualized treatment. Patients who characteristically require greater volumes of fluid than those estimated by the formulas include those with high-voltage electric injury, those with inhalation injury, those with delayed resuscitation, and those who are burned while drunk. Conversely, *volume-sensitive* patients who should receive the least possible resuscitation volume consistent with maintenance of organ function include those older than 50 years of age, those younger than 2 years of age, and those with pre-existing cardiopulmonary disease.

The use of concentrated salt solution for burn patient resuscitation has been recommended by some. Hypertonic salt solution may be of value in diminishing volume loading, off-loading of administered sodium, and promoting kaliuresis in volume-sensitive burn patients. However, there appear to be limits to both serum sodium concentration elevation (160 mEq./L.) and cellular dehydration (15%), which when reached interfere with cell, tissue, or organ function and necessitate that resuscitation be continued with more dilute fluids. In some reports those limitations appear to have been fortuitously avoided by allowing the patient access to hypotonic oral fluids. Calculation of the sodium content of the total fluid dose received by such patients approximated isotonicity. Moreover, in studies of a murine model with a 25% body surface area burn, the intravenous administration of a hypertonic saline solution containing 6% dextran-40 did not eliminate metabolic acidosis and markedly increased mortality when intraperitoneal resuscitation fluids were not administered.[95] Additionally, in a canine model, resuscitation using a solution of hypertonic saline and dextran-70 did not increase cardiac contractility and produced only a short-lived increase in cardiac output.[75] Finally, Huang and colleagues[40] have recently reported an association between use of hypertonic saline solution for resuscitation in burn patients and a startlingly high incidence of acute renal failure.

The goal of burn patient fluid resuscitation is the maintenance of vital organ function at the least immediate or delayed physiologic cost. This can be achieved by using only a balanced salt solution for fluid replacement during the first

24 hours post burn. The quantity to be infused in the adult, estimated by the commonly used formulas, ranges from 2 to 4 ml. per kg. of body weight per per cent burn. We recommend use of 2 ml. per kg. per per cent burn for the initial estimate to minimize volume loading and increase the infused volume only as necessary. The time-related changes in capillary permeability dictate administering, in the first 8 hours post burn, half of the volume calculated for infusion during the first 24 hours and giving the remaining half over the succeeding 16 hours. The volume actually infused is governed by the patient's response to his or her injury and resuscitation.

Moore and associates have reported that in a porcine model of burn injury, infusion in the first 2 hours post burn of one half of the first 24-hour resuscitation volume more rapidly returned cardiac index to 88% of baseline.[52] Infusion of such large volumes during the period when intravascular pressure is the predominant determinant of capillary filtration only serves to accentuate edema formation. Consistent with that possibility was those authors' observation that when the infusion rate of resuscitation fluid was thereafter decreased so that the remaining half of the calculated volume would be administered over the next 22 hours, the salutary effect on cardiac index promptly dissipated, and the hemodynamic indices became identical to those in animals that received resuscitation according to the standard clinical regimen. The administration of additional electrolyte-free water in the first 24 hours post burn appears to be unnecessary because evaporative water loss is, at most, modest during that period of hypovolemia and peripheral vasoconstriction, and because the balanced salt solutions commonly employed for burn patient resuscitation are hypotonic with respect to sodium. Since the endocrine response to burn injury commonly induces hyperglycemia, glucose-containing fluids should not be used for resuscitation in burned adults.

During the second 24 hours post burn, one should plan to replace any persistent plasma volume deficit by infusing colloid-containing fluids. The plasma volume deficit can be either measured directly or estimated as ranging between 0.3 and 0.5 ml. per kg. of body weight per per cent burn (0.3 ml.

in patients with 30% to 50% burns, 0.4 ml. in patients with 50% to 70% burns, and 0.5 ml. in patients with burns of more than 70% of the total body surface). The colloid-containing solution should be administered as a plasma equivalent, using salt-free albumin diluted to physiologic concentration in normal saline (5 gm. per 100 ml.). The administration of other colloid-free salt-containing fluids can usually be stopped. Even though a 10% pentastarch form of hydroxyethyl starch infused at the end of the first 24 hours has been reported to be as effective in expanding plasma volume as a 5% albumin solution, the prolongation of prothrombin time and plasma thromboplastin time following infusion of as little as 500 ml. of pentastarch speaks against use of larger volumes of that solution.[86] Electrolyte-free fluid, such as 5% dextrose in water, is infused in a volume sufficient to maintain urinary output while covering evaporative water loss and meeting metabolic needs.

There are different fluid needs for children younger than 15 years of age who have a larger surface area per unit body mass than adults. For such patients, use 3 ml. per kg. of body weight per per cent burn for calculating fluid needs for the first 24 hours. As in the adult, half of the volume calculated for infusion for the entire first 24 hours should be administered in the first 8 hours post burn, with the remaining half infused over the succeeding 16 hours. The administration of additional electrolyte-free water in the first 24 hours may be necessary in children, particularly small children with small burns. In such patients it is important that one administer sufficient fluid to meet maintenance fluid needs. The limited glycogen reserves and relatively small blood volume of the burned child who weighs less than 30 kg. mandate scheduled monitoring of blood glucose levels and the infusion of 5% dextrose in one-half normal saline solution to meet fluid maintenance needs not satisfied by the resuscitation fluids to prevent hypoglycemia.

In burned children the plasma volume deficit present at the beginning of the second 24 hours post burn should be corrected by infusing colloid-containing fluids as described for the adult. Electrolyte-free fluid such as 5% dextrose in water is infused in a volume sufficient to maintain urinary output and satisfy maintenance needs. In small children, hyponatremia and the associated risk of cerebral edema should be avoided by using 5% glucose in one-quarter normal saline to maintain urinary output during the second 24 hours post burn.

Monitoring of Fluid Resuscitation. Resuscitation fluids should be infused during the first and second post-burn day in amounts sufficient to maintain vital signs and an hourly urinary output of 30 to 50 ml. in the adult and 1 ml. per kg. per hour in children weighing less than 30 kg. The fluid infusion rate should be adjusted if the hourly urinary output falls below or exceeds the desired urinary output range by more than 33% for 2 to 3 hours. If a burn patient requires more than twice the estimated resuscitation volume during the first 12 hours post burn, and that need extends into the latter half of the first post-burn day, colloid-containing fluid should be administered. The remainder of the calculated first 24-hour electrolyte-containing fluid dose should be decreased by a volume of three times the amount of colloid infused to reduce the total volume of infusate.

Anxiety and restlessness may be early signs of hypovolemia and hypoxemia that require correction. Cuff blood pressure measurements in a burned limb can be misleading because the auditory blood pressure signal may be progressively attenuated as edema develops beneath the burn wound. Even blood pressure measurements obtained by the use of an intra-arterial cannula may be inaccurate in patients with extensive burns in whom markedly elevated circulating levels of catecholamines and other vasoactive materials cause severe vasospasm. If repeated arterial blood sampling is required, as may be necessary in patients with inhalation injury, an artery in the forearm should be cannulated.

Invasive monitoring of cardiac function should be reserved for those patients who do not respond to resuscitation in the anticipated manner. In these patients a Swan-Ganz catheter should be placed to measure pulmonary capillary wedge pressure to assess myocardial function and intravascular volume. If a burn patient continues to require significantly more than the estimated resuscitation volume, has no evidence of a significant blood volume deficit, and has a pulmonary capillary wedge pressure within or above the physiologic range, dobutamine or another inotropic agent can be used to improve myocardial function. Some patients with extensive burns may exhibit abnormally elevated systemic vascular resistance, leading to oliguria and reduced cardiac output. However, the use of early vasodilator treatment in these patients, in whom blood volume restoration may be incomplete, should be made with great caution lest cardiac output be further depressed by the unmasking of hypovolemia.

Since oliguria during the resuscitation period (first 48 hours post burn) is commonly due to inadequate resuscitation and is almost never an indication of acute renal failure, it should be treated by increased fluid administration, not by fluid restriction or administration of a diuretic. However, there are four categories of burn patients in whom administration of a diuretic may be necessary: those with high-voltage electric injury, those with associated mechanical soft tissue injury, those with particularly deep burns involving muscle, and those with extensive burns who remain oliguric in spite of receiving fluid volumes far in excess of estimated needs. Patients in the first three categories characteristically have heavy loads of hemochromogens in their urine and are prone to develop acute renal failure unless a brisk urinary output is maintained until the pigment concentration is reduced to insignificant levels. Fluid should be infused in such patients at the rate needed to achieve an hourly urinary output of 75 to 100 ml., but if the patient does not respond to increased fluid input with an increase in urine volume and clearing of the heme pigments, a diuretic should be given. One ampule (12.5 gm.) of mannitol is added to each liter of intravenous fluid until the desired level of urinary output is achieved and the pigment clears. Following administration of a diuretic, urinary output is no longer a reliable guide to the adequacy of resuscitation, and one should insert a Swan-Ganz catheter to monitor pulmonary capillary wedge pressure and cardiac function.

During the second post-burn day, the volume of fluids infused per hour should be arbitrarily reduced by 25% to 50%. If the urinary output remains satisfactory, that reduced rate of fluid infusion should be maintained over the next 3 hours, at which time the infusion volume should be further reduced in stepwise fashion.

A chest x-ray should be obtained at least daily during the resuscitation and edema resorption periods and later in the post-burn course if pneumonia or other pulmonary complications develop. Serum chemistries, blood urea nitrogen, blood glucose, arterial blood gases, and other baseline blood studies should be obtained on admission, and then as needed. The patient should be weighed on admission and daily thereafter as a means of monitoring fluid balance.

Escharotomy and Fasciotomy

Monitoring of the peripheral circulation and ventilatory exchange is required in those patients with circumferential full-thickness burns of the extremities or thoracic wall, respectively. The edema that forms beneath inelastic eschar may increase tissue pressure to a point at which it exceeds venous pressure, approaches arteriolar pressure, and severely impairs blood flow. The clinical signs of compromised limb blood flow include cyanosis, impaired capillary refilling, and progressive neurologic symptoms, particularly paresthesias and deep tissue pain. Absence of flow or progressive diminution of the flow signal on serial ultrasonic flowmeter examination of the palmar arch vessel in the upper limb or the posterior tibial artery in the lower limb are much more reliable indications of the need for escharotomy. Muscle compartment pressure can also be directly measured by insertion of either a slit catheter or wick catheter. A pressure above 30 mm. Hg is used as an indication for escharotomy. Edema formation in a burned limb and the need for escharotomy can be reduced by continuous elevation of the burned part and active motion of the part for 5 minutes every hour.

Escharotomy is performed as a ward procedure, and neither general nor local anesthesia is required, since only the insensate eschar is incised. The eschar on a circumferentially burned limb is incised in either the mid-lateral or mid-medial line. The incision should extend from the proximal to the distal margin of the burned area, should be carried across involved joints, and should be carried down through the eschar and the superficial fascia to a depth sufficient to allow the cut edges of the eschar to separate without incising other unburned subcutaneous tissues (Fig. 13–4). When the incision is performed in this manner, bleeding is minimal and can be controlled by electrocoagulation or a briefly applied compression dressing. If following one incision, distal flow is not restored, a second similar incision should be made in the contralateral midline of the limb. Mid-lateral escharotomy should also be performed on a circumferentially burned digit in which digital arterial flow is absent and the subeschar tissues are viable. If the digit is burned so severely as to be desiccated, such incisions are of no value. Rarely, mid-lateral line escharotomies may be needed for circumferential burns of the neck and a mid-dorsal escharotomy for a circumferential penile burn.

Impairment of ventilatory exchange by restriction of chest wall motion due to edema is an indication for a chest wall escharotomy. Chest escharotomies should be placed in the anterior axillary line bilaterally, extending from the clavicle to the costal margin. If the eschar involves the skin of the anterior abdominal wall, the anterior axillary escharotomies should be connected by a similar costal margin incision (Fig. 13–5).

Infrequently, escharotomy does not restore blood flow to

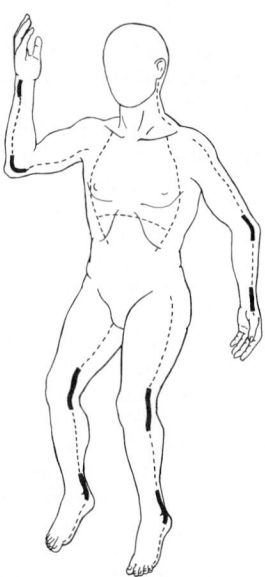

Figure 13–5. Diagram showing preferred sites of escharotomy incisions. Heavy portions of lines emphasize the necessity of extending escharotomy incisions across involved joints, where the vessels and nerves are readily compressed by subeschar edema.

unburned tissue, and fasciotomy is required. A muscle compartment requiring fasciotomy is characteristically stony hard to palpation. Patients who most often require fasciotomy are those in whom edema occurs beneath the investing fascia (i.e., those with high-voltage electric injury; those with associated soft tissue, long bone, or vascular injury; and those with burns involving muscle). Fasciotomy should be performed with the use of general anesthesia, and the fascia of all involved compartments must be adequately released. The anterior tibial compartment is the muscle compartment most frequently requiring fasciotomy in burn patients, and a single fasciotomy incision suffices to relieve the increased tissue pressure in that compartment. Hypesthesia of the skin of the first web space of the foot is an early sign of anterior tibial compartment compression, which, if untreated, causes anterior compartment necrosis. Autopsy studies of hands with full-thickness dorsal and palmar burns have revealed a high incidence of intrinsic muscle necrosis. On the basis of those findings, dorsal interosseous fasciotomies are performed in patients with such burns.

Inhalation Injury

Direct thermal injury of the tracheobronchial tree, except in the case of steam burns, is rarely encountered in clinical practice. Inhalation injury, a chemical tracheobronchitis and acute pneumonitis caused by the inhalation of smoke and other irritative products of incomplete combustion, is frequently present in patients admitted to burn centers (35% of patients treated at the United States Army Institute of Surgical Research during a recent 5-year period).[74]

Studies of inhalation injury in animal models suggest that inhaled smoke exerts deleterious effects on both the airways and the pulmonary vasculature. The inhalation of wood smoke has been reported to cause an increase in pulmonary vascular permeability,[59] and acrolein smoke appears to exert a toxic effect on peribronchial vessels.[32] Pulmonary vascular changes appear to represent local effects of absorbed toxic material since lung lesions are confined to the involved lung when only one lung is insufflated with smoke.[66]

The role of surfactant in the pathophysiology of inhalation

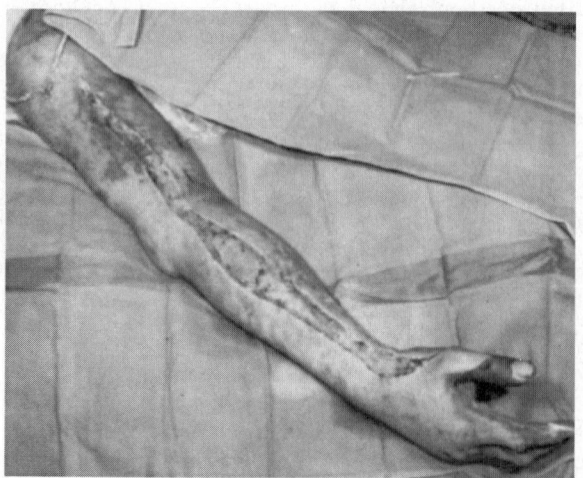

Figure 13–4. Escharotomy incision in the mediolateral line of a circumferentially burned arm. Note the separation of the incised edges of the eschar, particularly at the level of the wrist. Desiccation of distal phalanges indicates that escharotomies of the severely burned digits would be futile.

injury is uncertain and may be smoke-component specific. Other studies have implicated leukocytes, because leukopenia induced by preinjury nitrogen mustard treatment has been reported to attenuate significantly the vascular changes in the lung following smoke inhalation. Herndon and associates, on the basis of clinical experience, have recommended the administration of 50% more than the calculated resuscitation fluid volume to maintain cardiac output at normal levels to reduce neutrophil margination on the pulmonary capillaries of patients with inhalation injury.[38] Changes in the matching of ventilation and perfusion in an animal model indicate the predominance of airway damage in the pathogenesis of inhalation injury and the importance of ventilatory support.

Mortality in burn patients with inhalation injury is greater overall than in patients with burns of similar size who have no inhalation injury. The mortality-enhancing effect of inhalation injury is both age- and burn size–related, rising to a maximum increase in expected mortality of 20% in patients whose predicted mortality from burn injury alone would be 50% to 75%.[74] Maximal therapeutic effort should be directed to this group.

Inhalation injury should be suspected in any patient burned in a closed space or burned during a period of impaired mentation. Although head and neck burns and singeing of the nasal vibrissae are commonly present in patients with inhalation injury, these signs are nonspecific compared with frank inflammation of the oropharyngeal mucosa. Other signs of inhalation injury include a brassy cough, hoarseness and wheezing, bronchorrhea, unexplained hypoxemia, and the production of carbonaceous sputum, the last being specific. Unfortunately, carbon-stained bronchial secretions may be cleared from the airway by the time of admission, and the other signs may not be evident for 2 to 3 days following injury. Consequently, the diagnosis of inhalation injury is commonly delayed, and the second postburn day is the mean time of diagnosis on the basis of clinical signs.

The chest x-ray is notoriously insensitive in detecting even severe inhalation injury.[13] The use of two modalities enhances the timeliness and reliability of the diagnosis of inhalation injury: fiberoptic bronchoscopic examination and xenon-133 ventilation-perfusion pulmonary scintiphotography.

Fiberoptic bronchoscopy can be performed as a bedside procedure as soon as the burn patient suspected of having inhalation injury is hemodynamically stable. An appropriately sized endotracheal tube should be placed over the bronchoscope before performing the examination so that the tube can be placed during the course of the examination if the inflammatory reaction threatens airway patency. A topical anesthetic should be applied to the upper airway to provide for patient comfort and thereby facilitate the examination. The supraglottic airway is examined for signs of inflammation and for the presence and severity of glottic edema. If edema of the cords and upper airway threatens airway occlusion, the endotracheal tube should be placed immediately and the examination continued by passage of the bronchoscope through the tube into the lower airway.

Evidence of mucosal inflammation and ulceration of the infraglottic airway as well as deposition of carbon particles on the endobronchial mucosa indicate inhalation injury. The bronchoscopic examination of burn patients may be misleading, and both false-negative and false-positive results have been reported; the former are due to failure of inflammatory changes to develop in the hypovolemic patient with impaired mucosal perfusion, and the latter are due to pre-existing bronchitis.

Since the site of aerosol particle deposition within the airway is strongly influenced by particle size, it is possible for the large endoscopically visible airways to be relatively uninjured in the presence of significant terminal bronchiolar and alveolar inflammatory damage when the smoke particle mass median diameter is less than 0.05 μm. If a burn patient is suspected of having inhalation injury but has no or minimal inflammatory changes on bronchoscopic examination, a ^{133}Xe ventilation-perfusion lung scan should be performed after hemodynamic stability is achieved but before post-burn hyperventilation reaches significantly elevated levels (usually beyond 72 hours post burn). Serial scintiphotographs are obtained after injection of 10 μCi. of the insoluble gas into a peripheral vein. Unequal radiation density and retention of the gas in the lungs beyond 90 seconds post injection are considered positive indications of inhalation injury (Fig. 13–6). Both false-negative (5%) and false-positive (8%) lung scan results may be obtained: the former because the test was performed in the presence of pronounced hyperventilation, and the latter because of pre-existing bronchitis (common in heavy smokers).

Changes in various indices of pulmonary function are also produced by inhalation injury. An arterial oxygen tension of less than 70 mm. Hg and a peak flow rate of approximately 60% of predicted have been correlated with inhalation injury. When performed serially, maximum expiratory flow-volume curves are of prognostic value and can also be used to assess the effects of therapeutic agents such as isoproterenol. The necessity for full patient cooperation and the complexity of the equipment required for some of the pulmonary function tests severely limit their clinical usefulness in critically ill patients. The use of fiberoptic bronchoscopy and ^{133}Xe ventilation-perfusion lung scans permits the diagnosis of inhalation injury with 93% accuracy, the residual error being largely that of overdiagnosis.

The treatment of inhalation injury is guided by the severity of pulmonary insufficiency. In patients with mild disease, the administration of warm humidified oxygen-enriched air and the use of incentive spirometry may be adequate. Repeated bronchoscopy (using the rigid bronchoscope) may be needed for patients with extensive mucosal sloughing who are unable to clear their airway spontaneously. Progressive hypoxemia necessitates endotracheal intubation and the use of

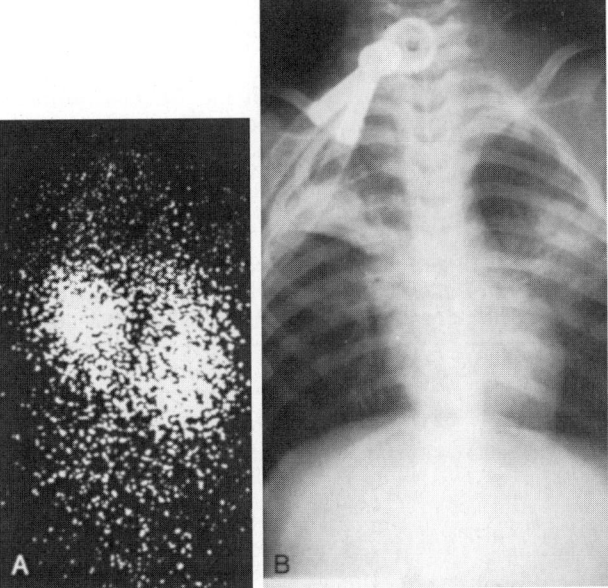

Figure 13–6. *A,* Scintiphotograph taken after injection of ^{133}Xe in a peripheral vein of a patient burned in a house fire. The initial standard chest roentgenogram was normal. Note the retention and focal increase in radiation density in both upper lung fields. *B,* Standard chest roentgenogram of the same patient showing subsequent development of pulmonary infiltrates in areas positive on the lung scan.

mechanical ventilatory assistance. The prophylactic use of high-frequency percussive ventilation as a means of minimizing airway collapse and atelectatic changes has been shown to reduce the incidence of pneumonia and mortality below that of historic controls.[12] Such treatment in patients with mild inhalation injury has reduced mortality by a factor of 4 and significantly decreased the mortality associated with moderate to severe inhalation injury (Table 13–5).[70] High-frequency ventilation also minimizes pulmonary barotrauma.[10] The prophylactic systemic administration of steroids has had no influence on the morbidity or mortality of patients with inhalation injury and, in fact, has been reported to increase the occurrence of infection.

Pulmonary infection is the most frequent cause of morbidity and mortality in patients with inhalation injury. At the first sign of pulmonary infiltrates on the chest x-ray, endobronchial cultures should be obtained and systemic antibiotic therapy begun as described for bronchopneumonia (see later).

Long-term morbidity of burn patients with inhalation injury who survive is related to both the severity of the airway injury and the treatment employed, particularly the use of invasive airway devices necessary to preserve respiratory function. In general, the sequelae of tracheotomy are more common and more severe than those associated with translaryngeal intubation. The duration of intubation, regardless of route, and the presence of a tracheal stoma are the most important etiologic factors in permanent airway damage such as granuloma formation and tracheal stenosis. Fiberoptic bronchoscopy is required to document airway lesions and should be performed on all patients in whom the duration of airway intubation has exceeded 10 days and evidence of airway compromise exists.

Other Considerations in Early Care

The almost universal occurrence of ileus during the immediate post-burn period necessitates insertion of a nasogastric tube to evacuate gastric contents and thereby prevent emesis and aspiration. Prophylaxis against stress ulcer complications should be initiated as described later in the chapter. The nasogastric tube should be removed as soon as gastrointestinal motility returns, usually on the third or fourth postburn day, at which time oral fluids should be started and the patient's diet advanced as tolerated.

Tetanus prophylaxis is dictated by the patient's immunization status as in other trauma patients. Those who have not undergone prior immunization should be given 250 to 500 units of human antitetanus globulin at one site, with an initial immunizing dose of toxoid administered at another site. Active immunization is thereafter completed using the routine dosage schedule.

Beta-hemolytic streptococcal infection prophylaxis is not employed by the authors, since such infections are now uncommon in burn patients and respond promptly to penicillin treatment if they do occur. Some physicians, those dealing principally with pediatric burn patients and those involved in the out-of-hospital treatment of patients with second-degree burns of 10% to 15% of the body surface, still employ penicillin prophylaxis, using 20,000 units per kg. of body weight per day in the child and 3 to 5 million units per day in the adult.

The severity of pain in the immediate postburn period is related to the depth of the burn. Second-degree burns may be very painful. Third-degree burns, on the other hand, because of coagulation necrosis of sensory nerve endings, are insensate. Analgesia in the immediate postburn resuscitation and edema-formation period is best achieved by the intravenous administration of small doses of morphine. Pain associated with second-degree burns abates when a serous crust forms on the burn surface, when an occlusive dressing is applied, or when the wound is covered with a biologic dressing. In such patients and in those with third-degree burns, wound pain is subsequently associated with wound manipulations such as cleansing, débridement, and dressing changes. Analgesics should be administered at an appropriate interval before wound manipulation to reduce pain and minimize pain-related stress.

Post-resuscitation Fluid Management

Fluid management after resuscitation is completed should permit excretion of the salt load infused during resuscitation, while permitting a daily loss of 10% to 12% of the weight gained during resuscitation, so that the patient returns to preburn weight by the eighth to tenth post-burn day. Any departure from that weight loss trajectory necessitates review of the patient's intake and output records and adjustment of fluid therapy. The development of secondary disturbances of fluid and electrolyte balance should also be prevented.

The modest hyponatremia present at the end of resuscitation, caused by infusion of large volumes of lactated Ringer's solution, which is hypotonic with respect to sodium, requires no treatment, since appropriate fluid management permits the increased evaporative water loss to correct that imbalance. Hyponatremia may persist or even be exaggerated in patients treated with 0.5% silver nitrate soaks. The administration of supplemental sodium chloride and sodium lactate prevents or corrects this complication. Inappropriate secretion of antidiuretic hormone is a rare cause of generally asymptomatic hyponatremia in burn patients and usually responds to reduction in the amount of administered electrolyte-free fluid. Early in the course of infection, modest hyponatremia may result from a reduction in free water clearance. In addition to adjusting the fluid therapy of such patients, the causative infection should be identified and controlled.

The most common post-resuscitation fluid and electrolyte disturbance is hypernatremia associated with dehydration due to inadequate replacement of insensible water loss. Burn injury destroys the water vapor barrier of the skin, and evaporative water loss from the burned area is markedly elevated. Fluid needs can be estimated on the basis of total insensible water loss, which is calculated as follows: insensible water loss (ml./hr.) = (25 + per cent of the body surface burned) × total body surface (m^2). The formula estimates water loss at the low end of the range of observed water losses, and the patient's body weight, serum sodium concentration, and serum osmolarity should be monitored on a

TABLE 13–5. Pneumonia Occurrence Rates and Mortality in Patients with Inhalation Injury Treated with High-Frequency Ventilation: 1985–1990

	Mild Injury	Moderate/Severe Injury
Number of Patients	85	245
Mean Age in Years	33.5	35.6
Average Extent of Burn (% of total body surface)	26.2	46.1
Number of Patients with Pneumonia	11 (13.1%)	115 (46.9%)
Deaths Observed	3 (3.6%)	94 (38.3%)
Deaths Predicted	14 (16%)	123 (50.4%)
95% CL	9–18	112–135

daily basis to assess the adequacy of hydration and the need to adjust fluid therapy. Other less-frequent causes of dehydration and associated hypernatremia include osmotic diuresis caused by glucosuria and increased urinary nitrogen, treated by dietary manipulation or therapy of underlying diabetes mellitus; diabetes insipidus, treated by the administration of vasopressin; and sepsis, treated by the control of infection.

The release of potassium from red blood cells and other tissues injured by the burn commonly produces a modest hyperkalemia during the resuscitation period that usually requires no specific therapy. If acidosis, due to inadequate resuscitation, supervenes, the serum potassium concentration may be elevated to symptomatic levels, necessitating rapid fluid infusion and specific therapy to reduce the potassium concentration.

Following resuscitation, hypokalemia may result from increased potassium loss. In patients treated with mafenide acetate (Sulfamylon) burn cream, the kaliuretic effect of that agent may accentuate those losses. Patients treated with 0.5% silver nitrate soaks, which exaggerate transeschar potassium losses, and patients with profuse diarrhea induced by enteral feeding may also become hypokalemic. In all burn patients, the serum potassium concentration and urinary potassium losses should be monitored and potassium supplements given to prevent or correct deficits.

Apparent hypocalcemia may be associated with the hypo-albuminemia resulting from dilution and the reprogramming of hepatic protein synthesis. In such cases, ionized calcium levels are commonly normal. True hypocalcemia may be produced by increased renal excretion resulting from the hypermetabolic increase in renal blood flow and the renal tubular effects of the carbonic anhydrase inhibition caused by mafenide acetate, increased transeschar losses in patients treated with 0.5% silver nitrate soaks, and as a consequence of sustained metabolic acidosis. Serum calcium levels should be monitored daily for the first postburn week and twice a week thereafter. An identified calcium deficiency should be corrected by administration of calcium.

Some degree of hypophosphatemia is often present in burn patients within the first post-burn week. Depression of phosphate levels has been reported to occur in association with elevated circulating levels of catecholamines; infusion of large volumes of glucose-containing solutions; respiratory alkalosis induced by the hyperventilation often present in burn patients, which can be exaggerated by the carbonic anhydrase inhibition caused by mafenide acetate; phosphate binding associated with antacid stress ulcer prophylaxis; and the initiation of high-calorie nutritional support. Circulating levels of phosphate should be monitored and a confirmed phosphate deficit corrected.

BURN WOUND CARE
Initial Treatment and Topical Therapy

Attention should be directed to the burn wound itself only after resuscitation has been initiated and hemodynamic and respiratory stability are being restored. The burn wound should be cleansed using a surgical detergent, all loose nonviable skin trimmed away, and all hair shaved from the burned areas and a generous margin of unburned skin. The initial débridement can best be performed in a shower-like area using a hand-held showerhead with the patient lying on a litter or, alternatively, with the patient lying on a slanted plinth suspended over (but not immersed in) a Hubbard or other physical therapy tank. Thereafter the burns are similarly cleansed each day in a tank or shower, or in the case of critically ill patients, at the bedside. Following cleansing and

débridement, the topical agent of choice is applied. In the case of patients treated with topical creams by the exposure technique, gauze sponges are used to remove the residual agent 12 hours after the initial exposure, following which a new coating of topical agent is applied to the entirety of the burn wound. In the case of patients treated with 0.5% silver nitrate soaks, the occlusive dressings are changed two or three times daily and kept moistened between dressing changes by application of additional 0.5% silver nitrate solution every 2 hours.

Both wound and microbial factors influence the rate of microbial proliferation in and penetration of the eschar. The burned tissue, which is rich in protein and moist by virtue of the transeschar movement of fluid and serum, serves as an excellent microbial culture medium. The avascularity of the burned tissue, resulting from thermal thrombosis, limits both the delivery of endogenous phagocytic cells and the effectiveness of systemically administered antibiotics. Wound maceration and pressure necrosis may also favor microbial proliferation and should be avoided by frequently changing the position of the patient. Later in the post-burn course, exposure and desiccation of granulation tissue may result in the formation of a neoeschar, which supports bacterial growth and proliferation. Systemic impairment of blood flow, as may occur with septic or hypovolemic shock, further predisposes the patient to invasive infection by reducing delivery of oxygen, energy substrates, and phagocytic cells to the viable tissue underlying the wound.

Microbial factors that influence the natural history of the burn wound and the likelihood of infection or systemic sepsis include density of organisms (invasion is uncommon unless the number of bacteria equals or exceeds 10^5 per gm. of tissue) and a variety of strain-specific factors. Relatively few organisms can be recovered from the burned surface immediately after injury, and those that are present are predominantly gram positive. The type and density of organisms present in the untreated burn wound change with time so that by the fifth post-burn day gram-negative organisms can be recovered from 60% of patients. By the middle of the second post-burn week, the burn wound organisms are predominantly gram negative and have increased to levels of 10^2 to 10^4 per sq. cm. of wound surface. Without topical therapy, the organisms penetrate the eschar down to the viable-nonviable tissue interface. At this site, further microbial proliferation commonly occurs and promotes lysis of denatured collagen and spontaneous slough of the eschar. In those patients with inadequate host defense capacity or those in whom topical therapy is ineffective, the subeschar organisms invade the underlying unburned tissue and may spread systemically.

The incidence of burn wound sepsis (defined as invasive burn wound infection associated with systemic sepsis) is related to burn depth, extent of burn, and patient age. Invasive infection is uncommon in partial-thickness burns. The incidence of burn wound sepsis is low in patients with burns of less than 30% of the body surface and rises as burn size increases above that level. Burn wound sepsis has been most common in children, less common in the elderly, and least common in young adults.

The use of clinically effective topical antimicrobial agents developed in the mid 1960s has significantly decreased the occurrence of invasive burn wound infection and burn wound sepsis, an effect that has been associated with the improved survival of burn patients. At the present time, even in patients with massive burns, the cause of death is seldom burn wound sepsis and is commonly infection at another site. The three clinically available topical agents, each with specific advantages and limitations, should be used selectively to meet the individual patient's wound care needs.

Mafenide acetate burn cream and 0.5% silver nitrate soaks were developed contemporaneously, and several years later silver sulfadiazine burn cream was formulated in an attempt to combine the good effects and reduce the side effects of the two agents developed earlier. All three agents have been found to be effective in the control of invasive burn wound infection and burn wound sepsis, although the silver nitrate soaks and silver sulfadiazine burn cream are most effective when begun immediately after burning, before significant microbial colonization has occurred.

Sulfamylon burn cream is an 11.1% suspension of mafenide acetate, which is bacteriostatic, is freely soluble, and readily diffuses through the eschar to establish an effective concentration at the nonviable-viable tissue interface. This agent also has the broadest spectrum of activity against *Pseudomonas* organisms in particular and gram-negative organisms in general. These characteristics make it the best agent for treating patients in whom a dense bacterial population has developed in the eschar or those whose prior wound care regimens have failed to control the bacterial proliferation in the wound. The principal limitations of mafenide acetate burn cream are the pain produced by its application to partial-thickness burns and its inhibition of carbonic anhydrase, which promotes wasting of bicarbonate by the kidney and accentuates postburn hyperventilation. Both of these derangements predispose the patient to the development of acidosis.

Silver sulfadiazine (Silvadene) burn cream, a 1% suspension of silver sulfadiazine, is bacteriostatic but poorly diffusible and penetrates the eschar to a lesser extent than mafenide acetate burn cream. This agent, in contradistinction to mafenide acetate burn cream, produces no pain when applied to partial-thickness burns and causes no electrolyte or acid-base disturbances. The principal limitations of this agent include development of neutropenia (the granulocyte count commonly returns to *normal* levels after change of topical agents and typically remains at those levels even if silver sulfadiazine is reinstituted) and ineffectiveness against certain gram-negative organisms (some *Pseudomonas* strains and virtually all *Enterobacter cloacae* species).

One-half percent silver nitrate solution has, as do the other agents, a broad spectrum of antibacterial activity. This agent, which is applied in the form of many-layered soaks, causes no wound pain, but the soaks impede motion of involved joints, and their removal at the time of dressing changes can cause pain. This agent does not penetrate the eschar, and, in fact, the silver ions are immediately precipitated on contact with any proteinaceous or other foreign material, a reaction responsible for the discoloration of the unburned skin of the patient, the skin of attending personnel, and virtually everything else in the environment. The principal limitations of this agent consist of the leaching of sodium, potassium, chloride, and calcium from the wound and the transeschar absorption of the aqueous vehicle, which may lead to mineral deficits, alkalosis, and water loading. Supplements of sodium and the other minerals must be administered to prevent or correct these electrolyte deficits, and fluid administration must be adjusted to prevent overhydration.

The microbial ecology of the burn wounds of the patients cared for in any burn unit changes with time, and alterations in the flora take the form of mini-epidemics with a succession of predominant organisms. In the 1960s, *Pseudomonas aeruginosa* was the most common cause of infection in severely burned patients; and since that time, mini-epidemics caused by *Providencia stuartii, E. cloacae, Klebsiella* species, and recrudescent *Pseudomonas* species have occurred. Since 1977, recovery of *Pseudomonas* species from the wounds and blood of patients treated at the United States Army Institute of Surgical Research has fallen precipitously. The virtual disappearance of invasive *Pseudomonas* burn wound infection has

occurred during a period in which the wounds were cleansed daily with chlorhexidine along with application of mafenide acetate burn cream and silver sulfadiazine burn cream alternately every 12 hours to minimize the side effects of each while taking advantage of the superior anti–gram-negative activity of the former and the superior anticandidal activity of the latter. In patients with sulfa drug allergy, 0.5% silver nitrate soaks are the treatment of choice.

Topical antimicrobial chemotherapy is utilized to limit microbial proliferation in the burn wound until the burned tissue can be surgically removed. Burn wound excision of even extensive burns should begin as soon after resuscitation as the patient's physiologic status permits. In patients whose wounds cannot be completely excised at a single sitting, topical chemotherapy is continued on the burn wounds that remain unexcised. In patients whose physiologic status does not permit early excision, topical chemotherapy is continued until excision can be carried out or until daily débridement removes the eschar.

Burn Wound Excision

Because of the increased fibrosis and greater likelihood of hypertrophic scarring associated with healing after 2 weeks, a 2-week period is allowed for spontaneous healing. As soon as it is clinically obvious that healing will not occur within 2 weeks, excision is scheduled.

The adverse effects of excision include the anesthetic risk and the operative stress associated with prodigious blood loss (amounts equal to or exceeding the blood volume) when excision of more than 20% of the total body surface is carried out as a single procedure. These effects speak for undertaking excision only when the patient's physiologic reserve has been re-established and for limiting an excision procedure to 20% of the total body surface or 2 hours of operative time. Other adverse effects include the susceptibility of the excised wound to infection from the microorganisms on adjacent unexcised burns; the sacrifice, when excision is at the level of the investing fascia, of viable skin in areas of partial-thickness burn that are intermixed with areas of full-thickness burn; and the uncertainty of graft take, particularly on fatty tissue that is exposed in a wound produced by tangential excision. Also limiting are the immunosuppressive effects of the transfusions needed to replace the blood loss caused by the excision.

The advantages of burn wound excision that have led to its acceptance and current widespread use include decreased hospital stay and associated lesser costs, an earlier return to work, a greater likelihood that the patient will return to work, a lesser incidence of invasive burn wound infection, and fewer complications. In patients with burns of more than 40% of the total body surface, burn wound excision has been credited with decreasing the duration and magnitude of injury-related physiologic stress by reducing the extent of the burn and recently with decreasing the degree of immunologic impairment. However, laboratory studies indicate that obliteration of post-burn hypermetabolism is achieved only when the entirety of the wound can be excised and completely closed by grafting immediately after burning.[19] Recent reports indicate improved survival as a result of such improved wound care, including early excision, as well as improved general care.

Since at least the mid-1950s, scalpel excision at the level of the investing fascia has been used to remove full-thickness burn wounds. A tourniquet can be used to reduce the blood loss associated with excision of burns on a limb. The carbon dioxide laser and standard electrocautery instruments have also been used for burn wound excision at the level of the investing fascia to reduce the associated blood loss. Use of the laser is attended by lesser blood loss than is the use of an electrocautery device, but the former is a more expensive instrument and the time required for excision has been reported to be longer. The take of immediately applied autograft skin is similar following the use of the scalpel, laser, or electrocautery device.

In the mid-1960s a technique, termed *tangential excision*, was introduced for the treatment of partial-thickness burns of generally limited extent. In recent years the technique has been applied to the treatment of patients with extensive partial-thickness and even full-thickness burns. Using a guarded skin knife or dermatome, successive thin layers of burned tissue are removed until all nonviable tissue is excised as indicated by uniformly dense capillary bleeding from the entire wound bed. The blood loss associated with this form of excision can be formidable (as much as 9% of the circulating blood volume/per cent of body surface excised), but the use of a tourniquet precludes capillary bleeding from the wound bed, which is used as the endpoint for the operative procedure. The loss of blood can be reduced by topical application of thrombin either as a spray or in moistened warm gauze sponges with or without epinephrine or by intravenous infusion or subeschar infiltration of vasopressin.

The wound produced by any form of excision must be closed by autografting or, if donor sites are limited, by application of a biologic dressing or skin substitute, as described later. If at the time of excision the adequacy of the excisional procedure is uncertain, as may occur when the level of excision is in the subcutaneous fat or if the excision is being done for the treatment of invasive burn wound infection, a biologic dressing can be applied to the wound bed. The patient is returned to the operating room 48 to 72 hours later, at which time the biologic membrane is removed and autografting accomplished if no residual nonviable tissue remains. If there is so much residual nonviable tissue present that extensive additional excision is required, the wound is again covered with a biologic dressing following re-excision. The patient is returned to the operating room every 48 to 72 hours until the sequential excisions produce a graftable wound bed.

The excision technique employed should be based on the depth and microbial status of the patient's burns. Scalpel or electrocautery excision at or below the level of the investing fascia should be employed in the treatment of full-thickness burns of limited extent, the débridement of high-voltage electrical injuries, and excision of areas of burn wound infection. Tangential excision is indicated in the treatment of deep partial-thickness burns of 20% or less of the total body surface (particularly burns involving the dorsum of the hand) and the staged excision of more extensive partial- and full-thickness burns.

In a group of 381 patients with burns of more than 30% of the total body surface treated at the United States Army Institute of Surgical Research during a 5½-year period, burn wound excision was carried out in all but 17 (7%) of the 235 surviving patients but was precluded by a complication in 75 (51%) of the 146 patients who died. The physiologic instability that either prevented movement of those 75 patients to the operating room or limited the patient's ability to withstand the operative stress was pulmonary insufficiency in 58, hemodynamic instability in 14, and sepsis with disseminated intravascular coagulation in 3. A temporary delay in excision may be necessitated by the need to control burn wound cellulitis or correct acid-base and electrolyte disturbances.

Nonexcisional Therapy

Burn wound care for those patients with superficial partial-thickness burns or deep partial-thickness and full-thickness burns that are not excised typically consists of daily cleansing and débridement with subsequent application of topical antimicrobial agents, as described earlier. As wound maturation proceeds, a membrane-like coagulum of serum, white blood cells, and topical agent forms over the surface of the wound. That membrane can be removed by serial applications of wet to dry soaks, following which the wound bed can be covered with a biologic dressing to hasten spontaneous healing. Analgesia may be necessary for daily cleansing and débridement, but anesthesia is not used for such procedures because of its adverse effects on gastrointestinal motility and appetite.

Treatment of the wound following daily cleansing depends on the maturity of the granulation tissue, the amount of residual necrotic debris, and the extent of the débrided area. If there is significant residual necrotic debris, the wound is covered with a topical antimicrobial agent. If there is less residual debris, only a small fully débrided area, or inadequate granulation tissue, the wound can be covered with a dressing soaked in an antimicrobial solution (5% mafenide acetate) that is changed two to three times per day and kept moist by applying additional antimicrobial solution every 2 hours between dressing changes. If there is little residual nonviable tissue and either granulation tissue over the base of a full-thickness burn or proliferating islands of epithelium on a partial-thickness burn, a biologic dressing can be applied.

Wound Closure

The goal of burn wound care is timely definitive closure. Those wounds ready for split-thickness autograft closure are those that have been excised or those treated by the nonexcisional methods that are characterized by absence of residual nonviable tissue and pooled secretions; firm, red, finely granular granulation tissue; a surface bacterial count of less than 10^5 organisms per sq. cm of wound surface; and absence of beta-hemolytic streptococci. Adherence of viable cutaneous allografts to the wound bed can be used as an index of the readiness for autografting of wounds, which for some reason have not been autografted. General adherence and vascularization of allograft skin are customarily associated with universal adherence of subsequently applied autograft skin (Fig. 13–7). Split-thickness autograft skin is applied directly to the areas from which the cutaneous allografts have been removed.

Autografts of 0.012 to 0.015 inch in thickness are generally

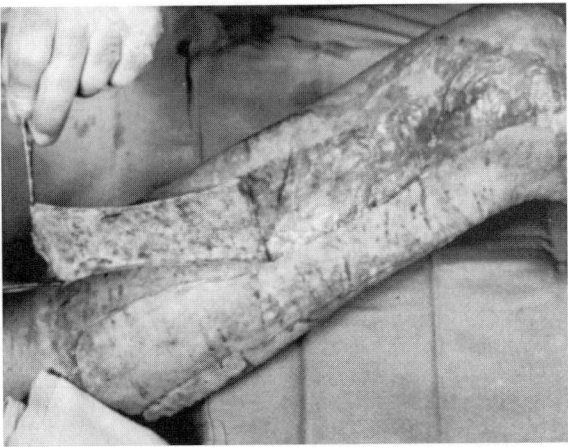

Figure 13–7. Removal, 5 days after application, of viable cutaneous allografts, which are generally adherent and free of subgraft suppuration. A mature, finely granular bed of fresh granulation tissue indicates that immediately applied autografts will invariably adhere.

used for initial skin coverage in patients with extensive burns. Donor sites are dressed with a single layer of fine-mesh gauze, and initial hemostasis of the donor site is obtained by application, in the operating room, of warm laparotomy packs over the fine-mesh gauze. Alternatively, any of a variety of pliable synthetic dressings that maintain better flexibility and elasticity can be applied to reduce donor site discomfort. Such dressings are held in place either by material that adheres to surrounding intact skin or by application of a light dressing. If fine-mesh gauze is applied to the donor sites, the laparotomy packs are removed when the patient returns to the recovery room or the ward and the donor site dressing is exposed to a heat lamp to hasten drying.

In patients with burns associated with an anticipated mortality of less than 50%, priority of skin grafting is given to burn wounds involving the hands, feet, face, and joints. In patients with more extensive burns, priority is given to coverage of flat planar surfaces such as the anterior and posterior trunk and the thighs, to reduce, as soon as possible, the extent of the total burn and the associated physiologic derangements. In patients with extensive burns and limited donor sites, the quality of skin graft harvested from donor sites overlying bony areas can be improved by the subcutaneous infiltration of saline, but this salt load must be taken into account in planning postoperative fluid management. The quality of skin grafts progressively declines with each subsequent harvest of a previously used donor site. Since the residual dermis is progressively thinner and the overlying epithelium is relatively immature, the grafts are typically thinner with each successive harvest. Treated as described, a donor site will heal in approximately 14 to 21 days, but the interharvest intervals should be as long as is consistent with skin graft coverage needs to permit maximal donor site maturation between harvests.

Scalp donor sites are characterized by rapid re-epithelization and freedom from hypertrophic scar formation, and the scalp can be used for repeated harvest of autograft skin with greater frequency than other areas. However, donor site alopecia has been reported following multiple reharvestings. Consequently, even on the scalp, when repeated harvesting is anticipated, each harvest should be of minimal thickness to reduce the risk of alopecia. When taking skin grafts from the scalp it is important to leave a fringe of hair at the anterior hair line so the donor site will not be extended onto the forehead.

Mesh grafts can be used to increase the extent of wound covered by donor skin. By use of the appropriate *carrier board* or mesh dermatome, it is possible to prepare grafts that can be expanded at ratios stated to be 1.5:1, 2:1, 3:1, 4:1, 6:1, and even 9:1, but the actual expansion is less than stated. Expansion ratios of 1.5:1 up to 4:1 appear adequate for virtually all needs. In general, mesh grafts should not be applied to the face or over joints, although unexpanded 1.5:1 mesh grafts that allow escape of serum and blood have been used to good effect after excision of burns of the dorsum of the hand. Use of the larger expansion ratios is associated with an excessive time for closure of the interstices and greater scar epithelium formation.

Mesh grafts are covered with occlusive dressings and kept wet with an antimicrobial solution such as 0.5% silver nitrate or 5% mafenide acetate to prevent desiccation of the interstices and limit microbial proliferation. Alternatively, sheets of cutaneous allograft or xenograft or sheets of the synthetic biologic dressing Biobrane can be applied over mesh grafts to prevent desiccation and protect them from dislodgment by shearing.

Biologic Dressings

Viable cutaneous allograft is the biologic dressing of choice, against which all other available materials must be evaluated (see Fig. 13–7). In the operating room using sterile technique, allograft skin is harvested from cadavers free of jaundice, cutaneous malignancy or infection, and viral disease. The harvested grafts are spread on fine-mesh gauze that is thinly impregnated with petrolatum, placed in sterile containers, and then refrigerated for up to 2 weeks. Alternatively, the tissue can be frozen using cryoprotective techniques. If refrigerated, such tissue performs better as a biologic dressing the sooner after harvest it is used.

Cutaneous allograft prevents wound desiccation; promotes maturation of granulation tissue; limits bacterial proliferation in the burn wound; prevents exudative protein and red blood cell loss; decreases wound pain, thereby facilitating movement of involved joints; diminishes evaporative water loss from the burn wound surface, thus decreasing heat loss; and serves to protect tendons, vessels, and nerves. If small areas of necrotic debris are covered, subgraft suppuration in those areas appears to effect more rapid débridement. When applied to superficial second-degree burns, cutaneous allografts accelerate re-epithelization and enhance the quality of healing. The limitations of cutaneous allografts (i.e., a finite shelf life, refrigeration requirements, potential transmission of viruses such as hepatitis virus and human immunodeficiency virus, and uncertain availability) have led to the use of other biologic dressings.

Lyophilized allograft skin has an indefinite shelf life and is easily reconstituted; however, it, too, is in limited supply, shows less adherence to the wound than viable allograft skin, and if harvested at too great a thickness, undergoes dermal-epidermal separation after application to the wound with subsequent desiccation of the exposed dermis. Cutaneous xenografts suffer from no shortage in supply but are less effective as physiologic dressings and allow survival of greater numbers of subgraft bacteria, presumably because such tissue is not vascularized by the host. Studies of porcine cutaneous xenografts have shown that biologic union is formed by the growth of fibrovascular tissue from the host into the dermis of the graft without vessel-to-vessel attachment. Such tissues are not rejected in the true sense of the word but slough following necrosis. Amnion is another physiologic dressing that is readily available and inexpensive. Since the amniotic tissue will desiccate and spontaneously separate from the wound bed if left exposed, it must be covered with occlusive dressings that preclude continuous observation of the dressing and underlying wound bed. Amnion, like cutaneous xenografts, is not vascularized by the host, and biologic union occurs by ingrowth of granulation tissue. Amniotic tissue carries the same risk of viral disease transmission as does cutaneous allograft.

Many studies have indicated that a bilaminate structure is required for a skin substitute to function effectively. The thin outer layer (epidermal analog) should have pores less than 5 μm. in diameter to permit passage of water vapor but no liquid water or bacteria. The thicker inner layer (dermal analog) should have pores at least 80 μm. in diameter that will permit ingrowth of fibrovascular tissue from the wound surface to form a satisfactory biologic union. Studies of a totally synthetic bilaminate membrane have demonstrated that when applied to clean wounds it functioned as well as cutaneous xenograft. When the membrane was applied to areas where nonviable tissue remained, purulent material generated by subgraft suppuration migrated through the skin substitute, indicating the need to remove or change the membrane. Used in that manner, the skin substitute will hasten débridement of limited areas of burn wound from which the bulk of the eschar has separated but on which nonviable tenaciously adherent dermis remains.

Clinical effectiveness has also been demonstrated for two collagen-based bilaminate skin substitutes. Biobrane consists of a collagen gel dermal analog and a Silastic epidermal analog. This material is indistinguishable from porcine cutaneous xenograft when applied to a freshly excised burn wound in terms of submembrane formation of granulation tissue, submembrane suppuration, wound adherence, conformation to the wound surface, and membrane pliability. When applied to the clean superficial partial-thickness burns of a child immediately following injury, Biobrane strikingly reduces wound pain. If submembrane suppuration does not occur, the Biobrane dressing need not be changed and will separate as the wound re-epithelializes. Another bilaminate skin substitute that has been used to provide immediate coverage of excised burn wounds consists of a Silastic epidermal analog and a dermal analog composed of collagen fibrils enriched with chondroitin 6-sulfate.[37] When the dermal analog of the skin substitute is adequately vascularized (3 to 4 weeks) by the ingrowth of granulation tissue, the Silastic membrane is removed and the wound closed by direct application of ultra-thin split-thickness skin grafts to the vascularized dermal analog. The residual exogenous tissue is apparently gradually resorbed and replaced by host tissue.

Signs of systemic sepsis following application of any biologic dressing or skin substitute dictate removal of such material and resumption of topical antimicrobial therapy. Particular care must be exercised when such membranes are placed on what are judged to be superficial second-degree burns, particularly in children in whom the initial appearance of the wound can be misleading. Application of these membranes to deep second- or third-degree burns may only serve to convert an open contaminated wound to a closed infected one and promote the development of invasive burn wound infection and systemic sepsis. Following initial application of a biologic dressing to other than a freshly excised wound, subgraft suppuration may be quite extensive within as brief a period as 24 hours. If this occurs, in the absence of signs of systemic sepsis, the membrane should be removed, the wound gently cleansed, and fresh biologic dressings reapplied. As the wound matures with such treatment, subgraft suppuration decreases and graft adherence increases. The frequency with which the biologic dressings must be changed likewise decreases. With the exception of patients in whom prolonged biologic dressing adherence is desirable, as in those patients with massive burns following excision, cutaneous allografts should be changed at least every 5 to 7 days to avoid the hazards of rejection or the need at the time of autografting to excise the foreign tissue, a procedure often associated with considerable blood loss. In the absence of submembrane suppuration and infection, cutaneous xenografts and synthetic skin substitutes need not be arbitrarily changed at a specific time post application.

Culture-Derived Epidermal Sheets

Biologic dressings provide only temporary wound coverage. Consequently, definitive coverage of the extensive burn wounds of a patient with a paucity of available donor sites represents a significant clinical problem. Sheets of cultured autologous keratinocytes have been used to close the wounds in such patients. Since it requires 3 to 4 weeks for a clinically useful amount of epidermal tissue to be produced by culture, the patient must survive that long for the epidermal sheets to be applied. Susceptibility to microbial lysis, low resistance to mechanical trauma, and the late occurrence of wound contraction and scar formation limit the clinical usefulness of the material. Research initiatives are under way to improve the usefulness of cultured epidermal sheets[76] and of dermal analogs.[34]

ELECTRIC INJURY

Electricity exerts its tissue-damaging effects by conversion to thermal energy. Tissue damage not only occurs at cutaneous contact sites but may also involve underlying tissues and organs along the route taken by the current. The heat generated in the conducting tissue is a function of current density (i.e., voltage drop and current flow per unit of cross-sectional area). This relationship accounts for the frequency of severe injury to the extremities and the rarity of significant injury to the trunk in high-voltage electric injury. At the points of electric contact (the sites of greatest current density), the skin is severely injured and charred (Fig. 13–8). When this occurs, resistance increases sharply with limitation of further passage of current and limitation of tissue heating, if the voltage is 1000 volts or less. At higher voltages, reduction of current flow does not occur, and tissue injury continues. When current flow stops, the deeper portions cool more slowly than the superficial portions; hence, the deeper tissues are more liable to severe injury.

As a consequence of these characteristics of electric injury, misleadingly small cutaneous lesions may overlie extensive areas of devitalized muscle that can liberate significant quantities of myoglobin and cause acute renal failure if an adequate urinary output is not maintained. Fluid estimates based on the limited cutaneous injury will lead to underresuscitation and further predispose the patient to acute renal failure. To avoid this complication, fluid management may have to be modified as described previously. Hyperkalemia may develop as a consequence of extensive tissue necrosis and require treatment based on its severity.

Both high-voltage electric injury and lightning injury can induce cardiopulmonary arrest, for which cardiopulmonary resuscitation must be initiated. Patients with high-voltage injuries who have lost consciousness or have an abnormal electrocardiogram should be monitored for at least 48 hours following injury even in the absence of arrhythmias and for 48 hours beyond the last electrocardiographic evidence of dysrhythmias if such are documented.

Patients who have sustained high-voltage electric injury may require operative treatment as soon as hemodynamic stability is achieved. Edema formation beneath the investing fascia may increase muscle compartment pressure to the point where it impairs the blood supply of distal unburned

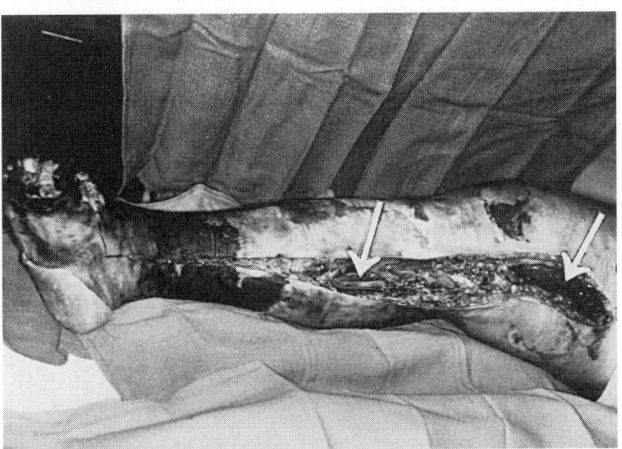

Figure 13–8. High-voltage electrical current (>1000 volts) vaporized the toes, metatarsal heads, and soft tissue at the forefoot contact site on this patient's right leg. Note the edematous dark muscle (right arrow) bulging above the fasciotomy incision in the medial thigh and the pallor of the "cooked" muscle (left arrow) visible in the base of the incision into the medial calf muscles. The severity of distal injury reflects the greater current density in that part of the limb with a lesser cross-sectional area.

tissue, in which case fasciotomy should be performed to prevent ischemic necrosis. Physical examination and several diagnostic modalities have been used to determine the need for fasciotomy and surgical exploration of extremities involved in high-voltage electric injury. Stony hard edema of muscle compartments should prompt fasciotomy and exploration, as should absence of peripheral pulses distal to the site of electric contact. In patients with contact sites on the hand, edema involving structures passing through the carpal tunnel can cause the patient to maintain the wrist and digits in a position of flexion, with marked discomfort noted on extension. Such symptoms and signs mandate performance of a forearm fasciotomy and a carpal tunnel release. The other noninvasive and invasive techniques used to assess the need for escharotomy as described previously can also be used to determine the need for fasciotomy.

Even if fasciotomy is not required, it may be necessary to débride nonviable tissue or even amputate a severely burned limb. Several diagnostic modalities have been used to assess the viability of muscle in a limb with high-voltage electric injury. Scintiphotographic findings after intravenous injection of technetium 99m pyrophosphate have been difficult to interpret. Arteriography may be helpful in determining the need for exploration of a limb in which clinical findings are equivocal. Narrowing of the arteries of an involved limb is used as an indication for exploration, and pruning of the nutrient vessels of muscle may also assist in determining the need for and the required level of amputation.

At the time of exploration of a limb that has been the site of high-voltage electric injury, all muscles, particularly those in the periosseous region, must be thoroughly explored, since even in the presence of viable superficial muscle, the underlying periosseous muscles may be necrotic. If amputation is necessary, the amputation wound is left open and covered with a light dressing. The patient is returned to the operating room in 24 to 48 hours for re-examination of the amputation site and any other débrided wounds. If no residual tissue necrosis is evident, the amputation wound may be closed. If further débridement is required, the wound should again be packed loosely open and dressed or covered with cutaneous allografts. The patient is returned to the operating room every 48 to 72 hours until all nonviable tissue has been removed, at which time the amputation wound is closed.

A variety of neurologic changes may occur in patients with high-voltage electric injury, ranging from immediate peripheral deficits due to the direct effects of the electrical current, from which recovery is rare, to relatively late-appearing deficits that may be a part of a polyneuritic syndrome involving remote nerves. In general, motor nerves appear to be more commonly affected than sensory nerves. Spinal cord function deficits can also be of immediate or delayed onset, with the delayed deficits taking the form of quadriplegia, hemiplegia, localized nerve deficits, ascending paralysis, transverse myelitis, or a syndrome resembling amyotrophic lateral sclerosis. Thrombosis of the nutrient vessels of nerve trunks or the spinal cord may play a role in the late-occurring spinal cord deficits, whereas the early onset deficits appear to be related to direct neuronal injury. Spinal cord deficits of late onset are more likely to be permanent, whereas those of immediate onset are more likely to be transient.

A complete neurologic examination should be performed on admission and at scheduled intervals thereafter to document the presence and time of occurrence of neurologic deficits in all patients following high-voltage electric injury. Physical therapy should be initiated on admission and continued thereafter to prevent contracture, particularly in those patients with paralyzed limbs in whom some return of nerve function is anticipated.

Although visceral injury is rare, liver necrosis, intestinal perforation, focal pancreatic necrosis, and focal gallbladder necrosis have all been reported in patients with high-voltage electric injury. An increased incidence of cholelithiasis has also been reported to occur within 2 years of electric injury. Compression fractures of the vertebrae may result from tetanic contractions at the time of electric contact, and fractures of the skull, spine, and long bones may result from falls occurring subsequent to the electric injury.

Late complications include delayed hemorrhage from even moderate-sized blood vessels. Such hemorrhage has been attributed by some to *arteritis* produced by the electric current, but it appears more commonly to be the result of inadequate wound débridement or exposure of the involved vessel. Cataracts may form early following electric injury or up to 3 or more years thereafter and have been frequent in patients in whom the electric contact has been on the head or neck.

An electric burn peculiar to children typically involves the commissure of the mouth and usually results from the child sucking on the end of a live extension cord or an electric outlet or biting an electric cord. The lesion typically has the pearly white appearance characteristic of a full-thickness burn, and bleeding from the labial artery is of sufficient frequency to justify at least initial in-hospital care. Although some authors favor early débridement and even excision, most prefer conservative treatment with delayed grafting if necessary. Even those injuries that initially appear to be of striking severity usually heal with minimal cosmetic sequelae, which can be repaired electively after spontaneous healing.

Cardiopulmonary arrest is common following lightning injury and must be treated by prompt cardiopulmonary resuscitation. Immediate post-injury coma and neurologic defects are also common but characteristically clear in a few hours or days. The lightning strike may rupture the tympanic membrane with resultant hearing loss. Myoglobinuria may also be a prominent feature in patients who have sustained lightning injury and is treated as previously described. Lightning burns are characteristically superficial and present with a spidery or arborescent pattern. Adequate fluid resuscitation has largely eliminated the cutaneous mottling and other signs of vasoconstriction that were formerly considered specific attributes of lightning injury. Contrary to popular belief, lightning injury is lethal in only about one third of patients.

Electric energy in the form of microwave radiation damages tissue by a heating effect. Microwave burns have been caused by malfunction of industrial equipment and home appliances and by intentional child abuse. Such injuries are treated like other burns.

CHEMICAL INJURIES

The reaction of a strong acid or base with tissue liberates damaging thermal energy. Other agent-specific mechanisms of local tissue damage include liquefaction necrosis caused by strong alkalis, delipidation caused by petroleum products, and vesicle formation caused by the vesicant gases. The severity of tissue damage from chemicals is related to the concentration of the agent, the amount of agent in contact with tissue, and the duration of contact. Thus, contrary to the case in all other burn patients, immediate wound care takes priority in patients with chemical injury, and initial treatment consists of removal of the offending material to preclude further tissue contact. This is best done by removing all clothing contaminated by the chemical agent (including gloves, shoes, and underclothing) and by immediate copious water lavage. The application of neutralizing agents has no advantage over copious water lavage and may even be counterproductive, since time may be lost searching for the agent, and the heat of reaction between the chemical and the neutralizing solution may accentuate tissue damage.

The inhalation of volatile chemical agents such as anhydrous ammonia, the ignition products of white phosphorus, and the vapors of strong acids, mustard gas, and chlorine can cause varying degrees of pulmonary insufficiency as a result of airway edema formation, mucosal desquamation, and bronchospasm. The pulmonary status of such patients must be frequently monitored, and pulmonary insufficiency is treated as described previously. A variety of chemical agents also exert systemic effects that may necessitate pharmacologic intervention and organ system support of variable duration.

Common pitfalls in the treatment of patients with chemical injury, in addition to the failure to remove all contaminated clothing and a delay in water lavage, include inadequate lavage and inaccurate assessment of tissue injury. Skin damaged by contact with strong acids may have a tanned appearance and a silky smooth texture. If such areas are mistaken for a *suntan* rather than the full-thickness tissue loss they represent, fluid needs will be underestimated, with resultant hypovolemia and oliguria. Wound irrigation should be carried out for at least 30 minutes; and, in the case of strong alkali injury in which rapid tissue penetration occurs, irrigation of even longer duration to restore a neutral pH may be necessary. Some authors recommended treating such patients under a continuous shower for 24 to 48 hours, but this is seldom needed. In patients in whom a strong alkali has been in prolonged contact with tissue, early excision may be necessary to limit extension of tissue damage.

There are several chemical agents for which more specific treatment is necessary. Hydrofluoric acid injury is an occupational hazard of petroleum refinery workers and those engaged in etching processes, the cleaning of air conditioning equipment, and certain chemical manufacturing processes. Contact with this agent is typically followed by a pain-free interval with subsequent focal pallor progressing to penetrating necrosis in association with severe tissue pain. Initial treatment consists of prolonged irrigation with benzalkonium chloride solution or application of calcium gluconate gel. If the pain does not relent or recurs, local injection of 10% calcium gluconate into the tissue damaged by hydrofluoric acid may afford prompt pain relief, but care must be taken not to compromise the circulation. Intra-arterial infusion of calcium gluconate has also been reported to limit tissue damage and relieve pain, but local excision with skin grafting may be necessary for definitive pain control and removal of damaged tissue. Hypocalcemia produced by extensive hydrofluoric acid injury is treated by intravenous infusion of calcium.

Burns caused by phenol should be treated by initial water lavage followed by washing of the entire area with a lipophilic solvent, such as polyethylene glycol, to remove residual phenol, which is only slightly soluble in water. If phenol burns are of such extent as to permit absorption of sufficient phenol, central nervous system depression, hypothermia, hypotension, intravascular hemolysis, and even death may occur.[56] In patients injured by contact with dry alkali powders or the condensate of anhydrous ammonia, any residual powder should be quickly brushed off the skin surface before lavage is instituted.

The injury caused by contact with white phosphorus is due to burning since white phosphorus ignites at 32° C. Systemic phosphorus toxicity is rarely a problem unless significant amounts of particulate phosphorus are retained within tissue. Most white phosphorus injuries have resulted from ignition of military munitions, and particles of phosphorus may be embedded in tissue because of the explosive force of the device. Such wounds should be irrigated with saline and then covered with a dressing moistened with water or saline to prevent ignition of retained particles. Use of a dilute 0.5% to 1% solution of copper sulfate as a wash followed by copious rinsing with water or saline results in the formation of a blue-gray cupric phosphide coating on the retained phosphorus particles that facilitates identification and impedes ignition. Avoid the use of more concentrated solutions and never apply a copper sulfate solution as a soak. Alternatively, retained particles of white phosphorus can be identified by virtue of their phosphorescence when exposed to ultraviolet light in a darkened operating room. Following removal, phosphorus particles should always be placed under water, lest they ignite and cause a fire.

Chemically injured eyes must be irrigated with water, saline, or phosphate buffer immediately (even before leaving the site of the accident) to minimize corneal damage. In the hospital, eye irrigation should be continued until the normal pH of the eye surface has been restored. Prolonged irrigation, 12 to 72 hours, is recommended for eyes injured by strong alkalis because of the rapidity with which such agents penetrate ocular tissue. Blepharospasm secondary to the injury makes irrigation difficult unless a modified scleral contact lens with irrigating sidearms is used. Following irrigation, a cycloplegic such as 1% atropine should be instilled on a scheduled basis to counteract iritis, and some authors recommend simultaneous instillation of a miotic agent as well. Corneal damage can be severe in spite of such treatment, presumably as a consequence of collagenase activation. Various authors recommend instillation of cysteine or edetic acid sodium, subconjunctival injection of autologous serum, and even removal of necrotic tissue with mucosal grafts used to cover the resulting defect. Xerophthalmia and symblepharon formation are late complications of severe alkali injury of the eye. The former is treated with variable results by the use of artificial tear solutions and bandage lenses, while the latter is treated by surgical release and repair after the acute process resolves. The results of corneal transplantation to restore vision in eyes severely damaged by alkali have been discouraging.

Tar and Bitumen Burns

Tar and bitumen injuries are actually contact burns. Immediate treatment consists of cooling the hot adherent material with cold water. Petroleum-based solvents should not be used to remove adherent bitumen since they may cause further tissue injury and even systemic toxic effects. After cooling, material adherent to blisters is removed when the blisters are débrided but that adherent to unblistered tissue should be covered with a petrolatum-based ointment and dressed. Daily reapplication of the ointment and dressing leads to emulsification and atraumatic removal of the bitumen, following which the burn is treated as is any other burn.

METABOLIC ALTERATIONS AND NUTRITIONAL SUPPORT

The metabolic response following burn injury increases in magnitude as the extent of burn increases. As formerly measured, that response appeared to be curvilinear; but recent measurements have defined a linear increase in metabolic rate, which rises to levels of twice normal in patients with burns of 75% and more of the total body surface (Fig. 13–9). Post-burn hypermetabolism is manifested by increased oxygen consumption, elevated cardiac output and minute ventilation, increased core temperature, wasting of lean body mass, and increased urinary nitrogen excretion. Thermoregulatory mechanisms are reset upward, and hypermetabolism

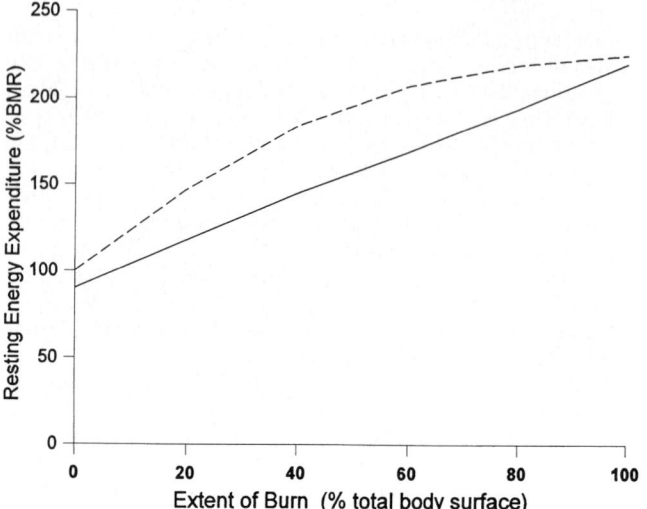

Figure 13–9. The curvilinear relationship between extent of burn and resting energy expenditure (expressed as percentage of expected normal basal metabolic rate) as measured in the 1970s (dashed line) has been transformed into the straight line relationship (solid line) by current techniques of burn care.

is temperature sensitive in patients with burns of more than 50% of the total body surface but is not temperature dependent. The core temperature, skin temperature, core-to-skin heat transfer, and metabolic rate remain elevated at and above thermal neutral temperature, but the metabolic rate in patients with burns of more than one-half of the body surface can be diminished by up to 10% by nursing such patients at ambient temperatures above 30° C.

Blood flow to the viscera likewise increases, although its fraction of the total flow remains unchanged or only slightly increased. Visceral oxygen utilization, although increased, remains an unchanged or only slightly elevated fraction of total-body oxygen consumption. By contrast, blood flow to the wound is markedly exaggerated in relationship to total body blood flow. In studies of patients with leg burns, blood flow to an injured extremity increased as the fraction of the limb surface involved by the burn increased and was significantly greater than the blood flow to the unburned contralateral limb of the patient. Blood flow to the muscle in the burned limb was not elevated above that to the muscle in the unburned limb, indicating that the increment in extremity blood flow was directed to the burn wound per se. These findings, in part, explain the direct influence of the burn wound on the post-injury hypermetabolic and cardiodynamic response.

The post-burn elevation in metabolic rate is associated with and appears to be mediated by increases in catecholamine (principally norepinephrine) release. These hormones influence the disposition and utilization of nutrients, both directly and as a result of their secondary effect on other hormones. Studies have identified a reciprocal relationship between thyroid hormone and catecholamine levels, with an initial depression of thyroid hormone levels followed by a gradual return to normal as catecholamine levels recede. In the early post-burn period, glucagon levels are elevated and insulin levels are absolutely or relatively decreased, resulting in marked lowering of the insulin-glucagon molar ratio that, in the absence of complications, gradually increases and returns to the normal value of 3 to 4 when the burn wound heals or is grafted and convalescence begins. Rather than being a secondary response to the early elevation of catecholamine concentrations, glucagon appears to be one of the primary mediators of the increase in catabolic biochemical pathways,

particularly those in muscle.[84] As a result of these hormonal changes, glucose flow rises, as does the glucose distribution space. Urinary urea nitrogen excretion increases as muscle protein is broken down to provide amino acid gluconeogenic precursors (principally alanine and glutamine), which are transported to the liver and gut, where they are deaminated and converted to glucose to provide the energy substrate needed to satisfy metabolic needs.

Infection, particularly gram-negative, may exaggerate metabolic needs but, when severe, impairs hepatic gluconeogenesis. This effect of sepsis can, in part, be counteracted by administration of exogenous glucose and insulin to maintain the necessary supply of nutrients to peripheral tissues.

Although post-burn hypermetabolism can be significantly reduced by beta-adrenergic blockade and pharmacologic doses of morphine, the hypermetabolic response appears in large part to be driven by the needs of the wound. As noted earlier, blood flow to the wound is significantly and disproportionately increased with respect to blood flow to the viscera and unburned soft tissues.[87] Glucose consumption and lactate production are significantly increased in the area of burn without a significant change in oxygen consumption, as compared with unburned tissue, and this metabolic milieu is characteristic of granulation tissue. Since pharmacologic attenuation of this response to injury might only diminish delivery of the nutrients and energy needed for wound healing, it appears physiologically sound to meet the elevated calorie and protein needs of the burn patient, rather than attempt to suppress the accelerated metabolic processes.

The nutritional needs of the burn patient can be measured by indirect calorimetry, predicted by use of any of several formulas and nomograms, or estimated (for adult patients with burns of over 70% of the total body surface) as being 2000 to 2200 calories and 12 to 18 gm. of nitrogen per m² of body surface per day. Since spontaneous nutritional intake at the usual mealtimes appears to be fixed at preinjury levels, it is commonly necessary to provide extensively burned patients with any of several liquid dietary supplements at scheduled intervals (usually every 2 hours) around-the-clock to meet their nutritional requirements. If the patient cannot or will not take adequate nutrients and has intact gastrointestinal function, the enteral route is preferred for nutritional supplementation. A weighted feeding tube should be positioned in the jejunum, either by spontaneous passage or by endoscopic or fluoroscopic guidance. In patients requiring long-term enteral feeding, the position of the tube should be verified weekly by an abdominal x-ray. If diarrhea or ileus precludes enteral feeding, or if the patient has lost more than 10% of his or her preburn weight and closure of the wounds will require more than an additional 7 to 10 days, parenteral nutrition should be initiated.

Nitrogen loss increases after burn injury, and 80% to 90% of the nitrogen appears in the urine as urea, which may exceed 40 gm. per day in patients with extensive burns who are being fed. Although the extent of nitrogen loss is proportional to the post-injury increase in energy expenditure, lipid stores, not the nitrogen-containing lean body mass, are the major source of metabolic fuel oxidized for energy. Over a wide range of metabolic response, body protein in burn patients contributes only 15% to 20% of the energy required to meet metabolic needs. Moreover, visceral proteins are quite labile and rapidly exhausted. Consequently, skeletal muscle is the primary source of nitrogen lost in the urine, and muscle proteolysis is reflected by increased excretion of creatinine and 3-methylhistidine. The intake of nitrogen spares protein and improves nitrogen balance in the burn patient.

Total protein intake appears to be more important than the form in which it is administered. Other investigators have demonstrated that protein intake improves the immunologic response and increases survival of burned children.[3] Branched chain amino acids have been reported to exert no beneficial effect on morbidity or mortality in severely stressed patients, at least in part because patients cannot effect their complete oxidation in muscle.[5, 9] Glutamine may have uniquely beneficial effects on total body nitrogen economy and organ function, particularly in the intestinal tract. After severe injury, the gut mucosa utilizes glutamine, thereby sparing glucose and allowing it to be utilized for tissues with an obligatory glucose requirement. Glutamine levels decrease in both tissue and plasma pools; and, in the absence of glutamine administration, the gut mucosa becomes atrophic. Addition of glutamine to the nutritional support regimen increases mucosal cellularity and decreases extremity glutamine efflux. The addition of glutamine to total parenteral nutrition after surgical stress spares glutamine in muscle, counteracts the fall in muscle protein synthesis, and improves nitrogen balance, suggesting that glutamine supplementation may be beneficial in the nutritional support of burned patients.[33]

The addition of nonprotein calories to the source of nitrogen further improves nitrogen balance and enables more calories to be utilized for the restoration of nitrogen equilibrium, as manifested by enhanced amino acid incorporation into protein and improved nitrogen balance. The optimal calorie to nitrogen ratio varies between 150:1 and 100:1. In the absence of exogenously administered calories, lipid stores are the major source of energy for meeting metabolic requirements, as reflected by the respiratory quotient, which is typically between 0.7 and 0.8.

In general, carbohydrate and fat can be used interchangeably as nonprotein calorie sources for patients with relatively small burns. However, as the hypermetabolic response becomes more pronounced in patients with more extensive burns, carbohydrate is more effective in maintaining body protein than fat when each food source is used alone.[29] If fat alone is administered parenterally as a long-chain triglyceride emulsion, the reduced nitrogen excretion is due to the glycerol in the emulsion. Studies have shown that emulsions of medium-chain triglycerides, in contrast to long-chain triglycerides, are much more effective in maintaining lean body mass. The medium-chain triglycerides demonstrate more rapid elimination kinetics and increased ketone production and are associated with less fat deposition in the tissues.[15] Unfortunately, available medium-chain triglyceride preparations commonly evoke a profuse diarrhea.

In practice, enteral intake is instituted on postburn day 3 and increased to meet predicted calorie requirements by postburn day 5. Any of the commercially available enteral formulas with an appropriate nitrogen-calorie ratio can be used. In patients who require parenteral nutrition, standard hypertonic glucose–amino acid solutions are used. Lipid emulsions are used only to prevent the development of essential fatty acid deficiencies. Five hundred to 1000 ml. of fat emulsion is administered twice a week. At this dose the fat overload syndrome rarely occurs. Blood sugar levels should be monitored frequently and kept below 200 mg. per 100 ml. Sudden intolerance of a previously well-tolerated glucose load is an early sign of sepsis and should prompt careful search for a source of infection. The high risk of cannula-related infection makes change of the intravenous cannula necessary every 72 hours. Total metabolic support of the burn patient also entails measures that minimize pain, maintain muscle activity to prevent disuse atrophy, permit timely diagnosis and prompt treatment of infection, and maintain a warm microenvironment to minimize cold stress. The efficacy of nutritional support regimens can be enhanced by use of specific pharmacologic agents, including human growth

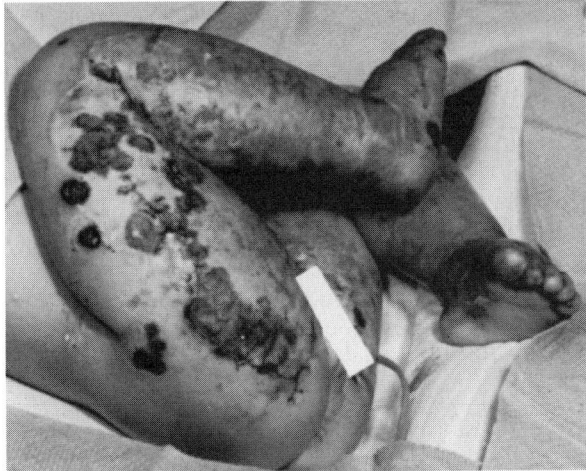

Figure 13–10. Focal hemorrhagic changes in burn wound characteristic of *Pseudomonas* burn wound sepsis. These lesions appeared on the tenth postburn day in this child aged 1 year and 4 months with burns over 25% of the total body surface. Note the edema and hemorrhagic change in the wound margin of the right buttock and extension of hemorrhage into unburned skin at the periphery of this lesion on the midlateral thigh.

hormone, insulin-like growth factor-1, beta-adrenergic agonists, and insulin administered with sufficient glucose to maintain euglycemia.

INFECTIONS AND SEPTIC COMPLICATIONS OF BURN PATIENTS

Diagnosis and Treatment of Burn Wound Infections

The available topical agents maintain the bacterial density in the burn wounds of most patients below the level of 10^5 organisms per gm. of tissue but do not sterilize the wound. Consequently, the bacteria in the burn wounds of any patients may escape from control and invade the underlying tissue. This complication occurs most commonly in patients with burns of more than 30% of the body surface, part or all of which have not been excised, or those in whom skin graft failure has occurred following initial excision. To identify invasive burn wound infection at the earliest possible time, it is mandatory that the entire burn wound be examined each day at which time any change in wound appearance is noted. Conversion of an area of partial-thickness burn to full-thickness necrosis and the appearance of focal areas of black or dark hemorrhagic discoloration are the most common changes indicative of burn wound infection (Fig. 13–10). If those or any of the other clinical signs of burn wound infection listed in Table 13–6 are identified, it is necessary to assess the microbial status of the burn wound to confirm the

---

TABLE 13–6. Clinical Signs of Burn Wound Infection

Conversion of second-degree burn to full-thickness necrosis
Focal dark brown or black discoloration of wound
Degeneration of wound with "neoeschar" formation
Unexpectedly rapid eschar separation
Hemorrhagic discoloration of subeschar fat
Erythematous or violaceous edematous wound margin
Crusted serrations of wound margin*
Metastatic septic lesions in unburned tissue†

---

*Characteristic of herpetic infections.
†Ecthyma gangrenosum characteristic of *Pseudomonas* burn wound sepsis.

diagnosis of invasive burn wound infection, since similar changes in wound appearance can be caused by hemorrhage due to local trauma or maceration.

Surface cultures of the burn wound may provide useful epidemiologic information but are not helpful in making the diagnosis of invasive infection. Even quantitative cultures of wound tissue are of limited usefulness. Quantitative counts of less than 10^5 organisms per gm. of biopsy tissue correlate well with the absence of invasive burn wound infection, but quantitative counts above that level correlate poorly with the presence of invasive infection.[49]

The histologic examination of a burn wound biopsy specimen is the most rapid and only reliable means of making the critical differentiation between microbial colonization of nonviable tissue, which is present in all burn wounds, and the presence of microorganisms in unburned viable tissue that is characteristic of invasive burn wound infection. By scalpel dissection, a 500-mg. lenticular tissue sample, including both eschar and underlying unburned tissue, is obtained from that area of the burn showing the most pronounced changes. The biopsy is carried out as a ward procedure, and hemostasis is seldom a problem. Blood loss is readily controlled by the brief application of direct pressure or by electrocoagulation. If local anesthesia is necessary, the anesthetic agent should be injected at the periphery of the intended biopsy site to minimize distortion of the morphologic characteristics of the tissue in the biopsy sample.

One half of the biopsy sample is submitted to the microbiology laboratory for culture identification of the organisms present and their antibiotic sensitivities. The other half of the specimen is submitted to the pathology laboratory, where histologic sections are prepared by rapid section technique requiring 3 to 4 hours or a frozen section technique requiring 30 minutes. A specimen originally processed by the frozen section technique should be subsequently processed by regular section technique to correct the 4% false-negative diagnosis rate of frozen sections. The pathologist examines the histologic preparations for the presence of microorganisms in unburned viable tissue, which confirms the diagnosis of invasive burn wound infection. The other histologic findings listed in Table 13–7 are not diagnostic of invasive burn wound infection but should raise the pathologist's index of suspicion and prompt him to search the specimen carefully for microorganisms in the unburned tissue.

The microbial status of a burn wound can be staged according to microscopic findings as noted in Table 13–8. If only colonization is evident in the first biopsy specimen obtained from a burn patient, no change in wound care is required. If examination of serially obtained biopsy specimens reveals evidence of microbial proliferation and penetration (i.e., progression from Stage IA to Stage IC), wound care should be altered. A histologic diagnosis of Stage II mandates prompt intervention as described below. Microscopically evident involvement of the microvasculature and lymphatics (Stage IIC) is associated with a high likelihood of hematogenous spread to remote tissues and mandates close monitoring of the lungs and the heart (Fig. 13–11).

TABLE 13–7. Histologic Criteria of Burn Wound Infection

Microorganisms in unburned tissue
Hemorrhage in unburned tissue
Heightened inflammatory reaction in adjacent viable tissue
Small vessel thrombosis or ischemic necrosis of unburned tissue
Perineural and intralymphatic migration of organisms*
Vasculitis with perivascular "cuffing" of organisms*
Intracellular viral inclusions

*Characteristic of invasive *Pseudomonas* infections.

TABLE 13–8. Histologic Staging of Microbial Status of Burn Wounds

Stage	Histologic Findings
I. Colonization	
A. Superficial	Microorganisms confined to surface of burn wound
B. Penetrating	Microorganisms extending into variable thickness of eschar
C. Proliferating	Variable density of microorganisms in subeschar space
II. Invasion	
A. Microinvasion	Microorganisms present in viable tissue
B. Deep invasion	Penetration of microorganisms deep into viable subcutaneous tissue
C. Microvascular invasion	Involvement of small blood vessels and/or lymphatics

Burn wound biopsy specimens can be misleading but are less commonly so than wound cultures. The limitations of burn wound biopsies are principally technical ones (i.e., sampling of a noninfected area, failing to include unburned tissue by sampling only the eschar, and erroneous histologic interpretation). Consequently, wound biopsy results should be interpreted in terms of the patient's hospital course. Negative biopsy results in the presence of clinical deterioration should prompt re-examination of the burns and biopsy sampling of other areas showing changes indicative of infection.

Histologic confirmation of invasive infection requires an immediate therapeutic response, with the treatment determined by both the extent and the depth of the septic process. If the infection is bacterial and one of the nondiffusible topical agents is being used, it should be stopped and topical therapy continued with mafenide acetate burn cream. Systemic antimicrobial therapy should be instituted based on the sensitivity patterns of the microbial flora resident in the burn center at that time, as determined by the microbial surveillance program. When culture and sensitivity results are available, systemic antimicrobial therapy should be adjusted accordingly.

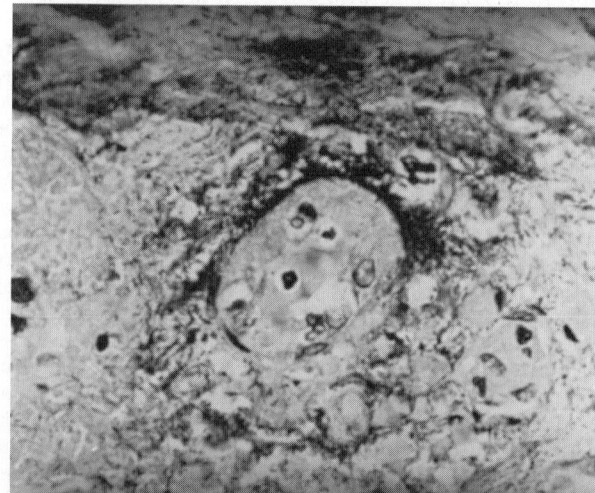

Figure 13–11. Photomicrograph of biopsy specimen obtained from a patient with invasive *Pseudomonas* burn wound sepsis. Note the perivascular cuffing of bacteria characteristic of *Pseudomonas* vasculitis. Even though the involved vessel is thrombosed in this area, such a finding makes hematogenous dissemination likely and mandates systemic antibiotic therapy.

The incidence of invasive burn wound infection has decreased markedly in recent years. Wound infections caused by *P. aeruginosa,* formerly very common, have become very rare, and those that do develop occur later in the postburn course and have a lesser comorbid effect than previously. Those invasive infections that are caused by *P. aeruginosa* most frequently occur in the pediatric age group in which wound maceration on dependent surfaces may be a contributory factor. Since such organisms are typically sensitive to high concentrations of broad-spectrum penicillins, one half of the daily dose of a broad-spectrum penicillin such as piperacillin suspended in 1000 ml. of normal saline should be immediately infused into the subeschar tissues beneath all infected areas of the wound using a No. 20 spinal needle to minimize the number of injection sites. The patient should be scheduled for excision of the infected tissue within the next 12 hours and a second subeschar antibiotic infusion carried out immediately before the excision to protect the patient from hematogenous dissemination of viable bacteria that may occur during the excision. Wide local excision, superficial to the fascia, is carried out if the process is confined to the subcutaneous tissue, as is commonly the case with bacterial infections. Excision of involved fascia and muscle is required for the treatment of deeper invasion.

As the incidence of bacterial wound infections has decreased over the past 30 years, the incidence of nonbacterial wound infections has increased. *Candida* species, the most common nonbacterial burn wound colonizers, seldom invade and typically remain confined to the burned tissue, and consequently require no specific treatment. Candidal infection may occur in the interstices of a mesh graft or an excised burn wound exposed by skin graft loss and requires treatment by twice-daily application of a topical antifungal agent such as clotrimazole cream or ciclopirox olamine cream. If such treatment is ineffective in preventing extension of this usually superficial infection, excision should be carried out and amphotericin-B administered systemically.

Filamentous fungi are much more aggressive burn wound invaders and may cause infections of grave consequence. *Aspergillus* species, the fungi that most often cause invasive burn wound infections, occur relatively late in the hospital course of patients with extensive burns who have undergone two or three excision procedures for which they received perioperative broad-spectrum antibiotics and still have ungrafted wounds. These fungi seldom traverse fascial planes and commonly remain confined to the subcutaneous tissues. The phycomycetes are the most aggressive true fungi, and these organisms spread rapidly along tissue planes, readily traverse fascia, and have a predilection to invade vessels. Infections caused by the phycomycetes are characterized by rapidly expanding soft tissue ischemic necrosis with a peripheral rim of subcutaneous edema and frequent hematogenous dissemination to remote tissues. The diagnosis of invasive fungal infection is best made by the histologic examination of a burn wound biopsy. Treatment of such infections consists of twice-daily topical application of an antifungal agent, systemic administration of amphotericin B, and prompt wide excision of the infected tissue. When a phycomycotic infection on a limb has traversed the investing fascia and involves significant amounts of underlying muscle, amputation is necessary to control the infectious process.

Viral burn wound infections are relatively uncommon and are caused most often by herpes simplex virus I. Herpetic infections occur most frequently in healing or recently healed partial-thickness burns, particularly those in the nasolabial area. Herpetic burn wound infection is most reliably diagnosed by the histologic examination of a biopsy or scrapings from the cutaneous lesions. Topical application of a 5% acyclovir ointment every 3 hours for 7 days has been reported to shorten the healing time, the duration of viral shedding, and the duration of pain of mucocutaneous herpetic lesions. Systemic herpesvirus infections involving multiple organs such as the liver, lungs, spleen, adrenals, and bone marrow may also occur and are typically fatal. Systemic signs of sepsis and unexplained hypotension in a burn patient with rapidly spreading cutaneous herpetic lesions should direct attention to the possibility of systemic herpes infection, which, if confirmed, is treated by systemic antiviral therapy using acyclovir. Cytomegalovirus infections may also occur in burn patients in whom diagnosis and treatment is the same as in other critically ill patients.

Other Septic Complications

Even though invasive burn wound infection has become uncommon, infection may occur in other organs and tissues as a reflection of the immunologic effects of both the injury and treatment. Infections in sites other than the burn wound have actually increased as principal causes of death because of the decrease in fatal invasive burn wound sepsis. As *Pseudomonas* species have decreased in importance, *S. aureus* has emerged as the most common organism recovered from infections in burn patients today, as exemplified by blood culture results in 1994 (Fig. 13–12).

Pneumonia. The most common site of infection in the burn patient is the lungs. In recent years pneumonia has been present in over 50% and considered to be the primary cause of death in one half of fatal burns treated at the United States Army Institute of Surgical Research. The reduction of invasive burn wound infection has been attended by a change in the predominant type of pneumonia from hematogenous to airborne pneumonia (bronchopneumonia). Bronchopneumonia in the burn patient, as in any other critically ill patient, is commonly caused by *S. aureus* and gram-negative opportunistic bacteria and occurs relatively early in the post-burn period (average onset tenth post-burn day). Atelectasis often precedes this complication, and the pneumonic process may first be evident on the chest x-ray as an ill-defined infiltrate of irregular outline. When such an infiltrate appears and the patient has clinical signs of pneumonia, the endobronchial secretions must be cultured and antibiotic treatment begun on the basis of the sensitivity of the treatment facility's resident flora as determined by the microbiologic surveillance program. Antimicrobial treatment is adjusted as necessary when the results of the patient's culture and sensitivity testing are obtained.

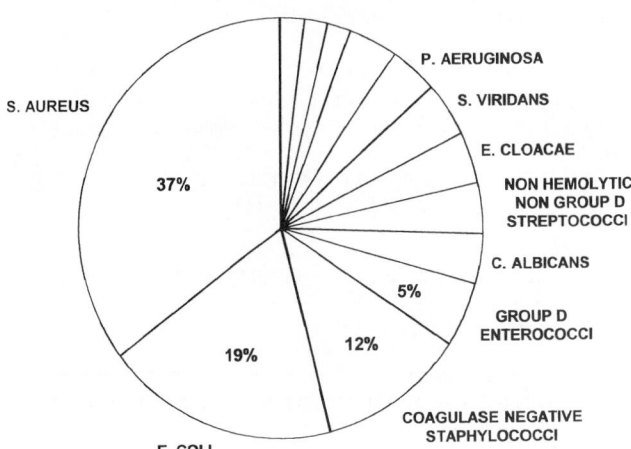

Figure 13–12. Frequency of blood culture isolates in 1994. Note that gram-positive organisms that do not exert the comorbid effects of gram-negative organisms were recovered from over 60% of positive blood cultures.

Hematogenous pneumonia commonly begins relatively late in the post-burn course (average time of diagnosis, seventeenth post-burn day) and is caused by microorganisms arising from a remote septic focus. The sudden appearance of a solitary rounded infiltrate on the chest x-ray may be the first manifestation of this pulmonary infection (Fig. 13–13). An infected wound or a vein harboring a focus of intraluminal suppuration is the source of infection in the vast majority (86%) of cases. The gastrointestinal tract and the prostate are rare sources of the microorganisms causing this infection. Examination of all possible sites must be carried out if such a characteristic pulmonary infiltrate appears. An identified source of infection must be removed or controlled and the pneumonic process treated by systemic administration of antibiotics active against the causative organism. Hematogenous pneumonia is more often associated with a fatal outcome than is airborne pneumonia, but as a reflection of its secondary nature it is less often the principal cause of death.

Suppurative Thrombophlebitis. Suppurative thrombophlebitis can occur in any previously cannulated peripheral or even central vein. The likelihood of occurrence increases with the duration of cannulation. Strict limitation of cannula residence to 3 days or less in burn patients has been associated with a reduction in the incidence of this complication from 4.3% to 2.5%. Because of the presence of an overlying burn and the immunosuppressive effect of the burn injury itself, local signs of this disease are present in less than half the patients so afflicted. The appearance of a pulmonary infiltrate characteristic of hematogenous pneumonia or the occurrence of septicemia in the absence of any other obvious source of infection should prompt ultrasonic flowmeter evaluation of all previously cannulated veins.

If occlusion is confirmed in a peripheral vein, that vessel should be promptly explored. The most frequent site of intraluminal suppuration is the area of the vein where the cannula tip resided, and that region must be examined before suppurative thrombophlebitis can be ruled out. Identification of purulent material within a vein mandates surgical removal of the entire length of vein involved in the suppurative process and the systemic administration of antibiotics to which the causative organism is sensitive. Failure of sepsis to clear following vein excision can be due to inadequate extent of the excision, suppuration within another vein, or hematogenous dissemination of the causative organism to other organs such as the heart or lungs before or during excision of the infected vein.

Acute Endocarditis. The incidence of acute endocarditis is relatively high in burn patients (1.3% of 1699 patients treated during a 6-year period) because of the frequent need for long-term intravenous infusions, the high incidence of suppurative thrombophlebitis, and the frequency of bacteremia associated with wound manipulation. Identification of characteristic murmurs is difficult in burn patients because of their hyperdynamic circulation. Two-dimensional echocardiographic examination may detect valvular lesions, but small vegetations may remain undetected. Although this infectious complication most frequently involves the right side of the heart, it may occur on either or both sides. *S. aureus* is the most common causative agent, and the presence of that organism in two or more blood cultures from a burn patient with sepsis and no other apparent infection should alert one to this diagnosis. When this complication is diagnosed, systemic maximum-dose antibiotic therapy should be started and continued for at least 3 weeks and longer as needed to clear the blood cultures.

Suppurative Sinusitis. Suppurative sinusitis is most likely to occur in patients who require long-term transnasal intubation, particularly those with tubes in both the airway and the gastrointestinal tract. Since this complication may be inapparent clinically, radiologic studies are required to confirm the diagnosis. Therapy is initiated with broad-spectrum antibiotics, but surgical drainage of the involved sinuses may be necessary if the infection is unresponsive to antibiotic therapy. A tracheostomy and/or gastrostomy should be considered if continued intubation of the airway and/or the gastrointestinal tract is required.

Bacteremia and Septicemia. To minimize the development of antibiotic resistance in the bacteria present on the burn wound and elsewhere, systemic antibiotics should not be given prophylactically but should be administered only on the basis of a secure clinical or laboratory diagnosis of infection. Wound care procedures may cause hematogenous dissemination of microorganisms. Studies in the 1970s indicated that one fifth of blood cultures obtained during burn wound manipulations were positive, with the recovery rate related to both the extent of the burn and the magnitude of the procedure. To minimize the seeding of remote tissues and organs due to such bacteremias, antibiotics against both gram-positive and gram-negative organisms have been administered perioperatively to patients undergoing surgical débridement or excision of the burn wound. Preliminary results from current studies indicate that the incidence of bacteremia associated with wound manipulation has decreased markedly, and the policy of perioperative systemic antibiotic prophylaxis is being reassessed.

In burn patients with septicemia, initial antibiotic therapy should be based on the results of the institution's microbial surveillance program and, if available, on the histologic findings of burn wound biopsy specimens or Gram-stained preparations of secretions and other infected material. Blood cultures should be obtained on a scheduled basis and the antibiotic regimen changed if necessary according to patient-specific culture and sensitivity test results. Blood cultures from critically ill, extensively burned patients may show growth of multiple organisms or growth of different organisms in serial cultures. Those culture results, reflecting the immunologic incompetence of such patients, should not be regarded as contaminants. Even though the survival of such patients is extremely low, they should be treated with antibiotics active against all of the organisms recovered.

Gastrointestinal Complications

Gastrointestinal complications of the burn patient are the same as those of other severely injured patients and include ulcerations of the gastrointestinal tract, acalculous cholecysti-

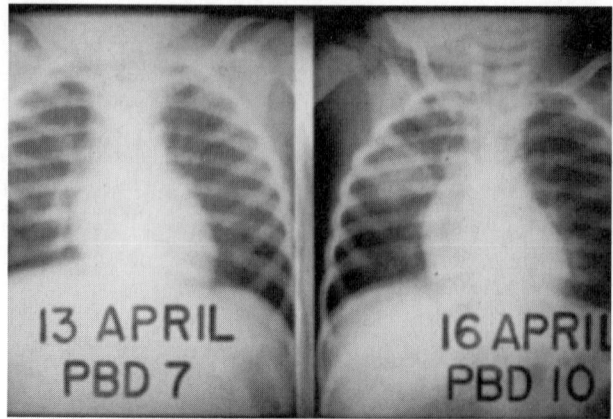

Figure 13–13. Chest roentgenograms documenting the sudden appearance, on the tenth post-burn day, of a nodular infiltrate characteristic of hematogenous pneumonia in the right lung. The patient died 2 days later, and the source of disseminated bacteria was found to be suppuration in a previously cannulated vein.

tis, and pancreatitis (usually associated with pre-existing alcoholism, sepsis, disseminated intravascular coagulation, or a posterior penetrating ulcer). Acute ulceration of the stomach and duodenum (Curling's ulcer), formerly the most frequent life-threatening gastrointestinal complication of burn patients, is now effectively controlled by prophylactic antacid or H_2 histamine receptor antagonist therapy. As a result of such prophylaxis, hemorrhage or perforation requiring surgical intervention is now vanishingly rare (six cases in a recent 18-year period). In the early post-burn period, when ileus is present, the quantity of antacid necessary to maintain gastric aspirate pH above 5 is instilled hourly through the nasogastric tube in all patients with burns of more than 30% of the body surface. Following return of gastrointestinal motility, similar doses of antacid are given orally until the burn has healed or been autografted. Alternatively, 400 mg. of cimetidine can be given parenterally every 4 hours during the period of ileus, with oral dosage of 300 mg. every 6 hours continued after the ileus abates. Occasionally, both forms of prophylaxis are necessary to maintain gastric aspirate pH above 5 in patients with extensive burns or patients with septic complications.

Although the neutralization of gastric acidity resulting from such prophylaxis has been implicated as a causative factor of the high incidence of bronchopneumonia in critically ill patients, a recent study at the United States Army Institute of Surgical Research has demonstrated that nonantacid prophylaxis with sucralfate provided adequate stress ulcer control but was associated with no lesser overall incidence of pneumonitis. The frequency and time of gram-negative colonization of the airway were comparable in the patients receiving sucralfate and those receiving antacid prophylaxis, and the incidence of pneumonia was higher in those receiving sucralfate who were intubated for mechanical ventilation.[11]

Acute dilatation of the colon may occur in burn patients who develop sepsis. Additionally, focal necrosis with acute ulceration of the colon has been identified in burn patients with severe complications, particularly those with sepsis-related episodes of hypotension. Certain of these lesions have penetrated the full thickness of the colonic wall to the level of the serosa, but only one free perforation of the cecum has been encountered. Healing of the more superficial of the ulcers of the large bowel can apparently occur when the underlying condition has been corrected, since distortion of the colonic mural architecture indicating healing of lesions of varying age has been noted in some burn patients who have died. Endoscopic examination should be performed if the colonic dilatation reaches significant proportions. The rectal stimulation of endoscopic examination and the placement of a rectal tube may provide nonoperative relief of the colonic dilatation in the burn patients who develop this form of Ogilvie's syndrome. If the dilatation of the colon does not relent with conservative therapy or if significant mucosal necrosis is endoscopically evident, operative intervention is indicated. Because of the increased risk of postoperative wound infection and dehiscence, retention sutures should be used in closing any abdominal incision in a burn patient.

In the recent past, necrosis involving a variable length of the small bowel has been noted in a few burn patients receiving hyperosmolar enteral feedings. Typically the small bowel necrosis begins at that point in the small bowel where the feeding tube tip resided and presents clinically as ileus with other signs and symptoms of an acute abdomen. Resection of the necrotic bowel and re-establishment of intestinal continuity is mandatory. At operation the necrotic small intestine has been found to be the same color as the tube feedings. Laparoscopic examination may be of use in identifying such intestinal discoloration and confirming the diagnosis of intes-

tinal necrosis preoperatively. Laparoscopic surgical techniques have also been utilized for the surgical treatment of acalculous cholecystitis in burn patients.

In patients with equivocal signs of an acute intra-abdominal process and in whom the findings of noninvasive diagnostic modalities are indefinite, peritoneal lavage has been used to identify the need for surgical intervention. Positive open lavage results (>500 white blood cells per cu. mm., >100,000 red blood cells, or a positive Gram stain) identified those patients requiring operation for the treatment of intestinal perforation and acalculous cholecystitis with 94% accuracy.[55]

Burn Scar Carcinoma

Burn scar carcinoma, or Marjolin's ulcer, is a rare neoplasm that occurs in the unstable scar of a full-thickness burn. This unstable scar, which is susceptible to trauma, continuously breaks down and reheals. The latent period for malignant change ranges from 1 to 75 years, with a mean of approximately 35 years. Although basal cell carcinomas have occurred in old burn scars, they are exceedingly rare, and most Marjolin's ulcers are squamous cell carcinomas. These tumors are highly invasive, and regional node metastases were present in 35% of 46 cases reported by Novick and associates.[61] Metastases are more frequent in patients with primary lesions located on the extremities than in patients with primary lesions on the trunk. All ulcerative lesions in burn scars should be examined by biopsy. If no tumor is found, the ulcerated area, with a 2-cm. margin, should be excised and the defect closed with a skin graft. If carcinoma is found, extirpation of the tumor must include all involved tissue, as verified by histologic examination of the wound margins.

Sun and Heat Overexposure

Overexposure to sunlight is a common cause of mild cutaneous burns but can also cause more severe injury. Erythema and pain from sunburn reaches a maximum at 10 to 24 hours after exposure and resolves within 72 to 96 hours.[73] Treatment is largely symptomatic, utilizing cooling showers, cold soaks, or topical analgesics to reduce pain; oral acetylsalicylic acid to reduce prostaglandin-mediated inflammation; and antihistamines or hydroxyzine to reduce histamine-mediated pruritus occurring on the second to fourth post-burn days. The patient should also be warned of possible postural hypotension. A severe sunburn with pain, erythema, and bullae should be treated like any other partial-thickness injury, as outlined previously.

Heat stroke usually occurs in the elderly during heat waves or in younger, otherwise healthy, individuals performing strenuous exercise in a hot environment. It represents a total loss of the body's thermoregulatory control, occurring because the demands for maintenance of blood pressure dominate the requirements for maintenance of body temperature. By definition, the core body temperature exceeds 40.6° C. (105° F.), with associated anhidrosis and central nervous system dysfunction.

Pathophysiologic changes commonly encountered include disorientation and bizarre behavior, hypovolemia, hemoconcentration, and hypotension. Variable disturbances of acid-base and electrolyte balance may occur, depending on the duration of heat exposure and the patient's compensatory response. Compensatory hyperventilation may cause respiratory alkalosis; but if hypovolemia is so severe as to impair tissue blood flow and cause shock, lactic acidosis results. Hypernatremia may be present with severe dehydration; but in unacclimated patients, hyponatremia may occur due to salt loss in sweat and can be exaggerated by intake of electrolyte-free water. Hypokalemia may result from the combined effect of respiratory alkalosis and hypovolemia-induced activation of renin, angiotensin, and aldosterone. Conversely, hyperkalemia may occur in those patients in whom acidosis develops or in whom heat stroke causes skeletal muscle necrosis. Mortality rates as high as 18% have been reported. The presence of coma, coagulopathy, hypotension, or renal failure, the need for intubation, and a high degree and long duration of hyperthermia are associated with a poor prognosis.

Vital to treatment is rapid cooling of the patient to a body temperature of 38.9° C. (102° F.) utilizing ice packs, cool water sprays, and intravenous administration of cold saline. Immersion in ice water can decrease body cooling because of cutaneous vasoconstriction and is therefore not recommended. During cooling, cardiac activity should be monitored continuously and any dysrhythmias treated as necessary. If hypotension does not resolve with cooling and intravenous saline, vasopressors may be necessary, but pure alpha-agonists should be avoided because of their peripheral vasoconstrictive effects. Metabolic acidosis should be corrected, as should any coagulopathy; but hypokalemia should be corrected only if acidosis is present. Hyperkalemia is treated as in other patients. Hyponatremia responds to administration of salt-containing fluids. Hypernatremia also responds to the infusion of cool lactated Ringer's solution. Intubation may be required to maintain adequate oxygenation. Administration of dantrolene, effective in the treatment of malignant hyperthermia, is controversial, with no proven efficacy in patients with heat stroke. On an empiric basis, seizure prophylaxis with phenytoin is recommended.

COLD INJURY

Exposure to cold environments can produce a spectrum of physiologic derangements, varying from direct tissue damage to severe total body hypothermia. The injury produced by exposure to cold depends on the degree of low temperature, the duration and time course of exposure, and environmental conditions that can influence the effects of low temperature. Although resembling heat injury in many ways, cold injury induces unique pathophysiologic alterations and requires a therapeutic approach distinct from that of heat injury. Always a concern in military populations, such injuries are now seen with increasing frequency as the popularity of winter sports rises, the elderly population grows, and the number of homeless individuals expands.

Frostbite

With frostbite, the skin and subcutaneous tissue of exposed body parts, especially the hands, feet, nose, and ears, are most often affected. The severity of the injury is enhanced by wet clothing, air movement (chill factor), peripheral vascular disease, and decreased level of consciousness. When less insulated parts of the body are exposed to below-freezing temperatures for prolonged periods of time, freezing begins distally at a relatively slow pace. Rarer and more devastating injuries follow contact with liquid petroleum products and metal surfaces at subfreezing temperature: subsequent tissue freezing is rapid, is often extensive, and can involve any part of the body.

Pathogenesis. Tissue necrosis following frostbite is related primarily to the mechanical effects of ice crystallization, loss of cellular water, and microvascular thrombosis (Table 13–9). With loss of heat, water freezes and forms crystals, which can appear within both the cells and the extracellular space in any tissue. Rapid lowering of tissue temperature causes supercooling, with tissue temperature reaching −10°

TABLE 13–9. Pathogenesis of Frostbite

Freezing

Intracellular ice crystallization
Cellular dehydration
Microvascular occlusion

Thawing

Extracellular loss of high-protein fluid
Vasospasm only in narrow border of frozen tissue
Surrounding vasodilation

---

to −15° C. before freezing occurs, and the formation of intracellular ice crystals, which irreversibly disrupt cellular architecture and cause cell death. Because of circulatory reflexes in response to cold, freezing usually is much slower, and ice crystals form primarily in the extracellular space with comparatively less structural damage to the cell. As freezing progresses, intracellular water shifts to the extracellular space and leads to intracellular dehydration, with an increase in the intracellular concentrations of electrolytes, proteins, sugars, and enzymes. The resulting hyperosmolarity leads to intracellular protein denaturation. Whereas skin is relatively resistant to these damaging effects, other tissues, including nerves and blood vessels, are quite sensitive.

At subzero environmental temperatures, the temperature in exposed tissue begins to decrease. Sensation in cooling skin is reduced and is finally abolished when tissue temperatures reach 10° C. During this phase, cutaneous vasculature exhibits vasoconstriction. If tissue temperatures stabilize at this level, the microcirculation displays alternating periods of vasoconstriction and vasodilation (hunting reaction, see later). However, with a further loss of heat, microvascular flow ceases and tissue temperature falls to below freezing.

The vascular system is particularly susceptible to freeze injury and appears to be the primary target organ of frostbite.[69] Although cooling increases viscosity and causes sludging of blood before tissue freezing, only after thawing do the detrimental vascular changes induced by freezing become evident. Endothelium is particularly vulnerable to cold injury, and microvascular permeability increases, with loss of plasma and hemoconcentration. Within minutes of thawing and restoration of blood flow, platelet aggregates form and begin to occlude venules.[93] Subsequently, red blood cells begin to aggregate and contribute to venous occlusion, which within 1 to 2 hours begins retrograde extension into capillary and arteriolar vascular beds of the damaged tissue. The net effect is decreased capillary flow in the thawed tissue. During this interval, arteriovenous shunts open, and while total blood flow to an injured body part characteristically rises above normal levels, flow in the damaged tissue remains compromised. If injury to the tissue is severe, arteriovenous shunt flow begins to fall after 24 to 48 hours and eventually ceases. This cessation of flow is followed by occlusion of major arteries and finally gangrene.

After thawing, high-protein, plasma-like fluid leaks from the injured capillary bed into the interstitial space in a manner similar to burn injury. Tissue pressure increases to some degree, promoting venous stasis and occlusion. Swelling is maximal in 2 to 6 hours and thereafter slowly subsides. Although the vessels in the thawed tissue retain the ability to constrict in response to adrenergic stimulation, the majority of vessels are dilated. Except in the narrow border zone surrounding the previously frozen tissue, persistent vasospasm of the nutritional vasculature is absent[93] and explains in part the ineffectiveness of therapeutic modalities designed to alleviate vasoconstriction. Blood viscosity changes following thawing are short-lived and relatively unimportant, and the use of antiviscosity agents would be expected to provide little benefit to microcirculatory blood flow.

Because of circulatory alterations that sacrifice core heat to keep peripheral structures warm, tissue freezing usually is a slow process. Maximal vasoconstriction occurs with tissue temperatures of approximately 15° C. As cooling falls below 10° C, vessels in peripheral tissues alternately constrict and dilate, often in a cyclic fashion. This cold vasodilation response, or *hunting reaction,* prevents or retards tissue freezing at the expense of body heat loss. If the individual is warm and well insulated, cold vasodilation is pronounced and exposed body parts are partially protected from the effects of low ambient temperatures. If the individual is cold and inadequately clothed, or if he or she is rapidly cooled, cold vasodilatation does not occur and tissues can freeze rapidly. Constricting clothing, peripheral vascular disease, and open wounds prevent these circulatory adaptations and increase the likelihood of tissue freezing.

Rapid freezing promotes supercooling and intracellular ice crystallization, both of which augment tissue destruction and blunt protective circulatory adjustments. Prolonged freezing increases both the depth and the extent of damage; by accentuating intracellular dehydration, very low temperatures are more injurious than higher sub-zero temperatures. Wet skin cools faster than dry skin and freezes at a higher ambient temperature. Air movement accelerates heat loss, and wind velocity determines what is called the wind chill factor. Thus, the chilling effect of a temperature of $-6°$ C. (20° F.) when the wind velocity is 45 miles per hour is equivalent to that of a temperature of $-40°$ C. ($-40°$ F.) when winds are calm. However, wind speed does not determine the final tissue temperature, which cannot fall below the ambient temperature. For freezing to occur, the ambient temperature must fall below $-2°$ to $-3°$ C. Nevertheless, increasing wind chill promotes nonfreezing cold injury and is a major contributing factor to body heat loss.

Epidemiology of Frostbite. In an excellent epidemiologic study, Urschel evaluated a large series of patients with severe frostbite.[83] Most patients were males who were poorly clothed during the winter months. Less than 20% displayed a normal mental status, and acute alcoholism and psychiatric illness were major predisposing factors leading to prolonged cold exposure. The arms and legs were involved with equal frequency. A past history of frostbite predisposed the patients to reinjury of the previously frostbitten body parts; and such areas more frequently required surgical therapy. The local environment and social conditions influence the presentation of severe frostbite. Occupational or recreational exposure often leads to injury in frigid climates, while the increasingly large homeless population of urban centers is subject to an escalating incidence of frostbite in more temperate environments.

Clinical Presentation. The depth of frostbite is classified into four levels of severity based on appearance after thawing. First-degree frostbite causes hyperemia, edema, and often very superficial freezing of the epidermis (frostnip). Necrosis is minimal, and vesicles do not form. Second-degree frostbite causes hyperemia, edema, and usually vesicle formation, resulting in a partial-thickness injury (Fig. 13–14). As in partial-thickness burns, cutaneous sensation remains intact. Third-degree frostbite causes necrosis of the entire skin thickness and extends to a variable depth into the underlying subcutaneous tissue. Vesicles formed with this severity of injury tend to be much smaller than those with second-degree injury. Fourth-degree frostbite results in full-thickness necrosis of the skin and extends into underlying muscle and bone. Such injuries commonly terminate with gangrene of the body part and require amputation.

Frozen tissue is usually cold to the touch and appears pale, gray, and bloodless. If frostbite is superficial, soft and pliable tissue can be palpated beneath the stiff frozen skin. The deeply frozen body part is stony hard. Although prediction of tissue loss is usually not possible for weeks following frostbite injury, the appearance of the tissue after thawing denotes the severity of tissue damage (Table 13–10). In mild injuries, capillary flow in the previously frozen tissue rapidly returns toward normal and total flow to the body part increases to supranormal levels as arteriovenous shunts open. The involved part, usually a hand or foot, becomes bright red and warm, and capillary pulsations may be visibly associated with throbbing pain. Paresthesias appear, and sensation and motor function return. Whereas swelling and edema rapidly develop a few hours following thawing, the underlying tissue does not become as tense as in a circumferential full-thickness burn. Large vesicles appear within a few hours, are filled with straw-colored fluid, and extend to the tips of

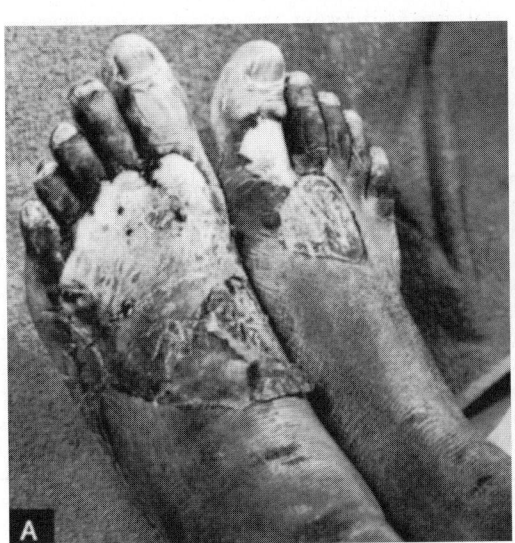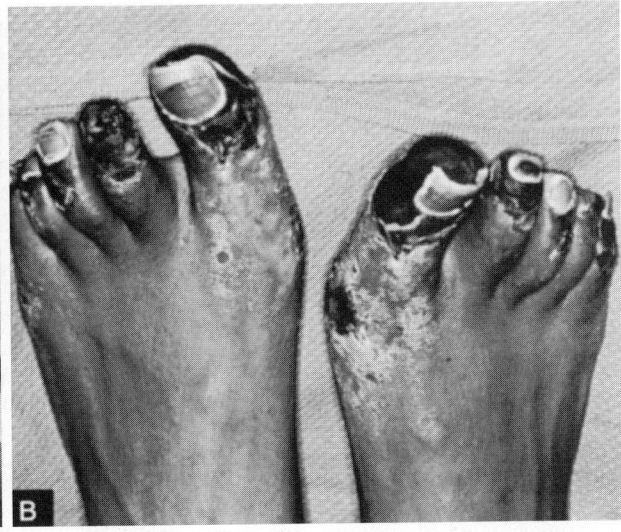

Figure 13–14. Frostbite of the feet. *A,* Thirteen days after injury. Bullae have desiccated and formed a crustlike eschar on each foot. *B,* At 70 days after injury. Clear demarcation of necrotic tissue is established. The distal phalanges of the toes were eventually amputated. Note that the final extent of tissue loss is considerably less than would have been estimated during the first weeks after injury. Unnecessary débridement was avoided and tissue loss was minimized by meticulous wound care that prevented maceration and infection.

TABLE 13–10. Signs and Symptoms of Frostbite

Mild Injury

Bright red and warm
Painful
Paresthesias
Rapid onset of edema
Large vesicles (early)
Superficial eschar (later)

Deep Injury

Deep purple and cool
Minimal pain
Small hemorrhagic vesicles
Slow onset of edema
Deep structures demarcate and mummify

affected extremities. Most of these changes resolve in 1 to 2 weeks with little or no tissue loss.

These blisters may form a black eschar, which eventually sloughs; the underlying regenerated skin is initially fragile and hypersensitive but later develops the characteristics of normal skin. After thawing of severely frostbitten tissue, blood flow remains depressed; while total flow to the injured part may transiently approach normal values, nutritional capillary flow is never restored. Because the majority of blood flow occurs through deep arteriovenous shunts, the injured area is cool to the touch and deep red to purple in appearance. Although sensation and distal muscle function are absent, the patient may still be able to move distal parts, since the tendons and proximal muscles remain intact. Blisters are small, dark, and hemorrhagic and may take weeks to form, if they occur at all. Except for very deep injury with primary arterial occlusion, edema formation is slow but extensive and may persist for months. Eventually, the nonviable skin and deep structures demarcate and mummify.

Most cases of frostbite fall between the two extremes described, and an involved extremity may display all degrees of freezing injury. Determination of tissue viability is all but impossible during the first several weeks following injury and often can be made only after the gangrenous tissue has demarcated and sloughed. Superimposed infection can amplify tissue loss. Since clinical signs and symptoms provide inaccurate guidelines for the estimation of potential tissue loss following frostbite, a number of laboratory procedures have been used to define nonviable tissue. Radionuclide scanning with ^{99m}Tc methylene diphosphonate accurately identifies nonviable bone, whereas Doppler ultrasonography and pulse volume plethysmography appear to be able to distinguish mild from severe frostbite soon after thawing. Angiographic techniques have been used primarily to evaluate chronic vascular abnormalities of freeze-injured tissue. These modalities may prove useful in evaluating the effectiveness of therapeutic interventions to increase tissue salvage following rewarming.

A rare form of cold injury may be encountered when liquid propane, butane, and other extremely low temperature liquids spill onto the skin. These cold injuries occur predominantly as an occupational accident in petroleum industry workers. Immediately after exposure, the cutaneous injury has the appearance of a relatively benign second-degree burn, displaying a pink color with no obvious evidence of deep-tissue necrosis. However, as this form of cold injury matures over the next 48 to 72 hours, the wound takes on the appearance of an eschar typical of a deep full-thickness burn. The clinical course also resembles that of a deep thermal injury, with early large fluid resuscitation requirements.

Wound care consists of topical antimicrobial agents and excision and grafting.

Treatment. Treatment of frostbite should begin as soon as feasible to decrease the duration of tissue freezing. All wet and constricting clothing, including socks, boots, and gloves, should be removed. Since frostbitten patients are often hypothermic to some degree, they should be wrapped in warm blankets and given hot fluids. Alcohol promotes further heat loss by causing vasodilatation and should not be used.

Rapid rewarming of the frozen part is the single most effective therapeutic maneuver for preserving potentially viable tissue. However, a frozen body part should not be thawed if refreezing of the injured extremity is possible. If it can be carried out expeditiously, transport to a medical facility is preferable before instituting rewarming procedures. The frozen part is placed in water at 40° C., which is circulated to prevent the formation of temperature gradients. Once the tissue is completely thawed, as reflected by the return of pink color and obvious perfusion, it should be removed from the heated water. Rewarming usually requires 20 to 30 minutes, and prolonged heating and the use of water temperatures above 42° C. decrease tissue salvage. Warmed water provides a well-regulated constant level of heat by virtue of its high heat capacity and thermal conductivity.

Rapid rewarming causes a rapid increase in the tissue temperature, prevents the long persistence of tissue temperature at a level just below freezing that occurs with euthermic conversion of ice to water, and promotes vasodilatation and a rapid return of tissue perfusion. Slow rewarming is not as effective in maintaining tissue viability and results in more extensive microvascular damage than that occurring with rapid rewarming. The use of dry heat, such as from a fire, is dangerous and not nearly as effective for rapidly thawing frozen tissue. The injured part lacks sufficient sensation to judge temperature, and a serious burn injury can result. The frozen part should not be rewarmed in ice water, rubbed with ice, or massaged. Such procedures invariably extend tissue damage. Refreezing thawed tissue further augments tissue loss, and if permanent thawing and subsequent treatment is not feasible, the frozen limb is best left alone until proper facilities and treatment are available. Before definitive treatment, less injury ensues from walking on a frozen foot than on one that has been thawed; local destruction of tissue and refreezing invariably occurs. The pain during and after rewarming is relieved by narcotics.

Local care is directed toward preserving damaged tissue and preventing infection. Unless infected or leaking, vesicles should be left intact and allowed to dry into a black eschar. The patient is placed at bed rest and the wounds are exposed to the air. Mechanical trauma from overlying bed sheets is prevented by a foot cradle, and lamb's wool is inserted between affected digits. Weight bearing on injured lower extremities is proscribed until complete healing has occurred. The wound is gently cleansed daily with an antibacterial solution in a whirlpool bath. The use of pressure dressings to decrease wound edema may cause extensive tissue destruction and is contraindicated. Smoking is not permitted.

Since assessment of tissue viability is difficult and often inaccurate, surgical intervention must be delayed until clear demarcation of dead tissue has occurred. Early débridement increases tissue damage and removes the protective covering of mummified tissue. Although *watchful waiting* for demarcation may take months, tissue loss is often much less than initial estimates (see Fig. 13–14). However, supervening infection with wet gangrene requires immediate surgical removal of the source of sepsis. The role of escharotomy and fasciotomy in the acute treatment of a previously frozen extremity is controversial, and these procedures probably should not be utilized in most situations. Since freezing directly damages blood vessels, the loss of circulation following thawing is more likely to be caused by primary vascular occlusion than by constriction of edematous tissues. Available studies document no benefit and suggest that such decompression procedures may increase tissue loss.

Tetanus prophylaxis is based on the patient's prior immunization status and the condition of the wound. Antibiotics are indicated when infection is evident or when an open wound was present before freezing. In the rare situation in which a large volume of tissue has been frozen, massive fluid loss into the injured tissues after thawing may require intravenous fluid resuscitation.

A number of controversial treatments have been employed in an attempt to promote survival of marginally viable tissue following thawing. Sympathectomy by nerve trunk section and more recently by intra-arterial injection of vasodilators has enjoyed considerable popularity based on the assumptions that resistant vasospasm in recently frozen tissue promotes ischemic tissue loss and that therapeutic sympathetic blockade induces vasodilatation and increased nutritional blood flow. However, histologic studies indicate that the vasculature in the freeze-injured wound is dilated, not constricted, and that inadequate perfusion is a consequence of endothelial injury and intravascular cellular platelet aggregation.[93] Vessels in the narrow border zone surrounding the injured tissue may initially be constricted but soon dilate as total blood flow increases. Sympathectomy may accentuate the damage of the freeze injury by diverting nutritional blood flow from the wound into arteriovenous channels. No rigorous studies to date have documented that the use of sympathetic blockade is better than rapid rewarming alone in promoting survival of recently thawed tissue. Although experimental studies have described beneficial tissue preservation effects from the use of heparin and low-molecular-weight dextran, especially if administered before the onset of freezing, no clinical studies have demonstrated clear evidence of increased tissue salvage. While rarely practical, low-molecular-weight dextran may be beneficial if administered before thawing. The efficacy of dimethyl sulfoxide, anti-inflammatory agents, and hyperbaric oxygen is unproved. Perhaps the most promising pharmacologic agents for treating frostbite are the antiprostanoid and antithromboxane agents. These drugs block the arachidonic acid cascade and appear in human studies to inhibit vasospasm and platelet aggregation responsible for the progressive ischemia in frostbite. In animal studies, intravenous administration of streptokinase, by reversing early thrombosis of damaged vessels, significantly reduced tissue loss following rewarming.

In contrast to acute frostbite, the use of sympathetic blockade is quite effective for the treatment of chronic postfrostbite sequelae. The most frequent complaints are hyperhidrosis, paresthesias, cool extremities, cold sensitivity, and edema, which are exacerbated by exposure to cold. These vasospastic sequelae must be differentiated from neuropathic sequelae, especially the intense constant burning pain of postfrostbite neuritis, which is unresponsive to and may be aggravated by sympathetic blockade. Angiography is useful for demonstrating vasospasm, which, if present, can be treated by the intra-arterial injection of reserpine, 0.25 mg. to 0.5 mg., into the brachial, femoral, or radial artery. A beneficial response is reflected by hyperemia and increased warmth in the distal extremity. Injection into the arterial inflow of an injured extremity allows the use of a small dose and minimizes systemic effects. Reserpine produces vasodilatation by causing vascular depletion of norepinephrine and provides prolonged relief from vasospastic symptoms. If these chronic symptoms recur after several injections of reserpine, surgical division of the regional sympathetic trunks provides long-term relief. Other postfrostbite sequelae, such as depigmenta-

tion and bone changes, are permanent. A rare long-term complication of deep frostbite injuries is squamous cell carcinoma in the frostbite scar. Clinical presentation, treatment, and prognosis are similar to that of Marjolin's ulcer in chronic burn scars. Wide local excision should be carried out after biopsy and histologic confirmation of squamous cell carcinoma.

Nonfreezing Cold Injury

Nonfreezing tissue injury on exposure to low environmental temperatures is more common than frostbite in both civilian and military settings. Tissue loss is usually not extensive and is due to microvascular injury with endothelial damage, capillary stasis, and eventual vascular occlusion. Trench foot and immersion foot occur after prolonged exposure to a wet and cold environment with ambient temperatures above freezing, and both conditions affect lower extremities that have been continuously immobile and dependent. Trench foot develops after 1 to several days' exposure to dampness at or near freezing. Immersion foot develops more slowly, after a few days to several weeks of immersion in cool or cold water at temperatures usually higher than those causing trench foot. The entire foot may turn black from superficial gangrene, but deep tissue destruction is unusual. Following rewarming, the injured limb is initially anesthetic and anhidrotic, and massive edema rapidly develops. Blood flow increases to above normal levels, and this hyperemia may persist for weeks. Paresthesias are common, and in deeper injuries ulceration, vesiculation, and occasionally gangrene may develop. Long-term sequelae are similar to those after frostbite and include paresthesias, cold sensitivity, muscle weakness, and pain on weight bearing. If persistent vasospasm is demonstrated, sympathetic blockade usually provides effective relief.

Pernio, or chilblain, is a less severe injury and develops after prolonged exposure to dry cold above freezing. It is more commonly seen in women and participants in certain winter sports, such as mountain climbers. Small superficial ulcers develop on chronically exposed body surfaces, especially the legs, and may be accompanied by hemorrhages, bullae, and areas of localized cyanosis.

Treatment of all three variations of nonfreezing cold injury is supportive and consists of rapid rewarming and meticulous local care described previously for frostbite. Shoes and wet clothing should be removed from the injured extremity. The local injuries should be protected from further trauma by soft dressings, and injured extremities should be elevated. Some patients develop acrocyanosis and persistently painful nodules in exposed areas, and these symptoms may respond to the calcium channel blocker nifedipine.[22]

Other nonfreezing cold injuries occasionally may be encountered. Extensor tenosynovitis may follow prolonged exposure of the hands to cold. Erythema, edema, and crepitation are present under the undamaged skin of the dorsum of the hand, and movement of the fingers produces pain along the extensor tendons. Treatment consists of warming and splinting the hand. If the pain and swelling do not resolve within 48 hours, aspirin and, if required, intrasynovial injection of corticosteroid produce prompt relief of symptoms.

Hypothermia

Because of a variety of social phenomena, total-body hypothermia resulting from prolonged exposure to low environmental temperatures is being encountered with increasing frequency. When the onset of hypothermia is rapid, as by immersion in near-freezing water, the signs and symptoms are obvious and should elicit prompt treatment. When the fall in body temperature occurs more slowly in environmental conditions that are temperate or only moderately cool, the more obvious clinical manifestations of hypothermia are often absent and the diagnosis is often overlooked. Unsuspected hypothermia particularly affects the elderly, whose ability to increase heat production and to decrease heat loss by vasoconstriction in response to cold is impaired.

The diagnostic hallmark of generalized hypothermia is a core temperature (clinically approximated by rectal temperature) below 34° C. Since standard clinical thermometers do not register below that level, special thermometers are required. An altered level of consciousness is the most constant symptom of hypothermia and ranges from confusion, poor judgment, and mood changes to severe agitation and coma. More than 90% of patients with rectal temperatures at or below 32° C. demonstrate these mental aberrations. Hypothermic patients often do not shiver, especially if heat loss has occurred slowly. In addition to low body temperature, the patient appears gray and cyanotic and is cool to the touch. Blood pressure, pulse rate, and respiratory rate are frequently decreased; a Doppler ultrasonic flowmeter is most useful in assessing the adequacy of circulation. However, vital signs correlate poorly with body temperature and ultimate recovery, and the absence of respiratory or cardiac activity early after exposure does not preclude recovery.

Prompt initiation of rewarming is the most important therapeutic intervention, and the patient's temperature and vital signs should be monitored during this process. All wet clothing is removed, and the patient, if alert, is given warm fluids to drink. Alcohol is never used. The choice of rewarming technique depends on the patient's response to his or her low body temperature and to the initial attempts at rewarming. Patients with mild hypothermia (32° C. to 35° C.) can be passively rewarmed by wrapping in warm clothes and blankets, drinking hot fluids, and allowing shivering to generate body heat. For moderately severe hypothermia (28° C. to 32° C.), passive rewarming is effective if shivering is present. Since the level of consciousness is usually depressed in such patients, warm fluids are administered intravenously. Active rewarming is necessary if passive rewarming fails to elevate body temperature faster than 1° C. to 2° C. per hour, if the initial body temperature is below 28° C., or if cardiac activity has ceased before or during rewarming treatment.

Active rewarming is most easily accomplished by placing the patient in a circulating water bath warmed to 40° C. This method of surface warming allows rapid gain of body heat, decreases shivering with its obligatory metabolic demands, and improves venous return and cardiac output by hydrostatic pressure, which may be beneficial to the hypovolemic patient. A heating blanket, although less efficient in heat transfer, may be used if a water bath is not available. The theoretical objection to surface rewarming is that external heat relieves peripheral vasoconstriction, thus accentuating hypovolemia and allowing cold blood and tissue metabolites to flow to the heart, which may cause subsequent ventricular fibrillation. However, this vasodilatory response may be mitigated by heat-induced cutaneous vasoconstriction and reflex opening of proximal arteriovenous anastomoses.[57]

Core heating with cardiopulmonary bypass, peritoneal dialysis, or mediastinal lavage has been advocated for active rewarming on the grounds that it directly warms the heart and avoids rewarming collapse; it may be indicated in the patient with cardiac arrest not responding to cardioversion. Cardiopulmonary bypass, if available, seems to be the most logical method, since it both supports the circulation and allows heating.[47] However, no available data indicate the superiority of core rewarming over surface rewarming, and

the complications of such procedures may outweigh any potential advantages.

The patient's vital functions must be appropriately supported during treatment. The hypothermic patient who is asystolic and apneic when brought to the hospital or who suffers cardiac arrest during therapy should be treated with intubation, closed chest massage, and rewarming. These efforts should be continued if necessary until the core temperature is over 30° C. Hypovolemia and electrolyte imbalance, usually hypokalemia, may be particularly severe if hypothermia was slow in onset and usually become evident during rewarming. Warmed balanced electrolyte solutions, with supplemental potassium as indicated by laboratory monitoring, provide adequate replacement of the depleted plasma volume. Most electrocardiographic abnormalities are supraventricular in origin, require no treatment, and revert to normal as body temperature increases. Occasionally, rhabdomyolysis and pancreatitis develop after rewarming and accentuate fluid requirements.

After the body temperature has been raised above 35° C., clinical assessment of the patient should be completed. Precipitating causes of hypothermia, such as sepsis, uncontrolled diabetes mellitus, pronounced malnutrition, neurologic disease, myxedema, drug overdose, and associated injuries, including frostbite, must be identified and treated. Signs of drug withdrawal may develop during hospitalization. The outcome of severe hypothermia is related to associated medical conditions and not to the method of rewarming. As such, the mortality is over 80% in the elderly and only 10% in otherwise healthy young individuals, who typically have no sequelae.

TREATMENT OF EXFOLIATIVE SKIN DISEASES

In recent years it has become evident that patients with toxic epidermal necrolysis and a variety of other exfoliative skin diseases in which the wounds resemble those caused by burns are best treated in burn centers. On receipt of a patient with cutaneous exfoliation, a wound biopsy specimen should be obtained to identify the plane of exfoliation and other histologic features that permit specific diagnosis. If a diagnosis of toxic epidermal necrolysis is made, the offending agent, most often a sulfonamide or phenytoin, should be stopped, as should any corticosteroid therapy begun before admission. The wounds should be gently cleansed, after which a biologic dressing should be applied. Systemic support measures should be used as necessary, oral and vaginal mucosal lesions should be treated symptomatically, and synechia formation should be prevented by elevation of the eyelids from the globe surface each day. Burn center care has significantly reduced the morbidity and mortality associated with toxic epidermal necrolysis. The treatment of other exfoliative dermatitides may require some modification of those general treatment themes.

SELECTED REFERENCES

Cioffi, W. G., Burleson, D. G., and Pruitt, B. A., Jr.: Leukocyte responses to injury. Arch. Surg., *128*:1260, 1993.
  The responses of the leukocytes to injury and infection are described in terms of both local and systemic effects. The effectiveness and limitations of therapeutic interventions are reviewed.

Herndon, D. N.: Total Burn Care. London, W. B. Saunders, 1996.
  This text, by authors selected on the basis of experience and skill, provides broad coverage of all aspects of burn care, including the prehospital, intensive care unit, convalescent, rehabilitation, and reconstructive phases.

Kelemen, J. J., III, Cioffi, W. G., McManus, W. F., et al.: Burn center care for patients with toxic epidermal necrolysis. J. Am. Coll. Surg., *180*:273, 1995.
  The applicability of burn wound care to the treatment of other skin diseases is

illustrated, and the reduction in morbidity and mortality of patients with exfoliative skin diseases treated at burn centers is documented.

Pruitt, B. A., Jr.: Burn wound. *In* Cameron, J. L. (Ed.): Current Surgical Therapy, 5th ed. St. Louis, Mosby–Year Book, 1995, p. 872.
The principles and techniques of burn wound care, including topical chemotherapy, burn wound excision, diagnosis and treatment of burn wound infections, and the use of biologic dressings are described.

Pruitt, B. A., Jr., and Cioffi, W. G.: Diagnosis and treatment of smoke inhalation. J. Intensive Care Med., 10:117, 1995.
This review relates the pathophysiologic characteristics of inhalation injury to the diagnosis, treatment, and outcome of the disease. Pharmacologic interventions and current techniques of ventilatory management are discussed.

Pruitt, B. A., Jr., McManus, A. T., and Kim, S. H.: Burns. *In* Gorbach, S. L., Bartlett, J. G., and Blacklow, N. R. (Eds.): Infectious Diseases. Philadelphia, W. B. Saunders, 1992.
The changing epidemiology and incidence of infections in burn patients are presented with extensive discussion of the pathogenesis, diagnosis, and treatment of infections in the burn wound and elsewhere.

Pruitt, B. A., and Mason, A. D.: Lightning and electric shock. *In* Weatherall, D. J., Ledingham, J. G. G., and Warrell, D. A. (Eds.): Oxford Textbook of Medicine, 2nd ed. Oxford, Oxford University Press, 1987, p. 6.126.
The clinical effects of electrical injury are related to the physical characteristics of electrical current and its interaction with tissue. The diagnosis and treatment of local injury as well as anatomically and temporally remote injuries are described.

Pruitt, B. A., Jr., McManus, W. F., and McDougal, W. S.: Surgical management of burns. *In* Nora, P. F. (Ed.): Operative Surgery: Principles and Techniques. Philadelphia, W. B. Saunders, 1990, p. 1283.
The surgical principles and techniques used in burn care are presented from the time of admission until wound closure.

Pruitt, S. K.: Burns. *In* D'Amico, T. A., and Pruitt, S. K. (Eds.): The Handbook of Surgical Intensive Care: Practices of the Surgical Residents at Duke University Medical Center, 4th ed. St. Louis, Mosby–Year Book, 1995, p. 418.
This concise outline provides the house officer with complete information on the resuscitation and early care of patients with burn injury and its complications.

Rue, L. W., III, and Pruitt, B. A., Jr.: Fluid and nutritional management of the burn patient. *In* Cameron, J. L. (Ed.): Current Surgical Therapy, 4th ed. St. Louis, Mosby–Year Book, 1992, p. 906.
This review of fluid management during and after resuscitation includes discussion of the principles and techniques of nutritional management of the burn patient.

REFERENCES

1. Alexander, J.: Alteration of opsonic activity after burn injury: Proceedings of the 40th Anniversary Symposium, U. S. Army Institute of Surgical Research, Fort Sam Houston, TX, 1989, p. 126.
2. Alexander, J., Gioanotti, L., Pyles, T., et al.: Distribution and survival of *Escherichia coli* translocating from the intestine after thermal injury. Ann. Surg., 232:558, 1991.
3. Alexander, J., MacMillan, B. G., Stinnett, J. D., et al.: Beneficial effects of aggressive protein feeding in severely burned children. Ann. Surg., 192:505, 1980.
4. Allen, R. C., and Pruitt, B. A., Jr.: Humoral-phagocyte axis of immune defense in burn patients: Chemiluminigenic probing. Arch. Surg., 117:133, 1982.
5. Aussel, C., Cynober, L., Lioret, N., et al.: Plasma branched-chain keto acids in burn patients. Am. J. Clin. Nutr., 44:825, 1986.
6. Burleson, D. G., Mason, A. D., Jr., and Pruitt, B. A., Jr.: Changes in lymphocyte surface antigen that precede infection in burned patients. F.A.S.E.B. J., 9(3):A520, 1995.
7. Burleson, D. G., Vaughan, G. M., Mason, A. D., Jr., et al.: Flow cytometric measurement of rat lymphocyte subpopulations after burn injury and burn injury with infection. Arch. Surg., 122:216, 1987.
8. Calvano, S. E., DeRiesthal, H. F., Marano, M. A., et al.: The decrease in peripheral blood CD4 + and T cells following thermal injury in humans can be accounted for by a concomitant decrease in suppressor-inducer CD4 + and T cells as assessed using anti-CD45R. Clin. Immunol. Immunopathol., 47:164, 1988.
9. Cerra, F. B., Mazuski, J. E., Chute, E., et al.: Branched chain metabolic support: A prospective, randomized, double-blind trial in surgical stress. Ann. Surg., 199:286, 1984.
10. Cioffi, W. G., deLemos, R. A., Coalson, J. J., et al.: Decreased pulmonary damage in primates with inhalation injury treated with high-frequency ventilation. Ann. Surg., 218:328, 1993.
11. Cioffi, W. G., McManus, A. T., Rue, L. W., III, et al.: Comparison of acid neutralizing and non-acid neutralizing acid stress ulcer prophylaxis in thermally injured patients. J. Trauma, 36:541, 1994.
12. Cioffi, W. G., Rue, L. W., III, Graves, T. A., et al.: Prophylactic use of high-frequency percussive ventilation in patients with inhalation injury. Ann. Surg., 213:575, 1991.
13. Clark, W. R., Bonaventura, M., and Myers, W.: Smoke inhalation and airway management at a regional burn unit: 1974–1983: I. Diagnosis and consequences of smoke inhalation. J. Burn Care Rehabil., 10:52, 1989.

14. Constantian, M. B.: Association of sepsis with an immunosuppressive polypeptide in the serum of burn patients. Ann. Surg., 188:209, 1978.
15. Cotter, R., Taylor, C. A., Johnson, R., et al.: A metabolic comparison of a pure long-chain triglyceride lipid emulsion (LCT) and various medium-chain triglyceride (MCT)—LCT combination emulsions in dogs. Am. J. Clin. Nutr., 45:927, 1987.
16. Damle, N. K., and Doyle, L. V.: IL-2-activated human killer lymphocytes but not their secreted products mediate increase in albumin flux across cultured endothelial monolayers. J. Immunol., 142:2660, 1989.
17. Deitch, E. A., Landry, K. N., and McDonald, J. C.: Postburn impaired cell-mediated immunity may not be due to lazy lymphocytes but to overwork. Ann. Surg., 201:793, 1985.
18. Demling, R. H., Kramer, G., and Harms, B.: Role of thermal injury–induced hypoproteinemia on fluid flux and protein permeability in burned and nonburned tissue. Surgery, 95:136, 1984.
19. Demling, R. H., and Lalonde, C.: Effect of partial burn excision and closure on postburn oxygen consumption. Surgery, 104:846, 1988.
20. Demling, R. H., Wong, C., Jin, L. J., et al.: Early lung dysfunction after major burns: Role of edema and vasoactive mediators. J. Trauma., 25:959, 1985.
21. Dong Y-L., Ko, F., Huang H-Q., et al.: Evidence for Kupffer cell activation by burn injury and *Pseudomonas* exotoxin A. Burns, 19:12, 1993.
22. Dowd, P. M., Rustin, M. H., and Lanigan, S.: Nifedipine in the treatment of chilblains. BMJ, 293:923, 1986.
23. Drost, A. C., Burleson, D. G., Cioffi, W. G., Jr., et al.: Plasma cytokines after thermal injury and their relationship to infection. Ann. Surg., 218:74, 1993.
24. Faist, E., Schinkel, C., Zimmer, S., et al.: Inadequate interleukin-2 synthesis and interleukin-2 messenger expression following thermal and mechanical trauma in humans is caused by defective transmembrane signaling. J. Trauma., 34:386, 1993.
25. Ferrara, J. J., Dyess, D. L., Luterman, A., et al.: The suppressive effect of subeschar tissue fluid upon in vitro cell-mediated immunologic function. J. Burn Care Rehabil., 9:584, 1988.
26. Fire/burn deaths and rates per 100,000 E890-899, E923-E925. National Center for Health Statistics Morality Data Tapes for Number of Deaths. Atlanta, Centers for Disease Control and Prevention, Division of Unintentional Injury Prevention, National Center for Injury Prevention and Control, 1991.
27. Gadd, M. A., Hansbrough, J. F., Hoyt, D. B., et al.: Defective T-cell surface antigen expression after mitogen stimulation: An index of lymphocyte dysfunction after controlled murine injury. Ann. Surg., 209:112, 1989.
28. Gennari, R., Alexander, J. W., Gianotti, L., et al.: Granulocyte macrophage colony-stimulating factor improves survival in two models of gut-derived sepsis by improving gut barrier function and modulating bacterial clearance. Ann. Surg., 220:68, 1994.
29. Gottschlich, M. M., and Alexander, J.: Fat kinetics and recommended dietary intake in burns. J. Parenter. Enterol. Nutr., 11:80, 1987.
30. Gough, D. B., Moss, N. M., Jordan, A., et al.: Recombinant interleukin-2 (rIL-2) improves immune response and host resistance to septic challenge in thermally injured mice. Surgery, 104:292, 1988.
31. Grbic, J. T., Mannick, J. A., Gough, D. B., and Rodrick, M. L.: The role of prostaglandin E_2 in immune suppression following injury. Ann. Surg., 214:253, 1991.
32. Hales, C. A., Barkin, P., June, W., et al.: Bronchial artery ligation modifies pulmonary edema after exposure to smoke with acrolein. J. Appl. Physiol., 67:1001, 1989.
33. Hammarqvist, F., Wernerman, J., Ali, R., et al.: Addition of glutamine to total parenteral nutrition after elective abdominal surgery spares free glutamine in muscle, counteracts the fall in muscle protein synthesis and improves nitrogen balance. Ann. Surg., 209:455, 1989.
34. Hansbrough, J. F., Boyce, S. T., Cooper, M. L., et al.: Burn wound closure with cultured autologous keratinocytes and fibroblasts attached to a collagen-glycosaminoglycan substrate. JAMA, 262:2125, 1989.
35. Harms, B. A., Bodai, B. I., Kramer, G. C., et al.: Microvascular fluid and protein flux in pulmonary and systemic circulations after thermal injury. Microvasc. Res., 23:77, 1982.
36. He, W., Fong, Y., Marano, M. A., et al.: Tolerance to endotoxin prevents mortality in infected thermal injury: Association with attenuated cytokine responses. J. Infect. Dis., 165:859, 1992.
37. Heimbach, D., Luterman, A., Burke, J., et al.: Artificial dermis for major burns: A multi-center randomized clinical trial. Ann. Surg., 208:313, 1988.
38. Herndon, D. N., Barrow, R. E., Linares, H. A., et al.: Inhalation injury in burned patients: Effects and treatment. Burns, 14:349, 1988.
39. Horgan, A. F., Mendez, M. V., O'Riordan, D. D., et al.: Altered gene transcription after burn results in depressed T-lymphocyte activation. Ann. Surg., 220:342, 1994.
40. Huang, P. P., Stucky, F. S., Dimick, A. R., et al.: Hypertonic sodiun resuscitation is associated with renal failure and death. Ann. Surg., 221:543, 1995.
41. Liu, X. S., Yang, Z. C., Luo, Z. H., and Li, A.: Clinical significance of the change of blood monocytic interleukin-1 production in vitro in severely burned patients. Burns, 20:302,1994.
42. Lund, T., and Reed, R. K.: Microvascular fluid exchange following thermal skin injury in the rat: Changes in extravascular colloid osmotic pressure, albumin mass, and water content. Circ. Shock., 20:91, 1986.
43. Lund, T., Wiig, H., and Reed, R. K.: Acute postburn edema: Role of strongly negative interstitial fluid pressure. Am. J. Physiol., 255:Hl069, 1988.

44. Maldonado, M. D., Venturoli, A., Franco, A., and Nunez-Roldan, A.: Specific changes in peripheral blood lymphocyte phenotype from burn patients: Probable origin of the thermal injury-related lymphocytopenia. Burns, 17:188, 1991.

45. Malloy, R. G., Nestor, M., Collins, K. H., et al.: The humoral immune response after thermal injury: An experimental model. Surgery, 115:431, 1994.

46. Mandrup-Poulsen, T., Wogensen, L. D., Jensen, M., et al.: Circulating interleukin-1 antagonist concentration are increased in adult patients with thermal injury. Crit. Care Med., 23:26, 1995.

47. Maresca, L., and Vasko, J. S.: Treatment of hypothermia by extracorporeal circulation and internal rewarming. J. Trauma, 27:89, 1987.

48. McIrvine, A. J., O'Mahony, J. B., Saporoschetz, I., et al.: Depressed immune response in burn patients: Use of monoclonal antibodies and functional assays to define the role of suppressor cells. Ann. Surg., 196:297, 1982.

49. McManus, A. T., Kim, S. H., McManus, W. F., et al.: Comparison of quantitative microbiology and histopathology in divided burn-wound biopsy specimens. Arch. Surg., 122:74, 1987.

50. Melikian, V., Laverson, S., and Zawacki, B.: Oxygen-derived free radical inhibition in the healing of experimental zone-of-stasis burns. J. Trauma, 27:151, 1987.

51. Minei, J. P., Williams, J. G., and Hills, S. J.: Augmented tumor necrosis factor response to lipopolysaccharide after thermal injury is regulated post-transcriptionally. Arch. Surg., 129:1198, 1994.

52. Moore, D. B., Rainey, W. C., Caldwell, F. T., Jr., et al.: The effect of rapid resuscitation upon cardiac index following thermal trauma in a porcine model. J. Trauma, 27:141, 1987.

53. Morganroth, M. L., Till, G. O., Schoeneich, S., et al.: Eicosanoids are involved in the permeability changes but not the pulmonary hypertension after systemic activation of complement. Lab. Invest., 58:316, 1988.

54. Moss, N. M., Gough, D. B., Jordan, A. L., et al.: Temporal correlation of impaired immune response after thermal injury with susceptibility to infection in a murine model. Surgery, 104:882, 1988.

55. Mozingo, D. W., Cioffi, W. G., Jr., McManus, W. F., et al.: Peritoneal lavage in the diagnosis of acute surgical abdomen following thermal injury. J. Trauma, 38:5, 1995.

56. Mozingo, D. W., Smith, A. A., McManus, W. F., et al.: Chemical burns. J. Trauma, 28:642, 1988.

57. Nagasaka, T., Hirata, K., Mano, T., et al.: Heat-induced finger vasoconstriction controlled by skin sympathetic nerve activity. J. Appl. Physiol., 68:71, 1990.

58. Napolitano, L. M., and Campbell, C.: Nitric oxide inhibition normalizes splenocyte interleukin-10 synthesis in murine thermal injury. Arch. Surg., 129:1276, 1994.

59. Nieman, G. F., Clark, W. R., Jr., Goyette, D., et al.: Wood smoke inhalation increases pulmonary microvascular permeability. Surgery, 105:481, 1989.

60. Nijsten, M. W., Hack, C. E., Helle, M., et al.: Interleukin-6 and its relation to the humoral immune response and clinical parameters in burned patients. Surgery, 109:761, 1991.

61. Novick, M., Gard, D. A., Hardy, S. B., et al.: Burn scar carcinoma: A review and analysis of 46 cases. J. Trauma, 17:809, 1977.

62. O'Riordan, M. G., Collins, K. H., Pilz, M., et al.: Modulation of macrophage hyperactivity improves survival in a burn-sepsis model. Arch. Surg., 127:152, 1992.

63. Ozkan, A. N., Hoyt, D. B., and Ninnemann, J. L.: Generation and activity of suppressor peptides following traumatic injury. J. Burn Care Rehabil., 8:527, 1987.

64. Peterson, M. W.: Neutrophil cathepsin G increases transendothelial albumin flux. J. Lab. Clin. Med., 113:297, 1989.

65. Pitt, R. M., Parker, J. C., Jurkovich, G. J., et al.: Analysis of altered capillary pressure and permeability after thermal injury. J. Surg. Res., 42:693, 1987.

66. Prien, T., Linares, H. A., Traber, L. D., et al.: Lack of hematogenous mediated pulmonary injury with smoke inhalation. J. Burn Care Rehabil., 9:462, 1988.

67. Pruitt, B. A., Jr.: The universal trauma model. Bull. Am. Coll. Surg., 70:2, 1985.

68. Pruitt, B. A., Jr., and Mason, A. D., Jr.: Epidemiological demographic and outcome characteristics of burn injury. In Herndon, D. N. (Ed.): Total Burn Care. London, W. B. Saunders, 1996, p. 5

69. Rubinsky, B., and Pegg, D. E.: A mathematical model for the freezing process in biological tissue. Proc. R. Soc. Lond. B Biol. Sci., 234:343, 1988.

70. Rue, L. W., III, Cioffi, W. G., Mason, A. D., et al.: Improved survival of burn patients with inhalation injury. Arch. Surg., 128:772, 1993.

71. Sakai, H., Daniels, J. C., Beathard, G. A., et al.: Mixed lymphocyte culture reaction in patients with acute thermal burns. J. Trauma, 14:53, 1974.

72. Schluter, B., Konig, W., Koller, M., et al.: Differential regulation of T- and B-lymphocyte activation in severely burned patients. J. Trauma, 31:239, 1991.

73. Schreiber, M. M.: Exposure to sunlight: Effects on the skin. Compr. Ther., 12:38, 1986.

74. Shirani, K. Z., Pruitt, B. A., Jr., and Mason, A. D., Jr.: The influence of inhalation injury and pneumonia on burn mortality. Ann. Surg., 205:82, 1987.

75. Suzuki, K., Ogino, R., Nishina, M., et al.: Effects of hypertonic saline Dextran 70 on cardiac functions after burns. Am. J. Physiol., 268:H864, 1995.

76. Suzuki, T., Ui, K., Shioya, N., et al.: Mixed cultures comprising syngeneic and allogeneic mouse keratinacytes as a graftable skin substitute. Transplantation, 59:1236, 1995.

77. Tabata, T., and Meyer, A. A.: Effects of burn injury on class-specific B-cell population and immunoglobulin synthesis in mice. J. Trauma., 35:750, 1993.

78. Tchervenkov, J. I., Epstein, M. D., Silberstein, E. B., et al.: Early burn wound excision and skin grafting postburn trauma restores in vivo neutrophil delivery to inflammatory lesions. Arch. Surg. 123:1477, 1988.

79. Teodorczyk-Injeyan, J. A., Sparkes, B. G., Mills, G. B., et al.: Impaired expression of interleukin-2 receptor (IL-2R) in the immunosuppressed burn patient: Reversal by exogenous IL-2. J. Trauma., 27:180, 1987.

80. Teodorczyk-Injeyan, J. A., Sparkes, B. G., Mills, G. B., et al.: Increase of serum interleukin 2 receptor level in thermally injured patients. Clin. Immunol. Immunopathol., 51:205, 1989.

81. Teodorczyk-Injeyan, J. A., Sparkes, B. G., Mills G. B., and Peters, W. J.: Immunosuppression follows systemic T lymphocyte activation in the burn patient. Clin. Exp. Immunol., 85:515, 1991.

82. Till, G. O., Guilds, L. S., Mahrougui, M., et al.: Role of xanthine oxidase in thermal injury of skin. Am. J. Pathol., 135:195, 1989.

83. Urschel, J. D.: Frostbite: Predisposing factors and predictors of poor outcome. J. Trauma, 30:340, 1990.

84. Vaughan, G. M., Becker, R. A., Unger, R. H., et al.: Nonthyroidial control of metabolism after burn injury: Possible role of glucagon. Metabolism, 34:637, 1985.

85. Warden, G. D.: Burn-related humoral immunosuppressants. Proceedings of the 40th Anniversary Symposium, US Army Institute of Surgical Research, Fort Sam Houston, TX, 1989, p. 134.

86. Waxman, K., Holness, R., Tominaga, G., et al.: Hemodynamic and oxygen transport effects of pentastarch in burn resuscitation. Ann. Surg., 209:341, 1989.

87. Wilmore, D. W., Goodwin, C. W., Aulick, L. H., et al.: Effect of injury and infection on visceral metabolism and circulation. Ann. Surg., 192:491, 1980.

88. Williams, G., and Giroir, B. P.: Regulations of cytokine gene expression: Tumor necrosis factor, interleukin-1, and the emerging biology of cytokine receptors. New Horizons, 3:276, 1995.

89. Wood, J. J., Rodrick, M. L., O'Mahony, J. B., et al.: Inadequate interleukin 2 production: A fundamental immunological deficiency in patients with major burns. Ann. Surg., 200:311, 1984.

90. Xiao, G. X., Chopra, R. K., Adler, W. H., et al.: Altered expression of lymphocyte IL-2 receptors in burned patients. J. Trauma, 28:1669, 1988.

91. Xu, D. Z., Deitch, E. A., Sitting, K., et al.: In vitro cell-mediated immunity after thermal injury is not impaired: Density gradient purification of mononuclear cells is associated with spurious (artifactual) immunosuppression. Ann. Surg., 208:768, 1988.

92. Yang, L., and Hsu, B.: The roles of macrophage (M0) and PGE-2 in postburn immunosuppression. Burns, 18:132, 1992.

93. Zacarian, S. A., Stone, D., and Clater, M.: Effects of cryogenic temperatures on microcirculation in the golden hamster cheek pouch. Cryobiology, 7:27, 1970.

94. Zapata-Sirvent, R. L., and Hansbrough, J. F.: Temporal analysis of human leukocyte surface antigen expression and neutrophil respiratory burst activity after thermal injury. Burns, 19:5, 1993.

95. Zapata-Sirvent R, L., Hansbrough, J. F., and Greenleaf, G.: Effects of small volume bolus treatment with intravenous normal saline and 7.5 percent saline in combination with 6 percent Dextran-40 on metabolic acidosis and survival in burned mice. Burns, 21:185, 1995.

96. Zhou, D., Munster A, M., and Winchurch, R., A.: Inhibitory effects of interleukin 6 on immunity: Possible implications in burn patients. Arch. Surg., 127:65, 1995.

CHAPTER 14

PRINCIPLES OF OPERATIVE SURGERY

Antisepsis, Technique, Sutures, and Drains

Julio Hochberg, M.D., and Gordon F. Murray, M.D.

Many surgeons have genius without industry; others have industry without genius; while many who have both are still deficient in judgment.

JOHN ABERNETHY

It is the wisdom of a nineteenth century surgeon that directs this revision of "Principles of Operative Surgery" toward the next 100 years of technical advances in surgical therapy. Brilliant development of surgical skills and instrumentation have provided a precise understanding of an operative intervention. Today, most surgical procedures are assessed by rigorous scientific methods, and such procedures become reproducible and predictable. Elaborate algorithms are available to calculate the requirement to replace or repair, to lengthen or shorten, to ablate or enhance, to drain or not. However, traditional axioms are often contravened. Urgent operations and insertion of foreign bodies are undertaken when one is confronted with acute sepsis; adhesives and staples are substituted for sutures; balloons challenge the bypass, and lasers, the scalpel. The essence of the modern surgeon is now, more than ever before, that quality called *judgment*—the ability to know what to use, when to use it, and for how long.

ANTISEPSIS AND ASEPSIS

The development of antisepsis in the late nineteenth and early twentieth centuries revolutionized health care.[25] The term *antisepsis* translates from the Greek and means "against putrefaction." In present use, *antisepsis* is the use of antimicrobial chemicals on human tissue, whereas disinfection is the employment of these agents on inanimate objects. Hygienic hand washing, preoperative preparation of the patient's skin, gloving and sterile draping during operative procedures, isolation precautions, autoclaving of instruments, and proper waste disposal are all examples of practices that are standard in modern medical institutions—the aseptic technique. Nevertheless, nosocomial infections seem to be one of the major preventable, iatrogenic complications of hospitalization.

Historical Aspects. In the latter half of the eighteenth century and early nineteenth century, the status of surgery as a specialty was bleak. Serious infections among hospitalized patients were rampant, and the morbidity and mortality were astounding. Nearly all traumatic and surgical wound healing was accompanied by inflammation and suppuration. Primary closure of wounds was infrequently performed, in anticipation of *laudable pus*. The concept of antisepsis arose from separate sources at about the same time in the mid-nineteenth century. In America, Oliver Wendell Holmes and, in

Vienna, Ignaz Philipp Semmelweis independently observed high mortality among women hospitalized with puerperal fever. Both observed the death of a fellow physician who had been infected during participation in the autopsy of an infected subject. The experience brought attention to the fact that infection was being transmitted directly, and both urged washing of hands and changing of clothing. This policy reduced maternal mortality from 11.4% in 1846 to 1.3% in 1848. Subsequently, Pasteur's discovery of a bacterium prompted Lister to recognize the role of bacteria in the development of wound infections. Lister published his first descriptions of the "antiseptic principles" in 1867. Later progress by German physicians enabled Kocher to report a 2.3% infection rate in clean wounds by 1899. This accomplishment remains an enviable standard for modern surgeons.

ASEPTIC PROCEDURES

The Operating Room. The operating room (OR) should provide an environment that is as free of bacterial contamination as possible. The minimum size recommended for an OR is usually 20 by 20 feet, which should allow space for gowning of the operative team, draping of the patient, and movement of the other personnel without contamination of sterile areas.[20] The concept of separating clean traffic from dirty traffic is theoretically sound but has not been shown to lower wound infection rates. Studies suggest that the redispersal of bacteria from the OR floor into the air is very low. Appropriate ventilation rapidly clears bacteria from the air, and the degree of floor contamination should not increase infection rates. The very low concentrations of airborne particulate matter and bacteria in most ORs are achieved by changing room air 20 to 25 times each hour and passing the inflow air through a high-efficiency particulate air (HEPA) filter, which efficiently removes bacteria and fungi but not viruses. The pattern of air inflow is designed to decrease turbulence at the operating table and prevent entrapment of air from the periphery. All OR doors should remain closed except as needed for passage of equipment, personnel, and the patient. Also, the pressure in the OR should be positive relative to the outside corridor for preventing particles and bacteria from entering the room. Only infrequently is the OR air implicated as a possible source of infection. Organisms recovered from the air often are not those that cause wound infection.

The absence of measurable benefit after efforts to diminish environmental sources of infection is probably related to the fact that the primary source of perioperative infection is the *patient* and the secondary sources are the *OR team*.

The Patient. The most important source of contamination

in the OR is the patient. Infections that develop from operations classified as clean-contaminated, contaminated, or dirty are primarily caused by bacteria already present in the operative field as a result of disease or the procedure performed. Wound infections that occur in clean operations are often caused by staphylococci or other bacteria from a source in the patient such as the skin or nares. The danger is especially evident in operations in which prosthetic devices are implanted. Preparation of the patient's skin before an incision is one of the most important methods of decreasing infection. It is effective to have the patient shower with an antibacterial preparation the night before elective procedures. Hair removal should be employed only when the hair may interfere with the performance of the procedure. Shaving the patient with a razor the night before the operation has been associated with a relatively high wound infection rate. The risk of infection is decreased by shaving the patient in the OR immediately before the procedure or in the same setting by using a depilatory cream or electric clippers.[10] The most commonly used antimicrobial agents for intact antisepsis are iodophors (e.g., Betadine). Iodine is recognized as a broad-spectrum antimicrobial with activity against fungi, viruses, and gram-positive and gram-negative bacteria. Highly complexed iodine compounds are very stable, do not stain, have no odor, and are considerably less irritating to tissues than tincture of iodine. After contact with the skin, such complexes release iodine slowly, causing prolonged activity. The most commonly accepted technique in cleansing the patient's skin is to begin with the area where the incision is to be made and to consider this as the cleanest portion of the area of operation. The contaminated sponge stick should never be returned to the cleansing solution. The skin is cleansed in ever-widening circles, and the surgeon never returns the cleansing sponge to the incision site from the periphery.

Intact skin can stand very strong disinfecting agents, whereas cells of a fresh surgical wound are very susceptible to further damage. Solutions containing iodophors and hexachlorophene are not safe for use in surgical wounds. Contaminated experimental wounds subjected to a topical treatment with these scrub solutions developed more infections than wounds subjected to 0.9% saline. In heavily contaminated wounds, high-pressure irrigation can help to decrease the number of bacteria and to clean the wound of small particulate matter and soil.

The patient has another role in the bacteria-versus-host relationship: the intrinsic resistance to contamination. Age, obesity, diabetes, cirrhosis, uremia, and connective tissue disorders as well as hereditary or induced immunodeficiency states have all been associated with increased infection rates. The general state of nutrition and nutritional effects on cell-mediated immunity are clearly linked to the rate of infection and mortality of patients undergoing surgical procedures.

The OR Team. The preparation and conduct of the OR team are of paramount importance in the aseptic treatment of the surgical patient. The OR team should scrub their hands and arms to the elbows with an antiseptic solution before each operation. Agents such as iodophors and chlorhexidine combined with a detergent have proved effective, and no significant difference in wound infection rate has been demonstrated between these agents.[10] In addition, no difference in wound infection rate has been noted between scrub times of 3 to 5 minutes and longer times or between use of a sponge and use of a brush for scrubbing.

During operative procedures, a face mask should cover the mouth and nose comfortably, yet snugly enough to alter the projectile effect introduced by talking and breathing. It is of interest that recent studies have questioned the utility of wearing a mask at all. A prospective randomized study from Sweden[35] found no difference in wound infection rates when

masks were eliminated (except for personnel with respiratory tract infection). Similarly, although they are commonly used, there is no good evidence that shoe covers are beneficial.[16] Gloves are commonly made of latex and are disposable. It should be appreciated that gloves perform a dual function: They protect the patient from the hands of the surgeon and protect the surgeon from potentially contaminated blood. The incidence of puncture holes developing may be as high as 50% to 70%, with as many as 40,000 organisms passing through a glove pinhole in a 20-minute period.[6] Most perforations in gloves (90.6%) are found after operations that last for more than 2 hours. The left (nondominant) index finger is the most common site for perforation (44%).[17]

A major current concern to the surgical team members is the acquired immunodeficiency syndrome, which can be transmitted in ways similar to those in which hepatitis B can be transmitted.[37] Changing gloves at intervals under 2 hours and reinforcing the nondominant index finger by double gloving are factors that can be considered for better protection of surgeons against contagious blood exposure.[17]

A sterile gown contains the skin flakes constantly shed by each member of the surgical team and thereby prevents the transmission of bacteria to the patient. The most important aspect of gown material is impermeability to moisture, because the wicklike effect of a wet gown transmits bacteria from one side of the material to the other. For procedures of small blood loss (less than 100 ml.) and of short duration (less than 2 hr.) a single-layer gown can be used. For procedures of 2 to 4 hours or 100 to 500 ml. of blood loss, or for any procedure in the abdominal or chest cavity, a reinforced gown should be used. For procedures lasting longer than 4 hours or with more than 500 ml. of blood loss, a plastic-reinforced and essentially impervious gown should be used.[29]

The primary function of the sterile drapes is to define and preserve the sterile field during operative procedures. Drapes should be made of reusable or disposable fabrics that have been shown to be nearly impermeable to bacteria, even when wet. In the draping process, the material should be held above waist level, in a compact position, draping from the operative site to the periphery. When placing drapes, the gloved hand should be protected by cuffing draping material over the hands. Once placed in position, sterile drapes should not be moved or lifted. The sterile field should be constantly monitored and maintained. Every team member should observe for events that may compromise the sterile field and initiate corrective action. All personnel moving within or around a sterile field should do so in a manner to maintain its integrity. Scrubbed surgical team members may move from sterile area to sterile area. If they must change positions, they should turn back to back or face to face, while maintaining a safe distance between one another. All cables, lines, and tubing for equipment should be secured onto the sterile field with a nonperforating clamp. Nonsterile equipment brought onto the field should be draped in a sterile envelope.

Instruments and equipment to be used at the operating table can be sterilized by steam heat, chemical solutions, dry heat, or gas methods. The method chosen usually depends on the characteristics of the material being sterilized. Autoclaves are often used in the operating suite to sterilize instruments that have become contaminated and are needed again quickly. Although flash sterilization is effective, contamination of flash sterilized items during transport poses a threat.[19]

Chemical sterilization is appropriate for disinfecting equipment that is not suitable for exposure to steam heat but can tolerate moisture. Two percent aqueous solutions of glutaraldehyde can be used with almost any form of rubber or plastic. Items that can tolerate heat but not moisture or that are not penetrated well by steam can be sterilized with dry heat. Gas methods are critical for sterilizing delicate instruments that might corrode and plastic or other nonmetal items that might melt.

Instruments should be passed deliberately so they arrive securely in the surgeon's hand in a functional position. When the maneuver is finished, the assistant should return the instrument to its proper place on the stand for future use.

SURGICAL TECHNIQUE

Surgeons must be very careful
When they take the knife!
Underneath their fine incisions stirs the culprit—life!

The poignant poetry of Emily Dickinson eloquently emphasizes the primacy of the surgical operative event. Whereas the surgeon must exhibit a capacity for compassionate interest and concern in all that illness implies to the patient and the patient's family, he or she must also devise an objective pattern for decision making in the most impersonal aspect of the operative procedure. The discipline is properly named: *surgery* is derived from its earlier name *chirurgery*, which means "hand work." Halstedian teaching emphasized gentle handling of the tissues, careful hemostasis, and appropriate irrigation of the wounds to enhance healing and prevent infection. These principles remain valid today.

Incisions. The principles of selecting an incision are simple and include ensurance of adequate exposure and good healing with an acceptable scar.[13] An incision is properly planned as to shape, direction, and size. In general, incisions are made along the normal skin lines. In reoperations, every attempt should be made to use the original incision. Countertraction, if properly applied, allows the surgeon to make a clean, precise scalpel incision. Skin incisions should be made with the stainless steel surgical scalpel, with care taken to ensure that the cutting edge does not drag or crush as it cuts. Often incisions are made with the No. 15 blade on a flat surface. Cutting with the tip of a blade makes it more difficult to control the depth of the incision. Incision of the skin made at an oblique angle may cause a *trapdoor* appearance. An incision should be beveled only to preserve the integrity of hair follicles.

Atraumatic Handling. Skin margins should be handled gently to minimize necrosis that may promote infection or delay healing. Adson toothed forceps are preferred for this purpose. Skin hooks are the least traumatizing instruments with which to hold or pull back skin borders.

Dissection. The least amount of trauma is accomplished in dissecting natural tissue planes. The surgeon's index finger readily dissects many lightly adherent normal tissue planes, creating a more bloodless division of the structures. Sometimes the tissue density and adherence require the use of a dampened gauze sponge or gauze instrument (Küttner pledget). Blunt-tipped scissors are excellent for opening tissue planes that are too dense for finger or sponge dissection. A sharp knife is needed for dissection whenever tissue is heavily scarred or very dense. Countertraction is one of the most important features of dexterous and smooth surgical dissection.

The newly developed tomoscope, for dissecting subcutaneous tissue under video monitoring, has opened a new frontier in plastic surgery. Delicate procedures can be performed through small incisions, with less tissue trauma, lower rate of infections, and minimal scars. The tomoscope has an acrylic capsule placed over the end of a regular video laparoscope, equipped with a window for visualization. A type of *windshield device,* the wedge-shaped acrylic tip works as a blunt dissector to undermine the subcutaneous tissue under monitor control.[9]

Débridement. Débridement is the most important single factor in the management of the contaminated wound. Débridement removes tissue heavily contaminated by bacteria or foreign bodies and protects the patient from the threat of invasive infection. In heavily contaminated wounds, high-pressure irrigation can clean the wound of small particulate matter and soil and decrease their amount. Determining the exact limits of devitalized tissue in wounds may be difficult. Color is of doubtful value in determining the viability of muscle; muscle is viable if it contracts after being stimulated. The viability of skin is usually easier to judge than that of muscle. Tissues such as dura, fascia, and tendon may survive without living cells if immediately covered by healthy vascularized flaps. In general, they should be left in the wound.

Hemostasis. The objectives of hemostasis are to minimize blood loss during and after operation and to prevent hematoma. Hematomas constitute a nidus for infection and prevent fibroblast migration and capillary formation. It is also imperative to maintain a clear, bloodless field during incision and dissection. A rhythm can be established whereby the assistant alternately blots the field and the surgeon dissects. If digital pressure is maintained for 15 to 20 seconds, small clots usually form in the ends of smaller vessels that have been divided, so that no further bleeding occurs. Definitive hemostasis of larger vessels is obtained by ligatures, suture ligatures, or metal clips. Unnecessary ligatures may cause excessive devitalization of living tissue with resultant poor healing or infection.

Wound Closure. The relationship between the number of viable bacteria in an open wound and the ability to close that wound successfully has been clearly demonstrated.[10] Wounds containing less than 10^5 bacterial organisms per gram of tissue nearly always heal primarily after closure, unless specific factors that impair host resistance are present. These quantitative wound relationships have been defined for almost all organisms but do not apply to the more virulent beta-hemolytic streptococci. A wound containing greater than 10^5 bacterial organisms per gram of tissue cannot be reliably closed, because the incidence of wound infection that follows is 50% to 100%. When the wound is contaminated by exceedingly large numbers of organisms (greater than 10^9), primary closure of the wound should be avoided. Delayed primary closure should be considered only on or after the fourth day after wounding, at which time the wound has gained considerable resistance to infection. When wounds involve vital structures that may be destroyed by exposure, however, flaps must be transposed immediately (Fig. 14–1).[38] Only well-vascularized flaps, such as muscle and myocutaneous flaps, are chosen. In wounds following irradiation-induced ischemic ulceration, closure can be accomplished only with pedicled flaps that bring in a new blood supply. Dead space in wounds allows fluid to collect and thus should be avoided. Such spaces should be collapsed by physiologic methods such as relaxing incisions, rotation of flaps, and splinting. The closure of dead space by sutures produces localized areas of wound ischemia and necrosis, and the presence of additional suture material may create infection. The suture tension adjustable reel (STAR), a new device for use in tensioned and nontensioned skin closures, is useful for preoperative and intraoperative tissue stretching in problem areas. Scars resulting after its use are remarkably better than those that can be expected with traditional closure (Fig. 14–2).[8] A more sophisticated skin-stretching device (Fig. 14–3) has been developed to harness the viscoelastic properties of the skin using incremental traction. The pins on the undersurface of the U-arms of the device abut against the intradermal needles, which in turn distribute the stretching force along most of the length of the wound margin. It is simple to use, even at bedside, and has been applied successfully in

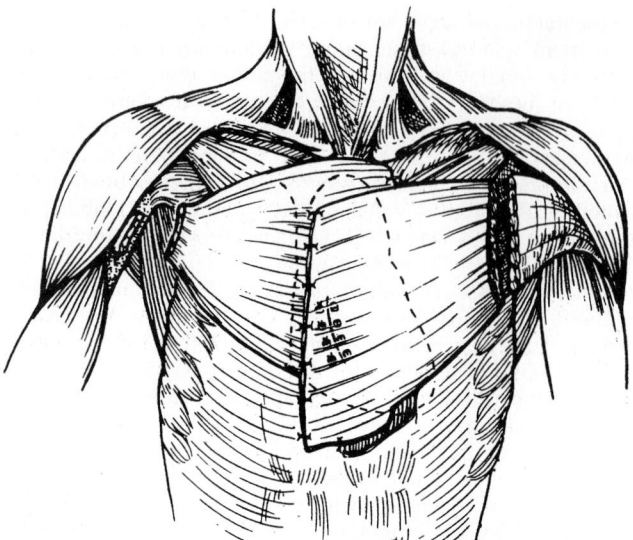

Figure 14–1. Bilateral pectoralis major muscle flaps are transposed to reinforce the cardiac repair and provide simultaneous chest wall reconstruction. (Reprinted with permission from Yuen, J. C., Hochberg, J., Cruzzavala, J., and Murray, G. F.: Immediate muscle flap coverage of cardiac rupture associated with mediastinitis. Ann. Plast. Surg., 27:358, 1991.)

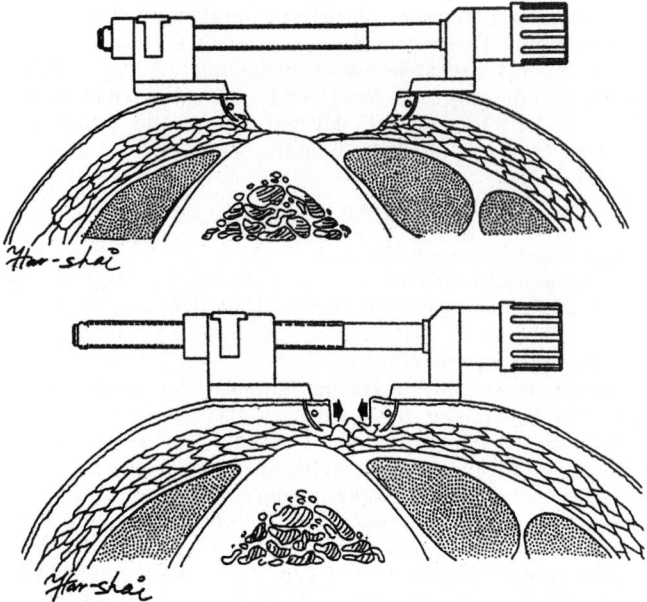

Figure 14–3. Wound edges are being drawn together by stretching of the skin and underlying subcutaneous tissue layer over the exposed bone without recourse to undermining. There is no tendency for the wound margins to become inverted because there is a tangential movement of the integument inward at the level of the deep fascia. (From Hirshowitz, B., Lindenbaum, E., and Har-Shai, Y.: A skin-stretching device for the harnessing of viscoelastic properties of skin. Plast. Reconstr. Surg., 92:260, 1993.)

difficult wounds of the abdomen, scalp, and lower and upper extremities.[21]

Suturing. Simple interrupted sutures are the most useful finishing stitches. They coapt the wound edges and correct any intervening gaps in the suture line or discrepancies in height between the two sides. The skin stitches are made to extend as little as possible from the wound edges. The passage of the needle should include deep dermis that is further removed from the cut margin of the skin. The result is slight elevation of the skin edges that is beneficial to postoperative healing. Closely placed, fine stitches create a stronger suture line than widely spaced heavy sutures. For a given closing force, perpendicular interrupted sutures exert the least tension.[31] Subcuticular sutures are an excellent choice when good cosmetic results are desired because they lower the tension on the skin margins and allow earlier removal to avoid hatchmarking. Subcuticular sutures should not be placed in the superficial dermis.

Running intradermal pull-out suture is most valuable in closing skin. It may be placed in the dermis close to the skin surface, because it is removed postoperatively. The suture material used must be strong and smooth, such as polypropylene or nylon.

Running cuticular suture is an easy and rapid method of skin closure and is readily removed postoperatively. However, it does not approximate skin as accurately as interrupted sutures and tends to cause ischemia of the skin margins. If a single knot unties, or if the suture breaks, the entire suture line undergoes dehiscence. Symmetrical continuous sutures require great tension. The advantages of continuous closure are achieved at the expense of increased tension.[31] If the suture remains in place too long, an unsightly scar may result.

Mattress sutures are frequently used to close abdominal or chest wall incisions. Vertical mattress sutures provide both a secure grasp of tissue and a good approximation of the skin margins. Unfortunately, permanent hatchmark scars result if the sutures are left in place for more than 5 to 7 days. With horizontal mattress sutures, partial necrosis of the skin margin can occur.

Both braided and monofilament sutures are at risk from surface damage. The surgeon must handle the sutures gently and avoid compressing suture between the needle holder jaws with teeth or any other surgical instrument with serration.

Dressing. Wound dressing, a major part of wound care, has a direct influence on the course of healing. Ideally, a dressing should protect wounds against mechanical trauma and bacterial invasion. Sterile dressing should be applied before surgical drapes are removed to avoid contamination of the incision. During the early postoperative period (48 hours), the fresh incision should be protected by dressings until epithelization is completed. A moist dressing speeds up epithelization tenfold. Draining and infected wounds require dressings that can absorb exudate and remove necrotic tissue remnants after surgical débridement. Wide-mesh cotton

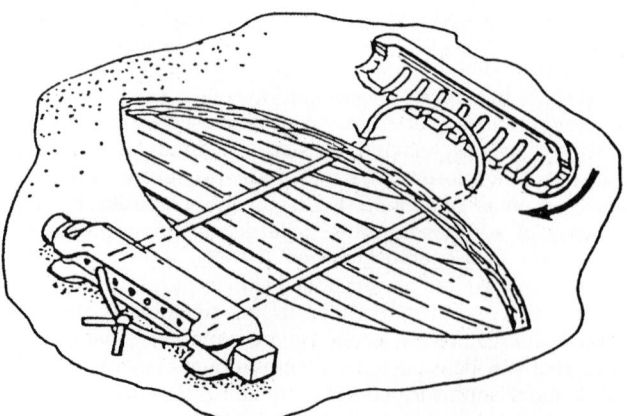

Figure 14–2. The suture is tied loosely across holes in the winder, and the inactive member is slipped under the exposed loop of suture material. (Reprinted by permission of the publisher from Cohen, B. H., and Cosmetto, A. J.: The suture tension adjustment reel: A new device for the management of skin closure. J. Dermatol. Surg. Oncol., 18:112, 1992. Copyright 1992 by Elsevier Science Inc.)

gauze applied to the wound surface traps necrotic debris and exudate, and these are removed when the dressing is changed. When skin loss is extensive, biologic dressings help achieve wound coverage and protection against bacterial invasion and evaporative loss. Allografts, xenografts, and various skin substitutes have been used.

Immobilization. When the site of any injury is immobilized, lymphatic flow is reduced, thereby minimizing the spread of the wound microflora. Moreover, immobilized tissue demonstrates more resistance to the growth of bacteria than nonimmobilized tissue. Elevation of the injured site limits the accumulation of fluid in the wound interstitial spaces. The wound with little edema proceeds more rapidly to complete rehabilitation.

Suture Removal. The proper timing for suture removal is determined by the amount of tension on the wound edges, nutritional status, prior radiation therapy, concurrent chemotherapy, exogenous steroid administration, the presence of sepsis, and cosmetic considerations. Percutaneous sutures create a sinus tract. Some of the cells may form keratin and inclusion cysts or a puncture scar. A typical railroad track appearance is the final result. In general, early suture removal (4 to 5 days) is possible in those areas with excellent blood supply. Distraction of the wound edges is greater with vertical incisions on the back and with large elliptical excision on an extremity due to greater tension.

Utmost care is needed in removing sutures. One must remember that dehiscence is likely to occur with injudicious provocation. The knot should be grasped with the forceps and the scissor tip used to cut the suture. Gentle pulling on the knot toward the incision line frees the suture.

Prophylactic Antibiotics. Prophylactic antibiotics are defined as those administered in the absence of or before infection and are distinguished from therapeutic antibiotics used to treat an established infection. Previous studies indicating that *a load of antibiotics should be on board* before operation apparently were not correct. Considerable experience has shown that antibiotics can be started intravenously when the need for antibiotic therapy appears during operation with just as good result as if prophylactic antibiotics were started before the surgical procedure.[4]

Antibiotics are recommended for operations that are associated with a high risk for infection (most alimentary tract operations, cesarean sections, hysterectomies, and selected biliary tract operations) and operations associated with life-threatening consequences if infection occurs (neurosurgical and cardiovascular procedures and operations involving implantable devices). Prophylactic orally administered antibiotics do not decrease the incidence of infection in patients with suture closure of simple lacerations. Only guarded recommendations can be made regarding the use of prophylactic antibiotics in procedures associated with a very low risk for serious infection.[23]

Electrocautery

Bovie discovered that high-frequency alternating current could be used to incise or coagulate tissue to obtain hemostasis. The technique was popularized by Cushing in the performance of neurosurgical procedures and subsequently extended to other operations.

A *unipolar* electrosurgical unit is used both for surgical dissection and for hemostasis. When undamped high-frequency electrical current is passed through tissue, the active electrode functions as a bloodless knife and the cells at the edges of the wound disintegrate. A mild thermal injury occurs away from the plane of cutting, and blood vessels thrombose. When the oscillations are dampened, hemostasis is accomplished without cutting. The cells experience a rapid

dehydration, and the vessels within the tissue coagulate. The damage to adjacent tissue may be extensive. The precise tip of the divided vessel is all that requires coagulation, and the power of the unit should be set at the lowest level possible.

The cutting cautery may be of significant value in saving operative time and diminishing blood loss during massive excisional surgery or when large flaps of skin or muscle are elevated. However, it creates an increased susceptibility to infection and seromas, compared with cold knife dissection. The grounding plate must be well secured at some appropriate point under the patient and kept as large as possible for dispersing the energy.

A *bipolar* cautery is more precise and confines the damage to the tissues between the tips of the cauterizing forceps. Notably, the bipolar instrument can be used in a wet environment.

In laparoscopic surgery, bipolar diathermy is safer and should be used in preference to monopolar diathermy, especially in anatomically crowded areas. Most injuries, not surprisingly, are caused by monopolar diathermy. The main causes of electrosurgical injuries in laparoscopy are inadvertent touching or grasping of tissue during current application; direct coupling between a portion of intestine and a metal probe that is touching the activated probe; insulation breaks in the electrodes; direct sparking to the intestine from the diathermy probe; and current passage to the intestine from recently coagulated, electrically isolated tissue. It seems prudent to use an all-metal cannula around the laparoscope.[36]

Finally, the *hemostatic scalpel* combines the advantages of a sharp knife with a heated blade for dissection. Heat seals small blood vessels as they are divided, and blood loss is minimized.

Argon Beam Coagulator

The argon beam coagulator (ABC) is a new device for hemostasis during and after operations of parenchymatous organs. The ABC allows unipolar coagulation in a nontouch technique. A needle electrode that is recessed inside a probe is activated, and the energy from the needle electrode is carried through space through a small plume of high-flow argon gas. This argon gas captures electrons from the needle electrode, and the energy is carried through space to impact on the tissue. The bolus of argon gas blows any oxygen away from the impact site, reducing smoke production, which is advantageous in laparoscopies. The gas plume also blows debris and blood away from oozing sites so that the coagulation effect is directly on the bleeding tissue. This gives less depth of penetration (usually no more than 2–3 mm) and more rapid, effective coagulation. The ABC has been effective in dissecting near the bowel, ureter, and bladder. In laparoscopic surgery it reduces the operating time because of the lack of smoke.

Potential complications may occur from ABC use with a laparoscope, such as the possibility of embolism of argon gas with high flow rates and accidental overdistention of the patient from failure to vent off the high inflow of argon gas.

Surgical Lasers

Surgical lasers are multipurpose tools that can cut, coagulate, vaporize tissue, weld, and selectively destroy pigmented pathologic tissues. Their use has permitted the development of therapeutic modalities that would have been otherwise impossible.

Argon Laser. Argon lasers result from the emission of a monochromatic beam of blue-green light (488 to 514 nm) that can be highly focused.[3] The energy is absorbed by red cell hemoglobin and transformed to heat, creating superficial thermal injury. Argon lasers have for years been the mainstay of ophthalmologic treatment and prevention of intraocular hemorrhage. Extensive experimental efforts support the potential benefits of laser fusion of tissue. The proposed advantages include speed, improved healing without the foreign body reaction associated with sutures, and reduction of intimal hyperplasia that is often seen in the region of sutured anastomoses. Exciting preliminary results have concluded that fusion of the vascular tissue with the argon laser is possible in humans. Reliable primary sealing of the vascular anastomosis is achieved. In addition, laser thermal arterial recanalization is an effective adjunct to balloon angioplasty.

CO₂ Laser. The CO_2 laser produces its effect through instantaneous heating of intracellular water to boiling, exploding cells in its pathway. It is used by some surgeons to cut tissue. Laser heating generates steam and carbonization of tissues. The laser creates a 0.1-mm. zone of histologic necrosis, which is equivalent to that of the scalpel. The superior hemostatic effect of the laser scalpel makes it especially suitable for massive surgical excision; electrosurgical excision has 1.67 times the blood loss of laser excision. Most comparative studies performed in the animal model as well as in the clinical setting prove that the CO_2 laser is *not* superior to electrosurgery in postoperative adhesion formation. The infection-potentiating effect of the laser scalpel militates against its use in incisional surgery.

Nd:YAG Laser. Forward penetration of the laser beam is least with the argon laser, intermediate with the CO_2 laser, and deepest with the neodymium:yttrium-aluminum-garnet (Nd:YAG) laser, with the Nd:YAG laser energy (1060 nm.) providing destructive coagulation effects on tissues. The Nd:YAG laser can direct light energy through a flexible quartz fiber, permitting the use of the fiberoptic endoscope in the paranasal sinuses and tracheobronchial tree.

Ho:YAG Laser. The holmium laser has a wavelength of 2.1 nm. and is highly absorbed by water. With this instrument one can vaporize, cut, coagulate, smooth, and sculpt tissue. This method is gaining wide acceptance among orthopedic surgeons as a useful arthroscopic surgical tool. It has a minimal amount of thermal necrosis and is able to cut and ablate tissues with great ease.[1]

Er:YAG Laser. The erbium laser has a wavelength of 2.94 nm. The wavelength is very strongly absorbed by the water component of tissue, and it can easily vaporize cartilage, fibrous tissue, and bone. It has a very shallow depth of penetration and affords extreme surgical precision.[1]

KTP Laser. The potassium-titanyl-phosphate (KTP) laser, with a wavelength of 0.532 nm., is a high-frequency pulsed laser. It can be transmitted by fiberoptics and can be used in an aqueous medium. The green light of KTP recognizes red and black pigments and is well absorbed by hemoglobin and melanin. It is considered a superficial photocoagulator (0.2 to 2 mm.), and it is useful for tissue cutting, coagulation, and disc ablation.[1]

Tunable Dye Laser. The modern tunable dye laser (577 nm.) provides excellent results in the difficult treatment of port-wine stains.

Cavitron Ultrasonic Surgical Aspirator

The Cavitron ultrasonic surgical aspirator (CUSA knife) is an ultrasound probe that functions as an acoustic vibrator. The instrument selectively fragments and aspirates tissue of high water and low collagen content (i.e., tumors), sparing other tissues such as blood vessels and nerves.[2]

The Cavitron aspirator was introduced into clinical use in 1967 for phacoemulsification of cataracts, and a more powerful version was approved for use in neurosurgery in 1976. The ability to remove a tumor without causing adjacent brain tissue trauma due to suctioning, coagulation, or manipulation has been greatly augmented with the development of the Cavitron. Advantages of reduced blood loss, reduced tissue injury, and improved visibility are significant compared with the scalpel or cautery. The main advantages of the Cavitron aspirator over the laser are the rapidity with which it can debulk large volumes of a tumor and the fact that it does not produce a char as it resects. This device is being used increasingly for a wide range of procedures, such as partial hepatectomy, pancreatectomy, nephrectomy, splenectomy, hemiglossectomy, mucosal proctectomy, vulvectomy, and cytoreduction of ovarian cancer, and in resection of spinal cord and brain stem tumors.[15]

SUTURES AND NEEDLES

Historical Aspects. The act of sewing is probably older than *Homo sapiens,* because Neanderthal man wore some sort of clothing. However, the overall priority for stitching probably should be credited to the ants, who had the idea long before man. *Oecophylla smaragdina* discovered a way to sew leaves with a triple combination of clamping, stitching, and gluing. Stitching of wounds among primitive man is exceptional. An ancient Egyptian scroll (3500 B.C.) alludes to sutures and suturing of wounds. Perhaps the world's oldest suture was placed by an embalmer on the belly of a twenty-first-dynasty mummy about 1100 B.C. In Sustruta's *Samhita* (600 B.C.) there is mention of suture material made from animal sinews, braided horsehair, leather strips, and vegetable fibers. *Suture* means "to sew" or "seam," and Hippocrates used the word in this sense circa 400 B.C. Celsus wrote about sutures in the treatise *De Medicina,* describing the suture of soft tissue with human hair. Galen, who was physician to Roman gladiators in the second century A.D., recommended the use of silk and hemp ligatures for hemostasis. Andreas Vesalius first advocated the suture of all fresh wounds as well as severed tendons and nerves.

During the Middle Ages, surgery regressed and sutures were forgotten until revived by Ambroise Paré (1510–1590). Paré revolutionized the treatment of wounds by substituting the ligation of blood vessels for cauterization. John Hunter (1728–1793) and Philip Syng Physick (1768–1837) were the early English and American exponents, respectively, of sutures and their routine use in surgery. Physick, first professor of surgery at the University of Pennsylvania, has been credited with the development in 1806 of absorbable ligatures using kid and buckskin. Joseph Lister (1827–1912) discovered that bacteria present in the suture strands, not the suture itself, caused wound infection. He obtained good results with wound healing by disinfecting the sutures with carbolic acid. Lister's use of sterile sutures made it possible to bury sutures in clean wounds without infection.

Selection of Suture Material. A wide choice of suture materials and suture/needle combinations is available today. The choice of suture for a particular procedure should logically be based on the known physical and biologic characteristics of the suture material and the healing properties of the sutured tissues. Adequate suture tensile strength is required for wound closure, but the finest suture that holds the tissues together safely should be used. A suture need be no stronger than the sutured tissues, and it is unwise to implant more foreign materials than is necessary. Unsecured knots allow slippage, a phenomenon that occurs to some degree with all knots. Factors that influence knot security are the material coefficient, the length of the cut ends, and the structural configuration. Regardless of the material employed, meticulous superimposition of squared knots is far superior to any other configuration. Multifilament or braided sutures are easier to handle and have better knot-holding properties.

Monofilament materials glide through tissue easily and are less reactive, but they are more difficult to handle or knot and are more likely to cut through tissue. The disadvantage of monofilament material is that the single filament, if partially fractured, may completely disrupt a continuous running suture. Coating of a multifilament suture with silicone or Teflon renders it serum-proof, with improved gliding characteristics. Unfortunately, the superior knotting quality of the suture is lost. All sutures should be avoided in dirty, contaminated, or infected wounds whenever possible. All sutures, as foreign bodies, clearly can impair the wound's ability to resist infection. When sutures are necessary in this setting, synthetic monofilament nonabsorbable sutures are recommended.

Needle and Needle Holder Selection. Surgical needles are designed to lead suture material through tissue with minimal injury. During the past two decades, major advances in surgical needle technology have markedly improved surgical wound repair. These advances include high nickel maraging stainless steels, compound curve needle, needle sharpening methods, laser-drilled holes for swages, needle suture ratio of 1:1, and silicone coating.[14]

The needle is selected according to the type of tissue to be sutured, the tissue's accessibility, and the diameter of the suture material. Surgical needles are composed of three anatomic parts: the eye, the body, and the point. The needle eye may be open, closed, or swaged. The open–French eye needle is easy to load with sutures of varying caliber but has additional bulk. Similarly, the eye of the closed-eye needle is wider than the needle body itself and it tends to spread the tissue. This disadvantage is resolved by the *swaged-on* needle, in which the suture is placed within the end of the needle. The body of the needle may be straight or curved. In cross section, the needle may be round, triangular, or flattened, and it is available in varying sizes and gauges. The needle point may be cutting, tapered, or blunt. The cutting point is used to cut through tough tissues, such as skin. The tapered point is used on soft, vulnerable tissue; and the blunt point is used in suturing friable tissues or in cannulating. The endothelial trauma at the site of microsurgical repairs has been minimized with the development of extremely fine needles (50 to 75 μm.). In contrast, arthroscopic meniscus repair has been made possible by the development of high-quality needles with the strength, sharpness, length (2 to 10 inches), and flexibility to pass smoothly through instruments and tissue. The use of percutaneous Keith needles attached to a strand of 2-0 Prolene (polypropylene) has greatly expedited the precise placement and fixation of synthetic mesh in laparoscopic hernioplasty.

The atraumatic needle holder ensures needle movement and compatibility of clamping movement. It has textured tungsten carbide jaw inserts, and its rounded needle holder jaw edges do not cause structural damage to either monofilament suture or needles.[14]

Available types of suture to be guided by surgical needles include a wide variety of materials. They may be absorbable or nonabsorbable, natural or synthetic, braided or monofilament, and clear or colored.

Absorbable Sutures

The term *absorbable suture* implies absorption and eventual disappearance of the suture from the tissue implantation site. The rate of absorption depends on the type of material used. Selecting a specific absorbable suture requires assessment of the length of time the material must be maintained and the strength it retains over that time. For example, plain catgut should not be used for major fascial repair with collagen deposition and maturation occurring at 7 to 42 days.

Catgut. The origin of the name *catgut* or *kittegut* is from a very delicate musical instrument called a kitte—a type of fiddle that required fine gut for its strings. At present, catgut is made from the intestines of cattle or sheep. The absorption rate of plain catgut is about 10 days. Chromic catgut has been treated with a chromium salt to retard its absorption by conditioning the surgical gut to resist digestion by the body; its absorption is delayed up to 20 days. Catgut acts as an active foreign body in the tissue and may interfere with wound healing. Plain catgut usually evokes a greater inflammatory reaction than chromic catgut. There is no evidence that catgut can produce an allergic response. Catgut is useful for tying off subcutaneous bleeding vessels and for closing the skin of the scrotum and perineum. The superiority of plain catgut over nonabsorbable sutures in elective surgical wound repair appears in avoidance of patient discomfort with suture removal, time spared for the surgeon and staff when absorbable suture material is used, and lower incidence of stitch marks. Repair with plain catgut is extremely helpful in children for whom the prospect of suture removal is frightening and often equated with the discomfort of suture placement. This repair is also helpful for patients who have to travel soon after the operative procedure.[18]

Polyglycolic Acid. An absorbable, braided, synthetic suture material, polyglycolic acid (Dexon) has a higher tensile strength than catgut. Total reabsorption by hydrolysis during wound healing occurs at 60 to 90 days postoperatively. Polyglycolic acid contains no collagenous protein, no antigens, and no pyrogens, thus causing minimal tissue reaction. It is useful in muscle, fascia, capsule, tendon, and subcuticular skin closure. Of the foregoing absorbable sutures, Dexon evokes the least inflammatory response and has significantly lower infection rates than either plain or chromic gut sutures.

Polyglyconate. A synthetic monofilament absorbable suture, sold commercially as Maxon, has the best *in vitro* knot security and tensile strength when compared with other synthetic absorbable sutures. It is indicated for use in all types of soft tissue wound closures, esophageal and intestinal anastomoses, and bronchial closures.[30]

Polyglactic Acid. Polyglactic acid (Vicryl) is a braided synthetic suture that is similar to polyglycolic acid in many respects. The tensile strength is very high (second to that of polyglycolic acid), and it is completely absorbed in 60 days. It is extremely useful as a completely buried suture to approximate wound edges until the wound has gained enough strength to keep the edges from separating. As noted earlier, these braided sutures may induce bacterial infection, and percutaneous sutures are contraindicated.

Polydioxanone. The synthetic polymer of polydioxanone suture (PDS) has the distinct advantage of being a monofilament absorbable suture with a long duration of absorbability and an extremely high tensile strength. It is, however, somewhat stiff and difficult to handle. The low reactive suture is able to maintain its integrity in the presence of bacterial infection and represents a major advance when used to close abdominal wounds.

Nonabsorbable Sutures

Silk. Silk is a protein filament obtained from the silkworm larva. The silk is dyed, treated with polybutilate, and braided. The suture has good tensile strength, is easy to handle, and has excellent knot characteristics. Although classified as nonabsorbable, silk does degrade in tissue at a variable rate and loses its tensile strength. Silk is a very comfortable suture for the patient when used as a premucosal suture in the mouth.

Polyester. Constructed of polyester fibers (Dacron), these braided sutures have superior strength and durability, which make them an excellent choice for fascial closure. The un-coated suture (Mersilene) tends to cut slightly when pulled through tissue; thus, Teflon (Tevdek), silicone (Tri-Cron), and polybutilate (Ethibond) have all been employed in its manu-facture. The material requires a minimum of five throw knots for knot security, compared with two throw knots for steel and three for silk, cotton, polyglactic, or polyglycolic acid sutures. Its knotting characteristics and the fact that it is braided and cannot be used in the presence of infection or contamination are its only disadvantages. Polibuster (No-vafil) is a special type of polyester suture. A monofilament suture, it is slippery and plastic like polypropylene, but ties like polyester. Polibuster induces very little inflammatory reaction when buried in tissue.

Nylon. A synthetic polyamide polymer, nylon is available in both monofilament and multifilament forms. It is very strong and smooth, but extra care must be taken in tying to prevent knot slippage. The suture is degraded and absorbed in about 2 years; thus, its tensile strength decreases signifi-cantly with time. Its smooth, monofilament composition en-sures facile passage through tissue and minimal reaction. Nylon sutures are the most commonly used sutures in cuta-neous operations—both percutaneous and subcuticular.

Polypropylene. A monofilament suture material, polypro-pylene (Prolene) provides smooth passage through tissues and minimal tissue reaction. A special manufacturing process tapers the end of the suture, so that it can be swaged to a needle of similar diameter, providing a hemostatic advantage for vascular anastomoses. Polypropylene sutures retrieved from vascular grafts at 2 to 6 years have shown no loss of tensile strength.[11] Easy removability renders polypropylene an ideal suture for a running intradermal stitch.

Stainless Steel. Stainless steel wire, made from low-carbon iron alloy, can be monofilament or multifilament. Wire is the strongest and least reactive suture. However, its handling characteristics are very poor, and great care must be taken to prevent kinking and cutting through tissue. Wire is used mainly in ligament, tendon, and bone operations. Although excellent in strength, wire is not particularly durable; and fatigue and fracture of the wire with time are not uncommon. Two considerable disadvantages of metal suture material are the linear artifacts caused by substances with high atomic number on computed tomographic images and the possible movement of metal suture during magnetic resonance im-aging. When stainless steel sutures are to be used in a patient with alleged *metal sensitivity,* a patch test for nickel sensitivity should be performed. The appearance or persistence of ante-rior chest wall pain weeks after median sternotomy may be caused by hypersensitivity to nickel in stainless steel suture material. Pain is relieved by removal of the wires.[12]

Staples

Historical Aspects. Surgical stapling was developed in 1908 by Humer Hultl in Austria. The original instrument was massive by today's standards, weighing 7.5 pounds. Modifications performed by Von Petz provided a lighter and simpler stapling device, and in 1934 Friedrich of Ulm de-signed an instrument that resembled the modern linear sta-pler. The next major advances came from Russia after World War II. In 1958, the instruments were brought to the United States by Ravitch, who, through research and development, refined the instruments to their current state and widespread use today. The most significant recent modification has been the introduction of absorbable staples (Lactomer). When these are used in gynecologic operations, morbidity related to infections, granulomas, and chronic dyspareunia has been diminished.

Contemporary devices include a great variety of skin and

internal stapling instruments: TA30, TA55, TA90, GIA, EEA, LDS, and skin and fascial staplers.

TA Instruments. The TA instruments place a linear everting (mucosa to mucosa) double line of staggered staples 30, 55, and 90 mm. long. Two staple sizes are available, 3.5 and 4.8 mm. depending on the thickness of the tissue stapled. The TA30 has, in addition, a special vascular cartridge (3.2 mm.) with closely spaced staples for closing vessels in such procedures as lobectomy and pneumonectomy.

GIA Instrument. The GIA instrument places two double-staggered rows of staples and, at the same time, divides the tissues between these pairs of staggered rows. The instru-ment was initially employed to form side-to-side intestinal anastomoses with serosal apposition. It is now used as an instrument for resection as well as other forms of anastomo-sis. Stapling of internal organs is faster than traditional hand-sewn efforts, reducing operation and anesthesia time, tissue trauma, blood loss, and eventual hospital stay.

EEA Instrument. The EEA instrument is employed for end-to-end and end-to-side minimally inverting anastomo-ses. The ends of the bowel to be anastomosed are secured with pursestring sutures about the central rod, the instru-ment is tightened, the central rings of tissue are stamped out by a circular knife, and the staples are applied in an encir-cling anastomosis. The EEA instrument and proximate ILS (Ethicon intraluminal stapling device) have become most popular in esophageal and rectal anastomoses. The ability to achieve a lower resection and end-to-end anastomosis of the bowel than previously possible has led to more sphincter-saving resections for rectal carcinoma and an improved qual-ity of life.

LDS Instrument. The LDS instrument places two metal clips of stainless steel on either side of a dividing blade. The instrument can be used in the simultaneous ligation and division of mesenteric, gastric, and omental vessels. The to-tally disposable powered instrument represents a quantum improvement over its relatively clumsy metal predecessor.

Skin Staples. The development of the disposable skin sta-pler has made this method of wound closure an increasingly popular technique. Numerous studies have confirmed the speed and efficacy of stapling compared with suture repair in wounds primarily in a postoperative environment. Staple closure also causes considerably less damage to wound de-fenses than closure with the least-reactive nonabsorbable su-ture. Suturing caused significantly more necrosis than sta-pling in myocutaneous flaps (Fig. 14–4).[22]

Skin Tapes

Ambroise Paré, the French military surgeon, introduced the use of stitched strips of linen adhesives to close saber wounds. Modern skin tapes are manufactured so that they are relatively nonocclusive and yet have excellent adhesive characteristics. The microporous surgical tapes with a back-ing of viscous rayon fibers coated with an adhesive copoly-mer are pervious to sweat but not to blood or purulent material. Skin tapes may be used in conjunction with subcu-ticular sutures and to secure skin grafts and also to decrease skin tension on a sutured skin wound in areas of motion. Application of the skin tapes minimizes the opportunity for wound dehiscence and allows earlier suture or staple re-moval. In addition, skin tapes may be reapplied to the wound for long periods of time to provide continuous support to the wound edges and may discourage scar expansion. In children, selection of skin tapes avoids the ordeal of suture replacement and removal. Significantly, skin tapes do not effectively evert the edges of the wound, and they readily loosen when wet by blood or serum. Wounds closed by adhesive tapes have less inflammatory reaction, a lower rate

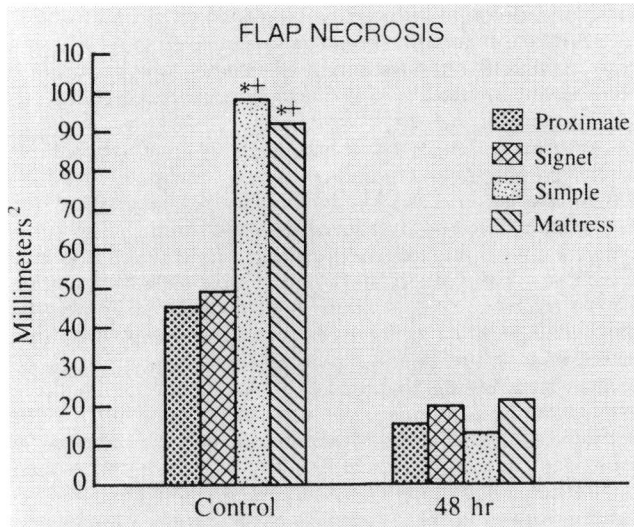

Figure 14–4. Flap necrosis in undisturbed (control) and disturbed (48 hr.) groups. Data for simple or vertical mattress suture control groups were significantly different (*) from Proximate or Signet stapling control groups and (+) from all disturbed groups at 48 hours after manipulation. (From Hochberg, J., Raman, M., Cilento, E., Kemp, K., Barrett, M., Thomas, R., and Reilly, F.: Development and evaluation of an in vivo mouse model for studying myocutaneous flap microcirculation and viability before and after suturing or stapling. Int. J. Microcirc., 14: 67, 1994; by permission of S. Karger AG, Basel.)

of wound infection, greater tensile strength, and better cosmetic results than sutured or stapled wounds. Needle puncture marks and suture canals are eliminated. Strangulation and necrosis of tissue are eliminated because of gentle handling of tissue. Foreign body granulomas and cellulitis are avoided. Sterile paper tape is a nonexpensive and convenient alternative with which to close wounds.[7, 27]

Surgical Adhesives

Autologous Fibrin Glue. Autologous fibrin glue is a biologic adhesive consisting of fibrinogen, factor XIII, fibronectin, thrombin, aprotinin, and calcium chloride. Fibrin glue works as an adhesive by emulating the exudative phase of wound healing. Animal and clinical studies have demonstrated its efficacy in stabilizing anastomoses of the esophagogastric system, small intestine, and nerves. It is also effective in obtaining hemostasis at skin graft donor sites. Fixation of skin grafts with excellent take and without requiring any sutures or pressure dressing is achieved. The preparation of the glue is easy and can be done on the morning of operation with approximately 200 ml. of autologous blood. Significantly increased stress, energy absorption, and elasticity values resulted from the use of a fibrin glue with a fibrinogen concentration of nearly 39 gm. per liter, a thrombin concentration of 200 to 600 units per ml., and no added factor XIII. The autologous fibrin glue is prepared from single donor human plasma, eliminating the danger of multidonor pools. Fibrin glue administered to tissue flaps of a mastectomy lessens the incidence of postoperative seromas. Sealing of pancreatic injuries, resections, and anastomoses with fibrin glue may help prevent formation of fistula after pancreatic operations.[24] Tissue adhesives may use the activity of growth factors to enhance healing in compromised wounds.[34] The advantages of fibrin glue are not adequately recognized by many surgeons.

Fibrin Seal Adhesive. Fibrin sealants are the most successful tissue adhesives to date.[32] Fibrin seal adhesive is a two-component system (Tissucol) derived from whole blood.

When mixed, the elements reproduce the final pathway of blood coagulation to form a viscous adhesive that maintains tissue approximation. The sealant, produced commercially only in Austria, is used both clinically and experimentally in Europe. In the United States, fibrin seal is available only for experimental use. Because fibrin seal is a blood product, its use may be associated with the transmission of human immunodeficiency virus or hepatitis, although this has not been substantiated.

Cyanoacrylate. Numerous encouraging experimental and clinical reports advocate the use of cyanoacrylate tissue adhesives for repair of organs or as hemostatic agents in emergency situations. However, when cyanoacrylate is applied to skin closure, the polymer acts as a barrier, prevents wound apposition, delays healing, and increases the infection rate. The adhesive has proved useful in fixating the articulating surface of artificial joints of the hip; but some problems exist, especially loosening of the adhesive over a period of time. In pulmonary resections butyl-2-cyanoacrylate glue (Histoacryl) is safe, offers protection to bronchial margins, and may be valuable in preventing bronchial stenosis after sleeve resections.

Protein Solder. To improve the welding strength of lasers, several protein solders are being evaluated. The solder is placed in a thin layer over the approximated tissue edges before application of the laser. Examples of protein solder are human albumin solution, dried albumin solution, fibrinogen solution, and fibrin glue and red blood cells.[28]

DRAINS

Historical Aspects. The use of drainage systems dates back to Hippocrates and may be divided into passive and active categories. Metal tubes, glass tubes, bone, gauze, wicking, and combinations of gauze and rubber were the initial means of providing *passive* drainage. The tapered lead and bronze tubes placed into the abdominal cavity by Celsus in the first century A.D. are the earliest examples of gravity drainage. Capillary attraction in small-bore tubes, the basis of all passive methods, was observed by Leonardo da Vinci, although the laws of hydrostatics explaining this phenomenon would only be elucidated three centuries later (1805) by Thomas Young, a physician and physicist. Such was still the state of the art when the familiar Penrose drain (1890) and later the cigarette drain (1897) were described. Heaton (1889) discovered air-vent suction, or *active*, drainage. Subsequently, Yates, in his 1905 classic article, concluded that "drainage of the general peritoneal cavity is physically and physiologically impossible," and the concept has not been seriously challenged.

Principles of Wound Drainage. The use of prophylactic drains for peritoneal contamination has been abandoned. Abdominal drains are quickly surrounded by omentum and bowel, which isolate the drains as ineffective sinus tracts. Soft tissue drains may help coapt tissue and prevent the collection of serum or blood underneath large undermined areas. However, drains must not be considered a substitute for hemostasis or a replacement for meticulous technique. For either prophylactic or therapeutic indications, the surgeon should select the form of drainage, either passive or active, that is best suited for the purpose intended. The drain must be appropriate to the demands of the viscosity or the volume of the expected drainage.

In general, prophylactic drainage may be best accomplished by the use of closed-wound suction drainage. As the volume or complexity of drainage increases and therapeutic drainage is indicated, passive and sump drains are more efficacious. Decreased drainage or the absence of drainage usually indicates that the drain may be withdrawn. The material of which the drain is made is of utmost concern: It should be soft to avoid injury; nonirritating to the tissue; firm, to remain in its intended place; resistant to decomposition; and smooth to allow easy removal. Four types of drains are used primarily: (1) the Penrose drain, (2) the closed-suction drain, (3) the sump drain, and (4) the closed-suction Penrose drain. Percutaneous catheter drainage represents a new method that is proving to be exceedingly valuable.

Penrose Drain. The Penrose drain is among the most efficient of contemporary drains. However, there is a significant risk of secondary infection.[5] The Penrose drain is a soft, flexible latex rubber wick ranging from 0.25 to 1 inch in diameter and is usually employed to drain purulent material, blood, or serum from a body cavity. Intra-abdominal drains should optimally be brought out through a stab wound in the flank and not through the abdominal incision itself. A drain tract coming through the suture line increases the risk of infection and is a potential source of weakness that may lead to a ventral hernia. The use of two drains is advantageous in allowing egress of fluid along the planes between the drains. The drains should be anchored to the skin with a nonabsorbable suture, and placement of a sterile safety pin prevents retraction of the drains into the wound. Management of the drains consists of either completely removing them or cracking and gradually withdrawing them several centimeters a day. The latter technique is designed to prevent the development of a fluid collection or abscess cavity deep to the drains. The length of time a Penrose drain is left in place varies with the initial indication for drainage, the presence of a foreign body, and the patient's overall status.

Closed-Suction Drain. The closed-suction drains have lower infection rates but clog and cease function early in the wound drainage process.[5] Closed-suction drains are firm, multiholed catheters made of polyvinyl chloride or silicone. The silicone material is softer, less irritating to the tissues, and less likely to cause infection. These drains are particularly effective under large skin flaps, such as those encountered after radical neck or breast dissections. Closed-suction drainage decreases the incidence of infection occurring secondary to contamination of the drain itself. When drainage diminishes, the tube may be removed directly, preferably within 24 to 72 hours.

Sump Drain. Sump drains are often large and bulky, and they rely on a continuous flow of air from outside the sump to work. This external air at the wound site predisposes to secondary infection.[5] Sump drains are available with double or triple lumens that allow irrigation and aspiration. Pressure in the catheter is maintained at atmospheric levels, and tissue occlusion of the drain is less likely. The sump drain is most useful in managing established enteric fistulas with high volumes.

Closed-Suction Penrose Drain. A combination of the closed-suction drain and the open Penrose drain that uses the capillary action of the Penrose design but maintains closed suction without bacterial contamination is the ideal drainage system.[5] Two tubes are included; while tails of the outer tube function by capillary action, the inner standard perforated tube sucks through a closed system.[5]

Catheter Drain. Through modern radiologic techniques, localized accumulations of fluid in different areas of the body can be diagnosed much earlier than in the past and confirmed by aspiration. In many instances adequate treatment can be instituted by means of percutaneous catheters inserted by radiologists guided by computed tomography or, less reliably, ultrasonography. Antibiotics are considered essential for success. Percutaneous catheter drainage is recommended for all postoperative trauma patients with accessible abdominal abscesses. Reoperation should be reserved for patients in whom safe access to the abscess is not available or if

percutaneous catheter drainage has failed to control the sepsis.[33] Surgical treatment should not be delayed even with the very ill patient, and exploration should be done promptly if there is any question as to the adequacy of percutaneous drainage of the abscess.[26]

Controversy. The continued use of drains in circumstances where experimental evidence suggests that they have no benefit or are detrimental is presumably a counsel of caution rather than perfection: "When in doubt, drain," and "It is better to have it and not need it than to need it and not have it." These concepts apparently are based on the assumption that there are no complications related to the use of drains. Drains left *in situ* are not innocuous: They may erode into the intestine or the blood vessels and thus promote the development of adhesions that lead to intestinal obstruction. Technical complications, such as hematoma, retraction of the drain into the wound, or herniation through the stab wound have been cited. Sutures can be inadvertently placed around or through drains, and drains may break off inside the body. Careful record keeping related to the number, type, and length of drains inserted and removed may avert the disastrous consequences of retained drains. For the benefit of wound drainage, the surgeon must consider the risk of contaminating the wound and increasing the incidence of infection. Accumulated wound fluids contain decreased levels of opsonizing proteins, making these fluids especially vulnerable to infection. It has been clearly documented that placing a drain in patients undergoing routine splenectomy increases the morbidity of the procedure. Similarly, researchers have demonstrated that children in whom Penrose drains were placed at operation for perforated appendicitis averaged nearly 4 more hospital days than those without drains. To drain or not, which drain, and for how long all remain unanswered questions, but the diversity of answers suggests that no single policy is necessarily correct.

SELECTED REFERENCES

Bates, T., Siller, G., Crathern, B. C., Bradley, S. P., Zlotnik, R. D., Couch, C. R. D. G., and Kaye, C. M.: Timing of prophylactic antibiotics in abdominal surgery: Trial of a preoperative versus an intra-operative first dose. Br. J. Surg., 76:52, 1989.
Previous studies indicating that "a load of antibiotics should be on board" before operation apparently were not correct. Considerable experience has been accumulated to show that antibiotics can be started intravenously when the need for antibiotic therapy appears during operative procedures with just as good results as if prophylactic antibiotics were started beforehand. Such data make it possible to reduce the use and expense of antibiotics in many patients.

Edgerton, M. T.: The Art of Surgical Technique. Baltimore, Williams & Wilkins, 1988.
This refreshing and detailed focus on "how to do it" is written by a plastic surgeon with years of experience in the broadest realms of reconstructive surgery. Edgerton is a master of the art of surgical technique. He provides a simple and basic description of operative techniques, the principles and details of which apply to all surgical procedures.

Lerner, R., and Binur, N. S.: Current status of surgical adhesives. J. Surg. Res., 48:165, 1990.
An extensive review is provided of the advances in the field of surgical adhesives, and the most common clinical applications in hemostasis for neurosurgery, plastic surgery, cardiovascular and thoracic surgery, and general surgery are presented. Genitourinary, gynecologic, orthopedic, ophthalmologic, ENT, and oral and maxillofacial use of these adhesives is described.

Nduka, C. C., Super, P. A., Monson, J. R. T., and Darzi, A. W.: Cause and prevention of electrosurgical injuries in laparoscopy. J. Am. Coll. Surg., 179:161, 1994.
Electrosurgical injuries occur during laparoscopy and are potentially serious. Most go unrecognized at the time of the electrical insult and commonly present 3 to 7 days afterward. This article reviews the physics of electrosurgery and provides the surgeon with insight into the mechanisms responsible in each type of injury. A comprehensive search of the world literature reviews all articles on the topic.

Wilmore, D. W., Brennan, M. F., Harken, A. H., Holcroft, J. W., and Meakins, J. L.: American College of Surgeons: Care of the Surgical Patient. Vol. 2, Elective Care. New York, Scientific American, 1989.
Care of the Surgical Patient is sponsored by the Pre- and Postoperative Care

Committee of the American College of Surgeons and is written by individuals who are recognized experts. The text represents their approaches to clinical problems and to other important issues in surgical practices. The content includes initial evaluation for elective surgery, perioperative care, and infections.

REFERENCES

1. Abelow, S. P.: Use of lasers in orthopedic surgery: Current concepts. Orthopedics, 16:551, 1993.
2. Adelson, M. D., Baggish, M. D., Seifer, D. B., Cassell, S. L., and Thompson, M. A.: Cytoreduction of ovarian cancer with the cavitron ultrasonic surgical aspirator. Obstet. Gynecol., 75:140, 1988.
3. Arndt, K. A., Noe, J. M., Northam, D. B. C., and Itzkan, I.: Laser therapy: Basic concepts and nomenclature. J. Am. Acad. Dermatol., 5:649, 1981.
4. Bates, T., Siller, G., Crathern, B. C., Bradley, S. P., Zlotnik, R. D., Couch, C. R. D. G., and Kaye, C. M.: Timing of prophylactic antibiotics in abdominal surgery: Trial of a preoperative versus an intra-operative first dose. Br. J. Surg., 76:52, 1989.
5. Berlin, R. B., and Javna, S. L.: Closed suction wide area drainage. Surg. Gynecol. Obstet., 174:421, 1992.
6. Brough, S. J., Hunt, T. M., and Barrie, W. W.: Surgical glove perforations. Br. J. Surg., 75:317, 1988.
7. Chao, T. C., and Tsaez, F. Y.: Paper tape in closures of abdominal wounds. Surg. Gynecol. Obstet., 171:65, 1990.
8. Cohen, B. H., and Cosmetto, A. J.: The suture tension adjustment reel: A new device for the management of skin closure. J. Dermatol. Surg. Oncol., 18:112, 1992.
9. Correa, M. A. F.: Video-endoscopic abdominoplasty. Plast. Surg. Forum, 27:167, 1994.
10. Cruse, P. J., and Foord, R.: The epidemiology of wound infection: A 10-year prospective study of 62,939 wounds. Surg. Clin. North Am., 60:27, 1980.
11. Dobrin, P. B.: Surgical manipulation and the tensile strength of polypropylene sutures. Arch. Surg., 124:665, 1989.
12. Eastridge, C. E., Mahfood, S. S., Walker, W. A., and Cole, F. H., Jr.: Delayed chest wall pain due to sternal wire sutures. Ann. Thorac. Surg., 51:56, 1991.
13. Edgerton, M. T.: The Art of Surgical Technique. Baltimore, Williams & Wilkins, 1988.
14. Edlich, R. F., Thacker, J. G., McGregor, W., and Rodeheaver, G. T.: Past, present, and future for surgical needles and needle holders. Am. J. Surg., 166:522, 1993.
15. Epstein, F. J., and Farmer, J-P.: Trends in surgery: Laser surgery, use of cavitron, and debulking surgery. Neurol. Clin., 9:307, 1991.
16. Garner, J. S.: Guideline for prevention of surgical wound infections, 1985. Public Health Service publication No. PB85-923403. Atlanta, Centers for Disease Control, 1985.
17. Greco, R. J., Wheatley, M., and McKenna, M.: Risk of blood contact through surgical gloves in aesthetic procedures. Aesthet. Plast. Surg., 17:167, 1993.
18. Guyurin, B., and Vaughan, C.: A comparison of absorbable and nonabsorbable suture materials for skin repair. Plast. Reconstr. Surg., 89:234, 1992.
19. Harris, M. H.: Flash sterilization. AORN J., 55:1547, 1992.
20. Health and Human Services: Requirements of Construction and Equipment for Hospitals and Medical Facilities. Publication No. HRS-M-HF-84-1. Rockville, MD, United States Department of Health and Human Services, 1984.
21. Hirshowitz, B., Lindenbaum, E., and Har-Shai, Y.: A skin-stretching device for the harnessing of viscoelastic properties of skin. Plast. Reconstr. Surg., 92:260, 1993.
22. Hochberg, J., Raman, M., Cilento, E., Kemp, K., Barrett, M., Thomas, R., and Reilly, F.: Development and evaluation of an *in vivo* mouse model for studying myocutaneous flap microcirculation and viability before and after suturing or stapling. Int. J. Microcirc., 14:67, 1994.
23. Hopkins, C. C.: Antibiotic prophylaxis in clean surgery: Peripheral vascular surgery, non-cardiovascular thoracic surgery, herniorrhaphy, and mastectomy. Rev. Infect. Dis., 13(Suppl. 10):869, 1991.
24. Kram, H. B., Clark, S. R., Ocampo, H. P., Yamaguchi, M. A., and Shoemaker, W. C.: Fibrin glue sealing of pancreatic injuries, resections, and anastomoses. Am. J. Surg., 161:479, 1991.
25. Larson, E.: Innovations in health care: Antisepsis as a case study. Am. J. Publ. Health, 79:92, 1989.
26. Levison, M. A., and Zeigler, D.: Correlation of APACHE II SCORE Drainage technique and outcome in postoperative intra-abdominal abscess. Surg. Gynecol. Obstet., 172:89, 1991.
27. Pepicello, J., and Yavorek, H.: Five year experience with tape closure of abdominal wounds. Surg. Gynecol. Obstet., 169:310, 1989.
28. Poppas, D. P., and Schlossberg, S. M.: Laser tissue welding in urologic surgery. Urology, 43:143, 1994.
29. Quebbeman, E. J., Telfors, G. L., Hubbard, S., Wadsworth, K., Hardman, B., Goodman, H., and Gottlieb, M. S.: In-use evaluation of surgical gowns. Surg. Gynecol. Obstet., 174:369, 1992.
30. Raffensperger, J. G., and Schwarz, D.: Polyglyconate suture in pediatric surgery. J. Pediatr. Surg., 26:82, 1991.
31. Rubenstein, C., and Russell, W. J.: Wound closure and suturing patterns: A vector analysis of suture tension. Aust. N. Z. J. Surg., 62:733, 1992.
32. Sierra, D. H: Fibrin sealant adhesive systems: A review of their chemistry, material properties and clinical applications. J. Biomater. Appl., 7:309, 1993.
33. Stylianos, S., Martin, E. C., Laffey, K. J., Bixon, R., and Forde, K. A.: Percutaneous drainage of intra-abdominal abscesses following abdominal trauma. J. Trauma, 29:584, 1989.
34. Toriumi, D. M., and O'Grady, K.: Surgical tissue adhesives in otolaryngology–head and neck surgery. Otolaryngol. Clin. North Am., 27:203, 1994.
35. Tuneval, T. G.: Surgical face mask: With or without? Presented at the 32nd World Congress of Surgery, Sydney, Australia, September 28, 1987.
36. Voyles, C. R., and Tucker, R. D.: Education and engineering solutions for potential problems with laparoscopic monopolar electrosurgery. Am. J. Surg., 164:57, 1992.
37. Wilmore, D. W., Behrman, M. F., Harken, A. H., and Holcroft, J. W.: Preparing the operating room. *In* American College of Surgeons: Care of the Surgical Patient. Vol. 2, Elective Care. New York, Scientific American, 1989.
38. Yuen, J. C., Hochberg, J., Cruzzavala, J., and Murray, G. F.: Immediate muscle flap coverage of cardiac rupture associated with mediastinitis. Ann. Plast. Surg., 27:358, 1991.

CHAPTER 15

SURGICAL INFECTIONS

I ——

SURGICAL INFECTIONS AND CHOICE OF ANTIBIOTICS

E. Patchen Dellinger, M.D.

During the second half of the nineteenth century many operations were developed after anesthesia was introduced by Morton in 1846, but advances were few for many years because of the high rate of infection and the high mortality that followed infections. Lister is generally recognized as one of the discoverers of the antiseptic principle after publication, in 1867, of his paper, "On the Antiseptic Principle in the Practice of Surgery," which revolutionized the practice of surgery. Application of antiseptic practices allowed infection rates for elective operations to drop from 90% to 10%. Other individuals whose work helped to introduce concepts of asepsis and antisepsis in surgical practice in this era include Louis Pasteur, Oliver Wendell Holmes, Ignaz Semmelweis, Theodor Kocher, and William S. Halsted. In addition, the practice of wearing gloves during operations became widespread around the turn of the century.

These basic principles of controlling infection set forth primarily between 1867 and 1900 set surgery free from the bonds of despair and disappointment, changing surgical therapy from a dreaded event, with infection almost universal and death to be expected, to one that alleviates suffering and prolongs life with close to universal success when carefully performed. Despite these gains, the large number of procedures performed every year leads to numerous postoperative surgical site infections. Patients who do develop infection have not only an increased morbidity but also a significant mortality. The cost of the care of postoperative wound infections alone in the United States is enormous, amounting to several billion dollars every year. For any given type of operation, the development of a wound infection will approximately double the cost of hospitalization. The introduction of antibiotic therapy in the middle of the twentieth century fostered hope that serious surgical infections would be eliminated. Unfortunately, this did not occur. Not only have postoperative wound and hospital-acquired infections continued, but widespread antibiotic therapy has often made prevention and control of surgical infections more difficult. The present generation of surgeons has seen increasing numbers of serious infections related to a complex combination of factors, including the performance of more complicated and longer operations; an increase in the number of geriatric patients with accompanying chronic or debilitating diseases; many new surgical procedures with implants of foreign materials; a rapidly expanding number of organ transplants requiring the use of immunosuppressive agents; and increased use of diagnostic and treatment modalities that cause greater bacterial exposures or the suppression of normal host resistance. Unfortunately, infections also result from laxity in aseptic technique, disregard for established surgical principles, and unwarranted reliance on prophylactic antibiotic therapy. The modern surgeon cannot escape the responsibility to deal with infections and must realize that knowledge of many aspects of microbiology, immunology, and pharmacology is an essential complement to surgical skills. Basic understanding of how the body defends itself against infection is essential to a rational application of surgical and other therapeutic principles to the control of infection.

CAUSES OF WOUND INFECTION

Infections of surgical wounds occur whenever the combination of microbial numbers and virulence in the wound is sufficiently large to overcome the local host defense mechanisms and establish progressive growth. Careful work performed in the 1960s demonstrated that essentially all clean operative wounds contain at least small numbers of bacteria at the end of the procedure, but only a small number develop infection.[5] The host defense interaction with potential pathogens is an extremely complex process and is beyond the scope of this presentation. However, certain factors need emphasis.

Bacterial Factors

The deposition and growth of bacteria within wounds is a prerequisite for the development of infection, and the kind and numbers of bacteria contribute significantly to the establishment of overt infection, or the lack of it. The development of infection is also affected by the toxins produced by the organism and the organism's ability to resist phagocytosis and intracellular destruction. Several bacterial species have surface components that contribute to their pathogenicity by inhibiting phagocytosis (e.g., the capsules of *Klebsiella* and *Streptococcus pneumoniae*). Gram-negative bacteria have surface components (endotoxin or lipopolysaccharide) that are toxic, and others, such as certain strains of clostridia and streptococci, produce powerful exotoxins. These exotoxins permit streptococci and clostridia to establish invasive infection after smaller inocula than other pathogens and to evolve much more rapidly. Thus, while most wound infections do not become evident clinically for 5 days or longer after the operation, infections due to streptococci or clostridia may become severe within 24 hours.

Careful studies of the bacterial flora of surgical wounds taken at the time of closure have shown that one or more types of organisms can be cultured from most wounds. Wounds classified as clean usually contain skin bacteria such as *Staphylococcus epidermidis* or diphtheroids. In traumatic wounds, the most likely organisms are *Staphylococcus aureus* and *Streptococcus pyogenes*. When a viscus is entered, the natural or disturbed resident flora become the expected potential pathogens. Because devitalized tissues and foreign materials are invariably present, far fewer organisms are necessary to cause infection in wounds than in normal tissues. Even so, overt infection is unusual unless cardinal surgical principles have been violated or exceptionally large numbers of organisms have been introduced into the wound. Studies of traumatic wounds in healthy subjects have shown that bacterial contamination with more than 10^5 organisms frequently causes infection, whereas contamination with less than 10^5 organisms usually does not. The normal defense mechanisms therefore are of great importance in preventing infection at its inception, but wound infection is inevitable if the bacterial inoculum is sufficiently large.

Local Wound Factors

In everyday practice, inhibition of local defense mechanisms for clearing bacteria is perhaps the most important cause of wound infections. Anything that interferes with the ability of phagocytic cells to contact directly and kill bacteria potentiates wound infection. The use of foreign bodies including sutures and drains, lack of accurate approximation of tissues, strangulation of tissue with sutures that are too tight, and the presence of any dead tissue, hematomas, or seromas all increase the risk of infection. Fortunately, most of these factors can be minimized by good surgical technique.

Patient Factors

Wound infections are more common in the very young and the very old, perhaps because of immature or senescent resistance mechanisms. Anything that reduces blood flow to the surgical incision—as may be found in vascular occlusive states, hypovolemic shock, or with the use of vasopressors or vasoconstrictors either locally or systemically—increases the incidence of infection. Local decrease in tissue oxygen tension, caused either by decreased blood flow or by systemic hypoxemia, increases the incidence and severity of infection. Furthermore, conditions that reduce vascular reactivity as in uremia, old age, or the use of high doses of corticosteroids and other drugs cause an increased susceptibility to infection. More complex problems leading to increased infection include cancer and trauma, both of which may be associated with complement activation and the generation of both tissue-derived and complement split product–derived inhibitors of cellular function, which influence both T-cell and phagocytic cell function. In many patients, these factors are believed to be primarily responsible for a decreased reactivity to delayed hypersensitivity antigens, creating an anergic state associated with an increased incidence of infectious complications.

PREVENTION OF WOUND INFECTION

Preventing infectious complications is far more practical than treating them once they have become established. Fortunately, strict adherence to the principles of wound care and application of knowledge concerning the pathogenesis of wound infections can prevent the vast majority of infectious complications in surgical practice. One of the most important factors in preventing wound infection is constant vigilance of the operating team, including the surgeon.

Avoidance of Bacterial Contamination

Environmental Factors. Engineering and architectural advances have helped limit airborne contamination in modern operating rooms to very low levels, but these have not been followed by substantial reductions in wound infection rates, because the two greatest sources of significant microbial contamination of operative wounds are exogenous contact from breaks in technique by the operating team and endogenous contamination from the patient's skin and various bacteria-containing tracts. Of the two, endogenous contamination causes a greater number of infections in all types of wounds except those classified as *clean* (Table 15–l). The use of ultraviolet light for decontamination of the operating room and laminar flow ventilation systems may be helpful in certain situations, such as insertion of prostheses for orthopaedic reconstruction. Perhaps as important are limiting traffic in and out of the operating room, providing positive pressure in the operating room, and limiting activity and talking within the operating room. With increasing numbers of people at the operating table, there is increased opportunity for breaks in sterile technique and increased dispersion of airborne bacteria. In addition to air handling, sterilization techniques must be strictly monitored.

Preoperative Preparation of the Patient. Many patients who are in the hospital for prolonged periods of time or who have substantial illness have increased numbers of resident organisms on the skin, especially in the groin and intertriginous areas. These and perhaps all patients, whenever able, should take a preoperative shower the night before operation using an antibacterial soap such as chlorhexidine or povidone-iodine.[14] Chlorhexidine seems to be the preferred material for reducing residual bacteria for a prolonged period. Whenever possible, all cutaneous infections should be controlled or cleared before the time of an elective operation. Presence of a distant-site infection at the time of an elective clean operation doubles the postoperative infection rate.

Hair Removal. When the operative area is shaved the night before the procedure, the injury of shaving itself promotes bacterial growth. This practice increases the infection rate about 100% compared with removing the hair by clippers at the time of the procedure or not removing it at all.[2] Therefore, the patient should not be shaved before an operation. Extensive removal of hair is not needed, and any that is done should be performed by electric clippers with disposable heads in the operating room at the time of the procedure.

Skin Preparation. The skin is an important source of organisms contaminating surgical wounds. Two methods can be recommended to prevent skin organisms from entering the wound. First, the time-honored technique is to scrub the entire operative area of the patient for 5 to 7 minutes with a germicidal detergent solution and then paint the region with an antimicrobial solution of either tincture of iodine, povi-

TABLE 15–1. Classification of Surgical Wounds According to Risk of Infection

Type	Definition
Clean	Nontraumatic
	No break in technique
	Respiratory, alimentary, or genitourinary tract not entered
Clean-contaminated	Gastrointestinal or respiratory tract entered without significant spillage
	Oropharynx, vagina, or noninfected genitourinary or biliary tract entered
	Minor break in technique
Contaminated	Major break in technique
	Traumatic wound
	Gross spillage from gastrointestinal tract
	Entrance into genitourinary or biliary tracts in presence of infected urine or bile

done-iodine, or chlorhexidine. An alternative way to isolate the skin from the wound is to use an antimicrobial incise drape applied to the entire operative area, with the incision made through the plastic.[1] Before the incise drape is applied, the skin should be scrubbed for 1 minute with a 70% solution of alcohol or a solution of 2% iodine in 90% alcohol to kill surface bacteria. When the incise drape is used, the skin should not be scrubbed with a detergent solution because it interferes with the ability of the incise drape to adhere to the skin; the effectiveness is lost when the drape lifts from the skin at the incision site. Thus, the *technique* of drape application, including cleansing of surface fat and debris from the skin and application only to a dry surface, becomes important for its success.

The Operating Room Team and Discipline

Contamination occurs easily from the operating room team, and this is, as an aggregate, one of the most important sources of organisms causing infection in clean cases. The operating team should wear clean scrub suits, caps that do not shed lint and completely cover the hair, and masks that effectively filter the exhaled air. Before each operation, the hands and forearms should be cleansed and scrubbed thoroughly with an antimicrobial soap for at least 5 minutes for the first case or after any dirty case and for 3 minutes for subsequent cases. The most popular antimicrobial scrubs are chlorhexidine and povidone-iodine. Careful gowning and gloving techniques should be used, and special attention should be paid to avoiding contamination when the patient is draped. It is perhaps during the gowning/gloving procedure and draping of the patient that the most breaks in technique occur in the modern operating room. Another frequent source of contamination is the use of sterile light handles, which become contaminated by the headgear of the operating team.

As many as 90% of an operative team puncture or tear their gloves at some time during a long operation. These gloves must be changed immediately to prevent bacterial contamination of the wound. Even though the numbers of organisms present after a surgical scrub are low, they increase with the length of the operation, and the numbers of organisms inside gloves at puncture sites increase remarkably when blood has gained entrance. The safest gloving practice is to wear two pairs of gloves, with one pair a half size larger than usual under the standard size. This practice has become popular to reduce the risk of getting the patient's blood onto the surgeon's hands, but it is equally effective in keeping the surgeon's bacteria out of the patient's wound. Two pairs of regular gloves are substantially more effective than a single pair of reinforced (*orthopaedic*) gloves.[20] Gowns worn by the operating room team may also be an important source of contamination, and the *contact areas* (i.e., sleeves and front of the gown) should be impervious to bacteria and fluids whether the gowns are disposable or reused.

Endogenous Contamination

Another very important but not always heeded source of bacterial contamination of the surgical wound is endogenous contamination at the time of transection of the gastrointestinal, respiratory, or genitourinary tract. Bacterial contamination occurs to varying degrees any time a hollow viscus is transected, but exceptional efforts to minimize the amount of contamination can keep the occurrence of bacterial infection low. Before a hollow viscus is entered, the operative area should be carefully isolated from the remainder of the operative field. A completely different set of instruments should be used for that portion of the operation until the hollow viscus is closed. At closure of the hollow viscus, all instruments, towels, and sponges that may have come into contact with the contaminated area must be removed from the operative field, and the gowns and gloves of the operative team should be changed. Strict observance of aseptic technique in clean-contaminated cases can markedly reduce the incidence of operative infections.

The Importance of Surgical Technique

As previously emphasized, infections in wounds associated with injury or planned operations increase morbidity and mortality. Gentle care of the tissues to minimize local damage is one of the most important ways to prevent wound infection. All devitalized tissues and foreign bodies should be removed from traumatic wounds. When complete débridement is not possible, the wound should not be closed, because foreign bodies left in a wound decrease the minimal infective dose of a bacterial inoculum 10,000-fold or more. More than a million viable staphylococci are necessary to produce a clinical infection when injected subcutaneously or intradermally into normal tissue, but as few as 100 of the same organisms introduced on a piece of silk suture material can produce a significant infection. Similar enhancement of clostridial infections by devitalized muscle and sterile foreign bodies is well known. Not only must all contaminated foreign bodies be removed from grossly contaminated wounds, but one should try to avoid the introduction of new foreign bodies such as prostheses, grafts, and suture materials. Experimental studies have shown that monofilament sutures are preferable to multifilament ones in contaminated wounds. Silk should not be used to tie or repair large blood vessels where there is a high potential for infection, because infection involving the suture can rupture the vessel and cause fatal hemorrhage. The best nonabsorbable sutures for use in contaminated wounds are polypropylene and nylon. The synthetic absorbable suture materials, such as polyglactin-910, polyglycolic acid, glycolide/lactide copolymer, polydioxanone, and polyglyconate, also have a low potential for increasing infection risk.

The presence of hematomas, seromas, or dead spaces favors bacterial localization and growth and prevents the delivery of phagocytic cells to such foci. When a large potential dead space occurs in an operative wound that is potentially contaminated but not yet infected and is not obliterated by fascial and dermal sutures, the best way to prevent fluid collection and infection is to provide a system of closed suction drainage. However, because any additional foreign body in a wound increases the risk of infection, the benefit of fluid removal and dead space obliteration must be balanced against the effect of the foreign body. Open drainage of wounds with Penrose-type drains increases rather than decreases the degree of contamination and the incidence of infection, so these should not be used to drain any wound that is not already infected.

In heavily contaminated wounds or in wounds in which all the foreign bodies or devitalized tissues cannot be satisfactorily removed, delayed primary closure minimizes the development of serious infection in most instances. With this technique, the subcutaneous tissues and skin are left open and *packed* loosely with gauze after fascial closure. The number of phagocytic cells at the wound edges progressively increases to reach a peak about 5 days after the injury. Capillary budding is intense at this time, and closure can usually be accomplished successfully even with heavy bacterial contamination because phagocytic cells can be delivered to the site in large numbers. Experiments have shown that the number of organisms required to initiate an infection in a surgical incision progressively increases as the interval of healing increases, up to the fifth postoperative day.

Systemic Factors

Host resistance is abnormal in a variety of systemic conditions and diseases, including leukemia, diabetes mellitus, uremia, prematurity, burn or traumatic injury, advanced malignancy, old age, obesity, malnutrition, and several diseases of inherited immunodeficiency. With surgical patients who have these or similar problems, extraordinary precautions should be taken to prevent the development of wound infections, including correction or control of the underlying defect whenever possible.

Malnutrition, even when subclinical, can significantly impair host defense mechanisms. Many surgical patients have some degree of malnutrition, especially when stress leads to hypermetabolism. This type of *insidious* malnutrition is probably the most important cause of acquired immunologic deficiencies leading to serious infection in surgical patients. Thus, one of the most important things a surgeon can do to prevent infection is to correct any underlying malnutrition before surgical therapy or as soon thereafter as possible. Alimentation by the oral route is preferable, when possible. Evidence indicates an increased requirement for protein and arginine in stressed patients.

Social Considerations

Traditionally, surgeons have monitored and recorded the incidence of postoperative surgical site infections long before the current enthusiasm for quality assessment and improvement. Several studies have now shown that accurate and continued surveillance for wound infection with feedback to the surgeon reduces its incidence by about 50%. This simple technique may be a powerful tool for controlling wound infection, because virtually every surgeon will increase his or her efforts to control infectious complications if they are perceived to be a problem. An unbiased observer (not the surgeon) should monitor infections, and infection should be diagnosed whenever there is discharge of any pus from the wound. Infection rates should be determined at 30 days postoperatively rather than at discharge because more than one half of the infections occur after discharge. This problem has become even more severe with the increasing number of operations being done on outpatients and the continuing trend to shorter hospital stays after operation. The logistics of survey for surgical site infections after discharge from the hospital are difficult, and few institutions have developed effective systems. With the surgical load in most hospitals and modern low infection rates, it is not possible to see a statistically significant difference in infection rates over intervals shorter than several months. Infection surveillance can, however, lead to a useful examination of surgical practices. Each infection that is noted should be discussed in the surgical complications meeting and should be categorized as apparently avoidable or apparently unavoidable.[16] If review of the case reveals that any of the known adjunctive measures that reduce wound infection risk were omitted (Table 15–2), then it is an apparently avoidable infection. The goal of surveillance and quality assurance should be to have no avoidable infections.

Immunotherapy

Active and passive immunization to prevent surgical infections has merit in only a few specific instances. Immunotherapy has had outstanding success in preventing tetanus. After a full course of active immunization (full childhood series or

TABLE 15–2. Important Factors in Preventing Wound Infection

Preoperative antimicrobial shower
Hair removal by clipping, not shaving, immediately before operation
Vigilance for breaks in aseptic technique by operating room team
Preventive antibiotics when indicated with therapeutic levels during the entire operative procedure
Limited use of electrocautery for dissection
Limit suture and ligatures
Use monofilament sutures
Closed suction rather than open drainage; no drainage if possible
Meticulous skin closure
High postoperative inspired oxygen
Surveillance of wound infection with review of preventive measures

three doses in adults), most persons are protected against tetanus for years, and many for a lifetime. A booster injection of toxoid invariably elicits protective levels of antibody for as long as 10 years. Adults should receive regular booster toxoid doses at 10-year intervals. When any wound is treated, a patient's immunization status should be reviewed and brought up to date. For those persons who do not have a reliable record of three prior toxoid injections or those who have not had a booster for 10 years, tetanus diphtheria toxoid (Td) should be given. If the wound is clean, no further immunization is needed. If that injection is not the third, then the patient should be scheduled to complete the entire series. Tetanus immune globulin (TIG) is not needed for a clean wound. For dirty or untidy wounds, Td should be given if it has been 5 or more years since the last booster. If the patient has had the complete immunization series in the past, then TIG is not needed. If the patient has not previously received a complete immunization, then TIG should be given at the same time as Td and administered in a different location. At the time of injury, 250 to 500 units of TIG should be administered intramuscularly, with the dose depending on the severity of the injury. If the patient is seen more than 24 hours after injury, the dose should be increased. TIG does not prevent infection with *Clostridium tetani,* but it does inactivate the toxin produced. Careful surgical débridement with removal of all devitalized tissue is the most important way to prevent infection. Administration of systemic antibiotics is of secondary importance and usually unnecessary.

Active and passive immunization for rabies is also highly effective in preventing the disease in exposed patients or those thought to be exposed. The currently available human rabies immune globulin and human diploid cell vaccine are very safe and effective. The use of pooled human gamma-globulin to prevent bacterial infections or treat bacterial infections is not warranted in surgical patients unless they have agammaglobulinemia or a dysgammaglobulinemia.

Reducing the Bacterial Load by Prophylactic Chemotherapy

The use of systemic prophylactic chemotherapeutic and antibiotic agents has been a controversial subject, mostly because of a lack of understanding of the basic principles involved. Experience has shown that the effectiveness of antibiotic treatment depends on the observance and practice of these principles. If they are ignored, the results are haphazard failures. There is little doubt that the administration of therapeutic doses of antimicrobial agents can prevent infection in wounds contaminated by bacteria highly sensitive to the agents. The decision to use prophylactic antibiotic therapy, however, must be based on the weight of evidence for possible benefit against the weight of evidence for possible adverse effects. Indiscriminate or blind use of antibiotics should be discouraged because it may lead to emergence of antibiotic-resistant strains of organisms or serious hypersensitivity reactions. Prolonged use of *prophylactic* antibiotics may also mask the signs of established infections, making diagnosis more difficult.

Prophylactic systemic antibiotics are clearly not indicated for most patients undergoing straightforward clean surgical operations in which no obvious bacterial contamination or insertion of a foreign body has occurred. When the incidence of wound infections is less than 1%, the potential for reducing this low infection rate does not justify the expense and side effects of antibiotic administration. Prophylactic antibiotic therapy is no substitute for careful surgical technique using established surgical principles, and its indiscriminate or general use is not in the best interest of the patient. Antibiotic agents can be used effectively only as adjuvants to adequate surgery.

In several clinical situations the administration of prophylactic systemic antibiotic therapy is usually beneficial. In principle, these situations almost always involve a brief period of contamination by organisms that can be predicted with reasonable accuracy. As examples, prophylactic systemic antibiotics reduce infection with clinical benefit in the following circumstances[13]:

1. High-risk gastroduodenal procedures. These include operations for gastric cancer, ulcer, obstruction, or bleeding; those operations when gastric acid production has been suppressed effectively; and gastric operations for morbid obesity.

2. High-risk biliary procedures. These include operations in patients older than 60 years old and those for acute inflammation, common duct stones, or jaundice and in patients with prior biliary tract operations or endoscopic biliary manipulation.

3. Resection and anastomosis of the colon or small intestine (see later)

4. Cardiac procedures through a median sternotomy

5. Vascular surgery of the lower extremities or abdominal aorta

6. Amputation of an extremity with impaired blood supply, particularly in the presence of a current or recent ischemic ulcer

7. Vaginal or abdominal hysterectomy

8. Primary cesarean section

9. Operations entering the oral pharyngeal cavity in continuity with neck dissections

10. Craniotomy

11. The implantation of any permanent prosthetic material

12. Any wound with known gross bacterial contamination

13. Accidental wounds with heavy contamination and tissue damage. In such instances, the antibiotic should be given intravenously as soon as possible after injury. The two best-studied situations are penetrating abdominal injuries and open fractures.

14. Injuries prone to clostridial infection because of extensive devitalization of muscle, heavy contamination, and/or impairment of blood supply

15. Presence of pre-existing valvular heart damage, to prevent the development of bacterial endocarditis

The administration of oral nonabsorbable antibiotics to suppress both aerobic and anaerobic intestinal bacteria before scheduled operations on the colon has also been successful in controlled trials. Neomycin plus erythromycin given only on the day before surgery, 19, 18, and 9 hours before the scheduled start of the procedure, is the most well-established combination at the present time.[8] Thorough mechanical cleansing of the intestinal tract is a critically important component of the oral regimen. Several reports demonstrate a reduced infection rate with the combination of oral nonabsorbable and intravenous antibiotics, and this is the most common practice among colorectal surgeons in the United States.[22]

Prophylactic antibiotic therapy is clearly more effective when begun preoperatively and continued through the intraoperative period, with the aim of achieving therapeutic blood levels throughout the operative period. This produces therapeutic levels of the antibiotic agents at the operative site in any seromas and hematomas that may develop. Antibiotics started as late as 1 to 2 hours after bacterial contamination are markedly less effective, and it is completely without value to start prophylactic antibiotics after the wound is closed. Failure of prophylactic antibiotic agents occurs in part through a neglect of the importance of the timing and dosage of these agents, which are critical determinants. For most patients with elective surgery, the first dose of prophylactic antibiotics should be given intravenously at the time anesthesia is induced. It is unnecessary and may be detrimental to start them more than 1 hour preoperatively, and it is unnecessary to give them after the patient leaves the operating room. A single dose, depending on the drug used and length of operation, is often sufficient. For operations that are prolonged, the prophylactic agent chosen should be given in repeated doses at intervals of one to two half-lives for the drug being used. It is almost never indicated to give prophylactic antibiotic coverage for more than 12 hours for a planned operation.

Many patients fail to receive needed prophylactic antibiotics because the system for their administration is complex at the time of multiple events just before a major operation. This problem has been made worse by the trend of admitting patients directly to the operating room for planned operations, which intensifies the pressures to accomplish a large number of procedures during a short interval before the operation. The possibility that prophylactic antibiotics will be unintentionally omitted can be minimized by establishing a system with a checklist. One member of the operative team (usually the preoperative nurse or a member of the anesthesia team) is responsible for initialing a portion of the operative record that states either that the patient received indicated prophylactic antibiotics or that the surgeon has determined that antibiotics are not indicated for the procedure.[13]

Many antibiotics effectively reduce the rate of postoperative surgical site infections when used appropriately for indicated procedures. No antibiotic has been reliably superior to another when each possessed a similar and appropriate antibacterial spectrum. The most important determinant is whether the planned procedure is expected to enter parts of the body known to harbor obligate colonic anaerobic bacteria (*Bacteroides* species). If anaerobic flora are anticipated, such as during operations on the colon or distal ileum or during appendectomy, then an agent effective against *Bacteroides* species, such as cefotetan, must be used. Cefoxitin is an alternative with a dramatically shorter half-life. If anaerobic flora are not expected, cefazolin is the prophylactic drug of choice. For patients who are allergic to cephalosporins or in settings where methicillin-resistant *S. aureus* is common, vancomycin can be used. If an intestinal procedure is planned, an agent with activity against gram-negative rods, such as aztreonam or an aminoglycoside, and an agent with activity against anaerobes, such as clindamycin or metronidazole, must also be used.

The use of topical antibiotics often effectively diminishes the incidence of infection in contaminated wounds. However, the combination of topical agents and parenteral agents is not more effective than either one alone, and topical agents alone are inferior to parenteral agents in complex gastric procedures. As a general rule, topical agents do not cause any harm if one adheres to the following rules: (1) do not use any agent in wounds or in the abdomen that would not be suitable for parenteral administration; and (2) do not use more of the agent than would be acceptable for parenteral administration. In considering the amount used, any drug being given parenterally must be added to the amount being placed in the wound. Topical agents used for burn wounds (discussed elsewhere) may be used in large open wounds in selected patients.

Prophylactic antibiotic therapy is generally ineffective in clinical situations in which continuing contamination is likely to occur. Examples are as follows: (l) in patients with tracheostomies or tracheal intubation to prevent pulmonary infections; (2) in patients with indwelling urinary catheters; (3) in patients with indwelling central venous lines; and (4) in most open wounds, including burn wounds.

NATURE, DIAGNOSIS, AND TREATMENT OF SURGICAL INFECTIONS

Surgical infections are distinguished from medical infections by the presence of an anatomic or mechanical problem that must be resolved by operation or other invasive procedure to cure the infection. Such procedures include, but are not limited to, incising and draining an abscess, opening an infected wound, removing an infected foreign body, repairing or diverting a bowel leak, and draining an intra-abdominal abscess with a percutaneous catheter. Antibiotic treatment of a surgical infection without this mechanical solution will not resolve the infection. The most important aspect of the initial approach to a surgical infection is the recognition that operative intervention is required.

Some broad generalizations can be made concerning typical differences between surgical and medical infections. In common community-acquired medical infections, such as primary pneumonia, general host defenses are usually intact. Some exceptions to intact host defenses occur in patients undergoing systemic treatment for malignancy or for transplant rejection and patients with human immunodeficiency virus (HIV) infection. Most surgical infections, in contrast, are the result of damaged host defenses, especially injury to the epithelial barrier that normally protects the sterile internal environment from endogenous and exogenous bacteria. Immunologic defects may be acquired, through either trauma (accidental or surgical) or tumor. Nonmechanical host defense defects are global, caused by nutritional deficiency and/or the systemic effects of trauma.

The pathogens found in medical infections are usually single and aerobic. They either derive from exogenous sources or are present only in a minority of asymptomatic normal hosts. Typically, they possess virulence properties, allowing them to infect invasively despite an intact epithelial barrier. Examples include beta-hemolytic streptococci, *S. pneumoniae*, *Shigella*, *Salmonella*, and *Vibrio cholerae*. The pathogens causing surgical infections, in contrast, are frequently mixed, involving aerobes and anaerobes, and usually originate from the patient's own endogenous flora. These pathogens are opportunistic, often depending on an acquired epithelial defect to cause infection.

Soft Tissue Infections. The distinction between surgical and medical infections in superficial tissues depends on the recognition of dead tissue in surgical infections. The most obvious example of a surgical infection is a subcutaneous abscess, an infectious process characterized by a necrotic center without a blood supply and composed of debris from local tissues, dead and dying white blood cells, components of blood and plasma, and bacteria. This semiliquid central portion (pus) is surrounded by a vascularized zone of in-

flammatory tissue. An abscess will not resolve unless the pus is drained and evacuated. It is recognized clinically as a localized swelling with signs of inflammation and tenderness. An abscess must be distinguished from cellulitis, which is a soft tissue infection with intact blood supply and viable tissue, marked by an acute inflammatory response with small vessel engorgement and stasis, endothelial leakage with interstitial edema, and polymorphonuclear leukocyte infiltration. Cellulitis resolves with appropriate antibiotic therapy alone if treatment is initiated before tissue death occurs.

An abscess may be mistaken for cellulitis when the central necrotic portion is located deep beneath overlying tissue layers and it cannot be readily detected by physical examination. It may also be disguised in anatomic locations where fibrous septa join skin and fascia, dividing subcutaneous tissue into compartments that limit the local expression of fluctuance while leading to high pressures that promote early tissue death. Examples of such infections include perirectal abscesses, breast abscesses, carbuncles on the posterior neck and upper back, and infections in the distal phalanx of the finger (felon).

Knowledge of the local anatomy and pathophysiology of these special abscesses helps provide optimal treatment. A perirectal abscess is often associated with a fistula communicating with the anus at a crypt. A fistula should be sought and, if found, unroofed at the time a perirectal abscess is drained. If a fistula is not found acutely, the surgeon should be alert for its occurrence in the postoperative period. A breast abscess is preferably drained by a circumferential incision in natural skin lines. A felon should be drained through a lateral incision to avoid a painful scar on the pressure-bearing distal pulp. At the time of incision and drainage for a felon, all fibrous septa in the infected pulp must be broken to resolve the infection.

Superficial abscesses on the trunk and head and neck are most commonly caused by *S. aureus*, often combined with streptococci. Abscesses in the axillae often have a prominent gram-negative component. Abscesses below the waist, especially on the perineum, are frequently found to harbor a mixed aerobic and anaerobic gram-negative flora.

Necrotizing Soft Tissue Infections. Necrotizing soft tissue infections, both clostridial and nonclostridial, are less common than subcutaneous abscesses and cellulitis but much more serious conditions whose severity initially may be unrecognized. These infections are marked by the absence of clear local boundaries or palpable limits. This lack of clear boundaries accounts both for the severity of the infection and for the frequent delay in recognizing its surgical nature. Anatomically, these infections are marked by a layer of necrotic tissue, which is not walled off by a surrounding inflammatory reaction and thus does not present a clear boundary. In addition, the overlying skin has a relatively normal appearance in the early stages of infection, and the visible degree of involvement is substantially less than that of the underlying tissues. A clostridial infection typically involves underlying muscle and is termed *clostridial myonecrosis* or *gas gangrene*. Most nonclostridial and some clostridial necrotizing infections spread in the subcutaneous fascia, between the skin and the deep muscular fascia. These infections have been described under a variety of labels but are most commonly called *necrotizing fasciitis* (Table 15–3).

Rapid progression of a soft tissue infection, a marked hemodynamic response to infection, or the failure to respond to conventional nonoperative therapy may be the earliest signs of a necrotizing soft tissue infection. An apparent cellulitis with ecchymoses, bullae, any dermal gangrene, extensive edema, or crepitus suggests an underlying necrotizing infection and mandates operative exploration to confirm the diagnosis and definitively treat the infection. The critical step in

TABLE 15–3. Comparison of Clostridial and Nonclostridial Infections

	Clostridial Myonecrosis	Nonclostridial Necrotizing Infections
Erythema	Usually absent	Present, often mild
Swelling/edema	Mild to moderate	Moderate to severe
Exudate	Thin	"Dishwater" to purulent
White blood cells	Usually absent	Present
Bacteria	Gram-positive rods ± others	Mixed ± gram-positive rods May be gram-positive cocci alone
Advanced signs	Hypesthesia Bronze discoloration Hemorrhagic bullae Dermal gangrene Crepitus	Hypesthesia Ecchymoses Bullae Dermal gangrene Crepitus
Deep involvement	Muscle > skin	Subcutaneous tissue ± fascia ± muscle (uncommon) > skin
Histology	Minimal inflammation Muscle necrosis	Acute inflammation Microabscesses Viable muscle

Physiology	Rapid onset of tachycardia, hypotension, volume deficit
	  ± intravascular hemolysis
		Variable—minimal to tachycardia, hypotension, and
		  volume deficit

Treatment		
General	Aggressive cardiopulmonary resuscitation	Aggressive cardiopulmonary resuscitation
Antibiotics	Penicillin G plus broad spectrum	Third-generation cephalosporin or ciprofloxacin plus antianaerobic agent
Hyperbaric oxygen	If it does not delay other treatment	No

Surgery	Aggressive removal of infected tissue; amputation of
	  extremity often required
		Débridement and exposure; not much removal required;
		  usually no amputation

Antitoxin	No	No

Adapted from Dellinger, E. P.: Crepitus and gangrene. *In* Platt, R., and Kass, E. H. (Eds.): Current Therapy in Infectious Diseases—3, 1990. Philadelphia, B. C. Decker. By permission of Mosby-Year Book, Inc.

diagnosis is to recognize the nonlocalized, necrotizing nature of the infection and the need for operative treatment. This is more important than applying a very specific diagnostic label to the process. Operative treatment requires excision of involved tissues for clostridial myonecrosis. On an extremity this may mean amputation. Nonclostridial infections can often be managed by wide incision and débridement and do not usually require amputation. In either case, all areas of necrotic tissue must be unroofed and débrided, which often produces large disfiguring wounds.

The most common organisms associated with clostridial infections are *Clostridium perfringens, C. novyi,* and *C. septicum.* Other bacteria are commonly found in association with the clostridial organisms. The only bacterium commonly reported as the sole cause of nonclostridial necrotizing soft tissue infections is beta-hemolytic *S. pyogenes.* This is the most common pathogen recovered when no prior injury or operation is the cause of the infection. Postoperative and postinjury cases of necrotizing soft tissue infection are most often caused by mixed bacterial species, including aerobic and anaerobic pathogens, both gram positive and gram negative, a very similar spectrum to that seen in intra-abdominal infections.

Intra-abdominal and Retroperitoneal Infections. Most serious intra-abdominal infections require surgical intervention for resolution. In this context, surgical intervention includes percutaneous drainage of intra-abdominal abscesses. The specific exceptions to the requirement for surgical intervention include pyelonephritis, salpingitis, amebic liver abscess, enteritis (e.g., *Shigella, Yersinia*), spontaneous bacterial peritonitis, some cases of diverticulitis, and some cases of cholangitis. However, all of these *exceptions* can be diagnosed presumptively with a rapid initial evaluation. If the diagnosis of one of these exceptions cannot be made, a patient with fever and abdominal pain should not be given antibiotics without a plan leading to operation or other drainage procedure. The administration of antibiotics in this setting before diagnosis

may obscure subsequent findings and delay diagnosis and will certainly delay definitive operative management. If the patient is too sick to go without antibiotic therapy, he or she is also too sick to avoid operative intervention and definitive diagnosis and treatment.

Despite modern antibiotics and intensive care, mortality from serious intra-abdominal or retroperitoneal infection remains high (5% to 50%) and morbidity is substantial. The systemic response to intra-abdominal or retroperitoneal infection is accompanied by fluid shifts similar to those seen in patients with major burns. Fever, tachycardia, and hypotension are common, and a severe hypermetabolic, catabolic response is universal. If a corrective operation and effective antibiotics are not employed promptly, the sequence of events termed *multiple-organ failure syndrome* may ensue and cause the death of the patient even after the primary focus of infection has been controlled. Regardless of the initial antibiotic choice and operative procedure there is a significant chance that a change in antibiotics may be required and that a reoperation may be necessary. The physician caring for a patient with intra-abdominal infection must be alert to these possibilities and diligent in following and re-examining the patient so this decision can be made at the earliest possible time.[7] Outcome is improved by early diagnosis and treatment. The risk of death and of complications increases with increased age, pre-existing serious underlying diseases, and malnutrition. The risk of death or failure to control the abdominal source of infection is also related to the normal homeostatic balance of the patient at the time of diagnosis and initiation of definitive therapy. This balance can be measured by scales designed to quantitate the number of physical findings and laboratory tests that are abnormal. One of the most widely used scales is the Acute Physiology And Chronic Health Evaluation (APACHE) scoring system.[10] The higher the score, the more abnormal tests and findings are present, and the greater the risk of death.

When a patient is diagnosed with intra-abdominal infec-

TABLE 15–4. Antibiotics with Predominantly Aerobic or Anaerobic Broad-Spectrum Activity

Aerobic Coverage

Gentamicin
Tobramycin
Amikacin
Netilmicin
Cefotaxime
Ceftizoxime
Ceftriaxone
Ceftazidime
Aztreonam
Ciprofloxacin

Anaerobic Coverage

Clindamycin
Metronidazole
Chloramphenicol

tion, initial treatment consists of cardiorespiratory support, antibiotic therapy, and operative intervention. In most cases, the responsible bacteria are not known for at least 24 hours, and sensitivity information is not available for 48 to 72 hours after cultures are obtained during the operative procedure. Because most intra-abdominal infections yield three to five different aerobic and anaerobic pathogens, specific, targeted antibiotic therapy is not possible at first and the initial choice must be empiric, designed to cover a range of possible organisms. In recent years, numerous new antibiotics have widened the available choices. For infections acquired in the community with a small likelihood of resistant gram-negative rods and for a patient not severely ill, empiric therapy can be initiated with cefoxitin, cefotetan, ticarcillin/clavulanate, or ampicillin/sulbactam. For the more severely ill, or a patient who has been in the hospital or has recently been treated with antibiotics, more comprehensive treatment is needed. Imipenem, piperacillin/tazobactam, or a combination chosen from Table 15–4 is useful, taking one antibiotic from the aerobic column and one from the anaerobic column (see later for discussion of specific antibiotics).[4] The choice of empiric antibiotic for other serious infections with a similar spectrum of pathogens, such as necrotizing soft tissue infections, is the same.

Operative Intervention for Intra-abdominal or Retroperitoneal Infection. The goal of operative intervention in patients with intra-abdominal infection is to correct the underlying anatomic problem that either caused the infection or perpetuates it. The cause of peritonitis must be corrected. Foreign material in the peritoneal cavity that inhibits white blood cell function and promotes bacterial growth (feces, food, bile, mucin, blood) must be removed. Large deposits of fibrin that entrap bacteria, allowing bacterial growth and preventing phagocytosis, should be removed.[15]

An intra-abdominal or retroperitoneal abscess requires drainage. In prior years this nearly always required an open operation. Computed tomographic scans provide precise localization of intra-abdominal abscesses, permitting selected abscesses to be drained percutaneously under radiologic or ultrasound guidance. If the abscess is single and has a straight path to the abdominal wall that does not transgress bowel (Fig. 15–1A), it can be drained percutaneously. This is accomplished by needle puncture with aspiration of a small sample of pus to confirm the location and diagnosis. Subsequently, a floppy guide wire is passed through the needle, which is then removed. The guide wire allows dilation of the tract, followed by placement of a drainage catheter. The progress of abscess closure can be followed by plain radiographs after instillation of contrast materials (Fig. 15–1B). If percutaneous drainage is not successful, an open operation may be required.[18]

If a patient has multiple abscesses or abscesses combined with underlying disease that requires operative correction, or if a safe percutaneous route to the abscess is not present, then open, operative drainage may be required. A single abscess in the subphrenic or subhepatic position may be drained by an extraperitoneal subcostal or posterior twelfth-rib approach, which provides open drainage without exposing the entire peritoneal cavity to the abscess contents. Likewise, most retroperitoneal abscesses should be drained from a retroperitoneal approach. However, most pancreatic *abscesses*, which, in reality, more often consist of diffusely infected, necrotic, peripancreatic retroperitoneal tissue, require transabdominal operation and débridement.[23] A pelvic abscess may be amenable to transrectal or transvaginal drainage. Retroperitoneal phlegmon (necrotizing cellulitis) is a rare condition, usually associated with extravasation of infected urine, which requires extensive débridement similar to that used to treat necrotizing fasciitis.

Postoperative Fever. Approximately 2% of all primary laparotomies are followed by an unscheduled operation for intra-abdominal infection, and roughly 50% of all serious intra-abdominal infections are postoperative.[11] Wound infections are more common but less serious. Postoperative fever occurs frequently and may be a source of concern to physician and patient. Fever is associated with infection, and the empiric

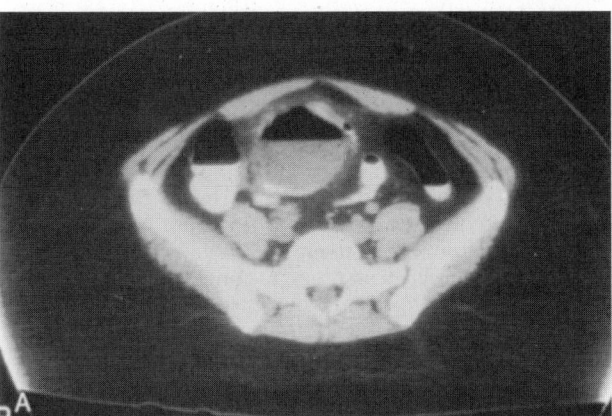
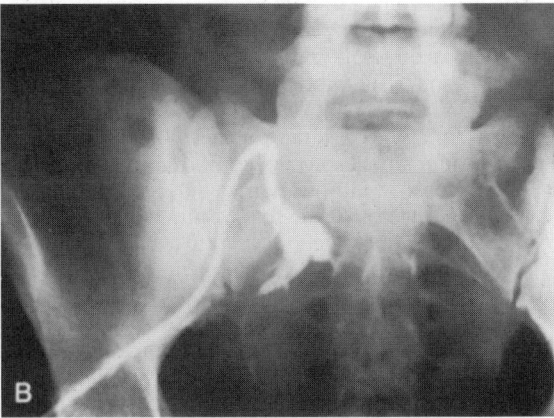

Figure 15–1. *A,* Computed tomographic scan demonstrating a right lower quadrant abscess containing gas, fluid, and barium in a young woman with 3 days of abdominal pain and fever and right lower quadrant tenderness. A mass was not palpable, probably because of marked obesity. *B,* A sinogram obtained after contrast injection into a percutaneous catheter placed 7 days earlier in the same patient.

prescription of antibiotics is a common response to this phenomenon. However, most febrile postoperative patients are not infected, and indeed a significant proportion of infected patients may not be febrile, depending on the definition of *fever*. Because fever is common in the absence of infection, it is important to consider causes of postoperative fever other than infection and to make a presumptive diagnosis before instituting antibiotic treatment.[9]

The most common nonsurgical causes of postoperative infection and fever, urinary tract infection, respiratory tract infection, and intravenous catheter-associated infection, are all readily diagnosed. The other important causes of postoperative infection and fever, wound infection and intra-abdominal infection, require operative treatment and are not properly managed with antibiotics in the absence of operative treatment. The most sensitive test for detecting infection and determining its location continues to be history taking and physical examination conducted by a conscientious physician. Supportive laboratory and x-ray evaluation, including white blood cell count, blood cultures, and computed tomography, can supplement the physical examination. Fever in the first 3 days after operation most likely has a noninfectious cause. However, when the fever starts 5 or more days postoperatively, the incidence of wound infections exceeds the incidence of undiagnosed fevers. Neither the prolongation of perioperative prophylactic antibiotics nor the initiation of empiric therapeutic antibiotics is indicated without a presumptive clinical diagnosis and a plan for operative intervention when needed.

Only two important infectious causes of fever are likely in the first 36 hours after a laparotomy. Both can be diagnosed readily if they are suspected and appropriate examinations are made. The first is an injury to bowel with intraperitoneal leak. This is characterized by marked hemodynamic changes—first tachycardia and then hypotension and a falling urine output. Fluid requirements are large, and physical examination reveals diffuse abdominal tenderness. The other early cause of fever and infection is an invasive soft tissue infection, beginning in the wound, caused either by beta-hemolytic streptococci or by clostridial species (most commonly *C. perfringens*). This event is diagnosed by inspection of the wound and Gram stain of wound fluid, which shows either gram-positive cocci or gram-positive rods. White blood cells are usually absent with streptococcal infections but may be absent in cases of clostridial infection.

Nonsurgical Infections in Surgical Patients. Postoperative patients are at increased risk for a variety of nonsurgical postoperative nosocomial infections.[12] The most common of these is urinary tract infection. Any patient who has had an indwelling urinary catheter is at increased risk for a urinary tract infection. Despite the benign course of most urinary tract infections, the occurrence of one in a surgical patient is associated with a threefold increase in death occurring during hospitalization. The best prevention is to use urinary catheters sparingly and for specific indications and to employ strict closed drainage techniques for those that are used.

Lower respiratory tract infections are the third most common cause of nosocomial infection in surgical patients and are the leading cause of death due to nosocomial infection. Diagnosis is usually relatively straightforward in a patient who is breathing spontaneously. However, a patient who is intubated and being ventilated because of adult respiratory distress syndrome presents an extremely difficult diagnostic problem. Patients with this syndrome commonly have abnormal chest x-ray findings, abnormal blood gas values, and elevated temperatures and white blood cell counts even in the absence of infection. Both false-positive and false-negative diagnosis of pneumonia is common. A surgeon faced with a postoperative patient with fever frequently considers pneumonia or atelectasis in the differential diagnosis. One should remember, however, that after an abdominal operation, one of the most common causes of lower lung field atelectasis and/or pleural effusion is an inflammatory process below the diaphragm.

Prosthetic Device–Associated Infections. As the ability to replace parts of the body has increased, so has the potential for infectious complications associated with these replacement parts. Some of the most significant complications associated with vascular grafts, cardiac valves, pacemakers, and artificial joints are caused by infections at the site of implantation. The presence of the foreign material (the prosthetic device) impairs local host defenses, especially polymorphonuclear leukocyte function. Accordingly, most such infections resist treatment short of removing the offending device. Morbidity and mortality associated with infection is high. Some success can be obtained by intensive antibiotic therapy, removal of the infected device under antibiotic cover, and replacement with a new uninfected device followed by prolonged antibiotic treatment. This approach is warranted when the device is life sustaining, as in the case of a cardiac valve.

PATHOGENS IN SURGICAL INFECTIONS

This discussion of pathogens commonly responsible for surgical infections is not intended to be a complete review. Rather, it focuses on some broad distinctions and classifications that help organize the vast body of data concerning the usual bacterial flora of different surgical infections and the antibiotic susceptibility patterns of these pathogens. Bacteria important in surgical infections are broadly divided into aerobic and facultative bacteria in one group and anaerobic bacteria in the other; into gram-positive and gram-negative bacteria; and into bacilli (rods) and cocci.

Gram-Positive Cocci. Gram-positive cocci of importance to surgeons include staphylococci and streptococci. Staphylococci are divided into coagulase-positive and coagulase-negative strains. Coagulase-positive staphylococci are *S. aureus* and are the most common pathogen associated with infections in wounds and incisions not subject to endogenous contamination. In the 1990s most coagulase-positive staphylococci should be assumed resistant to penicillin and require treatment by a penicillinase-resistant antibiotic. Extensive use of penicillinase-resistant beta-lactam antibiotics over the past two decades has encouraged the emergence of methicillin-resistant staphylococci. These organisms do not seem to have intrinsic pathogenicity greater than that of other staphylococci, but they are more difficult to treat because of antibiotic resistance. The prevalence of methicillin-resistant staphylococci varies considerably by geographic region. These organisms are especially common in cases of endocarditis associated with intravenous drug use. Methicillin-resistant staphylococci must be treated with vancomycin or a similar agent.

For many years, coagulase-negative staphylococci were considered contaminants and skin flora incapable of causing serious disease. However, in the correct clinical setting, coagulase-negative staphylococci can cause serious disease. This is most common in patients who have been compromised by trauma, extensive surgery, or metabolic disease and who have invasive vascular devices in place. Coagulase-negative staphylococci are the most common organisms recovered in nosocomial bacteremia and are frequently associated with clinically significant infections of intravascular devices. Coagulase-negative staphylococci are also found in endocarditis, prosthetic joint infections, vascular graft infections, and postsurgical mediastinitis. Most coagulase-negative staphylococci are methicillin resistant. Although most of these infections associated with intravascular devices are cured simply by removing the device, if empiric antibiotic therapy is indicated, vancomycin should be chosen.

The streptococcal species include beta-hemolytic streptococci, *S. pneumoniae*, and other alpha-hemolytic streptococci. These species used to be uniformly sensitive to penicillin G and almost all other beta-lactam antibiotics. Penicillin-resistant *S. pneumoniae* are now found in most urban communities. The beta-hemolytic streptococci alone, although not commonly recovered from soft tissue wounds, can cause life-threatening infections. *S. pneumoniae* is a common cause of community-acquired pneumonia but is a less common pathogen in hospitalized surgical patients. The other alpha-hemolytic streptococci or viridans streptococci rarely are significant pathogens in a surgical setting. They are commonly found on mucous membranes and skin and may be recovered from the peritoneal cavity after upper gastrointestinal perforations but are almost never found as the sole cause of significant surgical infections.

The precise significance of enterococci in surgical infections is controversial.[3] Enterococci are commonly recovered as part of a mixed flora in intra-abdominal infections. It is rare to recover enterococci alone from a surgical infection. In animal models of infection, enterococci clearly can increase the virulence of other bacteria. Enterococcal bacteremia in association with a surgical infection carries a grave prognosis. The occurrence of the bacteremia itself probably signals a profound compromise of host defenses. Enterococci clearly do cause significant disease in the urinary tract and the biliary tract and probably contribute to morbidity and mortality from intra-abdominal infections in high-risk patients with serious underlying diseases or protracted illnesses with impairment of host defenses. One recent report of patients with intra-abdominal infection found a significantly higher treatment failure rate in patients who had initial isolation of enterococci. The stimulus for discussing the pathogenic significance of enterococci derives from the relative resistance of these species to antibiotic therapy. No single antibiotic is reliably effective for eradicating deep-seated infections or bacteremia. The most effective antibiotic combination for treating enterococcal infections is gentamicin combined with either ampicillin (or another advanced-generation penicillin) or vancomycin. However, enterococci resistant to all known antibiotics including gentamicin and vancomycin have been isolated in increasing numbers in most major medical centers in the United States.

Aerobic and Facultative Gram-Negative Rods. A great variety of gram-negative rods are associated with surgical infections. Most fall into the family Enterobacteriaceae. These are all facultative anaerobic bacteria and include the familiar genera *Escherichia*, *Proteus*, and *Klebsiella*. These three genera (*easy* gram-negative rods) are considered together because they are relatively common in mixed surgical infections and because they are relatively sensitive to a broad variety of antibiotics, especially first- and second-generation cephalosporins. Other genera within the Enterobacteriaceae that are also common in surgical infections include *Enterobacter*, *Morganella*, *Providencia*, and *Serratia*. These genera (*difficult* gram-negative rods) commonly exhibit greater intrinsic antimicrobial resistance. Empiric antibiotic therapy directed at these organisms requires a third-generation cephalosporin, one of the expanded-spectrum penicillins, a monobactam, carbapenem, quinolone, or aminoglycoside. These organisms are more common in hospital-acquired and postoperative surgical infections. Gram-negative rods recovered from infections originating in the community, such as uncomplicated appendicitis, are less likely to involve antibiotic-resistant strains.

Obligate aerobic gram-negative rods that are often found in surgical infections include *Pseudomonas* species and *Acineto-*

bacter species. These organisms are most commonly found in hospital-associated pneumonias in surgical patients but may also be recovered from the peritoneal cavity or severe soft tissue infections. These species are often antibiotic resistant and require treatment with specific antipseudomonal antibiotics such as ceftazidime, aztreonam, imipenem, ciprofloxacin, an acylureido-penicillin, or an aminoglycoside. *Acinetobacter* species are resistant to aztreonam. A significant proportion of these species exhibit strains resistant even to the most effective antibiotics, and patients with such pathogens are probably best treated empirically with two antibiotics before *in vitro* susceptibility testing becomes available. Even after susceptibility data are known, critically ill patients may benefit from treatment with two effective agents. Bacteria from both of these genera have a tendency to develop resistance to antibiotics during therapy. Although using two agents may not reduce this process, it does leave the patient with at least one effective drug when it occurs.

Anaerobes. Anaerobic bacteria are the most numerous inhabitants of the normal gastrointestinal tract, including the mouth. The most common anaerobic isolate from surgical infections is *Bacteroides fragilis*. *B. fragilis* and *B. thetaiotaomicron* are two common anaerobic species with significant resistance to many beta-lactam antibiotics. The most effective antibiotics against these species are metronidazole, clindamycin, chloramphenicol, imipenem, and the combinations of a pencillin and a beta-lactamase inhibitor (ticarcillin/clavulanate, ampicillin/sulbactam, and piperacillin/tazobactam). Other anaerobic species commonly recovered from surgical infections but with less significant bacterial resistance patterns include *Bacteroides melaninogenicus* and most of the anaerobic cocci.

The other important genus of anaerobic bacteria found in surgical infections is *Clostridium*, previously mentioned in the discussion of necrotizing soft tissue infections. Although they can survive for variable periods while exposed to oxygen, they require an anaerobic environment for growth and invasion and for elaboration of the toxins that account for their dramatic virulence in soft tissue infections. The *Clostridium* species are all gram-positive, spore-forming rods. However, when present in human infections they do not form spores, so gram-stained material from a soft tissue infection shows gram-positive rods without spores. *C. tetani* is responsible for tetanus. The prevention of tetanus is accomplished solely through active and passive immunization, not through antibiotic administration.

Anaerobic bacteria have a special importance in relation to surgical infections. These strains grow only in settings with a low oxidation-reduction potential, which is incompatible with the survival of mammalian tissue. Thus, the recovery of anaerobes from a soft tissue infection or even from the blood implies their growth and multiplication in a focus of dead tissue. The predominant source of anaerobic bacteria is the gastrointestinal tract; thus, an anaerobic infection implies a defect in the anatomic integrity of the gastrointestinal tract. Both of these conditions require surgical correction, so the great majority of anaerobic infections (other than lung abscess) require surgical intervention. Certainly an anaerobic bacteremia should always prompt a search for an abscess or for an enteric lesion that requires surgical intervention.

Fungi. Fungi are infrequently the primary pathogens in deep-seated surgical infections. Pathogens from the *Candida* genus, however, may be seen frequently as an opportunistic invader in patients with serious surgical infections who have received broad-spectrum antibiotic treatment suppressing normal endogenous flora. These infections are best avoided through judicious use of systemic broad-spectrum antibiotics and through prophylaxis with oral nystatin or ketoconazole when broad-spectrum antibacterial therapy is required. *Can-*

dida species recovered from open wounds usually represent contamination, not true invasion. Recovery of *Candida* species from peptic ulcer perforations also does not usually require treatment. However, recovery of *Candida* from an established intra-abdominal abscess or from urine and sputum in an otherwise compromised patient may warrant therapy. Intra-abdominal *Candida* infections are more common in association with infections after severe pancreatitis. Therapy for *Candida* infections in this setting is commonly more successful with lower doses of amphotericin than the doses used for systemic medical fungal infections with pathogens such as *Cryptococcus, Blastomyces,* or *Histoplasma.* Surgical patients with fungal colonization of multiple sites or with fungi in well-drained abscesses have been managed successfully with total doses of amphotericin, ranging from 3 to 5 mg. per kg. administered over 10 to 14 days. Although there are fewer data regarding the efficacy of fluconazole in treating surgical *Candida* infections, there are reports of its successful use.

Viruses. Viruses do not cause any infections that require operation for resolution and thus are not discussed in any detail here. As a result of immune suppression to prevent rejection, transplant patients are at significant risk of viral infection, especially with cytomegalovirus. The viral infections of most relevance to routine surgical patients are the bloodborne viruses that may be transmitted through blood transfusion: the hepatitis B virus (HBV), the hepatitis C virus (HCV), and HIV. Transmission of HBV and HIV is unusual because of the use of accurate tests for screening infected units of blood. Previously, HCV was one of the most common viruses transmitted by transfusion in the medical setting, but a new serologic test for HCV has greatly reduced that risk. Cytomegalovirus is also commonly transmitted by transfusions. However, other bloodborne viruses (including hepatitis non-A, non-B) are likely to be described in the future. Therefore, it is good medical practice to limit blood transfusion to circumstances clearly requiring it.

ANTIBIOTICS

This discussion of antibiotics is not intended to be exhaustive. Rather, it focuses on the antibiotics that are most commonly indicated in the treatment of patients with surgical infections. Table 15–5 lists these antibiotics with their relative half-lives, important toxicities, and general antibacterial spectra. Several handy references are updated yearly and provide more detailed information regarding all commercially available antibiotics, including doses and dose ranges, pharmacokinetic data, sensitivity patterns, incompatibilities, and excretion data.[21] One of the largest and most versatile classes of antibiotics is the beta-lactam group. Penicillin G was the prototype of this group, which now includes the penicillins, the cephalosporins, the carbapenems, and the monobactams. All of these antibiotics possess the four-membered beta-lactam ring (Fig. 15–2). All but the monobactams have another ring attached and all have various side chains that determine their antibacterial activity, enzyme stability, and pharmacokinetic characteristics (see Fig. 15–2). All of this group act on bacteria by binding to one of several penicillin-binding proteins and interfering with bacterial cell wall synthesis.

Penicillins. The penicillins are broadly divided into those that are stable against staphylococcal penicillinase and all others. The antistaphylococcal penicillins are active against methicillin-susceptible staphylococcal species but have reduced activity against streptococcal species and essentially no activity against gram-negative rods or anaerobic bacteria. All the remaining penicillins are readily hydrolyzed by staphylococcal penicillinase and are therefore unreliable for treating staphylococcal infections. They all have excellent activity against other gram-positive cocci except for enterococci,

which are variably resistant. The major difference among these penicillins is in their spectrum of aerobic and facultative gram-negative rod activity. The more advanced acylureido-penicillins are very active against this group, including the *difficult* gram-negative rods.

Recently, various penicillins have been combined with one of the beta-lactamase inhibitors, clavulanic acid, sulbactam, or tazobactam. These combinations provide antibiotic compounds that retain their broad gram-negative activity while also acting against methicillin-sensitive staphylococci and anaerobes, facultative species, and aerobic bacteria that are resistant to the penicillins by virtue of beta-lactamase production. The beta-lactamases produced by some *Escherichia coli,* and by *Pseudomonas* species, *Enterobacter* species, *Citrobacter* species, and *Serratia* species, however, are not susceptible to these inhibitors, so these organisms are not susceptible to antibiotic combinations that rely on beta-lactamase inhibition unless they are susceptible to the antibiotic alone.

Cephalosporins. The cephalosporin class is the largest and most frequently used group of antibiotics. It is commonly divided into three *generations,* but there are also important differences between members within each generation. The first-generation cephalosporins have excellent activity against methicillin-susceptible staphylococci and all streptococcal species, but not against enterococci. No cephalosporin in any generation has reliable activity against enterococci, and indeed many cephalosporins seem to encourage enterococcal overgrowth. The first-generation cephalosporins also have modest activity against the *easy* Enterobacteriaceae, such as *E. coli, Proteus mirabilis,* and many *Klebsiella* species. The only important difference between members of the first generation is in half-life. Cefazolin, with its longer half-life, can be given every 8 hours rather than every 4 to 6 hours and maintains more reliable serum and tissue levels when used for prophylaxis than do the other members of this class.

The second-generation cephalosporins have expanded gram-negative activity when compared with the first generation but still lack activity against many gram-negative rods. They can be used when susceptibility patterns are known or when community-acquired infections with a low probability of antibiotic-resistant bacteria are being treated. This class of antibiotics is not reliable for empiric treatment of hospital-acquired gram-negative rod infections. The most important distinction within the second generation is between those antibiotics with good activity against anaerobes (cefoxitin, cefotetan, and cefmetazole) and those without important anaerobic activity (cefamandole, ceforanide, and cefonicid). Within each of these groups are antibiotics with relatively short half-lives (cefamandole and cefoxitin) and with relatively long half-lives (cefotetan, cefmetazole, ceforanide, and cefonicid).

The third-generation cephalosporins have greatly expanded activity against gram-negative rods, including many resistant strains, and rival the aminoglycosides in their coverage while having a much more favorable safety profile. In exchange for this gram-negative coverage, most members of this group have significantly less activity against staphylococci and streptococcal species than first- and second-generation cephalosporins. Anaerobic coverage is, generally, rather poor as well. The important distinction in the third-generation cephalosporins is between those with significant activity against *Pseudomonas* species (cefoperazone and ceftazidime) and those without (cefotaxime, ceftizoxime, and ceftriaxone).

Monobactams. Aztreonam is the only currently available member of the class of monobactams. It has gram-negative coverage, including most *Pseudomonas* species, similar to the aminoglycosides, and like the aminoglycosides lacks significant activity against gram-positive cocci and anaerobes. It also lacks activity against most *Acinetobacter* species. It has

TABLE 15–5. Characteristics of Antibiotics Used to Treat Surgical Infections

Drug Class and Name	Comment	Half-Life*	Toxicity	Antibacterial Spectrum
Penicillins				
Penicillin G	Prototype; hydrolyzed by all beta-lactamases	Short	Low, but rarely allergic reaction may be life threatening	Streptococcal species except enterococcus; *Neisseria* species, except lactamase-producing gonococci
Antistaphylococcal				
Methicillin	First antistaphylococcal drug	Short	Interstitial nephritis	Staphylococcal species (methicillin sensitive) and streptococcal species except enterococcus.
Oxacillin		Short	Interstitial nephritis	Narrow spectrum; usually used for staphylococcal infections
Nafcillin		Short	Interstitial nephritis	only
"Easy" gram-negative				
Ampicillin	Hydrolyzed by all beta-lactamases	Low	Diarrhea and rashes	Streptococcal species including many enterococcus, *Neisseria* species (non–lactamase producing),
Amoxicillin		Medium		*Haemophilus influenzae* (non–lactamase producing), some *Escherichia coli* and *Proteus mirabilis*
Expanded spectrum				
Carbenicillin	Hydrolyzed by all beta-lactamases	Short	High sodium load. Inhibition of platelet aggregation	Greatly expanded gram-negative spectrum while still active against streptococcal species including enterococcus. Moderate antianaerobe activity. May not be reliable as sole agent for established gram-negative rod infections.
Ticarcillin	Same	Short		Same, but less activity against enterococcus
Very advanced spectrum				
Mezlocillin	Hydrolyzed by all beta-lactamases	Short	Low	Same as expanded-spectrum penicillins with more activity against *Pseudomonas, Acinetobacter,* and *Serratia* species.
Piperacillin	Same	Short	Low	Same
Beta-Lactamase Inhibitor Combination				
Clavulanic acid plus			Low; same as constituent beta-lactam	Same as ticarcillin or amoxicillin plus *Staphylococcus* (methicillin sensitive), lactamase-positive *Haemophilus influenzae,* and some lactamase-producing gram-negative rods and anaerobes.
Ticarcillin		Short		
Amoxicillin	Oral only	Medium		
Sulbactam plus				
Ampicillin	Intravenous only	Short		Similar to cefoxitin with activity against enterococcus
Tazobactam plus				
Piperacillin		Short		Similar to piperacillin plus *Staphylococcus* (methicillin sensitive), some lactamase-producing gram-negative rods and anaerobes

Table continued on following page

TABLE 15–5. Characteristics of Antibiotics Used to Treat Surgical Infections *Continued*

Drug Class and Name	Comment	Half-Life*	Toxicity	Antibacterial Spectrum
Cephalosporins				
"First" generation				Streptococcal species except enterococcus, staphylococcal species (methicillin sensitive), and "easy" gram-negative rods
Short half-life				
Cephalothin	Prototype of class	Short	Low	
Cephapirin		Short	Low	
Longer half-life				
Cefazolin		Medium		
"Second" generation				Same as first-generation cephalosporins with expanded gram-negative activity not including *Pseudomonas, Acinetobacter,* or *Serratia*
Poor anaerobic activity				
Shorter half-life				
Cefamandole		Short	Low	
Cefuroxime		Medium	Low	
Longer half-life				
Ceforanide				
Cefonicid	Reduced antistaphylococcal activity			
Good anaerobic activity				Same as above, plus most anaerobes
Short half-life				
Cefoxitin		Short	Low	
Longer half-life				
Cefmetazole		Medium	Low	
Cefotetan		Long	Prolonged prothrombin times	
"Third" generation				Very active against most gram-negative rods except *Pseudomonas, Acinetobacter,* and *Serratia.* Poor against anaerobes. Less activity against streptococcal and staphylococcal species than first- and second-generation cephalosporins.
Poor *Pseudomonas* activity				
Short half-life				
Cefotaxime		Short	Low	
Ceftizoxime		Medium	Low	
Long half-life				
Ceftriaxone		Long	Low	
Good *Pseudomonas* activity				Same as above plus activity against many *Pseudomonas, Acinetobacter,* and *Serratia* species.
Cefoperazone		Medium	Low	
Ceftazidime		Medium	Low	
Monobactams				
Aztreonam	Safe for most patients with penicillin allergy	Short	Low	Excellent activity against most gram-negative organisms, including *Pseudomonas* and *Serratia.* Inactive against gram-positive cocci, anaerobes, and most *Acinetobacter* strains.
Carbapenems				
Imipenem	Provided combined with cilastatin to prevent renal breakdown and renal toxicity	Short	Low; seizures in certain high-risk patients	Extremely broad gram-positive and gram-negative aerobic and anaerobic. Modest activity against enterococcus. Inactive against *Stenotrophomonas* (formerly *Xanthomonas) maltophilia.*
Quinolones				
Norfloxacin	Oral only; urine levels only	Long	Low	Very broad gram-negative activity
Ciprofloxacin		Long	Interaction leads to accumulation of theophylline	Gram-positive and very broad gram-negative activity, including *Pseudomonas, Acinetobacter,* and *Serratia.*
Ofloxacin		Long		

Drug	Spectrum of Activity	Toxicity	Half-life*	Route
Aminoglycosides	Extremely broad coverage of gram-negative rods. Poor activity against streptococci. Some synergism with penicillin or vancomycin against enterococci. No activity against anaerobes.	Nephrotoxicity and eighth nerve toxicity, both auditory and vestibular	Medium	All have low ratio of therapeutic/toxic levels. All are frequently underdosed. All exhibit significant postantibiotic effect.†
Gentamicin	Most active against enterococci and *Serratia*.	See above	Medium	See above
Tobramycin	More active against *Pseudomonas*.	Statistically but questionably clinically significant decrease in nephrotoxicity	Medium	See above
Amikacin	Active against a significant number of gentamicin- and tobramycin-resistant organisms.	See above (aminoglycosides)	Medium	See above
Netilmycin	See above (aminoglycosides)	See above (aminoglycosides)	Medium	See above
Other				
Antianaerobes				
Chloramphenicol	Many gram-positive and easy gram-negative rods. *Haemophilus influenzae*, most anaerobes.	Dose-dependent, reversible bone marrow suppression Rare (1/25,000–40,000) irreversible bone marrow aplasia	Long‡	Oral or intravenous
Clindamycin	Streptococcal species except enterococci, staphylococci, most anaerobes. Inactive against gram-negative rods.		Long‡	Oral or intravenous
Metronidazole	Very active against most anaerobes. Inactive against facultative and aerobic bacteria. Active against protozoa (amebae and *Giardia*).	Disulfiram-type (Antabuse) reaction. Peripheral neuropathy with prolonged use	Long‡	Oral or intravenous
Glycopeptides				
Vancomycin	Streptococcal species, including many enterococci, staphylococci (including methicillin-resistant strains), *Clostridium* species. No activity against gram-negative rods.	Hypertension and histamine release phenomena (Redman syndrome) during infusion. Nephrotoxicity and ototoxicity	Long	
Macrolides				
Erythromycin	Most gram-positive *Neisseria, Campylobacter, Mycoplasma, Chlamydia, Rickettsia, Legionella*	Cholestasis with estolate (intravenous) form	Medium	Oral or intravenous
Tetracyclines				
Tetracycline	Many gram-positive, easy gram-negative rods, some anaerobes, *Rickettsia, Chlamydia, Mycoplasma*	Stain teeth of children	Long	Oral or intravenous
Doxycycline		Same	Very long	Oral or intravenous
Antifungal				
Amphotericin	Most fungi	Nephrotoxicity, fever and chills	Very long	Oral or intravenous
Ketoconazole	Most fungi		Long	Oral only
Fluconazole	Most fungi except *Candida krusei*.		Long	Oral or intravenous

*Drugs have been grouped into those with short, medium, and long half-lives. Short half-life drugs usually have a half-life of 1 hour or less and are commonly administered every 3 to 6 hours, depending on the severity of the infection and the sensitivity of the pathogen. Medium half-life drugs usually have half-lives of 1 to 2 hours and are administered every 6 to 12 hours, most commonly every 8 hours. Long half-life drugs have half-lives longer than 2 hours and are usually administered every 12 to 24 hours. Amphotericin with a half-life of approximately 24 hours can be administered every other day.

†Postantibiotic effect is the effect of certain antibiotics that results in inhibition of bacterial growth for several hours *after* the antibiotic levels have fallen below the minimal inhibitory concentration.

‡Chloramphenicol, clindamycin, and metronidazole all have half-lives greater than 2 hours but traditionally have been administered at 6- to 8-hour intervals.

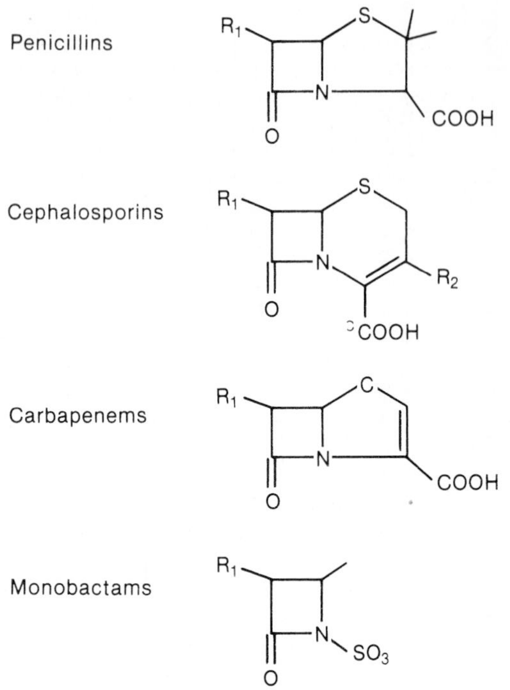

Penicillins

Cephalosporins

Carbapenems

Monobactams

Figure 15–2. The four-member beta-lactam ring. R_1, R_2, side chains.

the safety profile of other beta-lactam antibiotics but does not cross react in patients who are allergic to penicillins or cephalosporins.

Carbapenems. Imipenem is the first representative of the class of carbapenems. It has probably the broadest spectrum of antibacterial activity of any antibiotic currently available. It has excellent activity against all gram-positive cocci except for methicillin-resistant staphylococci and only modest activity against enterococci. It is very active against all anaerobic bacteria. It has broad activity against gram-negative rods, including most *Pseudomonas* species, but it is inactive against *Pseudomonas cepacia* and *Stenotrophomonas maltophilia* (formerly *Xanthomonas maltophilia)*, and strains of indole-positive *Proteus* are often resistant. As with all other antibiotics, *Pseudomonas* species have an unfortunate propensity to develop resistance during treatment. Imipenem is provided only in combination with the enzyme inhibitor cilastatin, which prevents its hydrolysis in the kidneys and resultant nephrotoxicity. The second carbapenem, meropenem, which is given without a renal enzyme inhibitor, has been released in Europe but not in the United States. Its spectrum of activity is similar to that of imipenem.

Quinolones. The quinolone class of antibiotics was long represented solely by nalidixic acid, useful only for urinary tract infections. More recently, a large number of newer fluoroquinolone antibiotics have been in development, with three currently available. As a class, the fluoroquinolones are marked by extremely broad activity against gram-negative rods, including *Pseudomonas* species. Most also have relatively broad activity against gram-positive cocci, including some methicillin-resistant staphylococci, although there is insufficient clinical information to recommend their routine use against methicillin-resistant staphylococci. Activity against anaerobes is mixed but generally not impressive. The currently available members of this class are norfloxacin, which has useful levels only in the urine, and ciprofloxacin and ofloxacin, which are effective against sensitive pathogens throughout the body. The fluoroquinolones are distinguished by excellent tissue penetration and comparable serum and tissue levels with either intravenous or oral administration.

Aminoglycosides. For many years the aminoglycoside class of antibiotics was the only reliable class of drugs for the empiric treatment of serious gram-negative infections. The availability of third-generation cephalosporins, advanced-generation penicillins, monobactams, carbapenems, and now fluoroquinolones has greatly reduced the instances when aminoglycosides must be used. As a class, aminoglycosides have very broad activity against aerobic and facultative gram-negative rods. They have relatively indifferent activity against gram-positive cocci but are an important component of synergistic therapy against enterococci when combined with a penicillin or vancomycin. Aminoglycosides have no activity against anaerobes or against facultative bacteria in an anaerobic environment.

Clinically, aminoglycosides are difficult to use because the ratio of therapeutic levels to toxic levels is low, approximately 2:3. The primary toxicities are nephrotoxicity and eighth nerve damage, both auditory and vestibular. Aminoglycosides distribute in interstitial fluid, a body compartment that varies significantly with disease and is greatly enlarged in patients with life-threatening infections. Therefore, aminoglycoside doses and intervals of administration need to be tailored to the individual patient, and the results must be confirmed by determination of serum levels. No nomogram or dosing scheme has been sufficiently reliable to recommend without this testing. In routine clinical practice it has been far more common to find inadequate levels of aminoglycosides than toxic levels. Because of these difficulties, many clinicians now reserve aminoglycosides for specific therapy for known resistant organisms or as part of a synergistic combination to treat serious enterococcal infections or certain gram-negative rod infections. More recent data suggest that once-daily administration of aminoglycosides is as effective as the more traditional twice or three times per day administration and is less toxic.[19]

Antianaerobes. The antibiotics with important antianaerobic activity are not logically grouped except by this characteristic. The oldest effective antianaerobe drug is chloramphenicol. It is still very active against most anaerobic pathogens by *in vitro* testing but is uncommonly used because of its potential for bone marrow toxicity. Clindamycin possesses excellent activity against most anaerobic bacteria as well as most gram-positive bacteria. Its complete lack of activity against gram-negative aerobic and facultative rods means that it must be used in combination with another antibiotic to cover the pathogens that commonly accompany anaerobes in clinical infections.

Metronidazole currently possesses the most complete activity against all anaerobic pathogens. However, it has no activity against any aerobic or facultative pathogens, either gram negative or gram positive, so it must always be combined with another antibiotic for complete coverage. Because it has no activity against the gram-positive cocci, as clindamycin does, its combination with aztreonam in the treatment of mixed aerobic and anaerobic infections leaves this potentially important group of pathogens uncovered. For this reason, metronidazole is theoretically better combined with a third-generation cephalosporin or a fluoroquinolone. Metronidazole is active against *Clostridium difficile.* Other antibiotics with important antianaerobic activity, including cefoxitin, cefotetan, the penicillin–beta-lactamase inhibitor combinations, and imipenem, are discussed elsewhere.

Macrolides. Erythromycin is a macrolide antibiotic with only modest antianaerobic activity in the concentrations that can be achieved systemically. It has found widespread use, however, as an oral agent (erythromycin base) used in combination with an aminoglycoside to reduce numbers of bacteria in the lumen of the bowel before operations on the colon. In the concentrations achieved within the lumen of the colon, it markedly suppresses anaerobic growth. Erythromycin is also active against most gram-positive cocci and *Neisseria* species. For this reason it is sometimes used as an alternate agent for patients allergic to penicillins. In addition, it has significant activity against mycoplasmas, *Chlamydia, Legionella* species, and *Rickettsia*. It is also an effective antibiotic against *Campylobacter jejuni*. Clarithromycin and azithromycin are two more recent macrolides with expanded antimicrobial spectra that are available only in oral formulations.

Tetracyclines. Tetracyclines have been an important class of antibiotics with significant antianaerobic activity. In addition to activity against anaerobes, tetracyclines possess modest activity against easy gram-negative rods and many gram-positive cocci. In the 1990s other agents are preferable as first and second choices for the overwhelming majority of surgical infections.

Glycopeptides. Vancomycin is the only glycopeptide antibiotic available. It is active against essentially all gram-positive cocci, especially the methicillin-resistant staphylococci, for which it is the only reliable antibiotic. It also has moderate activity against enterococci. Vancomycin is active against most *Clostridium* species, especially *C. difficile*, the primary pathogen responsible for antibiotic-associated diarrhea. However, it should not be used as a first-line agent against *C. difficile* diarrhea, owing to the risk that this will increase the incidence of vancomycin-resistant enterococci.[6]

General Principles

Whichever antibiotics are employed, the goal of therapy is to achieve levels of antibiotics at the site of infection that exceed the minimum inhibitory concentration for the pathogens present. For mild infections, including most that can be handled on an outpatient basis, this may be achievable with oral antibiotics when appropriate choices are available. For severe surgical infections, however, the systemic response to infection may make gastrointestinal absorption of antibiotics unpredictable and thus antibiotic levels unreliable. In addition, for intra-abdominal infections, gastrointestinal function is often directly impaired. For this reason, most initial antibiotic therapy for surgical infections is begun intravenously.

Each patient with a serious infection should be evaluated daily or more frequently to assess response to treatment. If obvious improvement is not seen within 2 to 3 days, one often hears the question, "Which antibiotic should we add/switch to?" That question is appropriate, however, only after the following question has been addressed: Why is the patient failing to improve? Likely answers include the following:

1. The initial operative procedure was not adequate.
2. The initial procedure was adequate but a complication has occurred.
3. A superinfection has developed at a new site.
4. The drug choice is correct, but not enough is being given.
5. Another or a different drug is needed.

The choice of antibiotics is not the most common cause for failure unless the original choice was clearly inappropriate, such as failing to provide coverage for anaerobes in an intra-abdominal infection.

As the patient improves, one must decide when to stop antibiotic therapy. For most surgical infections there is not a specific duration of antibiotics known to be ideal. Antibiotics generally support local host defenses until the local responses are sufficient to limit further infection. When an abscess is drained, the antibiotics prevent invasive bacterial infection in the fresh tissue planes opened in the course of drainage. After 3 to 5 days, the local responses of new capillary formation and inflammatory infiltrate provide a competent local defense. For deep-seated or poorly localized infections, longer treatment may be needed. A good guideline is to continue antibiotics until the patient has shown an obvious clinical improvement based on clinical examination and has had a normal temperature for 48 hours or more. Signs of improvement include improved mental status, return of bowel function, and spontaneous diuresis.

The white blood cell count may not have returned to normal when antibiotics are stopped. If the white blood cell count is normal, the likelihood of further infectious problems is small. If the white blood cell count is elevated, further infections may be detected but in most cases they will not be prevented by continuing antibiotics. Rather, a new infection requires drainage or different antibiotics for a new, resistant pathogen in a different location. In this case, the best approach is to stop the existing drugs and observe the patient closely for subsequent developments.[17]

Superinfection

A superinfection is a new infection that develops during antibiotic treatment for the original infection. Whenever antibiotics are used they exert a selective pressure on the endogenous flora of the patient and on exogenous bacteria that colonize sites at risk. Bacteria that remain are resistant to the antibiotics being used and become the pathogens in superinfection. Respiratory tract infections are common superinfections that occur during the treatment of intra-abdominal infection. The greater the severity of the abdominal infection and the greater the risk of poor outcome from it, the greater the risk of pneumonia as well.

Careful surveillance of hospitalized patients reveals superinfections in 2% to 10% of antibiotic-treated patients, depending on the underlying risk factors. The best preventive action is to limit the dose and duration of antibiotic treatment to what is obviously required and to be alert to the possibility of superinfections. The use of increasingly powerful and broad-spectrum antibiotics during the past two decades has also led to an increasing incidence of fungal superinfections.

Antibiotic-associated colitis is another significant superinfection that can occur in hospitalized patients with mild to serious illness. This entity is caused by the enteric pathogen *C. difficile* and has been reported after treatment with every antibiotic except vancomycin. *C. difficile* colitis can vary from a mild, self-limited disease to a rapidly progressive septic process culminating in death. The most important step in treating this disease is to suspect it. Diagnosis is by endoscopy, revealing the typical mucosal changes with inflammation, ulceration, and plaque formation; stool assay for the characteristic toxin; and stool culture to recover *C. difficile*. Treatment is supportive with fluid and electrolytes, withdrawal of the offending antibiotic if possible, and oral metronidazole to treat the superinfection. Vancomycin should be reserved for metronidazole failures. In rare instances when an overwhelming colitis does not respond to medical management, emergency colectomy may be required.

SELECTED REFERENCES

Fry, D. E. (Ed.): Surgical Infections. Boston, Little, Brown & Co, 1995.
This is an excellent and comprehensive book devoted entirely to surgical infections.

Howard, R. J., and Simmons, R. L. (Eds.): Surgical Infectious Diseases. East Norwalk, CT, Appleton & Lange, 1994.
This important text delineates the many problems of surgical infections. It is a well-written and comprehensive review of the entire field.

REFERENCES

1. Alexander, J. W., Aerni, S., and Plettner, J. P.: Development of a safe and effective one-minute preoperative skin preparation. Arch. Surg., 120:1357, 1985.

2. Alexander, J. W., Fischer, J. E., Boyajian, M., Palmquist, J., and Morris, M. J.: Influence of hair-removal methods on wound infections. Arch. Surg., *118*:347, 1983.

3. Barie, P. S., Christou, N. V., Dellinger, E. P., Rout, W. R., Stone, H. H., et al.: Pathogenicity of the enterococcus in surgical infections. Ann. Surg., *212*:155, 1990.

4. Bohnen, J. M. A., Solomkin, J. S., Dellinger, E. P., Bjornson, H. S., and Page, C. P.: Guidelines for clinical care: Anti-infective agents for intraabdominal infection. Arch. Surg., *127*:83, 1992.

5. Burke, J. F.: Identification of the source of staphylococci contaminating the surgical wound during operation. Ann. Surg., *158*:898, 1963.

6. Centers for Disease Control and Prevention: Preventing the spread of vancomycin resistance—a report from the hospital infection control practices advisory committee; comment period and public meeting; notice. Fed. Register, *59*(94):25758, 1994.

7. Christou, N. V., Barie, P. S., Dellinger, E. P., Waymack, J., et al.: Surgical Infection Society intra-abdominal infection study: Prospective evaluation of management techniques and outcome. Arch. Surg., *128*:193, 1993.

8. Clarke, J. S., Condon R. E., Bartlett, J. G., Gorbach, S. L., Nichols, R. L., et al.: Preoperative oral antibiotics reduce septic complications of colon operations: Results of prospective, randomized, double-blind clinical study. Ann. Surg., *186*:251, 1977.

9. Dellinger, E.: Approach to the patient with postoperative fever. *In* Gorbach, S., Bartlett, J., and Blacklow, N. R. (Eds.): Infectious Diseases in Medicine and Surgery. Philadelphia, W. B. Saunders, 1991, pp. 753–758.

10. Dellinger, E. P.: Use of scoring systems to assess patients with surgical sepsis. Surg. Clin. North Am., *68*:123, 1988.

11. Dellinger, E. P.: Surgery for intra-abdominal sepsis. *In* White, T. T., et al. (Eds.): Reoperative Gastrointestinal Surgery. New York, Appleton-Century-Crofts, 1989, pp. 63–73.

12. Dellinger, E. P.: Perioperative infection. *In* Meakins, J. L. (Ed.): Surgical Infections: Diagnosis and Treatment. New York, Scientific American, 1994, pp. 217–234.

13. Dellinger, E. P., Gross, P. A., Barrett, T. L., Krause, P. J., Martone, W. J., et al.: Quality standard for antimicrobial prophylaxis in surgical procedures. Clin. Infect. Dis., *18*:422, 1994.

14. Garibaldi, R. A.: Prevention of intraoperative wound contamination with chlorhexidine shower and scrub. J. Hosp. Infect., 2(Suppl. B):5, 1988.

15. Hau, T., Ahrenholz, D. H., and Simmons, R. L.: Secondary bacterial peritonitis: The biologic basis of treatment. Curr. Probl. Surg., *16*(10):1, 1979.

16. Lee, J. T.: Wound infection surveillance. Infect. Dis. Clin. North Am., *6*:643, 1992.

17. Lennard, E. S., Dellinger, E. P, Minshew, B. H., and Wertz, M. J.: Implications of leukocytosis and fever at conclusion of antibiotic therapy for intraabdominal sepsis. Ann. Surg., *195*:19, 1982.

18. Levison, M. A.: Percutaneous versus open operative drainage of intraabdominal abscesses. Infect. Dis. Clin. North Am., *6*:525, 1992.

19. Nicolau, D. P., Freeman, C. D., Belliveau, P. P., Nightingale, C. H., Ross, J. W., et al.: Experience with a once-daily aminoglycoside program administered to 2,184 adult patients. Antimicrob. Agents Chemother., *39*:650, 1995.

20. Quebbeman, E. J., Telford, G. L., Wadsworth, K., Hubbard, S., Goodman, H., et al.: Double gloving: Protecting surgeons from blood contamination in the operating room. Arch. Surg., *127*:213, 1992.

21. Sanford, J. P.: Guide to Antimicrobial Therapy. Dallas, Antimicrobial Therapy, 1995.

22. Solla, J. A., and Rothenberger, D. A.: Preoperative bowel preparation: A survey of colon and rectal surgeons. Dis. Colon Rectum, *33*:154, 1990.

23. Traverso, L. W.: Infections complicating severe pancre titis. Infect. Dis. Clin. North Am., *6*:601, 1992.

II

SURGICAL ASPECTS OF ACQUIRED IMMUNODEFICIENCY SYNDROME

Douglas Tyler, M.D., and H. Kim Lyerly, M.D.

Patients infected with human immunodeficiency virus type 1 (HIV-1) are susceptible not only to the usual surgical disorders that affect people of their given age but also to a host of other conditions related to their underlying immunodeficiency. As more experience has been gained in caring for HIV-1–infected patients, it is becoming clearer that there are several syndromes that will require surgical evaluation. It is, therefore, important for surgeons not only to understand the surgical problems associated with HIV-1 infection but also to appreciate how HIV-1–infected patients tolerate surgical procedures. In this section the various effects of HIV-1 infection on different organ systems are summarized, and several common clinical syndromes seen in HIV-1–infected individuals that may require surgical intervention are reviewed.

EVALUATION BY ORGAN SYSTEM

Esophagus. Esophageal complaints related to dysphagia, odynophagia, or retrosternal discomfort are relatively common in patients with HIV-1 infection, affecting 30% to 40% of patients at some time during the course of their disease.[1] These symptoms are usually the first manifestation that esophageal pathology is present. Candidal esophagitis is the most common cause of esophageal symptomatology, especially in patients with oral thrush. If shallow oral ulcers are present, then herpes simplex esophagitis is the most likely diagnosis. In general, most clinicians begin treatment empirically with an oral antifungal agent if *Candida* is suspected or use acyclovir if herpes esophagitis is suspected. If the patient does not respond after 1 to 2 weeks of initiating therapy, then upper endoscopy is recommended as the most cost-

effective diagnostic test.[2] Although barium swallow has been recommended by some, upper endoscopy offers the advantages of immediate biopsy and diagnosis. Specimens can be sent for viral, fungal, and bacterial cultures as well as put through special immunofluorescent staining procedures. Other common causes include cytomegalovirus (CMV), tuberculosis, and idiopathic HIV-1–associated esophageal ulceration. Other lesions that can involve the esophagus include Kaposi's sarcoma and lymphoma. These neoplastic lesions usually present as bleeding but can also cause dysphagia secondary to obstruction.[2]

Lungs and Heart. A wide variety of opportunistic pulmonary infections frequently occur in HIV-1–infected patients. *Pneumocystis carinii* pneumonia appears associated with an increased rate of pneumothorax presumably due to destruction of pulmonary parenchyma and visceral pleura. Treatment with tube thoracostomy is usually all that is required. Patients with persistent pulmonary air leaks after 8 to 10 days should undergo thoracotomy (or thoracoscopy) with excision of blebs and pleurodesis. According to one report, surgical intervention decreased mean hospital stays from 33 to 13 days.[3]

Advances in the work-up and diagnosis of the various HIV-1–related pulmonary processes usually can lead to a diagnosis in the hands of experienced individuals. Open lung biopsy is rarely required. Some potential indications for open lung biopsy include (1) a seropositive patient who has severe pulmonary disease and is deteriorating rapidly without a diagnosis after attempted bronchoscopy; (2) pulmonary disease persisting without a diagnosis in a seropositive patient despite one or two carefully performed bronchoscopic examinations that include transbronchial biopsy and bronchoalveolar lavage; and (3) a patient requiring mechanical ventilation in whom bronchoscopy with transbronchial biopsy and bronchoalveolar lavage has been nondiagnostic or cannot be performed.[4] Open lung biopsy is generally not useful in providing additional information when performed on patients whose conditions continue to deteriorate despite treatment for diseases, the diagnosis of which had been previously established bronchoscopically. Furthermore, two additional studies examining the role of open lung biopsy found that although the procedure was effective in diagnosing the underlying pulmonary process, only rarely was a successful therapeutic change made on the basis of the biopsy findings.[5, 6]

Myocarditis is the most common HIV-1–related cardiac problem identified in patients and can be caused by a wide variety of etiologic agents.[7] The clinical manifestations such as congestive heart failure, dilated cardiomyopathy, and cardiac arrhythmias are dependent on the magnitude of the inflammatory response. Endocarditis is also found occasionally in HIV-1–infected patients. In patients with the acquired immunodeficiency syndrome (AIDS) it is usually nonbacterial. Bacterial endocarditis, when found in HIV-1–infected patients, is usually related to intravenous drug abuse. The role of surgery in these individuals remains controversial. Some surgeons believe that patients with AIDS should not undergo cardiopulmonary bypass. For patients with asymptomatic HIV-1 infection, there is no evidence to support the contention that cardiopulmonary bypass accelerates HIV-1 disease progression to AIDS. Perioperative mortality for asymptomatic patients undergoing cardiopulmonary bypass for valvular surgery according to one report was 20%. This high figure was believed to be related more to the underlying condition of the intravenous drug abusers than to the HIV-1 infection itself.[8]

Stomach and Duodenum. HIV-1–related pathology that affects the stomach and duodenum usually presents with symptoms of either bleeding, abdominal pain, gastric outlet obstruction, and/or perforation. The most common cause of upper gastrointestinal bleeding in HIV-1–infected patients is Kaposi's sarcoma.[9] Although there have been occasional cases of gastric outlet obstruction secondary to lesions of Kaposi's sarcoma, they are usually asymptomatic.[10] Non-Hodgkin's lymphoma of the stomach also usually presents as bleeding, but obstruction and perforation can occur.[11] Gastritis as well as gastric and duodenal ulcers are usually secondary to various infectious causes. CMV is one of the more common pathogens, but others include *Cryptosporidium, Candida,* and herpesvirus.[12, 13] Upper endoscopy is the initial procedure in patients with gastrointestinal bleeding and in patients with persistent upper abdominal pain. Therapeutic as well as diagnostic interventions can be carried out. Operations are occasionally required for patients with persistent bleeding, gastric outlet obstruction, or gastric perforation and in some patients with localized gastric lymphoma.

Liver. The liver can be affected by both infectious and neoplastic sequelae of HIV-1 infection, but the need for surgical intervention to diagnose or treat these processes is uncommon.[14] Approximately 85% of HIV-1–seropositive patients have evidence of previous hepatitis B infection, with between 10% and 30% having detectable circulating surface antigen. Surprisingly, cases of primary hepatocellular carcinoma are very rare in patients with HIV-1.[15] The other types of viral hepatitis (A, C, and delta agent) are also very common in HIV-1–infected individuals. Several HIV-1–associated opportunistic infections, including those caused by *Mycobacterium avium-intracellulare, Mycobacterium tuberculosis,* CMV, *Cryptococcus neoformans, Histoplasma capsulatum, Candida albicans,* and *Coccidioides immitis,* can involve the liver, as can

neoplastic processes such as non-Hodgkin's lymphoma and Kaposi's sarcoma.[16] Clinical characteristics of liver involvement include constitutional symptoms such as fever, malaise, weight loss, and/or hepatomegaly. Liver function tests reveal mild to moderate elevations in enzyme levels. Alkaline phosphatase levels can be markedly elevated when granulomas or abscesses are present. Lymphoma usually causes a marked increase in the serum bilirubin level. It should be remembered that abnormalities in liver function tests are nonspecific findings, and results can also be elevated secondary to several medications that are frequently taken by HIV-1–infected individuals such as pentamidine, ketoconazole, and sulfa drugs. Diagnostic work-up usually involves a computed tomographic (CT) scan and/or a liver biopsy. Although most liver abscesses can be drained with percutaneous CT-guided catheters, surgical drainage is occasionally required.

Gallbladder and Biliary Tract. Biliary tract complications related to HIV-1 infection are being reported with increasing frequency. Although HIV-1–infected individuals are susceptible to biliary symptoms as a result of gallstones, a significant percentage of patients with gallbladder problems have acute acalculous cholecystitis.[14, 17] This cholecystitis is usually secondary to infection and subsequent gallbladder wall necrosis caused most commonly by *Cryptosporidium* and CMV. Cases secondary to *Candida* and *Campylobacter* have also been reported. Patients usually present with fever, fatigue, diarrhea, and right upper quadrant pain. Ultrasonography, the diagnostic test of choice, often demonstrates a thickened gallbladder wall, pericholecystic fluid, and a positive transducer-induced Murphy's sign. Despite the absence of stones, radionuclide scintigraphy is usually positive.[18] In patients with asymptomatic HIV-1 infection, cholecystectomy, performed laparoscopically if possible, is the preferred treatment and is usually well tolerated. The morbidity and mortality of cholecystectomy in patients with AIDS are much higher.[15] In this group of patients, consideration should be given to placement of a cholecystostomy tube to help defervesce the acute infection and allow time to optimize these patients' overall medical condition before subsequent surgical intervention.

Papillary stenosis and sclerosing cholangitis are also observed with surprising frequency in HIV-1–infected individuals. The cause of these changes appears to be either *Cryptosporidium* or CMV infection involving the bile ducts.[19, 20] Presenting symptoms include fever, nausea, vomiting, diarrhea, and right upper quadrant pain. Jaundice is only occasionally observed because biliary obstruction is rarely complete. Laboratory studies reveal most commonly a markedly elevated alkaline phosphatase level, a mildly elevated serum bilirubin value, and usually normal transaminase levels. Initial screening is performed with ultrasonography and/or CT scanning in an attempt to exclude extrinsic compression of the bile ducts secondary to lesions of Kaposi's sarcoma, lymphadenopathy, or lymphoma. Endoscopic retrograde cholangiopancreatography is preferable to transhepatic cholangiography and can help define the anatomy of the intrahepatic and extrahepatic bile ducts. In patients with papillary stenosis, prompt relief of abdominal pain is usually obtained when endoscopic sphincterotomy is performed.[14] Despite the bile ducts' remaining patent after successful sphincterotomy, serum alkaline phosphatase levels frequently stay the same or increase, presumably owing to ongoing intrahepatic duct disease or parenchymal infiltration of the liver. Patients with sclerosing cholangitis are best treated with balloon dilatation and stenting, especially when areas of localized stricture are present.[15] Surgical intervention is best reserved for lesions causing extrinsic compression and for patients in whom endoscopic sphincterotomy fails.

TABLE 15–6. Various Infectious Causes of Abdominal Pain in HIV-1–Infected Individuals

Bacterial	Nonbacterial
Salmonella	Entamoeba histolytica
Shigella	Giardia lamblia
Campylobacter	Cryptosporidium
Neisseria gonorrhoeae	Isospora belli
Treponema pallidum	Candida albicans
Mycobacterium avium-intracellulare	Cryptococcus neoformans
Mycobacterium tuberculosis	Histoplasma capsulatum
Listeria monocytogenes	Cytomegalovirus
	Herpes simplex virus

Pancreas. Symptomatic pancreatitis unrelated to alcohol, gallstones, or hyperlipidemia is uncommon in HIV-1–infected individuals. Interestingly, asymptomatic hyperamylasemia is relatively common, especially in patients with AIDS. Although pancreatic inflammation can occur as a result of opportunistic infections (especially CMV, Cryptococcus, Toxoplasma gondii, or M. avium-intracellulare) or secondary to neoplastic involvement by Kaposi's sarcoma or lymphoma, the majority of cases have no clear etiology.[21] Research involving a simian immunodeficiency virus has led to the theory that HIV-1 infection may lead to the reactivation of other pancreatitis-causing viruses, such as adenoviruses, that are latent within the host.[22] Pancreatitis has also been associated with a number of medications frequently taken by HIV-1–infected individuals such as dideoxyinosine, pentamidine, and trimethoprim-sulfamethoxazole.[23] Treatment of pancreatitis in the setting of HIV-1 infection is identical to that of patients not infected with HIV-1. Generally supportive care and discontinuing potentially exacerbating medications are all that is required. Concurrently, an evaluation for infectious etiologies as well as non–AIDS-related causes should be undertaken.

Intestine. Both neoplastic and infectious processes related to HIV-1 infection can occur in the small intestine. Non-Hodgkin's lymphoma and Kaposi's sarcoma are the most common neoplasms affecting the intestine in seropositive individuals. Lymphomas associated with AIDS are usually high-grade B-cell lymphomas that are symptomatic, presenting with signs of pain, fever, night sweats, weight loss, jaundice, ascites, obstruction, bleeding, and/or perforation.[24] Usually the diagnosis can be made with CT scanning, and CT therefore is the test of choice. Occasionally, additional information can be obtained from barium studies. Surgical therapy is usually required in cases that present with obstruction, hemorrhage, or perforation. Because several cases of perforation secondary to postchemotherapy tumor lysis have been reported, resection of localized disease before chemotherapy has been advocated.[11] Intestinal lesions of Kaposi's sarcoma are present in 40% to 50% of patients with cutaneous Kaposi's sarcoma lesions but are usually asymptomatic.[11] Rarely, they present with bleeding or obstruction requiring surgical intervention. In general, the prognosis for patients with intestinal Kaposi's sarcoma is poor, and treatment is directed more toward the underlying HIV-1 infection.

Infections involving the small intestine most often cause crampy abdominal pain and diarrhea. More than half of HIV-1–infected patients will develop diarrhea at some time during their illness. Common infectious causes are shown in Table 15–6. Complications of these infections may on occasion require surgical intervention. There are numerous reports of intestinal perforation secondary to CMV.[25] Despite surgical exploration and segmental bowel resection, morbidity and mortality remain high owing to the underlying condition

of the patients. Treatment with ganciclovir appears to help stabilize or improve gastrointestinal disease caused by CMV and should be tried in these patients. Several organisms can cause an inflammatory response in the terminal ileum mimicking regional enteritis or appendicitis and lead to surgical exploration.[26, 27] The most common of these organisms are Yersinia, Campylobacter, Shigella, Salmonella, and M. avium-intracellulare. Diagnosis can be difficult because the presence of these organisms in the patient's stool does not imply that they are the cause of the abdominal pain. Laparoscopy may prove useful in the evaluation of abdominal pain in this group of patients.

Appendix. Although appendicitis may occur in HIV-1–infected individuals by means of the same mechanisms through which it occurs in seronegative patients, there are several reports of appendiceal obstruction and subsequent appendicitis secondary to AIDS-related neoplasms such as Kaposi's sarcoma and non-Hodgkin's lymphoma.[28] In addition, appendicitis tends to be more difficult to diagnose in HIV-1–infected individuals because these patients frequently have chronic abdominal complaints.[28, 29] In a series of HIV-1–infected patients with appendicitis, increasing abdominal pain and diarrhea were common symptoms. Fever and leukocytosis were unreliable findings. Because the classic presentation was less common in HIV-1–infected patients, there tended to be a more frequent delay in diagnosis and a higher incidence of perforated appendicitis at the time of exploration, especially in patients with AIDS. Aggressive use of ultrasonography and/or laparoscopy can be helpful in diagnosing appendicitis in this patient population.

Colon. Colonic problems related to HIV-1 infection are usually infectious. The more common causes of infectious colitis are shown in Table 15–6. When the colon, as opposed to the small bowel, is the predominant site of infection, the diarrhea is more likely to be bloody and contain mucus. Patients frequently complain of lower abdominal pain. The diagnosis can usually be made by stool culture with examination for ova and parasites. Colonoscopy is performed if the diagnosis is unclear or resistant to therapy. CMV colitis is associated with cases of perforation that necessitate surgical intervention.[30] This clinical entity can occur early in AIDS and tends to involve predominantly the right colon and rectosigmoid region with frequent sparing of the transverse colon. Signs and symptoms are often nonspecific, and colon-

TABLE 15–7. Infections and Lesions of the Anorectum in HIV-1–Infected Individuals

Infections	Lesions
Neisseria gonorrhoeae	Anal fissure
Syphilis	Anal fistula
Lymphogranuloma venereum	Perirectal abscess
Chlamydia trachomatis	Hemorrhoids
Herpes simplex	Lymphoma
Herpes zoster	Kaposi's sarcoma
Campylobacter	Condylomata acuminata
Cytomegalovirus	Rectal ulcers
Mycobacterium avium-intracellulare	Trauma-induced lesions
Mycobacterium tuberculosis	Squamous cell carcinoma
Histoplasma	
Giardia lamblia	
Shigella	
Isospora belli	
Cryptosporidium	
Entamoeba histolytica	
Clostridium difficile	
Candida albicans	
Vibrio parahaemolyticus	

oscopically the colonic mucosa can appear normal, with the diagnosis being made only by mucosal biopsy. On rare occasions infectious colitis is so severe that diagnostic exploration (laparoscopy or laparotomy) is performed because of the presence of peritoneal signs.

Anus and Rectum. Anorectal problems are common in HIV-1–infected individuals, especially homosexuals and AIDS patients.[31] Symptoms usually include pain, ulceration, discharge, incontinence, bleeding, mass, and/or tenesmus. Several infectious agents as well as a wide variety of pathologic processes, both benign and malignant, can cause these symptoms (Table 15–7). It is important to remember that HIV-1–infected individuals are at increased risk of developing both rectal and anal cancers.[32, 33] Therefore, when one is evaluating anorectal lesions, anoscopy and sigmoidoscopy should be performed with rectal swabbing for ova and parasites, bacteria, and viruses. Biopsies of any suspicious mass or ulcer should be obtained.

In general, the management of anorectal problems in HIV-1–infected patients is similar to that in uninfected individuals, with conservative measures being attempted initially.[34, 35] Chemotherapy and/or irradiation is used for lymphoma, squamous cell carcinoma, and Kaposi's sarcoma involving the anorectal region. Anal condylomas can be treated with topical chemicals, cryosurgery, excision, or fulguration. Larger lesions usually require surgical excision with close follow-up so that any recurrent disease can be treated early. Ulcers of the anorectal lesions frequently have an infectious etiology, with CMV, herpes simplex virus, *Chlamydia, Treponema pallidum, Haemophilus ducreyi,* and *Mycobacterium* being the most common offenders. Treatment of the ulcers can be challenging because not uncommonly no cause can be found and the lesion does not respond despite appropriate drug therapy. Corticosteroid injections to diminish the inflammatory reaction or saucerization with or without mucosal flap advancement has been advocated for persistent ulcers.

Although patients with asymptomatic HIV-1 infection appear to tolerate anorectal surgery well based on recent reports, patients with AIDS appear to have significant perioperative morbidity and mortality. In one study that reviewed 73 anorectal procedures (23 biopsies, 16 incision and drainage procedures, 14 fistulotomies, 8 sphincterotomies, 8 excisions, 3 colostomies, and 1 hemorrhoidectomy) in 52 patients with AIDS, an 88% incidence of poor wound healing and an 18% perioperative mortality rate were found.[36] A second study of 18 anorectal procedures in 17 patients with AIDS found a similiar 16% perioperative mortality, but most wounds appeared to heal uneventfully.[35] Although caution is recommended for most anorectal problems, certain lesions, such as perirectal abscesses, should still be regarded as emergencies, with expedient definitive therapy being carried out in the operating room.

EVALUATION BY CLINICAL SIGN OR SYMPTOM

Abdominal Pain. Although it is difficult to estimate, most large group studies suggest that between 10% and 15% of patients infected with HIV-1 will develop problems with abdominal pain at some point during the course of their disease.[37, 38] Abdominal pain affecting these patients is more commonly seen in late-stage disease (AIDS), and its occurrence appears associated with reduced patient survival. Although it is uncommon for operations to be needed in this patient population, surgeons are frequently consulted to evaluate these patients when their abdominal pain develops. As experience has accumulated, it appears that there are four clinical syndromes of abdominal pain that affect patients with HIV-1 infection.[37, 38] These syndromes, their differential diagnosis, and their proposed work-up are summarized in Table 15–8.

The first abdominal pain syndrome is that of epigastric

TABLE 15–8. Clinical Syndromes of Abdominal Pain in HIV-1–Infected Individuals, Their Potential Etiology, and Recommended Work-up

Clinical Syndrome	Potential Etiology	Work-up
Epigastric pain with or without esophageal symptoms	CMV esophagitis CMV gastritis CMV duodenitis Peptic ulcer Pancreatitis Gastric lymphoma, Kaposi's sarcoma	Endoscopy Barium swallow Chest radiograph
Right upper quadrant pain with or without jaundice	Acute cholecystitis Sclerosing cholangitis Papillary stenosis Hepatic lymphoma, Kaposi's sarcoma Gastric lymphoma, Kaposi's sarcoma Acute hepatitis Hepatic abscess	Ultrasonography Hepatoiminodiacetic acid scan Endoscopic retrograde cholangiopancreatography if jaundice
Right iliac fossa pain	Acute appendicitis Crohn's ileitis MAI enteritis Irritable bowel syndrome	Ultrasonography Laparoscopy/laparotomy
Diffuse abdominal pain	CMV enteritis/colitis *Shigella* colitis Intestinal lymphoma Giardiasis Cryptosporidiosis Irritable bowel syndrome MAI enteritis Nodal mycobacteria	Chest radiograph Colonoscopy CT scan

CMV, cytomegalovirus; MAI, *Mycobacterium avium-intracellulare*; CT, computed tomography.

pain with or without esophageal symptoms. The differential diagnosis includes HIV-1–related diseases such as esophagitis, gastritis or duodenitis, and gastric malignancy (Kaposi's sarcoma or lymphoma) as well as non–HIV-1–related disease processes such as peptic ulcer disease and pancreatitis. After initial screening with laboratory studies, chest radiography, and abdominal films, if the diagnosis is still in question, then upper endoscopy should be performed. Endoscopy allows direct visualization of upper abdominal pathology as well as permits biopsy of any lesions that may be seen. On occasion, barium studies may help further define upper abdominal problems, especially if malignancy is suspected.

The second abdominal pain syndrome is right upper quadrant pain with or without jaundice. Pain in this region can be related to inflammatory processes, obstructive processes, or cancer. Ultrasonography is the first test of choice after initial blood work, chest radiography, and abdominal films. Ultrasonography should allow the diagnosis of acute cholecystitis, bile duct obstruction, and lesions within the liver such as tumors or abscesses. If acute cholecystitis is suspected, a hepatoiminodiacetic acid scan can confirm the diagnosis. This scan is usually positive even though most of the cases of acute cholecystitis in this patient population are acalculous. If the patient has jaundice or has dilated bile ducts, then endoscopic retrograde cholangiopancreatography should be performed. This usually demonstrates papillary stenosis and/or sclerosing cholangitis.

The third abdominal pain syndrome is right iliac fossa pain. This is usually secondary to either acute appendicitis or inflammation of the distal small bowel secondary to Crohn's disease or infection. After preliminary blood tests and plain chest films, ultrasonography is usually recommended as the first procedure to try when evaluating the appendix. If ultrasonography does not provide useful information, then the patient can be observed with serial examinations or undergo laparoscopy. Laparoscopy is becoming more popular for evaluating this problem because one can get immediate feedback and intervene therapeutically if necessary.

The fourth abdominal pain syndrome is characterized by diffuse abdominal pain. It is usually related to an infectious etiology. An operation is rarely required unless hemorrhage, obstruction, perforation, or peritonitis is present. In the absence of free air on initial work-up, colonoscopy is usually the first test of choice to evaluate these patients. Colonoscopy can identify many of the infectious lesions in the colon as well as visualize any malignancies. Although CT scans are frequently obtained, studies have found that they rarely give a definitive answer as to the cause of the abdominal pain. CT scans are best reserved for those HIV-1–positive patients in whom the cause of the abdominal pain is unclear after colonoscopy or as an adjunct for staging malignancy.

Thrombocytopenia. Thrombocytopenic purpura is a common hematologic problem in HIV-1–infected individuals, with approximately 11% of patients having platelet counts less than 100,000 per cu. mm.[39] Cases for which no obvious etiology can be determined other than coexisting HIV-1 infection have been diagnosed as HIV-1–associated thrombocytopenia. It has been suggested that this thrombocytopenia is secondary to the presence of cross-reactive antibodies between HIV-1 and platelet glycoproteins or high levels of platelet-bound IgG and circulating immune complexes.[40] The failure to find a unifying mechanism for all cases of HIV-1–associated thrombocytopenia suggests that this syndrome may have several different causes.

Clinically, HIV-1–associated thrombocytopenia is a syndrome that does not appear to be associated with progression of HIV-1 to AIDS-related complex or AIDS and is characterized by a spontaneous remission rate of between 10% and 30%.[41] Interestingly, although platelet counts may frequently

drop below 20,000 per cu. mm., episodes of life-threatening bleeding have rarely been reported. The development of a widely agreed upon treatment approach to this syndrome has been difficult because of its relatively indolent course, high spontaneous remission rate, and unclear etiology.

Corticosteroids were initially the treatment of choice in managing HIV-1–associated thrombocytopenia because they led to an increase in the platelet count in 60% to 90% of patients in whom they were tried.[42] Enthusiasm for corticosteroids has diminished, however, because increases in platelet counts are rarely maintained when these agents are withdrawn. Not wanting to chronically immunosuppress individuals whose underlying problem is immunodeficiency has led physicians to try other treatment options. Marked short-term improvement in platelet counts after splenectomy has led some researchers to propose this operation as a first-line therapy. However, although 75% of patients still have platelet counts above 100,000 per cu. mm. 1 year after splenectomy, platelet counts continue to fluctuate markedly.[43, 44] Patients should be given presplenectomy pneumococcal vaccination and postoperative oral antibiotic prophylaxis. Long-term evaluation of splenectomy suggests that it does not accelerate disease progression.

There are several reports, including prospective placebo-controlled studies, demonstrating that zidovudine leads to prolonged increases in circulating platelet counts in patients with HIV-1–associated thrombocytopenia.[45, 46] Approximately 70% of patients respond with platelet counts starting to rise within the first week of therapy. The mean time for partial or complete normalization of platelet counts is 12 weeks. Several mechanisms have been proposed for why zidovudine works, but because there are fewer theoretical risks for an individual taking zidovudine as compared with corticosteroids, most physicians recommend using this drug as initial therapy for HIV-1–associated thrombocytopenia. Corticosteroids and splenectomy are reserved for those individuals who are refractory to or cannot tolerate zidovudine. The algorithm in use at Duke University Medical Center for the treatment of HIV-1–associated thrombocytopenia is shown in Figure 15–3.

Gastrointestinal Bleeding. Gastrointestinal bleeding is an unusual occurrence in HIV-1–infected individuals, but when it does occur it is usually related to a complication of HIV-1 infection.[47] A review of gastrointestinal bleeding in 37 patients at San Francisco General Hospital over a 2-year period included 13 patients with upper gastrointestinal tract bleed-

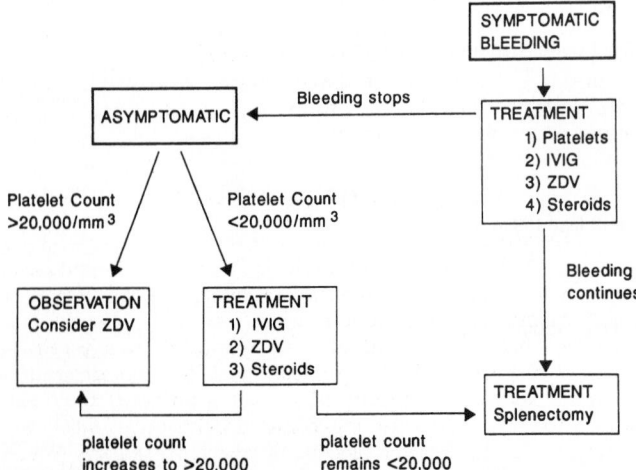

Figure 15–3. Algorithm used at Duke University Medical Center for treatment of HIV-1–associated thrombocytopenia. ZDV, zidovudine; IVIG, intravenous immunoglobulin.

ing and 24 patients with lower gastrointestinal tract bleeding.[9] The causes of upper gastrointestinal bleeding included 4 patients bleeding from Kaposi's sarcoma lesions, 2 bleeding from gastric lymphoma, and 2 from CMV-induced ulcerations. The remaining 5 patients were bleeding from non–HIV-1–related lesions. Evaluation of the 24 patients with lower gastrointestinal tract bleeding revealed most to have distal rectal lesions, the majority of which were related to their HIV-1 infection. The most common of these lesions was a localized colitis found in 14 patients, the cause of which included CMV (5 patients), bacteria (4 patients), herpes simplex virus (2 patients), and idiopathic ulcerative disease (2 patients). Other lesions responsible for lower gastrointestinal tract bleeding in this group included idiopathic proctitis (2 patients), hemorrhoids (4 patients), and Kaposi's sarcoma (2 patients). This study concluded that gastrointestinal bleeding should be treated aggressively in HIV-1–infected individuals who are not terminally ill because specific therapy exists for 75% of the precipitating lesions. Evaluation of upper gastrointestinal tract bleeding usually begins with endoscopy. Lower gastrointestinal tract bleeding is evaluated initially with colonoscopy in the stable patient, and with either nuclear scintigraphy and/or angiography in the patient who appears to be actively bleeding. The nature of the lesion and condition of the patient usually dictate what therapeutic intervention (medical, endoscopic, angiographic, or surgical) is chosen.

Lymphadenopathy. Generalized lymphadenopathy is a relatively common finding in patients with HIV-1 infection. Before recognition that HIV-1 was the etiologic agent of AIDS, lymph node biopsy was frequently used in an attempt to diagnose the syndrome. Although there are no characteristic histologic patterns pathognomonic of AIDS, the finding of Kaposi's sarcoma, B-cell lymphoma, or specific opportunistic infections can be diagnostic.

With the development of accurate serologic testing for antibodies to HIV-1 toward the end of 1985, the role of lymph node biopsy in HIV-1–infected individuals became unclear. Three prospective studies examining lymph node biopsies in patients with persistent generalized lymphadenopathy found that biopsy altered clinical management in only 2 of 71 patients.[48–51] All three studies suggested that the routine use of lymph node biopsy in HIV-1–infected individuals with uncomplicated persistent generalized lymphadenopathy was unnecessary. Their conclusion was that lymph node biopsy should be reserved for those individuals who have lymphadenopathy in the setting of constitutional symptoms, splenomegaly, cytopenia, oral candidiasis, or hilar adenopathy. In addition, a solitary lymph node enlarged disproportionally in relation to other lymph nodes should be removed for examination. This selective use of lymph node biopsy would increase the likelihood of diagnosing a specific infection, lymphoma, or other disease process that could alter the clinical management of the patient.

OTHER CONSIDERATIONS

Perioperative Course. The perioperative morbidity and mortality of HIV-1–infected individuals appear to depend on the patient's underlying immunocompetence and the nature of the underlying illness requiring an operation. Asymptomatic HIV-1–infected individuals undergoing elective surgical procedures do not exhibit significantly more problems with wound healing and infection than their uninfected counterparts.[10] Debate continues regarding the healing ability of patients with AIDS after elective surgical procedures. One study reviewing elective anorectal surgical procedures in patients with AIDS and AIDS-related complex described a high incidence of complications and poor wound healing.[36] Other studies suggest that AIDS patients appear to tolerate elective abdominal operations reasonably well, especially if surgical therapy is for an illness unrelated to HIV-1 infection.[26] Surgical intervention in this patient population, however, has been reported to occasionally exacerbate underlying HIV-1 infection.[52] Extremely high morbidity and mortality have been reported in two studies examining emergent abdominal operations in AIDS patients, attesting to the serious nature of surgical infections in immunocompromised hosts.[27, 53, 54] There are no reliable laboratory parameters that can accurately stratify or quantify the increase in operative risk as patients progress from asymptomatic HIV-1 infection to AIDS.[55]

Trauma. Surgeons also frequently encounter HIV-1 infection in managing trauma victims. In 1987, a report from Johns Hopkins Hospital revealed that 3% of 203 severely injured or critically ill patients initially evaluated in the emergency department were seropositive for HIV-1.[56] Interestingly, all 6 seropositive individuals in this study were trauma victims between the ages of 25 and 34 and represented 16% of this age group. Of more concern was the finding that all 6 patients were actively bleeding at the time of presentation and all required multiple invasive procedures in the emergency department.

A follow-up study, done by the same group, of all patients presenting to the Johns Hopkins Hospital emergency department who had blood drawn during a 6-week period in 1987 found that 4% (92 of 2275 patients) had unrecognized HIV-1 infection.[57] The highest seroprevalence in the study was 11.4%, found among black males between the ages of 30 and 34 years old. The only clinical presentation associated with an increased seroprevalence rate (13.6%), independent of other known predictors of infection, was penetrating trauma.

These studies emphasize the need for surgeons managing trauma patients to be knowledgeable about HIV-1 infection. Unfortunately, as these two studies have demonstrated, there is no clinical indicator that allows identification of seropositive patients with any certainty. Although rapid determination tests for detection of antibodies to HIV-1 within 5 minutes exist,[58] their use has been restricted by HIV-1 testing laws. As a result, a policy of universal blood and body fluid precautions should be followed by all health care workers regardless of whether HIV-1 status is known. Using universal blood and body fluid precautions should help keep the already small risk of occupationally acquired HIV-1 infection as low as possible.

SELECTED REFERENCES

Bonacini, M.: Hepatobiliary complications in patients with human immunodeficiency virus infection. Am. J. Med., 92:404, 1992.
This paper is another excellent review that focuses on hepatic and biliary tract disorders in HIV-1–positive patients. It is complete and well referenced. Emphasis is placed on differential diagnosis and work-up.

Cappell, M., and Geller, A. J.: The high mortality of gastrointestinal bleeding in HIV-seropositive patients: A multivariate analysis of risk factors and warning signs of mortality in 50 consecutive patients. Am. J. Gastroenterol., 87:815, 1992.
An analysis of 59 episodes of gastrointestinal bleeding in 50 patients gives a good overview of the problem plus multivariate analysis and helps assess prognosis and identify those patients who will benefit from aggressive diagnostic evaluation.

Parente, F., Cernuschi, M., Antinori, S., Lazzarin, A., Moroni, M., Fasan, M., Rizzardini, G., Rovati, V., Morandi, E., Molteni, P., and Bianchi Porro, G.: Severe abdominal pain in patients with AIDS: Frequency, clinical aspects, causes, and outcomes. Scand. J. Gastroenterol., 29:511, 1994.
This recent overview of abdominal pain in a busy AIDS clinic from Milan characterizes the various abdominal disorders well and discusses the various clinical syndromes along with their etiology in depth.

Wilcox, C. M.: Esophageal disease in the acquired immunodeficiency syndrome: Etiology, diagnosis, and management. Am. J. Med., 92:412, 1992.
This manuscript is a comprehensive overview of esophageal disease in patients with AIDS. Emphasis is placed on diagnosis and management. A clear algorithm is provided.

REFERENCES

1. Wilcox, C. M.: Esophageal disease in the acquired immunodeficiency syndrome: Etiology, diagnosis, and management. Am. J. Med., 92:412, 1992.
2. Baehr, P., and McDonald, G. B.: Esophageal infections: Risk factors, presentation, diagnosis, and treatment. Gastroenterology, 105:509, 1994.
3. Horowitz, M. D., and Oliva, H.: Pneumothorax in AIDS patients: Operative management. Am. Surgeon, 59:200, 1993.
4. Fitzgerald, W., Bevelaqua, F. A., Garay, S. M., et al.: The role of open lung biopsy in patients with the acquired immunodeficiency syndrome. Chest, 91:659, 1987.
5. Bonfils-Roberts, E. A., Nickoderm, A., and Nealon, T. F.: Retrospective analysis of the efficacy of open lung biopsy in acquired immunodeficiency syndrome. Ann. Thorac. Surg., 49:115, 1990.
6. McKenna, R. J., Mountain, C. F., and McMurtrey, M. J.: Open lung biopsy in immunocompromised patients. Chest, 86:671, 1984.
7. Aclerno, A. J.: Cardiac complication in acquired immune deficiency syndrome (AIDS): A review. J. Am. Coll. Cardiol., 13:1144, 1989.
8. Aris, A., Pomar, J. L., and Saura, E.: Cardiopulmonary bypass in HIV-positive patients. Ann. Thorac. Surg., 55:1104, 1993.
9. Cello, J. P., and Wilcox, C. M.: Evaluation and treatment of gastrointestinal hemorrhage in patients with AIDS. Gastroenterol. Clin. North Am., 17:639, 1988.
10. Macho, J. R.: Gastrointestinal surgery in the AIDS patient. Gastroenterol. Clin. North Am., 17:563, 1988.
11. Friedman, S. L.: Gastrointestinal and hepatobiliary neoplasms in AIDS. Gastroenterol. Clin. North Am., 17:465, 1988.
12. Tyms, A. S., Tayor, D. L., and Parkin, J. M.: Cytomegalovirus and the acquired immunodeficiency syndrome. J. Antimicrob. Chemother., 23(A):89, 1989.
13. Wilcox, C. M., and Schwartz, D. A.: Symptomatic CMV duodenitis: An important clinical problem in AIDS. J. Clin. Gastroenterol., 14:293, 1992.
14. Bonacini, M.: Hepatobiliary complications in patients with human immunodeficiency virus infection. Am. J. Med., 92:404, 1992.
15. Schneiderman, D. J.: Hepatobiliary abnormalities of AIDS. Gastroenterol. Clin. North Am., 17:615, 1988.
16. Schneiderman, D. J., Arenson, D. M., Cello, J. P., Margaretten, W., and Weber, T. E.: Hepatic disease in patients with the acquired immune deficiency syndrome (AIDS). Hepatology, 7:925, 1987.
17. Margulis, S. J., Honig, C. L., Soave, R., et al.: Biliary tract obstruction in the acquired immunodeficiency syndrome. Ann. Intern. Med., 105:207, 1986.
18. Adolph, M. D., Bass, S. N., Lee, S. K., Blum, J. M., and Schreiber, H.: Cytomegaloviral acalculousis cholecystitis in acquired immunodeficiency syndrome patients. Am. Surgeon, 58:679, 1993.
19. Bouche, H., Moosett, C., Dumount, J. L., Carrot, F., Menu, Y., Aveline, B., Belghiti, J., Boboc, B., Erlinge, S., Berthelot, P., and Pol, S.: AIDS-related cholangitis: Diagnostic features and course in 15 patients. J. Hepatol., 17:34, 1993.
20. Forbes, A., Blanshard, C., and Gazzard, B.: Natural history of AIDS related sclerosing cholangitis: A study of 20 cases. Gut, 34:116, 1993.
21. Kotler, D. P.: Intestinal and hepatic manifestations of AIDS. Intern. Med., 34:43, 1989.
22. Letvin, N. L., Eaton, K. A., and Aldrich, W. R.: Acquired immunodeficiency syndrome in a colony of macaque monkeys. Proc. Natl. Acad. Sci. USA, 80:2178, 1983.
23. Barone, J. E., Gingold, B. S., Nealon, T. F., et al.: Abdominal pain in patients with acquired immune deficiency syndrome. Ann. Surg., 204:619, 1986.
24. Cappell, M. S., and Botros, N.: Predominantly gastrointestinal symptoms and signs in 11 consecutive AIDS patients with gastrointestinal lymphoma: A multicenter multiyear study including 763 HIV-seropositive patients. Am. J. Gastroenterol., 89:545, 1994.
25. Soderlund, C., Bratt, G. A., Engstrom, L., Grutzmeier, S., Nilsson, R., Sjunnesson, M., and Sandstrom, E.: Surgical treatment of cytomegalovirus enterocolitis in severe human immunodeficiency virus infection. Dis. Colon Rectum, 37:63, 1994.
26. Wilson, S. E., Robinson, G., Williams, R. A., et al.: Acquired immunodeficiency syndrome: Indications for abdominal surgery, pathology and outcome. Ann. Surg., 210:4, 1989.
27. LaRaja, R. D., Rothenberg, R. E., Odom, J. W., et al.: The incidence of intra-abdominal surgery in acquired immunodeficiency syndrome: A statistical review of 904 patients. Surgery, 105:175, 1989.
28. Whitney, T. M., Macho, J. R., Russell, T. R., Bossart, K. J., Heer, F. W., and Schecter, W. P.: Appendicitis in acquired immunodeficiency syndrome. Am. J. Surg., 164:467, 1992.
29. Binderow, S. R., and Shaked, A. A.: Acute appendicitis in patients with AIDS/HIV infection. Am. J. Surg., 162:9, 1991.
30. Dieterich, D. T., and Rahmin, M.: Cytomegalovirus colitis in AIDS: Presentation in 44 patients and a review of the literature. J. Acquir. Immune Defic. Syndr., 4(S1):S29, 1991.
31. Safavi, A., Gotlesman, L., and Dailey, T. H.: Anorectal surgery in the HIV positive patient: Update. Dis. Colon Rectum, 34:299, 1991.

32. Daling, J. F., Weiss, N. S., Klopfenstein, L. L., Cochran, L. E., Chow, W. H., and Daifuku, R.: Correlates of homosexual behavior and the incidence of anal cancer. JAMA, 247:1988, 1982.
33. Daling, J. R., Weiss, N. S., Hislop, T. G., Maden, C., Coates, R. J., Sherman, K. J., Ashley, R. L., Beagrie, M., Ryan, J. A., and Corey, L.: Sexual practices, sexually transmitted disease, and the incidence of anal cancer. N. Engl. J. Med., 317:973, 1987.
34. Lorenz, H. P., Wilson, W., Leigh, B., Crombleholme, T., and Schecter, W.: Squamous carcinoma of the anus and HIV infection. Dis. Colon Rectum, 34:336, 1991.
35. Barone, J. E., Wolkomir, A. F., Muakkassa, F. F., et al.: Abdominal pain and anorectal disease in AIDS. Gastroenterol. Clin. North Am., 17:631, 1988.
36. Wexner, S. D., Smithy, W. B., Milson, J. W., et al.: The surgical management of anorectal diseases in AIDS and pre-AIDS patients. Dis. Colon Rectum, 29:719, 1986.
37. Thuluvath, P. J., Connolly, G. M., Forbes, A., and Gazzard, B. G.: Abdominal pain in HIV infection. Q. J. Med., 78:275, 1991.
38. Parente, F., Cernuschi, M., Antiori, S., Lazzarin, A., Moroni, M., Fasan, M., Bizzardin, G., Rouati, V., Morandi, E., Molteni, P., and Bianchiporro, G.: Severe abdominal pain in patients with AIDS: Frequency, clinical aspects, causes, and outcomes. Scand. J. Gastroenterol., 29:511, 1994.
39. Rossi, G., Gorla, R., Stellini, R., et al.: Prevalence, clinical, and laboratory features of thrombocytopenia among HIV-infected individuals. AIDS Res. Hum. Retroviruses, 6:261, 1990.
40. Bettaieb, A., Fromont, P., Lovache, F., Oksenhendles, E., Vainchenker, W., Dvedari, N., and Bierling, P.: Presence of cross-reactive antibody between human immunodeficiency virus (HIV) and platelet glycoproteins in HIV-related immune thrombocytopenic purpura. Blood, 80:162, 1992.
41. Walsh, C. M., Nardi, M. A., and Karpatkin, S.: On the mechanism of thrombocytopenic purpura in sexually active homosexual men. N. Engl. J. Med., 311:635, 1984.
42. Walsh, C. M., Krigel, K., Lennette, E., and Karpatkin, S.: Thrombocytopenia in homosexual patients: Prognosis, response to therapy, and prevalence of antibody to the retrovirus associated with the acquired immunodeficiency syndrome. Ann. Intern. Med., 103:542, 1985.
43. Tyler, D. S., Shaunak, S., Bartlett, J. A., et al.: HIV-1 associated thrombocytopenia: The role of splenectomy. Ann. Surg., 211:211, 1990.
44. Oksenhendler, E., Bierling, P., Chevret, S., Delfraissy, J. F., Laurian, Y., Clauvel, J. P., and Seligmann, M.: Splenectomy is safe and effective in human immunodeficiency virus–related immune thrombocytopenia. Blood, 82:29, 1993.
45. Oksenhendler, E., Bierling, P., Ferchal, F., Chauvel, J. P., and Seligmann, M.: Zidovudine for thrombocytopenic purpura related to human immunodeficiency viral (HIV) infection. Ann. Intern. Med., 110:365, 1989.
46. Rarick, M. V., Espina, B., Montgomery, T., Easley, A., Allen, J., and Levine, A. M.: The long-term use of zidovudine in patients with severe immune-mediated thrombocytopenia secondary to infection with HIV. J. Acquir. Immune Defic. Syndr., 5:1357, 1991.
47. Cappell, M. S., and Geller, A. J.: The high mortality of gastrointestinal bleeding in HIV-seropositive patients: A multivariate analysis of risk factors and warning signs of mortality in 59 consecutive patients. Am. J. Gastroenterol., 87:815, 1992.
48. Godley, J. M.: AIDS and lymphadenopathy. Br. J. Surg., 73:170, 1986.
49. Farthing, C. F., Henry, K., Shanson, D. C., et al.: Clinical investigations of lymphadenopathy, including lymph node biopsies, in 24 homosexual men with antibody to the human T-cell lymphocytotropic virus type III (HTLV-III). Br. J. Surg., 73:180, 1986.
50. Scott, H. J., Glynn, M. J., Lane, I. F., et al.: Strategy for lymph node biopsy in homosexual men suspected of having LAV/HTLV-III related disease. Br. J. Surg., 73:186, 1986.
51. Rashleigh-Belcher, H. J. C., Carne, C. A., Weller, I. V. D., et al.: Surgical biopsy for persistent generalized lymphadenopathy. Br. J. Surg., 73:183, 1986.
52. Ferguson, C. M.: Surgical complications of human immunodeficiency virus infection. Am. Surg., 54:4, 1988.
53. Burack, J. H., Mandel, M. S., and Bizer, L. S.: Emergency abdominal operations in the patient with acquired immunodeficiency syndrome. Arch. Surg., 124:285, 1989.
54. Robinson, G., Wilson, S. E., and Williams, R. A.: Surgery in patients with acquired immunodeficiency syndrome. Arch. Surg., 122:170, 1987.
55. Binderow, S. R., Cavallo, R. J., and Freed, J.: Laboratory parameter as predictors of operative outcome after major abdominal surgery in AIDS- and HIV-infected patients. Am. Surg., 59:754, 1993.
56. Baker, J. L., Kelen, G. D., Siverston, K. T., et al.: Unsuspected human immunodeficiency virus in critically ill emergency patients. JAMA, 257:2609, 1987.
57. Kelen, G. D., Fritz, S., Qaqish, B., et al.: Unrecognized human immunodeficiency virus infection in emergency department patients. N. Engl. J. Med., 318:1645, 1988.
58. Kemp, B. E., Rylatt, D. B., Bundensen, P. G., et al.: Autologous red cell agglutination assay for HIV-1 antibodies: Simplified test with whole blood. Science, 241:1352, 1988.

CHAPTER 16

BITES AND STINGS

Elaine E. Nelson, M.D., and Paul S. Auerbach, M.D., M.S.

SNAKEBITES

Epidemiology

An estimated 50,000 to 100,000 individuals die each year worldwide from venomous snakebites. The population at greatest risk includes agricultural workers and hunters living in tropical countries.[39] In the United States, approximately 45,000 snakebites occur annually, and poisonous snakes are responsible for some 8000 bites, of which 9 to 15 are fatal.[32] Venomous species indigenous to the United States can be found in all states except Alaska, Maine, and Hawaii. Most snakebites occur on the extremities of males.[32] Accidentally stepping near a snake can cause bites to the lower extremity, whereas purposeful handling of a snake produces bites to the upper extremity. Snakes are poikilothermic, explaining the high incidence of bites during July and August.[32]

Species

In the United States, the rattlesnakes, copperheads, and cottonmouths of the Crotalidae (pit viper) family account for 99% of medically significant bites; the coral snakes of the Elapidae family are responsible for less than 1% of bites.[18] Colubrid (rear-fanged) snakes also account for less than 1%. Several characteristics distinguish pit vipers from nonvenomous snakes. Pit vipers have triangle-shaped heads, elliptic pupils, heat-sensing pits, and a single row of subcaudal scales. Nonpoisonous snakes have rounded heads with round pupils, no fangs, and a double row of subcaudal scales (Fig. 16–1). Coral snakes have a red, black, and yellow band pattern similar to that of many nonpoisonous snakes. The unique placement of red bands next to yellow bands identifies the coral snake. Snakes brought in for identification

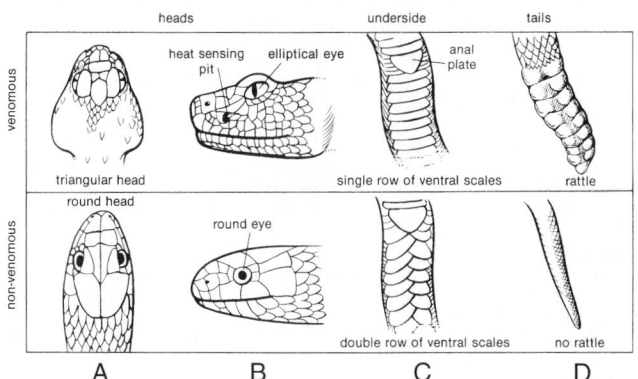

Figure 16–1. Identification of venomous pit vipers. *A*, Triangular head. *B*, Elliptic eye; heat-sensing facial pits on sides of head near nostrils. *C*, Single row of ventral scales leading up to anal plate. *D*, Rattles on tail. (From Sullivan, J. B., Wingert, W. A., and Norris, R. L.: North American venomous reptile bites. *In* Auerbach, P. S., [Ed.]: Wilderness Medicine: Management of Wilderness and Environmental Emergencies, 3rd ed. St. Louis, Mosby-Year Book, 1995, p. 684.)

should be handled cautiously, because a bite reflex may still be present.

Toxicology

Chemically, venom is quite complex, consisting of many enzymes and peptides. Damage to the endothelium by peptides increases vascular permeability, which may lead to edema and hypovolemic shock. The enzymes include proteases and L-amino acid oxidase, which cause tissue necrosis; hyaluronidase, which facilitates the spread of venom through tissues; and phospholipase A_2, which damages erythrocytes and muscle cells. Other enzymes include endonucleases, alkaline phosphatase, acid phosphatase, and cholinesterase.[18, 31] Besides causing local injury, these components also have deleterious effects on the cardiovascular, pulmonary, renal, and neurologic systems.[14] Other components of the venom profoundly affect coagulation, fibrinolysis, platelet function, and vascular integrity, sometimes producing either hemorrhagic or thrombotic sequelae.[22]

Clinical Manifestations

Local. Approximately 20% of bites by pit vipers do not cause envenomation.[36] These may appear as puncture wounds and lacerations associated with minimal pain only. Inoculation with venom produces burning pain within minutes, followed by edema and erythema. Edema progresses over the next few hours, with development of ecchymoses and hemorrhagic bullae. Involvement of the lymphatic system is common, causing lymphangitis and lymphadenopathy.[18, 35] Without treatment, the patient may develop severe extremity necrosis.

Systemic. Patients typically complain of weakness, nausea, vomiting, perioral paresthesias, metallic taste, and fasciculations.[35, 42] Continuing capillary leak leads to pulmonary edema, hypotension, and eventually shock. Victims of significant bites can develop coagulopathy within an hour, manifested as spontaneous bleeding from the gingivae, the bite site, venipuncture areas, and recent wounds. If untreated, progression to fulminant disseminated intravascular coagulation (DIC) can occur.[22] Acute renal failure secondary to direct nephrotoxins, circulatory collapse, and consumption coagulopathy is possible. Laboratory abnormalities include hypofibrinogenemia, thrombocytopenia, prolonged prothrombin and partial thromboplastin times, increased fibrin split products, creatinine and creatine phosphokinase, proteinuria, hematuria, and anemia or hemoconcentration.[22, 42]

Coral snakes produce primarily a neurotoxic venom. Local injury is generally minimal or absent. Systemic signs of coral snake bites, including cranial nerve dysfunction and loss of deep tendon reflexes, may progress to respiratory depression and paralysis over several hours.[14, 18] The differences in therapy make it important to distinguish between Elapidae and Crotalidae bites.

Management

Field Treatment. The patient should be placed at rest in an area away from the snake's territory. The wound should be cleansed and immobilized below the level of the heart. Cryotherapy, incision and suction, tourniquets, and electric shock therapy are not recommended and have, in certain circumstances, proved to be harmful.[18] Suction syringe devices now on the market successfully extract venom from the bite site if applied within 5 minutes and continued for at least 30 minutes.[18] A constriction band should be used, especially if a delay in treatment is anticipated. The band is applied 5 cm. above the bite, tight enough to occlude only lymphatic flow, and removed after antivenin therapy has been initiated.[18] Distal pulses and venous return should not be interrupted. These measures should not delay transport to the nearest hospital.

Hospital Management. A detailed history of the incident, type of snake, field management, and prior antivenin therapy is important. A rapid physical assessment should emphasize vital signs, wound appearance and size, and neurologic examination. Necessary laboratory analyses include a complete blood count (CBC), DIC panel, electrolytes, blood urea nitrogen, creatinine, creatine phosphokinase, urinalysis, and electrocardiogram. If the patient remains asymptomatic 6 hours after a pit viper bite or 24 hours after a coral snake bite, it is unlikely that envenomation occurred, so discharge is acceptable.[14]

Antivenin Therapy. Antivenin can neutralize venom at the bite site, making it the primary treatment modality. However, this therapy is not benign; severe hypersensitivity reactions can occur. In one study, 23% of the patients suffered acute anaphylaxis, and 50% suffered delayed serum sickness.[24] The use of antivenin for minor envenomation is controversial. Skin testing predicts hypersensitivity in most patients; this is performed by administering 0.02 ml. of 1:10 dilution of antivenin with 0.9% sodium chloride intradermally. Options for patients demonstrating hypersensitivity reactions or with known allergy to horse serum include premedication with diphenhydramine hydrochloride (25 to 50 mg. intravenously) and an epinephrine drip (2 to 20 μg. per minute) during antivenin administration in an intensive care setting.

Best results are achieved when an adequate amount of antivenin is administered within 4 hours of the bite.[18] Antivenin doses are determined by the severity of the envenomation (Table 16–1) and are administered over a 2- to 4-hour period. The patient's clinical condition should be re-evaluated every 2 hours, and, if necessary, a repeat dose of antivenin should be recalculated and given. Persistent hemodynamic instability and coagulopathy indicate inadequate antivenin dosage. Blood products are needed only if the antivenin is ineffective. Some experts recommend that in children, the dose of antivenin be increased by 50% because of the higher ratio of venom to body mass.[14, 18] Pregnancy is not a contraindication to antivenin therapy.[18]

A separate antivenin is available for coral snakes, excluding snakes from Arizona. Administration is similar to that of Crotalidae antivenin except that therapy should be initiated even when a coral snake bite is only strongly suspected because there are frequently no local manifestations. Poison control centers and zoos can provide information regarding the occasional exotic snakebite.

Wound Care. The wound should be cleansed thoroughly and the extremity splinted. Soaking the affected area in Burow's solution (1:20 aluminum acetate) three times a day is recommended.[18] Surgical débridement should be performed as necessary. Tetanus toxoid and tetanus immune globulin should be administered as indicated. Both gram-negative and -positive rods have been cultured from snakes' mouths and bite abscesses; therefore, a broad-spectrum antibiotic is recommended for 3 to 5 days after the bite.

Fasciotomy. Most snakebites cause subcutaneous deposition of venom. Clinically, differentiating true compartment syndrome from these local reactions is difficult, requiring the measurement of compartment pressures. Fasciotomies should be performed only if compartment pressures are over 30 mm. Hg.[18] Compartment syndrome in areas too small to measure pressures, such as the digits, can be diagnosed by pricking the skin of the affected extremity. Dark venous blood flow indicates increased pressure.[38] Routine fasciotomies to prevent compartment syndrome have not proved to be beneficial.[16]

MAMMALIAN BITES

Epidemiology

Many victims with minor injuries from animal bites do not present for treatment, so the actual incidence is unknown. Worldwide, thousands of people are killed each year, primarily by large animals such as lions and tigers. Death from animal bites is rare in the United States. Dogs are responsible for most animal bites, followed by cats and humans. In the United States, an estimated 1 to 2 million dog bites occur annually, accounting for 1% of emergency department visits.[8] Animal bites occur primarily on the upper extremities in adults and on the head in children.[26]

Treatment

Evaluation. Patients, especially children, attacked by animals are at risk for blunt and penetrating trauma. Animals can produce blunt injuries by striking with their extremities, biting with powerful jaws, and crushing with their body

TABLE 16–1. Degrees of Crotalid Envenomation and Antivenin Guidelines

Degree	Description	Antivenin Dose (Vials)
No envenomation	Fang marks only	0
Minimal	Fang marks, local swelling and pain only	0–5
Moderate	Fang marks, swelling beyond bite site, nausea, vomiting, paresthesias, mild coagulation abnormalities, hemoconcentration	10–20
Severe	Fang marks, marked swelling and ecchymosis, severe symptoms, disseminated intravascular coagulopathy, proteinuria, hematuria	20 or more

Data from Sullivan, J. B., Wingert, W. A., and Norris, R. L.: North American venomous reptile bites. *In* Auerbach, P. S. [Ed.]: Wilderness Medicine: Management of Wilderness and Environmental Emergencies, 3rd ed. St. Louis, Mosby-Year Book, 1995, pp. 680–709.

weight. Teeth and claws can puncture body cavities, including the cranium, and amputate extremities. These patients should be treated as trauma victims, with special attention to wound management (see later). Useful laboratory tests include a hematocrit when blood loss is of concern, and cultures when an infection is present. X-rays should be obtained to diagnose suspected fractures, joint penetration, severe infections, and foreign bodies such as teeth. Serious bites to the extremities and to the cranium, especially in children, warrant radiologic studies. Tetanus prophylaxis should be current.

Wound Care. Local wound management prevents infection and maximizes functional and aesthetic outcomes. Wound cleansing is the most important therapy for preventing infection.[8] Intact skin surrounding dirty wounds can be scrubbed with a sponge and normal saline or 1% povidone-iodine solution. Contamination of the wound with skin flora should be prevented. Copious irrigation of the wound with normal saline using a 19-gauge needle and syringe significantly decreases the likelihood of infection.[8] Alternatively, a 1% povidone-iodine solution can be used, providing the wound is irrigated afterward with normal saline. Studies suggest that irrigating with topical antibiotics such as penicillin or a cephalosporin is more effective in preventing infection than using normal saline alone.[8] Scrubbing the wound can increase tissue damage and infection and thus should be avoided. Wounds that are dirty or contain devitalized tissue benefit from débridement.[1, 7]

Options available for repair include primary, delayed, and secondary closure. The appropriate method is determined by the anatomic location of the bite, the source of the bite, and the type of injury. Contrary to past beliefs, primary closure of selected bites produces the best outcome for patients without increasing the risk of infection.[7, 8] This is especially true for head and neck wounds, where aesthetic results are more important. Maxillofacial surgeons recommend primary closure for facial wounds presenting within 12 hours.[1, 26] Severe human bites and avulsion injuries of the face requiring flaps have been successfully repaired with primary closure; however, this technique remains controversial.[1, 37] Healing by secondary intention generally produces unacceptable scars.

The primary goal in repairing bite wounds to the hand is to maximize functional outcome. Approximately one third of dog bites to the hand become infected even with adequate therapy.[7] Healing by secondary intention is recommended for most hand lacerations.[8] All tendon and nerve injuries should be managed by delayed repair.[27] After a thorough exploration, irrigation, and débridement, the hand should be immobilized, wrapped in a bulky dressing, and elevated. A common human bite wound associated with high morbidity is the clenched fist injury. Regardless of the history obtained, injuries over the dorsum of the metacarpophalangeal joints should be treated as clenched fist injuries resulting from striking another person's mouth. The extensor tendon retracts when the hand is opened, so evaluation needs to be done with the hand in both the open and the clenched positions. Minor injuries should be irrigated, débrided, and left open. Potentially deeper injuries and infected bites presenting after 24 hours require exploration and débridement in the operating room and administration of intravenous antibiotics.[4, 27]

The method of repair used for bite wounds to other body parts depends on the risk factors associated with the particular injury (Table 16–2). Healing by delayed repair or secondary intention should be considered for high-risk bites, whereas primary closure can be performed safely in low-risk bites.[8] Puncture wounds have an increased incidence of infection and should not be sutured. Deep irrigation of small puncture wounds and wide excision have not proved to be

TABLE 16–2. Animal Bite Risk Factors for Infection

High Risk

Location
  Hand, wrist, or foot
  Scalp or face in infants (high risk of cranial perforation; skull x-ray mandatory)
  Over a major joint (possible perforation)
  Through-and-through bite of cheek
Type of wound
  Puncture (difficult to irrigate)
  Tissue crushing that cannot be débrided
  Carnivore bite over vital structure (artery, nerve, joint)
Patient
  Older than 50 years
  Asplenic
  Chronic alcoholic
  Altered immune status
  Diabetic
  Peripheral vascular insufficiency
  Chronic corticosteroid therapy
  Prosthetic or diseased heart valve or joint
Species
  Domestic cat
  Large cat (deep punctures)
  Human (hand bites)
  Primates
  Pigs

Low Risk

Location
  Face, scalp, ears, or mouth
Type of wound
  Large clean lacerations that can be thoroughly irrigated
Species
  Rodents

From Callaham, M., French, S. P., Tetlow, P., and Rees, P.: Bites and injuries inflicted by mammals. *In* Auerbach, P. S. (Ed.): Wilderness Medicine: Management of Wilderness and Environmental Emergencies, 3rd ed. St. Louis, Mosby-Year Book, 1995, pp. 943–1009.

beneficial. Larger puncture wounds can benefit from irrigation and débridement.[7, 8] Sterile, dry dressings should be placed over all wounds. Early wound checks are mandatory.

Microbiology. Given the large variety and concentration of bacteria in mouths, it is not surprising that wound infection is the main complication of bites, occurring in 5% to 15% of dog bites and 15% to 50% of cat bites.[13, 40] Infections are usually polymicrobial, with both aerobic and anaerobic bacteria (Table 16–3). *Staphylococcus* and *Streptococcus* species and anaerobes are present in most infections. *Pasteurella multocida* is the primary microorganism responsible for infections in cat bites and occasionally dog bites, whereas *Eikenella corrodens* has been isolated from human bites.[8, 13, 40] Many micro-organisms that are present locally can progress to systemic disease. Atypical pathogens and organisms from unusual sources of bites are presented in Table 16–4.

Antibiotics. Prophylactic antibiotics are recommended for patients with high-risk bites (see Table 16–2).[7, 8, 13] Initial antibiotic choice and route should be based on the type of animal and the severity and location of the bite. Cat bites often cause puncture wounds that require antibiotics. Penicillin and dicloxacillin adequately cover expected pathogens, including *Pasteurella*.[8] Patients with low-risk dog bites do not benefit from prophylactic antibiotics unless the hand is involved. Antibiotics recommended for dog bites at high risk of infection and for most other animal bites include dicloxacillin or cephalexin because the incidence of *Pasteurella* is low.[8] Trimethoprim-sulfamethoxazole is an alternative for both cat and dog bites in patients allergic to penicillin. Human bites, which may carry *Eikenella corrodens*, can be treated with a

TABLE 16–3. Common Bacteria Found in Animals' Mouths

Actinobacillus spp.	*Fusobacterium* spp.
Peptococcus spp.	*Peptostreptococcus* spp.
Propionibacterium spp.	*Veillonella parvula*
Bacteroides spp.	*Escherichia coli*
Micrococcus spp.	*Moraxella* spp.
Leptotrichia bacillus	*Staphylococcus epidermidis*
Staphylococcus aureus	*Acinetobacter* spp.
Streptococcus spp.	*Enterobacter* spp.
Bacillus spp.	*Serratia marcescens*
Corynebacterium spp.	*Proteus mirabilis*
Eubacterium spp.	*Aeromonas hydrophila*
Pasteurella aerogenes	*Pasteurella dagmatis, canis*
Pseudomonas spp.	*Pasteurella multocida*
Eikenella corrodens	*Haemophilus aphrophilus*
Neisseria spp.	*Klebsiella* spp.
Clostridium perfringens	*Capnocytophaga canimorsus*
Brucella canis	*Bordetella* spp.
Haemophilus haemolyticus	

Data from Callaham, M., French, S. P., Tetlow, P., and Rees, P.: Bites and injuries inflicted by mammals. *In* Auerbach, P. S. (Ed.): Wilderness Medicine: Management of Wilderness and Environmental Emergencies, 3rd ed. St. Louis, Mosby-Year Book, 1995; and Dire, D. J.: Emergency management of dog and cat bite wounds. Emerg. Med. Clin. North Am., *10(4)*:719, 1992.

second- or third-generation cephalosporin or a combination of dicloxacillin and ampicillin.[8] Patients allergic to penicillin can receive ciprofloxacin or erythromycin.[8] Cefuroxime or amoxicillin-clavulanic acid is acceptable for all bites, although these drugs are usually more expensive. Patients presenting 24 hours after a bite without signs of infection usually do not need prophylactic antibiotics. Antibiotics should be administered early and, in serious bites, be given parenterally. Routine cultures of uninfected wounds have not proved useful and should be reserved for infected wounds that fail antibiotic therapy.[7, 8, 13]

Rabies. Worldwide, 20,000 to 30,000 people die from rabies annually, with dogs being the major source. Immunization of pets against rabies has decreased the number of cases to approximately one a year in the United States,[8] where skunks, raccoons, and bats are the most common sources.[19] Rabies is caused by a rhabdovirus found in the saliva of animals and is transmitted through bites or scratches. Patients contracting rabies develop acute encephalitis and usually die. The three phases of rabies include a prodromal phase, with nonspecific complaints and possibly pain or paresthesias at the bite site; an acute neurologic phase, manifested as dysphagia, hydrophobia, and hallucinations; and finally a clinical phase, with dysrhythmias, autonomic motor system dysfunction, and coma.[19]

The decision to administer rabies prophylaxis depends on the animal species and the nature of the event. Wild animals should be considered rabid. A bite from a healthy-appearing domestic animal does not require prophylaxis if the animal can be observed for 10 days. The local health department can help determine the risk for rabies in patients bitten by livestock or domestic animals that are not captured. Birds, rodents, and reptiles are unlikely to carry rabies. Unprovoked attacks are more likely to occur by rabid animals.[8, 13, 19]

Adequate wound care and postexposure prophylaxis can prevent the development of rabies. Washing the wound with soap and water may kill the virus.[13] If suspicion is high for a rabid bite, consider leaving the wound open. Both passive and active immunization should be given. Passive immunization consists of administering 20 I.U. per kg. of rabies immune globulin, half intramuscularly and half into the wound. Active immunization consists of administering 1 ml. of human diploid cell vaccine intramuscularly in the deltoid in adults and in the anterior thigh in children on days 0, 3, 7, 14, and 28. Patients with pre-exposure immunization do not need passive immunization and need active immunization only on days 0 and 3.

ARTHROPOD BITES

Black Widow Spiders

Black widow (*Latrodectus*) spiders are found throughout the world. At least one of five species inhabits all areas of the United States except Alaska.[6] The typical female black widow responsible for human envenomation is 1 to 4 cm., with shiny black coloration and a distinctive red ventral marking, usually in the shape of an hourglass (Fig. 16–2). Variations in color occur among the species, with some appearing brown or red and without the ventral marking. This nocturnal spider bites defensively, especially when trapped against the victim's skin.

Toxicology. The black widow spider produces a neurotoxic venom with minimal local properties. The primary action of the venom occurs at the presynaptic terminal, enhancing neurotransmitter release. Excess acetylcholine at the neuromuscular junction causes muscle spasm. Additionally, release of norepinephrine produces adrenergic stimulation.[41]

Clinical Manifestations. Initially the bite may be painful and slightly red and may appear as two small puncture wounds.[6, 9] It is not uncommon for the bite to go unnoticed. In such cases the patient generally presents with only systemic complaints, delaying diagnosis. Neuromuscular symptoms that occur as early as 30 minutes after envenomation include severe pain and spasms of large muscle groups.

TABLE 16–4. Atypical Organisms Associated with Bite Wounds and Unusual Sources

Source	Pathogen*
Alligator	*Aeromonas hydrophila*
Bear	Similar to dogs
Cat	*Afipia felis* (cat-scratch disease?)
	Rochalimaea (bacillary angiomatosis)
	Cowpox
Cat family (wild)	*Pasteurella* spp.
Coyote	*Francisella tularensis*
Human	Syphilis
	Tuberculosis
	Herpes
	Hepatitis B and C
	HIV (?)
Lion	*Pasteurella* spp.
Livestock	*Brucella* (brucellosis)
	Pasteurella spp.
Opossum	*Pasteurella* spp.
Platypus	Venomous bites
Primate	*Eikenella corrodens*
	Simian herpes B virus
Rabbit	*Francisella tularensis*
Rodent	*Streptobacillus moniliformis, Spirillum minus* (rat-bite fever)
	Pasteurella spp.
	Yersinia pestis (plague)
Short-tailed shrew	Venomous bites
Squirrel	*Francisella tularensis*

*In addition to organisms listed in Table 16–3 and excluding rabies.
Data from Callaham, M., French, S. P., Tetlow, P., and Rees, P.: Bites and injuries inflicted by mammals. *In* Auerbach, P. S. (Ed.): Wilderness Medicine: Management of Wilderness and Environmental Emergencies, 3rd ed. St. Louis, Mosby-Year Book, 1995; and Weber, D. J., and Hansen, A. R.: Infections resulting from animal bites. Infect. Dis. Clin. North Am., *5(3)*:663, 1991.

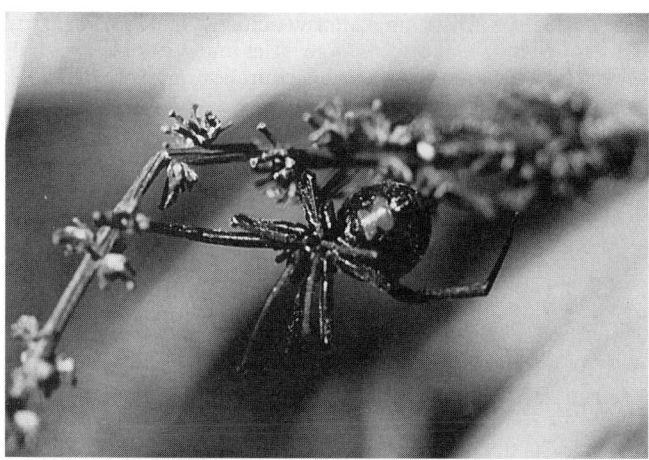

Figure 16–2. Female black widow spider with characteristic hourglass marking. (Courtesy of Paul Auerbach.)

Abdominal cramps and rigidity occasionally mimic an acute abdomen. Dyspnea can result from chest tightness. Adrenergic stimulation produces hypertension, diaphoresis, and tachycardia. Other symptoms include fasciculations, nausea and vomiting, headache, paresthesias, fatigue, and salivation.[6, 9, 30] Acute symptoms typically peak at several hours and resolve in 1 to 2 days. Mild pain and nonspecific symptoms, primarily neurologic, can persist for several weeks. Death is unusual from black widow spider bites.

Treatment. Mild envenomation is managed with local wound care, including cleansing, applying ice, and administering tetanus prophylaxis. The possibility of delayed, severe symptoms mandates an observation period of several hours. The optimal therapy for severe envenomation is controversial. Intravenous calcium gluconate, previously recommended as a first-line drug for black widow spider bite, has recently been challenged as a therapeutic agent.[6, 9] Relief of symptoms occurs in only a small percentage of patients treated with this medication and is usually transient. Alternatives include narcotics and benzodiazepines to relieve muscular pain.

Antivenin derived from horse serum is available. Its use should be reserved for severe envenomation, because anaphylaxis and serum sickness can occur. Antivenin is currently recommended for pregnant women, children under 16 years, individuals over 60 years, and patients with severe reactions such as uncontrolled hypertension, respiratory distress, and seizures.[6, 30] Skin testing may detect individuals who are allergic to antivenin and should receive pretreatment with diphenhydramine. The initial recommended antivenin dose is one vial, repeated as necessary. Studies have demonstrated that antivenin can decrease a patient's hospital stay, with discharge occurring as early as several hours after administration.[9] Treatment with antivenin can also prevent the development of persistent vague symptoms.

Brown Recluse Spiders

Envenomation by the brown recluse (*Loxosceles*) spider is termed *necrotic arachnidism* or *loxoscelism*. These arthropods primarily inhabit North and South America, Africa, and Europe. Several species of *Loxosceles* are found throughout the United States, with the greatest concentration in the Midwest. Most significant envenomations in the United States occur from the species *Loxosceles reclusa*. These spiders are varying shades of brownish-gray, with a characteristic dark brown violin-shaped marking over the cephalothorax—hence the

name violin spider (Fig. 16–3). Unlike other spiders, the brown recluse has three pairs of eyes, enabling identification. Both male and female spiders bite, usually when threatened.

Toxicology. Although several enzymes have been isolated from the venom, sphingomyelinase is the main dermonecrotic factor.[6, 15] This enzyme is a phospholipase that interacts with the cell membranes of erythrocytes, platelets, and endothelial cells and causes hemolysis, coagulation, and platelet aggregation. Necrosis is most severe in fatty areas such as the abdomen and thigh.[23, 41] Functioning polymorphonuclear neutrophils in the host may be necessary for the venom to have effect.[15]

Clinical Manifestations. Symptoms range from mild irritation to severe necrosis with ulceration. The patient may be unaware of the bite or may complain of stinging. Within several hours, a few patients develop local ischemia, causing pain, itching, swelling, and erythema. This progresses to formation of a blister. With a more severe bite, the center area turns purple secondary to thrombosis. Vasoconstriction can create a pale peripheral border. Over the next few days, the widening necrosis is replaced by eschar. The eschar separates, leaving an ulcer that usually heals within 2 months but occasionally requires grafting.[6, 23]

Systemic features can include headache, nausea and vomiting, fever, malaise, arthralgias, and maculopapular rash.[6] Possible additional findings include thrombocytopenia, DIC, hemolytic anemia, coma, and, rarely, death. Renal failure can result from intravascular hemolysis.[15, 23] Necessary laboratory tests include CBC, platelet count, urinalysis, electrolytes, and, if indicated, DIC panel and total bilirubin. Systemic involve-

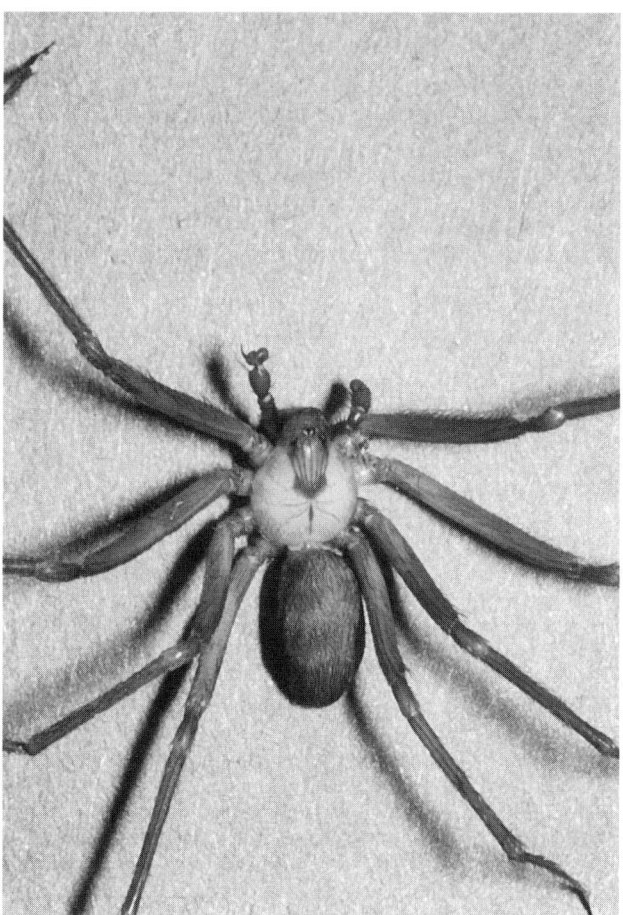

Figure 16–3. Brown recluse spider with fiddle-shaped marking on the cephalothorax. (Courtesy of Sherman Minton, Indiana University.)

ment (loxoscelism) is more common in children and can occur with minimal to absent local findings.[6]

Treatment. The recommended management has changed in the past few years and remains controversial. The bite site should be elevated and an ice compress applied. Cold therapy potentially inhibits venom activity and decreases inflammation and ulcer formation, whereas heat application enhances necrosis and ulcer development.[6, 41] A lipophilic antibiotic should be administered and tetanus status made current. Brown recluse bites that do not develop necrosis within 72 hours usually heal well and require no additional therapy.

Studies have shown that more severe lesions may benefit from dapsone administration if given during the first few days after envenomation.[25] Dapsone may reduce local inflammation by inhibiting neutrophil function. The recommended adult dose is 100 mg. per day. Dapsone is contraindicated in patients with glucose-6-phosphate dehydrogenase deficiency, and it can cause methemoglobinemia. The effects of systemic steroid administration on local wound healing are questionable, so this therapy should be reserved for patients with intravascular hemolysis only. Early surgical intervention, recommended previously, has proved to be controversial. Proponents argue that the venom burden is reduced; opponents argue that wound edges are compromised and do not heal well.[6] Pyoderma gangrenosum, presenting as nonhealing ulcers and failure of skin grafts, occurs more often in patients undergoing early excision and débridement, possibly secondary to the rapid spread of venom.[15] In 1 to 2 weeks, after the eschar margins are defined, débridement can be performed as necessary. In severe cases, wide excision and split-thickness skin grafting are necessary while dapsone therapy is continued.[41] Antivenin is not currently available in the United States.

Scorpions

Significant scorpion envenomations occur worldwide by species belonging to the Buthidae family. The genus *Centruroides* is responsible for most stings that occur in the United States. Approximately 7000 scorpion stings are reported yearly in the United States, with one third of these occurring in Arizona. *Centruroides,* a yellow to brown crablike arthropod, can measure up to 5 cm. in length. Scorpions tend to be nocturnal, stinging when threatened.

Clinical Manifestations. Reactions from scorpion stings vary from mild, local irritation to death. *Centruroides exilicauda,* the scorpion responsible for the rare deaths occurring in the United States, produces a neurotoxin that can prevent sodium channel closure. When stung, a patient typically experiences local paresthesias and burning. Systemic manifestations include cranial nerve and neuromuscular dysfunction, potentially causing respiratory distress.[10, 17] Patients may develop signs of adrenergic stimulation, accompanied by nausea and vomiting. Stings by other species of scorpions in the United States usually cause local pain and swelling only.

Treatment. All patients should receive tetanus prophylaxis if indicated, ice pack therapy to the bite site, and analgesics for pain. Patients with signs of systemic envenomation require supportive care, with close monitoring of cardiovascular and respiratory status in an intensive care setting. Antivenin therapy for these patients is controversial. Administration of antivenin can reverse cranial nerve and neuromuscular symptoms, but it may be accompanied by anaphylaxis and delayed serum sickness. In one study, administration of antivenin to children completely reversed neurologic and cardiopulmonary complications within hours, allowing discharge from the emergency department.[5] No child developed anaphylaxis, although a large percentage

developed serum sickness. Antivenin is available from Iatric Laboratories in Phoenix, Arizona. The initial dose is one vial, which should be preceded by skin testing. Patients with positive skin tests should be pretreated with diphenhydramine. Pain control may still be necessary.

Ticks

Several potentially serious diseases occur from tick bites. Timely and adequate removal of the tick is important. Common tick removal remedies, including application of gasoline, methylated spirits, and fingernail polish, are typically ineffective. Removal by forceps using a rotating technique has been found to be more effective than straight-pulling extraction.[12] Crushing the tick should be avoided, because this releases potentially infectious agents into the wound. After extraction, the wound should be cleansed. Prophylactic antibiotics are not recommended for the prevention of Lyme disease and other diseases. Tetanus immunization should be current. Occasionally, a granulomatous lesion requiring surgical excision may develop at the tick bite site a few weeks after the incident.

Hymenoptera

Most arthropod envenomations occur by species belonging to the order Hymenoptera, which includes bees, wasps, and ants. Bees and wasps are located throughout the United States, whereas fire ants inhabit primarily the southeastern region. The Africanized honeybee, characterized by mass attacks, has recently migrated to the southern United States.

Envenomation. Hymenoptera sting primarily defensively, especially if the nest is disturbed. The stingers of ants and wasps, attached to venom sacs located on the abdomen, can be used repeatedly. Some bees, however, have barb-shaped stingers, preventing detachment from the victim. Venom from bees and wasps is similar and complex.[43] Vasoactive compounds such as histamine and serotonin are responsible for the local reaction and pain. Peptides, such as mellitin, and enzymes, primarily phospholipases and hyaluronidases, have been identified as allergens that elicit an IgE-mediated response. Fire ant venom consists primarily of nonallergenic alkaloids that release histamine and cause necrosis. Allergenic proteins constitute only 0.1% of fire ant venom.

Clinical Reactions. A Hymenoptera sting in a nonallergic individual produces immediate pain followed by a wheal and flare reaction. Fire ants characteristically produce multiple pustules from repetitive stings at the same site. Multiple stings can produce a toxic reaction, including vomiting, diarrhea, generalized edema, cardiovascular collapse, and hemolysis, which can be difficult to distinguish from a systemic allergic reaction.[34]

Large local reactions develop in approximately 17% of envenomed subjects.[43] These reactions present as erythematous, edematous, painful, and pruritic areas larger than 10 cm. in diameter and may last 2 to 5 days. They represent a combination of IgE-mediated, cell-mediated, and possibly an Arthus-type reaction. Patients developing large local reactions are at risk for repeat episodes with future stings. However, there does not appear to be an increased risk of developing a systemic allergic reaction.[43]

Bee-sting anaphylaxis develops in 0.3% to 3% of the general population, causing approximately 40 reported deaths annually.[34, 43] Fatalities occur more often in adults and within 1 hour of the sting. Symptoms occur within minutes, ranging from mild urticaria and angioedema to respiratory arrest secondary to airway edema and cardiovascular collapse. A positive IgE-mediated skin test to Hymenoptera extract helps predict an allergic sting reaction. Unusual reactions to Hymenoptera venom include late-onset allergic reaction (more than 5 hours after the sting), serum sickness, renal disease, neurologic complaints such as Guillain-Barré syndrome, and vasculitis.[33] The etiology of these reactions is thought to be immunologic.

Treatment. Local therapy includes removing the stinger by gentle scraping, avoiding compression of the venom sac. Blisters from fire ant stings should be left intact. The bite site should be cleansed and ice applied. Topical or injected lidocaine can decrease pain from the sting, as can a solution of vinegar and salt. Antihistamines administered orally or topically can decrease pruritus. Treatment of a large, local envenomation includes the aforementioned therapy in addition to elevation of the extremity and analgesics. A 5-day course of prednisone (1 mg. per kg. per day) is also recommended.[43] Isolated local reactions do not require epinephrine or immunotherapy.

Mild anaphylaxis can be treated with 0.3 ml. of 1:1000 subcutaneous epinephrine (0.01 ml. per kg. in children, up to 0.3 ml.) and an oral or intravenous antihistamine. Severe cases may require intravenous fluids, vasopressors, oxygen, bronchodilators, and endotracheal intubation. Prolonged reactions may benefit from steroid administration. These patients should be observed closely in a monitored environment.

Venom immunotherapy effectively prevents anaphylaxis from subsequent stings in certain patients with positive skin tests.[34] All persons with previous severe systemic allergic reactions to Hymenoptera stings or who develop serum sickness should be referred for immunotherapy. This therapy is also recommended for adults with anaphylactic dermal reactions only, such as hives. Studies have demonstrated that children with isolated skin manifestations of anaphylaxis are at relatively low risk for repeat episodes with subsequent stings.[34] Desensitization, a therapy with its own complications, is not indicated for this subgroup. Patients with anaphylaxis secondary to Hymenoptera stings should carry injectable epinephrine and antihistamines.

MARINE TRAUMA AND ENVENOMATION

Four fifths of all living creatures reside underwater.[3] Hazardous marine animals are located primarily in temperate or tropical seas. Increased human exposure to marine life through recreation, research, and industry has led to more frequent encounters with aquatic organisms. Injuries generally occur through bites, stings, punctures, or envenomation.

Therapeutic Considerations

Initial Assessment. Injuries from marine organisms can range from mild local complaints to systemic collapse from major trauma or severe envenomation. Several aspects unique to marine trauma make the treatment of these patients challenging. Immersion in cold water predisposes patients to hypothermia and near drowning. Rapid ascent after an encounter with a marine organism can cause air embolism or decompression illness in a scuba diver. Anaphylactic reaction to venom further complicates an envenomation. Late complications include unique infections caused by a wide variety of aquatic microorganisms.

Microbiology. Most marine isolates are gram-negative rods.[3] *Vibrio* species are of primary concern. *Staphylococcus* and *Streptococcus* species are also frequently cultured from infections. The laboratory should be notified that cultures are sent from aquatic-acquired infections.

General Management. Initial management is focused on airway, breathing, and circulation. Patients with extensive blunt and penetrating injuries should be treated as major trauma victims. Patients with severe envenomation should receive specific intervention directed against a toxin (discussed separately, according to marine creature) in addition to general supportive care. Antivenins can be administered if available. Tetanus status should be updated for all bites, cuts, and stings. Radiographs should be obtained to locate foreign bodies and fractures.

Selection of antibiotics is tailored to marine bacteriology. Third-generation cephalosporins provide adequate coverage for the gram-positive and gram-negative microorganisms found in ocean water, including the *Vibrio* species.[3] Ciprofloxacin, cefoperazone, gentamicin, and trimethoprim-sulfamethoxazole are acceptable antibiotics. Outpatient regimens include ciprofloxacin, trimethoprim-sulfamethoxazole, or doxycycline.[3] Patients with large abrasions, lacerations, puncture wounds, or hand injuries, as well as immunocompromised patients, should receive prophylactic antibiotics. Infected wounds should be cultured.

Wound Care. Meticulous wound care is necessary to prevent infection and to optimize aesthetic and functional outcome.[21] Wounds should be irrigated with normal saline. Débridement of devitalized tissue can decrease infection and promote healing. Large wounds should be explored in the operating room. The decision to close a wound primarily must balance the cosmetic result against the risk of infection. Wounds should be loosely closed and drainage provided. Primary closure should be avoided in distal extremity wounds, punctures, and crush injuries.

Antivenin. Antivenin is available for several envenomations, including those from the box jellyfish, sea snake, and stonefish.[2] Patients demonstrating severe reactions to these envenomations benefit from antivenin. Skin testing should be performed if time permits before antivenin is administered to determine which patients would benefit from pretreatment with diphenhydramine and/or epinephrine. Serum sickness is a complication of antivenin therapy and can be treated with corticosteroids. Regional poison control centers can assist in locating antivenins.

Injuries from Nonvenomous Aquatic Animals

Sharks. Approximately 50 to 100 shark attacks occur annually. However, these attacks cause fewer than 10 deaths each year.[20, 21] The tiger, great white, and bull sharks are responsible for most attacks.[21] Most incidents occur at the surface of shallow water within 100 feet of shore.[20] Sharks locate prey by detecting motion and sensing body fluids through smell and taste. Most sharks strike the victim and then leave.[20, 21] Most injuries occur to the lower extremities.

Powerful jaws and sharp teeth produce crushing, tearing injuries. Hypovolemic shock and near drowning are life-threatening consequences of an attack.[21] Other complications include soft tissue and neurovascular damage, fractures, and infection.[20] Massive transfusions are frequently necessary, predisposing the patient to DIC. Most wounds require exploration and repair in the operating room (see the section on wound care). Occasionally, "bumping" by sharks can produce abrasions, which should be treated as second-degree burns.[3]

Moray Eels. Morays are savage bottom dwellers, residing in holes or crevices. Eels bite defensively, producing multiple small puncture wounds. The hand is most frequently bitten. Occasionally the eel remains attached to the victim, requiring decapitation of the animal for release. Puncture wounds and bites to the hand from all animals, including eels, are at high risk for infection and should not be closed primarily.[3]

Alligators and Crocodiles. Crocodiles can attain a length of more than 20 feet and travel at speeds of 20 miles per hour in water and on land. Like sharks, alligators and crocodiles attack primarily in shallow water. These animals can produce severe injuries by grasping victims with their powerful jaws and dragging them underwater. Injuries from alligator and crocodile attacks should be treated like shark bites.

Miscellaneous. Other nonvenomous animals capable of attacking include the barracuda, giant grouper, sea lion, and needlefish. Except for the needlefish, which spears victims with its elongated snout, these animals bite.

Envenomation by Invertebrates

Coelenterates. The phylum Coelenterata consists of hydrozoans, which include fire coral, hydroids, and Portuguese man-of-wars; scyphozoans, which include jellyfish and sea nettles; and anthozoans, which include sea anemones. Coelenterates carry venomous stinging cells called nematocysts.[29]

Mild envenomations, typically inflicted by fire coral, hydroids, and anemones, produce skin irritation.[2] The patient notices immediate stinging followed by pruritus, paresthesias, and throbbing pain with proximal radiation. The involved area develops edema and erythema, followed by blisters and petechiae. This can progress to local infection and ulceration.

Severe envenomations are caused by anemones, sea nettles, and jellyfish.[2] Patients have systemic symptoms in addition to the local manifestations. An anaphylactic reaction to the venom may contribute to the pathophysiology of envenomation. Patients can develop fever, nausea, vomiting, and malaise. Any organ system can be involved, and death is attributed to hypotension and cardiorespiratory arrest. One of the most venomous sea creatures, found primarily in northern Australia, is the box jellyfish, *Chironex fleckeri*. More deaths have been attributed to this creature than to sharks.

Therapy consists of detoxification of nematocysts and systemic support. The wound should be rinsed in sea water and gently dried.[2] Fresh water and vigorous rubbing can cause nematocysts to discharge. Dilute (5%) acetic acid (vinegar) can inactivate the toxin and should be applied for 30 minutes or until the pain is relieved.[2] This is critical with the box jellyfish. Isopropyl alcohol should be used only as a last resort. Baking soda may be more effective than acetic acid for inactivating the toxin of U.S. eastern coastal Chesapeake Bay sea nettles.[2] After the wound is irrigated with the appropriate solution, remaining nematocysts must be removed. One method is to apply shaving cream or a flour paste and shave the area with a razor. The affected area should again be irrigated, dressed, and elevated. Medical care providers should wear gloves for self-protection. Cryotherapy, local anesthetics, antihistamines, or steroids can relieve pain after the toxin is inactivated. Prophylactic antibiotics are usually unnecessary.

Sponges. Two syndromes occur after contact with sponges.[2] The first is an allergic plantlike contact dermatitis characterized by itching and burning within hours of contact. This can progress to soft-tissue edema, vesicle development, and joint swelling. Large areas of involvement can cause systemic toxicity with fever, nausea, and muscle cramps. The second syndrome is an irritant dermatitis after penetration of the skin with small spicules. Sponge diver's disease is actually caused by anemones that colonize the sponges rather than by the sponges themselves.

Treatment consists of washing the affected area and drying gently. Dilute (5%) acetic acid (vinegar) should be applied for 30 minutes three times daily.[2] Remaining spicules can be removed with adhesive tape. A steroid cream can be applied to the skin after decontamination. Occasionally, systemic steroids and diphenhydramine are required.

Echinodermata. Starfish, sea urchins, and sea cucumbers are members of the phylum Echinodermata. Starfish and sea cucumbers produce venoms that can cause contact dermatitis.[29] Sea cucumbers occasionally feed on coelenterates and secrete nematocysts; therefore, local therapy for coelenterates should also be considered. Sea urchins are covered with venomous spines capable of producing local and systemic reactions similar to those from coelenterates.[29] First aid consists of soaking the wound in hot, but tolerable, water. Residual spines can be located with soft-tissue x-rays or magnetic resonance imaging. They should be removed only if they are easily accessible or if they are closely aligned to joints or critical neurovascular structures. Reactive fusiform digit swelling attributed to spines near the metacarpal bones may be alleviated by high-dose corticosteroids given in an oral 14-day taper.

Mollusks. Octopuses and cone snails are the primary envenoming species in the phylum Mollusca. Most harmful cone snails are found in Indo-Pacific waters. Envenomation occurs from a detachable tooth injected into the victim.[2, 29] Blue-ringed octopuses can bite and inject tetrodotoxin, a paralytic agent. Both species can produce local symptoms such as burning and paresthesias. Systemic manifestations are primarily neurologic. Management of the bite site is controversial. Options include pressure and immobilization to contain the venom. Treatment of systemic complications is supportive.

Envenomation by Vertebrates

Stingrays. Rays are bottom dwellers ranging from a few inches to 12 feet long. Venom is stored in whiplike appendages. Stingrays attack defensively by thrusting spines into a victim, producing puncture wounds and lacerations. Local damage can be severe, with occasional penetration of body cavities.[11] This is worsened by vasoconstrictive properties of the venom, producing cyanotic-appearing wounds. The venom is often myonecrotic. Systemic complaints include weakness, nausea, diarrhea, headache, and muscle cramps. The venom can cause vasoconstriction, cardiac arrhythmias, respiratory arrest, and seizures.[28]

The wound should be irrigated and then soaked in non-scalding hot water (up to 45° C) for an hour.[2, 28] Débridement, exploration, and removal of spines should occur during or after hot water soaking. Immersion cryotherapy is detrimental. The wound should not be closed primarily. Lacerations should heal by secondary intention or be repaired by delayed closure. The wound should be dressed and elevated. Pain should be relieved locally or systemically. Radiographic studies should be obtained to locate remaining spines.

Miscellaneous Vertebrate Envenomations. Other fish that can produce injuries similar to those of stingrays include lionfish, scorpionfish, stonefish, catfish, and weeverfish. Each can produce envenomation, puncture wounds, and lacerations, with spines transmitting venom. Clinical manifestations and therapy are similar to those pertaining to stingrays.

Sea Snakes. Sea snakes of the family Hydrophiidae appear similar to land snakes. They inhabit the Pacific and Indian Oceans. Venom produces neurologic signs and symptoms, with possible death from paralysis and respiratory arrest. Local manifestations can be minimal or absent. Therapy is similar to that for coral snake (Elapidae) bites. The pressure-immobilization technique is recommended in the field. Antivenin should be administered if any signs of envenomation develop.[2, 28] The initial dose is one ampule, repeated as needed.

SELECTED REFERENCES

Auerbach, P. S. (Ed.): Wilderness Medicine: Management of Wilderness and Environmental Emergencies, 3rd ed. St. Louis, Mosby-Year Book, 1995.

This textbook is an in-depth review of wilderness medicine. Bites and stings by many organisms are discussed in detail by experts from each field. Many recent, pertinent studies are reviewed.

Dire, D. J.: Emergency management of dog and cat bite wounds. Emerg. Med. Clin. North Am., 10(4):719, 1992.
This is a comprehensive and practical review of dog and cat bites. The author discusses the epidemiology, bacteriology, and management of these injuries. A concise section on rabies is included.

Gold, B. S., and Wingert, W. A.: Snake venom poisoning in the United States: A review of therapeutic practice. South. Med. J., 87(6):579, 1994.
This monograph is a concise, practical review of snake venom poisoning. Current controversies regarding the management of snake bite victims are presented. Field and hospital treatments are thoroughly discussed.

Reisman, R. E.: Stinging insect allergy. Med. Clin. North Am., 76(4):883, 1992.
The reactions to Hymenoptera stings are well organized in this practical monograph. The natural history of stinging insect allergy is reviewed. Therapeutic considerations are discussed.

Wilson, D. C., and King, L. E.: Spiders and spider bites. Dermatol. Clin., 8(2):277, 1990.
This is a thorough review of spider bites. Current aspects of managing spider bites are presented. Several recent studies are discussed, addressing controversies in treating spider bites.

REFERENCES

1. Agrawal, K., Mishra, S., and Panda, K. N.: Primary reconstruction of major human bite wounds of the face. Plast. Reconstr. Surg., 90(3):394, 1992.
2. Auerbach, P. S.: Marine envenomation. *In* Auerbach, P. S. (Ed.): Wilderness Medicine: Management of Wilderness and Environmental Emergencies, 3rd ed. St. Louis, Mosby-Year Book, 1995, p. 1327.
3. Auerbach, P. S., and Halstead, B. W.: Injuries from nonvenomous aquatic animals. *In* Auerbach, P. S. (Ed.): Wilderness Medicine: Management of Wilderness and Environmental Emergencies, 3rd ed. St. Louis, Mosby-Year Book, 1995, p. 1303.
4. Basadre, J. O., and Parry, S. W.: Indications for surgical debridement in 125 human bites to the hand. Arch. Surg., 126:65, 1991.
5. Bond, G. R.: Antivenin administration for *Centruroides* scorpion sting: Risks and benefits. Ann. Emerg. Med., 21:788, 1992.
6. Boyer-Hassen, L. V., and McNally, J. T.: Spider bites. *In* Auerbach, P. S. (Ed.): Wilderness Medicine: Management of Wilderness and Environmental Emergencies, 3rd ed. St. Louis, Mosby-Year Book, 1995, p. 769.
7. Callaham, M.: Prophylactic antibiotics in common dog bite wounds: A controlled study. Ann. Emerg. Med., 9:410, 1980.
8. Callaham, M., French, S. P., Tetlow, P., and Rees, P.: Bites and injuries inflicted by mammals. *In* Auerbach, P. S. (Ed.): Wilderness Medicine: Management of Wilderness and Environmental Emergencies, 3rd ed. St. Louis, Mosby-Year Book, 1995, p. 943.
9. Clark, R. F., Wethern-Kestner, S., Vance, M. V., and Gerkin, R.: Clinical presentation and treatment of black widow spider envenomation: A review of 163 cases. Ann. Emerg. Med., 21:782, 1992.
10. Connor, D. A., and Seldon, B.: Scorpion envenomations. *In* Auerbach, P. S. (Ed.): Wilderness Medicine: Management of Wilderness and Environmental Emergencies, 3rd ed. St. Louis, Mosby-Year Book, 1995, p. 847.
11. Cooper, M. N. K.: Stone fish and stingrays—some notes on the injuries that they cause to man. J. R. Army Med. Corps, 137:136, 1991.
12. De Boer, R., and Van Den Bogaard, A. E. J. M.: Removal of attached nymphs and adults of Ixodes ricinus. J. Med. Entomol., 30(4):748, 1993.
13. Dire, D. J.: Emergency management of dog and cat bite wounds. Emerg. Med. Clin. North Am., 10(4):719, 1992.
14. Forks, T. P.: Evaluation and treatment of poisonous snakebites. Am. Fam. Physician, 50(1):123, 1994.
15. Futrell, J. M.: Loxoscelism. Am. J. Med. Sci., 304(4):261, 1992.
16. Garfin, S. R., Castilonia, R. R., Mubarak, S. J., Hargens, A. R., Akeson, W. H., and Russell, F. E.: Role of surgical decompression in treatment of rattlesnake bites. Surg. Forum, 30:502, 1979.
17. Gateau, T., Bloom, M., and Clark, R.: Response to specific *Centruroides sculpturatus* antivenom in 151 cases of scorpion stings. Clin. Toxicol., 32(2):165, 1994.
18. Gold, B. S., and Wingert, W. A.: Snake venom poisoning in the United States: A review of therapeutic practice. South. Med. J., 87(6):579, 1994.
19. Groleau, G.: Rabies. Emerg. Med. Clin. North Am., 10(2):361, 1992.
20. Guidera, K. J., Ogden, J. A., Highhouse, K., Pugh, L., and Beatty, E.: A case study of the injury and treatment: Shark attack. J. Orthop. Trauma, 5(2):204, 1991.
21. Howard, R. J., and Burgess, G. H.: Surgical hazards posed by marine and freshwater animals in Florida. Am. J. Surg., 166:563, 1993.
22. Hutton, R. A., and Warrell, D. A.: Action of snake venom components on the haemostatic system. Blood Rev., 7(3):176, 1993.
23. Ingber, A., Trattner, A., Cleper, R., and Sandbank, M.: Morbidity of brown recluse spider bites. Acta. Derm. Venereol. (Stockh.), 71:337, 1991.
24. Jurkovich, G. J., Luterman, A., McCullar, K., Ramenofsky, M. L., and Curreri, P. W.: Complications of Crotalidae antivenin therapy. J. Trauma, 28(7):1032, 1988.
25. King, L. E., and Rees, R. S.: Dapsone treatment of a brown recluse spider bite. JAMA, 251:889, 1983.
26. Lackmann, G., Wolfgang, D., Isselstein, G., and Tollner, U.: Surgical treatment of facial dog bite injuries in children. J. Craniomaxillofac. Surg., 20:81, 1992.
27. Martin, D., and Loth, T. S.: Bite wounds to the upper extremity. Orthopedics, 14(5):571, 1991.
28. McGoldrick, J., and Marx, J. A.: Marine envenomations. Part 1: Vertebrates. J. Emerg. Med., 9:497, 1991.
29. McGoldrick, J., and Marx, J. A.: Marine envenomations. Part 2: Invertebrates. J. Emerg. Med., 10:71, 1992.
30. Miller, T. A.: Latrodectism: Bite of the black widow spider. Am. Fam. Physician, 45(1):181, 1992.
31. Ownby, C. L.: Pathology of rattlesnake envenomation. *In* Tu, A. T. (Ed.): Rattlesnake Venoms. New York, Marcel Dekker, 1982.
32. Parrish, H. M.: Incidence of treated snakebites in the United States. Public Health Rep., 81:269, 1966.
33. Reisman, R. E.: Unusual reactions to insect venoms. Allergy Proc., 12(6):395, 1991.
34. Reisman, R. E.: Stinging insect allergy. Med. Clin. North Am., 76(4):883, 1992.
35. Russell, F. E.: Snake Venom Poisoning. New York, Scholium International, 1983.
36. Russell, F. E., Carlson, R. W., Wainschel, J., and Osborne, A. H.: Snake venom poisoning in the United States: Experiences with 550 cases. JAMA, 233(4):341, 1975.
37. Stucker, F. J., Shaw, G. Y., Boyd, S., and Shockley, W. W.: Management of animal and human bites in the head and neck. Arch. Otolaryngol. Head Neck Surg., 116:789, 1990.
38. Vigasio, A., Battiston, B., DeFilippo, G., Brunelli, G., and Calabrese, S.: Compartment syndrome due to viper bite. Arch. Orthop. Trauma Surg., 110:175, 1991.
39. Warrell, D. A., and Fenner, P. J.: Venomous bites and stings. Br. Med. Bull., 49(2):423, 1993.
40. Weber, D. J., and Hansen, A. R.: Infections resulting from animal bites. Infect. Dis. Clin. North Am., 5(3):663, 1991.
41. Wilson, D. C., and King, L. E.: Spiders and spider bites. Dermatol. Clin., 8(2):277, 1990.
42. Wingert, W. A., and Chan, L.: Rattlesnake bites in southern California and rationale for recommended treatment. West. J. Med., 148:37, 1988.
43. Wright, D. N., and Lockey, R. F.: Local reactions to stinging insects (Hymenoptera). Allergy Proc., 11(1):23, 1990.

CHAPTER 17

TRAUMA

Management of the Acutely Injured Patient

Gregory J. Jurkovich, M.D., and C. James Carrico, M.D.

The trauma surgeon is the lynchpin of modern trauma systems. This pivotal role mandates a working knowledge of all components of trauma care, including prevention, prehospital care, emergency room care, and rehabilitation, in addition to the surgeon's primary role of directing and providing acute care. The provision of acute care is not limited to recognition of injuries and operative repair. Acute care of the trauma patient encompasses the problems of shock, fluid resuscitation, blood transfusion, electrolyte imbalance, infections, pulmonary support, nutritional supplementation, and gastrointestinal problems unique to the surgical patient. Many of these topics are covered in other sections of this general surgery text. This chapter focuses on the acute management of specific injuries, and the development of trauma care systems.

INITIAL MANAGEMENT OF THE ACUTELY INJURED PATIENT

Priorities

Initial care of the injured patient necessitates two assumptions: that the patient may have more than one injury, and that the obvious injury is not necessarily the most important one. Successful resuscitation requires an approach predicated on prioritizing injuries. A simple method of prioritization includes four categories of injury:

1. Exigent—the most life-threatening conditions, requiring instantaneous intervention (e.g., laryngeal fracture with complete upper airway obstruction and tension pneumothorax)
2. Emergency—those conditions requiring immediate intervention, certainly within the first hour (e.g., ongoing hemorrhage and intracranial mass lesions)
3. Urgent—those conditions requiring intervention within the first few hours (e.g., open contaminated fractures, ischemic extremity, and hollow viscous injuries)
4. Deferrable—those conditions that may or may not be immediately apparent but will subsequently require treatment (e.g., urethral disruption and facial fractures)

Use of this scheme requires a deliberate and regimented approach to the resuscitation, while retaining the flexibility to reset the priorities depending on the diagnostic disclosures that arise during the resuscitation. The maintenance of this balance between a structured resuscitation protocol and the need to change direction properly generate the necessity for one person to be in charge of the entire resuscitation procedure.

Steps In The Initial Resuscitation

Airway. The crucial first step in managing an injured patient is securing an adequate airway. The mechanical removal of debris and the *chin lift* or *jaw thrust* maneuvers, both of which pull the tongue and oral musculature forward from the pharynx, are often useful in clearing the airway of less severely injured patients. However, if there is any question about the adequacy of the airway, if there is evidence of severe head injury, or if the patient is in profound shock, more definitive airway control is appropriate. In the vast majority of patients this involves endotracheal intubation. Unfortunately, control of the airway is sometimes more complex than simply placing an endotracheal tube. The presence of cervical spine injury in the unconscious patient is always a possibility, and injudicious movement of the neck in the process of endotracheal intubation can be devastating. The authors' approach to selecting the optimum airway control in these patients is outlined in Figure 17–1.

Endotracheal intubation, the most direct method for establishing an airway, requires that the head and neck be held in a neutral position to avoid exacerbation of potential cervical spine injury and that the spine be stabilized until an injury has been definitively ruled out. If the patient has no evidence of soft tissue or bony injury to the midface, and is breathing spontaneously, *naso*tracheal intubation is an acceptable alternative to *oro*tracheal intubation.

In a few patients, a surgical airway may be required. Although classic tracheostomy may be indicated in select patients, such as those with laryngeal injuries, cricothyroidotomy is generally the preferable emergency procedure. These surgical procedures may be preceded by needle cricothyroidotomy with jet insufflation to improve oxygenation and allow the surgical procedure to be performed in a more orderly fashion.

Breathing. If there is decreased respiratory drive or an unstable chest wall, assisted ventilation is usually necessary. The three most common reasons for ineffective ventilation following successful placement of an airway are malposition of the endotracheal tube, pneumothorax, and hemothorax. Therefore, palpation and auscultation of the chest are neces-

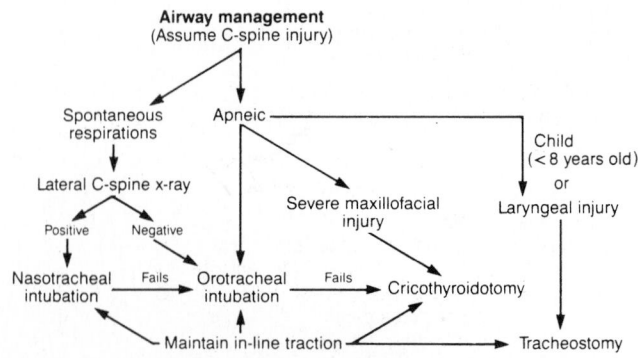

Figure 17–1. Algorithmn for airway management in the trauma patient. (From Maier, R. V.: Airway management. *In* Moore, E. E. [Ed.]: Early care of the injured patient, 4th ed. Toronto, B. C. Decker, 1990.)

sary diagnostic adjuncts at this point. A supine (anteroposterior [AP]) chest x-ray examination can validate the physical examination and better define chest wall and plural abnormalities. Although there is usually time to perform a chest radiograph prior to invasive therapeutic procedures, in the patient with profound hemodynamic instability and a high suspicion of tension pneumothorax, a needle catheter decompression can be both diagnostic and therapeutic. Under these circumstances decompression of the chest before the radiograph is appropriate.

Circulation. When possible, control of the hemorrhage precedes placement of the intravenous lines. This may be as simple as a compressive dressing over a bleeding wound or large vessel or may require broader compression, such as application of a pneumatic antishock garment in the patient who has an obvious pelvic fracture. Intravenous cannulas are usually placed percutaneously in the arm or groin. They should be large bore, and a minimum of two should be placed. Lines should not be inserted distal to extremity wounds with potential vascular injury. Alternatives are cutdown by either the antecubital or saphenous route, or intraosseus in children under the age of 3. With the exception of the use of the large (8 French) introducer catheter, subclavian venipuncture is not a rapid route for fluid administration and is best reserved for monitoring response to fluid therapy. Fluid resuscitation begins with a 1000-ml. bolus of lactated Ringer's solution for an adult, or 20 ml. per kg. for a child. Response to therapy is monitored by skin perfusion, urinary output, and central venous pressure readings when that line has been placed.

Disability/Neurologic Assessment. At this juncture, a brief examination to determine level of consciousness, pupillary response, and movement of extremities is a necessary prelude to the determination of severity of neurologic injury. In addition, this information becomes initial data in the computation of the Glasgow Coma Scale (GCS), which is a method of both following the evolution of neurologic disability and prognosticating future recovery[59] (Table 17–1). It is worth noting that pupillary response can still be assessed in the paralyzed patient. In recording the GCS in intubated and paralyzed patients, the authors have added the modifiers T and P (intubated and paralyzed, respectively) to signify that the score may be inaccurate.

Exposure for Complete Examination. By this point, most injuries that are either exigent or emergencies have been recognized and treated. The next step is to completely, but expeditiously, re-examine the patient to diagnose other injuries. Complete physical examination is typically done in a head-to-toe manner and includes ordering and collecting data from appropriate laboratory and radiologic tests. Data accumulated can then be used to reset priorities. This time period also allows for the placement of additional lines, catheters (nasogastric, Foley), and monitoring devices. When the patient is oxygenating, ventilating, and perfusing adequately, a priority plan should be established for subsequent treatment.

RECOGNITION AND MANAGEMENT OF SPECIFIC INJURIES
Cranium and Brain

Brain injury, either alone or in combination with other injuries, is the major determinant of survival and functional outcome in most cases of blunt trauma. Two principles guide the initial care of the patient with severe head injuries: (1) immediate and repeated assessment of injury severity, and (2) protection of the brain from further injury. The treatment approach depends on identifying the two fundamental varieties of head injury: focal or diffuse. Focal injuries consist of mass lesions (e.g., epidural or subdural hematoma) that cause neurologic dysfunction, largely by brain compression, and often require surgical evacuation. Diffuse brain injuries are equally frequent and cause prolonged coma without intracranial masses. These do not require specific surgical therapy but can be as devastating as focal injuries.

Initial Management

The ultimate outcome of brain injury is as much (or more) dependent on the early establishment of an airway, ventilation, control of hemorrhage, and restoration of perfusion as any other organ. The previous protocol proposed for resuscitation of the multiply injured patient is equally applicable to the patient with isolated brain injury. The airway should be secured immediately, taking care to remember that spinal cord injury is present in as many as 10% of head injury patients. The brain is extremely susceptible to lowered perfusion states following injury; consequently, it is critical that adequate arterial pressure, blood volume, and oxygenation be maintained. Resuscitation fluids and blood replacement should be administered to maintain perfusion while avoiding volume overload. It is worth emphasizing that brain injury per se rarely causes hypotension during the early period following trauma, and other causes and sources of blood loss should be sought out.

Assessment of Severity of Injury. The severity of brain injury can be rapidly estimated by determining three factors: *level of consciousness, pupillary function,* and *lateralized weakness* of the extremities.

Level of consciousness is best assessed by the GCS, a system that evaluates eye opening, best motor response, and verbal response (see Table 17–1). The GCS is determined by taking the best response in each category and totaling them; it ranges from 3 to 15.[59] Because of its repeatability, a difference of two signals a change in neurologic status; a decrease of three usually indicates an enlarging hematoma and demands prompt treatment. *Pupillary function* is assessed by the size, equality, and response to bright light. Whether or not there has been ocular injury, any pupillary asymmetry greater than 1 mm. must be attributed to intracranial injury unless proved otherwise. With few exceptions, the largest pupil is on the side of the mass lesion. The *lateralized extremity weakness* is detected by testing motor power in patients able to cooperate or by observing symmetry of movement in response to pain-

TABLE 17–1. The Glasgow Coma Scale

Eyes open	Never	1
	To pain	2
	To verbal stimuli	3
	Spontaneously	4
Best verbal response	No response	1
	Incomprehensible sounds	2
	Inappropriate words	3
	Disoriented and converses	4
	Oriented and converses	5
Best motor response	No response	1
	Extension (decerebrate rigidity)	2
	Flexion abnormal (decorticate rigidity)	3
	Flexion withdrawal	4
	Localizes pain	5
	Obeys	6
Total		3–15

ful stimulus. As the severity of injury becomes worse, lateralized weakness is more difficult to appreciate, and small differences may be important.

The GCS score should be assessed in the field or by the first responders, then reassessed after specific treatment interventions. Because intubation and paralyzing agents alter the ability to assess the components of the GCS, the presence of an endotracheal tube or the recent administration of paralytic agents is noted by the modifiers T and P, respectively, when computing the GCS score.

The presence of any of the following criteria suggest serious injury: (1) a GCS score of less than 10; (2) a decrease in the GCS score by 3 or more, regardless of the initial GCS score; (3) pupillary inequality greater than 1 mm. regardless of the GCS score; (4) lateralized extremity weakness regardless of the GCS score; (5) markedly depressed skull fractures; and (6) open cranial wounds with brain exposed.

Protection from Further Insult. Cerebral ischemia is present in more than 90% of patients who die from head trauma and is the most preventable complication. Most ischemic complications occur soon after injury, are much more common when multisystem trauma is present, and can be reversed in the early phases of care. In ischemia, fewer nutrients are reaching the brain than its metabolism demands; therefore, maximizing oxygen and glucose delivery to the brain can offset it. This requires ample blood flow to the brain and adequate concentration of oxygen and glucose in the blood. However, excess fluid resuscitation or blood pressure elevation must be avoided, because the cerebral vessels do not react normally after injury; they fail to constrict if subjected to elevated blood pressure. Invasive monitoring devices such as Swan-Ganz right heart catheterization and intracranial pressure (ICP) monitoring may be necessary to determine the appropriate fluid requirements and cerebral perfusion pressure.

Arterial oxygen content must be optimized, usually best accomplished by assisting ventilation. Prompt treatment of thoracic causes of hypoxia or hypoventilation (e.g., pneumothorax, hemothorax, and pulmonary contusion) are essential. Endotracheal intubation is often required for definitive treatment of head injuries. If urgent intubation is required, the same techniques that are used in the operating room should be applied. Failure to use paralytic agents, pharyngeal anesthesia, and barbiturate induction invites massive elevation of the ICP during intubation.

Even after relatively short periods of ischemia, the brain may respond to reperfusion in a pathologic fashion, with prompt and severe brain swelling and marked increases in intracranial pressure.[45] Elevated ICP can best be managed in the early phases of injury by decreasing the intravascular cerebral blood volume. Intravascular cerebral blood volume is best decreased by controlled hyperventilation, because the arterial carbon dioxide concentration is the most potent known regulator of cerebral vessel size. Decreasing brain water may also be beneficial and is accomplished with diuretics or hyperosmotic agents, the latter being more rapid. However, neither should be used in the underresuscitated patient in whom cerebral perfusion pressure is low.

Definitive Care

Definitive care begins with a definitive diagnosis, which is established exclusively by computed tomography (CT). Cranial CT has a high priority in the evaluation of a patient with altered level of consciousness or lateralizing neurologic signs. It should be performed as soon as cardiorespiratory stability has been achieved and a lateral cervical spine roentgenogram demonstrates no fracture or dislocation. Seriously injured

patients who are intubated should receive neuromuscular blockage during the study. A good quality CT scan identifies focal mass lesions and allows the diagnosis of the presence of diffuse brain injury. Focal injuries with significant mass effect require surgical evacuation; patients with these injuries go directly to the operating room. Patients with diffuse brain injury are managed in the intensive care unit. Monitoring devices for ICP are placed for on-line management of intracranial hypertension in both groups. Definitive care continues, with the principal effort directed toward controlling intracranial hypertension to keep the ICP within normal limits. Therapy is added as necessary to achieve this goal as follows: moderate hyperventilation (PCO_2 30 to 35 mm. Hg), diuretics (furosemide, 20 to 40 mg. three times per day), and finally, hyperosmolar therapy (20% mannitol to keep serum osmolality 295 to 305 mOsm). Although both barbiturates and glucocorticoids have been advocated in the management of severe head injury, clinical studies do not support their use. Systemic support must be vigorous to ensure continued cerebral oxygenation and to prevent infectious complication of prolonged coma.

Vertebrae and Spinal Cord

The incidence of spinal cord injury in the United States is approximately 50 cases per 1 million population per year. Motor vehicle accidents alone result in more than 500 people with quadriplegia per year. Approximately 6% of all injury hospitalizations are due to vertebrae injuries, and 1% are from spinal cord injuries.[105] Although these injuries represent a small proportion of the total injury-related hospitalizations, they result in significant physical and psychological changes, often requiring long-term and expensive medical treatment and rehabilitation. Average hospital charges for quadriplegic survivors cost $50,000 in 1988. Whereas brain and spinal cord injuries are the primary determinants of long-term disability, many spinal cord injuries are incomplete and, given proper care, may have a remarkable capacity for recovery. Many of the acute problems and complications that the patient with spinal cord injury faces have been identified, and there are effective procedures for preventing or limiting these problems. Rehabilitation programs for patients with spinal cord injuries have also been developed, which help the patient attain the highest possible functional level of recovery.

One review of 300 acute cervical fractures and dislocations reported that motor vehicle accidents (one third), falls (one third), and athletic injuries or missile wounds are the usual causes of injury to the cervical spine.[10] Other reports suggest that motor vehicle accidents are responsible for up to 60% of spinal cord injuries, falls for 20% to 30%, and diving accidents for 5% to 10%.[105] In Bohlman's series, one third of the patients were not diagnosed when first seen in the emergency department. He identified the following four specific categories of patients whose diagnoses were likely to be delayed: (1) patients with head injuries; (2) patients with multiple injuries, including fractures elsewhere; (3) patients with brain injuries and impaired consciousness; and (4) intoxicated patients. Careful follow-up examinations must be made during a traumatized patient's hospitalization if he or she complains of pain in the back or neck; if weakness, numbness, or loss of control of extremities or sphincters develops; or if only screening radiographs were obtained during the admission evaluation.

Initial Care

Proper care of the potentially unstable spine begins at the scene of injury and continues until the spine has been proved stable. Adequate help is essential. Gentle manual traction stabilizes the head, which can be turned to the midline if necessary to protect the airway and to correct gross deformity. The neck should be placed and maintained in a position of minimal extension and taped to a padded spine board or similar support during transportation. The lower spine is protected by taping the patient to the backboard above and below major joints. Sandbags on each side of the head in addition to a cervical collar provide additional stability when the patient is transported from one location to another. The forehead should be taped to the backboard.

The history should include information determining the mechanism and forces of injury, and the site and duration of any pain. Transient or persistent numbness, tingling, and weakness or other neurologic problems must be noted, as should any prior injuries or other difficulties involving the spine or spinal cord.

Physical examination should include notation of abrasions or contusions anywhere on the head or trunk. They provide clues to the mechanism of injury. Spinal deformity can occasionally be seen, but palpation of the spine processes is frequently more rewarding. The patient should be log rolled, and the dorsal spine palpated and checked for localized tenderness, swelling, rotational deformity, or the presence of a gap between the spinous processes (indicative of a rupture of the posterior ligaments with resultant instability).

If a neurologic deficit is present, the examination focuses on defining the neurologic level of injury and on determining whether or not there is sparing of some spinal cord function across this level. The patient with incomplete spinal cord injury has motor or sensory function below the injury level. Sacral sparing may be the only evidence that paralysis may not be complete. Therefore, sensation in the perineum, voluntary sphincter contraction, and toe flexion must be carefully examined. Most incomplete spinal cord injuries exhibit mixed motor and sensory sparing rather than a classic pattern of partial injury. The natural history of incomplete cord injuries is to improve. Well-documented evidence of deterioration is rare. If deterioration is observed, emergency diagnostic and surgical treatment is warranted. A complete spinal cord–injured patient has no distal motor or sensory function. It is essential that neurologic function be accurately recorded in the prehospital and emergency department notes to allow for later comparison. Unlike traumatic brain injury, steroids have been shown to play an important role in improving outcome in patients with complete or incomplete spinal cord injury. Methylprednisolone should be administered as an intravenous bolus of 30 mg. per kg., followed by a continuous infusion of 5.4 mg./kg./hr. for the next 23 hours, based on a double-blind, randomized, placebo-controlled multicenter study.[13]

A spinal cord injury is followed immediately by a transient period of disordered function, called *spinal shock*. During this time, no reflex or voluntary activity can be elicited distal to the level of the injury. When some reflex activity has returned, the spinal cord lesion can be deemed complete if there is no distal sensation or voluntary motor control. The normal sacral reflexes are the earliest to recover from spinal shock, usually within the first 24 hours. One such reflex is the bulbocavernosus reflex, contraction of the anal sphincter produced by compression of the glans or clitoris or by tugging gently on the Foley catheter. The other is the anal wink, or contraction of the anal sphincter in response to a pinprick adjacent to it. By following these reflexes during the early stages of spinal cord injury, valuable prognostic information can be obtained.

Good-quality roentgenograms are as essential as the history and physical examination in the thorough evaluation of the patient with spinal injury. Radiologic examination of the cervical spine must be accomplished before moving the neck of all blunt trauma patients, particularly those who are unconscious, obtunded, or complaining of neck pain. The initial screening view is a cross-table lateral of the supine patient, taken with the film just lateral to one shoulder, with both shoulders actively or passively depressed so the entire cervical spine is visualized from the occiput to the top of T1 (Fig. 17–2). The head is stabilized during this maneuver and not actively distracted away from the body, which can be disastrous in a severe C1–C2 ligamentous injury. Formal AP, lateral, and odontoid views should be obtained before the cervical spine is *cleared*, but flexion and extension radiograms are rarely indicated and are performed only if the preliminary films have shown no signs of instability and the patient is conscious and cooperative. The signs of impending spinal cord damage may be subtle. A small bony avulsion or slight malalignment of vertebrae may be the only suggestion of gross ligamentous instability. The physician who is seeking only fractures may ignore subluxations and even dislocations.

New-generation CT scanners greatly facilitate the evaluation of spinal trauma. Sagittal reconstructions can provide excellent portrayals of alignment, without the risk of positioning often required by conventional tomography or flexion and extension films. Retropulsion of bone fragments and occasionally of disc material can be demonstrated, clearly showing the amount of canal narrowing that results. Magnetic resonance imaging (MRI) can beautifully demonstrate detailed neuropathology, including disc herniation, ligamentous injuries, and spinal cord mass lesions. It often has a complementary diagnostic role to CT in spinal cord injuries.

Treatment of Specific Injuries

The injured spinal cord should be treated by prompt reduction of any dislocation or angular deformity that compromises the spinal canal. This can usually be achieved with traction (Gardner-Wells tongs or cranial halo) and the appropriate positioning of the patient. Frequent neurologic monitoring and radiographs are necessary to identify deterioration, overdistraction, or loss of alignment during reduction and when increased distraction weight is applied. If closed

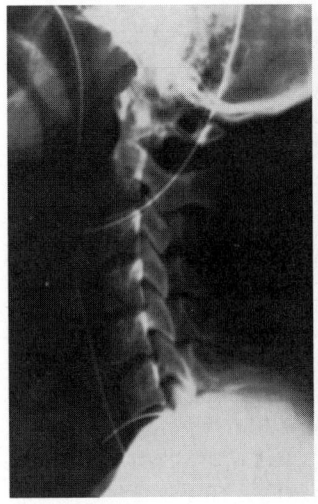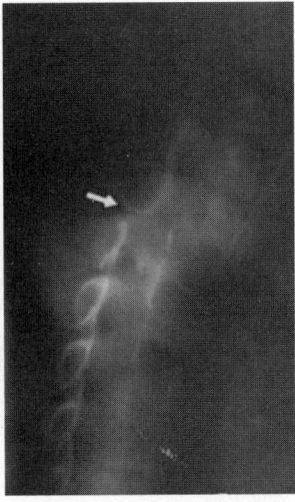

Figure 17–2. The importance of completely visualizing all seven cervical vertebrae in a cross-table lateral cervical spine radiograph is illustrated in these two photoradiographs. Inadequate cross-table lateral cervical spine radiograph (C7 not visualized) following blunt neck trauma is shown. Tomography was required for evaluation of the entire cervical spine, demonstrating subluxation of C7 on T1 (arrow). (From Jurkovich, G. J.: The neck. *In* Moore, E. E. [Ed.]: Early Care of the Injured Patient, 4th ed. Toronto, B. C. Decker, 1990, p. 129.)

means are not effective in restoring the spinal canal, or if an incomplete spinal cord lesion is deteriorating, emergency surgical treatment may be necessary. Experience with incomplete thoracic level paraplegia suggests that immediate or urgent posterior Harrington distraction instrumentation or anterior transthoracic decompression and fusion is preferable to posterior reduction or late anterior decompression, with improved neurologic function demonstrated in 90% of patients so treated.[68]

Neck

Although the neck is a unique trauma organ, with multiple vital structures concentrated in a small anatomic area, it is generally unprotected by bone or dense muscular covering. Whereas most significant neck injuries result from penetrating trauma, blunt neck trauma does occur and can be particularly difficult to manage because it often involves the airway, the first priority in trauma care. In addition, major blood vessel injury of the neck can result from cervical spine hyperextension, even in the absence of bony injury. Although the frequency of neck trauma is small (5% to 10% of all injuries), the consequences of this type of injury are great. Fatality rates for penetrating neck trauma range from 1% to 2% for stab wounds, 5% to 12% for gunshot wounds, and up to 50% for rifle or shotgun blasts. It is estimated that one half of these deaths are preventable with appropriate early care.[61]

The neck is classically divided into a number of anatomic triangles (Fig. 17–3). Two large triangles are important in discussing penetrating neck trauma. Penetrating wounds that enter through the sternocleidomastoid muscle or anterior triangle carry a high likelihood of significant vascular, airway, or esophageal injury. In contrast, wounds to the posterior triangle rarely involve the esophagus, airway, or major vascular structures, but, if directed inferiorly, intrathoracic injury can occur.

The anterior neck is further divided into three zones defined by horizontal planes (Fig. 17–4). Zone I represents the base of the neck and thoracic outlet. Injuries here carry the highest mortality because of the risk of major vascular and intrathoracic injury. Zone II represents the largest portion or midbody of the neck. Because of its relative size, Zone II injuries are most common but carry the lowest mortality. Significant injury is generally apparent, and exposure of vital structures is readily accomplished. Zone III is the part of the

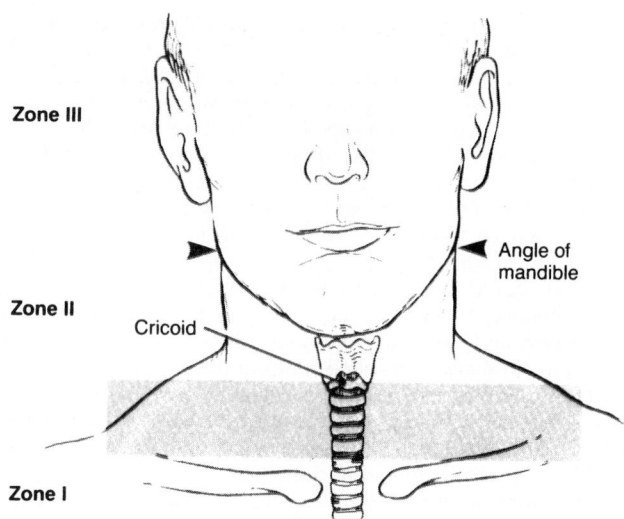

Figure 17–4. Zones of the neck. The junction of Zone I and Zone II is usually described as the cricoid cartilage or, alternatively, the top of the clavicles. (From Jurkovich, G. J.: The neck. *In* Moore, E. E. [Ed.]: Early Care of the Injured Patient, 4th ed. Toronto, B. C. Decker, 1990, p. 127.)

neck above the angle of the mandible. The risk of injury to the distal carotid artery, salivary glands, and pharynx is greatest in this zone, and exposure can be particularly difficult.

The other major anatomic landmark in the neck is the platysma muscle. This thin, broad muscle lies just beneath the skin and covers the entire anterior triangle and anteroinferior aspect of the posterior triangle. Wounds that fail to penetrate the platysma are considered superficial and do not warrant extensive evaluation. Wounds that do penetrate the platysma mandate hospital admission and further evaluation.

Selective Versus Mandatory Exploration

There continues to be controversy regarding management of neck wounds that penetrate the platysma muscle.[4] Two distinct schools of thought exist on this subject: one advocating mandatory surgical exploration of all such wounds and one favoring a more selective approach. Those favoring routine exploration justify their position by emphasizing the disastrous complications of missed injuries and the relative safety and short hospital course of a negative exploration. Authors favoring a more selective approach berate the high incidence of negative explorations and the fact that some injuries are missed in spite of a formal exploration. Merion and associates analyzed 27 series reported in the literature in which the clinical course of more than 4000 penetrating neck trauma patients was documented[80] (Table 17–2). Carducci and Dalsey re-examined these same series and determined that only 2.4% of initially observed patients required subsequent operation.[15] Both reviews emphasized the similar outcomes in these two approaches and argue that either approach can be justified.

Perhaps more significant than this controversy are the areas of uniform agreement. All patients with clinical signs of significant injury require prompt exploration (Table 17–3). All other patients (clinically silent) with wounds that penetrate the platysma should at least be admitted to the hospital and observed. The disagreement is whether patients *without* positive clinical findings should: (1) routinely undergo a surgical neck exploration; (2) undergo extensive diagnostic evaluation; or (3) simply be observed. The authors continue to

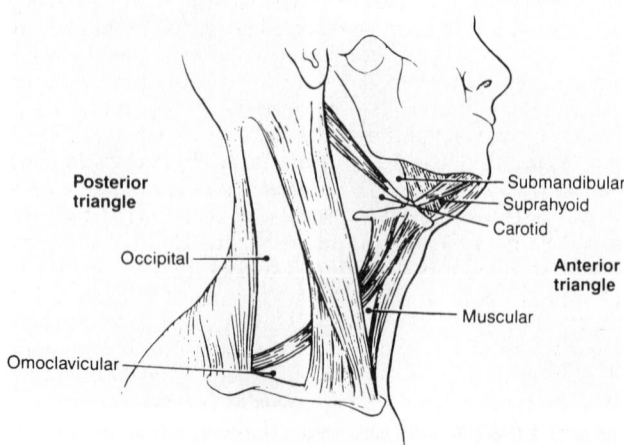

Figure 17–3. Anatomic triangles of the neck. The large *posterior triangle* is composed of the smaller occipital and omoclavicular triangles. The large *anterior triangle* is composed of the smaller suprahyoid, submandibular, carotid, and muscular triangles. (From Jurkovich, G. J.: The neck. *In* Moore, E. E. [Ed.]: Early Care of the Injured Patient, 4th ed. Toronto, B. C. Decker, 1990, p. 127.)

TABLE 17–2. Summary of 27 Collected Series of Mandatory Exploration Versus Selective Observation Policy for Penetrating Neck Trauma

	Selective Observation Policy (%) (13 Series, 2659 Patients)	Mandatory Exploration Policy (%) (14 Series, 1777 Patients)
Immediate operation	52.4	88.7
Injury requiring repair	67.0	61.3
Observed	47.6	11.3
Delayed operation/missed injury	2.4	7.8
Mortality		
Immediate operation group	9.2	8.3
Initially observed group	1.7	4.1
Delayed operation group	16.7	13.3

Adapted from Carducci, B., Lowe, R. A., and Dalsey, W.: Penetrating neck trauma: Consensus and controversies. Ann. Emerg. Med., *15*:208, 1986; and Merion, R. M., Harness, J. K., Ramsburgh, S. R., et al.: Selective management of penetrating neck trauma: Cost implications. Arch. Surg., *116*:691, 1981. Copyright 1981, American Medical Association.

recommend exploration of the majority of neck wounds that penetrate the platysma. More specifically, injuries to the base of the skull and thoracic outlet (Zones III and I) require angiography prior to, and occasionally in lieu of, exploration. Injuries to the mid-neck (Zone II) are generally managed by exploration without prior invasive diagnostic studies. Transcervical gunshot injuries represent a special category of neck wounds, with a greater than 80% likelihood of injury to cervical structures; surgical exploration is warranted in nearly all cases.[57]

Initial Management

Active airway management is critical in the patient with a serious neck wound and takes precedence over all other aspects of the evaluation and resuscitation. Emergency intubation is necessary if spontaneous respirations are inadequate, if blood or vomit obstructs the airway, or if progressive cervical swelling from hemorrhage threatens to occlude the airway. Procrastination converts a simple intubation into a difficult, bloody emergency tracheostomy. If the airway is not jeopardized, nasogastric and endotracheal intubation may be deferred to allow endoscopic evaluation of the larynx and hypopharynx. The remainder of the initial therapy follows the guidelines previously outlined, with particular attention

TABLE 17–3. Clinical Signs of Significant Injury in Penetrating Neck Trauma

Vascular

Shock
Expanding hematoma
External hemorrhage
Diminished carotid pulse

Digestive Tract

Subcutaneous air
Hemoptysis
Dysphagia/odynophagia

Airway

Stridor
Hoarseness
Dysphonia/voice change

Neurologic

Lateralized neurologic deficit
Altered state of consciousness
Brachial plexus injury

directed toward excluding cervical spine injury, providing adequate ventilation, and evaluating neurologic status.

Following initial resuscitation, a complete physical examination is performed to detect associated injuries and to better define the extent of neck trauma. The clinical signs that mandate neck exploration should be searched for (see Table 17–3). All patients should have a chest radiograph to rule out thoracic trauma. Stable patients should have soft tissue neck films to look for retropharyngeal hematoma, tracheal narrowing or deviation, retained missile fragments and pathways, and subcutaneous or retropharyngeal air. Neck CT is particularly helpful in blunt trauma to evaluate laryngeal structures. Patients sustaining blunt neck trauma, with a neurologic examination inconsistent with findings on head CT scan, should undergo four-vessel angiography. As previously mentioned, the need for further diagnostic testing (angiography, panendoscopy, and esophagography) versus immediate operative neck exploration is controversial.[6] The authors believe preoperative angiography is indicated in the hemodynamically stable patient with multiple wounds, or penetrating wounds to Zone III (because of the possible inaccessibility of internal carotid artery lesions) and Zone I (to identify injuries to the thoracic outlet vessels). Symptomatic isolated injuries to the mid-neck (Zone II) are generally explored without the aid of arteriography. Endoscopy is usually performed intraoperatively if pharyngeal or esophageal injury is suspected but cannot be found, and routinely if a nonoperative policy is selected. The sensitivity of endoscopy for esophageal injuries is reported to range from 29% to 83%.[135] The addition of esophagography increases the accuracy and should be considered a complimentary procedure.

Exploration should be performed in the operating room under general endotracheal anesthesia. A nasogastric tube is usually passed to ensure an empty stomach. Preparation and draping of the patient prior to induction of anesthesia allows control of hemorrhage if the patient starts to gag at the time of placement of the endotracheal tube. The chest is also auscultated before operation, and a chest x-ray examination is routinely performed. Wounds at the base of the neck (Zone I) may follow a downward path with pleural penetration. A pneumothorax may not develop until positive pressure ventilation is applied and may initially present as unexplained hypotension during anesthesia. The incision is planned to allow full exposure of the tract of the injury. Proximal and distal control of the major vessels must also be considered in the length and position of the incision, and the patient is always prepared for a possible median sternotomy. An oblique incision along the anterior border of the sternocleidomastoid muscle usually provides access to the vessels and other important cervical structures. If bilateral exposure is required, a transverse *collar* incision may be preferable. The tract of the injury is followed to its depth, systematically examining each structure in or near the tract.

Management of Specific Injuries

BLOOD VESSELS

Blood vessels are the most commonly injured structures in the neck, with major arterial injuries occurring in 18% of penetrating neck wounds and major venous injuries in 26%.[15] Blunt vascular injury accounts for perhaps only 3% of all carotid injuries, and, although the diagnosis is often difficult and delayed, it must be suspected in any patient with a direct blow or compression of the neck, particularly one who develops focal neurologic signs or symptoms after a latent interval.[25] The patient with the carotid artery injury can rapidly present with exsanguinating hemorrhage. The principles of operative repair of vascular structures in the neck are the same as those for other major blood vessels discussed later in the text. The topic of management of carotid artery injury and neurologic deficits has received considerable attention. The presence of shock, coma, or neurologic deficit certainly is an adverse prognostic indicator, but it is not a contraindication to carotid repair. Patients without a neurologic deficit and a carotid injury should have restoration of vascular continuity with little expected morbidity or mortality. Patients with all grades of neurologic deficits short of coma should also have primary vascular repair, because neurologic outcome and survival are improved with arterial reconstruction.[134] In comatose patients, neither repair nor ligation appears to influence a poor prognosis. The impact of prolonged ischemia and potential revascularization injury is not well defined. Ligation of the carotid artery is indicated in the comatose patient with no prograde flow, in the presence of uncontrollable hemorrhage, or when technical reasons prohibit repair. The role of extracranial-intracranial bypass in the patient requiring carotid artery ligation is in evolution.

TRACHEA AND LARYNX

Penetrating tracheal wounds are usually readily apparent and dramatic in their clinical presentation, with subcutaneous emphysema, crepitus, or hemoptysis as presenting signs. Early endotracheal intubation by field paramedics may, however, mask a high tracheal injury. Indications for primary surgical repair depend on the severity of the injury; hence, careful endoscopic or surgical evaluation is required. When repair is needed, the principles include débridement of devitalized cartilage, mucosal coverage of exposed cartilage, and closure of tracheal defects. Tracheostomy is not always required following a tracheal repair but certainly is useful if extensive edema or prolonged airway compression is anticipated.

Blunt laryngotracheal injuries are not always obvious and are easily overlooked in the multiple trauma victim.[44] These patients may initially appear deceptively normal, only to suddenly develop severe respiratory distress. Physical examination, flexible fiberoptic endoscopy, and CT may help access the neck for blunt laryngotracheal injury (Fig. 17–5). Equipment for emergency tracheostomy must always be readily at hand. If emergency airway is required, direct endotracheal intubation may be attempted if the laryngeal structures are well visualized, aided by passing the endotracheal tube over a flexible endoscope. However, even in the most experienced hands this may be impossible and may risk worsening the tracheal injury. Tracheostomy is therefore usually recommended as an emergency airway following blunt laryngotracheal injuries, even though it also carries risk of further

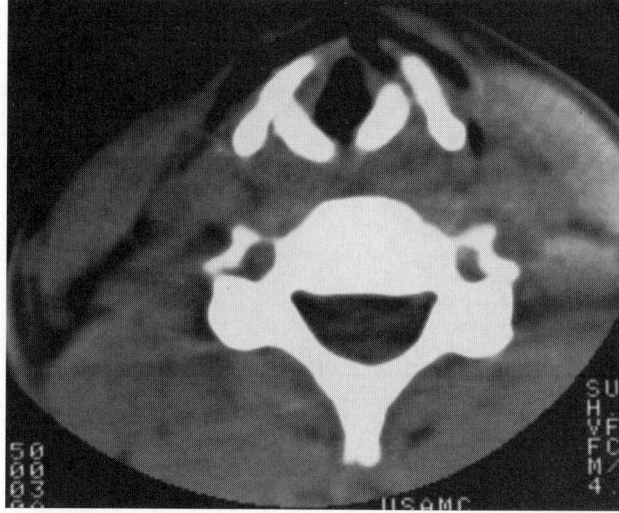

Figure 17–5. Computed tomography following blunt neck trauma. Subcutaneous emphysema, midline fracture, and diastasis of the thyroid cartilage, and posteriolateral displacement of the right cricoarytenoid complex are demonstrated. (From Jurkovich, G. J.: The neck. *In* Moore, E. E. [Ed.]: Early Care of the Injured Patient, 4th ed. Toronto, B. C. Decker, 1990, p. 126.)

injury.[115] The basic principles of repairing tracheal injuries are primary closure of mucosal lacerations and reduction of cartilaginous fractures. Mucosal repairs should be performed with fine absorbable suture. Simple lacerations of the subglottic trachea can generally be primarily repaired with simple nonabsorbable sutures. If the defect cannot be primarily closed, tracheal mobilization may bridge a gap of several tracheal rings. Controversial areas in the surgical care of laryngotracheal trauma patients include the timing of operation, the role of laryngeal stents, the use of steroids, indications for skin grafting, and the techniques of operative exposure of the larynx.[53]

PHARYNX AND ESOPHAGUS

Injuries to the esophagus are most difficult to diagnose. The sensitivity of esophagography in detecting esophageal injury varies from approximately 50% to 90%; the sensitivity of endoscopy varies from 29% to 83%.[25] These modalities should be considered complementary, and when combined, have an accuracy of nearly 100%. Operative exposure of the esophagus can be difficult. The morbidity and mortality of a missed esophageal injury demands a high index of suspicion, since virtually all reported deaths from cervical esophageal injuries are the result of a delayed or missed diagnosis. When injured, the structures may be repaired primarily in two layers using absorbable and nonabsorbable suture. It is important to drain all such wounds, because infection or salivary fistula is not an infrequent complication. If there is massive loss of tissue, as with a shotgun blast, it may be necessary to perform a cutaneous esophagostomy for feeding purposes and a cutaneous pharyngostomy for salivary drainage. A secondary reconstructive procedure is then required after the initial healing is complete. Most surgeons advocate primary repair of all esophageal injuries if accomplished early. Delays of greater than 12 hours significantly increase the risk of repair dehiscence, wound abscess, and death. Neck esophageal injuries diagnosed more than 24 to 48 hours after injury are best managed initially by diversion and drainage.

NERVES

A preoperative neurologic examination should be performed whenever possible. Brachial plexus, deep cervical plexus, phrenic nerve, and cranial nerves are systematically tested. The vagus nerve can be observed by examination of the vocal cords. A hypoglossal or spinal accessory nerve injury is particularly easy to miss unless a preoperative neurologic examination is performed. An associated head injury or drug intoxication frequently complicates the neurologic evaluation. Primary débridement and repair of all severed or lacerated nerves is preferred, using fine interrupted, nonabsorbable suture on the perineurium. If a motor nerve deficit is apparent, an expendable sensory nerve such as the great auricular may be interposed as a nerve graft to allow anastomosis without tension.

Maxillofacial

General Considerations

Maxillofacial injuries are among the most frequent injuries seen in the emergency department and carry a special significance to the patient, stemming from the human face's conspicuous location, aesthetic importance, and the psychological image of *self*. In addition, the face is the carrier of the senses of sight, smell, and taste, and is the center for the vital functions of speech and mastication. Optimal management of such injuries requires a skilled approach to establish both the nature and extent of injuries, to assess for associated injuries, and to initiate the appropriate treatment.

Diagnostic Techniques. CT has become an invaluable tool in the evaluation of significant maxillofacial trauma. The accuracy of defining specific fracture patterns with CT scanning is unsurpassed when compared with plain radiographs or tomography. CT scans are also helpful in diagnosing occult injuries that might otherwise have become apparent only during later stages of recovery and healing. In particular, the evaluation of injuries to the paranasal sinuses, orbits, and mandibular condylar heads is enhanced by the use of the CT scan. Fine-cut axial CT images with coronal reconstruction or direct fine-cut coronal scans can accurately define the extent of injuries, comminution of bony fragments, and degrees of displacement (Fig. 17–6). In addition, specific soft tissue involvement, such as medial or inferior herniation of the orbital contents through fracture lines, can be accurately diagnosed only by CT scanning. This information can be extremely useful to the surgeon in directing a treatment plan.

Airway Compromise. Preserving sight and speech and minimizing deformity are important goals but ones that occupy a relatively low priority in the care of the patient with multiple injuries. Rather, it is the fact that maxillofacial trauma is frequently associated with upper airway compromise that mandates its early attention in the resuscitation of the trauma victim. The initial approach to a patient with maxillofacial trauma is no different from the assessment of any patient with multiple trauma. Respiratory obstruction is often caused by the accumulation of blood, broken teeth, or other foreign substances. Certain constellations of facial and mandibular fractures are particularly prone to cause respiratory obstruction. Pulling the tongue or intact mandible anteriorly, suctioning the posterior pharynx, and passing an orotracheal, nasopharyngeal, or endotracheal tube often is necessary to re-establish the airway. In addition, laryngeal injuries should be suspected in all patients sustaining blunt facial trauma (see section on the neck).

The initial management of patients with combined facial trauma and a compromised airway is critical. Transoral endotracheal intubation is sometimes complicated by the possibility of cervical spine injury. Nasotracheal intubation is hazardous in patients with midface fractures resulting from possible disruption of the ethmoid and cribriform plate and the potential for injury to the base of the brain. In addition, derange-

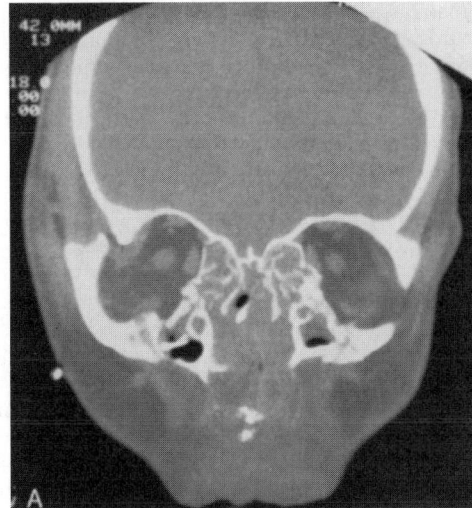

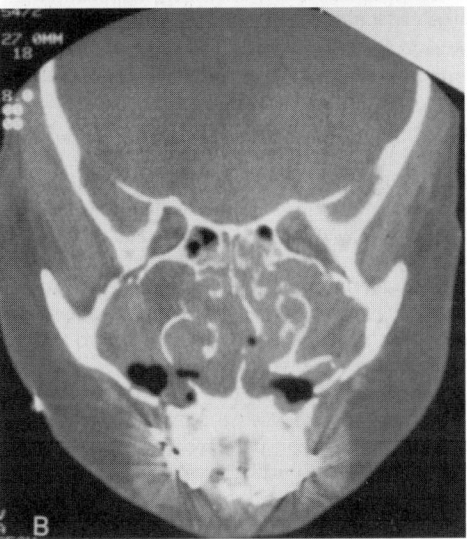

Figure 17–6. Computed tomography of the face. Coronal views (15-mm. separation) demonstrate the presence of a Le Fort III fracture of the right and a Le Fort II fracture of the left.

ment of the larynx may lead to a misdirected submucosal intubation and complete airway obstruction. Tracheostomy or cricothyroidotomy is therefore often required to secure the airway of a patient with significant facial injuries. If, however, the airway can be successfully managed preoperatively without tracheostomy, the need for subsequent postoperative tracheostomy, once considered routine, has decreased. The use of one-stage standard open reductions and rigid internal fixation of fractures using plates and screws has diminished the need for postoperative intramaxillary fixation along with the requirement for a postoperative tracheostomy for airway control.[50] However, some severe maxillofacial injuries still require postrepair tracheostomy airway control, including panfacial fractures involving both the midface and mandible, and complex facial fractures with severe soft tissue injury (e.g., gunshot wounds to upper and midface).

Hemorrhage. Severe hemorrhage in conjunction with a facial fracture usually occurs from the nasal or oral cavity and can usually be controlled by fracture reduction combined with pressure and packing. Bleeding from nasoethmoid and/or maxillary fractures may require placement of posterior nasopharyngeal packing in addition to anterior nasal packs. Hemorrhage not controlled by a standard nasal packing technique should arouse suspicion of laceration of one or both internal maxillary arteries or of basilar skull fracture with internal carotid artery involvement. If anatomic stabilization combined with anterior and posterior nasal and oropharyngeal packing fails to control hemorrhage, immediate angiographic evaluation and embolization is indicated and generally preferred over operative attempts at external carotid artery or selective branch ligation.

Treatment of Specific Injuries

EYES

Ocular trauma occurs in a remarkable 13.5% of trauma patients admitted to one regional trauma center, with motor vehicle injuries accounting for about one half of these injuries.[114] Major ocular injury (globe rupture, laceration, and a loss of sight) occurs in 2.5% of trauma victims. Ocular trauma reportedly accounts for 8% to 10% of all visual impairments and ranks second only to cataract disease as the cause of visual impairment requiring hospitalization.[114] The importance of visual function and the potential occult nature of ocular injuries therefore mandates eye examinations in any patient with upper facial trauma. Assessment of visual acuity by a standard eye chart; testing of the ocular muscles and their associated cranial nerve supply; and direct visualization of the cornea, anterior chamber, and retina should be routine. A more detailed ophthalmologic and slit-lamp examination may be indicated as directed by the severity of injury. As part of the initial assessment, one must suspect intraocular injury in patients with periorbital ecchymosis, edema, or lid lacerations. Frequently, the edema will be sufficiently severe to make direct examination of the eye difficult. Injuries such as anterior hyphema (blood in the anterior chamber), soft globe, loss of light perception, foreign bodies, and scleral laceration can be detected on an initial eye examination, which should be performed by all trauma surgeons. Impact injury to the optic nerve without concomitant facial fracture or penetrating wound can result in partial or complete loss of vision, a clinical entity known as *traumatic optic neuropathy*. Visual loss is permanent and is usually instantaneous with impact, although delayed visual loss has also been reported. This entity occurs in 0.5% to 5% of patients with closed head injury. There is no proven form of treatment, although high-dose steroids in doses similar to acute spinal cord injury regimens have been advocated.[126]

FACE

Upper Third of Face. Fractures of the upper third of the face may be accompanied by ocular or central nervous system (CNS) complications as well as by facial deformity. The facial bones are suspended from the base of the skull, and fractures of the superior facial region (e.g., the ethmoid sinuses) may readily extend into the cranial vault. Pertinent facial fractures in this region are those of the supraorbital ridge, orbital roof, frontal sinus, and nasoethmoid or orbital area. Fractures of the orbital roof are frequently associated with frontal sinus and nasoethmoid fractures but may occur as an isolated injury or as an extension of a low frontal skull fracture. The loss of upward gaze in association with this fracture indicates involvement of the superior rectus muscle and possibly superior oblique muscles. However, the most common cause of loss of upward gaze is due to orbital floor injury and associated entrapment or injury of the inferior rectus muscle. An important clinical sign of an orbital roof blow-in fracture is proptosis of the ocular globe. Blow-in fractures lead to a decrease in orbital volume and then proptosis, as opposed to orbital blow-out fractures, which lead to an increase in orbital volume and enophthalmos (sinking in of the eye). There is a much higher incidence of injury to the globe and periorbital contents with blow-in fractures. Occasionally, a fracture of the orbital roof may be so comminuted as to defy repair, and débridement with primary or delayed bone grafting may be necessary. Comminuted upper and midface fractures are best repaired primarily with immediate bone graft, as delayed grafting is more difficult and has a higher complication rate.[50]

Middle Third of Face. Patients with fractures of the middle third of the face may have aesthetic, CNS, ocular, and dental complications. The middle third of the face includes the maxilla, zygomas, orbits, and nose. In 1901 Professor Rene Le Fort published the results of his monumental experiments on human cadavers to determine the lines of least resistance in fractures of the face. The classification system proposed by Le Fort has great utility in describing the most common types of traumatic midface fractures. In a *Le Fort I fracture* (also known as *Guérin's fracture*, or *dentoalveolar dysjunction*), the fracture lines are transverse through the pyriform aperture above the alveolar ridge and run posteriorly to the pterygoid region (Fig. 17–7). The dental alveolar supporting bone and palate of the maxilla are involved as a single detached block. In addition, segmental fractures of the alveolar ridge and palate can also occur. The diagnosis of Le Fort I fracture may be suggested by the presence of upper lip lacerations, complaints by the patient of malocclusion, and mobility of the fracture fragment on digital manipulation of the incisor teeth by the examiner's thumb and index finger. Required treatment can vary from closed reduction with arch bars and intermaxillary fixation (e.g., intraosseous wiring or small plate osteosynthesis) to open reductions with internal fixation and, occasionally, bone grafting.

In *Le Fort II fractures* (pyramidal fracture of mid-face), the superior fracture lines are transverse through the nasal bones or through the articulation of the maxillary and nasal bones with the frontal bones. The fracture line extends laterally from that superior point into the medial orbital wall, through the lacrimal and ethmoid bones, and exits the orbital floor anteriorly at the medial to middle portions of the infraorbital rim (see Fig. 17–7). Occasionally, the right and left maxilla are completely separated at the midline of the hard palate, with each unit containing maxillary and palatal bones. This fracture line, or *palatal split*, may splay the maxillary alveolar ridge laterally and outside the occlusal arch of the mandible. The diagnosis is established by digital manipulation of the anterior maxilla and observation for mobility of the central triangle, consisting of the maxilla and nose. Treatment consists of reduction of the maxilla, repair of any nasoethmoid component, and fixation in the proper position—to the cranial base above and to the mandible below.

The *Le Fort III fracture* (craniofacial dysjunction fracture) is the highest level of midface injury. The central third of the face is literally displaced from its attachments to the cranial base. The transverse superior fracture line is similar to that of the Le Fort II fracture, but at the medial orbital wall it extends posteriorly or laterally, rather than anteriorly, and continues across the orbital floor to the inferior orbital fissure (see Fig. 17–7). From that point, the lines run through the lateral orbital wall and rim to the pterygoid fossa, zygomatic arch, and pterygoid process. An important component is a fracture line through the septum and the perpendicular plate of the ethmoid. This fracture may extend into the cribriform plate of the anterior cranial fossa and produce cerebrospinal fluid rhinorrhea, a finding that is deceptively common in patients with Le Fort II, Le Fort III, and nasoethmoid fracture.

The clinical diagnosis of Le Fort III fractures is not difficult. Massive facial edema and ecchymosis, an elongated face without normal projection, and mobility of the entire middle third of the face on digital manipulation of the maxilla establish the diagnosis. Occasionally, the midface may exhibit

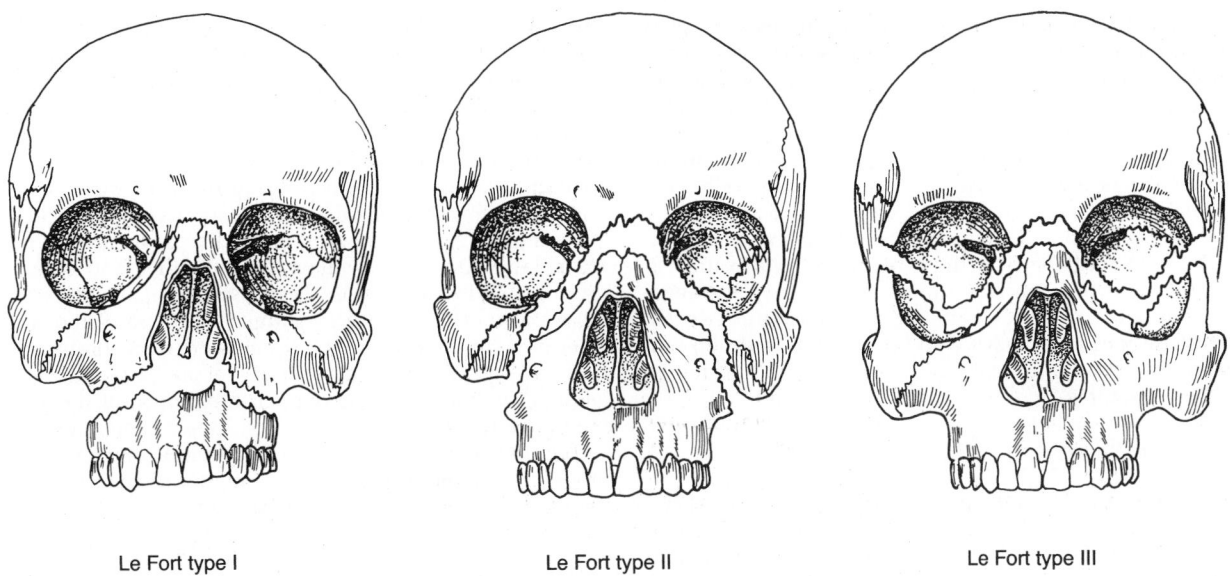

Le Fort type I   Le Fort type II   Le Fort type III

Figure 17–7. Le Fort I, II, and III fracture lines as seen in frontal view.

marked shortening of the midface and nasoethmoid region and loss of mobility of the midface on digital manipulation. A marked anterior open bite may be present. Management of Le Fort III fractures is usually deferred for stabilization and treatment of other injuries. Repairs and extensions of the principles outlined for the treatment of Le Fort I and II fractures, namely reduction and stabilization of the midface complex between the cranial base and mandible, and treatment of associated fractures still apply. Le Fort III fractures often require open reduction and internal fixation with interosseous wiring or plating of the frontal bone medially at the nasal root and laterally at the orbital rim, repair of the associated nasoethmoid-orbital component, suspension to the frontal bone, and intermaxillary fixation. Bone graft reconstruction of the orbital walls and floor is frequently required for the most severe cases.

The *zygoma* is also considered a structure of the middle third of the face, and its position and contour render it vulnerable to fracture. The zygoma fractures at four main articulations: the frontozygomatic suture at the superior-lateral rim; the zygomaticomaxillary suture at the infraorbital rim; the zygomaticotemporal suture at the midportion of the arch; and the zygomaticomaxillary buttress. The fracture line at the infraorbital rim is through the infraorbital foramen or, more laterally, at the zygomaticomaxillary suture and then continues laterally across the orbital floor at the juncture of the zygoma with the sphenoid bone and through the lateral orbital rim at the frontozygomatic suture line. Disruption of the orbital flood may allow prolapse and herniation of the orbital contents into the maxillary antrum. The loss of orbital fat and/or increase in orbital volume may produce a sunken or hollow appearance to the eye or an inferior displacement of the globe, again often obscured by early postinjury edema. Of particular importance is the simultaneous herniation of the inferior rectus and oblique muscles of extraocular motion. Incarceration or entrapment of these two muscles may prevent the eye from rotating downward and outward but more commonly acts as an impediment to upward rotation by the action of the superior rectus. This loss of upward gaze should be evident on examination and produces diplopia. Unilateral pain on closing the mandible may suggest depression of the zygomatic arch component. Medial displacement of the arch fragments may impinge on the coronoid process of the mandible and temporalis muscle and can prevent normal motion.

The zygomaticomaxillary buttress can be easily palpated intraorally at the maxillary buccal vestibule. Loss of sensation over the cheek, side of the nose, upper lip, gum, and teeth on the side of the fracture is a common finding. Damage to the infraorbital nerve from a direct blow or impingement at the infraorbital foramen and as the nerve traverses the orbital floor by bone fragments is responsible. The authors have generally adopted an aggressive treatment plan for zygomatic fractures that incorporates traditional orthopedic principles of open, direct reduction and internal fixation.

Lower Third of Face. The lower third of the face contains a single facial bone, the mandible. After the nasal bones, the mandible is the second most commonly fractured facial bone. The mandible does not articulate directly with the other facial bones but is suspended from the base of the skull at the temporomandibular joints. The location and direction of the fracture line are critically important in the degree of displacement of the fracture fragments and the success of maintenance of reduction. The sites of mandibular fractures are most commonly grouped anatomically: the regions of the coronoid process, the condyle, ramus, angle, body, parasymphysis, and symphysis (Fig. 17–8).

Patients may have little evidence of injury if they have sustained a single closed fracture of the condyle, although swelling, edema, and some pain on motion of the mandible are almost invariable with any fracture. Intraoral examination should focus on the occlusion, presence of lacerations, displaced mandibular fragments, and floor of mouth ecchymosis. The mandible may be gently manipulated bimanually to detect false motion or palpable fracture lines. The region of the condyles can be assessed by insertion of the examiner's

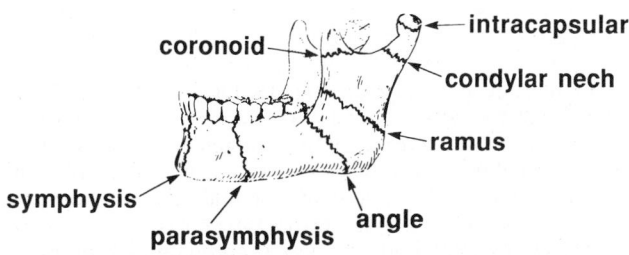

Figure 17–8. Anatomy of the mandible and common lines of fracture.

finger into each external auditory canal during movement of the mandible for detection of asymmetry and absence of the normally palpable condylar head. The clinical suspicion of the fractured mandible can be confirmed on radiographic examination.

Reduction and fixation of mandibular fractures should be accomplished as precisely and expeditiously as possible because malocclusion is a major long-term complication.[92] The risk of osteomyelitis and nonunion is enhanced by an extended period after injury without reduction and fixation. If a fracture line communicates intraorally, bacterial colonization of the bone continues until the fragments are reduced. For these reasons, antibiotics with coverage of common oral microflora are used in the interim between injury and reduction of the fractures.

Principles of Operative Care

The timing of operative repair of facial fractures is somewhat controversial. Advocates of *early* reduction and fixation argue that repair within 24 hours of injury is readily accomplished because of minimal edema formation and results in a shorter hospital stay and less patient discomfort. Proponents of a *staged* approach prefer to wait for resolution of facial edema, using the time for preoperative planning, more detailed radiographic analysis, and the production of operative aids such as acrylic interocclusal splints. In addition, many of these patients have significant associated injuries that require stabilization and treatment, and the facial fractures have a lower overall priority. The ideal window for staged facial fracture repair is generally between 3 and 14 days, depending on the amount of facial edema, associated injuries, and general status of the patient. The principles of repair of complex craniomaxillofacial injuries include (1) direct exposure of all fractures; (2) meticulous reduction and internal fixation, and (3) primary bone grafting of severely damaged or absent bone.[50] Early immediate repair is considered with severe soft tissue injury and large, open lacerations, which aids in the exposure of the fractures or if early neurosurgical repair is needed. A synchronous neurosurgical maxillofacial repair should always be attempted, as an asynchronous repair invariably disrupts the neurosurgical dural repair. Intracranial pressure monitoring during such procedures is required.

Thorax

One quarter of civilian trauma deaths are caused by thoracic trauma, and two thirds of these deaths occur after the patient reaches the hospital. Mortality rates of hospitalized patients with an isolated chest injury range from 4% to 8%; they increase to 10% to 50% when one other organ system is involved and rise to 35% when multiple additional organ systems are involved. Many of these deaths can be prevented with prompt diagnosis and correct management. Despite these high mortality rates, most thoracic injuries do not require a thoracotomy but rather simple lifesaving maneuvers of airway control and tube thoracostomy.

Mechanism of Injury

The life-threatening injuries incurred in penetrating trauma are distinctly different from those of blunt injuries. Penetrating thoracic injuries (e.g., stab wounds, gunshot wounds, and impalement on a foreign body) primarily injure the peripheral lung, producing both a hemothorax and pneumothorax. More than 80% of all penetrating chest wounds cause a hemothorax, and nearly all cause a pneumothorax. Penetrating injuries that enter or traverse the mediastinum must also be evaluated for potential cardiac, great vessel, or esophageal injury. Hemodynamically unstable patients with mediastinal entering or traversing wounds should be considered to have exsanguinating thoracic hemorrhage, pericardial tamponade, or tension pneumothorax. Preparation for immediate thoracotomy is indicated.

Blunt trauma can induce injury by three distinct mechanisms: a direct blow to the chest (e.g., rib fracture), deceleration injury (e.g., pulmonary or cardiac contusion and aortic tear), and compression injury (e.g., cardiac and diaphragm rupture). Rib fracture is the most common sign of blunt thoracic trauma. The less common fractures of the scapula, sternum, or first rib suggest massive force of injury and should invoke a thorough search for multisystem injury. In adults the bony thoracic cage absorbs much of the shock of blunt trauma. In children, the flexible cartilaginous thoracic structures allow the transmission of blunt force to the intrathoracic structures, resulting in a higher incidence of pulmonary contusion than of rib fractures.

Pathophysiology

The thorax is responsible for the vital cardiopulmonary physiology of delivering oxygenated blood to metabolically active tissues. Three pathologic consequences of thoracic injury, either alone or in combination, are responsible for inadequate oxygen delivery: hypoxemia, hypovolemia, and myocardial failure. Hypoxemia can result from any injury that disturbs the airway or ventilation, including airway obstruction, pneumothorax, flail chest, pulmonary contusion, tracheobronchial injury, or diaphragm rupture. Each of these injuries limits the physiologic function of air exchange. Hypovolemia from intrathoracic hemorrhage is second only to rib fractures as a sequel of thoracic trauma. Up to 40% of the circulating blood can accumulate in a hemothorax. Thoracic bleeding most frequently occurs from injuries to the lung parenchyma or intercostal vessels. Myocardial failure may be caused by either blunt or penetrating thoracic injuries. Cardiac contusion is a direct blow to the heart that is clinically manifested as dysrythmias and cardiac pump failure. Penetrating injuries resulting in direct cardiac injury and pericardial tamponade can rapidly compromise cardiac function. Other rare causes of cardiac pump failure include rupture of the ventricular septum, or valvular muscle and coronary air embolus. The initial management of patients with thoracic trauma must focus on both the mechanisms of injury and the pathologic consequences responsible for inadequate oxygen delivery.

Initial Treatment

The initial approach to the patient with thoracic trauma follows the basic tenets of resuscitation of all critically injured patients. The primary goal is to provide oxygen to vital organs. Airway control, adequate ventilation, and shock management are the top priorities. Some specific features of the initial management of thoracic trauma patients bear emphasis. Restlessness, confusion, and anxiety are the first signs of hypoxemia and should not be overlooked or ascribed to head injury or intoxication. Stridor and supraclavicular or intercostal muscle retractions are signs of airway obstruction; active airway control (endotracheal intubation or tracheostomy) may be required. Venting a major hemothorax or pneumothorax in the thoracic patient in extremis is an integral part of establishing adequate ventilation and should not await radiologic confirmation. Rapid tube thoracostomy reexpands the collapsed lung, tamponades lung parenchymal injuries against the chest wall, and allows the monitoring of ongoing blood loss. Large-bore needle insertion may alleviate

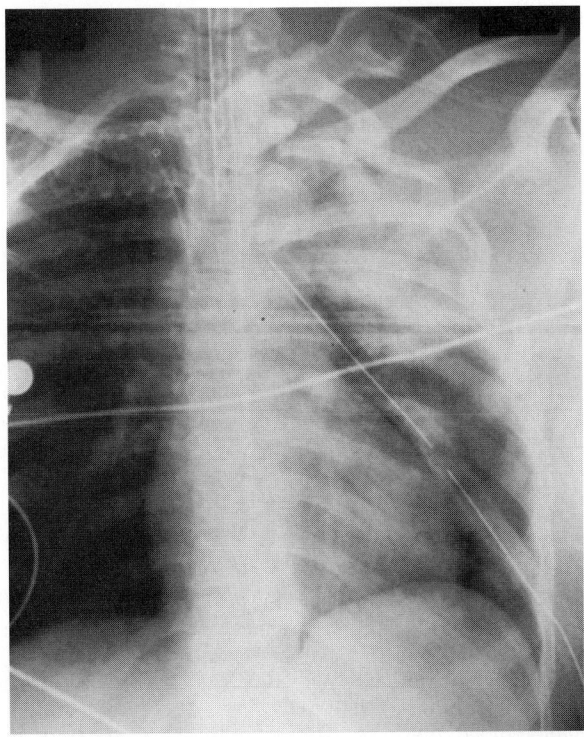

Figure 17–9. Flail chest over the left upper thoracic and shoulder girdle region and fracture displacement of ribs 1 through 4. Underlying pulmonary contusion is evident. No associated major vascular injury occurred.

a tension pneumothorax and obviate the need for *crash* intubation. Tube thoracostomy should always follow. Persistent shock despite adequate oxygenation and volume restoration in the thoracic trauma patient suggests significant ongoing hemorrhage or cardiogenic shock from tension pneumothorax, direct cardiac injury and tamponade, or coronary air embolism. The likelihood of these injuries must be rapidly determined and treatment immediately instituted. Physical examination and chest radiograph can usually differentiate among these etiologies, occasionally supplemented with central venous pressure monitoring, transthoracic ultrasound, or periocardiocentesis. Maximum attention should be given to these immediately life-threatening problems. The next echelon of management priorities is directed at assessing the patients' overall condition and at identifying other potentially lethal injuries. The treatment of specific thoracic injuries is detailed in the following section.

Treatment of Specific Injuries

CHEST WALL

Rib Fractures. Fracture of the ribs is the most common thoracic injury (Fig. 17–9). With simple fractures, pain on inspiration is the principal symptom. Localized pain, tenderness, and occasionally crepitus confirm the diagnosis. A chest x-ray should be obtained to exclude other intrathoracic injuries and not necessarily to identify a rib fracture. The use of narcotics in small amounts, intercostal nerve blocks, and muscle relaxants are usually adequate treatment. Hospital admission for pain relief, cough assistance, and endotracheal suction may be necessary for several days, particularly in elderly patients. Underestimating the pathophysiologic effect of simple rib fracture, particularly in the elderly patient, is one of the primary pitfalls in trauma care. Rib belts and adhesive taping, although once popular, should be avoided because the resultant limitation in motion increases the inci-

dence of retained secretions and atelectasis. Fracture of the upper ribs (1 through 3), clavicle, or scapula implies significant trauma, and associated major vascular injury must be suspected, although this exact association has been questioned. One report documents a 14% incidence of vascular injury in patients sustaining first rib fractures. All had associated absent pulse, brachial plexus injury, or a displaced fracture, implying that angiography may be selectively employed in this group of patients.[101]

Flail Chest. Unilateral fracture of four or more ribs anteriorly and posteriorly or bilateral anterior or costochondral fracture of four or five ribs produces enough instability that paradoxical respiratory motion results in hypoventilation of an unacceptable degree (see Fig. 17–9). Although usually visually apparent in the unconscious patient, because of splinting, the flail segment may not be readily apparent in the conscious patient. If severe and untreated, atelectasis, hypercapnia, hypoxia, accumulations of secretions, and ineffective cough occur. The pathophysiologic effects may be present immediately or may progress over several hours and present as late respiratory decompensation. Excellent pain relief and improved ventilation can often be provided by a segmental epidural anesthetic or serial intercostal rib blocks. Intrapleural anesthetic administration (usually via a previously placed chest tube) rarely provides adequate pain relief.

If spontaneous respirations prove inadequate, endotracheal intubation with the use of a volume respirator has largely supplanted attempts at stabilization of the chest wall. A respiratory rate of more than 40 breaths per minute and a PO_2 of less than 60 mm. Hg on 60% FIO_2 are indications for intubation and mechanical ventilation. The presence of pre-existing chronic lung disease, depressed level of consciousness, and concomitant intra-abdominal injuries are also relative indications for intubation. Only rarely is sternal fracture displacement or rib overlap and displacement severe enough to warrant open reduction and internal fixation.

Respiratory difficulty in flail chest injury is invariably aggravated by an underlying pulmonary contusion (Fig. 17–10; see also Fig. 17–9). Investigators have concluded that the major respiratory problem is the underlying pulmonary injury and that paradoxical movement is a minor factor.[118] These studies demonstrate a reduced need for mechanical ventilation if care is exercised in avoiding fluid overresuscitation. If intubation is required, positive end-expiratory pressure (PEEP) may be helpful in restoring functional residual

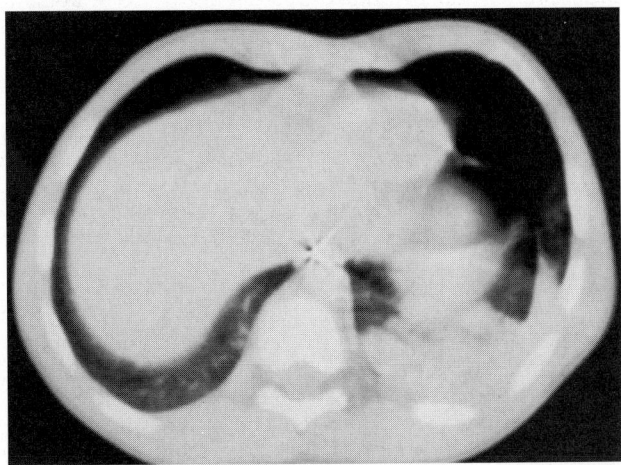

Figure 17–10. Chest computed tomography scan of 10-year-old patient following blunt chest trauma. Significant pulmonary contusion is evident. The chest anteroposterior radiograph is depicted in Figure 17–11.

capacity and reducing intrapulmonary shunts. Mechanical ventilation and a better understanding of the underlying pulmonary contusion have reduced the mortality of flail chest from 50% to less than 5%.

Open Pneumothorax. A defect in the chest wall provides a direct communication of the pleural space with the environment. A wound large enough to exceed the laryngeal cross-sectional area provides an alternative air pathway with less resistance than that of the normal tracheobronchial tree. Inability to generate negative intrathoracic pressure causes lung collapse and marked paroxysmal shifting of the mediastinum with each respiratory effort. The resultant hypoventilation and diminished cardiac output can become immediately life-threatening. Diagnosis is readily apparent, as each aspiration draws air into the interpleural space, causing the characteristic *sucking chest wound*. Treatment consists of prompt closure of the defect with a sterile dressing followed by venting of the chest with either a flutter valve or chest tube to treat the possibly resultant tension pneumothorax.

LUNGS

Pulmonary Contusion. As noted earlier, pulmonary contusion occurs in most patients with flail chest but can also appear without any evidence of rib fracture. Critical intrathoracic trauma may be present in the absence of skeletal injury, particularly in children, owing to the marked elasticity of the rib cage. Fluid and blood from ruptured vessels enter the alveoli, interstitial spaces, and bronchi and produce localized airway obstruction. As this process progresses, pulmonary compliance decreases and ventilation becomes more difficult. Pulmonary contusions are contrasted with localized lung hematomas, which result from local parenchymal injury and hemorrhage. Most hematomas resolve adequately with expectant treatment. Pulmonary contusion may be confused with the adult respiratory distress syndrome (ARDS) or may even be associated with it. Physical examination is usually unrewarding. Chest radiologic examination in ARDS eventually demonstrates patchy consolidation, from minimal to lobar, whereas x-ray examinations showing parenchymal consolidation immediately following injury are more suggestive of pulmonary contusion (Fig. 17–11; see also Fig. 17–10). In children, the relative elasticity of the thoracic cage makes

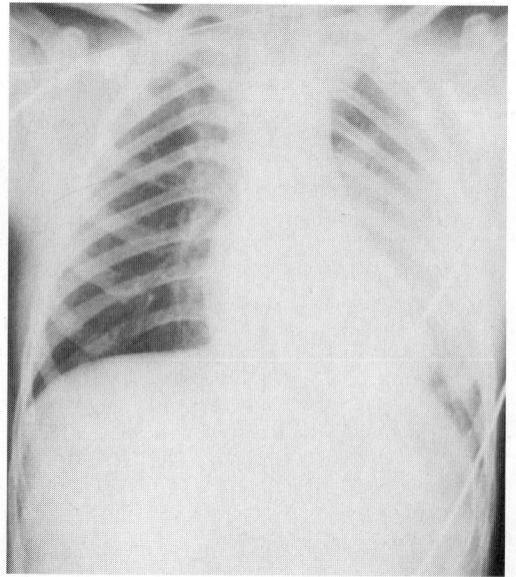

Figure 17–11. Chest anteroposterior radiograph of a 10-year-old boy involved in motor vehicle accident. Despite lack of rib fractures, significant pulmonary contusion is apparent (see Fig. 17–10).

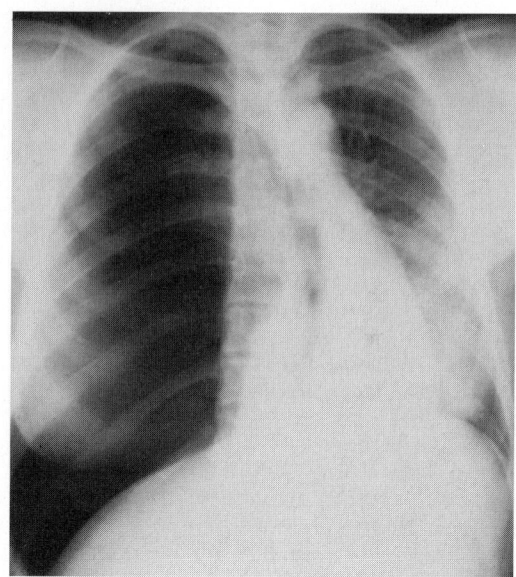

Figure 17–12. Right tension pneumothorax following stab wound to the chest.

pulmonary contusion likely even in the absence of rib fractures (see Fig. 17–11).

Management involves careful pulmonary support and clearing of secretions, with ventilatory support if arterial blood gas values cannot be maintained in a physiologic range. Fluid overload should be assiduously avoided. The use of albumin to maintain plasma oncotic pressure in this clinical setting is controversial. The hemorrhage and edema are self-limited and will clear if infection or other problems do not intervene. Although pulmonary contusion is usually a localized parenchymal defect, PEEP may be a useful adjunct in the management of those patients requiring ventilation, particularly if they have more generalized infiltration on chest x-ray examination.

Pneumothorax. Pneumothorax results from lacerations of the chest wall or lung, or rupture of an alveoli *(paper bag effect)* and can be caused by either penetrating or blunt trauma. Tension pneumothorax develops when a flap valve leak allows air to enter the pleural space but prevents its escape. Intrapleural pressure rises, causing total lung collapse and a shift of the mediastinum to the opposite side (Fig. 17–12). This pressure must be relieved immediately to avoid interference with ventilation in the opposite lung and impairment of cardiac function from impediment of venous return. Tension pneumothorax is a true surgical emergency, requiring immediate diagnosis and chest tube insertion. Subcutaneous emphysema, absent breath sounds, mediastinal shift, and acute respiratory distress warrant chest tube insertion without waiting for a chest x-ray examination. In contrast, a simple pneumothorax (without tension) of traumatic origin should also be managed by chest tube insertion, but only after documentation by chest x-ray examination. In many circumstances, 15 to 20 cm. water seal suction is all that is necessary. The temptation to watch a minimal pneumothorax should be resisted. Delayed increase in the volume of the pneumothorax may occur and become life threatening after the patient has been transferred from the critical care area. This is most likely to happen if the patient requires anesthesia, intubation, and a positive-pressure breathing system or if assisted mechanical ventilation is required.

Hemothorax. Hemorrhage into the pleural space occurs in some quantity in almost every patient with a diagnosable chest injury. Blood loss may vary from slight to extensive. Although an upright chest x-ray examination can diagnose an intrathoracic accumulation of more than 200 ml. of blood, a supine film may miss collections of up to 1 liter. Bleeding may be from any intrathoracic structure, although massive hemothorax generally signals a systemic arterial or major pulmonary vascular injury. Because the lung itself is a low-pressure system with an average pulmonary artery pressure of 15 mm. Hg, spontaneous hemostasis occurs for all but central injuries. Most often significant, persistent hemothorax is from intercostal arteries and, in penetrating wounds, the internal mammary artery is often the source (Fig. 17–13). Tube thoracostomy with a 32- to 36-French chest tube placed in the sixth or seventh intercostal space at the midaxillary line should be promptly performed. Note that this insertion point is somewhat lower than is required for pneumothorax, to allow for better sulcus drainage. Needle aspiration is not adequate. Early tube thoracostomy prevents clotted hemothorax or subsequent fibrothorax in most instances. When massive hemothorax is present, preparation for collection of the blood for autotransfusion should be made prior to the tube insertion. A sodium citrate solution can be added to the blood collection device to ensure anticoagulation and allow for possible autotransfusion.

In 85% of patients, tube thoracostomy is the only treatment required. Unrelenting hemorrhage following either penetrating or blunt thoracic trauma is an indication for immediate operating room thoracotomy. An initial thoracic blood loss greater than 1500 ml. (30% blood volume) or an ongoing loss of 250 ml. (5% blood volume) for 3 consecutive hours serves only as a practical guideline. The clinical situation and overall condition of the patient are the most influential factors. One study demonstrated that an acute hemothorax of 1500 ml. following penetrating trauma resulted in a surgically correctable lesion 85% of the time.[104] With blunt trauma, thoracotomy is less likely to demonstrate a discrete source of hemorrhage.

Pulmonary Parenchyma Injury. Although most pulmonary parenchyma injuries can be effectively managed nonoperatively, about 15% of penetrating lung injuries require thoracotomy for hemorrhage control. Various techniques for hemorrhage control have evolved, ranging from simple oversewing to anatomic resection. Approximately 80% to 90% of pulmonary injuries requiring operation can be managed by nonanatomic means, such as oversewing or stapling the injured segment of the lung, and only 10% to 20% require resection. Large trauma centers report the need for formal lobectomy following penetrating lung injuries in only 0.2%

to 0.5% of their patients.[74] Management of deep through-and-through injuries to a lobe of the lung with bleeding deep within the lung has been described using tractotomy with selective vascular ligation.[133] The possibility of pulmonary venous-systemic air embolism exists with these injuries and can be minimized with low peak inspiratory pressures and early hilar cross clamping. Emergent pulmonary pneumonectomy for massive thoracic injury is rarely effective; the sudden pulmonary hypertension and resultant hypoxia places an insurmountable physiologic load on the usually ischemic myocardium.

Trachea and Bronchus Injuries. Blunt tracheal or broncial injuries are often due to compression of the airway between the sternum and the vertebral column in decelerating *steering wheel* motor vehicle accidents with resultant shearing of the right main stem bronchus from the carina or transverse lacerations of the trachea. Alternatively, a blow-out injury to the membranous trachea may occur during chest wall compression with a closed glottis. Patients with tracheal injuries may present with mediastinal and deep cervical emphysema or pneumothorax with a massive air leak. Hemoptysis, hemopneumothorax, subcutaneous crepitance, and respiratory distress are frequent. When accompanied by acute airway obstruction, the immediate priority is establishment of an effective airway. If possible, this should be preceded by endoscopic evaluation of the injury prior to blind endotracheal intubation. Emergency treatment consists of inserting the endotracheal tube beyond the injury to facilitate ventilation and prevent aspiration of blood. Tube thoracostomy is clearly indicated in the presence of a hemothorax or pneumothorax. If endotracheal intubation is not possible, or if the anatomy is significantly distorted, surgical entry into the trachea for placement of a tracheostomy tube may be necessary.

The definitive diagnosis of tracheal or bronchial injury usually requires confirmation by bronchoscopy. When early diagnosis is made, the contralateral bronchus is intubated and primary repair is performed. Although small lesions may be managed initially without surgical treatment, delayed healing invites stricture formation, resulting in recurrent atelectasis, infection, and bronchiectasis, and parenchymal destruction will be the final result. For an early stricture, either resection or a bronchoplastic procedure may be performed. After permanent parenchymal damage, pulmonary resection should be performed.

HEART AND AORTA

Blunt Cardiac Injury. Blunt cardiac injury represents a spectrum of pathologic changes from a cardiac wall bruise (contusion) to ventricular, septal, or valvular rupture. The right ventricle is most frequently involved, presumably because of its proximity to the sternum (Fig. 17–14). Although most patients with rupture of the atrial or ventricular chambers do not reach a medical facility, survivors have been reported if vital signs can be maintained during transportation.[100] Myocardial contusion is a curious clinical entity whose definition, diagnosis, and significance have frustrated clinicians for several decades.[76] Cardiac contusion has occurred in up to 20% of all patients with blunt chest injuries and in an estimated 70% of multisystem trauma patients admitted to an intensive care unit. Fifty percent of autopsies performed on victims of fatal automobile accidents demonstrate significant trauma to the pericardium and heart. However, most clinicians believe these figures overly exaggerate the clinical significance of this entity. The true diagnosis can be made only pathologically, with findings of myocardial wall bruise or hematoma. There are no specific and practical laboratory findings, and specifically cardiac isoenzymes are of little or no value.[9] Perhaps many cardiac contusions are asymptomatic and go unrecognized. The clinically important

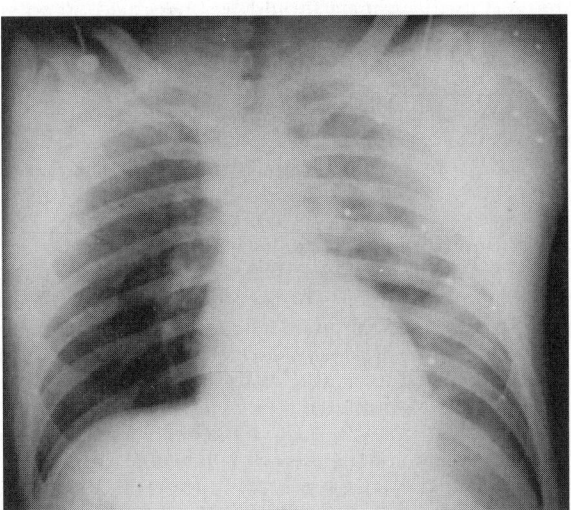

Figure 17–13. Massive hemothorax from a gunshot wound to the left chest.

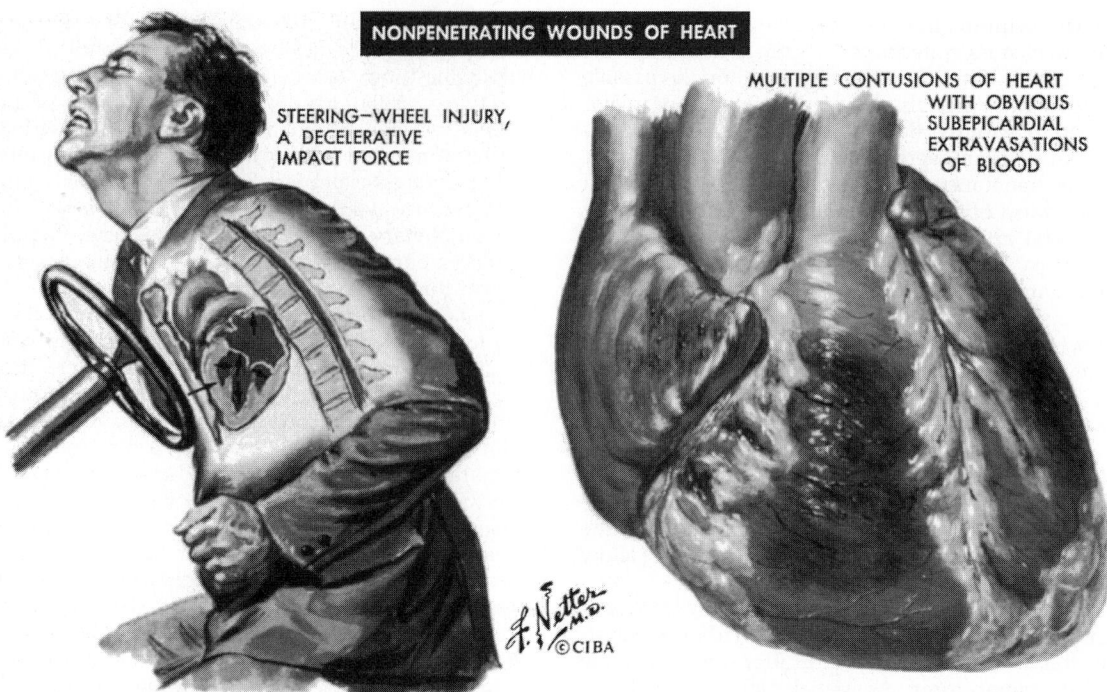

Figure 17–14. Mechanism for development of myocardial contusion with compression of the heart between the sternum and vertebral column. (Courtesy of CIBA Pharmaceuticals.)

sequelae of myocardial contusion are hypotension due to myocardial dysfunction and severe dysrhythmia. The clinical signs of myocardial contusions are conduction abnormalities on electrocardiogram (ECG) or wall motion abnormality on two-dimensional echocardiography, coupled with an appropriate mechanism of injury. All major thoracic trauma patients should therefore have an ECG performed early in their emergency care. The ECG changes are variable and may even indicate frank myocardial infarction. Multiple premature ventricular contractions, unexplained sinus tachycardia, atrial fibrillation, bundle branch block (usually right), and ST segment changes are the most common ECG findings. Elevated central venous pressure in the absence of obvious cause may indicate right ventricular dysfunction secondary to contusion. The injury event may have been precipitated by a true myocardial ischemic episode. Patients with myocardial contusion diagnosed by conduction abnormalities are at risk for sudden dysrhythmias and should have continuous ECG monitoring for 24 hours. Echocardiography may be helpful in diagnosing dysfunction of the ventricular wall and valve leaflets or in detecting blood in the pericardium. Following that interval, the risk of sudden dysrhythmia appears to decrease substantially.[81] The management of myocardial contusion is supportive and similar to that for acute myocardial infarction.

Tamponade. Cardiac tamponade is most frequently caused by penetrating thoracic injuries, but occasionally it is observed in blunt thoracic trauma from myocardial rupture, coronary artery laceration, or ascending dissection of an aortic tear. Accumulation of as little as 150 ml. of blood in the pericardial sack may impair diastolic filling enough to produce distended neck veins, shock, and cyanosis. Beck's classic diagnostic triad of distended neck veins, muffled heart sounds, and hypotension is present in only one third of patients with tamponade; pulsus paradoxus is even less frequently discernible. Pulseless electrical activity (formerly termed *EMD*) in the absence of hypovolemia and tension pneumothorax also suggests cardiac tamponade. Whereas volume resuscitation transiently improves cardiac output by increasing venous return (and can be used as a temporizing maneuver), treatment consists of evacuating even small amounts (15 ml. to 20 ml.) of blood followed by immediate repair of the underlying injury. This can most readily be accomplished by 18-gauge needle pericardiocentesis, which also provides the clinical diagnosis. However, approximately 15% of pericardiocenteses give false-negative results because of a clotted hemopericardium. Therefore, echocardiography is advisable to confirm the diagnosis if it can be promptly obtained, but it too has a small (<5%) false-negative rate. A subxiphoid pericardial window is an alternative method of diagnosing and evacuating pericardial blood, but it takes more time and is best performed in the operating room. If the result is positive, the incision can rapidly be converted to a median sternotomy for definitive cardiac repair. If the patient is in extremis, emergency thoracotomy with pericardiotomy and cardiac repair should be performed. Reports of successful emergency cardiorrhaphy for stab wounds vary from 15% to 80%.[3] Most patients with penetrating trauma to the heart do not require cardiopulmonary bypass. The presence of a postinjury cardiac murmur, suggesting valvular insufficiency or septal defect, should be an indication for echocardiography, cardiac catheterization, or angiography. Repair of these acquired lesions may involve valve replacement or repair or patch closure of septal lesions.

Aorta. Rupture of the thoracic aorta is the most lethal injury following blunt chest trauma, accounting for up to 40% of fatalities in motor vehicle accidents. The exact mechanism of injury is not fully understood, but the aortic arch at the descending aorta is believed to undergo flexion or torsion, disrupting the aortic wall at the ligamentum arteriosum immediately distal to the left subclavian artery. Occasionally, the ascending aorta at the root of the heart may be injured. Injuries to the innominate artery or the subclavian artery at the origin have also been reported. In addition, the descending thoracic aorta may be avulsed from one or several intercostal arteries.

Most patients with aortic rupture die immediately from exsanguination. However, in approximately 20% of these patients, the periaortic tissues in the pleura are able to contain the intravascular pressure, producing a traumatic aneurysm. In cases in which this occurs, almost all are located in the aortic isthmus. Typically, there is partial or complete circumferential tear of the aortic wall. The two ends retract from 1 to 2 cm. Survival is dependent on retention of the hematoma in the aorta adventitia until definitive repair can be performed. Time is of the essence. Historical data note that of those patients with a torn thoracic aorta who survive 1 hour, 15% will exsanguinate within 6 hours, and 25% within 24 hours.[96] Those few who survive the initial period develop a false aneurysm that slowly enlarges over a period of months to years. Calcification in the aneurysm wall usually appears. These types of aneurysms may span periods of 20 years or longer.

There may be no symptoms or findings to suggest aortic injury in those patients who do not demonstrate exsanguination immediately. Other lesions, such as intracranial trauma, chest wall injury, and a ruptured spleen or liver, explain most of the clinical findings. The most common abnormality observed is a widening of the mediastinal shadow on x-ray examination, although only 20% to 43% of patients with a widened mediastinum have aortic injury (Fig. 17–15).[52] Kirsh and Sloan have described the following 10 signs of aortic injury: (1) a mediastinum greater than 10 cm.; (2) loss of aortic contour; (3) shift of the endotracheal tube and trachea to the right; (4) elevation of the left main stem bronchus; (5) depression of the right main stem bronchus; (6) shift of the nasogastric tube to the left; (7) apical capping; (8) first rib fracture; (9) acute left-sided hemothorax; and (10) retrocardiac density.[67] Aortography is indicated if aortic injury is suspected based on the mechanism of injury and any of these suggestive findings (Fig. 17–16). Chest CT scanning has been evaluated as a possible tool for early diagnosis, but it has generally proven too insensitive and can only be considered useful in confirming the presence of mediastinal blood or hematoma suspected on initial plain chest radiograph. Transesophageal ultrasound has shown promise in diagnosing descending aortic injuries as well as cardiac tamponade, but it is unreliable for diagnosing other thoracic great vessel

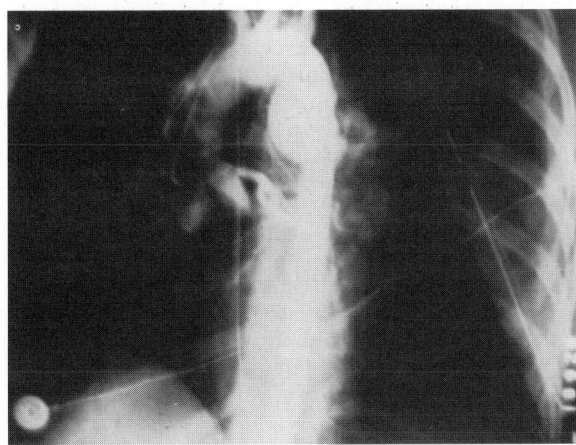

Figure 17–16. Aortogram of the patient in Figure 17–15 demonstrating rupture of the thoracic aorta to the left subclavian artery.

injuries and is highly operator dependent. At this time, retrograde aortography remains the standard of diagnosis.

Surgical repair should be performed immediately because of the risk with time of fatal hemorrhage. Several methods of partial bypass have been advocated and successfully used and are discussed in Chapter 50. Partial atrial-arterial bypass employing a nonheparinized centrifugal pump is the current preferred technique. Although the mandatory use of shunt or bypass is controversial, its main advantage is to protect the spinal cord from ischemia. End-to-end suture is occasionally feasible, but usually a short segment of woven Dacron graft must be interposed.

OTHER INJURIES

Diaphragm. Penetrating lacerations of the diaphragm outnumber blunt ruptures at least four to one. Both may result in herniation through the diaphragm, and therefore both require therapy. Herniation has been reported years following an initial small stab wound. Most blunt diaphragmatic ruptures result from motor vehicle accidents (Fig. 17–17). Rupture of the diaphragm may be either small or large and may involve almost any part of the diaphragm but is usually located radially. Herniation of the viscera may not occur immediately, delaying the diagnosis for an indefinite period. In one recent single institution review of 57 cases of blunt diaphragmatic injuries, 12% of diaphragmatic injuries were missed on initial evaluation, with recognition occurring 2 days to 3 months later.[54] In this report, the chest x-ray exami-

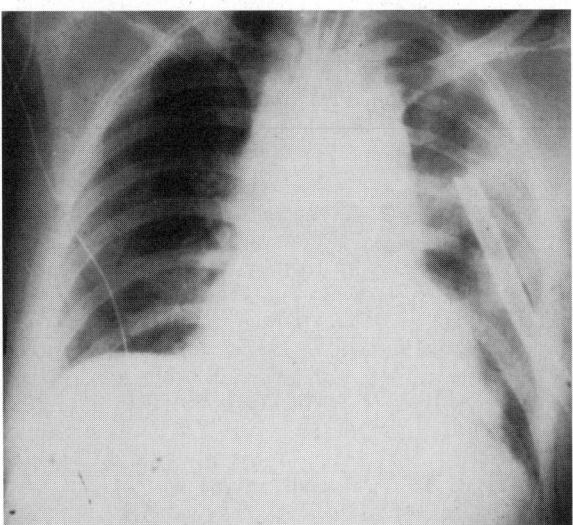

Figure 17–15. Chest x-ray status after a high-speed motor vehicle accident. Note that the mediastinum is >10 cm. across, there is loss of contour of the aortic knob, the endotracheal tube is displaced to the right, there is left apical capping, and there is left hemothorax. These signs are all highly suggestive of aortic disruption.

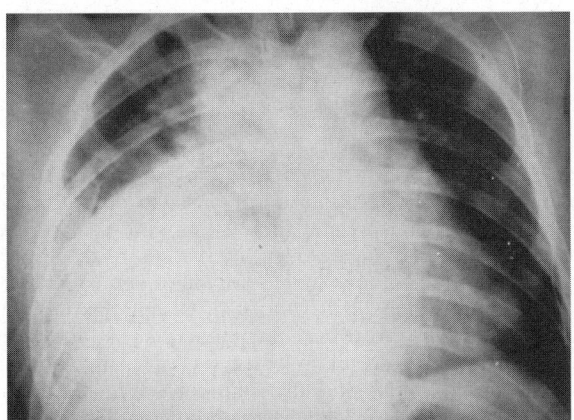

Figure 17–17. Opacification over the right lower lung field after placement of a right chest tube, which is highly suggestive of rupture of the right diaphragm.

nation was diagnostic in only 29 (51%) patients, whereas an early diagnosis was made at celiotomy in 21 (37%). Most patients with left diaphragmatic rupture have associated intra-abdominal injuries. With right-sided diaphragmatic rupture, this is less likely, and chest x-ray examinations may be normal in 30% of the patients. Although classically it has been observed that left-sided diaphragm injuries are more common than those on the right side, the more frequent use of CT scans and an awareness of the likelihood of this injury may explain some reports of a more equal distribution. If the diagnosis is made early, an abdominal approach is usually indicated to exclude associated injuries. If the diagnosis has been substantially delayed so as to exclude intra-abdominal injuries, repair may be preferred via a thoracic approach, particularly for right-sided injuries.

Esophagus. Blunt injury of the esophagus is rare, and penetrating injuries are rarely isolated. The most common symptom of esophageal perforation is extreme pain with the slow evolution of fever several hours later. Regurgitation of blood, hoarseness, dysphagia, or respiratory distress may also be present because of injuries to the trachea. Suspicious radiographic findings are mediastinal air and widening or presence of a foreign body. Pleural effusion or hydropneumothorax is frequently seen. All mediastinal traversing gunshot wounds or stab wounds near the posterior midline should be evaluated for possible esophageal injury. Both endoscopy and esophagography have reported sensitivities that vary from 50% to 90%.[135] Improvement of this accuracy can be obtained if the initial water-soluble contrast x-ray examinations are followed by barium studies. Endoscopy and esophagography should be considered complementary studies. Esophageal injury requires immediate débridement, suture closure, and drainage. Delays of 12 to 24 hours may preclude primary repair, and may mandate proximal diversion and distal feeding access.

RESUSCITATIVE THORACOTOMY

The initial rationale for emergency department thoracotomy and cardiac massage was the recognition that closed heart massage for cardiac arrest or pulseless electrical activity was ineffective in a hypovolemic patient. The technique was rapidly extended to include virtually all moribund trauma patients, regardless of etiology. Subsequently, it has become clearer which patients might stand to benefit from this dramatic technique.[35] Patients with *penetrating thoracic* injuries who arrive pulseless but with myocardial electrical activity are often reasonable candidates for immediate resuscitative thoracotomy, but the prognosis of patients sustaining *blunt* trauma who present with no signs of life is abysmal. The exact indications for emergency department resuscitative thoracotomy in patients who are in extremis, yet who have a measurable blood pressure, are ill defined and highly individual.

The technique consists of a left anterior thoracotomy in the fourth or fifth intercostal space with the patient supine to gain access to the left thoracic cavity; the incision can be extended across the mediastinum *(clam shell)* if more exposure is required. Restoration of intravascular volume is continued, and mechanical ventilation is essential. The therapeutic maneuvers that can be effectively accomplished with a resuscitative thoracotomy are evacuation of pericardial blood causing tamponade; direct control of exsanguinating intrathoracic hemorrhage; open cardiac massage; and cross-clamping of the descending aorta to diminish blood loss below the diaphragm and improve coronary and cerebral perfusion. With return of vital signs the patient is brought to the operating room for definitive surgical repair. Despite the value of these maneuvers, multiple reports confirm that emergency department thoracotomy for patients with blunt trauma and cardiac arrest is rarely effective.

Abdomen

Mechanisms and Diagnosis of Injury

The abdomen is the third most commonly injured body region, with injuries requiring operation occurring in about 20% of civilian trauma victims. Abdominal injuries can be particularly challenging, because it is often difficult to assess intra-abdominal pathology in the multiple-injured victim. *Blunt trauma* continues to be the most common mechanism of injury to the abdomen. This is in part related to the consequences of motor vehicle accidents, although falls, assaults, and industrial accidents contribute significantly. In children, automobile and pedestrian accidents, recreational activities (e.g., bicycling and falls), and child abuse are the leading causes of abdominal injury. In the urban setting, *penetrating trauma* is increasing in relative frequency. Knife wounds are more common than gunshot wounds and are generally less lethal (Fig. 17–18). After several decades of a generally accepted mandatory exploration policy for any penetrating abdominal wound, many trauma centers have again advocated a more selective approach to the management of penetrating wounds, particularly knife injuries. This is due, in part, to the large number of penetrating wounds evaluated at these institutions and to improved accuracy and availability of diagnostic techniques.

Current Diagnostic Techniques

In the awake, alert, responsive patient with isolated abdominal injury, the physical examination and history are quite accurate in predicting the presence of significant visceral injury. For this reason, additional laboratory, x-ray examination, and invasive procedures have a limited role as adjuncts to the physical examination in the patient with *isolated* abdominal injuries. However, in the multiple-injured patient with impaired ability to recognize abdominal pain, or hypotension not attributable to other injuries, additional diagnostic modalities may be of significant benefit. Two highly accurate diagnostic modalities—diagnostic peritoneal lavage (DPL) and CT—have been the mainstay in the United States. Ultrasound has been used extensively in Europe and Japan, although its role in the US is evolving.[111] Despite initial enthusiasm, diagnostic laparoscopy has shown a limited role in these patients. MRI has not proven useful in the initial evaluation of abdominal trauma.

In the early 1960s, needle pericentesis was incorporated

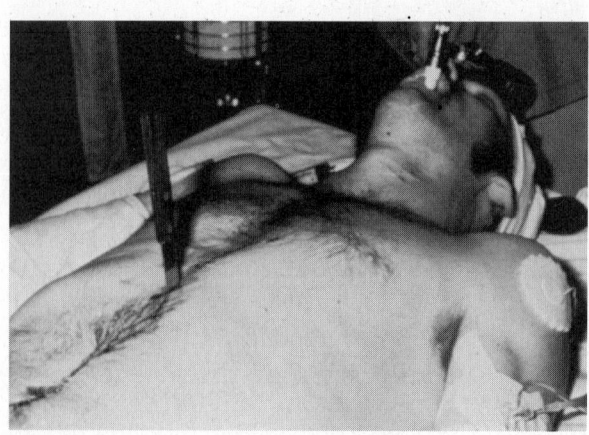

Figure 17–18. Butcher knife impaled in the epigastrium.

as a method of determining intraperitoneal hemorrhage in comatose patients. When positive, the test was highly predictive of significant intra-abdominal injury. Unfortunately, most of the early studies demonstrated a false-negative rate averaging 9.4% but ranging as high as 36% to 40%.[102, 109] Accordingly, in 1965 Root and associates attempted to improve these results by adding an infusion of 1 liter of normal saline to the technique of paracentesis, then retrieving and sampling the lavage effluent.[109] They called this technique *diagnostic peritoneal lavage*. In Powell's review of 31 collected series involving 10,358 patients in whom DPL was used to evaluate blunt trauma to the abdomen, the false-positive and false-negative rates were 1.4% and 1.3%, respectively.[102] Many other large reviews have confirmed an overall sensitivity of 95%, specificity of 98% to 99%, and accuracy of 97% for this technique. As a result, DPL remains the mainstay for diagnosis of intraperitoneal hemorrhage in unstable patients and those with penetrating abdominal trauma. An additional indication for its use is the patient in whom sequential abdominal examinations will be impossible (e.g., a patient undergoing extensive operative procedures such as multiple fracture fixations). In circumstances such as that, peritoneal lavage may be helpful in ruling out the possibility of intraperitoneal injury. The technical complication rate should be less than 2%.

CT scan was added to the surgeon's diagnostic armamentarium for blunt abdominal trauma in the early 1980s. Although initially widely criticized for its lack of sensitivity, the accuracy of CT scans in abdominal trauma has improved with experience and a better understanding of what constitutes abnormal findings. It has proved extremely valuable in assessing the retroperitoneum, an anatomic area of injury for which DPL is not helpful. CT should not be performed in unstable patients, who are best evaluated by exploratory laparotomy or DPL. Peitzman and colleagues[98] have listed five indications for abdominal CT scans in trauma victims: (1) a hemodynamically stable patient with an equivocal abdominal examination; (2) a patient with close head injury; (3) a patient with spinal cord injury; (4) hematuria in the stable patient; and (5) patients with pelvic fractures and significant bleeding. With these indications and a patient who is truly hemodynamically stable, the time required to perform CT does not delay surgical procedures, and experienced personnel are available for immediate interpretation of the results.

Controversy continues regarding the use of adjunctive diagnostic measures for patients who have penetration of the anterior abdominal wall fascia. The role of physical examination, local wound exploration, and quantitative peritoneal lavage in the management of stab wounds to the abdomen has been evaluated.[93] In the patient who is awake, alert, and responsive, physical examination with *positive* findings is highly predictive of intra-abdominal injury. The most common physical findings in patients with stab wounds to the abdomen are shock, peritonitis, and evisceration. When the physical examination results are *negative*, the wound is explored under local anesthesia with direct visualization for possible penetration of the fascia. If there is no penetration of the anterior fascia, the incidence of intra-abdominal injury is zero. In a patient who has a benign abdomen but positive fascial penetration, quantitative peritoneal lavage helps reduce the incidence of negative laparotomies while avoiding overlooked significant injuries. Using a lavage effluent count of greater than 1000 red blood cells per mm. as an indication for exploratory laparotomy, the overlooked injury rate is reduced to zero and the negative laparotomy rate is reduced to 10%. Other authors have advocated a less stringent lavage red blood cell count cut-off, but they sacrifice sensitivity.

Although certain investigators have suggested the use of lavage or even observation for gunshot wounds to the abdomen, the most current opinion is that because more than 90% of the time intra-abdominal injury is associated with gunshot wounds to the abdomen, abdominal exploration being the preferred approach of diagnosis.

Penetrating wounds to the back and flank present significant management dilemmas. Because neither physical examination nor peritoneal lavage is initially helpful in determining retroperitoneal colonic, duodenal, renal, or pancreatic injuries, many surgeons favor mandatory exploratory laparotomy for any penetrating wound to the back or flank. However, the incidence of significant intra-abdominal injury varies from only a 5%–10% for stab wounds to 50%–75% for gunshot wounds. Contrast-enhanced CT has been suggested as a method of noninvasively evaluating these patients, but the usefulness of this cumbersome technique remains controversial, since the incidence of the worrisome bowel injuries (retroperitoneal duodenum and colon) is so low.[78]

Some investigators have reported good success in both the diagnosis and treatment of solid organ injury with the use of visceral arteriography. However, because of the time and expense involved with arteriography and because of the lower false-positive and false-negative rates with peritoneal lavage, arteriography is not an alternative to peritoneal lavage at this time, but rather more useful for specific diagnostic and therapeutic procedures.

Ultrasonography for the diagnosis of intra-abdominal injuries has been slow to develop in the United States, perhaps primarily because of the wide availability of CT and the lack of training of surgeons in this operator-dependent technique. However, its noninvasive nature, coupled with its ability to detect hemoperitoneum and solid organ injuries, suggests it may supplant DPL in some circumstances. The rapid acceptance of laparoscopy as an elective surgical modality resulted in some initial enthusiasm for its use as a diagnostic and potentially therapeutic technique in trauma. The current requirement for general anesthesia, pneumoperitoneum, and incidence of missed injuries (particularly hollow viscus injuries) coupled with its limited therapeutic abilities, have dampened this enthusiasm. Its primary role now seems to be to exclude peritoneal penetration in a tangential or apparently superficial penetrating wound and thus avoid formal laparotomy.

Treatment of Specific Injuries

STOMACH

Most full-thickness gastric injury is due to penetrating trauma. Gastric rupture secondary to blunt trauma is rare; Yajko and colleagues[137] documented only 35 cases of gastric rupture secondary to blunt trauma in the literature from 1930 to 1972. Vigorous ventilation with an endotracheal tube misplaced in the esophagus, however, can cause iatrogenic gastric rupture in the trauma patient.

If vomitus or gastric aspirate is bloody, an injury to the stomach should be suspected. However, it is not unusual for small amounts of blood to be found in the gastric aspirate, even though laparotomy reveals no grossly apparent lesion. At laparotomy, if there is any reason to suspect a gastric injury, the gastrocolic omentum must be widely opened at operation so that the entire posterior surface of the stomach may be completely inspected. If there is any blood in the gastrohepatic ligament, the lesser curvature of the stomach must be closely examined.

Most gastric injuries can be treated simply with débridement and closure in layers. The healthy blood supply of the stomach allows gastric healing to occur readily but also predisposes gastric wounds to postoperative bleeding. Bleeding from the gastric submucosal vessels is more likely to occur postoperatively than from small bowel or colonic submucosal vessels, and it is especially important to repair gastric perforations with an inner row of continuous 3–0 Dexon or Vicryl suture and an outer seromuscular row of interrupted silk. If prolonged gastric decompression seems necessary and there is a strong likelihood that the patient will develop respiratory complications, a gastrostomy should be considered. Gastric diversion or resection is rarely necessary unless the amount of tissue destruction is extensive, such as with high-velocity gunshot or shotgun wounds.

DUODENUM

Approximately three fourths of duodenal injuries result from penetrating trauma, and one fourth are from blunt injuries. The most common mechanism producing blunt injury is a steering wheel blow to the abdomen in an unrestrained automobile driver. Penetrating injuries are usually readily diagnosed at operation, but the insidious nature of many blunt duodenal injuries makes the initial diagnosis difficult. In reviewing their experience with duodenal injury, Lucas and Ledgerwood[76] documented a delay in diagnosis of longer than 12 hours in 53% of their patients and a delay of longer than 24 hours in 28%. This delay markedly increases morbidity and mortality rates. The reported mortality rate was 40% among the patients in whom the diagnosis was delayed longer than 24 hours versus an 11% mortality rate in those patients operated upon in less than 24 hours.

In addition to maintaining a high index of suspicion in patients with appropriate injury mechanism, a serum amylase level should be initially obtained and if elevated, repeated at 6-hour intervals in patients with blunt abdominal trauma. Although hyperamylasemia can be diagnostically confusing (see pancreas section), a persistently elevated or rising amylase level may indicate pancreatic or duodenal injury and mandates further evaluation or operative exploration. The radiologic signs of duodenal injury on the initial plain abdominal or upright chest radiograph are subtle, showing only mild scoliosis, obliteration of the right psoas muscle, or retroperitoneal air that is difficult to distinguish from the overlying transverse colon. An early suspicion of retroperitoneal duodenal rupture is best confirmed (or excluded) by a Gastrografin upper gastrointestinal series or abdominal CT scan with oral and intravenous contrast enhancement. DPL is unreliable in detecting duodenal and other retroperitoneal injuries. Nevertheless, DPL may be useful in patients with duodenal injuries because approximately 40% have associated intra-abdominal injuries that would result in a positive peritoneal lavage and subsequent surgical exploration.

Factors that influence morbidity and mortality following duodenal trauma have also been reviewed by Snyder and colleagues.[125] In a review of 247 patients sustaining duodenal trauma, they reported an overall duodenal fistula rate of 7% and an overall mortality rate of 10%. These authors believed that the five factors listed in Table 17–4 most significantly correlate with the severity of duodenal injury and subsequent morbidity and mortality. Snyder and colleagues demonstrated that patients with *mild* duodenal trauma had 0% mortality and 2% duodenal fistula rates, as compared with 6% mortality and 10% fistula rates among those with *severe* duodenal injuries (see Table 17–4).

According to this classification system, approximately 80% to 85% of duodenal wounds can be primarily repaired safely. Approximately 15% to 20% are severe injuries that require more complex procedures. Débridement or segmental resection and primary anastomosis may be attempted in all but the second portion of the duodenum for wounds that involve the near-total circumference. An alternative is a Roux-en-Y jejunal limb anastomosis to the duodenal injury. Pancreatico-

TABLE 17–4. Determinants of Duodenal Injury Severity

	Mild	Severe
Determinants of Injury Severity		
Agent	Stab	Blunt or missile
Size	<75% wall	>75% wall
Duodenal site (no.)	3, 4	1, 2
Injury-repair interval (hr.)	<24	>24
Adjacent injury	No CBD	CBD
Outcome		
Mortality (%)	6	16
Duodenal morbidity (%)	6	14

CBD, common bile duct.
Adapted from Snyder, W. H. III, Weigelt, J. A., Watkins, W. L., and Bietz, D. S.: The surgical management of duodenal trauma: Precepts based on a review of 247 cases. Arch. Surg., *115*:422, 1980. Copyright 1980, American Medical Association.

duodenectomy is rarely required for duodenal injuries unless uncontrollable pancreatic hemorrhage or combined duodenal, ampullary, and/or intrapancreatic bile duct injuries are present.

Protection of a tenuous duodenal repair may be aided by the diversion of gastric contents. This is accomplished by a *Vaughn* pyloric exclusion and gastrojejunostomy, having generally replaced the more complete and anatomically disruptive *duodenal diverticulization* advocated by Berne[62] (Fig. 17–19). An alternative to gastric diversion is either lateral tube duodenostomy or duodenal drainage via a retrograde jejunostomy. Hasson and colleagues' review of the role of tube duodenostomy reports that the overall mortality with any type of tube decompression is 9%, compared with 19.4% without decompression.[56] The morbidity of duodenal fistula occurred in 2.3% of patients undergoing adjuvant tube duodenostomy, compared with an 11.8% fistula rate without decompression. They concluded that duodenal tube drainage should be performed either via stomach or retrograde jejunostomy, as these methods had the lowest fistula rate and less overall mortality than lateral tube duodenostomy. Stone and Fabian also appear to support this conclusion, reporting a duodenal fistula in only 1 of 232 patients with a variety of duodenal injuries, all treated by retrograde jejunostomy.[128]

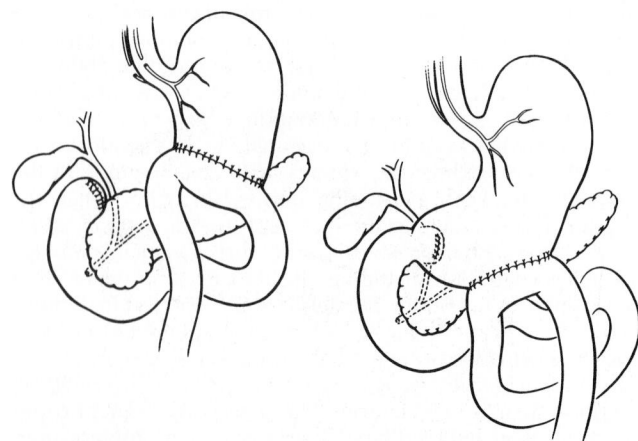

Figure 17–19. Illustration of Berne's *duodenal diverticulization (left)* and Vaughn's *pyloric exclusion* procedure *(right)* used as adjuncts to repair of severe duodenal or combined duodenal-pancreatic injury. Note that the Berne diverticulization includes vagotomy and antrectomy, whereas the Vaughn pyloroplasty is intended to be a temporary duodenal bypass. (From Jurkovich, G. J., and Carrico, C. J.: Management of pancreatic trauma. Surg. Clin. North Am., *70*:575, 1990.)

However, there has been no prospective or controlled analysis of the efficacy of either type of tube duodenal drainage or gastric diversion techniques in the management of duodenal wounds. On balance, the most effective and least morbid adjunctive procedure for *major* injuries is the Vaughn pyloric exclusion.

Duodenal hematoma usually does not require operative intervention. It can be diagnosed either by contrast-enhanced CT scan or upper gastrointestinal study. The initial Gastrografin examination should be followed by a barium study to provide greater detail needed to detect the so-called *coil spring* or *stacked coin* sign. Although characteristic of intramural duodenal hematoma, this finding is present in only approximately one fourth of patients with hematoma. Associated injuries should be excluded, with particular attention directed at the potential for pancreatic injuries. Continuous nasogastric suction should be employed and total parenteral nutrition begun. The patient should be re-evaluated with upper gastrointestinal contrast studies at 5- to 7-day intervals. Operative exploration and evacuation of the hematoma may be considered after 2 weeks of conservative therapy.

PANCREAS

Pancreatic trauma is relatively uncommon, accounting for less than 10% of all abdominal injuries. Although the pancreas is relatively protected in the retroperitoneum, the increasing frequency of high-speed motor vehicle accidents and large-caliber, high-velocity civilian gunshot wounds contribute to an increasing incidence of pancreatic injury. Several large series from urban trauma centers report that penetrating injuries account for 70% to 80% of pancreatic wounds. The mortality rates from several large series of pancreatic trauma patients range from 10% to 25%; major complications such as pseudocysts, abscesses, hemorrhage or pancreatic fistulas develop in 30% to 40% of patients surviving their initial injury.[62] This combined mortality and morbidity rate of approximately 50% emphasizes the significance of pancreatic injuries.

Because the pancreas is surrounded by major abdominal organs and blood vessels, associated injuries are common (Fig. 17–20). Overall, 90% of patients with pancreatic injuries have at least one associated injury, with an average of 3.5 associated intra-abdominal injuries per patient. The aorta, portal vein, or vena cava is injured in more than 75% of cases of penetrating pancreatic trauma, and injuries to the liver,

spleen, or hollow viscus of the gastrointestinal tract are equally common in blunt trauma. The significance of the associated injuries is highlighted by morbidity and mortality statistics. Intra-abdominal vascular injuries are responsible for one half of the overall mortality and nearly all the immediate deaths.[60] Infection and multiple organ failure account for most of the late deaths. Approximately 10% of deaths are directly attributable to the pancreatic injury. The key determinant of long-term outcome is the presence or absence of pancreatic duct injury, as most postoperative complications can be attributed to inadequate control of major duct disruption.[62] The implication of these observations is that the first priority in managing pancreatic trauma should be control of hemorrhage and repair of intestinal injuries to limit bacterial contamination. A diligent search for potential pancreatic injury should follow.

Preoperative Evaluation. The preoperative evaluation and management of patients with penetrating abdominal wounds and possible pancreatic injury are relatively straightforward. Unless injury to the intraperitoneal or retroperitoneal abdominal contents can be definitively ruled out, abdominal exploration is warranted. No further diagnostic test for pancreatic injury is required, as thorough intraoperative evaluation must be performed.

The evaluation of patients with possible blunt pancreatic injury is more complex and requires evaluation based on injury mechanism (e.g., steering wheel injury) and associated injuries. Since a significant proportion of pancreatic trauma patients have associated intra-abdominal injuries, clear-cut indications for laparotomy frequently exist (e.g., peritonitis, intra-abdominal hemorrhage, and positive DPL). These patients require no further preoperative evaluation to identify a possible pancreatic injury as a thorough, direct intraoperative pancreatic examination can be performed. In contrast, identifying a pancreatic injury in the absence of other indications for laparotomy is challenging. Patients with complete ductal transection have been reported to be asymptomatic for weeks to months following the initial injury, although the more typical presentation is abdominal pain that increases with time. Early identification of a subtle pancreatic injury therefore requires a high index of suspicion, a thoughtful diagnostic approach, and serial physical examinations.

Serum amylase determination has limited sensitivity or specificity for pancreatic injury. In Jones' review of pancreatic trauma, the serum amylase level was elevated in only 16% of the patients with penetrating pancreatic injuries and in only 61% of those who had blunt pancreatic trauma.[60] Even with complete transection of the pancreas, only 65% of the patients had elevated serum amylase levels.[60] Other reports have documented that as few as 8% of blunt abdominal injuries with hyperamylasemia had pancreatic injury. Isoamylase differentiation, initially hailed as an advance in diagnosing pancreatic injury, unfortunately has not increased the test's accuracy.[12] Nonetheless, an elevated serum or peritoneal lavage effluent amylase level does raise concern about pancreatic injury and mandates further evaluation. Persistent elevation or the development of abdominal symptoms are grounds for further evaluation or surgical exploration.

CT scan can be helpful in diagnosing pancreatic injury. Abdominal CT scans are currently reported as having sensitivity and specificity in excess of 80%, although the accuracy of this examination varies with interpreter experience and quality of the scanner.

Intraoperative Evaluation. Even at operation, the diagnosis of significant pancreatic injury may be difficult. A Kocher maneuver should be performed, with mobilization of the hepatic flexure and the third portion of the duodenum to the superior mesenteric vessels. This allows adequate inspection of the C loop of the duodenum and the posterior head of the

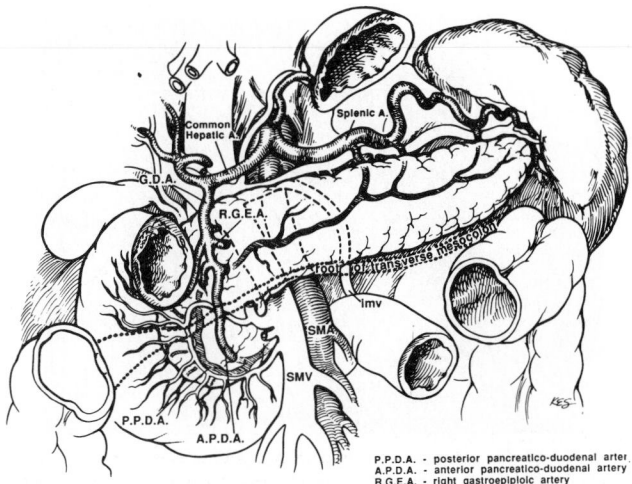

P.P.D.A. - posterior pancreatico-duodenal arter
A.P.D.A. - anterior pancreatico-duodenal artery
R.G.E.A. - right gastroepiploic artery
G.D.A. - gastro-duodenal artery

Figure 17–20. The blood supply to the pancreas and the pancreatic relational anatomy to other intra-abdominal organs. (From Jurkovich, G. J., and Carrico, C. J.: Management of pancreatic trauma. Surg. Clin. North Am., 70:575, 1990.)

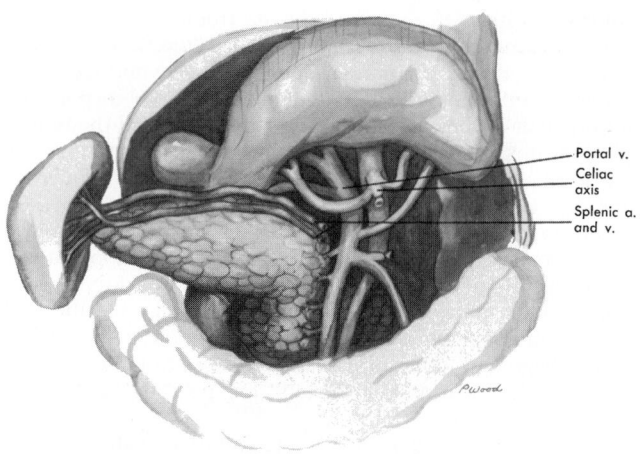

Figure 17–21. The spleen and pancreas have been dissected from the retroperitoneum and transferred into the right upper quadrant. Adequate mobility of the pancreas is essential to assess for potential posterior pancreatic injuries.

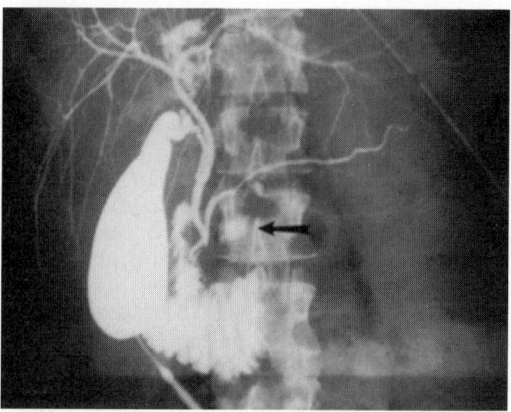

Figure 17–23. A cystocholangiogram demonstrating filling of the pancreatic duct, with extravasation in the proximal pancreatic duct, as depicted by the arrow.

pancreas. Inspection is continued by opening the lesser sac, allowing examination of the medial aspect of the duodenum and anterior surface of the pancreas, including its superior and inferior margins. When posterior injuries of the pancreas are suspected, mobilization of the spleen with elevation of the spleen and tail of the pancreas allows inspection of the posterior pancreas (Fig. 17–21).

Most (95%) of pancreatic injuries can be diagnosed by careful inspection following adequate exposure. The remaining 5% of injuries may require more elaborate investigative techniques to diagnose ductal injury. Intraoperative ultrasound and intraoperative endoscopic studies have been suggested as a possible means of identifying major ductal injuries. To date, the applicability and accuracy of these approaches have not been validated. Contrast studies through the biliary tree, ampulla, or tail of the pancreas are used when there is major concern about the integrity of the main pancreatic duct (Figs. 17–22 to 17–24). Skilled endoscopists may be of assistance in performing intraoperative endoscopic

retrograde pancreatography if the surgeon is reluctant to perform a duodenostomy or distal pancreatectomy. Routine performance of intraoperative pancreatography when proximal duct injury is strongly suspected has decreased the postoperative morbidity rate from 55% to 15% at one institution.[8]

Classification and Treatment. The classification system and management guidelines the authors favor are outlined in Table 17–5. This system addresses the key issues of parenchymal disruption and major pancreatic duct status by focusing on the anatomic location of the injury rather than the degree of injury itself. Although there is no anatomic distinction within the gland itself, the superior mesenteric vessels pass behind the pancreas at the junction of the pancreatic head and body; the pancreas to the patient's left is considered distal. The principles of managing pancreatic injuries are to control hemorrhage, débride devitalized pancreatic tissue, provide adequate drainage of injuries or resections, and preserve as much functional pancreatic tissue as possible. The difficult decisions in managing pancreatic trauma involve patients with parenchymal disruption and major duct injury. By focusing on the anatomic location of the duct and parenchymal injury (proximal versus distal), the proposed system provides a useful management guide.

Type I pancreatic injuries (no major duct involved) are the most common (80%), generally requiring only hemostasis

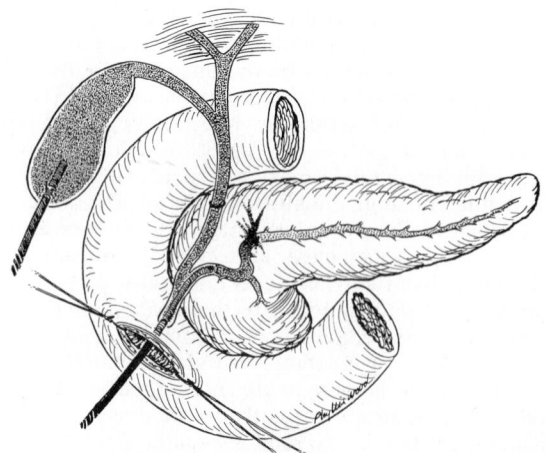

Figure 17–22. Opening of the duodenum at the level of the papilla of Vater, with direct cannulation of the pancreatic duct. This is best done after the intravenous administration of 70 units of secretin so that the pancreatic sphincter will relax and the tube will preferentially move into the pancreatic duct instead of the common bile duct. Two to 4 ml. of contrast material is injected by gravity flow only, demonstrating extravasation of the proximal pancreatic duct. Prior to the duodenotomy, the gallbladder is cannulated and a cholecystocholangiogram is always performed so that if reflux into the pancreatic duct occurs, a duodenotomy can be avoided.

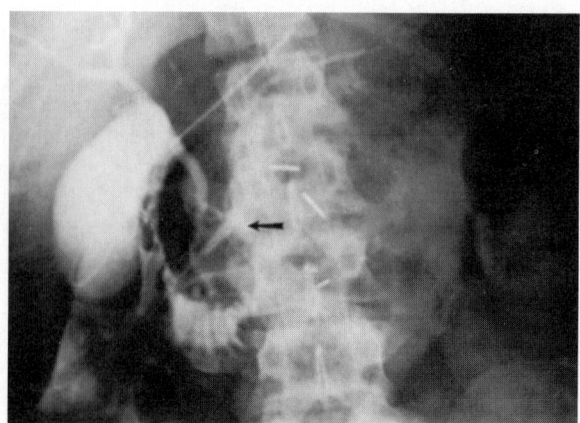

Figure 17–24. Simultaneous cholecystocholangiogram and cannulation of the pancreatic duct through a duodenotomy. The injection demonstrates extravasation in the proximal pancreatic duct at a position in such proximity to the common bile duct that had a subtotal pancreatectomy been performed, the common bile duct probably would have been injured. This use of intraoperative pancreatography demonstrated the need for a Whipple resection.

TABLE 17–5. Classification of Pancreatic Injuries

Injury Type	Injury Definition	Treatment*
I	Contusion and laceration *without* duct injury	External drainage Infrequent distal pancreatectomy
II	*Distal* transection and/or parenchymal injury with duct injury	Distal pancreatectomy
III	*Proximal* transection or parenchymal injury with probable duct injury	Distal pancreatectomy or Roux-en-Y pancreaticojejunostomy (see text)
IV	*Combined* pancreatic and duodenal injury Ampulla/blood supply intact	Repair/exclude duodenum (see text) Treat pancreas as per I, II, III
	Massive injury; ampulla destroyed; devascularization	Pancreaticoduodenectomy

*External drainage is necessary following any pancreatic resection, débridement, or repair.

and drainage. Type II pancreatic injuries (distal major duct injury) are best treated by distal pancreatectomy with or without splenectomy. If there is any concern regarding the status of the remaining proximal duct, intraoperative pancreatography can be performed through the open end of the proximal ducts. If the remaining proximal duct is normal, the transected duct and gland parenchyma are suture closed and external drainage is provided. Type III pancreatic injuries (proximal duct injury) require pancreatectomy distal to the duct injury, resulting in subtotal removal of the gland. If there is concern that the residual pancreatic tissue is inadequate to provide endocrine or exocrine function, preservation of the body and tail using a Roux-en-Y pancreaticojejunostomy is an option. If complete duct transection is not apparent clinically, confirmation by intraoperative pancreatography should be made before performing the formidable subtotal pancreatic resection. If the duct is spared, wide external drainage is usually adequate treatment.

The management of Type IV pancreatic injuries remains problematic. Because of the large number of combinations of injuries to the pancreas and duodenum that may occur, no single form of therapy is appropriate for all patients. In one review of 129 cases of combined pancreaticoduodenal injuries, 24% of the patients were treated with simple repair and drainage, 50% underwent repair and pyloric exclusion, and only 10% required a Whipple procedure.[41] Selecting the best treatment option for these combined injuries depends on the integrity of the distal common bile duct and the ampulla, and the severity of the duodenal injury. For that reason, any patient with a combined pancreaticoduodenal injury requires a cholangiogram, a pancreatogram, and evaluation of the ampulla.

When the common bile duct and ampulla are intact (as is the situation in most cases), the duodenum can be closed primarily and the pancreatic injury treated as previously described. If there is concern about the integrity of the duodenal closure, adjunctive techniques described in the previous section on duodenal injuries may be considered (see Fig. 17–19).

Rarely, in very massive injuries of the proximal duodenum and head of the pancreas, destruction of the ampulla and proximal pancreatic duct or distal common bile duct may preclude reconstruction. In this situation a pancreaticoduodenectomy may be required (Fig. 17–25). If confined to strict criteria, pancreaticoduodenectomy may be a viable option and can be performed for injury with less morbidity and mortality than described in resections done for treatment of cancer.

Postoperative Care. Although complications are frequent following pancreatic injury, some reports indicate that as many as one half of the postoperative complications could be avoided with careful inspection of the pancreas and accurate determination of the status of the main pancreatic duct.[60, 62] Pancreatic fistula occurs in as many as 35% of patients who have significant pancreatic injuries, but most of these cases resolve spontaneously if adequate external drainage is provided. Intra-abdominal abscess and wound infection occur nearly as frequently, but a true pancreatic abscess occurs in less than 5% of patients. Unlike controlled external fistulas, pancreatic abscesses require prompt surgical débridement and drainage. Pseudocyst formation and postoperative pancreatitis are less common complications, but these can greatly prolong the recovery time. Adequate nutritional support is essential throughout the postinjury period. Placement of a feeding jejunostomy (needle catheter or small feeding tube) at time of laparotomy for pancreatic trauma is often useful in supplying enteral nutrients in the early postoperative period. The low-fat, higher-pH elemental feeding formulas appear to cause less pancreatic stimulation than standard enteral formulas, and should be tried before committing the patient to total parenteral nutrition.

LIVER AND BILIARY TREE

Liver. The liver is the most commonly injured organ following penetrating trauma and the second most commonly injured organ following blunt trauma. Fortunately, the injury

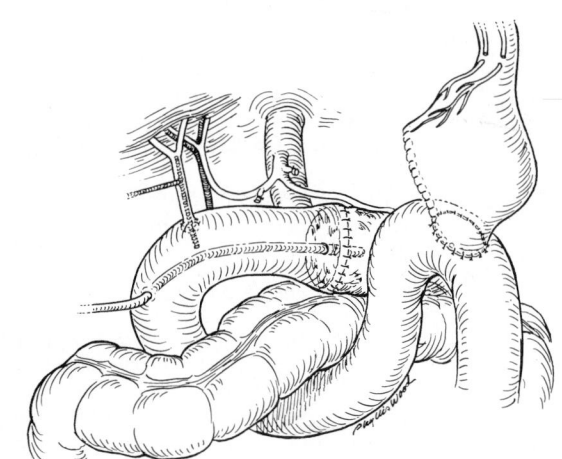

Figure 17–25. Surgical reconstruction following pancreaticoduodenectomy for trauma. The pancreaticojejunostomy is an end-to-end two-layer anastomosis over an indwelling stent. The choledochojejunostomy is an end-to-side anastomosis in a single layer with an indwelling stent, depending on the size of the common bile duct. The gastrojejunostomy is an end-to-side two-layer anastomosis. The pancreatic and bile duct stents are brought out through separate stab wounds on the abdominal wall.

is often minor and easily managed. In fact, 50% of all liver injuries are nonbleeding at the time of initial exploration, and an additional 20% can be managed either by direct suture ligation or by using hemostatic agents such as microfibrillar collagen. However, a severe liver injury, Grade III, IV, or V by the AAST organ injury severity classification system (Table 17–6), represents one of the true management challenges in trauma surgery. The high overall liver injury mortality rate of 11% and an overall morbidity rate of 22% are due to these severe injuries.[41]

Seven basic techniques are useful in operative management: (1) suture, (2) inflow occlusion, (3) packing, (4) hepatic artery ligation, (5) resection, (6) mesh hepatorrhaphy, and (7) atrial-caval shunting. The anatomy of the liver and the distribution of injuries permit separation of the role of each of these approaches.

When the liver is the only organ injured, half the lacerations are nonbleeding and do not require suture. In most lacerations that are bleeding, the source is within the substance of the liver, and control can be obtained by direct ligation. After obtaining adequate exposure, the depth of the wound can be explored in detail and significant vessels and biliary radicals individually suture ligated or secured with hemoclips. Digital compression and direct ligation are preferred over parallel vertical mattress sutures (which may be used if the entire cut surface of the liver is bleeding extensively). Traditional or argon-beam electrocautery, topical hemostatic agents, or biologic fibrin glue can be useful adjuncts in controlling oozing hemorrhage but are no substitute for direct ligation of bleeding vessels. If these measures are successful, closed drainage is usually established to control bile leakage, although drainage of liver laceration is controversial.[41]

With deeper lacerations, bleeding may initially be so significant as to prevent adequate exposure. Under these conditions, the next maneuver is that of inflow occlusion (*Pringle maneuver*). A noncrushing clamp is placed across the hepatoduodenal ligament, which occludes the common hepatic artery and the portal vein. This method often slows bleeding enough to provide adequate exposure to allow visualization and direct ligation of vessels and biliary radicals. Mobilization of the ventral attachments of the liver aid in exposure. Deep liver lacerations should not simply be sutured closed. This predisposes to liver abscesses and hemobilia. If hepatic inflow occlusion is used, some authors have advocated local hepatic hypothermia and systemic steroids,[94] although intentional hypothermia in the trauma victim may be ill advised.[63] Although the exact length of warm ischemia time tolerated by the human liver is not known, inflow occlusion for at least 20 minutes, and perhaps up to 1 hour, appears to be well tolerated.

If these techniques are unsuccessful in controlling hemorrhage, the surgeon is faced with deciding whether to simply tightly pack the liver with gauze pads or attempt direct repair. This is often an extremely critical decision point in hepatic trauma management, often complicated by associated injuries, hypothermia, and coagulopathy. Although perihepatic packing was once widely condemned, many experienced surgeons now prefer temporary packing, particularly in the cold or coagulopathic patient, followed by rewarming and resuscitation and re-exploration for pack removal.[38, 103] Angiography and embolization are also occasionally helpful if persistent hemorrhage is suspected after packing and rewarming. An alternative approach advocated by Pachter and associates involves extending the liver laceration to expose the bleeding vessels and control them. This usually involves a finger fracture hepatotomy along nonanatomic planes, a technique that requires some experience to perfect. Pachter and associates report using this technique in 121 patients with Grade III to Grade V liver injuries with a remarkably low mortality rate of 10.7%.[94] The relative merits of these two divergent techniques is a controversial topic, but both camps emphasize the high mortality rate (30% or more) and difficult management problems of these severe liver injuries.

The authors' experience with perihepatic packing and delayed reoperation is favorable, supporting the experience of the Ben Taub group in the management of complex liver trauma. As an adjunct in the presence of coagulopathy after

TABLE 17–6. Liver Injury Scale (1994 Revision)

Grade*		Injury Description	ICD-9	AIS90
I	*Hematoma*:	Subcapsular, <10% surface area	864.01	2
	Laceration:	Capsular tear, <1-cm. parenchymal depth	864.11	
			864.02	2
			864.12	
II	*Hematoma*:	Subcapsular, 10–50% surface area; intraparenchynal, <10-cm. diameter	864.01 864.11	2
	Laceration:	1–3 cm. parenchymal depth, <10-cm. long	864.03 864.13	2
III	*Hematoma*:	Subcapsular, >50% surface area or expanding; ruptured subcapsular or parenchymal hematoma; intraparenchymal hematoma >10 cm. or expanding		3
	Laceration:	>3-cm. parenchymal depth	864.04 864.14	3
IV	*Laceration*:	Parenchymal disruption involving 25–75% of hepatic lobe or 1–3 Couinaud's segments within a single lobe	864.04 864.14	4
V	*Laceration*:	Parenchymal disruption involving >75% of hepatic lobe or >3 Couinaud's segments within a single lobe		5
	Vascular:	Juxtahepatic venous injuries; i.e., retrohepatic vena cava/central major hepatic veins		5
VI	*Vascular*:	Hepatic avulsion		6

*Advance one grade for multiple injuries, up to Grade III.
ICD, International Classification of Diseases; AIS, abbreviated injury score.
From Moore, E. E., Cogbill, T. H., Jurkovich, G. J., et al.: Organ injury scaling: Spleen and liver (1994 revision). J. Trauma, *38*:323–324, 1995.

completion of hepatic repair, this approach led to a 34% survival rate in 41 patients, as reported by the Ben Taub group.[39] In contrast, there were no survivors if perihepatic packing was used as a final desperation technique in the setting of massive injury. Reed and colleagues' commentary on current hepatic trauma management tabulated 10 clinical reports in which hepatic packing was used in 230 hepatic trauma patients; packing mortality ranged from 10% to 58%, averaging 34%.[103] When the patient has a devastating injury or bilobular involvement and is cold, coagulopathic, and acidotic, or there is some question of the availability of blood resources, liver packing is preferred. Packing does not appear to be as effective for actively bleeding hepatic vein, retrohepatic caval injuries, or arterial bleeding. Arteriography and therapeutic embolization of hepatic arterial injury may be of benefit before re-exploration.

A preferred method of packing involves the use of gauze laparotomy pads in combination with a sterile plastic drape or an absorbable (Dexon) mesh at the liver surface to prevent tight adherence of the laparotomy pad to the exposed liver surface. Packs are removed in the operating room when the patient is rewarmed, the coagulopathy corrected, and fluid requirements stabilized. This generally occurs 24 to 72 hours after injury. Débridement of necrotic liver tissue and suture ligation of specific bleeding points are occasionally necessary. Closed-suction drains are always inserted when the packing is removed. The incidence of intra-abdominal abscess in survivors of liver packing is generally less than 15%.

After a brief period of enthusiasm for selective ligation of the right or left hepatic artery, it is now believed that it should be reserved for the occasional stab wound or the gunshot wound involving one lobe where exposure of the wound will require extensive incision of the liver. This should be necessary in less than 1% of all liver injuries.[24] The proper hepatic artery must never be ligated. Injudicious hepatic artery ligation may result in liver infarction, particularly if associated with portal vein injury (Fig. 17–26).[64]

Resection of hepatic parenchyma is unusual following liver injuries. In most circumstances, resection is performed to débride a segment or lobe that has been completely fractured or devitalized. Less commonly, resection is performed for vascular control of large stellate lacerations extending deep into the parenchyma and involving more than one segment. In a 5-year review of 1335 liver injuries treated at six trauma centers, hepatic resectional débridement was performed in only 36 patients (2.6%), hepatotomy and vessel ligation in 50

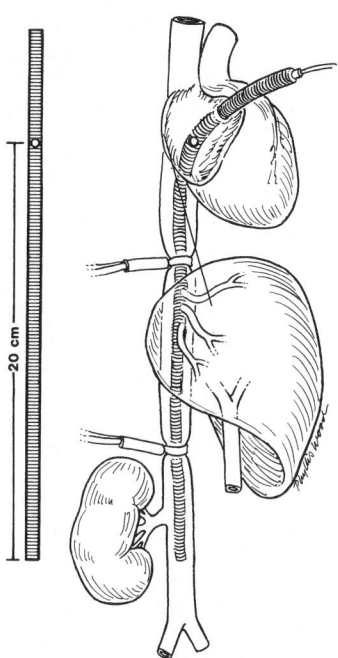

Figure 17–27. The atriocaval shunt placed through the auricular appendage. It has been guided to a position below the renal veins but above the iliac veins. In addition, as depicted, the retrohepatic vena cava has been isolated. A side hole has been cut to allow blood return to the right atrium. This allows total isolation of the venous outflow of the liver, so that when combined with inflow occlusion (clamping the porta hepatis), repair of hepatic veins can be obtained or the retrohepatic inferior vena cava can be properly exposed.

patients (3.7%), and segmentectomy in 18 patients (1.3%).[24] Formal hepatic lobectomy was performed in only 12 patients (0.9%). In conjunction with resection, the gallbladder must often be removed because of loss of blood supply from the cystic artery. Extensive drainage is indicated for all major hepatic resections. An 8% incidence of biliary fistula was noted in the 210 patients with significant injuries (Class III, IV, and V) reported in the foregoing review.

A new technique of compressive hemorrhagic control has been introduced, following the successful use of similar technique in splenic injuries. An absorbable mesh made of either polyglycolic acid or polyglactin has been used to wrap the liver compressively and achieve hemostasis.[103] Unlike splenic injuries, in which the entire spleen is encircled in the mesh (see Fig. 17–30), the liver must be wrapped one lobe at a time using the falciform ligament as a point of attachment for the wrap. A more complex technique involves creating a Y-shaped wrap, which is applied around the entire liver with the fork of the Y as an opening through which the inferior vena cava and porta hepatis can pass. Reed and colleagues reported using this technique in 14 patients, citing success in all cases except those patients with retrohepatic or juxtacaval hepatic vein injuries because these areas are excluded from the compression.[103] The mortality rate in hepatic trauma patients managed by mesh wrapping is 25% to 37.5%.

The final technique that may have a role in select cases of retrohepatic or juxtacaval injuries is placement of an atriocaval or Schrock shunt (Fig. 17–27). The purpose of this technique, combined with inflow occlusion (Pringle maneuver), is to divert all blood flow from the liver and allow resectional débridement or direct repair of these complex hepatic injuries. Placement of an atriocaval shunt requires that the liver injury first be tightly packed, a median sternotomy performed, and the diaphragm divided. This allows further mobilization of the liver so that the vena cava may be isolated superiorly within the pericardium and inferiorly above the

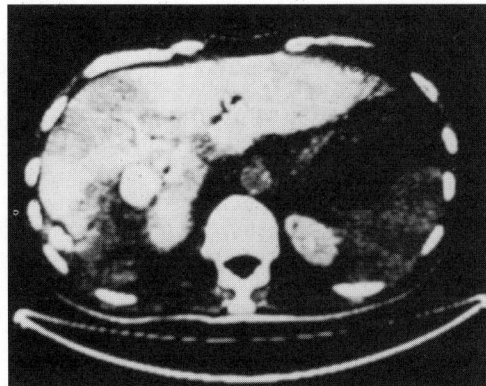

Figure 17–26. Computed tomography scan demonstrating infarction of both segments of the right lobe and part of the medial segment of the left lobe, with specific demarcation between infarcted and normal liver. In addition, the administration of intravenous contrast material has shown a connection between the arterial and biliary tree (hemobilia). The fracture site is evident along the posterior lateral aspect of the right lobe of the liver.

renal veins. Although many have debated the merit of this procedure, it may be indicated in that rare circumstance of hepatic vein or suprarenal caval injuries when vena cava occlusion and packing have already been attempted and the patient cannot be restored to a normovolemic state. Despite this technique, mortality for retrohepatic caval and intraparenchymal hepatic vein injuries exceeds 50%.

Porta Hepatis. Isolated penetrating or blunt injuries to the porta hepatis are uncommon. In a recent review from eight trauma centers, the incidence of portal triad injuries was only 0.07% of all trauma admissions.[64] Most of these unusual injuries follow penetrating trauma, although 30% of the porta hepatis injuries in the cited reference followed blunt trauma, primarily motor vehicle accidents. In this review of 99 patients with 118 portal structure injuries, there were 55 extrahepatic portal vein injuries, 28 extrahepatic arterial injuries, and 35 injuries of the extrahepatic bile ducts. Eighty-four patients had single porta hepatis structure injuries, and only 15 had combination injuries. Virtually all portal triad injuries occur in association with injury to the liver, duodenum, or other abdominal organs. Porta hepatis injuries pose difficult problems in management. The overall mortality rate is 50%, increasing to 80% in patients with combination injuries. Life-threatening hemorrhage and associated organ injury characterize the immediate concern, and sepsis, delayed stricture, or missed injuries of the common bile duct are the major factors in determining morbidity. Because most patients come to the emergency department in shock, the indication for operation usually is immediately established.

Unless there are associated injuries to the aorta and inferior vena cava (which take priority) noted at laparotomy, an immediate Pringle maneuver frequently allows isolation of the structures in the porta hepatis and determination of whether the injury involves the portal vein, hepatic arteries, or common bile duct. Repair of vascular injuries takes precedence over biliary structures.

Injuries to the portal vein have a 50% to 64% mortality rate. The portal vein supplies 80% of the total hepatic blood flow and 50% of the oxygen delivery. Techniques of portal vein repair are varied, but lateral venorrhaphy with 5–0 polypropylene suture is preferred if possible, and usually in tangential or partial lacerations. Alternatives for complete transection or large lacerations are ligation, resection with end-to-end anastomosis, interposition grafting, or portosystemic shunting. Although management of the portal vein injury by simple ligation alone is an attractive alternative, there is considerable controversy concerning this decision. It should not be a desperation maneuver but should be done immediately after determining that simple repair is impossible or impractical. Case reports have demonstrated that ligation is compatible with survival, but the surgeon must anticipate mesenteric venous congestion and massive fluid requirements. A *second-look* operation in 24 hours is advisable. Ligation in a patient with massive liver injury, hypotension, and multiple blood transfusions has an unacceptably high mortality rate. Interposition grafting with autogenous vein (jugular, splenic) is perhaps ideal, but a Gortex vascular graft is more expeditious and applicable. Portosystemic shunt is generally not an advisable alternative because, in a healthy patient with normal hepatic flow, it usually results in severe encephalopathy. In a recent multicenter review that included 55 patients with portal vein injuries, the mortality rate following primary repair was 42%, whereas ligation had a 90% mortality rate and the sole patient in whom interposition grafting was performed died.[64]

If injury to the porta hepatis involves a branch of the hepatic artery, ligation is preferred. If injury involves the proper hepatic artery, repair can be attempted, but if not easily accomplished, ligation should be performed. Mays has

demonstrated that hepatic arteries are not end-arteries, and that flow to a ligated hepatic artery is re-established within 24 hours through translobar and subcapsular collaterals.[77] However, in those patients with cirrhosis or severe pre-existing liver disease or even with prolonged periods of hypotension and crush hepatic injuries, hepatic artery ligation has been reported to result in hepatic infarction.[64] In such patients, efforts should be made to repair the hepatic artery if hemodynamic stability allows. If cystic artery inflow occlusion has occurred, cholecystectomy should be performed. When the patient has a combined injury of the hepatic artery and portal vein, after hemostasis has been obtained by the Pringle maneuver, it is advisable that the injured artery be ligated and attempts be made at portal vein repair.

The most important factor in determining how to manage the common bile duct injury is whether the duct is completely or incompletely transected. Attempts at primary repair or duct-to-duct anastomosis of complete transections or injuries involving more than 50% circumference of the bile duct wall result in a late stricture rate of more than 50%.[58] The late stricture rate declines to about 5% if biliary-enteric anastomosis is performed for similar injuries. If the duct has been only perforated or incompletely divided (<50%), primary repair can be successfully performed and is typically done over a T-tube or ureteral catheter stent. The T-tube should not be brought out through the repaired suture line. External drainage is provided in all circumstances. In an unstable patient, ligation of lobar or small biliary radicals is acceptable.[30] Duct ligation causes the affected liver parenchyma to atrophy and the remaining lobe to hypertrophy, as long as there is normal biliary flow from the residual 50% of the liver. Alternatively, T-tube drainage of the duct and perihepatic drainage are carried out, with definitive repair of the ductal injury performed later. Missed extrahepatic bile duct injuries occurred in nine patients in the recent multicenter review, with a 75% significant complication rate in those who survived.[64]

Gallbladder injury has been reported to occur after both penetrating and blunt trauma. Cholecystostomy is indicated in only a few patients and should be regarded as a temporary procedure. Even with minimal injury the gallbladder is nonfunctional and may become inflamed unless it is removed. Cholecystectomy is therefore the procedure of choice for severe contusion, avulsion, or perforating injuries to the gallbladder.

SPLEEN

The spleen is the most commonly injured intra-abdominal organ. Splenic injury must therefore be suspected in any patient with blunt abdominal trauma, particularly if associated with left lower rib fractures. The diagnosis is often suspected on physical examination but is generally confirmed by abdominal CT scan or exploratory celiotomy for hemoperitoneum. Although splenectomy was once considered the only management option for splenic injuries, trauma surgeons must now also consider splenic repair or nonoperative management as viable options in selected patients. These new options have been fostered by the recognition of the rare but highly lethal syndrome of overwhelming postsplenectomy sepsis. Indeed, perhaps more than 90% of pediatric splenic injuries are managed nonoperatively. However, it is also apparent that more splenic injuries have been diagnosed with the increased use of CT scanning in abdominal trauma.

Overwhelming Postsplenectomy Sepsis. The immunologic function of the spleen has been reviewed elsewhere.[70] Briefly, asplenic patients have impaired capacity for clearance of blood-borne particles, depressed phagocytic activity of alveolar macrophages, decreased antibody response to specific antigens, decreased levels of circulating opsins, diminished numbers of suppressor T cells, and altered levels of circulating immunoglobulins (such as decreased levels of IgM). After splenectomy there is a significant decrease in the primary immune response to bacterial capsular Type II polysaccharide antigens, which are the antigenic component of the capsule of the encapsulated bacteria such as *Streptococcus pneumoniae*, *Haemophilus influenzae*, and *Neisseria meningitides*. Many of these immunologic alterations in asplenic patients are transient, yet the risk of increased susceptibility to sepsis appears to be indefinite.

In 1952, King and Schumacher reported a postsplenectomy syndrome of severe, sometimes fatal meningitis and sepsis in four of five children splenectomized before the age of 6 months for congenital hemolytic anemia.[66] The term *overwhelming postsplenectomy infection* (OPSI) was coined by Diamond in 1969.[31] This syndrome is unlike fulminating bacteremias and septicemias in patients with normal splenic function. Rarely does a patient with an intact spleen with bacteremia deteriorate from good health to death in less than 24 hours, whereas the OPSI syndrome constitutes a distinct entity that often lasts only 12 to 18 hours. The onset is sudden, with nausea, vomiting, headache, and confusion, leading to coma. The infecting organism is *Pneumococcus* in just over half the patients, with *Escherichia coli*, *H. influenzae*, and *Meningococcus*, *Staphylococcus*, and *Streptococcus* organisms found in decreasing frequency. Disseminated intravascular coagulation is common. Severe hypoglycemia, electrolyte imbalance, and shock are often present. Of particular interest is the occasional presence of diplococci on peripheral blood smears. Blood culture reports in these patients indicate that there may be as many as 10^6 organisms per cu. mm., which clearly separates this syndrome from the bacteremia accompanying pneumonia and other ordinary infections.

Rapidity of course from onset until death with failure of antibiotic therapy is characteristic. The overall mortality rate has generally been reported to be as high as 50%, and even up to 80% for pneumococcal infections. However, Green and colleagues reported a much lower mortality of only 7% for postsplenectomy sepsis in a trauma population.[48] This discrepancy may be attributable to the universal use of polyvalent pneumococcal vaccine and close follow-up after trauma splenectomy in their patients.

The true incidence of overwhelming postsplenectomy sepsis is not well defined, although a commonly used estimation of the incidence of OPSI is 0.6% in children and 0.3% in adults,[71] which may be a low estimate.[70] In 1973, Singer attempted to establish the incidence of sepsis following splenectomy in nine categories of disease.[120] With specific reference to trauma, Singer reviewed the courses of 688 patients (388 children, 300 adults) who underwent splenectomy for injury to the spleen. Among these were 10 patients with sepsis (incidence of 1.45%), four of whom died, resulting in a mortality rate of 0.58%. When combined with four deaths from sepsis following splenectomy for trauma in a series of 342 children reported by Eraklis and Filler, the incidence rate of mortality from sepsis is 0.78%, for a total of 78 times the expected rate in the general population, as calculated by Singer.[34] Green and colleagues in the report cited in the previous paragraph estimated the risk of postsplenectomy septicemia, pneumonia, and meningitis to be 8.3% in trauma patients, or 166 times the 0.05% rate expected in the general population.[48] Only one patient of the 144 (0.7%) followed in that series died from a pneumococcal infection, and that single episode occurred 3 years after splenectomy. The longest follow-up of splenectomy patients is data compiled by Robinette involving 740 World War II veterans who underwent splenectomy between 1939 and 1945.[108] Six patients in this group (0.8%) died of pneumonia, whereas none of the 740 matched control patients had succumbed to this disease.

The most recent pneumococcal vaccine (Pneumovax 23, Merck; Pnu-Immune, Lederle) contains antibodies against 23 of the known 83 serotypes of pneumococci but covers about 90% of the serotypes responsible for significant pneumococcal infections. Most trauma surgeons recommend that splenectomy patients receive the most currently available polyvalent pneumococcal vaccine soon after splenectomy (prior to discharge), although the ideal time is unresolved. The initial polyvalent vaccine has been shown to be 80% effective in healthy volunteers with intact spleens, but it is unclear how effective or when it is effective in splenectomized patients, and protection has not been proved to correlate with antibody levels. The recent availability of *H. influenzae* type b conjugate and meningococcal polysaccharide vaccines have further confused the issue, and although the risk of these bacteria causing overwhelming postsplenectomy sepsis is extremely low, some clinicians also use these vaccines, particularly in the very young or very old.[37] The use of prophylactic antibiotics in asplenic patients is also unresolved, but even minor infections in this group should be treated with antibiotics.

Splenorrhaphy or Partial Resection. The segmental anatomy and blood supply of the spleen make splenic salvage a possibility. The splenic artery, which delivers 4% of the circulating blood volume per minute, divides into several segmental branches in the hilum, entering the spleen surrounded by the white pulp where they are known as *central arteries*. Leaving the white pulp, the blood passes through an ill-defined vascular space called the *marginal zone* before entering the venous sinuses of the red pulp. Most spleen injuries result in various degrees of transverse rupture of the spleen following the trabeculae and segmental blood supply (Fig. 17–28). The splenic organ injury grading scale is depicted in Table 17–7. This grading system is useful in describing and comparing injury severity and helping predict which injuries are more likely to be successfully managed nonoperatively.[23]

Reports of surgical procedures less than total splenectomy

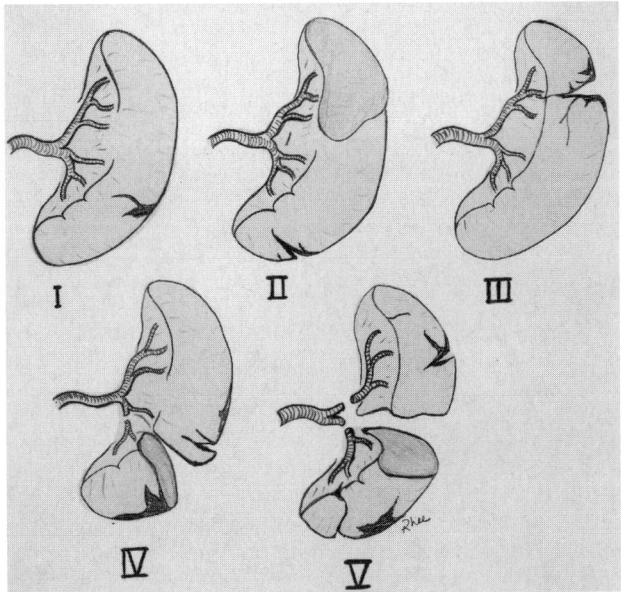

Figure 17–28. Common patterns of splenic injury, graded by the Organ Injury Scaling (OIS) Committee of the American Association of the Surgery of Trauma (see Table 17–7). I, superficial laceration; II, more extensive laceration or subcapsular hematoma; III, laceration >3 cm. involving trabecular vessels; IV, laceration involving segmental or hilar vessels; and V, shattered spleen.

TABLE 17–7. Spleen Injury Scale (1994 Revision)

Grade*		Injury Description	ICD-9	AIS90
I	*Hematoma*:	Subcapsular, <10% surface area	865.01 865.11	2
	Laceration:	Capsular tear, <1-cm. parenchymal depth	865.02 865.12	2
II	*Hematoma*:	Subcapsular, 10–50% surface area; intraparenchymal, <5-cm. diameter	865.01 865.11	2
	Laceration:	1–3 cm. parenchymal depth, that does not involve a trabecular vessel	865.02 865.12	
III	*Hematoma*:	Subcapsular, >50% surface area or expanding; ruptured subcapsular or parenchymal hematoma; intraparenchymal hematoma >5 cm. or expanding		3
	Laceration:	>3 cm. parenchymal depth or involving trabecular vessels	865.03 865.13	3
IV	*Laceration*:	Laceration involving segmental or hilar vessels producing major devascularization (>25% of spleen)		4
V	*Laceration*:	Completely shattered spleen	865.04 865.14	5
	Vascular:	Hilar vascular injury that devascularizes spleen		5

*Advance one grade for multiple injuries, up to Grade III.
ICD, International Classification of Diseases; AIS, abbreviated injury score.
From Moore, E. E., Cogbill, T. H., Jurkovich, G. J., et al.: Organ injury scaling: Spleen and liver (1994 revision). J. Trauma, *38*:323–324, 1995.

in the management of patients with splenic injury have appeared in the literature since the sixteenth century. A rent in the capsule may be conveniently treated by a mattress suture; this is also true of a puncture or stab wound. An absorbable suture is preferable and must be inserted with gentleness and tied with caution over cotton or Teflon pledgets (Fig. 17–29). For a laceration that does not involve the hilum of the spleen and that has adequate blood supply to all segments, the laceration is reapproximated with application of transverse mattress sutures over cut pledgets to reappose the cut surface of the spleen. More significant injuries may require partial resection or complete wrapping of the spleen in absorbable mesh compression bag (Fig. 17–30). Successful splenorrhaphy requires complete mobilization of the spleen (see Fig. 17–21). The splenic pedicle is approached through the gastrosplenic ligament, and the vessels in the hilus of the spleen supplying the injured portion of the spleen are ligated. Demarcation of the devascularized segment then becomes apparent, allowing accurate segmental resection of the injured tissue. Mattress sutures placed parallel to the cut

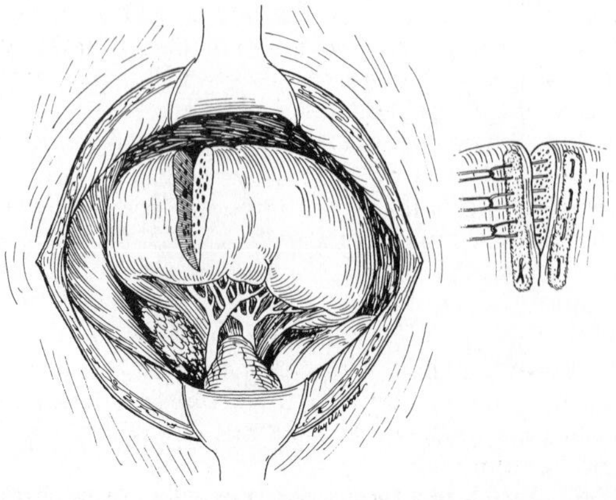

Figure 17–29. To perform a splenorrhaphy, the spleen must be properly mobilized into the operative field. The sutures are placed through the cotton pledgets so that when they are tied down, approximation of the parenchyma and capsule can occur without the sutures tearing through, as depicted in the inset.

surface of the spleen may be required to control bleeding. Alternatively, ligation of the individual bleeding points and the application of topical hemostatic agents may suffice. The relatively new technique of wrapping the spleen (or other injured solid organs) in an absorbable mesh compression envelope has value for extensive capsular avulsions and multiple shallow injuries but probably should not be relied on for control of deep parenchymal hemorrhage (see Fig. 17–30). Other adjuncts useful in obtaining splenic hemostasis include microfibrillar collagen, thrombin, fibrin biologic glues, and the argon beam cautery-coagulator. Although the reported success rate of splenic repair varies, most large urban trauma centers report splenic operative salvage rates between 40% and 60%. If one includes nonoperative management, splenic salvage rates approach 90% for both adults and children.[71, 117]

Total Splenectomy. Despite the segmental arrangement of the splenic arterial supply, the friability of the spleen often renders repair or partial resection impossible. The primary indications for splenectomy following trauma are hilar vascular injury, massive subcapsular hematoma, extensive fragmentation; total avulsion of the spleen; severe associated injuries requiring prompt attention; and continued bleeding after attempted splenic repair. In patients with multiple intra-abdominal injuries or extensive peritoneal contamination from visceral perforation, it is prudent to weigh the benefits of splenic salvage against the safer course of splenectomy. Most reserve splenic repair for patients in whom it is an isolated organ injury, who are normotensive, and do not have other bodily injuries of greater priority. In addition, splenic salvage is probably not warranted if only 50% or less of the splenic substance is to be preserved. The technique of implanting thin splenic fragments in an omental pouch (auto-transplantation) remains experimental and controversial but may provide significant long-term splenic function.

Nonoperative Management. The safety and effectiveness of nonoperative management of selected adult and pediatric patients with isolated splenic injuries have been confirmed by numerous reports.[22, 23, 117] The risk of delayed splenic rupture in these patients is small but must be considered, and the patient must be cautioned accordingly. Delayed rupture may be due to an enlarging subcapsular hematoma, rupture

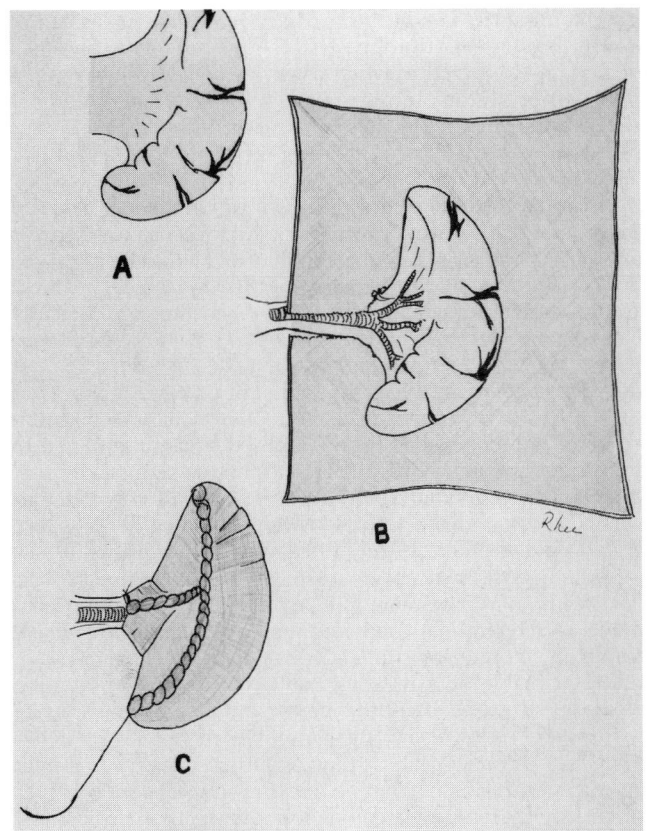

Figure 17–30. *A* to *C*, Technique of wrapping a shattered or complex-injury spleen with absorbable mesh. *B* depicts a key-hole cut into an appropriately sized, tightly meshed sheet of polyglycolic acid mesh. A running suture is used to secure the wrap, tight enough to control hemorrhage yet loose enough at the hilum to allow blood inflow.

of a traumatic arterial pseudoaneurysm, or simply recurrent or ongoing hemorrhage that is finally clinically inescapable. One recent review placed the incidence of delayed rupture of the spleen at 1.5%.[29] Another consideration in nonoperative management is the possibility of an unrecognized associated intra-abdominal injury. The risk of associated injuries was once considered to be as high as 12% to 22%, but a more recent report placed the incidence of occult injuries at a more reasonable 1.6% (1 of 56) of patients actually considered for observational management.[42] A multicenter retrospective review of 832 patients with blunt splenic trauma reported that 112 (13%) splenic injuries were intentionally managed nonoperatively.[23] Patients were considered candidates for nonoperative management if they were hemodynamically stable, if there were no serious associated abdominal organ injuries, and if no extra-abdominal injuries precluded assessment of the abdomen. Approximately two thirds of the patients were adults. In this select group of patients, nonoperative management was successful in 98% of the children and 83% of the adults. These authors suggested that patients with isolated splenic injuries of Grade I, II, and III (Table 17–7) who meet the above criteria are candidates for nonoperative management, although any patient meeting the hemodynamic stability requirement, regardless of CT image, is a potential observational management candidate. Although nonoperative management can be successful in highly selective patients, its injudicious administration to the generalized population could have unfavorable consequences. The long-term risk of splenectomy for isolated spleen injury (including the operative mortality and the long-term risk of OPSI) is probably a maximum of 1.5%. It seems rational that any

alternative to splenectomy for isolated splenic injury must not exceed this long-term risk.

An additional factor to be considered in weighing the risk of nonoperative management versus splenorrhaphy or splenectomy is the need for blood transfusion. Decisional analyses comparing the risks of surgical procedure, postsplenectomy sepsis, and blood transfusion–related infections have been conducted.[40, 73] They suggest that, because of the additional blood requirements of nonoperative management, *observation only* is associated with a *slightly* higher hospital survival but with more than a twofold increase in transfusion-related deaths. Based on these analyses, it would be wise to abandon nonoperative management if the observed patient requires any blood transfusion because of splenic injury.

SMALL INTESTINE

The incidence of small bowel injury secondary to blunt trauma ranges from 5% to 15% and approaches 50% for all penetrating abdominal injuries. Injuries to the small intestine following blunt trauma may be due to three mechanisms: (1) crush injury between the vertebrae and the anterior abdominal wall; (2) sudden increase in the intraluminal pressure; and (3) tears at the junction of a mobile and a fixed segment of bowel. Motor vehicle accidents, child abuse, bicycle accidents, and assorted falls account for most of these injuries. The sudden deceleration causes the mobile portion of the bowel to move away from its point of fixation (ligament of Treitz, ileocecal junction, sites of adhesions), causing a tangential tear. Rarely, adhesions involve a portion of the bowel in such a manner that during sudden compression of the abdomen a closed-loop phenomenon is created with a resultant blow-out of the area. Occasionally, direct trauma from a blow or seat belt may be responsible for the damage that occurs at the point of impact. The association of chance-type lumbar fracture with intestinal injuries in children and adults wearing only a lap belt restraining device has now been recognized with sufficient frequency as to require its exclusion.

Most patients with a perforated small intestine exhibit some evidence of peritoneal irritation and may have frank abdominal rigidity. Lacerations of the lower small bowel may be particularly deceptive, however, because surrounding loops may wall off the damaged area quickly and efficiently. In such cases, the patient may appear surprisingly well for days, demonstrating only mild localized tenderness. Free air may not be visible radiographically, and bowel sounds may persist. Such patients may eat and have bowel movements for a week or more before fever and other signs of intraperitoneal sepsis appear. Occasionally, damage may occur to the mesentery without involving the bowel. Minor tears are of little significance, but large hematomas may ultimately compress the adjacent mesenteric vessels and cause intestinal ischemia with later perforation.

Diagnostic peritoneal lavage is 95% accurate in identifying small bowel injury. Diagnostic errors are generally due to small intestinal perforations with minimal bleeding that have developed delayed signs of peritonitis. CT scanning is less precise and requires both oral and intravenous contrast agents and careful inspection for the presence of bowel wall thickening, mesenteric hematoma, or fluid of nonblood density pooling in the pelvis. The presence of any of these signs, particularly when combined with abdominal tenderness or absent bowel sounds, warrants further emergency evaluation or surgical exploration.

During any laparotomy for possible intra-abdominal injuries, the entire small bowel should be meticulously examined. Each tear, as it is encountered, should be clamped or quickly sutured to prevent further leakage and contamination of the peritoneal cavity during the remainder of the exploration. The wounds of entrance and exit on the abdominal wall cannot be used to predict the likely site of a small bowel injury because of the mobility of the small intestine and the variability of the patient's position at the time of injury.

Simple lacerations of the small bowel are sutured with a single layer of interrupted nonabsorbable Lembert sutures after removal of any tissue that is even questionably nonviable. Patients who have multiple additional injuries, shock, dilated small bowel, or a coagulopathy may benefit from a two-layer closure to ensure hemostasis. Care is taken to avoid excessive narrowing of the bowel by repair. Where damage to the bowel wall is extensive or where multiple tears are situated fairly close to one another, resection of the involved segment rather than repair of the individual perforations is preferred. Removal of the extensively damaged intestine is generally safer, provided that a sufficient length of viable bowel remains to permit adequate absorption of food.

COLON AND RECTUM

Colon. The colon is second only to the small bowel in frequency of abdominal organs injured from gunshot wounds, and third (liver, small bowel) following abdominal stab wounds. In most contemporary series, the infectious morbidity rate ranges from 25% to 35% and the mortality rate ranges from 3% to 12%. Major injuries to the rectum result in an even higher mortality, ranging from 4% to 22%. Most of the infectious morbidity following abdominal injury occurs as a consequence of delayed diagnosis or inadequate therapy for colon injuries.

Early diagnosis and treatment of colon wounds (within 2 hours of injury) dramatically reduce infectious complications. Since most colon injuries can only be definitively recognized at laparotomy, an aggressive approach to the management of penetrating abdominal trauma is warranted. Gunshot wounds to the abdomen generally require exploratory laparotomy. DPL can be beneficial in diagnosing intra-abdominal injury following stab wounds to the anterior abdomen. However, because considerable portions of the colon are retroperitoneal, DPL has limited value in identifying such injuries when the stab is to the flank or back. Many surgeons therefore advocate a policy of routine abdominal exploration for any penetrating wound to the back or flank, although some authors have suggested using intravenous, oral, and rectal contrast-enhanced CT to evaluate back and flank penetrating wounds.

In an effort to minimize the infectious wound complications, all people who sustain penetrating trauma to the abdomen who are at risk for a colon injury should receive preoperative antibiotics in the emergency department. In most patients with proven colon injuries requiring colon resection, primary closure of the skin and subcutaneous tissues is also avoided.

When a colon injury has been identified, a decision regarding management must be made. Because of a concern for infection following primary repairs, it has long been believed that the safest practice is to divert the fecal stream and anticipate a delayed colostomy closure. This concept has dominated modern management of colon wounds and can be traced to the experience of surgeons during World War II in which colostomy was credited with reducing the mortality rate from colonic injury to 37%, down from the World War I mortality rate of 60% for colon injuries treated by primary repair.[130] However, the need for uniform colostomy in civilian colon trauma has been challenged, the premise being that, unlike war injuries, most civilian colon wounds are due to low-velocity handguns or stab wounds. As a consequence, many trauma surgeons argue that more than half of all civil-

ian colon injuries can be treated by primary repair instead of exteriorization or colostomy. This change in practice has been documented by Nance, who has reviewed published reports from major trauma centers in the United States demonstrating the increasing incidence of primary repair versus colostomy for colon wounds over the last two decades (Table 17–8).[86]

Although the controversy between proponents of primary suture and colostomy continues, neither of these two schools of thought suggests that all colon injuries should be managed by one single technique. Instead, there seems to be agreement among most trauma surgeons that four techniques currently have a place in the management of colon injuries: primary repair, resection and primary anastomosis, exteriorization of repair, and colostomy. Exteriorization of primary repair, with subsequent delayed return of the repaired colon to its intra-abdominal domain, has been proposed as an alternative to colostomy or primary repair. This technique supposedly represents an intermediate between the two extremes of repair versus colostomy. The injured bowel is repaired but is exteriorized on the anterior abdominal wall to be dropped back into the abdomen in approximately 1 week. Several reports document an approximate failure rate of 50% with this technique, which requires attentive nursing care and occasionally results in colon obstruction.[14]

The available data indicate that primary closure of colon wounds without decompressive proximal colostomy can be performed selectively, using a number of criteria to determine in each patient which type of surgical treatment should be carried out. General guidelines that must be met to consider primary repair of a colon wound instead of a colostomy include operation within 4 to 6 hours of injury; less than 6 units of blood transfusion; no evidence of prolonged shock or hemodynamic instability; minimal soilage of peritoneal cavity; injury limited to one aspect of the colon; no associated colonic vascular injury; and no loss of abdominal wall or need for synthetic mesh repair. One report documented an anastomotic leak rate of 42% following primary colon repair if the patient had required massive (>6 units) blood transfusion or had underlying medical disease, compared with 3% leak rate in the absence of these two risk factors.[127] In addition, some would not perform primary repair in the face of associated renal pelvis or pancreatic injury, or when two or more other intra-abdominal organs have been injured. With these selective criteria, primary repair of either the right or left colon can be accomplished with minimum morbidity and mortality, a conclusion generally supported by prospective, randomized clinical trials.[20]

Although all these techniques are applicable to any segment of the colon, most surgeons treat the various anatomic components of the colon with some unique distinction. This is emphasized in a recent large review (727 patients) of colon trauma by Burch and colleagues from Ben Taub.[14] Ninety-seven per cent of the injuries were from penetrating wounds, and distribution among right, transverse, and descending colon was approximately equal. Primary repair was performed in 51.7% of the patients, a colostomy in 32.5%, exteriorization in 14.4%, and resection anastomosis in 1.4%. This experience demonstrates the general trend to primarily repair *right* colon injuries and *stab* wounds or *low-velocity* gunshot wounds. The right colon was primarily repaired in 78% of the injuries, the transverse colon in 62%, and the left colon in only 32%. Seventy per cent of stab wounds were primarily repaired, as opposed to 47% of gunshot wounds and 28% of blunt injuries.

The added morbidity rate involved in closing a colostomy is often considered in the operative decision to perform colostomy versus primary repair or exteriorization. Some series have reported significant morbidity related to the creation of

TABLE 17–8. Collected Series of Colon Repair Techniques

Reporting Institution	Colostomy		Primary Repair: No Colostomy	
	No. (%)	Mortality (%)	No. (%)	Mortality (%)
Charity Hospital, New Orleans, 1988 (347 patients)	202 (58)	16	145 (42)	6
Jefferson Davis (Ben Taub) Hospital, 1962 (272 patients)	52 (19)	33	220 (82)	6
Ben Taub Hospital, 1971 (406 patients)	182 (45)	21	224 (55)	8
Denver General Hospital, 1985 (228 patients)	83 (36)	2	110 (48)	1
Harlem Hospital, 1972 (138 patients)	49 (36)	18	85 (64)	5
Grady Memorial Hospital, 1979 (268 patients)	201 (75)	10	67 (25)	1
San Francisco General Hospital, 1977 (129 patients)	91 (71)	0	38 (29)	11
Total	860 (49)	13.7	890 (51)	5.6

Adapted from Nance, F. C.: Injuries to the colon and rectum. *In* Mattox, K. L., Moore, E. E., and Feliciano, D. V. (Eds.): Trauma. Norwalk, CT., Appleton & Lange, 1988, p. 495.

stomas, and rarely, the required closure of the stoma has resulted in death. Parks and Hastings' review of colostomy closures documented an overall complication rate from 9% to 49%; intra-abdominal complications occurred from 2% to 23%.[95] In this report, complications were less likely if the interval to colostomy closure was longer than 90 days. Thal and Yeary reviewed 137 patients who had colostomy closure following colostomies for trauma.[130] Of those patients, 14 had postoperative complications for an overall morbidity rate of 10.2%. There were no deaths in this series. Morbidity was lowest (4.8%) in those patients undergoing colostomy closure between 4 and 8 weeks after injury. They also concluded that colostomy closure in trauma patients appeared to be safer than in patients in whom colostomy was constructed for nontraumatic reasons.

Based on the foregoing data, the authors' general management plan for colon wounds is as follows. Small stab wounds or low-velocity gunshot wounds to the colon may undergo primary repair by adhering to the general guidelines just outlined. More significant penetrating injuries and most blunt injuries to the right colon are managed by right colectomy. Primary reconstruction via ileotransverse colostomy may be performed in a stable patient in whom there is an isolated injury with no evidence of shock or gross fecal contamination. Otherwise, a right colectomy is accompanied by the creation of an ileostomy and mucous fistula. The same guiding principles for primary repair of minor wounds can be followed for the left colon, although resection with primary anastomosis is generally not recommended because of the different vascularity, fecal consistency, and bacterial load. More extensive left colon injuries are usually treated by resection with proximal-end colostomy and distal mucous fistula or Hartmann's pouch. Stab wounds and low-velocity gunshot wounds of the transverse colon are considered for primary repair or exteriorized as loop colostomies. Major injuries, including most blunt injuries, are resected with the creation of an end colostomy and a mucous fistula.

Rectum. The same diagnostic modalities previously discussed for intraperitoneal colon injuries are used for rectal injuries, with the addition of two other procedures and one caveat: Abdominal x-ray films are obtained for the determination of retroperitoneal air, proctosigmoidoscopy is performed for either direct visualization of the injury or for evidence of hemorrhage, and transpelvic gunshot wounds should undergo celiotomy.[32] Primary closure of full-thickness rectal wounds above the dentate line are typically combined

with a diverting colostomy. The value of proximal diverting colostomy following rectal trauma was established during World War II. Although subsequent civilian reports have occasionally advocated primary closure without fecal diversion, the resultant mortality rate has been higher than 20%. In contrast, the management plan outlined in the following section for rectal trauma results in a less than 2% mortality rate.[132] For wounds occurring below the dentate line, débridement is accompanied by appropriate drainage and colon diversion is not performed routinely. For wounds above the levators with penetration of the pelvirectal space, treatment includes (1) closure, if possible, (2) proximal *diverting* colostomy, (3) presacral (retrorectal) drains, and (4) irrigation of the rectal stump with povidone-iodine. Rectal stump irrigation in this setting decreases the incidence of pelvic abscess, rectal fistulas, and sepsis.[119]

MAJOR ABDOMINAL VESSELS

The mortality rate from abdominal vascular trauma still ranges from 30% to 60% despite improvements in emergency resuscitation, transport, and trauma systems. As expected, most deaths are due to exsanguination. One third of abdominal vascular trauma patients arrive in the emergency department in shock. Rapid control of the injury is the primary management goal, and since most injuries are due to penetrating wounds, immediate triage to the operating room is simplified and must be encouraged.

Forty per cent of intra-abdominal vascular injuries involve two or more major vascular structures. Mortality is directly related to the number of vascular structures injured, the site of injury, and the mechanism of injury. Aortic wounds are associated with 40% to 80% mortality rate, highest from shotgun and gunshot wounds and highest with injuries in the suprarenal location. Vena caval injuries incur lower 10% to 40% mortality, suprarenal wounds again being the most difficult to repair. Iliac artery and vein injuries incur a 15% to 40% and 10% to 25% mortality, respectively. Superior mesenteric artery and vein injuries both have a 30% to 40% mortality rate.[97, 112, 121]

When the diagnosis is uncertain, peritoneal lavage may reveal intraperitoneal bleeding and present clear indications for exploration. Alternatively, CT in the hemodynamically stable patient may reveal an initially unsuspected mesenteric or retroperitoneal hematoma. If the patient is stable and uncertainty exists as to the need for exploration (e.g., in a patient with a stab wound or following blunt trauma), arteriography can confirm the diagnosis. Diagnostic studies, however, should never delay surgical exploration of the patient in shock. Absence of distal pulses and limb ischemia are difficult to interpret in hypotensive patients, and massive retroperitoneal bleeding may occur without being obvious.

Initial Management. Operative control of major vessel hemorrhage can be challenging. At the time of the exploration, any retroperitoneal hematoma should suggest the possibility of associated vascular injury. Central hematomas above the renal vessels suggest suprarenal aortocaval injuries, or injury to the celiac axis or superior-mesenteric artery or vein. Inferior central hematomas imply distal aortic or vena caval wounds. A lateral hematoma suggests renal artery or vein injury. Pelvic hematoma suggests iliac artery or vein injury.

The approach to the operative management of the patient suspected of having a major intra-abdominal vascular injury is different from that of the stable patient with penetrating or blunt abdominal injury. It is recommended that the approach be similar to that of managing a patient suspected of having a ruptured aortic aneurysm (i.e., these hemodynamically unstable patients are taken immediately to the operating room, and preparations completed as necessary; diagnostic maneuvers are interpreted, and additional lines are placed). The patient is prepared from the chin to midthigh. Warming blankets and blood warmers should be in place, as well as an autotransfusion device. The operating team is scrubbed and ready to intervene if there is sudden collapse. Anesthesia is not begun until just before the incision is to be made. With initiation of anesthesia, the blood pressure may fall suddenly as abdominal muscular relaxation occurs; then, fluid and blood replacement must be accomplished rapidly while bleeding is being controlled.

If a major arterial wound is suspected because of hypotension, a distended abdomen, or combined chest and abdominal penetration, some surgeons recommend entering the chest through the seventh interspace and obtaining control of the aorta before the distended abdomen is explored. This has not been the standard approach, because in most circumstances the abdominal aorta can be controlled at the level of the diaphragm. This approach is advocated for the hypotensive patient in which suprarenal aortic injuries are suspected by mechanism or projectile pathway. A retroperitoneal hematoma in this location obscures the gastrohepatic ligament and the diaphragmatic hiatus, making visual exposure of the abdominal aorta difficult.

If active hemorrhage is encountered on opening the peritoneum, it must be controlled before any other intraoperative maneuvers are performed. Injuries to solid organs with bleeding are usually rapidly packed, and standard techniques of vascular control are used to control the active hemorrhage. Proximal and distal control is needed for any major abdominal arterial injury. Direct digital or sponge compression at the site of injury is often required while obtaining such control. Major venous injuries, however, are often not amenable to proximal and distal clamping. Direct digital compression or compression with a sponge stick may secure adequate venous vascular control to repair tangential wounds with 4–0 or 5–0 polypropylene. If the patient has a contained retroperitoneal hematoma, the surgeon may have time to rapidly clamp or repair bowel injuries and thereby limit contamination. Specific approaches to individual intra-abdominal vessels depend on the location of the surrounding hematoma.

Exposure and Treatment of Specific Injuries. *Midline suprarenal hemorrhage* is perhaps the most difficult to control, as the aorta, celiac axis, mesenteric vessels, or vena cava may be responsible. In addition, with the usual penetrating wound, associated gastric, duodenal, or pancreatic injuries are likely.

Proximal aortic control may be attempted via direct aortic compression through the gastrohepatic sheaf, although a left anterolateral thoracotomy and thoracic aortic clamping may be necessary. Rotation of the colon, spleen, pancreas, and left kidney to the midline allows complete exposure of the aorta from the hiatus to the aortic bifurcation. The left diaphragmatic crux may be divided to provide even more proximal exposure. When control has been obtained and the aortic wound exposed, it is recommended that exploration be completed and the resuscitation be underway before definitive repairs are begun. In patients who have already experienced massive hemorrhage, continued bleeding, even at relatively low rates, from uncontrolled sources can result in significant blood loss. Autotransfusion can play a significant role in the resuscitation of these patients. In patients sustaining mesenteric vascular injuries, intestinal viability must be ensured at completion of the operation. A *second-look* procedure may be advisable in select patients.[121]

Suprarenal vena caval injuries are approached with an extended Kocher's maneuver, rotating the right colon and duodenum to midline and retracting the liver superiorly. Retrohepatic vena caval injuries are extremely difficult to control, and subsequently a retrohepatic caval shunt (Schrock shunt) has been developed (see Fig. 17–27). Modifications of this shunt allow its insertion through the saphenofemoral junction, or more commonly, through the cardiac atrial appendage. The survival rate, even with early use of this technique, remains dismal.

Midline infrarenal hematoma can usually be approached directly through the retroperitoneum or the base of the mesentery, and direct control with vascular clamps can be accomplished. The maneuvers used here are similar to those used to approach abdominal aortic aneurysms.

Lateral hematoma may be due to renal parenchymal or to vascular injury. If it is the result of blunt abdominal trauma, it is helpful if the preoperative evaluation includes an assessment of renal function. If the kidney is well perfused and the hematoma nonexpanding with no urine leak, no further exposure is required (see kidney section). In penetrating trauma, however, all lateral hematomas should be explored and the path of injury meticulously followed. Renal vascular control should first be obtained prior to opening Gerota's fascia. This step, though often unnecessary, clearly decreases the incidence of nephrectomy. The left renal vessels can generally be looped through direct exposure at the base of the mesocolon. The right renal vein, however, is more readily exposed after mobilizing the duodenum and unroofing the vena cava at its junction with the renal veins.

The approach to *pelvic hematomas* again depends on mechanism of injury. As discussed in the pelvic fracture section, blunt pelvic trauma can result in massive retroperitoneal pelvic hematomas. About 15% of these hematomas are the result of arterial injuries. Pelvic bone fixation and angiography with embolization play a role in managing these injuries, but direct operative exploration of the hematoma does not. Penetrating pelvic wounds, however, do require exploration of the projectile or stab pathway. Direct compression of active bleeding or an expanding hematoma precedes proximal and distal control. Proximal control of either the distal aorta or common iliac artery is obtained by eviscerating the small bowel and incising the retroperitoneum over the aortic bifurcation. Distal control is obtained just proximal to the inguinal ligament. Control of the internal iliac vessels is more problematic. Direct digital or sponge stick compression may be most efficacious while placing vascular loops about the common iliac bifurcation. Injuries to the common or external iliac artery should be repaired, if at all possible. In contrast, injuries to the internal iliac artery can be ligated with impunity, even if they occur bilaterally.[97, 112]

The general principles of vascular repair apply in abdominal vascular injuries. Débridement of devitalized tissue, tension-free anastomosis, and the preferential use of autogenous tissue to bridge extensive gaps are applicable to all vascular repairs. Lateral repair of the aorta or vena cava is often possible, even after local débridement. Removal of all damaged tissue is important, however, and should not be ignored to simplify the subsequent repair. If a lateral repair without vessel narrowing is not possible, patch graft angioplasty can be done. Occasionally, a limited resection and anastomosis can be performed, but mobility of the aorta and vena cava is not great, and it is better to interpose a graft than to compromise the repair by constructing it under excess tension.

Wounds to the inferior vena cava below the renal veins are generally easier to control than are aortic wounds. If the laceration involves only one wall, a partial occluding clamp such as a Satinsky may be properly positioned for doing the repair. Through-and-through injuries of the vena cava can be repaired by enlarging the anterior wound so the posterior injury can be sutured through the anterior wound. If greater mobility of the vena cava is required, a few lumbar veins or the gonadal vein may be ligated to allow rotation, although this is a more dangerous maneuver.

Ligation of the infrarenal cava should be considered if the cava is severely lacerated and requires complicated repair or graft interposition, or if repair poses a prohibitive risk in an unstable patient with multiple injuries; however, caval ligation is a distinctly unusual maneuver.[1, 47] If caval ligation is performed, it is important to maintain adequate intravascular volume and to keep both legs elevated and wrapped with elastic compression dressings for 5 to 7 days postoperatively. Ligation of the suprarenal vena cava should not be performed unless early reconstruction is planned. Alternatively, a segment of iliac vein or jugular vein can be used to reconstruct a segmental defect of the vena cava. In most cases, construction of such a venous graft is not required, and the time and effort involved unnecessarily increase the operative morbidity and mortality. Another option is to establish continuity of the inferior vena cava by interposing a vascular prosthesis (polytetrafluoroethylene) graft. Although such grafts may eventually clot, they can provide an expedient solution.

URINARY TRACT

Without gross hematuria, urologic injury is usually unsuspected. Because urologic injuries are frequently associated with other life-threatening trauma, their diagnosis may be delayed for hours or days until the patient is stabilized. A key tenet to be applied in diagnosing urologic trauma is to suspect injury by assessing the mechanism and forces involved. Urologic injury is particularly likely when there has been a crush injury of the upper abdomen or pelvis, direct forceful blow to the back or flank, or when the patient has sustained a severe accelerating or decelerating injury, such as in a fall from a height or in an automobile or auto-pedestrian accident. Signs of forceful injury include femur fracture, fracture of the pelvis, crush injury of the chest, severe bruising of the abdomen, and severe head trauma.

Specific signs of upper urologic tract injury include either gross or microscopic hematuria, fracture of the lower rib cage, or fracture of a lumbar process. The most telling signs of a lower urinary tract injury include the presence of blood at the urinary meatus, a *high-riding* or misplaced prostate that cannot be palpated on rectal examination, and urinary retention, bladder distention, and the desire to void but an inability to empty the bladder. The clinical signs of urinary tract injury may be initially absent, particularly in the rapidly transported multitrauma victim. Evaluation of possible uro-

logic trauma therefore must often be based on the mechanism and associated injuries.

Initial Evaluation. On presentation to the emergency department, every trauma patient should be asked to immediately produce a urine specimen. If he or she is unable to do so, catheterization may be necessary, particularly if the patient has experienced severe trauma. Under no circumstances should the patient be catheterized prior to urethrography if blood is present at the meatus of the penis or if the mechanism of injury suggests urethral injury. If there is resistance to catheterization, all efforts to catheterize the patient should cease and urologic consultation should be obtained. Inability to easily pass a Foley catheter into the bladder supports the possibility of a posterior urethral disruption, particularly when the patient has an associated pelvic fracture. If possible, the Foley catheter should never be passed until a rectal examination has been done. In men, the inability to palpate the prostate is highly suggestive of complete urethral transection (Fig. 17–31).

If upper or lower urinary tract injury is suspected, the initial evaluation depends in part on the patient's associated injuries and hemodynamic stability. If the patient requires emergent surgery, a limited *one-shot* intravenous pyelogram (IVP) may be performed in the emergency department or on the operating room table by the rapid intravenous injections of 60 ml. of high-density contrast medium followed by a flat plate radiograph of the abdomen and pelvis in 1 to 5 minutes. This study usually identifies the presence or absence of functioning kidneys but is an extremely limited study that may falsely fail to identify a renal outline in the presence of shock. In patients sustaining penetrating trauma, the entrance and exit wounds of the missile are marked with steel clips to determine the path of the bullet. The presence of pelvic crush injuries or blood at the urinary meatus suggests the need to perform retrograde cystourethrogram. Cystography is performed by filling the bladder to capacity with 200 to 300 ml. of contrast medium to maximally distend the bladder lumen. Films are obtained with the bladder distended and then emptied to demonstrate extravasation (Fig. 17–32).

The greatest diagnostic problem in blunt urologic trauma is recognition of renal pedicle injury. A high degree of suspicion is frequently the only mechanism to prevent the surgeon from overlooking this injury. No absolute amount of micro-

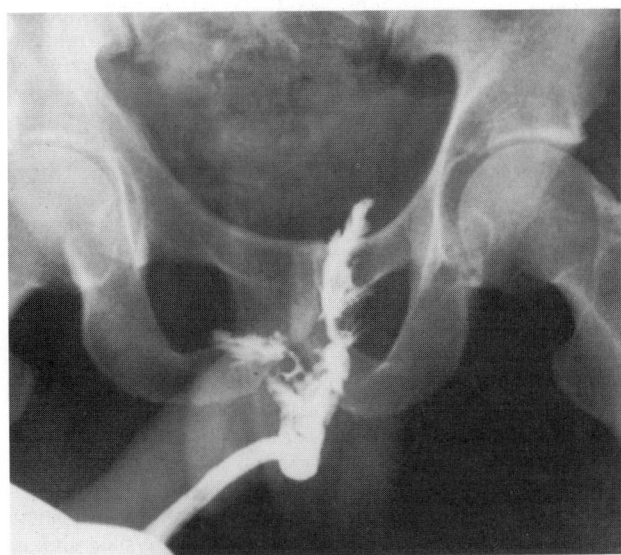

Figure 17–31. Retrograde cystourethrogram demonstrating complete disruption of the posterior urethra with extravasation of dye. Subsequent evaluation identified the tear just distal to the membranous urethra.

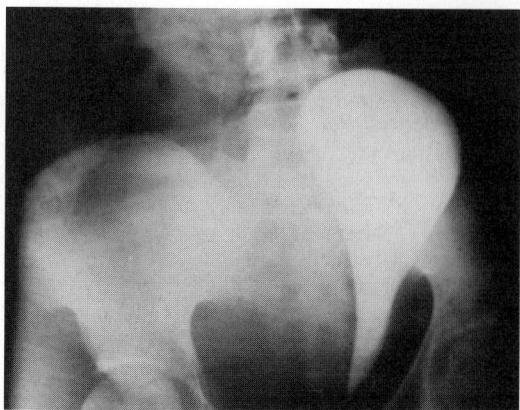

Figure 17–32. Cystogram demonstrating lateral displacement of the bladder secondary to a large pelvic hematoma.

scopic hematuria can accurately predict significant urinary tract injury. At one institution, all patients with gross hematuria or any degree of microscopic hematuria combined with associated abdominal injuries, shock, or a mechanism that suggests renal trauma undergo an evaluation to rule out the possibility of renal pedicle injury. In addition, all patients with penetrating wounds near the urinary tract system are either operatively explored or undergo radiographic evaluation.

Either IVP or CT with intravenous contrast agent is an effective method of evaluating the urinary tract, although CT scans provide more detailed information about both the urologic injury and the potential associated intra-abdominal and retroperitoneal injuries. IVP is also less accurate in the unprepared patient, and the dynamic phase of CT scan provides additional information regarding renal function. The degree of renal parenchymal injury identified on CT scans is also useful in classifying the injury and defining the management plan (see the following section). Demonstration by either CT scan or IVP of the apparent presence of a solitary kidney or a lack of function of a segment of the kidney is an indication for immediate arteriography.

Kidneys. Penetrating injury to the kidney may be secondary to a gunshot, stab wound, or impalement. Parenchymal injury caused by a low-velocity weapon is usually not life threatening and is generally easily treated with débridement and primary repair of the kidney with dependent drainage. Occasionally a partial nephrectomy may be necessary when the wound is in a polar position. High-velocity bullet wounds are different. Many nephrectomies and partial nephrectomies are performed in patients with high-velocity penetrating injury because of inability to control hemorrhage and accurately define the extent of the injury. In addition, injudicious rapid incision of Gerota's capsule with an extensive injury to the kidney may result in unnecessary nephrectomy. Preoperative arteriography is helpful in defining vascular disruption and may be therapeutic if embolization can be performed. Unfortunately, most patients are too unstable from other intra-abdominal injuries to warrant this time-consuming maneuver. A key operative technique is the proximal control of the renal pedicle before opening Gerota's fascia in any circumstance of kidney trauma. If the injury involves the hilum of the kidney, repair may be attempted in an isolated renal injury, but salvage of renal function is minimal in most circumstances, and associated organ injuries may take precedence. Any injury to the collecting system should be débrided and sutured in a watertight manner. Preservation of as much renal parenchyma as possible should be the rule.

Although virtually all patients with penetrating renal trauma undergo exploration because of the high incidence of associated intra-abdominal injuries (90% to 100% for gunshot wounds, 60% to 75% for stab wounds), many with blunt renal trauma can be managed nonoperatively.[18, 51, 113] Selection of patients for operative treatment of their renal lesion should be based on the overall clinical status and the necessity of surgical repair or resection, which in turn is based on the natural history of the lesion.[18, 151]

A classification system used to differentiate patients with minor renal trauma from those with major renal trauma is based on the principles illustrated in Figure 17–33. The key components of the classification system are: (1) the presence and extent of nonfunctioning renal segments; (2) the extent of perinephric hematoma; and (3) the degree of contrast extravasation. Eighty-five per cent of patients have minor renal injuries that may be managed expectantly. Patients with minor renal injuries have few serious sequelae. Approximately 10% of patients have immediately life-threatening renal injuries consisting of a shattered kidney, renal pedicle injury, or cortical laceration with disrupted fragments and extensive extravasation. These patients undergo surgical exploration and repair or resection, since the natural history of these lesions is such that the incidence of secondary nephrectomy, hypertension, abscess, and late bleeding managed nonoperatively is quite high. Additionally, approximately 15% of these patients have significant injury to other abdominal viscera.

Only about 5% of patients appear to have an intermediate degree of renal injury. Management may be either nonsurgical or surgical, depending on the clinical status of the patient

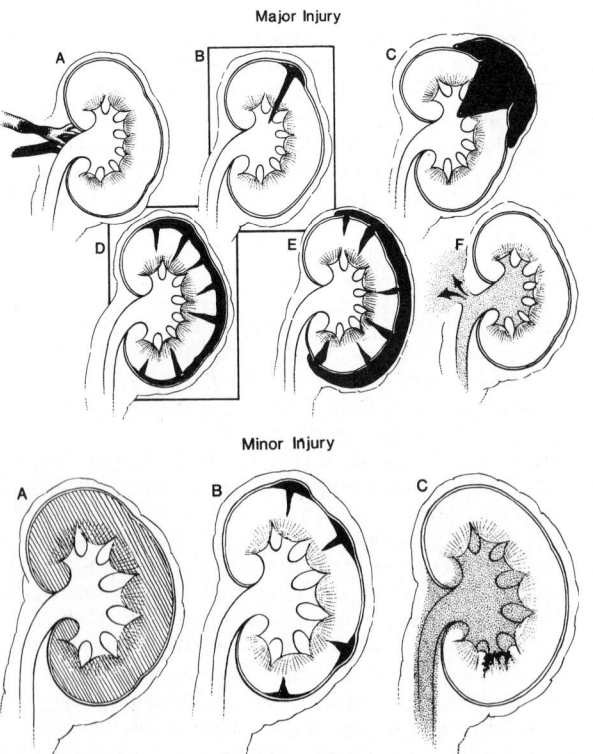

Figure 17–33. A system for classifying renal trauma. Six types of major injury are the following: *A*, renal pedicle injury; *B*, deep parenchymal injury with an intact capsule; *C*, deep parenchymal injury with a disrupted capsule; *D*, shattered kidney with an intact capsule; *E*, shattered kidney with a disrupted capsule; and *F*, ureteral or renal pelvis injury. Minor injury can be classified as *A*, contusion; *B*, shallow cortical laceration; and *C*, forniceal disruption. (From Guerriero, W. G.: Trauma to the kidneys, ureters, bladder, and urethra. Surg. Clin. North Am., *62*:1047, 1982.)

and the need for treatment of other associated injuries. Major cortical laceration with undisplaced fragments held in place by an intact renal capsule with minimal or no extravasation and the shattered functioning kidney with contained fragments are examples of this type. CT has been particularly helpful in identifying the extent of these injuries. If a significant hematoma is also demonstrated, angiographic evaluation and embolization can be successfully employed. In most cases, the kidney will heal in this situation, but sequelae such as hypertension are common.

Ureters. Injury to the ureter usually results from penetrating trauma. Fistula and stricture formation are the inevitable sequelae of undetected ureteral injury. Early detection and operative repair are preferred with a ureteral transection in which the blood supply of the ureter has not been injured and the injury is not far below the pelvic brim. The principles of ureteral repair are adequate débridement, tension-free repair, spatulated anastomosis, watertight closure, ureteral stenting, and drainage. Injuries in the upper and middle third of the ureter can usually be managed by primary ureteroureterostomy. Injuries to the distal third of the ureter should be treated with ureteroneocystostomy. The ureter should be stented with an indwelling polyvinyl Silastic catheter if there is associated vascular injury or if damage to the ureteral blood supply is suspected. Injury to the upper ureter may be stented with concomitant nephrostomy to drain urine away from the site of the injury. If primary repair is not immediately possible due to shock, associated injuries, or long segmental ureteral damage, diversion of the distal fistula with a percutaneous nephrostomy and secondary repair is the time-honored method of management. Alternatives to immediate diversion in the face of an extensive ureteral injury in the stable patient are transureteroureterostomy or autotransplantation.

Bladder. The bladder is the most commonly injured organ in association with pelvic fractures, with as many as 70% of patients with trauma to the bladder having associated pelvic fractures (see Fig. 17–32). The bladder may be contused, penetrated, or ruptured intraperitoneally or extraperitoneally. Large defects can be present despite a negative cystogram result, particularly if the cystogram is taken at a later date than the patient's initial examination, because blood clots, tissue, or peritoneal contents can fill the defect. False-negative cystogram results are common with penetrating injuries to the bladder. A postevacuation cystogram should always be obtained to see whether any possible extravasation has occurred on the oblique or lateral projections. CT cystograms are helpful in evaluating the more subtle bladder injury.

Treatment of bladder injuries is usually straightforward. Isolated extraperitoneal bladder ruptures can be treated by 10 days of Foley catheter drainage if no other operative intervention is planned.[27] However, most of the extraperitoneal bladder ruptures are associated with pelvic fracture, in which the anterior wall of the bladder has been perforated by a spicule of bone. The fracture should be reduced and stabilized away from the bladder, and the bladder wound should be débrided and closed in two layers. After the repair, the bladder should be tested for integrity by being filled with saline to a capacity of 400 ml. If the bladder can be made watertight and if the patient's other injuries are minimal, Foley drainage is adequate. If prolonged bed rest is expected or if there is a question of integrity of bladder closure, a suprapubic catheter should be placed.

Intraperitoneal rupture occurs in the posterior bladder wall when the patient has a compression injury of the abdomen with a full bladder, or it may be due to the penetrating trauma. Injuries of this type are repaired by developing the edge of the wound so as to mobilize the peritoneum off the ragged bladder tear and to permit a three-layer closure.

Catheterization of ureteral orifices may help protect the ureter during the closure of the bladder. The bladder should be inspected for watertightness, and a Foley catheter or suprapubic tube should be left in for drainage according to the principles just mentioned.

Pelvis and Perineum

Pelvic Fractures

Pelvic fractures are the third most common injury sustained in motor vehicle accidents. Although most constitute rather straightforward orthopedic problems, approximately 20% of pelvic fractures are complex injuries with a high likelihood of other major organ system trauma or significant pelvic hemorrhage. Crush injuries and open pelvic fractures exhibit mortality rates in excess of 50%, with morbidity ranging from 30% to 74%. The major cause of morbidity and mortality is associated organ system injury and uncontrolled blood loss. In one review of 538 consecutive patients with pelvic fracture, 92 patients (17%) required more than 6 units of blood.[82] Twenty-six per cent of this group died, one half from associated injuries and one half from recalcitrant bleeding or delayed pelvic sepsis. If injuries to the iliac or femoral vessels are present, mortality rates in excess of 80% have been reported. This contrasts with the overall reported mortality rate from pelvic fractures of approximately 5%, with 80% of deaths due to associated injuries and only 20% directly attributable to the pelvic fracture itself. Mucha and Farnell's review of 534 patients with pelvic fracture documented an overall mortality rate of 6.4%, although the pelvic fracture itself was directly responsible for less than 1% mortality, with the remainder due to associated head and torso injuries.[83]

Examination of the pelvis is begun by administering AP and lateral compression to assess for instability and pain. Digital rectal and vaginal examination should assess for blood, bony fragments, and mucosa lacerations. In men, particular attention should be directed at identifying the location of the prostate gland, as a high-riding or misplaced prostate indicates urethral disruption. Direct inspection of the urethral meatus is mandatory prior to insertion of a Foley catheter. The presence of meatal blood mandates retrograde urethrography prior to Foley insertion in men, because of the length of the male urethra and the possibility of converting a partial urethral tear into a complete disruption and false passage (see Fig. 17–31). The initial radiographic examination of the patient with blunt trauma should include an AP plain film of the pelvis. As time and the patient's condition allow, more select views such as the 40-degree inlet and outlet view may be indicated. CT scan is particularly helpful in identifying subtle fracture patterns (e.g., 50% of sacral fractures are missed on plain radiographs) and providing anatomic definition to complex pelvic and acetabular fractures. However, pelvic bone CT scanning can be time consuming and does not take precedence over the search for associated injuries.

The reporting of pelvic fractures is probably best done by simply describing each fracture line and the aspect of pelvic bone anatomy involved. Nonetheless, many attempts have been made at classifying pelvic fracture patterns. Pennal and associates originally championed a classification system based on three major *vectors of force:* AP compression, lateral compression, and vertical shear.[99] Gokcen and colleagues modified this system and added an additional category (*combined mechanisms injuries*) to take into account fractures that have features of more than one vector force pattern.[46] A commonly used pelvic fracture classification based on the anatomy of the fracture lines was described by Key and Conwell (modified by Kane), and is outlined in Table 17–9.[65]

TABLE 17–9. Kane's Modification of Key and Conwell's Pelvic Fracture Classification

Type	Criteria
I	*Individual bones not involving the pelvic ring.* Includes avulsion fractures of a single ramus and isolated fractures of the iliac wing.
II	*Single breaks in the pelvic ring.* Fractures occurring through (1) two ipsilateral rami or (2) one sacroiliac joint (rare) or (3) subluxation of the symphysis and pubis.
III	*Double breaks in the pelvic ring.* Fractures include three subsets: (1) the Malgaigne variants, also called the double-vertical or dimetric fractures; (2) bilateral double-ramus fractures, referred to as either straddle fractures or butterfly fractures; and (3) severe multiple or crushing fractures.
IV	*Acetabular fractures.* There are three types: (1) rim fractures; (2) central acetabular fractures; and (3) ischioacetabular fractures.

Modified from Kane, W. J.: Fractures of the pelvis. *In* Rockwood, C., and Green, D. P. (Eds.): Fractures. Philadelphia, J. B. Lippincott, 1975, p. 923.

The usefulness of any classification system lies in its ability to help direct treatment or predict morbidity. In Mucha and Farnell's review of pelvic fracture management, Kane's Type III and IV fractures had a significantly higher incidence of associated injuries, morbidity, and mortality rates.[83] Fractures involving the posterior ring are generally believed to have more associated injuries and complications, require more resuscitation fluid, and have a higher rate of mortality than do pure anterior fractures. The AP compression force fractures and the combined mechanism injury fracture patterns are also most frequently associated with morbidity and mortality. Unstable fracture patterns also may correlate best with higher blood loss. However, *any* pelvic fracture may have significant retroperitoneal hemorrhage.

The management objectives in a patient with a pelvic fracture are control of hemorrhage, skeletal fixation, and treatment of associated injuries. The initial objective is control of exsanguinating blood loss. Massive hemorrhage (≤20 units) can occur into the retroperitoneal space where it may be difficult to diagnose and control. Experimental evidence suggests that the pelvic retroperitoneal space can contain as much as 4000 ml. of blood under pressure equal to or lower than the pressure in the pelvic vessels[43]; this value increases with disruption of the posterior ring. The source of such significant blood loss can occur from pelvic arteries, veins, or the fracture line itself. Slatis and Huittinen have demonstrated that as much as 80% of bleeding is fracture surface and presacral venous plexus.[122] Extensive collateralization, difficult exposure, and release of the tamponade effect of the posterior peritoneum make surgical exploration of pelvic hematomas generally frustrating and fruitless. Application of a pneumatic antishock garment (PASG) or military antishock trousers (MAST) can serve as a temporizing agent, pending either immediate skeletal fixation or arteriographic evaluation and embolization. PASG should be removed as soon as definitive therapy is available, because of the danger of extremity compartment syndrome. Spica cast application (bilateral, long-leg) prevents motion of the pelvis and decreases fracture surface hemorrhage, although it challenges nursing care and limits abdominal observation, and complete patient immobility is associated with many other complications. Some studies have suggested that if pelvic hematoma–related blood requirements exceed 6 units, angiographic intervention

is indicated. However, because most of the bleeding associated with pelvic fractures is venous in origin, angiographic control may not be possible.[7] Immediate fixation of the unstable fracture, either by anterior external fixators or by newer posterior ring reduction clamps may be more helpful in this situation. Some centers are advocates of early (within 8 hours) open reduction and internal fixation of the unstable pelvic fracture, with retrospective data showing a lower complication rate and less blood loss.[69] Remarkably, there are no prospective comparative data to help determine which method or approach is superior, nor the exact indications for their use.

The search for associated intra-abdominal injuries in the patient with a pelvic fracture may require CT scan of the abdomen or DPL. CT scan is reserved only for the hemodynamically normal and stable patient, and peritoneal lavage is preferred as a screening tool. DPL should be performed in the supraumbilical location in patients with significant pelvic fractures to avoid entering the potentially blood-filled anterior abdominal preperitoneal space, an extension of Retzius' space between the bladder and the symphysis pubis. Gross blood on the initial aspirate is grounds for immediate exploratory celiotomy. Red blood cell count–only positive lavage is grounds for CT scanning of the abdomen (to provide better specificity) and an immediate search for other sources of blood loss (retroperitoneal space) in the hemodynamically unstable patient. This approach has resulted in a low 0.5% false-positive DPL rate at the authors' institution, compared with some literature reports of false-positive DPL rates ranging from 16% to 50% in patients with pelvic fractures.[79] Approximately 25% of patients with pelvic fracture have associated intra-abdominal injury.[82]

The hemodynamically unstable patient with a positive peritoneal lavage or with CT scan evidence of intra-abdominal injury, combined with a pelvic fracture and retroperitoneal hematoma, presents the trauma surgeon with a difficult challenge. The following management guidelines are suggested. A hemodynamically unstable patient with a grossly positive peritoneal lavage undergoes immediate exploratory celiotomy. Following repair of intra-abdominal injuries, either angiographic evaluation and embolization or skeletal fixation (or both) is performed, depending on the likelihood of an arterial source of the pelvic bleeding.[7] If exploratory celiotomy is not required, either immediate angiography or skeletal fixation is conducted if (1) 6 or more units blood transfusion have been required for pelvic hemorrhage; (2) presenting hematocrit is low (<25%) and blood loss is localized to the pelvis; or (3) ongoing blood loss is otherwise unexplained. If angiography is performed first, skeletal fixation should follow. Newer techniques of percutaneous screw fixation and posterior *C clamps* have made posterior ring stabilization achievable quickly and with less morbidity.[110] The authors apply these techniques in the angiography suite under fluoroscopic guidance and while preparing for angiography. The sequence of intervention commonly depends on the expertise and availability of support personnel. Although it is difficult to predict which individual patient is at risk for significant pelvic hemorrhage, the presence of posterior element fracture or *unstable open-book* pelvic fracture appears to correlate with significant arterial blood loss.

Perineal Wounds

Massive soft tissue injury of the perineum may occur in association with some pelvic fractures, or this injury may occur without bony pelvic injury. Selective use of descending colostomy to divert the fecal stream away from these injuries is advisable.[36] Early débridement and operative inspection of the wound are required. No attempt should be made to initially close the wound. Undermined skin flaps should be excised, necrotic muscle must be débrided, and deep space infections or pockets have to be eradicated. Repeat daily operating room inspections, débridement, and pulse irrigations should be planned. Eventual closure often requires skin grafting or rotational flaps.

Vaginal Injuries. Vaginal lacerations in association with pelvic fractures are less common (3.5%) but should be suspected when vaginal bleeding occurs in association with pelvic injury. The laceration should be carefully cleansed, débrided as necessary, and primarily closed if recognized early, within 8 to 12 hours.[91]

Extremity and Peripheral Vascular Injuries

Early Fracture Stabilization

Hemorrhage caused by massive disruption or transection of major blood vessels constitutes the only situation in which extremity injuries are immediately life-threatening. However, multiple long bone fractures have a strikingly adverse impact on survival following multiple trauma. Although specific treatments of fractures are not addressed in this chapter, the crucial role of early fracture fixation in the care of the multiply injured patient warrants comment. Early fixation of long bone fractures decreases the incidence of ARDS, fat embolization syndrome, and subsequent development of sepsis and multiple organ failure.[5, 11] The exact mechanism of this beneficial effect remains unknown but appears to be related to the *early* fracture stabilization with a subsequent diminished inflammatory response and an ability to mobilize the patient rapidly. Early patient mobilization lessens the likelihood of pneumonia, venous thrombosis, and pressure sores and seems to allow for better tolerance of feeding, factors that undoubtedly allow for earlier discharge from the intensive care unit. The argument that the patient is *too sick* for immediate fracture stabilization must be carefully weighed against the mounting evidence of the feasibility and global benefit of early fixation.

Soft Tissue Injuries

Although rarely immediately life threatening, extensive soft tissue wounds can present a difficult therapeutic challenge with significant morbidity and mortality, even in the face of optimal treatment. The principles of management of soft tissue injuries include débridement of devitalized tissue, restoration of adequate blood supply, and adequate coverage of vital structures including nerves, blood vessels, tendons, and other soft tissues subject to desiccation and infection.

All lacerations and penetrating injuries of the extremities should be cleansed and meticulously débrided. No maneuver contributes as much to the prevention of tetanus or gas gangrene infection as *complete débridement of all devitalized tissue*. Following initial débridement, if there is any question regarding the viability of remaining muscle or other soft tissue, re-exploration under anesthesia should be scheduled within the ensuing 24 hours. Rapidly spreading cellulitis, crepitus, erythema, or unexplained pain in an extremity is an indication for immediate surgical exploration and débridement.

Restoration of blood supply to an injured extremity receives high priority because as little as a few hours of ischemia may result in tissue necrosis and subsequent amputation. The classic signs of vascular compromise include *pain, pallor,* and *pulselessness,* although more subtle findings such as delayed capillary refill and venous congestion are signs of vascular compromise that may jeopardize healing of soft tissue wounds and invite secondary infection.

Adequate soft tissue coverage of exposed vital structures is essential to prevent dessication, secondary infection, and vascular suture line disruption. Although primary closure of native soft tissue is ideal, this is often impossible owing to the presence of untidy or ischemic tissue, infection, or large-area soft tissue defects. Early closure with autografts, allografts, or xenografts of skin can provide temporary coverage pending more elaborate soft tissue reconstructive maneuvers such as free muscle flaps and combined muscle and skin rotational flaps.

Primary Amputation. The decision to perform primary amputation of an injured extremity is predicated on the futility of attempted limb salvage. The combination of crush or avulsion soft tissue defects with complex fractures and neurovascular disruption, particularly avulsion or transection of nerves to weight-bearing surfaces, constitutes a nonsalvageable extremity. Early amputation of such mangled extremities can spare the patient the morbidity and expense of a long hospital stay with multiple surgical procedures, recurrent infections, pain, and vain attempts at rehabilitation for a useless appendage. Extremities with less severe combined injuries represent a more difficult challenge to the surgeon's judgment, and often age, associated medical problems, and concurrent injuries must also be considered.[55]

Tetanus. Tetanus, caused by toxins elaborated by the anaerobic organism *Clostridium tetani,* is characterized by local convulsive spasm of the voluntary muscles and a tendency toward episodes of respiratory arrest. It may occur as a complication of large or small wounds, including lacerations, open fractures, burns, abrasions, or even hypodermic injections. Regardless of the active immunization status of the patient, meticulous surgical care, including removal of all devitalized tissue and foreign bodies, should be provided immediately for all wounds. Such care is as essential for the prevention of tetanus as it is for the prevention of other types of wound infection. However, the fact that approximately one-third of patients seen with active tetanus have either no obvious wound or wounds considered to be insignificant emphasizes the problem of tetanus prophylaxis following unknown or minimal wounds and suggests that the disease will not be eliminated until universal active immunization has been achieved. The recommended prophylaxis schedule is outlined in Table 17–10.

The value of antibiotic agents in the prophylaxis of tetanus

TABLE 17–10. Immunization Schedule

Verify a history of tetanus immunization from medical records so that appropriate tetanus prophylaxis can be accomplished.

Td: Tetanus and diphtheria toxoids adsorbed (for adult use)
TIG: Tetanus immune globulin (human)

History of Adsorbed Tetanus Toxoid (doses)	Tetanus-Prone Wounds		Nontetanus-Prone Wounds	
	Td*	TIG	Td*	TIG
Unknown or fewer than 3	Yes	Yes	Yes	No
3 or more†	No‡	No	No§	No

*For children less than 7 years old: DTP (DT, if pertussis vaccine is contraindicated) is preferable to tetanus toxoid alone. For persons 7 years old and older, Td is preferable to tetanus toxoid alone.

†If only three doses of fluid toxoid have been received, a fourth dose of toxoid, preferably an adsorbed toxoid, should be given.

‡Yes, if more than 10 years since last dose.

§Yes, if more than 5 years since last dose. (More frequent boosters are not needed and can accentuate side effects.)

From Advanced Trauma Life Support Course Manual. Chicago, American College of Surgeons, 1989.

remains undetermined. There is no doubt that *C. tetani* is sensitive *in vitro* to penicillin and tetracycline, as well as to other antibiotics; but there seems to be some difficulty in delivering an adequate dose of antibiotics to the susceptible bacteria before they liberate toxin. The tetanus-prone wound characteristically has a decreased blood supply and contains necrotic tissue that may prevent high antibiotic levels from reaching the infecting bacteria. Antibiotic therapy is recommended to not be relied on as adequate prophylactic therapy in place of immunization. For patients with extensive necrotic wounds, particularly those in whom débridement has been delayed or compromised, penicillin and tetracycline have often been used as prophylaxis against other types of wound infection that occur, as well as for prophylactic action against tetanus.

Peripheral Vascular Injuries

Penetration, perforation, transection, and lateral lacerations are the usual forms of injury among patients with penetrating wounds, whereas fracture of the intima with obstruction and thrombosis is the usual type of arterial injury following blunt trauma. Both mechanisms may also induce significant arterial spasm in the vicinity of the injury which will diminish extremity blood flow, but will improve spontaneously. The trauma victim who has the classic clinical signs of arterial injury—loss of pulses, distal ischemia, active arterial bleeding, an expanding hematoma, or an arteriovenous fistula—rarely requires any diagnostic studies before operation. More commonly, however, the patient presents with *soft* signs of arterial injury, including diminished (but not absent) pulses, a history of *significant* bleeding, hypovolemic shock, or an injury in proximity to a major vessel. In such patients the yield from routine exploration is too low to justify the risks, expense, and morbidity. Contrast arteriography as a screening tool in such patients is therefore often used, but it too has high costs and some complications. More recently, some surgeons have reconsidered the merits of serial physical examination in such patients, generally supplemented with the noninvasive diagnostic techniques of Doppler arterial pressure measurement and duplex sonography. One recom-

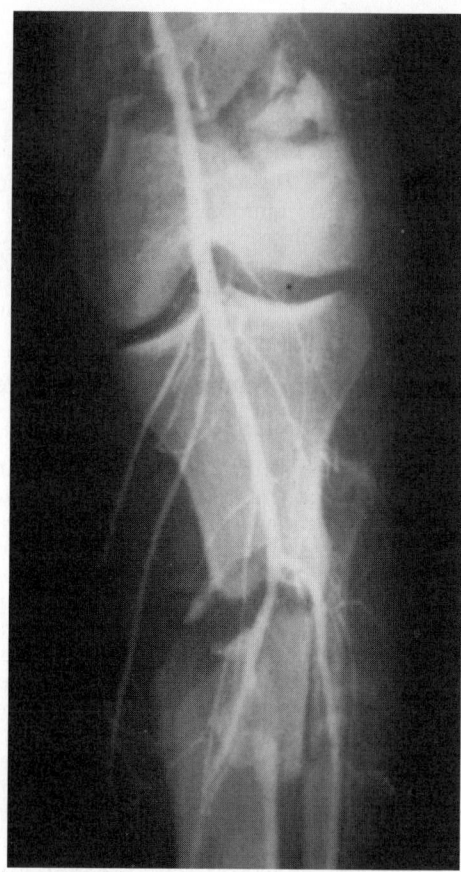

Figure 17–35. Vascular trifurcation injury in a patient with a *free-floating* knee from distal femur and proximal tibiofibular fractures.

mended diagnostic algorithm for the patient with potential extremity arterial injury is illustrated in Figure 17–34.

Arteriography remains a valuable adjunct in assessing the extent of damage, especially if multiple vascular injuries are involved. Additionally, if it is believed that the proposed exploration may not allow complete visualization of the vulnerable portions of the artery and vein, arteriogram may be helpful in planning the operative approach. If severe hemorrhage has occurred, it is often prudent to perform arteriography in the operating room where resuscitation and control of bleeding are usually easier. A patient hemodynamically unstable from extremity trauma should simply not be sent to the x-ray suite. Spontaneous cessation of bleeding is often only temporary and the sudden recurrence of severe hemorrhage is not uncommon.

In the distal part of the leg, vascular injuries are more commonly associated with long bone fractures or knee dislocation. More extensive diagnostic studies are often required in patients with these injuries. In particular, fracture, dislocation or even severe ligamentous disruption at the level of the knee is associated with popliteal artery and vein injuries, and arteriography should be routinely considered in patients with a *floating knee* or posterior knee dislocation (Fig. 17–35). Popliteal vascular trauma is particularly devastating, resulting in amputation more often than any other arterial injury, except the common femoral artery. In one report, 32% of patients with knee dislocations had arterial injuries, and the amputation rate was 86% in those limbs that were not revascularized within 8 hours.[49] When treated by simple ligation in World War II, 73% of these injuries resulted in amputation, and despite rapid transportation and improved vascular techniques, the amputation rate remained approximately

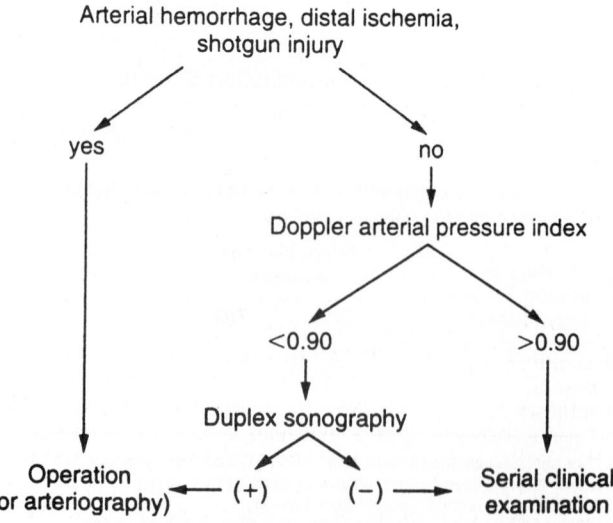

Figure 17–34. Diagnostic algorithm for the patient with potential extremity arterial injury using noninvasive Doppler and duplex sonography in the patient without obvious signs of arterial injury. (From Johansen, K.: Nonarteriographic assessment of penetrating vascular injuries. *In* Ernst, C., and Stanley, J. (Eds.): Current Therapy in Vascular Surgery. St Louis, C. V. Mosby, 1993, pp. 593–595.)

30% in Vietnam, and remains above 10% following civilian trauma.[124]

For fracture dislocations at the knee, a coordinated approach is necessary to allow early rigid fixation of the bony injury and restoration of perfusion as early as possible. External fixation is frequently advantageous. Temporary intraluminal plastic shunts positioned in the popliteal artery (and vein, if necessary) can be used to restore perfusion and to provide the time necessary for reduction and fixation of the bone. Following this, primary repair of the blood vessel is often possible. This approach is most applicable where there is extensive soft tissue and bony injury, and where immediate débridement and extensive extremity manipulation are required prior to bony fixation.

The principles of operative treatment of extremity vascular trauma are identical to those described in Chapter 50 for elective vascular repair. However, fasciotomy is much more often used in the trauma setting, and occasionally the operative field is contaminated. Fasciotomy is almost always necessary in situations in which there are combined popliteal artery and vein injuries, when the patients have extensive bony and muscular injury, following prolonged shock, or after 3 or 4 hours of extremity ischemia time. Current techniques allow routine and frequent measurements of compartment pressures, and accurately indicate those patients requiring fasciotomy. At compartmental pressures exceeding 45 mm. Hg, cell damage is more likely and decompression may be needed, regardless of distal arterial pressure. When fasciotomy is performed in this setting with these measurements, there is usually a prompt fall in pressure followed by a return of neuromuscular function. Percutaneous fasciotomy is not recommended, but rather four-compartment fasciotomy via either a single long lateral incision or a combined medial and lateral incision. Vein graft is generally preferred for bridging an arterial defect in a contaminated wound, although several authors support the use of polytetrafluoroethylene graft in this situation.[75]

Whether venous injuries are best treated by repair or by ligation is still controversial. Data compiled by the Vietnam Vascular Registry revealed a significant reduction in the morbid sequelae of lower extremity venous injuries treated by repair instead of ligation, especially when associated arterial injuries were present.[106] Civilian trauma experience supports this observation, and most trauma surgeons favor simple repair of major unpaired venous lacerations in the stable patient. The controversy relates to complex venous reconstruction in seriously injured patients who require extensive procedures for other injuries. In addition, the incidence of postrepair thrombosis is high, prompting the employment of a number of adjunctive techniques to maintain patency such as temporary distal arteriovenous fistula.[107] The sequelae of ligation or early thrombosis include diminished venous outflow and hence compromised arterial inflow, extremity edema, pulmonary embolism, venous stasis, and postphlebitic syndrome. Even transient patency of the venous repair allows time for the development of collateral circulation and improves arterial reperfusion. If ligation is performed, prolonged postoperative elevation and elastic extremity wrapping may reduce edema and decrease late morbidity.[84]

TRAUMA CARE SYSTEMS

Trauma is the leading cause of death in children and adults up to 44 years of age, and injuries kill more Americans aged 1 to 34 years than all diseases combined. Because trauma is often a disease of the young, it accounts for more productive years of life lost than cancer and all cardiovascular diseases combined. Each year, more than 140,000 Americans die from injuries, and one person in three has a nonfatal injury.[88] One

of every eight hospital beds is occupied by an injured patient. The cost of caring for these injuries is staggering. Direct and indirect health costs for trauma care in 1989 were an estimated $100 billion, and they continue to rise.[105]

In 1966 the National Research Council (NRC) presented a landmark report entitled "Accidental Death and Disability: The Neglected Disease of Modern Society," documenting how little progress had been made in explicating the scientific aspect of injury control and applying what was known.[5] In 1985, the NRC again reported on the status of trauma care in the United States in the report "Injury in America: A Continuing Health Problem."[88] Injury was once again identified as "the principal public health problem in America today," highlighted by the fact that over 2.5 million Americans had died from injuries since the 1966 report. These two sentinel reports acknowledged the need for a coordinated national approach to trauma care, suggesting that special emphasis be directed at six specific topics such as: data collection, injury prevention, biomechanics research, prehospital and hospital care, and rehabilitation. Regionalized trauma centers, integrated with public education, injury prevention, prehospital care, quality assurance, and rehabilitation, form the basis for a systems approach to trauma care.

Prevention and Injury Control

More than 50% of trauma deaths occur within seconds or minutes of injury, and virtually no organized trauma care system, no matter how sophisticated, can save these people. Most of these deaths, however, could be prevented. More than half of the motor vehicle related deaths in the United States involved intoxicated drivers; a staggering 80% of intentional penetrating trauma deaths occur in intoxicated individuals.[88] Cities and countries with fewer handguns have a significantly lower homicide rate.[123] The mandatory use of seatbelts in Australia resulted in a 27% reduction in motor vehicle fatalities.[131] Each of these statistics represents a potential area of injury control.

The field of injury control has progressed beyond the traditional limited focus on *accident prevention*. The injury itself should be considered as resulting from energy transfer to the individual that exceeds the threshold for tissue damage. This damage can be controlled by preventing the event itself from occurring (e.g., the motor vehicle crash), lessening the energy transfer to the individual (e.g., using seatbelts and airbags) or by limiting the extent of the injury once it has occurred (e.g., prompt emergency medical system [EMS] and trauma center care).

Concurrent with this broadening of the scope of injury control is the shift from active to passive approaches to prevention. Active strategies are those requiring the active, continued cooperation on the part of the individual to be protected. In contrast, passive strategies are effective without requiring any special response from the individual. Passive approaches or a combination of passive and active strategies, on the whole, have proved much more successful in reducing the toll from injuries than has sole reliance on active strategies. Motor vehicle occupant injuries can be prevented by the use of seatbelts or airbags, the latter being a much more effective option, particularly for teenagers and intoxicated drivers, because it works automatically, without requiring action by the individual. Tap water scalds to young children can be prevented by constant and close parental supervision for the first 5 years of the child's life; alternatively, the water heater temperature setting can be lowered to 125° F. or, better yet, preset to this temperature at the factory.

Legislation has also been used successfully in injury control. Motorcycle helmet laws are remarkably successful in increasing helmet use from approximately 50% to 95% or more. All 50 states have mandatory childseat restraint legislation, and more than half have mandatory seatbelt use laws for drivers and other passengers. These laws have increased seat restraint use more than 60% nationwide and have resulted in 9% to 12% reduction in occupant fatalities.[88] Many states have legislation requiring water heaters to be preset at 120 to 125° F. eliminating the risk of this type of burn in those states.

Many problems remain, however. For instance, the politically sensitive topic of firearm injuries is a major public health and trauma problem. Each year, more than 30,000 people lose their lives from gunshot wounds, either accidentally or as a result of suicide or homicide.[116] Approximately 10-fold more are injured and require hospital and surgical care. Substance abuse, particularly that from the use of alcohol, also makes an enormous contribution to the injury toll. Although the proportion of motor vehicle fatalities involving alcohol has decreased from 56% to 52% between 1981 and 1986, 77% of nighttime fatal crashes involve alcohol-intoxicated drivers.[87] The Surgeon General's Workshop on Drunk Driving has laid out a clear agenda for combating the problem, including administrative revocation of licenses, random breath testing, mandatory jail sentences, increased excise taxes, and lowered legal blood alcohol limits.[129]

Regional Organization of Trauma Care

The goal of a trauma care system is to decrease mortality and minimize disability and morbidity resulting from injury. Trauma deaths are often considered to follow a trimodal distribution: immediate, early, and late. As discussed in the preceding section, most immediate deaths (e.g., those from severe head injury and transected aorta) can be prevented only by public education and new insights into injury control. In contrast, patients dying an early death most often have severe, yet correctable, injuries such as epidural or subdural hematoma, hemopneumothorax, spleen or liver fracture, or blood loss from fractures and multiple injuries. The interval of time between injury and treatment and the quality of treatment are particularly critical in these patients. Trauma center hospitals and coordinated prehospital care impacts most directly on these patients. Those trauma victims dying late deaths generally succumb to infection, sepsis, and multiple organ failure, often as a consequence of initial management. It is argued that these patients, too, benefit from regionalized trauma care by concentrating the most difficult patients in centers specially equipped and staffed.

Incorporation of regionalized trauma care throughout the United States involves cooperation between governments, insurance agencies, hospitals, physicians, and other health care providers. Data have been provided by a number of currently functioning regional trauma care systems that clearly show a decrease in mortality and morbidity, at a reasonable cost.[16, 85] Regionalized trauma care ideally should incorporate all three phases of trauma care: prehospital, hospital, and rehabilitation.[33]

Prehospital Care

The vital components of prehospital care include a committed medical control, established lines of communication, tested triage criteria, effective transportation, and a cadre of prehospital providers well trained in specific field interventions. Although hospitals were first developed by the Romans for care of the military legions, prehospital or field care of the injured victim can be traced back to the Edwin Smith Papyrus (3000–1600 B.C.), and undoubtedly was provided in prehistoric times. Most of the ancient history of medicine involves the field care of the injured patient, consisting primarily of *first aid*. The beginning of modern EMS can perhaps be traced to 1962, when the Chicago Committee on Trauma and the Chicago Fire Department collaborated to develop a prehospital trauma school. In 1966 the National Highway Safety Act authorized the United States Department of Transportation to fund ambulance services, communication systems, and training programs to address the need of the trauma victim prior to reaching the hospital. In 1969 the United States Department of Transportation published the first manual for Emergency Medical Technician–Ambulance (EMT-A) training, based on the Chicago trauma school program, to which has subsequently been added training for paramedics (EMT-P).

Medical Control. An integral component of an EMS system is active physician involvement in establishing, directing, and monitoring emergency medical care. The 1973 Emergency Medical Services Systems (EMSS) Act authorized federal funding for EMSs that regionalized prehospital emergency care into a series of interrelated components and identified physician involvement as an essential element of this EMS. State and local governments have since assumed responsibility for EMS development and its medical control with variable enthusiasm and effectiveness. As a result, there is wide regional variability in the policies, procedures, and authority of medical control of EMSs. Nonetheless, the basic premise of medical control of an EMS remains the physician-directed assurance of quality emergency medical care. In caring for the trauma patient, such assurance requires that surgeons and other physicians involved and interested in and committed to quality trauma care be knowledgeable and active participants in the medical control of EMSs.

Triage. The term *triage* is derived from the French word *trier*, meaning "to sort or to cull out," originally used to describe the practice of sorting wool into various categories depending on its quality. Military triage involves prioritizing victims according to the severity of injury, likelihood of survival, and urgency of care. The goal of civilian prehospital triage in modern trauma systems is the rapid and accurate field identification of high-risk injured patients who would benefit from treatment in a trauma center. Since only 5% to 10% of all injured patients are believed to require high-level trauma center care, a second consideration of civilian triage is to limit the transport of the less severely injured victims to trauma centers, thereby preventing overburdening the trauma center and involving local or community hospitals.[33]

The accurate field identification of a patient with high risk of major injury is problematic. Assessment often must be made quickly, often under adverse conditions with limited resources. In addition, current schemes for identifying such high-risk patients are of limited accuracy. Many patients with severe injuries and at risk of dying can be identified at the scene of the accident by their abnormal physiology. A far more difficult problem in triage is the identification of high-risk patients whose physiologic status is normal at initial evaluation. A number of scoring systems, checklists, and criteria have been recommended to assist the EMS providers in this task of field triage and to aid hospitals and trauma systems in comparing outcomes.[19] Perhaps the most useful currently available system is that advocated by the Committee on Trauma of the American College of Surgeons, which assesses four components: physiologic response, injury anatomy, injury biomechanics, and comorbid factors (Fig. 17–36).[2]

Because the goal of a trauma system is to prevent unnecessary death, a certain degree of *overtriage* can be accepted, presuming that trauma centers can decrease the morbidity and mortality of injury as compared with nontrauma center care. *Undertriage* is therefore less desirable, because of the implication that an injured patient who would have benefited from trauma center care was misclassified and sent to a

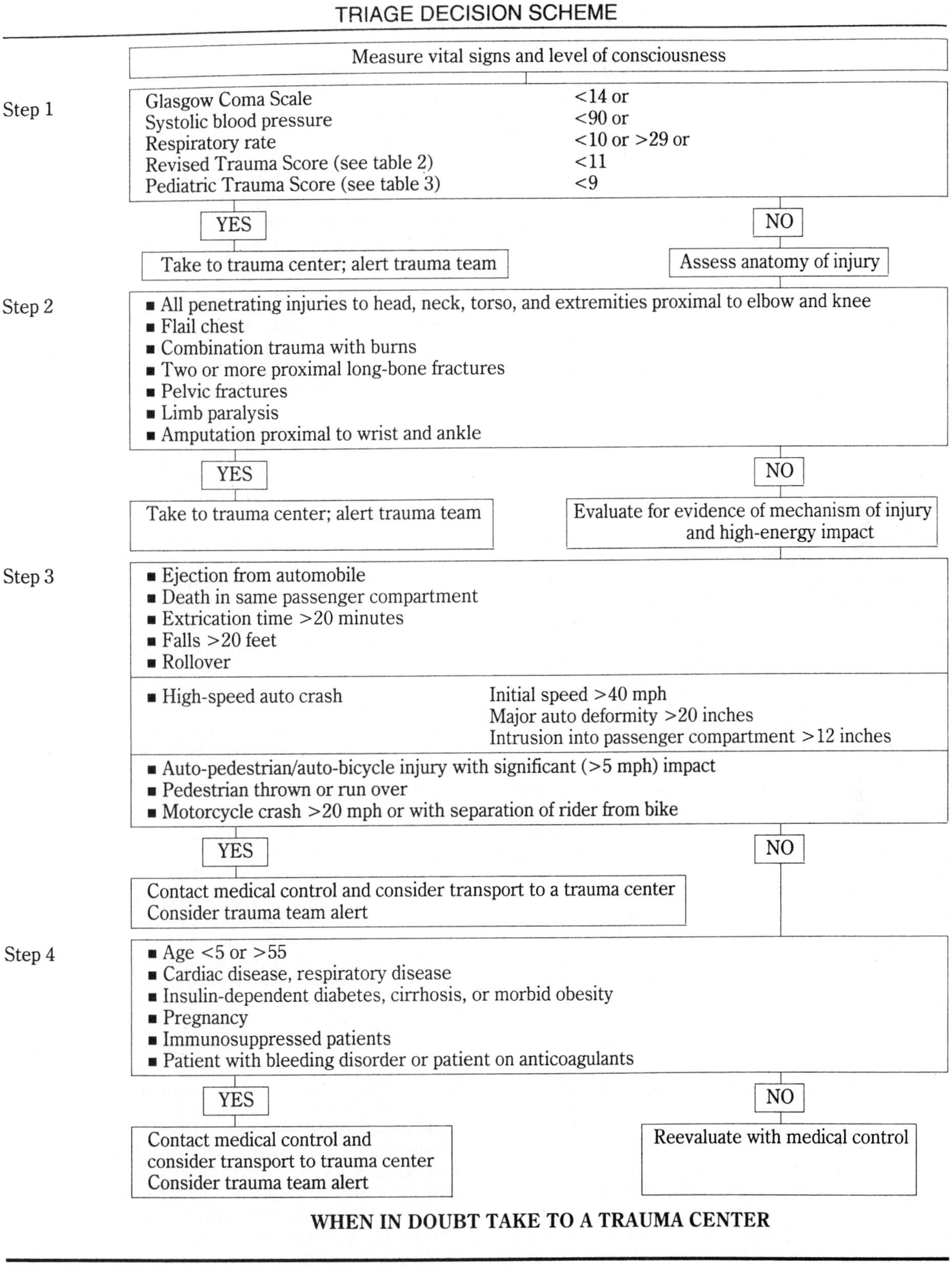

TRIAGE DECISION SCHEME

Measure vital signs and level of consciousness

Step 1

Glasgow Coma Scale	<14 or
Systolic blood pressure	<90 or
Respiratory rate	<10 or >29 or
Revised Trauma Score (see table 2)	<11
Pediatric Trauma Score (see table 3)	<9

YES → Take to trauma center; alert trauma team

NO → Assess anatomy of injury

Step 2

- All penetrating injuries to head, neck, torso, and extremities proximal to elbow and knee
- Flail chest
- Combination trauma with burns
- Two or more proximal long-bone fractures
- Pelvic fractures
- Limb paralysis
- Amputation proximal to wrist and ankle

YES → Take to trauma center; alert trauma team

NO → Evaluate for evidence of mechanism of injury and high-energy impact

Step 3

- Ejection from automobile
- Death in same passenger compartment
- Extrication time >20 minutes
- Falls >20 feet
- Rollover

- High-speed auto crash

| Initial speed >40 mph
| Major auto deformity >20 inches
| Intrusion into passenger compartment >12 inches

- Auto-pedestrian/auto-bicycle injury with significant (>5 mph) impact
- Pedestrian thrown or run over
- Motorcycle crash >20 mph or with separation of rider from bike

YES → Contact medical control and consider transport to a trauma center
Consider trauma team alert

NO →

Step 4

- Age <5 or >55
- Cardiac disease, respiratory disease
- Insulin-dependent diabetes, cirrhosis, or morbid obesity
- Pregnancy
- Immunosuppressed patients
- Patient with bleeding disorder or patient on anticoagulants

YES → Contact medical control and consider transport to trauma center
Consider trauma team alert

NO → Reevaluate with medical control

WHEN IN DOUBT TAKE TO A TRAUMA CENTER

Figure 17–36. An example of a field triage decision scheme, as advocated by the Committee on Trauma, American College of Surgeons. Note the four-step assessment of physiologic response, anatomic location, injury mechanism, and comorbid factors. (From Resources for Optimal Care of the Injured Patient. Chicago, American College of Surgeons, Committee on Trauma, 1993, p. 20.)

nontrauma center. Studies have suggested that an overtriage rate as high as 50% may be required to maintain a minimum level of undertriage. That is, 50% of patients brought to the trauma center did not constitute *major trauma victims*. The absolute number of patients overtriaged is small. A 1-year review of the Orange County, California, trauma center triage documented a 60% overtriage rate based on a definition of a major trauma victim as a patient with an injury severity score of 16 or higher, yet only 5.5% of all paramedic transports of trauma patients during that same year went to trauma centers.[136]

Field Interventions. The principles of field treatment of the trauma victim include (1) securing the area and preventing further injury; (2) determining the need for emergency treatment; (3) initiating treatment according to protocols or medical control direction; (4) communication with medical control; and (5) rapid transport of the patient to the appropriate trauma facility. The treatment rendered at the scene varies, depending on patient injury, local medical practices (as determined by medical control), and training and experience of prehospital providers. In general, the prehospital care and hospital destination of the trauma patient is much different from that of the medical arrest victim. Although advanced cardiac life support measures at the scene clearly improve survival for cardiac victims, the goal in prehospital trauma care is to deliver the patient to a hospital where definitive operative capabilities exist.

The role of advanced life support (ALS) interventions in the trauma victim is a topic of considerable debate, centering around the efficacy of immediate evacuation *(scoop and run)* versus scene resuscitation *(stay and play)*. Regions with highly trained and experienced paramedics often support the judicious use of prehospital ALS skills such as intravenous access and fluid administration, endotracheal intubation, and needle thoracentesis. Others argue that such interventions merely prolong field times and delay the definitive operative intervention and that fluid administration may in fact be deleterious in certain circumstances.

In contrast, few would argue that establishment of an effective airway and control of external hemorrhage are beneficial prehospital maneuvers. In some systems, the field resuscitation can mimic the emergency department maneuvers, short of diagnostic steps, and save emergency department time while not delaying transport. Over a 3-year period, the Seattle Medic One paramedic EMS transported 5761 injured patients to the same trauma center.[26] One hundred thirty-one of these patients required cardiopulmonary resuscitation, and 30 (23%) of the 131 patients survived. An endotracheal tube was successfully placed in 29 (97%) of 30 survivors, and two intravenous lines were successfully placed in all the survivors; 2200 ml. of lactated Ringer's solution was administered; and the transport time averaged 22 minutes. Such interventions were interpreted as effective in resuscitating the trauma victim, as evidenced by a statistically significant increase in blood pressure from the field to the trauma center. The Denver paramedic experience is similar.[28]

Transportation. The concept of rapid transportation of injured patients to a medical facility probably originated with Dominique Jean Larrey, the chief surgeon of Napoleon's French Army. Larrey is credited with developing horse-drawn carts, or *flying ambulances*, to transport the wounded as quickly as possible to medical care behind the battle lines. Until that time, wounded were left on the battle field until combat had ceased. By World War I the horse-drawn ambulance carts had been replaced by motorized vehicles, even though the first civilian use of a motorized ambulance was during the 1906 San Francisco earthquake, when trucks and milk wagons were pressed into service to help transport the injured. The Korean Conflict introduced helicopter transpor-

tation of the wounded, a technique that was expanded on and refined during the Vietnam War. Civilian aeromedical transport has been possible via military helicopters in the Military Assistance to Safety and Traffic program since 1970, and the first hospital-based aeromedical transport program in the United States was established in Denver in 1972.[21] The explosion of hospital-based aeromedical transport programs did not occur in the United States, however, until the early 1980s. According to the Association of Air Medical Services, in 1990 there were 180 hospital-based helicopter programs in the United States (personal communication, 1990).

The preferred method of transportation of the injured victim depends on the patient's condition, the distance to the regional trauma center, accessibility of the scene, and weather conditions. In the urban setting, ground ambulances usually afford the most efficient means of delivering the injured patient to a capable trauma center, although urban sprawl, traffic congestion, and natural barriers such as rivers may influence the decision to use helicopter transport. In rural areas, however, the time and distance to a regional trauma center may be long, and the prehospital care provider may be faced with the decision either to transport to a closer nontrauma center or to call for a remote aeromedical helicopter. Developing clear transportation guidelines is an integral component of regionalized trauma care. Such guidelines must account for regional variabilities in personnel, facilities, and geography. In general, helicopter transport may be beneficial if 15 to 20 minutes of prehospital time can be saved or when distance to the nearest trauma center is greater than 20 to 30 miles. If transport distances exceed 100 to 150 miles, fixed-wing aircraft is more useful.

Hospital Care

Hospital care consists of care provided in the emergency department, operating room, and acute care units. Trauma care is complex, having many confusing facets; a successful patient outcome demands concise thinking and practiced execution. The care of the multi-injured victim is best suited to a team approach, with help from nurses, aides, medical technicians, and consulting physicians. The importance of predesignated team members and preassigned duties cannot be overemphasized. Of equally vital importance is the predetermined selection of a single individual as the *team leader* or *captain*. It is critical that the team captain be willing to accept the responsibility of leadership and that other team members acknowledge and accept this person as the team captain. Ideally, the team captain is the most senior trauma surgeon available, although in some institutions an emergency physician assumes this role until the surgeon is available. Overall patient assessment and all management decisions are made by the team captain, but when possible, technical procedures should be delegated to other team members. This allows the team captain to oversee the resuscitation continually, ensuring that no details are neglected or overlooked and that the resuscitation is appropriately focused.

Other physician team members may include surgical house staff, emergency physicians, anesthesiologists, or primary care physicians experienced in trauma resuscitation. The available staffing clearly depends on the type of medical institution (i.e., community hospital versus university teaching hospital) and its resources, but sufficient personnel must be preassigned and available for trauma resuscitations. The primary role of the physician team members is to execute the therapeutic and diagnostic maneuvers ordered by the team captain, and they must refrain from independent clinical decision making. Emergency department nurses are also invaluable in trauma resuscitation. Their primary responsibilities include measuring and reporting vital signs, providing resuscitation fluids, and assisting in procedures, although myriad related activities are dependent on nursing organization and preparation. Documentation of resuscitation activities is an essential component of care and may require a single staff member's attention. The organized response and duties of aides, technicians (laboratory, radiology, and respiratory), and assistants should add efficiency, not chaos, noise, or confusion.

The emergency department is the portal of entry into the hospital's services, not the site of definitive care. Definitive care in trauma victims often requires a surgical operation, and considerable judgment must be exercised by the team captain in not delaying essential operative procedures by minor therapeutic efforts and nonessential diagnostic maneuvers.

Rehabilitation

Care of the disabled patient perhaps represents the most significant deficiency in trauma care in the United States today. Rehabilitation, too frequently ignored in regional plans, plays an integral role in returning the patient to a productive life. For each trauma-related death, two or three patients experience associated permanent or partial disabilities, annually accounting for 350,000 patients, yet only 1 in 10 newly disabled patients uses rehabilitation facilities. The cost of disability is staggering, accounting for an estimated annual $35 billion in lost wages and 570 million recuperating days off work.[105] Yet for every dollar spent on rehabilitation, several dollars are saved by state and federal governments in long-term support. The relatively low incidence and prevalence of neurologic, multiple orthopedic, and burn injuries simply fails to imply how important and costly the problems that result can be. Unfortunately, there are no aggregate statistics on the lifetime impact of these conditions.

With the exception of a few excellent spinal cord rehabilitation centers, insignificant effort has been expended on incorporating rehabilitation into regionalized trauma care systems. The efficacy of rehabilitation, however, has been well documented, at least for spinal cord injuries. Rehabilitation can provide deinstitutionalization for 85% of patients in spinal cord centers and decrease the incidence of complications and subsequent hospitalizations, while expending less than 10% of the cost of custodial care and repeated hospitalizations.[88] The spinal cord rehabilitation system should serve as a model of incorporating regionalized rehabilitation into the global trauma care system.

Research and Education

Identifying future directions in trauma care and injury research is also a requirement of regional centers. Research and education remain the mainstay of medical advances, and trauma care is no exception. Training providers of trauma care has historically been the province of surgery departments, with little emphasis placed on research into the epidemiology, biomechanics, rehabilitation, and prevention aspects of trauma care. Calls for improving trauma research expenditures have resulted in the formation of the Center for Injury Control (CIC) as a section of the Centers for Disease Control and Prevention and an increased focus on trauma care as a health and social issue. Support of research in the academic settings has been a goal of the CIC that will indirectly contribute to the care rendered and the training of future researchers. Adequate funding remains problematic in a time of restricted resources and multiple major federal commitments.

Summary

Idealized trauma care involves what has come to be known as the *systems approach* to trauma care. The key components of an idealized, well-functioning trauma care system begin with public education and injury prevention. Significant improvements in prehospital, hospital, and rehabilitative care can be accomplished by thoughtful organization and concentration of scarce and expensive resources. Many leaders in the field of trauma care argue that regionalization of care, increased funding for research, education, and prevention, and an equitable method of providing health care for the uncompensated or uninsured trauma victim are desperately required at this time.

REFERENCES

1. Allen, R., and Blaisdell, F.: Injuries to the inferior vena cava. Surg. Clin. North Am., *52*:699, 1972.
2. American College of Surgeons Committee on Trauma: Field categorization of trauma patients (field triage). Resources for Optimal Care of the Injured Patient. Chicago, American College of Surgeons Committee on Trauma, 1990.
3. Arreola-Risa, C., Rhee, P., Boyle, E., et al.: Factors influencing outcome in stab wounds of the heart. Am. J. Surg., *169*(5):553, 1995.
4. Asesnio, J., Valenziano, C., Falcone, R., et al.: Management of penetrating neck injuries: The controversy surrounding zone II injuries. Surg. Clin. North Am., *71*(2):267, 1991.
5. Behrman, S., Fabian, T., Kudsk, K., et al.: Improved outcome with femur fractures: Early versus delayed fixation. J. Trauma, *30*:792, 1990.
6. Beitsch, P., Weigelt, J., Flynn, E., et al.: Physical examination and arteriography in patients with penetrating zone II neck wounds. Arch. Surg., *129*(6):577, 1994.
7. Ben-Menachem, Y., Coldwell, D., Young, J., et al.: Hemorrhage associated with pelvic fractures: Causes, diagnosis, and emergent management. AJR, *157*:1005, 1991.
8. Berni, G., Bandyk, D., Oreskovich, M., et al.: Role of intra-operative pancreatography in patients with injury to the pancreas. Am. J. Surg., *143*:602, 1982.
9. Biffl, W., Moore, F., Moore, E., et al.: Cardiac enzymes are irrelevant in the patient with suspected myocardial contusion. Am. J. Surg., *169*:523, 1994.
10. Bohlman, H.: Acute fractures and dislocations of the cervical spine. J. Bone Joint Surg., *61A*:119, 1979.
11. Bone, L., Johnson, K., Weigelt, J., et al.: Early versus delayed stabilization of fractures: A prospective randomized study. J. Bone Joint Surg., *71A*:336, 1989.
12. Bouwman, D., Waver, D., and Walt, A.: Serum amylase and its isoenzymes: A clarification of their implication in trauma. J. Trauma, *24*:573, 1984.
13. Bracken, M., Shepard, M., Collins, W., et al.: A randomized, controlled trial of methylprednisolone or naloxone in the treatment of acute spinal cord injury. N. Engl. J. Med., *322*:1405, 1990.
14. Burch, J., Brock, J., Gevirtzman, L., et al.: The injured colon. Ann. Surg., *203*:701, 1986.
15. Carducci, B., Lowe, R., and Dalsey, W.: Penetrating neck trauma: Consensus and controversies. Ann. Emerg. Med., *15*:208, 1986.
16. Cales, R., and Trunkey, D.: Preventable trauma deaths: A review of trauma care systems development. JAMA, *254*:1059, 1985.
17. Carrico, C.: 1993 presidential address, American Association for the Surgery of Trauma: It's time to drain the swamp. J. Trauma, *37*(4):532, 1994.
18. Cass, A., and Luxenberg, M.: Which renal lacerations will heal satisfactorily with nonsurgical management? Urology, *33*:367, 1989.
19. Champion, H., and Sacco, W.: Trauma scoring. *In* Mattox, K., Moore, E. E., and Feliciano, F. V. (Eds.): Trauma. Norwalk, CT, Appleton & Lange, 1988, p. 63.
20. Chappuis, C., Frey, D., Dietzen, C., et al.: Management of penetrating colon injuries: A prospective, randomized trial. Ann. Surg., *213*(5):492, 1991.
21. Cleveland, H., Bigelow, D., Dracon, D., et al.: A civilian air emergency service: A report of its development, technical aspects, and experience. J. Trauma, *16*:452, 1976.
22. Coburn, M. C., Pfeifer, J., and DeLuca, F. G.: Nonoperative management of splenic and hepatic trauma in the multiply injured pediatric and adolescent patient. Arch. Surg., *130*(3):332, 1995.
23. Cogbill, T., Moore, E., Jurkovich, G., et al.: Nonoperative management of blunt splenic trauma: A multicenter experience. J. Trauma, *29*(10):1312, 1989.
24. Cogbill, T., Moore, E., Jurkovich, G., et al.: Severe hepatic trauma: A multicenter experience with 1335 liver injuries. J. Trauma, *28*:1312, 1988.
25. Cogbill, T., Moore, E., Meissner, M., et al.: The spectrum of blunt injury to the carotid artery: A multicenter perspective. J. Trauma, *27*(11):1221, 1994.
26. Copass, M., Oreskovich, M., Bladergren, M., et al.: Prehospital cardiopul-

monary resuscitation of the critically injured patient. Am. J. Surg., *148*:20, 1984.

27. Corriere, J., Jr., and Sandler, C.: Management of the ruptured bladder: Seven years of experience with 111 cases. J. Trauma, *26*:830, 1986.

28. Cwinn, A., Pons, P., Moore, E., et al.: Prehospital advanced life support for critical blunt trauma victims. Ann. Emerg. Med., *16*:399, 1987.

29. Dang, C., Schlater, T., Bui, H., et al.: Delayed rupture of the spleen. Ann. Emerg. Med., *19*:399, 1990.

30. Dawson, D., and Jurkovich, G.: Hepatic duct disruption from blunt abdominal trauma: Case report and literature review. J. Trauma, *31*(12):454, 1991.

31. Diamond, L.: Splenectomy in childhood and the hazard of overwhelming infection. Pediatrics, *43*:886, 1969.

32. DiGiacomo, J., Schwab, C., Rotondo, M., et al.: Gluteal gunshot wounds: Who warrants exploration? J. Trauma, *37*(4):622, 1994.

33. Eastman, A., Lewiss, F., Jr., Champion, H., et al.: Regional trauma system design: Critical concepts. Am. J. Surg., *154*:79, 1987.

34. Eraklis, A., and Filler, R.: Splenectomy in childhood: A review of 1413 cases. J. Pediatr. Surg., *4*:382, 1972.

35. Esposito, T., Jurkovich, G., Rice, C., et al.: Reappraisal of emergency room thoracotomy in a changing environment. J. Trauma, *31*(7):881, 1991.

36. Faringer, P., Mullins, R., Feliciano, P., et al.: Selective fecal diversion in complex open pelvic fractures from blunt trauma. Arch. Surg., *129*:958, 1994.

37. Fedson, D.: Adult immunization: Summary of the national vaccine advisory committee report. JAMA, *272*(14):1133, 1994.

38. Feliciano, D., Martin, T., Cruse, P., et al.: Management of combined pancreatoduodenal injuries. Ann. Surg., *205*:673, 1987.

39. Feliciano, D., Mattox, K., Burch, J., et al.: Packing for control of hepatic hemorrhage. J. Trauma, *26*:738, 1986.

40. Feliciano, P., Mullins, R., Trunkey, D., et al.: A decision analysis of traumatic splenic injuries. J. Trauma, *33*(3):340, 1992.

41. Feliciano, D., and Pachter, H.: Hepatic trauma revisited. Curr. Prob. Surg., *26*:459, 1989.

42. Flaherty, L., and Jurkovich, G.: Minor splenic injuries: Associated injuries and transfusion requirements. J. Trauma, *31*(12):1618, 1991.

43. Fox, M., and Fabian, T.: The pelvis. *In* Moore, E. E. (Ed.): Early Care of the Injured Patient, 4th ed. Toronto, B. C. Decker, 1990.

44. Fuhrman, G., Stieg, F., and Buerk, C.: Blunt laryngeal trauma: Classification and management protocol. J. Trauma, *30*(1):87, 1990.

45. Garcia, J.: Morphology of global cerebral ischemia. Crit. Care Med., *16*:979, 1988.

46. Gokcen, E., Burgess, A., Sigel, J., et al.: Pelvic fracture mechanism of injury in vehicular trauma patients. J. Trauma, *36*:789, 1994.

47. Graham, J., Mattox, K., Beall, A., Jr., et al.: Traumatic injuries of the inferior vena cava. Arch. Surg., *113*:413, 1978.

48. Green, J., Shackford, S., Sise, M., et al.: Late septic complications in adults following splenectomy for trauma: A prospective analysis in 144 patients. J. Trauma, *26*:999, 1986.

49. Green, N., and Allen, B.: Vascular injuries associated with dislocation of the knee. J. Bone Joint Surg., *59A*:236, 1977.

50. Gruss, J.: Complex craniomaxillofacial trauma: Evolving concepts in management. A trauma unit's experience—1989 Fraser B. Gurd lecture. J. Trauma, *30*(4):377, 1990.

51. Guerriero, W.: Trauma to the kidney, ureters, bladder, and urethra. Surg. Clin. North Am., *62*:1047, 1982.

52. Gundry, S., Williams, S., et al.: Indications for aortography in blunt thoracic trauma: A reassessment. J. Trauma, *22*:664, 1982.

53. Gussack, G. S., and Jurkovich, G. J.: Treatment dilemmas in laryngotracheal trauma. J. Trauma, *28*:1439, 1988.

54. Guth, A., Pachter, L., and Kim, U.: Pitfalls in the diagnosis of blunt diaphragmatic injury. Am. J. Surg., *170*:5, 1995.

55. Hansen, S. J.: Overview of the severely traumatized lower limb: Reconstruction versus amputation. Clin. Orthop., *24*:17, 1989.

56. Hasson, J., Stern, D., and Moss, G.: Penetrating duodenal trauma. J. Trauma, *24*:471, 1984.

57. Hirshberg, A., Wall, M., Johnston, R. J., et al.: Transcervical gunshot injuries. Am. J. Surg., *167*(3):208, 1994.

58. Ivatury, R., Rohman, M., and Nallathambi, M.: The morbidity of injuries of the extrahepatic biliary system. J. Trauma, *25*:967, 1985.

59. Jennett, B.: Prognosis of patients with severe head injury. Neurosurgery, *4*:243, 1979.

60. Jones, R.: Management of pancreatic trauma. Am. J. Surg., *150*:698, 1985.

61. Jurkovich, G.: The neck. *In* Moore, E. (Ed.): Early Care of the Injured Patient. Toronto, B. C. Decker, 1990, p. 126.

62. Jurkovich, G., and Carrico, G.: Management of pancreatic injuries. Surg. Clin. North Am., *70*:575, 1990.

63. Jurkovich, G., Greiser, W., Luterman, A., et al.: Hypothermia in trauma patients: An ominous predictor of survival. J. Trauma, *27*:1019, 1987.

64. Jurkovich, G., Hoyt, D., Moore, F., et al.: Portal triad injuries: A multi-institutional study. J. Trauma, *39*(3):426, 1995.

65. Kane, W.: Fractures of the pelvis. *In* Rockwood, C., and Green, D. (Eds.): Fractures. Philadelphia, J. B. Lippincott, 1975, p. 923.

66. King, H., and Schumacher, H.: Splenic studies: I. Susceptibility to infection after splenectomy performed in infancy. Ann. Surg., *136*:239, 1952.

67. Kirsch, M., and Sloan, H.: Blunt chest trauma. *In* General Principles of Management. Boston, Little, Brown & Company, 1977.

68. Krengel, W., Anderson, P., and Henley, M.: Early stabilization and decompression for incomplete paraplegia due to a thoracic-level spinal cord injury. Spine, *18*(14):2080, 1993.

69. Latenser, B., Getilleblo, L., Tarver, A., et al.: Improved outcome with early fracture fixation of skeletally unstable pelvic fractures. J. Trauma, *31*:28, 1991.

70. Llende, M., Santiago-Delpin, E., and Lavergne, J.: Immunobiological consequences of splenectomy: A review. J. Surg. Res., *149*:716, 1985.

71. Lucas, C. E.: Splenic trauma: Choice of management [see comments]. Ann. Surg., *213*(2):98, 1991.

72. Lucas, C., and Ledgerwood, A.: Factors influencing outcome after blunt duodenal injury. J. Trauma, *15*:839, 1975.

73. Luna, G., and Dellinger, E.: Nonoperative observation therapy for splenic injuries: A safe therapeutic option? Am. J. Surg., *153*:462, 1987.

74. Mansour, M., Moore, E., Moore, F., et al.: Exigent postinjury thoracotomy analysis of blunt versus penetrating trauma. Surg. Gynecol. Obstet., *175*(2):97, 1992.

75. Martin, L., McKenney, M., Sosa, J., et al.: Management of lower extremity arterial trauma. J. Trauma, *37*(4):591, 1994.

76. Mattox, K., Flint, L., Carrico, C., et al.: Blunt cardiac injury. J. Trauma, *33*(5):649, 1992.

77. Mays, E.: Demonstration of collateral arterial flow after interruption of hepatic arteries in man. N. Engl. J. Med., *290*:993, 1974.

78. McAllister, E., Perez, M., Albrink, M., et al.: Is triple-contrast computed tomographic scanning useful in the selective management of stab wounds to the back? J. Trauma, *37*(3):401, 1994.

79. Mendez, C., Gubler, K., and Maier, R.: Diagnostic accuracy of peritoneal lavage in patients with pelvic fracture. Arch. Surg., *129*(5):477, 1994.

80. Merion, R., Harness, J., Ramsburgh, S., et al.: Selective management of penetrating neck trauma: Cost implications. Arch. Surg., *116*:691, 1981.

81. Miller, F., Shumate, C., and Richardson, J.: Myocardial contusion: When can the diagnosis be eliminated? Arch. Surg., *124*:805, 1989.

82. Moreno, C., Moore, E., Majure, J., et al.: Hemorrhage associated with major pelvic fractures—a multispecialty challenge. J. Trauma, *26*:821, 1986.

83. Mucha, P. J., and Farnell, M.: Analysis of pelvic fracture management. J. Trauma, *24*:379, 1984.

84. Mullins, R., Lucas, C., and Ledgerwood, A.: The natural history following venous ligation for civilian injuries. J. Trauma, *20*:737, 1980.

85. Mullins, R., Veum-Stone, J., Helfand, M., et al.: Outcome of hospitalized injured patients after institution of a trauma system in an urban area. JAMA, *271*(24):1919, 1994.

86. Nance, F. Injuries to the colon and rectum. *In* Mattox, K., Moore, E., and Feliciano, D. (Eds.): Trauma. Norwalk, CT, Appleton & Lange, 1988, p. 495.

87. National Highway Traffic Safety Administration: Fatal accident reporting system. DOT HS 807 245 (March), 1988.

88. National Highway Traffic Safety Administration: Traffic Status Report, 1989.

89. National Research Council: Injury in America: A Continuing Public Health Problem. Washington, DC, National Academy Press, 1985.

90. National Research Council–National Academy of Sciences: Accidental Death and Disability: The Neglected Disease of Modern Society. Washington, DC, 1966.

91. Niemi, T., and Norton, L.: Vaginal injuries in patients with pelvic fractures. J. Trauma, *25*:547, 1985.

92. Olson, R. A.: Fractures of the mandible: A review of 580 cases. J. Oral Maxillofac. Surg., *40*:23, 1982.

93. Oreskovich, M., and Carrico, C.: Stab wounds of the anterior abdomen: Analysis of a management plan using local wound exploration and quantitative peritoneal lavage. Ann. Surg., *198*:411, 1983.

94. Pachter, H., Spencer, F., Hofstetter, S., et al.: Significant trends in the treatment of hepatic trauma. Ann. Surg., *215*(5):492, 1992.

95. Parks, S., and Hastings, P.: Complications of colostomy closure. Am. Surgeon, *149*:672, 1985.

96. Parmley, L., and Mattingly, T.: Nonpenetrating traumatic injury of the aorta. Circulation, *17*:1086, 1958.

97. Patel, K., Kulkarni, S., Semel, L., et al.: Abdominal vascular trauma. Contemp. Surg., *30*:13, 1987.

98. Peitzman, A., Makaroun, M., Slasky, B., et al.: Prospective study of computed tomography in initial management of blunt abdominal trauma. J. Trauma, *26*:585, 1986.

99. Pennal, G., Tile, M., Waddell, J., et al.: Pelvic disruption: Assessment and classification. Clin. Orthop., *151*:12, 1980.

100. Perchinsky, M., Long, W., and Hill, J.: Blunt cardiac rupture—the Emanuel Trauma Center experience. Arch. Surg., *130*(8):852, 1995.

101. Phillips, E., Rogers, W., and Gaspar, M.: First rib fractures: Incidence of vascular injury and indications for angiography. Surgery, *89*:42, 1981.

102. Powell, D., Bivins, B., and Bell, R.: Diagnostic peritoneal lavage. Surg. Gynecol. Obstet., *155*:257, 1982.

103. Reed, R., Merrell, R., Meyers, W., et al.: Continuing evolution in the approach to severe liver trauma. Ann. Surg., *216*(5):524, 1992.

104. Rene, G., Mattox, K., and Beall, A.: Recent advances in operative management of massive chest trauma. Ann. Thorac. Surg., *16*:52, 1973.

105. Rice, D., and MacKenzie, E.: Cost of injury in the United States: A report to congress. Institute for Health & Aging, University of California, and Injury Prevention Center, The Johns Hopkins University, 1989, p. 7.

106. Rich, N., Hughes, C., and Baugh, J.: Management of venous injuries. Ann. Surg., *17*:724, 1970.
107. Richardson, J., Jurkovich, G., Walker, G., et al.: A temporary arteriovenous shunt (Scribner) in the management of traumatic venous injuries of the lower extremity. J. Trauma, *26*:503, 1986.
108. Robinette, C.: Splenectomy and subsequent mortality in veterans of the 1939 to 1945 war. Lancet, *2*:127, 1977.
109. Root, H., Houser, C., McKinley, C., et al.: Diagnostic peritoneal lavage. Surgery, *57*:633, 1965.
110. Routt, M., Meier, M., Kregor, P., et al.: Percutaneous iliosacral screws with the patient supine technique. Op. Tech. Orthop. *3*:35, 1993.
111. Rozycki, G., Ochsner, M., Schmidt, J., et al.: A prospective study of surgeon-performed ultrasound as the primary adjuvant modality for injured patient assessment. J. Trauma, *39*(3):492, 1995.
112. Ryan, W., Snyder, W. III, Bell, T., et al.: Penetrating injuries of the iliac vessels: Early recognition and management. Am. J. Surgery, *144*:642, 1982.
113. Sagalowsky, A., McConnell, J., and Peters, P.: Renal trauma requiring surgery: An analysis of 185 cases. J. Trauma, *23*:128, 1983.
114. Sastry, S., Paul, B., Bain, L., et al.: Ocular trauma among major trauma victims in a regional trauma center. J. Trauma, *34*(2):223, 1993.
115. Schaefer, S.: The acute management of external laryngeal trauma. Arch. Otolaryngol. Head Neck Surg., *118*(6):551, 1992.
116. Schwab, C.: Violence: America's uncivil war. J. Trauma, *35*:657, 1993.
117. Shackford, S. R., and Molin, M.: Management of splenic injuries. Surg. Clin. North Am., *70*(3):595, 1990.
118. Shackford, S., Virgilio, R., and Peters, R.: Selective use of ventilator therapy in flail chest injury. J. Thorac. Cardiovasc. Surg., *81*:194, 1981.
119. Shannon, F., Moore, E., Moore, F., et al.: Value of distal colon washout in civilian rectal trauma-reducing gut bacterial translocation. J. Trauma, *28*:989, 1988.
120. Singer, D.: Post-splenectomy sepsis. Perspect. Pediatr. Pathol., *1*:285, 1973.
121. Sirinek, K., and Levine, B.: Traumatic injury to the proximal superior mesenteric vessels. Surgery, *98*:831, 1985.
122. Slatis, P., and Huittinen, V.: Double vertical fractures of the pelvis. Acta Chir. Scand., *138*:799, 1972.
123. Sloan, J., Kellerman, A., Reay, D., et al.: Handgun regulations, crimes, assaults, and homicide: A tale of two cities. N. Engl. J. Med., *319*:1256, 1988.
124. Snyder, W. I., Thal, E., and Perry, M.: Peripheral and abdominal vascular injuries. *In* Rutherford, R. (Ed.): Vascular Surgery. Philadelphia, W. B. Saunders, 1984, p. 460.
125. Snyder, W. III, Weigelt, J., Watkins, W., et al.: The surgical management of duodenal trauma: Precepts based on a review of 247 cases. Arch. Surg., *115*:422, 1980.
126. Steinsapir, K., and Goldberg, R.: Traumatic optic neuropathy. Surv. Ophthalmol., *38*(6):487, 1994.
127. Stewart, R., Fabian, T., Croce, M., et al.: Is resection with primary anastomosis following destructive colon wounds always safe? Am. J. Surg., *168*:316, 1994.
128. Stone, H., and Fabian, T.: Management of duodenal wounds. J. Trauma, *19*:334, 1979.
129. Surgeon General's Workshop on Drunk Driving Recommendations: Rockville, MD, Department of Health and Human Services, 1988.
130. Thal, E., and Yeary, E.: Morbidity of colostomy closure following colon trauma. J. Trauma, *20*:287, 1980.
131. Trunkey, D.: Issues in trauma care. *In* Davis, J. (Ed.): Clinical Surgery. St. Louis, C. V. Mosby Co., 1987, p. 2759.
132. Trunkey, D., Hays, R., and Shires, G.: Management of rectal trauma. J. Trauma, *13*:411, 1973.
133. Wall, M., Hirshberg, A., and Mattox, K.: Pulmonary tractotomy with selective vascular ligation for penetrating injuries to the lung. Am. J. Surg., *168*:665, 1994.
134. Weaver, F., Yellin, A., Wagner, W., et al.: The role of arterial reconstruction in penetrating carotid injuries. Arch. Surg., *123*:1106, 1988.
135. Weigelt, J., Thal, E., Snyder, W., et al.: Diagnosis of penetrating cervical esophageal injuries. Am. J. Surg., *154*:619, 1987.
136. West, J., Murdock, N., Baldwin, N., et al.: A method for evaluating field triage criteria. J. Trauma, *26*:655, 1986.
137. Yajko, R., Seydel, F., and Trimble, C.: Rupture of the stomach from blunt abdominal trauma. J. Trauma, *15*:177, 1975.

CHAPTER 18

SURGICAL COMPLICATIONS

A. R. Moossa, M.D., Marquis E. Hart, M.D., and David W. Easter, M.D.

Any deviation from the expected steady recovery after a surgical operation is defined as a complication. In general, most surgical complications can be traced to the operating room and are often related to the general health of the patient and to the magnitude of the operation. Each type of surgical procedure may present special problems. Some complications may be unavoidable, particularly after emergency operations, when time does not permit optimal preoperative preparation and investigation. When planning a surgical procedure, it is wise to "strive for the best but be prepared for the worst." Good perioperative care of surgical patients is designed to minimize the incidence and severity of complications:

Preoperatively: Review all surgical and anesthetic options and the associated hazards. Anticipate potential complications in each patient. Protect patients at risk with antibiotic and thromboembolic prophylaxis, and so forth.

Intraoperatively: Monitor vital functions. Use meticulous surgical technique with attention to detail. Avoid excessive operating time.

Postoperatively: Monitor to detect and correct abnormalities early. Prevent complications with physiotherapy, early ambulation, nutritional support, and so forth.

POSTOPERATIVE FEVER AND INFECTION

An elevated temperature often occurs during routine observation of postoperative patients but does not necessarily signal a serious complication or necessarily warrant an extensive diagnostic work-up. A specific cause is identified in less than 20% of patients with pyrexia during the initial 24 hours; in the remainder, it may be regarded as a normal response to surgical trauma. A comprehensive clinical examination is essential in the initial assessment of postoperative fever, although the timing and pattern of pyrexia may provide a clue to its origin.

Infective Causes of Postoperative Fever

The origin of contamination that leads to clinical infection directly influences subsequent prevention and treatment efforts. Community-acquired infections are initiated before a patient's contact with the hospital environment. Such pathogens pose less difficult management problems because they have not been exposed to the chronic selective pressures created by the antibiotic-laden atmosphere and to the concentration of critically ill patients in the hospital.

Most postoperative infections follow contamination at the time of operation, at the operation site itself, via the airway during general anesthesia, or from cannulas and catheters inserted in the operating room. Many are caused by hospital-acquired pathogens, which have often evolved through generations of antibiotic exposure and may have developed resistance to chemotherapeutic agents.

Local and systemic factors may compromise the ability of the host defense mechanisms to cope with contamination. The most important local factor is the adequacy of the blood supply. In devitalized tissue, necrotic areas provide an ideal environment for bacteria, where they are protected from circulating host defenses. Foreign bodies serve in a similar role, as do hematomas, in which hemoglobin is an additional potent adjuvant to bacterial proliferation.

Reduction in morbidity and mortality in patients with postoperative infection can be achieved only by a thorough understanding of prevention, early diagnosis, and definitive therapeutic intervention.

Since the mid-nineteenth century, a host of independent observations and studies has broadened understanding of the infection process. Semmelweis noted that contagion that passed from the physician to the patient was responsible for the dreaded childbed fever and for subsequent septic deaths of postpartum patients. Pasteur and Koch recognized bacteria as pathogens in human infection. Lister demonstrated the usefulness of antisepsis, which led to the evolution of asepsis, and emphasized the need for even more sophisticated efforts to control infection, which remains the most persistent enemy of the surgeon.

Clinical manifestations of postoperative infection generally cause either local or systemic signs and symptoms. Local signs of postoperative infection include the traditional cardinal signs of inflammation—namely, calor, dolor, rubor, and tumor. These signs, respectively, represent clinical evidence of the nonspecific inflammatory response (heat, pain, redness, and presence of mass) in surgical patients and should serve as significant indicators of emerging infection.

Systemic manifestations of postoperative infection are usually consequences of the host febrile response. Chills, rigors, and elevated core body temperature all represent systemic manifestations of the febrile response. A specific series of pathophysiologic events triggers this response. Agents that provoke fever are referred to as endogenous or exogenous pyrogens. In patients with postoperative fever, the exogenous pyrogens are usually bacterial organisms.

Numerous systemic factors increase vulnerability to infection. Neonates have inadequately developed host defenses, and elderly patients often experience a progressive decline in immunocompetence. The immune system may also be compromised in malnutrition, diabetes, hepatic disease, and disseminated malignancy and, of course, by immunosuppressant therapy, including corticosteroids.

Obesity increases the likelihood of infection, particularly in surgical and traumatic wounds, probably due to the relatively poor blood supply of large reservoirs of subcutaneous adipose tissue. Similarly, it appears that chronic or acute severe malnutrition predisposes to infection.

Many systemic illnesses are identified with increased rates of infection. Patients with disseminated malignancy are at increased risk, at least in part, owing to the cachectic influences of the primary neoplasm and the immunosuppressive influences of systemic chemotherapy. In addition, there is increasing evidence that a patient with an active infection is at increased risk of development of a second remote septic focus.

Moreover, selected medications and drugs contribute to increased frequency and severity of infection. Acute and chronic alcohol ingestion also appears to have an immunoinhibitory effect.

Diagnostic and therapeutic efforts in a patient with postoperative fever should be directed toward recognition and eradication of the primary source of exogenous pyrogens. Characteristics of the postoperative fever may be significant in determining its primary cause. Fever that begins within 24 hours after operation usually suggests atelectasis. Wound infections and, more rarely, abdominal abscesses are usually not identifiable until the fifth to tenth postoperative day or even later, although these patients often have fever beginning early in the postoperative course. Abscesses commonly have a recurrent, spiking pattern. Infections arising from environmental contamination during the postoperative period commonly show an antecedent period of no fever before temperature elevation. Foley catheter– and intravenous cannula–associated infections are commonly of this type.

A comprehensive physical examination is essential in the initial assessment of postoperative fever. Specific attention should be focused on identifying signs of inflammation, such as unusual wound tenderness. Rhonchi or rales on auscultation of the chest in the early postoperative period may point to a pulmonary cause of the fever.

Pulmonary infections are common in postoperative patients. Atelectasis frequently follows general anesthesia, and aspiration or, more rarely, contaminated ventilation equipment contributes to chest infections in the immediate postoperative period. Smokers and patients with nasogastric tubes are at particular risk. Urinary tract infections are usually associated with indwelling catheters, bladder outflow obstruction, or anorectal or urologic operations.

Postoperative suppurative parotitis is now a rare complication but is still occasionally observed in elderly or debilitated patients. Parotitis is associated with dehydration and poor oral hygiene; the time of onset is usually within 2 weeks of operation, and the organism is usually *Staphylococcus aureus*.

The operative site must always be considered a potential source of sepsis. The patient often has a fever beginning early in the postoperative course, although wound infections and intra-abdominal and intrathoracic abscesses are usually not identifiable clinically until at least the fifth postoperative day. Abscesses are typically associated with a recurrent, spiking fever. The pelvis and subphrenic spaces are the most common sites for intra-abdominal sepsis.

A rectal examination to exclude a pelvic collection is an essential part of any clinical examination in a febrile patient. Subphrenic collections may be associated with shoulder tip pain, tenderness on palpation of the subcostal region, or signs of a sympathetic pleural effusion with elevation of the diaphragm on clinical examination and chest films. However, there may be no localizing clinical features, and when intraperitoneal soiling is followed by a septic course, the subphrenic space should always be suspected.

Intravenous lines must also be considered as possible sites of infection, especially if blood cultures are positive. Infection at a peripheral cannulation site is usually obvious, with local cellulitis, which may be accompanied by inflammation along the course of the vein or by lymphangitis and regional lymphadenopathy. Central line sepsis, in contrast, is often clinically occult because it is usually due to an infected thrombus at the catheter tip, rather than sepsis at the site of skin puncture. Catheter-related sepsis is best diagnosed by culturing blood drawn through the line or the tip of the catheter following its removal.

Miscellaneous Causes of Postoperative Fever

Thrombophlebitis. Noninfective thrombophlebitis at an intravenous infusion site is a relatively common occurrence in patients receiving prolonged intravenous fluids or locally noxious drugs. Occasionally, bacterial contamination may be superimposed upon these primary chemical processes, causing suppurative infection within the vessel lumen. Unfortunately, unlike chemical thrombophlebitis, the treatment of septic thrombophlebitis involves more than simple removal of the intravenous catheter. Phlebitis is one of the most common causes of fever after the third postoperative day. Venous catheters should be removed at the first sign of redness, induration, or edema. Phlebitis is most frequent with cannulation of lower limb veins; thus, this route should be used only when upper extremity veins are unavailable. With suppurative phlebitis, the patient appears ill and, in addition to the local signs of inflammation, pus may be expressed from the venipuncture site. High fever and positive blood cultures are common. Treatment consists of excising the affected vein.

Postoperative Parotitis. Normal saliva from healthy patients has intrinsic bacteriostatic activity. This property makes spontaneous salivary gland infection very unusual in the absence of salivary duct obstruction, except in elderly and debilitated patients. Predisposing factors include poor oral hygiene, old age, avitaminosis, malnutrition, and malignancy. The time of onset is usually within 2 weeks after a major operation; the initiating factors are usually dehydration and poor oral hygiene. The infection is usually staphylococcal in origin. The diagnosis is usually evident by palpation of the swollen, tender parotid gland, and a drop of pus may be observed at the intraoral opening of Stensen's duct; there is normally a high fever and a leukocytosis. Prevention requires attention to those factors that predispose the patient to these infections, such as adequate oral hygiene, avoidance of dehydration, and attention to the use of anticholinergic drugs. When signs of acute parotitis appear, fluid from Stensen's duct should be cultured, and an appropriate antibiotic administered. If the disease progresses, incision and drainage become necessary, and care must be taken to avoid damage to the facial nerve.

Noninfective Causes of Postoperative Fever

Postoperative pyrexia is not necessarily infective in origin. It may be a manifestation of the underlying disease, as in a patient with disseminated malignancy. Transfusion or drug reactions may induce fever in the early postoperative period. A hematoma may elicit a mild febrile response, or fever may originate from inflammation around an intravenous catheter after the administration of irritant fluids or drugs. Deep vein thrombosis, with the risk of pulmonary embolism, may be associated with a mild pyrexia and usually presents after the fifth postoperative day.

Postoperative acute pancreatitis is an occasional complication after upper abdominal operations, and especially those involving the biliary tract and stomach. It probably occurs more often than the quoted 3% incidence, because mild attacks are difficult to detect. Severe episodes have a high mortality and present with persistent postoperative fever, abdominal pain, and distention due to ileus and may progress to multisystem failure. Serum amylase and lipase are usually elevated but are not diagnostic in the postoperative patient, and computed tomographic (CT) scanning is required to establish the diagnosis. There is no specific treatment other than intensive supportive care, although pancreatic collections and areas of necrosis may subsequently require drainage and débridement.

Metabolic causes of postoperative fever are rare but are life-threatening if untreated. Thyroid storm is an extreme manifestation of thyrotoxicosis with hyperpyrexia, tachycardia, arrhythmias, hypotension, and sweating precipitated by the stress of surgical intervention in a patient with unrecognized hyperthyroidism or thyroidectomy in an inadequately prepared patient with thyrotoxicosis. The immediate danger is tachyarrhythmia, and propranolol should be administered to control the heart rate. If still in progress, the operation should be terminated as soon as possible, and appropriate antithyroid therapy should be administered to block thyroid hormone synthesis.

Pheochromocytoma, a tumor derived from the adrenal medulla that produces catecholamines, may also be revealed by the stress of operation or anesthesia. It may present with fever associated with extremely labile hypertension and tachycardia, flushing, headaches, nausea, and vomiting. Treatment is to control the effects of catecholamine release with beta- and alpha-blockers, supplemented with a sodium nitroprusside infusion to control excessive fluctuations in blood pressure.

Malignant hyperthermia is a rare complication following the administration of muscle relaxants such as succinylcholine and inhalation general anesthetics and amide local anesthetics. It is due to a genetically determined defect in calcium release from the sarcoplasm of skeletal muscles and is manifest in approximately 1 in 50,000 adults but is more common in children. Blood creatinine phosphokinase is elevated in 70% of patients, but muscle biopsy is required to establish the diagnosis. It usually presents with high fever, tachycardia, rigidity, skin mottling, and cyanosis, usually within 30 minutes after induction of anesthesia, but occasionally with a delay of several hours. There is an associated metabolic acidosis and hyperkalemia. Treatment is to administer dantrolene, which blocks calcium release from the sarcoplasmic reticulum; to infuse sodium bicarbonate and dextrose and insulin to combat potentially lethal hyperkalemia; and to actively cool the patient. Early recognition and prompt treatment are essential in this condition, which is associated with mortality in excess of 30%.

WOUND COMPLICATIONS

All surgeons must be adept in managing the problem of wound complications. The incidence depends on the type of operation, the patient's disease and condition, and the technical proficiency and judgment of the surgeon. Most surgical services have an infection rate of 2% to 4% in clean wounds. Other complications such as dehiscence, hernias, and hematoma raise the complication rate in clean wounds to approximately 5%. In contaminated cases and in trauma surgery, the complication rate is higher. In emergency operations on unprepared bowel or an infected urinary tract, the rate of wound complications in reported series is as high as 50% to 60%. However, as noted by several investigators, these figures are higher than they should be for all categories.

With perfect foresight, serious wound complications would be rare, because techniques for their prevention are known. Wound healing is an exceptionally complicated process; however, there are four basic phases: inflammation, epithelialization, contraction, and collagen metabolism. These four phenomena occur in an ordered sequence and are interdependent. They may be altered by a number of factors that can ultimately lead to abnormal wound healing.

Hematoma and Seroma

A hematoma is a collection of blood in the wound, usually due to inadequate hemostasis. Patients being administered low-dose heparin or aspirin have a slightly higher risk, which is greater still in those who are fully anticoagulated or who have a coagulation disorder. Hypotension may cause vessel spasm during operation, and the wound may appear dry at the time of closure, only to develop a hematoma a few hours later when normal blood pressure is restored.

Hematomas cause fluctuant swelling and discomfort in the wound, and there may be local bruising or discharge between sutures. Large hematomas may collect after operations such as mastectomy, where the surrounding skin has been extensively undermined. Blood loss may be sufficient to cause tachycardia, hypotension, and a subsequent fall in hematocrit. Small hematomas may resorb, but they increase the incidence of wound infection. Treatment of larger collections requires evacuation of the clot under sterile conditions, ligation of bleeding vessels, and reclosure of the wound.

A seroma is a collection of fluid other than pus or blood. In small wounds, it usually follows liquefaction of necrotic fat. Large seromas are associated with operations that involve elevation of skin flaps and division of numerous lymphatic channels (e.g., mastectomy and axillary clearance or groin dissection). They can usually be prevented by placing closed suction drains beneath the flaps. Like hematomas, they provide an excellent culture medium for bacteria. Treatment consists of aspiration; if they reaccumulate, it may be necessary to insert more drains.

Wound Infection

A wound infection is a collection of pus in the wound. If there is no systemic disturbance and the complication is completely resolved by simple aspiration or discharge of pus, it can be considered a minor wound infection. A major wound infection is defined as one that makes the patient ill or delays discharge from the hospital.

The infection may be primary, when the initial collection is pus, or secondary, when a sterile hematoma, seroma, or area of fat necrosis is subsequently colonized by bacteria from the blood (bacteremia) or from the environment. An infection is endogenous if the source of the bacterial inoculum is from the patient and exogenous if the source is the environment.

As previously mentioned, modern surgical therapy was made possible by the work of Pasteur, who realized that sepsis was due to micro-organisms, and Lister, who introduced the concept of antisepsis. Previously, surgical procedures were generally complicated by exogenous infection with streptococci and staphylococci. Today, with the important exceptions of trauma and burns, exogenous infection is uncommon and usually indicates a break in aseptic technique or an excessively lengthy procedure. Most wound infections are endogenous, predominantly caused by enteric organisms.

Wound infection follows proliferation of micro-organisms in the wound. This requires:

1. Inoculation of the wound with the micro-organism. Experimental data indicate that an inoculum of a million or more viable staphylococci is required to produce a subcutaneous abscess in normal individuals. Almost all surgical wounds are contaminated with some microbes, but small numbers of micro-organisms can be eliminated by leukocytes and antimicrobials from the bloodstream.

2. A favorable environment for bacterial proliferation, such as blood or serous fluid, avascular or necrotic tissue, or foreign material that incites a tissue reaction. A wound hematoma provides an excellent culture medium for bacteria. Ischemia limits the access of host defenses from the blood, and bacteria can proliferate without hindrance if there is avascu-

lar necrotic tissue, clot, or foreign material in the wound. Wound infections develop in the subcutaneous adipose tissue, which has poor blood supply and is easily strangulated by sutures. Fat necrosis can also be caused by imprecise use of the diathermy coagulator. Many surgeons attempt to eliminate a potential dead space with fat sutures. This may be counterproductive. Skillful surgical technique, which minimizes tissue trauma, maintains the blood supply, produces good hemostasis with negligible local necrosis, and avoids foreign material (including sutures) in the adipose layer, yields the lowest incidence of wound infections.

If bacterial swabs are obtained from the viscera at the operative site during operation and from the wound before skin closure, wounds can be graded as *clean* if there is no growth from either swab, *potentially contaminated* if the visceral swab is positive, or *contaminated* if the wound swab is positive.

Clean wounds rarely become infected. Occasionally, a sterile collection or area of necrotic tissue becomes secondarily infected. In contrast, in 30% of contaminated wounds, a wound infection develops, even if prophylactic antibiotics are administered during the operation. Wounds that are only potentially contaminated have a much lower incidence of infection (approximately 10%), which suggests that direct inoculation of the wound during operation, rather than bacteremia, is the most important cause of wound infection.

Potentially contaminated wounds are usually associated with operations that involve opening a hollow viscus, and wound infection rates correlate with the bacterial load in the viscus. Thus, the greatest risk is in colonic operations, especially those involving the left colon and rectum. The bacterial count can be reduced by mechanical preparation with purgatives or enemas, but the colon cannot be completely sterilized even if nonabsorbable antibiotics are administered orally. Indeed, the efficacy of prophylactic oral antibiotics has been questioned, because they may merely lead to colonization of the bowel by resistant organisms.

The crucial element in the prevention of wound infection is a scrupulous surgical technique that avoids contamination of the wound. Occasionally, contamination is unavoidable, as in emergency laparotomy for generalized peritonitis. Wounds that are recognized as contaminated at the time of operation should be treated as infected from the outset and left open. If the wound is clean after at least 24 hours, a delayed primary closure can then be performed. Serious infections have resulted after failure to observe this important surgical principle.

The judicious use of prophylactic antibiotics has been demonstrated to reduce the incidence of wound infection in contaminated and potentially contaminated wounds. The principle is to have a high concentration of an appropriate antibiotic in the tissues and blood at the time of operation in order to eliminate any bacteria released into the operative field or bloodstream during the procedure. A single dose of antibiotic is probably sufficient unless the operation is prolonged, although two additional doses are frequently given postoperatively. Inappropriately extended administration of antibiotics intended for prophylaxis is condemned because it leads to the development of bacterial resistance. Similarly, prophylactic antibiotics should not be used as a remedy for poor aseptic technique in clean operations. It is important to distinguish prophylactic from therapeutic indications for antibiotics, because this will influence the duration of administration as well as the antibiotic selection. Appropriate antibiotics for these two distinct indications should be administered.

Unexplained fever in a postoperative patient always requires inspection of the wound, which may be painful and appear swollen, red, and indurated. A deep wound infection in an obese patient may not become evident for several days. The temperature usually subsides when pus is discharged.

The initial approach to an area of possible wound infection is to obtain a sample of pus or exudate for bacterial culture by needle aspiration using aseptic technique. The only definitive treatment for an infected wound is to drain it. Antibiotics are indicated only as an adjunct to surgical drainage if there is evidence of systemic infection. When wound infection is confirmed, the area should be opened to allow free drainage. Sutures or staples may need to be removed, and necrotic tissue in the wound may need to be débrided. Some irrigate the area with antiseptics to sterilize it, others pack it with gauze to keep it from closing, and others merely cover it with a pad to absorb the exudate. There is no evidence that any one of these measures is superior, provided free drainage is achieved.

Wound Failure

Wound failure is defined as partial or total disruption of any or all layers of the operative wound. There are two types of wound failure: early (wound dehiscence) and late (incisional hernia).

Dehiscence of chest wounds is rare, but when it occurs, it usually follows median sternotomy. Rupture of all layers of the abdominal wall with extrusion of the viscera is termed evisceration *(burst abdomen)*. Evisceration occurs in approximately 1% of laparotomy wounds and is associated with a mortality of approximately 20%. Infection is associated with more than half of wounds that rupture.

Factors that appear to interfere with wound healing and are associated with wound failure include malnutrition, sepsis, anemia, uremia, liver failure, diabetes, and corticosteroid therapy. Obesity, heavy coughing or retching, and the accumulation of ascites, which strain the wound during the postoperative period, also predispose to failure. However, even in these patients, dehiscence is an avoidable complication if the wound is closed securely.

The strength of a wound lies in the musculoaponeurotic layer (or bony layer in the case of a median sternotomy). In the early postoperative period, it depends on the sutures employed to close this layer of the wound. Wound dehiscence occurs because sutures break, stretch, or cut out of the tissues; because knots slip; or because an insufficient number of sutures are inserted. Thus, in closing a wound, the following factors must be considered:

1. *The tensile strength of the suture material.* Suture material may be absorbable or nonabsorbable, monofilament or braided, reactive or inert. Most surgeons use nonabsorbable sutures for wound closure because they retain tensile strength. Their disadvantage is that they persist as a foreign body in the wound and may provide a focus for infection and sinus formation, especially if made of a braided and reactive material such as silk. Absorbable sutures weaken with time, and the use of catgut, which is rapidly degraded, is associated with an unacceptable incidence of dehiscence in laparotomy wounds. The newer, relatively inert, longer-lasting absorbable materials, such as polydioxane, retain their strength during the initial weeks of wound healing and appear to be a satisfactory alternative to nonabsorbable materials.

2. *The stretching and knotting characteristics of the suture.* Braided materials, such as silk, have little plastic or elastic stretch and are easy to knot securely. However, they may predispose to wound infection because bacteria can lie harbored in the interstices of the material, which are difficult for leukocytes to penetrate. Monofilament materials, such as

nylon, require careful handling and knotting. They may stretch and lose strength if they are kinked or crushed with instruments. Some materials have *memory*, so that the loops used when knotting tend to straighten, causing a knot to slip. However, secure knots can be formed when a sufficient number of *throws* are used, when the knots are squared, and when friction knots or fishermen's knots are employed.

3. *The depth of bite and number of sutures used.* A suture will cut out if the fascia being sutured is weak, especially in patients with conditions associated with poor wound healing. Sutures should be placed at least 1 cm. from the wound edge. They should be tied sufficiently tightly to obtain secure apposition of the cut edges, but not so tightly as to cause strangulation. They should be placed no more than 1 cm. apart to prevent herniation of viscera between sutures. It is useful to use at least four times as much suture as the length of the wound. Continuous suture technique is frequently employed because of ease in performance. However, if the material should fail or cut out at a single point, the entire wound may be compromised. Interrupted suturing is more tedious to perform but is more reliable, particularly in the septic or debilitated patient.

4. *The site of the incision.* After a midline laparotomy incision, the linea alba can be closed as a single layer with secure, deep, bite sutures (mass closure). This is associated with a lower incidence of wound dehiscence than the standard paramedian incision, which requires separate suturing of the anterior and posterior rectus sheath, with shallower bites to avoid strangulating the rectus muscles. Incisional hernia appears to be more common after mass closure, perhaps because the longer lengths of the individual sutures stretch more and become apposition of the layers of the cut edges is less precise. A *near-far, far-near* technique may remedy this problem. A secure closure can be obtained with a lateral paramedian incision. This ensures wide separation of the incisions in the anterior and posterior sheaths with the rectus muscle, which reinforces the wound. However, unless a long incision is made, access to the abdomen may be impaired. Transverse incisions, which can be closed by either a mass or a layered technique, also have a good reputation for suture closure.

In wounds that are mending securely, a healing ridge (in the form of a palpable thickening about 0.5 cm. on each side of the incision) normally appears near the end of the first week after operation. This ridge is invariably absent from wounds that rupture. Usually, the first sign of an impending problem is a discharge of serosanguineous fluid from the wound, but in some cases, dehiscence presents as a sudden evisceration following an episode of coughing or retching (Table 18–1).

Evisceration is a harrowing experience for the patient. Immediate measures include calm reassurance, adequate analgesia, and covering of the viscera with a sterile moist towel. The wound can then be explored under general anesthesia. Devitalized tissues are excised, and the wound is closed with strong, nonabsorbable, nonreactive, interrupted sutures,

TABLE 18–1. Causes of Abdominal Wound Dehiscence

Imperfect technical closure
Increased intra-abdominal pressure from bowel distention, ascites, coughing, vomiting, or straining
Hematoma with or without infection
Infection
Metabolic diseases such as diabetes mellitus, uremia, Cushing's disease, and malignant disease with starvation
Tissues inadequate for strong closure

taking deep bites into healthy tissue. Near-far, far-near placement prevents long intraperitoneal bridges of suture that would threaten to erode into the viscera. If the wound has dehisced but not eviscerated, an alternative in a patient who might not tolerate a further anesthetic is to pack the wound, provide external support with a binder, and accept the hernia that inevitably follows.

Hernia formation is a relatively common complication of abdominal and flank wounds. Its incidence after primary healing is approximately 1%, rising to 10% for infected wounds and 30% after dehiscence and reclosure. Although there is evidence that fascial separation occurs in the early postoperative period in patients in whom incisional hernias develop, the defect may not become apparent for months or even years after the operation. Small abdominal hernias are often not noticed unless the patient increases intra-abdominal pressure by sitting up or coughing. Hernias with narrow necks may present acutely with incarceration, intestinal obstruction, or, if the blood supply is obstructed, strangulation.

Incisional hernias can be difficult to repair, with recurrence rates up to 40%. If possible, the repair should be delayed until the wound has healed, that is, for at least 6 months. Grossly obese patients rarely undergo successful repair unless they lose their excess weight.

RESPIRATORY COMPLICATIONS

Despite improvements in surgical and anesthetic techniques, pulmonary disorders remain the most frequent postoperative problem encountered in surgical patients. They are cited as the principal cause of death in 25% of surgical fatalities and as significant contributory factors in an additional 25%. Morbidity reported for chest complications depends on the diligence with which it is investigated. Research studies that subject all patients to postoperative blood gas analysis and chest radiographs reveal imperfections in lung function in over 50% of patients after general anesthesia for cholecystectomy. However, less than 20% have abnormal clinical signs, and perhaps 10% are considered to have a clinically significant chest complication.[18]

Several factors militate against normal respiratory function in the early postoperative period:

1. Effects of general anesthesia, mechanical ventilation, and postoperative analgesia, which depress the respiratory system and suppress reflexes such as coughing, which clears secretions, and periodic deep breathing and yawning, which expand collapsed alveoli
2. Depression of the immune system by trauma or sepsis
3. Progressive reduction in vital capacity by 50 to 70% during the initial 12 to 18 hours after thoracotomy and laparotomy.[7, 10]

Even with a 70% reduction in vital capacity, ventilatory reserve should be adequate to allow deep breathing and coughing unless a complication supervenes. Factors that predispose to chest complications include chronic restrictive or obstructive chest disease, smoking, obesity, prolonged general anesthesia, and the presence of a nasogastric tube.

Respiratory complications that occur in postoperative patients can be separated into two general categories: atelectasis/pneumonia and acute respiratory failure.

Atelectasis and Pneumonia

The terms *atelectasis* and *collapse* are often used synonymously, but strictly, atelectasis implies that the lung tissue has never expanded. It has, however, been used to describe the postoperative condition in which small airways and alveoli lose their patency and collapse. Atelectasis is the most common complication of operations performed under general anesthesia, with radiologic evidence in up to 70% of patients after thoracotomy and laparotomy.

If air passages are occluded by secretions, perhaps in association with bronchospasm, alveolar air is absorbed and the alveoli collapse. This is the most likely explanation for collapse that involves the entire segment or lobe of a lung, especially if the patient has thick, tenacious secretions. However, atelectasis is often patchy and diffuse, appearing as plates of collapsed tissue on chest films. Even during normal breathing, some alveoli collapse at the end of expiration but re-expand on inspiration. Re-expansion is facilitated by periodic deep breaths. Alveoli are able to re-expand because of surfactant, the release of which is stimulated by deep breathing, and which reduces surface tension as alveolar volume diminishes. Postoperatively, low tidal volumes and lack of periodic deep breaths inhibit release of surfactant and prevent the alveoli from re-expanding.

Therapy is directed toward prevention and early treatment. Smoking, bronchitis, prolonged general anesthesia, and nasogastric tubes all predispose to atelectasis; the incidence can be reduced if careful consideration is given to these risk factors. Smokers should be urged to abstain at their initial consultation, because at least 4 days are required for any benefit. Elective operations should be delayed so that intensive preoperative physiotherapy is allowed in patients with bronchitis. The incidence of chest complications is considerably reduced in such patients if operations such as hernia repair are performed under local anesthesia. Nasogastric tubes should be removed as soon as they are no longer required.

Radiologic signs of atelectasis (plate atelectasis) may occur in the absence of clinical evidence. Stasis in the airways is accompanied by an accumulation of secretions that are prone to infection, especially at the lung bases. Thus, the first clinical signs of atelectasis are rales, diminished breath sounds, and bronchial breathing, often accompanied by fever, tachycardia, and radiologic evidence of consolidation due to the associated pneumonia.

Treatment is directed toward clearing the secretions and re-expanding the alveoli. Physiotherapy with postural drainage and encouragement to expectorate is often effective in removing secretions. Suction is useful in patients unable to expectorate by coughing, either by the endotracheal route or via a thin, plastic cannula inserted percutaneously into the trachea (mini-tracheostomy). In patients with collapse of an entire lung segment or lobe, bronchoscopy may be required for visualizing and removing thick mucus obstructions from first- and second-degree bronchi.

Nebulized bronchodilators (e.g., salbutamol) should be used if there are wheezes characteristic of bronchospasm, and patients with thick secretions may also be helped by nebulized mucolytic agents (e.g., acetylcysteine). Antibiotics should be reserved for those patients with evidence of an established infection. The choice of antibiotic depends on sputum bacteriology.

When the airway has been cleared, re-expansion often follows with deep breathing exercises and early ambulation. Mechanical intermittent positive pressure breathing (IPPB) may be effective in the delivery of nebulized inhalations, but its ability to reinflate alveoli is countered by the possibility that secretions may be propelled into more distal air passages. On balance, it is not usually recommended.

Selection of the appropriate regimen of analgesia is crucial in patients with shallow breathing. Postoperative pain is one of the major causes of decreased tidal volume, but it is important to titrate the dose of analgesia to avoid depressing the respiratory center. Atelectasis is exacerbated by shallow respirations, and if the patient demonstrates evidence of respiratory insufficiency despite the measures outlined above, endotracheal intubation and intermittent mechanical ventilation (IMV), with positive end-expiratory pressure (PEEP) to reinflate the lung, are necessary, combined with frequent endotracheal suction.

Pulmonary Aspiration

Aspiration of material from the alimentary tract into the airway can lead to two distinct complications: aspiration pneumonitis, which is due to the chemical composition of the aspirate; and aspiration pneumonia, which is due to its bacterial content. The two can coexist, with aspiration pneumonia as a complication of aspiration pneumonitis.

Aspiration Pneumonitis. Aspiration pneumonitis is caused by the aspiration of gastric contents, which are normally sterile. The consequences depend on the nature of the aspirated material. If the pH of the aspirate is less than 2.5, it can cause a chemical burn to the airways. The syndrome was first described by Mendelson[12] in 1946 as a devastating complication of obstetric anesthesia. In addition to the effects of gastric acid, tiny particles of food cause an intense inflammatory reaction if they reach the distal air passages. Larger particles obstruct the airway, leading to collapse, and can rapidly cause hypoxic cardiac arrest if the trachea or main bronchi are occluded and not cleared rapidly.

Preventive measures minimize the risk of aspiration. The patient should take nothing orally for at least 6 hours before operation or, in an urgent situation, have had nasogastric drainage. As soon as muscle relaxants are administered during induction of anesthesia, the airway should be protected by cricoid pressure, followed by rapid intubation and inflation of a cuffed endotracheal tube. The development of Mendelson's syndrome may be reduced by pretreatment with antacids and H_2-antagonists.

The clinical features of dyspnea, cyanosis, and tachycardia usually appear within half an hour of aspiration, with rales and expiratory wheezes on auscultation. Chest films reveal interstitial pulmonary edema. Arterial blood gases demonstrate hypoxia and hypercapnia. The condition may rapidly deteriorate into respiratory failure and is associated with high mortality.

The supine posture and the absence of normal protective reflexes during general anesthesia predispose surgical patients to pulmonary aspiration. The risk is increased during pregnancy, in the elderly, in the obese, and in those with hiatal hernia, full stomach, or intestinal obstruction. Because the right main bronchus is more in line with the trachea than the left, the right lung is more often affected.

Aspiration usually occurs at the time of induction, when passive regurgitation occurs during the interim between administration of muscle relaxant and intubation, and following extubation, when active vomiting may occur as a side effect of narcotic analgesia.

Aspiration Pneumonia. Aspiration pneumonia is usually due to inhalation of contents from the oropharynx that are normally at physiologic pH but contain bacteria, particularly anaerobes. It is a common cause of postoperative pneumonia and is particularly associated with poor oral hygiene and the prolonged use of nasogastric and endotracheal tubes. The risk is also increased in patients with neurologic impairment and those with compromised upper airway defenses, including smokers, the elderly, and those with a chemically induced aspiration pneumonitis. It also has a predilection for the right lung. Unlike aspiration pneumonitis, however, the episode of aspiration is usually not observed, and clinical signs of pneumonia develop gradually, with fever, productive cough, rales, decreased breath sounds, and bronchial breathing. It may present as a lung abscess, which is classically associated with aspiration of purulent material and blood during dental extraction or tonsillectomy. A lung abscess presents with the production of large amounts of foul-smelling sputum or a characteristic cavity with a fluid level on chest films.

Pulmonary Edema

Pulmonary edema in a postoperative patient may be due to left ventricular failure following cardiac complications or to injury to the alveolar membrane as a result of sepsis, oxygen toxicity, and so forth, but it is generally the result of circulatory overload following excessive administration of intravenous fluids. Circulatory overload may also follow absorption of fluids used for irrigation of the peritoneum or hollow viscera such as the bladder, or it may occur during mechanical bowel preparation, especially in those with a history of cardiac disease.

Ordinarily, plasma oncotic pressure is sufficient to retain fluid in the capillaries during alveolar gas exchange; any fluid that escapes into the interstitial space is removed by lymphatic absorption. If capillary hydrostatic pressure rises after circulatory overload or left heart failure, fluid leaks out of the capillaries, overwhelms the lymphatic drainage, and enters the alveolar lumen. The situation is exacerbated if the plasma oncotic pressure is low, for example, following massive infusions of crystalloids, or when alveolar membrane permeability increases to permit the egress of plasma proteins with the edema fluid. Edema fluid predominates at the most dependent part of the lung, where hydrostatic pressure is greatest. Therefore, the typical clinical features include orthopnea and basal crepitations. As the condition progresses, the airways fill with pink, frothy fluid, which induces bronchospasm, and the patient becomes increasingly hypoxic.

Postoperative pulmonary edema can be avoided by careful attention to fluid balance, especially in patients with a history of cardiac problems. Auscultation of the chest and observation of the jugular venous pressure remain invaluable indicators of circulatory overload in postoperative patients receiving fluid therapy. If large fluid infusions are anticipated, a central venous or pulmonary artery line should be inserted preoperatively for monitoring the effects of fluid therapy.

Patients in the supine position are at particular risk of drowning in their edema fluid, and the immediate treatment of severe pulmonary edema is upright positioning of the patient, discontinuance of intravenous fluids, and provision of oxygen. An electrocardiogram (ECG) may demonstrate evidence of myocardial infarction or an arrhythmia requiring urgent treatment. Drug therapy includes diuretics to reduce circulatory volume, digoxin to increase cardiac output, and morphine, which is known to be effective, although the mechanism is unclear. If the condition is refractory to these measures, mechanical ventilation may be necessary for treating respiratory failure and phlebotomy or hemofiltration for correcting fluid overload.

Immediate Postoperative Respiratory Depression

Respiratory depression immediately following operation is usually due to the persistent effects of narcotic analgesia used during anesthesia, or to the sustained action of muscle relaxants. Narcotics depress the respiratory center in the brain stem and can usually be reversed by antagonists such as naloxone. Patients with emphysema who rely on an elevated $PaCO_2$ to drive their respiratory centers are particularly sensitive to narcotics, and respiratory efficiency may also be compromised by muscle weakness in elderly, malnourished, and septic patients.

Nondepolarizing muscle relaxants such as curare are relatively long acting. Their efforts can be potentiated by large doses of aminoglycoside antibiotics, particularly intraperitoneal irrigation with neomycin, which is readily absorbed. They can sometimes be reversed by an anticholinesterase such as neostigmine, administered in combination with atropine to prevent cholinergic bradycardia. Muscle relaxation with depolarizing agents such as neostigmine usually dissipates within about 10 minutes. The effects may be prolonged in patients taking anticholinesterase therapy for glaucoma and, more often, in those with atypical plasma cholinesterase. This is a congenital disorder with homozygous inheritance that affects 0.05% of the population. It may be suspected from the family history and can be confirmed by measuring the plasma cholinesterase activity.

If respiratory depression is refractory to the pharmacologic intervention outlined above, mechanical ventilation must be continued until the effects of the offending anesthetic agent disappear. It is important to be aware, however, that respiration may also be compromised in the immediate postoperative period because of aspiration, laryngeal edema, bronchospasm, massive atelectasis, pneumothorax (especially following insertion of a central venous cannula), pulmonary edema, and hypothermia. These must be sought separately and treated expeditiously, because they may not respond to, and may be exacerbated by, mechanical ventilation.

Acute Respiratory Failure

Acute respiratory failure is defined as a direct, life-threatening inability to maintain adequate gas exchange in the lungs.[17] Acute respiratory insufficiency is defined as a condition in which gas exchange in the lungs can be maintained at an acceptable level only at the expense of significantly increased work of the cardiopulmonary system.[1] The increased work cannot be maintained indefinitely, so unless the situation is improved, respiratory failure ensues. Although criteria for instituting mechanical ventilation require an assessment of arterial blood gases, ventilation, dead space, and muscle strength, in practice, respiratory failure is considered to be imminent if arterial partial pressure of oxygen (PaO_2) is less than 60 mm. Hg when one is breathing room air, or the arterial partial pressure of carbon dioxide ($PaCO_2$) is greater than 60 mm. Hg in the absence of metabolic alkalosis.[14]

Postoperative respiratory failure can be caused by one or a combination of pulmonary defects: hypoventilation, imbalance between ventilation and perfusion, and diminished alveolar oxygen diffusion. In addition, it may be aggravated by factors such as decreased cardiac output, anemia, and impaired oxygen-hemoglobin dissociation, which restricts oxygen delivery from the lungs to the tissues, or by sepsis, severe trauma, burns, and some formulations of intravenous nutrition that increase oxygen demand and carbon dioxide output.

Numerous etiologic features have been implicated in association with acute respiratory failure following trauma and surgical procedures (Table 18–2). Several associated syndromes have been described, many of which are synonymous, including acute respiratory distress syndrome, adult respiratory distress syndrome (ARDS), Da Nang lung, and shock lung. Essentially, however, they all refer to a lung injury that causes arterial hypoxemia and hypercarbia. Mechanisms suggested for the pathogenesis of the injury in the various syndromes described include bacterial injury, endotoxin, complement activation, autoimmunity, microemboli, ischemia, and oxygen toxicity.

Although the pathogenesis of the lesion is unclear, the site of injury in all these syndromes is at the interface between the alveoli and the pulmonary capillaries. Initially, inflam-

TABLE 18–2. Etiologic Factors Associated with Acute Respiratory Failure

Via the Airway

Aspiration
Oxygen toxicity
Smoke inhalation
Diffuse pneumonia
Lung contusion

Via the Blood

Sepsis
Transfusion
Fat embolism
Acute pancreatitis

Other

Head injury
Massive trauma
Radiation

matory cells and edema accumulate in the interstitial space, but as the lesion progresses, protein-rich fluid enters the alveoli. This leads to pulmonary edema and the development of hyaline membrane, which acts as a barrier to gas diffusion. Pulmonary vascular resistance increases, with a consequent rise in pulmonary artery pressure. The injury also leads to loss of Type II alveolar cells, which produce surfactant. Surfactant regulates surface tension in the alveolar membranes; without it, alveoli that collapse at the end of expiration are unable to re-expand, and compliance diminishes (the lungs become stiffer).

In terms of ventilatory parameters, the pathophysiology of acute respiratory insufficiency is characterized by a decrease in functional residual capacity of the lung, indicating that the amount of air within the lungs at the end of normal respiration is reduced. As the expiratory lung volume diminishes, an increasing number of small airways collapse at the end of normal tidal respiration. This leads to progressive atelectasis, with a diminished ventilation-perfusion ratio (intrapulmonary shunt) and a reduction in lung compliance.

The onset of acute respiratory insufficiency may be insidious. Clinically, there is a progressive increase in respiratory rate and effort due to a combination of hypoxemia and decreased lung compliance. Hyperventilation may initially induce a fall in $PaCO_2$.

In the early stages of the process, some patients may respond to an increased inspired concentration of oxygen delivered by a face mask. However, the mainstay of treatment is to provide ventilatory support with IMV and to reinflate collapsed alveoli with PEEP. It is important to understand that patients with hypoxemia are not improved by mechanical ventilation alone, because without PEEP, alveolar collapse occurs with each expiratory phase of the respiratory cycle. PEEP also permits the inspired oxygen concentration to be reduced, which is important in the context of oxygen toxicity.

The role of ventilatory support in these patients has altered the primary concern from one of providing adequate oxygenation to one of reducing the work in breathing. The rationale for IMV is to provide an intermediate support between 100% mechanical ventilation and spontaneous respiration that is tailored to the individual patient's requirement. The overall goal in postoperative respiratory failure is to provide early intervention with PEEP and IMV when hypoxemia and hypercarbia are detected, to avoid using continuous mechanical ventilation in an exhausted patient with noncompliant lungs and carbon dioxide retention.

Theoretically, PEEP should be administered in stepwise increments until adequate oxygenation, 70 mm. Hg, is obtained. There are, however, specific complications of PEEP therapy. Alveolar rupture, with the development of tension pneumothorax, occasionally occurs. More frequently, PEEP reduces cardiac output because intrathoracic pressure remains positive throughout the ventilatory cycle, inhibiting venous return to the heart. This is an indication for pulmonary artery catheterization and measurement of cardiac output in order to optimize the myocardial performance and to exclude other causes of diminished cardiac output.

Continuous positive airway pressure (CPAP) administered to a spontaneously breathing patient by a tight-fitting mask has been used as an alternative to PEEP therapy in patients who require intervention for hypoxemia, without hypercarbia or ventilatory insufficiency. CPAP has two advantages over PEEP: there is less effect on cardiac output, because negative intrathoracic pressures continue to be generated during spontaneous inspiration; and peak inspiratory pressures are lower, reducing the risk of pneumothorax. The disadvantage is that the patient is not relieved of the work of breathing, which increases oxygen consumption. Thus, a higher concentration of inspired oxygen must be delivered, which may exacerbate the lung lesion. This problem can be countered by delivering CPAP in conjunction with IMV to a spontaneously breathing but intubated patient.

Because of the contribution of pulmonary edema to the disease process, careful attention must be given to fluid balance, with particular care to avoid fluid overload and maintain colloid osmotic pressure. Pulmonary edema may be ameliorated by diuretics, but they should be used judiciously, because decreased vascular volume may aggravate the effect of PEEP on cardiac output.

In addition to ventilatory support, a careful search for an underlying disorder such as sepsis should be sought and treated appropriately.

SHOCK

Acute circulatory failure, commonly termed *shock*, may be defined as a life-threatening inability of the cardiovascular system to maintain adequate tissue perfusion. It is caused by a reduction in blood volume, a deterioration in cardiac output, or a combination of both. Shock can be divided into three categories according to etiology: hypovolemic, cardiogenic, and septic.

Hypovolemic Shock

Hypovolemic shock is caused by a fall in circulating blood volume and is the most frequent cause of postoperative shock. Seventy percent of circulating blood volume is in the venous system, with major venous reservoirs in the cutaneous, hepatic, and pulmonary vascular beds. An acute loss of approximately 30% of blood volume can be temporarily accommodated by compensatory mechanisms:

1. Catecholamine release activated by baroreceptors in the carotid sinus and aortic arch that stimulate the sympathetic nervous system and the adrenal medulla and inhibit vagal tone. This has a positive inotropic effect on the heart, accompanied by tachycardia, arterial vasoconstriction, and increased venomotor tone, causing a relative redistribution of blood from the venous system to the arterial system and from the skin, muscle, pulmonary, splanchnic, and renal beds to the heart and brain.

2. Fluid shift from the extravascular compartment into the circulation due to the reduction in hydrostatic pressure in the capillaries.

3. Increased sodium and water reabsorption from the kidney, mediated via the renin-angiotensin-aldosterone response and vasopressin release from the pituitary.

If acute blood loss exceeds approximately 40%, or shock is prolonged, there may be irreversible consequences:

1. Coronary hypoperfusion, with the risk of infarction, leading to cardiac failure and secondary cardiogenic shock.

2. Renal ischemia, causing acute tubular necrosis.

3. Metabolic acidosis due to a combination of deficient renal excretion of hydrogen ions and increased anaerobic metabolism, with lactate production by the tissues, which may further depress the myocardium.

4. Cerebral hypoperfusion, which is aggravated by the reduction in $PaCO_2$ associated with metabolic acidosis.

5. An initial increase in blood coagulability, which may progress to disseminated intravascular coagulation (DIC). Subsequently, clotting factors are diminished, both as a result of consumption and because of hepatic ischemia.

6. Depression of the reticuloendothelial system, in particular, the Kupffer cells in the liver, which detoxify portal blood from the bowel. This predisposes to the added insult of endotoxemia.

7. Ischemic injury to vascular endothelium following prolonged vasospasm, which increases capillary permeability, leading to generalized edema and *shock lung*.

Hypovolemia may reflect an uncorrected preoperative volume deficit, unreplaced blood or other fluid losses during the operation, or an inadequate postoperative fluid regimen. Continuing hemorrhage in the postoperative period must always be considered.

Tachycardia is the earliest sign of hypovolemia, followed by hypotension when compensatory mechanisms are overwhelmed. The mucous membranes are dry, there is loss of cutaneous elasticity, and the skin is pale, cold, and sweaty in response to catecholamine release. The respiratory rate increases in response to catecholamine release, baroreceptor reflexes, tissue hypoxia, and metabolic acidosis. Confusion is a sign of compromised cerebral blood flow.

Treatment is by rapid replacement of the volume deficit with intravenous fluids through one or more large-caliber intravenous cannulas and should be monitored by measurement of pulse rate, arterial and central venous or pulmonary artery pressures, urinary output, and return of skin blood flow (core-peripheral temperature). The choice of fluid used to correct hypovolemia is controversial and depends on the cause. Blood and colloid solutions may be used to maintain circulating volume during active hemorrhage but are not adequate to resuscitate a patient with a large extracellular or *third space* loss. Exteriorization of the viscera and extensive dissection of tissue planes are associated with loss of extracellular fluid through evaporation. Postoperatively, there is a redistribution of tissue fluids due to interstitial edema, and sequestration into the bowel. Optimal replacement is provided by fluids that are evenly distributed throughout the extracellular space, limiting the value of colloids and plasma expanders such as dextran, which are retained in the intravascular compartment alone. Maximal benefit is obtained with a combination of packed red cells to replace the red cell volume loss and a balanced electrolyte solution such as Hartmann's or Ringer's lactate to replace the extracellular fluid.

Resuscitation is adequate when the systolic blood pressure has returned to the preoperative level, with a central venous pressure (CVP) between 5 and 10 cm. H_2O or a pulmonary artery (PA) wedge pressure between 10 and 15 mm. Hg. The urinary output should exceed 30 ml. per hour. If this cannot be achieved or sustained, the likelihood of continuing hemorrhage must be considered. This may be obvious if copious amounts of blood appear from drainage tubes. However, bleeding from the operative site may be difficult to detect, especially after an abdominal operation, even when drains are present.

Hemorrhage in the immediate postoperative period (reactionary hemorrhage) is usually due to a single bleeding vessel, whereas delayed (secondary) hemorrhage is often associated with diffuse bleeding from an infected operative site. When a major transfusion has been required, a coagulation profile may reveal a hemorrhagic diathesis, which requires specific treatment with coagulation factors and platelets.

Cardiogenic Shock

Cardiogenic shock is usually secondary to myocardial ischemia or infarction with left ventricular failure or arrhythmia, causing inadequate cardiac output. Cardiac failure due to tamponade, mediastinal distortion, or compression can occur following cardiothoracic surgery. Cardiac failure may also complicate severe hypovolemic or septic shock and, conversely, may be induced by fluid overload, especially in the elderly or those with pre-existing heart disease.

Accurate diagnosis is essential, because treatment regimens for cardiogenic and hypovolemic shock are quite different. Even in the absence of ECG changes, cardiogenic shock is suggested on clinical examination by an elevated jugular venous pressure, gallop rhythm, and bilateral chest crepitations due to pulmonary edema, in addition to the features of poor peripheral perfusion.

Accurate evaluation and optimal therapy require invasive monitoring in an intensive care unit (ICU). The assessment of cardiac performance by CVP measurement is limited. The normal range of CVP is from 2 to 10 cm. H_2O, and values exceeding this range suggest a fluid overload or primary cardiac failure, as does an increase greater than 2 cm. H_2O above the control level in response to a 250-ml. fluid challenge. Pulmonary artery pressure measurements by means of a Swan-Ganz catheter allow more clear discrimination between inappropriate fluid replacement and pump failure. This balloon-tipped catheter, when wedged in a distal pulmonary artery, accurately reflects the left ventricular filling pressure and provides a sensitive guide to fluid loading when myocardial function is compromised. A pressure in excess of 15 mm. Hg indicates fluid overload, and a pressure below 10 mm. Hg suggests hypovolemia. In addition, cardiac output can be computed by means of thermodilution techniques if a thermistor-tipped catheter is used.

The accurate monitoring of fluid status and cardiac performance achieved by these methods allows fluid status to be carefully controlled to optimize filling of the heart (ventricular preload) in accordance with Starling's law; then attention can be directed to optimizing myocardial efficiency by means of inotropic vasoactive drugs.

A positive inotropic agent increases the force of myocardial contraction without increasing the heart rate. Conversely, some drugs (e.g., beta-blockers) and metabolic abnormalities, especially hypoxia and acidosis, have a negative inotropic effect, and their correction may be of paramount importance. Cardiac glycosides such as digoxin increase myocardial contractility and may improve cardiac output in cardiac failure, especially if there is associated cardiomegaly. However, their use is controversial, because they increase myocardial oxygen requirements, which may precipitate ischemia; they can induce serious arrhythmias; and digitalis toxicity is potentiated by electrolyte disturbances (hypokalemia and hypomagnesemia) and hypoxia in a metabolically unstable patient and by some anesthetic agents.

Catecholamines exert a positive inotropic effect through $beta_1$ receptors in the myocardium. In addition, vasoactivity may be mediated through alpha (vasoconstriction) and $beta_2$ (vasodilatation) receptors and renal dilatation through dopaminergic receptors. Epinephrine is the most potent inotrope, but its use is associated with a high incidence of arrhythmias; it increases myocardial oxygen consumption, and vasoactive effects redistribute blood to skeletal muscle and decrease diastolic pressure, which may reduce coronary blood flow. Norepinephrine, a powerful vasoconstrictor, has similar disadvantages and markedly increases heart rate (positive chronotropic effect) but can be beneficial in patients with bradycardia.

Dopamine and dobutamine are the two most frequently used catecholamines. Although similar to epinephrine at high doses (more than 5 μg. per kg. per minute), at lower doses, dopamine increases cardiac output without incurring the unwanted alpha-adrenergic effects that lead to peripheral vasoconstriction and decreased renal perfusion, and it improves renal function by stimulating dopamine receptors. Dobutamine is less potent as an inotrope, but it has the least effect on heart rate and arrhythmias and induces vasodilation without vasoconstriction, increasing myocardial blood flow. It is thus the agent of choice following myocardial infarction and is frequently used in combination with dopamine in patients in shock with poor renal perfusion.

If cardiac output remains inadequate despite optimal ventricular preload and contractility, vasodilators may help reduce ventricular afterload (peripheral resistance). They are indicated for severe hypertension, especially after cardiac operations and when there is poor peripheral perfusion due to high peripheral resistance. They may also relieve pulmonary edema associated with left ventricular failure or mitral incompetence. However, they can all cause profound hypotension and should not be used if blood pressure drops below approximately 90 mm. Hg. Sodium nitroprusside has a very rapid onset and offset of action, allowing fine control. It dilates venules as well as arterioles, reducing both preload and afterload. Hydralazine has a longer duration of action, but its effects are limited to the arterioles. Nifedipine is a calcium channel blocker, causing arteriolar dilatation.

If pharmacologic measures fail, an intra-aortic counterpulsation balloon pump may be considered. This is introduced via the femoral artery into the thoracic aorta just distal to the left subclavian artery. It is synchronized with the ECG and used to augment coronary flow by inflation during diastole and deflation during systole. The principal indications are to support patients after cardiac surgery until myocardial function is recovered and after myocardial infarction while consideration is given to coronary artery bypass.

Septic Shock

Small numbers (less than 10^3) of bacteria are commonly found in the blood (bacteremia) after minor procedures such as dental extraction. Septicemia is defined as the proliferation of bacteria in the bloodstream. This is accompanied by systemic manifestations of sepsis, including rigors, fever or hypothermia (characteristic of gram-negative septicemia with endotoxemia), leukocytosis or leukopenia (characteristic of profound septicemia or viremia), and tachycardia or circulatory collapse. Septicemia may be a direct complication of the surgical procedure (e.g., anastomotic leak), a complication of invasive investigations or monitors (e.g., infected CVP line), or secondary to another infective complication (e.g., chest or urinary tract infection). It may also complicate the late stages of hypovolemic shock due to intestinal ischemia and Kupffer cell failure.

The increasing incidence of septic shock may reflect the increasing numbers of patients who survive major operations and severe trauma, the development of antibiotic-resistant hospital organisms, or the more frequent use of invasive techniques. Elderly, malnourished, and immunocompro-

mised patients are at particular risk, as are those with a septic focus underlying their original disease. Any organism, including bacteria, fungi, rickettsiae, and viruses, may be involved, but gram-negative bacteria that produce endotoxin predominate. Improvements in culture techniques have yielded an increasing association with anaerobe infection.

Septic shock follows a combination of loss of vasomotor tone, increased capillary permeability, and myocardial depression. The pathogenesis of these lesions is still not completely clear. Platelets and white blood cells appear to be consumed in the process, and the vascular lesions may originate from an uncontrolled response of normal defense mechanisms to bacteria within the bloodstream, with dissemination of powerful vasoactive substances such as histamine, serotonin, and prostaglandins, which also increase capillary permeability. Complement activation causes white cell aggregates, and factors involved in phagocytosis by leukocytes, such as lysosomal enzymes and oxygen-derived free radicals, may be released, damaging capillary endothelium.

Gram-negative infections have a much worse prognosis than gram-positive infections, possibly because of an associated endotoxemia. However, the role of endotoxin, a complex lipopolysaccharide found in the cell wall of gram-negative bacteria, is unclear, because although it causes fatal shock in experimental animals, gram-positive bacteria can produce a similar syndrome.

Myocardial depression may also be due to the release of toxins from bacteria or phagocytic cells, or it may be secondary to lactic acid released from hypoxic cells. Pancreatic ischemia causes the release of a specific *myocardial depressant factor*.

Clinically, there are two patterns of septic shock:

1. *Warm shock* is characterized by tachypnea, rigors, fever spikes, and a hyperdynamic circulation. The periphery is warm to the touch and appears well perfused because of diffuse peripheral dilatation. The veins are dilated, which increases vascular capacitance and causes a reduction in effective blood volume.[10, 11]

2. *Cold shock* is characterized by peripheral vasoconstriction and is associated with hypovolemia, occurring most frequently in patients, who have extensive extracellular fluid losses following burns, peritonitis, or intestinal obstruction. A transition from the warm to the cold type may occur if circulating volume diminishes.

Uncontrolled sepsis leads to the development of multiple organ failure, with acute pulmonary failure (ARDS), acute renal failure, hepatic failure, gastrointestinal ulceration and hemorrhage, adrenal failure, and cerebral failure as potential additional manifestations. DIC is precipitated by the release of thromboplastin from damaged tissue into the circulation and consumption of clotting factors and platelets in the microcirculation. In addition, both cell-mediated immunity and antibody production are impaired, together with depression of the reticuloendothelial system. The patient is thus deprived of the essential mechanisms to combat the underlying sepsis and exposed to the added complication of opportunistic infection.

Therapy is directed toward supporting the cardiovascular and other compromised systems while the underlying septic focus is identified and treated aggressively.

Volume replacement is vital to prevent the transition from warm shock to cold shock, with its attendant high mortality. In severe sepsis, CVP correlates poorly with pulmonary wedge and left ventricular filling pressure, especially when there is an associated ARDS, and Swan-Ganz pressure monitoring is required. Under these conditions, optimal fluid replacement and inotropic and vasoactive support may be administered. Ideally, the choice of solution for volume expansion should reflect the underlying pathophysiologic abnormality. The relative hypovolemia due to increased vascular capacitance in warm shock requires volume supplementation with colloid. However, if increased capillary permeability is the prime concern, as in cold shock, infusion of large amounts of protein-rich fluid can aggravate fluid sequestration and protein accumulation in the interstitial space. This is of particular importance in the lungs, where colloidal solutions may enhance pulmonary edema and contribute to ARDS. Thus, some clinicians maintain that it is more appropriate to expand volume with a crystalloid such as a lactated Ringer's solution. Others maintain that crystalloids leak out of the circulation more rapidly than colloids, and the large volumes required produce osmotic abnormalities. Both views have merit, and in practice, a compromise is expedient, with infusion of crystalloid as the principal component for volume replacement, together with sufficient colloid to maintain plasma oncotic pressure.

It may be impossible to optimize ventricular filling or even to maintain a sufficient cardiac output to prevent renal failure without precipitating severe pulmonary edema. In these circumstances, it is essential to establish priorities. Acute renal failure is usually reversible, and a period of dialysis may have to be endured to allow optimal treatment of the life-threatening pulmonary complication. When renal failure develops, pulmonary edema is refractory to diuretics, but excess fluid can be removed by means of hemofiltration. In the hemofilter, arterial blood, flowing from an arterial cannula, passes over a membrane that is permeable to water and electrolytes but not to protein or cells, before being returned to the circulation by way of a venous cannula. The rate at which fluid is removed can be adjusted to optimize fluid balance. Hemofiltration is extremely useful in patients in renal failure who require precise control of fluid status and yet require intravenous nutrition—a mandatory requirement in severely septic patients.

The source of sepsis must be urgently sought and treated. Collections of pus or anastomotic leaks cannot be remedied by antibiotics and require surgical intervention. A localized accumulation of pus in a suitable anatomic location may be more appropriately drained by nonsurgical means with interventional radiologic techniques. When possible, blood and other specimen cultures should be obtained before antibiotic therapy. Until the offending organisms have been identified, broad-spectrum antibiotics active against common gram-positive and gram-negative bacteria and anaerobes should be administered. The antibiotic regimen is subsequently adjusted on the basis of bacteriologic reports, and unnecessary drugs must then be omitted to limit the development of resistant strains, opportunistic fungal infection, and pseudomembranous colitis.

The emergence of multiorgan system failure in the postoperative period serves as a clinical indicator of continued intra-abdominal infection, but ideally, the clinical situation should not be allowed to reach this advanced stage. Drainage is the only effective treatment for an abdominal abscess. Only by complete evacuation of the intra-abdominal purulence can clinical resolution be achieved. The most frequent sites of major pus collections in the abdomen are the subdiaphragmatic spaces, the pelvis, and the liver. The lateral gutters and pockets among adherent loops of bowel represent other sites.

The methods for drainage of abdominal abscess continue to be controversial, particularly in the current era of aggressive interventional radiologists. A limited abdominal exploration may be justified in a patient whose abscess is well localized by preoperative evaluation and who tolerates the clinical infection with relatively little difficulty. This limited approach prevents complications of inadvertent enterotomy and subsequent fistula formation. In the situation of a well-localized abscess, particularly if it is in the liver, there is good reason for insertion of a catheter under radiologic guidance by an experienced radiologist.

However, a patient without preoperative localization of the abscess cavity or a patient who is not tolerating the systemic manifestations of sepsis should have a complete exploratory operation of the abdomen. This approach avoids the possibility of overlooking multiple abscesses or inadequately drained established abscesses.

Subphrenic Abscess

The most common site of intra-abdominal abscess formation is beneath the diaphragm. Unfortunately, a large collection of pus may exist in either the right or the left subphrenic space with few localizing symptoms. However, when intraperitoneal soiling is followed by a septic course, and especially if lung infection or pelvic abscess has been nearly excluded, the subphrenic space should always be suspected. Hence the surgical dictum: "Pus somewhere; pus nowhere; pus under the diaphragm."

RENAL FAILURE

Acute renal failure (ARF) is defined as an abrupt reduction in excretion of waste products by the kidney that leads to a progressive rise in plasma creatinine and urea (azotemia). The onset is usually associated with oliguria, defined as a urinary output of less than 0.5 ml. per kg. per hour, which is equivalent to 35 ml. per hour for a 70-kg. man.

Acute renal insufficiency must be considered in any patient with oliguria after an operation. However, it must be remembered that operative procedures during anesthesia cause large increases in plasma vasopressin concentration,[9] and this may be potentiated by postoperative pain and by some narcotics. The antidiuretic effect of vasopressin is to reduce the flow and increase osmolality, whereas in ARF, concentrating ability is lost. Therefore, urine concentration as well as flow must be considered during the immediate postoperative period.

The cause of ARF can be grouped into three categories: prerenal, renal, and postrenal.

Prerenal failure implies an inadequate renal blood flow and is usually a direct result of diminished circulating blood volume. Cardiac failure, due to either inadequate cardiac output or vasoactive drugs, such as epinephrine used to support the failing myocardium, is occasionally responsible. In a hypovolemic patient, the catecholamine response to maintain systemic blood pressure constricts the renal arterioles. Arterial blood pressure may not, therefore, accurately reflect circulating blood volume or renal perfusion. Clinically, the patient may appear *dry*, but clinical assessment alone provides only an approximate guide to fluid status. If the urinary output does not rapidly improve after an intravenous fluid challenge with 500 to 1000 ml. of an isotonic saline solution administered over 30 to 60 minutes, a central venous or pulmonary artery catheter should be inserted so that fluid requirements can be accurately assessed.

Acute parenchymal renal failure usually follows uncorrected prerenal failure. The condition is frequently referred to as *acute tubular necrosis*, because this is the predominant lesion observed histologically. However, necrosis of renal tubules is a very variable feature and may not be present. Thus, some nephrologists prefer the term *vasomotor nephropathy* or *acute reversible intrinsic renal failure* (ARIRF), which defines the clinical condition more precisely. Although ischemic injury confined to the renal medulla usually recovers with appropriate therapy, cortical necrosis, which can be diagnosed only on biopsy, is more serious because it is irreversible.

Direct injury to the renal parenchyma can be caused by nephrotoxic drugs, in particular, aminoglycosides and intravenous radiocontrast agents; incompatible blood transfusions causing acute hemolysis and hemoglobinuria; and severe muscle injury with myoglobinuria. Renal failure may ensue, especially in dehydrated patients and those with previously compromised renal function. ARF is also observed postoperatively in jaundiced patients with hepatic edema. In these circumstances, it is essential to establish priorities. ARF is usually reversible and prevented by ensuring adequate hydration and diuresis throughout the perioperative period. The pathogenesis is unclear, but endotoxin has been implicated because the patient can be protected by measures to eliminate gram-negative bacteria, including antibiotics and mechanical bowel preparation using mannitol.

Postrenal failure is caused by obstruction of the urinary tract and usually presents with acute anuria. Obstruction should always be considered in a postoperative patient with poor or absent urinary output. It is most common in elderly male patients with prostatic enlargement and in patients with an obstructed urinary catheter. A more serious complication is accidental ligation of both ureters during abdominal or gynecologic surgery.

Accurate identification of the cause of postoperative renal failure is obviously important. Elementary problems such as bladder outflow obstruction and catheter blockage can easily be remedied. Prerenal failure and parenchymal renal failure are usually differentiated on the basis of clinical and laboratory features. Volume status, when assessed, should be rapidly corrected with appropriate intravenous fluid therapy. If adequate urinary output (more than 40 ml. per hour) is not achieved, an intravenous infusion of mannitol 25 mg., furosemide 250 mg. over 20 minutes, or a low-dose infusion of dopamine (2 to 5 μg. per kg. per hour) may be considered.

The use of diuretics is controversial, because clinical trials have failed to demonstrate their efficacy in preventing or reversing ARF[5] and, theoretically, they may aggravate the situation. Diuretics should never be administered to an oliguric patient until fluid status has been assessed and corrected, because although they may induce a reassuring diuresis, they only aggravate dehydration in a hypovolemic patient. Mannitol is an osmotic diuretic that is not metabolized and, if not excreted in the urine, can increase the osmolarity of the extracellular fluid as well as the blood, which could precipitate pulmonary edema. Therefore, if a single dose fails to produce a diuresis, it should not be repeated. Furosemide is a powerful loop diuretic that also increases cortical blood flow, but there is some evidence that it potentiates nephrotoxicity, at least in combination with some antibiotics. Dopamine may be a more effective alternative. In addition to its beta$_1$ receptor–mediated inotropic action on the heart, at low doses it improves renal perfusion via dopaminergic receptors in the renal arteries. The patient requires careful monitoring, however, because the effective renal dose may be near the higher dose that induces tachycardia, arrhythmias, and alpha receptor–mediated vasoconstriction.

Lack of response to the measures outlined suggests acute renal parenchymal or postrenal failure. The ratio of urine to plasma sodium, urea and osmolality, and the relative elevations in plasma urea (uremia) and creatinine concentrations may further differentiate renal from prerenal failure. If plasma sodium concentration is within the normal range, a urinary sodium of less than 20 mmol. per liter indicates increased renal conservation of sodium in association with reduced renal perfusion, whereas values greater than 40 mmol. per liter are consistent with acute parenchymal renal failure. Similarly, a urinary osmolality of greater than 500 mOsm. per liter indicates that the kidney is still able to concentrate urine, whereas formation of urine with a low specific gravity (approximately 1.010) and osmolality of less than 400 mOsm. per liter is evidence of a parenchymal injury. In prerenal failure, sodium conservation is associated with an increased renal reabsorption of urea, decreasing the urine-blood urea ratio from a normal 30:1 to less than 20:1. Creatinine, however, is not reabsorbed, and the rise in blood urea to plasma creatinine concentration is usually less than 10.

Before instituting an ARF regimen, the possibility of postrenal failure must be excluded. The index of suspicion varies with the operative procedure and is obviously highest following operations involving a retroperitoneal or pelvic dissection. Unilateral ureteric ligation is usually silent, because the remaining kidney can compensate for the loss. In contrast, bilateral ligation causes anuria. Obstruction to the outflow tract usually leads to hydronephrosis, which can be identified on ultrasound scan. If the kidney is able to excrete some urine, either because the ureters have been damaged but not ligated or because of bladder outflow obstruction, the anatomic site of the injury can be demonstrated on intravenous pyelography (IVP). Otherwise, cystography and retrograde pyelography are required. Renal isotope scans (renograms) may also be useful. Dynamic imaging with technetium-labeled diethylene tetramine pentacetic acid (DTPA) can be used to assess glomerular filtration by each kidney. Failure of renal concentration indicates renal ischemia, whereas progressive increase in renal concentration over 30 minutes indicates obstruction. Static imaging using technetium-labeled dimercaptosuccinic acid (DMSA) is useful in identifying and quantifying parenchymal damage, because DMSA is concentrated only by functioning renal tissue.

Untreated, acute renal failure leads to progressive electrolyte disturbance and metabolic acidosis, terminating in cardiac arrest from hyperkalemia. In postoperative patients, it is usually reversible, although it may require a prolonged period of support with dialysis. However, it is associated with a mortality of approximately 50% because of the underlying disorder, usually hypovolemic or septic shock.

Close attention to fluid balance is paramount. Initially, fluids are usually administered to optimize cardiac output, and thus renal perfusion, by increasing central venous or left atrial pressures. When it is clear that renal failure has become established, however, it is crucial to abandon aggressive fluid replenishment in order to avoid serious overload and to discontinue potassium. Changes in the patient's weight provide a useful guide to fluid balance and should be recorded daily. Fluid intake can be titrated to central venous or Swan-Ganz pressure, but an approximate guide to fluid intake is to replace urinary output and other measured losses plus approximately 500 ml., to replace insensible losses (which increase with pyrexia and tachypnea), and to adjust these in accordance with changes in weight and clinical signs of fluid overload (elevated central venous pressure, dependent edema, chest crepitations), or dehydration (dry skin and mucus membranes). Most postoperative patients with renal failure are in a highly catabolic state, and parenteral nutrition with glucose and essential amino acids or, if possible, a high-calorie, low-potassium diet provides optimal protein sparing. If the requirement for fluids associated with nutrition exceeds that dictated by fluid balance, hemofiltration or dialysis may be required.

The choice between hemodialysis and peritoneal dialysis depends on the feasibility of peritoneal dialysis, the availability of hemodialysis, the cardiovascular stability of the patient, and local preferences. The indications for dialysis include the following:

1. Plasma potassium greater than 6.5 mmol. per liter
2. Volume overload
3. Plasma urea greater than 35 mmol. per liter
4. Plasma creatinine greater than 900 μmol. per liter
5. Severe metabolic acidosis

Careful monitoring should allow severe electrolyte and acid-base disturbances to be anticipated and dialysis instituted to prevent, rather than correct, complications of renal failure. Hyperkalemic cardiac arrest is the most dangerous complication. In the urgent situation, dextrose and insulin or a calcium ion exchange resin can be used to rapidly reduce plasma potassium concentration.

If the underlying problem can be corrected, postoperative renal failure often resolves. Resolution is frequently heralded by polyuria, indicating the diuretic phase of acute renal failure. Again, this must be anticipated and may require frequent adjustments to the volume and electrolyte content of fluid regimens.

DEEP VEIN THROMBOSIS AND PULMONARY EMBOLISM

Thrombosis in the veins draining the lower limbs is an important cause of morbidity in surgical patients, both because of its frequency and because of the potentially fatal consequences should the clot become detached from the vein wall and embolize in the pulmonary arteries. Studies using radioactive fibrinogen scans indicate a prevalence of deep vein thrombosis (DVT) in excess of 40% in postoperative patients. One percent of general surgical patients die from pulmonary embolism.

Clinically, the classic features of DVT are calf swelling and tenderness, elevated temperature, and a positive Homans' sign (calf pain on dorsiflexion of the foot). Phlegmasia cerulea dolens (painful blue leg) represents the extreme situation caused by massive thrombosis involving the iliac veins and extending into the most distal venules in the leg; it is usually associated with an underlying malignancy (e.g., pancreatic cancer). However, clinical diagnosis of DVT is notoriously unreliable; only 50% of patients with evidence of DVT on venography have any clinical sign. Moreover, the majority of patients suffering fatal pulmonary embolism have no clinical features of venous thrombosis prior to sudden cardiovascular collapse.

The risk of DVT and pulmonary embolism is increased with age, obesity, oral contraception, cardiovascular disease, malignancy, leg trauma, and immobility. In addition, patients undergoing pelvic surgery or orthopedic operations on the hip are at increased risk. Immobility preoperatively, during a lengthy operation, or postoperatively is an important contributory factor.

Venous thrombosis begins in areas of stasis, particularly in the small calf veins or behind venous valve cusps. Hypercoagulability due to surgical stress and trauma, the effects of pooling and low venous flow in hypotonic limb muscles during anesthesia, and local vascular damage from extrinsic compression of the calf increase the risk of thrombosis.

Flanc and associates demonstrated that of the thrombi formed, spontaneous lysis occurs in one third.[4] Of the remaining two thirds, half of the emboli are localized in the calf, and the remainder move into the popliteal and femoral veins and may embolize. The clinical signs of DVT correlate poorly with the extent of the thrombosis.

Venography is the standard means of diagnostic investigation and is the assessment against which all new techniques are compared. Venography does not aggravate pre-existing thrombosis, nor does it predispose to embolization. The major disadvantages are the expense, invasive nature, and need to move the postoperative patient to a radiology suite for examination. Current interest centers on those procedures that may be performed expeditiously at the bedside, such as Doppler ultrasonography, ^{125}I-fibrinogen studies, and plethysmography. All have the advantage of being noninvasive and may be performed without moving the patient. Doppler ultrasonography provides an audible signal in response to blood flow. The normal venous flow is phasic with respiration and is augmented by calf compression; a Doppler sonogram detects any alteration in this pattern. Although its accuracy depends on the skill of the examiner, a sensitivity and specificity in excess of 90% can be achieved. The technique is most proficient in detecting major venous thrombosis and is least able to localize small vein thrombi.

[125]I-fibrinogen leg scanning measures local fibrinogen isotope activity as a percentage of the background cardiac fibrinogen activity. It is specific for fresh or recently formed thrombi and differentiates them from previous venous thrombosis. The technique is most effective in detecting small calf thrombi but lacks sensitivity above the midthigh level. Currently, its expense and time-consuming nature restrict its widespread application.

Plethysmography detects changes in limb volume in response to heartbeat or after the temporary occlusion of venous return. Various methods, including strain gauge, air, or impedance plethysmography, have been employed. Like ultrasonography, it is better designed to determine major venous thrombosis than small calf vein thrombi.[15]

Prophylaxis

Prophylactic measures to prevent deep vein thrombosis and, more important, fatal pulmonary embolism may be divided into mechanical devices that prevent venous pooling and stasis in the lower limbs and drugs that inhibit blood coagulation. The former group includes leg elevation, elastic compression or pneumatic stockings, and electrical stimulation of the calf muscles. However, with the possible exception of pneumatic calf compression devices, their efficacy has not been substantiated.

Anticoagulant drugs such as heparin, warfarin, and low-molecular-weight dextran and platelet inhibitors such as aspirin have been extensively studied, but all remain quite controversial. The objective is to prevent clotting in blood pooled in the lower limb veins without increasing the risk of perioperative hemorrhage. Low-dose heparin has been used as a prophylactic drug in general surgical patients but is flawed by the risk of sensitizing the patient to heparin and the development of DIC. Radiolabeled fibrinogen studies demonstrate a reduction in the incidence of deep vein thrombosis to below 10%,[8] and a subcutaneous regimen of 5000 units preoperatively and 12 units hourly thereafter until the patient is mobile does not appear to cause excessive bleeding. However, the subject remains controversial because heparin prophylaxis has not been conclusively proved to decrease the incidence of *fatal* pulmonary embolism.[6, 16]

In several large trials, although fewer deaths due to pulmonary emboli occurred in heparin-treated patients, the percentages were of debatable statistical significance and probably reflect the difficulties inherent in obtaining a sufficiently large patient population for study. Undoubtedly, certain groups are at greater risk. Ten percent of elderly patients who undergo repair of a fractured hip suffer a pulmonary embolus, compared with an incidence of 0.2% of the general surgical population older than 40 years of age. Currently, research is being directed toward development of an index that may define the high-risk group. Details of diagnosis and management of pulmonary emboli are discussed in Chapter 49.

FAT EMBOLISM

Approximately 5% of trauma patients suffer fat embolism, especially after long-bone fracture. Orthopedic patients are also at risk. Fat emboli probably originate from the bone marrow and enter the circulation through torn venules at the fracture site. Although direct occlusion of small blood vessels in the lungs, brain, and skin by fat droplets may cause ischemic injury, the pathogenesis of the syndrome probably involves generation of toxic free fatty acids by lipase in the lungs or platelet aggregation around the fat droplets, with release of vasoactive mediators such as serotonin.

The classic triad of the fat embolism syndrome consists of respiratory insufficiency, neurologic signs, and a petechial rash, although many patients exhibit only one or two of these features. Respiratory insufficiency is associated with dyspnea, inspiratory crepitations, and hypoxemia. Neurologic disturbance ranges from mild confusion to severe impairment of consciousness, which may be accompanied by focal neurologic signs. The petechial rash characteristically occurs in the distribution of the carotid and subclavian arteries, affecting skin, mucous membranes, and conjunctiva. Pyrexia, tachycardia, retinopathy, and oliguria due to renal embolization are additional features.

Laboratory investigations may reveal fat droplets in the blood, urine, or sputum; increased serum lipase and free fatty acid levels; decreased serum albumin and calcium levels; and decreased platelet count. However, none of these tests is specific for fat embolism syndrome, and a combination of clinical and laboratory features is required to establish the diagnosis.

No specific treatment is of proven benefit after fat embolism. Heparin, low-molecular-weight dextran, aprotonin, and alcohol have all been suggested on theoretic grounds, but they may add more risks than benefits. There is anecdotal evidence that high-dose steroids, which stabilize membranes and reduce the inflammatory response, may limit the pulmonary injury. Early immobilization of fractures is a logical preventive measure, and internal fixation may be the most effective method. Measures directed at the early identification and correction of hypoxia and avoidance of hypercarbia, which may exacerbate the neurologic injury, are currently the mainstays of treatment.

FLUID, ELECTROLYTE, AND pH IMBALANCE

Isotonic or hypertonic dehydration is common in patients requiring emergency abdominal operations and in those who undergo major surgical procedures without adequate fluid therapy. Special problems are encountered in patients with renal insufficiency, who are susceptible to fluid overload and hyperkalemia, and those with hepatic insufficiency, who are unable to achieve sodium homeostasis because aldosterone metabolism is impaired.

Several factors may contribute to a fluid deficit in surgical patients:

1. Preoperative fluid depletion, especially in patients with intestinal obstruction, diarrhea, or vomiting.
2. Intraoperative fluid loss. Considerable amounts of water may be lost by evaporation during laparotomy and thoracotomy because of the exposure of large areas of moist mesothelium.
3. Postoperative fluid loss. Fluid loss from nasogastric aspirates, drains, and fistulas can be measured. In addition, several liters of fluid may be sequestered into the *third space*, comprising the interstitial space, peritoneal or pleural cavities, and bowel lumen. Insensible fluid loss, principally via the respiratory tract, must also be considered and may contribute up to 1 liter per day in a hypermetabolic postoperative patient.

Clinical assessment can provide a guide to fluid status. Dry mucous membranes and loss of skin turgor are cardinal signs of dehydration, whereas an elevated jugular venous pressure and crepitations at the lung bases suggest fluid overload. However, in a patient at risk of severe fluid imbalance, the central venous or left atrial pressure must be measured.

Whenever possible, half of the estimated fluid deficit should be replaced during the first 2 hours, with the balance being corrected over the following 6 to 12 hours. Water lost by evaporation from mesothelial surfaces and as insensible loss from the lungs is best replaced with 5% dextrose in water (DW). Fluid from drains, nasogastric aspirates and fistulas, and third-space losses contain electrolyte concentrations similar to plasma and should be replaced with a balanced electrolyte solution such as Ringer's lactate. Urinary output must also be considered; a good, sustained urinary output of 1000 to 1500 ml. per day (40 to 60 ml. per hour) is required for excretion of the solute load created by the catabolic state.

Hyponatremia in the early postoperative period is frequently due to a stress-induced increase in antidiuretic hormone, causing retention of water in excess of sodium. Catabolism also aggravates hyponatremia by the release of water from glycogen, fat, or protein breakdown. Both of these effects resolve spontaneously. However, erroneous replacement of gastrointestinal losses with sodium-free fluids leads to dilutional hyponatremia requiring correction. Patients with dilutional hyponatremia may become waterlogged and are best treated with fluid restriction and diuresis until excess water has been eliminated by the kidneys, followed by careful sodium replenishment with isotonic saline. Severe cases, in which sodium levels may fall below 115 mmol. per liter, are often accompanied by neurologic disturbances, with confusion, headaches, and paroxysms. However, rapid correction with hypertonic saline solutions is potentially hazardous because of large alterations in the osmotic gradient across neuronal cell membranes.

Hypernatremia, which is an excess of sodium relative to water, is less common in the postoperative period. Most frequently it is iatrogenic, induced by sodium-rich parenteral alimentation or prolonged infusion of isotonic saline. Less often, hypernatremia may arise after inadequate replacement of insensible loss, which is hypotonic with respect to plasma. Correction should be made by infusion of balanced saline solutions. No attempt should be made to obtain rapid correction with salt-poor solutions, because this causes rapid movement of water into the intracellular compartment, leading to cell edema.

Potassium Imbalance

Hypokalemia in postoperative patients is most commonly associated with fluid loss from the gastrointestinal tract. This may be due to direct loss of potassium, as in diarrhea, or secondary to the metabolic alkalosis caused by vomiting or prolonged nasogastric aspiration, which promotes the renal excretion of potassium. Hypokalemia may also be induced by diuretic therapy. Muscle contractility and nerve conduction depend on the ratio of intracellular to extracellular potassium concentrations. Hypokalemia affects skeletal muscle, causing weakness and diminished tendon reflexes; smooth muscle, causing paralytic ileus; and cardiac muscle. A serum potassium below 2.5 mmol. per liter may be associated with U waves and flattened T waves on the ECG. Patients on digitalis derivatives are at a particular risk of ventricular ectopic beats and tachyarrhythmias.

Hyperkalemia is most frequently observed in patients with renal insufficiency, and particular care must be taken with potassium intake in postoperative patients with poor urinary output. Potassium is the principal intracellular cation, and plasma levels may be elevated after extensive tissue damage, particularly in trauma patients who have suffered a crush injury. Massive blood transfusion is another cause, due to release of potassium into the plasma from stored red cells. Hyperkalemia can induce spasm in the smooth muscle of the gastrointestinal tract, causing abdominal pain, diarrhea and vomiting, peaked T waves on the ECG, and the danger of cardiac arrest. A serum potassium level above 7 mmol. per liter constitutes a surgical emergency requiring aggressive treatment with intravenous glucose and insulin (100 ml. of 50% dextrose and 20 units of insulin), together with ion exchange resins (calcium resonium, 30 to 60 gm. orally or rectally). Diuretics combined with intravenous saline infusion promote potassium excretion in patients with normal kidneys, but dialysis may be needed in those with compromised renal function.

Acid-Base Imbalance

Acid-base imbalance in a postoperative patient is usually associated with respiratory insufficiency, renal impairment, or net loss of hydrogen ions or bicarbonate from the gastrointestinal tract. Marked deviations in blood pH compromise cellular metabolism, and the heart is especially vulnerable. Acidosis reduces myocardial contractility, whereas alkalosis is associated with decreases in serum potassium and ionized calcium that increase myocardial irritability. Cerebral vascular resistance is dependent on blood pH as well as carbon dioxide content. Acidosis increases cerebral blood flow and exacerbates cerebral edema associated with head injury.

A pure respiratory acidosis reflects inadequate pulmonary ventilation, with an increase in blood pH secondary to carbon dioxide retention. Diminished tissue oxygenation induces anaerobic glycolysis, increasing lactic acid production and creating a metabolic component to the acidosis. Abnormal bicarbonate losses in diarrhea or from biliary or pancreatic fistulas, or an increase in ketone or lactate production associated with diabetes or starvation, can produce a metabolic acidosis without any respiratory component. Any disturbance in blood pH stimulates compensatory responses. In respiratory acidosis, bicarbonate is retained by the kidneys; in metabolic acidosis, the respiratory rate rises, increasing carbon dioxide excretion.

Respiratory acidosis usually responds to improved ventilation, whereas metabolic acidosis may require correction with sodium bicarbonate infusion. Correction of a severe metabolic acidosis may lead to fluid overload and should be staged, directed initially toward one-half correction, followed by reassessment of the acid-base and fluid balance. Dialysis may be required in patients with renal insufficiency.

Respiratory alkalosis in the postoperative period, due to either spontaneous hyperventilation (frequently in response to pain) or excessive mechanical ventilation, usually responds to appropriate analgesia or readjustment of the ventilator settings. A metabolic alkalosis reflects depletion of extracellular hydrogen and potassium ions and is observed in gastric outlet obstruction or prolonged nasogastric aspiration. Fluid and potassium replacement usually enables the kidneys to restore normal pH through bicarbonate excretion. Acidifying agents such as arginine monohydrochloride or dilute hydrochloric acid are rarely, if ever, required.

ALIMENTARY TRACT DYSFUNCTION

After laparotomy, the normal propulsive activity of the gastrointestinal tract is temporarily depressed, a condition termed *postoperative ileus*. It probably follows trauma to the intestine if a laparotomy was performed or, in other procedures, increased sympathetic discharge from splanchnic nerves. The term *ileus* is misleading because small bowel motility rapidly returns, and feeding through a tube jejunostomy is often initiated within 24 hours. Gastric peristalsis returns 24 to 48 hours after operation, and colonic activity usually returns after 48 hours, beginning at the cecum and progressing caudally. This postoperative ileus leads to mild abdominal distention (primarily from a distended colon) and absent bowel sounds in the first 48 to 72 hours. Return of normal peristaltic activity is often noted by mild cramps, passage of flatus, and return of appetite.

Acute Gastric Dilatation

Acute gastric dilatation follows massive overfilling of the stomach by fluids and gas. It is more common in malnourished and chronically immobilized patients. Gastric outlet obstruction may cause gross distention of the stomach. Acute gastric dilatation is occasionally observed in asthmatics and young children in whom oxygen masks are used in the immediate postoperative period, which suggests excessive air swallowing as an initiating event. Gastric dilatation may also follow forceful insufflation of air during emergency resuscitation or during endoscopy. Surgical procedures in the vicinity of the stomach, such as fundoplication and splenectomy, may inhibit the intrinsic pacemaker of the stomach, and this is also the presumed mechanism in diabetics (diabetic gastroparesis).

As the stomach distends, it descends across the duodenum, producing a mechanical obstruction that exacerbates the problem. Increased intragastric pressure produces venous engorgement of the mucosa, causing fluid secretion and mucosal hemorrhage. If this is allowed to continue, ischemic necrosis and perforation result. The distended stomach pushes the diaphragm upward, causing collapse of the lower lobe of the left lung, rotation of the heart, and obstruction of the inferior vena cava. The acutely dilated stomach is also prone to gastric volvulus.

Clinically, the patient has severe pain and dyspnea, suggesting myocardial infarction. Frequently, however, the onset is insidious; the patient appears ill, experiences sweating and hiccups, is dehydrated, and has a hypochloremic metabolic alkalosis due to fluid and electrolyte loss into the stomach. The abdomen is distended, and the cardinal sign is a gastric splash.

Treatment consists of gastric decompression with a nasogastric tube and appropriate fluid replacement. In the late stages, gastric necrosis may necessitate gastrectomy.

Gastroduodenal Mucosal Hemorrhage

Hemorrhage from acute shallow ulcers in the stomach and duodenum is a well-recognized complication in severely ill and septic postoperative patients. It is associated with failure of multiple organ systems and is probably due to a defect in the protective gastric mucous layer, rendering the mucosa susceptible to acid injury. Histamine receptor antagonists have been recommended as prophylaxis in high-risk patients. Endoscopy usually reveals multiple erosions in the stomach or duodenum. Treatment with histamine receptor antagonists and antacids is usually effective, and surgical therapy, which may entail total gastrectomy, is now required infrequently.

Intestinal Obstruction

Intestinal obstruction in the early postoperative period may be the result of paralytic ileus or mechanical obstruction. Ileus may be prolonged in patients with metabolic disturbances (hypokalemia, uremia, diabetes), intraperitoneal or retroperitoneal inflammation or hematomas, and mesenteric vascular insufficiency and in those taking tricyclic antidepressant drugs. Acute colonic pseudo-obstruction (Ogilvie's syndrome) is a localized form of paralytic ileus affecting the large bowel, most frequently the proximal colon. It is observed in patients who have undergone surgical procedures not involving the abdomen, in particular, major orthopedic operations, when colonic activity appears to be impaired. Increasing abdominal distention develops, with risk of cecal perforation. Treatment is by colonoscopic decompression or, if this fails, laparotomy and tube cecostomy.

Mechanical intestinal obstruction is most often caused by postoperative adhesions or an internal hernia. The diagnosis may be difficult because the symptoms may first be attributed to paralytic ileus. The majority of postoperative patients with mechanical obstruction experience a short period of apparently normal recovery of intestinal function before manifestations of obstruction supervene. If plain films of the abdomen demonstrate air-fluid levels in loops of small bowel, mechanical obstruction is the likely diagnosis. Strangulation is uncommon, because the adhesive bands are broader and more pliable than in the case of late small bowel obstruction. Thus, initial treatment is conservative, with nasogastric decompression and careful observation. If the obstruction does not resolve spontaneously within 48 hours, or if tachycardia or increasing abdominal signs develop, laparotomy should be performed.

Postoperative Fecal Impaction

Fecal impaction after operative procedures is usually the result of colonic ileus and impaired rectal sensation. It is principally a disease of the elderly but may occur in younger patients who have predisposing conditions, such as paraplegia. The use of opiate analgesics and anticholinergic drugs may be an aggravating factor. Patients who have undergone anal surgical procedures such as hemorrhoidectomy may also be inhibited because of pain. Some patients complain of constipation, abdominal pain, distention, and anorexia, but diarrhea due to overflow of liquid feces around the impacted solid material is also a common presentation. In advanced cases, mechanical obstruction occurs and may progress to colonic perforation. The diagnosis is established by rectal examination. The impaction is manually removed, under general anesthesia if necessary, and enemas are given. A high-fiber diet and increased oral fluids should then be encouraged.

Constipation affecting principally the right colon often follows hardening of barium from an enema performed before operation, which is more difficult to clear than fecal impaction. Treatment is with laxatives and enemas.

Colitis

Return of bowel function following an abdominal operation is frequently heralded by the passage of liquid feces. Persistent postoperative diarrhea is occasionally due to pathogenic organisms such as *Shigella, Salmonella,* or *Campylobacter,* which should be identified from a fecal specimen. Patients treated with antibiotics are at risk of bacterial overgrowth with resistant staphylococci in the bowel, but a more serious consequence of antibiotic therapy is pseudomembranous colitis.

Pseudomembranous colitis is associated with *Clostridium difficile,* an anaerobic bacterium that releases a toxin. The condition can be induced by a variety of antibiotics, especially clindamycin and lincomycin. In addition to diarrhea, which may be the only symptom in mild cases, systemic illness with abdominal pain and fever may develop. Severe cases lead to colonic dilatation and perforation. Sigmoidoscopy reveals a characteristic yellow pseudomembrane associated with a friable rectal mucosa, and the diagnosis is con-

firmed by demonstrating the organism or its toxin in the feces or a rectal biopsy.

Anastomotic Leak

Anastomotic leakage is usually a technical complication. The cardinal principles of any gastrointestinal anastomosis are as follows:

1. Avoid tension across the anastomosis.
2. Ensure good blood supply to both ends of the bowel.
3. Achieve accurate and watertight apposition of the cut edges with inversion of the bowel edges to obtain serosa-to-serosa apposition.
4. Prevent sepsis or gross contamination.
5. Prevent distal obstruction.

Studies with radiographic contrast material following colorectal procedures indicate that most large bowel anastomotic leaks are well localized, and only a minority have any clinical sequelae. A pericolic abscess may form at the site of the leak, causing pyrexia, which resolves when the abscess discharges back into the bowel. This is frequently accompanied by an episode of diarrhea.

An enterocutaneous fistula results if the anastomotic leak discharges through the abdominal wound. If there is no persistent distal obstruction and the anastomosis was performed between healthy tissue, such fistulas heal, but a period of parenteral alimentation may be indicated to reduce the flow through the fistula.

Diffuse peritonitis is the most serious consequence of anastomotic disruption. The patient requires rapid resuscitation with intravenous fluids and nasogastric aspiration, followed by laparotomy. Because of their more tenuous blood supply, large bowel anastomoses are at greatest risk of leakage; because of the associated contamination, initial surgical management is to exteriorize both ends of the anastomosis. Leaks from proximal gastrointestinal anastomoses are less common and can often be managed by primary reconstruction of the anastomosis, preventing the substantial fluid losses that can follow a high gastrointestinal stoma or fistula.

Hepatobiliary Complications and Jaundice

Hepatic dysfunction leading to an elevated serum bilirubin follows 1% of surgical procedures performed under general anesthesia. As expected, the incidence of hepatobiliary complications is greatest after operations on the liver, biliary tract, and pancreas. Postoperative hyperbilirubinemia may be categorized as prehepatic, hepatocellular, or extrahepatic (obstructive).

Prehepatic jaundice is due to bilirubin overload, most often from hemolysis or the reabsorption of hematomas. Transfusion reactions, drugs, sepsis, and hypoxia in patients with hemoglobinopathies are common causes.

Hepatocellular insufficiency follows hepatic cell necrosis or extensive hepatic resection. Drugs, hypoxia, hypotension, and sepsis are among the injurious factors. Anesthetic agents, particularly halothane, have been implicated as a cause of potentially fatal postoperative hepatitis, especially after reexposure to the same agent. Posttransfusion hepatitis with hepatitis B, cytomegalovirus, and, in particular, hepatitis C has been reported in up to 10% of patients receiving blood transfusions. Although this usually has a long latent period, it may develop as early as the third postoperative week.

Extrahepatic obstruction is caused by direct surgical injury to the bile ducts, retained common bile duct stones, tumors, or pancreatitis. Acute acalculous cholecystitis is associated with jaundice in one third of cases. It is a disease largely confined to patients who have prolonged stays in the ICU, often requiring respiratory and other supports, including prolonged intravenous nutrition. Other associations include prolonged ileus and prolonged morphine administration. The pathogenesis appears to be gallbladder distention following deficient release of endogenous cholecystokinin-pancreozymin. Secondary mucosal injury and vascular thrombosis often lead to transmural necrosis and perforation of the gallbladder.

The diagnosis is often delayed, and an emergency cholecystectomy has a high mortality. Acute acalculous cholecystitis should always be suspected in a critically ill patient in whom an *unexpected septic pattern* develops. Ultrasonography of the gallbladder usually demonstrates a dilated gallbladder, with an edematous gallbladder wall, containing biliary sludge. In the early stage, a percutaneous cholecystostomy may be attempted. Generally, direct visualization of the gallbladder, accomplished through a small abdominal incision under local anesthesia, may be required to totally exclude or confirm the diagnosis. If the gallbladder appears normal, the mini-incision is closed. If the gallbladder appears inflamed and is surrounded by omentum, a standard cholecystectomy under general anesthesia is essential.

COMPLICATIONS OF MINIMAL-ACCESS SURGICAL PROCEDURES

The ongoing technical development of the laparoscope and associated instruments for minimal-access surgical procedures, coupled with patients' demands and the rapid general acceptance by the surgical profession, has led to a new series of complications. With the widespread use of laparoscopy, the incidence of many complications is increasing. However, as experience with the procedures is gained, techniques to minimize or eliminate these complications should evolve.[3, 13]

The complications of laparoscopic procedures can be broadly classified as those directly related to the performance of laparoscopy and those inherent in the performance of the actual procedure (e.g., cholecystectomy, Nissen fundoplication, appendectomy, bowel resection). Complications of laparoscopy include needle or trocar injury to a hollow viscus or a major vascular structure, as well as gas insufflation outside the peritoneal cavity due to improper placement of the Veress needle. Subcutaneous emphysema, mediastinal emphysema, pneumothorax, and gas embolism must all be considered if cardiovascular or respiratory problems occur during the procedure. This may necessitate abandoning the operation or conversion to an open procedure if major abdominal injuries cannot be excluded. These injuries invariably occur during the initial placement of the Veress needle to create a pneumoperitoneum or during the first insertion of a trocar. Patients with previous abdominal operations and peritoneal adhesions are most at risk. A recommended method of avoiding these *blind* or *stab* injuries is to use the *open* Hasson technique of introducing the initial needle and trocar under direct vision via a small *cut-down* incision in the fascia and peritoneum of the anterior abdominal wall. More recently, injury from the telescope itself has been reported. Moving the telescope through a wide arc may injure structures adherent to the anterior abdominal wall behind the viewing field of the scope. In addition, the tip of the telescope becomes hot, and inadvertent contact may further injure the tissue. The use of electrocautery or the laser may also seriously injure vital structures. Abdominal hernias have been reported at sites of main trocar insertion, and subumbilical wound infection at the telescope site has also been recognized.

Complications that can be directly attributed to the surgical procedure include hemorrhage, bile duct injury of varying degrees,[13] and bowel perforation leading to peritonitis and/

or localized abscess. The laparoscopic surgeon must be aware of all these dangers. Performing an operation through the laparoscope does not preclude attention to basic surgical principles of the operation. The surgeon should never operate in a *blind* manner without proper visualization and identification of structures. In difficult situations, the surgeon must never hesitate to convert a laparoscopic operation into an open one. It is always better to have an *elective* conversion (before causing a complication and anticipating it) than an *enforced* conversion (after recognizing the complication).

Postoperatively, one of the most widely accepted advantages of the laparoscopic operation is the relative freedom from pain. Hence, any patient with unusual amount of pain should be thought to have a complication of the operation until proved otherwise. Thus, early evaluation and, if indicated, early abdominal exploration are mandatory in these instances.

NEUROLOGIC COMPLICATIONS

Focal lesions in the central nervous system may occur as a direct result of operative trauma during operations on the brain or spinal cord, as a complication of spinal or epidural anesthesia, or as a consequence of focal ischemia, usually embolic in origin. Septic emboli may cause a brain abscess.

Peripheral nerves may also be inadvertently damaged during operative procedures. Examples include injury to the recurrent laryngeal nerve during thyroid or parathyroid surgery, to the facial nerve during parotidectomy, to the ilioinguinal nerve during inguinal hernia repair, and to the sciatic nerve during operations on the hip. Ischemic injury may also occur during prolonged use of a tourniquet used to obtain a bloodless field during orthopedic operations.

Prolonged Alteration of Consciousness

Patients subjected to general anesthesia undergo an induced loss of consciousness. Usually, this rapidly reverses after cessation of anesthesia. If the patient reacts to painful stimuli and all reflexes are present, with pupils that are of equal size and react to light, the prognosis for a rapid and complete recovery is favorable. Unfortunately, there are some patients who do not recover promptly, if at all.

The most common cause of delayed recovery is the excess or prolonged effect of the anesthetic agent. Elderly patients may be especially sensitive to anesthetic drugs, especially opiate analgesics; these can be specifically reversed with naloxone. Renal and hepatic insufficiency pose special problems for drug metabolism and elimination, and obese patients can absorb large amounts of a fat-soluble anesthetic agent that is slowly released from fat deposits postoperatively.

The major concern in patients who fail to recover consciousness after anesthesia is that they have suffered irreversible brain injury. In a patient with diabetes, this may be due to profound hypoglycemia following insulin therapy in a starved patient during anesthesia. However, the most devastating complication of general anesthesia is a hypoxic brain injury. Cerebral hypoxia may follow restricted oxygen supply during anesthesia (a complication that modern anesthetic monitoring equipment is designed to prevent), overdosage of narcotics in the postoperative period, various types of pulmonary insufficiency, or the reduced oxygen carrying capacity of the blood.

Brain damage may also be caused by diminished cerebral perfusion after a period of reduced cardiac output and hypotension during the operation or may follow a cerebrovascular accident. Cerebrovascular accidents occur most frequently in elderly patients with atherosclerosis who become hypotensive during operation. Severe hypertension, such as that experienced by patients with thyrotoxicosis or pheochromocytoma, and embolism from atherosclerotic plaques, blood clots, fat, or air are additional possible causes.

Prompt recognition and correction of the underlying cause are, of course, vital in hypoxic, hypotensive, or hypoglycemic patients. Individuals who sustain a mild brain injury may remain obtunded for 72 hours and then rapidly regain a normal state of consciousness without apparent sequelae. In contrast, those who sustain a severe brain injury commonly have abnormal limb reflexes, posture, and pupil size and may have convulsions or decerebrate rigidity. Although the prognosis is usually poor, even these severe manifestations of hypoxic damage are sometimes reversible if cerebral edema can be controlled with hyperventilation, mannitol, and steroids. Barbiturate therapy has also been advocated to protect the brain from further hypoxic damage.

Strokes occur in 1% to 3% of patients after carotid endarterectomy or other reconstructive operations on the extracranial portion of the carotid system. The outcome following perioperative strokes is as widely variable as it is in nonoperative stroke situations, ranging from complete recovery to serious or even fatal sequelae.

Convulsions

The previously mentioned cerebral injuries are capable of producing convulsions. Epilepsy or metabolic derangements may also lead to convulsions in the postoperative period. For unknown reasons, patients with complications of ulcerative colitis and Crohn's disease are particularly susceptible to convulsions with loss of consciousness in the postoperative period.

Therapy for convulsions in the postoperative period is no different from that for seizures in general. Close observation with maintenance of an adequate airway and oxygen administration is essential, because hypoxia may have an important role in the cause of this disorder. Moreover, because of residual anesthesia, reintubation and ventilation assistance may be required. Intravenous diazepam, barbiturates, or phenytoin may be required if the convulsions do not abate spontaneously. Complete laboratory analysis should be ordered immediately, and abnormalities such as hypoxia, hypomagnesemia, hypocalcemia, hypokalemia, and hypernatremia should be corrected appropriately. Excessive fluid overload should be treated by cautious diuresis and a reduction in maintenance fluids.

When the patient's condition is stable, a routine examination for epilepsy may be indicated. A decision can then be made whether maintenance therapy with phenytoin and phenobarbital is indicated to prevent the likelihood of further convulsions.

Postoperative Psychosis and Delirium

Anxiety and fear are normal in patients who undergo surgical procedures. Confusion is common in elderly patients who awake in strange surroundings in pain or under the influence of anesthetic and analgesic agents. Sleep deprivation, which is especially common in patients in ICUs, may cause disorientation and hallucinations. Alteration in body image is a major cause of morbidity in patients requiring a stoma, a mastectomy, or amputation. The ability to manage these stresses is largely determined by the patient's psychic strength. The boundary between these normal manifestations of stress and postoperative psychosis may be difficult to establish.

The incidence of postoperative psychosis is approximately 0.2% for general surgical patients but is much higher following open heart surgery, where postcardiotomy delirium is a well-recognized syndrome. Five specific criteria are necessary for the diagnosis of delirium[2]:

1. Diminished consciousness
2. Disturbance of perception, speech, sleep, or psychomotor activity
3. Disorientation and memory impairment
4. Rapid onset and fluctuating course of the illness
5. Identification of a specific organic factor related to the mental disturbance

Delirium in surgical patients was described in the nineteenth century as *interval psychosis*, referring to the lucid postoperative interval of days that may precede the onset of delirium.

Various factors predispose to postoperative delirium. Preoperative factors include age; chronic alcohol abuse; drug dependency; dementia; brain lesions such as tumors and infections; metabolic abnormalities, including uremia and hepatic insufficiency; and a previous history of delirium. Intraoperative and postoperative factors include hypotension, hypoxia, metabolic derangements, sepsis, and drugs. The duration of cardiopulmonary bypass may be related to the development of postcardiotomy delirium.

In general, psychiatric problems should be anticipated by the surgeon and the nursing staff in the elderly with chronic disease or in patients with other risk factors. Most overt psychiatric problems are observed after the third postoperative day. Some severe disturbances may be avoided by appropriate preoperative counseling of the patient by the surgeon.

Characteristically, delirium has a rapid onset, and symptoms may appear simultaneously in many areas of psychologic functioning. Typically, the patient is disorientated with respect to time, place, or person, but the severity of the disorientation may vary. The patient may show impaired perception, misidentifying shadows, sounds, and smells in a terrifying way. Hallucinations are characteristically visual and are exacerbated at night. Delirious patients who are agitated and combative may hurl themselves out of bed to escape imaginary assailants.

The distress and panic following disordered perception and thought require immediate symptomatic treatment until the delirium clears. Haloperidol, 1 to 5 mg. intramuscularly, is the drug of choice. Phenothiazines such as chlorpromazine are also effective and cause sedation but may cause hypotension. Benzodiazepines are, in general, contraindicated because they overly sedate the patient, are short-lived, and may not affect the psychotic symptoms. They may even aggravate the agitation and confusion. Fortunately, most psychiatric postoperative problems are of short duration and leave the patient without permanent disability.

SELECTED REFERENCES

Carey, L. (Ed.): Surg. Clin. North Am., 63, December 1983.
 This issue reviews the complications of the most common general surgical operations in a comprehensive manner.

Greenfield, L. J. (Ed.): Complications in Surgery in Trauma. Philadelphia, J. B. Lippincott, 1984.
 In this text, 67 authorities have contributed to all aspects of the complications of surgical therapy and trauma and their management.

Hardy, J. D. (Ed.): Complications in Surgery and Their Management, 4th ed. Philadelphia, W. B. Saunders, 1981.
 This extensive survey of surgical complications contains a wealth of information regarding the underlying pathophysiology and the appropriate treatment.

Moossa, A. R. (Ed.): Tumors of the Pancreas. Baltimore, Williams & Wilkins, 1980.
 This monograph provides the details of complications associated with pancreatic surgery and invasive investigations of the pancreas.

Moossa, A. R., Robson, M. C., and Schimpff, S. C. (Eds.): Comprehensive Textbook of Oncology, 2nd ed. Baltimore, Williams & Wilkins, 1990.

This text details all aspects, including complications, of the multidisciplinary approaches of the diagnosis and treatment of cancer.

REFERENCES

1. Braunwald, E., et al.: Principles of Internal Medicine, 11th ed. New York, McGraw-Hill, 1977.
2. Diagnostic and Statistical Manual of Mental Disorders, 3rd ed. Washington, D.C., American Psychiatric Association, 1980.
3. Easter, D., and Moossa, A. R.: Laser and laparoscopic cholecystectomy—a hazardous union? Arch. Surg., *126*:423, 1992.
4. Flanc, C., Kakkar, V. V., and Clarke, M. B.: Postoperative deep vein thrombosis—effect and intensive prophylaxis. Lancet, *1*:477, 1969.
5. Ganeval, D., Kleinknecht, D., and Gonzales-Duque, L. A.: High-dose furosemide in renal failure. Br. Med. J., *1*:244, 1974.
6. Greenfield, L. J.: Intraluminal techniques for vena caval interruption and pulmonary embolectomy. World J. Surg., *2*:4559, 1978.
7. Hamilton, W. K., et al.: Postoperative respiratory complications. Anesthesiology, *25*:607, 1964.
8. Kakkar, V. V., Corrigan, T. P., and Fossard, D. P.: International multicentre trial: Prevention of fatal postoperative embolism by low doses of heparin. Lancet, *2*:45, 1975.
9. Korde, M., and Warde, B. E.: Serum potassium concentrations after succinylcholine patients with renal failure. Anesthesiology, *36*:142, 1972.
10. Lee, A. B., et al.: Effects of abdominal operation on ventilation and gas exchange. J. Natl. Med. Assoc., *61*:164, 1969.
11. MacLean, L. D., Mulligan, W. B., MacLean, A. P. H., and Duff, J. H.: Patterns of septic shock in man: A detailed study of 56 patients. Ann. Surg., *166*:543, 1967.
12. Mendelson, C.: Aspiration of stomach contents during obstetric anesthesia. Am. J. Obstet. Gynecol., *52*:191, 1946.
13. Moossa, A. R., Easter, D., Van Sonnenberg, E., et al.: Laparoscopic injuries to the bile duct—a cause for concern. Ann. Surg., *215*:203, 1992.
14. Pontoppidan, H.: Treatment of respiratory failure in nonthoracic trauma. J. Trauma, *8*:938, 1968.
15. Strandness, D. E., Jr., and Summer, D. E.: Ultrasonic velocity detector in the diagnosis of thrombophlebitis. Arch. Surg., *104*:180, 1972.
16. Urokinase-streptokinase embolism trial and phase 2 results: A cooperative study. JAMA, *229*:1606, 1974.
17. Wilson, R., et al.: Acute respiratory failure: Diagnostic and therapeutic criteria. Crit. Care Med., *2*:293, 1974.
18. Wiren, F. E., Janson, L., and Hellekant, C.: Respiratory complications after upper abdominal surgery. Acta Chir. Scand., *147*:623, 1981.

CHAPTER 19

ACUTE RENAL FAILURE IN SURGICAL PATIENTS

Prevention and Treatment

R. Randal Bollinger, M.D., Ph.D., and Steve J. Schwab, M.D.

Acute renal failure (ARF) is a potentially lethal complication. Despite recent advances in dialysis and intensive care, almost half of patients in whom ARF develops in the postoperative period succumb. The severity of the trauma, the magnitude of the surgical procedure, the gravity of underlying medical conditions that predispose to ARF, and the high incidence of sepsis all contribute to multiorgan failure, which causes the high mortality rate. Prompt and effective treatment of each component of the multifaceted etiology of ARF can prevent the syndrome and offer the surgical patient the best likelihood of survival.

ARF is defined as an abrupt decline in renal function sufficient to cause retention of nitrogenous waste.[3] This definition of ARF does not depend on the urinary output of the patient. The emphasis is on the quality of the urine, rather than the quantity, because nonoliguric forms of ARF occur quite frequently.[4] Whether or not oliguria is present, a progressive rise in blood urea nitrogen (BUN) and serum creatinine concentration in the posttrauma or postoperative period should suggest the presence of ARF. Because ARF represents one of the few incidences of completely reversible severe organ failure, early intensive and continuing treatment is indicated.

THE LESSONS OF WAR

During World War I the problem of hypovolemic shock was observed among injured soldiers and civilians. The acute anuria that accompanied the hypovolemia responded to fluid replacement. Those patients with persistent ARF uniformly died. However, it was not until World War II that Bywaters and Beall described the new syndrome of renal shutdown following extensive crush injuries, particularly of the extremities.[21, 22] After the introduction by Kolff of the artificial kidney in the late 1940s, it was realized that the human kidney could recover from such a severe injury. Using the new technology of hemodialysis, Swan and Merrill of Boston achieved a 54% survival rate in 85 patients.[95] Both the incidence of ARF and the outcome were favorably affected by this improved treatment.

The first widespread application of the new dialysis technology occurred in the Korean War. The incidence of ARF among critically wounded soldiers decreased slightly from 42% to 35%. However, the mortality after combat injuries causing ARF declined from 90% in World War II to 53% in the later years of the Korean War.[90, 94] Better management of shock was largely responsible for this improvement, although dialysis became available near the end of the war. The Vietnam War experience demonstrated a significant beneficial effect of early dialysis. Conger reported in 1975 in a prospective trial of prophylactic dialysis in posttraumatic ARF

among United States combat casualties that rates of various septic, hemorrhagic, and neurologic complications tended to be lower in the more vigorously dialyzed patients. Survival was threefold better in those patients receiving more intensive dialysis.[26] Because of efficient evacuation by helicopter and rapid resuscitation, the incidence of ARF declined to 0.17% during the Vietnam War, but the mortality rate for those few patients in whom renal failure developed remained excessively high, at 77%.[37] The clear lesson from that war experience is that prevention of ARF in the surgical patient is much more effective than any treatment available.

CLASSIFICATION

When renal failure, defined as a decline in renal function sufficient to cause retention of nitrogenous waste, occurs abruptly, *acute* renal failure is present. When the azotemia develops gradually over many weeks or months, the renal failure is termed *chronic*. If a patient in renal failure presents with asymptomatic azotemia, the differentiation of acute from chronic disease may be difficult. Several aspects of the history and radiologic examination, particularly the presence of small *end-stage* kidneys, correctly classify the patient's disease as discussed subsequently.

Renal failure is termed *oliguric* if less than 400 ml. of urine is produced in 24 hours. Patients with *nonoliguric* renal failure void large volumes of isosthenuric urine but are unable to clear nitrogenous waste from their systems. Diuretic therapy may convert the oliguric form to the more easily managed nonoliguric form of renal failure.

ARF is conveniently classified according to its cause as prerenal, renal, or postrenal (Table 19–1). Each of these types may present in either the oliguric or nonoliguric form, and all are associated with rising BUN and serum creatinine levels. All the conditions that may impair renal function must be considered in the differential diagnosis of postoperative ARF. Foremost among the *prerenal* causes are volume depletion, heart failure, and abnormalities in the renal vasculature. Volume depletion may be the result of blood loss (either internally or externally), dehydration, or third-space sequestration in the gastrointestinal tract or other extravascular fluid spaces. Renal artery stenosis, renal artery emboli, and renal vascular thrombosis, although much less common than volume depletion, all can produce prerenal azotemia. The treatment for all prerenal conditions is correction of the internal environment toward the normal state by replacing the lost volume, improving cardiac function, removing sources of sepsis, and correcting abnormalities in the renal vasculature.

The intrinsic renal causes of ARF commonly observed in postoperative and posttrauma patients are acute tubular necrosis, pigment nephropathy from free myoglobin or hemo-

**TABLE 19–1. Common Causes of Surgical
Acute Renal Failure**

Prerenal
  Hypotension
  Hypovolemia
  Arterial occlusion or stenosis
  Cardiac failure

Intrarenal
  Toxins (radiographic contrast medium, endotoxin)
  Drugs (aminoglycosides, cyclosporine, amphotericin B,
    nonsteroidal anti-inflammatory drugs)
  Pigment nephropathy (myoglobin, hemoglobin)

Postrenal
  Ureteral obstruction or tear (stones, trauma, surgical injury)
  Bladder dysfunction (anesthetic, nerve injury, drugs)
  Urethral obstruction (trauma, benign prostatic hypertrophy,
    malignancy)

globin, nephrotoxicity from drugs or radiographic contrast material, sepsis, and acute interstitial nephritis. The common cause of acute tubular necrosis is shock, although any of the prerenal conditions already listed, as well as prolonged obstructive uropathy, may produce necrosis of the tubular lining. When ischemia becomes severe or prolonged, actual cortical necrosis, an irreversible condition, may develop. There are, of course, many other intrinsic renal diseases that may produce renal failure but are more closely associated with medical disease states than with the postoperative surgical patient and are not discussed in this chapter. Therapy for intrinsic renal causes of ARF is directed to support of the patient with hemodialysis or peritoneal dialysis until recovery of native renal function occurs.

Postrenal causes of ARF are obstructive uropathy and urinary extravasation. The obstruction can occur in the renal pelvis or ureter as the result of a stone, tumor, or clot. Injury to the ureter, sometimes iatrogenic, should be suspected when anuria develops after pelvic or retroperitoneal surgery or trauma. More distal obstruction in the urethra can be caused by a bladder stone, stricture, or benign prostatic hypertrophy. A common but easily corrected cause of obstructive uropathy in the postoperative period is an improperly placed or blocked Foley catheter. Urinary extravasation usually follows trauma that injures the bladder or urethra or, postoperatively, disruption of a cystotomy incision. Therapy for postrenal causes of ARF is directed to relief of the obstruction or repair of the urinary leak.

The difficult problem posed by surgical patients is in distinguishing a normal kidney attempting to function in an abnormal internal environment (prerenal failure) from a kidney that is no longer able to maintain the internal environment (renal failure). To differentiate the large number of possible disorders posed by a postoperative patient with diminished renal function, and to arrive at the correct conclusion and treatment, knowledge of the physiology of ARF is necessary.

PHYSIOLOGY OF ACUTE RENAL FAILURE

Normal Renal Physiology

The kidneys are paired organs that lie retroperitoneally along each side of the vertebral column between T12 and L3. Each kidney is supplied by a single renal artery that originates from the aorta at the level of L1. Occasionally, however, a single kidney is supplied by two or more main renal arteries that serve overlapping regions of the renal parenchyma. As the main renal artery enters the renal midsection,

it divides into the progressively smaller interlobar, arcuate, and interlobular arteries that branch into the afferent arterioles that supply each glomerulus. The glomerulus is a network of capillaries that are arranged around a mesangial matrix to form glomerular capillary tufts. After looping out and turning back on themselves, the capillaries rejoin to form an efferent arteriole, which exits the glomerulus at the vascular pole. After a short distance the efferent arteriole branches into another capillary bed that surrounds the renal tubules. These capillaries eventually coalesce to form venules, which ultimately join together as exiting renal veins. Functionally, therefore, the renal circulation is characterized by a number of progressively smaller arteries and two capillary beds in series: the glomerular capillary bed and the peritubular capillary bed. The afferent and efferent arterioles of the glomerulus are extremely active as variable resistance vessels and thus are important in autoregulating renal blood flow (RBF) and the glomerular filtration rate (GFR). This anatomic configuration of the individual nephron with its distinctive blood supply forms the basis of the current understanding of renal function and pathogenesis of vasomotor ischemic tubular injury (Fig. 19–1).

The glomerular capillary network is surrounded by a relatively impermeable epithelial capsule (Bowman's capsule), which forms a space that communicates directly with the lumen of the contiguous proximal tubule. Formation of urine begins with the filtration of plasma across the glomerular capillary wall and basement membrane into the lumen of Bowman's capsule. The passage of fluid across this filtration barrier depends primarily on the difference between the hydrostatic pressure within the capillary and the hydrostatic pressure that is in the surrounding Bowman's space. The hydrostatic pressure in Bowman's space is normally vented through the renal proximal tubule, so the variable that is normally responsible for the quantity of glomerular filtrate is the positive hydrostatic pressure within the glomerular capillary. Fixed oncotic forces due to plasma proteins in the capillary oppose filtration, as do the glomerular basement membrane and its cellular accouterment. Ischemic or chemical injury may decrease the formation of ultrafiltrate.[27]

The hydrostatic pressure in the glomerular capillaries depends on the difference in vascular resistance and pressure of the afferent and the efferent arterioles. Modulation of the afferent arteriolar resistance appears to be an intrinsic property of the arteriolar wall itself and is significantly influenced as well by renal sympathetic nerves, circulating catecholamines, angiotensin, and vasoactive prostaglandins and kinins.[9, 30, 73] Resistance of the efferent arteriole appears to be modulated primarily by angiotensin and norepinephrine but may be significantly influenced by prostaglandins and kinins under certain circumstances. Adjustments in these two resistances can maintain glomerular capillary pressure at a relatively constant level despite wide fluctuations in systemic and renal arterial pressure. For example, when systemic arterial blood pressure falls, glomerular capillary filtration pressure is still maintained by coordinated decreased resistance in the afferent arteriole and increased resistance in the efferent arteriole. The consequence of these changes in vascular resistance is to aid delivery of blood to the glomerular capillary system and hydrostatically force a greater fraction of the total glomerular blood flow per unit time across the capillary wall as filtrate. However, if the mean arterial blood pressure falls below a critical level, even this compensatory mechanism fails to maintain GFR. A corollary consequence of efficient arteriole vasoconstriction is reduction in peritubular blood supply; this relationship is depicted in Figure 19–2.

The principal functions of the kidney are to maintain the volume and ionic composition of the extracellular fluid (ECF) and to excrete the metabolic nitrogenous waste products.

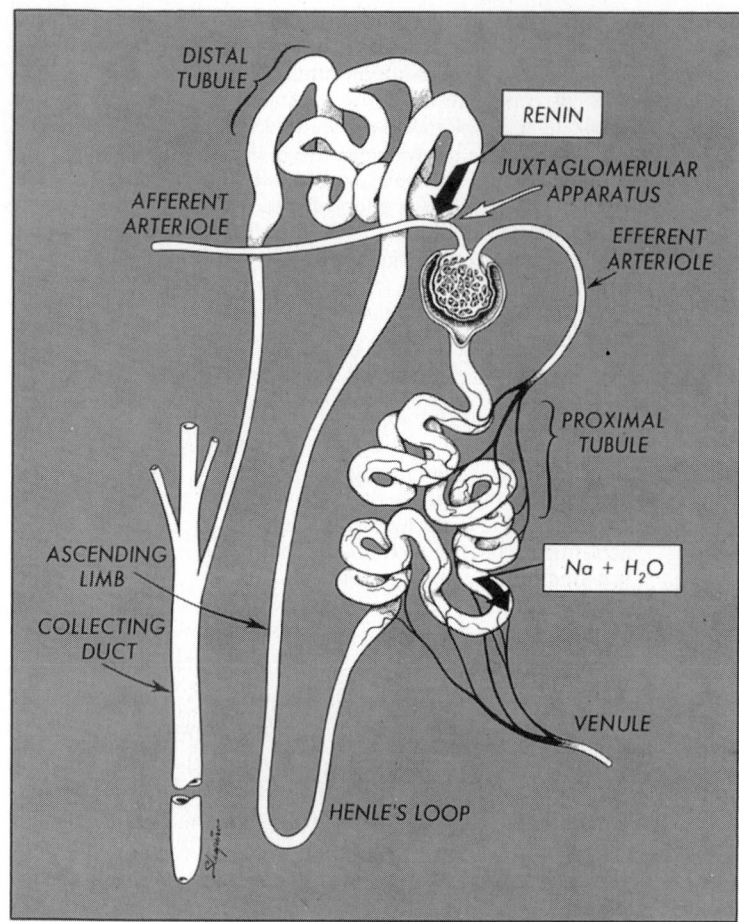

Figure 19–1. Principal structural features of the nephron and its blood supply. Blood enters the glomerulus through the afferent arteriole and exits through the efferent arteriole. Active dilation and constriction of these muscular vessels significantly modulate glomerular filtration. The tubule receives its blood supply primarily from the efferent arteriole. Renin is secreted by the juxtaglomerular apparatus in response to afferent blood flow and distal nephron urinary flow and composition.

Maintenance of ECF volume and composition is accomplished by tubular regulation of the secretion and reabsorption of solutes and water as the plasma filtrate flows through the renal tubule. The proximal tubule serves primarily to reclaim the bulk of glomerular filtrate, which is more than 150 liters of fluid per day. Thus, in the proximal nephron, large amounts of filtered sodium, chloride, potassium, calcium, bicarbonate, and phosphate are reabsorbed isotonically,

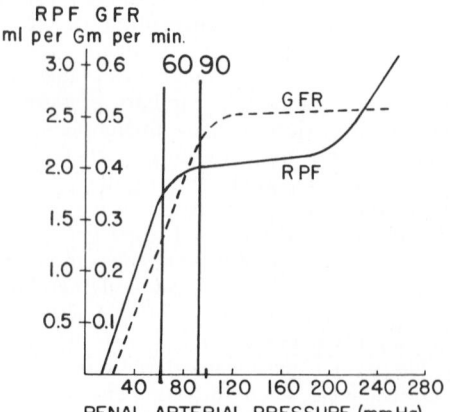

Figure 19–2. Autoregulation of renal plasma flow (RPF) and glomerular filtration rate (GFR) with varying arterial mean pressure. GFR and RPF are well maintained until mean pressure falls below 90 mm. Hg. GFR is reduced by approximately one half when pressure reaches 60 mm. Hg. (Adapted from Ochwadt, B.: The relation of renal blood supply to diuresis. Prog. Cardiovasc. Dis., *3*:501, 1961.)

together with glucose, amino acids, and other filtered solutes. Along the distal nephron and collecting duct, the chemical composition of the passing luminal fluid is more finely regulated. It is here that potassium secretion is modulated, acid is secreted, new bicarbonate is generated and delivered back into peritubular blood, sodium excretion is finely modulated, and water can be conserved or excreted. Proper performance of each of these precisely regulated functions requires sufficient blood flow to the glomeruli, sufficient filtration pressure, structurally intact tubules with operational metabolic systems, adequate flow of filtrate throughout the nephron, and adequate peritubular circulation. Disturbance or disruption of any one or all of these factors can cause tubular dysfunction and homeostatic failure in the chemical balance of the body fluids.

Excretion of nitrogenous wastes depends primarily on RBF and the rate of glomerular filtration. Urea is passively distributed across cellular membranes, so that its entry and passage through the nephron and excretion in the urine are entirely dependent on the GFR and the rate of urinary flow through the nephron. Creatinine is removed from the body primarily by filtration, and its accumulation in the blood is a reasonable reflection of glomerular filtration function. Other nitrogenous products such as uric acid are eliminated mainly through tubular secretion, which is dependent on blood flow.

Alterations in Acute Renal Failure

ARF with rapid deterioration of renal function and azotemia not due to extrarenal factors connotes acute tubular necrosis (ATN), which is actually a histologic diagnosis but represents the final common denominator in most forms of acute intrinsic renal failure. Acute suppression of urine formation (oliguria or anuria) generally occurs, but nonoliguric forms of renal failure are increasingly recognized where there is a marked disturbance in renal homeostatic and excretory function but a relatively high output of urine persists. *Azotemia* is a term that simply reflects the abnormal retention of nitrogen products in the blood; it is characterized by elevated serum concentrations of urea. Urea itself, however, is not a toxic compound and is not responsible for the symptoms of illness that accompany renal failure, although it serves as a reasonably good marker for other more toxic metabolites that are difficult to measure.[15]

Regardless of the initiating event or events that cause tubular injury, a number of factors function to perpetuate nephron dysfunction and delay renal recovery.[91] Thus, pathogenetic factors in ARF can be divided into those that initiate renal failure and those that maintain renal failure. The initiating event is a hemodynamic or nephrotoxic insult that causes tubular cellular injury. The extent of the tubular injury depends on various counterbalancing factors that obtain at the time of insult. These include the status of ECF volume and cardiac output, intrarenal blood flow and baseline renal vascular resistance, and urinary flow rate. Following tubular cell injury, a series of events are activated that maintain the renal dysfunction: (1) intratubular obstruction by cellular debris; (2) persistent renal vasoconstriction; (3) back-leakage of luminal fluid across the damaged tubular epithelia; and (4) possible alterations in glomerular membrane permeability.[45, 92]

INITIATION OF TUBULAR INJURY

Ischemia

As effective arterial volume or pressure declines, renal arterial blood flow is maintained through the vasomotor process of autoregulation, whereby afferent arteriolar tone diminishes and efferent arteriolar tone slightly increases. This process sustains GFR, but does so at the expense of decreased peritubular blood delivery. As mean systemic arterial pressure falls below 90 mm. Hg, hormonal and autonomic responses are evoked that cause the RBF and GFR to fall progressively, and intense renal vasoconstriction is demonstrated. The principal event is constriction of the afferent arteriole,[27] probably mediated by the combined action of circulating and sympathetically released norepinephrine and perhaps angiotensin.[45] These two agents probably couple to further increase efferent arteriole vasoconstriction. The result is a sharp reduction in glomerular and tubular blood flow and cellular hypoxia. The extent of cellular necrosis depends on the severity of blood flow restriction and the duration of ischemia.

Toxins

Tubular injury from nephrotoxins is initiated through different mechanisms, although there appears to be an element of vasoconstriction with each of the commonly encountered nephrotoxins.[45] With aminoglycosides, at least three mechanisms appear to be operative in the evolution of renal injury. Renal vasoconstriction is a dose-dependent feature that can be documented after a single dose as well as after chronic administration. Alterations in glomerular capillary permeability and direct tubular cell disruption, presumably from the intracellular accumulation of the drug, are also consistently observed.[83] Loss of luminal brush border membranes and intracellular vacuolization are observed histologically.[79] Myoglobinuric renal failure is accompanied by early vasoconstriction, accumulation of pigment casts in the proximal tubular lumen, and accumulation of hematin in the cells,

which is directly toxic to the cell when present in large amounts.[38] Dissociation of hematin from the pigment molecule is a pH-dependent event, which explains why injury is more likely in circumstances of acid urine pH. The almost immediate precipitation of myoglobin in the proximal tubule forms an obstruction that directly blocks filtration. Radiocontrast agents also are directly toxic to tubular cells and additionally induce prolonged vasoconstriction.[20, 70]

MAINTENANCE OF TUBULAR INJURY

In a number of experimental models of ARF there is evidence that intraluminal obstruction by cellular edema and accumulation of sloughed cellular debris and proteinaceous casts is an important factor in sustaining renal dysfunction.[91] Renal histology demonstrates edematous cells and intraluminal casts with obliteration of tubular lumina. Dilation of some proximal tubular lumina is an additional prominent histologic feature that is considered evidence of distal tubular obstruction (Fig. 19–3). Increased intratubular pressure in obstructed tubules is transmitted retrograde and opposes glomerular filtration.[91] This factor is considered critically important in the evolution of ischemic renal failure. Persistent intrarenal vasoconstriction is another important factor in the maintenance of ATN.[45]

Numerous experimental studies have also demonstrated that back-leakage of luminal fluid across damaged tubular epithelium may occur. Evidence supporting this hypothesis centers largely on observations in animals that a normally impermeable material, horseradish peroxidase, can pass paracellularly in areas of definite anatomic disruption of tubules; and observations in humans suffering from postsurgical ARF show that abnormal permeability to inulin exists.[29, 71] Back-leakage of filtrate is thus considered an important factor contributing to the sustained renal dysfunction observed in ischemic ARF. In addition, carefully performed micropuncture studies have documented that the glomerular barrier to filtration is directly altered by ischemic and aminoglycoside injury such that fluid filtration is impaired.[27, 83] The mechanism of this change is unknown.

ARF is most commonly initiated by a critical underperfusion of the kidney with consequent intense arteriolar vasoconstriction that causes ischemic tubular injury. In other circumstances, direct tubular cell damage is sustained from a toxin such as aminoglycoside or amphotericin. Myoglobin or hemoglobin pigment may cause direct tubular injury and intratubular obstruction when proteins coagulate. Iodinated contrast and nonsteroidal anti-inflammatory drugs (NSAIDs) may also be cellular toxins but are also powerful mediators of intrarenal vasoconstriction. When tubular damage is sustained, a number of factors converge to maintain the renal failure. These include back-leakage of filtrate across disrupted tubular barriers, intraluminal obstruction from cell swelling and sloughing, persistent vasoconstriction that might serve to perpetuate cellular ischemia, and changes in glomerular capillary membrane permeability (Fig. 19–4). Even in apparently intact renal tubular cells, the intracellular metabolism that supports the transport functions of the cell appears to be severely disturbed by hypoxia, free oxygen radical accumulation, and high levels of free ionized cytoplasmic calcium. The result is failure in the homeostatic maintenance of the ECF and failure to excrete accumulating toxic metabolic wastes.

BIOCHEMICAL ABERRATIONS IN ACUTE RENAL FAILURE

Retention of Nitrogenous Compounds

The progression of azotemia in ATN occurs at a rate that is largely determined by the degree of tissue catabolism

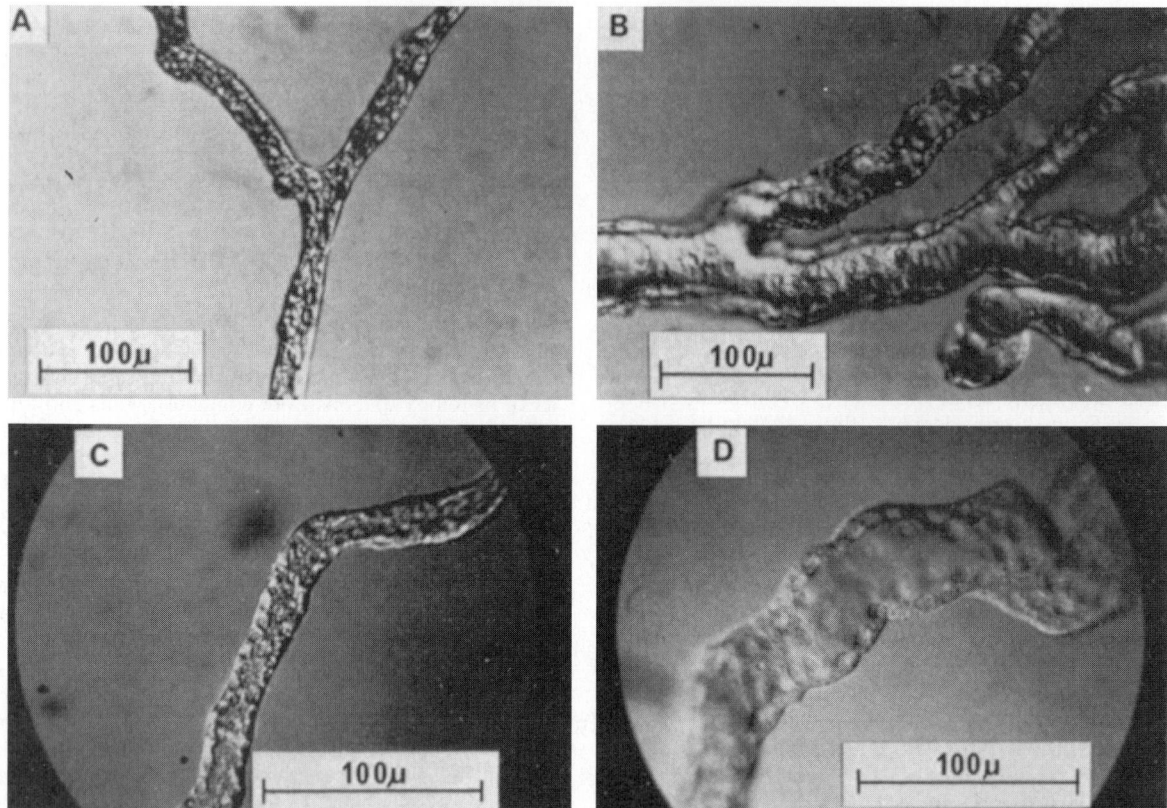

Figure 19–3. Microdissected tubules from ischemia-damaged kidneys showing tubular obstruction. *A,* Collecting and distal tubules from normal kidney. *B,* Collecting and distal tubules from kidney 1 day after temporary ischemia. Tubule lumina are distended and filled by a hyaline cast. Cells are swollen. *C,* Distal convoluted tubule from normal kidney. *D,* Distal convoluted tubule from kidney 5 hours after release of temporary artery occlusion. The lumen is distended and filled with material. Cells are swollen. (From Tanner, G. A., and Sophasan, S.: Kidney pressures after temporary renal artery occlusion in the rat. Am. J. Physiol., *230(4):* 1173, 1976.)

and protein breakdown. In the acutely ill patient who is hypercatabolic because of recent surgical intervention, trauma, or burn injury, the plasma urea nitrogen concentration may increase by as much as 40 mg. per dl. per day. In patients who are not excessively catabolic, the plasma urea nitrogen level may rise by only 10 to 20 mg. per dl. per day. Therefore, the rate of rise of urea can be used as an indication of severity of catabolism. It is important to bear in mind that for any specific level of plasma urea nitrogen or creatinine in the setting of ARF, the severity of clinical illness generally is more pronounced than that usually observed with comparable levels of azotemia in a patient with chronic renal insufficiency. This difference in the severity of the uremic state is probably related to the rapidity with which the abnormalities of fluid composition evolve in ARF. In the patient with

chronic renal failure, adaptive responses that attenuate the chemical derangements have had time to develop. In addition, in the setting of acute postoperative renal failure, tissue injury and cellular disintegration cause rapid liberation of intracellular products and their metabolites into the circulation; their accumulation is acute. In general, therefore, the severity of the acute uremia is closely correlated with the extent of associated catabolism, which is largely influenced by concurrent illness. Assessment of uremic symptoms and complications relies more on the clinical examination of the patient than on chemical indices.

Metabolic Acidosis

Plasma pH is maintained within extremely narrow limits by the concerted action of three mechanisms: (1) chemical buffering, which is provided by plasma bicarbonate, cellular membrane proteins, intracellular compounds (such as hemoglobin, cytosolic proteins, and phosphates), and bone buffers; (2) respiratory compensation, which is accomplished by altering arterial Pco_2; and (3) renal excretion of fixed acids and tubular regeneration of new bicarbonate. In postoperative patients with ARF, acid production is substantially increased from cellular catabolism and release of fixed acid equivalents such as sulfate, phosphate, and a number of organic compounds into the circulation. Chemical buffering occurs instantaneously and is manifested by a steady decline of plasma bicarbonate. The inability of the kidneys to excrete the accumulating acid load and regenerate new bicarbonate, however, causes a severe metabolic acidosis, for which respiratory compensation is usually inadequate.

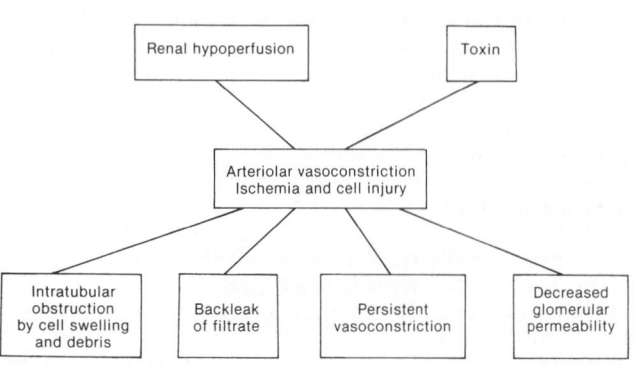

Figure 19–4. Evolution of acute renal failure.

Hyperkalemia

Serum potassium is also rigidly maintained within extremely narrow limits by precisely regulated secretion into the distal nephron. Acute reductions in RBF and acute tubular injury severely compromise potassium transport and its elimination. Moreover, because body tissues contain large quantities of potassium ions intracellularly (approximately 155 mEq. per liter), substantial amounts of potassium are liberated into the circulation if tissues are injured or necrotic. Because of oliguria or tubular injury, potassium released from the injured tissue cannot be effectively excreted into the urine, and dangerous hyperkalemia may evolve. Hyperkalemia is also a consequence of systemic acidosis because of redistribution of potassium ions from intracellular water to the ECF.

Hyponatremia

Hyponatremia is another commonly observed electrolyte disturbance in patients with acute oliguric renal failure. It is usually ascribable to the intravenous administration of salt-free water at rates that exceed the renal capacity for excretion. Metabolic water production from metabolism of nutrients and the liberation of intracellular water from tissue breakdown also contribute to the excess of free water. Undesirable consequences of hyponatremia include mental aberrations, convulsions, and cerebral edema.

Hyperphosphatemia and Hypocalcemia

Hyperphosphatemia evolves in patients with posttraumatic ARF because of inadequate excretion and excessive release from injured tissue. In patients with rhabdomyolysis, serum phosphate levels may exceed 12 mg. per 100 ml.[40, 62]

The untoward consequence of acute hyperphosphatemia is hypocalcemia, which tends to be especially severe in major rhabdomyolysis. Calcium and phosphate form an insoluble precipitate when the product of their respective serum concentrations exceeds 55 mg. per 100 ml. Injured tissue is usually the site of calcium phosphate deposition, but there is evidence that normal tissue can accumulate free calcium in the cytosol, causing cellular necrosis following activation of certain proteolytic enzymes.

Hypermagnesemia

The kidney is a major regulatory organ for magnesium balance. In renal failure, magnesium can accumulate rapidly owing to dietary intake and to the use of magnesium-containing antacids or cathartics. Symptomatic hypermagnesemia probably occurs only when patients with ARF are administered large amounts of these magnesium-containing antacids. For this reason, the clinician should choose aluminum hydroxide or aluminum carbonate when antacids are prescribed.

SURGICAL AND MEDICAL CONDITIONS THAT PREDISPOSE TO ACUTE RENAL FAILURE

ARF is a frequent complication of surgical procedures. The most common cause of ARF is ATN. Of the approximately 30 patients per year per million population who require dialysis for ARF, 20 have ATN, three fourths of these as a complication of surgical intervention.[51] Many factors cause this high incidence of ARF in the postoperative period. An important factor is the severity of underlying diseases, both medical conditions pre-existing in the patient before surgical therapy and the trauma or illness associated with the surgical procedure. Moreover, exposure to the risks of anesthetic agents and of incompatible blood transfusion, both possible causes of ARF, is a factor in the operative group. The most important factor, however, is hypovolemia from preoperative fluid restriction, surgical fluid loss, surgical blood loss, and gastric tube drainage of fluids.[5] The already ischemic kidney in the hypovolemic patient may be injured easily by nephrotoxic antibiotics and other drugs. The combination of toxic and ischemic damage to tubular epithelium is the direct cause of postoperative ARF. Prevention of this often fatal complication depends on recognition of predisposing conditions and correction of the physiologic disturbances for timely preservation of the sensitive renal tubular cells. The general physiologic disturbances confronted by many surgical patients are well illustrated by the trauma victim.

Trauma

Posttraumatic ARF was first described by Bywaters and Beall in the victims of crushing injuries during World War II.[21] They observed that hemorrhagic hypotension alone was rarely, if ever, associated with renal failure, whereas the combination of hypotension and crushing injuries frequently caused renal shutdown. The victim of severe trauma usually experiences some degree of hypovolemia. In addition to external acute blood loss, the patient may have internal hemorrhage, occult gastrointestinal bleeding, and gross hematuria. Extrarenal fluid loss in the form of vomiting and nasogastric suction contributes to volume depletion. Renal loss and excessive sweating with hyperpyrexia may further aggravate the hypovolemia. In the most severe case, the burn victim has a massive leak of fluid from the vascular bed into the wound during the first 6 to 8 hours after injury owing to dilatation and increased permeability of the damaged skin capillaries.

The kidney can normally withstand wide variations in renal perfusion pressure by the process of renal autoregulation, which maintains the RBF and GFR nearly unchanged. However, below a blood pressure of approximately 90 mm. Hg, the RBF is reduced and GFR decreases. Early in the course, the result is prerenal ARF. If trauma produces hemorrhage and other fluid losses sufficient to lower the blood pressure below the limit for autoregulation, immediate blood transfusion and fluid infusion are indicated before the ischemic injury progresses to ATN or, in the most severe and prolonged cases, acute cortical necrosis, which is irreversible. Rhabdomyolysis and myoglobinuria commonly accompany crush injury. Myoglobin pigment is prone to precipitate in the tubules during hypovolemic shock.

The requirement to transfuse the trauma and surgical patient has additional risks for ARF if mismatched blood is transfused. After transfusion of small amounts of incompatible blood, readily reversible ARF occurs as a consequence of intravascular hemolysis and hemoglobinuria. When 200 to 500 ml. has been transfused, ATN and a life-threatening hemorrhagic diathesis attributed to disseminated intravascular coagulation (DIC) may develop.

The trauma victim who requires surgical intervention is further subjected to the nephrotoxicity of anesthetic agents. Premedications, induction agents, and inhalational anesthetics all may impair renal function. For example, morphine may cause a reduction in urinary output and in solute excretion, as well as a reversible fall in the GFR and RBF. Urine volume, RBF, and the GFR fall transiently after barbiturate induction of anesthesia. It is likely that this reflects vasorelaxation and vascular pooling. The commonly used fluorinated inhalational anesthetic agents have been responsible for many cases of ARF following operation. Methoxyflurane has been particularly troublesome; toxicity from this agent is usually mild and consists of a transient decrease in the GFR and a concentrating defect. However, patients with more severe toxicity have been reported with a clinical course typical of ATN. It is generally believed that the fluoride ion, which is liberated from the fluorinated ether by the liver, is the true toxic metabolite. Fewer problems occur with enflurane and isoflurane; and the most commonly used agent, halothane, is an extremely uncommon cause of renal damage even after prolonged anesthesia.[5, 25]

The trauma victim who survives the initial resuscitation and anesthesia must still encounter several challenges to renal function. Severe plasma volume depletion may occur during the course of prolonged ileus. Peritonitis or acute posttraumatic pancreatitis causes the loss of additional fluid into the peritoneal cavity. The resulting severe hypovolemia may be further aggravated by the endotoxemia of sepsis, causing shock, ARF, and sometimes death.

Sepsis

When gram-negative bacteria invade the bloodstream, they produce the syndrome of septic shock. Common sources include urinary tract infections, biliary or intraperitoneal sepsis, colon surgery, and severe trauma, although the source is not always evident. The patient develops fever, chills, dyspnea, confusion, and hypotension. A frequent consequence is ARF. The offending agent for the multiple deleterious effects is lipid A, which is a fatty acid liberated from within the gram-negative bacterial wall. Endotoxin has numerous effects on cells throughout the body, the primary targets being the lung (shock lung), the liver (reticuloendothelial system blockade) the gastrointestinal tract (ulcers), and the kidneys (ARF).[97] Hypovolemic shock due to reduced cardiac output and capillary leaks, as well as diffuse intravascular coagulation, further damages the kidneys. The prerenal ARF induced by mild endotoxemia is readily reversed by improving renal perfusion.[5] Larger amounts of endotoxin cause severe vasoconstriction, local coagulation, and endothelial damage, which cause ATN. These patients create a therapeutic dilemma because nephrotoxic bactericidal antibiotics are used to treat gram-negative sepsis. It is sometimes impossible to know whether ARF is produced by the antibiotic or the massive release of endotoxin from killed bacteria, or both.[98]

Cardiopulmonary Bypass

In addition to the general risk of surgical procedures because of anesthesia, hypotension, blood transfusion, and the administration of numerous drugs, open heart surgery has an added risk for ARF. As many as 25% of patients undergoing open heart surgical procedures experience nonoliguric ARF, and another 5% have oliguric ARF.[2, 13, 100] While cardiac function is poor, prerenal ARF may develop from hypoperfusion of the kidneys. This condition is readily reversible if the cardiac output is increased by successful surgical therapy, but it progresses to ATN if allowed to continue for a protracted period. The kidneys are perfused at a volume of 200 to 500 ml. per minute during cardiopulmonary bypass. This relative underperfusion produces a markedly decreased GFR, which returns to normal in most patients with satisfactory cardiac output when the operation is completed.[5] Some patients, however, have persistent postoperative prerenal ARF continuing for several days. These patients have a low GFR following poor left ventricular function, low systemic blood pressure, and associated decreased RBF. The fall in GFR is disproportionately greater than the decrease in RBF. Myers and associates[72] have suggested that serum creatinine levels be monitored in these patients when vasodilator agents are used to reduce systemic vascular resistance, because a fall in blood pressure below the autoregulatory range may greatly reduce the GFR, causing a rise in creatinine. When the impairment in hemodynamics is prolonged and severe, ischemic ATN with back-leakage of glomerular filtrate through the damaged tubular epithelium occurs. Regeneration of the renal tubular lining requires days to weeks and may prolong the patient's recovery time.

Renal Transplantation

When a kidney transplant fails to function in the early postoperative period, several possible causes of ARF should be considered. A technical problem with the renal artery or renal vein may cause thrombosis in the vessels. Urinary flow may be obstructed by edema, clot, stenosis, or kinking of the ureter. Low intravascular volume may impair glomerular filtration. A lymphocele, hematoma, or urinoma may compress the kidney and its collecting system. ATN may be present because of ischemia in the donor prior to organ procurement, prolonged warm ischemia during the donor nephrectomy, or inadequate preservation during transportation of the kidney. In addition, hyperacute rejection, an uncommon but devastating complication causing nonfunction and destruction of the kidney, may be present. Pre-existing circulating humoral antibody is the usual cause of hyperacute rejection. If the kidney fails to become pink and have normal turgor despite a strong pulse and good renal vein outflow, biopsy should be undertaken at the time of operation. If thrombosis has occurred within the renal vessels and leukocytes are present in the interstitium and glomerular capillaries, immediate nephrectomy is indicated.

Measurements of central venous pressure and hematocrit suggest whether hypovolemia from bleeding is the cause of posttransplantation ARF. Early re-exploration to control the bleeding, relieve renal compression, and restore blood volume usually causes prompt return of renal function. Radionuclide renal scans and arteriography are helpful in the differential diagnosis of early posttransplantation ARF (discussed under radiographic studies). If the graft implantation site and ipsilateral leg become swollen and tender, iliac vein compression or thrombosis should be considered. A sonogram indicates whether a collection of blood, lymph, or urine is compressing the kidney and vein and whether dilatation of the collecting system indicative of ureteral obstruction is present. A more precise diagnosis can be made by needle aspiration or open exploration of the transplant wound. If the fluid collection proves on chemical analysis to be urine, immediate drainage is indicated. A Foley catheter prevents extravasation from a bladder or ureteroneocystostomy leak. If ureteral necrosis is suspected, the wound should be re-explored and a new ureteroneocystostomy, pyeloureterostomy, pyelocystostomy, or nephrostomy performed. Urine allowed to remain in and around the kidney usually becomes infected and leads to devastating complications, including death.

The differential diagnosis of ATN and rejection may be difficult in the early postoperative period. ATN should be suspected whenever there is prolonged hypotension in the donor, extensive warm ischemia time during the harvest procedure, or long cold preservation time. Because all cadaveric kidneys experience these problems to some extent, they are more susceptible to ATN from additional minor insults than are normally functioning native kidneys. ATN usually appears immediately or within 24 hours of transplantation and resolves within 3 weeks in most patients, although as long as 3 months may be required. If renal failure develops later after grafting, the likelihood of rejection increases. Oliguria, decreased creatinine clearance, and impaired function by renogram are evident. Graft tenderness, fever, edema, increase in weight, and hypertension may develop. On palpation, the graft may be swollen and tender. When ATN cannot be clearly differentiated from rejection, percutaneous needle biopsy of the kidney should be considered to establish the diagnosis, prognosis, and plan of immunosuppressive therapy. Biopsy is especially helpful in managing transplant patients receiving the effective but nephrotoxic drug cyclosporine. In conjunction with cyclosporine serum levels and measures of renal function, the degree and type of cellular infiltrate observed in the renal biopsy help differentiate ARF due to rejection from that due to drug toxicity.

Urologic Surgery

Most of surgically associated renal failure is due to ATN after trauma, sepsis, or gastrointestinal and cardiovascular surgery. Urologic procedures pose additional, special problems because of postrenal ARF produced by obstruction. Of 685 patients with ARF in one hospital series, 5% had urinary obstruction as the primary diagnosis.[51] Although obstruction is one of the most frequent causes of chronic renal failure, it is a relatively uncommon cause of ARF, because urinary flow must be suddenly and bilaterally interrupted for renal function to cease.[23] Postrenal ARF from obstruction is more likely to occur when only a single kidney is present owing to nephrectomy, congenital absence of a kidney, or more commonly, transplantation. Another important example that should never be overlooked is the patient with stable but moderately advanced intrinsic renal insufficiency. In these patients, a single renal stone, the most common cause of obstructive uropathy in the general population, or papillary necrosis may cause postrenal ARF. In patients with two functioning kidneys, bladder stones, bladder or urethral tumors, and commonly benign prostatic hypertrophy in men may cause postrenal ARF. Urethral obstruction in women may be caused by a retroverted gravid uterus, fibroids, ovarian cysts, obstetrical trauma, or neoplasms of the pelvic organs. In children, congenital problems such as urethral valves or urethral atresia can produce renal failure. A history of excruciating, colicky pain in the flank with radiation to the abdomen, passage of stones, hematuria, dysuria, or persistent backache suggests ureteric obstruction as the cause of oliguria. Infravesicular obstruction is suggested by decreased force of the urinary stream, frequency, urgency, postvoid dribbling, and overflow incontinence preceding anuria. Obstruction must be suspected any time anuria develops after surgical intervention or trauma to the pelvis or retroperitoneum. Numerous other causes of postrenal failure have been described.[23]

Persistent urinary obstruction eventually causes changes in renal morphology and metabolism. Reduced RBF and ischemia develop, and progressive interstitial fibrosis and tubular damage ensue which, after approximately 2 to 3 weeks of obstruction, become increasingly irreversible. Prompt diagnosis and treatment of the cause of obstruction lead to a rapid recovery of renal function. Postrenal failure should be considered whenever complete anuria develops suddenly or whenever intermittent oliguria occurs. It cannot be differentiated from other types of ARF by means of laboratory tests, but radiologic studies, including a plain film of the abdomen, sonograms, computed tomography (CT), renograms, and intravenous pyelography (IVP), may be quite helpful.

Liver Failure

Austin Flint observed in 1863 that some patients with cirrhosis and hydroperitoneum developed severe oliguria and died. In 1932 the term *hepatorenal syndrome* (HRS) was introduced to designate unexplained renal failure following biliary tract operations.[76] The term is now used to define any renal failure occurring in patients with parenchymal liver disease when no other known cause of renal failure can be found. In 1960 Kiley reported that the single most common operative procedure in civilian practice associated with acute postoperative renal failure was a complicated operation on the biliary tract.[54] The functional renal failure associated with icteric liver disease is indistinguishable from prerenal azotemia early in its course, except that it is only transiently responsive to volume expansion. In some patients there is progression to ATN, whereas in 10% to 20% of patients spontaneous remission occurs with improvement of liver function. Interestingly, the kidney from a patient with HRS functions normally when transplanted to a person without liver disease,[55] and successful transplantation of the liver in a patient with HRS also corrects the kidney failure.[47] In this syndrome, renal function is determined by the hepatic environment.

Patients with obstructive jaundice have a definite predilection to develop ATN. When renal failure occurs after biliary tract procedures, the possibility of HRS exists, but ATN occurs much more often. Other conditions observed in surgical patients that can mimic HRS are infections (sepsis, hepatitis B), shock, toxins, and pharmacologic agents (such as methoxyfluorane, halothane, tetracycline, streptomycin, sulfonamides), and metastatic neoplasms (such as renal cell carcinoma). In these situations, injury occurs simultaneously to both the liver and kidney, causing failure of both organs. These conditions should be distinguished from HRS so that treatment is efficiently directed to the underlying cause.

In the United States most patients who develop HRS have established alcoholic cirrhosis, but postnecrotic and idiopathic cirrhosis may also cause kidney failure.[99] In the patient with cirrhosis, kidney failure may be precipitated by surgical intervention, gastrointestinal bleeding, abdominal paracentesis, induced diuresis, or progression of jaundice, although no precipitating event is apparent in some cases.[12] The kidneys of these patients are perfectly normal without any evidence of identifiable primary renal disease by histology. However, the patient with fulminant hepatic failure, rather than cirrhosis, is likely to demonstrate ATN on microscopic examination of the kidneys. There is little evidence that bilirubin directly damages the kidney. However, bilirubin or bile acids may make the kidney more sensitive to ischemia, and jaundiced serum may contain materials other than bilirubin that increase vascular responsiveness to vasoconstrictor stimuli. In the early stages of HRS all the renal functional characteristics of a hypoperfused kidney are present, including concentrated urine and low urine sodium level. Further impairment of effective renal perfusion ultimately leads to ATN and renal failure. Treatment before and after surgical therapy should be directed to expansion of effective plasma volume, both to differentiate HRS from prerenal azotemia and as the most effective treatment for the renal functional impairment accompanying liver failure.

Vascular Disease

Grafting of an abdominal aortic aneurysm performed on an elective or on an emergency basis is a procedure early recognized to have substantial risk of renal failure.[54] The common factor in both is the placement of a clamp across the aorta just distal to the renal arteries. The probability that renal failure would occur postoperatively increases with the length of time that the aortic clamp remains in place. ATN occurs in 30% of patients when the aortic clamp is left in place for 100 minutes or longer. Occasionally, the aneurysm extends above the level of the renal arteries, necessitating total interruption of flow to the kidney for a portion of the grafting procedure. If the period is less than an hour and the patient does not have pre-existing renal ischemia or other renal disease, renal failure usually does not occur. Longer periods of interrupted RBF require preservation using hypothermia or temporary shunting of blood to the distal renal artery if ARF is to be prevented.

The operative manipulation required to mobilize and clamp the aorta stimulates the rich plexus of autonomic nerves surrounding the origin of the renal arteries, causing vasoconstriction and ischemia. Pharmacologic blockade of these nerves has offered significant protection to the kidneys in experimental studies. Atheromatous emboli to the kidneys may also follow manipulation and cross-clamping of the diseased aorta. The already ischemic kidneys are further damaged by washout acidosis as the lower body is reperfused.[95]

Atherosclerotic vascular disease produces not only aneurysms but also stenoses of the renal arteries. When a stenosis is high grade, renal ischemia results, and ARF may occur with levels of hypotension that would be tolerated by people with normal renal arteries. The stenosis may progress to renal arterial thrombosis and loss of functioning renal tissue. The kidney may also be destroyed by renal vein thrombosis, which may also cause renal arterial thrombosis. These events may be silent unless the patient has a solitary kidney or has already sustained a similar injury to the other kidney, in which case abrupt anuria and progressive azotemia occur.

Bilateral ureteral obstruction has been reported after aortic or iliac bypass operations.[23] The renal failure may occur weeks or even months after the operation because of obstruction produced by an organizing hematoma around the vascular anastomoses or ureteral strictures at sites of ureteric devascularization. Another complication of abdominal vascular injury or surgical intervention that can lead to ARF is postoperative hemorrhage. Even if intravascular volume is maintained, the rise in intra-abdominal pressure can lead to renal failure.[80] Polyuria and resolution of the ARF occur in response to operative decompression of the abdomen.

Hypotension and Hypovolemia

Mild hypovolemia and hypotension evoke a number of vasoactive responses in the kidney to maintain RBF and glomerular filtration.[88] Autoregulatory decrease in afferent arteriolar tone coupled with an increase in efferent arteriolar tone preserves glomerular flow and GFR. Intrarenal prostaglandin activity also increases, which mediates further vasodilation.[30] However, these preservative mechanisms are counterbalanced by vasoconstricting activities of circulating catecholamines and circulating angiotensin, which uphold central mean arterial pressure. A relative redistribution of RBF from outer cortical nephrons to inner cortical and juxtamedullary nephrons during mild hypotension also occurs. This redistribution of RBF is believed to follow vasoconstriction of the blood supply to the outer cortical nephrons and a relative vasodilation of the blood supply to the inner cortical nephrons, which is mediated by prostaglandin activity.[31] The renal tubular functional response is to conserve sodium and water. Because of diminished urinary flow rates, azotemia evolves. In this state, the kidney is particularly susceptible to further reduction in perfusion pressure or interference with the adaptive mechanisms. As long as the intrarenal adaptive mechanisms remain intact and the humoral vasoconstrictive responses to the hypotension do not override the autoregulatory capacity of the kidney, this condition does not in itself lead to ATN. However, persistence of hypovolemia makes the kidney quite vulnerable to other factors that might eventuate in renal damage, such as myo-

globinuria, hemoglobinuria, radiocontrast material, nephrotoxic antibiotics, and NSAIDs, which can severely compromise the intrarenal vasodilatory adaptation by interfering with vasodilating prostaglandin synthesis. In this clinical setting, there is a period in which restitution of effective ECF volume and elevation of blood pressure can prevent secondary insults and progression to ischemic tubular necrosis.

Cardiac Failure

ARF as a consequence of myocardial infarction and cardiogenic shock is rare, perhaps because survival is limited because of the usually massive cardiac injury. Nevertheless, in the patient with mild or moderate congestive heart failure, there is reduction in RBF, elevated serum renin and angiotensin levels, and increases in circulating catecholamines and intrarenal vasodilating prostaglandin compounds.[89] Like the kidney that is underperfused because of hypovolemia or hypotension, intrarenal blood flow and the GFR are precariously balanced. A further decrease in effective arterial volume and renal perfusion pressure from either overdiuresis or worsening congestive heart failure can cause further intrarenal vasoconstriction and ischemic renal damage. The tubule in this setting is again more likely to sustain toxic injury from pigment, drugs, or radiocontrast material.

Pre-existent Renal Disease

When the serum creatinine level is higher than 2 mg. per 100 ml. at baseline, there has already been an approximately 75% loss of nephron function. Whether the kidney is diseased because of diabetes mellitus and nephrosclerosis, chronic glomerulonephritis, or chronic tubular interstitial nephritis, it is predisposed to development of ARF from a variety of insults.[12] Autoregulatory capacity is compromised, so decreases in renal perfusion pressure can have a dramatic impact on the GFR and peritubular blood flow. Numerous prospective and retrospective studies have documented that pre-existent renal insufficiency is a major risk factor for radiocontrast-induced renal failure and nephrotoxic injury.[44, 96] Awareness of the predisposition for tubular injury in this setting is the primary requirement for successful prophylaxis. Dosages of antimicrobial agents must be altered and volume status carefully maintained. If a radiocontrast study is required, adequate hydration prior to the study and following the administration of the contrast material is essential. NSAIDs should probably be avoided in patients with renal insufficiency.

Radiographic Contrast Agents

ARF following the administration of radiocontrast agents occurs frequently.[10] It may range in severity from a nonoliguric, asymptomatic, and transient decline in renal function to fulminant oliguric renal failure requiring dialysis. The exact pathogenesis of renal injury is not well defined. A number of possibilities have been proposed, including prolonged vasoconstriction, direct cellular toxicity due to the iodinated compound with consequent degeneration and sloughing of cells, tubule obstruction by proteinaceous casts of cell debris and mucoprotein, and uric acid precipitates.[10] The incidence in patients without the well-recognized risk factor of pre-existent renal insufficiency appears to be very low.[20, 28, 44, 77, 85, 96] Available data indicate that the greater the level of pre-existing renal impairment, the greater the likelihood of nephrotoxicity from radiocontrast, regardless of underlying illness. It is generally agreed that susceptible patients who are at greater risk of developing radiocontrast-induced ARF should be adequately hydrated prior to the administration of the contrast. Advanced age, diabetes mellitus, congestive heart failure, and the amount of contrast agent administered are probably additional risk factors. Nonionic low osmolar contrast agents have fewer systemic side effects but have equal propensity to cause renal toxicity and should therefore also be used with caution.[28, 85]

Pigment Nephropathy

ARF associated with both myoglobinuria and hemoglobinuria has been recognized for many years. However, numerous studies indicate that neither myoglobin nor hemoglobin is a direct cellular toxin.[38] Only when the myoglobin and hemoglobin molecules are dissociated into ferrihemate (hematin) and the specific globin moiety of the macromolecule can tubular toxicity be demonstrated. This dissociation occurs at or below a urine pH of 5.6. There is now evidence that hematin is probably the toxic component of these globin pigments.[38] Many investigators believe that intratubular obstruction by the local precipitation of these pigments is a more important mechanism in pigment nephropathy. Thus, pigment-induced nephropathy appears to be a more severe problem during ECF volume depletion with low urinary flow and with acid urine. These observations have provided the basis for a therapeutic approach to the prevention and treatment of myoglobin- or hemoglobin-associated ARF. When myoglobinuria from rhabdomyolysis or hemoglobinuria from intravascular hemolysis occurs, it is recommended that the clinician (1) infuse saline or Ringer's solution with or without mannitol to enhance urinary flow, thereby flushing out the pigment and precluding its intratubular precipitation, and (2) infuse sodium bicarbonate to limit the generation of free hematin in acid urine (attempt to maintain urine pH >7). The clinician must be alert for the development of oliguric ARF. When this occurs, fluid infusion must be curtailed.

Drugs

Aminoglycosides are well known for their nephrotoxic potential. Even with carefully monitored serum levels in the therapeutic range, aminoglycosides are concentrated in the renal cortex and cause histologically noticeable cellular damage.[10, 79] Under the best of circumstances, the incidence of aminoglycoside nephrotoxicity is on average approximately 10% and is higher with gentamicin than tobramycin.[50, 58, 82] The duration of therapy, the daily quantity of drug administered, and the dosage schedule all influence aminoglycoside toxicity. Extracellular volume contraction, metabolic acidosis, and constant blood levels, rather than high peaks and low valleys, also predispose to nephrotoxicity. Amphotericin B and cyclosporine are also dose-dependent agents that cause tubular damage.[19, 68] Appropriate treatment is always reduction in the dose.[11]

NSAIDs operate by inhibiting prostaglandin synthesis. In the kidney that is hypoperfused, locally produced vasodilating prostaglandin hormones function critically to preserve intrarenal blood flow. Administration of an NSAID in this context can precipitate acute renal insufficiency by interfering with the prostaglandin-dependent vasodilatory adaptive response.[16] Conversely, in a patient already receiving NSAIDs, evolution of mild volume depletion might abruptly induce acute renal insufficiency because prostaglandin-mediated vasodilation is inoperative.

PREVENTION OF ACUTE RENAL FAILURE

Current knowledge of the pathophysiology of ARF and reflection on the surgical and medical conditions that predispose to it suggest several steps that help prevent ARF (Table 19–2). Any postrenal problem that is allowed to persist may

TABLE 19–2. Practical Guide to the Prevention of Postoperative Acute Renal Failure

Principle	Method
Monitor renal function	Serum creatinine
	Serum blood urea nitrogen
	Urinary output
Assess volume status	Physical examination
	Serial body weights
	Central venous pressure
	Pulmonary capillary wedge pressure
Control blood pressure	Intra-arterial monitoring
	Avoid hypotension (dopamine, isoproterenol)
	Reverse severe hypertension (nitroprusside)
Optimize cardiac function	Monitor cardiac output
	Afterload reduction
	Inotropic agents
Relieve urinary obstruction	Prompt radiographic diagnosis
	Catheter drainage
	Surgical correction
Avoid nephrotoxins	Limit radiologic contrast material, aminoglycosides, etc.
	Adjust drug dosages
Prevent sepsis	Catheter care
	Abscess drainage
	Isolation techniques
	Antibiotics
Consider diuresis	Mannitol
	Furosemide
	Dopamine

lead to ATN. Postoperative and trauma patients with a sudden onset of anuria should be considered to have mechanical obstruction of the ureters or lower urinary tract until this possibility has been excluded. Operative or traumatic injury of the urinary tract in the retroperitoneal or pelvic areas should be excluded whenever absolute anuria develops, because total anuria is rarely seen in the intrinsic renal and prerenal forms of ARF. The diagnosis can be established by cystoscopy, retrograde catheterization of the ureters, and radiographic techniques including ultrasonography, IVP, and CT scan of the abdomen.

The cystogram and urethrogram demonstrate traumatic rupture of the bladder and disruption of the urethra, respectively. These causes of acute postrenal ARF should be suspected in cases of pelvic fracture, particularly if the rectal examination reveals displacement of the prostate gland. Prompt recognition of the postrenal problem and surgical correction of the obstruction lead to complete recovery, whereas delayed recognition causes ARF.

Prerenal causes of ARF are prevented by optimizing volume status, cardiac function, and blood pressure, while avoiding nephrotoxins and infections. Extracellular volume can be estimated by physical examination in many instances. When it cannot be judged accurately, central venous pressure or pulmonary capillary wedge pressure must be measured. One of the most important means of evaluating the volume status in an oliguric patient is by fluid challenge. The intravascular volume is increased by infusing crystalloid or colloid until the wedge pressure is raised to 15 to 18 cm. H_2O. A brisk diuresis suggests a prerenal cause for the oliguria. If oliguria persists, an intrinsic renal problem is suspected.

The mean arterial blood pressure must be restored to normal levels and vasoconstriction reversed to maintain the GFR above 60 ml. per minute and avoid activation of the renin-angiotensin system. In patients who are oliguric after hypotension, the blood pressure should be monitored by means of an intra-arterial cannula. Blood pressure should be restored to a mean pressure of 80 mm. Hg and maintained at that level by adequate volume replacement. The extracellular volume replacement is adequate if urinary output is 40 ml. or more per hour and the central venous pressure is normal. If hypotension, oliguria, and renal vasoconstriction have persisted for more than a few hours, the kidney becomes progressively less responsive to volume replacement. During this stage of functional renal failure, the administration of furosemide or mannitol may facilitate the partial return of renal function in association with adequate volume replacement.

Treatment with a loop diuretic such as furosemide or an osmotic agent such as mannitol may reverse early ARF by flushing the tubules and reducing distal tubal oxygen consumption. This treatment may convert oliguric renal failure to the nonoliguric form, but it does not alter the course of ATN. High-output renal failure is easier to manage clinically and may have a better prognosis for survival.[3, 4] Although loop diuretics such as ethacrynic acid and furosemide are effective agents for increasing urinary flow in postoperative and posttrauma patients, they should not be used until the ECF volume has been restored to normal. Because furosemide is such an effective diuretic, it may induce a large urinary loss in a patient already volume depleted and whose oliguria is a normal response to the physiologic condition. Furosemide may convert homeostatic oliguria to ARF. To guard against the indiscriminate and dangerous use of loop diuretics, measurement of central venous or left atrial pressure should be made before administering these agents to an oliguric patient. When the ECF volume is proven normal, up to 200 mg. of furosemide or a single dose of 12.5 gm. of mannitol may be given intravenously for determining their efficacy. Alternatively, 5 μg. per kg. per min. of dopamine, a nonpressor dose, may be administered to increase RBF directly. If these measures fail to reverse the acute oliguria, further diuretic therapy will not help, and dialysis should be instituted as metabolic abnormalities or uremic symptoms develop.[36, 95] In cases of hemorrhagic or septic shock, diuretic therapy may be administered as part of the resuscitation. If the pulmonary capillary wedge pressure is normal or low, mannitol is an appropriate agent. If the wedge pressure is high, furosemide is better choice. Dopamine should be given with either regimen; but regardless of which agent is chosen, diuretic therapy is no substitute for adequate volume replacement. In fact, even dopamine administered alone can dehydrate critically ill patients.[36]

Specific disease states require specific steps to prevent ARF in the perioperative period. For example, when liver failure is present, most data indicate that the effective circulating volume of the patient is reduced. To prevent ARF under these circumstances, the vascular space should be cautiously expanded to achieve a central venous pressure of greater than 8 cm. H₂O. Moreover, any reduction in volume that reduces renal perfusion should be avoided. Diuretics must be used cautiously so that diuresis is slow and gradual (no more than 0.5 kg. daily). Paracentesis should be used only for essential diagnosis and therapy. Nephrotoxic drugs, radiographic contrast, and NSAIDs are particularly dangerous in the setting of kidneys prone to underperfusion and should be used only for clear and pressing indications.[75, 76]

DIAGNOSIS OF ACUTE RENAL FAILURE

Deterioration of renal function in the postoperative setting usually attracts attention because of oliguria and rising creatinine concentrations. A systematic approach to such a patient is of great importance. The physician must first consider and evaluate prerenal and postrenal causes of the deteriorating renal function before concluding that intrinsic renal tubular damage has occurred. Often, the distinction between prerenal failure and ischemic tubular necrosis is unclear. In these instances, assessing the patient's response to careful volume expansion and optimizing cardiac performance are essential. In the absence of a premorbid serum BUN or creatinine determination, as is often the case in the emergency patient admitted for reparative operation, it is essential to consider the possibility that volume contraction or compromised cardiac output, or some toxic insult is superimposed on preexisting chronic renal insufficiency. In this situation as well, the most important diagnostic test may be achieving volume restitution and improving the cardiac performance. In addition the surgeon is commonly confronted with critically ill patients whose multiple clinical problems and recent tissue injury provide reason for considering not only acute ischemic tubular necrosis but the concomitant presence of prerenal and postrenal compromises. Indeed, acute azotemia in the postoperative setting is commonly associated with combinations of volume depletion, third-spacing of body fluids, heart failure, and intrinsic tubular injury from ischemia and toxins and perhaps even an element of urinary tract obstruction. Failure to systematically consider and reasonably evaluate each of these possibilities for the declining renal function delays specific effective therapy and jeopardizes renal recovery.

Clinical Assessment

Evaluation should begin with a careful consideration of the clinical context, a review of the clinical course, and a physical examination with attention to blood pressure, heart rate, orthostatic changes if possible, and serial changes in body weight. Prerenal azotemia arises from inadequate perfusion of the kidneys. This must be considered in the patient with hemorrhage, an antecedent clinical history of congestive heart failure, a rapid diuresis induced by potent diuretic therapy, and loss of fluid by exudation from burned or otherwise traumatized tissue or by redistribution of intravascular fluid to a third space, such as in the patient with ascites, pleural effusions, or chest tube drainage. Detailed examination of intake and output is essential. Nasogastric fluid losses, diarrheal fluid losses, and fluid losses from drains all need to be counted in addition to the urinary output. Fluid intake should match these fluid losses both in quantity and in quality. For example, if blood losses or exudate fluid losses are replaced solely by protein-free crystalloid solutions, intravascular volume contraction evolves because only a fraction of administered pure crystalloid is retained in the intravascular space. Intravascular volume depletion can be suspected by the detection of orthostatic changes in blood pressure and heart rate and mucous membrane dryness. Heart failure is apparent by the finding of rales, distended jugular veins, and S₃ gallop, or sacral or lower extremity edema.

Specific clinical signs can aid in the diagnosis of obstructive ARF as well. Acute distention of the renal capsule causes flank pain, but this symptom is nonspecific and is also produced by pyelonephritis or renal infarction. Flank pain that radiates toward the groin may reflect ischemic necrosis and sloughing of renal papillae with obstruction or the presence of a stone. Disorders predisposing to renal papillary necrosis include chronic urinary tract obstruction with infection, diabetes mellitus, sickle cell disease, and analgesic overuse. Acute obstruction from nephrolithiasis is an unusual event but demands consideration in the patient who has known renal stones and is experiencing a deterioration in renal function. Obstruction of the ureter or the urethra from blood clots may occur in patients with urogenital trauma and gross hematuria or in patients who have recently undergone retrograde instrumentation as a diagnostic procedure. Edema accompanied by spasm at the ureterovesical junction is another complication from instrumentation that can impair urinary outflow. Finally, forced bed rest often eventuates in inadequate bladder emptying and urinary retention, particularly in the elderly person who might have an enlarged prostate or relaxed pelvic musculature. Complaints of suprapubic discomfort and the percussion of a distended tender bladder are signs of this problem. Simply inserting a Foley catheter and draining a large volume of retained urine can be a valuable diagnostic and therapeutic maneuver.

Acute tubular injury is suspected when the clinical history and examination allow exclusion of prerenal and postrenal causes of ARF and include data such as periods of hypotension, recent crush injury, and exposure to nephrotoxins. The patient may be in shock, with mottled cool skin and poor mentation, or may show signs of fluid overload and cardiac failure because of excessive fluid administration at a time when renal function is severely compromised. More specific diagnostic data are derived from laboratory studies.

The quantity of urine is helpful in the differential diagnosis. A 24-hour urine volume less than 100 ml. is most often associated with complete urinary tract obstruction, bilateral renal cortical necrosis from prolonged shock, or bilateral renal artery occlusion. If there is fluctuation in urinary flow from oliguria to polyuria, the physician should consider intermittent urinary tract obstruction. Prerenal states are most often associated with diminished urinary flows, because the kidney is hypoperfused and is attempting to maximally conserve salt and water. ATN, however, may present with oliguria or polyuria. Nonoliguric ARF from acute tubular injury is increasingly recognized and is believed to reflect a less severe form of tubular injury.

LABORATORY STUDIES
Urinalysis

Examination of the urine is an essential diagnostic test. A grossly cloudy urine suggests infection or crystalluria. Pink or red urine suggests the presence of either red blood cells, myoglobin, or free hemoglobin. A positive urine test for blood on the dip stick in the absence of red blood cells on microscopic examination is consistent with free hemoglobin or myoglobin. In patients with prerenal azotemia, the urine is usually concentrated and there may be numerous hyaline and finely granular casts. In patients with ATN, sloughed tubular cells, brown tubular cell casts, and numerous granular casts are common. In patients with urinary obstruction, the urine sediment is frequently unremarkable but may contain fragments of tissue, mucus, red blood cells, or numerous crystals of urate or calcium oxalate. Papillary necrosis is often associated with numerous red and white blood cells and small fragments of recognizable papillary tissue. In patients who have allergic interstitial nephritis from a drug reaction, leukocyturia and eosinophiluria are frequently noted. A number of diagnostic indices derived from urinary and serum chemistries have been developed to differentiate prerenal ARF from ATN. These are listed in Table 19–3 and are easily derived from simultaneously obtained spot urine and blood samples. Sodium, creatinine, urea, and osmolality levels should be measured on each sample.

Urine Osmolality

The urine in ATN is *isosthenuric*—that is, the urine osmolality is close to that of plasma. Thus, oliguric patients with a urinary osmolality near 300 mOsm. per liter are likely to have ATN, whereas patients with prerenal azotemia are likely

TABLE 19–3. Urine Diagnostic Indices

	Prerenal Azotemia	Tubular Injury	Obstruction
Urine osmolality (mOsm.)	>500	<350	Variable
U/P osmolality	>1.25	<1.1	Variable
U/P urea	>8	<3	Variable
U/P creatinine	>40	<20	<20
Urine sodium (m.Eq./l.)	<20	>40	>40
FE sodium	<1	>3	>3

U/P, urine to plasma ratio; FE, fractional excretion.

to have a more concentrated urine with osmolality greater than 500 mOsm. per liter. However, in actuality, many patients in either group have values between 300 and 500 mOsm. per liter, so that urine osmolality values do not provide precise discriminatory information. The ratio of urine to plasma osmolality, however, has been shown to be more discriminating than urinary values alone. Urine to plasma osmolality ratios less than 1:10 are consistent with ATN, whereas ratios greater than 1:25 are more consistently found in prerenal states.

Urinary Urea and Creatinine

Urine-to-plasma urea and urine-to-plasma creatinine ratios are more useful and widely used than osmolality ratios. A urine-to-plasma creatinine ratio below 20 is indicative of ATN, whereas a urine-to-plasma creatinine ratio above 40 indicates prerenal azotemia; values between 20 and 40 are nondiscriminatory. Likewise, a urine-to-plasma urea ratio less than 3 reflects tubular injury and a value greater than 8 is held to reflect prerenal azotemia. Again, values between 3 and 8 are nondiscriminatory. In patients with obstructive renal failure, decreased urine-to-plasma creatinine and urea ratios are found, but these tests are not helpful in this category of patient and can be misleading.

Urine Sodium

Much has been written concerning the usefulness of the urinary sodium concentration and the fractional excretion of sodium (FE_{Na}) as more precise diagnostic indices of the etiology of oliguria.[18, 32, 33, 74] The hypoperfused kidney is sodium avid, and a low urinary sodium concentration is characteristic of prerenal azotemia. However, when actual tubular injury has occurred, there is diminished renal sodium reabsorption. Thus, patients with established ATN or prolonged urinary obstruction usually have a higher urine sodium level—specifically above 40 mEq. per liter. Urinary sodium values between 20 and 40 mEq. per liter are nondiscriminatory and may reflect evolving tubular injury from a prolonged prerenal state. Because so many patients appear to be in the nondiagnostic zone, the urinary sodium concentration has not provided confident diagnostic discrimination between the two most frequently encountered causes of ARF: prerenal failure and ATN. Therefore, the FE_{Na}, which is that percentage of filtered sodium that escapes reabsorption, has been held as a more precise index of renal sodium handling and is generally believed to more effectively discriminate acute tubular injury from prerenal azotemia.[69] Calculation of the FE_{Na} requires simultaneous measurement of serum sodium and creatinine and urine sodium and creatinine levels. As shown in the following formulas, urine volume is not pertinent; therefore, the spot urine sample is sufficient.

$$FE_{Na} = \frac{\text{excreted Na}}{\text{filtered Na}}$$

$$FE_{Na} = \frac{U_{Na}V}{P_{Na} \times GFR}$$

$$FE_{Na} = \frac{U_{Na}V}{P_{Na}} \times \frac{Pcreat}{UcreatV}$$

$$FE_{Na} = \frac{U_{Na}}{P_{Na}} \times \frac{Pcreat}{Ucreat}$$

In prerenal azotemia the FE_{Na} is less than 1% of the filtered load. ARF from established tubular injury or obstruction is associated with FE_{Na} values above 3%. Although the FE_{Na} has become a widely used and credible diagnostic guide to the nature of the ARF, two exceptions to these rules have been well documented: (1) radiocontrast-induced ATN is often associated with FE_{Na} values below 1%,[34] and (2) occasional patients whose clinical course suggests the diagnosis of ATN have initial urine sodium values and FE_{Na} less than 10 mEq. per liter and 1%, respectively, but later become higher.[101] It is believed that these patients sustain tubular injury from prolonged hypotension or multiple episodes of such, so that they initially have less sodium in their urine. Additionally, diuretics administered within 12 hours prior to the test may alter these values.

Each of these diagnostic indices is useful and should routinely be employed; together, they can provide highly accurate diagnostic information. However, each test has known exceptions and should not be interpreted rigidly, particularly if it counters clinical judgment. Most important, regardless of the values of these renal failure indices, the patient should be examined carefully, and efforts should be directed toward improving circulatory hemodynamics, treating infection, relieving obstruction, and removing nephrotoxins. Following the clinical course while making these improvements may prove to be the most important diagnostic maneuver.

RADIOGRAPHIC STUDIES

The cause of ARF can usually be ascertained after eliciting a careful history, performing a thorough physical examination, and obtaining blood and urine tests as outlined. When the diagnosis is not clear after these steps, more sophisticated radiographic studies may be necessary. Radiologic techniques detect hydronephrosis; impairments in renal arterial or venous blood flow; abnormalities of size, shape, or location of the kidney; and certain abnormalities of the collecting system.

Plain Film of the Abdomen

The plain film of the kidneys, ureter, and bladder or tomography of the kidney is a simple and safe approach in demonstrating renal size and the presence of radiopaque stones. Longitudinal calcifications may suggest the presence of an abdominal aortic aneurysm.

Ultrasonography

In any patient with ARF, the possibility of obstruction should be considered. A safe and effective method of evaluating this possibility is provided by renal ultrasonography. The presence of the kidneys, their size, and the morphology of the collecting system can be defined. This completely noninvasive technique detects small renal calculi by their strong acoustic reflection at the surface of the stone and distal acoustic shadowing. Obstruction produces hydronephrosis, which is observed on the sonogram as a sonolucent *fluid-filled* area representing the dilated calices and renal pelvis surrounded by the echogenic renal parenchyma.

Radionuclide Scan

Radioisotopic renograms have been used to study both the perfusion and function of kidneys in patients with ARF.[8, 23, 87] The primary value of renal scans is to crudely assess perfusion of the kidneys. These examinations are most useful after major aneurysm repair and renal transplantation to assess patency of vessels. They are also useful in the evaluation of urine extravasation after pelvic trauma. Although the GFR can be calculated following injection of ^{99m}Tc-sodium pertechnetate or DTPA (diethylene-triamine-penta-acetic acid), the two most commonly used radiopharmaceuticals, this is rarely of clinical benefit in the acute evaluation of ARF.

Indiscriminate use of this expensive test should be discouraged. When assessment of renal perfusion is important, however, these scans remain useful. Arteriography is usually preferred to determine the cause and extent of most anatomic vascular obstruction and is essential if operation is being considered.

Intravenous Pyelography

In ARF, the need for a contrast study must be weighed carefully against the known risk of contrast-related nephrotoxicity and allergy. Twenty to 60 gm. of elemental iodine is commonly used in evaluating adults with azotemia.[8] The contrast agents are excreted by glomerular filtration; enter the tubules of the renal cortex to produce the nephrogram phase; and then are eventually excreted into the calices, pelvis, and ureter to produce the pyelogram phase. IVP is particularly valuable in the recognition of obstructive ARF because the level of obstruction may be identified. In fact, the absence of a diagnostic pyelogram suggests that obstruction is not the cause of the ARF. Patients with partial urinary tract obstruction filter the contrast agent and then reabsorb it in the tubules, thus speeding the development of the nephrogram and making it increasingly more dense. In obstructed patients with slow excretion into the collecting system, delayed films 12 to 24 hours after injection may be necessary to demonstrate the site of blockage. An immediate, dense, and persistent nephrogram is also characteristic of ATN. Retrograde pyelography is rarely used because it is painful, risks infection, and traumatizes the urinary tract, and the information it provides can now be obtained by less invasive techniques under most circumstances.[23]

Computed Tomography

CT scanning is a noninvasive, accurate procedure that can define kidney location and size as well as diagnose obstruction. The dilated renal collecting system can be visualized clearly without contrast media. In most patients with ARF, a sonogram or an IVP provides sufficient diagnostic data without need of the more expensive CT scan. However, when an aortic aneurysm, retroperitoneal fibrosis, or retroperitoneal malignancy is suspected as the cause of postrenal ARF, the CT scan not only discloses the obstruction but also may define the cause.

Arteriography

Arteriography is useful in selected patients when one suspects renal artery embolism (e.g., atrial fibrillation with history of mural thrombus), arteriosclerotic renal artery occlusion, abdominal aorta or renal artery aneurysm, or systemic vasculitis affecting the kidneys (e.g., polyarteritis nodosa). Radionuclide scans of the kidney can exclude renal artery thrombosis but cannot document the degree of renal artery stenosis. Digital subtraction arteriograms demonstrate the renal arteries while minimizing the exposure of the kidney to nephrotoxic contrast material. ARF due to bilateral renal vein thrombosis in dehydrated children is diagnosed with venography.[8]

BIOPSY

Biopsy is reserved for those cases of ARF where the diagnosis of ATN appears doubtful and where one or more intrinsic renal etiologies may be present, such as acute glomerular nephritis, acute interstitial nephritis, or acute vasculitis. When postrenal and prerenal causes of ARF have been excluded in surgical patients, most have ATN, and so renal biopsy has a *very* limited role in their management. An exception is the renal transplant patient with ARF, where biopsy has an important part in differentiating acute rejection from ATN, drug toxicity, and recurrent primary disease. Percutaneous needle biopsy of the kidney has some risk (e.g., a 9% complication rate in one series); therefore, it should be performed only for clear indications such as prolonged renal failure beyond 3 weeks and is contraindicated in the presence of bleeding diathesis or uncontrolled hypertension.[8, 56]

MANAGEMENT OF THE PATIENT WITH ESTABLISHED ACUTE RENAL FAILURE

When oliguria and/or an increase in BUN and creatinine levels supervene in the postoperative patient, the clinician should be alert to the possibility of evolving ARF. The clinician's attention at this time should be directed toward considering, seeking, and excluding specific reversible causes of the apparent deterioration of renal function. When the reversible factors have been corrected and the urinary indices have established tubular injury, a program of therapy should be immediately undertaken. The principles of therapy center on (1) anticipating the electrolyte and fluid balance problems that are known to be associated with ARF; (2) anticipating the consequences of various tests and fluid prescriptions so as to prevent electrolyte and volume disturbances from evolving; (3) correcting any existing biochemical and fluid balance aberrations; (4) preventing late systemic complications from the hypercatabolic state and uremia; and (5) adjusting the dosage of administered drugs to compensate for their impaired elimination (Table 19–4).

FLUID AND ELECTROLYTE MANAGEMENT
Hyperkalemia

Early attention must be given the fluid and electrolyte status of the patient, even while diagnostic information is being obtained. Of all the electrolyte abnormalities that might be encountered in ARF, hyperkalemia is the most serious and must be treated rapidly. The threat of hyperkalemia is cardiac arrest. The severity of hyperkalemia can be judged by the electrocardiographic (ECG) changes, which include peaked T waves, prolongation of PR intervals, loss of P waves, and widening of the QRS complex. These changes indicate diminished cardiac excitability and imminent cardiac standstill.

When significant ECG changes are apparent, emergent therapy is indicated. First, a calcium infusion with 1 to 2 gm. (ampules) of 10% calcium gluconate should be administered over 5 to 15 minutes to stabilize the cardiac membranes and reverse the toxic effects of hyperkalemia. This membrane-stabilizing action of calcium is immediate in onset but is relatively short-lived. It is often lifesaving, but other therapy must be instituted to actually lower the serum potassium level and remove the excess potassium from the body. These therapies include the administration of concentrated glucose and insulin and intravenous sodium bicarbonate therapy.

Glucose and insulin therapy is best administered as a 10% glucose solution ($D_{10}W$) with 20 to 30 units of regular insulin per liter. The rate of intravenous administration should be titrated according to serial serum potassium values but may be as rapid as 500 ml. per hour. The clinician might choose to initiate glucose-insulin therapy with a bolus of 50% glucose plus 10 units of regular insulin intravenously, followed by the drip infusion. The action of glucose and insulin begins within 10 minutes and may persist for as long as the drip is continued. It is essential that glucose and potassium levels be measured frequently.

Sodium bicarbonate can be administered either as a bolus over 5 to 10 minutes or diluted in 5% to 10% glucose in water and infused slowly. Both forms of therapy lower the serum potassium level by driving potassium into cells, rather than removing it from the body. Ultimately, therefore, enteral administration of cation-exchange resins such as sodium polystyrene sulfonate (Kayexalate) or dialytic therapy must be employed to remove the potassium from the body.

Each type of therapy has its limitations. With glucose-insulin infusion, water overload with progressive hyponatremia is a concern; and with large amounts of sodium bicarbonate, volume overload, pulmonary congestion, and hypernatremia are problems. Cation-exchange resins are most effective if administered orally with sorbitol. The presence of an ileus or intestinal injury precludes this mode of administration, and the less effective but still useful rectal route of administration is employed. In addition, precipitous reduction in serum potassium via hemodialysis can be associated with complex ventricular arrhythmias, particularly if other electrolyte disturbances coexist. Continuous ECG monitoring is mandatory.

Fluid Volume

Volume overload is another concern in the patient with ARF. Careful monitoring of fluid intake and output along with daily weights can prevent this undesirable situation. If the patient is oliguric, excessive salt and water input cause hypertension and pulmonary edema with their attendant complications. The clinician should restrict fluid intake to match actual fluid losses plus 500 to 700 ml. per day of insensible loss and 200 ml. per day per degree of fever. Quantitation of all fluid losses must be assessed regularly and often, because nasogastric drainage, wound drainages, stool losses, and urine flow vary from hour to hour. It is best that standing orders for a fixed amount of fluid per day not be written, because fluid administration must match fluctuating losses and represent necessary administration of blood products, antibiotics, nutrition, and so forth. Volume over-

TABLE 19–4. Management Priorities in the Patient with Acute Renal Failure

Initial
1. Review clinical setting, examine patient
2. Exclude/correct prerenal and postrenal factors
3. Analyze blood and urine for electrolyte emergencies, renal failure indices, sediment
4. Correct hyperkalemia, acidosis, volume

Ongoing
1. Monitor chemistries, fluid intake, output, daily weight
2. Match intake to output plus insensible losses
3. Initiate dialysis early; anticipate complications; individualize the prescription
4. Anticipate infection, sepsis, bleeding, volume problems
5. Initiate nutritional support early
6. Alter drug therapy
7. Anticipate and prevent additional injury

load in the oliguric patient can be treated successfully only with phlebotomy or some mode of dialysis.

Hyponatremia

Evolution of hyponatremia indicates that free water intake is exceeding free water elimination. Severe hyponatremia is often a contributing factor to the encephalopathy and propensity to convulsions that complicate ARF. This most often obtains when administered intravenous fluid is excessive and hypotonic. When hyponatremia begins to evolve, free water restriction must be prescribed. If the serum sodium concentration falls below 120 mEq. per liter, convulsions are imminent. Dialysis is the only maneuver that can correct the hyponatremia in this situation; hypertonic sodium chloride should not be administered in the oliguric patient with severe hyponatremia, because this patient is nearly always already in a fluid-overloaded state. Hyponatremia is best managed by being aware of how it might evolve and preventing it.

Metabolic Acidosis

Metabolic acidosis often accompanies ARF, especially in association with major surgical therapy, traumatic injury, or sepsis. In the hypercatabolic patient, acid production is substantially increased, and the markedly reduced renal function allows no means for excretion of the accumulating acid or the regeneration of consumed bicarbonate. There are a number of potentially harmful effects from the progressive metabolic acidosis. These include nausea, vomiting, and cerebral dysfunction, as well as cardiac depression, insulin resistance, and impaired cellular metabolism. Acidosis is also an important factor contributing to hyperkalemia. Metabolic acidosis is treated with oral administration of Shohl's solution, intravenous or oral sodium bicarbonate, or dialysis. Enough alkali must be administered not only to repair the already existing acidosis but to maintain arterial pH and bicarbonate reserves at a level that matches the daily endogenous acid production from catabolism. In the average resting adult, daily acid production is approximately 1 mEq. per kg. per day. Therefore, 70 to 100 mEq. of alkali would maintain acid-base balance. However, in the hypercatabolic patient who has tissue injury, has undergone a recent surgical procedure, or has sepsis, endogenous acid production can be two to three times this amount, which would require equal alkali administration. Care must be taken with administration of such large amounts of sodium bicarbonate. It expands extracellular volume, may precipitate pulmonary edema, and is often associated with hypernatremia because it is packaged as a hypertonic solution. If large amounts of sodium bicarbonate are required to maintain arterial pH, dialytic therapy must be initiated.

Hypocalcemia and Hyperphosphatemia

In an occasional patient, hypocalcemia and hyperphosphatemia may evolve. This occurrence is most common in the patient who has experienced tissue necrosis from a crush injury or a burn. When the serum phosphate exceeds 6 mg. per 100 ml., magnesium-free phosphate-binding antacids should be prescribed with meals to minimize elevations in the calcium-phosphate product and attenuate soft tissue deposition of calcium-phosphate crystals. Ionized calcium in ARF is usually near normal, owing to acidosis, uremic state, and hypoalbuminemia. Infusion of calcium is therefore unnecessary unless carpopedal spasm or tetany develops. If phosphate is not lowered, infusion of calcium causes soft tissue precipitation of calcium-phosphate. Ultimately dialysis may be required to control phosphate and calcium balance.

Use of Diuretics

The therapeutic value of diuretics in the patient with ATN has been extensively investigated, but there is no general agreement as to whether their use can influence the recovery of renal function or requirement for dialysis.[36, 61] Thus, at this time, it appears that high-dose diuretic use in patients with established ATN may increase urinary output and ease problems with fluid management. There is no certainty that it enhances renal recovery or diminishes the need for dialysis. It is generally agreed that diuretic use has no statistical influence on ultimate patient outcome or mortality. Multiple large doses of loop-blocking diuretics may cause transient or permanent nerve deafness and seizures in patients with renal impairment.

One cannot predict *a priori* which patient might be better served by a nonoliguric state. Higher urinary flow might obviate pulmonary congestion, ease blood product administration, and permit greater volumes of hyperalimentation solutions. Although these benefits might not be statistically quantifiable, they could be pivotal in an individual patient. Mortality in ARF is determined not so much by the renal failure itself but by supervening complications such as malnutrition, susceptibility to infection, bleeding, and cardiovascular events. To the extent that higher urinary flow might permit better management of these issues, then benefit from diuretic conversion to a nonoliguric state might accrue. Simultaneously, one must be aware of the ototoxic potential of the loop diuretics and of the necessity to follow any ensuing diuresis with appropriate volume replacement to avoid ECF volume contraction. Recently the use of continuous furosemide infusion has been prescribed as an adjunct to intermittent bolus therapy.[80a]

USE OF DIALYSIS IN ACUTE RENAL FAILURE

Dialysis should be initiated when there is life-threatening hyperkalemia, severe acidosis, volume overload, uremic encephalopathy, or uremic pericarditis (Table 19–5). However, dialysis is best initiated prophylactically before the occurrence of any of these life-threatening complications of ARF, rather than as an urgent procedure.

The goals of dialysis therefore are (1) to remove uremic nitrogenous metabolites and to ameliorate the uremic state; (2) to correct metabolic acidosis; (3) to remove excess fluid; (4) to normalize serum electrolyte concentrations; (5) to improve platelet and leukocyte function; and (6) to permit effective hyperalimentation.

There are currently three forms of renal replacement therapy available for patients in ARF. Hemodialysis, peritoneal

---

TABLE 19–5. Indications for Dialysis

Absolute indications (when unresponsive to conservative management)
1. Volume overload
2. Electrolyte abnormalities
3. Acidosis
4. Uremic signs and symptoms

Relative indications (when needed for improved patient management)
1. BUN >100 mg./dl. in patient with ARF
2. Need for enteral or hyperalimentation in patient with ARF
3. Need for multiple transfusions in patient with ARF
4. Hemorrhagic complications in patient with ARF
5. Drug intoxication with hemodialyzable substance

BUN, blood urea nitrogen; ARF, acute renal failure.

TABLE 19–6. Renal Replacement Therapy for Acute Renal Failure

Feature	Hemodialysis	Peritoneal Dialysis	Continuous Venovenous Therapy
Efficiency	High for toxin and electrolyte removal	Moderate for toxin and electrolyte removal	Moderate to high for toxin and electrolyte removal
Frequency	Intermittent 3–4 hr./day	Continuous 24 hr./day	Continuous 24 hr./day
Access	Venous catheter required	Abdominal catheter required	Venous and arterial catheters required
Cardiovascular strain	Significant	Limited	Limited
Anticoagulation	Not usually needed*	Not needed	Needed

*"No-heparin" or citrate regional anticoagulation.

dialysis, and continuous venovenous therapy each are available for use in a series of modifications. Each mode of therapy has its own advantages and disadvantages (Table 19–6). Usually one form of therapy is best for an individual patient. Consultation with a nephrologist to select and initiate renal replacement therapy is usually the best course of action.

Hemodialysis

For the hypercatabolic patient, hemodialysis is usually the treatment of choice because of its extreme efficiency. Early initiation of dialysis is now the practiced rule, because the demonstration that prophylactic dialysis initiated before the creatinine exceeds 8 to 10 mg. per 100 ml. and BUN exceeds 100 mg. per 100 ml. improves patient outcome. The frequency of dialysis depends on the severity of catabolism, the severity of uremia, the urgency of volume overload and serum electrolyte control, and certain accompanying clinical complications such as bleeding and sepsis. The dialysis prescription must be individualized and is best devised in cooperation with the consulting nephrologist. Recently it has been shown that the type of membrane employed can affect renal function recovery. The use of *biocompatible* membrane in both hemodialysis and continuous venovenous therapy is recommended.[43a]

In some postoperative patients, 4 to 5 hours of daily dialysis may be required to attenuate hypercatabolism and uremia; in others, a dialysis session 3 or 4 times per week may suffice. The degree of catabolism may be gauged by the interdialytic rise of BUN and fall in serum HCO_3 (bicarbonate). In general, dialyzing to maintain the BUN below 100 mg. per 100 ml. is a reasonable goal in this context.

The administration of blood products must be coordinated with the dialysis treatments. Removal of fluid by ultrafiltration during dialysis is controllable and can be increased to create the necessary *space* for the blood products. Banked blood often is a source of free potassium, owing to leakage from within the erythrocytes. Administration during dialysis can provide an exit for this exogenous potassium load. As a practical consideration, it is particularly stressful and expensive for the patient to undergo a 4-hour treatment in the morning, only to return to dialysis that night because of transfusions given in the day that caused pulmonary edema or hyperkalemia.

Hemodialysis efficiently clears certain antibiotics from the circulation. Aminoglycosides undergo approximately 50% clearance with a 4-hour dialysis, so their administration should be specifically ordered after each treatment, and the dosage should be gauged according to measured serum concentrations. Penicillins and cephalosporins also have high clearances, and their administration should coincide with the end of dialysis.

Vascular access for hemodialysis is usually provided by double-lumen venous dialysis catheters inserted percutaneously at the bedside in the jugular, subclavian, or femoral position. The continuous blood path made possible by the double-lumen design allows highly efficient toxin clearances and no-heparin dialysis techniques. The life of these catheters varies from 3 days for femoral insertion to 2 weeks for jugular and subclavian positions.[86] When dialysis dependence is prolonged, surgically inserted felt-cuffed dialysis catheters allow a longer use[86] (Fig. 19–5). Regardless of the catheter or site chosen, strict aseptic technique must be observed and regular maintenance care must be performed. These indwelling foreign bodies can be a source of secondary bacteremia and sepsis.

The advantages of hemodialysis rest almost exclusively with its highly efficient clearance of toxins and fluids. It remains the most efficient form of therapy readily available. New techniques and technology applied to hemodialysis have dramatically broadened the number of patients who can receive this therapy (Fig. 19–6). Hemodialysis can now be safely provided for the majority of unstable patients. Techniques for no-heparin dialysis[24, 81, 84] and citrate regional anticoagulation[41, 78] have eliminated the mandatory need for anticoagulation, minimizing dialysis-associated bleeding. Nonetheless, some significant disadvantages or complications remain; these also relate to the efficiency of the treatment.

Complications of Hemodialysis

Hypotension. Hypotension frequently accompanies acute hemodialysis in the critically ill patient.[60] It arises from a number of factors: First, there is an obligate extracorporeal blood volume of approximately 125 to 175 ml. This may be

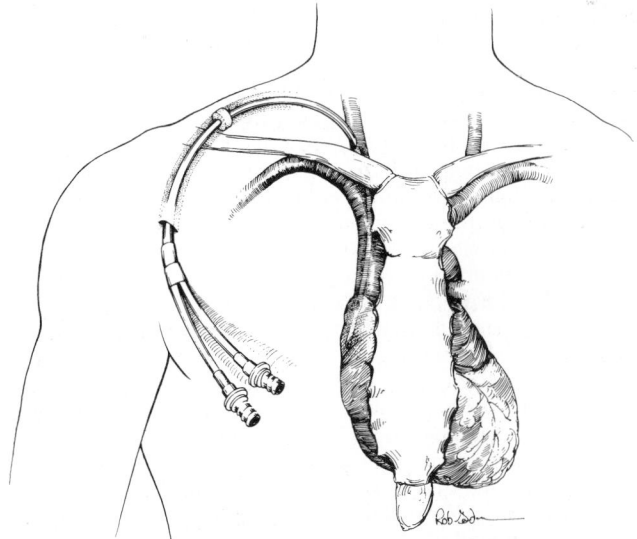

Figure 19–5. A Perma-Cath hemodialysis catheter inserted in the right internal jugular position. The felt cuff and subcutaneous tunnel reduce the frequency of catheter-mediated bacteremia. It has a longer use-life than standard subclavian dialysis catheters for treatment of acute renal failure. (From Schwab, S. J., et al.: Prospective evaluation of a Dacron-cuffed hemodialysis catheter for prolonged use. Am. J. Kidney Dis., *11:*167, 1988.)

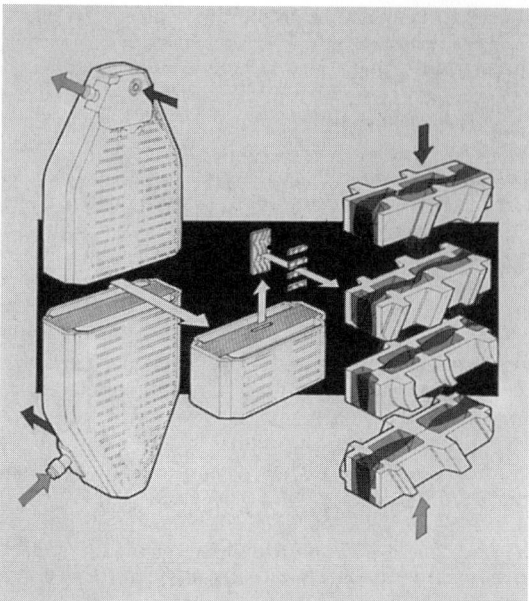

Figure 19–6. A cross-sectional view of one type of modern countercurrent flow dialyzer. Blood enters the dialyzer at the top through a central inlet, where it is evenly and symmetrically distributed to a number of parallel channels between pairs of membranes, and is then discharged at the bottom after treatment. The dialysis fluid flows against the current of the blood from bottom to top on the other side of the membranes to provide maximal gradients for solute diffusion. Constant changes in microchannel geometry create optimal conditions for solute transfer. (Diagram provided by Gambro AB, Lund, Sweden.)

sufficient intravascular depletion to cause a fall in blood pressure, particularly because coexistent acidosis, uremia, hypoxemia, and hyperkalemia may impair the cardiovascular reflex responses that might otherwise attenuate the hypotension. Routinely priming the patient with albumin, saline, or Ringer's solution should mitigate this problem. Second, as the dialysis proceeds, extracellular water and sodium are removed by ultrafiltration at a rate determined by dialyzer characteristics and transmembrane hydrostatic pressures. Hypotension caused by ultrafiltration or vascular unresponsiveness can be minimized by saline or blood product administration and modulation of the transmembrane pressures. The change in osmolarity of the blood as urea is removed is another important cause of hypotension because this is associated with shifts of plasma water into the intracellular compartment; it can be particularly troublesome if the patient already has low plasma oncotic pressure from hypoalbuminemia. Using high-sodium dialysate (140 to 144 mEq. per liter) and volumetric fluid removal or sequential ultrafiltration minimizes these problems. Use of acetate as the dialysate buffer is also associated with hypotension, particularly in the unstable patient, because of its action as a vasodilator. For this reason, bicarbonate is now used as the dialysate buffer in unstable patients. Blood oxygen saturation frequently decreases 5 to 10 mm Hg. in patients undergoing dialysis.[43] This can be hazardous in the marginal patient; therefore, oxygen should be administered or fraction of inspired oxygen increased in borderline hypoxic patients.

In summary, significant advances in dialysis technology have minimized hypotension so that this therapy can be offered to unstable patients from whom it was previously withheld. Nonetheless, hypotension remains a significant complication that must be respected and anticipated.

Bleeding. Despite the development of techniques for no-heparin dialysis[24, 81, 84, 93] and new methods of regional anticoagulation using citrate,[39, 78] postoperative patients in whom ARF develops are at risk of bleeding for many reasons. The incision has exposed many tiny vessels, which are apt to bleed if coagulation is not intact. Additionally, uremia is accompanied by a platelet defect that prolongs bleeding time and impairs clot formation. Blood loss and multiple transfusion might have depleted coagulation factors and impaired their cascade interaction because of the accompanying citrate, which complexes calcium ions. The convergence of these problems explains why hemorrhage is a major cause of death in postoperative patients with ARF. Effective dialysis improves the platelet defect. Administration of plasma or cryoprecipitate can restore coagulation factors with sometimes dramatic effectiveness. Administration of desmopressin acetate (DDAVP) and cryoprecipitate and intravenous administration of estrogens help correct the platelet defect of uremia.[48, 63, 64]

Disequilibrium Syndrome. The disequilibrium syndrome is a constellation of symptoms and signs experienced by intensively dialyzed patients that consists of nausea, vomiting, muscle twitching, lethargy, and confusion that may progress to coma and convulsions. It follows the rapid removal of solutes from ECF, paradoxical cerebrospinal fluid acidosis, and cerebral edema. The best management is prevention. The intensity of a dialysis session must be reduced at the first sign that disequilibrium is evolving; extracorporeal blood flow should be slowed, and the dialysis session should be shortened. Infusion of mannitol may effectively attenuate the osmolarity changes. Because of the problems that disequilibrium can create, initial dialysis sessions are usually conducted with slower blood flow rates and shorter durations. This may mandate more frequent sessions and is one principal reason for initiating dialysis early in the course of ARF.

Arrhythmias. Cardiac rhythm disturbances are not infrequent in patients with ARF undergoing hemodialysis. They have the risk of causing sudden death. Acute changes in serum potassium, calcium, pH, and perhaps sodium as well as the hypoxemia, hypocapnia, and release of catecholamines that accompany hemodialysis explain the risk. For this reason, continuous ECG monitoring is essential in the acutely uremic patient with electrolyte aberrations. Further into the course of renal failure, when serum electrolytes are stable between dialysis sessions, a more casual posture regarding continuous monitoring is permissible.

Peritoneal Dialysis

In a patient with severe coronary artery disease, acute myocardial infarction, advanced cardiac failure, and hypotension, or known cerebrovascular disease, hemodialysis may be deemed too hazardous. Similarly, a patient with dramatic or recurrent bleeding or multiple severe electrolyte abnormalities and advanced uremia may be harmed by the vigor of hemodialysis. In these situations, peritoneal dialysis may be safer than hemodialysis.

Peritoneal dialysis can accomplish removal of toxic metabolites, correction of electrolyte disturbances, and fluid removal by ultrafiltration at approximately one fifth the efficiency of hemodialysis. However, peritoneal dialysis is a 24-hour continuous therapy, so the apparent inefficiency is not as prohibitive as it appears initially. It is precisely for this reason that it might be preferable in the above-mentioned circumstances. For the patient with a fragile cardiovascular system, hypotension is avoided because fluid shifts are slower and there is no extracorporeal blood circulation. Solute shifts are also slower with peritoneal dialysis than with hemodialysis, which reduces the problems of disequilibrium and cardiac and neuromuscular irritability from rapid electrolyte changes. In addition, anticoagulants are not required for peritoneal dialysis.

In treating ARF with peritoneal dialysis, a small-lumen rigid *acute* catheter inserted by direct puncture may be used. The dialysis provided by this catheter is satisfactory, but peritonitis is an expected complication after more than 72 hours of use. The advantage of the acute catheter is that higher volumes (2 liters) of exchange are usually possible without leakage. Alternatively, a single-cuff Tenckhoff catheter can be placed either at the bedside or in the operating room. Sterile technique is essential, and a tunnel should be constructed to minimize fluid leaks and the likelihood of infection. Using a modern titanium tubing adaptor and single-bag technique that is employed for outpatient ambulatory dialysis, the dialysis procedure can be accomplished easily and aseptically. The Tenckhoff catheter is suitable for prolonged use, but initially lower volumes (1 liter per exchange) are required to minimize leaking around the catheter. When leaking occurs, volume of exchange should be reduced. If leaking continues, peritoneal dialysis should be temporarily discontinued to prevent peritonitis. Peritoneal dialysis should be performed with fluid continuously present in the abdomen and one to two hourly exchanges of the fluid with 1000 to 2000 ml. of dialysate. The larger the volume of dialysate and the more frequent the exchange of fluid, the more efficient the dialysis. The higher the glucose concentration, the more efficient the ultrafiltration.

One contraindication to peritoneal dialysis is the hypercatabolic patient. When the rate of ureagenesis is high, peritoneal dialysis may simply be inadequate. Peritoneal sclerosis, multiple intra-abdominal adhesions, and compartmentalization of the peritoneal cavity may preclude catheter insertion and cause inadequate fluid flow. Although peritoneal dialysis can be done in the postoperative abdomen, protruding drains, leaking incisions, and the presence of an enterostomy make this technique extremely hazardous in terms of infection and incomplete healing. Fresh vascular grafts in the abdomen are a relative contraindication to peritoneal dialysis because of the risk that peritonitis would lead to graft infection. Respiratory complications are not infrequent. The presence of 1.5 to 2 liters of fluid in the abdomen impairs ventilation and can cause hypoxia, atelectasis, and pneumonia. Communications between the pleural and peritoneal cavities are sometimes present, either congenital or acquired, and instilled peritoneal fluid may accumulate within the pleural space.

Continuous Therapies (Arteriovenous and Venovenous)

Hemofiltration is a technique of renal replacement therapy that uses the patient's own blood pressure to provide blood flow through a highly permeable artificial kidney (hemofilter). This technique requires a large-bore arterial line (usually femoral) and a large-bore venous return line (usually femoral). The higher the blood pressure, the better the blood flow; therefore, effectiveness improves. In cases of adequate blood pressure, a Scribner shunt can provide vascular access. When ultrafiltration alone is desired, the technique is termed *slow continuous ultrafiltration*. When ultrafiltrate is steadily replaced with a replacement fluid, the technique is termed *continuous arteriovenous hemofiltration*. When dialysate is dripped in a countercurrent manner as in hemodialysis, the technique is termed *continuous arteriovenous hemodiafiltration*.[7, 41, 42, 49, 57, 59, 65]

Venovenous continuous therapy is similar but has the advantage that an arterial line is not required. In this mode of therapy a blood pump is used to maintain extracorporeal blood flow. An additional advantage is that extracorporeal blood flow is not blood pressure dependent. Thus, continuous venovenous therapy is rapidly replacing arteriovenous therapy.[87a]

Continuous venovenous therapy can include continuous venovenous hemofiltration or continuous venovenous hemodialysis. When used in either mode, toxin removal may increase to levels similar to hemodialysis.

The advantages of this technique are similar to those of peritoneal dialysis. This technique provides smooth, continuous, moderately effective therapy. Demands on the cardiovascular system are minimal, hypotension is limited, and continuous fluid removal is allowed. The disadvantages include the need for some form of continuous anticoagulation, because flows are not rapid enough for no-heparin techniques, and 24 hours of citrate regional anticoagulation is difficult.

MANAGEMENT OF THE LATE COMPLICATIONS OF ACUTE RENAL FAILURE

Probably the one factor that determines patient survival in ARF more than any other single factor is the nature and severity of the associated illnesses. Nevertheless, in examining the primary causes of death in patients with ARF, it is apparent that the evolution of complications during the course of renal failure has a dramatic impact on patient prognosis. More than 50% of patients who die of ARF do so because of sepsis and pulmonary infections. Respiratory and cardiac failure represents another 25%, and severe bleeding is responsible for 10% to 15% of patient deaths. Malnutrition is a frequent concomitant and is probably a primary permissive factor. Therefore, when the postoperative patient with ARF is stabilized with regard to acute fluid and electrolyte complications and the intensity of the uremia is under control by an individualized dialysis prescription, attention must be directed toward preventing and managing these late complications (Table 19–7).

Nutrition

Adequate nutrition is a daily concern in any postoperative patient; in the context of ARF it assumes even greater importance. Acute uremia is a catabolic condition. The postoperative or trauma patient who cannot eat is also catabolic. Tissue catabolism in these patients releases potassium, acids, water, phosphorus, and nitrogenous products into the ECF. Such hypercatabolism not only contributes to the uremic problems that the patient is encountering but delays tissue healing, reduces immunity to infection, and weakens mucosal-epithelial barriers. Tissue breakdown and catabolic processes may be delayed by the administration of adequate calories and protein. However, the optimal amounts of calories and protein have not yet been precisely defined. Certainly, this varies in patients and is determined in part by age, body size,

TABLE 19–7. Complications of Acute Renal Failure

Early Complications	Late Complications
Hyperkalemia	Bleeding
Hyponatremia	Localized infections
Acidosis	Sepsis
Hypocalcemia, hyperphosphatemia	Malnutrition
Volume overload, pulmonary edema	Poor healing
Pericarditis	Cardiac failure
Arrhythmias	Somnolence, coma
Nausea, vomiting	
Convulsions, coma	

and associated illness and stress. The basal metabolic energy requirement for an adult is approximately 25 kcal. per kg. per day. When major surgical procedures, trauma, or renal failure supervenes, the number of calories required to neutralize tissue breakdown rises to approximately 40 to 50 kcal. per kg. per day.[54] The severely burned patient may require 60 to 75 kcal. per kg. per day. The relatively simple maneuver of supplying sufficient calories can markedly reduce endogenous protein catabolism and delay urea appearance in ARF, as was documented in 1949 and has since become the cornerstone of nutritional support.[17, 67] The other major thrust in nutritional support has been the use of high-quality protein feeding. Excessive protein intake simply increases the nitrogen load and ureagenesis. However, a limited high-quality protein intake can further improve nitrogen balance and net urea production over that achieved with carbohydrate support alone.[14] This observation has been documented and confirmed with elemental enteral feeding, as well as with elemental parenteral amino acid administration.[1, 35]

Accordingly, the following guidelines aid formulation of a nutritional plan for the surgical patient with ARF:

1. Supplemental nutrition should be initiated as early as possible to attenuate catabolism, support healing, and decrease uremia.

2. Approximately 30 to 50 kcal. per kg. per day should be administered either enterally or parenterally, or both; three fourths of the calories should be derived from carbohydrates.

3. Approximately 0.5 gm. per kg. ideal body weight (IBW) of high-quality protein should be supplied daily; it does not appear to be critical whether this is administered orally or parenterally. Patients receiving peritoneal dialysis or daily hemodialysis may require 1.0 gm. per kg. IBW more per day to replace dialysis losses.

4. A minimal volume of water should be used to administer these supplements to avoid volume overload and hyponatremia.

5. It is preferable to increase the frequency and intensity of dialysis so as to allow hyperalimentation rather than to spare its prescription if volume considerations become critical.

6. Insulin should be added to manage hyperglycemia; and potassium, sodium, chloride, calcium, magnesium, and phosphorus levels should be carefully monitored and their administration individualized to avoid electrolyte aberrations.

Infection

Infection is the most common late complication of established ARF and is estimated to occur in up to 90% of surgical or trauma patients with ARF.[46, 53, 66] Pulmonary infections and septicemia represent most of the cases. The primary reason for the high incidence of infection is the fact that the resistance of these patients is severely compromised. Uremia is associated with impaired white blood cell function, and the usual mechanical barriers to pathogen invasion are generally breached by indwelling venous and arterial catheters, arteriovenous shunts, endotracheal tubes, wounds, drains, and Foley catheters. To the extent possible, vascular lines should be minimized and eliminated, and those that are essential should be cleaned and dressed aseptically on a daily basis. At the first sign of cutaneous inflammation or infection, the line should be removed and the tip and skin area cultured. Foley catheters should be removed if the patient is oliguric. Routine use of prophylactic antibiotics in these patients is not indicated. No salutary effect has been demonstrated, and their use may even lead to an increased frequency of infection with resistant strains of bacteria. Infection surveillance should be a daily routine, and identified infections should be treated promptly with specifically directed antimicrobial therapy.

Bleeding

Gastrointestinal bleeding has been a particularly morbid complication in postoperative patients with ARF and may contribute to 20% of deaths.[53, 66] With early, aggressive prophylactic dialysis and the common use of antacids and H_2 histamine blockers, the incidence and severity have decreased.[66] Bleeding follows a number of factors, including irritated mucosa from nasogastric tubes, stress ulcerations, inadequate nutrition, depletion of coagulation factors from repeated transfusions, and a platelet defect associated with uremia. Management priorities include adequate dialysis with minimal heparin or no-heparin techniques or via the peritoneal route, maintenance of a neutral gastric pH, inclusion of fresh frozen plasma when numerous transfusions are being administered, and minimization of nasogastric tube suctioning. If bleeding is a threat or is not easily controlled, fresh cryoprecipitate may be beneficial. The platelet defect of uremia may be treated with DDAVP, cryoprecipitate, or conjugated estrogen.[48, 63, 64]

Drug Administration

Patients with ARF frequently require medications that are normally excreted by the kidneys. Digitalis and the penicillin, cephalosporin, and aminoglycoside families of antibiotics are common examples. Awareness of which drugs require dosage modifications is important in the management of these patients. The clinician should assume that each drug might require alteration in dosage and should consult the hospital pharmacist, nephrologist, infectious disease consultant, or appropriate literature references before prescribing potentially hazardous medication.[11]

PROGNOSIS OF ACUTE RENAL FAILURE

Untreated ARF in surgical patients rapidly causes death from fluid overload or hyperkalemia. When early resuscitation efforts are successful, infection becomes the overwhelming concern. Among published series reviewing mortality in patients with ARF, 50% to 80% of deaths are due to infections. In the Brigham Hospital series, for example, bronchopneumonia represented 27.5% and gram-negative septicemia 25% of deaths in patients with ARF.[95] Infections may arise from necrotic tissue in the operative site or from undetected abscess cavities. Particularly common are infections of the urinary tract and lungs, especially in patients with urethral catheters, endotracheal tubes, and intravenous lines. Anesthesia, surgical procedures, and uremia produce immune defects that contribute to this high incidence of infection. Renal transplant patients with ARF and drug immunosuppression might be expected to have an especially high mortality. The low mortality rate actually observed is probably due to the careful isolation techniques routinely employed in their care.

Despite advances in dialysis and nutrition, the mortality rate among surgical and trauma patients with ARF remains higher than that among medical patients, primarily because of their differing underlying diseases. Otherwise healthy patients in whom medical causes of ARF develop have only 3% mortality.[6] Patients who have severe, multisystem trauma, ruptured abdominal aortic aneurysms, or major surgical procedures for advanced cancer, abdominal catastrophes, or cardiovascular circulatory failure in addition to ARF have mortality rates higher than 50% in nearly every reported series.[95] The rate has decreased only modestly in the past 15 years, which emphasizes again the lesson of the wartime experience: Mortality due to ARF has been lowered primarily by a decrease in the incidence of ARF (42% in World War II versus 0.17% in Vietnam) after trauma and surgical therapy, rather than by improvements in the treatment of established ARF (90% fatality in World War II versus 77% fatality in Vietnam). An alternate explanation for the high mortality rate in surgical ARF is that patients with a higher percentage of multiorgan failure are surviving because of improved emergency department and intensive care unit support. Therefore, a much higher percentage of patients with multiorgan failure are surviving and thus subject to the development of ARF.

Recovery from Acute Tubular Necrosis

With early, aggressive, repeated dialysis to prevent the metabolic derangements associated with ARF and successful management of the late complications of bleeding, sepsis, and drug intoxication, most patients recover renal function after postoperative ARF. Among 353 patients who survived ATN, a spectrum of results was observed[52]: 30% to 40% of patients had normal renal function, 40% to 50% of patients had complete clinical recovery but persistent defects in glomerular or tubular function, 10% required medical management, and the remaining 10% to 20% required dialysis. Other studies demonstrate still lower likelihood of dialysis dependence in patients who survive ARF. Even after prolonged dialysis dependence (>1 month), recovery of renal function is the usual course. The regenerating tubular epithelium is particularly susceptible to further insult from ischemia, sepsis, and nephrotoxic drugs. Careful fluid management, not only during dialysis but also as urinary flow returns, is necessary to prevent volume depletion, hypotension, and return to another period of ARF. Accurate daily measurements of urine volume, electrolyte concentration, and patient weight with meticulous replacement of all fluid losses can prevent this frequently fatal complication. Initial recovery is indicated by an increase in urinary flow. However, dialysis must be continued for a few days to weeks until the nephrons regain their concentrating and excretory capabilities. Until the GFR and clearance return to normal and the kidneys can again maintain the integrity of the internal environment, the physician must continue to protect the patient from all the insults that might reinjure the recovering kidneys. Even during the recovery phase, *prevention* of ARF is much easier, more cost effective, and more successful than its treatment.

SELECTED REFERENCES

Bennett, W. M., Muther, R. S., Parker, R. A., Feig, P., Morrison, G., Golper, T. A., and Singer, I.: Drug therapy in renal failure: Dosing guidelines for adults. Ann. Intern. Med., *93*:62, 286, 1980.
This lengthy review provides important information on drug dosage modifications in the patient with renal failure. It is an essential reference for anyone caring for patients with impaired renal function.

Brenner, B. M., and Lazarus, J. B. (Eds.): Acute Renal Failure, 2nd ed. Philadelphia, W. B. Saunders Company, 1988.
This comprehensive monograph provides a complete review of medical and surgical aspects of acute renal failure. The section on differential diagnosis by Rudnick and associates is especially useful.

Nissenson, A., Fine, R. and Gentile, D. (Eds.): Clinical Dialysis. Norwalk, CT, Appleton & Lange, Publishers, 1995.
This text on dialysis provides extensive information on hemodialysis and peritoneal dialysis, including their complications.

Tilney, N. L., Morgan, A. P., and Lazarus, J. M.: Acute renal failure in surgical patients. *In* Tilney, N. L., and Lazarus, J. M. (Eds.): Surgical Care of the Patient with Renal Failure. Philadelphia, W. B. Saunders Company, 1982.
Diagnosis and care of previously healthy individuals in whom renal failure develops during the course of operation, trauma, or other catastrophes are admirably discussed according to clinical patterns of presentation.

REFERENCES

1. Abel, R. M., Beck, C. H., Abbott, W. M., Ryan, J. A., Barnett, G. O., and Fischer, J. E.: Improved survival from acute renal failure after treatment with intravenous essential L-amino acids and glucose. N. Engl. J. Med., *288*:695, 1973.
2. Abel, R., Buckley, J., Austen, W., Barnett, G., Beck, G., and Fischer, J.: Etiology, incidence, and prognosis of renal failure following cardiac operations. J. Thorac. Cardiovasc. Surg., *71*:323, 1976.
3. Anderson, R. J., and Schrier, R. W.: Clinical spectrum of oliguric and non-oliguric acute renal failure. *In* Brenner, B. M., and Stein, J. H. (Eds.): Acute Renal Failure. New York, Churchill Livingstone, 1980.
4. Anderson, R. J., Linas, S. L., Berns, A. S., Hinrich, W. L., Miller, T. R., Gabow, P. A., and Schrier, R. W.: Non-oliguric acute renal failure. N. Engl. J. Med., *296*:1134, 1977.
5. Andreucci, V.: Different forms of ischemic/toxic acute renal failure in humans. *In* Andreucci, V. (Ed.): Acute Renal Failure. Boston, Martinus Nijhoff, 1984.
6. Balslov, J. T., and Jorgensen, H. E.: A survey of 499 patients with acute anuric renal insufficiency: Causes, treatment, complications and mortality. Am. J. Med., *34*:753, 1963.
7. Bartlett, R. H., Mault, J. R., Dechert, R. E., Palmer, J., Swartz, R. D., and Port, F. K.: Continuous arteriovenous hemofiltration: Improved survival in surgical acute renal failure. Surgery, *100*:400, 1986.
8. Bast, C. P., Rudnick, M.E., and Narins, R. G.: Diagnostic approaches to acute renal failure. *In* Brenner, B. M., and Stein, J. H.: Acute Renal Failure. New York, Churchill Livingstone, 1980.
9. Baylis, C., and Brenner, B. M.: The physiologic determinants of glomerular ultrafiltration. Rev. Physiol. Biochem. Pharm., *80*:1, 1978.
10. Bennett, W. M., Luft, F., and Porter, G. A.: Pathogenesis of renal failure due to aminoglycosides and contrast media used in roentgenography. Am. J. Med., *69*:767, 1980.
11. Bennett, W. M., Muther, R. S., Parker, R. A., Feig, P., Morrison, G., Golper, T. A., and Singer, I.: Drug therapy in renal failure: Dosing guidelines for adults. Ann. Intern. Med., *93*:62, 286, 1980 (Parts I and II).
12. Better, O. S., and Berl, T.: Jaundice and the kidney. *In* Suki, W. N. (Ed.): The Kidney in Systemic Disease, 2nd ed. New York, John Wiley, 1981.
13. Bhat, J. G., Gluck, M. C., Lowenstein, J., and Baldwin, D. S.: Renal failure after open heart surgery. Ann. Intern. Med., *84*:677, 1976.
14. Blagg, C. R., Parsons, F. M., and Young, G. A.: Effect of dietary glucose and protein in ARF. Lancet, *1*:608, 1962.
15. Brenner, B. M., and Lazarus, J. M.: Acute Renal Failure. Philadelphia, W. B. Saunders Company, 1983.
16. Brezin, J. H., Katz, S. M., Schwartz, A. B., and Chinitz, J. L.: Reversible renal failure and nephrotic syndrome associated with non-steroidal anti-inflammatory drugs. N. Engl. J. Med., *301*:1271, 1979.
17. Bull, G. M., Joekes, A. M., and Lowe, K. G.: Conservative treatment of anuric uraemia. Lancet *2*:229, 1949.
18. Bull, G. M., Joekes, A. M., and Lowe, K. G.: Renal function studies in acute tubular necrosis. Clin. Sci., *9*:379, 1950.
19. Butler, W. T., Bennett, J. E., Alling, D. W., Wertlake, P.T., Utz, J. P., and Hill, G. J., II: Nephrotoxicity of amphotericin B: Early and late effects in 81 patients. Ann. Intern. Med., *64*:175, 1964.
20. Byrd, L., and Sherman, R. L.: Radiocontrast-induced acute renal failure: A clinical and pathophysiologic review. Medicine, *58*:270, 1979.
21. Bywaters, E. G. L., and Beall, D.: Crush injuries with impairment of renal function. Br. Med. J., *1*:427, 1941.
22. Bywaters, E. G. L.: Ischemic muscle necrosis. J.A.M.A., *124*:1103, 1944.
23. Canton, A. D., and Andreucci, V. E.: Acute obstructive renal failure (postrenal failure). *In* Andreucci, V. E. (Ed.): Acute Renal Failure. Boston, Martinus Nijhoff, 1984.
24. Casati, S., Moia, M., Graziani, G., et al.: Hemodialysis without anticoagulants. Int. J. Artif. Organs, *5*:233, 1982.
25. Coggins, C. H., and Fang, L. S. T.: Acute renal failure associated with antibiotics, anesthetic agents, and radiographic contrast agents. *In* Brenner, B. M., and Lazarus, J. M. (Eds.): Acute Renal Failure. Philadelphia, W. B. Saunders Company, 1983, p. 283.
26. Conger, J. D.: A controlled evaluation of prophylactic dialysis in post-traumatic acute renal failure. J. Trauma, *15*:1056, 1975.
27. Daughtry, T. M., Ueki, I. F., Mercer, P. F., and Brenner, B. M.: Dynamics of glomerular ultrafiltration in the rat. V. Response to ischemic injury. J. Clin. Invest., *53*:105, 1974.
28. Davidson, C., Hlatky, M., Morris, K., Schwab, S., and Bashore, T.: Cardiovascular and renal toxicity of non-ionic radiographic contrast following cardiac catheterization: A prospective trial. Ann. Intern. Med., *110*:119, 1989.
29. Donohoe, J. F., Venkatachalam, M. A., Bernard, D. B., and Levinsky, N. G.: Tubular leakage and obstruction after renal ischemia: Structural-functional relationships. Kidney Int., *13*:208, 1978.
30. Dunn, M. J., and Hood, V. L.: Prostaglandins in the kidney. Am. J. Physiol., *233*:F169, 1977.
31. Dunn, M. J., and Zambraski, E. J.: Renal effects of drugs that inhibit prostaglandin synthesis. Kidney Int., *18*:609, 1980.
32. Espinel, C. H.: The FE_{Na} test: Use in the differential diagnosis of acute renal failure. J.A.M.A., *236*:579, 1976.
33. Espinel, C. H., and Gregory, A. W.: Differential diagnosis of acute renal failure. Clin. Nephrol., *13*:73, 1980.
34. Fang, L. S. T., Sirota, R. A., Ebert, T. H., Lichtenstein, N. S.: Low fractional excretion of sodium with contrast media-induced acute renal failure. Arch. Intern. Med., *140*:531, 1980.

35. Feinstein, E. I., Blumenkrantz, M. J., Healy, M., Koffler, A., Silberman, H., Massry, S. G., and Kopple, J. D.: Clinical and metabolic responses to parenteral nutrition in acute renal failure. Medicine, 60:124, 1981.

36. Fink, M.: Are diuretics useful in the treatment or prevention of acute renal failure? South. Med. J., 75:239, 1982.

37. Fischer, R. P.: High mortality of post-traumatic renal insufficiency in Vietnam: A review of 96 cases. Am. Surg., 40:172, 1974.

38. Flamenbaum, N., Gehr, M., Gross, M., Kaufman, J., and Hamburger, R.: Acute renal failure associated with myoglobinuria and hemoglobinuria. In Brenner, B. M., and Lazarus, J. M. (Eds.): Acute Renal Failure. Philadelphia, W. B. Saunders Company, 1983, p. 269.

39. Flanigan, M. J., VonBrecht, J., Freeman, R. M., and Lim, V. S.: Reducing the hemorrhagic complications of hemodialysis: A controlled comparison of low-dose heparin and citrate anticoagulation. Am. J. Kidney Dis., 9:147, 1987.

40. Gabow, P. A., Kaehny, W. D., and Kelleher, S. P.: The spectrum of rhabdomyolysis. Medicine, 61:141, 1982.

41. Geronemus, R., and Schneider, N.: Continuous arteriovenous hemodialysis: A new modality for treatment of acute renal failure. Trans. Am. Soc. Artif. Intern. Organs, 30:610, 1984.

42. Golper, T. A., Ronco, C., and, Kaplan, A.: Continuous arteriovenous hemofiltration: Improvements, modifications and future directions. Am. J. Kid. Dis., 1:50, 1988.

43. Garella, S., and Chang, C. S.: Hemodialysis-associated hypoxemia. Am. J. Nephrol., 4:263, 1984.

43a. Hakim, R., Wingard, R. and Parker, R. Effect of the dialysis membrane in the treatment of patients with acute renal failure. N. Engl. J. Med., 20:1338, 1994.

44. Harkonen, S., and Kjellstrand, C.: Contrast nephropathy. Am. J. Nephrol., 7:69, 1987.

45. Hofstetter, T. H., Wilkes, B. M., and Brenner, B. M.: Renal circulatory and nephron function in experimental acute renal failure. In Brenner, B. M., and Lazarus, J. M. (Eds.): Acute Renal Failure. Philadelphia, W. B. Saunders Company, 1983, p. 99.

46. Hou, S. H., Bushinsky, D. A., Wish, J. B., Cohen, J. J., and Harrington, J. T.: Hospital-acquired renal insufficiency: A prospective study. Am. J. Med., 74:243, 1983.

47. Iwatsuki, S., Popoutzer, M. D., Corman, J. L., Ishikawa, M., Putnam, C. W., Katz, F. H., and Starzl, T. E.: Recovery from "hepatorenal syndrome" after orthotopic liver transplantation. N. Engl. J. Med., 289:1155, 1973.

48. Janson, P., Jubelirer, S., Weinstein, M., and Deykin, D.: Treatment of the bleeding tendency in uremia with cryoprecipitate. N. Engl. J. Med., 303:1318, 1980.

49. Kaplan, A. A., Longnecker, R. E., and Folkert, V. W.: Continuous arteriovenous hemofiltration. Ann. Intern. Med., 100:358, 1984.

50. Kaloyanides, G. J., and Pastoriza-Munoz, E.: Aminoglycoside nephrotoxicity. Kidney Int., 18:571, 1980.

51. Kasiske, B. L., and Kjellstrand, C. M.: Perioperative management of patients with chronic renal failure and postoperative acute renal failure. Urol. Clin. North Am., 10:35, 1983.

52. Kennedy, A. C.: Long term follow-up of renal function after recovery from acute tubular necrosis. In Andreucci, V. (Ed.): Acute Renal Failure. Boston, Martinus Nijhoff, 1984.

53. Kennedy, A. O., Burton, J. A., Luke, R. G., Briggs, J. O., Lindsay, R. M., Allison, M. E. M., Edward, N., and Dargie, H. J.: Factors affecting the prognosis in acute renal failure. Q. J. Med., 42:73, 1973.

54. Kiley, J. E., Powers, S. R., and Beebe, R. J.: Acute renal failure: Eighty cases of renal tubular necrosis. N. Engl. J. Med., 262:481, 1960.

55. Koppel, M. H., Coburn, J. W., Mims, M. M., Goldstein, H., Boyle, O. D., and Rubini, M. E.: Transplantation of cadaveric kidneys from patients with hepatorenal syndrome: Evidence for the functional nature of renal failure in advanced liver disease. N. Engl. J. Med., 280:1367, 1969.

56. Kourilsky, O., Morel-Maroger, L., and Richet, G.: Renal biopsy in acute renal failure: Its indications and usefulness. In Andreucci, V. (Ed.): Acute Renal Failure. Boston, Martinus Nijhoff, 1984.

57. Kramer, P., Wigger, W., Rieger, J., Matthaei, D., and Scheler, F.: Arteriovenous haemofiltration: A new and simple method for treatment of overhydrated patients resistant to diuretics. Klin. Wochenschr., 55:1121, 1977.

58. Kumin, G. D.: Clinical nephrotoxicity of tobramycin and gentamicin: A prospective study. J.A.M.A., 249:1808, 1980.

59. Lauer, A., Sacaggi, A., Ronco, C., Belledonne, M., Glabman, S., and Bosch, J. P.: Continuous arteriovenous hemofiltration in critically ill patients. Ann. Intern. Med., 99:455, 1983.

60. Lazarus, J. M.: Complications in hemodialysis: An overview. Kidney Int., 148:783, 1980.

61. Kevinsky, N. G., Bernard, D. B., and Johnston, P. A.: Mannitol and loop diuretics in acute renal failure. In Brenner, B. M., and Lazarus, J. M. (Eds.): Acute Renal Failure. Philadelphia, W. B. Saunders Company, 1983, p. 712.

62. Llach, F., Felsenfeld, A. J., and Haussler, M. E.: The pathophysiology of altered calcium metabolism in rhabdomyolysis-induced acute renal failure: Interactions of parathyroid hormone, 25-hydroxycholecalciferol, and 1,25-dihydroxycholecalciferol. N. Engl. J. Med., 315:731, 1981.

63. Liuio, M., Mannuccio, P., Vigano, G., Mingardi, G., Lombardi, R., Mecca, G., and Remuzzi, G.: Conjugated estrogens for the management of bleeding associated with renal failure. N. Engl. J. Med., 315:731, 1986.

64. Mannucci, P., Remmuzzi, G., Pusiweri, F., Lombardi, R., Valsechi, C., Mecca, G., Zimmerman, T.: Deamino-8-D-arginine vasopressin shortens the bleeding time in uremia. N. Engl. J. Med., 308:8, 1983.

65. Mault, J. R., Dechert, R. E., Lees, P., Swartz, R. D., Port, F. K., and Bartlett, R. H.: Continuous arteriovenous filtration: An effective treatment for surgical acute renal failure. Surgery, 101:478, 1987.

66. McMurray, S. D., Luft, F. C., Maxwell, D. R., Hamburger, R. J., Futty, D., Szwed, J. J., Lavelle, K. J., and Kleit, S. A.: Prevailing patterns and predictor variables in patients with acute tubular necrosis. Arch. Intern. Med., 138:950, 1978.

67. Michel, L., Serrano, A., and Matt, R. A.: Nutritional support for hospitalized patients. N. Engl. J. Med., 304:1147, 1981.

68. Mihatsch, M. J., Thiel, G., Basler, V., Ryffel, B., Landmann, J., von Overbeck, J., and Zollinger, H. U.: Morphological patterns in cyclosporine-treated renal transplant recipients. Transplant Proc., 17:101, 1985.

69. Miller, T. R., Anderson, R. J., Lina, S. L., Henrich, W. L., Berns, A. S., Gabow, P. A., and Schrier, R. W.: Urinary diagnostic indices in acute renal failure: A prospective study. Ann. Intern. Med., 89:47, 1978.

70. Mudge, G. H.: Nephrotoxicity of urographic contrast drugs. Kidney Int., 18:540, 1980.

71. Myers, B., Carrie, B. J., Yee, R. R., Hilberman, M., and Michaels, A. S.: Pathophysiology of hemodynamically mediated acute renal failure in man. Kidney Int., 18:495, 1980.

72. Myers, B. D., Hilberman, M., Carne, B. J., Spencer, R. J., Stinson, E. B., and Robertson, C. R.: Dynamics of glomerular ultrafiltration following open heart surgery. Kidney Int., 20:366, 1981.

73. Navar, L. G., and Rosivail, L.: Contribution of the renin-angiotensin system to the control of intrarenal hemodynamics. Kidney Int., 25:857, 1984.

74. Oken, D. E.: On the differential diagnosis of acute renal failure. Am. J. Med., 71:916, 1981.

75. Papper, S.: Hepatorenal syndrome. Contrib. Nephrol., 23:55, 1980.

76. Papper, S.. Hepatorenal syndrome. In Andreucci, V. (Ed.): Acute Renal Failure. Boston, Martinus Nijhoff, 1984.

77. Parfrey, P. S., Griffiths, S., Barrett, B., Paul, M., George, M., Withers, J., Farid, N., and McManamon, P.: Contrast material–induced renal failure in patients with diabetes mellitus, renal insufficiency or both. N. Engl. J. Med., 320:143, 1989.

78. Pinnick, R. V., Wiegmann, T. B., and Diederich, D. A.: Regional citrate anticoagulation for hemodialysis in the patient at high risk for bleeding. N. Engl. J. Med., 308:258, 1983.

79. Porter, G. A., and Bennett, W. M.: Nephrotoxic acute renal failure due to common drugs. Am. J. Physiol., 241:F1, 1981.

80. Richards, W. O., Scovill, W., Shin, B., and Reed, W.: Acute renal failure associated with increased intra-abdominal pressure. Ann. Surg., 197:183, 1983.

80a. Rudy, O., Voelker, J., Green, P., et al.: Loop diuretics for continuous renal insufficiency—a continuous infusion is more efficacious than bolus therapy. Ann. Intern. Med., 115:360,1991.

81. Sander, P. W., Taylor, H., and Curtis, J. J.: Hemodialysis without anticoagulation. Am. J. Kidney Dis., 5:32, 1985.

82. Schentag, J. J., Plaut, M. E., and Cerra, F. B.: Comparative nephrotoxicity of gentamicin and tobramycin: Pharmacokinetic and clinical studies in 201 patients. Antimicrob. Agents Chemother., 19:859, 1981.

83. Schor, N., Ichikawa, I., Rennke, H., and Brenner, B. M.: Pathophysiologies of ultraglomerular function in aminoglycoside-treated rats. Kidney Int., 19:288, 1981.

84. Schwab, S., Onorato, J., Sharar, L., and Dennis, P.: Hemodialysis without anticoagulation: Results of a one-year prospective trial in hospitalized patients at risk for bleeding. Am. J. Med., 83:405, 1987.

85. Schwab, S., Hlatky, M., Pieper, K., Morris, K., Davidson, C., and Bashore, T.: Contrast nephrotoxicity: A prospective randomized trial of a nonionic versus an ionic radiographic contrast agent. N. Engl. J. Med., 320:149, 1989.

86. Schwab, S., Buller, G., McCann, R., Bollinger, R., and Stickel, D.: Evaluation of a Dacron-cuffed jugular venous hemodialysis catheter for prolonged use. Am. J. Kidney Dis., 11:166, 1988.

87. Sherman, R. A., and Byun, K. J.: Nuclear medicine in acute and chronic renal failure. Semin. Nucl. Med., 12(3):265, 1982.

87a. Sigler, M., and Teehan, B.: Continuous renal replacement therapy in clinical dialysis. In Nissenson, A., Fine, R., and Gentile, D. (Eds.): Clinical Dialysis, 2nd ed. Norwalk, CT, Appleton & Lange Publishers, 1995.

88. Skorecki, K. L., and Brenner, B. M.: Body fluid homeostasis in man: A contemporary overview. Am. J. Med., 70:77, 1981.

89. Skorecki, K. L., and Brenner, B. M.: Body fluid homeostasis in congestive heart failure and cirrhosis with ascites. Am. J. Med., 72:323, 1982.

90. Smith, L. H., Jr., Post, R. S., Teschan, P. E., Abernathy, R. S., Davis, J. H., Gray, D. M., Howard, J. M., Johnson, K. E., Klopp, E., Mundy, R. L., O'Meara, M. P., and Rush, B. F., Jr.: Posttraumatic renal insufficiency in military casualties: II. Management, use of an artificial kidney, prognosis. Am. J. Med., 18:187, 1955.

91. Stein, J. H., Lifschitz, M. D., and Barnes, L. D.: Current concepts on the pathophysiology of acute renal failure. Am. J. Physiol., 234:F171, 1978.

92. Swan, R. C., and Merrill, J. P.: Clinical course of acute renal failure. Medicine, 32:215, 1953.

93. Swartz, R. D., and Port, F. K.: Preventing hemorrhage in high-risk hemodialysis: Regional versus low-dose heparin. Kidney Int., 16:513, 1979.

94. Teschan, P. E., Post, R. S., Smith, L. H., Jr., Abernathy, R. S., Davis, J. H., Gray, D. M., Howard, J. M., Johnson, K. E., Kiopp, E., Mundy, R. L., O'Meara, M. P., and Rush, B. F., Jr.: Posttraumatic renal insufficiency in military casualties: I. Clinical characteristics. Am. J. Med., 18:172, 1955.
95. Tilney, N. L., Morgan, A. P., and Lazarus, J. M.: Acute renal failure in surgical patients. In Tilney, N. L., and Lazarus, J. M. (Eds.): Surgical Care of the Patient with Renal Failure. Philadelphia, W. B. Saunders Company, 1982.
96. Van Zee, B. E., How, W. E., Talley, T. E., and Jaenike, J. R.: Renal injury associated with intravenous pyelography in nondiabetic and diabetic patients. Ann. Intern. Med., 89:51,1978.
97. Wardle, E. N.: Endotoxin and acute renal failure: A review. Nephron, 14:321, 1975.
98. Wardle, N.: Acute renal failure in the 1980s: The importance of septic shock and of endotoxemia. Nephron, 30:193, 1982.
99. Wong, P. Y.: The hepatorenal syndrome. Gastroenterology, 77:1326, 1979.
100. Yeboah, E. D., Petrie, A., and Pead, J. L.: Acute renal failure and open heart surgery. Br. Med. J., 1:415, 1972.
101. Zarich, S., Fang, L. S. T., and Diamond, J. R.: Fractional excretion of sodium: Exceptions to its diagnostic value. Arch. Intern. Med., 145:108, 1985.

CHAPTER 20

TRANSPLANTATION

I _____

HISTORICAL ASPECTS

R. Randal Bollinger, M.D., Ph.D., and Delford L. Stickel, M.D.

ANCIENT ACCOUNTS OF TRANSPLANTATION

Transplantation, the removal or partial detachment of a part of the body and its implantation to the body of the same or a different individual, has fascinated mankind for centuries. Legends of transplantation are recorded in the early written histories of both Eastern and Western cultures. Homer, in his *Iliad*, describes the monstrous Chimaera, a remarkable creature of transplanted animal parts created by the gods. This mythical hybrid animal had the heads of a lion, a goat, and a serpent. All three of its heads breathed fire.[35] The term *chimaera* is now used in transplantation to describe individuals who possess hybrid characteristics, such as the circulating cells of both donor and recipient after bone marrow transplantation.

A Chinese document written in approximately 300 B.C. contains this legendary account of transplantation: "One day two men, Lu and Chao, called on the surgeon Pien Ch'iao. He gave them a toxic drink and they were unconscious for three days. Pien Ch'iao operated and opened their stomachs and explored the heart; after removing and interchanging their organs he gave a wonderful drug and the two men went home recovered."[63]

The legend of Cosmas and Damian describes transplantation as one of the miraculous feats of these two medical martyrs. Born in Arabia in the third century A.D. and trained in medicine in Syria, Cosmas the physician and Damian the surgeon performed numerous miraculous healings until their martyrdom in 287 A.D. by decapitation. The miracle of the black leg is said to have occurred posthumously in approximately 348 A.D. While an elderly parishioner with a gangrenous, cancerous leg lay sleeping in the Basilica of Cosmas and Damian, the saints came to him and removed the diseased leg with a saw. They replaced the destroyed tissue with the fresh leg of a Moor buried that same day in the cemetery of Saint Peter. The new leg was attached at the thigh and ointment applied to the site. The parishioner awoke to find himself free of pain and able to walk on his new healthy black leg.[37] Attempts at transplantation during the Middle Ages did not always end so successfully. Tragically, in 1492 two boys were bled to death in a vain attempt to save the life of Pope Innocent VIII by means of transfusion of young blood.[63]

The oldest evidence of grafting that could have been of some therapeutic benefit is observed in the remains of trephined prehistoric skulls. The trephine holes were usually small, but in a Bronze Age skull a rather large defect evidently was filled by reimplanting the removed fragment.[30] In this specimen, the cut margin showed no sign of healing, so the operation may have been fatal. Recovery from primitive skull trephination is well documented, however, both archeologically and in studies of primitive peoples in modern times, and it is conceivable that such trephination was sometimes therapeutically effective.

Ancient Hindu surgeons described methods for repairing defects of the nose and ears using techniques of grafting similar to those used in modern times. The following technique for nasal reconstruction is quoted from a translation of the *Sushruta Samhita*, a document written about 700 B.C.[7]:

Now I shall deal with the process of affixing an artificial nose. First the leaf of creeper, long and broad enough to fully cover the hole or the severed or clipped off part should be gathered; and a patch of living flesh equal in dimension of the preceding leaf, should be sliced off from down upward from the region of the cheek and, after scarifying it with a knife, swiftly adhered to the severed nose. Then the cool-headed physician should steadily tie it up with a bandage decent to look at and perfectly suited to the end for which it has been employed. The physician should make sure that the adhesion of the severed parts has been fully effected and then insert two small pipes into the nostrils to facilitate respiration and to prevent the adhesioned flesh from hanging down. After that the adhesion part should be dusted with the powders of sappanwood, licorice-root and bayberry pulverized together; and the nose should be enveloped in cotton and several times sprinkled over with a refined oil of pure sesamum. . . . As soon as the skin has grown together with the nose, he cuts through the connection with the cheek.

This *Indian method* was lost to Western medicine until 1794 when English surgeons stationed in India described nasal reconstruction as they had seen it performed by an Indian surgeon, the technique quite similar to that described more than 1000 years earlier.[62]

A new Western tradition of transplantation surgery arose during the Renaissance in Bologna. The sixteenth century anatomist and surgeon Gasparo Tagliacozzi developed his technique for reconstruction using a flap of skin from the inner aspect of the upper arm. He carved the flap of skin in the shape of the patient's nose and then stitched it to the forehead and inner surface of the cheek, leaving a slender attachment to the arm to maintain blood supply until circulation was re-established from the face. After this painful procedure, the patient had to sit upright with the arm alongside the face and the head turned toward the arm for the next 3 weeks of healing; then the attachment to the arm was severed. Tagliacozzi was successful in replacing noses cut off in combat or for punishment or destroyed by syphilis. The technique is still in use and is known as the tagliacotian flap or the *Italian method*. In considering but discarding the idea of grafting tissue donated by another individual, Tagliacozzi made the following remarkable statement: "The singular character of the individual entirely dissuades us from attempting this work on another person. For such is the force and the power of individuality, that if anyone should believe that he could accelerate and increase the beauty of union, nay more, achieve even the least part of the operation, we consider him plainly superstitious and badly grounded in the physical sciences."[56]

EARLY EXPERIMENTS IN TRANSPLANTATION

The Scottish surgeon John Hunter (1728–1793) is known as the father of experimental surgery because of his pioneering research. Several of his experimental procedures involved transplantation, and some of his specimens are still preserved in the Hunterian Museum in London. Hunter revived the practice of transplanting teeth, which had been done in ancient Egypt, Greece, Rome, Arabia, and pre-Columbian America, as well as by Ambroise Paré of Paris in the sixteenth century.[46] With his crude techniques of transplanting tissues without primary revascularization and without antisepsis, Hunter was unable to distinguish allografts from autografts on the basis of graft survival. About this operation he wrote: "Success of this operation is founded on the disposition of all living substances to unite when brought in contact with one another, although they are of different structure and even though the circulation is carried in one of them."[10]

In other animal experiments he successfully autografted and allografted chicken testes and observed that the ends of severed Achilles tendons grew together after suturing. A variety of connective tissue transplant procedures were performed successfully for the first time during the eighteenth and nineteenth centuries. Foremost among these were skin grafts and corneal transplants.

Skin Grafts. The first well-documented report of successful free autografts of skin was in 1804 by Baronio, who experimented with sheep, although free autografts of human skin may have been used successfully centuries before.[10, 19, 46, 62] In 1822, Bunger reported successful use of a free full-thickness human skin autograft to repair a nasal defect. In 1870, Reverdin reported the observation that small grafts of epidermis on a granulating surface increased in size and grew out to coalesce with adjacent grafts. In 1886, Thiersch, in Germany, described the resurfacing of wounds with large sheets of split-thickness skin. Such grafts are still sometimes termed *Thiersch's grafts*, although essentially the same procedure was reported 14 years earlier by Ollier in France.

In 1863 Paul Bert, a student of Claude Bernard, reported that autografts, allografts, and xenografts behaved differently.[19, 62] The significance of these observations received little attention, however; nineteenth century authors (including Baronio and Reverdin) generally failed to observe that the results of allografts and autografts of skin were different. Skin allografts were used to some extent clinically, as illustrated in a story by Winston Churchill of his donating a small piece of skin to a wounded fellow officer in 1898.[19] There appear to have been three reasons for the mistaken belief that skin allografts grew permanently, a belief still widely held as late as the third decade of the twentieth century: (1) for a week or more skin allografts are indistinguishable from autografts; (2) it is difficult to distinguish between permanent survival of a small skin graft and ingrowth of adjacent host skin to cover the area of a sloughed graft; and (3) corneal allografts survive permanently.

Corneal Transplants. Corneal xenografts attempted early in the nineteenth century were unsuccessful. A successful corneal allograft between two gazelles was reported by Bigger in 1835[46, 62]; but the necessity of using a cornea from the same species was not recognized until the period 1872 to 1880, when successful corneal allografts were reported in animals and in man. Refinements of operative techniques, methods of preservation of grafts, and systems of graft procurement were subsequently developed. From 1925 to 1945, corneal transplantation emerged as a widespread and generally accepted therapeutic practice.[18, 46, 62]

TRANSPLANTATION IN THE TWENTIETH CENTURY

Although important developments in the last half of the nineteenth century, such as the use of ether and other general anesthetics and the acceptance of Lister's principles of antiseptic surgery, were important in the progress of transplantation, organ replacement is a development of the twentieth century. Transplantation of vascularized organs, including the kidney, liver, heart, lung, pancreas, and intestine, was first made possible when techniques for vascular anastomosis were developed.

The first long-functioning renal transplant was reported by Ullmann in March 1902. He transplanted kidneys into dogs using magnesium tube stents and ligatures to make the vascular anastomoses to the carotid artery and internal jugular vein in the neck.[59] That same year the French surgeon Carrel reported his new technique of suturing blood vessels together using triangulation and fine silk suture material (Fig. 20–1).[12] His revolutionary technique was rapidly applied to the problems of organ transplantation. Between 1902 and 1912, Carrel and Guthrie of Chicago performed a large series of animal transplantation experiments, including the transfer of blood vessels, kidneys, hearts, spleens, ovaries, thyroids, extremities, and even the head and neck. In 1905 in his preliminary communication entitled "The Transplantation of Organs" Carrel stated:

This operation consists of extirpating an organ with its vessels, of putting it in another region, and of uniting its vessels to a neighboring artery and vein. If the organ is replaced in the same animal from which it was removed the operation is called an *autotransplantation*. If it is placed in another animal of the same species it is called a *homotransplantation*, while if it is placed into an animal of a different species, the operation is called a *heterotransplantation*.[13]

Terminology. Although the terms defined by Carrel are still used occasionally, the preferred nomenclature is now *allotransplantation* (allograft) for transplants between nonidentical members of the same species and *xenotransplantation* (xenograft) for transplants between members of different spe-

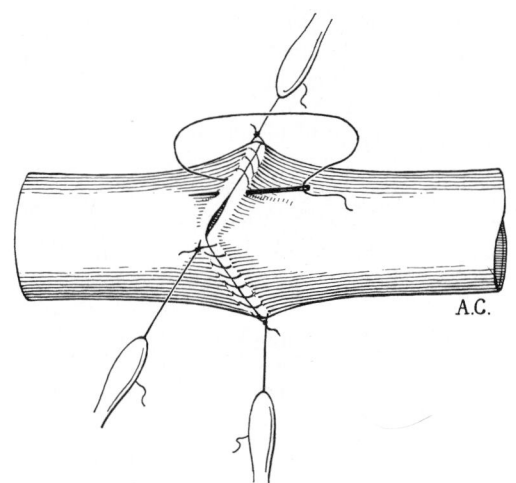

Figure 20–1. Carrel's technique of vascular anastomosis. Shortly after Alexis Carrel reported his new technique of suturing blood vessels together using triangulation and fine silk suture material, he applied the method to the transplantation of blood vessels, hearts, spleens, kidneys, and extremities. (From Carrel, A.: La technique opératoire des anastomoses vasculaires et la transplantation des viscères. Lyon Med., *98*:859, 1902.)

cies (Table 20–1). *Graft* is commonly used as a synonym for transplant and *host* as a synonym for recipient. The prefix *iso*- is ambiguous because it is used with two distinctly different meanings, as discussed by Gorer.[27] The term *isograft* as shown in Table 20–1 derives from geneticists' use of the term *isogeneic* in referring to genetically *identical* individuals, whereas for over 70 years immunologists have used *iso*- to refer to immunity to antigens of blood and tissues of genetically *dissimilar* individuals of the same species (e.g., isoimmune, isoantigen, isoantibody). Depending on the site of implantation, grafts are termed *orthotopic* if surrounded by the same type of tissues or located in the same part of the body after transplantation as previously; otherwise they are termed *heterotopic*. Heterotopic grafts are sometimes implanted into *privileged sites*, such as locations that protect the graft from rejection (e.g., the anterior chamber of the eye, the brain, the testes, or in a diffusion chamber).

Problem of Rejection. Carrel did not understand the biologic basis for differences in graft outcome among the various types of grafts he attempted, although by 1910 he recognized the problem of rejection:

Should an organ, extirpated from an animal and replanted into its owner by a certain technique, continue to functionate normally, and should it cease to functionate when transplanted into another animal by the same technique, the physiological disturbance could not be considered as brought about by the surgical factors. The changes undergone by the organ would be due to the influence of the host, that is, the biological factors.

Elucidation of the biologic factors hypothesized by Carrel required several decades and is, in fact, continuing today. A few of the milestones in transplantation immunology are cited.

Although the immunity theory of graft rejection was postulated by several authors during the first decade of the century, a number of other theories were held by prominent authorities, such as Loeb. The immunity theory was questioned largely because there was no direct evidence that circulating antibody—the traditional hallmark of immunity—was involved in the rejection process. Antibodies had been demonstrated in response to allografts of tumor but not allografts of normal tissues, and attempts to confer allograft immunity passively with serum were unsuccessful. The discovery of cellular immunity, histocompatibility antigens, and immunologic tolerance provided important steps in the understanding of transplant rejection.

Cellular Immunity. In 1914, Murphy reported lymphocytic infiltrates in host tissues surrounding rejecting transplanted tumors.[19, 62] He postulated that the small lymphocyte was responsible for that rejection, and he used radiation and treatment with benzene to modify the process. The role of *cellular immunity* (lymphocytes), as distinguishable from *humoral immunity* (circulating antibody), was not firmly established, however, until experiments were performed in which certain forms of immunity were observed to be transferable

to an unimmunized subject by lymphoid cells and not by serum.[62] By 1954, these *adoptive transfer* experiments were performed by Potter and then Mitchison for tumor allograft immunity in mice and by Landsteiner and Chase for delayed-type hypersensitivity reactions in man. In 1954, Billingham, Brent, and Medawar reported the use of lymphoid cells to transfer immunity to skin and other tissue grafts in mice. Only viable cells were capable of transferring the immunity, a phenomenon designated *adoptively acquired immunity* to distinguish it from passive immunity produced by injections of antibody.

The Second-Set Phenomenon. In 1903, Jensen observed that a second graft did not survive as long as the first when a mouse received two grafts of a tumor separated by an interval of several days, and he suggested that immunity was responsible for the difference. This effect of more rapid rejection of a second graft was not always observed with transplants of tumor, however. Under certain conditions survival of the second graft was prolonged. Casey, in 1932, termed the latter phenomenon *enhancement*, and Kaliss, in 1953, reported that enhancement is transferable to normal animals by injections of serum.[62] The effect was subsequently demonstrated to be due to an immunoglobulin, and enhancing or blocking antibodies have been used experimentally to prolong the survival of nonneoplastic as well as neoplastic tissues.

The second-set phenomenon in human skin graft recipients was observed by Holman while treating burn patients at the Johns Hopkins Hospital. He reported in 1924 that a second group of pinch grafts from the same donor were rejected more rapidly than the first and that "the destroying agency is specific for each set of grafts."[34] He postulated that each group of grafts developed its own antibody. In 1932, Shinoyi, in Japan, described the specificity of the second-set phenomenon. Gibson and Medawar, working in England in 1943, reported similar observations with burn patients, and use of the term *second set* dates to this report.[10, 19, 42, 62] In subsequent controlled experiments with rabbits, Medawar demonstrated the immunologic specificity of the phenomenon, which was observed uniformly only when the same donor was used for both the first set and the second set of grafts. Medawar also contrasted the histologic characteristics of first- and second-set rejections, the first-set rejection being predominantly a cellular event, whereas both cellular and humoral mechanisms are involved in the rejection of the second set of grafts.

Transplantation Antigens. When immunity, both cellular and humoral, had been established as the cause of graft rejection, study was focused on the antigens that both stimulated graft rejection and were the targets of the ensuing immune response. The antigens responsible for graft rejection and the genetic control of these antigens have been most extensively studied in the mouse. The influence of genetic factors was documented by Jensen, Tyzzer, and Little in the first two decades of the century.[46, 62] In 1948, Gorer, Lyman, and Snell described H-2 as a genetic locus controlling strong histocompatibility antigens in the mouse. Subsequently, this locus and numerous minor histocompatibility loci were characterized in great detail.

The definition of the major histocompatibility locus of man, HLA, is intertwined with the evolution of typing and cross-matching for human blood donor selection. The work of Landsteiner during the first four decades of this century with erythrocyte ABO and Rh antigens was necessary for blood banking and transfusion, which were done extensively during and after World War II. The development of blood transfusion contributed to progress with the problem of graft rejection in three respects. First, the A and B erythrocyte antigens are widely distributed in tissues and are transplantation antigens that must be considered in the selection

TABLE 20–1. Transplantation Terminology

Recent Nomenclature	Older Nomenclature	Relationship of Donor and Recipient of Graft
Autogeneic graft	Autograft	Same individual
Isogeneic graft	Isograft	Same species and genetically identical
Allogeneic graft	Homograft	Same species but not genetically identical
Xenogeneic graft	Heterograft	Different species

of tissue and organ donors. Second, by analogy with typing and crossmatching for blood donor selection, one of the major approaches to the problem of graft rejection has been tissue compatibility testing. Third, the sera of patients who have received multiple blood transfusions frequently contain antibodies to human leukocytes. It is now known that these are HLA antibodies, and sera from such patients were a principal source of antibodies in early studies of the HLA system.

The serologic identification of transplantation antigens began in 1952 when Dausset discovered a leukocyte antigen responsible for transfusion reactions.[11] Payne found in 1958 that antileukocyte antibodies were frequent in the sera of multiparous women, thus establishing a rich source of reagents for tissue typing. The new system of tissue matching was first used to select appropriate donors and recipients by Hamburger of Paris.[31] In 1964, Payne reported the first clear evidence that these leukocyte antigens segregated in families as a genetic system. Whereas the original serologic identification of transplantation antigens was done by leukoagglutination, Terasaki, in 1964, introduced a much more sensitive and specific microlymphocytotoxicity test.[57] Definition of the HLA system, the major histocompatibility gene complex of man, has followed a series of international workshops, the first of which was organized in 1964 by Amos at Duke University. A major advance that same year was the discovery that lymphocytes from potential donors and recipients, when mixed together in tissue culture, undergo a vigorous proliferative response. This reaction, termed a *mixed lymphocyte culture* (MLC), became, along with microlymphocytotoxicity, a major approach for histocompatibility testing.[11]

Immunologic Tolerance. The chimaera, an organism carrying living tissues of two or more genetically different individuals, exists not only as a creature of Greek mythology but also naturally in dizygotic cattle twins. Owen, in 1945, reported that each of such twins has two different types of erythrocytes, and he postulated that the marrow of each individual had become populated by cells of both *in utero* when the circulation of the two placentas was mixed.[45] Owen successfully exchanged skin grafts between the cattle twins, and in 1955 Simonson reported that kidneys as well as skin could be readily transplanted between them. In 1953, Dunsford discovered a human twin carrying both A and O erythrocytes, but the other member of the pair died in infancy. In 1959, Woodruff and Lennox reported successful exchange of skin grafts from dizygotic human twins showing blood chimaerism with types A and O.[42, 62] Allografts of skin placed on a chimaera from donors other than the chimaeric mate were rejected in the normal manner. Thus, a natural chimaera is specifically nonreactive to the tissue antigens of its chimaeric mate. Such nonreactivity specifically limited to particular antigens is termed *immunologic tolerance*. In contrast, *immunosuppression* is nonspecific suppression of immune responses to antigens generally. The most common example of naturally occurring tolerance is the normal state of nonreactivity to self antigens, that is, to the antigens of one's own body. Autoimmune diseases are the consequence of abnormal reactivity to self antigens. Burnet conceived recognition of self antigens as one of the aspects of embryologic maturation of the immunologic system.[42, 62]

The creation of states of *acquired tolerance* (i.e., induced specific immunologic tolerance) has been achieved largely by exposure of embryonic, fetal, or early postnatal hosts to grafts that the normal adult animal would reject. Before tolerance was defined immunologically, Murphy, in 1912, observed that rat sarcomas grew on chicken embryos but not in mature chickens, and he noted that the chick acquired the adult capacity to reject the tumor approximately 5 days after completion of shell life.[9, 62] In 1929, Danforth and Foster reported

successful skin grafts between newly hatched Rhode Island red and Plymouth Rock chicks (Fig. 20–2).[42] In 1950, Cannon and Longmire reported similar observations, but they noted additionally that the percentage of take was only 1% if the grafts were performed on chicks 3 days old and was nil at the age of 14 days.[42, 62] A landmark article in the understanding of transplantation immunology appeared on October 3, 1953, when Billingham, Brent, and Medawar reported their experiments on "actively acquired tolerance of foreign cells."[8] They systematically studied the phenomenon of actively acquired tolerance between inbred strains of mice of various ages before and after birth. It became clear that the barrier between self and non-self could be overcome if the exposure to alloantigens occurred in the neonatal period. Grafts established on the fetus survived permanently, and the host was tolerant of other grafts from the donor strain; grafts performed more than 1 or 2 days after birth were rejected, and the rejection of subsequent grafts from the donor strain was accelerated. These authors also reported *breaking* tolerance, that is, reversing tolerance and terminating the chimaeric state, by injecting lymphoid cells of normal adult host-strain mice into tolerant animals. The reversal of the tolerant state in these experiments was marked by the sloughing of long-established grafts of skin and other tissues from the donor strain.

Animals rendered tolerant prenatally or neonatally were normal except for being chimaeras and for being specifically nonreactive to antigens of the donor. Many subsequent studies have been directed toward the objective of inducing tolerance in the adult by methods that would be applicable to therapeutic transplantation in man. Lasting tolerance has been produced in adult mice that were temporarily immunosuppressed at the time of initial exposure to donor antigens, but tolerance is readily produced by this means only if the donor-recipient incompatibility is weak. Immunity, not toler-

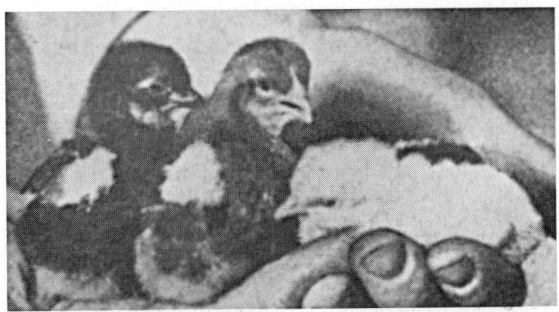

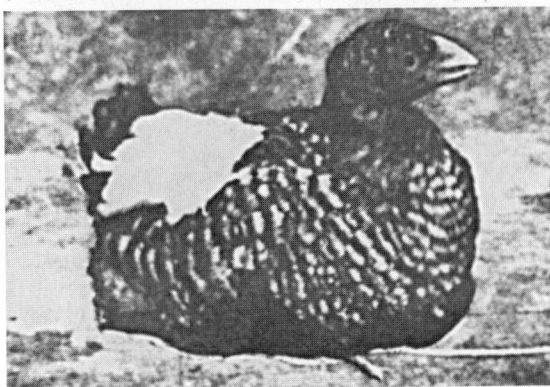

Figure 20–2. Tolerant chickens. In 1929 Danforth and Foster successfully transplanted skin between newly hatched Plymouth Rock (light) and Rhode Island red (dark) chickens. Such grafts take shortly after birth, but not 2 weeks later, and provide an example of actively acquired tolerance. (From Moore, F. D.: Give and Take: The Development of Tissue Transplantation. Philadelphia, W. B. Saunders, 1964.)

ance, usually results if the incompatibility is strong. Because a uniformly effective method of producing acquired tolerance to transplantation antigens in adult animals and humans has not yet been discovered, the progress of transplantation has depended on the development of methods of immunosuppression.

Immunosuppression. Total-body irradiation had been used extensively to prevent rejection of grafts in experimental animals before it was used in the first successful human allografts from living, related donors in Paris and in Boston.[42] However, in the 4 years between March 1958 and March 1962, of 12 potential recipients at the Peter Bent Brigham Hospital who were subjected to total-body x-irradiation with or without marrow infusion, only 1 survived. Although the one patient with a successful allograft lived for 25 years, irradiation as an immunosuppressive agent was judged "too blunt, nonspecific and unpredictable."[43] Schwartz and Dameshek[50] reported in 1959 that 6-mercaptopurine blocked the capacity of rabbits to form antibody. The animals could still react with proteins administered before or after the period of 6-mercaptopurine treatment, suggesting an element of specificity in the suppression. Calne and Zukoski independently used the drug successfully for canine renal transplants, and Hitchings and associates developed an imidazole derivative, azathioprine, in 1961 that could be administered conveniently and safely in an oral form. Murray, Hume, and Starzl reported clinical successes with the new drug that same year, thus initiating the modern era of transplantation.[43]

In the 1950s, numerous authors reported the efficiency of adrenocortical steroids in reversing the manifestations of various immunopathologic disease states. In 1963, Starzl reported that prednisone added to azathioprine produced good results in most patients. The following year, Marchioro and associates reported the successful use of prednisone to reverse established manifestations of renal allograft rejection. Antilymphocyte serum was demonstrated by Woodruff and Anderson in 1963 to prolong skin allograft survival in rats and was used clinically in 1966 by Starzl.[10, 43] The immunosuppressive properties of cyclosporine were discovered by Borel in 1972, used by him in animal studies in 1974, and used clinically by Calne in kidney transplantation trials in 1978.[9] Whereas the indiscriminate use of immunosuppression in the 1950s and 1960s employed modalities that affected cells and tissues in addition to the immunocompetent cells responsible for allograft rejection, cyclosporine and, subsequently, monoclonal antibodies allowed modulation of more defined populations of the involved cells. Although alloantigen-specific immunosuppression remained an elusive goal of transplantation research, cyclosporine markedly improved the results of liver, heart, and heart-lung transplantation, making them for the first time broadly applicable as therapies for end-stage organ failure.

THE ERA OF ORGAN REPLACEMENT

With the advent of chemical immunosuppression, the brief but exciting history of clinical transplantation began. For the first time, several vascularized organs were transplanted with regular success. Foremost among these was the kidney.

Kidney Transplantation. The technical barriers to kidney transplantation were overcome early in the twentieth century by Ullmann[59] and Carrel.[14] In 1908 Carrel wrote: "It is to be concluded that an animal which has undergone a double nephrectomy in the grafting of both kidneys from another animal can secrete almost normal urine with his new organs, and live in good health at least for a few weeks. This demonstrates that it is possible to re-establish sufficiently functions of transplanted kidneys."

In 1906, Jaboulay attempted two kidney xenografts from a pig and a goat to the extremities of patients with chronic renal failure. The kidneys failed after only 1 hour. In 1909, Unger attempted a monkey-to-human kidney transplant to save a girl dying in renal failure. The kidney was sutured to her thigh vessels, but no urine was produced.[32] The first human kidney allograft was performed in 1933 in the Ukraine by Voronoy. He transplanted a kidney donated from a head-injured victim to a patient with acute renal failure from mercuric chloride poisoning. Six hours were required to transplant the kidney to the recipient thigh vessels under local anesthesia, and the transplanted organ never functioned. Voronoy reported six unsuccessful human renal allograft attempts between 1933 and 1949. A kidney allograft to the arm vessels was performed by Hufnagel, Hume, and Landsteiner in Boston in 1946. The transplanted kidney functioned transiently until the patient's own kidneys recovered, and she eventually left the hospital fully recovered.[42] Between 1950 and 1953, human kidney allografts were attempted without immunosuppression in Paris and Boston.[32, 41] Most of these kidneys failed immediately, but one transplant recipient of Hume had life-sustaining renal function for several months. Living-related transplantation commenced in 1953 when Michon of Paris transplanted a kidney from a mother to her son, whose solitary kidney had been damaged in a road accident. The kidney functioned for 22 days before it was rejected.[32] In 1954, Murray performed the first renal transplant between monozygotic twins and achieved excellent, long-term function.[43] In March 1958, Murray, in Boston, and Hamburger, in Paris, each performed a series of human kidney allografts using total-body irradiation for immunosuppression.[32] The modern era of immunosuppression had begun, and the subsequent history of renal transplantation paralleled the development of immunosuppressive drugs.

Liver Transplantation. Canine liver grafts were shown to function after transplantation to the pelvis by Welch in 1955. Orthotopic liver transplantation in dogs was attempted by Cannon in 1956 and performed successfully by Moore in 1959. The first attempt at liver allotransplantation in man was made by Starzl at the University of Colorado on March 1, 1963.[52] The 3-year-old recipient with extrahepatic biliary atresia died of hemorrhage on the day of transplantation. Ensuing attempts in Denver, Boston, and Paris were unsuccessful until 1967, when the first extended survival of a human liver allograft recipient was achieved by Starzl. The addition of cyclosporine immunosuppression by Calne in 1978 and then combination therapy with cyclosporine and prednisone by Starzl in 1980, as well as better liver preservation and surgical techniques, improved the prospects for clinical liver transplantation.

Heart Transplantation. Carrel and Guthrie performed the first heart transplant in 1905 at the University of Chicago.[16] They transplanted a canine heart to the neck of another dog and observed rhythmic contraction for 2 hours until coagulation occurred in the cavities of the heart. Mann and associates, in 1933, transplanted canine hearts to the neck with more success.[40] One of their dogs survived 8 days, allowing them to be the first to recognize cardiac allograft rejection. The first clinical heart transplant was performed by Hardy in Jackson, Mississippi, in January 1964.[33] A 68-year-old patient in cardiogenic shock received a chimpanzee heart when the prospective human donor became unsuitable. The small animal heart proved inadequate to take the patient's venous return, and the recipient died after 1 hour. The first successful clinical transplant was performed on December 3, 1967, when Dr. Christiaan Barnard, at the University of Cape Town, transplanted the heart of a young man to a 54-year-old patient with a heart irreparably damaged by repeated myocardial infarction.[4] The recipient lived 18 days before dying of gram-negative pneumonia. The historical foundations of heart transplantation are reviewed by Griepp and Ergin.[28]

Lung Transplantation. In contrast to the success of cardiac allografts, clinical lung transplantation proved much more difficult. The first human lung transplant was performed by Hardy on June 11, 1963, in a patient with chronic lung disease and carcinoma of the left lung. The patient survived 18 days before dying of renal insufficiency. Because of the difficulty of finding suitable donors, bronchial anastomotic complications, and allograft rejection, only 38 lung transplants were performed in the first 15 years of clinical experience.[60] The longest survivor was a 23-year-old sandblaster with micronodular silicosis who lived 10 months after lung allotransplantation.[21] The tracheobronchial anastomotic complications were initially overcome by simultaneous transplantation of the lungs and heart, a procedure first performed by Reitz and associates at Stanford in 1981.[49] Single-lung and eventually double-lung transplantations without the heart were made possible by technical advances pioneered by Cooper and colleagues in Toronto.[58]

Pancreas Transplantation. The first clinical pancreatic transplant was performed by Williams.[23] His patient, a 15-year-old boy, died in coma 3 days later. Work in this area was sporadic and unsuccessful until 1922, when Banting and associates corrected the hyperglycemia of human diabetes mellitus by injection of bovine pancreatic extract.[3] However, clinical application of whole pancreas transplantation in a systematic manner was not to occur for more than 40 years. In 1970, Lillehei published the first cases in the extensive University of Minnesota series of clinical pancreatic allotransplants that began in 1966.[39] In the original 14 cases of pancreaticoduodenal transplantation, four patients and one graft survived more than 1 year, and one recipient was still alive in 1984. The same institution reported the first large series of human islet allografts in 1977. However, none of 20 islet allografts led to insulin independence, and only 3 of 10 islet autografts for chronic pancreatitis led to insulin independence.[44] The historical development of pancreatic islet transplantation is reviewed by Downing.[23]

During the short history of clinical pancreas transplantation, the difficult problem of eliminating or draining the pancreatic exocrine secretions was managed in several ways. Gliedman and associates attempted to anastomose the pancreatic duct to the ureter.[26] Duct ligation was attempted by the same group as well as by Groth in 1976.[29] The technique of injecting the pancreatic duct with a synthetic polymer to block exocrine function was reported by Dubernard and associates in 1978.[24] Free drainage of the duct into the peritoneal cavity was investigated by Sutherland and reported in 1979.[54] However, intractable ascites occurred in some patients, and an overall technical complication rate of 50% mandated reinvestigation of enteric drainage.[54] Bladder drainage, as popularized by Sollinger and associates,[51] produced improved results with combined kidney-pancreas transplants. With the use of the segmental technique and a pancreaticojejunostomy, living-related donor pancreas transplantation began in 1979.[55]

Intestine Transplantation. Although autotransplantation of the bowel is among the most frequently used and successful forms of organ transplantation (see Part XII in this chapter), intestinal allotransplantation has been generally unsuccessful. Clinical small intestinal allografting was attempted in several patients after 1967 for bowel infarction,[38] repeated sepsis on total parenteral nutrition,[1] and Gardner's syndrome with recurrent desmoid tumors of the bowel.[25] Even in the case of the HLA identical graft, which survived 76 days, minimal useful bowel function was observed. Rejection, graft-versus-host disease, infection, and high operative mortality historically diminished surgical enthusiasm for intestinal transplantation. The advent of cyclosporine immunosuppression and subsequent potent drugs have reawakened interest in the field.[20, 22, 47]

Xenotransplantation. When the techniques of vascular anastomosis were sufficiently well known to permit successful autotransplantation and allotransplantation, a number of xenogeneic transplants into humans were attempted. Between 1905 and 1910, several workers, including Jaboulay in France and Unger in Germany, performed xenografts but did not document graft function.[32] When the immunologic basis of rejection was established, renewal of interest in clinical xenotransplantation awaited the development of new immunosuppressive measures. After the efficacy of chemical immunosuppression with azathioprine, prednisone, and mitomycin-C was established, Reemtsma and associates, in 1963 and 1964, undertook xenografts in patients in renal failure using kidneys from nonhuman primates.[48] Several of these cases showed satisfactory immediate function, but all were eventually rejected within a few months. When cyclosporine became available for clinical use, human xenografting was again attempted in 1984.[2] A baboon heart was transplanted to a child born with a severe congenital malformation of the heart. Despite intensive immunosuppression, rejection developed and the infant died within weeks of transplantation.

Tissue and Organ Preservation. Along with the improved capability of transplanting tissues and organs, interest in preservation and storage of living tissue developed. The structural integrity and the viability of the graft had to be maintained during the interval from removal to implantation. Basically, two approaches were available: (1) methods that reduced or brought to a reversible standstill the need for oxygen and other metabolic requirements and (2) systems that supported active metabolism. Of the several methods that were tried to achieve long-term preservation, including freezing, only hypothermia and organ perfusion are in general use today. In addition, chemical inhibition of metabolism in the form of cardioplegia solution is used for cardiac transplantation and many other open-heart surgical procedures as discussed in Chapter 54.

In 1908, Carrel removed an artery from one animal, preserved it with hypothermia for days, and then successfully transplanted it to another animal.[15] The numerous other contributions of Carrel to tissue culture and ultimately organ perfusion were reviewed by Humphries and Dennis in their "Historical Developments in Preservation."[36] Using his newly developed media and culture techniques, Carrel was able to maintain chick embryo fibroblasts in continuous culture for more than 25 years! His attempts at organ culture were less successful. With the use of a pump and perfusion apparatus designed by Charles Lindbergh, organs were perfused for 20 to 40 days with normothermic serum. Although some cells remained viable, reimplantation of the organs was not undertaken to test the effectiveness of the preservation system. Maximal preservation of kidneys was approximately 2 days.[17]

A variety of solutions were used for continuous perfusion of organs. Humphries achieved 24-hour dog kidney preservation using continuous perfusion with dilute blood at 10° C. Plasma protein fraction, cryoprecipitated plasma, silicone-gel fraction of plasma, and albumin were all added to electrolyte solutions to improve preservation. Belzer and associates, in 1967, introduced a new pump and perfusate containing lipoprotein-free serum for continuous pulsatile perfusion at 10° C. that enabled him to consistently preserve kidneys for 72 hours.[5] Improved preservation solutions developed by him at the University of Wisconsin extended preservation times of the kidney and ultimately of the liver and pancreas as well.[7]

Hypothermia. At temperatures of 0° to 4° C., tissues remain viable in the absence of circulation 10 or more times longer than at normal body temperature. The simple method of hypothermia proved useful in preserving skin, cornea, kidney, liver, heart, pancreas, and blood. Flushing an organ with a cold perfusate, usually a balanced electrolyte solution, was used widely as a means of rapid cooling, within seconds, to temperatures that by surface cooling were achieved only after a number of minutes and at the expense of loss of viability. In 1960, Lapchinsky, of Moscow, reported successful reimplantation of dog kidneys and hind limbs after 24 to 28 hours of preservation using cold storage. He perfused the kidney or limb for 1 hour with cooled whole blood, then kept the organ cold at 2° to 4° C. until 1 hour before reimplantation, when he perfused the tissue again for 1 hour, this time with warm blood.[36] Collins and associates, in 1969, developed a flushing solution that mimicked intracellular fluid.[18] With this hyperkalemic and hyperosmolar solution, they flushed kidneys, kept them cold on ice, and obtained excellent function after 30 hours of iced storage. By removing the magnesium from Collins' solution, the EuroCollins solution, widely used by European transplant centers, was developed in 1976. EuroCollins and Sacks' solution, developed in 1978, successfully preserved human kidneys for 50 hours or more.[36] The use of preservation solutions to flush grafts and reduce their metabolism through hypothermia, hyperkalemia, hyponatremia, and hypocalcemia before cold storage should be distinguished from perfusion methods designed to support metabolism by simulating as fully as possible the normothermic internal environment of the organ. However, elements of the two approaches were often combined in the form of continuous perfusion at 4° to 10° C.

Organ-Sharing Networks. A natural outgrowth of the capabilities for organ preservation and tissue matching was the development of networks for sharing kidneys on the basis of histocompatibility. For example, in 1968, Hume, at the Medical College of Virginia, in cooperation with Amos, of Duke University, developed an organ-sharing plan to enlarge the potential recipient pool for each new kidney that became available so that better tissue matches between donor and recipient could be obtained. The resulting organization, named the Southeastern Organ Procurement Foundation (SEOPF), shared kidneys among nine institutions based on computer-assisted matching of all potential recipients in that region. The SEOPF network expanded to include 46 transplanting institutions and led in 1984 to the incorporation of the United Network for Organ Sharing (UNOS) to facilitate organ placement throughout the United States. Similar organ-sharing networks were developed in Europe, Scandinavia, the United Kingdom, and elsewhere. These regional networks began to cooperate in the sharing of human organs and tissues on an international scale.

SELECTED REFERENCES

Converse, J. M., and Casson, P. R.: The historical background of transplantation. *In* Rapaport, F.T., and Dausset, J. (Eds.): Human Transplantation. New York, Grune & Stratton, 1968.
  The authors present a history of the principal developments in transplantation from ancient to modern times, and they include some details not included in the other histories cited.

Griepp, R. B., and Ergin, M. D.: The history of experimental heart transplantation. Heart Transplant., 3:145, 1984.
  The authors present a brief, interesting, and well-illustrated summary of the development of heart transplantation.

Hamilton, D.: Kidney transplantation: A history. *In* Morris, P.J. (Ed.): Kidney Transplantation: Principles and Practice. London, Grune & Stratton, 1984.
  In this chapter written for the second edition of Kidney Transplantation, the author presents an interesting account of the evolution of human kidney transplantation from early European experiments to the modern era.

Moore, F. D.: Give and Take: The Development of Tissue Transplantation. Philadelphia, W. B. Saunders, 1964.

In this volume is presented a concise review of developments in basic biology and in medicine and surgery that apply to therapeutic renal transplantation. Interesting aspects of historic renal transplants in Boston are described by the author, who was there at the time and has communicated personally with scientists there and elsewhere who have made notable contributions. For the student, this book is an informative introduction to the subject of transplantation, and for the lay reader it is a readily understood account of some interesting developments in biology and medicine.

Starzl, T. E., Iwatsuki, S., Van Thiel, D. H., Garmer, J. C., Zitelli, B. J., Malatack, J. J., Schade, R. R., Shaw, B. W., Jr., Hakala, T. R., Rosenthal, J. T., and Porter, K. A.: Evolution of liver transplantation. Hepatology, 2:614, 1982.
  The researcher, physician, and author who has contributed the most to the development of liver transplantation provides an authoritative account of the development of the field.

Terasaki, P. I. (Ed.): History of Transplantation: Thirty-five Recollections. Los Angeles, UCLA Tissue Typing Laboratory, 1991.
  Personal reminiscences of pioneers who were involved in the initiation of clinical transplantation in the 1950s and 1960s are presented in unedited form.

REFERENCES

1. Alican, F., Hardy, J. D., Cayirli, M., Vamer, J. E., Moynihan, P. C., Turner, M. D., and Anas, P.: Intestinal transplantation: Laboratory experience and report of a clinical case. Am. J. Surg., 121:150, 1971.
2. Bailey, L. L., Nehlsen-Cannarell, S. L., Concepcion, W., and Jolley, W. B.: Baboon-to-human cardiac xenotransplantation in a neonate. JAMA, 254:3321, 1985.
3. Banting, F., Best, C., Gollip, J., Campbell, W., and Fletcher, A.: Pancreas extracts in the treatment of diabetes mellitus. Can. Med. Assoc. J., 12:141, 1922.
4. Barnard, C. N.: A human cardiac transplant: An interim report of a successful operation performed at Groote Schuur Hospital, Cape Town. S. Afr. Med. J., 41:1271, 1967.
5. Belzer, F. O., Ashby, B. S., and Dunphy, J. F.: Twenty-four-hour and 72-hour preservation of canine kidneys. Lancet, 2:536, 1967.
6. Belzer, F. O., Hoffman, R. M. and Southard, J. H. A new perfusate for kidney preservation. Transplantation, 33:322,1982.
7. Bhisragratna, K. K.: The Sushruta Samhita. An English translation based on the original Sanscrit text. Calcutta, 1907.
8. Billingham, R. E., Brent, L., and Medawar, P. B.: Actively acquired tolerance of foreign cells. Nature, 172:603, 1953.
9. Borel, J. F.: Cyclosporine: Historical perspectives. Transplant. Proc., 15 (Suppl. 1):2219, 1983.
10. Caine R. Y.: Renal Transplantation. London, Edward Arnold, 1967.
11. Carpenter, C. B.: Clinical histocompatibility testing: A brief historical perspective. Transplant. Proc., 13(Suppl. 1):55, 1981.
12. Carrel A.: La technique opératoire des anastomoses vasculaires et la transplantation des viscères. Lyon Med., 98:859, 1902.
13. Carrel, A.: The transplantation of organs: A preliminary communication. JAMA, 45:1645, 1905.
14. Carrel, A.: Transplantation in mass of the kidney. J. Exp. Med., 10:140, 1908.
15. Carrel, A.: Results of the transplantation of blood vessels, organs and limbs. JAMA, 51:1662, 1908.
16. Carrel, A., and Guthrie, C. C.: The transplantation of veins and organs. Am. Med., 10:1101, 1905.
17. Carrel, A., and Lindbergh, C. A.: The Culture of Organs. New York, Paul B. Hoeber, 1938.
18. Collins, G. M., Bravo-Shugarman, M., and Terasaki, P. I.: Kidney preservation for transportation. Lancet, 2:1219, 1969.
19. Converse, J. M., and Casson, P. R.: The historical aspects of transplantation. *In* Rapaport, P. T., and Dausset, J. (Eds.): Human Transplantation. New York, Grune & Stratton, 1968.
20. Craddock, G. N., Nordgren, S. R., Reznick, R. K., Gilas, T., Lossing A. G., Cohen, Z., Stiller, C. R., Cullen, J. B., and Langer, B.: Small bowel transplantation in the dog using cyclosporine. Transplantation, 35:284, 1983.
21. Dermon, F., Barbier, F., Ringoir, S., Versieck, J., Rolly, G., Berzsenyi, G., Venneire, P., and Vrints, L.: Ten-month survival after lung homotransplantation in man. J. Thorac. Cardiovasc. Surg., 61:835, 1971.
22. Diliz-Perez, H. S., McClure, J., Bedetti, C., Hong, H., de Santibanes, E., Shaw, B. W., Jr., Van Thiel, D., Iwatsuki, S., and Starzl, T. E.: Successful small bowel allotransplantation in dogs with cyclosporine and prednisone. Transplantation, 37:126, 1984.
23. Downing, R.: Historical review of pancreatic islet transplantation. World J. Surg., 8:137, 1984.
24. Dubernard, J. M., Traeger, J., Neyra, P., Touraine, J. L., Tranchant, D., and Blanc-Bruant, N.: A new method of preparation of segmental pancreatic grafts for transplantation: Trials in dogs and in man. Surgery, 84:633, 1978.
25. Fortner, J. G., Sichuk, G., Litwin, S. D., and Beattie, E. J., Jr.: Immunological responses to an intestinal allograft with HL-A-identical donor-recipient. Transplantation, 14:531, 1972.
26. Gliedman, M. L., Gold, M., Whittaker, J., Rifkin, H., Soberman, R., Freed, S., Tellis, V., and Veith, F. J.: Pancreatic duct to ureter anastomosis in pancreas transplantation. Am. J. Surg., 125:245, 1973.

27. Gorer, P. A.: Transplantese. Ann. N.Y. Acad. Sci., 87:604, 1960.
28. Griepp, R. B., and Ergin, M. A.: The history of heart transplantation. Heart Transplant., 3:145, 1984.
29. Groth, C., Lundgren, G., Arner, P., Collste, H., Hardstedt, C., Lewander, R., and Ostman, J.: Rejection of isolated pancreatic allografts in patients with diabetes. Surg. Gynecol. Obstet., 143:933, 1976.
30. Guthrie, D.: A History of Medicine. Philadelphia, J. B. Lippincott, 1946, p. 12.
31. Hamburger, J., Vaysse, J., Crosnier, J., Auver, J., M., and Hopper, J., Jr.: Renal homotransplantation in man after radiation of the recipient. Am. J. Med., 32:854, 1962.
32. Hamilton, D.: Kidney transplantation: A history. In Morris, P. J. (Ed.): Kidney Transplantation: Principles and Practice. London, Grune & Stratton, 1984.
33. Hardy, J. D., Chavez, C. M., Kurrus, F. D., Neely, W. A., Erasian, S., Turner, M. D., Fabian, L. W., and Labeckiz, T.: Heart transplantation in man: Developmental studies and report of a case. JAMA, 188:1132, 1964.
34. Holman, E.: Protein sensitization in isoskin grafting. Gynecol. Obstet., 38:100, 1924.
35. Homer: The Iliad, Book 6.
36. Humphries, A. L., and Dennis, A. J., Jr.: Historical developments in preservation. In Toledo-Pereyra, L. H. (Ed.): Basic Concepts of Organ Procurement, Perfusion and Preservation for Transplantation. New York, Academic Press, 1982, p. 1.
37. Kahan, B. D.: Cosmas and Damian revisited. Transplant. Proc., 15:2211, 1983.
38. Lillehei, R. C., Idezuki, Y., Feemster, J. A., Dietzman, R. H., Kelly, W. D., Merkel, F. K., Goetz, F. C., Lyons, G. W., and Manax, W. G.: Transplantation of stomach, intestine, and pancreas: Experimental and clinical observations. Surgery, 62:721, 1967.
39. Lillehei, R. C., Simmons, R. L., Najarian, J. S., Weil, R., Uchida, H., Ruiz, J. O., Kjellstrand, C. M., and Goetz, F. C.: Pancreaticoduodenal allotransplantation: Experimental and clinical experience. Ann. Surg., 172:405, 1970.
40. Mann, F. C., Priestley, J. T., Markowitz, J., and Yater, W. M.: Transplantation of the intact mammalian heart. Arch. Surg., 26:219, 1933.
41. Merrill, J. P.: Early days of the artificial kidney and transplantation. Transplant. Proc., 13(Suppl. 1):4, 1981.
42. Moore, P. D.: Give and Take: The Development of Tissue Transplantation. Philadelphia, W. B. Saunders, 1964.
43. Murray, J. E.: Remembrances of the early days of renal transplantation. Transplant. Proc., 13(Suppl. 1):9, 1981.
44. Najarian, J. S., Sutherland, D. E. R., Matas, A. J., Steffes, M. W., Simmons, R. L., and Goetz, F. C.: Human islet transplantation: A preliminary experience. Transplant. Proc., 9:233, 1977.
45. Owen, R. D.: Immunogenetic consequences of vascular anastomoses between bovine twins. Science, 102:400, 1945.
46. Peer, L. A.: Transplantation of Tissues. Baltimore, Williams & Wilkins, 1955.
47. Raju, S., Didlake, R. H., Gayirli, M., Turner, M. D., Grogan, J. B., and Achord, J.: Experimental small bowel transplantation utilizing cyclosporine. Transplantation, 38:561, 1984.
48. Reemtsma, K., McCracken, B. H., Schlegel, J. U., and Pearl, M.: Heterotransplantation of the kidney: Two clinical experiences. Science, 143:700, 1964.
49. Reitz, B. A., Wallwork, J. L., Hunt, S. A., Pennock, J. L., Billingham, M. E., Oyer, P. E., Stinson, E. B., and Shumway, N. E.: Heart-lung transplantation: Successful therapy for patients with pulmonary vascular disease. N. Engl. J. Med., 306:557, 1982.
50. Schwartz, R., and Dameshek, W.: Drug-induced immunological tolerance. Nature, 183:1682, 1959.
51. Sollinger, H. W., Pirsch, J. D., D'Alessandro, A. M., Kalayoglu, M., and Belzer, F. O.: Advantages of bladder drainage in pancreas transplantation: A personal view. Clin. Transplant., 4:32, 1990.
52. Starzl, T. E., Iwatsuki, S., Van Thiel, D. H., Gartner, J. C., Zitelli, B. J., Malatack, J. J., Schade, R., R., Shaw, B. W., Jr., Hakala, T. R., Rosenthal, J. T., and Porter, K. A.: Evolution of liver transplantation. Hepatology, 2:614, 1982.
53. Sutherland, D. E. R., Goetz, F. C., Elick, B. A., and Najarian, J. S.: Experiments with 49 segmental pancreatic transplants in 45 diabetic patients. Transplantation, 34:330, 1982.
54. Sutherland, D. E. R., Goetz, F. C., and Najarian, J. S.: Intraperitoneal transplantation of immediate vascularized segmental grafts without duct ligation: A clinical trial. Transplantation, 28:485, 1979.
55. Sutherland, D. E. R., Goetz, F. C., and Najarian, J. S.: Living related donor segmental pancreatectomy for transplantation. Transplant Proc., 12(Suppl. 2):19, 1980.
56. Tagliacozzi, G.: De curtorum chirurgia per instionem. Venice, 1597, p. 61.
57. Terasaki, P. I., and McClelland, J. D.: Microdroplet assay of human serum cytotoxins. Nature, 204:998, 1964.
58. The Toronto Lung Transplant Group: Unilateral lung transplantation for pulmonary fibrosis. N. Engl. J. Med., 314:1140, 1986.
59. Ullmann, E.: Experimentelle Nierentransplantation. Wien. Klin. Wochenschr., 15:281, 1902.
60. Veith, F. J.: Lung transplantation. Surg. Clin. North Am., 58:357, 1978.
61. Veith, F. J., Kamholz, S. L., Mollenkopf, F. P., and Montefusco, C. M.: Lung transplantation 1983. Transplantation, 35:271, 1983.
62. Woodruff, M. F. A.: The Transplantation of Tissues and Organs. Springfield, Ill., Charles C. Thomas, 1960.
63. Worshofsky, F.: The Rebuilt Man. New York, Thomas Y. Crowell, 1965.

II

THE IMMUNOLOGY OF TRANSPLANT ANTIGENS

Jeffrey L. Platt, M.D., and Pablo Rubinstein, M.D.

The history of transplantation immunology can be traced to the early years of the twentieth century. Ullmann and Carrel made the initial but unsuccessful attempts to transplant kidneys in 1902. In 1905, Floresco and also Carrel and Guthrie carried out technically successful renal allografts,[33] the best results being an orthotopic renal transplant performed by Floresco that functioned for 5 days. In 1906, Carrel and Guthrie transplanted both kidneys of one dog orthotopically into another dog, the native kidneys of which had been removed; the renal allograft functioned for 9 days. In 1907, Carrel performed a series of renal allografts into anephric cats; one recipient survived for 31 days, the others for 14 days or less.[6] In 1908, however, a renal autograft performed by Carrel maintained the life of the recipient for longer than 8 months. The experiments of Floresco, Carrel, and Guthrie were much acclaimed and were recognized to be landmarks in vascular surgery because they demonstrated for the first time that a kidney removed from its natural environment and reimplanted surgically would function, if only temporarily. Now these experiments might be viewed as the first demonstration of two fundamental principles of normal tissue transplantation: (1) that autografts are nearly always successful, whereas allografts in a random-breeding population of donors and recipients are always rejected, and (2) that rejection develops more rapidly than conventional immune responses. The immunologic basis for allograft rejection and the mechanisms that cause this immune response to be so rapid and intense are major themes of the sections that follow.

HISTOCOMPATIBILITY

Histocompatibility is the ability of a tissue or an organ to survive after grafting.[32] In the broadest sense, the term encompasses various immune and nonimmune factors that allow a graft to survive in a foreign environment. With the discovery that the fate of allografts is governed by the immune reaction of recipient against genetically determined cell surface structures in the donated organ, *histocompatibility* has more narrowly referred to the genetic determinants of graft rejection.

The concept that there is a genetic trait associated with histocompatibility can be traced to the work of Jensen, a Danish biologist who discovered that spontaneous tumors arising in an inbred mouse strain could be maintained by transplanting pieces of the tumor tissue into other members of the same strain. However, if the tumor was transplanted into a mouse of a different strain, it would grow only for a few days and then regress and disappear. If the tumor was transplanted into a mouse in which the tumor had previously regressed, it would not grow and would disappear almost immediately. Jensen speculated that regression of the tumor might be caused by immunity, and his observations sparked efforts in a number of laboratories to generate resistance to tumors by transferring serum from resistant mice. These efforts proved futile; indeed, Medawar, reflecting on this period, later commented that "nearly everyone who supposed that he was using transplantation to study tumors was in fact using tumors to study transplantation—not always to very good effect."[24]

Loeb, Jensen's contemporary, observed that spontaneous tumors often occurred in a partially inbred strain of Japanese "waltzing" mice, so named because of a neurologic defect that made them twirl when stimulated, which was appealing to mouse fanciers. Such tumors could be grafted and would grow in other waltzing mice but never in mice of other stocks. In 1906, Tyzzer made the fundamental observation that the F1 offspring of crosses between waltzing mice and other strains allowed the growth of a transplantable mammary adenocarcinoma originating in the waltzing strain, suggesting that a dominant trait governed acceptance of the tumor. If susceptibility to the tumor was conferred by a single genetic locus, then three fourths of the F2 generation and half of the offspring of the backcross of F1 to the resistant parent should be susceptible to the tumor. However, most F2 hybrids and offspring of backcrosses appeared as resistant as the nonwaltzing parent, and only a few accepted the graft. The explanation for this phenomenon—namely, that acceptance of the tumor requires the joint presence of many genes—was proposed by Little in 1914.

Little also suggested that the regression of tumor and normal tissue grafts might be governed by the same processes. Consistent with Jensen's observations, Little showed that a tumor transplanted within an inbred strain of mice would invariably grow and kill the recipient, whereas the same transplanted tumor would regress in outbred mice.[21] The F1 hybrid crosses of the inbred strain and outbred mice were always susceptible to the tumor, but, conversely, the parental strains were not susceptible to tumors that arose in F1 animals.[20] Tumors transplanted from the parental strain to F2 animals sometimes grew progressively but usually regressed. From a long series of experiments, Little concluded that susceptibility or resistance to tumor grafts depends on a number of independently segregating, codominant genes, each existing as multiple alleles. The presence of an allele of such a gene in the tumor and not in the recipient follows classical mendelian rules. Little's observations constitute the basis of our understanding of the genetics of transplantation.[32]

Little's work was continued by Snell, who devoted many years to the development of congenic *lines* of mice, that is, lines derived from hybrid mice that contain all the genes of one parental strain save for the allele at one locus, which is derived from the other parent. Snell used the congenic strains to examine in great detail the role of histocompatibility or H genes in the transplantation of strain-specific tumors. He demonstrated that the absence in the recipient of any one of the alleles of the donor strain genes determined the failure of such transplants. The speed of regression of the tumor varied in different congenic strains but was characteristically similar for all members of a given congenic strain. Thus, the *strength* of different H genes was a feature of the specific H gene. Snell's observations in mice paralleled observations by Bauer (1927) in human twins that skin grafts between human twins were accepted, whereas those between other relatives failed with regularity.

That the mechanism of the failure of tumor allotransplants is immunologic was proposed on general grounds by many investigators, including Jensen, but a formal demonstration was first provided in the 1930s by Gorer. Gorer studied the blood groups of the mouse using first a human anti-A serum and, later, rabbit antimouse antisera. The red cells of mice of the three strains available in Gorer's laboratory reacted with one rabbit reagent, designated antigen I, whereas the red cells of two of the three strains reacted with a second reagent, designated antigen II. Gorer established that the capacity of recipients to reject tumors was associated with the presence of antigen II in crosses involving a positive and a negative parent. The susceptibility to tumors from an antigen II–positive parent was inherited with the antigen, although there were also hybrid mice carrying the antigen and not growing the tumor, implying the need for additional genetic factors. That the tumor was immunologically rejected was surmised from the presence in the recipient's serum of antibodies reactive with the blood cells of the tumor donors. Gorer showed that these antibodies were directed against antigen II itself and that this antigen is present in both tumors and normal tissues. Gorer was thus able to declare that tumors and normal tissues contain inherited antigenic factors, which, if absent in a transplant recipient and present in the donor, produce an immune response that destroys the graft.

Further resolution was achieved by Gorer and Snell, who, together with the mouse geneticist Lyman, showed that antigen II segregated with the strongest of Snell's H antigens in linkage with the *fused* locus, a skeletal abnormality belonging to the IXth linkage group of the mouse. Thus, antigen II became H-2. The locus, which Snell called H-2, was considered a *strong* histocompatibility locus because tumors from animals disparate at H-2 would always regress, whereas transplants from donors disparate at H-2 would always be rejected and the rejection reaction would proceed rapidly. The strong histocompatibility locus was later found to be a complex of genes called the *major histocompatibility complex* (MHC). Transplants matched for major antigens might still undergo rejection, albeit at a slower tempo. This type of rejection was attributed to *weaker* histocompatibility antigens, later called *minor* antigens.

In 1958 Dausset discovered that patients who had received multiple transfusions of blood and who, as a result, were subject to transfusion reactions contained in their serum antibodies specific for leukocyte alloantigens. These antigens, ultimately called *human leukocyte antigens* (HLA), were shown to be the major histocompatibility antigens (MHC) in humans and were analogous to the murine H-2 antigens.

Since Jensen's report in 1903, the field of histocompatibility has attempted to address both the nature of the genetic determinants of tissue individuality and the factors that condition immune responses to foreign tissues as well as the mechanisms mediating those responses. One central question has been whether MHC antigens, like blood group antigens, function only as passive targets of immune responses or whether MHC antigens participate in some way in the physiology of the immune system.[8] Another question has been the mechanisms underlying the strong histocompatibility barrier provided by MHC antigens versus the weaker barrier posed by minor antigens. Yet another question concerned the nature of MHC genes and the proteins they encode that enable this system to confer distinctness to members of an outbred population. It is only very recently that detailed answers to these questions have emerged, permitting the study of the biologic role of histocompatibility determinants in initiating and regulating of immune responses in normal animals. In the intervening years, as these issues were addressed, histocompatibility has been an active contributor to, as well as a beneficiary of, the rapid advances in the fields of genetics, immunology, pathology, surgery, and cell biology.

HISTOCOMPATIBILITY AND THE PHYSIOLOGY OF CELLULAR IMMUNE RESPONSES

Transplantation of tissues and organs across MHC barriers elicits both humoral and cellular immune responses. The humoral response to allotransplantation, giving rise to antibodies specific for major histocompatibility antigens, allowed the genetic mapping of the MHC complex. Alloantibodies as such may also influence the course of the rejection reaction, sometimes for the worse, as in the case of hyperacute rejection, but sometimes for the better, as in the case of enhancement. However, the cellular immune response accounts for the characteristic manifestations of allograft rejection; and therefore the present discussion shall focus on the contribution of histocompatibility antigens to this type of response. The reader is referred to Part III in this chapter for a more comprehensive discussion of the mechanisms of immune responses to transplantation.

The normal immune response to any foreign antigen consists of two phases. The first involves the recognition of the foreign antigen in such a way that lymphocytes become *activated*. This activation leads to the second phase, which involves the effector action of lymphocytes and other cells recruited by activated lymphocytes into the reaction against the foreign organism or antigen. When a foreign organ or tissue is transplanted to an untreated recipient, the recognition of foreign antigens leads promptly into the second or *effector* phase, and thus to rejection of the graft. The immune response to allogeneic tissues and organs in this setting is nearly universal in its occurrence and customarily is quite rapid and powerful.

When a tissue or organ is transplanted into a recipient treated with immunosuppressive agents, recognition may occur much before the overt manifestations of rejection, which may not occur at all.

Immune Recognition. If the expression of histocompatibility antigens dictates susceptibility to rejection, the role of histocompatibility antigens in immune recognition is the preeminent issue in the pathogenesis of the rejection reaction. Immune recognition leading to allograft rejection involves the specific binding of receptors for antigens on the surface of T cells to major histocompatibility antigens bearing foreign peptides expressed on the surface of stimulator or target cells. The nature of this interaction has been elucidated by contributions of many laboratories in the fields of molecular immunology, cell biology, and genetics.

For most of this century, immune responses were considered to be exclusively humoral, the cellular elements involved resulting from nonspecific inflammatory responses engendered by antibodies and complement. Although the idea may have been proposed as early as 1926, by Murphy, that lymphocytes might mediate immune responses it was not formally demonstrated until the experiments of Landsteiner and Chase, who showed in 1944 that immunity leading to delayed-type hypersensitivity reactions could be transferred from one individual to another by the cells but not the serum of sensitized animals.[19] Mitchison later showed that transplantation immunity can be transferred by the cells and not by serum of a sensitized individual, suggesting that cells might be responsible for alloimmunity.[25] The mechanism by which these cells (later called T lymphocytes because of their origin in the thymus) recognize foreign tissues then became an issue of widespread interest.

Although recognition of foreign histocompatibility antigens by T lymphocytes offered one explanation for immunologic specificities, histocompatibility antigens proved at first very difficult to isolate; thus this idea remained for years untested. In the early 1970s, Doherty and Zinkernagel made an unexpected observation that revolutionized thinking about the cell biology of immune responses.[8] T cells, it seemed, could only recognize immunizing antigens if they were presented by cells that have one or more histocompatibility antigens in common with the T cells. For example, T cells from individual A infected by virus X thus could kill A cells bearing X antigen but not infected cells of individual B or C unless they had one or more histocompatibility antigens in common with A. This finding posed an obvious dilemma in the case of allogeneic responses; if the target and responder must share some MHC antigens, how could lymphocytes recognize cells that are totally MHC incompatible? Doherty and Zinkernagel proposed that foreign antigens might form a complex with *self* MHC molecules and that this complex might then be recognized as *altered self*. Such a model would allow allogeneic MHC molecules to serve as antigen or in their entirety as altered self.

Further progress in elucidating the relationship between MHC molecules and T-cell specificity emerged from various quarters. The existence of MHC Class I antigens was revealed by serology. Class II was revealed by the discovery that *HLA-D* defined originally on the basis of cellular responses was really made up of three series of genetic determinants (at least) whose distribution was for the most part limited to antigen-presenting cells. Studies in a number of laboratories during the 1970s and early 1980s led to characterization of the protein structure of histocompatibility antigens and to further mapping of the MHC complex. The elucidation of the crystal structure of MHC Class I molecules in 1987 and MHC Class II a few years later demonstrated that foreign peptides are physically complexed with the Class I and Class II molecules.[4, 5] The results of these observations, together with the more advanced understanding of structural features of the histocompatibility antigens brought about by the crystallographic analysis, have led to the discovery of the role of MHC molecules in generating antigenic stimulation for T cells and regulating immune homeostasis. Thus, histocompatibility antigens are no longer thought of as mere markers of individuality but rather as cellular tools for processing antigenic peptides and transmitting information between sets of functionally distinct immune cells. The function of MHC molecules in presentation of antigenic peptides is one element of the central role of MHC antigens in alloimmune responses.

The Role of T-Cell Receptors in the Recognition of Foreign Antigens. T cells recognize foreign antigens by means of a dimeric set of cell surface glycoproteins called the *T-cell antigen receptor* (TCR). The nature of the TCR emerged as a central question in immunology as the importance of cell-mediated immunity in delayed-type hypersensitivity and allograft rejection became apparent. The development of techniques by Kohler and Milstein for generating monoclonal antibodies provided the tool needed to identify the receptor. After immunizing mice with a single line of T cells, Mak made a series of monoclonal antibodies. Although most of the monoclonal antibodies bound to T cells in general, a few bound only to the line of T cells used to generate the antibodies and thus recognized an antigen exclusively expressed by a single clone of T cells—a specificity postulated to define this clone's TCR. Analysis of the protein recognized by these monoclonal antibodies as well as information derived later from the molecular cloning and sequencing of genes unique to the cloned T cells indicated that the *clonotypic* molecules belonged to the superfamily of immunoglobulin and MHC antigens. Although TCR are related structurally to immunoglobulins, they do not bind to *free* antigens as do immunoglobulins, but rather bind only to antigens that are associated with MHC Class I or Class II molecules. The TCR is a heterodimer consisting of alpha and beta chains, each 40 to 45 kd. The diversity of the alpha and beta chains is achieved through some of the same mechanisms that achieve diversity of the immunoglobulin repertoire. TCR genes are assembled by combining a constant region gene segment (C) with variable (V), diversity (D), and joining (J) gene segments in the case of beta chains and V and J segments in the case of alpha chains. Much of the diversity of the TCR repertoire is engendered by the inexact selection of the ends of the segments to be so spliced (i.e., from junctional diversity). The joining of V, D, and J segments to form a functional or rearranged T-cell antigen receptor gene yields, in theory, approximately 10^{12} to 10^{16} distinct combinations, a level of diversity comparable to that of immunoglobulin. A smaller repertoire of T cells, consisting of approximately 10^9 distinct TCRs, is selected in the thymus on the basis of ability to recognize altered self MHC to become part of the mature T-cell repertoire. Creation of the final T-cell repertoire in the thymus is also based on the general rule that the T cells that recognize peptides complexed with MHC Class II molecules express CD4 glycoproteins and that T cells that recognize MHC Class I molecules express CD8 glycoproteins. In addition, cells with high-affinity TCRs against self MHC antigens are clonally ablated.

Antigen Presentation. The first step in the recognition of foreign antigen by T cells and thus in the development of an immune response is *antigen processing and presentation.*[10] In this step, antigen taken up by an antigen-presenting cell is degraded to antigenic peptides, which in turn become associated with MHC molecules. Only antigens expressed on the cell surface in this manner can be recognized by T cells. In most cases, immune responses are initiated by helper T cells. Classically, the TCR on helper T cells recognizes foreign antigens complexed with MHC Class II molecules. The binding of the TCR to MHC Class II molecules is enhanced by the CD4 glycoproteins of helper T cells that adhere to MHC Class II molecules on opposing cells and serve as a marker for helper T cells. In some cases, helper T cells recognize antigen complexed with MHC Class I molecules; recognition by these helper T cells is enhanced by CD8 glycoproteins.

MHC Class II Molecules. MHC Class II molecules are heterodimers consisting of a 32-kd alpha chain and a 28-kd beta chain (Fig. 20–3). Class II molecules are expressed mainly by specialized, *professional,* antigen-presenting cells such as macrophages and dendritic cells. In humans, endothelial cells also constitutively express MHC Class II molecules. Other cells may express MHC Class II molecules after stimulation by cytokines or other inflammatory mediators. The structural organization of MHC Class II molecules includes four extracellular domains, a transmembrane region, and a cytoplasmic *tail.* This organization is related to the function of the molecules in peptide presentation. The tertiary structure of MHC Class II antigens provides a pocket or antigen-binding cleft between the two polypeptide chains.[5] Peptides of 12 to 24 amino acids may enter this cleft and become firmly bound. In taking up polypeptides, MHC antigens are relatively selective. Not only is the length of the peptide important, but certain amino acids at critical points

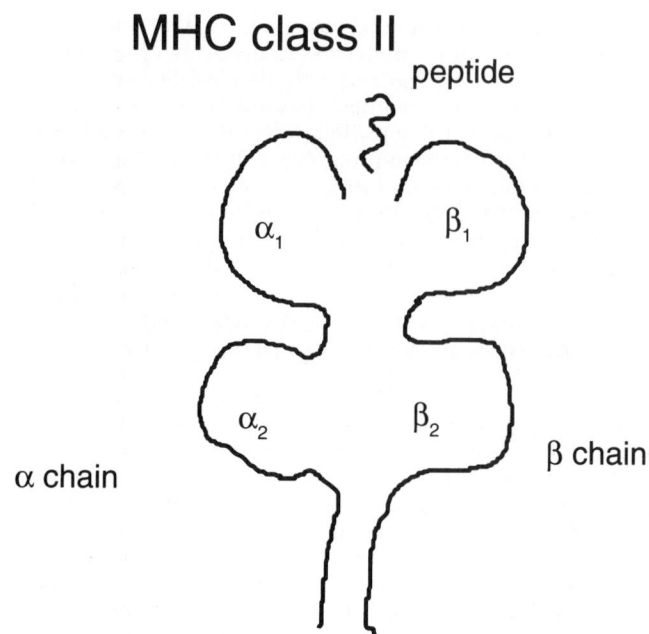

Figure 20–3. Schematic diagram of MHC Class II molecule.

in the peptide allow proper binding to the antigen-binding cleft.

The cellular events involved in antigen-processing and antigen-binding of the peptides to MHC Class II molecules and antigen presentation help regulate cellular immune responses. Foreign proteins are taken up by antigen-presenting cells into phagosomes where the proteins are denatured and cleaved by proteases. In a series of events yet to be fully elucidated, the phagosomes fuse with vesicles derived from the Golgi apparatus, which contain nascent MHC Class II molecules associated with an invariant, non-MHC membrane protein called the *Class II invariant chain peptide* (CLIP). CLIP occupies the antigen-binding cleft, stabilizing the complex and preventing premature binding of endogenous peptides to the Class II molecule. The partially degraded foreign peptide is then taken up by the MHC Class II molecules in exchange for the invariant membrane protein, and the vesicles fuse with the cell membrane, leading to cell surface expression of MHC Class II-peptide complexes. MHC Class II antigens that do not contain a peptide are not expressed on the cell surface, and cell surface MHC Class II antigens from which a peptide is lost are rapidly modulated away from the cell surface.[26] Thus, free MHC Class II antigens are not found on the surface of antigen-presenting cells, presumably ensuring that peptides in the extracellular environment are not inadvertently presented.

Expression of foreign peptides in association with MHC Class II molecules provides a target for T cells bearing TCR, which recognize the peptide plus the polymorphic $alpha_1$ and $beta_1$ domains of the Class II molecules (see Fig. 20–3). This interaction is enhanced by binding of CD4 to a nonpolymorphic domain of the Class II molecule. Whether the presentation of antigen in this way leads to activation of T cells depends on the probability that an antigen-presenting cell bearing a given peptide will encounter a T cell able to recognize the particular peptide-MHC complex; the density (molecules/cell) of those particular peptide-MHC complexes on the surface of the antigen-presenting cell; and the state of activation of the antigen-presenting cell. The probability of encountering a T cell of a given specificity is very low. For many foreign antigens the frequency of responder cells is 10^{-4} to 10^{-5}, and for some specificities only 10 or fewer T cells exist. The probability that members of a T-cell clone will encounter the antigen complex for which it has specificity is increased by the retention and concentration of antigens in draining lymph nodes and the continuous exposure of antigen-presenting cells to *recirculating* lymphocytes. Even if a T cell encounters an antigen-presenting cell possessing appropriate peptides, a certain number of TCRs on that T cell must bind to MHC-peptide complexes to generate a signal of sufficient magnitude to lead to activation of the T cell. Indeed, the activation of a T cell requires stimulation of 100 to 200 antigen receptors,[13] depending partly on the affinity of TCR for the MHC-peptide complex. Under normal circumstances, the occasional foreign proteins taken up by antigen-presenting cells compete with endogenous peptides for incorporation into MHC Class II antigens, making it unlikely that an antigen-presenting cell would express a sufficient number of MHC Class II peptide complexes to allow activation of a T cell able to recognize those peptides plus MHC. On the other hand, local trauma, infection, and inflammation activate antigen-presenting cells, increasing phagocytosis, antigen processing, and synthesis of MHC Class II molecules. If these changes occur in concert, antigen-presenting cells express higher concentrations of MHC molecules bearing foreign peptides. Activated antigen-presenting cells also exhibit greater motility, allowing them to enter the lymphatics through which they are carried to lymphoid organs where they can contact a dense population of resting T cells. All of these changes favor activation of T cells.

Another important mechanism controlling antigen presentation and T-cell activation is inherent in the structural constraints for the association of a peptide with MHC. Most of the peptides in an endocytic vesicle are unable to bind to MHC Class II; however, some peptides of appropriate size (12–24 amino acid residues) and correct amino acid sequences are especially likely to do so. The relatively stringent requirements for attachment to MHC molecules allow some peptides to compete favorably with others for binding to MHC Class II molecules. Thus, certain peptides derived from MHC molecules are preferentially taken up by MHC Class II antigens, and the propensity of MHC Class II antigens to take up MHC-derived peptides significantly contributes to the strength of alloimmune responses.

MHC Class I Molecules. Each MHC Class I molecule consists of a 45-kd alpha chain and beta$_2$-microglobulin, a 12-kd glycoprotein that is not encoded by the MHC complex (Fig. 20–4). The functional organization of Class I, like that of Class II, includes four extracellular domains, a transmembrane region, and a cytoplasmic tail. The physical association between Class I molecules and antigenic peptides, which was anticipated from the MHC restriction described previously, was directly demonstrated by analysis of the x-ray crystal structure of the Class I molecule HLA-A2.[4] On its surface the molecule is configured so as to make a groove that harbors an antigenic peptide, on which the correct folding of the Class I MHC proteins depends. The peptide and polymorphic regions of the alpha$_1$ and alpha$_2$ domains bind to the T-cell receptor. A nonpolymorphic region of the alpha$_3$ domain binds to CD8.

The types of peptides that bind to MHC Class I molecules and the mechanism by which these peptides are taken up distinguish MHC Class I from Class II molecules. The peptides presented by Class I are derived from molecules synthesized in the cell itself, not from the potentially vast array of foreign proteins taken up by phagocytosis. The peptides that associate with Class I are generated from antigenic molecules within the cytosol by proteasomes made up of low-molecular-weight proteins. The genes that code for at least some of these proteins are within the Class II region of HLA in close linkage with genes encoding the peptide transporters for

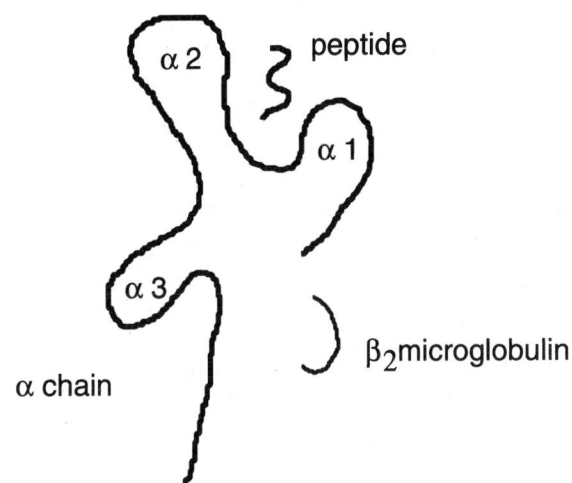

MHC class I

Figure 20–4. Schematic diagram of MHC Class I molecule.

both Class I and Class II molecules. These transporters, which appear to be the homologues of ATP-binding proteins in bacteria, carry the peptides into the endoplasmic reticulum, where the Class I assembly takes place. The major transporter of peptides destined to be associated with MHC Class I molecules is a protein called TAP (transporter associated with antigen processing). TAP mediates the transport of small peptides (8–11 amino acids) into the lumen of the endoplasmic reticulum. The ability of TAP to attach to a given peptide determines in part the immunogenicity of the peptide. In the endoplasmic reticulum the peptide associates with HLA-Class I alpha chains and beta$_2$-microglobulin, stabilizing the complex. MHC Class I molecules are retained in the microsomal fraction until assembly is complete, at which point they are carried in vesicle membranes to the cell surface.

T-Cell Activation. A second series of events in the development of immune responses involves the activation of T lymphocytes. Activation of T lymphocytes generally requires the delivery to a resting T cell of two types of signals, one provided by stimulation of the TCR by MHC-antigen complexes and one provided by accessory or *co-stimulatory* signals. Recent progress in the structural characterization of cell surface molecules involved in the stimulation of T cells has engendered current efforts in many laboratories to elucidate the signaling pathways that activate T cells.

Signals generated by the binding of TCR to MHC-peptide complexes are generated in part by CD3 molecules that consist of combinations of delta (25 kd), eta (20 kd), gamma (20 kd), and zeta (16 kd) chains that are noncovalently associated with TCR chains. CD3 chains anchor protein tyrosine kinases that, following stimulation of the TCR, initiate a cascade of signals. Other signals deriving from the binding of TCR to MHC-peptide complexes are owed to the CD4 and CD8 molecules, the cytoplasmic domains of which are associated with protein tyrosine kinases. Stimulation of the T-cell antigen receptor activates protein tyrosine kinases on CD3 and co-receptor molecules that phosphorylate various T-cell proteins. One consequence of this process is activation of phospholipase C, which catalyzes formation of inositol phosphates, yielding products that serve as second messengers to increase intracellular calcium and activate protein kinase C.

Although tight binding of the TCR stimulates the T cell, it is not usually sufficient to bring about T-cell activation. Activation of T cells requires the delivery of a second type of signal, called a *co-stimulatory* signal. In fact, binding of TCR without the delivery of co-stimulatory signals renders the T cell resistant to appropriate stimulation. This resistance, commonly called *anergy,* is an important mechanism that prevents inadvertent activation of T cells by innocuous antigens or autoantigens.[18] Co-stimulatory signals helping activate T cells may be generated when a T-cell surface glycoprotein, CD28, interacts with the corresponding ligands, B7-1 or B7-2, expressed by antigen-presenting cells (Fig. 20–5).

These signals together with the signals generated by stimulation of the TCR contribute to transcriptional activation of key T-cell genes such as interleukin-2 (IL-2). Expression of these genes causes the cell to undergo proliferation, leading to clonal expansion and to exert various effector functions discussed in Part III in this chapter. Although CD28–B7-2 interaction is thought to be of primary importance for many types of responses, signals generated by the action of cytokines and chemokines of the microenvironment may substitute for or amplify the signals generated by the CD28-B7 pathway.[16, 34] The mechanisms controlling availability of co-stimulatory signals determine the conditions in which activation of T cells occurs. B7-1 and B7-2 are expressed by professional antigen-presenting cells, and expression is increased in the course of inflammation. Other molecules such as the cytokines IL-2 and IL-1 can deliver co-stimulatory signals. These cytokines are not expressed constitutively but are synthesized in response to infection and inflammation. Furthermore, signals may downregulate the functions of T cells.[18] For example, interaction of the B7 glycoprotein with CTLA-4, a glycoprotein that is upregulated after activation of T cells, may inhibit T-cell responses despite antigen presentation. Exposure to prostaglandin E_2 may do likewise.[34] Thus, there is growing evidence that it is the constellation of signals provided to a T cell that directs the cell toward activation or anergy or else leaves the cell injured. Although pathways of activation and suppression have not been elucidated fully, they do suggest approaches that might inhibit alloimmune responses.

MHC Restriction and the T-Cell Repertoire. To contribute to host defense, T cells must be able to mount an immune response against the foreign proteins released by intracellular pathogens. At the same time, any tendency of T cells to respond to autoantigens or to other innocuous substances must be held in check. To achieve these conflicting goals, cellular immune responses are governed by two central rules. One is that foreign antigens are recognized only in association with self MHC molecules; that is, recognition by T cells is MHC restricted. MHC restriction limits the types of molecules that are recognized as antigens while ensuring that these antigens, when accessible, are presented stereotypically. A standardized mechanism of presentation involves an optimized array of interactive polymorphic molecules, all connected by MHC-TCR interactions, allowing stimulation of a maximum number of antigen-specific TCR. The second rule is that antigens of the T-cell host, even when incorporated into the clefts of MHC molecules, do not elicit T-cell responses. The second rule, generally referred to as *tolerance,* prevents autoimmunity. Mechanisms of tolerance are discussed in Part III of this chapter.

MHC restriction and tolerance occur partly through the processes involved in the development of the T-cell repertoire, which may be defined as the combined set of specificities of the T cells or as the set of distinct rearranged TCR genes expressed in a given individual. The development of the T-cell repertoire involves events that weed from a very large repertoire of precursor T cells those T cells that do not conform to the two rules stipulated previously. Most, or all, of this initial creation of the T-cell repertoire occurs in the thymus.

The thymus provides appropriate signals and a microenvironment that supports the maturation of a small proportion of the precursor T cells that it contains. The precursor cells with TCRs that recognize MHC antigens are *selected* for further maturation; the other more than 99% of precursor cells die without reaching maturity. This process is called *positive selection*[15, 17] and is the basis for MHC restriction. For any given foreign peptide and the few clones of T cells specific for that peptide, MHC restriction is stringent; that is, the T cells selected for survival recognize foreign peptides associated with a self MHC but not with an allogeneic MHC molecule. However, for reasons discussed later, the specificity of TCR recognition is sufficiently permissive that most T cells are able to recognize allogeneic MHC + peptide as if it were self-MHC + peptide.

Precursor T cells express both CD4 and CD8, and the synthesis of one of these proteins is downregulated in conjunction with maturation. Together with the generation of the definitive TCR repertoire, differentiation occurs such that T cells bearing TCR specific for MHC Class II antigens express CD4 and those specific for MHC Class I express CD8. The mechanism that coordinates the expression of the appropriate co-receptor with TCR specificity is thought also to involve positive selection, although the evidence is still not definitive.

The third step in the development of mature T cells is called *negative selection.* This step involves the elimination in the thymus of T cells that can recognize self MHC molecules associated with peptides derived from self MHC. Of course, this step must allow the survival of those T cells bearing TCR able to recognize foreign peptides. Overly efficient negative selection would cause immunodeficiency. Although inefficient negative selections would allow the emergence from the thymus of many autoreactive T cells, negative selection does not eliminate all potentially self-reactive T cells, because some self-proteins may not gain access to the thymus at this stage. Therefore, mechanisms must exist outside the thymus for suppressing or eliminating T cells that can be activated by autologous antigens. The mechanisms that contribute to

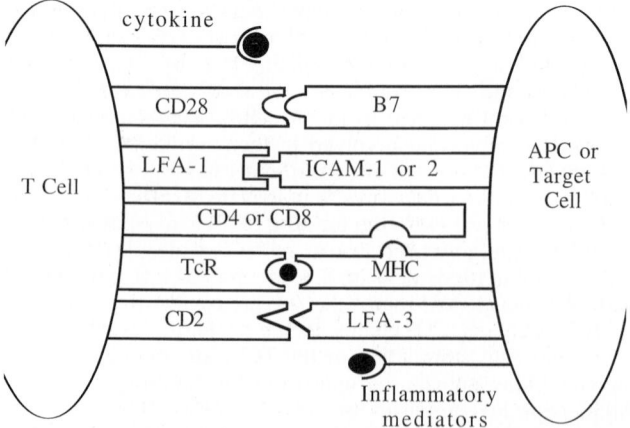

Figure 20–5. Mechanisms of interaction between T cells and antigen-presenting cells (APC). Interaction of the T-cell receptor (TcR) with MHC-peptide complex confers specificity on T-cell responses. Binding of CD4 or CD8 to MHC increases the affinity of the TcR-MHC interaction and generates signals in the T cell. In addition to this specific interaction, activation of T cells requires delivery of co-stimulatory signals brought about by the interaction of reciprocal pairs of cell adhesion molecules such as B7 on APC and CD28 on T cells, or by the action of cytokines. The ability of APC to stimulate T cells is augmented by various inflammatory mediators that activate the APC.

peripheral tolerance as such are described in Part III of this chapter.

THE IMMUNE RESPONSE TO ALLOANTIGENS AND ALLOGENEIC CELLS

Organ transplants between randomly bred individuals of the same species are invariably rejected, and the rejection proceeds so rapidly and powerfully that in the absence of immunosuppression an allograft would rarely function for longer than 2 weeks. The structural characteristics of transplantation antigens and the way in which they are presented account in part for the extraordinary speed and intensity of this response and thus for the apparently great immunogenicity of allografts. In general, in the absence of immunosuppression it is incompatibility of major histocompatibility antigens that produces rapid rejection of allografts and the incompatibility of minor histocompatibility antigens in combinations matched for major antigens that causes a more indolent course of rejection. However, the distinction between major and minor histocompatibility antigens reflects the physiology of cellular responses as much as it reflects the structure of the antigens.

Immunogenicity of Transplantation Antigens. The immunogenicity of transplantation antigens reflects in part their polymorphism: the amino acid sequences of these proteins (and hence, their peptides) differ among individuals in the population. Proteins bearing polymorphic domains that can produce an immune response in members of the same species are called an *allotype*. MHC Class I and MHC Class II genes are highly polymorphic; indeed, they are the most polymorphic genes known (see Table 20–1). So many alleles exist for each MHC locus that the likelihood for a donor and recipient selected at random to bear the same major histocompatibility antigens is very small.

In addition to polymorphism, certain structural features of Class I and Class II proteins contribute to their immunogenicity. Catabolized MHC Class I and Class II proteins form peptides of suitable length and composition to bind effectively to TAP and other transporters, causing incorporation into the peptide-binding clefts of MHC molecules. Analysis of the sequences of peptides occupying the binding clefts of MHC Class II molecules reveals that a significant proportion of the peptides derive from self MHC antigens. Although their structure accounts for the immunogenicity of MHC Class I and Class II proteins, it does not account for the extraordinary intensity and rapid tempo of alloimmune responses. Numerous bacterial proteins have similar structural properties without causing such responses. More important, attempts to induce immune responses by immunization with the extracts of allogenic cells may even fail totally to generate cellular alloimmunity and instead may cause secretion of antibodies that inhibit alloimmunity.

What, then, explains the special importance of MHC antigens as a barrier to allotransplantation? It derives in part from their localization on the surface of antigen-presenting cells and in part from their physiologic properties. Allogeneic antigen-presenting cells stimulate the activation of an extraordinarily high proportion of the T-cell repertoire. The high proportion of T cells activated in response to sensitization with allogeneic cells occurs because MHC antigens expressed by allogeneic cells are recognized *directly*, that is, as an intact structure on the allogeneic cell (Fig. 20–6). In some cases, the sequence of the endogenous peptide in the respective cleft contributes only nominally to recognition.[30] In other cases, multiple allogeneic peptides determine the overall specificity of the interaction.[14] The mechanisms allowing recognition of intact, allogeneic MHC antigens is inherent in the process that establishes the normal T-cell repertoire. All nor-

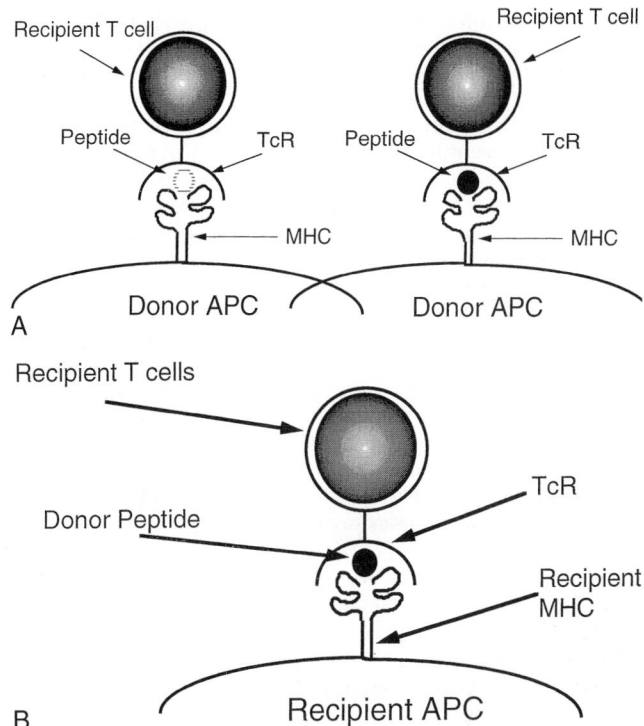

Figure 20–6. Mechanism of allorecognition. Direct recognition *(A)* involves the interaction of the recipient's T cells with donor antigen-presenting cells (APC). The specificity of this interaction may be dictated by the recognition of native structure of MHC (indicated by the light circle) or of the peptide (indicated by the dark circle) or both by the recipient's T-cell antigen receptors (TcR). Indirect recognition *(B)* involves the interaction of the recipient's T cells with recipient antigen-presenting cells expressing donor peptide in association with MHC. The specificity of indirect recognition is conferred by recognition of the donor peptide by recipient TcR.

mal T cells have TCRs that bind to MHC molecules that are *slightly different* from self MHC; thus, up to 1 in 10 T cells recognizes an allogeneic cell as slightly different from self, whereas only 1 in 10,000 to 1 in 100,000 T cells recognize foreign proteins complexed with self MHC.

Not only can a very large proportion of T cells recognize foreign MHC antigens directly on allogeneic cells, but, provided the allogeneic cells can deliver co-stimulatory signals, a very significant fraction of the T cells that encounter an allogeneic cell will be activated. One pathway contributing to the high *efficiency* of activating alloreactive T cells involves the high density of cell surface alloantigens. All of the MHC Class II molecules on allogeneic cells are potentially recognized by the recipient's T cells, and virtually every antigen-presenting cell is able to stimulate responses. In contrast, a given foreign peptide would occupy a small fraction of the MHC Class II molecules on the surface of only a small proportion of antigen-presenting cells. Thus, in each interaction with allogeneic antigen-presenting cells, a very large number of TCR molecules may be engaged; as a result, the threshold of avidity of TCR-MHC interactions needed to generate a biologic response is much lower than for other TCR interactions.

Another mechanism leading to the rapid recruitment of a large fraction of the alloreactive repertoire is related to the trafficking of antigen-presenting cells of donor origin. After organ or tissue transplantation, these cells enter the blood or lymphatic channels and are delivered rapidly and efficiently to the recipient's lymphoid organs. This process bypasses such events as phagocytosis, protein processing, and cell surface expression that must occur before presentation of foreign antigens under conventional circumstances and delivers the donor cells bearing alloantigens to sites where immune responses can be triggered.

Donor MHC molecules may also be taken up, degraded, and expressed as antigenic peptides in association with the recipient's MHC antigens. The presentation of donor antigens by antigen-presenting cells of the recipient is called *indirect recognition* (see Fig. 20–6). Although indirect recognition is thought to create less powerful responses than direct antigen recognition, the availability of many different foreign peptides may stimulate a multispecific, rapid, and intense response. Indirect presentation is thought to contribute to delayed immune responses to allotransplantation.[31]

Thus, the original conception of *major histocompatibility antigens* as antigens causing a rapid and powerful alloimmune response can be refined to a more precise definition: histocompatibility antigens that can be presented directly to allogeneic T cells. From this perspective, a minor histocompatibility antigen, originally defined as an alloantigen that provokes a slower, less intense response, might be defined functionally as an antigen giving rise to an alloimmune response through indirect presentation. A Class I or Class II alloantigen presented indirectly by responder cells may thus produce the more indolent response characteristic of a minor antigen.

THE HUMAN MHC: HLA

The HLA system is composed of a large number of genes that maintain important homologies with MHC genes of other species. These homologies refer to their reciprocal genetic relationships, to their chemical structure and molecular genetic organization, and to their functions.

HLA is located in chromosome 6 in the region bounded by the bands designated 6p21.31 and 6p21.33. The current genetic map of the human MHC was constructed by a combination of cytogenetics, segregation analysis in families, molecular cloning, and analysis of genomic DNA and spliced mRNA and population data. These methods allow a view of a system comprising three regions, each with well defined loci at the serologic, cellular, and biochemical levels. In addition to loci that code for the MHC Class I and Class II molecules discussed previously, MHC Class III loci code for specific serum complement components, enzymes, cytokines, and other nonalloantigenic proteins.

Recombination between MHC loci occurs regularly, although infrequently: the recombination fractions between the Class I loci encoding HLA-A and HLA-B and between HLA-B and the Class II gene HLA-DR are each about 1%. The recombination distance to the adjacent gene, GLO-1, is 5% to 10%. At this level of analysis, three Class I genes, HLA-A, HLA-B, and HLA-C, were recognized, almost solely by serologic testing through complement-mediated cytotoxicity. There are also three Class II markers: HLA-DR, DQ, and DP. These markers are recognized by a combination of techniques, including mixed lymphocyte culture (MLC) tests and variants thereof, and serologic and biochemical assays, mainly isoelectric focusing. Finally, the alleles of complement components mapping in the Class III region (factor B, C2, C4A, and C4B) are identified by immunoprecipitation and by isolectric focusing; loci coding for the two subunits of tumor necrosis factor were recognized more recently at the DNA level. Extensive polymorphism has been demonstrated for most Class I and Class II loci, the multiple alleles obstructing the efforts of transplant surgeons and facilitating those of immunogeneticists.

The most variable (allelic) domains in MHC molecules are clustered in the regions that circumscribe the peptide groove of the molecules. These domains have determinant influence on the specificity of the MHC-peptide interaction. It has

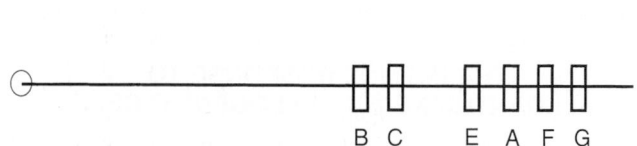

Figure 20–7. HLA Class I loci.

been speculated, therefore, that the evolution of the antigenic proteins of endemic and epidemic infectious organisms has driven the evolution of polymorphism in these domains, through selection for the capacity to bind peptides that are important in the antigenic homeostasis.

Current Understanding of HLA Complexity. The Class I region encodes more than 15 genes, including the classic transplant A, B, and C genes mentioned earlier as well as other expressible genes, HLA-E, F, and G and four pseudogenes, H, J, K, and L. Although their structures and association with beta$_2$-microglobulin are similar, E, F, and G are not highly polymorphic and are restricted to some tissues; only G appears on the cell surface and (thus far) only on cytotrophoblasts. The entire region is about 2 million base pairs long and is located at the telomeric end of the HLA gene complex. The organization of the Class I region is shown in Figure 20–7.

The Class II region, the organization of which is shown in Figure 20–8, contains more than 25 genes, including the loci for the alpha and beta chains of the Class II *professional* transplantation antigens DR, DQ, and DP. There are two other alpha genes, DMA and DNA, and two beta genes, DMB and DOB. DMA and DMB may function in the assembly of Class II-peptide complexes,[7] but the function of DOB, if any, is unknown. There are also the genes for the low-molecular-weight proteins (LMPs) LMP2 and LMP3 (involved in proteasome processing of antigens) and those for the transporter molecules TAP1 and TAP2. Other loci in this region include those for the collagen gene 11A2 and several genes of unknown function. The Class II region spans approximately 1 million base pairs.

In general, the loci contributing to the Class II HLA antigens are encoded by one alpha gene and one beta gene designated "A" and "B," respectively. However, the loci encoding the HLA-DR Class II antigens are DRA1, DRB1, and usually a second functional DR beta gene, most often DRB3, DRB4, or DRB5. Thus, each haplotype determines one alpha and one or (usually) two beta chains. Haplotypes in which DRB1 encodes the antigens DR3, 11, 12, or (some) 14 variants have an expressed DRB3 gene; those encoding for DR4, 7, or 9 possess DRB4; and DR1, 2, and 6 may carry DRB; but some variants of DR1 and 2 as well as DR8 do not have a second DRB gene. Each haplotype also carries one or more DRB pseudogenes. There are also two each, DQA and DQB as well as DPA and DPB loci, but only one of each is expressed. In contrast to DRA1, which is virtually invariant, DQA1 and DPA1 are both polymorphic.

The Class III region, occupying some 700 thousand base pairs between Class II and Class I regions, contains more

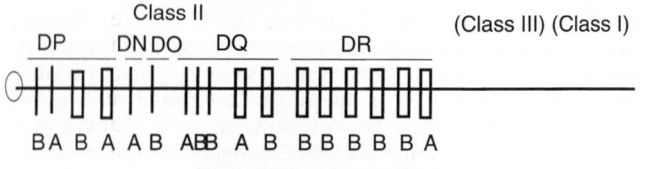

Figure 20–8. HLA Class II loci.

than 30 genes. The first to be identified were those encoding the complement components factor B, C2, and both C4 molecules. There are also the loci for tumor necrosis factor (TNF) genes and for the heat-shock proteins Hsp 1H and Hsp 70.2. The locus for the functional 21-hydroxylase gene, CYP21B, is immediate to C4B, whereas CYP21A, a 21-hydroxylase pseudogene, is next to C4A. Several additional genes are identified at the DNA level rather than by characterization of a gene product, including many (HLA-)B-associated transcripts (BATs).

To communicate effectively, it has been necessary to establish rules regarding the nomenclature of the many genes in the HLA complex and their many more alleles and to adhere strictly to these rules. Here some general principles are given concerning the logic of these designations, and the reader is invited to examine the listings of gene and allele designations published periodically by the World Health Organization Nomenclature Committee: "Nomenclature for Factors of the HLA System." *Haplotype* is a genetic term referring to the inheritance of all genes included in the HLA region of one chromosome. Barring genetic recombination, the haplotype is the unit of inheritance; as a result, the products of any one of the HLA genes in a parental HLA haplotype mark the whole haplotype and, when inherited by two siblings, suggest that the alleles of all the genes of that haplotype are common to both siblings. Thus 25% of the offspring of two parents will be "HLA-identical" and 50% will share one haplotype. This facilitates the search for HLA-identical sibling donors in transplantation, with the exception that 1% to 2% of the meioses are accompanied by intra-HLA recombinations due to crossing over.

The term *haplotype* is also used in a more restricted sense (e.g., the DR haplotype, the Class I haplotype) to mean a complex part of a whole HLA region, and care must be taken to prevent misunderstanding. Despite the existence of recombination, some haplotypes are very much more common than would be expected of the frequencies of the genes included in them. These haplotypes exemplify *linkage disequilibrium,* and their origin as well as the mechanism by which they remain in the population, sometimes in very high frequency, is not fully understood.

The polymorphism of HLA molecules reflects the existence of multiple alleles at one locus. Discerning alleles depends not only on the presence of such alleles but also on having methods that can disclose their differences. In HLA, both conditions are realized; of the common multiallelic systems, individual HLA loci are among the most variable and, as a system, the number of its variants outdistance all other systems by orders of magnitude. In addition to the complexity (the existence of multiple closely linked genes) and the extensive polymorphism, several highly discriminating methods have been applied to its study. Thus, besides the cytotoxicity test that is still the mainstay of Class I typing, there are cellular typing techniques and typing at the DNA level, including restriction fragment length polymorphisms, specific hybridization of amplified (by polymerase chain reaction) polymorphic regions, and even the determination of nucleotide sequence. The numbers of currently recognized alleles of the main HLA loci are listed in Table 20–2.

An interesting aspect of HLA genetics is that the sequences of discrete HLA alleles can be very different in different populations. The frequencies of the common haplotypes that maintain disequilibrium of linkage are even more variable, and haplotypes that are common in one population may be entirely absent in others. Obviously, this aspect of HLA population genetics has profound practical consequences for tissue and organ transplantation, particularly in hybrid populations: some individuals may have one haplotype common in one of the ancestral populations and restricted to it and

TABLE 20–2. Polymorphism of Some HLA Loci

Locus	No. of Alleles
HLA-A	50
HLA-B	97
HLA-C	34
HLA-E	4
HLA-G	5
DRA	5
DRB1	101
DRB3	2
DRB4	4
DRB5	5
DQA1	15
DQB1	26
DPA1	8
DPB1	59

another haplotype generally restricted to a second population. For such hybrid individuals, HLA-identical donors may only be found among the rare members of the same hybrid group, each parental population being able to provide only a single haplotype match.

Typing MHC Antigens and Outcome of Allografts. Exposure to allogeneic cells bearing foreign MHC antigens elicits the production of antibodies that have been used to characterize and map MHC allotypes. Multiparous women as well as patients who have received blood transfusions or organ transplants often have in their serum high titers of antibodies specific for allogeneic MHC antigens. Although such sera contain antibodies against a number of histocompatibility antigens, the sera can be used in conjunction with other sera to define an MHC *serotype*. The standard assay is conducted using multi-well plates, each well containing a small quantity of serum. Lymphocytes isolated from the patient's blood are added to the wells along with a sample of complement. Lysis of the cells in a well indicates that cells express an antigen recognized by the typing serum in that well. The results obtained with a panel of such typing sera are combined to indicate the patient's HLA type.

Clearly, HLA types defined serologically do not represent all possible polymorphisms but only those that produce antibody responses. Some of the variations in HLA antigens are not immunogenic, and some, although they are immunogenic, do not elicit antibodies that can be distinguished easily from antibodies against related HLA antigens. To overcome these limitations, several additional approaches to HLA typing have been developed that discriminate differences in HLA antigens based on the DNA or RNA sequences.

Cellular responses have also proved useful in defining and identifying HLA antigens. Lymphocytes exposed to allogeneic cells undergo proliferation and formation of blasts. Analysis of the specificity of such cellular responses allows typing of MHC Class II antigens.[2] As discussed earlier, MHC Class II antigens stimulate the activation and proliferation of helper T cells capable of discriminating antigenic differences that cannot be easily discriminated by serology.

In addition to the methods used to determine the histocompatibility type of the donor and recipient, a crossmatch test is generally performed to determine whether the potential recipient of an allograft has antibodies directed against the donor. The presence of such antibodies in the blood of a recipient of an organ graft could cause hyperacute or accelerated rejection. The test is performed by incubating donor cells labeled with chromium-51 with serum of the recipient and complement. If donor cells are killed, as deduced from the release of chromium-51, the crossmatch is considered positive. Even more sensitive methods, including flow cytometry, are in use in a number of laboratories.

The Impact of HLA Typing on the Outcome of Transplants. Despite the very large number of transplants performed every year, the importance of HLA typing for the outcome of allografts remains one of the oldest controversies in transplant immunology.[22, 23] In the absence of immunosuppression, experimental allografts between siblings matched for MHC antigens survive significantly longer than grafts between siblings mismatched for MHC. In clinical studies in which graft recipients are treated with immunosuppressive agents, the survival of renal allografts between HLA-matched siblings is about 90% at 1 year compared with about 80% for HLA-mismatched siblings. However, HLA typing is generally not conducted before cardiac or liver allotransplants are performed because there is not sufficient time; nevertheless the results of these transplants are better than the results of kidney transplants for which HLA typing is routinely performed. Still, retrospective analysis of matching for HLA-A, -B, and -DR does reveal a small but significant impact on survival of cardiac allografts.[27]

The importance of HLA matching can be considered in the context of the mechanisms of alloimmune responses. Mismatching of HLA antigens, producing direct presentation of donor antigens to T cells of the recipient, should have the greatest impact on cellular immune responses arising early after transplantation. If rejection is avoided for a period of time sufficient to allow depletion of donor antigen-presenting cells, then indirect antigen presentation should predominate and the pathophysiologic importance of MHC may then be as a source of antigenic peptides to be expressed in host MHC Class II molecules. This mechanism of antigen presentation may be associated with development of humoral responses to the graft as discussed in Part III of this chapter.

Analysis of mutant mice that lack both MHC Class I and Class II antigens led to the surprising observation that skin allografts from donors deficient in MHC Class I and Class II are rejected as rapidly and vigorously as allografts from donors expressing these antigens.[12] This observation would seem to contradict the importance of direct antigen presentation and to be consistent with the possibility that presentation of minor alloantigens by the indirect pathway can produce an intense alloimmune response.[12] Moreover, the observation might argue against the importance of MHC matching. In interpreting the results of these studies it is useful to consider alternative explanations.[12] For example, allorecognition of MHC antigens leads not only to destructive cellular immune responses but also to tolerance. The absence of MHC antigens vitiates the restraint that might be applied by veto or suppressor cells to rejection responses. Thus, the absence of MHC antigens in a donor is neither equivalent to nor, perhaps, preferable to MHC matching.

OTHER HISTOCOMPATIBILITY ANTIGENS

Although MHC antigens have overwhelming importance as a target of cellular immune responses, they are not the only immunologic barrier to allotransplantation. Other histocompatibility antigens may be targets of humoral responses, as discussed in Part III in this chapter. The following sections describe briefly these antigen systems; for more detailed discussion the reader is referred elsewhere.[28]

Blood Group Antigens and Histocompatibility. In the early years of this century, when Floresco, Carrel, and Guthrie began their experiments in renal transplantation, the discovery of blood groups provided potential explanation for immune reactions that might underlie the failure of allografts. However, studies by several investigators, mainly using skin transplants, failed to reveal any evidence that matching of blood types would improve the survival of tissue grafts. In the 1960s, as kidney transplantation entered the clinical arena, concepts concerning the importance of blood group antigens in allotransplantation changed again. Clinical analysis revealed that transplantation of ABO-incompatible kidneys conferred a 25% risk of immediate graft failure.[11] The cause of the failure was hyperacute rejection initiated by binding of anti-A or anti-B antibodies to blood group antigens expressed on donor endothelium. Even when hyperacute rejection did not occur, blood group incompatibility substantially increased the risk of early cellular rejection. The importance of blood group antigens stems in part from the expression of the antigens on endothelial cells. Thus, an allogenic organ, but not a neovascularized tissue such as skin, can serve as the target of a humoral reaction (see Part III in this chapter). Because of the significant risk of graft failure, and especially of hyperacute rejection, incompatibility of blood groups due to expression of A or B antigens on donor cells but not in the recipient has been viewed as an absolute contraindication to organ transplantation. More recently, studies at several centers have revealed that temporary removal of anti–blood group antibodies of an organ graft recipient may allow enduring survival of an ABO-incompatible organ graft even after those antibodies return to the circulation,[1, 3] a phenomenon termed *accommodation*.

OTHER ENDOTHELIAL ANTIGENS

Occasional cases of humoral rejection occur in patients who have no detectable antibodies against donor HLA or blood group antigens. Among the antigen systems apparently involved in these cases are alloantigens expressed only on endothelium, antigens expressed on endothelium and on monocytes, and antigens in the extracellular matrix. For example, individuals with Alport's syndrome, a hereditary disease associated with hearing loss and renal failure, have a genetic abnormality of type IV collagen. After transplantation, some of these individuals develop antibodies against the corresponding antigen in the transplanted organ, causing rapid, unremitting decline in renal function. The *rejected* organ contains recipient immunoglobulin and complement along glomerular capillary basement membranes in a pattern resembling the classic appearance of the Goodpasture syndrome.

Xenotransplantation Antigens. The critical shortage of donor organs has increased interest in using animal organs in lieu of human organs for clinical transplantation. Clinical attempts at xenotransplantation failed in the past because of severe and devastating humoral rejection reactions, triggered either by binding of the recipient's natural antibodies to the transplanted organ or by direct activation of complement on the foreign cells. The nature of these reactions has been characterized. The transplantation of nonprimate organs into primates leads to immediate rejection of the organ transplant caused by binding of naturally occurring antibodies. The natural antibodies involved in this process were recently shown to recognize a disaccharide, $Gal\alpha(1-3)Gal$, synthesized by the cells of nonprimate mammals and New World monkeys.[9] Binding of antibodies to this structure triggers activation of the complement system leading to tissue injury, as discussed in Part III of this chapter. In addition to the antibody-antigen reaction, susceptibility to humoral rejection is heightened by incompatibility of cell-associated complement regulatory proteins such as decay-accelerating factor, CD59, and membrane co-factor protein. These proteins ordinarily restrict the inadvertent activation of complement on autologous cells, allowing complement reactions to proceed on the surface of microorganisms. Because these proteins function more effectively against homologous complement than against heterologous complement, xenografts are especially susceptible to complement-mediated injury. Evidence for the importance of these biologic barriers to xenotransplantation has led to efforts to genetically modify pigs to decrease expression of Galα(1–3)Gal and confer expression of human complement-regulatory proteins. The latter goal has been achieved: hyperacute rejection has been avoided in a few cases in experimental xenotransplantation from pigs to non-human primates.[29]

SELECTED REFERENCES

Germain, R. N.: MHC-dependent antigen processing and peptide presentation: Providing ligands for T lymphocyte activation. Cell, 76:287, 1994.
The paper provides a contemporary review of the structure of MHC molecules and the events associated with the processing and presentation of antigens. The role of these events in the development of cell-mediated immunity is discussed.

Jenkins, M. K.: Activation of T-cell costimulation. Immunity, 1:443, 1994.
This paper reviews mechanisms by which T cells are activated and how T-cell activation is controlled.

Matas, A. J.: Is MHC matching as a primary criterion in kidney allocation justified? Nat. Genet., 5:210, 1993.
This paper and a companion one by Martin and Dyer take up the controversy of MHC matching in transplantation. Regardless of one's point of view, these papers offer current information about the incidence of rejection and the outcome of allografts.

Shoskes, D. A., and Wood, K. J.: Indirect presentation of MHC antigens in transplantation. Immunol. Today, 15:32, 1994.
This review provides a current perspective on the mechanisms by which alloantigens are presented and how those mechanisms determine the type of alloimmune responses that follow. The clinical implications of antigen presentation are discussed.

Snell, G. D., and Stimpfling, J.H.: Genetics of tissue transplantation. In Green, E. L., Coleman, D. L., Dagg, C. P., et al. (Eds.): Biology of the Laboratory Mouse. New York, Dover Publications, 1968, pp. 457–491.
This chapter provides an authoritative and detailed summary of immunogenetics of the mouse. The principles described apply as well to humans.

REFERENCES

1. Alexandre, G. P. J., Squifflet, J. P., De Bruyere, M., Latinne, D., Reding, R., Gianello, P., Carlier, M., and Pirson, V.: Present experiences in a series of 26 ABO-incompatible living donor renal allografts. Transplant. Proc., 19:4538, 1987.
2. Bach, F., and Hirschhorn, K.: Lymphocyte interaction: A potential histocompatibility test in vitro. Science, 143:813, 1964.
3. Bannett, A. D., McAlack, R. F., Raja, R., Baquero, A., and Morris, M.: Experiences with known ABO-mismatched renal transplants. Transplant. Proc., 19:4543, 1987.
4. Bjorkman, P. J., Saper, M. A., Samraoui, B., Bennett, W. S., Strominger, J. L., and Wiley, D. C.: Structure of the human class I histocompatibility antigen, HLA-A2. Nature, 329:506, 1987.
5. Brown, J. H., Jardetzky, T. S., Gorga, J. C., Stern, L. J., Urban, R. G., Strominger, J. L., and Wiley, D. C.: The three-dimensional structure of the human class II histocompatibility antigen HLA-DR1. Nature, 364:33, 1993.
6. Carrel, A.: Transplantation in mass of the kidneys. J. Exp. Med., 10:98, 1908.
7. Ceman, S., Rudersdorf, R. A., Petersen, J. M., and Demars, R.: DMA and DMB are the only genes in the class II region of the human MHC needed for class II-associated antigen processing. J. Immunol., 154:2543, 1995.
8. Doherty, P. C., and Zinkernagel, R. M.: A biological role for the major histocompatibility antigens. Lancet, 1:1406, 1975.
9. Galili, U., Clark, M. R., Shohet, S. B., Buehler, J., and Macher, B. A.: Evolutionary relationship between the natural anti-Gal antibody and the Gal α1-3Gal epitope in primates. Proc. Natl. Acad. Sci. USA, 84:1369, 1987.
10. Germain, R. N.: MHC-dependent antigen processing and peptide presentation: Providing ligands for T lymphocyte activation. Cell, 76:287, 1994.
11. Gleason, R. E., and Murray, J. E.: Report from kidney transplant registry: Analysis of variables in the function of human kidney transplants. Transplantation, 5:343, 1967.
12. Grushy, M. J., Auchincloss, H., Lee, R., Johnson, R. S., Spencer, J. P., Zulstra, M., Jaenisch, R., Papaioannou, V. E., and Glimcher, L. H.: Mice lacking major histocompatibility complex class I and class II molecules. Proc. Natl. Acad. Sci. USA, 90:3913, 1993.
13. Harding, C. V., and Unanue, E. R.: Quantitation of antigen-presenting cell MHC class II/peptide complexes necessary for T-cell stimulation. Nature, 346:574, 1990.
14. Heath, W. R., Kane, K. P., Mescher, M. F., and Sherman, L. A.: Alloreactive T cells discriminate among a diverse set of endogenous peptides. Proc. Natl. Acad. Sci. USA, 88:5101, 1991.
15. Hogquist, K. A., Jameson, S. C., Heath, W. R., Howard, J. L., Bevan, M. J., and Carbone, F. R.: T cell receptor antagonist peptides induce positive selection. Cell, 76:17, 1994.
16. Ihrcke, N. S., Wrenshall, L. E., Lindman, B. J., and Platt, J. L.: Role of heparan sulfate in immune system–blood vessel interactions. Immunol. Today, 14:500, 1993.
17. Janeway, C. A., Jr.: Thymic selection: Two pathways to life and two to death. Immunity, 1:3, 1994.
18. Jenkins, M. K.: The ups and downs of T cell costimulation. Immunity, 1:443, 1994.
19. Landsteiner, K., and Chase, M. W.: Experiments on transfer of cutaneous sensitivity to simple compounds. Proc. Soc. Exp. Biol. Med., 49:688, 1942.
20. Little, C. C.: The genetics of tissue transplantation in mammals. Cancer Res., 8:75, 1924.
21. Little, C. C., and Tyzzer, E. E.: Further experimental studies on the inheritance of susceptibility to a transplantable tumor, carcinoma (J.W.A.) of the Japanese Waltzing mouse. J. Med. Res., 33:393, 1916.
22. Martin, S., and Dyer, P. A.: The case for matching MHC genes in human organ transplantation. Nat. Genet., 5:210, 1993.
23. Matas, A. J.: Is MHC matching as a primary criterion in kidney allocation justified? Nat. Genet., 5:210, 1993.
24. Medawar, P. B.: The immunology of transplantation. Harvey Lectures Ser., 52:144, 1958.
25. Mitchison, N. A.: Passive transfer of transplantation immunity. Proc. R. Soc. Lond., 142:72, 1954.
26. Nelson, C. A., Petzoid, S. J., and Unanue, E. R.: Peptides determine the lifespan of MHC class II molecules in the antigen-presenting cell. Nature, 371:250, 1994.
27. Oplez, G., and Wujciak, T.: The influence of HLA compatibility of graft survival after heart transplantation. N. Engl. J. Med., 330:816, 1994.
28. Platt, J. L.: Antibodies in graft rejection. In Bach, F. H., and Auchincloss, H. (Eds.): Transplantation Immunology. New York, Wiley-Liss, 1995, in press.
29. Platt, J. L.: Hyperacute Xenograft Rejection. Austin, Tex., R. G. Landes Company, 1995.
30. Rotzschke, O., Falk, K., Faath, S., and Rammensee, H.: On the nature of peptides involved in T cell alloreactivity. J. Exp. Med., 174:1059, 1991.
31. Shoskes, D. A., and Wood, K. J.: Indirect presentation of MHC antigens in transplantation. Immunol. Today, 15:32, 1994.
32. Snell, G. D., and Stimpfling, J. H.: Genetics of tissue transplantation. In Green, E. L., Coleman, D. L., Dagg, C. P., et al. (Eds.): Biology of the Laboratory Mouse. New York, Dover Publications, 1968, pp. 457–491.
33. Ullmann, E.: Tissue and organ transplantation. Ann. Surg., 60:195, 1914.
34. Wrenshall, L. E., Cerra, F. B., Singh, R. K., and Platt, J. L.: Heparan sulfate initiates signals in murine macrophages leading to divergent biological outcomes. J. Immunol., 154:871, 1995.

III

MECHANISMS AND CHARACTERISTICS OF ALLOGRAFT REJECTION

Jeffrey L. Platt, M.D., and Pablo Rubinstein, M.D.

IMMUNOLOGIC BASIS OF ALLOGRAFT REJECTION AND TOLERANCE

The beginning of modern transplantation biology can be traced to World War II and to the collaboration between an experimental embryologist and a military surgeon. The embryologist, Peter Medawar, was invited by the surgeon, Thomas Gibson, to devise a strategy for dealing with burn wounds, which had become an increasing part of military medicine. Medawar believed that the best approach to treating such wounds was the grafting of normal skin onto the wound, because such grafts might limit the loss of plasma, the risk of infection, and the formation of contractures. The more extensive the burn, however, the more scarce would be the normal skin available to create a graft. Although skin might be obtained from other individuals, skin transplants other than autotransplants invariably lost viability after a period of days to weeks. The challenge Medawar perceived would be to discover why skin grafts between different individuals always failed and to develop approaches to overcome their failure.

Medawar and Gibson reasoned that the failure of skin grafts might result from one of three mechanisms.[20] First, there was the possibility that the loss of the graft was the consequence of blood group incompatibility and thus a reflection of the natural immunity of the host against the graft. This idea was not a new one and indeed was a favored explanation in the early decades of this century when blood groups and serotypes were considered to be the expression of genetic incompatibility between individuals. However, all attempts to demonstrate that anti–blood group antibodies mediate skin graft injury or improve graft outcome by careful blood typing had been unsuccessful.

A second mechanism for the failure of skin grafts was proposed by Leo Loeb.[18] Loeb postulated that the tissues of each individual have biologic properties unique to that individual; in a transplant, the incompatibility of donor and recipient tissues would have a toxic effect that calls forth lymphocytes and fibroblasts, which in turn would mediate injury to the graft. This theory might have set the stage for the discovery of cellular immunity except for a fundamental error in experimental design. To test whether graft loss was mediated by immunity, Loeb performed a series of allografts in which tissues from different donors were transplanted in sequence into one recipient. The second and third grafts did not fail more quickly or violently than the first grafts and so Loeb concluded that graft failure was not caused by an immune response and that the presence of lymphocytes in the graft was simply a reflection of tissue injury.

The third explanation for the failure of skin grafts was that the recipient of the foreign tissue develops immunity against the donor and that the immune reaction to donor tissue destroys the graft. This idea had been proposed as early as 1912 by Schoene and 1914 by Underwood, but it did not gain wide adherence because of the failure to demonstrate the existence of antidonor antibodies or evidence that such antibodies cause injury to transplants (before the discovery that lymphocytes mediate immunity directly, antibodies were considered the sole effectors of immune responses). Furthermore, skin grafts usually developed evidence of injury much sooner than would have been expected for a primary antibody response.

To distinguish between the various theories of allograft failure, Medawar and Gibson carried out a classic experiment in which a series of skin grafts were placed on a patient with extensive burns.[8] Some of the grafts were taken from the patient's own, uninvolved skin (i.e., autografts), and some were from another individual (i.e., allografts). All of the skin grafts healed and appeared healthy for a period of days. By the fifteenth day the allografts had begun to degenerate and they were completely destroyed by the twenty-third day, while the autografts showed no evidence of damage. A second set of autografts and allografts (from the same donor as the first set) was placed on the patient 15 days after the first. The second set of autografts healed normally and remained healthy, whereas the second set of allografts did not heal and was destroyed within a week. Medawar concluded that the hastened deterioration of the second set of allografts compared to a first set was caused by an immune reaction of the recipient against the graft. Subsequently in rabbits, as in the human, Medawar showed that second skin grafts from one donor to the same recipient are rejected in an accelerated fashion (second-set) and that the third and later grafts from that donor may not even become vascularized (white grafts).[21, 22] These studies demonstrated some of the basic principles of alloimmune responses. First, the reaction against tissue allografts engenders immunologic *memory*—the second-set response can be observed long after a first graft is destroyed. Second, the response is donor-specific—recipients sensitized to one donor reject that donor's skin very rapidly but simultaneously accord a first set reaction to a graft from another, *third party,* donor. Third, alloimmunity is systemic—the placement of a graft in one location sensitizes the recipient against a graft placed in another location.

In the meantime, from a very different perspective, came an observation that eventually revolutionized the whole of immunology. Ray Owen, a geneticist, undertook the study of the blood types of freemartins—fraternal twins in cattle.[25] Freemartins exhibit aberrant sexual behavior and infertility, making them rather a nuisance to own. In addressing the question of how the freemartin phenotype might arise, Owen discovered on the basis of blood typing that freemartins have two kinds of erythrocytes, some bearing the blood group antigens of autologous hematopoietic cells and the others the blood group antigens of the fraternal twin. Thus, freemartins were hematopoietic chimeras. The existence of chimerism was taken as evidence that the blood of the twin cattle containing hematopoietic precursor cells had been exchanged *in utero.* Owen suggested that chimerism resulted from the failure of the freemartin to mount an immunologic response against the blood cells of the twin and considered this failure, which was permanent, to be evidence of induced acceptance of a genetically distinct intrauterine graft of the kind that was later to be called *tolerance.* Owen's interpretation was confirmed experimentally by Billingham, Brent, and Medawar in mice, a few years later. Thus, the discrimination between self and non-self, long a dogma of immunology and particularly of transplantation, was *learned* or acquired and not merely inherited.

By 1945, then, there was evidence that the outcome of

grafts is influenced by several biologic systems. First, as discussed in Part II of this chapter, there was a phenotype determined by histocompatibility genes whose correspondence in donor and recipient would predict the survival or the rate of failure of a graft. Second, there was the immune system, which would actually cause the destruction of grafts between *incompatible* individuals. Third, there was a system, seemingly related to ontogeny, which would prevent the emergence of this immunologic reaction against the individual's own tissues or against tissues to which the individual is tolerant. Transplantation biology was thus inextricable from immunology and development. Yet, how the systems were interconnected, especially the mechanisms that related histocompatibility and immunity, were uncertain.

Perhaps the first clues about the immunologic mechanisms of graft rejection should have been found in the histology of the rejecting grafts. A skin graft placed on an allogeneic recipient is invaded by capillaries of the host after a period of 2 to 3 days and for the first 7 to 10 days appears outwardly normal. Despite this normal outward appearance, the blood vessels of the graft bed are surrounded by dense populations of lymphocytes, and microthrombi can be found.[21] Shortly thereafter, the altered capillaries develop focal disruption leading to microhemorrhage and tissue damage. As a cellular basis for immune responses had yet to be discovered, Medawar and others sought the mechanism of this reaction in the serum of skin graft recipients and tested for cytotoxic antibodies and for the ability of serum to transfer immunity against allogeneic tissues. The routine failure of these efforts supported persistent skepticism about the role of immunity in graft destruction. In the early 1950s, Simonsen and Dempster performed careful histologic analysis of allotransplanted kidneys in dogs.[7, 35] The major change observed in the first renal allografts from a given donor was infiltration of mononuclear cells; however, second kidney grafts from the same donor were rapidly rejected with histologic evidence of edema, hemorrhage, and thrombosis but little cellular infiltration. The historic features of the second graft were regarded as evidence that humoral immunity was the cause of graft failure; the role of mononuclear cells was still obscure.

One example of how humoral immunity might cause cellular infiltrates was the Arthus reaction. The orthodox Arthus reaction is brought about by repeated inoculation of a foreign antigen (originally horse serum) and is characterized by swelling, necrosis, and leukocyte influx at the site of inoculation. Like the allograft reaction, the Arthus reaction is systemic because it can be induced in sensitized subjects at any site where the antigen is administered. The Arthus reaction could be generated by passively transferring the serum of a hyperimmunized individual and then injecting the antigen subcutaneously or by systemic administration of the antigen and local inoculation of antibody. Thus, the presence of leukocytes in the lesion was clearly a secondary consequence of the antibody-antigen reaction. Medawar, Simonsen, and others postulated that antibodies might function similarly in allograft rejection, yet efforts to induce rejection by passive transfer of immune serum almost always failed and in some cases led to prolongation of survival of free tissue and tumor grafts.

Whereas nearly all immune responses were thought to be mediated by antibodies, one exception already characterized in the 1940s and 1950s was delayed-type hypersensitivity (DTH). DTH is typically observed in immune individuals after intracutaneous inoculation of a sensitizing antigen and in response to mycobacterial infection. Like the Arthus reaction, the DTH lesion contains infiltrating leukocytes, in this case predominantly mononuclear cells; however, unlike the Arthus reaction, the injection of immune serum fails to transfer immunity. Clearly DTH was mediated by something other

than antibodies. The nature of the DTH reaction was first revealed by Landsteiner and Chase, who demonstrated in 1942 that contact sensitivity in guinea pigs (a reaction similar to DTH) is transferable by peritoneal exudate cells.[16] In 1945, Chase showed in guinea pigs that DTH to tuberculin could also be transferred by peritoneal exudate and not by serum; and in 1949, Lawrence transferred DTH using mononuclear cells isolated from the blood of immune human subjects.[17]

A potential relationship between DTH and the allograft reaction was finally elucidated in 1954 by N. A. Mitchison. Mitchison showed that lymph node and spleen cells harvested from allograft recipients could *adoptively transfer* immunologic resistance to tumor allografts.[24] Mitchison's observations were supported by the work of Algire, who showed that allogeneic tissue encased in diffusion chambers, which would admit antibodies but not cells, are protected from injury.[1] Still the relative importance of cellular versus humoral responses as a cause of allograft failure was debated into the 1960s when observations on the outcome of clinical allografts suggested that cellular and humoral immune responses might cause distinct types of allograft rejection.[29] This concept was supported by rigorous analysis of experimental organ allografts. For example, Altman distinguished three types of allograft reactions in a canine renal allograft model.[2] The first type of response was primary allograft rejection, characterized by cellular infiltration leading to graft failure in 5 to 7 days. This response could be transferred with recipient lymphocytes but not with plasma. The second type of response was "accelerated cellular rejection," observed in recipeints that had been exposed previously to donor tissue or to whole blood. This response arose over 3 to 4 days but was otherwise like the primary response. The third type of response, which was also seen in presensitized recipients, led to destruction of the graft in minutes to hours and was probably like the response observed by Simonsen in sensitized recipients. This *hemorrhagic* response now referred to as hyperacute rejection was characterized by loss of vascular integrity, leading to interstitial hemorrhage, edema, and sometimes infiltration of neutrophils and it could be transferred to naive recipients by the serum of presensitized animals. With the development of potent immunosuppressive agents, which allow even more prolonged survival of allografts, other, chronic types of rejection have been observed. These chronic forms of graft injury are major causes of clinical allograft failure.

Table 20–3 summarizes the types of rejection observed in vascularized allografts. Much of the discussion that follows focuses on acute cellular rejection, about which more is known and which is the immunologic process that causes destruction of allografts in the absence of immunosuppressive therapy.

ACUTE CELLULAR REJECTION

An organ or tissue transplanted between unrelated individuals is almost invariably destroyed by acute cellular rejection manifest within 7 to 14 days of transplantation unless the recipient receives immunosuppressive therapy. Even if the recipient of an allograft is treated with immunosuppressive agents, acute cellular rejection is observed in about 50% of cases, although graft destruction is now infrequent. Acute cellular rejection in immunosuppressed recipients usually occurs within 6 months of transplantation and usually does not destroy the graft as in the unmanipulated recipient.

Although the manifestations of allograft rejection are hardly subtle, the diagnosis of rejection can be fraught with pitfalls. Some diagnostic indices of rejection have been proposed. These indices emphasize pathognomonic signs of

TABLE 20–3. Common Types of Graft Rejection*

Type of Rejection	Time of Onset After Transplantation	Type of Graft	Immunopathogenesis	Responses to Immunosuppression
Acute cellular rejection	Days–months	Free tissue, vascularized	Primary cellular immune response	Yes
Accelerated rejection	Days†	Free tissue, vascularized	Secondary or second-set cellular immune response; humoral plus cellular response	Sometimes
Hyperacute rejection	Hours	Vascularized	Antidonor antibodies + complement	No
White graft	Hours–days	Free tissue	Failure of vascularization	Not known
Acute vascular rejection	Days–months	Free tissue vascularized	Humoral + cellular response	Poor
Chronic rejection	Months	Vascularized, free tissue?	Persistent/recurrent cellular immune response; humoral response; nonimmunologic factors	No

*The types of rejection listed in the table and the nomenclature used reflect distinct pathogenetic entities. An alternative and more complex nomenclature, based on histologic features, may be used. The reader is referred to the literature for such classifications (Kidney Int, *44*:411, 1993).
†Immunosuppressive therapy may delay time of onset.

rejection rather than features reflecting the immunologic mechanisms, as shown in Table 20–3. In the clinical setting, the diagnosis of rejection is usually based on the finding of aberrant graft function, histologic changes, and absence of other problems; however, dense cellular infiltrates may be observed in experimental cardiac or renal allografts that function normally or nearly so.[31] Given the potential complications of immunosuppressive therapy, including infection, hypertension, and accelerated atherosclerosis, graft biopsy is often used as a means to avoid unnecessary immunosuppressive therapy rather than as a justification for such therapy.

The events leading to acute cellular allograft rejection are summarized in Figure 20–9. These events, which include sensitization leading to activation of alloreactive T cells and lymphocyte trafficking and graft injury caused by the effector functions of activated, donor-specific T lymphocytes, are discussed in the sections that follow.

Sensitization. The first event in the development of allograft rejection is sensitization, a process in which the interaction of donor cells with the recipient's immune system causes activation of alloreactive T cells of the recipient. Activation of alloreactive T cells leads to proliferation of the activated cells and manifestation of their effector functions. The cellular and molecular events involved in the activation of T cells are discussed in Part II in this chapter and the effector functions in a later section of this part.

Sensitization of the host to a graft consisting of *free tissue* such as the skin or the islets of Langerhans is thought to be initiated when donor cells enter the lymphatics that drain the graft bed and are carried to regional lymph nodes where they are brought into contact with T cells of the recipient. The importance of lymphatics was suggested by classic experiments in which skin pedicle grafts that were given a primary vascular supply but no lymphatic drainage were found to be rejected very slowly or not at all.[4]

Although lymphatics are undoubtedly important in the immune sensitization to free tissue grafts, other mechanisms must bring about sensitization in the case of primarily vascularized grafts such as the kidney or heart because the lymphatic circulation to such an organ graft is not primarily restored. One potential mechanism of sensitization after organ transplantation involves the entry of donor cells into the host circulation and the passage of those cells to the spleen and other lymphoid organs. Sensitization after organ transplantation may also involve the encounter of host T cells with donor endothelial cells or leukocytes in the graft.

The cells of donor origin that migrate to the recipient's lymphoid organs and trigger the host immune response have been designated *passenger leukocytes* because they are carried in the interstitium of transplanted tissues and organs and include antigen-presenting cells such as macrophages and dendritic cells. Experiments in rodents suggested that depletion of passenger leukocytes from free tissues such as the islets of Langerhans or from whole organs decreases the immunogenicity of a tissue or organ transplants.[15] Unfortunately, the depleting of passenger leukocytes before allotransplantation has not as yet shown a clear benefit in the clinical setting. One reason why depletion of passenger leukocytes might fail to prevent rejection of clinical allografts is that sensitization might be mediated by endothelial cells, which in humans but not in mice constitutively express MHC Class II and Class I antigens.

The ability of donor cells such as passenger leukocytes and endothelial cells to stimulate an immune response would be favored by a high level of expression of MHC Class I and Class II antigens and by expression of co-stimulatory molecules such as B7-1 and B7-2. Expression of these molecules is in turn favored by conditions of inflammation and perhaps by ischemia-reperfusion injury. Donor cells that express MHC Class I and Class II molecules can stimulate directly the activation of T cells of the recipient. As discussed in Part II of this chapter, this type of antigen presentation, called direct

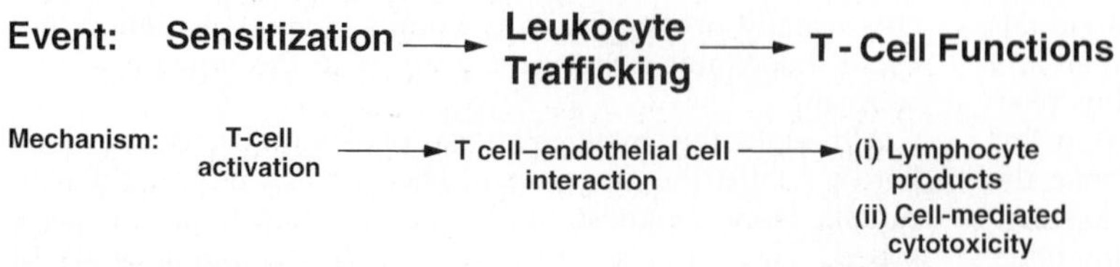

Event: Sensitization ⟶ Leukocyte Trafficking ⟶ T-Cell Functions

Mechanism: T-cell activation ⟶ T cell–endothelial cell interaction ⟶ (i) Lymphocyte products (ii) Cell-mediated cytotoxicity

Figure 20–9. Events contributing to acute cellular rejection. The mechanisms responsible for each event are shown.

presentation, can lead to activation of a high proportion of the host T-cell repertoire and is thought to account for the rapid tempo and great intensity of the cellular immune response to allografts.

After transplantation, the donor's passenger leukocytes that have exited the graft are replaced by the host's leukocytes and dendritic cells. These cells may take up and metabolize donor antigens and express immunogenic peptides in association with recipient MHC molecules. The presentation of foreign peptides in association with self MHC, called indirect presentation (see Fig. 20–6 in Part II of this chapter), usually contributes only a small fraction of the cellular immune response seen immediately after transplantation. However, under conditions in which direct antigen presentation does not occur, for example in experiments in which the donor is a mutant mouse lacking MHC Class I and Class II antigens, indirect presentation may lead to a rapid and vigorous alloimmune response.[3, 9] Furthermore, over time, antigen-presenting cells of the recipient become the major source of stimulation of host T cells. T cells stimulated by the indirect pathway are thought to be important in providing help for B-cell (humoral) responses against the donor and in mediating the more chronic forms of rejection that now are the major cause of graft loss.[34]

One issue of interest from a theoretical perspective is that T cells that are activated by the indirect pathway, thus recognizing donor antigens only in the context of self-MHC, should be unable to interact directly with donor cells unless the donor and recipient have one or more MHC alleles in common. This limitation might not affect free tissue grafts, which, after neovascularization, have endothelial cells of recipient origin that may take up, process, and present donor antigens. However, T cells activated by the indirect pathway should have less influence on whole organ grafts in which the endothelium remains that of the donor; in this case the presence of host antigen-presenting cells may be needed to allow immunologic recognition.

Leukocyte Trafficking. After triggering of the recipient's immune response, the next event in allograft rejection involves the migration of the recipient's T cells and mononuclear cells into the graft. This process is called leukocyte trafficking. The migration of activated lymphocytes from lymphoid organs into a graft is a signal event in rejection. Lymphocyte migration or homing to the graft depends, mechanistically, on metabolic changes that alter the motility and metabolism of the lymphocytes and on changes in the permeability of graft blood vessels. As just one example of this process, activated lymphocytes release enzymes that cleave cell-associated heparan sulfate proteoglycan and the loss of heparan sulfate renders endothelium susceptible to penetration by leukocytes.[11]

Migration of lymphocytes from lymphoid organs into the circulation and homing to inflamed tissues is also orchestrated by changes in the expression of adhesion molecules expressed on lymphocytes and on endothelium (Table 20–4).[36] The contribution of lymphocyte trafficking and its contri-

bution to allograft rejection have received much attention in recent years.[10] As one example, resting lymphocytes, and most other blood leukocytes, express L-selectin, a glycoprotein that binds to sialated oligosaccharides on specialized endothelial cells. The expression of L-selectin and other adhesion molecules causes resting lymphocytes in the circulation to stick to endothelium in lymphoid organs and to migrate through the vascular bed. T-cell activation is associated with the shedding of L-selectin and increased expression and function of certain glycoproteins of the integrin family. For example, expression of LFA-1 and VLA-4 by activated T cells promotes binding to intercellular adhesion molecule 1 (ICAM-1) and vascular cell adhesion molecule 1 (VCAM-1), reciprocal adhesion molecules expressed at high levels by activated endothelial cells. Cell adhesion molecules promote lymphocyte trafficking, and some adhesive interactions also promote lymphocyte activation, as discussed in Part II of this chapter.

Lymphocyte trafficking is also promoted and enhanced by the action of chemotactic cytokines or *chemokines.* Chemokines such as macrophage inflammatory protein-1 and RANTES (regulated upon activation, normally T cells expressed and secreted) are small peptides produced by macrophages and endothelial cells and tethered to cell surfaces by heparan sulfate proteoglycan.[38] Interaction of chemokines with T cells causes cell surface integrins to direct the migration of T cells into the tissue and causes changes in conformation of such molecules as LFA-1, promoting adhesion to the corresponding ligand.

Inflammation leads to the secretion of cytokines, chemokines, and other inflammatory mediators and triggers the activation and increased expression of cell adhesion molecules. These products of inflammatory cells promote increased synthesis of MHC molecules, stimulation of lymphocytes and differentiation of resting T cells into effector cells, and directed migration of leukocytes into the graft. Because of the importance of the molecules that promote the interaction of lymphocytes with endothelial cells, therapeutic strategies aimed at hindering these interactions are being developed for clinical use. For example, agents directed against P-selectin, a cell adhesion molecule expressed on platelets and endothelial cells, has proved to be effective in the treatment of reperfusion injury. Similarly, agents directed against ICAM-1 have shown some promise as adjuncts in treating or preventing reperfusion injury and graft rejection.[10]

Although it might be assumed that most of the lymphocytes infiltrating an allograft have antigen receptors specific for the donor, in fact, many infiltrating cells are not specific for donor antigens but rather they are innocent bystanders. One reason for the presence of such bystanders is that the events that lead to the influx of leukocytes depend on a loss of vascular integrity and on the interactions of cell adhesion molecules that are not immunologically specific. Thus, in tissues undergoing allograft rejection, the intensity of the cellular influx does not necessarily represent the intensity of the immune response directed against the donor.

Effector Mechanisms of Allograft Rejection. The third step in the rejection of allografts is the development of tissue injury caused by the recipient's leukocytes that have entered the graft. The pathologic picture of allograft rejection includes such features as interstitial edema, focal ischemia, thrombosis, and hemorrhage, suggesting that endothelial cells are the major target of the immune response. To be sure, there is also dysfunction of parenchymal cells; however, it is uncertain to which extent such dysfunction reflects direct immunologic injury to those cells or to which extent it is secondary to aberrant circulation caused by endothelial cell damage. Regardless of the pathophysiology of allograft rejection, there remains the fundamental question of whether

TABLE 20–4. Some Cell Adhesion Molecules That Control T-Cell–Endothelial Cell Interactions

T Cell	Endothelium
L-selectin	L-selectin ligand
LFA-1*	ICAM-1,* ICAM-2*
VLA-4*	VCAM-1*
MAC-1*	ICAM-1*

*Expression or function increased in activated cells.

injury to the graft is caused by the secreted products of helper T lymphocytes, T cell–mediated cytotoxicity, or both.[30] The helper and cytotoxic functions of T cells have been associated with the expression of CD4 and CD8 glycoproteins. It is now known that CD4 and CD8 molecules serve as adhesions for MHC Class II and Class I, respectively (see Part II of this chapter), and are not strictly related to effector functions. Nevertheless, most alloreactive helper cells are CD4 positive and most alloreactive cytolytic cells are CD8 positive.

The Role of Helper T Lymphocytes in Allograft Rejection. There is evidence for the concept that allograft rejection, like DTH, is mediated at least in part by the secreted products of T lymphocytes, particularly CD4-positive T cells. T lymphocytes that mediate immune reactions in this way are called *helper* T lymphocytes because the secreted products include cytokines such as interferon gamma that stimulate other cells to exert effector functions. Designation of these cells as helper cells should not obscure the fact that the secreted products may also contribute to tissue injury by acting directly on the graft.

The cellular events that might lead to the recruitment of donor-specific alloreactive helper T lymphocytes may be as follows. CD4-positive helper T cells, activated by interaction with MHC Class II-peptide complexes on allogeneic antigen-presenting cells proliferate and secrete interleukin-2 and other cytokines, which in turn contribute to the activation of other alloreactive cells, including cytolytic T cells and B cells. Driven to full maturation, the helper T cells migrate to the graft, where they release a variety of cytokines that further stimulate cytolytic T cells and activate macrophages and donor endothelial cells. Activated donor endothelial cells in turn express cell adhesion molecules that promote migration of leukocytes into the interstitium of the graft.

Work in mice, and more recently in humans, indicates that CD4-positive helper T cells can differentiate along one of two pathways. One pathway yields mature effector cells, called Th1 cells. Th1 cells produce interferon gamma, which stimulates the activation of endothelial cells and antigen-presenting cells, resulting in enhanced expression of MHC molecules; and they secrete large quantities of inerleukin-2, which promotes activation of T lymphocytes. Differentiation along the Th1 pathway is promoted by interleukin-12. DTH is considered to be an immune response prototypic of Th1 effector cells. The other pathway leads to mature effector cells called Th2 cells. Th2 cells release interleukin-4, a cytokine that promotes the maturation of B cells and the production of antibodies. Differentiation along the Th2 pathway is promoted by small amounts of interleukin-4 and inhibited by interleukin-12. Products of Th2 cells, interleukin-4 and interleukin-10, inhibit differentiation along the Th1 pathway. Although understood less fully, some CD8-positive T cells also release cytokines and function like Th1 or Th2 helper T cells.[32, 33] For example, under conditions in which a skin graft is transplanted into a congenic recipient bearing disparate MHC Class I antigen, CD8-positive cells capable of secreting interleukin-2 and interferon gamma, that is, Th1-like cells, are detected and found to be critical to the development of the rejection reaction. As one other example, CD8-positive T cells exposed to interleukin-4 lose cytotoxic function and, like CD4-positive Th2 cells, develop the ability to secrete interleukin-4.[33]

There is much interest in the paradigm that cellular rejection may be associated with selective maturation of cells through the Th1 pathway and tolerance or nonresponsiveness to an allograft by selective maturation along the Th2 pathway. If this model proves correct, then future therapeutic strategies may aim at selectively inhibiting Th1 or stimulating Th2 differentiation, rather than at nonspecific inhibition of all T cells.

Cytotoxicity and the Role of Cytolytic T Cells in Allograft Rejection. Although the initial concept concerning cell-mediated alloimmune responses focused on the relationship to DTH, the discovery that T cells can directly mediate lysis encouraged the view that alloimmunity might involve cytotoxicity and that in many cases CD8-positive T cells may be important effector cells in the rejection reaction. Cytolytic T cells target cells that bear antigen in the form of MHC-peptide complexes recognized by the TcR. Because all cells possess MHC class I antigens, all may potentially serve as targets of CD8-positive cytolytic T cells. Immunohistologic analysis of allograft biopsy specimens obtained early in the course of rejection often reveals CD8-positive T cells in greater numbers than CD4-positive T cells, suggesting that cytotoxic cells may contribute to the rejection reaction.[28] CD4-positive cytolytic T cells recognizing MHC Class II can also be detected under some circumstances and may contribute to some alloimmune responses. On the other hand, studies showing that CD8-positive T cells can exert helper functions make it difficult to exclude the possibility that these CD8-positive cells may participate in a DTH-like response.

T cells mediate cytotoxicity by two mechanisms.[5] One mechanism of T-cell–mediated cytotoxicity involves release of granules containing perforin and other cytotoxic substances. Perforin is a protein that polymerizes on target cell membranes leading to formation of membrane pores, which, like the polymerized C9 complement component, promotes ion flux and death of the target cells. A second mechanism by which T cells can mediate cytotoxicity involves the *FAS* pathway. This pathway is initiated by the interaction of target cell surface FAS with T-cell FAS ligand, leading to apoptosis of the target cell. The FAS system is thought to be involved in downregulating T cell functions, but it may also contribute to cytotoxic effector functions. Under some conditions, mice with targeted deletions of the perforin gene have an impaired ability to mount allograft rejection responses,[13] suggesting that perforin-mediated cytoxicity may be important in rejection.

An important aspect of cell-mediated cytotoxicity is the very high degree of specificity, which unlike DTH spares *innocent bystander* cells that do not have foreign antigen. The potential ability of cellular immunity to specifically destroy allogeneic target cells and the potential import for the rejection of allografts was suggested by studies on the fate of allografts in allophenic mice. Allophenic or tetraparental mice were developed by combining the embryonic cells from two embryos of different strains to produce a single blastocyst. After implantation into a pregnant female, the hybrid blastocyst develops into a chimera consisting of cells of the two strains. Mintz and Silvers used allophenic mice to make some fundamental observations in transplant immunology.[23] Skin from each parental strain transplanted onto an allophenic mouse was not rejected, indicating that rejection is not the result of biologic incompatibility between donor and recipient but requires an active immune process and this process is subject to tolerance. More to the point were the results of transplants of allophenic skin to the parental strains. These transplants did undergo rejection; however, rejection was restricted to the patches of skin or hairs derived from the other parental strain, while skin and hairs syngeneic to the recipient strain were spared. This result suggested that the rejection response can discriminate between adjacent cells. This observation suggests that rejection of the skin grafts was caused by T-cell–mediated cytoxicity rather than a mechanism such as DTH involving the secreted products of T cells. Such fine discrimination of alloimmune responses was suggested more recently by the studies of Sutton and colleagues,[37] in which after transplantation of a mixture of isogeneic and allogeneic islets of Langerhans only the allogeneic islets were destroyed while the isogeneic islets remained intact.

If cytotoxic T cells mediate allograft rejection, why is cell death not a major feature of early rejection lesions? One possibility is that cytotoxic T cells might mediate perturbations of target cell function rather than or in addition to cell death. For example, cytolytic effector cells might cause nonlethal changes in endothelial cells, leading to loss of endothelial integrity and control of vascular potency. As the allograft rejection lesion progresses, focal ischemia, thrombosis, and ultimately necrosis become more pronounced. Whether necrosis seen in more advanced cases of allograft rejection represents primary effects of cytolytic T cells on the graft or are secondary, nonspecific changes is unknown.

Accelerated Cellular Rejection. In some cases, despite administration of immunosuppressive therapy, cellular rejection proceeds more rapidly and aggressively than expected. Such responses may be observed in recipients who have been previously sensitized to donor antigens. Presensitization leads to the generation of a set of *memory* T cells able to respond more rapidly and intensely than the resting T cells of a naive recipient. Presensitization to donor antigens may also engender a humoral response, which in addition to causing the various types of *humoral rejection* discussed later, may result in a more aggressive form of cellular rejection, perhaps reflecting the activation of endothelial cells in the graft by the humoral reaction.

HUMORAL REJECTION

The reaction of recipient antibodies with a vascularized organ graft is associated with a spectrum of clinical and pathologic syndromes. Binding of antidonor antibodies to a newly transplanted organ may cause a *hyperacute* rejection, in which the function of the organ rapidly declines and ceases in minutes to hours. Antidonor antibodies can also cause more indolent forms of rejection. On the other hand, in some cases, antidonor antibodies appear to protect vascularized grafts against cell-mediated rejection, and indeed sometimes potential recipients are exposed to donor blood cells with the objective of generating such antibodies.

The influence of a humoral response on the outcome of an allograft depends on such factors as (1) whether the graft is a free tissue such as the skin or whether it is a vascularized organ; (2) whether antidonor antibodies are present in the circulation before transplantation or are elicited in response to the graft; (3) the isotype of the responding antibodies; and perhaps (4) the target antigen recognized by the humoral response.

Hyperacute Rejection. The clinical picture of hyperacute rejection was probably first observed in 1902 when Ullmann connected a goat kidney to the circulation of a patient with renal failure. The kidney issued a few drops of urine and then ceased functioning. The failure of the kidney was attributed to technical complications. In the early 1960s, as the number of clinical renal transplants was increasing, it was observed that on occasion a renal transplant would function very briefly or not at all. Although most cases seemed to result from technical problems or from acute tubular necrosis, the incidence of immediate graft failure seemed to be higher in recipients with antibodies against donor blood groups, suggesting that ABO incompatibility might be responsible.

In 1966, Kissmeyer-Nielsen observed a similar type of problem in kidneys transplanted into recipients who were matched for ABO blood groups but who had circulating antibodies against donor lymphocytes and kidney tissue.[14] This type of rejection, which was called hyperacute rejection, was soon recognized to be caused by antibodies against donor human leukocyte antigen (HLA) or antibodies against donor blood groups that existed in the patients' serum before transplantation.

Hyperacute rejection is defined as immune-mediated failure of a primarily vascularized graft within hours of initiation of transplantation. It is observed in approximately 80% of kidneys transplanted into recipients with circulating anti-HLA antibodies[26] and approximately 25% of kidneys transplanted into recipients with antidonor blood group antibodies. To minimize the risk of hyperacute rejection the serum of a potential recipient is routinely tested for the presence of antibodies against the donor using a *crossmatch* assay. A positive crossmatch is generally viewed as a contraindication to transplantation. Despite the wide application of sensitive crossmatch assays, hyperacute rejection occurs in approximately 0.4% of renal allografts. Some of these cases may be caused by antibodies directed against antigens expressed on donor endothelial cells but not on donor lymphocytes or erythrocytes.

The clinical picture of hyperacute rejection can be observed immediately on reperfusion of the organ graft. The graft, perhaps initially taking on a normal color, rapidly develops a mottled or beefy red appearance and swells. In concert with these changes, blood flow to the organ declines dramatically and organ function ceases within minutes to hours. The pathology of rejection is characterized by prominent evidence of platelet aggregation, interstitial hemorrhage, edema, and endothelial injury. In some cases, neutrophils are found to be attached to graft endothelium and infiltrating the interstitium. Immunopathologic studies reveal deposits of immunoglobulin and complement along the microvasculature and macrovasculature.

Hyperacute rejection is initiated by the binding of antidonor antibodies to the endothelial lining of graft blood vessels. Antibody binding triggers activation of the complement cascade, which in turn mediates tissue injury. Most cases of hyperacute rejection occur in recipients previously sensitized to donor HLA antigens by blood transfusion, prior allotransplantation, or pregnancy. The isotype of immunoglobulin involved in these cases is usually thought to be IgG; however, IgM antibodies may also be involved. Although prior exposure to donor HLA antigens increases the risk of hyperacute rejection, *third party* stimulation may also lead to the synthesis of antibodies capable of reacting with donor's antigens and mediating hyperacute rejection.

Although hyperacute rejection has not proven amenable to therapy, it has been prevented in some cases by depleting antidonor antibodies from the recipient before transplantation. For example, surgeons at some centers have successfully transplanted organs across ABO barriers using plasmapheresis or immunoaffinity columns to deplete anti–blood group antibodies. For reasons yet to be elucidated, the return of antidonor antibodies after successful transplantation does not necessarily cause rejection of the graft; instead the graft may continue to function despite the return of these antibodies, a condition called accommodation.

Hyperacute rejection can be understood as a condition in which the critical functions of endothelial cells are lost. Under the most extreme circumstances, loss of endothelial function may be caused by complement-mediated lysis of endothelial cells. Although lysis of endothelial cells is sometimes seen, noncytotoxic effects of complement on endothelial cells such as loss of heparan sulfate or alteration in shape of endothelial cells probably contributes to the pathogenesis in many cases. Endothelial cell lysis and noncytotoxic changes result in loss of barrier function of endothelium, which allows the rapid formation of interstitial edema and hemorrhage and the consequent interaction between extraendothelial tissue factor and the coagulation plasma proteins that promote clotting.

Acute Vascular Rejection. Acute vascular rejection is typically observed weeks to months after transplantation of an organ into a recipient treated with immunosuppressive therapy. Acute vascular rejection is characterized by swelling of endothelium, particularly in arterial vessels, by formation of fibrin thrombi, and sometimes by the influx of inflammatory cells into the blood vessel walls. This type of rejection usually resists conventional types of immunosuppression; however, responses to more heroic measures have been observed on occasion.

The pathogenesis of acute vascular rejection is not yet certain, but some clues have been obtained by the analysis of the outcome of renal and cardiac xenografts. Renal and cardiac xenografts exposed to antidonor antibodies over a period of days develop endothelial cell changes consistent with *activation* of the endothelial cells. Activation of endothelial cells in an allograft mediated by antidonor antibodies, complement, antibody-dependent cell-mediated cytotoxicity, or alloreactive cells causes endothelium to become procoagulant and proinflammatory.

Chronic Rejection. The most common cause of allograft failure is chronic rejection. Chronic rejection is observed months or years after transplantation and is characterized clinically by a slow decline in graft function that is unresponsive to immunosuppressive therapy.[27] The pathologic manifestations of chronic rejection vary with the type of organ transplanted. In the kidney, chronic rejection is characterized by progressive interstitial fibrosis, glomerulopathy, and a scant cellular infiltrate. In cardiac transplants, chronic rejection is manifest as accelerated atherosclerosis. Chronic rejection in the lung may be manifest as bronchiolitis obliterans. In liver transplants, chronic rejection is associated with loss of bile ducts.

The pathogenesis of chronic rejection is controversial. It may result from repeated episodes of acute cellular rejection or from persistent, incompletely treated cellular rejection. There is evidence that certain types of chronic rejection, particularly transplant glomerulopathy and accelerated atherosclerosis, might be caused by the effects of antidonor antibodies on the graft blood vessels. Metabolic or pathophysiologic changes in blood vessels and persistent viral infection have also been considered as potential causes of chronic allograft failure. Regardless of which one or more of these mechanisms causes this process there is no effective treatment for chronic rejection, and graft loss appears to be inevitable.

TOLERANCE

Tolerance is defined as a failure to respond immunologically to a particular antigen in the presence of a suitable challenge by that antigen. Tolerance to one's own antigens is a fundamental property of the immune system, and developing the means to induce tolerance to an allogeneic organ or tissue has been a central goal of transplantation immunology.[6] It was first thought that the failure to respond immunologically to self antigens was inherent and passive; thus, Ehrlich proposed that to avoid *horror autoxicus* there exists a constitutive mechanism that directs immunity toward foreign antigens and that at the same time does not allow immune responses to autologous antigens. It has been shown, however, that tolerance is not constitutive but rather learned. One way in which tolerance to self antigens is learned is through a process called central tolerance, which is brought about during the maturation of T cells in the thymus. As discussed in Part II of this chapter, the thymus *selects* those (~5%) few primitive T cells bearing TcR able to recognize self-MHC Class I or Class II antigens for continued maturation, while precursor T

cells that do not recognize self MHC die. This process, called positive selection, ensures that the T-cell repertoire will be able to recognize peptides expressed in the antigen-binding cleft of MHC molecules and not native proteins. A second process referred to as negative selection then eliminates those T cells that bind very tightly to self MHC and that as a result might be autoreactive. T cells that bind weakly to self MHC–bearing self peptides but that might bind more avidly to self MHC–bearing foreign peptides are allowed to finish maturation and eventually comprise the T-cell repertoire. The process involved in the maturation of T cells in the thymus underlies the phenomenon of neonatal tolerance as elucidated by Billingham, Brent, and Medawar. Allogeneic cells transplanted into the fetus or newborn may enter the thymus, causing deletion of T cells bearing TcR able to bind to those cells. As long as the transplanted cells continue to populate the thymus, each *generation* of T cells that arises after the newborn period is subjected to *negative* selection or deletion of T cells that might recognize the foreign cells. In a similar way, the injection of allogeneic bone marrow into an animal in which mature T cells have been depleted (to prevent rejection of the allogeneic cells) leads to establishment of a new T-cell repertoire tolerant to both the host and the bone marrow donor. Similarly, injection of allogeneic cells directly

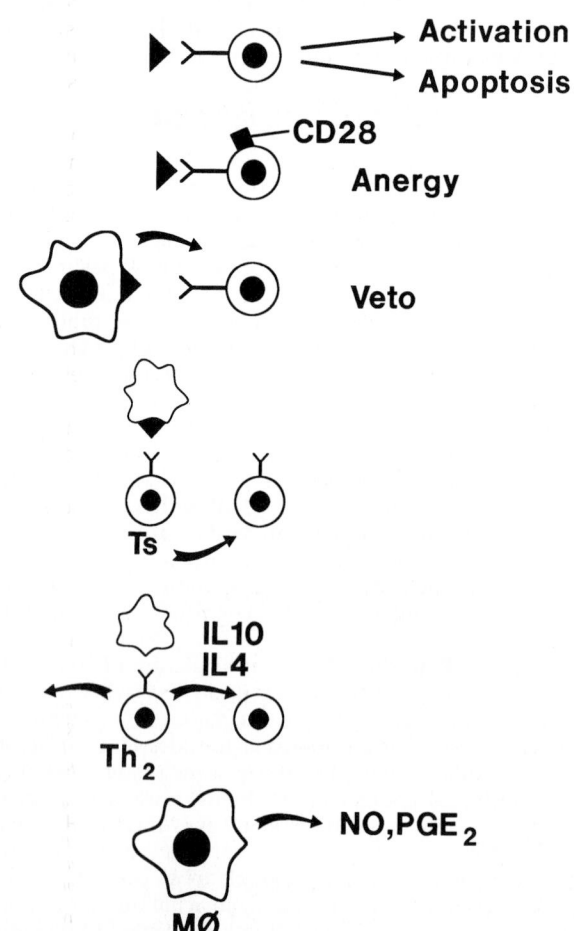

Figure 20–10. Mechanisms of peripheral tolerance. Some potential mechanisms contributing to peripheral tolerance are illustrated. Stimulation of the T cell may cause apoptosis rather than activation. Stimulation of the T-cell receptor (TcR) without co-stimulation (CD28) may cause anergy. Veto cells may kill and suppressor cells (Ts) may inhibit alloreactive T cells. T-cell responses may be inhibited by cytokines such as interleukin-10 and interleukin-4 secreted by Th2 cells or metabolites such as nitric oxide or prostaglandin E_2 secreted by macrophages.

into the thymus in conjunction with depletion of the mature T cells may sometimes lead to tolerance to the inoculum. Administration of donor bone marrow and intrathymic injection have been proposed as approaches to achieving tolerance for allotransplants.

Although central tolerance is clearly effective at preventing responses to MHC antigens, some antigens in peripheral tissues do not gain access to the thymus and thus might give rise to autoreactivity. Nonresponsiveness or tolerance to such peripheral antigens is mediated by peripheral tolerance, which through several mechanisms prevents mature T cells from responding to autoantigens (Fig. 20–10). Stimulation of the TcR under conditions in which co-stimulatory receptors such as B7-2 are unperturbed actually leads to inhibition of T-cell responses.[12] This process, termed *anergy*, presumably averts the development of cellular immune responses to *innocent* foreign antigens or to self antigens, the presentation of which is not associated with inflammation. On the other hand, even full stimulation of T cells under some conditions may lead to tolerance. For example, stimulation of a T cell may cause the T cell to undergo apoptosis (i.e., programmed cell death). Which factors determine whether T-cell apoptosis or activation occurs is an important subject of current investigation. Stimulation of T cells leading to differentiation along the Th2 pathway is associated with inhibition of Th1 responses and tolerance in experimental allograft models. This mechanism of tolerance may be mediated in part by the cytokines interleukin-4 and interleukin-10 synthesized by Th2 cells. Another mechanism of peripheral tolerance may involve the functions of suppressor T cells, that is, T cells that, after recognition of antigen, inhibit responses by other T cells against that antigen. Suppressor T cells, may in fact be *incompetent* T cells that interact with target cells and hinder access of mature, potentially competent effector T cells,[19] or they may be cells that secrete suppressor cytokines. Peripheral tolerance may be mediated by *veto* cells. Veto cells are leukocytes that kill T cells that recognize MHC antigens expressed by the veto cells. Peripheral tolerance might also be promoted by antigen-presenting cells and parenchymal cells that secrete substances such as prostaglandin E_2 and nitric oxide, which in turn inhibit immune responses.[11, 39]

One goal of transplantation is the development of methods that will allow the generation of allospecific tolerance. Existence of allospecific tolerance would allow a graft recipient to be free of immunosuppression and to fight against invasive microorganisms. Methods employing central and peripheral tolerance are being tested clinically.

SELECTED REFERENCES

Charlton, B., Auchincloss, H., Jr., and Fathman, C. G.: Mechanisms of transplantation tolerance. Annu. Rev. Immunol., *12*:707, 1994.
It has always been apparent that the physiology of the immune system must provide mechanisms that prevent immune-mediated injury to normal, autologous tissues yet allow generation of potent responses to infectious agents or foreign cells. The generation of tolerance, as such, to allografts has been a central goal in transplantation. This article provides a lucid and incisive review of this complex topic.

Heemann, U. W., Tullius, S. G., Azuma, H., Kupiec-Weglinsky, J., and Tilney, N. L.: Adhesion molecules and transplantation. Ann. Surg., *219*:4, 1994.
This article considers the role of cell adhesion molecules in the activation and migration of lymphocytes. These are two of the major events in the development of acute cellular rejection and potential targets for therapeutic intervention.

Porter, K. A.: Morphological aspects of renal homograft rejection. Br. Med. Bull., *21*:171, 1965.
Cellular and humoral immune responses cause a spectrum of pathologic changes in allotransplants. This article provides a detailed summary of those changes and some of the mechanisms responsible.

Rosenberg, A. S., and Singer, A.: Cellular basis of skin allograft rejection: An *in vivo* model of immune-mediated tissue destruction. Annu. Rev. Immunol., *10*:333, 1992.
A major question in transplantation is which of the many T cells that might be activated in the recipient of an allograft actually participates in the rejection

reaction. This article begins to address that issue by considering the relationship between the specificity and the function of T lymphocytes.

Sutton, R., Gray, D., McShane, P., Dallman, M. J., and Morris, P. J.: The specificity of rejection and the absence of susceptibility of pancreatic islet B cells to nonspecific immune destruction in mixed strain islets grafted beneath the renal capsule in the rat. J. Exp. Med., *170*:751, 1989.
This article provides a lucid discussion of the effector mechanisms that may be involved in allograft rejection.

REFERENCES

1. Algire, G. H., Weaver, J. M., and Prehn, R. T.: Studies on tissue homotransplantation in mice, using diffusion-chamber methods. Ann. N.Y. Acad. Sci., *64*:1009, 1957.
2. Altman, B.: Tissue transplantation: Circulating antibody in the homotransplantation of kidney and skin. Ann. R. Coll. Surg., *33*:79, 1963.
3. Auchincloss, H., Lee, R., Shea, S., Markowitz, J. S., Grusby, M. J., and Glimcher, L. H.: The role of "indirect" recognition in initiating rejection of skin grafts from major histocompatibility complex class II–deficient mice. Proc. Natl. Acad. Sci. USA, *90*:3373, 1993.
4. Barker, C. F., and Billingham, R. E.: The role of regional lymphatics in the skin homograft response. Transplantation, *5*:962, 1967.
5. Berke, G.: The CTL's kiss of death. Cell, *81*:9, 1995.
6. Charlton, B., Auchincloss, H., Jr., and Fathman, C. G.: Mechanisms of transplantation tolerance. Annu. Rev. Immunol., *12*:707, 1994.
7. Dempster, W. J.: Kidney homotransplantation. Br. J. Surg., *40*:447, 1953.
8. Gibson, T., and Medawar, P. B.: The fate of skin homografts in man. J. Anat., *77*:299, 1943.
9. Grushy, M. J., Auchincloss, H., Lee, R., Johnson, R. S., Spencer, J. P., Zulstra, M., Jaenisch, R., Papaioannou, V. E., and Glimcher, L. H.: Mice lacking major histocompatibility complex class I and class II molecules. Proc. Natl. Acad. Sci. USA, *90*:3913, 1993.
10. Heemann, U. W., Tullius, S. G., Azuma, H., Kupiec-Weglinsky, J., and Tilney, N. L.: Adhesion molecules and transplantation. Ann. Surg., *219*:4, 1994.
11. Ihrcke, N. S., Wrenshall, L. E., Lindman, B. J., and Platt, J. L.: Role of heparan sulfate in immune system–blood vessel interactions. Immunol. Today, *14*:500, 1993.
12. Jenkins, M. K.: The ups and downs of T cell costimulation. Immunity, *1*:443, 1994.
13. Kagi, D., Ledermann, B., Burki, K., Seiler, P., Odermatt, B., Olsen, K. J., Podack, E. R., Zinkernagel, R. M., and Hengartner, H.: Cytotoxicity mediated by T cells and natural killer cells is greatly impaired in perforin-deficient mice. Nature, *369*:31, 1994.
14. Kissmeyer-Nielsen, F., Olsen, S., Petersen, V. P., and Fjeldborg, O.: Hyperacute rejection of kidney allografts, associated with pre-existing humoral antibodies against donor cells. Lancet, *2*:662, 1966.
15. Lafferty, K. J., Prowse, S. J., and Simeonovic, C. J.: Immunobiology of tissue transplantation: A return to the passenger leukocyte concept. Annu. Rev. Immunol., *1*:143, 1983.
16. Landsteiner, K., and Chase, M. W.: Experiments on transfer of cutaneous sensitivity to simple compounds. Proc. Soc. Exp. Biol. Med., *49*:688, 1942.
17. Lawrence, H. S.: The cellular transfer of cutaneous hypersensitivity to tuberculin in man. Proc. Soc. Exp. Biol. Med., *71*:516, 1949.
18. Loeb, L.: Transplantation and individuality. Physiol. Rev., *10*:547, 1930.
19. Lombardi, G., Sidhu, S., Batchelor, R., and Lechler, R.: Anergic T cells as suppressor cells *in vitro*. Science, *264*:1587, 1994.
20. Medawar, P. B.: Notes on the problem of skin homografts. Bull. War Med., *4*:1, 1943.
21. Medawar, P. B.: A behaviour and fate of skin autografts and skin homografts in rabbits. J. Anat., *78*:176, 1944.
22. Medawar, P. B.: A second study of the behaviour and fate of skin homografts in rabbits. J. Anat., *79*:157, 1945.
23. Mintz, B., and Silvers, W. K.: Histocompatibility antigens on melanoblasts and hair follicle cells. Transplantation, *9*:497, 1970.
24. Mitchison, N. A.: Passive transfer of transplantation immunity. Proc. R. Soc. Lond., *142*:72, 1954.
25. Owen, R.: Immunogenetic consequences of vascular anastomoses between bovine twins. Science, *102*:400, 1945.
26. Patel, R., and Terasaki, P. I.: Significance of the positive crossmatch test in kidney transplantation. N. Engl. J. Med., *280*:735, 1969.
27. Petersen, V. P., Olsen, T. S., Kissmeyer-Nielsen, F., Bohman, S. O., Hansen, H. E., Hansen, E. S., Skov, P. E., and Solling, K.: Late failure of human renal transplants. Medicine, *54*:45, 1975.
28. Platt, J. L., LeBien, T. W., and Michael, A. F.: Interstitial mononuclear cell populations in renal graft rejection: Identification by monoclonal antibodies in tissue sections. J. Exp. Med., *155*:17, 1982.
29. Porter, K. A. Renal transplantation. *In* Heptinstall, R. H. (Ed.): Pathology of the Kidney, vol. 3. Boston, Little, Brown, & Co., 1992, pp. 1799–1933.
30. Rosenberg, A. S., and Singer, A.: Cellular basis of skin allograft rejection: An *in vivo* model of immune-mediated tissue destruction. Annu. Rev. Immunol., *10*:333, 1992.
31. Russell, P. S., Chase, C. M., Colvin, R. B., and Plate, J. M. D.: Kidney

transplants in mice: An analysis of the immune status of mice bearing long-term, H-2 incompatible transplants. J. Exp. Med., *147*:1449, 1978.

32. Sad, S., Marcotte, R., and Mosmann, T. R.: Cytokine-induced differentiation of precursor mouse CD8+ T cells into cytotoxic CD8+ T cells secreting Th1 or Th2 cytokines. Immunity, *2*:271, 1995.

33. Seder, R. A., and Gros, G. G.: The functional role of CD8 T helper type 2 cells. J. Exp. Med., *181*:5, 1995.

34. Shoskes, D. A., and Wood, K. J.: Indirect presentation of MHC antigens in transplantation. Immunol. Today, *15*:32, 1994.

35. Simonsen, M., Buemann, J., Gammeltoft, A., Jensen, F., and Jorgensen, K.: Biological incompatibility in kidney transplantation in dogs: Experimental and morphological investigations. Acta. Pathol. Microb. Scand., *32*:1, 1953.

36. Springer, T. A.: Traffic signals for lymphocyte recirculation and leukocyte emigration: The multistep paradigm. Cell, *76*:301, 1994.

37. Sutton, R., Gray, D., McShane, P., Dallman, M. J., and Morris, P. J.: The specificity of rejection and the absence of susceptibility of pancreatic islet B cells to nonspecific immune destruction in mixed strain islets grafted beneath the renal capsule in the rat. J. Exp. Med., *170*:751, 1989.

38. Tanaka, Y., Adams, D. H., and Shaw, S.: Proteoglycans on endothelial cells present adhesion-inducing cytokines to leukocytes. Immunol. Today, *14*:111, 1993.

39. Tineke, C. T. M., van der Pouw, K., Boeije, L., Smeenk, R., Wijdenes, J., and Aarden, L. A.: Prostaglandin-E$_2$ is a potent inhibitor of human interleukin 12 production. J. Exp. Med., *181*:775, 1995.

IV

RENAL TRANSPLANTATION

Clyde F. Barker, M.D., Ali Naji, M.D., Ph.D.,
James F. Markmann, M.D., Ph.D.,
and Kenneth L. Brayman, M.D., Ph.D.

HISTORICAL ASPECTS

Since animal donors were used for the first kidney tranplants attempted in humans (1902–1906), their rapid failure was inevitable.[31] The therapeutic possibilities of the procedure were defined soon after in a series of experiments between 1904 and 1910 by Alexis Carrel. He successfully transplanted kidneys and other organs into animals, utilizing this model to develop the technique of modern blood vessel surgery. This brilliant work resulted in a Nobel Prize in 1912 but was far ahead of its time and was not followed by clinical trials for 4 decades. In the early 1950s, Medawar's detailed description of rejection, and his discovery with Billingham and Brent that it could be prevented in mice by tolerance, stimulated surgeons to resume attempts at renal transplantation. Medawar's work was rewarded with a Nobel Prize in 1960. Some of the clinical trials that followed were technically successful, but because immunosuppressive drugs had not yet been discovered, the transplanted kidney allografts were all destroyed by rejection. However, transplants from identical twins in 1954 by Murray in Boston were successful. In the late 1950s, rejection was first circumvented in several patients by Murray and by Hamburger with the use of whole-body irradiation. Murray was awarded the Nobel Prize in 1990 for his role in these pioneering studies. When immunosuppressive drugs became available in the early 1960s, prolonged allograft survival became more common, though not yet consistent. Over the next 30 years, progress in histocompatibility typing, immunosuppressive therapy, and organ preservation, as well as the accumulation of clinical experience, all contributed to the present status of transplantation, which now allows successful long-term management of previously fatal renal disease in a majority of the more than 20,000 patients per year who receive renal allografts (Table 20–5).

RECIPIENT SELECTION AND MANAGEMENT

Indications

The two diseases most commonly leading to renal failure and treatable by kidney transplantation are glomerulonephritis and insulin-dependent diabetes mellitus, each accounting for about 30% of the total.[9] Other important causes include polycystic kidney disease, hypertensive nephrosclerosis, Alport's disease, IgA nephropathy, systemic lupus erythematosus, nephrosclerosis, interstitial nephritis, pyelonephritis, obstructive uropathy, and hypertensive nephrosclerosis, which is the most common of all causes of renal failure in blacks.

The best recipients are young individuals whose renal failure is not due to a systemic disease that will damage the transplanted kidney or cause death from extrarenal causes. With the increasing appreciation that the results of transplantation are superior to those of chronic dialysis, the indications for transplantation have been broadened. The presence of infection or malignancy that cannot be eradicated remains an absolute contraindication to transplantation, since immunosuppression encourages both microbial and tumor growth. Predicted noncompliance is also a contraindication, since careful adherence to immunosuppression is necessary. Advanced age and severe cardiovascular disease, such as unreconstructable coronary artery or aortoiliac disease, are also deterrents. However, even in such patients, the long-term cumulative risks of dialysis are at least as great as those of transplantation. Therefore, because of improvements in perioperative care and immunosuppression, many patients who would have previously been denied transplantation are now considered acceptable. For example, diabetics, once considered poor candidates, clearly do better with transplantation than with dialysis. In fact, both graft and patient survival for 1 to 2 years are reported to be as good in diabetics as in other patients; on chronic dialysis, only 18% of diabetics survive 5 years.[9] Even diseases in which the transplanted kidney may eventually be damaged by recurrent disease (e.g., lupus erythematosus, cystinosis, amyloidosis, diabetes, and some forms of glomerulonephritis) are often better palliated by transplantation than by dialysis. Indeed, the current results of transplantation mandate serious consideration of this therapy in virtually any patient with terminal renal disease. The quality of life is far better with transplantation than with dialysis, and since the mortality in the first year after transplantation is now less than 5%, survival is also superior. Unfortunately, however, the insufficient availability of donors keeps many appropriate transplant candidates on chronic dialysis. In fact, the number of patients awaiting transplantation is increasing more rapidly than the number of transplants done per year (Fig. 20–11).[11]

TABLE 20–5. Important Events in the Development of Kidney Transplantation

Year	Event
1902–06	First unsuccessful attempts at kidney transplantation in man (Ullmann, Jabouloy)
1904–10	Perfection of experimental kidney transplantation and vascular anastomoses (Carrel)
1946	Establishment of the principles of immunologic rejection (Medawar)
1953	Experimental demonstration of actively acquired tolerance of allografts (Billingham, Brent and Medawar)
1954–58	Successful identical twin transplant (Murray)
1959	First experimental immunosuppression with a drug, 6-mercaptopurine (Schwartz and Demeshek)
1960–62	6-Mercaptopurine and azathioprine shown to prolong dog kidney allograft survival (Calne, Zukowski and Hume, Hitchings)
1962–66	Introduction of tissue typing to select donors, recognition of importance of crossmatch test (Hamberger, Dansch, Terasaki, Kissmeyer-Nielsen, Starzl)
1963	Immunosuppressive effects of antilymphocytic serum described (Woodruff and Anderson)
1967	Preservation of kidneys for 3 days by continuous perfusion (Belzer)
1968	Brain death criteria proposed by ad hoc committee of Harvard Medical School
1973	Beneficial effect of pretransplant blood transfusions noted (Opelz and Terasaki)
1978	Introduction of cyclosporine (Borel, Calne); its release for general use (1984)
1981	Clinical use of monoclonal antibody OKT3 for antirejection therapy (Cosimi)
1986	As result of National Transplant Act, a mandated national organ procurement network takes shape (UNOS)
1987	University of Wisconsin solution extends survival of organs preserved by simple cooling (Belzer and Southard)
1990–95	Importance of persistent microchimerism suggested (Starzl) and new immunosuppressive agents developed (e.g., FK 506, MMF)

Recipient Evaluation and Preparation

The medical evaluation of all transplant candidates should include a history; physical examination; complete blood count; urinalysis; urine culture; cytomegalovirus antibody titer; creatinine clearance; serum electrolytes; serology for syphilis, HIV, and hepatitis B and C; evaluation of parathyroid status; chest x-ray; electrocardiogram; coagulation profile; Pap smear; ABO and histocompatibility typing; urologic evaluation (including a voiding cystourethrogram in selected patients to assess outlet obstruction and reflux); gastrointestinal evaluation, as warranted by history of ulcer, diverticulitis, or other symptoms; and psychiatric evaluation.

The proper timing of transplantation is a delicate decision, since the progression of renal dysfunction is variable, and premature imposition of the risks of transplantation is not justified. However, dialysis and/or transplantation should not be withheld until advanced uremic symptoms, such as pericarditis, cardiac failure, severe anemia, osteodystrophy, and neuropathy ensue, since some of these complications may become irreversible. Even when a donor is readily available, pretransplant dialysis is often necessary, at least briefly, to optimize the patient's general condition (nutrition, electrolyte balance, coagulation status). Careful attention must be given to eradication of all infections, including those of the urinary tract, lungs, teeth, and skin (especially at the site of the planned incision). Since cardiovascular complications are as common as infection as a cause of posttransplantation mortality, the patient's cardiovascular status should be carefully evaluated and optimized. In older patients and diabetics, this might require stress testing or even pretransplant coronary artery bypass.

Histocompatibility Typing and Crossmatching

Although opinions vary regarding the significance of histocompatibility testing for the selection of unrelated donors, its importance is unquestionable for the selection of the optimal donor within a family. Regardless of the donor source, compatibility for ABO blood groups and a negative leukocyte crossmatch are mandatory.

ABO Blood Groups. Because the major blood group antigens are not expressed by human leukocytes, it was initially assumed that they might be unimportant in transplant rejection. However, experimental and clinical evidence soon indicated that ABO antigens function as important histocompatibility antigens, probably because they are expressed on vascular endothelium.[5] Rapaport and Dausset demonstrated experimentally that prior exposure to erythrocytes from ABO-incompatible donors provoked accelerated rejection of skin grafts from donors of the same blood group. In the early days of renal transplantation, it was noted that ABO incompatibility often led to acute or hyperacute rejection, a finding that resulted in adherence to the rule of blood group compatibility. Because of the donor organ shortage and reports of some success with ABO-incompatible liver and heart allografts, attempts have been made at breaching the ABO barrier for kidney allografts. In 1982, Brynger and colleagues reported successful transplantation in blood group O recipients of kidneys from A_2 donors (who have a lower number of A antigenic determinants on their cells than A_1 donors).[5] Successful ABO-incompatible transplants have also been reported in recipients whose ABO isoagglutinins have been removed by plasmapheresis or immunoadsorption. Because isoagglutinins eventually reappear and the long-term outcome of these transplants is likely to be inferior, most centers

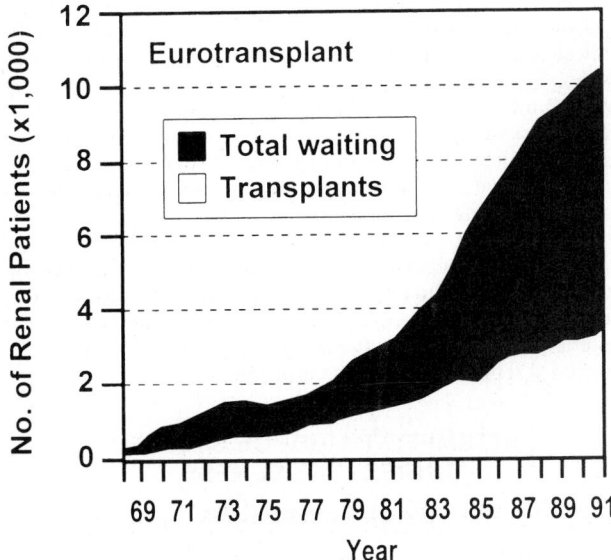

Figure 20–11. Because of the donor shortage, the number of patients awaiting renal transplants is increasing much more rapidly than the limited number of transplants that can be done. This is true both in Europe, as depicted in this figure, and in the United States. (From Cohen, C., and Persijn, G.: Twenty-five years of Eurotransplant. *In* Terasaki, P. I., and Cecka, J. M. [Eds.]: Clinical Transplants. Los Angeles, UCLA Tissue Typing Laboratory, 1992, p. 109.)

do not employ this strategy. However, it is an intriguing approach, especially for allowing the utilization of HLA-identical but ABO-incompatible family donors.

Lymphocytotoxic Crossmatching. Sensitization to HLA antigens, as indicated by the presence of lymphocytotoxic antibodies in the recipient's serum, may occur with pregnancy, blood transfusion, or prior renal transplantation. Presence of donor-reactive antibodies, detected by incubation of recipient serum with donor cells in the presence of complement (a positive crossmatch), is considered a contraindication to renal transplantation because of its strong association (80%) with hyperacute renal allograft rejection. Serum from patients awaiting cadaveric renal transplantation is periodically screened against a panel of randomly selected HLA-typed lymphocyte donors. Nonreactivity of a patient's serum to the panel cells indicates a high likelihood of obtaining a crossmatch-compatible donor, whereas uniform reactivity of a patient's serum with panel cells greatly reduces this probability. The number of highly sensitized patients on most transplant waiting lists is increasing, because less-sensitized patients receive transplants, sensitized individuals remain on the list, and those with failed renal allografts (frequently sensitized) are returned to the list.

Recently, it has been noted that successful transplantation can often be achieved despite positivity of certain types of crossmatches, a finding that allows transplantation of some apparently sensitized patients.[59] For example, lymphocytotoxic autoantibodies do not cause rejection. In some patients, the titer of bona fide lymphocytotoxic antibodies declines or disappears with time. In the past, it was a common practice to store serum from the period of peak sensitization for later use in crossmatching; if it was found to be positive, transplantation was denied, even if current serum was negative. Several reports now indicate that a positive crossmatch using peak serum may be disregarded with only a minimal risk of hyperacute rejection, as long as current serum is negative. The conditions that allow transplantation in a patient with a historic positive but current negative crossmatch are not clearly defined. Most centers require a certain interval (1 to 12 months) between the last positive serum and transplantation. There is controversy whether the most sensitive crossmatching methods such as antiglobulin and flow cytometry techniques should be used, since they may exclude donors who might have been used successfully. In addition, the clinical relevance of positive crossmatches to B lymphocytes (especially if performed in the cold) and those caused only by IgM antibodies is questionable. Attempts have also been made to define the role of antibodies against minor (non-HLA) specificities. For example, there is evidence that antibodies reactive to determinants on vascular endothelial cells can damage renal allografts.

To allow transplantation of sensitized patients, several methods have been tried to remove cytotoxic antibody, including thoracic duct drainage, total lymphoid irradiation, and plasmapheresis. Since none of these maneuvers has gained wide acceptance, the increasingly large sensitized patient pool remains a formidable problem.

ATTEMPTS TO INDUCE SPECIFIC UNRESPONSIVENESS

Blood Transfusions

In the first 2 decades of renal transplantation, transfusions were avoided whenever possible to minimize the formation of lymphocytotoxic antibodies, which might prevent transplantation or destroy the allograft. However, in 1973, Opelz and co-workers[35] made the surprising observation in a multi-institutional survey that renal allograft survival was actually 10 to 15% better in transfused than nontransfused recipients. This caused a worldwide policy of deliberate pretransplant blood transfusion, which was subsequently credited with a substantial improvement in the outcome of renal transplants that occurred over the next decade.

Reasons for this beneficial transfusion effect were unclear. Some thought that transfusions simply prevented *high-responder* patients from being transplanted by sensitizing them so that they were crossmatch-positive to most available donors. This would cause most kidneys to go instead to *low-responder* patients who remained crossmatch-negative despite transfusions and were likely to have a successful transplant, but for reasons unrelated to the transfusions. Another possible explanation was that transfusions had a true immunosuppressive effect, mediated through induction of suppressor T lymphocytes and/or enhancing alloantibodies.

Based on a rationale similar to that for random transfusions, some groups practiced deliberate transfusions of blood from a prospective living-related donor. Salvatierra credited this maneuver with improving graft survival of one-haplotype-matched related recipients from 56 to 91%.[46] However, this procedure was also associated with a 30% risk of inciting cytotoxic antibodies, thus precluding transplantation from the chosen donor. However, when azathioprine was given at the time of transfusion, the rate of sensitization decreased to only 8%, and graft survival remained better than 90%.[3]

With the improvement in graft survival that occurred when the new immunosuppressive agent cyclosporine became available in 1984, the need for blood transfusions was questioned. For a few years, there was disagreement whether cyclosporine-treated patients still benefited from transfusions, but within the ensuing 5 to 6 years, a consensus was reached that the transfusion effect had indeed been *lost*.[1] This was caused not by a decline in graft survival in transfused patients but rather by improved graft outcome in nontransfused recipients attributable to cyclosporine and other improvements in practice that also occurred during this era. In any case, the question has become moot, since the fear of transmission of infection (HIV and hepatitis) has become a major factor in patient nonacceptance of transfusions, and most transplant surgeons believe that whatever benefit might still be achieved is outweighed by the risk of sensitization, especially in previously transplanted or sensitized patients. Thus, deliberate preconditioning of transplant recipients with transfusions is no longer recommended by most groups.

Bone Marrow Conditioning

As enthusiasm for blood transfusions has waned, there has been an increasing interest in pretransplant conditioning with bone marrow from the organ donor. Although this procedure might act by the same (unexplained) mechanism as blood transfusions, an additional intriguing rationale is the self-replicating ability of bone marrow and the resultant potential for persistent microchimerism. For many years, animal experiments have shown that administration of donor bone marrow is an especially effective method of conditioning transplant recipients. Bone marrow was found by Billingham, Brent, and Medawar in the 1950s to be an ideal inoculum for the induction of neonatal tolerance. Monaco later found that donor bone marrow promotes skin allograft survival in adult rodents if combined with a brief course of antilymphocytic serum. In 1987, Barber and Diethelm initiated a randomized study in which cryopreserved donor bone marrow was administered 10 to 14 days after kidney transplantation to recipients who were treated with antilymphocyte serum and other standard immunosuppressive agents. Because the incidence of acute rejection was decreased, the early results were quite encouraging.[6] However, by the time the study was concluded in 1995, improvement in long-term patient and graft survival was less impressive and, disappointingly, chronic rejection was not prevented. This group and several others continue to explore the potential benefit of bone marrow conditioning.

Pretransplant Operations

Any necessary urinary tract reconstructions must be carried out prior to transplantation (e.g., lysis of posterior urethral valves, transurethral resection for obstructing prostatic hypertrophy). The patient's own bladder should be utilized for ureteroneocystostomy, even if this necessitates bladder reconstruction or augmentation of a small bladder by ileococcocystoplasty. Careful intermittent catheterization of a neurogenic bladder three to four times daily posttransplant is preferable to the use of an intestinal conduit. In the absence of an alternative strategy, ileal conduits should be constructed at least 6 weeks prior to the transplant operation to avoid risk of infection.

Bilateral nephrectomy of recipients was once routine, the rationale being that even if current urine was sterile, pyelonephritic kidneys would remain a dangerous focus of infection and glomerulonephritic kidneys, if retained, would be a stimulus for autoimmune destruction of the allograft. Since evidence to support these hypotheses was never forthcoming, bilateral nephrectomy is now performed only for special indications, such as recalcitrant urinary tract infections (especially in the presence of stones, reflux, or obstruction), uncontrollable hypertension, massive proteinuria, bilateral renal tumors, or large polycystic kidneys, especially if they are bleeding or infected.

Splenectomy was once widely practiced on an empiric basis for its nonspecific immunosuppressive effect. A large randomized study eventually indicated that the procedure modestly improved early but not late graft survival,[55] and other studies actually showed a detrimental effect on patient survival.[2] During the pre-cyclosporine era, a rationale for splenectomy was the resultant increase in white blood cell count, which allowed larger maintenance doses of azathioprine without leukopenia. Since cyclosporine does not cause leukopenia, there is now general agreement that splenectomy is rarely indicated.

SELECTION AND MANAGEMENT OF LIVING DONORS

For the prospective recipient, there are major advantages to obtaining a living donor, which obviates the discomfort, expense, and risks of prolonged dialysis while waiting for a cadaver kidney. Posttransplant morbidity is also minimized by decreasing the chances of acute tubular necrosis (ATN) or early rejection crises. Since the advent of cyclosporine therapy, short-term results of cadaveric transplantation in some centers now approach those with living-related donors. Nevertheless, because of better histocompatibility, long-term results of related donor transplantation remain superior to those of cadaveric grafts. Thus, most authorities believe that the use of living donors is still justified, and in the United States, they account for about 25% of kidney transplants.

Histocompatibility Considerations in Living Donor Selection

The HLA antigens are gene products of alleles at a number of closely linked loci on the short arm of chromosome 6 in humans. At least six (A, B, C, DQ, DP, DR) have been defined, and the existence of several others has been deduced from family studies and immunochemical findings. The extreme polymorphism of the HLA system, which is the basis of infinite genetic variability of the human species, plays a pivotal role in regulation of the immune response. The gene products of the HLA-A, -B, and -C loci are referred to as Class I major histocompatibility (MHC) antigens, and the products of the D region are Class II MHC antigens. MHC Class I antigens are expressed on all nucleated cells and can be readily detected serologically using lymphocytotoxicity assays. Class II MHC antigens are important in antigen presentation and are expressed on B lymphocytes, dendritic cells, endothelium, and activated T cells.

HLA antigens are inherited as co-dominant alleles, and because of the relatively low recombinant frequency, the HLA genes are usually inherited *en bloc* from each parent. In immediate families, inheritance of the HLA antigens, which is of overriding importance in transplant outcome, can be determined serologically and falls into four different combinations of haplotypes. Any two siblings have a 25% chance of being HLA identical (i.e., having inherited the same chromosome 6 [haplotype] from each parent), a 50% chance of sharing one haplotype, and a 25% chance of sharing neither haplotype. Parent-to-child donation always involves a one-haplotype identity.

The importance of matching HLA antigens in the selection of living-related donors for renal transplantation is well established. Excellent long-term graft survival (>95%) can be expected when a related donor and recipient are HLA identical. There is a progressively lower graft survival associated with one- or zero-haplotype matches, although even totally mismatched related living donor grafts have a significantly better outcome than cadaveric grafts.[10]

Risks to the Living Donor

Despite the major advantages of related donors, their use can be justified only because the risks to the donor are minimal. Nevertheless, it is important to present these risks frankly to the donor. In addition to discomfort and morbidity associated with any operation, there is an operative mortality of about 0.05%. Concern for even a small mortality has led to a traditional policy of accepting as donors only individuals between 18 and 55 years of age and in virtually perfect health. As donor age limits are extended, it will be important to exercise even greater care to avoid unacceptable risks.

Obviously, the donor must have two normal kidneys, as confirmed by standard renal function tests, intravenous pyelography, and arteriography. Despite the knowledge that unilateral nephrectomy is followed by compensatory hypertrophy of the remaining kidney, near normal renal function, and normal life expectancy, concern has been expressed regarding the long-term status of living donors.[17] This concern is based on the finding that ablation of renal tissue in the rat leads to hyperfiltration by the remaining kidney tissue and eventual functional deterioration due to sclerosis. Ten years after nephrectomy, some human donors were also noted to exhibit proteinuria and hypertension, but larger studies failed to confirm this.[33] Perhaps the most reassuring evidence that long-term sequelae are unlikely is that 98% of insurance companies require no increase in life insurance premiums for otherwise healthy individuals after kidney donation.

The identification of a donor from a family group is preferably based on histocompatibility factors, although selection of a less well matched donor by a well-informed family must be respected. It is important that potential candidates be protected from pressure to donate against their will, especially if they are minors. However, most family members willingly donate, and the psychologic benefits of doing so are often profound.

Living-Unrelated Donors

Until recently, unrelated volunteers were excluded from donation, since the outcomes were assumed not to be sufficiently advantageous, compared with cadaver grafts, to warrant the risk. The improvement in unrelated kidney allograft survival with cyclosporine and the shortage of cadaver donors have provoked re-examination of this issue. Although the use of paid donors is unlawful, genetically unrelated but emotionally related donors (especially spouses) are now considered acceptable by many centers and currently account for about 1% of all kidney transplants in the United States. Two hundred eighty-two such transplants reported to the United Network for Organ Sharing (UNOS) between 1987 and 1991 had a 1-year graft survival of 92%, which was significantly better than the survival of cadaveric transplants, even those in whom prompt function indicated little or no ischemic damage.[9] In view of the critical donor shortage, the use of such donors is currently advocated by many groups, although it remains the subject of ethical debate.

Techniques of Living Donor Nephrectomy

The left kidney is chosen, if possible, since its longer renal vein facilitates the recipient operation. However, if the arteriogram shows multiple renal arteries on one side, the kidney with a single artery is usually selected to facilitate the anastomosis. A flank incision is used. After Gerota's fascia is incised, the greater curvature of the kidney and the upper pole are mobilized, and the hilar structures are exposed. On the left side, the adrenal and gonadal veins are ligated so that the full length of the renal vein can be utilized. Traction on the renal artery should be avoided, since it causes spasm and decreased kidney perfusion, possibly compromising early function. The ureter should be mobilized, along with its blood supply and a generous amount of periureteric tissue. It is divided close to the bladder after ligating the distal end. If the donor is well hydrated, urine should be seen issuing from the proximal end of the divided ureter. Mannitol and furosemide are useful in promoting a diuresis. At this stage, attention is given to coordination with the recipient operation (which is performed simultaneously by a separate team). When the recipient iliac vessels have been prepared, the donor renal artery and vein are clamped and divided in that order. Blood is flushed from the kidney via the artery with 4° C. heparinized preservative solution, and the kidney is immersed in a basin of cold solution to protect it during the brief interval prior to transplantation. The donor blood vessels are oversewn, and the incision is closed without drainage.

SELECTION AND MANAGEMENT OF CADAVERIC DONORS

In the absence of a family donor, cadaveric renal transplantation is a satisfactory alternative. In most countries, acceptance of the concept of brain death allows removal of viable organs from donors whose hearts are beating, and cadaveric kidneys account for about 75% of transplants. Should the results of cadaveric transplants continue to improve because of better immunosuppression, the shortage of cadaver kidneys may eventually be the only justification for the use of living donors. However, at present, the results (especially long-term results) remain better with a family donor.

The donor shortage is an important limitation. Although in the United States the Uniform Anatomical Gift Act has been adopted in all 50 states, few cadaver kidneys are actually removed on the basis of donor cards alone without permission of the next of kin. Only about half of U.S. citizens currently consent to donation of organs from deceased relatives, and organs are recovered from less than 20% of potentially acceptable donors. Although in the United States it has been estimated that about 20,000 brain-dead patients per year are acceptable donors, only 8100 cadaveric kidney transplants were done in 1993—a number that has changed little over the last few years, despite continued increases in waiting lists.[9, 54] The donor shortage is similarly severe in Europe (see Fig. 20–11). It is important that primary physicians, neurosurgeons, and intensive care nurses identify potential donors. Procurement personnel (usually part of a regional team) are then available to help obtain permission from the family and coordinate removal and distribution of viable organs.

The best cadaveric donors are previously healthy subjects between 3 and 65 years of age who have sustained fatal head injuries or cerebrovascular accidents. Careful history, physical examination, and laboratory surveys should be carried out to uncover factors that are contraindications to organ donation, such as the presence of generalized infections (including occult ones such as HIV or hepatitis B and C), malignancy other than nonmetastasizing brain tumors, and known renal disease, hypertension, or advanced arteriosclerosis. Donors over 65 may also sometimes be suitable, but the likelihood of vascular disease makes them less attractive. The use of kidneys from infants is also possible, but technical aspects are exacting, and both kidneys may need to be implanted into a single recipient, a procedure that is associated with an increased incidence of technical complications. Because of the severe donor shortage, the use of older donors and cadaveric donors without a heartbeat is being practiced by some groups.

The use of cadaver donors raises the ethical and legal problems of defining brain death. Consideration of transplantation should never be allowed to influence the definition or declaration of death, which must always be the responsibility of the patient's primary physician or a neurologic consultant, with the full understanding and permission of the family. To avoid any conflict of interest, the transplant team must never be involved with care of the donor or with decisions regarding prognosis or therapy. Current criteria for brain death at the authors' hospital require two in-hospital examinations at least 12 hours apart by a neurologist or neurosurgeon documenting loss of function of the entire brain. The interval between examinations must be extended to 24 hours in case of anoxic-ischemic brain injury. Loss of cerebral function is documented by lack of response to painful stimuli or movement except for spinal reflexes. The loss of brain stem function is documented by fixed pupils; absence of corneal, oculovestibular, and oculocephalic reflexes; loss of gag reflex; and absence of movement or spontaneous respiration off the respirator for 3 minutes, a test that is done only after other criteria indicate no brain function. The declaration of brain death may be accelerated by 6 hours if a confirmatory test is performed, such as a flat electroencephalogram (EEG). Strict adherence to these criteria is not always possible. For example, EEG confirmation is not required to declare brain death in the presence of angiographic evidence of complete lack of blood flow to the brain, which may occur with severe brain swelling. The diagnosis of brain death should not be made in the presence of severe hypothermia, marked hypovolemia, or toxic levels of depressant drugs such as barbiturates, since these factors can produce an isoelectric EEG pattern that is reversible.

Donor Pretreatment

An interesting procedure that has been recommended but not widely accepted is donor pretreatment with immunosuppressive drugs, a strategy that can be employed only for cadaver donors.[16] The rationale is that interstitial cells of hematopoietic origin that are normally present in the transplant organ (*passenger* cells) contribute importantly to graft immunogenicity and that their removal is beneficial. Conflicting results of pretreatment of donors with such agents as methylprednisolone, cyclophosphamide, or cyclosporine emphasize that circulating passenger cells are not the only source of transplantation antigens within kidney allografts. Interstitial dendritic cells and vascular endothelial cells that cannot be removed are probably also important in antigen presentation. It is conceivable that more thorough eradication of passenger cells by vigorous, prolonged treatment of donors or treatment of the *ex vivo* kidney might be more beneficial. However, current attention is focused on the potential benefits of employing the opposite strategy, i.e., augmenting passenger cell transfer. This is based on the recent observation by Starzl that in many long-term successful organ transplant recipients, persistent donor lymphoid cells (especially dendritic cells) can be identified in various organs of the recipient (skin, thymus, brain).[52] It remains to be seen whether these cells are the cause of successful organ transplantation or merely accompany it. Several trials are under way to condition transplant recipients with donor bone marrow.

HLA Considerations in Cadaver Donor Selection

Although the benefit of matching for HLA-A and -B antigens in selection of family donors is well established, its value for cadaveric grafts remains controversial. For many years, reports from European centers indicated that matching has a beneficial effect.[41] Not only was there a significant difference between grafts fully matched and those totally mismatched for HLA-A and -B, but graded improvements in outcome could be related to the extent of the match. The value of HLA-A and -B typing has been confirmed by some reports from North America but not by others. The benefit of matching is more apparent in long-term than in short-term results.[58] Several possible explanations have been put forth for differences in American and European results, such as the greater genetic heterogeneity of the U.S. population and the uniformity of tissue typing, which in Europe is performed only in the select and highly experienced laboratories of Eurotransplant. Both in Europe and in the United States, Class II (HLA-DR) matching appears to be of greater benefit than Class I matching.[60] However, many authors, especially in the United States, believe that the improved survival of kidney allografts that occurred with the advent of cyclosporine largely overrides the effect of HLA matching, at least in first transplants. It appears that the DR matching is still important in selecting donors for previously transplanted patients.

Even in the United States, the benefits of six-antigen-matched (or zero-antigen-mismatched) kidney transplants are now uncontested, causing UNOS to mandate their sharing on a national basis.[56] Whether lesser degrees of matching are important is controversial (especially in the cyclosporine era) and is the central issue of an ongoing debate whether to change UNOS's point system for cadaveric kidney allocation, which currently emphasizes HLA matching.[34] Two recent analyses of the same data on the outcomes of over 30,000 renal transplants led to opposite conclusions. Takemoto and colleagues noted that HLA matching and transplant success were correlated,[57] whereas Held and co-workers, who stratified other risk factors, found little benefit and argued that the ischemic damage inherent in the transportation necessary for national sharing would outweigh the advantage of matching.[20] By their calculations, national sharing might increase the 5-year graft survival by only 2%. They also noted that totally unmatched, unrelated, living (and thus only briefly ischemic) kidneys have a 94% 1-year survival, whereas four-antigen-matched cadaveric grafts have only a 77% 1-year survival.

The recent advent of DNA typing raises the interesting possibility that with the more accurate matching these methods allow, there would be closer correlation between histocompatibility and success of cadaveric transplants. DNA typing can be done in several ways, including restriction fragment length polymorphism (RFLP) and allele-specific amplification via polymerase chain reaction (PCR-SSP).[36] RFLP testing takes 4 to 14 days and thus can be used only retrospectively for cadaveric donors. It has detected errors that were made in serologic typing of DR antigens and has shown that DR typing, if correct, is quite important. Since PCR-SSP can be done in about 2 hours, it could be used prospectively and is currently under evaluation as to correlation with outcome.

Operative Technique for Cadaveric Donors

After declaration of brain death, the donor is brought to the operating room and optimal respiration and circulation are maintained during the procedure. Before and during the operation, it is often necessary to administer large volumes of intravenous fluids because of diabetes insipidus or to restore blood volume, which may have been depleted during premortem attempts to decrease brain swelling and achieve neurologic recovery.

Prior to the widespread application of extrarenal transplantation, the technique of cadaver nephrectomy was similar to that described for related donors. As multiorgan recovery has now become almost routine, the following technique of *in situ* perfusion and *en bloc* dissection has evolved as the standard (Fig. 20–12). The peritoneal cavity is entered through a midline incision, usually extended to the suprasternal notch to facilitate heart, lung, and liver donation. After exploration for unsuspected neoplasia or infection, the small bowel is retracted and the posterior peritoneum incised in the midline up through the ligament of Treitz to expose the aorta and inferior vena cava. The peritoneal reflections around the cecum are incised and continued cephalad, allowing visualization of retroperitoneum. By retraction of the duodenum and pancreas superiorly, the proximal aorta and vena cava are exposed. Following dissection of the vascular structures of extrarenal organs to be recovered concomitantly (liver, pancreas, heart, lung), the aorta and vena cava are divided just above their bifurcations after proximal insertion of large-bore cannulas for retrograde *in situ* perfusion. Anticoagulation is achieved by intravenous heparin, and the aorta is clamped proximally (at the aortic arch for cardiac recovery, above the celiac axis for liver and pancreas, and just above the renal arteries if only the kidneys are to be removed). Infusion of cold (4° C.) preservation solution via the aortic cannula is initiated, along with simultaneous decompression via the caval cannula. The kidneys, which rapidly become pale and cold, are then mobilized, avoiding damage to the hilar structures or ureters. The divided distal aorta and vena cava are mobilized cephalad by securing the lumbar vessels between clips, and the aorta is divided above the renal arteries. The entire bloc of kidneys, ureters, aorta, and vena cava is transferred to a basin of cold solution, where careful dissection of the renal vessels is performed. The kidneys are then separated by division of the vena cava and aorta and packaged for cold storage to allow time for recipient selection, tissue typing, and transportation. Additional *bench surgery* for accurate dissection of the renal vessels

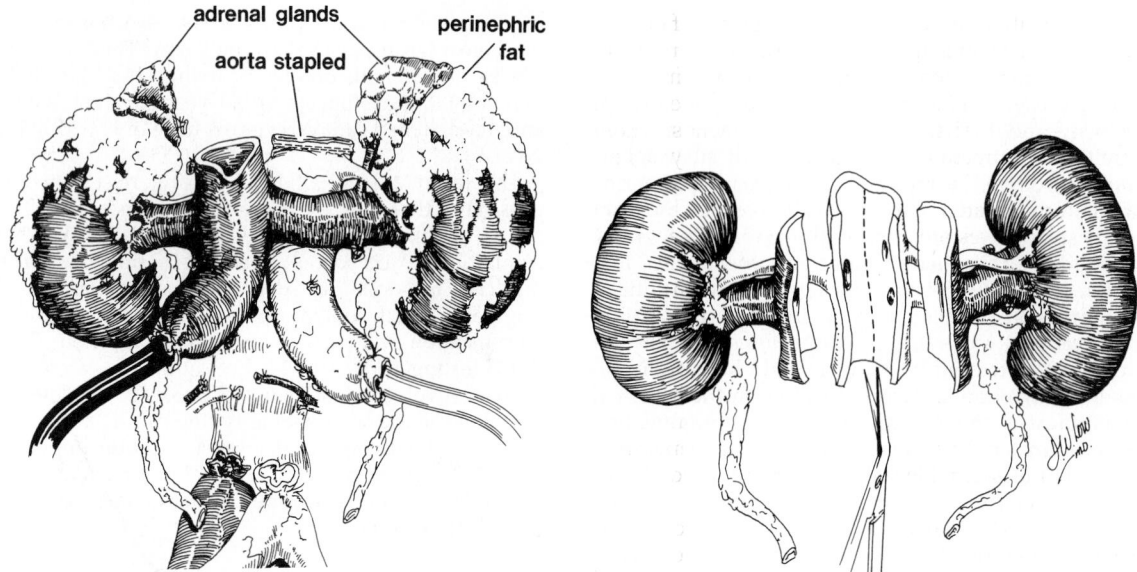

Figure 20–12. Dissection for cadaver kidney donation is depicted. Cannulas are placed in the aorta and vena cava for hypothermic perfusion to protect the kidneys during the terminal phases of the operation and for short-term storage. Segments of aorta and vena cava are left intact when the kidneys are separated. The use of a Carrel patch of aorta is especially helpful when there are multiple renal arteries.

and ureter is usually carried out later under continued hypothermic conditions just prior to transplantation.

Preservation of Cadaveric Kidneys

Two methods of kidney preservation (simple cooling and continuous pulsatile perfusion) have been widely utilized.[7] Both allow sufficient time for transportation of kidneys to distant transplant centers. Simple cooling is achieved by flushing the allograft with a cold iso-osmolar or hyperosmolar buffered solution followed by storage at 4 to 10° C. Additives to the solutions include various ratios of K^+, Na^+, Cl^-, citrate, PO_4^-, SO_4^-, glucose, sucrose, mannitol, bicarbonate, and magnesium. These solutions are used for short-term (<48 hours) preservation. Although some disagreement exists, it is generally held that if longer preservation of organs is necessary (48 to 72 hours), it requires the use of a pulsatile perfusion apparatus that circulates either cryoprecipitated homologous plasma or a preservation solution through the kidney.

In the late 1970s, there was a trend away from machine pulsatile preservation (which had previously been used by about two thirds of centers) and toward simple cooling, which is now employed at almost all centers. Responsible for the change were the greater costs and inconvenience of machine perfusion, including the need for a trained attendant during transportation to distant centers. In addition, it was shown that for short preservation times (<24 hours), pulsatile perfusion probably had little if any advantage. In 1987, Belzer introduced a solution (University of Wisconsin, or UW, solution) containing several new components (lactobionate, raffinose, hydroxyethyl starch) that substantially extended the storage period for liver and pancreas to 24 hours.[7] Although the solution is widely used by others for simple cold storage of kidneys, it has also been used by Belzer as a perfusate for machine preservation, with excellent results. Even with improved preservation solutions, however, simple cooling has a finite time limit, and it seems likely that major progress in preservation can come only from advances in perfusion techniques. Several groups that resisted the trend toward simple cooling and continue to use machine perfusion have reported an extremely low incidence of ATN. The additive adverse effects of ischemia and cyclosporine nephrotoxicity may eventually provoke a general return to pulsatile preservation.

XENOGENEIC (INTERSPECIES) GRAFTS

The growing shortage of human organs for transplantation has rejuvenated interest in using donors of other species. Although the success of cross-species organ grafts could revolutionize the field of transplant operation, uncertainty exists as to when, if ever, this will be feasible.[27] The xenograft barrier consists of three components—humoral, cellular, and physiologic. In the first two, experimental advances have been considerable in the last 5 to 10 years. Specific carbohydrate epitopes have been defined that serve as the dominant targets of the natural antibody response in the discordant primate antiporcine response. Progress has been made in preventing preformed and induced antibody-mediated graft damage by immunosuppressive regimens that blunt the induced response and by the novel strategy of inducing transgene encoded regulators of complement activation to avoid the attack of natural antibodies. The 30-hour survival in a baboon of a heart xenograft from a pig (genetically engineered to express human proteins on endothelial cells) is quite encouraging, since preformed antibody and complement activation destroy xenografts from normal pigs in 60 to 90 minutes.

Progress has also been made in defining and overcoming the cellular aspects of xenorejection. In fact, no specific evidence exists that, in the absence of a humoral response, the cellular response to xenografts would be substantially more formidable than that to allografts or any less susceptible to conventional immunosuppression. Although genetic engineering to delete donor antigens is intriguing, the indirect pathway of graft antigen presentation is a potential pitfall to this strategy.

Despite these experimental advances, recent experience with clinical xenografts is much less encouraging. About 40 whole-organ xenografts have been performed in man during this century. However, the longest functional survival (9 months) was a chimpanzee-to-human kidney xenograft performed by Reemstma more than 30 years ago. In the same year, 19 other primate-to-human kidney transplants failed in patients who were immunosuppressed with azathioprine and steroids. Careful studies done by Starzl in 1992, in which baboon livers were transplanted to two human patients, are the most informative.[53] These xenografts were transplanted with the optimal immunologic advantages of the day: a concordant donor species; the known relative resistance of the liver to antibody-mediated damage; and maximal modern immunosuppression. Despite the well-conceived nature of this trial, graft and patient survival were short-lived (25 and 70 days). Moreover, the development of graft dysfunction in the absence of significant histologic evidence of rejection raises serious concerns that some as yet undefined physiologic incompatibility existed between graft and recipient.

Considering that the outcomes obtained today with clinical xenografts might well be comparable to those with allografts of 40 to 50 years ago and that recent progress in experimental xenobiology has been considerable, one might predict that eventual clinical success is likely. In fact, limited success might be almost within reach now if primate donors were used. However, the shortage of these animals in most parts of the world, the difficulty of breeding them in captivity, and the ethical question of their use are major deterrents.

Another important cautionary note deserves mention—the possible danger of zoonoses.[30] The consequences of transferring micro-organisms from other species into immunosuppressed humans via organ xenografts are unknown. However, virologists believe that the probable origin of the HIV epidemic in man was transfer of a virus originating in nonhuman primates. A workshop on the benefits and risks of xenografts sponsored by the Institute of Medicine in June 1995 was influential in current deliberations by the Food and Drug Administration, which could impose government regulation of xenografts or a ban of further clinical trials.

THE RECIPIENT OPERATION

General anesthesia is usually employed, although spinal anesthesia is also satisfactory. Good relaxation is important during the vascular and ureteral anastomosis, but excessive use of muscle relaxants (especially succinylcholine) must be avoided, since low cholinesterase levels in dialysis patients may otherwise lead to prolonged apnea. The muscle relaxant atracurium can be used safely, since this agent has a short half-life, and its degradation is independent of renal and hepatic metabolism.

The iliac vessels are exposed retroperitoneally through an oblique incision just above the inguinal ligament (Fig. 20–13). The dissection is slightly easier on the right, but a more important consideration in selecting the appropriate side is avoiding sites of previous transplants, other operations (e.g., appendectomy, herniorrhaphy, bladder or ureteral operations), or peritoneal dialysis catheters. The least possible dissection is done to accomplish adequate exposure of planned anastomotic sites. Lymphatics that must be divided to expose the iliac vessels are ligated to prevent prolonged lymph drainage or lymphocele formation. Exposure of the bladder is facilitated by dividing the inferior epigastric vessels and, in females, the round ligament. Division of the spermatic cord should be avoided, since this may cause epididymitis, testicular ischemia, and atrophy.

Traditionally, vascular anastomoses were performed between the end of the donor renal artery and the proximal end of the recipient's divided internal iliac artery and between the end of the donor renal vein and the side of the external iliac vein. An end-to-side anastomosis of renal artery to external iliac artery is now used instead, especially if there is significant atheromatous disease in the internal iliac artery, as there often is in older or diabetic recipients, or if the contralateral

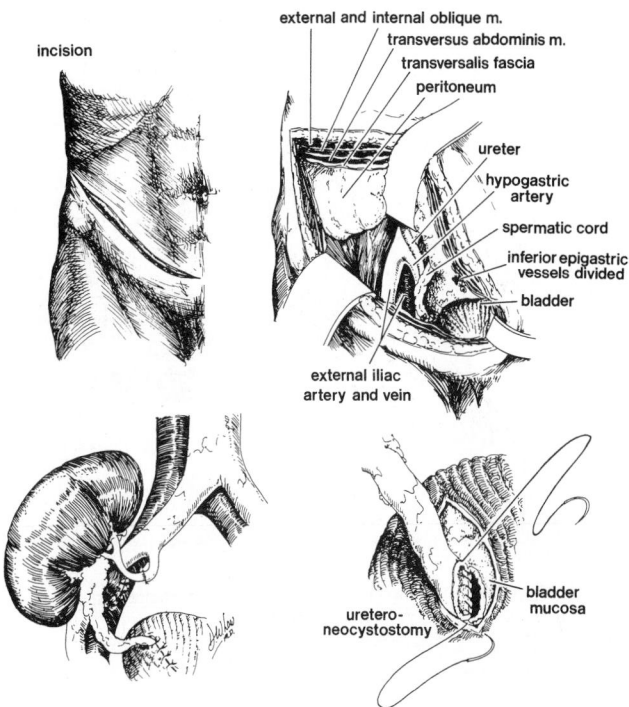

Figure 20–13. The recipient operation is done through a retroperitoneal incision using the iliac vessels to revascularize the kidney and a ureteroneocystostomy to establish urinary continuity.

internal iliac artery has been ligated during a previous transplant operation. Many transplant surgeons routinely favor the end-to-side procedure anyway, because exposure of the external iliac artery requires less dissection and stenosis at the anastomosis may be less likely, especially if a Carrel patch of donor aorta is used (as is usually the case for cadaveric but not living donors).

If there are multiple donor renal arteries that are not on an aortic cuff, the authors favor anastomosis of the end of the smaller renal arteries to the side of the largest renal artery. These anastomoses can be performed deliberately under magnification while the *ex vivo* kidney is protected by immersion in a basin of cold saline (Fig. 20–14). Revascularization in the recipient can then be accomplished rapidly by a single anastomosis. The sacrifice of even small accessory donor renal arteries should be avoided, since occlusion of these end arteries causes renal infarcts. Preservation of accessory arteries to the lower portion of the kidney is especially important, as they may constitute the blood supply of a segment of collecting system or ureter, and their ligation may lead to necrosis and urinary fistula. In 470 living-related donors studied at the University of Pennsylvania, multiple renal arteries were present in one kidney in 30% and bilaterally in 9%.[44] In 42 patients in which the type of *ex vivo* anastomosis described above was performed for multiple arteries, only one kidney was lost due to a technical complication; the 1-year survival of 76% was no different from that of single-artery kidneys in the pre-cyclosporine period. Venous collateral circulation is almost always adequate, so in instances of multiple renal veins (which are even more common than multiple arteries), only one large vein need be saved for anastomosis.

If a large adult kidney is to be transplanted into a small child, a transperitoneal approach is used to provide adequate room for the kidney, which is revascularized via the aorta and vena cava.

Urinary tract continuity is usually established by uretero-

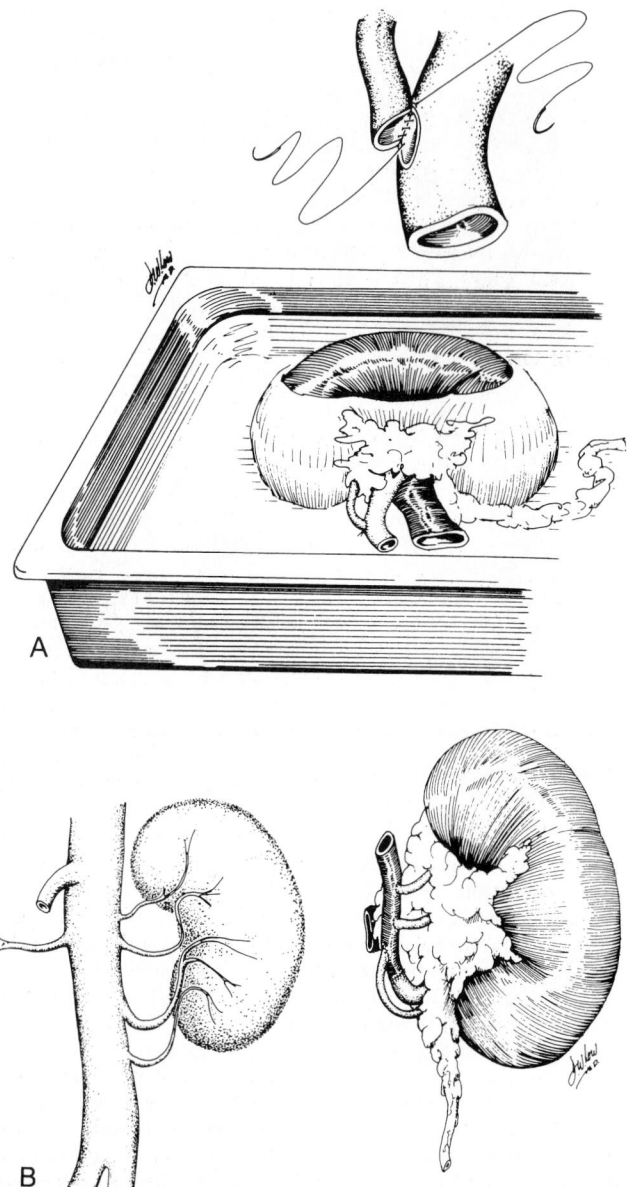

Figure 20–14. *A,* The smaller of two renal arteries is anastomosed to the larger one in an end-to-side manner while the *ex vivo* kidney is protected by submersion in cold (4° C.) electrolyte solution. *B,* With magnification and hypothermic protection, even complex *ex vivo* microvascular reconstructions can be performed safely. This donor kidney had four small renal arteries arising from the aorta. A short segment of autogenous saphenous vein was removed and under *ex vivo* hypothermia each of the four renal arteries was anastomosed separately into the vein. Revascularization in the recipient was then accomplished with only one anastomosis between the end of the saphenous vein graft and the recipient iliac artery.

neocystostomy. The ureter should pass beneath the spermatic cord to avoid obstruction. Ureteropyelostomy (anastomosis of the recipient's ureter to the pelvis of the donor kidney) is an alternative procedure that should be used in instances of transplant ureteral devascularization or injury. A few surgeons prefer this procedure to ureteroneocystostomy, but it is associated with a higher incidence of urinary fistula.

Meticulous technique and hemostasis are particularly important because of the coagulopathy and susceptibility to infection of uremic immunosuppressed patients. The authors prefer to close the wound without drains, but if hemostasis is suboptimal, closed suction catheters may be used.

POSTTRANSPLANT MANAGEMENT

If the transplanted kidney has not suffered ischemic damage, a brisk diuresis is likely to begin within minutes of revascularization. Responsible for the diuresis (which may reach 1000 ml. per hour) are osmotic factors secondary to uremia or high glucose concentrations in intravenous fluids, total body fluid and electrolyte overload secondary to chronic uremia, and mild proximal tubular damage resulting from allograft ischemia. Early in the postoperative period, mild diuresis is reassuring and should be encouraged by replacement of urine volumes and, if necessary, by diuretics. Initial underreplacement of fluid may lead to oliguria or impaired transplant function, interfering with diagnosis of vascular occlusion, urinary obstruction, or early rejection. Severe dehydration can be the outcome of inadequate replacement of losses during a massive diuresis, especially in children. During the first few days, there may also be a need for colloid or blood replacement because of losses into the wound.

Serious problems can also result from overreplacement of volume, especially if the transplant is not producing urine. Hyperkalemia is particularly dangerous in this setting and may necessitate administration of an ion exchange resin (Kayexalate 25 to 50 gm. orally or by enema). In more emergent circumstances, administration of intravenous glucose and insulin or prompt dialysis may be necessary to control hyperkalemia. Suggested replacement fluids include 0.45% saline solution with or without isotonic glucose, sodium bicarbonate (30 mEq per liter), and potassium (10 to 15 mEq per liter), depending on the status of the serum electrolytes and blood glucose. If diuresis continues, fluid replacement should lag behind the urine output, allowing gradual return to normal urine volumes over the next 12 to 24 hours.

Because of the retroperitoneal approach, the transplant operation is relatively nondisruptive to intestinal function, and medications and fluids can usually be given by mouth within 12 to 24 hours. Ambulation on the first postoperative day is beneficial. The Foley catheter can be removed within the first few days. Hypertension, which is common, should be managed conventionally with drugs such as hydralazine, beta-blockers, calcium channel blockers, or angiotensin-converting enzyme inhibitors. Antacids are given to prevent ulcer and nystatin for prophylaxis against monilial infections. Perioperative antibiotics (which should be given for no more than 48 hours) decrease the incidence of wound infection. Trimethoprim and sulfamethoxazole are used routinely by most centers for prophylaxis against urinary tract infections and *Pneumocystis carinii*. If rejection and other postoperative complications do not occur, the subsequent care is relatively simple, since the restoration of renal function is associated with a rapid return to normal health in patients previously suffering from single organ system failure.

Immunosuppression

Azathioprine and Steroids. In the late 1950s, prevention of rejection of human renal allografts was first attempted by whole-body irradiation. Although one irradiated patient retained his allograft for 25 years without ever receiving immunosuppressive drugs, 11 others died from infections due to the profound immunodepression caused by this treatment.[31] In 1959, Schwartz and Dameshek discovered that the antimetabolite 6-mercaptopurine inhibited humoral immunity in rabbits. Shortly thereafter, Calne and Zukowski and their associates found that the drug could prevent kidney allograft rejection in dogs.[31] This drug and its derivative, azathioprine, had more predictable, reversible, and safer action than radiation and were soon used with considerable success in human renal allograft recipients. In 1988, the Nobel

Prize was awarded to Gertrude Elion and George Hitchings for the development of these drugs.

The previously known immunosuppressive effects of adrenal corticosteroids, although not sufficient in themselves to prevent rejection, proved to be synergistic with those of azathioprine. The combination of azathioprine and steroids became standard therapy. Brief intensification of steroid therapy could sometimes abort *rejection crisis,* which usually ensued despite baseline immunosuppression. Thus rejection was recognized to be an episodic and potentially reversible process.[51]

Antilymphocytic Antibodies. In the 1960s, Woodruff, Medawar, Monaco, and others studied a new immunosuppressive agent, antilymphocyte serum (ALS), which was a more potent and more specific immunosuppressant than azathioprine.[65] ALS contained xenoantibody raised by repeated immunization of heterologous animals (e.g., rabbits, horses) with lymphoid cells of the prospective allograft recipient species. In rodents, small doses strikingly reduced the number of circulating lymphocytes and often completely prevented rejection of skin allografts. Although ALS also proved to be a potent immunosuppressant in man, several problems limited its usefulness. Even the purified globulin fraction (antilymphocyte globulin, ALG) of the foreign serum sometimes provoked allergic reactions. The therapeutic window of ALG was quite small, and large doses or prolonged therapy often led to leukopenia, thrombocytopenia, and serious infections, especially of viral origin (e.g., herpes, cytomegalovirus, varicella zoster). In addition, patients formed antibodies to the heterologous protein, further diminishing the feasibility of prolonged or repeated courses. Thus, ALS or ALG could be given for only a limited time, at marginal doses, and only as an adjunct to *conventional* immunosuppressive agents. Some investigators reported that routine prophylactic use of ALS to prevent rejection in the first few postoperative days improved outcomes of renal transplantation, but others were unconvinced of its usefulness as a prophylactic agent. Most randomized studies have failed to show a statistical benefit, and in the most recent UNOS registry analysis of all U.S. kidney transplants from 1988 to 1994, no benefit was found in the prophylactic use of either OKT3 or ALG.[9] However, in individual patients in whom cyclosporine is temporarily contraindicated (e.g., patients with posttransplant acute tubular necrosis [ATN]), these agents are helpful in delaying rejection episodes. ALS has been found to be very effective in reversing rejection crises, even those resistant to high-dose steroid therapy, and this has become its most common indication.[19]

The effectiveness of ALS was the rationale for the introduction by Cosimi and colleagues of monoclonal mouse antihuman anti-T-cell antibodies.[12] Monoclonal anti-T-cell antibodies induce rapid depletion of T lymphocytes from peripheral blood while having little detrimental effect on other populations such as red blood cells, platelets, or granulocytes, all of which are affected by cross-reacting antibodies present in the polyclonal ALG preparation. Because of lesser cost, greater availability, specificity, and standardization of the preparation, monoclonal antibodies such as OKT3 have largely replaced ALS and ALG in many centers. The structure recognized by OKT3, the CD3 antigen, is linked to the T-cell antigen receptor, which is critical for the activation of human T cells. *In vivo* depletion of T cells following exposure to OKT3 is believed to be mediated by mechanisms such as complement-mediated lympholysis or opsonization of cells. In the presence of bound OKT3, the CD3 T-cell receptor complex is internalized by the cell, further rendering the T-cell population inactive. Multi-institutional, randomized prospective trials revealed the efficacy of OKT3 in reversing acute rejection in 94% of cadaveric renal allograft rejections—a figure significantly better than that achieved with steroid treatment.[37]

Side effects associated with OKT3 therapy (particularly the initial doses) include fever, shaking chills, headache, nausea, vomiting, diarrhea, wheezing, and pulmonary edema. These phenomena are probably due to the release of cytokines, especially tumor necrosis factor (TNF), and have been termed the *cytokine release syndrome.* Fortunately, such side effects can often be ameliorated by pretreatment with methylprednisolone, acetaminophen, and antihistamines or, more recently, antibodies against TNF or its receptor. As with polyclonal ALG, the use of monoclonal antibody OKT3 may induce rapid sensitization to mouse antibody, causing the neutralization of OKT3 and the reappearance in the peripheral blood of CD3+ cells. Concomitant administration of azathioprine and steroids may delay the production of anti-OKT3 antibody and prolong its immunosuppressive effect. Beyond return of graft function, *in vivo* efficacy of OKT3 may be monitored by sequential analyses of the CD3+ T-cell populations in the peripheral blood and the circulating level of OKT3 and by measurement of human antibodies to the murine immunoglobulin.

Other monoclonal antibodies have been developed for the prevention or treatment of rejection and are the subject of clinical investigation. These include mouse antihuman monoclonal antibodies directed against the CD4 antigen (T-helper cells), the interleukin-2 (IL-2) receptor, adhesion molecules (e.g., anti-ICAM-1), and the T-cell receptor itself, among others. Also promising is the development of monoclonal antibodies in which the entire protein structure of the antibody molecule is replaced with corresponding human sequences, except for the idiotypic specific region. Such engineered molecules, termed *humanized* antibodies, appear to retain their *in vivo* efficacy for T-cell depletion but may have limited side effects (diminished cytokine release syndrome) and prolonged effectiveness, since their elimination through the development of human antimurine immunity is less.

Cyclosporine. Cyclosporine is credited with revolutionizing transplantation by facilitating successful extrarenal transplants and improving cadaver kidney graft survival by as much as 20%.[22] Some of the improvement in results that occurred in the 1980s was probably attributable to progress in other aspects of transplantation, but cyclosporine was undoubtedly a major factor. Cyclosporine is a fungal derivative first noted by Borel in 1974 to have immunosuppressive qualities. It appears to block T-lymphocyte production of the lymphokine IL-2 through inhibition of the production of its messenger RNA. Like azathioprine but unlike OKT3 and ALS, cyclosporine is most useful for prophylaxis rather than reversal of rejection. Calne, using it for single-drug immunosuppression in 1979, found it to be potent but also quite toxic at higher doses, and its administration was associated with infections, tumors, and renal failure. By reducing the dose of cyclosporine and combining it with small doses of prednisone, Starzl subsequently reported spectacular improvement in the outcome of liver and kidney allografts. Similarly, improved results were confirmed by multicenter randomized studies. After its release for general use in 1983, cyclosporine was adopted by virtually all centers. In 1996, it remains the basis of most immunosuppressive protocols.

Cyclosporine has the major advantage over azathioprine of lacking bone marrow toxicity but the disadvantage of nephrotoxicity, which is its major side effect. Nephrotoxicity may be manifest as a delay in function of a newly transplanted kidney or impairment of function of a well-established renal allograft. Although therapeutic drug monitoring and maintenance of blood levels in the therapeutic range are helpful, they do not eliminate the possibility of nephrotoxicity due to cyclosporine, which may occur even at subtherapeutic levels. Even after prolonged, stable, low-dose cyclo-sporine administration, elevated blood levels of the agent and toxicity may appear, especially during concurrent use of certain drugs (such as erythromycin, cimetidine, diltiazem, and ketoconazole) that increase bioavailability through inhibition of hepatic metabolism. Conversely, decreased blood levels may result from patient noncompliance or interactions with drugs such as phenobarbital, phenytoin, and trimethoprim-sulfamethoxazole, which activate the hepatic P-450 cytochrome system and increase conversion of the parent compound to immunologically less active metabolites. In addition to nephrotoxicity, other side effects attributable to cyclosporine include hypertension, hepatotoxicity, seizures, tremor, hypertrichosis, nausea, vomiting, and diarrhea. Delayed renal allograft function from ischemic damage of cadaveric kidneys may be accentuated by nephrotoxic drugs. Therefore, many centers avoid the use of cyclosporine until delayed function has resolved. A prophylactic course of ALG or OKT3 is advocated by some, along with steroids and azathioprine, to delay rejection until graft function allows institution of cyclosporine therapy. Even without initial ischemic renal damage, patients on cyclosporine tend to have persistently higher serum creatinine levels than azathioprine-treated patients and histologic changes of interstitial fibrosis in the kidney over the long term. Because of uncertainty regarding the risk of permanent renal damage from long-term cyclosporine therapy, most centers use lower doses of cyclosporine in combination with azathioprine and predni-sone (triple therapy). The risks of chronic renal damage appear to be outweighed by the substantial advantages of cyclosporine, including the possibility that in selected cyclosporine-treated patients, steroid therapy could eventually be minimized or completely withdrawn.

A typical cyclosporine-based triple-drug regimen currently used at the University of Pennsylvania calls for intraoperative administration of methylprednisolone (1 gm.) and aza-thioprine (10 mg. per kg.) intravenously (Fig. 20–15). On the first postoperative day, prednisone is begun at 1.5 mg. per kg. per day and tapered to 30 mg. per day by the end of the first week and eventually to a maintenance dose of 10 mg. per day. Azathioprine is rapidly tapered to 1 mg. per kg. per day. Patients whose transplants function promptly receive oral cyclosporine (10 to 14 mg. per kg. per day) on the first postoperative day, and subsequent daily doses are determined by trough levels in whole blood that are maintained at 100 to 200 ngm. per ml. (as determined by high-performance liquid chromatography). This regimen produces a lower incidence of nephrotoxicity than encountered in the early cyclosporine era, when higher doses were utilized without azathioprine.

Patient survival has also been improved by the introduction of cyclosporine, probably because of a decrease in the incidence and severity of infections. Many believe that histocompatibility matching is less important than in the pre-cyclosporine era, although this is controversial.[22] Disappointingly, the impact of cyclosporine on long-term results has not been nearly as favorable as its influence on early outcome. Both U.S. and European multicenter reports indicate a continuing attrition in late graft survival from chronic rejection that is not avoided by cyclosporine. It is even possible that the chronic nephrotoxicity of cyclosporine is additive to the effects of chronic rejection. Despite these shortcomings, the introduction of cyclosporine represented a major advance.

Since the absorption and bioavailability of cyclosporine are variable after oral administration, it is hypothesized that variable or low blood levels of cyclosporine initially after operation or over the long term may precipitate either nephrotoxicity or rejection. A microemulsion formulation of cyclosporine (Neoral) has recently been introduced. Its better

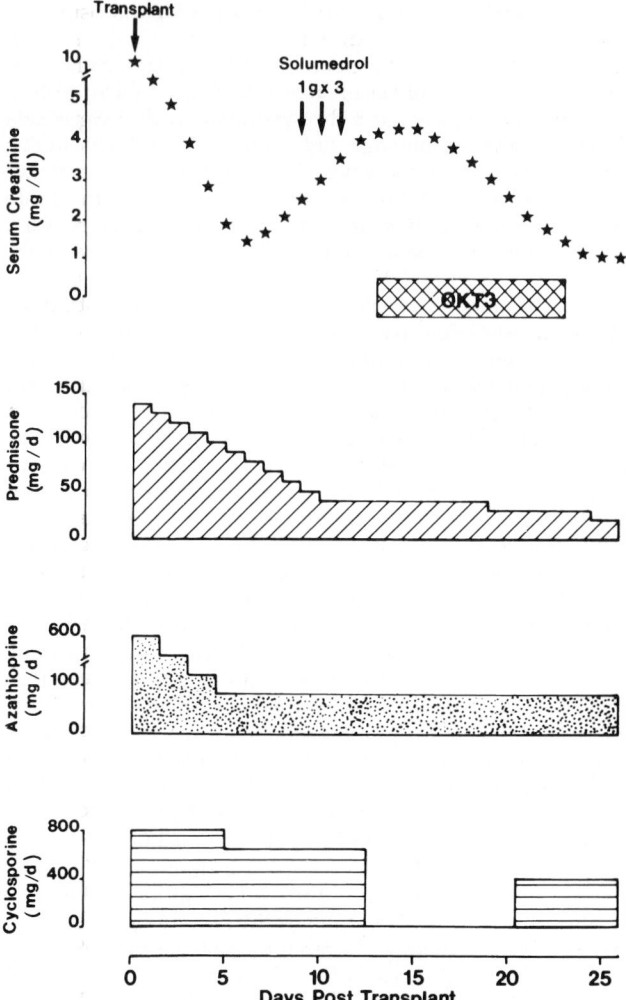

Figure 20–15. Clinical course of a renal allograft recipient under triple-drug immunosuppressive therapy. Rejection was ushered by a rising serum creatinine level that did not improve after high-dose steroid treatment. Because of the steroid-resistant nature of rejection, *rescue* treatment consisting of a 10-day course of monoclonal antibody OKT3 was employed. This was followed by complete resolution of the rejection crisis and a normal creatinine level. Note that cyclosporine was discontinued during OKT3 treatment so that excessive immunosuppression could be avoided.

absorption allows more consistent whole-blood levels, and it is hoped that it will improve the results of cyclosporine therapy.

Tacrolimus (FK 506). Tacrolimus has properties similar but perhaps superior to those of cyclosporine.[21] It was first described by Kino and colleagues in 1987, introduced clinically in the United States at the University of Pittsburgh in 1989, and approved for use in liver transplantation in 1995. It is about 100 times more potent as an anti–T-cell agent than cyclosporine (on a per-mg. basis). It appears to be particularly valuable in its ability to *rescue* grafts observed to be failing on cyclosporine-based immunosuppression. Its adverse effects are similar to those of cyclosporine: nephrotoxicity, neurologic problems (tremor, headache), and diabetes. Although it has not yet been used extensively in kidney transplant patients, the 1994 UNOS report indicates that patients treated with tacrolimus have a statistically better rate of graft survival than patients on any other immunosuppressive protocol.[9]

Mycophenolate Mofetil. Mycophenolate mofetil (MMF), the morpholinoethyl ester of mycophenolic acid (MPA) that *in vivo* is hydrolyzed to free MPA, the active immunosuppressive moiety, is a potent and specific inhibitor of *de novo* purine synthesis. MPA blocks the proliferation of both T and B lymphocytes by virtue of its action in inhibiting *de novo* purine biosynthesis. T and B lymphocytes lack a significant purine biosynthetic salvage pathway activity. MPA is further metabolized by conjugation to form a phenolic glucuronide conjugate (MPAG). MPA has proved promising both in prophylaxis of rejection and in treatment of refractory rejection crisis, which was reversed in about 70% of patients when the drug was used for graft salvage.[50] MMF lacks bone marrow toxicity. Its most common side effects involve the gastrointestinal tract. In 1995, it was approved for prophylaxis of renal rejection following transplantation.

Sirolimus (Rapamycin). Sirolimus, which is structurally similar to tacrolimus, was discovered in a search for novel antifungal agents. It is a macrocyclic triantibiotic produced by *Streptomyces hygroscropicus*, an actinomyces that was isolated from a soil sample collected from Rapa Nui (Easter Island).[23] The immunosuppressive activity of sirolimus is mediated through a mechanism distinct from that of tacrolimus or cyclosporine. The latter two agents inhibit T-cell stimulation through reduction of IL-2 production and IL-2 receptor expression. In contrast, sirolimus has little or no effect on these immunologic events but instead markedly suppresses IL-2- and IL-4-driven T-cell proliferation, thus acting at a later stage of the cell cycle than either cyclosporine or tacrolimus. Whereas cyclosporine and tacrolimus block T-cell activation induced by stimuli employing calcium-dependent pathways in the early G1 phase of the cell cycle, sirolimus inhibits proliferation and response to stimuli that induce calcium-dependent and -independent single-transduction pathways later in the G1 phase. *In vitro* and *in vivo* synergy studies have demonstrated that sirolimus potentiates the action of cyclosporine. Conversely, cyclosporine has been shown to augment the action of sirolimus, suggesting that these agents may be synergistic.

Deoxyspergualin. Deoxyspergualin (DSG) is an antibiotic that was isolated from culture filtrates of *Bacillus laterospores* in 1981. Its immunosuppressive mechanisms are completely different from those of cyclosporine, tacrolimus, MMF, or other conventional immunosuppressive drugs.[32] It does not inhibit the functions of macrophages or helper T cells but does inhibit proliferation and differentiation of cytotoxic T cells and antibody-producing B cells. In rats it prolongs heart, kidney, islet cell, pancreas, and liver graft survival, with only minor toxicity. The inhibitory effect of DSG on B-cell responses may also be applicable in the treatment of autoimmune diseases, in the prevention of rejection in presensitized recipients, and for ABO-incompatible allografts.

The long-term impact of these new agents on human renal allograft survival remains to be tested. It is encouraging, however, that potent new immunosuppressants are now being discovered with frequency, considering that the interval between the introduction of the first useful drug (azathioprine) and the second one (cyclosporine) was almost 25 years.

REJECTION

Considerable effort has been made to correlate allograft morphology with the clinical course of rejection. However, histologic study of a kidney biopsy can never provide more than a narrowly focused *snapshot* of the target of a complex systemic process that is in continuous evolution while also being modified by immunosuppression. Rejection is conveniently categorized as hyperacute, acute, or chronic, but there are overlapping features of and transitions between these categories. The introduction of newer potent immunosup-

pressives has also changed the classic histologic course of rejection. The outcome of an interventional conference in Banff was the proposal of new criteria for the semiquantitative analysis of rejection and the development of standardized nomenclature.[49]

Hyperacute Rejection

In the 1960s, there were several instances in which transplanted kidneys that initially seemed viable were rejected within minutes of revascularization, as evidenced by bluish discoloration of the kidney, deterioration of perfusion, and cessation of function. Histologically, extensive intravascular deposits of fibrin and platelets and intraglomerular accumulation of polymorphonuclear leukocytes, fibrin, platelets, and red blood cells, along with accumulation of polymorphonuclear cells in the peritubular and glomerular capillaries, were seen.[24] This process proved refractory to immunosuppressive or anticoagulant therapy and inevitably led to rapid destruction of the kidney. It soon became evident that the occurrence of hyperacute rejection was usually correlated with the presence of preformed circulating antibodies against donor antigens and that these could be identified by a pretransplant crossmatch. The classic form of hyperacute rejection has become rare, since transplants are no longer performed when the crossmatch is positive.

Acute Cellular Rejection

This type of rejection most commonly becomes evident during the early days or weeks following transplantation, although it occasionally occurs after months or years. The diagnosis of acute rejection is based on a constellation of findings that include clinical signs and symptoms, laboratory assays of blood and urine, radioisotope studies, and allograft biopsies. Classic signs and symptoms are malaise, fever, oliguria, hypertension, and tenderness from swelling of the allograft. However, these symptoms are rarely seen in patients receiving cyclosporine. Under the influence of this agent, rejection takes on a more subtle clinical picture in which fever and allograft swelling are absent and impaired renal function may be the only signal. Under these circumstances, a radioisotopic renal perfusion scan is usually obtained. This test cannot provide specific evidence of rejection but helps exclude several other conditions that can cause impaired renal function, such as vascular occlusion, ureteric obstruction, or urinary fistula.

Since the diagnosis of rejection on clinical grounds alone may be difficult, a biopsy is often performed when rejection is suspected. This procedure can be performed transcutaneously with little risk. Early microscopic signs of acute rejection include the adherence of lymphocytes to the endothelium of peritubular capillaries and venules, which then progresses to disruption of these vessels, tubular necrosis, and interstitial infiltrates. Cellular infiltration, which is the hallmark of rejection, is composed at first of small lymphocytes and later consists of a variety of cells, such as large lymphocytes and macrophages. As rejection proceeds toward irreversibility, there is greater involvement of the vascular elements of the graft. Swelling of the intima and focal fibrinoid necrosis of the media take place, followed by endothelial cell proliferation and obliteration of the lumina of small arteries by fibrin, platelets, and lymphoid cells.

In the Banff schema, glomerular, interstitial, tubular and vascular lesions are graded 0 to 3+, depending on whether they are absent (0), mild (1), moderate (2), or severe (3). Total reliance cannot be placed in a biopsy as the gold standard for diagnosing acute rejection. Not only are biopsies subject to sampling error, but lymphocytic infiltration in itself cannot be taken as conclusive evidence of rejection, since, for obscure reasons, even perfectly functioning renal allografts may exhibit some degree of mononuclear infiltration.

Distinguishing impairment of renal function due to rejection from cyclosporine nephrotoxicity is a challenging problem. Some authorities believe that biopsies can discriminate between these two entities, but others do not.[63] In cyclosporine nephrotoxic states, variable degrees of lymphocytic infiltration in the interstitium of the kidney have been observed. Careful attention to trends and fluctuations of cyclosporine blood levels may aid in decision making. Cyclosporine nephrotoxicity characteristically causes smaller increments in serum creatinine than rejection, and these are usually reversible within a few days following dose reduction. Arteriolar hyalinosis is another factor considered in the Banff criteria, since this is thought to be a feature of cyclosporine toxicity.

A particularly challenging clinical problem is the diagnosis of rejection in the setting of ATN. Under this circumstance, a biopsy may be the only aid to diagnosis. Unfortunately, however, even a skilled pathologist cannot always distinguish the histologic picture of rejection from that of ATN (or cyclosporine toxicity). Therefore, enthusiasm for repeated biopsies varies; some transplant surgeons are content in most instances to rely on their clinical judgment. At times, empiric antirejection therapy is employed as a diagnostic test for suspected rejection. In the presence of acute rejection (and the absence of ATN), this usually lowers the creatinine promptly.

When the diagnosis of acute rejection is made, prompt institution of antirejection therapy (steroids, ALS, OKT3) is necessary to prevent permanent damage to the allograft. This treatment is usually capable of reversing the process, although it may recur. Intravenous high-dose steroids (0.5 to 1.0 gm. methylprednisolone) are used as first-line therapy for rejection at most centers. About 65% of acute rejections usually respond to three to five doses. Steroid-resistant rejection may respond to ALG or OKT3 in an additional 30% of cases. Currently under intensive study is the possibility that rejection that is refractory to both steroid and antilymphocyte antibody therapy might still respond to treatment with newer agents such as tacrolimus or MMF.

It is important that antirejection therapy not be employed needlessly or for a prolonged period, since this is the cause of most morbidity and mortality. During the 1970s (prior to the introduction of cyclosporine), a progressive improvement in patient survival took place in most centers. This was probably the result of the realization that overly intense immunosuppression and repeated courses of antirejection therapy were unwise and dangerous and that better long-term results could be accomplished by more conservative therapy. Many groups adopted the policy of refusing to treat aggressively more than two episodes of acute rejection. Experience taught the important lesson that eventual loss of some grafts could not be avoided. Early recognition and acceptance of this eventuality, transplant nephrectomy, reinstitution of dialysis, and the chance of a later successful transplant were obviously preferable to pushing heavy immunosuppression to the point of serious infection and death. Employment of this philosophy has allowed us to reduce the 1-year mortality of cadaveric transplantation to less than 5% at the University of Pennsylvania.

Immunologic Monitoring

Because the clinical diagnosis of rejection is so frequently uncertain, attempts have been made to find an *in vitro* method of evaluating the recipient's response to the allograft as an early marker or even a predictor of rejection. Two types of assays have been used: those defining the level of specific antidonor activity, and those reflecting the general level of immunosuppression and thus presumably the risk of rejection. Assays of cellular and humoral immunity to donor antigens such as mixed lymphocyte reactions, donor-specific cytotoxic T lymphocytes, antibody-dependent cellular cytotoxicity, complement-dependent cytotoxicity, and donor-specific anti-B-cell antibodies have been evaluated, but none is reliably correlated with early rejection. Enthusiasm has also declined for utilizing T-lymphocyte subset ratios as an index of adequate immunosuppression or impending rejection. Unfortunately, a number of confounding factors, such as generalized lymphopenia and lymphocyte subset variations associated with bacterial and viral infections, limit the specificity and usefulness of such assays. Study of the phenotypic composition of the interstitial cellular infiltrate obtained directly from the allograft by means of fine-needle aspiration, although advocated by some authors, has also failed to gain popularity.

Chronic Rejection

The border between acute and chronic rejection is not always sharply defined, but the typical course of chronic rejection is gradual, progressive loss of renal function. It may begin after years of stable function but is more often seen in patients who have had multiple early and incompletely reversible episodes of acute rejection. Humoral injury (thought to be a more important factor in this condition than in acute cellular rejection) is manifested histologically by intimal fibroproliferative arterial lesions, which probably stem from repetitive cycles of immune injury to the endothelium, with focal thrombosis and incorporation of thrombus into the arterial wall. Also seen in chronic rejection are glomerular changes. Histologically, increased mesangial matrix and mesangial proliferation are seen. The glomerular basement membrane is thickened, and focal deposition of IgM, IgG, and complement may be identified along capillary walls and within the mesangium. Clinically, these are manifested by proteinuria, microscopic hematuria, and slowly deteriorating function. As with acute rejection, a semiquantitative analysis for assessing chronic rejection has been proposed under the Banff schema.[49]

In the presence of these morphologic vascular and glomerular changes, antirejection therapy is ineffective. Employment of high-dose steroid or ALS or OKT3 therapy in the hope of reversing the process should not be risked, since this will be of no benefit and may lead to opportunistic infection or other serious sequelae. An abrupt cessation of immunosuppression is also unwarranted early in the course of chronic rejection, since its progression may be slow, and significant periods of useful though diminishing transplant function are possible. However, immunosuppression should generally be reduced as renal failure progresses, since the additive immunodepressive effects of uremia and immunosuppressive drugs are particularly dangerous.

It is important to remember that acute cellular rejection is also occasionally encountered after years of stable transplant function, sometimes as the result of discontinuation of immunosuppression by a careless or noncompliant patient. This must be distinguished from chronic rejection, if possible, although a timely diagnosis of late acute rejection is usually fortuitous, since symptoms are uncommon. A prompt biopsy is warranted in cases of unexpected or precipitous deterioration in stable function, since late cellular rejection (unlike chronic rejection) can often be reversed if treated before severe damage occurs.

RECURRENT DISEASE IN TRANSPLANTED KIDNEYS

Since transplantation does not modify the underlying etiology of the renal disease, it is not surprising that the transplanted kidney is sometimes regarded by the host as an appropriate new target for destruction by the original disease process, especially in autoimmune or metabolic diseases.

Glomerulonephritis

In his earliest identical twin donor transplants, Murray recognized recurrent glomerulonephritic damage, which sometimes became apparent within only a few months. Late follow-up of 30 twin grafts indicated that 8 had failed from recurrent glomerulonephritis, making a strong case for the use of mild immunosuppression even in recipients of twin grafts.[62] Fortunately, recurrent disease is less common in allografts, but in this setting it is more difficult to diagnose, since its clinical manifestations and even histologic changes may be confused with those of chronic rejection. Recurrence occurs more commonly in glomerular than interstitial renal diseases, although glomerular damage of allografts is still much more likely to result from rejection than from recurrent disease. Recurrent disease is most likely in patients whose original disease process ran a rapid course. Recurrence appears to be most likely in twins and next most likely in recipients of closely matched related donor allografts.

In patients with glomerulonephritis, the incidence and severity of recurrence vary with the particular variety of glomerulonephritis.[28] For example, membranous nephropathy recurs in 10% of transplants. Type II mesangiocapillary glomerulonephritis can be expected to recur in 95%, and Henoch-Schönlein purpura recurs in 80%. However, the graft loss from recurrent glomerulonephritis appears to be quite low (2 to 4%), at least for the first several years. Thus the risk of recurrence is rarely a contraindication to transplantation, although the very long-term impact is not fully known at this time.

Collagen Diseases

Collagen diseases such as lupus erythematosus are possible but unlikely causes of recurrent damage and are often well palliated by transplantation.

Metabolic Diseases

Cystinosis causes intracellular deposition of cysteine crystals in various organs, usually leading to end-stage renal disease by age 10. Although recurrent renal deposition may occur after transplantation, its effects appear to be mild.

Oxalosis is likely to reappear and destroy transplanted kidneys very rapidly, although these changes may be delayed by prolonged pretransplant dialysis and posttransplant diuresis. However, hepatic transplantation that reverses the metabolic defect and concomitant renal transplantation is the ideal treatment, especially in patients with renal and other systemic oxalate damage.[64]

Diabetes, when it causes end-stage nephropathy, has become one of the most common indications for renal transplantation. Diabetic nephropathy is thought to be caused by protracted abnormal glucose homeostasis, which, of course, is not corrected by successful renal transplantation. Thus, in diabetic patients, it is not surprising that Kimmelstiel-Wilson lesions may be found on biopsies of the transplanted kidney within 2 years. However, since 10 to 20 years are probably required for these changes to cause functional deterioration, the threat of recurrence is certainly not a contraindication to renal transplantation, which gives diabetics a better chance of survival than does chronic dialysis. Successful pancreatic transplantation, if performed concomitantly with renal transplantation, prevents the early morphologic changes of diabetes in the transplanted kidney.[8]

COMPLICATIONS OF RENAL TRANSPLANTATION
Technical Complications

Complications occurring in the first few hours or days after transplantation are commonly related to technical problems in establishing vascular and urinary continuity or to damage that occurs during donor nephrectomy or preservation. Since rejection may also be an early event, its differentiation from various other causes of poor function may be difficult.

Vascular Complications. Arterial obstruction, although less common than ATN or urinary tract complications as a cause of early postoperative oliguria or anuria, should be considered promptly if an established diuresis suddenly ceases. A diseased hypogastric artery may thrombose and should never be used to vascularize the transplant. Instead, the usually more normal common or external iliac artery should be utilized. Partial occlusion of the transplant vessels may be caused by kinking from unfortunate positioning of the kidney. Although radioisotopic scanning and arteriography confirm suspected vascular occlusion, immediate reoperation without delay for diagnostic studies is usually the only chance for salvaging such a graft, since only a few minutes of total ischemia can be tolerated before damage becomes irreversible.

Hemorrhage. Imperfect operative hemostasis in the setting of uremic coagulopathy or anticoagulation during hemodialysis is the usual cause of early postoperative bleeding. Fracture or frank rupture of the transplanted kidney is an unusual cause of bleeding but may occur from rapid swelling of the transplant during acute rejection. Rupture is more common in kidneys from infant or child donors, in which the small organ is sometimes unable to tolerate adult levels of blood pressure and flow.

Bleeding from the arterial suture line, except in the early hours postoperatively, should bring to mind the strong possibility of infection. Resuturing of an infected suture line is futile, since recurrent disruption is virtually assured. The kidney should be removed, and the hypogastric artery securely ligated. If the anastomosis is in the common or external iliac artery, the problem is more serious. Even removal of the kidney necessitates a suture line to close the iliac arteriotomy. This then becomes a potential site of arterial disruption. Ligation of the iliac artery and extra-anatomic bypass (femorofemoral or axillofemoral) may be necessary.

Hypertension and Renal Transplant Artery Stenosis (RTAS). More than half of renal transplant recipients are hypertensive. Impaired allograft function, cyclosporine, and steroids are the major causes. In about 10%, the native kidneys may be the source, and alleviation can be accomplished by nephrectomy. A source of hypertension that is important to diagnose is renal transplant artery stenosis. This condition may be confused with rejection, since both may result in hypertension and diminished renal function. Although RTAS is a relatively unusual cause of decreased renal function (it is more commonly the result of rejection or cyclosporine toxicity), a high index of suspicion should be maintained, since it is correctable. Patients usually present with symptoms between 3 months and 2 years after transplant (peak, 6 months). The true incidence of RTAS is not known, but in patients suspected on clinical grounds of having RTAS, confirmation of the diagnosis by biplanar arteriography occurs in 4 to 12%. However, when 100 consecutive transplant patients were subjected to routine postoperative arteriography by Lacombe, a surprising prevalence of stenosis was found (23%).[25]

The etiology of RTAS is frequently technical, including improper anastomosis, injury of the intima of the renal artery during washout or perfusion, or kinking at the anastomotic site from redundancy or twisting of the arteries. Arteriosclerotic lesions of the donor or recipient vessels may be a contributing factor, especially as the donor shortage has mandated the use of older donors. An immunologic pathogenesis also seems likely, since intimal proliferation and subintimal fibrotic changes seen in RTAS are similar to small vessel changes caused by rejection. About 70% of the lesions are at the anastomotic site, but 20% are beyond the anastomosis in the transplant renal artery proper. Thus, even the use of a Carrel patch does not preclude this complication.

Fortunately, not all instances of RTAS are clinically relevant. Since the incidence of at least mild hypertension is as high as 50% in transplant patients, RTAS is by no means always its cause. Thus its correction cannot always be expected to be followed by normotension. A cautious trial of angiotensin-converting enzyme inhibitors may be useful in identifying those patients whose hypertension will respond to correction of the stenosis, since these patients often respond to these drugs with a sudden rise in creatinine and a dramatic fall in blood pressure.

Percutaneous transluminal angioplasty (PTA) is currently advocated in most instances of RTAS. Of 547 consecutive renal allograft recipients, 39 suspected of having RTAS because of refractory hypertension had the diagnosis confirmed by arteriography and underwent balloon dilatation.[15] Seventy-six percent of PTAs were successful, and only one graft was lost as a result. Three patients who were initially treated successfully developed recurrent stenosis, which was corrected operatively by patch angioplasty. Other groups have reported poorer initial success (58%) and high recurrence (16%).[43] Although some authors favor operation over PTA, surgical treatment is difficult and not always successful. In seven instances of RTAS in 369 renal grafts, operative treatment was successful in only four patients. Others have reported successful surgical treatment in 33 to 72% of cases. The long-term results of PTA and operation are probably roughly comparable, but because of its simplicity and patient acceptability, most surgeons advocate PTA as the initial approach, with operations reserved for persistent or recurrent stenosis.[13]

Venous Thrombosis. Occlusion of the transplant renal vein, although rare, can result from technical anastomotic errors or from kinking or compression. Iliofemoral thrombosis occasionally follows renal transplantation, presumably because of clamping of the vein or compression by the transplant. The thrombus rarely extends into the renal vein, and standard anticoagulant treatment is generally effective. In a few cases, therapy with urokinase has been successfully employed to lyse clots occluding the renal vein. If pulmonary embolus occurs despite adequate anticoagulation, caval interruption should be performed by standard techniques, such as a Greenfield filter, and rarely compromises transplant function.

Urinary Tract Complications. The most common cause of sudden cessation of urinary output in the immediate postoperative period is presence of a blood clot in the bladder or urethral catheter, which can be relieved by irrigation. Other more serious causes of urinary obstruction are unusual (2 to 5% in most series) and should be investigated simultaneously, with consideration of vascular occlusion, ATN, or rejection.[26] A ureteroneocystostomy may become occluded by a hematoma at the site of the submucosal tunnel in the bladder or by a technically unsatisfactory anastomosis. An adynamic ureter, or edema at the orifice in the bladder, can also cause temporary partial obstruction.

Devascularization of the ureter during donor nephrectomy is a more serious problem, which may lead to ureteral necrosis and fistula within the first few days or weeks. Mild ureteral ischemia is the probable cause of an occasional late distal ureteral stenosis, which may lead to partial or total occlusion (Fig. 20–16). Fluid obtained from wound drains or needle aspiration can be identified as urine by its urea content, which is several-fold higher than that of serum or lymph. Ultrasonography studies for fluid collections, radioactive scans, and cystograms (which, via reflux, may visualize the ureter) are also helpful. However, ureterography is usually necessary to define the status of the ureter and is best accomplished by percutaneous fine-needle puncture of the kidney and antegrade catheterization of the pelvis and ureter. Treatment must be individualized and may consist of either reconstruction of the ureteroneocystostomy (if it is not ischemic) or ureteropyelostomy using the patient's own ureter.

Acute Tubular Necrosis. Ischemia occasionally precipitates ATN in a related-donor transplant, but in cadaver transplants, the incidence is much higher. Despite the fact that almost all such kidneys are from heart-beating cadavers, ATN occurs in 5 to 30%. Therefore, in the absence of vascular or ureteral problems, initially nonfunctional cadaver kidneys may be assumed to suffer from ATN, especially if ^{131}I-technetium and iodohippurate scans demonstrate good blood flow and poor tubular function. At times, however, a kidney has adequate urine output briefly and then lapses into ATN. Estimating the true output of the transplanted kidney may be difficult if the patient's own kidneys are producing substantial amounts of urine.

Oliguria in the early transplant period should be treated with aliquots of fluid and colloid to exclude hypovolemia, while care is taken not to fluid overload the patient. Mannitol 12.5 to 25 gm. and furosemide 100 to 200 mg. intravenously in divided doses may be used to increase the output but are unlikely to alter the course of true ATN. The impact of ATN is definitely an adverse one. The latest UNOS registry indicates that grafts exhibiting delayed function have at least 10% less survival after 1 year than those that function promptly (Fig. 20–17).[9] Some kidneys that never produce urine (termed *primary nonfunction*) are no doubt lost because potentially reversible damage from ATN is compounded by undiagnosed rejection before function returns, with the result that antirejection therapy is delayed until immunologic dam-

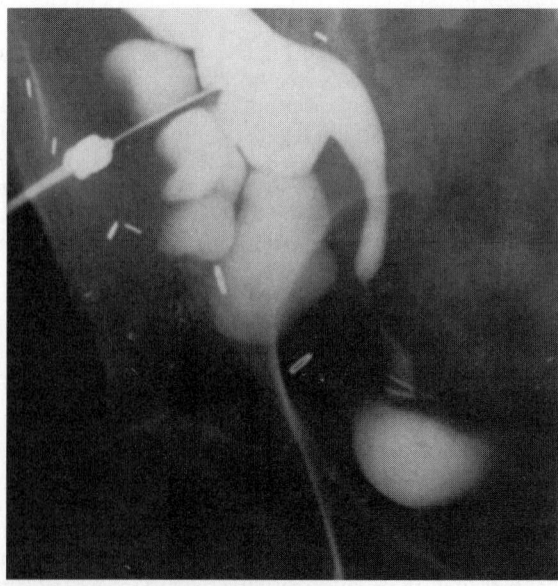

Figure 20–16. An antegrade percutaneous pyelogram of a renal allograft demonstrating obstruction of the distal ureter as it enters the bladder. Calyces are widely dilated and clubbed. (Courtesy of Mark Banner, M.D., Department of Radiology, University of Pennsylvania, Philadelphia.)

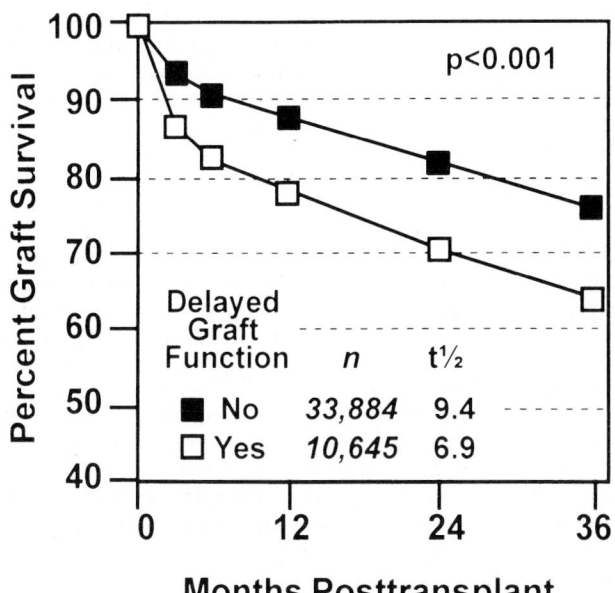

Figure 20–17. The substantial impact of delayed renal transplant function is depicted. This may be the result of difficulty in diagnosing and delay in treating rejection because of posttransplantation acute tubular necrosis. It is one of the arguments against extended periods of preservation necessitated by sharing with distant centers. (From Cecka, J. M., and Terasaki, P. I.: The UNOS scientific registry. *In* Terasaki, P. I., and Cecka, J. M. [Eds.]: Clinical Transplants. Los Angeles, UCLA Tissue Typing Laboratory, 1994.)

age progresses to an irreversible stage. In an attempt to avoid this sequence, many authors employ ALG or monoclonal anti-T-cell antibodies prophylactically in all instances of ATN. Since there is no specific treatment for ATN, the return of function (usually within 1 to 4 weeks) must be patiently awaited while adequate but safe immunosuppression and good general condition are maintained, if necessary, by dialysis. If there is reasonable clinical confidence in the diagnosis of ATN, it is best to minimize the use of invasive studies such as cystoscopy, arteriography, or biopsy, none of which will provide positive evidence of ATN. Serial renal scans to identify decreases in blood flow may be helpful in making the difficult diagnosis of rejection during ATN, but biopsy is often necessary for confirmation. Even in the absence of rejection, management of immunosuppression is difficult during ATN. The nephrotoxic potential of cyclosporine is particularly disturbing when renal function cannot be assessed. Blood levels of this agent should be carefully monitored during ATN. Many centers avoid cyclosporine entirely during ATN because of the additive damage of ischemia and cyclosporine toxicity.

Lymphoceles. Extensive mobilization of the iliac vessels during the transplant operation or failure to ligate lymphatics crossing them may predispose to lymphoceles, which have a variable reported incidence (0.6 to 18%). Possible manifestations that can occur weeks or months postoperatively are swelling of the wound; edema of the scrotum, labia, and lower extremity; and urinary obstruction due to pressure on the collecting system or ureter. Ultrasonography to identify a fluid-filled mass is the most useful diagnostic study. Aspiration of the cyst is of only temporary benefit, since lymph rapidly reaccumulates. External drainage should be avoided, since this places the kidney and vascular suture line at risk from infection. The treatment of choice is fenestration of the cyst into the peritoneal cavity. This can often be accomplished by laparoscopic technique. Another nonoperative treatment is percutaneous drainage followed by repeated instillation of tetracycline or povidone-iodine to sclerose and obliterate the cyst.

Nontechnical Complications

Infections. Factors predisposing to infection in transplant recipients include a major surgical operation involving the urinary tract, infection carried over from the donor, and indwelling catheters in the bladder, bloodstream, and peritoneal cavity. Because of these and the immunodepression associated with uremia and antirejection therapy, 30 to 60% of patients suffer some type of infection during the first transplant year; in half of the deaths that occur during the first year, infection is an important contributing feature. More cautious use of immunosuppression over the last decade and the recent introduction of cyclosporine have reduced the magnitude of this problem, but infection remains the most common and most lethal complication of renal transplantation.

Bacterial Infections. During the first month after transplant, conventional bacterial infections are the most common, and the urinary tract, respiratory system, and wound are the most prevalent sites. These infections usually respond to prompt vigouous conventional antibiotic therapy. Acute bacterial infections may have a clinical presentation that can be confused with rejection, including fever, malaise, swelling and tenderness of the wound, or even rising creatinine in the case of a urinary tract infection. It is especially important to exclude the possibility of infection prior to antirejection therapy, since during infection, immunosuppression should be decreased rather than intensified, even though this action may lead to acute rejection. The incidence of wound infections (reported to be anywhere from 1 to 10%) can probably be reduced by pre- or intraoperative prophylaxis with a cephalosporin, which should not be continued for more than 24 to 48 hours. Even more important, however, is meticulous surgical technique to avoid hematoma, urinary fistula, and lymphocele. Transplant recipients are subject to the usual respiratory infections that occur in normal or hospitalized individuals, and acute bacterial pneumonitis is a potentially lethal infection in these patients. The incidence of urinary tract infections, which are the most common bacterial infections in transplant recipients, can be decreased by 50% by using trimethoprim-sulfa antibiotics for the first 6 months after transplantation. This is also helpful in decreasing the incidence of *Pneumocystis carinii*.

Opportunistic Infections. The period 30 to 180 days after transplant, usually the time of the most intense immunosuppression, is also the most common for infection with opportunistic organisms, which rarely cause significant illness in normal individuals. In recent years, it has become evident that viral infections are even more important than bacterial ones in this regard in terms of prevalence, diagnostic and therapeutic difficulty, and immunologic and neoplastic ramifications. This epidemiologic change is probably due to cyclosporine therapy, which allows lower doses of azathioprine and steroids and has decreased the incidence of bacterial infections. At the same time, the use of antibodies against T lymphocytes, which cause seriously impaired antiviral defenses, has increased.

Cytomegalovirus (CMV), a member of the herpes family, is the most important viral pathogen. This ubiquitous agent infects most normal people at some point in their lives. Although CMV infections are either clinically silent or mild in healthy individuals, the presence of the latent virus and seropositivity persist for life. Following renal transplantation, previously seropositive patients usually excrete CMV and exhibit elevations of antibody titer, on the basis of either reactivation of latent virus during immunosuppression or transmission of virus latent in the donor tissues. Under these circumstances, symptomatic illness sometimes occurs (20%) and is usually mild, supporting the hypothesis that previous exposure and immunity to the virus confer protection.[45] However, seronegative recipients who receive a kidney from a seropositive donor are subject to a three times greater incidence of symptomatic illness; of affected patients, one fourth have severe disease. CMV disease (as distinguished from asymptomatic seroconversion) varies in severity from mild fever and malaise to a debilitating syndrome marked by leukopenia, hepatitis, interstitial pneumonia, arthritis, central nervous system changes, including coma, gastrointestinal ulceration and bleeding, renal insufficiency, bacterial or fungal infection, and even death.

Distinguishing CMV disease, which usually has its onset 4 to 6 weeks after transplant, from rejection can be especially difficult, since the viral infection can cause renal insufficiency. Seroconversion may not occur for an additional 3 to 6 weeks, and viral cultures consume several weeks. A diagnosis can be made in 48 hours by an indirect immunofluorescence test utilizing a monoclonal antibody directed at an early CMV antigen. Possible causes of renal malfunction during CMV infections include direct damage from the virus (glomerulopathy) and triggering of rejection.[45] This is a dilemma, since delay in institution of antirejection therapy may lead to irreversible renal damage, but intensification of immunosuppression may lead to lethal superinfection. In cases of decreasing renal function, a decision for or against antirejection therapy must often be based on clinical grounds, but biopsy should probably be done first if CMV is suspected, since it may distinguish rejection from CMV.

Since CMV disease has an adverse impact on morbidity, mortality, and graft loss, it is important to find ways of avoiding it. One obvious partial solution would be to avoid transplantation of all kidneys from seropositive donors to seronegative recipients. Although this might substantially improve graft survival as well as avoid morbidity in seronegative recipients, it would have the disadvantage of greatly reducing the donor pool for seronegative recipients, since most adult donors are CMV seropositive. Another possibility would be active immunization for CMV, since the most severe disease occurs in seronegative recipients. A live attenuated CMV vaccine was developed that, although not totally preventing infection after transplantation, strikingly reduced the incidence of symptomatic and severe illness.[42] However, it is not available commercially. Passive immunization with immune globulin has, however, proved similarly effective in decreasing the severity of CMV disease.[48]

Fortunately, both the incidence and the severity of CMV disease appear to be diminished in cyclosporine-treated patients. There is impressive evidence that prophylactic acyclovir decreases the incidence of CMV, although prolonged administration of large doses is necessary.[4] In established CMV disease, neither adenine arabinoside nor acyclovir has been effective, although both, and especially the latter agent, are effective for herpes zoster and herpes simplex. Recently, it has been demonstrated that ganciclovir (DHPG) is quite effective, even in established severe CMV infections;[47] it has also been used effectively in prophylaxis. However, it must be given intravenously, making its use in outpatients inconvenient.

Other opportunistic infections such as aspergillosis, blastomycosis, nocardiosis, toxoplasmosis, and cryptococcosis are particularly likely to occur in transplant patients. The protozoan Pneumocystis carinii, which has infected most individuals by age 10, is a pulmonary pathogen only in immunodepressed patients. It is the organism most commonly causing fatal pneumonia in this group. A prompt diagnosis by aggressive measures, such as bronchoscopic alveolar lavage and brushing or percutaneous transbronchoscopic or open lung biopsy, is important in cases of Pneumocystis, since effective treatment exists (trimethoprim and sulfamethoxazole). Pro-

phylaxis with the same agents is warranted in the early postoperative period and also reduces the incidence of bacterial urinary tract infections. Mycobacterial infections are unusual, but their potential lethality mandates constant vigilance.

Hyperglycemia. For reasons not entirely clear but generally attributed to intensive or persistent steroid administration, previously normoglycemic patients may become diabetic in the posttransplant period. Uncontrolled hyperglycemia may cause pseudorejection on the basis of interference with the laboratory determination for creatinine and increased serum osmolality, with resultant intra- and extracellular dehydration and impaired renal function. In this condition, control of the blood glucose promptly corrects the elevated creatinine.

Gastrointestinal Complications. Ulceration and perforation of the stomach, duodenum, and small and large intestine are relatively common following transplantation. The colon is especially vulnerable to ischemia and perforation, and in immunosuppressed patients, abdominal pain or signs of peritoneal irritation merit very close attention, if not immediate laparotomy.[39] Pancreatitis is also a recognized complication of both azathioprine and steroid therapy in transplant patients, in whom its course is frequently fulminating and fatal. Infectious gastrointestinal complications such as Candida stomatitis and esophagitis, pseudomembranous colitis, and CMV ulceration are also common. Symptoms and signs of these conditions may be masked by steroid therapy.

Hyperparathyroidism. Secondary hyperparathyroidism from chronic renal failure usually subsides after a successful transplant. However, its persistence (tertiary hyperparathyroidism) has been reported in 2.6 to 70% of patients, with the smaller number being closer to the true incidence. In cases in which significant hypercalcemia and elevated parathyroid hormone levels persist for more than 12 months after transplant despite normal renal function, the recommendation is total parathyroidectomy and autotransplantation of fragments from a portion of one gland into the muscle of the forearm, where they are easily accessible for further resection without neck exploration, should hypertrophy persist and recurrent hypercalcemia ensue. The sequelae of hyperparathyroidism, such as renal calculi, bone pain, and muscle weakness, are usually benefited by this procedure. In some unfortunate patients, a devastating complication of persistent hyperparathyroidism occurs, in which diffuse cutaneous vascular calcification leads to extensive ulceration and gangrene.[40] Despite total parathyroidectomy, most such patients never heal their ischemic ulcers, which eventually lead to sepsis and death. Common to these patients is persistent posttransplant elevation of serum calcium and radiographic evidence on xerography of extensive small and medium vessel calcification. Fortunately, this complication is uncommon, but in a patient with nonhealing ulceration in unusual areas such as the upper extremities, elevation of serum calcium, and increased parathyroid hormone levels, this diagnosis should be entertained.

Tumors. In the early days of transplantation, it was found that utilization of apparently uninvolved kidneys from donors with known cancer sometimes resulted in transmission of the malignancy. Since then, in occasional instances, tumors have inadvertently been transplanted from donors with unrecognized cancer. If this complication is recognized early, cessation of immunosuppression is sometimes followed by rejection of not only the transplanted kidney but also the allogeneic tumor. However, once the transplanted tumor becomes well established, it may continue to flourish and cause death, even in the absence of immunosuppression.

It has been known for many years that both naturally occurring and iatrogenic states of immune deficiency are accompanied by an increased risk of neoplasia. In renal transplant recipients, the reported incidence of 6% *de novo* malignant neoplasms represents a risk approximately 100 times greater than that in normal age-matched populations.[38] The increased incidence of tumors appears to be related to the degree of immunosuppression rather than to any particular agent. The incidence of tumor increases with the posttransplant duration, but the age of onset is unusually young, and the behavior of the malignancies is unusually aggressive. Cancers common in the general population (lung, breast, prostate, and colon) are not increased, but several uncommon neoplasms are extremely prevalent (lymphoma, lip cancer, Kaposi's sarcoma, carcinoma of the vulva and perineum). Carcinoma of the uterine cervix is also very common, although most of these are *in situ* lesions.

The most common tumors are squamous cell carcinomas of skin and lip, which are especially prevalent in sunny areas such as Australia and New Zealand, where their incidence is increased 21-fold. Patients from these countries who survive 15 years after transplantation have a striking 44% incidence of skin cancer. These cancers kill 5.1% of their victims.

Transplant recipients in all parts of the world have a disproportionately high incidence of lymphoma (350 times normal), which constitutes 20% of all tumors in this population. Extranodal involvement is unusually common (69%), and the transplanted kidney is often involved (23%). Twenty-two percent of these tumors are in the central nervous system—an unusual site for lymphoma. One hypothesis invoked to explain the prevalence of malignancies in immunosuppressed patients is a breakdown of normal immunologic surveillance mechanisms, which allows persistence of mutant malignant cells that would be recognized and destroyed by an intact immune system. It is theorized that such *forbidden clones* are particularly likely to go unrecognized in the brain, an immunologically privileged site. Other etiologic possibilities for the increased neoplasia are chronic immunologic stimulation of the lymphoreticular system by the transplant, direct carcinogenic action of immunosuppressive drugs, and oncogenesis by the viral pathogens whose growth is encouraged by immunosuppression. The latter possibility is supported by the finding that tumors in which a viral pathogenesis seems likely (lymphoma and skin, lip, and uterine cervix cancers) are especially prevalent in transplant patients.

De novo lymphomas may begin as lymphoproliferative lesions induced by viruses. Compelling evidence of this is the finding of Epstein-Barr virus (EBV) incorporated into the genome of lymphoma cells. These patients often have a syndrome resembling mononucleosis, with fever, pharyngitis, and diffuse lymphadenopathy. Polyclonal B-cell proliferation rather than true malignancy is the finding in these early lesions of a diversity of cellular immunoglobulins.[18] During the stage of polyclonality, cessation of immunosuppression may allow regression of the lesions. The use of the antiviral agent acyclovir, which blocks EBV-inhibited oropharyngeal shedding of the virus, has also been reported to contribute to remissions. Tumors that are initially polyclonal may eventually undergo a cytogenetic alteration, leading to malignant transformation and the monoclonality that is characteristic of true B-cell lymphomas. Monoclonal tumors do not regress following cessation of immunosuppression or acyclovir therapy. They are aggressive malignancies that can be treated only by surgical excision and irradiation, neither of which is very effective.

RESULTS OF RENAL TRANSPLANTATION

The outcome of each renal transplant depends on a number of complex and interrelated variables, the importance of which has been the subject of sometimes contradictory reports from individual centers. The cumulative influence of these variables is now analyzed annually by the UNOS Scientific Registry, which regularly receives data on all transplants performed in the United States. Since rejection is the chief deterrent to success, it is not surprising that histocompatibility has been the most consistently influential factor. This was clear from the earliest days of transplantation, when the success of HLA-identical sibling donor grafts was noted to be twice that of cadaveric transplants. Since then, the short-term results of cadaveric grafts have improved greatly and approach the success of HLA-identical sibling grafts at 1 year (84 versus 95%). However, when long-term survival is examined, the importance of histocompatibility remains obvious (Fig. 20–18). Even with the striking advances in immunosuppressive therapy that have occurred in the last decade, only 40% of cadaveric grafts can be expected to survive after 10 years, as compared with almost 80% of HLA-identical sibling grafts.[9]

Factors compromising transplant outcome include unusually young or old recipients or donors (<5 or >60 years); interracial grafts (especially black to white); broadly sensitized recipients, as identified by preformed antibodies against a panel of donor lymphocytes; previous transplants, especially if lost from early rejection; delayed transplant function, requiring dialysis; poor early function (serum creatinine >3 at the time of hospital discharge); poor histocompatibility; and certain disease states (e.g., hypertensive nephrosclerosis, oxalosis). Positive factors include youthful donors (especially 19 to 30 years old), good histocompatibility (especially HLA or DR identity, and living donors (even if not related to the recipient). Somewhat surprisingly, the particular immunosuppressive protocol employed was not found to be influential, although a slight advantage was detected in the relatively small group of patients treated with the new immunosuppressant tacrolimus. Omission of cyclosporine from the regimen had a negative influence, probably because it was necessary to omit this nephrotoxic agent in patients with delayed graft function, which in itself is a negative prognostic factor. Whether or not antilymphocytic antibodies were employed prophylactically was not found to be influential.

An important variable is the *center effect*, which is more influential than any single factor other than histocompatibility. The center effect is probably the sum of multiple factors, such as patient selection, the histocompatibility matching criteria used, individual expertise in operative technique, and postoperative management. Prior to cyclosporine, the best and worst results reported from centers in the United Kingdom differed by about 18%, and since cyclosporine by only 7%. In 1994, the UNOS data showed a greater than 13% difference between the best and worst centers for both 1-year and 3-year graft survival.

For HLA-identical sibling donors, better than 90% 1-year graft survival has been reported for more than 25 years[58] and is now 96%.[9] The 1-year graft survival of parental or one-haplotype sibling transplants has steadily improved during the last 20 years from about 70% to the current 90 to 93%.[9] Over this same period, the overall 1-year survival of first cadaveric grafts has gradually improved from 50% to almost 85% (Table 20–6). The 20% improvement that occurred between 1973 and 1984 was attributed to the policy of deliberate pretransplant blood transfusions. The additional 10 to 15% improvement since 1983 was due mostly to the introduction of cyclosporine. Cumulative experience and improvements in the art and science of transplantation undoubtedly also played a role in these progressively better short-term results.

One-year survival of patients who receive cadaveric grafts has improved even more dramatically than graft survival

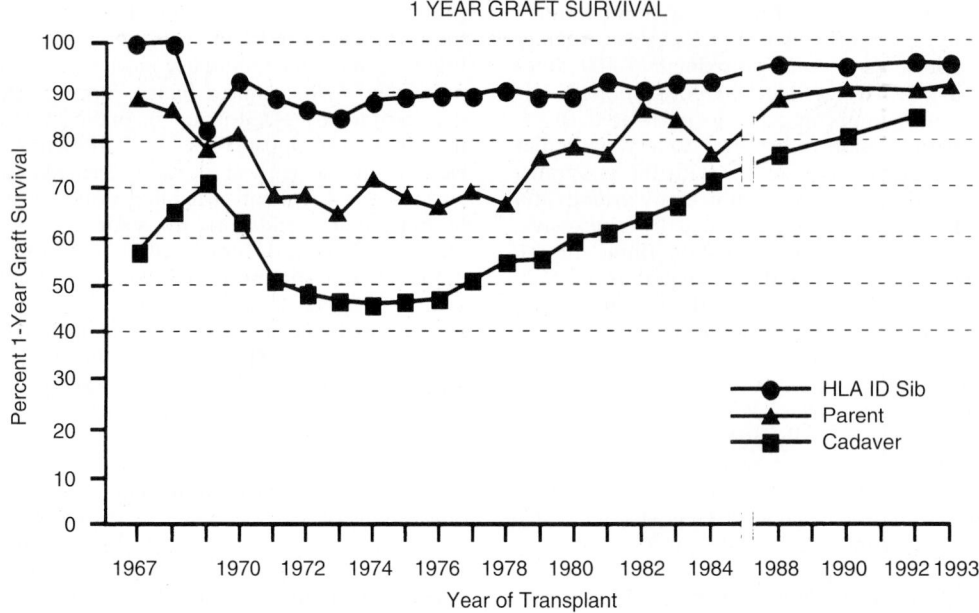

Figure 20–18. The 1-year survival of HLA-identical sibling transplants has been in the 90% range for more than 25 years. A decrease in the success of parental and cadaveric grafts noted in the early 1970s was attributed to withholding transfusions during that era. Subsequently, as deliberate transfusions were adopted, 1-year graft survival improved. The introduction of cyclosporine in 1984 led to further improvement, despite the loss of the transfusion effect. This composite figure depicts the survival of renal transplants in white patients as reported to the UCLA registry from 1968 to 1984 juxtaposed with data on all U.S. renal transplants as reported to the UNOS registry from 1987 to 1994. (Adapted from Terasaki, P. I.: Overview. *In* Terasaki, P. I. [Ed.]: Clinical Transplants. Los Angeles, UCLA Tissue Typing Laboratory, 1985; and Cecka, J. M., and Terasaki, P. I.: The UNOS scientific registry. *In* Terasaki, P. I., and Cecka, J. M. [Eds.]: Clinical Transplants. Los Angeles, UCLA Tissue Typing Laboratory, 1994.)

and now closely approaches that seen for recipients of related-donor grafts, at greater than 90%.[9]

One disappointing aspect of the results of renal transplantation is evident from examining long-term cadaveric

TABLE 20–6. One-Year Patient and Graft Survival Rates as Reported to UNOS for Recipients of Renal Transplants in the United States

Donor and Survival Type	One-Year Survival (%)					
	1988	*1989*	*1990*	*1991*	*1992*	*1993*
HLA-identical sibling donors						
Patient survival	97.5	97.7	98.3	98.9	97.8	97.5
Graft survival	95.0	94.7	94.5	96.9	95.9	95.7
Parental donors						
Patient survival	97.3	98.1	98.3	98.6	97.6	98.5
Graft survival	88.4	90.5	90.9	92.4	90.6	91.6
One-haplotype sibling donors						
Patient survival	95.5	97.8	98.2	97.9	98.0	97.6
Graft survival	85.5	92.0	93.6	92.9	91.7	93.4
Zero-haplotype sibling donors						
Patient survival	97.1	97.2	96.8	93.4	96.5	97.0
Graft survival	90.0	87.5	90.4	89.1	91.3	87.2
Living-unrelated donors						
Patient survival	100	98.2	100	98.6	99.0	97.0
Graft survival	94.2	91.3	96.9	95.9	86.6	89.8
First cadaveric donors						
Patient survival	91.9	92.5	92.9	94.5	93.6	93.8
Graft survival	77.4	79.9	80.8	84.3	84.2	83.9

Note that the patient survival for all types of renal transplants is over 90%. However, graft survival with cadaveric donors, although improved by more than 30% in the last 20 years, remains substantially poorer than survival of living donor grafts (even those from unrelated living donors).

Data for this table are taken from Cecka, J. M., and Terasaki, P. I.: The UNOS scientific renal transplant registry. *In* Terasaki, P. I., and Cecka, J. M. (Eds.): Clinical Transplants. Los Angeles, UCLA Tissue Typing Laboratory, 1994.

graft survival. Despite the dramatic short-term improvements in both patient and graft survival over the last 2 decades, there is a continuing attrition of cadaveric grafts after 1 year (Fig. 20–19). In fact, until 1988, this remained almost constant at about 7% per year, despite the introduction of cyclosporine.[61] Since then, the half-life of cadaveric grafts has improved to 9 years. Patients who received cadaveric grafts in 1967 had a 10-year graft survival of 23%; today, patients are still not expected to have a better than 44% 10-year graft survival, leaving considerable room for further improvement.[9]

SOCIOECONOMIC AND ETHICAL CONSIDERATIONS IN THE TREATMENT OF END-STAGE RENAL DISEASE

Transplantation is an expensive treatment, although not as expensive as chronic dialysis. The median charge for renal transplantation is $38,487 in 1988 dollars, including hospital charges, professional fees, and charges for the acquisition of donor organs.[14, 54] Second or subsequent kidney transplantations cost even more ($41,980). Although dialysis costs remain constant over the years, those for transplantation decrease to about $4000 after the first year, which is about one third the cost of dialysis. Thus, after 3 years, patients with functioning grafts represent a net savings to the Medicare program, which funds the treatment of end-stage renal disease in most patients. In addition to its cost-effectiveness and better survival, transplantation is superior to dialysis because it returns 75% of patients to work (as compared with 25 to 60% of dialysis patients), with substantial consequent savings in expenses for dialysis and welfare payments, not to mention the benefit to patients' families. Over the last decade, improved survival and other advantages of transplantation over dialysis have been widely recognized by the public and nephrologists, greatly increasing the demand for transplants. Only elderly or very poor-risk patients are now

FIRST CADAVER GRAFT SURVIVAL

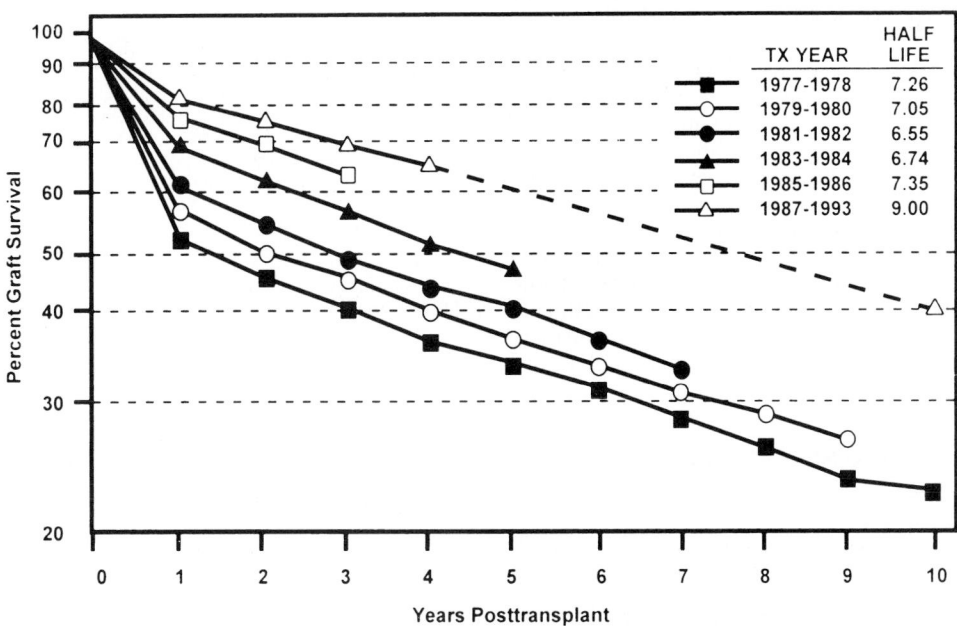

TX YEAR	HALF LIFE
1977-1978	7.26
1979-1980	7.05
1981-1982	6.55
1983-1984	6.74
1985-1986	7.35
1987-1993	9.00

Figure 20–19. Cadaver donor kidney grafting has shown progressive improvement in 1-year survival rates since 1977, but the subsequent rate of transplant loss was not affected between 1977 and 1986. When plotted on a natural logarithmic scale, the survival curves 1 year after transplantation were essentially linear. The half-life of 7.26 in 1977–78 was not different from the 7.35 half-life of transplants performed in 1985–86, despite the use of cyclosporine in about 90% of transplant patients during the latter period. The upper curve in which the estimated 4- to 10-year survival is represented by a dotted line was taken from the UNOS registry for transplants done beween 1987 and 1993. It is superimposed on the earlier data of the UCLA registry. It indicates the continued progressive attrition of cadaveric grafts despite a modest improvement in the half-life to 9.0 years. (Adapted from Terasaki, P. I.: An overview. *In* Terasaki, P. I. [Ed.]: Clinical Transplants. Los Angeles, UCLA Tissue Typing Laboratory, 1988; and Cecka, J. M., and Terasaki, P. I.: The UNOS scientific registry. *In* Terasaki, P. I., and Cecka, J. M. [Eds.]: Clinical Transplants. Los Angeles, UCLA Tissue Typing Laboratory, 1993.)

treated preferentially by dialysis rather than transplantation. Despite this, because of the donor shortage, the number of patients on dialysis continues to increase, and the number of cadaveric renal transplants performed remains relatively constant at about 8000 per year. Only those transplants from living donors have increased appreciably in the last 5 years (from 1656 to 2562 per year).[9]

Public interest in transplantation during the 1980s led to the appointment of a national task force to address issues such as the donor shortage, establishment of standards, and provision of transplant services to all citizens. As a result, the National Organ Transplant Act was passed by Congress, which mandated a national organ procurement and transplantation network (OPTN).[29] In 1986, a government contract to provide these services was awarded to UNOS, a private nonprofit organization formed by representatives of the majority of transplant centers in anticipation of these governmental actions.

UNOS's board of directors includes representatives of 11 regions in the United States and is composed of transplant surgeons and physicians, nurses, representatives of voluntary health organizations, transplant recipient families, lawyers, ethicists, theologians, and health care financing representatives. UNOS has established criteria for the accreditation of transplantation surgeons and centers, histocompatibility laboratories, and local organ procurement organizations. All patients awaiting transplants must now be registered with UNOS. A central computer and a point system based on medical criteria determine the assignment of kidneys, which local organ procurement organizations distribute first locally, then regionally, and then nationally. Because hospitals performing transplantation must be members of UNOS to be eligible for Medicare funding, the organization has assumed a powerful role. Each center must now submit outcome data on every transplant performed, and these data are published

regularly. Some ambivalence exists regarding federal control of transplantation, but since transplant professionals have had a major role in the development and leadership of the OPTN, most believe that the organization is necessary for achieving standardization and equity for patients and that it contributes to general progress in the field.

The National Organ Transplant Act was due for renewal in 1994, but as of mid-1995, Congress had still not enacted this important legislation. Issues prominent in congressional debates were budget recommendations, which vary from $2.45 million by the House Budget Committee to half this amount by the Senate Labor and Health Resources Committee; whether organ distribution should be based on a national or regional listing of patients; and how the performance of substandard organ procurement organizations can be improved with regard to the number of donors recovered in their region.

The severe donor shortage, which limits application of transplantation as a life-saving treatment, causes an ethical dilemma. Criteria for distribution of cadaveric kidneys are the subject of continuing debate. By law, age, race, and socioeconomic status cannot have a role. Should scarce organs go to high-risk patients, e.g., older, highly sensitized individuals whose need might be more pressing but who are unlikely to experience long-term benefits because of rejection or death? Or should younger, better-risk patients whose need is less acute be transplanted, since they will have a more lasting benefit? The sale of human organs has been condemned by the (International) Transplantation Society and is forbidden by law in most Western countries. It remains an issue, because needy individuals in many parts of the world are sometimes willing to sell one of their kidneys for the high price it will bring. Fortunately, rumors of kidnapping for forced donation or trafficking of organs appear to be entirely unfounded. Of great concern, however, are reports of the use of kidneys, corneas, and possibly other organs from executed criminals in China. These tarnish the image of transplantation.

The evolution of renal transplantation from an experimental curiosity to a highly successful therapy represents one of the remarkable medical achievements of the twentieth century. Terminal renal disease, an entity that was uniformly fatal 30 years ago, can now be treated with greater success than most cancers. The primary goal should be successful transplantation. Dialysis should be reserved for the maintenance of patients awaiting transplants or as a primary treatment in those patients who are unsuitable for transplantation because of age or other serious illness. Since most victims of end-stage renal disease are relatively young, the achievement of a successful transplant in this group is one of the most gratifying of all surgical therapies.

SELECTED REFERENCES

Morris, P. J. (Ed.): Kidney Transplantation: Principles and Practice. Philadelphia, W. B. Saunders, 1994.
This is the fourth edition of a comprehensive work that has become a standard. In addition to Morris, who is an expert in clinical renal transplantation and many of its scientific and experimental aspects, the authors of this 36-chapter, 569-page book include other well-known figures in all aspects of the field. The comprehensive bibliography helps make this the most authoritative text on the subject.

Proceedings of the XVth World Congress of the Transplantation Society. Transplant. Proc., 27:1, 1995.
The proceedings of the latest semiannual congress of this international society contains brief, up-to-date communications on virtually all aspects of research and clinical activity in transplantation as authored by the major authorities in the field.

Suthanthiran, M., and Strom, T. B.: Medical progress: Renal transplantation. N. Engl. J. Med., 331:365, 1994.
This concise reference discusses many of the current issues in renal transplantation and presents the opinions of one of the most experienced and respected transplantation nephrologists.

Terasaki, P. I. (Ed.): History of Transplantation: Thirty-five Recollections. Los Angeles, UCLA Tissue Typing Laboratory, 1991.
This volume contains fascinating autobiographical essays by the most important pioneers in transplantation. Their accomplishments chart the entire modern history of this field, which had its beginnings less than 50 years ago.

Terasaki, P. I., and Cecka, J. M.: Clinical Transplants. Los Angeles, UCLA Tissue Typing Laboratory, 1994.
For over 25 years, Terasaki, the foremost pioneer in histocompatibility testing, has maintained a worldwide registry of transplant patients, collecting data from more than 150 centers. He now also maintains the official U.S. registry for UNOS, to which outcome data on all U.S. transplants must be submitted. These results and other data collected from around the world are published annually, along with insightful commentaries by selected experts. These volumes constitute an invaluable record of progress in transplantation.

REFERENCES

1. Ahmed, Z., and Terasaki, P. I.: Effect of transfusions. *In* Terasaki, P. I., and Cecka, J. M. (Eds.): Clinical Transplants. Los Angeles, UCLA Tissue Typing Laboratory, 1991, p. 305.
2. Alexander, J. W., First, M. R., Majeski, J. A., Munda, R., Fidler, J. P., Morris, M. J., and Suttman, P.: The late adverse effect of splenectomy on patient survival following cadaveric renal transplantation. Transplantation, 37:467, 1984.
3. Anderson, C. B., Sicard, G. A., and Etheredge, E. E.: Pretreatment of renal allograft recipients with azathioprine and donor-specific blood products. Surgery, 92:315, 1982.
4. Balfour, H. H., Chace, B. A., Stapleton, J. T., Simmons, R. L., and Fryd, D. S.: A randomized, placebo-controlled trial of oral acyclovir for the prevention of cytomegalovirus disease in recipients of renal allografts. N. Engl. J. Med., 320:1381, 1989.
5. Bannett, A., Brynger, H., McAlack, R. F., Breimer, M., and Samuelson, B. (Eds.): ABO Incompatibility and Transplantation. New York, Grune & Stratton, 1987.
6. Barber, W. H., Mankin, J. A., Laskow, D. A., et al.: Long term results of a controlled prospective study with transfusion of donor specific bone marrow in 57 cadaveric renal allograft recipients. Transplantation, 51:70, 1991.
7. Belzer, F. O., and Southard, J. H.: Principles of solid organ preservation by cold storage. Transplantation, 45:673, 1988.
8. Bilous, R. W., Mauer, S. M., Sutherland, D. E. R., Najarian, J. S., et al.: The effects of pancreas transplantation on the glomerular structure of renal

9. allografts in patients with insulin-dependent diabetes. N. Engl. J. Med., 321:80, 1989.
9. Cecka, J. M., and Terasaki, P. I.: The UNOS scientific transplant registry. *In* Terasaki, P. I., and Cecka, J. M. (Eds.): Clinical Transplants. Los Angeles, UCLA Tissue Typing Laboratory, 1994, p. 1.
10. Cecka, J. M., and Terasaki, P. I.: The UNOS scientific transplant registry. *In* Terasaki, P. I., and Cecka J. M. (Eds.): Clinical Transplants. Los Angeles, UCLA Tissue Typing Laboratory, 1993, p. 1.
11. Cohen, C., and Persijn, G.: Twenty-five years of Eurotransplants. *In* Terasaki, P. I., and Cecka J. M. (Eds.): Clinical Transplants. Los Angeles, UCLA Tissue Typing Laboratory, 1992, p. 109.
12. Cosimi, A. B., Robert, B. C., Burton, R. C., Rubin, R. H., Goldstein, G., Kung, P. C., Hansen, W. P., Delmonico, F. L., and Russell, P. S.: Use of monoclonal antibodies to T-cell subsets for immunologic monitoring and treatment in recipients of renal allografts. N. Engl. J. Med., 305:308, 1981.
13. DeMeyer, M., Pirson, T., Dautrebande, J., Squifflet, J. P., et al.: Treatment of renal graft artery stenosis. Transplantation, 47:784, 1989.
14. Evans, R. W., Mannien, D. L., Dong, F. B., and McLynne, D. A.: Is transplant cost effective? Transplant. Proc., 25:1694, 1993.
15. Greenstein, S. M., Verstandig, J., McLean, G. K., Dafoe, D. C., Burke, D. R., Meranze, S. G., Naji, A., Grossman, R. A., Perloff, L. J., and Barker, C. F.: Percutaneous transluminal angioplasty (PTA): The procedure of choice in the hypertensive renal allograft recipient with renal artery stenosis. Transplantation, 43:29, 1987.
16. Guttmann, R. D., Morehouse, D. D., Meakins, J. L., Milne, C. A., and Knaack, J.: Donor pretreatment as an adjunct to cadaveric renal transplantation—update 1979. Transplant. Proc., 12:341, 1980.
17. Hakim, R. H., Goldszer, R. C., and Brenner, B. M.: Hypertension and proteinuria: Long term sequelae of uninephrectomy in humans. Kidney Int., 25:930, 1984.
18. Hanto, D. W., Gajl-Peczalska, K. J., Frizzera, G., Arthur, D. C., Balfour, H. H., McClain, K., Simmons, R. L., and Najarian, J. S.: Epstein-Barr virus (EBV) induced polyclonal and monoclonal B-cell lymphoproliferative diseases occurring after renal transplantation. Ann. Surg., 198:356, 1983.
19. Hardy, M. A., Nowygrod, R., Elberg, A., and Appel, G.: Use of ATG in treatment of steroid-resistant rejection. Transplantation, 29:162, 1980.
20. Held, P. J., Hahan, B. D., Hunsicker, L. G., et al.: The impact of HLA mismatches on the survival of first cadaveric kidney transplants. N. Engl. J. Med., 331:765, 1994.
21. Jordan, M. L., Shapiro, R., Vivas, C. A., et al.: FK506 "rescue" for resistance of renal allograft under primary immunosuppression. Transplantation, 57:860, 1994.
22. Kahan, B. D.: Cyclosporine: The Ten Year Experience. Norwalk, Conn., Appleton and Lange, 1994.
23. Kahan, B. D., Gibbons, S., Tejpol, N., et al.: Synergistic interactions of cyclosporine and rapamycin to inhibit immune performances of normal peripheral blood leukocytes in vitro. Transplantation, 51:232, 1991.
24. Kissmeyer-Nielsen, F., Olsen, S., Petersen, V. P., and Fjeldborg, O.: Hyperacute rejection of kidney allografts associated with preexisting humoral antibodies against donor cells. Lancet, 2:662, 1966.
25. Lacombe, M.: Arterial stenosis complicating renal allotransplantation in man. Ann. Surg., 181:283, 1975.
26. Loughlin, K. R., Tilney, N. L., and Richie, J. P.: Urologic complications in 718 renal transplant patients. Surgery, 95:297, 1984.
27. Markmann, J. F., and Barker, C. F.: Basic and clinical considerations in the use of xenograft. Curr. Probl. Surg., 31:385, 1994.
28. Matthew, T. H.: Recurrent disease after renal transplantation. Transplant. Rev., 5:31, 1991.
29. McDonald, J. C.: The national organ procurement and transplantation network. JAMA, 259:725, 1988.
30. Michaels, M. G., and Simmons, R. L.: Xenotransplant-associated zoonoses. Transplantation, 57:1, 1994.
31. Moore, F. D. (Ed.): Transplant: The Give and Take of Tissue Transplantation. New York, Simon and Schuster, 1972.
32. Morris, R. E.: 15-Deoxyspergualin: A mystery wrapped within an enigma. Transpl. Int., 5:530, 1991.
33. Najarian, J. S., Chavers, B. M., McHugh, L. E., and Matas, A. J.: Twenty years or more of follow-up of living kidney donors. Lancet, 340:807, 1992.
34. Opelz, G.: The benefit of exchanging donor kidneys among transplant centers. N. Engl. J. Med., 318:1289, 1988.
35. Opelz, G., Dharmendra, P. S., Sengar, D. P. S., Mickey, M. R., and Terasaki, P. I.: Effect of blood transfusions on subsequent kidney transplants. Transplant. Proc., 4:253, 1973.
36. Opelz, G., Mytilineos, J., Scherer, S., et al.: Survival of DNA-HLA-DR typed and matched cadaver kidney transplants. Lancet, 338:641, 1991.
37. Ortho Multicenter Transplant Study Group: A randomized clinical trial of OKT3 monoclonal antibody for acute rejection of cadaveric renal transplants. N. Engl. J. Med., 313:337, 1985.
38. Penn, I.: Occurrence of cancers in immunosuppressed organ transplant recipients. *In* Terasaki, P. I., and Cecka J. M. (Eds.): Clinical Transplants. Los Angeles, UCLA Tissue Typing Laboratory, 1994, p. 99.
39. Perloff, L. J., Chon, H., Petrella, E. J., Grossman, R. A., and Barker, C. F.: Acute colitis in the renal allograft recipient. Ann. Surg., 183:77, 1976.
40. Perloff, L. J., Spence, R. K., Grossman, R. A., and Barker, C. F.: Lethal posttransplantation calcinosis. Transplantation, 27:21, 1979.
41. Persijn, G. G., Cohen, B., Lansbergen, Q., D'Amaro, J., Selwood, N., Wing,

A., and VanRood, J. J.: Effect of HLA-A and HLA-B matching on survival of grafts and recipients after renal transplantation. N. Engl. J. Med., 307:905, 1982.

42. Plotkin, S. A., Starr, S. E., Friedman, H. M., et al.: Effect of Towne live vaccine on cytomegalovirus disease after renal transplantation: Controlled trial. Ann. Intern. Med., 114:525, 1991.

43. Roberts, J. P., Ascher, N. L., Fry, D. S., et al.: Transplant renal artery stenosis. Transplantation, 48:580, 1989.

44. Roza, A., Perloff, L. J., Naji, A., Grossman, R. A., and Barker, C. F.: Living-related donors with bilateral multiple renal arteries: A twenty year experience. Transplantation, 47:397, 1989.

45. Rubin, R. H., Cosimi, B., Tolkoff-Rubin, N. E., Russell, P. S., and Hirsch, M. S.: Infectious disease syndromes attributable to cytomegalovirus and their significance among renal transplant recipients. Transplantation, 24:458, 1977.

46. Salvatierra, O., Flavio, V., Amend, W. J. C., Garovoyk, M. R., Potter, D., and Feduska, N. J.: The role of blood transfusions in renal transplantation. Urol. Clin. North Am., 10:243, 1983.

47. Snydman, D. R.: Ganciclovir therapy for cytomegalovirus disease associated with renal transplants. Rev. Infect. Dis., 10(suppl. 3):S554, 1988.

48. Snydman, D. R., Werner, G. W., Tilney, N. S., Kirkman, E. L., Milford, S. I., et al.: Final analysis of primary cytomegalovirus disease prevention in renal transplant recipients with a cytomegalovirus-immune globulin: Comparison of the randomized and open label trials. Transplant. Proc., 23:1357, 1991.

49. Solez, K., et al.: International standardization of nomenclature for the histologic diagnosis of renal allograft rejection: The Banff working classification of kidney transplant pathology. Kidney Int., 44:411, 1993.

50. Sollinger, H. W., Deierhoi, M. H., Belzer, F. O., Diethelm, A. G., and Kaufman, R. S.: R561443: A phase one clinical trial and pilot rescue study. Transplantation, 53:428, 1992.

51. Starzl, T. E., Marchioro, T. L., and Waddell, W. R.: The reversal of rejection in human renal homografts with subsequent development of homograft tolerance. Surg. Gynecol. Obstet., 117:385, 1963.

52. Starzl, T. E., Demetris, A. J., Murase, N., Ilstad, S., Ricordi, C., and Trucco, M.: Cell migration, chimerism, and graft acceptance. Lancet, 330:1579, 1992.

53. Starzl, T. E., Valdivia, L. A., Murase, N., Demetris, A. J., Fontes, P., Rao, K. S., Manes, R., Marino, R., Todo, S., Thompson, A. W., and Fung, J. J.: The biological basis of and strategies for clinical xenotransplantation. Immunol. Rev., 141:213, 1994.

54. Suthenterian, M., and Strom, T. B.: Renal transplantation. N. Engl. J. Med., 331:365, 1994.

55. Sutherland, D. E. R., Fryd, D. S., So, S. K. S., Bentley, F. R., Ascher, N. L., Simmons, R. L., and Najarian, J. S.: Long-term effect of splenectomy versus no splenectomy in renal transplant patients. Transplantation, 38:619, 1984.

56. Takemoto, B. S., Terasaki, P. I., Cecka, J. M., Cho, Y. W., and Gjentson, D. W.: Survival of nationally shared HLA-matched kidney transplants from cadaveric donors. N. Engl. J. Med., 327:834, 1992.

57. Takemoto, B. S., Terasaki, P. I., Gjertson, D. W., Cecka, J. M.: Equitable allocation of HLA-compatible kidneys for local pools and minorities. N. Engl. J. Med., 331:765, 1994.

58. Takiff, H., Cook, D. J., Himaya, N. S., Mickey, M. R., and Terasaki, P. I.: Dominant effect of histocompatibility on 10 year kidney transplant survival. Transplantation, 45:410, 1988.

59. Taylor, C. J., Chapman, J. R., Ting, A., and Morris, P. J.: Characterization of lymphocytotoxic antibodies causing a positive crossmatch in renal transplantation. Transplantation, 48:953, 1989.

60. Taylor, C. J., Welch, K. I., Grey, C. M., Bunce, M., Boyne, A. M., Sutton, P. M., Gray, D. W. R., Ting, A., and Morris, P. J.: Clinical and socioeconomic benefits of serological HLA-DR matching for renal transplantation over 3 eras of immunosuppression regimens at a single center. In Terasaki, P. I., and Cecka, J. M. (Eds.): Clinical Transplants. Los Angeles, UCLA Tissue Typing Laboratory, 1993, p. 233.

61. Terasaki, P. I., Cecka, J. M., Takemoto, S., Yuge, J., et al.: An overview. In Terasaki, P. I., and Cecka, J. M. (Eds.): Clinical Kidney Transplants. Los Angeles, UCLA Tissue Typing Laboratory, 1988, p. 409.

62. Tilney, N. L.: Renal transplantation between identical twins: A review. World J. Surg., 10:381, 1986.

63. Verani, R. R., Flechner, S. M., vanBuren, C., and Kahan, B. D.: Acute cellular rejection of cyclosporine A nephrotoxicity? A review of transplant renal biopsies. Am. J. Kidney Dis., 4:185, 1983.

64. Watts, R. W. E., Caine, R. Y., Rolles, K., et al.: Successful treatment of primary hyperoxaluria type 1 by combined hepatic and renal transplantation. Lancet, 2:474, 1987.

65. Wolstenholme, G. E. W., and O'Connor, M. (Eds.): Antilymphocytic Serum. Boston, Little, Brown, 1968.

V

VASCULAR ACCESS PROCEDURES FOR RENAL DIALYSIS (INCLUDING PERITONEAL DIALYSIS)

Carl E. Haisch, M.D., and James Cerilli, M.D.

VASCULAR ACCESS

Indications

Hemoaccess by means of an arteriovenous fistula or a jump graft is appropriate when frequent access to the vascular system is required, when a high-flow system is needed, when the ability to withstand multiple needle punctures is required, or when highly sclerotic solutions are administered intravenously. The most common uses of arteriovenous shunts, fistulas, or grafts are hemodialysis for acute and chronic renal failure, administration of chemotherapeutic agents and other drugs, and hyperalimentation. Patients with hemophilia may also require a fistula for repeated infusions of factor VIII.[17]

Types of Angioaccess

External Shunts. The first successful shunt for repeated hemodialysis was the Scribner shunt, which employed a Teflon tip inserted into both the artery and the vein. Silastic tubing, attached to the Teflon tip, was placed through the skin through a skin incision, both ends were connected, and continuous blood flow was established (Fig. 20–20). These shunts are most commonly placed in the nondominant arm by use of the radial artery and an easily accessible (usually cephalic) vein. They are also inserted into the leg through the posterior tibial artery and the saphenous vein. If the radial artery is used, blood flow through the ulnar artery must be adequate. These shunts are still used in some select situations, such as when trauma patients require dialysis for acute renal failure.

The major complications of these shunts are thrombosis, infection, bleeding, erosion of the skin, and dislodgment. Acute thrombosis is a major complication particularly when there is injury to the vessel intima. Thrombosis occurs more often in patients with small or diseased arteries (i.e., small women, children, diabetics) and those with poor venous outflow, usually secondary to multiple prior intravenous punctures or previous subclavian catheter placements. Dislodgment can lead to death from exsanguination. Infection occurs with an incidence of 1 per 6.9 patient-months to 1 per 35 patient-months at the site of the Silastic tubing exiting the skin. This is usually caused by *Staphylococcus aureus* or *S. epidermidis* and can be minimized by aggressive and appropriate sterile techniques.[17]

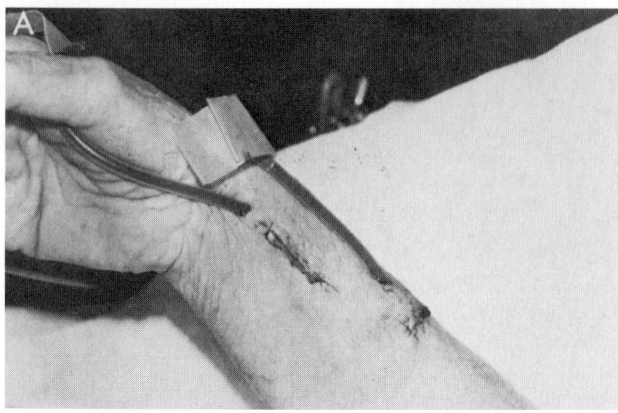

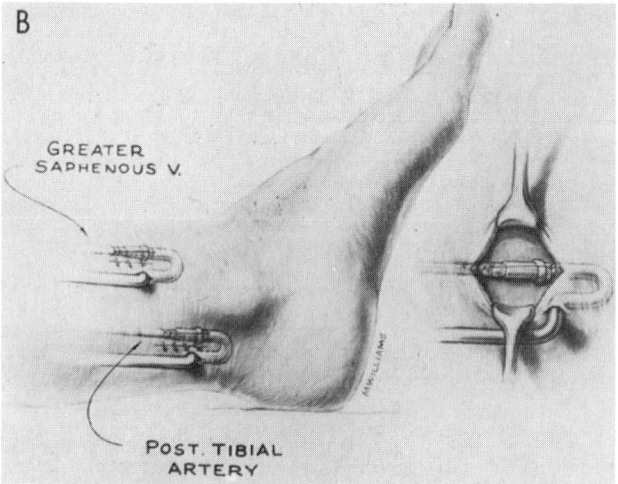

Figure 20–20. *A,* Shunt positioned in the forearm. *B,* The shunt is placed in the posterior tibial artery and the saphenous vein of the ankle. (From Ozeran, R. S.: Construction and care of external arteriovenous shunts. *In* Wilson, S. E., and Owens, M. L. [Eds.]: Vascular Access Surgery. Chicago, Year Book Medical Publishers, 1980; with permission of Mosby-Year Book, Inc.)

The patency of external shunts ranges from 2 to 14 months. Maintaining patients on low-dose aspirin (160 mg./day) decreased the number of thromboses with an external shunt from 72% in a placebo-treated group to 32% in an aspirin-treated group over a 5-month period. Warfarin therapy decreased the thrombosis rate from 1 per 3.6 patient-months to 1 per 13 patient-months.[17]

Access via Major Vessels. Short-term angioaccess for hemodialysis may be obtained by insertion of catheters into the subclavian, external jugular, internal jugular, or femoral vein. Single-lumen catheters, using a to-and-fro dialysis machine, give a higher percentage of recirculation than do double-lumen catheters. The single- and double-lumen catheters have an infection rate one fifth that of external shunts such as the Scribner. The advantage of external access using the subclavian vein is that the peripheral veins can be used to construct a fistula. However, these percutaneously placed catheters may make construction of an autogenous or internal arteriovenous fistula more difficult because up to 50% of the subclavian veins have a significant stenosis causing either clotting of the fistula or a swollen arm after fistula placement.[11] This complication may not be clinically evident because of collateral circulation, but a high-flow system such as a fistula will make the stenosis evident. While the patient is on dialysis, the fistula or graft may have a high venous pressure. Femoral catheters may be placed at the bedside; ideally after dialysis they are removed to prevent infection or venous thrombosis. Repeated use of these catheters may

cause iliofemoral thrombosis, local bleeding, or arterial puncture and injury.

Additional experience has been gained with dual-lumen, silicone rubber catheters. These are soft and therefore usually placed through a cutdown in the external jugular or internal jugular vein. Other catheters have introduction sheaths that allow percutaneous introduction of the soft catheters. These catheters have a low incidence of recirculation, because they are double lumen (Fig. 20–21). Uldall and colleagues have introduced a new catheter with a peel-away sheath that allows repeated insertions into the internal jugular vein. This catheter is compressible during insertion and allows blood flows of up to 400 ml. per minute, thus allowing high-flux dialysis.[44]

It is hoped that the use of silicone internal jugular catheters will decrease the incidence of subclavian stenosis. This stenosis has been treated with balloon dilatation and vascular stents. One group has found that angioplasty gave greater than 50% improvement in diameter, but 23% showed no improvement. There was a significant rate of recurrence of stenosis, with restenosis occurring within 8 months.[21] The preferred site for temporary access or placement of a long-term catheter is through the internal jugular vein.[12]

Some patients are not candidates for placement of a fistula or a polytetrafluoroethylene (PTFE) graft. In these cases a PermaCath (a double-lumen silicone catheter with a Dacron cuff) may be adequate. Mosquera and associates have shown that the PermaCath has a survival that is almost equivalent to placement of a fistula. The cumulative survival rates of the PermaCath were 74% at 1 year and 43% at 2 years. This compares with 65% and 58% at 1 and 2 years, respectively, for fistulas.[27] One of the major problems with these catheters is that they clot. The use of tissue plasminogen activator for opening the catheters has been discussed. This is safe and is nonallergenic. It may be expensive but may prolong catheter life.[31] The patency can be improved by maintaining the patient on aspirin and selected patients on warfarin.[43]

Internal Arteriovenous Fistulas. Prosthetic material, regardless of type, has a greater tendency toward thrombosis than autogenous tissue. For this reason, the development of arteriovenous fistulas by direct anastomosis without the use of intervening prosthetic material represented one of the major advances in the management of patients with end-

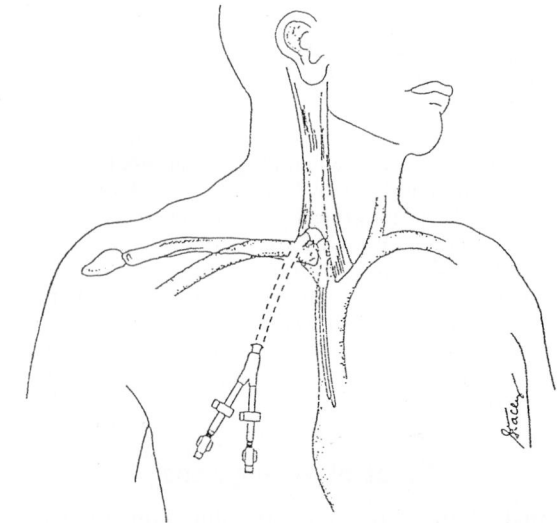

Figure 20–21. Position of a soft Silastic internal jugular catheter for dialysis. (From Uldall, R., DeBruyne, M, Besley, M., McMillan, J., Simons, M., and Francoeur, R.: A new vascular access catheter for hemodialysis. Am J. Kidney Dis., *21*:270, 1993.)

stage renal disease who are on hemodialysis. The fistula most frequently used and the standard by which all other fistulas are compared is the Brescia-Cimino fistula. An Allen test should be performed before operation to ensure adequate collateral flow from the ulnar artery so that the problem of hand ischemia is minimized. The artery and vein are isolated through a longitudinal incision, with care being taken to avoid the superficial branch of the radial nerve. The artery and vein can be anastomosed in a number of ways, including side to side, end artery to side vein, side artery to end vein, or end artery to end vein (Fig. 20–22). The anastomosis can be made larger with more options for blood flow in a side-to-side anastomosis.[8] This can cause venous hypertension in the hand, which can be corrected by ligation of the vein distal to the anastomosis. The end-to-end anastomosis appears to be accompanied by a somewhat higher initial thrombosis rate because there are fewer collateral channels. Dilatation of the artery and vein at the time of creation of the fistula by insertion of Fogarty balloon catheters seems to diminish the initial thrombosis rate of these anastomoses.

Types of Arteriovenous Fistulas. There are several different anastomotic possibilities for arteriovenous fistulas. In addition to the wrist fistula, other anastomoses include the snuff-box fistula, the ulnar artery to the basilic vein fistula (seldom used), the antecubital vein to brachial artery fistula, and the brachiobasilic fistula. The last calls for dissection of the basilic vein and moving it to a superficial position on the medial portion of the upper extremity (Fig. 20–23).[23] If at all possible, these options should be exhausted before nonautogenous material is considered for dialysis access.

The patency of these shunts depends on the anatomic type. The Brescia-Cimino arteriovenous wrist fistula has a patency at 2 years of between 55% and 89%. One analysis combined a collective series of over 1400 Brescia-Cimino fistulas and found an overall patency rate of 65% at 1 year.[23] An early failure rate of 10 to 15% is attributed to poor vessels, poor

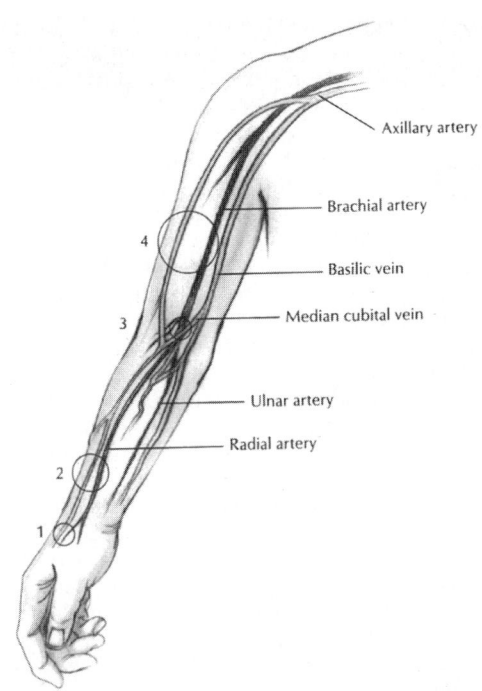

Figure 20–23. Four possible anastomotic sites for arteriovenous fistulas in the upper extremity. (Redrawn from Tilney, N. L., and Lazarus, J. M. [Eds.]: Surgical Care of the Patient with Renal Failure. Philadelphia, W. B. Saunders, 1982. As shown in Haisch, C. E.: Chronic vascular and peritoneal access. *In* Davis, J. H., et al. [Eds.]: Clinical Surgery. St. Louis, C. V. Mosby, 1987.)

venous outflow, excessive dehydration, or hypotension. The patency rate for brachiocephalic fistulas is approximately 80%.[17] All patients who are potential dialysis patients should have an arm vein preserved for future placement of dialysis access.

Complications of Internal Fistulas. Several complications occur with arteriovenous fistulas. The most common is stenosis at the proximal venous limb (48%). Aneurysms (7%) and thrombosis (9%) are the next most common complications.[23] Aneurysms from repeated needle punctures are more likely to occur when venous access is obtained repeatedly in the same location, causing localized weakening of the vessel wall. Heart failure can occur in those patients with a marginal cardiac reserve and a fistula flow rate of more than 500 ml. per minute. The placement of a Teflon band around the outflow track of the fistula until the blood flow is decreased below 500 ml. per minute may reverse the cardiac failure; occasionally, the fistula requires ligation. The arterial steal syndrome and its ischemia occur in about 1.6% of patients with arteriovenous fistulas. This problem is unusual in wrist fistulas (0.25%) but is relatively common in the more proximal type large brachiocephalic fistulas (approximately 30%).[16] The steal syndrome is caused by blood flowing from the anastomosed artery to the low-resistance vein, with additional blood flowing retrograde from the hand and forearm, creating ischemia. The complication of venous hypertension distal to the fistula results from high-pressure arterial blood flowing into the low-pressure venous system, causing venous hypertension with distal tissue swelling, hyperpigmentation, skin induration, and eventual skin ulceration similar to that seen in the legs of patients with venous stasis.[16] Both the steal syndrome and distal venous hypertension occur more frequently with side-to-side anastomosis. Ligation of the distal limb of a side-to-side shunt corrects the problem, but this often causes shunt occlusion because the proximal vein is usually at least partially occluded, so that the blood is redi-

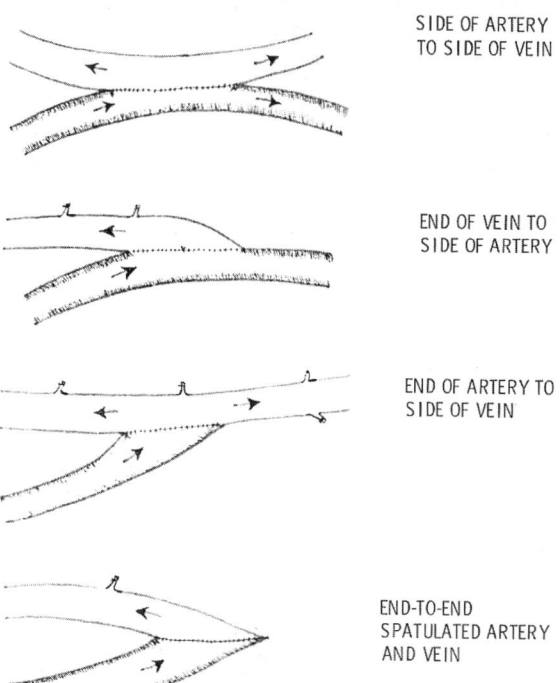

SIDE OF ARTERY TO SIDE OF VEIN

END OF VEIN TO SIDE OF ARTERY

END OF ARTERY TO SIDE OF VEIN

END-TO-END SPATULATED ARTERY AND VEIN

Figure 20–22. Four different anastomoses commonly constructed between the radial artery and cephalic vein. (From Ozeran, R. S.: Construction and care of external arteriovenous shunts. *In* Wilson, S. E., and Owens, M. L. [Eds.]: Vascular Access Surgery. Chicago, Year Book Medical Publishers, 1980; with permission of Mosby-Year Book, Inc.)

rected through the distal limb of the venous anastomosis. This proximal partial occlusion can be detected clinically by balloting the vein to feel a transmitted pulse wave in the proximal vein or by using duplex scanning to map the veins of the arm.[32, 42] Infection of a Brescia-Cimino arteriovenous fistula rarely occurs (less than 3%). Rarely, a patient develops neurovascular problems characterized by pain, weakness, paresthesias, and muscle atrophy. These can be reversed by closure of the fistula.[17]

Prosthetic Grafts for Vascular Access. The construction of vascular access using subcutaneously placed prosthetic material joining an artery to a vein is becoming increasingly necessary in patients with poor peripheral veins or previously failed arteriovenous fistulas. The material ideally should be easy to handle and suture, allow graft-host biocompatibility, and be minimally thrombogenic. It should be inexpensive, seal after repeated needle punctures, and allow tissue ingrowth.[17]

Several different prosthetic materials have been used for *jump* grafts in the past. PTFE is the most popular material. It permits ingrowth of tissue through the interstices of the graft, thus incorporating the graft in viable tissue. A neointima is formed in the graft, presumably lessening the likelihood of thrombosis. PTFE has a lower incidence of aneurysm formation than do bovine grafts and does not always have to be removed when it becomes infected.

Technique of Arteriovenous Jump Grafts. Successful creation of vascular access using prosthetic material requires good arterial inflow and venous outflow. Duplex scanning can help outline the arterial and venous vasculature.[42] Checking digital pressures and comparing these with the brachial pressure give information regarding the adequacy of small vessel inflow to the hand. The radial artery, especially in diabetic females, may be too small to provide good inflow necessary to keep a jump graft patent. Also, in patients who have had multiple venous punctures and subsequent venous stenosis, the site of the venous anastomosis must be chosen carefully so that it is proximal to these areas of obstruction. Rotation or pinching of the graft in its tunnel must be avoided. The graft must be large enough to readily permit needle puncture. The usual sizes used are a 6-mm. graft or a rapid-taper 4- to 7-mm. graft. The latter gives approximately 20% of the maximum flow that the straight 6-mm. graft can give at the same pressure and length. Dialysis can usually be performed relatively promptly after the graft has been placed; however, hematoma formation from bleeding at the puncture site is a serious complication because of the propensity for infection and pressure occlusion of the graft. Allowing the graft to mature for 1 to 2 weeks minimizes this problem by permitting tissue ingrowth, which facilitates sealing of the graft at the needle puncture site.

Several graft configurations have been developed for dialysis. Just as in natural arteriovenous fistulas, the nondominant arm should be used first and an attempt made to start as distal in the arm as possible. A graft between the radial artery at the wrist and the cephalic vein just below the elbow accomplishes this. This graft has the lowest patency rate of any of the configurations because of the low flow through the radial artery. A forearm loop is easily constructed, joining the brachial artery to the cephalic vein or the brachial vein at the elbow. In the upper arm, a brachial artery to axillary vein approach may be used. A loop between the axillary artery and axillary vein is also possible (Fig. 20–24). These upper-arm grafts have a very high flow rate and a low incidence of thrombosis. However, they do have a higher incidence of ischemia in the hand compared with other grafts because of preferential flow of arterial blood through the graft rather than to the peripheral circulation (Fig. 20–25). After placement, swelling is frequently seen secondary to surgical trauma and changes in venous outflow. Both of these problems usually resolve with elevation and time.

Interposition grafts in the lower extremity are used for patients without usable vessels available in the upper arms. A loop graft in the thigh (superficial femoral artery to saphenous vein) or a jump graft between the popliteal artery and the femoral vein are the two most common configurations. However, both of these grafts are associated with a high incidence of infection. They are an especially poor choice for diabetics and elderly patients who frequently have peripheral arterial insufficiency. A high mortality and amputation rate occur in patients who develop femoral triangle sepsis.[26]

In patients who have exhausted all previously described sites, other sites can be used for the creation of an arteriovenous jump graft. These possibilities include axillary artery to axillary vein across the chest, a loop on the anterior chest, axillary artery to iliac vein, or an arterial to arterial graft (Fig. 20–26). The latter requires narrowing the artery between the anastomoses with the prosthesis to allow adequate flow through the graft itself.[15]

Complications. Early hemorrhage can occur at the anasto-

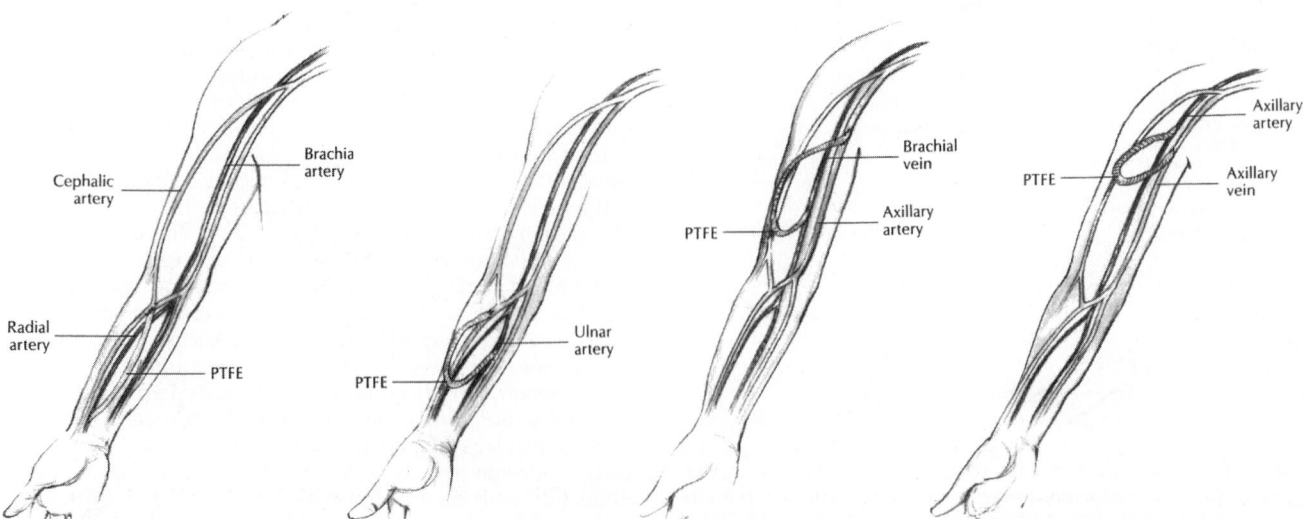

Figure 20–24. Four most common sites for placement of a jump graft in the upper extremity (From Haisch, C. E.: Chronic vascular and peritoneal access. *In* Davis, J. H., et al. [Eds.]: Clinical Surgery. St. Louis, C. V. Mosby, 1987.)

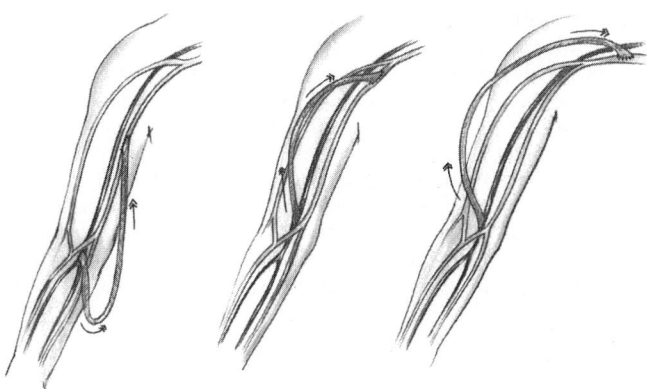

Figure 20–25. Three possible graft configurations for jump grafts in which standard sites have been used. (Redrawn from Tilney, N. L., and Lazarus, J. M. [Eds.]: Surgical Care of the Patient with Renal Failure. Philadelphia, W. B. Saunders, 1982. As shown in Haisch, C. E.: Chronic vascular and peritoneal access. In Davis, J. H. et al. [Eds.]: Clinical Surgery. St. Louis, C. V. Mosby, 1987.)

motic site, whereas late hemorrhage is usually secondary to needle puncture of the graft and bleeding into the perigraft space. Early thrombosis usually occurs for technical reasons, such as narrowing of inflow or outflow. Later thrombosis is secondary to venous intimal hyperplasia at or distal to the anastomosis.[17] Outflow stenosis or occlusion may be repaired by a patch graft, balloon dilatation of the strictured area, or a graft bypass of the obstruction. Several studies have used streptokinase to dissolve clot in the graft and then used balloon dilatation with 17 atm. of pressure in the balloon to dilate a venous stenosis. Additional experience has been gained in which over 250 patients had angioplasty performed for graft thrombosis, evidence of significant recirculation, or questions of venous stenosis. Balloon dilatation was performed with a balloon having a minimum of 17 atm. burst pressure. Lesions were dilated that were longer than 6 cm. The results indicated that this is a useful technique and showed success rates of 40% at 1 year.[3] Venous stents have been placed in patients with both central and peripheral stenoses.[2, 24] These have had early successes, but more time is needed to determine the exact place this technique will have in reducing problems in later access surgery.

Low blood pressure or excessive external pressure applied to the graft can contribute to the incidence of thrombosis. Thrombosis unaccompanied by narrowing of either inflow or outflow is often corrected by simple thrombectomy of the graft. Occasionally, there is no anatomic or blood pressure reason for a patient to have recurrent episodes of thrombosis. Prevention of thrombosis has been undertaken in a randomized, double-blind study. The results indicate that dipyridamole helps prevent thrombosis in patients with new PTFE grafts. However, neither aspirin nor dipyridamole has any beneficial effect in patients who have previously clotted a PTFE graft.[38]

Prevention of access thrombosis has led to an increased interest in the use of color Doppler ultrasonography in fistulas and PTFE grafts. This technology has been highly accurate in detecting stenoses and thrombosis. Color Doppler imaging can show a maximum constriction of the vascular access diameter. A 50% stenosis produced thrombosis of the graft within 6 months in 50% of the patients.[40] This technology is useful enough that Schwab has shown that prospective identification and correction of venous stenoses markedly decreases graft thrombosis.[36]

Infection is a major problem with prosthetic jump grafts. Local drainage and wound care may resolve the problem in

a number of grafts, if the suture line is not involved. In some cases, the infected area may be bypassed with a small local graft or covered with a skin flap.[25] The major reasons for removal are involvement of the suture line, tunnel infection, clotted graft, or lack of success with local wound therapy. The salvage rate of infected grafts is low—25% to 50%. In patients infected with the human immunodeficiency virus the leading complication is infection, with 32% of the grafts becoming infected within 30 days. The organisms are *Staphylococcus aureus* or coagulase-negative staphylococcal species.[28]

PTFE and other prosthetic materials are also associated with false aneurysms, usually secondary to laceration of the graft material with the dialysis needle; these can be bypassed. The hemodynamic complications of venous hypertension, congestive heart failure, vascular steal, and vascular access neuropathy may occur with jump grafts as they do with natural fistulas. These complications can be decreased with a rapid-taper 4- to 7-mm. graft. This decreases the flow rate in the graft and has been used in elderly and diabetic patients.[33] The steal syndrome is more likely to occur in upper-arm fistulas than in forearm fistulas.

Patency. The patency rate of jump grafts is less than that of autogenous arteriovenous fistulas. Marx and colleagues, in an evaluation of numerous articles, show that the 1-year patency rate for PTFE grafts is 80% and the 2-year rate is 69%.[23] This is approximately the same rate as for a natural fistula; however, most of the losses with natural fistulas are early; and the rate of loss decreases after the first 3 to 6 months. Therefore, a natural fistula should always be attempted if vessels are available. Raju has reported a 93% patency of PTFE at 1 year and a 77% patency at 2 years.[32] Munda and associates have analyzed their experience with PTFE and have shown that the location of the graft affects patency rates. In an upper-arm location, the patency rate was 60% at 12 months; a straight forearm graft produced a 35% patency rate at 12 months compared with a 78% patency for a forearm loop.[27a] Wilson and Owens show a 12-month patency rate of 80% for grafts in the thigh. Overall, the patency rate appears to be related to the magnitude of arterial inflow and the size and distensibility of the venous outflow.[17]

Physiology

The physiologic consequences of arteriovenous fistulas depend on the size of the proximal and distal arteries and veins, the collateral flow around the fistula, and the diameter of the fistula. The length of the fistula influences the flow very little when it is less than 20% of the arterial diameter or greater than 75% of the arterial diameter. Between these two

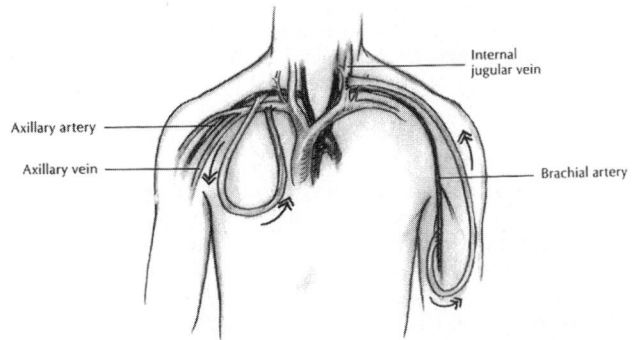

Figure 20–26. A graft from axillary artery to axillary vein with a loop on the chest. (Redrawn from Haimov, M.: Vascular access for hemodialysis: New modifications for the difficult patient. Surgery, *92*:109, 1982. As shown in Haisch, C. E.: Chronic vascular and peritoneal access. In Davis, J. H., et al. [Eds.]: Clinical Surgery. St. Louis, C. V. Mosby, 1987.)

values, however, small changes in the size of the fistula can change dramatically. Most clinical fistulas are constructed so that the fistula is larger than the arterial diameter, thus allowing some margin for error for subsequent stenosis.[13] Blood flow through a side-to-side or end vein-to-side artery wrist fistula is contributed by both the proximal and distal arteries, with as much as one third of the flow coming from the distal artery.[1]

A large functioning arteriovenous fistula may cause a fall in both systolic and diastolic blood pressure, an increase in cardiac output, an increase in venous blood pressure both proximal and distal to the fistula, an increase in pulse rate, and a slight increase in the size of the heart. There are also increases in blood volume in patients with chronic arteriovenous fistulas. These changes are all reversible with fistula closure.[13]

Platelets and fibrin may accumulate in a chronic fistula, with eventual closure of the lumen. With a larger fistula, there is usually progressive lengthening and dilatation of both the proximal artery and vein. The proximal artery elongates and dilates, and smooth muscle hypertrophy occurs. Eventually, smooth muscle atrophy develops, and additional elongation and dilation occurs. This produces an aneurysmal dilatation and a tortuous vessel. The outflow vein develops and increases in smooth muscle, fibrous tissue, and collagen and also enlarges significantly. There is increased blood flow around the fistula and a corresponding increase in temperature. However, blood flow distal to the fistula may be decreased, with resulting cool temperatures, particularly in the hand.[13]

Summary

The development of convenient vascular access revolutionized and made chronic long-term hemodialysis possible. Clearly, the three major improvements in the development of adequate vascular access were the development of the external shunt with prosthetic material penetrating the skin, the development of the arteriovenous wrist fistula, and the use of a subcutaneous prosthetic material to connect the artery and vein. These techniques have been associated with an increasing success rate and decreasing morbidity. However, for some patients, hemodialysis is still not clinically appropriate. For patients with these and other indications, peritoneal dialysis is now widely used.

PERITONEAL DIALYSIS

Physiology

The exact surface through which the fluid and solute exchange occurs is not known. The peritoneal surface approximates the total body surface area. However, the visceral peritoneum appears more crucial, although there are more capillary blood vessels in the parietal peritoneum. The exact route and mechanism by which solutes move across the peritoneal cell membrane are also unknown. Middle molecules (500 to 5000 daltons) such as vitamin B_{12} are cleared more rapidly in chronic ambulatory peritoneal dialysis (CAPD) than in hemodialysis; that is, the equivalent of 50 liters of serum is cleared of vitamin B_{12} per week for CAPD compared with 30 liters per week for hemodialysis (1008 liters per week for normal kidneys). This is not true for smaller molecules such as urea, the clearance rate of which is much lower in CAPD than in hemodialysis; that is, 84 liters per week of urea is cleared for CAPD compared with 135 liters per week for hemodialysis (604 liters per week for normal kidneys). These rates can be increased by increasing the volume of fluid exchange; however, this has certain prac-

tical limitations. Dialysis flow required for a urea clearance of 40 ml. per minute is 18 liters per hour.[29]

The evidence that peritoneal capillary blood flow is the major source of fluid and solute exchange is indirect and is based on the following: vasoconstrictors can decrease peritoneal clearance; vasodilators increase peritoneal clearance; and inflammation increases dialysate white blood cell counts. Peritoneal cavity clearance does not depend totally on capillary blood flow. Peritoneal dialysis can be used even when blood pressure is low. A urea clearance of 70% of normal levels can be obtained with patients in shock.[29]

Indications

Short-term peritoneal dialysis is usually used for acute renal failure until recovery is complete, while a hemoaccess site is maturing, or for insertion of chemotherapeutic agents in abdominal or hepatic malignancy.

CAPD places dialysis fluid into the peritoneal cavity, and solutes and fluids pass through the peritoneal membrane and are drained out of the peritoneum after a period of time. CAPD is indicated in patients (1) desiring home dialysis; (2) with no available sites for vascular access; (3) with repeated infections of vascular access sites; (4) with an unstable cardiovascular system; (5) with diabetes, who would benefit from a constant insulin infusion from the peritoneal cavity; (6) older than 65 years of age; (7) with bleeding difficulties in which heparin is contraindicated (i.e., duodenal ulcer); (8) who wish to avoid blood transfusions; (9) with the acquired immunodeficiency syndrome; and (10) who are small children. CAPD is frequently recommended and enthusiastically accepted by patients who wish to avoid the restriction of activity associated with hemodialysis.[41]

The number of absolute contraindications for the use of CAPD are few. If there is an obliterated peritoneal space from previous surgery or infection, CAPD cannot be used. If there is poor peritoneal clearance or lack of diaphragmatic integrity, then CAPD cannot be used.[30] In the latter case, this anatomic defect allows dialysate to move into the chest cavity, thereby causing pulmonary and cardiac compromise. Relative contraindications include respiratory insufficiency, because the increased abdominal volume compromises respiratory function; a diffuse peritoneal malignancy; a large hernia; or low back pain caused by degenerative disk disease.[29]

Technical Procedures

Several types of catheters are available for use in peritoneal dialysis today. The Tenckhoff catheter has been used for percutaneous bedside insertion as well as for surgical insertion. The percutaneous route is used for acute dialysis and the Silastic catheter most commonly has a single Dacron cuff. It is inserted aseptically below the umbilicus under local anesthesia and directed toward the pelvis.[34] The catheter is brought out through a subcutaneous tunnel to the side of the insertion site with the Dacron cuff placed in the tunnel at least 1 inch from the skin surface.

In a surgical approach with the use of local anesthesia, the Tenckhoff or curl tip catheter is placed by making a paramedian incision below the umbilicus longitudinally through the anterior rectus sheath and muscle and exposing the posterior fascia and peritoneum. A pursestring suture is placed, and the catheter is directed toward the pelvis with a metal guide. Care is taken to avoid bowel or bladder injury. The deep Dacron cuff is left in the muscle just above the posterior fascia and is sutured into place with the pursestring suture. The anterior fascia is closed, and the second cuff is placed in the subcutaneous tunnel with the catheter exiting distally. If

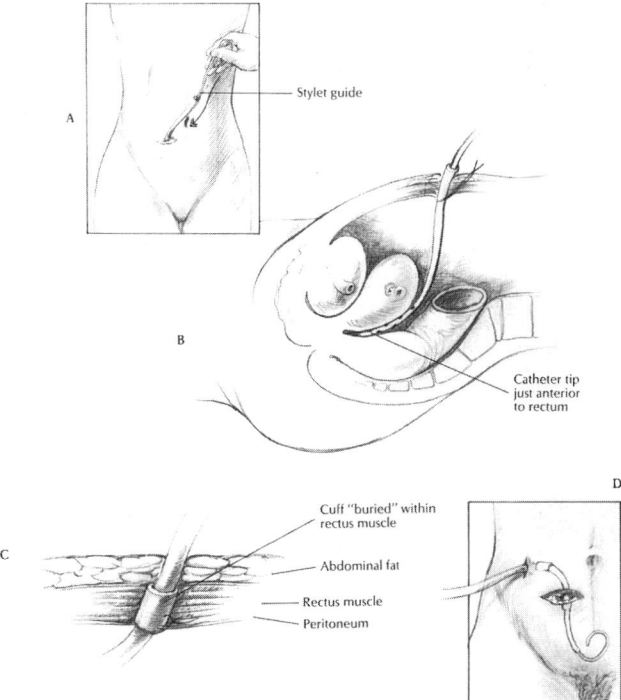

Figure 20–27. Location of the chronic ambulatory peritoneal dialysis (CAPD) catheter. *A*, Location of the surgical incision. *B*, Location of the catheter in the pelvis. *C*, Dacron cuff at the level of the posterior rectus sheath. *D*, Exit site shown with final placement. (Redrawn from Simmons, R. L. et al. [Eds.]: Manual of Vascular Access, Organ Donation and Transplantation. New York, Springer-Verlag, 1984. As shown in Haisch, C. E.: Chronic vascular and peritoneal access. *In* Davis, J. H., et al. [Eds.]: Clinical Surgery. St. Louis, C. V. Mosby, 1987.)

necessary, placement and fixation of the catheter in the pelvis under direct vision decrease the incidence of nonfunctioning straight catheters (Fig. 20–27). Omentectomy may also be necessary in some instances.[9]

The place of laparoscopy in peritoneal dialysis catheter placement is still being developed. One retrospective study using laparoscopy indicates that the catheter can be placed with a much better catheter survival rate at 2 years (84% vs. 30%) when compared with an open surgical procedure.[10] Peritoneoscopy also has a place for patients who have adhesions and need these divided[20] and for repositioning catheters that have migrated.[5]

Dialysis Fluids

Dialysis fluids vary in dextrose concentration. The lowest concentration, 1.5%, causes little removal of fluid (200 ml. per 2-liter exchange), whereas the greatest concentration, 4.5%, treats or prevents fluid overload (800 ml. per 2-liter exchange). The electrolytes are adjusted for the patient's needs. A typical exchange per day is 2 liters four times per day. This technique allows the patient to be at home and work with minimal disruption of activities. This approach to the management of chronic renal failure is gaining popularity because of the decreasing incidence of catheter infections, fewer cardiac complications, less anemia, and greater convenience than hemodialysis. Superb patient compliance is necessary.[29]

Complications

Complications can be divided into those related to surgical placement of the catheter and those occurring after place-

ment. Those related to placement include leakage of dialysate, intraperitoneal bleeding, bowel or bladder perforation, subcutaneous bleeding with hematoma formation from tunnel construction, and ileus. All of these except ileus can be prevented by close attention to technical details. Reflex ileus gradually resolves, and most patients eat within 24 hours of surgery.

The most significant complication after catheter placement is peritoneal infection, occurring approximately once every 16 to 18 months. There are five routes of infection: through the dialysis tubing and peritoneal catheter; tissue around the catheter; fecal contamination, such as diverticulitis; bloodborne infections; and ascending infection from the fallopian tubes in women.[46] Infections are most commonly caused by gram-positive organisms (75%), with gram-negative organisms being the second greatest cause (20%).[45] Uncommon causes are tuberculosis and fungus. The peritonitis is treated by peritoneal and parenteral antibiotics. If the Dacron cuff is involved, the catheter must be removed.

Catheter malfunction may be caused by a number of factors and is manifested by poor inflow or total obstruction. Poor inflow is caused by displacement, omental wrapping, or partial blockage of the catheter holes. Total obstruction is caused by kinking of the catheter, blockage of all catheter holes, or omental wrapping of the entire intra-abdominal portion of the catheter. If the catheter flips out of the pelvis, it can be repositioned under fluoroscopic guidance or with peritoneoscopy.[37] Other complications such as hernia formation, fluid loculation, or dialysate leaks can be detected using computed tomography peritoneography.[19]

Catheter Longevity

CAPD catheters function for 1 year in 85% of patients. However, diabetic patients have a significantly shorter catheter survival than do nondiabetics.[35] The leading reason why patients do not remain on CAPD is infection.

Cost Comparisons

More recent comparisons indicate that the costs of in-center hemodialysis and CAPD are approximately the same. However, inpatient admissions for peritonitis can raise the cost of CAPD above that of hemodialysis.[7, 22]

SUMMARY

Peritoneal dialysis has the advantage over hemodialysis of allowing the patient more freedom in activity and protein and fluid intake. The major complication is infection, which causes patients to switch to hemodialysis. The technique may not be usable for as long as hemodialysis in a number of patients. Because these techniques may produce uncertain results, transplantation is still the therapy of choice for suitable patients with end-stage renal failure.

SELECTED REFERENCES

Brescia, M. J., Cimino, J. E., Appel, D., and Harwich, B. J.: Chronic hemodialysis using venipuncture and a surgically created arteriovenous fistula. N. Engl. J. Med., 275:1089, 1966.
This article is the original description of the wrist fistula, which revolutionized dialysis and allowed patients long-term vascular access with fewer complications than occurred with external shunts. The article describes the fistula by which all other methods of vascular access for dialysis are measured.

Haimov, M., Baez, A., Neff, M., and Slifkin, R.: Complications of arteriovenous fistulas for hemodialysis. Arch. Surg., 110:708, 1975
A group of over 400 patients with slightly over 500 arteriovenous fistulas are reported. The 30 vascular complications are examined. Complications including ischemia, steals, gangrene, aneurysms, and venous hypertension are outlined, and

their incidence is noted. The therapy and outcome are discussed for these complications.

Henry, M. L., and Ferguson, R. M. (Eds.): Vascular Access for Hemodialysis III. Hong Kong, W.L. Gore and Associates, Inc. and Pluribus Press, Inc. 1993.
The results of a meeting on dialysis access held in 1992 are reported. The symposium reviewed some historical insights, physiologic changes, anesthetic techniques, and various types of access that can be used for patients with end-stage renal disease.

Marx, A. B., Landmann, J., and Harder, F. H.: Surgery for vascular access. Curr. Probl. Surg., 27:1, 1990.
This is a nice overview of vascular access surgery for nonuremic patients as well as those requiring dialysis. There are good diagrams and a good overview of results for both acute and chronic hemodialysis.

Nolph, K. D.: Peritoneal anatomy and transport physiology; and Mion, C. M.: Practical use of peritoneal dialysis. *In* Drukker, W., Parsons, F. M., and Maher, J. F. (Eds.): Replacement of Renal Function by Dialysis. Boston, Martinus Nijhoff, 1983.
These two chapters give an excellent overview of peritoneal physiology and anatomy and the practical uses and limitations of peritoneal dialysis. The chapter on physiology compares peritoneal dialysis to hemodialysis and gives its limitations. The chapter on the use of peritoneal dialysis includes sections on solutions and catheter insertion, complications, and catheter longevity.

REFERENCES

1. Anderson, C. B., Etheredge, E. E., Harter, H. R., Graff, R. J., Codd, J. E., and Newton, W. T.: Local blood flow characteristics of arteriovenous fistulas in the forearm for dialysis. Surg. Gynecol. Obstet., 144:531, 1977.
2. Antonucci, F., Salomonowitz, E., Stuckmann, G., Stiefel, M., Largiader, J., and Zollikofer, C. L.: Placement of venous stents: Clinical experience with a self-expanding prosthesis. Radiology, 183:493, 1992.
3. Beathard, G. A.: Percutaneous transvenous angioplasty in the treatment of vascular access stenosis. Kidney Int., 42:1390, 1992.
4. Brescia, M. J., Cimino, J. E., Appel, K., and Harwich, B. J.: Chronic hemodialysis using venipuncture and a surgically created arteriovenous fistula. N. Engl. J. Med., 275:1089, 1966.
5. Bruchner-Beyerlein, C., and Albert, F. W.: Endoscopic peritoneal dialysis catheter placement. *In* LaGreca, G., Olivares, J., Feriani, M., Passlick-Deetjen, J. (Eds.): CAPD—A Decade of Experience. Contrib. Nephrol., 89:28, 1991.
6. Bulgin, R. H.: Comparative costs of various dialysis treatments. Peritoneal Dial. Bull., 1:88, 1981.
7. Butt, K. M. H., Friedman, E. A., and Kountz, S. L.: Angioaccess. Curr. Probl. Surg., 13:1, 1976.
8. Cerilli, J., and Limbert, J. G.: Technique and results of the construction of arteriovenous fistulas for hemodialysis. Surg. Gynecol. Obstet., 137:922, 1973.
9. Cerilli, J., Walker, J., and Bay, W.: A new technique for placement of catheters for peritoneal dialysis. Surg. Gynecol. Obstet., 156:663, 1983.
10. Cruz, C, and Faber, M. D.: Peritoneoscopic implantation of catheters for peritoneal dialysis: Effect on functional survival and incidence of tunnel infection. *In* LaGreca, G., Olivares, J., Feriani, M., Passlick-Deetjen, J. (Eds.): CAPD—A Decade of Experience. Contrib. Nephrol., 89:35, 1991.
11. Davis, D., Petersen, J., Feldman, R., Cho, D., and Stevick, C. A.: Subclavian venous stenosis. JAMA, 252:3404, 1984.
12. DeMoor, B., Vanholder, R., and Ringoir, S.: Subclavian vein hemodialysis catheters: Advantages and disadvantages. Artif. Organs, 18:293, 1994.
13. Dow, P., and Hamilton, W. F.: Handbook of Physiology. Section 2. Circulation, Vol. III. Washington, D.C., American Physiological Society, 1965.
14. Friedman, E. A., Butt, K. M. H., Pascua, L. J., Hardy, M. A., Lawton, R. L., and Uldall, P. R.: Vascular access update. Trans. Am. Soc. Artif. Intern. Organs, 25:526, 1979.
15. Haimov, M.: Vascular access for hemodialysis: New modifications for the difficult patient. Surgery, 92:109, 1982.
16. Haimov, M., Baez, A., Neff, M., and Slifkin, R.: Complications of arteriovenous fistulas for hemodialysis. Arch. Surg., 110:708, 1975.
17. Haisch, C. E.: Access for dialysis. *In* Cerilli, G. J. (Ed.): Organ Transplantation and Replacement. Philadelphia, J. B. Lippincott, 1988.
18. Hertzer, N. R.: Circulatory access for hemodialysis. *In* Rutherford, R. B. (Ed.): Vascular Surgery. Philadelphia, W. B. Saunders, 1984.
19. Hollett, M. D., Marn, C. S., Ellis, J. H., Francis, I. R., and Swartz, R. D.: Complications of continuous ambulatory peritoneal dialysis: Evaluation with CT peritoneography. Am. J. Radiol., 159:983, 1992.
20. Kimmelstiel, F. M., Miller, R. E., Molinelli, B. M., and Lorch, J. A.: Laparo-

scopic management of peritoneal dialysis catheters. Surg. Gynecol. Obstet., 176:565, 1993.
21. Kovalik, E. C., Newman, G. E., Suhocki, P., Nelson, M., and Schwab, S. J.: Correction of central venous stenoses: Use of angioplasty and vascular Wallstents. Kidney Int., 45:1177, 1994.
22. Luvin, M., McGoldric, M. D., and McCoy, G. C.: Charges for in-hospital treatment of peritonitis in continuous ambulatory peritoneal dialysis. Clin. Res., 31:300A, 1983.
23. Marx, A. B., Landmann, J., and Harder, F. H.: Surgery for Vascular Access. Curr. Probl. Surg., 27:1, 1990.
24. Matthews, R., Clugston, R., Eisenhauer, A., Dake, M., Schatz, R., and Feinstein, E.: Balloon expandable stents to treat central venous stenoses in hemodialysis patients. Am. J. Nephrol., 12:451, 1992.
25. McKenna, P. J., and Leadbetter, M. G.: Salvage of chronically exposed Gore-Tex vascular access graft in the hemodialysis patient. Plast. Reconstr. Surg., 82:1046, 1988.
26. Morgan, A. P., Knight, D. C., Tilney, N. L., and Lazarus, J. M.: Femoral triangle sepsis in dialysis patients: Frequency, management and outcome. Ann. Surg., 191:460, 1980.
27. Mosquera, D. A., Sibson, S. P., and Goldman, M. D.: Vascular access surgery: A 2-year study and comparison with the PermaCath. Nephrol. Dial. Transplant, 7:1111, 1992.
27a. Munda, R., First, M. R., Alexander, J. W., et al.: Polytetrafluoroethylene graft survival in hemodialysis. JAMA, 249:219, 1983.
28. Nannery, W. M., Stoldt, H. S., and Fares, L. G.: Hemodialysis access operations performed upon patients with human immunodeficiency virus. Surg. Gynecol. Obstet., 173:387, 1991.
29. Nolph, K. D.: Peritoneal anatomy and transport physiology; and Mion, C. M.: Practical use of peritoneal dialysis. *In* Parsons, F. M., and Maher, J. F. (Eds.): Replacement of Renal Function by Dialysis. Boston, Martinus Nijhoff, 1983.
30. Nolph, K. D., Miller, L., Husted, F. C., and Hirszel, P.: Peritoneal clearances in scleroderma and diabetes mellitus: Effects of intraperitoneal isoproterenol. Int. Urol. Nephrol., 8:161, 1976.
31. Paulsen, D., Reisother, A., Aasen, M., and Fauchald, P.: Use of Tissue plasminogen activator for reopening of clotted dialysis catheters. Nephron, 64:468, 1993.
32. Raju, S.: PTFE grafts for hemodialysis access. Ann. Surg., 206:666, 1987.
33. Rosental, J. J., Bell, D. D., Gaspar, M. R., Movius, H. J., and Lemire, G. G.: Prevention of high flow problems of arteriovenous grafts: Development of a new tapered graft. Am. J. Surg., 140:231, 1980.
34. Rubin, J., Adair, C. M., Raju, S., and Bower, J. D.: The Tenckhoff catheter for peritoneal dialysis: An appraisal. Nephron, 32:370, 1982.
35. Sanderson, M. C., Swartzendruber, D. J., Fenoglio, M. E., Moore, J. T., and Haun, W. E.: Surgical complications of continuous ambulatory peritoneal dialysis. Am. J. Surg., 160:561, 1990.
36. Schwab, S. J.: Assessing the adequacy of vascular access and its relationship to patient outcome. Am. J. Kidney Dis., 24:316, 1994.
37. Siegel, R. L., Nosher, J. L., and Gesner, L. R.: Peritoneal dialysis catheters: Repositioning with new fluoroscopic technique. Radiology, 190:899, 1994.
38. Sreedhara, R., Himmelfarb, J., Lazarus, J. M., and Hakim R. M.: Antiplatelet therapy in graft thrombosis: Results of a prospective, randomized, double-blind study. Kidney Int., 45:1477, 1994.
39. Steinberg, S. M., Cutler, S. J., and Novak, J. W.: Report of the National CAPD Registry of the National Institutes of Health, January 1984.
40. Strauch, B. S., O'Connell, R. S., Geoly, K. L., Grundlehner M., Yakub, N., and Tietjen, D. P.: Forecasting thrombosis of vascular access with Doppler color flow imaging. Am. J. Kidney Dis., 19:554, 1992.
41. Tenckhoff, H.: Home peritoneal dialysis. *In* Massry, S. G., and Sellers, A. L. (Eds.): Clinical Aspects of Anemia and Dialysis. Springfield, Ill., Charles C Thomas, 1976.
42. Tordoir, J. H. M., de Bruin, H. G., Hoeneveld, H., Eikelboom, B. C., and Kitslaar, P. J. E. H. M.: Duplex ultrasound scanning in the assessment of arteriovenous fistulas created for hemodialysis access: Comparison with digital subtraction angiography. J. Vasc. Surg., 10:122, 1989.
43. Uldall, R., Besley, M. E., Thomas, A., Salter, S., Nuezca, L. A., and Vas, M.: Maintaining the patency of double-lumen Silastic jugular catheters for haemodialysis. Int. J. Artif. Organs, 16:37, 1993.
44. Uldall, R., DeBruyne, M., Besley, M., McMillan, J., Simons, M., and Fancoeur, R.: A new vascular access catheter for hemodialysis. Am. J. Kidney Dis., 21:270, 1993.
45. Vas, S. I.: Peritonitis. *In* Nolph K. D. (Ed.): Peritoneal Dialysis. The Hague, Marinus Nijhoff, 1983.
46. Wu, G., Khanna, R., Vas, S. I., Digenis, G., and Oreopoulos, D. G.: Continuous ambulatory peritoneal dialysis: No longer experimental. Can. Med. Assoc. J., 130:699, 1984.

VI _____

PRINCIPLES OF THERAPEUTIC IMMUNOSUPPRESSION

Angus W. Thomson, Ph.D., D.Sc., Suzanne T. Ildstad, M.D., and Richard L. Simmons, M.D.

Transplantation of solid organs has become the treatment of choice for end-stage renal, hepatic, cardiac, and pulmonary disease. The field has progressed rapidly in the past 3 decades primarily as a result of the development of safer and more effective immunosuppressive agents. After Carrel described a reliable technique for vascular anastomosis in the early 1900s, technical problems confronting surgeons seeking to replace diseased kidneys or other solid organs were largely resolved. However, the crucial advance that made clinical organ transplantation between unrelated individuals become feasible was the development of immunosuppressive drugs able to prevent or control rejection.[7, 18] The combination of azathioprine with corticosteroids, introduced in 1962, was the first effective clinical immunosuppressive regimen. It is still used in many patients today. The introduction in 1978 of cyclosporine, a specific and nonmyelotoxic immunosuppressant, changed heart and liver transplantation from research to service procedures and increased dramatically the success rates of renal transplantation.[28] Continued improvements in control of rejection at both the cellular and molecular levels have been possible, owing to increased understanding of the complexity of the immune system and of the events that constitute the rejection process.[3, 31] Because these events vary with the type of graft and the patient's clinical history, the choice of immunosuppression depends on as complete an understanding as possible of the interrelationship between host and graft.

CONCEPTUAL APPROACHES TO IMMUNOSUPPRESSIVE THERAPY

Lymphocytes have an essential, central role in the immune response and mediate its specificity.[1] The rejection reaction begins when T lymphocytes recognize foreign histocompatibility antigens present on cells of the transplanted tissue.[41] The foreign cell or antigen is thought to be presented directly to host lymphocytes by donor dendritic cells or, alternatively, to host macrophages, which phagocytose and then display the processed antigeneic epitope on their surface. Whatever the antigen-presenting cell (APC),[27] the ability to differentiate *self* from *non-self* resides with the lymphocytes. Early in the development of the body's immune system, groups or clones of lymphocytes are formed that have rather discrete target specificities. A lymphocyte, therefore, can recognize only one or a few closely related antigens. The range of possible antigen configurations is matched by a panoply of lymphocyte clones arrayed against them. Immune specificity is acquired during early development, and it is postulated that fully competent clones of small resting lymphocytes await immunologic stimulation by foreign antigens (Fig. 20–28). Among the vast variety of antigens that can be recognized are the foreign antigens, which are governed by the major histocompatibility complex (MHC).[37]

Stimulation of a resting lymphocyte by the antigen for which it is specific causes it to transform into a large active cell that secretes intercellular chemical communicators called *cytokines*. These are soluble proteins or glycoproteins (Table 20–7) that are effective across short distances and that, in turn, amplify the response and activate other cells.[2, 25] Before the antigen is disposed of, however, myriad cellular and subcellular events ensue; these are depicted in much simplified form in Figure 20–29. Interference with this complex series of events at one or more stages offers many opportunities for therapeutic intervention to suppress the rejection response.[46, 48] For the transplant patient, the encounter of the APC and the T lymphocyte is generally considered to be the first point of possible immunosuppressive attack. The earlier developmental steps leading to the antigen-specific clones of small lymphocyte have been completed *in utero* and are no longer susceptible to inhibition. Theoretically, there is a possibility of destroying all the host lymphoid tissue and forcing the individual to re-establish the self/non-self discrimination. This process has not yet proven to be a clinical possibility but is practiced routinely in rodents.

Once the lymphocyte has responded to foreign antigen and become activated, immunosuppressive therapy is less effective. Many cells and molecules are involved. Specific effectors, such as preformed antibodies and activated killer (cytotoxic) lymphocytes, as well as nonspecific agents such as platelets, neutrophils, complement, and coagulation factors, are difficult to suppress. The suppression of only one or two effectors is ineffective.[18]

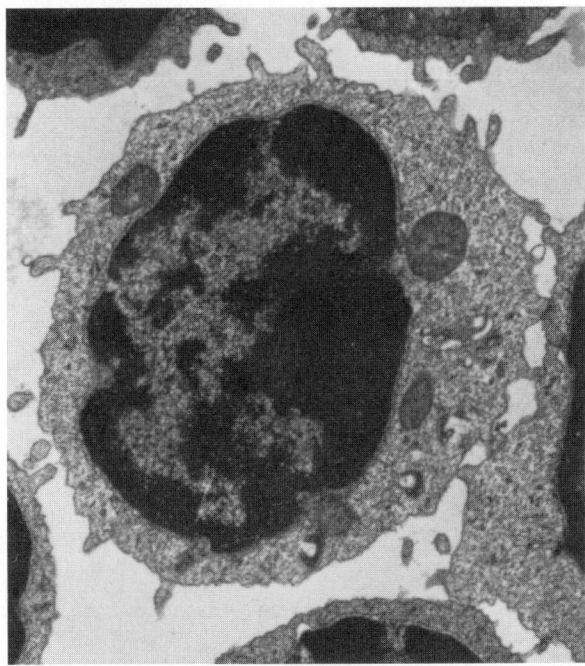

Figure 20–28. The morphology of this small lymphocyte is typical of mammalian peripheral small lymphocytes from the blood, thoracic duct, lymph nodes, or spleen. The dense, inactive nucleus occupies much of the intracellular volume. The rim of cytoplasm contains ribosomes, a few inclusion bodies, and occasional mitochondria. The small lymphocytes are resting cells, awaiting immunologic stimulation that transforms them into large active cells. If resting lymphocytes do not encounter antigen, they probably die within a few days or weeks ($\times$12,000).

TABLE 20–7. Properties of Various Cytokines

Cytokine	Alternative Name(s)	Source	Target Cell Type	Action
IFN-α and IFN-β	Type I interferon	Lymphocytes, endothelial cells, macrophages, fibroblasts, some epithelial cells	Activated T and B, NK, LAK	Induces antiviral state; antitumor activity; induces fever; increases Class I and II MHC expression; stimulates activated B-cell differentiation and proliferation and NK activity; inhibits T and LAK cell activity
IFN-γ	Immune interferon; type II interferon	Activated T cells, NK cells	T and B cells, NK, endothelial, macrophages, fibroblasts	Induces antiviral state; antitumor activity; induces fever; increases Class I and II MHC expression; stimulates activated B-cell differentiation and proliferation and NK and LAK activity; activates macrophages and endothelial cells; stimulates IgG2a isotype switch
TNF-α	Cachectin	Activated T cells, LAK cells, macrophages, fibroblasts	Resting T, activated T and B, plasma, stem, endothelial, eosinophil, fibroblast, macrophage	Induces antiviral state; antitumor activity; induces fever; increases Class I MHC expression; activates macrophages, granulocytes, eosinophils, endothelial cells; chemotactic and angiogenic activity
IL-1	Lymphocyte activating factor; endogenous pyrogen	Activated T and B cells, NK cells, endothelial cells, macrophages, dendritic cells, fibroblasts, smooth muscle cells	Resting T and B, activated T and B, plasma, stem, endothelial, eosinophil, fibroblast, macrophage	Induces antiviral state; antitumor activity; induces fever; stimulates activated B-cell differentiation and proliferation; activates and stimulates proliferation of T cells; activates granulocytes and endothelial cells; stimulates hematopoiesis
IL-2	T-cell growth factor	Activated T cells, LAK cells	T and B cells, NK, LAK, macrophage	Activates macrophages, T, NK, and LAK cells; stimulates differentiation of activated B cells; stimulates proliferation of activated B and T cells; induces fever
IL-3	Multi-CSF; mast cell growth factor	Activated T cells, mast cells, eosinophils	Stem, activated B, eosinophil, monocytes	Stimulates hematopoiesis, promotes B-cell proliferation, monocyte activation, and eosinophil activity
IL-4	B-cell stimulating factor-1	T cells, mast cells	Activated T, activated and resting B, plasma, LAK, macrophage, epithelial cells, fibroblasts	Activates macrophages, T and B cells; stimulates differentation of activated B cells; stimulates proliferation of activated B and T cells; induces IgE receptors on B cells; stimulates IgE and IgG1 isotype switch
IL-5	B-cell growth factor 2; eosinophil differentiation factor	Mast cells, T cells, eosinophils	Activated and resting B, plasma, eosinophil	Stimulates IgA isotype switch and eosinophil colony formation and differentiation
IL-6	B-cell stimulating factor-2; hepatocyte stimulating factor; interferon-β_2	T cells, B cells, endothelial cells, fibroblasts, macrophages, bone marrow stromal cells	Activated T, resting B, stem	Activates T cells; stimulates activated B-cell differentiation, activated T- and B-cell proliferation
IL-7	Lymphopoietin-1	Bone marrow, thymic stromal cells and spleen cells	B cells, T cells, monocytes, NK cells	Stimulates growth of progenitor B cells and T cells and mature T cells
IL-8	Neutrophil attractant/ activating protein	Lymphocytes, monocytes and multiple other cell types	Granulocytes	Stimulates granulocyte activity, chemotactic activity; potent angiogenic factor
IL-9	P40; mast cell growth-enhancing activity, T-cell growth factor III	Activated T_{H2} lymphocytes	T cells, mast cells, hematopoietic progenitors	Enhances proliferation of T cells, mast cell lines, erythroid precursors and megakaryoblastic cell lines
IL-10	Cytokine synthesis inhibitory factor	T_{H0} and T_{H2} subsets of mouse CD4-positive T cells, activated human T cells, B cells, mast cells, macrophages, keratinocytes	T_{H1} cells, macrophages, NK cells, thymocytes, B cells, mast cells	Inhibits activation of cytokine synthesis by T_{H1} cells, activated macrophages and NK cells; stimulates thymocyte, B-cell and mast cell proliferation
IL-11	Adipogenesis inhibitory factor	Fibroblasts, bone marrow stromal cell lines	Hematopoietic progenitors, mouse preadipocytes	Stimulates growth of hematopoietic multipotential and committed megakaryocytic and macrophage progenitors; stimulates growth of plasmacytomas; inhibits adipogenesis
IL-12	NK cell stimulatory factor; cytotoxic lymphocyte maturation factor	Macrophages, B cells, B lymphoblastoid cells	T_{H1} cells, NK cells	Induces IFN-γ production by T cells and NK cells; enhances NK and ADCC activity; stimulates proliferation and differentiation of T_{H1} cells

TABLE 20–7. Properties of Various Cytokines *Continued*

Cytokine	Alternative Name(s)	Source	Target Cell Type	Action
IL-13	P600 (mouse)	Activated T cells	Human (not mouse) B cells, macrophages	Inhibits cytokine and nitric oxide production by activated macrophages; induces B-cell proliferation; stimulates IgE and IgG isotype switching
IL-14	High-molecular-weight B-cell growth factor	T cells and some B-cell tumors	Activated B cells	Enhances proliferation of activated B cells; inhibits immunoglobulin synthesis
IL-15		Monocytes, epithelial cells and many other cell types	T cells, LAK cells	Enhances T-cell proliferation and cytolytic activity of T cells and LAK cells
G-CSF	CSF β	Endothelial cells, fibroblasts, macrophages, bone marrow stroma	Neutrophils and their precursors	Stimulates neutrophil growth and neutrophil activity, hematopoiesis
M-CSF		Macrophages	Macrophages	Activates macrophages
GM-CSF	CSF-α	Endothelial cells, fibroblasts, activated T cells, macrophages	Stem, granulocyte, macrophage, endothelial cells	Activates macrophages; stimulates granulocyte and eosinophil activity, hematopoiesis
TGF-β	Differentiation inhibiting factor	Most nucleated cell types	Most cells	Inhibition of cell growth; pleiotropic effects on tissue remodeling, wound repair, development, and hematopoiesis

Cytokines are secreted polypeptides that mediate autocrine and paracrine cellular communication but do not bind antigen. They include those compounds previously termed interleukins and lymphokines. ADCC, antibody-dependent cellular cytotoxicity; IFN, interferon; TNF, tumor necrosis factor; IL, interleukin; G, granulocyte; M, macrophage; CSF, colony-stimulating factor; NK, natural killer; LAK, lymphokine-activated killer; TFG-β, transforming growth factor-β.

From Balkwill, F. R., and Burke, F.: The cytokine network. Immunol. Today, *10*:299, 1989; Thomson, A. W.: The Cytokine Handbook, 2nd ed. San Diego, Academic Press, 1994; and Callard, R. E., and Gearing, A. J. H.: The Cytokine Factsbook. San Diego, Academic Press, 1994.

In the early days of organ transplantation, the major problem was suppression of allograft rejection. This can now be achieved, but its consequences and potential dangers are apparent. Immunosuppressive agents that are in widespread use today act largely *in a nonspecific manner* to suppress the entire immune response so that there is increased risk of opportunistic infections and malignancy. Effective general immunosuppression can cripple the host response to infections or suppress other proliferating cells (e.g., bone marrow and intestinal mucosal cells). Infections with agents such as cytomegalovirus and *Pneumocystis carinii*, which are not life threatening to normal individuals, frequently become lethal to the transplant recipient.

At present, clinical immunosuppression relies on three gen-

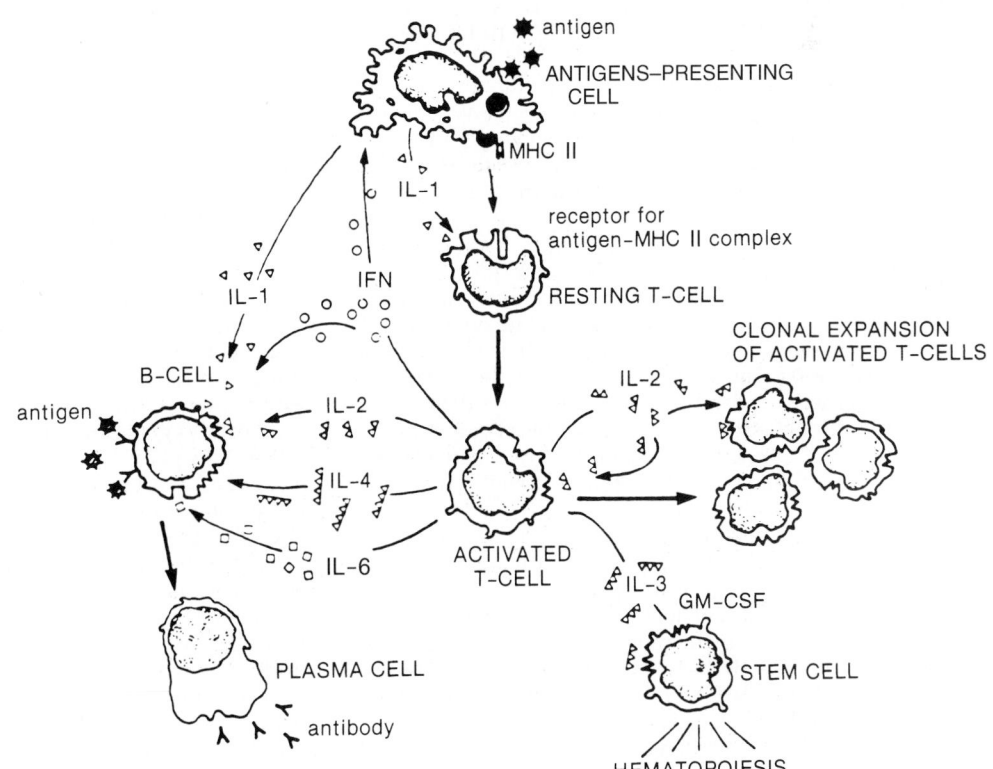

Figure 20–29. Roles of various cytokines produced during antigenic challenge. Beginning with the uptake of antigen by the macrophage, processed antigen is presented to the resting T cell with the histocompatibility molecule MHC Class II and interleukin-1 (IL-1). The T cell becomes an activated T cell, producing interferon gamma (IFN-γ), IL-2, IL-3, IL-4, and IL-6. The antigen also activates B cells through surface antibodies; and under the influence of INF-γ, IL-1, IL-2, IL-4, and IL-6, these cells become antibody-secreting plasma cells. Activated T cells also undergo clonal expansion under the influence of IL-2. IL-3 and granulocyte-macrophage colony-stimulating factor (GM-CSF), produced by the activated T cell, induce hematopoiesis by stimulating the marrow stem cells. (Adapted from Dinarello, C. A., and Mier, J. W.: Lymphokines. N. Engl. J. Med. *317*:940, 1987. Copyright 1987. Massachusetts Medical Society. All rights reserved.)

eral approaches. The first is to simply deplete circulating lymphocytes by destroying them with corticosteroids or anti-lymphocyte serum.[18, 23] The second uses an inhibitor of lymphocyte activation (cyclosporine or tacrolimus [formerly FK 506]) to interrupt the early event of antigen-induced T-lymphocyte activation and cytokine production crucial for the subsequent cascade of immunologic events leading to graft rejection.[42] The third is the use of various metabolic inhibitors (e.g., azathioprine) to interfere with lymphocyte proliferation essential to amplify the response.[22] These agents are biochemically specific but do not distinguish between dividing lymphocytes and other proliferating cells.

Future progress in immunosuppressive therapy concerns the successful implementation of an *antigen-specific approach* in which the goal is to induce long-lasting *donor-specific unresponsiveness (immunologic tolerance)* in the host while preserving general immunocompetence.[40] The full promise of transplantation will not be fulfilled until graft rejection can be specifically and safely prevented, while the integrity of the immune system as a whole is maintained. Such tolerance of the recipient to allografted organs without the requirement for nonspecific immunosuppression is the ultimate goal for transplantation.[40] Approaches to the achievement of this state are discussed later. Xenotransplantation of animal organs into humans represents a special case[4, 6] and poses difficult challenges for therapeutic immunosuppression that are not discussed here.

THE BIOLOGY OF ANTIGRAFT IMMUNITY
The Cells Involved

The development of the lymphoid system begins with a pluripotential stem cell in the liver and bone marrow of the fetus.[1, 11] As the fetus matures, the bone marrow becomes the primary site for lymphopoiesis. The cells migrate to the thymus, which becomes the primary lymphoid organ wherein the CD3+ T lymphocyte matures and becomes *educated*. Then it is released to populate the peripheral lymphoid tissues, lymph nodes, spleen, and gut. It is in the thymus that T lymphocytes acquire their cell surface subset differentiation markers (e.g., CD4+, CD8+, T-cell receptor [TCR]), which in turn permit their *specific* functions in the immune system.[1, 38] A second lymphocyte subpopulation that descends from the stem cell is the B-cell line.[13] The primary lymphoid organ that produces B cells in birds is the bursa of Fabricius. Evidence shows that the fetal liver or bone marrow may be the bursa equivalent in mammals.[13]

Macrophages, which also have an integral role in the immune response, are derived from the same pluripotential stem cell as intraepithelial cells, such as keratinocytes. They function to process antigen and present it to lymphocytes and produce various cytokines (*monokines*) that regulate the immune response.[27] The most potent APCs, however, are bone marrow–derived dendritic cells, which are distributed ubiquitously throughout the lymphoid and nonlymphoid tissues of the body.[5] Dendritic cells can migrate and convey antigen from nonlymphoid to lymphoid tissue where they present antigen to T cells.

Considerable progress has been made in dissecting the mechanisms of T cell maturation in the thymus. There is evidence that the thymic stromal cells produce two types of molecule that are important for T-cell maturation. The first are thymic hormones (e.g., thymopoietin, thymosin) and the cytokine interleukin-7 (IL-7, lymphopoietin-1) that regulate the functional differentiation of the peripheral T-cell system. The second are MHC molecules that may be important for selection of the T-cell repertoire. This repertoire, when mature, has two important fundamental properties: antigen rec-

ognition is self-MHC restricted and the mature T-cell repertoire is self-tolerant. The migration of cells from bone marrow, their maturation in the thymus, and their subsequent migration to peripheral lymphoid tissues occur *in utero*, and humans are fully immunocompetent for T-cell function before birth. Although the human thymus begins to atrophy before puberty, T-cell function is well established in the periphery and remains self-perpetuating. Only slight deterioration comes with age. The mechanism responsible for the self-renewal of T lymphocytes after atrophy of the thymus is not understood.[18]

The ontogeny of B-cell immunocompetence in mammals is also poorly understood, but it is postulated that humoral factors, similar to those secreted by the thymus, may have integral roles in the maturation and self-renewal of B cells. IL-7, produced by bone marrow stromal cells is a growth factor for pre-B cells, whereas IL-4, IL-5, and IL-6 are cytokines that stimulate the maturation and proliferation of primed B cells.[1, 13]

A behavioral difference between B and T cells reflects their functional abilities. B cells specialized to synthesize and secrete antibody that can interact with antigen at distant sites are relatively sessile cells within lymph nodes and spleen. The T cells that are responsible for cell-mediated immunity are of necessity more peripatetic and must migrate to the periphery to neutralize or eliminate foreign antigens. From the peripheral blood, T cells enter the lymph nodes or spleen through highly specialized regions in the postcapillary venules. After exiting lymphoid tissue through the efferent lymph, they percolate through the thoracic duct and return to the blood to begin recirculation in quest of antigen.[1] When an organ is transplanted, responsive clones of T cells are activated in the organ itself; in addition, donor dendritic cells leave the graft, home to host lymph nodes, and stimulate both host T cells and B cells therein. Activated T cells leave the node and can augment the cellular response in the graft. B cells send out antibody molecules within a few days that bind to antigens in the graft, mediating destructive reactions.

The T cells, B cells, and APCs have unique roles in orchestrating the immune response. It is a very tightly controlled network, with most communication being mediated by soluble factors (cytokines). B cells have the distinct capacity to synthesize antibody. Subpopulations of T cells have several different functional activities. Certain T-effector cells bearing the CD8+ molecule can directly lyse a foreign cell and become antigen-specific, cytotoxic cells. In addition, there are T-helper (CD4+) and T-suppressor (also CD8+) cells that function to activate or suppress, respectively, the response to a given antigen.[1, 38] Because each of these T-cell subpopulations expresses both the T-cell (CD3+) receptor plus its own unique antigenic molecule (CD4+ or CD8+), individual subpopulations can be selectively depleted, enriched, or modulated by the use of antiserum or monoclonal antibody (mAb) immunotherapy. OKT3, an mAb directed against the CD3/T-cell receptor (TCR) complex, is used clinically in episodes of acute solid organ graft rejection.[15]

The T helper (T_H) cell has a central role in response to alloantigen. Once antigen has been processed and presented in the context of cell surface MHC class II molecules on an APC, the T_H cell proliferates. The second stimulus is now thought to be provided by the B7 family of cell surface co-stimulatory molecules that stimulate CD4+ T cells via CD28 on their surfaces. This latter pathway also serves as a potential target for immunosuppressive therapy. The CD4+ T cell produces cytokines that amplify the immune response. Through direct effects and cytokines, the T_H cell functions to assist T precytotoxic cells to develop into mature effectors, stimulate macrophages to effect a nonspecific, delayed-type inflammatory response, and stimulate B cells to produce antibody (see Fig. 20–30).[2, 25, 38] The result is an assault on the graft by a variety of sensitized cells and antibodies.

Cell-to-Cell Interactions

Once confronted with an antigen, the response of the lymphocytes is complex (Fig. 20–29). Multiple cell-to-cell interactions are required to produce the immune response.[1, 24, 31] T cells, B cells, APCs, and cytokines all have a role. Critical to this response are the *professional* APCs, dendritic cells[5] and macrophages,[27] that act in a nonspecific manner to bind antigen and present it to T and B cells. Certain complex antigens may first need to be partially digested by phagocytic cells before the antigenic information can be presented to the lymphocyte for self and non-self recognition. In addition, activated macrophages produce and secrete interleukin-1 (IL-1), a cytokine that further amplifies the response and stimulates T- and B-lymphocyte activation.[1, 27]

Even the recognition of foreign cells is a complex process. One class of antigens on the surface of the graft cells stimulates certain T cells to divide.[1, 38] The proliferating cells do not destroy the graft; rather, they activate another group of T cells (cytotoxic), which in turn damages the graft. The first group of T cells, the CD4⁺ T helper (T_H) cells, are so-called because their proliferative and cytokine secretory responses are necessary for the development of cell-mediated and antibody-mediated cytolytic activity in a less frequently dividing T-cell population. T_H-cell proliferation is an important step mediating amplification of the immune response, and these actively dividing cells are particularly vulnerable to antimetabolites. The activities of the CD4⁺ T_H cells are thus one of the major targets of clinical immunosuppression using drugs or mAbs.[7, 32, 42, 48]

Studies on mouse helper CD4⁺ T cells have identified two functional subsets (Fig. 20–30) on the basis of their pattern of cytokine synthesis.[35] T helper-1 (T_{H1}) cells secrete IL-2 and interferon gamma (IFN-γ); T_{H2} cells secrete IL-4, IL-5, and IL-10; both types secrete cytokines such as IL-3 and granulocyte-macrophage colony-stimulating factor (GM-CSF). T_{H1} and T_{H2} cells regulate distinct biologic functions. T_{H1} cells induce macrophage activation producing delayed-type hypersensitivity (DTH) responses and killing of intracellular parasites; T_{H2} cells control antibody-mediated responses. An important feature of these CD4⁺ T_H cells is the ability of one subset to regulate the activities of the other. Thus, IFN-γ directly inhibits the proliferation of T_{H2} cells, whereas IL-10 (and IL-4) inhibits cytokine production by T_{H1} cells. Cross-regulation also occurs at the level of the effector cells triggered by these subsets. Thus IFN-γ inhibits IL-4–induced B-cell activation while IL-4 suppresses IL-2–induced T (and B) cell proliferation.

Another type of T cell, the suppressor cell, is able to suppress the immune response. This type of T cell is a subset of the CD8⁺ population of T cells and helps to regulate the immune response and prevent an overreaction to a given immunologic stimulus. Suppressor cells are currently the subject of much investigation and have been identified in a number of models of allograft tolerance.[1, 9, 18] Lymphocytes that apparently suppress antibody production have been generated experimentally both *in vivo* and *in vitro*. That suppressor cells might be able to inhibit the development of the immune response may open an avenue for clinical application in transplantation (see later). Stimulating an abundance of specific suppressor lymphocytes would, theoretically, be a way to produce effective immunosuppression without toxicity.[7, 18]

Subcellular Events

Mature small lymphocytes, both T and B cells, appear to be in a resting but immunologically *ready* state.[13, 38] Antigenic

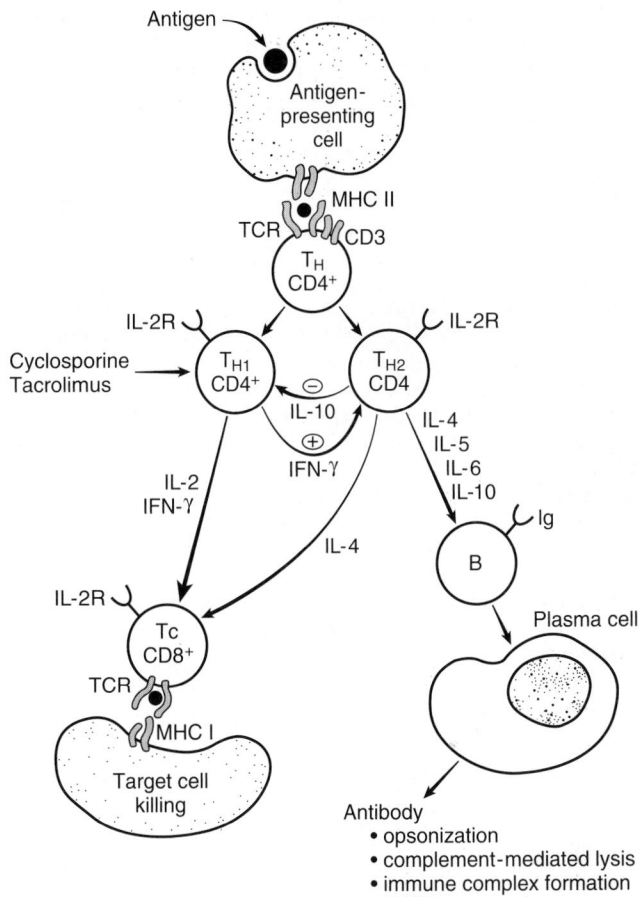

Figure 20–30. T-helper (CD4-positive) cells can be divided into functionally distinct subsets (T_{H1} and T_{H2}) based on their cytokine secretion profiles. Cytokines secreted by T_{H1} cells play a key role in cell-mediated immunity, whereas those produced by T_{H2} cells are important in B-cell stimulation and antibody production. An important feature of the T_{H1}/T_{H2} cell paradigm is that cross-regulation of function between T_{H1} and T_{H2} cells occurs. Thus, for example, IFN-γ stimulates T_{H2} cells, whereas IL-10 inhibits T_{H1} cells. Cyclosporine and tacrolimus (FK 506) are potent inhibitors of IL-2 and IFN-γ production by T_{H1} cells. There is evidence, however, that they may spare IL-10 (cytokine synthesis inhibitory factor) production by T_{H2} cells. ADCC, antibody-dependent cell-mediated cytotoxicity.

stimulation of a clone of these cells triggers a remarkable cellular transformation. Gene activation is followed by a rapid increase in RNA and protein synthesis. A host of membrane, cytoplasmic, and nuclear changes all occur within the first 2 hours. Over the succeeding hours, the small lymphocyte is transformed into a large, active cell, bulging with polysomes and organelles (Fig. 20–31). Included in the activation are the complex cellular changes of further differentiation and proliferation. Two aspects of these changes are of the greatest importance: (1) the T_H cells secrete *cytokines*,[2, 25, 47] which function as intercellular mediators to aid the maturation of effector T cells and B cells; and (2) both T cells and B cells begin to proliferate in response to the cytokines. *It is at this point that the lymphocyte becomes most vulnerable to several of the commonly used immunosuppressive agents.*

As lymphocytes transform from resting to dividing cells, they pass through distinct phases common to all cells (Fig. 20–32). Although the present subdivisions of the cell cycle are oversimplified, susceptibility to the commonly used immunosuppressive agents varies over the different phases of the cycle. The small lymphocyte is in the resting or G_0 phase. Antigenic stimulation activates the cell and moves it into the

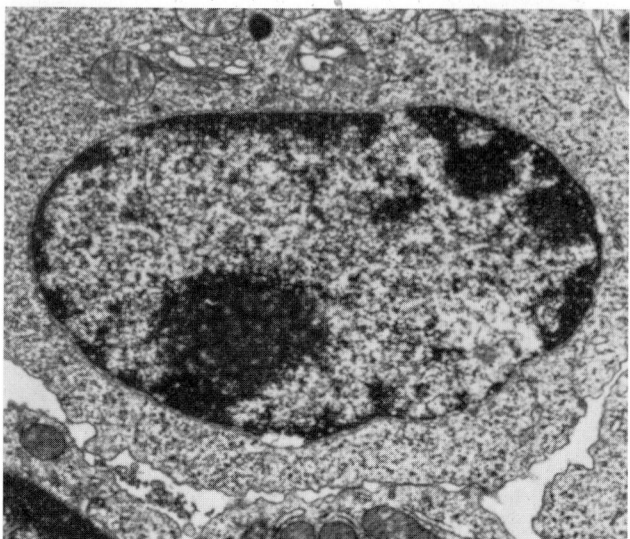

Figure 20–31. The transformed lymphocyte, 24 hours after stimulation, is a much larger, more active cell. The open nucleus is the site of increased RNA synthesis, and the enlarged cytoplasm contains abundant polysomes and mitochondria. Many subcellular changes take place in the conversion from resting to active lymphocytes. These biosynthetic events are vulnerable to the antimetabolites used to prevent allograft rejection. In addition, these cells begin to synthesize DNA at this time, increasing their susceptibility to antimetabolites, alkylating agents, and radiation ($\times$12,000).

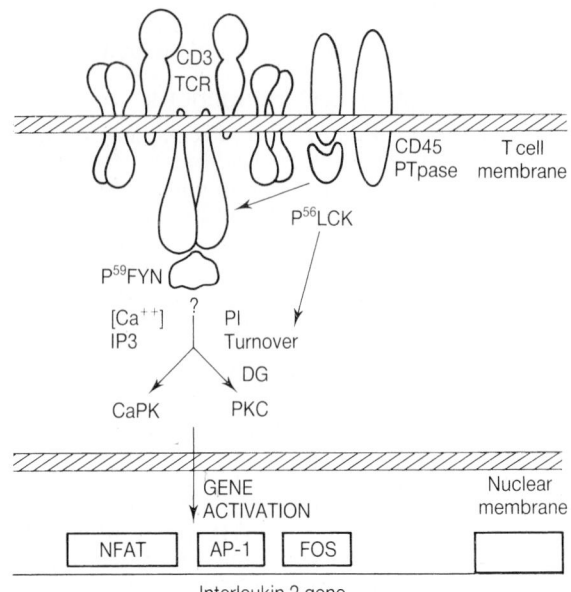

Figure 20–33. Intracellular signal transduction through the T-cell receptor (TCR). Stimulation of the TCR by HLA/peptide leads to turnover of membrane phospholipids (PI) with generation of second messengers such as diacylglycerol (DG). This pathway is dependent on dephosphorylation (Pt$_{pase}$) of the tyrosine protein kinase p56LCK, which is associated with CD4 or CD8. This leads to phosphorylation of the zeta chains of CD3. The tyrosine protein kinase p59FYN is also associated with the TCR. DG activates protein kinase C (PKC), and IP3 elevates intracellular calcium (from internal and external sources), which activates calcium/calmodulin-dependent protein kinases. PKC leads to the phosphorylation of CD3γ. By unknown mechanism, early activation genes (such as NFAT and c-*fos*) are transcribed. The proteins derived from these genes in association with other transcriptional regulators (such as AP-1) lead to the activation of more genes (such as the IL-2 gene). Pt$_{pase}$, protein tyrosine phosphatase; PI, phosphoinositol; CaPK, calcium-dependent protein kinase; PKC, protein kinase C. (From Lazarovits, A. I.: T cell responses to alloantigens. *In* Thomson, A. W., and Catto, G. R. D. [Eds.]: Immunology of Renal Transplantation. London, Arnold 1993, p. 59.)

first gap (or G$_1$) phase of the proliferative cycle. The complex G$_1$ phase includes the commitment to cell division, but whether this occurs early or late in G$_1$ is not known. After the cell becomes committed to divide, DNA synthesis (S phase) occurs. The gap (G$_2$) between S phase and the final mitosis (M phase) is relatively short. After mitosis has occurred, the cells enter into the G$_1$ phase again, and the cell cycle is complete.

Differentiation appears to progress with cell division; and, with each successive cycle, the cells become more and more able to eliminate the activating antigen. After successive divisions, B cells become plasma cells, which are the most efficient producers of specific antibody. A similar progression occurs among T cells. T-cell activation occurs through the TCR complex (CD3) (Fig. 20–33); secretion of IL-2 and expression of the IL-2 receptors (IL-2R) lead to expansion of T-cell numbers.[25] Briefly, activated T$_H$ cells secrete IL-2, a cytokine that functions as a T-cell growth factor (Fig. 20–34). The IL-2

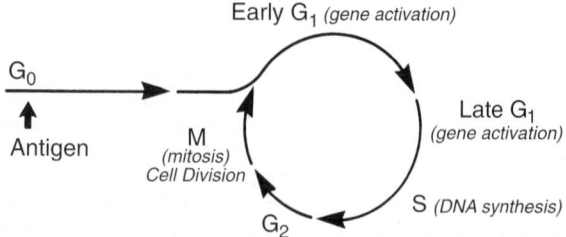

Figure 20–32. The phases of the cell cycle are depicted in this diagram. After stimulation by an antigen or another type of mitogen, small lymphocytes are activated. They are converted from the resting G$_0$ phase to the active G$_1$ phase. The G$_1$ phase lasts 10 hours or longer before DNA synthesis (S phase) begins. The S phase lasts about 10 hours and is followed by a short (2 to 4 hours) G$_2$ phase before mitosis (M phase). M phase is relatively brief, usually less than 2 to 3 hours, after which the cells are returned to the G$_1$ phase. The susceptibility of the cell to the immunosuppressive agents used in transplantation varies with the phase of the cycle. Periods of intense nucleic acid synthesis, particularly S phase, are most vulnerable to the antimetabolites. As discussed in the text, the resting G$_0$ lymphocyte is also susceptible to several of the clinically used immunosuppressive agents.

then binds to the IL-2R on resting T cells and stimulates DNA synthesis and cell mitosis by activation of the inositol phosphate pathway with protein kinase C. When the antigenic stimulus is no longer present, IL-2 is no longer produced and T-cell activation and proliferation cease. The presence of the IL-2R for activation suggests a hormone-receptor system with negative feedback control. An understanding of the activation of the T cell by means of the IL-2–IL-2R autocrine/paracrine pathway allows a more focused approach for targeted immunosuppression.

Much of the susceptibility of lymphocytes to immunosuppression follows from the cellular changes produced by immune stimulation. The many biosynthetic events that occur make the lymphocytes vulnerable to errors and inhibitions caused by structural analogs, termed *antimetabolites*.[7, 18] Alkylating agents such as cyclophosphamide and radiation produce cross-linkages and breaks in DNA strands that interfere with cell differentiation and division. The subcellular actions of steroids are also complex. The actions of the individual immunosuppressive agents are discussed in more detail in subsequent sections. The inhibitory effects of these diverse agents, except for cyclosporine, tacrolimus, (formerly FK 506), OKT3, and antilymphocyte globulin (ALG), are not specific for lymphocytes, and similar metabolic alterations are induced in other differentiating and dividing cells.

Graft Rejection

Graft rejection requires the participation of various combinations of immunologically specific and nonspecific cells.

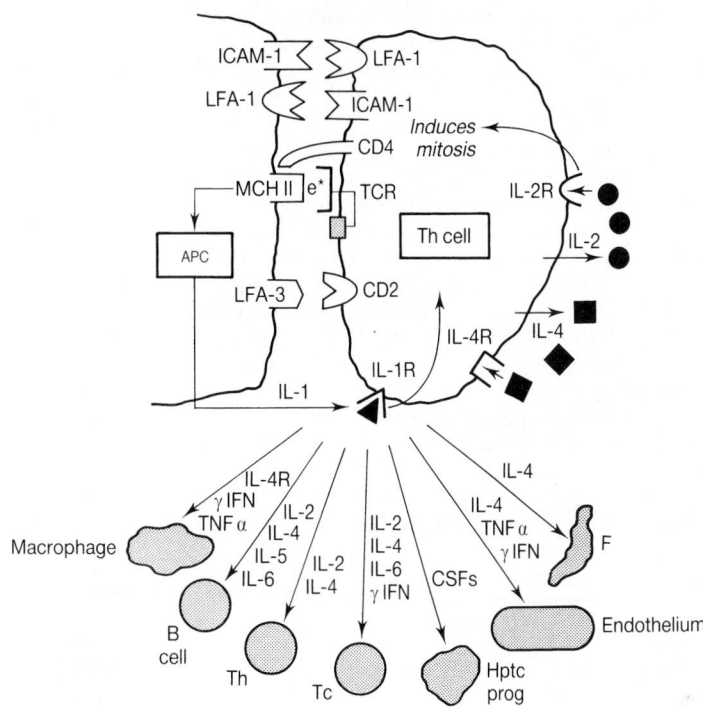

* e = peptide fragment of antigen

A

Figure 20–34. *A,* Activation and function of CD4-positive T-helper cells. Note key cell surface molecules and their respective ligands on the antigen-presenting cell and T cell. Note also the paracrine and autocrine actions of secreted cytokines. *B,* Activation and function of CD8-positive T-cytotoxic cells. Note key cell surface molecules and their respective ligands and the paracrine action of T-helper cell–derived cytokines (IL-2 and IL-4). (From Ritter, M.: T lymphocytes. *In* Neuberger, J., and Adams, D. [Eds.]: Immunology of Liver Transplantation. London, Arnold 1993, p. 3.)

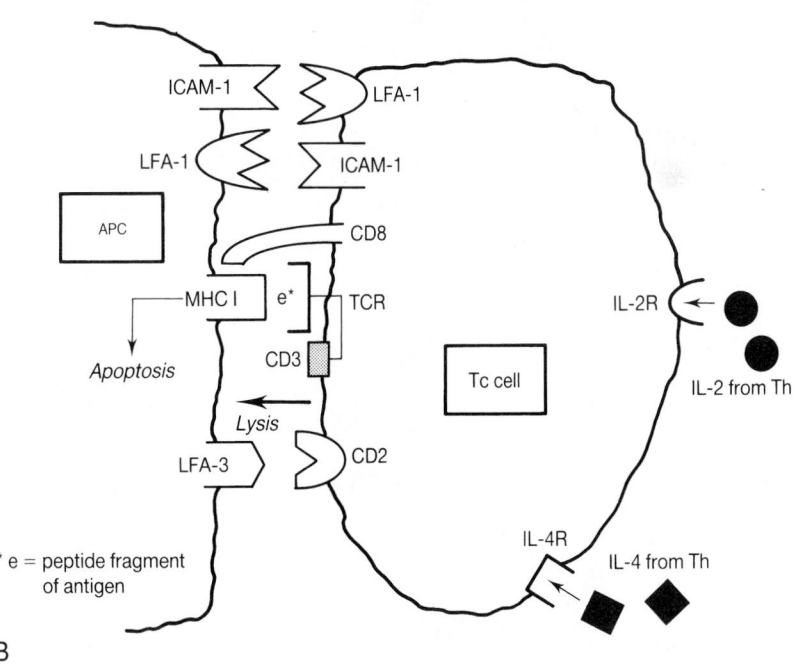

B

Three types of graft rejection are encountered. *Acute rejection* is the most common.[33] It is mediated primarily by T lymphocytes and first occurs between 1 and 3 weeks after solid organ transplantation. *Hyperacute rejection* occurs during the first 1 to 2 days after transplantation and is mediated primarily by preformed antibody. *Chronic rejection* occurs over months and is probably caused by both T- and B-cell–mediated responses.

T cells play the major role in most graft rejection processes.[1, 3, 12, 31] They can be directly cytotoxic to graft cells, be armed with specific antibodies and act as killer cells, help B cells to produce antigraft antibody, and recruit destructive *activated* macrophages. The T_H lymphocyte has a central role in the activation of other cells through the production of cytokines. The graft is infiltrated with a variety of inflammatory cells, including sensitized T_H cells, cytotoxic T cells, noncommitted lymphocytes, sensitized and nonsensitized B lymphocytes, macrophages, and polymorphonuclear lymphocytes. B cells produce antigraft antibodies, which attach to the graft cells. Damage follows the activation of the complement, coagulation, and kinin pathways triggered by the antigen-antibody complexes. Vasoactive peptides, chemotactic factors, and thrombus formation then directly produce the damage by occluding small vessels, causing microinfarcts in the parenchyma. Neutrophils, platelets, and macrophages are recruited to the scene and release their many proteolytic enzymes. Antibody-mediated damage appears to be particularly important to the arteritis and proliferation occlusion observed in the arteries of grafted organs.

The preceding, abbreviated description of the development of allograft immunity reveals *many vulnerable processes that may potentially be manipulated to suppress the immune response:* (1) destroying the immunocompetent cells that would otherwise react to donor antigen *before* transplantation; (2) minimizing histoincompatibility or making the antigen unrecognizable or even toxic to the reactive lymphocyte clones; (3) interfering with antigen processing and presentation by the recipient cells; (4) inhibiting antigen recognition by lymphocytes; (5) inhibiting production or release by macrophages or lymphocytes of the signal substances or cytokines involved in differentiating lymphocytes into cytotoxic or antibody-synthesizing cells; (6) suppressing clonal expansion of lymphocytes; (7) activating sufficient numbers of suppressor lymphocytes; (8) interfering with the binding of immunoglobulins to graft target antigens; (9) preventing tissue damage by the nonspecific cells and molecules that are activated by sensitized cells or antigen-antibody complexes; and (10) inducing donor-specific transplantation tolerance.[7, 46] Potential sites for regulation are shown in Figure 20–35 and are discussed in detail below.

CLINICAL IMMUNOSUPPRESSION

Until the advent of cyclosporine, clinical immunosuppression relied primarily on agents or procedures with antiproliferative activity.[7, 18] These include the antimetabolites, alkylat-

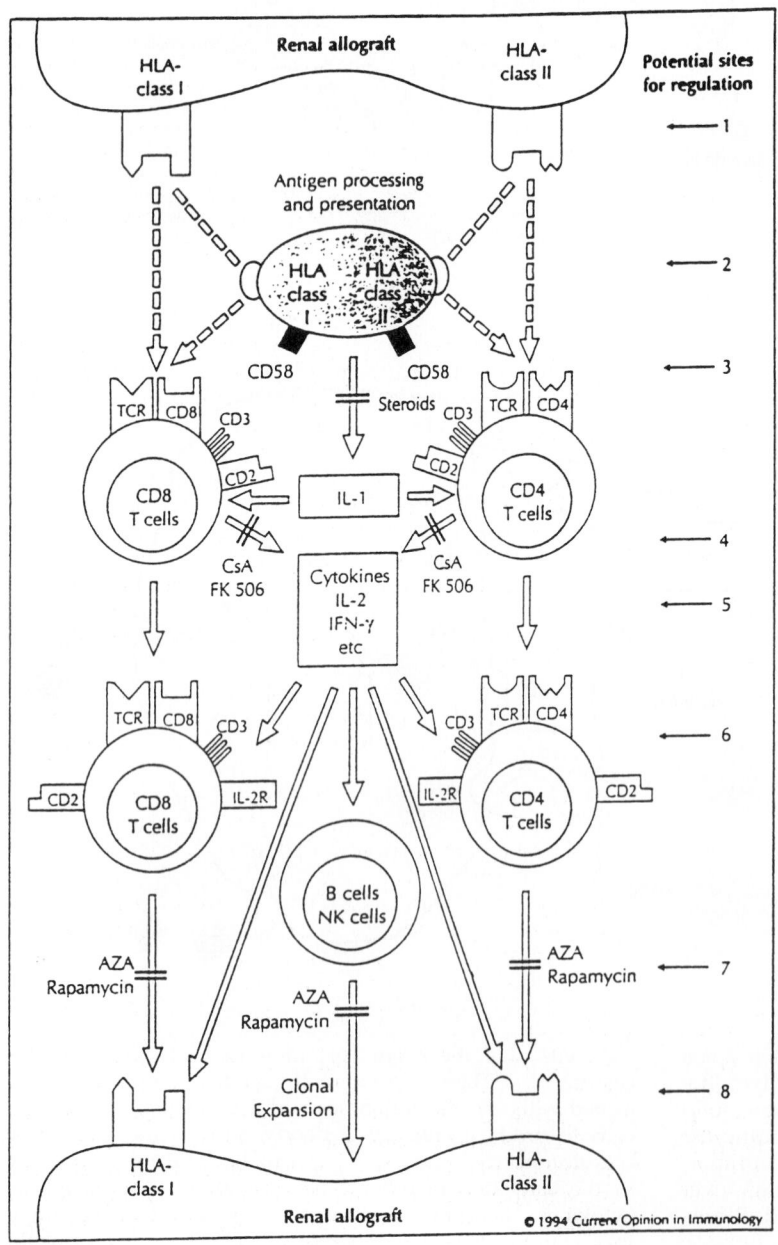

Figure 20–35. A schematic representation of the anti-allograft response showing HLA, which is the primary stimulus for the initiation of the anti-allograft response, the cell surface proteins participating in antigenic recognition and signal transduction, the contribution of the cytokines and cell types to the immune response, and the potential sites for the regulation of the anti-allograft response. *Potential sites for regulation are shown on the right. Site 1:* histoincompatibility between the recipients and the donor can be minimized (e.g., HLA matching); *site 2:* monokine production by antigen-presenting cells can be prevented (e.g., by corticosteroids); *site 3:* antigen recognition can be blocked (e.g., by OKT3 mAbs); *site 4:* T-cell cytokine production can be inhibited (e.g., by cyclosporine [CsA]); *site 5:* cytokine activity can be inhibited (e.g., by anti-IL-2 antibody); *site 6:* cell-cycle progression can be inhibited (e.g., by anti-IL-2 receptor antibody); *site 7:* clonal expansion can be inhibited (e.g., by azathioprine); and *site 8:* allograft damage can be prevented by masking target antigen molecules (e.g., antibodies directed at adhesion molecule sites). HLA Class I represents HLA-A, -B and -C antigens, and HLA Class II represents HLA-DR, -DP and -DQ antigens. (From Sharma, V. J., et al.: Which way for drug-mediated immunosuppression? Curr. Opin. Immunol., 6:784, 1994.)

ing agents, toxic antibiotics, and irradiation, all of which are used as cytoreductive agents in cancer chemotherapy. Thus, the only immunosuppressive agents generally available for transplantation until the early 1980s were azathioprine, corticosteroids, radiation, and antilymphocyte serum.[7, 18] The introduction of cyclosporine and OKT3 radically changed the principles of immunosuppression.

Modification of Antigen-Presenting Cells and Antigenicity by Donor and/or Graft Pretreatment

Modulation of donor organ immunogenicity through pretreatment of the donor or the allograft before transplantation has been investigated. Irradiation, cyclophosphamide, ALG, and mAb pretreatment have all been reported to decrease the immunogenicity of grafts in laboratory animals. However, clinical trials have not demonstrated a significantly better outcome for renal grafts, and further laboratory studies are required before this technique is considered for clinical application. Without continuous treatment, regeneration of MHC alloantigens occurs and the immunogenicity of the graft returns. It is well recognized that professional APCs of donor origin resident within grafts are important in stimulating alloantigenic immune responses *in vivo*.[5] These APCs express MHC Class II and provide co-stimulatory molecules for host CD4+ T$_H$ cells. Efforts to remove these *passenger leukocytes*[5] from grafts before transplantation using, for example, anti-MHC Class II or anti-CD45 (leukocyte common antigen) Ab + complement reduce the incidence and severity of rejection. In human organ transplantation, however, attempts to remove such cells have not proved useful. A possible explanation is that graft endothelial cells in humans may be able to provide co-stimulator functions that are sufficient to activate host T cells in the absence of passenger leukocytes.

Immunosuppressive Drugs

Adrenal Corticosteroids

Adrenal corticosteroids are the immunosuppressive agents most commonly used in clinical practice.[18, 23] Glucocorticoids have many diverse anti-inflammatory actions, which make them potent immunosuppressants (Fig. 20–36). A profound decrease in the blood lymphocyte count occurs within the first 6 hours of steroid administration. In humans, the decrease in peripheral blood lymphocytes reflects a redistribution of these cells out of the intravascular space into lymphoid depots. Recirculating lymphocytes (approximately two thirds of all lymphocytes) are mainly T cells, which travel back and forth between the intravascular compartment and lymphoid tissues such as the spleen, bone marrow, thoracic duct, and lymph nodes. Sessile lymphocytes, including some T and most B cells, stay within the lymphoid compartment. Glucocorticoids cause emigration of the recirculating T cells from the intravascular compartment to the lymphoid tissues, with less effect on the distribution of B cells. The mechanism of lymphocyte distribution is probably a cell surface alteration, promoting cell adhesion to vascular endothelium.[18, 23]

A major effect of corticosteroids appears to be the inhibition of cytokine gene transcription in and cytokine secretion (IL-1, IL-6, TNF) by macrophages. Corticosteroids also suppress the production and the effect of T-cell cytokines, which amplify the responses of lymphocytes and macrophages. Thus, IL-2 production and binding of IL-2 to its receptor is inhibited by glucocorticoids. Moreover, the ability of macrophages to respond to lymphocyte-derived signals such as migration inhibition factor (MIF) and macrophage activation

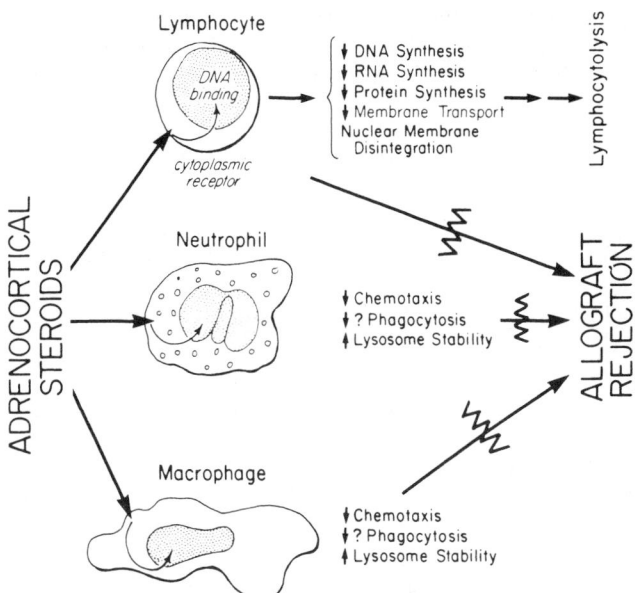

Figure 20–36. Adrenocortical steroids have an important role in clinical allograft immunosuppression. Many apparent sites of action have been located experimentally. These compounds bind to cytoplasmic receptors, and this complex combines with DNA. How this relates to the many functional consequences of steroids presented in this diagram is unclear. In the complex clinical transplantation setting it is not possible to determine whether the primary suppression of lymphocytes is more important than the anti-inflammatory effects on neutrophils and macrophages in the suppression of allograft rejection. Nevertheless, steroids produce a significant portion of the immunosuppressive effect of current clinical therapy.

factor (MAF) is blocked by corticosteroids. This may underlie the marked inhibition of delayed-type hypersensitivity reactions observed with these agents. An additional effect is the suppression of prostaglandin synthesis. Corticosteroids have little net effect on antibody production.

Some of the molecular mechanisms by which glucocorticoids exert their effect have been elucidated. Much activity is initiated at the subcellular level by means of hormone receptors. Unlike polypeptide mediators with receptors on the cell surface, steroids move freely through the cell membrane to bind receptors in the cytoplasm, producing a steroid-receptor complex. This complex then moves into the nucleus, where it attaches to the DNA. There it acts on gene promoter either to depress or activate part of the genome and causes transcription of specific messenger RNA. Thus, some protein synthesis is downregulated and other proteins are synthesized. These changes are the presumed effectors of glucocorticoid action.

Specific intracytoplasmic receptors for glucocorticoids have been identified in normal human lymphocytes, monocytes, neutrophils, and eosinophils. In addition, varying degrees of receptor density have been demonstrated in different lymphoid cell subpopulations. Presumably, the sensitivity of a particular subpopulation of lymphocytes relates to the relative density of the intracytoplasmic receptors for the corticosteroids. These messengers can inhibit DNA, RNA, and protein synthesis. Glucose and amino acid transport can also be affected.

The effectiveness of cortisone in suppressing allograft rejection was first recognized more than 40 years ago by its prolongation of skin graft survival in rabbits. In organ allografts, corticosteroids are not effective by themselves, but they are valuable in combination with such agents as azathioprine, nitrogen mustard, and ALG. Steroids, in high doses, are especially useful at interrupting ongoing rejection reactions in clinical practice, but their prolonged use leads to unacceptable side effects, such as hypertension, weight gain, peptic ulcers and gastrointestinal bleeding, euphoric personality changes, cataract formation, hyperglycemia that may progress to steroid diabetes, pancreatitis, muscle wasting, and osteoporosis with avascular necrosis of the femoral head and other bones. Susceptibility to pyogenic and opportunistic infections is a direct result of the suppression of phagocytic microbial killing by macrophages and neutrophils. Cushingoid features are the external signs of these dangerous processes. Clinical transplantation will be improved tremendously when more specific means of immunosuppression are developed and present corticosteroid dosages can be reduced substantially or eliminated.

Antiproliferative Agents

Antiproliferative agents inhibit the full expression of the immune response by preventing the differentiation and division of the immunocompetent lymphocytes after their encounter with antigen.[7, 22] They either structurally resemble essential metabolites or combine with certain cellular components, such as DNA, and thereby interfere with molecular function.

The antimetabolites, the former group, either inhibit enzymes that regulate a particular metabolic pathway or are incorporated during synthesis to produce *faulty* molecules. They include purine, pyrimidine, and folic acid analogs that are most effective against proliferating and differentiating cells. These drugs are given at the time of transplantation when the immunocompetent cells are first stimulated and for the life of the graft to interfere with the continuing response of the immune system.

Alkylating agents (e.g., cyclophosphamide) and certain antibiotics (e.g., dactinomycin) include those compounds that combine with DNA and other cellular components. Although these agents would be useful in the pretransplant period to reduce the number of effective immunocompetent cells in prospective graft recipients, and thereafter to prevent lymphocyte proliferation, their use has been limited to bone marrow transplantation and occasional substitution for azathioprine.

Purine Analogs. Until recently, the purine analog azathioprine was the most widely used immunosuppressive drug in clinical organ transplantation. Azathioprine is 6-mercaptopurine (6-MP) plus a side chain to protect the labile sulfhydryl group (Fig. 20–37). In the liver, the side chain is split off to form the active compound 6-MP. The mechanism of action of these two compounds is similar, although azathioprine appears to have the advantage of slightly lower toxicity.[7, 18]

Full metabolic activity occurs in the cell with the addition of ribose-S6-phosphate from phosphoribosyl pyrophosphate to form 6-MP ribonucleotide. The structural resemblance of this molecule to inosine monophosphate is obvious, and 6-MP ribonucleotide inhibits the enzymes that begin to convert inosine nucleotide to adenosine and guanosine monophosphate (see Fig. 20–37). In addition, the presence of 6-MP ribonucleotides slows the entire purine biosynthetic pathway by fraudulent feedback inhibition of an early step. The steric similarity to either adenosine or guanine nucleotides is not sufficient to allow significant incorporation into DNA or RNA and synthesis of faulty molecules. The result of inhibiting these several enzymes, however, is to block the synthesis of cellular DNA, RNA, certain co-factors, and other active nucleotides.

The biologic activity of azathioprine and 6-MP is greatest when nucleic acid synthesis is most required.[7, 18] These agents thus strongly inhibit the development of both humoral and cellular immunity by interfering with the differentiation and proliferation of the responding lymphocytes. When the expansion of fully immunocompetent cells is complete, nucleic acid synthesis is less important and the drug is less effective. An additional benefit of azathioprine is that it can also reduce neutrophil production and macrophage activation, effects that suppress the nonspecific inflammatory components of the immune reaction.

The toxicity of azathioprine derives from the same antimetabolite action.[7, 18, 22] The primary effect is bone marrow suppression, leading to leukopenia. Liver toxicity may also occur, possibly because of the high rate of RNA synthesis by hepatocytes. Because hepatic dysfunction does not appear to be dose related, the mechanism is unclear. Promising new purine biosynthesis inhibitors include mizoribine and mycophenolate mofetil (a derivative of mycophenolic acid); these agents have been used in place of azathioprine in recent kidney transplantation trials.

Pyrimidine Analogs. Although pyrimidine analogs have been studied extensively as immunosuppressants in the laboratory, they have had only limited clinical use. The pyrimidine analog cytarabine inhibits DNA synthesis and, therefore, the proliferative phase of the immune response. This molecule has an altered sugar moiety and can be mistaken for cytosine riboside. Experimentally, the immunosuppressive effect of cytarabine has been more easily demonstrated in inhibition of primary antibody responses than in cell-mediated reactions.[17] Clinically, it is used in preparing leukemic patients for bone marrow transplantation.[7, 18]

Folic Acid Antagonists. The immunosuppressive effect of a diet deficient in pteroylglutamic acid was originally noted by Little and led to the use of the folic acid antagonists aminopterin and methotrexate. Both drugs inhibit the enzyme dihydrofolate reductase and prevent the conversion of folic acid to tetrahydrofolic acid. This step is necessary for the synthesis of DNA, RNA, and certain coenzymes.[7, 18]

The therapeutic ratio of immunosuppression to toxicity has not justified the use of these drugs in clinical solid organ transplantation. The immune reactions that accompany bone marrow transplantation, however, are more difficult to control, and methotrexate can be used both to prevent and to reverse severe graft-versus-host (GVH) reactions.[17] The toxic effects of methotrexate can be difficult to identify. Megaloblastic hematopoiesis, mucosal breakdown with severe gastrointestinal bleeding, and liver damage appear to be related to methotrexate therapy. Even with high dosages of methotrexate, however, these effects can usually be prevented by folinic acid (citrovorum rescue). Obviously, depression of

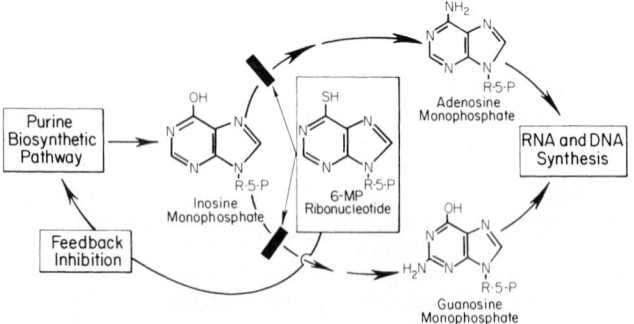

Figure 20–37. The mechanisms of action of the antimetabolites 6-mercaptopurine (6-MP) and azathioprine are similar. These molecules are converted in the cell to 6-MP ribonucleotide, which resembles inosine ribonucleotide in its steric configuration. Consequently, there is competition between these molecules in the pathways of adenosine monophosphate and guanosine monophosphate. Although 6-MP nucleotide is not extensively incorporated, it effectively inhibits the enzymes of these pathways, which reduces the precursors available for incorporation into RNA and DNA. In addition, 6-MP slows the purine biosynthetic pathway by feedback inhibition. The net effect of 6-MP and azathioprine is to greatly reduce RNA and DNA synthesis by their competitive activity.

the transplanted marrow may also follow the activity of methotrexate, although assigning the cause may be difficult in the complex clinical situation. In bone marrow transplantation, a combination of methotrexate with cyclosporine has afforded superior control of GVH disease with lower dosages of each drug.[17] As a result, the toxicities have also been reduced.

Alkylating Agents. The alkylating agents have highly reactive rings as part of their molecular structure. These unstable rings have electron-seeking points that combine with electron-rich nucleophilic groups, such as the tertiary nitrogens in purines and pyrimidines, or with —NH$_2$, —COOH, —SH, and —PO$_3$H$_2$ groups on a variety of molecules. The high-energy rings of alkylating agents break and combine with these constituents to form stable covalent bonds.[7, 18] Obviously, many cell components have such groups, including DNA, RNA, and the enzymatic and structural proteins. Alkylation of DNA is probably the most detrimental. If the DNA strands are not repaired, chromosomal replication will be faulty in proliferating cells. Both DNA and RNA can be alkylated at several points, but a common site appears to be N-7 of the guanine ring (Fig. 20–38). Mispairing of DNA during replication may be caused by the presence of the alkylating agent itself, the excision out of the alkylated guanine residue, or the cleavage of an alkylated guanine ring. Also, chain breaks and cross-linkages frequently interfere with chain replication.[7, 18]

The damage to DNA can be repaired. Thus the effects of these agents are time dependent. The administration of alkylating agents just before and during antigenic stimulation would interfere most with the ability of the immunocompetent cells to respond to that antigen. Continued use of alkylating agents would also suppress the proliferative response of these cells in the presence of a persistent antigenic stimulus. There are differences, however, in the responses of T and B cells. The B cell appears to be more susceptible to cyclophosphamide than is the T cell. This drug is a potent inhibitor of antibody formation, but its effect on skin or kidney allograft rejection is much less spectacular. The reason(s) for this apparent difference is unknown.[7, 18]

The usefulness of alkylating agents, which include nitrogen mustard, phenylalanine mustard, busulfan, and cyclophosphamide, is limited by their toxicity. However, cyclophosphamide has been used with good results in renal transplantation when liver toxicity prohibited the use of azathioprine. Cyclophosphamide is frequently used in clinical bone marrow transplantation to prepare recipients for transplantation. In this setting, it potentiates the effects of radiation and enhances the disruption of DNA. When cyclophosphamide is used, lower doses of radiation are required to deplete the recipient bone marrow population and provide space for donor cells. When leukemia is the indication for bone marrow transplantation, cyclophosphamide also helps destroy the leukemic cells. More recently, cyclophosphamide has been used experimentally in the generation of suppressor cell-like activity to alloantigens and is most effective when given 2 to 4 days after antigenic exposure. If given earlier, it has the opposite effect and enhances the immune reactivity.

Toxicity is high, however, and predictable reactions occur, principally to rapidly replicating cell populations. Stomatitis, nausea, vomiting, diarrhea, rash, anemia, and alopecia are all common reactions. The more specific effects of cyclophosphamide administration are prompt fluid retention, occasionally severe hemorrhagic cystitis, and cardiac toxicity; the cardiac and edema problems suggest that even nonreplicating cell populations are adversely affected by this drug.

Antibiotics. The immunosuppressive antibiotics include inhibitors of nucleic acid synthesis and chloramphenicol and puromycin, which interfere with cellular protein synthesis.[7, 18] Dactinomycin binds to the guanine residue of DNA, thereby sterically interfering with RNA synthesis. This potentially effective means of suppressing the development of immunity led to its use in reversing acute rejection of kidney grafts. The toxicity of dactinomycin has limited its overall clinical benefit, however, and it has been used less and less frequently.

Puromycin structurally resembles an amino acid–charged transfer RNA molecule and is accepted into the ribosome. There is no amino acid to be donated, however, and the peptide chain is prematurely terminated. Although protein synthesis is obviously central to immunologic expression, it is so general a requirement for other cells that toxicity is widespread. Chloramphenicol has also been investigated experimentally. It is most potent in prokaryotic (bacterial) cell systems, and its effects on mammalian cells may be due to inhibition of mitochondrial synthesis. Unfortunately, it is only weakly immunosuppressive, and potentially severe bone marrow toxicity precludes its use.

T-Cell–Directed Immunosuppressants

Cyclosporine. Borel's discovery, in 1972, of the immunosuppressive properties of cyclosporine, a fungal metabolite

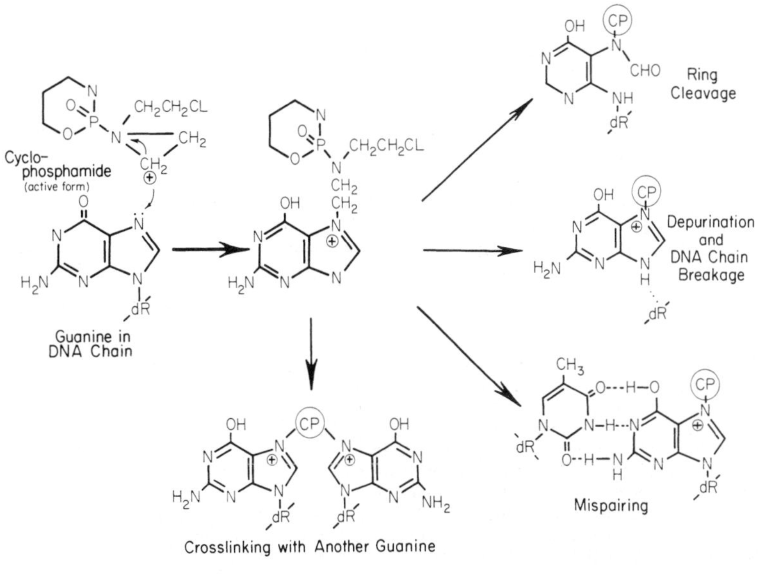

Figure 20–38. The alkylating agents have reactive rings that can combine with electron-rich points of a variety of molecules. The effect of the alkylating agents appears to be related to their DNA binding. Cyclophosphamide (CP), for example, binds extensively to guanine molecules within the DNA chain. The guanine-cyclophosphamide complex has several possible consequences for the DNA strand. The ultimate effect of the four examples shown is to interfere with accurate base pairing and DNA replication.

extracted from *Tolypocladium inflatum* Gams, contributed enormously to the rapid and successful growth of the field of clinical organ transplantation, especially of livers and hearts.[28] It represented a completely new class of clinically important immunosuppressive agents. Many of its selective, suppressive effects on T cells appear to be related to its selective inhibition of TCR-mediated activation events. It inhibits cytokine production by T_H cells *in vitro* and impairs the development of mature $CD4^+$ and $CD8^+$ T cells in the thymus. Cyclosporine is a cyclic peptide (11 amino acids; molecular weight 1202 daltons).

Cyclosporine was discovered to be immunosuppressive by its ability to suppress antibody production in mice. Other *in vivo* properties include inhibition of antibody plaque-forming cell production, GVH disease, skin graft rejection, delayed solid organ allograft rejection, and DTH reactions. Absence of myelosuppression was a major advance over other immunosuppressive agents and indicated that the mechanism of action was relatively specific for lymphocytes.[22, 28, 42, 46] Other inflammatory cells are much less sensitive to its inhibitory effects. Clinically, prophylactic administration of cyclosporine suppresses allograft rejection and GVH disease.

Analyses of the effect of cyclosporine on T lymphocytes have shown (1) inhibition of both IL-2–producing T lymphocytes and cytotoxic T lymphocytes, (2) inhibition of IL-2 gene expression by activated T lymphocytes, (3) no inhibition of activated T lymphocytes in response to exogenous IL-2, (4) inhibition of resting T-lymphocyte activation in response to alloantigen and exogenous lymphokine, (5) inhibition of IL-1 production, and (6) inhibition of mitogen (concanavalin A) activation of IL-2–producing T lymphocytes. The above T-lymphocyte responses involve both $CD4^+$ (T_H) and/or $CD8^+$ (T-cytotoxic/suppressor) lymphocytes, and the inhibition appears to occur at the level of activation, and perhaps even maturation, of the resting cell. In mice, maturation of T cells that occurs in the thymus is significantly suppressed by cyclosporine, thus enriching a population of immature and less responsive T cells.

A number of kidney and other solid organ transplantation trials have shown that cyclosporine induces potent immunosuppression without myelosuppression. The addition of steroids to cyclosporine permitted a lowering of the cyclosporine dosage and decreased nephrotoxicity (the principal clinical side effect of the drug). The introduction of cyclosporine into widespread clinical use in 1983 led to a substantial improvement in the outcome of cadaveric renal transplantation and permitted the widespread practice of heart and liver grafting.

The potential adverse effects of cyclosporine include nephrotoxicity, hypertension, hyperkalemia, hirsutism, gingival hyperplasia, tremor and other neurotoxicities, diabetogenicity, and hepatotoxicity. As with other immunosuppressive agents, cyclosporine therapy increases the risk of infection and malignancy but, by reducing steroid requirements, generally decreases infection rates.

Tacrolimus. Tacrolimus (formerly known as FK 506) is a potent new immunosuppressive agent isolated in 1984 in Japan from the soil fungus *Streptomyces tsukubaensis.* It is a macrocyclic lactone with a molecular weight of 822 daltons. Although structurally distinct from cyclosporine, it exhibits a very similar molecular action. Both drugs are now regarded as *pro-drugs.* Their antilymphocytic effects result from the formation of active complexes between the drug and its respective intracellular binding protein or *immunophilin*[42] (cyclophilin or FK 506 binding protein; FKBP) (Fig. 20–39). The drug-immunophilin complex blocks the phosphatase activity of calcineurin that is important in regulation of IL-2 gene transcription.[42, 46] The activity of tacrolimus *in vitro,* however, is approximately 100 times greater than that of

cyclosporine. Like cyclosporine, tacrolimus functions to inhibit (1) IL-2 gene expression and IL-2 production; (2) mixed lymphocyte culture cellular proliferation, which is mediated by T helper (T_H) cells; (3) the generation of cytotoxic T cells; and (4) the appearance of IL-2R on human lymphocytes. *In vivo,* tacrolimus prolongs the survival of MHC-disparate skin, cardiac, renal, hepatic, and small bowel allografts. It has recently been approved for the treatment of liver allograft rejection. Side effects of cyclosporine and tacrolimus are similar, although tacrolimus does not cause hirsutism or gum hypertrophy.

Sirolimus. Like tacrolimus, the experimental immunosuppressant sirolimus (also known as rapamycin) is a macrolide antibiotic. It is a close structural analog of tacrolimus and binds to the same cytoplasmic receptor (FKBP). Unlike tacrolimus or cyclosporine, however, sirolimus does not block T-cell cytokine gene expression but instead inhibits the transduction of signals from the IL-2R to the nucleus.[42, 46] Binding of sirolimus to FKBP inhibits P70S6 protein kinase activity, which is essential for ribosomal phosphorylation and cell cycle progression. Sirolimus potently inhibits experimental allograft rejection. Two additional, important properties of this drug are that it acts synergistically with cyclosporine and prevents chronic graft vessel disease in rat transplant models.[46] Combination of sirolimus with low-dose cyclosporine and use of sirolimus to prevent chronic rejection and atheromatous disease are important future clinical considerations. Promiscuity of the drug's inhibitory action on the response of hematopoietic cells to growth factors and poor oral bioavailability, however, are considered potential clinical limitations.

Eicosanoids

The *eicosanoids* are the largest class of lipid mediators. They are produced by all human cells except lymphocytes and possess a wide variety of biologic activities. The term includes the oxygenation products of long-chain polyunsaturated fatty acids, such as arachidonic acid and linolenic acid, *essential* fatty acids, and the compounds such as prostaglandins into which they are incorporated for synthesis. The immunomodulatory effects of the eicosanoids are mediated by direct actions on cells and also by indirect influences on the release of platelet activating factor, cytokines, and other substances.[1]

The antirejection eicosanoids (prostaglandin [PG] E_2 and PGD_2) inhibit T-cell proliferation by inhibition of IL-1, IL-2, and MHC Class II antigen expression on macrophages. Other prorejection eicosanoids (thromboxane A_2; leukotriene [LT] B_4 [LTB_4]; LTC_4; and LTD_4) enhance T-cell proliferation. Investigations are preliminary but promising, and potential clinical applications to control or prevent rejection by manipulating these agents await further study.

Lymphocyte Depletion Measures

Numerous clinically important immunosuppressive agents are effective because they deplete the host of lymphocytes. As the mechanism of action of these agents becomes better understood, a more sophisticated classification system may evolve; but for the present, antilymphocyte globulin, radiation, and mAb therapy appear to act by relatively nonselective lymphocyte depletion or inactivation.[7, 18]

Antilymphocyte Globulin (ALG). ALGs are produced when lymphocytes are injected into animals of a different species. Rabbit, goat, and horse antisera are commonly used.[18] The action of ALG appears to be directed mainly against the T cell; the use of thymocytes therefore creates the most potent sera. The suppression produced by ALG can at

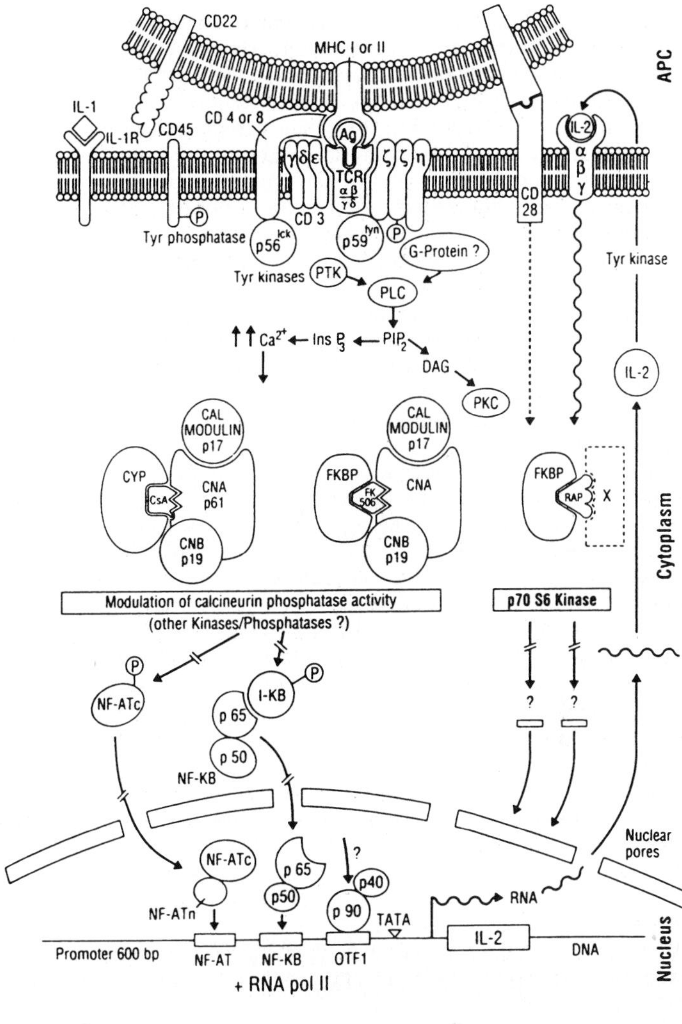

Figure 20–39. Signal transduction in activated T cells and the sites (center of figure) at which cyclosporine (CsA), tacrolimus (FK 506), and sirolimus (rapamycin [RAP]) are believed to act. CsA or FK 506 bound to their respective immunophilins (cyclophilin [CYP]) or FK 506 binding protein (FKBP) form pentameric complexes with calmodulin and calcineurin A (CNA) and B. Inhibition of the phosphatase activity of calcineurin is believed to inhibit translocation to the nucleus of the cytoplasmic component of the nuclear factor of activated T cells (NF-ATc) that is required for activation of the IL-2 gene. RAP, which also binds to FKBP, inhibits phosphorylation and activation of a 70-kd. ribosomal S6 protein kinase (p70S6), which normally occurs within minutes of cell activation by cytokine receptors. RAP also targets other kinases (not shown) that are essential for cell cycle progression. (From Schreier, M., et al.: Molecular basis of immunosuppression. Transplant. Sci., 3:185, 1993.)

least partially be reversed by T cells, but not by bone marrow cells. Thymectomy enhances the effect of ALG, and ALG decreases the number of circulating T cells. As would be expected, ALG administration interferes most with the cell-mediated reactions: allograft rejection, tuberculin sensitivity, and the GVH reaction. ALG can abolish pre-existing delayed hypersensitivity reactions, and larger doses prolong the survival of some xenografts. ALG has a definite, but lesser, effect on T-cell–dependent antibody production. Lymphocytes coated with ALG are either lysed or cleared from the blood by reticuloendothelial cells in the liver and spleen.

ALG may be administered prophylactically, during the early posttransplant period, or used effectively to reverse ongoing rejection. Favorable results depend on potent ALG and prolonged administration, rather than a single dose. The use of ALG is not confined to kidney transplantation, and beneficial results have also been reported in bone marrow transplantation. ALG pretreatment of the recipient is of value in suppressing the response to the donor cells and for enlarging the marrow space. In addition, ALG may be useful in preventing the GVH reactions that arise in these patients.

The toxicity of any heterologous serum prepared against human tissue depends on two factors: its cross-reactivity with other tissue antigens and the ability of the patient to make antibodies against the foreign protein. Anemia and thrombocytopenia can occur and are presumably caused by a reaction between the ALG and host erythrocytes and platelets. Although prior absorption with human platelets and red

cell stroma reduces its severity, some cross-reactivity with these cells persists in all ALG preparations.

Allergic reactions to the antiserum itself are the most common clinical problems associated with the use of ALG. Urticaria, anaphylactoid reactions, and serum sickness, including joint pain, fever, and malaise all follow development of immunity to the heterologous globulin. These reactions are reduced, however, in the presence of the other immunosuppressive drugs used in renal transplantation.

The major problem in producing a standardized antihuman ALG is the inability to develop a method of assaying its *in vitro* antilymphocytic potency. Unfortunately, individual laboratories make their own ALG preparations, and a standard method of assay has not been developed. Cytotoxic assays, the formation of cellular rosettes by antibody-coated cells, and animal assays for immunosuppressive activity have been employed, but a consistent test has not emerged. A suitable assay is necessary to identify the better ALG preparations, making their use increasingly beneficial.

Monoclonal Antibody (OKT3). In 1975, Kohler and Milstein developed the technology for somatic cell hybridization (*hybridoma formation*), which could establish immortalized cell lines that each secrete a single or *monoclonal antibody* in limitless supply.[1] Subsequently, monoclonal antibodies (mAbs) have been generated that react with T cells in general (OKT3, anti-CD3) and various T-cell subsets (OKT4, anti-CD4; OKT8, anti-CD8). Further information on newer experimental mAbs is found later in this chapter. OKT3, first used clinically in 1980, has become the most useful therapeutic mAb. It is used to treat established episodes of acute kidney, liver, heart, or heart-lung rejection. The prophylactic potency of regimens including OKT3 in renal transplantation has also been demonstrated. OKT3 binds to a site associated with the TCR (CD3) and functions to modulate the receptor and inactivate T-cell function (Fig. 20–40).[15, 19]

By engaging the TCR complex, OKT3 blocks not only the function of naive T cells but also the function of established cytotoxic T cells, thereby blocking cell-mediated cytotoxicity. OKT3 blocks the T-cell effector functions involved in allograft rejection. After intravenous administration, OKT3 opsonizes or binds to T cells. These are then removed by the reticuloendothelial cells that reside in liver and spleen. Circulating T cells decrease abruptly (30–60 min.) after the first OKT3 injection. Once OKT3 is stopped, CD3+ cells rapidly return to their normal levels.[19]

The major limitation to use of OKT3 is that it is immunogenic and can elicit immune reactions.[15] After prolonged use, OKT3 becomes less effective owing to the production of antibody that binds to and effects the removal of circulating OKT3. An acute systemic reaction secondary to polyclonal T cell activation by OKT3 and subsequent cytokine release is, in most cases, easily controlled. In addition, overimmunosuppression can occur with OKT3; treatment cannot be pursued for more than 2 weeks owing to the risk of infections and malignancies.

Radiation. The concept of using total lymphoid irradiation (TLI) is based on the profound immunosuppressive effects observed after TLI for treatment of Hodgkin's disease.[1] Preoperative TLI of allograft recipients is immunosuppressive when used alone or together with chemical immunosuppression. Immunologic monitoring after TLI and transplantation has confirmed a sustained and uniform reduction in CD4+ T_H cells and in the proliferative responses of these cells to mitogenic and allogeneic lymphoid stimulation during the first year after grafting. Other studies have shown an increase in numbers of CD8+ cytotoxic/suppressor cells in these patients, and some postulate that the immunosuppression observed follows the generation of endogenous suppressor cells. B cells probably also have a role in this effect, because they are relatively radiosensitive and are also affected by the radiation.

Radiation was probably the first agent used clinically to produce immunosuppression.[7, 18] Ionizing radiation (x-rays, alpha rays, beta rays) affects both nucleic acids and cellular proteins. Despite the fact that relatively small doses of irradiation may disrupt the secondary protein structure formed by hydrogen bonding and the tertiary conformation that results, biologically significant alterations of protein function appear to require very high dosages. Consequently, most of the immunosuppressive effects of x-radiation are caused by changes produced in nucleic acids. DNA is particularly vulnerable, as is cell replication. The most important of the several modes of damage is the production of scattered breaks in the deoxyribose-phosphate backbone of DNA. Disruption of either the carbon-to-carbon bonds of the deoxyribonucleotides or the bonds involving the phosphate groups produces breaks in one of the DNA strands. Occasionally, both strands are broken at the same point. Other sites of damage, such as the bases themselves, are even less frequent.

Repair mechanisms exist to mend the break, but insufficient time may be available in the dividing cell. Therefore, the effectiveness of radiation depends on the phase of the cell cycle. Cells in the M or G_2 phase are most sensitive to irradiation. Presumably, DNA breaks that occur during these phases cannot be repaired rapidly enough, and the synthetic events and precise apportionment of the cellular components that occur during mitosis may become scrambled. Conversely, the early G_1 phase and the latter part of S phase are the most resistant parts of the cell cycle. Although irradiation is generally most effective just before or during mitosis, lymphocytes represent a special case. For reasons that are not known, these cells are also sensitive in their resting, or G_0, phase, and lysis of lymphocytes follows radiation of sufficient doses.[7, 18]

Despite the complexity of the subcellular mechanism, the effect of irradiation on the immune response is predictable and depends greatly on its timing in relation to antigen exposure. The possibilities are best seen when a relatively simple response, antibody production against a defined antigen, is measured. When the antigen is given soon after irradiation, the immune response is inhibited because there is insufficient time for the immunocompetent cell population to recover before the antigen is encountered. If radiation is given during the time of maximal proliferation of the immunocompetent cell population to an antigen (soon after antigen administration), the response is strongly inhibited. However, if antigenic stimulation is delayed sufficiently for the precursor cells to recover from the radiation, augmentation of the response ensues. Radiation is also effective if initiated long after exposure to the antigen, when the mature population of antibody-synthesizing cells has been formed. Differentiated plasma cells and presumably cytotoxic lymphocytes are radioresistant. The timing of radiation must be carefully planned for the greatest immunosuppressive effect. X-radiation has had limited use in clinical transplantation.

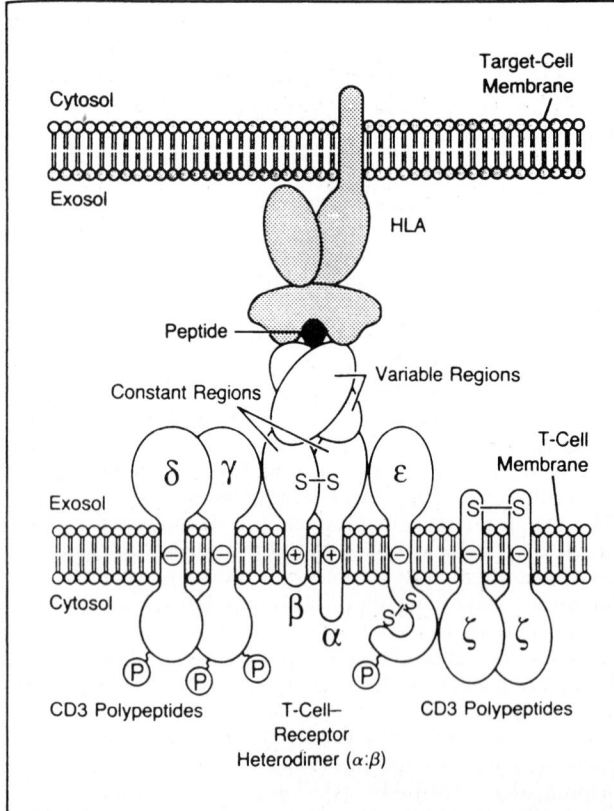

Figure 20–40. Interaction of the T-cell receptor (TCR) and the major histocompatibility complex (MHC). The alpha and beta polypeptide chains of the TCR form a heterodimer linked by a disulfide bond (S—S). This heterodimer binds to peptide associated with a MHC on the surface of a presenting cell. The nonpolymorphic CD3 polypeptides (gamma, delta, epsilon, and zeta) are assembled together with the TCR and are probably involved in signal transduction. P, phosphorylation site. (Reprinted by permission of *The New England Journal of Medicine* from Krensky, A. M., Weiss, A., Crabtree, E., et al.: T-lymphocyte–antigen interactions in transplant rejection. N. Engl. J. Med., 322:513, 1990, Copyright 1990, Massachusetts Medical Society.)

After transplantation, radiation of the graft may damage invading cells and produce nonspecific anti-inflammatory effects. Although proof of its benefit is lacking, some centers irradiate the kidney graft at the onset of a rejection reaction.

Total-body radiation is used as *cytoreductive therapy* to prepare patients for bone marrow transplantation. In theory, the radiation treatment creates *space* in the bone marrow to allow the grafting of new cells. The toxicity is predictable. The rapidly replicating cells in the skin and the gastrointestinal tract are universally affected, and nausea, vomiting, diarrhea, and skin changes occur. Late problems are also probably attributable to damage to the cellular genetic apparatus: growth retardation, vertebral deformities, sterility, cataracts, and an increased incidence of cancer.

Total Lymphoid Irradiation (TLI) Plus Bone Marrow Transplantation. This technique combines the use of radiation and donor bone marrow transplantation to promote acceptance of kidney or other organ grafts.[7, 40] It is still experimental. Potential graft recipients are given a fractionated course of approximately 3000 cGy (or a brief exposure to 600 cGy) to the lymphoid-bearing areas with shielding of the skull, ribs, lungs, and legs to preserve the bone marrow. After the irradiation is completed, both a bone marrow transplant and an organ graft are performed. Proliferation of the donor bone marrow cells causes a partial chimeric state that facilitates acceptance of the organ graft. By a process not yet well understood, the donor and host bone marrow cells both repopulate the periphery, producing a form of tolerance. Experimentally, the tolerant state is stable and may be due, in part, to the generation of large numbers of suppressor cells. In contrast to the situation after total-body irradiation (TBI), the bone marrow after TLI does not as readily cause GVH disease. Experimental success has prompted a few clinical trials. The logistic difficulty of administration of radiation and the uncertain interval between discontinuing the irradiation and performing cadaveric transplantation reduce the attractiveness of the procedure.

Thymectomy and Lymphoid Extirpation. Experimentally, immune reactivity can be delayed for brief periods by interrupting the lymphatic channels, by placing grafts in sites with poor lymphatic drainage, or by excising local lymphoid tissue. Excision of locally draining lymph nodes or the spleen, however, is also ineffective as an immunosuppressive technique.

Thoracic Duct Drainage. Cannulation and drainage of the thoracic duct can successfully deplete the body of a large proportion of its circulating T lymphocytes.[2, 9] This prolongs allograft survival and decreases antibody synthesis. Thoracic duct cannulation has been employed successfully to deplete patients' lymphocytes and to prolong allograft survival but is no longer used because patency of the cannula was difficult to maintain and prolonged hospitalization was required.

Other Immunosuppressive Approaches

Blood Transfusion. Many studies over the past 20 years have showed that multiple allogeneic blood transfusions before cadaveric kidney transplantation improved graft survival, and some form of transfusion protocol became part of the preparative regimen for most patients in renal failure who were awaiting a graft.[14, 18] There is also evidence that blood transfusion from a living-related donor induces a degree of specific immunologic hyporeactivity against graft antigens if administered several weeks before grafting. Some, though not all, studies in the past 5 years have shown that the beneficial effect of transfusion may no longer be present,[14] perhaps because of better immunosuppressive drug therapy. With the advent of erythropoietin to prevent anemia in dialysis patients, transfusion is also less necessary. The salutary

effects of transfusion have also been evident in nonrenal solid organ grafts. A retrospective analysis of cardiac transplant recipients showed a 13% improvement in 1-year graft survival. An important consideration is that 30% of uremic individuals and nearly all nonuremic patients receiving deliberate transfusions become allosensitized. To circumvent this problem, azathioprine or cyclosporine administered at the time of transfusion reduces the rate of sensitization substantially. Elective random or donor-specific blood transfusions also carry a risk of transmission of viruses, including human immunodeficiency virus and hepatitis virus. The exact mechanism(s) by which transfusions exert a beneficial effect is unknown, but the following have been suggested: clonal deletion or inactivation; the induction of suppressor cells; the presence of blocking antibodies or anti-idiotypic antibodies; and cross-reactivity.[14]

POTENTIAL NEW DIRECTIONS TO PREVENT REJECTION

Monoclonal Antibodies. The most important goals in the development of new immunosuppressive modalities for therapy for allograft rejection are to narrow the target cell population and to induce donor antigen-specific tolerance in the host. Monoclonal antibodies (mAbs) are uniquely suited to realize both of these goals because of their remarkable specificity.[32, 48] After transplantation of an allograft, only a small fraction of the entire T-lymphocyte pool is activated. The *ideal* mAb would select only this activated subpopulation for either elimination or modulation. Ideally, this would produce tolerance by the induction of clone-specific anergy. To date, the major emphasis in improving the selectivity of mAb therapy has been to identify suitable molecular targets expressed on the surface of the graft recipient's responding T cells. Anti-IL-2R mAbs are excellent examples of this type of approach. By blocking these receptors, the mAbs interfere directly with the ability of activated T cells to respond to normal growth/differentiation signals.

Anti-IL-2R mAbs. The IL-2R is a complex of several transmembrane polypeptide chains. Two IL-2 binding chains, alpha (CD25; p55) and beta (p70) have been characterized. Noncovalent association of these chains forms the high affinity binding site for IL-2. The alpha chain is present only on activated T cells and a subset of activated B cells and APC. Thus anti-CD25 mAb treatment targets a minor population of cells enriched for antigen-activated T cells. Several anti-CD25 mAbs have been shown to prolong allograft survival in rodents and nonhuman primates. In clinical studies, two anti-CD25 mAbs (anti-Tac and 33B3.1) have been used to prevent renal allograft rejection.[29, 43] Both antibodies were well tolerated. Rejection was also controlled with cyclosporine, azathioprine, and prednisone. Anti-Tac decreased the number of early rejection episodes and delayed the time to first rejection but no improvement, on patient or graft survival, was noted.[29]

In an effort to reduce the immunogenicity of rodent mAbs that causes rapid development of neutralizing human anti-mouse antibodies (HAMA), humanized mAbs have been produced. Anti-Tac-H is the best characterized of these. The immunogenicity of this molecule, as measured by *in vivo* circulating half-life and by the appearance of circulating anti-Tac-H antibodies is significantly reduced compared with murine anti-Tac.[10] Although certain limitations have been encountered with the function of humanized mAbs, these should be overcome by further customization (genetic remodeling) of the molecules.

Antiadhesion Molecule mAbs. Another potentially useful group of mAbs are those that block T-cell adhesion molecules, such as lymphocyte function associated antigen-1

(LFA-1) or very late appearing antigen-4 (VLA-4), or their endothelial cell ligands, such as intercellular adhesion molecule-1 (ICAM-1) and vascular cell adhesion molecule-1 (VCAM-1). These mAbs can prevent T cells *homing* into the allograft. ICAM-1 is constitutively expressed on about 20% of blood mononuclear cells and on vascular endothelium. It is readily induced on many cell types, including endothelial and epithelial cells, by cytokine-induced activation, and it functions as a ligand for LFA-1 that is expressed constitutively on T cells. Significantly, LFA-1–ICAM-1 interaction provides a co-stimulatory signal for T-cell activation that is synergistic to the signal delivered by the TCR/CD3 complex. After testing of anti-ICAM-1 for both prophylaxis and treatment of renal allograft rejection in monkeys, a Phase I trial of murine anti-ICAM-1 prophylaxis has been performed in a small group of cadaveric renal allograft patients at high risk for delayed graft function. The data suggest that anti-ICAM-1 treatment is well tolerated, and is efficacious in preventing human allograft rejection and, possibly, in reducing the severity of reperfusion injury.[26] A multicenter randomized, controlled trial is now under way to further evaluate the clinical potential of anti-ICAM-1.

Anti-T-Cell Subset Molecule mAbs. The CD4 and CD8 molecules are expressed on reciprocal subsets of CD3$^+$, $\alpha\beta$ TCR$^+$ T cells that are classified functionally as T$_H$ cells (CD4$^+$) or cytotoxic/suppressor T cells (CD8$^+$). CD4 and CD8 function to facilitate intercellular adhesion between T cells and APCs bearing Class II and Class I MHC-associated antigens, respectively. Both CD4 and CD8 have a role in TCR-CD3–mediated signal transduction via interaction with intracellular protein tyrosine kinase. Anti-CD4 mAbs have demonstrated the capacity to prolong allograft survival in rodents and nonhuman primates. Clinical studies are very limited,[34, 49] although both anti-CD4 and anti-CD8 mAb selectively deplete their target cells in renal allograft recipients.

Pretransplant Treatment with mAbs. The possibility of using mAbs in conjunction with donor-specific transfusion (DST) to help induce donor antigen-specific tolerance is being examined. This approach has potential application in the pretransplant conditioning of potential living-related or living-unrelated allograft recipients. The underlying principle is that DST can be used to elicit donor-specific activated T cells, which may then be eliminated by mAb directed against the IL-2R or other cell membrane molecules associated with T-cell activation.

Other Target Molecules. Attempts are being made at the experimental level to induce specific T cell clonal anergy by preventing T cells from receiving the appropriate co-stimulatory signals from APCs during their initial encounter with graft alloantigens. Potential targets include, in particular, CD28 and its homologue CTLA-4 on the T-cell surface. These molecules are involved, through their interaction with B7 family proteins on APCs, with the delivery of the crucial *second signal* (in addition to antigen) that is essential for T-cell activation. A soluble form of CTLA-4, the recombinant fusion protein CTLA4-Ig, has been administered to rodents to prevent the interaction of graft cell B7 molecules with host T-cell CD28 and prevent allograft rejection.[30] There is evidence that under these conditions, the T-cell IL-2 gene is not expressed and the cells become specifically unresponsive to donor alloantigens.

Immunotoxins. These are chemical conjugates between mAbs and either toxin moieties (e.g., ricin A chain) or radionuclides (e.g., ^{90}Y or ^{212}Bi) that selectively deliver a lethal *package* to specific target cells. These molecules are under development to treat cancer, autoimmune disease, or solid organ allograft rejection. Anti–pan-T cell (CD5) ricin A-chain immunotoxin has already been shown to be effective in steroid-resistant acute GVH disease. ^{90}Y-labeled murine anti-

Tac (CD25) is more effective than nonlabeled anti-Tac in prolonging primate xenografts, due presumably to highly effective killing of IL-2R$^+$ cells.

Fusion Proteins and Immunoligands. Unlike an immunotoxin, which is the product of biochemical fusion of payload toxin to mAb, a fusion protein is the translational product of fusion of the genes encoding the two protein elements. For example, various toxins are being genetically appended to antigen-binding domains of pre-existing mAbs. An example is the recombinant immunotoxin anti-Tac (Fv)-PE40, in which the antibody variable domains of the anti-Tac mAb are linked to *Pseudomonas* exotoxin. A second type of mAb fusion protein is one in which the antigen binding domains of the antibody are replaced with another targeting protein. An example is the bivalent molecule IL-2/Fc that possesses functional activity of both the incorporated human proteins. In principle, IL-2 directs specific binding of the construct to IL-2R bearing cells, while the Fc portion directs cytopathic immune effector functions against the target cells. Such immunoligands offer several potential advantages over antireceptor mAbs, including much greater target specificity and affinity.

Anticytokine mAbs. Other targets for mAb therapy are the leukocyte-derived cytokines that play important roles in intercellular signaling. Already there is evidence that anti-TNF-α and anti-TNF-β enhance cardiac allograft survival in rodents. Other potential cytokine targets include IL-1, IL-2, IL-6, and IFN-γ.

Local Immunosuppression

One approach toward reducing the drug-specific and general adverse consequences of systemic immunosuppression is the use of local drug administration systems to establish more selective presence of immunosuppressive agents in the transplanted organ. Experimental drug targeting approaches include intra-arterial drug infusion, implantable infusion pumps, controlled-release matrices, drug-impregnated polymer rods, liposomes, topical application (skin or cornea), and aerosol inhalation (lung). These diverse methods prevent rejection and reduce systemic toxicity in rodent and canine models and provide a basis for future clinical application. This topic has been reviewed.[21]

A CONVENTIONAL IMMUNOSUPPRESSIVE REGIMEN FOR KIDNEY TRANSPLANTATION

Before cyclosporine became generally available for clinical immunosuppression in 1983, most transplant surgeons used a combination of azathioprine and prednisone with or without ALG.[7, 18] At present, in most transplant centers, recipients of cadaveric and living-related donor kidneys (except HLA-identical recipients) receive cyclosporine and prednisone. Azathioprine is often added and tapered to a dose adjusted according to peripheral white blood cell counts, platelet levels, and renal function. Recipients of HLA-identical antigen matches receive prednisone plus cyclosporine or azathioprine. At some centers, ALG is given intravenously early postoperatively. The dosage is reduced if the platelet level is less than or equal to 50,000 per cu. mm. Treatment is continued for 7 to 14 days or until sensitivity to ALG appears.[7, 18, 22, 23]

First rejection episodes in patients receiving conventional immunosuppression are treated with increased corticosteroids (2 mg./kg.) with a subsequent rapid taper in dosage. In addition, ALG and/or OKT3 may be added. Subsequent rejection episodes are treated with increased steroids alone. Increasing corticosteroids is also the method of treatment for patients receiving cyclosporine immunosuppression.[7, 18, 23]

An important but unanswered question is how long immunosuppressive therapy should be continued when the kidney functions well without signs of rejection. Isolated successful instances of discontinuing medication have been reported, suggesting that some host-to-graft accommodation may occur. Rejection reactions do occur, however; and although there is some disagreement, it appears they are more numerous or intense than those encountered during therapy. Until more information is available, immunosuppressive therapy is considered a lifelong necessity.

CONSEQUENCES OF IMMUNOSUPPRESSION

In addition to the many specific immunologic and potentially toxic effects of immunosuppressive therapies, there are several additional clinically important consequences of immunosuppression (Table 20–8).

Infection. Infection remains the most common complication of immunosuppression and the most common cause of death in recipients of organ allografts. These patients are more prone to develop a wide variety of infectious diseases, many of which are not encountered in immunocompetent individuals. Infections due to viral pathogens (especially cytomegalovirus) are particularly common, and it has proved extremely difficult to prevent their occurrence. However, increased experience in prevention has both lowered the incidence of serious infection and delayed its occurrence. Infectious complications after transplant surgery have been reviewed.[16, 39]

Malignancy. The incidence of *de novo* malignancy is increased in recipients of organ transplants and is related to length of time on immunosuppressive therapy. Only certain tumors, however, grow more readily. Seventy-five percent of the cancers are either lymphoid or epithelial in origin. Use of potent antilymphocytic drugs and a role for potentially oncogenic viruses have been implicated. In transplant patients who develop cancer, the issue of change or even withdrawal of immunosuppressive therapy is an important one. Cancer and its management in transplant recipients has been reviewed.[36]

Effects on Growth. The antiproliferative effects of certain immunosuppressive drugs make satisfactory growth in pediatric allograft recipients unlikely. The growth response after transplantation is highly variable; although many children return to a normal growth rate, growth lost during the original illness is not regained.

Influence on Pregnancy. Many questions are raised concerning pregnancy and the birth of a normal child, when one parent is a transplant recipient. Antigrowth and possible mutagenic effects of certain immunosuppressants are accompanied by the specter of viral activation, infection, and the increased risk of cancer. In addition, the life expectancy of transplant recipients is decreased.

TABLE 20–8. Problems of Long-Term Immunosuppression in Humans

Failure to prevent and control chronic rejection
Failure to induce tolerance
Opportunistic infections
Spontaneous neoplasms
Metabolic alterations (e.g., hyperlipidemia, glucose intolerance)
Drug toxicities
Growth retardation

INDUCTION OF TRANSPLANTATION TOLERANCE

The cherished goal of transplant scientist and clinician alike is to create tolerance of transplantation without the need for exogenous immunosuppressants. Although tolerance can be achieved readily in small animals, it has proved very difficult to accomplish clinically. Nevertheless, rare instances of the establishment of drug-free unresponsiveness to organ allografts have occurred in humans who have discontinued immunosuppressive therapy for various reasons. Contemporary developments in our understanding of cellular and molecular immunology and of the basis of experimental tolerance induction hold promise for the development of clinically effective approaches. Authentic transplantation tolerance is antigen specific. It is induced as the result of prior exposure to antigen and does not depend on the continuous administration of exogenous antigen-nonspecific immunosuppressive agents. Over 40 years ago, in a seminal study, Billingham and associates[8] showed that specific unresponsiveness to donor alloantigens could be induced by the inoculation of adult allogeneic cells into fetal or neonatal mice. An important lesson from this experiment was that the acquired tolerance was due to the immunologic incompetence of the graft recipient and not to any alteration in the grafted tissue itself.

APPROACHES FOR THE CREATION OF TOLERANCE

Potential approaches for the creation of tolerance in *adult* individuals include (1) cell depletion protocols using irradiation (TBI or TLI) or depleting mAbs; (2) reconstitution protocols (using allogeneic bone marrow); (3) combination of 1 and 2; (4) cell surface molecule targeted therapy (e.g., use of anti-CD4 or anti-intercellular adhesion molecule mAbs); (5) immunosuppressive drugs (e.g., cyclosporine, rapamycin); and (6) donor-specific blood transfusion combined with drug or mAb therapy.

The principal hypotheses proposed for the cellular basis of transplantation tolerance are clonal deletion of antigen-reactive lymphocytes either in the thymus or peripherally; clonal anergy (or functional silencing) of lymphocytes, due to the delivery of the antigenic signal alone without co-stimulatory signals; and suppressor mechanisms (suppressor cells or suppressor *factors*). In the latter instance, suggested mechanisms are anti-idiotypic regulatory cells directed against the TCR idiotype of the responsive T lymphocytes, *veto* cells or suppressor cytokines, such as tumor growth factor-beta (TGF-β).

Antilymphocyte Antibody Plus Donor Bone Marrow. The induction of unresponsiveness with a combination of antilymphocyte serum and donor bone marrow has been documented in mice and also in dogs and monkeys. It is thought that under these circumstances, tolerance is induced by a naturally occurring regulatory cell (veto or suppressor cell) within the bone marrow inoculum. The development of these cells may be facilitated by appropriate growth factors, such as GM-CSF and IL-3. In a limited human study conducted by Barber and colleagues,[7a] transfusion of donor-specific bone marrow a week after a course of ALG was performed in cadaveric renal allograft recipients. These patients received conventional immunosuppressive drugs—cyclosporine, prednisone, azathioprine—and most subjects were also given cyclophosphamide starting at the time of marrow cell infusion. Although the number of rejection episodes and renal function were not affected, graft survival at 1 year was improved significantly.

Irradiation Plus Donor Bone Marrow. TLI plus donor bone marrow infusion of adult mice can cause tolerance induction. Its clinical application was discussed previously. Perhaps the best documented account of acquired immune tolerance in humans is the report by Strober and colleagues in 1989 of specific unresponsiveness in cadaver renal allograft recipients preconditioned with TLI plus a short course of ALG, together with low dose corticosteroids.[45a] Lethal irradiation (TBI) and reconstitution of mice with mixtures of T-cell–depleted syngeneic and allogeneic bone marrow (pioneered by Ildstad and Sachs) produces mixed bone marrow chimerism and donor-specific tolerance to skin grafts. Nonlethal preparative regimens, using anti-T-cell mAb in addition to sublethal TBI plus donor bone marrow, have more recently been shown to create tolerance in mice. However, several problems, including toxicity of TBI, GVH reactions, and the need for donor-host histocompatibility, must be resolved in relation to the mixed chimerism approach.

Bone Marrow Infusion Without Cytoreductive Therapy. Starzl and colleagues have observed long-lasting donor-cell chimerism in conventionally immunosuppressed human organ allograft recipients.[44] Augmentation of this *natural chimerism* by infusion of donor bone marrow at the time of organ transplantation is being performed in patients who do not receive any form of cytoreductive therapy. The procedure has been shown to be safe and effective in augmenting chimerism, but the chimerism is not yet accompanied by donor-specific tolerance.[20]

Suppressor Cells and Tolerance Induction. Suppressor cells have been implicated in a number of experimental models of tolerance induction.[9, 40] Thus, the existence of suppressor T cells generated in the presence of cyclosporine can be demonstrated by the adoptive transfer of tolerance from cyclosporine-treated organ graft recipients. It has not been possible, however, to show that cyclosporine can induce authentic tolerance in human organ transplantation. In experimental animals, donor-specific blood transfusion (DST) before transplantation induces antigen-specific unresponsiveness associated with dysregulation of IL-2 production and the generation of suppressor cells. DST together with cyclosporine has been shown clinically to reduce sensitization and improve renal allograft outcome.

Monoclonal Antibodies. A variety of mAbs to cell surface molecules, in particular anti-CD4, used alone or in combination with other immunosuppressive modalities, such as cyclosporine or TLI, induce tolerance in rodents.[32, 48] Targeting of adhesion molecules or of the CD28 molecule on T cells or B7 molecules on APC also seem important approaches to promoting tolerance induction.

Intrathymic Injection of Donor-Specific Cells. Within the last few years, intrathymic inoculation of allogeneic tissue (e.g., pancreatic islet cells or renal glomeruli) has been shown to induce antigen-specific tolerance to subsequent islet cell or renal allografts, respectively, in the rat. Clonal deletion, anergy, and/or suppressor cells have been postulated as underlying mechanisms.

Oral Tolerance. Another novel approach is the oral administration of MHC Class II allopeptides. In rats, this can prevent sensitization by skin allografts. Depending on the dose of antigen, regulatory cells secreting *suppressor* cytokines (IL-4, IL-10, TGF-β) or anergy have been implicated.

Antisense Oligonucleotides. Selective gene-targeted immunosuppressive therapy offers a new experimental approach to the prevention of allograft rejection. The use of antisense technology to prolong organ allograft survival in mice has been described.[45] ICAM-1 antisense oligonucleotides inhibited the rejection of murine cardiac allografts and, in combination with anti-LFA-1 mAb, induced donor-specific tolerance. There were no toxic effects of the oligonucleotide, which offered the additional advantage, compared with xenogeneic mAb, of not inducing an antigenic response.

SELECTED REFERENCES

Abbas, A. K., Lichtman, A. H., and Pober, J. S.: Cellular and Molecular Immunology, 2nd ed. Philadelphia, W. B. Saunders, 1994.
This is a standard and easily read textbook of immunology.

Halloran, P., Batiuk, T., and Goes, N.: An overview of the cytokines in transplantation. Transplant Sci., 3:69, 1993.
This article briefly reviews the cytokines involved in transplantation immunology.

Masroor, S., Schroeder, T. J., Michler, R. E., Alexander, J. W., and First, M. R.: Monoclonal antibodies in organ transplantation: An overview. Transplant. Immunol., 2:176, 1994.
Monoclonal antibodies directed to cell surface molecules have the potential to provide selective targets during immunosuppression.

Thomson, A. W. (Ed.): The Cytokine Handbook, 2nd ed. San Diego, Academic Press, 1994.
This book provides a thorough review of the cytokines identified before 1994.

Thomson, A. W., and Starzl, T. E. (Eds.): Immunosuppressive Drugs: Developments in Anti-Rejection Therapy. Boston, Little, Brown, & Co., 1994.
This book is a comprehensive review of clinically useful and developing drugs for clinical immunosuppression.

REFERENCES

1. Abbas, A. K., Lichtman, A. H., and Pober, J. S.: Cellular and Molecular Immunology, 2nd ed. Philadelphia, W. B. Saunders, 1994.
2. Arai, K., Lee, F., Miyajima, A., Miyatake, S., Arai, N., and Yokota, T.: Cytokines: Coordinators of immune and inflammatory responses. Annu. Rev. Biochem., 59:783, 1990.
3. Ascher, N. L., and Simmons, R. L.: Immunobiology of transplant rejection. In Cerilli, G. J. (Ed.): Organ Transplantation and Replacement. Philadelphia, J. B. Lippincott, 1988.
4. Auchincloss, H., Jr.: Xenografting: A review. Transplant Rev., 4:14, 1990.
5. Austyn, J. M., and Larsen, C. P.: Migration patterns of dendritic leukocytes: Implications for transplantation. Transplantation, 49:1, 1990.
6. Bach, F. H.: Xenotransplantation: Problems for consideration. Clin. Transplant., 5:595, 1991.
7. Bach, F. H., and Sachs, D. H.: Transplantation immunology. N. Engl. J. Med., 317:489, 1987.
7a. Barber, W. H., Mankin, J. A., Laskow, D. A., et al.: Long-term results of a controlled prospective study with transfusion of donor-specific bone marrow in 57 cadaveric renal allograft recipients. Transplantation, 51:70, 1991.
8. Billingham, R. E., Brent, L., and Medawar, P. B.: Actively acquired tolerance of foreign cells. Nature, 172:603, 1953.
9. Bloom, B. R., Salgame, P., and Diamond, B.: Revisiting and revising suppressor T cells. Immunol. Today, 13:131, 1992.
10. Brown, P. S., Jr., Parenteau G. L., Dirbas F. M., et al.: Anti-Tac-H, a humanized antibody to the interleukin 2 receptor, prolongs primate cardiac allograft survival. Proc. Natl. Acad. Sci. USA, 88:2663, 1991.
11. Butcher, E. C., and Weissman, I. L.: Lymphoid tissues and organs. In Paul, W. E. (Ed.): Fundamental Immunology, 2nd ed. New York, Raven Press, 1989.
12. Colvin, R. B.: Cellular and molecular mechanisms of allograft rejection. Annu. Rev. Med., 41:361, 1990.
13. Cooper, M. D.: Current concepts on B lymphocytes: Normal development and function. N. Engl. J. Med., 317:1452, 1987.
14. de Waal, L. P., and Van Twuyer, E.: Blood transfusion and allograft survival. Crit. Rev. Immunol., 10:417, 1991.
15. Demattos, A. M., and Norma, D. J.: OKT3 for treatment of rejection in renal transplantation. Clin. Transplant., 7:374, 1993.
16. Dunn, D. L., and Najarian, J. S.: Infectious complications in transplant surgery. In Shires G. T., and Davis J. (Eds.): Principles and Management of Surgical Infection. Philadelphia, J. B. Lippincott, 1990.
17. Ferrara, J. L. M., and Deeg, H. J.: Graft-versus-host disease. N. Engl. J. Med., 324:667, 1991.
18. Foker, J. E., Simmons, R. L., and Najarian, J. S.: Allograft rejection. In Najarian, J. S., and Simmons, R. L. (Eds.): Transplantation. Philadelphia, Lea & Febiger, 1972, pp. 63–145.
19. Goldstein, G.: Overview of the development of orthoclone OKT3: Monoclonal antibody for therapeutic use in transplantation. Transpl. Proc., 19:1, 1987.
20. Good, R. A.: Mixed chimerism and immunologic tolerance. N. Engl. J. Med., 388:801, 1993.
21. Gruber, S. A.: The case for local immunosuppression. Transplantation, 54:1, 1992.
22. Gruber, S. A., Chan, G. L. C., Canafax, D. M., and Matas, A. J.: Immunosuppression in renal transplantation: I. Cyclosporine and azathioprine. Clin. Transplant., 5:65, 1991.
23. Gruber, S. A., Chan, G. L. C., Canafax, D. M., and Matas, A. J.: Immunosuppression in renal transplantation: II. Corticosteroids, antilymphocyte globulin, and OKT3. Clin. Transplant., 5:219, 1991.
24. Hall, B. M.: Cells mediating allograft rejection. Transplantation, 51:1141, 1991.
25. Halloran, P., Batiuk, T., and Goes, N.: An overview of the cytokines in transplantation. Transplant Sci., 3:69, 1993.

26. Haug, C. E., Colvin, R. B., Delmonico, F. L., Auchincloss, H., Jr., Tolkoff-Rubin, N., Preffer, F. I., Rothlein, R., Norris, S., Scharschmidt, L., and Cosimi, A. B.: A phase I trial of immunosuppression with anti-ICAM-1 (CD54) mAb in renal allograft recipients. Transplantation, 55:766, 1993.

27. Johnson, R. B.: Immunology: Monocytes and macrophages. N. Engl. J. Med., 318:747, 1988.

28. Kahan, B. D.: Cyclosporine. N. Engl. J. Med., 321:1725, 1989.

29. Kirkman, R. L., Shapiro, M. E., Carpenter, C. B., et al.: A randomized prospective trial of anti-Tac monoclonal antibody in human renal transplantation. Transplantation, 51:107, 1991.

30. Lin, H., Bolling, S. F., Linsley, P. S., Wei, R.-Q., Gordon, D., Thompson, C. B., and Turka, L. A.: Long-term acceptance of major histocompatibility complex mismatched cardiac allografts induced by CTLA4Ig plus donor-specific transfusion. J. Exp. Med., 178:1801, 1993.

31. Mason, D. W., and Morris, P. J.: Effector mechanisms in allograft rejection. Annu. Rev. Immunol., 4:119, 1986.

32. Masroor, S., Schroeder, T. J., Michler, R. E., Alexander, J. W., and First, M. R.: Monoclonal antibodies in organ transplantation: an overview. Transplant Immunol., 2:176, 1994.

33. Miller, J., Esquenazi, V., Fuller, L., Zucker, K., Roth, D., Fernandez, J., Burke, G., and Nery, J.: The immunologic response to allografts: Acute rejection. Clin. Transplant., 5:477, 1991.

34. Morel, P., Vincent, C., Cardier, G., Panaye, C., Carosella, E., and Revillard, J. P.: Anti-CD4 monoclonal antibody administration in renal transplanted patients. Clin. Immunol. Immunopathol., 56:311, 1990.

35. Mosmann, T. R., and Coffman, R. L.: Heterogeneity of cytokine secretion patterns and functions of helper T cells. Adv. Immunol., 46:111, 1989.

36. Penn, I.: The problem of cancer in organ transplant recipients: An overview. Transplant Sci., 4:23, 1994.

37. Powis, S. H., and Trowsdale, J.: Major and minor histocompatibility antigens. In Thomson, A. W., and Catto, G. R. D. (Eds.): Immunology of Renal Transplantation. Boston, Little, Brown, & Co., 1993, p. 3.

38. Roger, H. D., and Reinherz, E. L.: T lymphocytes: Ontogeny, function and relevance to clinical disorders. N. Engl. J. Med., 317:1136, 1987.

39. Rubin, R. H.: Infections in patients after renal and liver transplantation. In Rubin, R. H., and Young, L. S. (Eds.): Clinical Approach to Infections in the Immunocompromised Patient, 2nd ed. New York, Plenum, 1988, p. 557.

40. Sachs, D. H.: Antigen-specific transplantation tolerance. Clin. Transplant., 4:78, 1990.

41. Sayegh, M. H., Watschinger, B., and Carpenter, C. B.: Mechanisms of T cell recognition of alloantigen: The role of peptides. Transplantation, 57:1295, 1994.

42. Sigal, N. H., and Dumont, F. J.: Cyclosporin A, FK 506 and rapamycin: Pharmacologic probes of lymphocyte signal transduction. Annu. Rev. Immunol., 10:519, 1992.

43. Soulillou, J. P., Cantarovich, D., Le Mauff, B., et al.: Randomized controlled trial of a monoclonal antibody against the interleukin-2 receptor (33B.1) as compared to rabbit antithymocyte globulin for prophylaxis against rejection of renal allografts. N. Engl. J. Med., 322:1175, 1990.

44. Starzl, T. E., Demetris, A. J., Murase, N., Ildstad, S., Ricordi, C., and Trucco, M.: Cell migration, chimerism and graft acceptance. Lancet, 339:1579, 1992.

45. Stepkowski, S. M., Tu, Y., Condon, T. P., and Bennett, C. F.: Blocking of heart allograft rejection by intercellular adhesion molecule-1 antisense oligonucleotides alone or in combination with other immunosuppressive modalities. J. Immunol., 153:5336, 1994.

45a. Strober, S., Dhillon, M., Schubert, M., et al.: Acquired immune tolerance to cadaveric renal allografts: A study of three patients treated with total lymphoid irradiation. N. Engl. J. Med., 321:28, 1989.

46. Thomson, A. W., and Starzl, T. E. (Eds.): Immunosuppressive Drugs: Developments in Anti-Rejection Therapy. Boston, Little, Brown, & Co., 1994.

47. Thomson, A. W.: The Cytokine Handbook, 2nd ed. San Diego, Academic Press, 1994.

48. Waldmann, H.: Manipulation of T-cell responses with monoclonal antibodies. Annu. Rev. Immunol., 7:407, 1989.

49. Wee, S. L., Phelan, J. M., Preffer, F. I., Colvin, R. B., and Cosimi, A. B.: Anti-Leu2a (anti-CD8) monoclonal antibody therapy: antibody-mediated cell clearance in vivo requires Fc-FcRII interaction. Transplant. Proc., 21:117, 1989.

VII

ORGAN PRESERVATION

Folkert O. Belzer, M.D., and James H. Southard, Ph.D.

Organ transplantation is a proven modality and the method of choice for treatment of end-stage organ diseases. Liver, kidney, pancreas, heart, lung, and small intestine transplants have become quite common in the surgeon's armamentarium. The successes of these procedures are due to the developments in *surgical skill*, availability of *immunosuppressive agents*, and *methods to preserve* the organs. Preservation is a necessary component of organ transplantation because for optimal use of cadaveric organs the organs must be transported to the recipient's hospital. This takes time, and preservation procedures buy the time necessary to maintain the viability of the organ until transplant. Most organs can be shared between donor and recipient hospitals within 24 to 36 hours. Currently, methods are sufficient to preserve the kidney, liver, and pancreas for this length of time. However, methods to effectively preserve the lung and heart for more than 4 to 6 hours have not been developed.

There are two methods of organ preservation: simple cold storage and continuous machine perfusion. Most organs are preserved by simple cold storage, which involves flushing the blood out from the organ with a cold (4° C.) solution and storage at 4° C. Some centers use continuous machine perfusion for kidneys (about one fifth of the kidneys are preserved by this method). Kidneys are initially harvested, flushed out with a cold solution to remove blood, and placed on a perfusion machine and continuously perfused at 5° C. to 8° C.

The success of organ preservation methods is due to three principles (Table 20–9). The first principle is hypothermia, which is a key to organ preservation. Although the ideal temperature is not known, it is commonly accepted that

about 4° C is suitable for most organs. The second principle is the use of an appropriate preservative (either for simple cold storage or machine perfusion). The appropriate preservative is one that satisfies two criteria. First, it must create a physical environment that maintains the viability of and interrelationship among the structural components of the tissue. Thus, components of the solution must counteract the tendency for cells to swell in the cold, provide an optimal pH, provide an appropriate concentration of electrolytes and osmotically active agents, and be well distributed throughout the tissue. Second, the ideal preservative maintains an appropriate biochemical environment for the organ. This environment is created by agents added to the preservative that will suppress unwanted reactions (i.e., use of metabolic inhibitors), suppress the breakdown of critically important metabolites, or provide the metabolites, substrates, and the like that will enhance the recovery of the organ on reperfusion. The optimal types and concentrations of biochemical factors necessary for high-quality long-term organ preservation are not fully known but make an important area for future research. Finally, another factor important in organ preservation is reperfusion injury—injury caused to ischemic or injured tissue when reperfused with blood. Blood reperfusion is thought to initiate a cascade of events, many of which have been defined, that lead to organ failure. Some of the events include formation of oxygen free radicals and destruction of tissue, induction of synthesis of vasoactive agents (constrictors) that lead to poor reflow to the organs and hypoxic or anoxic damage to the cells, recruitment and activation of circulating macrophages, and an inflammatory response that destroys tissue or causes metabolic depression in the tissue,

TABLE 20–9. Principles of Organ Preservation

I. Hypothermia (0° to 4° C.): slows down catabolic reactions that lead to tissue destruction
II. Preservative solution
  A. Physical environment: created by agents in the preservative
    1. Osmotically active agents—suppress cell swelling (i.e., lactobionate, gluconate, citrate, raffinose, glucose, histidine)
    2. Electrolytes—contribute to osmotic effect and help maintain structural integrity of tissue (i.e., Na, K, Ca, Mg)
    3. Hydrogen ion buffers—regulate extracellular (intracellular) pH at near neutrality (i.e., phosphate, histidine, HEPES)
    4. Colloid—large molecular mass compounds to facilitate initial vascular flushout and for continuous perfusion of organs (i.e., hydroxyethyl starch, albumin)
  B. Biochemical environment—created by agents in the preservative
    1. Metabolic inhibitors to suppress degradation of functionally and structurally important constituents of the tissue (i.e., allopurinol, quinacrine, antiproteases, chlorpromazine, eicosanoid synthesis inhibitors)
    2. Metabolites—to facilitate restoration of metabolism on reperfusion (i.e., adenosine, glutathione, fructose)
    3. Antioxidants—to suppress reperfusion induced oxygen free radical generation (i.e., vitamin E, desferyl [iron chelator], amino steroids)
III. Reperfusion injury—oxygen dependent and perfusion dependent injury
  A. Blood components interact with damaged vascular system
  B. Oxygen free radical production
  C. Membrane permeability alterations and altered calcium metabolism
  D. Depressed energy regeneration—cell swelling
  E. Uncontrolled generation of potentially cytotoxic agents (eicosanoids, cytokines, proteases, phospholipases)

leading to cell swelling and poor reperfusion of the injured organ. Suppression of reperfusion injury in organ preservation is an important topic and one that is actively being studied by many laboratories.

Often the question is raised whether individual organs require a specific preservation method or whether a universal preservative can be used for all organs. There is no satisfactory answer for this question at this time. One organ preservative (the University of Wisconsin solution [UW solution]) appears to be relatively effective for most organs, but this does not mean that it is ideal for all. The heart may require a method of preservation that is different from that of other organs.

This chapter presents a brief historical overview of organ preservation, discusses some of the basic concepts of organ preservation, and reviews current methods and outcome in specific organs. More detailed accounts of organ preservation methods, reperfusion injury, and comparison of method for clinical use can be found in the literature (see Selected References).

HISTORICAL OVERVIEW

After the successful demonstration of a living-related renal transplantation by Joseph Murray and colleagues in the early 1950s, an interest in transplantation of cadaveric organs de-

veloped. It was recognized that to use cadaveric organs, a method to preserve the viability of the organ *ex vivo* was necessary to allow time to transport the organ to the recipient's hospital. When removed from the donor, the organ is exposed to a period of ischemia (no blood flow, no oxygen or nutrients), and earlier studies demonstrated that the kidney's tolerance to ischemia could be extended by cooling the organs.[16, 17] Thus, hypothermic treatment of the cadaveric organ became a central principle for effective preservation. Methods to cool the kidney included surface cooling or vascular flushout with cold saline or blood. These methods increased the time of safe preservation, but only to 4 to 8 hours.

In 1967, Belzer and associates[1] reported successful 3-day preservation of the canine kidney by continuous machine perfusion. This group found that low-flow (0.6 to 1.0 ml./min.) and low-pressure (40 to 60 mm. Hg) pulsatile perfusion of the kidney with a perfusate consisting of cryoprecipitated plasma was effective. The plasma, frozen before use, was thawed, and the precipitate of lipid materials was removed by ultrafiltration. In the cold, lipoproteins and other lipids were unstable and coalesced, thus obstructing the glomerular capillaries. Removal of these materials before continuous machine perfusion was essential for successful preservation. This method rapidly became assimilated into renal preservation and remains in use today, although with a different perfusion solution. The original perfusion machine was large and difficult to transport; subsequently, a smaller version of the perfusion machine was developed that could be easily transported and was battery operated.

In 1969, Collins and associates[7] demonstrated successful 30-hour preservation of the canine kidney by a method of simple cold storage. The kidney was flushed out with a solution (Collins' solution) that contained a high concentration of potassium (115 mmol./L.), a low concentration of sodium (10 mmol./L.), phosphate (57.5 mmol./L.), and a large concentration of glucose (140 mmol./L.). This solution became known as an intracellular cold storage solution because the high concentration of potassium resembled the high intracellular concentration of this cation in the kidney. The high concentration of glucose was necessary to raise the osmolality of the solution and was a primary reason why this solution was effective. Glucose is relatively impermeable across the renal cell plasma membrane and suppresses hypothermia-induced cell swelling. This method of preservation quickly became favored among renal transplant surgeons because of its simplicity: a machine was not needed, nor was a trained technician. This method did not allow the quality or duration of preservation equivalent to machine perfusion, but because most kidneys could be transplanted within about 24 hours, this method became favored by transplant centers.

These methods of renal preservation were not particularly effective in preserving other organs. However, in the early 1970s the long-term survival of the liver, pancreas, and heart after transplant was not particularly good; and there was not a great interest in clinical transplantation of these organs. In the early 1980s, cyclosporine for immunosuppression became clinically available and changed organ transplantation. Now the liver, pancreas, and heart could be successfully transplanted with survival results nearly identical to those obtained with kidney transplantation.

METHODS OF ORGAN PRESERVATION

The general process of organ preservation is quite simple. Ideally, the time between the cessation of blood flow to the organ and the start of cooling by vascular flushing should be short. In multiorgan harvesting, the organs are usually cooled before they are removed. The cold-preservation solution flushes blood from the organ and cools the organ to the preservation temperature (0° C. to 5° C). The organ is stored in the preservation solution and kept at 0° C. to 5° C. Organs are preserved by either refrigeration storage (simple cold storage) or continuous machine perfusion.

HYPOTHERMIA AND CELL SWELLING

Two critical components of successful organ preservation are the maintenance of organ hypothermia (0° C. to 8° C.) and the suppression of cell swelling. Hypothermia is induced by flushing the vasculature of the organ with a cold solution (usually about 4° C.) that lowers the temperature of the organ to 4° C. within 5 to 15 minutes. The organ is then either stored at 0° C. to 4° C. on ice or machine perfused at 4° C. to 8° C. The value of hypothermia stems from the effect of temperature on metabolism (i.e., on enzyme activity). Arrhenius and van't Hoff showed that, in general, a 10° C. change in temperature produces about a twofold (1.5 to 2.5) change in enzyme activity.[17] An equation devised by van't Hoff shows that a decrease in temperature from 37° C. (normothermia) to an organ-storage temperature of 4° C. would theoretically decrease enzyme activity (metabolism) by 12 to 13 times. For a more concrete example, consider that a kidney can tolerate about 1 hour of warm ischemia (37° C.) before being irreversibly damaged, but if the kidney is flushed with cold blood (4° C.), tolerance to ischemia is increased to about 12 hours. The tolerance of other organs to ischemia is also increased by cold, although not always to the same extent as are kidneys. Clearly, then, hypothermia increases the time an organ can be preserved.

The inhibition of metabolism by the cold suggests that one mechanism by which ischemia damages organs is related to rates of enzymatically catalyzed changes in the tissue (i.e., degenerative changes in structural components [membranes] or the loss of essential metabolites). The primary benefit of hypothermia is, therefore, the reduction of metabolism, including the requirements for a continual supply of nutrients, oxygen, and energy (in the form of adenine nucleotides), and the suppression of hydrolytic enzymes (phospholipases, lysosomal enzymes, and proteases).

Hypothermia is essential for successful organ storage, but it is not without its detrimental effect on the organ. Hypothermia-induced cell swelling (Fig. 20–41) results from a decrease in the activity of membrane-bound ion pumps (particularly the sodium-potassium adenosine triphosphatase pump) and from a decrease in the rate of turnover of adenosine triphosphate (ATP); it is ATP that provides the energy for ion pump activity and for the control of cell volume. Normally the cell is bathed in a fluid that contains a high concentration of sodium and chloride, whereas the inside of the cell contains a high concentration of potassium and impermeants (proteins and anions) that have a high relative molecular mass. The cell must expend considerable energy (ATP) to keep sodium and chloride outside the cell. If the cell lacks sufficient energy, sodium diffuses down its concentration gradient and is exchanged with potassium. This exchange is not lethal to the cell; and when normal metabolism is re-established, sodium is pumped back out of the cell in exchange for potassium. However, when ion pump activity is suppressed for long periods, the membrane potential is lost and chloride diffuses down its concentration gradient. Furthermore, the colloids in the cell exert a colloidal osmotic pressure that pulls water into the cell. The result is cell swelling, organelle swelling, a disruption of the architecture of the cell (cytoskeleton), and a dilution of the intracellular milieu. Cell swelling can be tolerated for short periods, but eventually it causes irreversible damage.

Successful organ preservation has, therefore, depended on

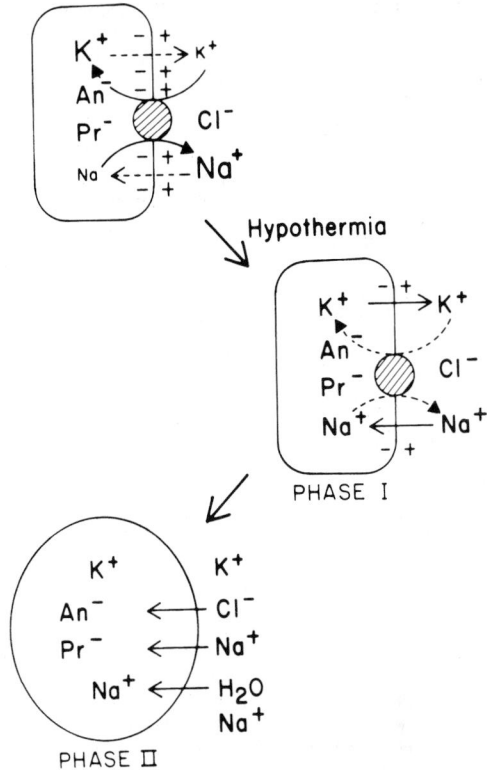

Figure 20–41. Schematic representation of hypothermia-induced cell swelling. A cell at normothermia (top) uses the sodium pump (hatched circle) to maintain a high intracellular potassium level and pump sodium out of the cell. This makes sodium an effective impermeant, which counteracts the oncotic pressure inside the cell derived from impermeable anions (An) and proteins (Pr). The sodium pump also generates a membrane potential (negative inside relative to the outside of the cell). When cooled (middle), the sodium pump activity decreases and there is a stoichiometric exchange of potassium and sodium derived by their chemical potentials (Phase I). This equilibration of cations is stoichiometric and does not cause the cell to gain water. However (Phase II, bottom), in the absence of membrane potential, chloride diffuses down its concentration gradient and the increased osmotic activity inside the cell (as well as the presence of impermeable colloids) pulls water into the cell, causing cell swelling.

the development of methods to suppress safely and effectively hypothermia-induced cell swelling. Agents that suppress cell swelling are termed *impermeants* (i.e., they are relatively unable to cross the plasma membrane). These impermeants exert sufficient osmotic force to counter the intracellular colloidal osmotic force. In general, cell swelling can be suppressed in cells that are metabolically depressed (due to hypothermia or the chemical inhibition of energy production) by including about 100 to 140 mmol. per liter of impermeant in a saline-based solution (140 mmol./L.) that increases the osmotic strength of the solution from 300 mOsm. per liter to 400 to 440 mOsm. per liter. Saccharides (glucose, mannitol, sucrose, and raffinose) commonly serve as impermeants, and other agents that can also suppress cell swelling include impermeant anions (phosphate, sulfate, glycerophosphate, gluconate, lactobionate, and citrate). It is the cell membrane's limited permeability to these substances that determines their effectiveness. The permeability properties of cell membranes are a function of the type of organ, and impermeants effective for some organs are not effective for others. For example, glucose and mannitol suppress cell swelling in the kidney, but they are not as effective for the liver, pancreas, and heart.

Organs can be well preserved for relatively long periods with preservation solutions that suppress cell swelling. However, even if cell swelling is prevented, organs and tissues stored at hypothermia eventually lose viability. Some other mechanisms must therefore also cause cell death during organ storage. Exactly what these mechanisms are is unclear, but some evidence indicates that oxygen-free radical injury, calcium-induced toxicity, the loss of energy-producing capabilities (mitochondrial injury, the loss of precursors to ATP resynthesis), the loss of phospholipids, and the activation of hydrolytic enzymes are involved in preservation injury. It is likely that several of these mechanisms are involved in the loss of organ viability during the long-term storage of organs.

KIDNEY PRESERVATION

The methods of preserving kidneys that were developed during the late 1960s by Collins[7] and Belzer[1] were quickly adopted for clinical use and had enormous impact on kidney transplantation. Successful storage methods greatly increased the number of cadaveric kidneys that were transplanted and the number of hospitals that performed kidney transplantations; they also eased the urgency of performing transplant operations and allowed time for tissue matching between donors and recipients. The success of these preservation methods is reflected in the fact that they have remained in use, essentially unchanged, for 30 years.

Collins and associates developed the method of simple cold storage for kidneys. Their preservation solution (Collins' solution; Table 20–10) was designed to mimic the intracellular milieu of the kidney and thus contains a high concentration of potassium and magnesium, phosphate as a hydrogen ion buffer, and glucose to raise the osmolality to that of kidney cells. Glucose, the primary impermeant in Collins' solution, suppresses cell swelling in the kidney. This solution successfully preserved dog kidneys for as long as 30 hours after simple vascular flushing and storage at 0° C. to 4° C. Collins' solution preserves ideally harvested kidneys for as long as 48 hours, and the modified version, EuroCollins' solution (without magnesium), is equally effective. EuroCollins' solution is used more than the original Collins' solution because magnesium forms an insoluble precipitate with phosphate.

Because cold storage is so simple, many transplant centers have favored this method over the more complex method of continuous machine perfusion (see later). Several types of cold storage solution have been tested, and the most successful and widely accepted, other than the Collins' solution, is the Ross-Marshall solution (Table 20–11). This solution uses citrate as an impermeant; although poorly buffered (hydrogen ions), it has preserved kidneys for 3 days.[23] Other cold storage solutions include Sacks' solution, which contains a high concentration of mannitol for osmotic support, and a phosphate-buffered sucrose solution that has preserved dog kidneys for 3 days (Table 20–12).[13]

A second method of preserving kidneys is continuous hypothermic perfusion. This method was developed by Belzer and associates, who discovered that cryoprecipitated plasma is a good perfusion fluid for the 3-day preservation of dog kidneys. The plasma is frozen, thawed, and filtered to remove lipoproteins that accumulate in the capillaries of the kidney and block effective perfusion. The perfusate is pumped through the renal artery at a pressure of 40 to 60 mm. Hg with a pulsatile pump (60 beats per minute) that produces a flow rate of 0.6 to 1.0 ml. per minute. This low pressure prevents the perfusion-induced vascular damage that occurs at higher perfusion pressures. The initial experiments were performed with the perfusate continuously oxygenated (membrane oxygenator), but subsequent work showed that continuous oxygenation is not necessary and that the perfusate contains sufficient oxygen (from equilibration with room air) to support low-level aerobic metabolism in the kidney at 4° C. to 10° C.

Other perfusates have been developed, including a silica gel–filtered fraction of plasma.[26] Silica gel removes lipid material from plasma, and this perfusate is about as effective as cryoprecipitated plasma. Saline-based solutions containing human serum albumin also successfully preserve kidneys for about 48 hours.

Both simple cold storage and machine perfusion have been used clinically, and during the early history of kidney preservation and transplantation there was debate over which method was most effective. Continuous machine perfusion has consistently provided longer and better kidney preservation both in the laboratory and in the clinic. However, most kidneys are transplanted within 20 to 30 hours after they are harvested and a comparison of short- and long-term graft survival shows that the two preservation methods are equally effective. One difference, however, is that 15% to 50% of kidneys preserved by cold storage need dialysis, compared with 5% to 15% of kidneys preserved by continuous machine perfusion.

Although simple cold storage and continuous perfusion were effective for kidney preservation, they were not particularly effective for the long-term preservation (more than 24 hours) of other organs. Moreover, neither method afforded successful preservation of kidneys for longer than about 3 days.

In the late 1970s and early 1980s, the authors' group studied methods of improving kidney preservation and devel-

TABLE 20–11. Composition of Citrate Solutions

Component	Hypertonic		Isotonic	
	gm./L.	mmol./L.	gm./L.	mmol./L.
K citrate	8.6	80	8.6	80
Na citrate	8.2	80	8.2	80
HCl (2 M)	0.26		0.26	
Mannitol	33.8	188	17.0	95
MgSO$_4$	10.0	35	10.0	35

Osmolality, 400 mOsm./L.; pH = 7.1 (hypertonic).
Na = 80 mmol./L.; K = 80 mmol./L.
Citrate = 55 mM.
Osmolality, 300 mOsm./L. (isotonic).

TABLE 20–10. Composition of Collins' C2 Solution

Component	gm./L.	mmol./L.
KH$_2$PO$_4$	2.05	15.0
K$_2$HPO$_4 \cdot$ 3H$_2$O	9.7	42.5
KCl	1.12	15.0
NaHCO$_3$	0.84	10.0
Glucose	25.0	139.0
MgSO$_4 \cdot$ 7H$_2$O	7.38	30.0

Na$^+$ = 10 mmol./L.; K$^+$ = 115 mmol./L.; PO$_4$ = 57.5 mmol./L.
Osmolality, 320 mOsm./L.; pH = 7.2.

TABLE 20–12. Composition of Phosphate-Buffered Sucrose

Component	gm./L.	mmol./L.
NaH$_2$PO$_4$	2.16	15.7
NaHPO$_4$	7.41	52.2
Sucrose	51.3	140.0

Osmolality, 320 mOsm.L.; pH = 7.2.

TABLE 20–13. Composition of UW Machine Perfusion Solution

Component	gm./L.	mmol./L.
Na gluconate	17.45	80
KH$_2$PO$_4$	3.4	25
Mg gluconate	1.04	5
Adenine	0.68	5
Ribose	0.75	5
Glutathione	0.922	3
CaCl$_2$	0.068	0.5
HEPES	2.38	10
Glucose	1.8	10
Mannitol	5.4	30
Penta starch	50	

Na$^+$ = 100 mmol./L.; K$^+$ = 25 mmol./L.
Osmolality, 310 mOsm./L.; pH = 7.4.

oped a synthetic kidney perfusion fluid (Table 20–13). This solution contained hydroxyethyl starch as a colloid, replacing serum albumin. Evidence shows that albumin causes endothelial injury during machine perfusion, and the search for effective colloids led to the discovery that hydroxyethyl starch is the most effective. Other colloids, such as Haemaccel,[18] may also be acceptable.

A colloid is essential with continuous machine perfusion to counteract the hydrostatic pressure produced by the perfusion pump. In addition to hydroxyethyl starch, the new perfusate contained gluconate as an impermeant anion to suppress cell swelling, adenosine and phosphate to stimulate ATP synthesis, glutathione to suppress damage due to lipid peroxidation and oxygen-free radicals, and other agents. This solution preserved dog kidneys for 3 days, and it has proved successful for the clinical preservation of kidneys. This perfusate has been modified by replacing the adenosine with adenine and ribose as precursors of ATP synthesis. Adenosine is catabolized during kidney perfusion and loses its ability to stimulate ATP synthesis. Adenine and ribose are not severely degraded during machine perfusion and consequently are able to keep ATP concentrations near normal during 5 days of preservation. It was also found that by including 0.5 mM. of calcium, kidneys could be successfully preserved for 5 days by machine perfusion.[15] This modified perfusion fluid is now being used in the clinic with excellent results.

PANCREAS PRESERVATION

Methods developed for kidney preservation proved unsuccessful for long-term pancreas preservation. The pancreas was difficult to preserve by continuous perfusion because it became edematous, so attention was turned to simple cold storage. Wahlberg and associates[28] experimented with different versions of the kidney perfusion solution that contained hydroxyethyl starch and found that a solution containing lactobionate prevented pancreatic edema during preservation and when the organ was reperfused. Lactobionic acid is the acid of the saccharide lactose (milk sugar), and it has a relatively large molecular weight (358 daltons) compared with chloride (58 daltons) and gluconate (180 daltons). The combination of lactobionate and raffinose (100 mmol./L. and 30 mmol./L., respectively) provided a preservation solution that effectively suppressed hypothermia-induced pancreas cell swelling. Wahlberg[27] used this solution for segmental pancreatic preservation in the autotransplant dog model; the results were consistent 3-day organ preservation and long-term animal survival. This solution (the University of Wisconsin [UW] solution) is very similar to the kidney perfusion

solution described previously; its composition is shown in Table 20–14.

The UW solution has provided excellent clinical pancreas transplantation and has extended pancreas preservation from about 6 hours to more than 29 hours.[8] This solution also appears to preserve the pancreas sufficiently well so that islets can be isolated and used for islet cell transplantation.[32] Although the UW solution was being developed, the Minnesota group obtained reasonably good pancreas preservation with a silica gel fraction of plasma that is similar to a kidney perfusate.[9] Both solutions appear to be clinically useful for preserving pancreases, but the silica gel fraction of plasma does not appear to be acceptable for the simple cold storage of livers and kidneys.

LIVER PRESERVATION

The two methods developed for kidney preservation were not as effective for long-term liver preservation. Collins' solution preserved dog livers for about 18 hours, but its safe clinical application was limited to only 6 to 10 hours. A plasma protein fraction also preserved dog kidneys for more than 12 hours, but it, too, was considered clinically safe for only about 6 to 10 hours of liver preservation. Early work on liver preservation has been reviewed elsewhere.[4]

Shortly after Wahlberg developed the method for successfully preserving pancreases, Jamieson and Sundberg and associates[11] used the same UW solution for 48-hour preservation in the orthotopic dog liver transplant model. Dog livers flushed with the UW solution and stored for 48 hours were 100% viable and showed a return of normal liver functions (bilirubin, serum enzymes, clotting factors) within about 2 to 3 days after transplantation. These studies prompted the clinical use of the UW solution for liver transplantation at the University of Wisconsin[12] and at other centers[25]; preservation times have been as long as 35 hours, and the results have been excellent.

Livers can be successfully preserved with simple cold storage, but recently an even better preservation of dog livers has been achieved with continuous machine perfusion.[20] A modified version of the UW kidney perfusion solution was used to preserve livers for 3 days. The modifications included reversing the ratio of cations (high potassium, low sodium) and adding calcium, 1.0 mmol. per liter. Although it is an excellent method of preserving livers, continuous perfusion has not been used in the clinic.

Not only is the UW solution effective for the simple cold storage of pancreases and livers, but it is also effective for the simple cold storage of kidneys. Ploeg and associates[22] used the UW solution to preserve dog kidneys for 3 days, and a recent report describes its clinical use for kidney pres-

TABLE 20–14. Composition of UW Solution

Component	gm./L.	mmol./L.
Penta starch (HES)	50	
Lactobionic acid	35.83	100
KH$_2$PO$_4$	3.4	25
MgSO$_4$ · 7H$_2$O	1.23	5
Raffinose	17.83	30
Adenosine	1.34	5
Glutathione	0.92	3
Allopurinol	0.136	1

Neutralized to pH 7.4 with NaOH:KOH.
Na$^+$ = 20 mmol./L.; K$^+$ = 140 mmol./L.
Osmolality, 320 mOsm./L.

ervation.[2] In a prospective, randomized European trial to compare the UW solution with EuroCollins' solution in kidney preservation, kidneys preserved with the UW solution functioned, initially, better than those preserved with EuroCollins' solution.[21] The UW solution therefore appears to be close to a universal preservation solution for all intra-abdominal organs.

HEART PRESERVATION

Currently, hearts can be preserved for only about 4 hours before being transplanted. The solutions used vary among transplant centers, but they are similar to those developed by the groups at Stanford University and St. Thomas Hospital. The heart, unlike other organs, must rapidly regain its maximal work capacity to support life and therefore must be optimally preserved. No heart has been optimally preserved for more than about 10 hours by simple cold storage, as tested in an orthotopic transplant model; and, consequently, heart surgeons understandably have a sense of urgency when performing a heart transplantation.

The UW solution, or some modification of it, may be effective for preserving hearts. Studies have shown superior results in laboratory models of heart preservation and transplantation when the UW solution is compared with other solutions.[30] Exactly what additions or subtractions must be made to the UW solution to produce ideal heart preservation are not yet known.

Although simple cold storage is a convenient method of organ preservation, successful heart preservation may require continuous perfusion, as suggested by the work of Collins and associates[31] and others. The longest successful preservation of hearts has been with continuous perfusion. Much additional work is needed to develop the optimal perfusate fluid and methods of perfusing the heart before these methods become clinically acceptable.

STATUS OF CLINICAL ORGAN PRESERVATION

Organs are preserved in the United States by simple cold storage, using either Collins' solution or the UW solution. Collins' solution is primarily used for kidneys, and the UW solution is used for kidneys, livers, and pancreases. Because of an increase in multiorgan donors and *in situ* vascular flushing, more organs are available now than in the past. Also, the longer preservation time provided by the UW solution allows organs to be more easily shipped between transplant centers, allows transplant surgery to be performed on an elective basis, and improves the quality of organs available for transplantation.

The main problems yet to be solved are how to prevent primary nonfunction in transplanted livers and kidneys and how to reduce the incidence of delayed graft function. Solutions to these problems may demand the development of a still better preservation solution and a greater understanding of the relationship between donor status and preservation quality. However, current methods of organ preservation appear satisfactory for most organs that are transplanted (except the heart, lungs, and intestine).

The goal of organ preservation research is to provide preservation of unlimited duration. This end may be accomplished only by cryopreservation (freezing), which has been discussed elsewhere.[31] In all probability, methods of hypothermic preservation (above freezing) have limits, but it is unlikely that those limits have been reached. The ability to preserve all organs for at least 1 week would make organ banks a reality. Organs could be transplanted on the basis of the best immunologic match and could be conveniently shipped throughout the world, and far fewer would be wasted. Long-term preservation may allow the immunoalteration of organs, reduce the recipient need for immunosuppressive drugs, and reduce the incidence of graft rejection. If livers could be preserved for longer than 1 week, they would be available for recipients who developed primary nonfunction and needed immediate retransplantation. Improved and long-term preservation will, however, require an understanding of the mechanisms of tissue damage caused by hypothermic preservation. When these mechanisms are understood, a rational approach to therapeutic intervention can be defined and better quality and long-term organ preservation will become a reality.

SELECTED REFERENCES

Bonventre, J. V., and Weinberg, J. M.: Kidney preservation *ex vivo* for transplantation. Annu. Rev. Med., 43:523, 1992.
   This is a comprehensive review of the mechanisms of renal injury as related to kidney preservation and transplantation. It is very well written by two investigators with an excellent background in ischemic injury that is not directly related to cold preservation. Thus, there is a new look at renal cold ischemia/reperfusion injury.

Clavien, P., Harvey, P. R. C., and Strasberg, S. M.: Preservation and reperfusion injuries in liver allografts: An overview and synthesis of current studies. Transplantation, 53:957, 1992.
   This is a comprehensive review of the mechanisms of injury to the transplanted liver. The authors have a long-standing interest in liver preservation and transplantation and develop their concepts on mechanisms of liver injury very well.

D'Alessandro, A. M., Southard, J. H., Love, R. B., and Belzer, F. O.: Organ preservation. Surg. Clin. North Am., 74:1083, 1994.
   This is a review of the University of Wisconsin solution from its development through its use in clinical organ preservation. The authors show how the UW solution has affected the results in clinical organ preservation and transplantation at the University of Wisconsin Hospitals.

Marshall, V. C., Jablonski, P., and Scott, D. F.: Renal preservation. *In* Morris, P. J. (Ed.): Kidney Transplantation: Principles and Practice. Philadelphia, W.B. Saunders, 1994, pp. 86–108.
   This is an update of current methods for renal preservation. In this chapter the discussion is focused on the clinical use of different preservatives, the mechanisms by which these solutions are effective, and the history of kidney preservation. This group has been involved with organ preservation from its earliest periods.

REFERENCES

1. Belzer, F. O., Ashby, B. S., and Dumphy, J. E.: 24- and 72-hour preservation for transplantation: Initial perfusion and 30 hour ice storage. Lancet, 2:536, 1967.
2. Benoit, G., Moukarzel, M., Bitker, M., Bensadoun, H., Hiesse, C., Charpentier, B., Jardin, A., and Fries, D.: Intérêt de la solution UW dans la preservation rénale en vue de transplantation. Presse Med., 27:1076, 1989.
3. Calne, R. Y.: Liver Transplantation. New York, Grune & Stratton, 1983.
4. Calne, R. Y.: Preservation of the liver. *In* Calne, R. Y. (Ed.): Liver Transplantation. New York, Grune & Stratton, 1983, pp. 17–24.
5. Calne, R. Y., Pegg, D. E., Pryse-Davies, J., and Leigh-Brown, F.: Renal preservation by ice cooling. Br. Med. J., 651, 1963.
6. Cecka, M. J.: Donor and preservation factors. *In* Terasaki, P. I. (Ed.): Clinical Transplants. Los Angeles, UCLA Tissue Typing Laboratory, 1989, pp. 399–408.
7. Collins, G. M., Bravo-Shugarman, M. B., and Terasaki, P. I.: Kidney preservation for transplantation: Initial perfusion and 30 hour ice storage. Lancet, 2:1219, 1969.
8. D'Alessandro, A. M., Stratta, R. J., Sollinger, H. W., Kalayoglu, M., Pirsch, D., and Belzer, F. O.: Use of UW solution in pancreas transplantation. Diabetes, 38(Suppl. 1):7, 1989.
9. Florack, G., Sutherland, D. E. R., Heil, J., Squifflet, J. P., and Marjarian, J. S.: Preservation of canine segmental allografts: Cold storage versus pulsatile machine perfusion. J. Surg. Res., 34:443, 1983.
10. Hernandez, L. A., and Granger, N. D.: Role of antioxidants in organ preservation and transplantation. Crit. Care Med., 16:543, 1988.
11. Jamieson, N. V., Sundberg, R., Lindell, S., Southard, J. H., and Belzer, F. O.: Preservation of the canine liver for 24–48 hours using simple cold storage with UW solution. Transplantation, 46:517, 1988.
12. Kalayoglu, M., Sollinger, H. W., Stratta, R. J., D'Alessandro, A. M., Hoffman, R. M., Pirsch, J. D., and Belzer, F. O.: Extended preservation of the liver for clinical transplantation. Lancet, 2:617, 1988.
13. Lam, F. T., Mavor, A. I. D., Potts, D. J., and Giles, G. R.: Improved 72 hour renal preservation with phosphate buffered sucrose. Transplantation, 47:767, 1989.
14. Lokkegaard, H., and Bilde, T.: Preselection and pretreatment of donor

kidneys. *In* Marberger, M., and Dreikorn, K. (Eds.): Renal Preservation. Baltimore, Williams & Wilkins, 1983, pp. 165–176.

15. McAnulty, J. F., Ploeg, R. J., Southard, J. H., and Belzer, F. O.: Successful five day perfusion preservation of the canine kidney. Transplantation, *47*:37, 1989.

16. Owens, T. C., Preuedel, A. E., and Swan, H.: Prolonged experimental occlusion of thoracic aorta during hypothermia. Arch. Surg., *70*:95, 1955.

17. Pegg, D. E.: The biology of cell survival *in vitro*. *In* Karow, A. M., Jr., and Pegg, D. E. (Eds.): Organ Preservation for Transplantation. New York, Marcel Dekker, 1981, pp. 31–52.

18. Pegg, D. E., and Green, C. J.: Renal preservation by hypothermic perfusion: IV. The use of gelatin polypeptide as the sole colloid. Cryobiology, *15*:27, 1978.

19. Pegg, D. E., and Karow, A. M., Jr. (Eds.): The Biophysics of Organ Cryopreservation. Nato ASI Series, vol. 147. New York, Plenum Press, 1987.

20. Pienaar, B. H., Lindell, S. L., van Gulik, T., Southard, J. H., and Belzer, F. O.: 72-hour preservation of the canine liver by machine perfusion. Transplantation, *49*:258, 1990.

21. Ploeg, R. J.: A clinical trial of the UW solution in organ preservation. Transplantation, in press.

22. Ploeg, R. J., Goossens, D., McAnulty, J. F., Southard, J. H., and Belzer F. O.: Successful 72-hour cold storage of dog kidneys with UW solution. Transplantation, *46*:191, 1988.

23. Ross, H., Marshall, V. C., and Escott, M. L.: 72-hour canine kidney preservation without continuous perfusion. Transplantation, *21*:498, 1978.

24. Schrier, R. W., Arnoud, P. F., Van Putten, V. J., and Burke, T. J.: Cellular calcium in ischemic acute renal failure: Role of carcinoma entry blockers. Kidney Int., *82*:313, 1987.

25. Todo, S., Nery, J., Yanaga, K., Podesta, R., Gordon, R., and Starzl, T. E.: Extended preservation of human liver grafts with UW solution. JAMA, *261*:711, 1989.

26. Toledo-Pereyra, L. H., Condie, R. M., Malmberg, R., Simmons, R. L., and Najarian, J. S.: A fibrinogen-free perfusate for preservation of kidneys for one hundred and twenty hours. Surg. Gynecol. Obstet., *138*:901, 1974.

27. Wahlberg, J. A., Love, R., Landegaard, L., Southard, J. H., and Belzer, F. O.: 72-hour preservation of the canine pancreas. Transplantation, *43*:5, 1987.

28. Wahlberg, J. A., Southard, J. H., and Belzer, F. O.: Development of a cold storage solution for pancreas preservation. Cryobiology, *23*:477, 1986.

29. Weiss, S. J., and LoBuglio, A. F.: Phagocyte-generated oxygen metabolites and cellular injury. Lab. Invest., *47*:5, 1982.

30. Wicomb, W. N., Collins, G. M., Wood, J., and Hill, J. D.: Improved cardioplegia using new perfusates. Transplant. Proc., *21*:1357, 1989.

31. Wicomb, W. N., Hill, J. D., Avery, J., and Collins, G. M.: Comparison of cardioplegic and UW solutions for short-term rabbit heart preservation. Transplantation, *47*:733, 1989.

32. Zucker, P. F., Bloom, A. D., Strasser, S., and Alyandro, R.: Successful cold storage preservation of canine pancreas with UW-solution prior to islet isolation. Transplantation, *48*:168, 1989.

VIII

LIVER TRANSPLANTATION

Pierre A. Clavien, M.D., Ph.D., and Allan D. Kirk, M.D., Ph.D.

INDICATIONS FOR TRANSPLANTATION

The specific indications for liver transplantation have become more standardized (Tables 20–15 and 20–16) owing to the better knowledge of the natural history of a number of liver diseases and concomitant improvement in short- and long-term results of orthotopic liver transplantation (OLT).[2, 6, 12] As with most aspects of this topic, however, significant controversy remains about several disease states leading to end-stage liver failure.

Cholestatic Liver Diseases. Cholestatic diseases, including primary biliary cirrhosis (PBC), secondary biliary cirrhosis, and primary sclerosing cholangitis (PSC), are the diseases most successfully treated by liver transplantation.[7, 25] Opera-

TABLE 20–15. Adult Indications for Orthotopic Liver Transplantations

Indication	Percentage Before 1991 n = 4833	Percent 1992 n = 2315
Primary cholestatic liver disease	23.7	19.1
Other cirrhosis	55.9	65.2
Alcoholic	17.5	21.1
Hepatitis C/ non-A, non-B	14.7	20.3
Autoimmune and other	16.5	18.7
Hepatitis B	7.2	5.1
Fulminant hepatic failure	7.0	5.5
Metabolic diseases	4.2	4.1
Malignant neoplasms	6.1	3.4
Benign neoplasms	0.5	0.5
Biliary atresia	0.6	0.4
Miscellaneous	2.0	1.8

Data from Belle, S. H., Beringer, K. C., and Detre, K. M.: Trends in liver transplantation in the United States. *In* Terasaki, P. I., and Cecka, J. M. (Eds.): Clinical Transplants. Los Angeles, UCLA Tissue Typing Laboratory, 1993.

TABLE 20–16. Pediatric Indications for Orthotopic Liver Transplantation

Indication	Percentage Before 1991 n = 1117	Percent 1992 n = 394
Biliary atresia	56.8	51.0
Fulminant hepatic failure	9.4	14.0
Metabolic diseases	13.0	12.2
Cirrhosis	7.8	7.4
Hepatitis B	0.4	0.5
Hepatitis C/ non-A, non-B	1.6	1.0
Alcoholic	0.0	0.0
Autoimmune and other	5.8	5.9
Malignant neoplasms	2.2	2.5
Primary cholestatic liver disease	2.2	1.5
Benign neoplasms	0.2	0.0
Miscellaneous	8.5	11.4

Data from Belle, S. H., Beringer, K. C., and Detre, K. M.: Trends in liver transplantation in the United States. *In* Terasaki, P. I., and Cecka, J. M. (Eds.): Clinical Transplants. Los Angeles, UCLA Tissue Typing Laboratory, 1993.

tive survival is greater than 90%, and 5-year survival is approximately 80%.[6] This rate is due mostly to the slow onset of illness, which allows for preoperative preparation of the recipient and appropriate timing of the procedure, as well as absence of recurrence of the disease in the graft. As a result of this success, cholestatic disease is one of the most frequent indications for transplantation, accounting for 22% of all transplants performed in the United States. Clearly, the timing of operation is critical, and a substantial literature has addressed the rate of disease progression.

The indications for transplantation in patients with PSC are based on refractory symptoms resulting from recurrent cholangitis or impaired synthetic function. The risk of cholangiocarcinoma, approximately 15% in these patients, is an additional relative indication for OLT. A current trend toward earlier intervention with liver transplantation in PSC is underway, with retrospective comparisons of transplant versus nontransplant therapy weighing heavily in favor of the transplant approach.[21] Clearly, however, some patients, particularly those with predominantly extrahepatic biliary strictures do well with conventional bypass[42] or endoscopic procedures.[30] Thus, timing remains a matter of clinical judgment, with most patients benefiting from allotransplantation.

Several models of survival have been established to predict outcome in patients with PBC.[7, 27] All prognostic scores are based in part on the rise in serum bilirubin. In general, transplantation is recommended when the bilirubin level exceeds 15 mg./100 ml., although earlier transplantation for severe associated symptoms such as pruritus or fatigue, refractory ascites, or variceal bleeding is appropriate. Although close monitoring of asymptomatic patients is reasonable, it is important not to delay intervention until the clinical status of the patient deteriorates, because OLT is the only definitive treatment.[7]

Alcoholic Liver Disease. Nineteen percent of all liver transplants performed in the United States have been for alcoholic cirrhosis.[6] Although the procedure was originally avoided because of fears of high postoperative recidivism and a tendency toward medical noncompliance, the national trend has been to transplant in this setting more frequently, and in 1993 it was the most common indication reported by the United Network for Organ Sharing (UNOS) registry. Experience has demonstrated that graft and patient survival are not significantly different from those of other favorable indications and that disease recurrence (return to heavy alcohol use) is approximately 12%.[29] Given these results, combined with the extraordinary prevalence of alcohol-related liver disease compared with other transplantable diseases (36,000 deaths per year), transplantation for alcoholic cirrhosis could easily exhaust the already scarce supply of donor organs. Selection is clearly needed to exclude comorbidities, alcohol-associated organ failure such as cardiomyopathy, and patients with continued dependence on alcohol. Even so, the need far outpaces the supply. Considerable philosophical debate addresses the use of scarce resources for individuals with self-inflicted disease. At this point, the decision to transplant should be based on a thorough preoperative medical evaluation supplemented by involvement in alcoholic rehabilitation and abstinence for at least 6 months. Patients presenting *too sick to drink* must be evaluated individually with an estimate of recidivism made to optimize long-term results. Palliative procedures are appropriate when possible. The recent development of the transjugular intrahepatic portosystemic shunt (TIPS) procedure has allowed many of these patients to be stabilized without extensive surgical intervention, for more thorough evaluation in a nonemergent setting.

Hepatitis C and Cryptogenic Cirrhosis. Another rapidly increasing indication for OLT is hepatitis caused by the hepatitis C virus (HCV). This is frequently discussed in tandem with cryptogenic cirrhosis. Transplantation is pursued for symptomatic infection only. Since the discovery of reliable methods for detecting HCV, this pathogen has been identified as the etiologic agent for liver failure in an increasing number of recipients.[5] In 1996, it was associated with more than 25% of transplants in most centers. Cryptogenic disease accounted for an additional 12%. Excellent short-term results have been achieved with a 3-year survival of 70% (63% nonretransplant survival). These results have been tempered, however, by reinfection at almost 90%, with active recurrent hepatitis at 50%. Recurrent hepatitis has led to few deaths, although a fourth of the reinfected patients have converted to a chronic state. More deaths from recurrent disease can be expected in this group, and longer follow-up is required to

determine whether results will remain acceptable. Disease recurrence has also been seen in cryptogenic cases, again suggesting a viral infection. Several treatments have been studied for HCV infection, with the most promising being parenteral therapy with interferon alfa.

Metabolic Diseases. Several metabolic diseases have been successfully cured with OLT, including alpha$_1$-antitrypsin deficiency, Wilson's disease, hemochromatosis, Crigler-Najjar syndrome, tyrosinemia, primary hyperoxaluria, and familial homozygous hypercholesterolemia. Survival is uniformly excellent. The recipient hepatectomy is usually simple, and the preoperative state of the patient is stable. Timing of transplantation should be such that secondary effects of the disease are not extensive.

Fulminant Hepatic Failure. In the absence of pre-existing liver disease, rapid loss of hepatic function culminating in jaundice and coma is termed *fulminant hepatic failure* (FHF). The etiologic agent can vary. The time course relates inversely to the prognosis, with those progressing to coma in less than 2 weeks having a 36% survival and those progressing in 2 to 8 weeks having a 7% survival. Despite the dramatic rate of progression of disease, these patients have very acceptable results from OLT (about 60% 5-year survival).[6, 37, 56] Predictably, survival after OLT improves with improved health of the patient at the time of transplant. Survival for all etiologies of FHF has doubled in the past decade, primarily due to great strides in supportive intensive care. Unlike chronic viral diseases, recurrence of disease for viral causes of FHF is unusual.

Care of patients with FHF is complex, and OLT should be considered early. Thus, prompt transfer to a liver transplantation center is critical. In patients with rapid deterioration, supportive care (e.g., hyperventilation, diuresis) should be supplemented with monitoring of intracranial pressure (ICP) for best results. Subdural ICP monitors have obviated the need for intraventricular devices and have thus reduced the bleeding risks of this approach. Perfusion pressures (mean arterial pressure minus ICP) of less than 40 mm. Hg, especially when combined with pupillary fixation, suggest that irreversible brain injury has occurred, and OLT should be avoided. Patient decompensation can be rapid and unpredictable. In the absence of a suitable donor, several aggressive maneuvers can successfully delay the onset of brain death from intracranial pressure. These include hepatectomy with end-to-side portacaval shunt, xenogeneic *ex vivo* perfusion, and bioartificial hepatic support (see later). Donor criteria may be liberalized to achieve timely hepatic replacement, and ABO incompatibility is acceptable.

Chronic Hepatitis B. Transplantation for chronic hepatitis B virus (HBV) cirrhosis remains a controversial topic.[39, 55] The discouraging reinfection rate of over 80% of recipients associated with a high rate of clinical hepatitis recurrence (60% at 1 year) and high related mortality (30% at 1 year and 52% at 5 years) raises questions about the procedure.[6, 14] Although generally contraindicated, transplantation may be appropriate in certain settings. Recent intense investigation in this area has identified several factors affecting reinfection. In general, the state of viral replication at the time of transplantation is critical in establishing reinfection. Identification of active viral replication (serum HBV DNA and HBeAg detection) at the time of transplantation clearly worsens the prognosis. Immunoprophylaxis with anti-HBV antibodies improves outcome for replication-negative patients, but long-term results for patients so treated remain to be seen. In general, OLT in the presence of HBV infection should be reserved for patients enrolled in specific viral prophylaxis protocols.

Intrahepatic Malignancy. Predictably, transplantation for primary and metastatic cancer has been associated with a high recurrence of tumor and a poor 5-year survival.[6, 40] Thus, there is little indication for OLT in a patient with known malignancy. Liver transplantation is no longer an accepted therapy for hepatic metastasis except perhaps in some patients with rare neuroendocrine tumors.[19] Today, liver transplantation is usually limited to patients with nonresectable hepatoma fulfilling the following criteria: asymptomatic hepatoma (i.e., not associated with recent weight loss, ascites, or constitutional symptoms); tumor less than 5 cm. in diameter; and fewer than or equal to three intrahepatic tumors. If feasible, liver resection should always be considered first. Extensive evaluation is required to exclude the presence of extrahepatic spread. Transplantation for cholangiocarcinoma is even more controversial and should probably be performed only under the guidance of specific protocols. The role of adjuvant chemotherapy or chemoembolization in patients undergoing transplantation for cancer remains unknown.

Pediatric Indications. The most common indication for liver transplantation in children is biliary atresia (see Table 20–16). This diagnosis accounts for 55% of the pediatric recipients in the UNOS registry.[6, 41] Although the creation of a portoenterostomy (Kasai procedure) remains the standard initial treatment, long-term survival without eventual hepatic failure is uncommon. Five-year survival remains under 50%. For this reason, many have proposed that early intervention with OLT be considered. The results of liver transplantation in infants have been somewhat better, with 5-year patient survival of 64%. Thus, a reasonable course of action appears to be neonatal nontransplant surgical intervention, with transplantation reserved for those children developing hepatic insufficiency despite a Kasai procedure.[38] The interim growth improves the donor pool substantially and decreases the technical difficulties inherent in the management of small children. Five-year survival improves to 74% at 3 to 5 years and 79% from 5 to 15 years. However, multiple reoperations and revisions after an initial portoenterostomy should be avoided because they rarely provide long-term disease-free survival and substantially hinder efforts to transplant the patient. The remaining usual indications for pediatric transplantation also occur in the adult population, with 13% performed for metabolic diseases (see above) and 10% associated with fulminant hepatic failure secondary to hepatitis of various etiologies.

SPECIFIC PATIENT SELECTION AND PREOPERATIVE CONSIDERATIONS

Patient Selection. The success of liver transplantation is closely related to the rational selection of patients most likely to benefit from the procedure. In fact, the single most important prognostic factor affecting survival is the medical condition of the recipient at the time of OLT (Fig. 20–42).[6] As with the recipients of other organs, patients should be without additional end-organ failure (other than that clearly related to hepatic insufficiency) and should be candidates for a major operative intervention. In general, dependence on alcohol or other harmful substances should be resolved for at least 6 months. Extrahepatic malignancy, sepsis, and diffuse mesenteric venous thrombosis represent absolute contraindications. Isolated portal vein thrombosis is a relative contraindication. The patient's liver function should be such that complications of dysfunction are emerging, with the predicted life span of the patient managed medically less than 2 years. With the improvements in survival after allotransplantation realized in the past decade, it is also appropriate to consider patients with metabolic diseases or moderately advanced liver disease with significant alterations in quality of life such as extreme fatigue, refractory pruritus, or encephalopathy.

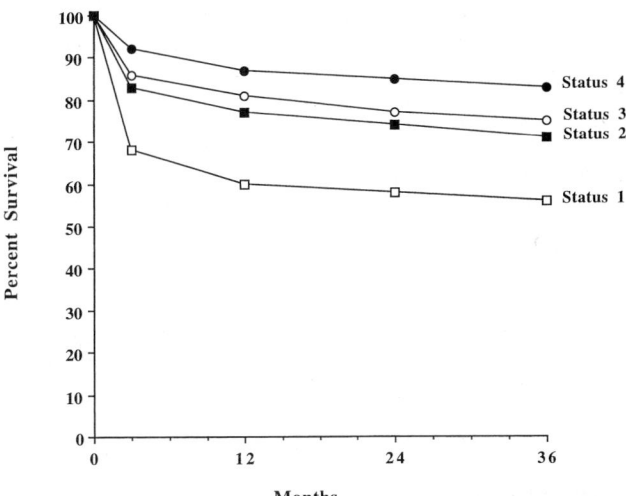

Figure 20–42. United Network for Organ Sharing (UNOS) status and survival after orthotopic liver transplantation (for definition of UNOS status, see text).

Preoperative Preparation. Once advanced liver disease is identified, efforts to proceed with transplantation should be initiated, because the preoperative health of the recipient greatly affects the chance for success. Early evaluation by a multidisciplinary team schooled in the specific requirements for liver transplantation is critical. In addition to surgical evaluation, the selection of appropriate candidates for transplantation should be based on input from medical colleagues, including a hepatologist and infectious disease specialist. Evaluation by a social worker and psychiatrist to establish the ability of the patient and family to manage themselves postoperatively is important. Immediate efforts should optimize the candidate's nutritional status and overall medical condition. Finally, education of the patient must be initiated early to ensure that complications of medical noncompliance are avoided postoperatively.

For all liver recipients, thorough preoperative evaluation to determine the antibody titer directed against hepatitis A, B, and C as well as cytomegalovirus, human immunodeficiency virus, Epstein-Barr virus, and herpes simplex is mandatory. In addition, viral antigen detection is required to identify active infection. The role of transplantation for primary viral hepatitis was discussed previously. Active infection with cytomegalovirus or herpesvirus requires clinical resolution before transplantation, but viral carriers can receive transplants given appropriate antiviral prophylaxis. Human immunodeficiency virus infection contraindicates OLT. In addition to the recipient's status, the donor's status for these viruses should be ascertained before implantation, again to allow for antiviral prophylaxis when indicated.

Several alternative therapies should be considered in the candidate for transplantation, not necessarily to obviate the need for transplantation but to improve the medical condition before transplantation. Patients with good synthetic function (normal bilirubin, normal coagulation, normal albumin), such as an individual with Child's A cirrhosis and recurrent variceal bleeding, may benefit from nontransplant surgical palliation such as a Warren shunt. The TIPS procedure is also a useful palliative step for refractory complications of portal hypertension. Stabilization of disease with these interventions gives more time to evaluate patients and optimize preoperative conditions. It allows for a more thorough evaluation of a patient's ability to comply with the posttransplant medical regimen, particularly alcoholic patients who present abstinent because they are *too sick to drink.* This compliance alone may stabilize the disease in an alcoholic patient with Child's A cirrhosis and avoid the need for transplantation. Reduction in the degree of portal hypertension may also minimize intraoperative bleeding during the recipient hepatectomy. Problems with these palliative procedures are frequent and require surveillance with particular attention to portal vein patency. Identified candidates should be treated at a center with transplant expertise to facilitate palliation that does not jeopardize future transplantation. Alternative treatment should not delay transplantation.

SELECTION OF DONORS

Immediate function of a transplanted liver is imperative. Unlike kidney, pancreas, or, to some extent, heart transplantation, no artificial means is readily available to support an anhepatic patient in the event of graft failure. Without a rapid restoration of synthetic function, death from bleeding or cerebral edema generally ensues within 72 hours. The single most important factor determining the early function of a liver allograft is the viability of the donor liver. Although this seems obvious, determining the state of the liver in a heart-beating cadaver remains imprecise, so careful attention to the conditions of the donor's death, the morphology and function of the organ before harvest, and the specifics of the extirpation is critical. Failure of a graft to function at all after a technically successful transplantation is known as primary nonfunction (PNF). The only treatment for PNF is retransplantation within 24 to 72 hours. Factors contributing to the development of PNF include parenchymal insufficiency unrecognized at the time of harvest, graft injury during the harvest or cadaver resuscitation, preservation injury or prolonged cold ischemia, prolonged rewarming time, and reperfusion injury after implantation.[15]

Several factors have been investigated to aid in the prediction of PNF. The most widely noted is the estimated parenchymal fat content.[18, 53] Donor liver biopsy specimens that show a 40% or greater parenchymal replacement by fat have a higher chance of PNF, and in some settings this is a reasonable indicator of the adequacy of a donor organ. This must, however, be balanced against the severity of the recipient's disease and the urgency of the planned operation. Other factors used to evaluate the donor's status include the age of the donor, the level of inotropic support, the mechanism of the donor's death, the level of hepatic or intra-abdominal trauma, the presence of hypernatremia, and the biochemical studies of liver function. No single parameter has been established absolutely governing the acceptance of a donor for organ harvest.[11, 50] Rather, combinations of risk factors are generally responsible for discarding a potential donor liver. In case of doubt about the quality of an organ, the personal inspection of the liver by an experienced transplant surgeon is often critical for decision about the use of an organ.

Donor use has been improved with the introduction of UW preservation solution as mentioned earlier. Until 1987 the outer limit for cold storage of the liver using EuroCollins solution was about 8 hours. Use of UW solution has extended the time to about 24 hours, allowing for better allocation of the organ and preparation of the recipient. The specifics of this and other preservation solutions are detailed in Part VII of this chapter.

The considerations of ABO typing and other immunologic concerns are discussed later. An additional issue is size compatibility. Smaller organs are easily adapted to a large recipient, but the converse is not true. One advance has been the use of reduced-size allografts, particularly in children. Usually the left lateral lobe (segments 2 and 3) or left lobe (segments 2, 3, and 4) is used, allowing up to 1/10 weight

mismatch. This has been the most important factor in the success of transplantation in small children. This technique is sometimes used in adults when an emergency transplantation is required. Finally, male recipients of female organs have 10% worse survival than other sex-match combinations, according to the 1994 UNOS registry.

OPERATION ON THE DONOR

Harvest of the donor organ should be performed by an experienced surgeon, with particular care taken to optimize the preharvest resuscitation of the heart-beating cadaver. Because immediate hepatic function after transplantation is required, there is no room for error. Errors in resuscitation include injudicious use of vasopressors, prolonged acidosis, and hypoperfusion from hypovolemia. Visual inspection and palpation of the liver with knowledge of the potential recipient's status and size aid in the assessment of the appropriateness of a donor liver.

The liver is generally procured through a midline incision from jugular notch to pubis, including median sternotomy (Fig. 20–43). Harvest is coordinated with the harvest teams for other organs. Complete mobilization of the liver is required, including division of both triangular ligaments and the falciform ligament. The hepatogastric ligament is divided. Particular attention is paid to the vascular supply, including preservation of aberrant hepatic arteries (20% aberrant right from the superior mesenteric artery, 15% aberrant left from the left gastric artery). Unlike the relative impunity associated with arterial ligation in nontransplanted livers, failure to complete the arterial revascularization due to an unrecognized arterial supply is poorly tolerated after cold storage.

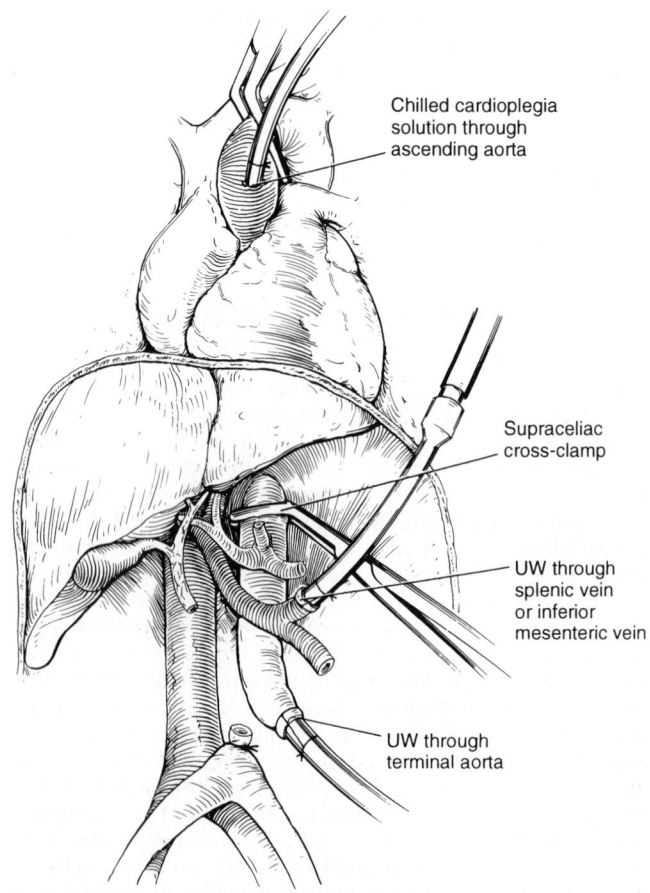

Chilled cardioplegia solution through ascending aorta

Supraceliac cross-clamp

UW through splenic vein or inferior mesenteric vein

UW through terminal aorta

Figure 20–43. The donor procedure. UW, University of Wisconsin.

PNF, late biliary stricture, or intrahepatic abscess may result. Additional care must be taken when simultaneous pancreas harvest is performed to avoid hepatic artery injury or portal vein transection. The suprahepatic vena cava should be preserved for the hepatic graft, and care should be taken to avoid caval injury during cardiac retrieval. The gallbladder is removed either *in situ* or after explantation.

Once mobilization is completed, perfusion with UW solution is initiated through the distal aorta or common iliac arteries with ligation of the supraceliac aorta. The inferior mesenteric vein or splenic vein is used for portal perfusion. When pancreatic harvest is performed, some surgeons prefer to use the portal vein for cold perfusion. UW solution is also flushed into the biliary tree. Topical slush is rapidly applied. Hepatic extirpation is performed after cardiopulmonary retrieval and before harvest of the pancreas and kidney. The iliac artery and vein should be harvested in the event that vascular reconstruction is required.

IMMEDIATE PREOPERATIVE MANAGEMENT

Patients awaiting liver transplantation are prioritized on a national waiting list based on severity of disease as defined by the UNOS. Status 4 patients are at home and functioning normally, status 3 patients can be at home but require continuous medical care. Status 2 patients are continuously hospitalized in an acute care unit for at least 5 days or are in the intensive care unit. Status 1 patients are in the intensive care unit because of acute or chronic liver failure with a life expectancy without a liver transplant of less than 7 days. Status 7 is reserved for patients taken from the active list for a temporary medical contraindication such as sepsis.[1] These patients can accrue points for time on the list despite not being able to accept an organ. Strict adherence to guidelines for proper categorization is required to allow for ethical allocation of organs. As soon as a donor is identified, the organ is paired with a potential recipient, who is called to the hospital for preoperative evaluation before organ harvest.

Appropriate perioperative management of a transplant recipient begins with a thorough preoperative physical examination (including rectal and dental examinations) to rule out the possibility of ongoing infection or malignancy. Routine screening includes a complete blood cell count, electrolyte and metabolic profile, urinalysis, and chest film. Blood is crossmatched. Intravenous lines, including arterial lines and pulmonary artery catheters, should be placed with strict attention to aseptic technique because cutaneous contamination with bacteria or fungi can cause serious postoperative complications in the transplant patient. Selective decontamination of the gut and mechanical preparation of the bowel are advocated at many centers, as is a shower with an antimicrobial soap.

For patients in the intensive care unit, supportive measures are continued as needed. Of specific concern is the potential for neurologic recovery in patients with advanced encephalopathy and cerebral edema. A recent advance has been the use of intracranial pressure monitoring in the perioperative period. This was once shunned as a prohibitive risk for cerebral bleeding in the coagulopathic fulminant hepatic failure patient, but routine assessment is now possible through minimally invasive techniques. Small-gauge catheter pressure monitors can be placed into the subdural space without the need for parenchymal puncture, thus decreasing the risk of the intervention substantially. Greatly elevated intracerebral pressures, especially in association with signs of transtentorial herniation in a Grade 5 coma patient, suggest an irreversible lesion that is unlikely to resolve after transplantation.

OPERATION ON THE RECIPIENT

Few surgical procedures require the fastidious attention to technical detail required in liver transplantation. Technical errors are translated directly into infectious complications or marginal biliary function. Thus, transplantation should be performed only by surgeons proficient in the procedure. In addition, the operative environment should include experienced nursing and ancillary support.

Intraoperative management by a knowledgeable anesthesiologist with experience in liver transplantation is critical for a successful technical result. The procedure presents the challenge of maintaining homeostasis of temperature, circulation (including oxygen-carrying capacity and coagulation competence), gluconeogenesis, and electrolyte concentration while establishing adequate anesthesia and paralysis with agents not requiring hepatic function for degradation. Intraoperative ICP monitoring is appropriate for patients with severe encephalopathy. In procedures using a venovenous bypass, a perfusionist is required, and procedures performed without bypass require adequate maintenance of preload during caval occlusion and correction of metabolic abnormalities after release of the congested portal circulation. After the initial function of the allograft, the most important factor predictive of technical success is the stability of the patient intraoperatively and his or her delivery to the intensive care unit normothermic with adequate circulatory competence.

Successful engraftment of the organ begins with a controlled recipient hepatectomy. This can be a formidable task in patients with severe portal hypertension and extensive collateral formation or in those with multiple operative interventions. In general, extirpation follows the basic surgical guidelines of establishing proximal and distal vascular control combined with lysis of all ligamentous attachments. Specific technical concerns include retaining maximal length on all vessels. Mobilization of the common bile duct depends on the planned biliary reconstruction (choledochocholedochostomy versus choledochojejunostomy). Care to avoid injury to the right adrenal vein during caval dissection is important. If venovenous bypass is planned, cannulation of the left axillary, femoral, and portal veins is performed.

The decision to place the recipient on bypass is routine at a number of centers; and liberal use of this technique, originally developed by Shaw and colleagues,[2, 3] has clearly led to improved operative mortality. Bypass avoids mesenteric congestion and minimizes the release of lactate and other by-products of hypoperfusion into the portal circulation. In addition, it improves venous return to the heart during implantation and thus improves hemodynamic stability during the period of caval occlusion. Bypass also diverts the portal flow during difficult recipient hepatectomies to minimize blood loss, particularly during dissection of the retrohepatic cava and bare spot.[11] Despite these benefits, it is now clear that many patients tolerate OLT without the additional manipulation required by bypass. It has thus become policy at many centers to employ this technique selectively after an intraoperative trial of portal vein and vena caval occlusion.

The implantation procedure (Fig. 20–44) begins with the suprahepatic vena caval anastomosis followed by the infrahepatic caval anastomosis. Alternatively, the donor vena cava can be anastomosed side to side with the recipient vena cava if it is left *in situ* during the recipient hepatectomy (piggyback technique). The operation then proceeds to the portal anastomosis. After all venous connections, the liver is reperfused with the suprahepatic vena cava temporarily occluded and the infrahepatic vena cava vented to allow washout of the hyperkalemic and adenosine-rich UW solution. The hepatic artery anastomosis is the final vascular step in the procedure.

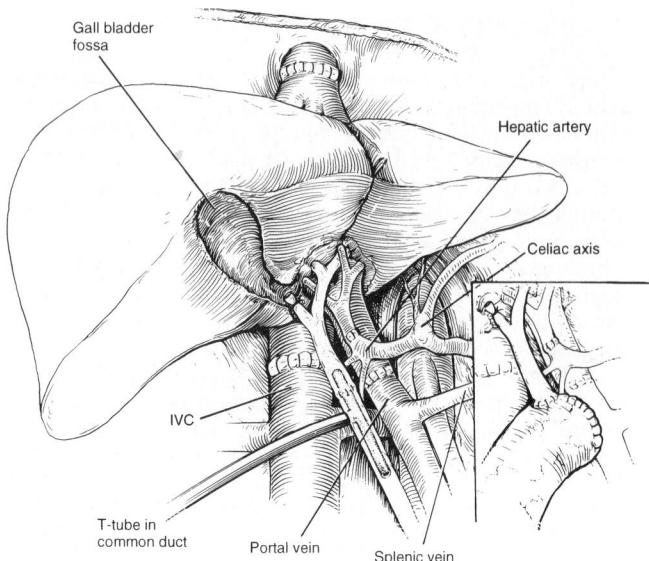

Figure 20–44. The recipient procedure.

Labels on figure: Gall bladder fossa · Hepatic artery · Celiac axis · IVC · T-tube in common duct · Portal vein · Splenic vein

Some groups perform simultaneous arterial and venous reperfusion.[43]

The biliary reconstruction remains an additional area of debate.[54] Options include choledochocholedochostomy with or without externalized T-tube stents. This has the advantage of easy access for subsequent biliary manipulations or evaluation of bile, as well as preservation of the sphincter mechanism. Unfortunately, the anastomosis is particularly sensitive to ischemic injury of the common duct, and complications of leak when the T tube is removed remain vexing.[31] The incidence of technical complications related to this method ranges from 12% to 50% in published series, with the cumulative average being 25%.[36] These problems are obviated for the most part by use of a Roux-en-Y choledochojejunostomy at the expense of convenient biliary access.[8] Leak or stricture is still observed in 4% to 30% of cases (mean 14%).[36] This method is frequently used in pediatric transplants. One report of 300 transplants performed with a side-to-side choledochocholedochostomy technique has reported a remarkable 2.2% technical complication rate.[36] This technique awaits confirmation in other centers.

POSTOPERATIVE MANAGEMENT

Management in the postoperative intensive care unit is similar to that after any major procedure. Ventilatory support and volume replacement are standard. Isolation is not required beyond standard universal precautions. No sedation is given until extubation. For unclear reasons, postoperative pain is usually mild, and any major discomfort should alert one for possible complications. Close monitoring of serologic liver enzymes is critical because increasing enzymes or a failure of enzyme values to correct rapidly suggests PNF or technical complications such as hepatic artery thrombosis. Liberal use of the Doppler ultrasonography and rapid return to the operating room are mandatory in these situations because early detection is the only factor separating a return to normal liver function from complete graft necrosis and patient death.

Use of drains and antibiotics is no different in this operation from that in any other major abdominal procedure. Closed-suction drains should be used and removed early after the threat of postoperative hemorrhage is over. Brief antibiotic prophylaxis is appropriate with an agent with adequate skin and biliary organism coverage. Prolonged use of prophylactic antibiotics is contraindicated. A protocol for decontaminating the small bowel can be used but is usually discontinued within a few weeks of transplantation. At Duke University Medical Center, decontamination (colistin, 100 mg./10 ml.; gentamicin, 80 mg./10 ml.; nystatin, 2×10^6/10 ml.) is discontinued at the time of normal enteral feeding, often within the first postoperative week).

If a T tube is used in the biliary reconstruction, a T-tube cholangiogram is obtained within a week with internalization contingent on a normal result. Patients are discharged when they are familiar with their medications. Patients living more than 2 hours from the transplant center generally stay in the vicinity for an additional 2 to 4 weeks. Close monitoring of hepatic function and medical compliance is continued twice a week for 4 weeks and weekly for an additional 4 weeks. After this outpatient evaluation, patients are returned to their referring community for chronic follow-up. It is important to establish open lines of communication between the community physician and the transplant center to ensure prompt recognition and referral of postoperative complications.

IMMUNOLOGIC MANAGEMENT

The liver must be considered separately from other solid organs with regard to immunologic management. Many well-established concepts of donor-host interaction after kidney or heart transplantation do not apply after hepatic transplantation, and failure to recognize the unique properties of this situation can lead to detrimental perioperative treatment.[35]

HLA Typing. HLA matching is not feasible before liver transplantation. However, because new techniques have been developed that allow donor HLA data to be provided in a timely manner, the future use of these data is pertinent. Although matching donors and recipients with regard to HLA type clearly improves outcome after kidney, heart, and pancreas transplantation, no such correlation exists with liver transplantation. Indeed, matching may, in fact, reduce overall survival.[33, 49] The reasons for this lie in the dualistic nature of HLA in the pathophysiology of liver disease. T-cell–mediated rejection of the organ is mechanistically the same as with other organs, so rejection is reduced with improved HLA compatibility. However, the physiologic role of HLA is to present viral peptides to T cells to initiate destruction of virally infected cells. Thus, HLA compatibility potentiates the inflammation during viral reinfection after transplantation for viral hepatitis and increases the chance for clinical recurrence of the original disease. Similarly, T-cell–mediated autoimmune diseases (e.g., PBC) are etiologically based on T-cell recognition of HLA presented peptides. Therefore, recurrence of autoimmune diseases may be potentiated as well. Further knowledge regarding specific disease states worsened by certain HLA matches may be useful in selective typing in the future.

Crossmatch and ABO Matching. The lymphocytotoxic crossmatch is not used prospectively before liver transplantation. Again, temporal concerns are most pressing; but in this case, the value of a positive crossmatch in predicting subsequent poor outcome from hyperacute rejection is minimal. Indeed, hyperacute rejection is rarely seen even in the face of documented preformed antibodies and ABO incompatibility.[22, 24, 49] The reasons for this remain controversial because hyperacute rejection can be readily produced experimentally.[28] Although preformed antibodies reduce long-term graft survival somewhat, early results appear to be minimally affected. Grafts unmatched for ABO antigens can cause antibody-mediated graft-versus-host disease with mild hemolytic anemia and fever occurring between postoperative days 5 and 12.[44] This is the result of intrahepatic B cells that secrete antibody directed against the recipient ABO antigens. Although it is usually self-limited, increased immunosuppression may be required. Alternatively, some groups suggest a decrease in immunosuppression to allow for a limited rejection of the offending B cells. It is preferred that rules for ABO compatibility be followed for elective transplantation. In the emergent setting, however, ABO-incompatible grafts can be used with acceptable results. The 5-year survival for grafts that are ABO incompatible is approximately 15% lower than that for grafts without ABO discrepancy.[6] This not only reflects some immune preference but also the patient population that receives ABO mismatched grafts, that is, emergent transplants for FHF and PNF.

Acute Rejection. As with other allografts, T-cell–mediated destruction of the liver is inevitable without immunosuppressive therapy. The primary targets for T-cell recognition are HLA antigens on the biliary epithelium and vascular endothelium. The characteristics of this rejection, termed *acute rejection,* are similar to those of kidney or heart in that it develops in most of the cases during the first 6 months after transplantation, usually within the first 4 postoperative weeks. More than half of patients develop at least one episode of rejection. Symptoms are nonspecific, often including mild intermittent fever and general malaise with alteration in liver tests. The diagnosis should be confirmed by liver biopsy. Most episodes are readily reversible (90%), given prompt recognition and initiation of antirejection therapy. This contrasts sharply to chronic rejection, discussed later.

Monitoring for acute rejection is a continuous process. Needle-core biopsy of the allograft is the best diagnostic test (Fig. 20–45). Histologically it appears as a predominantly T-cell and monocyte infiltrate in the portal tracts, with subendothelial (endotheliitis) and biliary epithelial aggregates. Eosinophils and polymorphonuclear leukocytes are present to a lesser degree but are more prevalent in hepatic rejection than in infiltrate seen in other organs. Although protocol biopsies are performed in some centers, most groups rely on monitoring of the liver function studies and/or the serum beta$_2$-microglobulin value, with biopsy used to clarify detected abnormalities. Because a primary target in acute rejection is biliary epithelium, it often presents initially as a cholestatic process with rapid increases in the alkaline phosphatase and bilirubin values. However, changes in hepatic biochemical parameters are nonspecific and can also indicate technical or infectious complications where alter-

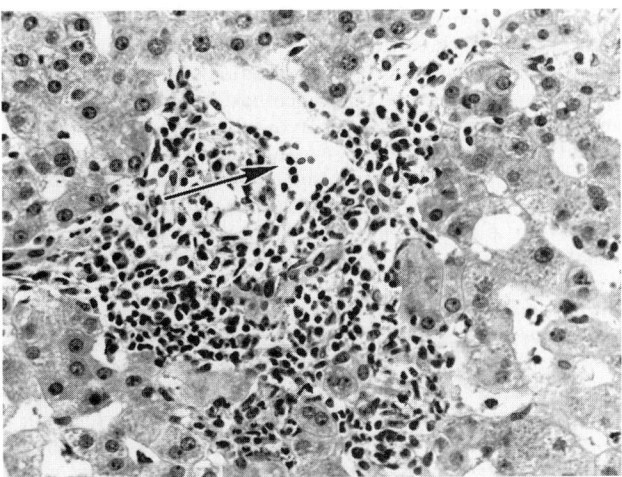

Figure 20–45. Acute rejection after liver transplantation. Portal tracts contain a mixed inflammatory infiltrate, with mononuclear cells and eosinophils. Bile duct damage is evident, and endothelium of a branch of the portal vein is disrupted and infiltrated by lymphocytes (arrow). Hematoxylin and eosin, original magnification ×325. (Courtesy of Kay Washington, M.D., Department of Pathology, Duke University Medical Center.)

ations in the immunosuppressive regimen would be ineffective or even detrimental. Thus, liberal use of biopsy and Doppler ultrasound evaluation of hepatic blood flow and bile duct integrity is critical. Once acute rejection is diagnosed, rescue immunosuppression is initiated as described later.

Chronic Rejection. The development of liver allograft dysfunction over a period of months to years is termed *chronic rejection* and, like other allografts, is controversial and multifactorial in its etiology, and is usually not reversible. Histologically it appears as a paucity of bile duct epithelium without conspicuous lymphocytic infiltration and has thus been described as the "vanishing bile duct syndrome" (Fig. 20–46). Additionally, an obliterative vasculopathy can occur with parenchymal fibrosis. The time course, histology, and refractory nature of chronic rejection suggest that direct cell-mediated destruction is not a primary mechanism. It is likely that the cumulative effects of mild subclinical immune recognition by several limbs of the immune system, and the resulting

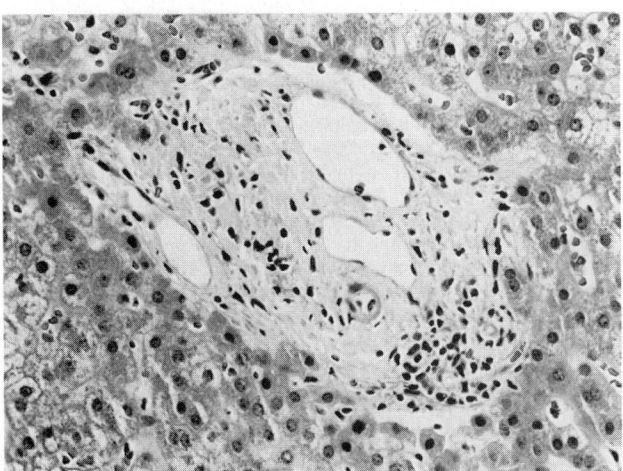

Figure 20–46. Vanishing bile duct syndrome as a manifestation of chronic rejection after liver transplantation. Portal inflammation diminishes as interlobular bile ducts disappear. There is no bile ductular proliferation. Hematoxylin and eosin, original magnification ×325. (Courtesy of Kay Washington, M.D., Department of Pathology, Duke University Medical Center.)

exposure to soluble factors including fibrogenic cytokines, eventually take their toll on the fragile epithelium. Chronic rejection often requires retransplantation.

Immunosuppressive Pharmacology. Manipulation of the immune system is required to avoid graft loss from rejection. Identifying a safe, effective, and minimally immunosuppressive regimen requires a careful balance aimed at reducing infectious and neoplastic complications without a resultant increase in allograft rejection and/or dysfunction. Thus, rational, selective use of several immunosuppressive agents is required to manage successfully the broad array of patients who are transplanted. Three general classifications of immunosuppression are used: (1) induction therapy, a relatively intense initial conditioning of the newly transplanted recipient; (2) maintenance therapy, drugs given at minimal doses required to maintain graft function; and (3) rescue therapy, heightened immunosuppression given to reverse an episode of acute rejection. Most transplant centers have specific protocols for each situation. For example, the Duke University liver transplant protocol is presented in Table 20–17.

Several issues specific to liver transplantation should be mentioned. Of major importance is that the liver appears to have less immunostimulatory antigenicity than other organs. The specifics of this perceived resistance remain somewhat controversial but may relate to several peculiarities of hepatic physiology. First, the portal circulation is exposed regularly to enteric pathogens and, more importantly, to absorbed peptides, which have potential antigenicity. A generalized perihepatic anergy has been postulated as protective in this setting to prevent vascular thrombosis and inappropriate hepatic inflammation. Clearly the reticuloendothelial system of the liver—the Kupffer cells—is important in establishing appropriate versus inappropriate presentation of portal antigen. Most of the Kupffer cells of the liver are replaced with those of recipient HLA type within a few weeks after transplantation. In addition, the Kupffer cells of the donor have been described as migrating to other recipient tissues and establishing a state of chimerism. Whether this chimerism creates specific tolerance or is the result of it remains to be seen. From a practical standpoint, maintenance immunosuppression after liver transplantation can be comparatively low, and many patients have been weaned to little or no immunosuppression for years. Also of importance in this regard, the liver can tolerate brief periods on immunosuppression withdrawal if it becomes necessary to combat a potentially lethal infection.

A recent issue of particular importance in liver transplant immunosuppressive pharmacology has been the development of the drug tacrolimus (FK 506). This agent has been suggested as having particular efficacy in the setting of liver transplantation, with truly remarkable results in early, uncontrolled trials performed at the University of Pittsburgh.[48] Tacrolimus has a mechanism of action similar to that of cyclosporin A and it has been used as a replacement for this drug. A possible benefit is the potential steroid-sparing effect of tacrolimus, exceeding that of cyclosporine. Single-drug maintenance therapy is being actively investigated. Multicenter, randomized, prospective trials comparing cyclosporine to tacrolimus are underway, with the initial 1-year follow-up demonstrating a significant reduction in rejection episodes and a lower need for rescue therapy with OKT3 in the tacrolimus group.[20, 52] No graft or patient survival advantage has been demonstrated. The side effect profile for tacrolimus differs from that of cyclosporine in that the cosmetic complications of hirsutism, acne, and gingival hyperplasia are not present but the potential for neurologic abnormalities, diabetes mellitus, and renal impairment appears to be more prevalent. An important consideration is that the combination of cyclosporine and tacrolimus drastically increases the incidence and severity of side effects. Thus, therapy must be limited to one or the other, and limiting the use of either in the early postoperative setting may benefit renal function. Clearly, both cyclosporine and tacrolimus have proven efficacy for maintenance immunosuppression after liver transplantation. The specific selection of either remains to be established by randomized investigation. As a rescue agent during established acute rejection, neither tacrolimus nor cyclosporine is particularly efficacious compared with glucocorticosteroids or antilymphocyte antibody preparations.

Another practical issue unique to liver transplant immunosuppression relates to the absorption of cyclosporine and, to a lesser degree, tacrolimus. Drug uptake depends on the availability of enteric bile salts. Thus, with decreased production of bile in the initial posttransplant period or during a rejection episode, or biliary diversion through a T tube, cyclosporine should be administered intravenously to maintain adequate plasma levels. A new cyclosporine formulation (Neoral), which is bile salt independent for absorption, is now available.

Antiviral Immunity and Immunosuppression. The importance of viral infection in liver transplant patients cannot be overstated. *De novo* infection or latent virus reactivation of pathogens, including cytomegalovirus, herpes simplex virus, and Epstein-Barr virus, and reinfection of hepatotropic viruses, including hepatitis B and C, remain serious sources of posttransplant morbidity and mortality and are directly re-

TABLE 20–17. The Duke University Immunosuppressive Protocol for Orthotopic Liver Transplantation

Induction Therapy

Methylprednisolone: Induction of anesthesia: 125 mg. IV
　　　　Postoperatively: tapered from 300 to 20 mg./
　　　　day on 5th postoperative day

Cyclosporine: Intraoperatively: continuous IV infusion (2 mg./kg./
　　　　day)
　　　　Postoperatively: continuous IV infusion (4 mg./kg./
　　　　day) on arrival in the surgical intensive care unit
　　　　On postoperative days 2–3: oral cyclosporine (Neoral)
　　　　is started at 5 mg./kg. q12h. The IV cyclo-
　　　　sporine is decreased according to serum levels.
　　　　(Targeting postoperative levels: 250–300 ng./ml.
　　　　[HPLC assay])

Azathioprine (1–1.5 mg./kg./day): Started as soon as the patient can
　　　　tolerate oral feeding, usually by
　　　　day 2 or 3

Maintenance Therapy

Prednisone: First 3 months: 20 mg./day
　　　　3–6 months: 15 mg./day
　　　　After 6 months: 5–10 mg./day

Cyclosporine: Targeted levels: initial 10 days: 250–300 ng./ml.;
　　　　10–30 days: 200–300 ng./100 ml.; 1–6 months:
　　　　150–200 ng./ml.; 6–12 months: 120–200 ng./ml.;
　　　　and after 1 year: 80–120 ng./ml.

Azathioprine: 1–2 mg./kg., usually discontinued within 9 months of
　　　　transplantation

Rescue Therapy for Biopsy-Proven Acute Cellular Rejection

First episode: 3-day recycling with IV methylprednisolone
　　　　500 mg./day

Second episode: repeated 3-day recycling with IV
　　　　methylprednisolone

Third episode: monoclonal antibody muromonab-CD3 (OKT3,
　　　　Orthoclone, Raritan, NJ) or antithymocyte globulin
　　　　(ATGAM, Upjohn, Kalamazoo, MI) is given for
　　　　10–15 days

Refractory rejection: cyclosporine (Neoral) is discontinued and
　　　　FK 506 (Prograf) (target levels 10–15 ng./ml.)
　　　　is initiated

lated to the intensity of the immunosuppressive regimen employed. In particular, the use of antilymphocyte antibody preparations, particularly OKT3, have been implicated in increasing the likelihood of viral infection and associated complications such as lymphoproliferative disorders. In response to this association, most transplant centers have incorporated antiviral prophylaxis into their immunosuppressive protocols, with the specific agents, duration of therapy, and dosages governed by the viral status of the recipient and the donor organ. The relationship between the pathophysiology of acute T-cell–mediated rejection and the physiologic function of T cells in viral immunity is underscored in the transplant patient on T-cell–directed immunosuppression.

OUTCOMES

Clearly, liver transplantation is the most significant advancement in the treatment of end-stage liver disease this century. Diseases treated by OLT are by definition terminal with few exceptions, and as such are lethal without hepatic replacement. Survival of a patient with no other hope for survival is the most obvious positive outcome. Operative survival now exceeds 90% for first grafts. Retransplant-free survival has improved steadily in the past 10 years and is now 73% at 1 year for all transplants reported to the UNOS registry. The 5-year survival reflecting transplantation before ganciclovir became available is approximately 60%, and improvements of 2% to 3% per year have been made each year since 1987. Predicted actuarial survival for transplants performed in 1995 is over 75%.

Survival and retransplant rates have been the principal, if not the only, measures of outcome in the transplant literature until recently. The technical issues of survival in the first decade of widespread transplantation have overshadowed other outcome measures to the point of their exclusion from the literature. Critical evaluation of costly health care interventions has become a fundamental priority in our society. Outcomes can be defined either from a physician's, patient's, payer's, or society's perspective. The medical perspective is in the traditional purview of the clinician and clinician investigator, who use objective and quantifiable medical parameters, whereas the patient's perspective involves a more subjective assessment of quality of life. Today, survival has become the norm after OLT, and thus the next decade should clearly define outcome with regard to each of these perspectives.

Medical Perspective. Despite the recent advances in all aspects of liver transplantation, the procedure remains one with considerable morbidity.[14] Most patients have some complications that deviate from an ideal recovery, and all patients accept the trade of their liver disease for the *disease* of immunosuppression. These negative outcomes are generally remedied by prompt recognition of problems and aggressive corrective intervention. It is, therefore, critical that the potential obstacles arising postoperatively are thoroughly understood. The authors have recently categorized negative outcomes under three headings: negative sequel, complications, and failure to cure.[16]

A *negative sequel* is an adverse effect inherent to the transplant procedure.[16] Transplantation in general carries with it the risk of lifelong immunosuppression. Patients must adapt their lifestyle to ensure that medications are taken as prescribed and that the immune system and organ function are monitored when necessary. The risk of opportunistic infection and malignancy that accompanies chronic immunosuppression persists for life. These factors, however, are less intrusive for liver transplant patients than for recipients of other solid organs because of their reduced need for immunosuppression, especially after the first transplant year.

Failure to cure refers to pre-existing conditions that remain unchanged or recur after the transplant procedure.[16] The likelihood of cure reflects the primary disease. Metabolic and cholestatic diseases are generally resolved, as are the physiologic disorders of alcoholic cirrhosis. Unfortunately, viral infections remain generally uncured by liver replacement. As mentioned earlier, clinically significant recurrence of hepatitis B and hepatitis C may limit long-term cure. The cure for these illnesses remains in more potent antiviral therapeutics. Practically, however, viral reinfection that creates a clinically insignificant carrier state is viewed as a cure by the patient. Obviously, no extrahepatic malignancy can be cured by OLT, and the potential for cure in patients with intrahepatic malignancy is solely related to the presence or absence of metastatic disease at the time of recipient hepatectomy.

A *complication* is any other negative outcome that does not fit clearly into the definition of negative sequel or failure to cure. Complications of some kind occur in almost all patients, but the significance of these setbacks varies greatly. For example, acute rejection must be considered a complication of sorts, but most episodes are treated without significant alteration of a patient's comfort or residual disability. Conversely, PNF at best leads to retransplantation and at worst to death. The lack of uniform reporting of complications makes interpretation of the results of OLT difficult.[14] The authors have presented a classification of complications stratified by severity[14] (Table 20–18). With the heightened requirement for outcomes-based research in the current economic environment, standardized evaluation of transplant programs with regard to complication rates will likely increase.

Several common complications, such as acute and chronic rejection, have been discussed. Some complications deserve particular attention because of their seriousness and requirement for prompt intervention. PNF presents as a complete lack of synthetic function from the time of reperfusion. The patient develops encephalopathy, increased intracranial pressure, coagulopathy, hyperbilirubinemia, and hypertransaminasemia. Aggressive supportive therapy and prompt retransplantation are required within 72 hours. Total transplant hepatectomy with portacaval shunt can improve the hemodynamic and metabolic status of the patient for 24 to 36 hours if a suitable liver is not found immediately.

Hepatic artery thrombosis remains a complication, especially in the pediatric population. This presents as a rapid rise in serum transaminase levels. The transplanted liver does not tolerate loss of arterial flow, and failure to restore flow produces graft loss. Hepatic artery stricture or stenosis generally presents as a lesser degree of metabolic change later in the postoperative course. An alternative presentation of dearterialization is bile leak resulting from hepatic duct necrosis. An additional vascular complication that is less frequent but equally devastating is early portal vein thrombosis. Given the rapid and serious but reversible nature of these vascular complications, any suspect change in hepatic function requires immediate evaluation of the hepatic vasculature by Doppler ultrasonography, followed by either re-exploration or a confirmatory arteriogram.

Biliary complications, which occur in 15% to 30% of patients, suggest vascular compromise.[54] Both leaks and strictures can occur regardless of the method of reconstruction. Percutaneous or endoscopic management is generally considered an acceptable first alternative, but reoperation should not be avoided for appropriate lesions at the expense of hepatic function or cholangitis.

Patient Perspective. Today, increasing emphasis is given to patient-oriented subjective outcomes such as quality of life and well-being. Subjective outcomes have inherent limitations, but they are arguably more relevant to individual pa-

TABLE 20–18. Classification of Common Complications of Liver Transplantation

Grade 1: An alteration from ideal postoperative course *with complete recovery* or which can *be easily controlled* and which fulfills the general characteristics, namely (1) not life threatening; (2) not requiring use of drugs other than immunosuppressive agents, analgesics, antipyretic, anti-inflammatory, and antiemetic, drugs required for urinary retention or lower urinary tract infection, arterial hypertension, hyperlipidemia or transient hyperglycemia; (3) requiring only therapies that can be performed at the bedside; (4) postoperative bleeding requiring ≤ 3 units of blood; and (5) never associated with a prolongation of the intensive care unit (ICU) stay ≥ 5 days or total hospital stay ≥ 4 weeks.

Examples:
Superficial wound infection treated without antibiotics
Bile leak treated conservatively
Corticosteroid-responsive acute rejection
Well-controlled arterial hypertension

Grade 2: Any complication that is *potentially life-threatening* or results in ICU stay ≥ 5 days or hospital stay ≥ 4 weeks, but that *does not cause residual disability or persistent diseases.*

Grade 2a Complications requiring only use of drug therapy or postoperative bleeding requiring ≥ 3 units of blood.

Examples:
Rejection requiring immunosuppressors not routinely used after induction therapy (e.g., OKT3 or other antilymphocyte drugs)
Bacterial, viral, or fungal infection requiring antibiotic, antiviral, or antifungal therapy
Primary graft dysfunction (opening aspartate transaminase [AST] ≥ 2000 or a transient increase in AST levels ≥ 1000 I.U./ L., or a persistent elevated prothrombin time > 20 over 3 days)

Grade 2b Complications requiring therapeutic interventions, reoperation, readmission in the ICU, or prolongation in the ICU stay ≥ 5 days but that do not result in residual disability.

Examples:
Primary graft dysfunction extending the ICU stay ≥ 5 days
Postoperative bleeding requiring laparotomy
Biliary problems requiring endoscopic or surgical procedures

Grade 3: Any complication with residual or lasting functional disability or development of malignant disease (except squamous and basocellular cutaneous malignancies).

Grade 3a Complication with lasting disability that shows no evidence of progression and that has a relatively low risk of graft failure and/ or death.

Examples:
De novo hepatitis C
Nonprogressive chronic rejection
Persistent bile duct stricture without evidence of progressive liver failure or recurrent cholangitis

Grade 3b Complications with lasting disability that are either difficult to control or have a significant risk of leading to graft failure and/or death.

Examples:
De novo hepatitis B
Development of malignancy (e.g., sarcoma, carcinoma, and lymphoma)
Persistent bile duct stricture not amenable to surgical or endoscopic treatment with progressive liver failure or recurrent cholangitis
Progressive chronic rejection

Grade 4: Complications that lead to retransplantation (Grade 4a) or death (Grade 4b)

Data from Clavien, P.-A., Camargo, C., Jr., Croxford, R., Langer, B., Levy, G., and Greig, P.: Definition and classification of negative outcomes in organ transplantation: Application in liver transplantation. Ann. Surg., 220:109, 1994.

tients. Well-being represents a composite of several different aspects, including mental, physical, and social criteria.

Due to the initial formidable technical issues of OLT, analyses of quality of life have been almost absent from the literature. With improved results these past few years, researchers in numerous centers are evaluating the effects of OLT on quality of life. Successful transplantation allows a return to an active lifestyle free from the metabolic and hematologic complications of hepatic failure or portal hypertension. Preliminary studies have already shown that self-image, functioning ability, and perception of health status are significantly improved after OLT.[32] Currently, about 60% of patients undergoing OLT return to work within the first year,[4] a figure that continues to increase long term.[32]

Payer's Perspective. Once therapy has been shown to be effective, it is necessary to determine whether the treatment is cost-effective in order to compare it with other competing technologies. Analysis of cost-effectiveness is difficult to apply to liver transplantation because there is no alternative therapy with which the results of the procedure can be compared. Thus, the cost issue becomes one of establishing a monetary value for one's life. There is no doubt that OLT is expensive. The total first-year expenses for a new liver average $200,000, with an additional $10,000 to $20,000 per year required thereafter. Cost for patients in the intensive care unit at the time of transplant are 3 to 5 times higher than those called in from home for the procedure. With current health care reform underway, these amounts are falling somewhat. In addition, consolidation of transplant centers in the United States is likely to improve efficiency and reduce costs. As new immunosuppressive agents are introduced, competition is also likely to drive the cost down. Nonetheless, the extent to which physicians should go to return patients to health and to work is a matter of great societal debate. As with all other aspects of liver transplantation, rational selection of patients is the most important factor affecting cost.

EMERGING TECHNIQUES

Split and Reduced-Size Transplantation. The remarkable ability of the liver to regenerate and support the metabolic needs of an individual despite major resection has allowed for correction of most conditions with partial hepatic transplantation.[10] This is useful for major size mismatches, especially in children, and can also help address the growing donor organ shortage.[41] Anatomic division of the lobes of the liver with preservation of hepatic venous and arterial, portal, and biliary branches has become increasingly successful but remains technically formidable. The anatomic boundaries are based on the segmental anatomic system of Couinaud and Bismuth.[17] Left lateral segments 2 and 3 or left lobe grafts (segments 2, 3, and 4) can be placed in recipients who are substantially smaller than the donor. Because of the anterior to posterior dimensions of the right lobe (segments 5 through 8), placement of this graft requires a recipient similar in size to the donor.

Several major centers have initiated protocols for split and reduced-size transplantation with excellent results. Predictably, biliary complications are increased in this procedure, but in children the problem of hepatic artery thrombosis is improved, owing to the comparatively large vasculature present in the graft when an adult liver is reduced for use in a child. Patient survival is as good as or better than full-size grafts in children. Use of reduced-size grafts has decreased the mortality of pediatric recipients on the waiting list to approximately 3%.

Living-Related Transplantation. Arising from the success of reduced-size grafting, living-related transplantation has been initiated at selected centers.[9, 57] This involves a reduced-size graft usually derived from a donor left lobe (segments 2 and 3 or 2, 3, and 4). Technically, this has been quite successful and has the benefits of reduced ischemic time, better HLA match, and better timing of transplantation, producing excellent graft survival. Because most of the transplants are performed for congenital anomalies, the negative aspects of HLA typing have not been problematic. The most pressing concern with this procedure is ethics. Although hepatic resection is generally safe, the mortality is not zero. One donor perioperative death has been reported, and many argue that with the success of reduced-size cadaveric allografts, a procedure that places a healthy parent at risk is not necessary. The concept of informed consent is difficult to establish because most parents disregard personal safety when the life of their child is at risk. One consensus hearing on the matter has approved this procedure, with the caveat that only centers with established success in reduced cadaveric grafts, pediatric transplantation, and adult hepatic surgery be involved.[10]

Heterotopic Liver Transplantation. Placement of an allograft in an anatomically altered site has the advantages of avoiding the recipient hepatectomy (often the most morbid portion of the procedure) and preserving the orthotopic position for future use in the event of graft failure.[51] Metabolic abnormalities are correctable by this approach. Obviously, however, disorders leading to portal hypertension are not amenable to this mode of therapy.

ALTERNATIVE THERAPIES

The development of artificial support devices has revolutionized perioperative management in all areas of transplantation except hepatic. Renal dialysis, ventricular assist and intra-aortic counterpulsation devices, total parenteral nutrition, and insulin have all helped optimize the condition of solid organ recipients to some degree, making emergent transplantation unusual for any organ other than the liver. The importance of preoperative condition is clear from the survival statistics presented in this chapter. Thus, great effort has been directed toward finding adequate hepatic replacement.

Xenogeneic Support. Xenotransplantation, the use of organs from other species, has many theoretical advantages. A renewable supply of organs subject to genetic manipulation available on an elective basis would greatly alter the course of patients with liver failure. In addition, the hepatotrophic viruses responsible for most hepatitis are generally specific for human hepatocytes, so the specter of reinfection would be abolished. Unfortunately, the immune barriers to transspecies transplantation remain formidable. Organs from discordant species, those phylogenetically distant animals to which preformed natural antibodies exist, are hyperacutely rejected. Organs from these animals also produce plasma proteins that are similar but not identical to their human homologues, thus raising the possibility of antigenic proteins subject to immune clearance. Concordant species, namely primates, are rejected in a more conventionally acute manner, but antibody-mediated rejection occurs. Although the immune barrier is less daunting, primates are slow-breeding animals that could quickly become extinct if widespread use were initiated. Of additional concern is the potential for introducing new viruses from primates to man.

Several efforts in xenogeneic organ use have been made in the past 5 years. Baboon livers were used to treat two patients with hepatitis B at the University of Pittsburgh.[46] Both livers functioned well enough to carry out the major physiologic functions of the liver. Interpretation of the immune implications of these procedures, however, is difficult because one patient was infected with the human immunodeficiency virus with an inverted T4:T8 ratio pretransplant and the other received a concurrent baboon bone marrow transplant. An orthotopic pig liver transplant performed at Cedars Sinai Hospital in Los Angeles was hyperacutely rejected (L. Makowka, personal communication, 1994).

Ex vivo perfusion with porcine livers has been successfully employed as a bridge to orthotopic allotransplantation by the authors' group.[13] Biochemical improvement in all measured parameters, including reversal of cerebral edema and reduction of coma, has been demonstrated by the authors' group and others.[3] This approach has the advantage of being reversible without requiring a surgical procedure. It is, however, logistically difficult and temporary.

Bioartificial Liver. The ability of porcine hepatocytes to perform many of the functions of human hepatocytes has been exploited by several investigators by development of an *ex vivo* apparatus for hepatic support consisting of porcine hepatocytes attached to a hollow-fiber dialysis cassette.[45] Early clinical trials have shown promise in reducing cerebral edema as well as mild improvement in biochemical parameters. Additional investigation in this field will determine whether the volume of the liver can be reproduced in cellular form and whether temporary support will allow recovery of hepatic function, thus avoiding transplantation for some patients with viral or toxin-induced acute liver failure.

SUMMARY

Liver transplantation has evolved in the past decade from an experimental procedure to an accepted, effective therapy for end-stage diseases of the liver. Extended survival of over 75% in appropriately selected patients is now commonplace with return to an excellent quality of life. Continued improvements in perioperative management and operative technique are being realized. The most important predictors of success are the state of the patient at the time of transplantation and the disease being transplanted. Early intervention once end-stage disease is diagnosed is preferable. A critical shortage of suitable donor organs remains the single most important barrier to transplantation

SELECTED REFERENCES

Advances in liver transplantation. Gastroenterol. Clin. North Am., 22:entire issue, 1993.
This is an excellent review written by experts in transplantation. Most clinical aspects of liver transplantation are critically discussed, including indications, immunosuppression, and management of short- and long-term complications.

Consensus conference on indications of liver transplantation. Hepatology, 2(Suppl.):entire issue, 1994.
Consensus conference held in Paris by a panel of medical and surgical experts thoroughly discussed indications for liver transplantation regarding both adult and pediatric diseases.

Neuberger, J., and Adams, D. (Eds.): Immunology of Liver Transplantation. London, Edward Arnold, 1993.
This excellent monograph covers most of the immunological aspects of liver transplantation, including mechanisms of rejection, immunosuppression, and viral prophylaxis. It is extremely well referenced.

REFERENCES

1. Annual Report of the U.S. Scientific Registry of Transplant Recipients and the Organ Procurement and Transplantation Network, 1994.
2. Consensus statement on indications for liver transplantation. Hepatology, 20:63, 1994.
3. Abouna, G., Fisher, L., Porter, K., and Andres, G.: Experience in the treatment of hepatic failure by intermittent liver hemoperfusion. Surg. Gynecol. Obstet., 137:141, 1963.
4. Adams, P., Ghent, C., Grant, D., and Wall, W.: Employment after liver transplantation. Hepatology, 21:140, 1995.
5. Ascher, N. L., Lake, J. R., Emond, J., and Roberts, J.: Liver transplantation for hepatitis C virus-related cirrhosis. Hepatology, 20:24, 1994.
6. Belle, S. H., Beringer, K. C., and Detre, K. M.: Trends in Liver Transplantation in the United States. *In* Terasaki, P. I., and Cecka, J. M. (Eds.): Clinical Transplants. Los Angeles, UCLA Tissue Typing Laboratory, 1993, p. 19.
7. Benhamou, J.-P.: Indications for liver transplantation in primary biliary cirrhosis. Hepatology, 20:11, 1994.
8. Bismuth, H., Castaing, D., Gugenheim, J., et al.: Roux-en-Y hepatojejunostomy: A safe procedure for biliary anastomosis in liver transplantation. Transplant. Proc., 19:2413, 1987.
9. Broelsch, C. E., Burdelski, M., and Rogiers, X.: Living donor for liver transplantation. Hepatology, 20:49, 1994.
10. Broelsch, C. E., Emond, J. C., Whitington, P. F., Thistlewaite, J. R., Baker, A. L., and Lichtor, J. L.: Reduced sized liver transplantation. Ann. Surg., 212:368, 1990.
11. Busuttil, R. W., Shaked, A., and Mills, J. M.: One thousand liver transplants: The lessons learned. Ann. Surg., 219:490, 1994.
12. Calne, R. Y.: Contraindications to liver transplantation. Hepatology, 20:3, 1994.
13. Chari, R., Collins, B. H., and Magee, J. C.: Treatment of hepatic failure with *ex-vivo* pig liver perfusion followed by liver transplantation. N. Engl. J. Med., 331:234, 1994.
14. Clavien, P.-A., Camargo, C., Jr., Croxford, R., Langer, B., Levy, G., and Greig, P.: Definition and classification of negative outcomes in organ transplantation: Application in liver transplantation. Ann. Surg., 220:109, 1994.
15. Clavien, P.-A., Harvey, P. R. C., and Strasberg, S. M.: Preservation and reperfusion injuries in liver allografts: Overview and synthesis of current studies. Transplantation, 53:957, 1992.
16. Clavien, P.-A., Sanabria, J. R., and Strasberg, S. M.: Proposed classification of complications of surgery with examples of utility in cholecystectomy. Surgery, 111:518, 1992.
17. Couinaud, C.: Le Foie: Études Anatomiques et Chirurgicales. Paris, Masson et Cie, 1957.
18. D'Alessandro, A. M., Kalayoglu, M., and Solinger, H. W.: The predictive value of donor liver biopsies on the development of primary nonfunction after orthotopic liver transplantation. Transplant Proc., 23:1536, 1991.
19. Dousset, B., Houssin, D., Soubrane, O., Boillot, O., Baudin, F., and Chapuis, Y.: Metastatic endocrine tumors: Is there a place for liver transplantation? Liver Transpl. Surg., 1:111, 1995.
20. European FK506 Multicentre Liver Study Group: Randomized trial comparing tacrolimus (FK506) and cyclosporin in prevention of allograft rejection. Lancet, 344:423, 1994.
21. Farges, O., Malassagne, B., Sebagh, M., and Bismuth, H.: Primary sclerosing cholangitis: Liver transplantation or biliary surgery. Surgery, 117:146, 1995.
22. Gordon, R. D., Iwatsuki, S., Esquivel, C. O., Tsakis, A., Todo, S., and Starzl, T. E.: Liver transplantation across ABO blood groups. Surgery, 100:342, 1986.
23. Griffith, B. P., Shaw, B. W., Hardesty, R. L., Iwatsuki, S., and Bahnson, H. T.: Venovenous bypass without systemic anticoagulation for transplantation of the human liver. Surg. Gynecol. Obstet., 160:271, 1985.
24. Gugenheim, J., Samuel, D., Reynes, M., and Bismuth, H.: Liver transplantation across ABO blood group barriers. Lancet, 336:519, 1990.
25. Harrison, J., and McMaster, P.: The role of orthotopic liver transplantation in the management of sclerosing cholangitis. Hepatology, 20:14, 1994.
26. Kalayoglu, M., Sollinger, W. H., and Stratta, R. J.: Extended preservation of the liver for clinical transplantation. Lancet, 1:617, 1988.
27. Klion, F., Fabry, T., Palmer, M., and Schaffner, F.: Prediction of survival in patients with primary biliary cirrhosis: Examination of the Mayo Clinic model on a group of patients with known endpoint. Gastroenterology, 102:310, 1992.
28. Knechtle, S. J., Kolbeck, P. S., Tsuchemntos A., et al.: Hepatic transplantation into sensitized recipients: Demonstration of hyperacute rejection. Transplantation, 43:8, 1987.
29. Krom, R. A. F.: Liver transplantation and alcohol: Who should get transplants? Hepatology, 20:28, 1994.
30. Lee, J., Schutz, S., England, R., Leung, J., and Cotton, P.: Endoscopic therapy of sclerosing cholangitis. Hepatology, 21:661, 1995.
31. Lerut, J., Gordon, R. D., Iwatsuki, S., et al.: Biliary tract complication in human orthotopic liver transplantation. Transplantation, 43:47, 1987.
32. Levy, M., Jennings, L., and Abouldoud, M.: Quality of life improvements at one, two, and five years after liver transplantation. Transplantation, 59:515, 1995.
33. Markus, B. H., Duquesnoy, R. J., Gordon, R. D., et al.: Histocompatibility and liver transplantation: Does HLA exert a dualistic effect? Transplantation, 46:372, 1988.
34. National Institutes of Health Consensus Development Conference Statement. Liver transplantation. Hepatology, 4(Suppl. 1):107, 1983.
35. Neuberger, J., and Adams, D. (Eds.): Immunology of Liver Transplantation. London, Edward Arnold, 1993.
36. Neuhaus, P., Blumhardt, G., Bechstein, W. O., Steffen, R., Platz, K.-P., and Keck, H.: Technique and results of biliary reconstruction using side-to-side choledochocholedochostomy in 300 orthotopic liver transplants. Ann. Surg., 219:426, 1994.
37. O'Grady, J. G., Schalm, S., and Williams, R.: Acute liver failure: Redefining the syndromes. Lancet, 342:273, 1993.
38. Otte, J.-B., Goyet, J. D. V. D., and Reding, R.: Sequential treatment of biliary atresia with Kasai portoenterostomy and liver transplantation: A review. Hepatology, 20:41, 1994.
39. Perrillo, R., and Mason, A.: Hepatitis B and liver transplantation: Problems and premises. N. Engl. J. Med., 329:1885, 1993.
40. Pichlmayr, R., Weimann, A., and Ringe, B.: Indications for liver transplantation in hepatobiliary malignancy. Hepatology, 20:33, 1994.
41. Piper, J. B., Whitington, P. F., and Woodle, E. S.: Pediatric liver transplantation at the University of Chicago Hospitals. *In* Terasaki, P. I., and Cecka, J. M. (Eds.): Clinical Transplants. Los Angeles, UCLA Tissue Typing Laboratory, 1992, p. 179.
42. Pitt, H., Thompson, H., Tompkins, R., and Longmire, W.: Primary sclerosing cholangitis: Results of an aggressive surgical approach. Ann. Surg., 196:259, 1982.
43. Post, S., Palma, P., Gonzalez, A., Rentsch, M., and Menger, M.: Timing of arterialization in liver transplantation. Ann. Surg., 220:691, 1994.
44. Clavien, P. A., Camargo, C. A., Cameron, R., Washington, M. K., Phillips, M. J., Greig, P. D., and Levy, G. A.: Kupffer cell erythrophagocytosis and graft-versus-host hemolysis in ABO-unmatched liver transplantation. Gastroenterology, 110:1891, 1996.
45. Rozga, J., Podesta, L., and LaPage, E.: A bioartificial liver to treat severe acute liver failure. Ann. Surg., 219:538, 1994.
46. Starzl, T., Fung, J., and Tzakis, A.: Baboon-to-human liver transplantation. Lancet, 341:65, 1993.
47. Starzl, T. E., Marchiaro, T. L., Von Kaulla, K., et al.: Homotransplantation of the liver in humans. Surg. Gynecol. Obstet., 117:659, 1963
48. Starzl, T. E., Todo, S., Fung, J., Demetris, A. J., Venkataramanan, R., and Jain, A.: FK 506 for human liver, kidney and pancreas transplantation. Lancet, 2:1000, 1989.
49. Steinhoff, G.: HLA/ABO matching. *In* Neuberger, J., and Adams, D. (Eds.): Immunology of Liver Transplantation. London, Edward Arnold, 1993, p 261.
50. Strasberg, S., Howard, T., Molmenti, P., and Hertl, M.: Donor evaluation of liver allograft. Hepatology, 20:829, 1995.
51. Terpstra, O., Schalm, S., Weimar, W., et al.: Auxiliary partial liver transplantation for end-stage chronic liver disease. N. Engl. J. Med., 319:1507, 1988.
52. The US Multicenter FK506 Liver Study Group: A comparison of tacrolimus (FK506) and cyclosporine for immunosuppression in liver transplantation. N. Engl. J. Med., 331:1110, 1994.
53. Todo, S., Demetris, A., VanThiel, D., Teperman, L., Fung, J., and Starzl, T. E.: Orthotopic liver transplantation for patients with hepatitis B virus–related liver disease. Hepatology, 13:619, 1991.
54. Vallera, R. A., Cotton, P. B., and Clavien, P.-A.: Biliary reconstruction for

liver transplantation and management of biliary complications: Overview and survey of current practices in the United States. Liver Transpl. Surg., 1:143, 1995.
55. van Thiel, D. H., Wright, H. I., and Fagiuoli, S.: Liver transplantation for hepatitis B virus–associated cirrhosis: A progress report. Hepatology, 20:20, 1994.

56. Williams, R., and Wendon, J.: Indictations for orthotopic liver transplantation in fulminant liver failure. Hepatology, 20:5, 1994.
57. Yamaoka, Y., Tanaka, K., and Ozawa, K.: Liver transplantation from living-related donors. In Terasaki, P. I., and Cecka, J. M. (Eds.): Clinical Transplants. Los Angeles, UCLA Tissue Typing Laboratory, 1993, p. 179.

IX

PANCREAS TRANSPLANTATION

Hans W. Sollinger, M.D., Ph.D., and Stuart J. Knechtle, M.D.

HISTORICAL ASPECTS

According to Erich Lexer, the first surgical step toward treating Type I diabetes mellitus by transplantation of the pancreas took place in 1891, 30 years before the discovery of insulin. An English surgeon, Williams, transplanted extracts of sheep pancreas into the abdominal wall of a comatose diabetic patient, and his early trial demonstrates that the concept of replacing nonfunctioning islets by transplanting vital endocrine tissue is a very old one. The first clinical pancreas transplant was performed by Kelly and Lillehei on December 17, 1966.[9] It was a segmental graft transplanted to the iliac fossa, with the pancreatic duct ligated. In 1973, Gliedman and associates[7] first suggested the use of the urinary tract for exocrine pancreatic drainage. Merkel and colleagues[10] reported end-to-side anastomosis of the pancreatic duct to the ureter, believing that this would obviate the need for native nephrectomy when transplantation is performed in a nonuremic patient. In the mid-1970s, the Stockholm group, headed by Groth, embarked on a larger series of enterically drained grafts.[8] A new method of handling exocrine secretions was suggested by Dubernard and associates,[6] who thought that exocrine secretions could be obliterated by injecting the pancreatic duct with a polymer. In 1982, Cook and Sollinger, from the University of Wisconsin, suggested channeling the exocrine secretions to the urinary bladder. In their initial clinical experience, the pancreatic duct of a segmental graft was sutured to the bladder mucosa. They then turned to whole pancreatic grafts, using the duodenal button technique and, later, to the duodenal segment method as described by Nghiem and associates.[12] Other techniques of managing exocrine pancreatic secretions are enterically drained pancreaticoduodenal grafts, paratopic grafting with exocrine drainage into the stomach,[4] and a variety of modifications of the bladder technique, such as skeletonizing the pancreatic duct before implantation into the bladder[15] or implanting the entire cut edge of the pancreas end-to-side into the bladder.

INDICATIONS

The indications for transplanting the pancreas remain controversial. It can be performed in three settings: alone in a preuremic patient, after successful kidney grafting, and simultaneously with a kidney transplant. Clearly, pancreas transplantation should be performed before the patient develops end-stage secondary complications, such as advanced retinopathy leading to blindness, disabling neuropathy, end-stage nephropathy, or extensive macrovascular and microvascular disease. In the authors' view, pancreatic transplantation in a preuremic patient is justified only in a setting where careful long-term monitoring of its potential effect on second-ary complications can be performed. The advantage of transplanting the pancreas after successful transplantation of the kidney is that the patient is already on immunosuppressive therapy. Unfortunately, the results of sequential grafting are worse than the results of combined transplantation of kidney and pancreas. For this reason, most pancreas transplants have been combined transplants. In this setting, only one surgical procedure is required, and the patient receives an immunosuppressive regimen similar to that of a patient undergoing a kidney transplant alone. Absolute contraindications for pancreas transplantation are similar to those for kidney transplantation and include the presence of malignancy and active infection. Patients with advanced cardiovascular disease, major amputation, and inability to understand the nature of the procedure are excluded in the authors' program. Of major importance is evaluation of the patient's cardiac status, because many diabetic patients, as a result of neuropathy, do not present with the classic symptoms of angina, even in the presence of advanced coronary artery disease. Therefore, preoperative evaluation requires thallium stress testing in all patients over age 30. If the thallium stress test suggests coronary artery disease, patients must undergo coronary angiography. Liberal use of coronary angiography is indicated.

DONOR SELECTION, ORGAN PROCUREMENT, AND PANCREAS PRESERVATION

Donor selection and organ procurement are of paramount importance to the success of pancreas transplantation. Age limits for donors range from 3 to 55 years. In older donors, the presence of significant atherosclerosis involving the celiac axis must be excluded. Absolute contraindications to pancreas donation include intra-abdominal contamination, acute pancreatitis, injury to the pancreas, and a history of diabetes in the donor. Donor blood glucose values and serum amylase levels do not reflect the quality of the graft. The pancreas can be procured either with the liver or alone. Many teams in the United States now routinely procure combined liver and pancreas, thus eliminating the controversy and competition between liver and pancreas transplant teams.[14] During the combined procurement of liver and pancreas, it is important that the portal flush is vented during the *in situ* flush, so that the pressure of the splenic vein does not become elevated, which could lead to significant pancreatic edema (Fig. 20–47). After both organs are removed, the pancreas and liver are separated and prepared for transplantation. In most instances, pancreatic arterial blood supply must be restored with an iliac artery Y-graft (Fig. 20–48). Safe preservation time for the pancreas in either University of Wisconsin (UW) solution (Viaspan, DuPont Pharmaceuticals) or Minnesota SGF solution is between 20 and 30 hours. The average preser-

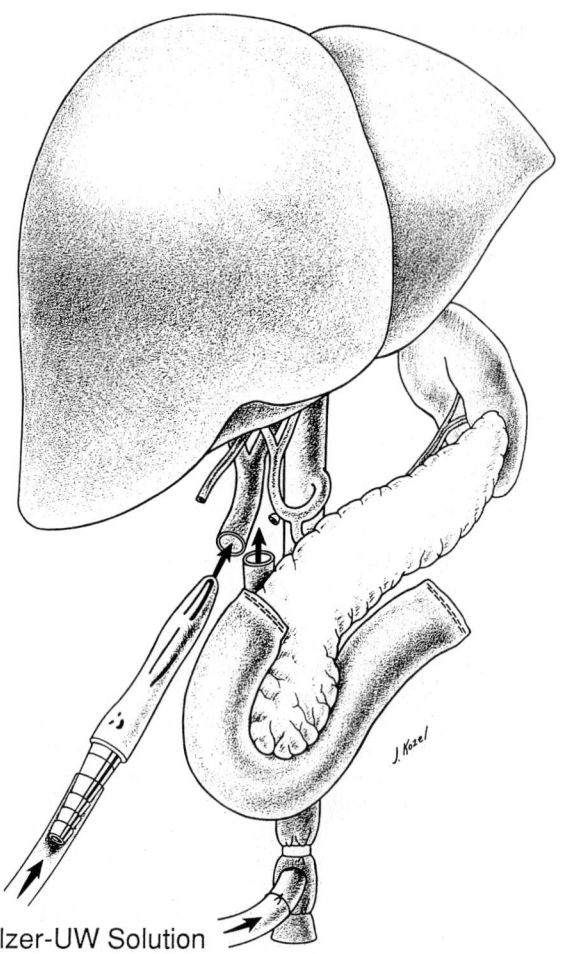

Belzer-UW Solution

Figure 20–47. Technique of combined liver-pancreas procurement. The portal vein is divided before the *in situ* flush is started. This maneuver prevents pancreatic edema.

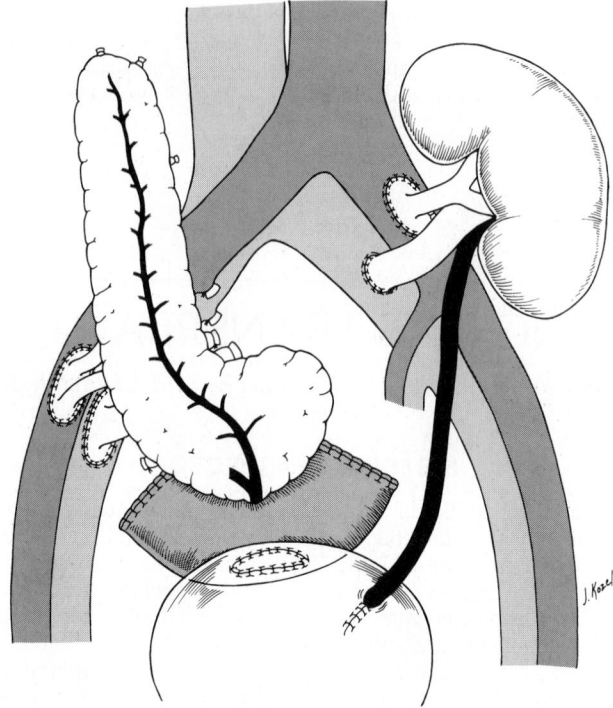

Figure 20–49. Pancreas transplantation with the duodenal segment technique.

vation time for pancreatic grafts at the authors' center is 16 to 18 hours. Recently, D'Alessandro and colleagues[5] demonstrated that pancreatic grafts can be procured successfully from non-heart-beating donors.

SURGICAL ASPECTS

Since transplantation of the pancreas was first performed in December 1966, a number of technical procedures have been used. Only in recent years have significant data been gathered on a national and international level so that the merits and disadvantages of these techniques can be evaluated. The pancreas can be transplanted as a whole graft, or a segment of the pancreas consisting of the tail and body can be transplanted as segmental grafts. Major controversy has surrounded the optimal management of exocrine pancreatic secretions. Possible approaches for managing the pancreatic duct include ligation of the pancreatic duct; leaving the pancreatic duct open, with drainage of exocrine pancreatic secretions into the peritoneal cavity; duct injection with polymer; enteric drainage into a Roux-en-Y loop; and anastomosis of the pancreatic duct to the bladder. When whole pancreas transplants are used, the duodenal segment can be sutured side-to-side to the bladder (Fig. 20–49), or side-to-side anastomosis to the small bowel can be performed.

Duct injection with neoprene or prolamine has been cham-

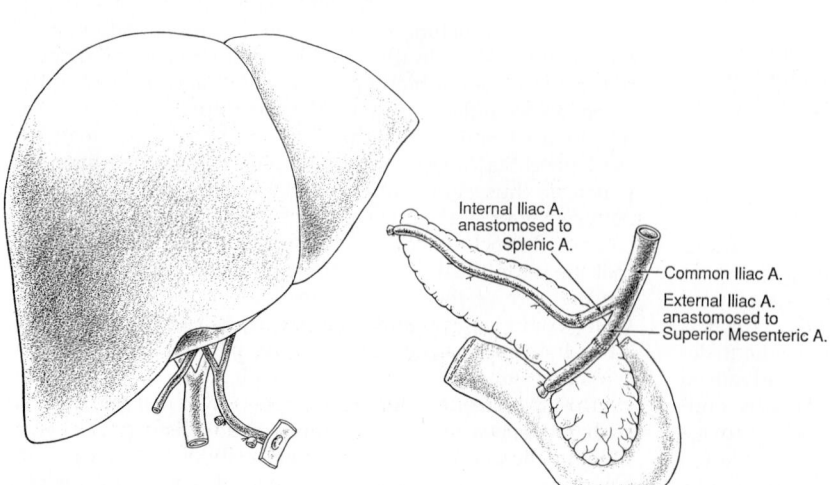

Internal Iliac A. anastomosed to Splenic A.

Common Iliac A.

External Iliac A. anastomosed to Superior Mesenteric A.

Figure 20–48. Reconstruction of the arterial blood supply of the pancreas after combined liver-pancreas procurement.

pioned by several European groups. In all cases, a segmental pancreatic graft was used. Although the surgical procedure is rather simple, because no anastomosis to the draining organ is required, the results of duct injection in the leading centers have remained inferior to the best results reported for enteric drainage and bladder drainage. A leading cause of graft loss with segmental grafts using duct injection is venous thrombosis, which occurs in 15 to 20% of all transplants (Table 20–19). In addition, fistula formation leading to peripancreatic infection is more common in grafts with duct injection than in other drainage procedures. Segmental pancreas transplantation with drainage of the pancreas into a Roux-en-Y loop was used extensively by the Stockholm group. Most recently, instead of a segmental graft, a whole pancreatic graft with the duodenal segment anastomosed side-to-side to the small bowel has been used for enteric drainage. Preliminary reports by the Stockholm group and the authors' experience demonstrate that this method is far safer than drainage of a segmental graft into a Roux-en-Y loop. The complication rate with the use of the whole pancreas and duodenal segment has been significantly reduced. Bladder drainage, at present the most popular technique, has the advantage of being technically simple and associated with a low infection rate. Because exocrine pancreatic secretions can be determined by measuring urinary amylase, this technique has the advantage of facilitating the diagnosis of rejection, which is particularly important in sequential or isolated pancreatic grafting. The disadvantages of the bladder technique include metabolic acidosis caused by bicarbonate loss into the urine; urinary problems such as hematuria, urethral stricture, or frequent urinary tract infections; and reflux pancreatitis. Surgical and urologic complications after simultaneous pancreas-kidney transplantation are listed in Table 20–20. Nevertheless, graft loss from technical complications with the use of the bladder technique has become a rare exception at the authors' center.

DIAGNOSIS OF PANCREATIC ALLOGRAFT REJECTION

Because rejection is the major cause of graft loss, the timely diagnosis and treatment of rejection are major obstacles to successful pancreas transplantation. These difficulties stem from the histologic sequence in which the rejection process occurs. Extensive studies by the Minnesota group have demonstrated that in the initial phase of rejection, mononuclear cell infiltration involves predominantly the acinar tissues, and vasculitis may occur before any islet cell changes. Only in the later stages of advanced rejection have infiltration of islets and islet damage been observed. Therefore, serum glucose may become elevated at an already irreversible stage of rejection. Fortunately, in combined kidney-pancreas transplantation, renal allograft rejection and a rise in serum creatinine precede pancreatic rejection in almost all instances. This

TABLE 20–19. Duct Injection with Prolamine: Reasons for Graft Loss—University of Munich

Reason	Number	Percentage
Venous thrombosis	8	15
Infected fistula	6	12
Bleeding	1	2
Rejection	8	16
Death	1	2

From Illner, W. D., Abendroth, D., Landgraf, R., and Land, W.: Pancreatic transplantation using the duct occlusion technique. In Terasaki, P. I. (Ed.): Clinical Transplants. Los Angeles, UCLA Tissue Typing Laboratory, 1988, p. 65.

TABLE 20–20. Complications After Simultaneous Pancreas-Kidney Transplantation

Complication	All SPK* (n = 237)
Surgical/Nontransplant Related	
Small bowel obstruction	11 (4.6%)
Reoperation for intra-abdominal bleeding	11 (4.6%)
Wound infection	11 (4.6%)
Wound dehiscence	10 (4.2%)
Incisional hernia	5 (2.1%)
Negative laparotomy	4 (1.7%)
Intra-abdominal abscess drainage	
Operative	5 (2.1%)
Percutaneous	3 (1.3%)
Enterocutaneous fistula repair	1 (0.4%)
Fasciitis	1 (0.4%)
Surgical/Transplant Related	
Lymphocele drainage	3 (1.5%)
Graft thrombosis	
Pancreas only	3 (1.3%)
Pancreas-kidney	4 (1.7%)
Renal artery stenosis	1 (0.4%)
Iliac artery stenosis	1 (0.4%)
Urologic/Related to Pancreas Transplant	
Hematuria	35 (14.8%)
Bladder/duodenal segment leak	35 (14.8%)
Reflux pancreatitis	24 (10.1%)
Recurrent urinary tract infection	24 (10.1%)
Urethritis	7 (2.9%)
Urethral stricture/disruption	7 (2.9%)

*Simultaneous kidney-pancreas transplant.

may be the most sensitive marker for pancreatic allograft rejection. Isolated rejection of a pancreas transplant without kidney rejection is a rare event.

In isolated or sequential pancreatic grafting, when the kidney cannot serve as a monitor, the early diagnosis of pancreatic allograft rejection remains difficult. Urinary amylase monitoring has been demonstrated to be the most useful clinical test. This explains the superiority of urinary-drained grafts over duct-injected and enteric grafts for nonsimultaneous transplants. Other clinically useful methods include technetium-DTPA perfusion scanning.

Characteristics of rejection include graft swelling, haziness of the pancreatic borders, and diminished visualization, especially in the tail of the pancreas. Ultrasonography and magnetic resonance imaging have not been uniformly accepted as reliable techniques for detecting pancreatic allograft rejection. In bladder-drained grafts, the pancreas and duodenum can be biopsied using cystoscopy; however, this requires general anesthesia and cannot be performed frequently. Percutaneous needle biopsy of the pancreas has recently been reported by Allen and associates[2] and, surprisingly, was associated with only minimal morbidity. If this experience can be confirmed by other centers in a larger series of patients, percutaneous needle biopsy might indeed become the standard for diagnosing pancreatic allograft rejection, and the value of all other methods can be correlated with the biopsy result.

IMMUNOSUPPRESSION AND POSTOPERATIVE MANAGEMENT

Current immunosuppressive strategies have evolved with an extrapolation of the experience gained with standard regimens in clinical renal transplantation (Table 20–21). Conventional immunosuppression (prednisone and azathioprine) has met with limited success in pancreas transplantation and

TABLE 20–21. Immunosuppressive Protocol in Pancreas Transplantation

Days 1–14:	ALG* 20 mg./kg. IV/day
	Prednisone 30 mg./day
	Cyclosporine 6–12 mg./kg./day
	Azathioprine 1–2 mg./kg./day
Days 15–60:	Prednisone 20–30 mg./day
	Cyclosporine 4–10 mg./kg./day
	Azathioprine 1–2 mg./kg./day

*OKT3 may be used instead of ALG for induction therapy. Rejection episodes are treated with a steroid bolus or OKT3.

has led to early trials of cyclosporine. Cyclosporine has had modest immunosuppressive effects in an allogeneic pancreas transplant system in a number of species; however, cyclosporine is not nearly as successful in preventing rejection of pancreatic allografts as it is with other organs. Most North American transplant centers have adopted the use of quadruple immunosuppressive therapy. This includes the use of OKT3 for 7 to 14 days after transplantation and maintenance therapy with cyclosporine, prednisone, and azathioprine. More than 95% of all rejection episodes can be successfully reversed with high-dose steroids, ALG, OKT3, or tacrolimus (FK 506) retreatment. More recently, several centers have used FK 506 for maintenance and rescue therapy.

The general guidelines for the postoperative management of recipients of pancreas or combined pancreas-kidney transplants follow those established in kidney transplantation; however, there are two specific considerations for pancreas transplant recipients. Because pancreas transplant recipients have a high thrombosis rate, many centers prefer to use anticoagulation with either heparin or a combination of heparin and dextran. In the authors' experience, this regimen has not helped prevent pancreatic allograft thrombosis and has led to a significantly higher incidence of postoperative bleeding episodes. Antibiotic coverage after pancreas transplantation must be broad spectrum to treat aerobic, anaerobic, and fungal organisms. In whole pancreas transplantation with the duodenal segment, the content of the duodenal segment is cultured at the time of transplantation, and antibiotics are adjusted on the basis of the culture result.

An infrequent but potentially fatal complication is the rapid development of adult respiratory distress syndrome after pancreas transplantation. This might be the result of preservation-induced pancreatitis, and patients experiencing this syndrome usually require intubation and maintenance on mechanical ventilation. Unfortunately, pulmonary damage is frequently extensive, and superimposed infections contribute greatly to long-term morbidity or death. If this syndrome occurs, immediate removal of the pancreas transplant should be considered.

Peripancreatic fluid collections as visualized by ultrasonography and computed tomography are frequent and need be addressed only if infection is suspected. Fine-needle aspiration of the fluid collections and culture of the fluid aid the diagnosis. If a peripancreatic abscess is diagnosed, catheter drainage or open drainage should be performed. Constant awareness of the possibility that the vascular anastomosis may be eroded by the infection is of paramount importance. If there is any suspicion that this is the case, such as an unexpected drop in hematocrit or blood from the fistula, immediate removal of the pancreas is mandatory.

EFFECT ON SECONDARY DIABETIC COMPLICATIONS

Following successful pancreas transplantation, normalization of carbohydrate metabolism occurs. Although freedom from insulin injections undoubtedly improves the patient's quality of life, it is not in itself the purpose of the procedure, since the patient is exposed to prolonged immunosuppressive therapy instead of insulin. The purpose of pancreas transplantation is to reverse or arrest secondary diabetic complications. The first evidence of the potential beneficial influence of pancreas transplantation on diabetic nephropathy was the observation that patients who receive a combined pancreas-kidney transplant do not develop diabetic nephropathy in the transplanted kidney.[3] These initial findings have recently been confirmed by the Minnesota group, which demonstrated a significant difference between mesangial volume of the transplanted kidney in patients who receive a kidney transplant alone and that in patients who receive a combined pancreas-kidney transplant. Many patients undergoing pancreas transplantation subjectively indicate improvement in neuropathy. Preliminary data from various centers indicate improvement in motor nerve conduction velocity in the upper and lower extremities and, in some patients, sensory conduction velocity.[16] Thermography, muscle oxygen tension measurements, and laser Doppler determination demonstrate a beneficial effect of pancreas transplantation on microcirculation.[1]

The influence of pancreatic transplantation on diabetic retinopathy remains controversial. In an initial report, the Minnesota group did not find any improvement in diabetic retinopathy within the first 2 years after pancreas transplantation in preuremic patients.[13] More recently, however, the same group reported that during a longer follow-up of between 3 and 4 years, a trend in favor of pancreas transplantation is now being observed. When diabetic retinopathy is advanced and patients have laser treatments or a vitrectomy, little improvement can be expected.

Quality of life after combined pancreas-kidney transplantation has been assessed by several centers in Europe.[11] Patients receiving combined pancreas-kidney transplants require less sickness pension than patients with kidney transplants alone, more patients have full-time employment, and lost workdays are reduced by 44%.

TRANSPLANTATION OF PANCREATIC ISLETS AND FETAL PANCREAS

Transplantation of isolated pancreatic islets and fetal pancreas offers the possibility of restoring normoglycemia without the patient's undergoing a surgical procedure. In addition, in animal experiments, the immunogenicity of islets has been reduced. Thus, it would be theoretically possible to transplant islets or fetal pancreatic tissue without the need for immunosuppressive therapy. Unfortunately, clinical transplantation of fetal pancreas and islets of Langerhans has met with very limited success. The problems associated with the transplantation of islets of Langerhans involve the difficulty in isolating a sufficient number of islets from one single adult pancreas to restore normoglycemia in the recipient. Numerous investigators since the 1970s have suggested a number of digestion and isolation procedures, and only recently have selected groups been successful in isolating a sufficient number of islets (300,000 to 500,000). The standard islet isolation techniques generally include mechanical separation of the gland combined with partial digestion, using collagenase to dissociate the islets from the endocrine tissue. The islets are then separated from the exocrine tissue by density-gradient centrifugation. Islets can be implanted beneath the renal subcapsular space, into the splenic parenchyma, or they can be injected into the portal vein for engraftment in the liver. Some studies have demonstrated significant levels of C peptides in patients undergoing injection of pancreatic islets into the portal vein. These patients also received a kidney allograft from the same donor and underwent conventional immunosuppression. Only a few patients became insulin independent for more than 1 year. Therefore, it is necessary to develop a better immunosuppressive strategy to ensure long-term graft survival of pancreatic islets. In addition, with the increasing number of pancreas transplants performed in the United States, pancreatic grafts suitable for islet isolation will be more difficult to obtain. Moreover, because only a few thousand pancreata are available in the United States each year for islet isolation, and since at least one pancreas is necessary to obtain a significant number of islets, this approach, even if successful is available for only a very small number of diabetic patients. Therefore, at least theoretically, the use of human fetal pancreas offers much more promise for the future.

The typical fetal pancreas used for transplantation is from a 16- to 20-week-old human fetus, is approximately 0.5 cm. long, and weighs 10 to 20 mg. A pancreas this size contains more than 50% endocrine tissue in isolated, immature beta cells and very little exocrine tissue. The immature beta cells release insulin in response to glucagon and theophylline, but not to increased glucose concentration. Nevertheless, human fetal pancreata grow and mature after transplantation and release a sufficient amount of insulin within 10 to 15 weeks after transplantation to cure a diabetic animal. Over 200 fetal pancreatic allografts have been performed worldwide, but success has been limited. Very few grafts ever demonstrated any evidence of function, either by increasing the C-peptide levels or by reducing or abolishing exogenous insulin requirements. Clinical trials using multiple donors and cultured fetal pancreata may provide more information about the effectiveness of this form of islet transplantation. However, ethical questions surrounding the use of fetal pancreatic tissue for transplantation remain.

SELECTED REFERENCES

Groth, C. G. (Ed.): Pancreatic Transplantation. Philadelphia, W. B. Saunders, 1988.
This is the first book entirely dedicated to the topic, and it covers a wide range of all aspects. More than 30 nationally and internationally renowned authorities in the field discuss technical aspects, indications, patient selection, and pathologic aspects of pancreatic graft rejection. Several chapters are dedicated to metabolic control after pancreas transplantation as well as its effect on the secondary complications of diabetes.

Stratta, R. J., Perlman, S. B., Kalayoglu, M., Belzer, F. O., and Sollinger, H. W.: The diagnosis of rejection and immunosuppressive strategies in vascularized pancreas transplantation. *In* van Schilfgaarde, R., and Hardy, M. (Eds.): Transplantation of the Endocrine Pancreas in Diabetes Mellitus. New York, Elsevier Science Publishers, 1988, p. 251.
This chapter describes in a comprehensive manner experimental and clinical studies directed at the diagnosis of pancreatic allograft rejection, providing a complete overview of the current status.

Sutherland, D. E. R., Dunn, D. L., Goetz, F. C., et al.: A 10-year experience with 290 pancreas transplants at a single institution. Ann. Surg., *210*:274, 1989.
The Minneapolis group not only performed the first pancreas transplant but also has the largest experience in pancreas transplantation worldwide. This group has applied every technique of transplantation of the pancreas in its own institution and is eminently qualified to compare these techniques. In addition, the Minneapolis group has championed the long-term follow-up of patients receiving transplants and has reported extensively on the effect of pancreas transplantation on diabetic retinopathy and neuropathy and the influence of pancreatic graft on diabetic nephropathy.

Sutherland, D. E. R., and Moudry-Munns, K.: Report of the International Pancreas and Islet Transplant Registry.
Sutherland has been responsible for collecting and analyzing the results of all pancreas transplants performed worldwide since 1966. This is the most comprehensive organ transplant registry in existence today. Reports of the International Pancreas Transplant Registry are published at regular intervals and are presented at major national and international meetings.

van Schilfgaarde, R., and Hardy, M. (Eds.): Transplantation of the Endocrine Pancreas in Diabetes Mellitus. New York, Elsevier Science Publishers, 1988.
This book is dedicated to the field of pancreas and islet transplantation. Surgical and other aspects are covered in detail by the foremost authorities in the field, such as the isolation of pancreatic islets, immunomodulation, and the autoimmune etiology of diabetes mellitus.

REFERENCES

1. Abendroth, D., Illhmer, V. D., Landgraf, R., et al.: Are late diabetic complications reversible after pancreas transplantation? A new method of follow-up of microcirculatory changes. Transplant. Proc., *19*:23, 1987.
2. Allen, R. D. M., Chapman, J. R., Deane, S. A., et al.: Combined pancreas and kidney transplantation: A pilot study. Transplant. Proc., *21*:3784, 1989.
3. Bohman, S. O., Wildzek, H., Tyden, G., et al.: Recurrent diabetic nephropathy in renal allografts placed in diabetic patients and protective effect of simultaneous pancreatic transplantation. Transplant. Proc. *19*:2290, 1987.
4. Calne, R. Y., McMaster, P., Rolles, K., et al.: Technical observations in segmental pancreas allografting: Observations on pancreatic blood flow. Transplant. Proc., *12*:51, 1980.
5. D'Alessandro, A. M., Hoffmann, R. M., Knechtle, S. J., et al.: Successful extrarenal transplantation from non-heart-beating donors. Transplantation, *59*:977, 1995.
6. Dubernard, J. M., Traeger, J., Neyra, P., et al.: New method of preparation of a segmental pancreatic graft for transplantation: Trials in dogs and in man. Surgery, *84*:634, 1978.
7. Gliedman, M. L., Gold, M., Whittaker, J., et al.: Pancreatic duct to ureter anastomosis for exocrine drainage in pancreatic transplantation. Am. J. Surg., *125*:245, 1973.
8. Groth, C. G., Collste, H., Lundgren, G., et al.: Successful outcome of segmental human pancreatic transplantation with enteric exocrine diversion after modifications in technique. Lancet, *2*:522, 1982.
9. Kelly, W. D., Lillehei, R. C., Merkel, F. K., et al.: Allotransplantation of the pancreas and duodenum along with the kidney in diabetic nephropathy. Surgery, *61*:827, 1967.
10. Merkel, F. K., Ryan, W. G., Armbruster, K., et al.: Pancreatic transplantation for diabetes mellitus. Ill. Med., *144*:477, 1973.
11. Nakache, R., Tyden, G., and Groth, C. G.: Quality of life in diabetic patients after combined pancreas-kidney or kidney transplantation. Diabetes, *38* (suppl. 1):40, 1989.
12. Nghiem, D. D., and Bentel, W. D.: Duodenocystostomy for exocrine drainage in total pancreatic transplantation. Transplant. Proc., *18*:1753, 1986.
13. Ramsay, R. C., Goetz, F. C., Sutherland, D. E. R., et al.: Progression of diabetic retinopathy after pancreas transplantation for insulin-dependent diabetes mellitus. N. Engl. J. Med., *318*:208, 1988.
14. Sollinger, H. W., Vernon, W. B., D'Alessandro, A. M., et al.: Combined liver and pancreas procurement with Belzer-UW solution. Surgery, *106*:685, 1989.
15. Tao, L., Sutherland, D. E. R., Cavallini, M., et al.: Duct drainage in the bladder for management of exocrine secretions of segmental pancreas grafts in dogs. Surg. Forum, *24*:376, 1983.
16. Van der Vliet, J. A., Navarro, X., Kennedy, W. R., et al.: The effect of pancreas transplantation on diabetic polyneuropathy. Transplantation, *45*:368, 1988.

X

CARDIAC AND CARDIOPULMONARY HOMOTRANSPLANTS

R. Morton Bolman III, M.D.

CLINICAL CARDIAC TRANSPLANTATION

Recipient Selection

Criteria for candidate selection for cardiac transplantation have evolved with improvements in techniques and outcomes. The acceptable age for transplant candidacy has expanded and now includes individuals from newborn age up to age 60 years routinely and age 65 years in unusual circumstances. Patients selected must experience symptoms that place them in Class IV of the New York Heart Association classification or must have angina pectoris that is severely limiting their lifestyle in a setting where revascularization is not an option. Certain individuals can be considered for transplantation before experiencing Class IV symptoms if they have life-threatening cardiac arrhythmias refractory to medical and surgical therapies. Patients undergo a careful screening process to ensure suitable extracardiac and psychosocial health status. Fixed, irreversible deficits in extracardiac organ function contraindicate transplantation, because they would not be expected to be corrected by improved cardiac function. Psychosocial screening is important to ensure a proper support structure for the patient and strict compliance with prescribed medical regimens both before and after transplantation.

Patients must have end-stage heart disease not amenable to conventional medical or surgical therapies. From a hemodynamic standpoint, the most critical predictor of operative risk at the time of transplantation is the pulmonary vascular resistance, defined as the difference between the mean pulmonary artery pressure and the pulmonary capillary wedge pressure, divided by the cardiac output. If the pulmonary vascular resistance is greater than 5 to 6 Wood units and cannot be pharmacologically reversed with manipulations in the catheterization laboratory that could be duplicated at the time of transplantation, orthotopic transplantation would pose a substantial risk. Other options can be considered in this setting as appropriate, including heterotopic transplantation to preserve the recipient right ventricle. Determinations and decisions involving the pulmonary vascular resistance are among the most difficult in the area of heart transplantation. In children, these values must be indexed to body size to allow rational decisions to be reached.

There must be no active malignancy or infection in a potential recipient. Active peptic ulcer is a contraindication, at least in programs in which corticosteroids form a part of the immunosuppressive regimen. Severe peripheral or cerebral vascular disease may pose a relative contraindication, as does insulin-dependent diabetes mellitus, although the author's program and others have demonstrated that these patients can undergo successful transplantation (Table 20–22).

Patients who received transplantation at the University of Minnesota and their diagnoses are shown in Figure 20–50. Among 308 patients, approximately equal numbers had coronary artery disease and idiopathic cardiomyopathy as their underlying cardiac diagnosis. These two diagnostic categories constitute the most frequent indications for cardiac transplantation. Approximately 40% of the author's transplant patients have had at least one previous cardiac operation, usually for coronary revascularization. Of note is the cate-

TABLE 20–22. Recipient Selection Criteria for Heart Transplantation

Age: newborn to 60 years
Irremediable cardiac disease—New York Heart Association
  Class IV
Normal function or reversible dysfunction of kidneys, liver,
  lungs, central nervous system
Pulmonary vascular resistance less than 6 to 8 Wood units
  or pharmacologically reversible
Absence of:
  Active malignancy or infection
  Recent pulmonary infarction
  Severe peripheral or cerebrovascular disease

gory of allograft coronary artery disease. Four patients in this series have required retransplantation for this problem, and in time this number is expected to increase.

Donor Selection

The donor should be a young person who has sustained brain death either through accidental or natural causes. Cardiac retrieval is performed as part of a multiple-organ retrieval and requires careful coordination for a successful outcome. Criteria for donor selection are outlined in Table 20–23. Individuals up to 55 and occasionally 60 years of age with demonstrable normal function of the heart and absence of severe coronary disease can be suitable donors. These individuals should be on low-dose pressor support (less than or equal to 10 μg. per kg. per minute of dopamine or an equivalent dose of dobutamine). They should have a negative cardiac history and, of course, negative serologic tests for hepatitis and human immunodeficiency virus infection. Useful

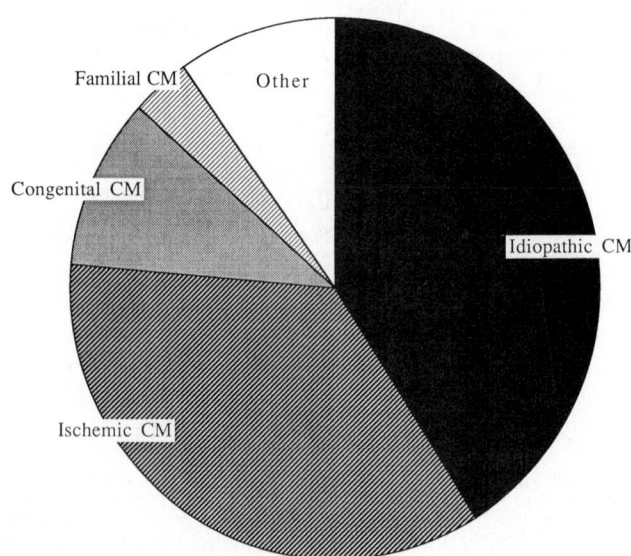

Figure 20–50. Indications for cardiac transplantations at the University of Minnesota in 308 patients receiving transplants between 1978 and 1995.

TABLE 20–23. Donor Selection Criteria for Heart Transplantation

Age younger than 60 years
Minimal pressor support
Negative cardiac history
Normal electrocardiogram
Normal echocardiogram
ABO compatibility
Size within 20% to 50% of recipient
Negative T-cell crossmatch if panel reactive antibodies 10% or greater
Negative human immunodeficiency virus and hepatitis B and C

screening tests include electrocardiography and echocardiography. The latter provides a readily available assessment of anatomic features and functional status and should be obtained whenever possible. Donor and recipient in all cases need to be ABO compatible, and a prospective crossmatch is not necessary provided the recipient is reactive to 10% or less of a panel of randomly selected HLA types (panel reactive antibodies less than 10%). Donor and recipient weight should be matched within 20% to 50%, depending on the pulmonary vascular resistance level in the recipient. Individuals with high pulmonary vascular resistance require transplantation with the heart of a donor of at least equal size to provide a large right ventricular mass better able to cope with the elevated pulmonary resistance.

Distant graft procurement is now routine, and approximately 80% of donor hearts are currently retrieved at a distance.[40] In the author's program, as far as 2020 km. (1300 miles) have been traveled with successful graft function. The limiting factor, of course, is ischemic time of the graft; with careful preservation, up to 4 hours of *ex vivo* ischemia is well tolerated. Donor hearts are preserved with 1 liter of crystalloid cardioplegia coupled with copious topical cooling.

Operative Technique

Coordination of the retrieval and implantation portions of the transplant procedure is critical to minimize cardiopulmonary bypass time and graft ischemia time and to optimize function of the graft. When the surgeon has visually inspected the donor heart, preparation of the recipient may proceed. The recipient is cannulated for cardiopulmonary bypass with an aortic cannula in the usual position and right-angle venous cannulas far posterior in the right atrium. In cases with one or more previous cardiac procedures, it is advisable to have a femoral artery and vein exposed such that expeditious femoral-femoral bypass can be instituted in the event of a misadventure on reopening the sternum or in mobilizing the recipient heart. The necessary dissection is completed such that the recipient heart can be removed expeditiously. The right atrium is divided at a level several centimeters anterior to the cannulas. The left atrium is entered just behind the aorta, and the interatrial septum is divided adjacent to the atrioventricular valves. The left atrium is transected to the plane of the coronary sinus and the left atrial appendage is excised, leaving a generous cuff of left atrium about the left pulmonary veins. The great vessels are transected at the level of the semilunar valves, and the aorta and pulmonary artery are separated using electrocautery. This completes preparation of the recipient mediastinum (Fig. 20–51A).

The donor heart is removed from its preservation container and tailored for implantation. The posterior wall of the left atrium is excised by connecting incisions in the pulmonary veins. The right atrium is incised from the inferior vena cava

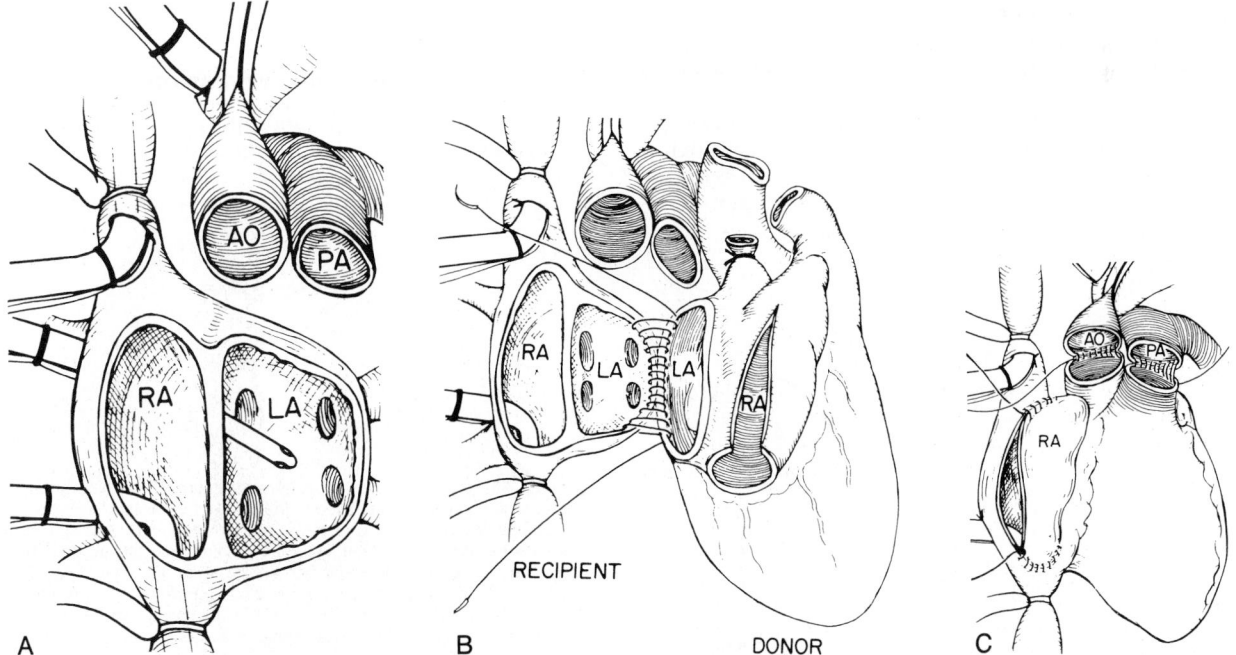

Figure 20–51. *A,* Appearance of the recipient mediastinum after excision of the diseased recipient heart. One can see the position of the arterial and venous cannulas for cardiopulmonarey bypass as well as the left ventricular vent catheter passing through the right superior pulmonary vein. Posterior cuffs of left and right atria, aorta, and pulmonary artery have been fashioned. *B,* The donor heart has been lowered into the operative field, and the lateral wall of the left atrial anastomosis is being fashioned. *C,* The medial aspect of the right atrial anastomosis has been completed, and the methods of the anastomosis of the aorta and pulmonary artery are illustrated. (From Bolman, R. M.: Cardiac transplantation: The operative technique. *In* Thompson, M. E. [Ed.]: Cardiac Transplantation. Philadelphia, F. A. Davis, 1990, pp. 136–144.)

orifice to the right atrial appendage, avoiding the sinoatrial node. Implantation begins with anastomosis of donor and recipient left atria. The anastomosis begins at the level of the left pulmonary veins and is completed at the level of the interatrial septum (see Fig. 20–51B). Timing of individual anastomoses at this point is determined by the elapsed ischemic time of the donor heart and the pulmonary vascular resistance of the recipient. Ideally, the order of anastomoses is left atrium, pulmonary artery, right atrium, aorta. However, in cases in which the ischemic time is already long and there is concern regarding donor right ventricular function because of elevated pulmonary vascular resistance in the recipient, it is prudent to perform the aortic anastomosis immediately after the left atrial anastomosis such that the cross-clamp can be released, thereby shortening the ischemic time and allowing earlier reperfusion of the donor heart (see Fig. 20–51C). A principle to be observed in anastomosing the great vessels is that the aorta should be left long and the pulmonary artery should be trimmed short so that there is no redundancy with resumption of cardiac dynamics. After at least 30 minutes of perfusion, during which hemostasis can be secured along the suture lines, the donor heart assumes the circulation. All patients receive an infusion of isoproterenol, and temporary atrial and ventricular pacing wires are routine. The chest is copiously irrigated with antibiotic solution and closed only when hemostasis is secured.[9]

The surgical technique of orthotopic cardiac transplantation has remained relatively unmodified since its initial description by Lower and Shumway. Recently, however, there has been renewed interest in procedures initially described in the 1950s employing individual caval and/or pulmonary venous anastomoses. This technique allows removal of virtually the entire diseased recipient right and/or left atrium. Sievers and associates,[37] employing bicaval versus conventional atrial anastomoses, and Blanche and co-workers,[8] employing both bicaval and pulmonary venous anastomoses, report lower incidence of tricuspid regurgitation, better preservation of atrial size, and reduced bradyarrhythmias postoperatively in patients receiving direct venous anastomoses. Although these techniques are not universally accepted, many groups are adopting the bicaval approach to standard cardiac transplantation.

In cases in which orthotopic transplantation is not feasible, a *piggyback* or heterotopic transplantation can be considered. Such instances include (1) a recipient with elevation of pulmonary vascular resistance that is fixed and cannot be reversed pharmacologically and (2) a small donor heart available for a large recipient who is critically ill. The completed procedure of heterotopic transplantation is depicted in Figure 20–52. Donor cardiectomy is similar to that for orthotopic transplantation with the exception that the entire superior vena cava is removed. In addition, a longer segment of aorta is retrieved to include the arch with ligated brachiocephalic vessels. The left-sided pulmonary venous orifices are opened widely and united in preparation for anastomosis with the left atrium of the recipient. The right-sided pulmonary veins are oversewn. The inferior vena cava is closed at its atrial junction, and the superior vena cava is ligated distally. An incision is made into the posterior portion of the superior vena cava with the venotomy extended 3 to 4 cm. onto the right atrial surface. The incision is positioned posteriorly to minimize risk of injury to the sinus node.

The recipient is placed on cardiopulmonary bypass, and the left atrium of the recipient is incised just posterior to the interatrial groove, similar to the approach for mitral valve surgery. The donor heart is positioned in the right chest anterior to the lung, and the common orifice to the left pulmonary veins is anastomosed to the recipient left atrium. A right lateral atriotomy is created in the recipient heart, and a continuous anastomosis is created between the cavoatrial opening in the donor and the atriotomy in the recipient. Donor aorta is anastomosed end-to-side to the recipient ascending aorta, which is controlled with a side-biting vascular clamp. The main pulmonary artery of the donor is generally of insufficient length to reach the recipient pulmonary artery. This gap can be bridged with the right pulmonary artery of the donor or a segment of donor aorta or prosthetic graft that has been preclotted. Donor and recipient pulmonary arteries are then joined. The patient is allowed to return to normal temperature and is separated from cardiopulmonary bypass.[19] The operative procedure of cardiac transplantation, whether orthotopic or heterotopic, must be performed with meticulous attention to technical detail and hemostasis. The morbidity after technical and bleeding complications is likely to be high.

Immunosuppression

Cyclosporine-based immunosuppression is performed using one of two protocols in most programs. Triple therapy, introduced by the author and his colleagues in 1983, consists of the combination of cyclosporine, azathioprine, and predni-

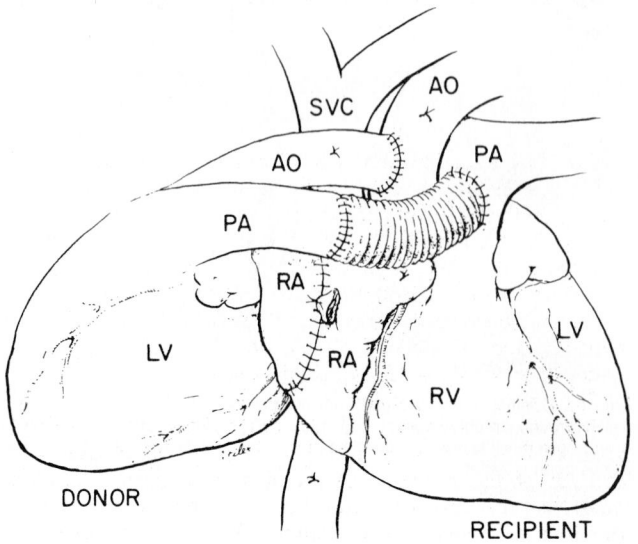

Figure 20–52. The completed procedure of heterotopic transplantation. The donor aorta is anastomosed directly to the side of the recipient ascending aorta. The donor pulmonary artery and recipient pulmonary artery have been joined with an interposed Dacron graft. Alternatively, this may be accomplished with interposition of a segment of donor descending aorta. The right atrial suture line is visible, as is the final orientation of donor and recipient hearts. (From Bolman, R. M.: Cardiac transplantation: The operative technique. *In* Thompson, M. E. [Ed.]: Cardiac Transplantation. Philadelphia, F. A. Davis, 1990, pp. 136–144.)

sone and remains the mainstay of immunosuppressive management in this program. Patients receive cyclosporine, 4 to 10 mg. per kg., as a preoperative dose and azathioprine, 2 to 3 mg. per kg., preoperatively. Methylprednisolone sodium succinate, 1 gm., is administered in the 24 hours surrounding the procedure, and then prednisone is administered on day 2 at 1 mg. per kg. per day in divided doses. Cyclosporine is targeted to a 12-hour trough level of 200 to 300 ng. per ml. and azathioprine to a white blood cell count of 4000 to 5000 per cu. mm. Prednisone is tapered to a level of 5 to 10 mg. per day by 3 to 6 months. This regimen has been associated with the lowest reported incidence of cardiac rejection and has yielded excellent rates of survival and a low incidence of infection.[10-13, 30]

The other cyclosporine-based protocol is one in which the monoclonal antibody OKT3 is used in conjunction with triple therapy (the *induction* regimen). This innovative approach, introduced by Bristow and associates, involves the administration of OKT3 for 2 weeks beginning on day 2, during which time patients receive corticosteroid therapy and azathioprine. Cyclosporine is initiated just before the discontinuation of OKT3 and is titrated to therapeutic levels when OKT3 is discontinued. Patients are then maintained on cyclosporine and azathioprine, and prednisone is tapered off over a 2-week period in those patients who do not reject the transplanted heart. This regimen has been associated with a significant portion of patients being able to successfully discontinue corticosteroid therapy, although the use of OKT3 has been associated with significant side effects.[14] Gay and colleagues and others have reported excellent results with this regimen, but reports of increased incidence of lymphoproliferative disorder after OKT3 in cardiac transplant recipients has raised significant concern about the safety of this agent.[38]

Although cyclosporine-based immunosuppression regimens remain the mainstay of anti-rejection therapy for cardiac allograft recipients, a new generation of immunosuppressive agents is emerging that promises to have a major impact on solid organ transplantation. Armitage and associates have reported on a clinical trial of FK 506 (tacrolimus) immunosuppression in adult cardiac transplantation. In this study, FK 506 provided immunosuppressive therapy that was at least as efficacious as cyclosporine in a group of 72 patients.[3] This drug has been employed also in trials of liver, kidney, and, most recently, lung transplantation. Another new agent, mycophenolate mofetil (RS-61443), is undergoing multicenter investigation as an adjunct to cyclosporine in heart transplant recipients. This drug appears to hold considerable promise for solid organ transplantation as well.[39]

Complications

Allograft Rejection. The diagnosis of cardiac rejection depends on an index of suspicion associated with new-onset cardiac arrhythmia, hypotension, or fever. Associated symptoms may include fatigue, malaise, and shortness of breath. The electrocardiogram is not routinely useful in the diagnosis of rejection, and confirmation depends on the endomyocardial biopsy. A useful adjunct is radionuclide ventriculography, which, if performed as a baseline study in all patients shortly after transplant, can constitute a very helpful study to follow both grade and severity of rejection hemodynamically and its course with treatment. The gold standard for diagnosis of allograft rejection of the heart is the endomyocardial biopsy. The diagnosis and grading of rejection has been standardized to some degree by a working group of transplant pathologists. The grading system has been described by Billingham and colleagues for the International Society for Heart and Lung Transplantation. This grading scheme characterizes the endomyocardial biopsy with respect

to distribution and characteristics of lymphocytic infiltration and damage to the myocytes.[7]

Infection. Several measures of prophylaxis against infection have proved highly useful in the management of these postoperative transplant recipients. All patients who are seronegative for cytomegalovirus before transplantation receive exclusively cytomegalovirus-negative blood and blood products postoperatively. All patients receive nystatin orally and high-dose acyclovir (800 mg. four times a day) for 3 months and trimethoprim-sulfamethoxazole indefinitely after the transplant operation. Perioperative wound prophylaxis consists of a second-generation cephalosporin and vancomycin coupled with copious intraoperative irrigation with a vancomycin solution. This regimen, coupled with the low incidence of rejection experienced with triple therapy, has caused a very low incidence of serious infection, and none of the author's patients has had mediastinitis or a sternal wound infection.[2] Miller and associates, reporting for the Cardiac Transplant Research Data Base Group, notes that infection remains the leading cause of death after heart transplantation. This is an excellent review of the current status of infection after cardiac transplantation.[27]

Transplant Coronary Artery Disease. A dreaded sequel of cardiac transplantation is that of transplant coronary artery disease. This entity continues to plague cardiac transplant recipients and is expected to become an increasing problem in time and with the increasing numbers of patients receiving transplants. Olivari and colleagues reported the experience at the University of Minnesota with this problem. When coronary artery disease is defined by any decrease in luminal diameter, 8% at 1 year and 24% at 2 years demonstrated findings of transplant coronary artery disease.[29] This incidence can be expected to increase with time. It is thought to represent a manifestation of chronic rejection in the form of immune complex disease directed at the intima of the major epicardial coronary vessels. Rickenbacher and associates, employing the new modality of intracoronary ultrasonography, have followed 174 heart transplant recipients from baseline up to 15 years after transplantation. This group demonstrated that intimal thickening progresses in patients over time. Furthermore, calcification supervenes, being present in 2% to 12% of patients at 5 years and up to 24% of patients at 6 to 10 years.[35] This new modality represents an important tool in the follow-up of patients for this long-term complication of cardiac transplantation. Close surveillance is required, and some cases have been treated with percutaneous transluminal coronary angioplasty. If the problem becomes severe and/or associated with significant or multiple myocardial infarctions, retransplantation may be the only option available.

Results

The 1994 report of the Registry of the International Society of Heart and Lung Transplantation documents that the explosive growth in heart transplantation that occurred in the late 1980s has plateaued. For each of the last 5 to 6 years, approximately 2500 heart transplants have been performed annually in the United States. Reporting on 26,704 heart transplantations from 251 centers worldwide, the Registry reports actuarial survival of 80% at 1 year, 64% at 5 years, and 45% at 10 years.[22] Figure 20–53 depicts actuarial survival in 308 patients undergoing transplantation at the University of Minnesota between 1978 and 1995. Actuarial patient survival of 77% at 5 years and 62% at 10 years attests to the efficacy of the methods of recipient and donor selection, operative management, and immunosuppression outlined previously. These outcomes contrast sharply to the life expec-

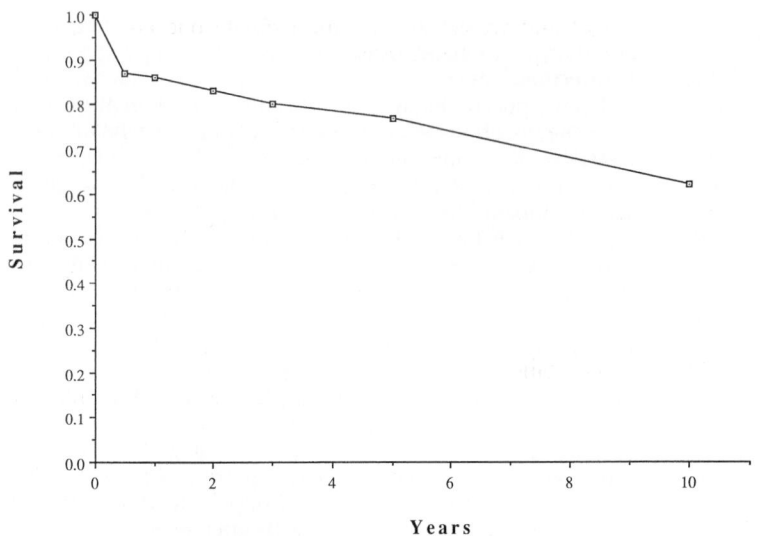

Figure 20–53. Actuarial survival in 308 patients receiving transplants at the University of Minnesota since the inception of triple-drug immunosuppression in 1983. Survival at 5 and 10 years is 78% and 65%, respectively.

tancy of individuals with end-stage heart failure who do not receive a heart transplant.

Rates of rejection, expressed as rejection-free survival, are demonstrated in Figure 20–54. Eighty-six percent of patients are free of rejection at 1 year after transplantation when treated with triple-therapy immunosuppression.[30] There is a very low incidence of serious and life-threatening infections in patients treated with this regimen. Because fewer patients require treatment for rejection, the total amount of immunosuppression received is less, and this is reflected in a decreased rate of infection. The routine administration of trimethoprim-sulfamethoxazole has proved very beneficial, because there have been no cases of *Pneumocystis* or *Nocardia* infection in these heart transplant recipients.[2]

Summary

Since its inception in 1967, cardiac transplantation has progressed steadily. Today this procedure represents an established treatment for end-stage heart disease. Improved patient selection and effective, safe immunosuppressive strategies have restored health to patients formerly destined for premature death. Serious problems remaining to be solved include a shortage of donor organs and the problem of transplant coronary artery disease, which currently is the number one factor limiting long-term survival. New surgical and immunosuppressive strategies promise to improve these outcomes further.

CARDIOPULMONARY TRANSPLANTATION
Recipient Selection

Certain individuals have disease of the heart and lungs that requires replacement of these organs. The dramatic advent of successful cardiopulmonary transplantation, introduced by Reitz and colleagues, has made this procedure a clinical reality.[34] Recipient selection criteria are outlined in Table 20–24. The most common indications for this procedure have been primary pulmonary hypertension and Eisenmenger's syndrome. Other less frequent diagnoses necessitating *en bloc* heart-lung replacement are cystic fibrosis, obstructive lung disease with cor pulmonale, and other end-stage lung diseases associated with severe right ventricular decompensation. With the development of successful lung transplantation, patients formerly thought appropriate for heart-lung transplantation are being treated with single or bilateral single lung transplants. Certain examples would be patients with primary pulmonary hypertension before the onset of severe right ventricular failure and also those with Eisenmenger's syndrome with relatively straightforward congenital heart defects (e.g., atrial septal defect, ventricular septal defect, patent ductus arteriosus). These individuals

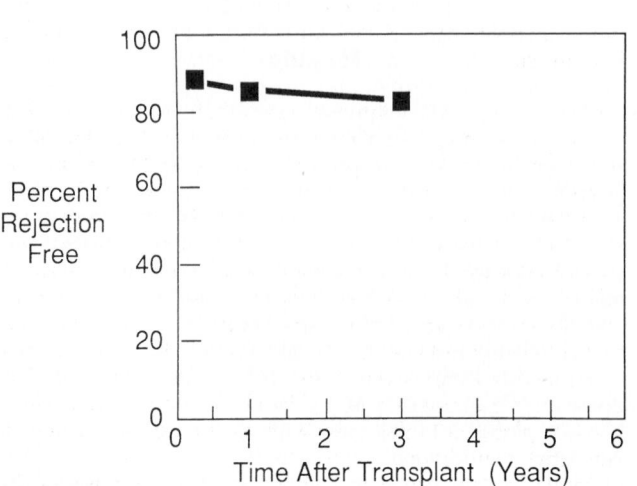

Figure 20–54. Incidence of acute allograft rejection in patients receiving transplants at the University of Minnesota since the inception of triple-drug immunosuppression in 1983.

TABLE 20–24. Recipient Selection Criteria for Cardiopulmonary Transplantation

Age: 50 years or younger
End-stage pulmonary vascular or parenchymal disease
  associated with end-stage cardiac decompensation
Absence of:
  Other nonreversible organ dysfunction or disease
  High-dose corticosteroid therapy
  Major prior thoracotomy or sternotomy (controversial)

could undergo single- or bilateral lung transplantation combined with repair of the congenital cardiac defect. Such procedures, if feasible, increase the number of patients who can receive transplants. Donor hearts can be used for patients in need of heart transplantation, and donor lungs for patients with parenchymal lung disease or pulmonary vascular disease (primary or secondary) with adequate preservation of cardiac function.

Prospective recipients should be severely limited by their disease and unable to work or attend school, and most are on supplemental oxygen therapy. Because of the marked scarcity of suitable donors, individuals should be considered for transplantation only when their lifestyle is seriously impaired and it is believed that they are in the final 12 to 24 months of natural life. These individuals must fulfill all the other criteria for transplantation as outlined in the section on heart transplantation; namely, they must demonstrate normal extrathoracic organ function and must possess sufficient psychosocial stability and support to withstand the rigors of the procedure and postoperative period.

Donor Selection

A small percentage of donors suitable for heart donation also have lungs that can be transplanted (10% to 20%). Increased awareness of the need as well as improved donor management can increase this percentage; however, lack of suitable donors continues to severely restrict the number of these procedures that can be performed. Criteria for suitable cardiopulmonary donors are depicted in Table 20–25. In addition to normal heart function, the heart-lung donor must have normal gas exchange with a PaO_2 greater than 400 mm. Hg on 100% inspired oxygen with peak airway pressures of 30 mm. Hg or less. The chest film should be normal and pulmonary secretions minimal. The presence of fungus in any amount or gram-negative bacteria in large numbers heralds increased risk of serious infection after transplantation and should contraindicate donation.

Donor and recipient are matched according to ABO type as well as on the basis of results of an HLA antibody screen. Size-matching is also important, and comparison of measurements made from standard portable roentgenograms is helpful in determining size compatibility. Donor and recipient

TABLE 20–25. Donor Selection Criteria for Cardiopulmonary Transplantation

Close size match—donor smaller than or same size as
  recipient
Satisfactory gas exchange—arterial PO_2 > 400 mm. Hg on
  FIO_2 of 1.0
Normal lung compliance—peak airway pressure of 30 mm.
  Hg with normal tidal volume
Clear chest radiograph
Absence of purulent pulmonary secretions

height and weight should approximate one another; however, height is a better indicator of relative lung volume than is weight.

Scrupulous attention to fluid management in the donor both before and during organ harvest is critical to avoid overload and compromise of suitability for transplantation. The donor should be maintained as dry as possible consistent with adequate function of the other organs being retrieved, and a central venous pressure of 5 cm. H_2O or less is desirable. Successful organ function has been repeatedly demonstrated after up to 4 hours of *ex vivo* preservation by means of either of two main techniques. The donor can be placed on cardiopulmonary bypass using a portable heart-lung machine. With this technique, the donor is cooled uniformly to a temperature of 15° C. to 18° C. and the heart-lung block is removed after the abdominal viscera are mobilized.[6] The other main technique in use is that of cardioplegic arrest of the heart, combined with pulmonary artery flushing with a modified EuroCollins solution in the amount of 50 to 100 ml. per kg. donor weight. Copious topical cooling with 4° C. saline is also employed, and the donor is ventilated with small tidal volumes of room air while the flush solution is being delivered. This method is preferred by most groups because of its simplicity and the fact that it is somewhat cumbersome to transport a cardiopulmonary bypass circuit to a distant donor hospital.[4]

Operative Technique

As with heart transplantation, careful coordination between donor retrieval and recipient preparation is essential for a satisfactory outcome. The recipient is brought to the operating room and lines are placed, such that the surgical procedure can begin immediately on receiving word that the donor organs are suitable for transplantation. Through a midline sternotomy, both pleural spaces are explored and any adhesions lysed before heparinization. This allows achievement of optimal hemostasis in the pleural spaces before the institution of cardiopulmonary bypass. The pericardium is then opened and the patient cannulated for bypass with standard aortic cannulation and bicaval cannulation through the posterior right atrium. Cardiopulmonary bypass is instituted, and the heart is removed much as described for heart transplantation. Employing electrocautery, an incision is made behind the phrenic nerve bilaterally from the level of the pulmonary artery to the diaphragm to create a window for passage of the donor lungs into the recipient pleural spaces. Care must be taken to avoid injury to the phrenic nerves, and the recurrent laryngeal nerve can be damaged if the dissection is carried above the pulmonary artery on the left. The lungs are removed individually. The inferior pulmonary ligaments are divided, and the respective pulmonary hila are stapled with a TA90 surgical stapler. The lungs are then removed. This technique has greatly simplified this portion of the operation and improves hemostasis. It is then necessary to incise the posterior left atrium vertically to allow the donor lung to pass posterior to the right atrium and phrenic pedicle. Figure 20–55 depicts several salient portions of the heart-lung transplant procedure. The trachea is mobilized between the aorta and superior vena cava, taking care to avoid devascularizing the supracarinal portion. The mainstem bronchi are mobilized, and the trachea is transected just above the carina. With the thoracic organs removed, meticulous hemostasis should be achieved, because the posterior mediastinum is very difficult to visualize after implantation of the donor heart-lung block. The donor heart-lung block is placed into the chest with each lung placed into its respective hemithorax.

The transplant procedure begins with anastomosis of do-

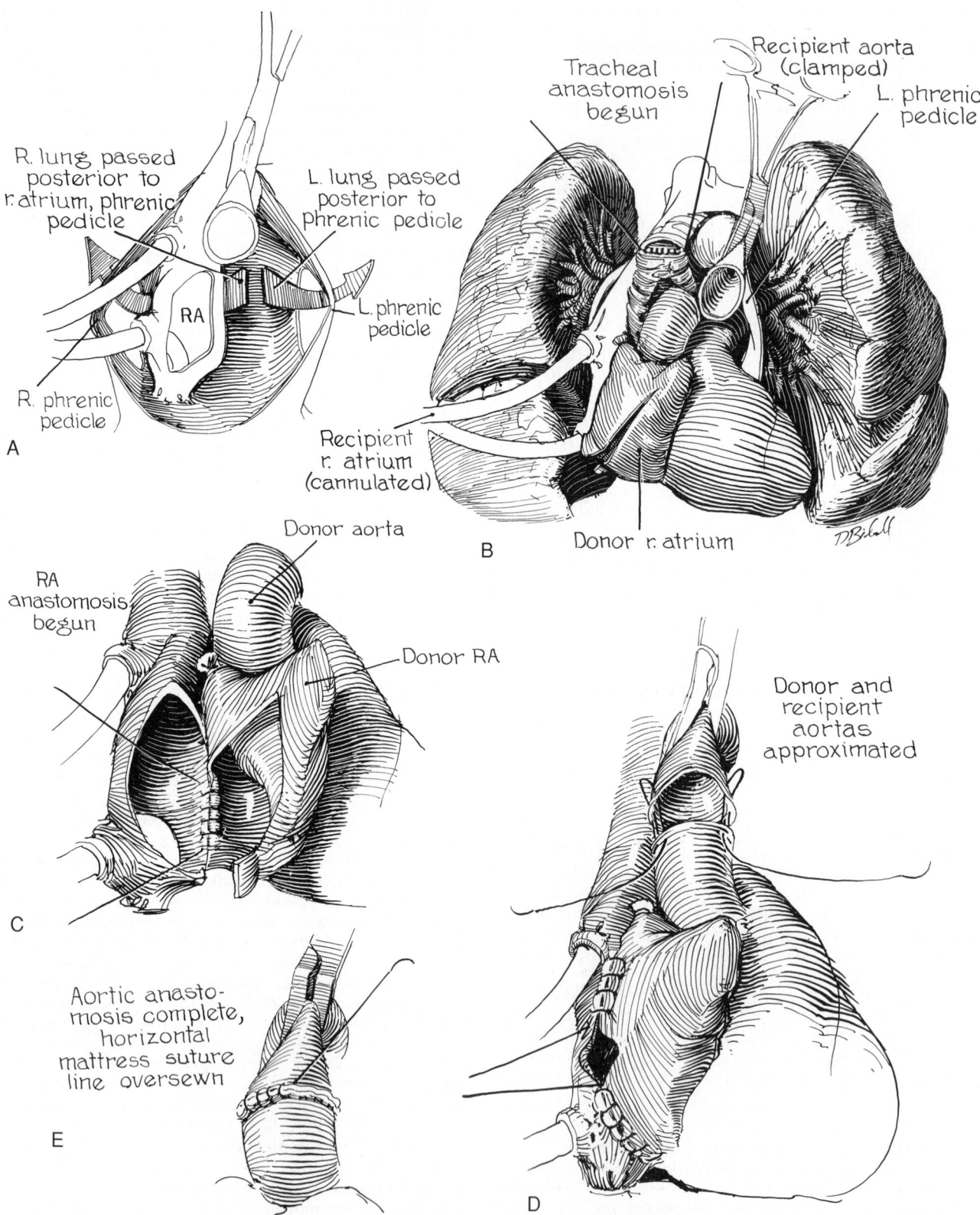

Figure 20–55. *A,* The schematic represents the prepared mediastinum with the diseased heart and lungs removed. *B,* The donor heart-lung bloc has been positioned in the chest with the respective lungs positioned behind their corresponding phrenic pedicles. The tracheal anastomosis is shown in progress. *C to E* depict the right atrial and aortic anastomoses that complete the procedure. (From Flye, M. W. [Ed]: Atlas of Organ Transplantation. Philadelphia, W. B. Saunders, 1995, p. 289.)

nor and recipient tracheas using a running suture technique with 3–0 monofilament suture. The donor trachea is transected two tracheal rings above the carina. When the tracheal anastomosis is completed, ventilation with low tidal volume and room air is initiated. Donor and recipient aortas and right atria are then anastomosed, completing the procedure. In the past 2 years, the author has adopted a bicaval technique of implanting the donor heart. The same benefits pertain as described for heart transplant recipients.

Another option is the *domino* heart-lung transplant procedure. This operation has been performed on two occasions at the author's institution. In this procedure, the recipient heart, which must be demonstrated to be suitable for transplantation, is removed and sent for implantation either in an adjacent operating room or in another transplant center. Individual caval anastomoses are necessary at the time of heart-lung implantation because the entire recipient right atrium is removed. Otherwise, the implant procedure is identical to that described in the preceding section.

Immunosuppression

Recipients of heart-lung allografts receive cyclosporine-based immunosuppression. Cyclosporine and azathioprine are administered preoperatively. Corticosteroids are administered beginning in the operating room and then continuously thereafter. Patients are maintained on triple-drug immunosuppression, consisting of cyclosporine, azathioprine, and prednisone, for the long term. Cyclosporine is targeted to a 12-hour trough level of 200 to 300 ng. per ml. Azathioprine is administered to tolerance determined by a white blood cell count of 4000 to 5000 per cu. mm. Prednisone is initiated at 0.5 mg. per kg. per day and tapered slowly over time.

Complications

Rejection. Most recipients experience an episode of rejection within the first 2 weeks. Heart and lungs do not necessarily reject synchronously; therefore, heart biopsy is not a reliable means of monitoring lung rejection. The diagnosis of lung rejection depends on clinical grounds, although recent experience with the transbronchial biopsy suggests that this procedure is very useful if coupled with a careful assessment of the patient's clinical status. Signs of graft rejection include a decrease in oxygenation, a new radiographic infiltrate, fever, and auscultatory findings of basilar rales. Symptoms may include breathlessness, malaise, and a feeling of anxiety. Treatment is with pulse corticosteroid therapy for a period of 3 days followed by reassessment.

Infection. Infection prophylaxis in the heart-lung recipient is identical to that described for the heart transplant recipient with the exception that recipients who are positive for cytomegalovirus, or who receive a cytomegalovirus-positive donor block, receive ganciclovir for 90 days after transplant. Most infections after heart-lung transplantation are, in fact, pulmonary. Any new radiographic abnormality, especially in the presence of fever, must be urgently evaluated by bronchoscopy with lavage. Broad-spectrum antibiotics are administered until specific culture data are available; at that time, all unnecessary antibiotics are discontinued. The use of trimethoprim-sulfamethoxazole routinely has prevented infections caused by *Pneumocystis* and *Nocardia* organisms in the author's heart and heart-lung recipient population.

Bronchiolitis Obliterans. One of the most serious complications in recipients of these procedures is that of bronchiolitis obliterans. This entity is thought to represent a form of chronic rejection analogous to transplant coronary artery disease in recipients of heart allografts. Indeed, in some autopsies of heart-lung recipients, both processes have been

identified in the same patient. Often appearing without any obvious radiographic abnormality, bronchiolitis obliterans is an insidious process, initially causing a decrement in the midexpiratory flow measurement (forced expiratory flow, 25% to 75%). There is then progression to breathlessness, and eventually the individual becomes severely limited. This occurs in 30% to 50% of heart-lung recipients and may appear at any time after the first several months after transplant. Attempts to reverse the course of this process in most cases prove futile, although in some cases the patient can be stabilized, albeit at a lower level of function. Approaches to treatment primarily involve increased immunosuppression. Studies in the author's laboratory have demonstrated the immunologic nature of this disorder. A large animal model has been created by tapering of immunosuppression after successful porcine lung allografting.[1]

Clinical Outcomes

The main impediment to progress in the field of cardiopulmonary transplantation has been the severe limitation in the numbers of available donors. Only a few centers in the United States have accrued a significant experience. Since the pioneering work of Reitz, subsequent investigators at Stanford have continued to develop the techniques of cardiopulmonary transplantation, including refined patient selection and improved posttransplant management. Comparing 30 patients transplanted between March 1981 and February 1986 with 32 patients transplanted subsequent to that period, this group was able to demonstrate improved in-hospital and long-term survival with a decreased incidence of bronchiolitis obliterans in the later group. Perioperative mortality decreased from 35% to 16%, 3-year survival improved from 43% to 65%, and the incidence of bronchiolitis obliterans decreased from 63% to 20% among hospital survivors. Survival at 3 years in the more recent group has paralleled that in heart transplants performed at Stanford during the same time span. The improved outcomes are attributed to the routine employment of triple-drug immunosuppression and more aggressive surveillance for rejection and infection, including the routine application of bronchoscopy with bronchoalveolar lavage and transbronchial biopsy.[26]

Since 1986 at the University of Minnesota, there have been 33 heart-lung transplants performed in patients ranging from 6 to 54 years of age. Two of these were domino procedures with the recipient heart being transplanted in another individual. The diagnoses for which these patients received heart-lung transplantation are listed in Table 20–26. Figure 20–56 demonstrates survival after heart-lung transplantation at the University of Minnesota up to 5 years. As is evident, these outcomes are very similar to those observed after heart transplantation.

TABLE 20–26. Indications for Heart-Lung Transplantation at the University of Minnesota, 1986–1995

Diagnosis	No. of Patients
Primary pulmonary hypertension	14
Eisenmenger's syndrome	12
Alpha₁-antitrypsin deficiency	3
Cystic fibrosis	2
Other	2
Total	33

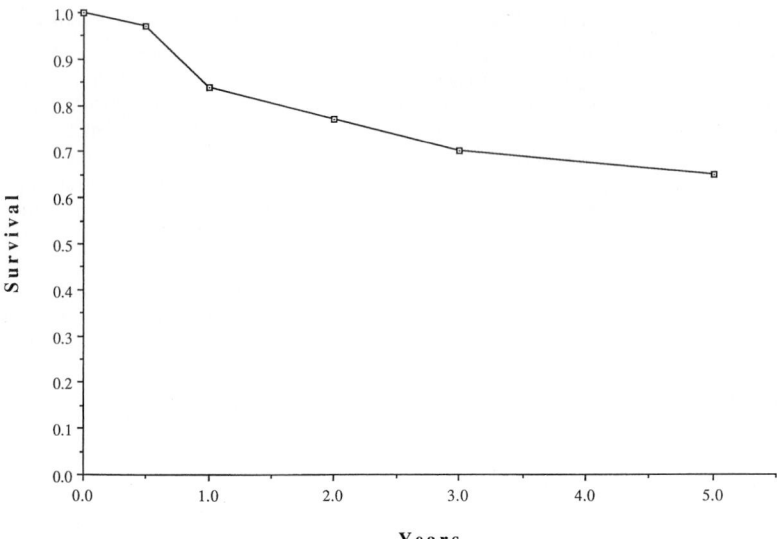

Figure 20–56. Actuarial survival in 33 recipients of heart-lung transplants at the University of Minnesota between 1986 and 1994. Survival at 5 years is 59%.

Summary

Owing to severe restrictions in donor availability, small numbers of these procedures have been performed in the United States each year. Despite this, the gratifying results achieved in transplanted individuals have inspired further efforts in this field. Cardiopulmonary transplantation remains a therapeutic option for selected individuals for whom no other conventional or transplant alternative is available. With the establishment of good therapy for patients with end-stage lung disease, heart-lung transplantation is now reserved only for individuals with disease of the heart and lungs. There remains a group of individuals for whom no other procedure is available. Work continues at the author's institution and elsewhere in the area of chronic rejection of allografted lung. Complications and decrements in pulmonary function due to bronchiolitis obliterans remain the greatest barriers to long-term survival in these patients.

SELECTED REFERENCES

Al-Dossari, G. A., Kshettry, V. R., Jessurun, J., and Bolman, R. M. III: Experimental large animal model of obliterative bronchiolitis after lung transplantation. Ann. Thorac. Surg., *58*:34, 1994.
This is the first time that a large animal model of bronchiolitis obliterans has been established. Porcine recipients of single lung allografts were tapered off immunosuppression and a pathologic lesion of bronchiolitis obliterans was observed, thereby confirming the immunologic nature of this lesion.

Bolman, R. M., Elick, B., Olivari, M. T., Ring, W. S., and Arentzen, C. E.: Improved immunosuppression for cardiac transplantation. J. Heart Transplant., *4*:315, 1985.
This is the first report demonstrating the usefulness of the combination of cyclosporine, azathioprine and prednisone in heart transplant recipients. The so-called triple therapy was to become the mainstay of immunosuppression for heart and, subsequently, lung and heart-lung transplantation until the present time.

Demikhov, V.P.: Experimental Transplantation of Vital Organs. New York, Consultants Bureau, 1962.
This work by a brilliant Russian investigator antedated many of the current techniques in cardiothoracic surgery. He first performed mammary artery implants, and his descriptions of techniques of transplantation of heart and heart-lung blocks before the availability of cardiopulmonary bypass were innovative. He performed experimental transplants of many other vital organs, but his work was overlooked for many years. Only recently has the importance of his work been realized.

Gay, W. A., O'Connell, J. G., Burton, N. A., et al.: OKT3 monoclonal antibody in cardiac transplantation: Experience with 102 patients. Ann. Surg., *208*, 287, 1988.
Experience with 102 patients undergoing cardiac transplantation under treatment with OKT3 monoclonal antibody is reported in this article. The results of this regimen are equal to those reported previously in cardiac transplantation in terms of survival, and the concept of steroid withdrawal was made possible by this regimen. This pioneered the application of this "induction" regimen using OKT3.

McCarthy, P. M., Starnes, V. A., Theodore, J., et al.: Improved survival after heart-lung transplantation. J. Thorac. Cardiovasc. Surg., *99*:54, 1990.
With the somewhat discouraging results experienced by many early pioneers in heart-lung transplantation, this excellent summary of 2 years in heart-lung transplantation at Stanford provides encouragement for continuing application in selected circumstances. The authors demonstrate an improved survival and decreased incidence of chronic rejection in the form of bronchiolitis obliterans. The improvements are attributed to the routine employment of triple-drug immunosuppression and aggressive posttransplant monitoring with frequent bronchoscopy, bronchoalveolar lavage, and transbronchial biopsy for diagnosis of infection and rejection.

Oyer, P. E., et al.: One year experience with cyclosporin A in clinical heart transplantation. Heart Transplant., *1*:285, 1982.
The Stanford group reports the initial experience with cyclosporine in heart transplantation. The increment in survival and decrease in serious infection reported in this paper served as inspiration to many programs in cardiac transplantation.

Reitz, B. A., Burton, N. A., Jamieson, S. W., et al.: Heart and lung transplantation, autotransplantation and allotransplantation in primates with extended survival. J. Thorac. Cardiovasc. Surg., *80*:360, 1980.
This excellent article reports successful transplantation of heart and lungs in primates, with long-term survival. This work clearly was the impetus for human clinical heart-lung transplantation and demonstrated conclusively that the denervated heart and lungs could function normally for long periods of time and support an entirely normal quality of life.

Reitz, B. A., Wallwork, J. L., Hunt, S. A., et al.: Heart-lung transplantation: Successful therapy for patients with pulmonary vascular disease. N. Engl. J. Med., *306*:557, 1982.
This landmark report of the first successful human heart-lung transplant is one of the most significant contributions in vital organ transplantation as well as cardiothoracic surgery. Successful laboratory investigations made clinical heart-lung transplantation a reality and served as an impetus for many future developments in this area, including single- and double-lung transplantation. This was the first demonstration that the transplanted airway could heal effectively.

REFERENCES

1. Al-Dossari, G. A., Kshettry, V. R., Jessurun, J., and Bolman R. M. III: Experimental large animal model of obliterative bronchiolitis after lung transplantation. Ann. Thorac. Surg., *58*:34, 1994.
2. Andreone, P. A., Olivari, M. T., Elick, B., Arentzen, C. A., Bolman, R. M., Simmons, R. L., and Ring, W. S.: Reduction of infectious complications following cardiac transplantation. J. Heart Transplant, *5*:13, 1986.
3. Armitage, J. M., Kormos, R. L., Shigeki, M., Fung, J., Marrone, G. C., Hardesty, R. L., Griffith, B. P., and Starzl, T. E.: Clinical trial of FK506 immunosuppression in adult cardiac transplantation. Ann. Thorac. Surg., *54*:205, 1992.
4. Baldwin, J. C., Frist, W. H., Starkey, T. D., et al.: Distant graft procurement for combined heart and lung transplantation using pulmonary artery flush and simple topical hypothermia for graft preservation. Ann. Thorac. Surg., *43*:670, 1987.
5. Barnard, C. N.: A human cardiac transplant: An interim report of a successful operation performed at Groote Schuur Hospital, Capetown. S. Afr. Med., J., *41*:1271, 1967.
6. Baumgartner, W. A., Williams, G. M., Frazer, C. C., et al.: Cardiopulmonary bypass with profound hypothermia: An optimal preservation method for multi-organ procurement. Transplantation, *47*:123, 1989.

7. Billingham, M. E., Cary, N. R., Hammond, M. E., Kemnitz, J., Marboe, C., McCallister, H. A., Snovar, D. E., Winters, G. L., and Zerbe, A.: A working formulation for the standardization of nomenclature in the diagnosis of heart and lung rejection: Heart rejection study group. J. Heart Transplant., 9:587, 1990.

8. Blanche, C., Czer, L. S., Valenza, M., and Trento, A.: Alternative technique for orthotopic heart transplantation. Ann. Thorac. Surg., 57:765, 1994.

9. Bolman, R. M.: Cardiac transplantation: The operative technique. Cardiovasc. Clin., 20:133, 1990.

10. Bolman R. M., Elick, B., Olivari, M. T., Ring, W. S., Arentzen, C. E.: Improved immunosuppression for cardiac transplantation. J. Heart Transplant, 4:315, 1985.

11. Bolman, R. M., Cance, C., Spray, T., et al.: The changing face of cardiac transplantation: Washington University program 1985–1987. Ann. Thorac. Surg., 45:192, 1987.

12. Bolman, R. M., Elick, B., Olivari, M. T., et al.: Improved immunosuppression for cardiac transplantation. J. Heart Transplant, 4:315, 1985.

13. Bolman, R. M., Olivari, M. T., Sibley, R., et al.: Current results with triple therapy for heart transplantation. Transplant Proc., 19:2490, 1987.

14. Bristow, M. R., Gilbert, E. M., Renlund, D. G., et al.: Use of OKT3 monoclonal antibody in cardiac transplantation: Review of the initial experience. J. Heart Transplant., 7:1, 1988.

15. Carrel, A., and Guthrie, C. C.: The transplantation of veins and organs. Am. J. Med., 10:1101, 1905.

16. Castaneda, A. R., Amar, O., Schmidt-Habelmann, P., et al.: Cardiopulmonary autotransplantation in primates. J. Cardiovasc. Surg., 37:523, 1972.

17. Demikhov, V. P.: Experimental Transplantation of Vital Organs. New York, Consultants Bureau, 1962.

18. Gay, W. A., O'Connell, J. G., Burton, N. A., et al.: OKT3 monoclonal antibody in cardiac transplantation: Experience with 102 patients. Ann. Surg., 208:287, 1988.

19. Griffith, B. P., Kormos, R. L., and Hardesty, R. L.: Heterotopic cardiac transplantation: Current status. J. Cardiac Surg., 2:283, 1987.

20. Haglin, J., Telander, R. I., Muzzall, R. E., et al.: Comparison of lung autotransplantation in the primate and dog. Surg. Forum, 14:196, 1963.

21. Heck, C. F., Shumway, S. J., and Kaye, M. P.: The Registry of the International Society for Heart Transplantation: Sixth Official Report–1989. J. Heart Transplant, 8:271, 1989.

22. Hosenpud, J. D., Novick, R. J., Breen, T. J., and Daily, O. P.: The Registry of the International Society for Heart and Lung Transplantation: Twelfth Official Report–1995. J. Heart Lung Transplant., 14(4), 1995.

23. Lillehei, C. W.: Discussion of Wildevuur, C. R. H., and Benfield, J. R.: A review of 23 human lung transplantations by 20 surgeons. Ann. Thorac. Surg., 9:489, 1970.

24. Lower, R. R., and Shumway, N. E.: Studies on the orthotopic homotransplantation of the canine heart. Surg. Forum, 11:18, 1960.

25. Marcus, E., Wong, S. N. T., and Luisada, A. A.: Homologous heart grafts: Transplantation of the heart in dogs. Surg. Forum, 2:212, 1951.

26. McCarthy, P. M., Starnes, V. A., Theodore, J., et al.: Improved survival after heart-lung transplantation. J. Thorac. Cardiovasc. Surg., 99:54, 1990.

27. Miller, L. W., Naftel, D. C., Bourge, R. C., Kirklin, J. K., Brozena, S. C.,

Jarcho, J., Hobbs, R. E., and Mills, R. M.: Infection after heart transplantation: A multiinstitutional study: Cardiac Transplant Research Database Group. J. Heart Lung Transplant., 13:381; discussion 393, 1994.

28. Neptune, W. B., Crookson, B. A., Bailey, C. P., et al.: Complete homologous heart transplantation. Arch. Surg., 66:174, 1953.

29. Olivari, M. T., Homans, D. C., Wilson, R. F., et al.: Coronary artery disease in cardiac transplant patients receiving triple-drug immunosuppressive therapy. Circulation, Suppl. III:III–111, 1989.

30. Olivari, M. T., Kubo, S. H., Braunlin, E. A., Bolman, R. M., and Ring, W. S.: Five-year experience with triple-drug immunosuppressive therapy in cardiac transplantation. Circulation, Suppl. IV:276, 1990.

31. Oyer, P. E., et al.: One year experience with cyclosporin A in clinical heart transplantation. Heart Transplant, 1:285, 1982.

32. Reitz, B. A.: The history of heart and heart-lung transplantation. In Baumgartner, W. A., Reitz, B. A., and Achuff, S. C. (Eds): Heart and Heart-Lung Transplantation. Philadelphia, W. B. Saunders, 1990, pp. 1–14.

33. Reitz, B. A., Burton, N. A., Jamieson, S. W., et al.: Heart and lung transplantation, autotransplantation and allotransplantation in primates with extended survival. J. Thorac. Cardiovasc. Surg., 80:360, 1980.

34. Reitz, B. A., Wallwork, J. L., Hunt, S. A., et al.: Heart-lung transplantation: Successful therapy for patients with pulmonary vascular disease. N. Engl. J. Med., 306:557, 1982.

35. Rickenbacher, P. R., Pinto, F. J., Chenzbraun, A., Botas, J., Lewis, N. P., Alderman, E. L., Valantine, H. A., Hunt, S. A., Schroeder, J. S., Popp, R. L., et al.: Incidence and severity of transplant coronary artery disease early and up to 15 years after transplantation as detected by intravascular ultrasound. J. Am. Coll. Cardiol., 25:171, 1995.

36. Sibley, R. K., Olivari, M. T., Ring, S. W., and Bolman, R. M.: Endomyocardial biopsy in the cardiac allograft recipient: A review of 570 biopsies. Ann. Surg., 203:177, 1986.

37. Sievers, H. H., Leyh, R., Jahnke, A., Petry, A., Kraatz, E. G., Hermann, G., Simon, R., and Bernhard, A.: Bicaval versus atrial anastomoses in cardiac transplantation: Right atrial dimension and tricuspid valve function at rest and during exercise up to thirty-six months after transplantation. J. Thorac. Cardiovasc. Surg., 108:780, 1994.

38. Swinnen, U., Costanzo-Nordin, M. R., Fisher, S. G., et al.: Increased incidence of lymphoproliferative disorder after immunosuppression with the monoclonal antibody OKT3 in cardiac-transplant recipients. N. Engl. J. Med. 323:1723, 1990.

39. Taylor, D. O., Ensley, R. D., Olsen, S. L., Dunn, D., Renlund, D. G.: Mycophenolate mofetil (RS-61443): Preclinical, clinical, and three-year experience in heart transplantation. J. Heart Lung Transplant., 13:S130, 1994.

40. Thomas, F. T., Szentpetery, S. S., Mammana, R. E., et al.: Long-distance transportation of human hearts for transplantation. Ann. Thorac. Surg., 26:344, 1978.

41. Webb, W. R., and Howard, H. S.: Cardiopulmonary transplantation. Surg. Forum, 8:313, 1957.

42. Wilson, L. G.: The development of cardiac surgery in Minnesota 1940–1960. In Wilson B.A. (Ed.): Medical Revolution in Minnesota: A History of the University of Minnesota Medical School. St. Paul, Minn., Midewiwin Press, 1989, pp. 481–528.

XI

LUNG TRANSPLANTATION

R. Sudhir Sundaresan, M.D., and Joel D. Cooper, M.D.

PATHOPHYSIOLOGY OF END-STAGE LUNG DISEASE

Four basic categories of pulmonary disease constitute the majority of indications for lung transplantation in most centers.

Obstructive Lung Disease. Obstructive lung disease affects about 10 million Americans, and chronic obstructive pulmonary disease (COPD) has been the fifth leading cause of death in the United States since the late 1970s.[1] Emphysema is the most common obstructive disorder treated by lung transplantation worldwide. An important subtype of emphysema is that related to alpha$_1$-antitrypsin deficiency, a congenital disease in which there is a lack of protection against neutrophil elastase in the distal airways. Multicenter trials have identified *age* and the *degree of airways obstruction*

(as reflected by the postbronchodilator forced expiratory volume in 1 second [FEV$_1$]) as important prognostic factors.[2]

Cystic Fibrosis (CF). CF is an inherited disease occurring in 1 in 2000 live births in the United States. It is the most common cause of end-stage obstructive lung disease in the first three decades of life.[3] In the lung, involvement of exocrine glands leads to copious thick secretions, which, along with poor ciliary clearance, lead to mucous plugging and chronic bronchiectasis. Although therapeutic advances have dramatically improved the outlook for CF patients, the majority die of respiratory failure in the third or fourth decade.[4]

Restrictive Lung Disease. Idiopathic pulmonary fibrosis (IPF) is the most common restrictive lung disease requiring lung transplantation. Excessive interstitial deposition of collagen causes loss of pulmonary compliance, associated with

TABLE 20–27. Lung Transplant Recipient Selection: General Guidelines

Clinically and physiologically severe lung disease
Limited life expectancy (12–24 months)
Other medical or surgical treatment ineffective, unavailable, or inappropriate, and prognosis poor without lung transplant
Ambulatory with rehabilitation potential
Satisfactory nutritional status
Appropriate mental state
   Satisfactory psychosocial profile and good support system
   Comprehends and accepts procedure, results, complications, future implications
   Well-motivated and compliant with treatment
Adequate financial resources for medications and follow-up
Absence of any contraindications

From Sundaresan, R. S.: Lung transplantation. *In* Makowka, L., and Sher, L. (Eds.): Handbook of Organ Transplantation. Austin, TX, R. G. Landes Company, 1995, pp. 133–171.

diminished lung volumes and expiratory flow rates, but usually with preservation of the FEV_1-forced vital capacity (FVC) ratio. Available data suggest that for patients with pulmonary fibrosis, median survival is less than 5 years from the time of diagnosis.[5]

Pulmonary Hypertension. This category includes primary pulmonary hypertension (PPH) and Eisenmenger's syndrome. PPH is the most common form of pulmonary hypertension requiring lung transplantation. This idiopathic process leads to luminal obliteration of small pulmonary arteries and a sustained elevation in pulmonary vascular resistance. It tends to affect young individuals, more often females. The National Institutes of Health PPH registry estimated the median survival to be 2.8 years.[6] Prolonged medical therapy is notoriously ineffective, although some patients benefit from continuous infusion of prostacyclin.

Miscellaneous Conditions. Other conditions treated by lung transplantation include sarcoidosis, lymphangioleiomyomatosis, pulmonary fibrosis from prior chemotherapy or radiotherapy, idiopathic bronchiectasis, and repeat lung transplantation.

RECIPIENT SELECTION

Crucial questions in the selection of recipients are: Which patients with end-stage lung disease should be transplanted?

TABLE 20–28. Contraindications to Lung Transplantation

Absolute	Relative
Acutely ill, unstable	Systemic diseases, possibly with involvement of nonpulmonary vital organs (e.g., renal, hepatic)
Significant disease of other organ systems, especially cardiac, renal, hepatic, central nervous system	Cardiac disease (coronary artery disease, ventricular dysfunction)
Uncontrolled sepsis (pulmonary, other)	Ongoing high-dose steroids
Uncontrolled neoplasm	Age >65 yr.
Still smoking	Unsatisfactory nutritional status (obesity, cachexia)
Psychologic or social problems, including drug or alcohol abuse	Osteoporosis
Noncompliant with treatment	Major prior cardiac or thoracic operation
Inadequate resources	

From Sundaresan, R. S.: Lung transplantation. *In* Makowka, L., and Sher, L. (Eds.): Handbook of Organ Transplantation. Austin, TX, R. G. Landes Company, 1995, pp. 133–171.

What is the ideal timing of the transplant procedure? Unfortunately, these questions cannot always be answered exactly. The general principle is to choose patients who are ill enough to require transplantation but who are well enough to undergo the procedure with acceptable mortality and morbidity.[7] One must subjectively determine an appropriate survival probability for the patient, given the natural history and prognosis of the underlying disease, and compare this with the survival probability after undergoing a lung transplant, which can be gleaned from registry data.[8]

General guidelines for selecting recipients for lung transplantation are presented in Table 20–27. Contraindications to lung transplantation are shown in Table 20–28. Guidelines for the timing of referral of patients for lung transplantation at the Washington University Medical Center have been summarized by Trulock[9] and are shown in Table 20–29. One must ensure that there are no other treatment options available that might delay or even obviate the need for transplantation. For example, the recent development of volume reduction of pulmonary tissue for emphysema has enabled the successful application of that option in a number of patients who had been on the transplant list.[10]

PREOPERATIVE EVALUATION AND MANAGEMENT OF POTENTIAL LUNG TRANSPLANT RECIPIENTS

Preoperative Evaluation for Lung Transplantation. The scheme for evaluating potential recipients is shown in Table 20–30.[9] Acceptance to the program follows review of the

TABLE 20–29. Guidelines for Timing Referral for Lung Transplantation

Chronic obstructive pulmonary disease and antitrypsin deficiency emphysema
   Postbronchodilator FEV_1 <30% predicted
   Resting hypoxia (Po_2 <55–60 mm. Hg)
   Hypercapnia
   Significant secondary pulmonary hypertension
   Clinical course
      Determine rate of decline of FEV_1
      Life-threatening exacerbations
Cystic fibrosis
   Postbronchodilator FEV_1 <30% predicted
   Resting hypoxia (Po_2 <55 mm. Hg)
   Hypercapnia
   Clinical course (extremely important)
      Increasing frequency and severity of exacerbations
      Weight loss
   Controversial issues regarding acceptability for transplantation
      Colonization with panresistant *Pseudomonas* species, *Aspergillus*, or mycobacteria
      Liver disease
Idiopathic pulmonary fibrosis
   VC, TLC <60% predicted
   Resting hypoxia
   Significant secondary pulmonary hypertension
   Clinical, radiologic, physiologic score >60 after 6 months of therapy
Primary pulmonary hypertension
   NYHA Class III or IV
   Mean right atrial pressure ≥10 mm. Hg
   Mean pulmonary arterial pressure ≥50 mm. Hg
   Cardiac index ≤2.5 L./min./sq. m.

FEV_1, forced expiratory volume in 1 sec.; VC, vital capacity; TLC, total lung capacity; NYHA, New York Heart Association.
From Trulock, E. P.: Recipient selection. Chest Surg. Clin. North Am., *3*:1, 1993.

TABLE 20–30. Scheme for Evaluation of Potential Lung Transplant Recipients

Medical history and physical examination
Chest radiograph, electrocardiogram, and routine blood tests
Other laboratory tests
  ABO blood type
  HLA type and panel of reactive antibodies (PRA)
  Serologic tests for hepatitis A, B and C; human immunodeficiency virus; cytomegalovirus
Pulmonary studies
  Standard pulmonary function tests and arterial blood gases
  Quantitative ventilation-perfusion lung scan
  Cardiopulmonary exercise test
  Computed tomography of chest*
Cardiovascular studies
  Radionuclide ventriculography
  Doppler echocardiography (with saline contrast*)
  Right heart catheterization
  Left heart catheterization with coronary angiography*
  Transesophageal echocardiography*
Rehabilitation assessment
  Six-minute walk test
  Determination of supplemental oxygen requirements (rest and exercise)
Psychosocial evaluation
Nutritional assessment
Additional appropriate studies to determine the status of any other medical problems

*In selected patients as indicated.
From Trulock, E. P.: Recipient selection. Chest Surg. Clin. North Am., 3:1, 1993.

resultant data by a multidisciplinary selection team. Potential recipients are then required to relocate within 6 to 9 months to the transplant center, along with their support persons. Patients with emphysema, pulmonary fibrosis, and septic lung disease must also participate regularly in a rigorous cardiopulmonary rehabilitation program.

Choice of Transplant Procedure. Both single lung transplantation (SLT) and bilateral lung transplantation (BLT) can be used to treat end-stage obstructive lung disease.[11, 12] Patients with CF or other septic lung disease must undergo BLT. An SLT procedure (with or without contralateral native lung pneumonectomy) would expose the patient to the risk of a number of serious septic complications. SLT is theoretically ideal in treating IPF, since the diminished compliance and elevated pulmonary vascular resistance of the native lung favor both ventilation and perfusion of the allograft, respectively. BLT has been employed occasionally in IPF when the recipient is large, especially if the lung volumes are normal. The ideal operation for PPH is still a matter of controversy. Although the traditional operation was combined heart-lung transplantation,[13] the scarcity of donor lungs has led to the employment of SLT, with excellent results. The disadvantage of this approach is that any significant late graft problem (for example, cytomegalovirus pneumonitis or chronic rejection) leads to severe functional ventilation-perfusion imbalance, which often proves fatal. Hence, several experienced groups have advocated using BLT in PPH, based on the notion that BLT provides these patients with more functional reserve in the long term.

Timing of Transplantation. Lung transplantation is not considered as an option until the patient's estimated life expectancy is 12 to 24 months. The average wait for a lung transplant in the United States is 13.5 months.[14] A potential consequence of this wait is that patients on the active list can undergo functional deterioration and even require ventila-

tory support. Inevitably, some patients die while waiting, the risk of which is highest with PPH, IPF, and CF and lowest with COPD.[9]

Other Important Issues. Approximate age limits are 55 years for BLT and 65 years for SLT. Mechanical ventilation is regarded as an absolute contraindication to lung transplantation, and ventilator-dependent patients are not accepted for evaluation. However, several patients have undergone successful lung transplantation after developing respiratory failure during their wait for suitable donors.[15]

Corticosteroid therapy was also traditionally regarded as a contraindication to lung transplantation on the basis of early experimental data showing it to have a prejudicial effect on bronchial anastomotic healing.[16] However, many patients with end-stage lung disease (especially COPD and IPF) are treated with steroids, and completely weaning such patients off these agents prior to lung transplantation may precipitate serious deterioration. A moderate clinical experience with lung transplantation in patients taking corticosteroids suggests that low-dose prednisone (less than 0.2 mg. per kg. per day) does not increase the risk of airway complications[17] and may actually enhance early bronchial circulation in the allograft.[18] Prior operation was formerly a relative contraindication due to concerns regarding the increased complexity of surgery and excess bleeding. A number of advancements in technique have decreased these risks, so that prior operation is no longer a contraindication.

CRITERIA FOR DONOR LUNG SUITABILITY

Only 20 to 25% of multiple organ donors have lungs that satisfy the traditionally rigorous donor criteria. Unfortunately, less than half of these are identified as lung donors, and this shortage of suitable donor lungs is the main impediment to more widespread application of lung transplantation. Most lung transplant centers recognize the traditional criteria for donor lung suitability presented in Table 20–31.[19] Recent strategies to overcome the donor lung scarcity include the

TABLE 20–31. Traditional Criteria for Donor Lung Suitability

Preliminary assessment
  Age <55 yr.
  ABO compatibility
  Chest roentgenogram
    Clear
    Allows estimate of size match
  History
    Smoking ≤20 pack-years
    No significant trauma (blunt, penetrating)
    No aspiration, sepsis
    Gram's stain and culture data if prolonged intubation
    No prior cardiac or pulmonary operation
  Oxygenation
    Arterial oxygen tension ≥300 mm. Hg, on inspired oxygen fraction of 1.0
    5 cm. H_2O positive end-expiratory pressure
    Adequate size match
Final assessment
  Chest roentgenogram shows no unfavorable changes
  Oxygenation has not deteriorated
  Bronchoscopy shows no aspiration or mass
  Visual/manual assessment
    Parenchyma satisfactory
    No adhesions or masses
    Further evaluation of trauma

From Sundaresan, R. S., Trachiotis, G. D., Aoe, M., et al.: Donor lung procurement: Assessment and operative technique. Ann. Thorac. Surg., 56:1409, 1993.

use of *marginal* donor lungs (that is, donor lungs that fail to meet all the traditional criteria) in carefully selected circumstances[20] and the use of living-related donors.[21]

TECHNIQUE OF DONOR LUNG PRESERVATION

The authors currently accomplish lung preservation using techniques shared by most other centers: bolus administration of prostaglandin E_1 before inflow occlusion and cross-clamp, pulmonary artery flush using 3 liters of cold (4° C.) EuroCollins solution, extraction of the lungs semi-inflated with 100% oxygen, transportation of the grafts under hypothermic conditions (0° to 1° C.), and protection during implantation by topical cooling with ice slush. The rationale for this approach is based on laboratory evidence that prostaglandin E_1 exerts a variety of beneficial effects, including potent pulmonary vasodilatation.[22] In addition, lung grafts appear to be capable of utilizing alveolar oxygen during the preservation interval to maintain a low level of aerobic metabolism until reperfusion.[23] Using preservation methods similar to the ones described above, we have achieved satisfactory lung function after ischemic intervals as long as 24 hours in a canine left lung allotransplant model.[24]

TECHNIQUE OF LUNG TRANSPLANTATION

Incision and Approach. SLT is accomplished through a posterolateral thoracotomy. For patients with Eisenmenger's syndrome secondary to atrial or ventricular septal defect, a median sternotomy can be used to accomplish cardiac repair along with transplantation of the right lung. When the thoracotomy approach is used, the ipsilateral groin is always prepped and draped within the field, so that femoral cannulation for cardiopulmonary bypass (CPB) can be performed if required. BLT is now accomplished through the bilateral transverse thoracosternotomy incision (*clamshell* approach), which provides exposure far superior to that afforded by median sternotomy (Fig. 20–57).[25]

Choice of Side. A general consideration in SLT is to try to avoid the side of a prior thoracotomy or pleurodesis if possible. Otherwise, in SLT performed for obstructive or restrictive lung disease, the approach is to transplant the side with the least function demonstrated by preoperative quantitative ventilation-perfusion lung scintigraphy. In SLT for PPH, the approach is to transplant the side with the best function so to minimize postoperative ventilation-perfusion mismatching.

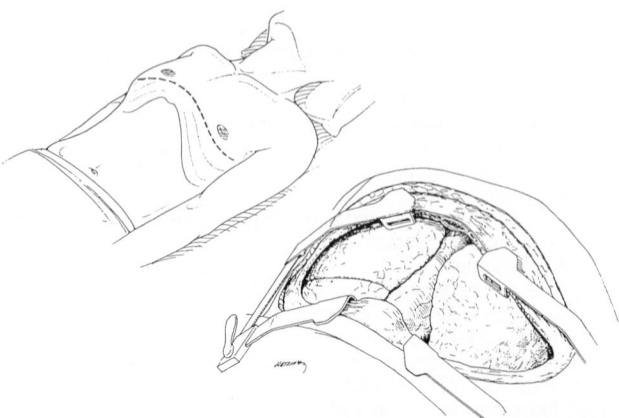

Figure 20–57. Clamshell incision used for bilateral lung transplantation. (Reprinted from Arcidi, J. M., and Patterson, G. A.: Technique of bilateral lung transplantation. *In* Patterson, G. A., and Couraud, L. [Eds.]: Current Topics in General Thoracic Surgery: An International Series, Vol. 3: Lung Transplantation; with kind permission from Elsevier Science—NL, Sara Burgerhartstraat 25, 1055 KV Amsterdam, The Netherlands.)

Bilateral lung replacement is accomplished using a bilateral sequential single lung technique, in which the side with the least function is transplanted first. If there is no discrepancy between sides, the approach is to reimplant the right lung first.

Conduct of the Operation and Use of Cardiopulmonary Bypass. Aside from lung transplants for pulmonary vascular disease, CPB is used in a selective fashion. In SLT, after initial dissection of hilar vessels, the ipsilateral pulmonary artery is temporarily occluded. The patient is then carefully observed, with attention being paid to the pulmonary artery pressure and right ventricular function, as judged by transesophageal echocardiography. If pulmonary artery occlusion is well tolerated, pneumonectomy is performed, followed by implantation of the graft. In BLT, CPB is also used in a selective manner (see below).

In general, CPB in lung transplantation is used for inadequate ventilation, oxygenation, and/or hemodynamics. CPB is routinely used for all transplants for pulmonary vascular disease and is instituted prior to extraction of the recipient lung. CPB is almost never required in SLT for emphysema but is occasionally required in SLT for IPF, especially if there is associated secondary pulmonary hypertension. In about 10 to 20% of bilateral sequential lung transplants, CPB is required to facilitate the implantation of the second lung, due to dysfunction in the first allograft implanted, resulting in unsatisfactory gas exchange and/or hemodynamics upon clamping of the pulmonary artery of the remaining native lung. When CPB is required in SLT, cannulation is usually performed in the chest, although another alternative is femoral cannulation. In BLTs, standard cannulation techniques are employed utilizing the right atrial appendage and ascending aorta.

In patients with PPH and severe hypoxemia, it is necessary to rule out the presence of a patent foramen ovale. This is usually identified during the pretransplant evaluation. However, a transesophageal echocardiogram bubble study is also performed after anesthesia induction. If a patent foramen ovale, significant enough to require closure, is identified, closure is performed immediately after institution of CPB. Subsequently, the right lung is excised and the allograft implanted. A similar order is followed in Eisenmenger's syndrome; that is, the patient is first placed on CPB, after which the cardiac defect is repaired. Then pneumonectomy is performed, and the allograft is implanted.

Technique of Lung Implantation. A technique originally described by Cooper and colleagues[26] or a modification of it is often used. The recipient pneumonectomy is begun after collapsing the lung and dividing the pulmonary ligament. The pulmonary artery and its first branch are then dissected, allowing temporary occlusion to be performed. If this is tolerated satisfactorily, the first branch of the pulmonary artery is divided between ligatures, and the remainder of the arterial trunk is divided between vascular staple lines. Pulmonary venous tributaries are divided between ligatures peripherally, leaving the venous stumps as long as possible. Both pulmonary veins are also fully mobilized intrapericardially. Finally, the main bronchus is transected (Fig. 20–58). In patients with end-stage lung disease, the bronchial circulation can be hypertrophied, and it is imperative to secure adequate hemostasis around the bronchus and in the subcarinal space prior to implantation.

Topical cooling of the graft during implantation is critical and is accomplished by wrapping the allograft in a gauze sponge soaked in ice slush. The bronchial anastomosis is performed first (Fig. 20–59), using a continuous 4-0 monofilament absorbable suture to approximate the membranous portion. The donor and recipient cartilaginous arches are approximated using a telescoping or intussuscepting technique, using interrupted figure-of-eight or horizontal mat-

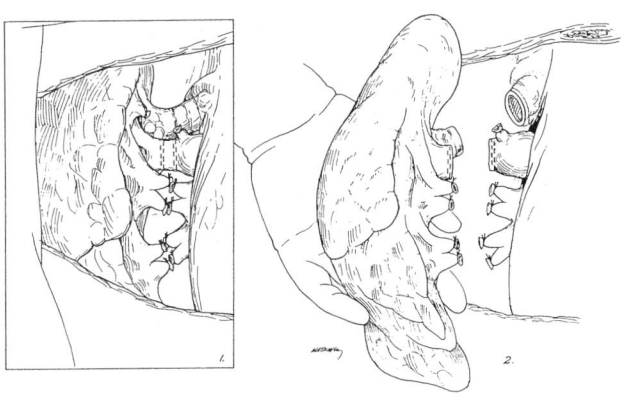

Figure 20–58. Technique of explantation of recipient (right) lung. (Reprinted from Arcidi, J. M., and Patterson, G. A.: Technique of bilateral lung transplantation. *In* Patterson, G. A., and Couraud, L. [Eds.]: Current Topics in General Thoracic Surgery: An International Series, Vol. 3: Lung Transplantation; with kind permission from Elsevier Science—NL, Sara Burgerhartstraat 25, 1055 KV Amsterdam, The Netherlands.)

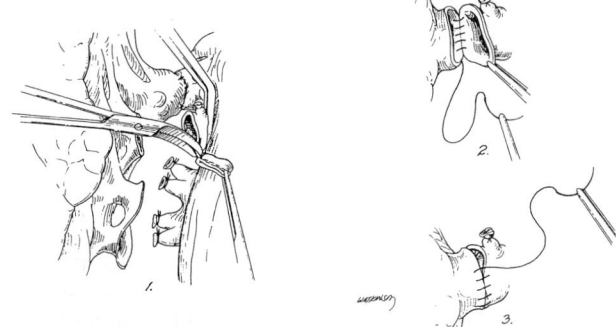

Figure 20–60. Technique of pulmonary artery anastomosis. (Reprinted from Arcidi, J. M., and Patterson, G. A.: Technique of bilateral lung transplantation. *In* Patterson, G. A., and Couraud, L. [Eds.]: Current Topics in General Thoracic Surgery: An International Series, Vol. 3: Lung Transplantation; with kind permission from Elsevier Science—NL, Sara Burgerhartstraat 25, 1055 KV Amsterdam, The Netherlands.)

tress sutures of a similar suture material, so that the smaller bronchus telescopes by about one cartilaginous ring within the larger bronchus. The loose peribronchial nodal tissue is then approximated to cover the anastomosis. The use of simple interrupted sutures to perform an end-to-end anastomosis, as originally described, is used only for small-caliber donor and recipient bronchi. Bronchial omentopexy is no longer employed. The pulmonary artery anastomosis is performed next by applying a vascular clamp centrally on the recipient artery and then trimming the donor and recipient arteries to appropriate lengths. An end-to-end anastomosis is then created using a continuous 5-0 monofilament nonabsorbable suture (Fig. 20–60). The left atrial anastomosis is performed last, after application of a Statinsky clamp centrally on the recipient left atrium. A large recipient atrial cuff is created by excising the pulmonary vein stumps and trimming them appropriately. The anastomosis is then created using a continuous 4-0 monofilament nonabsorbable suture (Fig. 20–61). Before restoring perfusion to the graft, 500 to 1000 mg. of methylprednisolone is administered. Gentle manual ventilation of the graft is commenced, and the graft is then de-aired both antegrade (by temporarily releasing the pulmonary artery clamp) and retrograde (by temporarily releasing the left atrial clamp). Full perfusion is then restored to the graft, ending the ischemic interval. Two chest

drains are inserted in the pleural space, and a standard closure is performed. Finally, the double-lumen endotracheal tube is exchanged for a regular single-lumen tube. Fiberoptic bronchoscopy is carried out through the tube to verify that the donor bronchial mucosa is pink and viable and to aspirate any blood and secretions from the donor and recipient airways.

POSTOPERATIVE MANAGEMENT

These strategies reflect the biases of the Washington University Lung Transplant Program.

Intensive Care Unit Monitoring. The recipient is admitted postoperatively to the intensive care unit, where monitoring includes the electrocardiogram, oximetry, and continuous monitoring of systemic and pulmonary arterial pressures. All patients undergo quantitative perfusion lung scintigraphy immediately after transplantation to document the percentage of overall pulmonary blood flow to the graft (in SLT) or to document the distribution between the two sides following BLT.

Pain Control. Pain relief is achieved with the use of an epidural catheter. This is removed after several days, and patient-controlled analgesia (PCA) is initiated.

Ventilation. Ventilatory management varies with the type of transplantation. In SLT for emphysema, no positive end-

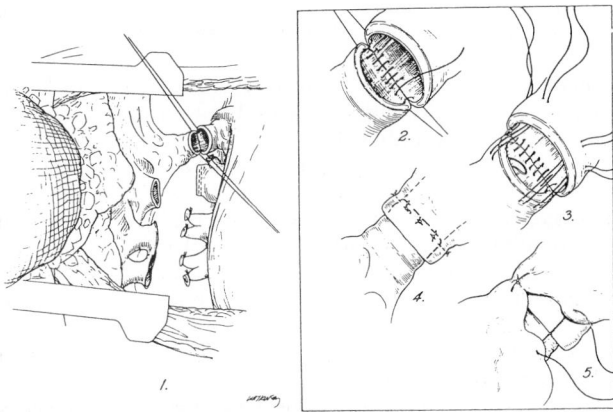

Figure 20–59. Telescoping technique used in the bronchial anastomosis. (Reprinted from Arcidi, J. M., and Patterson, G. A.: Technique of bilateral lung transplantation. *In* Patterson, G. A., and Couraud, L. [Eds.]: Current Topics in General Thoracic Surgery: An International Series, Vol. 3: Lung Transplantation; with kind permission from Elsevier Science—NL, Sara Burgerhartstraat 25, 1055 KV Amsterdam, The Netherlands.)

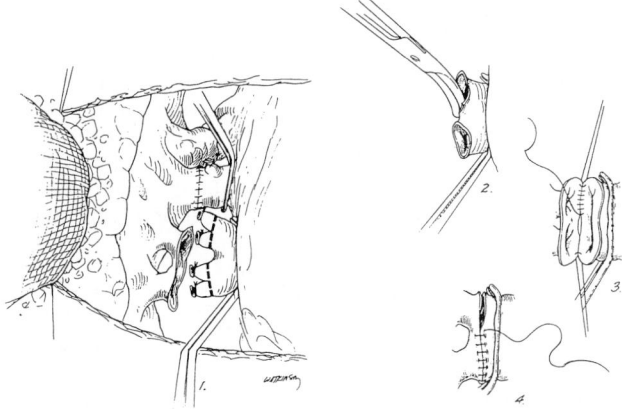

Figure 20–61. Technique of left atrial anastomosis. (Reprinted from Arcidi, J. M., and Patterson, G. A.: Technique of bilateral lung transplantation. *In* Patterson, G. A., and Couraud, L. [Eds.]: Current Topics in General Thoracic Surgery: An International Series, Vol. 3: Lung Transplantation; with kind permission from Elsevier Science—NL, Sara Burgerhartstraat 25, 1055 KV Amsterdam, The Netherlands.)

expiratory pressure (PEEP) is utilized, to avoid distention of the overly compliant native lung. Conversely, in SLT for PPH, we deliberately employ 10 cm. of water PEEP for at least 36 hours to minimize the development of edema in the hyperperfused allograft. In BLT or in SLT for IPF, standard ventilatory parameters are used, with 5 to 10 cm. of water PEEP. Oxygenation is optimized by minimizing fluid administration, the careful use of diuretics and PEEP, and aggressive chest physiotherapy and frequent bronchoscopies.

The approach to weaning and extubation is also somewhat variable. In SLT for IPF and emphysema and in BLT, we favor early weaning and extubation. However, in SLT for PPH, patients are maintained sedated and paralyzed (and therefore on full ventilatory support) for at least 36 hours after transplantation to avoid the development of pulmonary hypertensive crises.

Postural Drainage and Physiotherapy. Vigorous chest percussion and postural drainage are important to achieve maximum secretion clearance and early weaning and extubation. SLT recipients are maintained in the lateral position with the allograft side *up* for the first 24 hours, whereas BLT recipients are maintained supine as much as possible in the first 12 hours and rotated from side to side as tolerated. These aggressive maneuvers are withheld for the first 36 hours in single lung recipients for PPH.

Hemodynamics. Most patients are initially maintained on low-dose dopamine infusion (1 to 3 μg. per kg. per minute) to promote diuresis. Prostaglandin E_1 infusion (10 to 100 ng. per kg. per minute) to control the pulmonary artery pressure and pulmonary vascular resistance is also utilized. Recently, inhaled nitric oxide (at 40 to 80 parts per million) has been found to be useful in decreasing pulmonary artery pressures and improving oxygenation in patients with early allograft dysfunction.

Bronchoscopy. Bronchoscopy is necessary to clear airway secretions, inspect the integrity of the anastomosis, and obtain washings to guide antimicrobial therapy. It is performed at the conclusion of the transplant, on the first postoperative day, immediately prior to extubation, and whenever indicated by the clinical situation.

Pleural Drainage. Two drains are placed in each pleural space at the time of transplantation. An aggressive policy of early removal of these drains has been initiated as soon as there is no evident air leak and when fluid drainage is minimal.

Nutrition. Intravenous alimentation is started within 24 hours of the transplant. In most patients, an oral diet is started within 5 to 7 days of the procedure, but if prolonged ventilatory support is required, intravenous alimentation is stopped and an enteral feeding tube is placed.

Infection Control. In patients with chronic septic lung disease (for example, CF), initial antibiotics are directed at the recipient's organisms, based on preoperative culture and sensitivity data. Otherwise, initial antibiotic prophylaxis is guided by donor specimens (washings obtained at the donor bronchoscopy, and swabs from the donor bronchus at the time of implantation) and swabs from the recipient bronchus at the time of recipient pneumonectomy. If no organisms are identified, cefazolin 1 gm. intravenously every 8 hours is used for at least 3 or 4 days. If gram-positive organisms are identified, vancomycin 1 gm. every 12 hours is used. If gram-negative organisms are seen, ceftazidime 1 to 2 gm. intravenously every 8 hours is used. If pulmonary infiltrates progress despite the use of intravenous ceftazidime, imipenem 500 mg. intravenously every 6 hours is used. In documented bacterial infections, treatment is based on culture and sensitivity data. Herpes simplex prophylaxis is achieved with acyclovir 200 mg. twice a day for at least 2 years after the transplant. *Pneumocystis carinii* prophylaxis is achieved with

Septra-DS, 1 tablet orally twice a day on Monday, Wednesday, and Friday after oral intake starts. Oropharyngeal *Candida* prophylaxis consists of nystatin 500,000 units in the form of a mouthwash four times a day. For cytomegalovirus (CMV) prophylaxis, an attempt is made to match donor and recipient CMV serology. CMV infection is frequent and is most severe in CMV-negative recipients receiving lungs from CMV-positive donors. Therefore, CMV prophylaxis is employed when a CMV-positive graft is implanted into a CMV-negative recipient. The regimen begins on day 14 and consists of ganciclovir 5 mg. per kg. intravenously twice a day for 3 weeks, followed by ganciclovir 5 mg. per kg. intravenously daily for 8 to 9 weeks and ganciclovir 5 mg. per kg. intravenously three times weekly for 4 weeks.

Immunosuppression. Most programs use a triple-drug protocol that combines cyclosporine, azathioprine, and corticosteroids. The authors' current protocol is, pretransplant, azathioprine 2 mg. per kg. intravenously; posttransplant:

1. Cyclosporine 3 to 5 mg. per hour intravenously, later converted to an oral dose twice a day. The cyclosporine dose is adjusted based on the level as determined by a whole blood immunoassay.
2. Azathioprine 2 mg. per kg. intravenously daily (initially); later converted to 2 mg. per kg. orally daily.
3. Steroids: methylprednisolone 500 to 1000 mg. intravenously before reperfusion, then 0.5 mg. per kg. intravenously daily for 4 days; later converted to prednisone 0.5 mg. per kg. orally daily for 3 months, tapered to 15 mg. orally daily at 1 year.
4. Antithymocyte globulin (ATGAM, Upjohn, Kalamazoo, Michigan) 15 mg. per kg. intravenously over 8 to 24 hours for 1 week (usually from the first through eighth postoperative days).

POSTOPERATIVE SURVEILLANCE OF LUNG TRANSPLANT RECIPIENTS

Lung transplant recipients have an ongoing risk of acute and chronic rejection as well as septic complications. Therefore, routine surveillance (monitoring of clinically and physiologically stable patients) is necessary. Different lung transplant centers vary in their approach to surveillance, but the fundamental components include clinical follow-up, pulmonary function tests, chest radiograph, and fiberoptic bronchoscopy with transbronchial lung biopsy (TBLB).

The focus of pulmonary function tests has been mainly on the FEV_1. Frequent early spirometry allows a baseline value of the FEV_1 (the average of the two previous highest consecutive measurements taken 3 to 6 weeks apart) to be established.[27] Significant allograft dysfunction is then determined based on a fractional decline in the FEV_1 relative to this baseline value.[27] At the Washington University Lung Transplant Program, spirometry is carried out weekly in the first 3 months, then monthly between 3 and 12 months posttransplantation, and then every 2 to 3 months beyond 1 year.[28]

Fiberoptic bronchoscopy is performed liberally in the early postoperative period. Subsequently, surveillance bronchoscopies with TBLB are performed at 3 to 4 weeks postoperatively, at around 3 months, at around 6 months, at 1 year, and annually thereafter.[29] TBLB is also performed for clinical indications, including symptoms (dyspnea, cough), signs (fever, adventitious chest sounds), the presence of radiographic infiltrates, and the finding of declining spirometry and/or oxygenation. The practice for handling specimens is to send them in formaldehyde for routine hematoxylin and eosin staining. Gomori methenamine silver stains are routinely obtained to detect the presence of fungi or *Pneumocystis carinii*, and acid-fast staining is routinely done. Additionally, immunoperoxidase staining (for detection of CMV infection) and connective tissue stains (for detection of bronchiolitis obliterans) are obtained if clinically indicated. Occasionally, patients present with clinical and physiologic deterioration in whom fiberoptic bronchoscopy with TBLB is inconclusive. Under these circumstances, open lung biopsy may be necessary to clarify the underlying pathology (especially in documenting the presence of bronchiolitis obliterans).

REJECTION IN LUNG ALLOGRAFTS

Acute Rejection

Acute lung allograft rejection is a frequent clinical problem encountered any time from 3 to 5 days after the transplant to several years later. Experience indicates that nearly all patients have at least one acute rejection episode in the first 3 to 4 weeks after transplantation, and the subsequent risk seems to decrease with time.

Acute lung allograft rejection has numerous manifestations, but none is truly specific for rejection. The early manifestations (within the first month) can also differ substantially from those in the late phase (several months or even years after the transplant). In the first few weeks after lung transplantation, the usual indications of acute rejection are malaise, mild dyspnea, fever (more than 0.5° C. above the previous stable baseline), a drop in oxygenation (PO_2 dropping by more than 10 mm. Hg below the previous stable baseline), a slight drop in spirometry (FEV_1 dropping by more than 10% from the previous stable baseline), and a new or changing infiltrate on chest radiograph (in particular, a hilar or basal haziness). The differential diagnosis in the early postoperative period includes acute rejection, bacterial sepsis, and pulmonary edema (resulting either from reperfusion injury or from iatrogenic fluid overload). In the late posttransplantation period, acute rejection may result in a similar constellation of clinical features but without any chest x-ray abnormalities. At this stage, the main differential diagnosis is acute rejection, CMV infection, and chronic allograft rejection.

The clinical picture described here usually raises the suspicion of acute rejection. Formerly, antirejection therapy was begun solely on clinical grounds, so that the diagnosis was ascertained only in retrospect after observing an appropriate response. An aggressive approach for documenting acute rejection by fiberoptic bronchoscopy with TBLB is the current practice. Bronchoalveolar lavage (BAL) is usually done concomitant to TBLB but is useful mainly in identifying graft infection. The utility of TBLB in diagnosing acute lung allograft rejection in heart-lung transplant recipients is well established, with a sensitivity of 84% and a specificity of 100%.[30] The key histologic finding in acute lung allograft rejection is that of perivascular mononuclear cellular infiltrates.

The approach to the management of acute lung allograft rejection at Washington University has recently been summarized by Trulock[28] and is similar to that followed by most lung transplant programs. The basic components include:

1. High-dose corticosteroids, consisting of an intravenous bolus of methylprednisolone (500 to 1000 mg. daily for 3 days). This usually reverses most acute rejection episodes.

2. An increase in the maintenance prednisone dose to 1 mg. per kg. per day, then tapering back to the previous dose over 2 to 3 weeks. This approach has been found to be useful in treating severe acute rejection episodes, especially if the oral prednisone dose has been drastically diminished or actually discontinued.

3. In unusual acute rejection episodes refractory to steroids, options include the use of OKT3 monoclonal antibody (5 mg. per day for 10 to 14 days) or antithymocyte globulin (ATGAM, 10 to 20 mg. per kg. per day for 10 to 14 days).

Successful treatment of acute rejection as described above generally produces improvement in the clinical, radiographic, histologic, and physiologic parameters. Despite this, however, several investigators have furnished evidence that repeated or severe episodes of early acute rejection predispose lung transplant recipients to the later development of chronic lung rejection or bronchiolitis obliterans.[31]

Chronic Lung Allograft Rejection and Bronchiolitis Obliterans Syndrome

With the achievement of considerably better early survival in clinical lung transplantation, the entity of obliterative bronchiolitis (OB) has become recognized as the main impediment to prolonged survival. OB is an inflammatory disorder of the small airways and was first described in the lung transplant population in 1984.[32] It was originally thought to affect about 25 to 30% of long-term survivors of heart-lung transplantation, but OB is also being recognized after isolated single and bilateral lung transplantation. OB has no predilection for age, sex, or indication for transplantation. A recent retrospective review showed that OB appears to exhibit considerable latency (with an average of 15 months before onset) and that, if followed for a sufficient time interval, has a prevalence as high as 50%.[33]

This syndrome of chronic lung allograft dysfunction is associated with characteristic clinical, functional, and histologic features. Clinically, the patient may complain of dry or productive cough and dyspnea refractory to bronchodilators, along with generalized and progressive respiratory difficulty. The predominant functional abnormality is airflow obstruction, as evidenced by serial decline in the FEV_1. The characteristic histologic correlate of this form of graft dysfunction is OB, which consists of dense fibrosis and scar tissue that obliterates the bronchial wall and lumen, along with bronchiectatic widening of the peripheral as well as the central bronchi. At a 1993 meeting of representative members of the International Society for Heart and Lung Transplantation, the term bronchiolitis obliterans syndrome (BOS) was proposed to connote this graft dysfunction secondary to progressive airway disease for which there is no specific identifiable etiology.[27] It is now widely presumed (but not proved) that BOS is a manifestation of chronic lung allograft rejection.

To date, the fibrosis resulting from BOS is irreversible, and there is no satisfactory treatment once it is established. Since the true pathogenesis of BOS is unknown, the standard treatment in most centers has been empiric and consists of augmented immunosuppression,[34] similar to that described for acute lung rejection. Although a few patients stabilize with this treatment, most experience a steady progression of the disease and often succumb to it or to opportunistic infections induced by the augmented immunosuppression. Repeat transplantation has been attempted in some centers for severe BOS, with far less success than that achieved in primary lung transplantation.[8] Hence a strong research effort to elucidate the etiology and pathogenesis of BOS is vital if any hope of effective prophylactic or therapeutic intervention is to be entertained.

BRONCHIAL ANASTOMOTIC COMPLICATIONS IN LUNG TRANSPLANTATION

Failure of bronchial anastomotic healing in lung transplantation usually represents an ischemic complication. Although such complications were formerly frequent and a

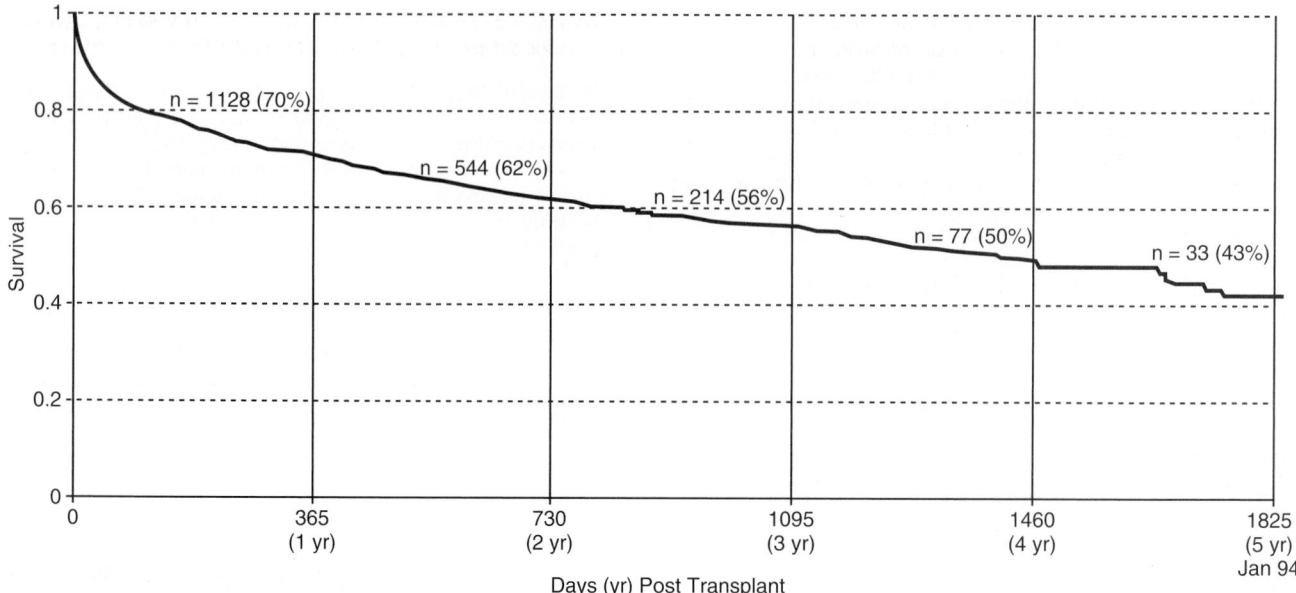

Figure 20–62. Five-year actuarial survival for total reported international experience. (From the St. Louis International Lung Transplant Registry, Courtesy of Dr. Joel D. Cooper.)

serious impediment to progress in the field, the incidence is now dramatically decreased. Most airway complications can be treated conservatively, with a combination of early drainage followed by bronchoscopic débridement and dilatation and/or stent placement. Schafers and his colleagues recently reported a successful experience in a small number of patients with bronchial strictures who underwent bronchoplasty.[35] Retransplantation is an option but is generally the last resort.

RESULTS OF LUNG TRANSPLANTATION

Until recently, success in lung transplantation was based on hospital survival rates. In recent years, early results have

steadily improved.[36, 37] The results of 131 consecutive lung transplants have been reported, and a 92% hospital survival has been achieved.[37] Therefore, in addition to analyzing early survival, a critical evaluation of the long-term survival rates and the functional results following lung transplantation must be made.

Survival Trends

The St. Louis International Lung Transplant Registry is a voluntary international registry.[8] It contains survival and other clinical data, and as of the September 1994 update, it represented a cumulative experience of over 2700 lung transplants from more than 121 programs worldwide. Actu-

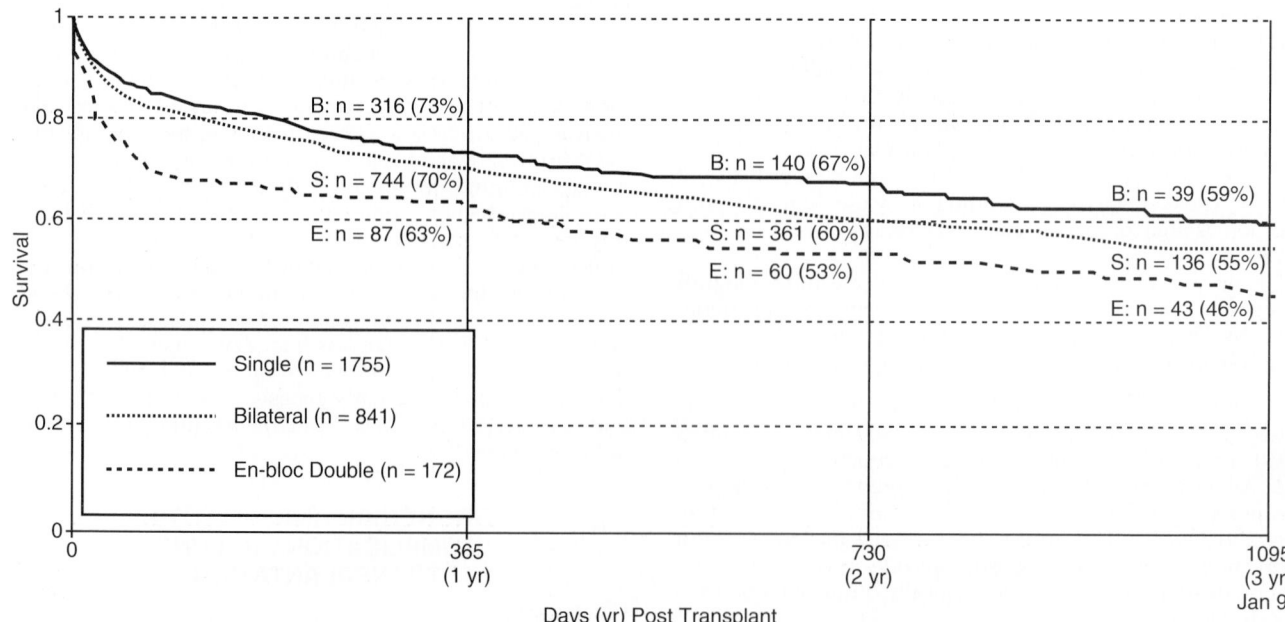

Figure 20–63. Three-year actuarial survival, by type of transplant, for reported international experience. (From the St. Louis International Lung Transplant Registry, Courtesy of Dr. Joel D. Cooper.)

arial survival data for the reported international experience is shown in Figure 20–62. One-year survival for all patients is 70%, and the 5-year survival is 43%. The 3-year actuarial survival by the *type of transplant* (Fig. 20–63) shows a slight (but not significant) survival advantage for patients undergoing bilateral compared with single lung replacement. Three-year actuarial survival *by diagnosis* is shown in Figure 20–64 and does not differ substantially among the different groups. The long-term results of lung transplantation can be expected to continue to improve in the future, since the vast majority of reported transplants (about 90%) were recorded over the past 4 years,[8] many from new centers that are still gathering experience.

Functional Results

In general, the functional outcome of lung transplantation has been excellent and sustained in all of the diagnostic groups. Two recent reports analyzed the functional outcome in single and bilateral lung transplantation for emphysema.[11, 12] The University of Toronto group reported improvement in FEV_1, PaO_2, and distance covered in the 6-minute walk test, all of which were significantly better following bilateral lung replacement compared with single lung replacement.[11] The Washington University study showed similar improvements but also a higher incidence of complications in the BLT group.[12] Both SLT and BLT are suitable operations for emphysema, in terms of both actuarial survival and functional improvement. BLT is a longer, more complex operation with a higher perioperative complication rate and is currently offered to patients under age 50 to 55. Furthermore, BLT provides more functional reserve in the event of a serious late graft complication (namely, chronic allograft rejection). Two obvious advantages of SLT for emphysema are that it is a shorter, simpler, less complicated operation and that it achieves more transplants from the same number of donors. Patients with emphysema over the age of 60 or who might otherwise represent a high risk are offered SLT.

Pasque and colleagues reported the initial Washington University experience with SLT for pulmonary vascular disease.[38] Based on a review of seven patients undergoing right SLT

TABLE 20–32. Causes of Transplant Recipient Deaths Occurring More Than 90 Days After Transplant (n = 407)

Cause of Death	Number of Deaths	% of Deaths > 90 Days	% of Total Transplants
Infection (other than CMV)	117	29	4
OB/rejection	112	28	4
Malignancy	26	6	<1
Respiratory failure	26	6	<1
CMV	18	4	<1
Hemorrhage	8	2	<1
Heart failure	9	2	<1
Other	84	21	3

CMV, cytomegalovirus; OB, obliterative bronchiolitis.
From the St. Louis International Lung Transplant Registry, Courtesy of Dr. Joel D. Cooper.

for PPH (two of whom had simultaneous closure of atrial septal defects), they noted the following: no operative mortality and significant right ventricular functional recovery, as evidenced by improvements in pulmonary artery systolic pressure, central venous pressure, pulmonary vascular resistance index, and right ventricular ejection fraction. All patients were in New York Heart Association (NYHA) Class I or II postoperatively, whereas all had been in NYHA Class III or IV preoperatively. Longer follow-up of more than 30 patients treated similarly showed that the dramatic improvements documented in the early report are sustained for as long as 3 years.

The ideal transplant procedure for CF patients is a subject of some controversy. Egan and associates recently reported the largest single-institution experience with BLT for CF patients.[39] There were no operative deaths and, as has been reported previously, functional results were outstanding. However, the Papworth and Harefield groups continue to advocate heart-lung transplantation with the domino procedure whenever possible.[40]

Pulmonary fibrosis, the condition for which isolated lung

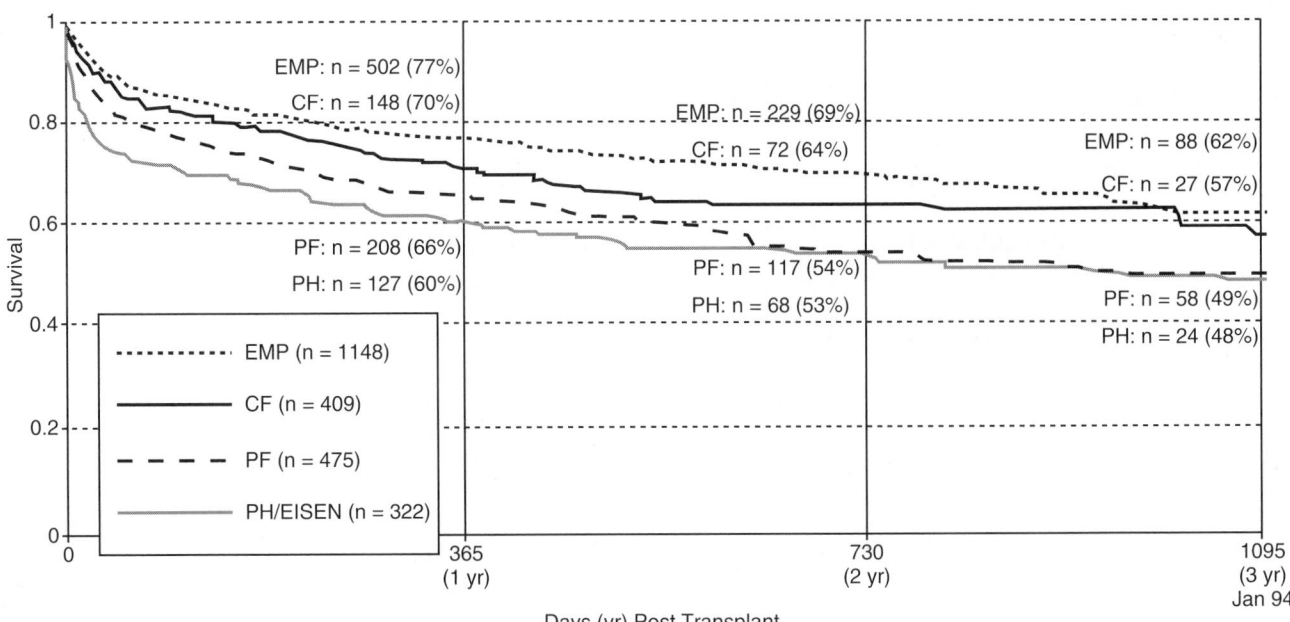

Figure 20–64. Three-year actuarial survival, by diagnosis, for international experience. (From the St. Louis International Lung Transplant Registry, Courtesy of Dr. Joel D. Cooper.)

transplantation was first successfully employed, represents a minority condition in most lung transplant programs. However, the functional results of SLT are excellent. Indeed, the longest surviving lung transplant recipient received a right SLT for IPF over 7 years ago and continues to do well.

Causes of Late Death

Table 20–32 shows data from the international registry and lists the major causes of death in lung transplant recipients occurring more than 90 days after transplantation. Although OB is listed as the second leading cause of death (at 28% of all late fatalities), the majority of fatal septic episodes and lymphoproliferative malignancies arise as a consequence of the heightened immunosuppression used to treat this entity. It is therefore quite clear that BOS in lung transplantation is the main factor limiting long-term survival (directly or indirectly) and that a better understanding of the immunologic and molecular mechanisms of this process is the main challenge facing clinical lung transplantation today.

SELECTED REFERENCES

Cooper, J. D., Patterson, G. A., Trulock, E. P., et al.: Results of single and bilateral lung transplantation in 131 consecutive recipients. J. Thorac. Cardiovasc. Surg., 107:460, 1994.
This recent paper provides an overview of an extensive single-center experience with isolated lung transplantation. The article discusses virtually all aspects of preoperative selection and postoperative care; analyzes the operative mortality and morbidity and the incidence of airway complications; and evaluates long-term survival in several different diagnostic groups. It also emphasizes the importance of acute and chronic allograft rejection in lung transplantation and the impact of cytomegalovirus infection.

Sundaresan, S., Trachiotis, G. D., Aoe, M., Patterson, G. A., and Cooper, J. D.: Donor lung procurement: Assessment and operative technique. Ann. Thorac. Surg., 56:1409, 1993.
This article provides an updated review of the traditional rigorous donor selection criteria. It also provides useful guidelines for management of the multiple organ donor from the standpoint of lung procurement, as well as a step-by-step description of the technique of donor lung extraction with pictorial accompaniments.

Toronto Lung Transplant Group: Unilateral lung transplantation for pulmonary fibrosis. N. Engl. J. Med., 314:1140, 1986.
This is one of the early reports describing the successful implementation of isolated single lung transplantation. The authors describe in detail their first two successful cases and summarize the history of lung transplantation as well as their own pioneering laboratory investigations in this field. This important article originated from the pioneering center in successful clinical lung transplantation.

Trulock, E. P.: Recipient selection. Chest Surg. Clin. North Am., 3:1, 1993.
This up-to-date article gives an excellent general overview of the pathophysiology of the various disease categories constituting the indications for transplantation. It provides an excellent summary of recipient selection criteria, indications and contraindications for lung transplantation, a scheme for pretransplant evaluation, and a summary of recent trends in lung transplant activity.

REFERENCES

1. Feinleib, M., Rosenberg, H. M., Collins, J. G., et al.: Trends in COPD morbidity and mortality in the United States. Am. Rev. Respir. Dis., 140:S9, 1989.
2. Anthonisen, N. R.: Prognosis in chronic obstructive pulmonary disease: Results from multicenter clinical trials. Am. Rev. Respir. Dis., 140:595, 1989.
3. Holsclaw, D. S.: Cystic fibrosis: Overview and pulmonary aspects in young adults. Clin. Chest Med., 1:407, 1980.
4. Kerem, E., Reisman, J., Corey, M., Canney, G. J., and Levison, H.: Prediction of mortality in patients with cystic fibrosis. N. Engl. J. Med., 326:1187, 1992.
5. Hay, J. G., and Turner-Warwick, M.: Interstitial pulmonary fibrosis. In Murray, J. F., and Nadel, J. A. (Eds.): Textbook of Respiratory Medicine. Philadelphia, W. B. Saunders, 1988, p. 1445.
6. D'Alonzo, G. E., Barst, R. J., Ayres, S. M., et al.: Survival in patients with primary pulmonary hypertension: Results from a national prospective registry. Ann. Intern. Med., 115:343, 1991.
7. Marshall, S. E., Kramer, M. R., Lewiston, N. J., Starnes, V. A., and Theodore, J.: Selection and evaluation of recipients for heart-lung and lung transplantation. Chest, 98:1488, 1990.
8. Pohl, M. S., and Cooper, J. D.: Results of the international registry. In Pat-

terson, G. A., and Couraud, L. (Eds.): Current Topics in General Thoracic Surgery. Vol. 3, Lung Transplantation. Amsterdam: Elsevier, 1995, p. 455.
9. Trulock, E. P.: Recipient selection. Chest Surg. Clin. North Am., 3:1, 1993.
10. Cooper, J. D., Trulock, E. P., Triantafillou, A. N., et al.: Bilateral pneumectomy (volume reduction) for chronic obstructive pulmonary disease. J. Thorac. Cardiovasc. Surg., 109:106, 1995.
11. Patterson, G. A., Maurer, J. A., Williams, T. J., et al.: Comparison of outcomes of double and single lung transplantation for obstructive lung disease. J. Thorac. Cardiovasc. Surg., 101:623, 1991.
12. Low, D. E., Trulock, E. P., Kaiser, L. R., et al.: Morbidity, mortality, and early results of single vs. bilateral lung transplantation for emphysema. J. Thorac. Cardiovasc. Surg., 103:1119, 1992.
13. Reitz, B. A., Wallwork, J., Hunt, S. A., et al.: Heart-lung transplantation: Successful therapy for patients with pulmonary vascular disease. N. Engl. J. Med., 306:557, 1982.
14. UNOS Update. September 1993.
15. Low, D. E., Trulock, E. P., Kaiser, L. R., et al.: Lung transplantation of ventilator dependent patients. Chest, 101:8, 1992.
16. Lima, O., Cooper, J. D., Peters, W. J., et al.: Effects of methyl prednisolone and azathioprine on bronchial healing following lung autotransplantation. J. Thorac. Cardiovasc. Surg., 83:418, 1982.
17. Calhoon, J. H., Grover, F. L., Gibbons, W. J., et al.: Single lung transplantation: Alternative indications and technique. J. Thorac. Cardiovasc. Surg., 101:816, 1991.
18. Inui, K., Schafers, H. J., Aoki, M., et al.: Bronchial circulation after experimental lung transplantation: The effect of long-term administration of prednisolone. J. Thorac. Cardiovasc. Surg., 105:474, 1993.
19. Sundaresan, S., Trachiotis, G. D., Aoe, M., Patterson, G. A., and Cooper, J. D.: Donor lung procurement: Assessment and operative technique. Ann. Thorac. Surg., 56:1409, 1993.
20. Sundaresan, S., Semenkovich, J., Ochoa, L., et al.: Successful outcome of lung transplantation is not compromised by the use of marginal donor lungs. J. Thorac. Cardiovasc. Surg., 109:1075, 1995.
21. Cohen, R. G., Barr, M. L., Schenkel, F. A., De Meester, T. R., Wells, W. J., and Starnes, V. A.: Living-related donor lobectomy for bilateral lobar transplantation in patients with cystic fibrosis. Ann. Thorac. Surg., 57:1423, 1994.
22. Novick, R. J., Reid, K. R., Denning, L., Duplan, J., Menkis, A. H., and McKenzie, F. N.: Prolonged preservation of canine lung allografts: The role of prostaglandins. Ann. Thorac. Surg., 51:853, 1991.
23. Date, H., Matsumura, A., Manchester, J. K., Cooper, J. M., Lowry, O. H., and Cooper, J. D.: Changes in alveolar oxygen and carbon dioxide concentrations and oxygen consumption during lung preservation: The maintenance of aerobic metabolism during lung preservation. J. Thorac. Cardiovasc. Surg., 105:492, 1993.
24. Date, H., Matsumura, A., Manchester, J. K., et al.: Evaluation of lung metabolism during successful twenty-four-hour canine lung preservation. J. Thorac. Cardiovasc. Surg., 105:480, 1993.
25. Pasque, M. K., Cooper, J. D., Kaiser, L. R., Haydock, D. A., Triantafillou, A., and Trulock, E. P.: Improved technique for bilateral lung transplantation: Rationale and initial clinical experience. Ann. Thorac. Surg., 49:785, 1990.
26. Cooper, J. D., Pearson, F. G., Patterson, G. A., et al.: Technique of successful lung transplantation in humans. J. Thorac. Cardiovasc. Surg., 93:173, 1987.
27. Cooper, J. D., Billingham, M., Egan, T., et al.: A working formulation for the standardization of nomenclature and for clinical staging of chronic dysfunction in lung allografts. J. Heart Lung Transplant., 12:713, 1993.
28. Trulock, E. P.: Management of lung transplant rejection. Chest, 103:1566, 1993.
29. Trulock, E. P., Ettinger, N. A., Brunt, E. M., Pasque, M. K., Kaiser, L. R., and Cooper, J. D.: The role of transbronchial lung biopsy in the treatment of lung transplant recipients: An analysis of 200 consecutive procedures. Chest, 102:1049, 1992.
30. Higenbottam, T., Stewart, S., Penketh, A., and Wallwork, J.: Transbronchial lung biopsy for the diagnosis of rejection in heart-lung transplant patients. Transplantation, 46:532, 1988.
31. Yousem, S. A., Dauber, J. A., Keenan, R., Paradis, I. L., Zeevi, A., and Griffith, B. P.: Does histologic rejection in lung allografts predict the development of bronchiolitis obliterans? Transplantation, 52:306, 1991.
32. Burke, C. M., Theodore, J., Dawkins, K. D., et al.: Post transplant obliterative bronchiolitis and other late lung sequelae in human heart-lung transplantation. Chest, 86:824, 1984.
33. Sundaresan, S., Trulock, E. P., Mohanakumar, T., Cooper, J. D., and Patterson, G. A.: Prevalence and outcome of bronchiolitis obliterans syndrome after lung transplantation. Ann. Thorac. Surg., 60:1341, 1995.
34. Paradis, I. L., Duncan, S. R., Dauber, J. H., et al.: Effect of augmented immunosuppression on human chronic lung allograft rejection. Am. Rev. Respir. Dis., 145:A705, 1992.
35. Schafers, H. J., Schafer, C. M., Zink, C., et al.: Surgical treatment of airway complications after lung transplantation. J. Thorac. Cardiovasc. Surg., 107:1476, 1994.
36. de Hoyos, A. L., Patterson, G. A., Maurer, J. R., et al.: Pulmonary transplantation: Early and late results. J. Thorac. Cardiovasc. Surg., 103:295, 1992.

37. Cooper, J. D., Patterson, G. A., Trulock, E. P., et al.: Results of single and bilateral lung transplantation in 131 consecutive recipients. J. Thorac. Cardiovasc. Surg., 107:460, 1994.
38. Pasque, M. K., Trulock, E. P., Kaiser, L. R., and Cooper, J. D.: Single lung transplantation for pulmonary hypertension: Three-month hemodynamic follow-up. Circulation, 84:2275, 1991.

39. Egan, T. M., Detterbeck, F. C., Mill, M. R., Thompson, J. T., et al.: Improved results of lung transplantation for end-stage cystic fibrosis. J. Thorac. Cardiovasc. Surg., 109:224, 1995.
40. Oaks, T. E., Aravot, D., Dennis, C., Wells, F. C., et al.: Domino heart transplantation: The Papworth experience. J. Heart Lung Transplant., 13:433, 1994.

XII

AUTOTRANSPLANTATION

R. Randal Bollinger, M.D., Ph.D.

Autotransplantation is the transfer of an organ, part of an organ, a tissue, or cells from one place to another in the same individual. Autotransplantation has several practical advantages over *allotransplantation* (transfer between individuals of the same species) or *xenotransplantation* (transfer between individuals of different species). Immunologic rejection does not occur, the donor is always readily available, and prolonged preservation is usually unnecessary in the case of autotransplants. Because of these advantages, autotransplantation was used earlier, more successfully, and more widely by all surgical specialties than other forms of transplantation.

The first well-documented autografting technique was the transfer of skin and subcutaneous tissue from the forearm to the face to form a new nose. The staged tubular pedicle graft technique was described in 1587 by Gasparo Tagliacozzi in his landmark textbook on plastic surgery, *De Cutorum Chirurgia per Insitionem (On the Surgery of Mutilation by Grafting)*. However, the earliest record of autogenous pedicle grafts antedates Tagliacozzi by more than 1000 years. The Sanskrit text of India, the *Sushruta Samhita*, describes restoration of mutilations of the nose, ear, and lip using pedicle grafts from the forehead, neck, and cheeks.[68] From its origin in the transfer of skin for reconstructive surgery, autotransplantation has grown to include muscle, bone, joint, nerve, artery, vein, composite tissue, endocrine gland, bone marrow, cardiac valve, kidney, ureter, bladder, and intestinal transfers.

SKIN AUTOGRAFTS

Skin grafts are used to cover wounds where insufficient skin is available to permit immediate (primary) or delayed (secondary) suture closure. All successful skin grafting was done on pedicles until 1804, when Giuseppe Baronio of Milan published the results of his experiments in sheep involving successful free transplantation of large pieces of skin from one site to another. The pinch graft introduced by Jacques Louis Reverdin in 1869 was followed by thin split-thickness grafts, which were introduced by Louis Ollier and more carefully studied and described by Carl Thiersch.[68] The modern, thicker split-thickness grafts were popularized by Brown and McDowell.[8]

Prior to the advent of free skin grafting, surgeons had no alternative to allowing open wounds to heal by contraction and epithelialization. Unfortunately, the epithelium that migrates from the cutaneous perimeter of the wound across the granulating surface develops no firm attachment to the underlying connective tissue. The rete pegs, which are closely interlocking ridges of dermis and epidermis found in normal skin, do not develop. The new epidermis is easily torn from the underlying tissue, causing such re-epithelialized wounds to break down frequently. In addition, wound contraction

during natural healing can cause contractures at joints and distortion of facial features. These unsatisfactory consequences of natural healing can be prevented by skin grafting.

A pedicle graft or one of several different types of free skin grafts may be selected, depending on the size of the site to be covered, the functional and cosmetic requirements of the recipient site, and the availability of donor sites. A *pedicle graft* is never separated from its blood supply, since revascularization at the recipient site is allowed to develop before the original blood supply is severed. Pedicle flaps, which include subcutaneous fat as well as skin, provide padding that prevents ulceration and are useful for wounds, such as decubitus ulcers, that sustain frequent trauma. Pedicle flaps should be used to cover wounds requiring later reoperation (e.g., for bone, tendon, or nerve repair) and in some cases in which appearance is an important consideration. Pedicle grafts can be *advanced* or moved to recipient sites far from their place of origin. The graft in the form of a flap is first created by making skin and subcutaneous incisions along three sides, leaving intact the side with the best blood supply. The flap is undermined and may then be sutured immediately to an adjacent area requiring the graft or may be delayed—that is, allowed to remain in its primary bed until its new blood supply is better established. In the form of a flap or a tube, the pedicle may be *walked* through a series of repeated divisions and reattachments until a distant recipient site is reached. The donor site may be closed by primary suturing or by covering with a split-thickness skin graft.

A *free graft* is completely separated from its vascular, nervous, and lymphatic connections during the transplantation procedure. A *full-thickness* skin graft is a free graft including the entire epidermis and dermis, whereas a *partial* or *split-thickness* graft includes all of the epidermis and a variable part of the dermis. *Anastomosed free grafts*, in which the small arteries and veins supplying a graft are reanastomosed to small vessels at the recipient site, have gained in popularity as microsurgical techniques have improved. Anastomosed free grafts are discussed further in the section on composite tissue autotransplantation.

Full-thickness skin grafts are used when pigment matching, resistance to contraction, or growth of a child are important considerations in the outcome of wound healing. Full-thickness grafts require a better blood supply for survival than do split-thickness grafts, because the graft vessels are cut below the level of their dermal branching. Relatively fewer cut vessels are available to absorb nutrients from the wound bed to meet the relatively greater nutritional needs of the thicker graft. Other disadvantages of full-thickness grafts include the limited area that can be covered, the need to surgically close the donor site, and their poor resistance to infection, which generally precludes use of these grafts on contaminated wounds. Full-thickness skin is best harvested from locations where the skin is thin, such as the eyelids, postauricular area, and supraclavicular area, or where it is loose and redundant, such as the flexor creases of the elbow, buttock, or groin. The grafts are cut freehand, using a template pattern made of the defect, and must be completely free of subcutaneous fat to be successful.

Split-thickness skin grafts are able to survive on compromised surfaces, such as granulating wounds contaminated with bacteria, because split-thickness skin is more richly supplied with open blood vessels on its underside. Split-thickness skin is used to cover wounds with precarious circulation and those with large areas of skin loss from burns or other traumatic injuries, as well as to cover large full-thickness skin donor sites. The skin is cut through a preselected level of the dermis. The dermis is approximately 20 times thicker than the epidermis in most areas of the body, permitting a wide latitude in graft thicknesses. Average grafts are between 12/1000 and 18/1000 of an inch thick (0.30 to 0.45 mm.), but thinner grafts must be taken from children, from the aged, and from certain areas of the face where the skin is thinner. Since only a part of the dermis is taken, the donor site heals spontaneously by epithelial outgrowth from the remaining epithelial islands, sweat glands, and hair follicles.[67]

Split-thickness grafts are cut using freehand knives, hand-driven drum dermatomes, or power dermatomes. Before the introduction of power and drum dermatomes, all skin grafts were cut with handheld knives. Since much skill and experience are required to cut grafts of uniform thickness, the freehand technique is now used primarily for covering small wounds requiring limited quantities of skin. The Goulian knife, which incorporates a guard, allows cutting of small split grafts that are far superior to the irregular, unsightly pinch graft. The Padgett and Reese instruments are drum dermatomes. Both require the skin to be fixed to the drum with an adhesive. When the drum and adherent skin are elevated, the calibrated knife blade slides back and forth on an axle to cut a long, wide graft of uniform thickness. The dermatome most often used to harvest split-thickness skin is the power-driven Brown. The rapidly vibrating knife (similar to barbers' clippers) is driven by an electric motor or gas turbine. The cutting width and depth are adjustable, much like a wood planer. The skin to be cut must be clean, well-lubricated with mineral oil, and locally anesthetized if the patient is not under general anesthesia. After the graft is cut, the donor site is dressed with fine mesh gauze and kept dry (e.g., with a hair dryer) until re-epithelialization is complete. The practical details of use for each type of dermatome are concisely described and clearly illustrated in the monograph by Rudolph and associates.[67]

Color match, texture, and scar visibility must be considered in choosing the donor skin, since grafted skin always maintains the epidermal specificity of its donor site. Split-thickness grafts are taken from broad, flat areas such as the abdomen, thigh, buttock, medial arm, or chest. However, in difficult cases such as extensively burned patients, any available skin can be used, and healed donor sites can be reused as often as necessary until coverage is complete. Split-thickness skin can be harvested from traumatically or surgically amputated tissue to close huge defects. Extra skin may be stored at 4° C. in normal saline with antibiotics for up to 4 weeks, then utilized in the same manner as fresh split-thickness skin.

A rich vascular supply is essential for support of a split-thickness graft. Skin does not survive when placed directly on bone, cartilage, or bare tendon. However, muscle, fascia, peritoneum, pleura, meninges, and vascularized fat, as well as bone débrided of its outer cortex to permit proliferation of granulation tissue, all support skin grafts. Exposed cartilage is best removed before grafting, and tendons are best

covered by full-thickness flaps. The wound to be skin grafted must be clean and free from bleeding. Surgical débridement and frequent dressing changes are employed to remove necrotic tissue, exudate, and all foreign material from the recipient site. When healthy granulation tissue, appearing pink or beefy-red from its many blood vessels, fills the wound and epithelial ingrowth begins from the margins, the wound is ready for grafting. The granulating bed with its rich supply of phagocytic cells is resistant to infection but is not sterile. Skin grafts generally survive when placed over beds containing less than 10^5 organisms per gram of tissue[58] unless the organisms are streptococci, which can rapidly dissolve transplanted skin. Further surgical débridement, administration of systemic antibiotics (e.g., penicillin) and topical antibacterials (e.g., silver sulfadiazine), and placement of pigskin xenografts or amnion allografts eliminate recipient site infections and promote healthy granulation tissue.

Hemostasis after débridement and at the time of grafting may be obtained by conservative electrocautery, temporary clamping, fine absorbable sutures, or direct pressure for 5 to 7 minutes. Topical hemostatic substances, such as oxidized cellulose or absorbable gelatin sponge, which create a diffusion barrier between the skin graft and its vascular bed, should be avoided. Meshing or perforation of the graft prevents serum accumulation beneath it. If the recipient site is free of debris and if bleeding is controlled and motion between the graft and its bed is prevented, the approximation necessary for fibrin adhesion and subsequent capillary invasion is achieved. A stable, firm pressure dressing or even splinting in plaster may be necessary to completely immobilize the graft. Cultured epidermal autografts are recent additions to the armamentarium of autotransplantation. In cases of extensive burns, especially in children, the ability to expand the available covering cells in culture may prove lifesaving.[13]

NERVE AUTOGRAFTS

Nerve autografts are used to repair unsuturable defects in major peripheral nerves. Wallerian degeneration occurs in the distal damaged nerve and the donor graft before reinnervation. The Schwann cells, endoneural tubes, and connective tissue survive in the form of conduits through which the axons may regenerate to reach viable end-organs. Axon regeneration progresses at a rate of 1 mm. per day in free grafts and 1.5 mm. per day in revascularized nerve grafts. As with autografted skin, one key to success is adequacy of the residual or acquired blood supply. Since free grafts of thick nerves usually undergo central ischemic necrosis, thin nerves are usually employed alone or in groups known as *cable grafts*. The grafted and recipient nerves must be of similar diameter and the ends carefully approximated. Microneural interfascicular reconstruction improves results.[48] The sural, brachial cutaneous, superficial radial, or lateral femoral cutaneous nerves can be used. The greater auricular nerve has been autotransplanted to replace the facial nerve in cases of facial paralysis. When the nerve gap is large, when the recipient bed is scarred, or when a thick nerve is needed, conventional nerve grafts frequently fail because of ischemia. Free vascularized nerve grafts of superficial radial nerve and the adjacent radial artery to supply blood have been utilized successfully in these adverse circumstances.[81] The combination of microneural and microvascular anastomoses provides hope for the future in an area of autotransplantation in which success is currently partial and unpredictable. Human muscle autografts that can provide long, large parallel arrays of basement membrane tubes to bridge large peripheral nerve gaps may also offer significant advantages over conventional techniques.[10, 54]

MUSCULOSKELETAL AUTOGRAFTS

Muscle. Nonvascularized muscle transplants rapidly undergo ischemic necrosis, resorption, and replacement by fibrous tissue. Transfer of an entire muscle group without division of its neurovascular supply has been used to restore function in the distribution of an adjacent damaged nerve, for example, radial nerve and muscle transfer for ulnar palsy. Microneurovascular free muscle transplantation of gracilis muscle from the leg to the forearm to re-establish finger flexion in a patient with severe Volkmann's ischemic contracture has been reported.[79] Free grafts of latissimus dorsi, gracilis, or extensor digitorum brevis muscle have been used to treat facial paralysis. Transplanted whole muscle can survive and be reinnervated 5 months after microneurovascular anastomosis. Muscle is frequently a component of composite tissue autografts, as described in a subsequent section.

Bone. Autografts of bone in the form of trephine defects with reinserted bone plugs have been found in a Bronze Age skull. In 1809, Merrem reported the healing of autotransplanted dog skull. Subsequent experiments have demonstrated that the bulk of the bone implanted as a conventional free autograft does not survive transplantation.[53] All but the most superficial cells of cortical grafts die of ischemia, causing bone resorption and replacement in a process termed *creeping substitution*. Larger numbers of cells survive in the case of cancellous bone, which has an open structure that facilitates diffusion of nutrients and ingrowth of osteoclasts and osteoblasts.[7] Local blood supply and recipient bed conditions are crucial to the success of conventional bone grafts. Broad contact with recipient bone and complete immobilization contribute to success. Infection, scarring, and irradiation of the tissues usually cause failure.

Bone grafts are used for the reconstruction of major skeletal defects produced by trauma, disease, or congenital malformation. The open reduction and internal fixation of some fresh fractures are supplemented with cancellous implants to promote healing. Barrel-stave autografts are used to achieve bony union in cases of pseudarthrosis or delayed healing of fractures. Cortical bone is used to supplement joint arthrodesis, and cancellous bone is used to fill cavities in other bones, such as the defect left after curettement of a unicameral bone cyst. Reconstruction of the jaw and face after radical cancer surgery or severe trauma often utilizes combined bone and other tissue grafts to re-establish function and contour.

Cancellous bone is usually obtained from the iliac crest, although it is also available from the metaphyseal ends of long bones. Cortical grafts are derived from the ribs, the central and proximal portions of the fibula, and the diaphysis of long bones. Vascularized, *living* bone grafts, in which the primary blood supply to the bone is preserved or immediately reconstituted, avoid resorption and maintain their original size and structural strength.[56] Vascularized grafts of ribs, fibula, and ilium are discussed in the section on composite tissue autografts.

Cartilage. Autotransplantation of cartilage has been used primarily in reconstructive surgery to rebuild nasal contours, to repair the pinna of the ear, and to fill defects in the bones of the face and skull. The cartilage graft heals to adjacent tissue by formation of a fibrous or fibrocartilaginous scar. Grafts from adults do not grow in their new position, and portions of the graft frequently undergo slow resorption. Most grafts are taken from the costochondral junction of the ribs, but nasal septum and articular cartilage have also been used. Interestingly, because of its avascular structure, few cells, and large amounts of uniform, amorphous collagenous matrix, cartilage is an immunologically privileged tissue.[26] Although all cartilage grafts tend to degenerate in time, allografts of cartilage last nearly as long as autografts.

Tendon. Autografts of tendon are used to replace damaged or destroyed tendons in the hands and feet in order to restore motion and strength. A strip of patellar tendon can be used to reconstruct the anterior cruciate ligament in the knee.[31] Free tendon grafts are taken from the palmaris longus, the flexor digitorum superficialis of the ring finger, the triceps, the plantaris, or the extensor digitorum communis tendons of the toes. A more detailed discussion of tendon grafting is contained in Chapter 42-X.

Other Connective Tissue. Fascia lata from the thigh has been autografted to the groin to reinforce a hernia repair, to the neck to cover the carotid artery after neck dissection, and to heart valves to replace damaged leaflets.[2] Autologous pericardium has been used to replace aortic valves.[18]

Hemijoints and whole joints have been autografted in animals and humans, with good early function but gradual destruction of the cartilaginous surface.[20] When small joints are transplanted on vascular pedicles, degenerative changes do not occur.[9]

Composite Tissue Autografts. Composite tissue transplantation involves the transfer of entire functional units rather than individual components of the musculoskeletal or other systems. Toe-digital transfers and the iliac rib or fibular osteocutaneous neurosensory flaps are examples of composite tissue autografts.[72] Successful one-stage hallux-to-thumb transplantation was first performed in humans by Cobbett in 1969.[41] In addition to fixation of the bone autograft with intermedullary wires and suturing of the flexor and extensor tendon autografts, the toe-digital arteries, dorsal veins, and digital nerves are all anastomosed to their hand counterparts to achieve a fully functional thumb. Osteocutaneous transplantation allows simultaneous reconstruction of both bone and skin defects, with provision of sensation in the transplanted skin. Conventional groin flap skin and subcutaneous tissue may be transplanted together with a segment of the underlying iliac bone, the origin of the sartorius and tensor fascia lata muscles, the superficial circumflex iliac artery and vein, and the lateral femoral cutaneous nerve.[80] This composite autograft can achieve a one-stage repair of bone, subcutaneous tissue, skin, and sensory defects following severe trauma. Similar grafts can be created from autogenous rib and fibula for reconstruction of the face and extremities, as described by Serafin and Buncke.[72] Objective monitoring of blood flow to the composite graft in the perioperative period is possible with laser Doppler flowmetry.[38]

VASCULAR AUTOGRAFTS

Arterial Replacement. Both autogenous arteries and veins are used to replace destroyed or obstructed sections of major arteries. Veins were the first to be used successfully, experimentally by Carrel in 1905 and clinically by Goyanes in 1906, and are currently the most commonly used substitutes for peripheral arteries.[15] Although femoral, popliteal, upper extremity, and neck veins have been used, the greater saphenous vein has proved to be the most satisfactory arterial replacement. The saphenous vein wall is sufficiently strong to withstand arterial pressures without becoming dilated or aneurysmal, yet it is flexible and easily sutured. The diameter is sufficiently great (minimum of 4 mm.) to avoid thrombosis, and nourishment is provided by the intraluminal blood flow. Saphenous vein is ordinarily harvested from the same leg for femoropopliteal bypass and from the opposite leg for repair of vascular trauma to the lower extremity. A groin incision over the saphenofemoral junction and one or more small longitudinal incisions over the course of the vein for ligation of tributaries permit removal of the vein as a continuous conduit. Alternatively, a single longitudinal incision can be used to remove the required length of saphenous vein. The vein segment is flushed with heparinized saline so that any leaks can be identified and repaired. Care is taken to avoid intimal damage, which would promote thrombosis. The vein is reversed to prevent obstruction by the valves and is sutured end-to-end for arterial replacement or end-to-side for arterial bypass. In cases of *in situ* saphenous vein bypass, the vein may be left in its bed, all branches ligated, all valves internally disrupted, and flow reversed by suturing the vein proximally to the femoral artery and distally to a tibial or peroneal artery.[40]

Autogenous saphenous vein is the material of choice for peripheral bypass procedures because it is the most resistant to clotting and infection. The smooth, natural endothelial lining is less thrombogenic than any known synthetic surface, particularly when placed across joints. Moreover, the lining surface heals itself and may sequester white cells to fight infection, unlike Dacron grafts, which provide a haven for infecting organisms in the interstices of their synthetic fibers. Autografts heal even when placed into the infected bed of a previous synthetic graft.

The versatility and ease of harvesting of greater saphenous vein grafts have led to their use in many locations. The subcutaneous crossover graft from a patent right femoral artery to an obstructed left femoral artery is performed in preference to an intra-abdominal aortofemoral bypass whenever age and associated diseases make the patient an unacceptable risk for major abdominal surgery. Saphenous vein is frequently used to bypass superficial femoral artery obstruction, by grafting from the proximal common femoral artery to either the popliteal artery or one of the smaller tibial arteries in the lower leg.[14] Visceral and cerebral ischemia has also been treated with saphenous vein bypasses from the thoracic or abdominal aorta. Patients with atherosclerotic coronary artery disease may have segmental occlusions bypassed with reversed saphenous vein grafts, a technique popularized by Favaloro in 1967.[55] Coronary artery bypass grafting is discussed more extensively in Chapter 54-XIV.

Saphenous vein is also used to create vascular patches for widening diseased arteries.[90] To prevent constriction at the site of a longitudinal arteriotomy, a diamond-shaped piece of vein may be inserted into the closure (Fig. 20–65). Whether used as a patch or as a tube graft, saphenous vein placed into the high-pressure, pulsatile arterial system undergoes

a variety of pathologic changes, which are described and illustrated in Chapter 50.

Intimal hyperplasia occurs in both autografted arteries and veins, but stenosis due to fibrosis of venous valve cusps could be avoided if other arteries were used for replacement of the diseased arteries. Unfortunately, it is uncommon to find a long uninvolved segment of artery in a patient with atherosclerosis severe enough to require autografting. Few dispensable large-diameter arteries are available, and more complicated operations than vein harvesting are required to obtain them. A variety of graft shapes can be created from the common, internal, and external iliac arteries. Certain dispensable arteries are anatomically situated in positions that allow relatively easy direct diversion to bypass obstructing lesions in more critical arteries. The internal mammary artery has been used increasingly as a preferred source of blood for partially occluded coronary arteries, and the splenic artery can be rotated down to the left renal artery to bypass proximal renal artery stenosis. In the Duke University renovascular hypertension clinical series, splenorenal arterial bypass achieved durable control of hypertension in 91% of patients. The radial artery has been used as a coronary artery bypass graft.[64]

Arterial autografts have been recommended for use in repairing fibromuscular dysplastic lesions of the renal artery and aneurysms of peripheral, renal, and visceral arteries. Arterial grafts are stronger and more flexible than synthetic grafts and are therefore especially useful in areas of extreme motion.[76] Infected prostheses, mycotic aneurysms, and infected arterial repairs can be successfully managed by excision and replacement with arterial autografts. Arterial and venous autografts are discussed further in Chapter 50-IV.

Venous Replacement. Autografting for repair of diseased or damaged veins has been much less successful than arterial replacement, primarily because of early graft thrombosis in low-pressure, low-flow venous systems. Autogenous vein remains the best replacement material, since no synthetic graft has consistently remained open except in the superior vena cava position.[36] The Vietnam War experience demonstrated that acute venous hypertension following interruption of major lower extremity veins increased the rate of amputation but was preventable if autogenous vein interposition grafts were used.[65] Edema was eliminated without the production of thrombophlebitis or pulmonary embolism. During the 1- to 2-week period after grafting, when a neointima is being formed, a distal arteriovenous fistula to increase flow through the graft and anticoagulation to diminish thrombosis may improve patency.[36]

ENDOCRINE AUTOGRAFTS

Autotransplantation of endocrine glands has had an indispensable role in the evolution of endocrinology. Berthold is acknowledged to be the father of experimental endocrinology for his studies in 1849 demonstrating that autotransplanted testes caused secondary sexual characteristics in castrated cocks.[39] Literally every endocrine gland has been experimentally autotransplanted, with identification of several technical requirements for success: delicate handling of the tissues, prevention of ischemia by cooling or placement in an appropriate medium, and implantation of small fragments. The oxygen and nutrients in interstitial fluid around a subcutaneous, intramuscular, or renal capsular implant maintain an endocrine graft until revascularization occurs if the fragments are no more than 1 mm. thick. Although thyroid,[78] pituitary,[39] ovary,[89] adrenal, testis, pancreas, and parathyroid have all been autografted in humans, only the last four are often transplanted therapeutically today. Excellent synthetic

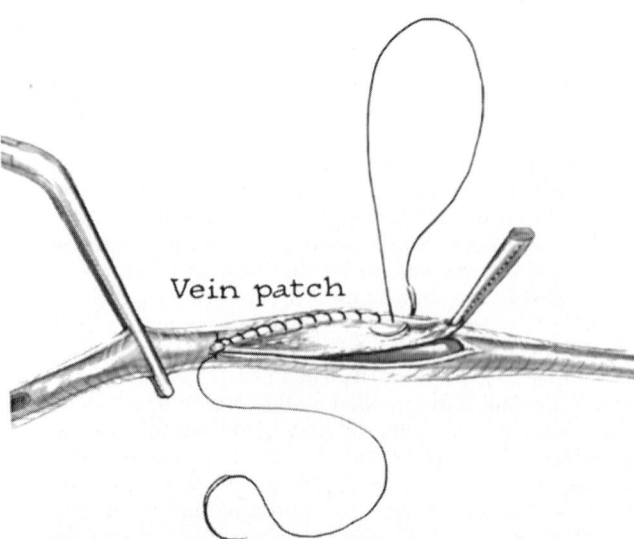

Figure 20–65. Application of a vein patch in closing an arteriotomy to avoid narrowing at the suture line. (From Wylie, E. J., Binkley, F. M., and Albo, R. J.: Femoropopliteal endarterectomy. Am. J. Surg., *108*:215, 1964.)

Vein patch

hormone replacement is available for thyroid, adrenal, and gonadal deficiency states.

Testis. Autotransplantation is the treatment of choice for an undescended testis.[27] The cryptorchid or ectopic testis must be removed from the abdomen and placed in a cooler location prior to age 6, and preferably at 1 year of age, for normal spermatogenesis to occur. Orchidopexy and repair of any associated hernia are performed as described in Chapter 37.

Pancreas. Pancreatic autotransplantations have been performed both as segmental grafts and as isolated islet cell grafts. Although it is clear that diabetes can be prevented when either type of graft is successful, each approach has its special problems that have limited its clinical usefulness. Segmental pancreas autografts contain large amounts of exocrine tissue with secretions that are difficult to manage. Despite occlusion of the pancreatic ductules by neoprene injection, all three autograft recipients in one series developed pancreatic fistulas but eventually recovered.[83] The tendency for venous thrombosis that causes ischemia and death of the tissue has been only partially relieved by creating a distal arteriovenous fistula between the splenic artery and vein.[45] Islets for autotransplantation have proved difficult to isolate in sufficient quantities from the fibrotic adult pancreas, particularly after chronic pancreatitis, and have often not prevented diabetes over the long term.[11, 51] Moreover, when dispersed islets are injected directly into the human portal vein, they have occasionally produced untoward effects such as disseminated intravascular coagulation, portal hypertension, and hepatic necrosis.[11, 82]

Pancreatic autotransplantation has been attempted most frequently in cases of total pancreatectomy for relief of the pain of chronic pancreatitis, but it has also been used after a modified pancreaticoduodenectomy for carcinoma of the head of the pancreas.[45] A report from the International Pancreas and Islet Transplant Registry[77] reveals that 13 of 17 segmental or total autograft recipients and approximately half of 79 islet autograft recipients do not require insulin. However, in cases in which less than a 95% pancreatectomy is performed, it is difficult to assess how much insulin is contributed by the pancreas left *in situ*.

Parathyroid. Survival of parathyroid autotransplants in humans was demonstrated histologically (Fig. 20–66) and biochemically by Wells in 1975.[87] Since parathyroid hormone replacement is not available and medical therapy for hypoparathyroidism is complicated, preservation and autografting of parathyroid tissue are essential to prevent the deficiency symptoms of tetany, psychologic disturbances, convulsions, coma, and death. Parathyroid glands removed during thyroid surgery should be cut into 1-mm. pieces and reim-

planted into pockets in the sternocleidomastoid muscle.[44] When all glands are removed for diffuse parathyroid hyperplasia, implantation of fragments into the forearm muscles facilitates subsequent removal of more tissue under local anesthesia if hyperparathyroidism persists.[88] Parathyroid tissue that has been cryopreserved functions normally when autografted to treat hypoparathyroidism. Parathyroid autografting is discussed more extensively in Chapter 25.

Adrenal. Hyperplastic human adrenal tissue has been successfully autotransplanted for many years.[17] Whole-gland autotransplantation with vascular anastomosis to the inferior epigastric vessels has been used to treat Cushing's disease.[91] The 1987 report of open microsurgical autotransplantation of adrenal medulla to the caudate nucleus of the brain for treatment of intractable Parkinson's disease awakened great interest in the topic.[42, 43] Subsequent multicenter trials demonstrated improvement, but not cure, of the disease and had substantial postoperative morbidity, so the technique is not recommended for widespread use.[28]

BONE MARROW AUTOGRAFTS

High-dose irradiation or intensive chemotherapy can produce severe bone marrow depression, leading to anemia, thrombocytopenic bleeding, and infection. Since 1956 it has been known that intravenous injection of bone marrow cells can restore hematopoiesis.[23] The responsible cells are hematopoietic stem cells, which occur at the low frequency of 4 per 1000 bone marrow cells but are capable of rapid replication and differentiation into myeloid, erythroid, megakaryocytic, and lymphoid cell series.[16] Bone marrow transplants are used to reconstitute the marrow of patients with acute leukemia and to speed bone marrow recovery in patients receiving high-dose myelosuppressive therapy for solid tumors.[32]

When marrow autografts are used, neither graft rejection nor the graft-versus-host reaction is a factor in transplantation success. Rather, outcome is determined by the number of leukemia cells in the remission marrow graft, the effectiveness of the antitumor therapy, and the number of stem cells that survive frozen storage. The hematopoietic marrow, obtained from a leukemia patient in remission or a patient with a solid tumor not involving the marrow, is harvested from the iliac crest and sternum by needle aspiration. The cells are mixed with a cryopreservative and cooled stepwise until frozen at $-192°$ C. The patient is given intensive, high-dose chemotherapy or *lethal* doses of irradiation, which destroy not only the malignancy but also the remaining marrow. The preserved marrow is then thawed and infused intravenously to reconstitute the hematopoietic system. This procedure has proved helpful in the treatment of non-Hodgkin's and

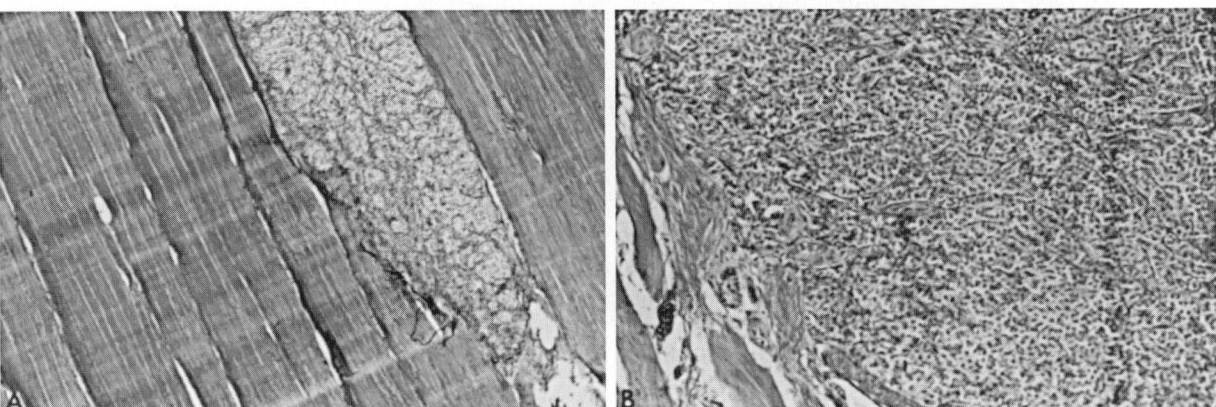

Figure 20–66. Histologic section of a parathyroidgraft within a muscle bed at magnification of 41× *(A)* and 100× *(B)*. (Courtesy of Samuel A. Wells, Jr., M.D.)

Burkitt's lymphomas, ovarian cancer, and Stage IV melanoma as well as acute leukemia.[16]

URINARY AUTOGRAFTS

Kidney. Renal autotransplantation and extracorporeal reconstruction permit salvage of some kidneys that cannot be repaired by conventional *in situ* operative techniques.[75] The approach was originally reported by Hardy, who used autotransplantation of the kidney to manage a very proximal ureteral injury.[35] Belzer added hypothermic pulsatile perfusion to improve preservation and permit *ex vivo* or *workbench* microvascular surgery on the kidney before reimplantation.[4] The kidney can be returned to its original site or grafted to the iliac vessels using the allotransplantation technique. The ureter can be reimplanted into the bladder or preserved intact during the autografting (Fig. 20–67).

In the case of a large high abdominal aortic aneurysm associated with a horseshoe kidney, hypothermic preservation and autografting to the Dacron aortic graft and vena cava were used to preserve renal function.[47] *Ex vivo* operations and renal autografting have been employed for extensive renovascular disease from fibrous dysplasia, atherosclerotic disease, or abdominal aortic aneurysms; for repair of traumatic arterial injuries; for excision of renal cell carcinoma involving both kidneys or a solitary kidney;[85] and for kidneys with diseased or damaged ureters that are too short for reimplantation.[62] Renovascular hypertension not amenable to correction by conventional surgical procedures responded to autotransplantation, with normalization of blood pressure and creatinine.[73] A remnant of renal pelvis can be anastomosed directly to the bladder following resection and autotransplantation for renal pelvic and high ureteric tumors.[58] Long-term renal function after autotransplantation with direct pyelocystostomy has been excellent.[63]

Ureter and Bladder. Synthetic prostheses and free grafts have generally failed as ureteral substitutes. Autotransplantation of the bladder in the form of a vesicopsoas hitch or a bladder flap is the treatment of choice for injury or disease in the distal third of the ureter.[6] Up to 18 cm. of distal ureter can be replaced with bladder by combining a tubular pedicle graft of bladder and the superior suturing (hitch) of posterior bladder to psoas tendon with chromic catgut. In cases in which a more proximal segment of ureter is lost or the entire bladder must be removed, autotransplantation of a segment of ileum currently provides the most successful replacement conduit (see Chapter 45). Alternative reconstructions include suturing one ureter to the other ureter (transureteroureterostomy), to the skin (cutaneous ureterostomy), or to the sigmoid colon (ureterosigmoidostomy). A contracted bladder from interstitial cystitis or partial resection can be enlarged by autotransplantation of a segment of ileum and cecum, an augmentation ileocecocystoplasty.[92]

GASTROINTESTINAL AUTOGRAFTS

The gastrointestinal tract is ideally suited for autotransplantation. The mesentery provides a long, natural vascular pedicle for attached grafts, and the vascular arcades provide easily anastomosed arteries and veins for free grafts. Small intestinal autografts are widely used to replace the colon after proctocolectomy for inflammatory bowel disease.[30] The principles of gastrointestinal autografting are well demonstrated by the replacement of the hypopharynx and esophagus with transplanted stomach, jejunum, colon, or free intestinal segments. These operations are performed most commonly following extirpation of carcinomas of the larynx, pharynx, or esophagus but may also be used to reconstruct strictures following ingestion of caustic substances and defects from severe trauma to the face and neck.

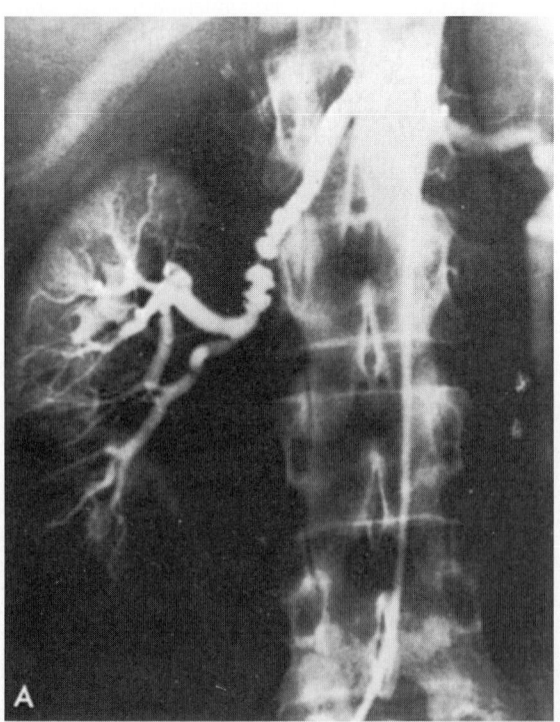

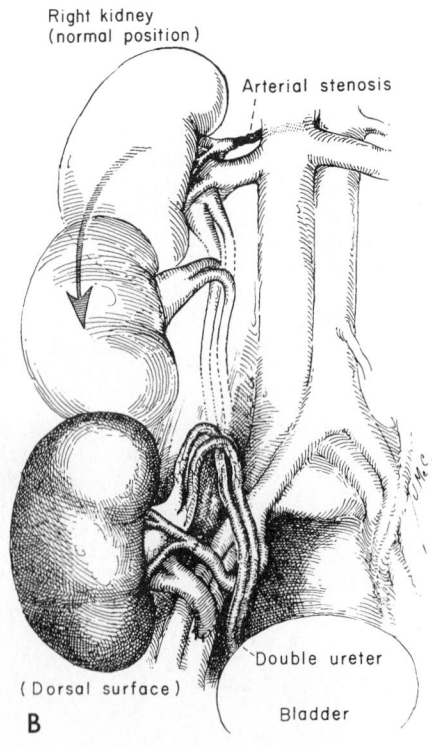

Figure 20–67. Ipsilateral renal autotransplant. A preoperative excretory urogram revealed a right complete ureteropelvic duplication, and an arteriogram *(A)* demonstrated medial fibroplasia involving the entire length of the right renal artery. The kidney was perfused extracorporeally while the renal artery was dissected. The organ was then rotated down into the iliac fossa *(B)* and rearterialized using the hypogastric artery without dividing the double collecting system. (*A* and *B* From Corman, J. L., et al.: Surg. Gynecol. Obstet., *137*:659, 1973. By permission of SURGERY, Gynecology & Obstetrics, now known as the JOURNAL OF THE AMERICAN COLLEGE OF SURGEONS.)

Stomach. Adams and Phemister reported the successful replacement of the lower esophagus with stomach after resection of an esophageal carcinoma in 1938.[1] To perform esophagogastrostomy, the stomach is mobilized by dividing all its ligamentous, nervous, and vascular attachments except the right gastric artery. After performance of a pyloroplasty or pyloromyomectomy to ensure drainage from the distal stomach, the stomach is passed through the esophageal hiatus and anastomosed to the proximal esophageal remnant in the chest. The stomach can even be transposed into the neck and sutured to the pharynx at the base of the tongue for reconstruction after pharyngolaryngectomy.[3] Problems associated with esophagogastrostomy include acid regurgitation esophagitis, intrathoracic gastric distention, distal graft ischemia, and the dumping syndrome characterized by diarrhea, colicky pain, and a rapid transit time for ingested food. Despite these shortcomings, stomach remains the most frequently used autograft for esophageal reconstruction after extirpative operation.[50] The procedure can be performed at low risk as a single-stage operation and achieves satisfactory long-term relief of dysphagia in at least 90% of patients.[19] The greater curvature of the stomach can also be formed into an isoperistaltic tube, as described by Beck and Carrel in 1905, or into an antiperistaltic one, popularized by Gavriliu and Heimlich, of sufficient length to reconstruct the entire esophagus. Gastric tubes, reviewed by Postlethwait,[61] have the advantages of a mucosal lining, a serosal covering, a natural opening into the stomach, and an excellent blood supply based on the gastroepiploic vessels.

Jejunum. Sections of jejunum with intact blood supply are most useful for replacing relatively short segments of the lower esophagus.[33] If a long graft is necessary, the jejunal arterial inflow and venous drainage may be tenuous at the proximal esophageal anastomosis. Careful section and positioning of the vascular pedicle (Fig. 20–68) are essential to

success. The autograft is brought behind the transverse colon and stomach, through the esophageal hiatus, and into the posterior thorax without tension. A pyloroplasty and temporary gastrostomy should be performed. If there is any question of jejunal viability, the proximal end can be left exposed in the neck for several days of observation before the cervical anastomosis is completed. Alternatively, the jejunal graft can be abandoned and replaced with a segment of large bowel.

Colon. The right colon, transverse colon, left colon, and ileocolon have all been used for autografts. The ileocecal valve continues to function as a partially competent valve after transplantation, thus preventing reflux up the ileal component of the graft. However, the left colon has a better diameter, a more muscular and less distensible wall, and a more dependable blood supply for total esophageal replacement than any other segment of large bowel.[34] Whether based on the left colic artery to produce an isoperistaltic graft or based on the middle colic artery to produce an antiperistaltic tube, the large marginal artery ensures adequate perfusion (Fig. 20–69). The colon can be placed through a posterior mediastinal, substernal, or subcutaneous tunnel to reach the neck. The last two routes are especially useful for bypassing nonresectable carcinomas in debilitated patients. A pyloroplasty and temporary gastrostomy should be performed, particularly if the vagus nerves are resected.

Free Jejunal Autografts. The first successful free intestinal autograft was reported by Seidenberg in 1959.[71] Although stomach, ileum, and colon have all been transplanted using microvascular techniques to re-establish their blood supply,[52] the jejunum just distal to the ligament of Treitz is currently the most frequently employed free graft.[45, 46] This segment of bowel has the largest vasculature and best matches the size of the hypopharynx and cervical esophagus. After an initial tracheostomy, laryngopharyngoesophagectomy is performed, with care taken to preserve the superior thyroid artery and a

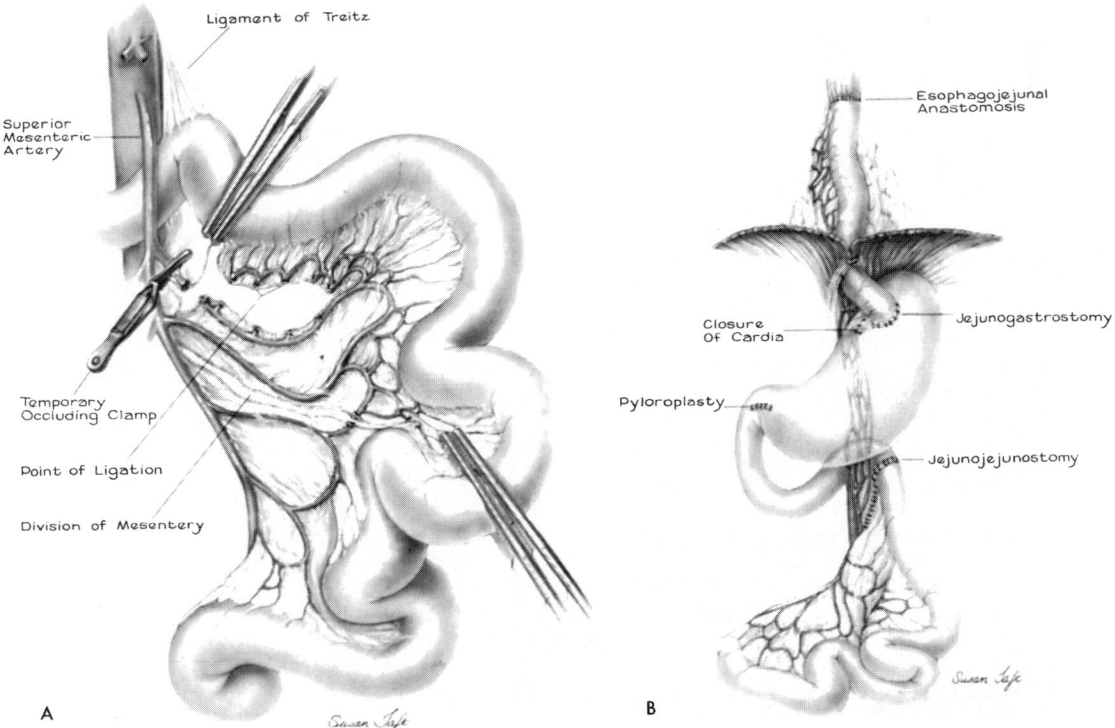

Figure 20–68. *A,* Preparation of the jejunal segment for interposition. The second artery in the jejunal mesentery has been divided after its temporary occlusion to ensure that the one remaining artery in the pedicle can adequately nourish the segment. *B,* The position of the jejunal transplant at completion of the procedure. During reconstruction of the esophageal hiatus, care is taken to avoid pressure on the vascular pedicle of the jejunal graft. (From Grimes, O. F.: Surgical reconstruction of the diseased esophagus. I. Interposition of the jejunum. Surgery, *61:*325, 1967.)

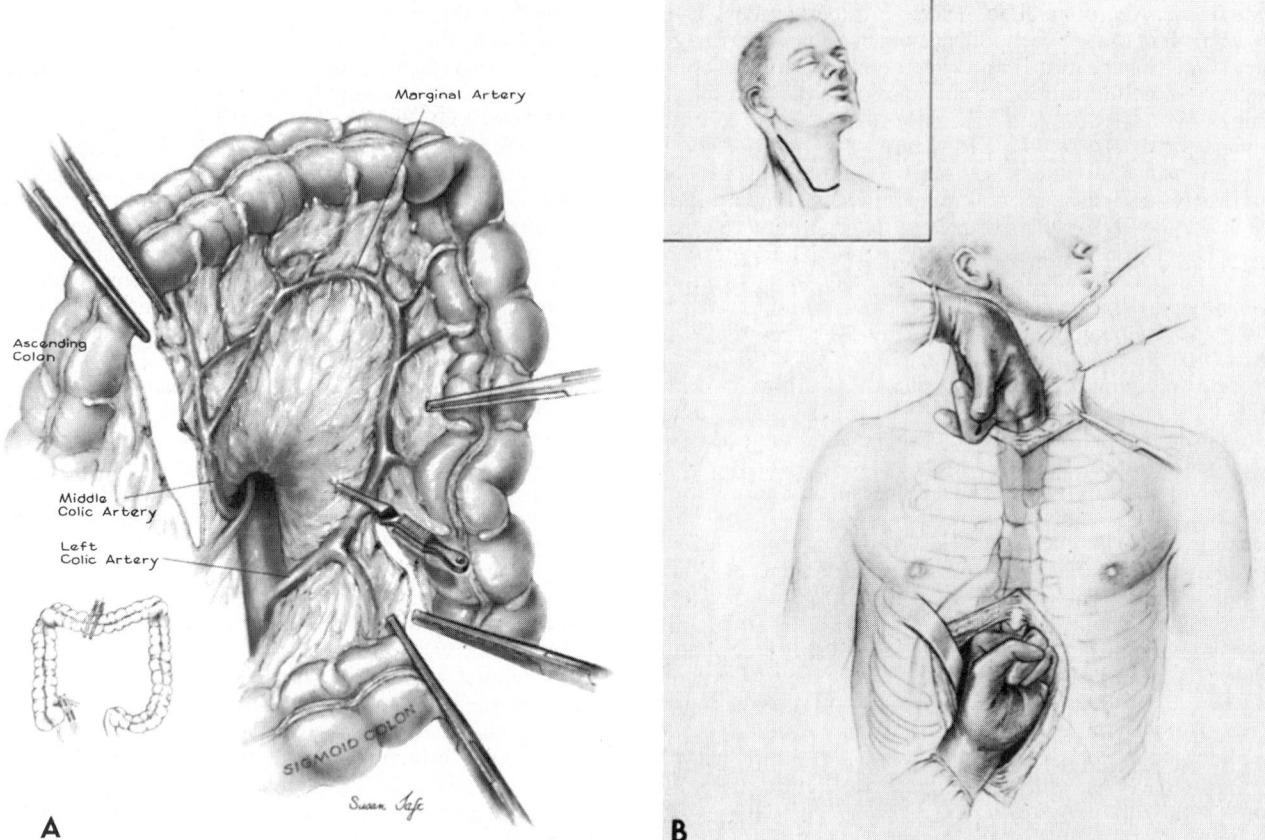

Figure 20–69. *A*, The middle colic or left colic artery used for blood supply to a left colon transplant. Note the rich collateral circulation via the marginal artery. *B*, A substernal tunnel is created by blunt dissection through which the colon transplant can be passed to the neck. (From Grimes, O. F.: Surgical reconstruction of the diseased esophagus. II. Interposition of the ileocolon and colon. Surgery, *61*:487, 1967.)

suitable vein as recipient vessels for the autograft.[19] If the parathyroid glands can be identified and safely separated from tumor, they can be transplanted as described in the section on parathyroid autografts. An appropriate length of proximal jejunum is then resected after careful delineation of its vascular pedicle. The graft is cooled by perfusion with cold saline or Ringer's or Sack's solution and insertion of an intraluminal cooling tube or an ice slush–filled condom. The vascular anastomoses are completed under the operating microscope. When graft color, peristalsis, and bleeding are normal, the double-layer visceral anastomoses are formed. Unlike the colon transplants, which act merely as conduits without peristalsis, manometric studies of free jejunal grafts from many patients in the Duke University series show coordinated waves of peristalsis passing through the implants. Equal success has been reported using the transverse colon as a free intestinal autograft for pharyngoesophageal reconstruction.[49]

OTHER AUTOGRAFTS

Many other tissues have found limited but effective use as autotransplants. The greater omentum was transferred as a vascularized graft to reconstruct the scalp after massive skin and subcutaneous tissue loss,[37] as a pedicle graft to relieve chronic lymphedema of the extremities,[29] and as a free graft to relieve the pain of constrictive, radiation-induced brachial plexus paralysis.[84] Autolipotransplantation has been used for restoration of the plantar fat pad.[12] However, free fat autografts are of questionable value because of unpredictable results due to variable graft survival and wide variations

in the final bulk of the autograft.[5] A combination of well-vascularized omentum and pectoralis major muscle flaps permitted successful reconstruction of infected median sternotomy incisions, with reduction of mortality from 10% to zero.[57] Spleen can be autotransplanted to preserve immunologic function after splenic trauma.[60] Hair was transferred to the scalp as punch grafts, even through split-thickness skin grafts.[53] Tongue was autotransplanted to reconstruct defects of the lips, and teeth were successfully autografted.[24] Bowel smooth muscle was autotransplanted as a sphincter replacement to create a continent colostomy.[70] Following pulmonary valve autograft replacement of diseased aortic valves, 40 of 43 patients in one series were reported to be well 2½ to 5 years after autotransplantation.[74] A pulmonary valve autograft has also been used to replace an aortic valve involved with a cardiac tumor in a neonate.[25] The entire heart was autotransplanted to permit removal of a large myxoma.[69]

Autotransplantation has proved to be a valuable research technique in experimental surgery. John Hunter successfully transplanted testis to the peritoneal cavity of an animal in 1771, and Berthold used autotransplantation in 1849 to demonstrate the endocrine function of cock testis.[39] Autotransplantation continues to be used experimentally today to study organ preservation, to develop and test new surgical techniques, and to evaluate the physiologic changes produced by denervation of organs—for example, erythropoietin production by the transplanted kidney and pulmonary blood flow in the transplanted lung. Single-lung autografts in dogs were demonstrated to provide adequate total respiratory function while carrying the entire pulmonary blood flow at tolerable arterial pressures without evidence of functional deterioration over more than 5 years.[86] Experimental auto-transplantation studies such as these have preceded and supported the ultimate feasibility of many allotransplantation procedures currently in clinical use.

SELECTED REFERENCES

Grimes, O. F.: Surgical reconstruction of the diseased esophagus. I. Interposition of the jejunum. II. Interposition of the ileocolon and colon. Surgery, 61:325, 487, 1967.
The important surgical considerations in the selection and use of an intestinal autograft as a substitute for the esophagus are reviewed in these two well-written articles.

Ochsner, J. L., and Mills, N. L.: Coronary Artery Surgery. Philadelphia, Lea & Febiger, 1978.
The most common thoracic autograft, the saphenous vein coronary artery bypass, is discussed in a concise and practical manner. The pathophysiology of coronary artery disease is related to angiographic findings to permit selection of the appropriate bypass procedure.

Rudolph, R., Fisher, J. C., and Ninnemann, J. L.: Skin Grafting. Boston, Little, Brown, 1979.
This book is a clearly written account of the biology and technique of modern skin grafting. The text progresses chronologically through the successive steps in skin grafting and is beautifully and profusely illustrated.

Serafin, D., and Buncke, H. J., Jr.: Mirrosurgical Composite Tissue Transplantation. St. Louis, C. V. Mosby, 1979.
This comprehensive monograph reviews the entire field of microsurgical composite tissue transplantation. Autografting of skin, various subcutaneous tissue flaps, muscle, omentum, intestine, and bone are covered.

REFERENCES

1. Adams, W. E., and Phemister, D. B.: Carcinoma of the lower thoracic esophagus: Report of a successful resection and esophagogastrostomy. J. Thorac. Surg., 7:621, 1938.
2. Bailey, C. P., Zimmerman, J., Hirose, T. T., Folk, F. S., and Bakst, A. A.: Reconstruction of cardiac valves with autologous tissue. Vasc. Surg., 30:99, 1976.
3. Baines, M. S., and Spiro, R. H.: Pharyngolaryngectomy, total extrathoracic esophagectomy and gastric transposition. Surg. Gynecol. Obstet., 149:693, 1979.
4. Belzer, F. O., Salvatierra, O., Palumbinskas, A., and Stoney, R. J.: Ex vivo renal artery reconstruction. Ann. Surg., 182:456, 1975.
5. Billings, E., and May, J. W.: Historical review and present status of free fat graft autotransplantation in plastic and reconstructive surgery. Plast. Reconstr. Surg., 83:368, 1989.
6. Boxer, R. J., Johnson, S. F., and Ehrlich, R. M.: Ureteral substitution. Urology, 12:299, 1978.
7. Boyne, P. J.: Autogenous cancellous bone and marrow transplants. Clin. Orthop., 73:199, 1970.
8. Brown, J. B., and McDowell, F.: Skin Grafting, 3rd ed. Philadelphia, J. B. Lippincott, 1958.
9. Buncke, H. J., Jr., Daniller, A. E., Schulz, W. P., and Chase, R. A.: The fate of autogenous whole joints transplanted by microvascular anastomoses. Plast. Reconstr. Surg., 39:333, 1967.
10. Calder, J. S., and Norris, R. W.: Repair of mixed peripheral nerves using muscle autografts: A preliminary communication. Br. J. Plast. Surg., 46:557, 1993.
11. Cameron, J. L., Mehigan, D. C., Broe, P. J., and Zuidema, G. D.: Distal pancreatectomy and islet autotransplantation for chronic pancreatitis. Ann. Surg., 393:312, 1981.
12. Chairman, E. L.: Restoration of the plantar fat pad with autolipotransplantation. J. Foot Ankle Surg., 33:373, 1994.
13. Coleman, J. J.: Cultured epidermal autografts: A life-saving and skin-saving technique in children. J. Pediatr. Surg., 27:1029, 1992.
14. Darling, R. C.: Peripheral arterial surgery. N. Engl. J. Med., 280:26, 1969.
15. Darling, R. C., Linton, R. R., and Razzuk, M. A.: Saphenous vein bypass grafts for femoropopliteal occlusive disease: A reappraisal. Surgery, 61:31, 1967.
16. Dicke, K. A., Lotzova, E., Spitzer, G., and McCredie, K. B.: Immunobiology of bone marrow transplantation. Semin. Hematol., 15:263, 1978.
17. Drucker, W. D., Localio, S. A., Becker, M. H., and Berman, B.: Autotransplantation of hyperplastic human adrenal tissue. Arch. Intern. Med., 120:185, 1967.
18. Duran, C. M., Gallo, R., and Kumar, N.: Aortic valve replacement with autologous pericardium: Surgical technique. J. Cardiac Surg., 10:1, 1995.
19. Ellis, H. F., Jr., and Gibb, P. S.: Esophagogastrectomy for carcinoma. Ann. Surg., 19:699, 1979.
20. Entin, A., Daniel, G., and Kahn, P.: Transplantation of autogenous halfjoints. Arch. Surg., 96:359, 1968.
21. Esser, E., Austermann, K. H., and Schmallenbach, H. J.: Lippenrotersatz durch gestielte Zungenlappen. Fortschr. Kiefer Gesichtschir., 2:31, 1978.
22. Flynn, M. B., and Acland, R. D.: Free intestinal autografts for reconstruction following pharyngolaryngoesophagectomy. Surg. Gynecol. Obstet., 149:858, 1979.
23. Ford, C. F., Hamerton, J. L., Barnes, D. W. H., and Loutit, J. F.: Cytological identification of radiation chimeras. Nature, 177:452, 1956.
24. Gardiner, G. T.: The autogenous transplantation of maxillary canine teeth: A review of 100 consecutive cases. Br. Dent. J., 146:382, 1979.
25. Giamberti, A., Giannico, S., Squitieri, C., Iorio, F. S., Amodeo, A., Carotti, A., Picardo, S., and Marcelletti, C.: Neonatal pulmonary autograft implantation for cardiac tumor involving aortic valve. Ann. Thorac. Surg., 59:1219, 1995.
26. Gibson, T., Davis, W. B., and Curran, R. C.: The long term survival of cartilage homografts in man. Br. J. Plast. Surg., 11:177, 1958.
27. Glenn, J. F., and Boyce, W. H. (Eds.): Urologic Surgery, 2nd ed. New York, Harper & Row, 1975.
28. Goetz, C. G., Olanow, C. W., Koller, W. C., Penn, R. D., Cahill, D., Morantz, R., Stebbins, G., Tanner, C. M., Klawans, H. L., Shannon, K. M., Comella, C. L., Witt, T., Cox, C., Waxman, M., and Gauger, L.: Multicenter study of autologous adrenal medullary transplantation to the corpus striatum in patients with advanced Parkinson's disease. N. Engl. J. Med., 320:337, 1989.
29. Goldsmith, H. S., De los Santos, R., and Beattie, E. J., Jr.: Relief of chronic lymphedema by omental transposition. Ann. Surg., 166:573, 1967.
30. Goligher, J. C. (Ed.): Progress symposium: Surgical treatment of inflammatory bowel disease. World J. Surg., 12:139, 1988.
31. Good, L., Odensten, M., and Gillquist, J.: Sagittal knee stability after anterior cruciate ligament reconstruction with a patellar tendon strip: A two-year follow-up study. Am. J. Sports Med., 22:518, 1994.
32. Graze, R. R., and Gale, R. P.: Autotransplantation for leukemia and solid tumors. Transplant. Proc., 10:177, 1978.
33. Grimes, O. F.: Surgical reconstruction of the diseased esophagus. I. Interposition of the jejunum. Surgery, 61:325, 1967.
34. Grimes, O. F.: Surgical reconstruction of the diseased esophagus. II. Interposition of the ileocolon and colon. Surgery, 61:487, 1967.
35. Hardy, J. D.: High ureteral injury: Management by autotransplantation of the kidney. JAMA, 184:97, 1963.
36. Hiratzka, L. F., and Wright, C. B.: Experimental and clinical results of grafts in the venous system. J. Surg. Res., 25:542, 1978.
37. Ikuta, Y.: Omental transplantation. In Serafin, D., and Buncke, R. J., Jr. (Eds.): Microsurgical Composite Tissue Transplantation. St. Louis, C. V. Mosby, 1979.
38. Jenkins, S., Sepka, R., and Barwick, W. J.: Routine use of laser Doppler flowmetry for monitoring autologous tissue transplants. Ann. Plast. Surg., 21:423, 1988.
39. Krohn, P. L.: Transplantation of endocrine glands. In Peer, L. A. (Ed.): Transplantation of Tissues. Vol. 2. Baltimore, Williams & Wilkins, 1959, p. 401.
40. Leather, R. P., Shah, D. M., Corson, J. D., and Karmody, A. M.: Instrumental evolution of the valve incision method of in situ saphenous vein bypass. J. Vasc. Surg., 1:113, 1984.
41. Littlor, J. W.: On making a thumb—one hundred years of surgical effort. J. Hand Surg., 1:35, 1976.
42. Madrazo, L., Drucker-Colin, R., Diaz, V., et al.: Open microsurgical autograft of adrenal medulla to the right caudate nucleus in two patients with intractable Parkinson's disease. N. Engl. J. Med., 316:831, 1987.
43. Madrazo, I., Drucker-Colin, R., Leon, V., and Toires, C.: Adrenal medulla transplanted to caudate nucleus for treatment of Parkinson's disease: Report of 10 cases. Surg. Forum, 38:510, 1987.
44. Matsuura, H., Sako, K., and Marchetta, F. C.: Successful reimplantation of autogenous parathyroid tissue. Am. J. Surg., 118:779, 1969.
45. McDonald, J. C., Rohr, M. S., and Tucker, W. Y.: Recent experiences with autotransplantation of the kidney, jejunum, and pancreas. Ann. Surg., 197:678, 1983.
46. McKee, D. M., and Peters, C. R.: Reconstruction of the hypopharynx and cervical esophagus with a microvascular jejunal transplant. In Serafin, D., and Buncke, R. J., Jr. (Eds.): Microsurgical Composite Transplantation. St. Louis, C. V. Mosby, 1979.
47. McLoughlin, M. D., Williams, G. M., and Stonesifor, G. L., Jr.: Ex vivo surgical dissection: Autotransplantation in renal disease. JAMA, 235:1705, 1976.
48. Millesi, R., Meissl, G., and Berger, A.: The interfascicular nerve grafting of the median and ulnar nerves. J. Bone Joint Surg. [Am.], 54:727, 1972.
49. Modica, L. A., and de Koos, P. T.: Free bowel autografts in pharyngoesophageal reconstruction: Colon revisited. Orolaryngol. Head Neck Surg., 9:73, 1988.
50. Mullen, D. C., Young, W. G., Jr., and Sealy, W. C.: Results of twenty years experience with esophageal replacement for benign disorders. Ann. Thorac. Surg., 5:481, 1968.
51. Najarian, J. S., Sutherland, D. E. R., Baumgartner, D., Burke, B., Rynasiewicz, J. J., Matas, A. A., and Goetz, F.: Total or near total pancreatectomy and islet autotransplantation for treatment of chronic pancreatitis. Ann. Surg., 192:526, 1980.
52. Nakayama, K., Yamamoto, K., Tamiya, T., Makino, H., Odaka, M., Ohwada, M., and Takahashi, R.: Experience with free autografts of bowel with new venous anastomosis apparatus. Surgery, 55:798, 1964.
53. Nordstrom, R. E.: Punch hair grafting under split skin grafts on scalps. Plast. Reconstr. Surg., 64:9, 1979.

54. Norris, R. W., Glasby, M. A., Gattuso, J. M., and Bowden, R. E. M.: Nerve repair in humans using muscle autografts: A new technique. J. Bone Joint Surg., 70:530, 1988.

55. Ochsner, J. L., and Mills, N. L.: Coronary Artery Surgery. Philadelphia, Lea & Febiger, 1978.

56. Ostrup, L. T., and Frederickson, J. M.: Distant transfer of a free living bone graft by microvascular anastomoses: An experimental study. Plast. Reconstr. Surg., 54:274, 1974.

57. Pearl, S. N., and Dibbell, D. G.: Reconstruction after median sternotomy infection. Surg. Gynecol. Obstet., 159:47, 1984.

58. Pettersson, S., Brynger, H., Henriksson, C., Johansson, S., Nilson, A. E., and Ranch, T.: Autotransplantation with direct pyelovesical anastomosis in renal pelvic and ureteric tumors, a new approach. Scand. J. Urol. Nephrol. Suppl., 60:45, 1981.

59. Phemister, D. B.: The fate of transplanted bone and regenerative power of its various constituents. Surg. Gynecol. Obstet., 19:303, 1914.

60. Pisters, P. W., and Pachter, H. L.: Autologous splenic transplantation for splenic trauma. Ann. Surg., 219:225, 1994.

61. Postlethwait, R. W.: Surgery of the Esophagus. New York, Appleton-Century-Crofts, 1979.

62. Putnam, C. W.: Renal autotransplantation and "bench work" surgery: Techniques and applications. In Rutherford, R. B. (Ed.): Vascular Surgery. Philadelphia, W. B. Saunders, 1977.

63. Ranch, T., Granerus, G., Henricksson, C., and Pettersson, S.: Renal function after autotransplantation with direct pyelocystostomy: Long-term follow-up. Br. J. Urol., 63:233, 1989.

64. Reyes, A. T., Frame, R., and Brodman, R. F.: Technique for harvesting the radial artery as a coronary artery bypass graft. Ann. Thorac. Surg., 59:118, 1995.

65. Rich, N. M., Collins, G. J., Anderson, C. A., and McDonald, P. T.: Autogenous venous interposition grafts in repair of major venous injuries. J. Trauma, 17:512, 1977.

66. Robson, M. C., and Krizek, T. J.: Predicting skin graft survival. J. Trauma, 13:213, 1973.

67. Rudolph, R., Fisher, J. C., and Ninnemann, J. L.: Skin Grafting. Boston, Little, Brown, 1979.

68. Saunders, J. B. de D. M.: A conceptual history of transplantation. In Najarian, J. S., and Simmons, R. L. (Eds.): Transplantation. Philadelphia, Lea & Febiger, 1972.

69. Scheld, H. H., Nestle, H. W., Kling, D., Stertmann, W. A., Langebartels, H., and Hehrlein, F. W.: Resection of a heart tumor using autotransplantation. Thorac. Cardiovasc. Surg., 36:40, 1987.

70. Schmidt, E., Bruch, H. P., Greulich, M., Rothhammer, A., and Romen, W.: Kontinente Colostomie durch freie Transplantation Autologer Dickdarmmuskulatur. Chirurg, 50:96, 1979.

71. Seidenberg, B., Rosenak, S., Surwitt, E. S., and Som, M. L.: Immediate reconstruction of the cervical esophagus by a revascularized isolated jejunal segment. Ann. Surg., 149:162, 1959.

72. Serafin, D., and Buncke, R. J., Jr. (Eds.): Microsurgical Composite Tissue Transplantation. St. Louis, C. V. Mosby, 1979.

73. Sicard, G. A., Valentin, L. I., Freeman, M. D., Allen, B. T., and Anderson, C. B.: Renal autotransplantation: An alternative to standard renal revascularization procedures. Surgery, 104:624, 1988.

74. Somerville, J., Ross, D., Sachs, G., Emanuel, R., and McDonald, L.: Long term results of pulmonary autograft replacement for aortic valve disease. Lancet, 2:730, 1972.

75. Stewart, B. R., Banowsky, L. R., Hewitt, C. B., and Straffon, R. A.: Renal autotransplantation: Current perspectives. J. Urol., 118:363, 1977.

76. Stoney, R. J., and Wylie, E. J.: Arterial autografts. Surgery, 67:18, 1970.

77. Sutherland, D. E. R.: Pancreas and islet transplant registry statistics. Transplant. Proc., 16:593, 1984.

78. Swan, H., Harper, F., and Christensen, S. P.: Autotransplantation of thyroid tissue in the treatment of lingual thyroid. Surgery, 32:293, 1952.

79. Tamai, S.: Experimental neuromuscular transplantation. In Serafin, D., and Buncke, R. J., Jr. (Eds.): Microsurgical Composite Tissue Transplantation. St. Louis, C. V. Mosby, 1979.

80. Tamai, S.: Osteocutaneous transplantation. In Serafin, D., and Buncke, R. J., Jr. (Eds.): Microsurgical Composite Tissue Transplantation. St. Louis, C. V. Mosby, 1979.

81. Taylor, G. I.: Vascularized nerve transfer. In Serafin, D., and Buncke, R. J., Jr. (Eds.): Microsurgical Composite Tissue Transplantation. St. Louis, C. V. Mosby, 1979.

82. Toledo-Pereyra, L. R., Rowlett, A. L., Cain, W., Rosenberg, J. C., Gordon, P. A., and MacKenzie, G. R.: Hepatic infarction following intraportal islet cell autotransplantation after near-total pancreatectomy. Transplantation, 38:88, 1984.

83. Tosati, E., Valente, U., Campisi, C., Barabino, C., and Pozzati, A.: Segmental pancreas autotransplantation in man following total or near total pancreatectomy for serious recurrent chronic pancreatitis. Transplant. Proc., 12:15, 1980.

84. Uhlschmid, G., and Clodius, L.: Eine neue Anwendung des frei transplantierten Omentums. Chirurg, 49:714, 1978.

85. van der Velden, J. J., van Bockel, J. H., Zwartendijk, J., van Krieken, J. H., and Terpstra, J. L.: Long-term results of surgical treatment of renal carcinoma in solitary kidneys by extracorporeal resection and autotransplantation. Br. J. Urol., 69:486, 1992.

86. Veith, F. J., and Montofusco, C. M.: Long term fate of lung autografts charged with providing total pulmonary function. Ann. Surg., 190:654, 1979.

87. Wells, S. A., Jr., Gunnells, J. C., Shelburne, J. D., Schneider, A. B., and Sherwood, L. M.: Transplantation of the parathyroid glands in man: Clinical indications and results. Surgery, 78:34, 1975.

88. Wells, S. A., Ross, A. J., Dale, J. K., and Gray, R. S.: Transplantation of the parathyroid glands: Current status. Surg. Clin. North Am., 59:167, 1979.

89. Woodruff, M. F. A.: The Transplantation of Tissues and Organs. Springfield, Ill., Charles C Thomas, 1960.

90. Wylie, E. J., Binkley, F. M., and Albo, R. J.: Femoropopliteal endarterectomy. Am. J. Surg., 108:215, 1964.

91. Xu, Y., Qiao, Y., Wu, P., Chen, Z., and Jin, N.: Adrenal autotransplantation with attached blood vessels for treatment of Cushing's disease. J. Urol., 141:6, 1988.

92. Zinman, L., and Libertino, J. A.: Technique of augmentation cecocystoplasty. Surg. Clin. North Am., 60:703, 1980.

CHAPTER 21

IMMUNOBIOLOGY AND IMMUNOTHERAPY OF NEOPLASTIC DISEASE; MELANOMA; SOFT TISSUE SARCOMAS; TUMOR MARKERS

I

IMMUNOBIOLOGY AND IMMUNOTHERAPY OF NEOPLASTIC DISEASE

H. Kim Lyerly, M.D., and Cohava Gelber, Ph.D.

Cancer is the second leading cause of death in the United States, and more than 340,000 Americans die of cancer every year. Although surgical excision remains the standard for the treatment of the primary cancer and is curative for a significant percentage of patients, many malignancies recur locally or, more commonly, at a distant site. Advances in the treatment of recurrent disease and metastases have been limited; thus, the prevention of recurrence and metastasis remains a major focus in surgical and medical oncology. Because cytoreductive chemotherapy and hormonal therapy have had limited success, a renewed interest in the role of immune-based therapies has emerged, in large part because of an increase in the understanding of how the immune system recognizes abnormal or malignant cells.[1-4] Immune-based therapy of cancer in the past has usually focused on the humoral component of the immune system, in which antibodies were required to recognize molecules that were expressed on the cell surface. This limitation on the types of molecules that could be recognized as well as the inherent limitations of murine antibodies in destroying neoplastic cells *in vivo* led to disappointing clinical results. Current antibody-based strategies using humanized antibodies, or antibodies linked to toxins, show some promise in certain clinical situations but are limited to external molecules expressed and disseminated on tumors. The recent growth of knowledge and understanding of how cytotoxic cells recognize neoplastic cells[2, 5] has led to an increase in enthusiasm for cellular-based strategies using adoptive and active immunotherapy.

IMMUNOLOGIC BASIS FOR CELLULAR IMMUNOTHERAPY

The underlying assumption of immune-based therapies directed at cancer is that tumor cells encode antigens (tumor-associated antigens [TAAs] and tumor-specific antigens [TSAs]), which are capable of being specifically recognized by components of the immune response that can eradicate the growing tumor.[6, 7] Several observations made in the past

cast serious doubts on the validity of this assumption and questioned the rationale of cancer immunotherapy. First, most human cancers were considered nonimmunogenic; that is, tumor-specific immune responses are not detected in the cancer patient. Some patients, however, such as melanoma or renal cancer patients, do exhibit weak antitumor immune responses that are generally considered ineffective in controlling tumor progression. Second, spontaneously arising rodent tumors are generally nonimmunogenic as judged by the fact that repeated *vaccinations* with irradiated tumor preparations do not affect the growth of a subsequent tumor challenge, nor do they elicit measurable tumor-specific immune responses. This is in great contrast to virally or chemically induced tumors in rodents that can be highly immunogenic. Third, the incidence of cancer is not elevated in patients with defects in their immune system, except for specific forms of cancers associated with a viral etiology. For example, patients recovering from bone marrow transplants are severely immunocompromised and may develop B-cell lymphomas (associated with Epstein-Barr virus); patients who have undergone solid organ transplant are maintained on immunosuppressive drugs and may develop B-cell lymphomas; and patients with the acquired immunodeficiency syndrome may develop B-cell lymphomas, as well as Kaposi's sarcoma (possibly associated with human herpesvirus)[8, 9] and invasive cervical carcinomas (possibly linked with human papillomavirus).[10] Taken together, these observations have suggested in the past that tumor cells of cancer patients do not encode TAA or TSA capable of inducing effective antitumor immune responses.

Yet another set of observations suggested otherwise. First, spontaneous regressions of tumors have been noted, especially among patients with metastatic melanoma and renal cell carcinoma, and clinical trials of tumor vaccination and adoptive immunotherapy have on occasion led to statistically significant responses. This suggests that effective antitumor immune responses may be generated either *de novo* or after some clinical intervention and that optimized immunization protocols could lead to improved clinical outcome. Second, compelling, although circumstantial, evidence that immune responses have an important role in surveillance in limiting tumor progression in cancer patients is provided from observations that tumors often downregulate major histocompatibility complex (MHC) Class I expression[11] or secrete high levels of immune suppressive factors such as transforming growth factor-beta.[12, 13] The inference is that tumors must have elaborated special means to evade an existing, and apparently effective, immune response. Finally, because most immunosuppressed patients in the past died of infections, which are now better controlled by antibiotic or immunoglobulin prophylaxis, an emerging awareness of increasing neoplastic and preneoplastic conditions in the immunocompromised patient has occurred.

The question of whether naturally occurring, as opposed to mutagen or virally induced, tumors express TAAs or TSAs has been controversial. The existence of such molecules on spontaneous human tumors has been confirmed by their direct identification. The first clue that TAAs or TSAs did exist in spontaneous tumors came in 1982, when van Pel and Boone demonstrated that a mutagenized form of a strictly defined, nonimmunogenic tumor of mouse origin was capable of inducing an immune response against the *nonimmunogenic* parental tumor.[14] The parental tumor in this instance failed to induce an immune response, not because it was devoid of antigen but rather because in its original form it was incapable of presenting the antigens to the immune system. Two years later, Key and colleagues made a similar observation showing that manipulation of a spontaneous nonimmunogenic tumor of guinea pig origin simply by admixing the tumor with bacille Calmette-Guérin could elicit an immune response against the parental tumor.[15] Amazingly, in both studies the block of the immune response was at the level of induction of T-cell responses and not during the recognition and target (tumor) cell killing phase. That is, the TAAs or TSAs were present and could be recognized on the tumor cells by the effector cells, but only after a high level of specific immune response was elicited.

Complementing these animal experiments was an understanding at the molecular level of how a cytotoxic T lymphocyte (CTL) recognizes an antigen on a cell.[15] It was long thought that CTLs recognize antigen expressed on the surface of the target cell destined to be killed, similar to the recognition of an antigen by an antibody. However, it was found that the mechanism of CTL recognition of antigens was fundamentally different from the mechanism of antibody recognition. CTLs can detect antigens derived from cell surface-associated proteins but in addition can recognize proteins that are normally in the cytoplasm or in the nucleus.[2] In fact, the normal location of the protein can be anywhere within the cell.

To understand how a CTL can recognize an antigen from a protein that is normally located within the cytoplasm or nucleus of the cell, investigators had to determine exactly what was being recognized by the CTL (Fig. 21–1). T cells were found to recognize short linear fragments of processed or even denatured protein. It was found that proteins that were endogenously synthesized were degraded within the cytoplasm into 9–10-amino acid-long peptides. These peptides were then transported to the endocytoplasmic reticulum and associated with newly synthesized MHC Class I molecules. Certain peptides could fit within the MHC Class I molecule and were then transported to the cell surface as a complex. It was this complex, consisting of a 9–10 amino acid peptide within a MHC Class I molecule that was presented to, and recognized by, CD8+ CTLs.[16] Alterations of normal genes leading to their overexpression, to the production of novel fusion proteins, or to simple amino acid substitutions in these peptides were sufficient to be recognized by

CTLs as foreign. Because it is now recognized that tumor cells do overexpress normal genes or express mutated genes, such as mutated oncogenes[17] or tumor suppressor genes,[18] tumor cells should express tumor-associated or tumor-specific proteins that can be recognized by CTLs as foreign and thus serve as targets to facilitate their elimination. In fact, methods to identify and isolate genes encoding for TAAs or TSAs recognized by CD8+ CTLs have been developed, proving that tumor cells do express genetically defined TAAs or TSAs. A list of these antigens is depicted in Table 21–1, and some of the major antigens that have been recently defined are briefly discussed here.

MAGE. *MAGE-1* was first isolated in 1992 by Boon and co-workers as encoding a gene product that was recognized by autologous cytotoxic T cell clones generated from patients with melanoma.[19, 20] Subsequent cloning of this gene led to the identification of a family of 12 closely related genes. With the exception of the testis, expression of these genes is not found in normal adult tissue. Six of the genes (i.e., *MAGE-1, -2, -3, -4, -6,* and *-12*) are expressed in a significant portion of human tumors of varied histologic types. Although *MAGE-1* was isolated from melanoma cells, preliminary reports suggested that a significant percentage of other human cancers, such as breast cancer, expressed *MAGE-1* as determined by detection of *MAGE-1* transcripts. The peptide antigen encoded by *MAGE-1* is presented to CTL in the context of a distinct human MHC allele (HLA-A1).

Further analysis of the family of *MAGE* gene expression in cancers suggested that although *MAGE-1* was expressed only by a fraction of melanoma cells, another member of the family, *MAGE-3*, was expressed by the majority of melanoma cells.[21] It was hoped that the widespread expression of *MAGE-3* in melanoma cells would be mimicked in other tumor types, allowing the development of a *universal* tumor vaccine. Unfortunately, *MAGE-3* expression has not been as widespread as originally hoped.

HER-2/neu. *HER-2/neu* is a proto-oncogene that encodes a 185-kd transmembrane protein with extensive homology to the epidermal growth factor receptor.[22] *HER-2/neu* is amplified and overexpressed in 20% to 40% of invasive breast and ovarian cancers, and its overexpression is thought to be associated with aggressive disease and poor clinical prognosis. Because *HER-2/neu* encodes a gene product (p185 neu) that is expressed during fetal development and is detectable in a number of normal adult tissues, there has been much speculation as to whether an overexpressed nonmutated protein could serve as a target for immunotherapy. Ioannides and colleagues have proposed that discrete determinants within the *HER-2/neu* protein may serve as targets for CTLs.[22] Similarly, Eberlein and colleagues have proposed the use of overexpressed *HER-2/neu*-derived peptides as targets for HLA-A2-restricted CTLs in ovarian and non–small cell lung cancer.[23] Cheever and colleagues reported the existence of T-cell and antibody reactivities against *HER-2/neu* in patients with breast cancer,[24] and Fisk reported that peptide analogs of *HER-2/neu* were capable of inducing HLA-A2-restricted CTLs *in vitro* using lymphocytes from normal healthy volunteers.[25] Collectively, these results amply document the potential immunogenicity of overexpressed *HER-2/neu* protein.

MUC-1. *MUC-1* encodes a mucopolypeptide polymer that is expressed in pancreatic and breast cancers and contains several repeats of carbohydrate and peptidic segments.[26] *MUC-1* has been shown to be recognized by the humoral and cellular immune system. Interestingly, cytotoxic T-cell recognition of the *MUC-1* gene product is non-MHC restricted. *MUC-1* is expressed on a variety of tumor types and is the subject of intense studies.[27] Currently, methods are being developed to generate non–MHC–restricted *MUC-1*-specific CTLs from the peripheral blood mononuclear cells

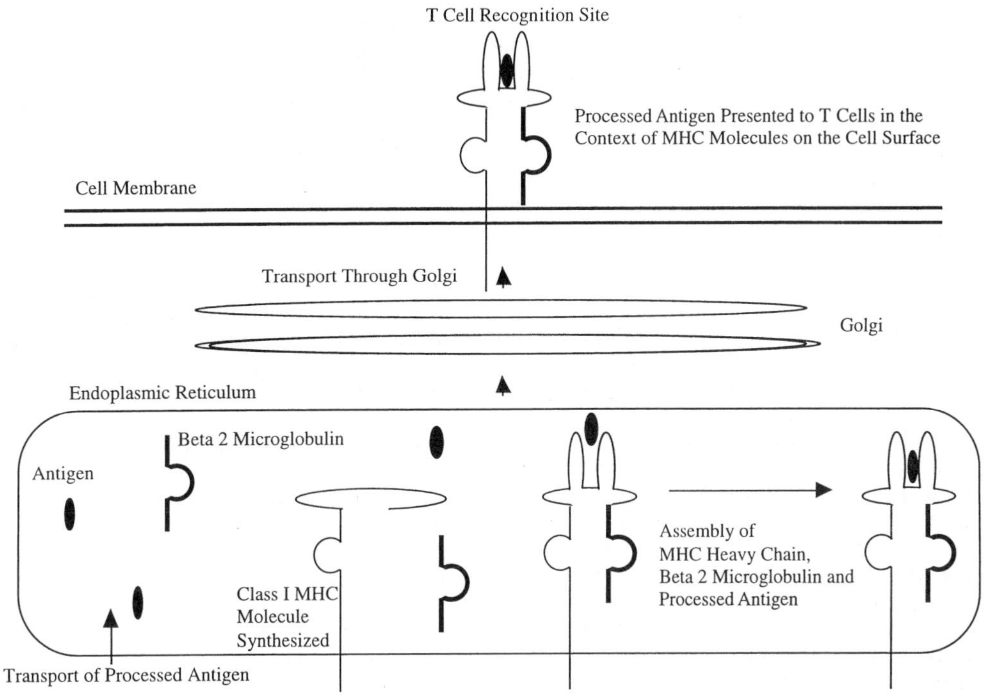

Figure 21–1. Class I MHC antigen processing and presentation. Class I MHC molecules associate with endogenously derived, processed antigen in the lumen of the endoplasmic reticulum. Peptide antigen is transported into the lumen of the endoplasmic reticulum. MHC molecules are synthesized within the lumen. Beta 2 microglobulin is present in excess. Fully folded trimerix complexes of class I MHC heavy chain, beta 2 microglobulin, and processed antigen are assembled and transported through the Golgi apparatus to the cell surface. Peptide antigen is then present on the surface of the cell and can interact with the T cell receptor in the context of MHC molecules and beta 2 microglobulin.

of patients using the peptidic segments and will allow investigators to explore the use of *MUC-1*-specific CTLs in clinical trials.

p53. The mutated form of the tumor suppressor gene *p53* is widely expressed among human cancers.[28] *p53* may be mutated at a variety of positions and is overexpressed in a significant fraction of cancers, suggesting that it is a likely

TABLE 21–1. Tumor-Specific Antigens Shared by Different Human Tumors

Gene	Normal Expression	MHC	Peptide
MAGE-1	Testis	HLA-A1	EADPTGHSY
		HLA-Cw16	SAYGEPRKL
MAGE-3	Testis	HLA-A1	EVDPIGHLY
		HLA-A2	FLWGPRALV
BAGE	Testis	HLA-Cw16	AARAVFLAL
GAGE-1,2	Testis	HLA-Cw6	YRPRPRRY
HER-2/neu	Ubiquitous (low levels)	HLA-A2	ELVSEFSRM
Tyrosinase	Melanocytes	HLA-A2	MLLAVLYCL
		HLA-A2	YMNGTMSQV
		HLA-B44	SEIWRDIDF
MART-1	Melanocytes	HLA-A2	(E)AAGIGILTV
		HLA-A2	ILTVILGVL
gp100	Melanocytes	HLA-A2	KTWGQYWQV
		HLA-A2	ITDQVPGSV
		HLA-A2	VLYRYGSFSV
CEA	Embryonic antigen gastro-intestine	HLA-A2	YLSGANLNL
Mutant p53	*	HLA-A2	
Mutant ras	†	HLA-DR	DILDTAGLEEYSAMRD

*Tumor suppressor gene; mutation is widely expressed among human cancer.

†Oncoprotein; mutation is expressed in various malignancies.

target for immune attack. Base substitutions have been documented in 90 different codons, although three *hot spot* codons (175, 248, and 273) account for a great majority of mutations. Mutant *p53* binds heat shock protein (hsp 70), thought to belong to a family of chaperones that facilitate directing peptides to the subcellular domains in which complexes of MHC and peptide are formed and transported to the cell surface. Thus, this interaction may enhance the overall immunogenicity of *p53*. Antibodies to *p53* can be demonstrated in a fraction of patients with breast tumors containing mutated forms of *p53*; however, they cross-react with wild type *p53* and therefore are not specific binding to the mutations. Reports have also described a CTL response against *p53*; however, the frequency of these effector reactivities in patients with different tumors is uncertain.[29]

Carcinoembryonic Antigen. Carcinoembryonic antigen (CEA) is an oncofetal protein, best known for its overexpression in gastrointestinal malignancies, but is also overexpressed in approximately 50% of breast cancers. Schlom and colleagues demonstrated that mice immunized with recombinant CEA–expressing vaccinia expression vectors were rendered capable of rejecting an otherwise lethal challenge of syngeneic tumor cells containing a human CEA gene.[30] Results of phase I clinical trials of CEA vaccination of patients with end-stage CEA expressing tumors showed minimal toxicity. No published data regarding the induction of CEA specific cellular immune reactivities from the patients in this trial are available.

MART. The *MART* gene encodes a transmembrane protein that is expressed in melanomas, melanocyte cell lines, and human retina. *MART-1* is expressed on over 90% of human melanomas and is recognized by tumor infiltrating lymphocytes (TILs) isolated from HLA-A2 patients.[31]

Tyrosinase and gp100. Melanoma-specific CTLs isolated from patients recognized common melanoma antigens in conjunction with HLA-A2 restriction element. Two of these common melanoma antigens were initially found to be derived from tyrosinase, an enzyme involved in the synthesis of melanin.[32] Several tyrosinase, HLA-A2–, HLA-A24–, and HLA-B44–restricted T-cell epitopes were identified.[33] A tyrosinase-derived antigen recognized by CD4+ T cells has been discovered. This antigen, presented by HLA-DR, was the first tumor antigen recognized by CD4+ cells to be characterized in humans. The presence of epitopes recognized by CD4+ and CD8+ T cells within the same protein might increase its immunogenicity. Pmel17 and gp100 are two almost identical melanocyte-specific proteins that were found to produce four distinct peptides recognized by HLA-A2–restricted TILs.[32]

The significance and importance of identifying TAAs or TSAs that are recognized by CTLs, as opposed to tumor antigens that are recognized by antibodies, is that CTL antigens are more likely to constitute effective tumor rejection antigens. Thus, elicitation of cellular immune response against such antigens produces elimination and control of the neoplastic growth. The implications for immune therapies is that strategies based on CTL antigens, as opposed to humoral antigens, are more likely to be therapeutically useful. The theoretical disadvantage of this approach at this time is that it is not clear that a TAA-specific immune-based therapy is sufficient for rejection of the entire tumor, which consists of a heterologous population of cells[34] or promotes the selection of tumor cells devoid of the specific antigen used in the vaccine. Nonetheless, the emergence of defined tumor antigens is an important consideration in designing new strategies for cancer immunotherapy.[5, 35]

Tumor antigens expressed on spontaneous malignancies may be auto or self antigens. For example, several of the identified melanoma-specific antigens such as MAGE and MART are also expressed in normal melanocytes and in other tissues. It is not altogether clear why, but the fact is that whereas tolerance is maintained to self antigens expressed on normal tissue they induce an immune response when expressed on tumor cells.[35] The immune response induced against the self antigen expressed on the tumor cells could very well cross-react with normal tissue expressing the same antigen and lead to autoimmunity. The concern is therefore that effective immune strategies against tumors could also lead to autoimmunity. Although clear manifestations of autoimmunity in animals treated with active or adoptive immunotherapy have not yet been observed or reported, it is suspected that development of increasingly potent immune therapy protocols may lead to autoimmune manifestations, and, as in other instances in clinical medicine, a risk/benefit assessment will be needed in each case.

In summary, the biologic basis of immune-based therapy against cancer has become strongly supported by basic research in defining how the cellular immune response identifies cells as foreign and the identification of TAAs or TSAs as discussed earlier. It appears that the lack of demonstrable immunity of most human forms of cancer may not reflect lack of TAAs or TSAs, but rather that tumors have elaborated mechanisms to prevent the induction of effective antitumor immune responses. It is therefore becoming increasingly clear that cellular responses, in particular CTL responses, may be highly effective in recognizing tumor cells and initiate a cascade of events that would lead to their eventual destruction. Indeed, animal studies support the notion that tumor-specific CTLs, and occasionally T-helper cells,[36, 37] constitute an important effector arm in the antitumor immune response. If so, the purpose of tumor immunotherapy would be to direct the immune system to the TAA capable of mediating tumor rejection, and the question then becomes how to achieve it most effectively. Two approaches that have received increasing consideration are *adoptive* and *active* immunotherapy.

ADOPTIVE IMMUNOTHERAPY

Adoptive immunotherapy refers to the adoptive transfer of specific immunologic components, usually cellular components, for the treatment of cancer. The principles, safety, and therapeutic efficacy of adoptive cell transfer for therapy for malignant diseases have previously been established in animal models but more recently have been explored as treatment of human disease.[38, 39] This type of immunotherapy is most readily recognized in the form of non–antigen-specific effectors, which include lymphokine activated killer (LAK) cells or TILs as established by Rosenberg and colleagues.[40, 41]

LAK cells, generated by short-term culture of peripheral blood lymphocytes in the presence of high concentrations of interleukin (IL)-2, lyse transformed target cells and have minimal lytic activity for most normal tissues. Up to 10^{11} *in vitro*–generated LAK cells have been administered in a single intravenous infusion to cancer patients. Treated patients experienced only minor constitutional symptoms and no pulmonary compromise, demonstrating the safety of systemically administering large numbers of *in vitro*–activated lymphocytes.[41] Therapeutic trials have also combined short courses of high-dose systemic IL-2 administration with LAK cell transfer to promote LAK function and viability with apparent enhanced efficacy. The shortcomings of LAK and IL-2 therapy included a larger degree of toxicity, including pulmonary, renal, and hepatobiliary, with a significant proportion of patients requiring intensive care unit admissions and a 2% to 5% treatment-related mortality. Despite this, the response rate remained relatively low, although demonstrating some promise in selected tumors.

In an effort to increase the efficacy of the cellular component of the therapy, more effective effector cells were sought. One such therapy using *in vitro*–expanded lymphocytes derived from a TIL has been evaluated in clinical trials. In humans, TIL cell lines have been generated by mincing tumor specimens and culturing eluted lymphocytes with high concentrations of IL-2. TIL lines can be expanded to 10^8 to 10^{11} cells over 3 to 8 weeks in culture, and some lines appear to function as T cells with lytic specificity for autologous but not allogeneic tumor targets, whereas others function as LAK cells and lyse both autologous and allogeneic tumor targets. Adoptive transfer of 5×10^{10} TIL alone has not been associated with significant toxicity, and administration of 5×10^{10} TIL cells with concurrent systemic IL-2 has caused toxicities that are attributable to the IL-2. Evaluation of the migration patterns of transferred TIL cells by infusion of indium-111–labeled cells has revealed initial localization of TIL cells in the lungs, liver, and spleen at 2 hours after intravenous infusion, followed by emigration and preferential localization at sites of metastatic tumor by 24 hours.[42] Partial and complete tumor regressions have been seen in patients after a single TIL cell infusion, demonstrating that these long-term cultured immune effector cells can mediate *in vivo* biologic effects. Nonetheless, response rates continued to remain relatively low, although demonstrating some promise in patients with melanoma and renal cell carcinoma. These clinical studies of adoptive immunotherapy relied on non–antigen-specific LAK and TIL cells, because specific TAAs recognized by the cytotoxic effector cells had not yet been identified. Nonetheless, they have established the feasibility and safety of this approach and demonstrated *in vivo* biologic effects of transferred effector cells. Other types of effector cells including cells from draining lymph nodes and *in vivo* primed cells have also been evaluated in the era before the clear elucidation of defined TAAs. The recognition and availability of defined TAAs will allow investigators to attempt to determine the usefulness of therapy using antigen-specific CTL, because they can be generated *in vitro* and their function specifically monitored *in vivo*.

ACTIVE IMMUNOTHERAPY

In addition to adoptive immunotherapy, active immunotherapy has emerged as another modality of immunotherapy and has received increasing attention. Specific active immunotherapy (SAI) differs dramatically from the nonspecific immune-based trials that have been previously used, in that the objective is not to generally stimulate the immune system or nonspecifically stimulate one component of the immune system. Rather, SAI refers to the specific induction of a component of the immune system that affects the rejection of a particular tumor type. Several different approaches in experimental animal studies in the 1970s formed the basis for human clinical trials of SAI against human cancers. Although several thousand patients have been injected with a variety of tumor cell preparations in this country and elsewhere during the past 25 years,[42a–63] the complexity of the studies has made it difficult to assess definitively the value of this approach to cancer therapy. Nonetheless, a number of clinical trials have suggested a therapeutic benefit of SAI.

The results of 81 trials of this type, many that involve the treatment of metastatic melanoma, have been summarized previously in a review by Livingston.[64] Of these 81 trials, which included more than 3000 patients, at least seven have had clinical responses in the 20% to 50% range, and two randomized adjuvant trials have shown prolongation of disease-free interval and survival. Most of these 81 trials have two features in common: (1) a therapeutic effect was not seen or, if seen, has not been confirmed independently; and (2) no acceptable information was provided regarding the presence of tumor antigens in the vaccines and the immune response of patients to these antigens. Skin tests for delayed-type hypersensitivity to whole tumor cells, cell extracts, or cell-mediated cytotoxicity assays were performed in a number of trials,[44] but the difficulty of defining specificity limits the usefulness of these assays. Therefore, a solid foundation for future progress has not been provided by most of these clinical studies. These studies suggest that a review of traditional response criteria is needed, and perhaps focus not on response rates but on disease stabilization, time to relapse, survival, and quality of life.

Because of the lack of clinical success in these trials, active immunotherapy remained confined to clinical trials, usually in melanoma and renal cell carcinoma. However, advances in gene transfer have steered to a new direction of active immunotherapy, based on gene modification of the tumor cells in an effort to enhance their ability to elicit a tumor-specific immune response.

ACTIVE IMMUNOTHERAPY USING GENETICALLY MODIFIED TUMOR CELLS

It is well recognized that soluble factors act as modulators of immune responses, which has led to their incorporation in experimental treatment protocols to augment antitumor immune responses in cancer patients. The limited efficacy of using IL-2 or other cytokines in the treatment of cancer is due in part to the toxicity associated with the administration of high doses of cytokines to the patient. Because most immunomodulators act as local hormones whose accumulation in the serum is prevented by their short half-life, it was suggested that local delivery of cytokines might have a more pronounced therapeutic benefit. An approach of approximating the physiologic conditions of cytokine delivery to sites where immune responses are generated would be to introduce genes encoding cytokines into tumor cells. In that case, the ectopically expressed cytokines are continuously expressed and secreted from the tumor cell and reach effective concentration in close proximity of the tumor and tumor antigens but not elsewhere in the body.

The initial premise that prompted investigators to consider the use of genetically modified tumor vaccines was to induce strong antitumor CTL responses. The interaction between the tumor cell and its cognate T cell is sufficient for tumor cell lysis by an activated CTL and may also be sufficient to reactivate memory CTLs. However, induction of CTL responses in the naive animal (i.e., activation of an unprimed CTL) was shown to require also the participation of antigen-specific MHC Class II–restricted CD4 T cells (T-helper cells).[36, 37] The CD4 T cells are believed to mediate their accessory role through the secretion of IL-2 and/or other cytokines that are required for the full activation and maturation of the CTL. Because most tumor cells express MHC Class I molecules but not MHC Class II molecules, it is postulated that some tumor cells are degraded, and released antigen is picked up by MHC Class II expressing antigen-presenting cells (APCs) such as macrophages or dendritic cells. The APCs would then present processed antigen to the CD4 T cells, leading to proliferation and production of cytokines, such as IL-2. It is hypothesized that providing IL-2 directly to unprimed CTL would augment the antitumor CTL response, possibly *short-circuiting* the need for APC presentation and CD4 T-cell activation.

The use of cytokine gene-modified tumor cells was first proposed and used by Bubenik and colleagues in 1988.[65] Watanabe and colleagues were the first to show that rejection of cytokine-secreting tumor cells was also accompanied by the induction of tumor-specific systemic immunity.[66] In close succession to Watanabe's studies, Fearon and colleagues using murine colon carcinoma cells transduced with an IL-2 gene,[67] and Gansbacher and colleagues, using mouse fibrosarcoma cells expressing IL-2 or interferon gamma, have reported that the cytokine-secreting tumor cells were promptly rejected and engendered tumor-specific immunity.[68]

The observation that cytokine gene-modified tumor cells are rejected and induce systemic immunity have been extended to other animal tumor model systems and other cytokines, including IL-4, IL-6, granulocyte-monocyte colony-stimulating factor (GM-CSF), and IL-7.[69–78] However, dependent on the tumor model and cytokine used (and probably dependent on the experimental conditions used in a particular study), cytokine-secreting tumor cells that were rejected did not always induce systemic immunity, nor were cytokine-secreting tumor cells rejected in every case. Nonetheless, these observations that genetically modified tumor cells were capable of inducing significant immune responses against parental nonimmunogenic tumors extends the initial findings of Van Pel and Boone that such *nonimmunogenic tumors* encode potent tumor rejection antigens that can be made accessible to the immune system on proper manipulation of the tumor cells. Collectively, these observations support the view that active immunization of cancer patients deserves consideration.

CLINICAL STUDIES WITH GENE-MODIFIED TUMOR VACCINES

It must be recognized that these animal studies merely provided *proof of principle* that genetically modified tumor could be potentially useful, and therefore improvements leading to better potency and therapeutic outcome are not unlikely. Animal studies use rapidly growing tumors that could mask the therapeutic benefit of immunization strategies that take time to develop. Although more recent animal studies have attempted to approximate as closely as possible the conditions prevailing in the human patient, animal models cannot accurately reproduce the complexity and variability exhibited among human patients, and therefore information obtained from such studies provides useful but only general guidelines for planning clinical studies in human patients. For example, animal models use tumor cell lines and clones that are vastly different from the tumor heterogeneity seen in freshly isolated human tumors. In addition, the tumor models used are often extremely sensitive to the tumor burden in the experimental animals, such that the success of a particular immunization strategy can be negated by increasing the tumor burden. Because the individual tumor burden may vary between subjects, the immunization strategies used may show variable results despite induction of similar levels of tumor-specific immunity. Another difference in the clinical studies is that the relative age of patients is much greater compared with the animals, which may have a significant impact on the ability of the host to mount a vigorous specific immune response. A particular concern with animal studies exploring immunotherapeutic strategies is the fact that treatment of recently established 3- to 7-day-old tumors in animals fails to take into account the fact that cancer patients would become candidates for immunotherapy after a long history of disease and treatments. The concern has been raised that such individuals may be in a state of generalized or tumor-specific immunosuppression, and therefore the question not addressed in animal studies is whether treatment with genetically modified tumor cells would also be able to reverse a possible state of unresponsiveness.

Simplified methods to introduce and express cytokine genes in primary tumor explants that are compatible with clinical procedures have been developed and improved. Retroviral vectors have so far been the method of choice to introduce and express genes in mammalian cells, including tumor cells.[72, 79] The major drawbacks of using retroviral vectors is their complexity and the fact that retroviral vectors require actively dividing cells for stable gene transfer. This represents a serious limitation in clinical studies because of difficulties in establishing even short-term cultures from many freshly obtained tumor specimens. Because stable and long-term expression of cytokines from tumor vaccines is not a prerequisite (because irradiated tumor vaccines are expected to persist in view for a limited period of time), alternative and simpler methods of gene transfer that would result in efficient, although transient, expression of cytokines from tumor cells may be also useful and would be preferable to the use of retroviral vectors. Two types of alternative gene-delivery systems can be considered.

The first alternative includes viral vectors that result in efficient, although transient, gene transfer and expression, such as vectors derived from poxviruses[80] or adenoviruses.[81, 82] In either case, cell division is not a prerequisite for viral infection and gene transfer. Adenoviruses or poxviruses are large viruses encoding a multitude of genes. The viral vectors consist of replication competent attenuated viruses or replication-incompetent defective viruses from which essential genes were deleted. In either case, many viral genes are still expressed in the transduced cell with the gene of interest. The potential drawbacks of using such vectors in immunotherapy are adverse effects on cellular metabolism and hence tumor antigen presentation; viral antigenic load that could mask or interfere with presentation of tumor antigen; pre-existence or induction of antiviral responses that may limit their use or secondary boosting; and safety concerns stemming from the use of attenuated or replication incompetent viruses in human patients, especially if they are immunodeficient.

A second alternative gene delivery system consists of *physical* gene delivery methods, in which plasmid DNA is delivered directly to the tumor cells. There is a long list of such nonviral or physical methods of gene delivery into mammalian cells, including calcium phosphate–mediated gene transfer, electroporation, use of liposomes[83, 84] as DNA carriers, receptor-mediated gene transfer, or even gene transfer by particle bombardment using a gene gun. Although on occa-

sion nonviral gene delivery can result in efficient gene transfer, persistence and expression in the transduced cells is invariably transient and waning within 2 to 3 days. However, if cells are growth arrested after gene transfer, the transduced gene will persist episomally and be expressed for an extended period of time, which could extend over 7 to 14 days. Because tumor vaccines will be used in an irradiated form, such transient and potentially efficient gene delivery systems may be adequate.

Given the potential of gene-modified tumor vaccines, it is next necessary to embark on the rational and systematic application of this approach to human tumors. Traditionally recognized immunologic targets such as melanoma and renal cell carcinoma are clearly candidates for this approach, yet they represent only a small fraction of the tumors seen annually. More important, it must be questioned if SAI with gene-modified tumor approach can be rationally applied to other common tumors or if only tumors considered *immunogenic* are candidates. As discussed earlier, animal studies suggest that active immunotherapy may be effective also against cancers that do not manifest intrinsic immunogenicity.

A more compelling concern for investigators may be in developing trials of efficacy in human tumors that are likely to show the benefit of SAI. It is clear that an important prerequisite of the ability of SAI to inhibit metastasis is the ability to reduce to a minimum the numbers of tumor cells in the animals by surgical cytoreduction. Therefore, it is possible that the efficacy of SAI in human tumors may only be demonstrated in patients in which no clinically detectable disease is present (i.e., only microscopic disease remains). In addition to selection of a tumor type and disease stage that would favor the demonstration of a clinical response in the application of SAI with gene-modified tumor vaccines, practical considerations such as the availability of tumor for gene modification must be considered. It does not appear justifiable to advocate complex or hazardous operations simply for the acquisition of tumor to be used for trials of SAI with gene-modified tumor.

Ideally, an effective vaccine would reduce the incidence and growth of metastasis and, most importantly, prolong patient survival. Initial studies with gene-modified tumor vaccines will concentrate on patients with established disease who may not demonstrate a measurable clinical response in spite of the induction of biologically detectable antitumor immune response. Because clinical end-points may lack the sensitivity to document an effective antitumor immune response, other parameters elicited by the gene-modified tumor vaccine are necessary. Other clinical parameters that may suggest that adequate levels of cytokine are being expressed to elicit an inflammatory response include delayed-type hypersensitivity reactions surrounding the vaccination sites and possibly inflammatory reactions surrounding non–gene-transduced sentinel lesions.[85] Nonetheless, neither of these responses are known to correlate with either clinical benefit or the appearance of biologically relevant immunologic responses.

Therefore, the design of the current phase I/II clinical trials attempts to provide information to address these areas in addition to providing safety and toxicity data. Specifically, the phase I/II clinical trials will focus on (1) risk assessment of the gene modification, especially by replication defective retroviral constructs in tumor modified by retroviral vectors; (2) local versus systemic toxicity from cytokine production; (3) effects on the patients' humoral and cellular immune response; (4) impact on the growth of established metastatic tumor nodules at other sites; and (5) patient survival.

Although animal studies have shown that genetically modified tumor vaccines have considerable potency, by no means do they signify a breakthrough in cancer immunotherapy. An optimistic view is that following additional research and development, some forms of cancer will eventually respond to such treatment.

NEW APPROACHES TO SPECIFIC ACTIVE IMMUNOTHERAPY

Whereas most animal studies have used genetically modified syngeneic tumor cells, an alternative strategy to gene-modified tumor vaccinations is to use allogeneic or even xenogeneic cells engineered to secrete specific cytokines, which are administered to the patient in a mixture with unmodified irradiated autologous tumor cells. This approach is based on the reasonable assumption that cytokines secreted from the genetically modified tumor cells function in a paracrine, and not autocrine, manner is most efficient in stimulating an immune response. For example, Tahara and colleagues have shown that syngeneic fibroblasts engineered to secrete IL-12 can suppress tumor growth and induce systemic immunity in a murine melanoma model.[86] The advantages of using a well-characterized, optimized, and universal cytokine-secreting cell line are obvious. The concern, however, is that expression of foreign and potentially immunogenic determinants from nonautologous cells could be detrimental to the generation of effective antitumor immune responses.

Fascination with genetic techniques should not preclude the consideration of more *conventional* non–gene therapy–based approaches. If paracrine secretion of cytokines is all that is needed, then perhaps controlled delivery devices such as pumps or biodegradable microspheres loaded with and secreting cytokines could be used to locally deliver cytokines in the vicinity of the autologous tumor vaccine. Indeed, Golumbek and colleagues have shown that GM-CSF–secreting microcapsules admixed with unmodified irradiated B16 melanoma cells were capable of inducing a protective immune response against a tumor challenge.[87] Whether this approach is comparable or superior to the use of genetically modified tumor vaccines and whether it would have therapeutic benefit in tumor animals as shown with GM-CSF gene-modified vaccines remains to be seen.

The past decade has witnessed quantum leaps in the understanding of immunologic phenomena and led to renewed interest in using immunologic modalities in clinical medicine. A major development that could shape the next generation of tumor vaccines is the emerging recognition that dendritic cells have a pivotal role in immune responses.[88] Dendritic cells, also known as Langerhans cells in the skin or veiled cell in lymph nodes, are derived from bone marrow and are present in low numbers in various tissues throughout the body.[89] Evidence is mounting that the bone marrow–derived dendritic cells are responsible for initiating all T-cell responses *in vivo*, including CD4 T-helper, as well as CD8 CTL responses, by the fact that dendritic cells, but not other cells in the body, are endowed with the unique capability of presenting antigen to naive T cells.[90] This means that an antitumor immune response is not initiated by the tumor that presents antigen directly to unprimed T cells but requires first the uptake and processing of tumor antigen to dendritic cells for presentation to T cells. Some indirect evidence in favor of this pathway in tumor immunity has been reported. The implication for vaccine design is that dendritic cells would be more potent than tumor cells as immunogens.

It is tempting to speculate that the next generation of tumor vaccines could be based on dendritic cells transduced with gene-encoding tumor CTL antigens or *pulsed* with corresponding peptides or proteins. Recently, investigators have treated patients with refractory B-cell lymphoma with dendritic cell–pulsed antigens corresponding to the unique idiotypic determinants on the B cell. Tumor-specific immune responses were documented, and some clinical responses were observed in this small study. Whereas isolation of dendritic cells from the blood is tedious and yields low numbers of cells, advances in generating dendritic cells from hematopoietic progenitors may result in simplified procedures and higher yields.

An astonishingly simpler alternate vaccination strategy was suggested in a report by Ulmer and colleagues, who have shown that injection of naked plasmid DNA encoding the influenza virus nucleoprotein (NP) gene into mice is capable of inducing NP-specific CTL responses and provides cross-protective immunity against challenges with lethal doses of influenza virus. This study has shown that a simple procedure, intramuscular injection of plasmid DNA, can lead to the generation of physiologically relevant CTL immunity, raising the possibility that injection of plasmid DNA encoding tumor rejection antigens into cancer patients would constitute a simple and effective method to induce effective antitumor protective immunity.

COMBINATIONS OF ACTIVE AND ADOPTIVE IMMUNOTHERAPY

Animal studies have also shown that genetically modified tumor cells are capable of inducing T-cell reactivity against tumors with no previous detectable intrinsic immunogenicity, even in instances when therapeutic benefit is not seen. This has tantalizing implications if such observations are demonstrated in tumor-bearing patients. First, it supports the hypothesis that nonimmunogenic forms of human cancer could also respond to immunologic intervention. Second, treatment of patients with genetically modified tumor preparations will provide a ready source of tumor-specific T-cell reactivities that can be further expanded *ex vivo* and reinfused into the patient. Whereas adoptive immunotherapy of cancer patients has been attempted and has shown some promise as discussed previously, a major factor is the limited availability of tumor-specific T-cell reactivities. If animal studies are any indication, then use of genetically modified autologous (irradiated) tumor cells will generate tumor-specific T-cell reactivities from a broader spectrum of cancers and provide the basis for a dual-modality immunologic treatment strategy of cancer patients: (1) active immunotherapy with the genetically modified tumor vaccines to induce antitumor immunity in the patient and (2) adoptive immunotherapy with *ex vivo* expanded T-cell reactivities generated by this treatment. It is not unreasonable to expect that passive and active immunotherapeutic protocols will complement each other and synergize to improve the therapeutic outcome for the patient.

REFERENCES

1. Houghton, A. N.: Cancer antigens: Immune recognition of self and altered self. J. Exp. Med., *180*:1, 1994.
2. Townsend, A., and Bodmer, H.: Antigen recognition by Class I–restricted T lymphocytes. Annu. Rev. Immunol., 7:601, 1989.
3. Wallack, M. K., Steplewski, Z., Koprowski, H., et al.: A new approach in specific, active immunotherapy. Cancer, *39*:560, 1977.
4. Fidler, I.: Critical factors in the biology of human cancer metastases: Twenty-eight G.H.A. Clowes Memorial Award Lecture. Cancer Res., *50*:6130, 1990.
5. Pardoll, D.: New strategies for enhancing the immunogenicity of tumors. Curr. Opin. Immunol., *5*:719, 1993.
6. Boon, T., Cerottini, J., Van den Eynde, B., et al.: Tumor antigens recognized by T lymphocytes. Annu. Rev. Immunol., *12*:337, 1994.
7. Stewart, T. H. M., Shelley, W. E., Willan, A. R., et al.: An evaluation of the role of tumor-specific antigens. Annu. Clin. Conf. Cancer, *28*:351, 1986.
8. Kempf, W., Adams, V., Hassam, S., Schmid, M., Moos, R., Briner, J., and Pfaltz, M.: Detection of human herpesvirus type 6, human herpesvirus type 7, cytomegalovirus and human papillomavirus in cutaneous AIDS-associated Kaposi's sarcoma. Pathology, *78*:260, 1994.

9. Razzaque, A., Williams, O., Wang, J., and Rhim, J. S.: Neoplastic transformation of immortalized human epidermal keratinocytes by two HH-6 DNA clones. Virology, 195:113, 1993.

10. Munoz, N., Bosch, F. X., de Sanjose, S., and Shah, K. V.: The role of HPV in the etiology of cervical cancer. Mutat. Res., 305:293, 1994.

11. Stern, P.: Natural history of HLA expression during tumour development. Immunol. Today, 14:491, 1993.

12. Fontana, A., Constam, D. B., Frei, K., Malipiero, U., and Pfister, H. W.: Modulation of the immune response by transforming growth factor beta. Int. Arch. Allergy Immunol., 99:1, 1992.

13. Arteaga, C. L., Hurd, S. D., Winnier, A. R., Johnson, M. D., Fendly, B. M., Forbes, J. T.: J. Clin. Invest., 92:2569, 1993.

14. Van Pel, A., and Boon, T.: Protection against a nonimmunogenic mouse leukemia by an immunogenic variant obtained by mutagenesis. Proc. Natl. Acad. Sci. USA, 79:4718, 1982.

15. Key, M., Brandhorst, J., and Hanna, M.: More on the relevance of animal tumor models: Immunogenicity of transplantable leukemias of recent origin in syngeneic strain 2 guinea pigs. J. Biol. Res. Modif., 3:359, 1984.

16. Monaco, J.: A molecular model of MHC class-I–restricted antigen processing. Immunol. Today, 13:173, 1992.

17. Geddel-Dahl, T., Spurkland, A., et al.: T cell epitopes encompassing the mutational hot spot position 61 of p21 ras. Promiscuity in ras peptide binding to HLA. Eur. J. Immunol., 24:410, 1994.

18. Yanuck, M., Carbone, D., Pendleton, C., Tsukui, T., Winter, S., Minna, J., and Berzofsky, J.: A mutant p53 tumor suppressor protein is a target for peptide-induced CD8+ cytotoxic T cells. Cancer Res., 53:3257, 1993.

19. Traversari, C., Van der Bruggen, P., Leescher, I. F., Lurquin, C., Chomez, P., Van Pel, A., De Plaen, E., Amar-Costesec, A., and Boon, T.: A nonapeptide encoded by human gene MAGE-1 is recognized on HLA-A1 by cytolytic T lymphocytes directed against tumor antigen MZ2-E. J. Exp. Med., 176:1453, 1992.

20. van der Bruggen, P., Szikora, J.-P., Boel, P., Wildman, C., Somville, M., Sensi, M., and Boon, T.: Autologous cytolytic T lymphocytes recognize a MAGE-1 nonapeptide on melanoma expressing HLA-Cw* 1601. Eur. J. Immunol., 24:2134, 1994.

21. Gaugler, B., Van den Eynde, B., van der Bruggen, P., Romero, P., Gaforio, J. J., De Plaen, E., Lethe, B., Brasseur, F., and Boon, T.: Human gene MAGE-3 codes for antigen recognized on a melanoma by autologous cytolytic T lymphocytes. J. Exp. Med., 179:921, 1994.

22. Ioannides, C. G., Fisk, B., Fan, D., Biddison, W. E., Wharton, J. T., and O'Brian, C. A.: Cytotoxic T cells isolated from ovarian malignant ascites recognize a peptide derived from the HER-2/neu proto-oncogene. Cell. Immunol., 151:225, 1993.

23. Yoshido, I., Peoples, G. E., Goedegebuure, P. S., Maziarz, R., and Erberlin, T. J.: Association of HER-2/neu expression with sensitivity to tumor-specific CTL in human ovarian cancer. J. Immunol., 152:2393, 1994.

24. Disis, M. L., Bernhard, H., Gralow, J. R., Hand, S. L., Emery, S. R., Calenoff, E., and Cheever, M. A.: Immunity to the HER-2/neu oncogenic protein. Ciba Found. Symp., 187:198, 1994.

25. Fisk, B., Chesak, B., Pollack, M. S., Wharton, J. T., and Ioannides, C. G.: Oligopeptides induction of a cytolytic T lymphocyte response to HER-2/neu proto-oncogene in vitro. Cell Immunol., 157:415, 1994.

26. Jerome, K. R., Barnd, D. L., Bendt, K. M., Boyer, C. M., Papadimitriou, J. T., McKenzie, I. F. C., Bast, Jr., R. C., and Finn, O. J.: Cytotoxic T-lymphocytes derived from patients with breast adenocarcinoma recognize an epitope present on the protein core of a mucin molecule preferentially expressed by malignant cells. Cancer Res., 51:2908, 1991.

27. Apostolopoulos, V., Pietersz, G. A., Xing, P. X., Lees, C. J., Michael, M., Bishop, J., and McKenzie, I. F.: The immunogenicity of MUC1 peptides and fusion protein. Cancer Lett., 90:21, 1995.

28. Cox, L. S., and Lane, D. P.: Tumor suppressors, kinases and clamps: how p53 regulates the cell cycle in response to DNA damage. Bioessays, 17:501, 1995.

29. Gohring, U. J., Scharl, A., Heckel, C., Ahr, A., and Crombach, G.: p53 protein in 204 patients with primary breast carcinoma: Immunohistochemical detection and clinical value as aprognostic factor. Arch. Gynecol. Obstet., 256:139, 1995.

30. Bei, R., Kantor, J., Kashmiri, S. V., Abrams, S., and Schlom, J.: Enhanced immune responses and antitumor activity by baculovirus recombinant carcinoembryonic antigen (CEA) in mice primed with the recombinant vaccinia CEA. J. Immunother. 16:275, 1994.

31. Kawakami, Y., Eliyahu, S., Sakaguchi, K., Robbins, P. F., Rivoltini, L., Yanneli, J. R., Appella, E., Rosenberg, S. A.: Identification of the immunodominant peptides of the MART-1 human melanoma antigen recognized by the majority of HLA-A2 restricted tumor infiltrating lymphocytes. J. Exp. Med., 180:347, 1994.

32. Kawakami, Y., Elyahu, S., Jennins, C., Sakaguchi, K., Kang, X., Southwood, S., Robbins, P. F., Sette, A., Appella, E., and Rosenberg, S. A.: Recognition of multiple epitopes in human melanoma antigen gp100 by tumor-infiltrating T lymphocytes associated with in vivo tumor regression. J. Immunol., 54:3961, 1995.

33. Wolfel, T., Van Pel, A., Brichard, V., Schneider, J., Seliger, B., Meyer zum Buschenfelde, K.-H., and Boon, T.: Two tyrosinase nanopeptides recognized on HLA-A2 melanoma by autologous cytolytic T lymphocytes. Eur. J. Immunol., 24:759, 1995.

34. McCune, C. S., Schapira, D. V., Henshaw, E. C., et al.: Specific immunotherapy of advanced renal carcinoma: Evidence for the polyclonality of metastases. Cancer, 47:1984, 1981.

35. Parmiani, G.: Tumor immunity as autoimmunity: Tumor antigens include normal self proteins which stimulate anergic peripheral T cells. Immunol. Today, 14:536, 1993.

36. Keene, J., and Forman, J.: Helper activity is required for the in vitro generation of cytotoxic T lymphocytes. J. Exp. Med., 155:768, 1982.

37. Kast, W., Bronkhorst, A., De Waal, L., and Melief, C.: Cooperation between cytotoxic and helper T lymphocytes in protection against lethal Sendai virus infection. J. Exp. Med., 164:723, 1986.

38. Greenberg, P.: Adoptive T cell therapy of tumors: Mechanisms operative in the recognition and elimination of tumor cells. In Dixon, F. (Ed.): Advances in Immunology, Orlando, Fla., Academic Press, 1991.

39. Riddell, S., and Greenberg, P.: Principles for adoptive T cell therapy of human viral diseases. Annu. Rev. Immunol., 13:545, 1995.

40. Rosenberg, S., et al.: Observation on the systemic administration of autologous lymphokine-activated killer cells and recombinant interleukin-2 to patients with metastatic cancer. N. Engl. J. Med., 313:1485, 1985.

41. Rosenberg, S., et al.: A progress report in the treatment of 157 patients with advanced cancer using lymphokine-activated killer cells and interleukin-2 or high-dose interleukin-2 alone. N. Engl. J. Med., 316:1310, 1986.

42. Fisher, B., Packard, B. S., Read, E. J., Carrasquillo, J. A., Carter, C. S., Topalian, S. L., Yang, J. C., Yolles, P., Larson, S. M., and Rosenberg, S. A.: Tumor localization of adoptively transferred indium-111 labeled tumor infiltrating lymphocytes in patients with metastatic lymphoma. J. Clin. Oncol., 7:250, 1989.

42a. Wallack, M. K., Bash, I., and Bartolucci, A.: Improvement in disease-free survival of melanoma patients in conjunction with serologic response in a phase 1a/1b Southeastern Cancer Study Group trial of vaccinia melanoma oncolysate. Am. Surg., 55:244, 1989.

43. Arroyo, P. I., Bash, J. A., and Wallack, M. K.: Active specific immunotherapy with vaccinia colon oncolysate enhances the immunomodulatory and antitumor effects of interleukin-2 and interferon-α in a murine hepatic metastasis model. Cancer Immunol. Immunother., 31:305, 1990.

44. Freedman, R. S., Edwards, C. L., Bowen, J. M., et al.: Viral oncolysates in patients with advanced ovarian cancer. Gynecol. Oncol., 29:337, 1988.

45. Furukawa, K., Lotzova, E., Freedman, R. S., et al.: Effect of virus-modified tumor cell extracts, autologous mononuclear cell infusions and interleukin-2 on oncolytic activity of effector cells of patients with advanced ovarian cancer. Cancer Immunol. Immunother., 30:126, 1989.

46. Ioannides, C. G., Platsoucas, C. D., O'Brian, C. A., et al.: Viral oncolysates in cancer treatment: Immunological mechanisms of action (Review). Anticancer Res., 9:535, 1989.

47. Ioannides, C. G., Platsoucas, C. D., Patenia, R., et al.: T-cell functions in ovarian cancer patients treated with viral oncolysates: I. Increased helper activity to immunoglobulin production. Anticancer Res., 10:645, 1990.

48. Wolfram, B., Schlag, P., Liebrich, W., et al.: Postoperative active specific immunization in colorectal cancer patients with virus-modified autologous tumor-cell vaccine (first clinical results with tumor-cell vaccines modified with live but avirulent Newcastle disease virus). Cancer, 66:1517, 1990.

49. Hollinshead, A., Elias, E. G., Arlen, M., et al.: Specific active immunotherapy in patients with adenocarcinoma of the colon utilizing tumor-associated antigens (TAA). Cancer, 56:480, 1985.

50. Hollinshead, A., Stewart, T. H. M., Takita, H., et al.: Adjuvant specific active lung cancer immunotherapy trials. Cancer, 60:1249, 1987.

51. Kurth, K. H., Marquet, R., Zwartendijk, L., et al.: Active, specific immunotherapy with autologous tumor cells and mixed with Corynebacterium parvum in patients with metastatic renal cell carcinoma. In: Klippel, K. F., and Macher, E. (Eds.): Proceedings of the International Symposium, Nonnweiler, Present Status of Non-toxic Concepts in Cancer, Basel, Karger, 1986, pp. 221–236.

52. Specific Immunotherapy of Cancer with Vaccines: Proceedings of a Conference, Washington, D.C., January 21–24, 1993. Ann. N.Y. Acad. Sci., 690:388, 1993.

53. Wiseman, C., Presant, C., Rao, R., and Smith, J.: Clinical responses to intralymphatic whole-cell melanoma vaccine augmented by in vitro incubation with alpha-interferon. Ann. N.Y. Acad. Sci. 690:388, 1993.

54. Hoon, D. S.: Morisaki, T., Uchiyama, A., Hayashi, Y., Foshag, L. J., Nizze, A. J., and Morton, D. L.: Augmentation of T-cell response with a melanoma cell vaccine expressing specific HLA-A antigens. Ann. N.Y. Acad. Sci., 690:343, 1993.

55. Wallack, M. K., and Sivanandham, M.: Clinical trials with VMO for melanoma. Ann. N.Y. Acad. Sci., 690:178, 1993.

56. Hersey, P.: Evaluation of vaccinia viral lysates as therapeutic vaccines in the treatment of melanoma. Ann. N.Y. Acad. Sci., 690:167, 1993.

57. Mitchell, M. S., Harel, W., Kan-Mitchell, J., LeMay, L. G., Goedegebuure, P., Huang, X. Q., Hofman, F., and Groshen, S.: Active specific immunotherapy of melanoma with allogeneic cell lysates: Rationale, results, and possible mechanisms of action. Ann. N.Y. Acad. Sci., 690:153, 1993.

58. Berd, D., Maguire, H. C., Jr., and Mastrangelo, M. J.: Treatment of human melanoma with a hapten-modified autologous vaccine. Ann. N.Y. Acad. Sci., 690:147, 1993.

59. Morton, D. L., Hoon, D. S., Nizze, J. A., Foshag, L. J., Famatiga, E., Wanek, L. A., Chang, C., Irie, R. F., Gupta, R. K. and Elashoff, R.: Polyvalent melanoma vaccine improves survival of patients with metastatic melanoma. Ann. N.Y. Acad. Sci., 690:120, 1993.

60. Galligioni, E., Francini, M., Quaia, M., Carbone, A., Spada, A., Sacco, C., Favaro, D., Santarosa, M., Carmignani, G., Di Donna, D., et al.: Randomized study of adjuvant immunotherapy with autologous tumor cells and BCG in renal cancer. Ann. N.Y. Acad. Sci., 690:367, 1993.

61. Schirrmacher, V., Schlag, P., Liebrich, W., Patel, B. T., and Stoeck, M.: Specific immunotherapy of colorectal carcinoma with Newcastle-disease virus-modified autologous tumor cells prepared from resected liver metastasis. Ann. N.Y. Acad. Sci., 690:364, 1993.

62. Ulsperger, E., Rainer, H., Locker, G., Vetterlein, M., Schiessel, R., and Hofbauer, F., Armbruster, C., Depisch, D., Politzer, P., Dinstl, K., et al.: Adjuvant vaccination in colorectal carcinoma. Ann. N.Y. Acad. Sci., 690:360, 1993.

63. Hanna, M. G., Jr., Ransom, J. H., Pomato, N., Peters, L., Bloemena, E., Vermorken, J. B., and Hoover, H. C., Jr.: Active specific immunotherapy of human colorectal carcinoma with an autologous tumor cell/bacillus Calmette-Guérin vaccine. Ann. N.Y. Acad. Sci., 690:135, 1993.

64. Livingston, P.: Active specific immunotherapy in the treatment of patients with cancer. Immunol. Allergy Clin. North Am., 11:401, 1991.

65. Bubenik, J., Perlmann, P., Indrova, M., Simova, J., Jandlova, T., and Neuwirt, J.: Growth inhibition of an MC-induced mouse sarcoma by TCGF (IL-2) containing preparation. Cancer Immunol. Immunother., 14:205, 1983.

66. Watanabe, Y., Kuribayashi, K., Miyatake, S., Nishihara, K., Nakayama, E., Taniyama, T., and Skata, T.: Exogenous expression of mouse interferon gamma cDNA in mouse neuroblastoma C1300 cells results in reduced tumorigenicity by augmented anti-tumor immunity. Proc. Natl. Acad. Sci., 86:9456, 1989.

67. Fearon, E., Pardoll, D., Itaya, T., Golumbek, P., Levitsky, H., Simons, J., Karasuyama, H., Vogelstein, B., and Frost, P.: Interleukin-2 production by tumor cells bypasses T helper function in the generation of an antitumor response. Cell, 60:397, 1990.

68. Gansbacher, B., Zier, K., Daniels, B., Cronin, K., Bannerji, R., and Gilboa, E.: Interleukin-2 gene transfer into tumor cells abrogates tumorigenicity and induces protective immunity. J. Exp. Med., 172:1217, 1990.

69. Gansbacher, B., Bannerji, R., Daniels, B., Zier, K., Cronin, K., and Gilboa, E.: Retroviral vector-mediated gamma-interferon gene transfer into tumor cells generates potent and long lasting anti-tumor immunity. Cancer Res., 50:7820, 1990.

70. Colombo, M., and Forni, G.: Cytokine gene transfer in tumor inhibition and tumor therapy: Where are we now? Immunol. Today, 15:48, 1994.

71. Tepper, R., and Mule, J.: Experimental and clinical studies of cytokine gene-modified tumor cells. Hum. Gene Ther. 5:153, 1994.

72. Gilboa, E., Lyerly, H., Vieweg, J., and Saito, S.: Immunotherapy of cancer using cytokine gene modified tumor vaccines. Semin. Cancer Biol., 23:8101, 1996.

73. Porgador, A., Tzehoval, E., Katz, A., Vadai, E., Revel, M., Feldman, M., and Eisenbach, L.: Interleukin 6 gene transfection into Lewis lung carcinoma tumor cells suppresses the malignant phenotype and confers immunotherapeutic competence against parental metastatic cells. Cancer Res., 52:3679, 1992.

74. Porgador, A., Bannerji, R., Watanabe, Y., Feldman, M., Gilboa, E., and Eisenbach, L.: Antimetastatic vaccination of tumor-bearing mice with two types of gamma-interferon gene inserted tumor cells. J. Immunol., 150:1458, 1993.

75. Porgador, A., Gansbacher, B., Bannerji, R., Tzehoval, E., Gilboa, E., Feldman, M., and Eisenbach, L.: Antimetastatic vaccination of tumor bearing mice with IL-2 gene inserted tumor cells. Int. J. Cancer, 53:471, 1993.

76. Connor, J., Bannerji, R., Saito, S., Heston, W., Fair, W., and Gilboa, E.: Regression of bladder tumors in mice treated with interleukin-2 gene-modified tumor cells. J. Exp. Med., 177:1127, 1993.

77. Dranoff, G., Jaffee, E., Lazenby, A., Golumbek, P., Levitsky, H., Brose, K., Jackson, V., Hamada, H., Pardoll, D., and Mulligan, R.: Vaccination with irradiated tumor cells engineered to secrete murine granulocyte-macrophage colony-stimulating factor stimulates potent, specific, and long-lasting anti-tumor immunity. Proc. Natl. Acad. Sci. USA, 90:3539, 1993.

78. Vieweg, J., Rosenthal, F., Bannerji, R., Heston, W., Fair, W., Gansbacher, B., and Gilboa, E.: Immunotherapy of prostate cancer in the Dunning rat model: Use of cytokine gene modified tumor vaccines. Cancer Res., 54:1760, 1994.

79. Jaffee, E., Dranoff, G., Cohen, L., Hauda, K., Clift, S., Marshall, F., Mulligan, R., and Pardoll, D.: High efficiency gene transfer into primary human tumor explants without cell selection. Cancer Res., 53:2221, 1993.

80. Carter, B. J.: Parvoviruses as vectors. In Tijssen, P. (Ed.): Handbook of Parvoviruses, vol. II. Boca Raton, Fla., CRC Press, 1990, pp. 247–284.

81. Berns, K. I., and Bohenzky, R. A.: Adeno-associated virus: An update. Adv. Virus Res., 32:243, 1987.

82. Muzyczka, M.: Use of adeno-associated virus as a general transduction vector for mammalian cells. Curr. Topics Microbiol. Immunol., 158:97, 1992.

83. Wang, C.-Y., and Huang, L.: pH-sensitive immunoliposomes mediate target-cell-specific delivery and controlled expression of a foreign gene in mouse. Proc. Natl. Acad. Sci. USA, 84:7851, 1987.

84. Felgner, P. L., Northrop, J. P., Ringold, G. M., and Danielsen, M.: A highly efficient, lipid-mediated DNA transfection procedure. Proc. Natl. Acad. Sci. USA, 84:7413, 1987.

85. Barth, A., Hoon, D. S. B., Foshag, L. J., Nizze, A., Famatiga, E., Okun, E., Morton, D. L.: Polyvalent melanoma cell vaccine induces delayed-type hypersensitivity and in vitro cellular immune response. Cancer Res., 54:3342, 1994.

86. Tahara, H., Zeh, H. J., III, Storkus, J., et al.: Fibroblasts genetically engineered to secrete interleukin 12 can suppress tumor growth and induce antitumor immunity to a murine melanoma in vivo. Cancer Res., 54:182, 1994.

87. Golumbek, P. T., Azhari, R., Jaffee, E. M., et al.: Controlled release, biodegradable cytokine depots: A new approach in cancer vaccine design. Cancer Res., 53:5841, 1993.

88. Steinman, R.: The dendritic cell system and its role in immunogenicity. Annu. Rev. Immunol., 9:271, 1991.

89. Romani, N., Gruner, S., Brang, D., Kampgen, E., Lenz, A., Trockenbacher, B., Konwalinka, G., Fritsch, P. O., Steinman, R. M., Schuler, G.: Proliferating dendritic cell progenitors in human blood. J. Exp. Med., 180:83, 1994.

90. Huang, A., Golumbek, P., Ahmadzadeh, M., Jaffee, E., Pardoll, D., and Levitsky, H.: Role of bone marrow–derived cells in presenting MHC Class 1–restricted tumor antigens. Science, 264:961, 1994.

II

MELANOMA

Craig L. Slingluff, Jr., M.D., and H. F. Seigler, M.D.

Melanoma is a neoplastic disorder produced by malignant transformation of the normal melanocyte. Melanocytes are the cells that produce the pigment melanin. During the first trimester of fetal life, precursor melanocytes arise in the neural crest. As the fetus develops, these cells migrate to areas including the skin, meninges, mucous membranes, upper esophagus, and eyes. In each of these locations, melanocytes have demonstrated a potential for malignant transformation, but the site most commonly associated with melanocytic transformation is the skin, where melanocytes reside at the dermal-epidermal junction. Melanoma represents 4% to 5% of all skin malignancies. Although malignant melanoma is only the eighth most common cancer diagnosis in the United States,[9] the large majority (80%) of melanoma patients present in the productive years from age 25 to 65. The mean age for diagnosis of melanoma is 48, which is substantially lower than that of patients with colon, lung, or prostate cancer. Melanoma ranks second behind leukemia as a cause of cancer deaths in U.S. males aged 15 to 34.[9]

The actual incidence of melanoma is increasing more rapidly than that of any other malignancy, with over 30,000 cases diagnosed each year in the United States. In the early part of this century, the lifetime risk of a Caucasian developing melanoma was approximately 1 in 1500. Currently this risk is approximately 1 in 100.[32, 53] Despite general physician awareness and excellent public education, this malignancy has an approximate 25% to 30% mortality in the United States.[9] The management of malignant melanoma involves prevention, early diagnosis, surgical extirpation, and management of metastatic disease. There is continued debate about the role of elective lymph node dissection (ELND). Recent trends in therapy have included aggressive surgical treatment of isolated distant metastases, hyperthermic limb perfusion, and application of experimental immunotherapeutic methods.

EPIDEMIOLOGY AND ETIOLOGY

Several demographic factors affect both the incidence and the outcome of melanoma. Individuals with Celtic ancestry appear to have the highest predilection for development of this disease. As Celtic people migrate to more temperate climates, the incidence of melanoma increases and exceeds that of non-Celtic subjects living in a similar area.[59, 67] This is particularly evident in Australia, where the highest per capita incidence of melanoma is found. In general, melanoma is far more common in Caucasians than in Asian and black populations. Reintgen and associates have reviewed the literature and suggest that a risk ratio of whites to blacks for melanoma is 20 to 1.[77] Women develop melanoma slightly more often than men, and their melanomas arise more commonly on the lower extremities. Women also have a better prognosis than men with equivalent lesions. These differences do not appear to be due to direct effects of estrogen, but the effects of gender on the development and progression of melanoma are significant. Although patients of any age may develop melanoma, it is extremely rare for melanoma to occur before puberty, and the median age for diagnosis is in the late forties.

The role of ultraviolet light as an etiologic factor in melanoma remains unresolved.[82] Malignant transformation is thought to require initiation of DNA damage, promoting factors, and altered stimulation for cell growth. Ultraviolet radiation is suspected to have a role in the development of skin cancers, including basal cell cancer, squamous cell cancer, and melanoma. Ultraviolet rays are divided into spectra according to the wavelength of the radiation: UVC (200–290 nm.), UVB (290–320 nm.), and UVA (320–400 nm.). UVC is probably completely absorbed by the ozone layer. UVB radiation is responsible for sunburn and for inducing melanin production in skin, causing tanning. UVA penetrates more deeply into the dermis and probably is responsible for most of the sun-induced changes of dermal connective tissue and loss of elasticity that characterize the aging process and skin wrinkling. It is thought, however, that both UVA and UVB radiation can be carcinogenic. Bodenham has suggested that both the incidence of melanoma and the subsequent mortality can be correlated with the degree of sunlight exposure.[8] Other reports are controversial. It has been reported that persons exposed chronically to the sun (e.g., maritime workers and farmers) are not at increased risk of melanoma, but that severe sunburns early in life correlate best with increased risk of melanoma.

At present, the only avoidable presumed risk factor for melanoma is sun exposure. Sun block is recommended, especially in fair-skinned children, to prevent severe burns, which may reduce the risk of developing melanoma. Because melanoma does occur in sites not exposed to the sun, such as mucous membrane sites, sun exposure is clearly not the only etiologic factor. It is likely that several factors are important in producing malignant transformation of the melanocyte. Age, hormonal status, genetic predisposition, environmental factors, injury, and other host factors probably contribute to various degrees. Other risk factors include sun exposure, dysplastic nevus syndrome, xeroderma pigmentosum, a history of nonmelanoma skin cancer, higher socioeconomic status, and family history of melanoma.[27, 29, 61] Increasingly, carcinogenesis is recognized as a multifactorial process, usually involving the presence of a genetic component and an environmental one. Abnormalities of chromosomes 1, 6, and 9 have each been implicated in melanoma patients.[2, 21, 72, 73] The

tumor suppressor gene *p16* (*MTS1*) has been linked to some familial melanomas.[1]

PRECURSOR LESIONS AND RISK FACTORS

Most melanomas occur in patients with a Celtic complexion (fair and freckled skin that burns easily, blond or red hair, blue eyes).[28] A pre-existing mole (nevus) at the site of primary cutaneous melanoma is common. One must, therefore, focus on precursor pigmented lesions that have a high potential for malignant transformation if early diagnosis and appropriate therapy are to be meaningful. Rhodes and Melsky have reported a cumulative risk of melanoma for individuals with small congenital nevi to be as high as 5%.[83]

The best-known clinical syndrome associated with melanoma is the dysplastic nevus syndrome (alternatively known as the B-K mole syndrome[19] or the atypical mole syndrome[52]). Clinically, dysplastic nevi tend to be large (6–15 mm.) and to have variations in colors and indistinct borders, but they usually remain macular.[40] Although the dysplastic nevus has been described in detail, opinions differ about its precise definition and about the definition and appropriate management of patients with the syndrome.[20, 88] There is general agreement that dysplastic nevi (DN) may be confused with melanomas by both the clinician and the pathologist, that they are associated with an increased risk of melanoma, and that any lesion that looks suspicious or has recently changed deserves careful examination and probable biopsy. Questions remain about optimal management of two groups of patients: those with numerous dysplastic nevi (e.g., > 100), and those with DN and a family history of melanoma.

Several approaches are taken by dermatologists and surgical oncologists, and individualization is indicated. Approaches include regular full-body photographs every 6 months to assess for and to document changes. This is an expensive but thorough approach. Another is to biopsy lesions that appear to change clinically, using physical examination but not routine photography. Other approaches include sequential excisional biopsies of all dysplastic nevi.

The probability that a single dysplastic nevus will become a melanoma is quite small, but in a patient with dysplastic nevus syndrome and a family history of melanoma, the risk of developing melanoma approaches 100%.[39, 54] A reasonable approach to the management of these patients, practiced in several major centers, is histologic verification of the diagnosis by excisional biopsy of representative lesions, screening and education of all family members, regular examinations by physician and patient, photographic surveillance, and biopsy of changing lesions.[40, 102]

Spitz nevi (spindle and epithelioid nevi) are commonly confused with melanoma,[113] both clinically and pathologically. This nevus usually demonstrates a pattern of rapid growth with differing pigmentation. The lesion is well circumscribed, is raised, and may vary in color from pink to dark brown, black, or blue-black. This lesion is most common in young adults. Simple but complete excision of the Spitz nevus is recommended. An experienced dermatopathologist is often required to distinguish between Spitz nevi and melanoma.

Giant congenital nevi occur in approximately 1 in 20,000 newborns. The consensus suggests that the risk of melanoma in these lesions is approximately 5% to 8%.[113] Malignant transformation may be observed during early childhood; therefore, it is recommended that these lesions be excised prophylactically, if possible. Although excision may require multiple procedures, the overall benefits usually outweigh the risks.

Melanoma may occur as a familial disease. Over 150 kindreds have been reported in the literature, with an average

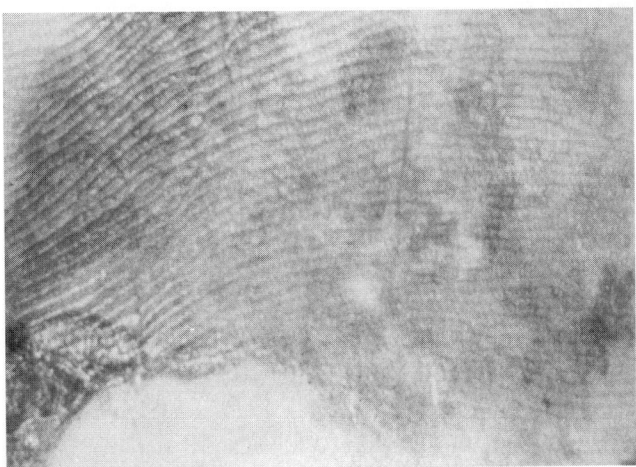

Figure 21–2. Clinical appearance of lentigo maligna melanoma.

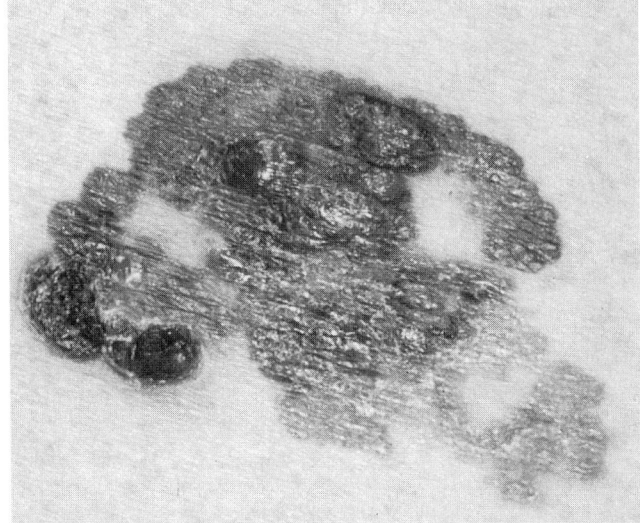

Figure 21–4. Superficial spreading melanoma with irregular borders, differing pigmentation, and nodular degeneration.

of 3 cases per family. Half of the families report an affected parent with one or more affected siblings. The kindred reported by Anderson and associates had 15 affected individuals.[1] All reported kindreds were of Caucasian descent, with Celtic extraction being the most prevalent.

CLINICAL FEATURES

Melanoma usually presents as a pigmented skin lesion that has recently changed. The lesions typically have irregular borders; variegated pigmentation ranging from pink to blue to black; and a raised, irregular surface. Advanced lesions present with itching and bleeding, presumably signs that the lesion has invaded into the cutaneous nerve plexus or superficial capillary bed. Advanced lesions also may be ulcerated.

Any change in a nevus is an important sign that the nevus may be malignant or may be undergoing malignant transformation. A change in color, a papule arising in the center of an existing nevus, bleeding, and ulceration, are each highly suspicious for malignant melanoma. Although melanomas arise *de novo* in most cases, they may arise from pre-existing nevi in 10% to 50% of cases.[18, 62] It is not unusual for a melanoma to present as a nevus present since childhood that has undergone malignant transformation. Unfortunately, patients often ignore these lesions, thinking that because the lesion is not new, it must be benign. This explains some

delays in diagnosis and treatment and identifies a place for education in the prevention of advanced disease.

Melanoma's typical characteristics usually include the following five features that can be remembered with the commonly cited mnemonic "ABCDE," whose letters stand for asymmetry, border irregularity, color variation, diameter greater than 6 mm., and elevation. Typical examples of malignant melanoma are seen in Figures 21–2 to 21–5. It is important to remember that melanoma can present in an atypical manner with only some of these features. In particular, it is preferable to diagnose melanomas in the absence of skin elevation and when the diameter is small, because those are most likely to be thin melanomas or melanomas *in situ*, associated with a very good prognosis.

In a minority of cases, malignant transformation of the melanocyte is associated with loss of pigment production; these patients present with amelanotic, or nonpigmented, melanoma. This presentation is particularly insidious and threatening to the patient. Patient and clinician alike expect a melanoma to have pigment, so a raised, skin-colored lesion may go unnoticed or untreated for an extended time. The absence of pigment may also indicate a more poorly differentiated state, which may be more aggressive.[49]

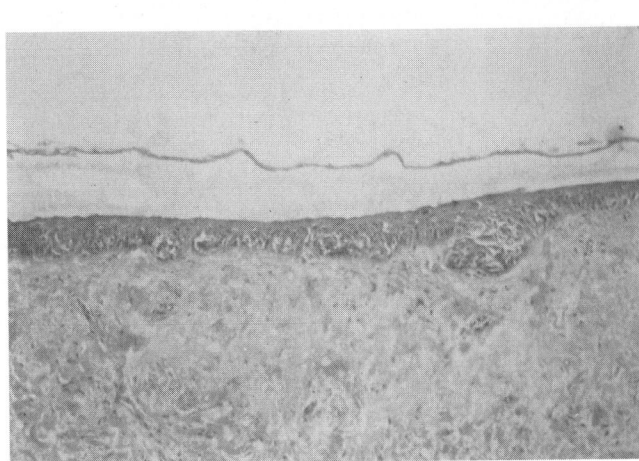

Figure 21–3. Histopathologic pattern of lentigo maligna melanoma.

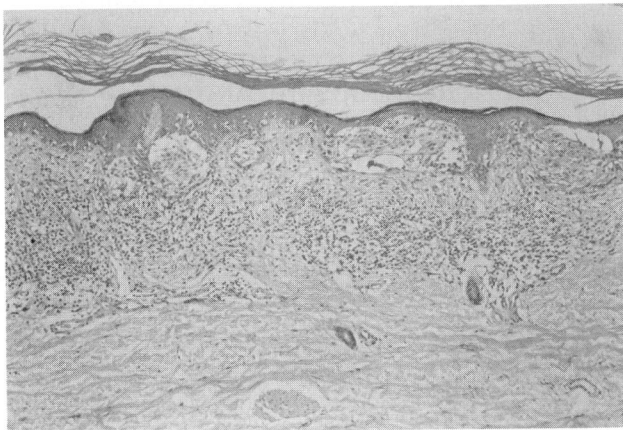

Figure 21–5. Histopathologic pattern of superficial spreading melanoma.

Unknown Primary Lesion

In approximately 3% to 5% of cases, patients present with evidence of metastatic disease but without evidence of a primary lesion. These circumstances may be associated with a history of an excised nevus for which pathology is no longer evaluable, or a history of a nevus that spontaneously blanched and resolved. The diagnosis of an unknown primary lesion is a diagnosis of exclusion and may be made only after carefully ruling out a primary lesion arising from the scalp, a volar or subungual site, a mucous membrane, or the eye. A patient presenting with metastatic melanoma without definitive evidence of a primary lesion usually has lymph node involvement. These patients can usually be managed by complete clearance of the involved lymph node basin, and the outcome is comparable to, or better than, that of patients with known primary lesions who have a similar extent of metastatic disease.[76, 99]

Noncutaneous Melanomas

Although melanomas arise most commonly from the skin, melanocytes are present in other tissues. These cells are of neural crest origin and undergo migration during embryologic development[58] and may be found in noncutaneous sites. Furthermore, although sun exposure is a primary etiologic factor for melanoma, it does not appear to be exclusive. Melanomas may arise, therefore, from sites not exposed to sunlight. These sites include mucous membranes, specifically the oral cavity and nasal sinuses, the genitalia, and the anorectum. Rarely, primary lesions of viscera (e.g., esophagus, lung, and adrenal gland) have been reported. These are rare enough that distinct prognostic information is not available. Esophageal lesions have been associated with melanocytic atypia, melanoma in situ, and melanosis,[42, 74] which strongly support the diagnosis of a primary melanoma rather than metastatic melanoma from an unknown primary lesion.

Ocular melanomas are the most common of the noncutaneous melanomas, accounting for approximately 4% of melanoma cases. The racial predilection for Caucasians persists in this subgroup. The lesions are usually located in the uveal tract (iris, ciliary body, and choroid), which contains melanocytes in the normal population.[26] The uveal tract lacks lymphatic drainage,[37] and it is uncommon for uveal melanoma to metastasize to regional nodes. The most likely site of recurrence is the liver.[26] Ocular melanoma is also associated with the longest intervals from diagnosis to recurrence (as long as 47 years).[22, 26] Treatment options include photocoagulation, partial ocular resection, or enucleation.[17, 31]

Mucous membrane melanomas are associated with aggressive behavior and high mortality rates.[101, 105, 115] Other unusual presentations include dural or meningeal melanomas.[45]

HISTOLOGIC FEATURES OF CUTANEOUS MELANOMA

Cutaneous melanoma is divided into four histopathologic types: lentigo maligna melanoma (LMM), superficial spreading melanoma (SSM), acral lentiginous melanoma (ALM), and nodular melanoma (NM). The first three groups have a junctional component, whereas NM is entirely subjunctional. Junctional melanomas proliferate in a horizontal direction initially along the dermal-epidermal junction, and this is referred to as the *radial growth phase*. In time, vertical growth appears, and this progression may be associated with both invasive features and metastatic capabilities.

LMM (see Fig. 21–2) is more commonly seen in individuals in their sixth, seventh, or eighth decade of life. On histologic examination (see Fig. 21–3), most of the spindle-shaped ma-

lignant cells are junctional in location. The lesion has prominent solar elastosis, with very atrophic epidermis. Pagetoid cells are usually not seen with this lesion. These often present as thin melanomas and are associated with a correspondingly good prognosis. This lesion is found on sun-exposed surfaces, especially the face. The characteristic histologic finding is solar elastosis. Typically it arises from a macular brown lesion, often large in diameter, which has been present for decades[66] (Hutchinson's freckle[48]).

Superficial spreading melanoma is the most common histologic type. It occurs on both sun-exposed and nonexposed areas of the body. Initially, the lesion demonstrates a radial growth phase, and, from a clinical standpoint, irregular margins with differing pigmentation are common (see Fig. 21–4). In time, although radial growth continues, a vertical growth phase usually appears. This lesion is characterized histologically by pagetoid cells with both junctional activity and upward growth that causes bulging of the epidermis. Solar elastosis is not a dominant feature. The epidermis is not atrophic; rather, it may demonstrate hyperplastic characteristics (see Fig. 21–5).

ALM has some of the histologic characteristics of LMM and SSM, with a prolonged radial growth phase. It most commonly arises on the glabrous skin of the palms and soles or in a subungual position (Figs. 21–6 and 21–7). This lesion is more common among blacks than are any of the other histologic types, and it tends to have a poor prognosis.[62] These lesions are devoid of pagetoid cells on histologic examination (Fig. 21–8). There is marked junctional proliferation with large atypical melanocytes with long dendritic processes. Both atrophic epidermal changes and solar elastosis are absent in this lesion. Subungual melanomas are often misdiagnosed as subungual hematomas, and plantar melanomas are often misdiagnosed as plantar warts. Thus, definitive biopsy is often delayed, and these lesions are diagnosed when they are already advanced. Mucous membrane presentation is most commonly seen on the vulva; however, the vagina, clitoris, penis, anus, nasopharynx, sinuses, and oral cavity are other sites of involvement (Figs. 21–9 and 21–10). Melanomas in these distinctive sites are generally associated with a 5-year survival rate of less than 20% (Fig. 21–11).[90]

NM does not express a junctional component; vertical

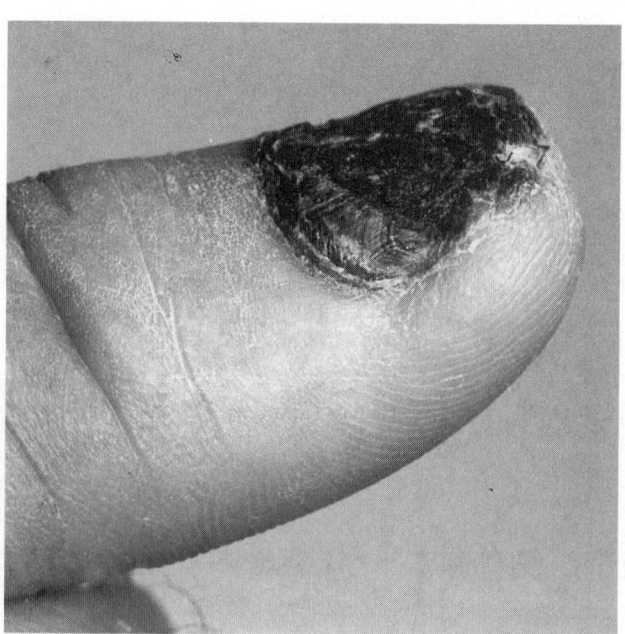

Figure 21–6. Subungual melanoma.

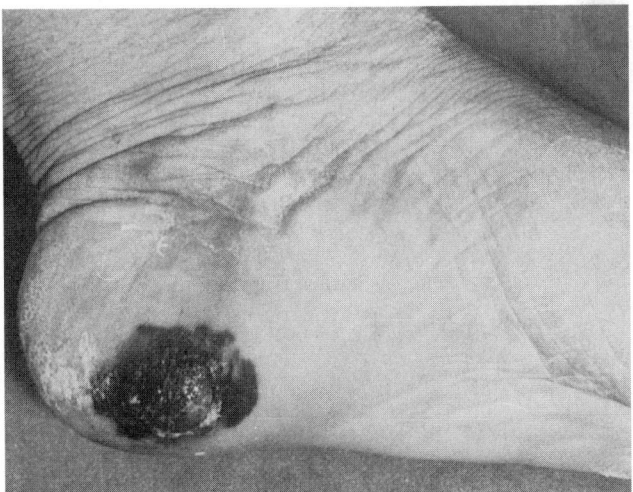

Figure 21–7. Plantar acral lentiginous melanoma.

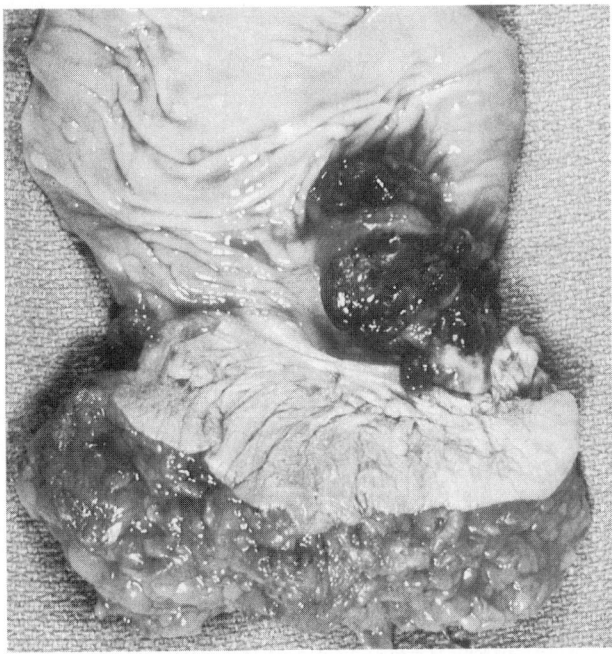

Figure 21–9. Anorectal melanoma.

growth predominates. The borders are usually well circumscribed, and pigmentation is generally uniform (Fig. 21–12). A variant of NM is the polypoid lesion. This exophytic lesion has a characteristic appearance (Fig. 21–13). The histologic demonstration of upward growth and absence of an intraepithelial component is characteristic (Fig. 21–14).

PROGNOSTIC FACTORS

In melanoma, as in other neoplastic diseases, the extent of malignancy at the time of diagnosis is the most important prognostic indicator. Patients with localized disease involving only the skin have a better prognosis than patients with disease involving first-order lymph nodes or tissue locations between the primary sites and the first-order lymph nodes (in-transit lesions). When nodal disease has occurred, the prognosis is based on the number of lymph nodes involved. Patients with distant metastases involving visceral organs, the skeleton, or the central nervous system have a very grave prognosis.

Identification of both clinical and pathologic features that accurately predict the biologic capability of the disease is an important concept. Many of these prognostic factors have been identified for cutaneous melanoma. The original paper by Clark and associates in 1969 documented the different histologic types of melanoma and the importance of the level of invasion; it continues today to be a major contribution to

the understanding of melanoma.[18] The levels of tumor invasion as described can be used to plan surgical management as well as any experimental adjuvant regimen. Clark's criteria for levels of tumor invasion are outlined in Table 21–2.

In 1970, Breslow noted that the tumor thickness itself (in millimeters) predicted the biologic behavior of cutaneous melanoma.[12] Although the Breslow thickness and the Clark level are well correlated, thickness is the best single prognos-

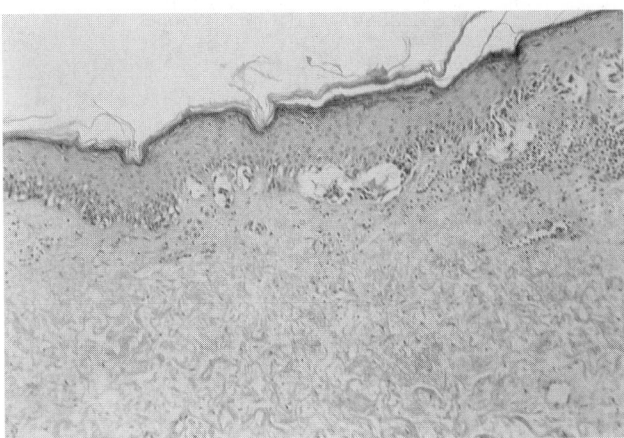

Figure 21–8. Histopathologic pattern of acral lentiginous primary lesion.

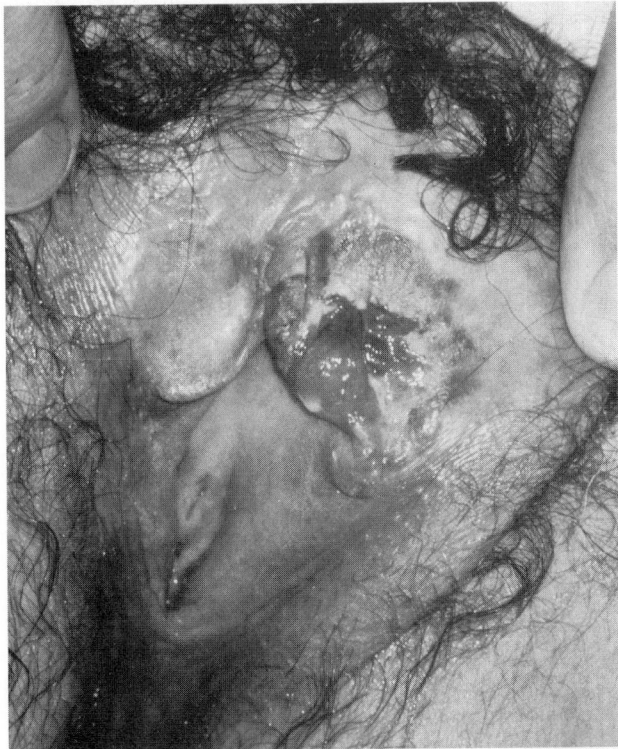

Figure 21–10. Acral lentiginous melanoma of the mucous membrane of labia majora.

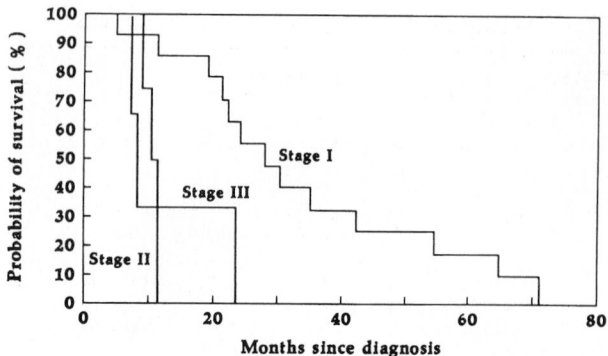

Figure 21–11. Kaplan-Meier survival curves for patients with anorectal melanoma in Stage I, II, or III. Nodal metastases defined Stage II disease, and distant metastases defined Stage III disease. Survival of patients with Stage I disease was prolonged relative to survival of patients with Stage II disease (p = 0.0003) and patients with Stage III disease (p = 0.022).

tic indicator for localized melanoma. Figure 21–15 depicts a schematic reflection of both the determination of tumor thickness and its correlation with patient survival.

A lesion less than 0.76 mm. thick is considered a *thin* melanoma. Breslow initially reported a series of 38 patients with thin melanomas, all of whom remained disease free at least 5 years.[12] Others have since reported recurrent disease and death in a small percentage of patients with thin melanomas (rate of recurrence 5% or less).[41, 68, 98] Lesions 0.76 to 4.0 mm. are generally considered intermediate thickness lesions, and lesions more than 4 mm. thick are considered thick.

The prognosis is markedly poorer for thicker lesions. Balch reported that the 10-year mortality rate is a function of the tumor thickness. Mortality rates associated with a 1-mm. lesion, a 3-mm. lesion, and a 6-mm. lesion would be approximately 10% to 20%, 45%, and 70%, respectively.[7] Breslow thickness is the principal prognostic factor described.[6] When correcting for thickness, Clark's level has secondary prognostic value. Other characteristics that have prognostic significance include ulceration, sex, age, race, primary site, and histology of the lesion.

STAGING

Two principal staging systems exist for melanoma. The system defined by the American Joint Committee on Cancer

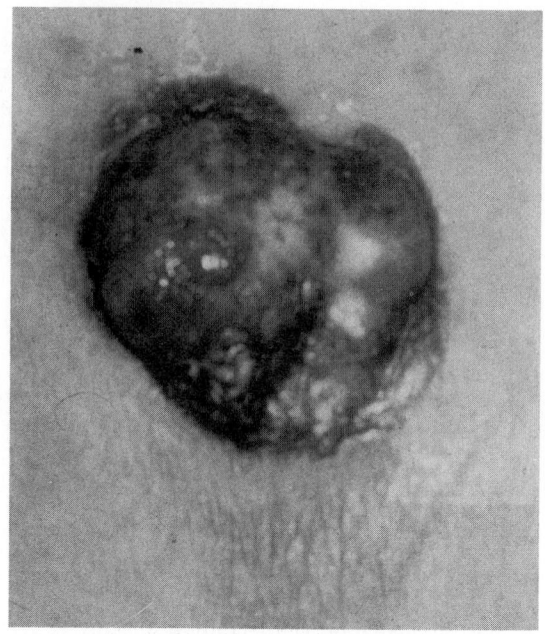

Figure 21–13. Polypoid variant of a nodular melanoma. The surface is typically ulcerated.

(AJCC) is a four-stage tumor, node, metastasis (TNM) system and is summarized in Table 21–3.[51] The older system, prevalent in the literature,[38] is a three-stage system:

I—localized, including local recurrences <5 cm. from the primary site
II—lymph node metastases or in-transit metastases
III—distant metastatic disease

Either system permits an estimation of outcome based on stage, but the AJCC staging is preferred. The advantage of the AJCC classification is that it takes into account the microstaging information available from the Breslow thickness of the primary tumor. It is important to compare patients in the context of the stage of disease. However, neither system includes all relevant prognostic factors. Because many relevant prognostic factors have been defined for melanoma, it is appropriate, when comparing or describing patient groups, not to limit information to stage alone.

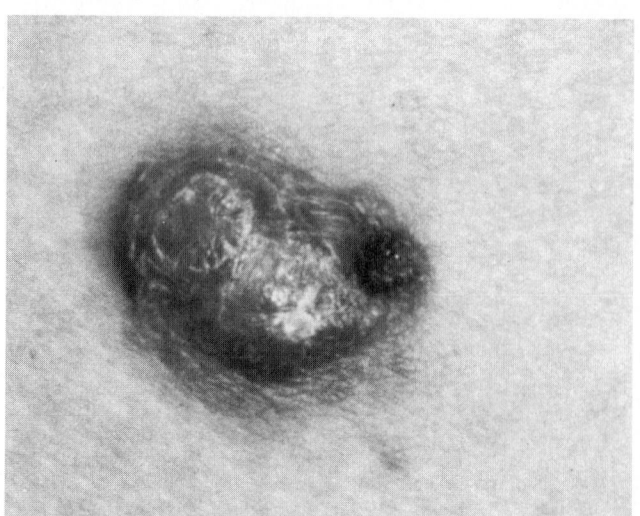

Figure 21–12. Clinical appearance of a nodular melanoma. The borders are well circumscribed, and the growth is in a vertical direction.

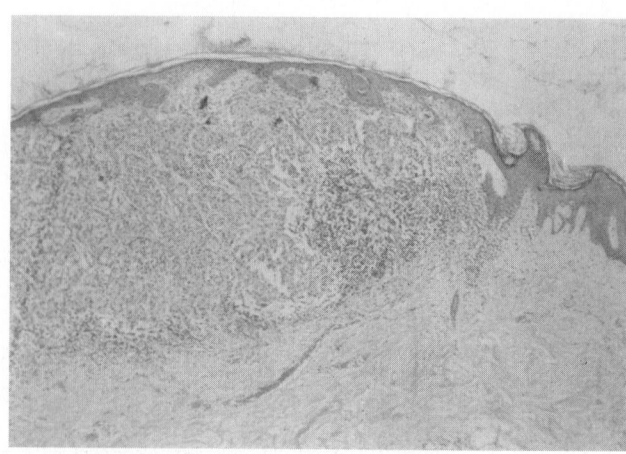

Figure 21–14. Histopathologic pattern of nodular melanoma.

TABLE 21–2. Clark's Levels of Tumor Invasion

Level	Description
1	All tumor cells above basement membrane
2	Invasion into loose connective tissue of papillary dermis
3	Tumors cells at junction of papillary and reticular dermis
4	Invasion into reticular dermis
5	Invasion into subcutaneous fat

TABLE 21–3. AJCC Staging for Melanoma

Stage*	Description
I	Localized <1.5 mm. thick
II	Localized >1.5 mm. thick
III	Nodal metastases involving only one regional nodal basin or 1–4 in-transit nodes
IV	Advanced regional metastases or any distant metastases

*Stage I is further subdivided into IA (<0.76 mm. thick) and IB (0.76–1.5 mm. thick), and Stage II is further subdivided into IIA (1.5–4 mm. thick) and IIB (>4 mm. thick). When Breslow thickness is not available, Stages IA, IB, IIA, and IIB can be defined by Clark Levels 2, 3, 4, and 5, respectively.[51]

CLINICAL MANAGEMENT: CHOICE OF BIOPSY

A comprehensive treatment plan for melanoma depends on accurate diagnosis and complete assessment of the histologic features that make up the prognostic indicators. Careful examination of the skin is a critical first step in diagnosis. Any lesion that has irregular borders, has variations in pigmentation, is black in color, or has an irregular surface, especially if it has undergone recent change, is raised, or has begun to itch or to bleed, should arouse suspicion. In order to make a diagnosis, a full-thickness biopsy should be performed. If the lesion is small, an excisional biopsy, including subcutaneous fat, should be performed. The lymph node basins draining the region of the lesion also must be examined carefully (Table 21–4).

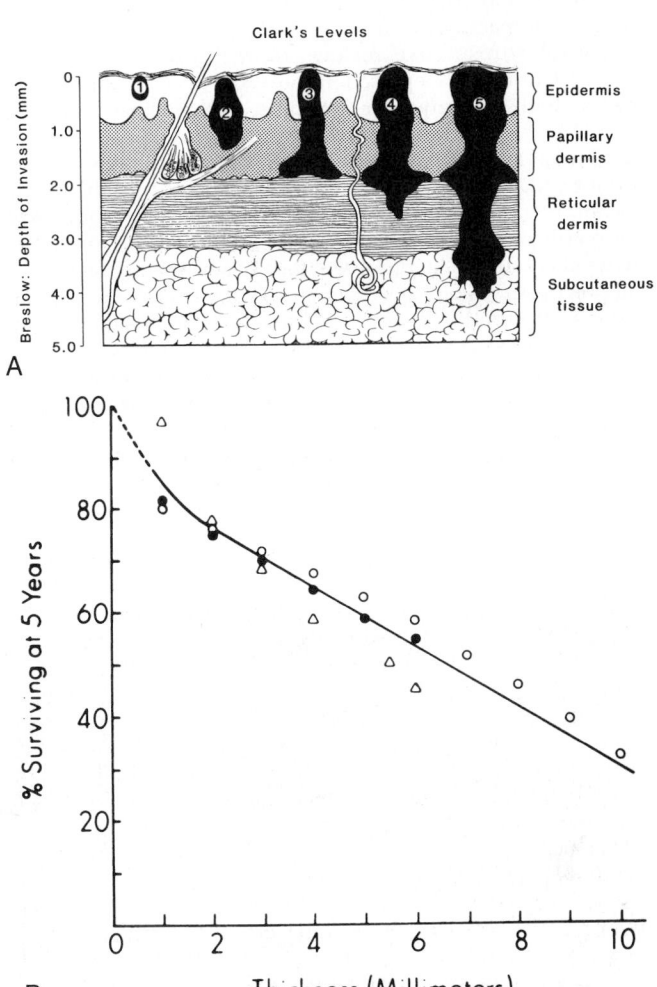

Figure 21–15. Schematic representation reflecting both the determination of tumor thickness (A) and its correlation to patient survival (B).

Although complete excisional biopsy is ideal, in some patients (e.g., those with large facial lesions), complete excision of a pigmented lesion would be unreasonably deforming. In those patients, partial excision is recommended for diagnosis, with full-thickness skin included in the specimen.[60] It may be reasonable to perform a punch biopsy that includes full-thickness skin in the most suspicious region of the nevus. It is preferable to include an area of transition to normal skin in the biopsy specimen. Patient outcome does not depend on whether the initial biopsy includes the entire specimen, as long as the excision is full thickness and an accurate diagnosis can be made. The outcome is the same for punch, incisional, excisional, or wide excisional biopsies.[57]

SURGICAL MANAGEMENT OF THE PRIMARY LESION

Once the diagnosis of melanoma has been made, a wide re-excision (wide local excision, or WLE) should be performed. The purpose of a WLE is to reduce the risk of local recurrence. The initial concept of a WLE for melanoma was proposed by Handley,[43] who found microscopic metastases in the skin up to 5 cm. away from a large primary melanoma. The frequent presence of satellite lesions, the aggressive and unpredictable nature of melanoma, and the observation of local recurrence after apparently adequate excision promoted the routine practice of a 5-cm. margin for melanoma excision. This margin, however, often requires skin grafting and, in some locations, can be very deforming. The current data and current practice, based on randomized, prospective comparisons, have shown that 5-cm. margins are excessive, and that 2- to 3-cm. margins or less usually suffice.[36] In a multicenter, randomized, prospective trial coordinated by the World Health Organization, patients with cutaneous melanomas less than 2 mm. in thickness were randomized to 1-cm. margins and >3-cm. margins of excision. There were 4 local recurrences among 612 patients (0.7%), and all occurred in patients with narrow excision of melanomas 1.1 to 2 mm.

TABLE 21–4. Draining Nodal Basins Based on Primary Site

Site of Primary Melanoma	Primary Nodal Basin(s)	Secondary Nodal Basin(s)
Upper extremity	Axillary	Subpectoral, supraclavicular
Lower extremity	Inguinal	Iliac
Head and neck	Cervical	Supraclavicular
Chest and upper back	Axillary, supraclavicular	Subpectoral, cervical
Abdomen and lower back	Inguinal axillary	Iliac

thick. The disease-free survival and overall survival after a mean follow-up of 90 months (7½ years), however, were no different for the two groups.[109] These data suggest that 1-mm. lesions can be safely treated with 1-cm. margins and that slightly larger margins are advised for 2-mm. lesions. Additional studies support this conclusion. Current practice in major centers is complete full-thickness excision with margins substantially less than 5 cm. for most primary lesions. Recommendations from several melanoma clinics are listed in Table 21–5. Margins of 5 mm. are recommended for melanoma *in situ* (level I) and 1-cm. margins are recommended for invasive melanomas up to 1-mm. thick. Beyond that, 2-cm. margins suffice for most lesions.

This type of surgical excision permits primary wound closure on most areas of the body. The excision can be accomplished on an outpatient basis using local anesthesia, thus lowering cost, morbidity, and the incidence of significant cosmetic deformity associated with wider excisions requiring skin grafts. Almost without exception, truncal melanomas can be closed by primary intention; only very large lesions with microscopic satellites require skin grafting. Melanomas of the extremities are treated in a manner similar to those on the trunk but may occasionally require grafting. Head and neck melanomas are a more difficult problem for surgical oncologists and reconstructive surgeons. In this area, optimal excision margins are sometimes sacrificed to avoid significant debility or deformity. Primary melanomas involving the mucous membranes, palmar and plantar surfaces, nail bed, and anorectal junction require special expertise.

Patients with mucosal melanomas usually have extensive primary disease, and their risk of mortality within 5 years approaches 100%. Local recurrence, especially in the pelvis, is a common initial site of failure. Only those patients with thin primary lesions are salvaged by simple surgical excision. Slingluff and associates recently reported 24 patients with anorectal melanoma with no survival beyond 6 years. Surgical options for these patients include wide excision or abdominoperineal resection. Abdominoperineal resection decreases local and regional recurrence but does not alter ultimate patient survival.[101]

The diagnosis of subungual melanoma is delayed in approximately 40% of patients.[71] These patients require amputation at the distal interphalangeal joint for finger primaries and at the interphalangeal joint for thumb primaries. This permits opposition and excellent functional characteristics. An overall 5-year survival rate of approximately 60% can be expected for patients with subungual lesions.[56, 100]

SURGICAL MANAGEMENT OF REGIONAL DISEASE

There is no question that a substantial number of patients survive long term after therapeutic resection of regional lymph nodes.[99] The therapeutic role of resecting clinically negative nodes (elective lymph node dissection [ELND]) remains unclear, however.[4, 15] ELND has long been in the armamentarium of surgeons managing melanoma. Because regional lymph nodes are the first sites of metastatic melanoma in over 60% of cases, it is rational to suspect that early resection of regional nodes might have therapeutic value. However, the operation can be associated with significant morbidity. Although some surgeons do not consider ELND to have a role in melanoma, others believe that it has a limited role, primarily in a patient who has an intermediate-thickness melanoma (1.5–4.0 mm.) without evidence of metastatic disease, a single nodal basin draining the site of the primary lesion, and no other contraindications to the procedure.[4] Relative contraindications to ELND include ambiguity of lymphatic drainage, morbid obesity, severe cardiopulmonary disease, and other contraindications to general anesthesia.

Thin melanomas have such a low risk of recurrence and mortality (up to 5% recurrence rate for lesions <0.76 mm. thick) that any potential benefit from ELND would have to be very small. Thick melanomas metastasize so frequently to distant sites that resection of clinically negative nodes is not considered likely to alter the risk of mortality.[3] There is documentation that ELND for lesions thicker than 4 mm. does not impact outcome.[23]

Several retrospective reviews from the major melanoma clinics worldwide reported improved survival among patients with intermediate-thickness melanomas receiving ELND.[5, 6, 18, 75] Despite these retrospective data, prospective randomized trials have failed to show any survival benefit from ELND.[95, 107, 108] These trials were performed by the World Health Organization and by the Mayo Clinic, but they have been criticized for not including well-matched or representative patient groups and not specifically addressing intermediate-thickness lesions. Another prospective randomized trial (Intergroup trial) is under way, but final results have not yet been reported. No improvement in survival has been described in preliminary reports, except for a borderline significance among males with intermediate-thickness trunk primaries. A recent review of the experience at a large American medical center found that ELND did not affect survival among patients well matched for melanoma prognostic factors, and some of the principles upon which ELND have been based were questioned.[97]

Because the benefit of ELND remains an issue of debate and its putative value is modest at best, it is reasonable to follow nodal basins clinically and to perform ELND only for palpable nodes. Issues other than outcome, however, may influence the decision about performing ELND. A patient's prognosis is substantially worse if an ELND reveals tumor-involved nodes, so the performance of an ELND has prognostic value. Since the likelihood of positive nodes with thin melanoma is very low, the prognostic value of ELND is also low. For thicker lesions, however, the risk of positive nodes increases, and the ELND has increased prognostic value. For patients who would not be available for close follow-up or for those patients being considered for experimental adjuvant therapy protocols who need pathologic staging of regional lymph nodes, ELND may be appropriate in selected cases.

Lymphoscintigraphy as a Guide to ELND

Lymphoscintigraphy (using technetium-99 antimony sulfur colloid) has been used to map the lymphatic drainage from

TABLE 21–5. Recommendations for Margins of Excision in the Definitive Management of Primary Cutaneous Melanoma, Based on Breslow Thickness

Author (Clinic)	Tumor Thickness (mm.)			
	<0.76	0.76–1.5	1.5–4	>4
Breslow[13]	1 cm.	—	—	—
Das Gupta[24]	1 cm.	1 cm.	1 cm. (<3 mm.)	—
Fisher[30]	1 cm.	1 cm. (<1.7 mm.)	2 cm. (1.7–3.6 mm.)	3 cm. (>3.6 mm.)
Seigler	1 cm.	2 cm.	2 cm.	2 cm.
Ross & Balch[87]	1 cm. (<1 mm.)	3 cm.	3 cm.	3 cm.
Ho & Sober[47]	1 cm. (<1 mm.)	1.5 cm. (1–1.5 mm.)	3 cm.	3 cm.
Summary	1 cm.	1–3 cm.	1–3 cm.	2–3 cm.

a primary site and therefore to determine the nodal basins for ELND.[33, 79, 94, 112] In several body sites, drainage may be to more than one nodal basin. Performing ELND in these cases without lymphoscintigraphy may involve excessive surgery on nodal basins that do not drain the primary site, or it may leave occult disease in a nodal basin that is not dissected. This is especially true of head, neck, shoulder, and trunk lesions. In a recent report reviewing 212 patients with lesions of the head, neck, shoulder, and trunk, lymphoscintigraphy altered therapy in 47% of cases, due to discordant scans. After 2.8 years, no lymph node metastasis appeared outside the nodal basins predicted by lymphoscintigraphy.[69, 70] Lymphoscintigraphy is not required in all patients but may be helpful in selected cases, when ELND is planned. Its future role depends on resolving the questions about the benefit of ELND.

The Sentinel Node

A novel approach to ELND is to identify the first node in the nodal basin to which the lesion will drain (sentinel node). This has been performed by intraoperative mapping with a vital blue dye, followed by selective node dissection.[70] Preliminary results suggest that it may have a role in the management of patients with clinical Stage I melanoma, but further follow-up and additional clinical experience at other institutions is needed to evaluate its place in the management of melanoma. It appears to permit accurate assessment of regional nodes by a procedure performed under local anesthesia, thus permitting improved staging with minimal morbidity.

SURGICAL CONSIDERATIONS FOR DISTANT METASTATIC DISEASE

Metastatic Patterns and Patterns of Failure

The natural history of melanoma is to grow locally and to metastasize by lymphatic and hematogenous routes. After excision of a primary lesion, the disease may recur locally, regionally, or systemically. Among those patients who develop recurrent or metastatic disease, the metastases are local in 16% of cases, nodal (lymphatic metastases) in 60%, and distant (hematogenous metastases) in 24%. Approximately 20% to 30% of patients with intermediate-thickness melanomas (1.5–4.0 mm. thick) develop recurrent or metastatic disease within 5 years,[25] and 30% to 40% recur within 10 years. The relative incidence of distant versus local or regional recurrences is higher for head and neck melanomas (30%) than for truncal (19%) and extremity (13%) melanomas.[81]

Local Recurrence

Local recurrence (<5 cm. from the primary site) is the manifestation of residual disease not excised with the primary tumor or may represent the outgrowth of satellite lesions, which are common with melanoma. The risk of local recurrence is a function of tumor thickness and the adequacy of excision. Although margins need not be as wide as once thought, adequate excision with a margin appropriate for the specific tumor remains important in preventing local recurrence. The risk of local recurrence reported by Urist and co-workers[106] is 0.2% for thin lesions (<0.76 mm.), 2% for low intermediate-thickness lesions (0.76–1.49 mm.), 6% for high intermediate-thickness lesions (1.5–3.99 mm.), and 13% for thick lesions (≥4 mm.).

Locally recurrent disease is usually defined as cutaneous or subcutaneous disease arising within 5 cm. of the primary site after complete excision of the primary lesion. These should be managed surgically. Whereas excision of primary lesions dicates 2-cm. margins, locally recurrent disease should probably be managed in a more aggressive manner.

Regional Recurrence

The most common manifestation of recurrent melanoma is involvement of lymph nodes. Lymph node metastases are usually found in draining nodal basins, according to the lymphatic drainage patterns defined by Sappey.[89] The major nodal basins draining several body sites are listed in Table 21–4. These are the basins that are most likely to become involved with tumor, which may be found in any or all of the draining nodal basins when more than one is implicated. When a patient presents with lymph node metastases, it is wise to restage the patient with computed tomography (CT) scans, because the risk of visceral metastases increases and may affect the treatment plan. If lymph node metastases are present in the absence of distant metastatic disease, radical resection of the involved lymphatic basin is advised. Fifty percent of patients with one tumor-involved node will survive 5 years,[99] and although the prognosis is poorer with increased nodal involvement, a substantial minority live long term after aggressive surgical treatment of regional nodal disease.

If the patient experiences in-transit disease between the primary lesion and the first-order lymph nodes, this should be managed by complete surgical removal, restaging, and consideration of systemic therapy. Radical amputation for extensive disease of the extremities is usually discouraged; experience has supported the conclusion that hemipelvectomy and forequarter amputation for melanoma are rarely indicated. Patients with such advanced disease generally demonstrate systemic manifestations of their disease, negating any possibility of meaningful disease-free interval or prolongation of survival. Occasionally, however, partial amputation of an extremity for bulkier diffuse recurrent disease proves to be palliative in a meaningful sense. Approximately 20% of the patients in this category experience an improved quality of life, with 5-year survivals being reported.[103]

Another option for patients with regionally recurrent extremity melanoma is hyperthermic limb perfusion. This involves surgical isolation of the arterial supply and venous drainage of the extremity, followed by perfusion of high-dose chemotherapy into the effected limb under hyperthermic conditions (usually 40–41° C.). Use of melphalan for this procedure is associated with greater than 80% response rates, and these responses are often complete. Toxicity can be so severe that amputation is necessary, but the treatment is usually well tolerated. Recent studies with hyperthermic limb perfusion have included using tumor necrosis factor, which may induce a response more rapidly than other therapeutic agents.

The theoretical fallacy of regional hyperthermic perfusion is that mortality results from distant metastases because regional therapy does not treat distant microscopic disease. Ghussen and colleagues reported, however, that 5-year disease-free survival after hyperthermic perfusion plus surgery was 90%, versus 50% for a prospectively randomized control group,[35] which suggests that a systemic effect may be observed, either directly or indirectly. The more obvious role of hyperthermic perfusion is to avoid amputation in patients with advanced regional disease in the absence of visceral metastases. The administration of hyperthermic regional perfusion requires experienced personnel, and its role as an adjuvant remains undefined. Patients with advanced, unresectable, regional disease are appropriate candidates for this therapy, and a response can be expected in most cases.

Distant Metastases

The most common sites of distant metastases are pulmonary and hepatic, but a first recurrence can present in any of numerous other sites, including distant skin, brain, bone, gastrointestinal tract, or other sites (Table 21–6). These may appear early or many years after diagnosis.[16, 22, 92] The predilection of melanoma for central nervous system (CNS) metastasis is well known and may be due to embryologic similarities between melanoma cells and neuronal tissue. Certainly, any focal neurologic change in a patient with a history of melanoma, regardless of how distant, should arouse suspicion of melanoma metastatic to the brain.

After the first recurrence, subsequent recurrences are more likely to be distant rather than local or regional. The second recurrence is distant in 56% of cases (Table 21–5). Once melanoma has metastasized to distant sites, it usually becomes so widely disseminated that at autopsy it can be found in virtually every organ.[101] The typical clinical course after the development of recurrent disease is progressive nodal disease and extension to visceral and distant skin sites. Commonly, CNS metastasis is the terminal event.

Although this unrelenting, progressive course is expected in patients with metastatic melanoma, some patients develop extensive local and regional recurrences without visceral involvement. Palliation of the local disease in such patients may be as difficult as preventing mortality or systemic disease. And some patients who develop isolated metastases or limited nodal disease survive for decades after resection of these lesions. Thus, although the prognostic factors for melanoma have been well studied, its behavior in any given case may not be consistent with the behavior expected.

Management of Visceral Metastases

Metastatic disease to the lungs is frequent in patients with melanoma. Pulmonary involvement reflects hematogenous metastasis, so the long-term prognosis is quite poor. If CT examination of the chest fails to demonstrate hilar adenopathy but verifies the presence of a single metastatic lesion, surgical management may be considered.[44] A conservative approach should be outlined by both a surgical oncologist and a medical oncologist, working in concert. Such patients should be placed on a chemotherapeutic regimen and observed over a 40-day interval. If additional metastatic lesions are not evident and the tumor doubling time suggests that the biologic growth rate of the tumor is slow, removal of the metastatic lesion with continuation of postoperative chemotherapy is associated with both an increased disease-free interval and prolonged survival. Patients with multiple metastatic lesions of the lung are best managed by systemic therapy and are not significantly benefited by surgical removal of metastatic deposits.

Approximately 10% of patients with melanoma experience metastatic disease to the skeleton. Most often the axial skeleton is involved. Bone pain is the usual presenting symptom, and a bone scan is the most sensitive study in terms of diagnosis. Architectural changes are outlined by routine roentgenograms. Because bone metastasis indicates a grave prognosis, with mean survival time of approximately 4 months, a conservative approach to treatment of pathologic fractures is recommended.[103] External fixation followed by radiation and chemotherapy is preferred. Occasionally, neurologic symptoms appear and can be improved by laminectomy. Unstable pathologic fractures of the long bones may also require internal fixation and radiation.

Hematogenous metastases from melanoma commonly affect the gastrointestinal tract. Branum and Seigler and Reintgen and co-workers reported this to be the malignancy most likely to metastasize to the gastrointestinal tract.[11, 80] In their series, the small intestine was involved in approximately one third of the patients with melanoma of the bowel, whereas the colon and stomach were less frequently involved. The polypoid masses involving the small bowel can cause occult bleeding or can act as the focal point for an intussusception, causing either intermittent or prolonged bowel obstruction. Ulcerating masses occasionally perforate. The endoscopic and radiographic findings are quite characteristic for this disorder. Although more than half of the patients with documented visceral metastases have other body sites affected, surgical intervention for symptomatic lesions should be considered. More than 90% of patients may gain relief of symptoms. In some cases, overall survival may be improved.

Metastatic melanoma to the adrenal gland appears also to be a favored site. Preoperative diagnosis was exceedingly rare before CT scanning was developed. Branum and colleagues recently reported 26 patients with metastatic melanoma to the adrenal gland.[10] Twenty-three of the 26 patients had unilateral disease. Survival in the patients resected for cure was approximately 5 years, whereas survival in the group resected for palliation only was approximately 1 year. The authors indicated that patients with metastatic melanoma to the adrenal gland who were resected for cure benefit from early detection and surgical intervention.

Metastatic melanoma involving the CNS occurs frequently and is a common cause of death. Clinical evidence of involvement of the CNS occurs in approximately one third of patients. This can be much higher in advanced disease, with more than 90% involvement in autopsy series. Patients with a solitary brain metastasis managed by surgical extirpation experience a 1-year survival rate of approximately 45%.[14, 34] Multiple lesions of the CNS are present in approximately half of the patients, however. Magnetic resonance imaging has improved the ability to document single or multiple lesions. The present recommendation for metastatic disease involving the brain includes surgical removal of solitary lesions followed by whole-brain radiation and adjuvant systemic therapy if disease involving other organ sites is not limiting or indicative of restricted survival time. Patients with multiple metastases involving the CNS are best managed by radiation, chemotherapy, and medication designed to control seizure activity.

HORMONAL ASPECTS OF MELANOMA

Prognostic studies indicate that women have better survival with malignant melanoma than men. Multivariate analyses reveal that women have a higher survival rate at each Clark's level of invasion and with each tumor thickness level.[93] A multivariate regression analysis confirms that gender remains a factor in the prognostic index after controlling for the input of factors such as histologic type, Clark's level, primary tumor thickness, and site of the lesion.[78] These re-

TABLE 21–6. Sites of First and Second Metastases

Site	First (%)	Second (%)
Local skin	15	19
Nodes	60	25
Distant skin	5	12
Lung	8	15
Liver	3	7
Central nervous system	3	10
Bone	1	4
Gastrointestinal	1	2
Other	4	6

sults suggest that there may indeed be a difference in the biologic behavior of melanoma in men and women. The presence of estrogen receptors on malignant melanocytes has been evaluated extensively. Some groups have reported estrogen receptor binding as well as detection of these receptors using immunofluorescent techniques.[50, 104] Others have questioned the presence of true estrogen receptors in malignant melanoma. All tumors in which estradiol binding was observed were melanin-producing lesions. Purified tyrosinase appears to mimic the estrogen binding detected in melanoma cells. Tyrosinase is an enzyme involved in the melanin synthetic pathway. It appears that the estradiol-binding component in melanoma most likely represents an artifact and that true estrogen receptors are absent from this tumor.[64, 116]

A practical question concerns the relationship of melanoma and pregnancy. Several reports since the 1950s have suggested that women diagnosed with melanoma during pregnancy had a particularly dismal prognosis. These results were largely anecdotal or were not controlled for risk factors that are now known to be important. More recent studies have failed to demonstrate a convincing difference in outcome when melanoma is diagnosed during pregnancy. Wong and associates reported on 66 patients with clinically localized melanoma diagnosed during pregnancy.[114] These patients were compared with 619 nonpregnant patients with melanoma in comparable disease status. No significant difference appeared between the pregnant population and the control population with respect to location of the primary tumor at diagnosis, Clark's level, mean depth of invasion, and histologic type. These authors concluded that women diagnosed with melanoma during pregnancy fare no worse than their nonpregnant counterparts. Slingluff and associates studied 100 patients with melanoma arising during pregnancy and compared them with an age-matched group of 86 female patients who were not pregnant at the time of diagnosis and who had similar disease status.[96] The pregnant patients had an increased incidence of lymph node metastases, but there was no significant difference in the time to development of distant metastatic disease nor any difference in long-term survival. Other studies have failed to demonstrate a difference in survival for patients who become pregnant subsequent to diagnosis of and treatment for melanoma. Also, there does not appear to be a significant association between parity and prognosis or incidence of melanoma.

SYSTEMIC TREATMENT FOR MELANOMA

Systemic chemotherapy for melanoma must be considered only a palliative measure and generally should be used only for disease beyond the first-order lymph nodes. The biologic growth rate and doubling time of malignant melanocytes suggest that this disease should be sensitive to chemotherapeutic agents. A multitude of clinical trials, however, reveals that single-drug response is approximately 20% at most. The single agent with greatest efficacy to date is dacarbazine (DTIC). Different combinations of drugs have been evaluated, and the most efficient appear to be multiple-drug regimens administered in a pulse manner. These regimens appear to be an effective palliative treatment for metastatic melanoma, with tumor response in approximately 40% of the patients being observed.[65, 91]

As mentioned above, chemotherapy can be administered for regional disease by isolated limb perfusion. This is not a trivial technique, and it is not available routinely at most institutions. Its appropriate role in the management of melanoma remains an area of continuing investigation. It is used most widely to treat unresectable regional disease in the absence of systemic disease. Some reports suggest a survival benefit of regional limb perfusion therapy in an adjuvant

setting after resection of primary melanoma,[35, 55] although the use of limb perfusion therapy in the adjuvant setting is not common.

In addition to cytotoxic chemotherapy, there has been increasing interest in biologic response modifiers, which, for the most part, are cytokines. Tumor necrosis factor, which has some effect in regional therapy, is lethal if given systemically at therapeutic doses. Interleukin-2 (IL-2) and alpha-interferon have been used systemically and continue to be investigated in experimental treatment programs. Alpha-interferon has been administered in the treatment of metastatic disease, but with minimal response rates. Recent investigations are focusing on its potential use in the adjuvant setting for patients with high-risk melanoma. Recent results show that high-dose alfa interferon reduces mortality when given in the adjuvant mode for patients who have had surgical clearance of nodal metastases (Stage III). As a result, alfa interferon was approved by the Food and Drug Administration for this use at the end of 1995.[51a]

High-dose recombinant IL-2, a T-cell growth factor, has been used to treat patients with metastatic melanoma. Partial tumor regressions have been reported in approximately 20% of patients.[63, 85] In a few patients, durable complete responses have been observed for as long as 8 years.[85] Rosenberg and colleagues used recombinant IL-2 in conjunction with adoptive cellular immunotherapy. Early studies used IL-2 with lymphokine-activated killer cells in patients with metastatic melanoma.[84] More recently, this group at the National Cancer Institute used IL-2 with tumor-infiltrating lymphocytes expanded *in vitro* from metastatic tumor deposits. This appears to give a greater response rate than IL-2 alone or IL-2 plus lymphokine-activated killer cells. The most recent reports suggest a response rate of 35%, including some complete responses. This is the single most effective immunotherapeutic regimen evaluated in humans to date.[86] This and other immunotherapeutic approaches for melanoma remain experimental. Monoclonal antibody therapy for melanoma has been evaluated but has not yet proved effective.

An area of intense interest is an immunotherapeutic approach using tumor vaccines intended to induce cellular immune responses against melanoma. This is described in more detail elsewhere in this text. Existing tumor vaccines have not been evaluated extensively in randomized prospective trials, but a recently completed randomized trial with a vaccinia melanoma cell oncolysate failed to demonstrate a therapeutic advantage.[111] Other tumor vaccine protocols appear to have survival benefit relative to historic controls in some patients.[99] Several investigators have shown positive correlations between immune responses to tumor vaccines and longer survival in immunized patients.[46, 110] Ongoing research into the nature of the immune response to melanoma and the nature of melanoma-associated antigens is ushering in a new era of gene therapy and purified peptide vaccine therapy, offering new hope for novel treatments.

SELECTED REFERENCES

Balch, C. M., Soong, S.-J., Shaw, H. M., and Milton, G. W.: An analysis of prognostic factors in 4000 patients with cutaneous melanoma. *In* Balch, C. M., and Milton, G. W., (Eds.): Cutaneous Melanoma: Clinical Management and Treatment Results Worldwide. Philadelphia, J. B. Lippincott, 1985, p. 321.
This is a comprehensive, classic review of prognostic factors in melanoma. It provides excellent information about prognosis for all stages of disease. Further follow-up is available in the second edition of this text, published in 1992.

Breslow, A.: Thickness, cross sectional areas and depth of invasion in the prognosis of cutaneous melanoma. Ann. Surg., 172:902, 1970.
Tumor thickness is the most reproducible prognostic factor for cutaneous melanoma. Disease-free interval and ultimate patient survival are in a linear relationship with tumor thickness measured in millimeters.

Clark, W. H. J., From, L., Bernadino, E. A., and Mihm, M. C.: The histogenesis and biologic behavior of primary human malignant melanoma of the skin. Cancer Res., 29:705, 1969.

This classic reference provides insight into the histologic aspects of melanoma and its relationship with the biologic behavior. The levels of invasion into the skin correlate with patient survival.

Slingluff, C. L., Jr., Stidham, K. R., Ricci, W. M., Stanley, W. E., and Seigler, H. F.: Surgical management of regional lymph nodes in patients with melanoma: Experience with 4682 patients. Ann. Surg., 219:120, 1994.

Lymph node metastases and their treatment by elective or therapeutic node dissections are described. Patterns of nodal metastasis and the outcome of elective node dissections are reviewed. The role of surgery for lymph node disease is discussed. In this large review, no therapeutic effect for elective lymph node dissection can be demonstrated.

Veronesi, U., and Cascinelli, N.: Narrow excision (1-cm margin): A safe procedure for thin cutaneous melanoma. Arch. Surg., 126:438, 1991.

This report on a prospective randomized trial shows narrow excisions of thin melanomas to be effective.

REFERENCES

1. Albino, A. P.: Genes involved in melanoma susceptibility and progression. Curr. Opin. Oncol., 7:162, 1995.
1a. Anderson, D. E., Smith, J. L., and McBride, C. M.: Hereditary aspects of malignant melanoma. JAMA, 200:741, 1967.
2. Balaban, G., Herlyn, M., Guerry, D. I. V., Bartolo, R., Koprowski, H., Clark, W. H., and Nowell, P. C.: Cytogenetics of human malignant melanoma and premalignant lesions. Cancer Genet. Cytogenet., 11:429, 1984.
3. Balch, C. M.: Surgical management of regional lymph nodes in cutaneous melanoma. J. Am. Acad. Dermatol., 3:511, 1980.
4. Balch, C. M.: The role of elective lymph node dissection in melanoma: Rationale, results, and controversies. J. Clin. Oncol., 6:163, 1988.
5. Balch, C. M., Soong, S. J., Milton, G. W., Shaw, H. M., McGovern, V. J., Murad, T. M., McCarthy, W. H., and Maddox, W. A.: A comparison of prognostic factors and surgical results in 1,786 patients with localized (stage I) melanoma treated in Alabama, USA, and New South Wales, Australia. Ann. Surg., 196:677, 1982.
6. Balch, C. M., Soong, S.-J., Murad, T. M., Ingalls, A. L., and Maddox, W. L.: A multifactorial analysis of melanoma. II. Prognostic factors in patients with stage I (localized) melanoma. Surgery, 86:343, 1979.
7. Balch, C. M., Soong, S.-J., Shaw, H. M., and Milton, G. W.: An analysis of prognostic factors in 4000 patients with cutaneous melanoma. *In* Balch, C. M., and Milton, G. W. (Eds.): Cutaneous Melanoma: Clinical Management and Treatment Results Worldwide. Philadelphia, J. B. Lippincott, 1985, p. 321.
8. Bodenham, D. C.: A study of 650 observed malignant melanomas in the south-west region. Ann. R. Coll. Surg. Engl., 43:218, 1968.
9. Boring, C. C., Squires, T. S., and Tong, T.: Cancer statistics, 1993. CA, 43:7, 1993.
10. Branum, G. D., Epstein, R. E., Leight, G. S., and Seigler, H. F.: The role of resection in the management of melanoma metastatic to the adrenal gland. Surgery, 109:127, 1991.
11. Branum, G. D., and Seigler, H. F.: Role of surgical intervention in the management of intestinal metastases from malignant melanoma. Am. J. Surg., 162:428, 1991.
12. Breslow, A.: Thickness, cross sectional areas and depth of invasion in the prognosis of cutaneous melanoma. Ann. Surg., 172:902, 1970.
13. Breslow, A., and Macht, S. D.: Optimal size of resection margin for thin cutaneous melanoma. Surg. Gynecol. Obstet., 145:691, 1977.
14. Bullard, D. E., Cox, E. B., and Seigler, H. F.: Central nervous system metastases in malignant melanoma. Neurosurgery, 8:26, 1981.
15. Cady, B.: "Prophylactic" lymph node dissection in melanoma: Does it help? J. Clin. Oncol., 6:2, 1988.
16. Callaway, M. P., and Briggs, J. C.: The incidence of late recurrence (greater than 10 years); and analysis of 536 consecutive cases of cutaneous melanoma. Br. J. Plast. Surg., 42:46, 1989.
17. Char, D. H.: Current treatments and trials in uveal melanoma. Oncology (Williston Park), 3:113, 1989.
18. Clark, W. H. J., From, L., Bernadino, E. A., and Mihm, M. C.: The histogenesis and biologic behavior of primary human malignant melanoma of the skin. Cancer Res., 29:705, 1969.
19. Clark, W. H., Jr., Reimer, R. R., Greene, M., Ainsworth, A. M., and Mastrangelo, M. J.: Origin of familial malignant melanomas from heritable melanocytic lesions. "The B-K mole syndrome." Arch. Dermatol., 114:732, 1978.
20. Cook, M. G., and Fallowfield, M. E.: Dysplastic nevi—an alternative view. Histopathology, 16:29, 1990.
21. Cowan, J. M., Halaban, R., Lane, A. T., and Francke, U.: The involvement of 6p in malignant melanoma. Cancer Genet. Cytogenet., 20:255, 1986.
22. Crowley, N. J., and Seigler, H. F.: Late recurrence of malignant melanoma: Analysis of 168 patients. Ann. Surg., 212:173, 1990.
23. Crowley, N. J., and Seigler, H. F.: The role of elective lymph node dissection in the management of patients with thick cutaneous melanoma. Cancer, 66:2522, 1990.
24. Das Gupta, T. K.: Results of treatment of 269 patients with primary cutaneous melanoma: A five-year prospective study. Ann. Surg., 186:201, 1977.
25. Day, C. L. J., Mihm, M. C. J., Lew, R. A., et al.: Prognostic factors for patients with clinical stage I melanoma of intermediate thickness (1.51–3.99 mm): A conceptual model for tumor growth and metastasis. Ann. Surg., 195:35, 1982.
26. Donoso, L. A., Song, Y., and Shields, J. A.: Clinical and immunohistological features of uveal melanomas. *In* Ferrone, S. (Ed.): Human Melanoma: From Basic Research to Clinical Application. Berlin, Springer-Verlag, 1990, p. 229.
27. Elder, D. E.: Human melanocytic neoplasms and their etiologic relationship with sunlight. J. Invest. Dermatol., 92(suppl):297S, 1989.
28. Elwood, J. M., Gallagher, R. P., Hill, G. B., Spinelli, J. J., Pearson, J. C. G., and Threlfall, W.: Pigmentation and skin reaction to sun as risk factors for cutaneous melanoma: Western Canada melanoma study. Br. Med. J., 288:99, 1984.
29. Evans, R. D., Kopf, A. W., Lew, R. A., Rigel, D. S., Bart, R. S., Friedman, R. J., and Rivers, J. K.: Risk factors for the development of malignant melanoma. I: Review of case-control studies. Derm. Surg. Oncol., 14:4, 1988.
30. Fisher, J. C.: Melanoma excision: How far? How deep? Contemp. Surg., 27:42, 1985.
31. Foulds, W. S.: Management of intraocular melanoma. Br. J. Ophthalmol., 74:559, 1990.
32. Friedman, R. J., Rigel, D. S., Silverman, M. K., Kopf, A. W., and Vossaert, K. A.: Malignant melanoma in the 1990s: The continued importance of early detection and the role of physician examination and self-examination of the skin. CA, 41:201, 1991.
33. Froelich, J. W., Swanson, D. P., Mast, C., et al.: Tc 99m HSA: The ideal agent for cutaneous lymphoscintigraphy. Radiology, 153:316, 1984.
34. Galichich, J. H., Sundaresan, N., Arbit, E., and Passe, S.: Surgical treatment of single brain metastases: Factors associated with survival. Cancer, 45:381, 1980.
35. Ghussen, F., Kruger, I., Groth, W., and Stutzer, H.: The role of regional hyperthermic cytostatic perfusion for melanoma of the extremities. Surg. Gynecol. Obstet., 140:339, 1975.
36. Goldman, L. I., and Byrd, R.: Narrowing resection margins for patients with low-risk melanomas. Am. J. Surg., 155:242, 1988.
37. Goldschmidt, L., and Char, D. H.: Immunobiology of ocular malignant melanoma. *In* Ferrone, S. (Ed.): Human Melanoma: From Basic Research to Clinical Application. Berlin, Springer-Verlag, 1990, p. 164.
38. Goldsmith, H. S.: Melanoma: An overview. CA, 29:194, 1979.
39. Greene, M. H., Clark, W. H. J., Tucker, M. A., Elder, D. E., Kramer, K. H., and Fraser, M. C.: High risk of malignant melanoma in melanoma-prone families with dysplastic nevi. Ann. Intern. Med., 102:458, 1985.
40. Greene, M. H., Clark, W. H. J., Tucker, M. A., Elder, D. E., Kramer, K. H., Guerry, D. I. V., Witmer, W. K., Thompson, J., Matozzo, I., and Fraser, M. C.: Acquired precursors for cutaneous malignant melanoma: The familial dysplastic nevus syndrome. N. Engl. J. Med., 312:91, 1985.
41. Gromet, M. A., Epstein, W. L., and Blois, M. S.: The regressing thin malignant melanoma. Cancer, 42:2282, 1978.
42. Guzman, R. P., Wightman, R., Ravinsky, E., and Unruh, H. W.: Primary malignant melanoma of the esophagus with diffuse melanocytic atypia and melanoma in situ. Am. J. Clin. Pathol., 92:802, 1989.
43. Handley, W. S.: The pathology of melanotic growths in relation to their operative treatment. Lancet, 1:927, 1907.
44. Harpole, D. H., Jr., Johnson, C. M., Wolfe, W. G., George, S. L., and Seigler, H. F.: Analysis of 945 cases of pulmonary metastatic melanoma. J. Thorac. Cardiovasc. Surg., 103:743, 1992.
45. Hartmann, L. C., Oliver, G. F., Winkelmann, R. K., Colby, T. V., Sundt, T. M., and O'Neill, B. P.: Blue nevus and nevus of Ota associated with dural melanoma. Cancer, 64:182, 1989.
46. Hersey, P., Edwards, A., Coates, A., Shaw, H., McCarthy, W., and Milton, G.: Evidence that treatment with vaccinia melanoma cell lysates (VMCL) may improve survival of patients with stage II melanoma: Treatment of stage II melanoma with viral lysates. Cancer Immunol. Immunother., 25:257, 1987.
47. Ho, V. C., and Sober, A. J.: Therapy for cutaneous melanoma: An update. J. Am. Acad. Dermatol., 22:159, 1990.
48. Hutchinson, J.: Senile freckles. Arch. Surg., 3:319, 1982.
49. Huvos, A. G., Shah, J. P., and Goldsmith, H. S.: A clinicopathologic study of amelanotic melanoma. Surg. Gynecol. Obstet., 135:917, 1972.
50. Karakousis, C. P., Lopez, R. E., Bhakoo, H. S., Rosen, F., Moore, R., and Carlson, M.: Estrogen and progesterone receptors and tamoxifen in malignant melanoma. Cancer Treat. Rep., 64:819, 1980.
51. Ketcham, A. S., and Balch, C. M.: Classification and staging systems. *In* Balch, C. M., and Milton, G. W. (Eds.): Cutaneous Melanoma: Clinical Management and Treatment Results Worldwide. Philadelphia, J. B. Lippincott, 1985, p. 62.
51a. Kirkwood, J. M., Strawderman, M. H., Ernstoff, M. S., et al.: Interferon alfa-2b adjuvant therapy of high-risk resected cutaneous melanoma: The Eastern Cooperative Oncology Group Trial EST 1684. J. Clin. Oncol., 14:7, 1996.
52. Kopf, A. W., Friedman, R. J., and Rigel, D. S.: Atypical mole syndrome. J. Am. Acad. Dermatol., 22:117, 1990.
53. Kopf, A. W., Rigel, D. S., and Friedman, R. J.: The rising incidence

and mortality rate of malignant melanoma. J. Dermatol. Surg. Oncol., 8:760, 1982.

54. Kraemer, K. H., Greene, M. H., Tarone, R., Elder, D. E., Clark, W. H., and Guerry, D.: Dysplastic naevi and cutaneous melanoma risk. Lancet, 2:1076, 1983.

55. Krementz, E. T., Carter, R. D., Sutherland, C. M., Muchmore, J. H., Ryan, R. F., and Creech, O., Jr.: Regional chemotherapy for melanoma: A 35-year experience. Ann. Surg., 220:520, 1994.

56. Krementz, E. T., Feed, R. J., Coleman, W. P., 3d., Sutherland, C. M., Carter, R. D., and Campbell, M.: Acral lentiginous melanoma: A clinicopathologic entity. Ann. Surg., 195:632, 1982.

57. Lederman, J. S., and Sober, A. J.: Does wide excision as the initial diagnostic procedure improve outcome in patients with cutaneous melanoma? J. Dermatol. Surg. Oncol., 12:697, 1986.

58. LeDouarin, N.: The neural crest. In Kissel, P., Andre, J. M., and Jacquier, A.: The Neurocristopathies. New York, Masson, 1981, pp. 19–38.

59. Lee, J. A. H., and Carter, A. P.: Secular trends in mortality from malignant melanoma. J. Natl. Cancer Inst., 45:91, 1970.

60. Lee, Y. N.: Diagnosis, treatment, and prognosis of early melanoma: The importance of depth of microinvasion. Ann. Surg., 191:87, 1980.

61. Lehmann, A. R., and Bridges, B. A.: Sunlight-induced cancer: Some new aspects and implications of the xeroderma pigmentosum model. Br. J. Dermatol., 122 (suppl 35):115, 1990.

62. Lopansri, S., and Mihm, M. C. J.: Clinical and pathological correlation of malignant melanoma. J. Cutan. Pathol., 6:180, 1979.

63. Lotze, M. T., Chang, A. E., Seipp, C. A., Simpson, C., Vetto, J. T., and Rosenberg, S. A.: High-dose recombinant interleukin 2 in the treatment of patients with disseminated cancer: Responses, treatment-related morbidity, and histologic findings. JAMA, 256:3117, 1986.

64. McCarty, K. S., Jr., Wortman, J., Stowers, S., Lubahn, D. B., McCarty, K. S., Sr., and Seigler, H. F.: Sex steroid receptor analysis in human melanoma. Cancer, 46:1463, 1980.

65. McClay, E. F., Mastrangelo, M. J., Sprandio, J. D., Bellet, R. E., and Berd, D.: The importance of tamoxifen to a cisplatin-containing regimen in the treatment of metastatic melanoma. Cancer, 63:1292, 1989.

66. McGovern, V. J.: The nature of melanoma: A critical review. J. Cutan. Pathol., 9:61, 1982.

67. McGovern, V. J., Lane Brown, M. M., and Sharpe, C.: Genetic predisposition to melanoma and other skin cancers in Australians. Med. J. Aust., 1:852, 1971.

68. Naruns, P. L., Nizze, J. A., Cochran, A. J., et al.: Recurrence potential of thin primary melanomas. Cancer, 57:545, 1986.

69. Norman, J. J., Cruse, W., Ruas, E., Beatty, E., Hymes, S., Espinosa, C., Clark, R., and Reintgen, D.: The expanding role of lymphoscintigraphy in the management of cutaneous melanoma. Am. Surg., 55:689, 1989.

70. Norman, J., Wells, K., Kearney, R., Cruse, C. W., Berman, C., and Reintgen, D.: Identification of lymphatic drainage basins in patients with cutaneous melanoma. Semin. Surg. Oncol., 9:224, 1993.

71. Papachristou, D. N., and Fortner, J. G.: Melanoma arising under the nail. J. Surg. Oncol., 21:219, 1982.

72. Pathak, S., Drwinga, H. L., and Hsu, T. C.: Involvement of chromosome 6 in rearrangements in human malignant melanoma cell lines. Cytogenet. Cell Genet., 36:573, 1983.

73. Pederson, M. I., Benett, J. W., and Wang, N.: Nonrandom chromosome structural aberrations and oncogene loci in human malignant melanoma. Cancer Genet. Cytogenet., 20:11, 1986.

74. Piccone, V. A., Klopstock, R., LeVeen, H. H., and Sika, J.: Primary malignant melanoma of the esophagus associated with melanosis of the entire esophagus: First case report. J. Thorac. Cardiovasc. Surg., 59:864, 1970.

75. Reintgen, D. S., Cox, E. B., McCarty, K. S., Jr., Vollmer, R. T., and Seigler, H. F.: Efficacy of elective lymph node dissection in patients with intermediate thickness primary melanoma. Ann. Surg., 198:379, 1983.

76. Reintgen, D. S., McCarty, K. S., Woodard, B., Cox, E., and Seigler, H. F.: Metastatic malignant melanoma with an unknown primary. Surg. Gynecol. Obstet., 156:335, 1983.

77. Reintgen, D. S., McCarty, K. S., Jr., Cox, E., and Seigler, H. F.: Malignant melanoma in the American black. Curr. Surg., 40:215, 1983.

78. Reintgen, D. S., Paull, D. E., Seigler, H. F., Cox, E. B., and McCarty, K. S., Jr.: Sex related survival differences in instances of melanoma. Surg. Gynecol. Obstet., 159:367, 1984.

79. Reintgen, D. S., Sullivan, D., Coleman, E., Briner, W., Croker, B. P., and Seigler, H. F.: Lymphoscintigraphy for malignant melanoma: Surgical considerations. Am. Surg., 49:672, 1983.

80. Reintgen, D. S., Thompson, W., Garbutt, J., and Seigler, H. F.: Radiologic, endoscopic, and surgical considerations of melanoma metastatic to the gastrointestinal tract. Surgery, 95:635, 1984.

81. Reintgen, D. S., Vollmer, R., Tso, C. Y., and Seigler, H. F.: Prognosis for recurrent stage I malignant melanoma. Arch. Surg., 122:1338, 1987.

82. Rhodes, A. R.: Public education and cancer of the skin: What do people need to know about melanoma and nonmelanoma skin cancer? Cancer, 75:613, 1995.

83. Rhodes, A. R., and Melsky, J. W.: Small congenital nevocellular nevi and the risk of cutaneous melanoma. J. Pediatr. 100:219, 1982.

84. Rosenberg, S. A., Lotze, M. T., Muul, L. M., Chang, A. E., Avis, F. P., Leitman, S., Linehan, W. M., Robertson, C. N., Lee, R. E., Rubin, J. T., et al.: A progress report on the treatment of 157 patients with advanced cancer using lymphokine-activated killer cells and interleukin-2 or high-dose interleukin-2 alone. N. Engl. J. Med., 316:889, 1987.

85. Rosenberg, S. A., Yang, J. C., Topalian, S. L., Schwartzentruber, D. J., Weber, J. S., Parkinson, D. R., Seipp, C. A., Einhorn, J. H., and White, D. E.: Treatment of 283 consecutive patients with metastatic melanoma or renal cell cancer using high-dose bolus interleukin 2 [see comments]. JAMA, 271:907, 1994.

86. Rosenberg, S. A., Yannelli, J. R., Yang, J. C., Topalian, S. L., Schwartzentruber, D. J., Weber, J. S., Parkinson, D. R., Seipp, C. A., Einhorn, J. H., and White, D. E.: Treatment of patients with metastatic melanoma with autologous tumor-infiltrating lymphocytes and interleukin 2. J. Natl. Cancer Inst., 86:1159, 1994.

87. Ross, M. I., and Balch, C. M.: The current management of cutaneous melanoma. Adv. Surg., 24:139, 1991.

88. Roth, M. E., Grant-Kels, J. M., Ackerman, A. B., Elder, D. E., Friedman, R. J., Heilman, E. R., Maize, J. C., and Sagebiel, R. W.: The histopathology of dysplastic nevi: Continued controversy. Am. J. Dermatopathol., 13:38, 1991.

89. Sappey, M. P. C.: Anatomie, physiologie, pathologie, des vaisseaux lymphatiques consideres chez l'homme et les vertebres. Paris: A. DeLahaye and E. Lecrosnier, 1894.

90. Scheistroen, M., Trope, C., Kaern, J., Pettersen, E. O., Abeler, V. M., and Kristensen, G. B.: Malignant melanoma of the vulva: Evaluation of prognostic factors with emphasis on DNA ploidy in 75 patients. Cancer, 75:72, 1995.

91. Seigler, H. F., Lucas, V. S., Pickett, N. J., and Huang, A. T.: DTIC, CCNU, bleomycin, and vincristine (BOLD) in metastatic melanoma. Cancer, 46:2346, 1980.

92. Shaw, H. M., Beattie, C. W., McCarthy, W. H., and Milton, G. W.: Late relapse from cutaneous stage I malignant melanoma. Arch. Surg., 120:1155, 1985.

93. Shaw, H. M., McGovern, V. J., Milton, G. W., Farago, G. A., and McCarthy, W. H.: Malignant melanoma: Influence of site of lesion and age of patient in the female superiority in survival. Cancer, 46:2731, 1980.

94. Sherman, A., and Ter-Pogossian, M.: Lymph node concentration of radioactive colloidal gold following interstitial injection. Cancer, 6:1238, 1953.

95. Sim, F. H., Taylor, W. F., Pritchard, D. J., et al.: Lymphadenectomy in the management of stage I malignant melanoma: A prospective randomized study. Mayo Clin. Proc., 61:697, 1986.

96. Slingluff, C. L., Jr., Reintgen, D. S., Vollmer, R. T., and Seigler, H. F.: Malignant melanoma arising during pregnancy: A study of 100 patients. Ann. Surg., 211:552, 1990.

97. Slingluff, C. L., Jr., Stidham, K. R., Ricci, W. M., Stanley, W. E., and Seigler, H. F.: Surgical management of regional lymph nodes in patients with melanoma: Experience with 4682 patients. Ann. Surg., 219:120, 1994.

98. Slingluff, C. L., Jr., Vollmer, R. T., Reintgen, D. S., and Seigler, H. F.: Lethal "thin" malignant melanoma: Identifying patients at risk. Ann. Surg., 208:150, 1988.

99. Slingluff, C. L., Jr., Vollmer, R., and Seigler, H. F.: Stage II malignant melanoma: Presentation of a prognostic model and an assessment of specific active immunotherapy in 1,273 patients. J. Surg. Oncol., 39:139, 1988.

100. Slingluff, C. L., Jr., Vollmer, R., and Seigler, H. F.: Acral melanoma: A review of 185 patients with identification of prognostic variables. J. Surg. Oncol., 45:91, 1990.

101. Slingluff, C. L., Jr., Vollmer, R. T., and Seigler, H. F.: Anorectal melanoma: Clinical characteristics and results of surgical management in twenty-four patients. Surgery, 107:1, 1990.

102. Slue, W., Kopf, A. W., and Rivers, J. K.: Total-body photographs of dysplastic nevi. Arch. Dermatol., 124:1239, 1988.

103. Stewart, W. R., Gelberman, R. H., Harrelson, J. M., and Seigler, H. F.: Skeletal metastases of melanoma. J. Bone Joint Surg. [Am.], 60:645, 1978.

104. Thompson, A. J., Cook, M. G., and Gill, P. G.: Immunofluorescent detection of hormone receptors in cutaneous melanocytic tumours. Br. J. Cancer, 43:644, 1981.

105. Trapp, T. K., Fu, Y.-S., and Calcaterra, T. C.: Melanoma of the nasal and paranasal sinus mucosa. Arch. Otolaryngol. Head Neck Surg., 113:1086, 1989.

106. Urist, M. M., Balch, C. M., and Milton, G. W.: Surgical management of the primary melanoma. In Balch, C. M., and Milton, G. W. (Eds.): Cutaneous Melanoma: Clinical Management and Treatment Results Worldwide. Philadelphia, J. B. Lippincott, 1985, p. 76.

107. Veronesi, U., Adamus, J., Bandiera, D. C., et al.: Stage I melanoma of the limbs: Immediate versus delayed node dissection. Tumori, 66:373, 1980.

108. Veronesi, U., Adamus, J., Bandiera, D. C., et al.: Delayed regional lymph node dissection in stage I melanoma of the skin of the lower extremities. Cancer, 49:2420, 1982.

109. Veronesi, U., and Cascinelli, N.: Narrow excision (1-cm margin): A safe procedure for thin cutaneous melanoma. Arch. Surg., 126:438, 1991.

110. Wallack, M. K., Bash, J. A., Leftheriotis, E., Seigler, H., Bland, K., Wanebo, H., Balch, C., and Bartolucci, A. A.: Positive relationship of clinical and serologic responses to vaccinia melanoma oncolysate. Arch. Surg., 122:1460, 1987.

111. Wallack, M. K., Sivanandham, M., Balch, C. M., Urist, M. M., Bland, K. I., Murray, D., Robinson, W. A., Flaherty, L. E., Richards, J. M., Bartolucci, A. A., and Rosen, L.: A phase III randomized, double-blind, multiinstitu-

tional trial of vaccinia melanoma oncolysate-active specific immunotherapy for patients with stage II melanoma. Cancer, 75:34, 1995.
112. Wanebo, H. J., Harpole, D., and Teates, C. D. Radionuclide lymphoscintigraphy with technetium 99m antimony sulfur colloid to identify lymphatic
drainage of cutaneous melanoma at ambiguous sites in the head and
neck and trunk. Cancer, 55:1403, 1985.
113. Weldon, D., and Little, J. H.: Spindle and epithelioid cell nevi in children
and adults. Cancer, 40:217, 1977.

114. Wong, J. H., Sterns, E. E., Kopald, K. H., Nizze, J. A., and Morton, D. L.:
Prognostic significance of pregnancy in stage I melanoma. Arch. Surg.,
124:1227, 1989.
115. Woolcott, R. J., Henry, R. J. W., and Houghton, C. R. S.: Malignant
melanoma of the vulva: Australian experience. J. Reprod. Med., 33:699,
1988.
116. Zava, D. T., and Goldhirsch, A.: Estrogen receptor in malignant melanoma: Fact or artifact? Eur. J. Cancer Clin. Oncol., 19:1151, 1983.

III

SOFT TISSUE SARCOMAS

Jonathan J. Lewis, M.D., Ph.D., and Murray F. Brennan, M.D.

Soft tissue sarcomas are rare and unusual neoplasms. The annual incidence in the United States is approximately 5000 to 6000, and this number has remained relatively constant. They account for 1% of adult malignancies and 15% of pediatric malignancies. Although these tumors may develop in any anatomic site, approximately 50% occur in the extremities. This chapter focuses on the biology and management of soft tissue sarcomas among adults (>16 years old).

PREDISPOSING FACTORS

In most patients, no specific etiologic agent is found. Multiple predisposing factors have been identified (Table 21–7). Genetic syndromes such as neurofibromatosis, familial adenomatous polyposis, and the Li-Fraumeni syndrome have all been shown to be associated with the development of soft tissue sarcoma.[4, 27, 28, 36] Ionizing radiation and lymphedema are well-established but uncommon antecedents to the development of soft tissue sarcoma.[7] The association with trauma is uncertain as a true causal factor. Chemical carcinogens have also been widely implicated, but the data to support their association are not well founded.[16, 25, 40]

Genetic factors play a role in the development of soft tissue sarcoma. Several cytogenetic and molecular abnormalities have been identified in association with these tumors (Table 21–8). Most sarcomas are characterized by recurrent chromosome translocations that are specific to histologic types.[17, 19, 24, 30, 37] Cytogenetics may also provide an essential adjunct to diagnostic surgical pathology. In addition, investigation of molecular changes of genes at the sites of chromosomal alterations has led to the identification of novel genes and the characterization of their mechanisms of deregulation. The tumor suppressor genes best studied in sarcomas are *p53* and *RB1*. Inactivation of both genes is involved in the tumorigenesis of several sarcomas.[10, 12, 37] The relevance of the *p53* gene to sarcoma tumorigenesis is underscored by the frequent occurrence of soft tissue sarcomas in the Li-Fraumeni syndrome; all families studied have *p53* germ line mutations.

HISTOLOGIC SUBTYPES

The histologic subtypes most commonly found are liposarcoma, malignant fibrous histiocytoma (MFH), and leiomyosarcoma (Fig. 21–16). Histopathology is anatomic site dependent: the common subtypes in the extremity are liposarcoma or MFH, whereas in retroperitoneal or visceral lesions, leiomyosarcoma or liposarcoma are found almost exclusively (Fig. 21–17). Age is also a factor in histopathology. In childhood, embryonal rhabdomyosarcoma is most common; synovial cell sarcoma is more likely to be seen in young adults (less than 35 years old); and there is an even distribution of liposarcoma and MFH as the predominant types in the older population. In general, a specific histologic diagnosis appears to be of secondary importance. However, this may be due

TABLE 21–7. Predisposing Factors for Sarcomas

Genetic Predisposition

- Neurofibromatosis (von Recklinghausen's disease)
- Li-Fraumeni syndrome
- Retinoblastoma
- Gardner's syndrome (familial adenomatous polyposis)

Radiation Exposure

- Ortho and megavoltage therapeutic radiation

Lymphedema

- Postsurgical
- Postradiation
- Parasitic infection (filariasis)

Trauma

- Postparturition
- Extremity

Chemical

- 2,3,7,8 tetrachlorodibenzodioxin (TCDD)
- Polyvinyl chloride
- Hemachromatosis
- Arsenic

TABLE 21–8. Cytogenetic and Molecular Abnormalities in Sarcomas

Histology	Cytogenetic Abnormality
Synovial sarcoma	t(X;18)(p11.2;q11.2)
Myxoid liposarcoma	t(12;16)(q13;p11)
Ewing's sarcoma	t(11;22)(q21–24;q11–14)
Alveolar rhabdomyosarcoma	t(2;13)(q35–37;q14)
Extraskeletal myxoid chondrosarcoma	t(9;22)(q22;q11–12)

Histology	Molecular Abnormality
Leiomyosarcoma	*RB1* point mutations or deletions
Malignant fibrous histiocytoma	
Malignant peripheral nerve sheath tumor	
Malignant fibrous histiocytoma	*p53* point mutations or deletions
Leiomyosarcoma	
Liposarcoma	
Rhabdomyosarcoma	

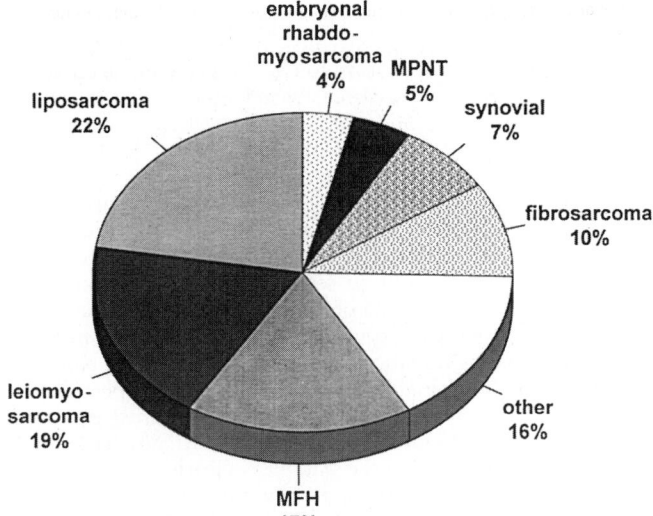

Figure 21–16. Histopathologic subtype distribution of 2457 patients with soft tissue sarcoma treated at Memorial Sloan-Kettering Cancer Center from 1982 through 1994. These data include extremity, trunk, visceral, and retroperitoneal tumors. MFH, malignant fibrous histiocytoma; MPNT, malignant peripheral nerve tumor.

partly to the paucity of histologic subtypes. Biologic behavior is currently best predicted based on histologic grade as determined by the mitotic index, cellularity, necrosis, and degree of nuclear anaplasia.[23] The difficulty in grading leiomyosarcoma and the impression that most of these tumors appear to be high grade may account for the suggested poorer prognosis of this histologic subtype. Increasing use of molecular and tissue-specific immunohistochemistry may better define this issue.

DIAGNOSIS

Patients with extremity sarcoma usually present with a painless mass, although pain is noted at presentation in up to 33% of patients. Delay in diagnosis is common, with the most common differential diagnosis for extremity and trunk lesions being a hematoma or a pulled muscle. Physical examination should include assessment of the size of the mass and its relationship to neurovascular and bony structures. Generally, in an adult, any soft tissue mass that is symptomatic or enlarging, any mass that is larger than 5 cm., or any new mass that persists beyond 4 weeks should be biopsied.[8] Biopsy technique is important. For any mass larger than 5 cm., an incisional biopsy is usually preferred, with a longitudinal incision (extremity lesions) to facilitate subsequent wide local excision. The incision should be centered over the mass in its most superficial location. No tissue flap should be raised, and meticulous hemostasis should be ensured to prevent cellular dissemination by hematoma. At the time of definitive resection, the previous scar should be excised *en*

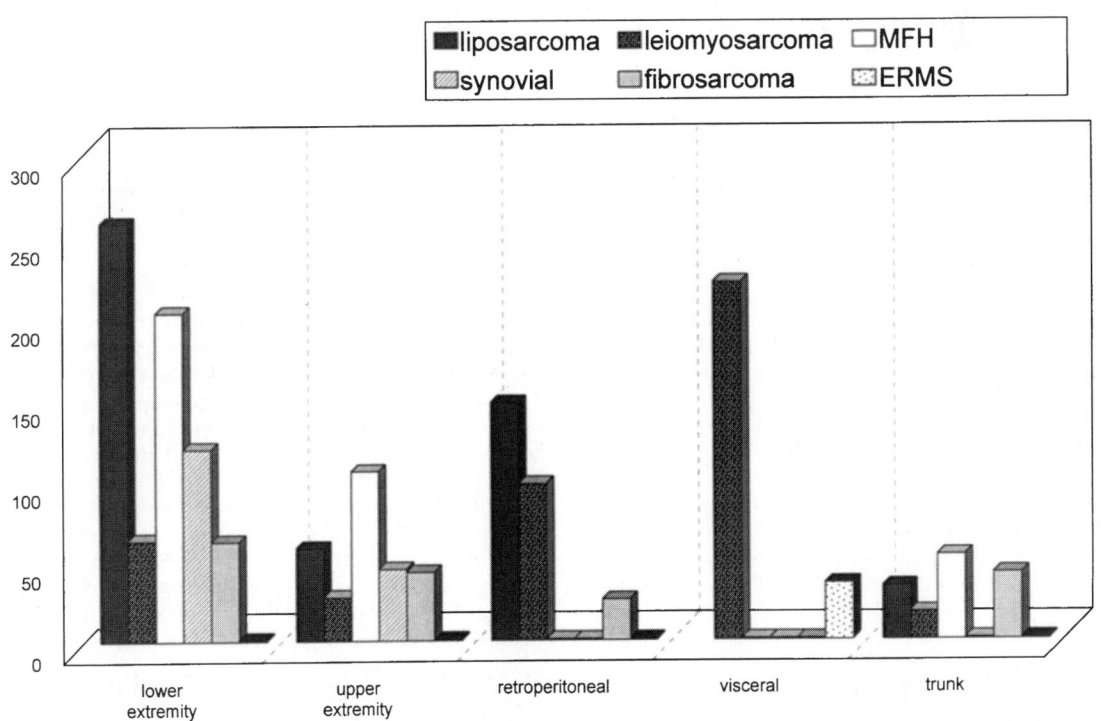

Figure 21–17. Site-specific histopathologic subtype distribution of 2457 patients with soft tissue sarcoma treated at Memorial Sloan-Kettering Cancer Center from 1982 through 1994. MFH, malignant fibrous histiocytoma; ERMS, embryonal rhabdomyosarcoma.

bloc, together with the tumor. Fine-needle aspiration biopsy has no role in diagnosing extremity soft tissue tumors. Tru-Cut core biopsies have been found to have an accuracy of 98% for diagnosing malignancy and 94% for diagnosing sarcoma.[3] Tumor type and grade are correctly identified in most patients. The ease of performance, low cost, and low complication rate make this technique attractive.

Patients with intra-abdominal or retroperitoneal sarcomas often experience nonspecific abdominal discomfort and gastrointestinal symptoms before diagnosis.[26] The diagnosis is usually suspected on finding a soft tissue mass on abdominal computed tomography (CT) or magnetic resonance imaging (MRI) scan. Fine-needle aspiration biopsy has no role in the routine diagnostic evaluation of these patients. Needle biopsy is indicated if abdominal lymphoma is strongly suspected as part of the differential diagnosis. In most patients, exploratory laparotomy should be performed and the diagnosis made at operation, unless the patient is clearly unresectable or will be undergoing preoperative investigational treatment.[26]

EVALUATION OF EXTENT OF DISEASE

All patients require a thorough history and physical examination. MRI examination is now regarded as the procedure of choice for imaging soft tissue masses.[13] MRI enhances the contrast between tumor and adjacent structures and provides excellent three-dimensional definition of fascial planes. The relative value of MRI over CT is currently the subject of a nationwide study. Once the diagnosis and grade are known, evaluation for sites of potential metastasis can be performed. Lymph node metastases occur in less than 3% of adult soft tissue sarcoma.[18] For extremity lesions, the lung is the principal site for metastasis of high-grade lesions;[20] for visceral lesions, the liver is the principal site.[22] Thus, patients with low-grade extremity lesions require a chest x-ray, and those with high-grade lesions require a chest CT scan. Patients with visceral lesions should have their livers imaged as part of the initial abdominal CT or MRI scan. The authors do not generally perform angiography because this adds few data that will change the management strategy.

PROGNOSTIC FACTORS

Current staging systems (Table 21–9) focus on histologic grade of the tumor, size of the primary tumor, and presence or absence of metastasis.[5, 21] Histologic grade is a major prognostic determinant and is based on degree of mitosis, cellularity, presence of necrosis, differentiation, and stromal content. Various grading systems exist, all of which should be considered as categories in a histologic spectrum. For therapeutic planning, the broad categories of low (Grades I or II) and high (Grades III or IV) grade suffice. Clearly such arbitrary decisions may be difficult, but they facilitate practical management of the patient. Low-grade lesions are assumed to have a low (<15%) risk of subsequent metastasis, and high-grade lesions have a high (>50%) risk of subsequent metastasis.

Size has historically been considered a less important determinant of biologic behavior, but large lesions can be associated with late recurrence. Unequivocal characterization of grade is difficult in large lesions, especially in tumors that can reach 2 or 3 kg. Conversely, very small, high-grade lesions less than 5 cm. in maximal diameter have limited risk for metastatic disease if treated appropriately at the first encounter. Re-evaluations of staging systems are currently being performed, with greater emphasis on combinations of grade and size, rather than making grade an absolutely arbitrary factor, particularly in very small lesions.[22]

TABLE 21–9. Current Staging Systems for Soft Tissue Sarcomas

American Joint Committee on Cancer Staging System

G   *Histologic Grade*

GX	Grade cannot be assessed
G1	Low grade
G2	Moderate grade
G3	High grade
G4	Undifferentiated

T   *Primary Tumor Site*

TX	Primary size cannot be assessed
T0	No evidence of tumor
T1	Tumor less than 5 cm.
T2	Tumor 5 cm. or greater

N   *Regional Nodes*

NX	Regional nodes cannot be assessed
N0	No regional lymph node metastasis
N1	Regional lymph node metastasis

M   *Distant Metastasis*

MX	Presence of distant metastasis cannot be assessed
M0	No distant metastasis
M1	Distant metastasis present

Staging Grouping

Stage IA	G1	T1	N0	M0
Stage IB	G1	T2	N0	M0
Stage IIA	G2	T1	N0	M0
Stage IIB	G2	T2	N0	M0
Stage IIIA	G3, G4	T1	N0	M0
Stage IIIB	G3, G4	T2	N0	M0
Stage IVA	Any G	Any T	N1	M0
Stage IVB	Any G	Any T	N1	M1

Memorial Sloan-Kettering Cancer Center Staging System

Prognostic Factors

	Favorable Factors	Adverse Factors
Size	<5 cm.	>5 cm.
Site	Superficial	Deep
Histologic grade	Low	High

Staging

Number of Adverse Factors	Stage
0	0
1	I
2	II
3	III
Metastasis	IV

MANAGEMENT

Algorithms for management are shown in Figures 21–18 and 21–19. Surgical excision remains the dominant modality of curative therapy for all soft tissue sarcomas.[8] Whenever possible, function- and limb-sparing procedures should be performed.[34] As long as the entire tumor is removed, less radical procedures have not been demonstrated to adversely affect local recurrence or outcome.[32, 35] The surgical objective should be complete removal of the tumor with negative margins and maximal preservation of function. When possible, tumors should be excised with 2 to 3 cm. of normal tissue, because of the propensity for local, unappreciated spread.[34] Conversely, deliberate sacrifice of major neurovascular structures can generally be avoided, provided the surgeon pays meticulous attention to dissection.[32, 39]

Adjuvant radiation has been demonstrated to improve local control.[9, 38] This includes using either brachytherapy for high-grade lesions[9, 31] or external beam radiation therapy for large (>5 cm.) high- or low-grade lesions.[9] Patients with

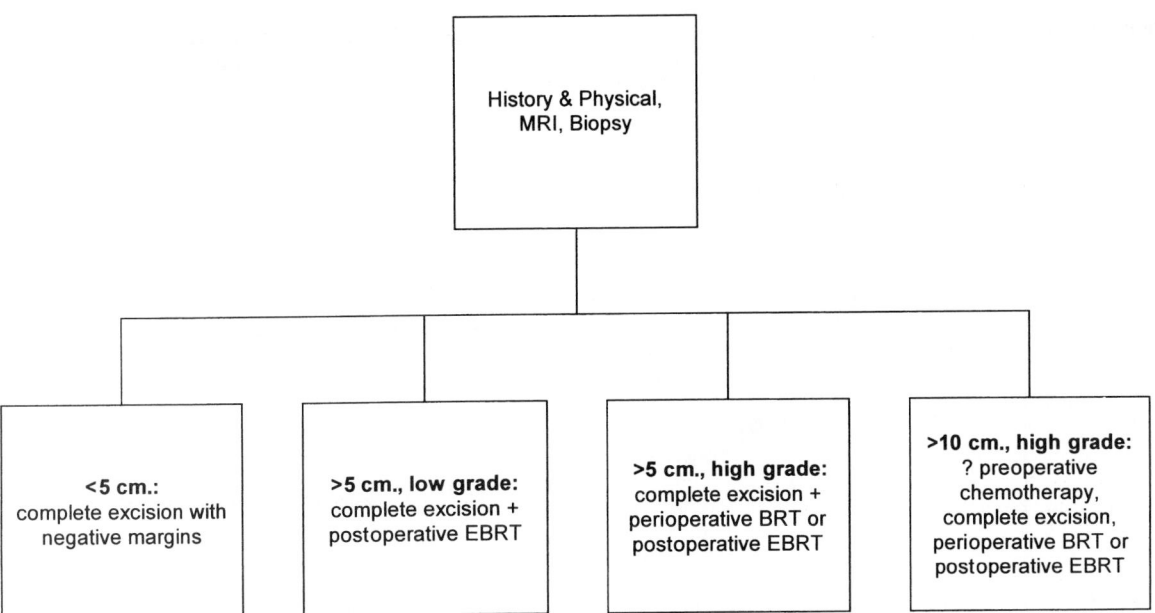

Figure 21–18. Algorithm for management of primary (with no metastases) extremity or trunk soft tissue sarcoma, using a biologic rationale (i.e., size and grade of tumor). MRI, magnetic resonance imaging; EBRT, external beam radiation therapy; BRT, brachytherapy.

small (<5 cm.) primary lesions have an inherently good prognosis, regardless of histologic grade, and are not appropriate candidates for adjuvant treatment, unless there is a recurrence.

Adjuvant chemotherapy has not proved to be efficacious, although some suggest that patients with large, high-grade lesions may benefit from a preoperative regimen.[11] Adjuvant chemotherapy for soft tissue sarcoma should be regarded as investigational and is rarely indicated, except in a clinical trial.[11, 29]

In retroperitoneal and visceral lesions, operation remains the dominant method of therapy[26] because of the apparent lack of benefit of chemotherapy and the inability, thus far, to deliver adequate doses of radiation without serious damage to normal tissue.[6] Current studies are re-evaluating the use of intraoperative radiation and preoperative chemotherapy in this setting.[15]

TREATMENT OF RECURRENT DISEASE

Despite optimal multimodality therapy, at least one third of patients develop recurrent disease, after a median disease-free interval of 18 months.[9] Local extremity recurrence presents as a nodular mass or series of nodules arising in the surgical scar. Patients with retroperitoneal recurrence usually present with nonspecific symptoms, often only after the lesion has reached a substantial size. After work-up to determine the extent of disease, patients with isolated local recurrence should undergo re-resection. The results of re-resection are good, and two thirds of these patients experience long-

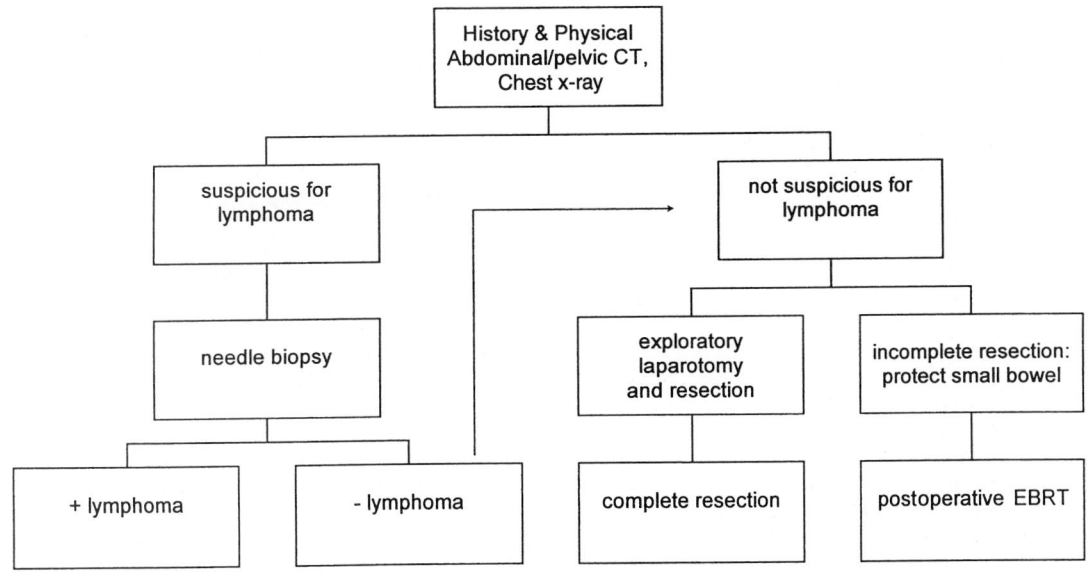

Figure 21–19. Algorithm for management of primary retroperitoneal or visceral soft tissue sarcoma. Fine-needle aspiration biopsy is not routinely used. CT, computed tomography; EBRT, external beam radiation therapy.

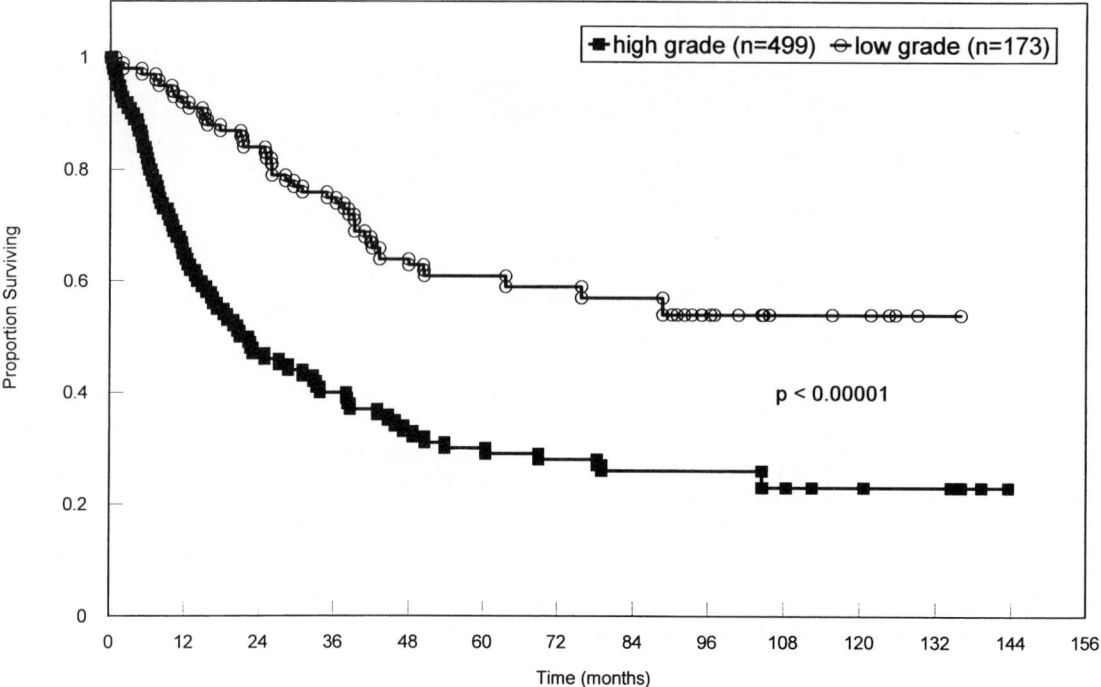

Figure 21–20. Overall survival of patients with retroperitoneal or visceral sarcoma from the date of first operation at Memorial Sloan-Kettering Cancer Center for patients with high-grade (n = 499) and low-grade (n = 173) sarcomas.

term survival. Adjuvant radiation therapy should be administered after surgery. The approach will depend on the method and extent of previous radiation.

For extremity lesions, the most common site of metastasis is the lung. It is the only site of recurrence in approximately half of all patients.[20] Extrapulmonary metastases are uncommon and occur as a late manifestation of widely disseminated disease. Patients whose primary tumors are controlled

or controllable, who have no extrathoracic disease, who are medically fit for thoracotomy, and in whom complete resection of all lung disease appears possible should undergo thoracotomy with the intent of resecting all disease.[20, 33] Patients with unresectable pulmonary metastases or extrapulmonary metastatic sarcoma have a uniformly poor prognosis and are best treated with systemic chemotherapy. Current active drugs that have significant response include doxorubi-

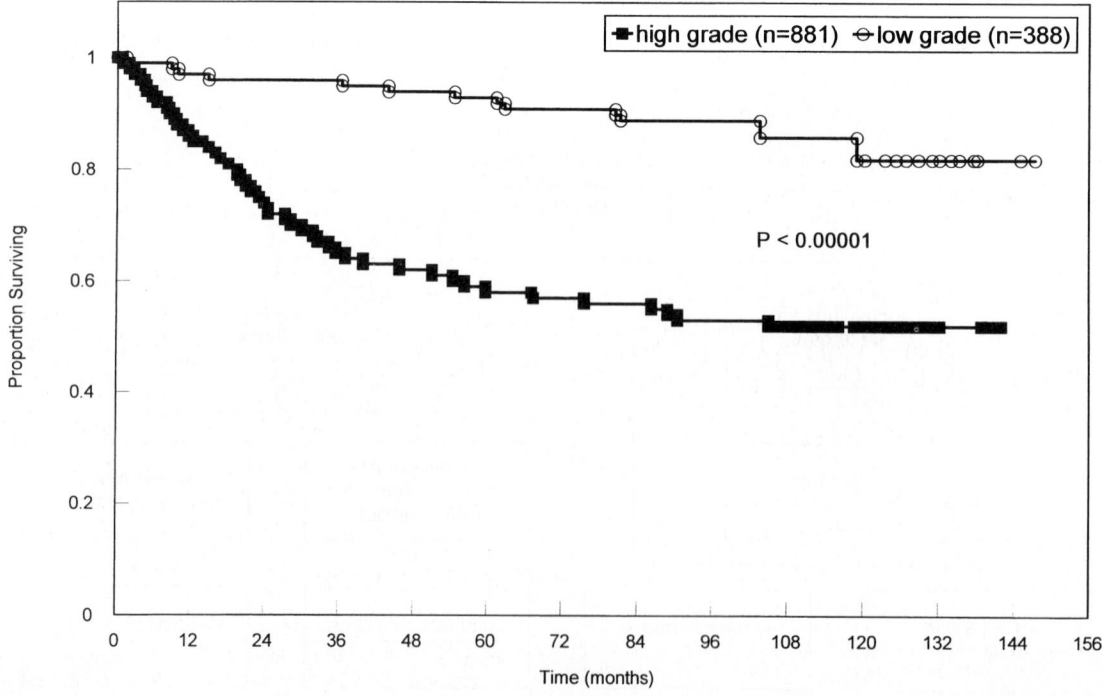

Figure 21–21. Overall survival of patients with extremity sarcoma from the date of first operation at Memorial Sloan-Kettering Cancer Center for patients with high-grade (n = 881) and low-grade (n = 388) extremity sarcomas.

TABLE 21–10. Prognostic Factors for Extremity Soft Tissue Sarcoma[21]

Outcome Variable	Factors Prognostic by Multivariate Analysis
Local recurrence	Presentation with recurrent disease
	Gross or microscopically positive surgical margin
Distant metastasis	High histologic grade
	Deep location
	Size ≥5 cm.
Postmetastasis survival	Age ≥60 yr.
	Time from presentation to metastasis
	Metastasis to sites other than single lung
Disease-specific mortality	High histologic grade
	Deep location
	Size ≥5 cm.

cin, ifosfamide, and dacarbazine (DTIC), but none has had a major impact on long-term survival.[1, 2] Recently, the combination of mesna, ifosfamide, doxorubicin, and dacarbazine (MAID) has been shown to have a 47% response rate and a 10% complete response rate.[14] Trials are currently under way to evaluate MAID and other ifosfamide-doxorubicin combinations with cytokine support.

RESULTS

Results are highly dependent on the presenting features and the prognostic factors previously described. Survival for patients treated with retroperitoneal sarcoma is depicted in Figure 21–20. Significant prognostic factors for extremity soft tissue sarcoma are summarized in Table 21–10. For patients with extremity sarcoma, the development of effective adjuvant strategies and the application of a multimodality approach allow most to retain a functional extremity, with 5-year survival rates that approach 60% to 90% (Fig. 21–21).

SUMMARY

Soft tissue sarcomas are relatively rare, with an annual incidence of 5000 to 6000 in the United States. Primary therapy is predicated on surgical resection with an adequate margin of normal tissue. For high-risk patients, local control is improved with postoperative adjuvant radiation. Local recurrence rates vary, depending on anatomic site. In extremity lesions, one third of patients develop locally recurrent disease, with a median disease-free interval of 18 months. Treatment results for extremity local recurrence may approach those for primary disease. Isolated pulmonary metastases may be resected with 20% to 30% 3-year survival rates. Patients with unresectable pulmonary metastases or extrapulmonary metastatic sarcoma have a uniformly poor prognosis and are best treated with systemic chemotherapy.

SELECTED REFERENCES

Brennan, M. F., Casper, E. S., Harrison, L. B., Shiu, M. H., Gaynor, J., and Hajdu, S. I.: The role of multimodality therapy in soft tissue sarcoma. Ann. Surg., 214:328, 1991.
This study describes the development of a prospective database incorporating more than 1600 patients. These data have produced several important observations that relate to biology and management. In addition, this is the first study to examine local recurrence and survival as a function of site or individual histopathologic diagnosis.

Gaynor, J. J., Tan, C. C., Casper, E. S., Colin, C., Friedrich, C., Shiu, M. H., Hajdu, S. I., and Brennan, M. F.: Refinement of clinicopathologic staging for localized soft tissue sarcoma of the extremity: A study of 423 adults. J. Clin. Oncol., 10:1317, 1992.
This study represents a comprehensive statistical analysis of the prognostic value of factors used in the clinicopathologic staging of extremity soft tissue sarcoma. The data demonstrate that tumor grade, depth, and size are crucial prognostic variables and that stage is defined according to the number of unfavorable characteristics.

Mazanet R., and Antman, K. H.: Adjuvant therapy for sarcomas. Semin. Oncol., 18:603, 1991.
This review summarizes studies of adjuvant chemotherapy for soft tissue sarcoma. The review of 12 randomized studies focuses on overall survival advantage. The authors discuss the investigational nature of adjuvant chemotherapy and outline populations for future randomized trials.

Shiu, M. H., and Brennan, M. F.: Surgical Management of Soft Tissue Sarcoma, 1st ed. Philadelphia, Lea & Febiger, 1989.
This book details the experience and approach of Memorial Sloan-Kettering Cancer Center, an institution with a vast experience managing patients with this uncommon disease. The contents include concepts and principles as well as the management of sarcoma in specific sites. Although the title is Surgical Management, *a multidisciplinary approach is emphasized.*

Sreekantaiah, C., Ladanyi, M., Rodriguez, E., and Chaganti, R. S. K.: Chromosomal aberrations in soft tissue tumors: Relevance to diagnosis, classification and molecular mechanisms. Am. J. Pathol., 144:1121, 1994.
This thorough review details the significant progress made in recent years in characterizing chromosomal changes associated with soft tissue sarcomas. In addition, recent molecular analyses of several sarcoma-associated translocations and the identification of novel genes and mechanisms of dysregulation are discussed. The role of cytogenetics and molecular changes, in the context of diagnosis and future investigation, is discussed.

REFERENCES

1. Antman, K. H.: Chemotherapy of advanced sarcomas of bone and soft tissue. Semin. Oncol., 19:13, 1992.
2. Antman, K. H., Ryan, L., Elias, A., Sherman, D., and Grier, H. E.: Response to ifosfamide and mesna: 124 previously treated patients with metastatic or unresectable sarcoma. J. Clin. Oncol., 7:126, 1989.
3. Ball, A. B., Fisher, C., Pittam, M., Watkins, R. M., and Westbury, G.: Diagnosis of soft tissue tumors by Tru-Cut biopsy. Br. J. Surg., 77:756, 1990.
4. Barken, D., Wright, E., and Nguyen, K.: Gene for von Recklinghausen neurofibromatosis is in the pericentromeric region of chromosome 17. Science, 236:1100, 1987.
5. Beahrs, O. H., Henson, D. E., Hutter, R. V. P., and Myers, M. H.: Manual for Staging of Cancer, 3rd ed. Philadelphia, J. B. Lippincott, 1988.
6. Bevilacqua, R. G., Rogatko, A., Hajdu, S. I., and Brennan, M. F.: Prognostic factors in primary retroperitoneal soft-tissue sarcomas. Arch. Surg., 126:328, 1991.
7. Brady, M. S., Gaynor, J. J., and Brennan, M. F.: Radiation-associated sarcoma of bone and soft tissue. Arch. Surg., 127:1379, 1992.
8. Brennan, M. F.: Management of extremity soft-tissue sarcoma. Am. J. Surg., 158:71, 1989.
9. Brennan, M. F., Casper, E. S., Harrison, L. B., Shiu, M. H., Gaynor, J., and Hajdu, S. I.: The role of multimodality therapy in soft tissue sarcoma. Ann. Surg., 214:328, 1991.
10. Cance, W. G., Brennan, M. F., Dudas, M. E., Huang, C. M., and Cordon Cardo, C.: Altered expression of the retinoblastoma gene product in human sarcomas. N. Engl. J. Med., 323:1457, 1990.
11. Casper, E. S., Gaynor, J. J., Harrison, L. B., Panicek, D. B., Hajdu, S. I., and Brennan, M. F.: Preoperative and postoperative adjuvant chemotherapy for adults with high grade soft tissue sarcoma. Cancer, 73:1644, 1994.
12. Cavenee, W. K., Hansen, M. F., Nordenskjold, M., Kock, E., Maumenee, I., Squire, J. A., Phillips, R. A., and Gallie, B. L.: Genetic origin of mutations predisposing to retinoblastoma. Science, 228:501, 1985.
13. Demas, B. E., Heelan, R. T., Lane, J., Marcove, R., Hajdu, S. I., and Brennan, M. F.: Soft-tissue sarcomas of the extremities: Comparison of MR and CT in determining the extent of disease. AJR Am. J. Roentgenol., 150:615, 1988.
14. Elias, A., Ryan, L., Eisner, J., and Antman, K. H.: Mesna, doxorubicin, ifosfamide, dacarbazine (MAID) regimen for adults with advanced sarcoma. Semin. Oncol., 17:41, 1990.
15. Engel, C. J., Eilber, F. R., Rosen, G., Selch, M. T., and Fu, Y. S.: Preoperative chemotherapy for soft tissue sarcoma of the extremities: The experience at the University of California, Los Angeles. Cancer Treat. Res., 67:135, 1993.
16. Fingerhut, M. A., Halperin, W. E., Marlow, D. A., Piacitelli, L. A., Horchar, P. A., Sweeney, M. H., Griefe, A. L., Dill, P. A., Steenland, K., and Suruda, A. J.: Cancer mortality in workers exposed to 2,3,7,8-tetrachlorodibenzo-p-dioxin. N. Engl. J. Med., 324:212, 1991.
17. Fletcher, J. A., Kozakewich, H. P., Hoffer, F. A., Loge, J. M., Weidner, N., Tepper, R., Pinkus, G. S., Morton, C. C., and Corson, J. M.: Diagnostic relevance of clonal cytogenetic aberrations in malignant soft-tissue tumors. N. Engl. J. Med., 324:436, 1991.
18. Fong, Y., Coit, J., Woodruff, J. M., and Brennan, M. F.: Lymph node metastasis from soft tissue sarcoma in adults: Analysis of data from a prospective database of 1772 sarcoma patients. Ann. Surg., 217:72, 1993.
19. Fountain, J. W., Wallace, M. R., and Bruce, M. A.: Physical mapping of a translocation breakpoint in neurofibromatosis. Science, 244:1085, 1989.

20. Gadd, M. A., Casper, E. S., Woodruff, J., McCormack, P. M., and Brennan, M. F.: Development and treatment of pulmonary metastases in adult patients with extremity soft tissue sarcoma. Ann. Surg., 218:705, 1993.

21. Gaynor, J. J., Tan, C. C., Casper, E. S., Collin, C., Friedrich, C., Shiu, M. H., Hajdu, S. I., and Brennan, M. F.: Refinement of clinicopathologic staging for localized soft tissue sarcoma of the extremity: A study of 423 adults. J. Clin. Oncol., 10:1317, 1992.

22. Geer, R. J., Woodruff, J., Casper, E. S., and Brennan, M. F.: Management of small soft-tissue sarcoma of the extremity in adults. Arch. Surg., 127:1285, 1992.

23. Hajdu, S. I.: Differential Diagnosis of Soft Tissue and Bone Tumors, 1st ed. Philadelphia, Lea & Febiger, 1986.

24. Harbour, J. W., Lai, S. L., Whang Peng, J., Gazdar, A. F., Minna, J. D., and Kaye, F. J.: Abnormalities in structure and expression of the human retinoblastoma gene in SCLC. Science, 241:353, 1988.

25. Hoar, S. K., Blair, A., Holmes, F. F., Boysen, C. D., Robel, R. J., Hoover, R., and Fraumeni, J. J., Jr.: Agricultural herbicide use and risk of lymphoma and soft tissue sarcoma. JAMA, 256:1141, 1986.

26. Jacques, D. P., Coit, D. G., Hajdu, S. I., and Brennan, M. F.: Management of primary and recurrent soft tissue sarcoma of the retroperitoneum. Ann. Surg., 212:51, 1990.

27. Li, F. P., and Fraumeni, J. F., Jr.: Soft-tissue sarcomas, breast cancer, and other neoplasms: A familial syndrome? Ann. Intern. Med., 71:747, 1969.

28. Li, F. P., Fraumeni, J. F., Jr., Mulvihill, J. J., Blattner, W. A., Dreyfus, M. G., Tucker, M. A., and Miller, R. W.: A cancer family syndrome in twenty-four kindreds. Cancer Res., 48:5358, 1988.

29. Mazanet, R., and Antman, K. H.: Adjuvant therapy for sarcomas. Semin. Oncol., 18:603, 1991.

30. Menon, A. G., Anderson, K. M., Riccardi, V. M., Chung, R. Y., Whaley, J. M., Yandell, D. W., Farmer, G. E., Freiman, R. N., Lee, J. K., Li, F. P., et al.: Chromosome 17p deletions and p53 gene mutations associated with the formation of malignant neurofibrosarcomas in von Recklinghausen neurofibromatosis. Proc. Natl. Acad. Sci. USA, 87:5435, 1990.

31. Pisters, P. W. T., Harrison, L. B., Woodruff, J. M., Gaynor, J. J., and Brennan, M. F.: A prospective randomized trial of adjuvant brachytherapy in the management of low grade soft tissue sarcomas of the extremity and superficial trunk. J. Clin. Oncol., 12:1150, 1994.

32. Rosenberg, S. A., Tepper, J., Glatstein, E., Costa, J., Baker, A., Brennan, M. F., DeMoss, E. V., Seipp, C., Sindelar, W. F., Sugarbaker, P., and Wesley, R.: The treatment of soft-tissue sarcomas of the extremities: Prospective randomized evaluations of limb-sparing surgery plus radiation therapy compared with amputation and the role of adjuvant chemotherapy. Ann. Surg., 196:305, 1982.

33. Roth, J. A., Putnam, J. B., Jr., Wesley, M. N., and Rosenberg, S. A.: Differing determinants of prognosis following resection of pulmonary metastases from osteogenic and soft tissue sarcoma patients. Cancer, 55:1361, 1985.

34. Shiu, M. H., and Brennan, M. F.: Surgical Management of Soft Tissue Sarcoma, 1st ed. Philadelphia, Lea & Febiger, 1989.

35. Sondak, V. K., Economou, J. S., and Eilber, F. R.: Soft tissue sarcomas of the extremity and retroperitoneum: Advances in management. Adv. Surg., 24:333, 1991.

36. Sorensen, S. A., Mulvihill, J. J., and Nielsen, A.: Long-term follow-up of von Recklinghausen neurofibromatosis: Survival and malignant neoplasms. N. Engl. J. Med., 314:1010, 1986.

37. Sreekantaiah, C., Ladanyi, M., Rodriguez, E., and Chaganti, R. S. K.: Chromosomal aberrations in soft tissue tumors: Relevance to diagnosis, classification and molecular mechanisms. Am. J. Pathol., 144:1121, 1994.

38. Suit, H. D., and Proppe, K. H.: Soft Tissue Sarcomas. New York, Pergamon Press, 1983.

39. Williard, W. C., Collin, C., Casper, E. S., Hajdu, S. I., and Brennan, M. F.: The changing role of amputation for soft tissue sarcoma of the extremity in adults. Surg. Gynecol. Obstet., 175:389, 1992.

40. Wingren, G., Fredrikson, M., Brage, H. N., Nordenskold, B., and Axelson, O.: Soft tissue sarcoma and occupational exposure. Cancer, 66:806, 1990.

IV

TUMOR MARKERS

Jeffrey A. Norton, M.D., and Douglas L. Fraker, M.D.

In specific types of cancer, circulating markers have greatly facilitated the treatment of patients by early diagnosis and accurate reflection of residual microscopic disease. A clinically useful marker was first identified by Gutman and Gutman in 1938 when they detected elevated levels of the enzyme acid phosphatase in the serum of patients with metastatic prostate carcinoma. Similarly, in 1965, Gold and Freedman showed that another fetal antigen, carcinoembryonic antigen (CEA), was present in extracts of tumors from the gastrointestinal tract and fetal gut tissue, but not in extracts of adult intestinal tissue. Subsequently, CEA was measured in the circulation of patients with cancer, but not in the circulation of patients with nonmalignant conditions.

Several scientific advances during the past 20 years were instrumental in the development of clinically useful tumor markers. First, Yalow and Berson developed the technique of radioimmunoassay (RIA), for which they later received the Nobel Prize. RIA allowed the reproducible, sensitive, and specific detection of minute amounts of substances in serum based on structural immunogenic characteristics of the marker, as opposed to more cumbersome and less specific assays based on bioactivity. Second, the description of hybridomas that secrete monoclonal antibodies has been applied to tumor antigens, greatly facilitating the detection and characterization of new tumor markers. Finally, with recently developed molecular biologic methods, tumor markers can be characterized at the gene level.

"IDEAL" TUMOR MARKER

Successes and inadequacies of initial investigations with tumor markers helped define the characteristics of an "ideal"

tumor marker. First, markers must be specific; that is, false-positive tests in the normal population or in patients with benign conditions are rare. Second, a reliable tumor marker must have a low false-negative rate or a high degree of sensitivity. All patients with a particular histologic type of cancer should test positive for an ideal tumor marker with minimal tumor burden. Third, the circulating level of an ideal tumor marker should correlate directly with the amount of viable tumor present. A correlation between marker level and tumor burden augments the utility of a marker as a prognostic means and as a yardstick to measure the response to therapy. Finally, sensitive and specific assays for tumor markers must be reproducible and widely available at a reasonable cost.

The potential utility of an ideal tumor marker covers a broad array of clinical problems, such as screening, diagnosis, prognosis, assessment of therapeutic efficacy, and detection of residual or recurrent disease. A successful screening test for the detection of cancer must have a high sensitivity for early lesions, so as to detect disease in asymptomatic patients with small curable tumor burdens. In that situation, early diagnosis by tumor marker screening may translate into therapeutic cure. Currently, the performance of available tumor markers as screening tests for curable malignancies has been unsatisfactory, owing to inadequate sensitivity, an inability to accurately detect small tumor burdens, and the occurrence of numerous false-positive results.[34] An exception to this generalization is patients who develop medullary thyroid carcinoma in familial settings. These cancers can be detected by provocative testing and measurement of plasma calcitonin level, and further studies now document that these individuals can be accurately identified by changes in the *RET* proto-oncogene.

Circulating tumor markers are also used as a diagnostic measure. The best examples of this application are the hormone markers of endocrine tumors. In these conditions, biologic activity of the elevated circulating hormone levels defines the clinical syndrome (i.e., carcinoid syndrome), and the level of circulating hormone (serotonin) or hormone degradation products (urinary 5-hydroxyindoleacetic acid [HIAA]) is the major diagnostic criterion for the disorder. The diagnosis depends on the measurement of the circulating marker or the staining of the tumor for the marker by immunohistochemistry.

A third application for measurement of tumor markers at the time of diagnosis is the ability of some markers to yield prognostic information. The presence or absence of a marker for a specific histologic type may be an independent prognostic variable. For example, patients with testicular cancer with normal serum marker levels respond better to therapy than do patients with markedly elevated ones.[11] In addition, the absolute serum level of tumor marker may predict outcome, as seen in patients with colorectal carcinoma, whose prognosis worsens with greater serum levels of CEA.

The final application for measurement of tumor markers, and the area in which tumor markers appear to have the greatest clinical utility, is as a reflection of treatment efficacy and in follow-up for recurrent disease. In these settings, alterations in tumor marker level may be the primary clinical variable influencing patient management decisions, such as continuing or discontinuing therapy or embarking on efforts to define the extent of disease by imaging studies or exploratory operation.

INADEQUACIES OF TESTING BY TUMOR MARKERS

Despite considerable technical advances and extensive clinical investigations, the actual benefits of any given tumor marker do not achieve the theoretical potential discussed. In other words, no ideal tumor marker exists at present. The characteristics of individual tumor markers, such as specificity, sensitivity, and correlation of marker level with tumor burden, define the actual clinical utility for each marker.

The measurement of tumor markers in serum must be integrated with other technical advances in medicine that relate to similar clinical questions. In this regard, the most important developments are the dramatic improvements in and the increased availability of new radiologic imaging techniques, such as computed tomography (CT), high-resolution ultrasonography, and magnetic resonance imaging (MRI), which are also used in the initial diagnosis and the detection of recurrent or metastatic disease. Data from measurement of serum markers must be interfaced with imaging results. For example, early studies evaluating serum CEA levels as a marker for recurrent colorectal cancer were done before the availability of CT scanners. Current strategy for the follow-up of patients with colorectal cancer should include both serum CEA levels and imaging techniques in a complementary manner. Another potential use of the relationship between tumor markers and radiologic imaging techniques is the ability to localize tumors not imaged by standard studies, such as selective venous sampling for hormone levels or the use of radiolabeled antibody to tumor antigens.

Another reflection of the inadequacy of serum tumor markers is the overlap between different markers and different tumors; that is, many different types of tumors have elevations of two or more serum markers to variable extents. For example, testicular tumors may produce elevations in serum levels of both alpha-fetoprotein (AFP) and beta-human chorionic gonadotropin (β-hCG). Conversely, a given serum marker may be elevated histologically in more than one tumor, such as AFP in both testicular tumors and hepatomas. This lack of specificity probably arises because many of the available tumor markers were developed from fetal tissue and not specific tumor tissues. As a reflection of the dichotomy, this chapter is divided into two sections. The first section is organized by tumor marker and describes the history, biochemistry, assay characteristics, and disease states in which individual markers are useful. The second section is organized by the type of neoplasm and describes the markers relating to that histologic type and the ways in which those markers are used.

TYPES OF TUMOR MARKERS

Circulating tumor markers can be categorized by functional and biochemical characteristics into tumor antigens, enzymes, hormones, oncogenes or gene products, and miscellaneous markers of tumor or host origin (Table 21–11).

Tumor antigens were identified and are defined by immunogenic structural characteristics. Enzymes and hormones are identified by bioactivity as catalysts of specific chemical reactions or effects from binding specific receptors. Although measurement was initially accomplished by bioassays using these activities, immunoassays now exist for essentially all enzymes and hormones used as tumor markers.

Tumor antigens can be subcategorized by historic, biochemical, and distributional features as oncofetal antigens and polyclonal- or monoclonal-defined antigens. Oncofetal antigens are compounds produced during normal development by the placental-fetal complex and are also produced by neoplastic tissue. This group contains the original and most prevalent tumor markers, including CEA, AFP, and β-hCG. A second and rapidly enlarging group of tumor markers consists of tumor-associated antigens detected by conventional immunologic techniques or by monoclonal antibodies directed against fresh tumor extracts or, more commonly, cell lines derived from human neoplasms. Tumor-associated antigens include the newer serum markers such as CA 125, CA 19–9, and CA 15–3. As they are further characterized, these markers typically satisfy the criteria stated earlier for oncofetal antigens, since they are present in specific fetal tissue as well as in neoplasms. The only real differences between these new cancer antigens (CA) and traditional oncofetal antigens is length of experience and familiarity with them.

Enzymes produced in excess amounts by a tumor or by the tumor-bearing host constitute another category of tumor markers and include neuron-specific enolase (NSE) and acid phosphatase. Hormones and hormone degradation products are specific and sensitive markers for a wide variety of endocrine tumors. Oncogenes or gene products have recently been defined and characterized. Some can serve as markers for specific tumors and predictors of prognosis. A miscellaneous group of tumor markers includes host products that increase in response to tumors, such as serum ferritin levels, cytokine levels, and lipids.

Carcinoembryonic Antigen

CEA is a glycoprotein (molecular weight 180 kd.) consisting of a single polypeptide chain with a variable carbohydrate content. Recent studies indicate that CEA is only one of a family of related molecules that share antigenic determinants. Other glycoproteins in the CEA family include nonspecific cross-reacting antigen (NCA) and biliary glycoprotein. The CEA family is a subset of the immunoglobulin gene superfamily, and CEA may have a role in cell recognition as

TABLE 21–11. Categorization of Tumor Markers

Type	Tumor Marker	Tumor Histologies
Tumor antigen		
Oncofetal	Carcinoembryonic antigen (CEA)	Colorectal, pancreatic, breast, lung, gastric
	Alpha-fetoprotein (AFP)	Hepatocellular carcinomas, testicular tumors
Polyclonal antibody-defined	Prostate-specific antigen (PSA)	Prostatic
	Tissue polypeptide antigen (TPA)	Breast, gynecologic tumors
Monoclonal antibody-defined cancer antigens	CA 15–3	Breast
	CA 19–9	Colorectal, pancreatic, gastric
	CA 50	Colorectal, pancreatic, gastric
	CA 242	Colorectal, pancreatic, gastric
	CA 125	Ovarian, other gynecologic tumors
Cytoskeletal filaments	CYFRA 21–1	Non-small-cell lung cancer
Enzymes	Neuron-specific enolase (NSE)	Neuroendocrine tumors (APUDomas) Small-cell lung cancer Medullary thyroid cancer Islet cell tumors, carcinoids
	Prostatic acid phosphatase (PAP)	Prostatic
Hormones	Beta-human chorionic gonadotropin (β-hCG)	Testicular tumors, trophoblastic gestational tumors
Oncogene	*erb B-2*	Breast, ovarian, stomach

an adhesion molecule.[9] Biliary glycoprotein is present in bile, and forms of NCA occur in normal lung, granulocytes, and epithelial cells. Differences in genetic and polypeptide sequences between CEA and related glycoproteins have recently been elucidated. Description of this family of related compounds has led to the discovery of unique epitopes on CEA, which may enable development of a more specific assay by eliminating false-positive results caused by shared epitopes with related glycoproteins in normal tissues.

CEA modulates intercellular adhesion[8] and, as an accessory adhesion molecule, expedites colon epithelial cell–collagen interactions. Because high concentrations of CEA are present in fetal tissues and tumors, it may disrupt the normally operative intercellular or cell-collagen adhesion forces, allowing more cell movement and the development of a less ordered tissue architecture and greater cell-cell interaction.

Various CEA immunoassay kits are available commercially. Normal serum values of CEA vary with different assays. In general, CEA serum levels less than 2.5 ng. per ml. are normal, and CEA levels greater than 5.0 ng. per ml. are elevated. Serum levels between 2.5 and 5.0 ng. per ml. are considered borderline. As with other tests, the normal range affects specificity and sensitivity of serum CEA determinations. If one attempts to increase sensitivity by indicating a lower level for normal CEA values, one loses specificity as a greater number of false-positive results are detected.

The serum half-life of CEA varies between 1 and 7 days, depending on hepatic function. Large glycoproteins such as CEA are cleared mainly by Kupffer cells and hepatocytes. Therefore, both cholestatic and hepatocellular disorders prolong the half-life of CEA.

CEA is a classic example of a tumor marker that, although widely used, is not an ideal marker because of low specificity and sensitivity. Both malignant and nonmalignant diseases may elevate serum CEA levels (Tables 21–12 and 21–13). Although CEA is associated primarily with colorectal cancer, serum levels may also be elevated in cancer of the pancreas, stomach, lung, breast, thyroid, and ovary (see Table 21–13). The lack of specificity is further evidenced by nonmalignant conditions that also may elevate serum CEA levels (see Table 21–12): gastrointestinal disorders (e.g., peptic ulcer disease, gastritis, pancreatitis, and inflammatory bowel disease), hepatobiliary diseases (e.g., cirrhosis, hepatitis, and obstructive

jaundice), and nonmalignant pulmonary disease (e.g., bronchitis and emphysema), as well as benign prostatic hypertrophy and renal failure. Because CEA is excreted and concentrated in the bile, some suggest that measurement of bile concentrations may be more sensitive for detecting occult metastases within the liver. A recent large series reported that biliary levels of CEA have low specificity and low sensitivity for occult hepatic disease and thus offer no advantages over serum levels of CEA.[30]

Alpha-Fetoprotein

AFP was the first oncofetal antigen discovered and is currently a useful tumor marker for primary hepatocellular carcinoma (HCC) and nonseminomatous germ-cell tumors of the testis. AFP is a single-chain glycoprotein (molecular weight 70 kd.) with alpha-globulin electrophoretic mobility characteristics that was originally described as a predominant circulating species during fetal development. AFP is synthesized by fetal yolk sac, hepatic parenchymal cells, and other endodermally derived gastrointestinal tissue. Peak serum levels of AFP (3 mg. per ml.) occur during the twelfth week of gestation; then serum AFP levels decline to approximately 0.1 mg. per ml. at birth and continue to decrease to normal adult levels (<10 ng. per ml.) by 1 year of age.

In 1963, Abelev and colleagues first described the presence of an alpha-globulin that was immunochemically identical to AFP in the serum of adult mice with transplantable, chemically induced hepatomas. The following year, AFP was measured in the serum of patients with hepatoma. Initially, investigators used low-sensitivity agar immunodiffusion assays (level of detection approximately 300 ng. per ml.) and were able to detect AFP in the serum of only 30% of patients with hepatoma. Development of a radioimmunoassay for AFP improved the sensitivity of detection several-fold (10 ng. per ml.) and correspondingly improved the clinical utility of the marker.

Several commercially available immunoassays for AFP, both radiometric and enzyme-linked, are available and reliably detect approximately 5 ng. per ml. of AFP in serum. The half-life of circulating AFP in the serum of patients is 4 to 6 days. Abnormal serum levels of AFP usually occur in malignant neoplasms but may occur in benign diseases of endodermally derived organs, including hepatitis, inflam-

TABLE 21–12. Serum Levels of Markers in Healthy Normal Controls and Other Nonmalignant Conditions

Marker	Mean Level	Upper Limit Normal	Controls with Abnormal Levels at Upper Limit Normal (%)	Nonmalignant Conditions Associated with Elevated Levels
CEA	1.9 ng./ml. nonsmokers 3.1 ng./ml. smokers	<2.5 ng./ml. <5.0 ng./ml. <10 ng./ml.	9–16 1–5 0–1	Hepatitis, cirrhosis, jaundice, COPD, peptic ulcer, pancreatitis, inflammatory bowel disease, renal failure
AFP	1–10 ng./ml.	<10 ng./ml. <40 ng./ml.	1–3 0	Chronic and active hepatitis, cirrhosis, pregnancy, inflammatory bowel disease
β-hCG	<1 unit/ml. men <3 units/ml. premenopausal women 3–4 units/ml. postmenopausal women	<3 units/ml. <8 units/ml.	<1 <1	Pregnancy
Prostate-specific antigen	1.1 ± 0.7 ng./ml.	<2.5 ng./ml.	1–3	Benign prostatic hypertrophy, prostatic massage or biopsy
Tissue polypeptide antigen	66 ± 16 units/L.	<100 units/L. <200 units/L.	5 <1	—
CA 15–3	13.3 ± 6 units/ml.	<22 units/ml. <25 units/ml. <30 units/ml.	9 5	Acute and chronic hepatitis, cirrhosis, benign breast disease
CA 19–9	10.8 ± 7 units/ml.	<35 units/ml. <37 units/ml	1.3 1 0–1	Acute and chronic hepatitis, cirrhosis, sclerosing cholangitis, other extrahepatic cholestatic diseases
CA 50	—	<17 units/ml.	0–1	Pancreatitis, cirrhosis, ulcerative colitis, sclerosing cholangitis
CA 242	—	<20 units/ml.	0–10	Pancreatitis, cirrhosis, ulcerative colitis, sclerosing cholangitis
CA 125	10–16 units/ml. (greater in women)	<35 units/ml. <65 units/ml.	1	Pancreatitis, jaundice, pregnancy, menstruation, endometriosis, PID, renal failure
Neuron-specific enolase	4.7–9.3 ng./ml.	<13 ng./ml.	<1	
Prostatic acid phosphatase	Enzymatic assay: 0.1–0.5 unit/L. Immunoassay: 1.2 + 0.5 ng. ml.	<0.8 unit/L. <2.1 ng./ml.	<1 1–3	Benign prostatic hypertrophy, dermatologic disorders
Ferritin	27–96 ng./ml.	<300 ng./ml.	0–1	Alcoholism, hepatocellular disease, hematologic diseases, chronic inflammation
CYFRA 21–1	1.2 ng./ml.	<3.3 ng./ml.	0–4	Benign lung conditions

CEA, carcinoembryonic antigen; AFP, alpha-fetoprotein; β-hCG, beta-human chorionic gonadotropin; COPD, chronic obstructive pulmonary disease; PID, pelvic inflammatory disease.

matory bowel disease, ataxia-telangiectasia, and hereditary tyrosinemia (Table 21–12). However, highly elevated serum levels of AFP (>500 ng. per ml.) are present almost exclusively in primary HCC and nonseminomatous testicular tumors.

Because cirrhosis due to chronic hepatitis is both a major risk factor for HCC and a cause of elevated AFP without HCC, using this marker for screening is difficult in this high-risk population. Recent studies show that AFP associated with HCC can be differentiated from AFP associated with hepatitis or cirrhosis on the basis of variability in carbohydrate side chains characterized by differential lectin binding.[35] As assay techniques to measure these different profiles of AFP become available, they may increase the utility of AFP as a potential screening tool.

Patients with other malignant tumors may also have elevated serum levels of AFP. Twenty per cent of patients with gastric or pancreatic cancer and 5% of patients with colorectal or lung cancer have significant elevations (>5 ng. per ml.) of serum AFP levels.

Human Chorionic Gonadotropin

hCG is a placental hormone that is also a tumor marker for gestational trophoblastic neoplasms and nonseminomatous testicular cancer. hCG is a glycoprotein consisting of two distinct noncovalently bound subunits. The alpha subunit of hCG (molecular weight 15 kd.) is identical to the alpha subunit of the pituitary hormones luteinizing hormone (LH), follicle-stimulating hormone (FSH), and thyroid-stimulating hormone (TSH). The beta subunit of these four glycoprotein hormones is distinct and defines the activity of each. In particular, the 29 amino acids on the carboxy-terminal end of the hCG beta subunit are unique to that hormone, but there is an 82% overall sequence homology between the beta subunit of LH and that of hCG. Further evidence of the structural similarity between hCG and LH is that these two hormones bind to a common cell surface receptor on gonadal tissues.

Assays for levels of hCG in serum and urine have been available since the 1930s. Elevations of this hormone in women diagnose pregnancy (see Table 21–12). Initial bioassays for hCG were based on the appearance of hemorrhagic follicles or changes in ovarian weight. Owing to structural similarities to other glycoprotein hormones, initial immunoassays lacked specificity for hCG: antibodies to intact hCG cross-reacted with the alpha subunit of TSH, FSH, or LH, and antibodies to the beta subunit of hCG cross-reacted with the beta subunit of LH. In 1972, Vaitukaitis and associates

significant; for patients with baseline levels greater than 4.0 ng. per ml., a PSA slope of greater than 0.40 ng. per ml. is considered significant.[40]

The focus of these recent studies of PSA relates primarily to its use for screening populations at risk for developing prostate cancer. Serum PSA is already a highly sensitive marker not only for detecting advanced disease (nearly 100% have elevated serum levels of PSA) but also for following patients after systemic, surgical, or radiation therapy. One innovative use of PSA is to assay for circulating cells expressing PSA mRNA by reverse transcriptase polymerase chain reaction (RT-PCR).[37] As this protein is tissue specific, any circulating cell expressing this RNA indicates metastatic spread, but even with the highly sensitive detection by RT-PCR, over half of patients with metastases have negative results.[37] Due to the specificity of PSA for the prostate and the greater appreciation for the magnitude of the problem presented by prostate cancer, intensive and innovative research like that discussed above makes PSA one of the most important tumor markers currently available.

CYFRA 21–1

A recently defined tumor marker identified as CYFRA 21–1 is circulating fragments of cytokeratin 19 (CK 19), which is evaluated primarily in non-small-cell lung cancer (NSCLC).[28, 32] The cytoskeleton of a cell is composed of actin, myosin, microtubules, and intermediate filaments. Cytokeratin is the predominant component of intermediate filaments, and over 20 different such structural proteins have been immunologically defined. CK 19 is an acidic, 40-kd. protein that is expressed only in unstratified epithelium, such as the bronchial tree. Immunohistochemistry studies show that CK 19 has increased expression in bronchogenic lung cancer.[32] Fragments of CK 19 can be measured by a double antibody sandwich immunoassay that is commercially available in both the United States and Europe.[28, 32] These CK 19 fragments are designated CYFRA 21–1.

The mean serum level in normal healthy volunteers is 1.2 ng. per ml. (see Table 21–12).[32] Patients with nonmalignant pulmonary disease have some elevation in serum levels, with a mean level of 2.95 ng. per ml. From the recent evaluation of over 1200 non-cancer-bearing individuals, a normal limit of 3.3 ng. per ml. has been established (see Table 21–12).[32]

CYFRA 21–1 is elevated in 41% of patients with NSCLC and 16% of patients with small-cell lung cancer.[32] Another study reports that it is elevated in 48% of patients with NSCLC.[28] For both studies, the histologic subgroup of squamous cell carcinoma had the highest sensitivity—63% and 69%, respectively. Direct comparisons of CYFRA 21–1 to NSE, CEA, and TPA demonstrate equivalent or improved sensitivity and specificity for NSCLC. Since an acceptable marker for this common solid tumor has not yet been identified, this new marker may become important in the near future.

CA 242

Another recent gastrointestinal tumor antigen defined by monoclonal antibody is CA 242.[26] This large glycoprotein was defined by raising a murine monoclonal antibody to the human adenocarcinoma cell line COLO 205—the same line used to develop CA 50.[16] The precise biochemical structure of this moiety is not yet defined.

The activity and utility of this marker parellel those of the similarly identified glycoproteins CA 19–9 and CA 50; that is, the upper limit of normal serum level is between 17 and 20 units per ml., and abnormal levels are seen in patients with gastrointestinal neoplasms, including colorectal, pancreatic, and gastric.[16] This marker has been best studied in patients with colorectal cancer. It was equivalent to CEA in one study[19] and slightly inferior to CEA but better than CA 50 in another study.[16] In both comparative studies, measurements of CEA and CA 242 were complementary, and using both tools significantly improved sensitivity in detecting colorectal cancer.[16, 19] The utility of CA 242 in pancreatic cancer has been recently reported and compared with that of CA 19–9.[18, 25] In both studies, CA 242 had a lower sensitivity but a higher specificity than CA 19–9. The improved specificity is due to the observation that CA 242 is rarely elevated above the established upper limit in benign gastrointestinal diseases such as pancreatitis, hepatitis, and cirrhosis.[18, 25]

Prostatic Acid Phosphatase

Gutman and Gutman's report over 50 years ago of elevated levels of acid phosphatase activity in the serum of patients with metastatic prostate cancer was the first identification of a circulating tumor marker. Initial clinical applications were limited by the enzymatic assays used to measure serum acid phosphatase levels. Currently, an RIA has improved the ability to measure low serum levels of specific prostatic acid phosphatase (PAP). A recent study of healthy men reported a mean PAP serum level of 1.2 ± 0.5 ng. per ml. and a normal range of less than 2.1 ng. per ml. Acid phosphatase activity detected by enzymatic assay ranges between 0.1 and 0.5 unit per liter in normal subjects, with the upper limit of normal less than 0.8 unit per liter (see Table 21–12).

PAP is not a useful circulating tumor marker in patients with prostatic cancer. Although the initial studies using immunometric assays for PAP reported advantages over enzymatic assays, subsequent studies document limitations of serum acid phosphatase measurements using either an immunoassay or a biochemical assay. Specifically, serum PAP level is not useful as a screening test because elevations frequently occur in patients with BPH, and serum levels are not usually elevated in patients with early prostatic cancer or small amounts of residual disease.

Neuron-Specific Enolase

NSE is an acidic isoenzyme of enolase. NSE was initially isolated from bovine brain and reported to be found exclusively in neural tissue. Subsequent studies indicated a high level of NSE in neuroendocrine tissues, the amine precursor uptake and decarboxylation (APUD) cells. NSE was then used as an immunohistochemical marker to identify and study the distribution and development of peripheral neuroendocrine cells.

The development of a specific RIA enabled measurement of NSE in the serum of normal subjects and patients with malignant disease originating from neuroendocrine tissues. Normal individuals have serum levels between 5 and 10 ng. per ml. (see Table 21–12). Study of patients with different neuroendocrine tumors demonstrated elevated serum levels of NSE in patients with pancreatic islet cell tumors, gut carcinoids, adrenal tumors, neuroblastomas, medullary cancer of the thyroid, and small-cell lung cancer. Because other more specific and sensitive tumor markers exist for most patients with endocrine tumors, serum NSE levels do not help in the management of these patients. However, one recent study suggests that circulating NSE levels may be a valuable marker for patients with small-cell lung cancer, since good alternative markers are not available.[17] Another potential application of serum NSE levels is for the management of patients with seminomas, because 73% of such patients have elevated levels.

TABLE 21–14. Genes That Are Possible Tumor Markers

Type of Genetic Change	Gene	Tumor
Gene amplification	c-erb B-2	Breast, ovary, stomach
	N-myc	Neuroblastoma
	c-myc	Lung
Gene mutation	ras	Pancreas, lung, colorectal, kidney
Loss of tumor suppressor gene	APC	Colorectal
	Rb-1	Retinoblastoma, breast
	p53	Lung, breast, colorectal

Ferritin

Ferritin is a large storage protein (molecular weight 450 kd.) composed of multiple identical subunits found in all tissues of the body, with highest concentrations in the liver, spleen, and bone marrow. Serum levels of ferritin directly correlate with total body iron stores. The normal range of serum ferritin levels is between 20 and 300 ng. per ml., with a mean level of 90 ng. per ml. (see Table 21–12). Serum ferritin levels are nonspecific and are elevated in a variety of malignant diseases, including lymphoma, leukemia, and colorectal, breast, pancreatic, and lung cancer. It is best used as a serum tumor marker in patients with hepatoma and reportedly is elevated in a high proportion of patients with normal serum levels of AFP. Recent studies suggest that a related, more acidic tumor-derived ferritin is present in patients with hepatoma. This may explain why ferritin is a good serum marker in patients with hepatoma.

Oncogenes

There are specific genes and gene products associated with cancer. Proto-oncogenes are cellular DNA sequences that are inappropriately overexpressed during tumorigenesis. Many proto-oncogenes exist in normal cells because they have a role in normal growth and development. If activation occurs outside these functions, cell transformation may result. Oncogenes affect cell function through expression of protein products called oncoproteins. Dominant oncogenes produce proteins that cause cellular growth, dedifferentiation, and transformation. Tumor suppressor genes produce proteins that inhibit cellular growth and transformation, and these genes are deleted, causing neoplasia. The involvement of oncogenes and their proteins in tumorigenesis has been studied using monoclonal antibodies, and these proteins may be useful tumor markers. Table 21–14 shows examples of abnormalities of oncogene expression and their products in various malignancies. Currently, the significance of oncogenes in tumor virulence and prognosis has been demonstrated in only a few tumors. For example, c-erb B-2 expression correlates with poor prognosis in patients with breast cancer. N-myc copy number is associated with extent of disease and prognosis in pediatric patients with neuroblastoma. C-ras mutations have been associated with a worse prognosis in patients with lung cancer. Some suggest that detection of amplification of oncogenes or oncogene products will be useful in future screening programs for colon and breast cancer.[31]

THE ROLE OF SERUM MARKERS IN SPECIFIC TUMORS

Hepatoma

HCC is one of the most malignant and common cancers. The estimated annual world incidence of HCC is 0.3 to 1.2 million, with an apparent rise in frequency in many parts of the world. One etiologic factor of HCC may be related to prior exposure to aflatoxin and other environmental and chemical agents, but the primary cause of the disease is chronic active liver infection with hepatitis B virus (HBV). In Taiwan, the chance of persons who are hepatitis B antigen (HBsAg) positive developing HCC is 233 times greater than for those who are HBsAg negative.[6] The use of AFP as a specific diagnostic marker for HCC and as a means of monitoring response to therapy in patients with HCC has been well established. However, not all patients with HCC have elevated serum levels of AFP, and nearly 40% of patients with HCC may have normal serum levels.

Early Diagnosis

In 1983, a case report was published in *Lancet* demonstrating the feasibility of screening a population at high risk for developing HCC with serial serum levels of AFP.[23] High rates of primary HCC have been reported in Alaskan natives (Eskimos, Indians, Aleuts), with the annual incidence being between 7.6 and 11.2 per 100,000 population. Sera from 24 members of a family with a strong history of HCC were screened every 6 months for HBV markers and AFP. The patient who eventually developed HCC was HBsAg positive and, on initial screening, had normal serum levels of AFP (<25 ng. per ml.) (Fig. 21–22). Two years later, serum levels of AFP rose to 104 ng. per ml., and 2 months later, levels increased to 667 ng. per ml. Preoperative imaging studies, including CT, ultrasonography, and selective arteriography, failed to image the 2-cm. primary HCC that was subsequently removed from the left lobe of the liver. Serum AFP level at discharge from the hospital was 25 ng. per ml., and subsequent follow-up measurements demonstrated a further decline of AFP levels to 5 ng. per ml.[23] This report demonstrates the feasibility of screening populations at risk for the

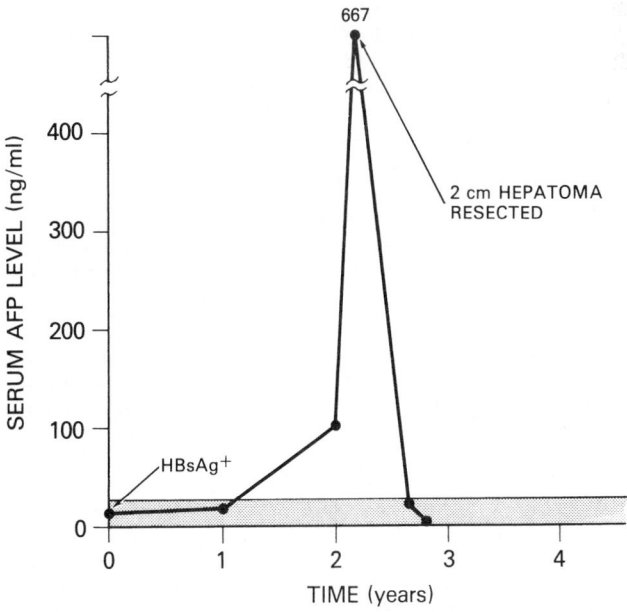

Figure 21–22. Alaskan native who was at risk for the development of hepatocellular carcinoma because of his family history and the fact that he was hepatitis B antigen (HBsAg) positive. He was followed with yearly serum alphafetoprotein (AFP) levels, which remained within the normal range (shaded area). After 2 years of follow-up, his serum AFP level was elevated at 104 ng. per ml.; repeat level 1 month later was further increased to 667 ng. per ml. Despite negative preoperative imaging, exploratory laparotomy demonstrated a 2-cm. hepatoma, which was resected. Postoperative serum levels of AFP declined to normal range.

development of HCC (patients who are chronic carriers of HBV). It also suggests that simple measurement of serum AFP levels can be a sensitive and specific screening method for the early detection of HCC at a stage when surgical intervention can increase survival or provide cure.

Other investigators have tried to use serum AFP levels to detect HCC in at-risk populations, with disappointing results. Serum AFP levels may be normal in 35 to 50% of patients with biopsy-proven HCC (Table 21–15). In a minority of patients with HCC, serum levels of AFP decline despite continued tumor growth, and other patients have elevated levels of AFP and nonmalignant diseases of the liver (see Table 21–15).

Because patients with cirrhosis of the liver are at risk for developing HCC, serum levels of AFP have been used in this group to diagnose HCC. Elevations of serum AFP levels are seen in approximately 85% of patients who have HCC within a cirrhotic liver. In patients with cirrhosis without HCC, only 5% have elevated serum AFP levels, but in one series, 40% of patients with this diagnosis had elevated levels. These false-positive results usually occur in patients with cirrhosis and chronic active hepatitis, a condition in which the need for distinction from HCC seldom arises. In a prospective study of the ability to detect HCC in 450 patients with cirrhosis, the sensitivity and specificity of results depended on the definition of normal serum AFP level. If a serum AFP level greater than 10 ng. per ml. was chosen as abnormal, the sensitivity was 86% and the specificity was 91%. If the abnormal level was defined as greater than 500 ng. per ml., sensitivity decreased to 62% and specificity increased to 100%. Thus, a serum AFP level greater than 500 ng. per ml. in the presence of cirrhosis was diagnostic for HCC.

Prognosis

Serum levels of AFP in patients with HCC may be of prognostic value. The subgroup of patients who have HCC and normal serum levels of AFP appears to have a relatively good prognosis. In these patients, the primary factor predicting better prognosis may be the absence of cirrhosis. Normal serum AFP levels are more common in patients without underlying cirrhosis. A rapid AFP doubling time is also associated with a poorer prognosis (see Table 21–15).

Recurrence of Tumor

Resection of HCC in patients with HCC and cirrhosis has produced 2-year survival of 60% and 5-year survival of 33%. Although the results after initial resection of patients with

HCC are improving because of AFP-directed earlier tumor detection, the long-term survival after resection needs additional improvement because of tumor recurrence. In 41 patients who underwent curative resection of HCC and subsequently developed recurrent HCC, serial serum measurement of AFP levels was the best detector of recurrent disease. It was the first measured abnormality in 34% of patients, and imaging studies, including ultrasound and CT, were less sensitive than serum AFP level—17% and 2%, respectively. However, in some patients who had elevated serum levels of AFP with their original HCC, postoperative levels of serum AFP were unreliable to detect recurrence. Five of 41 patients (12%) did not have elevated serum levels despite recurrent HCC.

Serial measurement of serum AFP level can be helpful before and after presumably curative surgical therapy in patients with HCC. However, the serum levels of this tumor marker do not always show the presence of recurrent HCC. HCC may be recurrent despite normal serum AFP levels. AFP synthesis varies in different parts of the same tumor. The ability of the tumor to secrete AFP may change with growth. It may be that tumor recurrences within the liver are really new primary tumors with different characteristics.

Following the Response to Treatment

In the absence of effective antitumor therapy, serum AFP levels rise exponentially, the doubling time being approximately 40 days (range, 6 to 120 days; tumors with a poorer prognosis have a more rapid AFP doubling time). Following complete resection of all hepatoma, AFP levels drop, with a half-life of 4 days, and should remain less than 10 ng. per ml. if all tumor has been removed (see Fig. 21–22). Spontaneous normalization of serum AFP level has been reported in some patients with HCC despite the persistence of tumor. This event is unusual but may occur in some patients (24%) with metastatic HCC in whom serum AFP levels are followed. Serum AFP levels also decline with the use of effective chemotherapy. This permits rapid *in vivo* testing of a particular chemotherapeutic regimen. If a given chemotherapy is effective, serum AFP levels fall continuously, indicating tumor regression and effective treatment. If serum AFP levels demonstrate a continued rise despite antitumor treatment, the tumor is resistant to the treatment, and an alternative regimen should be used. Monitoring of serum AFP levels in patients with HCC avoids prolonged ineffective use of potentially toxic chemotherapy.

Serial estimation of serum AFP level in patients with metastatic or recurrent HCC is valuable in monitoring response

TABLE 21–15. Role of Serum Markers in the Management of Patients with Hepatocellular Carcinoma (HCC)

Marker	Screening and Early Diagnosis	% of True-Positives	% of False-Negatives	Following Treatment	Comments
Alpha-fetoprotein (AFP)	Useful if positive, but may have false-negatives	80 (60–90)	20 (10–40)	Correlates with tumor response but may decline falsely	Serum levels vary inversely with prognosis Patients with cirrhosis and active hepatitis may have falsely elevated AFP; levels >500 ng./ml. diagnostic. False-negatives may approach 40%
PIVKA-II	Not useful	65	40	Correlates with tumor response	Elevated in some patients with HCC and normal serum AFP levels
Vitamin B$_{12}$ binding capacity	Not useful	55	50	Does not correlate with tumor response	May be useful only in fibrolamellar variant of HCC
CA 50	Not useful	64	40	No information	Experimental

to therapy (see Table 21–15). However, some patients may have spontaneous regression of serum AFP levels without tumor imaging changes, and others—especially those without underlying cirrhosis—may have normal serum AFP levels despite disease. AFP for HCC, like CEA for colon cancer, remains a good but not an ideal marker.

Other Markers

In patients with fibrolamellar HCC, serum levels of AFP may be normal and serum vitamin B_{12} binding capacity levels may be markedly increased and mirror progressive or regressive disease following treatment. In a study of patients with all types of HCC, 7 of 11 (64%) patients had elevated serum AFP levels, and 6 of 11 (55%) patients had elevated serum B_{12} levels, including elevated levels in 3 patients with normal AFP levels. However, in 4 patients with elevated serum B_{12} levels treated with chemotherapy, levels did not appear to reflect other parameters of disease status (see Table 21–15).

CA 50 is a carbohydrate antigen that is elevated in patients with cholangiocarcinomas, hepatocellular carcinomas, and metastatic carcinomas to the liver. In one recent study, circulating CA 50 levels were elevated in 14 of 22 (64%) patients with HCC. In a prospective comparison with AFP, serum levels of CA 50 antigen were elevated in 6 of 11 patients with HCC (55%), whereas AFP levels were elevated in 9 of the same 11 patients (82%). AFP appears to be a better marker than CA 50 for HCC (see Table 21–15).

Colorectal Cancer

CEA has been studied as a marker of colorectal tumors since the 1960s. Although CEA is not colorectal tumor–specific, the highest concentrations in tissue and serum are found in patients with colorectal carcinoma. Tissue CEA concentrations and presumably CEA production vary in different tumors by up to 800-fold. Even when colorectal tumors have high concentrations of CEA, serum values are not always raised, possibly because of poor access from the tumor to the circulation or rapid clearance.[7]

Early Diagnosis

Serum CEA determinations are not useful in screening normal populations of adults for colorectal cancer (Table 21–16). Elevated CEA levels occur in only 5% of patients with localized, surgically curable colon cancer and in 65% to 90% of patients with either distant or locally advanced disease (see Table 21–13), as well as in some patients with noncancerous conditions produced by cigarette smoking or pulmonary inflammation (see Table 21–12). Therefore, serum CEA levels are only marginally useful in detecting early-stage colon carcinomas, because benign unrelated conditions produce most of the elevated CEA levels detected.[7]

Screening of patients with conditions such as ulcerative colitis and polyposis coli that predispose to colorectal cancer has also been unsuccessful, because these diseases themselves can produce elevated serum levels of CEA. Although benign polyps may slightly elevate serum CEA levels, levels exceeding five times normal are consistent with carcinoma. Measurement of serum CEA levels in a patient who presents with a suspicious polypoid lesion has been recommended by some clinicians, but most prefer colonoscopy and biopsy to obtain a definitive diagnosis.

Prognosis

Several reports have indicated that the preoperative serum CEA concentration before definitive resection of primary co-

TABLE 21–16. Clinical Utility of Serum Carcinoembryonic Antigen (CEA) Levels in Patients with Colorectal Cancer

Question	Answer	Comment
Useful for early diagnosis?	No	Few patients (5%) with localized disease have elevated levels
Useful for prognosis?	Yes	Higher levels have poorer prognosis
Useful to detect recurrence?	Yes	67–79% of patients have elevated serum levels prior to or at the time of recurrence
Can second-look procedures be based on CEA?	Yes	All tumor can be removed in 60–70% of patients, for an overall 5-year survival of 30% Radioimmunolocalization with CEA antibodies possible
Useful to follow treatment response?	Yes	In 90% of patients, serum CEA levels accurately reflect disease progression or regression

lorectal cancer is an independent prognostic parameter of subsequent survival; that is, the higher the serum CEA level, the poorer the prognosis (Fig. 21–23). The prognostic significance of the preoperative serum CEA level was still evident when selected subgroups were stratified for resectability and extent of local tumor involvement. This information should

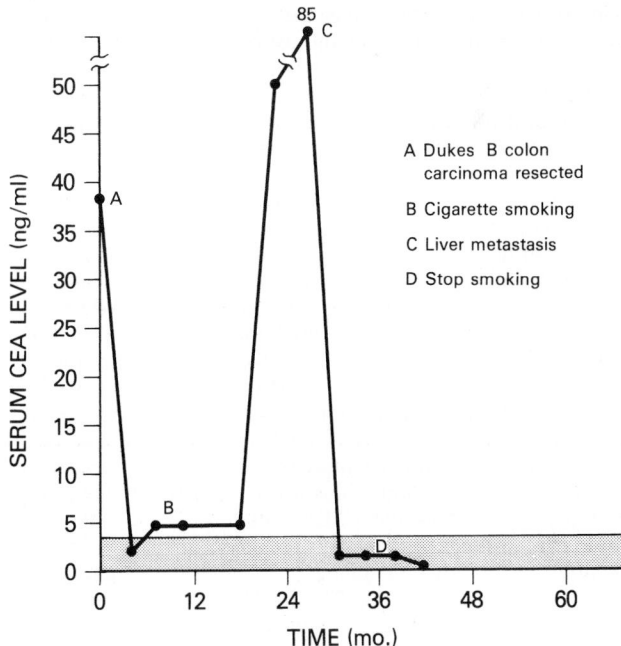

Figure 21–23. Patient who presented with a Dukes B colon carcinoma and an elevated serum level of carcinoembryonic antigen (CEA) (point A). The primary tumor was resected, and postoperative serum CEA levels dropped to the normal range (shaded area). The patient became a cigarette smoker, and levels increased to minimally abnormal levels (point B). Approximately 2 years following his primary resection, the patient developed markedly elevated serum levels of CEA. Computed tomography of the chest and abdomen demonstrated a solitary liver metastasis (point C). This lesion was resected, and the patient quit smoking. Postoperatively, serum CEA levels dropped to the normal range (point D).

be used when stratifying trials of adjuvant therapy after primary tumor resection and when suggesting which individual patients may benefit from adjuvant therapy (see Table 21–16).[7] The preoperative serum level of CEA and hepatic enzymes may also be used to determine whether to initiate imaging studies such as CT to detect liver metastases. If the serum level of CEA and liver function studies are normal, CT scan of the liver is not indicated, because the normal studies have a true negative predictive value of 97%.

Recurrence of Tumor

Surgical re-resection is the only method of treatment offering a significant chance of long-term survival to patients with recurrent colorectal cancer after apparently curative resection of the primary tumor. Elevated serum CEA levels indicate recurrent colorectal cancer usually 4 to 6 months before it is clinically evident. In one study of 171 patients who developed proven or suggested recurrence, 114 (67%) had a prior rise in the serum CEA level, and in another 21 patients (total of 135 patients, or 79%), the serum CEA level rose simultaneously with recurrence (see Table 21–16). The pattern or the magnitude of rising serum CEA levels was of no practical value in distinguishing localized from distant disease. In some studies, some patients have elevated serum CEA levels on a single determination that subsequently return to normal. Elevated serum CEA levels should therefore be verified by repeating the analysis on a second or third occasion. In general, serum CEA levels are elevated in approximately two thirds of patients before any other evidence of recurrent colon or rectal cancer. Serum CEA levels need not have been raised preoperatively to be elevated postoperatively as a marker of tumor recurrence following resection. Recent studies demonstrate that measurement of CEA levels in gallbladder bile may allow earlier detection of liver metastases from colorectal cancer. Each of 17 patients with documented colon cancer and liver metastases had CEA levels in bile greater than 10 ng. per ml., whereas none of 7 patients with morbid obesity had elevated levels. However, false-positive results may occur in patients with cholecystitis, cholangitis, and other hepatic malignancies such as hepatoma.[46] The results may not be clinically useful because a bile level of CEA in nonoperative patients is difficult to obtain.

If serial serum CEA levels rise following resection of primary colorectal carcinoma, the clinician is faced with the problem of how to treat a tumor that is not clinically evident. One study of patients in this category randomized them to chemotherapy with 5-fluorouracil and methyl CCNU versus follow-up and therapy when clinical indications arose. There were no significant differences between the two groups with respect to disease-free interval and overall survival, indicating that CEA-initiated chemotherapy was of no benefit. Because there is no dramatic effective therapy for colorectal carcinoma that cannot be imaged, second-look exploratory operation with resection of recurrent disease has been used by many groups. Results of CEA-initiated second-look procedures vary among different groups, with one group reporting the ability to remove all tumor in 70% of patients and others finding no benefit (see Fig. 21–23). This strategy of reoperation can cure a small percentage of patients (10% to 20%) and can document recurrent colorectal carcinoma in most patients (80%), who can then graduate to other therapies. In Martin and associates' large experience, second-look operation was initiated in approximately 20% of patients with colorectal cancer who were followed postoperatively with serial serum CEA levels; in nearly 60% of these patients, a complete surgical re-resection was possible, and the 5-year survival in this group was over 30%.[27a] Others have performed second-look procedures based on elevated serum CEA levels and found that the actuarial 5-year survival rate was 33% (see Table 21–16). Candidates most likely to benefit from second-look operations are those with isolated liver, pulmonary, and, less frequently, regional recurrences.[12]

Potential improvement in selection of patients and in results for CEA-initiated second-look procedures may be achieved through better preoperative demonstration of the location and extent of disease. A new method is the use of radiolabeled antibody to CEA and external scintigraphy to detect the exact location and extent of recurrent tumor. Patients with localized, resectable recurrent disease can then be selected for second-look operation. In initial reports, this method of radioimmunolocalization appears promising, and labeled monoclonal antibodies to tumor antigens are being developed to potentially image and treat tumors. Systemic preoperative imaging of patients with indium-labeled anti-CEA monoclonal antibody in one study detected 69% of primary tumors and 42% of liver metastases. Another study showed increased sensitivity and ability to accurately image colorectal hepatic metastases; 80% of lesions were imaged when 40 mg. of labeled anti-CEA monoclonal antibody was used. Although these results probably represent the best possible current data for imaging with CEA-directed monoclonal antibodies, these data do not sufficiently establish this technique as standard in the management of patients with colorectal cancer. However, future methodologic improvements are likely to upgrade monoclonal antibody imaging of tumor antigens, making it sensitive, specific, and cost-effective. Radioimmunoguided surgery using a gamma detecting probe has been used to localize surgically nonpalpable tumor deposits at the time of second-look surgery. This feature may improve the ability to detect and remove colorectal tumor during these operations. However, at present, it has been used in only a few centers, and it has not improved outcome or survival.[27]

Following the Response to Treatment

Serum CEA levels appear to correlate fairly well with disease extent in patients with colorectal cancer. Serum levels usually rise with progression and fall with disease regression, but once they are markedly elevated, they do not always correlate directly with tumor burden. Serum CEA levels have been used to follow the response to chemotherapy in patients with metastatic colorectal cancer. In patients with metastatic colorectal carcinoma who had elevated serum CEA levels and responded to chemotherapy, 89% showed a decrease in serum CEA level. In patients who had progressive disease despite chemotherapy, 90% had an increase in serum CEA level compared with pretreatment level (see Table 21–16). The survival of patients with colorectal carcinoma who had a decrease in CEA level during chemotherapy was also significantly longer. In patients with other gastrointestinal cancers, changes in CEA levels do not correlate as well with clinical response.

Other Markers

Recently developed tumor antigens have been used to monitor tumor response in patients with colorectal carcinoma. These newer antigens include TPA, CA 19–9, and CA 125. In cancerous colon tissues, levels of both CEA and CA 19–9 antigens are significantly greater than levels in normal tissues; however, there are no differences in CA 125 levels (which have been useful primarily in epithelial ovarian cancers). Direct comparison of these tumor markers in serum indicates that serum CEA levels are still the most useful clinical marker in patients with colorectal carcinoma. CEA has the greatest sensitivity to predict recurrent disease, and combinations of all markers do not increase sensitivity. Serum CEA level was the best individual predictor of recurrent colorectal cancer (sensitivity 90%) compared with TPA (sensitivity 60%) and CA 19–9 or CA 125 (sensitivity 20%). The specificity of serum CEA determinations was 78%, primarily because other benign and malignant processes (false-positives) can elevate serum CEA levels. The commercial availability of CEA plus its sensitivity makes it the marker of choice to monitor response of disease to therapy in patients with colorectal carcinoma.

Testicular Germ-Cell Neoplasms

Testicular cancers are relatively rare neoplasms, with an incidence of 2.2 per 100,000 population and constituting only 2% of malignant tumors in men.[1] These neoplasms do, however, affect young men in the prime of life, and testicular cancer is the most common cancer killer in men between the ages of 29 and 35.[1] The only known predisposing factor is a history of cryptorchidism, which increases the risk of developing testicular cancer from 10- to 1000-fold.[1] Diagnosis and histologic classification of testicular germ-cell neoplasms have been advanced by the development of sensitive and specific assays to quantitatively measure elevated serum levels of the tumor markers AFP and hCG and immunohistochemical techniques to detect their presence in tissue specimens.

Diagnosis

Seventy-five of 101 patients (75%) with proven nonseminomatous testicular germ-cell tumors had an increased serum AFP level (Table 21–17).[1] Most of these patients (75%) had serum AFP levels greater than 40 ng. per ml. and less than 2000 ng. per ml. Seventy-three of these patients also had elevated serum hCG levels. More recent studies indicate that the incidence of elevated serum levels of β-hCG in patients with nonseminomatous testicular neoplasms is lower, between 40 and 60%. In addition, approximately 10% of patients with pure seminoma also have elevated serum hCG levels.

If both markers are measured, 89% of patients with nonseminomatous testicular cancer have an elevation of one or both serum markers.[1] The determination of both marker levels is very important, since nearly half of these tumors secrete only one substance. In addition to the high rate of marker positivity, there have been very few cases of spuriously elevated serum levels of hCG or AFP in patients with testicular cancer.

The value of preoperative serum hCG or AFP level to guide initial surgical therapy in a patient with a testicular mass lesion is limited. The presence of an elevated serum hCG and/or AFP level before orchiectomy makes the diagnosis of testicular cancer likely. However, most seminomas and nearly one third of other testicular tumors are marker-nega-

tive; therefore, the absence of elevated serum markers does not alter the necessity of performing a biopsy. In addition, patients who are marker-positive and become marker-negative following orchiectomy cannot be presumed to be disease-free, because a small percentage still have positive retroperitoneal lymph nodes at lymphadenectomy. The decision whether to perform lymphadenectomy should not be based solely on marker status, but serum marker status is helpful in following patients after operation, both in detecting persistent or recurrent disease and in following response to therapy.

NSE may be a useful serum marker in patients with seminoma (see Table 21–17). Increased serum NSE activity was detected in 8 of 11 patients (73%) with metastatic seminoma, whereas only 6 of 40 patients (15%) with nonseminomatous testicular cancer had elevated levels. NSE is a new marker for patients with metastatic seminoma, and because it is shed into the bloodstream as tumor cells are lysed, it may be able to monitor response to therapy in these patients.

Prognosis

Since specific tumor markers such as hCG and AFP are secreted by distinct clones of cells, serum tumor marker levels may help identify biologically distinct categories of morphologically similar tumors, and marker levels may reflect tumor virulence. This hypothesis was supported by examining the outcome of patients treated with similar regimens based on pretreatment serum levels of either AFP or hCG. Complete remissions occurred in 92% of patients with normal levels of both hCG and AFP, in 26% of patients with elevated AFP only, in 46% of patients with elevated hCG only, and in 35% of patients (13 of 36) with elevations of both hCG and AFP. Patients with very high serum AFP or hCG levels responded very poorly to chemotherapy. Higher serum marker levels were seen in patients with larger tumor burdens, and the poor prognosis associated with elevated serum marker levels may simply represent extent of disease. Surgical therapy eliminated the correlation between the *poor prognostic factors* associated with specific marker elevations and could convert an incomplete response with chemotherapy alone to a complete response by resection of residual tumor.

When patients are categorized by amount of advanced metastatic testicular cancer, the proportion of favorable responders is greater in patients with normal serum markers (99%) than in patients with markedly elevated serum markers (58%). This finding in a separate group of patients stratified for extent and amount of disease also suggests that level of serum marker has a negative impact on prognosis.[11] Patients with similar tumor burdens and elevated serum hCG or AFP levels appear to do worse than patients with normal serum levels. This observation bears important prognostic information for individual patients and should be considered when clinical trials are designed. Therapeutic options in patients with testicular cancer should be modified based

TABLE 21–17. Serum Markers in the Diagnosis and Management of Testicular Cancer

Tissue Diagnosis	Precentage of Patients with				
	Elevated hCG Level	Elevated AFP Level	Elevated AFP or hCG Level	Neither hCG nor AFP Elevated	Elevated NSE Level
Nonseminomatous testicular cancer	40–60	75	89	10*	15
Seminoma	10	0	10	90	73

*Prognosis is better if neither serum hCG nor AFP is elevated.
hCG, human chorionic gonadotropin; AFP, alpha-fetoprotein; NSE, neuron-specific enolase.

on tumor histology, extent of disease on imaging studies, and presence or absence of serum tumor markers.[33] Studies have concluded that elevated serum levels of AFP predict a poor prognosis, especially when levels are greater than 500 ng. per ml. An elevated serum level of hCG predicts an even poorer prognosis. Individuals with hCG levels greater than 1000 ng. per ml. have a poor prognosis, and individuals with levels greater than 10,000 ng. per ml. have an extremely poor prognosis.[3]

Recurrence of Tumor and Following the Response to Treatment

The serial measurement of serum AFP and hCG levels by RIA appears to be useful in monitoring the effectiveness of therapy in patients with nonseminomatous germ-cell tumors. A small percentage of patients with metastatic testicular cancer have no response to chemotherapy, and the serum AFP and hCG levels progressively rise until death. In a larger percentage of patients, AFP and hCG serum levels drop into the normal range and remain there throughout the period of observation. These patients also have no tumor on imaging studies, and hCG and AFP serum levels accurately predict no tumor recurrence. In a small group of patients (6%), tumor masses do not regress during chemotherapy, but serum AFP and hCG levels decline to normal. Subsequent surgical resection of persistent mass lesions demonstrates tumor conversion to mature teratoma. The most interesting group is patients with no radiologic evidence of disease who have elevated serum levels of hCG or AFP. In one study, 28 of 34 patients had elevated serum marker levels following induction chemotherapy, and no patient had any radiographic evidence of persistent disease. Each patient had clinically documented recurrent testicular cancer within a 2- to 14-month period of observation.[1] Although false-negative hCG or AFP estimations of testicular cancer occur between 10 and 15% of the time, false-positive levels in patients followed with testicular cancer have not been noted. Approximately 22% to 35% of patients who develop recurrent disease while on surveillance have increased serum marker levels before radiographic recurrence. Once the elevated serum marker has been confirmed (false-positive result excluded), treatment should be instituted.[3] These studies indicate that serum levels of hCG and AFP are of great value in following the treatment of patients with testicular germ-cell neoplasms, especially patients without other evidence of disease. Newer urinary immunoassays for β-hCG may further enhance the utility of this marker and its use in different cancerous diseases.

Other Markers

The other markers for nonseminomatous testicular germ-cell neoplasms do not compare with hCG and AFP for sensitivity and specificity. In patients with known testicular cancer, 19 of 23 had elevated serum levels of hCG, AFP, or both, whereas only 6 of 20 had elevated serum neopterin levels.

In patients with pure seminomas of the testis, measurement of serum hCG and AFP levels is not helpful. However, approximately 10% of patients with seminoma have elevated serum levels of either hCG or AFP. If levels of these peptides are elevated, it indicates that the testicular tumor is not a pure seminoma. Serum NSE activity is abnormal in 73% of patients with metastatic seminoma, and levels return to normal following successful therapy. Only 15% of patients with metastatic nonseminomatous germ-cell neoplasms of the testis have elevated serum levels of NSE activity. Serum NSE activity is a new marker for patients with seminoma, and levels appear to accurately reflect response to therapy.

Epithelial Ovarian Cancer

Epithelial ovarian carcinomas are among the malignant diseases that respond to treatment with cytoreductive surgical therapy, radiotherapy, and cytotoxic chemotherapy. Monitoring the response to treatment has been difficult because these neoplasms often metastasize to peritoneal surfaces and form small metastatic nodules that cannot be detected by imaging studies. Medical oncologists have demanded restaging laparotomies that may be hazardous in the presence of tumor and multiple adhesions from prior surgical procedures. A glycoprotein antigen, CA 125, is associated with epithelial ovarian cancer and has been detected in the serum of patients with these neoplasms.

Early Diagnosis

Elevated serum CA 125 levels (>35 units per ml.) were detected in 50% to 96% of patients with nonmucinous epithelial ovarian carcinoma confined to the pelvis (Table 21–18). A patient has recently been identified in whom serum CA 125 levels were elevated 12 months before the clinical diagnosis of Stage II ovarian cancer. At diagnosis, 61% of patients with Stage I or II disease have serum levels greater than 35 units per ml., and 50% have levels greater than 50 units per ml.[4] This finding suggests that measurement of CA 125 in the serum may be useful in the diagnosis of an ovarian mass lesion detected by physical examination or pelvic ultrasound. Most studies demonstrate a sensitivity of 75% and a specificity of near 90% when serum levels of CA 125 are used to diagnose ovarian masses.[22] Elevated serum levels of CA 125 at the time of diagnosis of ovarian cancer portends a poor prognosis.[22] However, determination of CA 125 levels in the serum of patients with ovarian masses is not diagnostic for ovarian cancer.[2]

Ninety-nine per cent of normal subjects have serum levels of CA 125 less than 35 units per ml. Eighty-three per cent of patients with surgically proven ovarian cancer have elevated serum levels (see Table 21–18). Elevations have also been found in the serum of patients with carcinomas of the endometrium, endocervix, fallopian tube, pancreas, stomach, liver, bile duct, lung, breast, and colon. Elevations of serum CA 125 levels also have been found in benign conditions, including pregnancy, menstruation, endometriosis, pelvic inflammatory disease, pancreatitis, hepatitis, and renal failure (see Table 21–12).

Following the Response to Treatment and Monitoring Recurrent Disease

Approximately 25 studies from different cancer centers have reported the use of serum CA 125 levels to monitor the response of ovarian cancer to treatment and to detect recurrent disease following conclusion of treatment. The newer studies have confirmed the original report[5] that serum CA 125 levels are elevated in approximately 80% to 85% of patients with ovarian cancer. If abnormal, serum CA 125 levels have correlated with disease progression or regression in 80% to 95% of cases. New elevations of serum CA 125 levels have preceded clinical detection of recurrent ovarian cancer by a median time of 3 months. Elevation of serum CA 125 levels at the time of second-look procedures for ovarian cancer predicts that disease is present approximately 90% of the time. However, CA 125 levels may return to normal and second-look operation may still document the presence of residual disease in some cases. This finding of a high false-negative rate indicates that one cannot withdraw chemotherapy based on normalization of serum CA 125 level, because over half of these patients still have persistent disease at

TABLE 21–18. Other Serum Markers That Are Useful for the Diagnosis and Management of Cancer

Type of Malignancy	Marker	Percentage of Patients with Elevated Serum Levels	Comments
Ovarian cancer	CA 125	80–85	Changing levels correlate with tumor response; normalization of elevated levels does not allow discontinuation of therapy; 40% of patients with Stage I disease have normal serum levels
Granulosa-cell tumors of the ovary	Inhibin	100	Granulosa-cell tumors produce inhibin; serum levels reflect tumor size; useful as marker for primary as well as recurrent disease
Pancreatic cancer	CA 19–9	82–96	Able to distinguish benign from malignant disease of the pancreas and biliary tree with 78% sensitivity and 75% specificity
Breast cancer	CA 15–3	73	Correlates with extent of disease; not specific for breast cancer; cannot distinguish whether localized breast disease is benign or malignant

laparotomy.[22] However, if serum levels of CA 125 remain elevated during chemotherapy, there is a 90% chance that the patient has persistent disease, so additional therapy can be given without laparotomy.

CA 125 levels in peritoneal fluid washings may be more sensitive than serum levels, and results may remain elevated with smaller amounts of residual disease. Therefore, if serum levels become normal during treatment, peritoneal fluid levels may be able to distinguish the patients with persistent disease from those who are truly without disease. Peritoneal fluid levels in normal patients were less than 200 units per ml., whereas most patients with ovarian cancer have levels greater than 200 units per ml.

Another potential utility of CA 125 levels is the antigen's rate of decline in the serum of patients with treated ovarian cancer. If all tumor is removed, serum CA 125 levels decline, with a half-life of 4.5 days. In patients with elevated serum levels of CA 125, levels should decline to less than 35 units per ml. within 3 months of the initiation of treatment. Of patients whose serum CA 125 levels failed to drop below 35 units per ml. after 3 months of treatment or remained persistently elevated despite treatment, nearly all had documented disease at laparotomy.

Other Markers

CEA, hCG, and TPA have also been used to predict the extent or presence of disease in patients with epithelial ovarian cancer. Serum levels of neither CEA nor hCG have any usefulness as tumor markers in ovarian carcinoma. However, the utility of TPA and serum levels of CA 125 in monitoring ovarian cancer is confirmed. In one study, 86% of patients with active ovarian cancer had an elevation of serum CA 125 levels, and 76% of patients had an elevation of TPA levels. Moreover, for patients in clinical remission, the simultaneous measurement of TPA and CA 125 antigen in the serum revealed recurrent disease in more patients than either antigen alone, although CA 125 was the better marker.

Investigators have shown that a small population of subjects with nontrophoblastic gynecologic cancers have elevated serum levels of hCG, but only about 18% of women with epithelial ovarian cancer have elevated levels. A recent study measuring urinary hCG fragments and subfragments in patients with gynecologic malignancies demonstrated that 73% of patients with ovarian cancer had elevated levels of urinary gonadotropin fragments (UGF). By stage, 50, 62, 75, 86, and 100% of those patients with Stage I, II, III, IV, or recurrent disease, respectively, had elevated levels. The study suggests that UGF may be a promising new marker of ovarian and other gynecologic cancers.

With the technology of monoclonal antibodies directed toward cancer antigens, two specific new antigens, TAG 72.3 and CA 15–3, have been developed that may add to the efficacy of CA 125 alone as a tumor marker. In two independent studies of serum from patients with pelvic masses, determination of CA 125, TAG 72.3, and CA 15–3 in combination was more sensitive than the determination of CA 125 alone.[41] Simultaneous measurements of multiple antigens in cancer patients may improve results, compared with measurements of individual antigens alone. However, these results are preliminary, and, at present, CA 125 remains the marker of choice for epithelial ovarian cancer.

Granulosa-Cell Tumors of the Ovary

Inhibin is a peptide hormone that is normally produced by ovarian granulosa cells. It can be detected at peak levels in the serum of women during the follicular phase of the menstrual cycle, and it is undetectable in the serum of postmenopausal women. Peak serum levels in normal menstruating women are 770 units per liter. In patients with recurrent or persistent granulosa-cell tumor of the ovary, levels can exceed 3000 units per liter (see Table 21–12). It can become elevated in the serum before there are other clinical signs of detectable disease. After the tumor is removed, serum inhibin levels become normal. Levels of inhibin are more sensitive for detection of disease than are levels of estradiol, the other proposed hormonal marker for these tumors. Serum inhibin levels accurately reflect the amount of tumor and can be used as a circulating marker for primary as well as recurrent disease.

Gestational Trophoblastic Neoplasia and Germ-Cell Ovarian Cancer

With the rare exception of germ-cell tumors, hCG is generally produced by benign or cancerous trophoblastic cells. If pregnancy can be excluded, hCG is a specific and sensitive serum marker for trophoblastic tumors in women. Immunologic assays for hCG are very sensitive for the early detection of trophoblastic tumors. Only 10,000 tumor cells are required to produce a detectable level of hCG in serum.

Normalization of serum hCG levels has been used to confirm complete evacuation of benign gestational trophoblastic tumors, including molar pregnancy. An increase or abnormal elevation of serum hCG levels following evacuation of an apparently benign tumor, an abortion, or a termination of a normal pregnancy can indicate the presence of a malignant trophoblastic tumor. Absolute serum levels of hCG distinguish gestational cancers with good prognosis (<40,000 mIU.

per ml.) from those with poor prognosis (>40,000 mIU. per ml.). Serum inhibin levels have also been suggested as a useful marker for hydatidiform mole. Serum inhibin levels are generally much higher in women with hydatidiform moles than in women with normal pregnancies.

hCG is an excellent serum marker for the diagnosis and detection of germ-cell ovarian cancers, including choriocarcinomas and embryonal carcinomas. Sensitivity is approximately 50% for these tumors, and specificity nearly 100%. Serum AFP levels may be elevated in ovarian embryonal carcinomas but are not elevated in pure ovarian choriocarcinomas. Both serum AFP and hCG levels should be measured to document presence of tumor, to follow response to therapy, and to detect recurrence.

Following the Response to Treatment

With effective treatment of malignant gestational trophoblastic cancer, the serum half-life of hCG is 36 hours, and the levels should decrease by 20% to 25% following each treatment cycle. Any plateau or increase in serum hCG level demands alternative therapy. Three consecutive serum hCG levels less than 5 mIU. per ml. are diagnostic of complete remission. These levels should be obtained every month for 3 months before determining that complete remission has been achieved. The utility of hCG in the treatment of malignant gestational trophoblastic cancers is amplified because of the sensitivity of these tumors to aggressive chemotherapy. Recurrent elevations or plateau levels of serum hCG levels have prompted changes in chemotherapeutic agents. The availability of a sensitive, specific marker as well as effective chemotherapy has provided an 80% to 100% cure rate for patients with a previously uniformly fatal cancer.

Pancreatic Cancer

The incidence of pancreatic carcinoma is rising in the United States, with an estimated 20,000 new cases each year. Early diagnosis of pancreatic cancer has been a major problem. Imaging studies such as CT or endoscopic retrograde cholangiopancreatography have not improved detection of the disease. A specific blood marker may lead to earlier initiation of potentially curative treatment.

CA 19–9 is a circulating marker that has sensitivity and specificity for pancreatic carcinoma. Initial work indicated that CA 19–9 was undetectable in the serum of normal subjects and patients with extragastrointestinal tumors or nonmalignant diseases. Patients with colorectal, stomach, and pancreatic cancer may have high levels of CA 19–9 in the serum. Subsequently, studies have indicated that the marker has its greatest utility in the diagnosis and management of patients with pancreatic cancer (see Table 21–12).

Diagnosis

Eighty-two per cent of patients with pancreatic cancer have elevated serum levels of CA 19–9, whereas few patients with pancreatitis, gallstones, or sclerosing cholangitis have elevated levels.[20] The upper limit of normal is 37 units per ml. In addition, 89% of patients with carcinoma of the gallbladder and 100% of patients with carcinoma of the bile duct have elevated serum levels.[20] Another group demonstrated that serum levels of CA 19–9 were abnormally elevated in 5 of 121 patients with chronic pancreatitis (4%), 7 of 30 patients with acute pancreatitis (23%), and 82 of 99 patients with pancreatic cancer (85%). Measurement of the antigen in serum appears to reliably differentiate benign from malignant diseases of the pancreas and biliary tree (see Table 21–18).

In a direct comparison among CA 19–9, CA 125, and CEA as tumor markers for pancreatic cancer, CA 19–9 had the greatest sensitivity (78%), compared with approximately 50% for CA 125 and CEA. Each had comparable specificity of 78%. The addition of multiple tests (CA 19–9 and CA 125) increased the sensitivity by only 6%. This and other comparisons[20] show that the serum CA 19–9 level is currently the best marker for pancreatic cancer. Absolute serum levels of CA 19–9 may predict unresectability of pancreatic cancer. Levels greater than 1000 units per ml. have been associated with unresectability of disease in 96% of patients. Furthermore, in postoperative resected patients, serial measurement of CA 19–9 levels predict the development of tumor recurrence in most patients before detection of disease by radiographic or clinical findings.[43]

However, serum CA 19–9 levels may be elevated in patients with other cancers, including colorectal (15%), stomach (5%), bile duct (95%), hepatoma (7%), lung (13%), and ovary (2%). In addition, it may be elevated in some patients with benign gastrointestinal diseases, including pancreatitis (5%), hepatitis (1%), and cirrhosis (3%). Occurrence of these potential false-positive results explains why the specificity of this marker is 75% for the diagnosis of pancreatic cancer.

Following the Response to Treatment

Levels of the serum marker CA 19–9 in patients with pancreatic cancer appear to correlate with amount of disease and therefore can be used to follow the response to treatment. In one series, four patients with known resected pancreatic cancer who were being followed without clinical evidence of disease had serum levels less than 17 units per liter. Most patients with disease localized to the pancreas and without metastases had levels that were elevated (>120 units per liter) but were not as elevated as those with documented metastatic disease.[20] Because there is no effective treatment for pancreatic carcinoma, evaluation of the serum marker's ability to reflect response to treatment is impossible. Although it appears that serum CA 19–9 levels reflect extent of disease, better testing must await effective treatment modalities.

Monoclonal antibodies to the carbohydrate antigen CA 19–9 have been used to treat patients with pancreatic cancer. Preliminary results indicate minimal efficacy, and this method of treatment has been abandoned.

Other Markers

CEA has been measured in patients with pancreatic cancer, but it is not a useful marker because it is elevated in only 45% to 65% of patients with known cancer.[20] However, another recently identified carbohydrate antigen, CA 50, shows promise as a serum marker in patients with pancreatic cancer. If the upper limit of normal for the serum CA 50 level is defined as not exceeding 100 units per liter, 81% of patients with known pancreatic cancer have elevated levels, and similar percentages of patients with biliary cancers have elevated serum levels. In addition, like CA 19–9, serum levels of CA 50 discriminate benign from malignant diseases of the pancreas and biliary tree, because patients with pancreatitis, gallstones, and/or sclerosing cholangitis have normal serum levels of CA 50.[20] Serum CA 50 levels show results similar to those of serum CA 19–9 levels in the diagnosis of pancreatic and biliary cancers. Both markers are still under investigation, but more studies with CA 19–9 have already been performed. Studies demonstrate that CA 50 and CA 19–9 are comparable.[20] CA 242 is another new marker for pancreatic cancer with promising preliminary results.

Breast Cancer

Breast cancer is the second leading cause of death from cancer in women, ranking only below carcinoma of the lung. Each year, approximately 120,000 newly diagnosed cases of breast cancer occur in the United States, and nearly a third will be fatal. One in nine women in this country develops breast cancer. The mainstay of early diagnosis of breast cancer is self- or physician examination and mammography. Serum markers are being developed, but their current clinical utility is limited.

CEA and Gross Cystic Disease Fluid Protein

CEA serum levels are normal in 98% of patients with localized breast cancer and in 60% of patients with metastatic breast cancer. When serum levels are elevated and continue to rise on subsequent determination, nearly all patients (98%) with breast cancer have metastatic disease. Serum CEA levels are elevated in only 20% of patients with primary breast cancer, and the CEA-positive patients appear to have a significantly poorer prognosis. Serum levels of CEA and another marker, gross cystic disease fluid protein (CDP), can reflect increasing or decreasing tumor burden during therapy of metastic breast cancer. Serum levels of CDP in patients with metastatic breast cancer are elevated in only 40% of patients. Neither serum CEA nor CDP levels are clinically useful markers for breast cancer. Neither can help with the early diagnosis of a breast mass. Because of widespread availability, CEA levels may be helpful in following treatment response in patients with metastatic breast carcinoma who have elevated serum levels.

CA 15–3

CA 15–3 is a circulating antigen expressed by human breast carcinoma cells (see Table 21–18). Recent studies have determined the percentage of breast cancer patients with elevated serum levels of the antigen CA 15–3. Of 1050 normal subjects, serum from 99 (9%) had CA 15–3 antigen levels greater than 22 units per ml. In contrast, 115 of 158 patients (73%) with metastatic breast cancer had levels greater than 22 units per ml. Fifty per cent of patients with nodal metastases, 79% of patients with bone metastases, and 83% of patients with liver metastases had elevated serum levels of the antigen, so a greater percentage of patients with more advanced disease had elevated levels. Significantly, more patients in this population with breast cancer had elevated serum levels of CA 15–3 than of CEA. However, serum levels of CA 15–3 were elevated in some patients (20%) with benign breast lesions and in some patients with other cancers, including 4% of patients with gastrointestinal cancer, 71% with lung cancer, and 66% with epithelial ovarian cancer. Serum levels appear to correlate with and reflect either tumor progression or regression. These results indicate that although it is nonspecific, CA 15–3 may have potential as a serum marker for diagnosing and evaluating treatment response in patients with metastatic breast carcinoma.

Another study using a greater serum level of CA 15–3 (40 units per ml.) to define the normal range had fewer false-positive results (0% for control subjects, 1.5% for patients with benign breast disease, and 6.5% for those with other cancers) but, as expected, detected elevated circulating levels of the marker in fewer patients with localized disease (6% of patients with Stage II disease) and all of 22 patients with Stage IV breast carcinoma. Following therapy, serum CA 15–3 levels were significantly different in patients without evidence of disease, patients with stable disease, and patients with progressive disease. However, in some individual patients, serum antigen levels did not appear to follow clinical response, since 20 of 34 patients with objective responses had abnormally elevated serum levels, including patients with a complete response. The results indicate that CA 15–3 serum levels correlate with the stage of breast cancer and the response to therapy, but results in individual patients may differ from this general observation.

Finally, a third study corroborates the other two. CA 15–3 was not useful for early diagnosis, because only 16% of patients with Stage I breast cancer had elevated serum levels (>25 units per ml.). As the disease progressed, more and more patients had elevated serum levels of CA 15–3: 54% with Stage II disease, and 91% with Stage III and IV disease. In addition, 70 of 100 women with metastatic breast cancer and normal serum levels of CEA had elevated serum levels of CA 15–3. Serum levels of CA 15–3 have been shown to be useful in predicting relapse in patients with breast cancer following primary therapy. For this indication, numerous studies have shown a sensitivity between 45 and 77% and a specificity between 94 and 98%. There are few false-positives. The serum levels have been elevated from 1 to 18 months before the detection of recurrent disease by imaging studies or physical examination.[21]

CA 15–3 appears to be a promising recent advance for the management of patients with breast cancer. Most patients with metastatic breast carcinoma have elevated serum levels, and in most patients, serum levels accurately reflect response to therapy. However, it is not useful for the early diagnosis of breast cancer, because few patients with localized breast cancer have elevated serum levels, and some patients with benign breast disease have elevated levels. Finally, in some patients, despite documented metastatic breast carcinoma, serum levels of CA 15–3 are normal, and in some patients, serum levels do not accurately reflect disease response (or lack of it) to therapy.

C-erb B-2

The *c-erb B-2* gene encodes a protein with properties very similar to the epidermal growth factor receptor (EGFR). Both are membrane-bound proteins possessing protein kinase activity. Amplification of the *erb B-2* oncogene is found in approximately 20% to 30% of primary breast cancers. Amplification of this oncogene has been shown to be of poor prognostic significance. Slamon and colleagues demonstrated that *erb B-2* amplification has prognostic value equal to positive axillary lymph nodes in node-negative patients and is a stronger prognostic marker than progesterone receptor status, tumor size, and estrogen receptor status for both disease-free and overall survival.[38] However, measurement of gene amplification is relatively demanding and may not be suitable for routine clinical laboratories.

Lung Cancer

Non-Small-Cell Lung Cancer

Currently, there are no clinically useful circulating markers for the management of patients with bronchogenic carcinoma. In an older study of 100 patients with biopsy-proven NSCLC, serum markers including CEA, TPA, CA 19–9, and combinations had less than 56% sensitivity for the diagnosis. In addition, no marker had a diagnostic accuracy of 50%.[13] However, as mentioned previously, the recently defined tumor marker CYFRA 21–1 is elevated in between 41 and 48% of patients with NSCLC.[28, 32] Studies have demonstrated its superiority to other available markers. Because its sensitivity is low (<50%), it may not be a clinically useful marker. Future studies will need to determine its exact utility.

Mutations in the dominant oncogene *Ki-ras* are present in approximately a third of lung adenocarcinomas, mainly in smokers, and are associated with a poor prognosis for this group.[39] Detection of this oncogene product in the serum of patients at risk for the development of lung cancer may be useful as a screening strategy. A recent study following 46 patients with exposure to asbestos and silicosis showed that 7 of 11 patients (64%) who developed mesothelioma had elevated serum levels of the *ras* oncogene product. Six had detectable levels in serum prior to any evidence of disease. Future studies will be necessary to further substantiate these exciting findings.[44]

Small-Cell Lung Cancer

Among the various histologic types of lung cancer, small-cell lung cancer (SCLC) has a number of unique characteristics. It is a very malignant tumor that proliferates rapidly, with a clear tendency for early metastatic spread. Recent advances in chemotherapy and radiation therapy of SCLC have improved the outlook of patients with this tumor, and dramatic responses have been documented during therapy. However, durable complete remissions are rare. Early diagnosis of persistent or recurrent disease is desirable to either alter or intensify therapeutic regimens. The need for reliable, sensitive serum markers for SCLC is apparent, since they may be able to guide therapeutic decisions.

Neuron-Specific Enolase

Serum levels of NSE, a glycolytic enzyme produced by neuroendocrine cells of the peripheral and central nervous system (CNS), may be elevated in newly diagnosed patients with SCLC. In the original report, 15 of 38 patients (39%) with limited disease and 49 of 56 patients (87%) with extensive disease had elevated serum levels of NSE. Overall, 69% of all patients with proven SCLC had elevated serum levels of NSE, and serial measurements in 23 patients receiving combination chemotherapy demonstrated an excellent correlation between serum NSE levels and clinical response. Cell lines established from 10 of the patients in the study each expressed high levels of NSE. Additional studies indicate that between 80 and 98% of patients with extensive SCLC have elevated serum levels of NSE, and approximately 55% of patients with limited disease have elevated levels. In addition, elevated levels of NSE in the cerebrospinal fluid (CSF) appear to indicate either parenchymal CNS metastases or meningeal carcinomatosis. CSF levels of NSE were elevated in 54% of patients with brain parenchymal SCLC and 95% of patients with meningeal carcinomatosis. The only other CSF marker with comparable percentages was adrenocorticotropic hormone (ACTH), which was elevated in 85% of patients with CNS metastases in one study. Because as many as 50% of patients with SCLC present with CNS disease, CSF levels of markers may be helpful in documenting CNS disease.

At present, serum NSE levels appear to be the best serum marker for patients with SCLC. In comparison studies, it has the greatest sensitivity and specificity. It is elevated in nearly all patients with progressive, metastatic SCLC, and it appears to correlate well with response to therapy. However, its ability to establish with certainty the absence of residual disease is poor; in some studies, 50% to 70% of patients with minimal disease have normal serum NSE levels. Therefore, one cannot withdraw therapy based on a normal serum NSE level, but progressive serial elevation of serum NSE levels is fairly reliable evidence of poor response to treatment and the need to alter therapy.

TABLE 21–19. Serum Markers and Hormones in Patients with Known Small-Cell Lung Cancer

Marker or Hormone	Percentage of Patients with Elevated Serum Levels
NSE	67
Calcitonin	59
ACTH	27
ADH	65
Oxytocin	30
Gastrin	20
MSH	19
PTH	31
Insulin	5
Glucagon	11
Secretin	0
Growth hormone	9
VIP	0
Bombesin	7
CEA	44
TPA	55
Ferritin	52
AGP	90
LDH	59
CYFRA 21–2	16

NSE, neuro-specific enolase; ACTH, adrenocorticotropic hormone; ADH, antidiuretic hormone; MSH, melanocyte-stimulating hormone; PTH, parathyroid hormone; VIP, vasoactive intestinal polypeptide; CEA, carcinoembryonic antigen; TPA, tissue polypeptide antigen; AGP, alpha-acid glycoprotein; LDH, lactate dehydrogenase.

Other Markers

Many different hormonal peptides have been measured in the serum of patients with SCLC. The most common hormone markers in these patients include calcitonin, ACTH, antidiuretic hormone (ADH), melanocyte-stimulating hormone (MSH), oxytocin, parathyroid hormone–related protein (PTH-RP), insulin, gastrin, glucagon, secretin, vasoactive intestinal peptide (VIP), growth hormone, and bombesin. The percentage of patients with SCLC in whom serum levels of an individual hormone or marker were elevated is shown in Table 21–19. Serum calcitonin levels appear to be elevated in a significant percentage (59%) of patients with SCLC. Calcitonin levels in these patients do not increase with provocative agents such as pentagastrin or calcium. Inappropriate ADH levels have been associated clinically with lung cancer, and 65% of patients with SCLC have elevated serum levels of ADH. Serum ACTH levels are important in these patients, because some patients present with Cushing's syndrome. These lung tumors are the most common source of ectopic ACTH syndrome, and 27% of patients with SCLC have elevated serum ACTH levels. In addition, it should be recognized that most RIAs for ACTH will cross-react with MSH and vice versa, and some patients with elevated MSH levels (19% of patients with SCLC) may really have elevated ACTH levels. Finally, it is clear that because of the neuroendocrine origin of these tumors, they might secrete any hormone and potentially cause significant symptoms, but if the hormone is recognized, it can also produce a useful serum marker for a specific patient.

Other serum markers in patients with SCLC include alpha-acid glycoprotein (AGP), CEA, CYFRA 21–1, and lactate dehydrogenase (LDH). These markers are not specific and therefore have not been used to establish the diagnosis of SCLC. They may indicate the presence of disease and have been used to follow treatment response. Of these serum markers, AGP is the best. It was elevated in 54 of 60 patients (90%) with disease, whereas CEA and LDH were elevated in

TABLE 21–20. Serum and Urinary Markers for Diagnosis and Follow-up of Patients with Endocrine Neoplasms

Organ	Disease	Marker	Body Fluid	Special Test (Stimulation or Suppression)	Result	Diagnosis	Follow-up
Thyroid	Well-differentiated thyroid cancer	Thyroglobulin	Serum	None	Elevated levels indicate disease	Nonspecific, but used to diagnose malignancy in patients with radiation exposure	Useful for follow-up of patients following thyroidectomy or radioactive iodine ablation
	Medullary carcinoma*†	Calcitonin	Serum	Pentagastrin/ calcium test	Calcitonin levels increase	Sensitive, specific stimulation test	Sensitive, specific follow-up marker reflects tumor burden; RET oncogene better in MEN† syndromes
Parathyroid	Hyperpara-thyroidism	Calcium, PTH, cAMP	Serum and urine	None	Elevated calcium and PTH levels and elevated UcAMP level	Sensitive, specific	Carcinoma is rare, but PTH and UcAMP are sensitive markers of persistent or recurrent disease
Adrenal cortex‡	Adrenal cancer	Cortisol	Serum and urine	Dexamethasone suppression, CRH stimulation	No change in cortisol levels	Sensitive but not specific for cancer, must rule out other causes of Cushing's syndrome	Urinary 17 OHCS and free cortisol usually reflect disease, but some tumors dedifferentiate
Adrenal medulla	Pheochro-mocytoma*†	Norepinephrine, epinephrine, catecholamines, VMA, metanephrine	Serum and urine	Clonidine suppression	No change in serum epinephrine or norepinephrine with clonidine	Specific, sensitive	May be malignant; careful follow-up urinary catecholamines important
Pancreatic islet cell	Gastrinoma*§ (ZES)	Gastrin	Serum, stomach acid	Secretin test	Increased gastrin level; elevated acid output	Specific	Useful but may not accurately reflect tumor volume
	Insulinoma*§	Insulin	Serum	Fast	Insulin levels still elevated with hypoglycemia	Sensitive	Most benign; only 5% malignant
						Sensitive, specific	
	Glucagonoma*§	Glucagon	Serum	None	Elevated glucagon levels	Specific	Malignant
	VIPoma*§	VIP	Serum	None	Elevated VIP levels	Specific	Malignant
Pancreas, testis, ovary, bronchus, gastro-intestinal tract	Carcinoid*†§	Serotonin 5-HIAA	Urine	None	Elevated levels	73% sensitivity, 100% specificity	Levels reflect tumor mass

*Neuron-specific enolase is produced by nearly all neuroendocrine tumors and can be used as a serum marker.
†L-dopa decarboxylase and/or chromogranin A have been measured in tissue extracts of these tumors and may be useful as a circulating marker, although studies are currently ongoing and not completed.
‡Adrenal cortex carcinomas may secrete androgens or aldosterone, which, if elevated, serve as marker substances.
§Pancreatic polypeptide may be used as a serum marker in patients with pancreatic islet cell tumors, but its sensitivity is only 45%.
MEN, multiple endocrine neoplasia; PTH, parathyroid hormone; cAMP, cyclic adenosine monophosphate; CRH, corticotropin-releasing hormone; OHCS, hydroxy-corticosteroids; VMA, vanillylmandelic acid; ZES, Zollinger-Ellison syndrome; VIP, vasoactive intestinal polypeptide; HIAA, hydroxyindoleacetic acid.

only 52 and 59% of patients, respectively.[17] CYFRA 21–1 was elevated in only 16% of patients with SCLC. In addition, the pair of serum markers (AGP and LDH) has been used to correctly classify 37 patients in whom both serum measurements were obtained, including 4 patients who were incorrectly classified with AGP alone. Each of the markers correctly tracked the clinical response to therapy in two thirds of patients in whom an individual marker was elevated at diagnosis.[17]

Detection of CNS Involvement

With an increase in the median survival of patients with SCLC, there is an increase in the frequency of CNS metastases. Despite careful neurologic evaluation, cytologic and biochemical evaluation of CSF, and careful CT or MRI of the brain and spinal cord, 20% to 50% of parenchymal and meningeal metastases are not diagnosed until death and au-

topsy. More than 20% of 2-year survivors with SCLC develop meningeal carcinomatosis that is difficult to diagnose, because 50% of patients with this disease have negative CSF cytologic findings for cancer cells.

As previously mentioned, CSF levels of NSE is one proven method to document CNS involvement with SCLC, since 71% of individuals have elevated CSF levels. CSF levels of bombesin and calcitonin may also be helpful. CSF bombesin levels were detectable in 7% of SCLC patients without CNS involvement, 21% of patients with parenchymal involvement, and 78% of patients with meningeal carcinomatosis. In addition, 53% of patients with meningeal carcinomatosis and 48% with parenchymal SCLC had CSF calcitonin levels greater than 18 fmol. per ml., whereas only 7% without CNS disease had these levels. Sixty-seven per cent of all patients with CNS involvement by SCLC had elevated CSF levels of either bombesin or calcitonin. Thus, in SCLC patients, an elevated CSF level of calcitonin or NSE suggests CNS metastases, and an elevated bombesin level suggests meningeal carcinomatosis.

Endocrine Neoplasms

In general, endocrine neoplasms secrete hormones that serve as serum markers of the tumor. The hormones secreted are measured in the serum or urine by RIA, and elevated levels are diagnostic of specific tumors. A complete list of endocrine neoplasms and their marker serum hormones is given in Table 21–20. If an individual tumor is malignant and recurs or progresses, serum or urinary hormone levels reflect tumor burden and increase as tumor mass increases and decrease as tumor mass decreases. It is beyond the scope of this chapter to consider all endocrine tumors; rather, the reader is referred to Table 21–20 and other chapters for specific serum or urinary markers.

Chromogranin A is a 49-kd. protein that occurs in the secretory granules of most neuroendocrine cells. Detection of the protein in tumors and serum may serve as a marker for neuroendocrine tumors by immunoassay. Measurement of chromogranin A levels in tumor and/or serum may be useful in patients with any endocrine or neuroendocrine tumor that does not appear to produce any other functional hormone or peptide. Although the exact biologic function of chromogranin A is unknown, it appears to be a precursor molecule for a family of biologically active peptides. Levels of chromogranin A may be a new tool in managing patients with neuroendocrine tumors.[15]

SUMMARY

Serum markers have changed the diagnosis and management of patients with testicular, hepatocellular, trophoblastic, colonic, and endocrine neoplasms. New serum markers may have similar effects on patients with ovarian, pancreatic, breast, small-cell lung, and biliary cancer. Recent advances in technology may provide additional malignant tumor markers in the immediate future. This work updates the current status of available serum markers and provides the reader with the necessary background information to make decisions based on the results of individual markers in individual diseases and individual patients.

Acknowledgments

We would like to acknowledge the assistance of Dr. Michael Kahn and Dr. Mark Frisse, who reviewed the manuscript and contributed their expertise in the field of medical informatics.

SELECTED REFERENCES

Anderson, T., Waldmann, T. A., Javadpour, N., and Glatstein, E.: Testicular germ-cell neoplasms: Recent advances in diagnosis and therapy. Ann. Intern. Med., 90:373, 1979.

Although 17 years old, this paper describes the use of serum levels of alpha-fetoprotein (AFP) and human chorionic gonadotropin (hCG) in the management of patients with testicular germ-cell neoplasms. The authors have extensive experience in the management of these patients, and they describe the use of these serum markers to make treatment decisions. Serum levels of hCG and/or AFP are elevated in 5% to 90% of patients with nonseminomatous testicular cancer. Elevated serum levels reflect tumor presence and reliably indicate response to therapy.

Begent, R. H.: The value of carcinoembryonic antigen in clinical practice. Br. J. Hosp. Med., April:335, 1987.

This excellent article updates the use of serum carcinoembryonic antigen (CEA) levels in the management of patients with colorectal cancer. It suggests specific management questions in which serum CEA levels can be used in decision analysis. It also describes radioimmunolocalization of primary and metastatic tumor using isotopic scanning with radiolabeled CEA monoclonal antibodies.

Kanematsu, T., Matsumata, T., Takenaka, K., Yoshida, Y., Higashi, H., and

Sugimachi, K.: Clinical management of recurrent hepatocellular carcinoma after primary resection. Br. J. Surg., 75:203, 1988.

This article carefully documents the use of serum alpha-fetoprotein (AFP) levels to document recurrent hepatocellular carcinoma (HCC) following successful excision to remove the primary tumor in 121 patients with primary HCC. Sixty-six per cent of 41 patients with documented recurrent HCC had elevated serum AFP levels at the time of detection of recurrent disease. However, 12% of patients who had elevated serum AFP levels at the time of initial operation did not have elevated levels at the time of recurrence. Serum AFP levels are helpful to detect recurrent tumor in most, but not all, patients with recurrent HCC.

Partin, A. W., and Oesterling, J. E.: The clinical usefulness of prostate specific antigen: Update 1994. J. Urol., 152:1358, 1994.

Prostate-specific antigen (PSA) is a valuable marker to detect prostate cancer and follow the response to therapy. These authors provide the latest information about the clinical utility of PSA and a critical review of the current studies and information.

Perren, T. J.: c-erb B-2 oncogene as a prognostic marker in breast cancer. Br. J. Cancer, 63:328, 1991.

This editorial provides an excellent summary of the role of the c-erb B-2 oncogene as a prognostic factor for patients with breast cancer. This is important information for all surgeons and should be required reading. In the new age of management of patients with cancer, this is a true advance.

REFERENCES

1. Anderson, T., Waldmann, T. A., Javadpour, N., and Glatstein, E.: Testicular germ-cell neoplasms: Recent advances in diagnosis and therapy. Ann. Intern. Med., 90:373, 1979.
2. Barber, H. R.: Ovarian cancer: Cause, diagnosis and treatment. Compr. Ther., 13:25, 1987.
3. Bartlett, N. L., Freiha, F. S., and Torti, F. M.: Serum markers in germ cell neoplasms. Hematol. Oncol. Clin. North Am., 5:1245, 1991.
4. Bast, R. C., Jr., Hunter, V., and Knapp, R. C.: Pros and cons of gynecologic tumor markers. Cancer, 60:1984, 1987.
5. Bast, R. C., Jr., Klug, T. L., and St. John, E.: A radioimmunoassay using a monoclonal antibody to monitor the course of epithelial ovarian cancer. N. Engl. J. Med., 390:883, 1983.
6. Beasley, R. P., Hwang, L. Y., and Lin, C. C.: Hepatocellular carcinoma and hepatitis B virus: A prospective study of 22,707 men in Taiwan. Lancet, 2:1129, 1981.
7. Begent, R. H. J.: The value of carcinoembryonic antigen in clinical practice. Br. J. Hosp. Med., April:335, 1987.
9. Benchimol, S., Fuks, A., Jothy, S., Beauchemin, N., Shirota, K., and Stanners, C.: Carcinoembryonic antigen, a human tumor marker, functions as an intercellular adhesion molecule. Cell, 57:327, 1989.
10. Benson, M. C., and Olsson, C. A.: Prostate specific antigen and prostate specific antigen density. Cancer, 74:1667, 1994.
11. Birch, R., Williams, S., and Cone, A.: Prognostic factors for favorable outcome in disseminated germ cell tumors. J. Clin. Oncol., 4:400, 1987.
12. Bleday, R., and Steele, G., Jr.: Second-look surgery for recurrent colorectal carcinoma: Is it worthwhile? Semin. Surg. Oncol., 7:171, 1991.
13. Bucceri, G. F., Ferrigno, D., and Sartoris, A. M.: Tumor markers in bronchogenic carcinoma. Cancer, 60:42, 1987.
14. Cole, L. A., Wang, Y., and Elliott, M.: Urinary human chorionic gonadotropin free B-subunit and B-core fragment: A new marker of gynecological cancer. Cancer Res., 48:1356, 1988.
15. Deftos, L. J.: Chromogranin A: Its role in endocrine function and as an endocrine and neuroendocrine tumor marker. Endocr. Rev., 12:181, 1991.
16. Eskelinen, M., Pasanen, P., Kulju, A., et al.: Clinical evaluation of serum tumour markers CEA, CA 50 and CA 242 in colorectal cancer. Anticancer Res., 14:1427, 1994.
17. Ganz, P. A., Ma, P. Y., Wang, H. J., and Elashoff, R. M.: Evaluation of three biochemical markers for serially monitoring the therapy of small-cell lung cancer. J. Clin. Oncol., 5:472, 1987.
18. Haglund, C., Lundin, J., Kuusela, P., and Roberts, P. J.: CA 242, a new tumour marker for pancreatic cancer: A comparison with CA 19–9, CA 50 and CEA. Br. J. Cancer, 70:487, 1994.
19. Hall, N. R., Finan, P. J., Stephenson, B. M., Purves, D. A., and Cooper, E. H.: The role of CA 242 and CEA in surveillance following curative resection for colorectal cancer. Br. J. Cancer, 70:549, 1994.
20. Harmenberg, U., Wahren, B., and Wiechel, K. L.: Tumor markers carbohydrate antigens CA 19–9 and CA 50 and carcinoembryonic antigen in pancreatic cancer and benign diseases of the pancreaticobiliary tract. Cancer Res., 48:1985, 1988.
21. Hayes, D. F.: Tumor markers for breast cancer. Ann. Oncol., 4:807, 1993.
22. Hempling, R. E.: Tumor markers in epithelial ovarian cancer. Obstet. Gynecol. Clin. North Am., 21:41, 1994.
23. Heyward, W. L., Lanier, A. P., and Bender, T. R.: Early detection of primary hepatocellular carcinoma by screening for alpha-fetoprotein in high-risk families. Lancet, 2:1161, 1983.
24. Jager, W., Kissing, A., Cilaci, S., Melsheimer, R., and Lang, N.: Is an increase in CA 125 in breast cancer patients an indicator of pleural metastases? Br. J. Surg., 70:495, 1994.
25. Kawa, S., Tokoo, M., Hasebe, O., et al.: Comparative study of CA 242 and CA 19–9 for the diagnosis of pancreatic cancer. Br. J. Cancer, 70:481, 1994.

26. Kuusela, P., Haglund, C., and Roberts, P. J.: Comparison of a new tumour marker CA 242 with CA 19–9, CA 50 and carcinoembryonic antigen (CEA) in digestive tract diseases. Br. J. Cancer, 63:636, 1991.

27. LaValle, G. J., Chevinsky, A., and Martin E. W., Jr.: Impact of radioimmuno-guided surgery. Semin. Surg. Oncol., 167:170, 1991.

27a. Martin, E. W., Jr., Minton, J. P., and Carey, L. C.: CEA-directed second-look surgery in the asymptomatic patient after primary resection of colorectal carcinoma. Ann. Surg., 202:310, 1985.

28. Niklinski, J., Furman, M., Chyczewska, E., et al.: Evaluation of CYFRA 21–1 as a new marker for non-small cell lung cancer. Eur. J. Cancer Prev., 3:227, 1994.

29. Oesterling, J. E., Jacobsen, S. J., Chute, C. G., et al.: Serum prostate-specific antigen in a community-based population of healthy men. JAMA, 270:680, 1993.

30. Paganuzzi, M., Onetto, M., De Paoli, M., et al.: Carcinoembryonic antigen (CEA) in serum and bile of colorectal cancer patients with or without detectable liver metastases. Anticancer Res., 14:1409, 1994.

31. Pandha, H. S., Waxman, J., and Sikora, K.: Tumour markers. Br. J. Hosp. Med., 51:297, 1994.

32. Rastel, D., Ramaioli, A., Cornillie, F., and Thirion, B.: CYFRA 21–1, a sensitive and specific new tumour marker for squamous cell lung cancer: Report of the first European multicentre evaluation. Eur. J. Cancer, 15:601, 1994.

33. Richie, J. P., Sorinsky, M. A., and Fung, C. Y.: Management of patients with clinical stage I or II nonseminomatous germ cell tumors of the testis. Arch. Surg., 122:1443, 1987.

34. Roulston, J. E.: Limitations of tumour markers in screening. Br. J. Surg., 77:961, 1990.

35. Sato, Y., Nakata, K., Kato, Y., et al.: Early recognition of hepatocellular carcinoma based on altered profiles of alpha-fetoprotein. N. Engl. J. Med., 328:1802, 1993.

36. Scambia, G., Gadducci, A., Panici, P. B., et al.: Combined use of CA 125 and CA 15–3 in patients with endometrial cancer. Gynecol. Oncol., 54:292, 1994.

37. Seiden, M. V., Kantolf, P. W., and Krithivans, K.: Detection of circulating tumor cells in men with localized prostate cancer. J. Clin. Oncol., 12:2634, 1994.

38. Slamon, D. J., Clark, G. M., Wong, S. G., Levin, W. J., Ulrich, A., and McGuire, W. L.: Human breast cancer: Correlation of relapse and survival with amplification of the HER-2/neu oncogene. Science, 235:177, 1987.

39. Slebos, R. F. C., Kibbelaar, R. E., and Dalesio, O.: K-ras oncogene activation as a prognostic marker in adenocarcinoma of the lung. N. Engl. J. Med., 323:561, 1990.

40. Smith, D. S., and Catalona, W. J.: Rate of change in serum prostate specific antigen levels as a method for prostate cancer detection. J. Urol., 152:1163, 1994.

41. Soper, J. T., Hunter, V., and Tanner, M.: Use of CA 125, CA 72 and CA 15–3 to discriminate malignant from benign pelvic masses. Proc. Am. Assoc. Cancer Res., 28:205, 1987.

42. Stamey, T. A., Prestigiacomo, A. F., and Chen, Z.: Standardization of immunoassays for prostate specific antigen. Cancer, 74:1662, 1994.

43. Steinberg, W.: The clinical utility of the CA 19–9 tumor-associated antigen. Am. J. Gastroenterol., 85:350, 1990.

44. Szabo, E., Birrer, M. J., and Mulshine, J. L.: Early detection of lung cancer. Semin. Oncol., 20:374, 1993.

45. Takeshima, N., Shimizu, Y., Umezawa, S., et al.: Combined assay of serum levels of CA125 and CA19–9 in endometrial carcinoma. Gynecol. Oncol., 54:321, 1994.

46. Yeatman, T. J., Kimura, A. K., Copeland, E. M., and Bland, K. I.: Rapid analysis of carcinoembryonic antigen levels in gall bladder bile: Identification of patients at high risk for colorectal liver metastasis. Ann. Surg., 213:113, 1990.

CHAPTER 22

THE BREAST

J. Dirk Iglehart, M.D.

ANATOMY[10, 24]

Knowledge of the anatomy and embryology of the breast and the chest structures under it is required not only for the performance of surgical procedures but also in planning therapeutic radiation, predicting sites of locally recurrent disease, and assessing the adequacy of surgical procedures used in an increasing number of therapeutic trials. Embryologically, the human breast develops in the thickened portion of ectodermal tissue known as the *milk streak* coursing from the pubis to the axilla in early fetal life. Late in the first trimester, the milk streak atrophies, leaving only its pectoral portion, which continues to thicken and to form the nipple bud. The entire gland then forms as a dermally derived organ lying within the subcutaneous tissue in a manner similar to that of sweat gland development. The ductal system develops from the nipple bud by invasion and downgrowth of primitive ectodermal cells from the nipple surface. The mature breast parenchyma lies cushioned in fat between the layers of superficial pectoral fascia (Fig. 22–1). Between the deep layer of the superficial fascia and the fascial investment of the pectoralis major muscle, the breast rests on a thin layer of loose areolar tissue, the retromammary space, containing lymphatics and small vessels. When a total mastectomy is performed, the correct plane is found under the pectoral fascia and includes the retromammary space as emphasized by earlier surgeons and anatomists.

Deep to the pectoralis major muscle, the pectoralis minor muscle is enclosed in the clavipectoral fascia that envelopes it and extends laterally to fuse with the axillary fascia. In a standard modified radical mastectomy, dissection along the lateral border of the pectoralis minor muscle divides the axillary fascia and exposes the contents of the axilla. Within the loose areolar fat of the axilla, one finds a variable number of lymph nodes grouped as shown in Figure 22–2. The number of lymph nodes found in the axillary space of patients undergoing mastectomy varies depending on the extent of dissection and the diligence of methods used to identify these nodes. An upper limit is established by the work of Durkin and Haagensen using ethanol clearing. These investigators found an average of 50 nodes in 100 specimens obtained in the course of a Halsted-type radical mastectomy. The current approach to less radical procedures has reduced the number of nodes retrieved.

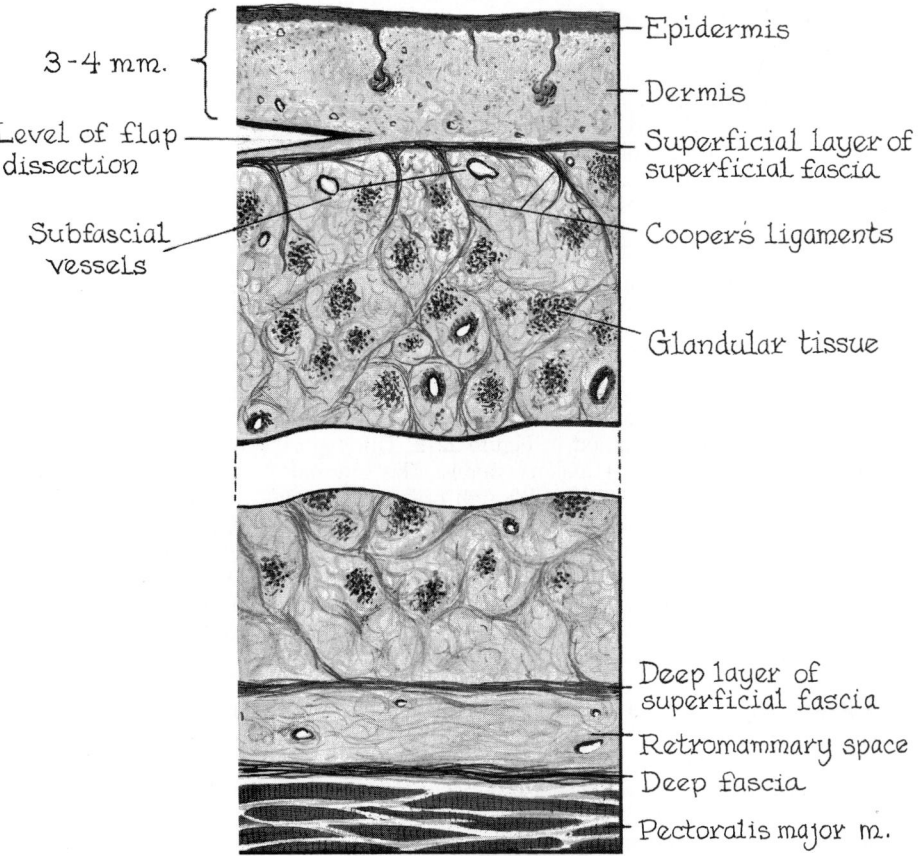

Figure 22–1. Diagrammatic cross-section of the breast showing its fascial relationships. Glandular tissue of the breast lies within a cushion of fat between the superficial and deep layers of the superficial pectoral fascia. Cooper's ligaments are fibrous continuations of the superficial fascia, which span the parenchyma of the breast coursing between the superficial and deep fascial layers. Dissection of the breast off the pectoralis major muscle usually includes the deep fascia. The clavipectoral fascia, not shown here, invests the pectoralis minor muscle and the undersurface of the pectoralis major muscle. (From Haagensen, C. D.: Diseases of the Breast, 3rd ed. Philadelphia, W. B. Saunders, 1986, p. 15.)

3-4 mm.

Level of flap dissection

Subfascial vessels

Epidermis

Dermis

Superficial layer of superficial fascia

Cooper's ligaments

Glandular tissue

Deep layer of superficial fascia

Retromammary space

Deep fascia

Pectoralis major m.

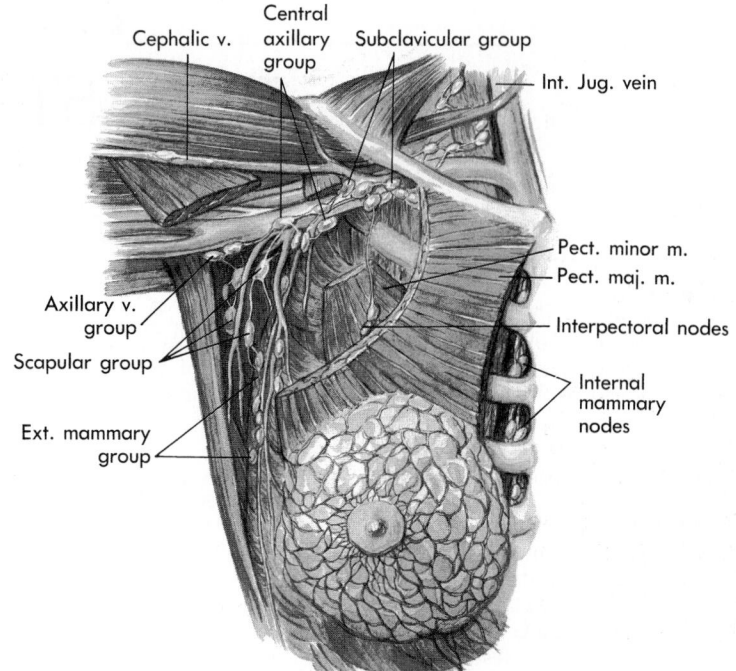

Cephalic v.

Central axillary group

Subclavicular group

Int. Jug. vein

Pect. minor m.
Pect. maj. m.

Interpectoral nodes

Internal mammary nodes

Axillary v. group

Scapular group

Ext. mammary group

Figure 22–2. Contents of the axilla. Five named groups of lymph nodes are generally contained within a complete dissection of the axillary contents. These groups tend to follow the course of the major veins that are encountered within the axilla. Lymphatic afferent channels course under the deep layer of the superficial fascia in the retromammary space. The first node groups in the circuit are the external mammary, axillary, and central nodal groups. Scapular and subclavicular nodes are also contained in the axillary chain. However, lymphatic afferents drain directly to internal mammary nodes. In addition, more distal groups at risk for involvement in more advanced progression are the interpectoral nodes (Rotter's nodes), subclavicular nodes high along the axillary chain, and supraclavicular nodes above the ipsilateral clavicle. (Illustration from Donegan, W. L., and Spratt, J. S.: Cancer of the Breast, 3rd ed. Philadelphia, W. B. Saunders, 1988, p. 19.)

To standardize the extent of axillary dissection, the axillary space is arbitrarily divided into three levels shown in Figure 22–3. Level I nodes are those in the external mammary, scapular, axillary vein, and central axillary groups, which lie lateral to the lateral border of the pectoralis minor muscle. Level II nodes are those in the central axillary group, which lie under the pectoralis minor muscle. The level III nodes are difficult to visualize and remove unless the pectoralis minor muscle is sacrificed or divided and include those subclavicular nodes medial to the minor muscle. The apex of the axilla is defined by the costoclavicular ligament (Halsted's ligament), at which point the axillary vein passes into the thorax and becomes the subclavian vein. Lymph nodes in the space between the pectoralis major and minor muscles are known as the interpectoral group, or Rotter's nodes, described by Grossman and Rotter. Unless this group is specifically exposed, they are not encompassed in surgical procedures that preserve the pectoral muscles.

The lymphatic drainage of the breast is rich, and appreciation of the major pathways allows one to predict the sites most commonly containing lymph-borne metastases. Lymphatic channels within the breast follow centrifugal pathways from the subareolar plexus along major lactiferous ducts and then along efferent veins to draining nodal beds. Three principal pathways are identified in Figure 22–2. The major site of drainage is to central axillary nodes. The internal mammary and interpectoral nodes, although primary routes of lymph flow, are rarely the sites of nodal metastasis from breast cancer in the absence of simultaneous axillary disease. Secondarily, the lymphatic spread of cancer is into the high axillary nodes in the subclavicular chain and henceforth into the supraclavicular fossa.

As the surgeon endeavors to remove the lymph nodes of the axilla, a keen knowledge of the nerve structures in the axilla is required to avoid their sacrifice. Coursing close to the chest wall on the medial side of the axilla is the long thoracic nerve, or the external respiratory nerve of Bell, which innervates the serratus anterior muscle. This muscle is important in fixation of the scapula to the chest wall during adduction of the shoulder and extension of the arm, and its

denervation results in the winged scapula deformity. For this reason, the long thoracic nerve is carefully preserved during standard axillary dissection. The second major nerve trunk encountered during axillary dissection is the thoracodorsal nerve to the latissimus dorsi muscle at the lateral border of the axilla. This nerve arises from the posterior cord of the brachial plexus and enters the axillary space under the axillary vein, close to the entrance of the long thoracic nerve, and then crosses the axilla to the medial surface of the latissimus dorsi muscle. The thoracodorsal nerve is usually preserved during dissection of axillary nodes, unless its sacrifice is required for complete removal of tumor-containing nodes.

Innervation of the pectoralis major muscle has gained the attention of some who emphasize the advantage of protecting these nerves during modified radical mastectomy. Loss of innervation results in a flaccid and atrophic muscle and a diminished tissue covering over the chest wall after amputation of the breast. These investigators have named the pectoral nerves according to their actual position as encountered during axillary dissection. The lateral pectoral nerve has a variable course, as depicted in Figure 22–4. In the majority of patients, the lateral pectoral nerve travels around the lateral margin of the pectoralis minor muscle and is in a vulnerable position during the division of the clavipectoral fascia and exposure of the axillary space. If possible, this branch can be saved without compromising the dissection.

The final nerves of interest to the surgeon are the large sensory intercostal brachial or brachial cutaneous nerves that span the axillary space and supply sensation to the undersurface of the upper arm and skin of the chest wall along the posterior margin of the axilla. Cutting these nerves, which is routinely done in removing the lymph node-containing tissues, causes cutaneous anesthesia in these areas. It is helpful to emphasize this to the patients before operation. Denervation of the areas supplied by these sensory nerves can cause chronic and uncomfortable pain syndromes in a small percentage of patients. Contemporary surgeons have advocated preservation of the most superior brachial cutaneous nerve, which crosses the central axilla to supply cutaneous sensation to the posterior upper arm. This nerve can be preserved

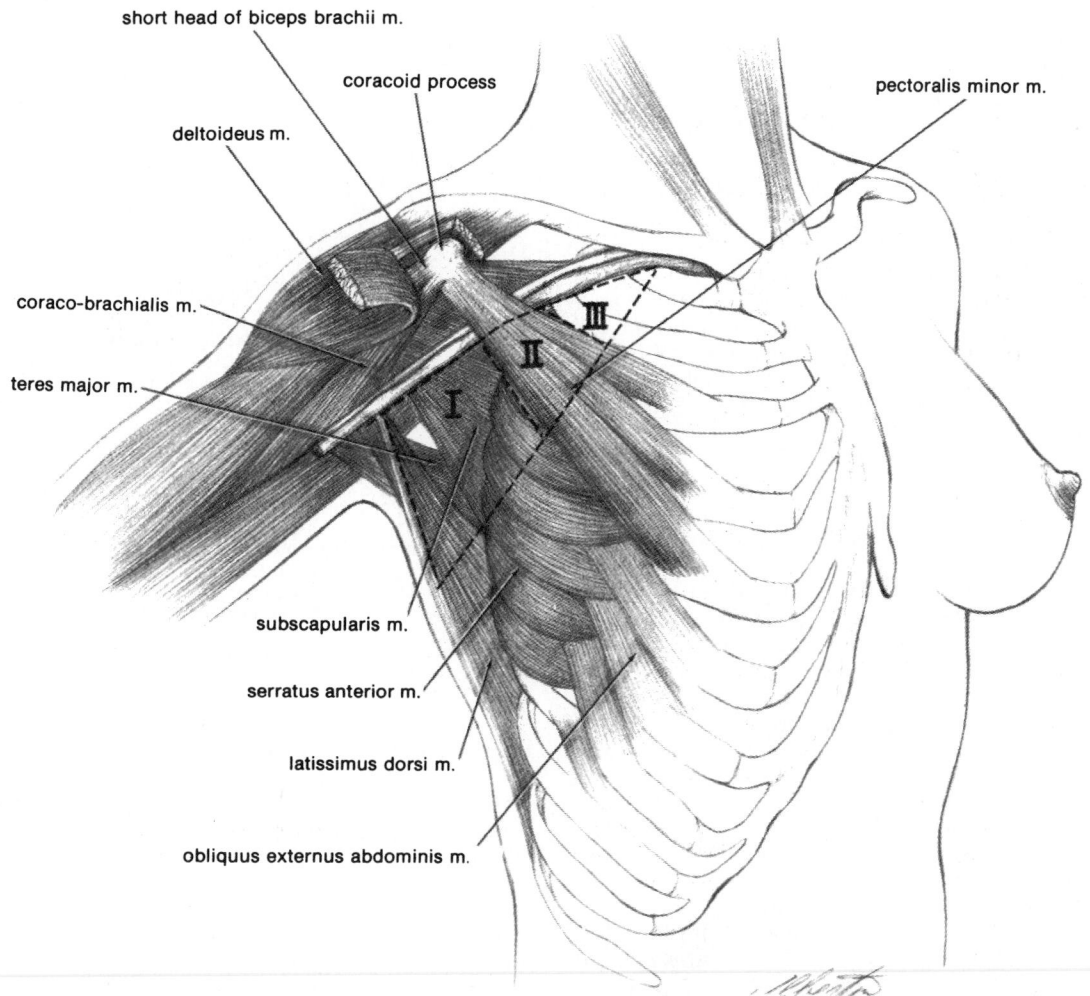

short head of biceps brachii m.

coracoid process

pectoralis minor m.

deltoideus m.

coraco-brachialis m.

teres major m.

subscapularis m.

serratus anterior m.

latissimus dorsi m.

obliquus externus abdominis m.

Figure 22–3. Standardized description of axillary nodal contents. The axillary nodes are divided into three groups defined by their position relative to the pectoralis minor muscle. Level I defines those nodes lateral to the pectoralis minor muscle. Level II nodes are those that lie under the pectoralis minor. The Level II nodes are located medial to the medial border of the minor muscle. In a normal patient, these nodes can be removed only after division or sacrifice of the minor muscle during a modified radical mastectomy or axillary dissection. They are routinely removed in a standard radical mastectomy. Operative notes should specify accurately the levels of axillary dissection. (From Donegan, W. L., and Spratt, J. S.: Cancer of the Breast, 3rd ed. Philadelphia, W. B. Saunders, 1988, p. 425.)

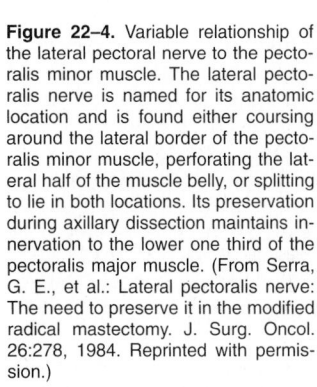

Figure 22–4. Variable relationship of the lateral pectoral nerve to the pectoralis minor muscle. The lateral pectoralis nerve is named for its anatomic location and is found either coursing around the lateral border of the pectoralis minor muscle, perforating the lateral half of the muscle belly, or splitting to lie in both locations. Its preservation during axillary dissection maintains innervation to the lower one third of the pectoralis major muscle. (From Serra, G. E., et al.: Lateral pectoralis nerve: The need to preserve it in the modified radical mastectomy. J. Surg. Oncol. 26:278, 1984. Reprinted with permission.)

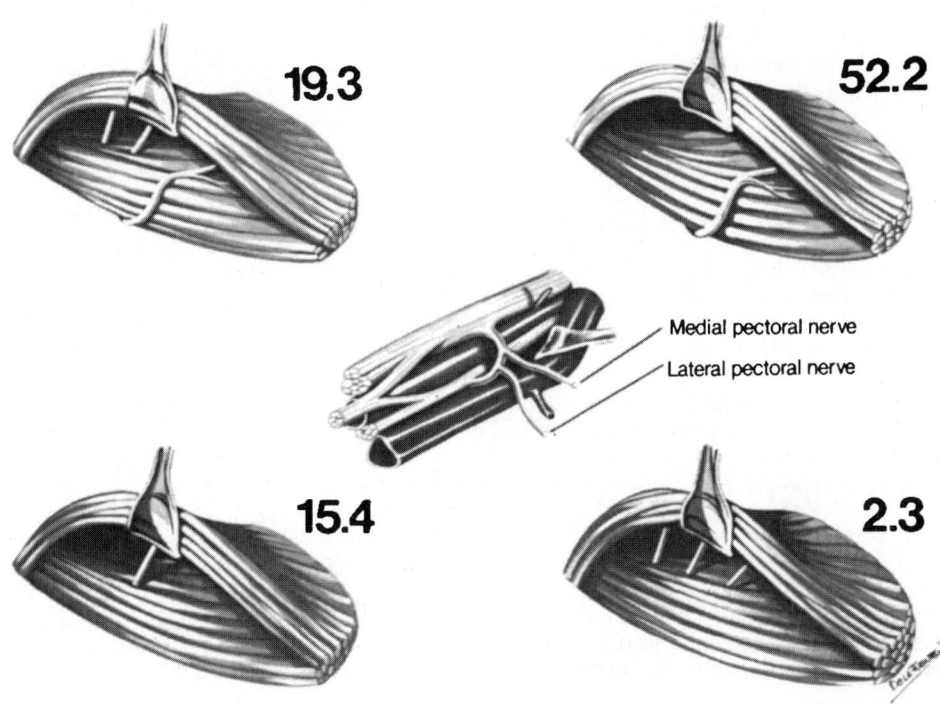

19.3

52.2

Medial pectoral nerve

Lateral pectoral nerve

15.4

2.3

without compromising the axillary dissection in many patients.

Microscopic Anatomy of the Breast[24, 38]

The mature breast is composed of three principal tissue types: epithelium, fibrous stroma and supporting structures, and fat. The relative amounts tend to vary with age, but there is even greater variability among individual women. In youth, the predominant tissues are epithelium and stroma, replaced by fat in the breast of older women. For this reason, mammography in women younger than 30 years of age, whose breast tissue is dense with stroma and epithelium, produces images without much definition that are rarely useful clinically. In contrast, fat absorbs relatively little radiation and provides a contrasting background that favors detection of small density lesions in the older patient. Throughout the fat of the breast, coursing from the overlying skin to the underlying deep fascia, strands of dense connective tissue provide shape and hold the breast upward. These strands, devoid of epithelial elements, are called Cooper's ligaments (see Fig. 22–1). Because they are anchored into the skin, tethering of these ligaments by a small scirrhous carcinoma commonly produces a dimple or subtle deformity on the otherwise smooth surface of the breast (see Fig. 22–8).

The glandular apparatus of the breast is composed of a branching system of ducts, roughly organized in a radial pattern, which spread outward and downward from the nipple-areolar complex (Fig. 22–5). These lactiferous ducts are so named because they carry the milk produced in the more distal lobular groupings. At the summit of the arborizing ductal system, the subareolar ducts widen to form the lactiferous sinuses, which then exit through 15 to 20 orifices on the nipple. These large ducts close to the nipple are lined with a low columnar or cuboidal epithelium that abruptly meets the squamous epithelium of the nipple surface, which invades the duct for a short distance. Awareness of this junction helps understand Paget's disease of the nipple, described later.

At the opposite end of the ductal system and after progressive generations of branching, the ducts end blindly in clusters of spaces that are called terminal ductules or acini. These are the milk-forming glands of the lactating breast and together with their small efferent ducts or ductules are known as the lobular units or lobules. As shown in Figure 22–6, the terminal ductules are invested in a specialized loose connective tissue that contains capillaries, lymphocytes, and

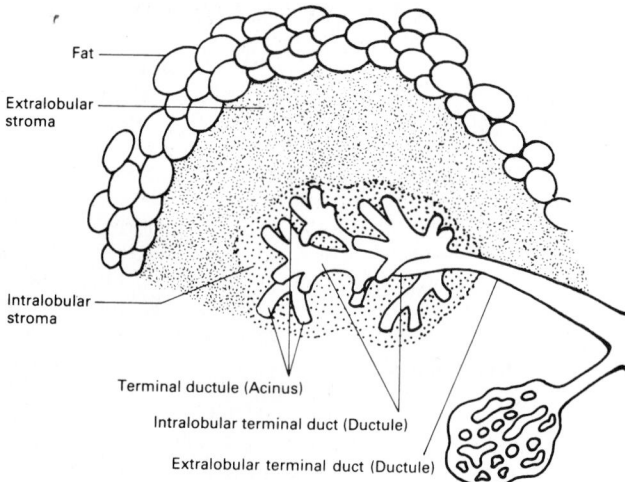

Figure 22–6. A mature resting lobular unit within the breast. The lobular unit consists of terminal ductules or acini surrounded by loose connective stroma and tiny efferent ductules referred to as extralobular terminal ducts. The surrounding intralobular stroma is denser and collagen rich. The efferent ductules coalesce to form larger ducts that course up to the nipple-areola complex. (From Page, D. L., and Anderson, T. J.: Diagnostic Histopathology of the Breast. Edinburgh, Churchill Livingstone, 1987. Reprinted with permission.)

other migratory mononuclear cells. This intralobular stroma is clearly distinguished from the denser and less cellular interlobular stroma and from the fat within the breast.

Under the luminal epithelium, the entire ductal system is surrounded by a specialized myoepithelial cell of ductal epithelial origin that has contractile properties and serves to propel secretion of milk toward the nipple. Outside the epithelial and myoepithelial layers, the ducts of the breast are surrounded by a continuous basement membrane containing laminin, type IV collagen, and proteoglycans. The basement membrane layer is extremely important in differentiating *in situ* from invasive breast cancer. Continuity of this layer around proliferations of ductal cells guarantees that progression to an invasive cancer has not yet occurred (Fig. 22–7).

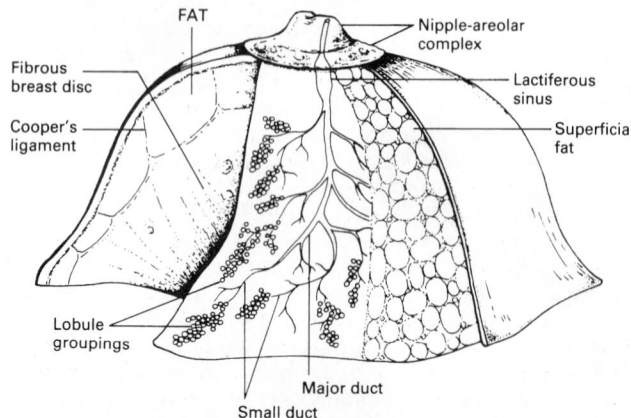

Figure 22–5. The mature breast, showing the organization of the ductal and lobular components and their relationship to the nipple-areola complex. (From Page, D. L., and Anderson, T. J.: Diagnostic Histopathology of the Breast. Edinburgh, Churchill Livingstone, 1987. Reprinted with permission.)

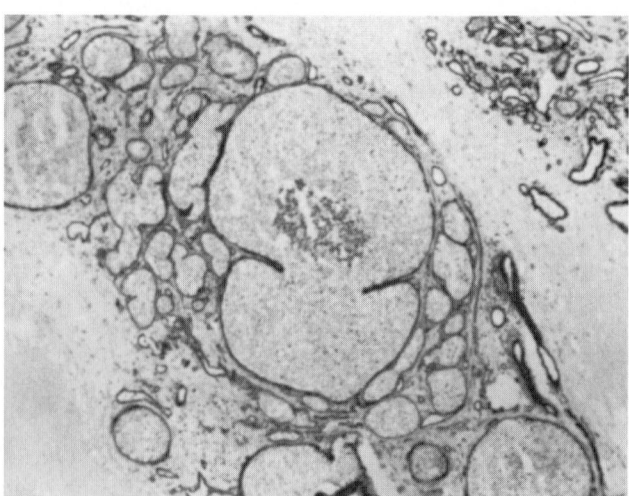

Figure 22–7. Integrity of the basement membrane around normal ducts and around intraductal neoplasm. Antibodies against collagen Type IV, a normal constituent of basement membrane, were reacted with fresh breast tissue from a case of *in situ* ductal carcinoma. Although greatly expanded and displaying central necrosis, the duct in the center of the illustration has an uninterrupted basement membrane highlighted by the immunohistochemical reaction. More normal ducts in the upper right are also contained by a continuous basement membrane.

BREAST DEVELOPMENT AND PHYSIOLOGY[24, 38]

In many mammalian species, full breast development requires the stimulation of copulation or pregnancy. Humans do not require either of these two events to initiate and complete breast maturation. Appreciation of the stages of breast development is necessary to understand many benign and even malignant states that come to clinical attention. During adolescence, the breast is composed primarily of dense fibrous stroma and scattered ducts lined with epithelium. In the United States, puberty begins at about 12 years of age, during which time there is hormone-dependent maturation of the genital organs. In the breast, this process entails increased deposition of fat, formation of new ducts by branching and elongation, and the first appearance of lobular units. This process of growth entails cell division and is under the control of estrogen, progesterone, adrenal hormones, pituitary hormones, and trophic effects of insulin and thyroid hormone. There is evidence that local growth factor networks are also important, including epidermal growth factor, which can replace estrogen as a developmental mammogen. The exact timing of these events and the coordinated development of both breast buds may vary from the average in individual patients. The term *prepubertal gynecomastia* refers to the symmetrical enlargement and projection of the breast bud in a young girl before the average age of 12, unaccompanied by the other changes of puberty. This process, which may be unilateral, should not be confused with neoplastic growth and should not be subjected to biopsy.

The mature or *resting* breast contains fat, stroma, lactiferous ducts, and lobular units. During phases of the menstrual cycle or in response to exogenous hormones, the breast epithelium and lobular stroma undergo cyclic stimulation. It appears that the dominant process is hypertrophy and alteration of morphology rather than hyperplasia. In the late luteal (premenstrual) phase, there is accumulation of fluid and intralobular edema that appears to correspond to the clinical complaint of breast engorgement, which may be painful.

On physical examination, and even by mammography, this may lead to increased nodularity and even be mistaken for development of a dominant tumor. Accordingly, ill-defined masses in premenopausal women are correctly observed through the course of one or two menstrual cycles. Finally, any alteration in the periodicity of the menstrual cycle, such as anovulatory cycles, can cause accentuation of engorgement, pain, and nodularity.

With pregnancy, there is diminution of the fibrous stroma to accommodate the hyperplasia of the lobular units. This formation of many new acini or lobules is termed the *adenosis of pregnancy* and is influenced by high circulating levels of estrogen and progesterone and by levels of prolactin that steadily rise during gestation. After birth, there is sudden loss of the placental hormones and the continued high level of prolactin. This may be the principal trigger for lactation. The actual expulsion of milk is under hormonal control and is caused by the contraction of the myoepithelial cells that surround breast ducts and terminal ductules. There is no evidence for innervation of the myoepithelial cells; their contraction appears to be in response to the pituitary-derived peptide oxytocin. Stimulation of the nipple appears to be the physiologic signal for continued pituitary secretion of prolactin and for the acute release of oxytocin.

When breast feeding ceases there is a fall in prolactin and no stimulus for release of oxytocin. The breast then returns to a resting state and to the cyclic changes induced when menstruation begins again. With the approach of menopause, phases of the menstrual cycle may not be as symmetrical and regular. This irregularity can induce functional nodularity and breast pain where there had been none in earlier years. Menopause is defined by a cessation in menstrual flow for a significant period of time (i.e., 6 months or more) and the variable appearance of constitutional systems such as diaphoresis, minor psychological disturbances, or even clinical depression. For the breast, menopause results in involution and a general decrease in the epithelial elements of the resting breast. These changes include increased fat deposition, diminished connective tissue, and the virtual disappearance of the lobular units. The persistence of lobules, hyperplasia of the ductal epithelium, and even cyst formation can all occur under the influence of exogenous ovarian hormones. Most commonly, hormones are administered to relieve the symptoms of menopause, to prevent demineralization of bone, or to slow the appearance of atherosclerosis. The surgeon evaluating patients at any age for breast disease should inquire about the menstrual history, establish the cessation of menses in postmenopausal women, and record the use of any exogenous hormones. It is important that the pathologist who is examining biopsy material also have this information.

Abnormal Physiology and Development

Gynecomastia. Hypertrophy of breast tissue in men is a common clinical entity for which there is frequently no identifiable cause. Haagensen distinguishes *pubertal hypertrophy*, occurring in young boys between the ages of 13 and 17 years, from *senescent hypertrophy*, which occurs in men older than 50. The enlargement in teenage boys is very common and is frequently bilateral but may be unilateral. Unless it is unilateral or painful, it passes unnoticed and regresses with adulthood. Pubertal hypertrophy is generally treated by reassurance and without operation. Surgical excision should be discussed only if the enlargement fails to regress and the breast is cosmetically unacceptable.

Hypertrophy in older men is also common and may regress spontaneously. It is frequently unilateral, although the contralateral breast may enlarge with passage of time. The discoid mass is smooth, firm, and symmetrically distributed beneath the areola. It may be tender, and patients occasionally complain of breast discomfort. A number of commonly used medications, such as digoxin, thiazides, estrogens, phenothiazines, and theophylline, may exacerbate senescent gynecomastia. In addition, gynecomastia may be a systemic manifestation of hepatic cirrhosis, renal failure, and malnutrition. There should be little confusion with carcinoma occurring in the male breast. Carcinoma is usually not tender, it is asymmetrically located either beneath or beside the areola, and may be fixed to the overlying dermis or to the deep fascia. As with pubertal hypertrophy, gynecomastia in older men is usually left untreated. A dominant mass suspected of carcinoma should be sampled or carefully observed.

Nipple Discharge. The appearance of a discharge from the nipple of a nonlactating woman is frequently frightening to the patient and misunderstood by the physician.[7, 11] Nipple discharge is very common and rarely associated with an underlying carcinoma. It is important to establish whether the discharge comes from one breast or from both breasts, whether it comes from multiple duct orifices or from just one, and whether the discharge is grossly bloody or contains blood. A milky discharge from both breasts is termed *galactorrhea*. In the absence of lactation or history of recent lactation, galactorrhea may be associated with increased production of prolactin. Radioimmunoassay for serum prolactin is diagnostic. However, true galactorrhea is very rare and is diagnosed only when the discharge is milky (contains lactose, fat, and milk-specific proteins).

Unilateral non-milky discharge coming from one duct orifice is surgically significant and warrants special attention. However, the underlying cause is rarely a breast malignancy. In one review of 270 subareolar biopsy results of discharges coming from one identifiable duct, and without an associated breast mass, carcinoma was found in only 16 patients (5.9%). In each of these cases, the fluid was either grossly bloody or tested strongly positive for occult hemoglobin. In another series of 249 patients, including both multiple-duct and single-duct discharges, breast carcinoma was found in 10 (4%). In 8 of these patients, a mass lesion coexisted with the discharge. Among 67 patients with breast cancer presenting with nipple discharge and studied by Leis and colleagues, only 8 (12%) had no palpable mass and 7 (10%) had a negative mammogram. To conclude, nipple discharge that comes from a single duct and contains blood must be investigated further. However, in the absence of a palpable mass or a suspicious mammogram, this symptom is usually not associated with cancer.

The most common cause of spontaneous nipple discharge from a single duct is a solitary intraductal papilloma in one of the large subareolar ducts directly under the nipple. Fibrocystic change, or cystic mastopathy, typically produces multiple-duct discharge and is another commonly associated finding. Subareolar duct ectasia, producing inflammation and dilatation of large collecting ducts under the nipple, is a common finding in the aging breast and usually produces multiple-duct discharge. In summary, nipple discharge that is bilateral and comes from multiple ducts is usually not a surgical problem. Discharge from single ducts is not commonly associated with carcinoma in the absence of detectable blood or a palpable mass. Bloody discharge from a single duct requires surgical biopsy to establish diagnosis. Intraductal papilloma is found in the majority of cases. If an occult cancer is found, it invariably is an early intraductal lesion.

Breast Pain. Painful breast tissue is an exceedingly common symptom but is usually of functional origin and very rarely a symptom of breast cancer. Haagensen[24] carefully recorded the symptoms of women presenting with breast carcinoma and found pain as an unprompted symptom in only 5.4% of patients. Although not a symptom of cancer, breast pain is a common reason for patients to seek medical attention. Breast pain appears to be aggravated by abnormal menstrual cycles and may be seen in young women with menstrual irregularity, as a premenstrual symptom, or when exogenous ovarian hormones are administered during and after the menopause. In addition, fibrocystic change, in its severest forms, may cause disabling breast pain. Although many observers find painful cystic mastopathy is aggravated by excessive intake of caffeine, nicotine, or commonly used antihistamines, other investigators disagree.

Fibrocystic Change (Cystic Mastopathy, Cystic Mastitis). Fibrocystic change, popularly referred to as *fibrocystic disease,* represents a spectrum of clinical and histologic findings and describes a loose association of cyst formation, breast nodularity, stromal proliferation, and epithelial hyperplasia.[34] Fibrocystic change appears to represent an exaggerated response of breast stroma and epithelium to a variety of circulating and locally produced hormones and growth factors. Clinically, patients with fibrocystic change have dense, firm breast tissue with palpable lumps and frequently gross cysts. This condition is commonly painful and tender to touch. Histologically, the lesion recognized as fibrocystic complex contains macrocysts, microcysts, stromal fibrosis, adenosis, and a variable amount of epithelial metaplasia and hyperplasia. All these changes can occur alone or in combination and to a variable degree in the normal female breast. Autopsy studies have questioned whether any of these changes, except perhaps macrocysts, are abnormal. In fact, all of these lesions occur commonly in the breasts of elderly patients and appear to have no particular pathologic potential. It appears preferable to describe each of the lesions separately and comment about the extent and severity of the process. The term *fibrocystic disease* should be abandoned in the absence of any well-defined clinical and pathologic syndrome.

As discussed later, there is no consistent association between fibrocystic complex and breast cancer. It is well established that women who have undergone breast biopsy for any reason, regardless of the underlying pathology, have a slightly higher risk of developing subsequent breast cancer. Moreover, the incidence of finding fibrocystic disease in autopsied breasts from women dying of causes other than breast cancer exceeds the incidence of these same changes in cancer-containing breasts. For those patients with fibrocystic changes, higher risk appears to concentrate in those whose biopsy specimens show abnormal ductal and lobular hyperplasia and, to a lesser extent, cyst formation. Therefore, the fibrocystic complex appears to be an exaggerated or abnormal response to otherwise physiologic stimuli in most patients and represents a health risk only in certain subsets.

Galactocele. A galactocele is a milk-filled cyst that is round, well circumscribed, and easily movable within the breast. It usually occurs after the cessation of lactation or when feeding frequency has been curtailed significantly. Haagensen states that it may occur up to 6 to 10 months after breast feeding has stopped. The pathogenesis of galactocele is not known for certain, but it is thought that inspissated milk within a large lactiferous duct is responsible. The tumor is usually located in the central portion of the breast or under the nipple. Needle aspiration produces thick, creamy material that may be tinged dark-green or brown. Although it appears purulent, the fluid is sterile. The treatment is needle aspiration. Withdrawal of thick milky secretion confirms the diagnosis, operation is reserved for those cysts that cannot be aspirated or that become superinfected.

Absent or Accessory Breast Tissue. Absence of breast tissue (amastia) or absence of the nipple (athelia) are very rare anomalies. Unilateral rudimentary breast development is much more common, as is adolescent hypertrophy of one breast with more normal development of the other. In contrast, accessory breast tissue (polymastia) and accessory nipples (supernumerary nipples) are both common. Supernumerary nipples are usually rudimentary and occur along the milk line from the axilla to the pubis in both males and females. They may be mistaken by the patient for a small mole. However, accessory nipples are removed only for cosmetic reason. True polythelia refers to more than one nipple serving a single breast and is very rare.

Accessory breast tissue is commonly located above the breast in the axilla. Rudimentary nipple development may be present, and lactation is possible with more complete development. Accessory breast tissue, which may present as an enlarging mass in the axilla during pregnancy, is treated by surgical removal if it is large, cosmetically deforming, or to prevent enlargement during future pregnancy.

DIAGNOSIS OF BREAST DISEASE

History and Physical Examination

History. For patients with benign breast conditions, the history is an exceedingly important part of the overall evaluation and frequently points to the underlying cause of the symptom or physical finding. For patients suspected of having cancer, the history directly aids in the approach to the patient, and the ultimate treatment if cancer is confirmed, and helps estimate the risk that cancer will be found. First, the examiner should determine the patient's age and obtain a careful menstrual history. The age of menarche, menstrual irregularities, and the age at menopause should be sought. Previous surgical procedures should be recorded, including hysterectomy and removal of the ovaries. Because hysterectomy is a common surgical procedure, accurate determination of menopause may be difficult. It is useful to inquire about menopausal symptoms in these patients. Determination of the menopausal status may be used as a deciding factor in recommending adjuvant therapy, and this information is required for entry into most therapeutic trials. In younger women, the history of pregnancy and lactation should be recorded. A careful accounting of drug use should pay particular attention to exogenous estrogen or progestins given for postmenopausal replacement or for contraception. As discussed later, the family history should be directed to cancer of the breast in primary relatives (mother, sisters, daughters).

In questioning the patient about the specific breast problem, it is worthwhile to inquire about breast pain, nipple discharge, and new masses in the breast. Obviously, if a mass is present, it helps to know how long it has been present, how it was found, and what has happened since its discovery. If cancer is likely, inquiry about constitutional symptoms, bone pain, weight loss, and similar clinical indications of metastatic disease may occasionally reveal unsuspected distant spread.

Risk Factors for Breast Cancer.[14, 22] Identification of factors responsible for increasing an individual's chance of acquiring breast cancer is important in daily clinical practice for clinicians who care for women. *Major* risk factors that are important in practice and *minor* risk factors that are less relevant clinically, although important to understanding mammary cancer, are listed in Table 22–1.

Gender is an important risk factor. Males are at risk for breast cancer, although the incidence in males is less than 1% of the incidence in females. Lumps in the male breast are much more likely to be benign and the result of gynecomastia (discussed earlier) or other noncancerous tumors. The age-adjusted incidence of breast cancer continues to increase with advancing age of the population. Breast cancer is exceedingly rare in persons younger than the age of 20, and cases in women younger than 30 generally constitute less than 2% of the total cases. Thereafter, the incidence rises to an annual frequency of greater than 300 cases per 100,000 in the eighth decade of life. Age is probably the most important risk factor that clinicians use in everyday clinical practice.

A history of mammary cancer in one breast increases the likelihood of a second primary cancer in the contralateral breast. In many studies, the relative risk (ratio of observed cases over expected cases) ranges between three and four. The magnitude of relative risks depends on age at diagnosis of the first primary cancer. For patients younger than 45, risk for the remaining breast is five or six times that of the general population. In older patients, this decreases to a twofold or less increased risk. In absolute terms, the actual risk varies between 1% per year in young patients to 0.2% in older patients.

Many studies have examined the relationship of family history and the risk of breast cancer. These studies can be summarized as follows: (1) There is a twofold to threefold excess risk of the disease in first-degree relatives (mothers, sisters, and daughters) of patients with breast cancer; (2) risk falls quickly with more distant affected relatives; and (3) the risk is much higher if affected first-degree relatives had premenopausal onset or bilateral breast cancer. In families with multiple affected members, particularly with bilateral and premenopausal cancers, the absolute risk to first-degree relatives approaches 50%, consistent with an autosomal dominant mode of inheritance in these particular pedigrees. It is important to realize that these families are rare and that high-penetrance genes are an uncommon cause of breast cancer. Because the disease is so common in North American and European populations, constellations of breast cancer in families are more often an expression of random occurrence than due to a genetic defect in these families. An often difficult question posed by high-risk patients concerns prophylactic surgical therapy, either subcutaneous or total mastectomy. Arguments can be made in favor of intervention for the young patient whose mother or sister(s) had bilateral cancer at an early age, in families with many affected women and a consistent pedigree, and in families linked to established genetic loci. In other situations, the recommendation is harder to justify. Useful tabulations of risk for various combinations of primary and secondary probands are now available to use in counseling families.

It is well known that women with fibrocystic complex and those who have undergone breast biopsy are at increased risk of subsequent mammary carcinomas. However, fibrocystic complex is a spectrum of pathologic changes that may include lobular and ductal epithelial proliferation, cyst formation, and stromal sclerosis. The excess risk of breast cancer in these patients concentrates in those whose specimens show abnormal breast epithelial proliferation and, to a lesser extent, cyst formation. Moreover, the addition of features such as history of breast cancer in first-degree relatives and age produces additional risk.

Dupont and Page have divided the proliferative lesions into those with atypical epithelial hyperplasia and those without atypia. The relative risk of cancer in women with atypical hyperplasia was 4.4 times the risk of developing breast cancer in a control population of women. The coexistence of a positive family history with atypia on biopsy increased the risk to nearly nine times the general population. These authors have tabulated the cumulative effects of hyperplasia, age, family history, and calcification on the risk of breast cancer in a clinically useful manner. Breast biopsy is a common surgical procedure providing important prognostic information. Clinicians should request complete pathologic descriptions and not accept unqualified reports such as *fibrocystic disease* or *cystic mastitis.*

Noninvasive breast carcinoma is listed as a major risk factor in Table 22–1. The current management of noninvasive lobular and ductal carcinoma is discussed later in greater depth. However, many patients with lobular carcinoma *in situ* and certain patients with ductal *in situ* lesions are treated by biopsy only. These patients are subject to a considerable risk of subsequent invasive cancer and should be followed carefully if breast preservation has been recommended (see later).

To assist medical counseling, a model for breast cancer risk has been developed from case-control data in the Breast Cancer Detection Demonstration Project by Gail and co-workers. By examination of multiple variables, these investigators were able to reject many factors that did not contribute

TABLE 22–1. Risk Factors for Breast Cancer

Major	Minor
Gender (female > male)	Early menarche
Age	Late menopause
Family history (mother, sister, or daughter with premenopausal or bilateral cancer)	Obesity
Personal history of contralateral breast cancer	Low-dose radiation
Noninvasive carcinoma (ductal or lobular carcinoma *in situ*)	
Benign proliferative changes with atypia	

to breast cancer risk. These included oral contraceptives, long-term menopausal estrogen use, modest alcohol consumption, and cigarette smoking. Factors that did contribute to risk in this model included age at menarche, number of previous breast biopsies, age at first live birth, and the number of first-degree relatives with breast cancer. Combined with current age in years, the Gail model for breast cancer risk was used in the design of the Breast Cancer Prevention Trial, which is currently randomizing women at high risk to receive tamoxifen versus a placebo.

Physical Examination. Breast examination should be done in a well-lighted room, preferably with an available indirect light source. Respect for privacy and patient comfort should always be considered. The examination begins with careful visual inspection for obvious masses, asymmetries, and skin changes. The nipples are inspected and compared for the presence of retraction, nipple inversion, or excoriation of the superficial epidermis in Paget's disease. Inspection should be done with the patient in the upright, sitting position. The use of indirect lighting can unmask subtle dimpling of the skin or nipple caused by the scirrhous reaction of a carcinoma placing Cooper's ligaments under tension (Fig. 22–8). Simple maneuvers such as stretching the arms high above the head, tensing the pectoralis muscles, or gently lifting the patient's breast may accentuate asymmetries and dimpling. It is a misconception to equate skin dimpling with advanced cancer. This sign is frequently found in very small, scirrhous tumors that do not produce a large mass effect. If carefully sought, dimpling of the skin or nipple retraction is a sensitive and specific sign of underlying cancer.

Edema of the skin, frequently accompanied by erythema, produces a clinical sign known as peau d'orange (Fig. 22–9). When combined with tenderness and warmth, these signs and symptoms are the hallmark of inflammatory carcinoma and may be mistaken for acute mastitis. Although these clinical signs are often dramatic, they can be overlooked in dark-skinned people or if a careful examination with proper lighting is not performed. The inflammatory changes and

edema are caused by obstruction of dermal lymphatic channels with emboli of carcinoma cells. Occasionally, a bulky tumor may produce obstruction of large lymph channels that results in overlying skin edema. This is not, strictly speaking, an inflammatory carcinoma in which the visible signs are out of proportion to the palpable mass. In 40 patients with inflammatory carcinoma treated by Haagensen, all cases presented with erythema and edema of the skin; a palpable mass or localized induration was present in 19; and in 21 patients no localized tumor was present.

Involvement of the nipple and areola is a common histologic finding in breasts removed for carcinoma. Direct involvement may accompany tumors originating in breast tissue under the areola and may result in retraction of the usually protruding nipple. Flattening or actual inversion of the nipple can be caused by fibrosis in certain benign conditions, especially subareolar duct ectasia. In these cases, the finding is frequently bilateral and the history confirms that the condition has been present for many years. Unilateral retraction or retraction developing over weeks or months is more suggestive of carcinoma. Centrally located tumors may directly invade and ulcerate the skin of the areola or nipple. More peripheral tumors may distort the normal symmetry of the nipples by traction on Cooper's ligaments.

The second clinical feature of carcinoma that directly involves the nipple was described by Sir James Paget in 1874 and named Paget's disease. Histologically, this disease is produced by intraductal carcinoma occurring in the large sinuses just under the nipple. Carcinoma cells invade across the epidermal-epithelial junction and enter the epidermal layer of the skin of the nipple. Clinically, this histologic variant produces a dermatitis that may appear eczematoid and moist or dry and psoriatic. It is usually confined to the nipple, although it can spread to the skin of the areola. Haagensen points out that benign skin conditions frequently begin on the areola, whereas Paget's disease originates on the nipple and secondarily involves the areola.

Palpation follows visual inspection. While the patient is

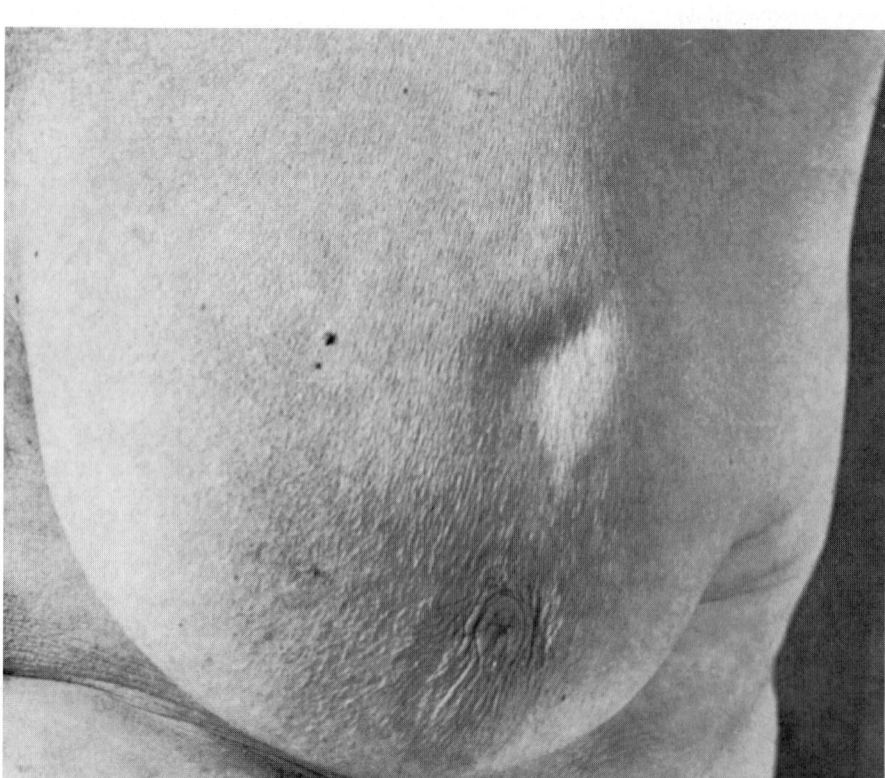

Figure 22–8. Dimple in the skin of the breast overlying a small carcinoma in the upper quadrant. The use of indirect lighting accentuates this subtle clinical finding, which might be overlooked if examined under poor lighting or without the subject sitting upright with the arm extended. (From Haagensen, C. D.: Diseases of the Breast, 3rd ed. Philadelphia, W. B. Saunders, 1986, p. 521.)

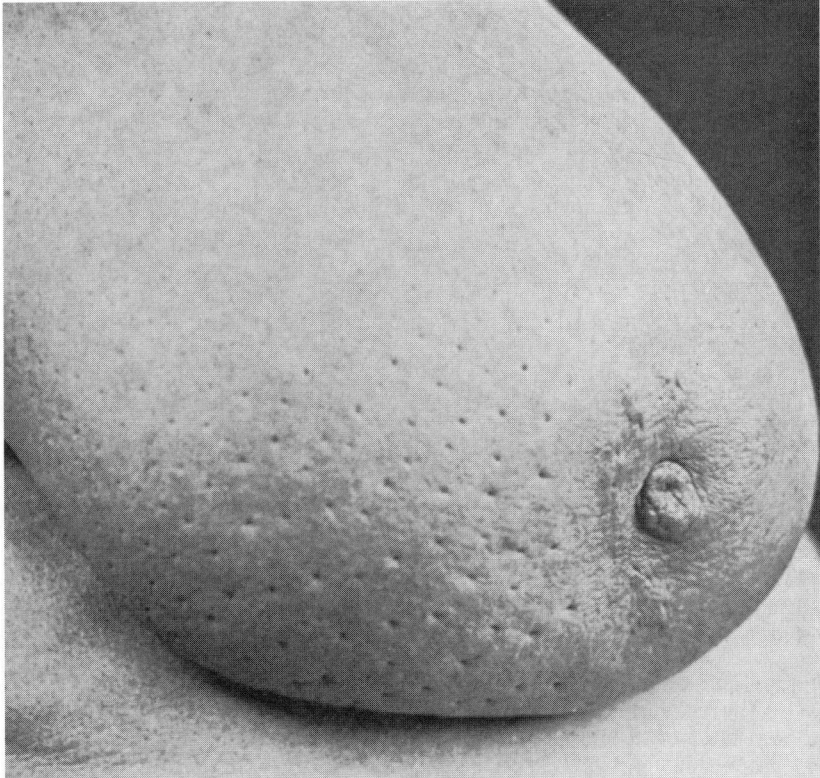

Figure 22–9. Edema of the skin in a breast with inflammatory carcinoma. Edema of the dermis produces the peau d'orange (orange peel) appearance of the skin. The pitting is caused by the tethering of the epidermis over the swollen dermis by small hair follicles. Erythema of the skin generally accompanies the peau d'orange change. (From Haagensen, C. D.: Diseases of the Breast, 3rd ed. Philadelphia, W. B. Saunders, 1986, p. 521.)

still in the sitting position, the examiner supports the patient's arm and palpates each axilla to detect the presence of enlarged axillary lymph nodes. The supraclavicular space is similarly palpated for enlarged nodes. Palpation of the breast is always done with the patient lying supine on a solid examining surface and with the arm stretched above the head. Palpation of the breast while the patient is sitting is insensitive and inaccurate. The examiner compresses the breast parenchyma against the chest wall, carefully palpating each quadrant and the tissue under the areola. Masses found during this examination are characterized according to their size, shape, consistency, and location. Benign tumors, such as fibroadenomas and cysts, can be as firm as carcinoma; however, these tumors are usually distinct, well-circumscribed, and movable. Carcinoma is typically firm but less circumscribed, and its movement produces a drag of adjacent tissue. Neither benign nor malignant tumors are usually tender; tenderness is rarely a helpful diagnostic sign. Generally, 75% of breast cancers produce palpable masses and 75% of palpable masses are discovered by patients during casual or intentional self-examination.

Fine-Needle Aspiration. Fine-needle aspiration has become a routine part of the physical diagnosis of breast masses.[13] It can be done with a 22-gauge needle, an appropriate size syringe, and an alcohol prep pad. Its main utility is the differentiation of solid from cystic masses, but it may be done whenever a new dominant, unexplained mass is found in the breast. This simple procedure is postponed only if mammography is necessary and there is worry that a small hematoma, resulting from needle puncture, might confuse the radiographic evaluation. Cyst fluid is usually turbid dark green or amber and can be discarded if the mass totally disappears and the fluid is not bloody. By using fine-needle aspiration in the routine examination of the breast, unnecessary open biopsy of cystic change is avoided. As a result of adding fine-needle aspiration to the routine examination of breast masses, a restating of criteria for open biopsy is help-

ful. Carcinoma will not be missed if a formal biopsy is done when (1) needle aspiration produces no cyst fluid and a solid mass is diagnosed, (2) the cyst fluid produced is thick and blood tinged, (3) fluid is produced but the mass fails to resolve completely, and (4) the mass reappears in the same area after more than two aspirations. Donegan adds rapid accumulation of fluid after initial aspiration (<2 weeks) to this last criterion.

If the mass is solid, and the clinical situation is consistent with carcinoma, a cytologic examination of the aspirated material may be helpful. The needle is repeatedly inserted into the mass while constant negative pressure is applied to the syringe. Suction is released and the needle is withdrawn. The scanty fluid and cellular material within the needle are submitted either in physiologically buffered saline (Normosol) or fixed immediately on slides in 95% ethyl alcohol. Most authors would not recommend definitive treatment based on a cytologic examination only. However, a positive result allows for informed discussion with the patient, definite plans for treatment can be made, and appropriate consultations or second opinions can be obtained.

Breast Imaging[2, 30]

The goal of any technique that seeks to image the breast is to extend the capability of physical examination to either detect smaller abnormalities or to provide more information about palpable abnormalities. Mammography is clearly the most sensitive and specific test that can be used to complement the physical examination of the breast. It is used either as a diagnostic modality that seeks to answer specific questions about the health of the breast or as a screening test that seeks to find any abnormality within the breast. A variety of other methods have been used to generate useful images of the breast. Of these, ultrasonography is the only one in common use today. Thermography, which images heat generated by the breast, was added to the Breast Cancer Detection

Demonstration Project (BCDDP) to evaluate its usefulness as a screening tool. However, because of a low overall yield, thermography was dropped from the project. Computed tomography (CT) has been used by some investigators with success but can require contrast medium enhancement, has limited ability to resolve small abnormalities, and requires a larger exposure of radiation. CT appears to be the best way to image internal mammary nodes and to evaluate the chest and axilla after mastectomy. Magnetic resonance imaging (MRI) is a technique that requires expensive equipment. The long times required to construct a suitable image are acceptable for diagnostic applications but prohibit MRI as a screening tool. MRI may have a role in evaluating breasts that are difficult to image or after prosthetic implantation. Digital imaging is an evolving hybrid technology that has found application in chest radiography and may be used to store radiographic information in a digital format or to directly produce images. This technology is improving and may have application in mammography.

Diagnostic Mammography. Film-screen mammography has replaced xeromammography as the standard breast imaging technology. Xeromammography was developed by the Xerox corporation and produced a blue image viewed in ambient reflected light. Modern film-screen mammography uses a combination of an enhancing screen and a molybdenum anode tube that produces low kilovolt electron photons. The enhancing screen converts and amplifies a low-energy radiation beam into high-energy photons that, in turn, expose a standard x-ray film. This technique uses compression of the breast between plexiglass plates to lessen the thickness of the tissue through which the radiation must pass and to separate adjacent structures and improve resolution. The image, like standard x-rays, is viewed using transmitted light and is a negative image. Film-screen mammography delivers an average glandular dose of radiation that is less than 100 mrad. (0.1 cGy. or 0.1 rad.). In comparison, the average dose to the center of the breast in patients undergoing barium swallow is more than 10-fold the dose of two-view mammography.

The mammographic features of malignancy can be broadly divided into density abnormalities (including masses, asymmetries, and architectural distortions) and microcalcifications. Each mammogram should also be assessed for the presence of abnormalities in the axillary nodes and for the presence of skin or nipple changes, such as thickening or retraction. These mammographic features can coexist in any one particular abnormality and may exist in the presence or absence of physical findings. In fact, integration of each of the radiographic features and the physical findings leads to a prediction of malignancy. An atlas of mammographic abnormalities has been compiled by Kopans and includes excellent narrative descriptions and a general review of breast imaging. Selected pictures of mammographic abnormalities are displayed in Figures 22–10 and 22–11, which illustrate common findings of malignancy.

Nonpalpable Mammographic Abnormalities.[31, 45] Mammographic abnormalities that cannot be detected by physical examination are classified in three broad categories: (1) lesions consisting of microcalcifications only, (2) density lesions (masses, architectural distortions, and asymmetries), and (3) those with both calcifications and density abnormalities. The incidence of malignancy after biopsy depends on the characteristics of the radiographic finding. The results from 179 patients at Duke University are shown in Table 22–2. Overall, the incidence of malignancy was 24%; this figure agreed with several similar studies reporting chances of malignancy of between 14% and 29%. Lesions with both microcalcifications and a mass effect, spiculated masses, and linear branching calcifications carry the highest probability of being malig-

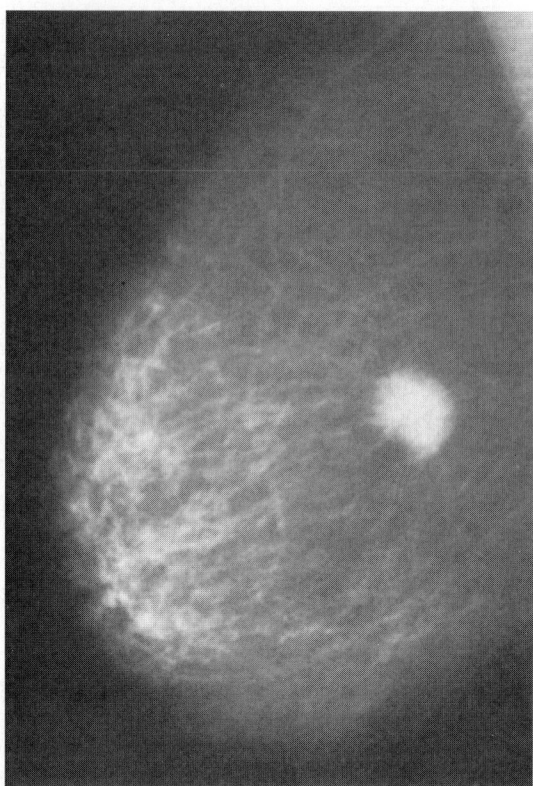

Figure 22–10. Mammographic features of malignancy: a stellate mass. The combination of a density, surrounding spiculations, and distortion of the breast architecture strongly suggest a malignancy in this mammogram.

nant. However, even well-defined densities can be malignant. To be certain, not every abnormality should undergo biopsy, and recommendations must be made by the surgeon in consultation with an experienced radiologist. For those patients not undergoing biopsy, interval mammograms must be done to ensure stability of the abnormality.

If a biopsy is performed, it is usually done after mammographic placement of a needle or hook wire. A newer alternative is automated stereotactic core-needle biopsy. This procedure requires a large and dedicated unit, which is expensive. The patient generally lies prone with the breast hanging through the table. A robotic arm and biopsy gun is positioned by computerized analysis of triangulated mammographic images. A small amount of local anesthesia is used at the point of core-needle entry into the breast. Firing the machine obtains a core biopsy through the abnormality. Many series containing hundreds of patients have shown good correlation between stereotactic biopsy and subsequent needle-placement open biopsy. For lesions with calcification, a specimen radiograph must be done to confirm the presence of the abnormality in the specimen. This is true for both stereotactic and open biopsy procedures. Cooperation is required between the radiologist, surgeon, and pathologist for the correct interpretation of biopsy material obtained by either technique. If stereotactic biopsy is available to the surgeon, judgment must be used to determine the optimal biopsy strategy. Because stereotactic biopsy does not remove the abnormality, a subsequent localization and open procedure will be required if a cancer is found and the patient wishes to attempt breast conservation. If the abnormality proves benign after stereotactic biopsy, follow-up mammography needs to be done if the lesion is indeterminate. The false-negative rate of stereotactic biopsy is low but finite.

Screening Mammography.[6, 20] The goals of screening mam-

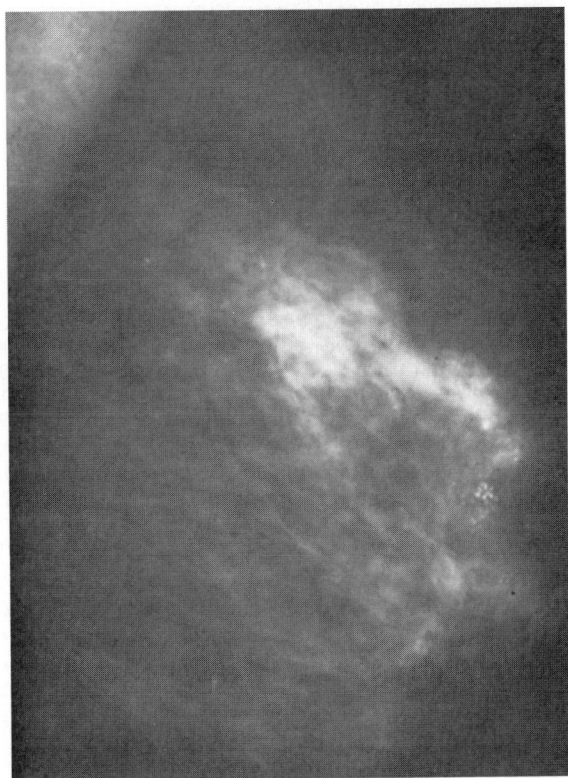

Figure 22–11. Mammographic features of malignancy: clustered microcalcifications. Fine, irregular, and branching forms suggest malignancy in this mammogram. Fine calcifications, <0.5 mm. in size, are more often associated with cancer than larger, coarse calcifications.

mography differ from those of diagnostic mammography. Screening studies seek to identify any abnormality, maximizing sensitivity and cost effectiveness. During the past three decades, there have been eight major randomized controlled

TABLE 22–2. Biopsy Results for Various Mammographic Features

Mammographic Feature*	Malignant	Benign	Per Cent Positive	
Asymmetric density†	6	25	19	
Architectural distortion	7	10	41	
Mass†	20	51	28	
Mass subtotals				
Stellate	6	2	75	
Irregularly defined	12	22	35	
Well defined	2	27	6	
Number of calcifications				
>10	14	27	34	
≤10	8	44	15	p = .07
Size of calcifications				
≥0.4 mm.	13	41	24	
<0.4 mm.	9	30	23	p > .25
Distribution of calcifications‡				
Clustered	9	37	20	
Scattered	9	15	38	p = .15

*The radiographic features are considered independently (i.e., lesions having both a soft tissue lesion and calcifications are included twice).

†Lesions not associated with an architectural distortion.

‡Lesions having more than five calcifications.

From Skinner, M. A., Swain, M., Simmons, R., et al.: Nonpalpable breast lesions at biopsy: A detailed analysis of radiographic features. Ann. Surg., 208:203, 1988.

trials that compared a screened population to women given usual care. Although screening intervals and mammographic techniques differed, each of these studies included mammography with or without clinical breast examination in the screened arms. In the United States, a single uncontrolled study was done to demonstrate the feasibility of a population-based screening program. The BCDDP screened 280,000 women annually in 29 centers throughout the United States. Each center offered free mammograms and a breast examination and taught breast self-examination. Participants in the BCDDP have been followed for 14 years, and survival data were published. Because this was not a controlled trial, comparison has been made to national statistics compiled by the Surveillance, Epidemiology, and End Results (SEER) program within the National Cancer Institute (NCI). Comparison of survival data 8 years after diagnosis of cancer in the BCDDP to corresponding data from the SEER program demonstrates improved survival in the screened population, which seems to be explained by a shift to earlier stage disease in the BCDDP.

In 1993, the NCI held an International Workshop on Screening for Breast Cancer that reviewed the world's most current data on screening women between the ages of 40 and 74. Tables 22–3 and 22–4 are derived from the summary of this conference. Table 22–3 presents selected characteristics of eight trials from North America and Europe that randomized nearly 500,000 women. Table 22–4 summarizes results expressed as the relative risk of breast cancer mortality in the screened cohort compared with the control group. After reviewing published and presented data, the NCI workshop concluded the following:

1. Randomized trials of women aged 40 to 49 are consistent in showing no statistically significant benefit in mortality after 10 to 12 years of follow-up.

2. Results from all trials confirm a significant benefit for women aged 50 to 69, which is approximately a 34% reduction in mortality from breast cancer.

3. Too few women over the age of 70 were included in randomized studies to draw valid conclusions regarding screening.

As a result of this review, the NCI has modified its recommendations regarding the routine use of screening in women younger than 50.

BENIGN BREAST TUMORS AND RELATED DISEASES

Breast Cysts.[24] Cysts within the breast are fluid-filled, epithelial-lined cavities that may vary in size from microscopic to large, palpable masses containing as much as 20 to 30 ml. of fluid. As discussed, cysts are generally discovered by physical examination and confirmed by ultrasound or needle aspiration. At least one woman in every 14 will develop a palpable cyst, and 50% of cysts are multiple or recurrent. Cysts occur as solitary abnormalities, called macrocysts or gross breast cysts, or as part of a generalized process of microscopic cyst formation. This latter disease process is frequently bilateral and the cystic transformation can be extensive. The pathogenesis of cystic formation is not well understood; however, cysts appear to arise from destruction and dilation of lobules and terminal ductules. Three-dimensional microscopic studies and extensive sectioning have shown that stricture and fibrosis at or near terminal branching of small ductules, combined with continued secretion by the distal lobule, result in expansion of a cavity containing fluid and lined by ductal epithelium.

Cysts are unquestionably influenced by ovarian hormones, a fact that explains their sudden appearance during the men-

TABLE 22–3. Selected Characteristics of the Design and Conduct of Eight Randomized Controlled Trials of Breast Cancer Screening

Study (Year Begun)	Age at Entry (yr.)	Periodicity (mo.)	Randomization	Sample Size Study	Sample Size Control
HIP (1963)	40–64	12	Individual	30239	30756
Sweden					
Two-county (1977)	40–74	24 (age >50 yr.) 33 (age ≥50 yr.)	Cluster: geographic	78085	56782
Malmö (1976)	45–69	18–24	Cluster: birth cohort	21088	21195
Stockholm (1981)	40–64	28	Cluster: birth cohort	39164	19943
Göteborg (1982)	40–59	18	Individual (age 40–49 yr.) Cluster (age 50–59 yr.)	20724	28809
Edinburgh (1976)	45–64	12	Cluster: physician	23226	21904
Canada NBSS1 (1980)	40–49	12	Individual: volunteers	25214	25216
Canada NBSS2 (1980)	50–59	12	Individual: volunteers	19711	19694

Adapted from Fletcher, S. W., Black, W., Harris, R., et al.: Report of the International Workshop on Screening for Breast Cancer. J. Natl. Cancer Inst., *85*:1644, 1993. All references to individual trials are included in the report.

strual cycle, their rapid growth, and their spontaneous regression with completion of the menses. Most women with new cyst formation present after the age of 35 and rarely before the age of 25 years. The incidence of cyst development steadily increases until the age of menopause and sharply declines after menopause (Fig. 22–12). Autopsy studies of women dying with clinically normal breasts generally confirm the age relationship of gross cyst development but do find that the breasts of older women can contain gross and microscopic cysts. New cyst formation detected clinically in older women commonly is explained by the use of exogenous hormone replacement.

When encountered during operation, cysts are frequently dark. These are often referred to as *blue dome cysts,* and they reflect the dark cyst fluid contained within. Grossly, they are usually unilocular and lined by a smooth and glistening surface, although larger cystic structures may be trabeculated and multiloculated. Histologically, cysts are frequently lined by a flattened epithelium. However, the epithelial layer may display apocrine metaplasia or may have papillary features. Intracystic carcinoma is exceedingly rare. Rosemond was able to report only three examples in over 3000 cyst aspirations (0.1%), and other investigators confirm this exceedingly low incidence. Regarding the risk of developing cancer for women with cystic disease, no studies demonstrate an increased risk in women with small or microscopic cysts. For

patients with large cysts, called gross cystic disease by Haagensen, there remains some controversy. Patey and Nurick found no increase in cancers subsequent to cyst aspiration. Of 810 cancers treated by Patey, only 10 had a previous history of gross cysts. Other recent reviews have emphasized that women with gross cysts have a risk of twofold to fourfold that of age-matched women without cysts. The studies of Page and associates and of Dupont and Page do not show a significant increase in cancers after long-term follow-up of over 2000 women who underwent biopsy of palpable cysts when compared with the slight increase borne by women who have had breast biopsy alone.

Fibroadenoma and Related Tumors. Fibroadenoma (adenofibroma) is a benign tumor composed of both stromal and epithelial elements in the breast.[38] After carcinoma, fibroadenoma is the second most common solid tumor in the breast and is the most common tumor in women younger than age 30 years. The benign nature of this lesion was recognized in 1840 by Cooper, who referred to the lesions as "chronic mammary tumors." Clinically, they present as firm, solitary tumors that may increase in size over several months of observation. They may be lobulated but will slip easily under the examining fingers. At operation, fibroadenomas appear to be well-encapsulated masses that may easily detach from the surrounding breast tissue. By history, fibroadenoma is favored over cyst in the adolescent or young adult (see Fig.

TABLE 22–4. Relative Risk for Death due to Breast Cancer in Eight Randomized Trials of Screening

Trial	Age at Entry (yr.)	Duration of Follow-up (yr.)	Relative Risk (95% Confidence Interval) All Ages	Relative Risk (95% Confidence Interval) Younger than 50 yr.
HIP (1963)	40–64	10	0.71 (0.55–0.93)	0.77 (0.50–1.16)
Sweden				
Kopparberg	40–74	12	0.68 (0.52–0.89)	0.75 (0.41–1.36)
Ostergotland	40–74	12	0.82 (0.64–1.05)	1.28 (0.76–2.33)
Malmö	45–69	12	0.81 (0.62–1.07)	0.51 (0.22–1.17)
Stockholm	40–64	8	0.80 (0.53–1.22)	1.04 (0.53–2.05)
Göteborg	40–59	7	0.86 (0.54–1.37)	0.73 (0.27–1.97)
All centers	40–74	7–12	0.74 (0.66–0.87)	0.87 (0.63–1.20)
Edinburgh	45–64	10	0.84 (0.63–1.12)	0.86 (0.41–1.80)
Canada				
NBSS1	40–49	7		1.36 (0.84–2.21)
NBSS2	50–59	7	0.97 (0.62–1.52)	

Adapted from Fletcher, S. W., Black, W., Harris, R., et al.: Report of the International Workshop on Screening for Breast Cancer. J. Natl. Cancer Inst., *85*:1644, 1993. All references to individual trials are included in the report.

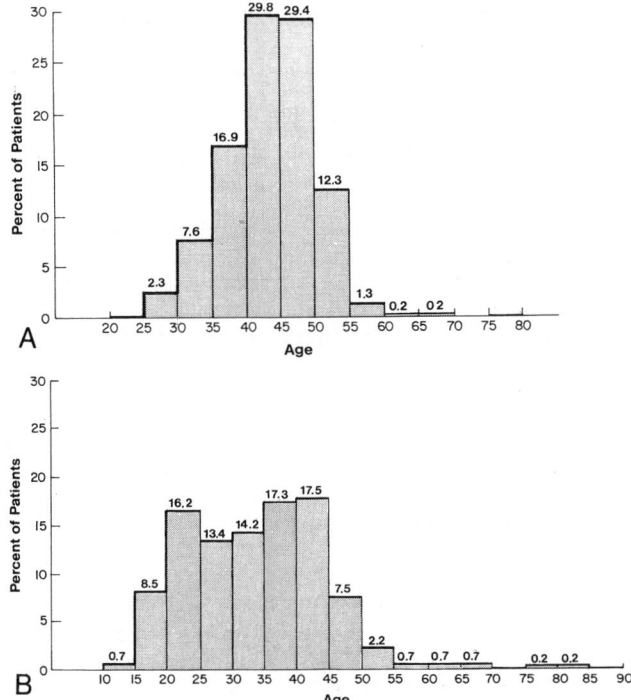

Figure 22–12. Age distribution of common benign breast tumors. In *A*, the age distribution of gross breast cysts is shown. The incidence is very low until the fourth decade of life, increases sharply until the age of menopause, and then declines sharply. In *B*, the age distribution of fibroadenoma is shown. In contrast to breast cysts, fibroadenoma can occur in young women after the menarche, but the incidence again declines sharply after menopause. (From Haagensen, C. D.: Disease of the Breast, 3rd ed. Philadelphia, W. B. Saunders, 1986, pp. 256, 268.)

22–12); and on examination, these tumors are distinguished from cysts by the needle aspiration that yields no fluid. Mammography is of little help in distinguishing between cysts and fibroadenomas; however, ultrasound usually clearly shows the cavity of a cyst. The gross appearance and histopathology are distinctive of fibroadenoma. Grossly, the tumor appears well encapsulated, with smooth borders that may be lobulated. Histologically, a variable proportion of epithelial and stromal proliferation is present, and the stroma may be quite cellular or replaced by acellular swirls of collagen. In older patients, the lesions may contain deposits of calcium within dense fibrosis. The epithelium can display the entire spectrum of proliferative changes seen elsewhere in the breast. Although fibroadenomas are not considered to have a malignant potential, the epithelial elements appear to be at risk for neoplasia just as epithelium elsewhere in the breast. More than 100 invasive and noninvasive carcinomas have been reported in preexisting fibroadenomas since 1985. Most of these (50%) have been lobular carcinoma *in situ*, 35% were infiltrating carcinomas, and 15% were intraductal carcinoma. The risk of cancer in a newly discovered fibroadenoma found in the breast of a young woman is obviously exceedingly rare and is not an issue that influences treatment. A modest risk of subsequent carcinoma in women who have previously been treated for fibroadenoma has been reported, but the magnitude is about two times the general population. This is only slightly higher than the reported excess risk for all women who have had a breast biopsy.

The treatment of fibroadenoma follows that for any unexplained solid mass within the breast. The great majority of patients in the United States are treated by excisional biopsy to remove the tumor and establish the diagnosis. It is worth recognizing that a different approach is taken by physicians

in other countries. A typical fibroadenoma is frequently left untreated by European physicians when the tumor is encountered in the breast of a young women. If excision is recommended, the approach to a young women with a typical fibroadenoma on examination should be very different than the approach in older women with indeterminate masses. Cosmetic incisions around the areola with a modest amount of tunneling to remove the lesion are commonly used techniques and are proper for the treatment of fibroadenoma. Emphasis should be placed on removing a minimum amount of breast tissue adjacent to a typical fibroadenoma. If the gross appearance is that of a fibroadenoma, frozen section is superfluous, the patient can be immediately reassured, and final diagnosis can be established by inspecting permanent sections.

Juvenile Fibroadenoma, Giant Fibroadenoma. Clinicians treating breast masses should be aware of these two terms, which are sometimes confusing. *Giant fibroadenoma* is a descriptive term that applies to a fibroadenoma that attains an unusually large size, typically greater than 5 cm. Haagensen calls these lesions "massive adenofibromas in youth" to denote their common occurrence in adolescent women. *Juvenile fibroadenoma* refers to the occasional large fibroadenoma that occurs in adolescents and young adults and histologically is more cellular than the usual fibroadenoma. Both these lesions overlap, and both may display remarkably rapid growth within the breast. Although alarming to the patient and physician, prompt surgical removal is always curative. The term *benign cystosarcoma phylloides* refers to a tumor that may be difficult to distinguish clearly from juvenile fibroadenoma. If the tumor has been completely removed, the diagnosis of benign cystosarcoma should reassure the surgeon and the patient that the risk of recurrence is low, particularly if the patient is an adolescent or a young adult. Malignant cystosarcoma phylloides is a distinctive and aggressive tumor discussed later.

Hamartoma and Adenoma. Although probably not of the same histogenesis as fibroadenoma, these tumors are benign proliferations of variable amounts of epithelium and stromal supporting tissue. The hamartoma is a discrete nodule that contains closely packed lobules and prominent, ectatic extralobular ducts. By physical examination, mammography, and gross inspection, the hamartoma is indistinguishable from fibroadenoma. The nodule is entirely benign, and removal is curative. The mammary adenoma or tubular adenoma has been a more elusive entity to define. Page and Anderson describe this tumor as a cellular neoplasm of ductules packed closely together and forming a sheet of tiny glands without supporting stroma. During pregnancy and lactation, these tumors may increase in size and histologic examination shows secretory differentiation. Malignancy is not a feature of tubular adenoma or lactating adenoma, but biopsy is required to establish the diagnosis.

Breast Abscess and Infections. Breast abscess commonly occurs in the subareolar breast tissue and may be recurrent and difficult to treat.[24] Although the exact cause is not known, subareolar duct ectasia and obstruction of major ducts may lead to proliferation of bacteria and subsequent abscess. Further destruction of the normal ductal openings leads to fistula formation and chronic recurrent abscess. Mammary duct ectasia, first named by Haagensen, is an inflammatory condition that causes distortion and dilation of the lactiferous sinuses under the nipple. It is a common entity and is frequently responsible for nipple inversion in older women. In understanding subareolar abscess and probably mastitis in general, it is useful to remember that the nipple and areolar complex contains secretory ducts that are exposed to the environment. Chronic inflammation, duct dilation, and obstruction may combine at the nipple to produce circumstances that favor bacterial invasion.

The treatment of acute abscess of periareolar tissue should be conservative if possible. Antibiotics with broad-spectrum coverage should be used initially. More severe infections may require hospitalization and intravenous antibiotics. A small incision with drainage is preferred if the process cannot be controlled by antibiotics alone. Needle aspiration may be attempted, but the abscess cavity is usually multiloculated. Recurrent infection is best treated by excision of the diseased subareolar ducts as described by Haagensen and others. However, recurrence is common and leads to chronic and recurring infection.

Mastitis describes a more generalized cellulitis of breast tissue that may involve a large area of the breast but may not form a true abscess. The etiology appears to be an ascending infection beginning in subareolar ducts and extending outward from the nipple. Occasionally, mastitis involves areas of cystic disease and may be sterile. Mastitis presents with erythema of the overlying skin, pain, and tenderness to palpation. There is induration of the skin and underlying breast parenchyma. Especially in young women, an apparent mastitis may develop that is dramatic in its presentation and responds poorly to antibiotics but resolves spontaneously. The etiology is unknown but may be related to menstrual cycle irregularity. More commonly, mastitis complicates lactation, possibly due to inspissation of milk, obstruction, and secondary infection. Local measures such as application of heat, ice packs, or use of a mechanical breast pump on the affected side have all been recommended. If conservative measures are not effective, administration of broad-spectrum antibiotics is usually indicated. In many situations, the differential diagnosis of acute mastitis includes inflammatory carcinoma. It is important to follow patients with mastitis and confirm that there has been a complete resolution of symptoms and signs. The erythema produced by an inflammatory carcinoma will not resolve with conservative measures and generally will worsen in a short period of follow-up.

Papilloma and Related Ductal Tumors.[24, 38] Solitary intraductal papillomas are true polyps of epithelial-lined breast ducts. Solitary papillomas are located under the areola in the majority of cases. In contrast, certain patients have multiple intraductal papillomas that Haagensen believes are more likely to be peripherally located and associated with an increased risk of cancer. Solitary papillomas may be located in peripheral ducts and can grow to large size, presenting as a breast mass. When papillomas attain a large size, they may appear to arise within a cystic structure, probably representing a greatly expanded duct. In general, these lesions are less than 1 cm. but can grow to as large as 4 or 5 cm.

Tumors under the nipple and areolar complex often present with a bloody nipple discharge. Less frequently, they are discovered as a palpable mass under the areola or as a density lesion on the mammogram. Treatment is total excision through a circumareolar incision. The surgeon must keep in mind that one of the most difficult areas in differential diagnosis is between a papilloma and invasive papillary carcinoma. Because these lesions can infarct, scar, and even develop squamous metaplasia, they can appear bizarre and disordered. Most pathologists urge evaluation on permanent sections for the majority of papillary lesions before more extensive surgery is undertaken.

It is also important not to confuse the commonly used term *papillomatosis* with either solitary or multiple papillomas. Papillomatosis refers to epithelial hyperplasia that commonly occurs in younger women or is associated with fibrocystic change. This lesion is not composed of true papillomas. Hyperplastic epithelium in papillomatosis may fill individual ducts like a true polyp but has no stalk of fibrovascular tissue

nor the frondlike growth. Solitary papillomas are entirely benign and do not predispose to development of cancer in the patients who have them. Page and Anderson state that the degree of subsequent risk for breast cancer in patients with either papillomatosis or with true papillomas, either solitary or multiple, relates to the degree of atypical epithelial proliferation associated with them.

Sclerosing Lesions[25]

Sclerosing Adenosis. Adenosis refers to an increased number of small terminal ductules or acini. It is frequently associated with a proliferation of stromal tissue producing a histologic lesion, sclerosing adenosis, which can simulate carcinoma both grossly and histologically. There may be deposition of calcium, which can be seen on mammography in a pattern indistinguishable from microcalcifications in intraductal carcinoma. In fact, sclerosing adenosis was the most common pathologic diagnosis in patients undergoing needle-directed biopsy of microcalcifications at Duke University. Sclerosing adenosis is frequently listed as one of the component lesions of fibrocystic disease; it is very common and has no malignant potential.

Radial Scar. Radial scar belongs to a group of related abnormalities known as complex sclerosing lesions. They are important to the surgeon and pathologist because they can simulate carcinoma mammographically and on physical examination. These lesions contain microcysts, epithelial hyperplasia, adenosis, and a prominent display of central sclerosis. The gross abnormality is rarely more than 1 cm. in diameter. The larger lesions form palpable tumors and appear as a spiculated mass with prominent architectural distortion on the mammogram. These tumors can even produce skin dimpling by traction on surrounding fibrous bands that become involved in the cicatrix. Biopsy is always recommended for tumors with these signs and symptoms. Aside from their confusing presentation, these lesions are benign.

Fat Necrosis. As with the other sclerosing abnormalities, fat necrosis can mimic cancer by producing a mass, a density lesion on mammography that can calcify, and surrounding distortion of the normal breast architecture. Fat necrosis typically occurs in pendulous fatty breasts; and although it may follow an episode of trauma, commonly there is no such history. Histologically, the lesion is composed of lipid-laden macrophages, scar tissue, and chronic inflammatory cells. This is not a lesion of epithelial tissue and has no malignant potential. It is usually sampled because of the signs it produces.

MALIGNANT TUMORS OF THE BREAST
Epidemiology

The likelihood of developing breast cancer is highly dependent on both age and the interval over which an individual is at risk.[24, 25] Although the lifetime risk of developing breast cancer is estimated at 10%, more than one half of patients with breast cancer are older than 65. Furthermore, the 10% figure is based on a hypothetical interval that extends from birth to age 110. A more realistic view considers risk starting at a particular age and extends over a finite period of time. For instance, the chance that a woman age 35 will develop breast cancer during the next two decades of her life, until age 55, is only 2.5%. A woman who is 50 has close to a 5% chance of developing cancer before she turns 75 and a 65-year-old woman has a 5.5% chance of getting breast cancer before she turns 85 years of age. These figures apply to white women in the United States; the same idealized African-American woman has a lifetime risk of breast cancer that is 7% or 8%.

The odds of dying of breast cancer over the ideal lifetime

of birth to 110 are about 3.6%. Although carcinoma of the lung has overtaken breast cancer as the leading cause of cancer-related death in American women, breast cancer remains far more common. Of 595,000 new cases of cancer among women in 1996, 186,000 occurred in the breast while 78,000 arose in the lung.

Several studies based on cancer registries in the SEER program of the NCI have reported an increasing attack rate for breast cancer in the United States. In Washington State there has been an annual estimated increase of 2.5%. A greater increase was apparent among black and low-income women. In the Connecticut Tumor Registry the overall annual incidence rose from 53 cases per 100,000 women during the years 1935 to 1939 to an average annual rate of 86.4 per 100,000 for the years 1975 to 1979. The annual rate of increase during 1980 to 1985 averaged 3%; during the past 5 years, this rate of increase has declined to about 1% per year. Data from other studies and from other western countries confirm the increase in the incidence of breast cancer. Despite this increased incidence, the age-adjusted death rate from carcinoma of the breast was stable until 1979 and may have decreased in the 5-year period between 1979 and 1984. Although it is tempting to speculate that this is a real improvement attributable to early diagnosis or improved therapy, no direct proof can be cited.

Genetics of Breast Cancer[29, 43]

Passage of genetic factors contributes to a small number of breast cancers, estimated to be about 5%, but may account for 25% of cases in women younger than 30 years of age. In 1988, a group led by Mary-Claire King provided evidence for transmission of a gene in high-risk families and by 1990 had identified a region on the long arm of chromosome 17 (17q21) that contained a susceptibility gene. This effort was made possible by the recognition that genetically determined breast cancer was more likely to occur in younger patients. The gene, BRCA1, was intensively sought by several international groups and finally discovered in the summer of 1994. Although it is inherited as a dominant genetic trait, BRCA1 acts like a tumor suppressor or recessive oncogene, which may provide a negative regulation of cell growth or perhaps is involved in recognition and repair of genetic damage or spontaneous mutation. Germ-line mutation that inactivates a single inherited allele precedes a somatic event, which occurs in at-risk breast epithelial cells, and eliminates the remaining BRCA1 allele. BRCA1 is a large gene with 24 exons, which makes genetic testing a technically difficult procedure. In addition, genetic testing for cancer susceptibility genes raises ethical, legal, and financial considerations just beginning to undergo intense research and scrutiny. These issues are challenging topics for clinical researchers in the future.

At the same time BRCA1 was identified, a second susceptibility locus was mapped to chromosome 13. This gene, known as BRCA2, accounts for up to 30% of familial breast cancer. Although BRCA1 predisposes to both breast and ovarian cancer in families, BRCA2 appears to be more restricted to breast cancer, and these families may have cases of male breast cancer. In the fall of 1995, BRCA2 was identified and cloned. Like BRCA1, it is a large and complex gene of unknown function. Together BRCA1 and BRCA2 account for about 75% of highly penetrant hereditary breast cancer. The unanswered questions are many but include the following:

1. What are the functions of these genes in normal breast cells?

2. Who should be tested and what should physicians and surgeons recommend to patients carrying mutations in these genes?

3. What can these genes teach us about the prevention of breast cancer?

Surgeons should be informed and play active roles in this rapidly evolving field of oncology that concerns genetic susceptibility.

Pathology of Breast Cancer[23, 38]

Modern classification of breast cancer attempts to recognize morphologic patterns that reflect both the histogenesis of the malignancy and its biologic behavior, or prognosis. As such, these classifications impose artificial divisions on diseases that are fundamentally poorly understood. As advances are made in our understanding of breast malignancies, the classifications presented today will be improved on by future generations of surgeons and pathologists. Malignancies of the breast are broadly divided into epithelial tumors of cells lining ducts and lobules and nonepithelial malignancies of the supporting stroma. A second important division of the epithelial tumors that recognizes their evolution is between noninvasive and invasive cancers. The noninvasive malignancies are proliferations of either ductal or lobular cells confined to the basement membrane. These are true carcinoma in situ. As in other organs, carcinoma in situ commonly coexists with invasive cancer. In the breast, this association is very frequent and argues for the progression of cancer through stages of noninvasive proliferation, disruption of the basement membrane, and invasion of the supporting stroma.

Most pathologists utilize the classification scheme proposed by the World Health Organization (WHO) and outlined in the fascicles of the Armed Forces Institute of Pathology. Historically, Foote and Stewart presented most of this material in 1945, including a recognition of noninvasive carcinoma and the differentiation between tumors originating in the breast lobule from those arising in the lactiferous ducts. Table 22–5 presents the WHO classification scheme for the major histologic types of both benign and malignant tumors in the breast. Figure 22–13 is a reproduction of examples provided by the WHO for illustrating some of the common morphologies of invasive breast cancers.

Ductal Carcinoma in Situ (DCIS), Intraductal Carcinoma. The concept of a purely noninvasive form of breast cancer and recognition of various subtypes have evolved slowly since the beginning of this century. DCIS was probably recognized first by surgeons who appreciated its favorable prognosis. Bloodgood, at the Johns Hopkins Hospital, impressed by the tumor of an early patient of Halsted, recognized a disease he termed "pure comedo tumor" that had an extremely favorable prognosis. Pathologically, breast ducts become swollen with proliferating malignant epithelium. In the solid or comedo type, the ducts can expand to visible proportions 1 or 2 mm. in diameter. The term pure intraductal carcinoma refers to the absence of detectable invasion of the basement membrane, illustrated by special stains in Figure 22–7. Devoid of blood supply, the center of the lesion undergoes necrosis and the intraductal spaces fill with necrotic cellular debris, as shown in Figure 22–14. The central detritus can undergo dystrophic calcification that is fine, focally clustered, and even linear and branching when seen on high-quality mammography (see Fig. 22–11). This process can locally produce a palpable mass if multiple ducts are involved.

Subtypes of DCIS are now well recognized and frequently reported pathologically. The solid or comedo type is most common and probably more virulent. This type, described previously and illustrated in Figure 22–14, is characterized by the closely packed cells within ductal spaces that are susceptible to central necrosis. Papillary or cribriform DCIS

TABLE 22–5. World Health Organization Classification of Breast Tumors

I. Epithelial Tumors	
A. Benign	
1. Intraductal papilloma	8503/0*†
2. Adenoma of the nipple	8506/0
3. Adenoma	8140/0
a. Tubular	8211/0
b. Lactating‡	
B. Malignant	
1. Noninvasive	
a. Intraductal carcinoma	8500/2
b. Lobular carcinoma *in situ*	8520/2
2. Invasive	
a. Invasive ductal carcinoma	8500/3
b. Invasive ductal carcinoma with a predominant intraductal component	8500/3 and 8500/2
c. Invasive lobular carcinoma	8520/3
d. Mucinous carcinoma	8480/3
e. Medullary carcinoma	8510/3
f. Papillary carcinoma	8503/3
g. Tubular carcinoma	8211/3
h. Adenoid cystic carcinoma	8200/3
i. Secretory (juvenile) carcinoma	8502/3
j. Apocrine carcinoma	8573/3
k. Carcinoma with metaplasia	
i. Squamous type	8570/3
ii. Spindle cell type	8572/3
iii. Cartilaginous and osseous type	8571/3
iv. Mixed types§	
l. Others	
3. Paget's disease of the nipple	8540/3¶

II. Mixed Connective Tissue and Epithelial Tumors	
A. Fibroadenoma	9010/0
B. Phyllodes tumor (cystosarcoma phyllodes)	9020/—†
C. Carcinosarcoma	8980/3
III. Miscellaneous Tumors	
A. Soft tissue tumors	
B. Skin tumors	
C. Tumors of hematopoietic and lymphoid tissues	
IV. Unclassified Tumors	8000/—†
V. Mammary Dysplasia/Fibrocystic Disease	74320
VI. Tumor-like Lesions	
A. Duct Ectasia	32100
B. Inflammatory pseudotumors	76820
C. Hamartoma	75500
D. Gynecomastia	71000
E. Others	

*These code numbers correspond to ICD-O and SNOMED morphology fields.
†Code behavior: /0, benign; /1, uncertain whether benign or malignant; /2, noninvasive; /3, malignant.
‡No specific code available for lactating adenoma.
§Code specific types.
¶Paget's disease plus invasive carcinoma is coded 8541/3.

are characterized by papillary projections of tumor cells into the ductal lumen or by the presence of a branching, cribriform pattern filling ducts. These types are less likely to form palpable masses and uncommonly calcify to produce a mammographic abnormality. However, it is important to emphasize that these subtypes can coexist and that DCIS is best described by the pathologist in terms of its extent, multicentricity, and involvement of the surgical margin. Confusion arises in a number of ways. First, the uninitiated may confuse the term *infiltrating ductal carcinoma* with the term *intraductal carcinoma*; the former is invasive disease and the latter is noninvasive disease. Second, these two stages of tumorigenesis usually coexist, particularly when they are carefully searched for in pathologic specimens. Finally, as discussed later, the treatment and outcome for patients with intraductal disease may depend on variables such as multifocality, multicentricity, and extent of disease in a way more demanding for the pathologists and surgeons than in the past.

Lobular Carcinoma *in Situ* (LCIS) or Lobular Neoplasia. This disease of the breast lobules or acini was first clearly delineated by Foote and Stewart in 1941, who gave it the name *lobular carcinoma* in situ. Haagensen first used the term *lobular neoplasia* to emphasize its more benign course. Pathologically, it is a proliferation of small round epithelial cells within lumens of multiple breast acini. The resulting picture is multiple clusters of epithelial cells forming islands of neoplastic cells but maintaining a lobular architecture. Although the ducts expand with proliferating cells, they usually do not reach the large size seen with DCIS. The typical lesion seen pathologically is shown in Figure 22–14.

Unlike DCIS, LCIS never forms a palpable mass by itself and is therefore not recognized on physical examination. In addition, there are no mammographic findings in LCIS. It does not form a density and rarely calcifies, both of which are typical for DCIS. Therefore, this is a disease that is recognized incidentally after biopsy for another abnormality that is producing a clinical or mammographic finding. The treatment of this incidental pathologic entity remains controversial and is reviewed later.

Infiltrating Ductal Carcinoma. This is the most common malignant tumor in the breast recognized after biopsy. The term *ductal carcinoma* refers to its origin from ductal epithelium; *infiltrating* describes its growth pattern and distinguishes this lesion from noninvasive carcinoma. Some add the terms *not otherwise specified* (NOS) and *no special type* (NST) to emphasize that this disease is diagnosed after the other, more distinctive histologies have been eliminated. The tumor infiltrates into a variable amount of stroma as cords or islands of malignant epithelium (see Fig. 22–13). It may form primitive glandular forms, but not to the extent of a pure tubular carcinoma. As discussed, and as reflected in the WHO classification, many infiltrating carcinomas display an *in situ* component. This fact reflects its ductal origin and may be used to prove a mammary origin of the tumor. The stromal *reaction* may be intense and has led to the older term *scirrhous carcinoma* of the breast.

Clinically, most infiltrating ductal carcinomas present as a mass found on physical examination or as a density lesion on the mammogram. Microcalcifications seen mammographically are commonly found in the necrotic centers of the intraductal component but may be seen in the infiltrating component as well. The treatment of infiltrating carcinoma is discussed later, and the approach taken is generally the same regardless of the morphologic appearance. However, there

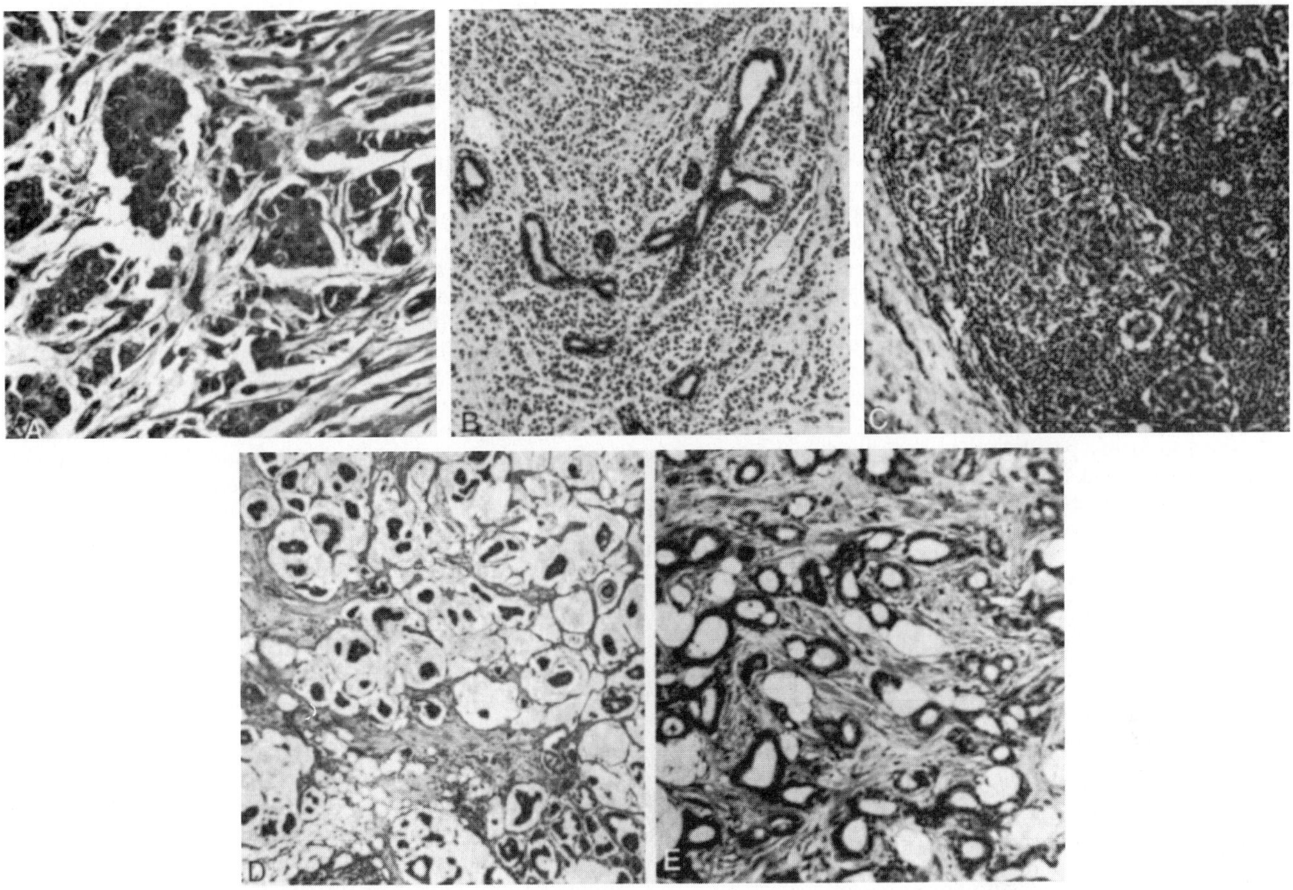

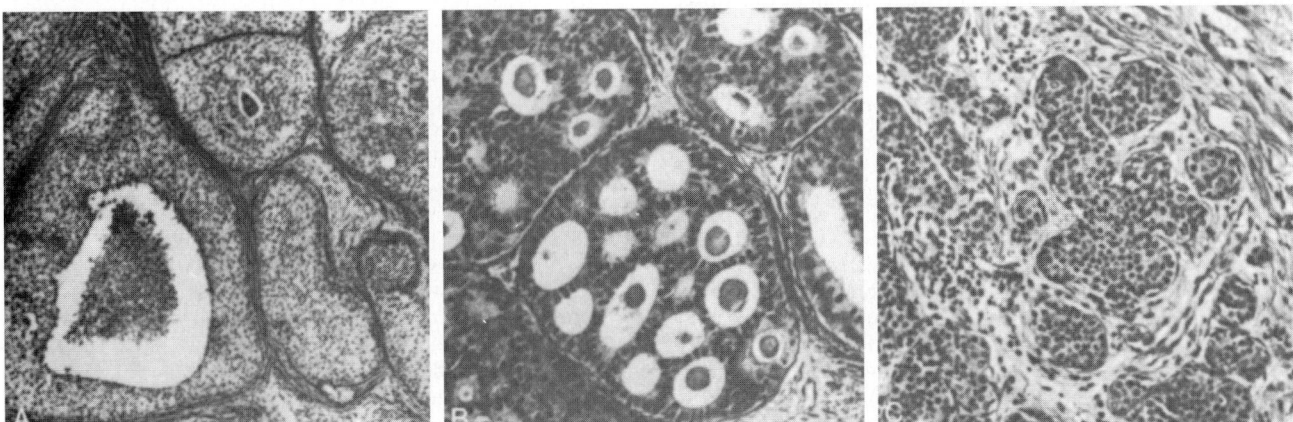

Figure 22–13. Histologic appearance of common breast tumors. *A,* Infiltrating ductal carcinoma, NOS. The tumor cells infiltrate the stroma without any distinctive morphologic pattern. *B,* Infiltrating lobular carcinoma. Small tumor cells infiltrate the stroma oriented in linear array known as an "Indian file" arrangement. *C,* Medullary carcinoma. Large and bizarre tumor cells are surrounded by a distinctive lymphocytic infiltrate. *D,* Mucinous carcinoma, also called colloid carcinoma. Well-differentiated tumor cells form islands within lakes of mucin. *E,* Tubular carcinoma. Small tubules are lined by well-differentiated, uniform tumor cells and infiltrate the stroma in a disorganized fashion. (Reprinted with permission from the World Health Organization, Geneva, Switzerland.)

is great biologic diversity among breast cancers; and after identification of an infiltrating ductal carcinoma, pathologists attempt to describe features that reflect the likely behavior of the tumor.

The evaluation of breast cancers should always specify the tumor size, the status of the surgical margin, and the content of estrogen and progesterone receptors. In addition, the nuclear and histologic grade is frequently reported and modern evaluation may include measurement of DNA content and estimation of the proliferating fraction, or S-phase. Vascular invasion, tumor necrosis, and the extent of the intraductal component are all used to make decisions about the primary

Figure 22–14. Noninvasive breast carcinoma or carcinoma *in situ* (CIS). *A,* Ductal carcinoma *in situ* (DCIS), solid or comedo growth pattern. Tumor cells fill and expand breast ducts and may undergo central necrosis. *B,* Ductal carcinoma *in situ* (DCIS), cribriform growth pattern. Papillary projections of tumor cells span the duct lumen to form a cribriform growth pattern. *C,* Lobular carcinoma *in situ* (LCIS). Tumor cells fill and distend the terminal ductules but preserve the architecture of the lobular unit.

or adjuvant treatment of patients with operable breast cancer. The dedicated breast surgeon must be acquainted with all of these parameters and their interpretation.

Invasive Lobular Carcinoma. This disease probably originates in the breast lobule. Invasive lobular carcinoma constitutes between 3% and 15% of all invasive breast cancers, depending on the series consulted. Histologically, the tumor is composed of small round cells that infiltrate surrounding stromal tissue in a peculiar *Indian file* fashion (see Figure 22–13B). Lobular carcinoma presents in an identical fashion as ordinary infiltrating ductal carcinoma and produces no distinguishing mammographic features. The treatment of lobular carcinoma is the same as for the more common ductal carcinomas and may carry a better prognosis. There may be a somewhat higher incidence of bilateral cancer or of second primary tumors in the contralateral breast. However, this is rarely used to justify prophylactic procedures in the contralateral breast in the absence of synchronous disease.

Less Common Forms of Ductal Carcinoma. These tumors, although heterogeneous, are all morphologic variants of common ductal carcinoma. In general, these less common variants have improved prognosis, reflecting their more differentiated phenotype. One exception to this rule is medullary carcinoma of the breast, which is pathologically characterized by bizarre and anaplastic tumor cells surrounded by a prominent lymphocytic infiltrate with a scant fibrous stroma (see Fig. 22–13C). Although the epithelial component is undifferentiated, this phenotype appears to enjoy a small but significant survival advantage when compared with infiltrating ductal carcinoma NOS. Mucinous carcinoma, also called colloid carcinoma, is characterized by well-differentiated epithelial cells surrounded by a large accumulation of extracellular and extraluminal mucin that is secreted by the carcinoma cells (see Fig. 22–13D). This histologic type enjoys a favorable prognosis in several published series. Although there are no definite clinical or mammographic signs of mucinous and medullary carcinoma, these tumor types are suggested by a well-circumscribed density with smooth borders that tend to be softer on physical examination. The final major histologic type that is distinctive and well differentiated is tubular carcinoma. This tumor is characterized by infiltrating tubular structures, lined by one cell layer, and with an open central space (see Fig. 22–13E). The tumor is characteristically small, is scirrhous, and has an excellent prognosis after treatment. The descriptions of these histologic variants refer to their predominant features. However, each may coexist with more undifferentiated infiltrating carcinoma of the usual type. In general, if the tumor is composed of definite infiltrating ductal carcinoma of poor differentiation, the final diagnosis reflects the poorest histologic pattern. Because tubular and mucinous variants are less likely to metastasize, some modern breast surgeons tailor their primary approach to these lesions by, for instance, omitting axillary node dissections for small and well-differentiated lesions.

Staging Breast Cancer

The most widely used system for staging primary breast cancer has evolved from classifications proposed by the International Union Against Cancer (UICC) and the American Joint Committee on Cancer (AJCC). Figure 22–15 presents the 1992 TNM classification system as it appears on a staging worksheet from the AJCC. This modern system is based on the description of the primary tumor (T), the status of regional lymph nodes (N), and the presence of distant metastases (M). Reports may contain numerical codes behind each letter, such as $T_2N_1M_0$, which refers to a tumor greater than 2 cm. but less than 5 cm. (T_2), the presence of movable homolateral axillary nodes (N_1), and the absence of distant metastases (M_0). These designations may be combined as outlined in the AJCC/UICC Stage Grouping (see Fig. 22–15) to give a summary staging category, in this example Stage IIA. This system can be used to determine clinical stage, based on physical examination and radiographic findings, or to determine pathologic stage after operation and histologic evaluation of the surgical material. Any staging system seeks to provide information about the prognosis of patients after treatment and to allow comparison of results within and between clinical trials. These divisions are imposed on a spectrum of cancer presentations and are useful only if they are interpreted with knowledge of their limitations.

Very few studies of the natural history of untreated patients with breast cancer are available. Furthermore, the growth rate of breast cancer and its biologic behavior is heterogeneous. The ability of tumors to metastasize is a variable that cannot as yet be predicted and differs among individual patients and tumors. Haagensen has presented a patient with a well-documented tumor in the right breast that slowly grew for 30 years before the patient died. Bloom collected a remarkable series of 250 patients with untreated breast cancer from the Middlesex Hospital cancer charity ward between 1805 and 1933. As shown in Figure 22–16, the median survival of these patients was 2.7 years, although 20% survived more than 5 years from presentation.

In the modern era of adjuvant therapy, it is helpful to review the natural history of patients with operable cancer treated with surgical therapy alone. In general, these are patients with Stage I or II breast cancer who underwent either radical or modified radical mastectomy before 1975, when adjuvant chemotherapy was first widely used. A cooperative Natural History Data Base was established at the National Cancer Institute in Milan, at the Royal Marsden Hospital, and at the M. D. Anderson Hospital that included 1971 patients carefully staged and followed for at least 10 years. Figure 22–17 displays the overall survival results by Kaplan-Meier estimation and shows the effect of tumor size (T) and nodal status (N). Nodal involvement is divided into those with one to three and four or more nodes pathologically containing cancer. Metastasis to ipsilateral axillary nodes predicts outcome after surgical treatment more precisely than any other prognostic factor. This relationship between nodal status and outcome is underscored by a survey of the management and survival of female breast cancer sponsored by the American College of Surgeons. Five-year end-results of absolute survival and recurrence were tabulated in this survey, according to the number of pathologically positive axillary nodes, and revealed an almost linear decrement in survival with increasing nodal involvement (Table 22–6).

The survival of patients presenting with locally advanced or metastatic disease who are nonoperated, operated for palliation, or with recurrent cancer is heterogeneous but very poor. This group includes patients with Stage IIIB and IV disease. In general, no more than 20% of patients presenting with locally advanced carcinoma will survive for 10 years. However, certain patients with locally advanced Stage III disease have been operated for cure, including those tumors larger than 5 cm. with negative nodes ($T_3N_0M_0$). Inclusion of these more favorable cases influences the reporting of results for this group. Division of stage III into more and less favorable categories reflects this heterogeneity. The median survival of patients with metastatic disease is in the range of 24 months from time of diagnosis but varies according to the principal site of disease involvement. It is helpful to recognize that staging systems that divide a given disease into four categories (Stage I–IV) should be designed to evenly distribute outcome from 100% to 0%.

Breast Carcinoma
Clinical TNM Classification and Staging

BREAST: ☐ **LEFT** ☐ **RIGHT**
TUMOR SIZE _____cm X_____ cm X_____cm
LYMPH NODES Total No._____ No. with metastases_____

PATIENT NAME _____

ACCESSION NUMBER _____

DEFINITIONS:
PRIMARY TUMOR (T)
☐ TX Primary tumor cannot be assessed
☐ T0 No evidence of primary tumor
☐ Tis Carcinoma in situ: Intraductal carcinoma, lobular carcinoma in situ, or Paget's disease of the nipple with no tumor
☐ T1 Tumor 2 cm or less in greatest dimension
  ☐ T1a 0.5 cm or less in greatest dimension
  ☐ T1b More than 0.5 cm, but not more than 1 cm in greatest dimension
  ☐ T1c More than 1 cm, but not more than 2 cm in greatest dimension
☐ T2 Tumor more than 2 cm, but not more than 5 cm in greatest dimension
☐ T3 Tumor more than 5 cm in greatest dimension
☐ T4 Tumor of any size with direct extension to chest wall or skin
  ☐ T4a Extension to chest wall
  ☐ T4b Edema (including peau d'orange) or ulceration of the skin of breast or satellite skin nodules confined to same breast
  ☐ T4c Both T4a and T4b
  ☐ T4d Inflammatory carcinoma

REGIONAL LYMPH NODES (N) *(Please refer to diagrams)*
The regional lymph nodes are: (1) Axillary (ipsilateral): interpectoral (Rotter's) nodes and lymph nodes along the axillary vein and its tributaries which may be divided into the following levels: (i)Level I (low axilla): lymph nodes lateral to the lateral border of pectoralis minor muscle. (ii) Level II (mid-axilla): lymph nodes between the medial and lateral borders of the pectoralis minor muscle and the interpectoral (Rotter's) lymph nodes. (iii) Level III (apical axilla): lymph nodes medial to the medial margin of the pectoralis minor muscle including those designated as subclavicular, infraclavicular, or apical. Note: Intramammary lymph nodes are coded as axillary lymph nodes. (2) Internal mammary (ipsilateral): lymph nodes in the intercostal spaces along the edge of the sternum in the endothoracic fascia. Any other lymph node metastasis is coded as a distant metastasis (M1), including supraclavicular, cervical, or contralateral internal mammary lymph nodes.

☐ NX Regional lymph nodes cannot be assessed (e.g., previously removed or not removed for pathologic study)
☐ N0 No regional lymph node metastasis
☐ N1 Metastasis to movable ipsilateral axillary lymph node(s)
  ☐ N1a Only micrometastasis (none larger than 0.2 cm)
  ☐ N1b Metastasis to lymph node(s), any larger than 0.2 cm
    ☐ N1bi Metastasis in 1 to 3 lymph nodes, any more than 0.2 cm and all less than 2 cm in greatest dimension
    ☐ N1bii Metastasis to 4 or more lymph nodes, any more than 0.2 cm and all less than 2 cm in greatest dimension
    ☐ N1biii Extension of tumor beyond the capsule of a lymph node metastasis less than 2 cm in greatest dimension
    ☐ N1biv Metastasis to a lymph node 2 cm or more in greatest dimension

☐ N2 Metastasis to ipsilateral axillary lymph nodes that are fixed to one another or to other structures
☐ N3 Metastasis to ipsilateral internal mammary lymph node(s)

DISTANT METASTASIS (M)
☐ MX Presence of distant metastasis cannot be assessed
☐ M0 No distant metastasis
☐ M1 Distant metastasis (includes metastasis to ipsilateral supraclavicular lymph node(s))

AJCC/UICC Stage Grouping

☐ Stage 0	☐ Tis	N0	M0
☐ Stage I	☐ T1	N0	M0
☐ Stage IIA	☐ T0	N1	M0
	☐ T1	N1	M0
	☐ T2	N0	M0
☐ Stage IIB	☐ T2	N1	M0
	☐ T3	N0	M0
☐ Stage IIIA	☐ T0	N2	M0
	☐ T1	N2	M0
	☐ T2	N2	M0
	☐ T3	N1	M0
	☐ T3	N2	M0
☐ Stage IIIB	☐ T4	Any N	M0
	☐ Any T	N3	M0
☐ Stage IV	☐ Any T	Any N	M1

Figure 22–15. Worksheet for determining TNM stage for breast cancer. This worksheet displays the definitions used to assign TNM classification and to determine overall stage. (From American Joint Committee on Cancer and the International Union Against Cancer, 1992.)

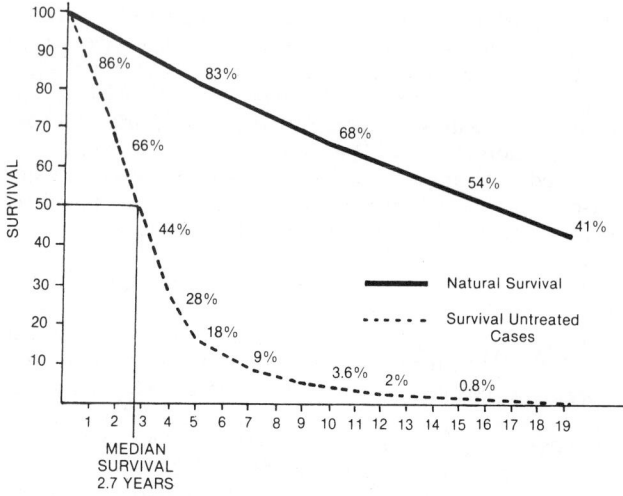

Figure 22–16. Length of survival in 250 patients with untreated breast cancer at the Middlesex Hospital between 1805 and 1933. (From Bloom, H. J. G., et al.: Natural history of untreated breast cancer (1805–1933). Br. Med. J., 2:213, 1962.)

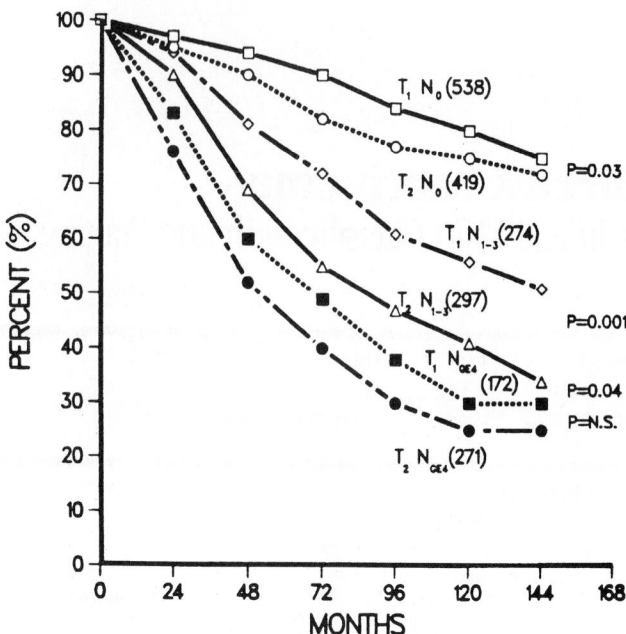

Figure 22–17. Survival by nodes and tumor size from a Natural History Data Base. The survival data from 1971 patients in whom follow-up was complete were collected from three hospitals to form a Natural History Data Base. These patients were treated by either radical or modified radical mastectomy; none of the patients received postoperative chemotherapy. (From Moon, T. E., et al.: Development of a natural history data base of breast cancer studies. In Jones, S. E., and Salmon, S. E. [Eds.]: Adjuvant Therapy of Cancer IV. Orlando, FL, Grune & Stratton, 1984.)

Modern Surgical Procedures for Invasive Breast Cancer

The surgical treatment of breast cancer, for the most part, concerns the treatment of potentially curable cancer that is confined to the breast and regional lymph nodes. For early stages of breast cancer, surgical removal provides a reasonable chance for cure. Although the approach to operable breast cancer has changed dramatically over the past century, so, too, has the clinical presentation of breast tumors changed. In 1894, Halsted presented his first 50 patients treated by the "complete operation," which became the radical mastectomy. Over the next 75 years, radical mastectomy was used to treat virtually every breast malignancy operated on for cure in the United States. Examination of Halsted's first cases found at least two thirds with locally advanced

disease and 60% with clinically evident axillary nodal metastases. By comparison, a 1980 survey by the American College of Surgeons found that 85% of patients presented with Stage I or Stage II disease. The frequency of cases with positive axillary lymph nodes was 40%, and the average tumor presenting to physicians in the 1970s measured 2 cm. or less. In addition to these fundamental changes, realization that 90% of treatment failures will be systemic or visceral recurrences has led surgical oncologists to explore alternatives to radical mastectomy as an initial approach to operable breast cancer.

Surgical Procedures Past and Present

In 1982, the American College of Surgeons investigated surgical practice in cases of operable breast cancer and compared results with practice in earlier years (Fig. 22–18). Clearly, a change in surgical practice occurred in the mid 1970s with an abrupt shift from radical mastectomy to modified radical mastectomy. Procedures that preserved the breast, as described later, were performed in only 7.2% of cases in this survey. Current estimates of conservative breast procedures range between 20% and 40%, and this procedure probably continues to increase in popularity. The following paragraphs describe procedures in widespread use now and in the past.

Radical and Extended Radical Mastectomy.[19, 24] In the radical mastectomy, the breast and underlying pectoralis muscles are sacrificed leaving a bare chest wall. Regional lymph nodes along the axillary vein up to the costoclavicular ligament (Halsted's ligament) are removed with the breast specimen. This procedure frequently requires a skin graft and uses incisions placed either vertically or obliquely. Prosthetic reconstruction is impossible unless muscle flaps are mobilized to cover the anterior chest defect. Cure of breast cancer can certainly be achieved by the application of this procedure alone, as shown earlier in Figure 22–17 from a natural history data base of surgically treated patients. Other studies docu-

TABLE 22–6. Five-Year End-Results (Absolute Survival, Cure, and Recurrence Rates) in 20,547 Patients with Breast Cancer According to Number of Pathologically Positive Axillary Nodes*

Number of Positive Axillary Lymph Nodes	Total Observed	Survival (%)	Cure (%)	Recurrence (%)
0	12,299	71.8	59.7	19.4
1	2012	63.1	48.4	32.9
2	1338	62.2	45.4	39.9
3	842	58.8	39.3	43.0
4	615	51.9	38.4	43.9
5	478	46.9	29.1	54.2
6–10	1261	40.7	23.0	63.4
11–15	562	29.4	14.8	71.5
16–20	301	28.9	13.3	75.1
21 +	225	22.2	9.8	82.2
All nodes or some nodes positive	614	40.4	26.9	58.6
Total, positive nodes	8248	50.9	35.0	49.2

*Excluding cases with distant metastasis.

From Nemoto, T., Vana, J., Bedwani, R. N., et al.: Management and survival of female breast cancer: Results of a national survey by the American College of Surgeons. Cancer, 45:2917, 1980. Copyright © 1980 American Cancer Society. Reprinted by permission of Wiley-Liss, Inc., a subsidiary of John Wiley & Sons, Inc.

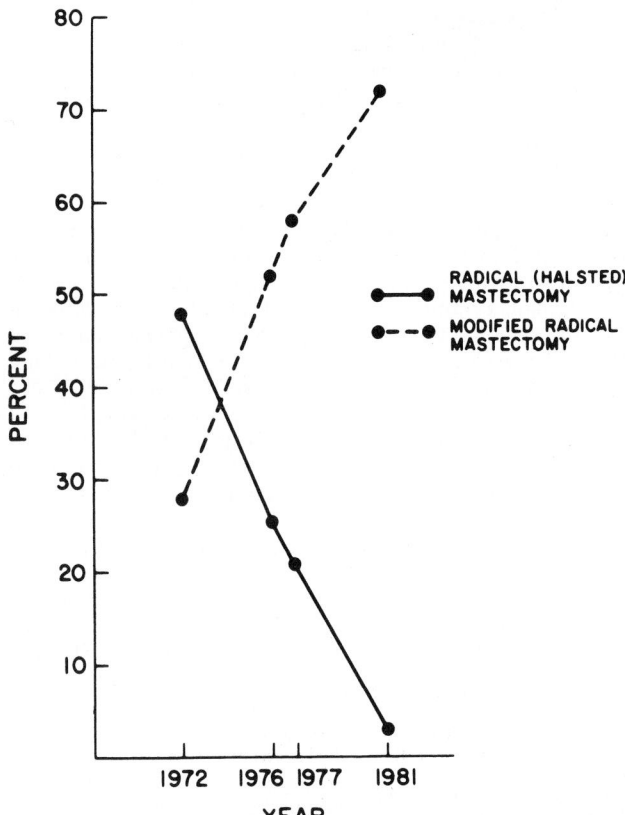

Figure 22–18. Trends in the procedures performed for operable breast cancer from 1972 to 1981. (From Wilson, R. E., et al.: The 1982 national survey of carcinoma of the breast in the United States by the American College of Surgeons. Surg. Gynecol. Obstet., *159*:309, 1984.)

ing a soft tissue covering over the chest wall and a normal-appearing junction of the shoulder with the anterior chest wall and avoiding the hollow defect inferior to the clavicle that accompanies the removal of the pectoralis muscle. The patient is left with intact musculature around the shoulder and a situation that is well suited to prosthetic reconstruction (discussed in Chapter 22-I). Two forms of the procedure are in use by surgeons: the Patey procedure and modifications described by Scanlon and the procedure described by Auchincloss.

Patey, at the Middlesex Hospital in London, developed a procedure that preserves the pectoralis major muscle and sacrifices the underlying pectoralis minor muscle to remove levels I, II, and III lymph nodes in the axilla. A large number of Patey procedures performed by Handley, who wrote extensively about this procedure, were reviewed independently and reported by Donegan and associates. The survival of patients with negative axillary nodes was 82% at 10 years with a local recurrence rate of 5%. For patients with positive nodes, the survival was 48%, very similar to results with radical mastectomy. Thus, preservation of the pectoralis major muscle did not appear to produce inferior results. Scanlon modified the Patey procedure by dividing but not removing the pectoralis minor muscle, allowing removal of apical (level III) nodes and preservation of the lateral pectoral nerves to the major muscle.

The procedure described by Auchincloss differs from the Patey procedure by not removing or dividing the pectoralis minor muscle. This modification limits the complete removal of high axillary nodes but is justified by Auchincloss, who calculated that only 2% of patients will potentially benefit by removal of the highest level nodes. It is probable that the Auchincloss mastectomy was the most popular procedure for breast cancer in the United States during the past decade.

Radical Versus Modified Radical Mastectomy.[35, 47] Radical mastectomy and modified radical mastectomy were directly tested in two randomized clinical trials in this country and in England. The first, from the Alabama Breast Cancer Project, was a community-based study that prerandomized patients according to birth date to receive modified radical mastectomy or radical mastectomy. Stage I and II and operable Stage III tumors were included. Those patients with histologically positive axillary nodes were further randomized to receive two different adjuvant chemotherapy programs. An update reported 10-year results for 175 patients undergoing modified radical mastectomy and 136 patients treated with radical mastectomy. No significant difference in overall survival rates was demonstrated. However, there was a significantly higher local recurrence rate (p = .04) in patients undergoing modified radical mastectomy compared with radical mastectomy. Moreover, patients with larger tumors and those with clinically positive nodes survived better after radical mastectomy (p = .05). A university-based study in England randomized 534 patients to radical mastectomy and modified radical mastectomy in a similar study design. This study was limited to patients with clinical Stage I and II disease. No significant differences in overall or event-free survival were seen. In addition, no consistent trends were seen in clinically or pathologically staged subgroups. These results, combined with the clear functional and cosmetic superiority of modified radical mastectomy, make this procedure the standard of care for nearly all patients with operable breast cancer.

Wide Local Excision and Primary Radiation Therapy. Excision of the primary tumor with preservation of the breast has been referred to by many names, including partial mastectomy, segmentectomy, tylectomy, or lumpectomy. *Wide local excision* seems to be the most descriptive term for the procedure, which removes the malignancy with a surrounding rim of grossly normal breast parenchyma. An even

ment both the strengths and weaknesses of maximal local therapy represented by this procedure. The personal series of Haagensen reports results from treatment of 1036 patients; 727 patients with clinically negative nodes (Stage A, Columbia clinical staging) had a survival of 72.4% at 10 years. In contrast, only 42.3% of clinically node-positive patients (Stage B) survived at 10 years. These figures were confirmed by the National Surgical Adjuvant Breast and Bowel Project (NSABP) early trial of adjuvant thiotepa. By 10 years, 76% of patients with histologically positive nodes suffered recurrence of breast cancer and one fourth of patients with negative nodes failed surgical treatment. In contrast, *local failure* rates have been extremely low since introduction of the Halsted radical mastectomy. Published figures are generally between 5% and 7% and provide the standard against which newer procedures are judged.

The extended radical mastectomy is a standard radical mastectomy to which en bloc removal of internal mammary nodes is added. This procedure was popularized in the United States by Urban, who reported a 35.5% 10-year survival in patients undergoing extended radical mastectomy. Other studies have resulted in abandonment of the extended procedure. A large prospective trial and several uncontrolled series have failed to provide evidence of improved clinical outcome after extended radical mastectomy.

Modified Radical Mastectomy.[13, 41] Modified radical mastectomy refers to a procedure combining total mastectomy with removal of axillary lymph nodes in continuity with the mastectomy specimen. This is the most widely used procedure to treat operable breast cancer and is the alternative to breast-sparing procedures described later. Modified radical mastectomy leaves the pectoralis major muscle intact, provid-

more aggressive local procedure designed to remove 1 to 2 cm. of adjacent breast and overlying skin is called *quadrantectomy*. In modern practice, these more limited surgical procedures are applied as part of a multidisciplinary approach to breast cancer and always include postoperative radiation therapy, giving at least 4500 cGy. to the whole breast and usually including a boost of radiation to the tumor bed. Axillary dissection is done through a separate incision in the majority of patients. Therefore, conservative breast surgery or breast preservation usually refers to wide local excision of the primary tumor, whole breast radiation, and a separate axillary dissection.

Surgical Trials of Local Therapy for Operable Breast Cancer

The gradual shift away from radical surgery and toward preservation of the breast and soft tissues was influenced by the results of several large trials of lesser surgical procedures. The Manchester and Alabama trials comparing radical to modified radical mastectomy, reviewed earlier, were important in establishing the place of modified radical mastectomy as the standard surgical approach to patients with operable breast cancer. Other trials that should be mentioned include the Capetown Trial comparing radical mastectomy with simple mastectomy and the Cardiff–St. Mary's Trial of modified radical mastectomy versus simple mastectomy with axillary node biopsy. Although there are deficiencies in both trials, they generally support the notion that alternative strategies for the treatment of operable breast cancer do achieve acceptable survival results.

NSABP Trial B-04 Comparing Radical Mastectomy to Alternatives.[18] In 1971, the National Surgical Adjuvant Breast and Bowel Project initiated a large prospective trial to examine widely disparate approaches to the local and regional control of breast cancer. Protocol B-04 used radical mastectomy as its control arm and randomized patients with and without clinically positive axillary lymph nodes to receive

alternative approaches to regional lymph nodes as shown in Figure 22–19. Patients with clinically negative nodes were randomized to one of three treatment regimens: Halsted radical mastectomy (362 patients), total mastectomy with radiation treatment of the ipsilateral nodes (352 patients), and total mastectomy alone with delayed axillary dissection if nodes became enlarged (365 patients). Clinically node-positive patients were randomly allocated to receive radical mastectomy (292 patients) or total mastectomy with radiation of the enlarged nodes (294 patients). This study has been widely referred to for its contribution to understanding the significance of axillary and regional nodal metastases, the effect of local and regional therapy on recurrence, and the validity of anatomic principles in the treatment of breast cancer. First results of the landmark study were published in 1977, and various aspects of the study have since been reported.

A final update of protocol B-04 was published in 1985 with complete 10-year follow-up for the entire study. No significant differences in either overall survival or disease-free survival were noted for 1079 clinically node-negative patients treated by random allocation with radical mastectomy, total mastectomy plus nodal radiation, or total mastectomy and delayed axillary dissection (Fig. 22–20). Likewise, for 586 clinically node-positive patients receiving either radical mastectomy or total mastectomy and nodal radiation, survival and recurrence statistics were identical (see Fig. 22–20). The only differences were local and regional failures experienced by clinically node-negative patients. Patients receiving radical mastectomy or total mastectomy plus regional radiation had local failures of less than 10%, whereas those treated by mastectomy plus delayed nodal dissection experienced about a 15% cumulative 10-year local recurrence rate. Several important conclusions have been reached as a result of this ground-breaking study:

1. Variations in local and regional treatments that involve total mastectomy do not alter the frequency or pattern of distant treatment failures. Although local treatment failures are influenced, overall survival is unaffected.

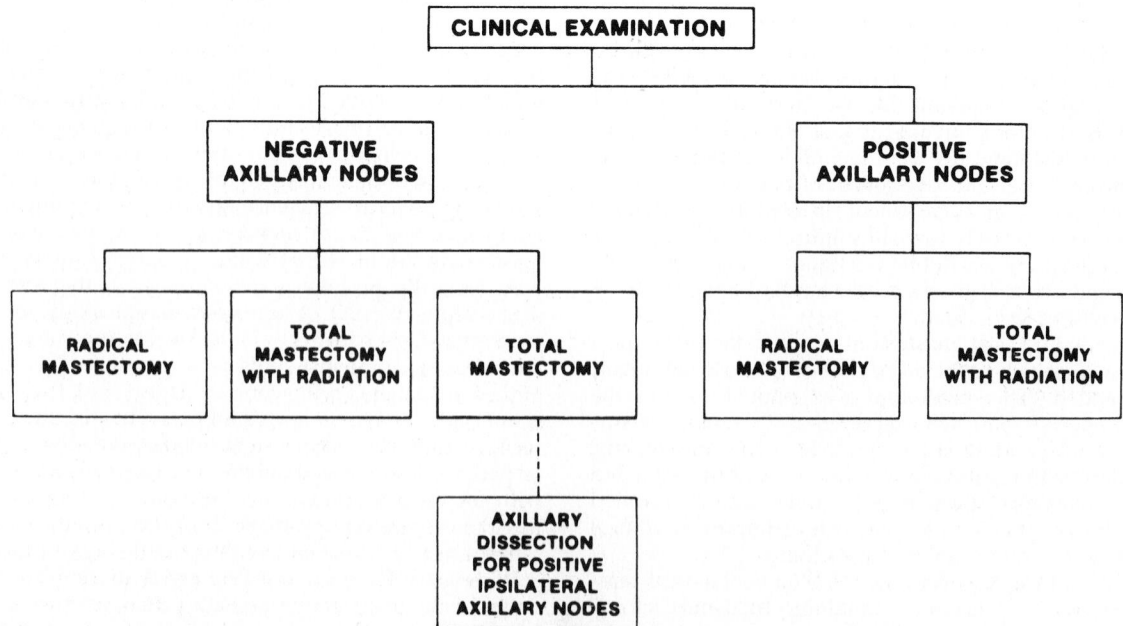

Figure 22–19. Randomization scheme for NSABP protocol B-04. Patients with clinically negative nodes were randomized to receive standard radical mastectomy, total mastectomy and radiation to undisturbed axillary nodes, or total mastectomy with axillary dissection reserved for patients developing delayed axillary node enlargement. Patients with clinically positive nodes were randomized to receive standard radical mastectomy versus total mastectomy with radiation to the involved nodes. (From Fisher, B., et al.: Findings from NSABP protocol No. B-04: Comparison of radical mastectomy with alternative treatments: II. The clinical and biologic significance of medial-central breast cancers. Cancer, *48*:1863, 1981.)

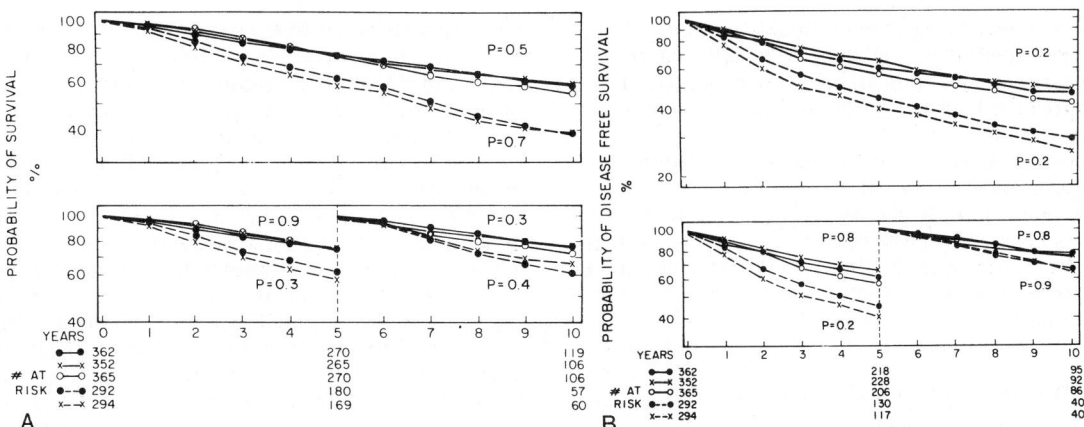

Figure 22–20. Tenth-year results of NSABP protocol B-04 comparing radical mastectomy with alternative treatments. Patients were randomly allocated to receive radical mastectomy (solid circle), total mastectomy and radiation to undisturbed axillary nodes (x), or total mastectomy alone with delayed axillary dissection only for patients developing clinically enlarged nodes (open circle). Patients with clinically negative nodes (solid line) and clinically positive nodes (broken line) were randomized. *A,* Top, Total survival of all groups through the tenth year. Bottom left, Survival through the fifth year. Bottom right, Survival during the next 5 years of all patients alive at the end of the first period. *B,* Top, Disease-free survival for the total study through 10 years. Bottom left, Survival free of disease during the first 5 years of study. Bottom right, Survival free of disease for patients free from disease at the end of the first period. (From Fisher, B., et al.: Ten-year results of a randomized clinical trial comparing radical mastectomy and total mastectomy with or without radiation. N. Engl. J. Med., *312*:674, 1985.)

2. The mode and time of treatment of axillary nodes does not alter outcome, either disease-free survival or overall survival. Immediate removal, delayed removal, or radiation all produced equivalent results. Removal of lymph nodes and enumeration of the number that are positive for cancer provides the best indication of eventual relapse.

3. Results of breast cancer treatment trials can reliably be assessed at 5 years; the frequency of new events occurring in the second 5 years of protocol B-04 were small and predictable. Patients with positive nodes who were free of disease at 5 years had about the same probability of remaining disease free as did the negative node group.

4. The location of the primary tumor in the breast does not influence outcome. Furthermore, there was no justification for irradiation of internal mammary nodes in patients with medial quadrant lesions.

The results of the NSABP B-04 protocol address treatment alternatives that all use total mastectomy. However, the experimental arms in this study represented significant departures from accepted local and regional treatment of operable breast cancer. The results of this study support the overriding importance of distant disease as the cause of breast cancer mortality even in early stage disease. The occurrence of distant disease was independent of local treatment across a wide range of strategies, particularly the surgical approach to axillary nodes. The question of whether procedures substituting breast conservation for mastectomy can be safely applied to treatment of operable breast cancer was first addressed in uncontrolled trials in European centers, by pioneering radiotherapists in the United States, and finally in randomized prospective trials (reviewed later).

Conservative Surgical Procedures for Operable Breast Cancer.[8, 25] Conservative procedures (e.g., breast-preserving surgery, breast conservation) refers to various treatment strategies that leave the breast largely intact, with or without postsurgical radiation therapy and with or without axillary dissection. The use of radiation only, leaving the tumor *in situ,* was reported in 1928 by Keynes, who was a surgeon at St. Bartholomew's Hospital in London. Calle and his colleagues at the Foundation Curie in France reported disease-free survival of 43% at 10 years for patients with tumors 3 cm. or larger treated initially by radiation only. These results were confirmed in large series of patients from France; however, many of these patients required secondary surgery for

persistent or recurrent disease (55% of Calle and colleagues' patients). There seems to be little justification for leaving invasive cancer in the breast unless it technically cannot be removed (as with locally advanced or inflammatory cancers) or unless the patient has documented metastatic disease that is considered more immediately threatening. There are no clinical trials that omit surgical excision of early stage breast cancers.

In contrast to radiation therapy alone, total extirpation of the tumor without further local treatment has been studied in retrospective and in prospective clinical trials. The NSABP has randomized patients with small tumors to receive either excision alone, excision plus tamoxifen, or excision plus radiation therapy. A trial of excision and tamoxifen, with or without radiation therapy, in older women is an NCI high-priority intergroup trial and is currently entering patients. Cope, Crile, Adair, and others demonstrated the possibility that excision alone of certain breast cancers did result in long-term cures. Patients treated with very limited surgery had local recurrence rates that generally exceeded 20% at intervals of 3 to 5 years. In a series of more than 800 patients treated without mastectomy at the Princess Margaret Hospital between 1958 and 1980, 177 were treated by excision without radiation. One hundred and four tumors treated in this fashion were small T_1 (less than 2 cm.) lesions. The majority of patients treated conservatively received postsurgical radiation to the breast, with or without radiation of regional nodal groups. At 5 years, there was an 8.7% relapse rate in the breast treated by excision plus radiation. Patients who underwent excision only, with no radiation, experienced an ipsilateral breast relapse rate of 24.9%. By 10 years, local failure had occurred in 13.3% and 28.3%, respectively, despite the preponderance of smaller tumors in the group excised without radiation. Significantly, distant relapse and overall survival were unaffected by the choice of local therapy. These early results were similar in magnitude and direction to more recent trials, including prospectively randomized trials.

The Princess Margaret Hospital has reported a prospective randomized trial of lumpectomy and axillary dissection with or without postoperative radiation therapy. The purpose of this study was to identify a subgroup of patients with node-negative breast cancer who might be spared breast irradiation after complete surgical excision of the ipsilateral breast cancer. Among 837 patients randomized, the ipsilateral breast failure was 25.7% in the patients who did not receive radiation and was reduced to 5.5% in the irradiated patients. There was no subgroup of patients with sufficiently low-risk breast cancers (e.g., small tumors, low histologic grade) identified that could be spared radiation and still maintain a relapse rate of less than 5%.

Noncontrolled Trials of Conservative Operations Plus Radiation Therapy.[21, 48] Early work leading to the modern use of radiation therapy in the treatment of primary breast carcinoma began in European centers more than 40 years ago. Mustakallio was encouraged by favorable result in clinical Stage I disease and was able to produce results comparable to radical mastectomy using tumor excision and radiation therapy. Calle reported similar favorable 10-year results at the Foundation Curie in Paris. For patients with tumors less than 3 cm. and without clinical involvement of axillary nodes, excision plus radiation therapy produced absolute survival, free of disease, of 85% and 75% at 5 and 10 years, respectively.

Early successes were duplicated in North America and in larger populations of patients. Montague treated patients at the M. D. Anderson Hospital between 1955 and 1980 and produced 10-year survivals in 80% and 65% of patients with Stage I and Stage II disease, respectively. Prosnitz reported results from a cooperative study of breast preservation and radiation therapy in early stage breast cancer treated at four university hospitals in the Northeast. Actuarial disease-free survival rates at 5 years were 91% and 60% in Stages I and II disease. Similar results were reported from the Joint Center for Radiation Therapy at Harvard, from the Princess Margaret Hospital, from the National Cancer Institute in Milan, and from the University of Pennsylvania.

Local failure in these studies, defined as ipsilateral in-breast recurrence of cancer, was between 8% and 20% at 10 years of follow-up. Risk for recurrence was relatively constant over time and translates for an individual patient to a risk estimate of between 1% and 2% chance of in-breast failure each year after treatment. In no published study do investigators find a difference in distant-site relapse rates or in overall survival when total mastectomy is compared with breast conservation. These studies were generally noncontrolled and retrospective; however, they provided sound evidence that tumor excision and modern radiation therapy offered an alternative treatment for certain patients with early stage breast cancer. Because of the inherent issue of patient selection, which tends to include more favorable pa-

tients in alternative treatment approaches, randomized prospective trials were necessary to provide the remaining proof.

Controlled Trials Comparing Breast Preservation with Mastectomy.[49] Seven prospective clinical trials have randomized more than 4500 patients to various surgical strategies, all of which include a mastectomy arm and a breast-preserving arm. These trials are listed in Table 22–7, which includes survival figures and rates of ipsilateral breast recurrences. References to updates of these trials are included in the table legend. Endpoints of these studies are local failure, distant failure, and survival. All studies except that of the NCI randomized trial required histologically negative margins for the lumpectomy specimen. Whole-breast radiation after surgical removal of the primary tumor was designed to deliver between 45 and 50 Gy. (4500–5000 rads.) in all of these trials. Six of seven trials used a boost to the tumor location; the NSABP gave 50 Gy. to the whole breast without boosting the primary site. All of the studies required axillary dissection, and adjuvant chemotherapy was prescribed for most node-positive patients. Follow-up times from 8 to more than 10 years have elapsed in all of these studies, allowing firm conclusions to be drawn. In 1990, a consensus conference of the National Institutes of Health was held and reviewed all of the available data regarding breast conservation. The conclusion of the conference was a clear statement of the superiority of wide excision and radiation therapy for women who desire preservation of their breast. The addition of radiation therapy to surgical excision is required for nearly all patients with invasive cancers of any size. Depending on many factors, including tumor size, breast size, location, and preference, patients can safely be offered modified radical mastectomy, modified radical mastectomy with delayed or immediate reconstruction, or wide excision to negative margins and postoperative radiation.

Certain comments should be made to assist the reader in interpreting results from the prospective trials tabulated in Table 22–7. The NSABP trial was by far the largest and randomized patients to receive mastectomy, tumor excision (lumpectomy) alone, or lumpectomy plus postoperative breast radiation. All patients underwent axillary dissection. Lumpectomy alone, without postoperative radiation therapy, was the assigned treatment for 565 patients. After 9 years of actuarial follow-up, about 45% of patients suffered ipsilateral breast recurrence even though gross and histologic margins were required. Even after complete surgical excision, radia-

TABLE 22–7. Modern Prospective Studies Comparing Mastectomy with Wide Excision and Radiation Therapy

Surgical Trial*	Total No. of Patients	Maximum Primary Tumor Size (cm.)	Systemic Therapy	Follow-Up (yr.)	Survival (%)		Local Recurrence (Irradiation) (%)
					Irradiation	*Mastectomy*	
1. National Surgical Adjuvant Breast Project	1219	4	Yes	8	76	71	10
2. National Cancer Institute (Milan)	701	2	Yes	10	79	78	4
3. Institut Gustave-Roussy	179	2	No	10	78	79	7
4. Danish Breast Cancer Group	905	None	Yes	6	79	82	4
5. National Cancer Institute (U.S.)	237	5	Yes	10	77	75	16
6. European Organization for Research and Treatment of Cancer	903	5	Not stated	8	71	73	13
7. Guy's Hospital Trial	399	4	Yes	Not stated	NS	NS	8

*Published sources (in order): 1. Fisher, B., et al.: N. Engl. J. Med., *320*:822, 1989; 2. Veronesi, U., et al.: Eur. J. Cancer, *26*:668, 1990; 3, Sarrazin, D., et al.: Radiother. Oncol., *14*:177, 1989; 4. Blichert-Toft, M., et al.: Acta Oncol., *27*:671, 1988; 5. Jacobson, J. A., et al.: N. Engl. J. Med., *332*:907, 1995; 6. van Dongen, J. A., et al.: Eur. J. Cancer, *28A*:801, 1992; 7. Habibollahi, F., et al.: Proc. Am. Soc. Clin. Oncol., *6*:A231, 1987.

NS, no significant difference in survival (numbers not specified).

tion should be recommended to the majority of patients. The NSABP trial allowed tumors as large as 4 cm. and included patients with palpable axillary adenopathy that was movable (Stage I and II). Most experts agree that the size of the tumor and the presence of grossly positive axillary nodes does not necessarily exclude patients from pursuing breast conservation. In May 1994, the *New England Journal of Medicine* published an account of fraud within the B-06 study involving a single institution. The elimination of data from this one site did not change the overall conclusions of the study and reaffirmed the equivalence of breast conservation to mastectomy in overall and disease-free survival (excluding ipsilateral breast failures). In addition, results from other randomized trials paralleled those from the NSABP B-06 study.

One such study was conducted by the NCI that was begun in 1979 and compared lumpectomy, axillary dissection, and postoperative radiation therapy to modified radical mastectomy. This study enrolled 237 patients with invasive breast cancer into its two arms and included patients with T_1 and T_2 primary tumors and with clinically N_0 or N_1 axillary nodes. The NCI study is a relatively small one that has the statistical power to detect a disease-free survival difference of 15% at 5 years. Results were presented in 1992 with a median follow-up of 67 months and updated in 1995 after a median follow-up of 10 years. No differences were seen in overall actuarial survival at 10 years (75% for patients receiving lumpectomy and 77% for patients in the mastectomy arm; Fig. 22–21*A*). There were no differences in the 10-year

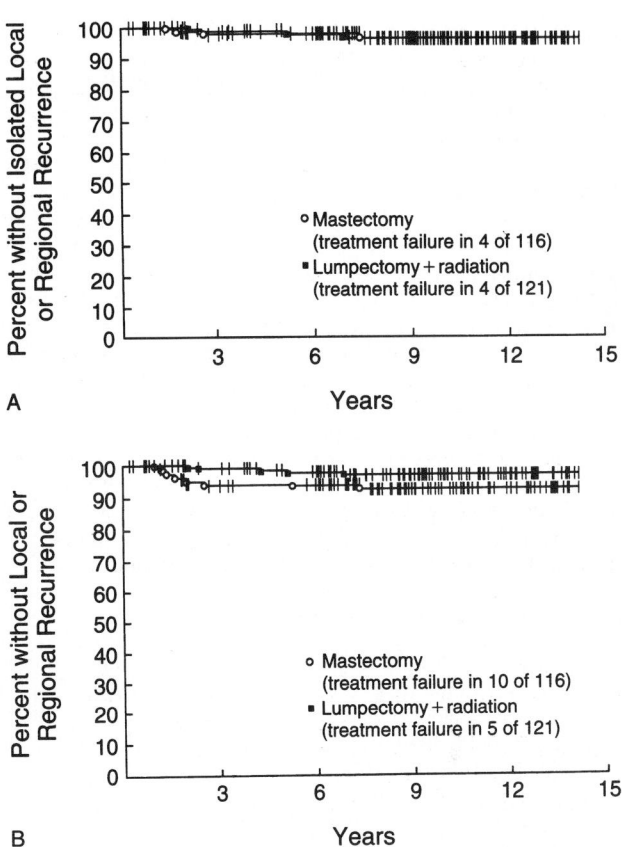

Figure 22–22. Local or regional recurrences as isolated first events *(A)* or as any component of a first event *(B)* in the two treatment groups. Data were censored on patients with recurrences confined to the ipsilateral breast and successfully treated. Tick marks indicate follow-up times for patients who had not had recurrences. (Reprinted by permission of *The New England Journal of Medicine* from Jacobson, J. A., et al.: Ten-year results of a comparison of conservation with mastectomy in the treatment of stage I and II breast cancer. N. Engl. J. Med., *332*:907, Copyright 1995, Massachusetts Medical Society.)

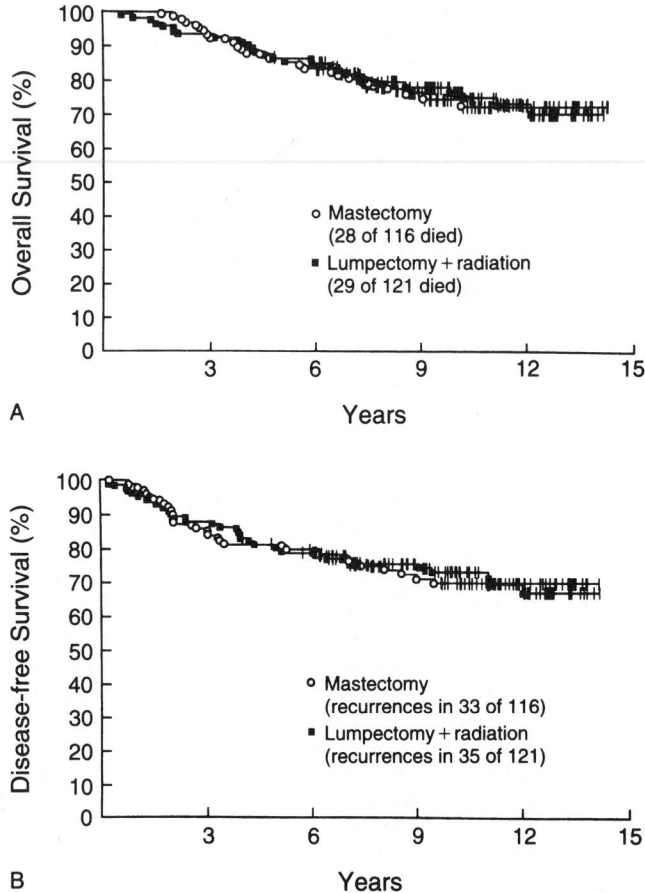

Figure 22–21. Overall survival *(A)* and disease-free survival *(B)* in the two groups. Tick marks indicate the lengths of follow-up for patients who had not died *(A)* or had a recurrence of disease *(B)*. Wider bars represent overlapping tick marks. (Reprinted by permission of *The New England Journal of Medicine* from Jacobson, J. A., et al.: Ten-year results of a comparison of conservation with mastectomy in the treatment of stage I and II breast cancer. N. Engl. J. Med., *332*:907, Copyright 1995, Massachusetts Medical Society.)

disease-free survival (72% for breast conservation patients and 69% for patients randomized to receive mastectomy; see Fig. 22–21*B*). For calculation of disease-free survival, patients in the breast conservation arm with an in-breast failure salvaged by mastectomy were not counted as treatment failures (events). This is the standard way in which event-free survival is presented in surgical trials of breast conservation but is different from the way in which the NCI presented their first report at 5 years. As predicted, most of the events in the conservation arm were breast failures after radiation and 6 of 10 patients with a local failure in the mastectomy arm also had concomitant distant failure (actuarial plots shown in Fig. 22–22). Overall, only 3 of 116 (2.6%) patients treated with mastectomy suffered local failure that was not associated with a regional or distant failure. The actuarial risk of in-breast relapse for the group treated by lumpectomy and radiation therapy was 18% at 10 years of follow-up and is shown in Figure 22–23. Nineteen patients have suffered a recurrence of breast cancer in the treated breast, of which 18 have been treated by salvage mastectomy. The risk of relapse in the treated breast appears constant over time and in the range of 1% to 2% per year after treatment. The majority of patients treated with radiation therapy rated their cosmetic result as excellent (63%), and the complication rate after breast radiation was low. Common complications were rib fracture, chest wall and breast pain, and a higher incidence of seroma formation in the axillary wound or breast lumpectomy site.

The results of this small study are analogous to other

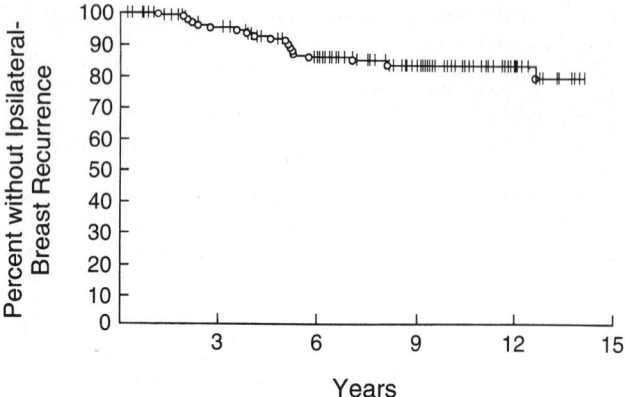

Figure 22-23. Actuarial risk of recurrence confined to the ipsilateral breast among 121 patients assigned to lumpectomy plus radiation. Nineteen patients had a recurrence (16%). Tick marks indicate follow-up times for patients without recurrences. (Reprinted by permission of *The New England Journal of Medicine* from Jacobson, J. A., et al.: Ten-year results of a comparison of conservation with mastectomy in the treatment of stage I and II breast cancer. N. Engl. J. Med., *332*:907, Copyright 1995, Massachusetts Medical Society.)

prospective and retrospective series of comparable patients treated in a similar way (see Table 22-7). Several guidelines for breast conservation will follow and represent a viewpoint that may not be held by all practitioners. In general, it is probably accurate to quote a 1% per year ipsilateral breast recurrence rate to candidates who are considering breast conservation. It is also fair to inform these women that their chance of surviving breast cancer is not affected by choosing either mastectomy or breast radiation therapy. Complication rates are low (between 2% and 5%) and consist of spontaneous rib fracture, transient pericarditis for left-sided cancers, some distortion of the breast and tissues around the wide excision, a higher incidence of seroma formation, and difficulty with wound healing. If an axillary dissection is performed, axillary radiation should not be routine unless there are many positive nodes or gross disease remains. If axillary dissection and radiation are combined, ipsilateral arm edema will be more common. Radiopaque clips should be placed within the lumpectomy defect to assist the radiotherapist in therapeutic planning. In general, no attempt should be made to approximate the deep tissues within the lumpectomy defect. If meticulous hemostasis is obtained, the wound will temporarily fill with serous fluid and slowly contract over a period of several weeks. The specimen that is removed should be oriented and ink applied before it is bisected. If a histologically positive margin is found, a reoperation to remove more tissue will frequently achieve a clear margin and allow conservation of the breast. Waiting for 2 or 3 weeks for healing and wound contracture makes the second operation technically easier and can be combined with the axillary dissection if indicated and not performed at the first operation. A gross or histologically positive margin is the only unerring contraindication to recommending breast conservation. Extensive intraductal carcinoma may be associated with a higher recurrence rate but does not negate lumpectomy and radiation therapy as long as a negative margin can be obtained.

Treatment of Locally Advanced and Inflammatory Breast Cancer[16, 26]

Locally advanced breast cancer is difficult to precisely define but generally refers to Stage IIIa and IIIb. Central to the concept is the notion that the disease is advanced on the chest wall (any T_3 or T_4 tumor) and/or in regional nodes (N_1 or N_2 in the 1992 TNM system), but without evidence for

distant metastases (M_0). In 1986, the AJCC specifically defined inflammatory carcinoma according to clinical criteria and assigned a new T code, T_{4d}, which falls under Stage IIIb disease. Confusion was compounded in older systems, which placed inflammatory carcinoma in Stage IV and placed large T_3 tumors without nodal metastases in Stage III. The revised TNM system segregates the uncommon T_3N_0 case to Stage IIb, reflecting its more favorable prognosis after standard therapy. Furthermore, metastases to homolateral supraclavicular nodes now are coded as distant metastasis (M_1) and designated as Stage IV disease. This leaves us with a more precise definition of locally advanced disease, which is composed of Stage III tumors in the 1986 AJCC TNM system and includes inflammatory carcinoma.

The treatment of noninflammatory Stage III tumors has been changing during the past two decades. The disease is heterogeneous and defies a uniform treatment approach. For large primary cancers and movable axillary nodes, mastectomy appears to be appropriate initial treatment. The use of breast-preserving procedures has not been specifically defined in these patients, but some authors believe excision and radiation therapy is appropriate in specific situations where the tumor can be excised with clear surgical margins, leaving a cosmetically acceptable breast. When operation is used alone, local relapse rates in the range of 30% to 50% can be anticipated and the long-term cure rates rarely exceed 30%. Similar results are reported when radiation therapy is the sole mode of local-regional treatment. These poor results have motivated trials using multiagent chemotherapy, particularly combinations that include doxorubicin (Adriamycin). Investigators at the National Cancer Institute in Milan pioneered the use of combination chemotherapy given before either radiation therapy or mastectomy and reported 3- and 4-year survivals in the range of 50%, which was better than historical controls. Response to primary chemotherapy is usually good. Substantial shrinkage of the local-regional disease is expected in 70% of patients, and local control is long lasting in the majority of patients. With combination chemotherapy before or after local treatment, improved survival and local control rates were reported by other groups. Although the optimum approach has not been found, the modern approach to patients with large locally aggressive breast cancer should include combination chemotherapy, given either before or after local treatment by mastectomy or intense radiation therapy or both.

Inflammatory breast cancer presents with a dramatic clinical picture, described earlier. The pathologic hallmark, dermal lymphatic permeation by tumor cells, may be present. However, most investigators accept a clinical picture of erythema and warmth that extends over a significant area of breast skin and may or may not be associated with a palpable mass. Diffuse invasion of lymphatic channels within the breast unifies the clinical picture, with or without dermal lymphatic invasion. Axillary nodal metastases are almost always present and distant disease should be sought using radiographic modalities such as bone scan and computed tomography. Recent treatment approaches emphasize the aggressive use of combined modality treatment, which can include combination chemotherapy, mastectomy, and radiation therapy. Inflammatory breast cancer was once a uniformly fatal disease that claimed its victims after a median survival of 9 to 12 months. Newer treatment protocols use intensive chemotherapy as the first modality. Objective responsive rates are in the range of 60% to 80%, and most patients are rendered free of disease after mastectomy and a limited nodal dissection. Recent authors have discouraged extensive surgical dissections of ipsilateral axillary nodes, preferring regional radiation therapy to address residual nodal disease. A reasonable approach to this disease that is practiced in many North American centers uses a sequence of chemotherapy, mastectomy, and radiation therapy to treat inflammatory breast cancer. For instance, results of combining these three treatment modalities produced a better relapse-free survival (50% at 5 years) compared with patients who received less treatment (7% at 5 years) in a single institution. The role of dose intensification using high-dose chemotherapy with hematopoietic and growth factor support is under investigation in many centers and may improve initial and long-term response rates.

The Management of Noninvasive (in Situ) Carcinoma

Special attention to the problem of *in situ* carcinoma is justified by the increasing frequency of its recognition and the controversy surrounding the proper treatment of noninvasive cancer of the breast. Treatment decisions require appreciation of the various types and stages of *in situ* disease and demand that the surgical oncologist understand this sometimes complicated disease process. Moreover, its relationship to invasive cancer is a fascinating biologic question. Understanding these early proliferative states should give investigators a clue to the underlying cause of breast cancer. Finally, finding early malignancy is the goal of population screening. It is hoped that the high cure rate after treatment of noninvasive breast carcinoma will someday contribute to a decline in mortality from this malignancy.

Ductal Carcinoma in Situ (DCIS) or Intraductal Carcinoma[32, 39, 44]

Before modern mammography, intraductal lesions presented as palpable tumors in 50% or more of patients. In the 1980s, more were recognized by the calcifications they produce, observable on mammograms, than by physical detection. The comedo or solid form fills small mammary ducts and is likely to undergo central necrosis. The central detritus within ducts undergoes dystrophic calcification, producing fine punctate and even linear calcification, which is seen first on mammography long before invasive disease develops into a palpable mass. Clearly, these are early lesions that can be approached in a different manner from that for usual invasive disease. Treatment recommendations for patients with intraductal carcinoma are based on consideration of several issues, including (1) occult invasive cancer coexisting with the *in situ* lesion, (2) multicentricity of intraductal carcinoma, (3) the occurrence of disease in the contralateral breast, and (4) the natural history after diagnosis by biopsy.

The incidence and the significance of occult foci of invasive disease have been difficult to determine. Rosen and associates from Memorial Hospital in New York found invasive disease in 12 (11%) of 110 patients undergoing mastectomy for DCIS. None of these patients had axillary nodal metastases. Carter and Smith examined mastectomy specimens from patients undergoing breast removal after a biopsy diagnosis of purely DCIS. Seven patients (18%) had residual invasive disease within the breast. Three patients with occult invasive disease had nodal metastases. Lagios and co-workers used specimen mammography and careful serial sectioning to examine breasts removed after a biopsy diagnosis of DCIS. Overall, a 21% incidence of residual invasive cancer was found. A similar trend was noted in studies by Silverstein and associates, who reviewed 208 cases of intraductal carcinoma treated by a variety of means. Patchefsky and associates emphasized the relation between microinvasion and a comedocarcinoma histology. These authors also found a higher incidence of microscopic invasion in lesions that presented with clinical signs (palpable mass, nipple discharge, or Paget's change). Table 22–8 summarizes data from three published series with more than 200 patients treated. It is important to realize that axillary and distant metastases can only come from the invasive breast cancer within the tumor, which may or may not be found histologically.

Axillary metastases are very rare in lesions that appear to be pure intraductal cancers. In the three studies just listed, a total of 316 intraductal carcinomas were studied. Axillary metastases were present in only 5 of these; in one case a second primary invasive cancer in the ipsilateral breast was present. Although not all patients underwent axillary dissection, there were no nodal recurrences during the follow-up of these patients. Significantly, all patients with positive nodes had large tumors, palpable tumors, or microscopic invasion (see Table 22–8). In a series of 227 patients reported by Silverstein with intraductal carcinoma selected for the absence of microscopic invasion, 163 axillary dissections were performed and all were negative. In patients with small mammographically detected *in situ* tumors, axillary dissection is definitely not required nor recommended. In larger tumors, particularly those that require mastectomy because of size and involved margins, a low nodal dissection (level I or less) can be added to guarantee the absence of metastasis.

Many authors who have written about intraductal carcinoma are influenced by the high incidence of multicentric, multifocal, and even bilateral disease. *Multifocal* is a term referring to disease within the vicinity or same quadrant as the dominant lesion. Multicentric refers to disease in distant sites or quadrants within the same breast. Bilateral implies the concurrent finding of disease in both breasts. The existence of multicentric disease has led many to favor mastectomy for the treatment of DCIS, and concerns about bilaterality have prompted the use of prophylactic procedures on the contralateral breast. The most widely reported figure for the incidence of multicentric disease within the ipsilateral breast is 33%, or one third of cases in which a biopsy discloses intraductal cancer as the predominant lesion. However, estimates vary depending on how extensively other quadrants of the breast are examined. For example, although a large review of NSABP material failed to find multicentric disease, only a single random section from remote quadrants was examined. In contrast, Schwartz reported an incidence of approximately 37% after examining four random sections from each remote quadrant and from under the areola. Other

TABLE 22–8. Incidence of Microinvasion and Node Metastases in a Composite Series of Intraductal Carcinoma

	No. of Tumors	Percentage with Occult Invasions (No.)	Percentage with Positive Nodes (No.)
Size (mm.)			
1–10	99	4 (4)	0
11–20	57	16 (9)	1.7 (1)
2.1–4.9	62	16 (10)	0
>5.0	43	37 (16)	2.3 (1)
Histology			
Cribriform	45	2.3 (1)	0
Solid	22	4.5 (1)	0
Micropapillary	33	18 (6)	3 (1)
Papillary	30	10 (3)	3.3 (1)
Comedo	124	27 (33)	0

Data for tumors of differing size from Silverstein, M. J., et al.: Cancer, *66*:102, 1990, and Lagios, M. D., et al.: Cancer, *50*:1309, 1982. Data for tumors of differing histology from Patchefsky, A. S., et al.: Cancer, *63*:731, 1989, and Silverstein, M. J., et al.: Cancer, *66*:102, 1990.

estimates range between the results of these two studies. The risk of multicentric disease appears to depend both on the histologic type of the intraductal tumor and on the size or extent of the primary cancer. In the study of Lagios and associates, 2 of 24 small tumors less than 2 cm. (8%) were associated with disease in other quadrants of the breast. In moderate size tumors, between 2 and 5 cm., 2 breasts of 16 examined (12.5%) had multicentric disease. In large tumors whose extent was greater than 5 cm., all 13 cases examined had disease in remote quadrants of the ipsilateral breast. The study of Patchefsky and colleagues examined multicentricity as a function of the histology of the primary tumor. In agreement with other authors, this series found that micropapillary pathology was associated with a high (80%) incidence of multicentric disease. An intermediate percentage (40%) of papillary and comedocarcinomas were associated with remote disease, and solid and cribriform types were lowest. Size was not noted in this study. Pathologic review of DCIS should include an estimate of size, a comment about pathologic margins, and assessment of multifocal disease within the surgical specimen. Histologic type should be noted and a statement made about the presence or absence of microscopic invasion.

A special note should be made about assessing the surgical margins in cases of both pure DCIS and when DCIS surrounds and approaches the margin of an invasive cancer. The undisturbed specimen is inked in pathology and grossly sectioned. Histologic evidence of ink touching tumor cells defines a positive microscopic margin. As shown in Figure 22–24, a close but negative margin for invasive disease is more certain than a close but technically negative margin for *in situ* cancers. This is because the inked perimeter of the specimen may divide the intervening stroma between malignant ducts, leading to a technically negative surgical margin. A close margin, particularly in several locations, implicates the presence of malignant ducts beyond the fringe of the specimen. A careful pathologic report should point this out and comment about whether the close margin is focal (in one spot) or is seen at other locations around the perimeter of the biopsy.

Treatment Trials (*see tables for references to literature*). Although there is no consensus on the treatment of intraductal carcinoma, recent publications provide a great deal of information and are altering the surgical approach to this vexing disease. Most of these studies are retrospective reviews; however, authors are increasingly stratifying patients according to tumor size, involvement of the surgical margin, and histology. The NSABP has published early results of a randomized trial comparing total excision of intraductal lesions to a negative surgical margin (lumpectomy) to lumpectomy plus postoperative breast radiation therapy. Treatment of pure DCIS by total mastectomy should produce a nearly complete cure, approaching 100% of patients. Collected results of the National Task Force for Breast Cancer in Italy (FONCAM) contained 210 patients with DCIS treated by mastectomy and followed for an average of 5.5 years (1259 patient-years at risk). There were three local recurrences for a 98.5% cure rate at about 5 years. A single institution review reported by Silverstein and associates included 98 mastectomies. These patients had a 98% actuarial disease-free survival at 7 years of follow-up; there was a 100% survival over the same interval.

Lesser procedures definitely result in higher rates of treatment failures. Tables 22–9 and 22–10 summarize the results of recent reports that examine two strategies for treating intraductal carcinoma. Both tables organize the studies by the length of their follow-up. Table 22–9 presents seven studies that have followed patients treated by excision only. Not all studies required negative margins or excluded tumors

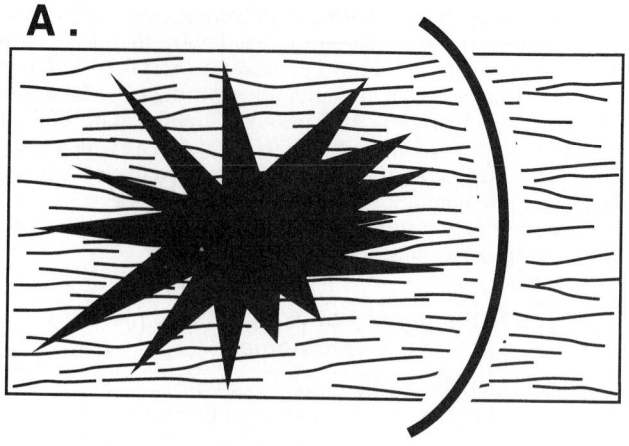

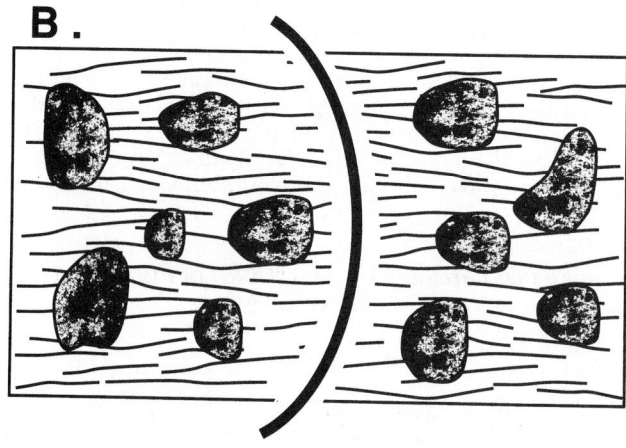

Figure 22–24. Significance of a negative surgical margin in invasive (*A*) compared with intraductal (*B*) carcinoma. If one strictly defines a positive margin as ink touching tumor cells on histologic section, it is possible to underestimate positive margins in an intraductal cancer because of its distinctive pattern of growth.

with microscopic invasion. Four studies contained 125 patients followed for more than 5 years. In these patients, there was a 25% recurrence rate (32 patients) in the treated breast and one half of these failures (18) were invasive cancer. Furthermore, there were five deaths among the 18 patients who failed local treatment of invasive disease. Although the results tend to discourage treatment of intraductal carcinoma by excision alone, patients in these reports are not typical of those with intraductal carcinoma found and treated in 1995. Patients today should have accurate histology, negative margins, tumors found by minimal mammographic change, and close follow-up. It is reasonable to treat a mammographically detected *in situ* cancer involving a small number of ducts and totally excised by biopsy or re-excision with observation and careful follow-up.

Local recurrence after excision of intraductal carcinoma can be reduced by application of radiation to the ipsilateral breast, similar to the case for invasive cancer. Local failure rates are reduced by a factor of about 50% over similar periods of follow-up (see Table 22–10). For example, four series are listed with average follow-up periods of 5 years or greater and in which 350 patients were treated by excision and radiation therapy. In the majority of these cases, clear margins were required for conservative treatment. A total of 36 patients experienced recurrence in the ipsilateral breast (10%) during this 5-year interval. This compares with the

TABLE 22–9. Treatment of Intraductal Carcinoma by Excision Without Postoperative Radiation Therapy

Study*	No. of Patients	Median Follow-Up (mo.)	Total No. of Recurrences (%)	No. of Invasive Recurrences (%)
1. Gallagher	13	100	5 (38)	3 (23)
2. Graham	53	97	14 (26)	7 (13)
3. NSABP B-06	21	85†	9 (43)	5 (24)
4. FONCAM	38	66†	4 (11)	3 (8)
5. NSABP	391	43†	64 (16)	32 (8)
6. Baird	30	39†	4 (13)	1 (3)
7. Silverstein	26	18	2 (8)	1 (4)

*Published sources (in order): 1. Gallagher, W. J., et al.: J. Clin. Oncol., 7:376, 1989; 2. Graham, M., et al. Eur. J. Surg. Oncol., 17:258, 1991; 3. Fisher, E. R., et al. J. Surg. Oncol., 47:139, 1991; 4. Ciatto, S., et al., Tumori, 76:552, 1990; 5. Fisher, B., et al. N. Engl. J. Med., 328:1581, 1993; 6. Baird, R. M., et al. Am. J. Surg., 159:479, 1990; 7. Silverstein, M. J., et al. Eur. J. Cancer, 28:630, 1992.
†Mean follow-up time (months).

25% failure in patients treated with excision only, although the patient groups are not strictly comparable. It is important to recognize that recurrence of intraductal cancer, whether treated by excision alone or with radiation therapy, can occur at any time during follow-up. Risk appears to remain constant over time and does not diminish. Actuarial local failure was studied in a cooperative series of 261 breasts treated by excision and radiation therapy at nine institutions in the United States and Europe. During 10 years of follow-up, there was a steady rate of breast failures reaching 16% in the 10th year; 13 of 28 breast failures occurred beyond 5 years of follow-up. Therefore, constant vigilance is required over the life-time of patients treated by breast-conserving strategies, whether or not they employ radiation.

In 1985, the NSABP began a randomized trial that compared the use of lumpectomy alone to lumpectomy plus 50 Gy. of postoperative radiation therapy. After a mean follow-up of 43 months, results were published in 1993. Five-year actuarial event-free survival was better in 399 patients who were treated by lumpectomy plus radiation therapy (84.4%) compared with 391 women treated by lumpectomy alone (73.8%). Considering just ipsilateral breast failures, there were 64 cases of breast cancer (16.4%) in the patients receiving just lumpectomy compared with 28 (7.0%) breast failures in those who received postoperative radiation therapy. Overall, there were only three deaths attributed to breast cancer and no significant differences in survival between the two arms of this study. The results are summarized in Figure 22–25, which separately displays the incidence of noninvasive and invasive cancers as the first events in women treated during the course of this trial. The third panel is the actuarial comparison of all other events, which includes second primary cancers, deaths of all causes, and distant metastases. Follow-up is not long enough to draw definite conclusions from the NSABP study. However, the numbers agree well with retrospective series and support the conclusion that radiation reduces the number of local relapses in the breast but does not affect distant disease or survival. This study did require negative surgical margins, and the majority (80%) of tumors were mammographically detected and not clinically apparent. Based on this randomized study, many oncologists believe that radiation should always be recommended after excision of intraductal carcinoma. Because mastectomy was not compared in this protocol, it remains an important option for treatment of well-informed patients.

In contrast to LCIS, discussed next, DCIS does not convey increased risk to the contralateral breast over and above the risk inherent for any woman who has had one breast cancer. An average risk of contralateral cancer in the range of 0.5% to 1% per year is a reasonable figure to quote in counseling patients with either invasive cancer or DCIS, even when the noninvasive cancer is diffuse and multicentric. As discussed earlier, age and family history are important modifiers of this risk estimate. For the vast majority of patients with DCIS, arguments for procedures on the opposite breast are hard to support. Identification of patients with contralateral disease should be based on careful follow-up and high-quality mammography for the majority of women with intraductal carcinoma.

Lobular Carcinoma in Situ (LCIS)[24]

Lobular carcinoma *in situ* is a relatively uncommon disease that occurs predominantly in younger, premenopausal women. As noted earlier, this disease is rarely diagnosed before biopsy, does not form a palpable mass, and rarely calcifies. Haagensen has collected the largest series of patients, all of whom were identified by review of biopsy material. In this review, LCIS was found in 3.6% of more than 5000 biopsies done for benign disease. Haagensen prefers the term *lobular neoplasia* to emphasize that this pathologic entity predisposes to subsequent carcinoma after a long latency

TABLE 22–10. Treatment of Intraductal Carcinoma by Excision Plus Radiation Therapy

Study*	No. of Patients	Median Follow-Up (mo.)	Total No. of Recurrences (%)	No. of Invasive Recurrences (%)
1. Solin	172	84	16 (9)	7 (4)
2. Bornstein	38	81	8 (21)	5 (13)
3. FONCAM	37	66†	2 (5)	2 (5)
4. Silverstein	103	62	10 (10)	5 (5)
5. Cutuli	34	56	3 (9)	1 (3)
6. NSABP	399	43†	28 (7)	8 (2)

*Published sources (in order): 1. Solin, L. J., et al.: Cancer, 71:2532, 1993; 2. Borstein, B. A. et al.: Cancer, 67:7, 1991; 3. Ciatto, S., et al.: Tumori, 76:552, 1990; 4. Silverstein, M. J., et al.: Eur. J. Cancer, 28:630, 1992; 5. Cutuli, B., et al.: Eur. J. Cancer, 28:649, 1992; 6. Fisher, B., et al.: N. Engl. J. Med., 328:1581, 1993.
†Mean follow-up (months).

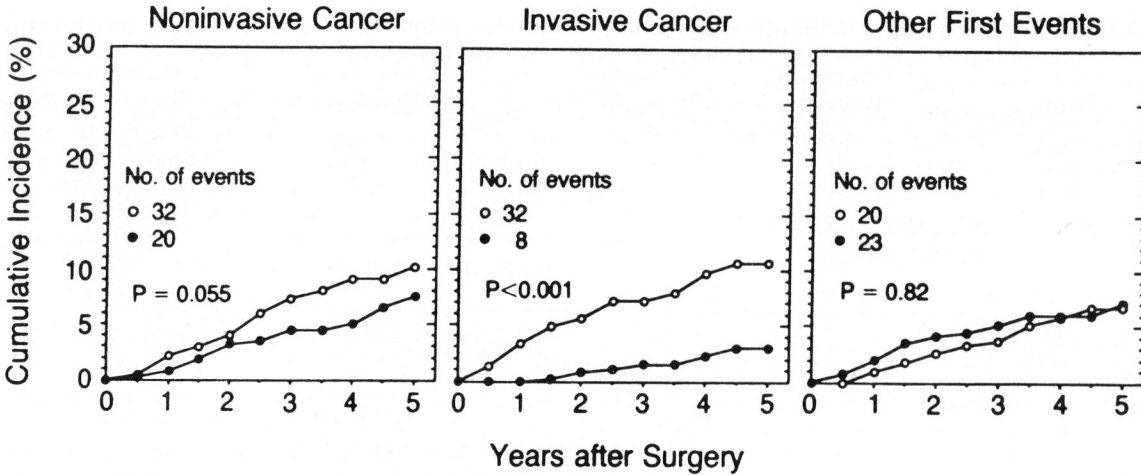

Figure 22–25. Cumulative incidence of noninvasive and invasive ipsilateral breast cancers and of all other first events in women treated by lumpectomy (open circle) or lumpectomy and radiation therapy (solid circle); p values are for the comparisons of average annual incidence rates between treatment groups. (From Fisher, B., et al.: Lumpectomy compared with lumpectomy and radiation therapy for the treatment of intraductal breast cancer. N. Engl. J. Med., *328*:1581, 1993.)

period. However, in a review of 297 patients with LCIS (lobular neoplasia) treated by biopsy and careful observation, Haagensen determined the actuarial probability of developing carcinoma at the end of 35 years was 21.4%. Compared with the Connecticut Tumor Registry data, a risk ratio (observed to expected cases) of 7:1 was calculated. Significantly, 40% of the carcinomas that subsequently developed were purely *in situ* lesions and one half of all subsequent carcinomas occurred in the contralateral breast. Haagensen preferred a practice of close observation after a biopsy diagnosis of LCIS. Similar data have led others to express doubts about the need for mastectomy. These authors have recommended a conservative policy of close observation after a biopsy diagnosis of LCIS or lobular neoplasia.

A contrary position has been supported by Rosen, who reviewed the experience of the Memorial Hospital Breast Service. In a series of 99 patients with LCIS treated by biopsy alone, subsequent carcinomas developed in 37% of patients followed for an average of 24 years. Consistent with Haagensen's data, recurrences were divided equally between the affected and contralateral breast. Comparison to the Connecticut Tumor Registry produced a risk ratio for development of subsequent breast carcinoma of 9:1 in patients with a biopsy diagnosis of LCIS. Although similar in magnitude to the calculations of Haagensen, in the past these investigators recommended total mastectomy with low axillary node dissection.

Although no direct survey of surgical practice has been done, a conservative approach to LCIS is probably more commonly practiced than mastectomy. Certainly, a policy of close observation is widely recognized as standard care. However, patients must be informed that LCIS predisposes to subsequent carcinoma and that their risk is life long and increases over passage of time. In selected patients, particularly young patients with significant family history of invasive breast cancer, mastectomy may be an appropriate choice for a well-counseled patient to make. Because the risk of subsequent breast cancer is equal for both breasts, biopsy of the opposite breast adds little useful information. Subcutaneous mastectomy, or glandular mastectomy, preserving the cosmetic appearance of the breast would be an ideal procedure and could be done on both sides. Unfortunately, this procedure will not remove all tissue at risk and is an unproven method of cancer prevention. Total mastectomy remains the procedure of choice for those who elect surgery in preference to observation; however, bilateral mastectomy is

theoretically the only means to significantly diminish subsequent risk.

Male Breast Cancer[1, 24]

Breast cancer occurring in the mammary gland of males is infrequent, accounting for no more than 1% of the incidence in women. It generally occurs at an older age. The average age at diagnosis is 10 years older in men than in women. Probably because the breast tissue is scant in men, breast tumors in males involve the pectoralis major muscle more commonly. Delay in diagnosis also must play a role in the more advanced presentation of male breast cancer. Histologically, tumors of the male breast are most commonly infiltrating ductal carcinomas that are similar in appearance to their counterparts in females. Lobular carcinoma, both invasive and noninvasive, is rarely seen in males. Interestingly, male breast cancer very often contains steroid hormone receptors. Gupta found that 84% of tumors arising in male mammary glands contain estrogen receptor, and other studies support the high incidence of receptors and the frequent hormone sensitivity of male breast tumors.

The treatment of carcinoma in the male breast depends on the stage and local extent of the tumor. If the underlying pectoral muscle is involved, radical mastectomy is the procedure of choice. Alternatively, modified radical mastectomy with excision of the involved portion of muscle is adequate treatment. There seems to be little reason to practice breast preservation, but there are no studies to the contrary and no *a priori* reason for excluding men from treatment by local excision and radiation if technically feasible and preferred by the patient. For smaller tumors, which are movable across the chest wall, modified radical mastectomy appears to be the procedure of choice. Because of the local aggressiveness of these tumors, some authors have advocated the use of postoperative radiation therapy.

The presence of nodal metastases appears to have at least the same prognostic power in men as in women. A large review of male breast cancer at Memorial Hospital reported survival in node-negative cancer similar to that in women. However, node-positive disease portended a worse prognosis in men than in women. There is little experience with adjuvant chemotherapy or hormonal therapy in male breast cancer. Because the majority of these tumors are hormone sensitive, the use of adjuvant tamoxifen for node positive and high-risk node-negative patients seems logical. Bagley and colleagues at the NCI have used combination chemotherapy with cyclophosphamide, methotrexate, and 5-fluorouracil (CMF) in node-positive men according to dose scheduling used in women. The 5-year survival of more than 80% of men treated with adjuvant therapy appeared to be a significant improvement over historical controls.

Adjuvant Chemotherapy for Operable Breast Cancer

Perhaps no single aspect of modern cancer therapy has been so well studied as the use of adjuvant systemic treatment after definitive local therapy for breast cancer. A fundamental assumption that underlies the addition of systemic therapy to the local treatment of breast cancer by surgery or radiation emphasizes the importance of metastatic disease as the principal cause of death in this disease. Indeed, the vast proportion of patients who benefit from chemotherapy or hormonal therapy do so because metastasis is prevented, cured, or delayed. The first prospective trials of systemic treatment combined oophorectomy to radical mastectomy. As we shall see, these treatments were effective in certain patients. Since these early trials, well over 100 randomized studies of systemic therapy have been published one or more times in the medical literature. One analysis of worldwide randomized trials in which any form of systemic therapy was compared with surgery alone in early breast cancer found 75,000 women, estimated to be 90% of those ever randomized. Interpreting the results of these many studies requires a basic knowledge of descriptive and analytical statistics.

Interpreting Results of Clinical Trials. Survival curves are the most familiar way in which groups of patients are compared in randomized trials of different therapies. To estimate the survival curve for any group of people, investigators use the life-table method (also called the actuarial method). A popular modification of these general methods that suit clinical trials was proposed by Kaplan and Meier, and the resulting curves are often called Kaplan-Meier curves. This method tabulates the number of patients surviving as a proportion of the total number of patients reaching the interval of time in question after entering the trial. The curve is generated by plotting data for each interval of time. Survival or death is only one outcome that can be expressed in actuarial terms. Disease-free survival, event-free survival, or freedom from local failure (to list a few) can all be expressed in actuarial terms. Comparisons between survival or freedom from event curves can be described in several ways, each of which has limitations and ambiguities. The simplest way is to measure the absolute difference in survival at an interval, usually a specific time or the last interval. Other ways to express the difference include citing the proportional reduction in mortality (the difference in survival at an interval divided by the percent of patients dead in the control group in the same interval). For the same proportional reduction in mortality, the absolute difference in survival varies greatly and is generally larger in groups of patients with higher risks of dying (node-positive versus node-negative patients). The proportional increase in survival divides the absolute difference between the control and experimental curves in a specified interval by the total surviving in the experimental group (assuming it is larger). For groups with poor survival, small absolute differences lead to larger estimates of the percentage increase in survival.

Finally, the median survival time is the length of survival until an event occurs in 50% of the patients. It is useful to consider the differences in median survival times between treated and control patients, even though overall survival percentages are similar. Extension of life, if it is of good quality, is an important treatment endpoint and may be overlooked if one only considers the proportion of patients surviving.

Adjuvant Chemotherapy for Lymph Node-Positive Patients.[3, 4, 17, 50] The first trials of prolonged postoperative chemotherapy in operable breast cancer were begun by the NSABP in 1972 and by the National Cancer Institute of Italy (NCI-Milan) in 1973. Only patients with positive axillary nodes were chosen for study. The NSABP protocol B-05 compared oral L-phenylalanine mustard (L-PAM, Melphalan) with a placebo in patients receiving radical mastectomy. The NCI-Milan studied a combination of cyclophosphamide, methotrexate, and 5-fluorouracil (CMF) versus no treatment after either radical mastectomy or extended radical mastectomy. Neither study allowed the use of postoperative radiation therapy or hormone therapy. Both studies stratified patients into a group younger than 50 years of age (commonly denoted premenopausal) and into a group older than age 50. Nodal involvement was divided in both studies into a group with one to three positive nodes and a group with four or more positive nodes.

The results from these two trials are similar and convincingly positive for women treated with chemotherapy who are younger than 50 and who have one to three positive nodes. In both studies, the magnitude of difference in this subgroup was relatively large and statistically significant. A trend toward prolongation of survival was seen in young women with four or more positive nodes, but this group was more heterogeneous. In contrast to the positive effect of chemotherapy in younger patients, women older than 50 years of age did not significantly benefit, as a whole, from the use of adjuvant cytotoxic chemotherapy. Subsequent studies have shown that combination chemotherapy is generally better than the use of single agents, and 20-year follow-up of the initial NCI-Milan CMF combination has shown very few complications.

Twenty-year results from the NCI-Milan trial continue to show significant overall benefit from adjuvant CMF chemotherapy. Table 22–11 shows the outcome of treatment for all subgroups of patients in the trial. With the exception of postmenopausal patients with four or more nodes, all subgroups of women benefited by the use of adjuvant chemotherapy. In the analysis of the Milan trial, the question of dose intensity was investigated as a determinate of effectiveness of chemotherapy. The outcome of patients receiving greater than 85% of their calculated chemotherapy dose was significantly better than patients who received less than 65% of their scheduled dose. Because of protocol requirements in this study, dose intensity was generally less in postmenopausal women, particularly those older than age 60. Authors of the Milan study argue that this fact explains the difference between results in premenopausal and postmenopausal women.

In the first NCI-Milan study of CMF, adjuvant therapy was given over 1 year postoperatively. In the NSABP study of oral melphalan, the drug was continued for 2 years after surgery. The effectiveness of shorter durations of postoperative treatment was demonstrated in the second Milan CMF study and in several other trials. Figure 22–26 shows 14-year results comparing 12 cycles of CMF to 6 cycles of adjuvant treatment. Newer strategies rely on doxorubicin containing regimens and have cut treatment times to less than 6 months and 4 cycles of therapy.

The question of dose intensity has been formally addressed in two important national cooperative trials initiated by the Cancer and Leukemia Group B (CALGB). The first was a randomized trial of different dose levels of chemotherapy given to women with node-positive (stage II) breast cancer after curative surgery (mastectomy or conservation with radi-

TABLE 22–11. Relapse-Free and Overall Survival at 20 Years in Two Groups of Patients, According to Their Characteristics at Entry in the Study

Characteristic	Percentage of Total		Relapse-Free Survival* (%)		Overall Survival† (%)	
	Control Group (N= 179)	CMF Group (N= 207)	Control Group	CMF Group	Control Group	CMF Group
Premenopausal	48	50	26	37	24	47
Postmenopausal	52	50	24	26	22	22
Tumor size‡						
≤2.0 cm.	54	50	28	33	22	36
>2.0 cm.	46	50	21	31	26	31
No. of involved nodes						
1–3	70	68	29	37	24	38
4–10	25	23	18	26	27	27
>10	5	9	0	0	0	17

*In the analysis of relapse-free survival, second primary cancers and deaths due to other causes were not considered events. The rate of relapse-free survival was 25% in the control group as a whole and 32% in the CMF group as a whole.

†The rate of overall survival was 23% in the control group as a whole and 34% in the CMF group as a whole.

‡Tumor size on pathologic analysis.

Adapted from Bonadonna, G., Valagussa, P., Moliterni, A., et al.: Adjuvant cyclophosphamide, methotrexate, and fluorouracil in node-positive breast cancer. N. Engl. J. Med., *332*:901, 1995.

ation). Three arms in this study received escalating dose intensity (by varying both duration and total dose) of cyclophosphamide, doxorubicin, and fluorouracil (CAF). With a relatively short follow-up time (median of 3.4 years), women treated with either high- or moderate-dose intense CAF had a significantly longer disease-free and overall survival. To extend the question of dose and intensity of treatment, a national cooperative group trial of high-dose chemotherapy with autologous marrow support has accrued several hundred patients. In this study, all women with 10 or more positive nodes entered receive adjuvant chemotherapy with doses that do not require marrow support followed by marrow harvest and high-dose therapy in one arm and compared with a strategy of observation in the second arm. In Milan, high-dose chemotherapy for women with 10 or more positive lymph nodes has produced a 2-year disease-free survival of 93%. Results from the CALGB study are not yet available. Importantly, modern dose-intense treatments include the use of hematopoietic growth factors to both accelerate recovery of peripheral white blood cell count after treatment and to stimulate the production of circulating hematopoietic cells for harvest and autologous transplantation. This technical advance has allowed medical oncologists to use far higher doses of adjuvant therapy in standard clinical practice, particularly in node-positive patients at high risk for relapse.

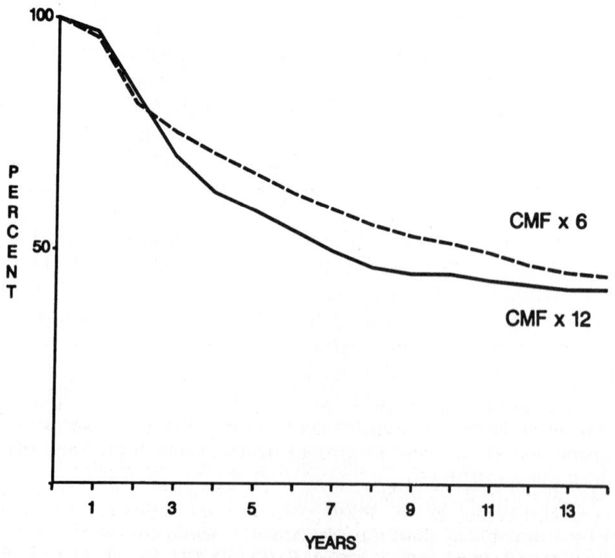

Adjuvant Chemotherapy for Node-Negative Patients.[9, 40] A smaller fraction of node-negative patients suffer recurrence of cancer after primary therapy. In the Natural History Data Base, shown in Figure 22–17, the absolute survival at 10 years for Stage T_1 or T_2 disease in patients with negative lymph nodes is between 75% and 80%. As discussed earlier, even if the magnitude of reduction in recurrence is similar between node-positive and node-negative patients, the absolute difference is much smaller in the node-negative groups. It is likely that certain characteristics of the primary tumor are associated with a greater chance of metastasis and treatment failure. In addition, other characteristics of the tumor may predict a greater chance of responding to systemic therapy. Poor prognostic signs include (1) tumor size greater than 2 cm., (2) poor histologic and nuclear grade, (3) absent hormone receptors, (4) high proliferative fraction (S-phase), (5) aneuploid DNA content, and (6) content of certain oncogenes such as *erbB-2* (*HER2/neu*), *p53,* and the epidermal growth factor receptor. Most studies of adjuvant chemotherapy in node-negative women have restricted enrollment to those patients with tumors possessing some markers of poor prognosis.

Survival statistics from large series of node-negative patients undergoing mastectomy without postoperative systemic therapy support a selective approach to adjuvant treatment. Rosen and associates reviewed survival statistics from Memorial Sloan-Kettering for patients treated by operation alone between 1964 and 1970, allowing a long follow-up. For node-negative patients with tumors 1 cm. or less, the likelihood of remaining free of disease at 10 years was 91%. In contrast, for tumors between 1.1 and 2.0 cm., the chance of remaining free of disease fell to 78%. Other groups of node-negative patients suffer even higher relapse rates, as noted earlier. Several trials of postoperative systemic therapy have addressed node-negative patients. Because of a general trend toward a more favorable outcome in patients treated with postoperative chemotherapy, the NCI issued a clinical alert

Figure 22–26. Second CMF program. Comparative relapse-free survival at 14 years. There were no significant differences between CMF given for 12 compared with 6 months' duration. (From Bonadonna, G.: Evolving concepts in the systemic adjuvant treatment of breast cancer. Cancer Res., *52*:2127, 1992.)

TABLE 22–12. Representative Studies Comparing Adjuvant Systemic Therapy to No Treatment After Surgery for Node-Negative Breast

Study	No. of Patients	Tumor Size	ER Status	Therapy	Median Follow-Up (mo.)	Survival			
						Relapse-Free		Overall	
						Cont.	Treat. (p Value)	Cont.	Treat. (p Value)
Milan	90	$T_1–T_{3a}$	Negative	CMF	80	42	85 (<.001)	58	86 (.006)
NSABP B-13	737	Any	Negative	MF	60	66	78 (<.001)	84	95 (.09)
NSABP B-14	2844	Any	Positive	TAM	60	72	82 (<.001)	90	90
Intergroup	425	Any	Both*	CMFP	54	61	83 (<.001)	80	86 (.31)
IBCSG	1275	$T_1–T_{3a}$	Both	CMF	60	68	74 (.02)	85	88 (.31)

*Any ER-negative, ER-positive tumors ≥3 cm.
ER, estrogen receptor; C, cyclophosphamide; M, methotrexate; F, fluorouracil; P, prednisone; TAM, tamoxifen; IBCSG, International Breast Cancer Study Group; Cont., control groups; Treat., treatment groups.
All studies are included in the Consensus Development Conference on the Treatment of Early Breast Cancer. J. Natl. Cancer Inst. Monogr, vol. 11, 1992.

in 1988 urging consideration of adjuvant systemic therapy in many node-negative patients. Five randomized postoperative trials influenced the NCI then and continue to show benefit for groups of node-negative patients. Since that time, several more trials enrolling node-negative patients have been started. Results from the five trials are summarized in Table 22–12.

In 1992, the NCI issued a report from its Consensus Conference on the Treatment of Early Breast Cancer. Panelists agreed that evidence supported a reduction in recurrence and fatality for patients treated with adjuvant polychemotherapy or tamoxifen. However, the panel report acknowledged the generally good survival for many women with node-negative breast cancer. Entry onto clinical trials was favored for most women. For those who were not candidates for such trials, the panel supported individualizing recommendations. These tailored recommendations should take into consideration quality of life, patient desires, and established prognostic factors. It is likely in 1995 that most premenopausal women with tumors larger than 1 cm. and negative lymph nodes are offered adjuvant chemotherapy. Women who are postmenopausal with hormone receptor–positive tumors and negative lymph nodes are likely to receive tamoxifen for tumors larger than 1 cm.

Hormonal Therapy for Breast Cancer[25, 27]

The effect of steroid hormones on sensitive tissues has been the subject of important basic and clinical efforts. Surgeons have participated in this research from its beginning. Beatson, surgeon to the Glasgow Cancer Hospital, was the first to demonstrate that bilateral oophorectomy can lead to regression of metastatic breast cancer. Surgical castration became the first effective means to control advanced breast cancer, producing a beneficial regression in 25% to 40% of premenopausal patients. Huggins reemphasized oophorectomy and demonstrated the effectiveness of adrenalectomy in the treatment of metastatic breast cancer. Hypophysectomy, which deprives the patient of pituitary polypeptide hormones, causes palliative remissions of metastatic breast cancer in up to 40% of patients. This procedure, which carries an operative mortality between 2% and 9% and results in diabetes insipidus in a significant number of patients, is not widely used. Endocrine organ ablation has been replaced by estrogen and antiestrogen therapy in the majority of patients during the past decade. Oophorectomy has been compared with tamoxifen in two controlled clinical trials of patients with metastatic breast cancer. Results are equivalent in both the surgically treated and drug-treated groups. Aminoglutethimide, which blocks a number of steroid hydroxylation

steps in the adrenal and peripherally, appears capable of replacing adrenalectomy in the treatment of advanced disease. Overall, tamoxifen is at least as effective as every form of endocrine ablative therapy to which it has been compared. Understanding the cellular and molecular mechanism underlying the trophic effect of estrogen and progesterone represents one of the major advances in the treatment of breast cancer and has allowed physicians to predict patient responses to hormone manipulation.

Steroid Hormone Receptors.[13, 25] Specific accumulation of estradiol in the reproductive organs of animals suggested the presence of receptors for sex steroids. Availability of tritiated estradiol enabled investigators to demonstrate and measure specific, high-affinity protein receptors first for estrogen and later for progesterone. Numerous studies have demonstrated specific receptors for both estrogen and progesterone in tumor tissue from mammary origin. These receptor proteins are probably located in the cell nucleus and are activated when occupied by their specific ligand. Activation of the estrogen receptor leads to the induction of numerous cellular genes, including those that may encode critical enzymes and secreted peptide growth factors (Fig. 22–27). Clinically, the

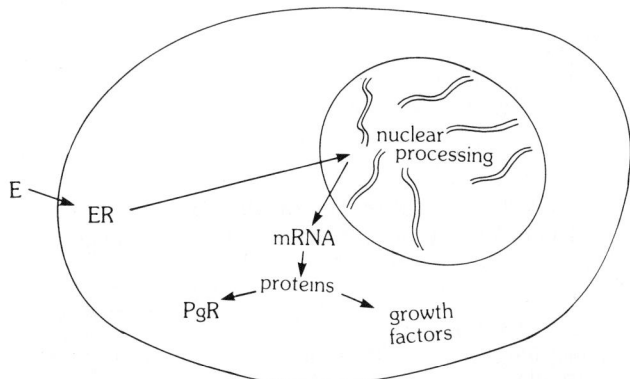

Figure 22–27. Mechanisms of estrogen action in breast cancer cells containing functional estrogen receptor. Lipid-soluble estrogen molecules (E) passively diffuse through the cell membrane where they bind to estrogen receptors (ER), most of which are located in the cell nucleus. The hormone-receptor complex interacts with specific sites on cellular DNA to stimulate transcription of mRNA and synthesis of cellular proteins. A predominant product in stimulated cells is the receptor for progesterone (PgR). Presence of PgR implies an intact estrogen-sensitive pathway. Cellular proliferation may depend on syntheses of certain polypeptide growth factors, such as the transforming growth factors (TGF-alpha and -beta) and insulin-like growth factors. By interacting with their specific receptors, these "second messengers" may close the loop and result in cellular division. (From Osborne, C. G: Receptors. In Harris, J. T., et al. [Eds.]: Breast Diseases. Philadelphia, J. B. Lippincott, 1987.)

most important protein induced by the estrogen receptor is the receptor for progesterone. Therefore, progesterone receptor may serve as an indicator for the presence of a functional estrogen receptor. This relationship explains clinical observations that relate the presence of functional receptors to response to hormone manipulation.

The quantity of receptor is expressed as a binding capacity in femtomoles (10^{-15} moles) of labeled steroid bound per milligram of protein. In this assay format, levels less than 3 fmol. per mg. protein are considered negative and indicate a slim chance of hormone responsiveness. Levels above 10 fmol. per mg. are clearly positive and indicate a high probability of hormone responsiveness. Newer assay formats are based on immunohistochemistry or enzyme-linked immunoassays and are increasing in popularity. The majority of human breast tumors contain detectable amounts of either estrogen receptor or progesterone receptor or both. As shown in Table 22–13, postmenopausal patients are more likely to have estrogen receptor–positive tumors than younger, premenopausal women. In contrast, the relationship between age and progesterone receptor is not as significant.

The observation that the presence and the amount of estrogen receptor was a positive marker for tumors likely to respond to endocrine therapy has been confirmed by many clinical investigators. The presence of estrogen receptor predicts clinical response to all types of endocrine therapies, both additive and ablative. Furthermore, because progesterone receptor expression is induced by estrogen binding to estrogen receptor, the presence of progesterone receptor correlates with response to endocrine therapy. The presence of both receptors in a tumor is associated with almost an 80% chance of favorably responding to hormone addition or blockade (Table 22–14).

Hormonal manipulation for the treatment of breast cancer has been simplified dramatically by the introduction of tamoxifen and related compounds. Tamoxifen is a weak estrogen agonist. In molar excess, tamoxifen acts like a competitive antagonist of estrogen activity in the breast, but not in other estrogen-sensitive tissues. Both the beneficial and unfavorable actions of tamoxifen in tissues other than the breast are due to its estrogen-like actions. Regardless of its exact mode of action, tamoxifen can effectively replace oophorectomy in premenopausal women with metastatic cancer. Tamoxifen is as effective as either ablative or additive therapies in treating hormone-sensitive cancers; it is considered the first drug of choice when hormonal manipulation is employed. Response rates in metastatic disease are approximately 50% when the tumor is estrogen receptor or proges-

TABLE 22–13. Distribution of Steroid Receptors in Tumor Biopsy Specimens According to Patient Endocrine Status*

Receptor Status of Tumor Biopsy Specimen	Endocrine Status of Patient	
	Premenopausal (%)	Postmenopausal (%)
ER$^+$, PgR$^+$	222 (45)	520 (63)
ER$^+$, PgR$^-$	58 (12)	128 (15)
ER$^-$, PgR$^-$	136 (28)	137 (17)
ER$^-$, PgR$^+$	72 (15)	41 (5)
Total	488	826

*Fifty-five years of age was chosen as an age at which virtually every woman may be considered postmenopausal.
From Wittlift, J. L.: Steroid hormone receptors in breast cancer. Cancer, 53:630, 1984. Copyright © 1984 American Cancer Society. Reprinted by permission of Wiley-Liss, Inc., a subsidiary of John Wiley & Sons, Inc.

TABLE 22–14. Relationship Between Steroid Receptor (ER, PgR) Status of Breast Tumor and Patients' Objective Response to Endocrine Therapy

Steroid Receptor Status*			
ER$^+$, PgR$^+$	ER$^+$, PgR$^-$	ER$^-$, PgR$^-$	ER$^-$, PgR$^+$
135/174 (78%)	55/164 (34%)	17/165 (10%)	5/11 (45%)

*Number of patients responding to treatment/number of women with receptor status designated.
Based on the collective paper presented at the NIH Consensus Development Conference on Steroid Receptors in Breast Cancer (Proceedings of the NIH Consensus Development Conference, 1980).
From Donegan, W. L., and Spratt, J. S. (Eds.): Cancer of the Breast. Philadelphia, W. B. Saunders, 1988.

terone receptor positive and falls to 10% for receptor-negative tumors. Tamoxifen has been carefully tested as an adjuvant after surgery or radiation therapy for primary breast cancer. It is being tested as a chemopreventive agent in 16,000 American women who are at increased risk to develop their first breast cancers.

Adjuvant Hormonal Therapy for Operable Breast Cancer.[5, 28, 37] Early trials of endocrine manipulation after breast cancer operation employed ovarian irradiation or surgical oophorectomy. The first modern trial of adjuvant tamoxifen was begun in Copenhagen in 1975. This study compared tamoxifen with placebo in premenopausal women. Three treatment arms in postmenopausal women were tamoxifen, diethylstilbestrol (DES), or placebo. Disease-free and overall survival were improved by the use of tamoxifen (or DES in postmenopausal women) compared with control arms. However, these differences reached significance only for postmenopausal patients in whom disease-free survivals at 5 years were 71% for DES-treated patients, 68% for adjuvant tamoxifen, and 49% for postmenopausal patients in the control arm.

In 1977, the Nolvadex Adjuvant Trial Organization (NATO) enrolled 1285 patients age 75 or younger into a two-arm study of tamoxifen versus observation after surgery for operable breast cancer. Premenopausal women with positive axillary nodes and postmenopausal women with or without positive nodes were eligible. Treatment with tamoxifen was continued for 2 years or until relapse resulted in withdrawal from study. Nearly one half (49%) of tumors were assayed for estrogen receptor content. At 5 and 8 years of follow-up, moderate and statistically significant prolongation in disease-free and overall survival was noted in the tamoxifen-treated patients compared with untreated controls. Overall, 34% fewer fatalities were observed in the treatment arm compared with the control group. Because tamoxifen was given for only 2 years, investigators looked for a rebound in relapses after stopping treatment. Benefit from 2 years of adjuvant treatment persisted after the drug was discontinued. Furthermore, the advantage of tamoxifen was independent of menopausal status, stage of cancer, and the estrogen receptor status in those patients whose tumors were analyzed. Similar findings were reported at 5 years from the Cancer Research Campaign in England who treated Stage I and II breast cancer patients with 20 mg. of tamoxifen daily for 2 years.

The second major trial of adjuvant tamoxifen in operable breast cancer was conducted in Scotland and began in 1978, one year after the NATO trial opened. The Scottish trial randomized 1312 patients 80 years of age or younger who had negative lymph nodes or who were postmenopausal and had positive axillary nodes. The trial differed from the NATO study by using 5 years of adjuvant tamoxifen and by treatment of first relapses in the control arm with tamoxifen by trial design. More tumors (57%) were analyzed for their estrogen receptor content in the Scottish trial. When assessing survival data, it is necessary to remember that 93% of patients suffering relapse in the control arm were treated with therapeutic tamoxifen. Therefore, the survival prolongation by use of adjuvant tamoxifen is determined by comparison to a policy of delayed tamoxifen after first relapse.

Moderate reduction in both recurrence and fatality was observed in the tamoxifen-treated patients. In the control arm, 38% of patients suffered a recurrence and 23% had died by 1987. In the tamoxifen-treated arm, there were recurrences in 24% of patients and 18% died of disease. The results of these trials in the United Kingdom have been confirmed by 24 other randomized comparisons of adjuvant tamoxifen to a no-treatment control arm. In all but one of these trials, tamoxifen has shown a trend toward improved disease-free survival and most trials also show a modest survival benefit. These results have been combined into a large meta-analysis, which also confirms the benefits of adjuvant tamoxifen.

The International Overview of Adjuvant Therapy for Breast Cancer[15]

The benefits of adjuvant systemic therapy for operable breast cancer are modest and in the range of a 20% to 30% reduction in the odds of recurrence or death for patients receiving postoperative treatment compared with those who did not. Although these differences are clinically worthwhile, their detection requires large trials with a high degree of statistical power. For this reason, it is helpful to combine results of randomized clinical trials and ask simple questions that average large numbers of heterogeneous patients. For instance, the question asked might be "Is adjuvant tamoxifen capable of improving overall survival of breast cancer patients, at any age or stage, compared with no treatment?" An international collaboration was begun in 1985 that sought primary data from any randomized trial of adjuvant systemic therapy of breast cancer begun before that same year. Data

from over 75,000 patients was collected and covered adjuvant chemotherapy, ovarian ablation, immunotherapy, and tamoxifen trials. In this overview, adjuvant tamoxifen resulted in a 17% reduction in the annual hazard rate for survival (2p<.00001). However, none of the 42 tamoxifen trials analyzed had the statistical power alone to detect a 17% difference in mortality and 36 of the 42 trials yielded nonsignificant survival differences.

Adjuvant Chemotherapy. In this phase of the overview analysis, information from 11,000 women in 31 trials was collected. These patients were randomized to receive long-term (more than just a perioperative dose) polychemotherapy (more than one agent) and were compared with a no-treatment arm. Overall results for all treated patients versus controls are shown in Figure 22–28. For recurrence-free survival, the main effect is seen by 5 years and there is an absolute difference of 9.2% in the number of recurrences. This translates to a highly significant reduction in the annual hazard rate for recurrence of 28%. For survival, the beneficial effect continues to accrue beyond 5 years. The absolute difference in surviving patients doubles to 6.3% at 10 years of follow-up. This translates to a 16% reduction in the odds of dying during each year after treatment and is highly significant. It is important to realize that this overview is an average of many different chemotherapy regimens and addresses the simple question of whether chemotherapy in general is biologically capable of improving outcome.

Subgroup analysis is possible in an overview provided the data are present and the groups are uniformly defined. Figure 22–29 subdivides the overview according to nodal status: those with positive nodes and those with negative nodes. Absolute benefits appear greater for node-positive patients than for node-negative patients. However, the reduction in annual odds of recurrence is 26% for node-negative patients and 30% for all node-positive women. Reductions in the odds of death from any cause is 18% and identical for both node-positive and node-negative patients. This relationship is a good example of the principle, discussed earlier, that a

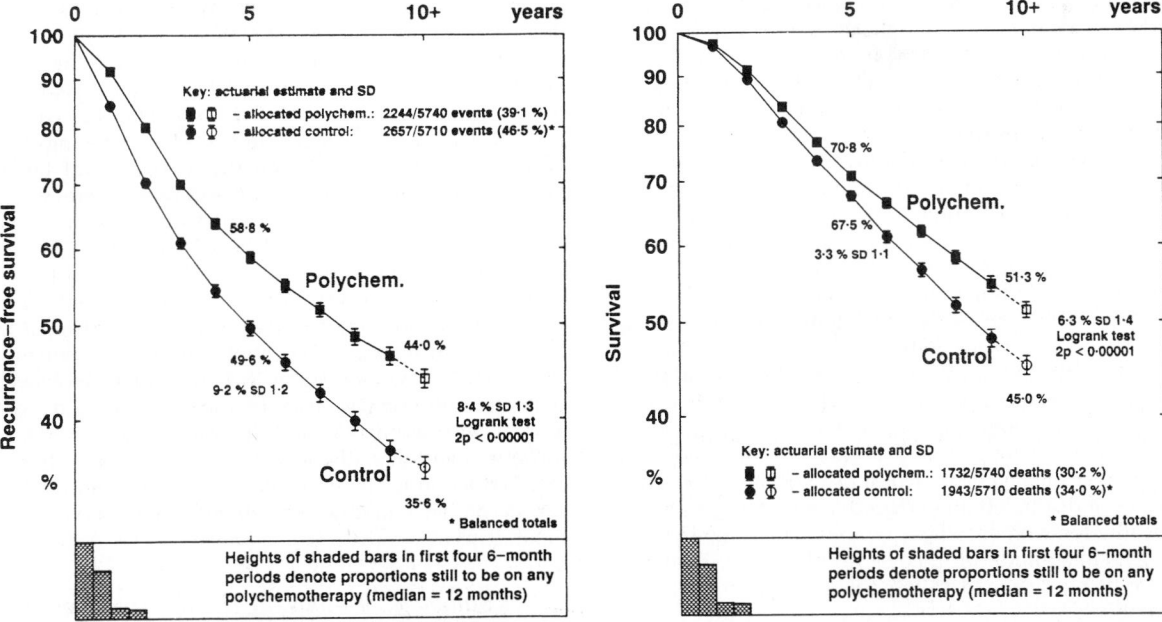

Figure 22–28. Ten-year outcome in polychemotherapy trials: overall results for all 11,000 randomized women. The left panel shows recurrence in all polychemotherapy trials for women of all ages; the right panel shows survival for all ages in polychemotherapy trials. Because the rates after year 10 are based on small numbers, combination of the data for years 5–9 and 10+ yields annual rates in years 5+ that favor active treatments. The shaded bars at the bottom of the graph show, just for those with a first event in each year, the proportions who, if allocated active treatment, would have been scheduled to still be on polychemotherapy: the median (and the mean) scheduled polychemotherapy duration was 1 year. (From the Early Breast Cancer Trialists' Collaborative Group. Lancet, 339:71, 1992. © by the Lancet Ltd., 1992.)

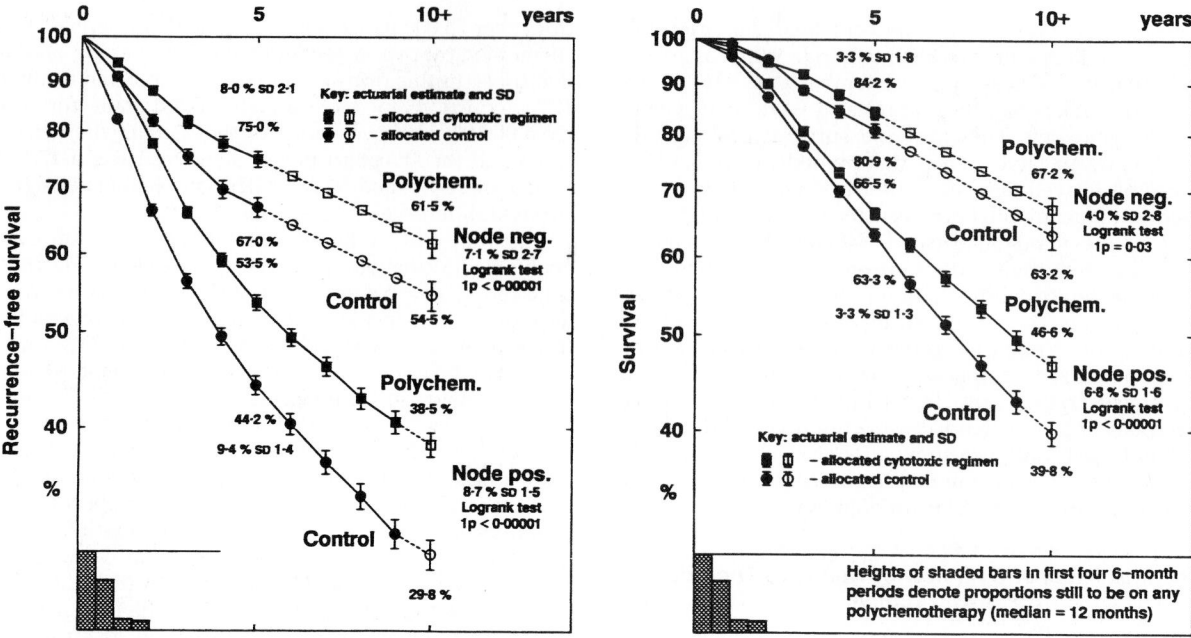

Figure 22–29. Ten-year outcome in polychemotherapy trials, subdivided by nodal status. The odds reduction for deaths due to cancer and other causes in node-negative patients was 15%, p=.04. The absolute difference in overall mortality was only 4% for all node-negative patients of any age. (From the Early Breast Cancer Trialists' Colllaborative Group. Lancet, *339*:71, 1992. © by the Lancet Ltd., 1992.)

constant reduction of the odds of recurrence or death leads to larger differences in absolute benefits for groups with an inherently higher event rate. The same subgroup analysis was applied to women younger than 50 or to those 50 and older. In general, the proportional reduction of odds for both survival and recurrence is greater in younger women compared with those 50 or older. However, polychemotherapy is still beneficial in women aged 60 to 69, producing a 20% delay of recurrence that remains highly statistically significant.

Immunotherapy. There were 6300 women randomized in 24 immunotherapy trials that involved bacille Calmette-Guérin (BCG), levamisole, and other forms of immunotherapy. There were no benefits noted in any single trial, and no benefits were discovered in the meta-analysis for immunotherapy as an adjuvant to surgery for the treatment of breast cancer. In fact, BCG administration resulted in a significantly adverse effect compared with control in the overview that was only recognized as a trend in individual trials.

Adjuvant Ovarian Ablation. One surprising result of the overview process was to rekindle interest in ovarian ablation as an effective treatment of operable breast cancer in premenopausal women. Ten trials were reviewed that accomplished ovarian ablation by oophorectomy, ovarian irradiation, and by certain drugs (other than tamoxifen). Results were strikingly positive for women younger than 50 years of age who were premenopausal. Overall survival was improved by 25% in women younger than 50 who received ovarian ablative therapy. Consideration of node-negative women younger than 50 who died of breast cancer, excluding other causes of death, left an odds reduction of 47% in breast cancer deaths for women whose ovaries where removed or ablated. This magnitude of biologic effect was so great that studies are being designed to test this effect in modern cohorts of patients.

Adjuvant Tamoxifen in Operable Breast Cancer. The overview looked at 30,000 women randomized in 40 trials to receive tamoxifen or no treatment. Statistically significant benefits for both node-positive and node-negative women were discovered, as shown in Figure 22–30. Interestingly, the

benefits gained by taking tamoxifen for 1 to 5 years (average duration of treatment was about 2 years in the overview) were felt during later years and after treatment had ceased. For recurrence, the curves are parallel past 5 years. For survival, the benefits gained during years of treatment continue to grow steadily after treatment has been stopped.

The proportional reduction in the odds of recurrence or death are almost identical for node-positive (28% reduction in recurrence, 18% reduction in odds of death) and node-negative women (26% for recurrence, 17% for survival). However, there is a steady trend toward improved benefits with longer durations of treatment (<1 year vs. 2 years vs. >2 years). For instance, reduction in the annual odds of recurrence is 16% for treatment times of 1 year or less but increases to 39% for treatment longer than 2 years. There is also a significant improvement in benefits for women who are 50 years of age or older compared with younger patients. However, there are still statistically significant benefits for young women as well. As an example, there was a 12% reduction in the chance of recurrence for women younger than 50 compared with a 29% benefit in women 50 and older; both were statistically highly significant benefits. Finally, there was a trend toward improved responses to tamoxifen in women whose tumors tested positive for estrogen receptor compared with those with estrogen-receptor–poor tumors or those whose receptor status was unknown. However, even patients with estrogen receptor–poor tumors did experience a small but significant benefit from tamoxifen, particularly those women older than the age of 50. Overall, there was a 39% reduction in the odds of developing a contralateral cancer in patients taking tamoxifen compared with no-treatment arms.

Summary of Adjuvant Therapy for Operable Breast Cancer[9, 36]

Guidelines for adjuvant therapy after primary treatment of breast cancer have evolved toward extending the recommendation to wider groups of patients. In fact, investigators are now attempting to identify groups of women who do not

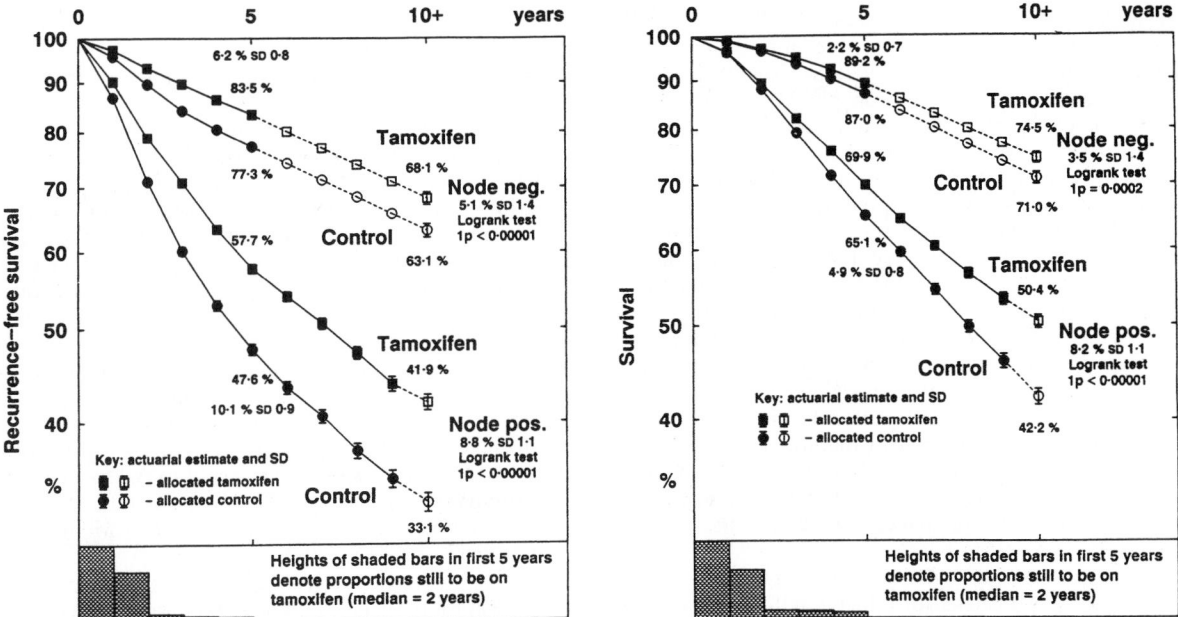

Figure 22–30. Ten-year outcome in tamoxifen trials, subdivided by nodal status. The odds reduction for deaths due to cancer and other causes in node-negative patients was 19% in the tamoxifen-treated patients, p = .0001. The absolute difference in overall mortality was only 3.5% for all node-negative patients of any age. (From the Early Breast Cancer Trialists' Collaborative Group. Lancet, *339*:71, 1992. © by the Lancet Ltd., 1992.)

benefit from some form of systemic treatment. This is because both adjuvant chemotherapy and adjuvant tamoxifen are likely to benefit nearly all patients groups with invasive breast cancers. *There is no proven benefit for any form of systemic therapy given to women with noninvasive breast cancer.* For patients with positive lymph nodes, additional therapy is of proven benefit. This is certainly the case for premenopausal women, but benefits extend to women well into their seventh

TABLE 22–15. Recommendations for Adjuvant Treatment Outside Clinical Trials

Menopausal Status	Axillary Nodes	Tumor Characteristics*	Recommended Treatment
Premenopausal	Positive	Favorable or unfavorable	Combination chemotherapy†
Premenopausal	Negative	Favorable	No data to support adjuvant therapy
Premenopausal	Negative	Unfavorable	Combination chemotherapy acceptable
Postmenopausal	Positive	Favorable	Tamoxifen ± chemotherapy
Postmenopausal	Positive	Unfavorable	Chemotherapy ± tamoxifen
Postmenopausal	Negative	Favorable	No data to support adjuvant therapy
Postmenopausal	Negative	Unfavorable	No data to support adjuvant therapy

*Favorable tumor characteristics include size <2 cm., ER- or PgR-positive, nuclear and histologic grade good (1 or 2). Unfavorable tumor characteristics include size >2 cm., ER- or PgR-negative, nuclear and histologic grade poor (3).

†Combination chemotherapy is usually CMF × 6 months (9 cycles).

decade of life (up to age 70). Because toxicity is related to other illnesses and to age, therapy may be less well tolerated with advancing age and declining health. Combination chemotherapy regimens are superior to single agents, and CMF is probably the polychemotherapy mixture of choice. Newer combinations, particularly for women with more advanced cancer, include doxorubicin. Chemotherapy administered for 4 to 6 months is just as effective as longer courses of treatment. Lymph-node negative patients receive a benefit from therapy whose magnitude appears to be equal to the benefits imparted to node-positive women. However, patients with very favorable tumors (<1 cm. or good histologies up to 2 or 3 cm., such as tubular or mucinous cancers) may not derive benefits that outweigh side effects.

Adjuvant tamoxifen is given for a minimum of 3 years and is remarkably free from toxicity. A slightly increased incidence of endometrial cancer, venous thrombosis, and ophthalmologic complications are the major toxicities of tamoxifen. Therapy in excess of 5 years or doses larger than 20 mg. per day are unproven and not recommended outside clinical trials. Women whose tumors test positive for hormone receptors, either estrogen receptor or progesterone receptor, are likely to derive more benefit from tamoxifen than women with hormone receptor–negative tumors. Tamoxifen should not be routinely recommended for receptor-negative tumors. Table 22–15 summarizes recommendations distilled from published data and from two National Institutes of Health Consensus Conferences held in 1985 and 1990. These recommendations change constantly as ongoing trials mature, toxicities improve, and new therapies reach clinical application.

TREATMENT OF METASTATIC DISEASE[25, 26, 46]

Once breast cancer has spread outside the confines of the breast and regional axillary lymph nodes it is not curable. The median life expectancy of patients with newly diagnosed stage IV breast cancer is about 24 months. However, although not curable, metastatic breast cancer can be controlled and patients can be offered palliative therapy. Occasional patients, particularly those with skeletal disease or disease in soft tissues and those whose tumors are hormone sensitive, can survive many years with advanced disease. Newer therapies such as autologous bone marrow transplantation after dose-intense chemotherapy offer the chance for improvement in survival and perhaps, someday, long-term remission or cure.

Chemotherapy for stage IV breast cancer is generally based on the use of two drugs, cyclophosphamide and doxorubicin, frequently in combination with other agents. Cyclophosphamide is a prototype alkylating agent that has been extensively studied in breast cancer and is used in the majority of combination programs. Doxorubicin is an anthracycline antibiotic that is the most active single agent in advanced breast cancer. Response rates in more than 50% of patients who have not been previously treated have been reported. In the absence of investigational protocols, combinations of cyclophosphamide, fluorouracil, and methotrexate (CMF) or cyclophosphamide, doxorubicin (Adriamycin), and fluorouracil (CAF) offer response rates of up to 50%. These combinations are standard care for patients with the first relapse of breast cancer.

As discussed earlier, one of the most important discoveries that has improved the outlook for patients with breast cancer is the identification of hormone receptors in tumor tissue. Response rates to endocrine treatment in metastatic disease for patients whose tumors harbor hormone receptors is in excess of 50%. The success rates for endocrine therapy are at least as good as those reported for cytotoxic therapy. However, the time required for measurable response is frequently longer for hormone manipulation than for chemotherapy. Furthermore, chemotherapy is more predictable and less dependent on the presence of hormone receptor content. These judgments depend on knowledge of the estrogen and progesterone receptor status of the tumor, the age of the patient, menopausal status, overall health, and determination of how life-threatening the metastatic disease is at diagnosis. For patients with life-threatening metastases in visceral organs, those patients whose tumors are estrogen receptor and progesterone receptor negative and those patients who are able to tolerate the side effects of cytotoxic drugs, combination chemotherapy is the first choice and a central entry in the algorithm. For older patients, patients with hormone-sensitive tumors, or for those patients whose disease sites are in bone, soft tissues, or other nonthreatening locations, endocrine manipulation can be tried first. Tamoxifen appears to be the agent of first choice for most of these patients.

NONEPITHELIAL BREAST TUMORS[38]

Cells comprising the connective tissue investments of the breast can give rise to both benign and malignant tumors. Generally, these tumors are sarcomas and can be categorized according to existing schemes describing sarcomas that originate in other body sites. An exception to this rule is the phylloides tumor or cystosarcoma phylloides, which is peculiar to the mammary gland. There are three principal tumor types discussed under the category of nonepithelial tumors: angiosarcoma, cystosarcoma phylloides, and other primary stromal sarcomas.

Angiosarcoma.[4, 33] This is an exceedingly malignant tumor, perhaps related to benign hemangiomas that can occur in the breast. It generally presents as a spongy, ill-defined mass that is composed of numerous dilated vascular channels. Hemorrhage, either spontaneous or complicating biopsy, is not uncommon. Necrosis, which never occurs in hemangiomas, is characteristic of angiosarcoma. The tumor characteristically achieves a large size by the time of presentation, usually larger than 5 cm. and the average age of patients with this malignancy is 10 to 15 years younger than for patients with usual ductal carcinomas. Metastases to regional nodes is extraordinarily rare; the usual mode of spread is hematogenous to the lungs, brain, bone, abdominal viscera, and even the contralateral breast.

The treatment of angiosarcoma is total mastectomy in the vast majority of cases. There seems to be agreement that axillary dissection is not necessary nor helpful. Because radiation therapy is of benefit in the treatment of related sarcomas in other body sites, some authors recommend postoperative radiation therapy to the chest wall. There have been only anecdotal reports of chemotherapy in angiosarcoma. Most regimens that are reported to have activity in this tumor contain either dactinomycin or doxorubicin. The role of adjuvant chemotherapy is even less well studied, but for high-grade lesions it seems to be logical and offers the only chance to alter the natural history of this tumor.

Survival seems to depend on the histologic grade of tumor. High-grade lesions (grade 3) are said to be the most lethal of all primary breast cancers. The survival rate of grade 3 lesions was only 11% of patients treated at Memorial Sloan-Kettering Hospital. In contrast, low-grade lesions are more likely to be cured after total mastectomy. However, some of these lesions may be confused with benign hemangiomas. As pointed out by Page, size is a valuable means to differentiate benign hemangiomas from angiosarcoma. Benign lesions are frequently found histologically and are rarely large enough to form palpable lesions. In contrast, angiosarcomas are usually large palpable masses that invade breast parenchyma. This fact, and the presence of mitoses and necrosis, will usually differentiate the malignant vascular tumors from the benign ones.

Cystosarcoma Phyllodes (Phyllodes Tumor).[33] This tumor is the most common neoplasm of nonepithelial origin in the breast. It is also a unique neoplasm that occurs exclusively in the female breast and appears in no other site in the body. The term *phyllodes* comes from the Greek word *phyllon*, which means "leaf." This descriptive terminology refers to a bulky tumor whose cut surface is embossed with a leaflike appearance. The term *cystosarcoma* refers to the microscopic cystlike spaces lined with a low epithelium and are reminiscent of fibroadenoma. The inclusion of sarcoma in the terminology may be confusing because the majority of these lesions are considered to be benign. For this reason, the WHO classification of breast tumors uses the term *phyllodes tumor*, which carries no implication of biologic potential. A diagnosis of phyllodes tumor (or cystosarcoma) should be qualified by indication of its malignancy, of its benignity, or whether it has indeterminate characteristics, a so-called borderline lesion.

The majority of tumors are sharply demarcated and freely mobile with a smooth contour. These tumors can be any size but frequently are large with a median size of 4 to 5 cm. They can occur in patients at any age, although the median age is generally in the fifth decade of life, at least a decade older than the average age of patients presenting with fibroadenoma. Mammographically, they present as round densities with a smooth border that are indistinguishable from fibroadenoma. The diagnosis is suggested by their larger size, history of rapid growth, and occurrence in older patients. The diagnosis is usually made by excisional biopsy followed by careful pathologic review.

The clinical behavior of this tumor is difficult to predict with accuracy. Some low-grade tumors do have the potential to metastasize, a fact that dictates the surgical approach to most of these tumors. Wide local excision seems appropriate for those that appear *benign* histologically, but patients must be carefully followed because of the risk for local recurrence and metastases. Excision with a rim of normal tissue seems most appropriate for these lower-grade tumors. When the histologic picture suggests malignancy or when their size is large, total mastectomy appears to be warranted. In a review of seven series reporting 332 patients, axillary metastases were present in 3 (0.9%) of the patients. Formal axillary dissection seems to be unnecessary, but removal of low axillary lymph nodes cannot be criticized.

Most recurrences of phyllodes tumors are local recurrences in the site of excision. For these patients, total mastectomy is most appropriate. Metastatic disease is commonly seen in the lung, mediastinum, and skeleton. The optimal treatment of metastatic phyllodes tumors has not been found. Most authors have used cyclophosphamide or doxorubicin-containing combinations. Three patients with metastatic tumors have been treated with cisplatin and etoposide combination chemotherapy. Effective palliation was achieved by this combination in two patients, and radiation to symptomatic metastases was helpful in all three. The tumors of two of these patients contained either estrogen or progesterone receptor, although hormone manipulation was ineffective.

REFERENCES

1. Bagley, C. S., Wesley, M. N., Young, R. C., et al.: Adjuvant chemotherapy in males with cancer of the breast. Am. J. Clin. Oncol., 10:55, 1987.
2. Basset, L. W.: Breast imaging: Current status and future directions. Radiol. Clin. North Am., 1992.
3. Bonadonna, G.: Evolving concepts in the systemic adjuvant treatment of breast cancer. Can. Res., 52:2127, 1992.
4. Bonadonna, G., Valagussa, P., Moliterni, A., et al.: Adjuvant cyclophosphamide, methotrexate, and fluorouracil in node-positive breast cancer. N. Engl. J. Med., 332:901, 1995.
5. Breast Cancer Trials Committee, Scottish Cancer Trials Office (MRC), Edinburgh: Adjuvant tamoxifen in the management of operable breast cancer: The Scottish trial. Lancet, 2:1, 1987.
6. Byrne, C., Smart, C. R., Chu, K. C., et al.: Survival advantage differences by age: Evaluation of the extended follow of the breast cancer detection demonstration project. Cancer, 74(Suppl. 1):301, 1994.
7. Chaudary, M. A., Millis, R. R., Davies, G. C., et al.: Nipple discharge: The diagnostic value of testing for occult blood. Ann. Surg., 196:651, 1982.
8. Clark, R. M., McCulloch, P. B., Levine, M. N., et al.: Randomized clinical trial to assess the effectiveness of breast irradiation following lumpectomy and axillary dissection for node-negative breast cancer. J. Natl. Cancer Inst., 84:683, 1992.
9. Consensus Development Conference on the Treatment of Early Breast Cancer, J. Natl. Cancer Inst. Monogr., vol. 11, 1992.
10. Danforth, D. N., Jr., Findlay, P. A., McDonald, H. D., et al.: Complete axillary lymph node dissection for stage I-II carcinoma of the breast. J. Clin. Oncol., 4:655, 1986.
11. Devitt, J. E.: Management of nipple discharge by clinical findings. Am. J. Surg., 149:789, 1985.
12. Devitt, J. E.: Benign disorders of the breast in older women. Surg. Gynecol. Obstet., 162:340, 1986.
13. Donegan, W. L., and Spratt, J. S.: Cancer of the Breast, 3rd ed. Philadelphia, W. B. Saunders, 1988.
14. Dupont, W. D., and Page, D. L.: Risk factors for breast cancer in women with proliferative breast disease. N. Engl. J. Med., 312:146, 1985.
15. Early Breast Cancer Trialists' Collaborative Group: Systemic treatment of early breast cancer by hormonal, cytotoxic, or immune therapy (133 randomised trials involving 31,000 recurrences and 24,000 deaths among 75,000 women). Lancet, 339:1 and 71, 1992.
16. Fein, D. A., Mendenhall, N. P., Marsh, R. D. W., et al.: Results of multinodality therapy for inflammatory breast cancer. Am. Surgeon, 60:220, 1994.
17. Fisher, B., Osborne, C., Margolese, R., and Bloomer, W.: Neoplasms of the breast. In Holland, J. F., Frei, E. III., Bast, R. C. Jr., Kufe, D. W., Morton, D. L., and Weichselbaum, R. R. (Eds.): Cancer Medicine, 3rd ed. Philadelphia, Lea & Febiger, 1993.
18. Fisher, B., Redmond, C., Fisher, E. R., et al.: Ten-year results of a randomized clinical trial comparing radical mastectomy and total mastectomy with or without radiation. N. Engl. J. Med., 312:674, 1985.
19. Fisher, B., Slack, N., Katrych, D., et al.: Ten year follow-up results of patients with carcinoma of the breast in a cooperative clinical trial evaluating surgical adjuvant chemotherapy. Surg. Gynecol. Obstet., 140:528, 1975.
20. Fletcher, S. W., Black, W., Harris, R., et al.: Report of the international

21. workshop on screening for breast cancer. J. Natl. Cancer Inst., 85:1644, 1993.
21. Fowble, B., Solin, L. J., Schultz, D. J., et al.: Ten year results of conservative surgery and radiation for stage I and stage II breast cancer. Int. J. Radiat. Oncol., 21:269, 1991.
22. Gail, M. H., Brinton, L. A., Byar, D. P., et al.: Projecting individualized probabilities of developing breast cancer for white females who are being examined annually. J. Natl. Cancer Inst. 81:1879, 1989.
23. Gallager, H. S.: Pathologic types of breast cancer: Their prognoses. Cancer, 53:623, 1984.
24. Haagensen, C. D.: Diseases of the Breast, 3rd ed. Philadelphia, W. B. Saunders, 1986.
25. Harris, J. R., Hellman, S., Henderson, I. C., and Kinne, D. W.: Breast Diseases, 2nd ed. Philadelphia, J. B. Lippincott, 1991.
26. Hortobagyi, G.: Multidisciplinary management of advanced primary and metastatic breast cancer. Cancer (Suppl.), 74:416, 1994.
27. Ingle, J. N., Krook, J. E., Green, S. J., et al.: Randomized trial of bilateral oophorectomy versus tamoxifen in premenopausal women with metastatic breast cancer. J. Clin. Oncol., 4:8, 1986.
28. Jordan, V. C.: A current view of tamoxifen for the treatment and prevention of breast cancer. Br. J. Pharmacol., 110:507, 1993.
29. King, M. C., Rowell, S., and Love, S. M.: Inherited breast and ovarian cancer: What are the risks? What are the choices? JAMA, 269:175, 1993.
30. Kopans, D. B.: Breast Imaging. Philadelphia, J. B. Lippincott, 1989.
31. Kopans, D. B.: Review of stereotaxic large-core needle biopsy and surgical biopsy results in nonpalpable breast lesions. Radiology, 189:665, 1993.
32. Lagios, M. D., Westdahl, P. R., Margolin, F. R., et al.: Duct carcinoma in situ: Relationship of extent of noninvasive disease to the frequency of occult invasion, multicentricity, lymph node metastases, and short-term treatment failures. Cancer, 50:1309, 1982.
33. Lichter, A. S., and Lippman, M. E.: Special situations in the treatment of breast cancer. In Lippman, M. E., Lichter, A. S., and Danforth, D. N. (Eds.): Diagnosis and Management of Breast Cancer. Philadelphia, W. B. Saunders, 1988.
34. Love, S. M., Gelman, R. S., and Silen, W.: Fibrocystic "disease" of the breast—A nondisease? N. Engl. J. Med., 307:1010, 1982.
35. Maddox, W. A., Carpenter, J. T., Laws, H. L., et al.: Does radical mastectomy still have a place in the treatment of primary operable breast cancer? Arch. Surg., 122:13, 1987.
36. National Institutes of Health Consensus Development Panel on Adjuvant Chemotherapy and Endocrine Therapy for Breast Cancer: Introduction and conclusions. NCI Monogr., 1:1, 1986.
37. Nolvadex Adjuvant Trial Organization: Controlled trial of tamoxifen as single adjuvant agent in management of early breast cancer. Lancet, 1:836, 1985.
38. Page, D. L., and Anderson, T. J.: Diagnostic Histopathology of the Breast. Edinburgh, Churchill Livingstone, 1987.
39. Patchefsky, A. S., Schwartz, G. F., Finkelstein, S. D., et. al: Heterogeneity of intraductal carcinoma of the breast. Cancer, 63:731, 1989.
40. Rosen, P. P., Groshen, S., Saigo, P. E., et al.: A long-term follow-up study of survival in stage I ($T_1N_0M_0$) and stage II ($T_1N_1M_0$) breast carcinoma. J. Clin. Oncol., 7:355, 1989.
41. Scanlon, E. F., and Caprini, J. A.: Modified radical mastectomy. Cancer, 35:710, 1975.
42. Seidman, H., Mushinski, M. H., Gelb, S. K., et al.: Probabilities of eventually developing or dying of cancer—United States, 1985. CA, 35:36, 1985.
43. Shattuck-Eidens, D., McClure, M., Simard, J., et al.: A collaborative survey of 80 mutations in the BRCA1 breast and ovarian cancer susceptibility gene. JAMA, 273:535, 1995.
44. Silverstein, M. J., Waisman, J. R., Gamagami, P., et al.: Intraductal carcinoma of the breast (208 cases): Clinical factors influencing treatment choice. Cancer, 66:102, 1990.
45. Skinner, M. A., Swain M., Simmons, R., et al.: Nonpalpable breast lesions at biopsy: A detailed analysis of radiographic features. Ann. Surg., 208:83, 1988.
46. Triozzi, P. L.: Autologous bone marrow and peripheral blood progenitor transplant for breast cancer. Lancet, 344:418, 1994.
47. Turner, L., Swindell, R., Bell, W. G. T., et al.: Radical versus modified radical mastectomy for breast cancer. Ann. R. Coll. Surg. Engl., 63:239, 1981.
48. Vicini, F. A., Recht, A., Abner, A., et al.: Recurrence in the breast following conservative surgery and radiation therapy for early-stage breast cancer. Monogr. Natl Cancer. Inst., 11:33, 1992.
49. Winchester, D. P., and Cox, J. D.: Standards of breast-conservation treatment. CA, 42:134, 1992.
50. Wood, W. C., Budman, D. R., Korzun, A. H., et al.: Dose and dose intensity of adjuvant chemotherapy for stage II, node-positive breast carcinoma. N. Engl. J. Med., 330:1253, 1994.

I

RECONSTRUCTIVE AND AESTHETIC BREAST SURGERY

Gregory S. Georgiade, M.D.

The introduction of new, improved surgical techniques has allowed surgeons to be increasingly innovative. Patient satisfaction has increased because of improvement in the aesthetic results. Familial, congenital, and developmental breast abnormalities, such as hypermastia, hypomastia, breast asymmetry, breast ptosis, and postmastectomy deformities, all affect a patient's self-image and confidence, and patients want to improve these deformities. The psychologic impact on a woman who has undergone ablative breast operations for breast cancer cannot be underestimated. Reconstruction of the breast mound produces positive results in the patient's self-image by the restoration of a more normal body contour.

MAMMARY HYPERPLASIA

Breast hypertrophy can limit physical activity and cause back, neck, and shoulder pain, accompanied by skin excoriations in the inframammary area. A reduction mammoplasty in this group of woman can be performed at any age, on an outpatient basis or with a short hospitalization.

Reduction in breast volume and correction of the usually accompanying ptosis can be accomplished by a number of techniques. Many of the concepts in the management of the problems are predicated on the use of the nipple-areola and dermal pedicle flaps (Fig. 22–31).[9, 13, 32, 34]

The surgical design can be based on the resection of an inferior wedge of triangular breast tissue or the vertical excision of breast tissue.[27] A third concept, often utilized, involves maintenance of a central core of breast tissue with the associated nipple-areola complex and resection of the excess breast tissue in the medial, superior, and lateral positions.[3] The technique for minimizing the inferior areolar vertical scar and the inframammary scar should be incorporated in the reduction technique whenever possible.[23] In the author's experience, the most versatile technique utilizes a pyramidal-based breast flap with an inferior dermal nipple-areolar pedicle.[13] A large reduction mammaplasty with resection of up to 3000 gm. of tissue from each breast can also be done with this technique with excellent aesthetic results and improved functional aspects.

Reduction mammaplasty by liposuction alone has been reported by Courtiss.[8] Liposuction has been used as an adjunct in vertical mammaplasty reduction by Le Jour.[22]

Massive breast hyertrophy of over 3000 gm. usually necessitates utilization of a breast amputation technique with immediate free nipple-areola grafting.[30]

HYPOMASTIA

The correction of hypomastia is designed to produce satisfactory volume, contour, and softness of the breast mound.

Prostheses

The availability of breast prostheses has been heavily regulated by the Food and Drug Administration since 1992. At this time, silicone gel prostheses are available only for utilization in patients undergoing breast reconstruction or in those individuals having replacement of their old silicone gel prostheses.

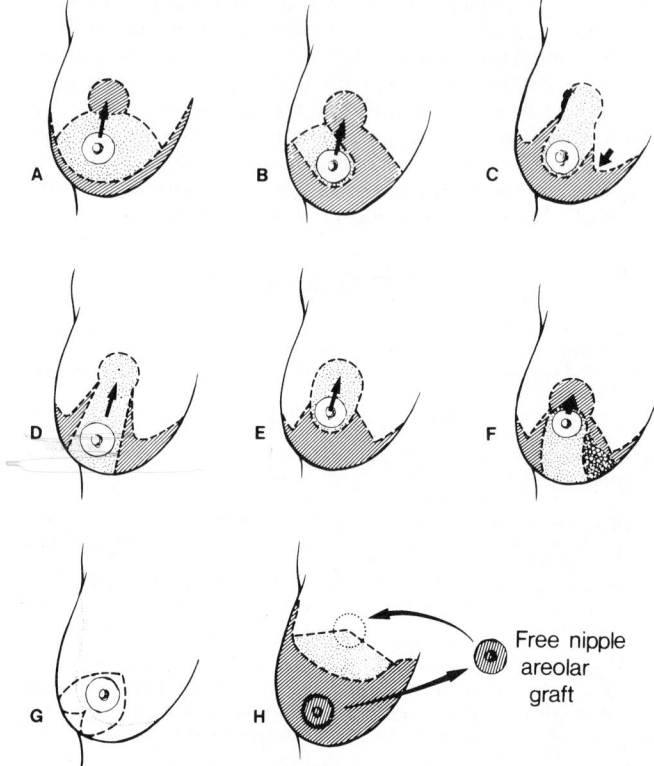

Figure 22–31. Multiple possible types of dermal flaps supporting the nipple areola. *A,* Horizontal (Strömbeck, 1960). *B,* Lateral dermal pedicle (Skoog, 1963). *C,* Superior medial dermal (Orlando, 1975). *D,* Verticle bipedicle dermal (McKissock, 1972). *E,* Superior dermal (Cramer, 1971). *F,* Inferior dermal (Robbins, 1977). *G,* Oblique wedge (Dufourmentel, 1961). *H,* Amputation—dermal with free nipple areola graft (Rubin, 1970).

Saline-filled Silastic envelope breast implants with a smooth or microtextured surface are available for both aesthetic and reconstructive utilization. They are produced in a variety of sizes and shapes to meet individual patient's needs.

Surgical Techniques

Breast augmentation can be performed through a number of differently placed incisions. An inframammary incision approximately 5.5 cm. in length is the most popular surgical approach and perhaps the safest, although a small scar remains in the inframammary crease. Postoperatively, this is usually acceptable. A circumareolar incision or transareolar incision is also used frequently, particularly in patients with a large areola, where the incision can easily be placed within the areola.[21] The axillary approach described by Hoehler[18] has the advantage of producing a breast augmentation without creating any visible scars on the breast. A 4-cm. incision is made in the anterior axillary line in the shadow of the pectoralis muscle. The dissection is then made either over the pectoral fascial plane or beneath the pectoralis major musculature.

There has been increased interest in performing the dissection and placement of the prosthesis with the aid of endoscopic visualization. Axillary endoscopic augmentation has been described by Chajchir et al.[6] Johnson and Christ[20] reported on endoscopic breast augmentation utilizing a transumbilical incision. An endoscopic inframammary approach can also be used. This technique provides excellent hemostasis and better prosthesis placement.

Regardless of the surgical approach used for breast augmentation, a decision to place the prosthesis in the subpectoral position versus the submammary position must be weighed carefully, because there are several potential problems. The decision to place the prosthesis subpectorally is usually based on the clinical observation that the patient has a limited amount of breast tissue. In the subpectoral position, the appearance of the breast mound may be altered and often distorted by contracture of the pectoralis musculature in such positions as abduction of the arm in lifting weights.[4] Those patients who indulge in varied athletic pursuits should be advised of this possible undesirable effect.

Complications and Untoward Effects

Hematoma occurs infrequently, usually within the first 48 hours, although it can occur as late as 7 days postoperatively. The patient must always be advised to report any sudden occurrence of tightness developing in the augmented breast postoperatively. Abstinence from aspirin products 10 days prior to operation should be the practice. When a hematoma is recognized, the prosthesis should be removed as soon as possible, and the hematoma should be carefully evacuated. All bleeding points should be identified and coagulated. The prosthesis can usually be safely replaced and the operative incision carefully closed in layers. A supportive bulky dressing is applied, and the patient is examined 24 hours later for further bleeding into the operative areas.

Extrusion of the breast prosthesis is encountered infrequently but can occur when too large a prosthesis has been inserted into too small a pocket, creating excessive tension on the surrounding tissues. Usually this can be remedied by removal of the prosthesis and subsequent creation of a larger pocket or the insertion of a smaller prosthesis.

The occurrence of a firm breast mound after an augmentation mammaplasty occurs with sufficient frequency (up to 25%) to be of concern to surgeons. Smooth-walled prostheses have been found to create a linear scar, which is more likely to contract. Recent investigative and clinical observations have led to the development of microtextured outer wall prosthesis coverings that redirect the scar formation into irregular contour, thus minimizing the possibility of linear contracture of any consequence. When the contracture is clinically severe, an open capsulectomy should be carried out and the same or a new prosthesis inserted.

Infection occurs infrequently, but when it does occur, it should be treated vigorously with appropriate antibiotics determined by sensitivity tests. The prosthesis is usually removed, and the infection is controlled. The prosthesis is replaced 3 to 4 months later.

Severe capsular contracture can also occur secondary to *Staphylococcus epidermidis*, which causes a low-grade infection with an inflammatory response that produces excessive scar formation. Removal of the prosthesis with resterilization and capsulectomy is necessary. This is followed by irrigation of the operative pocket with bacitracin and a povidone-iodine solution, after which the prosthesis can be replaced. The patient is then maintained on appropriate antibiotic therapy for at least 10 days.

BREAST PTOSIS

Ptosis of the breast is an aesthetic problem. The severity of the ptosis is determined by the relationship of the nipple to the inframammary line and is categorized as Stage A, B, or C ptosis, with Stage C being the most severe. In a minimally ptotic patient, the ptosis can be corrected by the insertion of a prosthesis alone. In those with more severe deformity, a combination of augmentation mammaplasty and elevation of the nipple-areola complex is performed simultaneously.[5, 28] These procedures can usually be performed under local anesthesia with intravenous sedation on an outpatient basis. More extensive ptosis can be corrected using the Benelli-type subcuticular areolar approximation technique.[2]

MAMMOGRAPHY

After breast augmentation, the sensitivity of mammography can be reduced by the inability to visualize the peripheral areas of the breast. This is more of a problem when prostheses are placed in the subglandular position. For this reason, patients who have undergone breast augmentation require specialized mammographic views for adequate evaluation.[33]

RECONSTRUCTION OF THE BREAST AFTER MASTECTOMY
Immediate

Reconstructive surgery at the time of modified radical mastectomy has generally been accepted as an excellent procedure.[4, 11] If early reconstruction is considered, the feasibility of the procedure is determined by a team consisting of a surgical oncologist, a plastic surgeon, and a pathologist on the basis of clinical and pathologic evaluation of the size of the primary tumor, the tumor grade, lymph node status, and location. A thorough discussion with the patient as to her desires, expectations, and possible complications should follow. The expected number of operative procedures to fulfill these requirements is also discussed with the patient. The age of the patient is probably of minimal importance, because this procedure can be performed at any age.

When the decision to perform an immediate breast reconstruction has been made, incision planning should be a joint venture of the surgical oncologist and the plastic surgeon. A modified radical mastectomy with an *en bloc* removal of the axillary node is performed.

Reconstruction is initiated, using a 6-cm. horizontal, slightly curved incision at the level of the sixth rib through the serratus muscle. A pocket is created beneath the serratus and pectoralis major muscles, extending medially to the perforating internal mammary vessels and inferiorly beneath the fascial insertion of the rectus abdominis muscle (Fig. 22–32). At this point, a determination is made whether to insert a permanent prosthesis or a tissue expander, to be filled with small increments of saline at a later date. The tightness of the skin closure and the desired eventual size of the mammary mound determine the type of prosthesis utilized. A suction drain is inserted into the subpectoral pocket and also into the axillary dissection area. The serratus muscle is closed with 4-0 nylon sutures, followed by 4-0 Vicryl or Dexon sutures in the dermis. A 4-0 Prolene subcuticular pullout suture is then inserted, followed by Steri-Strips for the skin closure.

If a tissue expander has been inserted, the subsequent expansion of the breast mound can be initiated approximately 3 weeks after the initial operation.[35] Up to 100 ml. of saline can usually be inserted in the prosthesis via the reservoir at one time (Fig. 22–33). This procedure can be repeated

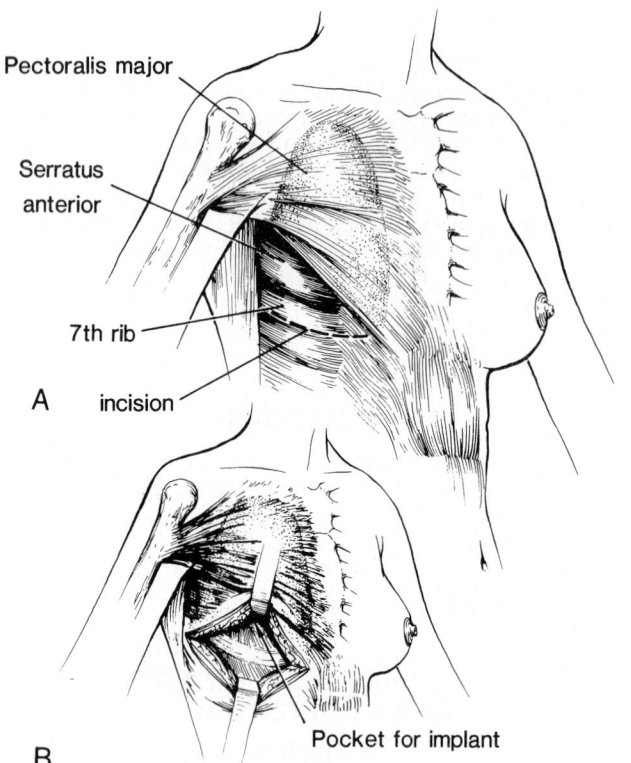

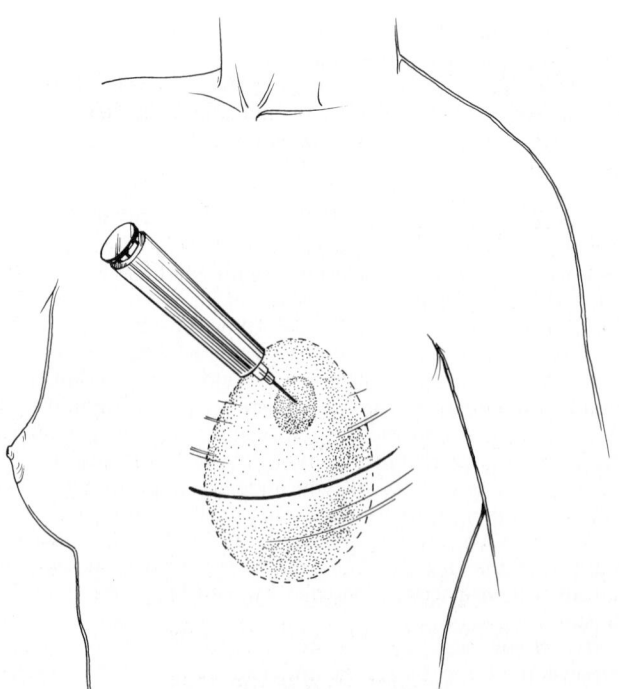

Figure 22–32. *A*, Location of the incision over the sixth or seventh rib. *B*, Undermining of the serratus anterior and pectoralis major muscles and, beneath, fascial insertion of the rectus abdominis muscle.

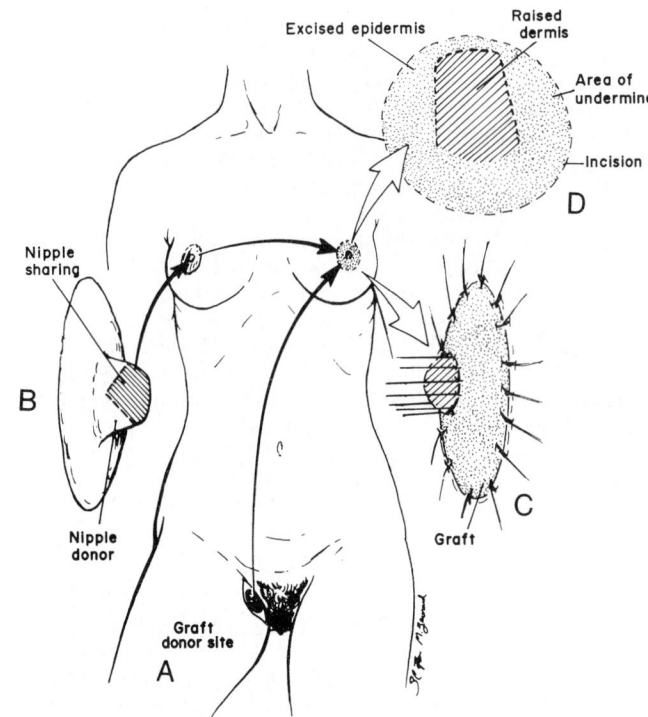

Figure 22–34. Possible sites and various techniques for constructing the nipple *(B and D)* and the areola *(A and C).*

at 2-week intervals until an overexpansion of approximately 150 ml. has been accomplished and maintained for 2 months. At this time, the expander can be removed, and the final prosthesis can be inserted. The outer covering may be micro-

textured, if desired, to minimize the capsular contracture. The final procedure, nipple-areolar reconstruction, on an outpatient basis, involves the utilization of a full-thickness groin (inner thigh) skin graft to reconstruct the areola. Simultaneously, the nipple is reconstructed either by using a portion of the opposite nipple as a composite graft or by elevating a skin fat flap from the breast mound itself and subsequent tattooing of this new nipple at a later date (Fig. 22–34).[12]

In the author's experience over the past 15 years, immediate breast reconstruction has had no adverse effect on the natural course of the patient's breast cancer. Psychologically, patient satisfaction has been extremely good in this series of over 500 patients who have undergone immediate breast

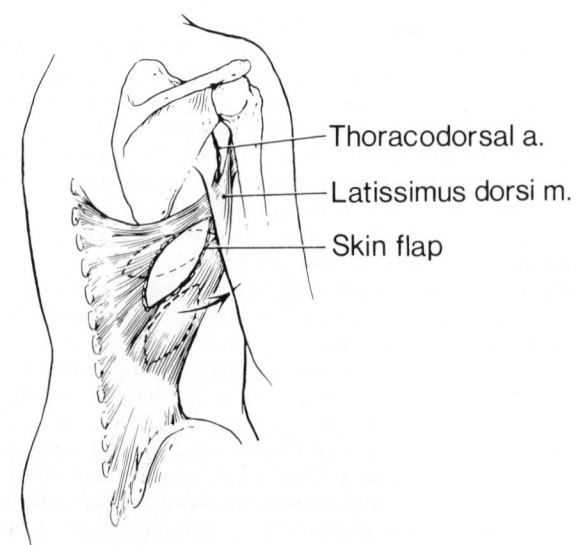

Figure 22–33. The location of the injection port of an inflatable prosthesis is shown.

Figure 22–35. Various locations of the latissimus dorsi myocutaneous flap.

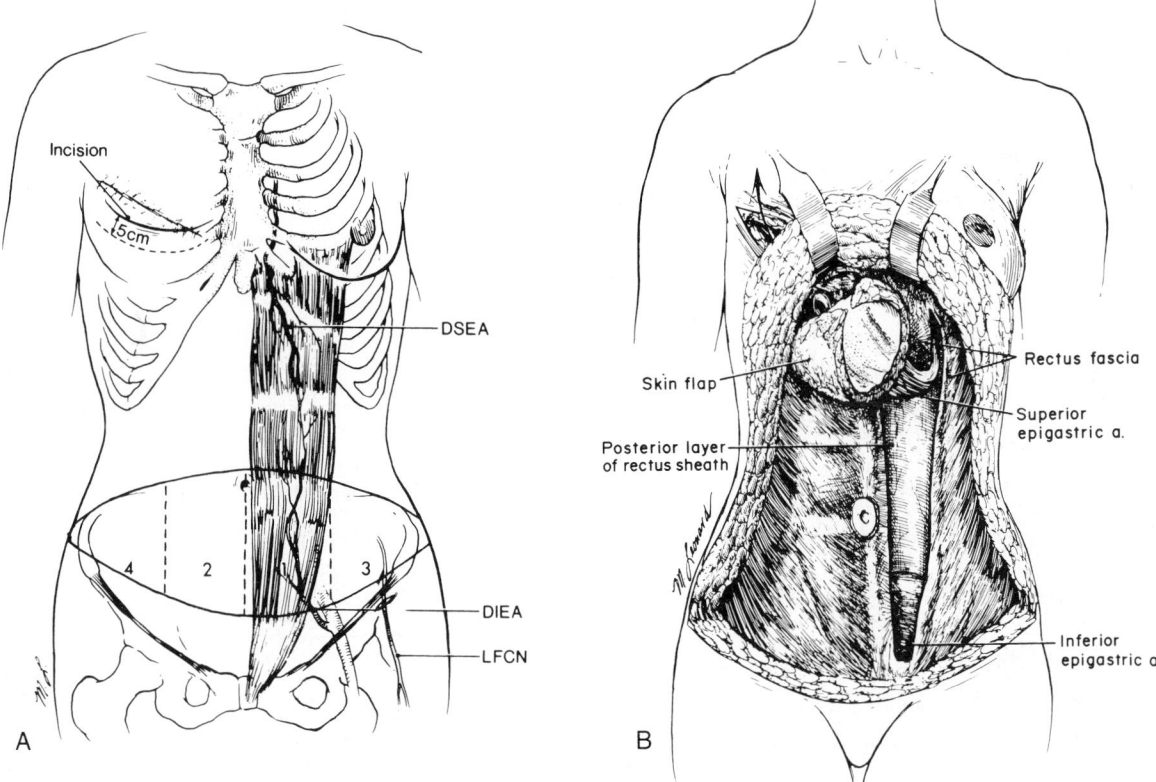

Figure 22–36. *A,* Location and design of the rectus abdominis myocutaneous flap using the contralateral rectus flap. *B,* Rectus abdominis flap being transferred on the rectus muscle pedicle.

reconstruction. The use of this transverse rectus abdominis muscle (TRAM) flap for immediate reconstruction has gained increasing popularity.[1] It allows for breast mound reconstruction with autologous tissue, alleviating the need for a prosthesis.

Delayed

Reconstruction can be initiated postoperatively after the completion of adjuvant chemotherapy or radiation therapy. In this situation, it is not advisable to perform reconstructive surgery until this treatment phase has been completed and an adequate recovery period has been attained.[7]

The most commonly used procedure, when there is sufficient skin and pectoralis muscle present, is insertion of a tissue expander into the subserratus-subpectoral pocket as previously described for immediate breast reconstruction.[4, 11, 35] If either the chest skin or the pectoralis major muscle is of insufficient quantity and quality, tissue must be brought into the area via remote skin and muscle flaps.

A latissimus dorsi musculocutaneous flap transferred on its blood supply via the thoracodorsal artery and vein is commonly used.[4, 24] This yields a large composite flap of skin and muscle that is easily transferred from the back to allow the construction of a large breast mound augmented by a saline-filled prosthesis placed beneath the latissimus dorsi flap at the time of its insertion (Fig. 22–35). The nipple-areola reconstruction is performed at a later date when the breast mound is of stable size and contour, in a manner similar to immediate breast reconstruction.

Extensive postmastectomy defects necessitate the use of a large musculocutaneous flap.[14, 17, 28] Also, when the patient wants to avoid the use of an implant, the rectus abdominis flap is the procedure of choice. The flap can be raised on the contralateral rectus abdominis muscle as shown in Figure 22–36, or both rectus muscles can be utilized. In selected patients, the use of the *free* rectus abdominis or other myocutaneous flaps has become increasingly popular.[7] The thoracodorsal or anterior serratus vessels can usually be anastomosed to the inferior epigastric vessels of the rectus abdominis flap.[16]

MANAGEMENT OF THE OPPOSITE BREAST IN PATIENTS WITH UNILATERAL BREAST CANCER

In many patients, some alteration in the shape of the contralateral breast may be required to produce adequate symmetry. This usually includes ptosis correction or breast reduction. This should be carried out only after a thorough oncologic evaluation of the contralateral breast with mammography and physical examination.

SUMMARY

Breast reconstruction initiated at the time of ablative surgery has increased in frequency and now represents approximately 40% of all breast reconstructions. The choice of timing for breast reconstruction and the techniques utilized are based on a multivariable analysis of the individual patient and her desires and concerns. The opposite breast is treated on an individual basis. As the final step, the nipple-areola complex is constructed. Quite often, tattooing of the new nipple is necessary for appropriate color matching.

SELECTED REFERENCES

Bohmert, H. H., Leis, H. P., and Jackson, I. T.: Breast Cancer: Conservative & Reconstructive Surgery. Stuttgart and New York, Georg Thieme Verlag, 1989.

This excellent textbook presents information on the treatment of breast cancer and reconstructive breast surgery by international authorities in the field.

Bostwick, J.: Aesthetic and Reconstructive Breast Surgery. St. Louis, Quality Medical Publishing, 1990.
This is an excellent textbook encompassing various aspects of aesthetic and reconstructive surgery.

Georgiade, N. G., Georgiade, G. S., and Riefkohl, R.: Aesthetic Breast Surgery, Philadelphia, W. B. Saunders, 1990.
This well-illustrated book is a compilation of the various surgical procedures for all aspects of aesthetic breast surgery by authorities in the field from many countries of the world.

Georgiade, G. S., Georgiade, N. G., Riefkohl, R., and Barwick, W. J.: Textbook of Plastic, Maxillofacial and Reconstructive Surgery. Philadelphia, W. B. Saunders, 1992.
This book includes details about breast surgery.

Noone, R. B.: Plastic and Reconstructive Surgery of the Breast. Philadelphia, B. C. Decker, 1991.
This is an excellent comprehensive text on breast surgery.

REFERENCES

1. Baldwin, B. J., Schusterman, M. A., Miller, M. J., Kroll, S. S., and Wang, B.: Bilateral breast reconstruction: Conventional versus free TRAM, Plast. Reconstr. Surg., 93:1410, 1994.
2. Benelli, L.: The Benelli periareolar mammaplasty: The round block technique. *In* Georgiade, N. G., Georgiade, G. S., and Riefkohl, R. (Eds.): Aesthetic Breast Surgery. Philadelphia, W. B. Saunders, 1990, p. 747.
3. Bolger, W., Seyfer, A., and Jackson, S.: Reduction mammaplasty using the inferior glandular "pyramid" pedicle. Plast. Reconstr. Surg., 80:75, 1987.
4. Bostwick, J.: Aesthetic and Reconstructive Breast Surgery. St. Louis, C. V. Mosby, 1983.
5. Brink, R.: Management of true ptosis of the breast. Plast. Reconstr. Surg., 91:657, 1993.
6. Chajchir, A., Benzaquen, I., Spagnolo, N., and Lusicic, N.: Endoscopic augmentation mastoplasty. Aesthetic Plast. Surg., 18:377, 1994.
7. Codner, M. A., Bostwick, J., Nahai, F., Bried, J. T., and Eaves, F. E.: TRAM flap vascular delay for high-risk breast reconstruction. Plast. Reconstr. Surg., 96:1615, 1995.
8. Courtiss, E.: Reduction mammaplasty by suction alone. Plast. Reconstr. Surg., 92:1276, 1993.
9. Cramer, L., and Chong, J.: Unipedicle cutaneous flap: Areola-nipple transposition or an end-bearing, superiorly based flap. *In* Georgiade, N. G. (Ed.): Reconstructive Breast Surgery. St. Louis, C. V. Mosby, 1976, p. 143.
10. Dufourmentel, L., and Mouly, R.: Plastie Mammairie par la methode oblique. Ann. Chir. Plast., 6:45, 1961.
11. Georgiade, G. S., Georgiade, N., McCarty, K., Jr., and Seigler, H.: Rationale for immediate reconstruction of the breast following modified radical mastectomy. Ann. Plast. Surg., 8:210, 1982.
12. Georgiade, G. S., Riefkohl, R., and Georgiade, N. G.: To share or not to share. Ann. Plast. Surg., 14:180, 1985.
13. Georgiade, G., Riefkohl, R., and Georgiade, N.: Inferior pyramidal reduction mammaplasty: 10 years experience. Ann. Plast. Surg., 23:40, 1989.
14. Georgiade, G. S., Voci, V., Riefkohl, R., and Scheflan, M.: Potential problems with the transverse rectus abdominis myocutaneous flap in breast reconstruction and how to avoid them. Br. J. Plast. Surg., 37:121, 1984.
15. Georgiade, N., Serafin, D., Georgiade, G., and McCarty, K., Jr.: Subcutaneous mastectomy: An evolution of concept and technique. Ann. Plast. Surg., 8:8, 1982.
16. Grotting, J. C., Urist, M., Maddox, W. A., and Vasconez, L. O.: Conventional TRAM flap versus free microsurgical TRAM flap for immediate breast reconstruction. Plast. Reconstr. Surg., 83:828, 1989.
17. Hartrampf, C. R.: Breast reconstruction with a transverse abdominal island flap: A retrospective evaluation of 335 patients. Perspect. Plast. Surg., 1:123, 1987.
18. Hoehler, H.: Breast augmentation: The axillary approach. Br. J. Plast. Surg., 26:373, 1973.
19. Jarrett, J. R., Cutler, R. G., and Teal, D. F.: Subcutaneous mastectomy in small large or ptotic breasts with immediate submuscular placement of implants. Plast. Reconstr. Surg., 62:702, 1978.
20. Johnson, G. W., and Christ, J. E.: The endoscopic breast augmentation: The transumbilical insertion of saline-filled breast implants. Plast. Reconstr. Surg., 92:801, 1993.
21. Jones, F. R., and Tauras, A. A. P.: A periareolar incision for augmentation mammaplasty. Plast. Reconstr. Surg., 51:641, 1973.
22. Le Jour, M.: Vertical mammaplasty and liposuction of the breast. Plast. Reconstr. Surg., 94:100, 1994.
23. Marchac, D., and DeLoarte, G.: Reduction mammaplasty and correction of ptosis with a short mammary scar. Plast. Reconstr. Surg., 69:45, 1982.
24. McCraw, J. B., Papp, C., Edwards, A., and McMellin, A.: The autogenous latissimus breast reconstruction. Clin. Plast. Surg., 21:279, 1994.
25. McKissock, P. K.: Reduction mammaplasty with a vertical dermal flap. Plast. Reconstr. Surg., 49:245, 1972.
26. Orlando, J., and Guthrie, R.: The superomedial dermal pedicle for nipple transposition. Br. J. Plast. Surg., 28:42, 1975.
27. Pitanguy, L.: Surgical treatment of breast hypertrophy. Br. J. Plast. Surg., 20:78, 1967.
28. Regnault, P.: Breast ptosis: Definition and treatment. Clin. Plast. Surg., 3:193, 1976.
29. Robbins, T. A.: A reduction mammaplasty with the nipple areola based on an inferior dermal pedicle. Plast. Reconstr. Surg., 55:64, 1977.
30. Rubin, L. R.: The surgical treatment of the massive hypertrophic breast. *In* Georgiade, N. G. (Ed.): Reconstructive Breast Surgery. St. Louis, C. V. Mosby, 1976.
31. Scheflan, M., and Dinner, M. I.: The transverse abdominal island flap: Indications, contraindications, results and complications. Ann. Plast. Surg., 10:24, 1983.
32. Skoog, T.: A technique of breast reduction. Transposition of the nipple on a cutaneous vascular pedicle. Acta Chir. Scand., 126:453, 1963.
33. Steinbach, B. G., Hardt, N. S., and Abbitt, P. L.: Mammography: Breast implants—types, complications and adjacent breast pathology (Review). Curr. Probl. Radiol., 22:43, 1993.
34. Strömbeck, J. O.: Mammaplasty: Report of a new technique based on the two pedicle procedure. Br. J. Plast. Surg., 13:79, 1960.
35. Ward, J., Cohen, I., Knaysi, G., and Brown, P.: Immediate breast reconstruction with tissue expanders. Plast. Reconstr. Surg., 80:559, 1987.

THE THYROID GLAND

I

PHYSIOLOGY

H. Kim Lyerly, M.D.

The thyroid gland functions primarily to produce thyroid hormone for development and regulation of metabolism. A constant supply of thyroid hormone is necessary for growth, for brain development, and for maintenance of metabolism and functional activity of most organs. Thyroid hormone production is under the regulation of the anterior pituitary hormone thyrotropin, or thyroid-stimulating hormone (TSH), and by a system of autoregulation within the thyroid gland. The thyroid hormones are iodinated amino acids, thyroxine (T_4) and 3,5,3'-triiodothyronine (T_3). In the thyroid they are an integral part of thyroglobulin, in which they are synthesized and stored. In the plasma, they circulate as free amino acids in reversible equilibrium with the thyroid hormone-binding proteins; however, they have an effect on metabolism only when they are in the free form. Free thyroid hormones are able to penetrate cells to induce and stimulate oxygen consumption; increase body heat and the rates of metabolism of carbohydrates, fats, and proteins; and stimulate the feedback mechanism with the pituitary gland.[8]

THYROID HORMONE SYNTHESIS

Iodine is necessary for the synthesis of thyroid hormones. In the normal American diet, about 200 to 500 μg. of iodine is ingested daily, mainly in drinking water, sea fish, salt, milk, and eggs. The inorganic iodine is reduced to iodide ion in the gut, where most is absorbed from the small intestine and is cleared from plasma by the thyroid to provide the normal thyroid requirement of 50 to 100 μg. or is excreted by the kidney. Approximately 150 to 500 mg. per day is excreted in the urine. Iodide clearance is dependent on the glomerular filtration rate (GFR) and increases and decreases with enhancement or reduction of GFR. Thyroid hormone synthesis incorporates a complex sequence of processes (Fig. 23–1).[71] The thyroid actively transports and concentrates iodide in the thyroid follicular cell and the colloid at a rate of about 2 μg. per hour.[14] A concentration gradient of 20-fold to 40-fold is established that may be increased 20-fold by TSH stimulation, low dietary levels of iodide, and pharmacologic interference with thyroid hormone formation. Iodide remains free only briefly before being oxidized to a highly reactive form that binds to tyrosine residues in thyroglobulin. Thyroglobulin is a dimeric glycoprotein with a molecular weight of 660,000 and contains approximately 120 tyrosyl units, of which about 30% undergo iodination. After its synthesis and intracellular transport, exophytic vesicles discharge their content into the follicle, and thyroglobulin accumulates in the lumen.[45] The colloid, which fills the follicle lumen, is almost exclusively composed of iodinated thyroglobulin. The iodination reaction of thyroglobulin is catalyzed by thyroid peroxidase (TPO). This is the step interrupted by the thiocarbamide

group of drugs (such as propylthiouracil), which causes a large concentration of unbound iodide to remain in the thyroid.[45] After being bound to tyrosine residues in thyroglobulin, iodide proceeds to be part of T_4 and T_3 via monoiodotyrosine (MIT) and diiodotyrosine (DIT). By this complex coupling mechanism, two molecules of DIT combine to form T_4, and one molecule of DIT plus one molecule of MIT form T_3.

Thyroglobulin breakdown and thyroid hormone release occur when the colloid is engulfed by the apical pole, forming endocytotic vesicles that fuse with lysosomes and form phagolysosomes. Proteases within these vesicles then hy-

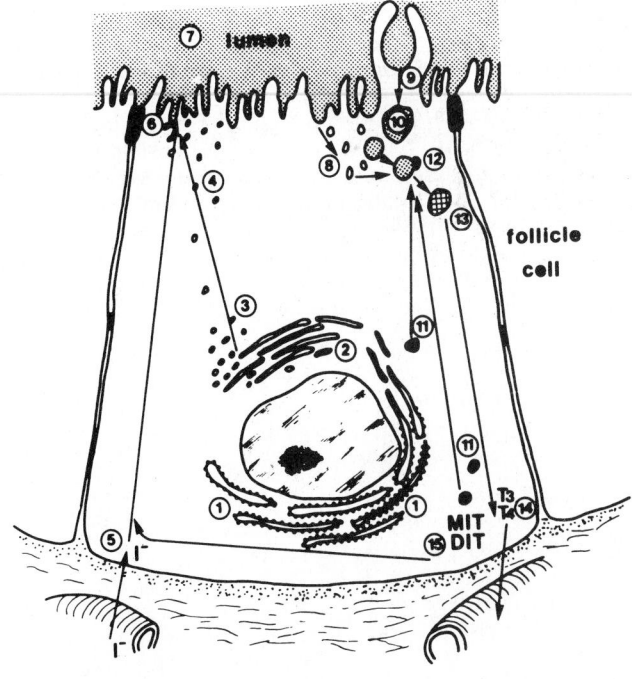

Figure 23–1. Diagrammatic scheme of thyroid hormone formation and secretion. 1, Thyroglobulin and protein synthesis in the rough endoplasmic reticulum. 2, Coupling of the thyroglobulin carbohydrate units in the smooth endoplasmic reticulum and Golgi apparatus. 3, Formation of exocytotic vesicles. 4, Transport of exocytotic vesicles with noniodinated thyroglobulin to the apical surface of the follicle cell and into the follicular lumen. 5, Iodide transport at the basal cell membrane. 6, Iodide oxidation, thyroglobulin iodination, and coupling of iodotyrosyl to iodothyronyl residues. 7, Storage of iodinated thyroglobulin in the follicular lumen. 8, Endocytosis by micropinocytosis. 9, Endocytosis by macropinocytosis (pseudopods). 10, Colloid droplets. 11, Lysosome migrating to the apical pole. 12, Fusion of lysosomes with colloid droplets. 13, Phagolysosomes with thyroglobulin hydrolysis. 14, T_3 and T_4 secretion. 15, Monoiodotyrosine (MIT) and diiodotyrosine (DIT) deiodination.

drolyze the thyroglobulin to iodothyronines, which are secreted. Free iodotyrosines formed by hydrolysates are deiodinated into tyrosine and iodide, which may be recycled to form new thyroid hormone molecules. Some thyroglobulin molecules are not hydrolyzed and escape into the bloodstream.

The normal thyroid contains approximately 8000 μg. of iodine, only about 1% being inorganic iodide. T_4 constitutes approximately 35% of the total amount of thyroid hormone; T_3, 5%; DIT, 25%; and MIT, 25%. Approximately 1% of the hormone in the thyroid store is released to the circulation each day after being separated in the cell by acid proteases and peptide enzymes. Eighty to 100 μg. of T_4 and 26 to 39 μg. of T_3 are produced each day. T_4 has a half-life of 6 days, and T_3 has a half-life of 1 to 3 days. The thyroid gland has a storage reserve of approximately 3 weeks. The concentration of total thyroxine is 30 to 50 times the concentration of T_3. However, only 0.03% of the total serum T_4 and 0.3% of the total serum T_3 is present in the unbound or biologically active form (Fig. 23–2). The major serum thyroid hormone-binding proteins are thyronine-binding globulin (TBG), thyroxine-binding prealbumin, and albumin.[33, 58]

Hormone-binding proteins are the principal intravascular factors influencing total hormone concentration, which is normally maintained at a level appropriate for the concentration of carrier proteins to maintain a constant free hormone level. Various factors may cause changes in the concentration of TBG (Table 23–1).[2, 4, 10, 12, 26, 29, 48, 49, 51, 57, 62, 69] Because alterations in TBG may alter the total hormone concentration independent of the metabolic status of the body, free hormone, rather than the total hormone, is a more accurate indicator of the thyroid hormone-dependent metabolic state.

Although T_4 is the principal secretory product of the thyroid gland, the principal active hormone in metabolic regulation is T_3 (Fig. 23–3). T_3 is produced by deiodination of T_4 by the enzymes T_4 5'-deiodinase (5'-D) Types I and II. Type I T_4 5'-D is found predominately in the liver and the kidneys. Its action is responsible for the production of two thirds of the total T_3 in the body. Type II T_4 5'-D is responsible for most of the T_3 found in the pituitary, the brain, and brown fat. T_3 enters the cell or is locally produced and then transported into the nucleus. Transcriptionally active forms of thyroid hormone receptors includes monomers, homodimers, and heterodimers with nuclear protein partners, such as the retinoid X receptor.[63] The T_3-receptor complex interacts with

TABLE 23–1. Conditions Associated with Alterations in Thyronine-Binding Globulin (TBG) Concentration

	Increased TBG	Decreased TBG
Genetic	Inherited elevated TBG	Inherited absent or low TBG
Acquired	Acute intermittent porphyria Acute and chronic active viral hepatitis Primary biliary cirrhosis Hepatocellular carcinoma Myeloma Collagen disease Hypothyroidism	Major illness Protein calorie malnutrition Galactosemia Nephrotic syndrome Hepatic cirrhosis Acromegaly Protein-losing enteropathy Hyperthyroidism
Pharmacologic	Perphenazine Heroin and methadone Clofibrate 5-Fluorouracil	
Hormonal	Estrogens Hyperestrogenemic state (pregnancy, newborn, molar pregnancy, tumors)	Androgens Anabolic steroids Glucocorticoids L-asparaginase

specific sequences in deoxyribonucleic acid (DNA) regulatory regions and modifies gene expression. T_3 causes both increases and decreases in gene expression and may also influence the stability of messenger ribonucleic acid (RNA).

By control of the expression of genetic information, all other activities of the cell may be controlled. The diversity of thyroid hormone effects may be observed as the logical consequence of controlling the expression of specific sets of genetic information within the various tissue types, in concert with other regulatory factors.[22] This regulation could also be dependent on the organism's development, thus explaining why certain effects are observed only when the hormone is administered or removed at certain times in the organism's developmental cycle. Thyroid hormone appears to have both generalized actions on RNA and protein synthesis and specific actions in the transcription of particular proteins.[19, 22, 55]

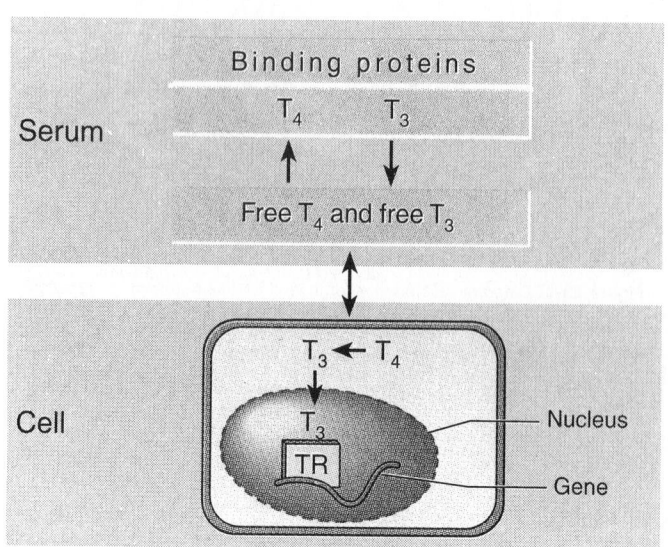

Figure 23–2. Thyroid hormone transport in serum and hormone action. The binding proteins include thyroxine-binding globulin, transthyretin, and albumin. Drugs may alter the production or clearance of a binding protein or inhibit the binding of thyroxine (T_4) and triiodothyronine (T_3) to the protein. TR, thyroid receptor. (Reprinted by permission of *The New England Journal of Medicine* from Surks, M. I., and Sievert, R.: Drugs and thyroid function. N. Engl. J. Med., *333*(25):1688–1693, 1995. Copyright 1995, Massachusetts Medical Society.)

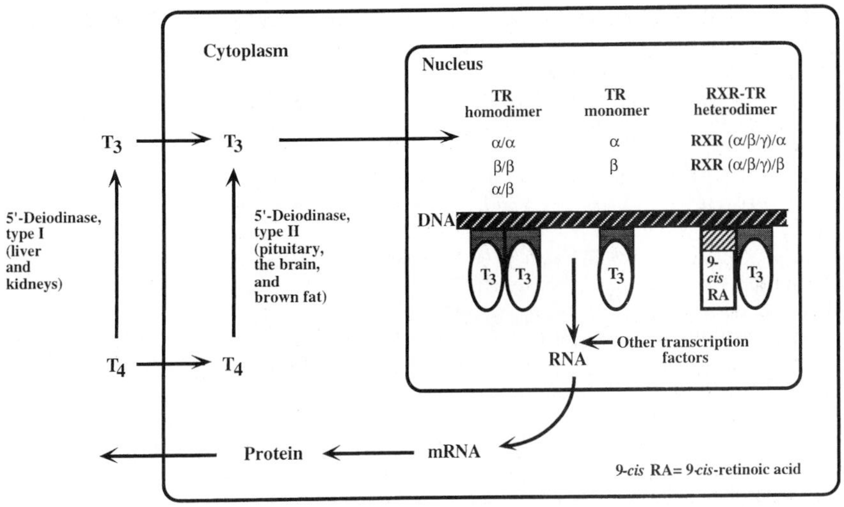

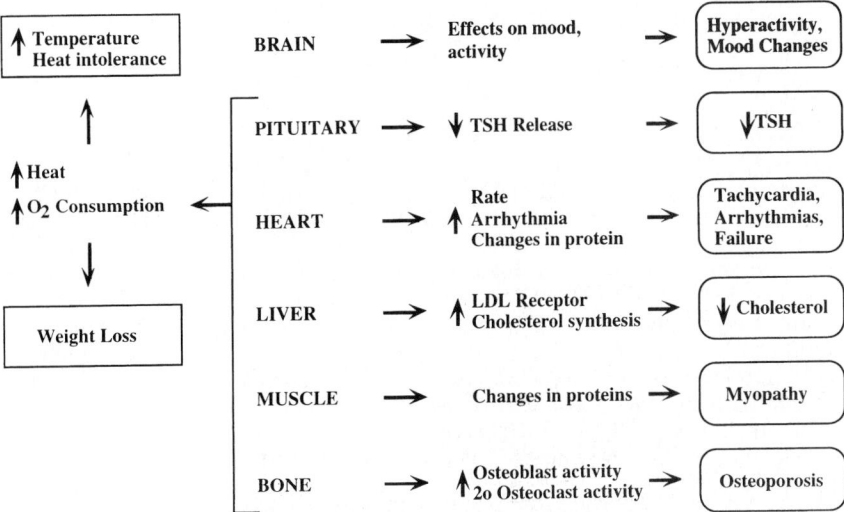

Figure 23–3. Cellular and molecular events involved with thyroid hormone function. T_4 is converted in the periphery and in the cytoplasm of the cell into T_3. T_3 travels to the nucleus, where it binds to the thyroid hormone receptor, either homodimer, monomer, or heterodimer. Thyroid hormone receptor binding leads to RNA transcription in association with other transcription factors, with expression of mRNA that is then translated to protein.

Thyroid hormones have numerous metabolic effects (Fig. 23–4). Enhancement of the basal metabolic rate (BMR) as reflected by increased oxygen consumption is one of the classic actions of thyroid hormone. An optimal amount is necessary for balanced growth and maturation, and many of the effects of thyroid hormones on carbohydrate metabolism appear permissive with respect to the effects of other hormones. Thyroid hormone stimulates both lipogenesis and lipolysis. Thyroid hormone characteristically lowers the level of serum cholesterol by enhanced excretion in the feces and conversion of cholesterol to bile acids. Hypothyroidism is associated with altered lipoprotein metabolism, including an increase in serum concentrations of intermediate density lipoprotein and low-density lipoprotein cholesterol. The generalized metabolic response increases the demand for vitamins and cofactors, and there is a magnified catecholamine effect produced by excess thyroid hormone.

T_3 has both direct and indirect effects on cardiac ventricle proteins.[27] Patients receiving doses of T_4 that suppress thyrotropin secretion have an increase in the left ventricular mass index as well as left ventricular contractility.[42, 59]

The syndrome of resistance to thyroid hormone is characterized by diffuse goiter, varying manifestations of hypothyroidism, elevated serum concentrations of T_3 and T_4, and normal or elevated serum thyrotropin levels. Attention deficient disorder is found in as many as 60% of affected children. Resistance to thyroid hormone is associated with abnormalities in the T_3 receptor β gene.[28]

MECHANISMS OF THYROID REGULATION

The principal regulatory mechanisms of the thyroid gland are the hypothalamic-pituitary-thyroid control system and the intrathyroidal autoregulatory system (Fig. 23–5). The former is represented by the pituitary thyrotropin TSH, which stimulates many aspects of thyroid activity, particularly thyroid hormone synthesis and secretion, and thyroid hormones inhibit the secretion of TSH by the pituitary.[43]

Thyroid-Stimulating Hormone

TSH is a glycoprotein hormone that, like luteinizing hormone, follicle-stimulating hormone, and human chorionic gonadotropin, has α and β subunits.[34] The α subunits of these hormones are identical, and the β subunits are responsible for their biologic and immunologic specificities. TSH is required for the normal production and secretion of thyroid hormone; in its absence, the thyroid gland releases a reduced

Figure 23–4. Systemic and physiologic effects of thyroid hormone action. The effects of hyperthyroidism are demonstrated above, with the systemic effects noted in the left column. The middle columns represent specific effects on organ systems. The clinical manifestations are noted in the right column. TSH, thyroid-stimulating hormone; 2o, secondary.

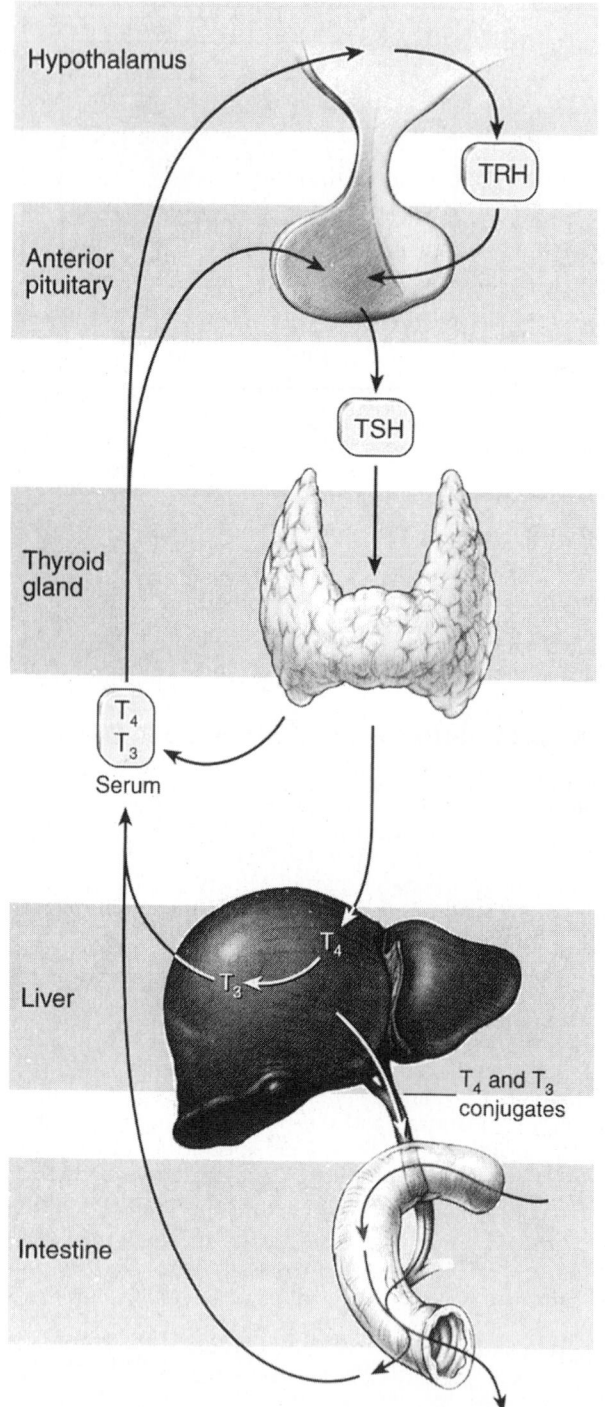

Figure 23–5. The hypothalamic-pituitary-thyroid axis and extrathyroidal pathways of thyroid hormone metabolism. Triiodothyronine (T_3) and thyroxine (T_4) inhibit the secretion of thyrotropin (thyroid-stimulating hormone [TSH]) both directly and indirectly, by inhibiting the secretion of thyrotropin-releasing hormone (TRH). TSH stimulates the synthesis and secretion of T_4 and T_3 by the thyroid gland. T_4 is converted to T_3 in the liver (and many other tissues) by the action of T_4 monodeiodinases. Some of the T_4 and T_3 is conjugated with glucuronide and sulfate in the liver, excreted in the bile, and partially hydrolyzed in the intestine; the T_4 and T_3 formed there may be reabsorbed. Drug interactions can occur at any of these sites. (Reprinted by permission of *The New England Journal of Medicine* from Surks, M. I., and Sievert, R.: Drugs and thyroid function. N. Engl. J. Med., *333*(25):1688–1693, 1995. Copyright 1995, Massachusetts Medical Society.)

amount of thyroid hormone. TSH secretion is most profoundly influenced by tonic stimulation by hypothalamic thyrotropin-releasing hormone (TRH) and feedback inhibition by thyroid hormone.[28, 73] T_3 regulates the transcription of the genes for both subunits of TSH, and elements from the region of each gene involved in this regulation have been identified.

The normal serum concentration of TSH is 0.5 to 4.5 μU. per ml. when assayed. The normal daily production and degradation is 40 to 150 μU. TSH secretion has a circadian rhythm, and the levers rise approximately 2 hours after sleep to peak between 2 and 4 A.M.[20]

An initial effect of TSH is in iodide transport, which is reflected by an acute increase in the efflux. Other effects of TSH include activation of iodide binding to thyroglobulins, increased coupling of MIT and DIT to form T_3 and T_4, activation of exocytosis and transfer of protein in the lumen of the follicle, and secretion of thyroid hormone.

It is generally accepted that TSH has a major role in thyroid growth. Iodide deficiency and excessive treatment of hyperthyroidism with blockers of iodide binding to thyroglobulin lead to increased TSH secretion and thyroid enlargement. In situations in which TSH action is lacking, such as hypophysectomy and inactive TSH, the thyroid exhibits a decrease in size, whereas prolonged administration of TSH leads to an increase in thyroid weight. Chronic stimulation of the thyroid gland by TSH causes the proliferation of capillaries and fibroblasts, rather than follicle cells.

Thyrotropin-Releasing Hormone

TRH is a tripeptide (pyroglutamyl-histidylproline amide), and it was the first hypothalamic hormone to be isolated. It is produced by the supraoptic and paraventricular nuclei of the hypothalamus and passes down their axons to the median eminence, where it is stored. Following secretion into the hypophyseal portal blood vessels, TRH travels to the pituitary and binds to specific receptor sites. TRH action on the pituicytes includes stimulation of TSH secretion and synthesis, as well as the stimulation of prolactin release and synthesis.[41, 54, 64]

The primary role of TRH appears to be tonic stimulation of TSH-producing cells within the pituitary, because the normal secretion of TSH and thyroid hormone is dependent on hypothalamic stimulation. The primary clinical use of this hormone had been in the diagnosis of thyroid disease. A dose-response relationship between TRH and TSH is found in humans with intravenous bolus doses between 6.5 and 400 μg. In hyperthyroid patients, there is no peak in TSH after TRH administration because of autonomous thyroid function. In hypothyroidism due to primary thyroid disease, there is an exaggerated rise in TSH after TRH. In pituitary disease the TRH test is less useful, because a rise in TSH may still be observed in the presence of a low circulating T_4 concentration. The TRH stimulation test is costly and can cause hypertensive and arrhythmic episodes in the elderly. It has been largely replaced by the third-generation TSH assay.

Autoregulation of Thyroid Function

Although TSH is the primary regulator of the activity of the thyroid gland, the gland has intrinsic ability to alter the production and release of thyroid hormone. This autoregula-

tory ability is most prominent in adaptation to conditions of iodine deficiency or excess.

In humans, the Wolff-Chaikoff block (acute block of iodide binding) is induced by an elevation of the plasma iodide concentration to approximately 25 μg. per dl. As iodide levels in plasma increase, there is an increase in the amount taken up and bound by the thyroid gland. After a critical amount of iodide accumulates, there is a progressive inhibition of iodide binding to tyrosyl residues in thyroglobulin.

In addition to the Wolff-Chaikoff block, administration of potassium iodide to a patient with Graves' disease or a normal subject causes a prompt reduction in the release of iodine-containing compounds from the gland and a prompt decrease in serum thyroid hormone levels (Fig. 23–6). Moreover, there is a reduction of the hypervascularity and hyperplasia characteristic of Graves' disease. Conversely, exposure to large quantities of iodine can also induce hyperthyroidism. Although this was believed to occur in iodine-deficient areas, it has also been recognized as responsible for nodular goiter in patients from iodine-sufficient areas.

Monovalent anions including thiocyanate, perchlorate, and nitrate inhibit iodide uptake. Thiocyanate and perchlorate both stimulate discharge of free iodide from the thyroid gland, and thiocyanate also inhibits iodide binding and iodotyrosine coupling. Lithium is concentrated in the thyroid by the same mechanisms as iodide and induces goitrous hypothyroidism in susceptible people.[7, 66]

Thionamides such as methimazole and propylthiouracil are commonly used antithyroid medications. They impair the covalent binding of iodine to thyroglobulin and iodotyrosine coupling and appear to inhibit the thyroid iodide peroxidase. Propylthiouracil and, to a lesser degree, methimazole also inhibit the peripheral tissue deiodination of T_4 to T_3.

Glucocorticoids influence thyroid function at multiple levels, including reducing the secretion of TSH. Estrogens may decrease serum TSH on an acute basis but chronically enhance the TSH response to TRH. They also increase the concentration of TBG and consequently increase total serum T_4 and T_3, although free T_4 and T_3 do not change. Similarly, pregnancy is associated with several important alterations in thyroid function.[13] During the first trimester, there is a doubling of the serum TBG concentration, leading to an increase in the total serum T_4 and T_3 levels but normal free thyroid hormone levels. TSH levels are normal or slightly elevated and have an exaggerated response to the administration of TRH.

In infants, the normal range for serum T_4 remains approximately 25% higher than for adults but progressively declines during childhood.[25] In healthy elderly men, the T_4 turnover rate is decreased, BMRs are lower, and the uptake of radioactive iodine by the thyroid gland is diminished.[65, 78]

Multiple alterations in thyroid physiology have been noted in the presence of other disease. Whereas basal TSH levels and the response to TRH are increased by iodine administration to normal subjects, this alteration is reduced or absent in sick patients. In patients with reduced thyroid levels and severe illness, there has been observed a rise in TSH levels during the recovery period, followed by a later rise in serum T_4 levels.

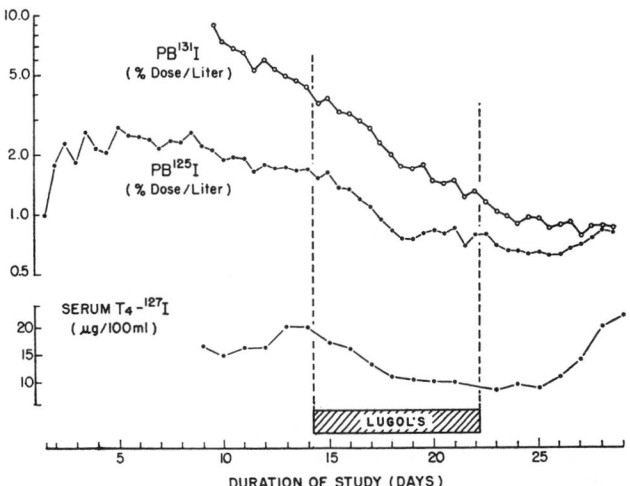

Figure 23–6. Iodide inhibition of thyroid hormone release. A patient with thyrotoxicosis was administered inorganic ^{125}I as a marker for newly synthesized iodoproteins and several days later was administered ^{131}I-T_4 to monitor the rate of clearance of thyroid hormone. Iodine was then administered in the form of Lugol's solution. Serum protein-bound ^{125}I (PB ^{125}I) and ^{131}I (PB ^{131}I) and nonradioactive T_4 (T_4-^{127}I) were measured serially. The decline in serum T_4 while peripheral ^{131}I-T_4 degradation remained stable indicates decreased release of hormone from the thyroid gland during iodine administration. (Redrawn from Wartofsky, L., Ransil, B. J., and Ingbar, S. H.: Inhibition by iodine of the release of thyroxine from the thyroid glands of patients with thyrotoxicosis. J. Clin. Invest., 49:78, 1970, copyright by the American Society for Clinical Investigation.)

THYROID FUNCTION TESTS AND EFFECTS OF DRUGS ON THYROID FUNCTION

The fundamental issues in the evaluation of thyroid disease are the metabolic status of the patient, the etiology of the disease process responsible for the hormonal imbalance, and the etiology of the thyroid gland abnormality in the euthyroid patient.[9, 47] Figure 23–7 demonstrates the relationships between TSH, T_4, and cholesterol in a patient through progressive stages of hyperthyroidism, hypothyroidism, and

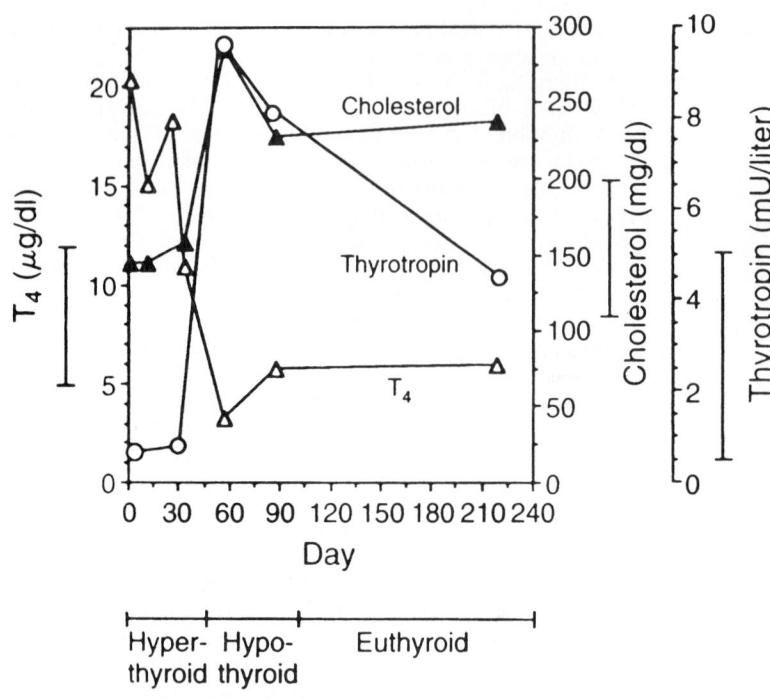

Figure 23–7. Serial measurements of serum total thyroxine (T_4), cholesterol, and thyrotropin in a man with subacute thyroiditis. The graph shows the bidirectional relationship between serum T_4 and both serum cholesterol and thyrotropin throughout the hyperthyroid and hypothyroid phases of the illness, in the absence of treatment. The I bars show the normal ranges. To convert values for thyroxine to nmol. per liter, multiply by 12.87; to convert values for cholesterol to mmol. per liter, multiply by 0.02586. (Reprinted by permission of *The New England Journal of Medicine* from Brent, G. A.: The molecular basis of thyroid hormone action. N. Engl. J. Med., *331*(13):847–853, 1994. Copyright 1994, Massachusetts Medical Society.)

euthyroidism. These specific tests are discussed in detail in the following sections.

Tests of Thyroid Gland Activity and Hormone Synthesis

Thyroid-Stimulating Hormone. Currently the most effective measure of thyroid activity is the third-generation TSH assay.[74] This newer generation is different from previous TSH assays in that it can discriminate degrees of TSH suppression. Thus, TSH levels produced by normal circardian variation, in which the peak concentration occurs before sleep, are detected but not found to be outside the normal range. TSH status is independent of the level of TBG, which is known to vary in conditions such as pregnancy and can alter T_4 measurements. Moreover, the ultrasensitive TSH test has made the TRH stimulation test (previously used to monitor TSH suppression in patients with primary hypothyroidism) almost obsolete. A diagnostic algorithm using the ultrasensitive TSH test is depicted in Figure 23–8. The disadvantage of the current TSH assay is that some clinically euthyroid patients are found to have abnormally low TSH levels. In some patients TSH is immunologically active but biologically inactive, and the result is a spuriously high TSH level. In addition, TSH levels can take as long as 6 months to normalize after treatment is initiated, so that it may not be ideal for monitoring thyroid disease. Use of dopamine and corticosteroids can suppress TSH levels.

Free T_4 and T_3. Free T_4 is the metabolically active form of T_4 and is a better indicator of thyroid status than total T_4.[44] Free T_4 can be measured by the free T_4 index, radioimmunoassay techniques, and equilibrium dialysis.[79] The accuracy of free T_4 measurements by radioimmunoassay varies with the type of assay used and can be influenced by serum levels of drugs, lipids, or proteins. Equilibrium dialysis is highly sensitive and specific and is considered the most reliable of assays. Because of its cost, it is usually used for the diagnosis of euthyroid sick syndrome.

Serum T_3 determinations are not as useful as other tests in the diagnosis of hypothryoidism. In the early stages of hypothyroidism, T_3 values may be normal because of TSH-induced hyperstimulation of T_3 initially.[67] In contrast, T_3 concentrations are below normal in patients who have a debilitating illness, because their ability to convert T_4 to T_3 in the peripheral tissue is diminished.[39] These patients are euthyroid, even though T_3 values are decreased.

Total Thyroxine (TT_4). The usual concentration of TT_4 in adults ranges from 5 to 11.5 μg. per dl. TT_4 measures both the protein-bound and free T_4 and is not affected by iodine-containing drugs but can be altered by changes in TBG level.

Resin T_3 Uptake (RT_3U). RT_3U measures the unoccupied thyroid hormone binding sites on TBG by measuring the competitive binding for radioactive T_3 between TBG and a resin and provides an indirect measure of free T_4.[68] The radioactive T_3 added to the system is bound preferentially by the resin if the thyroid hormone binding sites on TBG are occupied by T_4. The resin uptake of T_3 is directly proportional to the fraction of free T_4 in the serum and inversely related to the unoccupied TBG binding sites. RT_3U is high in thyrotoxicosis and low in hypothyroid states. Depending on the method used, typical normal values of RT_3U are 25% to 35%. The test serves as an indirect measurement of the unbound fraction of T_4 and is valuable because it is simpler to perform than other measurements of T_4.

Thyroid Radioiodide Uptake (RAIU). After oral ingestion of ^{123}I (which has a short half-life and is associated with minimal radiation, compared with ^{131}I), the thyroid uptake is near its peak at 24 hours. A dose of 400 pCi. is usually administered orally, and the quantity accumulated by the thyroid gland at various intervals is measured by counting with a γ scintillation counter. Normal values for 24-hour RAIU in most parts of North America are approximately 15% to 30%. Disease states leading to excessive production and release of thyroid hormone are most often associated with an increased thyroid RAIU, and those causing hormone underproduction are associated with a decreased RAIU.[31]

Pertechnetate-Technetium 99m (^{99m}Tc) Uptake Measurement. Because thyroid uptake in the early period after administration of radioiodine reflects mainly trapping activity, ^{99m}Tc may be used to assay thyroid trapping. In euthyroid patients, thyroid trapping is maximal at about 20 minutes and is approximately 1% of the administered dose.

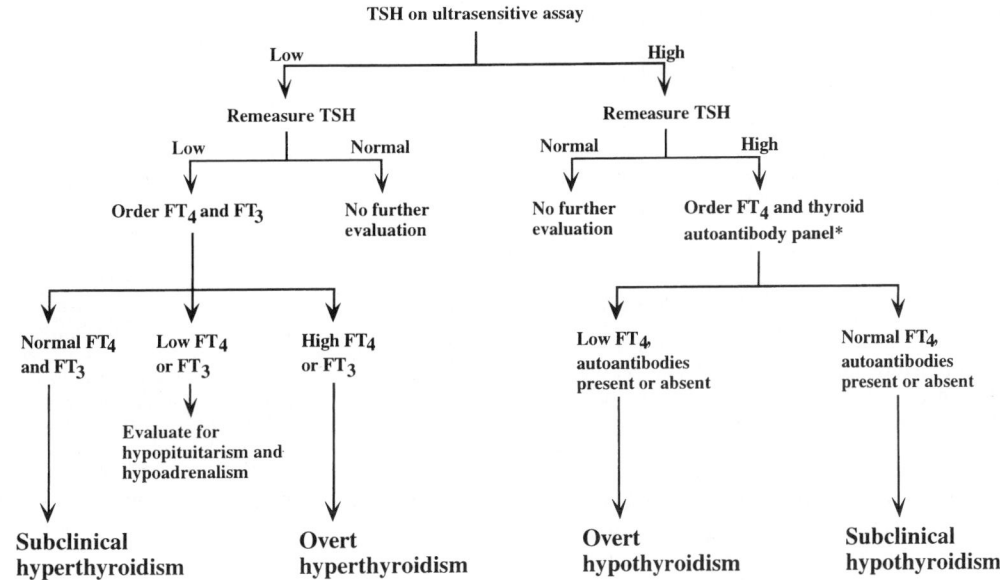

Figure 23–8. Flow diagram demonstrating the evaluation of hypothyroidism based on an abnormal thyroid-stimulating hormone assay.

Other Thyroid Tests

Serum Thyroglobulin. Thyroglobulin is present in normal serum at a low concentration (5 to 10 ng. per ml.), which reflects normal thyroid secretion. Radioimmunoassay methods are now used routinely for measurement of thyroglobulin in serum.[51] Elevated serum levels are present in patients with goiter, hyperthyroidism, thyroiditis, and thyroid tumors. Serum thyroglobulin is suppressed in factitious thyrotoxicosis, a feature that helps differentiate this condition from subacute thyroiditis.[50] The major clinical application of serum thyroglobulin levels is in the management of thyroid carcinoma.[5, 70] Because thyroglobulin levels are increased in both benign and malignant tumors, thyroglobulin determination cannot be used to differentiate these disorders; however, determination of serum thyroglobulin levels is helpful in following patients with thyroid cancer after thyroidectomy. Serum thyroglobulin levels should revert to normal or undetectable levels if metastatic disease is absent. Most patients who have a recurrence of a tumor or metastatic disease demonstrate an increase in serum thyroglobulin levels.

Serum Calcitonin. Calcitonin is a hormone secreted by the parafollicular cells of the normal thyroid. It functions to reduce the resorption of calcium from bone, lowering serum calcium in opposition to parathormone. It is released in response to hypercalcemia, gastrin, and cholecystokinin but is not governed by the anterior pituitary. Radioimmunoassays are now available that distinguish the normal range of plasma calcitonin from elevated levels. Plasma calcitonin is elevated in association with a number of conditions. Clinically, the most important has been medullary thyroid carcinoma (MTC).[75]

Plasma calcitonin levels are elevated in most patients with MTC. In some patients with MTC, the basal serum calcitonin level is normal. The diagnosis of MTC in these patients can be made by documenting an increase in the serum calcitonin level in response to provocative testing with calcium or pentagastrin.[38] Recent advances in the genetic basis of MTC have led to genetic testing for those at risk, as discussed in the following paragraphs.

RET **Proto-oncogene.** Twenty per cent of MTCs are associated with familial patterns of occurrence. These include those occurring in the setting of multiple endocrine neoplasia (MEN) types 2A and 2B and less commonly, familial non-

MEN medullary thyroid carcinoma (FMTC). Each syndrome is inherited in a mendelian dominant fashion and is characterized by near-complete penetrance. MTC is the most common cause of death in patients with MEN 2 and occurs early in life. The primary management goal in MEN 2 is to provide early treatment of affected presymptomatic people.[76]

The most commonly used method of screening people within afflicted kindred for the presence of MTC or premalignant C-cell hyperplasia was until recently the measurement of plasma calcitonin levels following calcium and pentagastrin stimulation as discussed earlier. Although this method of screening can be effective in diagnosing MTC, as many as 10% have metastatic disease at the time of diagnosis. In addition, this method of testing is associated with discomforting symptoms reducing compliance with annual screening and requires life-long testing for all members of a kindred. In 1987, the gene for MEN 2A (and subsequently for MEN 2B and FMTC) was localized by genetic linkage analysis to the centromeric region of chromosome 10. Recent studies have identified mutations in the *RET* proto-oncogene (which resides in this region of chromosome 10) in afflicted people in more than 90% of kindred with MEN 2A and MEN 2B and approximately 70% of those with FMTC.[23] *RET* is a tyrosine kinase receptor that is expressed in normal human thyroid tissue, MTC, and pheochromocytoma.

These genetic findings have dramatically altered the approach to presymptomatic people within MEN 2 and FMTC kindred. People related to patients with MTC in whom a mutation in the *RET* proto-oncogene has been detected all are screened for the *RET* mutation. Asymptomatic family members who carry the *RET* mutation are then offered prophylactic thyroidectomy. Thyroidectomy in children identified to be carriers of the *RET* mutation is recommended at 5 years of age or at any time thereafter, once the diagnosis is established. People who by mutational analysis are negative for the *RET* mutation are considered to have essentially the same risk as the general population for MTC and thus warrant no further evaluation.

Tests Assessing the Effects of Thyroid Hormone on Body Tissues

Thyroid hormone activity has numerous metabolic effects that can be measured, as seen in Figure 23–4. The BMR is a

measure of oxygen consumption under basal conditions by allowing the person to breathe into a closed system, under presumably basal conditions of overnight fasting and rest from mental and physical exertion. It can be estimated from the oxygen consumed over a timed interval by analysis of samples of expired air. In addition to BMR, deep tendon reflex time, cardiovascular function, and serum cholesterol levels can also be measured to reflect hypothyroidism and hyperthyroidism.

Evaluation of the Hypothalamic Pituitary Thyroid Axis

Thyrotropin Stimulation Test. This test is employed to differentiate primary thyroid failure from thyroid hypofunction caused by inadequate TSH stimulation.[11] If an increase in RAIU of 10% or more or a rise in T_4 of at least 2 µg. per 100 ml. can be demonstrated, it is likely that the thyroid can respond to exogenous TSH stimulation. Thyrotropin is administered in a dose of 5 to 10 units intramuscularly for assessment of primary thyroid insufficiency or diminished thyroid reserve. Increased amounts of TSH may be necessary in the presence of pituitary failure (Table 23–2).[56]

TRH Stimulation Test. The TRH test measures the increase of pituitary TSH in serum in response to the administration of synthetic TRH.[72] The magnitude of the TSH response to TRH is modulated by the thyrotropic response to active thyroid hormone and is thus inversely proportional to the concentration of free thyroid hormone in serum. The standard test dose is a single TRH dose of 400 µg. per 1.73 sq. m. of body surface area. Serum is collected at intervals, and in normal subjects there is a prompt increase in the serum TSH level, with a peak level at 20 to 40 minutes, which is on average five times the basal level. The test provides a unique method of distinguishing between secondary and tertiary hypothyroidism. A TSH response is indicative of a hypothalamic disorder, and a failure to respond is compatible with intrinsic pituitary dysfunction.

Thyroid Suppression Test. This test is based on the principle that the administration of thyroid hormone does not suppress the patient's thyroid function when normal homeostatic mechanisms are disrupted. After an initial RAIU test, T_3 is administered in a dose of 100 µg. daily for 7 days. Evidence for thyrotropin suppression is present if follow-up RAIU is less than 20%. Values above 20% in 24 hours indicate a disturbance of homeostatic control, which might be present in hyperthyroidism or in the presence of thyroid hormone–secreting tumors.

Anti-thyroid Antibodies

The primary indications for measuring antithyroid antibodies include diagnosis of Hashimoto's disease and identi-

TABLE 23–2. Classification of Hypothyroidism by Level of Lesion

	Hypothalamus	Primary Pituitary	Thyroid
Serum TSH	Low	Low	High
Serum TSH after TRH stimulation	Increase	No response	Exaggerated increase
Thyroid response to exogenous TSH*	Increase	Increase	No response

*In thyroid radioiodine uptake and serum thyroxine.
TSH, thyroid-stimulating hormone; TRH, thyrotropin-releasing hormone.

TABLE 23–3. Drugs that Can Affect Thyroid Function Test Results

Drug	Type of Effect
Aluminum hydroxide	Decreases T_4 absorption
Amiodarone hydrochloride	Induces hypothyroidism and hyperthyroidism by interfering with T_4 metabolism (lowers or raises TT_4 and free T_4)
Aminoglutethimide	Decreases thyroid hormone secretion
Androgens	Decrease serum TBG concentration, lowers TT_4
Carbamazepine	Lowers TT_4 and free T_4
Cholestyramine	Decreases T_4 absorption
Dopamine hydrochloride	Suppresses TSH
Estrogens, tamoxifen	Increase serum TBG concentration, increases TT_4
Ferrous sulfate	Decreases T_4 absorption
Glucocorticoids	Suppress TSH; block conversion of T_4 to T_3 (lower TT_4 and free T_4)
Iodine and iodinated cough medications	Induce hypothyroidism by inhibiting thyroid hormone synthesis or release (TT_4 and free T_4)
Lithium	Blocks secretion of T_4 and T_3 (lowers total and free T_4 and T_3); elevates TSH
Octreotide	Suppresses TSH
Phenytoin sodium	Decreases TT_4 by interfering with binding of T_4 to plasma proteins
Propanolol hydrochloride	Inhibits conversion of T_4 to T_3 (lowers TT_3 and free T_3)
Salicylates	Decreases TT_4 by interfering with binding of T_4 to plasma proteins
Slow-release nicotinic acid	Decreases serum TBG concentration, lowers TT_4
Sucralfate	Decreases T_4 absorption

T_3, triiodothyronine; T_4, thyroxine; TT_4, total thyroxine; TBG, thyronine-binding globulin; TSH, thyroid-stimulating hormone; TT_3, total triiodothyronine.

fication of those patients with Graves' disease who, by having antibodies, are particularly susceptible to hypothyroidism after subtotal thyroidectomy. In Hashimoto's disease, antibodies may be detected against thyroglobulin, usually in a titer of more than 1:100, and to microsomes in the thyroid cell in a titer of more than 1:32. Other antibodies that may be detected include those against another colloid antigen (second colloid antigen), which is of no value in the diagnosis of Hashimoto's disease, those to cell-surface antigen (which has an unestablished value), and those to TSH receptors on thyroid cells. The latter are thyroid-stimulating immunoglobulins, also called *long-acting thyroid-stimulating substance protector*, and are found in patients with Graves' disease and in patients with Graves' disease after thyroidectomy.

Factors Affecting Thyroid Function Tests

A large number of compounds may affect thyroid function and economy (Table 23–3).[40, 77]

ANATOMIC AND TISSUE DIAGNOSIS

Radioactive Scanning. This long-established test using radioisotopes of iodine (^{131}I) or ^{99m}Tc remains useful.[60] A ^{99m}Tc thyroid scan can be obtained almost immediately, and the dose required is quite small.[53] A ^{131}I scan must be delayed

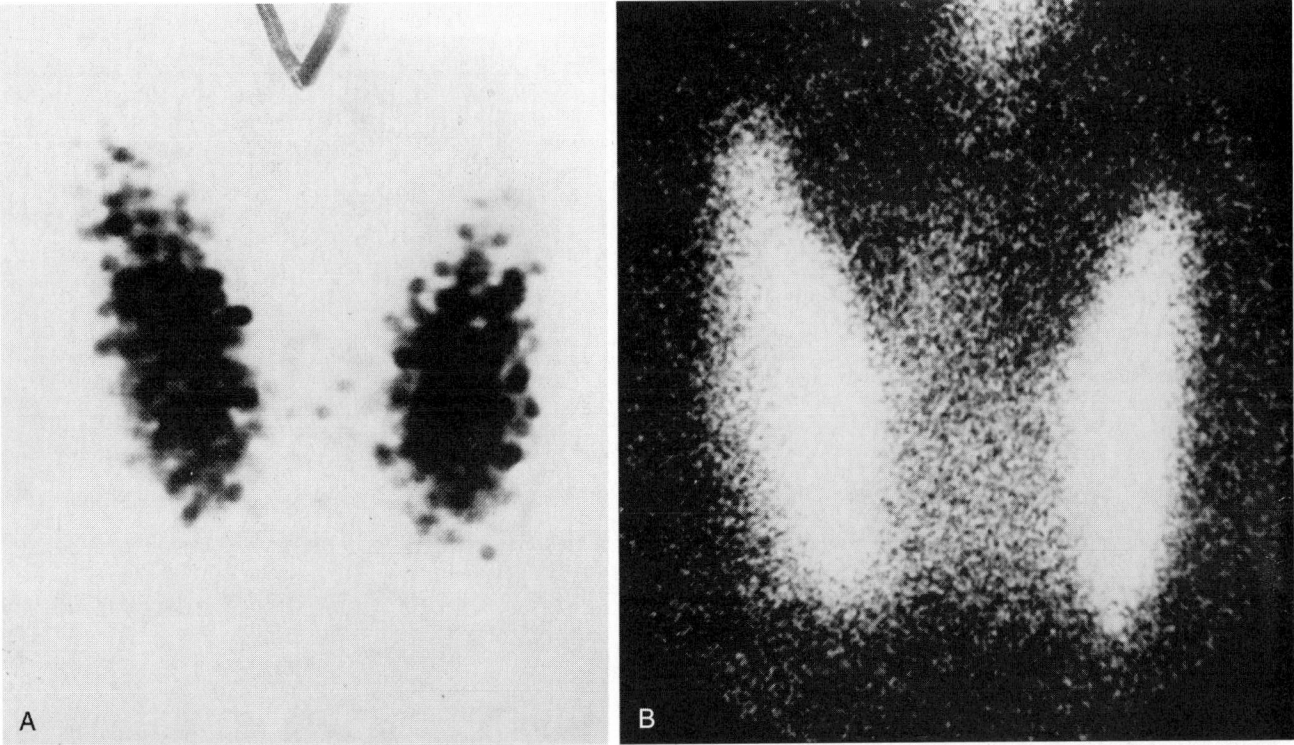

Figure 23–9. *A,* Normal ¹²³I rectilinear thyroid scan in a 24-year-old woman with a history of head-and-neck irradiation as a child. The scan itself is characterized by a 1:1 size relationship with the thyroid, which is advantageous for anatomic marking. *B,* ⁹⁹ᵐTc scintillation camera pinhole collimator image of the same patient, demonstrating the higher data density, higher spatial resolution, and lack of tomographic effect, which is seen with rectilinear scanning. In this patient, it resulted in a much better delineation of the right-sided pyramidal lobe. (From Price, D. C.: Radioisotopic evaluation of the thyroid and the parathyroids. Radiol. Clin. North Am., *31*[5]:991, 1993.)

for at least 24 hours and requires a larger dose, but the uptake reflects the nodule's ability to both trap and incorporate iodine, whereas the uptake of ⁹⁹ᵐTc measures only the trapping function. Malignant tissue should neither trap nor incorporate iodine, so it should appear nonfunctioning, or cold, on an uptake scan (Figs. 23–9 through 23–11) The true functional status of a nodule can be misclassified if normally functioning tissue overlies a nonfunctioning nodule. In one large review study, malignant tumors were found in 16% of cold nodules compared with 9% of warm nodules and 4% of hot nodules.

Radioactive scanning is useful in distinguishing a solitary nodule from a multinodular goiter. In a multinodular goiter, the normal activity pattern is absent and uptake is distributed throughout the gland in a haphazard manner. An intrathoracic or retrosternal goiter extends the haphazard uptake

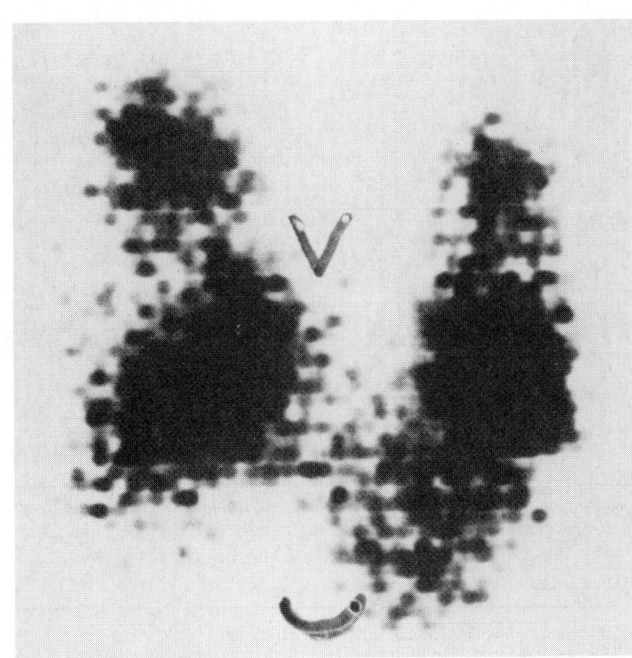

Figure 23–10. Typical ¹²³I rectilinear scan of a toxic multinodular goiter in a 71-year-old woman who had elevated radioiodine uptakes of 38% at 4.5 hours and 57% at 24 hours. The scan is characterized by moderate thyroid enlargement and multiple foci of increased uptake, these foci being palpable nodules in the markedly irregular gland. (From Price, D. C.: Radioisotopic evaluation of the thyroid and the parathyroids. Radiol. Clin. North Am., *31*[5]:991, 1993.)

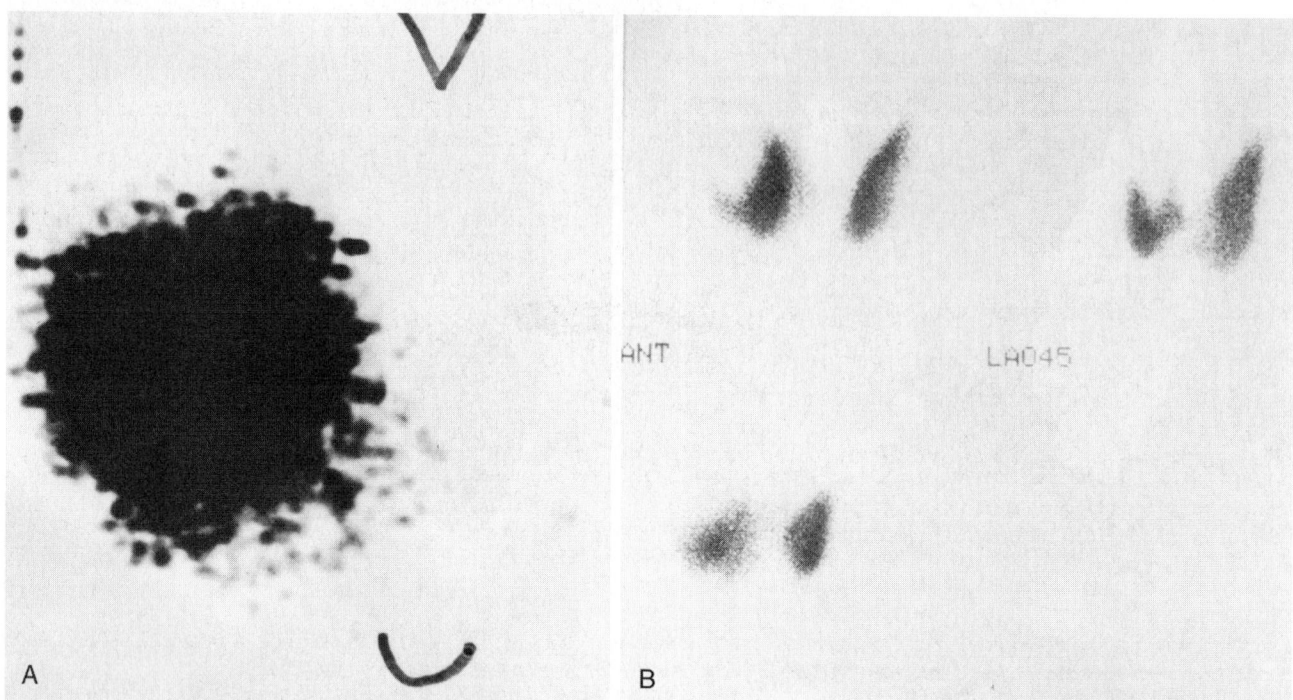

Figure 23–11. *A,* [123]I rectilinear scan in a 61-year-old man with mild thyrotoxicosis, A large palpable right thyroid nodule demonstrated slightly elevated radioiodine uptakes of 19% at 5 hours and 35% at 24 hours. Because of thyroid-stimulating hormone (TSH) suppression, there is virtually no uptake in the rest of the right lobe or the left lobe. *B,* Approximately 1.5 years after 38.7 mCi. [131]I therapy for the toxic right nodule in the same patient, the TSH level has returned to normal, and the left and remaining nonnodular right lobe demonstrate normal ^{99m}Tc visualization. The right nodule is still palpable and now appears cold after therapy. (From Price, D. C.: Radioisotopic evaluation of the thyroid and the parathyroids. Radiol. Clin. North Am., *31*[5]:991, 1993.)

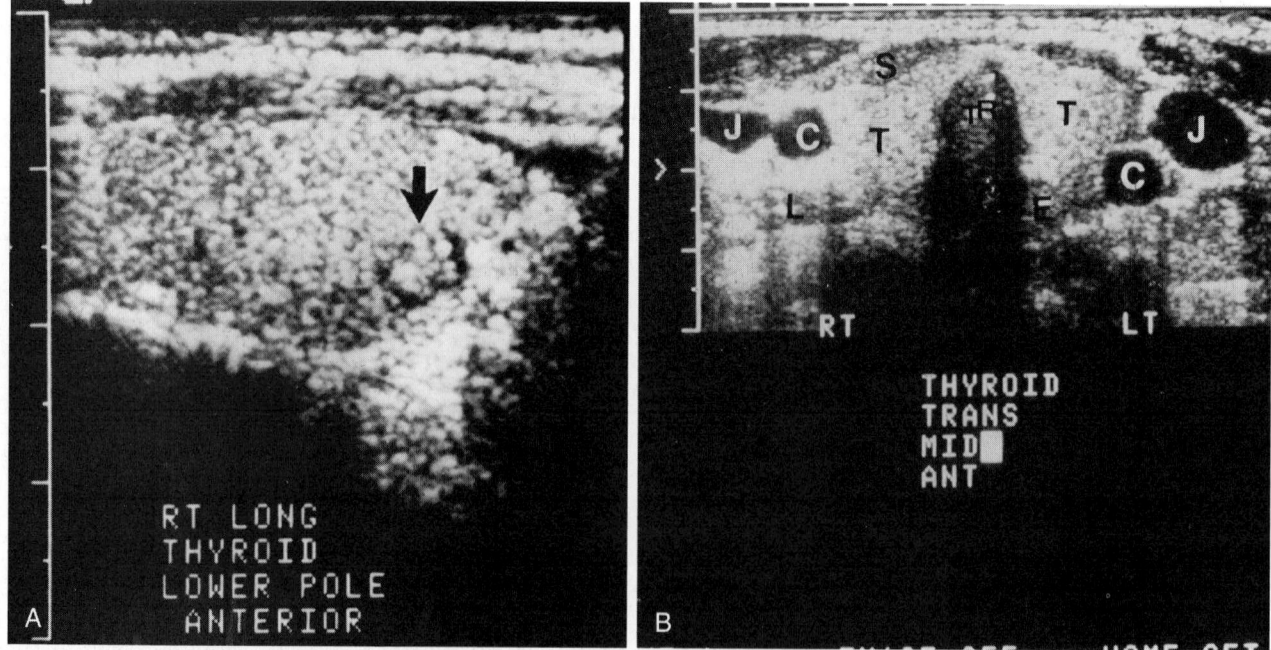

Figure 23–12. *A,* A longitudinal 7-MHz. sonogram of the thyroid in a patient with primary hyperparathyroidism shows an inferior solid lesion with calcification (arrow), which on aspiration was proved to be a benign thyroid mass. *B,* A transverse 7-MHz. sonogram in dual imaging shows normal thyroid. J, jugular vein; L, longus colli; C, carotid artery; S, strap muscle; TR, trachea; E, esophagus; T, thyroid. (From Gooding, G. A. W.: Sonography of the thyroid and parathyroid. Radiol. Clin. North Am., *31*[5]:967, 1993.)

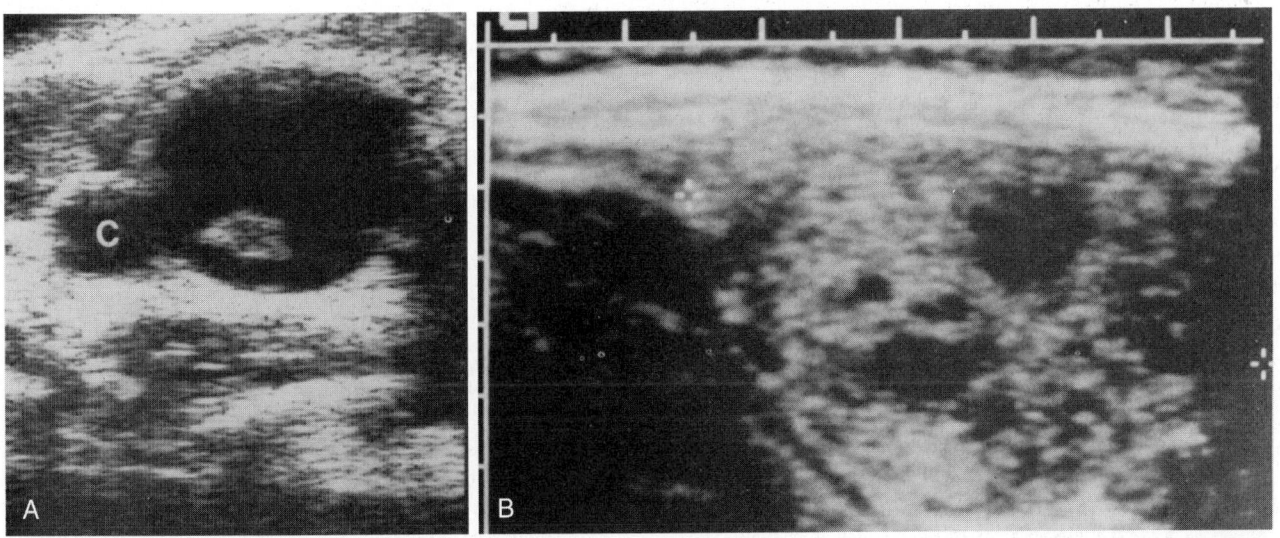

Figure 23–13. *A,* A transverse 10-MHz. sonogram of the thyroid shows a cystic thyroid mass with an inferior solid component that proved to be papillary thyroid cancer. C, carotid. *B,* A transverse sonogram shows a large complex thyroid mass in a patient who has primary hyperparathyroidism. (From Gooding, G. A.: Sonography of the thyroid and parathyroid. Radiol. Clin. North Am., *31*[5]:967, 1993.)

of a multinodular goiter down into the chest, but not all intrathoracic goiters appear to take up radioactive tracer. Radioactive scanning is useful in localizing aberrant thyroid tissue in the tongue and in the line of the thyroid's descent in the midline of the neck. [131]I scanning is also useful for the surveillance and treatment of patients with thyroid cancer.[16]

Ultrasound Scanning. Ultrasonography can be used in children and in pregnant women because it does not use ionizing radiation.[32, 37] Ultrasonography can be used to detect and measure the volume of a thyroid nodule, and B-mode ultrasonography can distinguish among solid, cystic, and mixed solid and cystic lesions, which is a distinction that cannot be made by radioactive scanning (Figs. 23–12 and 23–13).[15] Although most cystic lesions are benign, ultrasonography cannot distinguish between a solid benign lesion and a carcinoma. In one large review 69% of nodules were solid, 19% cystic, and 12% mixed. Of the surgically resected nodules, 21% of the solid lesions, 7% of the cystic lesions, and 12% of the mixed nodules were malignant.

Computed Tomography (CT) and Magnetic Resonance Imaging (MRI). CT scans provide useful information on the location and architecture of the thyroid gland as well as its relationship to surrounding tissues. An important application is the assessment and delineation of mediastinal tumors. MRI scans may also be useful in the evaluation of mediastinal tumors. Both CT and MRI scans are also useful in the evaluation of exophthalmos to exclude retro-orbital mass lesions.

Fine-Needle Aspiration Biopsy. Fine-needle aspiration biopsy is the diagnostic procedure of choice in solitary thyroid nodules.[30, 35, 36, 46, 52] Success of this procedure is dependent on the experience of the clinician performing the aspiration, which involves cells being aspirated into a syringe barrel and then smeared onto a glass slide.[1, 17, 24]

Results of fine-needle aspiration include benign, malignant, and indeterminate. In one review of 641 patients undergoing fine-needle aspiration, 436 (68%) had benign cytologic findings, and only 5 (0.7%) were found to be false negative. Of the 26 (4%) patients with cytologic findings of malignancy, the false-positive rate was 0%.

In about 20% of cases, results of fine-needle aspiration are indeterminate. In a study of 253 patients with indeterminate cytologic findings who had surgical resection, malignant lesions were found in 61 (24%) patients. Of 123 patients who underwent radionuclide scanning, 21 (17%) had hot nodules

and a malignant thyroid tumor was found in 2 (2%) patients at operation.

These techniques can also be helpful in diagnosing thyroiditis, anaplastic carcinoma, and malignant lymphoma.[18] Analysis of DNA content in aspirated cells may also be helpful in delineating benign from malignant lesions.[3]

SELECTED REFERENCES

Duh, Q. Y., and Grossman, R. F.: Thyroid growth factors, signal transduction pathways, and oncogenes. Surg. Clin. North Am, *75*(3):421, 1995.
A comprehensive review of the modern concepts of thyroid growth and intracellular signaling.

Brent, G. A.: The molecular basis of thyroid hormone action. N. Engl. J. Med., *331*(13):847, 1994.
A comprehensive review of the modern concepts of thyroid hormone action and its consequences in thyroid physiology and pathology.

Gharib, H.: Fine-needle aspiration biopsy of thyroid nodules: Advantages, limitations, and effect. Mayo Clin. Proc., *69*(1):44, 1994.
An updated review of fine-needle aspiration of thyroid nodules.

Gooding, G. A.: Sonography of the thyroid and parathyroid. Radiol. Clin. North Am., *31*(5):967, 1993.
An excellent review of the state of the art of thyroid ultrasound with many clinical scenarios with corresponding figures.

Price, D. C.: Radioisotopic evaluation of the thyroid and the parathyroids. Radiol. Clin. North Am., *31*(5):991, 1993.
An excellent review of the state of the art of radioisotopic evaluation of the thyroid with many clinical scenarios with corresponding figures.

REFERENCES

1. Al-Sayer, Z. M., Krukowski, Z. H., Williams, V. M. M., and Matheson, N. A.: Fine-needle aspiration cytology in isolated thyroid swelling: A prospective two-year evaluation. Br. Med. J., *290*:1490, 1985.
2. Azizi, F., Vagenakis, A. G., Portnay, G. L., et al.: Thyroxine transport and metabolism in methadone and heroin addicts. Ann. Intern. Med., *80*:194, 1974.
3. Backdahls, M., Wallin, G., Lowhagen, T., et al.: Fine-needle biopsy cytology and DNA analysis. Surg. Clin. North Am., *67*:197, 1987.
4. Barbosat J. Seal, U. S., and Doe, R. P.: Effects of anabolic steroids on hormone-binding proteins, serum cortisol, and serum nonprotein-bound cortisol. Clin. Endocrinol. Metab., *32*:232, 1971.
5. Barsano, C P., Skosey, C., DeGroot, L J., and Refetoff, S.: Serum thyroglobulin in the management of patients with thyroid cancer Arch. Intern. Med., *142*:763, 1982.
7. Bochm, T. M., Burman, K. D., Barnes, S., and Wartofsky, I.: Lithium and iodine combination therapy for thyrotoxicosis. Acta Endocrinol., *94*:174, 1980.
8. Brent, G. A.: The molecular basis of thyroid hormone action. N. Engl. J. Med., *331*(13):847, 1994.

9. Brody, M. B., and Reichard, R. A.: Thyroid screening: How to interpret and apply the results. Postgrad. Med., 98(2):54, 1995.

10. Burgi, H., Wimpfheimer, C., Burger, A., et al.: Changes of circulating thyroxine, triiodothyronine, and reverse triiodothyronine after radiographic contrast agents. J. Clin. Endocrinol. Metab., 43:1203, 1976.

11. Burke, G.: The thyrotrophin stimulation test. Ann. Intern. Med., 69:1127, 1968.

12. Burr, W. A., Ramsden, D. B., and Hoffenberg, R.: Hereditary abnormalities of thyroxine-binding globulin concentration. Q. J. Med., 49:295, 1980.

13. Burrow, G. N., Fisher, D. A., and Larsen, P. R.: Maternal and fetal thyroid function. N. Engl. J. Med., 331(16):1072, 1994.

14. Clark, D. E., Moe, R. H., and Adams, E. E.: The rate of conversion of administered inorganic radioactive iodine into protein-bound iodine of plasma as an aid in the evaluation of thyroid function. Surgery, 26:331, 1949.

15. Clark, O. H., Greenspan, F. S., Coggs, G. C., and Goldman, L.: Evaluation of solitary cold thyroid nodules by echography and thermography. Am. J. Surg., 130:206, 1975.

16. Colacchio, T. A., LoGerfo, P., Colacchio, D. A., and Feind, C.: Radioiodine total body scan versus serum thyroglobulin levels in follow-up of patients with thyroid cancer. Surgery, 91:42, 1982.

17. Crill, G., Jr.: The danger of surgical dissemination of papillary carcinoma of the thyroid. Surg. Gynecol. Obstet., 102:161, 1956.

18. Crill, G., Jr., Esselstyn, C. B., and Hawk, W. A.: Needle biopsy in the diagnosis of thyroid nodules appearing after radiation. N. Engl. J. Med., 301:997, 1979.

19. Damante, G., and Di Lauro, R.: Thyroid-specific gene expression. Biochim. Biophys. Acta, 1218(3):255, 1994.

20. DeCostre, P., Buhler, U., DeGroot, L. J., and Refetoff, S.: Diurnal rhythm in total serum thyroxine levels. Metabolism, 20:782, 1971.

21. DeGroot, L. J., Rue, P., Robertson, M., et al.: Triiodothyronine stimulates nuclear RNA synthesis. Endocrinology, 101:1690, 1977.

22. Duh, Q. Y., and Grossman, R. F.: Thyroid growth factors, signal transduction pathways, and oncogenes. Surg. Clin. North Am., 75(3):421, 1995.

23. Eng, C., Smith, D. P., Mulligan, L. M., Nagai, M. A., Healey, C. S., Ponder, M. A., et al.: Point mutation within the tyrosine kinase domain of the RET proto-oncogene in multiple endocrine neoplasia type 2b and related sporadic tumours. Hum. Mol. Genet., 3:237, 1994.

24. Engzell, U., Espoti, P. L., and Rubio, C.: Investigation on turnout spread in connection with aspiration biopsy. Acta Radiol. (Stockh.), 10:385, 1971.

25. Fisher, D. A., and Klein, A. H.: Thyroid development and disorders of thyroid function in the newborn. N. Engl. J. Med., 304:702, 1981.

26. Franklyn, J. A., Davis, J. R., Gammage, M. D., et al.: Amiodarone and thyroid hormone action. Clin. Endocrinol., 22:257, 1985.

27. Fnedman, M. J., Okada, R. D., Ewy, G. A., et al.: Left ventricular systolic ment and diastolic function in hyperthyroidism. Am. Heart J., 104:1303, 1982.

28. Furmaniak, J., Nakajima, Y., Hashim, F. A., et al.: The TSH receptor: Structure and interaction with autoantibodies in thyroid disease. Acta Endocrinol., 115(Suppl. 281):166, 1987.

29. Garnick, M. B., and Larsen, P. R.: Acute deficiency of thyroxine-binding globulin during L-asparaginase therapy. N. Engl. J. Med., 301:252, 1979.

30. Gharib, H.: Fine-needle aspiration biopsy of thyroid nodules: Advantages, limitations, and effect. Mayo Clin. Proc., 69(1):44, 1994.

31. Cluck, F. B., Nusynowitz, M. L., and Plymate, S.: Chronic lymphocytic thyroiditis, thyrotoxicosis, and low radioactive iodide uptake: Report of four cases. N. Engl. J. Med., 293:624, 1975.

32. Gooding, G. A.: Sonography of the thyroid and parathyroid. Radiol. Clin. North Am., 31(5):967, 1993.

33. Gordon, A. H., Gross, J., O'Connor, D., and Pitt-Rivers, R.: Nature of circulating thyroid hormone–plasma protein complex. Nature, 169:19, 1952.

34. Griswold, M. D., Heckert, L., and Linder, C.: The molecular biology of the FSH receptor. J. Steroid Biochem. Molec. Biol., 53:215, 1995.

35. Hamburger, B., et al.: Fine-needle aspiration biopsy of thyroid nodules: Impact on thyroid practice and cost of care. Am. J. Med., 73:381, 1982.

36. Harsoulis, P., Leontsini, M., Economou, A., Gerasimidis, T., and Smbarounis, C.: Fine-needle aspiration biopsy cytology in the diagnosis of thyroid cancer: Comparative study of 213 operated patients. Br. J. Surg., 73:461, 1986.

37. Hegedus, L., Perrild, H., Poulsen, L. R., et al.: The determination of thyroid volume by ultrasound and its relationship to body weight, age, and sex in normal subjects. J. Clin. Endocrinol. Metab., 56:260, 1983.

38. Hennessy, J. F., et al.: A comparison of pentagastrin injection and calcium infusion as provocative agents for the detection of medullary carcinoma of the thyroid. J. Clin. Endocrinol. Metabol., 39:487, 1974.

39. Hollander, C. S., Stevenson, C., Mitsuma, T., et al.: T3 toxicosis in an iodide-deficient area. Lancet, 2:1276, 1972.

40. How, A. S. M., Khir, A. N., and Bewsher, P. D.: The effect of atenolol on serum thyroid hormones in hyperthyroid patients. Clin. Endocrinol., 13:299, 1980.

41. Jackson, L. M. D.: Thyrotropin-releasing hormone. N. Engl. J. Med., 306:145, 1982.

42. Klein, L., and Levey, G. S.: New perspectives on thyroid hormone, catecholamines, and the heart. Am. J. Med., 76:167, 1984.

43. Larsen, P. R.: Thyroid-pituitary interaction: Feedback regulation of thyrotropin secretion by thyroid hormones. N. Engl. J. Med., 306:23, 1982.

44. Lehotay, D. C., Weight, C. W., Seltman, H. J., et al.: Free thyroxin: A comparison of direct and indirect methods and their diagnostic usefulness in nonthyroidal illness. Clin. Chem., 28:1826, 1982.

45. Lissitzky, S: Deiodination of iodotyrosomes. In Remwein, D., and Klein, E. (Eds.): Diminished Thyroid Hormone Formation: Possible Causes and Clinical Aspects. Stuttgart, Schattauer Verlag, 1982, pp. 49–61.

46. Lowhagen, T., Willems, J. S., Lundell, G., Sundblad, R., and Granberg, P. O.: Aspiration biopsy cytology in diagnosis of thyroid carcinoma. World J. Surg., 5:61, 1981.

47. Martinez, M., Derksen, D., and Kapsner, P.: Making sense of hypothyroidism: An approach to testing and treatment. Postgrad. Med., 93(6):135, 1993.

48. McKerron, C. G., Scott, R. L., Asper, S. P., and Levy, R. L.: Effects of clofibrate (Altromid-S) on the thyroxine-binding capacity of thyroxine-binding globulin and free thyroxine. J. Clin. Endocrinol. Metab., 29:957, 1969.

49. Malkasian, G. D., and Mayberry, W. E.: Serum total and free thyroxine and thyrotropin in normal and pregnant women, neonates, and women receiving progestogens. Am. J. Obstet. Gynecol., 108:1234, 1970.

50. Mariotti, S., Martino, E., Cupini, C., et al.: Low serum thyroglobulin as a clue to the diagnosis of thyrotoxicosis factici. N. Engl. J. Med., 307:410, 1982.

51. Martino, E., Safran, M., Aghini-Lombardi, F., et al.: Environmental iodine intake and thyroid dysfunction during chronic amiodarone therapy. Ann. Intern. Med., 101:28, 1984.

52. Miller, M. J., Hamburger, J. B., and Kini, S.: Diagnosis of thyroid nodules: Use of fine-needle aspiration and needle biopsy. JAMA, 241:4812, 1979.

53. MIRD: Dose estimate report no. 5: Summary of current radiation dose estimates to humans from 123I, 130I, 131I, and 132I as sodium iodide. J. Nucl. Med., 16:857, 1975.

54. Morley, J. E.: Neuroendocrine control of thyrotropin secretion. Endocrinol. Rev., 2:396, 1981.

55. Narayan, P., Liaw, C. W., and Towle, H. C.: Rapid induction of a specific nuclear mRNA precursor by thyroid hormone. Proc. Natl. Acad. Sci. U S A, 81:4687, 1984.

56. Nelson, J. C., Johnson, D. E., and Odell, W. D.: Serum TSH levels and the thyroidal response to TSH stimulation in patients with thyroid disease. Ann. Intern. Med., 76:47, 1972.

57. Oltman, J. E., and Fnedman, S.: Protein-bound iodine in patients receiving perphenazine. JAMA, 185:726, 1963.

58. Oppenheimer, J. H.: Role of plasma proteins in the binding, distribution, and metabolism of the thyroid hormones. N. Engl. J. Med., 278:1153, 1968.

59. Parisi, A. F., Hamilton, B. P., Thomas, C. N., et al.: The short cardiac pre-ejection period: An index to thyrotoxicosis. Circulation, 49:900, 1974.

60. Price, D. C.: Radioisotopic evaluation of the thyroid and the parathyroids. Radiol. Clin. North Am., 31(5):991, 1993.

61. Refetoff, S., and Lever, E. G.: The value of serum thyroglobulin measurement in clinical practice. JAMA, 250:2352, 1983.

62. Ruiz, M., Rajatanavin, R., Young, R. A., et al.: Familial dysalbuminemic hyperthyroxinemia: A syndrome that can be confused with thyrotoxicosis. N. Engl. J. Med., 306:635, 1982.

63. Ribeiro, R. C., Apriletti, J. W., West, B. L., Wagner, R. L., Fletterick, R. J., Schaufele, F., and Baxter, J. D.: The molecular biology of thyroid hormone action. Ann. N.Y. Acad. Sci., 758:366, 1995.

64. Sachson, R., Rosen, S. W., Cuatrecasas, P., et al.: Prolactin stimulation by thyrotropin-releasing hormone in a patient with isolated thyrotropin deficiency. N. Engl. J. Med., 287:972, 1972.

65. Sawin, C. T., Chopra, D., Azizi, F., et al.: The aging thyroid: Increased prevalence of elevated serum thyrotropin levels in the elderly. JAMA, 242:247, 1979.

66. Segal, R. L., Rosenblatt, S., and Eliasoph, L.: Endocrine exophthalmos during lithium therapy of manic-depressive disease. N. Engl. J. Med., 289:136, 1973.

67. Sterling, K., Refetoff, S., and Selenkow, H. A.: T3 toxicosis: Thyrotoxicosis due to elevated serum triiodothyronine levels. JAMA, 213:571, 1970.

68. Sterling, K., and Tabachnick, M.: Resin uptake of 131I-triiodothyronine as a test of thyroid function. J. Clin. Endocrinol. Metab., 21:456, 1961.

69. Surks, M. I., and Sievert, R.: Drugs and thyroid function. N. Engl. J. Med., 333(25):1688, 1995.

70. Van Herle, A. J., and Uller, R. P.: Elevated serum thyroglobulin: A marker of metastases in differentiated thyroid carcinoma. J. Clin. Invest., 56:272, 1975.

71. Van Herle, A. J., Vassart, G., and Dumont, J. E.: Control of thyroglobulin synthesis and secretion (11). N. Engl. J. Med., 301:307, 1979.

72. Wartofsky, L., Dimond, R. C., Noel, G. L., et al.: Effect of acute increases in serum triiodothyronine on TSH and prolactin responses to TRH, and estimates of pituitary stores of TSH and in normal subjects and in patients with primary hypothyroidism. J. Clin. Endocrinol. Metab., 42:443, 1976.

73. Wartofsky, L., Ransil, S. L., and Ingbar, S. H.: Inhibition by iodine of the release of thyroxine from the thyroid glands of patients with thyrotoxicosis. J. Clin. Invest., 49:78, 1970.

74. Wehman, R., Rubenstein, H. A., Pufeat, M. A., and Msula, S. C.: Extended clinical utility of a sensitive and reliable radioimmunoassay of thyroid-stimulating hormone. South. Med. J., 76:969, 1983.

75. Wells, S. A., Williams, M. D., Dilley, W. G., et al: Early diagnosis and treatment of medullary thyroid carcinoma. Arch. Intern. Med., 145:1248, 1985.

76. Wells, S. A., and Donis-Keller, H.: Current perspectives on the diagnosis

and management of patients with multiple endocrine neoplasia type 2 syndromes. Endocrinol. Metab. Clin. North Am., 23:215, 1994.

77. Wenzel, K. W.: Pharmacological interference with *in vitro* tests of thyroid function. Metabolism, 30:717, 1981.

78. Westgren, U., Burger, A., Ingemansson, S., et al.: Blood levels of 3,3',5'-

triiodothyronine and thyroxine: Differences between children, adults, and elderly subjects. Acta Med. Scand., 200:493, 1976.

79. Witherspoon, L. R., Suler, S. E., Garda, M. M., and Zollinger, L. A. An assessment of methods for the measurement of free thyroxine. J. Nucl. Med., 21:529, 1980.

II

HYPERTHYROIDISM

H. Kim Lyerly, M.D.

Hyperthyroidism is caused by increased levels of thyroid hormone with a loss of the normal feedback mechanism controlling the secretion of thyroid hormone. Common types of hyperthyroidism, including diffuse toxic goiter (Graves' disease, named after the Dublin physician Robert Graves [1796–1853] who described it in 1835 but known since its original description by Parry in 1786 and described by von Basedow in 1840) and toxic adenoma or toxic multinodular goiter (Plummer's disease).[57] Uncommon causes include thyrotoxicosis factitia, functioning metastatic thyroid carcinoma, trophoblastic tumors that secrete human chorionic gonadotropin having thyroid-stimulating properties, inappropriate secretion of thyrotropin by pituitary tumors, struma ovarii, iodide-induced hyperfunction, and thyroiditis.[34, 40, 70, 75, 76]

One must distinguish between hyperthyroidism due to Graves' disease or to single or multiple adenomas of the thyroid. Graves' disease is a systemic autoimmune syndrome with variable expression that includes goiter with hyperthyroidism, exophthalmos, pretibial myxedema, and acropachy.[21] Any or all of these features may be present because Graves' disease reflects disturbances of immunity not yet clearly defined. In contrast, an adenoma may be viewed as benign neoplasia associated with excess secretion of thyroid hormone and is thus a localized disease.

GRAVES' DISEASE

Epidemiology

Investigators at the Mayo Clinic established the incidence of Graves' disease in Rochester, Minnesota, and its neighboring county from 1935 to 1967. Approximately 36 females and 8 males per 100,000 of female and male population developed Graves' disease annually during that period.[25] The relative incidence of adenomatous hyperthyroidism and Graves' disease varies geographically, although precise assessment is complicated by differing diagnostic criteria. In a retrospective study of patients with hyperthyroidism in two clinics—one in Cardiff and the other in Toronto—the incidence of Graves' disease was 70%; toxic multinodular goiter and toxic adenoma occurred more frequently in Cardiff (25% versus 8%), whereas thyroiditis predominated in Toronto (17% versus 1%).[2, 87, 96]

Pathogenesis

A hereditary component of Graves' disease has been recognized; one of the first analyses was by Bartels.[3] Further evidence of genetic factors associated with Graves' disease include the increased incidence of clinical thyroid disorders and thyroid antibodies in families with Graves' disease.[35] Graves' disease may be found with other autoimmune conditions in the same individual and within families. These conditions include Type I diabetes mellitus, Addison's disease, pernicious anemia, myasthenia gravis, rheumatoid arthritis, Sjögren's syndrome, vitiligo, idiopathic thrombocytopenic purpura, and chronic hepatitis.[19] There are also several pairs of homozygous twins, one of whom has Graves' disease and the other, Hashimoto's disease. There is an increased frequency of specific human leukocyte antigens (HLAs) associated with Graves' disease, including B8 and DR3 in white populations, Bw35 in Japanese populations, and Bw46 in Chinese populations.[13, 64, 78] Graves' classic article described six patients, all of whom were recently pregnant women. In one patient, he noted, "the emotional disturbances preceded the onset of tachycardia by several weeks." His observation is of interest because clinicians describing the disease have been consistently impressed with the emotional component. Parry's original description included a *psychic trigger* to the illness. The precise cause-and-effect relationship between emotional disturbance and thyrotoxicosis is not always easy to establish.[33] Susceptibility to the development of thyrotoxicosis in response to emotional upheaval appears to vary widely. It has not been possible to predict such susceptibility, but there is little doubt that thyrotoxicosis does not develop in most of those who experience emotional upheavals pronounced enough to produce thyrotoxicosis in susceptible people.[11, 63]

Consumption of iodide in excess of that normally available and use of thyroid hormone have also been implicated as activators of hyperthyroidism in various reports.[88]

Although the origin of Graves' disease remains obscure, current evidence suggests it is an autoimmune disorder caused by thyroid-stimulating immunoglobulins (TSIs) that have been produced against an antigen in the thyroid. These polyclonal immunoglobulins appear to be directed to thyroid-stimulating hormone (TSH) receptors and can be detected by sensitive and specific radioreceptor assays. Graves' disease may also follow defective immune surveillance.[71] In 1956, Adams and Purvis made the initial observation that led, during the next 8 years, to the recognition that in many instances of Graves' disease there is a circulating thyroid-stimulating immunoglobulin (IgG) that can be measured by an *in vivo* mouse bioassay; this is the substance known as the long-acting thyroid stimulator.[1, 46] It is now known not to be the cause of Graves' disease. As assays were developed to detect and quantify TSI, two basic assay procedures were developed, involving either inhibition of the binding of ^{125}I-TSH to its receptor or the direct stimulation of a thyroid preparation. TSH-binding inhibition (TBI) is nonspecific, in that there are many recognized instances in which the IgG that inhibits TSH binding may not stimulate the thyroid gland. TSI determination is specific for thyroid stimulation; and although not all laboratories report identical results, TSI is present in more than 90% of patients with active Graves' disease and is now considered to be the probable cause of

Graves' disease.[59] TSI levels are sensitive and specific and correlate with the activity of hyperthyroidism, having been reported to decrease to normal in approximately 50% of patients treated with antithyroid medications or radioactive iodine and in 83% of patients after successful subtotal thyroidectomy.[98]

The pathogenesis of ophthalmopathy is less well understood than that of hyperthyroidism.[43] Possibilities include a pituitary exophthalmos-producing substance, circulating antibodies that bind specifically to eye muscle antigens, circulating lymphocytes sensitized to an antigen in the extraocular tissue, and a complex of thyroglobulin and antithyroglobulin antibody formed in the blood that is bound by the external orbital muscles.[37, 42, 91, 97]

Clinical Features

The symptoms and signs of hyperthyroidism are well known and are depicted in Table 23–4. Graves' disease is usually not difficult to diagnose clinically, because the history of irritability, weight loss, heat intolerance, and emotional instability is quite distinctive when joined with the physical findings of goiter, exophthalmos, and other eye signs. These features may be more subtle in the elderly or chronically ill.[23, 62]

The eye features of Graves' disease include a continuum from mere stare and lid lag to complete visual loss from corneal or optic nerve involvement. Diagnostic difficulty arises when the ophthalmopathic process occurs in a patient who is euthyroid or who has minimal or unrecognized symptoms or signs of hyperthyroidism, especially if the eye involvement is unilateral; the diagnosis then becomes one of exclusion of all other potential causes, particularly retrobulbar space-occupying lesions.[30]

Laboratory examinations are available to confirm the diagnosis; however, no single laboratory test is consistently superior to the others, because occasionally a test may yield results in the diagnostic range in one thyrotoxic patient but remain in the upper limit of normal in another.[27] Hyperthyroidism is usually confirmed by measuring circulating thyroid hormone concentrations of total thyroxine (TT_4). Resin uptake of ^{125}I-triiodothyronine (T_3) is concomitantly assessed for determining the free T_4 index, because the increased TT_4 may reflect a familial increase in thyroid-binding globulin or be secondary to estrogen, as in pregnancy or the use of oral contraceptives. As discussed in Chapter 23-I, free T_4 may also be directly determined. Serum concentration of T_3 is almost always enhanced in conjunction with an elevated T_4 level; however, the frequency of hyperthyroidism due to excess T_3 with a normal concentration of T_4 is sufficient to warrant measurement of T_3 in all those in whom clinical suspicion of hyperthyroidism remains despite a normal value of T_4.

The most effective measure of thyroid activity is the third-generation TSH assay. This newer generation is different from previous TSH assays in that it can discriminate degrees of TSH suppression; thus, low TSH levels are found in patients with hyperthyroidism.[74]

Measurement of thyroid uptake of radioiodine (^{131}I) is not routinely performed; however, it may be useful if the T_3 and T_4 levels are not clearly elevated but are at the upper limit of normal. If the radioactive iodine uptake (RAIU) is elevated, that result may be diagnostic for hyperthyroidism; however, if the patient has been taking appreciable amounts of iodine, either in the diet or in medication, the RAIU may be capriciously low.[8] A thyroid suppression test can then be used to diagnose hyperthyroidism, because an autonomously functioning thyroid should not be suppressible.

Treatment

Hyperthyroidism in Graves' disease is managed with a number of strategies. The thyroid hypersecretion can be controlled by reducing the functional mass of thyroid tissue by surgical removal of a large part of the gland or by destruction of most of the gland with ^{131}I. Thyrotoxicosis can also be controlled with antithyroid drugs to reduce the secretion of thyroid hormone and by drugs that block beta-adrenergic receptors. Most methods cause a reduction of the net secretion of thyroid hormone to euthyroid levels, and features of each are summarized in Table 23–5. Because each method has specific advantages and specific contraindications, the surgeon must choose the most appropriate treatment for each patient with Graves' disease. Between 1984 and 1991, the approach to treating hyperthyroid disease changed substantially among physicians in the United States, with a shift toward ^{131}I and away from antithyroid drugs.

Antithyroid Drugs. Thyrotoxicosis is effectively controlled by antithyroid drugs, and trials with antithyroid drugs are used in most patients to control signs and symptoms. They have relatively mild and infrequent side effects, are easy to use, have predictable therapeutic actions, and are inexpensive. In most patients, thyroid function returns to normal within several weeks to several months. Unfortunately, these agents may succeed in inducing a permanent remission in only a few adults and in approximately 20% of children (Fig. 23–14).[73, 90] In addition, prolonged use of these agents is limited due to toxic side effects such as rash, liver dysfunction, neuritis, arthralgia, myalgia, lymphadenopathy, psychosis, and the occasional development of irreversible agranulocytosis (<1 in 200). Therefore, antithyroid drugs are used primarily in patients in whom a remission is expected, such as younger patients with small goiters, and are administered for 18 to 24 months for maintaining a euthyroid state.[29] Factors predicting remission include a small toxic goiter, mild elevation of serum T_4 and T_3, rapid remission with antithyroid medication, and decrease in gland size following initiation of therapy.[16, 51] Beta-receptor blockade, even though it effectively controls some of the major effects of thyrotoxicosis, has not been effective as a sole means of therapy.[45, 52] Beta-receptor blockade improves cardiovascular and central nervous complications such as the pulse rate, tremor, and anxiety, but hypermetabolism and weight loss continue. Important roles for beta blockade in the treatment of hyperthyroidism include treatment of tachycardia that has not resolved with adequate antithyroid drug therapy and treatment in conjunction with iodide for the preoperative management of patients allergic or resistant to antithyroid drugs. Contraindications include significant myocardial disease, because beta-receptor blockade may precipitate heart failure, and asthma.

Radioiodine. ^{131}I has been used to treat hyperthyroid dis-

TABLE 23–4. Symptoms and Signs of Hyperthyroidism

Symptoms	Signs
Irritability, emotional lability	Tremor
Sweating, heat intolerance	Warm, moist skin
Palpitations	Tachycardia, atrial fibrillation
Shortness of breath	Heart failure
Fatigue, muscle weakness	Myopathy
Prominent eyes	Lid retraction, lid lag
Increased appetite, weight loss	
Diarrhea	
Goiter with or without bruit	
Hair loss and pruritus	
Menstrual irregularities	

TABLE 23–5. Management of Hyperthyroidism

	Antithyroid Drugs	Radioiodine	Subtotal Thyroidectomy
Success in control	Yes	Yes	Yes
Recurrence	<72%	<10%	<10%
Side effects	Agranulocytosis	Permanent hypothyroidism in 40–70% at 10 years	Postoperative hypothyroidism <15%
	Peripheral neuritis		Rarely, permanent hypoparathyroidism and damage to recurrent laryngeal nerve
	Hepatitis arthralgia		
	Myalgia		
	Lymphadenopathy		
	Psychosis		
Contraindications	Allergy	Pregnancy	—
	Toxicity		

ease for almost 50 years. [131]I therapy may be considered as therapy for nearly all patients with thyrotoxicosis, except newborns and pregnant females, or when it is precluded by a low iodine uptake.[5, 55] Treatment is highly effective, although hypothyroidism requiring thyroid replacement is common. Potential complications of radiation therapy, including thyroid carcinoma and congenital abnormalities in future offspring, have not been demonstrated; however, there is still reluctance to treat children and women of childbearing age with [131]I.[9, 12, 15, 31, 32, 67, 72, 93] The gonadal radiation dose from ^{131}I to treat Graves' disease has been estimated to range from 0.8 to 1.4 rem., a value not different from that associated with commonly used radiographic procedures such as abdominal computed tomography and barium enema.

Symptoms improve in most patients in 6 to 8 weeks, and most parameters of hyperthyroidism return to normal by 10 to 12 weeks. Because of the inherent delay in achieving a therapeutic response with ^{131}I, ancillary treatment with a beta-adrenergic blocking drug is often desirable. The primary drawback of ^{131}I treatment is the high incidence of subsequent hypothyroidism. Depending on the therapeutic strategy, permanent hypothyroidism occurs in as many as 50% to 80% of patients.[22, 48]

Subtotal Thyroidectomy. Although most patients with Graves' disease are treated with ^{131}I or antithyroid drug therapy, a significant percentage of patients require surgical therapy. Indications for subtotal thyroidectomy for Graves' disease include (1) intolerance or noncompliance with antithyroid drug therapy and (2) contraindications to ^{131}I therapy. Conditions in patients who undergo subtotal thyroidectomy include Graves' disease occurring in children and adolescents, in women who are potential mothers, in patients younger than 20 years of age unlikely to undergo remission because of a large goiter, and in those who do not experience a remission as indicated by persistent thyromegaly or the need for continued antithyroid medication beyond 1 or 2 years.[24, 41]

Surgical management of hyperthyroidism is directed to removal of sufficient thyroid tissue to render the patient euthyroid and is accomplished in 95% to 97% of patients.[84] Control of hyperthyroidism is immediate, and the need for drug therapy and the genetic hazards associated with ^{131}I therapy are avoided. Surgical risks are minimal but include recurrent laryngeal nerve injury, hypoparathyroidism, and permanent hypothyroidism.

Preoperative Preparation. Subtotal thyroidectomy should be performed after thyrotoxicosis is controlled medically. Restoration of euthyroidism improves nutritional status and provides the patient with normal homeostatic mechanisms and responses to the stress of operation. Propylthiouracil is used to inhibit thyroid hormone synthesis and limit peripheral conversion of T_4 to T_3. Absence of symptoms, a pulse lower than 100 beats per minute, and normal precordial activity indicate euthyroidism, which can be confirmed by a normal thyroid function test. The most common causes of failure to control hyperthyroidism are inadequate drug dose and lack of compliance; therefore, dosage should be adjusted if hyperthyroidism persists after 2 weeks of therapy. Agranulocytosis should be considered in patients with rash, fever, or sore throat, and a white blood cell count should be obtained. Drug therapy may be changed to methimazole if toxicity is present. Thyroidectomy performed immediately after control of thyrotoxicosis is associated with a risk of thyroid crisis, and it is preferable to wait approximately 2 months after a patient is euthyroid.

Thyrotoxic patients are usually treated with iodide and iodine (Lugol's solution, which is a combination of potassium

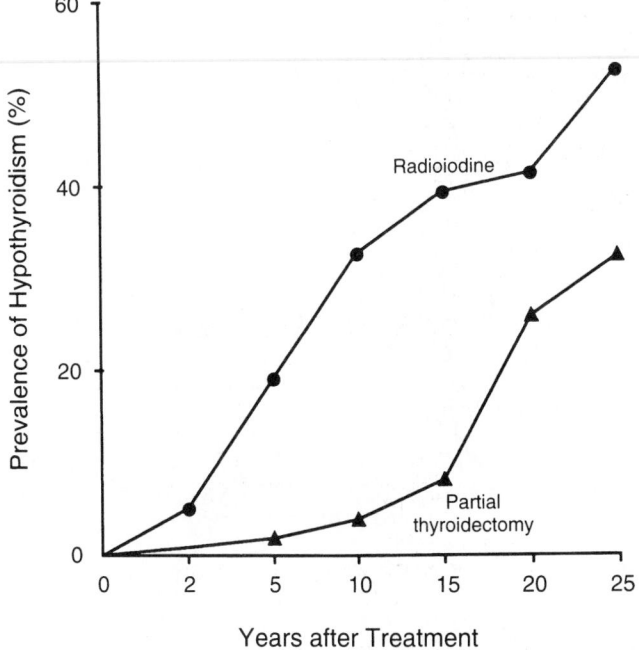

PATIENTS FOLLOWED						
Radioiodine						
1119	1119	1119	1119	513	281	118
Thyroidectomy						
295	295	295	295	285	239	121

Figure 23–14. Prevalence of hypothyroidism after treatment with radioiodine therapy or after partial thyroidectomy. The numbers of patients followed at each time point are shown below the figure. (Adapted from Franklyn, J.A., et al.: Long-term follow-up of treatment of thyrotoxicosis by three different methods. Clin. Endocrinol. [Oxf.], *34*:71, 1991.)

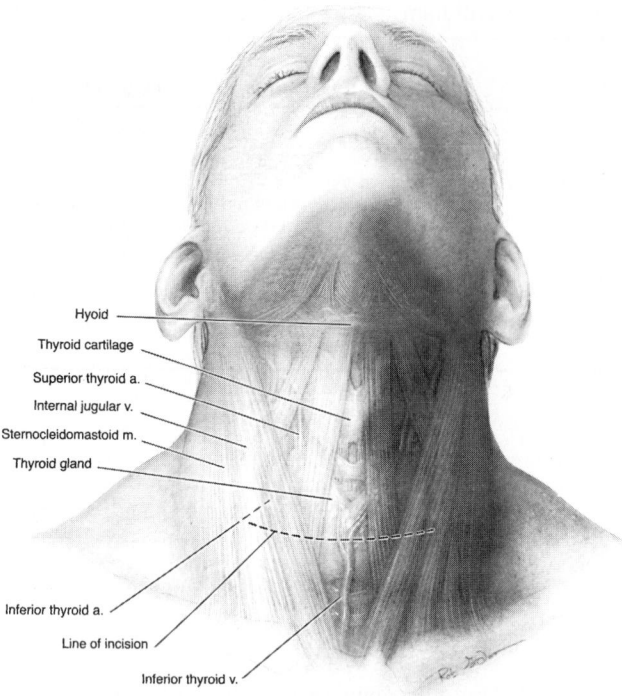

Hyoid

Thyroid cartilage

Superior thyroid a.

Internal jugular v.

Sternocleidomastoid m.

Thyroid gland

Inferior thyroid a.

Line of incision

Inferior thyroid v.

Figure 23–15. Proper positioning of the patient on the operating table is critical for achieving optimal exposure of the thyroid gland. Hyperextension of the neck, which moves the thyroid from under the manubrium, is accomplished by placing a rolled sheet under the patient and parallel to the spine. This allows the patient's shoulders to fall posteriorly while the head is supported on a foam rubber pad to prevent motion. The incision must be carefully planned so that it is positioned to give optimal access to the entire thyroid gland. The optimal site is dependent on the patient's anatomy and thyroid pathology; in general, an area approximately 2 fingerbreadths above the clavicular heads is selected. The incision should conform to Langer's lines, and a more prominent skin fold is selected if it is properly positioned. The incision should be symmetric, extending for equal distances from the midline, and should have a gentle upward curve. (From Sabiston, D. C., Jr. [Ed.]: Atlas of General Surgery. Philadelphia, W. B. Saunders, 1995.)

iodide, 10 gm. per 100 ml., and iodine, 5 gm. per 100 ml.) for 10 days before operation to decrease the vascularity of the gland.[49] Preoperative preparation with Lugol's solution without propylthiouracil to control the thyrotoxicosis is now uncommon, and operation must be scheduled before thyroid escape from iodine control occurs after 10 days of treatment.[50] Thyroid hormone, rather than iodine, can also be used to reduce the vascularity of the gland treated with propylthiouracil, because adequate doses of thyroid hormone suppress the TSH increase associated with propylthiouracil and decrease the thyroid vascularity stimulated by that mechanism.

Beta-adrenergic blockade alone has been prescribed for preoperative preparation but is more commonly used as an adjunct to thioamides, particularly if the patient at the time of operation is not euthyroid. Propranolol may be used alone or in conjunction with Lugol's solution in the preparation of the patient who is intolerant of antithyroid drugs or is noncompliant.[20] Propranolol administered in conjunction with Lugol's solution allows a patient to be prepared for thyroidectomy within 10 to 14 days. Propranolol is continued throughout the operation and then postoperatively for several days.

Preoperative evaluation of patients undergoing surgical treatment for thyrotoxicosis includes a thyroid scan and fine-needle aspiration biopsy if there is asymmetry of the gland or reason to suspect neoplasm. Serum calcium and phosphorous levels are determined to indicate baseline parathyroid gland function. A chest film is helpful to evaluate possible mediasti-

nal extension of the goiter. Laryngoscopy to assess vocal cord and recurrent laryngeal nerve function is advocated by some.

Surgical Technique. Knowledge of the anatomy of the thyroid gland and its surrounding structures is crucial for the surgeon performing thyroid procedures (Fig. 23–15).[82] The recurrent laryngeal nerve, the external motor branch of the superior laryngeal nerve, and the parathyroid glands are intimately located near the thyroidectomy dissection; therefore, awareness of the fine details of surgical anatomy is necessary if they are to be spared injury.[38, 81]

A curvilinear skin incision is made 2 cm. above the suprasternal notch and the clavicles, extending laterally to the sternocleidomastoid muscle. The platysma muscle is divided, and superior and inferior skin flaps are developed beneath it (Fig. 23–16). The midline raphe between the strap muscles is divided longitudinally. The surgeon may elect to divide the strap muscles horizontally to improve surgical access in patients with large goiters. A plane is developed between the strap muscles and the capsule of the thyroid gland, avoiding the small branches of the thyroid veins present on the surface of the gland.

Subtotal resection is performed in cases of toxic multinodular goiter, nontoxic multinodular goiter, or Graves' disease.[4, 7] The principle of the resection is excision of most of each lobe, with division and ligation of the superior thyroid vessels, the middle thyroid vein, and the inferior thyroid vein. The anterolateral aspect of each lobe, the isthmus, and the pyramidal lobe, when present, are excised, and the thyroid remnant of each lobe should weigh approximately 3 to 4 gm. The inferior thyroid arteries, the recurrent laryngeal nerves, the external laryngeal branch of the superior laryngeal nerve, and the parathyroid glands are left intact (Figs. 23–17 through 23–26).

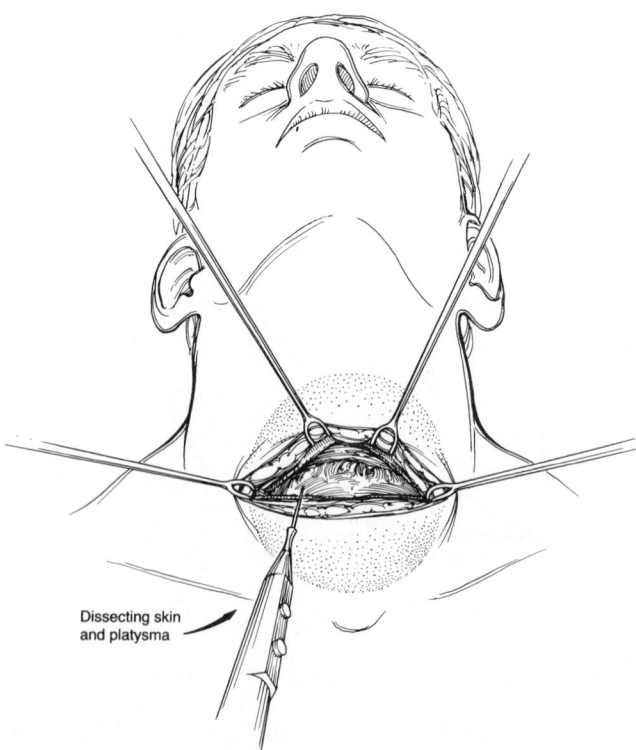

Dissecting skin
and platysma

Figure 23–16. The incision extends through the subcutaneous tissues, and the platysma muscle is divided with the cutting cautery. Flaps are then mobilized superiorly and inferiorly, dividing with the cautery the tissues just deep to the platysma muscle. The superior flap is taken to the level of the thyroid cartilage while the dissection is extended inferiorly to the clavicular heads and suprasternal notch. (From Sabiston, D. C., Jr. [Ed.]: Atlas of General Surgery. Philadelphia, W. B. Saunders, 1995.)

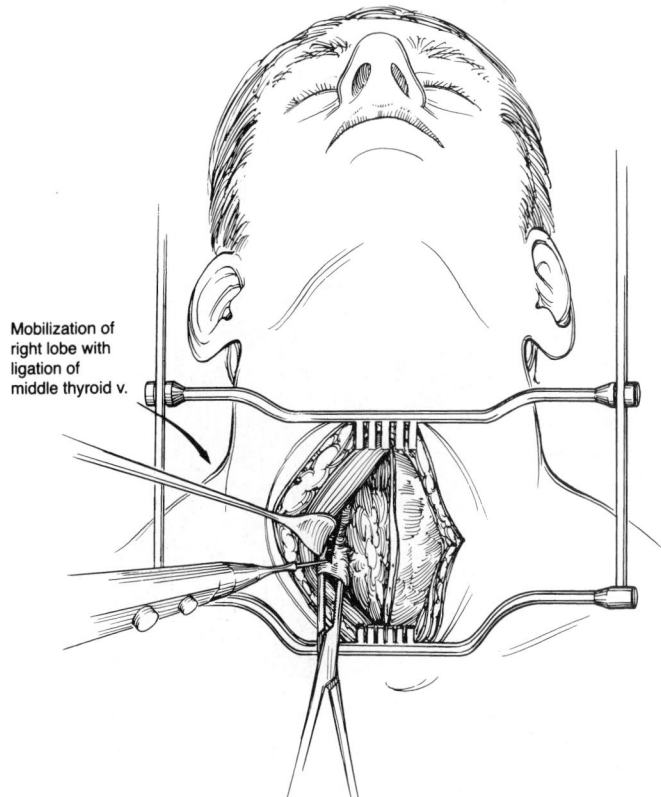

Figure 23–17. A Mahorner retractor is inserted, and towels (not shown) are placed, so that only the incision is exposed. The strap muscles (sternohyoid and sternothyroid) are then separated by dividing the tissues in the avascular midline plane from the thyroid cartilage to the suprasternal notch. The thyroid lobe is exposed by mobilizing the strap muscles away from the lobe by means of lateral retraction on the muscles and blunt dissection with a Kuettner *peanut* dissector. The middle vein is exposed, divided, and ligated. (From Sabiston, D. C., Jr. [Ed.]: Atlas of General Surgery. Philadelphia, W. B. Saunders, 1995.)

The recurrent laryngeal nerve lies adjacent to the posteromedial aspect of the thyroid (see Fig. 23–17). It contains the motor fibers innervating the abductor muscles of the true vocal cords.[44] Immediate hoarseness occurs if it is divided unilaterally, and the voice never recovers its timbre and focus, even though effective phonation can eventually be achieved.[58, 60, 69, 95] Bilateral recurrent nerve injury with acute paralysis of both vocal cords may obstruct the airway and require emergency tracheostomy, because the true vocal cords are adducted. Permanent debilitating hoarseness follows bilateral recurrent nerve injury.

As important as sparing the recurrent laryngeal nerve from operative injury is preservation of the parathyroid glands. Normal parathyroid glands are brownish yellow, distinct from adjacent fat and from lymph node tissue, with which they are sometimes confused. Parathyroids and their blood

Text continued on page 620

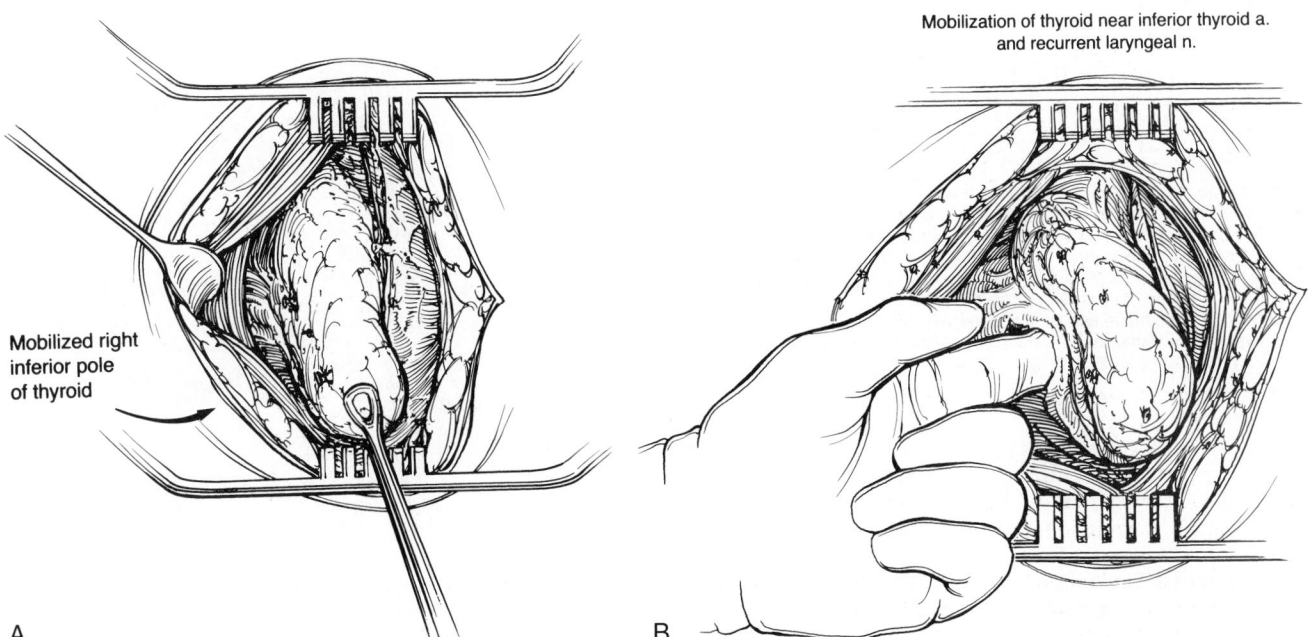

Figure 23–18. *A* and *B,* Babcock clamps are applied to inferior and superior (not shown) aspects of the thyroid lobe to facilitate medial retraction on the gland. This exposes the area where the parathyroid glands and recurrent laryngeal nerve are located. (From Sabiston, D. C., Jr. [Ed.]: Atlas of General Surgery. Philadelphia, W. B. Saunders, 1995.)

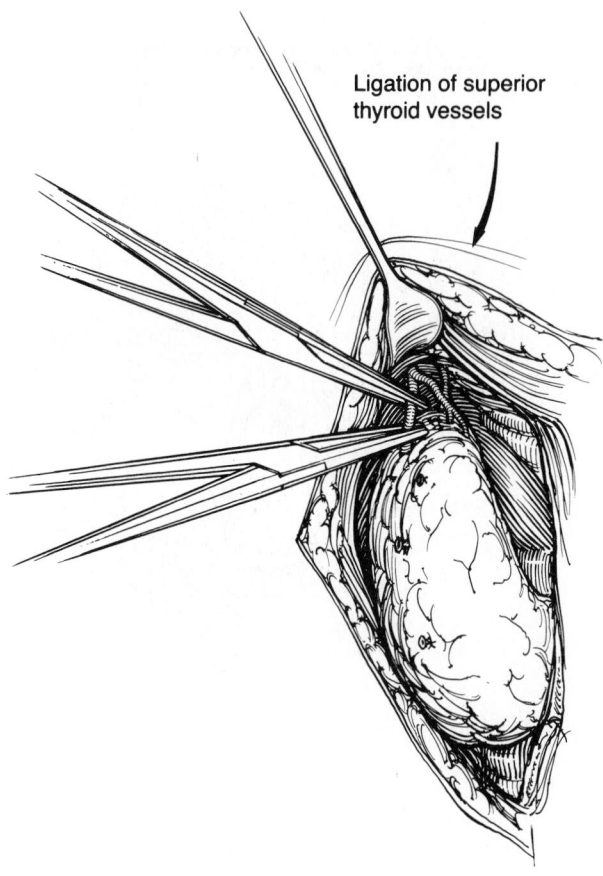

Ligation of superior
thyroid vessels

Figure 23–19. Downward traction on the superior Babcock clamp exposes the superior pole vessels, including the branches of the superior thyroid artery. The external laryngeal nerve courses along the cricothyroid muscle just medial to the superior pole vessels. To avoid injury to this nerve, which controls tension of the vocal cords, the superior pole vessels are divided individually as close as possible to the point where they enter the thyroid gland. (From Sabiston, D. C., Jr. [Ed.]: Atlas of General Surgery. Philadelphia, W. B. Saunders, 1995.)

Figure 23–20. As the thyroid is retracted medially, gentle dissection with a Hoyt clamp is used to expose the parathyroid glands, inferior thyroid artery, and recurrent laryngeal nerve. The recurrent nerve usually passes behind the inferior thyroid artery but occasionally lies anterior to it. It is best found by careful dissection just inferior to the artery. The nerve can then be traced upward, and its position in relation to the thyroid can be determined. Parathyroid glands that lie on the thyroid surface can be mobilized with their vascular supply and thus preserved. (From Sabiston, D. C., Jr. [Ed.]: Atlas of General Surgery. Philadelphia, W. B. Saunders, 1995.)

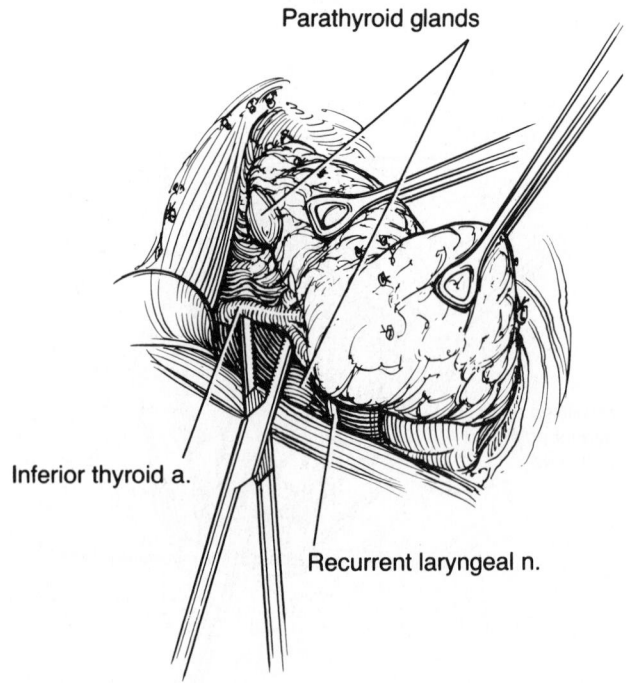

Parathyroid glands

Inferior thyroid a.

Recurrent laryngeal n.

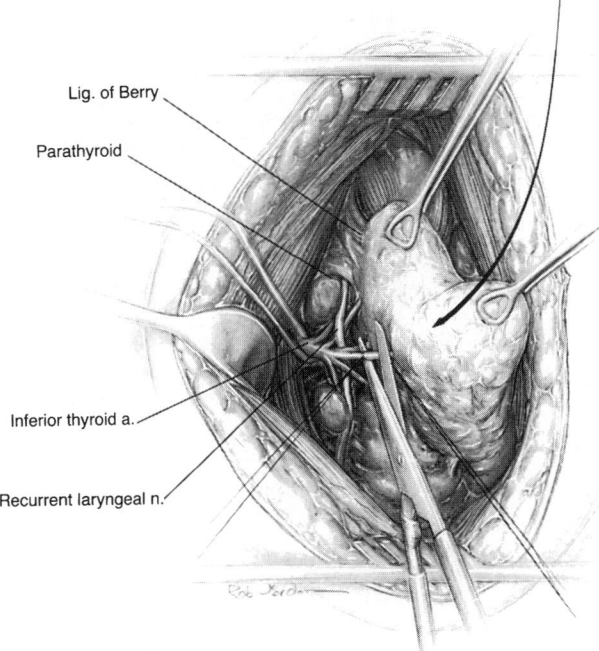

Ligation and division of distal branches of inferior thyroid a.
for **total thyroidectomy**

Lig. of Berry

Parathyroid

Inferior thyroid a.

Recurrent laryngeal n.

Figure 23–21. To perform total lobectomy, the branches of the inferior thyroid artery are divided at the surface of the thyroid gland. The inferior thyroid veins can now be ligated and divided. Superiorly, the connective tissue (ligament of Berry), which binds the thyroid to the tracheal rings, is carefully divided. There are usually several small accompanying vessels, and the recurrent nerve is closest to the thyroid and most vulnerable at this point. Division of the ligament allows the thyroid to be mobilized medially. (From Sabiston, D. C., Jr. [Ed.]: Atlas of General Surgery. Philadelphia, W. B. Saunders, 1995.)

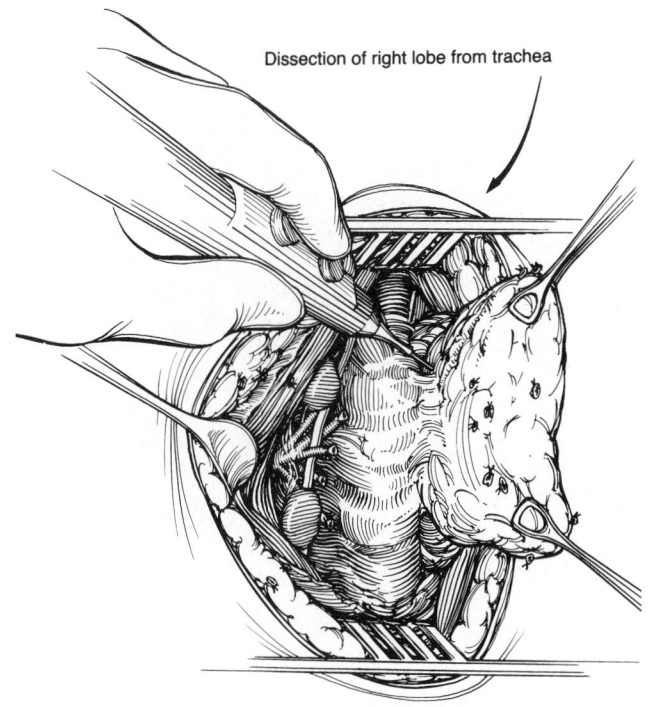

Dissection of right lobe from trachea

Figure 23–22. The dissection of the thyroid from the trachea can be performed with the cautery by division of the loose connective tissue between these structures. Dissection is extended under the isthmus, and the specimen is divided, so that the isthmus is included with the resected lobe. The pyramidal lobe also should be included if present. (From Sabiston, D. C., Jr. [Ed.]: Atlas of General Surgery. Philadelphia, W. B. Saunders, 1995.)

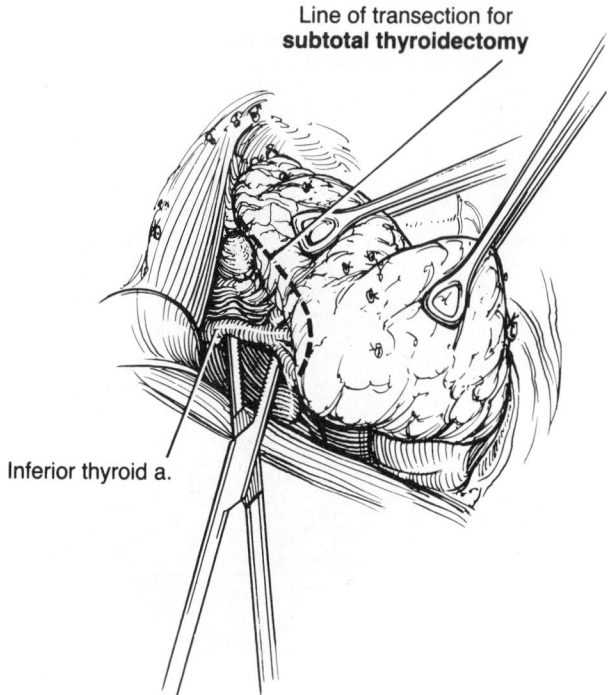

Line of transection for
subtotal thyroidectomy

Inferior thyroid a.

Figure 23–23. Subtotal lobectomy necessitates identification of the parathyroid glands' inferior thyroid artery, and recurrent laryngeal nerve, as previously described. The line of resection is selected to preserve the parathyroid glands and their blood supply and to protect the recurrent laryngeal nerve. It should be based on the inferior thyroid artery or its major branches. (From Sabiston, D. C., Jr. [Ed.]: Atlas of General Surgery. Philadelphia, W. B. Saunders, 1995.)

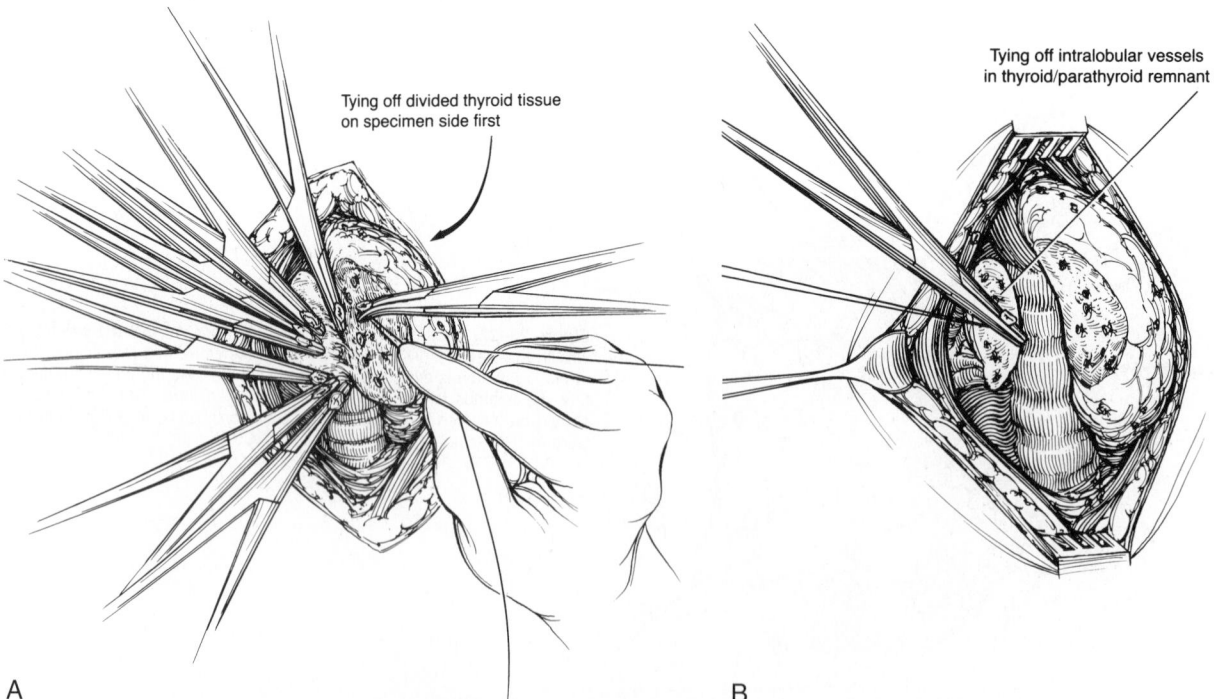

Tying off divided thyroid tissue
on specimen side first

Tying off intralobular vessels
in thyroid/parathyroid remnant

A

B

Figure 23–24. A and B, Clamps are placed along the line of resection, and the thyroid gland is divided. The divided tissue is ligated or suture-ligated with 3-0 silk. The dissection is extended to the trachea. (From Sabiston, D. C., Jr. [Ed.]: Atlas of General Surgery. Philadelphia, W. B. Saunders, 1995.)

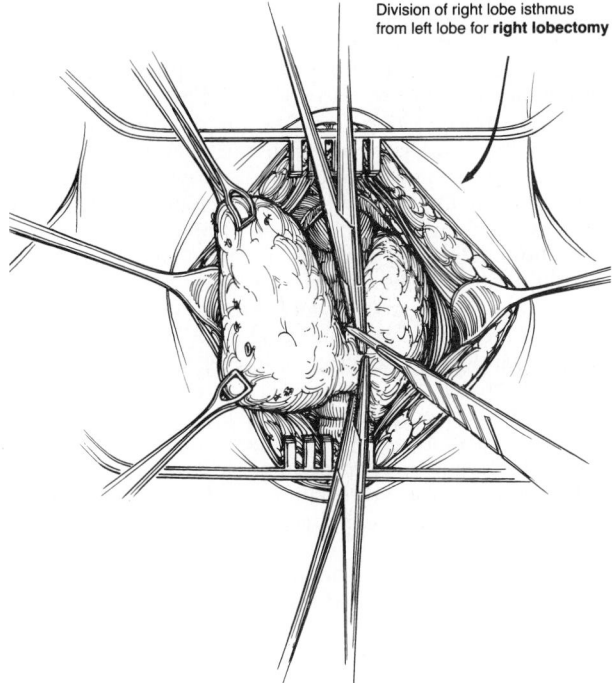

Division of right lobe isthmus
from left lobe for **right lobectomy**

Figure 23–25. The thyroid can now be divided so that the isthmus is included in the specimen. A running 2-0 silk suture is used to secure the line of division along the remaining thyroid lobe. (From Sabiston, D. C., Jr. [Ed.]: Atlas of General Surgery. Philadelphia, W. B. Saunders, 1995.)

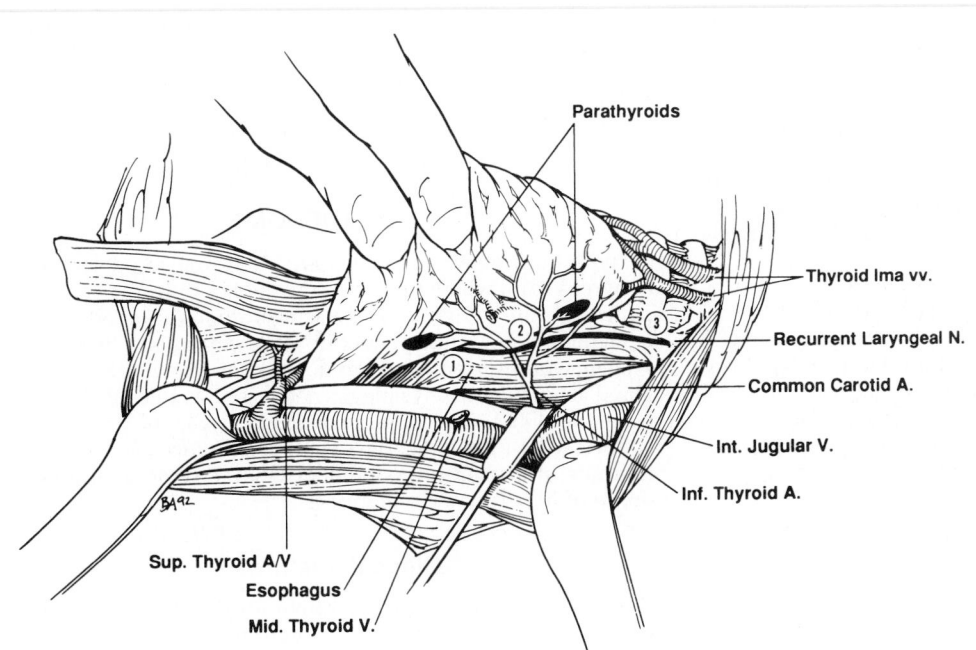

Parathyroids

Thyroid Ima vv.

Recurrent Laryngeal N.

Common Carotid A.

Int. Jugular V.

Inf. Thyroid A.

Sup. Thyroid A/V

Esophagus

Mid. Thyroid V.

Figure 23–26. During thyroidectomy, the recurrent laryngeal nerve is at greatest risk for injury (1) at the ligament of Berry, (2) during ligation of branches of the inferior thyroid artery, and (3) at the thoracic inlet. (From Kahky, M. P., and Weber, R. S.: Intraoperative problems: Complications of surgery of the thyroid and parathyroid glands. Surg. Clin. North Am., *73*[4]: 307, 1993.)

supply are fragile and easily injured, and injury can lead to infarction of the glands.[56] The inferior parathyroids can usually be found by following the origin of their arterial blood supply from the inferior thyroid artery. There is less variability in the location of the superior parathyroids, which may be found posteromedial to the inferior portion of the superior pole of the thyroid gland. There are usually four parathyroid glands, but there may be as many as seven. The inferior parathyroids originate from the third pharyngeal pouch, from which the thymus also arises, and the inferior parathyroids may descend long distances into the anterior mediastinum, within or adjacent to the thymus gland.

The external branch of the superior laryngeal nerve is also vulnerable to injury during thyroidectomy.[18, 54] The consequences of superior laryngeal nerve injury are more subtle than those following recurrent laryngeal nerve injury. The external branch of the superior laryngeal nerve contains the motor fibers to the cricothyroid muscle, which functions to maintain the tone of the true vocal cord. When the cricothyroid is paralyzed, the voice loses its timbre and focus.[39] Although many can compensate for such a tendency by spacing the conversational use of the voice, in some crucial situations such as in opera singers, this is not possible. Injuries to the superior laryngeal nerve have been overlooked in the past because voice fatigue and loss of timbre have been ascribed to tracheitis and chronic laryngitis following thyroidectomy.

Other complications of thyroid surgery include infection, bleeding, air embolism, and thyroid storm, which are rare in modern surgical practice.

Results. Subtotal thyroidectomy effectively and immediately controls thyrotoxicosis. The incidence of recurrent disease is inversely related to the incidence of hypothyroidism and is 1% to 5%.[86]

Within 1 to 2 years, hypothyroidism may develop in 5% to 50% of patients, with a slight additional increase in subsequent years. The incidence of hypothyroidism can be related to the estimated weight of the thyroid remnant. The incidence is 45% or higher with a remnant weight of 2 to 4 gm., compared with an incidence of less than 20% when a remnant weighs 8 to 10 gm.[90] The autoimmune nature of the disease also influences the overall rate of hypothyroidism. Patients with high titers of antibodies and lymphocytic infiltration of the thyroid tissue are more likely to develop postoperative hypothyroidism. Postoperative hypothyroidism is effectively treated with thyroid replacement.

The mortality rate of the subtotal thyroidectomy with adequate preoperative preparation using modern anesthetic agents and performed by an experienced thyroid surgeon approaches 0%. The associated rate of morbidity, related primarily to damage to the recurrent laryngeal nerves and parathyroid glands, is estimated to be 0.5% to 3%.[59] No reliable information is available concerning the incidence of damage to the external branch of the superior laryngeal nerve.

Thyroid Storm

An important feature of thyrotoxicosis treated by any modality is thyroid crisis or thyroid storm. Although thyroid storm is usually milder with preoperative control of thyrotoxicosis, it continues to occur not only in patients after operation for thyrotoxicosis but also in those with undiscovered hyperthyroidism and in thyrotoxic patients with active infection.[17, 83]

The manifestations of thyroid storm include hyperthermia, tachycardia, intense irritability, profuse sweating, hypertension, extreme anxiety, and eventual prostration, hypotension, and death—all of which are impressive adrenergic phenomena, and each of which has been produced experimentally

by either epinephrine or norepinephrine administration. It is pertinent that clinical hyperthyroidism and experimentally administered thyroid hormone excess both greatly augment many actions of catecholamines.

It is believed that thyroid storm is an acute adrenergic outburst in an organism tremendously sensitized to the effects of the adrenergic amines by thyroid hormone induction of additional myocardial catecholamine receptors. Sympatholytic treatment has been the most effective. Reserpine and guanethidine have been used to dissipate the thyroid crisis gently and effectively. Beta-adrenergic blockade is used to control the tachycardia, tremor, and anxiety.[14] Oxygen is delivered, as well as liberal amounts of intravenous glucose. Intravenous sodium or potassium iodide (1 to 2.5 gm.) is also recommended. Large doses of adrenal steroids have been advised, because cortisol breakdown is accentuated by excess thyroid hormone.

Ophthalmopathy

Although exophthalmos frequently occurs in hyperthyroidism, most patients require no heroic measures for a condition that is self-limiting and one that to a variable degree regresses. Treatment is directed to reducing periorbital swelling and safeguarding against infection. Malignant exophthalmos is fortunately rare, but sight may be endangered from optic nerve pressure or from corneal inflammatory involvement. Medical treatment includes high-dose systemic corticosteroid therapy or retrobulbar injection of a depot of corticosteroid.[80] Failure of medical therapy is a serious problem and is an indication for surgical intervention to relieve pressure on orbital contents.[16, 61] Alternative therapy is irradiation of retro-orbital tissue, and radiation therapy combined with steroid administration may be especially useful. Rarely, cryosurgical destruction of the pituitary may be indicated. Plasma exchange therapy and administration of immunosuppressive therapy such as cyclosporine and azathioprine have provided favorable results in some patients; however, these modalities must be considered investigational at present.[36, 92] The infiltrative edema that occurs in the orbital tissues may also involve those in the periorbital region, and occasionally pretibial myxedema is an accompanying finding.

TOXIC ADENOMA

Hyperfunctioning adenomas are often first recognized on a thyroid scan, where they appear as hot nodules.[26] Often the patient is still euthyroid, because even though the adenoma is hypersecreting independently of the pituitary feedback system, suppression of thyroid secretion from the normal gland maintains a physiologic net secretion rate of thyroid hormone. Only when the normal gland can no longer be suppressed and the adenoma continues to increase its secretion rate of thyroid hormone does laboratory or clinical evidence of hyperthyroidism appear.[68]

Clinical Features

The clinical features of hyperthyroidism due to toxic adenoma may be compared with those due to Graves' disease, and many points of difference are discernible. In adenomatous disease these include a slower rate of recognition of symptoms; the older age group affected, especially in multinodular disease; and the more common predominance of cardiac symptoms. However, the only clinical aspect that clearly differentiates one from the other is the presence of ophthalmopathy, pretibial myxedema, or acropachy in patients with Graves' disease. The correct diagnosis may rest with the character of the goiter. When there is a toxic adenoma, paranodular tissue and the contralateral lobe are functionally suppressed and are usually minimally, if at all, palpable. If the adenoma has developed in a multinodular goiter or if there are multiple adenomas, the clinical character of the goiter may be no different from that of the diffuse hyperplasia of Graves' disease being superimposed on preceding irregular enlargement. A diagnosis of toxic adenoma becomes unlikely if there is a family history of Hashimoto's or Graves' disease, extrathyroidal features of Graves' disease, or thyroid antibodies in the blood.

The diagnosis is suggested by thyroid scanning after administration of ^{131}I; and when the diagnosis is in doubt, a suppression test can be useful. The autonomous nodule has persistent, elevated RAIU, whereas normal thyroid tissue RAIU is suppressed. Confirmation of the diagnosis is commonly performed by a repeat uptake and scan after administration of TSH. In the presence of an autonomous nodule, TSH stimulates suppressed thyroid tissue to accumulate ^{131}I, so that the entire thyroid, including the autonomous nodule, is visualized on the scan.

Treatment

There is no evidence that drugs such as propylthiouracil exert a direct, permanent effect on thyroid function so that cessation of therapy inevitably is followed by relapse. Ablation of the neoplasm or neoplasms by surgery or ^{131}I is the only course to be offered these patients.[26, 27, 41, 47] Thyroid nodules of various forms require a clear understanding for treatment, and these features are discussed in Chapter 23-IV. For purposes of control of hyperthyroidism, eventual or achieved, surgical excision of the thyroid lobe containing the hyperfunctioning adenoma is simple, safe, and effective. If the patient is in a clinically hyperthyroid state, preoperative control with antithyroid drugs, using the same principles as previously discussed, is wise. The risk of posttreatment hypothyroidism is low. Whichever form of ablation is chosen, the para-adenoma tissue becomes active and maintains the patient in a euthyroid state, at least for several years.

APATHETIC HYPERTHYROIDISM

Attention should be directed to various forms of hyperthyroidism in elderly patients in whom the diagnosis is not suspected because of the insidious onset of the disease, which can be quite atypical. Diffuse myopathy, myocardial failure, and cachexia without adequate explanation all may be found to have occult hyperthyroidism as their basis, especially in older patients. The various thyroid function tests may be invaluable in establishing the diagnosis. The principles of treatment are the same as in Graves' disease, and it is expected because of their age that more patients will be found suitable for radioactive iodine treatment.

HYPERTHYROIDISM IN PREGNANCY

There is an increase in thyroid-binding globulin in pregnancy, and for this reason, serum T_4 levels tend to be elevated. Awareness of this and measurement of both serum T_3 and displacement of resin-bound T_3 are therefore most helpful in the establishment of the diagnosis of hyperthyroidism in the pregnant patient.[28] The management of such patients with hyperthyroidism is controversial. Radioactive iodine is absolutely contraindicated because destruction of the fetal thyroid would follow its use. Antithyroid drugs in conventional doses have a risk of development of fetal goiter that may obstruct the fetal airway at birth. Minimal-dose antithyroid drug therapy reduces this risk. The cause-and-effect relationship of mental retardation in the newborn and anti-

thyroid medication in the mother has been suggested but is difficult to substantiate.[11, 53]

In the middle trimester of pregnancy, subtotal thyroidectomy after a short course of antithyroid drugs and propranolol has been effective. So far as can be determined, the risks to the mother and to the fetus from the operation are comparable to those of nonoperative treatment.

SELECTED REFERENCES

Franklyn, J. A.: The management of hyperthyroidism. N. Engl. J. Med., 330(24):1731, 1994.
A comprehensive and updated review of the pathophysiology and management of hyperthyroid disease, with emphasis on medical therapy, radioisotope therapy, and surgical therapy.

Giuffrida, D., and Gharib, H.: Controversies in the management of cold, hot, and occult thyroid nodules. Am. J. Med., 99(6):642, 1995.
A review of management strategies for hyperfunctioning thyroid nodules.

Kahky, M. P., and Weber, R. S.: Complications of surgery of the thyroid and parathyroid glands. Surg. Clin. North Am. 73(2):307, 1993.
A recent update of surgical complications in thyroid surgery.

Klein, I., Becker, D. V., and Levey, G. S.: Treatment of hyperthyroid disease. Ann. Intern. Med., 121(4):281, 1994.
A comprehensive and updated review of the pathophysiology and management of hyperthyroid disease, with emphasis on medical therapy, radioisotope therapy, and surgical therapy.

Tietgens, S. T., and Leinung, M. C.: Thyroid storm. Med. Clin. North Am. 79(1):169, 1995.
A comprehensive and updated review of the pathophysiology and management of thyroid storm.

REFERENCES

1. Adams, D. D., and Purvis, H. D.: Abnormal responses in the assays of thyrotropin. Proc. Univ. Otago Med. School, 34:11, 1956.
2. Barker, D. J. P., and Phillips, D. L. W.: Current incidence of thyrotoxicosis and past prevalence of goitre in 12 British towns. Lancet, 2:567, 1984.
3. Bartels, E. D.: Heredity in Graves' Disease. Copenhagen, Monksgaard, 1941.
4. Beahrs, O. H., Ryan, R. F., et al.: Surgical thyroidectomy in the management of exophthalmic goiter. Arch. Surg., 96:512, 1968.
5. Becker, D. V., McConahey, W. M., Dobyns, B. M., et al.: The results of radioiodine treatment of hyperthyroidism: A preliminary report of the thyrotoxicosis therapy follow-up study. In Fellinger, K., and Hofer, R. (Eds.): Further Advances in Thyroid Research. Vienna, Verlag der Wiener Medizinischen Akademie, 1971, p. 603.
6. Brabant, G., Peter, H., Schwarzrock, R., et al.: Cyclosporin in infiltrative eye disease. Lancet, 1:515, 1984.
7. Bradley, E. L., DiGirolamo, M., and Tarcan, Y.: Modified subtotal thyroidectomy in the management of Graves' disease. Surgery, 87:623, 1980.
8. Braverman, L. E., Woeber, K. A., and Ingbar, S. H.: Induction of myxedema by iodide in patients euthyroid after radioiodine or surgical treatment of diffuse toxic goiter. N. Engl. J. Med., 281:816, 1969.
9. Bremner, W. F., McDougall, I. R., and Greig, W. R.: Results of treatment 297 thyrotoxic patients with [125]I. Lancet, 2:281, 1973.
10. Burger, A., Dinichert, D., Nicod, P., et al.: Effects of amiodarone on serum triiodothyronine, reverse triiodothyronine, thyroxime, and thyrotropin. J. Clin. Invest., 58:255, 1976.
11. Burrow, T. N.: The management of thyrotoxicosis in pregnancy. N. Engl. J. Med., 313:562, 1985.
12. Cevalos, J. L., Hagen, G. A., et al.: Low-dosage ^{131}I therapy of thyrotoxicosis (diffuse goiters): A five-year follow-up study. N. Engl. J. Med., 290:141, 1974.
13. Chan, S. H., Yeo, P. P. B., Lui, K. F., et al.: HLA and thyrotoxicosis (Graves' disease) in Chinese. Tissue Antigens, 12:109, 1978.
14. Das, G., and Krieger, M.: Treatment of thyrotoxic storm with intravenous administration of propranolol. Ann. Intern. Med., 70:985, 1969.
15. DeGroot, L. J., and Paloyan, E.: Thyroid carcinoma and radiation: A Chicago endemic. JAMA, 225:487, 1973.
16. DeSanto, L. W.: Surgical palliation of ophthalmopathy of Graves' disease: Transantral approach. Mayo Clin. Proc., 47:989, 1972.
17. Dobyns, B. M.: Prevention and management of hyperthyroid storm. World J Surg., 2:293, 1978.
18. Durham, C. F., and Harrison, T. S.: The surgical anatomy of the superior laryngeal nerve. Surg. Gynecol. Obstet., 118:38, 1964.
19. Faird, N. R.: Immunogenetics of autoimmune thyroid disorders. Endocrinol. Metab. Clin. North Am., 16:229, 1987.
20. Feek, C. M., Sawyers, J. S. A., Irvine, W. J., Beckett, G. J., Ratcliffe, W. A., and Toh, A. D.: Combination of potassium iodide and propranolol in preparation of patients with Graves' disease for thyroid surgery. N. Engl. J. Med., 302:883, 1980.

21. Feliciano, D. V.: Everything you wanted to know about Graves' disease. Am. J. Surg., 164(5):404, 1992.
22. Fish, L. H., Schwartz, H. L., Cavanaugh, M. D., et al.: Replacement dose, metabolism, and bioavailability of levothyroxine in the treatment of hypothyroidism. N. Engl. J. Med., 316:764, 1987.
23. Forfar, J. C., and Toft, A. D.: Thyrotoxic atrial fibrillation: An underdiagnosed condition? Br. Med. J., 285:909, 1982.
24. Franklyn, J. A.: The management of hyperthyroidism. N. Engl. J. Med. 330(24):1731, 1994.
25. Furszyfer, J., Kurland, L. T., McConahey, W. M., et al.: Epidemiologic aspects of Hashimoto's thyroiditis and Graves' disease in Rochester, Minnesota (1935–1967), with special reference to temporal trends. Metabolism, 21:197, 1972.
26. Giuffrida, D., and Gharib, H.: Controversies in the management of cold, hot, and occult thyroid nodules. Am. J. Med., 99(6):642, 1995.
27. Goldstein, R., and Hart, L. R.: Follow-up of solitary autonomous thyroid nodules treated with [131]I. N. Engl. J. Med., 309:1473, 1983.
28. Goluboff, L. G., Sisson, J. L., and Hamburger, J. L.: Hyperthyroidism associated with pregnancy. Obstet. Gynecol., 44:107, 1974.
29. Greer, M. A., Kammer, H., and Bouman, D. J.: Short-term antithyroid drug therapy for the thyrotoxicosis of Graves' disease. N. Engl. J. Med., 297:173, 1977.
30. Grove, A. S., Jr.: Evaluation of exophthalmos. N. Engl. J. Med., 292:1005, 1975.
31. Halnan, K. E.: Risks from radioiodine treatment of thyrotoxicosis. Br. Med. J., 286:1821, 1983.
32. Hayek, A., Chapman, E. M., and Crawford, J. D.: Long-term results of I–131 treatment of thyrotoxicosis in children. N. Engl. J. Med., 283:949, 1970.
33. Hermann, H., and Quarton, G.: Psychological changes and psychogenesis in thyroid hormone disorders. J. Clin. Endocrinol. Metab., 25:327, 1965.
34. Hershman, J. M., and Higgins, H. P.: Hydatidiform mole—a cause of clinical hyperthyroidism. N. Engl. J. Med., 284:573, 1971.
35. Howell-Evans, A. W., Woodrow, J. C., McDougall, C. D. D., et al.: Antibodies in the families of thyrotoxic patients. Lancet, 1:636, 1967.
36. Howlett, T. A., Lawton, N. F., Fells, P., et al.: Deterioration of severe Graves' ophthalmopathy during cyclosporin treatment. Lancet, 2:1101, 1984.
37. Jacobson, D. H., and Gorman, C. A.: Endocrine ophthalmopathy: Current ideas concerning ecology, pathogenesis, and treatment. Endocrinol. Rev., 5:200, 1984.
38. Kahky, M. P., and Weber, R. S.: Complications of surgery of the thyroid and parathyroid glands. Surg. Clin. North Am., 73(2):307, 1993.
39. Kark, A. E., Kissin, M. W., Auerbach, R., and Meikle, M.: Voice changes after thyroidectomy: Role of the external laryngeal nerve. Br. Med. J., 289:1412, 1984.
40. Kempers, R. D., Dockerty, M. B., Hoffman, D. L., et al.: Struma ovarii—associated, hyperthyroid and asymptomatic syndromes. Ann. Intern. Med., 72:883, 1970.
41. Klein, I., Becker, D. V., and Levey, G. S.: Treatment of hyperthyroid disease. Ann. Intern. Med., 121(4):281, 1994.
42. Kriss, J. P.: Pathogenesis and treatment of pretibial myxedema. Endocrinol. Metab. Clin. North Am., 16:409, 1987.
43. Kriss, J. P., Knoishi, J., and Herman, M.: Studies on the pathogenesis of Graves' ophthalmopathy (with some related observations regarding therapy). Recent Prog. Homm. Res., 31:533, 1975.
44. Lahey, F. H.: Routine dissection and demonstration of recurrent laryngeal nerve in subtotal thyroidectomy. Surg. Gynecol. Obstet., 66:775, 1938.
45. Lee, T. L., Coffey, R. J., Machn, J., et al.: The use of propranolol in surgical treatment of thyrotoxic patients. Ann. Surg., 177:643, 1975.
46. Lipman, L. M., Green, D. E., Snyder, N. J., et al.: Relationship of long-acting thyroid stimulator to the clinical features and course of Graves' disease. Am. J. Med., 43:486, 1967.
47. Livadas, D., Psarras, A., and Koutras, A.: Malignant cold thyroid nodules in hyperthyroidism. Br. J. Surg., 33:726, 1976.
48. Mandel, S. J., Brent, G. A., and Larsen, P. R.: Levothyroxine therapy in patients with thyroid disease. Ann. Intern. Med., 119(6):492, 1993.
49. Marigold, J. H., Morgan, A. K., Earle, D. J., et al.: Lugol's iodine: Its effect on thyroid blood flow in patients with thyrotoxicosis. Br. J. Surg., 72:45, 1985.
50. Martino, E., Aghini-Lombardi, F., Manotti, S., et al.: Treatment of amiodarone associated thyrotoxicosis by simultaneous administration of potassium perchlorate and methimazole. J. Endocrinol. Invest., 9:201, 1986.
51. McGregor, A. M., Rees-Smith, B., Hall, R., et al.: Prediction of relapse in hyperthyroid Graves' disease. Lancet, 1:1101, 1980.
52. McLarty, D. G., Brownlie, B. E. W., Alexander, W. D., et al.: Remission of thyrotoxicosis during treatment with propranolol. Br. Med. J., 2:332, 1973.
53. Momotani, N., Noh, J., Oyanagi, H., et al.: Antithyroid drug therapy for Graves' disease during pregnancy: Optimal regimen for fetal thyroid status. N. Engl. J. Med., 315:24, 1986.
54. Moosman, D. A., and DeWeese, M. S.: The external laryngeal nerve as related to thyroidectomy. Surg. Gynecol. Obstet., 127:1011, 1968.
55. Nofal, M. M., Beierwaltes, W. H., and Patno, M. E.: Treatment of hyperthyroidism with sodium iodide I-131. JAMA, 197:605, 1966.
56. Parfitt, A. M.: The incidence of hypoparathyroidism tetany after thyroid operations: Relationship to age, extent of resection, and surgical experience. Med. J. Aust., 1:1103, 1971.
57. Parry, C. H.: Collections from the Unpublished Medical Papers of the Late Caleb Hillier Parry, M.D., F.R.S. Vol. 2. London, Underwoods, 1825, p. 111.
58. Peters, L. L., and Gardner, R. J.: Repair of recurrent laryngeal nerve injury. Surgery, 71:865, 1972.
59. Rapoport, B., Greenspan, F. S., Filetti, S., et al.: Clinical experience with a human thyroid cell bioassay for thyroid-stimulating immunoglobulin. J. Clin. Endocrinol. Metab., 58:332, 1984.
60. Riddell, V. H.: Injury to recurrent laryngeal nerves during thyroidectomy. Lancet, 2:638, 1956.
61. Riley, F. C.: Surgical management of ophthalmopathy in Graves' disease: Transfrontal orbital decompression. Mayo Clin. Proc., 47:986, 1972.
62. Rodbard, D., Fujita, T., and Rodbard, S.: Estimation of thyroid function by timing the arterial sounds. JAMA, 201:206, 1967.
63. Safran, M., Paul, T. L., Roti, E., and Braverman, L. E.: Environmental factors affecting autoimmune thyroid disease. Endocrinol. Metab. Clin. North Am., 16:327, 1987.
64. Sasazuh, T., Kohno, Y., Iwamoro, L., et al.: HLA B-D haplotypes associated with autoimmune disease in Japanese populations. Tissue Antigens, 10:218, 1977.
65. Sawin, C. T., Surks, M. L., London, M., et al.: Oral thyroxine: Variation in biologic action and tablet content. Ann. Intern. Med., 100:641, 1984.
66. Schernthaner, G., Schleurener, H., Kotulla, P., et al.: Prediction of relapse of long-term remission in hyperthyroid Graves' disease. Lancet, 2:323, 1981.
67. Shapiro, S. J., Fnedman, N. B., et al.: Incidence of thyroid carcinoma in Graves' disease. Cancer, 26:1261, 1970.
68. Silverstein, G. E., Burke, G., and Cogan, R.: The natural history of the autonomous hyperfunctioning thyroid nodule. Ann. Intern. Med., 67:539, 1967.
69. Simon, M. M.: Recurrent laryngeal nerve in thyroid surgery. Am. J. Surg., 60:212, 1943.
70. Smallridge, R. C., and Smith, C. E.: Hyperthyroidism due to thyrotropin-secreting pituitary tumors. Arch. Intern. Med., 143:503, 1983.
71. Smith, B. R., and Hall, R.: Thyroid-stimulating immunoglobulins in Graves' disease. Lancet, 2:427, 1974.
72. Smith, R. N., Munro, D. S., and Wilson, G. M.: Two clinical trials of different doses of radio-iodine ^{131}I in the treatment of thyrotoxicosis. In Fellinger, K., and Hofer, R. (Eds.): Further Advances in Thyroid Research. Vienna, Verlag der Wiener Medizinischen Akademie, 1971, p. 611.
73. Solomon, B. L., Evaul, J. E., Burman, K. D., et al.: Remission rates with antithyroid drug therapy: Continuing influence of iodine intake. Ann. Intern. Med., 107:510, 1987.
74. Spencer, C. A., Lai-Rosenfield, A. O., Guttler, R. B., et al.: Thyrotropin secretion in thyrotoxic and thyroxine-treated patients: Assessment by a sensitive immunoezymometric assay. J. Clin. Endocrinol. Metab., 63:349, 1986.
75. Steigbigel, N. H., Oppenheim, J. J., Fishman, L. M., et al.: Metastatic embryonal carcinoma of the testis associated with elevated plasma TSH-like activity and hyperthyroidism. N. Engl. J. Med., 271:345, 1964.
76. Sung, L. C., and Cavalien, R. R.: T₃ thyrotoxicosis due to metastatic thyroid carcinoma. J. Clin. Endocrinol. Metab., 36:215, 1973.
77. Tamai, H., Nakagawa, T., Osako, N., et al.: Changes in thyroid functions in patients with euthyroid Graves' disease. J. Clin. Endocrinol. Metab., 50:1089, 1980.
78. Tamai, H., Uno, H., Hirota, Y., et al.: Immunogenetics of Hashimoto's and Graves' diseases. J. Clin. Endocrinol. Metab., 60:62, 1985.
79. Temple, R., Berman, M., Carlson, H. E., et al.: The use of lithium in Graves' disease. Mayo Clin. Proc., 47:872, 1972.
80. Thomas, I. D., and Hart, J. K.: Retrobulbar repository corticosteroid therapy in thyroid ophthalmopathy. Med. J. Aust., 2:484, 1974.
81. Thompson, N. W., and Harness, J. K.: Complications of total thyroidectomy for carcinoma. Surg. Gynecol. Obstet., 131:861, 1970.
82. Thompson, N. W., Olsen, W. R., and Hoffman, G. L.: The continuing development of the technique of thyroidectomy. Surgery, 73:913, 1973.
83. Tietgens, S. T., and Leinung, M. C.: Thyroid storm. Med. Clin. North Am., 79(1):169, 1995.
84. Toft, A. D.: Thyroid surgery for Graves' disease. Br. Med. J., 286:740, 1983.
85. Toft, A. D.: Thyroid enlargement. Br. Med. J., 290:1066, 1985.
86. Toft, A. D., Irvine, W. J., Sinclair, I., McIntosh, D., Seth J., and Cameron, E. H. D.: Thyroid function after surgical treatment of thyrotoxicosis. N. Engl. J. Med., 298:643, 1978.
87. Turnbridge, W. M. G., Evered, D. C., Hall, R., et al.: The spectrum of thyroid disease in a community: The Whickham Survey. Clin. Endocrinol., 7:481, 1977.
88. Vagenakis, A. G., Wang, C.-A., Burger, A., et al.: Iodide-induced thyrotoxicosis in Boston. N. Engl. J. Med., 287:523, 1972.
89. Van Onwerkerk, B. M., Wijugaarde, R., Hennemann, G., et al.: Radiotherapy of severe ophthalmic Graves' disease. J. Endocrinol. Invest., 8:241, 1985.
90. Wartofsky, L.: Low remission after therapy for Graves' disease: Possible relation to dietary iodine with antithyroid therapy results. JAMA, 226:1083, 1973.
91. Warthin, A. S.: The constitutional entity of exophthalmic goiter and so-called toxic adenoma. Ann. Intern. Med., 2:553, 1928.
92. Weetman, A. P., McGregor, A. M., Ludgate, M., et al.: Cyclosporin improves Graves' ophthalmopathy. Lancet, 2:486, 1983.
93. Weidinger, P., Johnson, P. M., and Werner, S. C.: Five years' experience with iodine-125 therapy of Graves' disease. Lancet, 2:74, 1974.

94. Werner, S. C.: Classification of the eye changes of Graves' disease. J. Clin. Endocrinol. Metab., 29:982, 1969.
95. Williams, A. F.: Recurrent nerve lesions. Surgery, 43:435, 1958.
96. Williams, L., Ankrett, V. O., Lazarus, J. H., et al.: Etiology of hyperthyroidism in Canada and Wales. J. Epidemiol. Commun. Health, 37:245, 1983.
97. Winand, R. J., and Kohn, L. D.: The binding of (3H) thyrotropin and a ³H-labeled exophthalmogenic factor by plasma membranes of retro-orbital tissue. Proc. Natl. Acad. Sci. U S A, 69:1711, 1972.
98. Zakanja, M., McKenzie, J. M., and Banovac, K.: Clinical significance of assay of thyroid-stimulating antibody in Graves' disease. Ann. Intern. Med., 93:28, 1980.

III

THYROIDITIS

H. Kim Lyerly, M.D.

The term *thyroiditis* refers to the infiltration of the thyroid gland by inflammatory cells, caused by a diverse group of infectious and inflammatory disorders.[28, 29] Inflammation of the thyroid may be organ specific or part of a multisystem process, and it may be acute and self-limiting or chronic and progressive.

AUTOIMMUNE THYROIDITIS

The term *autoimmune thyroid disease* defines a group of conditions characterized by the presence of circulating thyroid antibodies and immunologically competent cells capable of reacting with certain thyroid constituents.[17] However, it does not imply that these antibodies or cells necessarily have any causal relationship to the thyroid disease. These autoimmune thyroid diseases are Hashimoto's disease (lymphocytic thyroiditis); primary myxedema; and juvenile, fibrous, focal, and painless varieties of thyroiditis.

Hashimoto's Disease (Lymphocytic Thyroiditis)

Hashimoto's disease was first described in Japan by Hawkin Hashimoto in 1912 and is the most well known of the immunologic thyroid diseases. It is the most common cause of goitrous hypothyroidism in adults and sporadic goiter in children.[30] The incidence is 0.3 to 1.5 cases per 1000 population per year and is 10 to 15 times more common in women than men, with the highest incidence in the age group of 30 to 50 years.[8] Over the last 50 years, the number of new cases of Hashimoto's thyroiditis identified each year in the United States has risen exponentially. In Hashimoto's disease, thyroid tissue damaged by immunologic factors is replaced by lymphocytes, plasma cells, and fibrosis. Antithyroid antibodies are present in the serum of patients with Hashimoto's disease, being first discovered in 1957 by Doniach and associates.[6, 7] These antibodies have subsequently been demonstrated to be directed against elements in the thyroid cell or colloid such as thyroglobulin, a second colloid antigen (other than thyroglobulin), microsomes, and perhaps to a cell-surface antigen.[3, 21, 34] No antibodies to the thyroid-stimulating hormone (TSH) receptor of the cell surface (as seen in Graves' disease) have been associated with Hashimoto's disease.[23]

Patients with Hashimoto's disease usually have detectable antithyroid antibodies at some time in the course of their disease. The important cytotoxic effects of microsomal antibodies are increasingly recognized, and further studies on the exact prevalence of growth-modulating immunoglobulins will undoubtedly establish their role. T-cell–mediated factors may also be important, as it has been observed that lymphocytes from patients with Hashimoto's disease secrete lymphokines and undergo blast transformation when exposed to thyroid cells *in vitro*.[2, 25] The mechanism leading to antithyroid antibody formation and cell-mediated immune reactivity has not been fully established. Experiments in animal models point toward antibody-dependent cell-mediated cytotoxicity, antibody-dependent complement-mediated cytotoxicity, and direct T-cell killing as relevant mechanisms; however, their role in human disease is less clear. Hashimoto's thyroiditis has been linked to other autoimmune diseases, including Sjögren's syndrome, pernicious anemia, lupus erythematosus, and idiopathic thrombocytopenic purpura.

Clinical Features. Symptoms of hypothyroidism in association with a painless, firm goiter are frequent presenting complaints; however, patients may be euthyroid. The thyroid may be two to three times normal size and firm, and as the lobules become more prominent, finely nodular on palpation. In some, the gland is frankly nodular rather than diffusely enlarged. Tenderness is uncommon. Large goiters may be associated with pressure symptoms in the neck and rarely with superior vena caval obstruction. In an atrophic form of the disease, thyroid size is normal, and patients seek medical attention for symptoms of hypothyroidism.

The diagnosis of Hashimoto's disease begins by documenting hypothyroidism with thyroid function tests. Serum TSH is also measured and is invariably raised. A normal serum TSH level in the presence of low thyroxine (T_4) and triiodothyronine T_3 levels excludes primary thyroid failure. Although Hashimoto's disease is usually associated with hypothyroidism, thyroid function may change during the course of the disease.[9, 16, 31] Some patients with a previous diagnosis of Hashimoto's disease, goiter, and hypothyroidism have symptoms that suggest hyperthyroidism. This is believed to result from clones of lymphocytes that produce stimulatory anti-TSH antibodies, creating a hyperthyroid state known as *hashitoxicosis*. If the patient is receiving thyroid hormone therapy, the differential diagnosis for hyperthyroidism includes overreplacement of thyroid hormone and development of hashitoxicosis.

Routine tests for thyroglobulin and microsomal antibodies should be performed to confirm the diagnosis of Hashimoto's disease, because the presence and the titer of these antibodies correlate with the severity and extent of the autoimmune process. The titer regarded as positive varies in different laboratories and with the particular method and reagents used. Hypothyroidism associated with a goiter but negative thyroid antibodies suggests use of goitrogen, a dyshormonogenetic goiter, or an endemic goiter.

If thyroid neoplasia is suspected clinically owing to asymmetry of the goiter, cervical lymphadenopathy, pressure symptoms, hoarseness, or enlargement of the goiter despite adequate thyroid replacement, fine-needle aspiration or open biopsy of the suspicious area should be performed. There is a strong relationship between thyroiditis and malignant thyroid lymphoma.[12] This tumor is rare, but the risk of thyroid lymphoma is greatly increased in patients with Hashimoto's disease, in comparison with the general population.

Pathology. The enlarged thyroid is pale, firm, and pale yellow, with a finely nodular surface. Adjacent lymph nodes may be enlarged. Histologically, there is diffuse infiltration of the gland by lymphocytes and plasma cells, with formation of lymphoid follicles and germinal centers. The thyroid follicles are disrupted, and the follicular basement membrane is damaged. Some epithelial cells are enlarged and show a characteristic oxyphilic change in the cytoplasm (Askanazy cells).[15]

Treatment. There is no specific treatment for Hashimoto's disease. Patients are usually followed medically, and replacement therapy with T_4 is begun in patients with hypothyroidism that is symptomatic or associated with a goiter that is causing pressure symptoms. Early initiation of thyroid hormone therapy has been recommended by many clinicians to prevent further thyroid enlargement and reduce the risk of myxedema, especially in postpartum patients.

Surgical reduction of goiter should be performed if severe pressure symptoms that have not responded to corticosteroid therapy are present.[18] This usually consists of subtotal thyroidectomy. Biopsy to exclude malignancy in nodules suspicious for thyroid carcinoma (usually papillary) or lymphoma is indicated.[13, 17, 28] If carcinoma is suspected, a lobectomy should be performed; and if frozen section demonstrates carcinoma, a subtotal or total thyroidectomy should be performed.[9, 27, 28]

Painless Thyroiditis

The syndrome known as *painless thyroiditis*, increasingly described over the past decade and referred to as *silent thyroiditis* but most accurately as *lymphocytic thyroiditis* with spontaneous resolving hyperthyroidism, is now recognized as a distinct entity.[22, 26, 35] It presents either sporadically or in the postpartum period. Clinical features mimic those of subacute thyroiditis (SAT) but without the neck pain. Hyperthyroidism, which is usually self-limiting, develops abruptly in a patient in whom the thyroid is painless and only slightly enlarged, has low radioactive iodine uptake, and histologically demonstrates lymphocytic infiltration without the characteristic giant cell and granulomatous changes seen in SAT. Differentiation from SAT appears worthwhile, because with long-term follow-up, it is clear that whereas few patients with SAT have a recurrence or progress to permanent thyroid disease, this is not the situation with the painless thyroiditis syndrome. Silent thyroiditis has three clinical stages that mirror those of SAT. In Stage I, abrupt onset of thyrotoxic symptoms such as tachycardia, palpitations, nervousness, and weight loss occurs. Physical examination reveals a small, nontender goiter in about 50% of patients. This phase usually resolves in a few weeks, although about 40% of patients enter Stage II, demonstrating a drop in T_3 and T_4 to subnormal levels. Clinical transient hypothyroidism may develop, but in 4 to 16 weeks, normal thyroid function is usually recovered, and patients enter Stage III. Antithyroid antibodies, particularly thyroid microsomal antibody, are found in 50% to 80% of patients.

Treatment of silent thyroiditis is generally limited to reassurance and monitoring for recovery of thyroid function. Release of preformed T_3 and T_4 is the cause of hyperthyroidism, so that propylthiouracil and methimazole are not helpful. Beta blockers can be used for symptoms. Long-term follow-up is required because 6% of patients may have persistent hypothyroidism. Postpartum patients have an increased risk of recurrent episodes of silent thyroiditis with subsequent pregnancies.

DE QUERVAIN'S (SUBACUTE OR GIANT-CELL) THYROIDITIS

SAT represents approximately 1% of all cases of thyroid disease, is much less common than Hashimoto's thyroiditis, and has only one eighth the incidence of Graves' disease. It is the most common cause of an anterior neck mass and pain in the thyroid gland. It is uncommon in children, being most frequent in the third to fifth decades, with a female-to-male ratio of 5:1. Although a causative agent is rarely demonstrated, it often follows upper respiratory tract infections, suggesting that it is caused by a viral infection.[5, 10, 33]

Clinical Features. The course of SAT consists of several clinical stages, the first of which is a viral prodrome that brings myalgia, lassitude, low-grade fever, and sore throat. Stage I begins with acute pain in the thyroid gland that often develops rather suddenly, often with radiation to the jaw and ears, and may be associated with marked tenderness and dysphagia. The gland is generally moderately enlarged and tender and contains ill-defined nodules. The skin overlying the thyroid is erythematous. Compression of the esophagus may occur, and the patient has dysphagia or odynophagia. No fever or leukocytosis is noted.

Hyperthyroidism is observed in this first stage of the disease and is caused by the sudden disruption of the follicular structure with discharge of large quantities of thyroid hormone into the circulation. The syndrome lasts for several weeks to months.

The general laboratory findings include an increased erythrocyte sedimentation rate (ESR), a generalized increase in immunoglobulins; however, a marked elevation in granulocytes is usually not noted. The changes in thyroid function are quite characteristic, with an early thyrotoxic stage due to a sudden discharge of preformed T_4 and T_3 into the circulation. The thyroid radioactive iodine uptake (RAIU) and TSH level are characteristically reduced. Testing for thyroglobulin is sensitive but not specific. A normal thyroglobulin level essentially excludes the diagnosis.

Graves' disease and the thyrotoxic phase of SAT are differentiated by thyroid scan: patients with Graves' disease have diffuse increased uptake, whereas patients in the thyrotoxic phase of SAT demonstrate diffuse decreased uptake. SAT differs from Hashimoto's disease in that SAT is not consistently associated with antithyroid antibodies. Hypothyroidism may be observed after 2 to 4 weeks in those with SAT that progresses to thyroid failure. In addition, thyroid function returns to baseline after a period of months. Goiter associated with discrete nodularity of the gland is an indication for fine-needle aspiration or biopsy to differentiate SAT from colloid nodules or thyroid cancer.

Pathology. There is generally moderate thyroid enlargement, which may be asymmetric. The inflammatory reaction involving the thyroid may lead to adherence of the gland to the capsule and immediate extrathyroid tissues. Histologic features include desquamation of the follicular cells and disturbance and loss of colloid material. There is invasion of the thyroid by polymorphonuclear leukocytes, lymphocytes, and foreign-body giant cells. The most characteristic feature is the granuloma that consists of giant cells clustered around foci of degenerating thyroid follicles.[22]

Treatment. This condition remits spontaneously after a few days to a few months and relapses occasionally before the disease remits permanently. The treatment consists of analgesics such as aspirin and ibuprofen in mild cases. Steroids are effective in controlling symptoms in the more severe cases. Prednisone is usually initiated and tapered over a period of months. Twenty per cent of patients experience rebound swelling when it is discontinued. Medical therapy for the transient thyrotoxic phase is indicated; however, antithyroid drugs such as propylthiouracil and methimazole are ineffective because the thyroid hormone that is released is preformed rather than synthesized. Spontaneous recovery is observed in more than 90% of patients after 3 to 6 weeks; however, as many as 30% of patients progress to Stage II, a hypothyroid phase resulting from extensive destruction of follicular cells. Thyroid function must be carefully monitored during this phase. Most of these patients enter Stage III and regain normal thyroid function in 4 to 6 weeks, but in as many as 10% of patients hypothyroidism is permanent.

ACUTE SUPPURATIVE THYROIDITIS

Acute suppurative thyroiditis is a rare condition of the thyroid gland that is usually due to bacterial infection.[1, 11] Common pathogens include *Streptococcus*, *Staphylococcus*, and *Pneumococcus*, and rarely *Salmonella* or *Bacteroides*. Other extremely rare causes of a more indolent infection include tuberculosis, actinomycoses, echinococcosis, aspergillosis, and syphilis. Normal thyroid glands are susceptible to infection, as are those with underlying disorders. Infections usually arise from lymphatic drainage of adjacent structures such as the oropharynx and the lymph nodes or from congenital abnormalities such as a persistent thyroglossal duct or fistula; however, infection can also occur via hematogenous spread or after direct trauma.

Clinical Features. Symptoms occur with an acute onset and characteristically include tenderness, enlargement, warmth, erythema, and neck pain exacerbated by neck extension and swallowing. Septicemia or direct extension to the neck or chest may occur. The presence of blood-tinged sputum with the acute onset of symptoms suggests tracheal involvement. Fifty per cent of patients have pre-existing thyroid disease.

Thyroid function is usually normal, as is the RAIU, although should an abscess develop, it is observed as an area of decreased uptake on the thyroid scan. Transient hyperthyroidism may occur if thyroid hormone is released from inflamed follicles. Ultrasonography may demonstrate a partially cystic mass within the thyroid. Fine-needle aspiration may be diagnostic when polymorphonuclear leukocytes and organisms are observed.

Although the clinical characteristics of acute suppurative thyroiditis are usually straightforward, differentiation from de Quervain's thyroiditis is important. The latter is characterized by less severe pain and lack of involvement of adjacent neck tissues, a markedly elevated ESR, a markedly depressed RAIU, and a greater likelihood of transient hyperthyroidism. Acute thyroiditis may have leukocytosis with a left shift.

Patients with chronic suppurative thyroiditis usually present with a slowly growing neck mass that is suspected of being a cyst or adenoma, and only on biopsy or surgical exploration is the correct diagnosis made.

Pathology. Histologic examination of the gland reveals a marked polymorphonuclear leukocyte and lymphocytic infiltrate in the acute phase, which may be associated with frank thyroid necrosis and abscess formation. Fibrosis occurs with healing.

Treatment. Primary treatment of suppurative thyroiditis consists of appropriate antibiotics against the causative organism. Measurable improvement is usually observed within 48 to 72 hours, and complete resolution occurs in 2 to 4 weeks. Thyroid abscesses should be drained, and cysts communicating with the pyriform sinus or trachea recur and require excision.

RIEDEL'S THYROIDITIS

Riedel's thyroiditis is a rare inflammatory condition, being reported in only 20 of 42,000 surgical specimens of the thyroid at the Mayo Clinic. The most common ages of presentation are 30 to 60 years, and women are more frequently affected than men.[8] The cause of invasive fibrous thyroiditis remains uncertain. There is little evidence to support the formerly popular view that this condition represents a late stage of either autoimmune thyroiditis or SAT. There are reports linking it to extracervical fibrosclerosis, which includes retroperitoneal and mediastinal fibrosis, fibrosing cholangitis, pseudotumor of the orbit, and fibrosis of the lacrimal gland. It appears likely that the invasive fibrous thyroiditis represents one aspect of a generalized process that is not specifically related to the thyroid gland.

Clinical Features. The patient generally presents with a history of rapid increase in thyroid size, which is frequently associated with symptoms of tracheal and/or esophageal compression. The gland is often described as *woody* in texture; is generally uniformly enlarged, nontender, and strikingly hard on palpation; and is often mistaken for thyroid carcinoma. There are usually no other clinical features, although the disease may be associated with retroperitoneal fibrosis and other disorders.

There are no characteristic laboratory findings except that there are absent to low titers of antithyroid antibodies. In late stages of disease, hypothyroidism may be present. The diagnosis can be confirmed only by biopsy.

Pathology. The gland is involved wholly or in part by a dense, invasive fibrosis that extends to involve the surrounding tissues, so that the capsule and anatomic margins of the gland cannot be precisely defined. There is no lymphocytic infiltrate in the tissue, but lymphocytic perivasculitis is observed in most patients.

Treatment. Medical therapy includes thyroid replacement if hypothyroidism is present. Surgical treatment is indicated if pressure symptoms in the neck require relief, and partial thyroidectomy is required in most of these patients. The operation requires meticulous dissection because fibrosis may involve surrounding structures such as the trachea, the carotid sheath, and the recurrent laryngeal nerve. Although in most patients the fibrous process is confined to the neck and the disease is relatively benign, a few patients develop multifocal fibrosis as long as 10 years later, which may be life threatening.[32, 36]

SELECTED REFERENCES

Cady, B., and Rossi, R. L.: Surgery of the Thyroid and Parathyroid Glands, 3rd ed. Philadelphia, W. B Saunders, 1991.
    A comprehensive and authoritative monograph that discusses the modern management of thyroid disease, including thyroiditis.

Schubert, M. F., and Kountz, D. S.: Thyroiditis—a disease with many faces. Postgrad. Med., *98*(2):101, 1995.
    A straightforward, up-to-date, and practical guide to the management of thyroiditis.

REFERENCES

1. Altemeier, W. A.: Acute pyogenic thyroiditis. Arch. Surg., *61*:76, 1950.
2. Aoh, N., and DeGroot, L. J.: Lymphocyte blastogenic response to human thyroglobulin in Graves' disease: Hashimoto's thyroiditis and metastatic thyroid cancer. Clin. Exp. Immunol., *38*:523, 1979.
3. Burek, C. L., Hoffman, W. H., and Rose, N. R.: The presence of thyroid autoantibodies in children and adolescents with autoimmune thyroid disease and their parents. Clin. Immunol. Immunopathol., *25*:395, 1982.
4. Crile, G., Jr., and Hazard, J. B.: Incidence of cancer in struma lymphomatosa. Surg. Gynecol. Obstet., *115*:101, 1962.
5. de Quervain, F.: Die akute, nicht eitenge thyroiditis. Mitt. Grenzgeb. Med. Chir. 2(5uppl.):1, 1904.
6. Doniach, D., Hudson, R. V., and Roitt, L. M.: Human autoimmune thyroiditis: Clinical studies. Br. Med. J., *1*:365, 1960.

7. Doniach, D., Bottazzo, G. F., and Russell, R. C. G.: Goitrous autoimmune thyroiditis (Hashimoto's disease). Clin. Endocrinol. Metab. 8:63, 1978.
8. Furszyfer, J., Kurland, L. T., and Woolner, L. B., et al.: Hashimoto's thyroiditis in Olmstead County, Minnesota, 1935–1967. Mayo Clin. Proc., 45:586, 1970.
9. Gluck, F. B., Nusynowitz, M. L., and Plymate, S.: Chronic lymphocytic thyroiditis, thyrotoxicosis, and low radioactive iodide uptake. N. Engl. J. Med., 293:634, 1975.
10. Greene, J. N.: Subacute thyroiditis. Am. J. Med., 51:97, 1971.
11. Hagan, A. D., Goffinet, J., and Dans, J. W.: Acute streptococcal thyroiditis. JAMA, 202:829, 1969.
12. Hamberger, J. L., Miller, J. M., and Kini, S. R.: Lymphoma of the thyroid. Ann. Intern. Med., 99:685, 1983.
13. Holm, L. E., Blomgren, H., and Lowhagen, T.: Cancer risks in patients with chronic lymphocytic thyroiditis. N. Engl. J. Med., 312:601, 1985.
14. Hurley, D. L., and Gharib, H.: Detection and treatment of hypothyroidism and Graves' disease. Geriatrics, 50(4):41, 1995.
15. Knecht, H., and Hedinger, C. E.: Ultrastructural findings in Hashimoto's thyroiditis and focal lymphocytic thyroiditis with reference to giant cell formation. Histopathology, 6:511, 1982.
16. Larsen, P. R.: Serum triiodothyronine, thyroxine, and thyrotropin during hyperthyroid, hypothyroid, and recovery phases of subacute thyroiditis. Metabolism, 23:467, 1974.
17. Levine, S. N.: Current concepts of thyroiditis. Arch. Intern. Med., 143:1952, 1983.
18. Linden, M. C., Jr., and Clark, J. L. L: Indications for surgery in thyroiditis. Am. J. Surg., 118:829, 1969.
19. Mandel, S. J., Brent, G. A., and Larsen, P. R.: Levothyroxine therapy in patients with thyroid disease. Ann. Intern. Med., 119(6):492, 1993.
20. Martinez, M., Derksen, D., and Kapsner, P.: Making sense of hypothyroidism: An approach to testing and treatment. Postgrad. Med., 93(6):135, 1993.
21. McLachlan, S. M., McGregor, A. M., Rees Smith, B., and Hall, R.: Thyroid autoantibody synthesis by Hashimoto thyroid lymphocytes. Lancet, 1:162, 1979.
22. Mizukami, Y., Michigishi, T., Kawato, M., and Matsubara, F.: Immunohistochemical and ultrastructural study of subacute thyroiditis, with special reference to multinucleated giant cells. Hum. Pathol., 18:929, 1987.
23. Mulhern, L., M., Masi, A. T., and Shulman, L. E.: Hashimoto's disease: A search for associated disorders in 170 clinically detected cases. Lancet, 2:508, 1966.
24. Nikolai, T. F., Brosseau, J., Kettrick, M. A., et al.: Lymphocytic thyroiditis with spontaneously resolving hyperthyroidism (silent thyroiditis). Arch. Intern. Med., 140:478, 1980.
25. Okita, N., Kidd, A., Row, V. V., and Volpe, R.: Sensitization of T-lymphocytes in Graves' and Hashimoto's disease. J. Clin. Endocrinol. Metab., 51:316, 1980.
26. Papapertrou, P. D., and Jackson, L. M. D.: Thyrotoxicosis due to "silent" thyroiditis. Lancet, 1:361, 1975.
27. Rudman, L., Novota, O. J., and Keener, R. L.: Complications of Hashimoto thyroiditis surgery. Arch. Surg., 83:822, 1961.
28. Sakiyama, R.: Thyroiditis: A clinical review. Am. Family Physician, 48(4):615, 1993.
29. Schubert, M. F., and Kountz, D. S.: Thyroiditis: A disease with many faces. Postgrad. Med., 98(2):101, 1995.
30. Tunbridge, W. M. G., Evered, D. C., Hall, R., et al.: The spectrum of thyroid disease in a community: The Whickham survey. Clin. Endocrinol., 7:481, 1977.
31. Tunbridge, W. M. G., Brewis, B. M., French, J. M., et al.: Natural history of autoimmune thyroiditis. Br. Med. J., 1:258, 1981.
32. Turner-Warwick, R., Nabarro, J. D. N., and Doniach, D.: Riedel's thyroiditis and retroperitoneal fibrosis. Proc. R. Soc. Med., 59:596, 1966.
33. Volpe, R., Row, V. V., and Ezrin, C.: Circulating viral and thyroid antibodies in subacute thyroiditis. J. Clin. Endocrinol. Metab., 27:1275, 1967.
34. Weetman, A. P., and McGregor, A. M.: Autoimmune thyroid disease: Developments in our understanding. Endocrinol. Rev., 5:309, 1984.
35. Woolf, P. D., and Daly, R.: Thyrotoxicosis with painless thyroiditis. Am. J. Med., 60:73, 1976.
36. Woolner, L. B., McConahey, W. M., and Beahrs, O. H.: Invasive fibrous thyroiditis. J. Clin. Endocrinol., 17:201, 1957.

IV

NODULAR GOITER AND BENIGN AND MALIGNANT NEOPLASMS OF THE THYROID

George S. Leight, Jr., M.D.

The normal thyroid gland is a homogenous structure that weighs about 20 gm. (Fig. 23–27). The commonly accepted definition of a goiter is a thyroid gland that is at least twice its normal size. Goiter can also be described as a diffuse enlargement of the thyroid gland (diffuse goiter) or enlargement by one or more nodules (nodular goiter), and it can be further classified as endemic, sporadic, or compensatory. The classification system for goiter of the American Thyroid Association is represented in Table 23–6.

NODULAR GOITER

Incidence. Worldwide, nodular goiter remains a problem of enormous magnitude, although exact data on incidence are unavailable. The World Health Organization estimated in 1958 that goiter was present in 200 million persons, which represented 7% of the world's population at that time.[13] *Endemic goiter* refers to a situation in which more than 10% of the local population have goiter, usually because of low iodine intake. In some endemic goiter areas, the incidence of goiter may exceed 85%. Marine, in 1917, popularized the use of iodized salt in North America to prevent endemic goiter.[14] The incidence rates of goiter throughout the United States have diminished sharply as adequate dietary iodine has become available in all geographic areas. Comprehensive population surveys have demonstrated that the prevalence of palpable thyroid nodules in the adult U.S. population is approximately 4%. In the Framingham study, there was an overall 4.2% incidence of nodular thyroid disease, and the incidence was higher in women (6.4%) than in men (1.5%).[28] Nodular thyroid disease, however, is more prevalent than these studies would suggest, as demonstrated by autopsy surveys that have documented an even higher incidence of nodular goiter. In a thorough autopsy study of 821 patients whose thyroid glands had been considered normal clinically, 50% were found to have nodules with 75% of the glands multinodular, and 25% containing single nodules.[17] Ultrasonographic studies of the thyroid have revealed nodules in as high as 50% of the population older than 50 years of age.[11]

Etiology. The mechanisms by which the normal homogenous thyroid gland changes to become the enlarged nodular structure characteristic of multinodular goiter have been difficult to characterize. Nodular enlargement of the thyroid gland results from excessive replication of thyroid epithelial cells that form new follicles with variable morphology and function. In endemic goiter, the usual mechanism is a deficiency in production of thyroid hormone because of a deficiency of iodine in the diet. This leads to increased thyroid-stimulating hormone (TSH) secretion, which accelerates the goitrogenic process. In iodine-replete areas, many goitrogenic

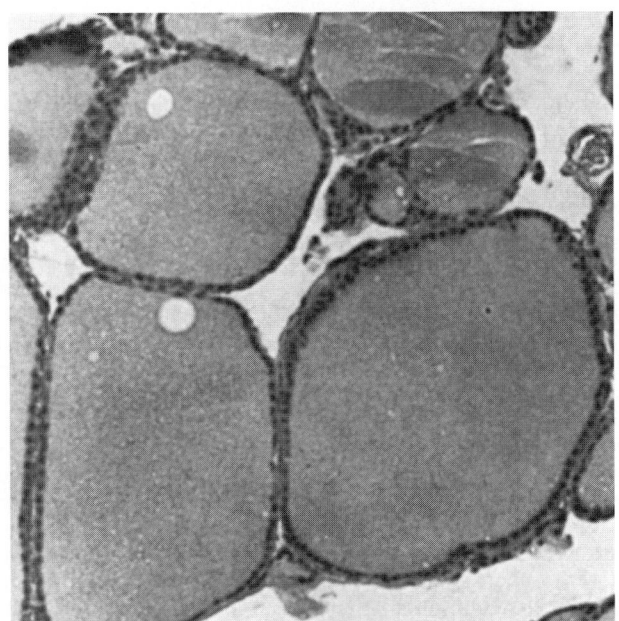

Figure 23–27. Photomicrograph of normal thyroid showing follicles of uniform size replete with colloid. Hematoxylin and eosin, ×100. (From LiVolsi, V. A. [Ed.]: Surgical Pathology of the Thyroid. Philadelphia, W. B. Saunders, 1990.)

agents may play a role in the etiology of nodular goiter, including dietary goitrogens, medications, malnutrition, inherited defects in thyroid hormone synthesis, ionizing radiation, and growth-stimulating antibodies. Most of these agents interfere with thyroid hormone synthesis, causing goiter formation by increasing TSH production. However, growth-stimulating antibodies can cause thyroid growth in the absence of TSH, as happens in Graves' disease, in which thyroid-stimulating antibodies are the goitrogenic agents. In many patients, similar growth-stimulating antibodies may be present in lower concentrations, acting as cofactors that stimulate intrinsic goitrogenic mechanisms, just as TSH does.[23]

The mechanisms by which TSH and other growth factors produce nodular goiter have been described by Studer and colleagues.[24] Most mature thyroid follicular cells are capable of entering the mitotic cycle, although the rate at which replication occurs varies widely from cell to cell. Cells with a high growth propensity also respond more vigorously to growth factors such as TSH. Over an extended period, these

growth factors tend to amplify the heterogeneous growth potential of various cell populations, promoting the appearance of nodular areas within the thyroid. Within a growing nodule with its many different populations of cells, the production of new follicular cells, the fundamental process of goitrogenesis, occurs in numerous areas throughout the growing tissue. The newly generated follicular cells contribute to nodular growth by forming new follicles or by enlarging existing follicles. The growth of these cellular cohorts occurs in successive bursts, with intervening quiescent intervals. The molecular events that cause some cells to replicate more often than others remain unknown. Whether this may be regulated by growth-controlling genes is currently under investigation.

Secondary events also play a role in the formation of nodular goiters. Necrosis of single follicles or entire areas of new follicles may occur as a consequence of an inadequate blood supply to these developing areas. This results in fibrous scars throughout the thyroid that form an inflexible network, producing a nodular growth pattern.

Pathology. The thyroid gland in patients with multinodular goiter may be slightly to massively enlarged and has a characteristic nodular external surface (Fig. 23–28). Cut section shows multiple nodules that vary in size and consistency from solid follicular lesions to colloid-rich nodules or degenerative cystic structures. Variable amounts of normal thyroid tissue, fibrous tissue, and calcification are seen interspersed among the nodules. Areas of hemorrhage and cysts are also often seen. Microscopically, one sees normal to hyperplastic foci of thyroid tissue, large areas of colloid, hemorrhage, fibrosis, and calcification. Variable amounts of lymphocytic infiltrate can also be seen.

Natural History. Diffuse and nodular sporadic goiters represent different stages of a single thyroid disease. Although a goiter may appear to be diffuse by palpation, histologic or autoradiographic studies usually reveal its micronodular structure. In an adult population presenting with goiter, 90% will be found to have nodular goiter.[2] The prevalence of sporadic nodular goiter increases from 1% in patients younger than 20 years of age to about 5% in patients older than 60 years of age.[21] The peak incidence of endemic goiter occurs between 10 and 50 years of age and decreases thereaf-

---

TABLE 23–6. Classification of Nontoxic Goiter

Nontoxic Diffuse Goiter

Endemic
   Iodine deficiency
   Iodine excess
   Dietary goitrogens
Sporadic
   Congenital defect in thyroid hormone biosynthesis
   Chemical agents (e.g., lithium, thiocyanate, p-aminosalicylic acid)
   Iodine deficiency
Compensatory following subtotal thyroidectomy

Nontoxic Nodular Goiter Due to Above

Uninodular or multinodular
Functional, nonfunctional, or both

From Burrow, G. N.: Nontoxic goiter—diffuse and nodular. *In* Burrow, G. N., Oppenheimer, J. H., and Volpe, R. (Eds.): Thyroid Function and Disease. Philadelphia, W. B. Saunders, 1989.

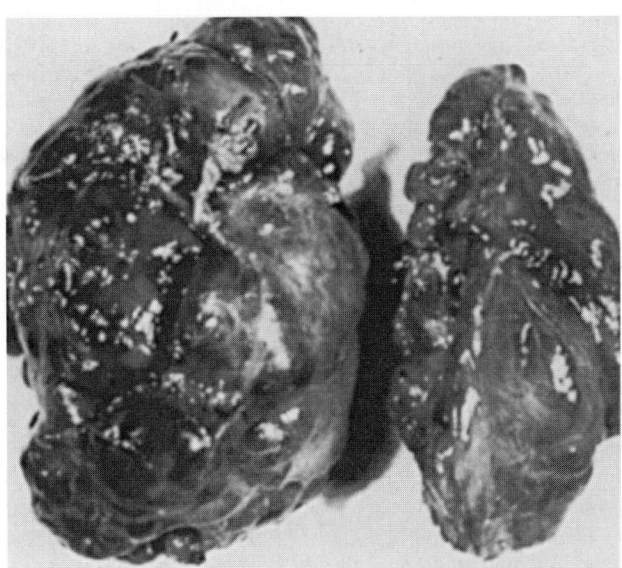

Figure 23–28. Multinodular goiter demonstrating asymmetric size of the two lobes and multiple nodules. (From LiVolsi, V. A. [Ed.]: Surgical Pathology of the Thyroid. Philadelphia, W. B. Saunders, 1990.)

ter. A high incidence of childhood goiter in an area correlates with an increased likelihood that the goiter will persist into adult life with the eventual appearance of nodularity. In all age groups, there is a threefold to sixfold higher incidence of thyroid dysfunction and goiter in women as compared with men. The pattern of growth of nodular goiter is unpredictable, ranging from slow, steady growth extending over decades to rapid growth of one or more nodules within a multinodular goiter.

With continued growth, nodular goiters come to clinical attention for a variety of reasons. Outside of endemic goiter areas, nodular goiter is usually found during routine physical examination or is noticed by the patient as a neck mass. Patients are usually unaware of nodules smaller than 2 cm., although rapid growth or hemorrhage into the nodule that produces pain may bring the nodule to attention. Even though large multinodular goiters rarely cause symptoms, the enlarging goiter can cause compression of neck structures such as the trachea and esophagus, resulting in dysphagia, cough, respiratory compromise, or a feeling of fullness in the neck. Symptoms related to compression are more common with goiters located substernally because of the limited space for expansion and the proximity of critical structures. Radiographs may show deviation and occasionally compression of the trachea by the enlarging goiter. This can be documented more precisely by computed tomographic (CT) scan of the neck structures. Peak inspiratory and expiratory flow rates can be used to document the diminished flow rates diagnostic of upper airway obstruction. This is a situation that should be viewed with concern because further airway compromise from a foreign body or tracheitis with edema could quickly produce a respiratory emergency or arrest. Other clinical problems presented by a goiter include hypothyroidism or the emergence of autonomous hyperfunctioning nodules with accompanying hyperthyroidism. Thyrotoxicosis may be difficult to recognize in the elderly, and periodic laboratory studies of thyroid function are mandatory in these patients.

The risk of underlying malignancy must also be considered in patients with nodular goiter. The presence of a multinodular goiter is usually considered to be associated with a low risk of malignancy of approximately 0.5%; the reports that indicate a 4% to 17% incidence of carcinoma in surgically treated multinodular goiters are believed to be the result of selection of these patients.[3] If there is a nodule within a multinodular gland that appears different from the other nodules or has undergone recent change or growth, the possibility of malignancy must be considered. Although fine-needle aspiration biopsy (FNAB) has been most useful in the management of single thyroid nodules, it can also be used effectively in the evaluation of specific nodules within a multinodular gland.

Treatment. In geographic areas where the soil has a low iodine content, people may not ingest more than the 50 mg. of iodine required to replace the iodine excreted in the urine. Although dietary goitrogens and genetic factors may contribute to endemic goiter formation, iodine deficiency represents the major cause of endemic goiter worldwide. In most developed countries, adequate amounts of dietary iodine are provided by the addition of iodine to salt or its use as a preservative in bread. Iodination of the water supply is effective if the entire population uses a particular water supply. In less-developed areas an injectable form of iodized oil provides goiter prophylaxis for as long as 3 years. Iodine is more effective in preventing the development of goiter than in causing actual regression of an established goiter. Early diffuse goiters may undergo involution, but an established multinodular goiter, with its areas of fibrosis and scarring, is unlikely to diminish in size. A possible complication of iodine therapy in these patients is thyrotoxicosis, although this is generally transient and self-limited.

Treatment of sporadic goiter by TSH-suppressing doses of thyroid hormone remains a controversial issue. Thyroid hormone administration may decrease the size of the goiter or block further increase in its size. Without such therapy, prolonged TSH stimulation of the thyroid gland makes it likely that the goiter will progress. Patients receiving replacement therapy with thyroxine T_4 must be monitored carefully because autonomous areas of the goiter may not be suppressible and the addition of exogenous hormone to that produced endogenously may result in thyrotoxicosis. In patients with nodular goiter caused by dyshormonogenesis or reduced thyroid hormone action, T_4 supplementation is indicated and may be used to avoid operation. If the goiter remains stable and the patient is asymptomatic, management can be continued in this manner; however, long-term medical treatment for nodular thyroid disease is not considered as acceptable by some authors.[18]

Surgical treatment for multinodular goiter becomes necessary when compressive symptoms begin to develop. The most common symptoms result from tracheal compression. Once these symptoms occur, it is extremely unlikely that medical therapy will produce a favorable result, and 18% of untreated patients eventually present with acute respiratory distress.[20] Prolonged airway compression may also result in tracheomalacia. The goal of surgical therapy is to remove all the abnormal nodular thyroid tissue, because all nodules potentially contain autonomously growing cells with the potential to cause recurrence of the goiter. Nodules that grow in spite of adequate T_4 therapy are autonomous and are associated with a higher incidence of malignancy. Needle biopsy should be performed in this situation, and when cytology indicates malignancy, surgical treatment should be employed. Cosmetic problems, recurrent laryngeal nerve paresis, and toxic nodules in a large multinodular goiter are also indications for surgical management. In patients with recurrent goiter or in those not considered to be good surgical candidates because of age or coexisting illness, radioiodine treatment may be a useful alternative to reduce goiter volume. This would be beneficial only in those situations where the symptomatic elements of the goiter consist of functionally active thyroid tissue with sufficient radioiodine uptake. In selected cases, this treatment may improve respiratory obstructive symptoms and dysphagia.

Substernal Goiter

Downward growth of the enlarged thyroid through the thoracic inlet into the mediastinum causes substernal goiter in 0.2% to 21% of patients with cervical goiter. The intrathoracic extension is located in the anterior mediastinum in approximately 75% to 90% of patients; the remainder descend into the posterior mediastinum.[5] In most cases substernal goiter is part of a cervical goiter, although isolated retrosternal goiters have been described.

The same complications that can occur in cervical goiters, such as thyrotoxicosis and malignancy, can also occur in substernal goiters. The potential for significant tracheal deviation or obstruction is perhaps greater with substernal goiter because of the limited space for expansion of the goiter. Obstruction of the superior vena cava with resulting dilated cervical and facial veins is a complication limited to substernal goiter. Some patients present with an asymptomatic mediastinal mass seen on a chest radiograph.

Because substernal goiter almost never regresses with thyroid hormone treatment and because tracheal compression can lead to serious respiratory embarrassment, resection of intrathoracic goiter is indicated unless significant medical contraindications are present. Progressive enlargement usually occurs, and resection becomes more difficult with time. In patients who have not had prior thyroid or mediastinal operations, most substernal goiters can be removed through a standard cervical incision. This approach facilitates control of the thyroid blood supply, allows identification of the recurrent laryngeal nerve and parathyroid glands, and permits resection of the cervical goiter. The arterial supply is controlled by ligation of the inferior and superior thyroid arteries on the affected side prior to blunt dissection of the goiter from the mediastinal structures (Fig. 23–29). The gland is delivered through the thoracic inlet into the cervical incision. When substernal goiters obstruct venous return, significant venous bleeding may occur until the goiter is mobilized out of the mediastinum, relieving the venous obstruction and bleeding. The recurrent laryngeal nerve is usually displaced posteriorly by the goiter, but if it can be identified before delivery of the goiter into the cervical incision, it should be carefully protected during this process. In some instances when the size of the goiter prevents delivery through the thoracic inlet, the capsule of the goiter can be opened, with removal of colloid and seminecrotic material allowing delivery into the neck. Median sternotomy is rarely necessary to remove an anterior substernal goiter. For posterior mediastinal goiter, initial cervical exploration with an attempt to mobilize and deliver the goiter is indicated. The patient should be positioned for simultaneous thoracotomy, should a combined approach be necessary, to accomplish safe and adequate mobilization of the goiter.[21]

BENIGN NEOPLASMS

Thyroid adenomas are benign neoplasms arising from follicular tissue. Histologically, these lesions can be classified as

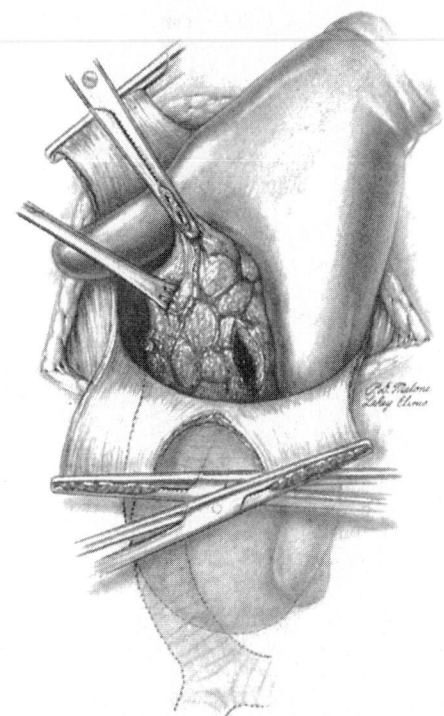

Figure 23–29. Removal of substernal goiter through a cervical incision. The gland is freed from the mediastinal structures by careful blunt dissection before its delivery through the thoracic inlet. Occasionally it may be necessary to enter the thyroid capsule and remove enough tissue to decompress the gland so that it will pass through the thoracic inlet and into the operative field. (From Sedgwick, C. E.: Surgery of the thyroid gland. *In* Sedgwick, C. E., and Cady, B. [Eds.]: Surgery of the Thyroid and Parathyroid Glands. Philadelphia, W. B. Saunders, 1980.)

TABLE 23–7. Benign Neoplasms of the Thyroid

Adenoma
   Follicular
      Colloid variant
      Embryonal
      Fetal
      Hürthle cell variant
   Papillary
   Atypical
Teratoma

the more common follicular adenoma and the rare papillary adenomas and teratomas (Table 23–7). Most papillary tumors are considered malignant, and the diagnosis of papillary adenoma should be made with great caution. Thyroid adenomas are usually considered distinct etiologically from the multiple adenomas that occur in multinodular goiter. Recently, it has been suggested that true adenomas may be the product of clones of follicular cells with high individual growth rates.[5]

Follicular adenomas are well circumscribed, solitary, homogenous lesions that are usually surrounded by a capsule separating them from the adjacent normal thyroid tissue (Fig. 23–30). Follicular adenomas are subdivided according to their architecture, cellularity, and amount of colloid into fetal (microfollicular), colloid (macrofollicular), embryonal (trabecular), and Hürthle (oxyphil) cell types. Colloid adenomas are similar histologically to the multiple nodules found in multinodular goiter. Microscopically, these lesions have large colloid-filled follicles within an incomplete capsule (Fig. 23–31). These are classified by some pathologists as colloid nodules, suggesting a focal process that is different from the development of a true adenoma.

Fetal adenoma is composed entirely of small follicles, whereas embryonal adenomas are composed of cells arranged in solid cords (Fig. 23–32). The individual cells in these lesions resemble those in normal thyroid tissue. Hürthle cell lesions contain cells that are markedly eosinophilic and whose cytoplasm contains abundant mitochondria when examined by electron microscopy (see Fig. 23–31). Some pathologists prefer the term *Hürthle cell tumor* because of the difficulty in establishing malignant potential of these lesions using histologic criteria.

Some pathologists classify all papillary lesions as malignant, although others consider selected papillary tumors to

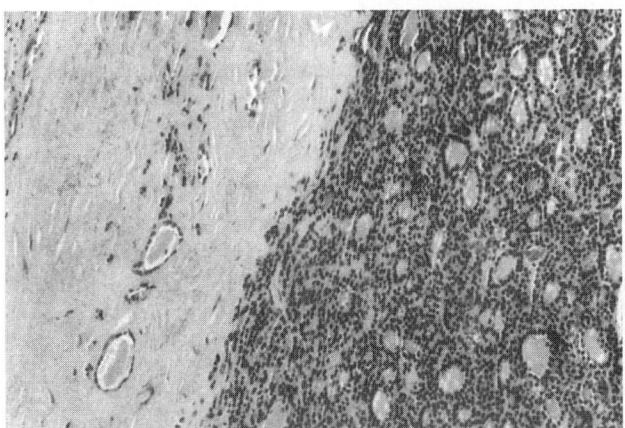

Figure 23–30. Photomicrograph of follicular adenoma with intact capsule and no evidence of invasion. Follicles in the capsule are considered to be trapped rather than representing invasion. ×100. (From LiVolsi, V.A. [Ed.]: Surgical Pathology of the Thyroid. Philadelphia, W. B. Saunders, 1990.)

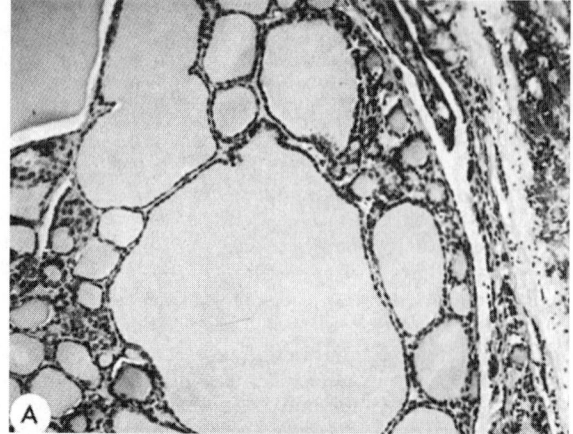

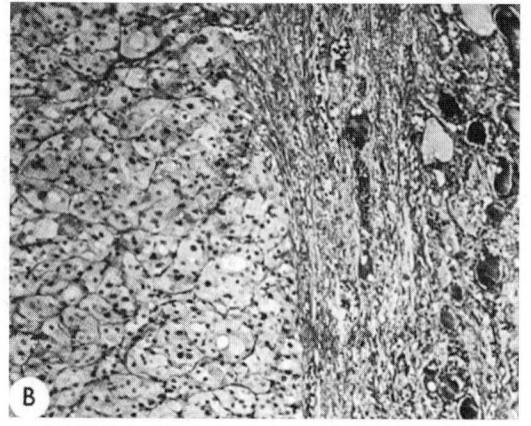

Figure 23–31. *A,* Colloid nodule demonstrating large follicles and minimal capsule. *B,* Hürthle cell adenoma. (From DeGroot, L. J., Larsen, P. R., Refetoff, S., and Stanbury, J. B.: The Thyroid and Its Diseases. New York, John Wiley and Sons, 1984.)

be benign adenomas. Teratomas of the thyroid are rare, and, although most are benign, malignant teratomas may also occur.

Clinical Features. Adenomas usually grow slowly, remain undetected for years, and are typically asymptomatic. They are usually discovered incidentally by the patient or the physician; rarely, they may present with local compressive symptoms or pain. Adenomas may undergo hemorrhagic necrosis, calcification, or cystic degeneration. Hemorrhage into the adenoma may cause pain, tenderness, and an increase in size, all of which draw attention to the nodule.

Approximately 70% of adenomas do not accumulate radioactive iodine and are thus *cold* on scan; 20% demonstrate uptake roughly equivalent to the remaining normal thyroid tissue and are therefore designated *warm.* Five per cent to 10% of adenomas are hyperfunctional and may produce thyrotoxicosis, particularly when the lesion exceeds 3 cm. in diameter.

Adenomas occasionally develop microinvasion, which is an indication of malignant degeneration. Colloid adenomas have no potential for microinvasion, but the cellular adenomas, including those of microfollicular, Hürthle cell, and embryonal types, demonstrate the potential for microinvasion. Approximately 5% of microfollicular and Hürthle cell tumors show capsular or vascular invasion, which is considered to be a definite indication of malignancy. The only method for differentiating these benign lesions from malignant ones is careful study of multiple tissue sections for evidence of capsular or vascular invasion.

Treatment. The most important factor in the management

of most thyroid adenomas is their differentiation from malignant thyroid lesions (see the following discussion on management of thyroid nodules). Once it can be established by aspiration cytology or other biopsy techniques that a nodule is a benign adenoma, the patient is usually followed closely. In the past, most of these patients have been placed on thyroid hormone suppressive therapy, but this has remained controversial, with recent studies showing that suppressive therapy has no significant effect on nodule size.[8] Adenomas that continue to enlarge progressively, cause compressive symptoms, or lead to thyrotoxicosis should be considered for surgical resection.

Management of Thyroid Nodules

Palpable thyroid nodules are common, with an incidence in the adult population of the United States of 4% to 7%. When detection is based on ultrasonographic or autopsy series of asymptomatic adults, the prevalence of thyroid nodules is 30% to 50%.[3, 17] A solitary thyroid nodule is described as a clinically discrete nodule in a normal size or a diffusely enlarged gland. A dominant nodule is a large nodule in a thyroid with other smaller nodules; multiple palpable nodules of similar size and consistency are designated as *multinodular goiter.* This classification based on physical examination underestimates the incidence of multiple nodules, which are found by histologic examination in two thirds of patients with thyroid malignancy. A solitary nodule (4.7%) or a dominant nodule in a multinodular gland (4.1%) has a higher risk of being malignant than the multiple palpable nodules of a

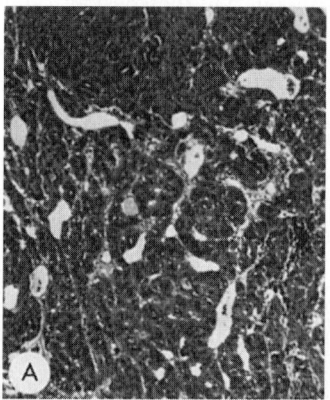

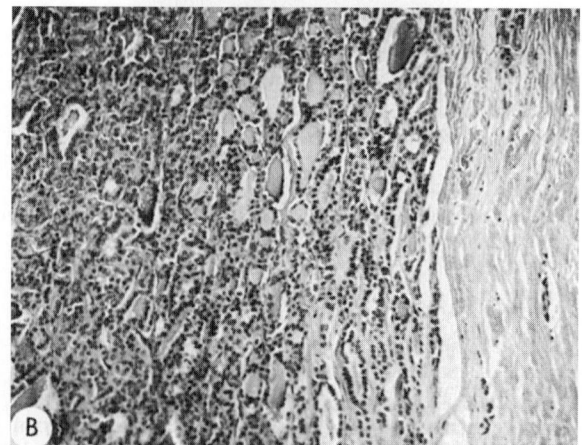

Figure 23–32. *A,* Embryonal adenoma showing cells arranged in solid cords. *B,* Fetal adenoma composed entirely of small follicles. (From DeGroot, L. J., Larsen P. R., Refetoff, S., and Stanbury, J. B.: The Thyroid and Its Diseases. New York, John Wiley and Sons, 1984.)

multinodular gland (1%).[8] The challenge to the clinician is to select from this large group of patients with thyroid nodules the 5% of patients whose nodules harbor thyroid cancer.[7]

A wide range of thyroid problems can present as a thyroid nodule (Table 23–8). Evaluation begins with a careful history and physical examination that may provide important information about the risk of malignancy. Age is a significant factor because thyroid nodules occurring in children or in the elderly are more likely to be malignant. Thyroid nodules are more common in women, but when they occur in men they are more likely to be malignant. If a patient has a family history of medullary or papillary thyroid carcinoma, it increases the likelihood that the thyroid nodule in this patient is malignant. A history of exposure of the thyroid to low-dose therapeutic radiation increases the risk of the development of thyroid carcinoma.

Historical information concerning the pattern of growth of the nodule may be important. A stable nodule that has existed for many years suggests a benign process, although a slowly growing malignancy cannot be excluded. A rapid progressive pattern of growth raises the level of concern about malignancy; very sudden enlargement in hours or days and frequently accompanied by pain is more likely associated with hemorrhage into a benign tumor or cyst. Dyspnea, dysphagia, vocal cord paralysis, or Horner's syndrome may indicate local tissue invasion from a thyroid malignancy, although large benign lesions can also cause these problems.

Physical examination characteristics of a nodule that suggest malignancy include a firm texture, irregularity, fixation to surrounding structures, and enlarged ipsilateral cervical lymph nodes. The presence of clinically positive lymph nodes is the most reliable physical examination indicator of malignancy because all the other findings can be associated with benign lesions. Consistency of the nodule is of limited diagnostic importance, because calcification of a benign adenoma may cause it to be quite hard, whereas soft nodules may occasionally be malignant. The most important function of physical examination, however, is the detection of the thyroid nodule rather than the determination of its benign or malignant status.

Noninvasive Evaluation. Studies of thyroid function are of little value in establishing the benign or malignant nature of a thyroid nodule. Thyroid function is usually normal in patients with thyroid carcinoma. Serum TSH level is usually the only biochemical test that may be needed in patients who have no clinical manifestations of hyperthyroidism or hypothyroidism. Serum calcitonin determination should be sought only when medullary thyroid carcinoma is suspected.[15]

Although not an essential element in the evaluation of thyroid nodules, ultrasonographic study of the thyroid may be useful in several specific situations. Ultrasonography permits the classification of a nodule as solid, cystic, or mixed solid and cystic. High-resolution ultrasonography can detect lesions as small as 1 mm. and can demonstrate multiple small nodules in as many as 40% of patients with clinically solitary nodules.[22] Although ultrasonography demonstrates high sensitivity for detection of thyroid nodules, there are no specific ultrasonographic criteria that are pathognomonic for malignancy. Benign nodules are frequently isoechoic, well defined, and homogeneous, whereas malignant lesions are more likely to be hypoechoic with a cystic component or calcification.[29] Ultrasonography is perhaps most useful for screening high-risk patients, assessing change in size of thyroid nodules in patients receiving thyroid-suppressive therapy, and characterizing anatomically a palpable nodule remaining after cyst aspiration.

Thyroid scintiscans have been the most widely used screening procedure in the evaluation of thyroid nodules since it was determined more than 45 years ago that thyroid carcinomas concentrated less radioactive iodine than did normal thyroid tissue. The most commonly used isotopes are radioiodine (^{123}I and ^{131}I), and technetium-99m pertechnetate. Uptake of technetium results from its trapping by thyroid follicular cells, whereas radioiodine uptake is a more sophisticated function, requiring both trapping and organification. Thyroid nodules are classified as cold (hypofunctional), warm (normally functional), or hot (hyperfunctional). Because malignant thyroid nodules usually do not organify iodine, hypofunctional nodules are more likely to be malignant than functioning nodules, and hyperfunctional nodules are rarely found to be malignant. The main limitation of radionuclide scanning is that it does not clearly differentiate benign from malignant lesions. In a large review of more than 5000 patients, nodules were classified as cold in 84%, warm in 10.5%, and hot in 5.5%.[1] Carcinomas were found in 16% of cold nodules, 9% of warm nodules, and 4% of hot nodules. Thus, when the scan showed a cold nodule, this test alone had a sensitivity of 87% and a specificity of 30%. For these reasons, most studies have shown that it is not cost effective to scan all patients with thyroid nodules. The most prevalent strategy is to limit the use of scans to those patients whose needle aspiration cytologic study suggests a follicular neoplasm. When such lesions are cold on scan, thyroid lobectomy is usually advised.

Thyroid hormone suppression has been used as a therapeutic and diagnostic tool for nodules thought to be benign by clinical criteria. Exogenous thyroid hormone suppresses the release of TSH and thus decreases the growth stimulation of normal and neoplastic thyroid cells. The rationale has been that benign nodules are more likely to be dependent on TSH for maintaining growth than are malignant nodules, which would continue their pattern of autonomous growth. Although many trials have examined the usefulness of this approach, the interpretation of results has been limited by imprecise and subjective criteria for response and adequacy of suppression. In addition, well-differentiated thyroid carcinomas may respond occasionally to suppressive therapy. In a randomized, prospective trial of suppressive therapy for benign thyroid nodules, more nodules in the thyroxine-treated patients decreased in size, although some nodules in patients receiving placebo also decreased in size, so that no significant difference was found.[9] In a review of 10 series consisting of more than 600 patients treated with thyroid

TABLE 23–8. Differential Diagnosis of a Solitary Thyroid Nodule

Cyst
    Simple cyst
    Mixed cystic-solid (complete)
Thyroid adenoma
    Autonomously functioning (hot)
    Nonfunctional or hypofunctional
Colloid nodule
Thyroiditis
Infection
    Granulomatous disease
    Abscess
Developmental abnormalities
    Unilateral lobe agenesis
    Cystic hygroma
    Dermoid
    Teratoma
Carcinoma
    Primary thyroid
    Metastatic to thyroid
Thyroid lymphoma

hormone suppression, the sensitivity of the suppressive therapy test was 83% with a specificity of 33% when defining a positive result as no change or growth of the nodule. When the nodule grew during suppressive therapy, the specificity of this test was 96%, although sensitivity decreased to 33%.[27] In patients followed on thyroid hormone suppressive therapy for nodules believed to be benign by biopsy and other clinical criteria, growth of the nodule is a strong indication for thyroidectomy.

Needle Biopsy. Needle biopsy is accepted as the most precise diagnostic screening procedure for differentiating benign from malignant thyroid nodules (Fig. 23–33). Because it is safe, inexpensive, and accurate, needle aspiration biopsy is used routinely as the initial diagnostic technique in the management of thyroid nodules. Several different techniques for performing needle biopsy have been described. FNAB, using a 21- to 25-gauge needle, provides a specimen for cytologic study. Large-needle biopsy and cutting-needle biopsy provide tissue for histologic study. The FNAB procedure has emerged as the most widely used technique, because it provides reliable information, has few complications, and is well tolerated by patients. The important factors for a satisfactory test include a representative specimen from the nodule and an experienced cytologist to interpret the findings. An unsatisfactory specimen occurs in 7% to 18% of patients in reported series; when repeated, 50% of these aspirates are diagnostic.[15] Sampling errors occur more frequently with lesions larger than 4 cm., lesions smaller than 1 cm., hemorrhagic nodules, or multinodular glands. These problems can be minimized by making multiple passes into the nodule or by using ultrasound-guided FNAB.

Results of FNAB are classified cytologically as benign (75%), suspicious or indeterminate (20%), and malignant (5%).[7] In a review of eight series consisting of 13,071 patients who underwent FNAB and operation, thyroid carcinoma was found in 22 of 848 patients with benign cytologic findings, a false-negative rate of 2.6%. In 484 patients with suspicious or malignant cytologic findings, 246 carcinomas were found, with seven false positive results.[1] Analysis of additional series demonstrated a false-negative rate of 2.4% and a false-positive rate of 3.3%. Sensitivity of FNAB was calculated to be 92% with a specificity of 74%. When patients were selected for operation based on suspicious or malignant cytology, the yield of cancer at thyroidectomy was 45%, with only 2.5% missed carcinomas.[27]

In the group of FNAB specimens interpreted as indeterminate or suspicious, most are found to be follicular or Hürthle cell neoplasms. The diagnosis of follicular or Hürthle cell carcinoma requires the histologic identification of invasion of the capsule or vascular structures. An FNAB specimen from such a lesion cannot provide the information about capsular or vascular invasion necessary to make the diagnosis of malignancy. When cytology is suggestive of a follicular or Hürthle cell neoplasm and the lesion is cold by scan, surgical resection is indicated. Approximately 20% of these lesions are found to be malignant.[7]

Although FNAB is the best method available for diagnosing thyroid carcinoma, false-negative diagnoses do occur. It is therefore mandatory that patients with an initial benign FNAB have adequate followup, with repeat periodic aspiration for those with persistent thyroid nodularity. Benign lesions continue to show consistently benign cytology; once identified, cytologically suspicious or indeterminate lesions should be removed surgically. Despite these limitations, the use of FNAB has reduced the number of patients requiring surgery while increasing the yield of malignancy in excised nodules.

Another advantage of FNAB is the therapeutic aspiration of thyroid cysts. Most simple cysts are benign, and aspiration alone is adequate treatment in 70% of cases.[4] Cyst fluid should be subjected to cytologic examination. Cysts that recur after repeated aspirations, or those with suspicious cytology, should be surgically removed. Complex cysts containing both cystic and solid components have a higher risk of malignancy. When a complex cyst is encountered, the solid component should be aspirated after the cystic fluid has been removed. A diagnostic approach for management of thyroid nodules based on FNAB is shown in Figure 23–34.[12]

THYROID CARCINOMA

Thyroid carcinomas are a heterogeneous group of tumors that show considerable variability in biologic behavior, histologic appearance, and response to therapy (Table 23–9). Although benign thyroid nodules are common, clinically detectable thyroid carcinoma is rare, representing approximately 1% of all malignancies. Thyroid carcinoma occurs with an incidence of 25 to 40 cases per million population per year. In the United States more than 11,000 patients per year are treated for carcinoma of the thyroid.[19] These tumors are rare in children and increase in frequency with increasing age; the female-to-male ratio is 2.5:1. The autopsy incidence of thyroid carcinoma in the United States has been reported to be in the range of 0.9% to 13%. It is likely that many thyroid carcinomas detected in these studies are not clinically significant and do not play a role in the clinical course of the patient. The annual mortality from thyroid carcinoma in the

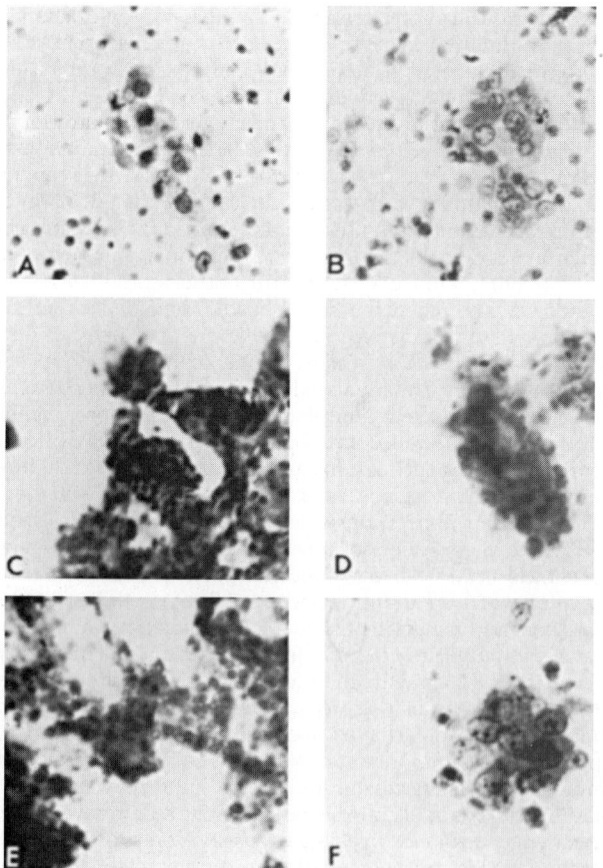

Figure 23–33. Cytologic patterns from fine-needle aspiration biopsy of thyroid nodules. *A,* Colloid nodule with benign-appearing thyroid epithelial cells and colloid. *B,* Hashimoto's thyroiditis with benign-appearing epithelial cells and lymphocytes. *C,* Follicular adenoma. *D,* Follicular carcinoma. *E,* Papillary carcinoma demonstrating papillary projections of malignant cells. *F,* Anaplastic carcinoma.

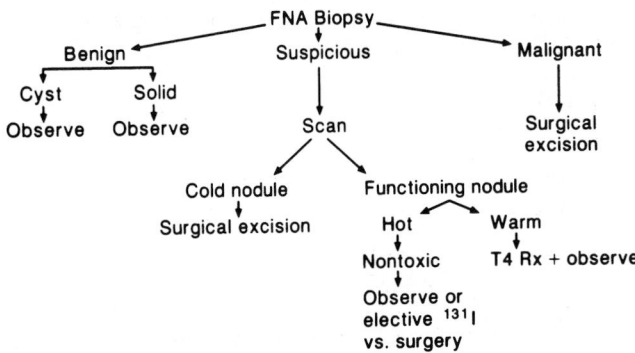

Figure 23–34. Management of thyroid nodule based on fine-needle aspiration biopsy as the initial diagnostic test. (From Gharib, H., and Goellner, J. R.: Evaluation of nodular thyroid disease. Endocrinol. Metab. Clin. North Am. *17*[3]:511, 1988.)

United States is only 6 per 1 million population, or approximately 1050 patients per year. This discrepancy between incidence and mortality rate presumably reflects the favorable prognosis for most thyroid carcinomas, although these tumors are capable of aggressive behavior, with metastatic disease and ultimately death.

Etiology. The cause of thyroid carcinoma has not been established, although recent advances in molecular genetics have improved understanding in this area. In papillary carcinoma, two dominantly acting fusion oncogenes have been identified on chromosomes 10q11-q12 and 1q32-q41. The *RET/D10S170* fusion gene is specific for papillary carcinoma and is believed to represent a primary event in the pathogenesis of this tumor. Activation of the *RET* oncogene has been observed in 19% of papillary thyroid carcinomas, and it is likely that other oncogenes are involved in the remaining cancers. In fact, increased expression of other oncogenes such as c-*myc*, c-*fos*, c-*ras*, and c-*erb* B2/*neu* has been reported in papillary thyroid carcinomas. The development of follicular thyroid carcinoma appears to involve multiple stages in which an activated *ras* gene mutation is involved in the progression from a normal follicular epithelial cell to a follicular adenoma. Inactivation of a tumor-suppressor gene on 3p then facilitates the progression of the follicular adenoma

TABLE 23–9. Malignant Thyroid Neoplasms

Well-Differentiated Neoplasms

Papillary adenocarcinoma
    Pure papillary
    Mixed papillary—follicular carcinoma
    Follicular variant of papillary carcinoma
    Encapsulated variant
Follicular adenocarcinoma
    Minimally invasive, encapsulated follicular carcinoma
    Widely invasive, angioinvasive follicular carcinoma
Hürthle cell carcinoma
Medullary carcinoma

Undifferentiated Neoplasms

Spindle and giant cell carcinoma
Small cell carcinoma

Miscellaneous Neoplasms

Lymphoma
Squamous cell carcinoma
Microepidermoid carcinoma
Teratoma
Sarcoma
Metastatic

to follicular carcinoma.[25] These advances may ultimately help establish the pathogenesis of these tumors.

The importance of irradiation as an etiologic factor in the development of thyroid carcinoma in humans is well documented. The major biologic effects on the thyroid are induction of neoplasia and loss of replicative ability. External irradiation therapy was widely used from the 1920s through the 1950s for various benign conditions of the head and neck region, predominantly in infants and children. Conditions such as enlarged thymus, tonsils, or adenoids as well as hemangiomas and acne, were frequently managed with external irradiation therapy. It was not until 1950 that Duffy and Fitzgerald reported an association between radiation therapy and thyroid carcinoma in children with a history of radiation exposure to the head and neck.[6] It is now known that approximately 30% of those exposed develop thyroid nodules, and approximately 30% of those nodules will be malignant. Radiation is more likely to cause neoplasia in children, and age at the time of radiation exposure is inversely correlated with risk; however, an increased risk for the development of thyroid carcinoma exists for patients as old as 50 years of age at the time of irradiation. Radiation-associated thyroid cancer usually begins to appear about 5 years after exposure, and the incidence peaks between 10 to 25 years following irradiation. Whether the increased risk persists for the entire lifetime of the irradiated subject or whether it decreases with time remains uncertain, although some studies suggest that the risk declines after 40 years. There is a linear increase in risk for both benign thyroid nodules and thyroid carcinoma with increasing radiation exposure from 0.07 to 15 Gy. of absorbed thyroid dose. The frequency of thyroid carcinoma decreases in patients after exposure to more than 20 Gy., but exposure of up to 60 Gy. is associated with a higher risk of thyroid carcinoma. At these higher dose levels the loss of replicative capacity is the dominant effect, and hypothyroidism frequently develops.[25]

The thyroid carcinomas seen in patients exposed to external irradiation are usually in the well-differentiated category, and most lesions are papillary carcinomas. A characteristic difference of the radiation-associated tumors is the presence of tumor multicentricity, which has been documented in 26% to 54% of patients. Despite this observation, the natural history of radiation-associated thyroid carcinoma is basically the same as in nonirradiated patients in the same age group.

The administration of ^{131}I for the treatment of hyperthyroidism has not been associated with a subsequent increase in risk of thyroid carcinoma. The usual dose of radiation to the thyroid gland in these patients is approximately 90 Gy., resulting in ablation of thyroid epithelium rather than potentiation of induction of neoplasia.[12]

Prognosis. The prognosis in most patients with well-differentiated thyroid carcinoma is quite favorable, although several factors that influence recurrence and survival have been identified. Some of these factors are related to the host (age and sex), some are intrinsic to the tumor (histologic type and grade), and others reflect the relationship between the host and the tumor (size, extent of invasion, local or distant metastases). The importance of identifying risk factors is to use the information to determine the extent of the operation required and to select appropriate postoperative therapy.

Several prognostic index systems have been devised in which multivariate analysis of the various prognostic factors is used to define groups of patients having different overall risks. Hay and colleagues developed the AGES prognostic scoring system based on patient *a*ge, tumor *g*rade, *e*xtent (local invasion and distant metastases), and *s*ize.[10] These factors were then weighted and combined to give a prognostic score. In 1500 patients who underwent surgical treatment for papillary thyroid carcinoma between 1945 and 1985, AGES criteria were used to separate the patients into four groups. Those with a score less than 3.99 had a 20-year mortality from papillary thyroid cancer of only 1%; mortality rates rose with increasing AGES scores to 20%, 67%, and 87% in the remaining groups. This system has subsequently been modified and designated MACIS, because it includes five variables abbreviated by *m*etastasis, *a*ge, *c*ompleteness of resection, *i*nvasion, and *s*ize (Table 23–10). Using this system the mortality rate after 20 years for patients with a total score of less than 6 is approximately 1%. When the score is greater than 8, overall mortality from tumor at 20 years was 76%. The AMES system was developed for follicular and papillary thyroid carcinoma based on *a*ge, distant *m*etastases, *e*xtent of primary tumor, and *s*ize.[3a] Age was the single most important variable, but additional information could be determined by the other factors. Other staging systems, including the tumor node, metastasis (TNM) system, the EORTC study, and the DeGroot classification, support the findings from Hay and Cady regarding the significance of prognostic factors for differentiated carcinoma of the thyroid gland. Approximately 85% to 90% of patients are in a low-risk category with a favorable prognosis.

Other prognostic indicators that may predict aggressive thyroid cancer behavior include deoxyribonucleic acid (DNA) ploidy, adenylate cyclase response to TSH stimulation, epidermal growth factor receptor status, multifocal tumors, and the presence of oncogenes and tumor-suppressor gene mutations.[12] Although DNA aneuploidy has been identified as an indicator of poor prognosis, the predictive value of DNA analysis is somewhat inconsistent in some series of patients. All these factors await further studies to define more precisely their importance in determining prognosis.

Strategies in Treatment

Papillary Carcinoma. Although the primary management of papillary thyroid carcinoma is surgical excision, the extent of resection and the indications for regional lymph node dissection remain controversial. In the absence of randomized, prospective studies, recommendations for therapy must be based on retrospective studies that have been conducted in an uncontrolled fashion. The controversy is also propagated by the observation that approximately 80% of these patients do well regardless of the extent of operation and that the more extensive thyroid resections carry a higher morbidity rate. There is consensus that the minimum operation for documented or suspected papillary carcinoma is a total lobectomy and isthmusectomy. Partial lobectomy or excision of the nodule itself is associated with a higher recurrence rate if lesion proves to be malignant. Because a benign diagnosis on frozen section may later be changed to malignant on permanent section, total lobectomy enables the surgeon to avoid reoperating on the side of a previous partial lobectomy, which can be technically difficult. For tumors of the isthmus, wedge resection with a 1 cm. margin of normal thyroid tissue is acceptable. In patients with a history of head and neck irradiation, total thyroidectomy should be performed because of the high incidence of multifocal neoplasms. Those patients undergoing thyroidectomy for Graves' disease or other benign conditions who are found to

have occult (<1 cm.) papillary carcinoma have an excellent prognosis and do not require more extensive operative procedures.

Surgical options include lobectomy, near-total thyroidectomy (ipsilateral total lobectomy and contralateral subtotal lobectomy), and total thyroidectomy. As the extent of thyroidectomy increases, the risk of complications such as recurrent nerve injury and hypoparathyroidism also increases. Because of this and the observation that prognosis is good with less aggressive procedures in patients categorized as low risk with tumors limited to one lobe, some experienced surgeons advocate lobectomy and isthmusectomy for these patients. Other surgeons recommend total thyroidectomy for all patients with papillary carcinomas greater than 1.5 cm. in diameter when this operation can be performed safely. Proponents of this approach offer several reasons to support total thyroidectomy as the preferred procedure.[12] Following total thyroidectomy radioactive iodine can be used to identify and treat local or distant metastases. Residual normal thyroid tissue has a much greater affinity for iodine than papillary carcinoma, thus limiting the effectiveness of ^{131}I when a large amount of normal thyroid tissue is not resected. Serum thyroglobulin level is more effective as a marker of recurrence when all normal thyroid tissue is removed. Patients undergoing lobectomy have a recurrence rate of 7% in the contralateral lobe and half of these patients die of thyroid cancer. The overall recurrence rate is lower in patients undergoing total thyroidectomy (11%) compared with subtotal resection (22%). This is a significant concern because approximately one half of patients with recurrent thyroid carcinoma eventually die of this disease.[12]

That total thyroidectomy can be performed by experienced surgeons with minimal morbidity has become accepted as this procedure has been refined and developed. In centers where total thyroidectomy is the procedure of choice, complication rates compare favorably with those for lobectomy or near-total thyroidectomy. In most current series the incidence of permanent hypoparathyroidism is approximately 1% to 2%, occurring primarily in patients with extensive lymph node involvement with metastatic tumor in the perithyroid area. Permanent recurrent laryngeal nerve injuries have been reported in fewer than 1% of patients. Whether these excellent results can be reproduced in the surgical community at large remains to be determined. The extent of thyroidectomy for papillary carcinoma should be determined by the individual surgeon based on training, experience, and the clinical findings, including risk factors, in the patient undergoing operation.

Patients with papillary thyroid carcinoma frequently have metastatic involvement of regional lymph nodes. Occult lymph node metastases have been reported in as many as 80% of patients undergoing prophylactic neck dissection for papillary thyroid carcinoma; however, the impact of nodal metastases on survival remains controversial. Some studies suggest that the presence of positive lymph nodes does not adversely affect survival. The possible explanation for these conclusions revolves around the age of the patient populations studied. Almost 80% of patients younger than 20 years of age have palpable nodal metastases, although their prognosis remains quite good because of their young age. In contrast, only 20% of older patients have clinically palpable nodes at presentation, but they have a less favorable prognosis as a function of age. Lymph node metastases at the time of presentation probably do increase the risk of recurrence in the neck but have only a minor detrimental effect on survival.[12]

When total thyroidectomy is performed for papillary thyroid carcinoma, the central neck nodes, including those in the ipsilateral tracheoesophageal groove, pretracheal area,

TABLE 23–10. Prognostic Index for Papillary Carcinoma

MACIS Score	Local or Distant Metastases at 10 Years (%)	PTC Mortality at 20 Years (%)
<6	3	1
6–6.9	18	13
7–7.9	40	45
8 +	60	76

along the recurrent laryngeal nerve and inferior thyroid veins, and in the anterior mediastinum, are removed with the operative specimen. Prophylactic lymph node dissection of nonpalpable nodes lateral to the carotid sheath is not recommended by most authors. In patients with palpably enlarged lateral cervical nodes, most surgeons believe that their removal by modified radical neck dissection is indicated. The procedure includes resection of the entire jugular chain of nodes and the spinal accessory nodes with preservation of the sternocleidomastoid muscle, jugular vein, and spinal accessory nerve unless they are directly invaded by tumor. A suprahyoid dissection is usually not necessary because nodes in this area rarely contain metastases. This procedure avoids the cosmetic and functional problems associated with standard radical neck dissection, and the results are equivalent to those achieved with the radical procedure.

Follicular Carcinoma. The incidence of follicular carcinoma has steadily decreased in the United States as the intake of dietary iodine has increased so that it now accounts for only 10% of new thyroid carcinomas. These tumors occur more in older patients than papillary carcinomas, with a peak incidence in the fifth decade of life. Follicular carcinoma usually presents as a solitary mass in the thyroid. This tumor has a marked propensity for vascular invasion but is less likely to invade lymphatic channels, and lymph node metastases are much less common than in papillary carcinoma. Follicular carcinoma frequently disseminates hematogenously, with bone, lung, liver, and the central nervous system as the most frequent sites of metastases. The incidence of distant metastases is as high as 33% although cervical lymph node involvement occurs in only 10% of patients. Factors that portend a less favorable prognosis include extensive angioinvasion, older patient age, and the presence of distant metastases. Pathologically, two types of follicular carcinoma are recognized and designated as the *low-grade encapsulated (microinvasive) follicular carcinoma* and the *high-grade angioinvasive* (macroinvasive) *follicular carcinoma.*

The microinvasive follicular carcinoma resembles a follicular adenoma with a well-defined capsule (Fig. 23–35); the diagnosis is based on the microscopic demonstration of invasion of the capsule, invasion through the capsule, or invasion into veins in or beyond the capsule. These lesions are rarely multicentric, rarely metastasize, and generally are associated with an excellent prognosis. Most patients being initially treated for follicular carcinoma have this minimally invasive type of tumor. The difficulty in managing these patients is

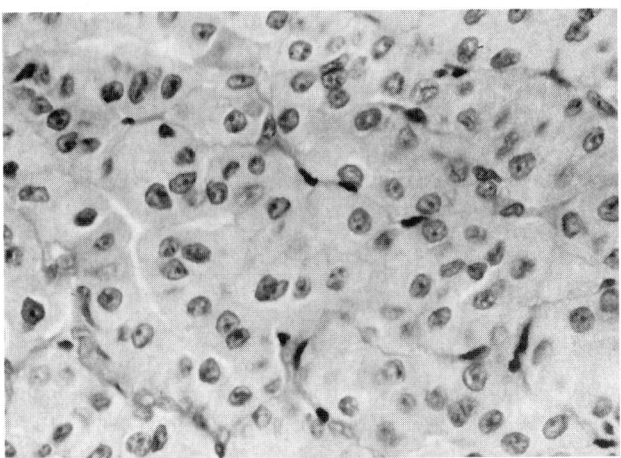

Figure 23–36. Hürthle cell tumor. Photomicrograph showing large polygonal cells with abundant granular cytoplasm and uniform nuclei. ×400. (Courtesy of Sudha R. Kini, M.D., from the book GUIDES TO CLINICAL ASPIRATION BIOPSY: THYROID, Igaku-Shoin Medical Publishers, New York, NY, 1987.)

that the diagnosis of microinvasive follicular carcinoma is usually made only after study of multiple permanent section slides following total lobectomy and isthmusectomy. Some experienced surgeons attempt to minimize this occurrence by performing total thyroidectomy in all patients with lesions larger than 4 cm., which are found to be follicular neoplasms by frozen-section analysis.[26] If an unequivocal diagnosis of follicular carcinoma can be made by frozen section at the time of operation, total thyroidectomy should be performed for lesions larger than 1 cm. Whether complete thyroidectomy should be done as a second-stage operation when permanent sections show microinvasive follicular carcinoma remains controversial. Some surgeons advocate complete thyroidectomy for tumors greater than 1 cm. with angioinvasion or more than minimal capsular invasion; others have elected to follow patients with smaller follicular carcinomas diagnosed only by microinvasion.[12]

High-grade angioinvasive follicular carcinomas are usually large and frequently show extension through the thyroid capsule into surrounding structures. This lesion is the most aggressive of the well-differentiated thyroid cancers, and those patients with high-risk follicular carcinoma have a 5-year survival of 47% and 20-year survival of 8%. Because of these factors, patients who present with locally aggressive tumors or who have proven metastatic disease are best treated with total thyroidectomy, which optimizes the effectiveness of ^{131}I treatment for metastatic disease.

Hürthle Cell Carcinoma. The Hürthle cell is derived from follicular epithelium and is characterized morphologically by its larger size and eosinophilic, granular cytoplasm produced by abundant mitochondria filling the cell. These cells are found in a nonencapsulated distribution in a variety of benign conditions, and this is believed to represent a metaplastic phenomenon with no malignant potential. True Hürthle cell neoplasms are solitary, encapsulated lesions composed of Hürthle cells in a follicular or solid pattern (Fig. 23–36). Despite similarities to follicular carcinoma, Hürthle cell carcinomas differ in that they rarely take up ^{131}I, are sometimes bilateral and multiple, and commonly metastasize to cervical lymph nodes.

The differentiation between Hürthle cell adenoma and carcinoma has been controversial in the past. More recently, studies have shown that when there is no microscopic evidence of capsular invasion or blood vessel invasion, cancer will develop in fewer than 1% of patients classified as having Hürthle cell adenomas. Thyroid lobectomy and isthmusec-

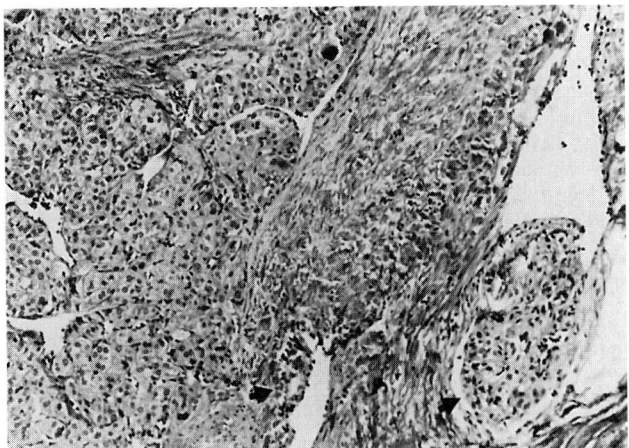

Figure 23–35. Photomicrograph of minimally invasive follicular carcinoma with vascular invasion (arrow). ×160. (Courtesy of Sudha R. Kini, M.D., from the book GUIDES TO CLINICAL ASPIRATION BIOPSY: THYROID, Igaku-Shoin Medical Publishers, New York, NY, 1987.)

tomy is considered adequate treatment for these patients. For patients with Hürthle cell carcinoma, total thyroidectomy and ipsilateral central neck dissection should be performed; a modified neck dissection should be performed in patients with enlarged jugular nodes.

Medullary Thyroid Carcinoma. See Chapter 23-V.

Undifferentiated Thyroid Carcinoma. Undifferentiated or anaplastic carcinomas (Fig. 23–37) are the most aggressive of all thyroid malignancies and fortunately constitute only about 5% of thyroid cancers in the United States. This is a disease of older patients, with a peak incidence in the seventh decade of life. This tumor occurs more commonly in iodine-deficient areas. The usual clinical presentation is a rapidly enlarging, symptomatic neck mass in a patient who frequently has a history of previously recognized goiter. Because of its aggressive growth pattern, the trachea and other vital neck structures are invaded, producing dyspnea or dysphagia. The tumors are typically quite large, and 50% have clinically positive cervical lymph nodes; approximately 30% have distant metastases at the time of presentation, with lung as the most common site. By the time of diagnosis most of these anaplastic lesions have spread locally to vital neck structures, precluding surgical resection. The small number of patients in whom operative resection is possible usually have evidence of disease of limited extent on physical examination. Current treatment protocols use diagnosis with FNAB followed by combination chemotherapy and radiation therapy. CT scanning is used to determine the extent and potential operability of the tumor; extensive growth into the mediastinum is usually an indication that operation should be avoided. Tracheostomy may be required for maintenance of the airway because of the propensity for invasion of the trachea. Prognosis is predictably quite poor, with mean survival in the 3- to 6-month range and 1-year survival of 5% to 15%.[16]

Lymphoma. Primary malignant lymphoma of the thyroid is a rare malignancy that typically presents as a rapidly enlarging, firm, painless mass in older women. This entity frequently arises in glands with evidence of chronic lymphocytic thyroiditis. Usually, the diagnosis can be made by FNAB or cutting-needle biopsy, although surgical resection is occasionally undertaken because the diagnosis cannot be established with certainty with needle biopsy techniques. It is critical that this lesion be distinguished from anaplastic carcinoma, which it frequently resembles in clinical presentation, because successful therapeutic options are available for lymphoma. Following diagnosis, appropriate staging should be performed to determine the extent of disease. Patients with local disease are treated with radiation therapy because this lesion is quite radiosensitive. In patients in whom lymphoma is discovered at the time of surgical therapy, survival is unaffected by the extent of operation, even if only biopsy is obtained. When there is extrathyroidal extension, the surgical procedure should be limited to obtaining a diagnostic specimen because more aggressive procedures may cause increased morbidity without improving survival time. Patients with more extensive disease or who relapse are treated with chemotherapy.[26]

Postoperative Treatment. The role of radioactive iodine in the postoperative management of patients with well-differentiated thyroid cancer remains controversial, partly because the mortality rate is so low in this disease. However, numerous convincing studies have demonstrated that the lowest recurrence and death rates are found in patients who have received both ^{131}I and thyroid hormone suppression. Radioactive iodine is more effective in treating microscopic foci of neoplastic thyroid tissue than it is in ablating macrometastases; this suggests that ^{131}I should be used prophylactically after total thyroidectomy when no tumor is clinically apparent, rather than therapeutically when gross tumor is detectable. Most experts recommend that patients with well-differentiated thyroid cancer lesions larger than 1.5 cm. receive postoperative radioactive iodine. Beneficial effects of radioactive iodine are less certain in patients younger than 40 years of age, and some authors do not routinely perform ablation in younger patients who have tumors smaller than 1.0 cm. unless there is a history of irradiation exposure. For the radioactive iodine to be most effective, however, normal thyroid tissue must first be removed, because it accumulates the isotope more avidly than do thyroid cancers.

Postoperative ^{131}I scans are usually performed 1 to 3 months following operation for well-differentiated thyroid cancer. A 2- to 4-week period without thyroid hormone replacement should precede the scan to achieve maximal concentration of endogenous TSH, which stimulates uptake of ^{131}I by any remaining thyroid tissue and metastatic lesions. Optimally, TSH levels should be determined before the scan, and patients should be advised to restrict iodine intake in preparation for the scan. Patients with significant residual functioning tissue and those with metastatic disease are candidates for radioactive iodine ablation. Ablation of residual thyroid tissue can usually be accomplished with one dose of 30 mCi of ^{131}I; patients with metastatic deposits in the neck are given 75 to 100 mCi and those with distant metastases are given 150 to 200 mCi. Radioiodine scan and treatment is then repeated at 6- to 9-month intervals until tumor uptake of the isotope is abolished or adverse effects of radioiodine are encountered. Female patients should always be carefully screened for pregnancy prior to ^{131}I treatment because damage to the fetus can occur.

Essentially all patients who undergo operations for well-differentiated thyroid carcinoma should receive thyroid hormone. This may be necessary to prevent hypothyroidism in many patients. In addition, there is abundant evidence that TSH can stimulate growth of differentiated thyroid carcinoma, and thyroid hormone given in adequate doses suppresses TSH. Recurrence rates of both papillary and follicular carcinoma are lower in patients treated postoperatively with thyroid hormone. All patients receive thyroid hormone doses that restore euthyroidism and maintain TSH suppression. Serum thyroglobulin measurements are helpful in determining the presence of recurrent disease in patients who have undergone ablative therapy of all thyroid tissue. Thyroglobulin is produced only by thyroid tissue and increasing levels in these patients is suggestive of disease recurrence.

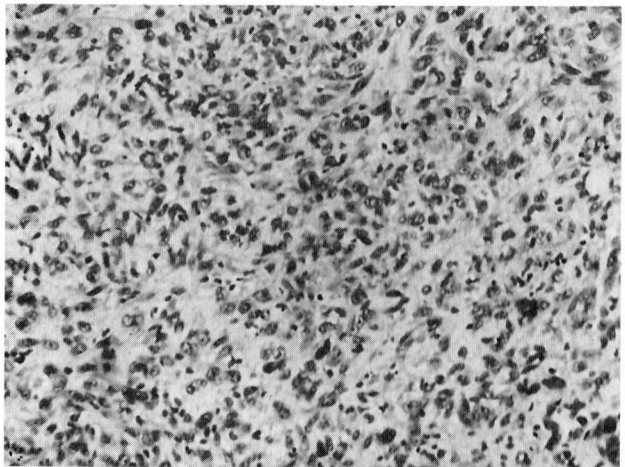

Figure 23–37. Anaplastic carcinoma. Photomicrograph showing spindle cell pattern. ×160. (Courtesy of Sudha R. Kini, M.D., from the book GUIDES TO CLINICAL ASPIRATION BIOPSY: THYROID, Igaku-Shoin Medical Publishers, New York, NY, 1987.)

External Radiation. External radiation has a limited role in the management of well-differentiated thyroid carcinoma, because these tumors are relatively radioresistant. It may be useful for the palliative treatment of patients with unresectable cancers that do not take up radioiodine and has a primary role in the treatment of lymphoma and undifferentiated thyroid carcinomas.

Chemotherapy. Chemotherapy is the third line of therapy for those thyroid malignancies that are not adequately controlled by surgery and radiation. Numerous chemotherapeutic agents have been tried, although the most widely used agents are doxorubicin, 5-fluorouracil, methotrexate, actinomycin D, and cyclophosphamide. Doxorubicin alone or in combination with other agents produces reponse rates in the range of 30% to 40%; a longer survival time is seen in patients whose tumors respond to chemotherapy. The usefulness of these single agents and multidrug combinations remains uncertain pending results of well-conducted studies comparing various drugs.

SELECTED REFERENCES

Studer, H., Gerber, H., Zbaeren, J., and Peter, H. J.: Histomorphological and immunohistochemical evidence that human nodular goiters grow by episodic replication of multiple clusters of thyroid follicular cells. J. Clin. Endocrinol. Metab. 75:1151, 1992.

A comprehensive summary regarding the basic process of goitrogenesis including recent studies on cellular mechanisms that allow growth of human goiter nodules. Conclusions are presented concisely, leading to a coherent overview of this difficult area.

Gharib, H., Goellner, J. R., and Johnson, D. A.: Fine-needle aspiration cytology of the thyroid: A 12-year experience with 11,000 biopsies. Clin. Lab. Med., 13:699, 1993.

This is a review of a large clinical series of patients with thyroid nodules evaluated by FNAB. Diagnostic criteria are thoroughly reviewed. Advantages and limitations of FNAB are emphasized. The importance of FNAB in the management of thyroid nodules is discussed.

Jossart, G. H. and Clark, O. H.: Well-differentiated thyroid cancer. *In* Wells, S. A. (Ed.): *Current Problems in Surgery*, Vol. 31. St. Louis, Mosby-Year Book, 1994, pp 933–1024.

This excellent review of diagnosis and current management of the well-differentiated types of thyroid carcinoma contains a wealth of information concerning risk assessment and surgical management. It also has an excellent section on postoperative management.

Thakker, R. V., Dynford-Thomas, D., Fierro-Renoy, J. F., and DeGroot, L. J.: Etiology of thyroid cancer. *In* Wheeler, M. H., and Lazarus, J. H. (Eds.): *Diseases of the Thyroid: Pathophysiology and Management.* London, Chapman & Hall Medical, 1994, p. 281.

A summary of the current state of knowledge regarding the molecular basis of thyroid carcinomas. Basic concepts in this area are reviewed. Specific information concerning the thyroid epithelial cell carcinomas is also presented in detail.

REFERENCES

1. Ashcraft, M. W. and Van Herle, A. J.: Management of thyroid nodules: I. History and physical examination, blood tests, x-ray tests, and ultrasonography. II. Scanning techniques, thyroid suppressive therapy, and fine needle aspiration. Head Neck Surg., 3:216, 297, 1981.
2. Berghout, A., Wiersinga, W. M., Drexhage, H. A., Smits, J. J. and Touber, J. L.: Comparison of placebo with L-thyroxine alone or with carbomazole for treatment of sporadic non-toxic goiter. Lancet, 193:336, 1990.
3. Brander, A., Virkinkoski, P., Nierels, J., and Kivisaari, L.: Thyroid gland: Ultrasound screening in a random adult population. Radiology, 181:603, 1991.
3a Cady, B., and Rossi, R.: An expanded view of risk-group definition in differentiated thyroid carcinoma. Surgery, 104:947, 1988.
4. Clark, O. H., Okerlund, M. D., Cavalieri, R. R., and Greenspan, F. S.: Diagnosis and treatment of thyroid, parathyroid, and thyroglossal duct cysts. J. Clin. Endocrinol. Metab., 48:983, 1979.
5. DeAndrade, M. A.: A review of 128 cases of posterior mediastinal goiter. World J. Surg., 1:789, 1977.
6. Duffy, B. J., Jr., and Fitzgerald, P. J.: Cancer of thyroid in children: A report of twenty-eight cases. J. Clin. Endocrinol., 10:1296, 1950.
7. Gharib, H.: Fine-needle aspiration biopsy of thyroid nodules: Advantages, limitations, and effect. Mayo Clin. Proc., 69:44, 1994.
8. Gharib, H., Goellner, J. R., and Johnson, D. A.: Fine-needle aspiration cytology of the thyroid: A 12 year experience with 11,000 biopsies. Clin. Lab. Med., 13:699, 1993.
9. Gharib, H., James, E. M., Charboneau, J. W., et al.: Suppressive therapy with levothyroxine for solitary thyroid nodules: A double-blind controlled clinical study. N. Engl. J. Med., 317:70, 1987.
10. Hay, I. D., Grant, C. S., Taylor, W. F., and McConahey, W. M.: Ipsilateral lobectomy versus bilateral lobar resection in papillary thyroid carcinoma: A retrospective analysis of surgical outcome using a novel prognostic scoring system. Surgery, 102:1088, 1987.
11. Horlocker, T. T., Hay, J. E., James, E. M., et al.: Prevalence of incidental nodular thyroid disease detected during high-resolution parathyroid ultrasonography. *In* Medeiros-Neto, G., and Gaitan, E. (Eds.): Frontiers in Thyroidology. New York, Plenum Medical, 1986, p. 1309.
12. Jossart G. H., and Clark, O. H.: Well-differentiated thyroid cancer. *In* Wells, S. A., (Ed.): Current Problems in Surgery, St. Louis, Mosby-Year Book, 1994, p. 933.
13. Kelly, F. C., and Snedden, W. W.: Prevalence of distribution of endemic goiter. Bull. WHO, 18:5, 1958.
14. Marine, D.: Etiology and prevention of simple goiter. Medicine, 3:453, 1924.
15. Mazzaferri, E. L.: Management of a solitary thyroid nodule. N. Engl. J. Med., 328:553, 1993.
16. Mazzaferri, E. L.: Undifferentiated thyroid carcinoma and unusual thyroid malignancies. *In* Mazzaferri, E. L., and Samaan, N. A. (Eds.): Endocrine Tumors. Boston, Blackwell Scientific, 1993, p. 378.
17. Mortensen, J. D., Woolner, L. B., and Bennett, W. A.: Gross and microscopic findings in clinically normal thyroid glands. J. Clin. Endocrinol. Metab., 15:1270, 1955.
18. Pickardt, C. R., and Scriba, P. C.: Multinodular goiter: Diagnosis and management. *In* Wheeler, M. J., and Lazarus, J. H. (Eds.): Diseases of the Thyroid. London, Chapman and Hall, 1994, p. 219.
19. Rossi, R. L., and Cady, B.: Differentiated Carcinoma of Thyroid Gland. *In* Cady, B., and Rossi, R. L. (Eds.): Surgery of the Thyroid and Parathyroid Glands, 3rd ed. Philadelphia, W. B. Saunders, 1991, p. 139.
20. Shaha, A.: Surgery for benign thyroid disease causing tracheoesophageal compression. Otolaryngol. Clin. North Am., 23:391, 1990.
21. Shahrian, D. M.: Surgical treatment of intrathoracic goiter. *In* Cady, B., and Rossi, R. L. (Eds.): Surgery of the Thyroid and Parathyroid Glands, 3rd ed. Philadelphia, W. B. Saunders, 1991, p. 215.
22. Solbiati, L. Volterrani, L., Rizzatto, G., et al.: The thyroid gland with low uptake lesions: Evaluation by ultrasound. Radiology, 155:187, 1985.
23. Studer, H., and Gerber, H.: Pathogenesis of nontoxic diffuse and nodular goiter. *In* Braverman, L. E., and Utiger, R. (Eds.): Werner's and Ingbar's The Thyroid, 6th ed. Philadelphia, J. B. Lippincott, 1992, p. 1107.
24. Studer, H., Gerber, H., Zbaeren, J., and Peter, H.: Histomorphological and immunohistochemical evidence that human nodular goiters grow by episodic replication of multiple clusters of thyroid follicular cells. J. Clin. Endocrinol. Metab., 75(4):1151, 1992.
25. Thakker, R. V., Dynford-Thomas, D., Fierro-Renoy, J. F., and DeGroot, L. J.: Etiology of thyroid cancer. *In* Wheeler, M. H., and Lazarus, J. H. (Eds.): Diseases of the Thyroid: Pathophysiology and Management, London, Chapman and Hall Medical, 1994, p. 281.
26. Thompson, N., Backdahl, M., et al.: Clinical features and management of thyroid cancer. *In* Wheeler, M. H., and Lazarus, J. H. (Eds.): Diseases of the Thyroid: Pathophysiology and Management, London, Chapman and Hall Medical, 1994, p. 367.
27. Van Herle, A. J., Rich, P., Ljung, B. E., et al.: Thyroid nodule. Ann. Intern. Med., 96:221, 1982.
28. Vander, J. B., Gaston, E. A., and Dawber, T. R.: The significance of nontoxic thyroid nodules: Final report of a 15-year study of the incidence of thyroid malignancy. Ann. Intern. Med., 69:537, 1968.
29. Watters, D. A., Ahuja, A. T., Evans, R. M., et al.: Role of ultrasound in the management of thyroid nodules. Am. J. Surg., 164:654, 1992.

V

MULTIPLE ENDOCRINE NEOPLASIA SYNDROMES

Terry C. Lairmore, M.D., and Samuel A. Wells, Jr., M.D.

Tumors of the endocrine system most often develop within a single gland. Some genetic disorders, however, are characterized by a predisposition to develop neoplasms in multiple endocrine glands. In these disorders, which are usually familial, the endocrine tumors may be benign or malignant and may develop either synchronously or metachronously. The pathologic change in affected glands is characteristically multicentric and may occur as hyperplasia, adenoma, or carcinoma.

The multiple endocrine neoplasia (MEN) syndromes are distinct genetic entities that are expressed in several specific patterns of involvement. In its full expression, MEN 1 is characterized by the concurrence of parathyroid hyperplasia, pancreatic islet cell neoplasms, and adenomas of the anterior pituitary gland. MEN 2A is characterized by the concurrence of medullary thyroid carcinoma (MTC), pheochromocytomas, and parathyroid hyperplasia, whereas MEN 2B consists of MTC, pheochromocytoma, mucosal neuromas, and a distinctive *marfanoid habitus*. These syndromes may occur *de novo* (especially MEN 2B) and are transmitted as mendelian autosomal dominant traits.

MULTIPLE ENDOCRINE NEOPLASIA TYPE 1

Genetic Studies and Pathogenesis

The mendelian autosomal dominant inheritance pattern of the trait for MEN 1 has been clearly established. Genetic linkage studies and studies using deletion mapping in tumor deoxyribonucleic acid (DNA) have localized the MEN 1 locus to the long arm of chromosome 11. In a classic study by Larsson and colleagues[16] in 1988, the MEN 1 locus was localized to chromosome 11 by simple but important observations that compared constitutional and tumor tissue genotypes from a pair of brothers with insulinomas who had inherited MEN 1 from their mother. These studies took advantage of polymorphic restriction enzyme recognition sites that are detected by recombinant DNA probes. In this original report, the MEN 1 locus was regionally mapped to chromosome 11 based on the location of the deletions, as well as genetic linkage to the human muscle glycogen phosphorylase gene. In addition, these investigators made the important observation that the deletions in the tumor tissue eliminate the wild-type allele (from the unaffected parent).

This pattern of allelic deletion is consistent with a two-mutational model of oncogenesis, in which *two hits* are required to inactivate both copies of a tumor suppressor gene, as demonstrated for other inherited neoplasms (notably retinoblastoma). According to this model, the first mutation is inherited in the germline and confers susceptibility to neoplastic change in the involved tissues. Elimination of the remaining normal allele through a second somatic mutational event, or *second hit* (such as a gene deletion), causes the development of neoplasia. The occurrence of multiple second hits would then cause multiple clones of neoplastic cells and the multicentric involvement characteristically observed in affected endocrine tissues.

One group has reported presence of a circulating factor with parathyroid mitogenic activity in plasma from patients with familial MEN 1, which they suggest may have a caus-

ative role in the development of hyperparathyroidism.[3] It is most likely that the parathyroid, pancreatic islet, and pituitary neoplasms all result from a single mutated locus on chromosome 11q13. Recent work[5, 10] using fine scale genetic mapping and tumor deletion studies has further refined the localization of the MEN 1 locus; however, at the time of this writing the specific MEN 1 mutation(s) has not been identified.

Clinical Features and Management

The clinical expression of MEN 1 most often develops in the third or fourth decade of life, with the onset of symptoms being rare before age 10 years. Males and females are affected equally, as predicted by the autosomal dominant inheritance pattern. MEN 1 has been described in many geographic regions and in many ethnic groups, and no racial predilection has been demonstrated.

The MEN 1 trait is transmitted with near 100% penetrance, but with variable expressivity, such that each affected person may exhibit some but not necessarily all of the components of the syndrome. The most common abnormality in MEN 1 is parathyroid hyperplasia, which occurs in virtually all affected people, followed by pancreatic islet cell neoplasms and pituitary adenomas. The distribution of endocrine involvement varies according to the method of study and the patient population, but approximately 90% to 97% of patients have biochemical evidence of hyperparathyroidism, whereas pancreatic islet cell neoplasms are manifested in 30% to 80%, and pituitary tumors occur in 15% to 50%.[4] If followed long enough, most affected patients eventually develop involvement of several endocrine tissues, and one study of MEN 1 patients at necropsy detected pathologic involvement in all three endocrine tissues in more than 90% of patients.[18]

The clinical manifestations of patients with MEN 1 depend on the endocrine tissue involved and, particularly in pancreatic islet and pituitary neoplasms, the overproduction of a specific hormone. Symptoms may also derive from the tumor mass itself. In a classic review of 85 patients by Ballard and associates[1] in 1964, the most frequent mode of clinical presentation was peptic ulcer disease or its complications. Manifestations of hypoglycemia represented the second most common presenting feature, whereas symptoms of hyperparathyroidism or complaints referable to pituitary dysfunction (headaches, visual field defects, and secondary amenorrhea) least often led to the diagnosis. However, the mode of clinical presentation did not actually indicate the incidence of involvement of the various endocrine tissues.

Parathyroid Glands. The most common endocrine abnormality in patients with MEN 1 is hyperparathyroidism, occurring in more than 90% of patients. Most affected people exhibit generalized parathyroid hyperplasia with involvement of all four glands. In contrast, fewer than 20% of patients with sporadic primary hyperparathyroidism have multiglandular involvement. Although there has been some debate among pathologists with respect to the occurrence of multiple adenoma versus asymmetric or nodular hyperplasia in MEN 1, most agree that generalized chief cell hyperplasia is the characteristic pathologic lesion.

Hyperparathyroidism is usually the first biochemical abnormality detected in patients with MEN 1 and this may precede the clinical onset of an islet cell or pituitary neoplasm by several years. The symptoms in the setting of MEN 1 are similar to those of patients with sporadic primary hyperparathyroidism. Asymptomatic hypercalcemia may be present in many patients over a long period of observation. Symptomatic patients may develop renal or ureteral lithiasis, nephrocalcinosis, or both. Skeletal complications of hyperparathyroidism occur but are uncommon. In general, hyperparathyroidism in MEN 1 has an earlier age of onset and usually causes a milder hypercalcemia than that observed in primary sporadic hyperparathyroidism. The diagnosis is made by measuring serum calcium and parathyroid hormone levels.

Patients with MEN 1 and parathyroid hyperplasia have most often been managed by subtotal (3½ gland) parathyroidectomy in an attempt to render them normocalcemic. The incidence of recurrent hyperparathyroidism postoperatively has been as high as 40%,[25] whereas the incidence of permanent hypoparathyroidism has been approximately 25%.[35] For these reasons, total parathyroidectomy with autotransplantation of parathyroid tissue into an ectopic site such as the forearm muscle has been advocated for patients with multiglandular hyperplasia.[42] The potential advantages of this technique include a lower incidence of hypocalcemia and the feasibility of managing recurrent hyperparathyroidism, should it develop, by excision of a portion of the grafted parathyroid tissue under local anesthesia (obviating the morbidity of repeat neck exploration).

Pancreas. The second most frequent expression of MEN 1 is neoplasia of the pancreatic islet cells. The pathologic change is typically multicentric, and diffuse hyperplasia and microadenoma formation may be present in areas of the gland distant from grossly evident tumor. Either single or multiple islet cell tumors may be present within the wall of the duodenum or in extrapancreatic sites.

The most common clinical pancreatic islet cell lesion in patients with MEN 1 is gastrinoma. These patients present with a severe peptic ulcer diathesis resulting from autonomous gastrin hypersecretion. Gastrinomas associated with MEN 1 comprise 20% of all cases of the Zollinger-Ellison syndrome (ZES).[37] Gastrinoma is diagnosed by the documentation of gastric acid hypersecretion (>15 mEq. per liter in patients without operation and > 5 mEq. per liter in patients with prior ulcer surgery) and elevated fasting levels of serum gastrin (>100 pg. per ml). The diagnosis can be confirmed by an abnormal secretin test. A test result is positive when serum levels of gastrin rise more than 200 pg. per ml. following the intravenous administration of secretin (2 U. per kg.).

Gastrinomas that develop in patients with MEN 1 are multicentric and usually malignant, as indicated by the presence of regional or distant metastases. Because of the multicentricity and small size of these neoplasms, the true gastrinoma may not be localized preoperatively by computed tomographic (CT) scanning, angiography, or portal venous sampling with measurement of gastrin levels.

Previously, the accepted surgical therapy for this disease was total gastrectomy to remove the end-organ responsible for the hyperacidity. However, H_2-receptor antagonists and proton pump inhibitors such as omeprazole effectively control acid hypersecretion and its attendant complications, and now gastrectomy is rarely indicated. In patients with MEN 1 who have the ZES and hyperparathyroidism, parathyroidectomy greatly facilitates medical control of the gastric acid hypersecretion. Operation is rarely curative in patients with MEN 1 and gastrinomas. Resection of the islet cell tumors may be attempted if the tumor is identifiable on CT or angiogram and measures 2 to 3 cm. Operation is recommended to control the tumoral process, because 50% of tumors this size are malignant with lymph node or hepatic metastases. Although the gastrinoma in patients with MEN 1 is frequently malignant, the disease progression is indolent in many patients. With aggressive medical management and operation to limit tumor progression, affected people may enjoy relatively long survival.

The second most common pancreatic islet cell neoplasm in patients with MEN 1 is insulinoma. These are usually small (< 2 cm.) and usually multiple, in contrast with those that occur sporadically, where approximately 80% are solitary. Patients commonly present with recurrent symptoms of neuroglycopenia: sweating, dizziness, confusion, or syncope. The diagnosis of insulinoma is made by documenting symptomatic hypoglycemia concomitant with inappropriately elevated plasma levels of insulin and C-peptide during a supervised 72-hour fast. Because no medical therapy for insulinoma is ideal, these lesions are most often treated by surgical resection (either enucleation of the tumor or partial pancreatectomy). Often, patients become asymptomatic and normoglycemic following resection of the tumor. Approximately 10% of insulinomas occurring in patients with MEN 1 are malignant. Patients with a disseminated or diffuse carcinoma may respond to treatment with streptozotocin, and some control of hypoglycemia may be achieved by the administration of either diazoxide or octreotide.

Other pancreatic islet cell neoplasms, such as glucagonoma, somatostatinoma, and tumors secreting vasoactive intestinal peptide or pancreatic polypeptide, occur rarely in association with MEN 1.

Pituitary Gland. Pituitary neoplasms occur in 15% to 50% of patients. Most of these tumors are prolactin-secreting adenomas. Pituitary tumors cause symptoms either by hypersecretion of hormones or compression of adjacent structures. Large adenomas may cause visual field defects by pressure on the optic chiasm or manifestations of hypopituitarism through compression of the adjacent normal gland. Prolactin-secreting tumors cause amenorrhea and galactorrhea in women or hypogonadism in men. Approximately 30% of patients exhibit acromegaly resulting from growth hormone overproduction.[1] Much less commonly, corticotropin-producing tumors cause Cushing's disease.

Pituitary tumors, either functioning or nonfunctioning, may require surgical ablation or irradiation. Bromocriptine, a dopamine agonist and an inhibitor of prolactin secretion, has been used to treat prolactinomas medically.

Other Tumors. As many as 40% of patients with MEN 1 develop adrenocortical lesions, including adenomas, but adrenocortical hyperfunction is rare. Benign follicular adenomas of the thyroid or colloid nodules occur in as many as 15% of patients. Rarely, multiple subcutaneous or visceral lipomas and bronchial or gastrointestinal carcinoid tumors may occur in association with the MEN 1 syndrome.

MULTIPLE ENDOCRINE NEOPLASIA TYPE 2A and 2B

Genetic Studies and Pathogenesis

The demonstration that the genetic mutations associated with MEN 2A, MEN 2B, and familial medullary thyroid carcinoma (FMTC) each map to the centromere region of chromosome 10[15, 19, 24, 29] was followed by the advent of DNA-based predictive testing to identify patients who have inherited the mutation before they manifest clinical or biochemical evidence of MTC.[20]

Recent work has identified germline mutations in the *RET* proto-oncogene, which encodes a receptor tyrosine kinase signal transduction molecule, in patients with the MEN 2A, MEN 2B, and FMTC syndromes (Fig. 23–38). Mulligan and

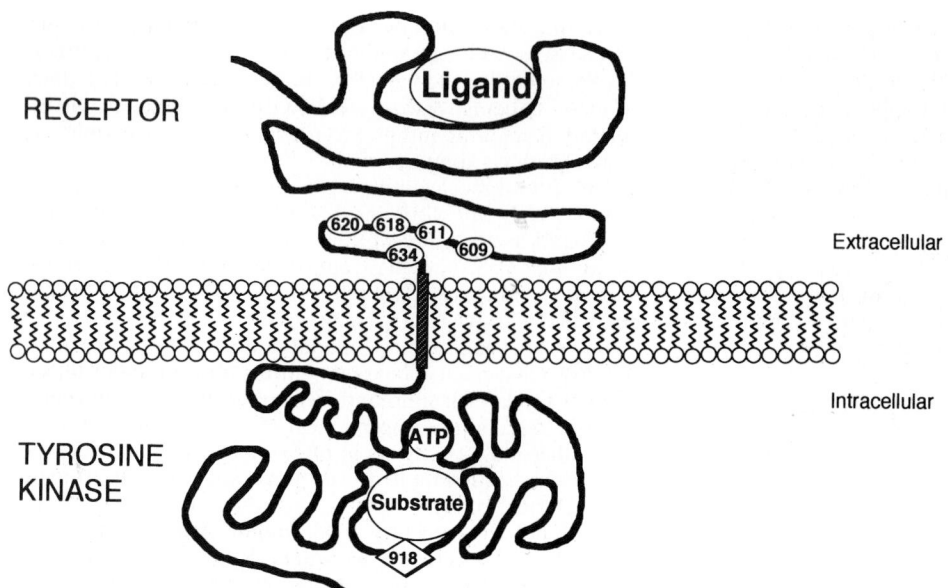

Figure 23–38. Schematic representation of the *RET* proto-oncogene structure. The locations of the MEN 2A and familial medullary thyroid carcinoma mutations that affect conserved cysteine residues in the portion of the extracellular domain immediately adjacent to the transmembrane segment are indicated by numbers in the oval-shaped circles. The single MEN 2B mutation that replaces methionine with threonine in a critical position with the tyrosine kinase catalytic domain is indicated by the number in the diamond-shaped box. The numbers within the symbols indicate the codon number. (Courtesy of Dr. David Chi, Washington University School of Medicine.)

coworkers[23] identified missense mutations in patients from 20 of 23 families with MEN 2A. Similarly, Donis-Keller and coworkers[7] identified 12 different mutations in the germline DNA and tumor DNA from patients with MEN 2A and FMTC. The *RET* proto-oncogene mutations in patients with MEN 2A and FMTC involve one of five codons specifying conserved cysteine residues within the portion of the extracellular domain immediately adjacent to the transmembrane segment of the protein. The amino acid substitution presumably confers conformational changes in the receptor portion of the molecule. In contrast with the allelic heterogeneity in MEN 2A and FMTC, a single point mutation in the tyrosine kinase catalytic domain of *RET*, which replaces methionine with threonine, has been identified in all patients with familial or sporadic MEN 2B who have been studied.[6, 13]

The ligand for the *RET* protein tyrosine kinase is currently not known. More important, the reason for the specific pattern of endocrine tissue involvement resulting from this germline mutation (which is present in every cell in the body) has not been elucidated. In contrast to the *two-hit* model of tumorigenesis in MEN 1, there is no evidence of consistent allelic deletions involving the portion of chromosome 10 containing *RET* in tumor DNA from patients with MEN 2. Patients with MEN 2A (as well as MEN 2B) have been found to be heterozygous (i.e., retain one normal allele) for *RET* missense mutations in both germline *and* tumor DNA. For this reason, it appears that *RET* acts as a dominant oncogene in the development of neoplasia in tissues derived from the neural crest. The altered *RET* alleles are transforming genes in NIH 3T3 cells as a consequence of constitutive activation of the *RET* tyrosine kinase.[27]

The *RET* receptor tyrosine kinase appears to have a pivotal role in regulating cellular growth and proliferation in tissues derived from the neural crest. The *RET* product is highly expressed in MTC, pheochromocytoma, and neuroblastoma tumors and is expressed at lower levels in normal human thyroid tissue. Schuchardt and co-workers[28] have demonstrated that mice homozygous for a targeted deletion in *RET* develop severe defects in the kidney and the enteric nervous system and die shortly after birth. In addition to the allelic *RET* mutations responsible for the MEN 2A, MEN 2B, and FMTC syndromes, some cases of familial Hirschsprung's disease have been associated with mutations that result in gene activation or abrogation of the functional *RET* product.[10, 26]

Finally, in approximately 25% of papillary thyroid carcinomas, an activated oncogene sequence is believed to result from the rearrangement of a novel amino-terminal sequence with the tyrosine kinase catalytic domain of the *RET* proto-oncogene.[11]

Clinical and Pathologic Features

The MEN 2A and MEN 2B syndromes are inherited in an autosomal dominant pattern; however, MEN 2B in particular may occur sporadically or arise as a new mutation with autosomal dominant transmission in subsequent generations. As is the case for MEN 1, the traits for MEN 2A and MEN 2B are transmitted with near 100% penetrance but with variable expressivity. Bilateral MTC occurs in nearly every affected person with MEN 2A and MEN 2B. In addition, patients with MEN 2A may have associated pheochromocytomas (approximately 50%) or parathyroid hyperplasia (approximately 25%).

MTC occurs in the rarer MEN 2B syndrome in association with pheochromocytoma, mucosal neuromas, diffuse ganglioneuromas of the gastrointestinal tract, skeletal abnormalities, and a *marfanoid* habitus. Patients with MEN 2B have a characteristic physical appearance (Fig. 23–39*A* to *C*), and affected persons are often recognizable at birth or in early infancy. Significantly, the MTC in patients with MEN 2B occurs earlier (sometimes before 2 years of age) and is a much more aggressive neoplasm biologically than its counterpart in patients with MEN 2A. Patients with MEN 2B may die from widespread metastatic MTC at an early age, underscoring the need for total thyroidectomy in affected patients as soon as the diagnosis is made. Owing to the aggressive nature of the disease, kindreds with MEN 2B are characteristically small, encompassing only two or three generations.

Medullary Thyroid Carcinoma. MTC constitutes 5% to 10% of all thyroid malignancies. Approximately 80% of these represent sporadic cases of MTC. Twenty per cent of MTC cases occur in a familial setting, either in association with MEN 2A or MEN 2B, or less commonly as FMTC.[9]

MTC is usually the first abnormality expressed in both MEN 2A and MEN 2B, and in most patients MTC is diagnosed either before or concurrently with pheochromocytoma. The peak incidence of MTC in the setting of MEN 2A or

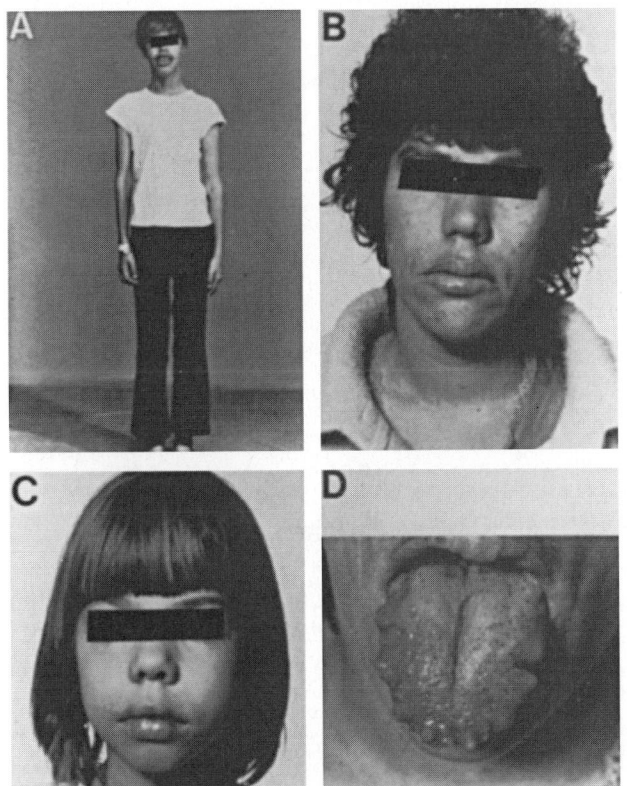

Figure 23–39. *A* to *C*, Characteristic phenotypic appearance of three patients with MEN 2B. *D*, Multiple neuromas on the tongue and oral mucosa in a patient with MEN 2B.

MEN 2B is in the second or third decade of life, compared with the fifth or sixth decade in patients with sporadic MTC.

Sporadic MTC is nearly always unilateral. In patients with MEN 2A or MEN 2B, MTC virtually always occurs as bilateral, multicentric foci of tumor in the middle and upper portions of each thyroid lobe. A diffuse premalignant proliferation of C-cells in the thyroid gland of patients with familial MTC has been described and is termed *C-cell hyperplasia*. Parafollicular clusters of increased numbers of C-cells represent the early manifestation of hyperplasia or microinvasive carcinoma that progresses to multifocal MTC. The presence of bilateral MTC or microscopic evidence of C-cell hyperplasia in areas of the thyroid adjacent to macroscopic foci of MTC strongly suggests the presence of familial disease.

MTC appears grossly as a circumscribed, gritty, whitish-tan nodule.[2] Microscopically it consists of nests or sheets of uniform round or polygonal cells separated by variable amounts of fibrovascular stroma. Less commonly, MTC may occur in a carcinoid-like trabecular pattern, or it may have a predominance of oval or spindle-shaped cells. Material with the staining properties of amyloid is frequently present in the stroma of MTC. This amyloid-like material is composed of an aggregate of a prohormone for calcitonin synthesized by the tumor cells.[32] Although the presence of an amyloid-like material in a thyroid neoplasm is a distinctive feature of MTC, it is not present in all tumors. MTC can be diagnosed immunohistochemically by demonstrating calcitonin within the MTC cells.

MTC cells are capable of great biosynthetic activity and have been reported to secrete (in addition to calcitonin) corticotropin, prostaglandins, melanin, and serotonin. However, the most important product of MTC cells is calcitonin, which is a sensitive tumor marker for the presence of MTC whether in preoperative screening or postoperative evaluation. Although it is uncommon, patients with MTC may present with any of several paraneoplastic syndromes, including Cushing's syndrome or the carcinoid syndrome. Diarrhea, which occurs in as many as 30% of these patients, is attributed to increased jejunal water and electrolyte secretion stimulated by high plasma calcitonin levels. Patients with clinically evident MTC most commonly present with a palpable thyroid nodule or multinodular thyroid gland. Enlarged, firm cervical lymph nodes suggest metastatic disease. Patients with locally advanced disease may present with hoarseness, dysphagia, respiratory difficulty, or signs of distant metastases (e.g., lung, liver, and bone).

MTC may also exhibit distinctive radiographic features. Plain films of the cervical region often reveal irregular dense calcifications, owing to the propensity of primary and metastatic MTC lesions to undergo degenerative calcification. Similarly, chest radiographs may reveal large calcified hilar or mediastinal nodes corresponding to calcified deposits of metastatic MTC.

Pheochromocytoma. The pheochromocytomas in patients with MEN 2A and MEN 2B appear in the second or third decade of life. Approximately 60% to 80% of these tumors are bilateral, compared with 10% of sporadic pheochromocytomas. Most tumors are diagnosed concurrently or a few years subsequent to the detection of MTC, and pheochromocytoma is infrequently the initial presenting feature. The pheochromocytomas are nearly always limited to the adrenal medulla, and they are nearly always benign. The histologic appearance of the tumor cells is similar to that observed in pheochromocytomas that occur in a nonfamilial setting.

Patients with MEN 2A or MEN 2B develop hyperplasia of the adrenal medulla before the development of pheochromocytomas. A spectrum of disease including nodular or asymmetric hyperplasia, multiple small pheochromocytomas, or a diffuse thickening of all adrenal medullary tissue may be observed. This pattern of adrenal involvement is comparable to the finding of C-cell hyperplasia in the thyroid of patients with MEN 2A or MEN 2B.

The pheochromocytomas in patients with MEN 2A and MEN 2B may be either clinically silent or associated with dramatic clinical symptoms such as severe pounding frontal headaches, episodic diaphoresis, palpitations, and vague feelings of anxiety. Hypertension, if present, may be sustained or episodic.

Parathyroid Glands. Hyperfunction of the parathyroid glands in patients with MEN 2A is the most variable component of the syndrome. Many patients are asymptomatic, and recognition of the parathyroid lesions may stem from the finding of hypercalcemia during routine laboratory studies. However, it is not uncommon to find one or more enlarged parathyroid glands at the time of thyroidectomy for MTC in a patient who is normocalcemic. The most common symptom of altered calcium homeostasis in patients with MEN 2A is the presence of asymptomatic or symptomatic renal stones. More advanced signs of hyperparathyroidism, such as osteitis fibrosa cystica and nephrocalcinosis, are unusual.

The parathyroid lesions in patients with MEN 2A consist primarily of generalized chief cell hyperplasia, and typically there is multiple gland enlargement.

Although some investigators have reported equivocal histologic abnormalities or increased numbers of chief cells in the parathyroid glands of patients with MEN 2B, hyperparathyroidism rarely, if ever, occurs in this syndrome.

Non-endocrine Manifestations of MEN 2B. In addition to MTC and pheochromocytoma, patients with MEN 2B develop abnormalities of the musculoskeletal and nervous systems. Unlike patients with MEN 1 or MEN 2A, these patients have a characteristic phenotype, including a tall, thin marfanoid body habitus (see Fig. 23–39A to C). Multiple neuromas develop on the lips, tongue, and oral mucosa (Fig. 23–39D). Slit-lamp examination of the eyes often reveals hypertrophied corneal nerves. Patients may develop diffuse ganglioneuromatosis of the gastrointestinal tract, characterized microscopically by hypertrophy and nerve fiber disarray of the myenteric and submucosal plexuses. A history of chronic constipation or recurrent crampy abdominal pain may be present because of the disordered motility of the gut. Contrast studies may reveal evidence of colonic dilatation or megacolon. There is also a high incidence of skeletal anomalies, including congenital dislocation of the hip, pes planus or cavus, pectus excavatum, and kyphosis.

Diagnosis

It is unusual for one to diagnose and treat cancer accurately when it is clinically occult. It is possible to detect minimal elevations of calcitonin in plasma using sensitive immunoassays. Because MTC occurs in nearly 100% of patients with MEN 2A and MEN 2B and is usually the first abnormality expressed, diagnosis of the disease in kindred members at risk may be accomplished by biochemical screening for the presence of the thyroid tumor.

In 1970, Tashjian and associates[33] first described the measurement of human calcitonin by radioimmunoassay and documented that nearly all patients with clinically detectable MTC have elevated plasma calcitonin levels. In normal subjects, basal plasma calcitonin levels are either very low or less than 200 pg. per ml. Patients with clinically palpable MTC generally have plasma calcitonin levels greater than 1000 pg. per ml. With extensive disease, basal plasma values may exceed 2000 to 3000 pg. per ml.

Subsequently, Melvin and colleagues[21] documented that

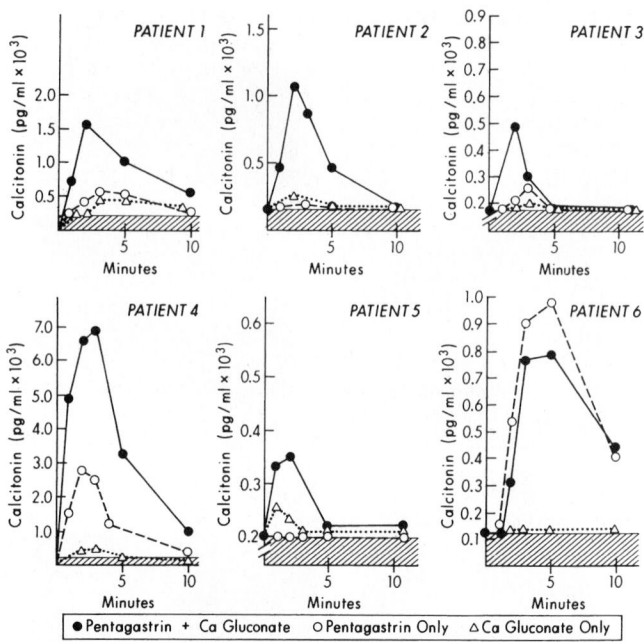

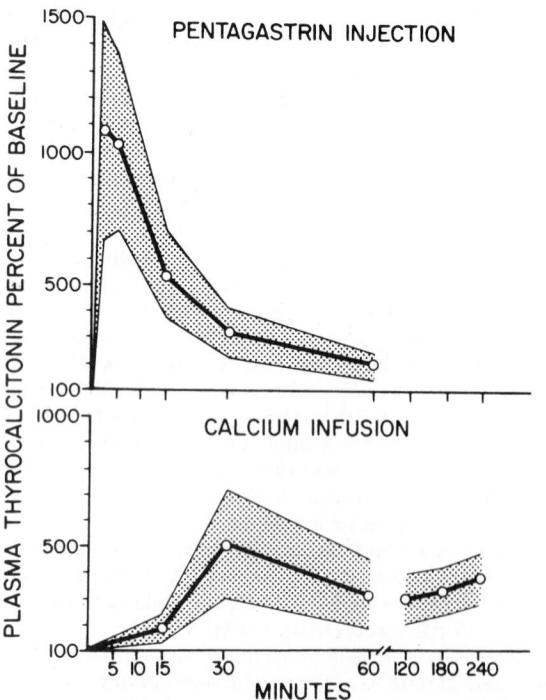

Figure 23–40. Combined responses of seven patients with elevated baseline levels of plasma calcitonin to pentagastrin injection and calcium infusion. Each patient received both tests on separate days, pentagastrin injection being the initial test in four of the patients and calcium infusion the initial test in three. Open circles and solid lines represent the mean responses, and the shaded areas indicate the range of the standard errors. (From Hennessy, J. C., et al.: A comparison of pentagastrin injection and calcium infusion as provocative agents for the detection of medullary carcinoma of the thyroid. J. Clin. Endocrinol. Metabol., 39:487, 1974.)

Figure 23–41. Plasma calcitonin levels following the administration of pentagastrin (0.5 μg per kg. over 5 seconds), calcium gluconate (2 mg. per kg. over 1 minute), and a combination of the two in six patients with familial medullary thyroid carcinoma. (From Wells, S. A., Jr., et al.: Provocative agents and the diagnosis of medullary carcinoma of the thyroid gland. Ann. Surg., 188:139, 1978.)

patients with clinically occult MTC may have minimally elevated plasma calcitonin levels. These researchers also demonstrated that such patients frequently have normal basal plasma calcitonin levels that markedly increase after a calcium infusion (15 mg. per kg. over 4 hours). The presence of MTC was correctly diagnosed in 11 patients whose only indication of disease was an elevated plasma calcitonin level either basally or after a calcium infusion. At thyroidectomy, these patients had small medullary carcinomas.

The peptide pentagastrin subsequently proved to be more potent than the standard 4-hour calcium infusion in stimulating calcitonin secretion from MTC cells.[12] After a bolus intravenous injection of pentagastrin (0.5 μg. per kg. over 5 seconds), peak plasma calcitonin levels were two to three times higher, and they occurred within 1 to 5 minutes after injection (Fig. 23–40). Later, it was demonstrated that the sequential intravenous administration of calcium gluconate (2 mg. per kg. over 1 minute), followed by a bolus injection of pentagastrin (0.5 μg. per kg. over 5 seconds), stimulated higher peak plasma levels of plasma calcitonin than did either agent alone (Fig. 23–41).[50]

Provocative testing with calcium gluconate and pentagastrin and measurement of plasma calcitonin by radioimmunoassay is an extremely sensitive way to detect MTC when it is clinically occult and was the method of choice for screening kindred members at risk for MEN 2A before the identification of mutations at the DNA level. Stimulated plasma calcitonin levels greater than 300 pg. per ml. are highly suggestive of MTC, and the diagnosis is virtually assured in patients with stimulated plasma calcitonin levels exceeding 1000 pg. per ml. Patients with MEN 2A whose MTC is diagnosed by provocative testing are younger, have smaller primary tumors, and have a lower incidence of regional lymph node and distant metastases when compared with patients whose MTC is detected clinically.[39] Also, the number of patients cured by total thyroidectomy, a parameter easily determined by measuring stimulated plasma calcitonin levels postoperatively, is significantly higher in the former group (Fig. 23–42). The disadvantages of provocative testing are the need for ongoing venipuncture and annual testing to detect new increases in plasma calcitonin and transient unpleasant side effects commonly experienced during infusion of the secretagogues. Measurement of the tumor marker calcitonin by sensitive immunoassay after calcium-pentagastrin stimulation remains the most important method for detecting persistent or recurrent MTC postoperatively.

The diagnosis of pheochromocytoma in patients with MEN 2A and MEN 2B can be made biochemically by measurement of the urinary excretion of catecholamines and catecholamine metabolites. Patients with symptoms characteristic of pheochromocytoma should have a 24-hour urine collection for measurement of total urinary catecholamines, epinephrine, norepinephrine, metanephrines, and vanillylmandelic acid. It is imperative that patients with MEN 2A and MEN 2B have pheochromocytoma excluded before undergoing thyroidectomy. This is particularly important because the pheochromocytoma may be unsuspected clinically. If a patient with MTC is found to have a pheochromocytoma, adrenalectomy

should be performed, followed by thyroidectomy 1 to 2 weeks later.

If the 24-hour urinary excretion rates of catecholamines and metabolites are equivocal and if there is any question about the presence of a pheochromocytoma, CT of the abdomen should be performed to exclude the presence of adrenal enlargement. Lesions 1 cm. or larger can be identified, and rarely adrenal hyperplasia is suggested. Beierwaltes and associates[31, 43] have used ^{131}I-metaiodobenzylguanidine (^{131}I-MIBG) scintigraphy in a large number of patients to visualize pheochromocytomas. This agent is structurally similar to norepinephrine and is taken up and stored in adrenergic vesicles. The normal adrenal glands are not visualized at 24 to 48 hours. ^{131}I-MIBG is specific for pheochromocytomas, and positive identification of these adrenal tumors has been possible in 90% of patients. There have been fewer than 5% false-positive test results. This technique provides functional and anatomic localization of hyperfunctioning chromaffin tissue and has been useful in demonstrating intra-adrenal and extra-adrenal pheochromocytomas, as well as adrenal medullary hyperplasia. This agent has proved particularly useful in patients who have ectopic pheochromocytomas that had not been found at prior operation.

The diagnosis of hyperparathyroidism rests on the finding of hypercalcemia (serum calcium >10.5 mg. per dl.) and an inappropriately elevated parathyroid hormone level.

DNA Testing and Prophylactic Thyroidectomy in Patients with MEN 2A. Before the advent of genetic testing, the early diagnosis of MEN 2A was made by biochemical testing for the presence of MTC. Although very sensitive and specific, annual provocative testing is expensive and labor intensive and is associated with bothersome side effects that have caused some kindred members to refuse repetitive testing. Mapping of the MEN 2A locus to the centromere region of chromosome 10[19, 29] by genetic linkage led to the development of predictive DNA testing. This analysis is based on following the inheritance pattern of the disease phenotype in relation to anonymous genetic markers that are closely linked to the disease locus. Using highly polymorphic markers and haplotype analysis, accurate predictions of the inheritance of the disease mutation can be made, but the analysis requires a suitable pedigree structure and collection of DNA from affected and unaffected kindred members for genotyping.

The recent identification of germline mutations in the *RET* proto-oncogene in patients with MEN 2A, MEN 2B, and FMTC has made direct DNA testing the preferred method of screening kindred members at risk.[41] Direct genetic testing may be performed at any age, requiring collection of a single peripheral blood sample for rapid preparation of a small amount of genomic DNA. The mutations associated with the disease phenotypes are detected by polymerase chain reaction amplification of specific *RET* exons, followed by digestion with restriction endonucleases or direct sequencing to detect the known mutations. The ability to detect mutations at the base-pair level has simplified the management of these patients by allowing the performance of prophylactic thyroidectomy in kindred members at risk who have inherited a disease-specific mutation, and by identifying those persons who do not require further testing. Because MTC develops in essentially all patients with MEN 2 and is the only component of the syndrome that is uniformly malignant, it can be argued that a patient, regardless of age, becomes a candidate for thyroidectomy as soon as an *RET* mutation is identified. Evidence suggests that this approach is curative or preventative of MTC in almost all patients. In a study by Lips and colleagues[17] comparing the accuracy of biochemical screening and DNA analysis, 8 of 14 patients with a positive DNA test result but normal plasma calcitonin levels had small foci of medullary carcinoma at thyroidectomy. In a report by Wells

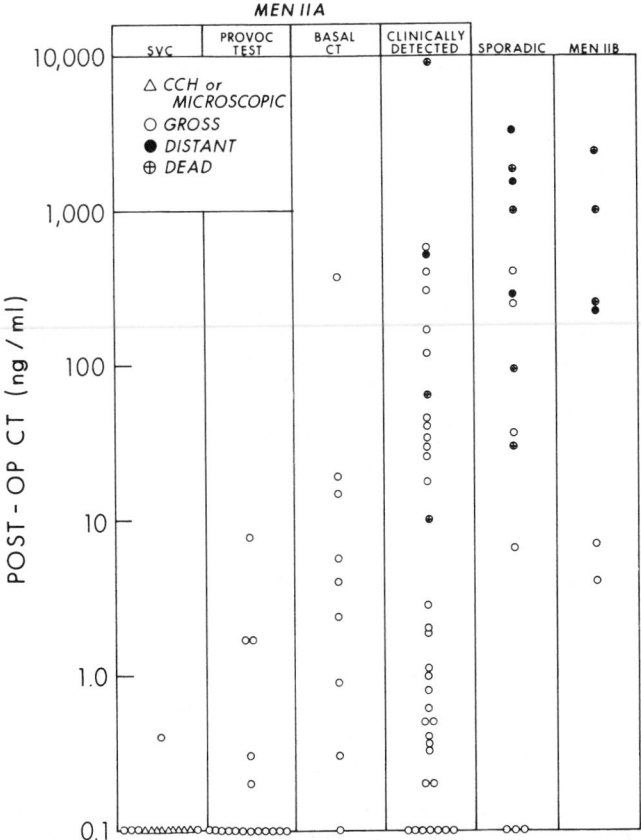

Figure 23–42. Postoperative stimulated plasma calcitonin (CT) levels in patients with MEN 2A diagnosed by selective venous catheterization with provocative testing (SVC; n = 14); documentation of increased plasma CT levels in peripheral plasma following provocative testing (Provoc Test; n = 17); documentation of elevated basal CT in peripheral plasma (Basal CT; n = 9); and palpation of the neck (Clinically Detected; n = 36). Postoperative CT values are also shown in patients with sporadic MTC and those with MEN 2B. The incidence of residual or recurrent MTC postoperatively (as indicated by an elevated plasma CT [>300 pg. per ml.] after provocative testing) increases as the method of diagnosis becomes less sensitive (i.e., residual or recurrent disease is much lower in patients diagnosed by SVC than in those diagnosed by physical examination). Patients presenting with sporadic medullary thyroid carcinoma or MEN 2B are rarely cured by thyroidectomy, regardless of the method of diagnosis, (From Wells, S. A., Jr., et al.: Early diagnosis and treatment of medullary thyroid carcinoma. Arch. Intern. Med., *145*:1248–1252, 1985. Copyright 1985, American Medical Association.)

and co-workers[41] of 13 patients (ages 6 to 20 years) undergoing early thyroidectomy based on the results of direct DNA testing for MEN 2A, only 4 had macroscopic evidence of MTC, and the remaining 9 had microscopic MTC, C-cell hyperplasia, or both. There were no metastases to regional lymph nodes, and postoperative stimulated plasma calcitonin levels were normal. Based on these data, the authors have recommended thyroidectomy for patients as young as 5 years of age with disease-specific mutations.

Surgical Management

Medullary Thyroid Carcinoma. The operative treatment of familial or sporadic MTC is total thyroidectomy. Meticulous removal of all thyroid tissue should be undertaken at the initial operation because MTC in the setting of MEN 2A or MEN 2B is nearly always multicentric and bilateral and it metastasizes early to cervical lymph nodes. The nodes in the central compartment of the neck (between the jugular veins and from the hyoid bone to the sternal notch) should be dissected in all patients with either clinically evident or occult MTC. Patients with macroscopic lymph node metastases should undergo ipsilateral modified neck dissection in addition to total thyroidectomy. Postoperatively, residual or recurrent MTC can be readily detected by calcium-pentagastrin stimulation and measurement of plasma calcitonin levels.

MTC often has an indolent biologic course, and although early metastases to cervical lymph nodes may occur, it may remain confined to the neck for many months or years. Tisell and colleagues[34] have reported the results of reoperation in 11 patients with persistently elevated plasma calcitonin levels after initial total thyroidectomy and central zone lymphadenectomy for MTC. Meticulous superior mediastinal and bilateral lymph node dissection under magnification with intent to remove all tumor in the neck resulted in normalization of postoperative plasma calcitonin levels in 4 (36%) patients. Moley and co-workers[22] reported the results of reoperation and lymph node microdissection in 32 patients with persistently elevated plasma calcitonin levels after primary thyroidectomy and achieved biochemical cure with normalization of stimulated plasma calcitonin levels in 9 (28%) patients and a decrease in postoperative stimulated plasma calcitonin levels of 40% or more in an additional 13 (41%) patients. In general, patients with distant metastatic disease are not candidates for reoperation.

Pheochromocytoma. Patients with macroscopic or radiographic evidence of bilateral pheochromocytomas should have both adrenal glands removed. The operative management of unilateral pheochromocytoma in patients with MEN 2A or MEN 2B is controversial. Some surgeons recommend empirical bilateral adrenalectomy in these patients even though there may be a macroscopic pheochromocytoma in only one gland.[36] This rationale is based on the arguments that adrenal medullary hyperplasia is nearly always bilateral, that there is a significant risk of subsequent development of pheochromocytoma in the opposite gland, and that the risk of complications from the anadrenal state should be low. Other surgeons advocate a more selective approach and perform unilateral adrenalectomy when macroscopic evidence of pheochromocytoma appears in only one gland. This surgical philosophy emphasizes that the risk of developing a pheochromocytoma in the opposite gland must be weighed against the need for life-long hormone replacement and potential risk of serious complications from the permanent addisonian state after bilateral adrenalectomy. In a study[14] of 58 patients with MEN 2A or MEN 2B and pheochromocytoma(s), 23 patients with macroscopic evidence of pheochromocytoma in a single gland were initially treated with unilateral adrenalectomy. A pheochromocytoma developed in the remaining adrenal gland in 12 (52%) of patients, with a mean interval of 11.9 years after the primary adrenalectomy. In the interval after unilateral adrenalectomy, no patient developed a hypertensive crisis related to undiagnosed pheochromocytoma. Conversely, 10 (23%) of 43 patients having bilateral adrenalectomy developed at least one addisonian crisis during the follow-up period, including one patient who died during a bout of influenza. The authors believe that unilateral adrenalectomy is the treatment of choice for patients with MEN 2A or MEN 2B and a unilateral pheochromocytoma, because only half of such patients develop a contralateral pheochromocytoma if followed longer than 10 years, the occurrence of malignant pheochromocytomas is rare, the development of a second pheochromocytoma is readily detected by serial biochemical and radiographic evaluation, and there is substantial morbidity and mortality associated with the addisonian state.

Preoperatively, patients with pheochromocytomas should be hospitalized to receive alpha-adrenergic blockade with phenoxybenzamine. They should be expected to develop postural hypotension. Beta-adrenergic blockade may be necessary if tachycardia or arrhythmia develops after phenoxybenzamine is administered. Beta-adrenergic blockade without prior alpha-adrenergic blockade is dangerous because patients are subjected to unopposed vasoconstriction. Intraoperative control of hypertension occurring with manipulation of the tumor is most effectively achieved with sodium nitroprusside or phentolamine. Laparoscopic adrenalectomy is a reasonable choice for excision of small pheochromocytoma(s) adequately localized by preoperative imaging studies.

Hyperparathyroidism. The characteristic parathyroid lesion in patients with MEN 2A is hyperplasia with involvement of all four glands. In patients with documented hypercalcemia, one can expect to find enlarged parathyroid glands at operation. However, grossly enlarged parathyroid glands may be found during thyroidectomy for MTC in a patient in whom hyperparathyroidism has never been documented. Although some surgeons perform a subtotal (3½ gland) parathyroidectomy in patients with parathyroid hyperplasia and MEN 2A, the authors perform total parathyroidectomy with autograft of parathyroid tissue into the forearm musculature. In patients without hypercalcemia undergoing thyroidectomy for MTC, grossly normal parathyroid glands should be left in place.

Prognosis

The course of MEN 2A and MEN 2B is essentially that of the thyroid lesion. MTC generally has an intermediate grade of malignancy, as compared with the more malignant anaplastic thyroid carcinomas or the less malignant papillary or follicular carcinomas. However, MTC exhibits variable biologic aggressiveness within the different MEN syndromes and sometimes from kindred to kindred. The MTC in the setting of MEN 2B is aggressive, and patients may die at a young age. MTC in patients with MEN 2A is usually indolent and progresses slowly. In some patients the disease has a more aggressive course.

Bigner and associates[2] evaluated resected tissue from 72 patients with MEN 2A who had undergone total thyroidectomy. They found that metastases to regional lymph nodes and residual MTC postoperatively, as indicated by increased plasma calcitonin levels, were significantly higher in patients who had larger primary thyroid malignancies (>1.5 cm. in diameter) than in patients who had smaller lesions (<0.5 cm. in diameter). Wells and associates[39] evaluated 92 patients with familial MTC to determine if the stimulated plasma calcitonin level was of prognostic significance. Patients whose preoperative peak stimulated plasma calcitonin levels

TABLE 23–11. Plasma Calcitonin (CT) Levels and Prognosis

Group	Preop. CT (pg./ml.)	RLNM* (%)	Postop. CT* (%) (>300 pg./ml.)	DM (%)	DTH (%)
1	250–1000 (n = 25)	1 (4)	1 (4)	0	0
2	1000–5000 (n = 36)	3 (8.3)	6 (16.7)	0	0
3	5000–10,000 (n = 8)	2 (25)	1 (12.5)	0	0
4	>10,000 (n = 23)	13 (57)	14 (61)	4 (17)	2 (8.7)

*Group 1 or Group 2 versus Group 4, p < 0.001.
Preop CT, preoperative stimulated plasma CT level; Postop CT, postoperative stimulated plasma CT level; RLNM, regional lymph node metastases; DM, distant metastases; DTH, death.

were less than 1000 pg. per ml. had a much better prognosis than patients whose peak calcitonin levels were greater than 10,000 pg. per ml. Specifically, metastases to regional lymph nodes, residual MTC postoperatively, distant metastases, and death were significantly less frequent in the former group than in the latter (Table 23–11).

Patients whose MTC is diagnosed biochemically have a more favorable pathologic stage than do patients whose tumor is diagnosed clinically. The authors' group[38] has divided patients into three categories: those with no clinical evidence of MTC and undetectable basal plasma calcitonin levels that become elevated following provocative testing with calcium or pentagastrin (Group 1), patients with no clinical evidence of MTC but elevated basal plasma calcitonin levels (Group 2), and patients with clinically evident MTC (Group 3). Regional lymph node metastases were present less frequently in cases diagnosed biochemically (5/28; Groups 1 and 2) than in those where there was clinically evident disease (15/24; Group 3, p <.02). In addition, the incidence of residual MTC after thyroidectomy, as evidenced by persistently elevated stimulated plasma calcitonin levels postoperatively, was less frequent in cases diagnosed biochemically (6/34; Groups 1 and 2) than in those patients with clinically evident MTC (17/26; Group 3, p<.002).

The ideal treatment of nonresectable metastatic MTC is unclear. MTC is relatively resistant to radiation therapy, and studies evaluating treatment with various chemotherapeutic agents have infrequently demonstrated significant responsiveness. It is imperative that the family with hereditary MTC be identified by an aggressive screening program because with early diagnosis and early thyroidectomy MTC is curable in a large percentage of patients.

SELECTED REFERENCES

Larsson, C., Skogseid, B., Oberg, K., Nakamura, Y., and Nordenskjöld, M.: Multiple endocrine neoplasia type I gene maps to chromosome 11 and is lost in insulinoma. Nature, 332:85, 1988.
This is the original report that maps the MEN 1 gene to chromosome 11 by genetic studies. Important observations of allelic loss on chromosome 11 in tumor DNA from a pair of brothers with MEN 1 and insulinoma also demonstrate that oncogenesis in MEN 1 is consistent with a two-hit *model that involves inactivation of both copies of a tumor-suppressor gene.*

Mulligan, L. M., Kwok, J. B. J., Healey, C. S., Elsdon, M. J., Eng, C., Gardner, E., Love, D. R., Mole, S. E., Moore, J. K., Papi, L., Ponder, M. A., Telenius, H., Tunnacliffe, A., and Ponder, B. A. J.: Germ-line mutations of the RET proto-oncogene in multiple endocrine neoplasia type 2A. Nature, 363:458, 1993.

Donis-Keller, H., Dou, S., Chi, D., Carlson, K. M., Toshima, K., Lairmore, T. C., Howe, J. R., Moley, J. F., Goodfellow, P. and Wells, S. A., Jr.: Mutations in the RET proto-oncogene are associated with MEN 2A and FMTC. Hum. Mol. Genet., 2:851, 1993.

These papers report the identification of missense germline mutations in the RET proto-oncogene that are associated with MEN 2A. The mutations produce amino acid substitutions affecting one of several conserved cysteine residues in the extracellular ligand-binding domain of RET, a tyrosine kinase receptor. These reports allowed the introduction of direct DNA testing to identify patients who have inherited a mutation for MEN 2A.

Wells, S. A., Jr., Chi, D., Toshima, K., Dehner, L. P., Coffin, C. M., Dowton, S. B., Ivanovich, J. L., DeBenedetti, M. K., Dilley, W. G., Moley, J. F., Norton, J. A., and Donis-Keller, H.: Predictive DNA testing and prophylactic thyroidectomy in patients at risk for multiple endocrine neoplasia type 2A. Ann. Surg., 220:237, 1994.

The investigators used direct DNA testing to identify patients who had inherited a mutation for MEN 2A and performed prophylactic thyroidectomy in 13 patients. C-cell hyperplasia with or without medullary thyroid carcinoma was present in the resected thyroid gland from each patient. There were no metastases to cervical lymph nodes, and postoperative plasma calcitonin levels were normal. This article reports the use of preventative surgical treatment based on direct DNA testing for germline mutations in this familial cancer syndrome.

REFERENCES

1. Ballard, H. S., Frame, B., and Hartsock, R. J.: Familial multiple endocrine adenoma–peptic ulcer complex. Medicine, 43:481, 1964.
2. Bigner, M. L., Mendelsohn, G., Wells, S. A., Jr., Cox, E. B., Baylin, S. B., and Eggleston, J. C.: Medullary carcinoma of the thyroid in the multiple endocrine neoplasia IIa syndrome. Am. J. Surg. Pathol., 5:459, 1981.
3. Brandi, M. L., Aurbach, G. D., Fitzpatrick, L. A., Quarto, R., Spiegel, A. M., Bliziotes, M. M., Norton, J. A., Doppman, J. L., and Marx, S. J.: Parathyroid mitogenic activity in plasma from patients with familial multiple endocrine neoplasia type 1. N. Engl. J. Med., 314:1287, 1986.
4. Brandi, M. L., Marx, S. J., Aurbach, G. D., and Fitzpatrick, L. A.: Familial multiple endocrine neoplasia type 1: A new look at pathophysiology. Endocr. Rev., 8:391, 1987.
5. Byström, C., Larsson, C., Blomberg, C., Sandelin, K., Falkmer, U., Skogseid, B., Öberg, K., Werner, S., and Nordenskjöld, M.: Localization of the MEN 1 gene to a small region within chromosome 11q13 by deletion mapping in tumors. Proc. Natl. Acad. Sci. U S A, 87:1968, 1990.
6. Carlson, K. M., Dou, S., Chi, D., Scavarda, N., Toshima, K., Jackson, C. E., Wells, S. A., Jr., Goodfellow, P. J., and Donis-Keller, H.: Single missense mutation in the tyrosine kinase catalytic domain of the RET proto-oncogene is associated with multiple endocrine neoplasia type 2B. Proc. Nat. Acad. Sci. U S A, 91:1579, 1994.
7. Donis-Keller, H., Dou, S., Chi, D., Carlson, K. M., Toshima, K., Lairmore, T. C., Howe, J. R., Moley, J. F., Goodfellow, P., and Wells, S. A., Jr.: Mutations in the RET proto-oncogene are associated with MEN 2A and FMTC. Hum. Mol. Genet., 2:851, 1993.
8. Edery, P., Lyonnet, S., Mulligan, L. M., Pelet, A., Dow, E., Abel, L., Holder, S., Nihoul-Fekete, C., Ponder, B. A. J., and Munnich, A.: Mutations of the RET proto-oncogene in Hirschsprung's disease. Nature, 367:378, 1994.
9. Farndon, J. R., Leight, G. S., Dilley, W. G., Baylin, S. B., Smallridge, R. C., Harrison, T. S., and Wells, S. A., Jr.: Familial medullary thyroid carcinoma without associated endocrinopathies: A distinct clinical entity. Br. J. Surg., 73:278, 1986.
10. Fujimori, M., Wells, S. A., Jr., and Nakamura, Y.: Fine-scale mapping of the gene responsible for multiple endocrine neoplasia type I (MENI). Am. J. Hum. Genet., 50:399, 1992.
11. Fusco, A., Grieco, M., Santoro, M., Berlingieri, M. T., Pilotti, S., Pierotti, M. A., Della Porta, G., and Vecchio, G.: A new oncogene in human thyroid papillary carcinomas and their lymph-nodal metastases. Nature, 328:170, 1987.
12. Hennessy, J. F., Wells, S. A., Jr., Ontjes, D. A., and Cooper, C. W.: A comparison of pentagastrin injection and calcium infusion as provocative agents for the detection of medullary carcinoma of the thyroid. J. Clin. Endocrinol. Metab., 39:487, 1974.
13. Hofstra, R. M. W., Landsvater, R. M., Ceccherini, I., Stulp, R. P., Stelwagen, T., Luo, Y., Pasini, B., Hoppener, J. W. M., Ploos van Amstel, H. K., Romeo, G., Lips, C. J. M., and Buys, C. H. C. M.: A mutation in the RET proto-oncogene associated with multiple endocrine neoplasia type 2B and sporadic medullary thyroid carcinoma. Nature, 367:375, 1994.
14. Lairmore, T. C., Ball, D. W., Baylin, S. B., and Wells, S. A., Jr.: Management of pheochromocytomas in patients with multiple endocrine neoplasia type 2 syndromes. Ann. Surg., 217:595, 1993.
15. Lairmore, T. C., Howe, J. R., Korte, J. A., Dilley, W. G., Aine, L., Aine, E., Wells, S. A., Jr., and Donis-Keller, H.: Familial medullary thyroid carcinoma and multiple endocrine neoplasia type 2B map to the same region of chromosome 10 as multiple endocrine neoplasia type 2A. Genomics, 9:181, 1991.
16. Larsson, C., Skogseid, B., Öberg, K., Nakamura, Y., and Nordenskjöld, M.: Multiple endocrine neoplasia type 1 gene maps to chromosome 11 and is lost in insulinoma. Nature, 332:85, 1988.
17. Lips, C. J. M., Landsvater, R. M., Höppener, J. W. M., Geerdink, R. A., Blijham, G., Jansen-Schillhorn van Veen, J. M., van Gils, A. P. G., de Wit, M. J., Zewald, R. A., Berends, M. J. H., Beemer, F. A., Brouwers-Smalbraak, J., Jansen, R. P. M., Ploos van Amstel, H. K., van Vroonhoven, T. J. M. V., and Vroom, T. M.: Clinical screening as compared with DNA analysis in

families with multiple endocrine neoplasia type 2A. N. Engl. J. Med., *331:*828, 1994.

18. Majewski, J. T., and Wilson, S. D.: The MEN-I syndrome: An all-or-none phenomenon. Surgery, *86:*475, 1979.

19. Mathew, C. G. P., Chin, K. S., Easton, D. F., Thorpe, K., Carter, C., Liou, G. I., Fong, S. L., Bridges, C. D. B., Haak, H., Nieuwenhuijzen Kruseman, A. C., Schifter, S., Hansen, H. H., Telenius, H., Telenius-Berg, M., and Ponder, B. A. J.: A linked genetic marker for multiple endocrine neoplasia type 2A on chromosome 10. Nature, *328:* 527, 1987.

20. Mathew, C. G. P., Easton, D. F., Nakamura, Y., Ponder, B. A. J., and Group, T. M. I. C.: Presymptomatic screening for multiple endocrine neoplasia type 2A with linked DNA markers. Lancet, *337:* 7, 1991.

21. Melvin, K. E. W., Miller, H. H., and Tashjian, A. H., Jr.: Early diagnosis of medullary carcinoma of the thyroid gland by means of calcitonin assay. N. Engl. J. Med., *285:*1115, 1971.

22. Moley, J. F., Wells, S. A., Dilley, W. G., and Tisell, L. E.: Reoperation for recurrent or persistent medullary thyroid cancer. Surgery, *114:*1090, 1993.

23. Mulligan, L. M., Kwok, J. B. J., Healey, C. S., Elsdon, M. J., Eng, C., Gardner, E., Love, D. R., Mole, S. E., Moore, J. K., Papi, L., Ponder, M. A., Telenius, H., Tunnacliffe, A., and Ponder, B. A. J.: Germ-line mutations of the *RET* proto-oncogene in multiple endocrine neoplasia type 2A. Nature, *363:*458, 1993.

24. Norum, R. A., Lafreniere, R. G., O'Neal, L. W., Nikolai, T. F., Delaney, J. P., Sisson, J. C., Sobol, H., Lenoir, G. M., Ponder, B. A. J., Willard, H. F., and Jackson, C. E.: Linkage of the multiple endocrine neoplasia type 2B gene (MEN 2B) to chromosome 10 markers linked to MEN 2A. Genomics, *8:*313, 1990.

25. Prinz, R. A., Gamvros, D. I., Selly, D., and Lynn, J. A.: Subtotal parathyroidectomy for primary chief cell hyperplasia in the multiple endocrine neoplasia type I syndrome. Ann. Surg., *193:*26, 1981.

26. Romeo, G., Ronchetto, P., Luo, Y., Barone, V., Seri, M., Ceccherini, I., Pasini, B., Bocciardi, R., Lerone, M., Kaarlainen, H., and Martucciello, G.: Point mutations affecting the tyrosine kinase domain of the *RET* proto-oncogene in Hirschsprung's disease. Nature, *367:*377, 1994.

27. Santoro, M., Carlomagno, F., Romano, A., Bottaro, D. P., Dathan, N. A., Grieco, M., Fusco, A., Vecchio, G., Matoskova, B., Kraus, M. H., and Di Fiore, P. P.: Activation of *RET* as a dominantly transforming gene by germline mutations of MEN 2A and MEN 2B. Science, *267:*381, 1995.

28. Schuchardt, A., D'Agati, V., Larsson-Blomberg, L., Costantini, F., and Pachnis, V.: Defects in the kidney and enteric nervous system of mice lacking the tyrosine kinase receptor. Ret. Nature, *367:*380, 1994.

29. Simpson, N. E., Kidd, K. K., Goodfellow, P. J., McDermid, H., Myers, S., Kidd, J. R., Jackson, C. E., Duncan, A. M. V., Farrer, L. A., Brasch, K., Castiglione, C., Genel, M., Gertner, J., Greenberg, C. R., Gusella, J. F., Holden, J. J. A., and White, B. N.: Assignment of multiple endocrine neoplasia type 2A to chromosome 10 by genetic linkage. Nature, *328:*528, 1987.

30. Sipple, J. H.: The association of pheochromocytoma with carcinoma of the thyroid gland. Am. J. Med., *31:*163, 1961.

31. Sisson, J. C., Frager, M. S., Valk, T. W., Gross, M. D., Swanson, D. P., Wieland, D. M., Tobes, M. C., Beierwaltes, W. H., and Thompson, N. W.: Scintigraphic localization of pheochromocytoma. N. Engl. J. Med., *305:*12, 1981.

32. Sletten, K., Westermark, P., and Natvig, J. B.: Characterization of amyloid fibril proteins from medullary carcinoma of the thyroid. J. Exp. Med., *143:*993, 1976.

33. Tashjian, A. H., Jr., Howland, B. G., Melvin, K. E. W., and Hill, C. S., Jr.: Immunoassay of human calcitonin: Clinical measurement, relation to serum calcium and studies in patients with medullary carcinoma. N. Engl. J. Med., *283:*890, 1970.

34. Tisell, L. E., Hansson, G., Jansson, S., and Salander, H.: Reoperation in the treatment of asymptomatic metastasizing medullary thyroid carcinoma. Surgery, *99:*60, 1986.

35. van Heerden, J. A., Kent, R. B., Sizemore, G. W., Grant, C. S., and ReMine, W. M.: Primary hyperparathyroidism in patients with multiple endocrine neoplasia syndromes: Surgical experience. Arch. Surg., *118:*533, 1983.

36. van Heerden, J. A., Sizemore, G. W., Carney, J. A., Grant, C. S., ReMine, W. H., and Sheps, S. G.: Surgical management of the adrenal glands in the multiple endocrine neoplasia type II syndrome. World J. Surg., *8:*612, 1984.

37. Vieto, R. J., Hickey, R. C., and Samaan, N. A.: Type 1 multiple endocrine neoplasias. Curr. Probl. Cancer, *7:*1, 1982.

38. Wells, S. A., Jr., Baylin, S. B., Gann, D. S., Farrell, R. E., Dilley, W. G., Preissig, S. H., Linehan, W. M., and Cooper, C. W.: Medullary thyroid carcinoma: Relationship of method of diagnosis to pathologic staging. Ann. Surg., *188:*377, 1978.

39. Wells, S. A., Jr., Baylin, S. B., Leight, G. S., Dale, J. K., Dilley, W. G., and Farndon, J. R.: The importance of early diagnosis in patients with hereditary medullary thyroid carcinoma. Ann. Surg., *195:*595, 1982.

40. Wells, S. A., Jr., Baylin, S. B., Linehan, W. M., Farrell, R. E., Cox, E. B., and Cooper, C. W.: Provocative agents and the diagnosis of medullary carcinoma of the thyroid gland. Ann. Surg., *188:*139, 1978.

41. Wells, S. A., Jr., Chi, D., Toshima, K., Dehner, L. P., Coffin, C. M., Dowton, S. B., Ivanovich, J. L., DeBenedetti, M. K., Dilley, W. G., Moley, J. F., Norton, J. A., and Donis-Keller, H.: Predictive DNA testing and prophylactic thyroidectomy in patients at risk for multiple endocrine neoplasia type 2A. Ann. Surg., *220:*237, 1994.

42. Wells, S. A., Jr., Farndon, J. R., Dale, J. K., Leight, G. S., and Dilley, W. G.: Long-term evaluation of patients with primary parathyroid hyperplasia managed by total parathyroidectomy and heterotopic autotransplantation. Ann. Surg., *192:*451, 1980.

43. Wieland, D. M., Wu, J., Brown, L. E., Mangner, T. J., Swanson, D. P., and Beierwaltes, W. H.: Radiolabeled adrenergic neuron-blocking agents: Adrenomedullary imaging with (^{131}I) iodobenzylguanidine. J. Nucl. Med., *21:*349, 1980.

CHAPTER 24

THE PARATHYROID GLANDS

Gerard M. Doherty, M.D., and Samuel A. Wells, Jr., M.D.

HISTORICAL ASPECTS

In 1880, a Swedish student, Ivar Sandstrom, first described the parathyroid glands in several animals, including man.[45] His discovery went unnoticed until 1891, when the glands were rediscovered by Gley, who demonstrated that their removal led to tetany.[25] MacCallum and Voegtlin subsequently noted a decrease in blood calcium levels of thyroparathyroidectomized animals and found that the tetany that ensued could be corrected by the infusion of calcium salts.[31]

In the same year as Gley's discovery, von Recklinghausen described a characteristic disease of bone that later was found to be caused by hyperparathyroidism.[54] The first to describe the association of bone disease and parathyroid neoplasia was Askanazy, who in 1904 studied a woman with pain in the extremities and spontaneous fractures.[6] At autopsy, she was found to have both the generalized osteitis fibrosa cystica described earlier by von Recklinghausen and "incidental" tumor lateral to the thyroid gland. In 1907, Erdheim studied several patients who had died of osteomalacia and correctly concluded that the marked parathyroid hyperplasia observed was secondary to the bone disease.[22] Thereafter, the theory evolved that all parathyroid tumors, single as well as multiple, arose to compensate for various osseous abnormalities. Schlagenhaufer, in 1915, argued that it was unlikely for compensatory hypertrophy to involve only a single gland and suggested that some parathyroid tumors were primary and caused secondary changes in the skeleton.[47] Mandl confirmed this hypothesis 10 years later when he excised an enlarged parathyroid gland from a Viennese streetcar conductor who was admitted to the hospital clinic with hypercalcemia, hypercalciuria, roentgenographic changes of von Recklinghausen's bone disease, and a broken leg.[32] After surgical therapy, the calcium levels in the blood and urine decreased, the bones became more dense and pain free, and the patient became ambulatory. Within 6 years, however, his disease recurred and became progressively worse, ultimately causing death. At the time of recurrence, he underwent a second neck exploration, but no abnormal parathyroid tissue was found then or at necropsy 3 years later.

The first parathyroid exploration in the United States was performed in 1926 at the Massachusetts General Hospital on a merchant mariner with severe bone disease, Captain Charles Martell.[41] Unfortunately, the abnormal gland was not found until his seventh operation in 1932; he subsequently died in tetany during a ureterolithotomy. The first successful parathyroidectomy was performed at Barnes Hospital in St. Louis in 1929 and was reported by Barr and Bulger,[8] who first proposed the term *hyperparathyroidism*. In 1934, Albright and colleagues noted an association of osteitis fibrosa cystica with renal stones and subsequently identified a group of patients with hyperparathyroidism who had calculi or nephrocalcinosis but no bone disease.[2]

Biologically active parathyroid extracts were first prepared by Collip in 1925.[16] Parathyroid hormone (PTH) was isolated and purified by Rasmussen and Craig[39] and Aurbach[7] in 1959. In 1963, Berson and associates developed a radioimmunoassay for PTH.[9]

EMBRYOLOGY

Phylogenetically, the parathyroids appear relatively late, being first seen in the Amphibia. In man, the superior parathyroids arise from the fourth pharyngeal pouch and the inferior parathyroids arise from the third pharyngeal pouch (Fig. 24–1). During the branchial complex stage, the glands are intimately associated with the derivatives of their respective pouches—the inferior parathyroids with the thymus and the superior parathyroids with the lateral thyroid complex. As the embryo matures and the thymus cord descends, the inferior parathyroids migrate caudad. Typically, the separation of these glands from the thymus becomes complete when they lie posterior to the lower pole of the thyroid lobe. This migration is extremely variable; as a result, the inferior glands are more likely to be found in an ectopic location than the superior glands. At one extreme the parathyroids may be found embedded in the pharyngeal mucosa, or, at the other, they may be found in the thoracic cavity, usually adherent to the thymus gland. Rarely, the parathyroids become completely enclosed within the thyroid parenchyma during migration of the lateral thyroid complex.

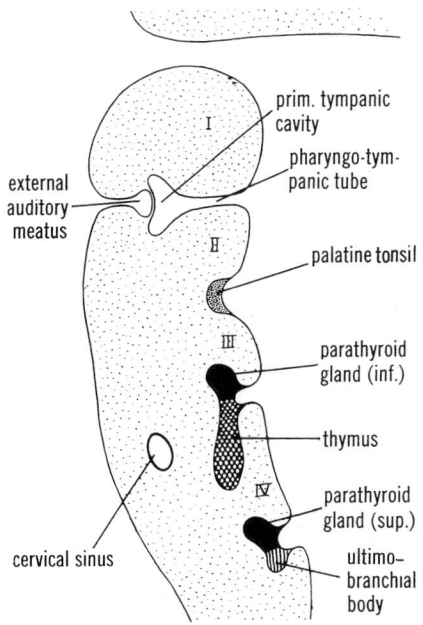

Figure 24–1. Schematic representation of the development of the pharyngeal pouches. The inferior parathyroid arises from the third pouch in conjunction with the thymus; the superior arises from the fourth in conjunction with the developing thyroid or ultimobranchial body. (From Langman, J.: Medical Embryology, 3rd ed. Baltimore, Williams & Wilkins, 1975, p. 266.)

ANATOMY

Typically, there are four parathyroid glands. In Alveryd's series of 354 adults studied at autopsy, 90.6% had four glands, 3.7% had five glands, 5.1% had three glands, and 0.6% had two glands.[4] In only 1 of Alveryd's 18 patients with three identified parathyroids was the combined weight of the glands sufficiently high to suggest that none had been overlooked.

Akerstrom and associates performed autopsy studies on 503 cadavers and found four parathyroid glands in all but 18 cadavers (3%).[1] In 421 cases, there were four glands; however, more than four glands were detected in 64 cases (13%). Most often, the supernumerary gland was located in the thymus. The anatomic location of the parathyroid glands demonstrated considerable constancy and is shown in Figure 24–2. In each of the two patients with renal osteodystrophy, eight parathyroid glands were identified.

In the 109 cases of Norris[35] and the 35 cases of Boyd[13] in which parathyroids were identified by studying serial sections of embryos, at least four parathyroid glands were found in every specimen. Norris considered supernumerary glands the result of the separation of parathyroid remnants when the glands pulled away from the pouch structures during the branchial complex phase.

The vascular supply to the parathyroid glands is usually from the inferior thyroid artery, but it can arise from the superior thyroid artery, the lowest thyroid artery (thyroid ima), and arteries in the larynx, trachea, esophagus, or mediastinum or from anastomoses between these vessels. The inferior, middle, and superior thyroid veins drain the parathyroid glands.

About 50% of all parathyroids are found adjacent to the area where the inferior thyroid artery enters the thyroid parenchyma. The superior parathyroid glands are usually embedded in fat and located on the posterior surface of the middle or upper portion of the thyroid lobe close to the point where the recurrent laryngeal nerve enters the larynx. The lower parathyroid glands are more ventral, close to the lower pole of the thyroid gland and the *thyrothymic ligament.* In 1% to 5% of patients, an inferior parathyroid gland is located in the deep mediastinum. The normal glands tend to be flat and ovoid; but on enlargement, they become globular. Nor-

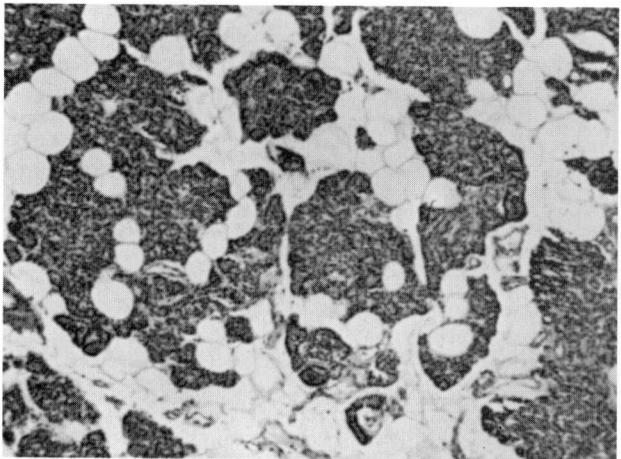

Figure 24–3. Normal adult parathyroid, composed of approximately 50% parenchymal cells and 50% stromal fat.

mally, they measure 5 to 7 mm. by 3 to 4 mm. by 0.5 to 2 mm. The combined weight of the parathyroid glands is 90 to 200 mg., and the upper glands are generally smaller than the lower. In adults, the parathyroids are usually red-brown to yellow, whereas in the newborn they are gray and semitransparent.

HISTOLOGY

The parathyroid glands consist of a parenchyma containing chief and oxyphil cells and a stroma composed primarily of adipocytes (Fig. 24–3). The chief and oxyphil cells are arranged in trabeculae or islands. The main cell of primate glands and the only cell of many lower species is the chief cell. Through infancy and early childhood the glands are composed almost entirely of chief cells. Normally present but few in number are the polygonal water-clear cells, which are glycogen-laden chief cells with little visible cytoplasm. Acidophilic, mitochondria-rich oxyphil cells appear near puberty and increase in number with age. The functional significance of the various cell types remains unclear. The water-clear and oxyphil cells are derived from chief cells and apparently remain capable of secreting PTH.

PHYSIOLOGY

Mineral Metabolism

Calcium is a constituent of all animal fluids and is involved in a variety of physiologic processes, from blood coagulation and bone formation to milk production. It represents a major cellular messenger and is critical in both muscle contraction and membrane repolarization. It constitutes about 2% of the adult body weight, and almost all is contained in the skeleton. Plasma calcium measures 9.0 to 10.5 mg. per 100 ml. (4.5 to 5.2 mEq. per liter) and is approximately equally divided between an ionized and a protein-bound phase. Five percent is bound to organic anions. Approximately 80% of the bound calcium is complexed to albumin. The amount of protein and the body fluid pH are the two most important factors regulating the distribution of calcium in plasma. Hydrogen ion competes with calcium for the same binding sites for all the calcium binding proteins in plasma. In general, for each 1 gm. per 100 ml. alteration in the total protein there is a similar 0.8 mg. per 100 ml. change in the total serum calcium level. Of greatest importance is the ionized calcium, which is the form most immediately related to the activity of the parathyroid glands.

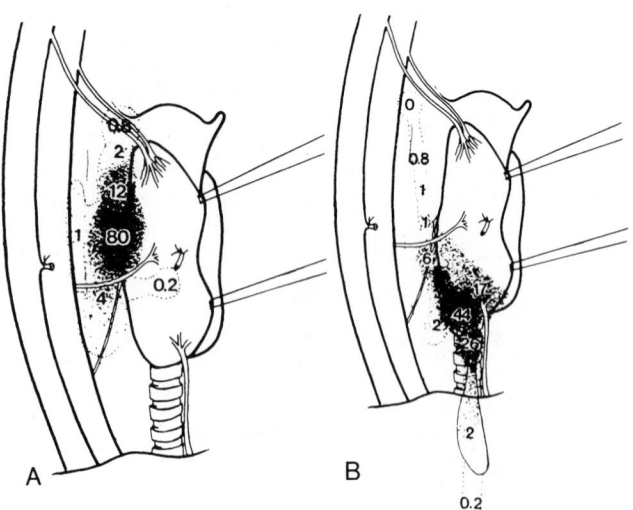

Figure 24–2. Locations of the superior *(A)* and inferior *(B)* parathyroid glands. The more common locations are indicated by the darker shading. The numbers represent the percentages of glands found at the different locations. (From Akerström, G., Malmaeus, J., and Bergstrom, R.: Surgical anatomy of human parathyroid glands. Surgery, *95:*17, 1984.)

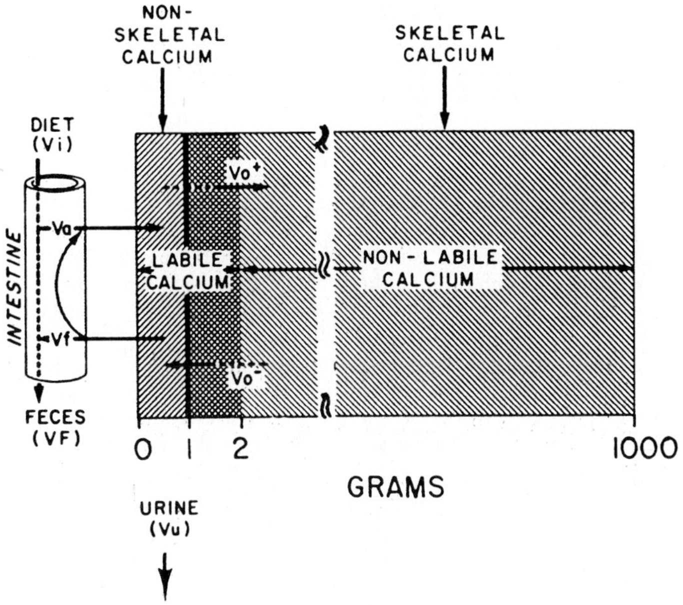

Figure 24–4. Schematic representation of calcium distribution and exchange. The skeletal calcium is denoted by all of the area to the right of the heavy vertical line. Of the 2 gm. of labile calcium in the body, approximately one half is skeletal and one half nonskeletal. Vi, dietary calcium intake; VF, fecal calcium; Va, calcium absorption; Vf, endogenous fecal calcium; Vo+, bone calcium accretion; Vo–, bone calcium release; Vu, urinary calcium excretion. (From Bringhurst F. R.: Calcium and phosphate distribution, turnover, and metabolic actions. In DeGroot L. J. [Ed.]: Endocrinology, 3rd ed. Philadelphia, W. B. Saunders, 1995, pp. 1015–1043.)

Calcium, in the inorganic form, is absorbed in the upper small intestine. On a regular diet, approximately 1 gm. is ingested daily. The calcium in the extracellular fluid is constantly being exchanged with that in the exchangeable bone, the intracellular fluid, and the glomerular filtrate, 99% of which is reabsorbed by the normal kidney (Fig. 24–4).

The adult body contains about 700 gm. of phosphate, most being located in the bones and teeth. Plasma phosphate measures 2.5 to 4.3 mg. per 100 ml. The plasma levels of calcium and phosphate vary inversely with one another. Normally, the relationship is such that the product of plasma calcium and phosphate (measured in milligrams per 100 ml.) is constant and between 30 and 40. On a regular diet, approximately 1500 mg. is ingested daily.

Magnesium, the fourth most abundant metal in mammals and the second most prevalent intracellular cation, is located primarily in the mineral phase of bone. Magnesium is important in the activation of enzymes necessary for intermediary metabolism and phosphorylation, in protein and nucleic acid synthesis, and in mitochondrial regulation. Approximately 300 mg. is ingested daily.

Regulation of Calcium Metabolism

The primary agents responsible for regulation of calcium metabolism are PTH, vitamin D, and calcitonin. Their major actions are summarized in Table 24–1.

Parathyroid Hormone. PTH is synthesized within the parathyroid as a larger precursor, pre-proparathyroid hor-

mone, which is cleaved in the parathyroid first to proparathyroid hormone and then to the final 84-amino acid PTH. The hormone is secreted and then metabolized in the liver into hormonally active N-terminal and inactive C-terminal fragments. PTH secretion is inversely related to the serum calcium level and also to the levels of 1,25-dihydroxyvitamin D. It has direct effects on the kidney and skeleton and indirect effects on the gastrointestinal tract through vitamin D.

In the skeleton, PTH promotes a release of calcium in two phases. The first is by an active transport process, and the second is by a process that requires lysosomal enzymes and the synthesis of hydrolytic enzymes. PTH inhibits osteoblasts and stimulates osteoclasts.

In the kidney, PTH causes a decrease in calcium clearance at any specific concentration of extracellular fluid calcium. Calcium is cleared linearly with sodium, and it appears that these two ions share a common transport mechanism. The hormone also causes an increased excretion of renal phosphate by inhibiting its reabsorption in the renal tubule. Enhanced bicarbonate secretion is also promoted by PTH. PTH stimulates hydroxylation of 25-hydroxyvitamin D to 1,25-dihydroxyvitamin D in the kidney, and it is the latter metabolite that then causes enhanced absorption of calcium from the intestine.

Vitamin D. The major D vitamins are vitamin D_2 and vitamin D_3. The most important physiologically is vitamin D_3, which is derived from ultraviolet activation of 7-dehydrocholesterol in the skin. The bulk of commercially prepared vitamin D is vitamin D_2. It is derived from ergosterol and is

TABLE 24–1. Actions of Major Calcium-Regulating Hormones

	Bone	Kidney	Intestine
Parathyroid hormone	Stimulates resorption of calcium and phosphate	Stimulates reabsorption of calcium and conversion of 25(OH)D_3 to 1,25 (OH)$_2D_3$; inhibits reabsorption of phosphate and bicarbonate	No direct effects
Vitamin D	Stimulates transport of calcium	Inhibits reabsorption of calcium	Stimulates absorption of calcium and phosphate
Calcitonin	Inhibits resorption of calcium and phosphate	Inhibits reabsorption of calcium and phosphate	No direct effects

the major form of vitamin D used clinically in the treatment of certain skeletal diseases. Vitamin D increases the intestinal absorption of calcium, and secondarily phosphate, and increases the mobilization of calcium and phosphate from bone to blood. Vitamin D appears to exert a growth-promoting effect that is not explained by mineral retention.

Calcitonin. Calcitonin inhibits bone resorption and produces hypocalcemia when administered to experimental animals. The hormone also induces the urinary excretion of calcium and phosphate. Several secretagogues for calcitonin have been identified, including beta-adrenergic catecholamines, glucagon, and cholecystokinin, but the most potent appear to be calcium and pentagastrin.

The activity of PTH and calcitonin appears to be mediated by cyclic 3′5′-adenosine monophosphate (AMP) produced through specific hormonal activation of the enzyme adenyl cyclase in bone and kidney. Calcitonin has not been demonstrated to be important in the control of serum calcium in man.

In summary, the serum calcium level is closely regulated by the action of PTH. A reduction in the amount of serum ionized calcium increases secretion of PTH, which secondarily stimulates production of 1,25-dihydroxyvitamin D_3. Conversely, a rise in serum calcium inhibits both PTH secretion and the formation of active calciferol.

DISORDERS OF THE PARATHYROID GLANDS

Hyperparathyroidism

The cause of spontaneous hyperfunction of the parathyroid glands is unknown and, as with many endocrine neoplasms, overactivity is recognized not because of anatomic enlargement but because of the peripheral effects of excess hormone. Primary hyperparathyroidism occurs when the normal feedback control by serum calcium is disturbed and there is increased production of PTH. Secondary hyperparathyroidism occurs most commonly in patients with renal disease but also compensates for the true hypocalcemia associated with some diseases of the gastrointestinal tract, bone, or other endocrine organs. There is a defect in mineral homeostasis leading to a compensatory increase in parathyroid gland function and size. Occasionally with prolonged compensatory stimulation, a hyperplastic gland develops autonomous function. This state is referred to as tertiary hyperparathyroidism.

Primary Hyperparathyroidism

Formerly thought to be a relatively rare condition associated with advanced renal or bone disease, primary hyperparathyroidism has been detected with increasing frequency in recent years, probably as a result of the widespread use of automated technology for determining serum calcium concentration.

The incidence of hyperparathyroidism is approximately 25 per 100,000 in the general population, and approximately 50,000 new cases occur annually. The incidence of the disease increases markedly with age, and it is especially common in postmenopausal women; in women older than 65 years of age the incidence is 2.5 per 1000. The gender and age of 250 patients with primary hyperparathyroidism studied at the University of California, San Francisco (UCSF), are shown in Figure 24–5.[51] Christensson, in a study of 15,903 individuals undergoing a "health checkup" in Sweden, found the prevalence of hyperparathyroidism to be 5 per 1000.[14] No cause could be found for the substantially higher incidence in that country.

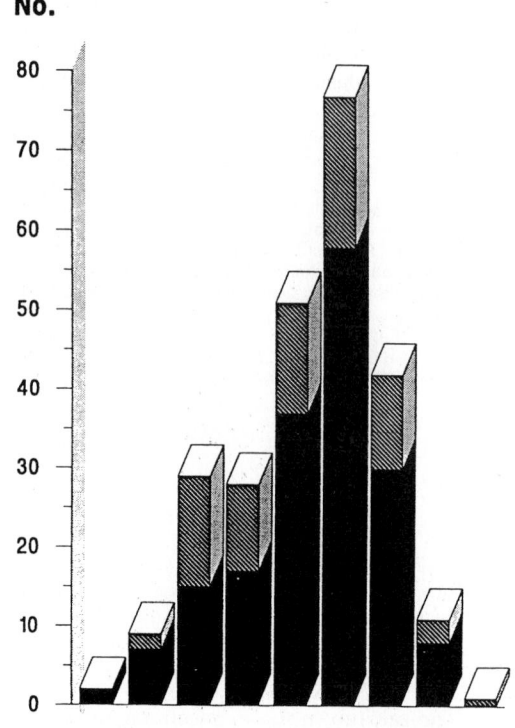

Figure 24–5. Age and gender distribution of 250 patients studied between 1980 and 1990 with surgically proven primary hyperparathyroidism. (From Uden P., Chan A., Duh Q.-Y., Siperstein A., and Clark O. H.: Primary hyperparathyroidism in younger and older patients: Symptoms and outcome of surgery. World J. Surg., *16*:791, 1992.)

ETIOLOGY

The cause of hyperparathyroidism is unknown and probably varies with the underlying pathologic condition. Single-gland or adenomatous disease is more consistent with a mechanism involving spontaneous hyperfunction, whereas multiglandular disease suggests the presence of some exogenous stimulus or underlying genetic defect. Recent studies have challenged the concept of complete parathyroid autonomy. An alteration in the set point, the sensitivity of the glands to suppression by calcium, appears more consistent with the present data. It has been proposed that a renal leak of calcium, if sufficient, may lead to hypocalcemia, thus stimulating PTH secretion and ultimately hyperfunctional parathyroid glands. Loss of renal function with age is associated with increased plasma levels of PTH as well as increases in nephrogenous cyclic AMP and decreases in renal phosphate clearance. This suggests increased biologic effects of PTH. The role that either the renal calcium leak or the increased plasmic levels of PTH with age has in the etiology of hyperparathyroidism is unclear.

Genetic studies of parathyroid adenomas have identified a subset with overexpression of the PRAD1 oncogene, which may be one step toward neoplasia.[5] Overexpression of PRAD1 allows cell cycle progression from the G1 phase to the S phase, thus promoting growth and cell division.

Several investigators have reported an increased incidence of hyperparathyroidism in patients exposed to low-dose ionizing irradiation, usually in childhood. In the study by Christensson, 8 (14%) of 58 individuals found to have hyperparathyroidism had received ionizing irradiation to the neck at a young age.[15] Nine of 58 normal subjects matched for age and sex had not been previously irradiated. Several other investigators have confirmed an association of radiation exposure to the neck and hyperparathyroidism.

Recent data on the etiology of hyperparathyroidism in multiple endocrine neoplasia Type 1 (MEN 1), discussed in Chapter 24 in greater detail, may have significance for sporadic disease as well. Friedman and associates have identified chromosome 11 deletions, including a gene locus previously associated with MEN 1, in 10 of 16 parathyroid tumors in patients with known MEN 1.[24] Similar losses were demonstrated in 11 of 34 sporadic adenomas. This may indicate a relationship between the deletions in MEN 1 and the losses in sporadic adenomas. However, the deleted areas in sporadic adenomas do not always include the 11q13 locus thought to contain the MEN 1 gene. Thus there may be other important genes on chromosome 11 contributing to the growth of sporadic adenomas.

CLINICAL PRESENTATION (SIGNS AND SYMPTOMS)

Since the advent of routine screening for calcium and phosphate, hyperparathyroidism has been detected with increasing frequency. Although in the past most patients presented with severe bone or renal disease, an increasing percentage of patients today are asymptomatic. For example, in the series from UCSF, less than one third of patients had a serious complication that could directly be attributed to parathyroid disease.[51] However, when carefully questioned, many of these patients describe symptoms or associated conditions that can be related to hyperparathyroidism, and their symptoms improved after parathyroidectomy in more than 80% of patients.[51]

The most frequent symptoms in 100 consecutive patients at the time of diagnosis are shown in Table 24–2.[58] The usual symptomatic patient with hyperparathyroidism is in the chronic phase of disease with signs and symptoms from secondary changes in the genitourinary system and skeleton. The earliest complaints, such as muscle weakness, anorexia, nausea, constipation, polyuria, and polydipsia, occasionally cause the patient to seek medical advice; often the examining physician does not suspect hyperparathyroidism.

Renal Complications. Renal complications are generally the most severe clinical manifestations of hyperparathyroidism. Many patients have only frequency, nocturia, and polydipsia, but usually the presenting symptoms are related to nephrolithiasis, which occurs in 25% to 30% of cases. Conversely, 5% to 10% of previously unscreened patients presenting with nephrolithiasis have hyperparathyroidism. Patients complain of back pain, hematuria, and the passing of renal calculi, most of which are composed of calcium phosphate or calcium oxalate. Nephrocalcinosis represents calcification within the parenchyma of one or both kidneys; it occurs in only 5% to 10% of patients with primary hyperparathyroidism. It is very unusual for nephrolithiasis and nephro-

calcinosis to occur simultaneously. Although renal stones can be removed surgically or treated with extracorporeal shock wave lithotripsy, there is little that can be done for nephrocalcinosis; even after definitive treatment of hyperparathyroidism there is rarely improvement of this condition. Renal damage is much more common in patients with nephrocalcinosis, but it can occur in the absence of renal calcification. If renal impairment is severe preoperatively, it tends to remain unchanged or to become progressively worse postoperatively; mild degrees of renal damage are usually functional and reversible. Careful evaluation of renal function reveals some degree of abnormality in 80% to 90% of patients with hyperparathyroidism.

The incidence of hypertension in patients with hyperparathyroidism was about 70% in Hellstrom and Ivemark's series of 139 patients, although other authors have reported a much less marked association[26]; hypertension is more frequent in older than younger patients.[51] Hypertension, with its associated clinical complications (heart failure, cerebral hemorrhage, and renal insufficiency), was responsible for death in 30% of the patients in whom it persisted after parathyroid surgery. Hellstrom and Ivemark's investigation demonstrated in a striking manner the importance of this complication in hyperparathyroidism and the urgency of early diagnosis and treatment if the late cardiovascular and renal sequelae are to be minimized. Various mechanisms have been proposed to explain this relationship of hyperparathyroidism with hypertension; it appears to be most closely correlated with the degree of renal impairment. Despite this, Diamond and associates found that parathyroidectomy led to a substantial fall in both systolic and diastolic pressures in 54% of hypertensive subjects unrelated to improvements in renal function.[19] Unfortunately, such improvement does not always occur.

Bone Disease. The early descriptions of hyperparathyroidism were of patients who had severe bone disease characterized by osteitis fibrosa cystica generalisata, a condition with a unique x-ray picture that is pathognomonic of hyperparathyroidism. Although the incidence of bone disease in patients with primary hyperparathyroidism reported in earlier studies was as high as 50% to 90%, the reported incidence in more current series is 5% to 15%.

Skeletal involvement is most readily demonstrated by radiographs of the hands (Fig. 24–6). Subperiosteal resorption, pathognomonic of hyperparathyroidism, is usually evident on the radial aspect of the middle phalanx of the second or third fingers. In more advanced cases, cysts are present, and there is tufting of the distal phalanges. The skull is the second most commonly affected skeletal site and presents a mottled appearance often associated with diffuse granularity and cystic lesions (Fig. 24–7A). With advanced disease, osteoclastomas, or *brown tumors*, may be present (Fig. 24–8). With the use of more sophisticated and sensitive technology, such as x-ray spectrophotometry and phosphate absorptiometric analysis, subtle derangements in bone density can be detected; the incidence of *bone disease* in patients with hyperparathyroidism has been shown to be relatively common. Although the significance of subtle bone loss has been questioned, Kochersberger and associates have demonstrated an increased prevalence of vertebral fractures in patients undergoing parathyroidectomy, compared with an otherwise matched group of patients undergoing cholecystectomy.[28]

Lloyd evaluated 138 consecutive patients with primary hyperparathyroidism and classified them into three groups: (1) those with bone disease only, (2) those with kidney disease (stones) only, and (3) those with neither bone disease nor kidney disease.[30] Twelve with bone disease had previously suffered from renal stones and were not classified. Comparing patients with bone disease only with those with kidney disease only, the mean plasma calcium was higher (13 versus

TABLE 24–2. Presenting Symptoms in 100 Patients with Primary Hyperparathyroidism

Symptom	Percentage of Population
Nephrolithiasis	30
Bone disease	2
Peptic ulcer disease	12
Psychiatric disorders	15
Muscle weakness	70
Constipation	32
Polyuria	28
Pancreatitis	1
Myalgia	54
Arthralgia	54

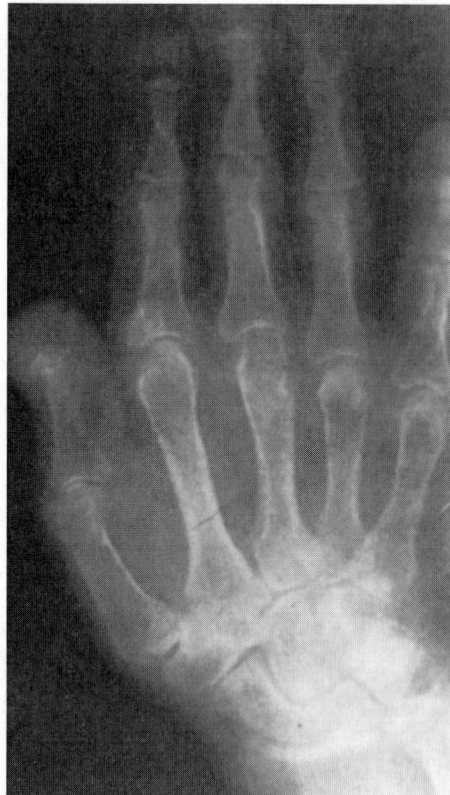

Figure 24–6. Hand radiograph. Note the uniform demineralization with concomitant soft tissue clubbing, severe erosion of distal phalanges, and cyst at base of middle phalanx of index finger. Subperiosteal cortical resorption is best shown along the metacarpal shaft of the fifth digit.

11.6 mg. per 100 ml.; p<.001), the mean tumor weight was greater (5.9 versus 1.05 gm.; p<.001), and the duration of symptoms was shorter (3.6 versus 6.8 years; p<0.001). On the basis of this observation, Lloyd proposed that there were two different types of parathyroid tumors: one growing rapidly, being highly active, and causing overt bone disease, and the other growing slowly, being of low activity, and causing kidney stones. There was no characteristic tumor histology associated with either type of disease, and the basis for this clinical variability remains unexplained.

Gastrointestinal Manifestations. An increased incidence of peptic ulcer disease in patients with primary hyperparathyroidism was first reported by Rogers in 1946.[42] Most subsequent studies have confirmed this association. The association appears logical because the induction of hypercalcemia experimentally in normal subjects is associated with increased gastric acid secretion and hypergastrinemia. In an experimental animal model, Bolman and associates clearly demonstrated that infusion of PTH into the gastroepiploic artery supplying the gastric antrum caused hypergastrinemia, even though blood calcium levels were not increased, which demonstrated the effect of PTH on gastric secretion.[12] Although some investigators have demonstrated significant reductions in serum gastrin levels and gastric acid secretion after the surgical correction of hyperparathyroidism, others have not. At present, it appears that the relationship of hyperparathyroidism to peptic ulcer disease is unclear.

The association of pancreatitis and hyperparathyroidism was first reported by Smith and Cooke in 1940.[49] Even though an increased incidence of pancreatitis was reported from various clinics in the subsequent two decades, there were no carefully controlled studies evaluating the relationship. Rosin screened the records of 1000 patients with hyperparathyroid-

ism between 1962 and 1972 from 26 hospitals in Great Britain and found pancreatitis in less than 1%.[43] A similar incidence was reported in the study of Bess and associates in their analysis of 1153 cases.[10] In the majority of the cases reported in the latter study, the presence of gallstone disease or alcoholism was also detected. Reeve and Delbridge have evaluated the concentration of serum amylase in 86 patients undergoing neck exploration for hyperparathyroidism.[40] Postoperative hyperamylasemia (>300 I.U.) occurred in 35% of the group, and clinically significant pancreatitis (serum amylase of >1000 I.U. associated with abdominal pain) occurred in eight of the patients (9%). Such an association has not been reported by other investigators and awaits confirmation. Pancreatitis also occurs in other conditions producing hypercalcemia.

There also appears to be an increased incidence (25% to 35%) of cholelithiasis in patients with hyperparathyroidism. This is presumably due to a high concentration of calcium in

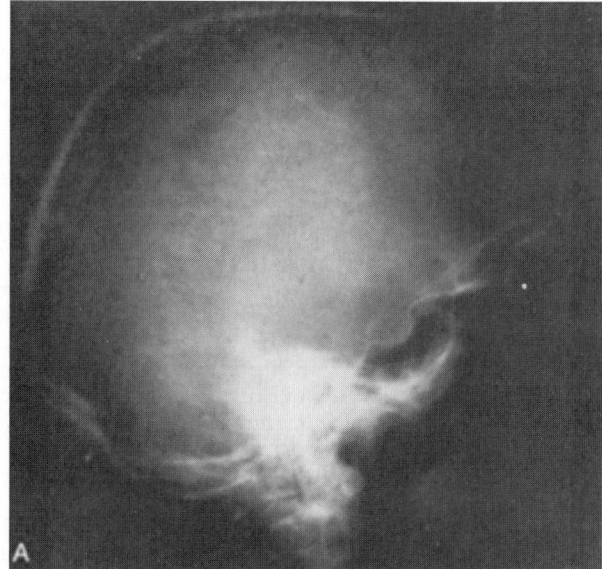

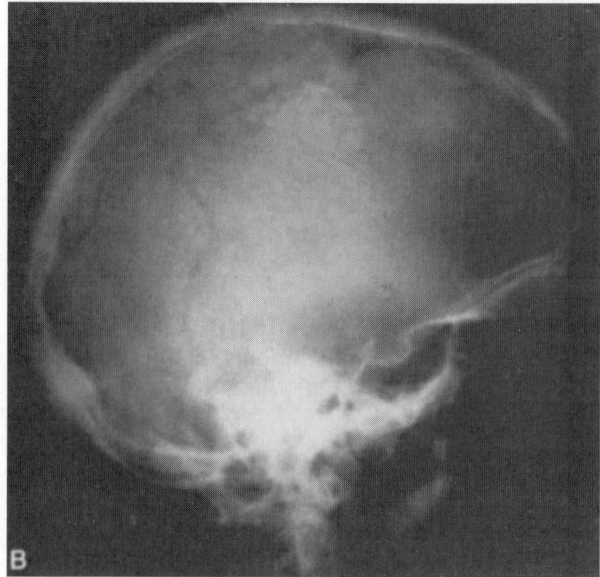

Figure 24–7. *A,* Skull film of a patient with hyperparathyroidism. There is demineralization, which imparts a salt-and-pepper texture to the calvarium with obliteration of the normal vascular grooves of the inner table. The cortex of the ascending ramus and alveolar ridge of the mandible are severely demineralized. *B,* Two years after removal of parathyroid adenoma there is restoration of normal bone mineralization.

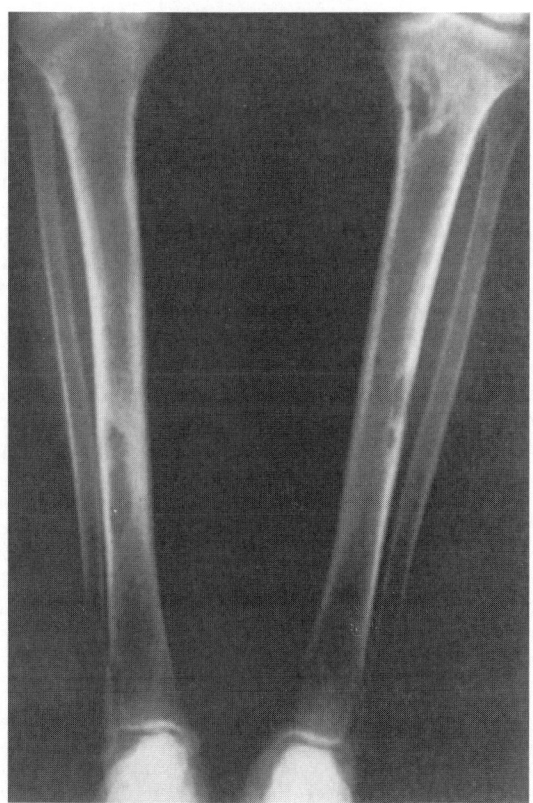

Figure 24–8. Lower leg radiograph. Multiple bone cysts (brown tumors) are present. The cortical location and sharp margins are characteristic.

the bile, which leads to the formation of calcium bilirubinate stones.

Emotional Disturbances. Patients with hypercalcemia of any cause may develop neurologic or psychiatric disturbances ranging from depression or anxiety to psychosis or coma. Most of the mental derangements associated with hyperparathyroidism are subtle. Petersen performed psychiatric examinations on 54 patients with hyperparathyroidism and detected mental disturbances in more than half of them.[37] Four patients had acute organic psychosis that returned to normal after surgical therapy. Most often, however, such severe disturbances are not correctable by parathyroidectomy. Joborn and associates examined monoamine metabolite levels in 48 such patients and found subnormal levels that improved after parathyroidectomy.[27] Similar abnormalities have been associated with endogenous depression. Many patients after parathyroidectomy experience a sense of well-being and relief of fatigue and dullness that often was not fully appreciated preoperatively.

Articular and Soft Tissue Manifestations. There is an increased prevalence of chondrocalcinosis and pseudogout in patients with hyperparathyroidism, the incidence being 3% to 7%. Characteristically, one can see radiographic evidence of calcium pyrophosphate deposition in the articular cartilages and menisci. Vascular and cardiac calcification, skin necrosis, and band keratopathy of the cornea have all been reported in patients with hyperparathyroidism. The latter usually occur, however, only in association with decreased renal function and hyperphosphatemia.

Neuromuscular Complications. It is well recognized that muscular weakness, fatigue, and even mental aberrations may occur in patients with hyperparathyroidism. Most commonly, the weakness is in the proximal muscle groups. In a study by Patten and associates, 14 (87.5%) of 16 patients with primary hyperparathyroidism demonstrated weakness, easy fatigability, and muscle atrophy.[36] There were sensory abnormalities in 50% of the patients, and muscle biopsies demonstrated atrophy of Type II muscle fibers most consistent with a neuropathic lesion and not a primary myopathy. The etiology of these findings remains unclear.

PHYSICAL FINDINGS

The diseased parathyroid glands are rarely palpable in patients with hyperparathyroidism, and a palpable mass in the neck should suggest the presence of a thyroid nodule.

LABORATORY DIAGNOSIS

The diagnosis of hyperparathyroidism is dependent on the documentation of an elevated serum calcium concentration usually in conjunction with an elevated serum PTH. The serum calcium level is best determined by atomic absorption spectrophotometry. Each laboratory should determine its own normal range, but values usually are from 8.5 to 10.5 mg. per 100 ml. Theoretically, one should be concerned with the serum ionized or free fraction of serum calcium rather than that portion bound to protein or organic anions. The measurement of ionized calcium is possible by means of a calcium-sensitive flow-through electrode. In evaluating 19 patients with subtle hyperparathyroidism and intermittent, minimal elevations of serum calcium, McLeod and associates obtained 151 concurrent preoperative measurements of total calcium and ionized calcium.[33] Only 46 (30.5%) of the total calcium measurements were elevated, whereas 134 (88.7%) of the ionized calcium determinations were increased. Hyperparathyroidism was confirmed at operation, and postoperatively the values of total and ionized calcium returned to normal.

It might appear that the most efficient method of diagnosing hyperparathyroidism would be to document an increased concentration of PTH in plasma. Owing to the heterogeneity of the circulating forms of PTH, most of the early studies using radioimmunoassay techniques reported conflicting results. The methodology has been greatly refined, however, and currently has wide clinical use. The finding of an elevated plasma level of PTH does not in itself establish the diagnosis of hyperparathyroidism. One must evaluate the PTH level as a function of the serum calcium concentration. Subjects with increased serum concentrations of both calcium and PTH generally have hyperparathyroidism (Fig. 24–9).

After secretion, PTH is very rapidly cleaved into an amino-terminal fragment and a carboxy-terminal fragment. The intact molecule and the biologically active amino-terminal fragment have half-lives of minutes, whereas the inactive carboxy-terminal fragment has a half-life of hours. Generally, antibodies directed against the carboxy-terminal fragment have been more useful in radioimmunoassay to establish the diagnosis of hyperparathyroidism.

The concentration of serum phosphate varies between 2.5 and 4.5 mg per 100 ml. Approximately half the patients with primary hyperparathyroidism have hypophosphatemia. However, in the presence of significant renal impairment, serum phosphate levels may be considerably elevated.

The serum concentration of alkaline phosphatase is normally below 110 I.U. per 100 ml. Ten to 40% of patients with hyperparathyroidism have increased levels. In such patients, there is almost always some degree of bone disease; after surgical therapy, the serum calcium concentration may fall more rapidly to lower levels, compared with that of patients whose serum alkaline phosphatase levels are normal (*bone hunger*). The alkaline phosphatase level is not helpful in diagnosing hyperparathyroidism, because it is also very often elevated with other causes of hypercalcemia.

Because of the effect of PTH on bicarbonate excretion in

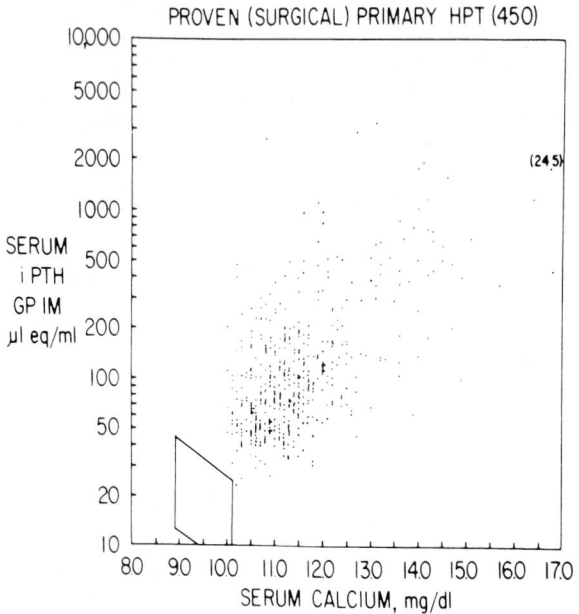

Figure 24–9. Serum iPTH values in 450 patients with surgically proven primary hyperparathyroidism as a function of serum calcium concentration. Serum iPTH was measured with a radioimmunoassay using GP Im antiserum. The area enclosed by the solid lines represents the normal range ± 2 SD for serum iPTH and serum calcium. Note that there is a 10% overlap of serum iPTH with the normal range but that greater than 95% of normal sera and all hyperparathyroid sera have measurable iPTH. Formal discriminative analysis of serum iPTH and serum calcium separates 100% of hyperparathyroid patients from normal subjects. (From Arnaud, C. D., et al.: Excerpta Medica International Congress Series, No. 270, 1973, p. 281.)

the kidney, patients with hyperparathyroidism often have a hyperchloremic metabolic acidosis at the time of diagnosis. Lind and Ljunghall have evaluated the serum calcium, chloride, albumin, and phosphorus levels in 86 patients with surgically confirmed primary hyperparathyroidism and in 53 patients with hypercalcemia due to malignancy.[29] They found that a modified chloride-phosphate ratio [(chloride − 84) × (albumin − 15)/phosphate, where the units for chloride and phosphate are mmol./100 ml. and the unit for albumin is gm./L.] could differentiate hyperparathyroidism from humoral hypercalcemia of malignancy in over 95% of cases. A value greater than 500 suggests primary hyperparathyroidism, while a value less than 400 suggests another cause. The chloride-phosphate ratio may have value in patients in whom the differential diagnosis of hypercalcemia is difficult.

The serum concentration of magnesium is below normal in only 5% to 10% of patients with hyperparathyroidism. If there is concomitant hypocalcemia and hypomagnesemia after parathyroidectomy, it is difficult to correct the hypocalcemia until the serum magnesium concentration has been returned to normal.

The serum concentrations of calcium, phosphate, alkaline phosphatase, and chloride, as well as the chloride-phosphate ratio, in 100 consecutive patients with primary hyperparathyroidism are depicted in Figure 24–10.

Nephrogenous Cyclic AMP. The interaction of PTH with specific receptors in the renal tubule causes activation of adenylate cyclase and an increase in cyclic AMP inside the cell. Because the cyclic AMP leaks into the tubular fluid, increased concentrations of cyclic AMP are present in the urine of patients with hyperparathyroidism. When measured as a function of creatinine clearance (nephrogenous cyclic AMP), it has been demonstrated that 90% of patients with hyperparathyroidism have increased urinary levels of this substance. The measurement of nephrogenous cyclic AMP

has been useful in the differential diagnosis of hyperparathyroidism, although it may be elevated in cases of malignancy-associated hypercalcemia caused by a tumor secreting PTH-related protein. This test is rarely used.

Urinary Calcium. In hyperparathyroidism, urinary calcium excretion is almost always elevated. This differentiates hyperparathyroidism from familial hypercalcemic hypocalciuria.

Bone Biopsy and Densitometry. Iliac crest bone biopsy and photon beam bone scanning can detect subtle changes when conventional radiographs are negative. These findings may help to establish the diagnosis in equivocal cases and may document the need for intervention in patients with hyperparathyroidism who are otherwise asymptomatic.

Other Hormones. Primary hyperparathyroidism is a component of the multiple endocrine neoplasia syndromes (MEN) Type 1 and 2A. Farndon and associates examined the utility of testing for other components of these syndromes in a group of 100 patients undergoing surgical therapy for primary hyperparathyroidism.[23] Measuring serum gastrin, calcitonin, and prolactin both preoperatively and postoperatively, they did not identify any patient with either type of multiple endocrine neoplasia. They concluded that laboratory measurements are not indicated in the absence of a family history or other clinical indications.

Less Common Manifestations

Familial Hyperparathyroidism. Hyperparathyroidism is a component of MEN Type 1 and MEN Type 2A. MEN Type 1 is characterized by the association of parathyroid hyperplasia, pituitary adenomas, pancreatic islet cell neoplasia, and, in some patients, tumors of the thyroid or adrenal cortex. MEN Type 2A is represented by medullary thyroid carcinoma, pheochromocytoma, and parathyroid hyperplasia.

Hyperparathyroidism in Pregnancy. Primary hyperparathyroidism in pregnancy is rare and is associated with neonatal tetany, stillbirth, and abortion. The risk of fetal complications appears to be higher if the hyperparathyroidism is untreated. When the diagnosis is made, the mother should undergo operation, if possible during the second trimester.

Neonatal Primary Hyperparathyroidism and Familial Hypercalcemic Hypocalciuria. These rare conditions are caused by a defect in the gene coding for the calcium-sensing receptor.[38] Homozygote infants present with hypotonia, poor feeding, constipation, and respiratory distress (neonatal severe hyperparathyroidism). The 1-year survival in symptomatic untreated patients is less than 50%, and total parathyroidectomy with autotransplantation is the treatment of choice. A more conservative approach may be justified in the absence of symptoms. People who have one normal gene copy have familial hypercalcemic hypocalciuria. This benign condition presents as an elevation in the calcium set-point. The patients have elevated serum calcium and mildly elevated serum PTH levels but no complications of primary hyperparathyroidism. This disease can be distinguished from primary hyperparathyroidism by the normal 24-hour urine calcium level.

Parathyroid Carcinoma. Parathyroid carcinoma is rare and probably represents less than 1% of patients with hyperparathyroidism. Parathyroid carcinoma usually presents in a manner different from that of benign hyperparathyroidism. In about one half of patients with parathyroid carcinoma, the involved parathyroid gland is palpable, a finding rarely observed in patients with benign hyperparathyroidism. Most patients with parathyroid carcinoma are symptomatic at the time of diagnosis and complain of nausea, vomiting, polyuria, generalized weakness, and weight loss. Moreover, both kidneys and skeleton are commonly affected in this disease, often in the same patients, a finding distinctly different from

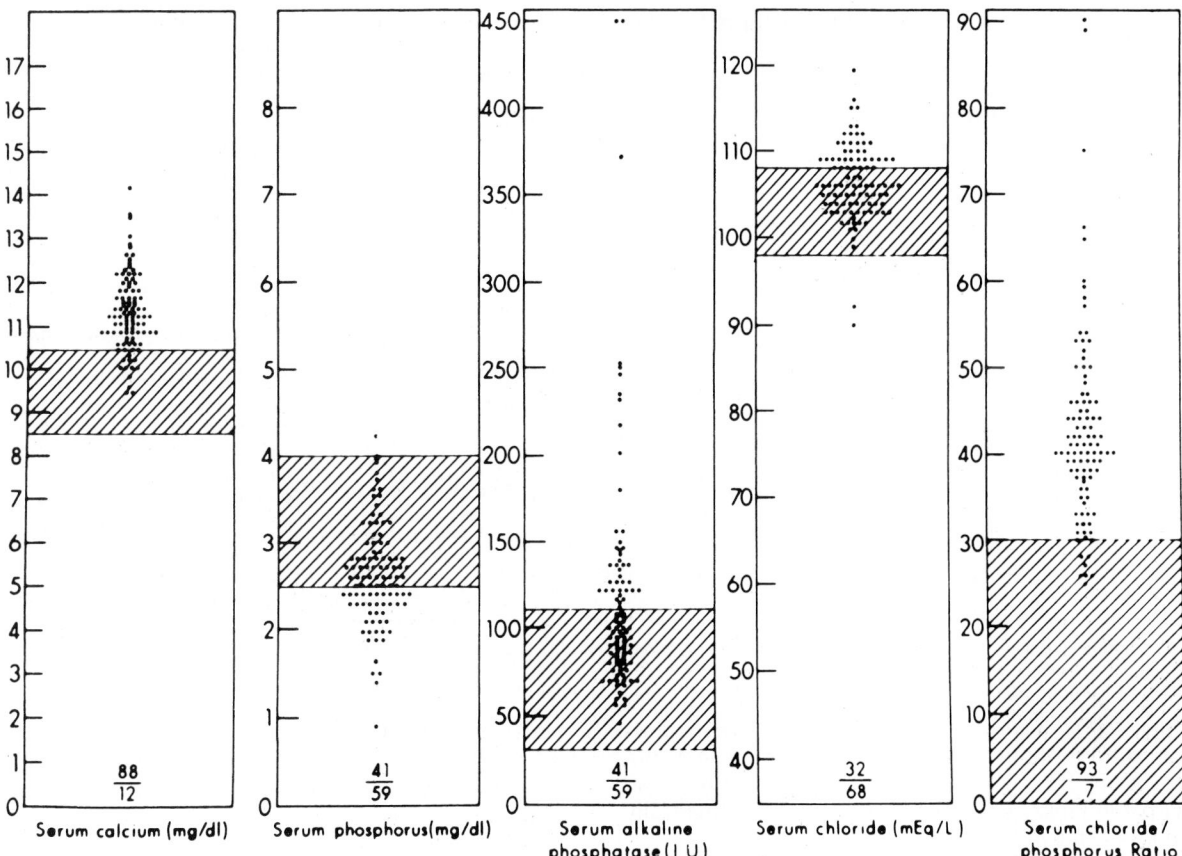

Figure 24–10. The serum concentrations of calcium, phophorus, alkaline phosphatase, and chloride in 100 consecutive patients with surgically proven hyperparathyroidism. The ratio of serum chloride to phosphorus is also shown (extreme right). The fractions at the bottom of each bar represent the number of abnormal values over the number of normal values. The laboratory values shown represent the determinations made at the time of hospital admission for parathyroidectomy. Even though 12 patients had serum calcium concentrations in the normal range, all had been demonstrated to be hypercalcemic on several preoperative determinations. (From Wells, S. A., Jr., Leight, G. S., and Ross, A. J.: Primary hyperparathyroidism. Curr. Probl. Surg., *17*:358, 1980.)

that observed in benign hyperparathyroidism. The diagnosis is most accurately made on histologic examination when there is local invasion of surrounding tissues or metastases to regional lymph nodes or distant sites. However, some pathologists believe that the diagnosis can be made when there is histologic evidence of vascular invasion, frequent mitotic figures, and capsular invasion of the parathyroid gland. Flow cytometry may be useful for equivocal cases. Characteristically, the serum concentrations of calcium, PTH, and alkaline phosphatase are markedly increased, compared with concentrations in patients with benign hyperparathyroidism.

It is important to recognize the disease at the initial neck exploration, because radical resection of the malignant parathyroid gland, the ipsilateral thyroid lobe, and involved adjacent soft tissue and regional lymph nodes offers the only possibility for cure. If the disease recurs, reoperation is indicated (including resection of pulmonary and liver metastases) because patients, if untreated, succumb to uncontrolled hypercalcemia. The long-term prognosis is poor; the opportunity for survival depends on complete initial resection.[55]

Hyperparathyroid Crisis

Most patients presenting with hyperparathyroidism are chronically ill with symptoms referable to the kidneys or the skeleton. Rarely, however, patients may become acutely ill with urgent symptoms that sometimes prove fatal. The terms *acute hyperparathyroidism* and *hyperparathyroid crisis* have been used to describe this clinical dilemma. The onset is usually characterized by rapidly developing muscular weakness, nausea and vomiting, weight loss, fatigue, drowsiness, and confusion. Males and females are affected equally. The serum calcium concentration is almost always elevated (16 to 20 mg. per 100 ml.), and azotemia is usually present. This clinical pattern not only is associated with hyperparathyroidism but also is observed in patients with acute hypercalcemia accompanying other diseases. The offending parathyroid gland(s) is usually large; and in about one third of the patients, a tumor is palpable in the neck preoperatively. The genesis of the condition appears to involve uncontrolled PTH secretion followed by hypercalcemia, polyuria, dehydration, and reduced renal function worsening the hypercalcemia.

Although the definitive therapy is resection of the hyperfunctioning parathyroid tissue, it is unwise to proceed with neck exploration until the patient has been prepared and the calcium concentration lowered, if possible. The cornerstone of therapy is diuresis, preferably with 0.9% sodium chloride in sufficient amounts to maintain urinary output above 100 ml. per hour. When urinary output becomes satisfactory, potassium chloride should be administered. The diuretic furosemide increases the renal excretion of sodium and calcium but should not be used until the patient is well hydrated. If the serum calcium level remains elevated with adequate sodium infusion and hydration, other agents that are known to lower the serum calcium concentration should be adminis-

TABLE 24–3. Agents Used in the Treatment of Hypercalcemia

Agent	Dosage	Administration	Comment
Calcitonin	2–6 MRC units/kg. 10–20 MRC units	Subcutaneous, every 6–8 hr. Intravenous, hourly	Nausea and vomiting are side effects. Allergy is the only contraindication. Onset of calcium-lowering effect is rapid.
Mithramycin	25 μg./kg.	Intravenously over 1 hr. in 100 ml. 0.9% saline or 5% dextrose	Contraindications are renal or hepatic dysfunction. Calcium-lowering effect occurs within 24 hr. Drug is useful when diuretic and intravenous saline are contraindicated. Nausea and vomiting are side effects.
Glucocorticoids	Prednisone, 40–50 mg./day Prednisolone phosphate, 40 mg.	Oral Intramuscularly or intravenously every 8 hr.	Lag period may be 7–10 days. Glucocorticoids are safe for short-term use. Alternate-day oral program may be used for long-term use.
Orthophosphate	1–2 gm./24 hr.	Oral	Dose adjustment for renal impairment. Soft tissue calcification may occur. Intravenous phosphate is not recommended.
Gallium nitrate	200 mg./m.²/day × 5 days	Intravenous	Inhibits bone resorption. Can have nephrotoxicity.

Modified from Purnell, D. C., and van Heerden, J. A.: Management of symptomatic hypercalcemia and hypocalcemia. World J. Surg., *6*:702; 1982.

tered (Table 24–3). If a diagnosis of hyperparathyroidism is in doubt, an ultrasound examination or a computed tomographic scan of the neck may be useful in identifying an enlarged parathyroid gland. The disease can be dramatically reversed by operative therapy.[11]

Secondary Hyperparathyroidism (Renal Osteodystrophy)

Since the initiation of maintenance dialysis and renal transplantation, the lives of patients with chronic renal failure have been prolonged. Secondary hyperparathyroidism develops as a result of the metabolic alterations occurring in chronic renal failure. Phosphate retention and hyperphosphatemia in conjunction with a decrease in the renal production of 1,25-dihydroxyvitamin D_3 reduce the serum calcium producing secondary hyperparathyroidism. Also, aluminum present in the dialysate water and in oral phosphate binder medications accumulates in bone and contributes substantially to the osteomalacia component of the disease. The pathogenesis of renal osteodystrophy is depicted in Figure 24–11. Therapy should be directed toward controlling the serum phosphate level by dietary restriction and phosphate-binding gels, maintaining adequate calcium intake, administering vitamin D sterols, and reducing aluminum in the dialysate bath and the diet.

In some patients a chronically stimulated parathyroid gland gains autonomous function and produces hypercalcemia after renal transplantation (tertiary hyperparathyroidism).

Differential Diagnosis

Many diseases are associated with hypercalcemia (Table 24–4). They must be excluded before subjecting a patient with suspected hyperparathyroidism to operation. The biochemical diagnosis of hyperparathyroidism should be established by the demonstration of an inappropriately elevated serum PTH level with hypercalcemia before undertaking neck exploration. In equivocal cases, 24-hour urine calcium measurement and the chloride-phosphate ratio may help establish the diagnosis.

Of the more common alternative causes of hypercalcemia, hyperthyroidism, the milk-alkali syndrome, hypervitaminosis D or A, and immobilization can be excluded by a careful history and physical examination. In patients with sarcoidosis or multiple myeloma, the serum globulin levels are usually elevated and there are characteristic radiographic findings, as there are also in patients with Paget's disease of

TABLE 24–4. Diseases Causing Hypercalcemia

Hyperparathyroidism
Malignancy
  Hematologic
  Solid (PTHrP producer)
Hyperthyroidism
Multiple myeloma
Sarcoidosis and other granulomatous diseases
Milk-alkali syndrome
Vitamin D intoxication
Vitamin A intoxication
Paget's disease
Immobilization
Thiazide diuretics
Addisonian crisis
Familial hypocalciuric hypercalcemia
Neonatal severe hyperparathyroidism

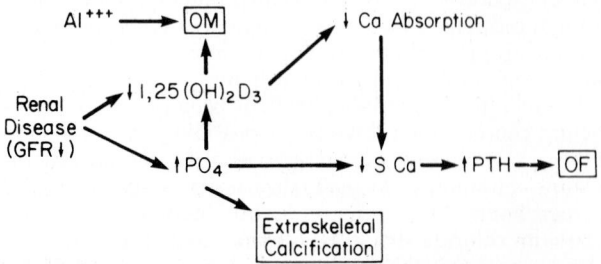

Figure 24–11. Scheme showing the proposed pathogenesis of secondary hyperparathyroidism and osteomalacia in renal failure. GFR, glomerular filtration rate; OM osteomalacia; OF osteitis fibrosa; SCa, serum calcium. (From Coburn, J. W.: Renal osteodystrophy. *In* Clinical Disorders of Bone and Mineral Metabolism. Amsterdam, Excerpta Medica, 1983, p. 250.)

the bone. If patients with hypercalcemia are taking thiazide diuretics, the drug should be discontinued and, if this is responsible, the calcium returns to normal within a few weeks.

Hypercalcemia and Malignancy. In hospitalized patients, malignancy rather than hyperparathyroidism is the most common cause of hypercalcemia; and, generally, patients can be divided into two groups: (1) those with hematologic malignancies (25%) and (2) those with solid tumors.

Patients in the hematologic malignancy group include those with multiple myeloma, those with some lymphomas or leukemias, and a subset of breast cancer patients. These patients have lytic bone metastases and histologically demonstrate increased osteoclast bone resorption adjacent to tumor cells. The cause of the hypercalcemia in these patients is local cytokine release (mainly interleukin-1β and tumor necrosis factor-β) stimulating osteoclasts to resorb bone. These patients have elevated serum levels of calcium and phosphate and low urine levels of cyclic AMP.

Patients in the solid tumor group most commonly have carcinoma of the breast, lung, kidney, or pancreas. These patients have elevated serum levels of calcium, but low serum phosphate and high urinary cyclic AMP levels, in contrast to the hematologic malignancy group. Their hypercalcemia is now known to be caused by tumor production of PTH-related protein, which mimics the effects of PTH and produces hypercalcemia. The focal bone metastases that many of these patients have as a part of their advanced disease are not thought to contribute significantly to the hypercalcemia.[50]

Localization

Approximately 95% of patients with primary hyperparathyroidism are cured at initial neck exploration performed by an experienced surgeon. This must be borne in mind in evaluating the need for methods to localize the site of hyperfunctioning parathyroid tissue. No study has yet demonstrated that preoperative localization reduces either the duration of the operation or the incidence of complications, and most surgeons believe that localization techniques should be reserved for the patient undergoing reexploration after a failed initial procedure. In this situation, glands are frequently found in ectopic locations and the normal tissue planes may be obscured. Generally, invasive techniques, such as arteriography and venography, have no place in localization before the initial operation for hyperparathyroidism. Noninvasive methods with greater utility include high-resolution, real-time ultrasonography; computed tomography; magnetic resonance imaging; and technetium-sestamibi scanning.

High-resolution, real-time ultrasonography differs from conventional ultrasound scanning in that the emitted sound waves are of higher frequency (10 MHz.), permitting resolution of structures less than 1 mm. but limiting the depth of visualization to 4 or 5 cm. from the skin. In an evaluation of 100 consecutive patients undergoing neck exploration at the Mayo Clinic, the radiologic accuracy was 76%; however, the success rate of identifying the parathyroid lesion at operation was the same with (96%) or without (97%) the utilization of ultrasound.[52] Similar results have been reported by others. The usefulness of this technique in patients with hypercalcemic crisis has previously been mentioned. Ultrasound-guided fine-needle aspiration with cytology and immunostaining for PTH may be helpful in confirming the localization if necessary.

In most recent studies, computed tomography appears to be equally as effective as ultrasonography. It is more expensive but is less operator-dependent than ultrasonography.

Computed tomography appears to be superior for identifying ectopically located glands, particularly those in the mediastinum. Magnetic resonance imaging appears to be equally sensitive.

Sestamibi is a radionuclide agent developed for cardiac imaging that has been discovered to concentrate in parathyroid tissue, thereby visualizing them on delayed scans. The single nuclide nature and short half-life, high-energy profile of this agent have provided advantages over thallium-technetium subtraction scanning. Thus, sestamibi imaging appears to be an improvement over thallium-technetium scan, although its appropriate use is still reserved for the reoperative setting.

Treatment

With the use of automated technology for determining the serum concentration of calcium, the diagnosis of hyperparathyroidism is made more often in asymptomatic patients. Whether all patients with hyperparathyroidism should undergo operation has been questioned, and some physicians have proposed that asymptomatic patients be followed intermittently without operative intervention. There are no definitive data on which to base an opinion for all asymptomatic patients, although some authors have attempted to address this issue. One study by Scholz and Purnell followed a group of 142 asymptomatic patients without operation.[48] After 10 years, more than 20% of patients had required operation for a serum calcium level above 11 mg. per 100 ml. or for specific complications. Another 20% were lost to follow-up. The remainder either died of apparently unrelated illness or remained asymptomatic. Because of the large proportion (greater than 40%) of patients who required operation or were lost to follow-up, the authors could not reliably recommend nonoperative management.

A National Institutes of Health Consensus Development Conference reviewed the available data on this subject in 1990.[17] The panel agreed that operation is indicated for all patients with symptoms. The indications for operation in asymptomatic patients (Table 24–5) were outlined, and the panel mandated semiannual follow-up for patients not operated on. In addition, operation was recommended for patients in whom medical surveillance was neither desirable

---

TABLE 24–5. Indications for Operative Treatment of Asymptomatic Patients with Primary Hyperparathyroidism

On initial evaluation:
- Markedly elevated serum calcium
- History of an episode of life-threatening hypercalcemia
- Reduced creatinine clearance
- Presence of kidney stone(s) detected by abdominal radiograph
- Markedly elevated 24-hour urinary calcium excretion
- Substantially reduced bone mass as determined by direct measurement

During monitoring of an asymptomatic patient, these developments:
- Typical symptoms of the skeletal, renal, or gastrointestinal systems
- Sustained serum calcium > 1.0–1.6 mg./100 ml. above normal
- Significant decline in renal function (>30% decline in creatinine clearance)
- Nephrolithiasis or worsening calciuria
- Significant decline in bone mass (to less than 2 SD below age/gender/racial matched mean)
- Significant neuromuscular or psychologic symptoms
- Inability or unwillingness of patient to continue medical surveillance

nor suitable, as when the patient requests surgical therapy, consistent follow-up is unlikely, coexistent illness complicates management, or if the patient is younger than 50 years of age.

Definitive resolution of this question will require a randomized, controlled trial. The only curative treatment for primary hyperparathyroidism is parathyroidectomy, and it is successful and uncomplicated in more than 95% of patients. Medical management should be reserved for patients who are either extremely debilitated or who have another life-threatening illness. Before subjecting a patient to operation, the surgeon should be confident of the diagnosis and have adequate experience to systematically explore the neck, recognizing in the process the normal and abnormal parathyroid glands. The patient should be made fully aware of the complications associated with the neck exploration, including potential damage to the superior and recurrent laryngeal nerves and the development of hypocalcemia with associated symptoms of tetany. In the asymptomatic patients, the alternative of nonoperative or medical management should be presented. The possibility of an unsuccessful parathyroid search should be mentioned, and the patient should be made aware that repeat operation, including a mediastinal exploration, may be required if the planned operation is unsuccessful. Although the likelihood of these complications is small, it is best to discuss them before the initial neck exploration.

A second exploration of the neck because of failure to locate the lesion at the initial procedure is very difficult and should be avoided by meticulous primary operation. If reoperation is required, not only is parathyroid tissue more difficult to identify, but damage to the recurrent laryngeal nerve is also more likely.

General anesthesia is used, and the neck is opened through a transverse cervical incision (Figs. 24–12 and 24–13). After the strap muscles are separated in the midline (Fig. 24–14), a chosen lobe of the thyroid gland is elevated and rotated medially. The tissues inferior to the thyroid lobe are cleaned

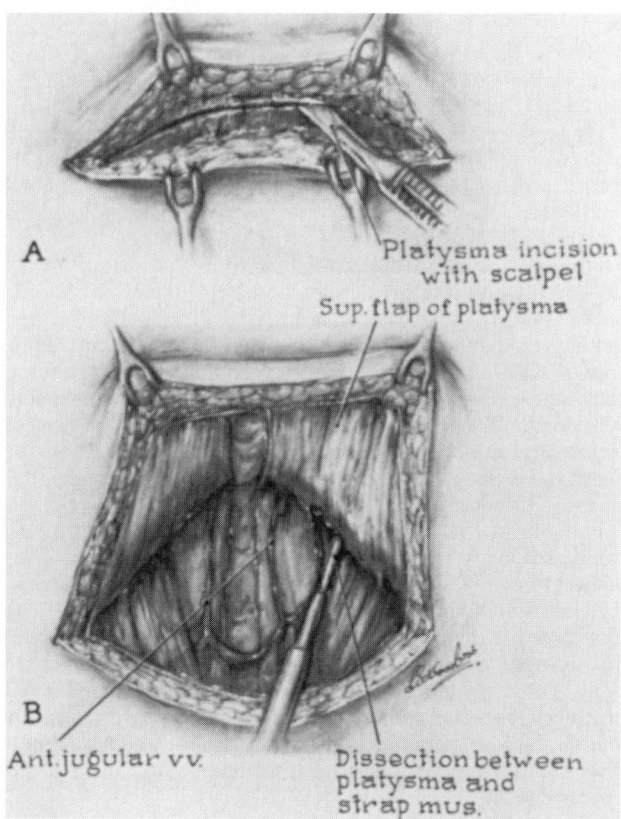

Figure 24–13. After incision of the platysma *(A)*, superior and inferior flaps are developed *(B)*. (From Wells, S. A., Jr., Leight, G. S., and Ross, A. J.: Primary hyperparathyroidism. Curr. Probl. Surg., *17*:358, 1980.)

down to the trachea to expose the recurrent laryngeal nerve and the inferior thyroid artery. In most patients, the nerve lies in the tracheoesophageal groove; less commonly, it is lateral to the trachea; and rarely it is anterolateral to the trachea, where it is especially vulnerable to injury. A laryngeal nerve may be given off directly in the neck without the usual looping around the right subclavian artery. The external branch of the superior laryngeal nerve is the most im-

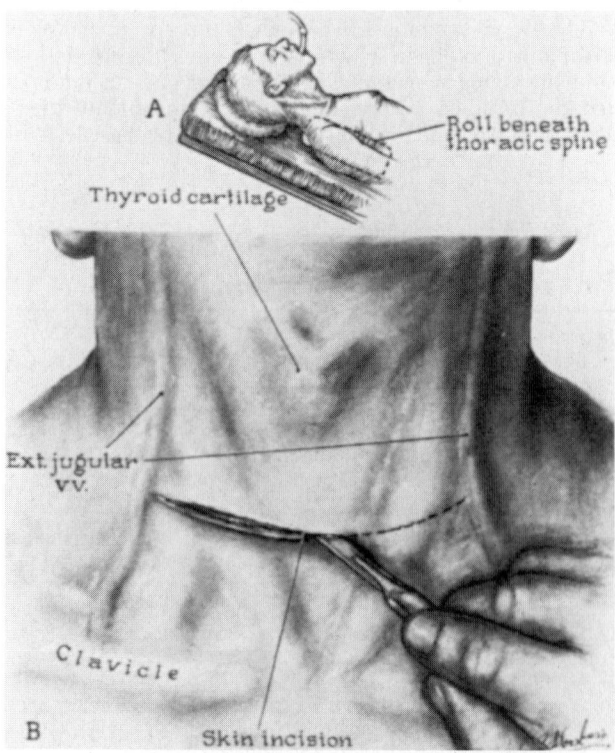

Figure 24–12. The cervical incision is usually made two fingerbreadths above the sternal notch. (From Wells, S. A., Jr., Leight, G. S., and Ross, A. J.: Primary hyperparathyroidism. Curr. Probl. Surg., *17*:358, 1980.)

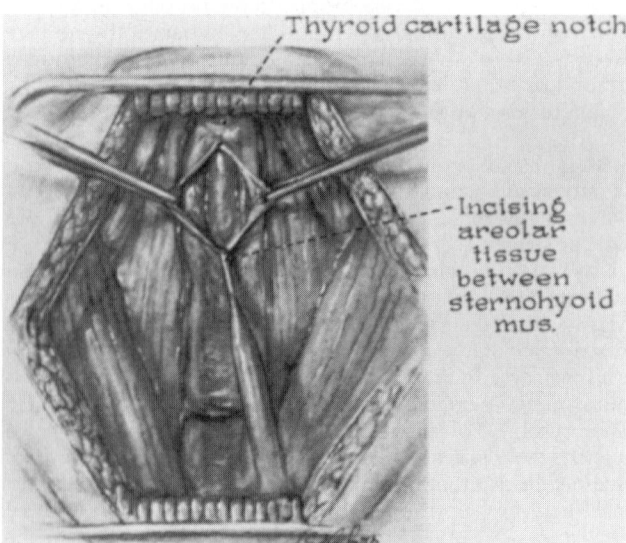

Figure 24–14. Separation of the pretracheal fascia and strap muscle. (From Wells, S. A., Jr., Leight, G. S., and Ross, A. J.: Primary hyperparathyroidism. Curr. Probl. Surg., *17*:358, 1980.)

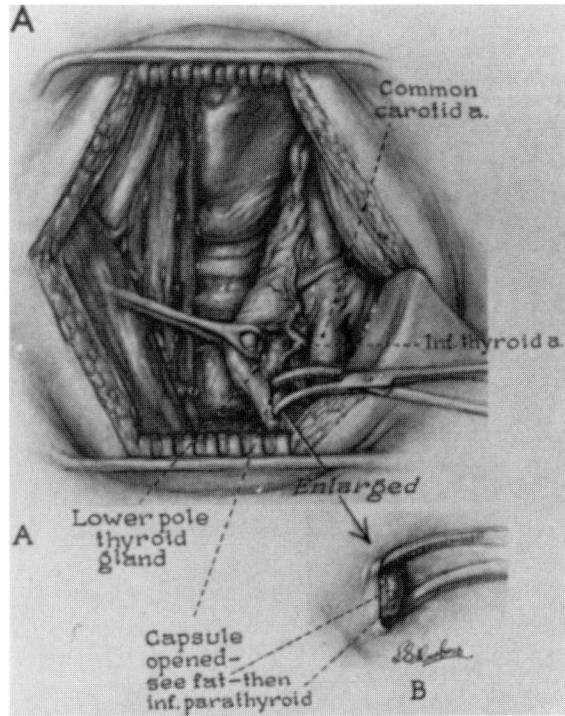

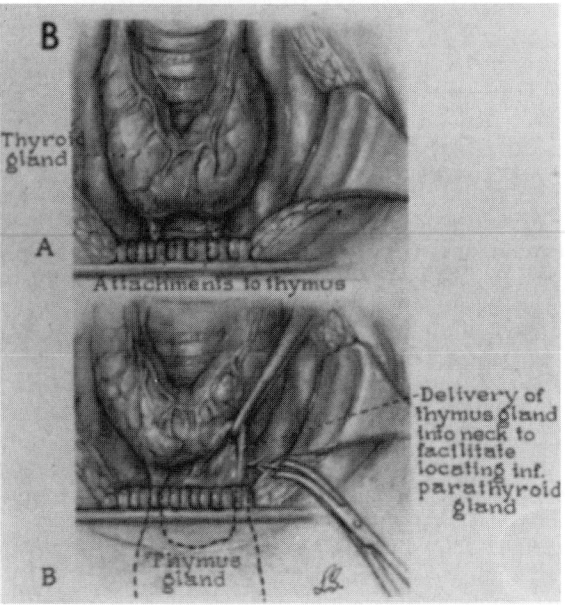

Figure 24–15. *A,* Identification of left lower parathyroid gland. *B,* Elevation of the thymus gland into the cervical incision. (From Wells, S. A., Jr., Leight, G. S., and Ross, A. J.: Primary hyperparathyroidism. Curr. Probl. Surg., *17*:358, 1980.)

portant tensor of the vocal cords, and it usually lies immediately adjacent and medial to the vascular pedicle of the superior thyroid lobe. With mobilization of the lobe, care must be taken not to injure this nerve. Four or more parathyroid glands may be present and abnormal, and the reconnaissance of the neck area requires great patience. The help of an experienced pathologist is required, because frozen-section identification of the parathyroid glands is helpful. The upper parathyroid glands are more easily found and are usually located far dorsally on the surface of the thyroid lobe at the level of the upper two thirds of the gland. The lower glands (Fig. 24–15A) are larger than the upper glands and less constant in location, being normally distributed from well above

the upper half of the thyroid to well within the mediastinum. The lower glands are usually more anterior than the upper glands. If the upper glands are identified (Fig. 24–16), the thymus pedicle on the side of the unfound gland should be carefully examined (see Fig. 24–15B) and removed. Most parathyroid adenomas located in the mediastinum can be removed through the cervical incision.

Weller termed the inferior parathyroid gland the *parathymus* to indicate the frequent association of the two structures.[56] In approximately half of normal subjects, the inferior parathyroid glands are adherent to or embedded in the cord of the thymus that extends out of the mediastinum and thoracic inlet to the inferior pole of the thyroid gland, the *thyrothymic ligament.* Edis and associates emphasized the clinical importance of the variable descent of the inferior parathyroid gland in seven patients with hyperparathyroidism, six of whom required a repeat neck operation for identification of the lesion (Fig. 24–17).[21]

If no parathyroid tissue is found after the thymus pedicle is removed, the surgeon should mobilize, examine, and palpate both lobes of the thyroid gland, because occasionally a parathyroid is completely encapsulated within the thyroid parenchyma. Removal of a thyroid lobe on the side where a parathyroid gland is not found is occasionally indicated as a last resort but should by no means substitute for a meticulous search for parathyroid tissue. It is also helpful to follow the branches of the inferior thyroid artery, especially if one is enlarged, because these often lead to an abnormal parathyroid gland or adenoma. Because of the possibility of multiple-gland involvement, every effort must be made to identify all four parathyroids. To ensure that one has actually identified parathyroid tissue, small biopsy specimens of the suspected glands should be obtained. The organs must be handled with extreme care, however, because they are delicate structures and their blood supply is easily damaged.

The operative management depends on the number of enlarged parathyroid glands. The incidence of single- and multiple-gland enlargement in 100 consecutive patients with hyperparathyroidism is depicted in Table 24–6. If one gland is large and the remaining three are of normal size, resection of the enlarged gland is curative in nearly all patients. In the event that two or three parathyroid glands are enlarged, most surgeons resect them, leaving the normal-sized glands undisturbed except for a biopsy. The question of whether these represent multiple adenomas or primary hyperplasia

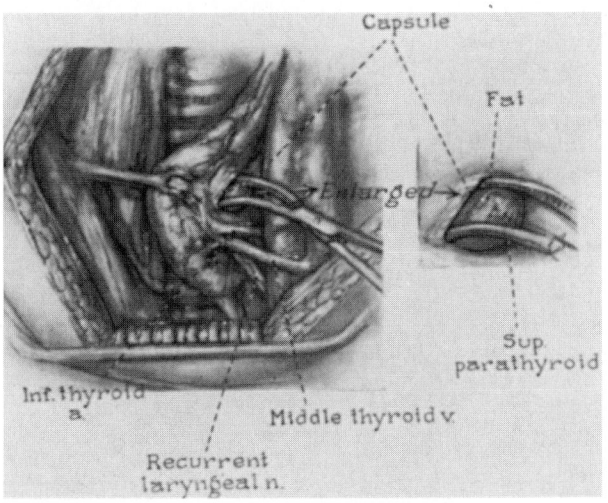

Figure 24–16. Identification of left superior parathyroid gland. (From Wells, S. A., Jr., Leight, G. S., and Ross, A. J.: Primary hyperparathyroidism. Curr. Probl. Surg., *17*:358, 1980.)

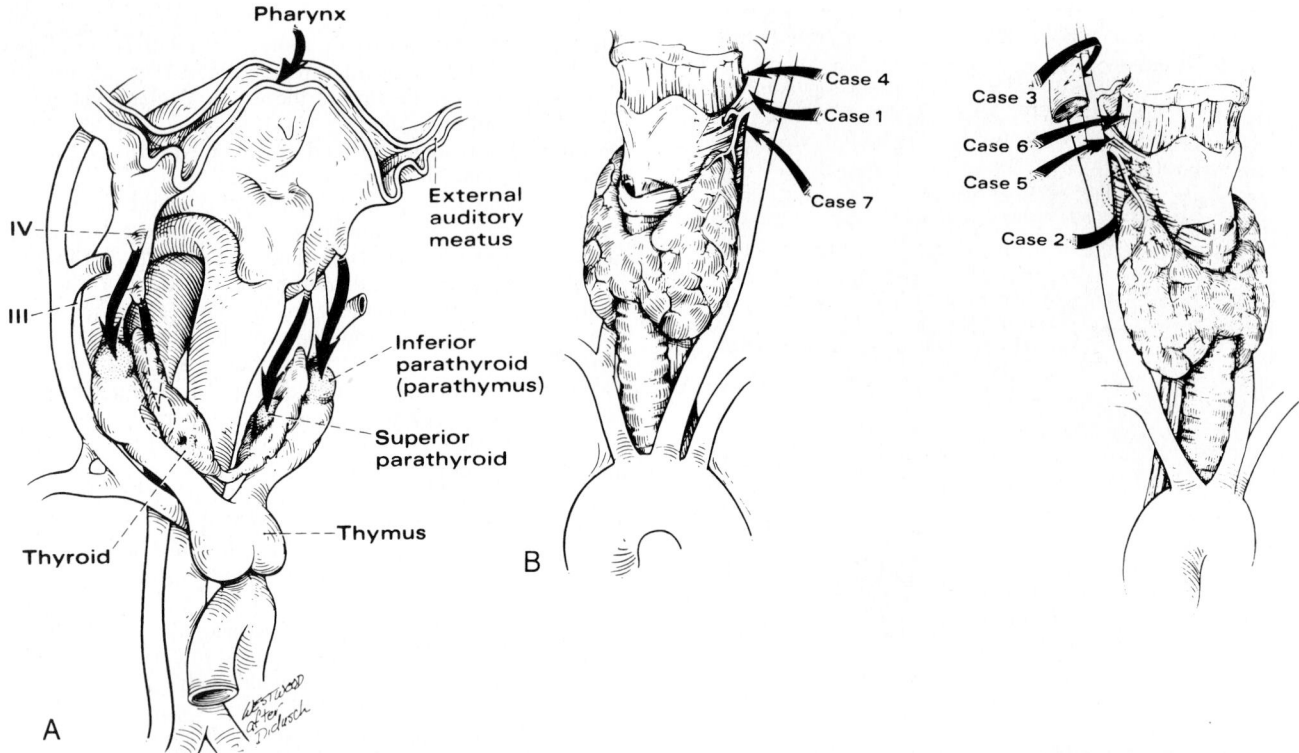

Figure 24–17. *A,* Inferior parathyroid glands and thymus have a common embryologic origin from the third branchial pouch and are closely related during caudal descent, hence the term parathymus. Arrested descent leads to undescended parathymus. Superior parathyroid glands arise from the fourth pouch and are thereafter more closely associated with thyroid. *B,* Locations of adenomas of undescended parathymus glands in 7 patients. (From Edis, A. J., Purnell, D. C., and van Heerden, J. A.: The undescended "parathymus." Ann. Surg., *190*:64, 1979.)

has not been resolved. Of 76 patients treated in such a manner and followed for 12 to 140 months postoperatively, 8 (10.5%) had recurrent hypercalcemia.[59] This recurrent disease tended to be mild, and it was concluded that the described management is generally acceptable. In patients with generalized (glandular) enlargement or parathyroid hyperplasia, the surgical management is much more difficult and the postoperative results less satisfactory.

Parathyroid Hyperplasia (Generalized [Four-Gland] Parathyroid Enlargement). This phenomenon occurs in two forms: water-clear cell hyperplasia and chief cell hyperplasia. Albright and associates described water-clear cell hyperplasia in 1934.[3] Clinically it is indistinguishable from the hyperparathyroidism associated with single-gland disease, but the gross appearance at operation is characteristic. All four glands are diffusely enlarged and dark brown with uneven surfaces and numerous pseudopods. The cut surface appears cystic. Microscopically the glands are composed almost entirely of water-clear cells.

TABLE 24–6. Gland Enlargement in 100 Patients with Primary Hyperparathyroidism

No. of Glands Enlarged	No. of Patients
1	65
2	15
3	10
4	10

From Wells, S. A., Leight, G. S., and Ross, A. J.: Primary hyperparathyroidism. Curr. Prob. Surg. *17*:358, 1980.

Primary chief cell hyperplasia was first described by Cope and colleagues in 1958.[18] There may be a great difference in the size of the glands, with the superior frequently being larger than the inferior. The glands are often nodular and red-brown and grossly are characterized by the presence of fibrous septa within the parenchyma. Histologically, chief cells predominate, but there are also nests of water-clear and oxyphil cells. In Cope's original series, several patients had associated endocrine disturbances, including insulin-producing and non–insulin-producing pancreatic islet cell adenomas, pituitary tumors, adrenal hyperplasia, and thyroid adenomas. It is now known that chief cell hyperplasia is the pathologic entity most commonly associated with familial hyperparathyroidism, particularly MEN Types 1 and 2A.

The standard therapy for patients with hyperparathyroidism and generalized parathyroid enlargement has been radical subtotal (three and one-half-gland) parathyroidectomy. In patients with nonfamilial parathyroid hyperplasia, the reported incidence of recurrent hypercalcemia is 0% to 16%. The incidence of permanent hypoparathyroidism is 4% to 5%. Patients with MEN Type 1, however, have a recurrent hypercalcemia rate of 26% to 36% with long-term follow-up. One institution that has reported a lower rate of recurrence also reports a high rate of permanent hypoparathyroidism (25%).[53]

Because of the relatively increased incidence of postoperative hypoparathyroidism and hyperparathyroidism in patients with *parathyroid hyperplasia,* particularly in patients with familial disease, the authors have elected to manage these patients by total parathyroidectomy and heterotopic autotransplantation. This operation has the advantage of allowing reexploration for recurrent hyperparathyroidism to take place in the nondominant forearm, rather than the neck.

In either operation, parathyroid tissue should be viably cryopreserved for later autografting if the patient has persistent hypoparathyroidism.

If after diligent search in the neck, including exploration of the upper mediastinum, retroesophageal area, carotid sheaths, and thyroid gland, no enlarged parathyroid gland has been found, a decision must be made regarding mediastinotomy. Most surgeons favor delay of this procedure, reasoning that the blood supply to the hyperfunctional gland may have been damaged during manipulation or that the pathologist may find the abnormal gland on further sectioning of the submitted tissues. Others have favored mediastinotomy at the time of the negative cervical exploration. Mediastinotomy is indicated in only about 1% of patients. If this procedure is elected, it should be done 2 to 4 weeks after the neck operation, if serum calcium values remain elevated. Delay of mediastinal exploration also allows localization studies to be performed in the interim. This can permit angiographic ablation in the few patients in whom this is indicated.[20]

In mediastinal exploration, a vertical incision is made from the center of the cervical incision to the xiphoid. The sternum is completely divided in the midline and a retractor is inserted. The remaining thymus tissue is first isolated and examined, because an adenoma may be associated with this structure located in front of the great vessels. In parathyroid adenomas that are true mediastinal organs, the blood supply is often from the mediastinal vessels and not the inferior thyroid artery. If the anterior mediastinal exploration is negative, the posterior mediastinum is next examined, especially posterior and lateral to the trachea (Fig. 24–18).

It should be mentioned that although the pathologist can readily distinguish parathyroid tissue from other tissue by frozen section, it is often difficult to discriminate between parathyroid *adenomas* and *hyperplasia*. In one study, three pathologists were asked to review 50 slides of parathyroid tissue and their diagnoses were compared with those made by the surgeon at the time of operation.[57] A specific diagnosis of adenomas was correct in only 60%. The most reliable index of abnormality is the surgeon's determination of gland size by visual observation.

Operation for Persistent or Recurrent Hyperparathyroidism. In the patients who remain hypercalcemic after neck exploration, approximately 60% have a missed parathyroid tumor. Inadequately excised hyperplastic tissue is another common cause of recurrent disease. Less commonly, late local recurrence of adenoma or carcinoma as a result of tissue that had inadvertently spilled from a broken gland and implanted at the time of initial operation occurs. In most cases, review of the original operative notes and pathologic report provides clues as to the position of undetected glands. The location of parathyroids missed at the initial operation but found on subsequent exploration in one large series is shown in Figure 24–19.

The diagnosis of hyperparathyroidism must be reconfirmed before reexploration, and urinary calcium should be measured to investigate familial hypercalcemic hypocalciuria. Patients should have clear indications for surgical management of their disease before reexploration. These can include serum level of calcium greater than 11.5 mg. per 100 ml. or complications of hypercalcemia, such as renal stones or osteopenia.

In contrast to initial operation, most surgeons agree that

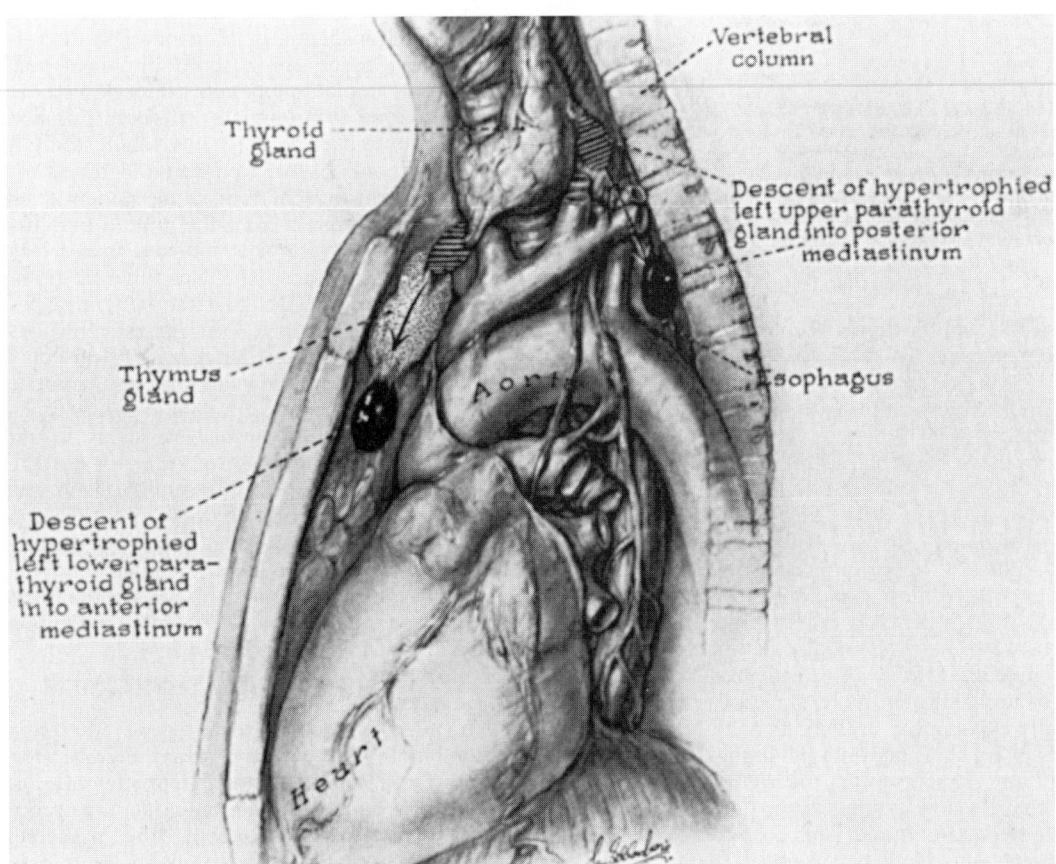

Figure 24–18. Ectopically located inferior parathyroid glands are most often located anteriorly in association with the thymus gland. Ectopically displaced superior parathyroid glands are usually located posteriorly in the tracheoesophageal groove or the posterior mediastinum. (From Wells, S. A., Jr., Leight, G. S., and Ross, A. J.: Primary hyperparathyroidism. Curr. Probl. Surg., *17*:358, 1980.)

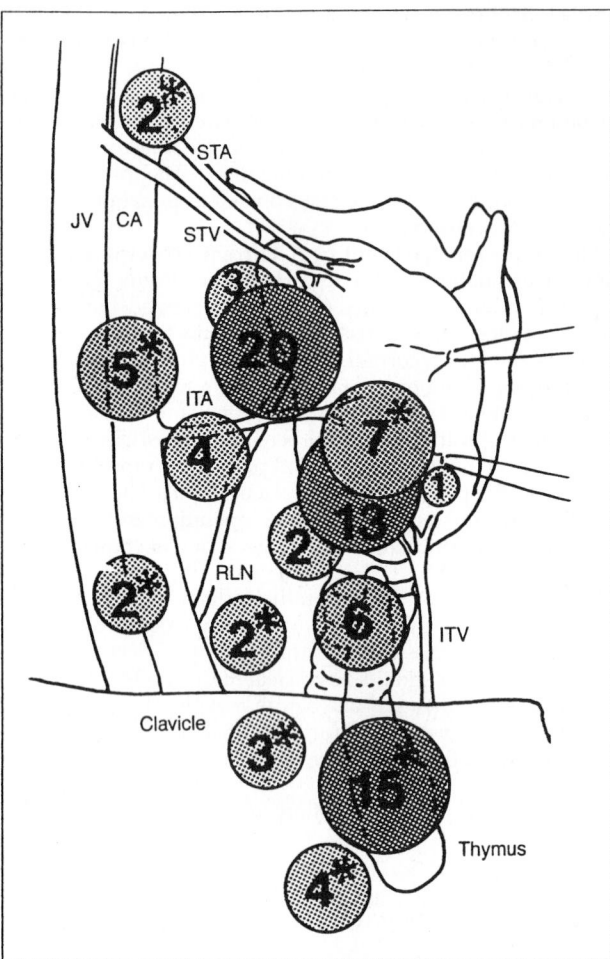

Figure 24–19. The locations of 89 parathyroid tumors at reoperation. The drawing shows a right anteriolateral view of the dissected neck with the thyroid lobe retracted medially. STA: superior thyroid artery; STV: superior thyroid vein; ITA: inferior thyroid artery; ITV: inferior thyroid vein; CA: carotid artery; JV: jugular vein; RLN: recurrent laryngeal nerve. (From Levin, K. E., Clark, O. H.: The reasons for failure in parathyroid operations. Arch. Surg., *124*:911, 1989. Copyright 1989, American Medical Association.)

localization studies should be performed before reexploration. A combination of the noninvasive studies described earlier should be used. If these are unsuccessful, selective angiography and venous sampling for PTH are useful.

Venous sampling for PTH, angiography, and intraoperative ultrasonography have been helpful in reevaluating patients in experienced centers. In a series from the National Institutes of Health, invasive studies identified the abnormal parathyroid gland in 41 of 43 patients who had negative or equivocal noninvasive studies.[46] Importantly, false-positive results, which could lead to fruitless exploration, were uncommon. These studies, although very accurate in centers with demonstrated expertise, also have potentially significant risks, such as transverse myelitis, stroke, and death from angiography. They should be applied carefully by skilled vascular radiologists specifically experienced in these techniques.

All patients who have parathyroid tissue removed at a reexploration for persistent or recurrent hypercalcemia should have tissue viably cryopreserved for reimplantation if they become hypoparathyroid. This is of particular importance in patients who have had multiple explorations or multiple glands identified and manipulated at an initial operation.

Management of Secondary Hyperparathyroidism. Indica-

tions for parathyroidectomy in patients with secondary hyperparathyroidism include the following: (1) persistent and symptomatic hypercalcemia in prospective renal transplant patients; (2) bone pain or pathologic fractures; (3) ectopic calcification, and (4) intractable itching. These patients can be managed by subtotal (three-and-one-half-gland) parathyroidectomy or total parathyroidectomy with heterotopic (forearm) autotransplantation. As in other forms of hyperplasia, reexploration for recurrent hyperparathyroidism is simplified by autotransplantation to the nondominant forearm. A randomized, prospective trial has been reported for patients with secondary hyperparathyroidism, comparing subtotal parathyroidectomy to total parathyroidectomy with autotransplantation.[34] Because of improved clinical parameters (less pruritus and muscle weakness), improved radiologic parameters, and the need for no reoperations compared with 20% with indications for reoperation after subtotal resection, the total parathyroidectomy with autotransplantation was judged the procedure of choice.

Parathyroid Transplantation. There are certain clinical situations in patients with hyperparathyroidism in which it would be preferable to reduce the total parathyroid mass and still have a portion of parathyroid tissue to maintain the patient in normal calcium homeostasis. As previously mentioned, parathyroid hyperplasia, either primary or secondary, has been the malady most frequently treated by subtotal parathyroidectomy. If patients develop hypercalcemia after a subtotal parathyroidectomy operation, a second neck exploration with all its attendant risks is usually required. It has been demonstrated in animals that parathyroid glands could be transplanted as autografts or as allografts if the hosts were immunosuppressed. It has also been demonstrated in humans that normal parathyroid glands will function as autografts when immediately implanted into muscle. The success of the transplantation depended on the freshly removed parathyroid tissue being sliced into very small pieces for subsequent implantation into a muscle bed. This technique has been applied in patients with both primary and secondary parathyroid hyperplasia. A total parathyroidectomy is performed, and 20 to 25 parathyroid pieces are autografted to the forearm musculature. If the patient subsequently develops hypercalcemia from the grafted parathyroid tissue, a few of the pieces can be removed under local anesthesia. The fact that the transplanted parathyroid tissue functions is documented by the fact that the patient remains normocalcemic with the grafted tissue as the only source of PTH. Moreover, large concentrations of PTH are detectable in the antecubital vein draining the graft bed, compared with normal PTH levels in the contralateral antecubital vein.

Parathyroid glands can also be viably frozen in dimethyl sulfoxide and in autologous serum for as long as 12 to 18 months. This capability offers the surgeon great versatility, because when there is uncertainty about the amount of parathyroid tissue in a patient undergoing reoperation, a portion can be frozen viably to await the postoperative course. If the patient becomes hypocalcemic, parts of the frozen autologous parathyroid tissue can be reimplanted under local anesthesia.

HYPOPARATHYROIDISM

The most common cause of hypoparathyroidism is damage to the parathyroid glands during a thyroid procedure, and it occurs more commonly with total thyroidectomy. It is not unusual for patients undergoing operative procedures on the thyroid gland to experience a drop in the serum calcium level after operation. This probably represents bruising or compromise of the blood supply of the parathyroids, and the hypocalcemia is transient. In patients with significant hyperparathyroidism and bone disease, there may be significant skeletal calcium deposition, so-called bone hunger. The serum calcium level reaches its lowest level in 48 to 72 hours and returns to normal 2 to 3 days thereafter. The sooner after operation the drop in serum calcium level occurs and the longer it persists, the greater likelihood that all parathyroid glands have been damaged and the poorer the prognosis for recovery. The major signs and symptoms of hypocalcemia are directly attributable to the reduction of plasma ionized calcium, which leads to increased neuromuscular excitability. Clinically, the earliest manifestations are numbness and tingling in the circumoral area, the fingers, and the toes. Mental symptoms are common, and patients are anxious, depressed, or occasionally confused. Tetany may develop, characterized by carpopedal spasms, tonic-clonic convulsions, and laryngeal stridor, which may prove fatal. On physical examination, contraction of the facial muscles is elicited by tapping on the facial nerve anterior to the ear (Chvostek's sign). This sign is present in a small number of normal individuals. Trousseau's sign is elicited by occluding blood flow to the forearm for 3 minutes. The development of carpal spasm indicates hypocalcemia.

A far less common cause of hypoparathyroidism is idiopathic lack of function. Approximately 150 cases have been reported, most of which occurred in childhood and some of which appeared to be familial. Hypoparathyroidism in newborns frequently follows prenatal suppression of fetal parathyroid glands by the hyperparathyroid mother. In DiGeorge's syndrome there is congenital absence of the parathyroid glands and the thymus. In addition to hypocalcemia, these children suffer from absence of the thymus-dependent lymphoid system.

The treatment of acute hypocalcemia is intravenous administration of calcium gluconate or calcium chloride. Vitamin D and oral calcium are used for long-term management.

SELECTED REFERENCES

The first three references on this list are from the National Institutes of Health Consensus Development Conference on Diagnosis and Management of Asymptomatic Primary Hyperparathyroidism held at the NIH from October 29 to 31, 1990.

Consensus Development Conference Panel: Diagnosis and management of asymptomatic primary hyperparathyroidism: Consensus Development Conference statement. Ann. Intern. Med., 114:593, 1991.
This report contains the conclusions of the expert panel which reviewed the data addressing the indications for surgery in patients with asymptomatic hyperparathyroidism, and to set standards for monitoring those patients who are followed without surgery.

Clark, O. H., Wilkes, W., Siperstein, A. E., and Duh, Q-Y.: Diagnosis and management of asymptomatic hyperparathyroidism: Safety, efficacy, and deficiencies in our knowledge. J. Bone Miner. Res., 6:S135, 1991.
Dr. Clark reviews his clinical experience to address the incidence of patients who were truly asymptomatic in his referral practice, and the safety of parathyroidectomy for hyperparathyroidism.

Wells, S. A.: Surgical therapy of patients with primary hyperparathyroidism: Long-term benefits. J. Bone Miner. Res., 6:S143, 1991.
This review addresses the evidence for long-term benefit from parathyroidectomy for hyperparathyroidism, with respect to the effect on bone, renal, neuromuscular and neuropsychiatric disease.

Nussbaum, S. R.: Pathophysiology and management of severe hypercalcemia. Endocrinol Metab. Clin. North Am., 22:343, 1993.
This article reviews the differential diagnosis of severe hypercalcemia and the pathophysiology of each, as well as the acute therapy of the hypercalcemia in detail. 90 references.

Parisien, M., Silverberg, S. J., Shane, E., Dempster, D. W., and Bilezekian, J. P.: Bone disease in primary hyperparathyroidism. Endocrinol Metab. Clin. North Am., 19:19, 1990.
This review covers normal bone remodeling, the changes in hyperparathyroidism, and the available modalities for measuring the bone alterations in this disease.

REFERENCES

1. Akerström, G., Malmaeus, J., and Bergstrom, R.: Surgical anatomy of human parathyroid glands. Surgery, 95:14, 1984.

2. Albright, F., Baird, P. C., Cope, O., and Bloomberg, E.: Studies in the physiology of the parathyroid glands: Renal complications of hyperparathyroidism. Ann. J. Med. Sci., 197:49, 1934.

3. Albright, F., Bloomberg, E., Castleman, B., and Churchill, E. D.: Hyperparathyroidism due to diffuse hyperplasia of all parathyroid glands rather than adenoma of one: Clinical studies on three such cases. Arch. Intern. Med., 54:315, 1934.

4. Alveryd, A.: Parathyroid glands in thyroid surgery. Acta Chir. Scand., 389:1, 1968.

5. Arnold, A.: Molecular mechanisms of parathyroid neoplasia. Endocrinol. Metabol. Clin. North Am., 23:93, 1994.

6. Askanazy, M.: Über Ostitis deformans ohne Osteoides gewebe. Arb. Geb. Path. Anath. Inst. Tubingen, 4:398, 1903.

7. Aurbach, G. D.: Isolation of parathyroid hormone after extraction with phenol. J. Biol. Chem., 234:3179, 1959.

8. Barr, D. P., and Bulger, M. A.: The clinical syndrome of hyperparathyroidism. Ann. J. Med. Sci., 179:449, 1930.

9. Berson, S. A., Yalow, R. S., Aurbach, G. D., and Potts, J. T.: Immunoassay of bovine and human parathyroid hormone. Proc. Natl. Acad. Sci. USA, 49:613, 1963.

10. Bess, M. A., Edis, A. J., van Heerden, J. A.: Hyperparathyroidism and pancreatitis: Chance or a casual association? JAMA, 243:246, 1980.

11. Bilezikian, J. P.: Management of acute hypercalcemia. N. Engl. J. Med., 326:1196, 1992.

12. Bolman, R. M., Cooper, C. W., Garner, S. C., Munson, P. L., Wells, S.A.: Stimulation of gastrin secretion in the pig by parathyroid hormone and its inhibition by thyrocalcitonin. Endocrinology, 100:1014, 1977.

13. Boyd, J. D.: Development of thyroid and parathyroid glands and thymus. Ann. R. Coll. Surg. Engl., 7:455, 1950.

14. Christensson, T.: Familial hyperparathyroidism. Ann. Intern. Med., 85:614, 1976.

15. Christensson, T.: Hyperparathyroidism and radiation therapy. Ann. Intern. Med., 89:216, 1978.

16. Collip, J. B.: The extraction of a parathyroid hormone that will prevent or control parathyroid tetany and which regulates the level of blood calcium. J. Biol. Chem., 63:293, 1928.

17. Consensus Development Conference Panel: Diagnosis and management of asymptomatic primary hyperparathyroidism: Consensus development conference statement. Ann. Intern. Med., 114:593, 1991.

18. Cope, O., Keynes, W. M., Roth, S. I., and Castleman, B.: Primary chief cell hyperplasia of the parathyroid glands: A new entity in the surgery of hyperparathyroidism. Ann. Surg., 148:375, 1958.

19. Diamond, T. W., Both, J. R., Wing, J., Meyers, A. W., and Kalk, W. J.: Parathyroid hypertension: A reversible disorder. Arch. Intern. Med., 146:1709, 1986.

20. Doherty, G. M., Doppman, J. L., Miller, D. L., et al.: Results of a multidisciplinary strategy for management of mediastinal parathyroid adenoma as a cause of persistent primary hyperparathyroidism. Ann. Surg., 215:101, 1992.

21. Edis, A. J., Purnell, D. C., van Heerden, J. A.: The undescended parathymus: An occasional cause of failed neck exploration of hyperparathyroidism. Ann. Surg., 190:64, 1979.

22. Erdheim, J.: Über Epithelkorperchenbefunde bei Osteomalacie. S. B. Akad. Wiss. Math. Naturw. Cl., 116:311, 1907.

23. Farndon, J. R., Geraghty, J. M., Dilley, W. G., Handwerger, S., and Leight, G. S.: Serum gastrin, calcitonin, and prolactin as markers of multiple endocrine neoplasia syndromes in patients with primary hyperparathyroidism. World J. Surg., 11:252, 1987.

24. Friedman, E., Sakaguchi, K., Bale, A. E., et al.: Clonality of parathyroid tumors in familial multiple endocrine neoplasia type I. N. Engl. J. Med., 321:213, 1989.

25. Gley, E.: Sur les fonctions du corps thyroide. C. R. Soc. Biol., 43:841, 1891.

26. Hellstrom, J., Ivemark, B. I.: Primary hyperparathyroidism. Acta Chir. Scand., 194:1, 1962.

27. Joborn, C., Hetta, J., Johanson, H., et al.: Psychiatric morbidity in primary hyperparathyroidism. World J. Surg., 12:476, 1988.

28. Kochersberger, G., Buckley, N. J., Leight, G. S., et al.: What is the clinical significance of bone loss in primary hyperparathyroidism? Arch. Intern. Med., 147:1951, 1987.

29. Lind, L., and Ljunghall, S.: Serum chloride in the differential diagnosis of hypercalcemia. Exp. Clin. Endocrinol., 98:179, 1991.

30. Lloyd, H. M.: Primary hyperparathyroidism: An analysis of the role of the parathyroid tumor. Medicine, 47:53, 1986.

31. MacCallum, W. B., and Voegtlin, C.: On the relation of tetany to the parathyroid glands and to calcium metabolism. J. Exp. Med., 11:118, 1909.

32. Mandl, F.: Therapeutischer Versuch bei einem Falle von Ostitis fibrosa generalisata mittels Exstirpation eines epithelk orperchen Tumors. Zentrabl. Chirurg, 5:260, 1926.

33. McLeod, M. K., Monchik, J. M., and Martin, H. F.: The role of ionized calcium in the diagnosis of subtle hypercalcemia in symptomatic primary hyperparathyroidism. Surgery, 95:667, 1984.

34. Miller, D. L., Doppman, J. L., Krudy, A. G., et al.: Localization of parathyroid adenomas in patients who have undergone surgery. II: Invasive procedures. Radiology, 162:138, 1987.

35. Norris, E. H.: The parathyroid glands and the lateral thyroid in man: Their morphogenesis, histogenesis, topographic anatomy and prenatal growth. Contrib. Embryol., 26:247, 1937.

36. Patten, B. M., Bilezikian, J. P., Mallette, L. E., Prince, A., Engel, W. K., and Aurbach, G. D.: Neuromuscular disease and primary hyperparathyroidism. Ann. Intern. Med., 80:182, 1974.

37. Petersen, P.: Psychiatric disorders in primary hyperparathyroidism. J. Clin. Endocrinol. Metab., 28:1491, 1968.

38. Pollak, M. R., Brown, E. M., Chou, Y-HW, et al.: Mutations in the human Ca-sensing receptor gene cause familial hypocalciuric hypercalcemia and neonatal severe hyperparathyroidism. Cell, 75:1297, 1993.

39. Rasmussen, H., and Craig, L. C.: Purification of the parathyroid hormone by use of countercurrent distribution. J. Am. Chem. Soc., 81:5003, 1959.

40. Reeve, T. S., and Delbridge, L. W.: Pancreatitis following parathyroid surgery. Ann. Surg., 195:1581, 1982.

41. Richardson, E. P., Aub, J. C., and Bauer, W.: Parathyroidectomy in osteomalacia. Ann. Surg., 90:730, 1929.

42. Rogers, H. M.: Parathyroid adenoma and hypertrophy of the parathyroid glands. JAMA, 130:22, 1946.

43. Rosin, R. D.: Pancreatitis and hyperparathyroidism. Postgrad. Med. J., 52:95, 1976.

44. Rothmund, M., Wagner, P. K., and Schark, C.: Subtotal parathyroidectomy versus total parathyroidectomy and autotransplantation in secondary hyperparathyroidism: A randomized trial. World J. Surg., 15:745, 1991.

45. Sandstrom, I.: On a new gland in man and several mammals (gladulae parathyroideae). Upsala. Lak. Foren. Forh., 15:441, 1879.

46. Saxe, A., Raile, R., Tesluk, H., and Toreson, W.: The role of the pathologist in the surgical treatment of hyperparathyroidism. Surg. Gynecol. Obstet., 161:101, 1985.

47. Schlagenhaufer, F.: Zwei Faller von Parathyreoideatumoren. Wien. Klin. Wochenschr., 28:1362, 1915.

48. Scholz, D. A., and Purnell, D. C.: Asymptomatic primary hyperparathyroidism: 10 year prospective study. Mayo. Clin. Proc. 56:473, 1981.

49. Smith, F. B., and Cooke, R. T.: Acute fatal hyperparathyroidism. Lancet, 2:650, 1940.

50. Strewler, G. J., and Nissenson, R. A.: Hypercalcemia in malignancy. West J. Med., 153:635, 1990.

51. Uden, P., Chan, A., Duh, Q-Y., Siperstein, A., and Clark, O. H.: Primary hyperparathyroidism in younger and older patients: Symptoms and outcome of surgery. World J. Surg., 16:791, 1992.

52. van Heerden, J. A., James, E. M., Caselle, P. R., et al.: Small part ultrasonography in primary hyperparathyroidism. Ann. Surg., 195:774, 1982.

53. van Heerden, J. A., Kent, R. B., Sizemore, G. W., Grant, C. S., and Remine, W. H.: Primary hyperparathyroidism in patients with multiple endocrine neoplasia syndromes. Arch. Surg., 118:533, 1983.

54. von Recklinghausen, F. D.: Die Fibrose oder deformierte Ostitis, die Osteomalacie und die Osteoplastische carnose in ihren gegenseitigen Beziehungen. Festschr. Rud. Virchow, 1:89, 1891.

55. Wang, C., and Gaz, R. D.: Natural history of parathyroid carcinoma: Diagnosis, treatment, and results. Am. J. Surg., 149:522, 1985.

56. Weller, G. L.: Development of the thyroid, parathyroid and thymus glands in man. Contrib. Embryol., 24:95, 1932.

57. Wells, S. A., Jr., and Cooper, J. D.: Closed mediastinal exploration in patients with persistent hyperparathyroidism. Ann. Surg., 214:555, 1991.

58. Wells, S. A., Jr., Leight, G. S., and Ross, A. J. III: Primary hyperparathyroidism. Curr. Probl. Surg., 17:398, 1980.

59. Wells, S. A., Jr., Leight, G. S., Hensley, M., and Dilley, W. G.: Hyperparathyroidism associated with the enlargement of two or three parathyroid glands. Ann. Surg., 202:533, 1985.

CHAPTER 25

THE PITUITARY AND ADRENAL GLANDS

John A. Olson, Jr., M.D., Ph.D., and Samuel A. Wells, Jr., M.D.

PITUITARY GLAND

Embryology

The pituitary has dual embryonic origin. The anterior pituitary arises from embryonic ectoderm (Rathke's pouch) and includes the pars distalis, pars intermedia (vestigial in humans), and pars tuberalis. The neural portion of the gland arises from the diencephalon and includes the neural stalk, infundibulum, and posterior lobe. Embryonic defects in invagination and obliteration of the pharyngeal extent of Rathke's pouch may lead to craniopharyngiomas or hormonally active ectopic pituitary adenomas.

Anatomy

The pituitary sits within the sella turcica (*Turkish saddle*). This fossa is bordered anteriorly, posteriorly, and inferiorly by the sphenoid bone and laterally by the cavernous sinus. The floor of the sella forms the roof of the sphenoidal sinus. The carotid arteries and cranial nerves III, IV, and VI traverse the cavernous sinus lateral to the sella (Fig. 25–1). Nearby structures also include the optic nerves and chiasm, the mamillary body, and the median eminence of the hypothalamus. The diaphragma sellae, a thick reflection of dura mater, covers the roof of the sella and closely encircles the pituitary stalk in 50% of individuals. In remaining individuals, the diaphragma sellae incompletely surrounds the stalk and may permit superior extension of pituitary tumors.

The arterial supply to the hypothalamic-pituitary region is complex and arises from three sources. The inferior hypophyseal artery, a branch of the carotid artery, supplies the posterior pituitary. The superior hypophyseal arteries branch from the circle of Willis to supply the median eminence. The middle hypophyseal arteries are of variable origin and supply the pituitary stalk. Capillary portions of the superior hypophyseal arteries drain from the hypothalamus, the median eminence, and the superior portions of the pituitary stalk. These vessels drain into the hypophyseal portal system, which forms a secondary venous plexus in the anterior pituitary and ultimately empties into the cavernous sinus. This portal venous system constitutes the principal blood supply to the anterior pituitary and serves as the medium through which releasing hormones from the hypothalamus reach the pituitary.

The average adult pituitary measures 10 × 15 × 5 mm. and weighs between 0.4 and 0.9 gm. The gland is oval, bilaterally symmetrical, and brownish red. The pituitary is approximately 20% larger in females than in males and it enlarges about 10% in females during pregnancy.

The adenohypophysis, or anterior pituitary, comprises 80% of the gland and, together with the posterior lobe, it fills approximately three fourths of the sellar space (Fig. 25–2). The pars tuberalis lies above the diaphragma sellae in proximity to the median eminence.

Histology

Previous nomenclature distinguished acidophil, basophil, and chromophobe cell types based on reactions of fixed and

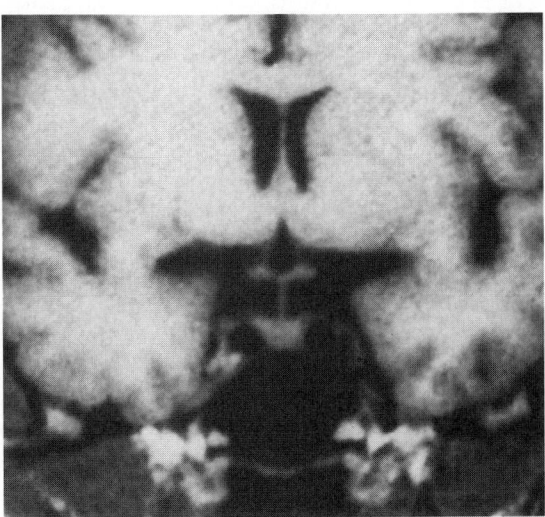
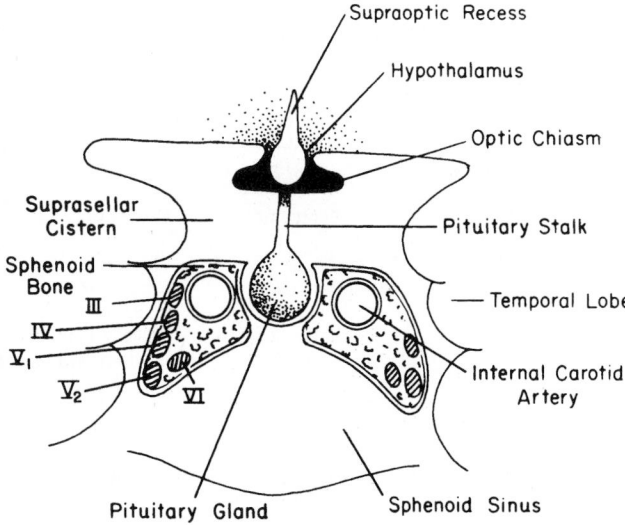

Figure 25–1. MR image (left) and schematic diagram (right) of the normal pituitary fossa. The pituitary is bordered laterally by the cavernous sinus, which contains the internal carotid artery and cranial nerves III, IV, V₁, V₂, and VI. The optic chiasm lies immediately above the pituitary gland. (From Lechan, R. M.: Neuroendocrinology of pituitary hormone regulation. Endocrinol. Metab. Clin. North Am., *16*:475, 1987.)

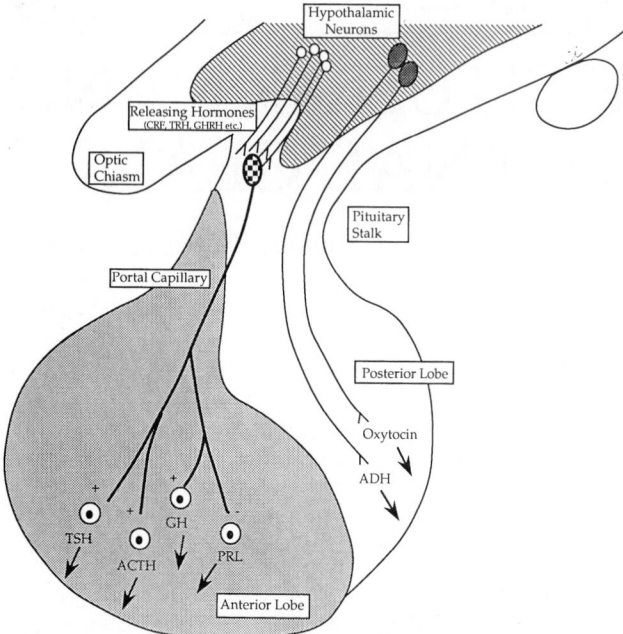

Figure 25–2. Schematic representation of hypothalamic-pituitary region. Releasing hormones synthesized by hypothalamic neurons reach the adenohypophysis via the hypothalamic-pituitary portal blood system. Cells of the anterior lobe include lactotrophs, which produce prolactin (PRL); somatotrophs, which produce growth hormone (GH); corticotrophs, which produce adrenocorticotropin (ACTH); thyrotrophs, which produce thyroid-stimulating hormone (TSH); and gonadotrophs, which produce follicle-stimulating hormone (FSH) and luteinizing hormone (LH). The neurohypophysis contains antidiuretic hormone (ADH) and oxytocin synthesized by neurons of the hypothalamus.

sectioned specimens with dyes. Cell types of the anterior pituitary are now classified by their secretory products: lactotrophs produce prolactin (PRL), somatotrophs produce growth hormone (GH), adrenocorticotrophs produce adrenocorticotropic hormone (ACTH), thyrotrophs produce thyroid-stimulating hormone (TSH), and gonadotrophs produce follicle-stimulating hormone (FSH) and luteinizing hormone (LH). Pituitary cells may, however, have plurihormonal potential, and some pituitary tumors secrete several hormones concurrently. The five pituitary cell types are regionally distributed within the gland. Lactotrophs and gonadotrophs are widely distributed, somatotrophs reside peripherally within two lateral wings of the gland, thyrotrophs are anteromedi-

ally located, and corticotrophs are found within a central median wedge.[53]

The neurohypophysis, or posterior pituitary, includes the posterior lobe, the pituitary stalk, and the median eminence. Antidiuretic hormone (ADH) and oxytocin are synthesized in supraoptic and paraventricular nuclei of the hypothalamus and are transported through axons from these nuclei to the posterior pituitary where the active hormones are released into the capillary circulation.

Physiology

Regulation of anterior pituitary hormone secretion is complex and is controlled by the arcuate and other anterior nuclei of the hypothalamus. Axons from these hypothalamic nuclei terminate in the median eminence next to portal capillaries where they release hormones into the hypothalamic-pituitary portal circulation to inhibit or stimulate cells of the anterior pituitary (Table 25–1).

The anterior pituitary secretes three groups of hormones: (1) Propiomelanocortin (POMC)-derived ACTH and beta-lipotropin (β-LPH); (2) the related hormones GH and PRL; and (3) the glycoprotein hormones LH, FSH, and TSH. ACTH controls glucocorticoid production by the adrenal cortex; GH regulates growth and intermediary metabolism; PRL is necessary for lactation; TSH regulates the thyroid; and LH and FSH together control the gonads in males and females. Target gland hormones, in turn, participate in feedback control of the pituitary and hypothalamus (Fig. 25–3).

ACTH. Adrenocorticotropic hormone is produced by corticotrophs of the anterior pituitary. This 39-amino acid peptide is part of the 241-amino acid precursor POMC, encoded by a gene on chromosome 2.[73] Tissue-specific processing of POMC occurs at the posttranslational level to form several biologically active polypeptides, including ACTH, β-LPH, a joining peptide, and a NH₂ terminal peptide (Fig. 25–4).[60] The biologic activity of ACTH resides in its initial 18-amino acid sequence, and a stable synthetic ACTH (1–24 amino acids) is available for diagnostic use. ACTH and β-LPH have melanocyte-stimulating activity, which may explain the increased skin pigmentation seen with corticotroph hyperactivity in patients with Addison's disease and Nelson's syndrome.

Corticotropin-releasing hormone (CRH) regulates ACTH release under normal conditions through receptor-mediated cyclic adenosine monophosphate production in corticotrophs. Stress of major surgery, burns, fever, or hypoglycemia may elicit large (2-fold to 10-fold) increases in ACTH and corti-

TABLE 25–1. Hypothalamic and Pituitary Hormones and Their Actions

Hypothalamic Hormone	Type of Effect	Hormone or Organ Affected	Ultimate Peripheral Action
Corticotropin-releasing hormone	Stimulatory	Corticotropin	Stimulates adrenal secretion of cortisol and androgens
Thyrotropin-releasing hormone	Stimulatory	Thyrotropin	Stimulates thyroid hormone secretion
	Stimulatory	Prolactin	Stimulates production of breast milk in women
Dopamine	Inhibitory	Prolactin	—
Gonadotropin-releasing hormone	Stimulatory	Follicle-stimulating hormone, luteinizing hormone	Stimulates estradiol and progesterone secretion, folliculogenesis and ovulation in women; stimulates testosterone secretion and sperm production in men
Growth hormone–releasing hormone	Stimulatory	Growth hormone	Stimulates insulin-like growth factor-1 production
Somatostatin	Inhibitory	Growth hormone	—
Vasopressin	Stimulatory	Kidney	Stimulates free-water reabsorption in renal collecting ducts
Oxytocin	Stimulatory	Uterus, breast	Stimulates uterine contraction and milk ejection

Adapted from Vance, M. L., N. Engl. J. Med., 1994, 330, 1651. Copyright 1994. Massachusetts Medical Society. All rights reserved.

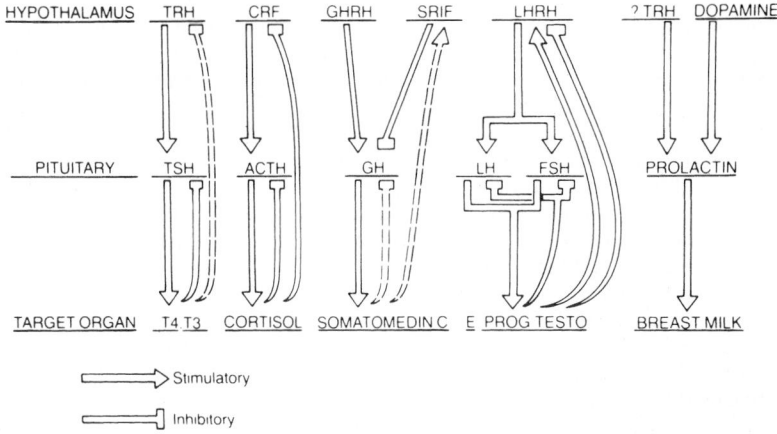

Figure 25–3. Hypothalamus-pituitary-target tissue interaction. (From Caldwell, B. V., and Kayne, R. D.: Normal endocrine function of the pituitary. *In* Goodrich, I., and Lee, K. J. [Eds.]: The Pituitary. Amsterdam, Elsevier, 1987, p. 30.)

sol.[113] A substantial component of stress-induced ACTH release is immune mediated by the cytokines interleukin-1, interleukin-2, and interleukin-6.[6]

ACTH stimulates cortisol production by the adrenal gland. Secretion of both hormones is normally pulsatile and follows a circadian rhythm. Plasma ACTH and serum cortisol levels are lowest between 10 P.M. and 2 A.M. and are highest at approximately 8 A.M. Glucocorticoids exert negative feedback at several levels, including hypothalamic CRH release, POMC transcription and processing, and CRH-stimulated ACTH release. In addition, ACTH exerts *short loop* negative feedback to hypothalamic CRH release.

Opioids. Cleavage of the β-LPH sequence of POMC releases the endogenous opioids beta-endorphin and met-enkephalin. Opioids stimulate opiate receptors in brain and spinal cord to produce analgesia. The endogenous opioids are released from many central nervous system sites during periods of stress, shock, or hypoglycemia.[50]

Prolactin and Growth Hormone Family. Prolactin, human GH, and human placental lactogen (hPL) comprise a related family of hormones sharing a common ancestral gene. Within the human PRL-GH family, a single PRL gene is present on chromosome 6 and five GH-related genes are located on chromosome 17.[98] Only PRL and GH seem relevant to pituitary function.

Prolactin. Prolactin is secreted by lactotrophs, which constitute 10% to 30% of the cells of the normal pituitary and 70% of cells in females during pregnancy.[26] PRL circulates as a 23,000-molecular-weight monomeric polypeptide, and normal baseline levels are less than 20 μg. per liter women and less than 10 μg. per liter in men. Synthesis and release of PRL by lactotrophs are under tonic inhibition by hypothalamic dopamine.[71] Suckling of the breast is the principal physiologic stimulus for PRL release under normal conditions and causes a 10- to 100-fold increase in PRL within 30 minutes of stimulation. No PRL-releasing factor has been conclusively identified, although thyrotropin-releasing hormone (TRH) and vasoactive intestinal peptide (VIP) are candidates.[92]

PRL binds to specific receptors in the breast to initiate and sustain lactation. Physiologic hyperprolactinemia suppresses gonadotropin-releasing hormone (GnRH) and transiently depresses the hypothalamic-pituitary-gonadal axis during lactation. This effect may explain the often observed, though unreliable, phenomenon of decreased fertility in lactating women. Dopamine, L-dopa, and the ergot alkaloid bromocriptine inhibit PRL release and lactation. Metoclopramide, haloperidol, chlorpromazine, and reserpine can interfere with release of dopamine into the pituitary portal circulation, enhance PRL secretion, and cause galactorrhea.

Growth Hormone. Growth hormone is a 191-amino acid peptide secreted by somatotrophs. These cells constitute about 50% of cells in the normal anterior pituitary. Plasma GH levels are normally less than 5 ng. per ml. in adults, and GH circulates bound to a GH-binding protein that is identical to the extracellular domain of the GH receptor.[7] The function of GH-binding protein is unclear.

Secretion of GH is normally under complex physiologic control. GH is regulated positively by growth hormone–releasing hormone (GH-RH) and negatively by somatostatin. GH-RH is a 44-amino acid peptide that binds to G protein–coupled receptors to stimulate adenyl cyclase. Somatostatin binds to separate receptors and inhibits adenyl cyclase.[51] Stress, exercise, hypoglycemia, protein depletion, and administration of glucagon and arginine can stimulate secretion of GH. Acute hyperglycemia suppresses GH secretion.

GH stimulates longitudinal growth of the skeleton and regulates several metabolic processes. Most GH effects are indirect and are mediated by the insulin-like growth factors (IGF-1 and IGF-2) produced by GH target organs. GH directly antagonizes insulin effects on sugar uptake and fatty acid release in peripheral tissues but complements the anabolic effect of insulin on amino acid uptake. GH also stimu-

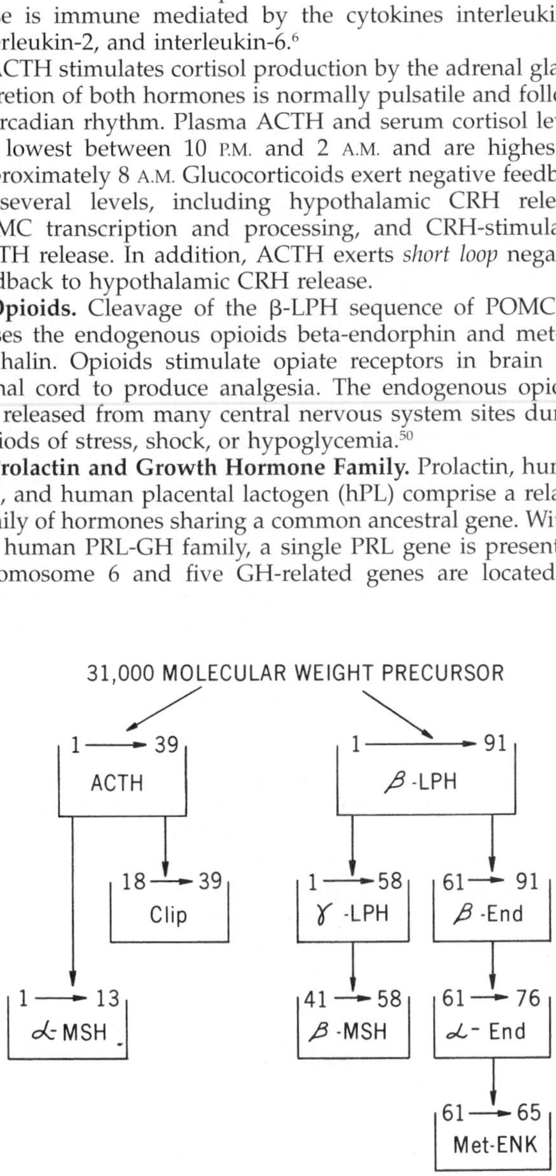

31,000 MOLECULAR WEIGHT PRECURSOR

Figure 25–4. High-molecular-weight precursor of ACTH and several other peptides secreted by the anterior pituitary. Clip, Clip peptide; MSH, melanocyte-stimulating hormone; LPH, lipotropin; end, endorphin; Met-ENK, met-enkephalin.

lates insulin secretion by the pancreas and directly stimulates hepatocyte growth and adipocyte metabolism. GH promotes anabolism in burn patients and has been shown to prevent corticosteroid-induced catabolism.[52, 133]

Glycoprotein Hormones. The glycoprotein hormones of the anterior pituitary, TSH, FSH, and LH, are each composed of two subunits. A 92-amino acid alpha subunit is encoded by a gene on chromosome 6q21.1-q23 and is identical among these three hormones.[37] The beta subunit is unique for each hormone and confers specificity.[102]

Thyroid-Stimulating Hormone. TSH is produced by thyrotrophs, which constitute about 5% of cells in the anterior pituitary. TSH is a 28,000-molecular-weight glycoprotein composed of an alpha subunit and a unique beta subunit encoded by a gene on chromosome 1p22.[32] TSH secretion is pulsatile and follows a circadian pattern in response to thyrotropic stimulation by the hypothalamic tripeptide TRH.[106] TSH binds to receptors on thyroid epithelium, which activates adenyl cyclase, stimulates iodide transport and thyroglobulin proteolysis, and stimulates thyroid hormone release. TSH also increases the size and vascularity of the thyroid gland. The thyroid hormones, triiodothyronine (T_3) and thyroxine (T_4), exert negative feedback on TSH release by the pituitary.[69] TSH also inhibits hypothalamic release of TRH by a short loop negative feedback (Fig. 25–5). Somatostatin, dopamine, and glucocorticoids also decrease TSH release.[75]

Luteinizing Hormone and Follicle-Stimulating Hormone. LH and FSH are produced by gonadotrophs, which constitute about 10% of anterior pituitary cells. Both hormones have the glycoprotein alpha subunit, and specificity is dictated by their distinct beta subunits. The LH beta gene is located on chromosome 19q13.32, and the FSH beta gene is located on chromosome 11p13.[37, 130]

In males, LH stimulates Leydig cells to produce testosterone, whereas FSH binds to receptors on the Sertoli cells to promote spermatogenesis. Testosterone and the gonadotropins influence both the rate and numbers of germ cells that ultimately differentiate into mature sperm. Testosterone and its metabolite, dihydrotestosterone, stimulate growth of the penis and scrotum; promote development of facial, axillary, and pubic hair; and influence states of libido and aggressiveness.

In females, LH and FSH regulate cyclic ovarian function. FSH stimulates maturation of the graafian follicle and its production of estradiol. A midcycle surge of LH causes follicular rupture, ovulation, and establishment of the corpus luteum. LH maintains luteal function until either pregnancy or luteolysis. In general, sex steroids exert negative feedback on release of LH and FSH by the pituitary. Over a 24- to 36-hour interval before ovulation, however, estradiol and progesterone transiently stimulate LH secretion and, to a lesser extent, FSH secretion. A gradual increase in plasma estradiol to levels above 300 pg. per ml. for a duration of 5 to 7 days followed by a rise in plasma progesterone from 0.5 to 1.5 ng. per ml. enhances release of LH and FSH and leads to ovulation.[64]

GnRH stimulates gonadotropin secretion from the pituitary. In the adult male, FSH and LH secretion is inhibited by androgens and by estradiol converted from testosterone in peripheral tissues. Androgens suppress GnRH from the hypothalamus, while estradiol inhibits GnRH-induced LH release from the pituitary. Sertoli cells release the peptide inhibin, which suppresses release of FSH but not LH.

Neurohypophyseal Hormones. Antidiuretic hormone (ADH, also known as vasopressin) and oxytocin are the two principal hormones secreted by the posterior pituitary. These hormones both contain nine amino acids and are derived from a common ancestral hormone, vasotocin. Both oxytocin and vasopressin are synthesized and released in conjunction with carrier proteins known as neurophysins.

Antidiuretic Hormone. Antidiuretic hormone is synthesized by the pituitary and is released into the circulation in conjunction with neurophysin II. ADH circulates to the kidney, where it stimulates sodium and chloride reabsorption by epithelial cells of the medullary thick ascending loop of Henle. In addition, ADH enhances permeability to water within the collecting ducts of the medulla.

Primary stimuli for ADH release include a rise in plasma osmolality above 285 mOsm. or a decrease in circulating blood volume by 5% or more. ADH is also secreted in response to catecholamines, angiotensin, opiates, and other analgesic or anesthetic agents. Drugs such as phenytoin, alcohol, and lithium suppress release of ADH.

Oxytocin. Oxytocin and its carrier protein neurophysin I are released by neural pathways during distention of the vagina or uterus or by suckling of the nipples. Oxytocin stimulates uterine contraction during labor and elicits milk ejection by myoepithelial cells of the mammary ducts during lactation.

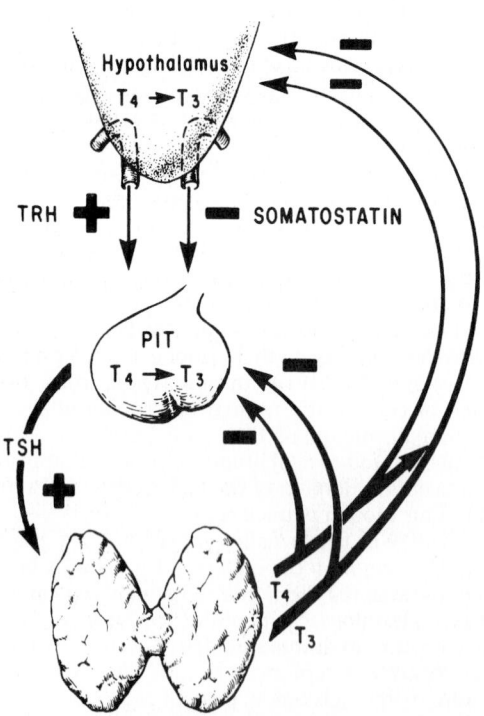

Figure 25–5. Schematic representation of hypothalamic-pituitary-thyroid gland axis. Hypothalamic thyrotropin-releasing hormone (TRH) regulates secretion of thyrotropin (TSH) by the pituitary, which in turn stimulates thyroid production of thyroid hormones, triiodothyronine (T_3) and thyroxine (T_4). Thyroid hormones feed back to inhibit TRH and TSH in the hypothalamus and pituitary, respectively. In addition, there is a "short loop" by which TSH feeds back at the hypothalamic level to inhibit TRH. (From Wilson, J. D., and Foster, D. W. [Eds.]: Williams Textbook of Endocrinology, 8th ed. Philadelphia, W.B. Saunders, 1992, p. 169.)

Evaluation and Diagnosis of Pituitary Disease

Pituitary tumors account for 10% to 15% of intracranial neoplasms and are classified as microadenomas (diameter <10 mm.) or macroadenomas (diameter >10 mm.). Pituitary tumors produce symptoms related to endocrine dysfunction or to mass effects of an enlarging pituitary. Prolactinomas, nonsecreting adenomas, and GH-producing adenomas are the most frequent pituitary tumor types. ACTH-producing adenomas, gonadotroph adenomas, and TSH-producing adenomas are uncommon.[117] Other sellar or parasellar tumors include craniopharyngiomas, germ cell tumors, and metastatic lesions.

Clinical Manifestations of Pituitary Endocrine Dysfunction. Hyperpituitarism associated with pituitary tumors may be suspected on clinical grounds. Prolactinomas cause galactorrhea and hypogonadism (e.g., amenorrhea and infertility in women and impotence in men). GH-secreting tumors cause gigantism in children and acromegaly in adults. ACTH-producing tumors produce signs and symptoms of hypercortisolism (Cushing's syndrome). Glycoprotein hormone (LH, FSH, and TSH)–producing adenomas cause infertility and sexual dysfunction. Conversely, patients may develop total or selective hypopituitarism from untreated pituitary adenomas, from pituitary radiation or surgery, or from head injury. Although variation occurs, the progressive loss of pituitary function generally occurs in the following order: LH/FSH, GH, TSH, then ACTH. The most common symptoms, sexual dysfunction in men and amenorrhea and infertility in women, are caused by hypogonadotropic hypogonadism. GH deficiency is generally clinically silent in adults but causes growth retardation in children. TSH deficiency causes secondary hypothyroidism with weight gain, fatigue, depression, and cold intolerance. ACTH deficiency leads to symptoms of adrenal insufficiency, although mineralocorticoid production is spared and hyperpigmentation is not observed.

Clinical Manifestations of Structural Abnormalities. Sellar masses may produce headache as well as signs and symptoms related to compression of nearby cranial nerves. Headache from pituitary tumors is variable, and its pathogenesis is unknown. Pituitary neoplasms enlarge superiorly toward the optic chiasm and may produce visual field changes. The classic defect, bitemporal hemianopsia, is variable, and other visual defects occur. Extraocular muscle movements can be limited secondary to compression of cranial nerves III, IV, and VI in the cavernous sinus. Funduscopic examination may reveal pallor of the optic disc, yet papilledema is most unusual. Spontaneous cerebrospinal fluid (CSF) rhinorrhea occurs rarely (0.5% of patients), but a pituitary tumor is the most common cause of this symptom.

Diagnosis of Suspected Anterior Pituitary Disease

Historically, patients had large pituitary lesions and presented with well-characterized endocrine and neuro-ophthalmologic abnormalities. Today, most pituitary tumors are diagnosed early in patients who present with syndromes of endocrine hypersecretion. These syndromes are diagnosed by careful history and physical examination followed by baseline determination of specific pituitary and target hormones. Dynamic testing to evaluate pituitary reserve should complement baseline studies. Patients with endocrine dysfunction and visual symptoms should receive a comprehensive neuro-ophthalmologic evaluation, including formal visual field testing. Pituitary tumors are best visualized by sellar magnetic resonance imaging (MRI) or computed tomography (CT), while inferior petrosal sinus sampling may be used to definitively localize tumors not seen radiographically.

Biochemical Testing of Anterior Pituitary Function. Biochemical assessment of anterior pituitary function generally includes measurement of basal plasma levels of a hormone under standard conditions (Table 25–2). Therefore, screening for pituitary dysfunction most often involves drawing a single blood sample for evaluation of basal pituitary and target hormone levels.[123] Dynamic testing of pituitary reserve using individual provocative or suppression tests may occasionally be required when basal levels are equivocal. Pituitary *batteries* using multiple releasing hormones have little diagnostic utility[14] but may guide replacement therapy after pituitary surgery or radiation. Careful consideration of time of day and stress factors must be made because even the discomfort associated with blood drawing may stimulate pituitary hormone secretion.

ACTH. Direct ACTH measurement with two-site immunoradiometric assay (IRMA) is now the preferred test to identify ACTH-dependent causes of Cushing's syndrome.[38] Normal levels are above 5 pg. per ml., while lower levels suggest ACTH-independent hypercortisolism. Levels above 10 to 20 pg. per ml. indicate pituitary or ectopic ACTH overproduction as the cause of Cushing's syndrome.

Prolactin. A random serum PRL level is sufficient to accurately diagnose prolactinoma in the majority of cases. A level above 300 μg. per liter is virtually always associated with a prolactinoma, and a level of 150 μg. per liter in a nonpregnant patient is usually caused by a prolactinoma.[68] Moderately elevated levels (25 to 100 μg. per liter) should be repeated to exclude stress-induced hyperprolactinemia. PRL deficiency may be diagnosed by measurement of subnormal serum PRL 15 minutes after intravenous administration of 200 μg. of TRH.

Growth Hormone. Random serum GH levels are extremely variable and are not helpful in the diagnosis of GH excess. Instead, serum IGF-1 is a useful screening test for this disor-

TABLE 25–2. Pituitary Hormone Evaluation

Pituitary Hormone	Basal Test	Dynamic Test—Hyperfunction	Dynamic Test—Hypofunction
PRL	Random Serum PRL	None	TRH stimulation
GH	Serum IGF-1	Glucose suppression	Insulin-induced hypoglycemia
ACTH	Urine free cortisol* ACTH IRMA	Low-dose DST* High-dose DST† Metyrapone† IPS-CRH†	ACTH stimulation
FSH/LH (also nonfunctioning adenoma)	Fasting PRL, LH, FSH, TSH, IGF-1, glycoprotein alpha subunit, testosterone	None	GnHRH stimulation
TSH	Serum T$_4$, Free T$_4$ index TSH IRMA	None	TRH stimulation

PRL, prolactin; GH, growth hormone; ACTH, adrenocorticotropin; FSH, follicle-stimulating hormone; LH, luteinizing hormone; TSH, thyroid-stimulating hormone; IPS-CRH, inferior petrosal sinus sampling—corticotropin-releasing hormone test; GnHRH, gonadotropin-releasing hormone; IGF-1, insulin-like growth factor-1; T$_4$, thyroxine; IRMA, immunoradiometric assay.
*Establishes hypercortisolism (Cushing's syndrome).
†Localizes cause of hypercortisolism to the pituitary (Cushing's disease).
See text for details of testing.

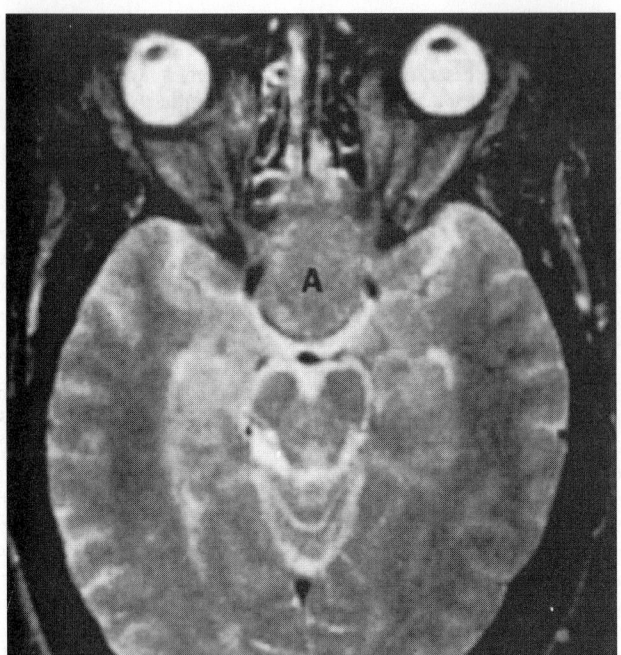

Figure 25–6. Axial spin-echo T2-weighted MR image of a large pituitary adenoma (A) that occupies the suprasellar cistern. (Courtesy of F. J. Wippold, M.D., Mallinckrodt Institute of Radiology, Washington University School of Medicine, St. Louis, Missouri.)

der and for monitoring patients after treatment.[68, 82] Conversely, testing for GH deficiency is performed by measurement of serum GH 30, 60, and 120 minutes after insulin-induced hypoglycemia (0.1 U. per kg. regular insulin).

Thyroid-Stimulating Hormone. Sensitive TSH IRMA is used in conjunction with serum T_4 or free T_4 index to evaluate central hypothyroidism. If T_4 and free T_4 levels are low and the TSH level is not elevated, then central hypothyroidism is likely. Failure of TRH to stimulate TSH secretion will confirm central hypothyroidism, but this test is not crucial for diagnosis.

Luteinizing Hormone/Follicle-Stimulating Hormone. Women with normal menses and men with normal testosterone levels and sperm counts have normal levels of gonadotropins and do not need to be tested. Estrogen-deficient premenopausal women and testosterone-deficient men with low-normal basal gonadotropin levels likely have gonadotropin deficiency that is confirmed by GnRH stimulation testing.

Diagnosis of Suspected Posterior Pituitary Disease

The syndrome of inappropriate antidiuretic hormone secretion (SIADH) is characterized by euvolemic hyponatremia with an inappropriately concentrated urine. SIADH is generally a diagnosis of exclusion after other causes of euvolemic hyponatremia, including hypothyroidism and adrenal insufficiency, have been excluded.

Deficiency of antidiuretic hormone (diabetes insipidus) is suggested by prolonged polyuria and polydipsia, and it is confirmed by a combination of high plasma osmolality (>285 mOsm.) and low urine osmolality (<200 mOsm.) after water deprivation. Correction of diabetes insipidus after exogenously administered ADH differentiates central versus nephrogenic diabetes insipidus.

Neuro-ophthalmologic Evaluation

All patients with visual complaints and suspected pituitary lesions should have neuro-ophthalmologic evaluation. Bed-

side testing with confrontation may detect gross field cuts only. Quantitative visual field examination with kinetic Goldmann perimetry or an automated method is necessary to detect subtle field defects and should be performed in patients before and after treatment for macroadenomas.

Diagnostic Imaging and Localization

High-resolution MRI with intravenous gadolinium contrast is the diagnostic modality of choice for radiologic localization of pituitary disease. MRI visualizes the optic chiasm, pituitary gland, pituitary stalk, cavernous portion of the internal carotid, and cavernous sinus with excellent detail (Figs. 25–6 through 25–8). MRI detects microadenomas with a sensitivity approaching 100%, although very small microadenomas, as in Cushing's disease, may be missed.[78] MRI also reliably identifies macroadenomas and pituitary apoplexy (hemorrhage into a macroadenoma), as well as most other pituitary pathology. MRI is superior to CT in assessing the dimensions of the sella turcica and in identifying pathologic processes in juxtasellar regions.[70]

When MRI is not available or is contraindicated, fine-section (1.5 mm.) coronal CT with intravenous contrast enhancement is an acceptable alternative. Coronal views best demonstrate the relationship of the sella to surrounding structures, the dimensions of the sella, the contour of the diaphragma sellae, and the sellar floor. A pituitary microadenoma characteristically appears as a well-circumscribed, variably dense, non-midline lesion on CT.[27] A hypolucent lesion greater than 2 mm. with erosion of the adjacent portion of the sella is also highly suggestive of a tumor. However, up to 40% to 50% of microadenomas are isodense with surrounding tissues or are not large enough to be resolved with present CT scanning techniques.[27]

Inferior petrosal sinus sampling assists in the evaluation of patients with acromegaly or Cushing's syndrome by localizing ACTH-secreting pituitary tumors that are undetectable by MRI or CT. Measurement of basal and corticotropin-releasing hormone (CRH)–stimulated ACTH levels reliably

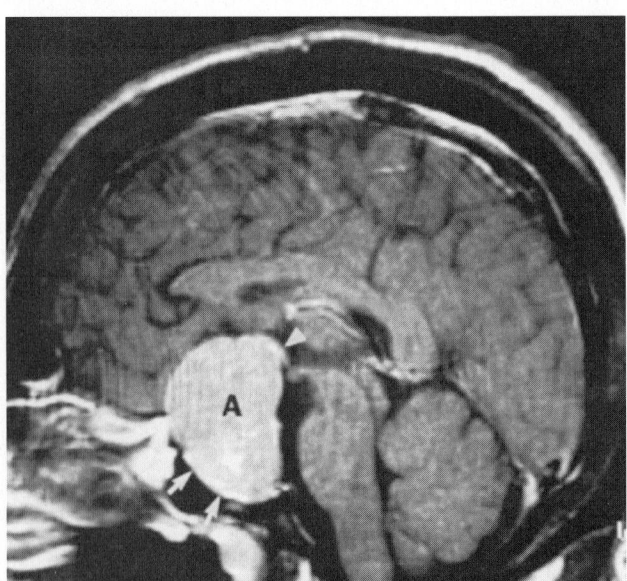

Figure 25–7. Sagittal spin-echo T1-weighted MR image of a pituitary adenoma after Gd-DTPA enhancement. The enhancing adenoma (A) fills an expanded sella turcica (white arrows) and extends into the suprasellar cistern. The mass indents the third ventricle (white arrowhead). (Courtesy of F. J. Wippold, M.D., Mallinckrodt Institute of Radiology, Washington University School of Medicine, St. Louis, Missouri.)

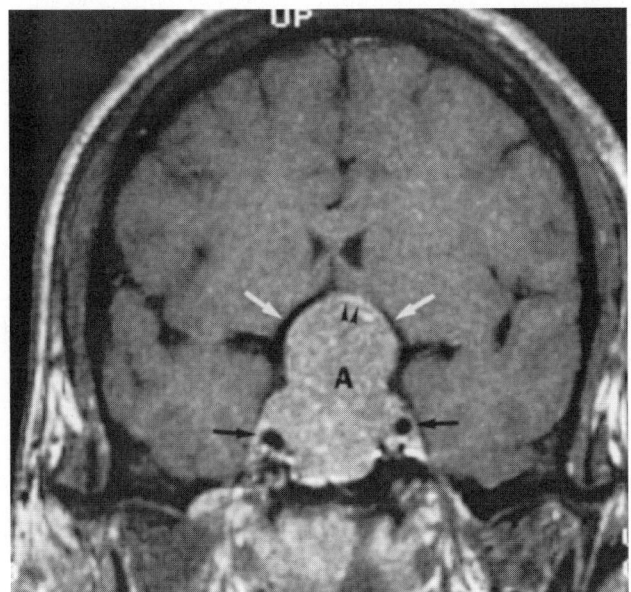

Figure 25–8. Coronal spin-echo T1-weighted MR image of a pituitary adenoma after Gd-DTPA enhancement. The adenoma (A) enhances, therefore increasing its signal. The tumor displaces the carotid arteries laterally (black arrows). Note that the A1 segments of the anterior cerebral arteries (white arrows) and the chiasm (arrowheads) drape over the mass. (Courtesy of F. J. Wippold, M.D., Mallinckrodt Institute of Radiology, Washington University School of Medicine, St. Louis, Missouri.)

differentiates pituitary from peripheral causes of Cushing's syndrome.[96] Angiography, particularly when performed with digital subtraction techniques, can detect abnormal carotid siphon anatomy, identify the positions of segments of the circle of Willis, and detect aneurysms or vascular malformations. Plain skull films, sellar tomograms, and pneumoencephalography have been supplanted by CT and MRI and are of little utility in the diagnosis of pituitary pathology.

General Approach to Management of Pituitary Disorders

Medical Therapy. Medical management of pituitary disease includes primary or adjuvant treatment for select functioning tumors and hormone replacement for hypopituitarism. Primary medical treatment of functioning pituitary tumors is generally limited to bromocriptine for the treatment of prolactinomas. Adjuvant medical treatment with bromocriptine or octreotide may also be beneficial in select cases of acromegaly following unsuccessful surgical treatment. Pituitary hormone replacement is mandatory for either selective or panhypopituitarism.[123] The goal of replacement therapy is to restore circulating hormone levels within the normal range. Adrenal insufficiency is treated with twice-daily hydrocortisone, hypothyroidism with once-daily thyroxine, and hypogonadism with daily oral estrogen and progesterone in women and depot testosterone biweekly in men. GH replacement may be beneficial in adults but is not approved for this use in the United States.

Surgical Therapy. The indications for surgical therapy for pituitary disease include pituitary adenomas other than prolactinoma, pituitary apoplexy, and tumors unresponsive to medical therapy.

Transsphenoidal pituitary microsurgery begins with an incision in the gingival mucosa beneath the upper lip followed by dissection through the nasal cavity and sphenoidal sinus to the sella turcica (Fig. 25–9). Intraoperative microscopy and image-intensification fluoroscopy facilitate maximal visualization of the operative field. The exposure provided by this approach allows selective removal of pituitary tumors as small as 2 mm. with preservation of surrounding normal pituitary tissue. The advantages of this technique, including low morbidity and mortality, a hidden incision within the oral cavity, and excellent exposure have made it the procedure of choice for the treatment of pituitary microadenomas as well as for small tumors remaining predominantly in the sella or for those tumors growing inferiorly.

The transfrontal approach is used for larger pituitary tu-

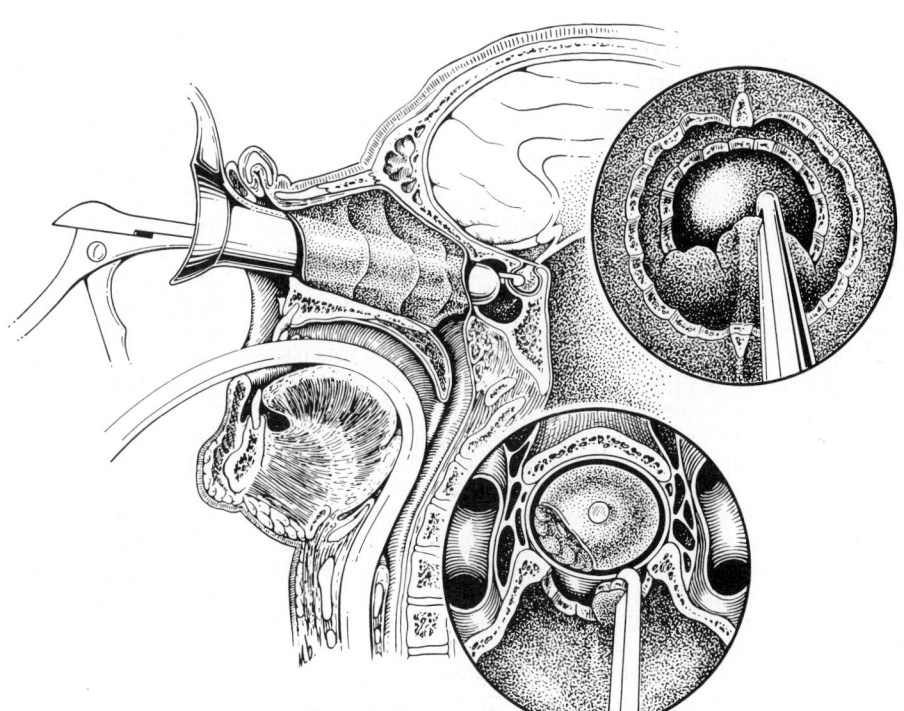

Figure 25–9. Endonasal transsphenoidal resection of a pituitary tumor. *Top Insert,* Removal of the sella floor with small rongeurs. *Bottom Insert,* Exposed inferior aspect of a pituitary adenoma. (Reproduced from Tindall, G. T., and Barrow, D. L.: Disorders of the Pituitary. St. Louis, C. V. Mosby Co., 1986, with permission.)

mors that have transgressed the diaphragma sellae into the subarachnoid space. Tumors that grow into the suprasellar cistern or laterally into the cavernous sinus and cause distortions of neural and vascular structures are also better approached transfrontally. Under some circumstances, however, even these tumors may be initially treated by the transsphenoidal approach.[138]

Results of operations for pituitary adenomas are generally good and reflect the expertise of the surgeon, the size of the tumor, and previous therapy.[120] Transsphenoidal resection of microadenomas that cause Cushing's disease, acromegaly, and hyperprolactinemia results in rapid reversal of hormone overproduction in up to 95% of cases. Recurrence, however, is common. Transsphenoidal resection of macroadenomas is curative in only 50% to 70% of cases. However, the visual field abnormalities produced by these large tumors are improved in 80% of cases and are stabilized in 16% of patients after resection.[119]

Complications of surgery for pituitary disease are uncommon.[137] Mortality rates from transsphenoidal resection are less than 1%, and morbidity rates are generally less than 5%. Complications most often involve CSF rhinorrhea, cranial nerve palsy, and vision loss. Permanent panhypopituitarism, defined by unremitting diabetes insipidus, is observed in less than 0.1% of operations performed for microadenoma and occurs in about 1% to 2% of operations for macroadenoma.

Radiation Therapy. Radiation therapy for pituitary neoplasms includes conventional treatment with 4500 rads over 5 weeks, focused high-dose radiation therapy in a single session (gamma knife), and heavy-particle therapy. These modalities are effective at controlling tumor growth but act slowly and are thus unsatisfactory for acute management of hypersecreting tumors. In properly selected cases, approximately 70% of patients respond to radiation therapy, although the full effects of radiation may not be realized for several years. The principal complication of all types of radiation therapy for treatment of pituitary lesions is panhypopituitarism, which occurs in up to 50% of cases.[20] Thus, the current role of radiation is largely adjunctive in patients with residual tumor after incomplete resection, in patients who refuse operation, or in those who are at unacceptable surgical risk.[46]

Diagnosis and Management of Specific Pituitary Disorders

Prolactinoma

Prolactinomas are the most common functioning pituitary tumors, representing 30% to 60% of all pituitary neoplasms. Prolactinomas are the most common cause of nonphysiologic hyperprolactinemia and produce hypogonadism, galactorrhea, or both.[91] Several medical conditions and medications may cause hyperprolactinemia (Table 25–3), and most are discernible by history, physical examination, and routine laboratory studies.[88] A pregnancy test is mandatory in all female patients with hyperprolactinemia.

Eighty-five per cent of pituitary prolactinomas are diagnosed in women, two thirds of which are discovered in the microadenoma stage. Microadenomas are diagnosed in 10% to 40% of women with amenorrhea alone and are found in 30% of women with amenorrhea and galactorrhea.[26] Oral estrogens may cause galactorrhea, but prolactinoma should be suspected if amenorrhea and galactorrhea persist more than 6 months after discontinuing oral contraceptive use.[91] Men with prolactinomas usually present with macroadenomas and experience symptoms of a space-occupying lesion of the sella. A minority of men with prolactinomas present with symptoms of hyperprolactinemia such as impotence,

TABLE 25–3. Causes of Hyperprolactinemia

Pituitary disease	**Other**
Prolactinoma	Pregnancy
Acromegaly	Hypothyroidism
Empty sella syndrome	Chronic renal failure
Lymphocytic hypophysitis	Cirrhosis
Cushing's disease	Pseudocyesis
Pituitary stalk section	
	Idiopathic
Hypothalamic disease	
Craniopharyngioma	**Medications**
Meningioma	Phenothiazines
Dysgerminoma	Haloperidol
Other tumors	Monoamine-oxidase inhibitors
Sarcoidosis	Tricyclic antidepressants
Eosinophilic granuloma	Reserpine
Neuraxis irradiation	Methyldopa
Vascular	Metoclopramide
	Amoxepin
Neurogenic	Verapamil
Chest wall lesions	
Spinal cord lesions	
Breast stimulation	

Reproduced, with permission, from the **Annual Review of Medicine,** Volume 40, © 1989, by Annual Reviews Inc.

infertility, or galactorrhea. Prolactinomas occur in up to 40% of individuals with multiple endocrine neoplasia Type 1.

Measurement of plasma PRL levels is central to the diagnosis of a PRL-secreting tumor, and the degree of hyperprolactinemia correlates roughly with tumor size.[68, 88] Basal PRL levels above 200 to 250 ng. per ml. in males and in nonpregnant females are almost invariably due to macroprolactinoma. Prolactin levels between 100 and 200 ng. per ml. suggest either a microprolactinoma or pituitary stalk compression by an adenoma with disruption of dopamine transport to the anterior pituitary (pseudoprolactinoma).[8] Most medications do not cause plasma PRL levels above 100 ng. per ml.

Most asymptomatic microprolactinomas remain stable over time and require only observation. Symptomatic microprolactinomas and macroprolactinomas require treatment. Therapeutic goals include amelioration of the tumor mass effects and correction of the endocrinopathy. Although surgery has been previously recommended for this disorder, bromocriptine is now the primary treatment of both microprolactinomas and macroprolactinomas. In several reported series, women with hyperprolactinemia who were treated with bromocriptine had return of PRL levels to normal in 64% to 100% of cases and experienced improvement of galactorrhea and return of menses and ovulation in 57% to 100% of cases.[124] Patients must realize that costly lifelong medical therapy is likely, and many therefore choose operation as primary therapy.[88] Surgical therapy should also be considered when medical therapy is ineffective. Pseudoprolactinomas should be treated surgically.[8]

Transsphenoidal resection of microprolactinomas results in normal serum PRL levels and restores menses in 80% of patients.[105] Many women with microadenomas treated by this approach are rendered fertile. However, intermediate range follow-up has indicated that at least 15% to 20% of patients with normal plasma PRL levels after surgery relapse and require bromocriptine. Surgical treatment of macroprolactinomas is less effective, and only 40% or less of patients treated surgically will achieve normal postoperative serum PRL levels.[35] Furthermore, recurrence is common, ranging from 16% to 80%.[108] Bromocriptine is now the preferred treatment for large, invasive prolactinomas because more than 90% of these lesions respond to this therapy.[89, 129] Radiation therapy is not recommended as primary treatment of prolactinoma because of slow response rates and a significant risk of panhypopituitarism.

Pregnant patients with known or suspected prolactinomas require special consideration because estrogens may stimulate prolactinoma growth. One percent of microprolactinomas and 15% of macroprolactinomas enlarge during pregnancy and produce symptoms.[89] All women with macroprolactinomas should have quantitative visual field testing before pregnancy and must be observed closely. Bromocriptine is considered safe during pregnancy and may be used to treat patients with symptomatic enlargement of the pituitary during this time. Surgical debulking of the tumor through the transsphenoidal approach may be required.

Nonfunctioning Adenoma

Clinically nonfunctioning adenomas, formerly termed *chromophobe adenomas*, are the second-most common pituitary tumor, representing 30% to 40% of surgically removed lesions.[111] Nonfunctioning adenomas occur predominantly in men and in postmenopausal women. These tumors are diagnosed when they cause mass-effect symptoms, including loss of vision, headache, hydrocephalus, and fifth or sixth nerve palsies. Many so-called nonfunctioning adenomas in fact secrete very low levels of LH, FSH, and glycoprotein hormone alpha subunit.[3] Partial or panhypopituitarism may occur; patients with macroadenomas most often have GH deficiency while those with microadenomas have hypogonadism.[123]

Evaluation of these patients includes measurement of basal PRL, IGF-1, LH, FSH, TSH, and alpha subunit levels. Abnormally high levels may identify an adenoma subtype, while low levels suggest hypopituitarism. Visual field testing should be performed and anatomic evaluation should include MRI or CT.

Transsphenoidal resection is the primary treatment of nonfunctioning adenomas. Patients with large tumors that traverse the diaphragma sellae and who present with visual impairment may require transfrontal resection. Postoperative irradiation is required in this group to prevent tumor regrowth. Visual field improvement occurs in 60% to 75% of patients treated surgically.[111] Radiation therapy and medical therapy with either bromocriptine or octreotide are reserved for adjuvant therapy after incomplete resection or to treat primary or recurrent tumors not amenable to resection.

Growth Hormone–Producing Adenoma

GH-producing adenomas are the third most common pituitary adenoma and cause acromegaly, a disease of bone and soft tissue overgrowth. Acromegaly has an estimated incidence of three to four cases per million and occurs most frequently in middle age. The diagnosis is often delayed 10 or more years owing to the slow progression of symptoms and physical changes. Gigantism results when GH excess occurs before epiphyseal plate closure in children and is much less common than acromegaly. Over 99% of cases of acromegaly are due to a primary pituitary adenoma.[116]

Clinical features of acromegaly are listed in Table 25–4. Physical findings include coarsening of facial features; enlargement of hands, feet, and tongue; carpal tunnel syndrome from soft tissue growth; frontal bossing; protruding jaw; hypertrophic osteoarthropathy; and kyphosis. The liver, spleen, kidney, and heart may also enlarge. Colorectal carcinoma has been observed more frequently in patients with acromegaly than in control populations and may correlate with the presence and number of skin tags.[57] GH-induced insulin resistance and glucose intolerance is frequent, yet only 10% to

TABLE 25–4. Clinical Features of Acromegaly

Features	Prevalence (%)
Acral enlargement	98
Hyperhidrosis	70
Menstrual disturbance	69
Headache	59
Weakness	59
Glucose intolerance	40
Skin tags	38
Impotence	34
Visual field abnormality	28
Goiter	25
Hypertension	23

Modified from Melmed, S., et al.: UCLA Conference: Pituitary tumors secreting growth hormone and prolactin. Ann. Intern. Med., *105*:245, 1986.

20% of patients with acromegaly are overtly diabetic. Amenorrhea is common in women with GH-producing adenomas and may be caused by tumor compression of normal surrounding pituitary tissue with hyposecretion of FSH and LH. In other cases, compression of the pituitary stalk may disrupt dopaminergic pathways and lead to hyperprolactinemia with inhibition of gonadotropins. Patients with untreated acromegaly experience chronic, debilitating symptoms and often die prematurely of cardiovascular and respiratory sequelae of GH excess.

The diagnosis of a GH-producing tumor formerly relied on demonstration of elevated basal GH levels by radioimmunoassay. Currently, measurement of serum IGF-1 concentration is the best screening test for acromegaly.[68, 82] Definitive testing with glucose suppression of GH release should follow. GH concentration at 60 and 120 minutes after oral administration of 100 gm. of glucose is less than 2 μg. per liter in normal persons and is greater than 2 μg. per liter (frequently over 10 μg. per liter) in patients with acromegaly. Positive biochemical testing should prompt MRI or CT of the sella. If these studies are negative, bilateral inferior petrosal sinus sampling may be performed.[78] If these studies still do not localize the tumor, then ectopic sources of GH production from a carcinoid or from an islet cell tumor should be considered. Conventional evaluation has included abdominal and chest CT, although newer ^{111}In-diethylenetriamine pentetic acid (DTPA)-octreotide scintigraphy has emerged as an effective localizing technique.[68] Plasma GH-RH may be measured to exclude rare (< 1%) hypothalamic lesions or ectopic sources of GH-RH production.[116]

Treatment goals in acromegaly include normalization of serum GH and IGF-1, alleviation of mass effects (headache, vision abnormalities), and preservation of anterior pituitary function. These goals are achieved most rapidly by transsphenoidal excision of the adenoma. Criteria for cure include basal plasma levels of GH less than 5 μg. per liter, GH levels less than 2 μg. per liter after oral glucose challenge, and normalization (< 2.2 U. per ml.) of IGF-1 levels in the plasma.[82, 84] Transsphenoidal surgery for microadenomas results in near-normalization of GH levels (< 5 μg. per liter) in 60% to 100% of cases, although stricter criteria using glucose suppression and IGF-1 levels show somewhat less favorable results. Surgical cure of macroadenomas is considerably lower.[82, 117]

The somatostatin analog octreotide has advanced the medical management of acromegaly considerably.[83] Octreotide persistently lowers GH and IGF-1 in 97% of patients with acromegaly and normalizes these levels (GH < 5 μg. per liter, IGF-1 < 2.2 U. per ml.) in 47% and 65% of patients, respectively.[34] Preoperative octreotide therapy may shrink large tumors and improve surgical outcome.[5] The role of octreotide as primary therapy is presently unclear, and the best therapy for acromegaly remains surgical in most cases.[83] Octreotide may be recommended after incomplete resection of macroadenomas and for reducing tumor size before surgical resection. Octreotide promotes gallbladder sludge that, if present, requires close observation with ultrasound and consideration of prophylactic laparoscopic cholecystectomy.[83]

Corticotropin-Producing Adenoma

Hypercortisolism, or Cushing's syndrome, is characterized by central obesity, moon facies, purple striae, proximal myopathy, amenorrhea, fatigue, and psychiatric abnormalities. Corticotropin-producing pituitary adenomas (Cushing's disease) cause up to 75% of cases of Cushing's syndrome and are diagnosed in the microadenoma stage in 90% of cases.

The diagnosis of Cushing's disease depends on biochemical demonstration of pituitary-dependent hypercortisolism. Laboratory evaluation of hypercortisolism is described subsequently in the adrenal section and is summarized in Figure 25–13. Radiologic evaluation includes MRI or high-resolution CT of the sella, although many microadenomas are less than 5 mm. and may not be detected by these modalities.[38, 120] Bilateral inferior petrosal sinus sampling with CRH stimulation may be required in these cases to localize the pituitary source of ACTH.[96] Rare patients with biochemical evidence of a pituitary source may instead have a bronchial or thymic carcinoid, a pancreatic islet cell tumor, or a pheochromocytoma, which should be sought with chest and abdominal CT.

Transsphenoidal resection of corticotroph microadenomas is the preferred management for Cushing's disease. Surgery is successful in 75% to 90% of cases, although recurrence rates may be as high as 10% to 20%.[120] Transsphenoidal resection of macroadenomas is less successful, and recurrence is more common.[120] Hypopituitarism occurs infrequently after transsphenoidal resection if the tumor has not replaced the entire sella. Patients in whom the tumor cannot be completely removed at operation require adjuvant radiation therapy.[126] Up to 90% of patients so treated experience remission. All patients undergoing pituitary resection for Cushing's disease require administration of stress-dose corticosteroids both perioperatively and chronically until the hypothalamic-pituitary-adrenal axis returns to normal.

Medical treatment of Cushing's disease is used for short-term reduction of serum cortisol before surgery or if surgical therapy fails. Medical adrenalectomy may be attempted with agents such as metyrapone, mitotane, aminoglutethimide, and ketoconazole. These drugs variably inhibit corticosteroid biosynthesis, have numerous side effects, and are thus not indicated as primary therapy in Cushing's disease. Radiation therapy for Cushing's disease is successful in 80% of children and in 20% of adults but is not recommended secondary to a high risk of hypopituitarism. Pituitary radiation after bilateral adrenalectomy for Cushing's disease was advocated to prevent Nelson's syndrome.

Bilateral adrenalectomy was performed previously in patients with pituitary lesions that caused bilateral adrenocortical hypertrophy and hypercortisolism. This operation has a 5% to 10% perioperative mortality and morbidity, with an even higher long-term mortality.[76] This operation is now rarely practiced as primary therapy for Cushing's disease. Adrenalectomy may still be indicated for patients who fail treatment with hypophysectomy, radiation, and medical therapy. Adrenalectomy may also be preferred in patients with severe forms of the disease as the surest means of reducing cortisol production.

Gonadotropin-Producing Adenoma

Gonadotroph adenomas occur most commonly in middle-aged men and usually produce symptoms of an enlarging sellar mass (headaches or visual abnormality). These tumors may secrete low levels of FSH, LH, or alpha subunit but usually cause no sexual dysfunction. Diagnosis of these tumors requires biochemical measurement of FSH, LH, alpha and beta subunits, as well as testosterone. Anatomic localization is performed with MRI or CT. Transsphenoidal resection is the treatment of choice for gonadotroph adenomas, and radiation therapy is indicated when surgical resection is incomplete or medically contraindicated. Medical treatment of gonadotroph adenomas is not proven.

Thyrotropin-Producing Adenoma

These tumors are the rarest pituitary adenomas ($< 1\%$) and produce symptoms of an enlarging sellar mass as well as hyperthyroidism secondary to elevated TSH levels. Treatment of thyrotroph adenomas is transsphenoidal resection.

Other Tumors and Conditions

Craniopharyngioma. Craniopharyngiomas represent 3% to 5% of intracranial neoplasms and arise from either sellar or extrasellar remnants of Rathke's pouch. These tumors usually affect children and produce symptoms of increased intracranial pressure (headache, vomiting, somnolence) as well as visual disturbances. Patients with craniopharyngioma frequently have a variable degree of hypopituitarism.[123] Evaluation of suspected craniopharyngioma includes biochemical determination of pituitary function, visual field testing, and imaging with CT. Calcification within the tumor is readily seen on CT, and it occurs in 70% to 90% of children and 40% to 60% of adults with this tumor.[117] Transfrontal resection is the treatment of choice for craniopharyngioma. Morbidity and mortality is high, and tumors recur frequently. Craniopharyngiomas are generally resistant to radiation therapy.

Pituitary Apoplexy. Pituitary apoplexy follows sudden hemorrhage into or infarction of a pituitary tumor. Symptoms occur suddenly due to expansion of blood within the sella and include severe headache, stiff neck, loss of vision, and extraocular nerve palsies. Secondary adrenal insufficiency may lead to hypotension and shock. Pituitary apoplexy most often occurs in an undiagnosed pituitary tumor but can appear during radiation therapy for pituitary tumors, during anticoagulation, or after closed-head trauma.[123] Symptomatic hemorrhage is observed in as many as 9% of patients with pituitary adenomas, and unrecognized hemorrhage is detected at operation or at autopsy in an additional 6% of patients.[127] Acute pituitary apoplexy is a neurosurgical emergency that requires acute transsphenoidal decompression of the sella.

Sheehan's Syndrome. Pituitary necrosis may occur rarely after postpartum hemorrhage and hypovolemia. The degree of subsequent hypopituitarism reflects the extent of pituitary necrosis and may include adrenal insufficiency, hypothyroidism, and amenorrhea. An inability to breast feed postpartum due to destruction of oxytocin-containing neurons of the posterior pituitary is an early clue to this diagnosis.

Empty Sella Syndrome. An empty sella turcica results from arachnoid herniation through an incomplete diaphragma sellae. This syndrome may occur in the absence of a recognized pituitary tumor and is either primary due to a congenital diaphragmatic defect or secondary due to an injury to the diaphragm by pituitary surgery, radiation, or infarction.[123]

Primary empty sella syndrome occurs in obese, multiparous, hypertensive women who experience headaches but have no underlying neurologic disorders. Pituitary function is usually normal, but occasionally PRL is increased and GH reserve is reduced. Secondary empty sella syndrome is observed in patients with otherwise benign CSF hypertension and in patients with a loss of pituitary function due to apoplexy or surgical therapy. Abnormal GH, PRL, or ACTH secretion may persist in such patients. The diagnosis is confirmed with MRI or CT. No treatment is necessary for the primary condition, while correction of the underlying cause is necessary for the secondary form.

ADRENAL GLAND

History

The anatomy of the adrenal gland was first described by Eustachius in 1563, yet evidence for a physiologic role of the adrenal was incomplete until 1855 when Addison described clinical features present in patients with adrenal disease identified at autopsy.[2] Brown-Séquard later conclusively demonstrated a vital role of the adrenals by performing experimental adrenalectomy in several animal species. A physiologic role of adrenal cortical derivatives was identified in the 1930s and was followed shortly thereafter by the successful use of adrenal cortical extracts in patients with adrenal insufficiency. Individual adrenal steroids were subsequently isolated, synthesized, and applied to the treatment of adrenal insufficiency and rheumatoid arthritis.

Syndromes of adrenal dysfunction have been characterized over the past century. Cushing described the clinical features of hypercortisolism in 1912, but the role of adrenal tumors in this syndrome was not understood until 1934.[128] Primary hyperaldosteronism was described by Conn in 1955.[19] Virilization of a female pseudohermaphrodite, now thought to be the first description of congenital adrenal hyperplasia, was reported in 1865, although adrenal pathology was not implicated in this condition until 1939.[28] Pheochromocytoma was first described by Frankel in 1886.

Embryology

Each adrenal is composed of two functionally distinct endocrine glands contained within a single capsule. The adrenal cortex and the medulla each have distinct embryologic, anatomic, histologic, and functional characteristics. The adrenal cortex arises from coelomic mesoderm adjacent to the urogenital ridge between the fourth and sixth gestational weeks. The gland then differentiates into a thin outer *definitive cortex* and a thick inner *fetal cortex* by the eighth week. The fetal cortex actively produces fetal steroids during gestation but involutes rapidly after birth. The definitive cortex persists and develops into the functional adrenal cortex, which has distinct zonae glomerulosa and fasciculata at birth. The zona reticularis develops later, during the first year of life. Aberrant adrenocortical tissue may be found near the kidney or in the pelvis along the path of migration of structures arising from the urogenital ridge. Adrenocortical tissue may also be found in locations that are not explained by normal patterns of migration of fetal tissues (Fig. 25–10).

The adrenal medulla and sympathetic nervous system develop together. During the fifth gestational week, neural crest cells migrate to the para-aortic and paravertebral regions and along the adrenal vein toward the medial aspect of the developing adrenal fetal cortex. Most extra-adrenal chromaffin cells regress. However, some cells remain and form the organ of Zuckerkandl, which is located generally to the left of the aortic bifurcation near the origin of the inferior mesenteric artery. Extra-adrenal chromaffin tissue may persist anywhere along the path of neural crest cell migration (Fig. 25–10).

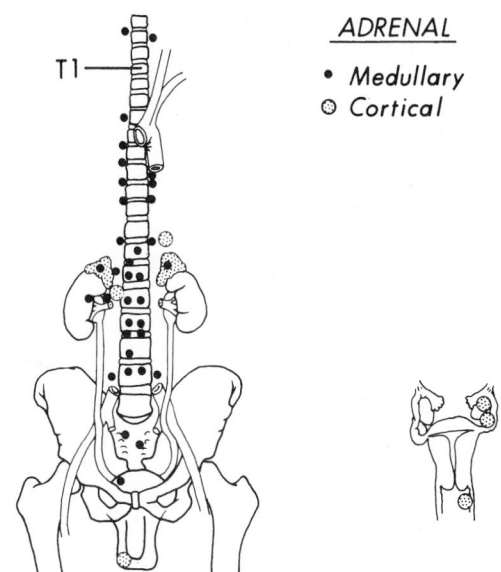

ADRENAL
• Medullary
⊙ Cortical

Figure 25–10. Sites of extra-adrenal cortical and medullary tissues.

Anatomy

The adrenal glands are bilateral retroperitoneal organs located on the superior medial aspect of the upper pole of each kidney. Each gland weighs approximately 4 gm. The pyramid-shaped right adrenal lies close to the inferior vena cava and frequently abuts the right diaphragmatic crus and the bare area of the liver. The left adrenal is larger and flatter and is found between the kidney and aorta near the tail of the pancreas and the splenic artery. The adrenal glands are firmer than the surrounding perirenal fat and can be palpated as distinct structures. The normal adrenal cortex is bright yellow and thicker than the red-brown medulla.

The adrenal glands are highly vascular and derive their blood supply from branches of the inferior phrenic artery superiorly, the aorta medially, and the renal artery inferiorly. The primary blood supply of the right adrenal comes from the superior and inferior adrenal arteries, while the left adrenal is supplied primarily by the middle and inferior adrenal arteries. Additionally, numerous small arterial branches enter the perimeter of the gland. Microvasculature within each adrenal integrates function of the cortex and medulla. A number of small vessels pass directly through the cortex to the medulla, but the majority enter the cortical plexus and form cortical sinusoids that empty into medullary sinusoids. Cortisol-rich venous effluent flows from the cortex to the medulla where cortisol stimulates the synthesis and activity of phenylethanolamine-N-methyl transferase (PMNT), leading to the conversion of norepinephrine to epinephrine. Extra-adrenal chromaffin tissues lack this regulatory mechanism and thus secrete predominantly norepinephrine.

Venous effluent from the right adrenal gland drains to the inferior vena cava through a wide but short central vein. The left adrenal vein empties primarily into the left renal vein but may occasionally drain directly to the vena cava. Lymphatic plexuses within the subcapsular portion of the adrenal cortex and the adrenal medulla drain to the adjacent para-aortic subdiaphragmatic and renal lymph nodes. The adrenal cortex has no known direct innervation, although the adrenal medulla is richly supplied by preganglionic sympathetic nerves from the greater splanchnic nerve, the celiac ganglion, and from other plexuses. Parasympathetic nerves to the medulla have not been identified.

Histologically, the adult adrenal cortex is composed of

three zones: an outer zona glomerulosa, a middle zona fasciculata, and an inner zona reticularis. Cells of the zona fasciculata are large, appear foamy secondary to many lipid inclusions, and constitute 75% of the cortex. Cells of the zona reticularis have compact cytoplasm and few lipid inclusions. ACTH stimulation causes cells of these two inner zones to enlarge due to increased storage of lipid and proliferation of mitochondria and endoplasmic reticulum. Cells of the zona glomerulosa are small, have an intermediate number of lipid inclusions, and constitute about 15% of the cortex.

The adrenal medulla is smaller than the cortex and contributes approximately 10% of the total gland weight. Adrenal medullary cells are polyhedral, are arranged in cords, and contain catecholamines that precipitate chromium salts (thus the name chromaffin cells). Core vesicles containing epinephrine and norepinephrine are apparent on electron microscopy.

Adrenal Steroid Biochemistry and Physiology

Three major biosynthetic pathways lead to the production of glucocorticoids, mineralocorticoids, and adrenal androgens. These pathways are compartmentalized within the adrenal gland and reflect the enzymatic capabilities of each

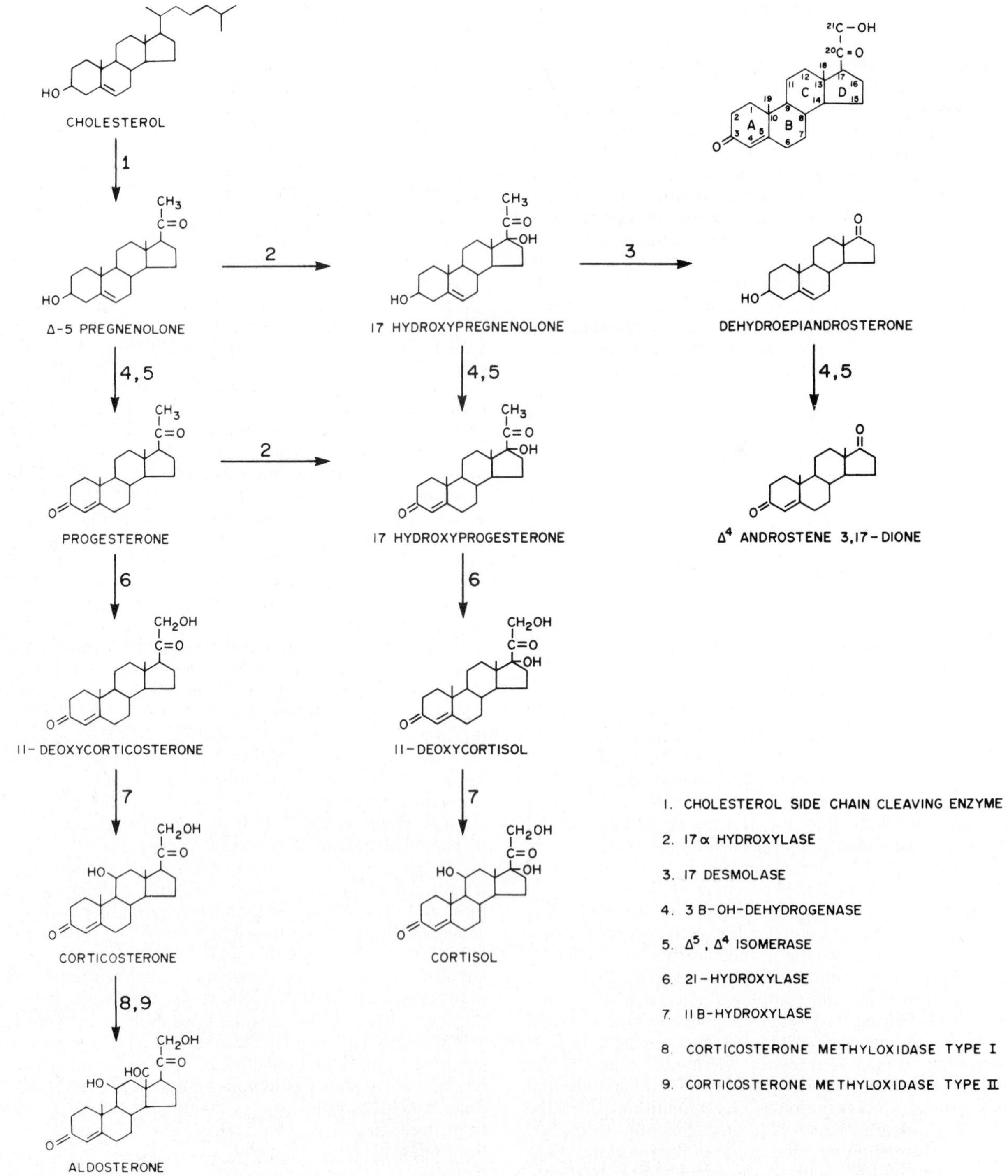

Figure 25–11. Biosynthetic pathways of adrenal corticosteroids.

zone. Mineralocorticoids are synthesized in the outer zona glomerulosa, while glucocorticoids and adrenal androgens are synthesized in the inner zonae fasciculata and reticularis. All adrenal steroids have either 19 or 21 total carbon atoms and share a common 17-carbon structure composed of three hexane rings and a single pentane ring. The androgenic C-19 steroids have methyl groups at positions 18 and 19 on the basic structure. Glucocorticoids and mineralocorticoids have an additional two-carbon side chain (C-20, 21) attached at position 17.

Adrenocortical hormones are synthesized from cholesterol that is either extracted from plasma or manufactured locally within the adrenal cortex. The parent compound cholesterol is cleaved during a series of enzymatic degradations within the cristae of the adrenal cell mitochondria to form delta-5 pregnenolone, the common precursor for glucocorticoids, mineralocorticoids, and androgenic steroids. After leaving the mitochondrion, pregnenolone enters the smooth endoplasmic reticulum where it is shunted to the divergent biosynthetic pathways (Fig. 25–11). In the zonae glomerulosa and reticularis, 17-alpha hydroxylase oxidizes pregnenolone and progesterone at C-17 to form 17-hydroxypregnenolone and 17-hydroxyprogesterone, respectively. Three-beta-hydroxydehydrogenase and delta-5, delta-4-isomerase convert 17-hydroxypregnenolone to 17-hydroxyprogesterone and then 21-hydroxylase converts this molecule to 11-deoxycortisol. Finally, 11-beta-hydroxylase adds a hydroxyl group at C-11 to form cortisol. Mineralocorticoid biosynthesis follows a parallel pathway in the zona glomerulosa but does not undergo initial hydroxylation at C-17 owing to absence of 17-alpha-hydroxylase activity in this zone. Additionally, corticosterone undergoes hydroxylation of C-18 to form aldosterone. Congenital absence of enzymes involved in any one of these pathways shunts pregnenolone derivatives through unaffected pathways and causes specific clinical syndromes.

Glucocorticoids

Cortisol is the principal glucocorticoid in man. Cortisol production remains constant as a function of body size (12 mg./sq. m. of body surface area) during all phases of life and a normal adult secretes 10 to 30 mg. of cortisol each day. Adrenal cortisol production is regulated by pituitary-derived ACTH under most conditions.

In plasma, 75% of cortisol is bound to corticosteroid binding globulin (transcortin), 15% is bound to albumin, and 10% to 15% is unbound and active. Plasma transcortin levels increase during pregnancy and by pharmacologic doses of estrogen. Alterations in transcortin or albumin concentrations in plasma can alter total plasma cortisol concentration without affecting its free concentration. Conversely, excessive cortisol production may exceed transcortin- and albumin-binding capabilities and lead to sharp increases in free cortisol.

The plasma half-life of cortisol is approximately 90 minutes. Cortisol is cleared predominantly by the liver, where it is transformed to the inactive metabolites dihydrocortisol and tetrahydrocortisol. These metabolites are conjugated to glucuronate and excreted in the urine, where they may be measured as 17-hydroxycorticosteroids. A small fraction of unmetabolized cortisol can be measured in the urine.

Steroid hormones exert their effects by binding to specific soluble intracellular cytosolic receptors. The activated steroid-receptor complex then moves to the nucleus, binds to DNA, and activates transcription of target genes. The diverse physiologic actions of glucocorticoids center upon intermediary metabolism, immune modulation, and regulation of intravascular volume.

Cortisol regulates the intermediary metabolism of carbohydrates, proteins, and lipids (Fig. 25–12). Cortisol stimulates

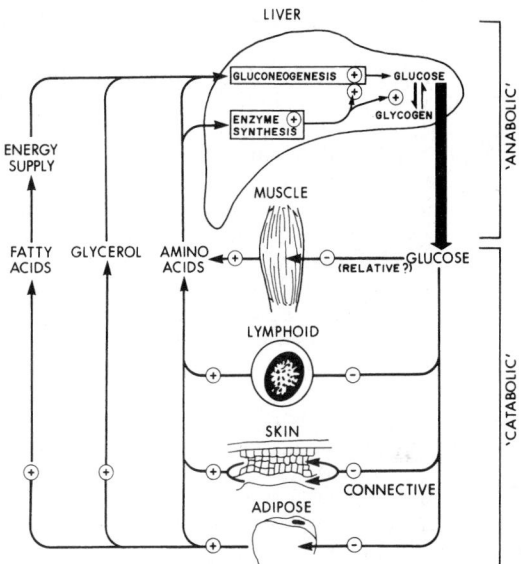

Figure 25–12. Glucocorticoid effects on carbohydrate, lipid and protein metabolism. Plus signs indicate stimulation and minus signs indicate inhibition. (From Baxter, J. D., and Rousseau, G. G.: Glucocorticoid hormone action: An overview. *In* Baxter, J. D., and Rousseau, G. G. [Eds.]: Glucocorticoid Hormone Action. New York, Springer-Verlag, 1979, p. 1.)

release of glucagon, and together these substances raise blood glucose by antagonizing insulin-stimulated glucose uptake by peripheral tissues and also by stimulating hepatic gluconeogenesis. Cortisol also decreases peripheral protein synthesis and amino acid uptake, thereby increasing glycogenic amino acid delivery to the liver. Cortisol also stimulates peripheral lipolysis. Thus, glucocorticoids function anabolically in vital tissues such as liver and brain but catabolically in skin, muscle, lymphoid tissues, and adipocytes. Prolonged administration of exogenous corticosteroids leads to a catabolic state with negative nitrogen balance, proximal muscle weakness, and insulin-resistant diabetes mellitus. Additionally, a redistribution of body fat occurs that results in truncal obesity and peripheral depletion.

Glucocorticoids possess profound anti-inflammatory and immunosuppressive properties.[80] These steroids suppress interleukin-2 production and inhibit lymphocyte activation and both monocyte and neutrophil migration to areas of inflammation. Cortisol inhibits histamine release and histamine-induced lysosomal degranulation by mast cells. Corticosteroids also modulate humoral immunity by regulating T-cell activation of B cells and, at high doses, by directly inhibiting B-cell activation and proliferation. Cortisol maintains intravascular volume by retarding entry of free water into cells, by decreasing capillary permeability to water, and by a weak mineralocorticoid effect. Cortisol also maintains blood pressure through stimulation of angiotensinogen release and by inhibition of prostaglandin I_2, a potent vasodilator. Glucocorticoids retard wound healing by impairing collagen formation and fibroblast activity, produce osteopenia by inhibiting osteoblast bone formation, and promote early closure of epiphyseal plates in children and adolescents. Other effects of chronic corticosteroid excess include emotional and psychologic disturbances, cataracts, and corneal ulcers.

Mineralocorticoids

Aldosterone is the major mineralocorticoid in man. Approximately 100 to 150 mg. of aldosterone is secreted from the zona glomerulosa into the bloodstream each day where it is bound to transcortin (20%) and albumin (40%), with the remainder circulating free. The plasma half-life of aldosterone is approximately 15 minutes, and 90% is cleared from the plasma after a single pass through the liver. Metabolic degradation of aldosterone occurs in the liver by enzymatic reduction and conjugation with glucuronic acid before excretion by the kidney. Only minute amounts of free aldosterone are excreted in the urine.

Aldosterone regulates fluid and electrolyte balance by stimulating sodium retention and potassium and hydrogen ion secretion by the distal convoluted tubule of the kidney. Aldosterone also promotes sodium absorption by a variety of epithelia, including sweat glands, gastrointestinal mucosa, and salivary glands. High levels of circulating mineralocorticoid thus tend to expand intravascular volume. Glucocorticoids appear to independently influence the glomerular filtration rate through effects on the microvasculature of the nephron and may also be necessary for the kidney to maximally dilute and concentrate the urine. Aldosterone and the adrenal glucocorticoids therefore act in concert to regulate sodium, potassium, and volume homeostasis of the extracellular and intravascular body spaces.

Aldosterone secretion is governed by multiple factors with complex interactions. The renin-angiotensin system and plasma potassium are the principal regulators of aldosterone. ACTH, plasma sodium, and POMC-derived peptides and others are minor contributors.[104]

Activation of the renin-angiotensin system begins with release of renin from juxtaglomerular cells of the kidney in response to a decrease in renal blood flow, to sympathetic nervous system stimulation, or to a decrease in plasma sodium. Renin enzymatically cleaves angiotensinogen to produce the decapeptide angiotensin I, which is then cleaved by angiotensin-converting enzyme (ACE) in the lung to form the active octapeptide angiotensin II. Angiotensin II directly stimulates aldosterone biosynthesis and release from the adrenal through receptor-mediated activation of phospholipase C.[104] Angiotensin II is also a potent vasoconstrictor and directly elicits a marked increase in arterial blood pressure. Factors that decrease renal arterial blood flow such as hemorrhage, dehydration, upright posture, or renal artery stenosis stimulate the renin-angiotensin system. Restoration of blood volume and pressure, as well as high levels of aldosterone, inhibit release of renin and angiotensin.

A reciprocal relationship exists between serum potassium and aldosterone. An increase of serum potassium level by as little as 0.1 mEq. per liter increases aldosterone secretion by 35%, whereas a fall in serum potassium by 0.3 mEq. per liter decreases aldosterone secretion by 50%. Hypokalemia blunts the aldosterone response that would otherwise be observed in a number of clinical settings, and restoration of the serum potassium level restores this response.

ACTH plays a comparatively minor role in aldosterone regulation. In fact, the zona glomerulosa does not atrophy after hypophysectomy, unlike the zona reticularis and fasciculata. ACTH may acutely stimulate aldosterone hypersecretion, although prolonged ACTH exposure ultimately leads to diminished aldosterone response. Other pituitary factors including POMC-derivatives and ADH stimulate aldosterone secretion. Sodium intake regulates aldosterone indirectly through changes in renin secretion and through modulation of the sensitivity of the zona glomerulosa to angiotensin II.

Adrenal Sex Steroids

In cells of the zona reticularis, pregnenolone is converted to 17-hydroxypregnenolone and subsequently to dehydroepiandrosterone (DHEA). DHEA is the major C-19 sex steroid produced by the adrenal cortex, although the sulfated derivative of DHEA and delta-4-androstenedione are also formed.

DHEA and androstenedione are weak androgens and exert their effect on peripheral tissues after local conversion to testosterone. Only minute amounts of testosterone or estrone are synthesized under normal circumstances, and the gonads are the primary source of these sex steroids. Adrenal androgen release is stimulated by ACTH and not by the gonadotropins.

Adrenal androgens promote development of male secondary sexual characteristics and cause virilization in women. During fetal life, circulating androgens influence development of the male external genitalia, the male ductal structures such as vas deferens, epididymis, and seminal vesicles, and the prostate. Absence of androgens prenatally prompts development of female genitalia and the vagina. Normally, the gonads are the principal source of sex steroids in males and females. During puberty, androgens contribute to growth of the phallus, muscle mass, and body hair in the male. Estrogens promote growth and maturation of the breast, uterus, and vagina in the female. Excessive production of adrenal sex steroids either prenatally or postnatally results in disorders of sexual development.

Diseases of the Adrenal Cortex

Cushing's Syndrome

Background. In 1932, Harvey Cushing described eight patients with central obesity, glucose intolerance, hypertension, plethora, hirsutism, osteoporosis, nephrolithiasis, menstrual irregularity, muscle weakness, and emotional lability.[25] He noted basophilic adenomas of the pituitary in six of these patients, but the relationship to adrenocortical hyperplasia and hypercortisolism was not appreciated. It is now known that this collection of signs and symptoms, termed *Cushing's syndrome*, is attributable to chronically elevated levels of plasma cortisol.

Cushing's syndrome is rare, with an incidence of 10 per million population. Today, the most common cause of this syndrome is iatrogenic due to chronic administration of synthetic corticosteroid for other disorders. Endogenous hypercortisolism in all cases is due to increased adrenal production of cortisol, which may be ACTH dependent or independent (Table 25–5).[97]

Cushing's syndrome is ACTH dependent in 80% to 90% of cases; and of the ACTH-dependent cases, most (80% to 90%) are due to an ACTH-secreting pituitary adenoma (Cushing's disease). Ectopic ACTH-producing nonendocrine tumors constitute the remaining 10% to 20% of cases of ACTH-dependent Cushing's syndrome. Hypothalamic or ectopic CRH oversecretion is uncommon. All causes of ACTH-

TABLE 25–5. Causes of Cushing's Syndrome

Diagnosis	%
ACTH-dependent	
Cushing's disease	68
Ectopic ACTH syndrome	12
Ectopic CRH syndrome	<1
ACTH-independent	
Adrenal adenoma	10
Adrenal carcinoma	8
Adrenal cortical hyperplasias	1
Pseudo-Cushing's syndrome	
Major depression	1
Alcoholism	<1

Adapted from Orth, D. N., N. Engl. J. Med., 1995, 332, 791–803. Copyright 1995. Massachusetts Medical Society. All rights reserved.

dependent Cushing's syndrome produce bilateral adrenal hyperplasia.

ACTH-independent Cushing's syndrome occurs in 10% to 20% of cases and is due to primary adrenal pathology including an autonomously hypersecreting adenoma, an adrenal carcinoma, or bilateral adrenal cortical hyperplasia. Patients with major depression and chronic alcoholism not infrequently have abnormally high cortisol secretion and may appear to have clinical and biochemical features of Cushing's syndrome. The pseudo-Cushing's syndrome produced by these disorders rapidly disappears with remission of the primary disorder.

Signs and Symptoms. Clinical features of Cushing's syndrome are listed in Table 25–6.[55] Centripetal obesity and the *orange on toothpicks* habitus are present in almost every patient. Excessive accumulation of fat around the head and neck is responsible for the characteristic *moon facies* and *buffalo hump*. Patients usually appear plethoric, and purple striae are most often observed on the abdomen and extremities. Purpura and easy bruisability are often evident, and acne with superficial skin infections is common. Hirsutism may be a striking feature in women. Menstrual abnormalities are present in most women, and impotence often occurs in men. High blood pressure is common and is usually moderate, although malignant hypertension has been observed. Volume expansion and sodium retention both contribute to an elevation in diastolic blood pressure. Hypertension and atherosclerosis contribute significantly to morbidity and mortality. Muscle weakness and bone pain, particularly backache, are also common. Weakness is due in part to proximal muscle wasting but also to hypokalemia. Bones demineralize, and pathologic fractures are observed in advanced cases. Neurologic symptoms, including headache, emotional lability, depression, and even psychosis may be observed. Glucose intolerance is common but can often be managed by alterations in diet alone. In 50% of patients, the white blood cell count is approximately 10,000 cells per cu. mm. and the red blood

TABLE 25–6. Clinical Features of Cushing's Syndrome

Clinical Feature	Reported Incidence (%)
Centripetal obesity	79–97
Weakness/proximal myopathy	29–90
Hypertension	74–87
Skin changes	
Thin skin/bruising	23–84
Acne, greasy skin	26–80
Hirsutism	64–81
Plethora	50–94
Abdominal striae	51–71
Infection (e.g., tinea versicolor)	30
Pigmentation	4–16
Psychiatric changes	31–86
Oligo/amenorrhea	55–80
Impotence	55–80
Osteoporosis	
Backache	40–50
Vertebral collapse	40–50
Pathologic fracture	40–50
Thirst/polyuria	25–44
Glucose intolerance	39–90
Ankle edema	28–60
Renal calculi	15–19
Exophthalmos	0–33
Headache	0–47
Abdominal pain	0–21

From Howlett, T. A.: Cushing's syndrome. Clin. Endocrinol. Metab., *14*:916, 1985.

cell count is above 5 million cells per cu. mm. Hypercalciuria may be present, but the serum calcium level is normal unless hyperparathyroidism and multiple endocrine neoplasia Type 1 are present. The serum potassium level is often low secondary to the weak mineralocorticoid properties of cortisol.

Diagnosis of Cushing's Syndrome. Hypercortisolism insensitive to suppression by administration of exogenous glucocorticoid is the *sine qua non* of Cushing's syndrome.[97] However, no single test is absolutely reliable in establishing this diagnosis. Cortisol is normally secreted episodically, and plasma cortisol levels may demonstrate considerable diurnal variation. Therefore, a single random plasma cortisol level is not helpful in establishing a diagnosis of Cushing's syndrome.[118]

Measurement of cortisol in two to three consecutive 24-hour collections of urine is the best screening test for Cushing's syndrome. Collections should be carefully timed and include concurrent creatinine measurement to ensure adequacy of collection. A 24-hour urinary free cortisol level greater than 100 μg. is diagnostic of Cushing's syndrome. Obese individuals may have elevated free urinary cortisol levels without having Cushing's syndrome because cortisol production is proportional to body mass. A ratio comparing urinary steroid content to urinary creatinine content may eliminate false-positive results.

The low-dose dexamethasone suppression test, originally devised by Liddle, continues to be a valuable confirmatory test in patients with suspected Cushing's syndrome and mildly elevated urinary cortisol excretion. Dexamethasone, a synthetic glucocorticoid, is more potent than cortisol in suppressing ACTH release from the pituitary and does not cross-react in standard cortisol radioimmunoassays. An overnight variation of the original Liddle test, in which 1 mg. of dexamethasone is administered orally at 11 P.M. and plasma cortisol is obtained at 8 A.M. the following day, is now preferred. In this test, the plasma cortisol level is suppressed to less than 3 to 5 μg. per 100 ml. in normal individuals, whereas very few individuals with Cushing's syndrome demonstrate suppression of plasma cortisol to below 3 μg. per 100 ml.[38] False-positive test results occur in 10% to 15% of cases with the overnight test and occur especially in patients with obesity, alcoholism, or those taking estrogens or phenytoin.[17]

Once the diagnosis of Cushing's syndrome is established, subsequent testing is directed toward identifying and localizing the underlying cause. Initial testing should discern ACTH-dependent (pituitary or ectopic source) from ACTH-independent (primary adrenal) causes. Determination of basal ACTH by IRMA is the best test to make this distinction.[38] Plasma ACTH levels are normally between 10 and 100 pg. per ml., and diurnal ACTH variations precede those of cortisol by 1 to 2 hours. Suppression of the absolute level of ACTH below 5 pg. per ml. is nearly diagnostic of adrenocortical neoplasms, which secrete high levels of cortisol and inhibit ACTH release by the pituitary. Patients with pituitary neoplasms and secondary bilateral adrenocortical hyperplasia have ACTH levels that may range from the upper limits of normal (15 pg. per ml.) to 500 pg. per ml. Highest plasma levels of ACTH (more than 1000 pg. per ml.) have been observed in patients with ACTH-producing nonendocrine tumors. These tumors are clinically evident in most patients. In patients with occult tumors, the cause of hypercortisolism must be deduced through other tests.

Although 80% to 90% of patients with ACTH-dependent Cushing's syndrome have Cushing's disease, standard high-dose dexamethasone suppression testing is required to exclude ectopic ACTH syndrome. This test is based on the principle that hypercortisolism due to ACTH-secreting pituitary adenomas will be suppressed at least partially by high-dose dexamethasone, while that due to adrenal tumors and ectopic ACTH-producing tumors will not. The standard test employs 2 mg. dexamethasone given orally every 6 hours over 2 days, with a 24-hour urine collection for free cortisol taken during the second day. Urine free cortisol is suppressed by 90% in 60% to 70% of patients with pituitary adenomas. Failure to suppress supports a diagnosis of an ectopic ACTH-producing tumor, an adrenal neoplasm or primary bilateral nodular hyperplasia. An overnight high-dose suppression test (8 mg. at midnight) and an intravenous test (1 mg. per hour for 7 hours) are available and have similar diagnostic accuracy.

The metyrapone stimulation test has traditionally been used to assay pituitary ACTH-secretory reserve and is useful in distinguishing subsets of patients with Cushing's syndrome.[55] Metyrapone inhibits the enzyme 11-hydroxylase and blocks conversion of 11-deoxycortisol to cortisol and conversion of 11-deoxycorticosterone to corticosterone and aldosterone. A resultant fall in plasma cortisol elicits a compensatory rise in ACTH secretion by the pituitary, signaling the adrenal cortex to produce increased quantities of cortisol precursors. Administration of metyrapone to normal individuals increases 24-hour urine levels of 17-hydroxycorticosteroids (17-OHCS). Plasma ACTH and 11-deoxycortisol are also measured. Patients with pituitary adenomas and little overall pituitary suppression respond with increased plasma ACTH and 11-deoxycortisol and increased urinary 17-OHCS. Patients with adrenal neoplasms or ectopic ACTH sources have marked pituitary suppression so that plasma ACTH, 11-deoxycortisol, and urinary 17-OHCS levels do not change.

Biochemical testing of suspected Cushing's syndrome is complemented by appropriately selected radiologic studies. Pituitary adenomas are best visualized with gadolinium-enhanced MRI of the sella turcica. Sensitivity of MRI approaches 100%, although small pituitary microadenomas may be missed.[96] High-resolution CT may miss up to two thirds of pituitary adenomas in Cushing's disease.[16] Patients with ACTH-independent Cushing's syndrome require thin-section CT or MRI of the adrenal. High-resolution CT or MRI identifies adrenal abnormalities with over 95% sensitivity. MRI may also provide evidence of adrenocortical carcinoma or unsuspected ACTH-producing pheochromocytoma.[101] CT or MRI of the chest may identify a source of ectopic ACTH and should be undertaken in patients with elevated ACTH and hypercortisolism that cannot be suppressed by high-dose dexamethasone.

Despite the accuracy of biochemical testing and radiographic localization, a pituitary versus ectopic source of ACTH sometimes cannot be determined. In these cases, bilateral inferior petrosal sinus sampling has emerged as the best test to settle this issue. Simultaneous bilateral petrosal sinus and peripheral blood samples are obtained before and after peripheral intravenous injection of 1 µg. per kg. of CRH. An inferior petrosal sinus to peripheral plasma ACTH concentration ratio of 2.0 at basal stimulated or of 3.0 after CRH administration is 100% sensitive and specific for pituitary adenoma.[96] Comparison of right and left inferior petrosal sinus ratios may also lateralize the adenoma. This is a technically difficult procedure with risks inherent to invasive procedures and may not be available in all centers.

The laboratory approach to the diagnosis of Cushing's syndrome is summarized in Figure 25–13.[97] It is worthwhile to re-emphasize that a careful history and physical examination form the basis for suspecting this condition. Urinary free cortisol measurement and the low-dose dexamethasone suppression test provide initial evidence for the diagnosis. Plasma ACTH determination, a high-dose dexamethasone suppression test, and the metyrapone test are then used to identify the cause of excess cortisol production by the adrenal

cortex. Imaging studies corroborate and in some cases clarify the cause of Cushing's syndrome suggested by biochemical testing.

Etiologies of Cushing's Syndrome. Treatment of Cushing's syndrome involves removing the cause of cortisol excess, either a primary adrenal lesion or ectopic and pituitary lesions secreting excessive ACTH. Approaches to this goal are individualized according to etiology.

Cushing's Disease. Pituitary causes of hypercortisolism are discussed in the preceding section on the pituitary. The treatment of choice for Cushing's disease is transsphenoidal resection of the pituitary tumor, which is successful in 80% or more of cases. Irradiation and medical therapy are adjunctive treatments.

Ectopic ACTH Syndrome. Approximately 12% of patients with ACTH-dependent endogenous Cushing's syndrome have a lesion secreting ACTH from a site other than the pituitary (Table 25–7). Small cell carcinoma of the lung is the most common cause of the ectopic ACTH syndrome, although bronchial, gut, and thymic carcinoids, endocrine pancreas tumors, pancreatic cystadenomas, medullary carcinoma of the thyroid, and pheochromocytomas have all been reported.[137] Ectopic production of CRF is rarely a cause of Cushing's syndrome, and described sources include medullary carcinoma of the thyroid and carcinoma of the prostate. Patients with ectopic ACTH syndrome usually appear cushingoid, but they more often present with signs of an advanced malignancy such as weakness and weight loss. These patients often have a severe metabolic alkalosis with hypokalemia. A presumptive diagnosis of ectopic ACTH hypersecretion is made on the basis of (1) increased urinary free cortisol, (2) increased plasma ACTH, and (3) failure to suppress ACTH and hypercortisolism with high-dose dexamethasone.

Treatment of ectopic ACTH syndrome involves removal of the primary lesion. Debulking of unresectable primary lesions or recurrences with or without bilateral adrenalectomy may provide palliation in some patients. Medical adrenalectomy with metyrapone, aminoglutethimide, and mitotane has been used to suppress production of corticosteroid in inoperable cases. Bilateral adrenalectomy may be beneficial in select patients with uncontrollable hypercortisolism or after unsuccessful localization of the ectopic ACTH source.[59]

Adrenal Adenoma and Adrenocortical Hyperplasia. Ten to 25% of patients with endogenous Cushing's syndrome have a primary adrenal cause. A solitary adrenal adenoma is present in 80% to 90% of these patients and is often associated with atrophy of both adjacent and contralateral adrenocortical tissue. Nodular cortical hyperplasia of both glands occurs in the remaining cases of primary adrenal Cushing's syndrome. Although nodular hyperplasia represents a diffuse process, one or more distinct nodules may simulate adenomas.

The majority of patients with apparent primary adrenocortical hyperplasia have hyperplasia that is pituitary-dependent secondary to an occult pituitary adenoma (Cushing's disease). A small subset of patients with bilateral nodular hyperplasia have a pituitary-independent cause, either autoimmune pigmented micronodular cortical dysplasia or gastric inhibitory peptide sensitive macronodular dysplasia.[67] Pituitary-dependent forms of nodular hyperplasia demonstrate increased urinary 17-OHCS excretion on day 1 or day 2 following metyrapone stimulation. Pituitary-independent forms show no change in urinary 17-OHCs with metyrapone.[55]

Removal of the adrenal tumor and affected gland is the primary approach to primary adrenal causes of Cushing's syndrome. Adrenal adenomas are cured by adrenalectomy, and prognosis is good following resection.[30, 121] Small lesions, less than 6 cm. in diameter, may be resected by the posterior

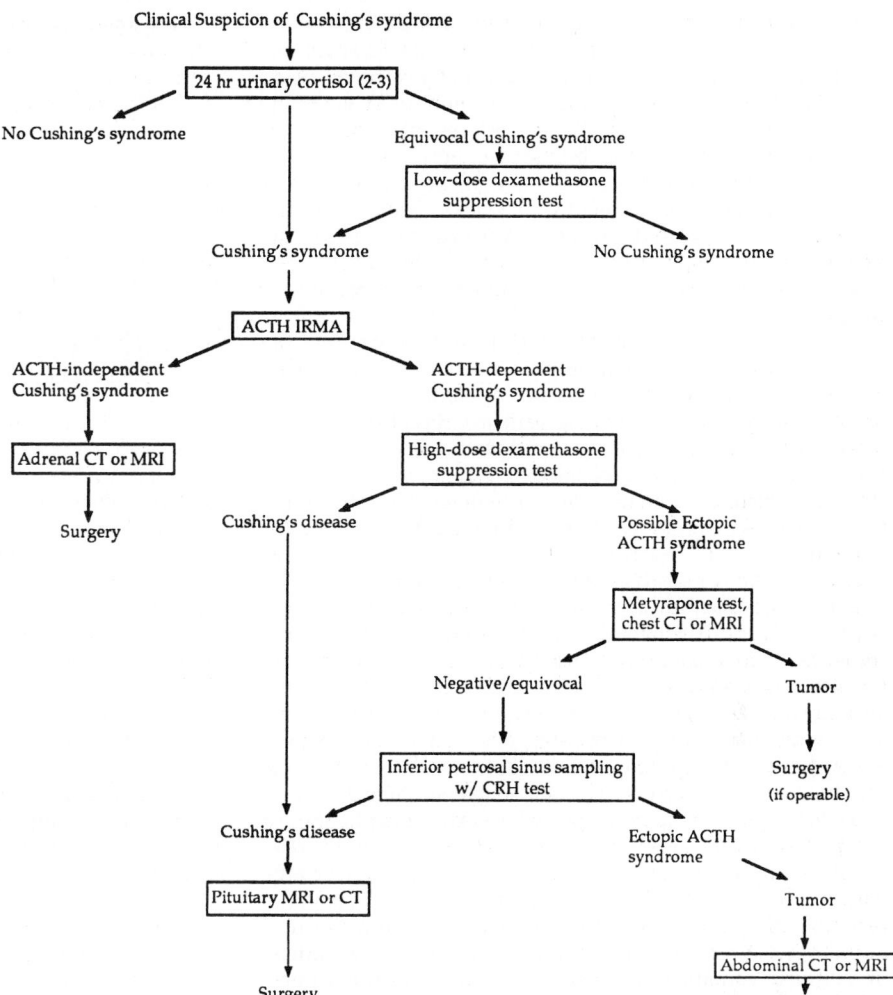

Figure 25–13. Diagnostic approach to Cushing's syndrome. ACTH, adrenocorticotropin; IRMA, immunoradiometric assay; CT, computed tomography; MRI, magnetic resonance imaging; CRH, corticotropin-releasing hormone. (Adapted from Orth, D. N., N. Engl. J. Med., 1995, 332, 791–803. Copyright 1995. Massachusetts Medical Society. All rights reserved.)

approach or laparoscopically.[45] Lesions larger than 6 cm. or those suspicious for carcinoma on T-2–weighted MRI require an anterior approach.[101] Micronodular pigmented hyperplasia and macronodular adrenal hyperplasia involve both adrenal glands and are cured only by bilateral adrenalectomy.[136] Medical adrenalectomy with mitotane or agents interfering with cortisol production is not currently recommended.

TABLE 25–7. Sources of Ectopic ACTH in 100 Cases

Tumor	Number
Carcinoma of lung	52
Carcinoma of pancreas (including carcinoid)	11
Thymoma	11
Benign bronchial adenoma (including carcinoid)	5
Pheochromocytoma	3
Carcinoma of thyroid	2
Carcinoma of liver	2
Carcinoma of prostate	2
Carcinoma of ovary	2
Undifferentiated carcinoma of mediastinum	2
Carcinoma of breast	1
Carcinoma of parotid gland	1
Carcinoma of esophagus	1
Paraganglioma	1
Ganglioma	1
Primary site uncertain	3

All patients who undergo adrenalectomy for primary adrenal causes of Cushing's syndrome require perioperative and postoperative glucocorticoid replacement, since the contralateral gland is suppressed. Replacement therapy with hydrocortisone, 12 mg. per sq. m. per day, may be required as long as 2 years postoperatively.[30] Adequacy of replacement is monitored clinically. Inadequate replacement results in signs of adrenal insufficiency, whereas overreplacement results in features of Cushing's syndrome. The duration of replacement therapy is guided by normalization of the ACTH stimulation test.[30]

Adrenocortical Carcinoma. Patients with this rare but aggressive malignancy may present with Cushing's syndrome. An acute and rapidly progressive course of Cushing's syndrome, virilization, and elevated urinary levels of 17-ketosteroids and dehydroepiandrosterone sulfate (DHEAS) strongly suggest adrenocortical carcinoma. This contrasts to the more gradual onset of symptoms experienced by patients with an adrenal adenoma. Adrenocortical carcinoma requires aggressive surgical resection, although cure is infrequent. Details of the management of adrenocortical carcinoma are discussed subsequently.

Cushing's Syndrome in Children. Adrenocortical neoplasia is the most common cause of hypercortisolism in children. Girls are affected three times as often as boys. The majority of lesions in patients younger than 15 years of age are malignant. Cushing's disease is relatively uncommon in children, and ectopic production of ACTH from malignant neoplasms is rare. As in adults, the predominant feature of Cushing's syndrome in children is obesity. Striae, plethora, headaches, hypertension, ecchymoses, osteoporosis, hypercalciuria, and impaired carbohydrate tolerance are also present. Virilization associated with hirsutism and acne is a frequent finding.

Children with Cushing's disease are best managed by transsphenoidal resection of the microadenoma. Although pituitary irradiation is frequently beneficial, some endocrinologists have expressed concern regarding the long-term effects of irradiation in children.

Surgical adrenalectomy is the treatment of choice for a child with Cushing's syndrome secondary to an adrenocortical neoplasm. Review of 18 children ranging in age from 18 months to 18 years with Cushing's syndrome revealed that eight patients had adrenal neoplasms, including five adenomas and three carcinomas.[115] One patient with adrenocortical carcinoma died of recurrent disease, but the other two were well 11 and 20 years after adrenalectomy. Eight other patients underwent bilateral adrenalectomy for hypercortisolism. Complications of adrenalectomy were common in this group; five of six children who reached adult stature were significantly stunted, and four of six who had Cushing's disease developed Nelson's syndrome 2 to 12 years after adrenalectomy.

Complications of Bilateral Adrenalectomy: Nelson's Syndrome. In 1960, Nelson and associates described a patient who developed a pituitary tumor 3 years after bilateral adrenalectomy for Cushing's disease.[93] The patient had progressive skin pigmentation, amenorrhea, and visual field disturbances from a functioning pituitary tumor. High plasma concentrations of ACTH and melanocyte-stimulating hormone (MSH) were demonstrated by bioassay. This phenomenon, hence termed *Nelson's syndrome*, was subsequently observed in approximately 10% of patients who underwent bilateral adrenalectomy for Cushing's disease. Combined approaches using surgical therapy and/or irradiation were successful in selected patients, but these tumors were often insensitive to radiation and recurred locally after transsphenoidal resection. This complication has become rare because bilateral adrenalectomy is no longer routinely performed for Cushing's disease.

Aldosteronism

Background. In 1955, Jerome Conn described a 34-year-old woman with hypertension, generalized weakness, and polyuria. Her electrolyte analysis revealed hypokalemia, and surgical exploration of the patient's abdomen revealed a right adrenal cortical adenoma, which was resected. The patient's blood pressure and metabolic abnormalities normalized within 2.5 weeks after operation, which led Conn to hypothesize that these abnormalities were due to secretion of aldosterone by the adenoma.

Aldosteronism is a syndrome of hypertension and hypokalemia caused by hypersecretion of the mineralocorticoid aldosterone. Aldosteronism may be primary, due to an autonomously functioning adrenal neoplasm with suppressed plasma renin, or may be secondary, as a result of elevated plasma renin (Table 25–8). Primary aldosteronism is twice as common in women as in men, and it usually occurs between the ages of 30 and 50.

An aldosterone-producing adrenal adenoma (Conn's syndrome) is the cause of primary aldosteronism in two thirds of cases.[56] Conn's syndrome is one of the few surgically correctable causes of hypertension, although it represents less than 1% of cases of hypertension. Idiopathic bilateral adrenal hyperplasia causes 30% to 40% of cases of primary aldosteronism.[11] Adrenocortical carcinoma is a rare cause of primary aldosteronism. Autosomal dominant glucocorticoid-suppressible aldosteronism is ACTH-dependent aldosteronism

TABLE 25–8. Causes of Hyperaldosteronism

Primary Aldosteronism
Aldosterone-producing adenoma (65%–70%)
Idiopathic bilateral adrenal (30%)
Hyperplasia
Adrenal carcinoma (<1%)
Glucocorticoid-suppressible (<1%)
Aldosteronism
Secondary Aldosteronism
Renal artery stenosis
Congestive heart failure

Modified from Melby, J. C.: Diagnosis of hyperaldosteronism. Endocrinol. Metab. Clin. North Am., 20:248, 1991.

corrected by administration of exogenous glucocorticoids. This rare disorder occurs secondary to fusion of the ACTH-responsive 11-beta-hydroxylase gene promoter to the aldosterone synthase gene.[72] ACTH-induced overexpression of this chimeric gene by cells of the zona fasciculata results in aldosteronism.

Secondary aldosteronism is a physiologic response of the renin-angiotensin system to renal artery stenosis, cirrhosis, congestive heart failure, and normal pregnancy. The adrenal functions normally and secretes aldosterone in response to the elevated plasma renin and angiotensin caused by these conditions. Secondary aldosteronism responds to treatment of the underlying cause.

Signs and Symptoms. Clinical manifestations of primary aldosteronism are varied and nonspecific; however, all are attributable to hypersecretion of aldosterone by the adrenal. Aldosterone-mediated retention of sodium and excretion of potassium and hydrogen ion by the kidney causes moderate diastolic hypertension. Edema is characteristically absent. Hypokalemia occurs spontaneously in 80% to 90% of patients with primary aldosteronism and is easily provokable in the remaining patients. In fact, 40% to 50% of hypertensive patients with spontaneous hypokalemia have primary aldosteronism.[81] Potassium depletion frequently causes symptoms of muscle weakness and fatigue, polyuria and polydipsia, as well as impaired insulin secretion and fasting hyperglycemia in 25% of cases.[135] Primary aldosteronism should be suspected in hypertensive patients with spontaneous hypokalemia (serum concentration < 3.5 mEq. per liter), moderate hypokalemia (serum potassium concentration < 3.0) during diuretic therapy despite concomitant use of oral potassium or potassium-sparing diuretics, or refractory hypertension without explanation. Criteria for diagnosis of primary aldosteronism are (1) diastolic hypertension without edema; (2) hyposecretion of renin in the face of volume depletion; and (3) hypersecretion of aldosterone that fails to suppress with intravascular volume expansion.

Diagnosis. Diagnostic evaluation must establish primary aldosteronism, discern surgically correctable adrenal adenoma from medically treatable idiopathic hyperplasia, and localize an adrenal tumor. Before evaluation, patients need to be potassium repleted and have an adequate sodium intake. Antihypertensive medication should be withheld for at least 4 weeks before study.

The biochemical diagnosis of primary aldosteronism requires demonstration of hypokalemia, inappropriate kaliuresis, and elevated aldosterone with normal cortisol levels (Fig. 25–14). A serum potassium value less than 3.5 mEq. per liter and urinary potassium excretion greater than 30 mEq. per day support a diagnosis of primary aldosteronism. Upright plasma renin activity less than 3 ng. per ml. per hour corroborates the diagnosis, although a few spontaneously hyperten-

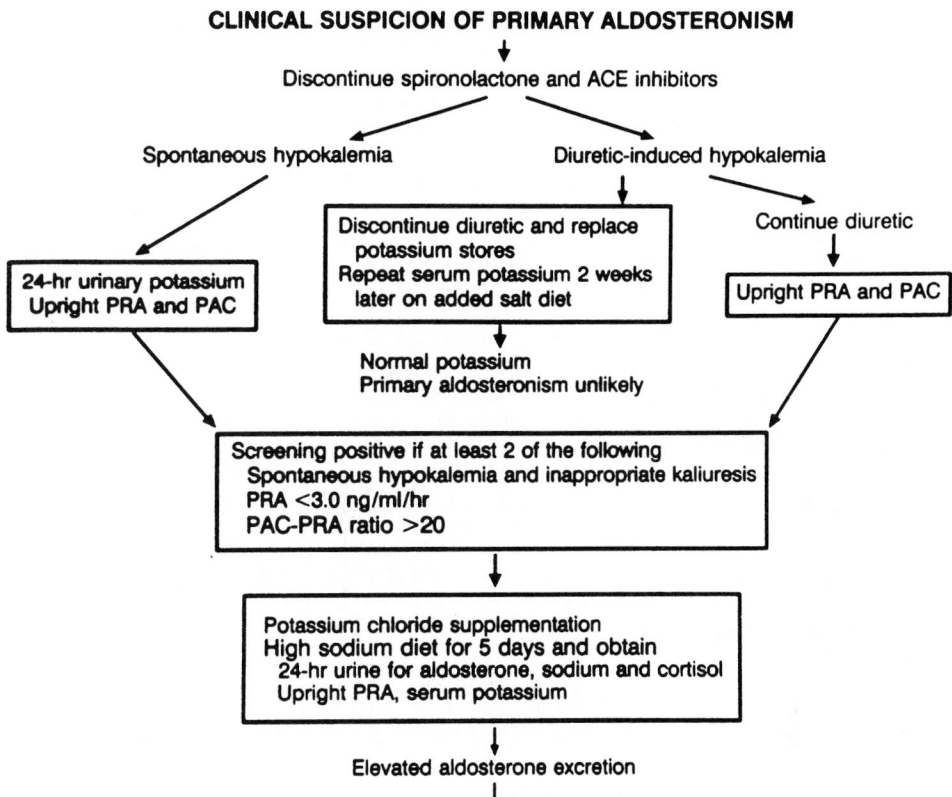

CLINICAL SUSPICION OF PRIMARY ALDOSTERONISM

↓

Discontinue spironolactone and ACE inhibitors

Spontaneous hypokalemia → Diuretic-induced hypokalemia

Discontinue diuretic and replace potassium stores
Repeat serum potassium 2 weeks later on added salt diet

Continue diuretic

24-hr urinary potassium Upright PRA and PAC

Upright PRA and PAC

Normal potassium
Primary aldosteronism unlikely

Screening positive if at least 2 of the following
Spontaneous hypokalemia and inappropriate kaliuresis
PRA <3.0 ng/ml/hr
PAC-PRA ratio >20

↓

Potassium chloride supplementation
High sodium diet for 5 days and obtain
** 24-hr urine for aldosterone, sodium and cortisol**
Upright PRA, serum potassium

↓

Elevated aldosterone excretion

↓

PRIMARY ALDOSTERONISM CONFIRMED

Figure 25–14. Screening and diagnostic confirmation of primary aldosteronism. ACE, angiotensin-converting enzyme; PAC, plasma aldosterone concentration; PRA, plasma renin activity. (From Young, W. F., Hogan, M. J., Klee, G. G., et al.: Primary aldosteronism: Diagnosis and treatment. Mayo Clin. Proc., 65:99, 1990.)

sive patients will have plasma renin activity suppressed to this level. Demonstration of an elevated plasma aldosterone concentration (PAC) in the setting of suppressed plasma renin activity (PRA) increases its diagnostic significance; a PAC/PRA ratio of greater than 20 strongly supports a diagnosis of primary aldosteronism.[135]

Confirmation of primary aldosteronism involves determination of serum potassium, plasma renin activity, and a 24-hour urine collection for sodium, cortisol, and aldosterone after 5 days of a high sodium diet. Twenty-four-hour urinary excretion of aldosterone reliably estimates endogenous aldosterone production, which is inversely proportional to sodium secretion, and should be less than 14 μg. per 24 hours. after a high-salt diet.[11] Patients with primary hyperaldosteronism do not demonstrate aldosterone suppressibility after salt loading. Serum potassium levels must be at least 3.0 mEq. per liter for this test to be accurate.

An intravenous saline infusion test is a shorter and reliable method to confirm primary hyperaldosteronism. Patients who have followed a low sodium diet for 3 days are given 2 liters of normal saline over 4 hours while supine, and a concurrent 24-hour urine collection for aldosterone and sodium is started. Plasma aldosterone may also be measured and will be greater than 10 μg. per ml. in patients with primary aldosteronism; however, this test is not nearly as reliable as the 24-hour measurement of urine aldosterone excretion, which should be less than 14 μg. per 24 hours. This intravenous test may precipitate congestive heart failure in patients with limited cardiac reserve and should be used judiciously. The captopril test and the plasma aldosterone-to-renin ratio test are other useful tests to define the appropriateness of the plasma renin activity for a given level of aldosterone.

After the diagnosis of primary aldosteronism is made, distinction must be made between an aldosteronoma and

idiopathic adrenal hyperplasia. Diagnosis is based on the observation that aldosteronomas are ACTH sensitive and secrete aldosterone with a diurnal variation, while aldosterone secretion from idiopathic adrenal hyperplasia is sensitive to small changes in circulating angiotensin. Two laboratory tests are useful in this regard (Fig. 25–15). The first test measures aldosterone, cortisol, plasma renin activity, and potassium in blood collected at 8 A.M. from a patient who has been supine overnight. Laboratory studies are repeated 4 hours later after the patient has been upright. Patients with an aldosteronoma show diurnal variation in plasma aldosterone that parallels cortisol and is unaffected by postural changes. The physiologic nadir of cortisol must be observed at 8 A.M., or the test may be invalid. Conversely, in patients with idiopathic adrenal hyperplasia, plasma aldosterone levels do not exhibit diurnal variation and are elevated 33% or more by postural changes. A second test measures serum levels of 18-hydroxycorticosterone and differentiates aldosteronoma from adrenal hyperplasia in 82% of cases: patients with aldosteronomas have supine 8 A.M. 18-hydroxycorticosterone levels greater than 100 ng. per 100 ml., whereas patients with adrenal hyperplasia have 18–hydroxycorticosterone levels less than 100 ng. per 100 ml.[135] A combination of posture and 18-hydroxycorticosterone studies may improve diagnostic accuracy.

High-resolution adrenal CT should be the initial step in localization of an adrenal tumor. CT localizes an aldosterone-producing adenoma in 90% of cases overall,[33] and the presence of a unilateral adenoma greater than 1 cm. on CT and supportive biochemical evidence of an aldosteronoma are generally all that is needed to make the diagnosis. Functional lesions larger than 3 cm. may harbor carcinoma. CT cannot discern an aldosterone-producing adenoma from adrenal hyperplasia in patients with multiple bilateral adrenal nodules.[31] MRI is less effective and more costly but may be useful

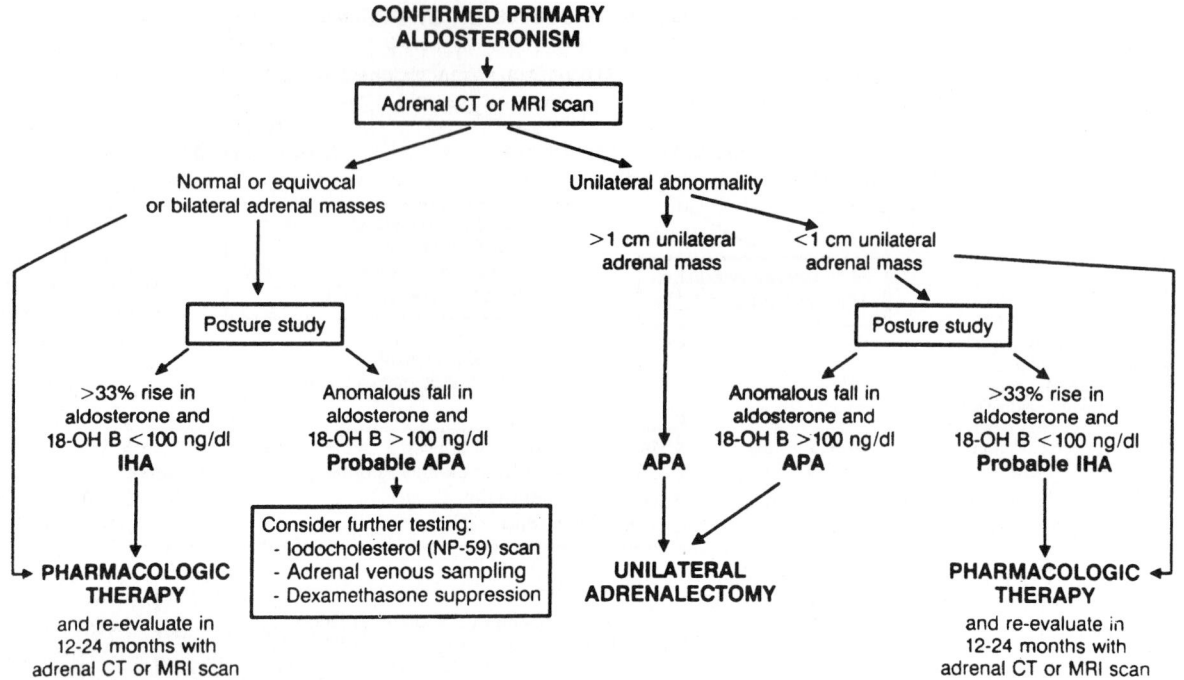

Figure 25–15. Diagnostic differentiation between aldosterone-producing adenoma (APA) and bilateral idiopathic hyperaldosteronism (IHA). CT, computed tomography; MRI, magnetic resonance imaging; 18-OH B, 18-hydroxycorticosterone. (From Young, W. F., Hogan, M. J., Klee, G. G., et al.: Primary aldosteronism: Diagnosis and treatment. Mayo Clin. Proc., *65*:101, 1990.)

during pregnancy or in situations in which intravenous contrast medium injection is undesirable or contraindicated. Imaging studies with CT and MRI may identify adrenal abnormalities that must be interpreted in the context of biochemical studies to avoid false-positive results. NP-59 scintigraphy identifies functional tumors and discriminates aldosteronoma from adrenal hyperplasia with an overall accuracy of approximately 72%.[135] Pretreatment with dexamethasone to suppress ACTH and endogenous cortisol synthesis is required. Sensitivity of this test correlates with the size of the adenoma, and it is unlikely to provide additional diagnostic information if the CT scan is normal. Absence of tracer uptake is seen with adrenocortical carcinoma.

Uncertainty regarding aldosteronoma versus idiopathic adrenal hyperplasia after biochemical testing and noninvasive localization may be definitively settled by bilateral adrenal venous sampling for aldosterone and cortisol.[44] Percutaneous transfemoral cannulation of both adrenal veins is performed and intravenous ACTH is administered. Simultaneous adrenal vein blood samples for aldosterone and cortisol are taken, and their ratios are determined. The ratio of aldosterone to cortisol is greater than 4:1 for a diagnosis of aldosteronoma or less than 4:1 for idiopathic adrenal hyperplasia. Comparison of cortisol samples ensures bilateral adrenal vein cannulation. This study is greater than 90% accurate but is technically difficult and may be unsuccessful in 25% of patients.

Management of Primary Aldosteronism

Adrenal Adenoma. Surgical removal of an aldosterone-secreting adenoma results in immediate cure or substantial improvement of hypertension and hyperkalemia in over 90% of patients.[112] Long-term cure rates average 70% to 90%.[135] Preoperative spironolactone and potassium are given to replete potassium stores and correct alkalosis before anesthesia. Blood pressure response to spironolactone in patients with primary hyperaldosteronism also predicts outcome after operation; a significant fall in blood pressure with spironolactone often predicts a successful outcome after adrenalectomy. Response to adrenalectomy is also influenced by the duration and severity of hypertension and by the presence of histo-

logic changes in the kidney.[85] Age greater than 50, male sex, and the presence of multiple nodules within the adrenal is also associated with a poor response to surgery.[95]

The preferred surgical technique for removal of an adrenal aldosteronoma almost always involves either a posterior approach or the newer laparoscopic approach. Morbidity and mortality following these procedures are almost negligible.

If an aldosterone-producing carcinoma is suspected, a transabdominal approach is used to permit assessment of local extension and metastasis to liver and other abdominal sites. Bilateral adrenalectomy for adenomas is not recommended because the resulting adrenal insufficiency is more difficult to treat than is the hypertension caused by the aldosteronism.[11] Patients do not require perioperative glucocorticoid coverage but may require treatment with synthetic mineralocorticoids when oral intake resumes. Selective hypoaldosteronism generally resolves within 3 months of aldosteronoma resection.

Idiopathic Adrenal Hyperplasia and Glucocorticoid-Suppressible Aldosteronism. Management of idiopathic adrenal hyperplasia is medical, because fewer than 20% to 30% of patients with this disease are cured by adrenalectomy.[11, 135] Idiopathic adrenal hyperplasia is treated with spironolactone, triamterene, amiloride, or nifedipine; adrenalectomy is indicated only when symptomatic hypokalemia is refractory to medical therapy.

Treatment of glucocorticoid-suppressible aldosteronism includes dexamethasone, 0.5 to 1.0 mg. per day. Glucocorticoids are used in small doses to avoid Cushing's syndrome. A combination of spironolactone, triamterene, or other potassium-sparing diuretic regimens may be helpful in reducing corticosteroid requirements.

Adrenogenital Syndromes

Congenital Adrenal Hyperplasia. The congenital adrenal hyperplasias are the most common adrenal disorders of infancy and childhood. These syndromes result from inherited defects of one or several of the enzymes necessary for cortisol biosynthesis (Table 25–9). Cortisol deficiency leads to ACTH overproduction and secondary hyperplasia of the adrenal cortex with shunting of cortisol precursors into adrenal androgen pathways. Peripheral tissues convert the excess adrenal androgens to testosterone, which causes virilization of the patient.

Prenatal adrenal virilization in females produces ambiguous external genitalia (female pseudohermaphroditism). Inappropriately elevated androgen levels *in utero* cause prenatal hypertrophy of the clitoris, fusion of the labioscrotal folds, and a urogenital sinus that may appear as a phallic urethra. The müllerian structures (ovaries, fallopian tubes, uterus) are not influenced by androgens and develop normally. Surgical correction of the external anomalies and control of the endocrine defect may allow these females to ultimately bear children.[132]

Postnatal congenital adrenal hyperplasia causes virilization of females and isosexual precocity of males. Females develop hirsutism, polycystic ovaries, and irregular menses. Male patients exhibit hypertrophy of the phallus, a well-developed muscle mass, and an increase in body hair by age 2 or 3. Males subsequently have accelerated growth of body hair and secondary sexual attributes, although their fertility is often impaired. Both sexes experience rapid somatic growth, an advanced bone age, early closure of epiphyses, and short stature. Hyperpigmentation may also occur from high levels of circulating POMC derivatives.

21-Hydroxylase Deficiency. Most cases (>90%) of congenital adrenal hyperplasia are secondary to deficiency of 21-hydroxylase. The incidence of this disorder in the general white population varies between 1 in 5000 to 1 in 15,000 live births, and a much higher incidence (approximately 1 in 700) is observed in certain Alaskan Eskimo populations. Mutations of the 21-hydroxylase gene, located within the HLA locus on the short arm of chromosome 6, cause the various forms of 21-hydroxylase deficiency.[132] Without 21-hydroxylase, progesterone and 17-hydroxyprogesterone cannot be converted to 11-deoxycortisol and 11-deoxycorticosterone, respectively, and both cortisol and aldosterone are decreased. Two forms of this deficiency are recognized that reflect partial or complete absence of the enzyme. The complete form is characterized by androgen excess at birth, salt-wasting in the urine and stool, diarrhea, hypovolemia, hyponatremia, hyperkalemia, and hyperpigmentation. The partial form is characterized by virilization only, which may occur at birth or perhaps not until late childhood or puberty. Increased levels of ACTH may be capable of driving cortisol and aldosterone production into their normal range; therefore, salt wasting, hypovolemia, and hyperpigmentation may be mild or absent.

The laboratory diagnosis of 21-hydroxylase deficiency is straightforward, because elevation of plasma 17-hydroxyprogesterone is the most characteristic abnormality found. Untreated patients with 21-hydroxylase deficiency also have variable deficiencies in both plasma cortisol and 24-hour free urinary cortisol excretion. Comparison of baseline and stimulated levels of 17-hydroxyprogesterone after ACTH stimulation testing can identify complete forms of the disorder.[132]

Treatment of 21-hydroxylase deficiency consists of glucocorticoid and mineralocorticoid replacement. Adequacy of therapy is documented by correction of plasma androgen and 17-hydroxyprogesterone levels. Female patients with ambiguous genitalia require surgical correction, which is best undertaken between the second and eighteenth months of life.

11-Beta-hydroxylase Deficiency. Eleven-beta-hydroxylase deficiency is the second-most common congenital adrenal hyperplasia syndrome and constitutes about 5% of cases. The incidence of this deficiency approaches 1 in 100,000 live births in the white population. This deficiency is inherited as an autosomal recessive trait, and the defective gene is located on chromosome 8q21.[18] Without 11-beta-hydroxylase, 11-deoxycorticosterone and 11-deoxycortisol cannot be converted to corticosterone or cortisol, and the elevated levels of the mineralocorticoid 11-deoxycorticosterone lead to hypertension and hypokalemia. Virilization and hyperpigmentation are also present.

Deficiency of 11-beta-hydroxylase is diagnosed by demonstrating elevated urinary excretion of 17-hydroxyprogesterone, androgens, and 17-ketosteroids. Treatment includes glucocorticoid replacement and surgical correction of the external genitalia in affected female infants.

3-Beta-hydroxydehydrogenase. Three beta-hydroxydehydrogenase deficiency reduces glucocorticoid, mineralocorticoid, and androgen synthesis, which causes 17-hydroxypregnenolone and the weak androgen dehydroepiandrosterone to accumulate. Females are mildly virilized, while males are incompletely virilized and are born with hypospadias. Marked salt wasting is usually present, and affected infants most often do not survive the first days of life. The responsible gene has been mapped to chromosome 1p13.[90]

17-Hydroxylase Deficiency. Seventeen-hydroxylase deficiency causes decreased cortisol and androgen production. A compensatory rise in ACTH stimulates synthesis of aldosterone and deoxycorticosterone. Thus, hypertension and hypokalemia are prominent in patients with this deficiency, who present as incompletely masculinized males or infertile females. The responsible gene has been mapped to chromosome 10q24.3.[36] Treatment involves corticosteroid and androgen replacement.

Congenital Adrenal Lipoid Hyperplasia. Congenital lipoid adrenal hyperplasia is the most severe form of congenital adrenal hyperplasia and is due to a deficiency of cholesterol desmolase (side-chain cleaving enzyme). All adrenal and gonadal synthetic pathways for steroid biosynthesis are inhibited; hence, all affected patients are phenotypic females with a severe salt-losing syndrome that is most often fatal despite replacement therapy. The gene for this disorder has not been definitively localized.

Adrenal Neoplasms Associated with Excess Sex Steroids

Virilizing Adrenal Tumors. Excess production of adrenal androgens by an adrenal adenoma or carcinoma can produce virilizing features. Often, other adrenal hormones are concurrently overproduced, which leads to a *mixed* virilizing and Cushing's syndrome. Girls prematurely develop clitoral enlargement and pubic hair. Boys prematurely develop hirsutism and macrogenitosomia praecox, but the testes remain small, and there may be inhibition of spermatogenesis. Development of an adrenal virilizing tumor in women causes hirsutism and masculinization. Males with these tumors may go unnoticed until signs and symptoms of tumor enlargement or distant metastases develop. Virilizing tumors secrete inordinately large amounts of androgen precursor, dehydroepiandrosterone, which can be measured either directly in plasma or in urine as a 17-ketosteroid. Abdominal CT is subsequently used to localize the lesion.

Resection of tumor and involved adrenal gland is the primary treatment for patients with adrenal virilizing tumors. Histologically, it may be difficult to determine whether a specific tumor is benign or malignant, although the presence of either local invasion or distant metastases makes the diagnosis obvious. Tumor recurrence is detectable by return of virilization and by detection of increased 17-ketosteroids in the urine. Aminoglutethimide or mitotane may be useful in controlling signs and symptoms in patients with metastatic disease.

TABLE 25–9. Defects of Adrenal Steroidogenesis*

Deficiency	Syndrome	Ambiguous Genitalia	Postnatal Virilization	Salt Metabolism	Steroids Increased	Steroids Decreased	Enzyme	Chromosome	Frequency†
Cholesterol desmolase	Lipoid hyperplasia	Males	No	Salt-wasting	None	All	P450scc	?	Rare
3β-OH-steroid dehydrogenase	Classic	Males and ? females	Yes	± Salt-wasting	DHEA, 17-OH-pregnenolone	Aldo, cortisol, T	3β-OH-steroid dehydrogenase	1p13	Rare
	Nonclassic	No	Yes	Normal	DHEA, 17-OH-pregnenolone		3β-OH-steroid dehydrogenase	1p13	? Frequent
17-Hydroxylase		Males	No	Hypertension	DOC, corticosterone	Cortisol, T	P450c17	10	Rare
17,20-Lyase		Males	No	Normal		DHEA, T, androstenedione	P450c17	10	Rare
21-Hydroxylase	Salt-wasting	Females	Yes	Salt-wasting	17-OHP, androstenedione	Aldo, cortisol	P450c21	6p (HLA)	1/10,000
	Simple virilizing	Females	Yes	Normal	17-OHP, androstenedione	Cortisol	P450c21	6p (HLA)	1/20,000
	Nonclassic	No	Yes	Normal	17-OHP, androstenedione		P450c21	6p (HLA)	0.1–1% (3% in European Jews)
11-Hydroxylase	Classic	Females	Yes	Hypertension	DOC, 11-deoxycortisol	Cortisol, ± aldo	P450c11	8q21	1/100,000
	Nonclassic	No	Yes	Normal	11-deoxycortisol, ± DOC		P450c11	8q21	? Frequent
Corticosterone methyl oxidase II		No	No	Salt-wasting	18-OH-corticosterone	Aldo	P450c11	8q21	Rare (except in Iranian Jews)

*Deficiency of 17,20-lyase is expressed in the gonads but is included here because it apparently involves the same gene as 17-hydroxylase deficiency.

†"Rare" denotes a syndrome accounting for less than 1% of reported cases of congenital adrenal hyperplasia, which has an overall frequency of about 1 in 5000 births. "? Frequent" syndromes may occur at frequencies similar to that of nonclassic 21-hydroxylase deficiency, but prevalence data are not available.

DHEA, dehydroepiandrosterone; DOC, deoxycorticosterone; 17-OHP, 17-hydroxyprogesterone; aldo, aldosterone; T, testosterone.

Reprinted by permission of The New England Journal of Medicine from White, P. C., New, M. I., and DuPont, B.: Congenital adrenal hyperplasia. N. Engl. J. Med., 316:1580, 1987, Copyright 1987, Massachusetts Medical Society.

Feminizing Adrenal Tumors. Feminizing adrenal neoplasms are extremely rare. Most of these tumors occur in adult males during the second through the fourth decades of life. Impotence is common, and both gynecomastia and testicular atrophy are frequent findings. In young males, the association of bilateral gynecomastia, rapid growth, and advanced bone age should suggest a feminizing adrenal tumor. Usually, urinary 17-ketosteroids and estrogens are elevated. Girls who develop feminizing adrenal tumors experience precocious puberty with breast enlargement, development of a female escutcheon, and early onset of menses. Approximately 50% of patients have a palpable abdominal mass at the time of diagnosis. Diagnosis depends on biochemical demonstration of elevated urinary levels of estrogens and 17-ketosteroids. Surgical resection is the treatment of choice for feminizing adrenal neoplasms. Generally, patients with benign adenomas experience a normal survival, whereas the prognosis is poor in patients with adrenocortical carcinoma.

Adrenocortical Carcinoma

Background. Adrenocortical carcinoma is a rare but aggressive malignancy that represents 0.05% to 0.2% of all cancers. The age distribution of adrenocortical carcinoma is bimodal, with peaks in the first and fifth decades. Females are affected more commonly than are males (1.4–2:1). The etiology of adrenocortical carcinoma is unclear; however, genetic alterations including tumor-specific loss of heterozygosity on chromosome 11p15 have been described.[134]

Most patients (70% to 76%) with adrenocortical cancer present with advanced Stage III or IV disease (Table 25–10).[103, 139] Syndromes of adrenal hormone overproduction occur in 36% to 60% of adult patients and may include hypercortisolism, hyperaldosteronism, or virilization. Functional tumors occur more often in females. Nonfunctioning adrenocortical carcinomas present most commonly as abdominal pain, increased abdominal girth, weight loss, weakness, anorexia, and nausea. Approximately 50% of patients have a palpable abdominal mass, and 25% have hepatomegaly. The right adrenal is involved as often as is the left.[74]

Diagnosis. An adrenocortical carcinoma should be suspected in patients with rapidly progressive Cushing's syndrome or in patients with both cushingoid and virilizing features. Large (> 6 cm.) adrenal masses that extend to nearby structures on CT scanning likely represent carcinomas. Adrenocortical carcinoma is also suggested by a unilateral adrenal tumor, with a T2-weighted MRI intensity as bright or brighter than liver.[94] Contrast-enhanced CT of the abdomen and chest is important to preoperatively diagnose local tumor invasion and metastatic lesions as well as to confirm a functioning contralateral kidney. A preoperative bone scan is obtained to evaluate for bony metastases.

Definitive diagnosis of adrenocortical carcinoma requires

TABLE 25–10. Staging of Adrenocortical Carcinoma

Stage	T,N,M	Criteria	% of Cases
I	T_1, N_0, M_0	<5 cm.; confined to adrenal	2
II	T_2, N_0, M_0	>5 cm.; confined to adrenal	19
III	T_31, N_0, M_0 $T_1/T_2, N_1, M_0$	Local invasion or positive nodes	18
IV	$T_3/T_4, N_1, M_0$ Any T/N, M_0	Local invasion and positive nodes, or metastases	61

Modified from Pommier, R. F., and Brennan, M. F.: Management of adrenal neoplasms. Curr. Probl. Surg., *28*:684, 1991.

operative and pathologic demonstration of nodal or distant metastases. Although there are exceptions, any adrenal neoplasm weighing more than 100 gm. should be considered malignant.[94] Tumor necrosis, hemorrhage, and local invasion are gross pathologic evidence of carcinoma, while cells with large, hyperchromatic nuclei and more than 20 mitoses per high-power field are histopathologic features of malignancy.

Management. The prognosis for patients with adrenocortical carcinoma is poor, with an overall 5-year survival rate of 16% to 23%.[103] Complete surgical resection of locally confined tumor is the only chance for cure of this malignancy. In two series, patients with Stage I and II disease had a mean survival of 24 and 25 months, with a 50% and 10% 5-year survival after resection, repectively.[9, 49] However, spread to local structures including the peritoneum, retroperitoneum, and lymph nodes is evident in 65% of cases and only about 80% of patients are able to undergo attempted resection for cure.[74] Treatment then involves *en bloc* resection of locally invasive, Stage III disease. In one series, mean disease-free interval for Stage III disease after *en bloc* resection was 12 months, and overall 5-year survival was 22%.[74]

Many patients with adrenocortical carcinoma present with metastatic disease, most often involving the lung, lymph nodes, liver, or bone. Surgical debulking of locally advanced or metastatic adrenocortical carcinoma may provide these patients with symptomatic relief from some slow-growing, hormonally productive cancers.[58] Close biochemical and radiologic follow-up is required after resection, because recurrent or metastatic disease is best treated by reoperation.[58, 103]

Chemotherapy for adrenocortical carcinoma usually includes mitotane. Partial, unsustained responses are noted in less than 15% to 34% of patients, and survival is unchanged.[58, 103] Although anecdotal reports of long-term survivors after mitotane exist, no controlled studies have established efficacy of mitotane in this disease.[74] Adjuvant chemotherapy with mitotane after complete resection for adrenocortical carcinoma is controversial, and most oncologists reserve its use for recurrent, unresectable or metastatic disease.[94] Other chemotherapeutic regimens have been ineffective.

Adrenal Insufficiency

Background. In 1855, Thomas Addison described 11 patients with primary adrenal insufficiency, including 5 patients with tuberculous destruction of the adrenal glands.[2] Today, adrenal insufficiency is estimated to occur in 1 of 4500 to 6250 hospitalized patients in the United States, indicating that it is a relatively rare disease. Adrenal insufficiency is most commonly diagnosed in the third to fifth decades of life, with a male to female ratio between 1.08:1 and 3.74:1.[29]

The most common causes of primary adrenal insufficiency are autoimmune adrenalitis, infection, and metastatic disease (Table 25–11).[131] Autoimmune adrenalitis represents 65% to 85% of cases and may occur alone or as a component of the polyglandular autoimmune syndromes Types I and II.[131] Tuberculosis, formerly the cause of adrenal insufficiency in 80% to 85% of cases, now causes 30% of cases.[29] Acquired immunodeficiency syndrome (AIDS) and AIDS-associated infections, including infection with cytomegalovirus and *Mycobacterium avium*, are increasing causes of primary adrenal insufficiency. Metastatic tumor infiltration of the adrenal may also produce adrenal insufficiency. As many as 58% of breast tumors, 50% of melanomas, 42% of lung cancers, 25% of malignant lymphomas, and 16% of gastric cancers metastasize to the adrenal.[66] Although overt adrenal insufficiency is not common, an insidious onset of symptoms and signs of adrenal insufficiency may be present in up to 20% to 30% of patients with bilateral adrenal metastatic lesions detected by

TABLE 25-11. Causes of Adrenal Insufficiency

Primary Adrenal Insufficiency

Autoimmune
  Polyglandular autoimmune syndromes I and II
Infections
  Tuberculosis, fungal, CMV, HIV-associated
Adrenal hemorrhage
  Waterhouse-Friderichsen syndrome, coagulopathy

Secondary Adrenal Insufficiency

Exogenous steroid use
Pituitary disease
  Tumor, hemorrhage
Surgery
  Following transsphenoidal removal of a pituitary tumor
  Following removal of a functioning adrenal tumor
Metastatic disease
  Lung, gastric, breast, melanoma, lymphoma
Drugs
  Mitotane, metyrapone, aminoglutethimide

Modified from Werbel, S. S., and Ober, K. P.: Acute adrenal insufficiency. Endocrinol. Metab. Clin. North Am., *22*:303, 1993.

CT scan. These patients are recognized by their weak responses to ACTH stimulation testing. Intra-adrenal hemorrhage and acute adrenal insufficiency may occur in a number of conditions, including trauma, shock, and coagulopathy. Spontaneous adrenal hemorrhage occurring during fulminant meningococcal, gram-negative, or pneumococcal septicemia is known as Waterhouse-Friderichsen syndrome. Exogenous steroid use, surgical resection of cortisol-producing adrenal tumors, and ACTH-producing pituitary tumors are important causes of secondary adrenal insufficiency.

Signs and Symptoms. Symptoms of adrenal insufficiency are variable and result from glucocorticoid and mineralocorticoid deficiencies. Acute adrenal insufficiency is an emergency and should be suspected in stressed patients with a history of either adrenal insufficiency or exogenous steroid use. Signs and symptoms include fever, nausea, vomiting, severe hypotension, and lethargy (Table 25–12). Chronic adrenal insufficiency presents more subtly, and diagnosis is often delayed. Most frequent chronic symptoms include fatigue, weight loss, anorexia, nausea and vomiting, abdominal pain, and diarrhea.

Diagnosis. Characteristic laboratory findings of adrenal insufficiency include hyponatremia, hyperkalemia, azotemia, and fasting or reactive hypoglycemia. Hypercalcemia may also be present. The peripheral blood smear may demon-

strate eosinophilia in 15% to 20% of patients. Adrenal calcifications may be visible on plain abdominal radiographs in 15% of cases.

The rapid ACTH stimulation test is the best test of adrenal insufficiency. Synthetic ACTH (250 μg.) is administered intravenously, and plasma cortisol levels are measured at 0, 30, and 60 minutes later. Normal peak cortisol response should exceed 20 μg. per 100 ml. Subnormal stimulation should be confirmed by the standard, prolonged ACTH infusion test. Measurement of ACTH by IRMA is then used to distinguish primary from secondary and tertiary adrenal insufficiency. High plasma concentration of ACTH (> 200 pg./100 ml.) and low plasma cortisol (< 10 mg./100 ml.) are diagnostic of primary adrenal insufficiency in a patient with characteristic symptoms and signs. Low levels of plasma ACTH indicate secondary (pituitary) or tertiary (hypothalamic) causes that can be differentiated by CRH stimulation testing.

Management. The management of adrenal crisis is outlined in Table 25–13. Treatment must be based on clinical suspicion before laboratory confirmation is available. Intravenous volume replacement with normal or hypertonic saline and dextrose is essential, as is immediate intravenous steroid replacement therapy with 4 mg. dexamethasone. Extreme states of hyponatremia should not be corrected too rapidly. Subsequent recognition and treatment of the underlying cause, particularly if it is infectious, usually resolves the crisis.

A rapid ACTH stimulation test is performed to establish the diagnosis of adrenal insufficiency after resuscitation and corticosteroid replacement. Hydrocortisone acetate is detected by laboratory assay for cortisol and so dexamethasone should be given until ACTH testing is complete. Thereafter, 100 mg. of hydrocortisone is administered intravenously ev-

TABLE 25-13. Treatment of Suspected Acute Adrenal Insufficiency (Adrenal Crisis)

Emergency Measures

1. Establish intravenous access with a large-gauge needle.
2. Draw blood for immediate serum electrolyte and glucose assays and routine measurement of plasma cortisol and ACTH. Do not wait for laboratory results.
3. Infuse 2 to 3 L. of 154 mmol./L. NaCl (0.9% saline) solution or 50 gm./L. (5%) dextrose in 154 mmol./L. NaCl (0.9% saline) solution as quickly as possible. Monitor for signs of fluid overload by following central or peripheral venous pressure and listening for pulmonary rales. Reduce infusion rate if indicated.
4. Inject 4 mg. of dexamethasone sodium phosphate intravenously. Intravenous hydrocortisone (100 mg. immediately and every 6 hr. thereafter) may also be used but will interfere with measurement of plasma cortisol during the short ACTH stimulation test. Mineralocorticoids are unnecessary at this time.
5. Use supportive measures as needed.

Subacute Measures After Stabilization of the Patient

1. Continue intravenous 154 mmol./L. NaCl (0.9% saline) solution at a lower rate for next 24 to 48 hr.
2. Search for and treat possible infectious precipitating causes of the adrenal crisis.
3. Perform a short ACTH stimulation test to confirm the diagnosis of adrenal insufficiency if patient does not have known adrenal insufficiency.
4. Determine the type of adrenal insufficiency and its cause if not already known.
5. Taper glucocorticoids to maintenance dosage over 1 to 3 days if precipitating or complicating illness permits.
6. Begin mineralocorticoid replacement with fludrocortisone (0.1 mg. by mouth daily) when saline infusion is stopped.

TABLE 25-12. Symptoms and Signs in Acute Adrenocortical Insufficiency ("Crisis")

Symptoms/Signs (Clinical Deterioration Without Obvious Cause)	Prevalence (100%)
Fever	70%
Nausea and vomiting	64%
Abdominal pain	46%
Hypotension	36%
Abdominal distention	32%
Obtundation/lethargy	26%
Hyponatremia	45%
Hyperkalemia	25%

Modified from May, M. E., Vaughan, E. D., Jr., and Carey, R. M.: Adrenocortical insufficiency: Clinical aspects. *In* Vaughan, E. D., Jr., and Carey, R. M. (Eds.): Adrenal Disorders. New York, Thieme, 1989, p. 176.

From Wilson, J. D., and Foster, D. W. (Eds.): Williams Textbook of Endocrinology, 8th ed. Philadelphia, W. B. Saunders, 1992.

ery 6 to 8 hours and is tapered to standard replacement doses as the patient's condition stabilizes. Mineralocorticoid replacement is not required until intravenous fluids are discontinued and oral intake resumes. Chronic adrenal insufficiency requires corticosteroid and mineralocorticoid replacement. The average adult requires 12 mg. per sq. m. of hydrocortisone, or its equivalent, each day, administered in divided doses along with 0.05 to 0.10 mg. of the mineralocorticoid fludrocortisone.

Patients who have known adrenal insufficiency or have received supraphysiologic doses of corticosteroid for at least 1 week in the year preceding surgery should receive perioperative stress-dose corticosteroids. If in doubt, rapid ACTH stimulation testing may be performed during the preoperative evaluation of the patient. Corticosteroid replacement should approximate the known capacity of the normal adrenal to secrete up to 300 mg. per day of cortisol under maximal stress. An accepted regimen includes administration of 100 mg. hydrocortisone the evening before and the morning of major surgery followed by 100 mg. of hydrocortisone every 8 hours during the perioperative 24 hours. If high-dose corticosteroids are administered for less than 72 hours, they can be rapidly tapered to replacement levels as the patient's condition permits. A rapid taper is desirable to minimize corticosteroid-related wound complications and infection.

Physiology of the Adrenal Medulla

Cells of the adrenal medulla secrete several biologically active amines, including dopamine, norepinephrine, and epinephrine. These catecholamines are synthesized in the brain, in sympathetic neurons, and in chromaffin cells of the adrenal medulla. Catecholamines are also produced by the organ of Zuckerkandl and by other extra-adrenal tissues derived from embryonic neural crest.

The catecholamine biosynthetic pathway converts tyrosine to active catacholamines by the sequential action of four enzymes: (1) tyrosine hydroxylase, which converts tyrosine to L-dihydroxyphenylalanine (dopa); (2) aromatic L-amino acid decarboxylase, which converts dopa to dopamine; (3) dopamine-beta-hydroxylase, which converts dopamine to L-norepinephrine; and (4) phenylethanolamine-*N*-methyltransferase (PNMT), which converts L-norepinephrine to L-epinephrine. PNMT is localized exclusively in cells of the adrenal medulla and the organ of Zuckerkandl. Thus, with rare exceptions, epinephrine-secreting tumors arise only in these two tissues. Epinephrine represents approximately 80%, norepinephrine represents 20%, and dopamine is a minute fraction of stored catecholamines in the adrenal medulla.

Regulation of catecholamine biosynthesis is complex. Splanchnic nerve activation dramatically increases the rate of catecholamine synthesis in the adrenal medulla. The metabolic milieu within the adrenal medulla also greatly influences tyrosine hydroxylase activity: glucocorticoids, phospholipids, cyclic adenosine monophosphate, adenosine triphosphate, protein kinase, and magnesium increase activity of PNMT and decrease catecholamine negative feedback.

Catecholamines and their associated matrix proteins, chromogranins, are stored in chromaffin granules of adrenal medullary cells. Excitation of these cells stimulates discharge of the granules and release of catecholamines into the circulation. These neurotransmitters profoundly alter the cardiovascular system, smooth and skeletal muscle activity, metabolism, and blood flow within the liver, spleen, lung, and brain. Catecholamines modulate endocrine functions of several organs through specific adrenergic receptors in the microcirculation and parenchymal cells of these organs.

Three pathways govern clearance of catecholamines from the circulation: specific uptake by sympathetic neurons, non-specific uptake and degradation by peripheral tissues, and excretion in the urine. Catecholamines are metabolized in liver and kidney by two enzymes, monamine oxidase (MAO) and catechol-O-methyl transferase (COMT). In these tissues, MAO and COMT convert epinephrine or norepinephrine to methoxyhydroxyphenylglycol (MHPG), vanillylmandelic acid (VMA), normetanephrine, and metanephrine (Fig. 25–16). These inactive metabolites are renally cleared and are measurable in the urine either as free compounds or as conjugates of glucuronide or sulfate.

Pharmacologic distinction of adrenergic receptors relies on their relative responsiveness to natural and artificial bioamines: alpha receptors have highest affinity for norepinephrine, less for epinephrine, and least for isoproterenol. Beta receptors are most responsive to isoproterenol and least to norepinephrine (Table 25–14). In addition, specific antagonists recognize each receptor class: alpha receptors are antagonized by phentolamine and phenoxybenzamine, and beta receptors are blocked by propranolol. Beta-receptor subtypes have been identified and characterized and have had their DNAs cloned: beta$_1$ receptors are present in cardiac muscle, adipose tissue, and small intestine, while beta$_2$ receptors are found in vascular, tracheal, and uterine smooth muscle, skeletal muscle, and liver. Alpha receptors have been similarly subdivided: alpha$_1$-receptors mediate vasoconstriction, pupillary dilatation, and uterine contraction, whereas alpha$_2$-receptors modulate presynaptic norepinephrine release and platelet aggregation. Dopaminergic receptors have also been identified, characterized, and cloned. Dopamine receptor activation causes positive inotropic and chronotropic effects on cardiac muscle, induces mild peripheral vasoconstriction, and dilates renal arterioles.

Diseases of the Adrenal Medulla

Pheochromocytoma

Background. Pheochromocytomas are functional adrenal tumors that arise from neuroectodermal cells of the adrenal medulla or in certain extra-adrenal sites. The term *pheochromocytoma* is derived from the Greek words *phaios* (dusky) and *chroma* (color). The term was introduced in 1912 by Pick, who noted that these tumors stain a deep rust color when treated with chromium salts. The first description of a pheochromocytoma is credited to Frankel, who reported finding bilateral adrenal tumors in an 18-year-old woman who died precipitously in 1886. Roux and Mayo independently reported the first successful resections of pheochromocytomas in 1926 and 1927, respectively.[79, 110] In the early 1950s, von Euler and associates demonstrated large quantities of catecholamines in the urine from patients with these tumors. Subsequently, other investigators identified the catecholamine metabolites VMA and normetanephrine in the urine along with their parent compounds epinephrine and norepinephrine.

Pheochromocytomas are rare tumors, occurring in 0.005% to 0.1% of persons.[22] These tumors are found with increased frequency in screened hypertensive populations and in individuals with multiple endocrine neoplasia Types 2a and 2b, von Recklinghausen's neurofibromatosis, and von Hippel-Lindau disease. The peak incidence of pheochromocytoma occurs during the fourth and fifth decades of life, and males and females are affected about equally. The *rule of tens* has been applied to pheochromocytoma: tumors are bilateral in 10%, extra-adrenal in 10%, familial in 10%, multicentric in 10%, malignant in 10%, and occur in children in 10% of cases.

Pheochromocytomas arise from neuroendocrine cells of the adrenal medulla or of extra-adrenal chromaffin tissue within ganglia near the heart, aorta, or urinary bladder. These tu-

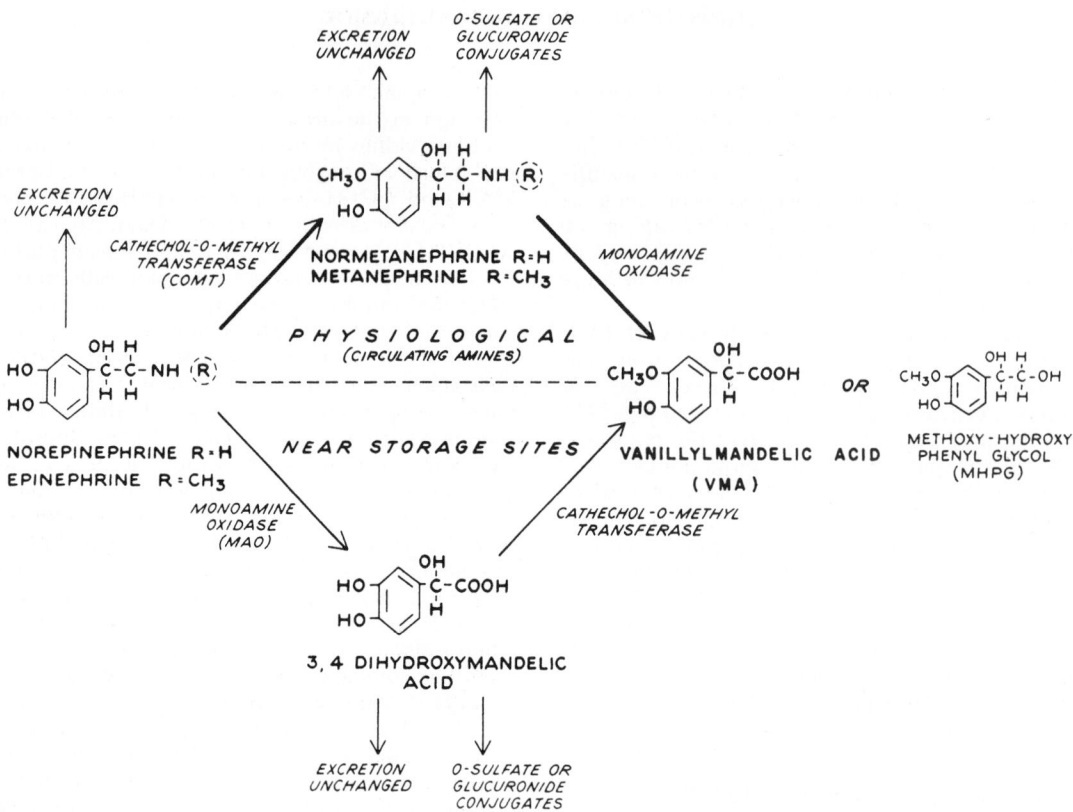

Figure 25–16. Biochemical pathways of catecholamine metabolism. (From Melmon, K. L.: Catecholamines and the adrenal medulla. *In* Williams, R. H. [Ed.]: Textbook of Endocrinology, 6th ed. Philadelphia, W. B. Saunders, 1981.)

TABLE 25–14. Classification of Adrenergic Receptors by Agonist and Antagonist Selectivity

Receptor	Agonist Potency Sequence	Agonist		Antagonist	
		Selective	*Nonselective*	*Selective*	*Nonselective*
Alpha$_1$	NE>E>ISP	Methoxamine Phenylephrine		Prazosin Terazosin Doxazosin Trimazosin	
			Epinephrine Norepinephrine Isoproterenol		Phenoxybenzamine Phentolamine
Alpha$_2$	E>NE>ISP	Clonidine Guanfacine Guanabenz		Yohimbine	
Beta$_1$	ISP>E≅NE	Dobutamine		Metoprolol Atenolol Acebutolol Esmolol	
			Isoproterenol Epinephrine Norepinephrine	Betaxolol	Propranolol Nadolol Timolol Oxprenolol Sotalol Alprenolol Pindolol Carteolol Penbutolol Labetalol
Beta$_2$	ISP>E>NE	Metaproterenol Terbutaline Salbutamol Pirbuterol Bitolterol		Butoxamine	

E, epinephrine; NE, norepinephrine; ISP, isoproterenol.
From Bravo, E. L., and Gifford, R. W., Jr.: Pheochromocytoma. Endocrinol. Metab. Clin. North Am., *22:*329, 1993.

TABLE 25–15. Symptoms of Pheochromocytoma

Symptom*	Approximate Percentage	
	Paroxysmal (37 Patients)	Persistent (39 Patients)
Headaches (severe)	92	72
Excess sweating (generalized)	65	69
Palpitations ± tachycardia	73	51
Anxiety or nervousness (± fear of impending death; panic)	60	28
Tremulousness	51	26
Pain in chest and/or abdomen (usually epigastric) and or lumbar regions and/or lower abdomen and/or groin	48	28
Nausea ± vomiting	43	26
Weakness, fatigue, prostration	38	15
Weight loss (severe)	14	15
Dyspnea	11	18
Warmth ± heat intolerance	13	15
Visual disturbances	3	21
"Dizziness" or faintness	11	3
Constipation	0	13
Paresthesias or pain in arms	11	0
Bradycardia (noted by patient)	8	3
Grand mal	5	3

*Symptoms presumably due to excess catecholamines and/or hypertension.
From Manger, W. M., and Gifford, R. W.: Pheochromocytoma. New York, Springer-Verlag, 1977, p. 89.

mors occur in the adrenal medulla in 90% of cases and are found more often in the right gland than in the left. The organ of Zuckerkandl is the most common extra-adrenal site of pheochromocytoma. The etiology of pheochromocytomas is unclear, although familial occurrence of this neoplasm suggests a genetic component. Indeed, loss of genetic material from chromosomes 1p (42%), 3p (16%), 17p (24%), and 22q (31%) has been shown in both familial and sporadic forms of this disease.[63]

Signs and Symptoms. All symptoms of pheochromocytoma are attributable to excessive circulating catecholamines (Table 25–15). Elevation of the blood pressure, which may range from mild hypertension to a dramatic hypertensive crisis, is the most consistent manifestation of this disorder. This hypertension is sustained in roughly half of patients, is paroxysmal in one third, and is absent in one fifth.[13] Other symptoms include palpitations, anxiety, and tremulousness. Cardiovascular complications frequently include myocardial infarction, cardiac dysrhythmias, and stroke. Orthostatic hypotension is common and results from diminished plasma volume and blunted autonomic reflexes. Gastrointestinal motility is also depressed and can cause severe ileus, obstipation, and sometimes megacolon. Asymptomatic patients with functioning tumors are rare, and nonfunctioning tumors are distinctly uncommon. Sudden death has been reported in patients with known or unsuspected pheochromocytomas who have undergone surgical procedures for other indications.

Diagnosis. Demonstration of increased urinary excretion of catecholamines and their metabolites is the *sine qua non* for the diagnosis of pheochromocytoma. Analysis of catecholamines and their metabolites in a single 24-hour urine collection is the best test to make or exclude this diagnosis because more than 90% of patients with pheochromocytomas have distinctly elevated urine levels of catecholamines, metanephrine, and VMA (Fig. 25–17).[114] Urinary VMA is the least specific assay, because false-positive findings result from ingestion of coffee, tea, raw fruits, or drugs such as alpha-

methyldopa. Nonetheless, all three assays are highly sensitive when performed under controlled conditions.[10] Measurement of plasma catecholamines is not as useful in distinguishing patients with pheochromocytoma from those with essential hypertension, because plasma catecholamine levels are usually elevated in both conditions (Fig. 25–18).[10, 12] Measurement of plasma chromogranin A has a 74% diagnostic specificity and is a poor diagnostic but potentially helpful confirmatory test.[10]

Occasionally the results of baseline testing do not definitively differentiate a low catecholamine-producing pheochromocytoma from essential hypertension with high sympathetic tone. This ambiguity may be resolved by stimulation testing designed to provoke catecholamine secretion from a tumor or by suppression testing designed to inhibit central sympathetic outflow in essential hypertension. Glucagon stimulation testing is useful when pheochromocytoma is clinically suspected and the blood pressure and plasma catecholamine levels are nearly normal. In a closely monitored setting, a 1.0- to 2.0-mg. intravenous bolus of glucagon is administered, which elicits at least a threefold increase in plasma catecholamines, or an absolute plasma level above 2000 pg. per ml. if a pheochromocytoma is present. Conversely, a clonidine suppression test may be used in normotensive or mildly hypertensive patients with elevated plasma catecholamine levels (1000–2000 pg. per ml.). An oral 0.3-mg. dose of clonidine suppresses centrally mediated release of catecholamines to less than 500 pg. per ml. within 2 to 3 hours but does not affect release of catecholamines by a pheochromocytoma (Fig. 25–19). The test must be performed in well-hydrated patients, and all adrenergic antagonists must be discontinued for at least 2 days before the test. Only assays that measure free plasma catecholamines should be used, otherwise false-positive results may be encountered.

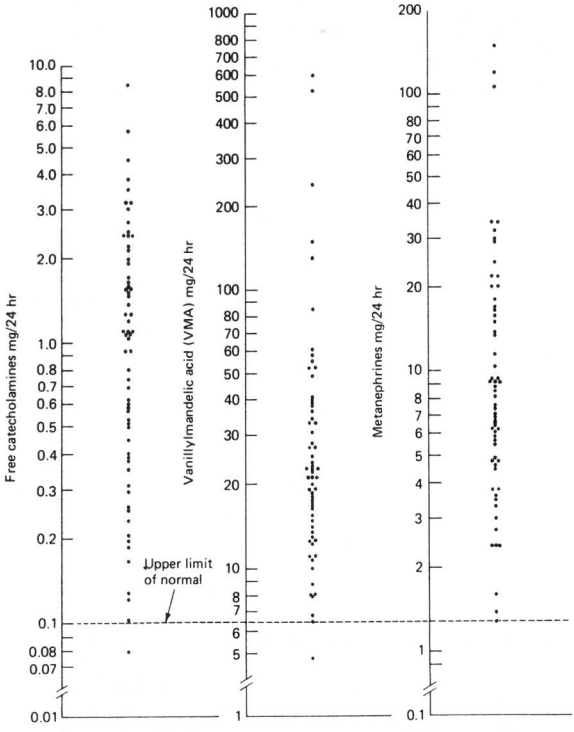

Figure 25–17. Levels of epinephrine, norepinephrine (free catecholamines), vanillylmandelic acid (VMA), and metanephrines in 24-hour urine samples obtained from 64 patients with proven pheochromocytoma. (From Sjoerdsma, A., et al.: Pheochromocytoma: Current concepts of diagnosis and treatment. Ann. Intern. Med., *65*:1036, 1966.)

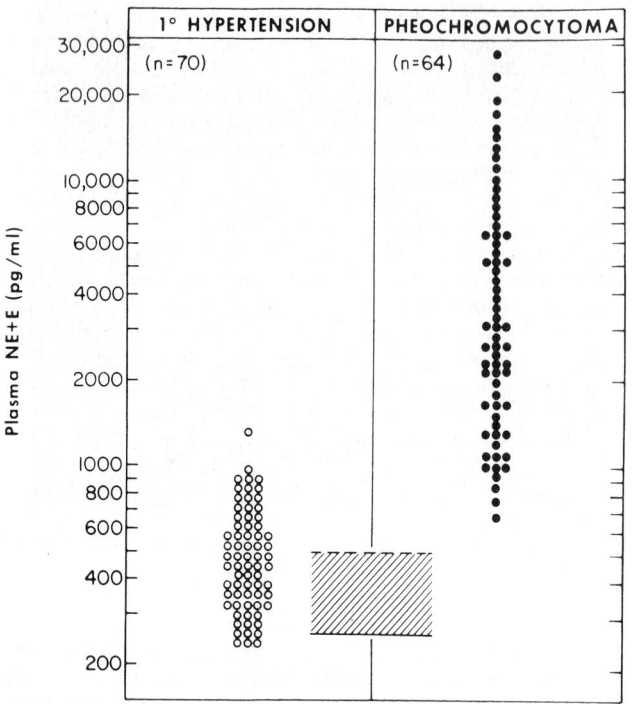

Figure 25–18. Supine resting plasma catecholamine values in patients with essential hypertension or pheochromocytoma. The cross-hatched area represents the mean (260 pg. per ml.) + 2 S.D. (500 pg. per ml.) of values in 47 normotensive healthy adults with an age and sex distribution similar to that of the two patient groups. For subjects with essential hypertension, the mean + 2 S.D. was 516 + 950 pg. per ml.; four patients with pheochromocytoma had levels that fell within the range of values in patients with essential hypertension. NE + E, norepinephrine plus epinephrine. (Reprinted by permission of *The New England Journal of Medicine* from Bravo, E. L., and Gifford, R. W.: Pheochromocytoma: Diagnosis, localization and management. N. Engl. J. Med., *311*:1298, 1984, Copyright 1984, Massachusetts Medical Society.)

Combined glucagon and clonidine testing has high sensitivity (97%) and specificity (100%).[10]

Radiologic localization of biochemically confirmed pheochromocytoma is obtained before operation because of the variable location of these tumors. Up to 98% of pheochromocytomas are found in the abdomen, 2% to 3% in the thorax, and 1% in the neck.[10] CT and MRI are the two radiologic modalities of choice to localize pheochromocytomas. CT readily detects tumors 1 cm. and larger and has sensitivity of 87% to 100% in several studies.[125] MRI is similarly sensitive, and a T2-weighted image brightness three times greater than liver is highly specific for pheochromocytoma (Fig. 25–20). MRI may evolve into the study of choice for localizing pheochromocytoma.[100] Adrenal arteriography and venography are no longer indicated.

Functional nuclear imaging with iodine-131-metaiodobenzylguanidine (^{131}I-MIBG) is another important technique used to localize pheochromocytoma. ^{131}I-MIBG selectively accumulates in chromaffin tissues and accumulates more rapidly in pheochromocytoma than in normal tissue. Multi-institutional experience with this technique has demonstrated an overall sensitivity of 77% to 87% and a specificity of 96% to 100%.[125] This test may be superior to CT and MRI in detecting small functional foci of tumor located outside the adrenal.

Management. When the diagnosis of pheochromocytoma has been established and localization studies are completed, preoperative preparation of the patient centers on blood pressure control and optimization of fluid balance. Blood pressure control is obtained through alpha-adrenergic blockade with phenoxybenzamine, starting at 10 mg. twice a day and increasing 10 to 20 mg. per day until blood pressure returns

to normal or to nearly normal levels. The drug is usually administered for 1 to 3 weeks before operation. Alpha blockade can also be accomplished with oral phentolamine (50 mg. every 4 hours) although gastrointestinal side effects and response to this drug are less satisfactory than with phenoxybenzamine. Side effects of alpha blockade include postural hypotension, reflex tachycardia, nasal congestion, and an inability to ejaculate. Preoperative alpha blockade also reverses the relative hypovolemia that is usually present in patients with pheochromocytoma and also prevents severe blood pressure swings during intraoperative manipulation of the tumor.

Beta-adrenergic blockade with propranolol is indicated in patients who develop tachycardia greater than 140 beats per minute, who have history of arrhythmia, or who harbor tumors that secrete primarily epinephrine. Propranolol may enhance pressor response to endogenous norepinephrine and thus should not be given until adequate alpha blockade has been established. Propranolol can also produce profound bradycardia, myocardial depression, and congestive heart failure. Cardiac asystole and death after propranolol administration have been reported in patients with pheochromocytoma. Newer drug regimens to manage hypertension in pheochromocytoma include selective alpha$_1$-adrenergic antagonists (terazosin and doxazosin) and calcium channel blockers (nifedipine and nicardipine).

Patients with pheochromocytoma can be expected to have blood pressure volatility and high intravascular volume requirements during and immediately after surgery. Elderly

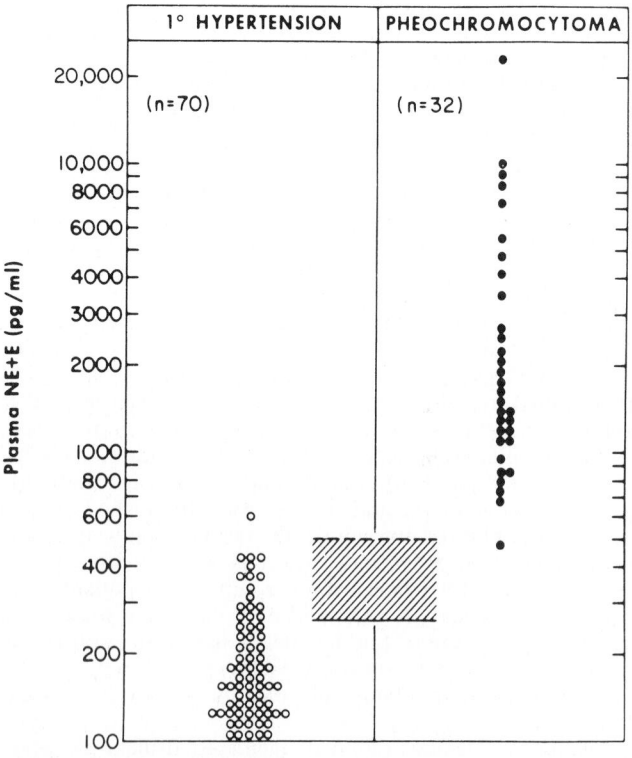

Figure 25–19. Effect of oral clonidine (0.3 mg.) on plasma catecholamine values in patients with essential hypertension or pheochromocytoma. Values shown represent the lowest levels reached (at either 2 or 3 hours) after administration of clonidine. The cross-hatched areas represent the mean + 2 S.D. of basal values in normotensive control subjects. All but one patient with pheochromocytoma had values above 500 pg. per ml. after clonidine administration. One patient with essential hypertension had a value above 500 pg. per ml. NE + E, norepinephrine plus epinephrine. (Reprinted by permission of *The New England Journal of Medicine* from Bravo, E. L., and Gifford, R. W.: Pheochromocytoma: Diagnosis, localization and management. N. Engl. J. Med., *311*:1298, 1984, Copyright 1984, Massachusetts Medical Society.)

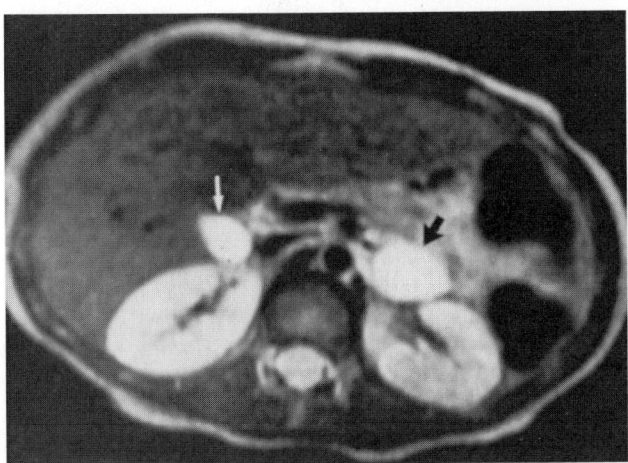

Figure 25–20. Magnetic resonance tomogram, T2-weighted image, of a left-sided pheochromocytoma (heavy arrow). The gallbladder (light arrow) has a high signal intensity, because of its high water content. Pheochromocytoma, adrenocortical carcinomas, and metastatic lesions to the adrenal demonstrate this high signal intensity, possibly because of their high water content. (Courtesy of J. Heiken, M.D., Mallinckrodt Institute of Radiology, Washington University School of Medicine, St. Louis, Missouri.)

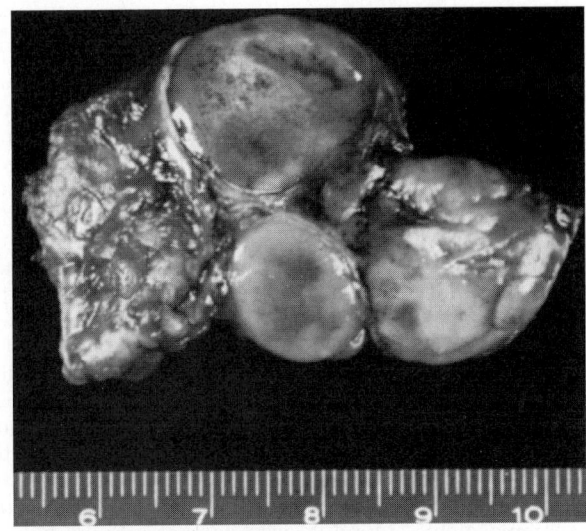

Figure 25–21. Multiple pheochromocytomas in a single adrenal gland resected from a patient with multiple endocrine neoplasia, Type 2a.

patients or those with history of heart disease require preoperative Swan-Ganz catheter insertion and hemodynamic optimization the night before surgery. The morning of the operation, an arterial line is placed for careful monitoring of blood pressure and arterial pH, and a right atrial pressure monitor is placed unless Swan-Ganz monitoring is used.

Anesthetic agents may trigger the release of catecholamines from pheochromocytomas. The anesthetic plane is now considered more important than the choice of agent, and both enflurane and isoflurane have been used successfully. Intraoperative hypertension is best treated with a sodium nitroprusside drip, and cardiac arrhythmias are best managed with short-acting beta blockers (esmolol) or lidocaine. Morphine and phenothiazines may precipitate hypertensive crisis and should be avoided preoperatively.[10]

Formerly, an anterior approach through either a midline or bilateral subcostal incisions was used exclusively to resect pheochromocytomas. This approach facilitates complete abdominal exploration and was necessary to evaluate possible extra-adrenal locations, metastases, and multifocal lesions. Today, CT, MRI, and nuclear scans permit preoperative localization of tumor in 95% or more of cases, so that the surgical approach may be more directed using either a posterior or a laparoscopic approach.[41] Regardless of approach, important common principles include minimal handling of the tumor, early isolation of the adrenal vein, and avoidance of capsular rupture.

The danger of pheochromocytoma does not immediately end with resection of the tumor. Patients can develop profound hypotension during intraoperative and postoperative periods as a result of the vasodilatation that occurs after tumor resection. These patients are usually admitted to an intensive care unit after the operation, where arterial blood pressure, central venous pressure, and urine output should be monitored continuously during the first 24 hours after operation.

Special Issues in Pheochromocytoma

Multiple Endocrine Neoplasia 2 (MEN 2). The MEN-2a syndrome is a hereditary, autosomal dominant predisposition to medullary carcinoma of the thyroid, pheochromocytoma, and parathyroid hyperplasia. Nearly all affected individuals develop medullary carcinoma of the thyroid, whereas only one fourth to one half develop pheochromocytoma or para-

thyroid hyperplasia.[15, 54] Patients with MEN-2a develop bilateral and often multiple pheochromocytomas (Figs. 25–21 and 25–22). As with medullary carcinoma and C-cell hyperplasia of the thyroid, hyperplasia of the adrenal medulla is observed before the appearance of pheochromocytoma.[15] The MEN-2b syndrome is much less common than the MEN-2a syndrome and affected patients have medullary carcinoma of the thyroid and pheochromocytoma. In addition, these patients often develop multiple mucosal neuromas, ganglioneuromatosis, and a characteristic facies and body habitus.

It is imperative that patients with medullary carcinoma of the thyroid be screened for pheochromocytoma, especially if there is a family history of either medullary carcinoma of

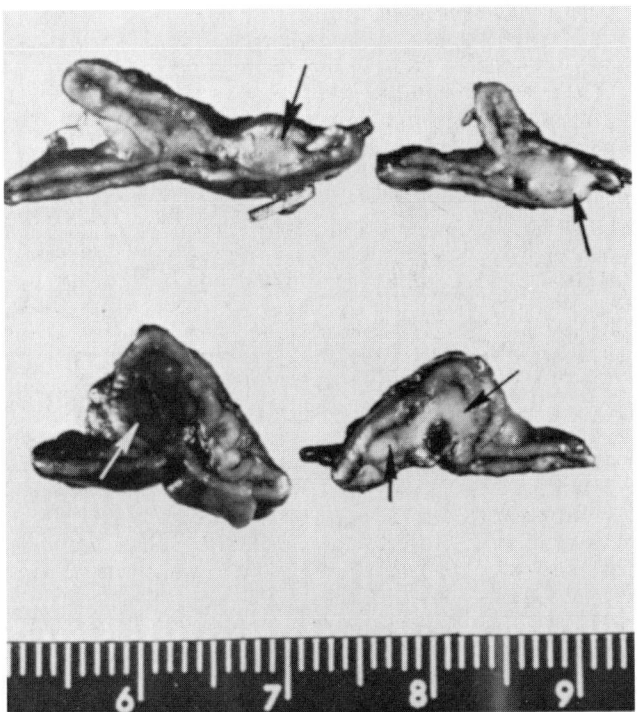

Figure 25–22. A small pheochromocytoma (arrow) and adrenal medullary hyperplasia (two arrows) are noted in the lower adrenal glands. Adrenal medullary hyperplasia (arrows) is demonstrated in the adrenal glands above.

the thyroid or pheochromocytoma. Approximately 10% of patients with MEN 2a present with symptoms of pheochromocytoma before those of medullary thyroid carcinoma.[15] Relatives of these patients should be screened for associated endocrinopathies even if they are asymptomatic. Screening strategies are more thoroughly discussed in Chapter 24.

Neuroectodermal Dysplasias. Von Recklinghausen's neurofibromatosis is diagnosed in 5% to 10% of patients with pheochromocytoma, although less than 1% of patients with von Recklinghausen's disease develop pheochromocytoma. Other neuroectodermal dysplasia syndromes associated with pheochromocytoma include tuberous sclerosis, Sturge-Weber syndrome, and von Hippel-Lindau disease.

Malignant Pheochromocytoma. Ten to 20% of sporadically occurring pheochromocytomas prove to be malignant. Females are three times more likely than are males to harbor such a malignancy. It is controversial whether such lesions in children are more or less likely to be malignant than in adults.[61] There is much stronger evidence, however, that pheochromocytomas found in extra-adrenal sites are two to three times as likely to be malignant as those of adrenal origin.[107] Hypertension associated with malignant pheochromocytomas is sustained and is rarely paroxysmal. The diagnosis of malignant pheochromocytoma is often difficult to make either by preoperative criteria or by inspection of the resected specimen. On gross examination, many benign tumors penetrate the capsule and may even invade the veins draining the gland. Microscopic examination of both benign and malignant lesions may reveal cellular pleomorphism, mitoses, and atypical nuclei. Therefore, a diagnosis of malignant pheochromocytoma is established only by demonstrating invasion of adjacent structures or by documenting nodal or distant metastases. Pheochromocytoma may spread to bone, liver, lymph nodes, lungs, and the central nervous system. Less common sites are pleura, kidney, omentum, and pancreas. Recurrences usually appear within 5 to 10 years after resection of the primary lesion but may be detected as many as 20 years later. There are no clear differences in

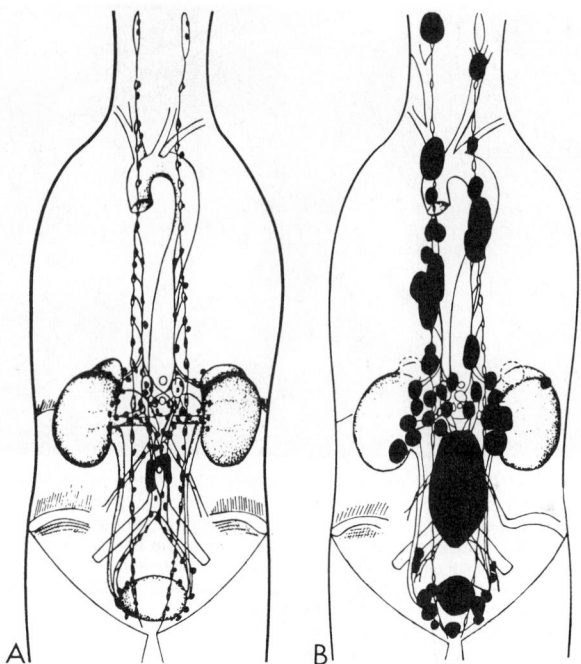

Figure 25–24. *A,* Distribution of extra-adrenal chromaffin tissue in the newborn. *B,* Distribution of extra-adrenal pheochromocytomas reported since 1965. (From Coupland, R.: The Natural History of the Chromaffin Cell. Essex, Longmans, Green and Company, 1965.)

secretion rates of the different catecholamines to distinguish benign from malignant lesions.

The treatment of malignant pheochromocytoma involves resection of metastases and medical control of hypertension. Radiation therapy may be helpful to ameliorate pain from bony metastases. Ablative therapy with ^{131}I-MIBG may produce partial responses,[65] and combination chemotherapy with cyclophosphamide, vincristine, and dacarbazine may also be effective.[4, 62] Overall 5-year survival is 36% to 60%.[122]

Extra-adrenal Pheochromocytoma. Approximately 10% of pheochromocytomas are extra-adrenal, although most (98%) are still located within the abdomen (Fig. 25–23). Extra-adrenal pheochromocytomas can occur at any site in the abdomen where chromaffin tissue is located and have been found in the paravertebral ganglia, the organ of Zuckerkandl, and the urinary bladder (Fig. 25–24). Pheochromocytomas that arise in the organ of Zuckerkandl can become large enough to press on adjacent vascular or genitourinary structures and can be quite vascular and difficult to resect. Pheochromocytomas located in the bladder can cause hypertensive episodes during micturition. Thoracic and cervical pheochromocytomas have also been identified in sympathetic ganglia of the posterior mediastinum, the carotid body (*chemodectomas*), the heart, and the jugular bulb.

Pheochromocytoma in Pregnancy. Nearly 130 cases of pheochromocytoma requiring management during pregnancy have been reported.[40] Although antenatal diagnosis is made in less than half of the patients, it significantly reduces maternal and fetal mortality at the time of delivery.[40] Pheochromocytoma may be suspected in pregnant women who experience preeclampsia, paroxysmal hypertension, or unexplained hyperpyrexia after delivery. Unfortunately, it may be diagnosed after sudden shock and death of the mother at the time of anesthesia and delivery. The period of greatest hazard occurs from the onset of labor until 48 hours postpartum.

If pheochromocytoma is diagnosed during the first or second trimester of pregnancy, surgical resection is recom-

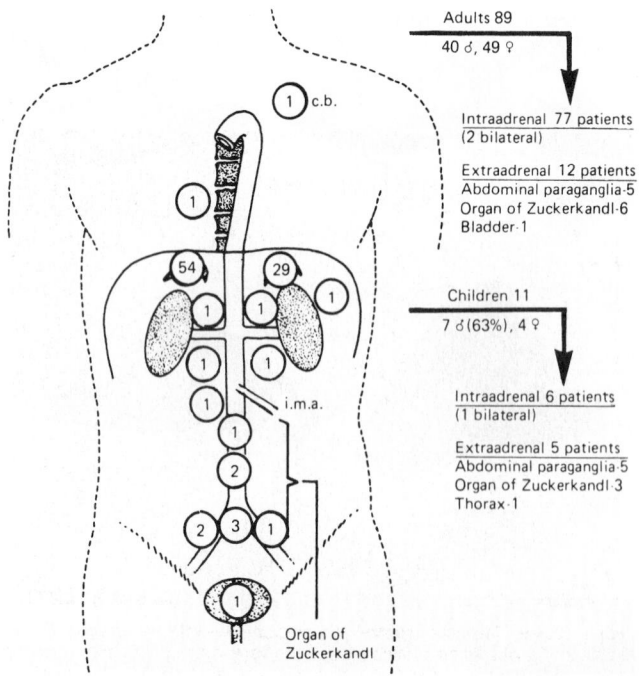

Figure 25–23. Locations of 107 pheochromocytomas in 100 patients. (From Manger, W. M., Gifford, R. W., and Melicow, M. M.: Pheochromocytoma. New York, Springer-Verlag, 1977, p. 45.)

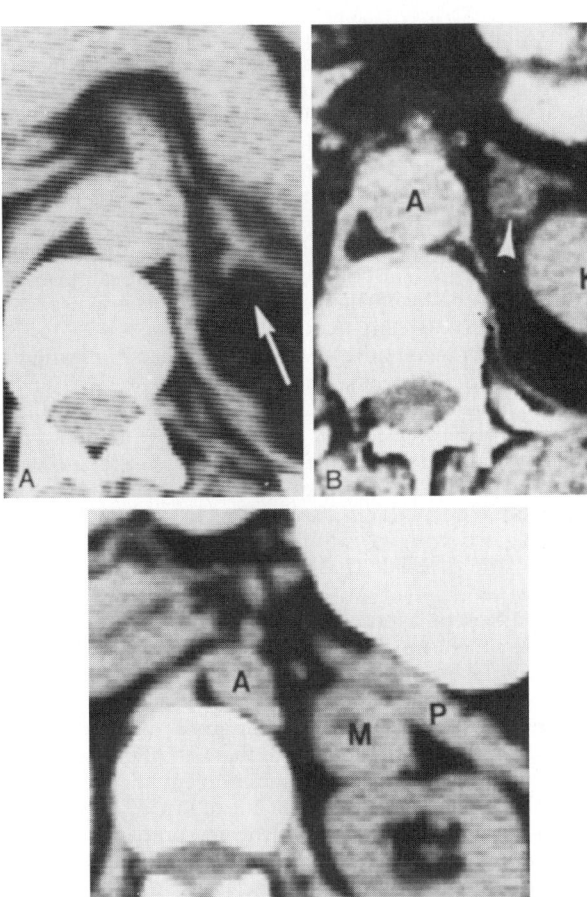

Figure 25–25. Computed tomography of the adrenal glands. *A,* Normal adrenal gland (arrow). *B,* Adrenal cortical adenoma 1.5 cm. in diameter (arrowhead) arising between the limbs of the left adrenal gland. A, aorta; K, upper pole of the left kidney. *C,* Pheochromocytoma (M) 2.5 cm. in diameter in the left adrenal gland. A, aorta; P, tail of pancreas. (Courtesy of M. Korobkin, M.D., Duke University Medical Center, Durham, North Carolina.)

neoplasms detected by CT varies between 0.6% and 1.3% and is somewhat lower than the estimated prevalence of 1.9% and 8.7% based on unselected autopsy data.[1]

The evaluation and management of incidental adrenal masses is controversial. Decisions may be guided by reports of pathologic findings in resected incidentalomas. A recent review of 171 such cases reported that 25.7% were cortical adenomas, 4.1% were metastases from other primary cancers, 4.7% were adrenocortical carcinomas, and 0.06% were pheochromocytomas, with the remainder unspecified.[43] Epidemiologic data indicate that up to 6.5% of incidentalomas are pheochromocytoma, 7% produce aldosterone, 0.035% produce cortisol, and 0.06% are carcinoma.[109]

Because disorders associated with adrenal masses are rare, evaluation decisions must weigh the prevalence of adrenal tumor types and the consequences of a missed diagnosis. Pheochromocytoma has a comparatively high prevalence, and the consequence of a missed diagnosis may be great; therefore, all patients with incidental adrenal masses should be screened by measurement of 24-hour urine levels of catecholamines, metanephrine, and VMA. Hypertensive patients with incidental masses should undergo serum potassium determination. If hypokalemia is present, then tests for aldosterone should follow. Six series of adrenal carcinoma indicate that carcinoma is present in roughly 92% of adrenal masses greater than 6 cm., while adenomas 6 cm. or greater were infrequent (0.025%).[21] Based on these data, it is estimated that fewer than 1 in 10,000 adrenal lesions less than 6 cm. harbor carcinoma,[109] so that adrenalectomy is recommended for lesions greater than 6 cm. Routine biochemical screening for hypercortisolism and hyperandrogenism in patients with incidental adrenal masses is not indicated and should be reserved for patients with clinical features suggestive of these disorders. The CT and MRI appearance of normal adrenal (CT), adrenal adenomas (CT/MRI), and pheochromocytoma (CT) are shown in Figures 25–25 and 25–26. Additional possibilities for adrenal masses, including simple cysts, myolipomas, and adrenal hemorrhage, can usually be distinguished by CT characteristics.

Masses that appear cystic may be aspirated under CT guidance. Fine-needle aspiration biopsy may be of value in patients with known extra-adrenal malignancy; however, it is not indicated in the evaluation of primary adrenal neo-

mended as soon as pharmacologic alpha blockade can be established. In the third trimester of pregnancy, the patient may be managed medically and undergo combined cesarean section and removal of the pheochromocytoma.[40] There is no direct evidence that short-term use of phenoxybenzamine is harmful to the fetus, although few patients have been studied and the long-term effects of the drug are unclear.

Pheochromocytoma in Childhood. Approximately 10% of pheochromocytomas occur in individuals younger than 20 years of age. Among children, prepubertal boys are most commonly affected. Symptoms are similar to those in adults but sustained hypertension, sweating, visual symptoms, weight loss, polydipsia, and polyuria are more common.[61] Multiple, bilateral, and extra-adrenal tumors are more common in children than in adults and occur in 25% to 40% of pediatric cases.[22] Familial pheochromocytomas with and without associated endocrinopathies are more common in children.

The Incidental Adrenal Mass

The increased availability and use of abdominal CT has led to the detection of incidental adrenal masses with rising frequency. The estimated prevalence of incidental adrenal

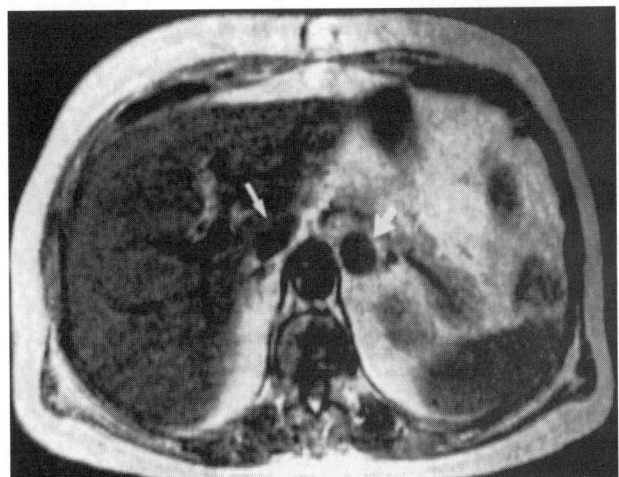

Figure 25–26. Magnetic resonance tomogram, T2-weighted image, of a left adrenal cortical adenoma (thick arrow). The vena cava is outlined on the right (thin arrow) just anterior to the normal right adrenal gland. The homogeneous nature of the adenoma is apparent. (Courtesy of J. Heiken, Mallinckrodt Institute of Radiology, Washington University School of Medicine, St. Louis, Missouri.)

plasms and is contraindicated if pheochromocytoma is suspected. A summary of the evaluation and management of the incidental adrenal mass is shown in Figure 25–27.

ADRENALECTOMY

Surgical approaches to the adrenal glands include the anterior transabdominal approach, a combined thoracoabdominal procedure, the posterior flank approach, and laparoscopic adrenalectomy. Either adrenal may be removed using any of these approaches, and the choice of approach depends on the suspected pathology and size of the adrenal lesion. Small tumors that are localized with confidence by radiologic imaging and are likely benign may be resected using a posterior or laparoscopic approach.[41, 42, 45] Large masses and those that may harbor malignancy should generally be resected using an anterior approach to adequately explore the entire abdomen and gain sufficient exposure for safe resection. Very large adrenocortical carcinomas, usually 10 to 15 cm., often require a thoracoabdominal approach for *en bloc* resection with involved adjacent structures.

Anterior Approach. The anterior approach for adrenalectomy begins with positioning the patient in reverse Trendelenburg position with elevation of the right flank. A midline or bilateral subcostal incision allows access to both adrenals and facilitates exploration of the abdomen. The abdomen is opened and explored for evidence of metastatic disease, including biopsy or excision of suspicious lesions. Resection of the right adrenal proceeds with mobilization and anteromedial retraction of the right hepatic lobe. Subsequently, the hepatic flexure and transverse colon are mobilized and are retracted medially. A Kocher maneuver of the duodenum is performed to uncover the inferior vena cava, the right kidney, and the right adrenal. The retroperitoneal space is entered behind the liver to expose the adrenal. Dissection of the gland proceeds from its superomedial aspect, where small feeding arteries are individually clipped and divided. The vena cava is carefully dissected along its posterolateral border, which allows identification of the right adrenal vein where it drains directly into the inferior vena cava from the medial aspect of the gland. The adrenal vein is ligated with a 2-0 silk tie and divided close to the vena cava. The adrenal vein is isolated early during an operation for a pheochromocytoma to avoid catecholamine surges and blood pressure fluctuations during manipulation of the gland. Once the adrenal vein is ligated, arterial feeding vessels are clipped and divided sequentially, beginning at the superolateral aspect of the gland and continuing medially.

Resection of the left adrenal gland requires mobilization of the spleen and left colon. The left colon is freed from its peritoneal attachments and is reflected inferiorly. The spleen is then delivered from the left upper quadrant medially, and the splenocolic ligament is divided. The spleen, stomach, and pancreatic tail are retracted medially *en bloc* to expose the left kidney and adrenal (Fig. 25–28). The left adrenal vein is isolated, ligated with 2-0 silk tie at its junction with the left renal vein, and divided. The gland is dissected and the arterial vessels are clipped and divided sequentially, beginning at the superolateral aspect of the gland and continuing medially. At the conclusion of the operation, a nasogastric tube or gastric tube is usually placed. A chest tube is placed if a thoracoabdominal incision is used.

Posterior Approach. A posterior approach is most suitable for small adrenal tumors for which there is little suspicion of malignancy. This approach is better tolerated, causes less postoperative pain, and allows faster return of bowel function and quicker postoperative recovery compared with the anterior approach. A posterior approach becomes increasingly more difficult as tumor size increases and is not recommended for excision of large pheochromocytomas, adrenal tumors greater than 6 cm., or adrenal carcinoma.

The patient is placed prone on the operating table and

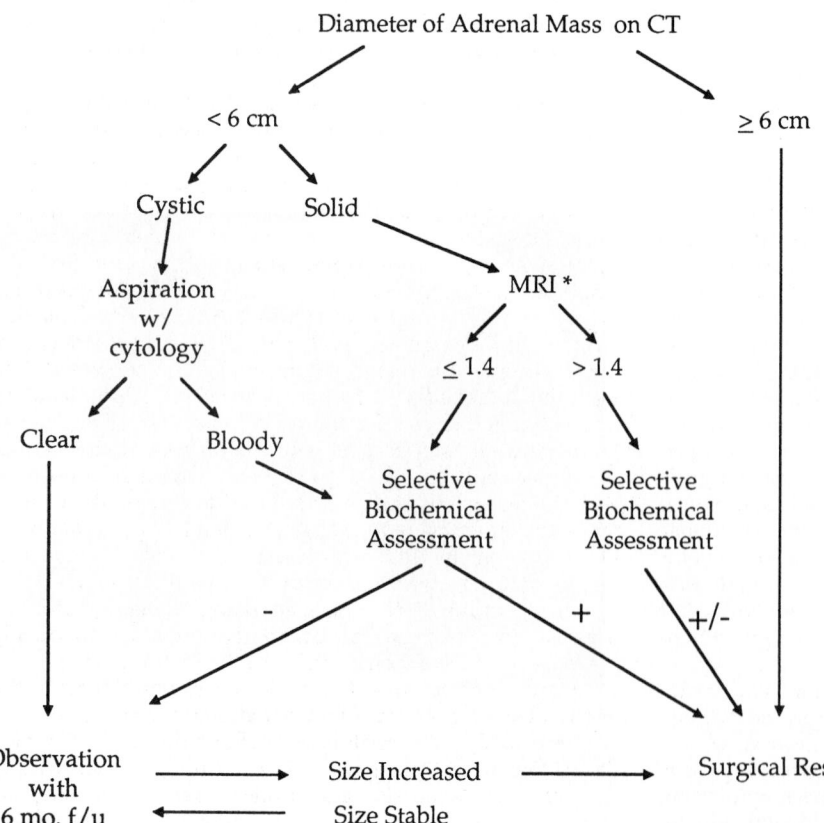

Diameter of Adrenal Mass on CT

Figure 25–27. Evaluation and management of an incidental adrenal mass. Asterisk indicates T2-weighted image intensity compared with liver. (Modified from Copeland, P. M.: The incidentally discovered adrenal mass. Ann. Intern. Med., *98*:940, 1983; and Norton, J. A., Levin, B., and Jensen, R. T.: Cancer of the endocrine system: The adrenal gland. *In* DeVita, V. T., Jr., Hellman, S., and Rosenberg, S. A. [Eds.]: Cancer: Principles and Practice of Oncology, Vol. 2. Philadelphia, J. B. Lippincott, 1993, p. 1352.)

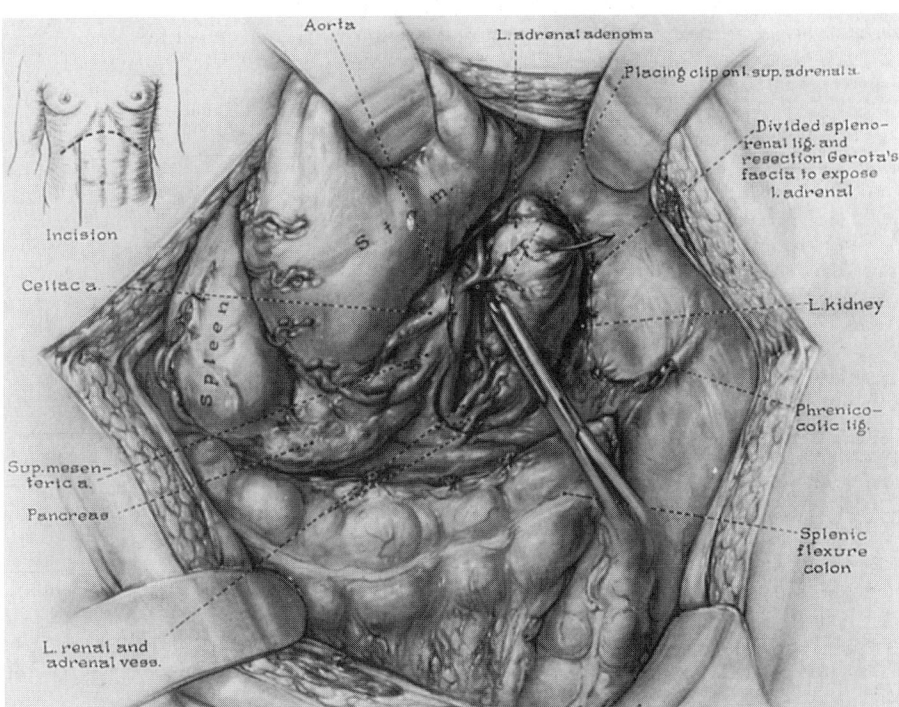

Figure 25–28. Transabdominal approach to the left adrenal gland.

flexed at the waist, which allows the abdominal contents to fall away from the retroperitoneum. A curvilinear skin incision is made from the midline at the tenth rib and is extended inferiorly and laterally to the superior border of the posterior iliac crest (Fig. 25–29A and B). Dissection is continued through the subcutaneous fat and latissimus dorsi muscle to the lumbodorsal fascia. This fascia is incised longitudinally, and the underlying sacrospinalis muscle is retracted medially. Intercurrent lumbar vessels and cutaneous nerves are sacrificed. The sacrospinalis muscle is retracted medially, and the twelfth rib and vascular bundle are resected as far medially as possible. The twelfth intercostal nerve is gently retracted superiorly. The retroperitoneum is entered to expose retroperitoneal fat and Gerota's fascia. The diaphragm is bluntly elevated from Gerota's fascia, the pleura is separated from the diaphragm, and the diaphragm is then divided. Gerota's fascia is incised, and the kidney is retracted inferiorly to expose the adrenal gland. The arterial blood supply is controlled first by clipping and ligating numerous arterial vessels, which course posteriorly. The adrenal vein, located deep to the arteries, is ligated as it is encountered. On the right, careful identification of the adrenal vein is required as it exits from the medial aspect of the gland and courses to the inferior vena cava. The vein is ligated with 2-0 silk ties, and the gland is then freed circumferentially from its lateral to medial aspect. The inferior border of the gland is dissected last to maintain attachment to the kidney and inferior retraction of the gland. The operation concludes with repair of the diaphragm and any incidental pleural defects, reapproximation of the lumbodorsal fascia, and closure of the skin.

Laparoscopic Adrenalectomy. Laparoscopic adrenalectomy is a recent addition to the list of minimally invasive surgical procedures.[41, 42, 45] Enthusiasm for this approach is based on the expectation of decreased postoperative pain, shorter postoperative ileus, faster rehabilitation, and more cosmetically acceptable incisions. Laparoscopic adrenalectomy is most suitable for small adrenal masses in an otherwise normal gland. This approach may become the procedure of choice for patients with aldosteronomas and may also be acceptable for resection of small cortisol-producing adeno-

mas and hereditary pheochromocytomas.[41, 42, 45] Importantly, expertise in open adrenalectomy is absolutely necessary for the laparoscopic surgeon to convert to an open procedure and promptly rectify any intraoperative laparoscopic complications. Experience with laparoscopic adrenalectomy is limited, and traditional open approaches are clearly indicated for most adrenal lesions. Adrenalectomy for a nonfamilial pheochromocytoma requires exploration of the entire abdomen, which is best conducted by direct palpation and visualization. Similarly, excision of large malignant tumors with potential invasion of nearby structures can be safely accomplished only by open adrenalectomy.

Laparoscopic adrenalectomy begins with induction of general anesthesia, placement of a urinary catheter and nasogastric tube, and positioning of the patient in the lateral decubitus position with the affected side facing superiorly. Surgeon and assistant stand at the patient's back and front, respectively. Monitors, the camera apparatus, video cassette recorder, and insufflation equipment are then connected. An insufflator is placed within the peritoneal cavity under direct vision, and the abdomen is insufflated with carbon dioxide gas. Under videoscopic monitoring, three intraperitoneal instrument ports are placed equidistantly in a transverse line from the lateral edge of the rectus sheath to the midaxillary line between the costal margin and iliac crest (Fig. 25–30). Four-quadrant exploration of the peritoneal cavity is first performed with the videoscope through the medialmost port, and the videoscope is then transferred to the middle port. A fan retractor is placed through the medial port to retract the viscera medially, anteriorly, and superiorly. Exposure is facilitated by hyperextension of the operating table at the waist. Operating instruments, grasping forceps, dissecting forceps, and an irrigation/suction apparatus are alternately placed within the abdomen through the lateral port.

Laparoscopic adrenalectomy then continues similar to the open anterior approach. Right adrenalectomy proceeds with entrance to the retroperitoneum behind the liver, at which time a fourth and final port is placed at the posterior axillary line into the retroperitoneum under direct vision. Hepatic attachments are dissected, and the right lobe of the liver is

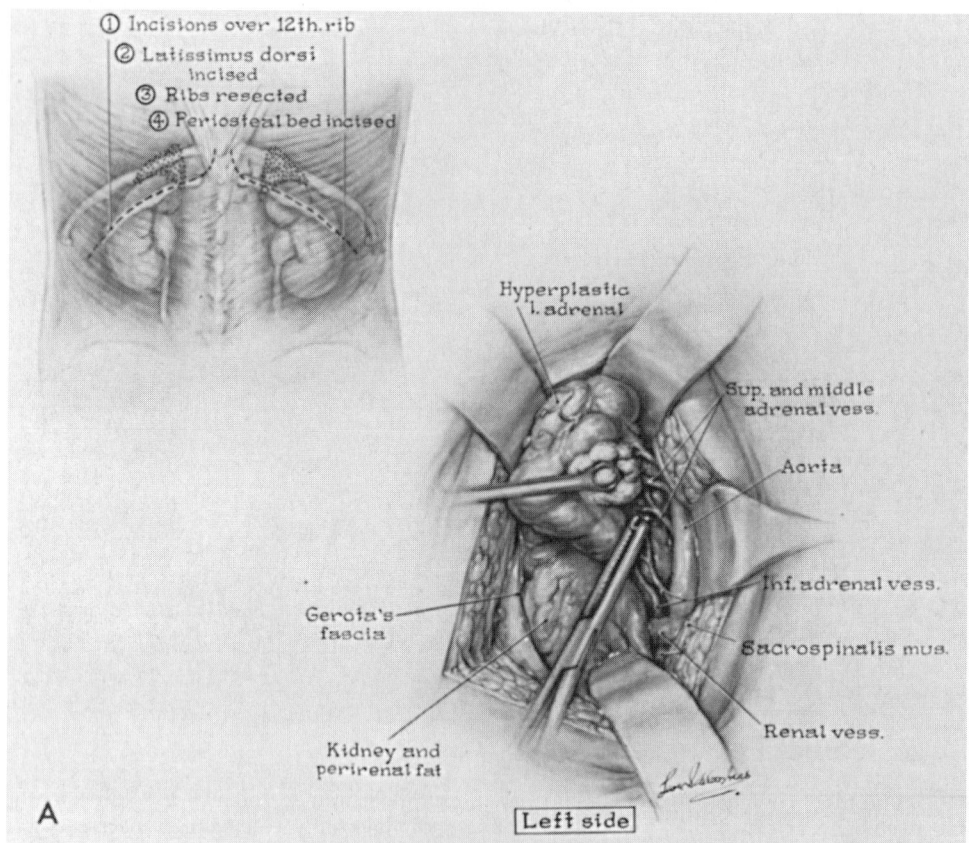

① Incisions over 12th. rib
② Latissimus dorsi incised
③ Ribs resected
④ Periosteal bed incised

Hyperplastic l. adrenal

Sup. and middle adrenal vess.

Aorta

Inf. adrenal vess.

Gerota's fascia

Sacrospinalis mus.

Renal vess.

Kidney and perirenal fat

Left side

A

Figure 25–29. *A,* Posterior approach to the left adrenal gland. *B,* Posterior approach to the right adrenal gland.

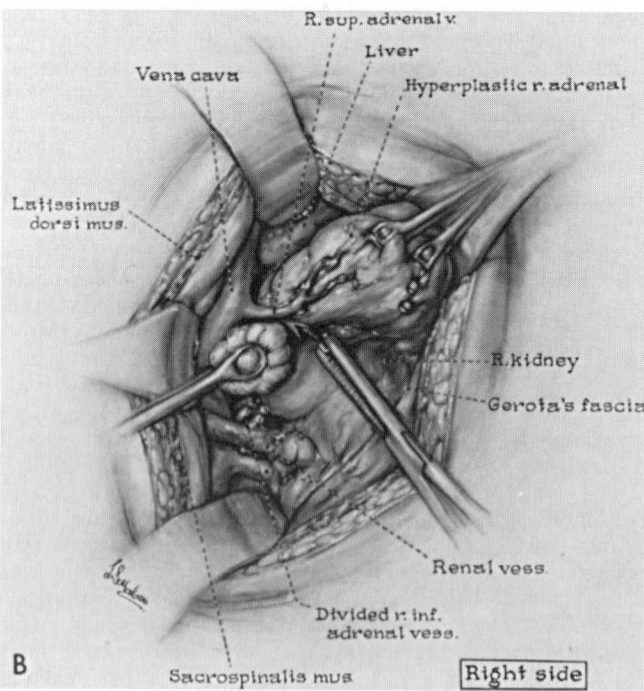

R. sup. adrenal v.

Liver

Vena cava

Hyperplastic r. adrenal

Latissimus dorsi mus.

R. kidney

Gerota's fascia

Renal vess.

Divided r. inf. adrenal vess.

B

Sacrospinalis mus

Right side

retracted anteriorly and medially with the fan retractor. The hepatic flexure of the large bowel is mobilized, allowing the colon to fall medially and anteriorly, away from the retroperitoneum. The adrenal gland is then identified posterolateral to the inferior vena cava and superior to the kidney. The right adrenal is dissected from its attachments using blunt dissection, and the feeding arteries are sequentially clipped and ligated. The right adrenal vein is carefully doubly clipped and ligated. The adrenal gland is carried out the lateral port with grasping forceps under videoscopic guidance. The adrenal bed is checked for hemostasis, and the retractor, instruments, and videoscope are withdrawn. The operation concludes with closure of the fascial and skin defects.

Left adrenalectomy is performed similarly, although patient position and port placement are opposite. Dissection

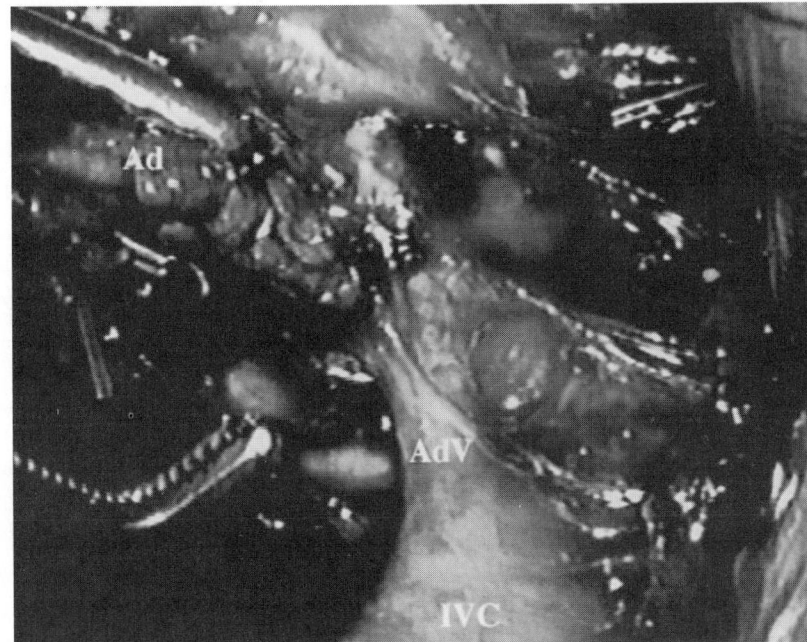
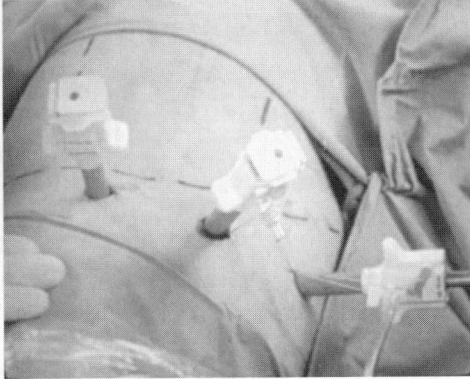

Figure 25–30. Laparoscopic approach to the right adrenal gland. Ad, adrenal; AdV, adrenal vein; IVC, inferior vena cava. *Inset,* Patient positioning and port placement for laparoscopic adrenal resection. (Courtesy of M. Brunt, M.D., Department of Surgery, Washington University School of Medicine, St. Louis, Missouri.)

begins with mobilization of the spleen and retraction of the spleen, tail of the pancreas, and stomach anteriorly and superiorly with the fan retractor. The splenic flexure of the colon is then mobilized, allowing the left colon to fall inferiorly and anteriorly, away from the retroperitoneum. The rest of the procedure is performed identically to a laparoscopic right adrenalectomy.

SELECTED REFERENCES

Pituitary

Thorner, M. O., Vance, M. L., Horvath, E., and Kovacs, K.: The anterior pituitary. *In* Wilson, J. D., and Foster, D. W. (Eds.): Williams Textbook of Endocrinology. Philadelphia, W. B. Saunders, 1992, p.221.
Comprehensive and well written, this textbook covers the history, presentation, diagnosis, and management of anterior pituitary disorders.

Adrenal

Bravo, E. L.: Evolving concepts in the pathophysiology, diagnosis and treatment of pheochromocytoma. Endocrinol. Rev., 15:356, 1994.
This is an up-to-date review by a leader in the field of adrenal disease.

Orth, D. N.: Cushing's syndrome. N. Engl. J. Med., 332:791, 1995.
A recent and thorough review of Cushing's syndrome is provided.

Pommier, R. F., and Brennen, M. F.: Management of adrenal neoplasms. Curr. Probl. Surg., 28:663, 1991.
This monograph presents the senior author's experience in diagnosis and treatment of adrenal neoplasms.

Werbel, S. S., and Ober, K. P.: Acute adrenal insufficiency. Endocrinol. Metab. Clin. North Am., 22:303, 1993.
A comprehensive review of the history, epidemiology, diagnosis. and treatment of adrenal insufficiency is presented. The issue in which this review is found is devoted entirely to endocrine emergencies.

Young, W. F., Jr., Hogan, M. J., Klee, G. G., Grant, C. S., and van Heerden, J. A.: Primary aldosteronism: Diagnosis and treatment. Mayo Clin. Proc., 65:96, 1990.
A thorough review is presented of the diagnosis and treatment of primary aldosteronism.

REFERENCES

1. Abecassis, M., McLoughlin, M. J., Langer, B., et al.: Serediptous adrenal masses: Prevalence, significance and management. Am. J. Surg., 149:783, 1985.
2. Addison, T.: On the Constitutional and Local Effects of Disease of the Suprarenal Capsules. London: Highly, 1885.
3. Asa, S. L., Cheng, Z., Raymar, L., et al.: Human pituitary null cell adenomas and oncocytomas *in vitro:* Effects of adenohypophysiotropic hormones and gonadal steroids on hormone secretion and tumor cell morphology. J. Clin. Endocrinol. Metab., 74:1128, 1992.
4. Averbach, S. D., Steakly, C. S., Young, R. C., et al.: Malignant pheochromocytoma: Effective treatment with a combination of cyclophosphamide, vincristine and dacarbazine. Ann. Intern. Med., 109:267, 1988.
5. Barkan, A. L., Lloyd, R. V., Chandler, W. F., et al.: Preoperative treatment of acromegaly with long-acting somatostatin analogue SMS 201-995: Shrinkage of invasive pituitary macroadenomas and improved surgical remission rate. J. Endocrinol. Metab., 67:1040, 1986.
6. Bateman, A., Singh, A., Kral, T., et al.: The immune-hypothalamic-pituitary-adrenal axis. Endocr. Rev., 10:92, 1989.
7. Baumann, G.: Molecular variants of human growth hormone in serum and circulating growth hormone binding proteins. *In* Frisch, H., and Thorner, M. O. (Ed.): Hormonal Regulation of Growth: Serono Symposia Publications, Vol. 58. New York, Raven Press, 1989, p. 175.
8. Besser, M.: Criteria for medical as opposed to surgical treatment of prolactinomas. Acta Endocrinol., S1:27, 1993.
9. Bodie, B., Novick, A. C., Pontes, J. E., et al.: The Cleveland Clinic experience with adrenal cortical carcinoma. J. Urol., 141:257, 1989.
10. Bravo, E. L.: Evolving concepts in the pathophysiology, diagnosis, and treatment of pheochromocytoma. Endocr. Rev., 15:356, 1994.
11. Bravo, E. L.: Primary aldosteronism: Issues in diagnosis and management. Endocrinol. Metab. Clin. North Am., 23:271, 1994.
12. Bravo, E. L., and Gifford, R. W., Jr.: Pheochromocytoma: Diagnosis, localization and management. N. Engl. J. Med., 311:1298, 1984.
13. Bravo, E. L., and Gifford, R. W. J.: Pheochromocytoma. Endocrinol. Metab. Clin. North Am., 22:329, 1993.
14. Burke, C. W.: The pituitary megatest: Outdated. Clin Endocrinol., 36:133, 1992.
15. Cance, W. G., and Wells, S. A., Jr.: Multiple endocrine neoplasia type IIa. Curr. Probl. Surg., 22:1, 1985.
16. Carpenter, P. C.: Diagnostic evaluation of Cushing's syndrome. Endocrinol. Metab. Clin. North Am., 17:445, 1988.
17. Chrousos, G. P., Vingerhoeds, A., Brandon, D., et al.: Primary cortisol resistance in man: A glucocorticoid receptor-mediated disease. J. Clin. Invest., 69:1261–1269, 1982.
18. Chua, S. C., Szabo, P., Vitek, A., et al.: Cloning of cDNA encoding steroid 11-beta hydroxylase (P450C11). Proc. Natl. Acad. Sci. USA, 84:7193, 1987.
19. Conn, J. W.: Presidential Address: 1) Painting background. 2) Primary aldosteronism. J. Lab. Clin. Med., 45:661, 1955.
20. Constine, L. S., Woolf, P. D., Cann, D., et al.: Hypothalamo-pituitary dysfunction after radiation for brain tumors. N. Engl. J. Med., 328:87, 1993.
21. Copeland, P. M.: The incidentally discovered adrenal mass, diagnosis and treatment. Ann. Intern. Med., 98:940, 1983.
22. Cryer, P. E.: Pheochromocytoma. Clin. Endocrinol. Metab., 14:203, 1985.

23. Cushing, H.: Partial hypophysectomy for acromegaly. Ann. Surg., 50:1002, 1909.
24. Cushing, H.: Acromegaly from a surgical standpoint. BMJ, 2:48, 1927.
25. Cushing, H.: The basophil adenomas of the pituitary body and their clinical manifestations (pituitary basophilism). Bull. Johns Hopkins Hosp., 50:137, 1932.
26. Daniels, G. H., and Martin, J. B.: Neuroendocrine regulation and diseases of the anterior pituitary and hypothalamus. In Braunwald, E., and Fauci, A. S. (Ed.): Harrison's Principles of Internal Medicine. New York, McGraw-Hill, 1994, p. 1891.
27. Davis, P. C., Hoffman, J. C. J., Tindall, G. T., et al.: Prolactin-secreting pituitary microadenomas: Inaccuracy of high resolution CT imaging. AJR, 144:151, 1985.
28. De Chrecchio, L.: Sopra un caso di apparenzi virili in una donna. Morgagni, 7:151, 1865.
29. Derosa, G., Corsello, S. M., Cecchini, L., et al.: Clinical study of Addison's disease. Exp. Clin. Metab, 90:232, 1987.
30. Doherty, G. M., Nieman, L. K., Cutler, G. B., et al.: Time to recovery of the hypothalamic-pituitary-adrenal axis after curative resection of adrenal tumors in patients with Cushing's syndrome. Surgery, 108:1085, 1990.
31. Doppman, J. L., Gill, J. R. J., Miller, D. L., et al.: Distinction between hyperaldosteronism due to bilateral hyperplasia and unilateral aldosteronoma: Reliability of CT. Radiology, 184:677, 1992.
32. Dracopoli, N. C., Rettig, W. J., Whitfield, G. K., et al.: Assignment of the gene for the beta subunit of thyroid-stimulating hormone to the short arm of human chromosome 1. Proc. Natl. Acad. Sci. USA, 83:1822, 1986.
33. Dunnick, N. R., Leight, G. S. J., Roubidoux, M. A., et al.: CT in the diagnosis of primary aldosteronism: Sensitivity in 29 patients. Am. J. Radiol., 160:321, 1993.
34. Ezzat, S., Snyder, P. J., Young, W. F., et al.: Octreotide treatment of acromegaly: A randomized multicenter study. Ann. Intern. Med., 117:711, 1992.
35. Fahlsbusch, R., and Buchfelder, M.: Present status of neurosurgery in the treatment of prolactinomas. Neurosurg. Rev., 8:195, 1985.
36. Fan, Y. S., Sasi, R., Lee, C., et al.: Localization of the human CYP17 gene (cytochrome P450(17 alpha)) to 10q24.3 by fluorescence in situ hybridization and simultaneous chromosome banding. Genomics, 14:1110, 1992.
37. Fiddes, J. C., and Talmadge, K.: Structure, expression, and evolution of the genes for the human glycoprotein hormones. Recent Prog. Horm. Res., 40:43, 1984.
38. Findling, J. W., and Doppman, J. L.: Biochemical and radiologic diagnosis of Cushing's syndrome. Endocrinol. Metab. Clin. North Am., 23:511, 1994.
39. Fröhlich, A.: Ein Fall von Tumor der Hypophysis cerebri ohne Acromegalie. Wien Klin. Rondsch., p. 47, 1901.
40. Fudge, T. L., McKinnon, W. M. P., and Geary, W. L.: Current surgical management of pheochromocytoma during pregnancy. Arch. Surg., 115:1224, 1980.
41. Gagner, M., Lacroix, A., and Bolte, E.: Laparoscopic adrenalectomy in Cushing's syndrome and pheochromocytoma (Letter). N. Engl. J. Med., 327:1033, 1992.
42. Gagner, M., Lacroix, A., Prinz, R. A., et al.: Early experience with laparoscopic approach for adrenalectomy. Surgery, 114:1120, 1993.
43. Gajraj, H., and Young, A. E.: Adrenal incidentaloma. Br. J. Surg., 80:422, 1993.
44. Geisinger, M. A., Zelch, M. A., Bravo, E. L., et al.: Primary hyperaldosteronism: Comparison of CT, adrenal venography, and venous sampling. AJR, 141:299, 1983.
45. Go, H., Takeda, M., Tomoyuki, T., et al.: Laparoscopic adrenalectomy for Cushing's syndrome: Comparison with primary aldosteronism. Surgery, 117:11, 1995.
46. Grigsby, P. W., Simpson, J. R., Emami, B. N., et al.: Prognostic factors and results of surgery and postoperative irradiation in the management of pituitary adenomas. Int. J. Radiat. Oncol. Biol. Phys., 16:1411, 1989.
47. Guiot, G., and Thebaul, B.: L'Extirpation des adenomes hypophysiares par voie transsphenoidale. Neurochirurgie, 1:133, 1959.
48. Hardy, J.: L'Exeres des adenomes hypophysaires par voie trans-sphenoidale. Union Med. Can., 91:933, 1962.
49. Henley, D. J., van Heerden, J. A., Grant, C. S., et al.: Adrenal cortical carcinoma: A continuing challenge. Surgery, 94:926, 1983.
50. Holaday, J. W., Long, J. B., Martinez-Arizala, A., et al.: Effects of TRH in circulatory shock and central nervous system ischemia. Ann. N.Y. Acad. Sci., 553:370, 1989.
51. Holl, R. W., Thorner, M. O., and Leong, D. A.: Intracellular calcium concentration and growth hormone secretion in individual somatotropes: Effects of growth hormone-releasing factor and somatostatin. Endocrinology, 122:2927, 1988.
52. Horber, F. F., and Haymond, M. V.: Human growth hormone prevents the protein catabolic side effects of prednisone in humans. J. Clin. Invest., 86:265, 1990.
53. Horvath, E., and Kovaks, K.: Fine structural cytology of the adenohypophysis in rat and man. J. Electron. Microsc. Tech., 8:401, 1988.
54. Howe, J. R., Norton, J. A., and Wells, S. A. J.: Prevalence of pheochromocytoma and hyperparathyroidism in multiple endocrine neoplasia type 2A: Results of long-term follow-up. Surgery, 114:1070, 1993.
55. Howlett, T. A., Rees, L. H., Besser, G. M., et al.: Cushing's syndrome. Clin. Endocrinol. Metab., 14:911, 1985.
56. Irony, I., Kater, C. E., Biglieri, E. G., et al.: Correctable subsets of primary aldosteronism: Primary adrenal hyperplasia and renin-responsive adenoma. Am. J. Hypertension, 3:576, 1990.
57. Ituarte, E. M., Petrini, J., and Hershman, J. M.: Acromegaly and colon cancer. Ann. Intern. Med., 101:627, 1984.
58. Jensen, J. C., Pass, H. I., Sindelar, W. F., et al.: Recurrent or metastatic disease in select patients with adrenocortical carcinoma: Aggressive resection vs chemotherapy. Arch. Surg., 126:457, 1991.
59. Jex, R. K., van Heerden, J. A., Carpenter, P. C., et al.: Ectopic ACTH syndrome. Am. J. Surg., 149:276, 1985.
60. Jones, M. T., and Gillham, B.: Factors involved in the regulation of adrenocorticotropic hormone/beta-lipotropic hormone. Physiol. Rev., 68:743, 1988.
61. Kaufman, B. H., Telander, R. L., van Heerden, J. A., et al.: Pheochromocytoma in pediatric age groups: Current status. J. Pediatr. Surg., 18:879, 1983.
62. Keiser, H. R., Goldstein, D. S., Wade, J. L., et al.: Treatment of malignant pheochromocytoma with combination chemotherapy. Hypertension, 7:1, 1985.
63. Khosia, S., Patel, V. M., Hay, I. D., et al.: Loss of heterozygosity suggests multiple genetic alterations in pheochromocytomas and medullary thyroid carcinomas. J. Clin. Invest., 87:1691, 1991.
64. Knobil, E.: The neuroendocrine control of the menstrual cycle. Recent Prog. Horm. Res., 36:53, 1980.
65. Krempf, M., Lumbroso, J., Mornex, R., et al.: Use of 131I iodobenzylguanidine in the treatment of malignant pheochromocytoma. J. Clin. Endocrinol. Metab., 72:455, 1991.
66. Kung, A. W., Pun, K. K., Lam, K., et al.: Addisonian crisis as presenting feature in malignancies. Cancer, 65:177, 1990.
67. LaCroix, A., Bolte, E., Tremblay, E., et al.: Gastric inhibitory peptide-dependent cortisol hypersecretion: A new cause of Cushing's syndrome. N. Engl. J. Med., 327:974, 1992.
68. Lamberts, S. W. J., de Herder, W. W., Kwekkeboom, D. J., et al.: Current tools in the diagnosis of pituitary tumours. Acta Endocrinol., S1:6, 1993.
69. Larsen, P. R.: Thyroid-pituitary interaction. N. Engl. J. Med., 306:23, 1982.
70. Lee, B. C. P., and Deck, M. D. F.: Sella and juxtasellar lesion detection with MRI. Radiology, 157:143, 1985.
71. Leong, D. A., Frawley, L. S., and Neill, J. D.: Neuroendocrine control of prolactin secretion. Annu. Rev. Physiol., 45:109, 1983.
72. Lifton, R. P., Dluhy, R. G., Powers, M., et al.: A chimeric 11 beta-hydroxylase/aldosterone synthase gene causes glucocorticoid-remediable aldosteronism and human hypertension. Nature, 355:262, 1992.
73. Owerbach, D., Rutter, W. J., Roberts, J. L., et al.: The proopicortin (adrenocorticotropin/beta-lipoprotein) gene is located on chromosome 2 in mice. Somat. Cell. Genet., 7:359, 1981.
74. Luton, J.-P., Cerdas, S., Billaud, L., et al.: Clinical features of adrenocortical carcinoma, prognostic factors, and the effect of mitotane therapy. N. Engl. J. Med., 322:1195, 1990.
75. Manger, J. A.: Thyroid-stimulating hormone: Biosynthesis, cell biology and bioactivity. Endocrine Rev., 11:354, 1990.
76. Manolas, K. J., Farmer, H. M., Wilson, H. K., et al.: The pituitary before and after adrenalectomy for Cushing's syndrome. World J. Surg., 8:374, 1984.
77. Marie, P.: Sur deux cas d'acromegalie, hypertrophie singul iérieure, non congenitale, des extrémités supérieures, inférieures, etc. céphalique. Rev. Med., 6:297, 1886.
78. Maroldo, T. V., Dillon, W. P., and Wilson, C. B.: Advances in diagnostic techniques of pituitary tumors and prolactinomas. Curr. Opin. Oncol., 4:105, 1992.
79. Mayo, C. H.: Paroxysmal hypertension with tumor of retroperitoneal nerve. JAMA, 89:1047, 1927.
80. McPartland, R. P.: Metabolic and pharmacologic actions of glucocorticoids. In Mulrow, P. J. (Ed.): The Adrenal Gland, Amsterdam, Elsevier, 1986.
81. Melby, J. C.: Diagnosis of hyperaldosteronism. Endocrinol. Metab. Clin. North Am., 20:247, 1991.
82. Melmed, S.: Acromegaly. N. Engl. J. Med., 322:966, 1990.
83. Melmed, S.: Medical management of acromegaly—what and when? Acta Endocrinol., S1:13, 1993.
84. Melmed, S., et al.: Pituitary tumors secreting growth hormone and prolactin (UCLA conference). Ann. Intern. Med. 105:238, 1986.
85. Milsom, S. R., Espiner, E. A., Nicholls, M. G., et al.: The blood pressure response to unilateral adrenalectomy in primary aldosteronism. Q. J. Med., 61:1141, 1986.
86. Mohr, R.: Tumor of the pituitary body. Wochenschr. Ges. Heilk., 6:565, 1840.
87. Molitch, M. E.: Pregnancy and the hyperprolactinemic woman. N. Engl. J. Med., 321:1364, 1985.
88. Molitch, M. E.: Management of prolactinomas. Annu. Rev. Med., 40:225, 1989.
89. Molitch, M. E., Elton, R. L., Blackwell, R. E., et al.: Bromocriptine as primary therapy for prolactin-secreting macroadenomas: Results of a prospective multicenter study. J. Clin. Endocrinol. Metab., 6:698, 1985.
90. Morrison, N., Nickson, D. A., McBride, M. W., et al.: Regional chromosome assignment of human 3-beta-hydroxy-5-ene steroid dehydrogenase to 1p13.1 by non-isotopic in situ hybridization. Hum. Genet., 87:223, 1991.
91. Nabarro, J. D. N.: Pituitary prolactinomas. Clin. Endocrinol., 17:129, 1982.

92. Nagy, G., Mulchahey, J. J., and Neill, J. D.: Autocrine control of prolactin secretion by vasoactive intestinal peptide. Endocrinology, *122*:364, 1988.

93. Nelson, D. H., Meakin, J. W., and Thorn, G. W.: ACTH-producing pituitary tumors following adrenalectomy for Cushing's syndrome. Ann. Intern. Med., *52*:560, 1960.

94. Norton, J. A., Levin, B., and Jensen, R. T.: Cancer of the endocrine system: The adrenal gland. *In* De Vita, V. T. J., Hellman, S., H., and Rosenberg, S. A. (Eds.): Cancer: Principles and Practice of Oncology, Vol. 2. Philadelphia, J. B. Lippincott, 1993, p. 1352.

95. Obara, T., Ito, Y., Okamoto, T., et al.: Risk factors associated with postoperative persistent hypertension in patients with primary aldosteronism. Surgery, *112*:987, 1992.

96. Oldfield, E. H., Doppman, J. L., Nieman, L. K., et al.: Petrosal sinus sampling with and without corticotropin-releasing hormone for the differential diagnosis of Cushing's syndrome. N. Engl. J. Med., *325*:897, 1991.

97. Orth, D. N.: Cushing's syndrome. N. Engl. J. Med., *332*:791, 1995.

98. Owerbach, D., Rutter, W. J., Cooke, N. E., et al.: The prolactin gene is located on chromosome 6 in humans. Science, *212*:815, 1981.

99. Paulesco, N. C.: L'Hypophyse du Cerveau. Paris, Vigot Frères, 1908.

100. Peplinski, G. R., and Norton, J. A.: The predictive value of diagnostic tests for pheochromocytoma. Surgery, *116*:1101, 1994.

101. Perry, R. R., Nieman, L. K., Cutler, G. B., et al.: Primary adrenal causes of Cushing's syndrome. Annals of Surgery, *210*:59, 1989.

102. Pierce, J. G., and Parsons, T. F.: Glycoprotein hormones: Structure and function. Annu. Rev. Biochem., *50*:465, 1981.

103. Pommier, R. F., and Brennan, M. F.: Management of adrenal neoplasms. Curr. Probl. Surg. *28*:659, 1991.

104. Quinn, S. J.: Regulation of aldosterone secretion. Annu. Rev. Physiol., *50*:409, 1988.

105. Randall, R. V., Laws, E. R. J., Abboud, C. F., et al.: Transsphenoidal microsurgical treatment of prolactin-producing pituitary adenomas. Mayo Clin. Proc., *58*:108, 1983.

106. Reichlin, S.: TRH: Historical aspects. Ann. N.Y. Acad. Sci., *553*:1, 1989.

107. Remine, W. H., Chong, G. C., van Heerden, J. A., et al.: Current management of pheochromocytoma. Ann. Surg., *179*:740, 1974.

108. Rodman, E. F., Molitch, M. E., Post, K. D., et al.: Long-term follow-up of trans-sphenoidal selective adenectomy for prolactinoma. JAMA, *252*:921, 1984.

109. Ross, N. S., and Aron, D. C.: Hormonal evaluation of the patient with an incidentally discovered adrenal mass. N. Engl. J. Med., *323*:1401, 1990.

110. Saegesser, F.: Cesar Roux (1857–1934) et son epoque. Rev. Med. Suisse Romande, *104*:403, 1984.

111. Sassolas, G., Trouillas, J., Treluyer, C., et al.: Management of nonfunctioning pituitary tumors. Acta Endocrinol., *S1*:21, 1993.

112. Shenker, Y.: Medical treatment of low-renin aldosteronism. Endocrinol. Metab. Clin. North Am., *18*:415, 1989.

113. Sheridan, R. L., Ryan, C. M., and Tompkins, R. G.: Acute adrenal insufficiency in the burn intensive care unit. Burns, *19*:63, 1993.

114. Sjoerdsma, A., Waldman, T. A., Cooperman, T. A., et al.: Pheochromocytoma: Current concepts of diagnosis and treatment. Ann. Intern. Med., *65*:1302, 1966.

115. Thomas, C. G., Smith, A. T., Griffith, J. M., et al.: Hyperadrenalism in childhood and adolescence. Ann. Surg., *199*:538, 1984.

116. Thorner, M. O., Frohman, L. A., Leong, D. A., et al.: Extrahypothalamic growth-hormone-releasing factor (GRF) secretion is a rare cause of acromegaly: Plasma GRF levels in 177 acromegalic patients. J. Clin. Endocrinol. Metabol., *59*:846, 1984.

117. Thorner, M. O., Vance, M. L., Horvath, E., et al.: The Anterior Pituitary. *In* Wilson, J. D., and Foster, D. W. (Eds.): Williams Textbook of Endocrinology. Philadelphia, W. B. Saunders, 1992, p. 221.

118. Tourniaire, J., Chalandar, D., Rebattu, B., et al.: The 24-h cortisol secretory pattern in Cushing's syndrome. Acta Endocrinol., *112*:230, 1986.

119. Trautmann, J. C., and Laws, E. R. J.: Visual status after transsphenoidal surgery at the Mayo Clinic 1972–1982. Am. J. Ophthalmol., *96*:200, 1983.

120. Tyrrell, J. B., and Wilson, C. B.: Cushing's disease: Therapy of pituitary adenomas. Endocrinol. Metab. Clin. North Am., *23*:925, 1994.

121. Valimaki, M., Pelkone, R., Porkka, L., et al.: Long-term results of adrenal surgery in patients with Cushing's syndrome due to adrenocortical adenoma. Clin. Endocrinol., *20*:229, 1984.

122. Van Heerden, J. A., Steps, S. G., Hamberger, B., et al.: Pheochromocytoma: Current status and changing trends. Surgery, *91*:367, 1982.

123. Vance, M. L.: Hypopituitarism. N. Engl. J. Med., *330*:1651, 1994.

124. Vance, M. L., Evans, W. S., and Thorner, M. O.: Drugs five years later: Bromocriptine. Ann. Intern. Med., *100*:78, 1984.

125. Velchick, M. G., Alavi, A., Kressel, H. Y., et al.: Localization of pheochromocytoma: MIBG, CT and MRI correlation. J. Nucl. Med., *30*:328, 1989.

126. Vincenti, A., Estrada, A., de la Cuerda, C., et al.: Results of external pituitary irradiation after unsuccessful transsphenoidal surgery in Cushing's disease. Acta Endocrinol., *125*:470, 1991.

127. Wakai, S., Yamakawa, K., Manaka, S., et al.: Spontaneous intracranial hemorrhage caused by brain tumor: Its incidence and clinical significance. Neurosurgery, *10*:437, 1982.

128. Walters, W., Wilder, R. M., and Kepler, E. J.: The suprarenal cortical syndrome with presentation of ten cases. Ann. Surg., *100*:670, 1934.

129. Wass, J. A. H., Williams, J., Charlesworth, M., et al.: Bromocriptine in management of large pituitary tumors. BMJ, *284*:1908, 1982.

130. Watkins, P. C., Edy, R., Beck, A. K., et al.: DNA sequence and regional assignment of the human follicle-stimulating hormone beta-subunit gene to the short arm of human chromosome 11. DNA, *6*:205, 1987.

131. Werbel, S. S., and Ober, K. P.: Acute adrenal insufficiency. Endocrinol. Metab. Clin. North Am., *22*:303, 1993.

132. White, P. C., New, M. I., and Dupont, B. O.: Congenital adrenal hyperplasia. N. Engl. J. Med., *316*:1519, 1987.

133. Wilmore, D. W., Moylan, J. A. J., Bristow, B. F., et al.: Anabolic effects of human growth hormone and high caloric feedings following thermal injury. Surg. Gynecol. Obstet., *138*:875, 1974.

134. Yano, T., Linehan, M., Anglard, P., et al.: Genetic changes in human adrenocortical carcinomas. J. Natl. Cancer Inst., *81*:518, 1989.

135. Young, W. F., Hogan, M. J., Klee, G. G., et al.: Primary aldosteronism: Diagnosis and management. Mayo Clin. Proc., *65*:96, 1990.

136. Zeiger, M. A., Neiman, L. K., Cutler, G. B., et al.: Primary bilateral adrenocortical causes of Cushing's syndrome. Surgery, *110*:1106, 1991.

137. Zeiger, M. A., Pass, H. I., Doppman, J. D., et al.: Surgical strategy in the management of non-small cell ectopic adrenocorticotropic hormone syndrome. Surgery, *112*:994, 1992.

138. Zervas, N. T.: Surgical results for pituitary adenomas: Results of an international survey. *In* Black, P. M., Zervas, N. T., Ridgeway, E. C., and Martin, J. B. (Eds.): Secretory Tumors of the Pituitary gland: Progress in Endocrine Research and Therapy. New York, Raven, 1984.

139. Zografos, G. C., Driscoll, D. L., Karakousis, C. P., et al.: Adrenal adenocarcinoma: A review of 53 cases. J. Surg. Oncol., *55*:160, 1994.

CHAPTER 26

THE ESOPHAGUS

I

HISTORICAL ASPECTS AND ANATOMY

Mark B. Orringer, M.D.

HISTORICAL ASPECTS

The modern surgical treatment of esophageal disease is the product of refinements in both anesthetic and operative techniques as well as methods of assessing normal and abnormal anatomy and physiology. The earliest esophageal operations were limited to cervical procedures, primarily for removal of foreign bodies. Semeleder (1863) used a forceps with spoon-shaped blades to view the upper esophagus. Rigid esophagoscopy was first used successfully in 1868 both by Waldenberg, who examined the cervical esophagus, and by Kussmaul, who used a modified urethroscope to diagnose a carcinoma of the thoracic esophagus. An esophagoscope with a distal electric light source was described by Mikulicz in 1881, and one fitted with an incandescent light was developed by Einhorn in 1902. The same year, Killian reported the first case of removal of a foreign body through an esophagoscope. Subsequent refinements in the optical system used in rigid esophagoscopy, as well as the development of flexible fiberoptic esophagoscopy by LoPresti and Hilmi in 1964,[24] have produced a procedure that is now performed almost universally in the evaluation of patients with esophageal symptoms. The pioneering clinical work of Chevalier Jackson established guidelines for proper rigid endoscopic technique that remain valid after almost 50 years.[14]

Safe operations on the thoracic esophagus awaited the development of anesthetic techniques that would permit the chest to be opened. Resection of the cervical esophagus for carcinoma was first performed successfully by Billroth (1871) and Czerny (1877). Mikulicz first resected and reconstructed the cervical esophagus with a skin tube (1886). In 1915, Torek performed the first successful resection of the intrathoracic esophagus for carcinoma without esophageal reconstruction.[36] Janeway and Green first reported a combined thoracoabdominal incision for carcinoma of the distal esophagus in 1910.[16]

Denk performed blunt transmediastinal esophagectomy without thoracotomy in cadavers and experimental animals using a vein stripper to avulse the esophagus from the posterior mediastinum in 1913. The British surgeon Turner performed the first successful transmediastinal blunt esophagectomy for carcinoma in 1933 and established continuity of the alimentary tract with an antethoracic skin tube at a second stage.[37] However, with the advent of endotracheal anesthesia and the ability to resect the esophagus under direct vision, the technique of transhiatal esophagectomy without thoracotomy was used infrequently. Ohsawa (1933) performed the first successful transthoracic distal esophagogastrectomy and intrathoracic esophagogastric anastomosis for esophageal carcinoma.[27] This feat was accomplished in the United States by Marshall (1937)[25] and Adams and Phemister (1938).[1] Sweet (1945) and Garlock (1946) were pioneers of esophageal resection in America.[10, 34] Lewis (1946) popularized the right-sided

transthoracic approach to carcinoma of the esophagus.[22] As methods of esophageal resection became refined, techniques of visceral esophageal substitution with stomach, jejunum, and colon were likewise developed.

Initially, surgery for most benign esophageal disease was empiric and directed toward abnormal anatomy rather than deranged physiology. In 1943, Haight first reported successful primary repair of esophageal atresia and division of the associated tracheoesophageal fistula in infancy.[11] This monumental achievement was to convert a condition that carried a 100% mortality to one that is now successfully repaired in 95% of infants. A pharyngoesophageal diverticulum was first resected successfully in 1886.[41] For the next 50 to 60 years, controversy centered on the advisability of one-stage versus two-stage procedures for resection of these pouches rather than on the abnormal cricopharyngeal motor function responsible for their formation. Similarly, in discussing the treatment of pulsion diverticula of the thoracic esophagus, Allen and Clagget (1965) and Belsey (1966) emphasized the need to perform an esophagomyotomy at the time of resection of the pouch.[2, 4] They pointed out that elimination of the cause of the diverticulum (i.e., the elevated intraesophageal pressure due to motor dysfunction) was more important than operating on the diverticulum itself.

Willis used ordinary esophageal bougienage to treat achalasia in 1674. Forceful dilation with disruption of the lower esophageal sphincter using pneumatic dilators,[6, 21] hydrostatic dilators,[28] and expanding metal dilators[30] was subsequently reported. A number of distal esophageal operations were used in the early 1900s to treat achalasia, but the origin of the currently used esophagomyotomy is credited to Heller (1913). The operation initially described by Heller consisted of two cardioesophagomyotomies, one on either side of the distal esophagus, performed transabdominally. Zaaijer (1923) modified the operation to a single esophageal incision,[42] and Ellis and associates established the merits of transthoracic esophagomyotomy in the treatment of achalasia.[7]

Early *hiatal hernia* surgery also emphasized anatomy rather than physiology, and initially reported series included both traumatic diaphragmatic hernias as well as hernias through the diaphragmatic hiatus. Emphasis was placed on correction of the anatomic defect and closure of the diaphragmatic hiatus, and this approach influenced the surgical therapy of hiatal hernias for more than two decades. Allison first coined the term *reflux esophagitis* in 1951 and clearly established gastroesophageal reflux as a cause for many of the symptoms experienced by patients with hiatal hernias.[3] He also emphasized anatomic correction of the hernia rather than correction of the abnormal distal esophageal sphincter mechanism in these patients. Several hiatus hernia operations were described over the next few years, culminating in the reports by Nissen[26] in 1961 and Skinner and Belsey[31] in 1967 of the use of fundoplication to create an intra-abdominal esophageal valve mechanism to control gastroesophageal reflux. These latter operations ushered in the era of true *antireflux* operations designed to restore a functional lower esophageal sphincter mechanism.

In the past 40 years, with refinements of manometric techniques[35, 39] and the ability to document gastroesophageal reflux with the intraesophageal pH electrode,[19, 38] operations for esophageal motor disorders and gastroesophageal reflux have become more of a science based on objective data. Tuttle and Grossman (1958) developed the intraesophageal pH electrode for the direct intraluminal assessment of gastroesophageal reflux.[38] Skinner and Booth (1970) popularized the standard acid reflux test (SART), in which 300 ml. of 0.1 N hydrochloric acid is placed in the stomach, a pH electrode is fixed 5 cm. above the lower esophageal sphincter, and the number of pH drops below 4 during standardized reflux provocative maneuvers is documented.[32]

The development of prolonged lower esophageal pH monitoring introduced by Spencer (1969)[33] and Pattrick (1970)[29] was an effort to circumvent the relatively artificial nature of the standard acid reflux test. Johnson and DeMeester (1974) first used normal controls in their evaluation of patients with abnormal gastroesophageal reflux, with 24-hour distal esophageal pH monitoring.[18] They subsequently classified their patients into upright, supine, and combined (upright and supine) refluxers. Since then, 24-hour monitoring of distal esophageal pH has become the gold standard for objectively diagnosing gastroesophageal reflux.[15]

The acid perfusion test developed by Bernstein and Baker (1958) was proposed as a simple test for differentiating patients with chest pain of cardiac origin from those with esophagitis.[5] Experience with this test has shown that a positive Bernstein test indicates *only* that the patient has an acid-sensitive esophagus and *not* that there is esophagitis or gastroesophageal reflux present. Similarly, measurement of the potential difference of esophageal mucosa was initially thought to be of value in the assessment of patients with reflux disease.[12] This study, however, is technically difficult to perform and evaluate and has thus not gained widespread use. Radionuclide scanning using technetium-99m sulfur colloid to detect gastroesophageal reflux was first reported by Fisher and associates (1976),[9] and although the test is clearly more sensitive than either standard radiology or short-term pH monitoring in diagnosing reflux,[20, 40] it has not replaced 24-hour distal pH monitoring as the most valuable diagnostic tool.

Within the past decade, the technique of long-term 24-hour ambulatory esophageal manometry has been developed to overcome the diagnostic difficulties in attempting to document the intermittent and unpredictable motor disturbances and symptoms in patients with esophageal motility disorders.[8, 17] Esophageal manometry and intraesophageal pH reflux testing have become basic tools in the preoperative assessment of most patients with benign esophageal disease and are used extensively to objectively assess the operative results of procedures designed to treat abnormal gastroesophageal reflux and esophageal motor function.

ANATOMY

The esophagus is a hollow tube of muscle that is approximately 25 cm. (10 inches) in length and extends from the pharynx to the stomach. It is arbitrarily divided into four segments: pharyngoesophageal, cervical, thoracic, and abdominal. The length between the laryngopharynx and cervical esophagus is the *pharyngoesophageal segment.* The pharyngeal musculature includes the superior, middle, and inferior constrictors, as well as the stylopharyngeus muscles. The inferior pharyngeal constrictor, or thyropharyngeus muscle,

passes obliquely and superiorly from its origin on the thyroid cartilage to its posterior insertion in the median raphe (see Fig. 26–34). The esophageal introitus (the cricopharyngeus muscle, or upper esophageal sphincter) is the most inferior portion of the inferior pharyngeal constrictor and is clearly identifiable by the transverse direction of its fibers. The transition between the oblique fibers of the thyropharyngeus muscle and the transverse fibers of the cricopharyngeus muscle creates a point of potential weakness in the pharyngoesophageal segment, which is the site of origin of a pharyngoesophageal (Zenker's) diverticulum as well as a common site of perforation during esophagoscopy (see Fig. 26–47). The cricopharyngeal sphincter is unique to the gastrointestinal tract because it does not consist of a circular ring of muscle but rather a *bow* of muscle connecting the two lateral borders of the cricoid cartilage. The cricopharyngeus muscle fibers blend into the longitudinal and circular muscle of the *cervical esophagus,* a 5- to 6-cm. long segment that extends to the beginning of the first thoracic vertebra. Although the cervical esophagus is a midline structure positioned posteriorly to the trachea, it tends to course more to the left of the trachea (Fig. 26–1) and is therefore more readily approached surgically through a left neck incision. The cervical esophagus lies just anterior to the prevertebral fascia and can normally be separated from its loose fibrous posterior attachments by blunt finger dissection of the prevertebral space. The *thoracic esophagus* passes into the posterior mediastinum, narrowing slightly behind the aortic arch and great vessels and curving somewhat to the left of the trachea as it passes behind the left mainstem bronchus. It then deviates slightly to the right for several centimeters in the subcarinal area, gradually returning to the left of midline and anterior to the thoracic aorta as it proceeds behind the pericardium to about the level of the seventh thoracic vertebra. At this point, the esophagus deviates farther to the left and anteriorly, entering the esophageal diaphragmatic hiatus at the level of the eleventh thoracic vertebra. The lateral boundaries of the thoracic esophagus are the right and left parietal pleurae, which are easily injured during esophageal operations.

The diaphragmatic esophageal hiatus is a sling of muscle fibers that arise from the *right* crus in approximately 45% of patients. At times, however, both the left and right crura contribute to the hiatus. The *abdominal esophagus* varies in length from 1 to several centimeters, extending from the esophageal hiatus to the point at which it joins the stomach, the so-called cardia, or esophagogastric junction. The precise location of the esophagogastric junction is a matter of considerable controversy, because this area has been defined in at least three different ways: (1) the junction of esophageal squamous and gastric columnar epithelium; (2) the point at which the tubular esophagus joins the gastric pouch; and (3) the junction of the esophageal circular muscle layer with the oblique sling fibers of the stomach (the loop of Willis or the collar of Helvetius). Each definition has its merit as well as its shortcomings. Clinically, however, the squamocolumnar epithelial junction (the ora serrata or Z-line), as identified endoscopically, is the most practical definition of the gastroesophageal junction, provided that the patient does not have a columnar-lined lower esophagus (Fig. 26–2). The *phrenoesophageal membrane* is a fibroelastic sheet of tissue that extends circumferentially from the muscular margins of the diaphragmatic hiatus to the esophagus. It is a misnomer to refer to this tissue as the phrenoesophageal *ligament,* because such terminology erroneously implies strong fibrous bands that connect bones or supporting viscera. The majority of the phrenoesophageal membrane arises from the endoabdominal fascia and inserts into the esophagus for a distance of 2 to 3 cm. above the hiatus and 3 to 5 cm. above the mucosal junction. Fibrous strands from the upper surface of the dia-

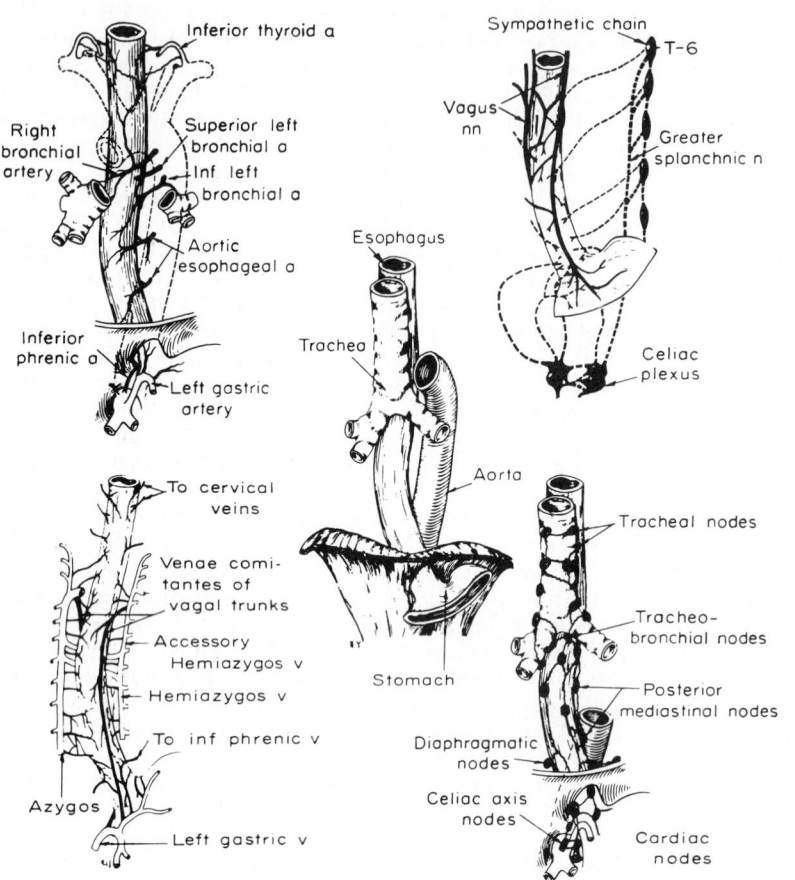

Figure 26–1. Anatomy of the esophagus: arterial supply (upper left), innervation (upper right), lymphatic drainage (lower right), and relationship of esophagus to trachea, aorta, and diaphragm.

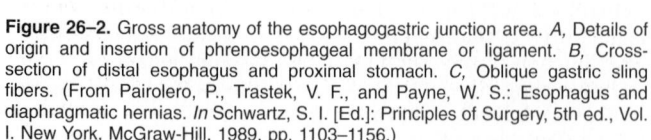

Figure 26–2. Gross anatomy of the esophagogastric junction area. *A,* Details of origin and insertion of phrenoesophageal membrane or ligament. *B,* Cross-section of distal esophagus and proximal stomach. *C,* Oblique gastric sling fibers. (From Pairolero, P., Trastek, V. F., and Payne, W. S.: Esophagus and diaphragmatic hernias. *In* Schwartz, S. I. [Ed.]: Principles of Surgery, 5th ed., Vol. I. New York, McGraw-Hill, 1989, pp. 1103–1156.)

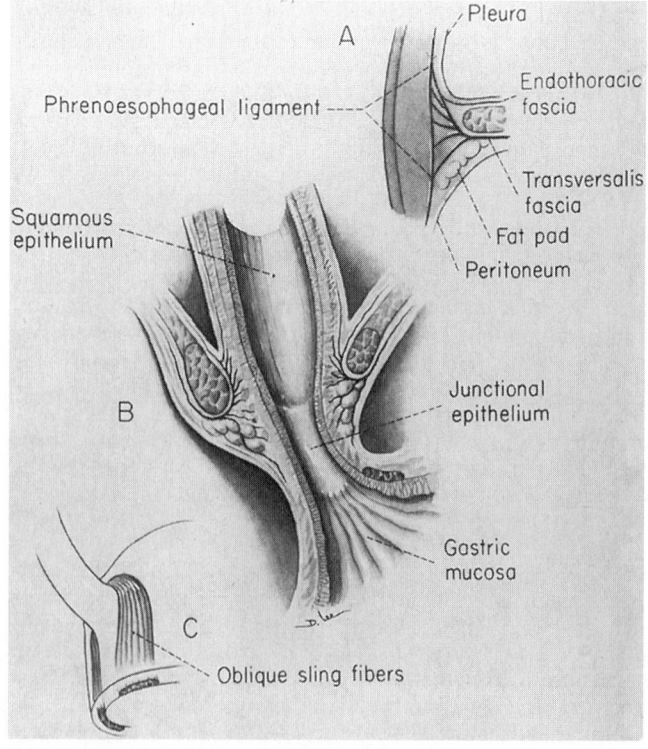

phragm (fascia of Laimer) contribute to the phrenoesophageal membrane. The functional significance of the phrenoesophageal membrane remains undetermined. However, it is now clear that this tissue lacks sufficient strength to *reliably* anchor the esophagogastric junction in the abdomen when performing an antireflux operation.

The esophagus has three distinct areas of naturally occurring anatomic narrowing (Fig. 26–3). The *cervical constriction* occurs at the level of the cricopharyngeus sphincter, the narrowest point of the gastrointestinal tract, typically measuring 14 mm. in diameter. The *bronchoaortic constriction* (15 to 17 mm.) is located at the level of the fourth thoracic vertebra behind the tracheal bifurcation where the left mainstem bronchus and aortic arch cross the esophagus. The *diaphragmatic constriction* (16 to 19 mm.) occurs where the esophagus traverses the diaphragm. The esophagus between these three areas of constriction has a wider caliber, which is termed the *superior* and *inferior dilatations,* respectively. The normal adult thoracic esophagus has a maximum diameter of approximately 2.5 cm. on barium swallow examination.

The esophagus is a mucosal-lined muscular tube that lacks a serosa. It is surrounded by adventitia or mediastinal connective tissue, a layer of loose fibroareolar tissue. Beneath the adventitia is a coat of longitudinal muscle that overlies an inner layer of circular muscle. Between the two muscular layers is a thin intramuscular septum of connective tissue that contains fine blood vessels and ganglion cells of Meissner's and Auerbach's plexuses. Both the longitudinal and circular muscle layers of the upper third of the esophagus are striated, whereas in the lower two thirds, they are nonstriated. The fatty and relatively thick submucosa permits considerable mobility of the esophageal mucosa, a point of particular importance in constructing anastomoses. The submucosa contains the mucus glands, blood vessels, Meissner's neural plexus, and an extensive lymphatic network. The esophageal mucosa consists of squamous epithelium except for the distal 1 to 2 cm., which are junctional columnar epithelium. Occasionally, islands of ectopic gastric mucosa may be found through the length of the esophagus.

The notorious *poor* blood supply of the esophagus is more of an excuse for complications of poor surgical technique than actual fact. Although it has a segmental blood supply, the esophagus is nourished by a number of arteries. The cervical esophagus receives blood from the superior thyroid artery as well as the inferior thyroid artery of the thyrocervical trunk, with both sides communicating through collateral vessels. The major blood supply of the intrathoracic esophagus is from four to six aortic esophageal arteries, supplemented by collateral vessels with the inferior thyroid, intercostal and bronchial, inferior phrenic, and left gastric arteries. Elegant anatomic studies of the aortic esophageal arteries indicate that these vessels terminate in fine capillary networks before actually penetrating the esophageal muscle layer.[23] Therefore, if in the process of transhiatal esophageal mobilization the dissection is kept close to the esophageal wall, the risk of serious hemorrhage from a sizable vessel is minimal. After penetrating and supplying the muscular layers of the esophagus, the esophageal capillary network runs longitudinally in the submucosa. The extensive venous drainage of the esophagus includes the hypopharyngeal, azygos, hemiazygos, intercostal, and gastric veins.

The esophagus has both sympathetic and parasympathetic innervation. In the neck, the superior laryngeal nerves arise from the vagus nerves and divide into the external and internal laryngeal branches. The external laryngeal nerve innervates the cricothyroid muscle and also, in part, the inferior pharyngeal constrictor. The internal laryngeal nerve is the sensory nerve of the pharyngeal surface of the larynx and the base of the tongue. The recurrent laryngeal branches of the vagus nerves provide parasympathetic innervation to the cervical esophagus as well as innervation to the upper esophageal sphincter. Thus injury to the recurrent laryngeal nerve may cause not only hoarseness but also upper esophageal sphincter dysfunction with secondary aspiration on swallowing. In the thorax, the vagus nerves send fibers to the striated muscle as well as parasympathetic preganglionic fibers to the smooth muscle. The sympathetic innervation consists of fibers to the cervical esophagus from the superior and inferior cervical sympathetic ganglia, to the thoracic esophagus from the upper thoracic and splanchnic nerves, and to the intra-abdominal esophagus from the celiac ganglion. In addition, Meissner's and Auerbach's plexuses provide an intrinsic autonomic nervous system within the esophageal wall. Meissner's plexus of nerves is located in the submucosa, while Auerbach's plexus is in the connective tissue between the circular and longitudinal muscle layers. The two vagus nerves lie along either side of the thoracic esophagus and form two large nerve plexuses supplying the esophagus and the lungs. Two to 6 cm. above the esophageal hiatus, the esophageal vagus plexuses coalesce and become single trunks, the left vagus coming to lie anterior to the esophagus and the right vagus posterior at the diaphragmatic hiatus.

The esophagus has an extensive lymphatic drainage that consists of two lymphatic plexuses, one arising in the mucosa and the other in the muscular layer. Mucosal lymphatic capillaries may pierce the muscular layer and drain to regional lymph nodes. Alternatively, these lymphatic capillaries may run longitudinally in the esophageal wall before exiting

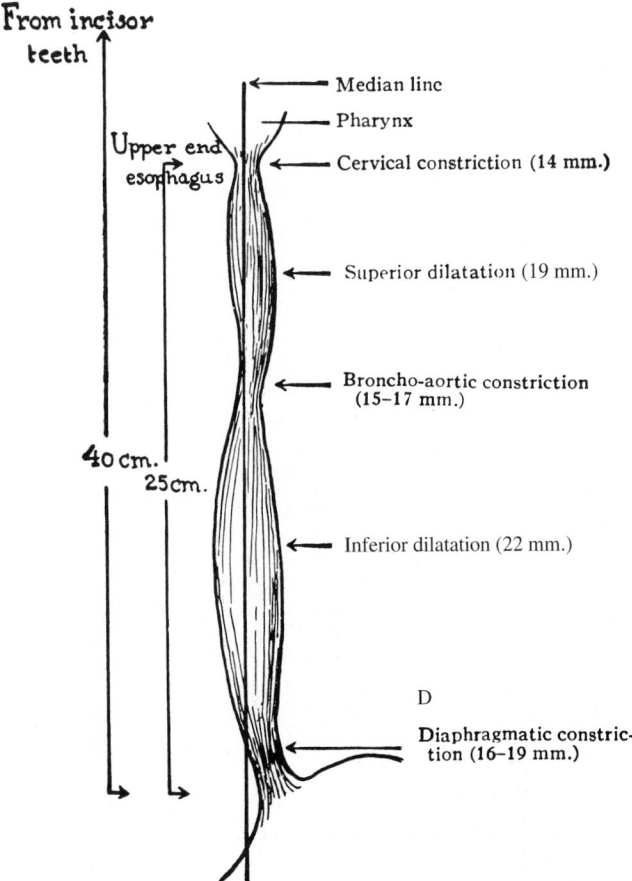

Figure 26–3. Normal esophageal constrictions, dilatations, and measurements. (From Shackelford, R. T.: Surgery of the Alimentary Tract, 2nd ed. Philadelphia, W. B. Saunders, 1978, p. 9.)

through the muscle into adjacent lymph nodes. In general, the flow of lymphatics of the upper two thirds of the esophagus tends to be upward, whereas that of the distal third tends to be downward. Thus, esophageal carcinomas may metastasize to internal jugular nodes in the neck, paratracheal nodes in the superior mediastinum, subcarinal nodes in the mid chest, paraesophageal nodes in the lower mediastinum, and inferior pulmonary ligament, perigastric, and left gastric artery lymph nodes.

THORACIC DUCT ANATOMY

The proximity of the thoracic duct to the esophagus makes it vulnerable to injury during esophageal surgery. It is therefore appropriate to emphasize this relationship. The thoracic duct forms at the confluence of the cisterna chyli at a level between the twelfth thoracic and second lumbar vertebrae and to the right side of the abdominal aorta. The duct enters the posterior mediastinum through the aortic hiatus at the level of T10 to T12 and continues cephalad on the anterior surface of the vertebral column between the aorta and the azygos vein and behind the esophagus. At the T4 to T5 level, the duct crosses to the left of the spine, under the aortic arch, and continues along the left side of the esophagus, ascending into the neck posterior to the left subclavian artery. In the neck, the duct lies anterior to the vertebral artery and vein, thyrocervical trunk, and phrenic nerve, and it enters the venous system at the junction of the left subclavian and left internal jugular veins. Operations on the thoracic esophagus, particularly after previous surgery or radiation therapy that have produced periesophageal fibrosis, may result in a chylothorax due to thoracic duct injury.

SELECTED REFERENCES

Elmslie, R. G.: Perspectives in the development of esophageal surgery. *In* Jamieson, G. G. (Ed.): Surgery of the Oesophagus. New York, Churchill Livingstone, 1988, pp. 3–7.
  This is a concise historical accounting of the evolution of esophageal surgery and contains a list of classic references representing the milestones in this specialty.

Liebermann-Meffert D., and Duranceau, A.: Anatomy and embryology. *In* Orringer, M. B., and Zuidema, G. D. (Eds.): Shackelford's Surgery of the Alimentary Tract, 4th ed., Vol. 1, The Esophagus. Philadelphia, W. B. Saunders, 1996, pp. 3–38.
  Perhaps one of the most authoritative available references on the subject, this comprehensive reference correlates esophageal anatomy and histology. There is an excellent discussion of the arterial blood supply of the esophagus that is based on Liebermann-Meffert's elegant corrosion cast technique of arterial system reconstruction from cadaver specimens (Liebermann-Meffert, D., Luscher, V., Neff, V., et al.: Esophagectomy without thoracotomy: Is there a risk of intramediastinal bleeding? A study on blood supply of the esophagus. Ann. Surg., 206:184, 1987).

Naef, A. P.: The story of thoracic surgery—milestones and pioneers. Toronto, Hogrefe and Huber Publishers, 1990, pp. 61–72.
  Within this modern, concise accounting of the relatively young specialty of thoracic surgery, the highly respected European thoracic surgeon, Andreas Naef of Lausanne, Switzerland, recounts the milestones in the surgical treatment of esophageal disease.

Skandalakis, J. E., Gray, S. W., and Skandalakis, L. J.: Surgical anatomy of the oesophagus. *In* Jamieson, G. G. (Ed.): Surgery of the Oesophagus. New York, Churchill Livingstone, 1988, pp. 19–35.
  This is an excellent discussion of esophageal anatomy related to operative considerations: endoscopy, diverticulum formation, surgical approaches, hiatal hernia regions, and lymphatic drainage of carcinoma.

REFERENCES

1. Adams, W. E., and Phemister, D. B.: Carcinoma of the lower thoracic esophagus: Report of successful resection and esophagogastrostomy. J. Thorac. Surg., 7:621, 1938.
2. Allen, T. H., and Clagget, O. T.: Changing concepts in the surgical treatment of pulsion diverticula of the lower esophagus. J. Thorac. Cardiovasc. Surg., 50:455, 1965.
3. Allison, P. R.: Reflux esophagitis, sliding hiatal hernia, and the anatomy of repair. Surg. Gynecol. Obstet., 92:149, 1951.
4. Belsey, R.: Functional diseases of the esophagus. J. Thorac. Cardiovasc. Surg., 52:164, 1966.
5. Bernstein, L. M., and Baker, L. A.: A clinical test for esophagitis. Gastroenterology, 34:760, 1958.
6. Browne, D. C., and McHardy, G.: A new instrument for use in esophagospasm. JAMA, 113:1963, 1939.
7. Ellis, F. H., Jr., and Olsen, A. M.: Major Problems in Clinical Surgery. Vol. 9, Achalasia of the Esophagus. Philadelphia, W. B. Saunders, 1969.
8. Eypasch, E. P., Stein, H. J., DeMeester, T. R., et al.: Ambulatory 24 hour esophageal motility monitoring: A new technique to define and clarify esophageal motor disorders. Am. J. Surg., 159:144, 1990.
9. Fisher, R. S., Malmud, L. S., Roberts, G. S., and Lobis, I. F.: Gastroesophageal (GE) scintiscanning to detect and quantitate GE reflux. Gastroenterology, 70:301, 1976.
10. Garlock, J. H.: Re-establishment of esophagogastric continuity following resection of esophagus for carcinoma of middle third. Surg. Gynecol. Obstet., 78:23, 1944.
11. Haight, C., and Towsley, H. A.: Congenital atresia of the esophagus and tracheo-esophageal fistula: Extrapleural ligation of the fistula and end-to-end anastomosis of esophageal segments. Surg. Gynecol. Obstet., 76:672, 1943.
12. Helm, W. J., Schlegel, J. F., Code, C. F., and Summerskill, W. H. J. Identification of the gastroesophageal mucosal junction by transmural potential in healthy subjects and patients with hiatal hernia. Gastroenterology, 48:25, 1965.
13. Ingelfinger, F. J.: Esophageal motility. Physiol. Rev., 38:533, 1959.
14. Jackson, C., and Jackson, C., Jr.: Bronchoesophagology. Philadelphia, W. B. Saunders, 1950.
15. Jamieson, J. R., Stein, H. J., DeMeester, T. R., et al.: Ambulatory 24 hour esophageal pH monitoring: Normal values, optimal thresholds, specificity, sensitivity, and reproducibility. Am. J. Gastroenterol., 87:1102, 1992.
16. Janeway, H. H., and Green, N. W.: Cancer of the oesophagus and cardia. Ann. Surg., 52:67, 1910.
17. Janssens, J., Vantrappen, G., and Chillibert, G.: 24-Hour recording of esophageal pressure and pH in patients with non-cardiac chest pain. Gastroenterology, 90:178, 1986.
18. Johnson, L. F., and DeMeester, T. R.: Twenty-four hour pH monitoring of the distal esophagus. Am. J. Gastroenterol., 62:325, 1974.
19. Kantrowitz, P. A., Corson, J. G., Fleischli, D. J., and Skinner, D. B.: Measurement of gastroesophageal reflux. Gastroenterology, 56:666, 1969.
20. Kaul, B., Peterson, H., Grettle, K., Erichsen, H., and Myrvold, H. E.: Scintigraphy, pH measurement and radiography in the evaluation of gastroesophageal reflux. Scand. J. Gastroenterol., 20:289, 1985.
21. Kurlander, D. J., Radkin, H. F., Kirsner, J. B., and Palmer, W. L.: Therapeutic value of the pneumatic dilator in achalasia of the esophagus: Long-term results in sixty-two living patients. Gastroenterology, 45:604, 1963.
22. Lewis, I.: The surgical treatment of carcinoma of the esophagus: With special reference to a new operation for growths of the middle third. Br. J. Surg., 34:18, 1946.
23. Liebermann-Meffert, D. M. I., Luescher, U., Neft, V., Ruedi, T. P., and Allgower, M.: Esophagectomy without thoracotomy: Is there a risk of intramediastinal bleeding. Ann. Surg., 206:184, 1987.
24. LoPresti, P. A., and Hilmi, A. M.: Clinical experience with a new foroblique fiberoptic esophagoscope. Am. J. Dig. Dis., 9:690, 1964.
25. Marshall, S. F.: Carcinoma of the esophagus: Successful resection of lower end of esophagus with re-establishment of esophagic gastric continuity. Surg. Clin. North Am., 18:643, 1938.
26. Nissen, R.: Gastropexy and fundoplication in surgical treatment of hiatal hernia. Am. J. Dig. Dis., 6:954, 1961.
27. Ohsawa, T.: The surgery of the oesophagus. Arch. Jpn. Chir., 10:605, 1933.
28. Olsen, A. M., Harrington, S. W., Moersch, H. J., and Andersen, H. A.: The treatment of cardiospasm: Analysis of a twelve-year experience. J. Thorac. Cardiovasc. Surg., 22:164, 1951.
29. Pattrick, F. G.: Investigation of gastroesophageal reflux in various positions with a two lumen pH electrode. Gut, 11:659, 1970.
30. Schindler, R.: Observations on cardiospasm and its treatment by brusque dilatation. Ann. Intern. Med., 45:207, 1956.
31. Skinner, D. B., and Belsey, R. H. R.: Surgical management of esophageal reflux and hiatus hernia. J. Thorac. Cardiovasc. Surg., 53:33, 1967.
32. Skinner, D. B., and Booth, D.: Assessment of distal esophageal function in patients with hiatus hernia and/or gastroesophageal reflux. Ann. Surg., 172:627, 1970.
33. Spencer, J.: Prolonged pH recording in the study of gastroesophageal reflux. Br. J. Surg., 54:912, 1969.
34. Sweet, R. H.: Transthoracic resection of esophagus and stomach for carcinoma: Analysis of postoperative complications, causes of death, and late results of operation. Ann. Surg., 121:272, 1945.
35. Texter, E. C., Jr., Smith, H. W., Moeller, H. C., et al.: Intraluminal pressures from the upper gastrointestinal tract: I. Correlations with motor activity in normal subjects and patients with esophageal disorders. Gastroenterology, 32:1013, 1957.
36. Torek, F.: The operative treatment of carcinoma of the oesophagus. Ann. Surg., 61:385, 1915.
37. Turner, G. G.: Excision of thoracic esophagus for carcinoma with constriction of extrathoracic gullet. Lancet, 2:1315, 1933.
38. Tuttle, S. G., and Grossman, M. I.: Detection of gastroesophageal reflux by simultaneous measurement of intraluminal pressures and pH. Proc. Soc. Exp. Biol. Med., 98:225, 1958.

39. Vantrappen, G., Liemer, M. D., Ikeya, J., et al.: Simultaneous fluorocinematography and intraluminal pressure measurements in the study of esophageal motility. Gastroenterology, 35:592, 1958.
40. Velasco, N., Pope C. E., Gamnan, R. M., Roberts, P., and Hill, L. D.: Measurement of esophageal reflux by scintigraphy. Dig. Dis. Sci., 29:977, 1984.
41. Wheeler, W. I.: Pharyngocele and dilatation of pharynx with existing diverticulum at lower portion of pharynx lying posterior to the esophagus, cured by pharyngotomy, being the first case of the kind recorded. Dublin J. Med. Sci., 82:349, 1886.
42. Zaaijer, J. H.: Cardiospasm in the aged. Ann. Surg., 77:615, 1923.

II

PHYSIOLOGY

Mark B. Orringer, M.D.

The esophagus is a muscular tube that begins proximally with the upper esophageal sphincter (UES) or cricopharyngeus muscle and ends distally with the lower esophageal sphincter (LES). Its basic function is to transport swallowed material from the pharynx into the stomach. Secondarily, retrograde flow of gastric contents into the esophagus is prevented by the LES and entry of air into the esophagus with each inspiration is prevented by the UES, which normally remains closed as a result of tonic contraction of the cricopharyngeus muscle. Much of our current knowledge of esophageal physiology is based on relatively recent developments in manometric techniques that permit recordings of intraesophageal pressure phenomena, such as the amplitude and length of the UES and LES, the extent and duration of relaxation of these sphincters with swallowing, and the characteristics of peristaltic activity in the body of the esophagus. In clinical practice, such recordings are most commonly obtained today from small swallowed catheters bonded together with terminal openings at different levels. The catheters are constantly perfused with small volumes of water, and intraluminal pressures generated by esophageal contractions or the sphincters are transmitted through strain gauges to recording equipment. Patterns of normal and abnormal esophageal motor function have been well established.[1, 8] The standard motility catheter is a triple-lumen, constantly perfused system of polyethylene or polyvinyl tubing with either an open-end or a lateral orifice (Fig. 26–4).

More recently, the availability of micropressure transducers has allowed measurement of esophageal pressures more simply and without the need for a water-perfused system. These microtransducers, fastened directly to the swallowed end of the recording catheters, are extremely accurate and more sensitive to pressure changes within the esophagus than the water-perfused system. However, the multitransducer catheters are relatively expensive and difficult to maintain and repair, and they have, therefore, not gained as widespread popularity in clinical use as the constantly perfused systems. Whereas esophageal motility studies have become a basic diagnostic tool in the evaluation of disorders of esophageal motor function, dysphagia, chest pain of undetermined origin, and gastroesophageal reflux, it must be realized that a multitude of factors affect the pressures recorded from patient to patient and from one laboratory to another. These variables include catheter size,[18, 19, 21] the character of the swallowed bolus (e.g., hot vs. cold liquid, dry vs. wet swallow), and resting time between swallows.[10, 20–23] It would seem most prudent to recognize that the quantitative values obtained from esophageal manometry are *not* absolute and that this study provides but one additional bit of corroborative information to be used along with the history, barium swallow, and endoscopic findings in the assessment of esophageal function.

Swallowing normally involves both voluntary and involuntary muscle function. It begins with voluntary movement of the tongue. This initiates an involuntary peristaltic wave that rapidly traverses the pharynx and reaches the UES, producing a brisk, coordinated relaxation that is followed by a postdeglutitive contraction (Fig. 26–5). Pharyngeal swallowing is a complex, rapidly occurring series of events that has been divided radiologically into six phases.[7] The rapidity of these events and the difficulty quantitating them with a standard water-perfused system prompted Doddes and associates to study pharyngeal motor function using an intraluminal strain gauge system.[6] Others have corroborated the difficulty in precisely measuring pharyngeal function.[2, 17] Concerned that variable sphincter pressure values were a function of movement proximal or distal to the recording orifice, Dent developed a 5-cm.-long perfused sleeve that records the highest pressure at any point over its length and therefore more reliably reflects LES pressure despite movement of the gastroesophageal junction.[5] The sleeve manometric catheter has an oval cross section that orients itself more consistently within the slitlike UES lumen than the traditional round motility catheters.[15, 16] The UES is 2.5 to 4.5 cm. in length and has a basal resting pressure that ranges from 16 to 118 mm. Hg (mean, 42 mm. Hg). Its duration of relax-

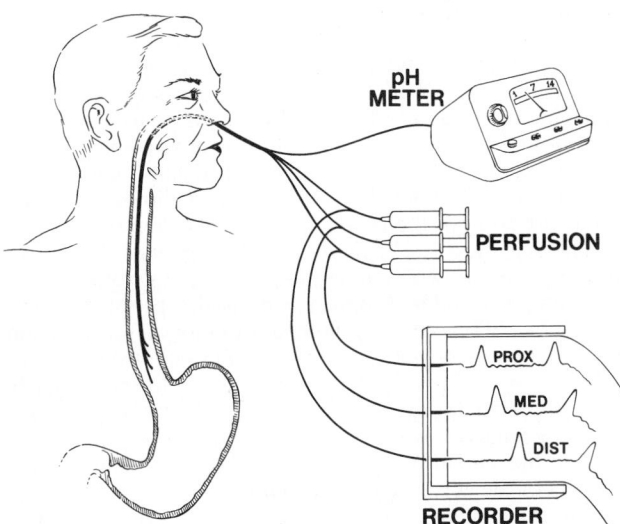

Figure 26–4. Schematic representation of combined manometric–pH recording system used in the evaluation of esophageal function. The triple-lumen perfused recording catheter measures intraluminal pressures from three levels in the esophagus, each separated from the next by 5 cm. Measurements are made in terms of centimeters from the nostrils to the proximal opening of the recording catheter (PROX). The medial catheter (MED) records pressures 5 cm. distal to the proximal opening, and the distal catheter (DIST), 5 cm. below this. The intraesophageal pH electrode is used to document gastroesophageal reflux.

UPPER ESOPHAGEAL SPHINCTER-NORMAL

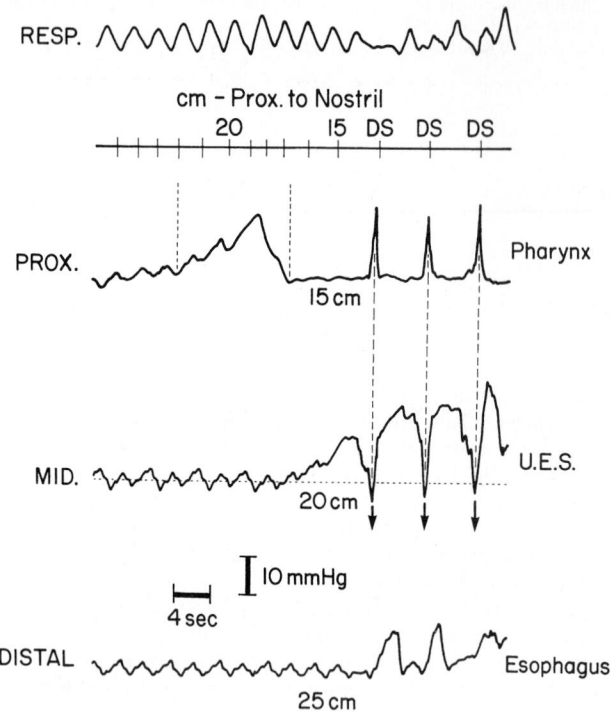

Figure 26–5. Motility tracing showing relaxation of the upper esophageal sphincter (UES). As the triple lumen recording catheter is withdrawn through the upper esophagus, the most proximal recording port first passes through the upper esophageal high pressure zone, which corresponds to the cricopharyngeal sphincter mechanism. Withdrawal of the catheter is stopped when the middle port is within the UES. Each time the patient swallows, pharyngeal contraction (proximal catheter), cricopharyngeal relaxation (middle catheter, arrows), and the peristaltic wave propagated by the swallow (distal catheter) are observed.

ation with swallowing is 0.5 to 1.2 seconds. Contraction of the UES after the relaxation phase produces intraluminal pressures that are often twice as high as resting pressures and last 2 to 4 seconds.

Three types of contractions are seen in the esophageal body. *Primary peristalsis* is progressive and is triggered by voluntary swallowing. *Secondary peristalsis* is also progressive but is generated by distention or irritation, not by voluntary swallowing. *Tertiary contractions* are nonprogressive (simultaneous) contractions that may occur either after voluntary swallowing or spontaneously between swallows. As the swallowed bolus enters the esophagus from the pharynx, a *primary* peristaltic wave is activated, traversing the esophageal body at a speed of 2 to 5 cm. per second and normally propelling the swallowed material from the pharynx into the stomach in 4 to 8 seconds in an orderly, progressive manner (Fig. 26–6). Normally a progressive peristaltic contraction (primary wave) follows 97% of all wet swallows.[8] Pressure within the body of the esophagus is a reflection of negative intrathoracic pressure, being maximally negative (-5 to -10 mm. Hg) during deep inspiration, and highest (0 to 5 mm. Hg) during expiration. Esophageal peristaltic pressure ranges from 20 to 100 mm. Hg, with a duration of contraction between 2 and 4 seconds.[8, 11] If the entire swallowed bolus of food does not empty from the esophagus into the stomach, *secondary* peristaltic waves are initiated. These contractions, like the primary waves, are progressive and sequential but begin in the smooth muscle segment of the esophagus (near the level of the aortic arch) and continue until retained intraesophageal contents are emptied into the stomach. Thus, unlike the primary wave, the secondary contraction is not initiated by a voluntary swallow but rather by local distention of the esophagus. *Tertiary* contractions are simultaneous, nonprogressive, nonperistaltic, monophasic or multiphasic waves that can occur throughout the esophagus and represent incoordinated contractions of the smooth muscle that are responsible for the classic "corkscrew" appearance of esophageal spasm on barium swallow examination. In-

creased resting pressures within the body of the esophagus and abnormal motor function are seen with either mechanical or functional obstruction.

The term *lower esophageal sphincter* implies the presence of an anatomic sphincter such as the pylorus or the anus. Although no such *anatomic* LES has been demonstrated, manometry has defined an elevated distal esophageal resting pressure that is 3 to 5 cm. in length, serves as the barrier against abnormal regurgitation of gastric contents into the esophagus, and represents a *functional* sphincter (Fig. 26–7). Thus, the LES is more accurately referred to as the LES *mechanism* or the *distal esophageal high-pressure zone* (HPZ). The factors responsible for maintaining competence of the LES are poorly understood, but the presence of an intraabdominal segment of distal esophagus, under the influence of positive intra-abdominal pressure, seems important to the success of most antireflux operations.

Normal resting pressure within the HPZ ranges from 10 to 20 mm. Hg, but there is *no absolute HPZ value per se that indicates either competence or incompetence of the LES mechanism.* Patients with no gastroesophageal reflux may have an extremely *low* HPZ amplitude on manometric recordings, whereas others with massive reflux may have seemingly high distal pressures. This inconsistency is a reflection of both HPZ variation due to individual body habitus as well as the radial asymmetry of the LES that results in varied readings during *pull-through* determinations, depending on the orientation of the catheter recording port. Mean HPZ pressures less than 6 mm. Hg or overall sphincter length less than 2 cm. are likely to be associated with incompetence of the LES and gastroesophageal reflux.

The distal HPZ is located in the region of the diaphragmatic hiatus. With standard pull-through studies, the distal portion of the sphincter demonstrates respiratory variations like those in the abdomen—increased pressure with inspiration, decreased pressure with expiration (see Fig. 26–7). In the proximal portion of the HPZ, however, there is an intrathoracic pattern of respiratory variation, namely, negative

PROGRESSIVE PERISTALSIS

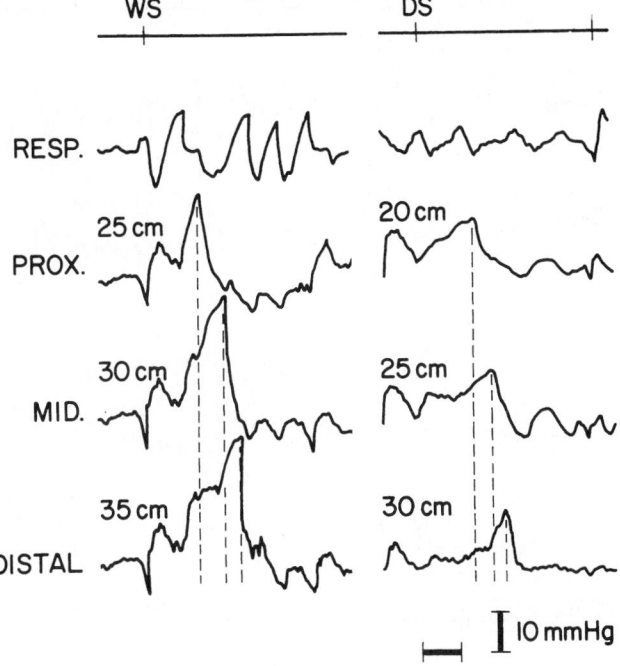

Figure 26–6. Motility tracing showing normal peristalsis. With each swallow, a progressive esophageal contraction is generated, passing first by the proximal recording port, then the middle, and finally the distal port. (WS, wet swallow; DS, dry swallow.)

NORMAL HPZ

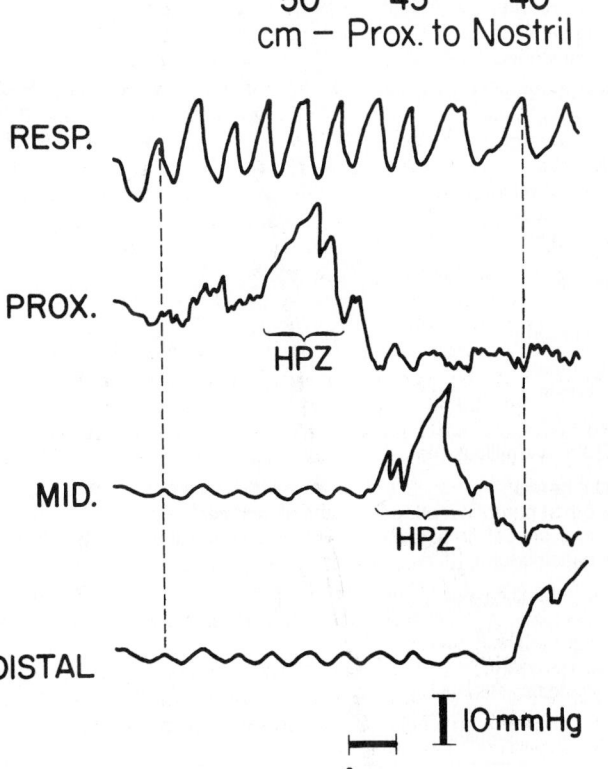

Figure 26–7. Motility tracing showing normal distal sphincter mechanism or high-pressure zone (HPZ). As the recording catheter is withdrawn from the stomach into the esophagus, the HPZ is identified sequentially in each catheter. Mean basal pressure within the thoracic esophagus is lower than that within the stomach (below the diaphragm). Below the diaphragm, within the stomach, a positive deflection is seen during respiratory excursions at the peak of inspiration (when the diaphragm is lowest). Conversely, in the esophagus, at the peak of inspiration, intrathoracic pressure is maximally negative and a negative deflection during inspiration is observed (dotted lines).

RELAXATION OF HPZ WITH SWALLOWING

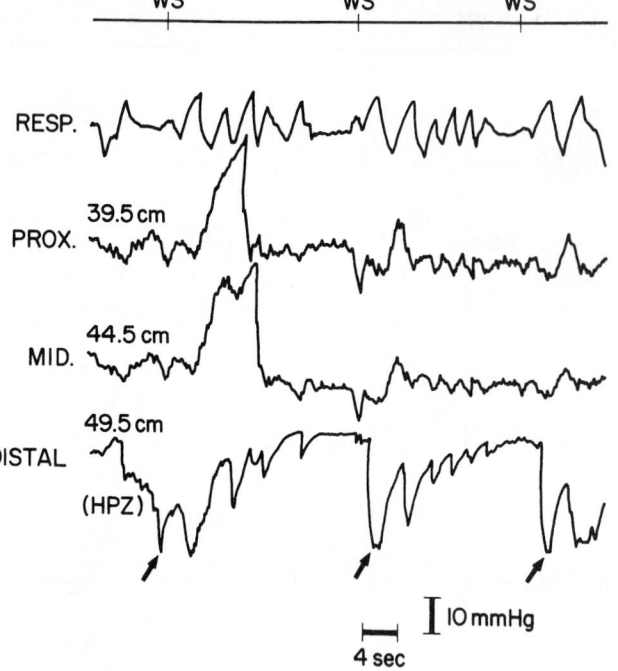

Figure 26–8. Motility tracing showing normal relaxation of the distal HPZ with swallowing. The distal recording port is within the HPZ (49.5 cm. from the nostrils). Each swallow normally results in relaxation of the HPZ (arrows) followed by a sustained postdeglutitive contraction, after which pressure again returns to basal level. (HPZ, high-pressure zone; WS, wet swallow.)

TABLE 26–1. Factors Affecting Distal High-Pressure Zone (HPZ) Tone

Factors	Increased HPZ Tone	Decreased HPZ Tone
Hormonal	Gastrin Motilin Prostaglandin $F_{2\alpha}$ Bombesin	Secretin Cholecystokinin Glucagon Progesterone Estrogen Prostaglandins E_1, E_2, A_1

Drugs	Caffeine
	Alpha-adrenergic agents
	  Norepinephrine
	  Phenylephrine
	Anticholinesterase
	  Edrophonium
	Cholinergic agents
	  Bethanechol (Urecholine)
	  Methacholine (Mecholyl)
	Betazole
	Metoclopramide
		Alpha-adrenergic blockers
		  Phentolamine
		Anticholinergics
		  Atropine
		  Theophylline
		Beta-adrenergic blockers
		  Isoproterenol
		Ethanol
		Epinephrine
		Nicotine
		Nitroglycerin

Foods	Protein meal	Fatty meal Chocolate
Myogenic	Normal resting muscle tone	? Aging ? Diabetes mellitus
Mechanical	Anti-reflux operation	Hiatal hernia Abnormal phrenoesophageal ligament insertion Short or absent intra-abdominal distal esophageal segment Nasogastric tube
Miscellaneous	Gastric alkalinization Gastric distention	Gastric acidification Gastrectomy Hypoglycemia Hypothyroidism Amyloidosis Pernicious anemia Epidermolysis bullosa

Modified from Hurwitz, A. L., Duranceau, A., and Haddad, J. K.: Disorders of Esophageal Motility. Philadelphia, W. B. Saunders Company, 1979, p. 120.

pressure with inspiration and positive pressure with expiration. The terms *point of respiratory reversal* or *pressure inversion point* (PIP) are used to designate the site at which this transition in respiratory pattern occurs on manometric tracings. In patients who totally lack a distal HPZ, the PIP is used as a reference point that is indicative of the cardia, 5 cm. above which the pH electrode can be positioned for acid-reflux testing (see Fig. 26–29). Within 1.5 to 2.5 seconds after a swallow is initiated, distal HPZ relaxation occurs and lasts 4 to 6 seconds (Fig. 26–8). A postdeglutitive contraction then occurs, generating pressures of 25 to 35 mm. Hg for 7 to 10 seconds, after which HPZ tone returns to resting levels.

Distal HPZ pressure varies continually in everyone, being influenced by a host of neural, hormonal, myogenic, mechanical, and environmental factors (Table 26–1).[12] Much more direct than esophageal manometry in determining esophageal exposure to gastric juice through an incompetent LES mechanism is 24-hour monitoring of intraesophageal pH by means of an indwelling pH probe positioned 5 cm. proximal to the upper extent of the distal HPZ.[4, 9, 14] Twenty-four-hour pH monitoring of esophageal exposure to pH less than 4[3] documents six components:

1. Total time pH less than 4 (normal <4%)
2. Total time pH less than 4 when upright (normal <8%)
3. Total time pH less than 4 when supine (normal <3%)
4. Total number of reflux episodes (normal <47)
5. Number of episodes greater than 5 minutes (normal <3)
6. Duration of longest reflux episode (normal <20 minutes)

A pH score incorporating the result of these six components into one expression of overall esophageal acid exposure below a pH threshold is calculated by using the standard deviation of the mean of each of the six components measured in 50 normal subjects as a weighing factor.[13]

Esophagoscopy, the barium swallow examination, and the acid perfusion (Bernstein) test remain unreliable and inconsistent indicators of gastroesophageal reflux.

SELECTED REFERENCES

Castell, J. A., and Dalton, C. B.: Esophageal manometry. *In* Castell, D. O. (Ed.): The Esophagus. Boston, Little, Brown Co, 1992, pp. 143–160.
This is a current and comprehensive review of manometric techniques used to assess esophageal function. The discussion of the manometric evolution of the esophageal sphincters and peristalsis within the body of the esophagus is excellent and enhanced by representative illustrative tracings.

DeMeester, T. R., and Stein, H. J. Physiologic diagnostic studies. *In* Orringer, M. B., and Zuidema, G. D. (Eds.): Shackelford's Surgery of the Alimentary Tract, 4th ed. Vol. I, The Esophagus. Philadelphia, W. B. Saunders, 1996, pp. 120–153.
This outstanding treatise on physiologic diagnostic studies used to assess esophageal function is highlighted by a current review of the senior author's sentinel work on 24-hour manometry and 24-hour esophageal pH monitoring.

Duranceau, A., and Liebermann-Meffert, D.: Physiology of the esophagus. *In* Orringer, M. B., and Zuidema, G. D. (Eds.): Shackelford's Surgery of the Alimentary Tract, 4th ed. Vol. I, The Esophagus. Philadelphia, W. B. Saunders, 1996, pp. 39–49.
This is an authoritative discussion of esophageal physiology that contains clear and understandable manometric tracings of sphincter relaxation and peristaltic activity.

Kahrilas, P. J.: Functional anatomy and physiology of the esophagus. *In* Castell, D. O. (Ed.): The Esophagus. Boston, Little, Brown Co, 1992, pp. 1–27.
This is a detailed, well-written discussion of normal esophageal physiology that contains excellent illustrative manometric tracings, many of which are from the author's well-known work in this field.

REFERENCES

1. Castell, J. A., and Dalton, C. B.: Esophageal manometry. *In* Castell, D. O. (Ed.): The Esophagus. Boston, Little, Brown, 1992, pp. 143–160.
2. Castell, J. A., Dalton, C. B., and Castell, D. O.: Pharyngeal and upper esophageal sphincter manometry in humans. Am. J. Physiol., *21*:G173, 1990.
3. DeMeester, T. R., and Stein, H. J.: Physiologic diagnostic studies. *In* Orringer, M. B., Zuidema G. D. (Eds.): Shackelford's Surgery of the Alimentary Tract, 4th ed. Vol. I, The Esophagus. Philadelphia, W. B. Saunders, 1996, pp. 120–153.
4. DeMeester, T. R., Wang, C. I., Wernly, J. A., et al.: Technique, indications, and clinical use of 24-hour esophageal pH monitoring. J. Thorac. Cardiovasc. Surg., *79*:656, 1980.
5. Dent, J.: A new technique for continuous sphincter pressure measurement. Gastroenterology, *71*:263, 1976.
6. Dodds, W. J., Hogan, W. J., Lydon, S. B., Steward, E. T., Stef, J. J., and Arndorfer, R. C.: Quantitation of pharyngeal motor function in normal human subjects. J. Appl. Physiol., *39*:692, 1975.
7. Donner, M. W., Bosma, J. F., and Robertson, D. L.: Anatomy and physiology of the pharynx. Gastrointest. Radiol., *10*:196, 1985.
8. Duranceau, A. C., DeVroede, G., Lafontaine, E., and Jamieson, G. G.: Esophageal motility in asymptomatic volunteers. Surg. Clin. North Am., *63*:777, 1983.
9. Emde, C., Garner, A., and Blum, A.: Technical aspects of intraluminal pH-metry in man: Current status and recommendations. Gut, *23*:1177, 1987.
10. Funch-Jensen, P., and Jacobsen, E.: Esophageal peristalsis before, during, and after food intake in healthy people. Scand. J. Gastroenterol., *16*:209, 1981.
11. Henderson, R. D.: Normal esophageal motor activity: Function and control. *In* The Esophagus—Reflux and Primary Motor Disorders. Baltimore, Williams & Wilkins, 1980, pp. 11–21.
12. Hurwitz, A. L., Duranceau, A., Haddad, J. K., et al.: Normal esophageal motility. *In* Disorders of Esophageal Motility. Philadelphia, W. B. Saunders, 1979, pp. 14–26.
13. Johnson, L. F., and DeMeester, T. R.: Development of 24-hour intraesophageal pH monitoring composite scoring. J. Clin. Gastroenterol., *8*:52, 1986.
14. Johnson, L. F., and DeMeester, T. R.: Twenty-four hour pH monitoring of the distal esophagus: A quantitative measurement of gastroesophageal reflux. Am. J. Gastroenterol., *62*:325, 1974.
15. Kahrilas, P. J., Dodds, W. J., Dent, J., Hogan, W. J., and Arndorfer, R. C.: A method for continuous monitoring of upper esophageal sphincter pressure. Dig. Dis. Sci., *32*:121, 1987.
16. Kahrilas, P. J., Dodds, W. J., Dent, J., Hogan, W. J., and Arndorfer, R. C.: The effect of sleep, spontaneous gastroesophageal reflux and a meal on UES pressure in normal human volunteers. Gastroenterology, *92*:466, 1987.
17. Kahrilas, P. J., Logemann, W. A., Lin, S., and Ergun, G. A.: Pharyngeal clearance swallow: A combined manometric and video fluoroscopic study. Gastroenterology, *103*:128, 1992.
18. Kaye, M. D., and Showalter, J. P.: Measurement of pressure in the lower esophageal sphincter: The influence of catheter diameter. Am. J. Dig. Dis., *19*:860, 1974.
19. Lydon, S. B., Dodds, W. J., Hogan, W. J., and Arndorfer, R. C.: The effect of manometric assembly diameter on intraluminal esophageal pressure recording. Am J. Dig. Dis., *20*:968, 1975.
20. Meyer, G. W., and Castell, D. O.: In support of the clinical usefulness of lower esophageal sphincter pressure determination. Dig. Dis. Sci., *26*:1028, 1981.
21. Pope, C. E.: Is measurement of lower esophageal sphincter pressure clinically useful? Dig. Dis. Sci., *26*:1025, 1981.
22. Stef, J. J., Dodds, W. J., Hogan, W. J., Lineham, J. H., and Stewart, E. T.: Intraluminal esophageal manometry: An analysis of variables affecting recording fidelity of peristaltic pressures. Gastroenterology, *67*:221, 1974.
23. Winship, D. H., Viegas de Andrade, S. R., and Zboralske, F. F.: Influence of bolus temperature on human esophageal motor function. Clin. Invest., *49*:243, 1970.

III _____

DISORDERS OF ESOPHAGEAL MOTILITY

Mark B. Orringer, M.D.

Disorders of esophageal motility are *functional* disorders—conditions that interfere with the normal act of swallowing or produce dysphagia without any associated intraluminal organic obstruction or extrinsic compression.[5] Although a cine-esophagogram and a skilled radiologist may diagnose disordered esophageal motility, the information obtained from esophageal manometry in these patients is much more precise. Early achalasia and diffuse esophageal spasm (DES), for example, may be indistinguishable radiologically, although each condition has its specific manometric characteristics. The differentiation is more than academic: a distal esophagomyotomy for achalasia may not relieve the symptoms of esophageal spasm. As a general rule, a barium swallow, esophagoscopy, and esophageal function tests, including manometry and intraesophageal pH reflux testing, constitute the basic evaluation of the patient with a suspected disorder of esophageal motility.

UPPER ESOPHAGEAL SPHINCTER DYSFUNCTION

Various terms have been used to define abnormal function of the upper esophageal or cricopharyngeal sphincter, such as *cricopharyngeal chalasia, achalasia,* and *spasm.* These terms have little validity, however, because in most patients, standard esophageal manometric techniques have been unable to demonstrate either true hypotonicity or hypertonicity of the upper esophageal sphincter (UES) or failure of the UES to relax with swallowing (achalasia). This is because of the limitations of standard perfused low-compliance infusion systems in recording the rapid sequence of events that occurs with normal deglutition in a unique asymmetrical sphincter that changes position with laryngeal excursions during swallowing.[14] Efforts to circumvent the characteristics of UES function that render manometric recordings in this area so difficult have included use of an eight-lumen perfused manometry catheter,[56] the flat, more flexible Dent sleeve manometry catheter,[12] and the newest circumferential sphincter microtransducer catheter.[6] The terms *oropharyngeal dysphagia*[15] or *cricopharyngeal dysfunction*[38] perhaps best describe the symptom-complex that occurs when there is difficulty propelling liquid or solid food from the oropharynx into the upper esophagus. The causes of this difficulty include abnormalities of the central and peripheral nervous systems, metabolic and inflammatory myopathy, gastroesophageal reflux, and other currently undefined factors (Table 26–2).

Additional causes of upper esophageal dysphagia but with an *anatomic* basis, such as carcinoma, caustic stricture, cervical vertebral bone spurs, thyromegaly, and trauma, should always be excluded. The designation of *globus hystericus,*

TABLE 26–2. Causes of Oropharyngeal Dysphagia

I. Neurogenic
  A. Central nervous system disease
    1. Neurologic disorders
      a. Amyotrophic lateral sclerosis
      b. Multiple sclerosis
      c. Spinocerebellar degeneration
      d. Syringobulbia
      e. Bulbar poliomyelitis
      f. Progressive bulbar paralysis
      g. Parkinson's disease
      h. Huntington's chorea, Sydenham's chorea
      i. Tabes dorsalis
      j. Congenital and degenerative disorders
      k. Dysautonomia
    2. Vascular lesions
      a. Cerebrovascular accident
      b. Basilar artery thrombosis
      c. Aneurysm and brain-stem compression
    3. Tumors
      a. Brain stem
      b. Base of the skull
    4. Operations
    5. Trauma
II. Myogenic
  A. Motor end-plate disease
    1. Myasthenia gravis
    2. Tetanus
  B. Skeletal muscle disease
    1. Muscular dystrophy
      a. Oculopharyngeal
      b. Myotonic
    2. Inflammatory
      a. Polymyositis
      b. Dermatomyositis
    3. Metabolic myopathy
      a. Thyrotoxicosis
      b. Hypothyroidism

III. Structural Causes
  A. Idiopathic: without pharyngoesophageal (Zenker's) diverticulum
  B. With pharyngoesophageal diverticulum
IV. Mechanical Causes
  A. Endoluminal
    1. Inflammatory disease
    2. Foreign body
    3. Webs
    4. Benign tumors
    5. Malignant tumors
  B. Extraluminal
    1. Thyromegaly
    2. Lymphadenopathy
    3. Skeletal hyperostosis
    4. Cervical spine osteophytes (dysphagia psittaca)
    5. Cervical lordosis
    6. Congenital vascular abnormalities (dysphagia lusoria)
    7. Hypertrophied or tortuous aorta (dysphagia aortica)
    8. Heart disease
    9. Pericarditis and mediastinitis
V. Iatrogenic Causes
  A. Neck surgery
    1. Laryngectomy
    2. Thyroidectomy
    3. Parathyroid exploration
    4. Tracheostomy
  B. Thoracic surgery: lung, mediastinal or esophageal surgery with recurrent laryngeal nerve trauma
  C. Irradiation
VI. Gastroesophageal reflux

Modified from Duranceau, A. C., Lafontaine, E., and Taillefer, R.: Oropharyngeal dysphagia. *In* Jamieson, G. G. (Ed.): Surgery of the Oesophagus. Edinburgh, Churchill-Livingstone, 1988, pp. 416–417.

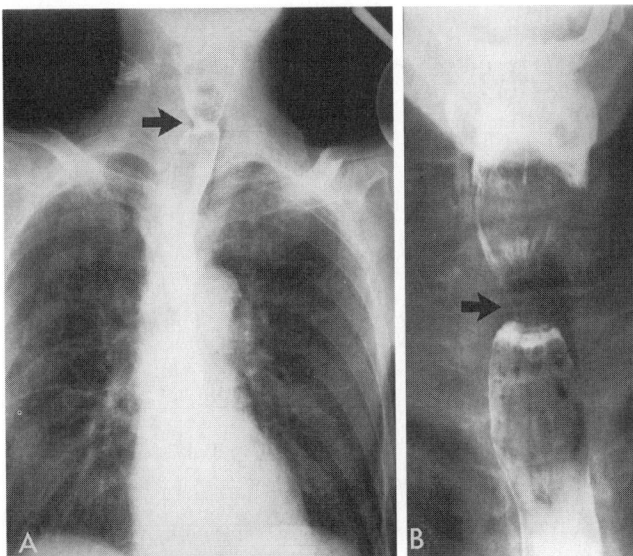

Figure 26-9. *A,* Prominence of the cricopharyngeal sphincter (arrow) in a patient with cervical dysphagia and symptomatic gastroesophageal reflux. *B,* Detail of cervical esophagus (arrow). (From Orringer, M. B.: Extended cervical esophagomyotomy for cricopharyngeal dysfunction. J. Thorac. Cardiovasc. Surg., *80*:669, 1980. Reprinted with permission from the Society of Thoracic Surgeons.)

occurs with cricopharyngeal dysfunction. The inferior pharyngeal constrictor muscle, of which the cricopharyngeal sphincter is a part, may affect the vocal cords in two ways. First, contraction of the inferior pharyngeal constrictor adducts or approximates the alae of the thyroid cartilage, lengthening and tensing the vocal cords. Second, by pulling the cricoid cartilage posteriorly, the cricopharyngeal muscle acts with the lateral cricothyroid muscle to stretch the vocal cords. Thus, there is adequate physiologic explanation for the association between symptoms of cervical dysphagia and hoarseness in the patient with cricopharyngeal dysfunction, and the patient who has these two complaints is seldom malingering. *Weight loss* secondary to impaired caloric intake completes the diagnostic symptom-complex of cricopharyngeal dysfunction. Symptoms of gastroesophageal reflux occur in 30% to 90% of patients with cricopharyngeal dysfunction, and it is unclear whether refluxed gastric acid is actually causing local irritation of the UES in these patients or whether distal esophageal reflux is triggering reflex incoordination of the pharyngoesophageal junction.[6, 28, 38]

The barium esophagogram in patients with cricopharyngeal dysfunction may be normal, particularly in those with intermittent symptoms, or demonstrate a spectrum of hypertonicity of the UES, a typical posterior cricopharyngeal bar, or a pharyngoesophageal (Zenker's) diverticulum (Figs. 26–9 to 26–11). A complete esophagogram, not one that focuses only on the cervical esophagus, should be obtained to rule out other significant esophageal pathology, particularly a hiatal hernia with gastroesophageal reflux or a distal tumor, which may produce symptoms that are referred to the cervical esophagus. Similarly, although esophagoscopy may provide little helpful information, it rules out neoplasm and reflux esophagitis, both of which can result in cervical dysphagia.

Esophageal function studies (manometry and acid reflux testing) should be performed whenever possible. Incoordination of the temporal relationship between pharyngeal contraction and cricopharyngeal relaxation has been reported to be responsible for the development of pharyngoesophageal diverticula.[17, 33] Abnormalities of thoracic esophageal peristalsis may be found in one third of patients with cricopharyngeal dysfunction, suggesting that the cervical esophageal complaints are only a manifestation of more generalized disordered esophageal motor function. Perhaps the most im-

indicating a purely psychological basis for a complaint of cervical dysphagia, is a diagnosis of exclusion made only after ruling out significant esophageal disease. After careful evaluation, few patients complaining of cervical dysphagia should have their symptoms ascribed to *nerves.*

Despite the variety of neurogenic and myogenic conditions involving the pharyngoesophageal junction, the resulting oropharyngeal dysphagia has a remarkably constant clinical presentation.[38] The patient complains of *cervical dysphagia,* which is localized between the thyroid cartilage and the suprasternal notch, a *lump in the throat,* a constriction around the neck, or occasionally pain radiating to the jaw and ears. *Expectoration of excessive saliva* is common in patients who are unable to swallow normally the 1 to 1.5 liters of saliva produced each day. Concomitant *intermittent hoarseness* often

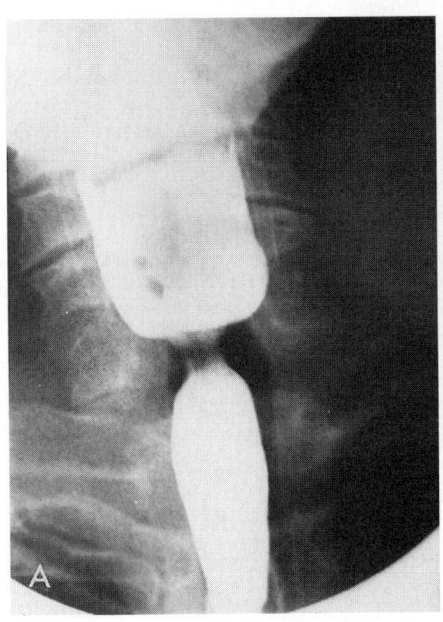
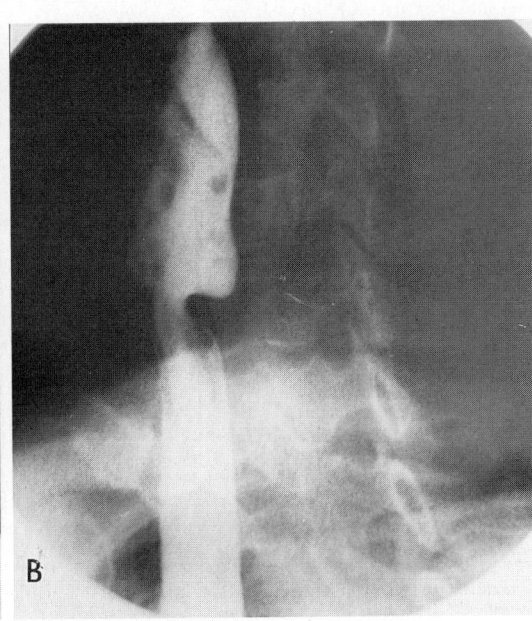

Figure 26-10. *A,* Typical appearance of hypertrophic cricopharyngeal sphincter (anteroposterior view). *B,* Lateral view showing posterior cricopharyngeal bar. (From Orringer, M. B.: Extended cervical esophagomyotomy for cricopharyngeal dysfunction. J. Thorac. Cardiovasc. Surg., *80*:669, 1980. Reprinted with permission from the Society of Thoracic Surgeons.)

portant information gained from esophageal function tests in these patients is the assessment with the intraesophageal pH electrode of distal high pressure zone competence. If a cervical esophagomyotomy for cricopharyngeal dysfunction is ultimately considered, knowledge of pre-existing gastroesophageal reflux allows appropriate postoperative positioning and reflux precautions.

In view of its multiple causes, the treatment of cricopharyngeal motor dysfunction must be individualized. Medical or surgical treatment of gastroesophageal reflux may eliminate secondary cervical complaints.[28] However, patients with severe cervical dysphagia but minimal or no reflux symptoms from their incompetent lower esophageal sphincter (LES) may be treated successfully with a cervical esophagomyotomy and institution of medical antireflux therapy without the need for an antireflux operation.[29, 38] Cervical dysphagia, a common presentation of myasthenia gravis, is relieved when the disease is under good medical control. Intermittent outpatient esophageal bougienage to the range of 54- to 56-French dilator may produce dramatic temporary relief of incapacitating cervical dysphagia in the patient with polymyositis, Parkinson's disease, or the residua of a midbrain (basilar artery) cerebrovascular accident. Alternatively, in the presence of incapacitating cervical dysphagia and aspiration and a radiographically or manometrically documented abnormal UES, a cervical esophagomyotomy is a relatively low-risk operation that may produce gratifying relief.

A cervical esophagomyotomy for cricopharyngeal dysfunction in the absence of Zenker's diverticulum is performed through a 5- to 8-cm. oblique left cervical incision centered at the level of the cricoid cartilage and paralleling the anterior border of the sternocleidomastoid muscle (Fig. 26–12). The sternocleidomastoid muscle and carotid sheath and its contents are retracted laterally, and the trachea is retracted medially. Care is taken to avoid placement of retractors on the tracheoesophageal groove and subsequent injury to the recurrent laryngeal nerve. The dissection proceeds directly posteriorly through the cervical fascial layers to the prevertebral fascia. The esophagus is immediately anterior to the preverte-

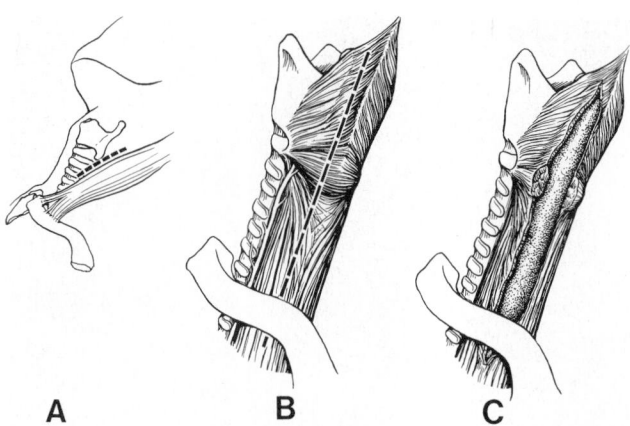

Figure 26–12. Cervical esophagomyotomy for cricopharyngeal dysfunction. *A,* A 5-cm. oblique skin incision anterior to the sternocleidomastoid muscle and centered over the cricoid cartilage. *B,* With a 40-French bougie within the esophagus, the esophagomyotomy is performed on the left posterolateral aspect of the esophagus to avoid injury to the recurrent laryngeal nerve, seen in the tracheoesophageal groove. *C,* Completed esophagomyotomy extends from the level of the superior cornu of the thyroid cartilage inferiorly to 1 to 2 cm. behind the clavicle. (From Orringer, M. B.: Extended cervical esophagomyotomy for cricopharyngeal dysfunction. J. Thorac. Cardiovasc. Surg., *80*:669, 1980. Reprinted with permission from the Society of Thoracic Surgeons.)

bral fascia. With a 40-French bougie within the esophagus, the cervical esophagomyotomy is performed on the posterolateral esophageal wall. The incision extends from the level of the tip of the superior cornu of the thyroid cartilage inferiorly to 1 to 2 cm. behind the clavicle and is 7 to 10 cm. long. This "extended" cervical esophagomyotomy is recommended to ensure division of all incoordinated UES muscle fibers. A cervical esophagomyotomy is successful in relieving cervical dysphagia from cricopharyngeal motor dysfunction in 65% to 85% of patients undergoing operation.[28, 38]

MOTOR DISORDERS OF THE BODY OF THE ESOPHAGUS

The esophageal motor disorders are best viewed as a continuum, with hypomotility (achalasia) at one extreme and hypermotility (diffuse spasm) at the other. Between these extremes are conditions such as vigorous achalasia, which has elements of both achalasia and esophageal spasm, as well as a variety of less well-characterized examples of neuromotor dysfunction. One of these latter conditions, *curling,* represents tertiary contractions of the esophagus that give rise to the *corkscrew* esophagus seen on barium swallow examination (Fig. 26–13). This abnormality may be seen in patients with DES or in those who are totally asymptomatic, particularly elderly patients who have an associated small, sliding hiatal hernia.

Nonspecific neuromotor esophageal dysfunction, that is, loss of generally progressive peristalsis and the appearance to varying degrees of simultaneous, weak-to-absent esophageal contractions after swallowing, is seen in numerous conditions, such as those characterized by peripheral neuropathy (diabetes, alcoholism), collagen vascular diseases (scleroderma, dermatomyositis), myasthenia gravis, multiple sclerosis, and amyotrophic lateral sclerosis. In none of these conditions is an absolutely diagnostic esophageal motor disturbance present, but, rather, an alteration of normal sequential peristaltic contractions with swallowing is often seen. As a muscular tube, the esophagus is limited in its response to these various neuromotor diseases. Thus, in the presence of distal obstruction from either tumor or a benign stricture, tertiary esophageal contractions may be seen in the body of

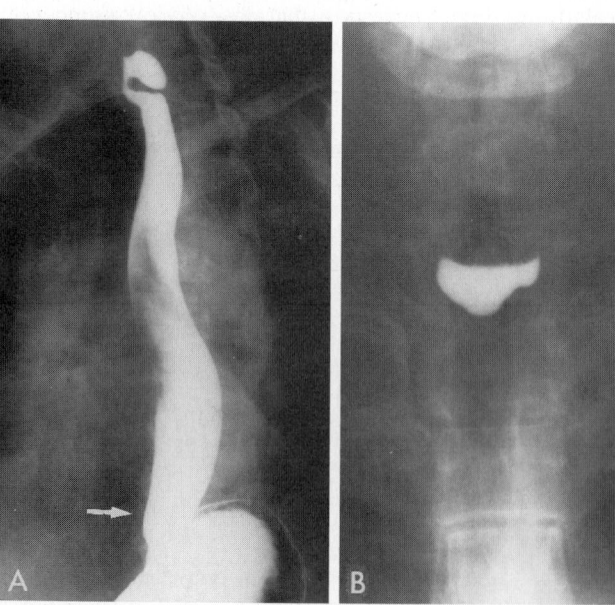

Figure 26–11. *A,* Zenker's diverticulum in a patient with an associated "patulous cardia" (arrow) and asymptomatic gastroesophageal reflux without esophagitis. *B,* Residual barium in the 2.5-cm. pouch (anteroposterior view). (From Orringer, M. B.: Extended cervical esophagomyotomy for cricopharyngeal dysfunction. J. Thorac. Cardiovasc. Surg., *80*:669, 1980. Reprinted with permission from the Society of Thoracic Surgeons.)

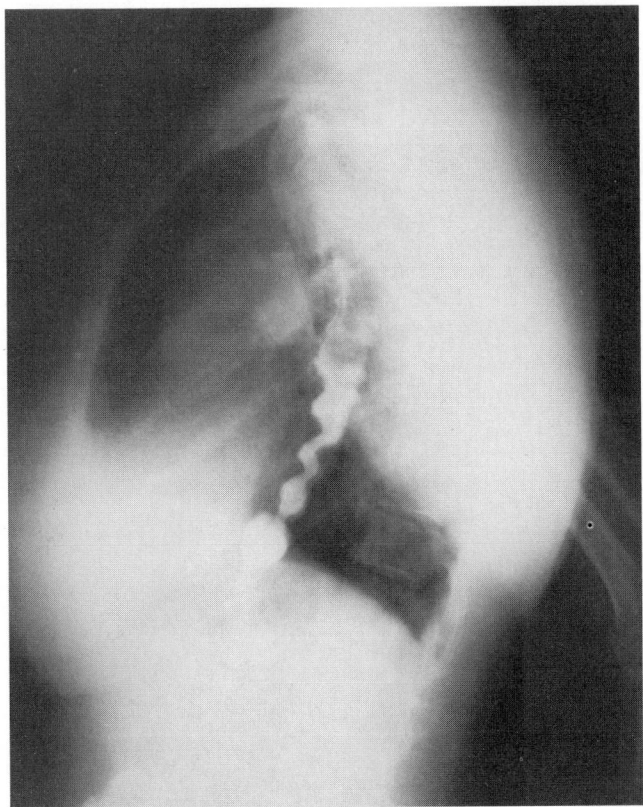

Figure 26–13. Esophagogram showing tertiary contractions of the circular muscle responsible for the characteristic *corkscrew* esophagus of diffuse esophageal spasm. This pattern may also be seen in totally asymptomatic individuals.

the esophagus, both radiographically and with motility studies. It must be remembered, therefore, that despite the emphasis on the need for esophageal function tests in assessing patients with neuromotor disorders of the esophagus, esophageal motility studies are only *one* facet of the total evaluation, and they should be interpreted in the light of the particular clinical situation, as well as the barium swallow and endoscopic findings.

ACHALASIA

The term *achalasia* is of Greek derivation and literally means "failure or lack of relaxation." Although this condition was originally described by Willis in 1674, the term was first coined by Hurst in 1915 as a reference to the failure of the LES in this disease to relax normally with swallowing. The name achalasia focuses on the distal sphincter, but the condition involves the entire esophageal body.

The etiology of achalasia is unknown, but the characteristic clinical, radiographic, and manometric findings have occurred following a variety of situations, including severe emotional stress, major physical trauma, Chagas' disease in South America, and drastic weight reduction in some markedly obese dieting patients. In Chagas' disease, caused by parasitic infestation by the leishmanial forms of *Trypanosoma cruzi*, the smooth muscle ganglionic cells of Auerbach's plexus are destroyed, resulting in motor dysfunction and progressive dilation not only of the esophagus but also of the colon, ureters, and other viscera. Histologic studies of autopsy and surgical specimens of the esophageal wall obtained at the time of esophagomyotomy have documented a loss of ganglion cells in the myenteric plexus as well as neuronal degeneration in patients with achalasia unrelated

to Chagas' disease. Various animal models suggest a relationship between either central or peripheral vagal nerve dysfunction and the development of achalasia, an achalasia-like picture being induced experimentally in dogs by vagal nerve injury and in cats by ablation of the dorsal motor nucleus of the vagus. Others have shown that in achalasia, cholecystokinin octapeptide produces a paradoxical rise in LES pressure from direct esophageal smooth muscle stimulation, suggesting that the underlying pathophysiology is loss of nonadrenergic, noncholinergic inhibitory nerves.[13] Except in Chagas' disease, the exact cause of the denervation is unknown. Although the exact mechanism remains unclear, the multiple conditions, including infections and physical and emotional stress, that seem to *trigger* achalasia seem to share a common pathway of altering either the central or peripheral vagal innervation of the esophagus or the ganglion cells of Auerbach's plexus.

The classic triad of presenting symptoms in achalasia includes dysphagia, regurgitation, and weight loss. Low retrosternal *hesitancy* or *sticking* of both solid food and liquids is typical, but the dysphagia is occasionally localized to the suprasternal notch. Stress or the ingestion of cold liquids may aggravate the symptoms. Patients with achalasia eat slowly, use large volumes of water to wash food into the stomach, and may contort their bodies, twisting the upper torso and elevating the chin and extending the neck, or may walk about the room in an effort to force down food. As more water is swallowed, the weight of the fluid column in the esophagus increases, along with the sensation of retrosternal fullness, until the LES is forced open, and sudden relief is felt as the esophagus empties. Retrosternal pain on swallowing (odynophagia) is *not* characteristic of achalasia but may occur in the early stages of the disease. Effortless regurgitation after eating, particularly on bending forward or reclining, is usually not associated with a sour taste of the undigested food in contrast to acid regurgitation in gastroesophageal reflux. With marked esophageal dilatation, eructation of foul-smelling stagnating intraesophageal contents may occur. Weight loss may be appreciable and is common.

Achalasia often results in recurrent respiratory symptoms due to aspiration pneumonitis, which may cause lung abscess, bronchiectasis, hemoptysis, or asthma (Fig. 26–14). Marked distention of the dilated esophagus may produce pronounced shortness of breath and dyspnea owing to displacement of adjacent intrathoracic organs (Fig. 26–15). Patients who give a history of soiling the pillow at night with regurgitated intraesophageal contents are invariably experiencing nocturnal tracheobronchial aspiration. Bleeding in achalasia is rare, and although it may be associated with retention esophagitis (discussed later), it is generally an ominous sign indicative of carcinoma. Achalasia is a premalignant esophageal lesion with carcinoma developing as a late complication in 1% to 10% of patients who have this condition an average of 15 to 25 years.[51] This is likely the result of mucosal irritation and subsequent metaplasia induced by the retention esophagitis. Esophageal carcinoma in achalasia tends to arise in the middle third of the organ, below the point at which the air-fluid level is most often seen on barium swallow examination and mucosal irritation is believed to be most pronounced. These tumors, usually squamous cell histologically, generally grow to a large size, unnoticed by the patient with a dilated esophagus and chronic dysphagia, and are hopelessly incurable unless detected fortuitously during surveillance esophagoscopy.

The radiographic appearance of achalasia varies with the extent of the disease, with the barium esophagogram showing mild dilation in the early stages and massive dilation, tortuosity, and a sigmoid shape in the later stages. Retained intraesophageal contents are typically seen. Peristalsis is dis-

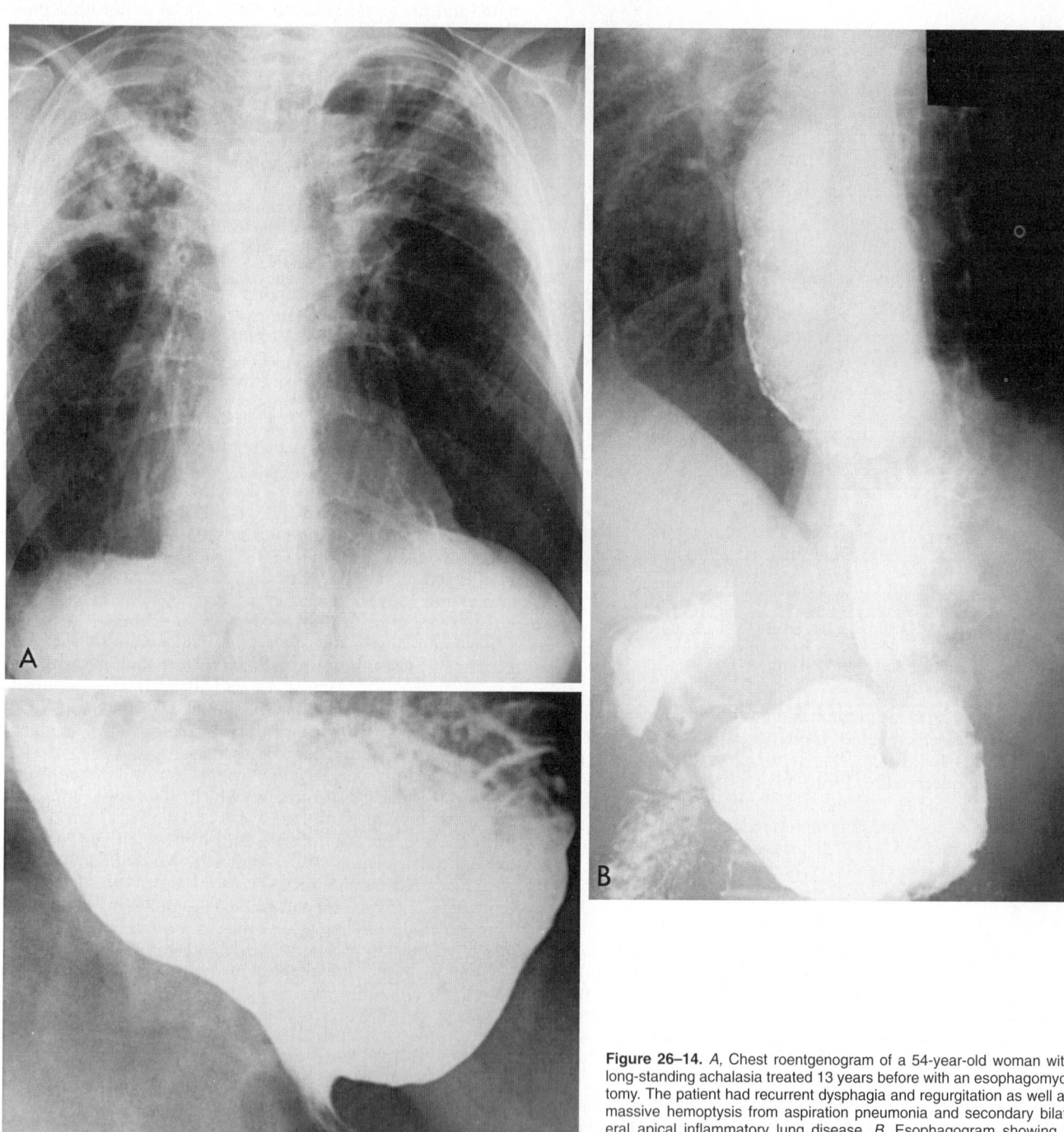

Figure 26–14. *A,* Chest roentgenogram of a 54-year-old woman with long-standing achalasia treated 13 years before with an esophagomyotomy. The patient had recurrent dysphagia and regurgitation as well as massive hemoptysis from aspiration pneumonia and secondary bilateral apical inflammatory lung disease. *B,* Esophagogram showing a megaesophagus with retained secretions in this patient. *C,* Detail of esophagogastric junction showing characteristic bird-beak taper of achalasia.

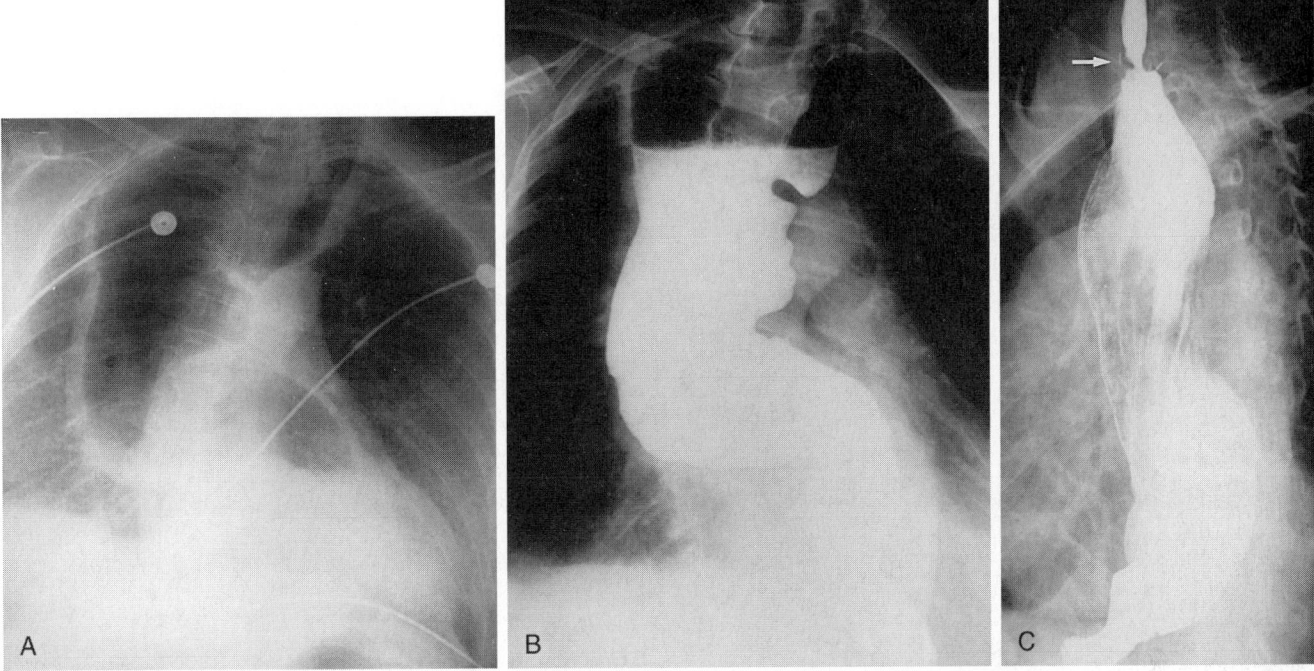

Figure 26–15. *A*, Chest roentgenogram of a 58-year-old woman who presented with respiratory distress and displacement of the trachea by a bulging cervical mass. A huge abnormal collection of air is seen in the mid thorax. *B*, Posteroanterior view from esophagogram showing an enormously dilated megaesophagus of achalasia that was responsible for the tracheal displacement and respiratory symptoms. *C*, Esophagogram after transhiatal esophagectomy without thoracotomy showing the esophageal substitute (stomach) within the posterior mediastinum in the original esophageal bed. Silver clip markers (arrow) indicate level of cervical esophagogastric anastomosis.

ordered in the early stages and totally lacking in the later stages. The roentgenographic hallmark of achalasia on barium swallow examination is the distal *bird-beak* taper of the esophagogastric junction (Fig. 26–16). The characteristic appearance of a *double mediastinal stripe* throughout the length of the chest on a posteroanterior view of the standard chest roentgenogram and a posterior mediastinal air-fluid level on a lateral view in a patient with typical symptoms are diagnostic of achalasia (Fig. 26–17).

The manometric criteria of achalasia are failure of the LES to relax reflexively with swallowing and lack of progressive peristalsis throughout the length of the esophagus. As the manometric recording catheter is withdrawn from the stomach into the esophagus, often there is absence of the normal fall in mean intraesophageal pressure below mean intragastric pressure as the thorax is entered, the pressure in the esophagus being higher than that below the diaphragm (Fig. 26–18). In the early stages of achalasia, contractions after swallowing may be of normal amplitude, but they are synchronous and simultaneous (Fig. 26–19). Later, contractions are either totally absent or weak and simultaneous (Fig. 26–20). Distal esophageal high pressure zone pressure is generally normal or somewhat elevated, but the marked hypertonicity of the spastic esophagus is not seen. Thus, the term *cardiospasm* is inappropriate when referring to achalasia. With mild esophageal dilation on the esophagogram, it may be difficult to differentiate early achalasia from diffuse spasm or scleroderma. Manometrically, however, administration of a mild vagomimetic agent (e.g., bethanechol [Urecholine]), produces marked elevation of intraesophageal pressure and increased amplitude and frequency of simultaneous esophageal contractions that correspond with the patient's complaint of chest pain (Fig. 26–21). This response does not occur in scleroderma but is common both in DES and achalasia. However, the patient with intermittent DES, unlike someone with achalasia, usually has some degree of progressive peri-

stalsis on standard manometric evaluation, and the LES shows reflex relaxation with swallowing. In their early stages, therefore, these two conditions can be differentiated manometrically.

Esophagoscopy is indicated in achalasia to rule out severe retention esophagitis, the possibility of associated carcinoma, a tumor of the cardia mimicking achalasia,[52] or a distal esophageal stricture from reflux esophagitis that may have followed prior forceful dilations or an esophagomyotomy that damaged the LES mechanism. Retention esophagitis in advanced achalasia is quite different endoscopically from reflux esophagitis. With chronic esophagitis due to reflux, the distal esophagus often appears whitish and fibrotic, with superficial mucosal ulceration. When there is prolonged retention esophagitis from achalasia, however, the irritating effects of putrifying food on the esophageal mucosa may induce severe edema, with reddish purple discoloration and marked friability. When performing esophagoscopy in the evaluation of achalasia, the presence of retained fluid and food in the dilated esophagus, even after an overnight fast, may complicate the procedure, and additional efforts to protect the airway are indicated (see Part V in this chapter).

Because this condition is incurable, and the derangement in esophageal motor function never returns to normal, the treatment of achalasia is purely palliative. Both the nonsurgical and surgical treatments of achalasia are directed toward relieving the obstruction caused by the nonrelaxing LES. In the early stages of the disease, before esophageal dilation occurs, sublingual nitroglycerin before or during meals, longacting nitrates, and calcium-channel blocking agents may improve swallowing. These drugs are most useful in the short-term treatment of achalasia before more definitive therapy or in elderly patients who are not candidates for other methods of treatment. Passage of mercury-weighted bougies in the 48- to 54-French range may relieve the dysphagia for several days or weeks but is seldom a satisfactory long-term

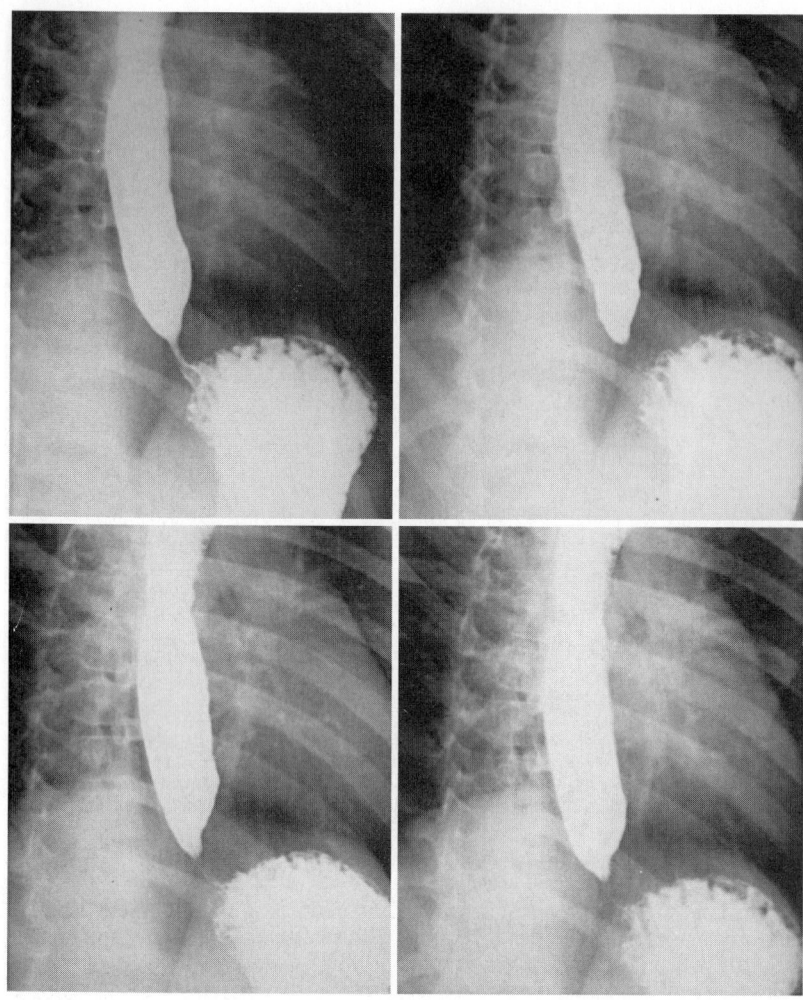

Figure 26–16. Multiple views from cine esophagogram in a patient with early achalasia showing a persistent *bird-beak* taper at the esophagogastric junction and impaired esophageal emptying.

solution. The most recent novel pharmacologic treatment of achalasia is intrasphincteric botulinum toxin injected into the LES through the flexible esophagoscope.[45] This potent neurotoxin inhibits release of acetylcholine from nerve endings and has been used with good results in a number of diseases characterized by muscle spasm (e.g., strabismus and various dystonias). Encouraging early results have been reported, but longer follow-up in patients with achalasia is needed before the efficacy of botulinum toxin can be established.

The two most widely used and analyzed methods of therapy for achalasia are forceful dilation, either pneumatic or hydrostatic, and esophagomyotomy. The comparative results of esophagomyotomy versus forceful dilatation for achalasia in 899 patients treated at the Mayo Clinic are shown in Table 26–3. Not only is esophagomyotomy safer than dilation (perforation occurs four times more often with dilatation, 4% vs. 1%), but it is also more reliable, providing good to excellent relief of dysphagia in 85% of patients, compared with 65% in patients treated with hydrostatic dilation. The late results of esophagomyotomy are also significantly better than those for forceful dilation.[37] Of the patients treated by hydrostatic dilation, 82% were treated once, 16% required two dilations, and 2% were dilated three times or more. Whereas the clearly superior results of esophagomyotomy make a strong argument for this approach as the preferred treatment of achalasia[11] the fact that 65% of patients undergoing forceful dilation have a good or excellent result cannot be ignored, particularly because both approaches are palliative, and the mortality for each is low. Gastroesophageal reflux secondary to disruption of the incoordinated LES is a potential compli-

cation of both methods of treatment. The Mayo Clinic data indicate no increased morbidity in patients undergoing esophagomyotomy after prior hydrostatic dilations. Others have also substantiated the effectiveness of forceful balloon dilation in achalasia, reporting good or excellent results in 77% of their patients so treated[4, 55] and an incidence of perforation ranging from 1% to 5%.[21, 53] When a perforation does occur after balloon dilation, it can usually be managed by having

TABLE 26–3. Comparison of Results of Hydrostatic Dilation and Esophagomyotomy (1949–1975)

Factors	Dilation (431 pts.)	Esophagomyotomy (466 pts.)
Mortality	2 (0.5)%	1 (0.2%)
Esophageal perforation	19 (4%)	5 (1%)
Requiring operation	10	3
Follow-up	311 (72%)	456 (97%)
Duration	1–18 yr	1–17 yr
Result		
Excellent	28 ⎫	50 ⎫
Good	37 ⎬65*	35 ⎬85*
Fair	16 ⎭	9 ⎭
Poor	19	6

*Significantly different (P <.001)
From Okike, N., Payne, W. S., Neufeld, D. M., et al.: Esophagomyotomy versus forceful dilation for achalasia of the esophagus: Results in 899 patients. Reprinted with permission from the Society of Thoracic Surgeons (The Annals of Thoracic Surgery, *28*:119, 1979).

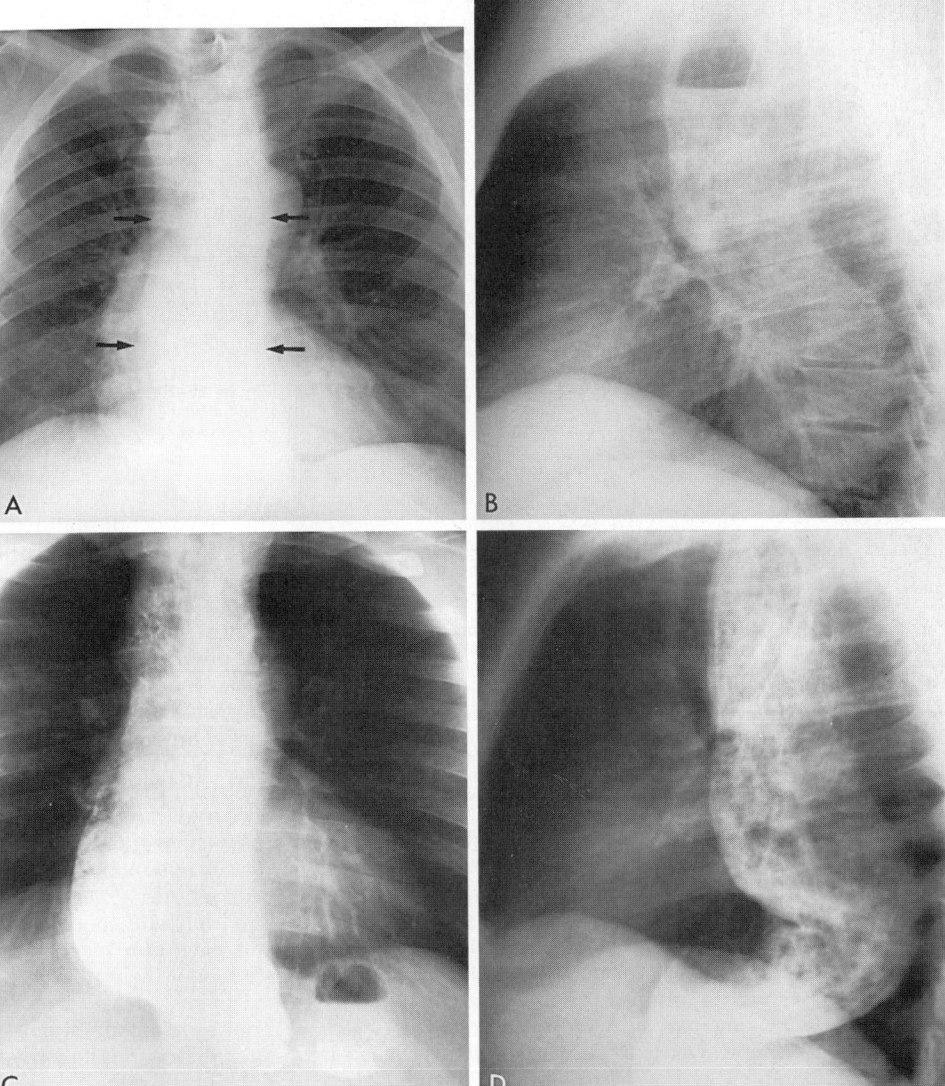

Figure 26–17. Posteroanterior (A) and lateral (B) chest roentgenograms in a patient with dysphagia, regurgitation, and weight loss. Note the double mediastinal stripe (arrows) on the posteroanterior view and the air-fluid level on the lateral view representing a dilated megaesophagus with retained secretions. These roentgenograms are virtually diagnostic of a megaesophagus of achalasia, which was confirmed with a barium esophagogram (posteroanterior [C] and lateral [D] views).

the patient refrain from eating for 1 to 3 days and by administering antibiotics and occasionally parenteral nutrition. Other significant complications of pneumatic dilation are infrequent, and late gastroesophageal reflux and esophagitis seem to occur in fewer than 1% of patients. Relative contraindications to balloon dilatation for achalasia include an extremely poor overall medical condition that would preclude repair if a perforation should occur, extremely young age (infants and small children); a tortuous sigmoid esophagus; a previous esophagomyotomy; and the presence of a concomitant sliding hiatal hernia. This list of contraindications has been revised and shortened as greater experience with balloon dilatation has been obtained, and pneumatic dilation has emerged as the most reasonable initial treatment for achalasia, while esophagomyotomy is reserved for those who fail to respond to dilation therapy.

The traditional transthoracic distal esophagomyotomy for achalasia is performed through a left thoracotomy and involves a 7- to 10-cm.-long vertical incision through the longitudinal and circular esophageal muscle layers, from the level of the inferior pulmonary vein superiorly down and across the lower sphincter inferiorly (Figs. 26–22 and 26–23). Transthoracic esophagomyotomy is a modification of the original transabdominal operation for achalasia described by the

German surgeon Heller in 1913, which involved an esophagomyotomy on both the anterior and posterior walls of the esophagogastric junction. In 1923 Zaaijer modified Heller's operation by performing the myotomy on only the anterior wall of the esophagus. Distal esophagomyotomy for achalasia has subsequently been performed successfully through either the abdominal or the thoracic routes.

Unresolved technical questions concern the distal extent of the esophagomyotomy and the need for a concomitant antireflux procedure.[22] Ellis has argued against an antireflux procedure at the time of esophagomyotomy, advocating a *short* esophagomyotomy carried onto the stomach only far enough to ensure complete division of the distal esophageal musculature but not to induce incompetence of the LES mechanism. With this approach he reports a late incidence of postoperative gastroesophageal reflux of 8%.[20] Similar results have been reported by others.[25] There are also reports that indicate an incidence of gastroesophageal reflux after an esophagomyotomy ranging from 3% to 50%.[8, 36] And many surgeons believe that complete relief of the obstruction caused by the incoordinated LES can be achieved only by rendering it incompetent, that is, intentionally carrying the esophagomyotomy onto the stomach for 1 to 2 cm.[8, 36] They stress that because the patient with achalasia has distal esophageal

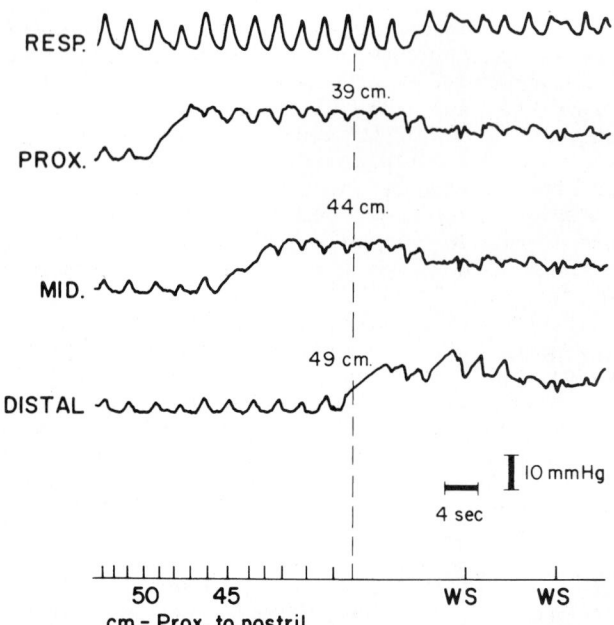

Figure 26–18. Motility tracing of the distal high pressure zone (HPZ) in achalasia. In contrast to the normal findings on withdrawing the recording catheter from the stomach into the esophagus (see Fig. 26–7) basal intraesophageal pressure is *greater* than that within the stomach. Furthermore, when the distal recording port is positioned in the HPZ and the patient swallows, there is neither reflex relaxation of the HPZ nor propagation of a progressive peristaltic contraction. WS, wet swallow.

obstruction, unless the incoordinated LES fibers are completely divided, dysphagia may not be relieved. Attempts by some to perform a *limited* esophagomyotomy without an antireflux procedure have resulted in an 8.3% incidence of reflux and a 20.8% incidence of inadequate relief of the distal esophageal obstruction.[32, 49] The majority of esophageal surgeons now carry out a complete esophagocardiomyotomy for achalasia with some type of fundoplication to prevent the subsequent development of gastroesophageal reflux. Whereas some have advocated a very loose, short 360-degree Nissen fundoplication, others have cautioned that the combination of a total fundoplication and an atonic esophagus may pro-

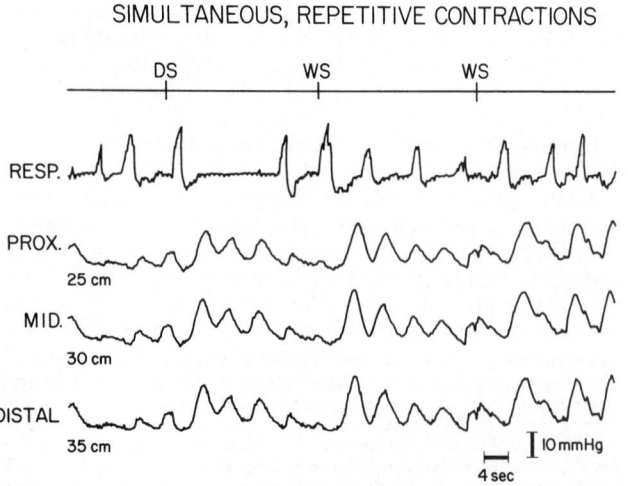

Figure 26–19. Motility tracing in early achalasia with minimal esophageal dilation on barium esophagogram. Esophageal contractions after swallowing are of normal amplitude, but they are simultaneous, multiphasic, and nonprogressive. DS, dry swallow; WS, wet swallow.

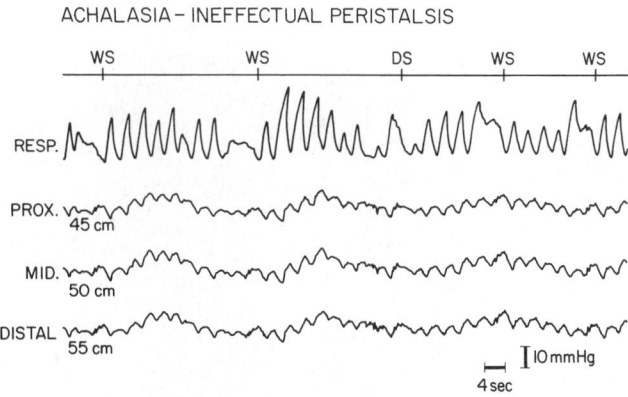

Figure 26–20. Motility tracing in advanced achalasia with megaesophagus contractions on barium esophagogram. Virtually no esophageal contractions are generated by swallowing. DS, dry swallow; WS, wet swallow.

duce obstruction that becomes more evident with long-term follow-up.[16] A partial fundoplication of the Belsey[5] or Dor types[24, 26, 48, 54] seems more satisfactory in controlling gastroesophageal reflux after an esophagomyotomy for achalasia, because these procedures provide good reflux control without producing an overcompetent LES that produces relative distal esophageal obstruction. Excellent long-term results suggest that a distal esophagomyotomy combined with a partial fundoplication may be the surgical approach of choice in achalasia. But even when this approach has been taken, gradual further deterioration of esophageal function over time and the late development of gastroesophageal reflux and esophagitis may jeopardize the late result.[35] More recently, minimally invasive video-assisted techniques have been used to accomplish an esophagomyotomy, both laparoscopically and thoracoscopically.[1, 2, 46, 51] Sufficient experience and long-term follow-up are not yet available to judge the efficacy of these newer approaches in achalasia.

Patients with recurrent esophageal obstruction following a prior esophagomyotomy or a reflux-induced peptic stricture after either esophagomyotomy or forceful dilation pose a difficult dilemma for the surgeon. Only two thirds undergoing a repeat esophagomyotomy benefit from the operation, and even poorer results occur after a fundoplication for reflux symptoms.[18] A more reliable approach may be esophageal

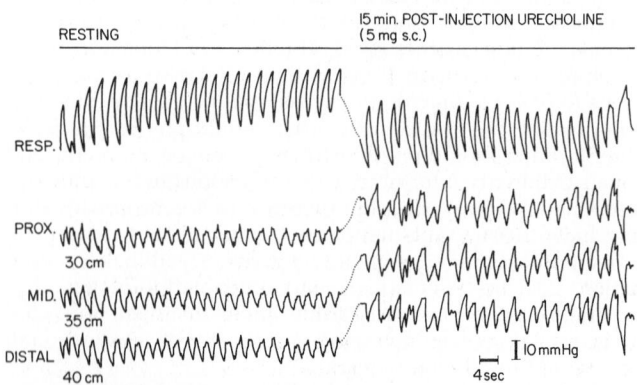

Figure 26–21. Motility tracing showing characteristic manometric response of achalasic esophagus to administration of cholinergic drug, in this case, bethanechol (Urecholine), 10 mg. subcutaneously. An elevation of the resting pressures in all recording catheters as well as an increase in the frequency and amplitude of spontaneous simultaneous esophageal contractions are seen. Chest pain and regurgitation may also be experienced by the patient. Both the symptoms and the manometric changes are reversed by administering atropine, 0.4 mg., intravenously. Similar findings are seen in the patient with diffuse esophageal spasm, but not in scleroderma.

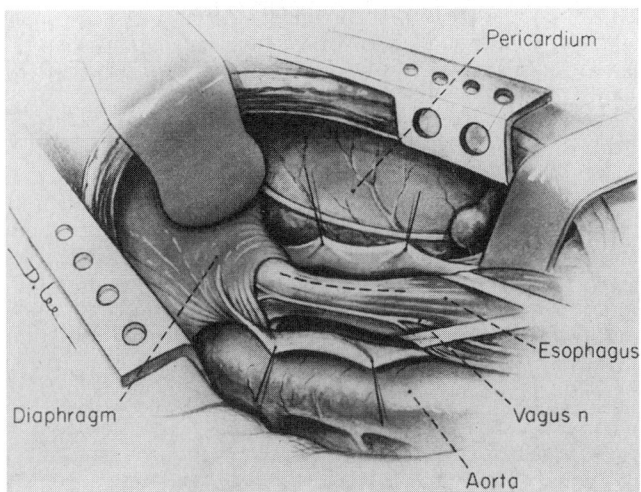

Figure 26–22. Transthoracic exposure of the distal esophagus for esophagomyotomy. After dividing the inferior pulmonary ligament and retracting the lung superiorly, the mediastinal pleura is opened and the esophagus and vagus nerves are encircled with a rubber drain. (From Ellis, F. H., Jr., Kaiser, J. C., Schlegel, J. F., Earlam, R. J., McVey, J. L., and Olsen, A. M.: Esophagomyotomy for esophageal achalasia: Experimental, clinical, and manometric aspects. Ann. Surg., *166*:640, 1967.)

resection and visceral esophageal substitution, preferably with stomach, which provides definitive treatment of the esophageal abnormality, eliminates the late risk of carcinoma, and can be accomplished transhiatally without opening the thorax. This approach is being used with increased frequency in patients with failed prior operations for achalasia or in those with advanced achalasia and a megaesophagus that may fail to empty adequately even after an esophagomyotomy (see Fig. 26–15).[9, 44, 47]

DIFFUSE ESOPHAGEAL SPASM AND RELATED HYPERMOTILITY DISORDERS

Diffuse esophageal spasm is a poorly understood and equally poorly treated hypermotility disorder in which patients experience chest pain and/or dysphagia as a result of repetitive, simultaneous, high-amplitude esophageal contractions. The etiology of DES is unknown. The patient with DES is typically anxious and complains of chest pain inconsistently related to eating, exertion, and position. The character of the chest pain may mimic that of angina pectoris due to coronary artery disease, often being described as squeezing, oppressive, retrosternal pressure that has a variable intensity and radiates toward the jaw, down the arms, and frequently straight through to the intrascapular region of the back. Symptoms are often greatest during periods of emotional stress, but the occasional association of dysphagia with the chest pain suggests an esophageal rather than a cardiac abnormality. Although patients may experience slow emptying of the esophagus, obstructive symptoms are uncommon, and regurgitation of food is unusual. Many patients, however, experience regurgitation of intraesophageal saliva (phlegm or foam) during bouts of the esophageal colic. Ingestion of cold liquids or foods may aggravate DES, as can gastroesophageal reflux. Most patients with DES, however, do *not* have associated gastroesophageal reflux. A history of irritable bowel syndrome, pylorospasm, spastic colon, or other functional gastrointestinal complaints is common; and gallstones, peptic ulcer disease, and pancreatitis can all trigger DES.

The initial evaluation of the patient with DES is essentially the same as that of the patient with chest pain of undetermined etiology: chest roentgenogram and standard electro-

cardiogram. In the cardiac-oriented Western society, despite a normal electrocardiogram, stress electrocardiogram, and dipyridamole thallium cardiac scan in a patient with recurrent chest pain, a cardiac catheterization in search of coronary artery disease is frequently considered before less invasive evaluation of the esophagus with a contrast study and esophageal function tests. By the time an esophageal evaluation is undertaken, significant coronary artery disease often has already been ruled out with a cardiac catheterization or the patient has even undergone coronary artery bypass but still has persistent chest pain.

A careful history is among the most important aspects of the diagnosis of DES, and causative intra-abdominal pathology (e.g., gallstones, gastritis, or peptic ulcer disease) should be excluded. The roentgenographic findings of DES are frustratingly variable (Fig. 26–24). At times, classic *curling* or a corkscrew esophagus caused by segmental contractions of the circular muscle may be apparent; but not infrequently, little if any impairment of peristalsis or even a distal beaklike taper, suggesting early achalasia is seen. An esophageal wall thickness of more than 5 mm. on a barium swallow examination suggests esophageal muscular hypertrophy in the patient with symptoms of DES. A hiatal hernia and/or gastroesophageal reflux may be seen. The finding of an esophageal pulsion diverticulum, particularly in a patient with anginalike symptoms, is virtually diagnostic of DES. Esophagoscopy should be performed in the patient with DES, because a distal esophageal obstructing lesion may produce proximal tertiary esophageal contractions that are confused with DES on barium study, and an infiltrating tumor, esophageal fibrosis, or esophagitis causing radiographic distal esophageal narrowing should be ruled out.

Although diagnosed with esophageal manometry, DES is typically characterized by *intermittent* episodes of spasm, and unless the patient is experiencing spasm at the time of the manometric study, just as with the barium esophagogram, the results may be entirely normal. The evaluation of the patient with DES is difficult because some of the radio-

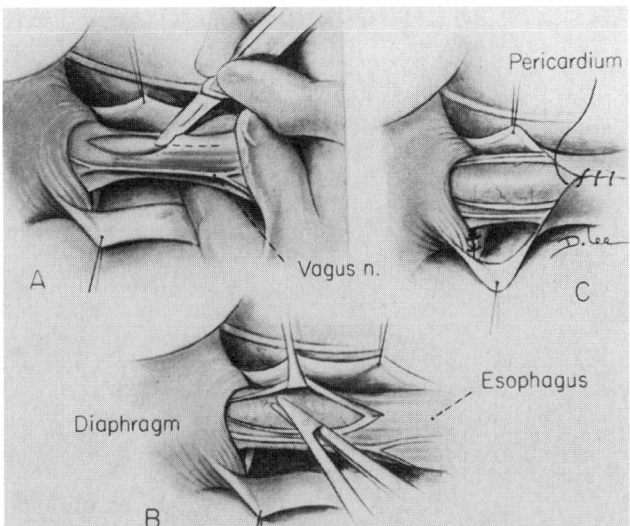

Figure 26–23. Technique of transthoracic esophagomyotomy. *A,* The longitudinal and circular esophageal muscle fibers are incised from beyond the esophagogastric junction to the level of the inferior pulmonary vein. *B,* The muscle layers of the esophagus are dissected away from the mucosa and submucosa for at least 50% of the circumference. *C,* When the esophagomyotomy is completed, the esophagogastric junction is restored to an intra-abdominal location after addition of a modified Belsey fundoplication, and the crura are approximated posterior to the esophagus. (From Ellis, F. H., Jr., Kaiser, J. C., Schlegel, J. F., Earlam, R. J., McVey, J. L., and Olsen, A. M.: Esophagomyotomy for esophageal achalasia: Experimental, clinical, and manometric aspects. Ann Surg., *166*:640, 1967.)

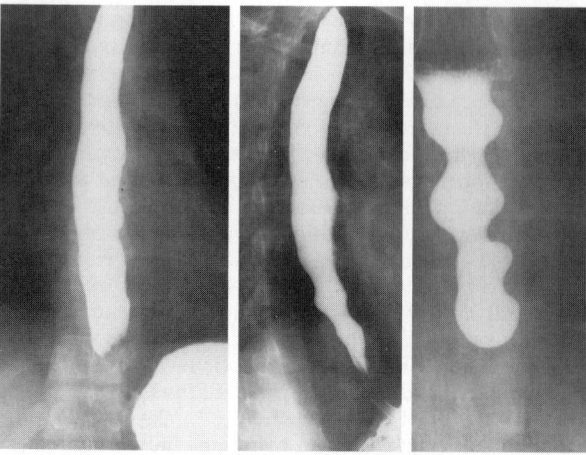

Figure 26–24. Three views from barium esophagograms in the same patient with intermittent diffuse esophageal spasm showing wide variability of roentgenographic findings in this condition, from a virtually normal appearance (left), to a distal esophageal taper suggesting achalasia (center), to a typical *corkscrew* esophagus (right). Esophageal manometry is essential for establishing a diagnosis in such a patient.

and providing reassurance is therapeutic and a great source of relief. Those complaining of dysphagia should avoid stress during meals as well as *trigger* foods or drinks. Psychiatric family counseling may be useful. If symptoms of gastroesophageal reflux are present, or if gastroesophageal reflux is documented with esophageal function tests, medical treatment of reflux should be instituted. Antispasmodics are occasionally helpful. The response of DES to sublingual nitroglycerin is variable but may be dramatic. Patients in whom sublingual nitroglycerin administered before meals is effective for intermittent bouts of pain or dysphagia may find more sustained relief with long-acting nitrates. Calcium channel blockers (e.g., nifedipine and diltiazem) may also be of benefit. Esophageal dilation with Hurst-Maloney bougies (50 to 60 French) may relieve dysphagia and chest pain from

graphic and manometric criteria of this disorder are seen in asymptomatic patients and the factors responsible for producing esophageal pain in these patients have not been established. The issue is further confounded by the inclusion of a variety of related hypermotility disorders, such as *nutcracker esophagus,* hypertensive LES, nonspecific esophageal motility disorders, and vigorous achalasia under the generic heading *diffuse esophageal spasm.* These conditions, however, are best defined by precise manometric criteria, an understanding of which provides an objective rationale for differentiating them in the evaluation of the patient with chest pain of esophageal origin (Table 26–4). The classic manometric criteria of DES are simultaneous, multiphasic, repetitive, often high-amplitude contractions that occur after a swallow and spontaneously in the smooth muscle portion of the esophagus (Fig. 26–25). Occasional progressive peristalsis may be seen but is most often present in the upper third of the esophagus. UES and LES resting pressures and relaxation with swallowing are usually normal, although a hypertensive LES with sustained contractions after swallowing may be seen. When standard manometry fails to demonstrate DES, evocative maneuvers using ice water or hydrochloric acid intraesophageal infusions or the administration of bethanechol, pentagastrin, or ergonovine may induce the motility disorder. The diagnostic hallmark of DES is the correlation of subjective complaints with objective evidence of spasm on manometric tracings (Fig. 26–26).

Because of the general lack of understanding of the etiology of this condition, it is not surprising that the treatment of DES is far from satisfactory. Many patients with esophageal spasm have an underlying psychiatric abnormality. The gut has long been known to be sensitive to emotional stimuli, and the striking clinical similarities between esophageal spasm and irritable bowel syndrome seem far from coincidental. Both the esophageal and colonic abnormalities, for example, are manifested by stress or reflex-induced spastic contractions, both occur predominantly in women, and both are associated with psychiatric disturbances. Documented psychiatric disorders, including depression, psychosomatic complaints, and anxiety, have been reported in more than 80% of patients with esophageal manometric contraction abnormalities.[10]

For many patients with DES, simply establishing an esophageal etiology for their previously unexplained chest pain

TABLE 26–4. Manometric Criteria of Primary Esophageal Motility Disorders

Normal

1. LES pressure 15–25 mm. Hg (never > 45 mm. Hg) with normal relaxation with swallowing
2. Mean amplitude of distal esophageal peristaltic wave 30–100 mm. Hg (never > 190 mm. Hg)
3. Simultaneous contractions occurring after < 10% of wet swallows
4. Monophasic waveforms (with not more than two peaks)
5. Duration of distal esophageal peristaltic wave: 2–6 seconds
6. No repetitive contractions

Primary Motility Disorders

Achalasia

1. Aperistalsis in esophageal body
2. Partial or absent LES relaxation with swallowing
3. LES pressure normal or > 45 mm. Hg
4. Intraesophageal basal pressure > intragastric

Diffuse Esophageal Spasm (DES)

1. Simultaneous (nonperistaltic) contractions
   a. Repetitive (at least three peaks)
   b. Increased duration (> 6 seconds)
2. Spontaneous contractions
3. Intermittent normal peristalsis
4. Contractions may be of increased amplitude

Nutcracker Esophagus

1. Mean peristaltic amplitude (10 wet swallows) in distal esophagus > 180 mm. Hg
2. Increased duration of contractions (> 6 seconds) frequent
3. Normal peristaltic sequences

Hypertensive LES

1. LES pressures > 45 mm. Hg but with normal relaxation
2. Normal esophageal peristalsis

Nonspecific Esophageal Motility Disorders

1. No or decreased amplitude of peristalsis
   a. Normal LES pressure
   b. Normal LES relaxation
2. Abnormal peristalsis, including any of the following:
   a. Abnormal waveforms
   b. Isolated simultaneous contractions
   c. Isolated spontaneous contractions
   d. Normal peristalsis sequence maintained
   e. LES normal

Vigorous Achalasia

1. Repetitive simultaneous contractions in body of esophagus (as with DES)
2. Partial or absent LES relaxation (as with achalasia)

Modified from Khan, A. A., and Castell, D. O.: Primary diffuse esophageal spasm and related disorders. *In* Jamieson, G. G. (Ed.): Surgery of the Oesophagus. Edinburgh, Churchill-Livingstone, 1988, pp. 483–488.

DIFFUSE ESOPHAGEAL SPASM

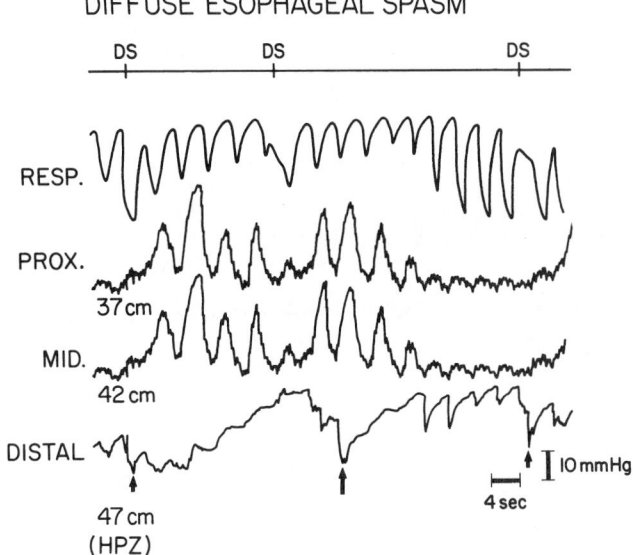

Figure 26–25. Motility tracing in diffuse esophageal spasm. This condition is characterized by simultaneous, nonprogressive, multiphasic esophageal contractions occurring both spontaneously and after swallowing. Unlike achalasia, however, reflex relaxation (arrows) of the distal sphincter with swallowing is still apparent. DS, dry swallow; HPZ, distal high-pressure zone.

DES for weeks to months and can be repeated on an outpatient basis as required. The use of pneumatic dilatation to treat DES is not generally advised because of concern that forceful dilatation of a hypertonic, spastic esophagus may result in a major tear.

Although thoracic esophagomyotomy has been advocated by some in the treatment of DES,[19, 23, 55] the results are much less reliable and favorable than in achalasia, with variable success being achieved in perhaps only 50% to 60% of patients. Despite apparent improvement in the manometric and radiographic indicators of DES after esophagomyotomy, patients may continue to complain of chest pain and slow emptying of the esophagus. When the spasm is secondary to gastroesophageal reflux, and LES competence is restored with an antireflux operation, relief of both reflux symptoms and those due to spasm may be gratifying. Unfortunately, however, *long-term* relief from the pain of DES is seldom achieved, and pain may persist despite a competent LES, multiple esophagomyotomies, and even total thoracic esophagectomy with visceral esophageal substitution.[42] Therefore, only in the most *extenuating circumstances,* when a patient is virtually incapacitated by chest pain or dysphagia, or in the presence of a pulsion diverticulum of the intrathoracic esophagus (to be discussed), should an esophagomyotomy be performed for DES.

The long esophagomyotomy for DES originally advocated by Ellis in 1960 differed from that used in achalasia in that its superior extent was the level of the aortic arch. It was proposed that the proximal extent of esophageal spasm on manometric evaluation dictates the level of the superior extent of the esophagomyotomy at operation. However, it is impossible to extrapolate with precision in the operating room esophageal manometric findings. Therefore, Henderson and Pearson favored a thoracic esophagomyotomy extended as high as possible, if necessary, under the aortic arch and into the superior mediastinum to the level of the thoracic inlet.[31] If only the distal two thirds of the esophageal circular muscle is divided, high retrosternal chest pain and dysphagia may persist because of residual spasm in the upper third of the esophagus. As is the case with achalasia, controversy

exists regarding the need to extend the myotomy entirely through the LES and onto the stomach, rather than limiting its distal extent to avoid the development of subsequent gastroesophageal reflux. However, because the potential for bouts of uncorrected spasm and obstruction exists so long as the distal circular esophageal muscle fibers remain undivided, the author endorses Belsey's view that the incision should be carried onto the stomach for at least 1 cm. to ensure that all circular esophageal muscle fibers have been divided. The incompetent LES mechanism thereby created should then be reconstructed with a modified Belsey-Mark IV operation.[5] A poorly contracting esophagus after an esophagomyotomy contraindicates a 360-degree fundoplication for reflux control in these patients, just as is the case with achalasia.

The *nutcracker* or *super-squeeze* esophagus is a hypermotility disorder characterized by extremely high-amplitude (up to 225 to 430 mm. Hg) progressive peristaltic contractions, often of prolonged duration. Symptoms of chest pain, dysphagia, and odynophagia are like those of DES, and treatment considerations are similar. Some patients develop clinical and manometric findings with elements of both achalasia and DES and are characterized as having vigorous achalasia. As in patients with achalasia, dysphagia and regurgitation are common in these patients, but chest pain typical of DES also occurs. Segmental spasm, rather than esophageal dilation, is often seen on barium swallow examination. Esophageal manometry demonstrates failure of normal LES relaxation (as in achalasia), lack of progressive peristalsis, and powerful, simultaneous, and repetitive esophageal contractions after swallowing (as in DES).

SCLERODERMA

Esophageal motor disturbances occur in several of the collagen vascular diseases, such as dermatomyositis, polymyositis, and lupus erythematosus, but particularly in scleroderma. Scleroderma, or systemic sclerosis, is a disease of unknown etiology that is characterized by induration of the skin, fibrous replacement of the smooth muscle of internal organs, and progressive loss of visceral and cutaneous function. Disruption of normal esophageal peristalsis is so common in scleroderma that it is recognized as a major diagnostic sign of the disease, particularly in acrosclerosis, the type of scleroderma associated with Raynaud's phenomenon but without the typical skin changes. As fibrous replacement of esophageal smooth muscle progresses, the distal esophageal

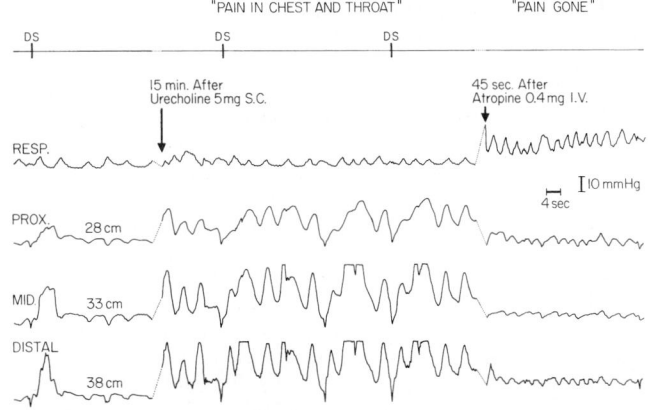

Figure 26–26. Motility tracing showing positive Urecholine test in diffuse esophageal spasm. The vagomimetic drug results in the development of both manometric and symptomatic esophageal spasm, both of which are eliminated within seconds of administering atropine, 0.4 mg., intravenously. DS, dry swallow.

SCLERODERMA – LACK OF HPZ

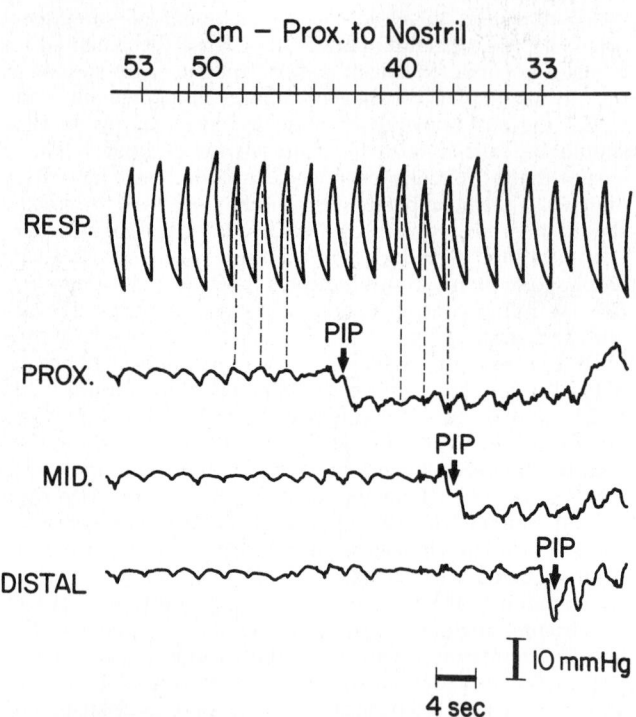

Figure 26–27. Motility tracing showing the resting-pressure profile of the gastro-esophageal junction in scleroderma. As the recording catheter is withdrawn from the stomach into the esophagus there is virtual lack of a distal esophageal high-pressure zone (HPZ). Distal to the pressure inversion point (PIP), there is an intra-abdominal pressure pattern, with peak intraluminal pressures occurring at the height of inspiration. Proximal to this point, within the thorax, intraesophageal pressures are negative at the peak of inspiration. For subsequent acid reflux testing (see Fig. 26–28), the intraesophageal pH probe is positioned 5 cm. proximal to the PIP. (From Orringer, M. B., Dabich, L., Zarafonetis, C. J., and Sloan, H.: Gastroesophageal reflux in esophageal scleroderma: Diagnosis and implications. Reprinted with permission from the Society of Thoracic Surgeons [The Annals of Thoracic Surgery, 22:120, 1976].)

high pressure zone loses its tone and normal response to swallowing and gastroesophageal reflux occurs (Figs. 26–27 and 26–28). In the distal two thirds to three quarters of the esophagus, normal progressive peristalsis gives way to weak, simultaneous, nonpropulsive contractions (Fig. 26–29). Patients initially complain of slow emptying of the esophagus, requiring large amounts of water to wash food into the stomach. Heartburn and gastroesophageal reflux are often severe. The prolonged duration of contact between refluxed gastric acid and the esophageal mucosa that occurs because

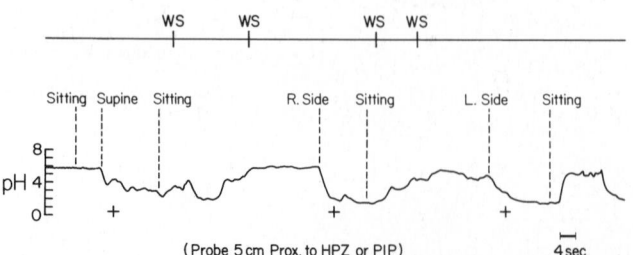

Figure 26–28. Strongly positive (3+) acid reflux test in the same patient with scleroderma as in Figure 26–27. Gastroesophageal reflux (+), indicated by drops in intraesophageal pH below 4, occurs whenever the patient assumes a supine position or lies on either side. WS, wet swallow; HPZ, distal high-pressure zone; PIP, pressure inversion point. (From Orringer, M. B., Dabich, L., Zarafonetis, C. J., and Sloan, H.: Gastroesophageal reflux in esophageal scleroderma: Diagnosis and implications. Reprinted with permission from the Society of Thoracic Surgeons [The Annals of Thoracic Surgery, 22:120, 1976].)

SCLERODERMA – APERISTALSIS

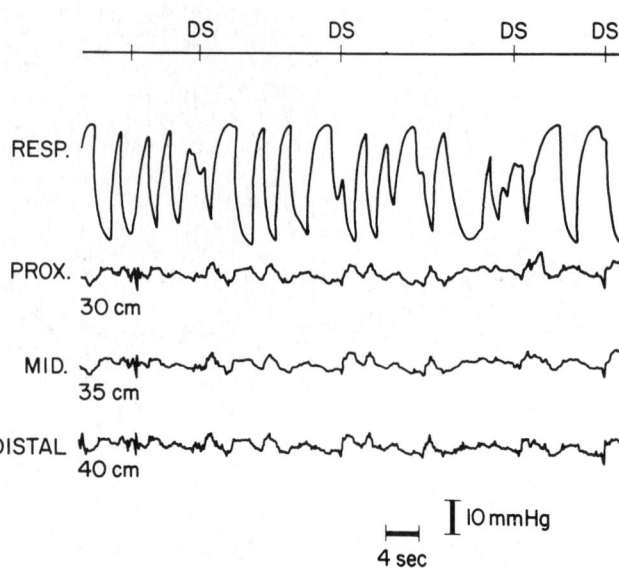

Figure 26–29. Motility tracing showing aperistalsis in esophageal scleroderma. There is a lack of effective peristalsis with swallowing in the distal esophagus. DS, dry swallow. (From Orringer, M. B., Dabich, L., Zarafonetis, C. J., and Sloan, H.: Gastroesophageal reflux in esophageal scleroderma: Diagnosis and implications. Reprinted with permission from the Society of Thoracic Surgeons [The Annals of Thoracic Surgery, 22:120, 1976].)

of impaired ability of the atonic lower esophagus to clear refluxed gastric contents back into the stomach results in accelerated reflux esophagitis (Fig. 26–30).[40] The barium esophagogram is a relatively crude early indicator of esophageal pathology in these patients, and esophageal manometry and acid reflux testing with the intraesophageal pH electrode are the most sensitive means of defining both the motility disorder and abnormal gastroesophageal reflux. At esophagoscopy, ulcerative distal esophagitis, with or without significant stricture formation, is common.

Although death from cardiac, renal, and pulmonary involvement is common, with proper medical management, 5-year survival from the time of the initial diagnosis of scleroderma varies from 33% to 70%. A standard antireflux medical regimen with the addition of H_2-blockers (e.g., cimetidine or ranitidine) and, more recently, omeprazole, generally controls the reflux symptoms and esophagitis associated with scleroderma esophageal involvement. In patients with intractable symptoms or persistent ulcerative esophagitis, however, surgical control of gastroesophageal reflux should be considered. Despite inferences about poor general wound healing in scleroderma based on the well-known chronicity of fingertip ulcerations that so commonly occur in association with Raynaud's phenomenon, sclerodactyly, and poor peripheral circulation, these patients can successfully undergo antireflux operation without an increased rate of complications.[30, 43] Use of the combined Collis gastroplasty-fundoplication procedures (Figs. 26–31 to 26–33) instead of the *standard* antireflux operations—the Hill, Belsey, or Nissen—has particular merit in the patient with scleroderma who typically has severe esophagitis, stricture formation, and fibrinoid degeneration and atrophy of distal esophageal smooth muscle that jeopardize the long-term success of the traditional operations. In selected patients with advanced esophageal scleroderma manifested by either marked dilation on a barium esophagogram or a severe reflux stricture that is refractory to dilatation and medical therapy, transhiatal esophagectomy without thoracotomy and construction of a cervical esophagogastric anastomosis may effectively eliminate reflux esophagitis and restore the ability to swallow comfortably.[39]

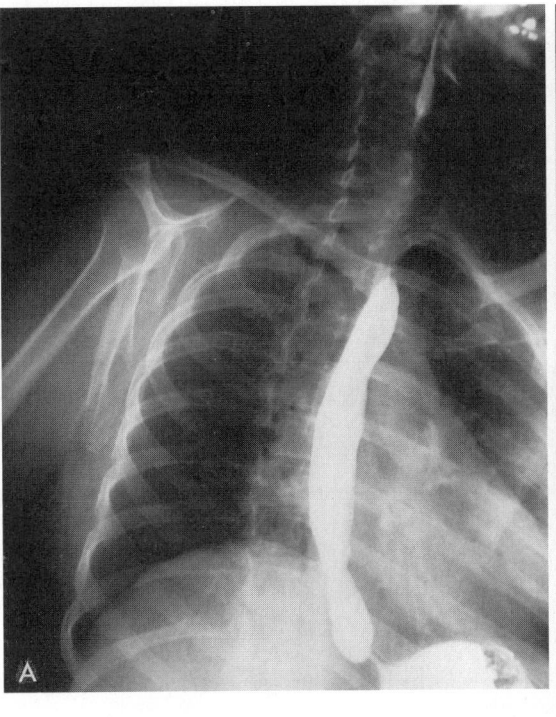
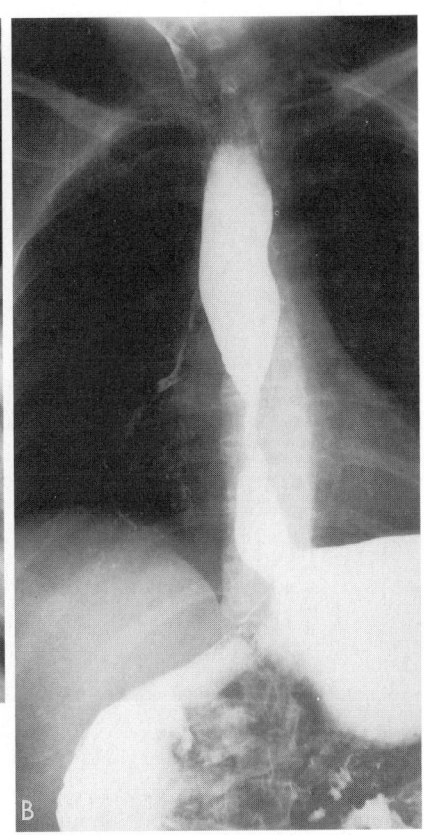

Figure 26–30. Progression of reflux esophagitis in scleroderma. *A,* Normal esophagogram at the time scleroderma was diagnosed (1969). *B,* Same patient (1974) with esophageal dilation proximal to a stricture and aspiration of barium in the right middle lobe secondary to the obstruction. (From Orringer, M. B., Dabich, L., Zarafonetis, C. J., and Sloan, H.: Gastroesophageal reflux in esophageal scleroderma: Diagnosis and implications. Reprinted with permission from the Society of Thoracic Surgeons [The Annals of Thoracic Surgery, *22*:120, 1976].)

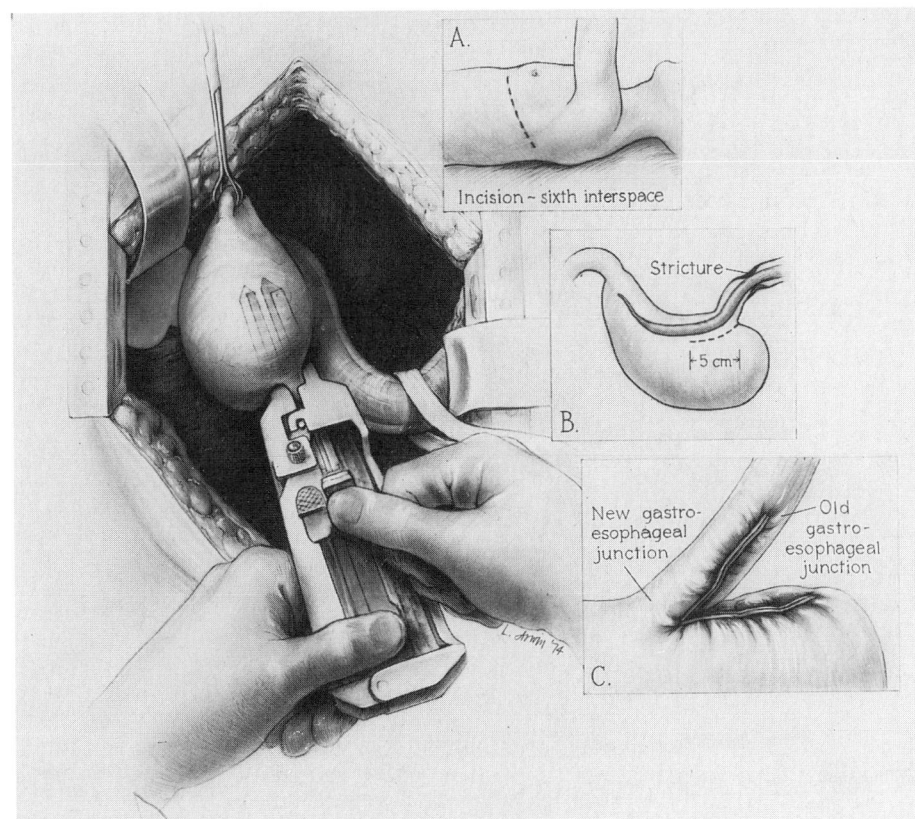

Figure 26–31. Construction of the Collis gastroplasty tube with the GIA surgical stapler. *A,* Mobilization of the esophagus and gastric fundus is performed through a lateral thoracotomy in the sixth or seventh left intercostal space. *B,* A 54- or 56-French Maloney dilator is passed through the esophagogastric junction and displaced against the lesser curvature of the stomach, and the stapler is applied. The knife assembly is advanced (main illustration), and the stapler is removed. The staple suture line is oversewn with a running 4-0 Prolene Lembert stitch. *C,* The result is a 5-cm. long gastric tube extension into the esophagus. (From Orringer, M. B., and Sloan, H.: Collis-Belsey reconstruction of the esophagogastric junction: Indications, physiology, and technical considerations. J. Thorac. Cardiovasc. Surg., *71*:295, 1976.)

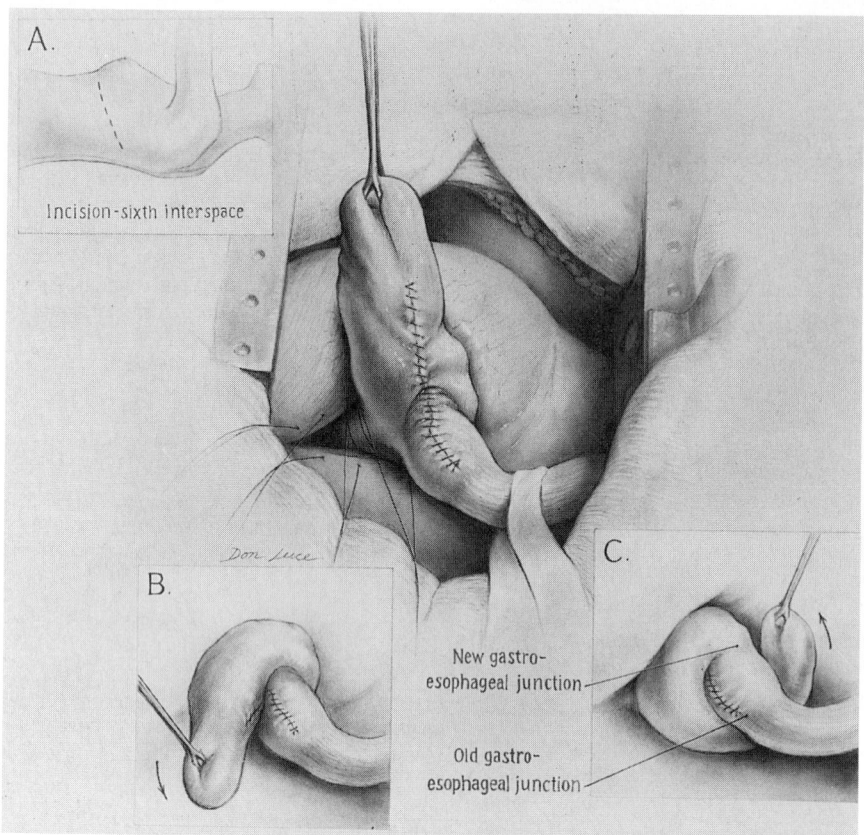

Figure 26–32. The combined Collis-Nissen reconstruction of the esophagogastric junction. Main drawing illustrates the elongated, narrowed gastric fundus available for fundoplication after completion of the Collis procedure. Inset *A* shows the placement of the left thoracotomy. Insets *B* and *C* show the gastric fundus being wrapped around the gastroplasty tube and adjacent stomach. The posterior crural sutures are placed but left untied until the fundoplication is reduced below the diaphragm. (From Orringer, M. B., and Sloan, H.: Combined Collis-Nissen reconstruction of the esophagogastric junction. Reprinted with permission from the Society of Thoracic Surgeons [The Annals of Thoracic Surgery, *22*:120, 1976].)

Figure 26–33. Completion of the combined Collis-Nissen procedure, with fundoplication limited to 3 cm. in length. *A,* Four seromuscular 2-0 silk sutures placed 1 cm. apart (main illustration) are used to construct the fundoplication around the gastroplasty tube. *B,* The fundoplication reduced beneath the diaphragm. In scleroderma patients who have impaired esophageal motility, the fundoplication must be performed loosely to minimize postoperative obstructive symptoms. (From Stirling, M. C., and Orringer, M. B.: The combined Collis-Nissen operation for esophageal reflux strictures. Reprinted with permission from the Society of Thoracic Surgeons [The Annals of Thoracic Surgery, *45*:148, 1988].)

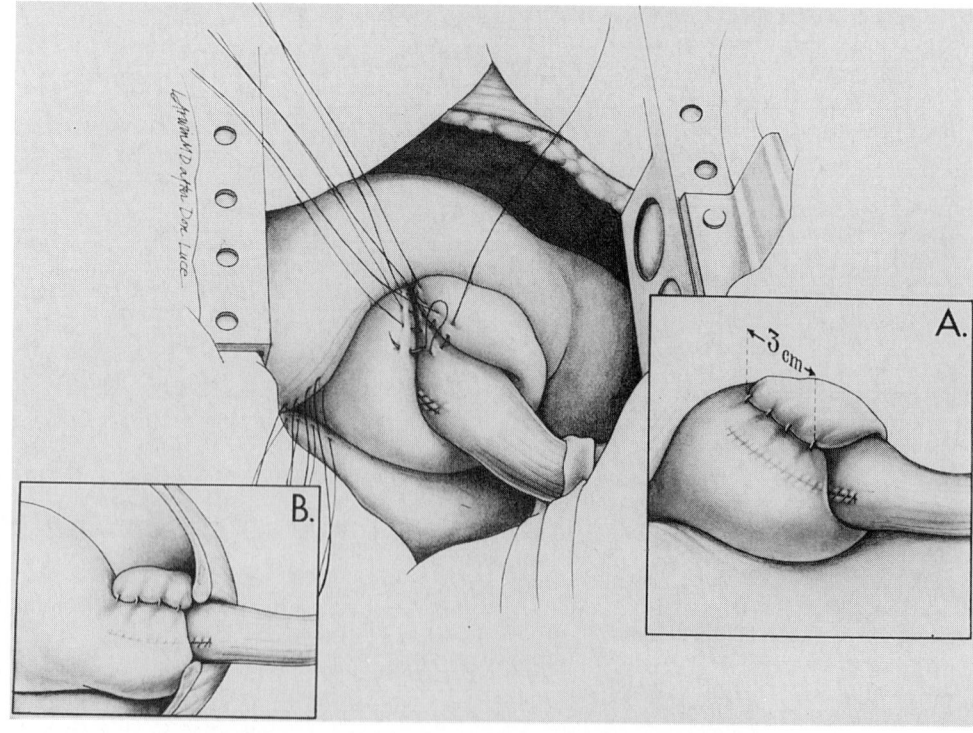

MISCELLANEOUS ESOPHAGEAL MOTOR DISORDERS

Hypertensive Lower Esophageal Sphincter. Some patients complain of low retrosternal chest pain, occasionally aggravated by swallowing, and are found to have unusually elevated, hypertensive LES pressures on manometric evaluation. Manometry shows elevated LES pressure, but normal relaxation with swallowing still occurs, and normal progressive peristalsis is preserved. Patients with Zollinger-Ellison syndrome have normally relaxing hypertensive sphincters but usually no dysphagia. Because gastroesophageal reflux may induce intermittent LES hypertonicity, this condition should be ruled out with pH reflux testing in these patients. Patients with a hypertensive LES may respond to intermittent bougienage but occasionally require esophagomyotomy for relief of symptoms.

Hypotensive Lower Esophageal Sphincter. It must be emphasized repeatedly that *hiatal hernia* and *gastroesophageal reflux* are not synonymous terms and that each may occur in the absence of the other. There are some patients who have an incompetent LES mechanism but no apparent associated hiatal hernia on barium esophagogram. A patient with symptoms of gastroesophageal reflux but normal results on barium swallow examination merits further evaluation with esophageal function tests. Manometry may demonstrate distal high-pressure zone pressures of less than 5 mm. Hg, but this finding *per se* does not prove the presence of abnormal gastroesophageal reflux. Acid reflux testing should be performed using the intraesophageal pH electrode. An incompetent LES in the absence of a hiatal hernia may follow operations on the lower sphincter (esophagomyotomy, vagotomy) or may occur in scleroderma. Therapy for the hypotensive LES is that of gastroesophageal reflux and is discussed in Part VIII of this chapter.

Postvagotomy Dysphagia. Dysphagia occurring after truncal vagotomy has been recognized for many years and occurs in 1% to 3.6% of patients undergoing this operation, primarily as a denervation injury of the distal esophagus. Selective vagotomy is associated with a slightly higher (4% to 12%) incidence of dysphagia.[3] Dysphagia after an antireflux operation may be a function of both local denervation as well as a fundoplication that is too tight. Whereas in some patients with postvagotomy dysphagia, manometric studies have demonstrated lack of distal esophageal sphincter relaxation with swallowing and abnormal distal esophageal peristalsis, in others,[34] acute periesophageal inflammation has been believed to be the cause of the problem. Patients with postvagotomy dysphagia usually experience difficulty swallowing once oral intake of solid food is begun, and the barium esophagogram shows poor esophageal emptying and a tapered distal esophagus, suggesting spasm. At times, the patient will experience referred cervical dysphagia or hiccoughs as food passes slowly through the distal esophagus. In most cases reassurance and maintenance of a soft diet for several days is adequate treatment. If dysphagia continues to be a problem, passage of 46- to 50-French tapered Maloney dilators at the bedside generally relieves the problem. No distal resistance to the passage of the dilators is usually encountered, and in most patients, the dysphagia resolves with one to three dilatations during the first several postoperative weeks.[27] If resistance to the passage of dilators is encountered, the problem is likely mechanical (e.g., a too-tight fundoplication, a too-narrow hiatus, or periesophageal fibrosis) and alternative, more direct therapy is required.

Dysmotility After Esophageal Atresia Repair. Long-term follow-up of patients who have undergone repair of esophageal atresia in infancy (with or without division of a tracheoesophageal fistula) has documented esophageal manometric abnormalities persisting into adult life.[41] Pressure tracings typically reveal weak or absent contractions in the body of the esophagus as well as a hypotensive LES. The motor abnormality appears to be a developmental failure of innervation rather than the result of surgical denervation during the repair. The incidence of gastroesophageal reflux in these patients is directly related to the length of distal esophageal mobilization and hence upward traction on the gastroesophageal junction required to achieve the primary repair. The combination of abnormal motility and concomitant gastroesophageal reflux predisposes to the development of reflux esophagitis. Parents of children who have undergone successful repair of esophageal atresia in infancy must be cautioned about the potential for reflux and its complications, and as these patients enter adulthood, careful monitoring for reflux esophagitis is warranted.

SELECTED REFERENCES

Duranceau, A. C., Lafontaine, E., and Taillefer, R.: Oropharyngeal dysphagia. In Jamieson, G. G. (Ed.): Surgery of the Oesophagus. Edinburgh, Churchill Livingstone, 1988, pp. 413–433.
This comprehensive review of pharyngoesophageal innervation, function, and disordered motility is richly illustrated with manometric tracings, representative radiographs, and scintigrams. The reported results of cricopharyngeal myotomy in patients with a variety of causes for their oropharyngeal dysphagia are nicely tabulated for the reader.

Ferguson, M. K.: Achalasia: Current evaluation and therapy. Ann. Thorac. Surg., 52:336, 1991.
This article provides a current and extensive review of the etiology, diagnosis, and treatment (pharmacologic, dilatation, and operative) of achalasia. The relative efficacy and risks of pneumatic dilatation versus esophagomyotomy are outlined. Controversial areas such as the operative approach (abdominal vs. thoracic), the extent of the distal myotomy, and the need for a concomitant antireflux procedure are thoroughly discussed.

Katz, P. O.: Disorders of increased esophageal contractility. In Castell, D. O. (Ed.): The Esophagus. Boston, Little, Brown & Co, 1992, pp. 261–275.
This is an excellent discussion of the esophageal hypermotility disorders—diffuse spasm (DES), nutcracker esophagus, hypertensive lower esophageal sphincter, and nonspecific esophageal motility disorders (NEMDs). The clinical features and radiographic and manometric findings in each are presented. Appropriate nonoperative therapy, which is the mainstay of treatment for these patients, is outlined.

Little, A. G.: Functional disorders of the esophagus. In Orringer, M. D., and Zuidema, G. D. (Eds.): Shackelford's Surgery of the Alimentary Tract, 4th ed. Vol. I, The Esophagus. Philadelphia, W. B. Saunders, 1996, pp. 269–284.
This is a well-written summary of the diagnosis and treatment of esophageal motility disorders. The sections on esophageal involvement in scleroderma, postvagotomy dysphagia, and long-term sequelae of repair of congenital tracheoesophageal fistula and esophageal atresia provide less widely known information about disturbances of esophageal motor function.

Pearson, F. G., Deslauriers, J., Ginsberg, R. J., Hiebert, C. A., McKneally, M. F., and Urschel, H. C., Jr. (Eds.): Esophageal Surgery. New York, Churchill Livingstone, 1995, pp. 425–457.
This authoritative textbook contains outstanding chapters on primary esophageal motor disorders (pp. 425–442) and Chagas' disease (pp. 443–457). In the former, Sugarbaker and associates present radiographic and manometric depictions of the various esophageal motor disorders and schematic illustrations of the operative approaches, particularly esophagomyotomy combined with a modified Belsey repair. The chapter by the Brazilian surgeon Ximenes-Netto is based on his vast personal experience with Chagas' disease and provides a unique perspective for those who are unfamiliar with this infectious cause of achalasia.

REFERENCES

1. Ancona, E., Anselmino, M., Zaninotto, G., et al.: Esophageal achalasia: Laparoscopic versus conventional open Heller-Dor operation. Am. J. Surg., 170:265, 1995.
2. Ancona, E., Peracchia, A., Zaninotto, G., et al.: Heller laparoscopic cardiomyotomy with antireflux anterior fundoplication (Dor) in the treatment of esophageal achalasia. Surg. Endosc., 7:459, 1993.
3. Andrup, E., Andersen, D., and Hostrup, H.: The Aarthus County vagotomy trial: I. An interim report on primary results and incidences of sequelae following parietal cell vagotomy and selective gastric vagotomy in 748 patients. World J. Surg., 2:85, 1978.
4. Barnett, J. L., Eisenman, R., Nostrant, T. T., and Elta, G. H. Witzel pneumatic dilation for achalasia: Safety and long-term efficacy. Gastrointest. Endosc., 36:482, 1990.
5. Belsey, R.: Functional diseases of the esophagus. J. Thorac. Cardiovasc. Surg., 52:164, 1966.

6. Bonavina, L., Khan, N. A., and DeMeester, T. R. Pharyngoesophageal dysfunctions: The role of cricopharyngeal myotomy. Arch. Surg., 120:541, 1985.

7. Castell, J. A., Dalton, C. B., and Castell, D. O.: Effects of body position and bolus consistency on the manometric parameters and coordination of the upper esophageal sphincter and pharynx. Dysphagia, 5:179, 1990.

8. Castrini, G., and Pappalardo, G.: Our experience in the surgical treatment of achalasia. In DeMeester, T. R., and Skinner, D. B. (Eds.): Esophageal Disorders: Pathophysiology and Therapy. New York, Raven Press, 1985, pp. 423–426.

9. Ceconello, I., DaRocha, J. M., Pollara, W., Zilberstein, B., and Pinotti, H. W.: Long-term evaluation of gastroplasty in achalasia. In Siewart, J. R., Holscher, A. H. (Eds.): Diseases of the Esophagus. Berlin, Springer-Verlag, 1988, pp. 975–979.

10. Clouse, R. E., and Lustman, P. J.: Psychiatric illness and contraction abnormalities of the esophagus. N. Engl. J. Med., 309: 1337, 1983.

11. Csendes, A., Velasco, N., Braghetto, I., and Henriquez, A.: A prospective randomized study comparing forceful dilatation and esophagomyotomy in patients with achalasia of the esophagus. Gastroenterology, 80:789, 1981.

12. Dent, J.: A new technique for continuous sphincter pressure measurement. Gastroenterology, 71:263, 1976

13. Dodds, W. J., Dent, J., Hogan, W. J., Patel, G. I. F., Toouli, J., and Arndorfer, R. C.: Paradoxical lower esophageal sphincter contraction induced by cholecystokinin-octapeptide in patients with achalasia. Gastroenterology, 80:327, 1981.

14. Dodds, W. J., Kahrilas, P. J., Dent, J., and Hogan, W. J. Considerations about pharyngeal manometry. Dysphagia, 1:209, 1987.

15. Duranceau, A. C., Lafontaine, E., and Taillefer, R.: Oropharyngeal dysphagia. In Jamieson, G. G. (Ed.): Surgery of the Oesophagus. Edinburgh, Churchill Livingstone, 1988, pp. 413–434.

16. Duranceau, A., LaFontaine, E., and Vallieres, B.: Effects of total fundoplication on function of the esophagus after myotomy for achalasia. Am. J. Surg., 143:22, 1982.

17. Duranceau, A., Rheault, M. J., and Jamieson, G. G.: Physiologic response to cricopharyngeal myotomy and diverticulum suspension. Surgery, 96:655, 1983.

18. Ellis, F. H., Jr., Crozier, R. E., and Gibb, S. P.: Reoperative achalasia surgery. J. Thorac. Cardiovasc. Surg., 92:859, 1986.

19. Ellis, F. H., Jr., Schlegel, J. F., Code, C. F., et al.: Surgical treatment of esophageal hypermotility disturbances. JAMA, 188:862, 1964.

20. Ellis, F. H., Watkins, E., Gibb, S. P., and Heatley, G. J.: Ten to 20-year clinical results after short esophagomyotomy without an antireflux procedure for esophageal achalasia. Eur. J. Cardiothorac. Surg., 6:86, 1992.

21. Elta, G. H., Nostrant, T. T., and Wilson, J. A. P.: Treatment of achalasia with the Witzel pneumatic dilator. Gastrointest. Endosc., 2:101, 1987.

22. Ferguson, M. K.: Achalasia: Current evaluation and therapy. Ann. Thorac. Surg., 52:336, 1991.

23. Flye, W. W., and Sealy, W. C.: Diffuse spasm of the esophagus. Ann. Thorac. Surg., 19:677, 1975.

24. Gerzic, A., Knezevic, J., Milicevic, M., Rakic, S., Dunjic, M., and Randjelovic, T.: Results of transabdominal cardiomyotomy with Dor partial fundoplication in the management of achalasia. In Siewart, J. R., and Holscher, A. H. (Eds.): Diseases of the Esophagus. Berlin, Springer-Verlag, 1988, pp. 970–974.

25. Goulbourne, I. A., and Walbaum, P. R.: Long-term results of Heller's operation for achalasia. J. R. Coll. Surg. Edinb., 30:101, 1985.

26. Gozzetti, G., Mattioli, S., Spangaro, M., Pilotti, V., Bassi, F., Felice, V., Conci, A., and Lerro, F.: Results of surgical therapy of achalasia with three different techniques. In Siewart, J. R., and Holscher, A. H. (Eds.): Diseases of the Esophagus. Berlin, Springer-Verlag, 1988, pp. 950–952.

27. Guelrud, M., Zambrano-Rincones, V., Simon, C., et al.: Dysphagia and lower esophageal sphincter abnormalities after proximal gastric vagotomy. Am. J. Surg., 149:232, 1985.

28. Henderson, R. D.: Disorders of the pharyngoesophageal junction. In The Esophagus: Reflux and Primary Motor Disorders. Baltimore, Williams & Wilkins, 1980, pp. 223–247.

29. Henderson, R. D., and Marryatt, G.: Cricopharyngeal myotomy as a method of treating cricopharyngeal dysphagia secondary to gastroesophageal reflux. J. Thorac. Cardiovasc. Surg., 74:271, 1977.

30. Henderson, R. D., and Pearson, F. G.: Surgical management of esophageal scleroderma. J. Thorac. Cardiovasc. Surg., 66:686, 1973.

31. Henderson, R. D., and Pearson, F. G.: Reflux control following extended myotomy in primary disordered motor activity (diffuse spasm) of the esophagus. Ann. Thorac. Surg., 22:278, 1976.

32. Hiebert, C. A.: Long-term follow-up of patients with achalasia treated by myotomy and partial fundoplication. In Siewart, J. R., and Holscher, A. H. (Eds.): Diseases of the Esophagus. Berlin, Springer-Verlag, 1988, pp. 962–965.

33. Knuff, T. E., Benjamin, S. B., and Castell, D. O.: Pharyngo-esophageal (Zenker's) diverticulum: A reappraisal. Gastroenterology, 82:734, 1982

34. Mazur, J. M., Skinner, D. B., Jones, E. L., and Zuidema, G. D.: Effect of transabdominal vagotomy on the human gastroesophageal high pressure zone. Surgery, 73:818, 1973.

35. Malthaner, R. A., Todd, T. R., Miller, L., and Pearson, F. G.: Long-term results in surgically managed esophageal achalasia. Ann. Thorac. Surg., 54:1343, 1994.

36. Moraldi, A., Bruscoli, A., Schillaci, A., and Stipa, S.: Results of achalasia of the esophagus. In Stipa, S., Belsey, R. H. R., and Moraldi, A. (Eds.): Medical and Surgical Problems of the Esophagus. London, Academic Press, 1981, pp. 293–295.

37. Okike, N., Payne, W. S., Neufeld, D. M., et al.: Esophagomyotomy versus forceful dilation for achalasia of the esophagus: Results in 899 patients. Ann. Thorac. Surg., 28:119, 1979.

38. Orringer, M. B.: Extended cervical esophagomyotomy for cricopharyngeal dysfunction. J. Thorac. Cardiovasc. Surg., 80:669, 1980.

39. Orringer, M. B.: Transhiatal esophagectomy for benign disease. J. Thorac. Cardiovasc. Surg., 90:649, 1985.

40. Orringer, M. B., Dabich, L., Zarafonetis, C. J., et al.: Gastroesophageal reflux in esophageal scleroderma: Diagnosis and implications. Ann. Thorac. Surg., 22:120, 1976.

41. Orringer, M. B., Kirsh, M. M., and Sloan, H.: Long-term esophageal function following repair of esophageal atresia. Ann. Surg., 186:431, 1977.

42. Orringer, M. B., and Orringer, J. S.: Esophagectomy: Definitive treatment for esophageal neuromotor dysfunction. Ann. Thorac. Surg., 24:237, 1982.

43. Orringer, M. B., Orringer, J. S., Dabich, L., et al.: Combined Collis-gastroplasty-fundoplication operations for scleroderma reflux esophagitis. Surgery, 90:624, 1981.

44. Orringer, M. B., Stirling, M. C.: Esophageal resection for achalasia: Indications and results. Ann. Thorac. Surg., 47:340, 1989.

45. Pasricha, P. J., Ravich, W. J., Hendrix, T. R., Sostre, S., Jones, B., and Kalloo, A. N.: Intrasphincteric botulinum toxin for the treatment of achalasia. N. Engl. J. Med., 322:744, 1995.

46. Pellegrini, C., Wetter, L. A., Patti, M., et al.: Thoracoscopic esophagomyotomy: Initial experience with a new approach for the treatment of achalasia. Ann. Surg., 216:291, 1992.

47. Pinotti, H. W., and Bettarello, A.: Chagasic mega-oesophagus. In Jamieson, G. G. (Ed.): Surgery of the Oesophagus. Edinburgh, Churchill-Livingstone, 1988, pp. 471–481.

48. Pinotti, H. W., Nasi, A., Cecconello, I., Zilberstein, B., and Pollara, W.: Chagas' disease of the esophagus. Dis. Esophagus, 1:65, 1988.

49. Possati, L., Bragaglia, S., Mattioli, M., Spangaro, M., Bortolotti, M., and Bassi, F.: Surgical management of achalasia of the esophagus. In Stipa, S., Belsey, RHR, and Moradi, A. (Eds.): Medical and Surgical Problems of the Esophagus. London, Academic Press, 1981, pp. 279–280.

50. Postlethwait, R. W.: Surgery of the Esophagus. Norwalk, CT, Appleton-Century-Crofts, 1979, p. 93.

51. Rosati, R., Fumagalli, U., Bonavino, L., Segalin, A., Montorsi, M., Bena, S., and Peracchia, A.: Laparoscopic approach to esophageal achalasia. Am. J. Surg., 169:424, 1995.

52. Sandler, R. S., Bopzymski, E. M., and Orlando, R. C.: Failure of clinical criteria to distinguish between primary achalasia and achalasia secondary to tumor. Dig. Dis. Sci., 27:209, 1982.

53. Slater, G., and Sicular, A.: Esophageal perforations after forceful dilatation in achalasia. Ann Surg., 2:186, 1981.

54. Torres, A. J., Suarez, A., Hernandez, F., Ruiz, A., Cuberes, R., Lapena, L, Fernandez, R., Villacorta, J., and Balibrea, J. L.: Importance of antireflux mechanism of typical achalasia of the cardia. In Siewart, J. R., and Holscher, A. H. (Eds.): Diseases of the Esophagus. Berlin, Springer-Verlag, 1988, pp. 936–941.

55. Vantrappen, G., and Hellemans, J.: Treatment of achalasia and related motor disorders. Gastroenterology, 79:144, 1980.

56. Winans, C. S.: The pharyngoesophageal closure mechanism: A manometric study. Gastroenterology, 63:768, 1972.

IV _____

DIVERTICULA AND MISCELLANEOUS CONDITIONS OF THE ESOPHAGUS

Mark B. Orringer, M.D.

DIVERTICULA

Esophageal diverticula are epithelial-lined mucosal pouches that protrude from the esophageal lumen. Almost all of them are acquired and occur predominantly in adults. Esophageal diverticula are classified according to their (1) site of occurrence, (2) wall thickness, and (3) mechanism of formation. They commonly occur at three distinct sites and are designated as *pharyngoesophageal* when they occur at the junction of the pharynx and esophagus, *parabronchial* (mid-esophageal) when they are located near the tracheal bifurcation, and *epiphrenic* (supradiaphragmatic) when they arise from the distal 10 cm. of esophagus. A *true* diverticulum contains all layers of the normal esophageal wall, including mucosa, submucosa, and muscle, whereas a *false* diverticulum consists primarily of only mucosa and submucosa. *Pulsion diverticula* arise because elevated intraluminal pressure forces the mucosa and submucosa to herniate through the esophageal musculature; therefore, they are false diverticula. *Traction diverticula* are the result of external inflammatory reaction in adjacent mediastinal lymph nodes that adhere to the esophagus and pull the entire wall toward them as they heal and contract; they are true diverticula. Pharyngoesophageal and epiphrenic diverticula are pulsion diverticula that typically arise as a result of abnormal esophageal motility. Parabronchial diverticula are generally of the traction variety and include all layers of the esophageal wall.

Pharyngoesophageal Diverticula. A pharyngoesophageal diverticulum was first described as an autopsy finding by Ludlow in 1769.[25] In 1878, Zenker reported 22 cases from the literature and added five of his own,[45] and his name subsequently became associated with this entity. The pharyngoesophageal diverticulum is the most common esophageal diverticulum, generally occurring in patients between 30 and 50 years of age and therefore believed to be acquired. The diverticulum characteristically arises within the inferior pharyngeal constrictor, between the oblique fibers of the thyropharyngeus muscle and the more horizontal fibers of the cricopharyngeus muscle, the upper esophageal sphincter (UES) (Fig. 26–34). The transition in the direction of these muscle fibers (Killian's triangle) represents a point of potential weakness in the posterior pharynx and is the site of formation of the pharyngoesophageal diverticulum. Due to the unique characteristics of the UES and the speed with which neuromotor events in this area occur during deglutition, precise documentation of the exact abnormality in pharyngoesophageal motor function in patients with Zenker's diverticula is extremely difficult to obtain. Ellis and associates first reported manometric abnormalities of the UES in these patients, namely, incoordination in the swallowing mechanism, with pharyngeal contraction occurring after cricopharyngeal closure, and resting pressures *lower* than in controls.[16] As indicated previously (see Part III in this chapter), the unique anatomic configuration of the UES—its asymmetry and change in position with laryngeal excursions—has prompted the development of a variety of recording devices to study UES function, and it is not surprising that the originally described manometric abnormalities of the UES in these patients have not been found consistently by other investigators. Regardless of the limitations of existing recording equipment in defining the underlying motor abnormality, however, a pulsion diverticulum would not occur unless there were *some* abnormality distal to it, generating usually elevated pharyngeal pressures. Thus, the swallowed bolus exerts pressure within the pharynx, and mucosa and submucosa herniate through the anatomically weak area proximal to the cricopharyngeus muscle. With time, the diverticulum enlarges, drapes over the cricopharyngeus, and dissects inferiorly in the prevertebral space behind the esophagus, occasionally into the superior mediastinum.

Pharyngoesophageal diverticula are usually associated with complaints of cervical dysphagia, effortless regurgitation of undigested particles of food or pills sometimes consumed hours earlier, a gurgling sensation in the neck on swallowing, choking, and recurrent aspiration. Weight loss and dysphagia suggest an esophageal malignancy may occur when the pouch is large and the obstruction becomes severe (Fig. 26–35). A barium esophagogram establishes the diagnosis. Surgical therapy in symptomatic patients is indicated in most cases, regardless of the size of the pouch, and, it is hoped, before complications occur. A patient with a 5-mm. Zenker diverticulum may be equally or even more symptomatic than a patient with a 3-cm. pouch. It is the degree of cricopharyngeal muscle dysfunction, *not the absolute size of the diverticulum,* that determines the relative severity of cervical dysphagia. Therefore, the proper surgical treatment of the pharyngoesophageal diverticulum, like that of *every* pulsion diverticulum, must be directed toward the underlying motor abnormality responsible for formation of the pouch and not at the pouch *per se.*

The history of the surgical management of the pharyngoesophageal diverticulum includes a variety of innovative operations.[20, 33] The morbidity and mortality of the initially

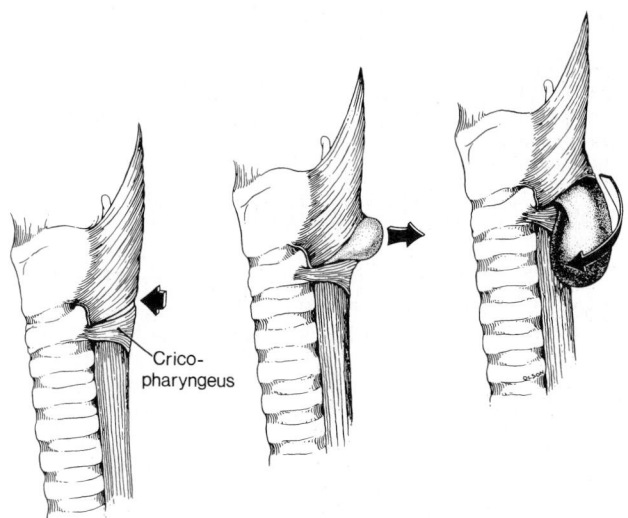

Figure 26–34. Formation of pharyngoesophageal (Zenker's) diverticulum. *Left,* Herniation of the pharyngeal mucosa and submucosa occurs at the point of transition (arrow) between the oblique fibers of the thyropharyngeus muscle and the more horizontal fibers of the cricopharyngeus muscle. *Center* and *right,* As the diverticulum enlarges, it dissects toward the left side and downward into the superior mediastinum in the prevertebral space.

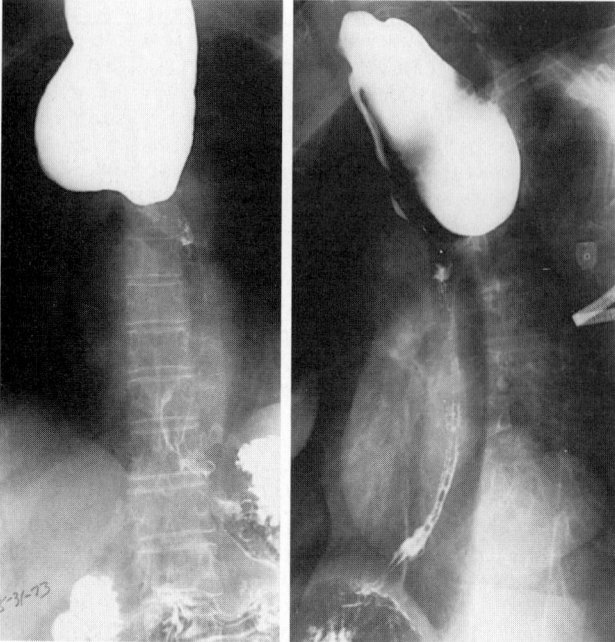

Figure 26–35. Posteroanterior *(left)* and oblique *(right)* views from barium esophagogram showing a huge 15-cm. pharyngoesophageal diverticulum in an elderly woman who presented with cervical dysphagia, a 40-lb. weight loss, and a right superior mediastinal paratracheal "mass" (the diverticulum) on standard chest roentgenogram and who was thought to have esophageal carcinoma. She was treated with diverticulectomy and cervical esophagomyotomy.

described one-stage resections, however, were prohibitive, with wound infection and sepsis from esophageal suture-line disruption being the primary complications. As a result, the concept of a two-stage procedure emerged. At the first operation, the pouch was isolated and suspended by suturing it to the skin so that it could empty through its now-dependent mouth and develop surrounding adhesions that would prevent later spreading cellulitis and mediastinitis. After 2 to 3 weeks, the pouch was resected. This approach gained widespread popularity and was championed by Lahey, who subsequently reported a series of 365 patients, with only two deaths and 12 recurrences.[21] As the two-stage approach was being developed, Jackson attacked the problem of infection following one-stage diverticulum resection by first aspirating the contents of the pouch through an esophagoscope.[19] Others adopted this approach; and in 1956, Sweet reported 77 patients treated with one-stage resection with no deaths, one fistula, and one recurrence.[38] This approach was adopted at the Mayo Clinic, where 888 patients were treated from 1944 to 1978 with a 1.2% mortality rate and a 3.6% recurrence rate.[32]

Alternative surgical approaches to pharyngoesophageal diverticula have not gained as widespread use as the currently most popular operation—cervical esophagomyotomy and resection. Diverticulopexy—simply mobilizing the pouch, inverting it, and suspending it from adjacent tissues so that the mouth is dependent—combined with a cricopharyngeal myotomy has its advocates.[2, 13] Invagination of the diverticulum has been utilized alone or combined with a cervical esophagomyotomy. Endoscopic division of the common wall between the diverticulum and esophagus (internal pharyngoesophagotomy, the Dohlman procedure) has been used with success primarily by otolaryngologists.[11, 40] In one of the largest such series, van Overbeck and Hoeksema (1982) have reported 211 patients with good results in 91.5% and a 5% incidence of esophageal perforation.[40]

Regardless of the surgical approach, operations directed primarily at the diverticulum without dealing with the underlying incoordinated cricopharyngeal sphincter responsible for the development of increased pharyngeal pressure and formation of the pouch leave the potential for recurrence of the diverticulum and suture-line disruption. Elevated pharyngeal pressure proximal to the cricopharyngeus cannot occur if this muscle is divided, and this is the basis for the most popular current surgical approach to the incoordinated UES.[29] The operation is performed through an oblique left cervical incision that parallels the anterior border of the sternocleidomastoid muscle or a transverse cervical incision centered over the cricoid cartilage. The sternocleidomastoid muscle and carotid sheath and its contents are retracted laterally, and the thyroid and the trachea are retracted medially. The inferior thyroid artery, an important anatomic landmark in this operation, is identified and usually divided. The diverticulum is consistently located beneath this vessel. With a 40-French bougie within the esophagus, the pouch is dissected to its base, and an extramucosal esophagomyotomy is performed in either vertical direction from the base of the pouch for several centimeters to ensure that all cricopharyngeal muscle fibers are divided (Fig. 26–36). Most pouches between 1 and 2 cm. in diameter simply *disappear* and blend into the exposed mucosa and submucosa after the cervical esophagomyotomy. Some surgeons, in fact, terminate the operation at this point without resecting the diverticulum, regardless of its size.[15] Most, however, advocate excising larger pouches using a surgical stapler. Cricopharyngeal myotomy, with or without diverticulectomy, is an extremely effective means of treating cricopharyngeal muscle dysfunction in these patients, carries a very low morbidity, and is justified in all patients undergoing surgery for a Zenker diverticulum.

Midesophageal (Traction) Diverticula. Traction diverticula of the midesophagus are typically associated with mediastinal granulomatous disease (e.g., tuberculosis, histoplasmosis).[26] They are characteristically small, with a blunt, tapered tip that points upward to the adjacent subcarinal and parabronchial lymph nodes to which they are adherent, and quite different from larger, round, relatively narrow-mouthed pulsion diverticula (Fig. 26–37). These diverticula are usually seen as incidental findings on a barium esophagogram. They rarely cause symptoms or require treatment. Occasionally, however, inflammatory necrosis of the granulomatous process results in a fistulous communication between the esophagus and the respiratory tract that requires division of the fistula and interposition of adjacent normal tissues. Rarely,

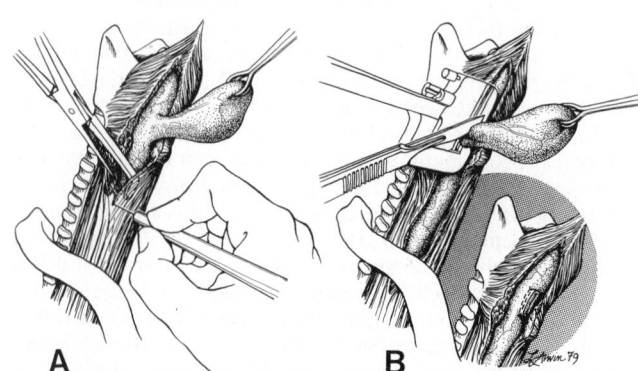

Figure 26–36. Cervical esophagomyotomy and concomitant resection of a pharyngoesophageal diverticulum. *A,* After mobilization of the diverticulum, the esophagomyotomy is performed in either direction from the base of the pouch for the same distance as described in Figure 26–37. *B,* After the esophagomyotomy is completed, the base of the diverticulum is crossed with a TA-30 stapler and amputated. (From Orringer, M. B.: Extended cervical esophagomyotomy for cricopharyngeal dysfunction. J. Thorac. Cardiovasc. Surg., *80:*669, 1980.)

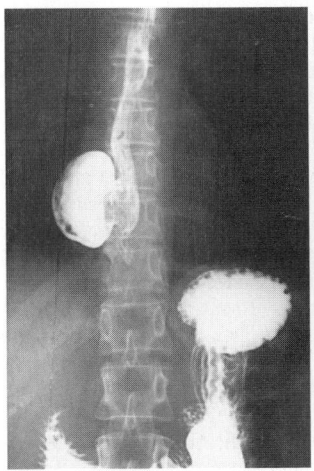 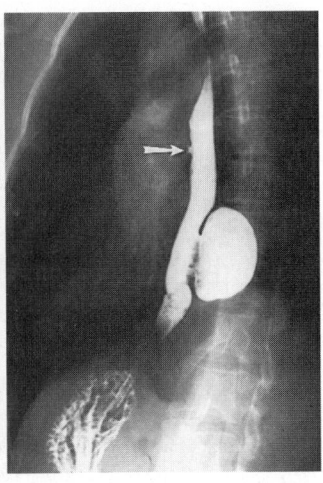

Figure 26–37. Posteroanterior *(left)* and oblique *(right)* views from barium esophagogram showing both a typical pulsion diverticulum of the junction of the mid and distal esophagus and a small traction diverticulum (arrow) of the mid-esophagus.

erosion of an adjacent mediastinal blood vessel can result in massive upper gastrointestinal bleeding. Midesophageal traction diverticula are to be differentiated from pulsion diverticula, which may occur in this location in association with neuromotor esophageal dysfunction,[4, 34] just as with epiphrenic diverticula.

Epiphrenic Diverticula. Epiphrenic or supradiaphragmatic diverticula generally occur within the distal 10 cm. of the thoracic esophagus and are pulsion diverticula that arise either because of esophageal motor dysfunction or a mechanical distal obstruction (see Fig. 26–37).[1, 5, 9] As with pharyngoesophageal diverticula, abnormally elevated intraluminal pressure is responsible for a blowout of mucosa and submucosa through the muscle of the esophagus. Many patients are asymptomatic when their epiphrenic diverticulum is diagnosed on barium esophagogram. In others, symptoms are difficult to differentiate from the frequently associated esophageal lesions—hiatal hernia, diffuse esophageal spasm, achalasia, reflux esophagitis, and carcinoma. Dysphagia and regurgitation are common symptoms, as is retrosternal pain from associated diffuse esophageal spasm. Although the diagnosis is readily apparent on barium esophagogram, esophageal function studies should be performed if possible to define the associated motor disturbance or the presence of an incompetent lower esophageal sphincter (LES) mechanism. Mildly symptomatic patients with pouches smaller than 3 cm. often require no treatment, whereas those with progressively severe dysphagia and chest pain or an anatomically dependent or enlarging pouch are surgical candidates. As with pharyngoesophageal diverticula, unless there is an associated distal esophageal stricture or tumor, it must be inferred that abnormally elevated intraesophageal pressure responsible for the pouch is caused by a motor disturbance, which can frequently be documented manometrically. Therefore, the operation, performed through a left thoracotomy, involves not only resection of the diverticulum but also a long extramucosal thoracic esophagomyotomy from beneath the aortic arch to the esophagogastric junction (Fig. 26–38). An associated hiatal hernia or incompetent LES should also be repaired during the same operation. So long as an esophagomyotomy is performed, suture-line disruption and recurrence after resection of the diverticulum are rare (Fig. 26–39). As is the case when performing an esophagomyotomy for achalasia, the question of the distal extent of the muscle incision and the need for a concomitant antireflux operation arises. Ellis

has maintained that the LES should not be disturbed if preoperative esophageal function tests show that it is normal.[14] On the other hand, Belsey has emphasized the need to eliminate completely the distal esophageal obstruction and routinely divides the LES, carrying the muscle incision 1.5 cm. onto the stomach.[2] When carrying out an antireflux procedure on a myotomized esophagus, a partial fundoplication of the Belsey type, rather than a 360-degree Nissen fundoplication, is less likely to produce functional obstruction on long-term follow-up.[12] Although generally viewed as a procedure of relatively low morbidity and mortality, diverticulectomy and esophagomyotomy at the Mayo Clinic has been associated with a 9% operative mortality,[3] and in view of this, operative intervention for a minimally symptomatic epiphrenic diverticulum is discouraged.

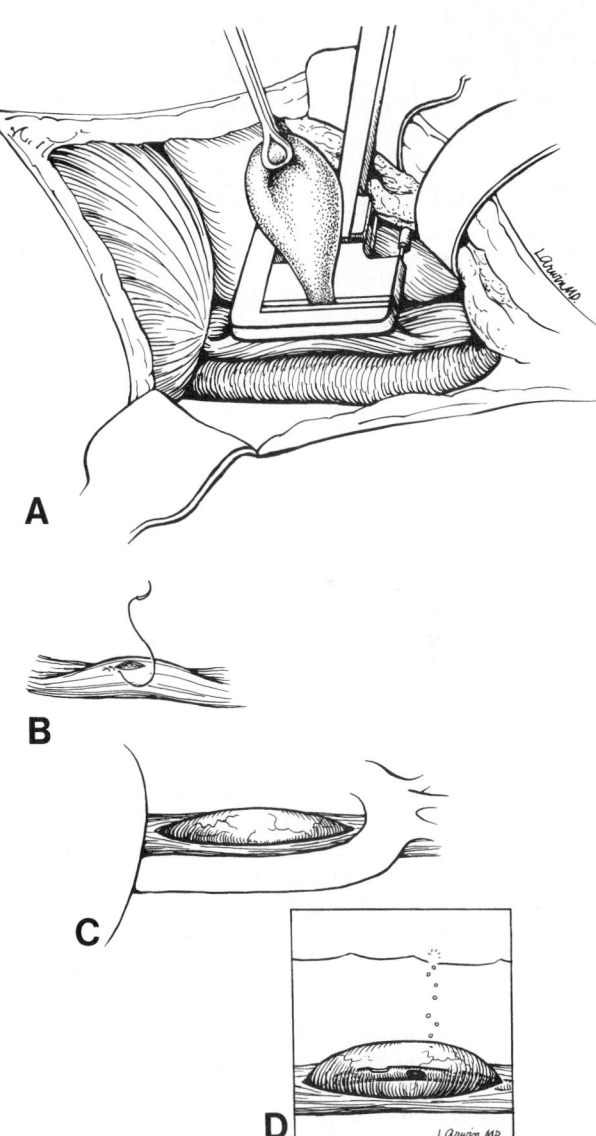

Figure 26–38. Technique of resection of epiphrenic diverticulum and concomitant thoracic esophagomyotomy. *A,* After the diverticulum is mobilized to its base, it is amputated with a TA-30 surgical stapler. *B,* The staple suture line is oversewn by approximating adjacent muscle. *C,* A long esophagomyotomy from the esophagogastric junction to the aortic arch is performed on the opposite wall of the esophagus. *D,* Air is insufflated through an intraesophageal nasogastric tube with the esophagus immersed under saline so that any disruption of the mucosa can be identified and repaired. (From Orringer, M. B.: Complications of esophageal surgery and trauma. *In* Greenfield, L. J. [Ed.]: Complications of Surgery and Trauma, 2nd ed. Philadelphia, J. B. Lippincott, 1990, pp. 302–325.)

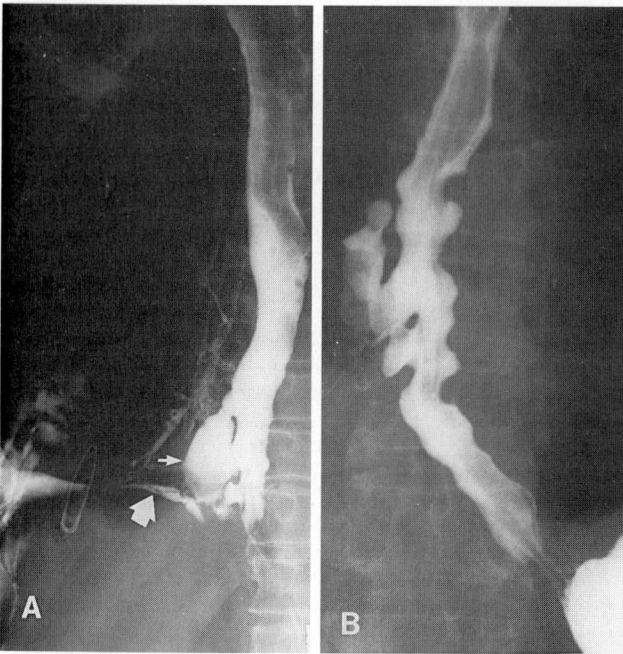

Figure 26–39. *A,* Esophagogram showing esophagopleural cutaneous fistula (large arrow) and a recurrent epiphrenic diverticulum (small arrow) in a patient who had undergone prior resection of the diverticulum without an esophagomyotomy. *B,* The patient's underlying esophageal neuromotor problem is evident in this view from the same esophagogram, showing a typical *corkscrew* esophagus. The relative distal esophageal obstruction secondary to intermittent spasm had not been relieved when the diverticulum was resected, hence disruption of the suture line with fistula formation and recurrence of the diverticulum followed. (From Orringer, M. B.: Complications of esophageal surgery and trauma. *In* Greenfield, L. J. [Ed.]: Complications of Surgery and Trauma, 2nd ed. Philadelphia, J. B. Lippincott, 1990, pp. 302–325.)

MISCELLANEOUS CONDITIONS OF THE ESOPHAGUS

Sideropenic Dysphagia (Plummer-Vinson or Patterson-Kelly Syndrome). Sideropenic dysphagia refers to the development of cervical dysphagia in patients with iron-deficiency anemia. These patients are usually edentulous women older than the age of 40 years. They have atrophic oral mucosa with glossitis and brittle spoon-shaped fingernails (koilonychia). The cause of the dysphagia is usually a cervical esophageal web (Fig. 26–40), but abnormal pharyngeal and esophageal motility may also play a role.[8] Treatment consists of esophageal dilation and correction of the nutritional deficiency. This syndrome has a high incidence in Scandinavia and Great Britain and is regarded as a premalignant lesion, because approximately 10% of patients so affected develop squamous cell carcinoma of the hypopharynx, oral cavity, or esophagus.[44] Kelly and Patterson described this condition in England in 1919. In the United States, the syndrome was reported by Plummer (1914) and by Vinson (1922).

Distal Esophageal Web (Schatzki's Ring). Distal esophageal webs are commonly seen radiographically at the esophagogastric junction in patients with a sliding hiatal hernia. They appear as annular strictures that project into the lumen at a right angle to the long axis of the lower esophagus (Fig. 26–41). Originally described by Templeton (1944), Schatzki and Gary (1953) and Ingelfinger and Kramer (1953) were the first to attribute symptoms to the lesion. The incidence of Schatzki's ring is impossible to determine, because most patients with this abnormality are asymptomatic. Intermittent dysphagia may occur when the ring size is 20 mm. or less, but the critical ring diameter at which dysphagia invariably occurs is 13 mm. or less. The etiology of the Schatzki ring

has not been established. When it was in vogue to resect those rings that were associated with dysphagia, the web was typically found 1 to 2 cm. above the junction of the tubular esophagus and the saccular stomach and involved only the mucosa and submucosa, not the esophageal muscle. Microscopically, squamous epithelium covered the upper surface of the ring and columnar epithelium covered the lower surface. There was only a slight amount of associated increased submucosal fibrosis.[42] Schatzki's ring, therefore, occurs precisely at the squamocolumnar epithelial junction and is seen radiographically on a barium esophagogram only because the squamocolumnar junction is above the diaphragm (i.e., because there is a hiatal hernia). The presence of a ring indicates that there is a hiatal hernia, but it does *not* indicate that there is either gastroesophageal reflux or esophagitis. Differentiation of this mucosal prominence at the esophagogastric junction from a localized peptic stricture owing to gastroesophageal reflux may be difficult. Many patients with symptomatic rings have no reflux symptoms and have an excellent response to intermittent esophageal bougienage. Others who have dysphagia as well as reflux symptoms may do well with periodic dilatations and an antireflux medical regimen. In those with refractory dysphagia or very symptomatic gastroesophageal reflux that fails to respond adequately to medical therapy, intraoperative dilation in association with an antireflux procedure effectively relieves symptoms so long as reflux control is maintained by the operation. Resection of the ring alone, without repair of the associated hiatal hernia, should not be performed. It has been suggested that there may be an inordinately high

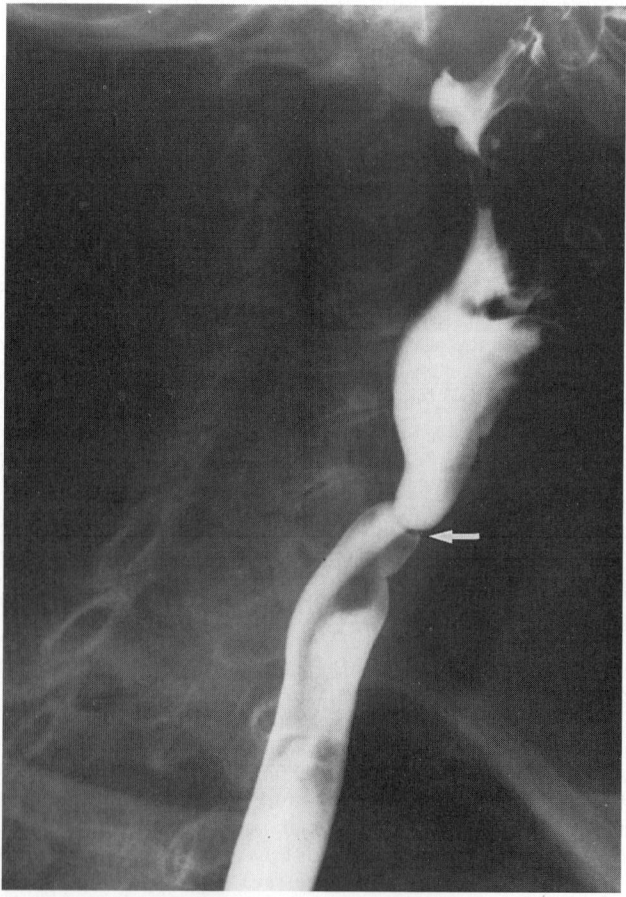

Figure 26–40. Esophagogram showing a cervical web (arrow), which is differentiated roentgenographically from a prominent cricopharyngeal sphincter by its location on the anterior esophageal wall.

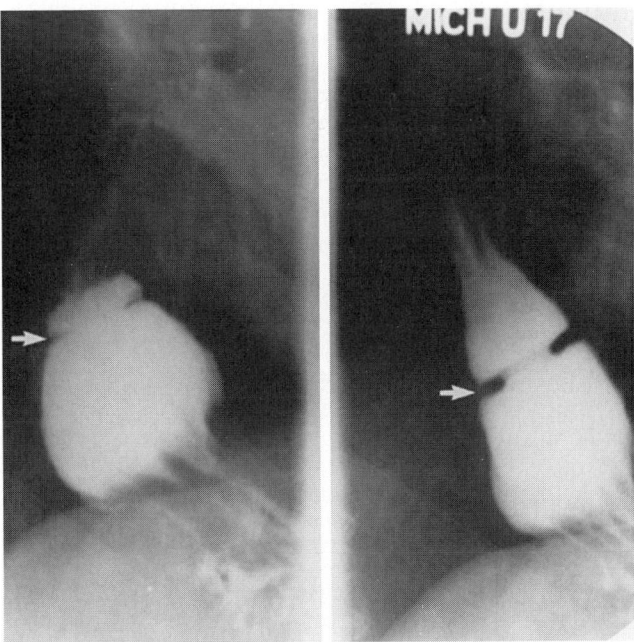

Figure 26–41. Esophagogram showing a distal esophageal (Schatzki) ring (arrows), which is always seen at the esophagogastric junction above a sliding hiatal hernia.

incidence of recurrent hiatal hernia in patients undergoing dilatation of the ring and an antireflux procedure.[31]

Mallory-Weiss Syndrome (Emetogenic Mucosal Laceration). During the act of extremely forceful emesis against a closed glottis, the rapid increase in intra-abdominal pressure is transmitted to the esophagus, where either a mucosal laceration at the esophagogastric junction (Mallory-Weiss syndrome) or a transmural esophageal tear (Boerhaave's syndrome) can occur. A history of emesis followed by either melena or hematemesis suggests the possibility of a Mallory-Weiss mucosal tear at the cardia. However, the diagnosis may not be considered because of the clinical settings in which this condition may occur: alcoholism, pregnancy, peptic ulcer disease, cirrhosis, bowel obstruction, drug withdrawal, or food poisoning.[6, 28, 37] A barium contrast study is rarely diagnostic, although it may rule out other potential causes of the bleeding. Selective celiac arteriography may at times demonstrate the site of bleeding if the volume of blood loss is brisk enough at the time of the study. Esophagoscopy may establish the diagnosis, but in this study, too, the site of bleeding is often not definitely seen. In more than 90% of cases the bleeding stops in response to nasogastric decompression, iced saline gastric lavage, and correction of blood loss. If massive hemorrhage continues, however, the upper abdomen should be explored and a long proximal gastrotomy performed for inspection of the cardia. After evacuation of clots from the stomach, the mucosal tear is identified and oversewn. The results of surgical treatment of Mallory-Weiss syndrome are excellent, and recurrence of bleeding is rare.

INFECTIOUS ESOPHAGITIS

Infectious esophagitis is encountered clinically in the setting of chronic debilitation, immunosuppression, or extended use of antibiotics. Although *Candida albicans* is the most common cause of infectious esophagitis, with the proliferation of the acquired immunodeficiency syndrome, esophageal infections due to other fungi (*Torulopsis* and *Histoplasma*), viruses (cytomegalovirus, herpes simplex, human immunodeficiency,

and Epstein-Barr), mycobacteria, and protozoa (*Cryptosporidium* and *Pneumocystis*) are now being reported.[41]

Candidal Esophagitis. *Candida albicans* is a fungus that is normally a commensal inhabitant of the human mouth, oropharynx, and gastrointestinal tract. The fungus may become pathogenic in severely debilitated or immunosuppressed patients. The incidence of candidal esophagitis is increasing because of the growing number of organ transplants, the use of chemotherapeutics in oncology, and potent broad-spectrum antibiotics.[17, 30, 35] Typically, in acute candidal esophagitis with oropharyngeal involvement, the patient complains of painful swallowing. Because the infection involves the thoracic esophagus, primary and secondary peristaltic waves are decreased in frequency and amplitude and spasm may occur. With progression of the disease and before frank mucosal ulceration, as inflammation and edema of the submucosa occur, the so-called cobblestone pattern of luminal nodularity is seen on the barium swallow. With advanced acute candidal esophagitis, ulceration of the mucosa and an irregular, shaggy-appearing, narrowed esophageal lumen due to mucosal and submucosal edema as well as pseudomembrane formation are seen radiographically. At endoscopy the esophageal mucosa initially appears erythematous and nonulcerated, with an overlying whitish, cheesy exudate or pseudomembrane. As the disease progresses, the mucosa becomes more granular and friable as the inflammatory reaction extends into the wall of the esophagus and the fungus invades the mucosal, submucosal, and muscle layers. If such extensive panmural esophagitis can be controlled by antifungal therapy and if the patient survives the underlying disease, healing of the inflamed esophagus may result in a chronic stricture. Strictures resulting from candidal esophagitis tend to occur in the upper half of the thoracic esophagus, where the esophageal submucosal glands predominate. Inflammation of these glands from infection, stasis, or distal obstruction can produce dilation and outpouching termed *intramural esophageal pseudodiverticulosis*, a pattern seen in many patients with candidal strictures (Fig. 26–42).

Acute candidal esophagitis should be detected promptly in debilitated, postoperative, and immunosuppressed patients. Treatment is dictated by the patient's immune status and extent of the infection. For mild cases in minimally compro-

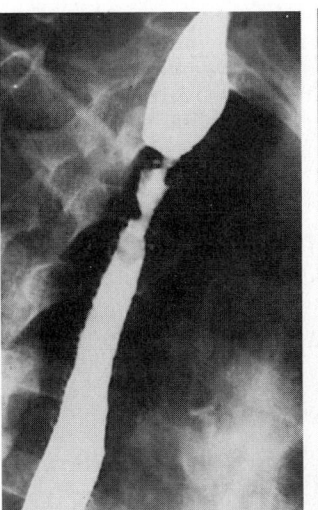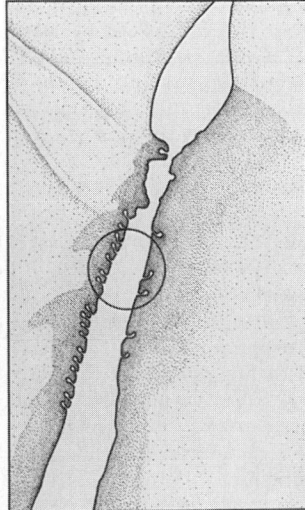

Figure 26–42. Esophagogram and line interpretation of irregular upper thoracic esophageal stricture from candidal esophagitis. The associated intramural pseudodiverticulosis represents dilated submucosal esophageal glands. (From Orringer, M. B., and Sloan, H.: Monilial esophagitis: An increasingly frequent cause of esophageal stenosis? Ann. Thorac. Surg., 26:364, 1978. Reprinted with permission of the Society of Thoracic Surgeons.)

mised patients, treatment with oral nystatin, 1 to 3 million units of the suspension every 6 hours, or clotrimazole, 100 mg. three to five times a day, generally arrests the infection within 7 to 10 days. This therapy should be continued for 1 to 3 weeks. Alternative drugs include oral amphotericin B lozenges, ketoconazole, or fluconazole. In more advanced cases or infections in more immunocompromised patients (e.g., those with the acquired immunodeficiency syndrome), high doses of fluconozole (100–200 mg. orally once daily) and ketoconazole (400–800 mg. orally once a day) are necessary. In granulocytopenic patients, intravenous fluconazole or amphotericin B may be required.[27] Because postinflammatory mural fibrosis can occur, patients recovering from severe acute candidal esophagitis should have several follow-up barium swallow examinations during the first year to ensure the earliest possible recognition of a developing stricture and institution of bougienage therapy.

Viral Esophagitis. Viral esophagitis is surpassed only by *Candida* as the most frequent form of infectious esophagitis. In patients infected with human immunodeficiency virus, cytomegalovirus is the most common viral pathogen, while in transplant patients taking immunosuppressive therapy, herpes simplex virus is more frequent.[41] Mucosal ulceration in viral esophagitis results in dysphagia and odynophagia, the common presenting symptoms, and is seen as discrete lesions on the barium esophagogram. Esophageal ulcers due to cytomegalovirus tend to be large, while those from herpes simplex virus are typically smaller than 1.5 cm. The diagnosis requires biopsy, brushings, and washings for histology, cytology, and viral culture.

Rare Esophageal Pathology. Crohn's disease of the esophagus is now a well-recognized entity, with dyspepsia, dysphagia, chest pain, and weight loss being common presenting symptoms.[24, 39] Aphthous ulcerations throughout the esophagus are the earliest manifestations, and symptoms respond rapidly to corticosteroid therapy. Various dermatologic conditions, such as pemphigus vulgaris and epidermolysis bullosa, may also involve the esophageal epithelium and produce dysphagia from esophagitis and stricture formation.[36] In certain situations, unusual causes of dysphagia may have to be considered in the differential diagnosis of patients with swallowing complaints. Dysphagia has been reported in patients with marked cardiac enlargement, hepatomegaly impinging the esophagus against the diaphragmatic hiatus, and tortuosity of the thoracic aorta.[10, 18, 22, 23] Cervical dysphagia may also be caused by esophageal compression by thyroid or parathyroid tissue or by cervical vertebral body osteophytic spurs (Figs. 26–43 and 26–44). Such exostoses typically involve the fifth, sixth, and seventh cervical vertebral interspaces and displace the esophagus from behind.[7] Esophagos-

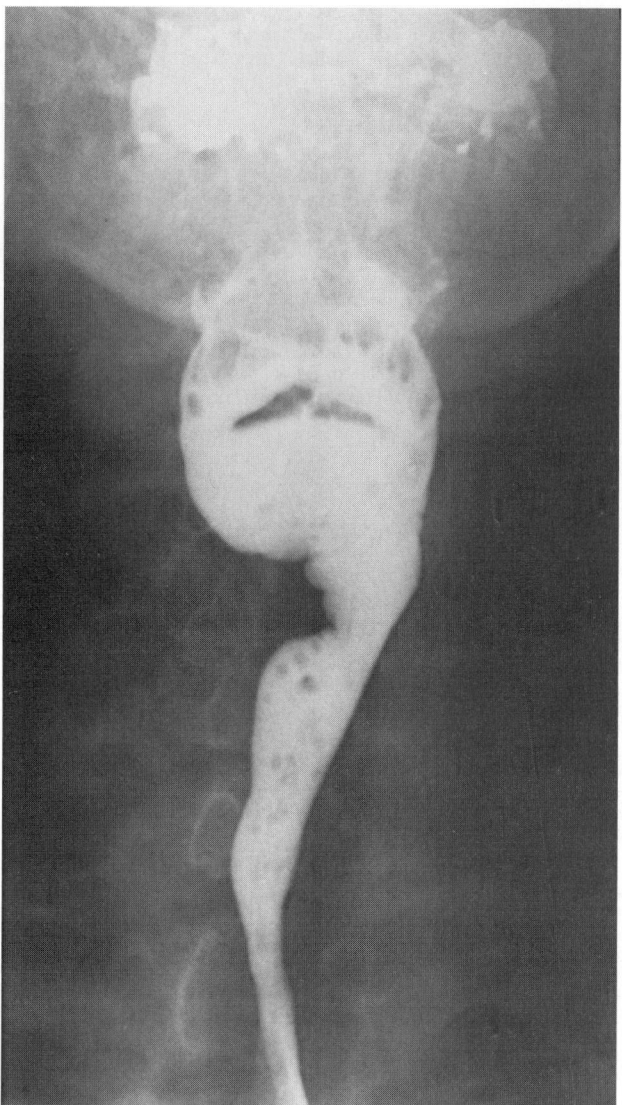

Figure 26–44. Cervical esophagogram showing extrinsic right lateral mass. This patient with dysphagia had an aberrant location of the right lobe of the thyroid gland, which was found at operation to be posterolateral to the esophagus. A right thyroid lobectomy was performed and resulted in relief of the patient's dysphagia.

copy is obviously more dangerous in the presence of exostoses and should be performed with a pediatric flexible fiberoptic esophagoscope to rule out carcinoma in these patients with dysphagia. The flexible esophagoscope, however, does not eliminate the risk of esophageal perforation in these patients.[43] Although removal of osteophytes may relieve the dysphagia, associated cricopharyngeal motor dysfunction, which is more easily treated, should be ruled out, and simple gentle dilation with a Maloney bougie may be therapeutic.

SELECTED REFERENCES

Duranceau, A. C.: Diverticula of the oesophageal body. *In* Jamieson, G. G. (Ed.): Surgery of the Oesophagus. Edinburgh, Churchill Livingstone, 1988, pp. 489–500.
  This chapter presents the radiographic manometric, endoscopic, and clinical features of the variety of esophageal diverticula (Zenker's, traction, epiphrenic) and discusses the results of surgical treatment of each.

Jamieson, G. G. (Ed.): Surgery of the Oesophagus. Edinburgh, Churchill Livingstone, 1988, pp. 435–459.
  Within this authoritative textbook are excellent well-illustrated chapters on the pharyngoesophageal (Zenker) diverticulum—its mechanism of formation, clinical

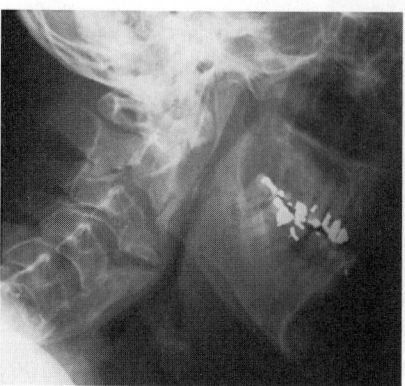 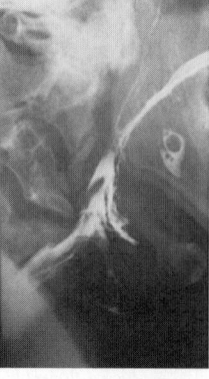

Figure 26–43. Cervical osteophytes displacing the esophagus anteriorly. *Left*, Soft tissue film of neck. *Right*, Displacement of barium-filled esophagus.

presentation, and treatment (pp. 435–443) and the surgical techniques of diverticulectomy and esophagomyotomy (pp. 445–452), cricopharyngeal myotomy and diverticulum suspension (pp. 453–456), and internal pharyngoesophagomyotomy (the Dohlman procedure) (pp. 457–459) used for this condition. The reported results with each of these approaches are well reviewed, and the reader can gain an appreciation of the spectrum of therapeutic options available for the treatment of Zenker's diverticula.

Pegram, P. S.: Esophagitis in the immunocompromised host. *In* Castell, D. O. (Ed.): The Esophagus. Boston, Little, Brown & Co, 1992, pp. 643–668.
This is a comprehensive modern reference source on the subject that reviews in depth the esophageal infections that most commonly afflict patients with human immunodeficiency virus infection or cancer as well as transplant recipients (including bone marrow transplant recipients). Excellent clinical descriptions of these conditions, their diagnosis, complications, current therapeutic recommendations for each, and an extensive bibliography are provided.

Wilkins, E. W., Jr.: Rings and webs. *In* Pearson, F. G., Deslauriers, J., Ginsberg, R. J., Hiebert, C. A., McKneally, M. F., and Urschel, H. C., Jr.: Esophageal Surgery. New York, Churchill-Livingstone, 1995, pp. 283–291.
This concise, well-written chapter reviews the anatomic and histologic morphology, diagnosis and treatment of lower-esophageal (Schatzki's) rings and esophageal webs, providing a scholarly, clear discussion of a topic that, surprisingly, seems to confuse many medical students and young surgical house officers.

REFERENCES

1. Allen, T. H., and Clagett, O. T.: Changing concepts in the surgical treatment of pulsion diverticula of the lower esophagus. J. Thorac. Cardiovasc. Surg., 50:455, 1965.
2. Belsey, R.: Functional disease of the esophagus. J. Thorac. Cardiovasc. Surg., 52:164, 1966.
3. Benacci, J. C., Deschamps, C., Trastek, V. F., et al.: Epiphrenic diverticulum: Results of surgical treatment. Ann. Thorac. Surg., 55:1109, 1993.
4. Borrie, J., and Wilson, R. L. K.: Oesophageal diverticula: Principles of management and appraisal of classification. Thorax, 35:759, 1980.
5. Bruggeman, L. L., and Seman, W. B.: Epiphrenic diverticula: An analysis of 80 cases. Am. J. Roentgenol., 119:266, 1973.
6. Bubrick, M. P., Lundeen, J. W., Onstad, G. R., and Hitchcock, C. R.: Mallory-Weiss syndrome: Analysis of 59 cases. Surgery, 88:400, 1980.
7. Carlson, M., Stauffer, R. N., and Paynes, W. S.: Ankylosing vertebral hyperostosis causing dysphagia. Arch. Surg., 109:567, 1974.
8. Dantos, R. O., and Villanova, M. G.: Esophageal motility impairment in Plummer-Vinson syndrome: Correction by iron treatment. Dig. Dis. Sci., 38:968, 1993.
9. Debas, H. T., Payne, W. S., Cameron, A. J., and Carlson, H. C.: Physiopathology of lower esophageal diverticulum and its implications for treatment. Surg. Gynecol. Obstet., 151:593, 1980.
10. Dines, D. E., and Anderson, M. W.: Giant left atrium as a cause of dysphagia. Ann. Intern. Med. 65:759, 1966.
11. Dohlman, G., and Mattsson, O.: The endoscopic operation for hypopharyngeal diverticula: A roentgencinematographic study. Arch. Otolaryngol., 77:744, 1960.
12. Duranceau, A., Cardin, J. L., and Taillefer, R.: Long-term effects of total fundoplication on the myotomized esophagus. *In* Siewert, J. R., and Holscher, A. H. (Eds.): Diseases of the Esophagus. Berlin, Springer-Verlag, 1988, pp. 1206–1209.
13. Duranceau, A., Rheault, M. J., and Jamieson, G. G.: Physiological response to cricopharyngeal myotomy and diverticulum suspension. Surgery, 94:655, 1983.
14. Ellis, F. H., Jr.: Surgical management of esophageal motility disturbances. Am. J. Surg., 139:752, 1980.
15. Ellis, F. H., and Crozier, R. E.: Cervical esophageal dysphagia: Indications for and results of cricopharyngeal myotomy. Ann Surg., 194:279, 1981.
16. Ellis, F. H., Jr., Schlegel, J. F., Lynch, V. P., et al.: Cricopharyngeal myotomy for pharyngoesophageal diverticulum. Ann Surg., 170:340, 1969.
17. Gundry, S. R., Borkon, A. M., McIntosh, C. L., and Morrow, A. G.: *Candida* esophagitis following cardiac operations and short-term antibiotic prophylaxis. J. Thorac. Cardiovasc. Surg., 80:661, 1980

18. Hanna, E. A., and Derrick, J. R.: Dysphagia caused by tortuosity of the thoracic aorta. J. Thorac. Cardiovasc. Surg., 57:134, 1969.
19. Jackson, C., and Shallow, T. A.: Diverticula of the esophagus, pulsion, traction, malignant and congenital. Ann. Surg., 83:1, 1926.
20. Jamieson, G. G., Duranceau, A. C., and Payne, W. S.: Pharyngo-oesophageal diverticulum. *In* Jamieson, G. G. (Ed.): Surgery of the Oesophagus. Edinburgh, Churchill-Livingstone, 1988, pp. 435–493.
21. Lahey, F. H., and Warren, K. W.: Esophageal diverticula. Surg. Gynecol. Obstet., 98:1, 1954.
22. Lambert, A.: Surgical correction of esophageal obstruction due to tortuosity of the aorta. J. Thorac. Cardiovasc. Surg., 62:973, 1971.
23. LeRoux, B. T., and Williams, M. A.: Dysphagia megalatriensis. Thorax, 24:603, 1969.
24. Levine, M. S.: Crohn's disease of the upper gastrointestinal tract. Radiol. Clin. North Am., 25(1):79, 1989.
25. Ludlow, A.: Obstructed deglutition, from a preternatural dilatation of, and bag formed in, the pharynx. Med. Soc. Phys., 3:85, 1769.
26. MacCarty, R. L., Dukes, R. J., Strimlan, C. V., Dines, D. E., and Payne, W. S.: Radiographic findings in patients with esophageal involvement by mediastinal granuloma. Gastrointest. Radiol., 4:11, 1979.
27. McDonald, G. B.: Esophageal disease caused by infection, systemic illness, medications, and trauma. *In* Sleisenger, M. S. (Ed.): Gastrointestinal Disease, 5th ed. Philadelphia, W. B. Saunders, 1993, p. 427.
28. Michel, L., Serrano, A., and Malt, R. A.: Mallory-Weiss syndrome: Evolution of diagnostic and therapeutic patterns over two decades. Ann. Surg., 192:716, 1980.
29. Orringer, M. B.: Extended cervical esophagomyotomy for cricopharyngeal dysfunction. J. Thorac. Cardiovasc. Surg., 80:669, 1980.
30. Orringer, M. B., and Sloan, H.: Monilial esophagitis: An increasingly frequent cause of esophageal stenosis? Ann. Thorac. Surg., 26:364, 1978.
31. Ottinger, L. W., and Wilkins, E. W., Jr.: Late results in patients with Schatzki's ring undergoing destruction of the ring and hiatus herniorrhaphy. Am. J. Surg., 139:591, 1980.
32. Payne, S. W., and King, R. M.: Pharyngoesophageal (Zenker's) diverticulum. Surg. Clin. North Am., 63:815, 1983.
33. Postlethwait, R. W.: Surgery of the esophagus. Norwalk, CT, Appleton-Century-Crofts, 1979, pp. 126–127.
34. Rivkin, L., Bremner, C. G., and Bremner, C. H.: Pathophysiology of midoesophageal and epiphrenic diverticula of the oesophagus. S. Afr. Med. J., 66:127, 1984.
35. Sheft, D. J., and Shrago, G.: Esophageal moniliasis: The spectrum of the disease. JAMA, 213:1859, 1972.
36. Shererzt, E. F., and Jorizzo, J. L.: Cutaneous disease of the esophagus. *In* Castell, D. O. (Ed.): The Esophagus. Boston, Little, Brown & Co, 1992, pp. 793–799.
37. Sugawa, C., Benishek, D., and Walt, A. J.: Mallory-Weiss syndrome: A study of 224 patients. Am. J. Surg., 145:30, 1983.
38. Sweet, R. H.: Excision of diverticulum of the pharyngoesophageal junction and lower esophagus by means of the one-stage procedure. Ann. Surg., 143:433, 1956.
39. Tishler, J. M. A., and Helman, C. A.: Crohn's disease of the esophagus. J. Can. Assoc. Radiol., 35:28, 1984.
40. van Overbeck, J. J. M., and Hoeksema, P. E.: Endoscopic treatment of the hypopharyngeal diverticulum—211 cases. Laryngoscope, 92:88, 1982.
41. Wilcox, M. C.: Esophageal disease in the acquired immunodeficiency syndrome: Etiology, diagnosis, and management. Am. J. Med., 92:412, 1992.
42. Wilkins, E. W., Jr.: Rings and webs. *In* Pearson, F. G., Deslauries, J., Ginsberg, R. J., Hiebert, C. A., McKneally, M. F., and Urschel, H. C., Jr. (Eds.): Esophageal Surgery. New York, Churchill Livingstone, 1995, pp. 283–287.
43. Wright, R.: Upper esophageal perforation with flexible endoscopy secondary to cervical osteophytes. Dig. Dis. Sci., 25:66, 1980.
44. Wynder, E. L., Hultberg, S., Jacobsson, F., et al.: Environmental factors in cancer of the upper alimentary tract: A Swedish study with special reference to Plummer-Vinson (Paterson-Kelly) syndrome. Cancer, 10:470, 1957.
45. Zenker, F. A.: Diseases of the oesophagus. *In* von Ziemssen, II (Ed.): Cyclopedia of the Practice of Medicine, Vol. 8. New York, William-Wood, 1878, pp. 1–214.

V

ESOPHAGOSCOPY

Mark B. Orringer, M.D.

Esophagoscopy, which permits direct evaluation of the interior of the esophagus, is among the most vital diagnostic tools in the assessment of the patient with esophageal symptoms from any cause. With technical advances in flexible fiberoptic esophagogastroscopy, the number of these procedures being performed has increased greatly. However, as esophagoscopy has become a more commonly performed operation, a rather cavalier attitude toward this procedure has emerged. It should be kept in mind that esophagoscopy, particularly with dilatation of a stricture, is one of the most dangerous operations performed, the horrendous complications of a perforation being all too familiar to those called on to treat patients with esophageal disruption. Rigid adherence to basic principles of esophagoscopy is consistently rewarded by fewer complications.

INDICATIONS AND CONTRAINDICATIONS

Esophagoscopy is indicated in a variety of diagnostic and therapeutic situations.[5] Diagnostically, features of dysphagia, odynophagia, reflux that persists or recurs despite adequate therapy, occult blood loss, hematemesis, and atypical chest pain most often warrant esophagoscopy.[1] Esophagoscopy is also useful in assessing established esophageal pathology—esophagitis, Barrett's mucosa, neuromotor dysfunction, caustic injury, or tumors. Definition and confirmation of radiologic abnormalities—stricture, hiatal hernia, suspected esophagitis, diverticula, varices, and extrinsic compression—are common indications for esophagoscopy. Finally, esophagoscopy is of great diagnostic value in the assessment of postoperative problems—anastomotic stricture, tumor recurrence, bleeding, dysphagia, or recurrent gastroesophageal reflux. From a therapeutic standpoint, dilation and biopsy of strictures, removal of foreign bodies, placement of endoluminal prostheses, sclerotherapy, endoscopic myotomy (Dohlman's procedure), and laser photocoagulation for bleeding or tumor debulking are the usual indications for esophagoscopy. Esophagoscopy is *not* indicated to assess reflux symptoms that respond to medical management, an uncomplicated sliding hiatal hernia, or a previous demonstrated benign stricture (not associated with Barrett's mucosa). It cannot be overemphasized that safe esophagoscopy demands a well-trained endoscopist, properly functioning equipment, and resuscitative support in the event that a cardiorespiratory complication occurs. Esophagoscopy should not be performed in a struggling, uncooperative, agitated patient. Additional relative contraindications include a recent myocardial infarction, severe cervical spine deformities, and a large thoracic aortic aneurysm.

GENERAL CONSIDERATIONS

Safe esophagoscopy requires familiarity with normal esophageal anatomy, particularly the three areas of constriction and the course of the esophagus through the thorax (see Part I in this chapter). As a general rule, and certainly in the case of rigid esophagoscopy, elective esophagoscopy should be preceded by a barium esophagogram, which ideally should be displayed in view of the endoscopist during the procedure. Knowledge of existing esophageal pathology that is readily visible on a barium esophagogram is extremely important, so that the endoscopist does not begin the *journey* down the esophagus without a *road map*. Perforating a pharyngoesophageal diverticulum, for example, cannot be condoned just because the surgeon was unaware of its presence before esophagoscopy.

Before performing esophagoscopy, it is helpful to relate pathology seen on the barium swallow examination to certain anatomic landmarks and then to extrapolate from this assessment the approximate level within the esophagus at which the abnormality should be seen. The cricopharyngeus sphincter, for example, is located on the barium esophagogram at the level of the seventh cervical or first thoracic vertebral bodies, or approximately 15 cm. from the upper incisor teeth at esophagoscopy. Topographically, the angle of Louis (the sternomanubrial junction) on the anterior chest wall aligns with the tracheal bifurcation, which can usually be seen in most barium esophagograms at about the level of the fourth thoracic vertebra, and corresponds to a point 25 cm. from the incisors on esophagoscopy. The esophagogastric junction is typically seen endoscopically 40 cm. from the upper incisors approximately at the level of the eleventh or twelfth thoracic vertebrae.

Until refinements and wide availability of the flexible esophagogastroscopes in the 1970s, rigid esophagoscopy was most commonly used for endoscopic assessment of the esophagus. Its disadvantages included the frequent need for general anesthesia and the danger of introduction of the instrument in a patient with cervical spine disease. The greater comfort and ease of flexible endoscopy have now made this the procedure of choice in most patients requiring esophagoscopy. However, there are definite situations in which rigid esophagoscopy has distinct advantages, and the endoscopist should ideally have available both rigid and flexible instruments, which should be viewed as complementary, not mutually exclusive. The rigid esophagoscope is best for evaluating lesions at or just below the cricopharyngeal sphincter, removal of foreign bodies, dilatation of certain high-grade stenoses, obtaining larger and more adequate biopsy specimens, and significant esophageal bleeding.

FLEXIBLE ESOPHAGOSCOPY

Preoperative Preparation. As with every elective operation, a thorough discussion with the patient of the indications for the procedure and its potential complications is warranted. Patients with a history suggesting increased bleeding tendencies should have an initial coagulation profile. Initial vital signs are recorded, and during the procedure, the electrocardiogram and oxygen saturation (with pulse oximetry) are monitored continuously.

Bacteremia during upper gastrointestinal endoscopy has been well documented, occurring with an average incidence of 0% to 10%, which rises as high as 50% during esophageal dilation or endoscopic sclerotherapy.[3, 36] The standard prophylactic antibiotic regimen recommended by the American Heart Association—ampicillin and gentamicin parenterally 30 to 60 minutes before the endoscopy—should be administered to patients with a prosthetic cardiac valve, systemic to pulmonary artery shunt, or a history of endocarditis. Vancomycin is used in those with a penicillin allergy.[27] Patients should avoid eating for 6 to 8 hours before the procedure.

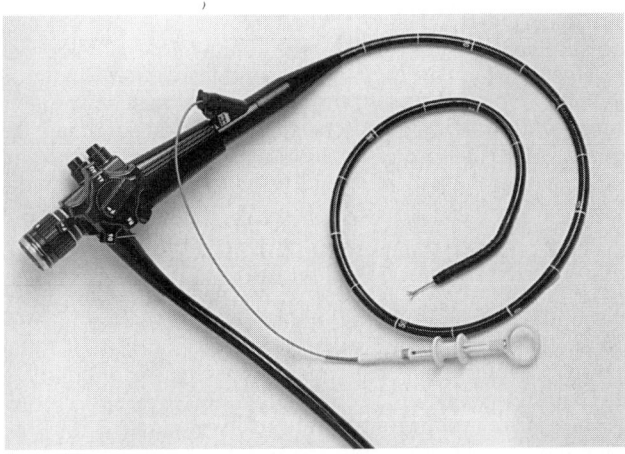

Figure 26–45. A flexible upper gastrointestinal endoscope with a biopsy forceps inserted through the instrumentation channel and protruding from the tip of the scope. This endoscope has a flexible tip, the movement of which (up, down, or side to side) is directed by the two control wheels.

Topical anesthesia of the posterior pharynx is achieved with benzocaine or 2% to 4% lidocaine spray, and intravenous sedation is obtained with either diazepam or midazolam, often administered in combination with meperidine. It is foolhardy to persist with attempts at esophagoscopy in an anxious, combative, or uncooperative patient, and general anesthesia is the safer choice in such cases.

Equipment. The flexible esophagogastroduodenoscopes in widest use today vary in outer diameter from 7.9 to 12.6 mm. and have instrument channels ranging in diameter from 2 to 3.7 mm. (Fig. 26–45). This permits passage of a variety of biopsy forceps, cytology brushes, and irrigation catheters (Fig. 26–46). Movement of the distal 8 cm. of the instrument is manually controlled by wheels near the eyepiece, and range of motion includes 210 degrees upward, 90 degrees downward, and 100 degrees to either side. The newer fiberoptic scopes are equipped to permit video recording and still photography. Proper cleaning and disinfection of fiberoptic scopes is extremely important to minimize the risk of cross-contamination, particularly with the human immunodeficiency virus.[2]

Technique. If only esophagoscopy and a limited examination of the stomach are to be performed, the patient may be positioned either in the usual left lateral position (which facilitates visualization of the pylorus and intubation of the duodenum) or in the sitting position (to minimize potential pulmonary complications of aspiration). A bite block is used to avoid damage to the scope from the patient's teeth. Before introduction of the scope, proper functioning of the suction, insufflation, and irrigation controls should be confirmed. The scope is introduced along the base of the tongue and into the posterior pharynx, and the esophagus is intubated as the patient swallows. Intubation of the esophagus is most often done blindly, but some prefer to advance the instrument through the pharynx and upper sphincter under direct vision.

As the instrument is advanced, gentle air insufflation maintains a patent lumen; and as is the case with rigid endoscopy as well, the scope should not be advanced unless a lumen ahead is clearly visible. Mucosal color, architectural abnormalities, and muscular contractions in the esophageal wall are assessed continually. The location of contiguous esophageal strictures is readily seen: left anterolateral indentation between 23 and 25 cm. from the upper incisors to the aortic arch; just distal to this, diagonal indentation anteriorly from superomedial to inferolateral from the left mainstem bron-

chus; and the pulsation from left atrial contractions on the anteromedial esophagus just beyond. In the distal esophagus, evidence of reflux esophagitis and Barrett's mucosa is carefully sought. The precise location of the squamocolumnar epithelial junction (in centimeters from the upper incisors), the *anatomic* esophagogastric junction (where the tubular esophagus ends and the mucosal folds of the stomach begin), and the level of the diaphragmatic hiatus are identified and recorded. The latter is visualized by having the patient sniff, which causes the crura to indent the esophagus at the level of the hiatus. The fundus and gastric side of the cardia are visualized by retroflexing the tip of the scope. Esophageal biopsies and brushings for cytologic evaluation as indicated are obtained after inspection of the length of the esophagus has been completed. The largest possible biopsy specimens, preferably with 8-French forceps, are harvested, carefully identifying their site of origin in centimeters from the upper incisors.

RIGID ESOPHAGOSCOPY

Preoperative Preparation. The considerations for preoperative preparation of the patient for rigid esophagoscopy are initially the same as for flexible instrumentation, including antibiotic prophylaxis for endocarditis when appropriate.

Equipment. Rigid esophagoscopes range in length from 29 cm. (the *short scope* for evaluation of only the upper esophagus) to 45 cm. (the length used in women) or 50 cm. (the length most often used in male patients). The tips are beveled and blunted. They have outer diameters of approximately 12 mm. for round tubes or 16 mm. for the oval Jesberg scopes. The light source is typically a long light-carrier, which is inserted in a channel that runs the length of the scope. Optical telescopes can be used for forward (0 degrees), angled (30 degrees), and side (90 degrees) viewing. The cup biopsy forceps introduced through the rigid esophagoscope obtains specimens that are considerably larger and deeper than those obtained through the flexible esophagoscope instrument channel.

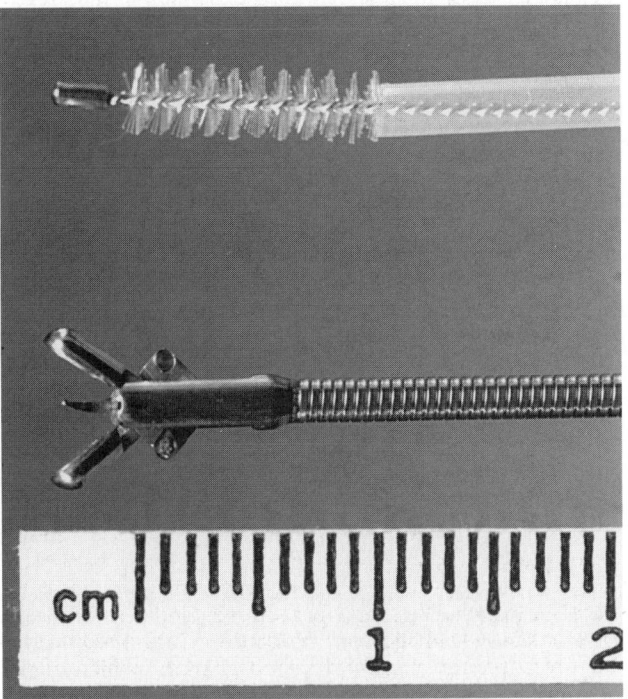

Figure 26–46. Biopsy forceps and cytology brush used in flexible fiberoptic endoscopy.

Technique. Rigid esophagoscopy is most commonly performed with the patient under general anesthesia, but with proper sedation and topical anesthesia, endoscopy with the patient in the sitting position is readily achieved.[37] After induction of general anesthesia, the patient's eyes are padded, taped closed, and covered with a folded towel to prevent inadvertent injury during the procedure. The endotracheal tube is displaced to the left side of the mouth and secured with tape.

The lubricated rigid esophagoscope is introduced into the right side of the posterior pharynx, displacing the tongue and the endotracheal tube to the left. The epiglottis is elevated by the tip of the advancing esophagoscope, which is introduced into the esophagus behind the right arytenoid cartilage into the narrow opening seen between the larynx and the posterior wall of the pharynx. This is the most critical step of rigid esophagoscopy. Because of the natural *pull* of the cricopharyngeus muscle against the cricoid cartilage, making this the narrowest point of the gastrointestinal tract, unless upward displacement of the larynx by the advancing esophagoscope is maintained, a posterior perforation by the instrument can occur, typically just proximal to the sphincter (Fig. 26–47). This is the most common mechanism of endoscopic esophageal injury. The esophageal lumen must be kept in view at all times. If the opening of the upper sphincter is not readily apparent, gentle introduction of a 12- or 14-French gumtipped Jackson dilator as a guide or *follower* through the upper sphincter facilitates entry of the esophagoscope into the upper esophagus. Because introduction of the rigid esophagoscope is performed under direct vision, in contrast to flexible esophagoscopy, the posterior pharynx and esophageal introitus are routinely examined as part of the procedure.

As the thoracic esophagus is traversed, the patient's head should be turned, raised, or lowered as necessary so that the lumen remains central and in view at all times. Once the tip of the esophagoscope is beyond the level of the aortic arch, the neck is extended and the head gradually lowered and rotated to the right as the instrument is advanced, because as the distal esophagus is approached, the esophagus normally deviates to the left and anteriorly as it leaves the thorax

and joins the stomach. After visualization of the mucosa, measurement of the level of the esophageal pathology in centimeters from the upper incisors, biopsy, and obtaining brushings for cytologic evaluation, the esophagoscope is slowly withdrawn, again concentrating on maintaining the lumen within the center of the visual field at all times and manipulating the patient's head to achieve this as required.

COMPLICATIONS OF ESOPHAGOSCOPY

Esophagoscopy can result in either relatively minor complications (laceration of the lips or tongue, fracture or dislodgment of teeth, and pharyngeal lacerations) or catastrophic events (massive tracheobronchial aspiration or esophageal perforation). Whereas the morbidity and mortality rates from esophagoscopy are relatively low,[9, 26, 35] a considerable number of complications of esophagoscopy do occur as a result of the large number of these procedures being performed. Most minor complications are a function of poor technique and failure to adequately protect the gums, lips, and teeth during the procedure. By far, the leading and most serious complication of esophagoscopy, with or without dilation of a stricture, is perforation, which occurs in less than 1% of patients, even in the hands of the most experienced endoscopist. The cervical esophagus is perforated in 40% of cases, the midesophagus in 25%, and the distal esophagus in 35%.[34] It is a basic tenet of esophageal surgery that pain or fever after esophageal instrumentation represents an esophageal perforation until proven otherwise and is an indication for an immediate esophagogram.[30] Because the mortality and morbidity of an esophageal perforation is directly related to the time interval between the occurrence of the injury and its diagnosis and repair or drainage, an extremely aggressive position toward diagnosing a perforation after endoscopy must be adopted. A contrast study with both a water-soluble agent (Gastrografin) as well as dilute barium if no perforation is seen should be obtained, because a perforation may be overlooked on roentgenographic evaluation when only Gastrografin is used (Fig. 26–48). The treatment of esophageal perforation is discussed elsewhere in this chapter (see Part VII). Sizable perforations proximal to obstructing esophageal lesions are unlikely to heal primarily if repaired and may be treated very effectively by emergent esophagectomy and esophageal substitution using stomach.[31]

Clinically significant bleeding complicating esophagoscopy is rare and occurs in 0.02% to 0.04% of patients.[35] It is typically a function of persistent bleeding from a biopsy site, varices, or a Mallory-Weiss tear from retching during endoscopy. Massive regurgitation and aspiration with hypoxemia and cardiorespiratory arrest are ever-present threats during esophagoscopy, particularly in the patient with gastroesophageal reflux or a megaesophagus of achalasia (see later). Proper positioning of the patient, constant availability of resuscitative equipment, and arterial oxygen saturation monitoring are safeguards but do not substitute for vigilance and the surgeon's awareness of the general condition of the patient, not simply the video image from the endoscopy.

SPECIFIC PATHOLOGY FOR THE SURGICAL ENDOSCOPIST

Reflux Esophagitis and Barrett's Mucosa

One of the most common indications for esophagoscopy is the assessment of the presence and extent of esophagitis associated with gastroesophageal reflux. The traditional designations of mild, moderate, and severe endoscopic esophagitis have inherent wide variations in meaning among observers. The consistent use of a standardized grading system

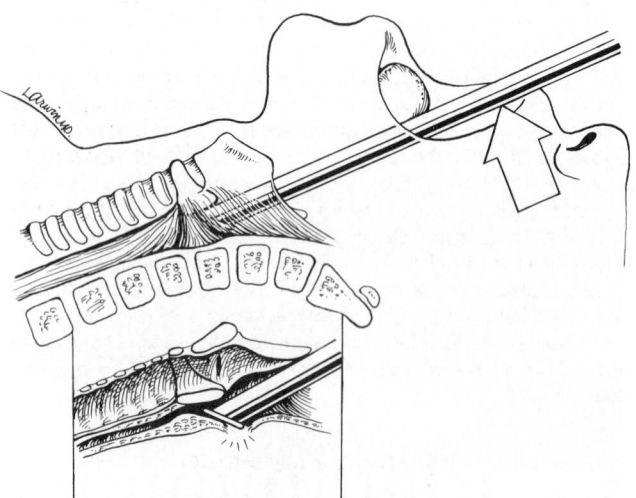

Figure 26–47. Mechanism of endoscopic cervical esophageal perforation. In performing rigid esophagoscopy, it is essential that a gentle, steady lifting force (arrow) be exerted to obtain forward displacement of the larynx and cricoid cartilage. Failure to overcome the natural pull of the upper esophageal sphincter against the cricoid cartilage results in a typical posterior perforation (inset). (From Orringer, M. B.: Complications of esophageal surgery and trauma. *In* Greenfield, L. J. [Ed.]: Complications of Surgery and Trauma, 2nd ed. Philadelphia, J. B. Lippincott, 1990, pp. 302–325.)

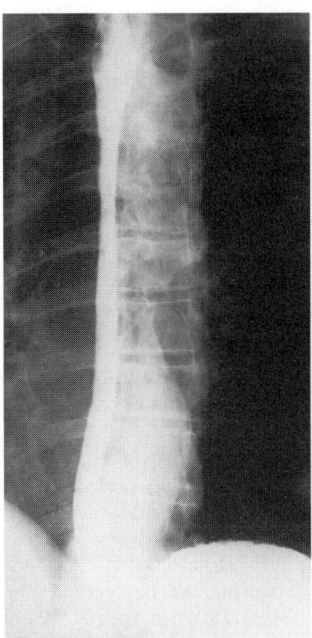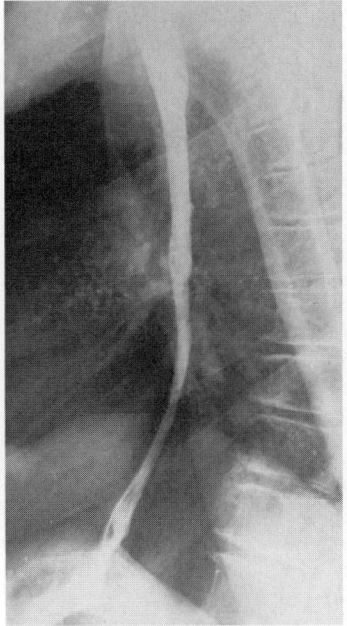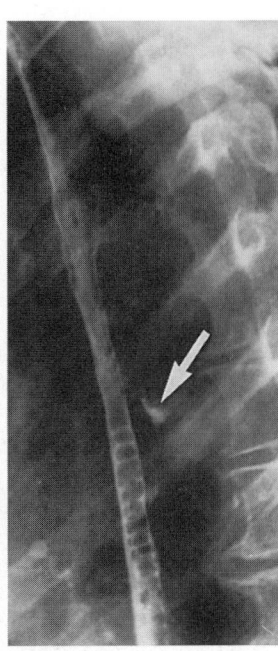

Figure 26–48. Failure of water-soluble contrast material to demonstrate esophageal perforation. Posteroanterior *(left)* and lateral *(center)* views from meglumine diatrizoate (Gastrografin) esophagogram of a patient with an acute caustic burn that was dilated prematurely within 10 days of ingestion of Drano. Despite the development of fever and chest pain, no perforation was seen in this study. A barium esophagogram *(right)* demonstrated a perforation (arrow) in the middle third of the thoracic esophagus. (From Orringer, M. B.: Complications of esophageal surgery and trauma. *In* Greenfield, L. J. [Ed.]: Complications of Surgery and Trauma, 2nd ed. Philadelphia, J. B.: Lippincott, 1990, pp. 302–325.)

for endoscopic reflux esophagitis provides a more objective description of the gross pathologic changes seen and permits a more meaningful evaluation of patients at different times and by different endoscopists. Unfortunately, uniform consensus on this topic has not been reached, and a number of systems for grading reflux esophagitis are in use. Two of the more popular classifications of reflux esophagitis are those of Skinner and Belsey (1967)[38] and Savary and Miller (1990).[29]

Classification of Endoscopic Grades of Esophagitis

Skinner and Belsey's Classification of Esophagitis

Grade I: Distal esophageal mucosal erythema (which may obscure the esophagogastric squamocolumnar junction)

Grade II: Mucosal erythema with superficial ulceration, typically linear and vertical and with an overlying fibrinous membranous exudate that is easily wiped away, leaving a bleeding surface (often misinterpreted as *scope trauma* by the inexperienced endoscopist)

Grade III: Mucosal erythema with superficial ulceration and associated submucosal fibrosis on biopsy—a dilatable *early* stricture

Grade IV: Extensive ulceration and fibrous luminal stenosis—may represent irreversible panmural fibrosis

Savary and Miller's Classification of Esophagitis

Grade I: Single erosive or exudate lesion, oval or linear, involving only one longitudinal fold

Grade II: Noncircular multiple erosions or exudate lesion involving more than one longitudinal fold, with or without confluence

Grade III: Circular erosive or exudative lesion

Grade IV: Chronic lesions: ulcer(s), stricture(s), or short esophagus isolated or associated with lesions of Grades I, II, or III

Grade V: Islands, fingerlike forms or circumferential distribution of Barrett's epithelium isolated or associated with a lesion of Grades I through IV.

Regardless of which classification is used, the endoscopist should have such an orderly method of defining the changes of reflux esophagitis seen at the time of esophagoscopy.

Barrett's mucosa—metaplastic replacement of normal esophageal squamous mucosa by columnar epithelium—is of particular importance in this context, because esophagoscopy with biopsy is the most sensitive and specific diagnostic test for this condition, and periodic surveillance is mandatory to detect progression of premalignant dysplastic change.[19] Because the squamocolumnar epithelial junction may normally be found within 2 to 3 cm. of the anatomic esophagogastric junction, by convention, the diagnosis of Barrett's mucosa requires the histologic identification of the metaplastic columnar epithelium 3 cm. or more proximal to the junction of the tubular esophagus with the stomach. Normal esophageal squamous epithelium has a pearly white (pinkish gray) color, in contrast to the reddish salmon-pink velvety metaplastic columnar mucosa. The location of the Z-line or squamocolumnar epithelial junction in centimeters from the upper incisors, the anatomic esophagogastric junction, and the level of the diaphragmatic hiatus should be recorded. Beginning at the esophagogastric junction, at least three biopsy specimens from different sites of the esophageal circumference should be taken at 2-cm. intervals, progressing proximally. Normal-appearing squamous mucosa proximal to the Z-line should also be sampled to confirm the endoscopist's impression of the extent of the Barrett's mucosa. For the patient whose squamocolumnar junction in a Barrett's esophagus is at 24 cm. and the esophagogastric junction at 35 cm. proximal to a hiatal hernia, two or more specimens may be required. Because the detection of significant dysplasia is a function of the adequacy of surveillance biopsies, although a tedious process, there is no better alternative to proper assessment and evaluation of the patient with Barrett's mucosa.

Esophageal Strictures

Two questions must be answered about every esophageal stricture identified with a barium swallow examination: (1) is the stricture benign or malignant, and (2) if benign, can the stricture be dilated? Both of these questions are answered by esophagoscopy, which is a mandatory part of the evaluation of every stricture. The caliber of the stenosis on the barium study does not correlate with the resistance that is encountered when dilators are passed through the stricture,

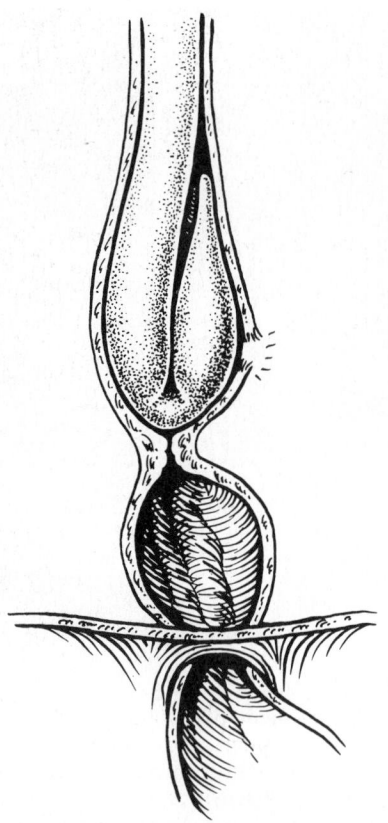

Figure 26–49. Attempt to dilate a tight esophageal stricture by "blind" passage of a dilator has resulted in curling of the bougie proximal to the stenosis and disruption of the esophagus as the dilator is advanced. (From Orringer, M. B.: Complications of esophageal surgery and trauma. In Greenfield, L. J. [Ed.]: Complications of Surgery and Trauma, 2nd ed. Philadelphia, J. B. Lippincott, 1990, pp. 302–325.)

steady gentle pressure with the esophagoscope. Specimens from within the stricture increase the yield in detecting malignancy. After obtaining specimens and withdrawing the scope, dilation of strictures can generally be carried out by segmental blind passage of lubricated tapered Hurst-Maloney dilators through the mouth. Some advocate never dilating a stricture more than three successive dilator sizes during one session (rule of threes) as a means of avoiding perforation.[10] The author has not found this to be practical and views both the amount of resistance encountered with passage of the dilators and experience as the best guides to dilation.

To obtain comfortable swallowing, dilation of the stricture to at least a 46-French caliber is the goal. Alternatively, if the initial evaluation of the stricture indicates that it is dense and rigid, a dilator passed blindly may curl proximal to the nonyielding stenosis and a perforation may occur (Fig. 26–49). In such cases, the Savary-Gilliard bougies present a safe and effective means of instrumentation.[20] The metallic guide wire is passed through the instrumentation channel of the flexible esophagoscope and is guided through the stenosis under direct vision. The scope is then removed, leaving the guide wire in place across the stricture, and the smooth, noncompressible Savary tapered dilators are threaded over the guide wire and advanced through the stricture (Figs. 26–50 and 26–51).

In the occasional difficult patient or one with a very eccentric or fibrotic *hard* stricture, rigid esophagoscopy under general anesthesia may be required. A mild stricture can be dilated directly with the rigid esophagoscope, and after specimens and brushings of the stenosis are obtained, tapered Maloney dilators may be passed as described earlier. A high-grade hard stenosis, however, requires gentle probing and evaluation with gum-tipped bougies passed under direct vision through the stenosis (Fig. 26–52). Once the course of the lumen is identified, the Savary-Gilliard system can be used to achieve adequate dilation. In an alternative method of dilation used by the author in such difficult cases, the standard rigid esophagoscope is removed and replaced with a special-order 45-cm. long, rigid esophagoscope (Pilling Company, Fort Washington, PA), which will accommodate up to a 50-French bougie (Fig. 26–53). After introducing this esophagoscope to the level of the stricture, progressively larger dilators, beginning with a 28-French dilator, are passed under direct vision through the stenosis. Virtually all reflux strictures that can be dilated either directly per os or through the esophagoscope to at least a 40-French bougie can be

with some of the tightest-appearing strictures being readily dilatable. Dilation of an esophageal stricture is among the most dangerous operations performed, and a consistent, organized operative approach is mandatory before it is begun. Most strictures are now evaluated initially using a flexible fiberoptic esophagogastroscope. Biopsy specimens of areas of mucosal abnormality as well as brushings for cytology should be obtained to exclude carcinoma. A stenosis with a relatively large-bore lumen may be traversed by applying

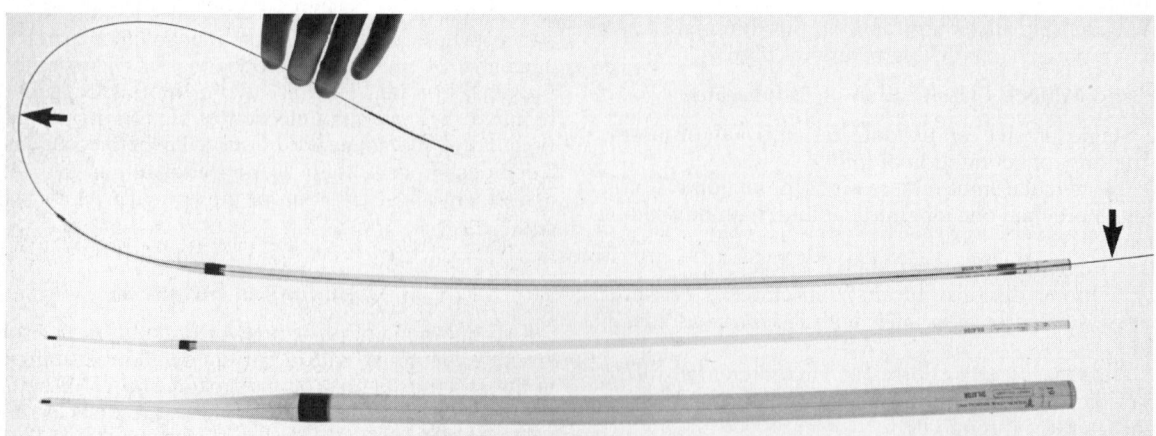

Figure 26–50. Savary-Gilliard esophageal bougies. These polyvinylchloride bougies are 100 cm. in length and have a 1.8 mm. in diameter central lumen that permits them to slide along the metallic guide wire (arrows). The bougies are smooth, noncompressible, and flexible in the longitudinal axis and provide a very safe means of dilating strictures (see Fig. 26–51).

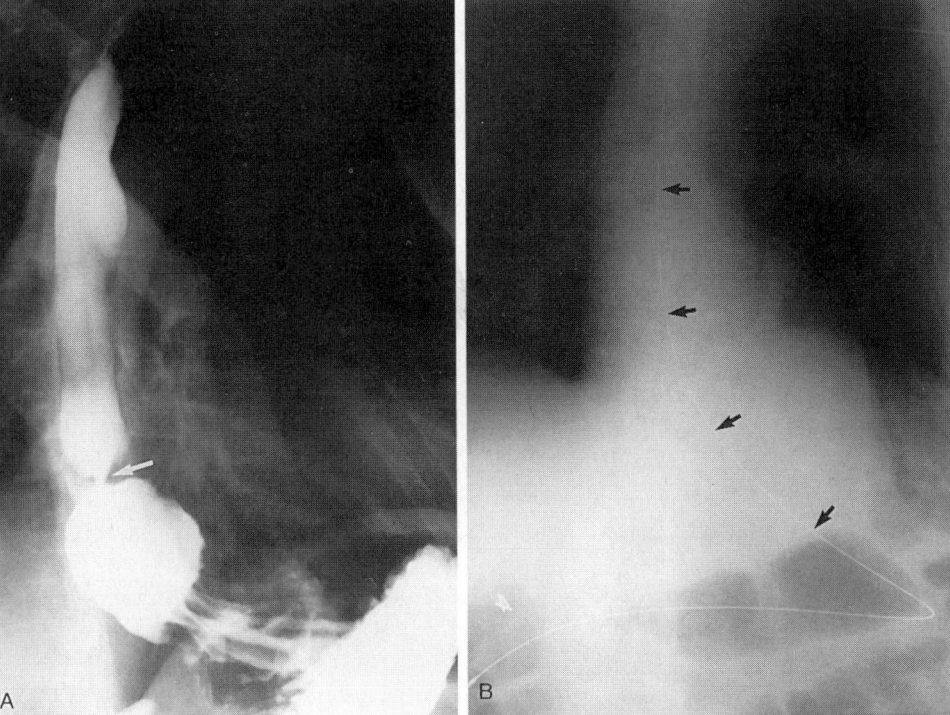

Figure 26–51. *A,* High-grade distal esophageal reflux stricture (arrow) proximal to a sliding hiatal hernia. *B,* Position of guide wire (arrows) through stricture and into stomach confirmed on portable chest roentgenogram before passage of Savary-Gilliard dilators. The stricture was successfully dilated up to a size 51-French bougie.

dilated intraoperatively to the 56- to 60-French bougie range at the time of an antireflux operation. Those strictures that will not accept a 40-French bougie may represent advanced, irreversible panmural fibrosis, which requires esophageal resection for relief of the obstruction.

Other instrumentation for dilating esophageal strictures is available. The Eder-Puestow system uses graded metal olive-tipped dilators passed over a guide wire placed endoscopically or fluoroscopically. It has a higher complication rate than the rubber dilators and has declined in popularity as a result. The American Endoscopy dilator system resembles the Savory-Gilliard system described earlier except for its shorter tip and radiopaque dilators.[10] Hydrostatic balloon dilators are the newest devices being used for dilation of esophageal strictures and have a reported success rate of 85%.[15] These inflatable balloons inserted through the flexible esophagogastroscope are constructed of a polymer that can be dilated only to a specified size, above which rupture of the balloon occurs. They range from 18 to 54 French. Balloon dilation of esophageal stenosis does not provide as effective

or lasting relief of dysphagia as simple passage of Maloney mercury-filled tapered dilators and has the added disadvantage of the requirement for sedation and endoscopy or fluoroscopy with their increased cost. The mercury-filled tapered dilators remain the safest, most efficient and widely used system for dilating the majority of esophageal strictures.[11, 17, 39]

Advanced Achalasia with Megaesophagus

Esophagoscopy in the patient with a megaesophagus is extremely dangerous and merits particular mention. In advanced achalasia, the esophagus may have a capacity of 1 to 2 liters, and disastrous massive tracheobronchial aspiration may follow attempts to introduce a flexible esophagoscope in the conscious but sedated patient on a casual outpatient basis. The routine preendoscopic instructions of giving nothing by mouth after midnight are entirely inadequate in this situation. The patient with a megaesophagus should be placed on a clear liquid diet for 48 hours before endoscopy or a scheduled esophageal operation. Just before the endos-

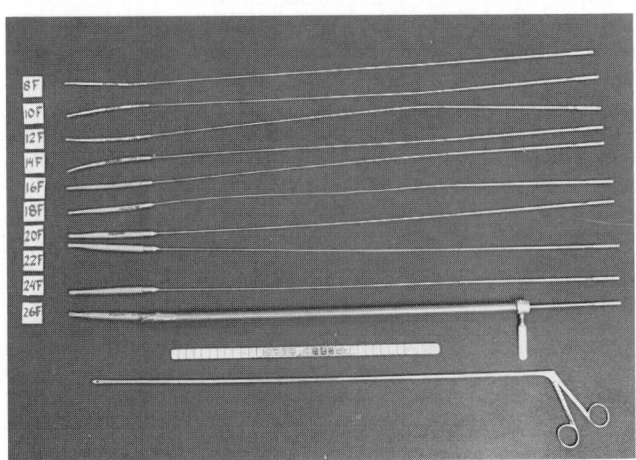

Figure 26–52. Jackson gum-tipped dilators, ruler, and biopsy forceps required for evaluating an esophageal stricture using the rigid esophagoscope. The stricture should be localized precisely (in centimeters from the upper incisor teeth), and brushings from the stricture as well as biopsy samples should be obtained. The dilators are gently manipulated through the stenosis and permit evaluation of the extent and pliability of the obstruction. The 26-French Jackson dilator is the largest one that will pass through the standard 45-cm. rigid esophagoscope shown. (From Orringer, M. B.: Complications of esophageal surgery and trauma. *In* Greenfield, L. J. [Ed.]: Complications of Surgery and Trauma, 2nd ed. Philadelphia, J. B. Lippincott, 1990, pp. 302–325.)

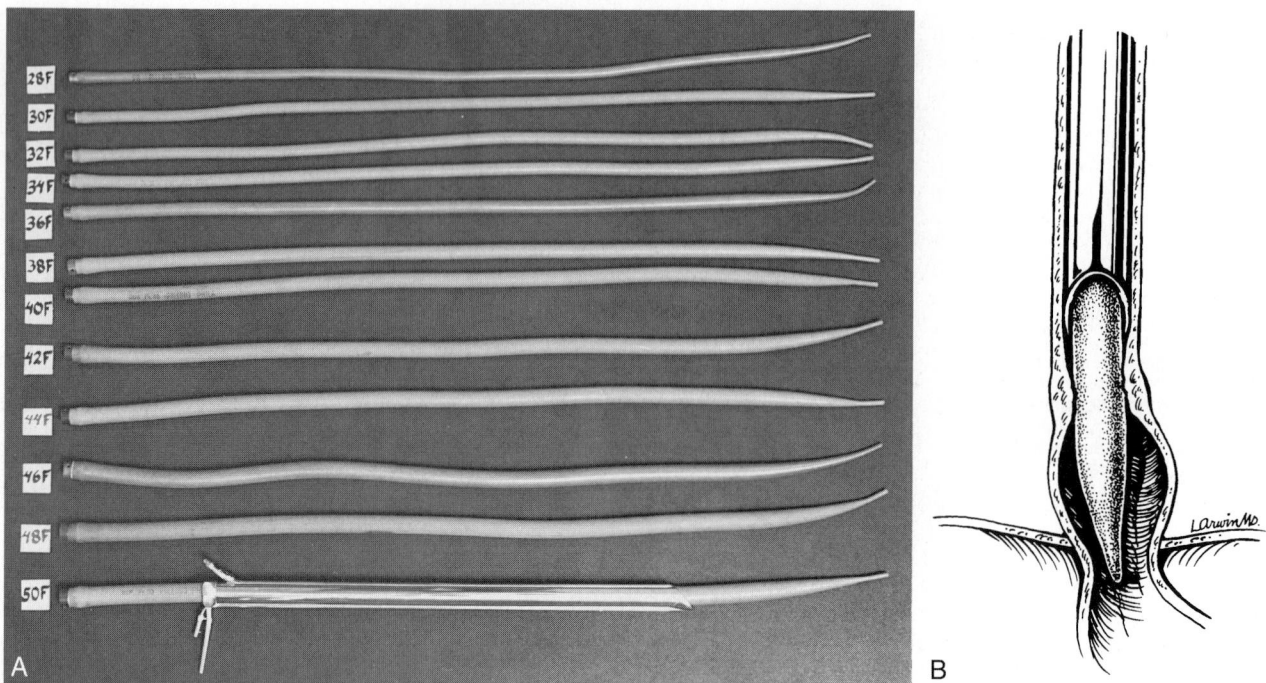

Figure 26–53. *A,* Tapered Maloney esophageal dilators and a 45-cm. Pilling esophagoscope, which accommodates up to a 50-French bougie, thus permitting progressive dilation of severe strictures under direct vision. *B,* Using a special-order large esophagoscope that accommodates up to a 50-French dilator, the stricture can be visualized directly for dilation. (From Orringer, M. B.: Complications of esophageal surgery and trauma. In Greenfield, L. J. [Ed.]: Complications of Surgery and Trauma, 2nd ed. Philadelphia, J. B. Lippincott, 1990, pp. 302–325.)

copy, with the patient in the upright position, an 18-French or larger nasogastric tube is passed orally into the esophagus, and intraesophageal contents are removed as thoroughly as possible by suctioning the tube at various levels and irrigating the esophagus with water as required. Once the esophagus is emptied, the endoscopy is performed. In such patients undergoing an esophagomyotomy or esophagectomy for achalasia, the esophagus is emptied as described earlier and the endotracheal tube is inserted using either an awake endotracheal intubation technique or a *crash* induction, maintaining constant backward pressure on the cricoid cartilage against the cervical spine to prevent regurgitation through the upper sphincter. Once the airway is protected by the inflated endotracheal tube balloon, the rigid esophagoscope is inserted into the esophagus and evacuation of intraesophageal contents is performed with large suction tubing. The mucosa can then be evaluated before operation. Standard flexible esophagoscopy is not ideal in the evaluation of the patient with a megaesophagus. Retained intraesophageal debris in these patients simply cannot be evacuated adequately through the flexible instrument, and a sedated patient with a megaesophagus undergoing a *standard* outpatient fiberoptic esophagoscopy may experience life-threatening pulmonary complications if regurgitation and aspiration occur when the cough reflex is suppressed. Equipment for endotracheal intubation and suctioning must always be available for these patients.

ADVANCES IN ESOPHAGOSCOPY

Vital Staining. Squamous cell carcinoma of the esophagus is seldom diagnosed at its earliest stages—carcinoma *in situ* (intraepithelial carcinoma) or microinvasive carcinoma—which may present at esophagoscopy as flat nondescript-appearing lesions (leukoplakia or erythroplakia).[8, 21, 22] Vital staining of the esophageal mucosa with either Lugol's

solution or toluidine blue through the esophagoscope offers the ability to diagnose these lesions and hence detect esophageal cancer at an earlier, more readily treatable stage. Three percent Lugol's solution, a negative tumor marker, stains normal glycogenic esophageal mucosa brown, while pathologic mucosa (early carcinoma, esophagitis, Barrett's mucosa) remains unstained.[16, 24, 41] The mucosa is easily evaluated using this technique by means of a swab of the solution applied through a rigid esophagoscope. Biopsy of nonstaining pathologic areas can then be obtained to establish a tissue diagnosis. A 1% aqueous solution of toluidine blue may also be used as a vital stain. It is a metachromatic stain with an affinity for cell nuclei; thus tissues with a high cellular density and nucleus/cytoplasm ratio take up the stain quickly and retain it for approximately 1 hour.[13, 23] With this later staining technique, again using rigid esophagoscopy, the esophageal mucosa is first washed with 1% acetic acid to remove excess mucus and food particles, 1% toluidine blue is applied for 1 minute, and the stain is washed away with 1% acetic acid. Those areas of the mucosa that remain stained are sampled and are likely to be neoplastic.[22]

Endoscopic Ultrasonography. Endoscopic ultrasonography has been used since the early 1980s in Japan and Northern Europe for the staging of cancer and assessment of a variety of esophageal disorders. Now into fourth- and fifth-generation models, existing instruments still have suboptimal optics that permit only side-viewing, but the ultrasound probes themselves have been significantly refined so that cervical, mediastinal, and upper abdominal anatomical detail is greatly enhanced. Now approximately 11 mm. in diameter, the esophageal ultrasound lacks an instrument channel and has a tip that houses the ultrasound emitter-receiver. The instrument is passed just as a flexible esophagoscope, and ultrasonograms showing esophageal wall anatomy, periesophageal, perigastric and celiac adenopathy are obtained. The five layers of the esophageal wall—mucosa, lamina propria, submucosa, muscularis propria, and adventitia—are identified. Criteria for the depth of penetration of primary carcinomas have been developed, and mediastinal lymph nodes involved with metastatic tumor have been identified with nearly 90% accuracy.[12, 25, 42, 43] Endoscopic ultrasonography provides better definition of benign tumors, specifically leiomyomas, than has been possible previously[40, 42, 44] and can be used to follow small asymptomatic intramural esophageal masses that meet criteria of benign lesions. The detection and assessment of esophageal varices by ultrasound has also been reported.[4]

Therapeutic Laser Endoscopy. Several types of lasers have proven to be applicable in the treatment of esophageal cancer. That in most common usage is the neodymium:yttrium-aluminum-garnet (Nd:YAG) laser, which is readily adaptable to flexible fiberoptic esophagoscopes and has been used to vaporize unresectable bulky intraluminal carcinomas, thereby providing variable palliation of dysphagia. With the prograde approach, the esophagoscope is advanced to the proximal extent of the tumor, and intermittent photocoagulation at 80 W. and a pulse duration of 0.5 to 1 second is used to destroy the tumor. Treatments are repeated at 2-day intervals, proceeding farther into the esophagus each day, until the majority of the obstructing tumor has been removed. An average of two to three sessions per patient is required to achieve an adequate lumen.[7]

A retrograde method of Nd:YAG photocoagulation was reported in 1985.[6] This procedure involves initial dilation of the tumor using Savary dilators until the endoscope can be advanced through it. The tumor is then treated beginning at its distal extent and working proximally. One treatment session is the goal of this approach, which involves more vigorous débridement than the prograde approach. With the availability of the contact laser sapphire probes in 1988, a lower wattage (15 W.) and continuous mode of energy delivery have decreased the risk of perforation and allowed more tumor to be removed per session.[18, 32, 33] Contact laser probes have also been used to treat some early esophageal carcinomas that have been localized by vital staining.[14, 28]

SELECTED REFERENCES

Miller, L. S.: Endoscopy of the esophagus. *In* Castell, D. O. (Ed.): The Esophagus. Boston, Little, Brown & Co, 1992, pp. 89–142.
This treatise on esophagoscopy contains excellent illustrative color photographs of virtually every type of pathologic process encountered at endoscopy. The various endoscopic grading systems for reflux esophagitis are listed. This is a fine general reference for every endoscopist. Its extensive bibliography is comprehensive.

Savary, M., and Monnier, P.: Esophagoscopy. *In* Pearson, F. G., Deslauriers, J., Ginsberg, R. J., Hiebert, C. A., McKneally, M. F., and Urschel, H. C., Jr. (Eds.): Esophageal Surgery. New York, Churchill Livingstone, 1995, pp. 105–117.
This is an excellent authoritative chapter on the subject, which includes descriptions of both rigid and flexible esophagoscopes, the indications for use of each, and proper positioning of the patient. The methodologies for vital staining, biopsying, obtaining endoscopic hemostasis, and photodynamic therapy are well described.

Skinner, D. B., and Belsey, R. H. R.: Endoscopy, instruments, anesthesia, and techniques. *In* Skinner, D. B., and Belsey, R. H. R. (Eds.): Management of Esophageal Disease. Philadelphia, W. B. Saunders, 1988, pp. 65–80.
This is a well-illustrated, concise review of the techniques of both flexible and rigid esophagoscopy that emphasizes the need for adequate anesthesia and illustrates the superior laryngeal nerve block. Endoscopic landmarks to be identified and common complications are discussed.

REFERENCES

1. American Society for Gastrointestinal Endoscopy: Appropriate use of gastrointestinal endoscopy. Manchester, MA, 1992.
2. American Society for Gastrointestinal Endoscopy: Infection control during gastrointestinal endoscopy. Gastrointest. Endosc., 34:375, 1988.
3. Botoman, V. A., and Surawicz, C. M.: Bacteremia with gastrointestinal endoscopic procedures. Gastrointest. Endosc., 32:342, 1986.
4. Caletti, G. C., Bolondi, L., Zani, L., Brocchi, E., Guizzardi, G., and Labo,

G.: Detection of portal hypertension and esophageal varices by means of endoscopic ultrasonography. Scand. J. Gastroenterol., 21(suppl. 123):74, 1986.
5. Castell, D. O., and Johnson, L. F.: Esophageal function in health and disease. *In* Castell, D. O., and Johnson, L. F. (Eds.): Clinical Topics in Gastroenterology. New York, Elsevier, 1983.
6. Dyer, R. M.: Single session palliation of obstructing esophageal cancer. Laser Surg. Med., 3:172, 1983.
7. Fleischer, D., and Sivak, M. U., Jr.: Endoscopic Nd-YAG laser therapy as palliation for esophagogastric cancer: Parameters affecting initial outcome. Gastroenterology, 89:827, 1985.
8. Froelicher, P., and Miller, G.: Esophageal cancer limited to the mucosa and submucosa in Europe. *In* DeMeester, T. R., and Skinner, D. B. (Eds.): Esophageal Disorders: Pathophysiology and Therapy. New York, Raven Press, 1985, pp. 355–357.
9. Gilbert, D. O., Silverstein, F. E., and Tebsco, F. J.: National ASGE survey on upper gastrointestinal bleeding complications. Endoscopy Dig. Dis. Sci., 26:555, 1981.
10. Graham, D. Y.: Treatment of benign and malignant strictures of the esophagus. *In* Silvas, S. E. (Ed.): Therapeutic Gastrointestinal Endoscopy. New York, Igaku-Shoin, 1990, pp. 1–41.
11. Harrison, M. E., and Sanowski, R. A.: Mercury bougie dilation of benign esophageal strictures. Hepatogastroenterology, 39:497, 1992.
12. Heyder, N.: Endoscopic ultrasonography of tumors of the oesophagus and the stomach. Surg. Endosc., 1:17, 1987.
13. Hix, W. R., and Wilson, W. R.: Detection of occult carcinoma of the esophagus by toluidine blue staining in high risk patients. *In* Siewart, J. R., and Holscher, A. H. (Eds.): Diseases of the Esophagus. Berlin, Springer-Verlag, 1988, p. 118.
14. Joffe, S. N.: Contact neodymium-YAG laser surgery in gastroenterology: A preliminary report. Lasers Surg. Med., 6:155, 1986.
15. Kozarek, R. A.: Hydrostatic balloon dilation of gastrointestinal stenoses: A national survey. Gastrointest. Endosc., 32:15, 1986.
16. Mandard, A. M., Tourneux, J., Gignaux, M., Blanc, L., Segol, P., and Mandard, J. C.: In situ carcinoma of the esophagus: Macroscopic study with particular reference to the Lugol test. Endoscopy, 12:51, 1980.
17. Marks, R., and Richter, J. E.: Peptic strictures of the esophagus. Am. J. Gastroenterol., 88:1160, 1993.
18. Miller, J. I., Jr.: Laser therapy. *In* Pearson, F. G., Deslauries, J., Ginsberg, R. J., Hiebert, C. A., McKneally, M. F., and Urschel, H. C., Jr. (Eds.): Esophageal Surgery. New York, Churchill Livingstone, 1995, p. 755.
19. Miller, L. S.: Endoscopy of the esophagus. *In* Castell, D. O. (Ed.): The Esophagus. Boston, Little, Brown & Co, 1992, pp. 93–95.
20. Monnier, P., Hsieh, V., and Savary, M.: Endoscopic treatment of esophageal stenosis using Savary-Gilliard bougies: technical innovations. Acta Endosc., 15:119, 1985.
21. Monnier, P., Savary, M., and Anani, P.: Endoscopic morphology of *early* esophageal carcinoma. *In* DeMeester, T. R., Skinner, D. B. (Eds.): Esophageal Disorders: Pathophysiology and Therapy. New York, Raven Press, 1985, pp. 333–345.
22. Monnier, P., Savary, M., and Pasche, R.: Contribution of toluidine blue to bucco-pharyngo-oesophageal cancerology. Acta Endosc. 11:299, 1981.
23. Monnier, P., Savary, M., Pasche, R., and Anani, P.: Intraepithelial carcinoma of the oesophagus: Endoscopic morphology. Endoscopy, 13:185, 1981.
24. Mori, M., Adachi, Y., Matsushima, T., et al.: Lugol staining patterns and histology of esophageal lesions. Am. J. Gastroenterol., 88:701, 1993.
25. Murata, Y., Muroi, M., Yoshida, M., et al.: Endoscopic ultrasonography in the diagnosis of esophageal carcinoma. Surg. Endosc., 1:11, 1987.
26. Nashef, S. A. M., and Pagliero, K. M.: Instrumental perforation of the esophagus in benign disease. Ann. Thorac. Surg., 44:360, 1987.
27. Neu, H. C., and Fleischer, D.: Recommendations for antibiotic prophylaxis before endoscopy. Am. J. Gastroenterol., 84:1488, 1989.
28. Ohyama, M.: Treatment of head and neck tumors by contact Nd-YAG laser surgery. Auris Nasus Larynx, 12(2):138, 1985.
29. Ollyo, J. B., Lang, F., Fontolliet, C., and Monnier, P. H.: Savary's new endoscopic grading of reflux-oesophagitis: A simple, reproducible, logical, complete and useful classification. Gastroenterology, 89:A100, 1990.
30. Orringer, M. B.: Complications of esophageal surgery and trauma. *In* Greenfield, L. J. (Ed.): Complications in Surgery and Trauma, 2nd ed. Philadelphia, J. B. Lippincott, 1989, pp. 302–325.
31. Orringer, M. B., and Stirling, M. C.: Esophagectomy for esophageal disruption. Ann. Thorac. Surg., 49:35, 1990.
32. Passe, H. I., and Reed, E. E.: Lasers in the management of upper aerodigestive malignancies. *In* Devita, V. T., Hellman, S., and Rosenberg, S. A. (Eds.): Important Advances in Oncology. Philadelphia, J. B. Lippincott, 1990, p. 159.
33. Pietrafitta, J. J., and Dyer, R. M. New laser techniques for the treatment of malignant esophageal obstruction. J. Surg. Oncol., 35:157, 1987.
34. Sarr, M. G., Pemberton, J. H., and Payne, W. S.: Management of instrumental perforations of the esophagus. J Thorac. Cardiovasc. Surg., 84:211, 1982.
35. Shahmir, M., and Schuman, B. M.: Complications of fiberoptic endoscopy: Esophagoscopy and gastroscopy. Gastrointest. Endosc., 26:86, 1980.
36. Shoruon, P. J., Eykyn, S. J., and Cotton, P. B.: Gastrointestinal instrumentation, bacteraemia, and endocarditis. Gut, 24:1078, 1983.
37. Skinner, D. B., and Belsey, R. H. R.: Endoscopy: instruments, anesthesia, techniques. *In* Skinner, D. B., and Belsey, R. H. R. (Eds.): Management of Esophageal Disease. Philadelphia, W. B. Saunders, 1988, pp. 65–80.

38. Skinner, D. B., and Belsey, R. H. R.: Surgical management of esophageal reflux and hiatus hernia. J. Thorac. Cardiovasc. Surg., 53:33, 1967.
39. Stoddard, C. J., and Simms, J. M.: Dilation of benign oesophageal strictures in the outpatient department. Br. J. Surg., 7:752, 1984.
40. Strohm, W. D., and Classen, M.: Benign lesions of the upper GI tract by means of endoscopic ultrasonography. Scand. J. Gastroenterol., 21 (suppl. 123):41, 1986.
41. Sugimachi, K., Kitamura, K., Baba, K., et al.: Endoscopic diagnosis of early carcinoma of the esophagus using Lugol's solution. Gastrointest. Endosc., 38:657, 1992.

42. Tio, T. L., and Tytgat, G. N. J.: Atlas of Transintestinal Ultrasonography. Aalsmeer, The Netherlands, Drukkerij Mur. Kostuerloren, B. V., 1986.
43. Tio, T. L., and Tytgat, G. N. J.: Endoscopic ultrasonography in the assessment of intra- and transmural infiltration of tumors in the oesophagus, stomach, and papilla of vater and in the detection of extra-oesophageal lesions. Endoscopy, 16:203, 1984.
44. Yasuda, K., Nakajima, M., and Kawai, K.: Endoscopic ultrasonography in the diagnosis of submucosal tumor of the upper digestive tract. Scand. J. Gastroenterol., 21 (suppl. 123):59, 1986.

VI

TUMORS OF THE ESOPHAGUS

Mark B. Orringer, M.D.

BENIGN ESOPHAGEAL TUMORS AND CYSTS

Benign tumors of the esophagus are rare, constituting only 0.5% to 0.8% of all esophageal neoplasms.[32] They may be classified broadly into two groups—mucosal and extramucosal (intramural)—but a more useful classification is that proposed by Nemir and associates (Table 26–5).[23] Approximately 60% of benign tumors and cysts of the esophagus are leiomyomas, 20% are cysts, and 5% are polyps. The remaining benign lesions occur with an incidence of less than 2%.

Leiomyomas. Leiomyomas are the most common benign tumors of the esophagus. They are intramural, typically occur between 20 and 50 years of age, have no clear-cut gender preponderance, and are multiple in 3% to 10% of patients.

TABLE 26–5. Classification of Benign Esophageal Tumors

I. Epithelial Tumors
  A. Papillomas
  B. Polyps
  C. Adenomas
  D. Cysts
II. Nonepithelial Tumors
  A. Myomas
    1. Leiomyomas
    2. Fibromyomas
    3. Lipomyomas
    4. Fibromas
  B. Vascular Tumors
    1. Hemangiomas
    2. Lymphangiomas
  C. Mesenchymal and other tumors
    1. Reticuloendothelial tumors
    2. Lipomas
    3. Myxofibromas
    4. Giant cell tumors
    5. Neurofibromas
    6. Osteochondromas
III. Heterotopic Tumors
  A. Gastric mucosal tumors
  B. Melanoblastic tumors
  C. Sebaceous gland tumors
  D. Granular cell myoblastomas
  E. Pancreatic gland tumors
  F. Thyroid nodules

From Nemir, P., Jr., Wallace, H. W., and Fallahaejad, M.: Diagnosis and surgical management of benign disease of the esophagus. Curr. Probl. Surg., 13:1, 1976.

More than 80% occur in the middle and lower thirds of the esophagus; they are rare in the cervical region. Calcification may occur within a leiomyoma, and this possibility must be considered in the differential diagnosis of a calcified mediastinal mass. Histologically, the tumors consist of interlacing bundles of smooth muscle cells. They vary greatly in size but seldom cause symptoms when less than 5 cm. in diameter. Larger tumors cause dysphagia, vague retrosternal pressure, and pain. Most reported leiomyomas have been found incidentally at autopsy and were asymptomatic. Obstruction and regurgitation may occur when these tumors virtually encircle the esophageal lumen, and bleeding is a more common symptom of the malignant form of the tumor, leiomyosarcoma. The potential for malignant degeneration of benign leiomyomas is apparently quite low. In the lower esophagus and cardia of the stomach, large confluent leiomyomas may occur. Another variation is leiomyomatosis, a condition in which multiple leiomyomas occur throughout the esophageal smooth muscle.

The characteristic appearance of an esophageal leiomyoma on barium swallow examination is a smooth concave defect with intact mucosa and sharp borders and abrupt sharp angles where the tumor meets the normal esophageal wall (Fig. 26–54). Typically, half the tumor appears to lie within and half outside the esophagus. As with every esophageal tumor, esophagoscopy is indicated to rule out carcinoma, but if a leiomyoma is suspected, a biopsy of the mass should *not* be performed so that subsequent extramucosal resection is not complicated by scarring at the biopsy site. Endoscopically, these tumors are mobile with intact overlying mucosa; and although they protrude into the esophageal lumen, they can be displaced and passed with the esophagoscope.

As a general rule, excision of symptomatic leiomyomas or those greater than 5 cm. is advised. Asymptomatic or smaller tumors discovered incidentally on a barium swallow examination can be observed and followed with periodic barium esophagograms. Whereas excision of the esophageal tumor provides the only absolute proof that it is not malignant, leiomyomas have such a characteristic radiographic appearance, generally slow growth rate, and low risk of malignant degeneration that periodic follow-up of some of these lesions is reasonable. The advent of esophageal ultrasonography has provided yet another means of diagnosing leiomyomas, which appear as hypoechogenic homogeneous areas beneath intact mucosa.[45] When resection is indicated, tumors of the middle third of the esophagus are approached through a right thoracotomy; those in the distal third are approached through a left thoracotomy. The tumor is located, and the overlying longitudinal esophageal muscle is split in the direc-

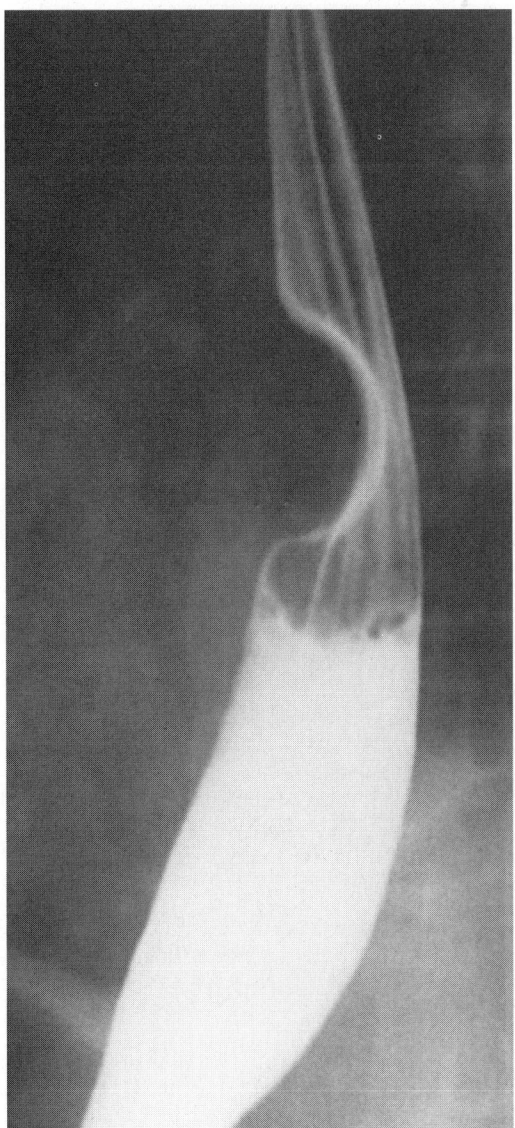

Figure 26–54. Esophagogram showing a typical leiomyoma.

are located along the right side of the esophagus. Esophageal duplication cysts, like other foregut cysts, are often associated with vertebral anomalies (e.g., Klippel-Feil deformity or spina bifida) and abnormalities of the spinal cord.

More than 60% of congenital esophageal cysts present in the first year of life with either respiratory or esophageal symptoms. The upper-third esophageal cysts tend to present in infancy, while the lower-third lesions may be asymptomatic initially and present later in childhood. Adults typically remain asymptomatic until bleeding or infection within the cyst causes enlargement, and then dysphagia, choking, or retrosternal pain (Fig. 26–56). Perforation may result in the rare cyst that contains ectopic gastric mucosa. Diagnostically, the cysts may cause displacement of the trachea on a posteroanterior chest roentgenogram or appear as a retrocardiac posterior mediastinal mass on a lateral chest film. The barium esophagogram shows a smooth extramucosal esophageal mass lesion and, very rarely, communication between the esophageal lumen and the cyst. Computed tomography demonstrates the location of the cyst relative to adjacent mediastinal structures. Spinal x-ray films should be obtained before surgery on a suspected duplication cyst in the event that its origin is the notochord.[44] Because of the potential for bleeding, ulceration, perforation, or infection, excision of these cystic esophageal lesions is recommended. This can

tion of its fibers, revealing the mass. The tumor is then gently dissected away from contiguous tissues and underlying submucosa, a relatively simple procedure. Once the tumor has been enucleated, the longitudinal muscle may be reapproximated, although large extramucosal defects may be left without complication. Esophageal resection may be required for either giant leiomyomas of the cardia that involve the adjacent stomach (Fig. 26–55) or for leiomyomatosis, although multiple enucleations may be performed if possible for the latter condition. The results of resection of leiomyomas are excellent, and recurrence has not been reported.

Esophageal Cysts. Esophageal cysts arise as diverticula of the embryonic foregut.[32] During its embryonic development, the esophagus is initially lined by simple columnar ciliated epithelium, which is eventually replaced by stratified squamous epithelium. Esophageal cysts contain both of these types of epithelium as well as fat and smooth muscle. A variation of the foregut cyst, the esophageal duplication cyst extends along the length of the thoracic esophagus, is lined by squamous epithelium, and has submucosal and muscle layers, the latter of which may interdigitate with the outer longitudinal muscle layer of the normal esophagus. Three fourths of duplication cysts present in childhood. Over 60%

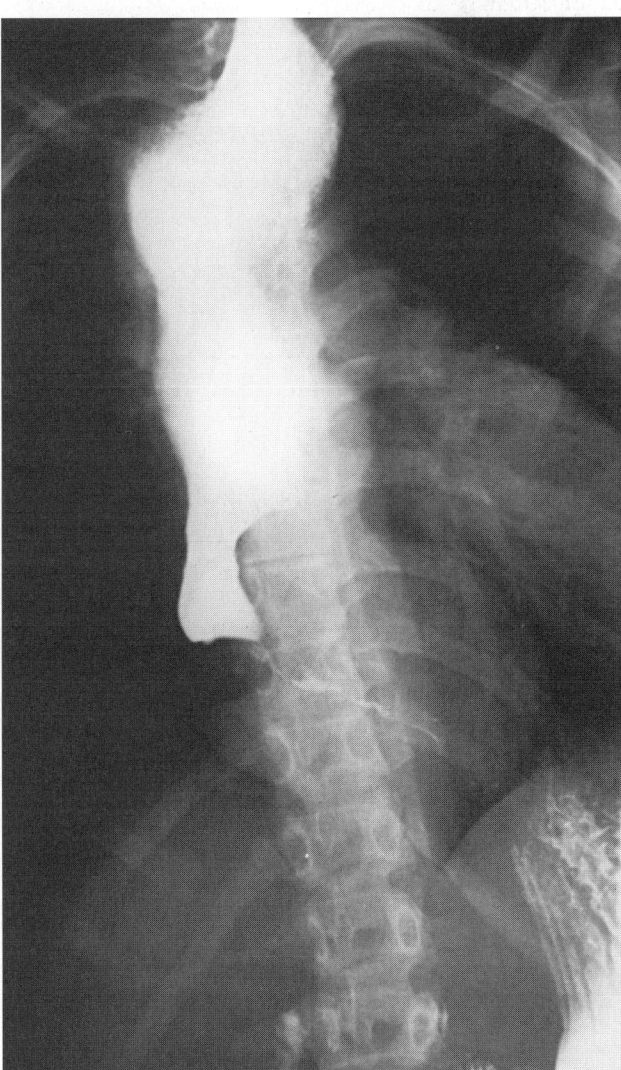

Figure 26–55. Esophagogram showing a giant leiomyoma involving the distal half of the esophagus and requiring an esophagectomy for resection.

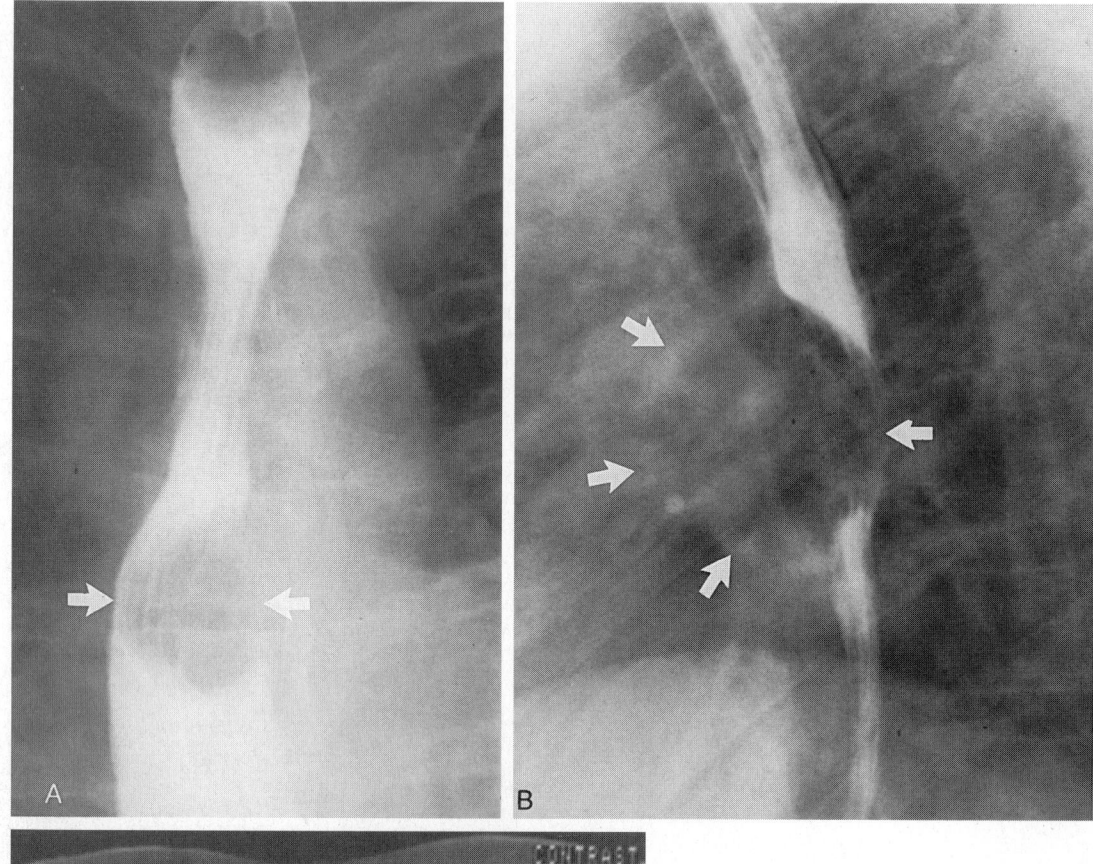

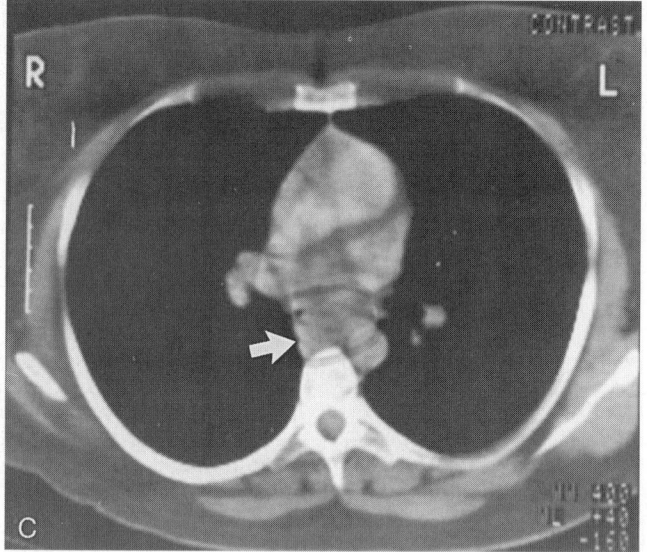

Figure 26–56. Duplication cyst. Posteroanterior *(A)* and lateral *(B)* views from barium esophagogram showing round extramucosal esophageal mass (arrows) below the level of the carina. *C,* CT scan showing the subcarinal mass of fluid density (arrow). This proved to be an esophageal duplication cyst that was successfully resected extramucosally through a right thoracotomy.

generally be achieved with low morbidity by means of an extramucosal resection. If the wall of the cyst cannot be separated from the common esophageal wall, it may be left behind, but the mucosa of the cyst must be stripped away to prevent recurrence. Marsupialization of the cyst and internal drainage and cauterization of the mucosa are not optimal methods of management. The long-term results of resection are excellent, and recurrence is rare if the initial excision is complete.

Pedunculated Intraluminal Tumors (Polyps) of the Esophagus. Benign esophageal polyps are rare but dramatic in their presentation, generally arising in the cervical esophagus, gradually developing progressively longer pedicles, and intermittently extruding into and even out of the mouth.

The majority of these polyps have occurred in older men, frequently attached to the cricoid cartilage. They cause intermittent dysphagia, but hematemesis or melena may occur if the overlying mucosa becomes ulcerated. The polyps are typically solitary and often long and cylindrical, producing marked esophageal dilation (Fig. 26–57). They are composed of vascular fibroblastic tissue with varying degrees of associated fat. The barium swallow examination may be nondiagnostic if the polyp is not seen, or a huge polyp may be misdiagnosed as carcinoma, a foreign body, or even as achalasia if it has caused marked esophageal dilation. Esophagoscopy similarly may fail to demonstrate the polyp, particularly if the pedicle is not seen and the mucosa overlying the polyp is normal. Although esophageal polyps have been removed

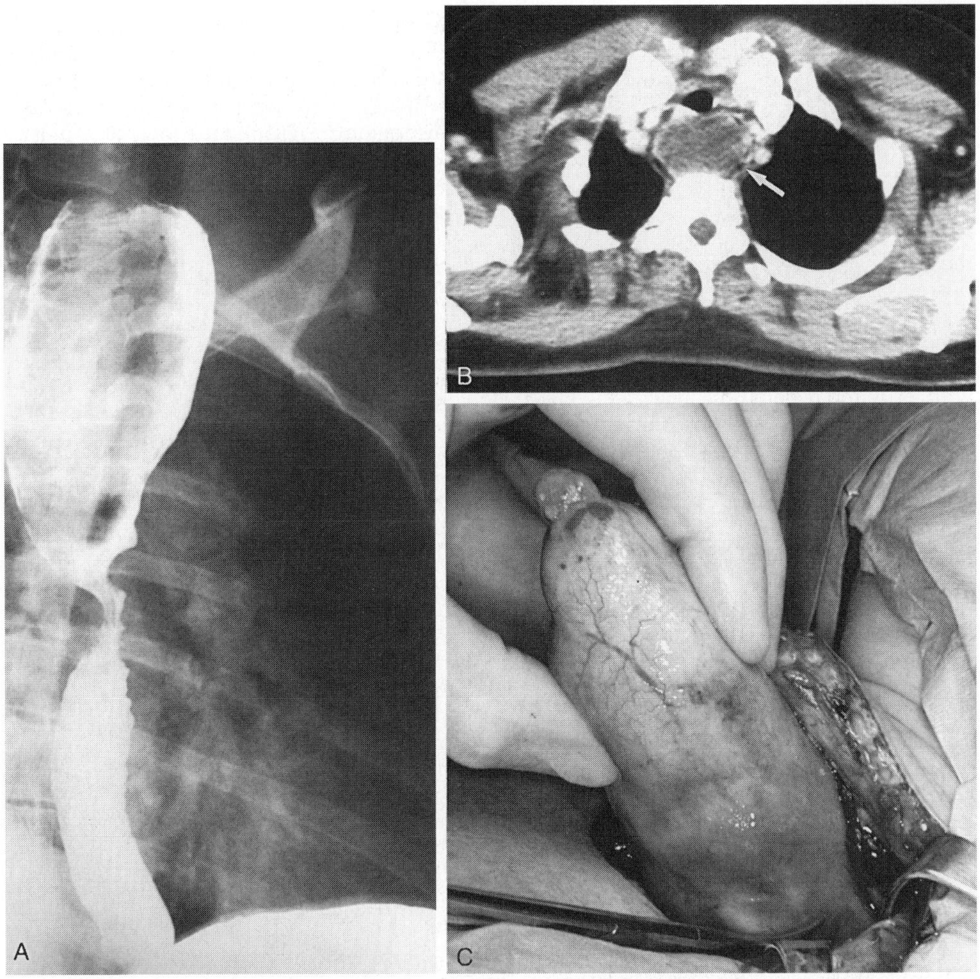

Figure 26–57. Giant benign fibroepithelial polyp. *A,* Barium esophagogram in a 37-year-old woman with progressive dysphagia. A large intraluminal mass is distending the cervical and upper thoracic esophagus. *B,* CT scan shows large intraluminal esophageal mass (arrow). *C,* Operative photograph showing a giant benign fibroepithelial polyp delivered out of the esophagus through a left cervical incision. The patient's head is toward the right. The mucosal base of the polyp was elliptically excised and the polyp removed.

endoscopically by electrocoagulating the pedicle, the preferred approach is resection through a lateral cervical esophagomyotomy, delivering the polyp from the esophagus, and resecting the mucosal origin of the pedicle under direct vision.

Granular Cell Myoblastomas. Granular cell myoblastomas are unusual rare benign tumors that most likely arise from Schwann cells rather than muscle as their name implies. They are found primarily in the breast, tongue, skin, mouth, upper respiratory tract, and gastrointestinal tract. About one third of gastrointestinal granular cell tumors are located in the esophagus and 50% to 80% in the distal third, and they vary from 0.5 to 4.0 cm. Patients are generally about 40 years of age and present with dysphagia, retrosternal or epigastric distress, nausea, and vomiting. The endoscopic diagnosis may be difficult, because these lesions are submucosal and have a grayish yellow appearance. Biopsy specimens may erroneously be mistaken for squamous cell carcinoma, because the overlying mucosa typically shows histologic pseudoepitheliomatous hyperplasia. Symptomatic tumors are effectively treated by local excision.

Hemangiomas. Esophageal mucosal hemangiomas constitute 2% to 3% of benign tumors, and although usually asymptomatic, may cause intermittent gastrointestinal bleeding, or even less commonly, massive and fatal hematemesis. Hemangiomas that have bled require treatment, while asymptomatic lesions discovered incidentally during esophagoscopy may be followed with periodic endoscopy. Although resection of symptomatic hemangiomas has been the standard approach, newer laser technology offers the potential for effective endoscopic therapy of this mucosal lesion.

Miscellaneous Benign Tumors. Benign esophageal tumors other than leiomyomas and polyps are rare. Papillomas are benign, sessile lobulated tumors that are covered by squamous mucosa and have a fibrous core. Most occur in the distal esophagus and are associated with some degree of esophageal obstruction. The significance of papillomas has not been established, and they have been postulated to represent localized epithelial hyperplasia or to be premalignant lesions. Occasionally they warrant esophageal exploration to rule out malignancy, and local excision is adequate. Esophageal adenomas, carcinoid tumors, and inflammatory pseudotumors have been reported but are so rare as to be only curiosities.

MALIGNANT TUMORS OF THE ESOPHAGUS AND CARDIA

Malignant tumors of the esophagus and cardia are among the most dismal of visceral tumors, owing to their generally advanced stage at the time of diagnosis. Accordingly, survival rates after treatment of these tumors have not changed appreciably in more than two decades.

Incidence. In the United States, the incidence of esophageal carcinoma averages 6 cases per 100,000 men per year, with approximately 4 cases per 100,000 white men per year and 12 cases per 100,000 black men per year.[50] Esophageal carcinoma is of epidemic proportion in northeastern Iran, the Transkei of South Africa, the Linxian County in Henan Province in northern China, certain areas of southern Russia, India, the Middle East, and Singapore.[7] In Henan Province of China, the prevalence of esophageal carcinoma is 0.9% in the population older than 30 years of age, and this extraordinary incidence in humans is matched in the poultry population in the same area. Epidemiologic studies have suggested that the cause in both instances is the presence of a large amount of carcinogenic nitrosamines in the soil of this region and contamination of foods by fungi, most often *Geotrichum candidum,* and yeast, which produce mutagens. In Northeast Iran, where more than 180 new cases of esophageal cancer per 100,000 population are recorded each year, primarily in the poorest social stratum, the use of opium, which contains pyrrolysates, and ingestion of very hot tea are believed to injure the esophageal mucosa and lead to malignant degeneration. In India, Pakistan, and Sri Lanka, the high incidence of esophageal cancer has been linked to chewing tobacco with or without betel nut, betel leaf, slaked lime, or a resin from the acacia. In Singapore, drinking *burning hot* beverages and the use of Chinese tobacco and wine are believed to be etiologic factors in the development of esophageal carcinoma. The South African Bantus and Zulus have a high incidence of esophageal carcinoma that is thought to be related to the high nitrosamine content of their soil as well as contamination of their food by molds, especially the *Fusarium* species, which can produce carcinogens. Alcohol consumption and cigarette smoking seem to be the most consistent risk factors in the populations from Normandy, Brittany, and other places in Europe with the highest incidence of esophageal cancer. Basically, esophageal squamous cell carcinoma is a disease of men (it occurs two to five times more frequently in men than in women) in the sixth and seventh decades of life, but carcinomas of the hypopharynx and cervical esophagus occur almost as often or even more frequently in women than in men. This may be related to the greater incidence of Plummer-Vinson syndrome in women. In Sri Lanka, however, esophageal carcinoma is primarily a disease of women and is the most commonly encountered malignancy of the gastrointestinal tract.

Etiology. The etiology of esophageal carcinoma is unknown, but as indicated earlier, certain nutritional factors and potential carcinogens have been incriminated: alcohol, tobacco, zinc, nitrosamines, malnutrition, vitamin deficiencies, anemia, poor oral hygiene and dental caries, previous gastric surgery, and chronic ingestion of hot foods or beverages. There is an increased incidence of esophageal carcinoma in patients with familial keratosis palmaris et plantaris (tylosis), which is inherited as an autosomal dominant trait. A number of esophageal lesions are premalignant, associated with an increased incidence of late carcinoma: achalasia, reflux esophagitis, and hiatal hernia, Barrett's (columnar epithelial-lined) esophagus,[37, 42] irradiation esophagitis,[38] caustic burns, Plummer-Vinson syndrome, leukoplakia, esophageal diverticula, and ectopic gastric mucosa.

Pathology. Histologically, approximately 95% of esophageal cancers worldwide are squamous cell carcinomas. In areas of China where the disease is endemic and mass screening using esophageal brush cytology for detection of early carcinomas is economically and medically justifiable, several macroscopic varieties of early esophageal cancer have been defined. These early forms of esophageal cancer have been variously termed carcinoma *in situ*, superficial spreading carcinoma, and intramucosal carcinoma, constitute less than 5% of all resected cases, are asymptomatic, and may take 3 to 4 years to progress to invasive squamous cell carcinoma. Endoscopically, carcinoma *in situ* most often presents as a slightly raised, granular, reddish plaquelike lesion, although superficial erosions or papillary lesions less than 3 cm. in diameter may also be seen. Microscopically, early esophageal carcinoma is either intraepithelial (carcinoma *in situ*), intramucosal (no deeper than the lamina propria), or invading submucosa; varying degrees of dysplastic change are seen.

Unfortunately, the vast majority of esophageal carcinomas are diagnosed at an advanced stage involving the muscular wall and often extending to adjacent tissues. Squamous cell esophageal cancer occurs least frequently in the cervical esophagus (8%) and most often in the upper- and mid-thoracic segments (55%) and the distal third (10 cm.) of the esophagus (37%).[8] The common growth patterns seen are the fungating (60%), ulcerative (25%), and infiltrative (15%) forms.

Esophageal cancer is notorious for its aggressive biologic behavior, infiltrating locally, involving adjacent lymph nodes, and metastasizing widely by hematogenous spread. Lack of an esophageal serosal layer tends to favor local tumor extension. Upper- and middle-third tumors tend to involve the tracheobronchial tree, aorta, and left recurrent laryngeal nerve as it loops around the aortic arch, whereas lower-third tumors may invade the diaphragm, pericardium, or stomach. The extensive mediastinal lymphatic drainage, which communicates with cervical and abdominal collateral vessels, is responsible for the finding of mediastinal, supraclavicular, or celiac lymph node metastases in at least 75% of patients with esophageal carcinoma. Cervical esophageal cancers drain to the deep cervical, paraesophageal, posterior mediastinal, and tracheobronchial lymph nodes. Lower esophageal tumors spread to paraesophageal, celiac, and splenic hilar lymph nodes. Distant spread to liver and lungs is common. The prognosis of invasive squamous cell carcinoma is poor, the overall 5-year survival for treated tumors being 5% to 12%.[8] Extraesophageal tumor extension is present in 70% of cases at the time of diagnosis, and the 5-year survival is only 3% when lymph node metastases are present, compared with 42% when there is no lymph node spread.

Adenocarcinomas constitute 2.5% to 8% of primary esophageal cancers, although this frequency is increasing dramatically in the United States at a rate surpassing that of any other cancer.[3, 17] They occur most commonly in the distal third of the esophagus, in the sixth decade of life, and with a male-to-female ratio of 3:1. Esophageal adenocarcinoma may have one of three origins: (1) malignant degeneration of metaplastic columnar epithelium (Barrett's mucosa), (2) heterotopic islands of columnar epithelium, or (3) the esophageal submucosal glands. Gastric cancer may also involve the esophagus secondarily. Patients with a columnar-lined lower esophagus (Barrett's metaplasia) are 40 times more likely to develop adenocarcinoma than the general population.[4, 42] Although the true incidence of Barrett's esophagus in the general population is unknown, it has been estimated that adenocarcinoma arises in 8% to 15% of patients with a columnar-lined esophagus.[15, 37] The finding of dysplasia in Barrett's mucosa is an ominous prognostic sign of impending malignant degeneration,[34] with severe dysplasia being virtually synonymous with carcinoma *in situ* and being an indication for resectional therapy.

As is the case with squamous cell carcinoma, adenocarcinoma of the esophagus exhibits an aggressive behavior, with frequent transmural invasion and lymphatic spread. Because many of these tumors arise in the distal esophagus, spread to paraesophageal, celiac axis, and splenic hilum lymph nodes is common. Metastases to the lung and liver are most frequent. The 5-year survival for esophageal adenocarcinoma is only 0% to 7%, with the presence of lymph node metastases exerting a significant negative effect on survival.

Several other rare types of esophageal malignant tumors occur. Anaplastic small cell (oat cell) carcinoma, apparently arising from the same argyrophilic cells that give arise to this tumor in the lung, can occur in the esophagus. Like their pulmonary counterparts, they demonstrate neurosecretory granules on electron microscopy. They tend to be very aggressive tumors and are commonly associated with distant spread at the time of diagnosis, with survival beyond 1 year being unusual. Adenoid cystic carcinoma typically occurs as a middle-third esophageal tumor, is discovered late in its course, metastasizes widely, and is associated with a median survival of only 9 months.[9] Malignant melanoma may present as a primary esophageal tumor, generally occurring as a large polypoid mass and associated with an average survival of 13.4 months and a 5-year survival of 4.2%.[6] Carcinosarcoma of the esophagus is a tumor with histologic elements of both squamous cell carcinoma and malignant spindle cell sarcoma. These typically polypoid tumors most often occur in the distal two thirds of the esophagus, grow to huge size (10 to 15 cm.), and are associated with only a 2% to 6% 5-year survival.[49]

Clinical Presentation and Diagnosis. Esophageal carcinoma typically occurs in the sixth or seventh decades of life, and a history of excessive use of tobacco and alcohol is common. Symptoms from esophageal carcinoma may be of insidious onset, beginning as nonspecific retrosternal discomfort or indigestion. As the tumor enlarges, the initially intermittent dysphagia becomes progressive and the predominant symptom, with weight loss, odynophagia, chest pain, and occasionally hematemesis following. Because dysphagia is the presenting complaint in 80% to 90% of patients with esophageal carcinoma,[10] any adult who complains of progressive dysphagia warrants both a barium esophagogram and esophagoscopy to rule out carcinoma. The combination of esophageal biopsy and brushings for cytologic evaluation establishes a diagnosis of carcinoma in 95% of patients with malignant strictures.[47, 48] The barium esophagogram, particularly using air contrast radiographic technique, has enabled the demonstration of lesions as small as 5 to 15 mm. in early detection programs.[39] Tumors this small, however, are seldom encountered among Western cultures, where the majority of patients present with irregular mucosal filling defects, distortion of the esophageal lumen, or annular constrictions on barium studies (Figs. 26–58 and 26–59). Despite these

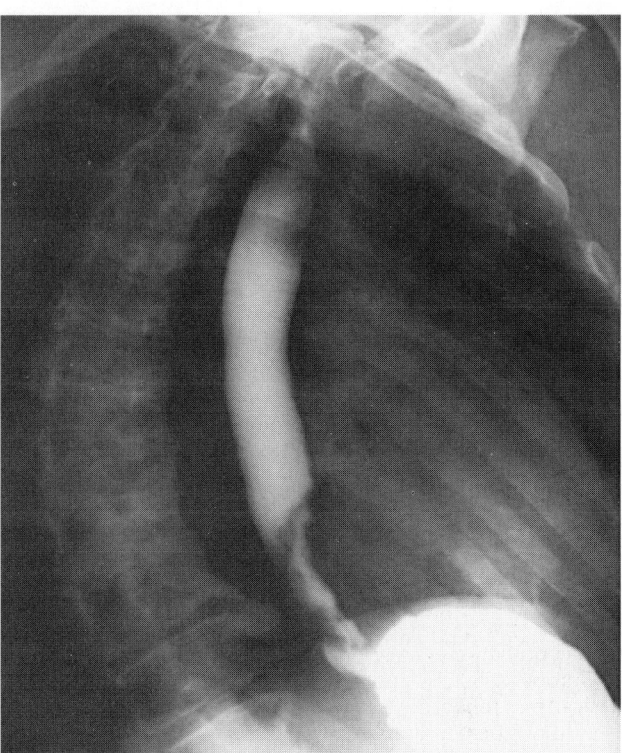

Figure 26–59. Esophagogram showing a distal esophageal carcinoma presenting as a typical "apple core" constricting lesion.

radiographic characteristics of esophageal malignancy and, conversely, the smooth, tapered radiographic stricture that generally signifies benign disease, esophagoscopy and biopsy to establish the diagnosis are mandatory in every patient with an esophageal stenosis (see Part V in this chapter). Unfortunately, programs for early detection of esophageal carcinoma using mass screening of patients with barium esophagograms, flexible fiberoptic esophagoscopy, and exfoliative cytology are not cost effective in Western cultures, where the incidence of this disease is relatively low (approximately 6 per 100,000 men in the United States).

Evaluation. Once the diagnosis of esophageal carcinoma has been established histologically after esophagoscopy and biopsy, staging of the tumor is the next critical step in determining which therapeutic option is appropriate. Since 1980, endoscopic ultrasound has been available to define the depth of mural invasion of esophageal carcinoma and to assess associated paraesophageal lymph nodes. The use of endoscopic ultrasound in these patients is limited if there is an obstructing tumor that cannot be traversed by the ultrasound probe. But in those in whom the probe can be positioned within the esophageal lumen involved by tumor, this procedure has an 86% accuracy in defining involved mediastinal lymph nodes.[22, 43] The barium swallow examination should be the first study in the patient with dysphagia because it provides information regarding the location and length of the tumor and the degree of associated obstruction (see Part V in this chapter). The plain chest radiograph is abnormal in only 50% of patients with esophageal cancer, with findings such as an air-fluid level in the obstructed esophagus in the posterior mediastinum, a dilated esophagus, abnormal mediastinal soft tissue representing adenopathy, a pleural effusion, or pulmonary metastases being most common. The chest film, however, may be deceivingly normal even with advanced disease. The most widely used and now standard radiographic means of staging esophageal

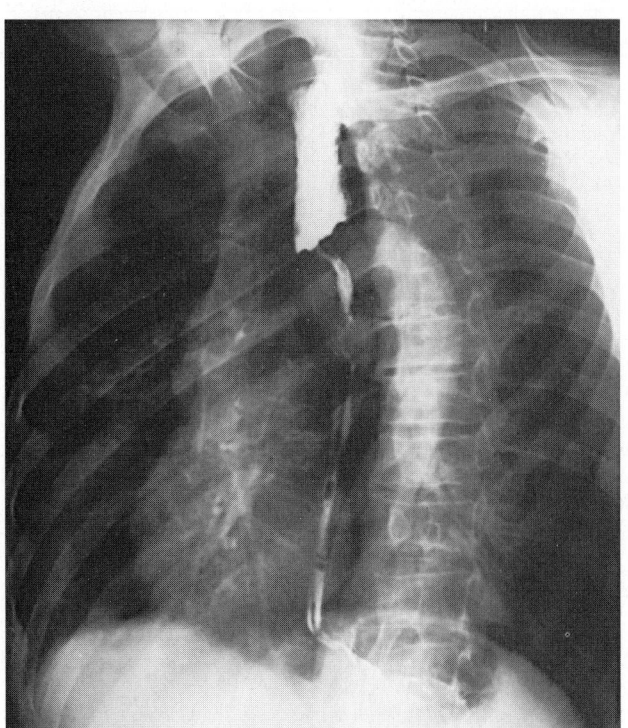

Figure 26–58. Esophagogram showing an upper esophageal carcinoma at the level of the aortic arch. There is mucosal irregularity and a "shelf" representing the tumor protruding into the esophageal lumen.

cancer is computed tomography of the chest and upper abdomen. CT permits evaluation of the esophageal wall thickness (which normally should not exceed 5 mm.), assessment of direct mediastinal invasion by the tumor and the presence of regional lymphadenopathy and pulmonary, liver, adrenal, and distant nodal metastases. Regional adenopathy that can be resected with the esophagus does not preclude esophagectomy. However, histologically documented distant metastatic (Stage IV) esophageal carcinoma (e.g., liver, pulmonary, or supraclavicular lymph node) contraindicates esophagectomy, since the expected survival is only 6 to 12 months. Although CT criteria of invasion of mediastinal structures have been well described in the literature, the only absolute indication of unresectability is the operative findings of such, and many esophageal carcinomas deemed unresectable on the basis of a CT scan are found to be resectable at surgery.[33]

Bronchoscopy is an integral part of the evaluation of esophageal carcinomas, which are in proximity to the trachea or mainstem bronchi (i.e., upper- and middle-third tumors), because endoscopic evidence of invasion of the airway precludes a safe esophagectomy. Additional studies such as magnetic resonance imaging to evaluate mediastinal structures, bone and brain scans to detect metastatic disease, or staging mediastinoscopy are not performed routinely unless indicated by specific symptoms or findings.

TNM Classification for Staging Esophageal Cancer. A standardized system for staging esophageal carcinoma permits assignment of patients to groups with similar prognosis, helps determine if local or systemic treatment is indicated, and allows comparison of results of treatment between programs. The most recent iteration of the TNM classification for esophageal cancer divides the esophagus into four sections: (1) the cervical (from the lower border of the cricoid cartilage to the thoracic inlet, 15 to 18 cm. from the upper incisor teeth); (2) the upper thoracic (from the thoracic inlet to the level of the carina at approximately 24 cm.); (3) the middle thoracic (from the carina to half the distance to the esophagogastric junction, or approximately 32 cm.); and (4) the lower (to the esophagogastric junction at approximately 40 cm.).[1]

The current TNM classification, in which "T" defines the depth of invasion of the primary tumor, "N" defines regional lymph involvement, and "M" defines the presence or absence of distant metastases, is shown in Table 26–6. Regional lymph nodes for tumors of the cervical esophagus are cervical and supraclavicular nodes; those for the thoracic esophagus are the mediastinal and perigastric nodes along the lesser curvature, fundus, and left gastric artery. The TNM categories are grouped into stages, which have been shown to reflect the prognosis of the tumors, the 5-year survival for Stage I esophageal carcinoma being approximately 60% while that for Stage IV disease is 5% or less.

Treatment. Therapy for esophageal carcinoma is influenced by the knowledge that *in the vast majority of these patients, local tumor invasion or distant metastatic disease precludes cure.* Single-agent chemotherapy has been used to treat many patients with esophageal carcinoma who present with distant disease at the time of diagnosis, with cisplatin, mitomycin, and 5-fluorouracil achieving reported response rates of approximately 35%.[36] Combination chemotherapy with regimens such as cisplatin, bleomycin, and vindesine or methotrexate; cisplatin, mitoguazone, and vindesine or vinblastine; and cisplatin and 5-fluorouracil have been used for metastatic or unresectable esophageal carcinoma, with reported response rates of 11% to 55% for 3 to 9 months,[36] but there are no data proving that combination chemotherapy alone provides either improved survival or palliation in these patients. Unfortunately, partial responses of the tumors to these agents, not long-term remission, is the rule. Combination chemotherapy has also been used preoperatively in a com-

---

TABLE 26–6. Tumor-Node-Metastasis (TNM) Staging System for Esophageal Carcinoma

Definition of TNM

Primary Tumor (T)

T_X Primary tumor cannot be assessed (cytologically positive tumor not evident endoscopically or radiographically)
T_0 No evidence of primary tumor (e.g., after treatment with radiation and chemotherapy)
T_{is} Carcinoma *in situ*
T_1 Tumor invades lamina propria or submucosa, but not beyond it
T_2 Tumor invades muscularis propria
T_3 Tumor invades adventitia
T_4 Tumor invades adjacent structures (e.g., aorta, tracheobronchial tree, vertebral bodies, pericardium)

Regional Lymph Nodes (N)

N_X Regional nodes cannot be assessed
N_0 No regional node metastasis
N_1 Regional node metastasis

Distant Metastasis (M)

M_X Presence of distant metastasis cannot be assessed
M_0 No distant metastasis
M_1 Distant metastasis

Stage Grouping

Stage 0	T_{is}	N_0	M_0
Stage I	T_1	N_0	M_0
Stage IIA	T_2	N_0	M_0
	T_3	N_0	M_0
Stage IIB	T_1	N_1	M_0
	T_2	N_1	M_0
Stage III	T_3	N_1	M_0
	T_4	Any N	M_0
Stage IV	Any T	Any N	M_1

Adapted from American Joint Committee on Cancer: *In* Beahrs, O. H. Henson, D. E. Hutter, R. V. P., and Kennedy, B. J. (Eds.): Manual for Staging Cancer, 4th ed. Philadelphia, J. B. Lippincott, 1992.

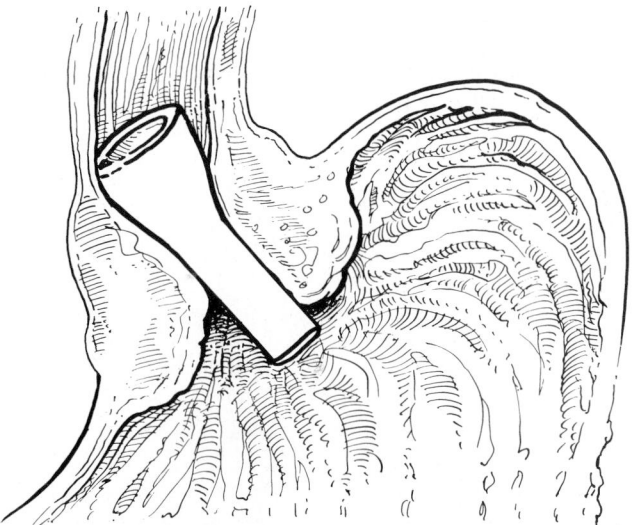

Figure 26–60. Intubation of unresectable distal esophageal carcinoma with a Celestin tube. (From Payne, W. S., and Olsen, A. M.: The Esophagus. Philadelphia, Lea & Febiger, 1974, p. 250.)

bined modality approach to esophageal cancer in hopes of controlling occult metastatic disease and improving the resectability rate.[10, 35] Postoperative radiation therapy, chemotherapy, and radiochemoimmunotherapy have also been used in an attempt to improve survival.[5, 24, 51] Again, however, no data substantiate the efficacy of these approaches.

Although squamous cell carcinoma is radiosensitive, radiation therapy as a single modality of treatment seldom achieves cure in patients with esophageal carcinoma.[46] Radiation therapy is used in the treatment of esophageal carcinoma with one of three theoretical objectives: palliation, cure, or as an adjunct to esophagectomy. Approximately one half of patients with advanced carcinoma and severe dysphagia are able to swallow sufficiently to nourish themselves after receiving a palliative course of radiation to the primary tumor in a dose range of 4000 to 5000 cGy over a 3- to 4-week period. Supervoltage radiation therapy delivers larger doses (5000 to 7000 cGy) over a 5- to 7-week period with *curative* intent, utilizing rotational and oblique ports to avoid spinal cord injury. Unfortunately, 5-year survival after this treatment ranges only from 3% to 9%. Either the local tumor is not controlled by radiation or, if it is, a stricture is left in its place; or, as is most often the case, continued progression of tumor outside the field of irradiation causes the patient's death. Similarly, surgical therapy, which most effectively relieves the obstruction to swallowing, generally fails to cure the patient with esophageal carcinoma. The explanation is all too apparent: esophageal carcinoma in Western cultures is almost uniformly a systemic disease when it is diagnosed; and local therapy, be it with radiation or operation, is simply unable to eradicate this malignancy. This fatalistic attitude toward esophageal carcinoma is born of the knowledge that the 5-year survival rate in Western countries from esophageal carcinoma treated by either radiation or surgery is generally less than 10%; more than 80% of the patients die within 1 year of diagnosis.[16, 41] Consequently, until very recently, the primary aim of therapy for esophageal carcinoma has been palliation, that is, restoring the patient's ability to swallow comfortably in the most simple and expeditious manner possible.

Endoscopic laser therapy and transoral intubation of esophageal carcinomas, using a variety of available tubes (Souttar—1924, Mackler—1954, Mousseau—1956, Fell—1966,

and Celestin—1969) and, most recently, the Wilson-Cook and self-expanding stents, have been used to provide palliation by re-establishing a passage for saliva (Fig. 26–60).[2] These tubes are divided into two types: *pulsion* tubes, which are pushed through the tumor from above (through the mouth) with the aid of an esophagoscope, and *traction* or pull-through tubes, which are pulled into place by downward traction through a gastrotomy. Unfortunately, although conceptually simple, transoral esophageal intubation carries an overall reported mortality that ranges from 3% to 15% and a complication rate of approximately 20%, largely the result of perforation of the esophagus, migration of the tubes, or obstruction of the tubes by food or tumor overgrowth. Although the ability of the patient to handle saliva is improved by intubation of the esophageal tumor, oral intake must be restricted to foods of a consistency compatible with passage through the rigid, indwelling esophageal conduits, and palliation is therefore not optimal (Fig. 26–61). The average survival after palliative intubation for esophageal carcinoma is less than 6 months. This method of therapy seems best suited to patients with malignant tracheoesophageal fistula, in whom an intraesophageal tube may both occlude the esophageal side of the fistula and permit oral alimentation for the several months of remaining life. Endoscopic laser therapy similarly improves dysphagia, but multiple treatments are required and long-term benefit is seldom achieved.

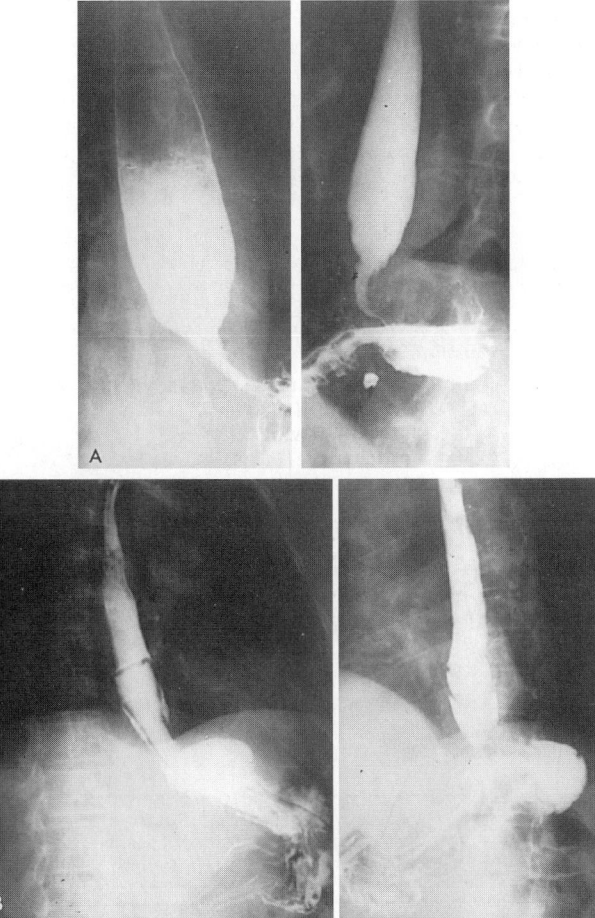

Figure 26–61. Esophageal intubation for palliation of unresectable carcinoma. *A,* Smooth, tapering, distal esophageal obstruction initially erroneously interpreted as esophageal spasm. This proved to be an unresectable carcinoma. *B,* Esophagogram after placement of a Celestin tube. Although the esophageal lumen was clearly no longer obstructed, this patient experienced excruciating pain from distal esophageal spasm in the region of the tube and died after 3 months. Satisfactory palliation was not achieved.

The concept of palliative internal bypass of incurable malignancies of the gastrointestinal tract has been applied to tumors of the stomach, biliary tract, pancreas, and large and small bowel. Bypass of unresectable esophageal carcinomas with a long segment colonic interposition has been advocated as a method of palliation (Fig. 26–62). This procedure, however, is of considerable magnitude. A cervical and two intra-abdominal anastomoses are required, and inadequate arterial blood supply to or venous drainage from the colonic graft may result in graft necrosis and anastomotic leak.[31] The mortality rate for colon interposition for esophageal carcinoma is approximately 20%. Gastric tubes to replace or bypass the esophagus have been constructed from the greater curvature of the stomach based on either the left gastroepiploic vessels (the reversed gastric tube)[13] or the right gastroepiploic vessels in an isoperistaltic manner. These tubes, however, require the construction and healing of a long gastric suture line, and the T formed at the cervical esophagogastric anastomosis frequently produces local ischemia and anastomotic disruption. Retrosternal gastric bypass of the excluded or internally drained unresected esophagus containing a carcinoma has been proposed as a method of achieving palliation (Fig. 26–63). Unfortunately, the mortality rate of retrosternal gastric bypass for esophageal carcinoma is 25% to 40%, the incidence of postoperative anastomotic disruption is high, and survival in these patients again averages less than 6 months.[27]

For most patients with localized esophageal carcinoma, resection, if possible, provides the best palliation. No current data irrefutably demonstrate the superiority of one operative approach for esophageal carcinoma over another. Despite

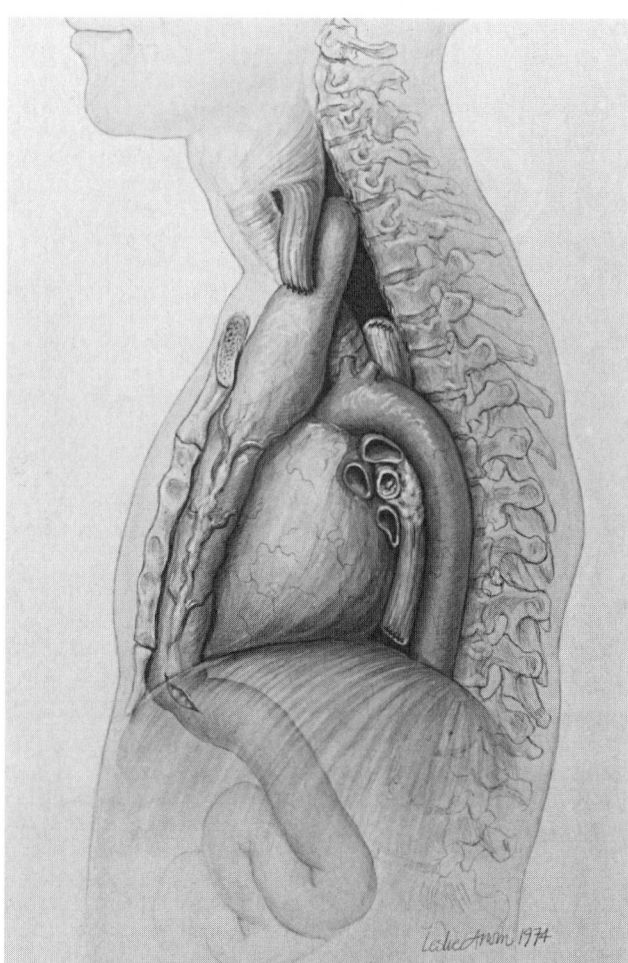

Figure 26–63. Lateral view showing substernal gastric bypass of the excluded thoracic esophagus. The gastric fundus is suspended from the cervical prevertebral fascia, the anastomosis is on the anterior gastric wall, and the esophagus with its unresectable tumor is excluded in the posterior mediastinum. This technique is now seldom used, because complications from the excluded thoracic esophagus are appreciable and survival after bypassing such an unresectable tumor averages only 6 months. (From Orringer, M. B., and Sloan, H.: Substernal gastric bypass of the excluded thoracic esophagus for palliation of esophageal carcinoma. J. Thorac. Cardiovasc. Surg., 70:836, 1975.)

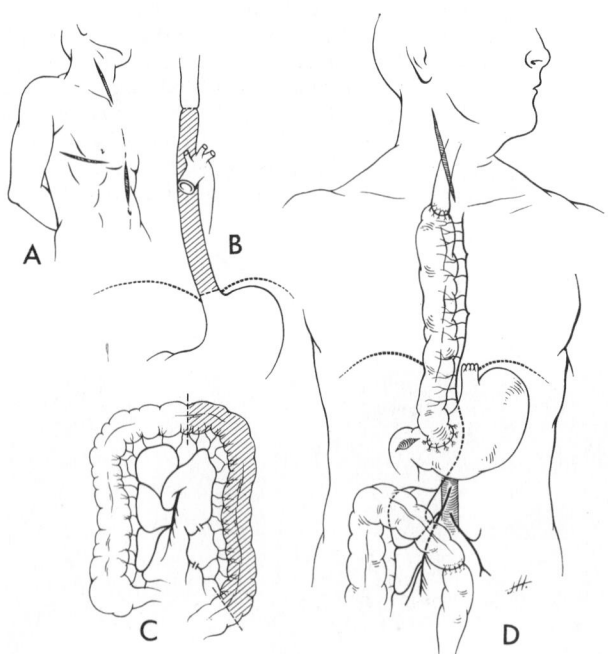

Figure 26–62. Use of the colon for esophageal replacement or bypass. A, Incisions: cervical, right thoracic, and abdominal. B, Length of esophagus resected (shaded area). If resection of the tumor is not possible, the cervical esophagus can be divided as shown and the distal end oversewn in preparation for a substernal colonic bypass. C, Segment of left colon mobilized for esophageal replacement (shaded area). The ascending, transverse, or descending colon may be used, depending on the adequacy of the blood supply to the mobilized segment. D, Completed operation. The colon may be positioned retrosternally if the esophagus is unresectable or in the posterior mediastinum in the original esophageal bed if resection is possible. A gastric drainage procedure is performed to prevent postvagotomy pylorospasm. (From Payne, W. S., and Ellis, F. H., Jr.: Esophagus and diaphragmatic hernias. In Schwartz, S. I. [Ed.]: Principles of Surgery. New York, McGraw-Hill Book Company, 1979, pp. 1081–1125.)

improvements in preoperative evaluation, anesthetic and operative techniques, and postoperative care, esophageal resection and reconstruction remain formidable operations in patients whose nutritional and pulmonary status have been compromised by impaired swallowing. The long-accepted traditional surgical approach to distal esophageal carcinoma has been a left thoracoabdominal incision (Fig. 26–64). The distal esophagus, proximal stomach, and adjacent lymph node-bearing tissues are resected, and an intrathoracic esophagogastric anastomosis is performed. For higher thoracic esophageal tumors, either a thoracoabdominal or separate thoracic and abdominal incisions are used, and a high intrathoracic esophagogastric anastomosis is performed (Fig. 26–65). In either case, a gastric drainage procedure (pyloromyotomy or pyloroplasty) is recommended to prevent subsequent postvagotomy gastric outlet obstruction due to pylorospasm. Unfortunately, standard transthoracic esophagectomy has significant drawbacks. A combined thoracic and abdominal operation in a debilitated patient may lead to respiratory insufficiency due to postoperative incisional pain and inability to breath deeply, requiring prolonged mechanical ventilatory assistance and often causing death.[11] Disruption of an intrathoracic esophageal anastomosis is the most dreaded

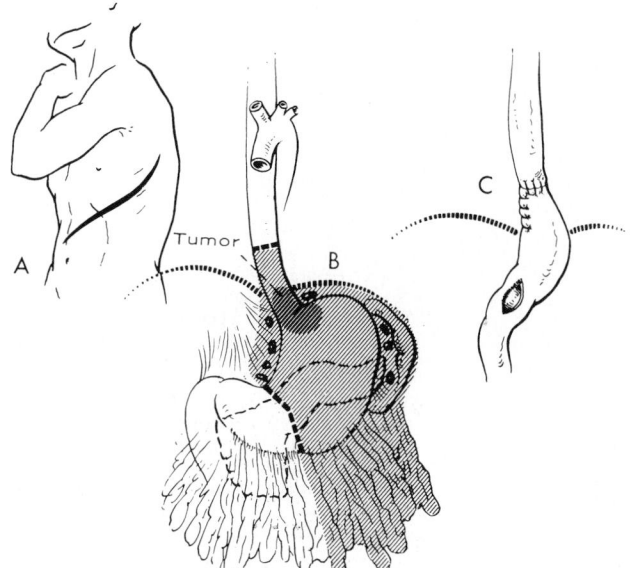

Figure 26–64. Standard thoracoabdominal esophagogastrectomy for lesions of the distal esophagus and cardia. *A,* Incision. *B,* Tissue to be resected (shaded area). *C,* Completed reconstruction with intrathoracic esophagogastric anastomosis and either pyloromyotomy or pyloroplasty to prevent postvagotomy pylorospasm. (From Ellis, F. H., Jr.: Treatment of carcinoma of the esophagus and cardia. Mayo Clin. Proc., *35*:653, 1960.)

complication of this type of surgical treatment. It results in mediastinitis and sepsis and is fatal in 50% of the patients in whom it occurs. The physiologic insult of a combined thoracoabdominal operation and the disastrous results of disruption of an intrathoracic esophageal anastomosis are thus major contributing factors to the morbidity and mortality rates of this type of esophageal resection and reconstruction and are responsible for reported operative mortality figures, which have ranged from 15% to 40% and averaged 30%.[10, 30] In the past decade, however, improvements in perioperative care, monitoring, and enteral and parenteral nutrition have reduced postoperative mortality associated with esophageal resection by 50%.[19, 21] Although there are a few reported series of transthoracic esophageal resection and reconstruction for carcinoma with operative mortality less than 3%,[20] these are exceptions, not the rule. An additional disadvantage of the intrathoracic esophageal anastomosis is inadequate long-term relief of dysphagia due to either anastomotic suture-line tumor recurrence or the development of reflux esophagitis above the anastomosis. Esophageal carcinoma is notorious for its ability to spread in the submucosal lymphatics well beyond the gross extent of the tumor, and the maximum proximal and distal margins of resection beyond gross tumor are therefore desirable to minimize the possibility of recurrent tumor at the anastomotic suture line. For a patient to undergo a major esophageal resection and reconstruction only to have dysphagia recur from tumor at the suture line within several months is a miserable failure of the operation as a palliative procedure. Finally, intrathoracic esophagogastric anastomoses are almost invariably associated with the development of reflux esophagitis, which follows resection of the lower esophageal sphincter mechanism. This not only can produce severe pyrosis and reflux symptoms but also can result in dysphagia from benign stenosis.

In the past two decades the technique of transhiatal esophagectomy without thoracotomy has gained popularity because of its potential for minimizing the aforementioned factors responsible for the major morbidity and mortality of standard esophageal resection and reconstruction.[29] In this

operation, regardless of the level of the tumor, the entire thoracic esophagus is resected and replaced whenever possible with the stomach, which is anastomosed to the remaining cervical esophagus above the level of the clavicles. This procedure, performed through an upper-midline abdominal and a cervical incision, involves resection of the thoracic esophagus through the diaphragmatic hiatus and the neck. The stomach is mobilized by dividing the left gastric and left gastroepiploic vessels, preserving the right gastric and right gastroepiploic arcades (Fig. 26–66). A pyloromyotomy and feeding jejunostomy are performed routinely. The entire thoracic esophagus from the level of the clavicles to the cardia is resected, while carefully monitoring intra-arterial blood pressure to avoid prolonged hypotension from cardiac displacement during the transhiatal esophageal dissection (Figs. 26–67 and 26–68). The stomach is then transposed to the posterior mediastinum, positioned in the original esophageal bed, and anastomosed to the cervical esophagus (Fig. 26–69). For distal-third esophageal tumors localized to the cardia, the high lesser curvature of the stomach is resected 4 to 6 cm. beyond the gross tumor, preserving that point on the high greater curvature that reaches cephalad to the neck (Figs. 26–70 and 26–71). Again, the entire thoracic esophagus is resected, and a cervical esophagogastric anastomosis is performed. Even relatively large intrathoracic esophageal carcinomas have been resectable through the hiatus; if necessary, the tumor can be fractured away from the prevertebral fascia or other adjacent mediastinal structures. For tumors of the upper-thoracic esophagus, the addition of a partial upper sternal split facilitates dissection of the esophagus from the trachea under direct vision (Fig. 26–72),[26] and, after this, the transhiatal esophagectomy can be completed as described previously. In performing a transhiatal esophagectomy, accessible cervical, intrathoracic, and intra-abdominal lymph nodes are removed for the purpose of staging, but no attempt is made to perform an *en bloc* resection of the esophagus and its adjacent lymph node-bearing tissue. The advantages of this approach are as follows: (1) a thoracotomy is avoided, thus minimizing the physiologic insult of the operation; (2) an intrathoracic esophageal anastomosis is avoided, and if a

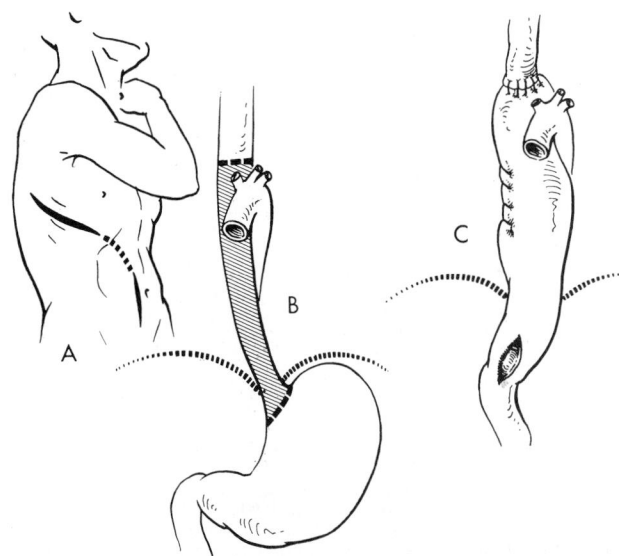

Figure 26–65. Standard thoracoabdominal Ivor-Lewis esophagogastrectomy for lesions of the lower and middle third of the thoracic esophagus. *A,* The continuous thoracoabdominal incision and the separate thoracic or abdominal incisions that may be used. *B,* Portion of the esophagus to be resected (shaded area). *C,* Completed reconstruction with high intrathoracic esophagogastric anastomosis and gastric drainage procedure. (From Ellis, F. H., Jr.: Treatment of carcinoma of the esophagus and cardia. Mayo Clin. Proc., *35*:653, 1960.)

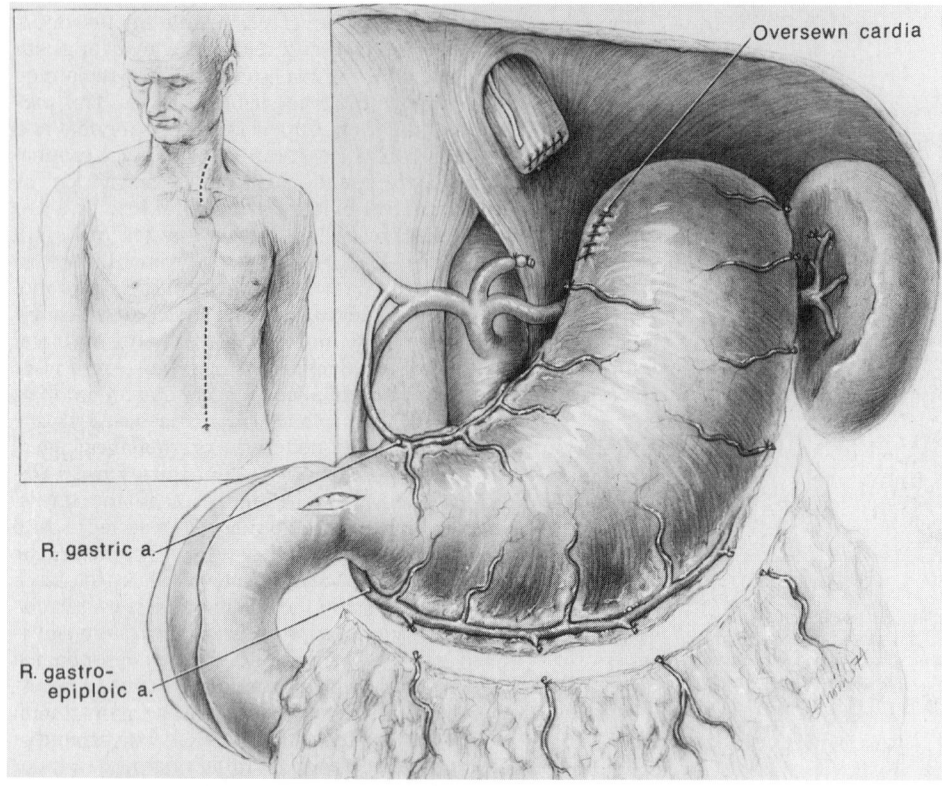

Figure 26–66. Mobilization of the stomach for either substernal gastric bypass or esophageal replacement after transhiatal esophagectomy. The gastric and right gastroepiploic vessels are preserved, a Kocher maneuver and pyloromyotomy are performed, and the divided cardia is stapled and oversewn. (From Orringer, M. B., and Sloan, H.: Substernal gastric bypass of the excluded thoracic esophagus for palliation of esophageal carcinoma. J. Thorac. Cardiovasc. Surg., *70*:836, 1975.)

cervical leak does occur, it is more easily managed, rarely causes mediastinitis, and is rarely fatal; (3) there are no intraabdominal or intrathoracic gastrointestinal suture lines, in contrast to the situation with colonic or jejunal interposition, or various gastric tubes; and (4) clinically significant gastroesophageal reflux seldom occurs after a cervical esophagogastric anastomosis. Critics of this operation object to its

limited exposure of the intrathoracic esophagus and its blood supply and therefore the risk of uncontrollable hemorrhage and the inability to carry out a complete mediastinal lymph node dissection for purposes of staging and potential cure.

Among 423 patients with carcinoma of the thoracic esophagus and cardia reported by the author, transhiatal esophagectomy was possible in 417 (97%).[29] The location of the 417

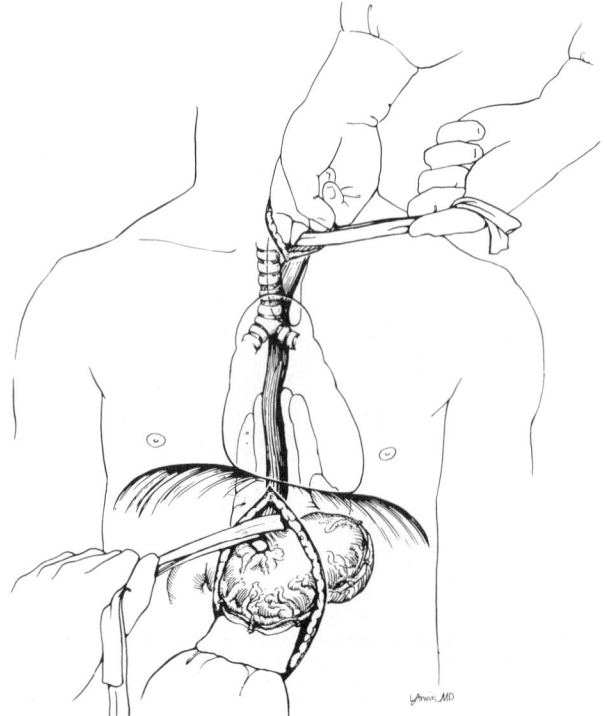

Figure 26–67. Transhiatal dissection of the lower esophagus through the diaphragmatic hiatus is achieved through an upper midline abdominal incision. Penrose drains around either end of the esophagus are used for traction during the dissection. The upper thoracic esophagus is mobilized through a limited cervical incision. (Modified from Orringer, M. B., and Sloan, H.: Esophagectomy without thoracotomy. J. Thorac. Cardiovasc. Surg., *76*:643, 1978.)

transhiatal esophagectomy whenever possible for resectable esophageal carcinomas. If an assessment of the tumor through the diaphragmatic hiatus indicates invasion of contiguous structures that precludes a transhiatal dissection, this approach should be abandoned for the traditional transthoracic esophagectomy. Those who criticize transhiatal esophagectomy without thoracotomy because it denies a formal lymph node dissection to patients with potentially curable tumors have yet to demonstrate that the number of lymph nodes resected has any effect on survival in these patients. When the results of radical transthoracic esophagectomy with *en bloc* dissection of contiguous lymph node-bearing tissues[40] are compared with those of transhiatal esophagectomy and no formal lymph node dissection, no significant difference in 3-year actuarial survival is apparent (Table 26–7). As has been demonstrated with carcinoma of the breast, it appears that survival after resection of esophageal carcinoma is more a function of tumor biology and host resistance than the extent of the resection performed. As a general rule, the stomach is preferred over all other organs as a visceral esophageal substitute, being far more resilient than either the colon or jejunum, and easily reaching to the neck to replace the entire thoracic esophagus. Colonic interposition is a relatively great operative undertaking in patients with esophageal carcinoma and should be used only when the stomach is not suitable for esophageal replacement.

In acknowledgment of the fact that most patients with esophageal carcinoma have systemic or locally invasive dis-

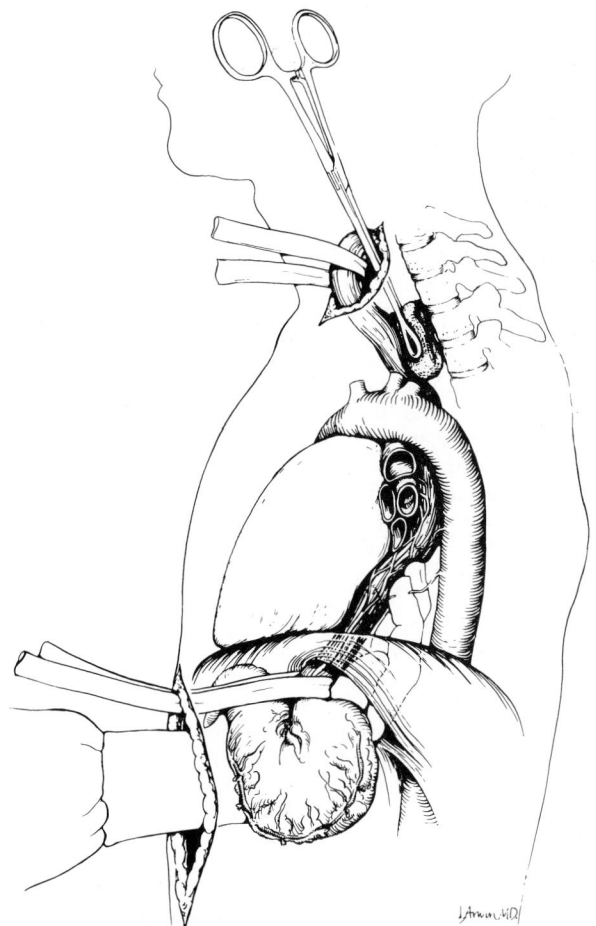

Figure 26–68. A "sponge-on-a-stick" inserted through the cervical incision is used to dissect the upper esophagus away from the trachea and adjacent mediastinal structures in performing a transhiatal esophagectomy without thoracotomy. As the hand inserted through the diaphragmatic hiatus dissects the esophagus free, careful monitoring of the intra-arterial blood pressure is required to prevent prolonged hypotension, which may result from cardiac displacement. (Modified from Orringer, M. B., and Sloan, H.: Esophagectomy without thoracotomy. J. Thorac. Cardiovasc. Surg.,*76*:643, 1978.)

tumors resected by transhiatal esophagectomy was the upper third in 23 patients (5%), middle third in 115 patients (28%), and lower third in 279 patients (67%). One hundred and forty-eight of the tumors (35%) were squamous cell carcinomas, and 256 (62%) were adenocarcinomas. Stomach was used to replace the esophagus in 408 (98%), and colon was used in nine patients who had undergone prior gastric resections for peptic ulcer disease. *The normal stomach readily reaches to the neck in every patient.* Postsurgical tumor-node-metastasis (TNM) staging of the 417 carcinomas based on histologic evaluation of the resected specimen indicated that 200 (48%) were either transmurally invasive or metastatic beyond regional lymph nodes (Stage III or IV tumors). In only 42 (10%) was the tumor confined to the mucosa (Stage I). There was one intraoperative death from mediastinal hemorrhage. Intraoperative blood loss averaged less than 1000 ml., the hospital mortality rate was 5%, and 89% of these patients left the hospital able to swallow within 3 weeks of operation (77% within 2 weeks). The overall 2-year survival was 41%, and the 5-year survival was 27%. These survival data are no better nor worse than those achieved by most series of transthoracic resections, but they were accomplished with less postoperative morbidity and mortality.

On the basis of this experience the author advocates a

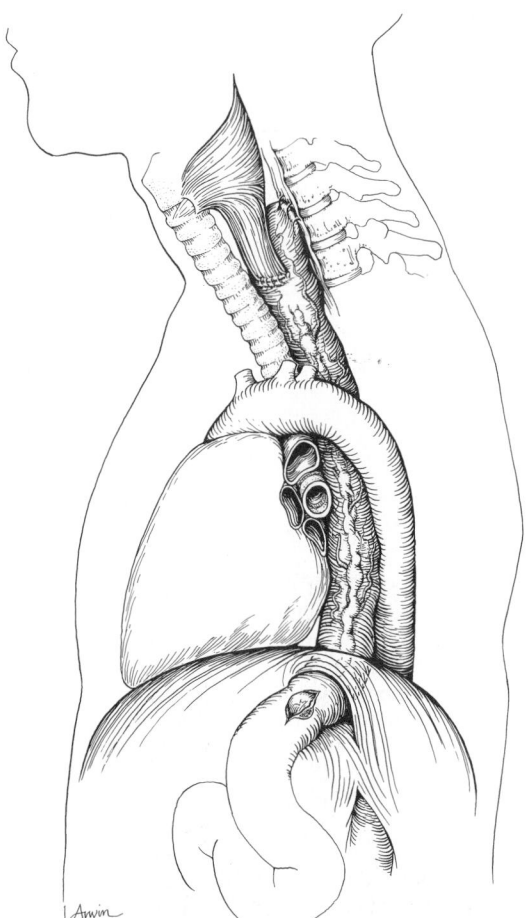

Figure 26–69. After transhiatal esophagectomy and pyloromyotomy, the stomach is mobilized through the posterior mediastinum, the fundus is sutured to the cervical prevertebral fascia, and an end-to-side esophagogastrostomy is performed. (From Orringer, M. B., and Sloan, H.: Esophagectomy without thoracotomy. J. Thorac. Cardiovasc. Surg., *76*:643, 1978.)

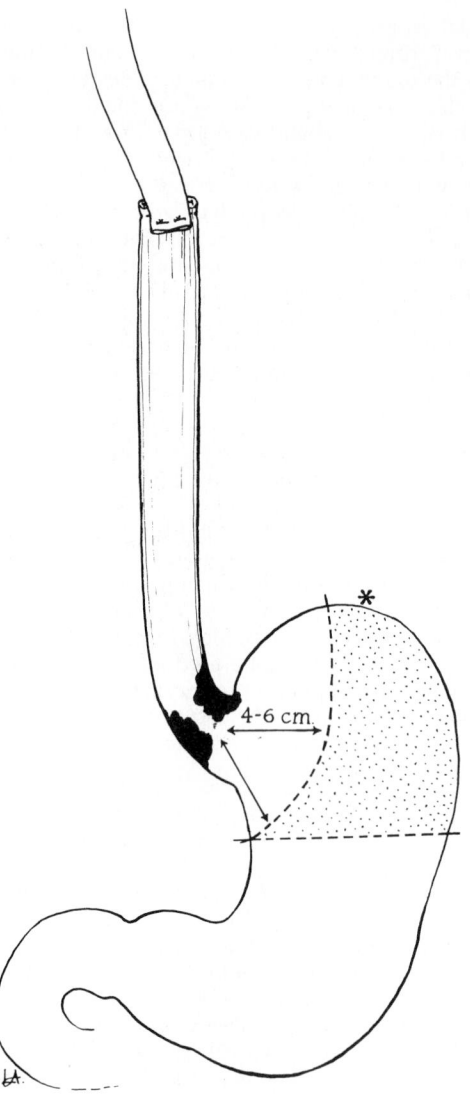

Figure 26–70. Total thoracic esophagectomy and proximal partial gastrectomy performed for adenocarcinoma limited to the esophagogastric junction and adjacent stomach. Such tumors may be resected with a 4- to 6-cm. gastric margin, thereby preserving the entire greater curvature aspect of the gastric fundus and that point (*) that reaches most cephalad to the neck. A proximal hemigastrectomy for such a tumor wastes valuable stomach (stippled area) that can be used for esophageal replacement and contributes little to the "cancer operation." (From Orringer, M. B., and Sloan, H.: Esophagectomy without thoracotomy. J. Thorac. Cardiovasc. Surg., 76:643, 1978.)

definite improvement over the 14-month median survival time with transhiatal esophagectomy alone; all complete responders were alive and tumor free. Most recently, with a 78.7-month median follow-up, the 5-year survival of all 43 patients is 34%, and that of the complete responders, a gratifying 60%.[12] Skinner and associates,[41] applying more stringent criteria to their use of radical esophagectomy for carcinoma, have reported their results in 31 additional patients, one half with squamous cell and one half with adenocarcinoma. They report an overall 1- and 2-year survival of 65% and 32%, respectively, which compares with the overall 1- and 2-year survival of 72% and 60%, respectively, in the 43 patients reported earlier who underwent chemotherapy, radiation therapy, and then transhiatal esophagectomy. It would thus appear that multimodality therapy provides better local-regional control of the tumor than can be achieved by radical resection of the esophagus alone. These exciting preliminary results add further support to the growing notion that the natural history of esophageal cancer can be altered and that long-term survival, not just palliation, may be achievable in many patients with this disease. The results of a recently completed randomized prospective Phase III trial undertaken at the University of Michigan in an attempt to substantiate the value of such multimodality therapy in the treatment of esophageal carcinoma are now being analyzed.

Carcinomas involving the cervicothoracic esophagus (and frequently the larynx) either primarily or secondarily pose the unique problem of esophageal reconstruction after laryngopharyngectomy. Concomitant radical neck dissection is often required because of regional lymph node involvement. Resection of these tumors, which may involve the high retrosternal trachea, is facilitated by removal of the anterior breast plate and construction of a mediastinal tracheostomy.[14, 25] Although replacement of the pharynx and cervical esophagus is possible with skin tubes, myocutaneous flaps, and isolated

ease that precludes cure at the time of diagnosis, during the past decade there have been a number of reported efforts to improve survival with multimodality therapy.[10] Stimulated by the Wayne State University experience with combined preoperative radiation therapy and chemotherapy,[18] as well as reports of preoperative chemotherapy and postoperative adjuvant radiation therapy,[5] a trial of combined preoperative chemotherapy and radiation therapy before transhiatal esophagectomy was carried out at the University of Michigan.[28] Forty-three patients (21 with adenocarcinoma and 22 with squamous cell carcinoma) received 3 weeks of chemotherapy with cisplatin, vinblastine, and 5-fluorouracil concurrent with 4500 cGy. radiation therapy before planned transhiatal esophagectomy 3 weeks later. The resectability rate in these patients was 91%, and 10 (24%) had no residual tumor in the resected specimen (i.e., were complete responders—$T_0N_0M_0$). At a mean follow-up of 36 months, the median survival for all 43 patients was 29 months (Kaplan-Meier estimate), a

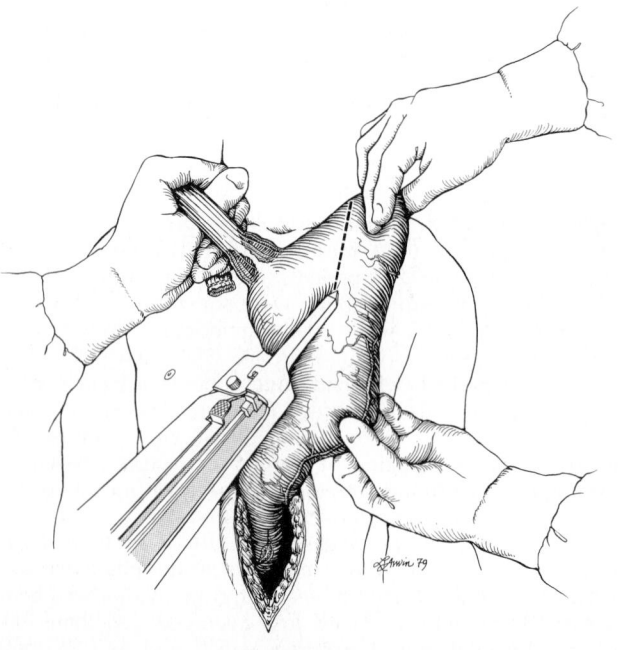

Figure 26–71. After completing the transhiatal esophagectomy for a localized distal third carcinoma, the surgical stapler is used to fashion a gastric tube from the greater curvature, resecting as much stomach as possible distal to gross tumor. The remaining stomach is then positioned in the posterior mediastinum in the original esophageal bed and is anastomosed to the cervical esophagus. (From Orringer, M. B., and Sloan, H.: Esophageal replacement after blunt esophagectomy. In Nyhus, L. M., and Baker, R. J. [Eds.]: Mastery of Surgery. Boston, Little, Brown & Co., 1984.)

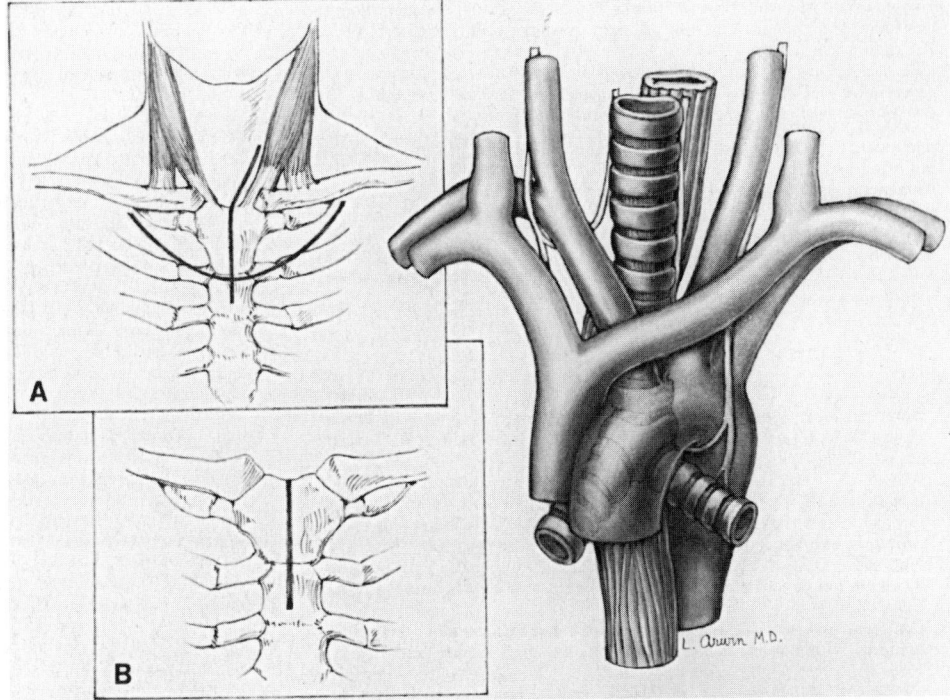

Figure 26–72. A partial upper median sternotomy permits direct dissection of cervical and upper thoracic esophageal carcinomas to the level of the carina. Inset *A* shows the usual oblique left cervical skin incision extending onto the anterior chest in the midline and the occasionally used curved anterior thoracic incision, which avoids a scar in the lower anterior neck. Inset *B* shows the sternotomy incision, which extends from the suprasternal notch, through the manubrium, and across the angle of Louis, which is approximately at the level of the carina. (From Orringer, M. B.: Anterior approach to the upper thoracic esophagus. J. Thorac. Cardiovasc. Surg., *87*:124, 1984.)

segments of jejunum anastomosed to a cervical arterial blood supply and venous drainage using microvascular technique, these operations are frequently multistaged, prolonged, and fraught with technical problems. In the author's experience, laryngopharyngectomy for cervicothoracic tumors and concomitant transhiatal esophagectomy without thoracotomy provide the maximum distal esophageal margin beyond the tumor and permit restoration of continuity of the alimentary tract using stomach, which generally reaches cephalad to the remaining pharyngeal margin. A one-stage resection and reconstruction of these carcinomas is as desirable as it is for tumors of the thoracic esophagus, avoiding staged procedures, multiple intestinal anastomoses, and prolonged hospitalization in patients with limited life expectancy.

Preoperative Preparation for Esophagectomy. Patients with esophageal carcinoma are typically cigarette smokers and often have had some degree of tracheobronchial aspiration from their esophageal obstruction. Therefore, rigid adherence to a regimen of vigorous pulmonary physiotherapy before operation is consistently rewarded by fewer postoperative complications. Abstinence from cigarette smoking and use of an incentive inspirometer for at least 2 weeks before operation should be routine. Antibiotics for associated pneumonitis may be required. In patients in whom severe cachexia has not occurred, relatively little time is spent with preoperative nutritional build-up. On the other hand, if the patient is dehydrated or the esophageal obstruction is tight, endoscopic dilation of the malignant stricture and insertion of a nasogastric feeding tube for enteral nutrition is performed so that an intake of approximately 2000 calories per day can be ensured. Intravenous hyperalimentation is seldom indicated, because it rarely provides as satisfactory nutrition as enteral feedings and is associated with more septic and metabolic complications. Oral hygiene is often neglected in patients with esophageal carcinoma, and carious teeth should be removed or repaired preoperatively to minimize the severity of an infection that may result from anastomotic disruption and swallowed oral bacteria. If there is a history of prior gastric operations that may preclude the use of the entire stomach as an esophageal substitute, a barium enema examination should be done to assess the suitability of the colon for esophageal replacement, and the colon should be prepared in the event that a colonic interposition is required.

SELECTED REFERENCES

Ferguson, M. K., and Skinner, D. B.: Carcinoma of the esophagus and cardia. *In* Orringer, M. B., and Zuidema, G. D. (Eds.): Shackelford's Surgery of the Alimentary Tract, 4th ed. Vol. I, The Esophagus. Philadelphia, W. B. Saunders, 1996, pp. 305–332.
This is a current comprehensive review with excellent illustrative radiographs and computed tomographic scans, well-illustrated schematics of techniques of esophagectomy, and a good overview of alternative therapy for esophageal cancer. The bibliography is extensive.

Forastiere, A. A., Orringer, M. B., Perez-Tamayo, C., et al.: Preoperative chemoradiation followed by transhiatal esophagectomy for carcinoma of the esophagus: Final report. J. Clin. Oncol., *11*:1118, 1993.
This is an encouraging report of a phase II trial of combination chemotherapy (cisplatin, 5-fluorouracil, and vinblastine) concurrent with radiation before transhiatal esophagectomy in 43 patients with esophageal cancer, approximately equally divided between adenocarcinoma and squamous cell carcinoma. The median survival of 29 months for all 43 patients and the 34% overall 5-year survival rate represents considerable improvement over the 14-month survival rate in historical controls treated with transhiatal esophagectomy alone. Ten patients (23%) were complete responders (T_0N_0), and of these, 60% were alive at 5 years.

TABLE 26–7. Effect of Extent of Esophageal Resection for Carcinoma on Three-Year Actuarial Survival

Esophageal Tumor Site	Radical Esophagectomy with En Bloc Lymph Node Dissection*	Transhiatal Esophagectomy Without Formal Lymph Node Dissection†
Middle third	14% (29)	17% (40)
Lower third	33% (37)	31% (47)

*Data from Skinner, D. B.: En bloc resection for neoplasms of the esophagus and cardia. J. Thorac. Cardiovasc. Surg., *85*:59, 1983.
†Data from Orringer, M. B.: Transhiatal esophagectomy without thoracotomy for carcinoma of the esophagus. Ann. Surg., *200*:282, 1984.

Orringer, M. B., Marshall, B., and Stirling, M. C.: Transhiatal esophagectomy for benign and malignant disease. J Thorac. Cardiovasc. Surg., *105*:265, 1993.
This is the latest University of Michigan report of 583 patients undergoing transhiatal esophagectomy for diseases of the intrathoracic esophagus. The operative and perioperative morbidity are thoroughly discussed, and survival data as well as detailed functional results of esophageal substitution are presented.

Postlethwait, R. W., and Lowe, J. E.: Benign tumors and cysts of the esophagus. *In* Orringer, M. B., and Zuidema, G. D. (Eds.): Shackelford's Surgery of the Alimentary Tract, 4th ed. Vol. I, The Esophagus. Philadelphia, W. B. Saunders, 1996, pp. 369–386.
This is a comprehensive authoritative and well-illustrated review of benign tumors and cysts of the esophagus with an extensive bibliography compiled by the senior author (R. W. P.) over the course of a professional lifetime, which has focused on surgical diseases of the esophagus.

REFERENCES

1. American Joint Committee on Cancer and Beahrs, O. H., Henson, D. E., Hutter, R. V. P., and Kennedy, B. J. (Eds.): Manual for Staging of Cancer, 4th ed. Philadelphia, J. B. Lippincott, 1992.
2. Barnett, J. L.: Esophageal carcinoma: Palliation with intubation and laser. *In* Zuidema, G. D., and Orringer, M. D. (Eds.): Shackelford's Surgery of the Alimentary Tract, 4th ed. Vol. I, The Esophagus. Philadelphia, W. B. Saunders, 1996, pp. 358–368.
3. Blot, W. J., Devesa, S. S., Kneller, R. W., and Fraumeni, J. F., Jr.: Rising incidence of adenocarcinoma of the esophagus and gastric cardia. JAMA, *265*:1287, 1991.
4. Cameron, A. J., Ott, B. J., and Payne, W. S.: The incidence of adenocarcinoma in columnar-lined (Barrett's) esophagus. N. Engl. J. Med., *313*:857, 1985.
5. Carey, R. W., Hilgenberg, A. D., Wilkins, E. W., Choi, N. C., Mathisen, D. J., and Grillo, H.: Preoperative chemotherapy followed by surgery with possible postoperative radiotherapy in squamous cell carcinoma of the esophagus: Evaluation of the chemotherapy component. J. Clin. Oncol., *4*:697, 1986.
6. Chalkiadakis, G., Wihlm, J. M., Morand, G., Weill-Bousson, M., and Witz, J. P.: Primary malignant melanoma of the esophagus. Ann. Thorac. Surg., *39*:472, 1985.
7. Duranceau, A.: Epidemiologic trends and etiologic factors of esophageal carcinoma. *In* Delarue, N. C., Wilkins, E. W., Jr., and Wong, J. (Eds.): International Trends in General Thoracic Surgery. Vol. 4, Esophageal Cancer. St. Louis, C.V. Mosby, 1988, pp. 3–10.
8. Enterline, H., and Thompson, J.: Pathology of the Esophagus. New York, Springer-Verlag, 1984.
9. Epstein, J. I., Sears, D. L., Tucker, R. S., and Eagan, J. W.: Carcinoma of the esophagus with adenoid cystic differentiation. Cancer, *53*:1131, 1984.
10. Ferguson, M. K., and Skinner, D. B.: Carcinoma of the esophagus and cardia. *In* Orringer, M. D., and Zuidema, G. D. (Eds.): Shackelford's Surgery of the Alimentary Tract, 4th ed. Vol. I, The Esophagus. Philadelphia, W. B. Saunders, 1996, pp. 305–332.
11. Fok, M., Law, S. Y. K., and Wong, J.: Operable esophageal carcinoma: Current results from Hong Kong. World J. Surg, *18*:355, 1994.
12. Forastiere, A. A., Orringer, M. B., Perez-Tamayo, C., et al.: Preoperative chemoradiation followed by transhiatal esophagectomy for carcinoma of the esophagus: Final report. J. Clin Oncol., *11*:1118, 1993.
13. Gavriliu, D.: The replacement of the oesophagus by gastric tube. *In* Jamieson, G. G. (Ed.): Surgery of the Oesophagus. Edinburgh, Churchill Livingstone, 1988, pp. 765–775.
14. Grillo, H. C., and Mathisen, D. J.: Cervical exenteration. Ann Thorac. Surg., *49*:401, 1990.
15. Haggitt, R. C., and Dean, P. J. Adenocarcinoma in Barrett's epithelium. *In* Spechler, S. J., Goyal, R. K. (Eds.): Barrett's Esophagus: Pathophysiology, Diagnosis, and Management. New York, Elsevier, 1985, pp. 153–166.
16. Hennessy, T. P. J., and Keeling, P.: Adenocarcinoma of the esophagus and cardia. J. Thorac. Cardiovasc. Surg., *94*:64, 1987.
17. Hesketh, P. J., Clapp, R. W., Doos, W. G., and Spechler, S. J.: The increasing frequency of adenocarcinoma of the esophagus. Cancer, *64*:526, 1989.
18. Leichman, L., Steiger, Z., Seydel, H. G., et al.: Preoperative chemotherapy and radiation therapy for patients with cancer of the esophagus: A potentially curative approach. J. Clin. Oncol., *2*:75, 1984.
19. Mathisen, D. J.: Ivor Lewis procedure. *In* Pearson, F. G., Deslauriers, J., Ginsberg, R. J., Hiebert, C. A., McKneally, M. F., and Urschel H. C., Jr. (Eds.): Esophageal Surgery. New York, Churchill Livingstone, 1995, pp. 669–676.
20. Mathisen, D. J., Grillo, H. C., Wilkins, E. W., Moncure, A. C., and Hilgenberg, A. D.: Transthoracic esophagectomy: A safe approach to carcinoma of the esophagus. Ann. Thorac. Surg., *45*:137, 1988.
21. Muller, J. M., Erasmi, H., Stelzner, M., et al.: Surgical therapy of oesophageal carcinoma. Br. J. Surg., *77*:845, 1990.

22. Murata, Y., Muroi, M., Yoshida, M., et al.: Endoscopic ultrasonography in the diagnosis of esophageal carcinoma. Surg. Endosc., *1*:11, 1987.
23. Nemir, P., Jr., Wallace, H. W., and Fallahaejad, M.: Diagnosis and surgical management of benign disease of the esophagus. Curr. Probl. Surg., *13*:1, 1976.
24. Nishihira, T., Nakano, T., and Mori, S.: Adjuvant therapies for cancer of the thoracic esophagus. World J. Surg., *18*:388, 1994.
25. Orringer, M. B.: Partial median sternotomy: Anterior approach to the upper thoracic esophagus. J. Thorac. Cardiovasc. Surg., *87*:124, 1984.
26. Orringer, M. B.: Anterior mediastinal tracheostomy with and without cervical exenteration. Ann Thorac. Surg., *54*:628, 1972.
27. Orringer, M. B.: Substernal gastric bypass of the excluded esophagus: Results of an ill-advised operation. Surgery, *96*:467, 1984.
28. Orringer, M. B., Forastiere, A. A., Perez-Tamayo, C., et al.: Chemotherapy and radiation therapy before transhiatal esophagectomy for esophageal carcinoma. Ann. Thorac. Surg., *49*:348, 1990.
29. Orringer, M. B., Marshall, B., and Stirling, M. C.: Transhiatal esophagectomy for benign and malignant disease. J. Thorac. Cardiovasc. Surg., *105*:265, 1993.
30. Postlethwait, R. W.: Complications and deaths after operations for esophageal carcinoma. J. Thorac. Cardiovasc. Surg., *85*:827, 1983.
31. Postlethwait, R. W.: Oesophageal bypass using the colon. *In* Jamieson, G. G. (Ed.): Surgery of the Oesophagus. Edinburgh, Churchill Livingstone, 1988, pp. 727–738.
32. Postlethwait, R. W., and Lowe, J. E.: Benign tumors and cysts of the esophagus. *In* Orringer, M. B., and Zuidema, G. D. (Eds.): Shackelford's Surgery of the Alimentary Tract, 4th ed. Vol. I, The Esophagus. Philadelphia, W. B. Saunders, 1996, pp. 369–386.
33. Quint, L. E., Glazer, G. M., Orringer, M. B., et al.: Esophageal carcinoma: CT findings. Radiology, *155*:171, 1985.
34. Riddel, R. H.: Dysplasia and regression in Barrett's epithelium. *In* Spechler, S. J., and Goyal, R. K. (Eds.): Barrett's Esophagus—Pathophysiology, Diagnosis, and Management. New York, Elsevier, 1985, pp. 143–153.
35. Roth, J. A.: Multimodality therapy of cancer arising from Barrett's epithelium. World J. Surg., *19*:205, 1995.
36. Roth, J. A., Lichter, A. J., Putnam, J. B., and Forastiere, A. A.: Cancer of the Esophagus. *In* Devita, V. T., Hehman, S., and Rosenberg, S. A. (Eds.): Cancer: Principles and Practice of Oncology, 4th ed. Philadelphia, J. B. Lippincott, 1993, p. 776.
37. Sarr, M. G., Hamilton, S. R., Marrone, G. C., and Cameron, J. L.: Barrett's esophagus: Its prevalence and association with adenocarcinoma in patients with symptoms of gastroesophageal reflux. Am. J. Surg., *149*:187, 1985.
38. Sherrill, D. J., Grishkin, B. A., Galal, F. S., Zajtchuk, R., and Graeber, G. M.: Radiation associated malignancies of the esophagus. Cancer, *54*:726, 1984.
39. Shirakabe, H., Yamaki, G., Maruyama, T., and Nishizawa, M.: Radiologic patterns of early esophageal cancer. *In* Delarue, N. C., Wilkins, E. W., Jr., and Wong, J. (Eds.): International Trends in General Thoracic Survey. Vol. 4, Esophageal Cancer. St. Louis, C. V. Mosby, 1988, pp. 19–24.
40. Skinner, D. B.: En bloc resection for neoplasm of the esophagus and cardia. J. Thorac. Cardiovasc. Surg., *85*:59, 1983.
41. Skinner, D. B., Ferguson, M. K., Soriano, A., Little, A. G., and Staszak, V. M.: Selection of operation for esophageal cancer based on staging. Ann. Surg., *204*:391, 1986.
42. Spechler, J. S., Robbins, A. H., Robbins, H. B., Vincent, M. E., Heeren, T., Doos, W. G., Colton, W. G., and Schimmel, E. M.: Adenocarcinoma and Barrett's esophagus: An overrated risk? Gastroenterology, *87*:927, 1984.
43. Sugimachi, K., Ohno, S., Fujishima, H., et al.: Endoscopic ultrasonographic detection of carcinomatous invasion and of lymph nodes in the thoracic esophagus. Surgery, *107*:336, 1990.
44. Thurston, S. E., and Lenn, N. J.: The association and spinal and gastroesophageal anomalies. Clin. Pediatr., *23*:652, 1984.
45. Tio, T. L., and Tytgat, G. N. J.: Atlas of Transintestinal Ultrasonography. Aalsmeer, The Netherlands, Drukkerij Mur-Kostuerloren B.V., 1986.
46. Turrisi, A. T.: Esophageal cancer: The role of radiation. *In* Zuidema, G. D., and Orringer, M. B. (Eds.): Shackelford's Surgery of the Alimentary Tract, 4th ed. Vol. I, The Esophagus. Philadelphia, W. B. Saunders, 1996, pp. 333–348.
47. Tytgat, G. N.: Non-radiological investigation of the oesophagus. *In* Watson, A., and Celestin, L. R. (Eds.): Disorders of the Oesophagus: Advances and Controversies. London, Pitman, 1984, pp. 24–36.
48. Vinayeh, R, and Levin B.: Endoscopic diagnosis. *In* DeMeester, T. R., and Levin, B. (Eds.): Cancer of the Esophagus. New York, Grune & Stratton, 1985, pp. 43–55.
49. Xu, L., Sun, C., Wu, L., Chang, Z., and Liu, T.: Clinical and pathological characteristics of carcinosarcoma of the esophagus: Report of four cases. Ann. Thorac. Surg., *37*:197, 1984.
50. Yang, P. C., and Davis, S.: Incidence of cancer of the esophagus in the U.S. by histologic type. Cancer, *61*:612, 1988.
51. Zieren, H. U., Muller, J. M., Jacobi, C. A., et al.: Adjuvant postoperative radiation therapy after curative resection of squamous cell carcinoma of the thoracic esophagus: A postoperative randomized study. World J. Surg., *19*:444, 1995.

VII

PERFORATION OF THE ESOPHAGUS

André Duranceau, M.D.

The initial report on postemetic esophageal perforation was by Boerhaave in 1704. It was only two centuries later that the first successful attempt at repairing such a condition was reported. Barrett, after producing a careful review of the literature on this topic, became the first surgeon to report the survival of a patient who was treated for a ruptured esophagus.[7, 8] Over the following five decades the etiology and management of esophageal perforation have evolved. New effective antibiotics, improved caloric intake, and better monitoring and life support systems have helped in the development of new strategies that have allowed better management and overall improvement in results (Fig. 26–73). Despite these improvements, esophageal perforation remains one of the major therapeutic challenges for the general and the thoracic surgeon.

ETIOLOGY AND PATHOPHYSIOLOGY

Esophageal perforations are classified in Table 26–8. Iatrogenic esophageal disruptions account for 58% of all perforations. Spontaneous perforation and external esophageal traumas are responsible individually for 15% to 20% of all esophageal ruptures. Pathologic lesions affecting the esophageal wall are responsible for the other perforations.

Iatrogenic Perforations. Development of endoscopy and of endoscopic manipulation of esophageal conditions has become the first cause of esophageal perforations. Fiberoptic endoscopy results in a 0.09% incidence of perforation, whereas if endoscopy is performed with a rigid instrument, the incidence of perforations is 0.07%. Esophageal wall disruption increases immediately to 0.25% when dilatation is added. Direct manipulations such as sclerosis of varices and hydropneumatic dilatations for motor disorder are associated with perforations for 1% to 5% of patients.

The area most at risk of being injured is the pharyngoesophageal junction, where a rigid neck, kyphosis, or promi-

TABLE 26–8. Causes of Esophageal Perforation

Iatrogenic

Instrumental

Endoscopy
Dilatations
Esophageal intubation
Variceal sclerosis
Laser

Intraoperative

Endotracheal intubation
Minitracheostomy
Thyroid resection
Anterior spine surgery
Mediastinoscopy
Pneumonectomy
Vagotomy

Radiation Therapy

Traumatic

Blunt trauma
Penetrating trauma
Accidental pneumatic rupture
Caustic injury
Foreign body

Spontaneous

Postemetic
Others

Esophageal Disease

Carcinoma
Barrett's esophagus
Infectious esophagitis

nent arthrosis spurs may render introduction of the endoscope more difficult. Mid and distal instrumental perforations result from attempts at biopsies to document malignancies or from dilatations. The anterior angulation toward the left of the intra-abdominal esophagus favors posterior wall perforation with frequent communication with the lesser sac. Difficult endotracheal intubation, blind installation of a minitracheostomy, staging and definitive operations for lung cancer, and blind dissection of the abdominal esophagus for vagotomy are all responsible for perforations or fistula formation. Operations on the cervical spine and thyroidectomy may result in esophageal damage. Palliative intubation or laser destruction of esophageal tumors also account for a significant number of perforations.

Spontaneous Perforations. Boerhaave's syndrome, an esophageal rupture induced by straining, represents the most typical example of this condition. Even if it refers usually to a postemetic rupture, straining in other situations may end with the same results. Childbirth, defecation, lifting heavy objects, or any acute rise in intra-abdominal pressure against a closed glottis have been reported as a cause for esophageal rupture. The pressure changes usually result in an esophageal tear on the left lateral wall, just above the diaphragm.[33] In most patients there is no esophageal wall pathology. Watts defined how the presence of a hiatal hernia could influence the site of the lesion.[36] Postemetic ruptures are located on the esophageal wall and rarely associated with a hernia. Retching

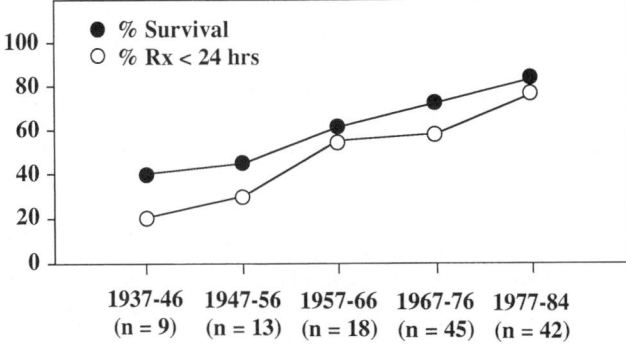

Esophageal Perforation

TRENDS IN SURVIVAL

% of total population

- ● % Survival
- ○ % Rx < 24 hrs

	1937-46	1947-56	1957-66	1967-76	1977-84
	(n = 9)	(n = 13)	(n = 18)	(n = 45)	(n = 42)

Year interval

Figure 26–73. Trends in frequency, early diagnosis, and survival in patients with esophageal perforation. (From Bladergroen, M. R., Lowe, J. E., and Postlethwait, R. W.: Diagnosis and recommended management of esophageal perforation and rupture. Reprinted with permission from the Society of Thoracic Surgeons [The Annals of Thoracic Surgery, *42*:235, 1986].)

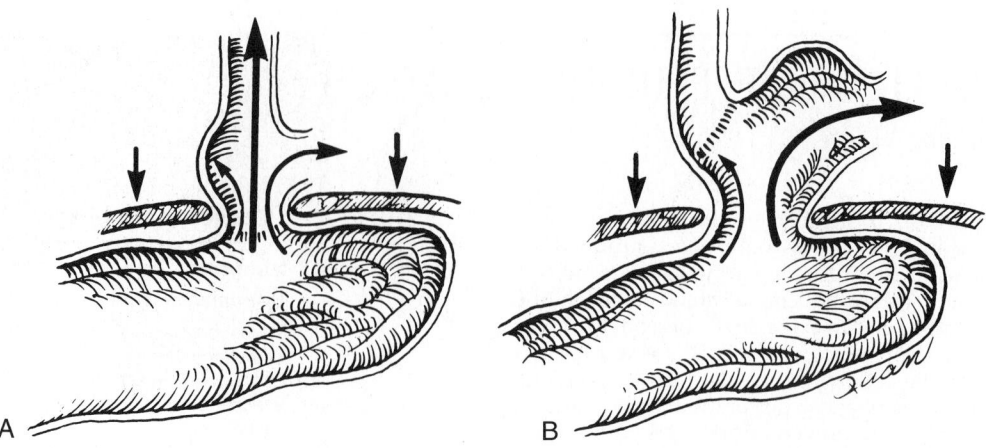

Figure 26–74. *A,* Postemetic rupture of the esophagus usually results from an acute pressure rise in the esophagus with a closed glottis and in the absence of esophageal wall pathology. *B,* When a sliding hernia is present, retching efforts predispose to gastroesophageal wall lacerations (Mallory-Weiss) or perforations.

in the presence of a hernia predisposes to a combined gastro-esophageal rupture or tears the gastric wall (Fig. 26–74). Forceful ejection of gastric contents into the mediastinum results in major contamination with subsequent infection and necrosis. Late diagnosis of the rupture is frequent.

Trauma to the Esophagus. Esophageal perforations from penetrating or blunt trauma are frequently overshadowed by associated injuries. This probably explains why chest trauma received during war produced few reported perforations. Civilian injuries, however, mostly neck, chest, and abdominal trauma, produce a significant incidence of esophageal injuries that carry the same poor prognosis if they go unrecognized.[15, 28] Foreign bodies and even carbon dioxide released from carbonated beverages or from compounds used during double-contrast radiography have been responsible for esophageal ruptures. Self-induced esophageal lesions by alkali or acid may cause extensive necrosis and esophageal destruction.

Esophageal Disease. The most severe forms of gastro-esophageal reflux disease, those with esophageal stricture or when extensive columnar-lined esophagus has replaced the squamous mucosa, are associated with more frequent esophageal perforations. Penetrating and bleeding ulcers are feared complications. Candidal, herpetic, and human immunodeficiency infections also cause pathologic perforations. Invasion and destruction of the esophageal wall by carcinoma may end in free mediastinal or pleural communications.

CLINICAL PRESENTATION

Symptoms and signs vary with the cause and location of the perforation (Table 26–9). They are influenced by the time delay between damage and consultation. Pain is the most consistent symptom. It is present in 70% to 90% of patients

TABLE 26–9. Symptoms and Signs of Esophageal Perforation

Symptoms	Signs
Vomiting	Tachycardia
Pain	Fever
Hematemesis	Subcutaneous emphysema
Dysphagia	Chest hypersonarity/dullness
Dyspnea	Cardiac *crunch*

and is usually related to the site of disruption. Neck ache and stiffness is suggestive of esophageal wall trauma after endoscopy. In the abdomen, dull epigastric pain irradiating to the back may be recorded if the disruption is posterior and communicates with the lesser sac. The sudden appearance, after straining, of excruciating chest pain is identified in 70% to 95% of postemetic ruptures. Blood-tinted vomitus or hematemesis is present in up to 30% of these patients. This pain pattern often results in a misdiagnosis of dissecting aortic aneurysm, spontaneous pneumothorax, or myocardial infarction. The acuteness of pain and its frequent epigastric location often suggest a perforated ulcer or acute pancreatitis. Dysphagia and odynophagia are reported more rarely. Dyspnea appears late and is usually related to a thoracic perforation. On examination, tachycardia and tachypnea are documented in 50% to 70% of patients. Hypotension and shock are present when sepsis or significant liquid losses have occurred. Subcutaneous emphysema is seen more frequently (50%) when the perforation is cervical. When associated with a thoracic perforation (30%) or with an abdominal disruption (10%), it is usually a late sign. Dyspnea with chest findings of dullness suggests a hydropneumothorax. The beating heart surrounded by mediastinal emphysema may produce a sound suggesting a *crunch* on auscultation.

DIAGNOSIS

The plain chest roentgenogram is diagnostic in 90% of patients with perforation. When obtained early after disruption, the chest film may be normal. Mediastinal emphysema may take more than an hour to appear, and air diffusion in the mediastinum is favored by intact pleura (Fig. 26–75A). Mediastinal edema and pleural effusion usually take many hours to appear. Still, pneumomediastinum, subcutaneous emphysema, mediastinal widening, or a mediastinal air-fluid level must prompt investigation to rule out esophageal perforation. Hydropneumothorax on the left, or occasionally on the right, is seen mostly with perforations of the middle and distal third esophagus. (see Fig. 26–75B and C).

The definitive diagnosis is obtained by contrast studies. The esophagogram reveals the primary site or area of leakage (see Fig. 26–75E and F). It shows if the leak is confined to the mediastinum or if it communicates freely with the pleural or peritoneal cavities. Esophageal opacification is usually obtained using a water-soluble contrast medium. The medium is hypertonic but causes no histologic reaction. If the study is negative, a thin barium solution is used to improve

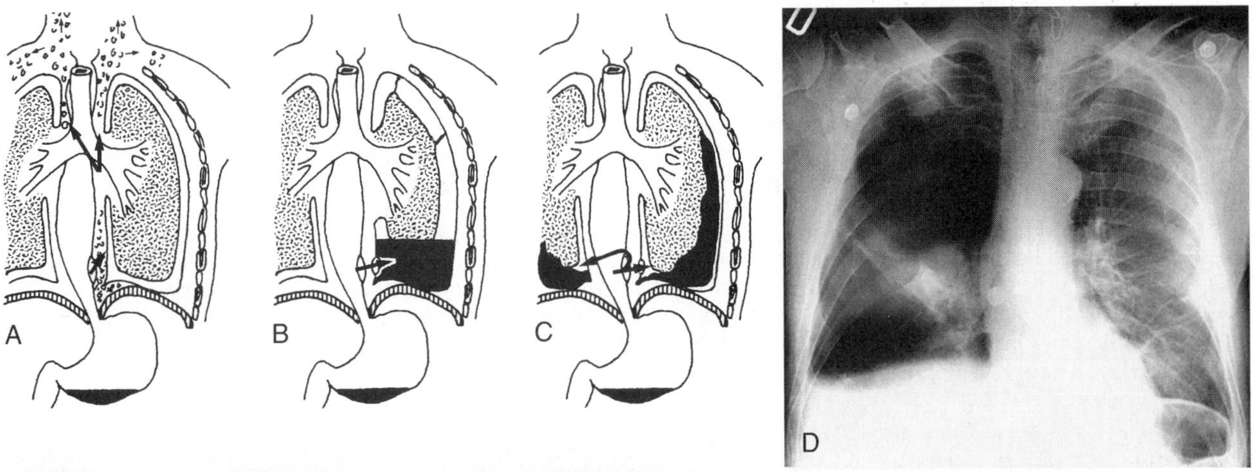

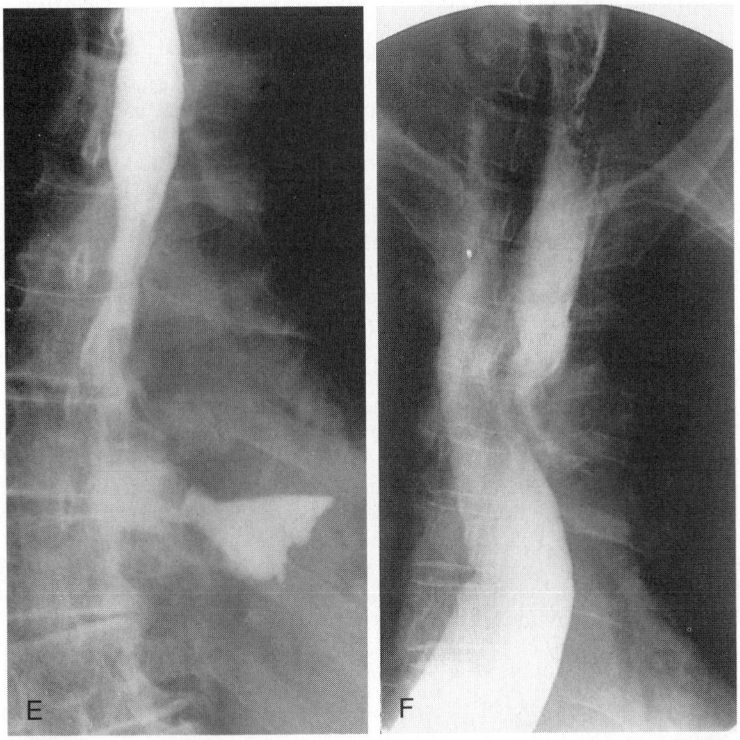

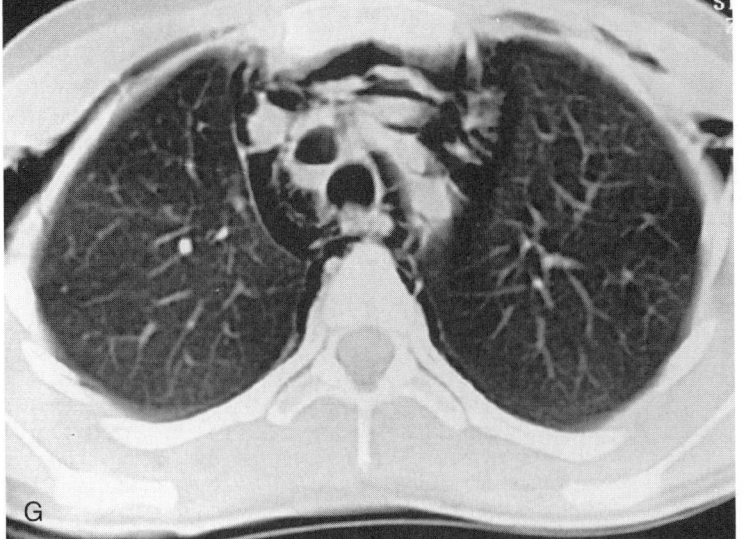

Figure 26–75. *A* to *C,* Chest roentgenogram findings suggestive of esophageal perforation. *D,* Right hydropneumothorax 5 days after vomiting efforts. *E,* Perforation of the esophagus is documented first by contrast studies. *F,* Large perforation diagnosed immediately after endoprosthesis installation. The contrast material is contained by mediastinal tissues. *G,* Computed tomography is used mostly in atypical presentation of esophageal perforations to document related complications such as periesophageal and pleural abscess cavities.

localization of more subtle perforations. False-negative esophagograms may be as high as 10%, usually because of a rapid transit in a standing position or when the rent is small (see Fig. 26–75C).

Computed tomography of the chest is used when the presentation is atypical, when signs and symptoms are vague or misleading, or when perforation involves the lesser sac (see Fig. 26–75D). In these circumstances, help is provided by computed tomography to identify the exact site of the perforation and related complications. The use of contrast material during the examination enhances the diagnostic value of the technique.[5] Esophagoscopy is rarely needed to diagnose a perforation. Pleural fluid analysis and laboratory findings are rarely helpful to establish the diagnosis. When suggestive, they always orient to a more specific radiologic investigation.

TREATMENT

There are three factors affecting management of esophageal perforation: etiology, location, and delay between rupture and treatment. Postemetic perforation is still considered the most morbid, with poorer survival due to late diagnosis. In contrast, iatrogenic and traumatic injuries are diagnosed earlier, resulting in less morbidity and mortality. Pharyngeal perforation rarely ends in fatality. Morbidity and mortality increases as soon as the perforation extends into the esophagus.[14] Eighty-five percent of patients with cervical esophageal perforations survive, whereas thoracic disruptions result in a 65% to 75% cure rate and 90% of patients survive after repair of an abdominal esophageal disruption. The time factor, regardless of etiology and location, still has the most significant influence in management results. Any delay is interpreted as being the reason for a significant increase in morbidity and mortality. In several studies poorer survival was observed when the perforation was diagnosed more than 24 hours after the onset of symptoms.[1, 3, 9, 37] Nesbitt and Sawyers[26] and Gouge and associates[19] observed no substantial worsening of results until treatment delay has reached 48 hours. A limit of 72 hours has been proposed by Gouge and associates to influence treatment philosophy of esophageal perforations. A rational approach based on this experience is described in Figure 26–76.

The early reports of Derbes and Mitchell[13] and Blichert-Toft[10] show a 60% to 100% mortality when conservative management or no treatment is offered. These results are from an era when antibiotics and means of management were less available. They must be taken in perspective with more recent reviews in which a 22% to 38% mortality is observed for medical treatment of selected groups of patients.[18, 22, 23] The difficulty with nonoperative management is prospective determination of which perforation will remain contained and those that will cause continued contamination with subsequent uncontrolled infection. For these reasons, the criteria set by Cameron and colleagues[11] remain appropriate: *a well-contained leak in a stable patient without evidence of sepsis and without communication with the pleural or peritoneal cavity* suggests a patient who has already defended himself against the perforation. The perforation must drain back easily into the esophagus.

Surgical treatment remains the mainstay of management in esophageal perforation. An early operative repair provides the best chances of survival. Sepsis, shock, pneumothorax, pneumoperitoneum, mediastinal emphysema, and respiratory failure are all absolute indications to intervene rapidly. Signs and symptoms of sepsis during conservative management indicate immediate surgical treatment.

Perforation with Early Diagnosis. Primary repair of the perforation is the first choice of therapy. The goals of the operation include extensive débridement of all nonviable tissue in the mediastinum and around the esophagus. Edema and necrotic tissue may be extensive even if the esophageal damage is recent. Decortication of trapped lung tissue may be necessary. Failure of repairs is often due to poor identification of the perforation itself. The esophagus and, if needed, the esophagogastric junction must be dissected completely to identify the site of the disruption. The muscularis may be edematous and necrotic while the mucosa usually remains normal. Myotomy is often necessary to visualize the full extent of mucosal injury. Nonviable muscle tissue is débrided, and primary repair is completed only if the edges of the perforation have been well identified (Fig. 26–77A). The technique of repair may be a single-layer or a double-layer suture closure (see Fig. 26–77B). Gayet and associates[16] have

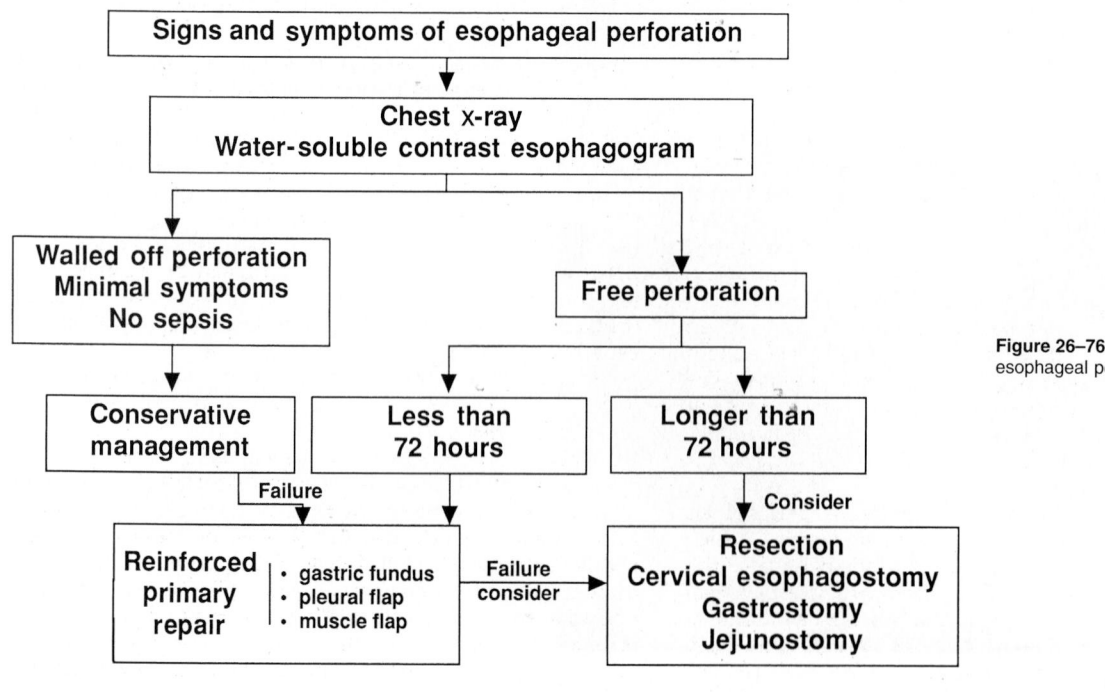

Figure 26–76. Algorithm for treatment of esophageal perforation.

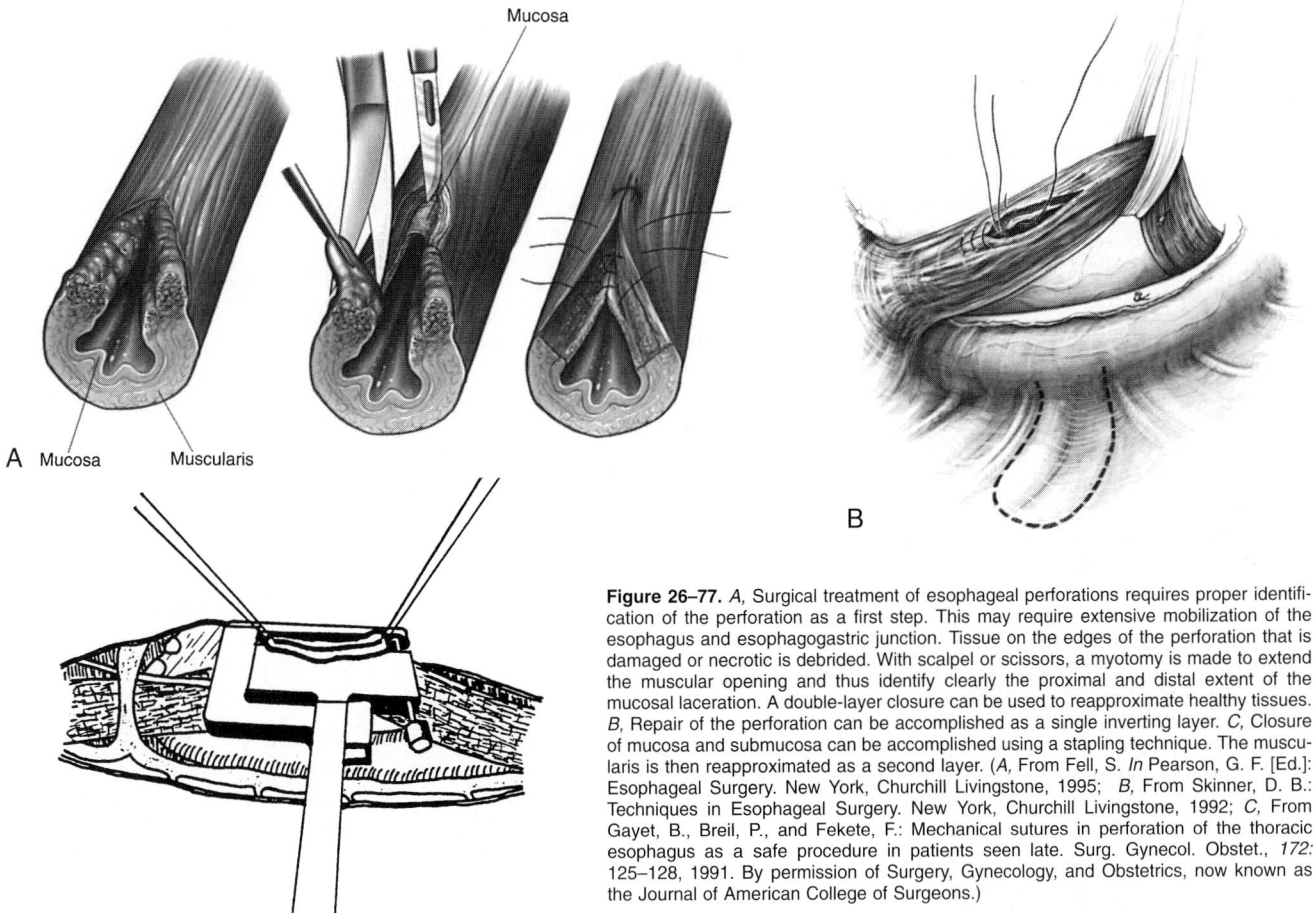

Figure 26–77. *A,* Surgical treatment of esophageal perforations requires proper identification of the perforation as a first step. This may require extensive mobilization of the esophagus and esophagogastric junction. Tissue on the edges of the perforation that is damaged or necrotic is debrided. With scalpel or scissors, a myotomy is made to extend the muscular opening and thus identify clearly the proximal and distal extent of the mucosal laceration. A double-layer closure can be used to reapproximate healthy tissues. *B,* Repair of the perforation can be accomplished as a single inverting layer. *C,* Closure of mucosa and submucosa can be accomplished using a stapling technique. The muscularis is then reapproximated as a second layer. (*A,* From Fell, S. *In* Pearson, G. F. [Ed.]: Esophageal Surgery. New York, Churchill Livingstone, 1995; *B,* From Skinner, D. B.: Techniques in Esophageal Surgery. New York, Churchill Livingstone, 1992; *C,* From Gayet, B., Breil, P., and Fekete, F.: Mechanical sutures in perforation of the thoracic esophagus as a safe procedure in patients seen late. Surg. Gynecol. Obstet., *172:* 125–128, 1991. By permission of Surgery, Gynecology, and Obstetrics, now known as the Journal of American College of Surgeons.)

proposed the use of a linear stapler to close the lacerated mucosa after a meticulous exposure of the proximal and distal limits of the rent (see Fig. 26–77C).

Even early primary repairs have a significant morbidity and mortality.[19, 22, 24, 26, 29] Larsen and Pettersson[24] and Pate and associates[29] observed a mortality of 33% to 43% in patients with a postemetic rupture, even if diagnosed and treated less than 24 hours after perforation. For these reasons, it is safe to suggest that primary repairs should be buttressed with well-vascularized autologous tissue. A well-mobilized gastric fundus provides the best protection when fashioned as a partial or total fundoplication around perforations of the distal esophagus (Fig. 26–78A). A Thal patch may be used if the perforation extends above the diaphragm (see Fig. 26–78B). Thoracic esophageal perforation repairs can be offered added protection by an autologous pleural flap (see Fig. 26–78C)[19, 21] or by pedicled muscle flaps from the diaphragm, intercostal muscles, or chest wall musculature.[30] Bladergroen and coworkers[9] report a 92% survival after early repair with no deaths during the last 6 years of their experience. The experience reported by Gouge and associates[19] and by Wright emphasize excellent survival when patients are treated with a buttressed repair within 72 hours of the perforation (Table 26–10).

Perforation with Late Diagnosis. Esophageal perforations with late presentation or delayed diagnosis result in more contamination and more extensive mediastinal tissue damage. Ideal repair of well-identified layers of the esophageal wall becomes more difficult and failures are more frequent. A sharp rise in morbidity and mortality is seen with delay in the initiation of operative therapy.[3, 9, 19, 30, 32]

Primary reinforced repair remains the first choice of operative therapy as long as the principles of primary repair can be respected. Gouge and associates[19] report that their 12 patients treated with the added protection of a pleural flap all survived, despite two patients who had a documented fistula. Gayet and associates,[16] after buttressing their stapled repair with pleural flaps or gastric fundus, also reported excellent results. They recognize that these results might be influenced by more extensive débridement, better exposure of the wound, the use of inert sutures, and coverage by autologous well-vascularized tissue. Both these reports conclude that even late perforations can be treated by primary repair as long as it is reinforced. In reviewing 10 large series (see Table 26–10), Gouge and associates[19] emphasized that the incidence of fistula (13%) and mortality (6%) is significantly less than when patients are treated by a simple primary repair without the added protection of covering tissue (fistula, 39%, mortality, 25%). Infectious complications are usually responsible for failures.

Alternative procedures have been proposed for late disruptions. They are esophageal exclusion, T-tube drainage, and esophageal resection (Fig. 26–79).

Exclusion of the perforated esophagus by division at the cardia and into the neck has been modified to offer a number of variations allowing partial or total exclusion of the perforated organ (see Fig. 26–79).[26, 34] Most of these operations involve débridement with suture of the perforation and wide drainage of the contaminated space. The rationale for this operation has been questioned because retained peristalsis in the excluded esophagus with stagnant secretions within the esophageal lumen would favor bacterial overgrowth and en-

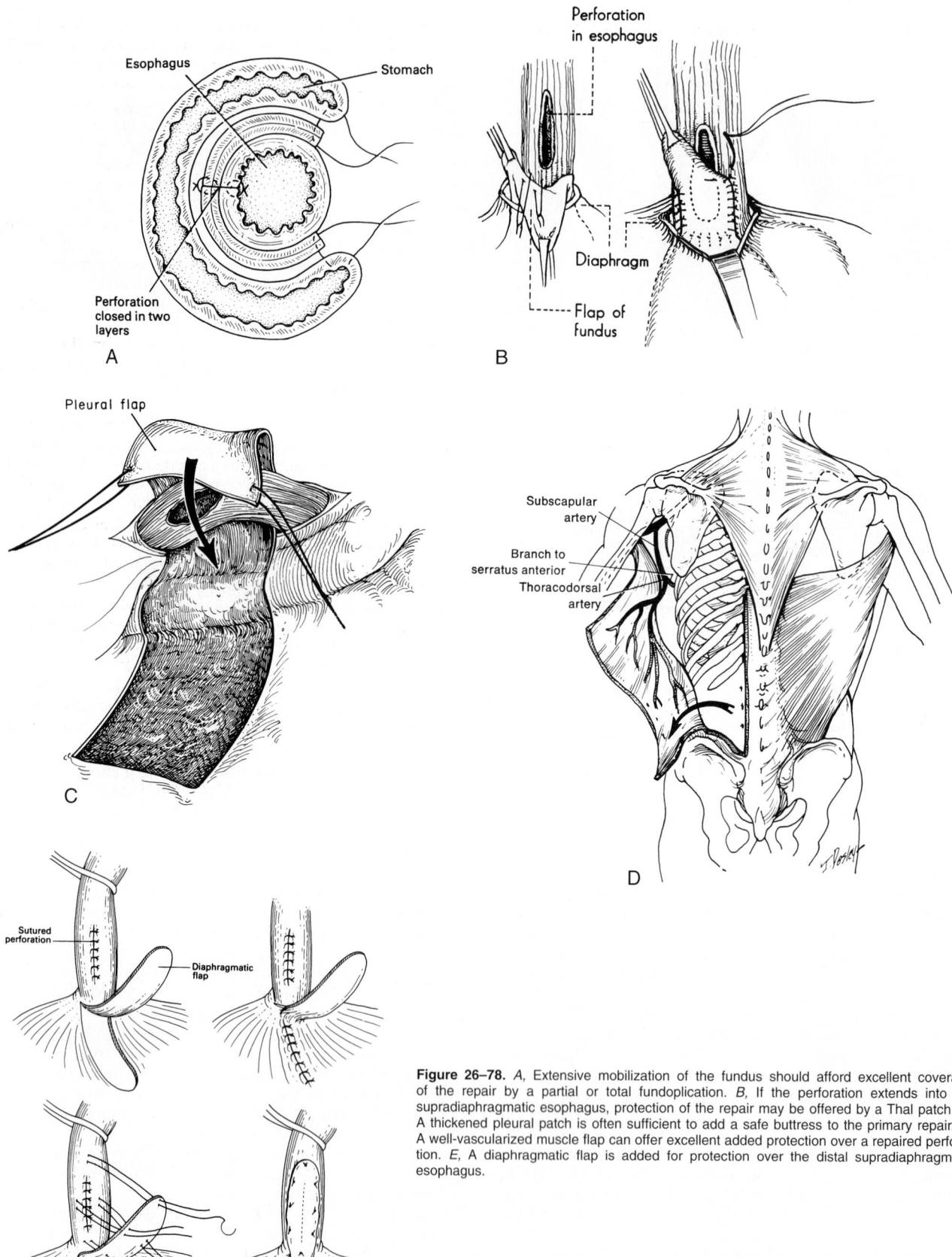

Figure 26–78. *A,* Extensive mobilization of the fundus should afford excellent coverage of the repair by a partial or total fundoplication. *B,* If the perforation extends into the supradiaphragmatic esophagus, protection of the repair may be offered by a Thal patch. *C,* A thickened pleural patch is often sufficient to add a safe buttress to the primary repair. *D,* A well-vascularized muscle flap can offer excellent added protection over a repaired perforation. *E,* A diaphragmatic flap is added for protection over the distal supradiaphragmatic esophagus.

TABLE 26–10. Results of Treatment Using Primary Repair

Method	No. of Patients	Fistulas (%)	Mortality (%)
Simple Repair	158	39	25
Repair with autogenous tissue buttress	99	13	6

From Gauge, T., Depan, H. J., and Spencer, F. C.: Experience with the Grillo pleural wrap procedure in 18 patients with perforation of the thoracic esophagus. Ann. Surg., *209*:612, 1989.

hance prolonged drainage of mucus and bacteria through the perforation. Moreover, free reflux from stomach has not been documented. One of the major disadvantages of this approach is the commitment to a second major operation. To avoid this, Bardini and colleagues[6] have proposed the use of resorbable staplers that allow repermeation of the esophageal lumen after a few weeks. Five of the 49 patients treated with this technique by Urschel[35] died. In the 10 reports studied by Gouge and associates,[19] the mortality was 35% in 58 patients, while Giudicelli,[17] looking at 78 exclusions, observed 33 deaths (42%). Richardson and colleagues[30] and Attar and coworkers[4] report dismal results with this approach.

T-tube drainage of the perforation is expected to result in a controlled esophagocutaneous fistula (see Fig. 26–79).[2] Larsson and coworkers[25] have suggested this technique for late esophageal perforations or as a secondary treatment after failed primary repair. Feared complications are related to continuous leakage with progression of mediastinal and pulmonary sepsis. The reported mortality with this approach varies from 36% to 50%.

Resection is indicated when a significant pathologic process exists in the esophageal wall or when extensive damage has resulted from the perforation. If extensive mediastinitis and sepsis are present with poor chances of survival from continued contamination, resection of the esophagus must be considered, with delayed reconstruction usually preferable in patients debilitated by sepsis and major surgery (Fig. 26–80). Fear of creating an obstruction distal to the repair or the extent of damage after failed previous attempts at repair are other indications for resection. In Gouge and associates' experience and review of patients undergoing other types of treatment than primary repair with buttressing beyond the limit of 72 hours, an uneventful recovery has never occurred, and the mortality was 75%. For these reasons in perforations older than 72 hours or perforations with extensive damage, resection must be considered with cervical esophagostomy, jejunostomy, and gastric decompression (see Fig. 26–80). As for other treatment modalities in esophageal perforation, a resection undertaken earlier favors an uneventful recovery. A resection undertaken late or after previous attempts at closure increases morbidity and mortality.[9, 12, 27, 32]

Perforation with Underlying Disease. Idiopathic motor disorders, when treated with hydrostatic dilatation, cause a 4% to 5% incidence of perforation after treatment. In this situation, repair of the perforation is completed first, followed by myotomy of the esophagogastric junction. A partial Belsey type of fundoplication is fashioned to cover both the repair and the myotomy area. A comparable evolution to patients undergoing an elective myotomy is observed in these patients.[31] When long-standing reflux disease has resulted in a stricture, or when a perforated ulcer complicates a columnar-lined esophagus, esophageal resection must be considered unless a safe repair can be accomplished without any obstruction distal to the repair.

If the underlying pathologic process is esophageal carcinoma, conservative therapy shows a high mortality.[38] Conservatism in this situation reflects the reluctance to institute major operations in elderly patients considered to be in poor shape and presenting with a poor prognosis or inoperable tumors. Esophagectomy and immediate reconstruction are indicated if the patient is otherwise operable and has suffered instrumental or spontaneous perforation of the tumor. If perforation has occurred during attempts at palliative intubation, efforts at proper endoluminal positioning of the prosthe-

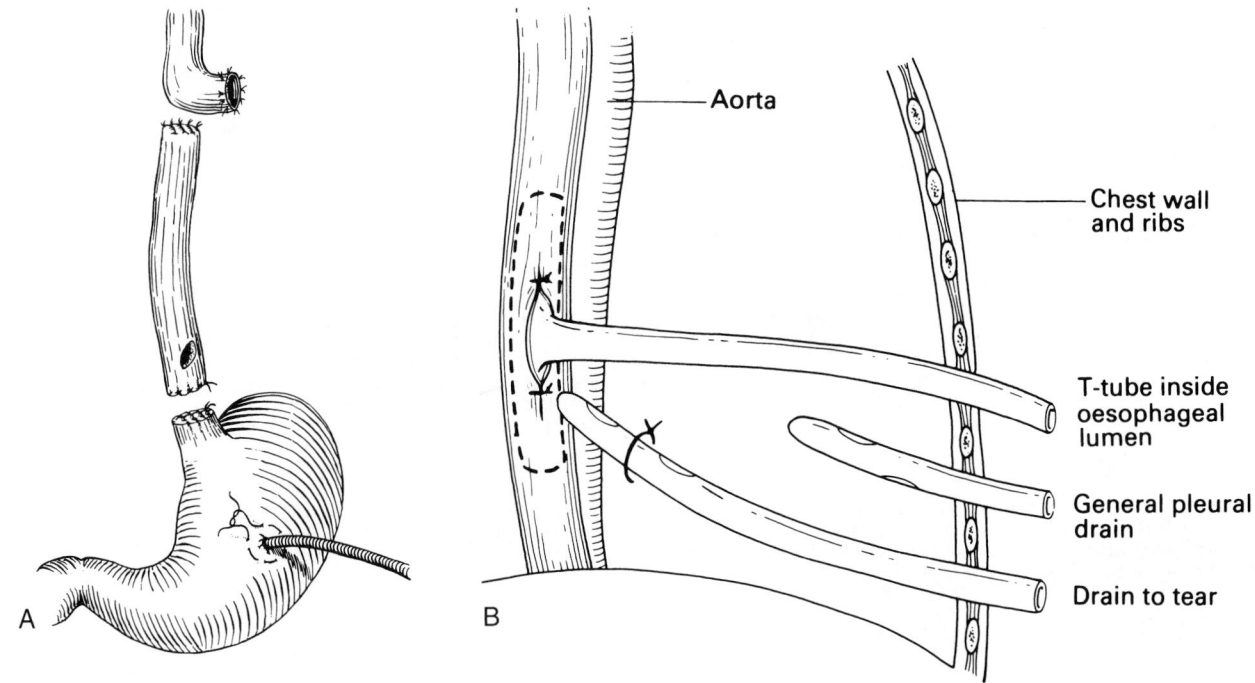

Figure 26–79. *A,* Exclusion of the perforated esophagus by closure or division at the cardia and into the neck. *B,* T-tube drainage of the esophageal perforation with pleural drainage.

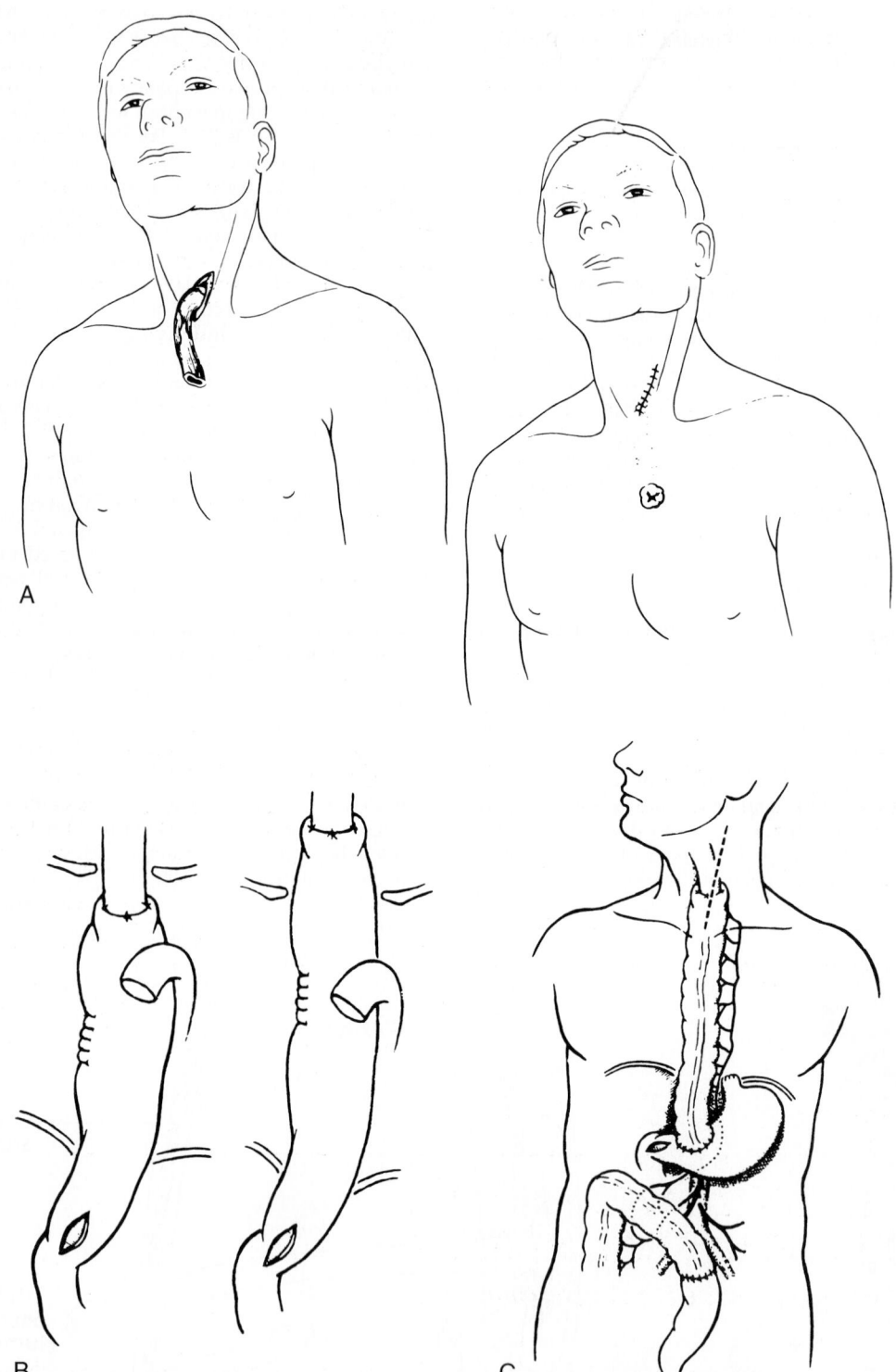

Figure 26–80. *A,* Uncontrolled sepsis with mediastinitis suggests esophagectomy, extensive mediastinal débridement, esophagostomy, gastrostomy, and jejunostomy. When creating the esophagostome, preservation of the longest proximal esophageal segment available is useful. It allows for easier care of an anterior chest wall esophagostome and easier subsequent reconstruction. *B,* Gastric interposition with anastomosis in the apex of the right chest or in the neck. *C,* Isoperistaltic long colon interposition with anastomosis in the neck.

sis are in order, using a push-through or a pull-through technique with the hope of sealing the perforation while antibiotics and chest drainage are added. If a perforation occurs in association with a carcinoma, Griffin and associates[20] have reported a total mortality of 30% in these patients, all from respiratory failure. In Giudicelli's review,[17] the overall mortality was 55% in 40 patients who required a resection.

REFERENCES

1. Aagaard, J., and Kjaergaard, H.: Treatment of iatragenic oesophageal perforation: Diagnosed with delay. Ann. Chir. Gynaecol., 80:346, 1991.
2. Abbott, O. A., Mansour, K. A., Logan, W. D., Hatcher, C. R. Jr., and Symbas, P. N.: Atraumatic so-called spontaneous rupture of the esophagus: A review of 47 personal cases with comments on a new method of surgical therapy. J. Thorac. Cardiovasc. Surg. 59:67, 1970.
3. Ajalat, G. M., and Mulder, D. G. Esophageal perforations. Arch. Surg., 119:1318, 1984.
4. Attar, S., Hankins, J. R., Suter, C. M., Coughlin, T. R., Sequeira, A., and McLaughlin, J. S.: Esophageal perforation: A therapeutic challenge. Ann. Thorac Surg., 50:45, 1990.
5. Backer, C. L., LoCicero, J., Hartz, R. S., Donaldson, J. S., and Shields, T.: Computed tomography in patients with esophageal perforation. Chest, 98:1078, 1990.
6. Bardini, R., Bonavina, L., Pavanello, M., Asolati, M., and Peracchia, A.: Temporary double exclusion of the perforated esophagus using absorbable staples. Ann. Thorac. Surg., 54:1165, 1992.
7. Barrett, N. R.: Spontaneous perforation of the oesophagus: Review of the literature and report of three new cases. Thorax, 1:48, 1946.
8. Barrett, N. R.: Report of a case of spontaneous perforation of the esophagus successfully treated by operation. Br. J. Surg., 35:216, 1947.
9. Bladergroen, M. R., Lowe, J. E., and Postlethwait, R. W.: Diagnosis and recommended management of esophageal perforation and rupture. Ann. Thorac. Surg., 42:235, 1986.
10. Blichert-Toft, M.: Spontaneous oesophageal rupture. Scand. J. Thorac. Cardiovasc. Surg., 5:111, 1971.
11. Cameron, J. L., Kieffer, R. F., Hendrix, T. R., Mehigan, D. G., and Baker, R. R.: Selective non-operative management of contained intrathoracic esophageal disruptions. Ann. Thorac. Surg., 25:346, 1971.
12. DeMeester, T. R.: Perforation of the esophagus. Ann. Thorac. Surg., 42:231, 1986.
13. Derbes, V. J., and Mitchell, R. E.: Rupture of the esophagus. Surgery, 39:688, 1956.
14. Dolgin, S. R., Wykoff, T. W., Kumar, N., and Maniglia, A. J.: Conservative medical management of traumatic pharyngoesophageal perforations. Ann. Otol. Rhinol. Laryngol., 101:209, 1992.
15. English, G. M., Hsu, S. F., Edgar, R., Gibson-Eccles, M., and Eccles, M.: Oesophageal trauma in patients with spinal cord injury. Paraplegia, 30:903, 1992.
16. Gayet, B., Breil, P., and Fekete, F.: Mechanical sutures in perforation of the thoracic esophagus as a safe procedure in patients seen late. Surg. Gynecol. Obstet., 172:125, 1991.
17. Giudicelli, R.: Oesophageal perforations: Results of a national survey. Ann. Chir. Thorac. Cardiovasc., 46:183, 1992.
18. Goldstein, L. A., and Thompson, W. R.: Esophageal perforations: A 15-year experience. Am. J. Surg., 143:495, 1982.
19. Gouge, T., Depan, H. J., and Spencer, F. C.: Experience with the Grillo pleural wrap procedure in 18 patients with perforation of the thoracic esophagus. Ann. Surg., 209:612, 1989.
20. Griffin, S. C., Desai, J., Townsend, E. R., and Fountain, S. W.: Oesophageal resection after instrumental perforation. Eur. J. Cardiol. Thorac. Surg., 4:211, 1990.
21. Grillo, H. C., and Wilkins, E. W., Jr.: Esophageal repair following late diagnosis of intrathoracic perforation. Ann. Thorac. Surg., 20:387, 1975.
22. Jones, W. G., and Ginsberg, R. J.: Esophageal perforation: A continuing challenge. Ann. Thorac. Surg., 53:534, 1992.
23. Larsen, K., Skovjensen, B., and Axelsen, F.: Perforation and rupture of the esophagus. Scand. J. Thorac. Cardiovasc. Surg., 17:11, 1983.
24. Larsen, K., and Pettersson, G.: Advisability of concomitant immediate surgery for perforation and underlying disease of the esophagus. Scand. J. Thorac. Cardiovasc. Surg., 18:275, 1984.
25. Larsson, S., Pettersson, G., and Lepore, V.: Esophagocutaneous drainage to treat late and complicated esophageal perforation. Eur. J. Cardiol. Thorac. Surg., 5:579, 1991.
26. Nesbitt, J. C., and Sawyers, J. L.: Surgical management of esophageal perforations Am. Surgeon, 53:183, 1987.
27. Orringer, M. B., and Stirling, M. C.: Esophagectomy for esophageal disruption. Ann. Thorac. Surg., 49:35, 1990.
28. Pass, L. J., LeNarz, L. A., Schreiber, J. T., and Estrera, A. S.: Management of esophageal gunshot wounds. Ann. Thorac. Surg., 44:253, 1987.
29. Pate, J. W., Walker, W. A., Cole, F. H., Owen, E. W., and Johnson, W. H.: Spontaneous rupture of the esophagus: 30 year experience. Ann. Thorac. Surg., 47:689, 1989.
30. Richardson, J. D., Martin, L. F., Burzotta, A. P., and Polk, H. C.: Unifying concepts in treatment of esophageal leaks. Am. J. Surg., 149:157, 1985.
31. Schwartz, H. M., Cahow, C. E., and Traube, M.: Outcome after perforation sustained during pneumatic dilatation for achalasia. Dig. Dis. Sci., 38:1409, 1993.
32. Skinner, D. B., Little, A. G., and DeMeester, T. R.: Management of esophageal perforation. Am. J. Surg., 139:760, 1980.
33. Tidman, M. K., and John, H. T.: Spontaneous rupture of the oesophagus. Br. J. Surg., 54:286, 1967.
34. Urschel, H. C., Razzuk, M. A., and Wood, R. E.: Improved management of esophageal perforation: Exclusion and diversion in continuity. Ann. Surg., 179:587, 1974.
35. Urschel, H. C. Discussion. In Gouge, T., Depan, H. J., and Spencer, F. C.: Experience with the Grillo pleural wrap procedure in 18 patients with perforation of the thoracic esophagus. Ann. Surg., 209:618, 1989.
36. Watts, H. D.: Lesions brought on by vomiting: The effect of hiatus hernia on the site of injury. Gastroenterology, 71:683, 1976.
37. White, R. K., and Morris, D. M.: Diagnosis and management of esophageal perforations. Am. Surgeon, 58:112, 1992.
38. Wilde, P. H., and Mullany C. J.: Oesophageal perforation: A review of 37 cases. Aust. N.Z. J. Surg., 57:743, 1987.
39. Wright, C. O., Mathisen, D. J., Wain, J. C., et al.: Reinforced primary repair of thoracic esophageal perforation. Ann. Thorac. Surg., 60:245, 1995.

VIII

HIATAL HERNIA AND GASTROESOPHAGEAL REFLUX

André Duranceau, M.D., and Glyn G. Jamieson, M.D.

Earlier texts on the esophagus emphasized the anatomic abnormalities of hiatal hernias and discussed as a separate entity the obstructive nature of esophageal strictures. At a time when radiology and rigid endoscopy were the mainstay of esophageal investigation, Barrett[4] and Allison,[2] through their observations, suggested the term *reflux esophagitis* after linking the reflux of gastric contents with the presence of a sliding hiatal hernia. Early operations emphasized restoration of the stomach to a normal abdominal position, with reapproximation of the pillars of the esophageal hiatus. Although these repairs led to initial success, longer-term results were disappointing, with a high incidence of reflux and esophageal mucosal damage.[1] During the past three decades, investigation of hiatal hernias and reflux disease has focused on the physiologic abnormalities responsible for reflux, with improved management and better results.

When sought assiduously, hiatal hernias are found in nearly half of the adult population. Symptomatic gastroesophageal reflux is also common, with daily heartburn reported by 11% of a large study population and an added 12% and 15% of persons, respectively, reporting weekly or monthly symptoms Although the vast majority of such persons do not require active treatment, reflux disease with or without hiatal hernias is certainly a common problem.

Although speculative, the increased prevalence and incidence of adenocarcinomas of the distal esophagus in industrialized societies may be related to an increased incidence of columnar-lined esophagus in this population. Gastroesophageal reflux is also important in another and often ignored aspect of our society. In the field of medical liability, 37% of liability problems in relation to the esophagus are brought about because of treatment of hiatal hernia and gastroesophageal reflux. Furthermore, these conditions are responsible for 50% of the costs for liability problems in esophageal surgery.

All of this emphasizes the importance of hiatal hernia and reflux disease as common and serious clinical problems in society. These conditions require a logical and well-planned approach for all forms of treatment.

EMBRYOLOGY AND ANATOMY OF THE ESOPHAGOGASTRIC JUNCTION

By the seventh week of embryologic life, the endoderm has formed the primitive foregut. It is surrounded by mesoderm, which provides the necessary material to form connective tissue, muscle layers, and periesophageal tissue. At this stage the esophagus is short, extending from the tracheal groove to the dilatation of the foregut, which becomes the future stomach.

The shape of the distal esophagus and the gastroesopha-geal junction develops from an increase in size of the greater curve of the stomach. This growth occurs from an increased mitotic activity within the greater curve, resulting in a fundus and an angle of His becoming better defined (Fig. 26–81A). The cardia is held in place by its dorsal attachments. All supporting and anchoring structures develop from the mass of mesodermal tissue (Fig. 26–81B). Around the distal esophagus, the septum transversum forms the diaphragm and the phrenoesophageal membrane differentiates from the same tissue mass (Fig. 26–81C). The longitudinal and circular muscular layers develop from the mesodermal cell mass and adopt their final arrangement at the 90-mm. stage. Neuroblasts from the neural crest give rise to ganglia, which form a periesophageal neural network around the circular muscle layer before the longitudinal muscle layer differentiates.

The muscle of the distal esophagus is arranged in two muscle layers. The inner layer is circular and formed from incomplete muscle bundles that overlap. At the gastroesophageal junction, the circular layer's fibers are asymmetrically thickened accounting for the high-pressure zone recorded by esophageal manometry (Fig. 26–82A). The outer longitudinal layer parallels the axis of the esophagus and its fibers continue through the esophagogastric junction, joining with the longitudinal gastric musculature. In this area of the esophagus all the musculature at the junction is smooth muscle. The submucosa is a strong layer, connecting muscle coat and

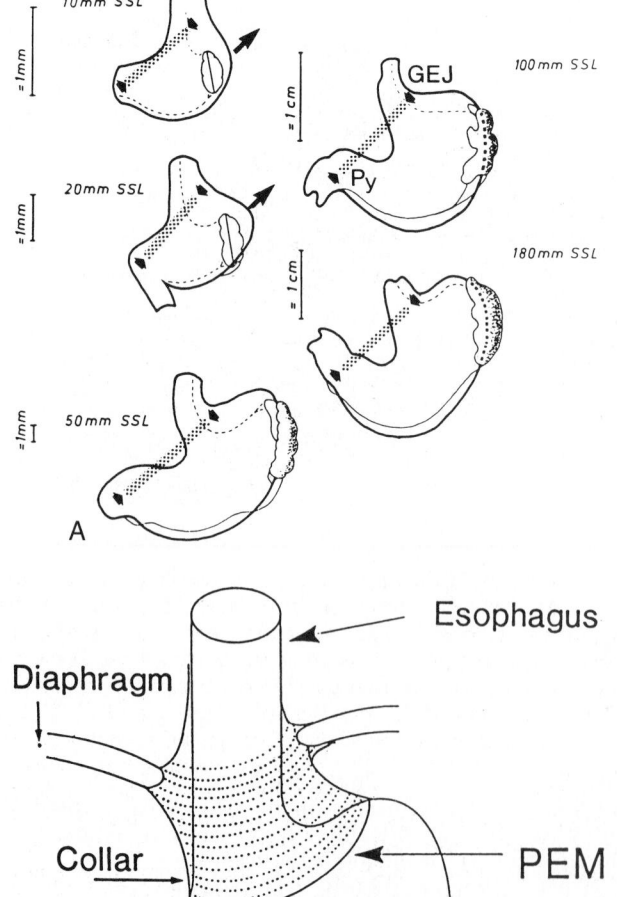

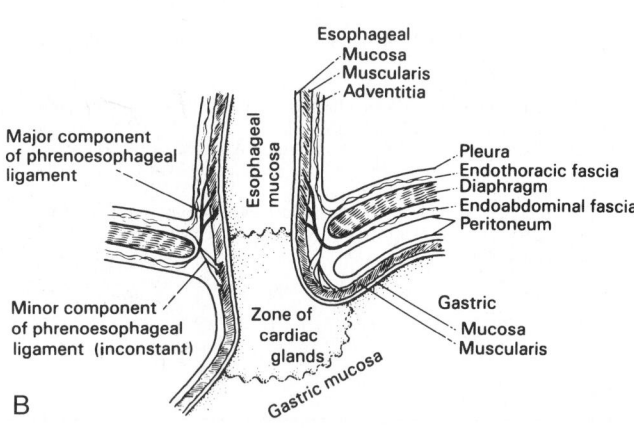

Figure 26–81. *A*, Increased mitotic activity of the greater curve of the stomach defines the shape of the gastroesophageal junction (GEJ). *B*, Supporting and anchoring structures holding the cardia in place develop from mesodermal tissue. *C*, Diaphragm and phrenoesophageal membrane (PEM) differentiate from the mesoderm.

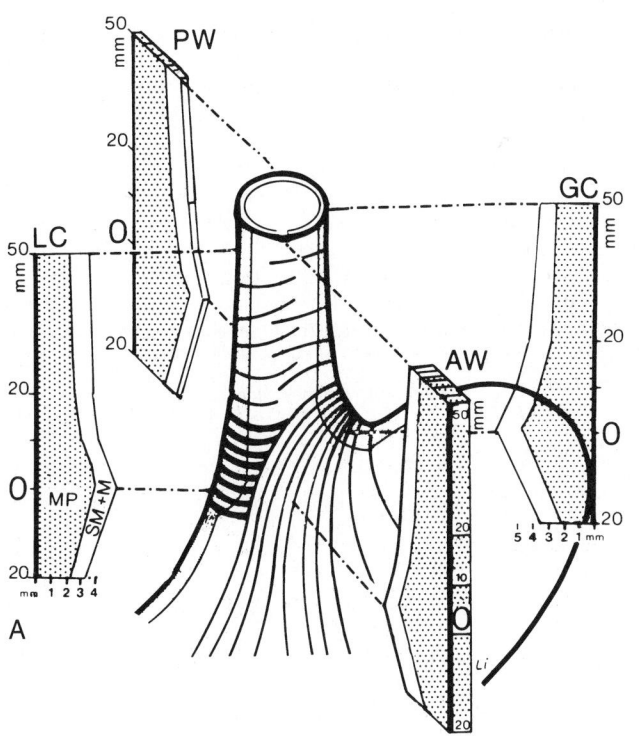

A

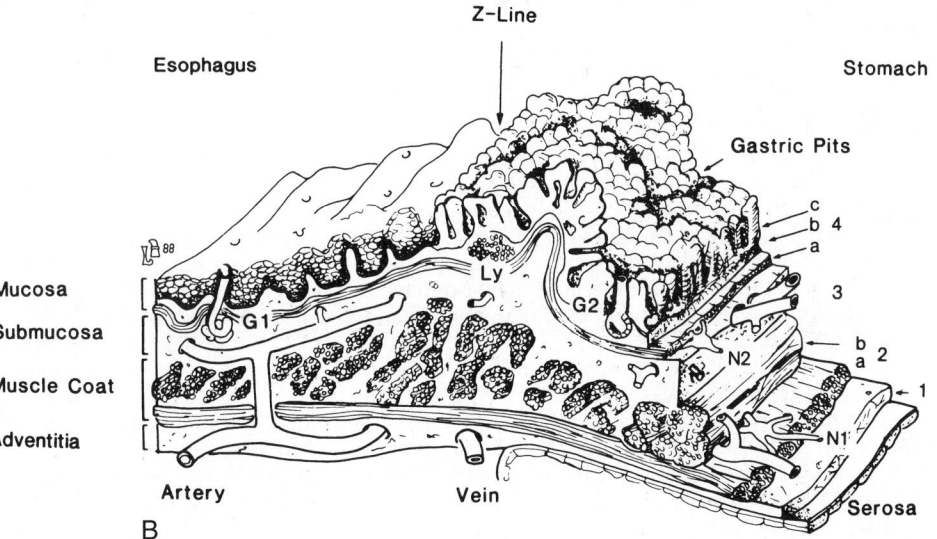

B

Figure 26–82. *A,* The asymmetry of the high pressure zone at the gastroesophageal junction is explained by the configuration and thickness of the muscle organization. *B,* Tissue organization of the esophagogastric junction.

mucosa. It is composed of elastic and collagenous fibers and contains a network of vessels and nerves. Deep esophageal glands penetrate the muscularis mucosa to extend into the submucosa. The mucosa of the distal esophagus is a multilayered squamous epithelium with a basal layer lying on the tunica propria. The squamous epithelium changes to a columnar epithelium approximately 2 cm. above the anatomic junction. The serrated aspect of this junction is called the Z line (Fig. 26–82*B*).

The vascular supply to the gastroesophageal junction comes from the left gastric artery, which gives two to six branches to the lower esophagus, the anterior aspect of the cardia, and the proximal lesser curve of the stomach. The splenic artery supplies the posterior esophageal wall and the posterior proximal stomach.

The innervation to the esophagus comes from the vagal nerves, which form a plexus around the lower esophagus before forming the right and left main vagal trunks.

The esophageal hiatus is an elliptical opening in the muscular part of the diaphragm. Posteriorly, the arms of the hiatus are formed by the diaphragmatic crura. The crura arise from the anterior surface of the L1 to L4 vertebrae on the right and from the first two lumbar vertebrae on the left. They insert anteriorly into the transverse ligament of the central tendon of the diaphragm. Configuration of the esophageal hiatus is variable. In 50% of individuals, both arms of the hiatus are formed from the right crus. In 44% of patients, the left arm originates from the right crus while the right arm originates from both crura (Fig. 26–83). The structure of the crura is musculotendinous, but they are more tendinous near their vertebral origin, an important technical consideration because sutures to repair a widened hiatus must be placed deep to include both the pleura and the tendinous portion of the crura.

The gastroesophageal junction is held in place in the diaphragmatic hiatus by the phrenoesophageal membrane (Fig.

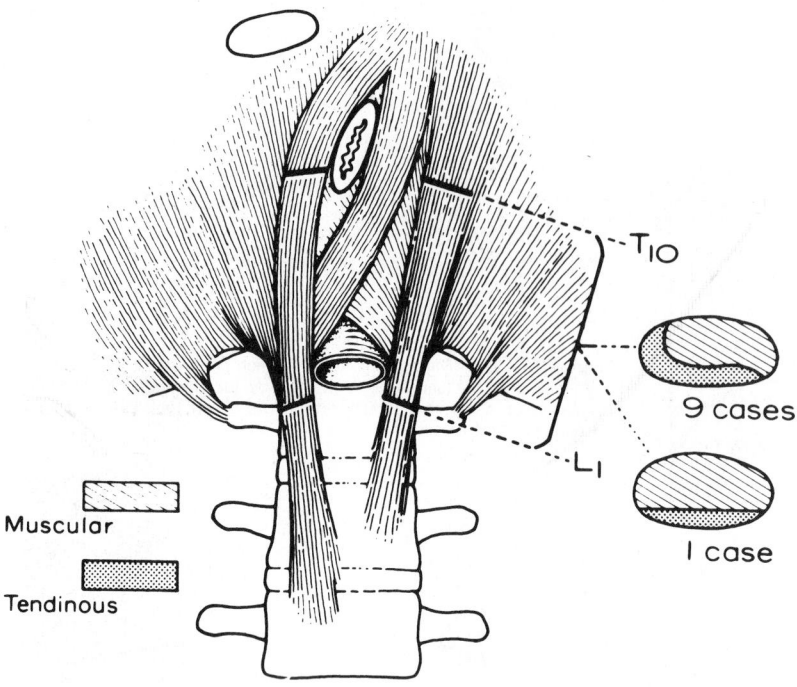

Figure 26–83. The arms of the esophageal hiatus and their musculotendinous individual organization. In 50% of individuals, both arms originate from the right crus. They are more tendinous near their vertebral origin.

T10

9 cases

L1

1 case

Muscular

Tendinous

26–81C). From its diaphragmatic origin, this membrane splits into two layers to attach cranially 2 to 4 cm. above the hiatus to the esophageal submucosa, and it attaches caudad to the gastric serosa, the gastrohepatic ligament, and the dorsal gastric mesentery. The space between the split layers of the phrenoesophageal ligament is filled by the precardial fat pad. This ligament is best seen in infants. With age, the ligament becomes less definite and fat infiltrates between the proximal and distal fibers. The ligament is virtually nonexistent in patients with long-standing hiatal hernia.[38] Thus, the anchoring tissue maintaining the esophagus in the hiatus consists of pleura, subpleural endothoracic fascia, phrenoesophageal proximal fascia, transversalis endoabdominal fascia, and peritoneum (Fig. 26–81B).

The thoracic duct usually lies posterior and to the right, away from the gastroesophageal junction. However, when a large hiatal hernia is present, the cysterna chyli lie near the right crus of the diaphragm on the bodies of the L1 and L2 vertebrae, so that chylothorax occasionally results from division of large lymph vessels, which are tributaries of the thoracic duct.

NORMAL FUNCTION OF THE ESOPHAGOGASTRIC JUNCTION

Voluntary deglutition causes a sweeping pharyngeal contraction to traverse and then close the upper esophageal sphincter area, and the swallowing wave then continues into the cervical esophagus to start the primary wave of peristalsis (Figs. 26–84A and 26–85A). Secondary peristalsis is an esophageal wave not preceded by swallowing. It is stimulated by distention of the esophagus and also by factors that may be regarded as esophageal irritants (e.g., acid). It represents an efficient defense mechanism of the esophagus for emptying itself of its content. Tertiary contractions are nonpropulsive contractions in the esophageal body, and they are either spontaneous or may follow deglutition (Fig. 26–85A, B, and C). Spontaneous tertiary contractions are frequent and may be stimulated by a large number of factors. They do not necessarily represent abnormality. If tertiary contractions occur after voluntary deglutition of a water bolus, this may

mean that an underlying pathologic process is present (Fig. 26–85B and C).

Primary peristalsis traverses both the striated and smooth muscle of the esophagus as a continuous wave. There is a pressure trough at the junction of the proximal and middle third, where striated and smooth muscle meet. The esophageal contraction waves travel at a speed of approximately 3.5 cm. per second over the distal half of the esophagus, slowing immediately above the lower esophageal sphincter (LES). When pressure waves are measured by intraluminal transducers, contraction pressure amplitude varies between 90 and 109 mm. Hg,[36] and their mean duration is around 5 seconds (Fig. 26–84B).

The esophagogastric junction, as recorded by manometry, is a high-pressure zone of 3 to 4 cm. in length located just above the junction of the esophagus with the stomach. The muscle arrangement at this level creates a radial asymmetry, with the highest pressures measured in the left posterior area (Fig. 26–84C). The LES is composed of smooth muscle and is under noncholinergic and nonadrenergic control mechanisms. The sphincter is maintained in a contracted state, mostly from intrinsic myogenic activity, but its resting tone is affected by numerous neural and hormonal factors (Table 26–11). The absolute resting pressures in the LES of one adult control group was 24.8 mm. Hg, with a resting intragastric pressure of 7.3 mm. Hg. This means there was a gradient of 17.5 mm. Hg between the esophagus and the stomach. Richter and coworkers[36] recorded pressures of 24.4 mm. Hg with a stationary pull-through and of 29 mm. Hg with a rapid pull-through method. The tone of the sphincter increases in response to increased intra-abdominal pressures and during gastric contractions. The LES relaxes at the same time as a peristaltic wave approaches it. Esophageal peristalsis pushes a bolus in the esophageal lumen toward the gastric cavity. The bolus then traverses the relaxed sphincter, which closes once the bolus has passed through. Closing pressures of the sphincter are about double the resting values in the sphincter (Fig. 26–84C). Pressure within the sphincter then returns to resting levels. LES relaxation occurs similarly with secondary peristalsis. After meals, when the stomach is full, transient LES relaxations unrelated to peristalsis occur, and these relax-

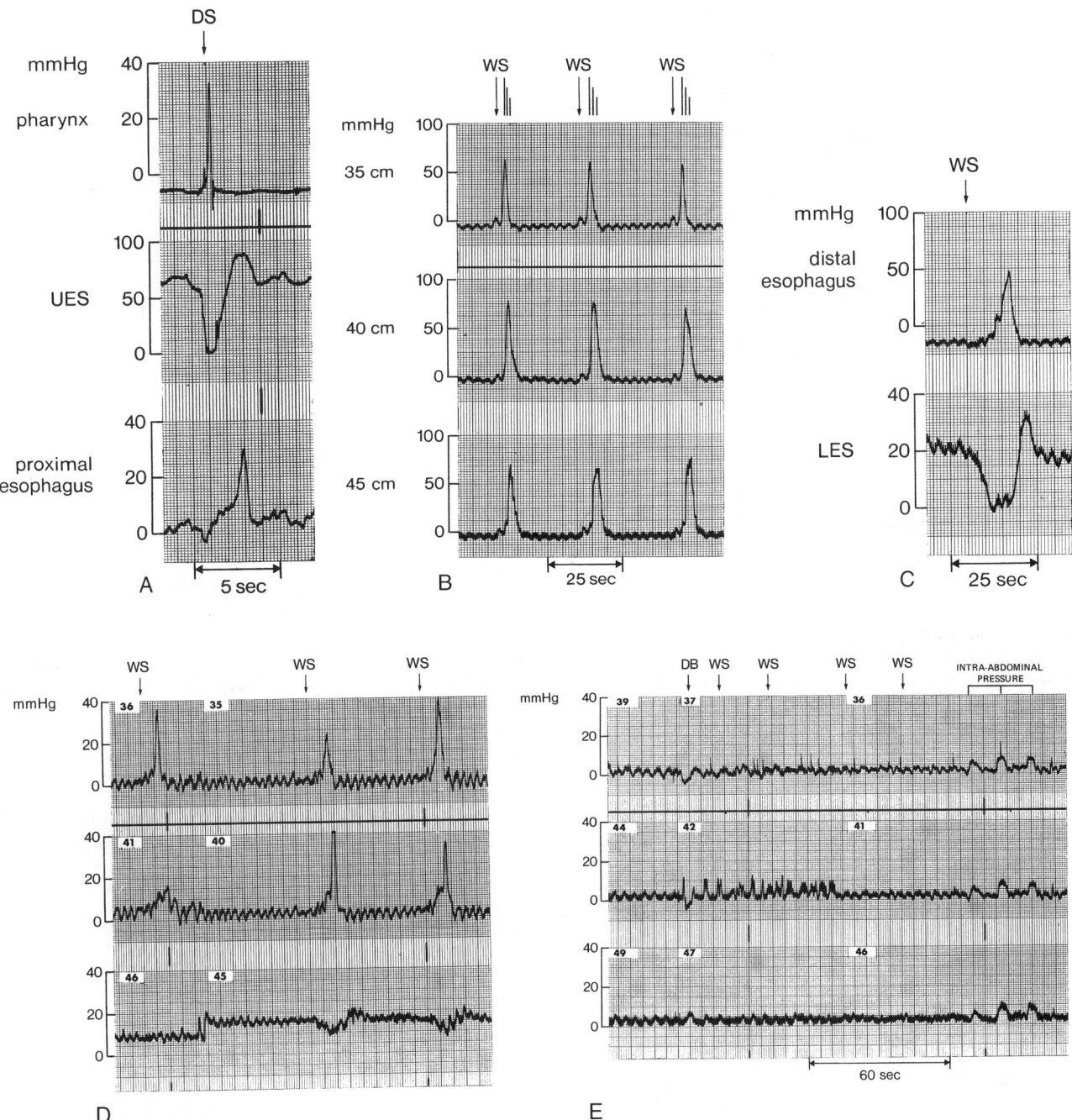

Figure 26–84. *A,* Voluntary deglutition is normally followed by a contraction that sweeps the pharynx, traverses the pharyngoesophageal sphincter and continues into the cervical esophagus. *B,* Primary peristalsis traverses both the striated and smooth muscle of the esophagus as a continuous wave. *C,* The high-pressure zone recorded at the esophagogastric junction (LES) opens in response to swallowing. Once the bolus has passed into the stomach, the passing wave closes the sphincter to return it to its normal resting tone. Transient relaxations of the LES, unrelated to peristalsis, occur mostly after meals. *D,* A poor LES tone suggests the possibility of reflux. *E,* When the LES is weaker than 6 mm. Hg, abnormal reflux is probable. When there is nonmeasurable sphincter tone, pathologic reflux is usually present. WS, wet swallow; DB, deep breathing; DS, dry swallow; UES, upper esophageal sphincter.

ations last from 5 to 30 seconds. It is during such transient relaxations that much reflux occurs, both in normal individuals and in patients with reflux disease.[8]

A number of factors other than intrinsic LES tone also play a role in preventing gastroesophageal reflux. Saliva functions as a weak base and is capable of neutralizing acid. Helm and associates[12] observed that stimulation of salivary flow led to more rapid clearance of acid from the esophagus and that a decrease in salivary secretion prolongs acid clearance. The capacity of the esophagus to empty itself of its content varies among normal subjects. It is influenced by position, by con-

sistency of the bolus, and by pH in the esophagus.[18] The squamous epithelium of the esophagus is normally impermeable to hydrogen ion. Exposure to acids, especially if mixed with bile salts and pancreatic enzymes, causes loss of mucosal resistance, and back-diffusion of acid through the mucosa may then occur.

The muscular organization of the sphincter, the length of the intra-abdominal esophagus, the acute angle of entry of the esophagogastric junction and its valve action, and the integrity of the supporting structures to maintain proper positioning of the junction within the hiatus all play a role

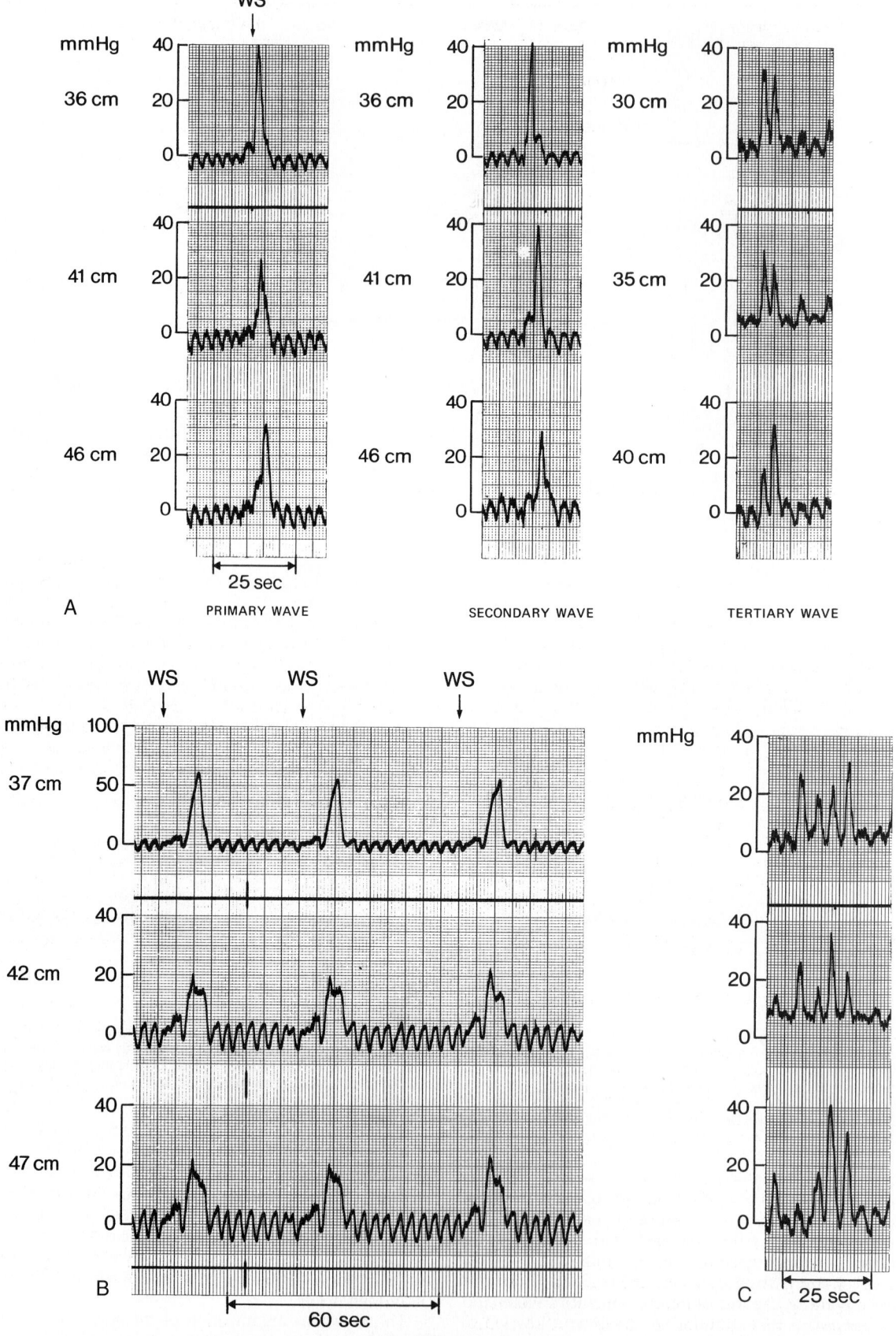

Figure 26–85. *A,* The three types of contraction seen in the esophagus. An organized peristaltic wave normally follows voluntary deglutition. Secondary peristalsis is a normal contraction stimulated by distention or irritation. Tertiary contractions are nonpropulsive. *B,* Tertiary contractions in response to deglutition. *C,* Spontaneous tertiary contractions. WS, wet swallow.

TABLE 26–11. Substances Influencing Lower Esophageal Sphincter Pressure

Substance	Increase Pressure	Decrease Pressure
Hormones	Gastrin Motilin Substance P	Secretin Cholecystokinin Glucagon Somatostatin Gastric inhibitory polypeptide Vasoactive intestinal polypeptide Progesterone
Neural agents	α-Adrenergic agonists β-Adrenergic antagonists Cholinergic agonists	α-Adrenergic antagonist β-Adrenergic agonists Cholinergic antagonists
Foods	Protein	Fat Chocolate Ethanol Peppermint
Medication	Histamine Antacids Metoclopramide Domperidone Prostaglandin $F_{2\alpha}$	Theophylline Prostaglandins E_2 and I_2 Serotonin Meperidine Morphine Dopamine Calcium channel blockers Diazepam Barbiturates

in the prevention of gastroesophageal reflux. Until recently, little documentation existed for the role of the diaphragm in maintaining competence of the gastroesophageal junction. Mittal and colleagues[24] have observed that the crural diaphragm has a special ability to squeeze that helps increase pressures at the esophagogastric junction, especially during inspiration and when increased intra-abdominal pressure occurs. The loss of this squeeze ability when the hiatus is widened in hiatal hernia may predispose to reflux episodes, particularly when there is a loss of sphincter tone.

PATHOPHYSIOLOGY OF REFLUX DISEASE

As mentioned earlier, normal individuals have daily physiologic reflux. These reflux episodes cause neither symptoms nor histologic changes. When reflux episodes cause symptoms, either by an increase in amount or change in composition or increase in frequency, then the pathologic entity of gastroesophageal reflux disease is present.

Lower Esophageal Sphincter Function

The association of hiatal hernias with the reflux of gastric content and the resulting esophagitis was first noted by Allison[2] and Barrett.[4] Subsequently, LES abnormalities were documented in patients with hiatal hernias and symptomatic reflux. When comparing patients with hiatal hernia and reflux to a control group, all but one patient showed poor LES tone. In the control group, all but one patient had normal basal LES pressure. These observations corresponded to the development of new manometric techniques, and a number of contradictory observations at that time emphasized the inaccuracies of early recording systems. Perfused catheters, noncompliant perfused systems, and intraluminal microtransducers subsequently improved the precision of recording the physiology of the esophagus and its sphincters. Perfused manometry with pH probe assessment of reflux episodes has been used to compare a group of free-reflux patients to a group of induced-reflux patients and a control population. The group with free reflux had the lowest basal LES tone, while patients with induced episodes showed a

higher LES pressure, and the control population had the highest values of all. Patients with resting pressures in the LES lower than 6 mm. Hg showed excellent correlation with their symptoms. They also showed good correlation between a normal LES resting pressure and the absence of symptoms. It was noted that finding histologic evidence of esophagitis was increased when the LES tone was weaker. A poor LES tone at the lower limits of normal (6 to 10 mm. Hg) suggests the possibility of reflux (see Fig. 26–84D and E). When the LES is weaker than 6 mm. Hg, abnormal reflux is probable; and when there is no measurable sphincter tone, significant pathologic reflux is usually present.

Esophageal Body Function

Primary and secondary peristalsis represent the most useful defense mechanism of the esophagus. Abnormal motility affecting the esophageal function is observed in patients with symptomatic hiatal hernias, whereas only a minority of patients with reflux disease presented with failure of peristalsis. There is, however, a significant increase in failed peristalsis and a loss of peristalsis strength with increasing mucosal damage. When extensive circumferential columnar-lined esophagus is present, there is an increase in failed peristalsis and an increase in the incidence of tertiary contractions in response to deglutition. Such loss of function suggests that there will be more prolonged exposure to any refluxate with an impaired clearance and emptying capacity from the esophagus. Significant functional abnormalities can be detected when both acid and alkaline reflux were responsible for the esophageal damage. When the esophageal emptying capacity in reflux patients is measured, normal individuals took a mean of 2 swallows (range, 1 to 9) to clear their esophagus of a solid bolus while patients with documented reflux took a median of 5 swallows (range, 1 to 30) to achieve the same results.

Other Factors Affecting Reflux

Type of Refluxate. In experiments with various liquids to induce esophagitis, unaltered gastric juice caused esophageal inflammation and ulceration. Bile alone did not cause esophagitis, but bile and pancreatic juice together caused significant damage. If hydrochloric acid is infused, erosive esophagitis can be produced, but the mucosal damage is increased when pepsin is added. Hydrochloric acid causes further damage when mixed with bile and bile salts. The digestive enzymes mixed with acid and bile salts induce loss of impermeability in the squamous epithelium. Back-diffusion of the hydrogen ion causes damage at the level of the middle and basal layers of the mucosa. Clinically, a mix of acid and bile is present in the more severe forms of reflux disease.[3, 11, 42] Patients with reflux esophagitis and the presence of Barrett's metaplasia show a greater exposure to both acid and alkaline reflux than patients with simple esophagitis.

Gastric Emptying. A significant number of patients with gastroesophageal reflux show abnormal liquid and/or solid emptying pattern. If delayed gastric emptying is a causative factor it is probably through the mechanism of prolonged fundal distention, which increases the frequency of transient LES relaxations.

Anatomic Alteration of the Gastroesophageal Junction. Previous operations at the gastroesophageal junction may have altered supporting structures at the hiatus. Although surgical alterations of the diaphragm or the phrenoesophageal membrane do not alter the physiologic characteristics of the gastroesophageal junction, they may expose the intra-abdominal esophagus and the hiatal structures to a modified response when intra-abdominal conditions are altered. Although the presence of a hiatal hernia in itself does not produce pathologic reflux, acute increases in intra-abdominal pressures, especially in obese patients, can decrease the gastroesophageal junction resistance, favoring reflux when the LES barrier is weakened.

Resection of the esophagogastric junction is always followed by reflux esophagitis, especially when reanastomosis of esophagus and stomach is completed in the lower chest. Similarly, when total gastrectomy is not reconstructed with the use of a Roux-en-Y reconstruction to exclude biliary and pancreaticoduodenal secretions, esophageal mucosal damage invariably occurs. Myotomy of the distal esophagus and esophagogastric junction in the treatment of motor disorders decreases substantially the muscle tone of the LES, and this also favors gastroesophageal reflux and its complications.

There is a widespread belief among clinicians that obesity is associated with abnormal reflux, despite a paucity of evidence implicating obesity in reflux damage. The delayed gastric and esophageal emptying reported in these patients, with possible changes in the gastroesophageal resistance by the resulting intra-abdominal conditions, may represent major factors leading to reflux symptoms and esophageal mucosal damage. Moreover, since the incidence of reflux episodes is directly related to the size of the diaphragmatic hiatus, herniation of the stomach with impairment of the circumferential squeeze ability of the crural diaphragm in these patients possibly facilitates reflux.[24]

Social Habits and Medication. Food is a frequent culprit, causing significant decrease in LES pressures with resulting heartburn. The list of these substances is described in Table 26–11. Fatty food, chocolate, and peppermint have all been shown to reduce LES tone. Proteins tend to increase basal LES pressures, while alcohol decreases resting pressures in the LES as well as the strength of contractions in the esophagus. Decreased esophageal clearance develops with longer exposure to the refluxate. Tobacco smoking causes a significant decrease in LES resting pressures. All medication affecting smooth muscle contraction, such as calcium channel blocking agents, nitrates, oxazepam, diazepam, and morphine derivatives, have been shown to affect LES pressures and esophageal contractions (see Table 26–11).

INVESTIGATION AND STAGING OF HIATAL HERNIAS AND GASTROESOPHAGEAL REFLUX DISEASE

Hiatal hernias and gastroesophageal reflux disease are measurable conditions, and they should be staged objectively to assess severity and degree of reflux.

Signs and Symptoms. There are three categories of clinical features in patients with reflux disease (Table 26–12). Typical symptoms are those of heartburn and/or regurgitation, made worse when the patient lies down or bends over. This category is by far the most common. A second category relates to complications of reflux disease. Mild dysphagia is often seen in the absence of any stricture, but more severe grades of dysphagia are usually caused by mechanical or functional obstruction from reflux damage. Odynophagia refers to painful swallowing and usually implies severe disease. Chest pain arising from the esophagus is probably a variant of the pain of heartburn. However, very occasionally it can be severe enough to mimic cardiac pain. Hematemesis and melena are rarer complications arising from esophagitis, and they indicate the presence of extensive mucosal damage and also suggest the possibility that columnar-lined mucosa is present. A third category sometimes associated with reflux disease includes oropharyngeal dysphagia, asthma, recurrent chest pain problems, recurrent hoarseness, and pharyngitis. These problems, before being considered a result and a complication of reflux disease, must be assessed and related to esophageal damage. In a similar fashion, features such as halitosis, waterbrash, acidic taste in the mouth, or dental problems must be considered nonspecific if unassociated with objective esophageal changes. Most of the time patients with regurgitation and heartburn have uncomplicated gastroesophageal reflux disease. However, typical heartburn has been shown to result from stomach or duodenal problems in 22% of patients, so heartburn cannot always be assumed to arise from the esophagus. Even in cases in which the esophagus is the cause of symptoms, the pathogenesis is not necessarily reflux. Because of this lack of specificity of clinical features, they must not be used as a guide to therapy but as a guide to investigation and documentation of the condition.[6]

Features present with larger hernias are caused mostly by the volume occupied by the hernia in the mediastinum. Postprandial fullness, substernal and parasternal discomfort, or pain and vomiting may occur after eating. Acute dysphagia with severe epigastric or chest pain is ominous and suggests intermittent volvulus and the danger of strangulation. Unexplained anemia is sometimes seen with these large hernias.

Radiology. Radiologic examination plays a major role in

TABLE 26–12. Signs and Symptoms of Gastroesophageal Reflux

Most Common

Regurgitations
Heartburn

Related to Complications of Reflux Disease

Dysphagia
Odynophagia
Hematemesis
Melena

Unrelated to Esophageal Damage

Oropharyngeal dysphagia
Asthma
Chest pain

defining the anatomic abnormalities present when hiatal hernia and reflux disease coexist. A hiatal hernia is the protrusion of an organ, usually the stomach, from the abdomen through the esophageal hiatus into the mediastinum and the thorax. Four types of hiatal hernia have been defined (Fig. 26–86 and Table 26–13).

When a patient presents with typical reflux symptoms and no anatomic defect at the esophagogastric junction (H^0) is found, this implies that physiologic abnormalities at the gastroesophageal junction are responsible for the symptoms (Fig. 26–86A). Patients with scleroderma may also present with the radiologic findings of a patulous cardia without a hernia but with variable mucosal damage. Twenty-five percent of patients with reflux symptoms but without a hiatal hernia may present with ulcerative esophagitis.

A sliding hernia is defined as one in which a viscus makes up part of the wall of the hernial sac. Because of the absence of peritoneum on the upper posterior part of the stomach, when the gastroesophageal junction and proximal stomach move through the hiatus, then a true sliding hernia is present. This is called a Type I hiatal hernia (H^1) (Fig. 26–86B). The hiatus may be widened, and there is a peritoneal sac anterior and lateral to the stomach; and the stomach forms part of the posterior wall of the hernia sac. The incidence of these hernias in the radiology literature ranges from 2.3% to 73%, and the incidence increases with age. The problem with diagnosing a hiatal hernia arises from the criteria used to make the diagnosis. The intra-abdominal portion of the esophagus when it moves upward into the chest loses its tubular appearance and easily mimics a small hiatus hernia. Ott and coworkers[27] observed gastric mucosal folds above the diaphragm in 59% of normal subjects. These hernias

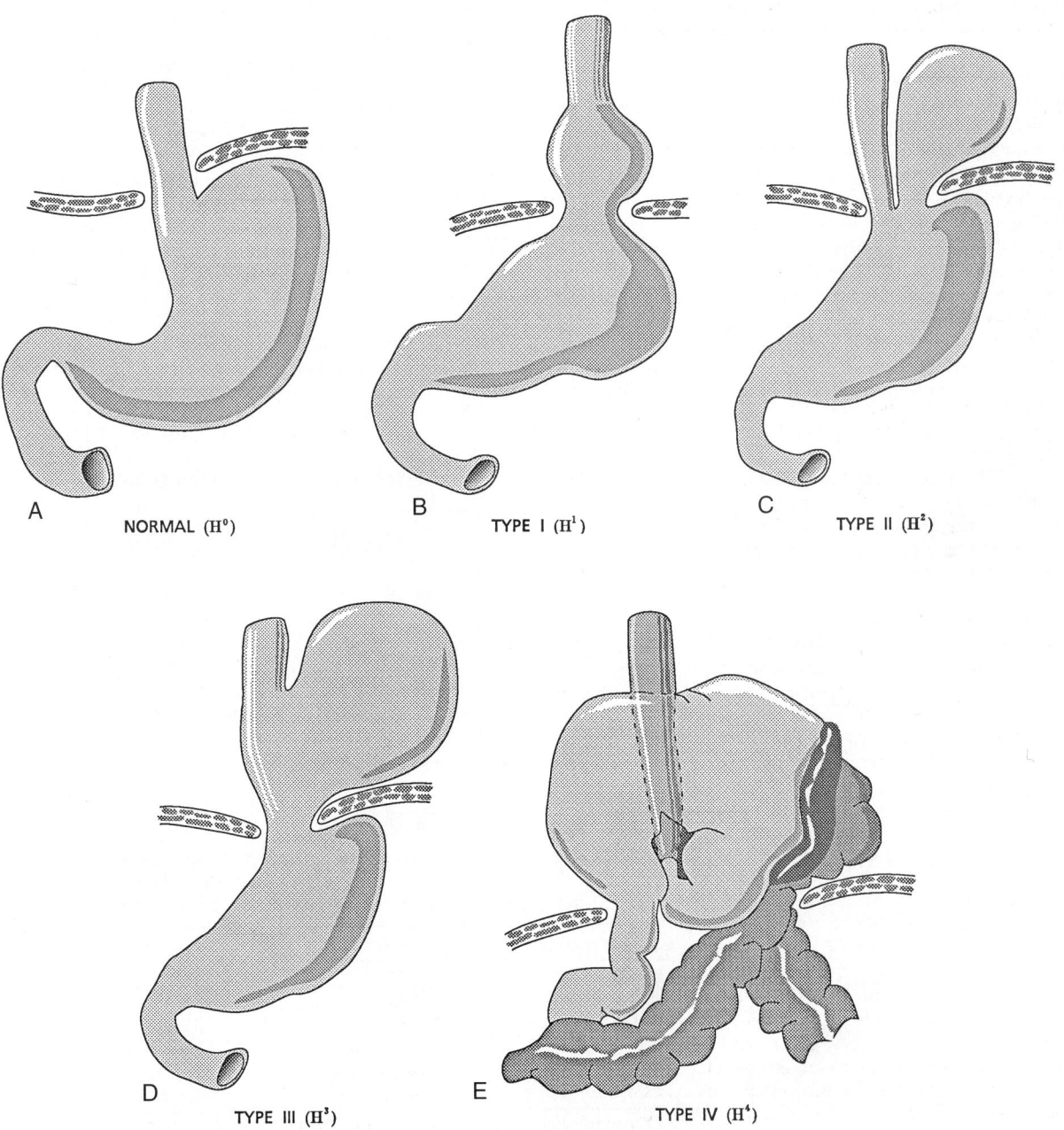

A   NORMAL (H^0)   B   TYPE I (H^1)   C   TYPE II (H^2)

D   TYPE III (H^3)   E   TYPE IV (H^4)

Figure 26–86. *A,* Normal position of the gastroesophageal junction. A defective sphincter is present when pathologic reflux occurs. *B,* Small sliding hiatal hernia (Type I). *C,* Type II hernias show an esophagogastric junction in a normal position with a hernia alongside the esophagus in the mediastinum. *D,* Type III hernias are paraesophageal with the esophagogastric junction in the chest. *E,* Type IV hernias are the massive herniation of stomach and of another abdominal organ into the distal mediastinum.

TABLE 26–13. Types of Hiatal Hernia

Type	Description
H⁰	No hiatal hernia
H¹	Sliding hernia
	Gastroesophageal junction above diaphragm
H²	Normal position of gastroesophageal junction
	Protrusion of the stomach alongside the esophagus
H³	Components of sliding and paraesophageal hernias
	The gastroesophageal junction is in the chest. The stomach rolls through the hiatus in a paraesophageal position.
H⁴	Large hiatal defect with components of the sliding and/or paraesophageal hernia accompanied by another abdominal organ (colon, spleen, pancreas, small bowel)

TABLE 26–14. Endoscopy

Equivocal Evidence of Esophagitis

E^0 = normal
E^1 = erythema

Unequivocal Evidence of Esophagitis

E^2 = erosions and ulceration
E^3 = stricture or columnar-lined esophagus

See text and Figure 26–87 for explanation of MUSE classification.

comprise 90% of all hiatal hernias and usually cause no esophageal symptoms. If symptoms are present, the aim of the investigation is to document reflux disease.

Type II hernias (H²) are those in which the gastroesophageal junction and phrenoesophageal ligament are maintained in their normal position but a peritoneal sac protrudes through the hiatus into the mediastinum alongside the esophagus (Fig. 26–86C). The fundus of the stomach and sometimes the body and antrum ascend through this defect to lie in a paraesophageal position. Progressive enlargement of such hernias often occurs, and the whole stomach may roll into the mediastinum, so that the pylorus is positioned near the cardia. These *pure* Type II hernias with an upside-down stomach are very uncommon, representing approximately 2% of all hernias. If a patient presents with symptoms attributable to such a hernia, this repair is strongly indicated to prevent strangulation, gangrene, and perforation. Somewhat surprisingly, these hernias are sometimes discovered as a coincidental finding, because they are easily seen on a chest x-ray film. Management then may become controversial, especially when the patients are elderly and frail.

Type III (H³) hernias are the combination of a sliding and a rolling hernia (Types I and II) (Fig. 26–86D). The esophagogastric junction is in the thoracic cavity, and this entity probably represents the evolution of an enlarging hiatus with an increase in size of either an initially sliding hernia or a paraesophageal hernia. Patients with this hernia are frequently overweight. Symptoms tend to be similar to those of the original hernia (i.e., Type II or Type III). However, these hernias behave like Type II hernias and so should be repaired.

Type IV (H⁴) hernias are massive hiatal hernias that have the special characteristic of the presence of another abdominal organ alongside the herniated stomach (Fig. 26–86E).

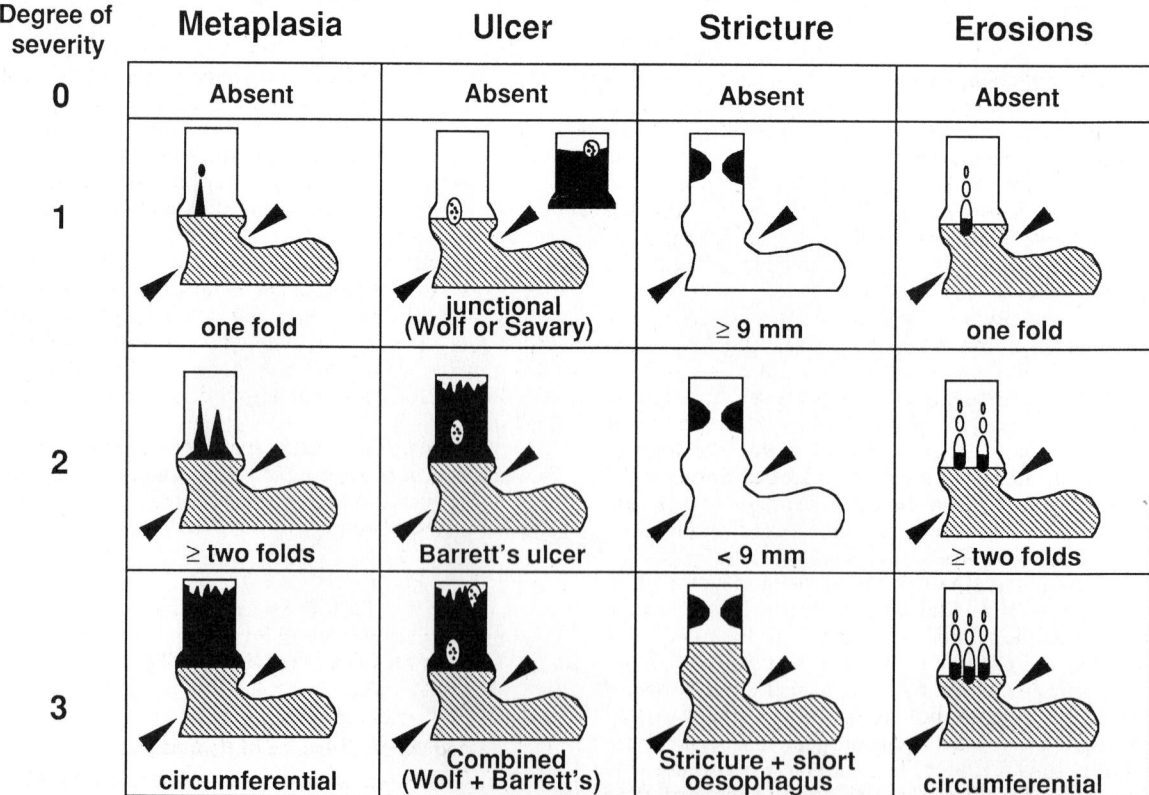

Figure 26–87. The MUSE classification of esophageal mucosal damage in which M = metaplasia, U = ulcer, S = stricture, and E = erosions. See Table 26–14 for staging of severity of endoscopy findings.

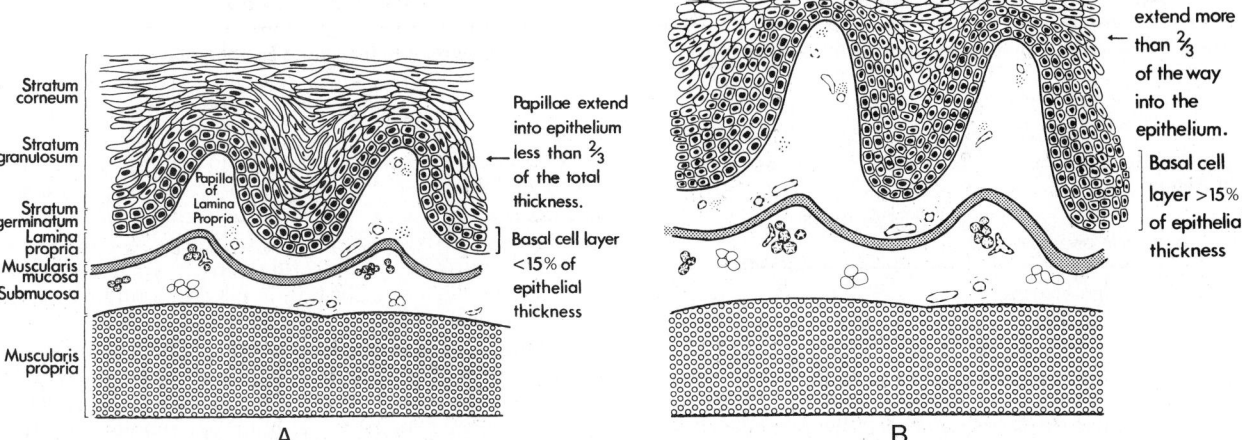

Figure 26–88. *A*, Normal esophageal mucosa. The basal cell layer is less than 15% of the epithelial thickness. *B*, Minimal esophageal mucosal manifestation of abnormal reflux. The thickness of the basal cell layers is increased. Papillae extend nearer the surface of the epithelium.

Colon, small bowel, spleen, and pancreas, along with the stomach, may find their way into the large hernia sac.

The radiologic examination also aims at documenting the mucosal alterations and esophageal wall complications present with reflux disease. Although the presence of moderate or severe acute esophagitis is demonstrated with a frequency of 98%, the observation of reflux of barium into the esophagus by itself does not mean that gastroesophageal reflux disease is present. When normal individuals are compared with endoscopic esophagitis patients, free radiologic reflux is seen in 20% of controls and in 25% of patients with documented esophagitis. The columnar-lined mucosa of Barrett's esophagus is suspected when gastric-like folds ascend into the chest with a slight narrowing identified in a high position. Strictures may be detected when adequate esophageal distention can be obtained during the examination.[27]

Esophagoscopy. Since the early description of endoscopic esophagitis, many classifications have become available to provide uniform reporting of visual damage. The absence of mucosal changes or minor degrees of inflammation usually causes significant interobserver variations. In these situations there is lack of correlation between symptoms and mucosal changes. When severe esophagitis is present, the endoscopic findings cause fewer objectivity problems. Ulceration, stricture, and Barrett's esophagus usually correlate well with the observations of different endoscopists.

The MUSE classification encompasses all aspects of mucosal damage, describing the changes of metaplasia (M), ulcers (U), strictures (S), and erosions (E). No place is given to minimal degrees of mucosal alteration as those suggested by hyperemia. Each category of mucosal damage can be scored on its own for a more objective quantification of lesions. The MUSE classification represents an effort to improve the objectivity of recording visual mucosal damage, and its use should lead to more accurate and standardized reporting of endoscopic findings (Fig. 26–87 and Table 26–14).

Esophageal Biopsies. The normal esophagus has a squamous epithelium with a basal layer supported by a lamina propria and a muscularis mucosa. The cells of the basal layer usually form less than 15% of the thickness of the epithelium. The lamina propria contains papillae, which extend toward the surface of the mucosa, but the papillae usually do not extend for more than two thirds into the thickness of the epithelium (Fig. 26–88). The initial events leading to mucosal damage involve an increase of the basal layer to form more than 15% of the epithelial thickness (Fig. 26–88). The papillae from the lamina propria penetrated over more than two thirds of the epithelial thickness and come to lie in close proximity to the esophageal lumen. These changes, however, are distributed at random over the distal 8 cm. of the esophagus, and similar changes have also been observed in 20% of normal controls.

The change in the lamina propria considered to be the best indicator of reflux damage is the presence of neutrophils and eosinophils. These inflammatory cells increase in proportion to the mucosal damage. Progression of damage results in epithelial destruction with erosions and ulcerations. These acute changes can then progress to chronic changes in the lamina propria and submucosa. Acute inflammatory changes rarely penetrate deeper than the submucosa.

When ulceration is present, granulation tissue with inflammation and fibrosis is part of the repair process ending with re-epithelialization. Repeated insults, especially by a refluxate containing acid, bile, and pancreatoduodenal enzymes, may result in ulcers becoming covered by a columnar mucosa growing in a cephalad direction. This epithelium is abnormal in function and may show three types of columnar cells: gastric, junctional, or intestinal (specialized). The junction between squamous and columnar epithelium is usually denuded of mucosa, with inflammation and granulation tissue being present.

The mucosal damage is classified according to the pathology found in the biopsy specimens. Basal cell hyperplasia should be regarded as equivocal evidence for mucosal damage. Acute inflammation, erosion, ulceration, a fibrotic stricture, and the columnar-lined mucosa of Barrett's epithelium are all unequivocal documentation of reflux damage (Table 26–15).

Motility Studies. Studies quantifying motor function of the esophagus provide the best evidence for the presence or absence of the physiologic abnormalities associated with gastroesophageal reflux disease (Table 26–16). As discussed

---

TABLE 26–15. Histology

Equivocal Evidence of Esophagitis

H^0 = normal
H^1 = basal cell hyperplasia

Unequivocal Evidence of Esophagitis

H^2 = acute epithelial or subepithelial inflammation and/or ulceration
H^3 = fibrosis or columnar-lined esophagus

TABLE 26–16. Manometry

Equivocal Evidence of Functional Abnormality Associated with Reflux

M^0 = normal esophageal motility, LES >10 mm. Hg
M^1 = normal esophageal motility, LES 6–10 mm. Hg

Unequivocal Evidence of Functional Abnormality Associated with Reflux

M^2 = normal esophageal motility, LES <6 mm. Hg
M^3 = aperistaltic esophagus, LES <6 mm. Hg

LES, lower esophageal sphincter.

previously, low LES basal pressures are associated with free-reflux episodes and the incidence of esophagitis is increased when the LES tone is very low. Increasing reflux damage is associated with weaker LES pressures. The lowest sphincter pressure (often absence of tone) tends to be found in patients with a stricture or columnar-lined esophagus.

Esophageal body peristalsis is usually normal when reflux episodes are associated with minimal wall damage. Active esophagitis, however, alters function in a manner proportional to damage severity. Patients with severe esophagitis have an increased incidence of failed peristalsis and weak peristaltic contractions. Patients with a columnar-lined esophagus again tend to show the worst functional changes. The events leading to the poor esophageal function remain unclear.

Motility studies offer prognostic information when physiologic damage is present. Normal function in the esophageal body with an LES pressure gradient above 6 mm. Hg remains equivocal evidence of the dysfunction leading to reflux damage. A sphincter gradient when absent or lower than 6 mm. Hg identifies patients at significant risk for reflux and with a poorer prognosis for long-term medical therapy (Fig. 26–84).

Absent peristalsis and absent LES tone usually accompany the worst categories of reflux disease as seen in the patient with scleroderma and the patient with end-stage esophagitis.

Monitoring of Acid and Bile Reflux. Twenty-four-hour pH monitoring is the most precise measure of the presence of acid in the esophageal lumen. The amount, frequency, and time of acid exposure are documented by a glass or antimony electrode placed 5 cm. above the LES. Multiple probes can be placed at various levels in the esophagus. These objective measurements, when technically adequate, measure and correlate acid reflux episodes with typical esophageal symptoms. Atypical chest pain, asthma episodes, and oropharyngeal symptoms must show close correlation with reflux episodes and mucosal damage before being attributed to reflux disease. When direct measurement of bile reflux is needed, the information is obtained by a new fiberoptic probe, which recognizes bilirubin and allows quantification of bile exposure on the gastric and on the esophageal mucosa.[46] It should be noted, however, that neither pH nor bile measurements are direct measures of which one is injurious to the mucosa. In the case of pH, the hydrogen ion concentration is measured, and this is not a measure of the amount of acid present. It is presumed that the greater the amount of acid, the greater the mucosal damage. Similarly, measurement of bile does not correlate necessarily with bile salts and pancreatic enzyme, both of which are the likely cause of damage in duodenogastroesophageal reflux.

Normal acid exposure in the esophagus is suggested to vary between 4.2% and 7%.[7] The acid contact time as measured by 24-hour pH monitoring is an excellent indication of possible reflux injury. Mattioli[22] reported that patients with nonconfluent erosive esophagitis had an acid exposure dur-

ing 12% of the recording time. Parilla[28, 29] reported 15% of acid exposure in their esophagitis group and 26% exposure for their columnar-lined esophagus patients. Stein[43] reported similar observations, suggesting that alkaline exposure in addition to acid exposure resulted in more extensive mucosal damage.

The staging of severity in regard to acid pH parameters is noted in Table 26–17. An acid exposure during less than 7% of total recording time is by itself only equivocal evidence of reflux disease. Exposure to acid between 7% and 12% suggests the probability of mucosal damage, while acid reflux of greater than 12% of recording is usually found in the more severe form of reflux disease. Although currently regarded as the most objective methods for diagnosing reflux, both endoscopy and 24-hour pH monitoring fall far short of being gold standards. Thus, 10% to 20% of patients with endoscopic esophagitis have negative 24-hour pH monitoring studies, and probably even a larger proportion of patients showing pH studies above 7% acid exposure have normal endoscopic findings.

Final Staging Process. The four objective methods that help quantify gastroesophageal reflux disease are (1) endoscopic documentation of mucosal damage, (2) histologic proof of pathologic changes in the mucosa and submucosa, (3) recording of an abnormal exposure to an acid and/or alkaline refluxate for the esophageal mucosa, and (4) recording of the functional abnormalities leading to reflux disease. The height and weight ratio might also be added to categorize patients, as well as the presence or absence of a hernia.

When all four tests are negative, this means that reflux disease has not been demonstrated (Stage 0). When the recording methods all show equivocal documentation of reflux, again clinically significant reflux has not been demonstrated (Stage 1). In both these groups, although patients may complain of being severely symptomatic, causes for their symptoms should be sought elsewhere. When physiologic abnormalities and pH documentation of reflux disease are present, but without the mucosal damage, this represents Stage 2 disease. When all objective methods of investigation document reflux damage the esophagus shows Stage 3 disease. The worst category of functional and histologic damage is seen with Stage 4 disease (Table 26–18).

TREATMENT

Medical Treatment

Gastroesophageal reflux disease is the most frequent problem seen in an esophageal clinic or esophageal investigational laboratory. The great majority of patients seen with small hiatal hernias and occasional reflux symptoms require symptomatic treatment only with advice on modifications of some life-style habits. For more intensive therapy, treatment should always be based on accurate staging of the disease as defined earlier. When gastroesophageal reflux disease has been well documented, medical treatment is always the first

TABLE 26–17. pH Monitoring

Equivocal Evidence of Reflux

R^0 = no reflux or <4%
R^1 = reflux 4–7%

Unequivocal Evidence of Reflux

R^2 = reflux 7–12%
R^3 = reflux >12%

TABLE 26–18. Staging of Severity in Gastroesophageal Reflux

Stage	Endoscopy				Histology				pH Monitoring				Manometry			
	0	1	2	3	0	1	2	3	0	1	2	3	0	1	2	3
0	X				X				X				X			
1		X				X				X				X		
2		X				X					X	X			X	X
3			X	X			X	X			X	X			X	X
4	Stricture formation and/or columnar-lined esophagus															

approach to control both symptoms and reflux damage (Table 26–19).

Life-style modification is inexpensive and seems to make common sense. However, although logical, none of these recommendations has been established scientifically as useful. Especially in societies affected with overeating and obesity, the first logical step is to aim at weight reduction to attain a normal height/weight ratio. A diet rich in proteins with decreased fats and glucose should help to improve LES resting pressures while reducing caloric intake. Moderate exercise is usually advised as well. Substances known to decrease sphincter pressures (mint, chocolate, alcohol, tobacco) should be avoided.

Patients with reflux are advised to elevate the head of the bed to obtain an oblique lying position during the night. This position, with the help of gravity, does not stop the reflux from occurring but helps the emptying and reduces the refluxate exposure time on the esophageal mucosa. Drugs known to negatively affect esophageal function and LES pressures should be avoided if possible (see Table 26–11).

Antacids are often self-administered as first-line treatment. They usually provide immediate relief of symptoms, but their action on documented esophagitis is not clearly established, although they are known to increase LES pressures. Alginic acid, which is frequently mixed with antacids, reacts with saliva to form a viscous solution that floats on gastric content, with the aim of protecting the esophageal mucosa when reflux episodes occur. Cytoprotectives are believed to protect the mucosa by forming a viscous film that binds to the protein exudate in areas of ulcers and inflammation. The cytoprotectives do not alter acid production or motor function.

TABLE 26–19. Medical Treatment of Gastroesophageal Reflux

Modify Life-Style

Reduce weight
Diet
  Increase proteins
  Reduce fat, sugar
Avoid alcohol, tobacco, mint, chocolate, and medications affecting
  function

Protect Esophageal Mucosa

Antacids, alginates, cytoprotective agents
H₂ receptor antagonists
Proton pump inhibitors

Improve Function

Esophageal
  Cisapride
  Metoclopramide
  Bethanechol
Gastric
  Domperidone
  Metoclopramide
  Cisapride

Cimetidine, ranitidine, famotidine, and nizatidine are H_2 receptor antagonists that provide a substantial decrease in gastric acid production. They have a proven effect on symptoms and provide healing of esophagitis in over 50% of patients after 6 to 12 weeks of treatment. They are probably more useful in lesser degrees of reflux disease. When compared with patients with a duodenal ulcer, patients with esophagitis require more acid suppression for longer periods to obtain successful results.

Omeprazole and lansoprazole are proton pump inhibitors and are used when esophagitis is severe and resistant to H_2 receptor antagonists. They provide a prolonged and highly effective inhibition of basal and stimulated acid secretion. They reduce esophageal acid exposure without modification of esophageal motor function or LES pressures. Relief of symptoms and healing of esophagitis is afforded more rapidly than with the H_2 receptor antagonists. These agents have underlined the importance of acid on the cause of symptoms and mucosal damage, and they have been extremely effective in the treatment of reflux disease. However, there are several problems in regard to their use. First is the fact that they do not address the problem, so that when therapy is stopped, symptoms tend to recur almost immediately. Thus, patients will need to take the drug throughout life if they wish to remain free of symptoms. Second, these drugs do not stop regurgitation, and in patients in whom this is the main problem, these drugs are less likely to be useful. And third is their cost. If patients are to take such agents over a lifetime, there is a substantial cost involved for the patient and for the society that provides for such agents. Although there is no reason to think that there will be dangers in taking the drug over many years, it must also be acknowledged that it is not known whether long-term administration will have any adverse effects. For instance, experimental evidence[20] suggests that modification of the pH environment favors the development of intestinal metaplasia as a repair process in the esophagus. Therefore, whether the treatment is medical or surgical, it is important to reinvestigate and restage the esophageal mucosa on a long-term basis.

Lieberman,[16] when comparing two groups of reflux esophagitis–treated patients, observed that those with extremely low LES pressures had a more severe degree of reflux and a poor prognosis on long-term medical therapy.

Esophageal function improvement may be provided by prokinetic agents. Bethanechol has been documented to increase LES pressure and esophageal emptying, but it also stimulates gastric secretions and it has not entered clinical practice. Metoclopramide, by stimulating gastrointestinal smooth muscle, causes increased LES pressure, better esophageal contractions, and improved gastric emptying. The side effects of this agent are frequent, especially the neurologic extrapyramidal symptoms, and limit its use. Domperidone, by improving gastric emptying, may improve esophageal symptoms by helping to prevent reflux. Both of these agents have been disappointing, despite their theoretical advantages. Cisapride exerts its action by increasing the availability of acetylcholine from postganglionic nerve endings of the myenteric plexus. The end-result is a stimulation of esophageal peristalsis, an increase in LES tone, and an improvement in gastric emptying. The combination of a prokinetic such as cisapride with H$_2$-blocker medication seems to improve healing in patients with esophagitis.[10] None of these agents, or combination of them, has proven as effective as the proton pump inhibitors omeprazole or lansoprazole in clinical practice, however.

Surgical Treatment

Antireflux Operations for Early-Stage Reflux Disease. The treatment of uncomplicated reflux by operation falls into the category of discretionary operation, which is one reason why it is very important to document abnormalities in patients before embarking on surgical therapy. The subjective indication for operative therapy in symptomatic disease is symptoms that are spoiling a patient's enjoyment of life. Before the laparoscopic and proton pump inhibitor era, operations were usually only undertaken when medical therapy was deemed to have failed. Nowadays, however, proton pump inhibitors render the great majority of patients either asymptomatic or relatively so. And yet, as mentioned earlier, there are several reasons why lifelong therapy with proton pump inhibitors is not an attractive option for many patients and in many societies. Therefore, antireflux operations today in uncomplicated cases are often undertaken in patients in whom medical therapy has been very successful. Because of the relative newness of both proton pump inhibitors and laparoscopic surgical procedures, these indications are somewhat controversial.

Indications for surgical treatment of complications of gastroesophageal reflux disease do not fall into the realm of discretionary operations and so are much less controversial. Complications should be categorized on the basis of the staging process described earlier (see Tables 26–14 to 26–18). Symptoms, in the absence of physiologic abnormalities and of proven endoscopic or mucosal damage (Stage 0 and Stage 1), should never be indications for an antireflux operation. The surgeon should be cautious in offering an operation to patients who are overweight and who appear to have a strong emotional overlay to their symptoms, because medicolegal information shows that these patients tend to be dissatisfied with the outcome. Patients with an incompetent LES accompanied by increased gastroesophageal reflux on 24-hour pH monitoring but without mucosal damage (Stage 2 disease) should always undergo a well-supervised period of medical management of at least 6 months to a year. At the end of this period, patients and their physicians will usually choose whether to continue medical therapy or undergo antireflux operation. Patients with esophagitis and defective function of the LES (Stage III disease) also should undergo intensive medical therapy, with the patient trying to lose weight during this period. As in Stage II disease, a decision is made at the end of a 6- to 12-month period in regard to further therapy. Patients showing severe complications of reflux disease, such as stricture with esophagitis or circumferential columnar-lined esophagus, should be treated surgically. Antireflux surgical treatment is indicated in such patients to correct the functional defects and limit progression of damage.

The most frequently used operations for reflux disease are total fundoplication or partial fundoplication. Their aim is to restore normal anatomy, by restoring an intra-abdominal segment of esophagus, re-creating an appropriate high-pressure zone at the esophagogastric junction, and maintaining this repair in a normal position. These operations are preferred for patients presenting at the first three stages of esophagitis, where there is usually no shortening or periesophageal inflammation with the reflux damage. The strictured esophagus or the esophagus with significant periesophagitis may prevent the resaturation of an adequate intra-abdominal length of esophagus without undue tension on the repair. This usually results in a significant failure rate.[13, 25] In this situation, techniques that elongate the esophagus are preferred.

Total Fundoplication. Complete mobilization of the abdominal esophagus is undertaken, and both vagi are protected. There are two methods of total fundoplication that are widely practiced in both the open and the laparoscopic settings. The first involves ligation of the gastrosplenic ligament and the last four or five short gastric vessels. This frees the fundus, enabling a loose wrap to be performed around the distal esophagus with a large (greater than 44 French), bougie within the esophageal lumen. The pillars of the diaphragmatic hiatus are usually closed behind the esophagus (Fig. 26–89A). The second technique is essentially similar except only the anterior wall of the stomach is used for the wrap and the short gastric vessels are not divided. It has never been established that there is any difference in outcome between these two types of fundoplication (Fig. 26–89B and C). These operations increase LES resting pressures.[7, 42] There is also an increase in the remaining basal tone of the relaxed sphincter, suggesting a permanent incomplete relaxation imposed by the fundoplication. The fundoplication prevents fundic distention, reduces transient sphincter relaxation, and increases gastric emptying. pH monitoring studies usually show an abolition of acid exposure in the esophagus.[21] Good to excellent results are reported in 84% to 94% of operated patients. Dysphagia, inability to belch or vomit, and postprandial fullness are side effects that occur commonly in the early postoperative period. Most of these symptoms get better with time, although postprandial fullness and bloating are often lifelong accompaniments to fundoplication. Among the small percentage of patients in whom surgical therapy fails, more than half experience problems because of recurrent reflux from breakdown of the fundoplication. In the remainder, problems usually arise from dysphagia, either due to making the wrap too tight or the hiatus too tight. Sometimes, the longitudinal muscle of the esophagus pulls the stomach through the fundoplication, causing what is frequently called a slipped Nissen. At other times, the fundoplication is actually placed around the upper stomach—a situation in which the operation always fails. Fortunately, if a reoperation has to be carried out, the results are generally good.

Partial Fundoplication. The Belsey-Mark IV operation is created by a left chest approach (Fig. 26–90A and B). A partial (240 degree) posterolateral fundoplication is created by completing two succeeding rows of mattress sutures between the fundus and esophageal wall. The second row is anchored through the diaphragm, ensuring an intra-abdominal esophageal length of 4 to 5 cm. Other partial fundoplication operations have been proposed in which the fundus is applied against the posterior distal esophagus (Fig. 26–90C). Hill's repair (see Fig. 26–90D) fixes and calibrates the anterior and posterior seromuscular leaves of the lesser curvature at the cardia to the median arcuate ligament. The Dor operation (Fig. 26–90E) first accentuates the angle of the esophagogastric junction and then anchors the fundus onto the anterior wall of the esophagus, creating an anterior hemifundoplication.

Results of partial fundoplication operations have been reported by their respective authors to be as good as total fundoplication. In one study in which treatment was randomized to either a partial or a total fundoplication, it was found that the partial Belsey fundoplication caused restora-

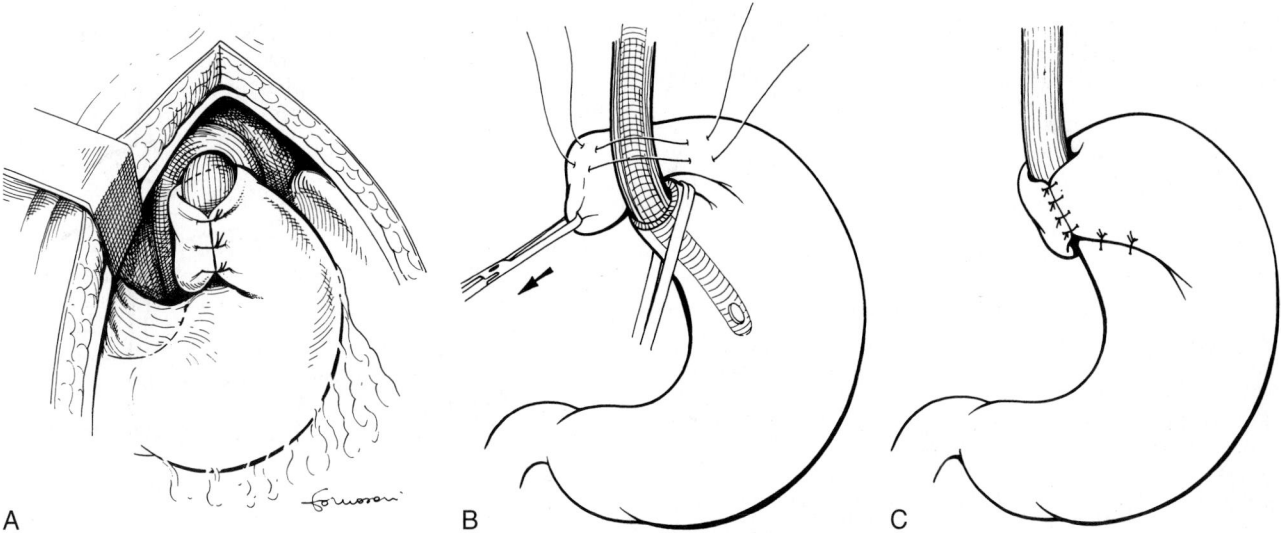

Figure 26–89. *A,* Loose total fundoplication with full mobilization of the gastric fundus. *B* and *C,* Total fundoplication using the anterior wall of the stomach.

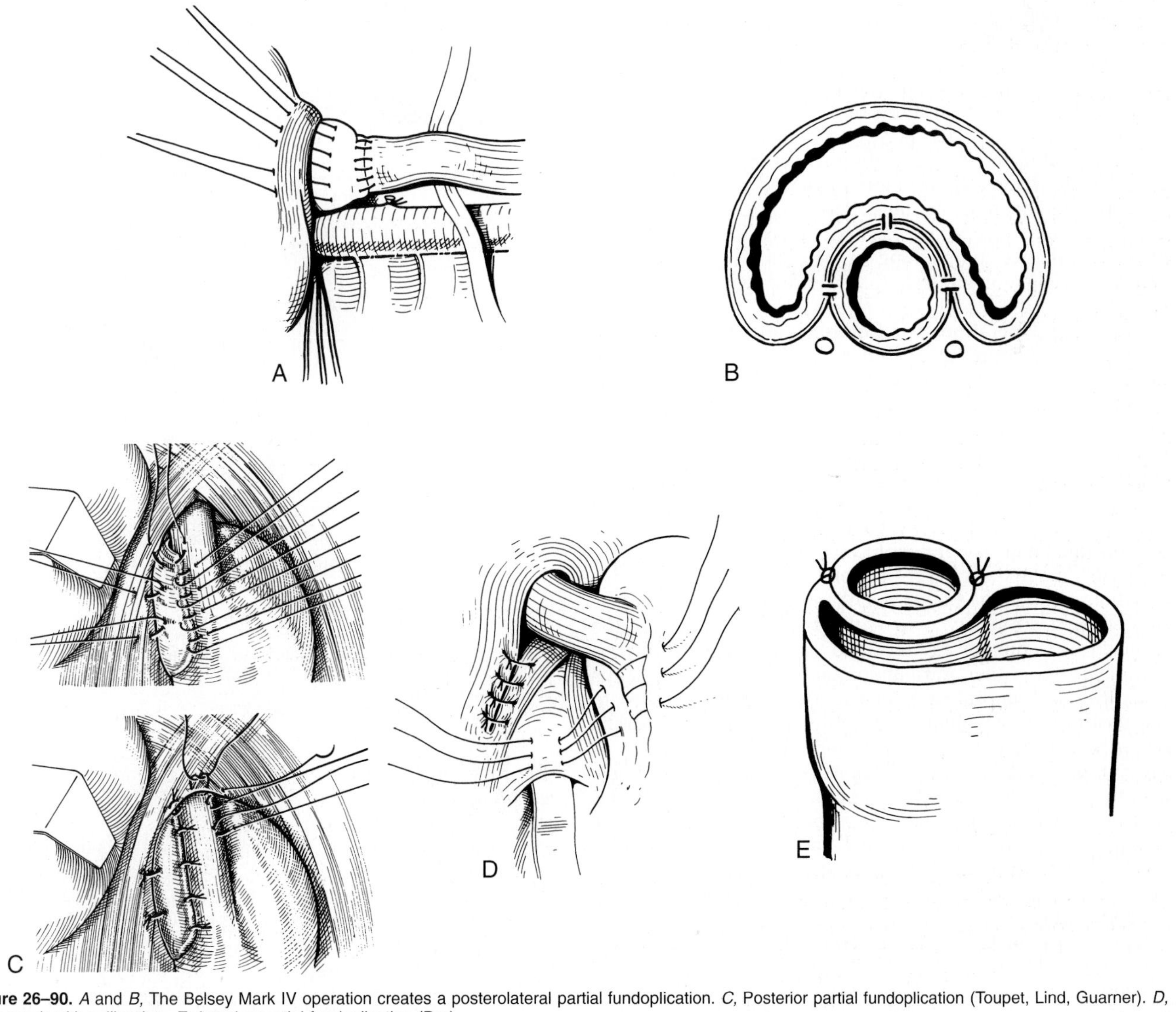

Figure 26–90. *A* and *B,* The Belsey Mark IV operation creates a posterolateral partial fundoplication. *C,* Posterior partial fundoplication (Toupet, Lind, Guarner). *D,* Hill's repair with calibration. *E,* Anterior partial fundoplication (Dor).

tion of an adequate high-pressure zone, but episodes of reflux occurred over time more frequently. Nevertheless, other randomized studies have shown similar results at 3 years for both partial and total fundoplication. Behar and associates[5] reported in a randomized study that the Belsey partial fundoplication created a significantly higher resting pressure than preoperative measurements at sphincter level and that the higher pressure persisted over time. In their medically treated group of patients, no change was seen in the LES pressures over time. Long-term follow-up of this operation has shown overall good results in 80% of the patients with progressive increase in the failure rate with the passage of time.[13, 25]

The Hill posterior gastropexy is associated with good to excellent results in 81% of patients undergoing operation when successful intraoperative calibration of the cardia is obtained. Hill and colleagues[14] reported a 15- to 20-year follow-up of over 400 patients, suggesting good to excellent subjective results in 82% of the population. The posterior partial fundoplication of Guarner and Lind also shows good reflux control at 5 to 10 years with fewer episodes of dysphagia and less inability to belch or vomit, when compared with the total fundoplication. It seems, from the existing literature, that most fundoplications result in good symptomatic results with low morbidity and mortality. Surgical treatment for gastroesophageal reflux, when looked at prospectively, results in superior control of the disease when compared with medical management.

All antireflux operations can be performed laparoscopically, but it is not yet known whether the operations prove as durable done in this way compared with the open approach. Factors influencing recurrence of symptoms or progression of damage are actually poorly documented and usually based on retrospective evaluation. Stricture formation and Barrett's esophagus signify more advanced disease and may logically lead to more failures. Poor gastric emptying may affect recurrent symptoms. Scleroderma is known to result in more patients complaining of persistent symptoms and recurrent reflux, even if a total fundoplication has been used.[35]

Antireflux Operations for Complications of Reflux Disease. Standard antireflux operations fail in a large proportion of cases when a stricture is present. In this situation, the esophagus, narrowed from long-term reflux or damaged with extensive columnar epithelium replacement, is frequently affected by periesophagitis and shortening. Even after extensive esophageal mobilization and freeing of the esophagogastric junction, a 4- to 5-cm reduction of an intra-abdominal segment of esophagus may be difficult to achieve, and a tension-free repair is not possible. The high failure rate (45%) when using standard partial or total fundoplications in this situation dictates the use of lengthening procedures such as the Collis gastroplasty, where the lesser curvature of the stomach is fashioned as a tube to elongate the esophagus and obtain a proper intra-abdominal length of esophagus (Fig. 26–91). A partial or a total fundoplication is added to the gastroplasty to obtain the antireflux function, and the repair is reduced without tension under the diaphragm.[26, 31, 34] These repairs are considered esophageal sparing operations, and they provide satisfactory results for patients with significant reflux damage to their esophagus. The intrathoracic fundoplications reported by Thal[45] and Maher[19] may offer good reflux control, but they are not used extensively because of dangers that have been reported for supradiaphragmatic fundoplications.

Operations for Correction of Hiatal Hernias. Type II, III, and IV hiatal hernias (Fig. 26–86C to E) all show a large portion of the stomach herniated into the mediastinum. Symptoms are mostly related to the size of the hernia and to

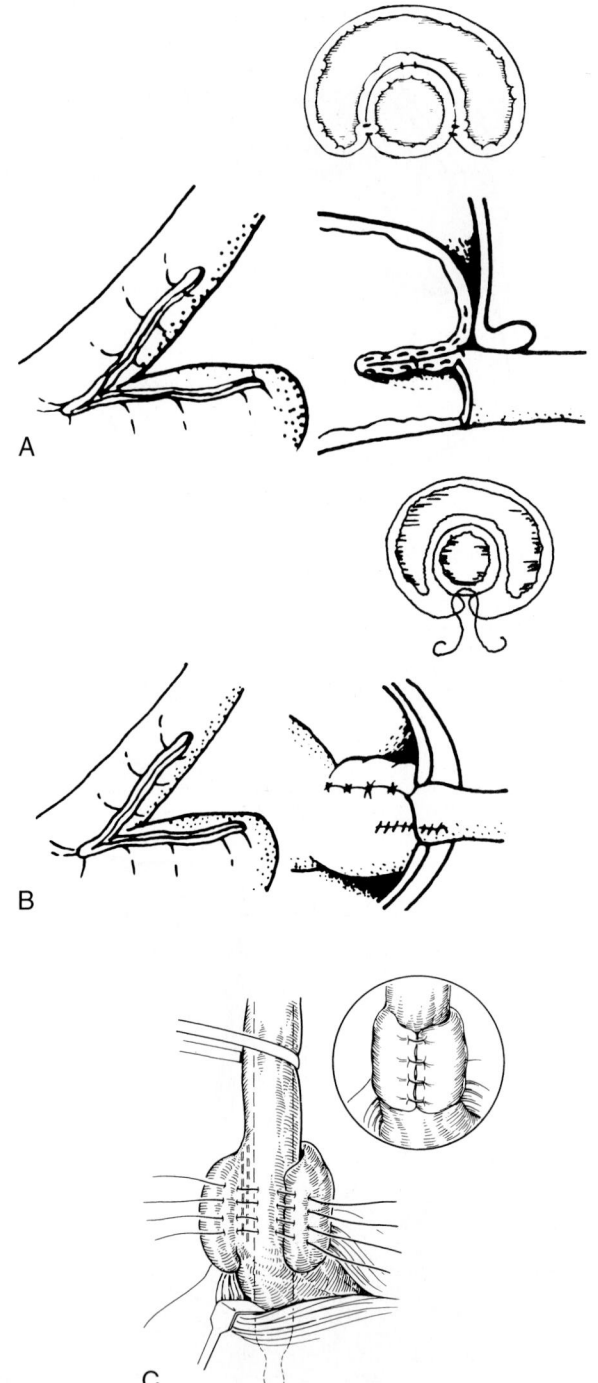

Figure 26–91. *A*, Cut Collis gastroplasty and partial fundoplication. *B*, Cut Collis gastroplasty with total fundoplication. *C*, Uncut Collis gastroplasty with total fundoplication.

the functional obstruction created by the angulation of the esophagogastric junction. Substernal or left lower chest pain, epigastric discomfort, early satiety, and shortness of breath often occur immediately after meals. Dysphagia and bleeding are ominous signs when these types of hernia are present. They suggest massive incarceration and warrant early repair. Often chronic anemia may be the laboratory abnormality bringing the patient to investigation.

In general, these massive hernias are indications for surgical treatment if the patient is a good surgical candidate. The risks of performing an operation are much less than the risks of nonoperative treatment or the risks of performing an operation in a patient with acute volvulus or perforation.[9, 30, 48] The repair principles are the same as those for sliding hernias and antireflux operations. Standard repairs with correction of a large hiatus may give satisfactory results. The large hernias frequently show shortening of the esophagus with apparent tension on the completed repair.[39] An elongation gastroplasty doubled of an antireflux repair is necessary in this situation.

SELECTED REFERENCES

Armstrong, D., Monnier, P. A., Nicolet, M., and Savary, M.: Endoscopic assessment of oesophagitis. Gullet, 1:63, 1991.
The authors classify and quantify mucosal disease in gastroesophageal reflux in an effort to improve objectivity for more accurate recording and reporting.

Bremner, R. M., Bremner, C. G., and De Meester, T. R.: Gastroesophageal reflux: The use of pH monitoring. Curr. Probl. Surg., 32:429, 1995.
This is the most recent review on a technique responsible for more objective documentation of reflux events and their relation with esophageal mucosal damage.

Castell, D. O., Richter, J. E., and Boag-Dalton, C.: Esophageal Motility Testing. New York, Elsevier, 1987.
This is an update on normal function and abnormalities in human esophageal motility with a solid perspective on dysfunction and reflux disease.

Jamieson, G. G., and Duranceau, A.: Gastroesophageal Reflux. Philadelphia, W.B. Saunders, 1988.
This monograph was planned as a text that would remain a solid reference book over the years. It is comprehensive and covers all aspects of the disease. It contains all earlier references mentioned in the present chapter that could not be included with the present list because of space restrictions.

Spechler, S. J.: Comparison of medical and surgical therapy for complicated gastroesophageal reflux disease in veterans. N. Engl. J. Med., 326:786, 1992.
This article is a prospective evaluation of treatment in gastroesophageal reflux disease.

REFERENCES

1. Allison, P. R.: Hiatus hernia: A 20-year retrospective survey. Ann. Surg., 178:273, 1973.
2. Allison, P. R.: Reflux esophagitis, sliding hiatal hernia and the anatomy of repair. Surg. Gynecol. Obstet., 92:419, 1951.
3. Atwood, S. E. A., Ball, C. S., Barlow, A. P., Jenkinson, L., Norris, T. L., and Watson, A.: Role of intragastric and intraoesophageal alkalinisation in the genesis of complications in Barrett's columnar lined lower oesophagus. Gut, 34:11, 1993.
4. Barrett, N. R.: Chronic peptic ulcer of the oesophagus and oesophagitis. Br. J. Surg., 38:175, 1950.
5. Behar, J., Biancani, P., Spiro, H. M., and Storer, P. H.: The effect of an anterior fundoplication on lower esophageal sphincter competence. Gastroenterology, 67:209, 1974.
6. Costantini, M., Crookes, P. F., Bremmer, R. M., Hueft, S. F., Ehsan, A., Peters J. H., Bremnor, C. G., and De Meester, T. R.: Value of physiologic assessment of foregut symptoms in a surgical practice. Surgery, 114:780, 1993.
7. De Meester, T. R., Bonavina, L., and Albertucci, M.: Nissen fundoplication for gastroesophageal reflux disease: Evaluation of primary repair in 100 consecutive patients. Ann. Surg., 204:9, 1986.
8. Dent, J. Dodds, W. J., Friedman, R. H., Sekiguchi, T., Hogan, W. J., Arndorfer, R. S., and Petrie, D. J.: Mechanism of gastroesophageal reflux in recumbent asymptomatic human subjects. J. Clin. Invest., 65:256, 1980.
9. Ellis F. A., Crozier, R. E., and Shea, J. A.: Paraesophageal hiatus hernia. Arch. Surg., 121:416, 1986.
10. Galmiche, J. P., Branstatter, G., Evreux, M., et al.: Combined therapy with cisapride and cimetidine in severe reflux oesophagitis: A double-blind controlled trial. Gut, 29:675, 1988.
11. Gillen, P., Keeling, P., Bryne, P. J., et al.: Barrett's oesophagus: pH profile. Br. J. Surg., 74:774, 1987.
12. Helm, J. F., Dodds, W. J., Pelc, L. R., Palmer, D. W., Hogan, W. J., and Teeter, B. C.: Effect of esophageal emptying and saliva on clearance of acid from the esophagus. N. Engl. J. Med., 310:284, 1984.
13. Hiebert, C., and O'Mara, C.: The Belsey operation for hiatal hernia: A 20-year experience. Am. J. Surg., 137:532, 1979.
14. Hill, L. D., Aye, R. W., and Ramel, S.: Antireflux surgery: A surgeon's look. Gastroenterol. Clin. North Am., 19:745, 1990.
15. Kahrilas, P. J., Dodds, W. J., Hogan, W. J., Kern, M., Arndorfer, R. C., and Reece, A.: Esophageal peristaltic dysfunction in peptic esophagitis. Gastroenterology, 91:897, 1986.
16. Lieberman, D. A.: Medical therapy for chronic reflux esophagitis. Arch. Intern. Med., 147:1717, 1987.
17. Maddern, G. J., and Jamieson, G. G.: Oesophageal emptying in patients with gastro-oesophageal reflux. Br. J. Surg., 73:615, 1986.
18. Maddern, G. J., Slavotinek, J. P., Collins, P. J., and Jamieson, G. G.: Effect of posture and pH on solid and liquid oesophageal emptying. Clin. Physiol., 5:425, 1985.
19. Maher, J. W.: Intrathoracic fundoplication for shortened esophagus. In Jamieson, G. G. (Ed.): Surgery of the Oesophagus. London, Churchill Livingstone, 1988, pp. 321–326.
20. Martin, C. J., Shaw, M., Ewing, H. P., and Machet, D.: Pancreatic reflux produces intestinal metaplasia in experimental columnar lined oesophagus. Presented before the Sixth World Congress, Milan, International Society for Diseases of the Esophagus, 1995, abstract volume, p. 225.
21. Martinez de Haro, L. F., Ortiz, A., Parilla, P., Garcia Marcilla, J. A., Aguayo, J. L., and Morales, G.: Long-term results of Nissen fundoplication in reflux esophagitis without strictures. Dig. Dis. Sci., 37:523, 1992.
22. Mattioli, S., Pilotti, V., Spangaro, M., Grigioni, W. F., Zannoli, R., Felice, V., Conci, A., and Gozzetti, G.: Reliability of 24 hr. home esophageal pH monitoring in diagnosis of gastroesophageal reflux. Dig. Dis. Sci., 34:71, 1989.
23. Mercer, C. D., Wren, S. F., Da Costa, L. R., and Hill, L. D.: Gastroesophageal pressure gradients and lower esophageal sphincter pressures in severely obese patients. Gastroenterology, 82:1129, 1982.
24. Mittal, R. K., Chowdhry, N. K., and Liu, J.: Is the sphincter function of crural diaphragm impaired in patients with reflux esophagitis. Gastroenterology, 1995, in press.
25. Orringer, M. B., Skinner, D. B., and Belsey, R. H.: Long term results of the Mark IV operation for hiatal hernia and analysis of recurrences and their treatment. J. Thorac. Cardiovasc. Surg., 53:25, 1972.
26. Orringer, M. B.: Evaluation and treatment of hiatal hernia and gastroesophageal reflux: Reflux stricture and short esophagus. In Orringer, M. B. (Ed.): Surgery of the Alimentary Tract. Vol. I, The Esophagus. Philadelphia, W.B. Saunders, 1991, pp. 210–228.
27. Ott, D. J., Gelfand, D. W., Chen, Y. M., Wu, W. C., and Munitz, H. A.: Predictive relationship of hiatal hernia to reflux esophagitis. Gastrointest. Radiol., 10:317, 1985.
28. Parilla, P., Ortiz, A., Martinez de Haro, L. F., et al.: Evaluation of the magnitude of gastroesophageal reflux in Barrett's oesophagus. Gut, 31:964, 1990.
29. Parilla, P., Martinez de Haro, L. F., Ortiz, M. A., et al.: Correlation between endoscopic and pH metric findings and motor oesophageal alterations in reflux oesophagitis. Dig. Surg., 8:210, 1991.
30. Pearson, F. G., Cooper, J. D., Ilves, R., et al.: Massive hiatal hernia with incarceration: A report of 53 cases. Ann. Thorac. Surg., 35:45, 1983.
31. Pearson, F. G., Cooper, J. D., Patterson, G. A., et al.: Gastroplasty and fundoplication for complex reflux problems. Ann. Surg., 206:473, 1987.
32. Pera, M., and Duranceau, A.: Malignant degeneration of Barrett's esophagus: Epidemiology of Barrett's esophagus and esophageal adenocarcinoma. Dis. Esophagus, 8:86, 1995.
33. Pera, M., Cardesa, A., Bombi, J. A., et al.: Influence of esophagoduodenostomy on the induction of adenocarcinoma of the distal esophagus in Sprague-Danley rats by the subcutaneous injection of 2,6-dimethylnitrosomorpholine. Cancer Res., 49:6803, 1989.
34. Pera, M., Deschamps, C., Taillefer, R., and Duranceau, A.: The uncut Collis-Nissen gastroplasty: Early functional results. Am. Thorac. Surg., 60:915, 1995.
35. Poirier, N. C., Taillefer, R., Topart, P., and Duranceau, A.: Antireflux operations in patients with scleroderma. Ann. Thorac. Surg., 58:66, 1994.
36. Richter, J. E., Wu, W. C., Johns, D. N., Blackwell, J. N., Nelson, J. L., Castell, J. A., and Castell, D. O. Esophageal manometry in 95 healthy volunteers: Variability of pressures with age and frequency of abnormal contractions. Dig. Dis. Sci., 32:583, 1987.
37. Singh, P., Taylor, R. H., Collin-Jones, D. G.: Esophageal motor dysfunction and acid exposure in reflux esophagitis are more severe if Barrett's metaplasia is present. Am. J. Gastroenterol., 89:349, 1994.
38. Skandalakis, J. E., Gray, S. W., and Skandalakis, L. J.: Surgical anatomy of the oesophagus. In Jamieson, G. G. (Ed.): Surgery of the Oesophagus. London, Churchill Livingstone, 1988, pp. 19–35.
39. Skinner, D. B., and Belsey, R. H.: Management of Esophageal Disease. Philadelphia, W. B. Saunders, 1988.
40. Sloan, S., and Kahrilas, P. J.: Impairment of esophageal emptying with hiatal hernia. Gastroenterology, 100:596, 1991.
41. Stipa, S., Fegiz, G., Iascone, C., Paolini, A., Moraldi, A., De Marchi, C., and Chieco, P. A.: Belsey and Nissen operations for gastroesophageal reflux. Ann. Surg., 210:583, 1989.
42. Stein, M. J., Barlow, A. P., De Meester, T. R., and Hinder, R. A.: Complications of gastroesophageal reflux disease: Role of the lower esophageal sphincter, esophageal acid/alkaline exposure and duodenogastric reflux. Ann. Surg., 216:35, 1992.
43. Stein, H. J., Hoeft S., and De Meester, T. R.: Reflux and motility pattern in Barrett's esophagus. Dis. Esophagus, 5:21, 1992.
44. Stein, H. J., and De Meester, T. R.: Indications, techniques and clinical use of 24 hours esophageal motility monitoring in a surgical practice. Ann. Surg., 217:128, 1993.
45. Thal, A. P.: A unified approach to surgical problems of the esophagogastric junction. Ann. Surg., 168:542, 1968.
46. Vaezi, M. F., La Camera, R. G., and Richter, J. E.: Validation studies of Bilitec 2000: An ambulatory duodenogastric reflux monitoring system. Am. J. Physiol., 107:749, 1994.

47. Vaezi, M. F., and Richter, J. E.: Synergism of acid and duodenogastric reflux in complicated Barrett's esophagus. Surgery, 117:699, 1995.
48. Walther, B., De Meester, T. R., Lafontaine, E., Courtney, J. V., Little, A. G., and Skinner, D. B.: Effect of paraesophageal hernia on sphincter function and its implication on surgical therapy. Am. J. Surg., 147:111, 1984.
49. Zacchi, P., Mearin, F., Humbert, P., Formiguera, X., and Malagelada, V. R.:

Effect of obesity on gastroesophageal resistance to flow in man. Dig. Dis. Sci., 36:1473, 1991.
50. Zaninotto, G., De Meester, T. R., Bremner, C. G., Smyrk, T. C., and Cheng, S. C.: Esophageal function in patients with reflux-induced strictures and its relevance to surgical treatment. Ann. Thorac. Surg., 47:362, 1989.

IX

CORROSIVE STRICTURES OF THE ESOPHAGUS

James L. Talbert, M.D.

Despite an enhanced public and legislative awareness, caustic ingestions remain a significant health threat in the United States, affecting between 5000 and 26,000 citizens annually.[17, 18, 21, 33] The incidence is bimodal in age distribution, with over 75% of injuries involving children younger than 5 years and a much lower, secondary peak occurring in late adolescence and early adult life.[29] The ingestion is almost always accidental in the young child who all too frequently has been enticed by chemical solutions that have been carelessly placed in familiar soft drink containers or by crystalline caustics that resemble sugar or candy exposed in jars or cans. Instances of caustic ingestion in adolescents and adults usually represent an intentional suicide attempt by an emotionally disturbed or psychotic individual and often involve intake of relatively large volumes of toxic substances with a proportionately greater potential for inflicting serious injury.[18, 21, 29]

ETIOLOGY

The most common chemicals implicated in corrosive burns of the esophagus include the alkaline caustics, acid or acid-like corrosives, and household bleaches. Hydrochloric, sulfuric, nitric, and phosphoric acids are contained in automobile battery acids, soldering fluxes, and a variety of commercial cleaners. The alkaline caustics consist of sodium or potassium hydroxide (the active ingredients of household lye and drain cleaners), sodium carbonate (washing soda), sodium metasilicate (dishwashing detergent), and ammonia water (household cleaners). Severe localized esophageal burns can also result from the ingestion of Clinitest tablets, which contain significant amounts of anhydrous sodium hydroxide, or from swallowing the small disk-shaped (button) alkaline batteries commonly used in calculators, cameras, hearing aids, and watches.[4, 25, 30] In the 40 years preceding 1965, most of the caustics ingested in the United States were flakes or solid pellets of sodium hydroxide. However, the introduction at that time of concentrated liquid drain cleaning products such as Liquid Plumr, containing 35% sodium hydroxide solution, heralded a relative epidemic of more severe and extensive injuries of the upper gastrointestinal tract that regressed in the early 1970s only after enforcement of federal legislation limiting the concentration of these agents and requiring the use of child-proof containers.[6, 21] As one threat subsided another emerged: in response to increasing concern for environmental pollution, phosphate dishwashing detergents of relatively mild toxicity were replaced by highly alkaline nonphosphate compounds containing sodium silicate, sodium carbonate, sodium metasilicate, and sodium borate, which presented an increased risk of injury to small children

in the home.[21] Subsequent modifications in the formulation of the nonphosphate detergents have diminished their potential toxicity, although they may still produce transient, severe respiratory distress when inhaled.[7] Moreover, our modern environment continues to offer a seemingly never-ending array of hazards for young children, as exemplified by more recent reports of accidental ingestions of concentrated alkaline solutions used on dairy farms to clean pipelines in milk houses, and orofacial burns induced by inquisitive applications of newly introduced products such as oven cleaning pads.[6, 29, 38]

Corrosive burns from ingested caustic agents may involve the oropharynx, larynx, esophagus, stomach, and even the small intestine and colon. The site and severity of injury depend primarily on the character, quantity, and concentration of the ingested substance. Household bleaches such as Clorox are ingested with relative frequency but rarely produce permanent damage unless swallowed in large amounts.[18, 21, 26] Solid lye substances tend to lodge in the oropharynx or upper esophagus, and concentrated liquid caustics not only present an increased potential for esophageal injury but may also damage the stomach and distal intestinal tract, especially in young children.[29] The ingestion of crystals of lye causes pain, and most children attempt to spit out the caustic material immediately on tasting it. This defense mechanism is absent in the case of liquid caustics, which are often colorless and odorless and may produce serious damage even in concentrations of less than 10%. Because caustic injury relaxes the lower esophageal sphincter, the resultant tendency for gastroesophageal reflux may promote prolonged exposure of the distal lumen to the injurious agent.[29] In instances of acid ingestion, the esophagus may escape injury because of the relative resistance of the squamous epithelium and the briefness of contact as the liquid rapidly traverses the extent of its lumen. However, on reaching the stomach the acid usually induces immediate pylorospasm, which pools the destructive chemical in the distal antrum and produces a severe gastritis that may progress within 24 to 48 hours to full-thickness necrosis and perforation.[24] The presence of food in the stomach limits the extent and severity of this process. The immediate pain experienced on ingestion makes the consumption of large quantities of acid less common than with alkaline poisoning, but an intent, emotionally disturbed person may swallow a significant volume, thereby producing the characteristic clinical picture.

As in the case of external body burns, caustic injuries of the gastrointestinal tract are categorized as superficial or deep on the basis of histologic appearance and clinical behavior, although at the time of endoscopy differentiation can sometimes prove difficult.[15, 21] Characteristically, superficial burns of the mucosa are manifest by erythema, edema, blister formation, or small, isolated ulcers. Deep burns are exemplified by circumferential ulcerations and may extend through the full thickness of the esophageal wall into adjacent mediastinal tissues, penetrating the pleural and peritoneal cavities and even occasionally producing tracheoesophageal or aortoenteric fistulae.[3, 39] Sites that appear especially susceptible to injury because of a relative delay in transit include the upper esophagus in the area of the cricopharyngeus, the midesophagus where the aorta and left mainstem bronchus may impinge on the lumen, and the distal esophagus immediately proximal to the lower sphincter. After superficial injuries, re-epithelialization of the esophageal mucosa is usually complete by the sixth week but, with full-thickness injury, scarring and contracture may progress for a period of months. Similarly, gastric outlet obstruction may be a late sequela of major acid injury to the stomach as a consequence of progressive antral scarring.[5, 24]

PROPHYLACTIC TREATMENT

The most important element in successfully managing a corrosive burn of the esophagus is immediate verification of the etiologic agent and accurate assessment of the depth and extent of injury. Subsequent treatment of the patient must be individualized on the basis of these findings. It is essential to seek the container from which the caustic material was obtained to confirm the type and to determine the pH. Alkaline solutions with a pH of less than 11.5 are considered relatively safe, but those with a pH exceeding this level possess a proportionately increasing potential for injury.[7, 18, 21] First-aid treatment of these patients by administration of antidotes is probably ineffective because the corrosive action is largely completed within a time span of seconds, and ipecac-induced vomiting poses a threat of compounding the original injury by re-exposing tissues to the offending agent.[18] Indeed, previous reports have emphasized an increased incidence of severe laryngeal and esophageal injury after vomiting of ingested caustic substances.[24]

The accidental ingestion of a small disk or *button* battery represents a special threat to the small child and demands prompt attention.[25, 30] Severe local damage to the esophagus may ensue within only 4 to 6 hours as a consequence of the separate or combined effects of generated electrical current, pressure necrosis, and leakage of the highly corrosive contents, either as a result of deterioration of the case or damage sustained during endoscopic retrieval. There is universal agreement that esophageal entrapment of a disk battery is an indication for its immediate extraction, although once the object has attained the stomach, spontaneous passage throughout the remainder of the gastrointestinal tract can be anticipated with an extremely low incidence of complications.[18, 25] Although use of a Foley balloon catheter under fluoroscopic guidance has been advocated for retrieval of these and other esophageal foreign bodies, in this circumstance, endoscopic extraction of disk batteries is preferred because of the importance of identifying any associated injury and, when confirmed, performing a concomitant bronchoscopy to exclude coexistent tracheal damage.

Caustic injury is manifest by the symptoms of oral pain, drooling, excessive salivation, and inability or refusal to swallow or drink. When there is a history of ingestion, the mucosa of the lips, tongue, and oropharynx, as well as the skin of the face, hands, and neck, must be carefully inspected for evidence of erythema, edema, blistering, or ulceration. Substernal and back discomfort or abdominal pain and rigidity may signify mediastinal or peritoneal perforation. Hoarseness, stridor, and dyspnea suggest laryngeal edema or actual epiglottic and laryngeal destruction through aspiration of the chemical agent. However, the absence of symptoms or visible evidence of oropharyngeal burns does not exclude the possibility of esophageal injury because in reported series, 10% to 30% of patients with no external evidence of burn have been subsequently confirmed by esophagoscopy to have sustained damage.[18, 27, 29] At the same time, as many as 70% of patients with evidence of oropharyngeal burns escape associated esophageal injury.[12] It is essential, therefore, that, as soon as an appropriate period of time has elapsed to allow gastric emptying and stabilization of the patient, esophagoscopy be performed expeditiously, preferably within the first 12 to 24 hours, and no later than the first 48 hours, to confirm the extent and severity of the burn.[12, 21] In children this procedure is best accomplished using general anesthesia to avoid undue emotional trauma and minimize the risk of incurring any serious secondary injury that might be induced by the movement of a struggling patient. The only exceptions to proceeding with early endoscopy are instances in which esophageal or gastric perforation or impending airway obstruction are suspected.

Any evidence of significant pharyngeal or laryngeal damage, either as identified by direct laryngoscopy or as suggested by symptoms of hoarseness, stridor, or dyspnea, demands immediate hospitalization and observation because the period of maximal edema and danger may be delayed for 6 to 24 hours. Esophagoscopy may be contraindicated in these situations because of its potential to compound the original injury. Blood gases should be monitored serially, and endotracheal intubation or a tracheostomy should be performed if the airway obstruction or respiratory distress appears progressive. Chest x-rays should be studied for evidence of pulmonary infiltrate or free perforation into the mediastinum or pleural or peritoneal cavities. In the absence of such findings, a barium esophagogram should be obtained to confirm the integrity of the upper gastrointestinal tract and to assess the extent of injury. Although some authors have noted that the initial barium swallow may appear falsely normal in as many as 30% of patients with significant caustic burns, others have found cine-esophagographically visualized abnormalities, especially disordered motility, to help predict the severity of injury and outcome.[23, 34]

The most reliable method for confirming the presence or absence of a caustic burn and estimating its severity is direct visualization. Although some authors have suggested that early endoscopy might prove misleading because of insufficient time for the burn wound to mature enough to permit accurate visual verification, recent clinical experience has refuted this concern.[21] In the past, the endoscopist has also been cautioned against passing a rigid esophagoscope beyond the proximal point of injury because of the potential danger of perforation.[15] However, the advent of the flexible pediatric fiberoptic scope has increased the relative safety of this procedure; and when liquid caustics or acids have been ingested, it is especially important to assess the status of the stomach because of the potential of these agents to produce gastric injury, even in the absence of an identifiable esophageal burn.[21, 27]

The depth of burn, as evaluated on the basis of superficial or deep involvement, is an important prognostic guide. In patients who have sustained only superficial injuries as manifest by erythema, edema, or blistering, the prognosis appears excellent, even in the absence of any specific treatment. However, the identification of ulcerations, especially when circumferential, warrants concern because of the inherent high potential for stricture formation.[21] In the presence of a validated injury, the status of the esophagus should be serially assessed by contrast studies repeated at intervals of 3 weeks, 3 months, and, again, between 6 months and 1 year to exclude the possibility of late stricture formation. In the acute phase of severe injury, the esophagus may appear atonic and dilated, rigid and persistently narrowed, or excessively irritable.[23] Although roentgenographic studies of the stomach during the first 1 to 2 weeks after acid ingestion may show only prominent mucosal folds, serial examinations frequently demonstrate progressive gastric outlet obstruction or the development of either an hourglass or linitis plastica–like appearance.[10]

In general, two treatment options have been advocated for prevention of stricture: maintenance of an esophageal lumen by mechanical means or pharmacologic modification of wound healing. Unfortunately, the continually changing spectrum of ingested caustics over the past 30 years involves a variety of substances with differing potentials for injury and the absence of any large, multi-institutional, randomized, well-controlled series of patients comparable to that used nationally for coordinated evaluations of childhood cancer treatment. Management of these injuries has remained controversial, with advocates espousing both forms of treatment, separately or in combination.[10, 21] Regardless of the mode of management, clinical reports have increasingly emphasized that in the presence of a full-thickness esophageal injury there is an inherent high potential for stricture formation.[2, 26]

Pharmacologic management of esophageal burns has been predicated on the use of corticosteroids to modify the inflammatory response to the burn injury and of antibiotics to control secondary bacterial infection. Experimental studies by Spain and colleagues in 1950 first suggested that early administration of cortisone produced an anti-inflammatory effect that would inhibit fibroplasia in wound healing.[32] These findings were subsequently applied to the treatment of experimental esophageal burns in animals, and the beneficial effects of corticosteroids in reducing the incidence of postinjury stricture appeared to be confirmed when antibiotic coverage was added to control secondary suppurative complications.[12, 13, 17] However, a report by Anderson and colleagues of a controlled trial involving 60 children treated over an 18-year period failed to substantiate any statistical benefit of corticosteroid administration in preventing stricture formation.[2] This study re-emphasized the potential for deep esophageal injuries to induce strictures regardless of mode of management, although a question persists as to whether prior corticosteroid treatment may facilitate subsequent mechanical dilation. Because the reflux of acidic gastric secretions may injure the esophageal mucosa and further increase the likelihood of stricture formation, either prophylactic use of H_2-blockers or administration of therapeutic doses of antacids has been recommended for 6 to 8 weeks.[29]

Corticosteroid treatment is clearly contraindicated in cases of severe caustic burns shown by clinical or roentgenographic evidence to have perforated the esophagus or produced necrosis of the stomach. Concentrated liquid lye preparations are especially likely to produce these complications.[3, 39] The use of corticosteroids is also of questionable value in the treatment of acid ingestion, because it may not only mask evidence of peritonitis but also increase the potential for gastric ulceration and bleeding. In contrast, patients with signs of dyspnea, hoarseness, or stridor may benefit from immediate administration of corticosteroids and antibiotics to relieve airway obstruction; and esophagoscopy is usually contraindicated in such circumstances.

The use of bougienage for early treatment of corrosive esophageal burns was introduced by Salzer in 1920 and characteristically has been performed blindly, with tapered bougies.[31] A graduated program is established in which esophageal dilation is performed daily for several weeks, and then every other day for 2 to 3 weeks, and finally once a week for many months. Previously, it was believed that early bougienage prevented intraluminal adhesions in the injured esopha-

gus, but experimental observations have suggested that this treatment may actually form cicatrix and increase the risk of perforation.[13, 22] Certainly in young children, the group most susceptible to caustic burns, prophylactic esophageal bougienage appears to add psychologic and physical hazards that are unwarranted when the potential benefit of the procedure is highly questionable.

Because stricture frequently forms in severe esophageal caustic injuries, an alternative to the bougienage technique has been increasingly advocated that involves mechanical modification of wound healing through placement of intraluminal Silastic stents.[21] The stent prevents obliteration of the esophageal lumen by either adhesions or scar contracture and provides a template for epithelial ingrowth. Whether used with or without systemic antibiotics and corticosteroids, the stents have successfully decreased the incidence of stricture formation, even with severe, circumferential esophageal mucosal injury, when left in place for a minimum of 3 weeks or until re-epithelialization has been completed. However, because a gastrostomy may be required for stent insertion and, depending on the type and configuration of the stent, prolonged hospitalization with intense monitoring may also be necessary, this treatment may not always be feasible to implement.[21]

MANAGEMENT OF CORROSIVE STRICTURES

The most frequent complication of caustic burns of the esophagus is stricture formation, which usually develops between 3 and 8 weeks after the initial injury but sometimes requires a much longer period for evolution. In some instances, these lesions are mild and immediately respond to dilation without subsequent recurrence. All too often, especially when concentrated liquid corrosives have been ingested, lye burns cause extensive full-thickness damage, eventually producing multiple areas of stricture throughout the extent of the esophagus (Fig. 26–92). When ultimate stenosis can be anticipated based on the severity of the original injury, early passage of a string or small catheter through the patient's nose into the stomach facilitates bougienage.[15] In some instances, a gastrostomy may be necessary to maintain satisfactory gastrointestinal alimentation and to facilitate subsequent esophageal dilation. Cases of multiple tight strictures are probably best handled by this approach, with retrograde esophageal dilation performed with rubber tapered-tip Tucker bougies guided by the string or catheter previously passed from above.

The complication of tracheoesophageal fistula may result from an extensive corrosive burn of the esophagus, and it is suggested by progressive pneumonia, choking, coughing with feedings, or aspiration of bile-stained mucus from the airway. These characteristic symptoms usually appear within the first few weeks after injury. The diagnosis can be confirmed by a contrast study using thin barium or propyliodone (Dionosil); use of water-soluble gastrointestinal contrast media should be avoided because they are highly irritating when exposed to the bronchi and lungs. Direct operative attack on the fistula has frequently been fraught with disaster because the extensive friability and necrosis of the tissues prevent them from holding sutures, patches, or muscle flaps. Instead, successful management entails bipolar exclusion of the esophagus by proximal and distal division and closure in the neck and abdomen along with a cervical esophagostomy and gastrostomy. A tracheostomy helps control aspiration while the trachea and defunctionalized esophagus heal, usually with complete scarring and obliteration of the latter.[3]

When full-thickness necrosis of the esophagus and stomach occurs, through ingestion of concentrated solutions of alkalis

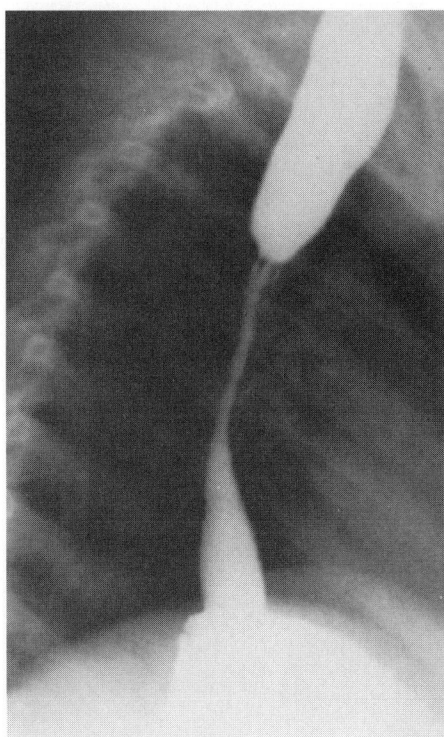

Figure 26–92. A characteristic extensive esophageal stricture in a child resulting from lye (Liquid-Plumr) ingestion.

or acids, an emergency gastrectomy and/or transhiatal blunt esophagectomy may be indicated to prevent lethal complications such as overwhelming sepsis or aortoenteric fistula.[11, 39] If a gastrostomy is required, it should be positioned on the stomach wall so that a gastric tube can be formed subsequently from the greater curvature, in the event this procedure proves necessary for esophageal reconstruction.[1] It is also important that the antrum and pylorus of the stomach be inspected carefully when a gastrostomy is performed, because a stricture may not be visible from the serosal side, and careful intraluminal palpation may be necessary to identify a circumferential thickening. If destruction by the ingested chemical has involved the stomach and pylorus with extensive necrosis and edema, a feeding jejunostomy may be employed as an alternate route for maintaining enteral alimentation.[39]

Although the safest approach to esophageal dilation is probably retrograde with Tucker bougies passed through a gastrostomy, this method is not necessarily required for all cases. Alternative approaches include antegrade dilation by Sabary-Guillard plastic bougies threaded over a previously positioned guide wire.[37] Another method of dilation especially helpful in managing isolated or persistent strictures in children uses the Gruntzig-type inflatable balloon catheter, which was originally devised for transluminal angioplasty. Even in small children with narrow, tortuous strictures, a flexible wire can usually be inserted endoscopically, over which a balloon catheter can be subsequently advanced and optimally positioned under fluoroscopic guidance. As the balloon is inflated with dilute contrast media under radiographic monitoring, the predominant force is focused outward at the site of esophageal scarring and constriction, thereby minimizing the potentially disruptive shearing effect produced by the passage of bougies.[26, 35] Chronic cases with minimal or moderate esophageal strictures can also be treated adequately in adults by swallowed mercury-filled

Maloney- or Hurst-type bougies when the patient is cooperative.

In cases of localized strictures that extend less than 1.5 cm. in length and fail to respond to bougienage alone, local injection of corticosteroids under direct vision through an esophagoscope into the four quadrants of the circumferential esophageal scar has proven beneficial.[8, 14] This technique first successfully achieved regression of cutaneous hypertrophic scars and burn contractures through local infiltration of triamcinolone diacetate. The corticosteroid injection is followed by bougienage, and the treatment course may be repeated if necessary. In some instances, failure of a stricture to respond to dilation may result from associated gastroesophageal reflux; if this diagnosis can be confirmed, an antireflux procedure is indicated.[8, 33] Clinitest tablets and disc batteries appear especially prone to produce localized esophageal strictures, and if these lesions fail to respond to dilation, resection and esophageal anastomosis are often feasible.[4]

Surgical reconstruction of the esophagus may be indicated by a continuing need to frequently dilate extensive or multiple strictures for longer than 6 months; by failure or refusal of the patient to follow a regimen of regular dilation; by the presence of a fistula between the esophagus and the tracheobronchial tree; or by iatrogenic perforation of the esophagus in the course of an attempted dilation.[26] Prolonged unsuccessful attempts at dilation not only expose the patient, frequently a child, to unnecessary physical and psychological trauma but also may impede normal growth and development. Use of the right colon with an attached segment of terminal ileum, tunneled through the retrosternal space into the neck, has proved eminently satisfactory in all patients older than 1 year with extensive esophageal scarring (Fig. 26–93).[1, 26, 28, 36] The inclusion of a short segment of terminal ileum for anastomosis to the proximal esophagus in the neck decreases the bulk of tissue and avoids obstruction at the thoracic inlet, previously a frequent problem in young children undergoing this procedure. Preservation of the ileocecal valve has also decreased the aspiration associated with regurgitation from the patulous substernal colonic segment into the proximal esophagus and oropharynx. Moreover, incorporation of a pyloroplasty or pyloromyotomy has diminished the incidence of colitis induced by reflux of acidic secretions from the contiguous stomach.[28, 36] An alternative method for colonic interposition is the technique of Waterston, in which transverse and descending colon is brought through the left pleural cavity in an isoperistaltic manner and interposed between the proximal esophagus and the stomach.[9] When the colon proves unsuitable for esophageal substitution because of an aberrant blood supply or an anatomic abnormality, such as associated imperforate anus, the gastric tube technique may be used.[1] This procedure most frequently employs a reversed, antiperistaltic gastric tube that is based proximally on the greater curvature of the stomach and receives its blood supply from the left gastroepiploic artery. The gastric tube is then passed through a retrosternal tunnel and is anastomosed to the cervical esophagus. Although the preceding techniques when used in children have provided excellent long-term function and allowed normal growth and development, the alternative procedure of gastric transposition has gained favor for adults and has also been applied increasingly in children for esophageal reconstruction.[1, 28, 33]

Successful management of acid ingestion frequently demands surgical intervention, in some instances entailing emergency cervical esophagostomy, esophagogastrectomy, and even duodenectomy.[24, 39] Coexistent esophageal injury is probably much more frequent than previously appreciated, and esophageal strictures have been reported in 6% to 20% of patients.[40] In a review of 27 patients with gastric injury as a result of acid ingestion, 23 eventually required surgical

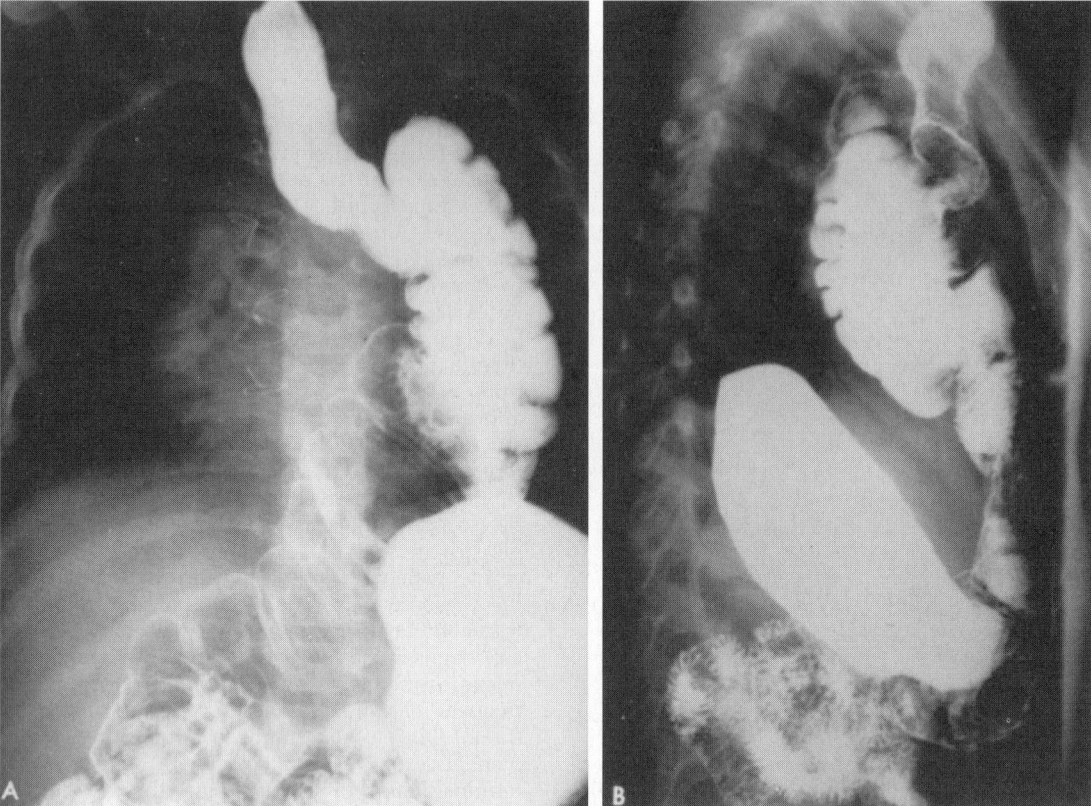

Figure 26–93. Anteroposterior *(A)* and lateral *(B)* views of a retrosternal pull-through of terminal ileum and right colon for bypass of an extensive esophageal lye stricture in a child.

correction of pyloric stenosis, with gastric resection performed in 17.[24] Gastric outlet obstruction as a result of progressive antral scarring may develop within 3 to 8 weeks or may be delayed for as long as 6 years.[5] Because of the documented incidence of carcinoma occurring in the gastric wall previously subjected to acid injury, subtotal gastrectomy with a Billroth I type of reconstruction is treatment of choice whenever feasible.[24] Prolonged inanition is inevitably encountered in patients sustaining severe gastrointestinal injuries as a result of caustic ingestion, and either total parenteral nutrition or placement of a feeding jejunostomy has been important in successful management.[40]

LATE COMPLICATIONS

A late complication of corrosive burns of the esophagus that has not been widely recognized is the development of a hiatal hernia between 25 and 69 years after injury.[19] Apparently, the fibrotic esophagus contracts and pulls the stomach into the chest. The patient then develops esophagitis and peptic stricture in an already narrowed esophagus secondary to gastroesophageal reflux. Dilation of the esophageal stricture in such cases is pointless because it increases the reflux, and the fibrotic stricture becomes tighter. An acquired form of achalasia has also been reported as a consequence of extensive intramural fibrosis.

A final, long-term complication of esophageal scarring and stricture formation is malignant degeneration.[20] It has been estimated that the incidence of esophageal carcinoma in patients who have previously suffered lye stricture is at least a thousand-fold greater than in the general population. A patient with a chronic lye stricture, especially one of more than 16 years' duration, with any change in symptoms should immediately receive radiographic and esophagoscopic exam-

ination. Inability to dilate a chronic stricture that has previously responded to treatment or late radiographic evidence of progressive stenosis strongly suggests malignant change. Biopsies performed through the esophagoscope can easily miss the tumor in such cases, because the carcinoma may be located distal to the area of stenosis and be inaccessible to the biopsy forceps. In these circumstances, therefore, negative biopsy specimens must be considered inconclusive. Fortunately, those carcinomas that develop in scar tissue appear to behave less aggressively than the usual esophageal cancer, possibly because the enveloping scar inhibits outward invasion and the resultant intraluminal proliferation produces early obstructive symptoms.[16] Resection of a strictured esophageal segment is indicated in any patient with a chronic lye stricture in whom the aforementioned changes have occurred. Identification of the tumor gives the patient an excellent chance of being cured of a lesion that ordinarily carries a dismal prognosis. Although transhiatal blunt esophagectomy can be performed concomitant with esophageal reconstruction, a dearth of reports of cancer occurring in defunctionalized, retained segments suggests that the increased operative risk may not be justified.[33]

SELECTED REFERENCES

Haller, J. A., Jr., Andrews, H. G., White, J. J., and Cleveland, W. W.: Pathophysiology and management of acute corrosive burns of the esophagus: Results of treatment in 285 children. J. Pediatr. Surg., *6*:579, 1971.
   This paper represents the classic reference on the physiologic rationale and clinical justification for corticosteroid and antibiotic treatment of esophageal caustic burns.

Kuhns, D. W., and Dire, D. J.: Button battery ingestions. Ann. Emerg. Med., *18*:293, 1989.
   This comprehensive review article focuses on the newest, relatively common source of potentially severe esophageal caustic injury—small disk battery ingestions.

Maull, K. I., Scher, L. A., and Greenfield, L. J.: Surgical implications of acid ingestion. Surg. Gynecol. Obstet., *148*:895, 1979.

This paper reviews the treatment of acid ingestion and emphasizes the significant dissimilarities that exist in the early management, late complications, and surgical therapy between cases of acid and alkali ingestion.

Rothstein, F. C.: Caustic injuries to the esophagus in children. Pediatr. Clin. North Am., 33:665, 1986.
This publication presents a comprehensive, current review of the subject of corrosive injuries of the esophagus in children.

Wason, S.: The emergency management of caustic ingestions. J. Emerg. Med., 2:175, 1985.
This review article emphasizes the controversial issues involved in the emergency management of caustic ingestions and attempts to resolve them relative to the formulation of an optimum treatment regimen for the individual patient.

REFERENCES

1. Anderson, K. A., Noblett, H., Belsey, R., and Randolph, J. G.: Long-term follow-up of children with colon and gastric tube interposition for esophageal atresia. Surgery, 111:131, 1992.
2. Anderson, K. D., Rouse, T. M., and Randolph, J. G.: A controlled trial of corticosteroids in children with corrosive injury of the esophagus. N. Engl. J. Med., 323:637, 1990.
3. Burrington, J. D., and Raffensperger, J. G.: Surgical management of tracheo-esophageal fistula complicating caustic ingestion. Surgery, 84:329, 1978.
4. Burrington, J. D.: Clinitest burns of the esophagus. Ann. Thorac. Surg., 20:400, 1975.
5. Cochran, S. T., Fonkalsrud, E. W., and Gyepes, M. T.: Complete obstruction of the gastric antrum in children following acid ingestion. Arch. Surg., 113:308, 1978.
6. Edmonson, M. B.: Caustic alkali ingestions by farm children. Pediatrics, 79:413, 1987.
7. Einhorn, A., Horton, L., Altieri, M., Ochsenschlager, D., and Klein, B.: Serious respiratory consequences of detergent ingestions in children. Pediatrics, 84:472, 1989.
8. Gandhi, R. P., Cooper A., and Barlow B. A.: Successful management of esophageal strictures without resection or replacement. J. Pediatr. Surg., 24:745, 1989.
9. German, J. C., and Waterston, D. J.: Colon interposition for the replacement of the esophagus in children. J. Pediatr. Surg., 11:227, 1976.
10. Goldman, L. P., and Weigert, J. M.: Corrosive substance ingestion: A review. Am. J. Gastroenterol., 79:85, 1984.
11. Gossott, D., Sarfati, E., and Celerier, M.: Early blunt esophagectomy in severe caustic burns of the upper digestive tract. J. Thorac. Cardiovasc. Surg., 94:188, 1987.
12. Haller, J. A., Jr., Andrews, H. G., White, J. J., and Cleveland, W. W.: Pathophysiology and management of acute corrosive burns of the esophagus: Results of treatment in 285 children. J. Pediatr. Surg., 6:579, 1971.
13. Haller, J. A., and Bachman, K.: The comparative effect of current therapy on experimental caustic burns of the esophagus. Pediatrics, 34:236, 1964.
14. Holder, T. M., Ashcraft, K. W., and Leape, L.: The treatment of patients with esophageal strictures by local steroid injection. J. Pediatr. Surg., 4:646, 1969.
15. Holinger, P. H.: Management of esophageal lesions caused by chemical burns. Ann. Otol. Rhinol. Laryngol., 77:819, 1968.
16. Hopkins, R. A., and Postlethwait, R. W.: Caustic burns and carcinoma of the esophagus. Ann. Surg., 194:146, 1981.
17. Howell, J. M., Dalsey, W. C., Hartsell, F. W., and Butzin, C. A.: Steroids for the treatment of corrosive esophageal injury: A statistical analysis of past studies. Am. J. Emerg. Med., 10:421, 1992.
18. Howell, J. M.: Alkaline ingestions. Ann. Emerg. Med., 15:820, 1986.
19. Imre, J., and Kopp, M.: Arguments against long-term conservative treatment of esophageal strictures due to corrosive burns. Thorax, 27:594, 1972.
20. Isolauri, J., and Markkula, H.: Lye ingestion and carcinoma of the esophagus. Acta Chir. Scand., 155:269, 1989.
21. Kikendall, J. W.: Caustic ingestion injuries. Gastroenterol. Clin. North Am., 20:847, 1991.
22. Knox, W. G., Scott, J. R., Zintel, H. A., Guthrie, R., and McCabe, R. E.: Bougienage and steroids used singly or in combination in experimental corrosive esophagitis. Ann. Surg., 166:930, 1967.
23. Kuhn, J. R., and Tunell, W. P.: The role of initial cine-esophagography in caustic esophageal injury. Am. J. Surg., 146:804, 1983.
24. Maull, K. I., Scher, L. A., and Greenfield, L. J.: Surgical implications of acid ingestion. Surg. Gynecol. Obstet., 148:895, 1979.
25. Litovitz, T., and Schmitz, B. F.: Ingestion of cylindrical and button batteries: An analysis of 2382 cases. Pediatrics, 89:747, 1992.
26. Moazam, F., Talbert, J. L., Miller, D., and Mollitt, D. L.: Caustic ingestion and its sequelae in children. South. Med. J., 80:187, 1987.
27. Previtera, C., Giusti, F., and Guglielmi, M.: Predictive value of visible lesions (cheeks, lips, oropharynx) in suspected caustic ingestion: May endoscopy reasonably be omitted in completely negative pediatric patients? Pediatr. Emerg. Care, 6:176, 1990.
28. Rodgers, B. M., Talbert, J. L., Moazam, F., and Felman, A. H.: Functional and metabolic evaluation of colon replacement of the esophagus in children. J. Pediatr. Surg., 13:35, 1978.
29. Rothstein, F. C.: Caustic injuries to the esophagus in children. Pediatr. Clin. North Am., 33:665, 1986.
30. Rumack, C. M., and Rumack, B. H.: Battery ingestions. Pediatrics, 89:771, 1992.
31. Salzer, H.: Early treatment of corrosive esophagitis. Wien Klin. Wochenschr., 33:307, 1920.
32. Spain, D. M., Malomert, N., and Haber, A.: The effect of cortisone on the formation of granulation tissue in mice. Am. J. Pathol., 26:710, 1950.
33. Spitz, L., and Lakhoo, K.: Caustic ingestion. Arch. Dis. Child., 68:157, 1993.
34. Stannard, M. W.: Corrosive esophagitis in children: Assessment by the esophagogram. Am. J. Dis. Child., 132:596, 1978.
35. Taub, S., Rodan, B. A., Bean, W. J., Koerner, R. S., Mullin, D. M., and Feng, T. S.: Balloon dilatation of esophageal strictures. Am. J. Gastroenterol., 81:14, 1986.
36. Touloukian, R. J., and Tellides, G: Retrosternal ileocolic esophageal replacement in children revisited. J. Thorac. Cardiovasc. Surg., 107:1067, 1994.
37. Tytgat, G. N. J.: Dilation therapy of benign esophageal stenoses. World J. Surg., 13:142, 1989.
38. Vilogi, J., Whitehead, B., and Marcus, S. M.: Oven-cleaner pads: New risk for corrosive injury. Am. J. Emerg. Med., 3:412, 1985.
39. Wu, M. H., and Lai, W. W.: Surgical management of extensive corrosive injuries of the alimentary tract. Surg. Gynecol. Obstet., 177:12, 1993.
40. Zargar, S. A., Kochhar, R., Nagi, B., Mehta, S., and Mehta, S. K.: Ingestion of corrosive acids. Gastroenterology, 97:702, 1989.

CHAPTER 27

LAPAROSCOPIC SURGERY

Steve Eubanks, M.D., and Philip R. Schauer, M.D.

The modern era of laparoscopic surgery has evoked remarkable changes in approaches to surgical diseases. The trend toward minimally invasive surgery has prompted general surgeons to scrutinize nearly all operations for possible conversion to laparoscopic techniques. The rate at which such drastic changes have occurred is unprecedented in surgical history. The inauspicious origins of modern laparoscopic surgery combined with the rapid dissemination of reports in the lay media led to a problem-filled infancy for this field of surgery.[1-15] *Laparoscopic cholecystectomy* had become a widely recognized term before its report in a peer-review journal. The validity of the claims of dramatic patient benefits were verified and serve as the basis by which laparoscopy has survived and flourished despite such an unusual beginning.

The adolescence of laparoscopic surgery has included the addition of numerous respected surgical investigators who have begun to establish the basic science foundation essential for the endurance of this rapidly advancing type of surgery. The pendulum of surgical opinion continues to swing with gradually decreasing sweeps as the appropriate application of laparoscopy to specific diseases and operations is established. Laparoscopy is certain to maintain an important place in the armamentarium of the general surgeon. The integration of laparoscopic training into the conventional surgical residency has provided the foundation for the safe propagation of minimally invasive surgery.

The goals of this chapter are to familiarize the reader with the extraordinary development of this field and to describe the fundamental physiologic principles of laparoscopic surgery that justify its existence. Additional goals are to define the current status of the art, to discuss complications specific to laparoscopic surgery, and to identify special issues regarding laparoscopic training. Discussion of specific laparoscopic procedures has been integrated into subsequent chapters corresponding to the respective organ systems.

Historical Aspects. Mühe performed the first totally laparoscopic cholecystectomy in 1985 and presented his work for the first time at the Congress of the German Surgical Society in 1986. His initial report was largely ignored. However, by the following year he had accumulated a personal experience of 94 cases.[16] In 1987, Mouret performed a laparoscopic cholecystectomy and a few months later showed a videotape of his technique to Dubois in Paris.[2] Within a year leaders in Europe, including Dubois, Perissat, Cuschieri, Nathanson, and in the United States, including McKernan, Saye, Reddick, and Olsen, perfected the technique and are responsible for the unprecedented and rapid worldwide expansion of this procedure. In just the United States, laparoscopic cholecystectomy grew from a few operations in 1988 to nearly half a million by 1993 (Fig. 27–1).[17]

The explosive success of laparoscopic cholecystectomy initiated a revolution within general surgery. At present, nearly every abdominal operation has been performed laparoscopically. Other specialty fields, including thoracic surgery, pediatric surgery, gynecology, urology, orthopedics, plastic surgery, and otorhinolaryngology, are now applying these advances in endoscopic techniques to their respective fields.

Major challenges and unresolved issues have arisen from this revolution. Ongoing clinical studies are being performed to determine which laparoscopic procedures have significant benefit over conventional procedures, particularly regarding the cost/benefit ratio. Unanticipated complications such as bile duct injuries during laparoscopic cholecystectomy[18] and esophageal perforations during laparoscopic Nissen fundoplication[19] have arisen that have provoked serious debate regarding appropriate training for this new technology.

The history of laparoscopy has been characterized by constant integration of new technology into the clinical arena. This technology has largely been developed outside medicine and only through critically important collaborative efforts between physicians and industry have these major gains been achieved. The relationships between industry and medicine will increase in importance and must do so in a manner that does not threaten academic freedom.

LAPAROSCOPIC TECHNOLOGY: THE ESSENTIAL EQUIPMENT

A discussion of the fundamental aspects of laparoscopic surgery is incomplete without mention of the equipment required. Laparoscopic surgery is technology dependent. Three new categories of equipment are necessary for the performance of laparoscopic surgery. The categories are optics, abdominal access, and specialized laparoscopic instruments (Table 27–1). This equipment not only distinguishes laparoscopic surgery from open surgery but also is required to safely and effectively perform laparoscopic techniques. Equipment malfunction during a laparoscopic procedure may occur and result in significant delays or complications if not addressed rapidly and appropriately. Therefore, it behooves the laparoscopic surgeon to be familiar with the specialized equipment and learn to quickly identify and correct common problems.

PHYSIOLOGIC CONSEQUENCES OF LAPAROSCOPIC SURGERY

The fundamental advantage of laparoscopic surgery over open surgery is that it reduces the postoperative morbidity and perhaps mortality that is specifically related to the adverse physiologic responses to surgery. Multiple clinical studies have compared open cholecystectomy with laparoscopic cholecystectomy and have clearly demonstrated a significant reduction in postoperative pain, hospital stay, perioperative morbidity, and convalescence.[20, 21] Surgeon scientists have begun to investigate the physiologic responses that account for the improved clinical outcome. Studies of the physiologic changes of laparoscopic surgery substantiate the benefits of laparoscopic surgery and contribute to the understanding of the fundamental relationship between injury and recovery.

Fundamental Differences Between Open and Laparoscopic Surgery. The major differences in technique between open and laparoscopic surgery may account for the different biologic responses observed when comparing the two ap-

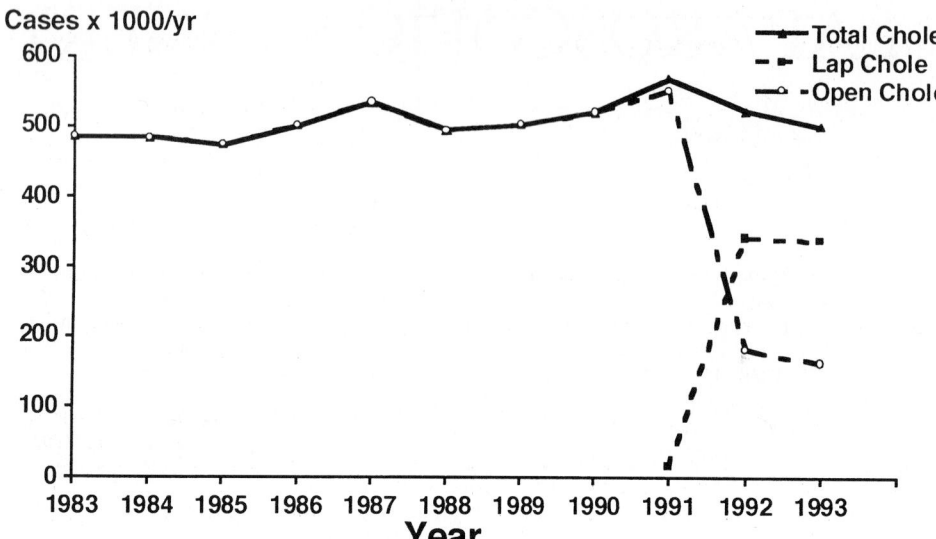

Figure 27–1. Total number of cholecystectomies performed in short-stay hospitals in the United States (exclusive of military and Veterans Administration facilities) from 1979 to 1993 according to method (traditional "open" vs. laparoscopic). By 1992, only 4 years after the introduction of the laparoscopic method, laparoscopic cholecystectomy had surpassed open cholecystectomy as the most common procedure for removal of the gallbladder. (Adapted from National Center for Health Statistics: Detailed diagnoses and surgical procedures for patients discharged from short-stay hospitals, United States, 1983–1993, DHHS publication No. [PHS] 94–1779. Hyattsville, MD, U.S. Government Printing Office, October, 1995.)

proaches (Table 27–2). The major differences between open and laparoscopic surgery are the method of access, carbon dioxide (CO_2) pneumoperitoneum, and the degree of tissue injury. Although other gases and gasless methods of laparoscopic access exist, currently CO_2 pneumoperitoneum is the standard and is used by the vast majority of laparoscopic surgeons. Two factors, reduced tissue injury and CO_2 pneumoperitoneum, most likely account for the important beneficial as well as adverse physiologic changes associated with laparoscopy. Reduced retraction and manipulation of abdominal viscera may be important secondary factors, especially with respect to postoperative gastrointestinal function. In general, the physiologic effects of CO_2 pneumoperitoneum are detrimental and occur transiently during the intraoperative period. Conversely, the beneficial response to reduced tissue injury affects the entire period from injury to complete recovery. The balance of these physiologic responses to the laparoscopic method should serve as the foundation for the overall benefit of laparoscopic surgery.

Physiologic Changes Associated with Laparoscopic Access

Insufflation of the abdomen with CO_2 has been the dominant method of laparoscopic access for many decades.[22] The advantage of CO_2 over other gases that have been used is that it does not support combustion, it is relatively inexpensive, and it is rapidly absorbed. Air (80% nitrogen), oxygen, nitrous oxide, nitrogen, helium, and argon are gases that have been used to create a pneumoperitoneum. Gas embolism is a potentially lethal complication of any gas used to produce pneumoperitoneum. A rapidly absorbed gas such as CO_2 is less likely to result in a persistent air-lock obstructing right ventricular outflow. The main disadvantage of CO_2 is that it readily dissolves into solution and becomes biologically reactive, potentially producing many adverse effects. Nitrous oxide is the second most commonly used gas. It is less preferred because it supports combustion more than room air or CO_2. The leakage of nitrous oxide into the operating room may also adversely affect operating room personnel.

A variety of adverse effects of CO_2 pneumoperitoneum ranging from minor nuisances to potentially lethal complications have been identified. These adverse effects, along with possible mechanisms, are listed in Table 27–3. Some adverse effects may be considered sequelae that are predictable physiologic responses. The adverse effects listed as complications are unusual or rare events. Studies of the hemodynamic effects of laparoscopy with pneumoperitoneum were performed in the 1970s primarily on young healthy women undergoing laparoscopic tubal ligations of 30 minutes' duration.[23, 24] The adverse effects of laparoscopy elucidated from these studies were either clinically insignificant or well compensated by this group of patients. Patient populations and operative environments have changed significantly since the early days of gynecologic laparoscopy. Major abdominal operations are now performed by means of the laparoscopic

TABLE 27–1. Essential Equipment for Laparoscopic Surgery

Optic Equipment

    Laparoscope 10 mm., 0 and 30 degree
    Computer chip video camera
    Light source
    Video monitors
    Video recorder

Abdominal Access Equipment

    Pneumoperitoneum
        Insufflator/pressure monitor
        Gas tank (carbon dioxide or alternate)
        Trocar cannulas (with air-tight one-way valves)
    Gasless laparoscopy
        Abdominal wall lifting device
        Trocar cannulas (air-tight not required)

Laparoscopic Instruments

    Atraumatic graspers/clamps
    Dissectors
    Scissors
    Suction/irrigator
    Clip applier
    Staplers
    Specimen retrieval bags
    Sutures/needles
    Needle holders

TABLE 27–2. Factors That May Account for Different Physiologic Responses Between Open and Laparoscopic Cholecystectomy

Factor	Open Cholecystectomy	Laparoscopic Cholecystectomy
Anesthesia	Equivalent	Equivalent
Patient position	Supine	Reverse Trendelenburg
Access method	"Open" surgery	CO_2 pneumoperitoneum
Surgical injury		
External: abdominal wall	Significant: 20-cm. incision through skin, muscle, fascia	Minimal: A 1.5-cm. and three 0.5-cm. trocar incisions
	Retraction with static retraction apparatus	Stretching from pneumoperitoneum
Internal: Triangle of Calot, hepatic fossa	Equivalent	Equivalent
Intra-abdominal visceral retraction/manipulation	Significant (using hands, metal retractors, and sponge packing)	Minimal (retraction of viscera rarely necessary for exposure)
Tissue desiccation	Moderate (open environment promotes evaporation)	Minimal (closed environment)
Body temperature reduction	Moderate (multifactorial—evaporation, cool irrigation fluids)	Moderate (multifactorial—circulating nonheated gas, cool irrigation fluids)

TABLE 27–3. Complications and Adverse Physiologic Effects of CO_2 Pneumoperitoneum

Complication/Adverse Effect	Possible Mechanism(s)	References
Cardiac-Hemodynamic		
Sequelae		
Tachycardia	Sympathetic response to impaired venous return, hypercarbia	26–28
Hypertension	Sympathetic response to impaired venous return, hypercarbia	26–28
Increased vascular resistance	Sympathetic response to impaired venous return, hypercarbia	26–28
Increased myocardial O_2 demand	Sympathetic response to impaired venous return, hypercarbia	26–28
Decreased cardiac output	Reduced venous return, increased afterload, impaired contractility from hypercarbia	26–28, 30
Complications		
Bradycardia	Vasovagal reaction to peritoneal stretching/irritation	30–32, 3
Cardiac arrhythmias	Hypercarbia, hypoxia, catecholamine response	22, 30–33
Hypotension	Venacaval compression	22, 31
Tension pneumothorax	Diaphragm injury, dissection near esophageal hiatus, barotrauma	22, 31
Pneumomediastinum	Defect in diaphragm	31
CO_2 gas embolus	Absorption of CO_2 through injured blood vessels	22, 31, 32
Myocardial infarction	Inadequate perfusion to meet increased demand	33
Severe hypertension	Sympathetic response to impaired venous return, hypercarbia	30, 31
Metabolic acidosis	Inadequate tissue perfusion from reduced cardiac output	22, 31
Pulmonary		
Sequelae		
Reduced lung compliance	Reduced lung volume	22, 38, 40
Increased airway resistance	Increased intrathoracic pressure from transmitted IIAP	40
Mild $\dot{V}/\dot{Q}$ mismatch	Reduced lung volume from mechanical effect of IIAP	22, 31, 32
Mild hypercarbia/acidosis	CO_2 retention	38
Atelectasis	Lung bases collapsed against diaphragm	38, 39
Complications		
Hypoxia	Atelectasis and reduced lung volume	22, 38, 39
Hypercarbia	CO_2 retention	31, 38
Respiratory acidosis	Hypercarbia	21, 38
Aspiration	Increased risk of regurgitation of gastric contents from IIAP	38
Renal failure	Impairment of renal blood flow by IIAP and/or hypercarbia	27, 34–37
Venous stasis	Impaired lower extremity venous return and endothelial damage from IIAP	77, 104–108
Deep venous thrombosis		
Pulmonary embolism		
Hypothermia	Cooling from irrigation fluid, CO_2 gas, lengthy procedures	38
Other problems		
Gas leakage	Inadequate seal at trocar sites	22
Monitoring artifacts	Falsely elevated central venous pressure from transmitted IIAP	29
Subcutaneous emphysema	Insufflation into preperitoneal space	31
Shoulder pain	Stretching/irritation of the diaphragm	31, 38

$\dot{V}/\dot{Q}$, ventilation/perfusion; IIAP, increased intra-abdominal pressure.

technique on elderly and critically ill patients. The potential adverse cardiopulmonary effects of CO_2 pneumoperitoneum pose significant risks for all patients undergoing laparoscopic surgery and especially for those with cardiopulmonary disease. Therefore, all surgeons performing laparoscopic surgery must be aware of the potential adverse effects of pneumoperitoneum to avoid devastating complications.

The physiologic mechanisms that account for the hemodynamic effects of CO_2 insufflation are complex and not fully understood at this time. CO_2 pneumoperitoneum may affect hemodynamics by entirely different mechanisms. The two dominating mechanisms involve the mechanical effects of increased intra-abdominal pressure and the physiologic effects of absorbed CO_2. Increased intra-abdominal pressure may impair venous return, thus reducing preload and leading to a reduced cardiac output. The reduction in cardiac output may vary with the magnitude and duration of the operation as well as the patient's hydration status. Distinct from pressure effects, the CO_2 may be absorbed systematically and lead to hemodynamic changes related to hypercarbia. CO_2 absorption/excretion may be affected by a variety of factors, including patient pulmonary function and ventilator settings. Factors other than pneumoperitoneum coexist during laparoscopic surgery that may significantly alter hemodynamic responses. These factors include the placement of the patient in Trendelenburg or reverse Trendelenburg positions, the patient's volume status, the patient's cardiac and pulmonary function, obesity, and the type and dose of anesthetic agents. A variety of methods of determining cardiac output (e.g., thermodilution, electrical impedance, and transesophageal echocardiography) have been used to evaluate hemodynamic effects of CO_2 pneumoperitoneum. The reliability of the latter two methods, especially in association with pneumoperitoneum, has not been adequately demonstrated. The disparity between methods used for the assessment of hemodynamics and the lack of an ideal animal model for pneumoperitoneum have contributed to the existing controversies surrounding the physiologic mechanisms.

Most clinical studies indicate that the hemodynamic effects of CO_2 pneumoperitoneum result in an increase in heart rate, mean arterial pressure, systemic vascular resistance, and central venous pressure, and a decrease in cardiac output.[25-28] Increases in measured central venous pressure are artifactual and related to transmitted increases in intra-abdominal pressure.[29] True preload is actually decreased because of impaired venous return. Although rare, potentially lethal dysrhythmias may result from hypercarbia or abdominal pressure effects.[30-32] Increases in cardiac workload may predispose patients with coronary disease to myocardial infarction.[33] Other studies regarding the effects of CO_2 pneumoperitoneum suggest that intra-abdominal organ perfusion may be reduced because of increased vascular resistance related to elevated abdominal pressure or vasoconstrictive effects of absorbed CO_2.[34, 35] These findings are consistent with studies that implicate increased intra-abdominal pressure as a cause of renal failure.[36, 37] These hemodynamic changes are usually transient and return to baseline levels after desufflation.

The effect of CO_2 insufflation on pulmonary function is less controversial. Impairments in oxygenation result from reduced lung volume and associated atelectasis due to cephalad displacement of the diaphragm.[38, 39] For similar reasons, ventilation may be impaired. Reduced pulmonary compliance and increased airway resistance are other untoward effects of pneumoperitoneum.[40] Anesthesiologists must often employ high concentrations of oxygen and use hyperventilation to compensate for impaired oxygenation and excess absorbed CO_2. The compensatory effects of these interventions may be limited by underlying pulmonary disease. The Trendelenburg position, required for lower abdominal laparo-

scopic surgery, exacerbates the adverse pulmonary effects of CO_2 pneumoperitoneum.[38]

Strategies to prevent complications of CO_2 insufflation have been based on identifying patients at risk who may not tolerate these physiologic responses. Fortunately, the majority of patients who undergo laparoscopic cholecystectomy can tolerate small reductions in cardiac output (0%–30%) associated with CO_2 pneumoperitoneum. Therefore, special considerations in young healthy patients are probably not necessary. Conversely, reduction in cardiac output may be a major concern in a patient with underlying cardiopulmonary disease. Intraoperative monitoring of high-risk patients with a Swan-Ganz catheter or transesophageal echocardiography may be helpful in determining dangerously low cardiac outputs.[33] Hemodynamic compromise may then be corrected by release of pneumoperitoneum or pharmacologic manipulation before severe consequences result.[41] In some patients, preoperative hydration effectively attenuates the reduction in preload caused by the pneumoperitoneum.

Alternatives to CO_2 pneumoperitoneum include other gases and gasless laparoscopy. Gases such as helium and argon have been studied and may potentially eliminate the adverse hemodynamic and metabolic effects of CO_2 absorption.[42, 43] Alternative gases, however, do not eliminate those adverse effects related to elevated abdominal pressure. Gasless laparoscopy involves obtaining exposure for laparoscopy by placing an internal retracting device through a small incision and lifting the anterior abdominal wall.[44] This method avoids both the adverse effects of CO_2 absorption and increased abdominal pressure of pneumoperitoneum.[45] Gasless methods of access have not received wide application, owing to inadequate exposure for many laparoscopic procedures. Investigation of the potential of these methods to circumvent adverse hemodynamic changes is underway in multiple centers. Refinements in abdominal wall lifting technology have improved exposure of the peritoneal cavity.

Laparoscopic surgery involving CO_2 pneumoperitoneum can lead to adverse hemodynamic effects and significant complications. As more abdominal operations are being performed laparoscopically, it is imperative that surgeons become informed of these adverse effects and take appropriate measures to avoid the potential complications related to CO_2 pneumoperitoneum.

Physiology of Reduced Tissue Injury

Modification of the Biologic Response to Injury—Pharmacologic Manipulation vs. Minimal Invasion. The biologic response to injury is the same whether the injury is accidental trauma or caused by elective surgery. The nature of the biologic response is primarily dependent on the magnitude of the insult and the host's ability to recover. Although teleologically the biologic response is adaptive, in many instances it is, in fact, maladaptive. Because elective surgery is a form of trauma, albeit well controlled, operative morbidity and mortality can be ascribed to either a technical failure or to a maladaptive physiologic response to surgical injury (Table 27–4). Historically, strategies to reduce operative mortality and morbidity related to the stress response have been aimed at countering the ill effects of surgery with perioperative nutrition, antibiotics, pulmonary toilet, early ambulation, anticoagulants, and so on. Laparoscopists attempt to reduce operative mortality and morbidity by minimizing the negative effects of surgery.

Many investigators have studied the merit of pharmacologically blocking or reducing the response to injury. Kehlet and coworkers demonstrated that general and regional anesthesia positively modify the stress response.[46, 47] The acute-phase response to injury may be attenuated with peri-

TABLE 27–4. Physiologic Responses to Laparotomy and Their Clinical Consequences

Mechanism	Adverse Effects	Surgical Complications
Stress response	Hypermetabolism	Catabolic state
	Increased myocardial O_2 demand	Myocardial ischemia/infarction
	Increased pulmonary workload	Respiratory failure
	Increased renal workload	Renal failure
	Impaired gut function–motility	Ileus, malabsorption
	Impaired immune function	Infectious complications
		Increased tumor growth
	Hypercoagulable state	Venous thrombosis
		Pulmonary embolus
Impaired pulmonary mechanics	Alveolar collapse	Atelectasis
		Hypoxia
		Pneumonia
Local wound effects	Increased metabolic demand of wound healing	Catabolic state
	Impaired barrier to infection	Wound infection
	Fascial injury	Wound dehiscence, hernia

operative corticosteroids, intrathecal neural blockade, and postoperative cyclooxygenase inhibitors, and thereby reduce postoperative fatigue scores.[48] Although promising, pharmacologic manipulation has inherent limitations related to its inability to completely block the stress response. There are also complications associated with delivering the agents and documented adverse effects of the agents. A fundamentally more logical approach is to minimize the magnitude of surgical injury. Minimally invasive surgery exploits the advantages of reduced tissue injury and the subsequent decrease in maladaptive host responses.

Laparoscopic surgeons focus on reducing abdominal wall trauma. For example, cholecystectomy could be considered two operations: the laparotomy and the gallbladder removal. Each aspect of the operation has its own specific local complications, such as incisional hernia or bile leak. However, both aspects contribute to the risk of systemic complications, such as deep venous thrombosis, ileus, and atelectasis. The potential adverse consequences of removal of the gallbladder must be risked to achieve the desired outcome of the removal of a diseased organ. Unfortunately the patient has traditionally been subjected to the risks inherent to the laparotomy without direct benefit from this portion of the operation. Because of the advances in minimally invasive techniques, major abdominal operations can now be accomplished with techniques that markedly decrease the unnecessary injury to the abdominal wall as compared with traditional surgical techniques. Consequently, the reduction in the biologic response to that injury is manifested by a reduction in postoperative morbidity.

Neuroendocrine and Metabolic Consequences of Surgery. The classic hypermetabolic stress response is the dominant physiologic response to injury. This response directly or indirectly affects all other organ systems and therefore has the largest impact on the duration and success of convalescence. In brief, the stress response is classically divided into early catabolic and late anabolic phases.[49, 50] Hypermetabolic changes of catabolism appear to be initiated by tissue damage and are characterized by increased fat oxidation and marked proteolysis, causing an increased loss of nitrogen in the urine. Postoperative lipolysis provides abundant quantities of free fatty acid as an additional energy source. Skeletal muscle proteolysis provides amino acid precursors for gluconeogenesis and hepatic protein synthesis at the expense of consumption of lean body mass. The catabolic phase begins with the onset of injury (the skin incision) and generally lasts 24 to 48 hours for a major abdominal operation. The anabolic phase begins 3 to 6 days after a major abdominal operation and persists for 4 to 6 weeks. This phase is characterized by

positive nitrogen balance and weight gain. In late anabolism, the patient reaches nitrogen equilibrium but positive carbon balance, and deposition of body fat resumes. It has long been established that the extent, degree, and duration of these metabolic changes that follow tissue injury depend on the severity of that injury.[51, 52] The relatively smaller injury sustained by the host during the laparoscopic operation accounts for the absent or attenuated hypermetabolic stress response. Factors other than tissue damage, such as volume loss, underperfusion, starvation, and invasive infection, may also significantly influence the biologic response to surgery.

Mediation of the Injury Response. The injury response begins in the wound and is primarily mediated by the central nervous system (CNS), which receives stimuli from three distinct sources: (1) afferent nerve fibers; (2) volume receptors, pressure receptors, and chemoreceptors; and (3) circulating substances. Afferent sensory nerve fibers from the wound relay the pain signal to the hypothalamus-pituitary-adrenal axis and initiate the adrenocortical response to injury. The hormones cortisol, glucagon, and catecholamines, among others, are released in high concentration and play a pivotal role in mediating the stress response. Fluid loss from the vascular compartment causes stimulation of volume and pressure receptors, which initiate a series of CNS-mediated cardiovascular adjustments aimed at redistribution of blood to vital organs. Chemoreceptors stimulated by acid-base disturbances resulting from regional hypoperfusion and anaerobic metabolism provide afferent input to vasomotor and respiratory centers where compensatory changes are initiated. Circulating substances such as cytokines are released locally at or near the wound and may directly or indirectly stimulate the CNS or may initiate their own effects independently.

The neuroendocrine and cytokine responses to injury have been evaluated through measured serum catecholamine, cortisol, and glucose levels in patients who underwent either open or laparoscopic cholecystectomy (Figs. 27–2 and 27–3).[53] Increases in each of these stress indicators were significantly less and returned to baseline quicker after laparoscopic cholecystectomy compared with open cholecystectomy. Because both groups had equal access to pain medication, and postoperative analgesic usage was similar, this attenuated response could not be attributed to differences in narcotic usage. This study suggests that the laparoscopic approach, at least in the immediate perioperative period, results in an attenuated neuroendocrine response to surgical trauma. Other studies of the effect of laparoscopic cholecystectomy on the neuroendocrine response have shown mixed results.[54–57] Studies specifically addressing the cytokine and acute phase response, however, have more consistently demonstrated a

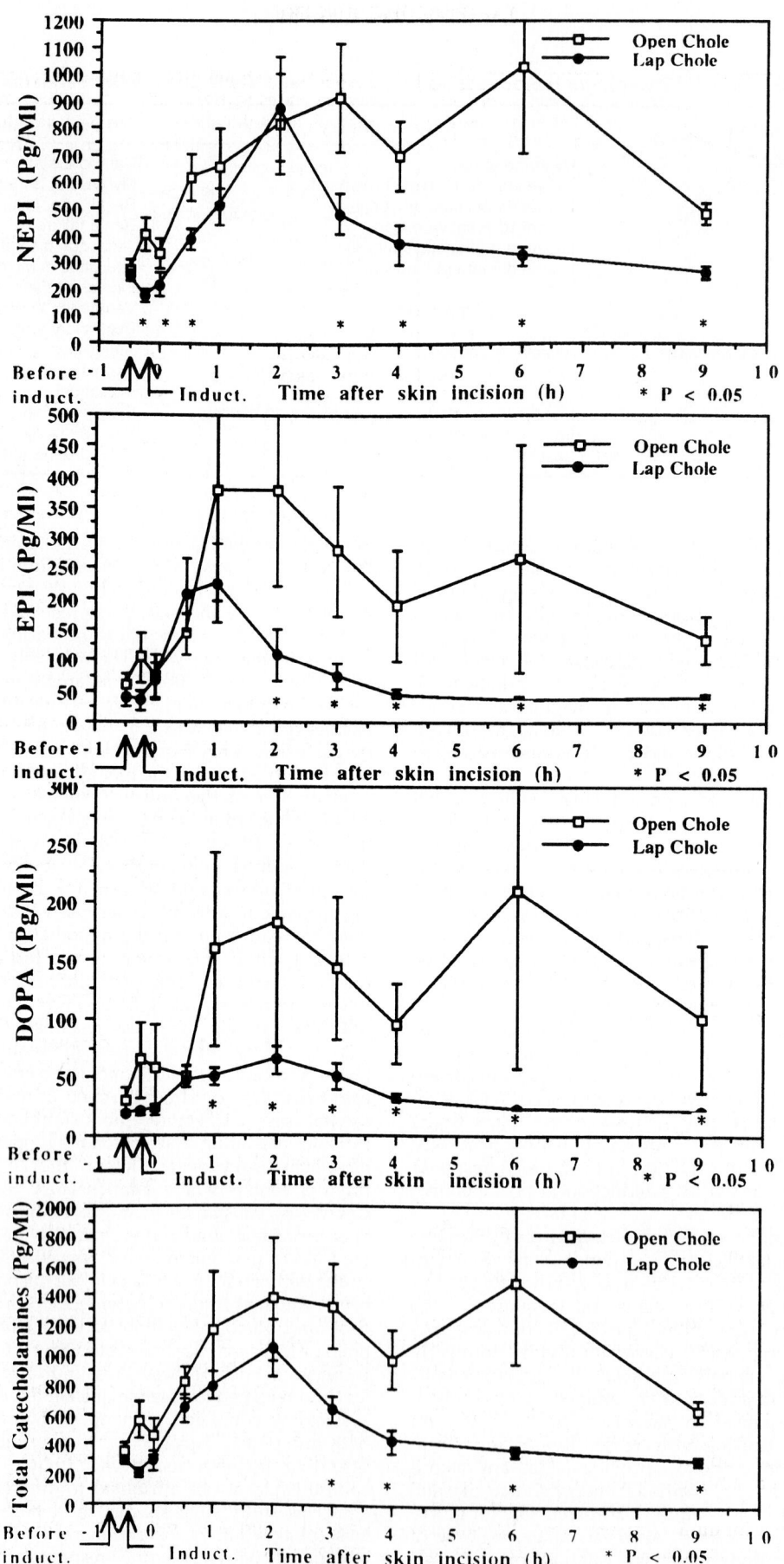

Figure 27–2. Changes in plasma catecholamines (mean ± SEM) after open and laparoscopic cholecystecomy. NEPI, norepinephrine; EPI, epinephrine; DOPA, dopamine. (From Schauer, P. R., and Sirinek, K. R.: The laparoscopic approach reduces the endocrine response to elective cholecystectomy. Am. Surg., 61:106, 1995.)

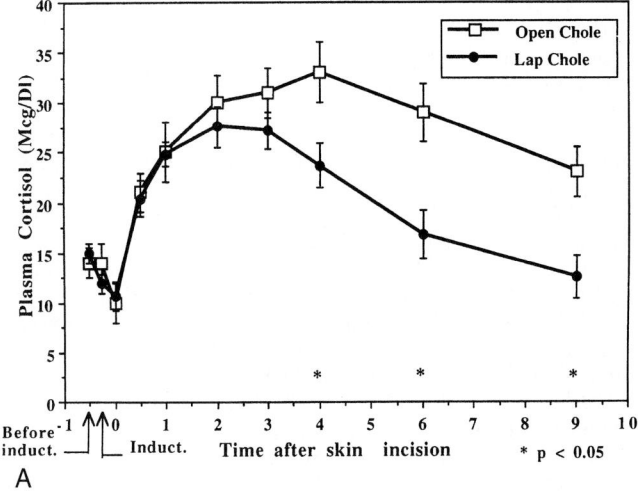

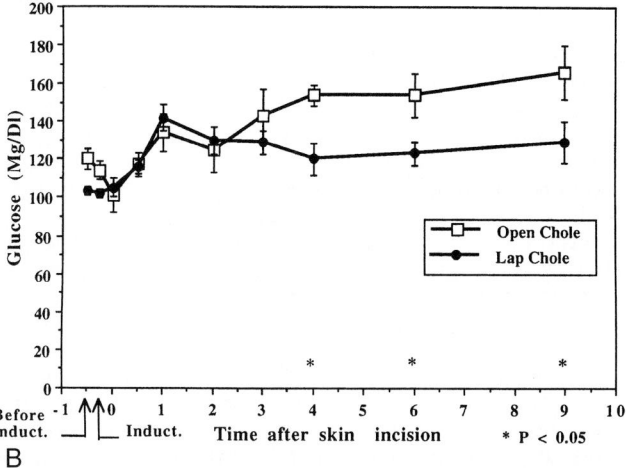

Figure 27–3. Changes in plasma cortisol *(A)* and glucose *(B)* concentrations (mean ± SEM) after open and laparoscopic cholecystecomy. (From Schauer, P. R., and Sirinek, K. R.: The laparoscopic approach reduces the endocrine response to elective cholecystectomy. Am. Surg., *61*:106, 1995.)

reduced maladaptive response to laparoscopic cholecystectomy compared with open cholecystectomy. Indicators of the cytokine response, such as interleukin-6 and C-reactive protein, leukocytosis, and erythrocyte sedimentation rate, have all been shown to be less after cholecystectomy by the laparoscopic method compared with the open method.[54–60] Collectively, these studies suggest that in the immediate perioperative period the laparoscopic method results in an attenuated neuroendocrine response and cytokine response compared with open techniques.

Perioperative Immune Function. Factors that may adversely alter immune function in the postoperative period include age, underlying disease, sepsis, malnutrition, splenectomy, immunosuppressive medications, blood transfusions, anesthetic agents, and injury.[61] The one factor that affects all surgical patients is the operation itself. Surgeons are aware that immunosuppression is an expected sequelae of surgical intervention. Multiple defects in the immune system have been described after operations and trauma.[62] Major components of cellular immunity are depressed after surgical procedures.[63–65] Response to antibody also appears to be adversely affected by surgery and trauma.[66] Other factors that contribute to general immunosuppression after surgery include increased circulating immunosuppressive agents such as prostaglandins and cytokines.[61] The clinical relevance of

impaired postoperative immune function is the subject of intense investigation, and many believe that this impairment may be a significant contributing factor to postoperative immune-related complications such as infectious complications and tumor growth.

Controversy still exists regarding the mechanisms by which surgery and trauma induce immunosuppression. The hypothesis that has received the greatest attention is that trauma or stress generates or liberates immunosuppressive factors that directly or indirectly suppress the normal immune response. Mediators of the stress response as described earlier appear to be the mediators of impaired immune function. Recent work has identified stress hormone release after injury as a potential mediator of impaired immune function. In a series of experiments involving healthy volunteers, the effect of stress hormones on cellular function of neutrophils and lymphocytes was evaluated.[67] Cortisol was found to suppress lymphocyte blastogenesis. Epinephrine and norepinephrine inhibited neutrophil chemotaxis. Glucagon impaired neutrophil chemotaxis and bactericidal activity. Factors such as prostaglandin E_2, endotoxin, tumor necrosis factor, proteolysis factor, and interleukin-1, among others, have been implicated as potential mediators of the immunesuppressed state after trauma or stress.[68–70] It is generally accepted that the extent of the injury is directly related to the magnitude of the immunosuppression as well as the magnitude of the overall stress response.

Because the laparoscopic method reduces tissue injury, investigators have begun to study the effects of reduced tissue trauma with laparoscopy on perioperative immune function.[27] Bessler and associates[71] evaluated the effect of laparoscopic versus open colon resection on postoperative T-cell–related immune function, as measured by delayed-type hypersensitivity using a swine model. Results of skin antigen testing showed that the group of pigs that underwent laparoscopic resection had a 20% greater response as determined by a 20% larger diameter of skin induration compared with the open group. This same group of investigators demonstrated that rats undergoing CO_2 insufflation had no differences in response to keyhole-limpet hemocyanin (KLH) and phytohemagglutinin (PHA) antigens from control animals (no procedure performed) at 24 and 48 hours after insufflation but that animals that underwent laparotomy had a significantly diminished postoperative response to the same antigens.[72] This group also demonstrated the clinical relevance of the preserved immune response after laparoscopic surgery by showing that tumor growth in mice after laparoscopy was less than after laparotomy.[73] These animal studies support the hypothesis that reduced surgical injury reduces the impairment of postoperative immune function specifically related to cell-mediated immunity.

Evidence of preserved immune function after laparoscopic surgery exists in humans as well. Interleukin-6 and white blood cell counts measured at 1 and 6 days postoperatively were not significantly changed after laparoscopic cholecystectomy, whereas significant increases occurred on postoperative day 1 for the patients who underwent open cholecystectomy.[74] Delayed-type hypersensitivity as determined by response to PHA was significantly reduced on postoperative day 1 for the patients who underwent open cholecystectomy but was preserved for patients who underwent laparoscopic cholecystectomy. In addition, the HLA-DR expression on monocytes, known to be important in antigen presentation, showed a significant reduction in the open cholecystectomy group but was preserved in the laparoscopic group. These changes occurred despite the fact that the operative time was twice as long for the laparoscopic group. Significant decreases in the monocyte and neutrophil release of superoxide anion, neutrophil chemotaxis, tumor necrosis factor, and white blood cell count have been demonstrated in laparoscopic patients when compared with patients undergoing open cholecystectomy.[75] Both the animal and human studies provide preliminary and complementary evidence that immune function after laparoscopic surgery is less impaired than after open surgery.

The findings of preserved immunocompetence are particularly noteworthy considering studies that suggest an increased occurrence of tumor implantation in the wounds after laparoscopic surgery compared with open surgery.[76] Although the mechanism of tumor implantation is not clear, these data supporting preserved immune function after laparoscopic surgery suggest that a technical mechanism may account for tumor implantation. Excessive tumor manipulation or shedding of tumor cells during specimen removal have been discussed as potential technical errors leading to tumor metastasis. The overall clinical benefit of preservation of postoperative immune function as related to tumor metastases remains to be determined.

Cardiac Function After Laparoscopic Surgery. There is no direct evidence that the stress of elective surgery impairs cardiac function. In healthy patients, cardiac performance, regulated by the sympathetic response, improves in the postoperative period to meet increased metabolic demands. The increase in cardiac work as a response to the hypermetabolic state, however, is detrimental to patients with compromised cardiac function. The added stress in patients with ischemic heart disease may lead to myocardial infarction. Cardiac complications remain the most common cause of death after cholecystectomy.[77] Thus, the potential for laparoscopic approach to reduce cardiac morbidity is of significant concern. A study in a single institution compared the outcome of evenly matched patients undergoing 1107 laparoscopic cholecystectomies to that of 1283 open cholecystectomies performed 10 years previously. There was a significant decrease in cardiac complications in the laparoscopic group (0.06% vs. 1.4%).[78] The minimally invasive approach is responsible for the reduced postoperative cardiac morbidity. However, because the study was noncontemporaneous, other factors such as improved perioperative care may have accounted for the reduction in cardiac morbidity. The potential benefit of the laparoscopic approach on postoperative cardiac function must be weighed against the detrimental intraoperative effects of CO_2 pneumoperitoneum on cardiac output.

Pulmonary Function After Laparoscopic Surgery. Significant impairment of pulmonary function after abdominal surgery and general anesthesia have been well documented.[79] General anesthesia typically produces transient impaired gas exchange as a result of decreased lung volumes, shunting, and changes in lung mechanics.[80] The effect of an upper abdominal operation on pulmonary function is more pronounced and of longer duration. Pulmonary impairment may frequently last up to 10 days after operation. A restrictive pattern characterized by a 50% reduction in vital capacity and a 30% decrease in tidal volume and functional residual capacity occurs after major abdominal procedures.[81, 82] Forced expiratory volume in 1 second decreases as a result of decreased lung volume rather than airway obstruction.[82] These changes become clinically significant when they contribute to pathologic conditions such as atelectasis, hypoxemia, and pneumonia.[83]

Pulmonary function is the most thoroughly studied of all the physiologic changes associated with the laparoscopic approach. Frazee and coworkers showed, in a nonrandomized, controlled study, that on the first postoperative day the reductions in forced vital capacity and forced expiratory volume in 1 second were 20% less after laparoscopic cholecystectomy than after open cholecystectomy.[84] Similar studies have also demonstrated benefits in immediate postoperative spirometry.[85, 86] Laparoscopic cholecystectomy results in improvements in postoperative spirometry, better oxygen saturation, reduced analog pain scores, and reduced narcotic consumption when compared with the *minilap* cholecystectomy.[87]

Patients undergoing laparoscopic cholecystectomy have a significant improvement over open cholecystectomy patients in postoperative spirometry, maximum voluntary ventilation, total lung capacity, and oxygen saturation (Fig. 27–4).[88] Pulmonary function returns to baseline 4 to 10 days sooner in the laparoscopic group. Lower rates of pulmonary complications, including atelectasis and hypoxia, are a result of less impairment of pulmonary function when the laparoscopic approach is used (Fig. 27–5). Many large laparoscopic cholecystectomy series have reported pulmonary complication rates less than 0.5%,[89, 90] compared with a rate of 2% for contemporary open cholecystectomy.[91]

The reduction in postoperative pain likely plays a role in accounting for decreased pulmonary dysfunction after the laparoscopic procedure. Pain resulting from deep inspiration contributes to the cascade of events resulting in chest wall splinting, reduced functional residual capacity, tachypnea, and shallow breathing, which are ultimately thought to lead to atelectasis. Atelectasis is considered to be the forebear of most postoperative pulmonary complications. In addition, minimal disruption of the abdominal wall musculature, which is a component of the ventilatory pump, probably accounts for some reduction in pulmonary impairment as well.

Intestinal Function After Laparoscopic Surgery. Postoperative ileus is a predictable consequence of many abdominal and extra-abdominal procedures. Ileus is often the major factor in prolonging the hospital stay. The cause of postoperative ileus is thought to be a sympathetically mediated inhibition of motility that most significantly affects the colon.[92, 93] Other proposed inhibitory mechanisms include bowel manipulation, stress-related hormones other than catecholamines (e.g., vasopressin), and postoperative narcotic usage. Gastrointestinal myoelectric studies have identified a consistent pattern of recovery after major abdominal operations.[94] Recovery begins with the return of small bowel motility within 24 hours, followed by return of stomach motility within 24 to 48 hours, and is complete with the recovery of colonic motility within 3 to 6 days.

Many clinical studies have demonstrated an earlier return of bowel function after laparoscopic procedures compared with conventional open operations.[89, 95, 96] A rapid return of colonic electrical activity and lack of postoperative impairment in small bowel motility after laparoscopic cholecystectomy has been demonstrated using a canine model.[97] However, gastric emptying was significantly delayed postoperatively compared with baseline. No differences in motility of the small or large bowel in dogs after open or laparoscopic cholecystectomy were found in one study that suggested that the observed clinical reduction in ileus after laparoscopic cholecystectomy may be explained by reduced narcotic intake rather than any direct benefit from reduced tissue injury.[98] In a similar study in dogs, a significant reduction was noted in time to occurrence of myoelectric activity of the small intestine after laparoscopic cholecystectomy compared with open cholecystectomy (5.5 hr. vs. 46.5 hr.).[99] Measured gastrointestinal transit time in dogs undergoing laparoscopic colectomy versus laparoscopic-assisted colectomy versus open colectomy revealed that laparoscopic colectomy caused less delay in gastrointestinal transit than laparoscopy-assisted or open colectomy in the canine model.[100] In a small human study (n = 6), however, no differences in myoelectric activity were determined after open versus laparoscopic colectomy. Yet, clinical indicators of bowel function, such as flatus and

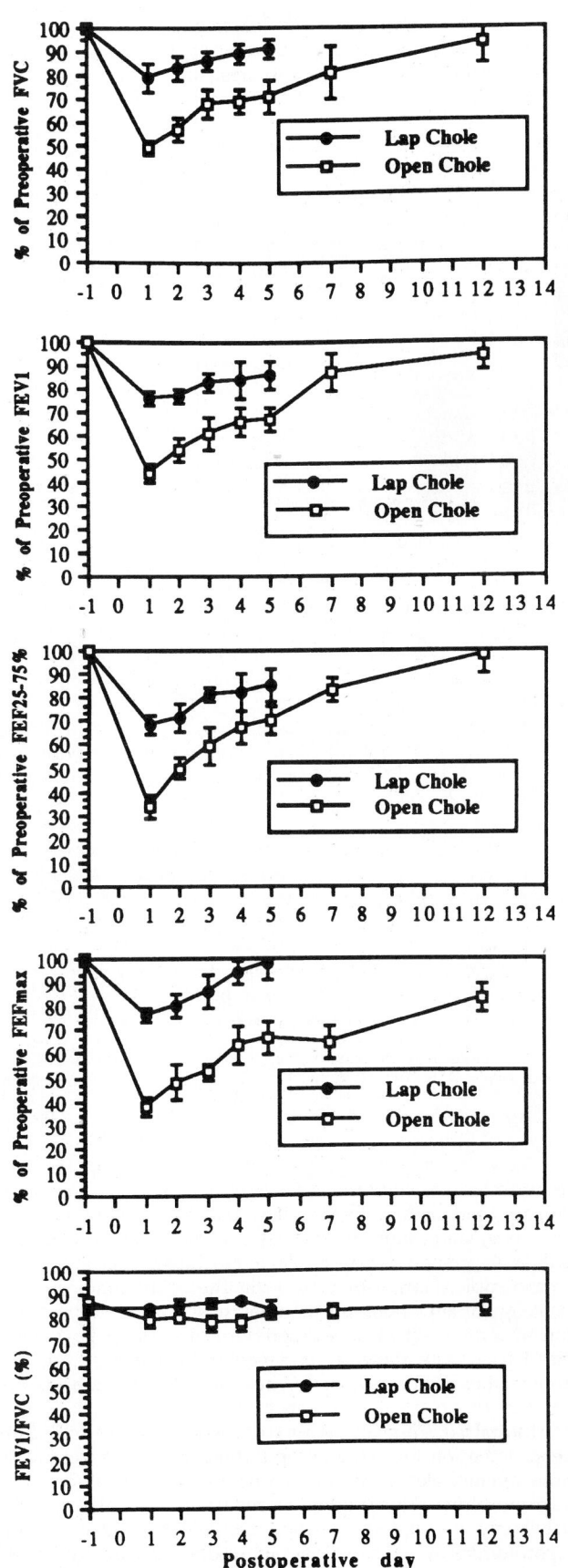

Figure 27–4. Postoperative spirometry after laparoscopic vs. open cholecystectomy. FVC, forced vital capacity; FEV1, 1-second forced expiratory volume; FEF25–75% and FEFmax, forced expiratory flow. (From Schauer, P. R., Luna, J., Ghiatas, A., Glen, M. E., Warren, J. M., and Sirinek, K. R.: Pulmonary function after laparoscopic cholecystectomy. Surgery, *114*:389, 1993.)

bowel movement, have been shown to return sooner after laparoscopic than after open cholecystectomy (10 and 36 hours vs. 60 and 96 hours, respectively).[102] Similar findings of rapid return of gastrointestinal function are consistently demonstrated with most laparoscopic procedures.

Thrombosis and Coagulation After Laparoscopic Surgery. Despite advances in prevention, deep venous thrombosis (DVT) and pulmonary embolism contribute significantly to perioperative morbidity and mortality. The incidence of DVT after general surgical procedures has been reported to be 14% to 33%.[103] The risk of pulmonary embolus after DVT formation is 1% to 2%. The incidence of DVT and pulmonary embolus after open cholecystectomy is less: 7% to 10% and 0.4%, respectively.[103] Isolated reports of DVT and pulmonary embolus occurring after laparoscopic cholecystectomy have been published.[77, 104, 105] The risk of DVT and pulmonary embolus as a complication of laparoscopic cholecystectomy cannot be accurately determined from currently available studies.

Several factors specific to the laparoscopic method may increase or decrease the risk of DVT associated with laparoscopic cholecystectomy (Table 27–5). The increased intra-abdominal pressure of the pneumoperitoneum can result in reduced venous flow in the lower extremities. Reduced flow during pneumoperitoneum has been demonstrated by reduced peak flow velocities and pulsatility in the common femoral veins.[106] Intermittent sequential pneumatic compression reverses significant reductions in common femoral vein peak flow velocity.[107] The majority of North American surgeons use prophylactic measures against DVT during laparoscopic operations (Table 27–6). Pneumoperitoneum may potentially cause venous distention by impairing venous return from the lower extremities, resulting in endothelial damage that has been shown experimentally to promote thrombosis.[108] The reverse Trendelenburg position required for laparoscopic cholecystectomy has been shown to increase intraoperative venous stasis.[109] Operative time is frequently longer for laparoscopic procedures. The more challenging cases such as laparoscopic cholecystectomy for acute cholecystitis may require significant increase in operative time as compared with open cholecystectomy. The length of the operation has been demonstrated to be a risk factor for postoperative thrombosis and, therefore, the laparoscopic method in this regard enhances the potential for venous thrombosis.[110]

The thrombosis-promoting factors associated with the lap-

TABLE 27–5. Laparoscopic Cholecystectomy and Postoperative Venous Thrombosis

Factor	Consequence
Pneumoperitoneum (15 mm. Hg)	Promotes venous stasis by decreasing lower extremity venous flow
	May promote venous distention and consequent endothelial damage
Reverse Trendelenburg position	Promotes venous stasis by reducing lower extremity venous flow
Increased operative time*	Increases effect of all operative factors that may promote thrombosis
Reduced postoperative immobility	Reduces venous stasis
Reduced postoperative hypercoagulability	May reduce associated risk of thrombosis although this has not been adequately studied

*Applies particularly to difficult cases (e.g., acute cholecystitis) or advanced laparoscopic surgery.

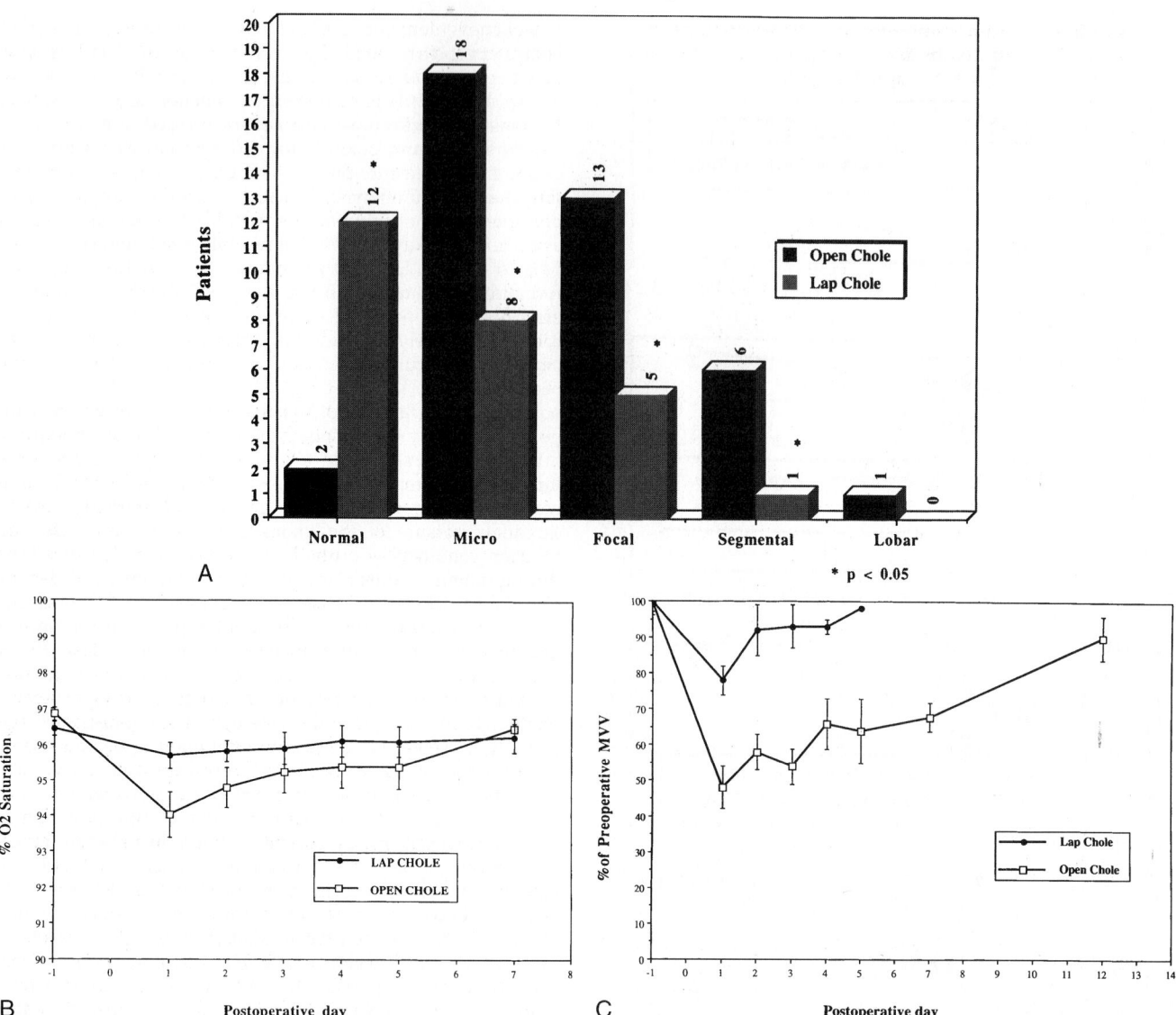

Figure 27–5. Postoperative atelectasis *(A)* and hypoxia *(B and C)* after laparoscopic cholecystectomy vs. open cholecystectomy. MVV, maximum voluntary ventilation. (From Schauer, P. R., Luna, J., Ghiatas, A., Glen, M. E., Warren, J. M., and Sirinek, K. R.: Pulmonary function after laparoscopic cholecystectomy. Surgery, *114*:389, 1993.)

aroscopic method may be at least partially negated by specific benefits of this modality. Patients are usually ambulatory within a few hours after laparoscopic cholecystectomy, while it may take several days for patients to become fully ambulatory after open cholecystectomy. Thus, enhanced mobility after laparoscopic procedures may reduce venous stasis and the risk of thrombosis. Hypercoagulability after an operation may be diminished by the reduced stress response associated with laparoscopic procedures. This condition is thought to be regulated by various cytokines of the acute-phase response, such as interleukin-6. These acute-phase mediators may stimulate the release or activation of the direct mediators of the coagulation and fibrinolytic system such as fibrinogen, von Willebrand factor, plasminogen activator, and plasminogen activator inhibitor-1.[111, 112] Attenuation of the acute-phase response after laparoscopic cholecystectomy suggests that the postoperative hypercoagulable state may be attenuated as well. However, no statistical differences in plasma concentrations of interleukin-6 or various mediators of coagulation-fibrinolysis were demonstrated between two evenly matched groups of patients undergoing open or laparoscopic cholecys-

tectomy.[112] In a similar study, coagulability increased after laparoscopic cholecystectomy compared with the preoperative state, suggesting that the laparoscopic method does not obliterate postoperative hypercoagulability.[113] Whether the laparoscopic method may to some degree attenuate the hypercoagulable response of the operation remains to be determined. The effect of laparoscopic procedures on postoperative hypercoagulability thus deserves further investigation, and prophylactic measures against venous thrombosis are advised.[114]

Abdominal Adhesion Formation After Laparoscopic Surgery. Adhesion formation after abdominal and pelvic operations remains extremely common and is a source of considerable morbidity. The incidence of intra-abdominal adhesions in clinical and autopsy studies of patients who had prior laparotomies was 70% to 90%.[115] Adhesions are the most common cause of small bowel obstruction in Western countries and account for approximately one third of all intestinal obstructions. Pelvic adhesions account for 20% to 25% of infertility.[116] Adhesions may also cause chronic abdominal and pelvic pain that may severely impair a person's quality

TABLE 27–6. Recommendations for Prevention of Venous Thromboembolism in Patients Undergoing Laparoscopic Surgery

Risk Category*	Recommended Modality
Low risk (Age < 60, no predisposing factors†)	Graduated compression stockings
Moderate risk (two to four predisposing factors)	Intermittent pneumatic compression or low-dose heparin
High risk (more than four predisposing factors)	Intermittent pneumatic compression and low-dose heparin

*All patients undergoing laparoscopic surgery should be considered "moderate risk" unless they are younger than 40 with no predisposing factors.

†Includes age > 60, immobility > 72 hours, history of deep venous thrombosis or pulmonary embolism, varicose veins, obesity, myocardial infarction, chronic obstructive pulmonary disease, cardiovascular accident, operation >2 hours, venous stasis disease, malignancy, pregnancy, severe sepsis, known hypercoagulable state.

Adapted from Caprini, J. A., Arcelus, J. J.: Prevention of postoperative venous thromboembolism following laparoscopic cholecystectomy. Surg. Endosc., 8:741, 1994.

of life. Abdominal adhesions account for major dangers of reoperative abdominal operations, including visceral damage and intestinal perforation. Despite a century of effort, little progress has been made in preventing or treating this challenging problem.

Multiple etiologic factors contribute to adhesion formation including mechanical trauma, thermal injury, infection, tissue ischemia, and foreign material. The pathophysiology of adhesion formation begins with the creation of an inflammatory vascular response to foreign material or ischemic tissue.[116, 117] This localized area of inflammation is rich in fibrinogen exudate, which forms *sticky* fibrin clots. Adherence to adjacent structures occurs, followed by the formation of granulation tissue composed of fibroblasts, macrophages, and new blood vessels within the fibrin network. Fibrinolysis acts to absorb newly developed fibrinous attachments in well-vascularized injured tissue. Ischemic tissue or foreign bodies inhibit fibrinolysis, thus allowing for permanent adhesions to develop.

Most surgeons have a clinical impression that laparoscopy produces fewer intra-abdominal adhesions. However, few studies have adequately addressed this issue. No adhesion formation was noted after laser injuries to the peritoneum and uterine horn were made laparoscopically in a rabbit model, but all animals had adhesions after the injuries were made through a laparotomy incision.[118] A prospective, randomized study in humans demonstrated that patients who underwent laparotomy for the management of ectopic pregnancy had significantly more adhesions at second-look laparoscopy than patients who initially underwent laparoscopy.[119]

The mechanism by which laparoscopic procedures reduce adhesions is not well established. Major factors include a reduction in the inciting event, tissue injury, and surrounding ischemia. Visceral injury as well as abdominal wall injury is less during laparoscopic operations because wound retractors, packing, and bowel handling are avoided. The laparoscopic method also reduces foreign body contamination from glove talc or particulate matter that may enter the wound during an open procedure. A reduction in the systemic inflammatory response elicited by the abdominal wound may also contribute to reduced adhesion formation.

Wound Healing. Complications related to abdominal wound healing such as hematomas, seromas, infection, dehiscence, and hernia contribute significantly to short- and long-term postoperative morbidity. Wound complications

dramatically increase medical costs. The causes of wound complications are generally related to technical failure, preexisting diseases, inhibitory drugs, or infection. The size of the wound itself is another major factor that may predispose to wound complications. Laparoscopic trocar incisions commonly range from 5 to 12 mm. Wounds of this size rarely result in complications even in high-risk patients. Multiple large series of laparoscopic cholecystectomies report overall wound-related complications much lower than expected for open cholecystectomy.[78, 90] Early laparoscopic series reported hernias occasionally occurring at trocar sites. Hernias at trocar sites can usually be avoided by full-thickness closure of all trocar sites 10 mm. or greater. Thus, the laparoscopic method has virtually eliminated the dreaded complications of large incisional hernias as well as wound dehiscence and evisceration.

Overall Morbidity and Mortality After Laparoscopic Surgery. Although there is much more to be learned regarding the physiologic response to laparoscopic surgical procedures, increasing evidence supports the concept that reduced surgical injury results in reduced morbidity and mortality. Several large series have clearly demonstrated a significant reduction in overall morbidity with the laparoscopic techniques. The morbidity rates remain improved with laparoscopy despite the early reports of increased bile duct injury.[77, 78, 90] A single-institution review of morbidity and mortality from elective cholecystectomy in high-risk patients (ASA Class III or greater) from 1982 to 1993 demonstrated a 50% reduction in overall morbidity with the introduction of laparoscopic cholecystectomy.[120] Although there was no statistically significant decrease in mortality from open cholecystectomy compared with laparoscopic cholecystectomy (1.2% vs. 0%, respectively), a significant decrease in cardiopulmonary morbidity was realized. In a similar study, a 50% reduction in major complications for patients undergoing elective cholecystectomy (7.5% vs. 3.1%) and a significant reduction in mortality for patients with acute cholecystitis (2.3% vs. 0%) after the introduction of laparoscopic cholecystectomy was reported.[78] A statewide study of 67,537 Maryland residents undergoing open and laparoscopic cholecystectomy from 1985 to 1992 demonstrated a 30% reduction in mortality associated with the laparoscopic technique.[121] The net reduction in physiologic stress from this minimally invasive procedure accounts for the observed improvement in overall morbidity and mortality.

The physiologic and clinical information gained from study of laparoscopic cholecystectomy suggests that minimizing abdominal wall trauma is clearly beneficial to patients. Thus, the abdominal wall should be considered as an organ system with its own local and systemic response to injury. It is now understood that most of the morbidity of open cholecystectomy is attributed to the abdominal incision and not the gallbladder dissection. These physiologic benefits translate into faster recovery for most patients and reduced major morbidity and mortality for high-risk patients.

CURRENT STATUS OF LAPAROSCOPIC SURGERY

The role of laparoscopic techniques in the management of surgical diseases remains the focus of heated debate. Laparoscopic cholecystectomy has been clearly established as the *gold standard* for the surgical treatment of calculus biliary disease.[122] Laparoscopic techniques have been used for the performance of pancreaticoduodenectomy, but this is considered to be an ill-advised application of laparoscopy.[123] Between these extremes exist numerous surgical procedures that have received varying degrees of acceptance by the surgical community.

The list of laparoscopic procedures that are deemed acceptable by the surgical community undergoes frequent revision (Table 27–7). Laparoscopic general surgical procedures may be categorized as those that are widely, although rarely unanimously, accepted as the gold standard or as a reasonable alternative technique. A second category includes those procedures that have been proven technically feasible but have yet to achieve widespread acceptance. Finally, the third category includes those operations not accepted within the surgical community.

The list of operations listed as *Accepted* is somewhat arbitrary and is based primarily on the opinions of the authors. These are operations that have an established foundation of literature support, are frequently performed, or warrant acceptance on the basis of common sense. Some of the operations listed as *Accepted* lack multiple supporting studies but adhere to proven laparoscopic techniques. The small numbers of patients benefiting from these less-invasive options in certain procedures are certain to eventually comprise an adequate number to draw a definitive conclusion without the need for extrapolation from higher-volume reports.

A discussion of *Accepted* procedures should begin with laparoscopic cholecystectomy. Throughout the history of general surgery, perhaps no single general surgical procedure has had as much impact as has the introduction of laparoscopic cholecystectomy.[124] Within 2 years of its introduction, laparoscopic cholecystectomy enjoyed widespread acceptance among surgeons. Within 5 years of its introduction, few general surgical procedures had escaped the attempts of the laparoscopist to perform these operations in a less invasive fashion. Had laparoscopy been applied to the repair of hernias or the removal of the spleen as the initial general surgical procedure, these techniques would have been unlikely to have received significant attention. Laparoscopic cholecystec-

tomy was the perfect introductory procedure, owing to the drastic differences in postoperative pain, recuperative time, length of hospital stay, and economic advantages.

Diagnostic laparoscopy predates the introduction of laparoscopic cholecystectomy yet has failed to achieve broad acceptance or significant attention until the commencement of laparoscopic cholecystectomy. Diagnostic laparoscopy is now almost unanimously accepted as the preferred approach to many disease processes. This technique averts many unnecessary laparotomies and often preempts other costly and time-consuming noninvasive studies. The opportunities for direct visualization with the potential for immediate definitive treatment has placed diagnostic laparoscopy in an early position in the management algorithm for many abdominal complaints. In the hands of a properly trained laparoscopist, diagnostic laparoscopy can be performed rapidly, safely, and with minimal sequelae.

The role of laparoscopy in the staging of malignancy has become of vital importance to the surgical oncologist. In a 1911 report,[125] Jacobaeus indicated that by using a laparoscope, diagnoses of metastatic tumors could be confirmed. However, it would be approximately 80 years before the concepts advanced by Jacobaeus would be widely acknowledged and applied by surgeons.[126] The benefits of laparoscopy as compared with laparotomy in the staging of pancreatic cancer,[127] hepatic tumors,[128] metastatic melanoma,[129] and Kaposi's sarcoma[130] have been documented. The application of laparoscopic techniques for the staging of Hodgkin's lymphoma is conceptually appealing and has been successfully performed in a limited number of patients. Further studies are required before recommendations can be made regarding patient selection, sensitivity, and specificity with laparoscopic staging for Hodgkin's lymphoma.

Laparoscopic colon resection is technically feasible in many patients with benign and malignant diseases of the colon. Many questions exist regarding the prudence of using the laparoscopic approach for the definitive treatment of colon cancer. Anecdotal reports of implantation of metastatic colon cancer at trocar sites after laparoscopic colon resection[131, 132] have markedly diminished enthusiasm for this application of laparoscopy. Multi-institutional clinical trials and numerous animal studies are underway in an attempt to define the mechanisms and magnitude of this problem of tumor implantation. The use of laparoscopy in the surgical treatment of benign diseases of the colon or small intestine is an appropriate option for the surgeon experienced with advanced laparoscopic procedures.

Laparoscopic appendectomy is for many surgeons the transitional procedure between simple diagnostic laparoscopy and more advanced procedures. Most surgeons learn basic laparoscopic skills during laparoscopic cholecystectomies and diagnostic procedures. Appendectomy is a commonly performed operation by the general surgeon. The laparoscopic procedure for the removal of the appendix requires the surgeon to operate with two-handed techniques and to manipulate the intestines with laparoscopic instrumentation. This operation serves the basic laparoscopist as training for more advanced procedures while simultaneously delivering improved patient care.

The patient benefits from laparoscopic appendectomy as compared with the traditional open approach are not as evident as those witnessed with the laparoscopic removal of the gallbladder. The primary improvements documented from laparoscopic appendectomy include decreased wound complications, slightly shorter length of hospital stay, decreased postoperative pain, and more rapid resumption of normal activities.[133]

The laparoscopic treatment of gastroesophageal reflux disease has received widespread attention and broad acceptance

TABLE 27–7. Current Status of Laparoscopic Procedures

Accepted

Cholecystectomy
Diagnostic laparoscopy
Staging for malignancy
Colon resection (benign disease)
Appendectomy
Antireflux operations
Small bowel resection
Adhesiolysis
Hernia repair
Splenectomy
Lymphadenectomy
Liver biopsies

Technically Feasible—Possible Future Acceptance

Colon resection (malignancy)
Adrenalectomy
Distal pancreatic resection
Gastrojejunostomy
Cholecystojejunostomy
Operations for ulcer disease
Esophagomyotomy
Gastric resection
Treatment of rectal prolapse
Office based/emergency department procedures
Exploration for trauma (hemodynamically stable)

Not Currently Accepted

Whipple procedure (pancreaticoduodenectomy)
Major hepatic resection
Bypass of aortoiliac occlusive disease
Exploration in the hemodynamically unstable patient

by surgeons, gastroenterologists, and patients. This minimally invasive operation compares favorably with medical treatment of gastroesophageal reflux. The surgical treatment of gastroesophageal reflux can be performed laparoscopically in a manner identical to the open operation but without the morbidity of the abdominal wall incision.

Laparoscopic removal of the spleen, lymph node retrieval, liver biopsies, and small wedge resections of the liver have become common operations in the hands of those with extensive training and experience in advanced laparoscopic procedures.

The laparoscopic repair of hernias is the focus of much controversy among surgeons. Many surgeons now accept laparoscopic herniorrhaphy as an optional, if not preferred, technique for the simultaneous repair of bilateral inguinal hernias. The application of laparoscopic techniques is also widely accepted for the repair of the recurrent inguinal hernia that was initially repaired through a traditional anterior approach. This topic is covered in detail in Chapter 37.

The list of procedures deemed as *Accepted* is certain to undergo continued modification. Long-term follow-up, multi-institutional trials, economic factors, and complication rates are among the factors that will impact the role of specific procedures.

A second category of procedures are those that have been categorized by the authors as *Technically feasible—possible future acceptance.* The reasons that cause a procedure to be categorized in this group are one or more of the following: (1) oncologic concerns, (2) small numbers of patients have successfully undergone this operation, (3) cost-effectiveness has not been demonstrated, and (4) technical complexity limits widespread application.

Laparoscopic colon resection exemplifies the type of operation for which its technical feasibility is well established. However, disturbing reports of trocar site implantation raise questions regarding increased metastases resulting from the laparoscopic environment.[131, 132] A government-sponsored multi-institutional trial is underway to evaluate laparoscopic colon resection for malignant disease. Basic science evaluation of the cause of trocar site tumor implantation has initially revealed a permissive effect on tumor establishment and growth in open operations in a murine model as compared with a peritoneal insufflation group.[73] It would be premature to count laparoscopic colon resection for curative removal of malignancy as accepted until proof of oncologic adequacy has been established.

Laparoscopic adrenalectomy, distal pancreatic resection, gastrojejunostomy, cholecystojejunostomy, operations for ulcer disease, esophagomyotomy, gastric resection, and treatment of rectal prolapse are minimally invasive procedures that have been successfully performed by several skilled, highly experienced laparoscopic surgeons. Many of these operations are performed but a few times each year by surgeons outside of referral centers. The relative infrequency with which these operations are performed makes standardization of approaches and enrollment of patients into studies difficult. It is likely that several years will pass before definitive statements can be made with regard to the appropriate role of laparoscopy in these operations.

Cost-effectiveness of all treatment modalities is under increasing scrutiny. Reimbursement policies have not been consistently established for many new minimally invasive procedures. Although technology and skills exist for office-based diagnostic and minor laparoscopic procedures, it remains extremely challenging to obtain reimbursement for operations outside the traditional settings. Care maps and algorithms, which include laparoscopic procedures in lieu of costly and time-consuming radiologic diagnostic procedures, will facilitate the resolution of reimbursement dilemmas.

Capitation in the setting of managed care magnifies the benefits of cost-effective laparoscopic operations.

The fourth reason for categorizing a laparoscopic operation as *Technically feasible—possible future acceptance* is technical complexity, which limits widespread acceptance. Laparoscopic adrenalectomy is an operation that presents the surgeon with the challenges of difficult exposure, tedious dissection, a friable organ, and potential for serious complications, including massive blood loss. Procedures of this nature should be undertaken only by surgical teams with large, successful experience with advanced laparoscopic operations. Several of the more complex laparoscopic operations will not be performed by all general surgeons.

Laparoscopy for the trauma patient warrants specific attention. Berci and colleagues[134] reported the successful application of diagnostic laparoscopy in trauma patients. This report predated the modern era of laparoscopic surgery. More recently, other authors[135–137] have demonstrated the efficacy of diagnostic laparoscopy in the trauma setting. Studies are needed to demonstrate superior sensitivity, specificity, and time efficiency for laparoscopy as compared with diagnostic peritoneal lavage and computed tomography before diagnostic laparoscopy for the evaluation of the injured patient is widely accepted.

Almost every operation performed by the general surgeon has undergone evaluation for the potential of a less invasive alternative. There are some operations that are unlikely to be performed by laparoscopic techniques in the foreseeable future. The Whipple procedure or pancreatoduodenectomy is one such operation. This operation includes the accomplishment of multiple, precise anastomoses. The complexity of these technical feats combined with the oncologic concerns and relative infrequency with which most surgeons perform this operation makes the acceptance of a laparoscopic approach unlikely.

Major hepatic resection illustrates another facet of an operation that is unlikely to be regularly performed laparoscopically. The removal of a large specimen requires morcellation, fracturing, or destruction of the specimen. Fracturing solid organs within a bag, such as spleens removed for hematologic disorders, poses no problems for the pathologist. However, hepatic resections are usually performed for malignancies, and identification of surgical margins on an intact specimen is of oncologic significance. Current techniques do not allow for the removal of an intact solid organ without an incision of significant size.

The use of laparoscopy in the surgical management of major vascular disease is undergoing evaluation in a limited fashion. It would be a misrepresentation to categorize laparoscopic vascular surgery in any way except currently unaccepted by general and vascular surgeons. There is little doubt that many vascular disorders will eventually be managed by minimally invasive techniques. Most of these techniques will use a transluminal approach. Laparoscopy will in all likelihood have a limited and transient role in the treatment of vascular abnormalities.

The procedures categorized in Table 27–7 are not intended as comprehensive, but rather as representative, lists. These lists are formed entirely by the opinions of this chapter's authors and not by credentialing or governing bodies. Table 27–7 should be used by the reader for the purposes of education or debate.

COMPLICATIONS

One cannot equate the term *minimal invasion* with minimal risk. Laparoscopic operations carry many of the same inherent risks as their traditional open counterparts. Additionally, there are risks that are attributable to the laparoscopic

TABLE 27–8. Complications Specific to Laparoscopy

Abdominal Wall Complications

Trocar site bleeding
Trocar site hernia
Trocar site infection
Trocar site fistula (e.g., biliary, enterocutaneous)

Visceral or Vascular Injuries

Thermal injuries
Trocar/Veress needle injuries
Visceral/vascular puncture
Instrument trauma (e.g., serosal tear of bowel from grasper)

Retained Foreign Bodies

Inorganic: instrument parts, clips, needle or suture material
Organic: lost gallstones, tissue fragments, blood clots

Pneumoperitoneum (Access)–Related Complications

Cardiopulmonary
Renal failure
Hypothermia
Venous thrombosis
Minor (e.g., subcutaneous emphysema)

TABLE 27–10. Conditions That May Precipitate Complications of Laparoscopy

Prior abdominal surgery
Obesity
Generalized peritonitis
Minor bleeding disorder
Uncontrolled coagulopathy
Pregnancy
Acute and chronic inflammation
Bowel obstruction with massively dilated bowel

method (Table 27–8). Awareness of these potential complications and the limitations of the laparoscopic method (Table 27–9) are the first steps toward preventing them. Awareness of conditions that may increase the risk of complications is equally important (Table 27–10). Although contraindications to a laparoscopic approach at present are few, many of these conditions were once regarded as contraindications and still demand careful consideration.

TRAINING AND CREDENTIALING ISSUES

The rapid evolution of laparoscopic surgery beginning with laparoscopic cholecystectomy has created unprecedented challenges in training and credentialing within this field.[138–140] The highly successful and time-honored method of training surgeons within a structured residency program was not applicable to practicing general surgeons who had completed a residency training program before the laparoscopic cholecystectomy era. Consequently, postgraduate courses of varying quality sprang up in an effort to meet the demand for training. Because of inherent limitations of these

weekend courses and the fact that the technique for laparoscopic cholecystectomy had not been perfected, many surgeons received inadequate training. As a result, the incidence of complications related to laparoscopic cholecystectomy, especially bile duct injuries, was inordinately high in the first few years after its introduction. Surgical societies such as the Society of American Gastrointestinal and Endoscopic Surgeons have taken the lead and responded by creating practical and well-thought-out guidelines for teaching, credentialing, and privileging within laparoscopic surgery (Table 27–11). The primary emphasis has been patient safety. These guidelines will undoubtedly be modified as new laparoscopic procedures and training methods develop.

Laparoscopic surgery has affected training within surgical residency programs in similarly profound ways.[141] Many operations in the prelaparoscopic era, such as appendectomy, cholecystectomy, and herniorrhaphy, were the primary teaching operations for junior residents. Due to the technical challenges of the laparoscopic method, these procedures have been delegated to more senior residents, leaving few procedures for junior residents to acquire basic surgical skills. Recently, however, in many surgical residency programs laparoscopic procedures are beginning to "trickle down" to junior residents as the faculty and senior residents become more experienced. In addition, there has been concern that residents will not acquire sufficient experience with open procedures to be able to adequately handle, for example, the difficult cholecystectomy that must be performed in an open fashion. These issues and others will undoubtedly occupy the attention of surgical educators as laparoscopic surgery finds its place within surgical residency training.

TABLE 27–9. Inherent Features of Laparoscopy That May Precipitate Complications

Altered Visibility

Two-dimensional view
Limited depth of view
Magnified view
Limited field of view
Limited angle of view (improved somewhat with angled scopes)
Laparoscopic "blind spots" of abdomen
Cautery smoke accumulation
Fogged lens or lens soilage
Equipment failure (light source, camera, monitor)

Reduced Sensation

Inability to manually dissect (e.g., periesophageal dissection during open Nissen fundoplication)
Inability to manually diagnose disease (e.g., intraluminal tumors of colon, intraparenchymal tumors of liver)

Limited Instrument Movement

Fulcrum effect of operating ports

TABLE 27–11. Guidelines for Privileges in Laparoscopic Surgery

1. Completion of a residency or fellowship that includes structured experience in laparoscopic surgery
2. Alternatively, demonstration of proficiency and clinical judgment equivalent to that obtained in a residency or fellowship program. Documentation of competence and verification by experienced colleagues is required.
3. For the surgeon lacking either of the above requirements the following basic minimum requirements are recommended:
   a. Completion of a residency in general surgery
   b. Privileges in diagnostic laparoscopy
   c. First-assisting in laparoscopic operations performed by an experienced surgeon
   d. Proctoring by an experienced laparoscopic surgeon until proficiency is observed and documented in writing

Adapted from Society of American Gastrointestinal Endoscopic Surgeons (SAGES) Publication No. 14: Granting of Privileges for Laparoscopic (Peritoneoscopic) General Surgery; May 1990, originally Publication No. 5 [published in American Journal of Surgery 161:324–325], January 1990. Revised October 1992 [Surgical Endocscopy 7:1 (Jan, Feb/93), pp. 67–68]. SAGES WWW Address: http://www.sages.org/sages.html.

SELECTED REFERENCES

Complications of laparoscopy: Strategies for prevention. *In* Soper, N. J., Odem, R. R., Clayman, R. V., and McDougall, E. M. (Eds.): Essentials of Laparoscopy. St. Louis, Quality Medical Publishing, 1994, p. 215.

In this chapter of a well-written textbook of laparoscopy the authors present a comprehensive yet concise discussion of complications related specifically to laparoscopy. The chapter also provides practical information regarding measures to prevent their occurrence and strategies to manage complications once they occur.

Davis, C. J., and Filipi, C. J.: A History of Endoscopic Surgery. *In* Arregui, M. E., Fitzgibbons, R. J., Katkhouda, M., McKernan, J. B., and Reich, H. (Eds.): Principles of Laparoscopic Surgery: Basic and Advanced Techniques. New York, Springer-Verlag, 1995, p. 3.

The authors present a history of the principal developments in laparoscopic surgery from ancient times through the modern age. Many details not found in other reviews are cited.

Deziel, D. J.: Complications of cholecystectomy: Incidence, clinical manifestations, and diagnosis. Surg. Clin. North Am., 74:809, 1994.

This article is a comprehensive review of complications of open and laparoscopic cholecystectomy. It provides a particularly detailed analysis of bile duct injuries resulting from both methods. The relative incidence of other technical and nontechnical complications is reviewed.

Meyers, W. C., Branum, G. D., and Farouk, M.: A prospective analysis of 1518 laparoscopic cholecystectomies. N. Engl. J. Med., 324:1072, 1991.

This is a landmark article that was the first prospective study to clearly demonstrate the safety and efficacy of laparoscopic cholecystectomy in a large group of patients. This study has probably been cited more than any other single study in modern laparoscopic literature.

Peters, J. H., and DeMeester, T. R. (Eds.): Minimally Invasive Surgery of the Foregut. St. Louis, Quality Medical Publishing, Inc., 1994, pp. 23–27.

This chapter defines many of the important physiologic issues of laparoscopic surgery. It reviews in significant detail the pathophysiology of increased intra-abdominal pressure and hypercarbia related to CO_2 pneumoperitoneum. It also reviews the effect of laparoscopic surgery on pulmonary function, the stress response, organ perfusion, and immune function. Helpful diagrams are included.

Steiner, C. A., Bass, E. B., Talamini, M. A., Pitt, H. A., and Steinberg, E. P.: Surgical rates and operative mortality for open and laparoscopic cholecystectomy in Maryland. N. Engl. J. Med., 330:403, 1994.

This is an important study that specifically addresses the effect of the introduction laparoscopic cholecystectomy on rates of cholecystectomy as well as mortality. The study involved over 67,000 patients over a 7-year period (1985–1992). The authors noted a 28% increase in the total rate of cholecystectomy and a 33% reduction in overall operative mortality per procedure since the adoption of laparoscopic cholecystectomy in Maryland. The total number of cholecystectomy-related deaths, however, did not fall, presumably because of the increase in the number of cases performed.

REFERENCES

1. Nitze, M.: Eine neue Beobachtungs und Untersuchungsmethode für Harnröhre, Harnblase und Rectum. Wien Med. Wochenschr., 24:649, 1879.
2. Davis, C. J., and Filipi, C. J.: A history of endoscopic surgery. *In* Arregui, M. E., Fitzgibbons, R. J., Katkhouda M, McKernan, J. B., and Reich, H. (Eds.): Principles of Laparoscopic Surgery: Basic and Advanced Techniques. New York, Springer, 1995, p. 3.
3. Kelling, G.: Ueber Oesophagoskopie, Gastroskopie und Kolioskopie. Munch. Med. Wochenschr., 1:21, 1902.
4. Ott, D.: Illumination of the abdomen (ventroscopy) (in Russian). J. Akush. I. Zhensk. Boliez., 15:1045, 1901.
5. Jacobaeus, H. C.: Ueber die Moglichkeit die Zystodkopie bei Untersuchung seroser Hohlungen anzuwenden. Munch. Med. Wochenschr., 57:2090, 1910.
6. Jacobaeus, H. C.: Kurze Ubersicht uber meine Erfahrungen mit der Laparo-thorakoskopie. Munch. Med. Wochenschr., 58:2017, 1911.
7. Orndoff, B. H.: The peritoneoscope in diagnosis of diseases of the abdomen. J. Radiol., 1:307, 1920.
8. Bernheim, B.: Cytoscopy of the abdominal cavity. Ann. Surg., 53:764, 1911.
9. Goetze, O.: Die Rontgendiagnostik bei gasgefulter Bauchhohle eine neue Methode. Munch. Med. Wochenschr., 65:1275, 1918.
10. Veress, J.: Instrument zur Ausfuhrung von Brustoder Bauchpunktionen und Pneumothoraxbehandlung. Dtsch. Med. Wochenschr., 64:1480, 1938.
11. Semm, K.: History. *In* Sanfilippo, J. S., and Levine, R. L. (Eds.): Operative Gynecologic Endoscopy. New York, Springer, 1989, p. 1.
12. Ruddock, J. C.: Peritoneoscopy. Surg. Gynecol. Obstet., 65:623, 1937.
13. Hopkins, H. H., and Kapany, N. S.: A flexible fiberscope, using static scanning. Nature, 173:39, 1954.
14. Hopkins, H. H.: The modern urological endoscope. *In* Gow, J. G., and Hopkins, H. H. (Eds.): Handbook of Urological Endoscopy. Edinburgh, Churchill Livingstone, 1978, p. 20.
15. Filipi, C. J., Fitzgibbons, R. J., and Salerno, G. M.: Historical review: Diagnostic laparoscopy to laparoscopic cholecystectomy and beyond. *In*

Zucher, K. (Ed.): Surgical Laparoscopy. St. Louis, Quality Medical Publishers, 1991, p. 3.
16. Muhe, E.: Laparoskopische Cholezystekomie-Spatergebnisse. Langenbecks. Arch. Chir. Suppl. 416, 1991.
17. National Center for Health Statistics: Detailed diagnoses and surgical procedures for patients discharged from short-stay hospitals, United States, 1983–1993. DHHS publication No. (PHS) 94–1779. Hyattsville, MD, U.S. Government Printing Office, October 1995.
18. Davidoff, A. M., Pappas, T. N., Muray, E. A., et al.: Mechanisms of major biliary injury during laparoscopic cholecystectomy. Ann. Surg., 215:196, 1992.
19. Schauer, P. R., Meyers, W. C., Eubanks, S. W., Norem, R. F., Franklin, M., and Pappas, T. N.: Mechanisms of gastric and esophageal perforations during laparoscopic Nissen fundoplication. Ann. Surg., 223:43, 1996.
20. Gadacz, T. R.: U.S. experience with laparoscopic cholecystectomy. Am. J. Surg., 165:450, 1993.
21. Cuschieri, A., Dubois, F., Mouiel, J., et al.: The European experience with laparoscopic cholecystectomy. Am. J. Surg., 161:385, 1991.
22. Chantigian, R. C., and Chantigian, P. D. M.: Anesthesia for laparoscopy. *In* Corfman, R. S., Diamond, M. P., and DeCherney, A. (Eds.): Laparoscopy and Hysteroscopy. Oxford, Blackwell Scientific Publications, 1993, pp. 11–21.
23. Motew, M., Ivankovich, A. D., Bieniarz, J., Albrecht, R. F., Zahed, B., and Scommegna, A.: Cardiovascular effects and acid-base and blood gas changes during laparoscopy. Am. J. Obstet. Gynecol., 115:1002, 1973.
24. Versichelen, L., Serreyn, R., Rolly, G., and Vanderkerckhove, D.: Physiopathologic changes during anesthesia administration for gynecologic laparoscopy. J. Reprod. Med., 29:697, 1984.
25. Ho, H. S., Gunther, R. A., and Wolfe, B. M.: Intraperitoneal carbon dioxide insufflation and cardiopulmonary functions: Laparoscopic cholecystectomy in pigs. Arch. Surg., 127:928, 1992.
26. Mclaughlin, J. G., Scheeres, D. E., Dean, R. J., and Bonnell, B. W.: The adverse hemodynamic effects of laparoscopic cholecystectomy. Surg. Endosc., 9:121, 1995.
27. Ortega, A. E., and Peters, J. H.: Physiologic alterations of endosurgery. *In* Peters, J. H., and DeMeester, T. R. (Eds.): Minimally Invasive Surgery of the Foregut. St. Louis, Quality Medical, 1994, pp. 23–37.
28. Safran, D. B., and Orlando, R.: Physiologic effects of pneumoperitoneum. Am. J. Surg., 167:281, 1994.
29. Marathe, U. S., Lilly, R. E., Silvestry, S. C., Schauer, P. R., Pappas, T. N., Davis, J. W., and Glower, D. D.: Alterations in hemodynamics and left ventricular contractility during carbon dioxide pneumoperitoneum. Surg. Endosc. (in press).
30. Shantha, T. R., and Harden, J.: Laparoscopic cholecystectomy: Anesthesia-related complications and guidelines. Surg. Laparosc. Endosc., 1:173, 1991.
31. See, W. A., Monk, T. G., and Weldon B, C.: Complications of laparoscopy: Strategies for prevention. *In* Soper, N. J., Odem, R. R., Clayman, R. V., and McDougall, E. M. (Eds.): Essentials of Laparoscopy. St. Louis, Quality Medical Publishing, 1994, p. 215.
32. Carmichael, D. E.: Laparoscopy—cardiac considerations. Fertil. Steril., 22:69, 1971.
33. Safran, D., Sgambati, S., and Orlando, R.: Laparoscopy in high-risk patients. Surg. Gynecol. Obstet., 176:548, 1993.
34. Caldwell, C. B., and Ricotta, J. J.: Changes in visceral blood flow with elevated intraabdominal pressure. J. Surg. Res., 43:1, 1987.
35. Ishizaki, Y., Bandai, Y., Shimomura, K., Abe, H., Ohtomo, Y., and Idezuki, Y.: Changes in splanchnic blood flow and cardiovascular effects following peritoneal insufflation of carbon dioxide. Surg. Endosc., 7:420, 1993.
36. Richards, W. O., Scovill, W., Shin, B., and Reed, W.: Acute renal failure associated with increased intra-abdominal pressure. Ann. Surg., 197:183, 1983.
37. Iwase, K., Takenaka, H., Ishizaka, T., Ohata, T., Oshima, S., and Sakaguchi, K.: Serial changes in renal function during laparoscopic cholecystectomy. Eur. Surg. Res., 25:203, 1994.
38. Chui, P. T., Gin, T., and Oh, T. E.: Anaesthesia for laparoscopic general surgery. Anaesth. Intensive Care, 21:163, 1993.
39. Wittgen, C. M., Andrus, C. H., Fitzgerald, S. D., Baudendistel, L. J., Dahms, T. E., and Kaminski, D. L.: Analysis of the hemodynamic and ventilatory effects of laparoscopic cholecystectomy. Arch. Surg., 126:997, 1991.
40. Farouck, O., Saba, A., Fath, J., et al.: Increases in intra-abdominal pressure affect pulmonary compliance. Arch. Surg., 130:544, 1995.
41. Feig, B. W., Berger, D. H., Dougherty, T. B., et al.: Pharmacologic intervention can reestablish baseline hemodynamic parameters during laparoscopy. Surgery, 116:733, 1994.
42. Leighton, T. A., Liu, S., and Bongard, F. S.: Comparative cardiopulmonary effects of carbon dioxide versus helium pneumoperitoneum. Surgery, 113:527, 1993.
43. Eisenhauer, D. M., Saunders, C. J., Ho, H. S., and Wolfe, B. M.: Hemodynamic effects of argon pneumoperitoneum. Surg. Endosc., 8:315, 1993.
44. Smith, R. S., Fry, W. R., Tsoi E. K. M., et al.: Gasless laparoscopy and conventional instruments: The next phase of minimally invasive surgery. Arch. Surg., 128:1102, 1993.
45. Schauer, P. R., Eubanks, S. W., Pappas, T. N., and Meyers, W. C.: Cardiopulmonary effects of gasless laparoscopy, vs. CO_2 pneumoperitoneum. Surg. Endosc., 10:182, 1996.

46. Kehlet, H.: The modifying effect of general and regional anesthesia on the endocrine-metabolic response to surgery. Reg. Anesth., 7:38, 1982.

47. Birch, K., Jorgensen, J., Chraemmer-Jorgensen, B., Kehlet, H.: Effect of I.V. lignocaine on pain and the endocrine metabolic responses after surgery. Br. J. Anaesth., 59:721, 1987.

48. Schulze, S., Sommer, P., and Bigler, D.: Effect of combined prednisolone, epidural analgesia, and indomethacin on the systemic response after colonic surgery. Arch. Surg., 127:325, 1992.

49. Wilmore, D. W.: Homeostasis: Bodily changes in trauma and surgery. In Sabiston, D. C., Jr. (Ed.): Textbook of Surgery: The Biologic Basis of Modern Surgical Practice, 14th ed. Philadelphia, W. B. Saunders, 1991, p. 19.

50. O'Riordain, M., Ross, J. A., and Fearon, K. C. H.: The inflammatory and metabolic response to open surgery and minimally invasive surgery. In Patterson-Brown S, and Garden, J. (Eds.): Principles and Practice of Surgical Laparoscopy. London, W. B. Saunders, 1994, p. 7.

51. Stoner, H. B., and Frayn, K. N.: The relationship between plasma substrates and hormones and the severity of injury in 277 recently injured patients. Clin. Sci., 56:563, 1979.

52. Vaughan, G. M., and Becker, R. A.: Cortisol and corticotrophin in burned patients. J. Trauma, 22:263, 1982.

53. Schauer, P. R., and Sirinek, K. R.: The laparoscopic approach reduces the endocrine response to elective cholecystectomy. Am. Surg., 61:106, 1995.

54. Joris, J., Cigarini, I., Legrand, M., et al.: Metabolic and respiratory changes after cholecystectomy performed via laparotomy or laparoscopy. Br. J. Anaesth., 69:341, 1992.

55. Mealy, K., Gallagher, H., Traynor, O., and Hyland, J.: Physiological and metabolic responses to open and laparoscopic cholecystectomy. Br. J. Surg., 79:1061, 1992.

56. Targarona, E. M., Pons, M. J., Martinez, J., et al.: Neuroendocrine and acute phase response to laparoscopic cholecystectomy: A comparative study with open cholecystectomy. IHPBA Abstract Book. Boston, 1994, (F100)51.

57. Dominioni, L., Cuffari, S., Giudce, G., Carcano, G., Nicora, L., and Dionigi, R.: The acute phase response after laparoscopic cholecystectomy and after open cholecystectomy. HPB Surg., 6:65, 1993.

58. Roumen, R. M. H., van Meurs, P. A., Kuypers, H. H. C., Kraak, W. A. G., and Sauerwein, R. W.: Serum interleukin-6 and C-reactive protein responses in patients after laparoscopic or conventional cholecystectomy. Eur. Surg. Res., 158:541, 1992.

59. Cho, J. M., LaPorta, A. J., Clark, J. R., Schofield, M. J., Hammond, S. L., and Mallory, P. L.: Response of serum cytokines in patients undergoing laparoscopic cholecystectomy. Surg. Endosc., 8:1380, 1994.

60. McMahon, A. J., O'Dwyer, P. J., Cruikshank, A. M., et al.: Comparison of metabolic responses to laparoscopic and minilaparotomy cholecystectomy. Br. J. Surg., 80:1255, 1993.

61. Nohr, C.: Non-AIDS immunosuppression. In Wilmore, D. W., Brennan, M. F., Harken, A. H., Holcroft, J. W., and Meakins, J. L. (Eds.): American College of Surgeons Care of the Surgical Patient, Section VII. New York, Scientific American, 1993, pp. 1–18.

62. Jubert, A. V., Lee, E. T., Hersh, E. M., and McBride, C. M.: Effects of surgery, anesthesia and intraoperative blood loss on immunocompetence. J. Surg. Res., 15:399, 1973.

63. Slade, M. S., Simmons, R. L., Yunis, E., and Greenberg, L. J.: Immunodepression after major surgery in normal patients. Surgery, 78:363, 1975.

64. Deitch, E. A.: Infection in the compromised host. Surg. Clin. North Am., 68:181, 1988.

65. Christou, N. V., Mclean, A. P. H., and Meakins, J. L.: Host defense in blunt trauma: Interrelationships of kinetic of anergy and depressed neutrophil function, nutritional status, and sepsis. J. Trauma, 20:833, 1980.

66. Nohr, C. W., Latter, D. A., Meakins, J. L., and Christou, N. V.: In vivo and in vitro humoral immunity in surgical patients: Antibody response to pneumococcal polysaccharide. Surgery, 100:229, 1986.

67. Deitch, E. A., and Bridges, R. M.: Stress hormones modulate neutrophil and lymphocyte activity in vitro. J. Trauma, 27(10):1146, 1987.

68. Beutler, B.: Identity of tumor necrosis factor and the macrophage-secreted factor cachectin. Nature, 316:552, 1985.

69. Ninnemann, J. L., Stockland, A. E., and Condie, J. T.: Induction of prostaglandin synthesis-dependent suppressor cells with endotoxin: Occurrence in patients with thermal injuries. J. Clin. Immunol., 3:142, 1983.

70. Clowes, G. H.: Survival form sepsis: The significance of altered protein metabolism regulated by proteolysis inducing factor, the circulating cleavage product of interleukin-1. Ann. Surg., 202:446, 1985.

71. Bessler, M., Whelan, R. L., Halverson, A., Treat, M. R., and Nowygrod, R.: Is immune function better preserved after laparoscopic versus open colon resection? Surg. Endosc., 8:881, 1994.

72. Trokel, M. J., Bessler, M., Treat, M. R., Whelan, R. L., and Nowygrod, R.: Preservation of immune response after laparoscopy. Surg. Endosc., 8:1385, 1994.

73. Allendorf, J. D. F., Bessler, M., Kayton, M. L., Whelan, R. L., and Nowygrod, R.: Tumor growth after laparotomy or laparoscopy: A preliminary study. Surg. Endosc., 9:49, 1995.

74. Kloosterman, T., von Blomberg, M. B. E., Borgstein, P., Cuesta, M. A., Scheper, R. J., and Meijer, S.: Unimpaired immune function after laparoscopic cholecystectomy. Surgery, 115:424, 1994.

75. Redmond, H. P., Watson, R. W. G., Houghton, T., Condron, C., Watson,

R. G. K., and Bouchier-Hayes, D.: Immune function in patients undergoing open vs. laparoscopic cholecystectomy. Arch. Surg., 129:1240, 1994.

76. Nduka, C. C., Monson, J. R. T., Menzies-Gow, N., and Darzi, A.: Abdominal wall metastases following laparoscopy. Br. J. Surg., 81:648, 1994.

77. Deziel, D. J.: Complications of cholecystectomy: Incidence, clinical manifestations, and diagnosis. Surg. Clin. North Am., 74:809, 1994.

78. Williams, L. F., Chapman, W. C., Bonau, R. A., McGee, E. C., Boyd, R. W., and Jacobs, J. K.: Comparison of laparoscopic cholecystectomy with open cholecystectomy in a single center. Am. J. Surg., 165:459, 1993.

79. Bartlett, R. H.: Pulmonary pathophysiology in surgical patients. Surg. Clin. North Am., 60:1323, 1980.

80. Rehder, K., Sessler, A. D., and Marsh, H. F.: General anesthesia and the lung. Am. Rev. Respir. Dis., 112:541, 1975.

81. Latimer, R. G., Kickman, M., Dav, W. C., Gunn, M. L., and Schmidt, C. D.: Ventilatory patterns and pulmonary complications after upper abdominal surgery determined by preoperative and postoperative computerized spirometry and blood gas analysis. Am. J. Surg., 122:622, 1971.

82. Meyers, J. R., Lembeck, L, O'Kane, H., and Baue, A. E.: Changes in functional residual capacity of the lung after operation. Arch. Surg., 110:576, 1975.

83. Bartlett, R. H., Brennan, M. L., Gazzaniga, A. B., and Hanson, E. L.: Studies on the pathogenesis and prevention of postoperative pulmonary complications. Surg. Gynecol. Obstet., 137:925, 1973.

84. Frazee, R. C., Roberts, R. W., Okeson, G. C., Symonds, R. E., Snyder, S. K., Hendricks, J. L., and Smith, R. W.: Open vs. laparoscopic cholecystectomy: A comparison of postoperative pulmonary function. Ann. Surg., 213:651, 1991.

85. Peters, J. H., Ortega, A., Lehnerd, S. L., Campbell, A. J., Schwartz, D. C., Ellison, E. C., and Innes, J. T.: The physiology of laparoscopic surgery: Pulmonary function after laparoscopic cholecystecomy. Surg. Laparosc. Endosc., 3:370, 1993.

86. Putensen-Himmer, G., Putensen, C., Lammer, H., Lingnau, W., Aigner, F., and Benzer, H.: Comparison of postoperative respiratory function after laparoscopy or open laparotomy for cholecystectomy. Anesthesiology, 77:675, 1992.

87. McMahon, A. J., Russell, I. T., Ramsay, G., et al.: Laparoscopic and minilaparotomy cholecystectomy: A randomized trial comparing postoperative pain and pulmonary function. Surgery, 115:533, 1994.

88. Schauer, P. R., Luna, J., Ghiatas, A., Glen, M. E., Warren, J. M., and Sirinek, K. R.: Pulmonary function after laparoscopic cholecystectomy. Surgery, 114:389, 1993.

89. Litwin, D. E. M., Girotti, M. J., Poulin, E. C., Mamazza, J., and Nagy, A. G.: Laparoscopic cholecystectomy: Trans-Canada experience with 2201 cases. Can. J. Surg., 35:291, 1992.

90. Meyers, W. C., Branum, G. D., and Farouk, M.: A prospective analysis of 1518 laparoscopic cholecystectomies. N. Engl. J. Med., 324:1072, 1991.

91. Roslyn, J. J., Binns, G. S., Hughes, E. F. X., Kirkwood, K. S., Zinner, M. J., and Cates, J. A.: Open cholecystectomy: A contemporary analysis of 42,474 patients. Ann. Surg., 218:129, 1992.

92. Bollinger, S. H., and Quigley, E. M. M.: Disordered gastrointestinal motility. In Quigley, E. M. M., and Sorrell, M. F. (Eds.): The Gastrointestinal Surgical Patient: Preoperative and Postoperative Care. Baltimore, Williams & Wilkins, 1994, p. 157.

93. Livingston, E. H., and Passaro, E. P.: Postoperative ileus. Dig. Dis. Sci., 35:121, 1990.

94. Carmichael, M. J., Weisbrodt, N. W., and Copeland, E. M.: Effect of abdominal surgery on myoelectric activity in the dog. Am. J. Surg., 133:34, 1977.

95. Hoffman, G. C., Baker, J. W., Fitchett, C. W., and Vansant, J. H.: Laparoscopic-assisted colectomy: Initial experience. Ann. Surg., 219:732, 1994.

96. Senagore, A. J., Luchtefeld, M. A., Mackeigan, J. M., and Mazier, W. P.: Open colectomy versus laparoscopic colectomy: Are there differences? Am. Surg., 56:549, 1993.

97. Schmieg, R. E., Schirmer, B. D., Combs, M. J., Edwards, M., and Fariss, A.: Recovery of gastrointestinal motility after laparoscopic cholecystectomy. Surg. Forum, 44:135, 1993.

98. Ludwig, K. A., Frantzides, C. T., Carlson, M. A., and Grade, K. L.: Myoelectric motility patterns following open versus laparoscopic cholecystectomy. J. Laparoendosc. Surg., 3:461, 1993.

99. Schippers, E., Ottinger, A. P., Anurov, M., Polivoda, M., and Schumpelick, V.: Laparoscopic cholecystectomy: A minor abdominal trauma? World J. Surg., 17:539, 1993.

100. Davies, W., Tu, Q., Kollmorgen, C., et al.: Duration of postoperative ileus after laparoscopic and open segmental colectomy. Gastroenterology, 108(Suppl.):A1217, 1995.

101. Hotokezaka, M., Dix, J., Mentis, E. P., Minasi, J. S., and Schirmer, B. D.: Gastrointestinal recovery following laparoscopic versus open colon surgery (Abstract). Surg. Endosc., 9:215, 1995.

102. Garcia-Caballero, M., and Vara-Thorbeck, C.: The evolution of postoperative ileus after laparoscopic cholecystectomy. Surg. Endosc., 7:416, 1993.

103. Caprini, J. A., and Arcelus, J. I.: Prevention of postoperative venous thromboembolism following laparoscopic cholecystectomy. Surg. Endosc., 8:741, 1994.

104. Mayol, J., Vincent-Hamelin, E., Sarmiento, J. M., et al.: Pulmonary embolism following laparoscopic cholecystectomy: Report of two cases and review of the literature. Surg. Endosc., 8:214, 1994.

105. Strasberg, S. M., Sanabria, J. R., and Clavien, P.: Complications of laparoscopic cholecystectomy. Can. J. Surg., 35:275, 1992.

106. Beebe, D. S., McNevin, M. P., Crain, J. M., et al.: Evidence of venous stasis after abdominal insufflation for laparoscopic cholecystectomy. Surg. Gynecol. Obstet., 176:443, 1993.

107. Millard, J. A., Hill, B. B., Cook, P. S., Fenoglio, M. E., and Stahlgren, L. H.: Intermittent sequential pneumatic compression in prevention of venous stasis associated with pneumoperitoneum during laparoscopic cholecystectomy. Arch. Surg., 128:914, 1993.

108. Schaub, R. D., Lynch, P. R., and Stewart, G. J.: The response of canine veins to three types of abdominal surgery: A scanning and transmission electron microscopic study. Surgery, 83:411, 1978.

109. Acrelus, J. I., Caprini, J. A., Traverso, C. I., Size, G., and Hasty, J. H.: The role of elastic compression stockings to prevent venous dilatation induced by a reverse Trendelenburg position. Phlebology, 8:111, 1993.

110. Sripad, S., Antcliff, A. C., and Martin, P.: Deep venous thrombosis in two district hospitals in Essex. Br. J. Surg., 58:563, 1971.

111. Seyfer, A. E., Seaber, A., Dombrose, F. A., and Urbaniak, J. R.: Coagulation changes in elective surgery and trauma. Ann. Surg., 193:210, 1981.

112. Velpen, G. V., Penninckx, F., Kerremans, R., Van Damme, J., and Arnout, J.: Interleukin-6 and coagulation-fibrinolysis fluctuations after laparoscopic and conventional cholecystectomy. Surg. Endosc., 8:1216, 1994.

113. Caprini, J. A., Arcelus, J. I., Traverso, C. I., Vittum, D., and Adams, P.: Hypercoagulability after laparoscopic cholecystectomy. Thromb. Haemost., 65:1347, 1991.

114. Hoffman, K. N., Arcelus, J. I., Traverso, C. I., et al.: Prevention of venous thromboembolism: Results of a survey among North American surgeons. Thromb. Haemost., 69:622, 1993.

115. Ellis, H.: The causes and prevention of intestinal adhesions. Br. J. Surg., 69:241, 1982.

116. Drollette, C. M., and Badaway, S. Z. A.: Pathophysiology of pelvic adhesions: Modern trends in preventing infertility. J. Reprod. Med., 37:107, 1992.

117. Annibali, R., Camps, J., Nguyen, N., and Fitzgibbons, R.: Prosthetic materials and adhesion formation. In Arregui, M. E., Fitzgibbons, R. J., Katkhouda, N., McKernan, B., and Reich, H. (Eds.): Principles of Laparoscopic Surgery: Basic and Advanced Techniques. New York, Springer-Verlag, 1995, p. 426.

118. Luciano, A. A., Maier, D. B., Koch, E. I., Nulsen, J. C., and Whitman, G. F.: A comparative study of postoperative adhesions following laser surgery by laparoscopy versus laparotomy in the rabbit model. Obstet. Gynecol., 74:220, 1989.

119. Lundorff, P., Hahlin, M., Bjorn, K., Thorburn, J., and Lindblom, B.: Adhesion formation after laparoscopic surgery in tubal pregnancy: A randomized trial versus laparotomy. Fertil. Steril., 55:911, 1991.

120. Schauer, P. R., Page, C. P., Schwesinger, W. H., and Sirinek, K. R.: The effect of laparoscopic cholecystectomy on the morbidity and mortality of elective cholecystectomy in high risk patients (Abstract). Minimally Invasive Therapy, 4(Suppl. 1):3, 1995.

121. Steiner, C. A., Bass, E. B., Talamini, M. A., Pitt, H. A., and Steinberg, E. P.: Surgical rates and operative mortality for open and laparoscopic cholecystectomy in Maryland. N. Engl. J. Med., 330:403, 1994.

122. Soper, N. J., Stockmann, P. T., Dunnegan, D. L., and Ashley, S. W.: Laparoscopic cholecystectomy: The new 'gold standard'? Arch. Surg., 127:917, 1992.

123. Gagner, M., and Pomp, A.: Laparoscopic pylorus-preserving pancreaticoduodenectomy. Surg. Endosc., 8:408, 1994.

124. Bailey, R. W., and Flowers, J. L.: Complications of Laparoscopic Surgery. St. Louis, Quality Medical Publishing, 1995.

125. Jacobaeus, H. C.: Kurze ubersichtuber meine Erfahrungen mit der Laparoskopie. Munch. Med. Wochenschr., 58:2017, 1911.

126. Greene, F. L.: Laparoscopy in malignant disease. Surg. Clin. North Am., 72:1125, 1992.

127. Warshaw, A. L., Gu Zhuo-yun, Wittenberg, J., and Waltman, A. C.: Preoperative staging and assessment of resectability of pancreatic cancer. Arch. Surg., 125:230, 1990.

128. Eubanks, S.: The role of laparoscopy in diagnosis and treatment of primary or metastatic liver cancer. Semin. Surg. Oncol., 10:404, 1994.

129. Caldironi, M. W., Nitti, D., Schiavon, M., Rossi, C., Aldinio, M. T., and Azzena, B.: Laparoscopy in the abdominal staging of melanoma. Eur. J. Cancer. Clin. Oncol., 25:223, 1989.

130. Hasan, F. A., Jeffers, L. J., Welsh, S. W., et al.: Hepatic involvement as the primary manifestation of Kaposi's sarcoma in the acquired immune deficiency syndrome. Am. J. Gastroenterol, 84:1449, 1989.

131. Fusco, M. A., and Paluzzi, M. W.: Abdominal wall recurrence after laparoscopic-assisted colectomy for adenocarcinoma of the colon: Report of a case. Dis. Colon Rectum, 36:858, 1993.

132. Cirocco, W. C., Schwartzman, A., and Golub, R. W.: Abdominal wall recurrence after laparoscopic colectomy for colon cancer. Surgery, 116:842, 1994.

133. Attwood, S. E. A., Hill, A. D. K., Murphy, P. G., Thornton, J., and Stephens, R. B.: A prospective randomized trial of laparoscopic versus open appendectomy. Surgery, 112:497, 1992.

134. Berci, G., Sackier, J. M., and Paz-Partlow, M.: Emergency laparoscopy. Am. J. Surg., 161:332, 1991.

135. Fabian, T., Croce, M., Stewart, R., Pritchard, F. E., Minard, G., and Kudsk, K.: A prospective analysis of diagnostic laparoscopy in trauma. Ann. Surg., 217:557, 1993.

136. Gazzaniga, A., Stauton, W., and Bartlett, R.: Laparoscopy in the diagnosis of blunt and penetrating injury to the abdomen. Am. J. Surg., 131:315, 1976.

137. Ivatury, R., Simon, R., and Stahl, W.: A critical evaluation of laparoscopy in penetrating abdominal trauma. J. Trauma, 34:4, 1993.

138. Schrock, T. R., and Dent, T. L.: Teaching, Credentialling, and Privileging. In Arregui, M. E., Fitzgibbons, R. J., Katkhouda, M., McKernan, J. B., and Reich, H. (Eds.): Principles of Laparoscopic Surgery: Basic and Advanced Techniques. New York, Springer-Verlag, 1995, p. 3.

139. Dent, T. L.: Training, credentialing, and evaluation in laparoscopic surgery. Surg. Clin. North Am., 72:1003, 1992.

140. Forde, K.: Endosurgical training methods: Is it surgical training that is out of control? (Editorial). Surg. Endosc., 7:71, 1993.

141. Schauer, P., Page P., Stewart, R., Schwesinger, W., and Sirinek, K.: The effect of laparoscopic cholecystectomy on resident training. Am. J. Surg., 168:566, 1994.

CHAPTER 28

ABDOMINAL WALL, UMBILICUS, PERITONEUM, MESENTERIES, OMENTUM, AND RETROPERITONEUM

Kevin M. Sittig, M.D., Michael S. Rohr, M.D., and John C. McDonald, M.D.

ABDOMINAL WALL

The abdominal wall is a complex musculoaponeurotic structure that is attached to the vertebral column posteriorly, the ribs superiorly, and the bones of the pelvis inferiorly. It is derived embryonically in a segmental, metameric manner, and this is reflected in blood supply and innervation.

The abdominal wall protects and restrains the abdominal viscera, and its musculature acts indirectly to flex the vertebral column. The integrity of the abdominal wall is essential to the prevention of hernias, whether they be congenital, acquired, or iatrogenic. Additionally, the abdominal wall is the repository of the panniculus adiposus, which may reach considerable proportions in some members of the species afflicted with morbid obesity.

The abdominal wall is subject to a wide variety of pathologic processes that may be difficult to assess on physical examination. Computed tomography often delineates these abnormalities.[17]

Embryology. The abdominal wall begins to develop early in the embryo, but it does not achieve its definitive structure until the umbilical cord separates from the fetus at birth. Most of the abdominal wall forms during closure of the midgut and reduction in relative size of the body stalk. The primitive wall is called the somatopleure (ectoderm and mesoderm without muscle, blood vessels, or nerves). The somatopleure of the abdomen is secondarily invaded by mesoderm from the myotomes that develop on either side of the vertebral column. This mesodermal mass (hypomere) migrates ventrally and laterally as a sheet and the leading edges differentiate, while still widely separated from each other, into the right and left rectus abdominis muscles. The final apposition of these muscles in the anterior midline closes the body wall (Fig. 28–1).

Before the primordia of the rectus muscles fuse anteriorly, the mesoderm from the hypomere splits into three layers, which can be recognized by the seventh week of development. The inner sheet differentiates into the transversus abdominis muscle, the middle sheet becomes the internal oblique muscle, and the superficial sheet becomes the external oblique muscle and aponeurosis. Dorsally, the superior and inferior posterior serratus muscles develop from the superficial layer of the hypomere.

Approximation of the two rectus abdominis muscles in the midline proceeds from both the cranial and caudal ends and is complete by the twelfth week, except at the umbilicus. The final closure of the umbilical ring awaits the separation of the cord at birth, but the ring may remain open, in which case an umbilical hernia is present. Most such hernias gradually close spontaneously.

Anatomy, Innervation, and Lymphatic Drainage. The abdominal wall is composed of nine layers. From outward in, they are (1) skin, (2) tela subcutanea (subcutaneous tissue), (3) superficial fascia (Scarpa's fascia), (4) external abdominal oblique muscle, (5) internal abdominal oblique muscle, (6) transversus abdominis muscle, (7) endoabdominal (transversalis) fascia, (8) extraperitoneal adipose and areolar tissue, and (9) peritoneum. Each layer is discussed individually.

The *skin* of the abdomen is general body skin ordinarily unadorned by heavy hair growth. It may be involved in generalized dermatoses but is otherwise unremarkable. It is rarely the site of cutaneous neoplasia because it is usually protected from exposure to the sun.

The *tela subcutanea* contains a layer of soft adipose tissue that generally increases with age. It contains little fibrous connective tissue and affords little strength in closure of abdominal incisions. The tela subcutanea rests upon the superficial fascia (Scarpa's fascia), which is not to be confused with the investing fascia of the abdominal wall muscles.

Scarpa's fascia is a layer of fibrous connective tissue of modest thickness. The layer contains abundant adipose tissue. A discrete layer of the fascia ordinarily can be demonstrated in the lower abdominal wall, and the layer may be confused with aponeurosis of the external oblique muscle by inexperienced surgeons. The layer affords little strength in wound closure, but its approximation aids considerably in the creation of an aesthetic hairline scar.

The *muscular abdominal wall* is composed of three flat muscles that have broad origins. The muscular wall encloses the largest fraction of the circumference of the torso. Anteriorly, the three flat muscles give way to flat aponeuroses that fuse to form the investing fascia (sheath) of the rectus abdominis muscles.

The *external abdominal oblique muscle* (paired right and left) is the largest and thickest of the flat abdominal muscles. Its broad origin includes the last seven ribs, the thoracolumbar fascia (lumbodorsal aponeurosis), the external lip of the iliac crest, and the inguinal ligament that inserts into the pubic tubercle. The muscle belly gives way to a flat, strong aponeurosis at about the midclavicular line, and it inserts medially into the linea alba (Fig. 28–2). The aponeurosis of the external oblique passes anterior to the sheath of the rectus abdominis,

THE ANTERIOR BODY WALL

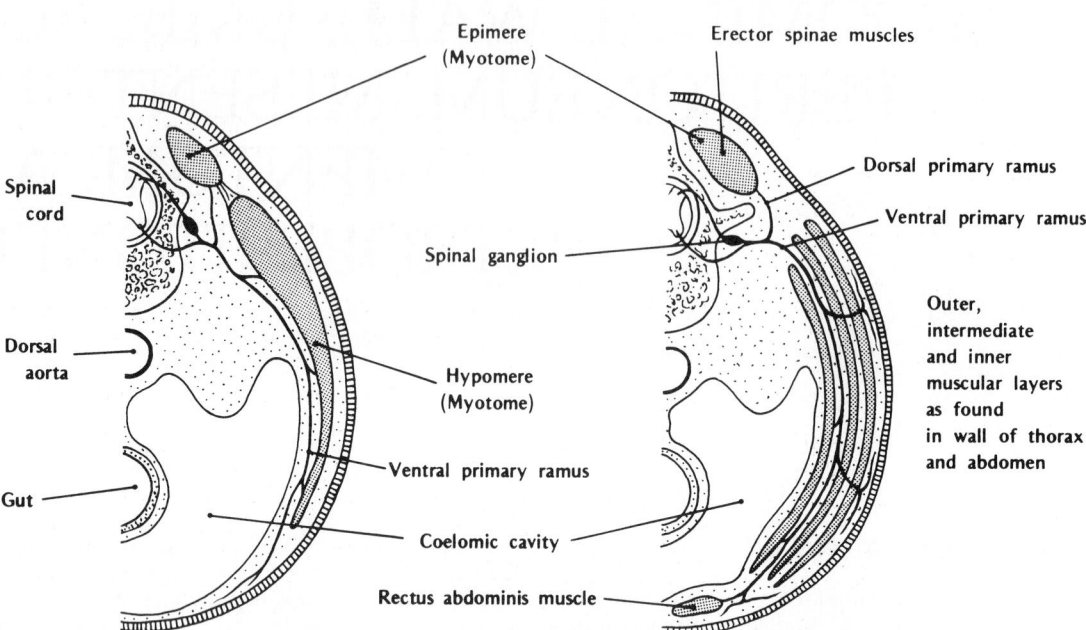

Figure 28–1. Schematic diagram showing the establishment of the primordia of the abdominal wall muscles. On the left, the relationship of the myotomes to the primitive central nervous system and coelomic cavity is shown. On the right, the differentiation of the hypomere to form the three layers of the abdominal wall musculature is depicted. (Modified from Langman, J.: Medical Embryology. Baltimore, Williams & Wilkins, 1969.)

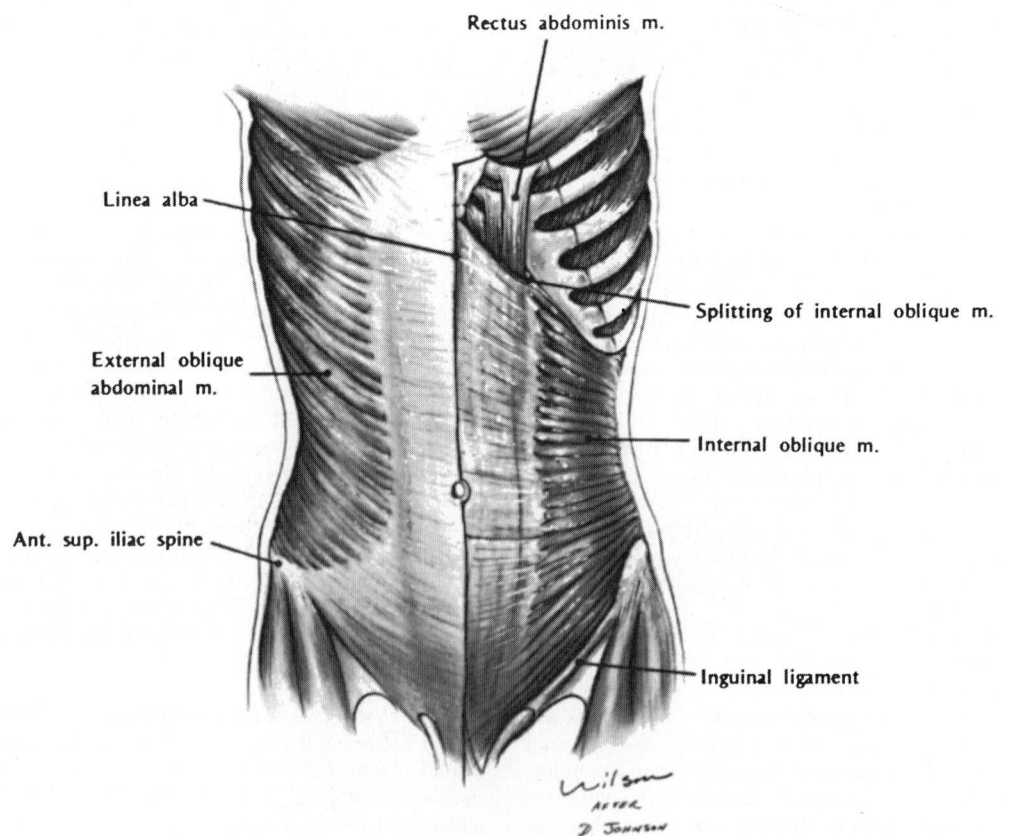

Figure 28–2. Schematic diagram of abdominal wall muscles showing the external oblique and the internal oblique abdominal muscles. The rectus muscles are seen near the midline. The right rectus muscle is covered by the rectus sheath. (Modified from Healey, J. E., Jr.: A Synopsis of Clinical Anatomy. Philadelphia, W. B. Saunders, 1969.)

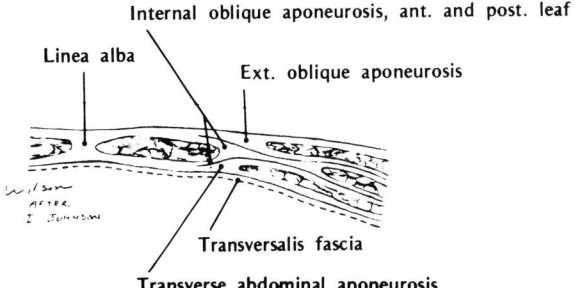

Figure 28–3. Schematic diagram of transverse section of upper abdominal wall muscles near the umbilicus. The aponeurosis of the internal oblique muscle splits to invest the rectus abdominis muscle. (Modified from Healey, J. E., Jr.: A Synopsis of Clinical Anatomy. Philadelphia, W. B. Saunders, 1969.)

and, with care, it can be dissected from it. In general, the fascicles of the external oblique muscle pass from superolateral to inferomedial. Thus, the direction of force generated by contraction of muscle is superolateral.

The *internal abdominal oblique muscle* originates from the last five ribs, the thoracolumbar fascia, the intermediate lip of the iliac crest, and the lateral half of the inguinal ligament. Its fibers course opposite the direction of those of the external oblique. The internal oblique muscle also gives way to a flat aponeurosis medially, which splits to enclose the rectus muscle. The aponeurosis reunites medial to the rectus and inserts into the linea alba (Fig. 28–3). The fibers that arise from the lateral half of the inguinal ligament pursue a downward course and insert into the os pubis between the symphysis and the tubercle. Some of the lower fibers of the internal oblique muscles are pulled into the scrotum by the testis as it passes through the abdominal wall. The latter fibers are called the cremasteric muscle of the spermatic cord. The cremasteric muscle is responsible for a superficial reflex

of the same name, in which the testis is retracted from the scrotum in the direction of the inguinal canal.

The *transversus abdominis muscle* is the smallest of the three flat muscles of the abdomen. Its origin is similar to that of the internal oblique muscle. It originates from the lower five ribs, the thoracolumbar fascia, the internal lip of the iliac crest, and the lateral one third of the inguinal ligament. The direction of its fibers is transverse, and they give way to a flat aponeurosis that inserts into the linea alba. The aponeurosis passes behind the rectus sheath in its upper two thirds. The fibers of the transversus abdominis that originate from the inguinal ligament pass downward to insert the os pubis, as do the fibers of the internal oblique muscle. Occasionally, the lower fibers of both muscles insert by means of a common tendon called the conjoint tendon (Fig. 28–4). Experience in the dissecting laboratory and operating room has led surgeons to believe that a true conjoint tendon occurs only infrequently. More often, the muscles insert into the os pubis as a *conjoint muscle*.

The plane between the internal oblique and transversus abdominis muscles can properly be considered a neurovascular plane because it contains the segmental arteries, veins, and nerves that supply the abdominal wall. The anterior primary rami of thoracic spinal nerves T7 to T12 and lumbar nerve L1 supply the abdominal wall in a segmental, sequential manner from above downward. The main trunks of the nerves are found in the neurovascular plane. The anterior cutaneous rami pierce the rectus sheath anteriorly to supply the anterior skin. The anterior cutaneous rami of T10 innervates a dermatome that includes the umbilicus. The lateral cutaneous rami of T7 through T9 supply skin of the thorax and lateral abdominal wall, and the lateral cutaneous rami of T12 and L1 supply the skin of the gluteal region.

The *transversalis fascia* is poorly named and often misunderstood. It more properly should be called the endoabdominal fascia, because it is a continuous lining of the abdominal

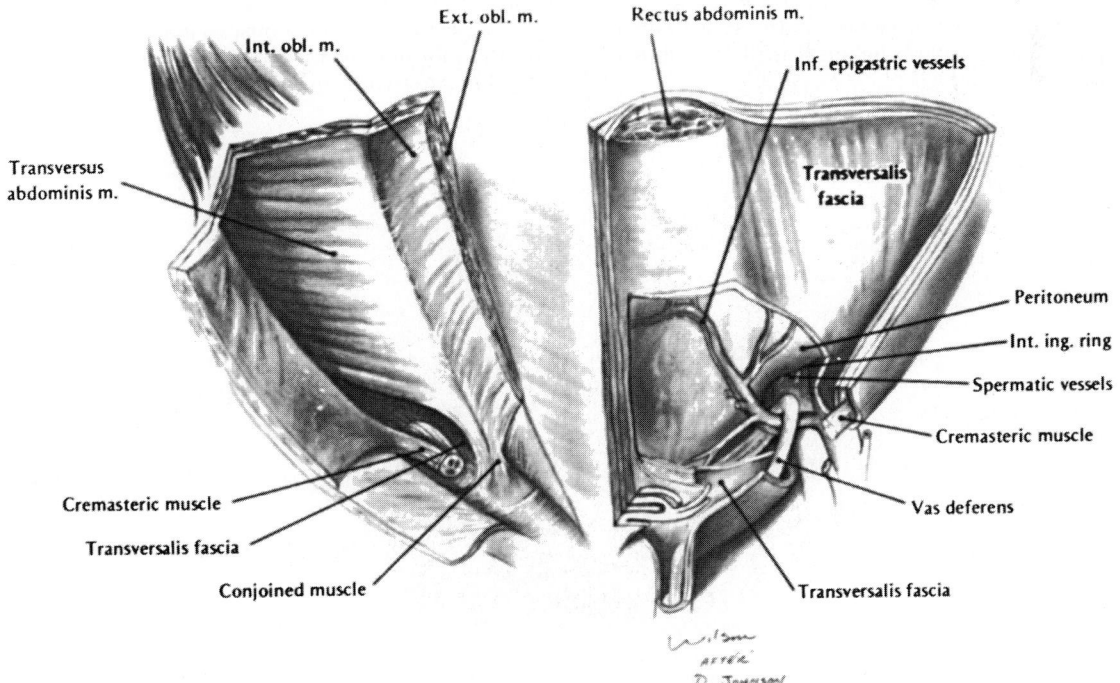

Figure 28–4. The lower abdominal wall and groin are depicted schematically. On the left, the external abdominal oblique and the internal abdominal oblique muscles are reflected, revealing the transversus abdominis muscle and its origin from the lateral half of the inguinal ligament. The cremaster muscle fibers can be seen originating from the lower part of the umternal oblique muscle. The important structures in the inguinal area are depicted. On the right, the transversalis fascia (with a window removed) is shown just superficial to the peritoneum. The inferior epigastric vessels are shown arising from the external iliac vessels. (Modified from Healey, J. E., Jr.: A Synopsis of Clinical Anatomy. Philadelphia, W. B. Saunders, 1969.)

cavity. Where this fascia is in direct relation to certain muscles, it is given a special name. Over the psoas muscle, it is called the *psoas fascia*. Where it lies deep to the transversus abdominis muscle, it is properly called the *transversalis fascia*. The integrity of the endoabdominal fascia is absolutely essential for the integrity of the abdominal wall. If this layer is intact, no hernia exists. A hernia may, in fact, be defined as a hole in the endoabdominal fascia or transversalis fascia. This definition applies to esophageal hiatus hernia, umbilical hernia, inguinal hernia, femoral hernia, and incisional hernia.

The transversalis fascia contains a thickened band, the iliopubic tract, which lies deep to the inguinal ligament. Like the inguinal ligament, the iliopubic tract extends from the anterior-superior spine of the iliac crest to the pubic tubercle. The iliopubic tract is of considerable importance in the repair of groin hernias.

The *extraperitoneal adipose and connective tissue layer* of the abdominal wall is surgically relatively unimportant. It is found between the endoabdominal fascia and the peritoneum. It contains a greater amount of adipose tissue in obese persons. It also contains the remains of four fetal structures and the inferior epigastric arteries and veins. The latter vessels course from the external iliac vessels upward and medial to the rectus sheath, where they supply the rectus abdominis muscle from below (Fig. 28–5). The obliterated umbilical arteries arise from the superior vesical arteries and course upward to the umbilicus. They raise a fold of peritoneum (visible from the inside of the peritoneal cavity) called the medial umbilical ligaments, which are paired right and left. In the midline, the obliterated urachus passes from the apex of the bladder to the umbilicus. It is a fibrous cord that represents the remnant of the allantoic stalk. Like the obliterated umbilical arteries, the obliterated urachus also raises a peritoneal fold, the median umbilical ligament.

Above the umbilicus, in the midline, the extraperitoneal adipose tissue projects deep between the two leaves of the falciform ligament of the liver. In the free margin of this sickle-shaped ligament is found the ligamentum teres hepatis and the obliterated umbilical vein, which courses from the umbilicus to the ligamentum venosum. The space between the two leaves of the falciform ligament is filled with extraperitoneal adipose tissue.

The *parietal peritoneum* is the innermost layer of the abdominal wall. It is a thin layer of dense, irregular connective tissue and is covered on the inside by a layer of simple squamous mesothelium. The peritoneal membrane is innervated from above downward in a sequential manner by spinal nerves T7 to L1. The peritoneum provides little strength in wound closure, but it affords remarkable protection from infection if it remains unviolated.

The rectus muscles and rectus sheath require special description. The muscles are paired right and left, and they extend from the fifth rib superiorly to the pubis inferiorly. They lie in apposition to each other, being separated only by the linea alba. Each muscle is a long, flat triangular ribbon, being wider above than below. Each muscle is composed of long, parallel fascicles interrupted by three tendinous inscriptions (Fig. 28–6). The rectus muscles serve to support the abdominal wall and to flex the vertebral column. Each muscle is contained within a fascial sheath, the rectus sheath, which is derived from the aponeuroses of the three flat abdominal muscles. Unfortunately for ease of understanding, the relationship of the aponeuroses of the flat muscles is not constant throughout the course of the rectus muscle. The relationship is different above and below the semicircular line of Douglas, which is about halfway between the umbilicus and pubic symphysis (see Fig. 28–6). Above the semicircular line, the rectus sheath is strong posteriorly. Here the posterior sheath is composed of fascia from the internal oblique muscle, the transversus abdominis muscle, and the transversalis fascia. Anteriorly, above the semicircular line, the rectus sheath is composed of the external oblique aponeurosis and the anterior lamella of the internal oblique aponeurosis.

Below the semicircular line, which is the point at which the inferior epigastric artery enters the rectus sheath, the posterior rectus sheath is lacking because the fasciae of the flat muscles pass anterior to the rectus muscle. The muscle, below the semicircular line, is covered posteriorly by a thin layer of transversalis fascia, which is usually transparent when viewed from the inside at operation.

The rectus abdominis muscles are held close together near the anterior midline by the *linea alba*. The linea alba itself has an elongated triangular shape and is based at the xiphoid

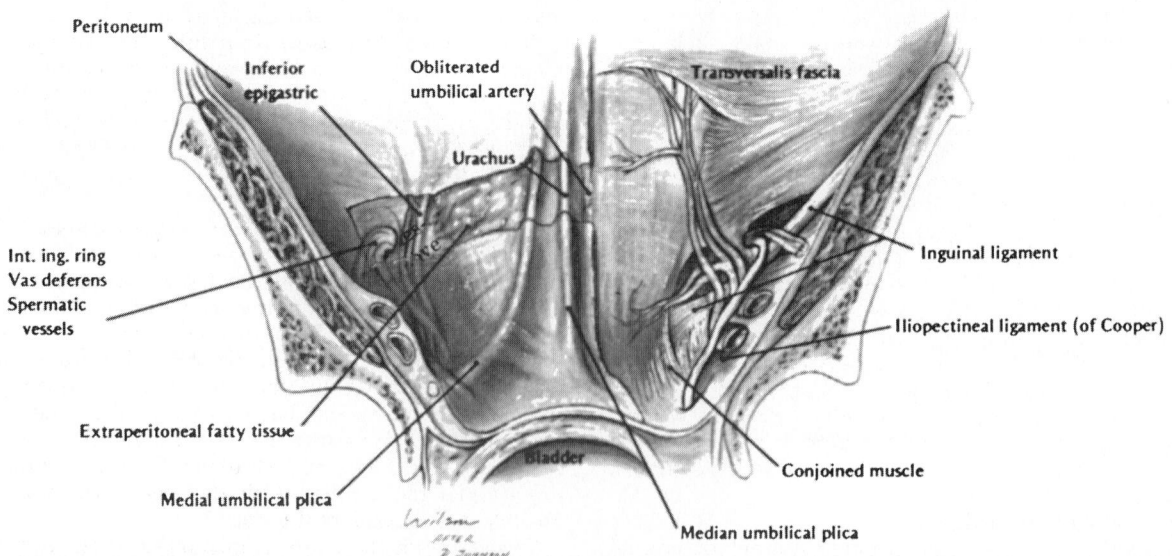

Figure 28–5. Schematic diagram of the lower abdominal wall as seen from the inside. On the left, the median and medial umbilical folds are apparent. On the right, the peritoneum has been removed, revealing the transversalis fascia. (Modified from Healey, J. E., Jr.: A Synopsis of Clinical Anatomy. Philadelphia, W. B. Saunders, 1969.)

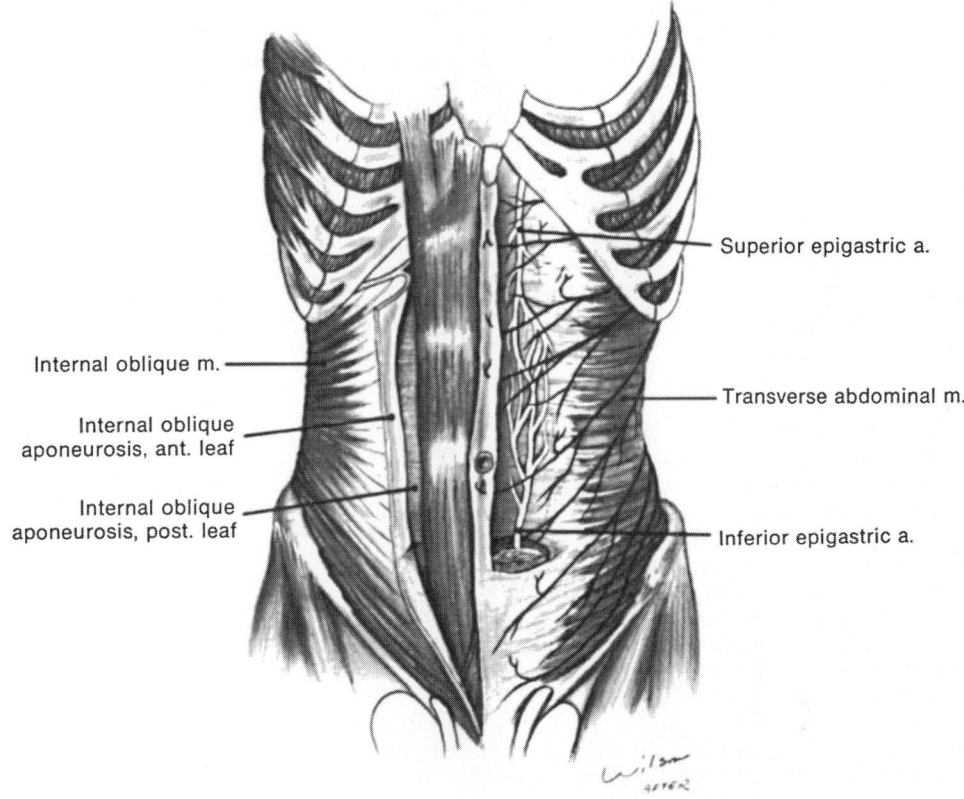

Figure 28–6. Schematic diagram of abdominal wall, demonstrating the rectus sheath as seen from an anterior dissection. On the right, the blood supply and innervation of the rectus abdominis muscle are depicted. (Modified from Healey, J. E., Jr.: A Synopsis of Clinical Anatomy. Philadelphia, W. B. Saunders, 1969.)

Internal oblique m.

Internal oblique aponeurosis, ant. leaf

Internal oblique aponeurosis, post. leaf

Superior epigastric a.

Transverse abdominal m.

Inferior epigastric a.

process of the sternum. The linea alba narrows considerably below the umbilicus so that the medial edge of one rectus muscle may actually overlap the other.

The linea alba is so called because it is a white line. However, it may take on dark pigmentation in pregnant women. It is then properly called the *linea nigra.* It never loses its dark pigmentation thereafter.

The lymphatic supply of the abdominal wall follows a simple pattern (Fig. 28–7). Above the umbilicus, the lymphatic pathways drain into the ipsilateral axillary lymph nodes. Below the umbilicus, they drain into the ipsilateral superficial inguinal lymph nodes. Basically, the superficial lymphatics parallel the superficial veins, which above the umbilicus drain into the axillary vein and below it into the femoral vein.

The arterial supply of the abdominal wall arises from several sources. Above, the superior epigastric arteries enter the rectus sheaths. The superior epigastric artery is a terminal branch of the internal thoracic artery. It has extensive collateral branches within the rectus muscle and the inferior epigastric artery. The inferior epigastric artery rises from the external iliac artery just before the external iliac artery passes into the thigh. The skin and subcutaneous tissues of the lower abdominal wall are supplied bilaterally by several small arteries arising from the femoral artery, which pass upward from the femoral triangle. They are, from medial to lateral, the superficial external pudendal artery, the superficial epigastric artery (misnamed because it really supplies the hypogastrium), and the superficial and deep circumflex iliac arteries.

Congenital Abnormalities

Abdominal Wall. The most common variant of normal anatomy seen in the abdominal wall is diastasis recti. This consists of an upper midline protrusion of the abdominal wall between the right and left rectus abdominis muscles. This abnormality represents a weakness of the linea alba and

does not require treatment unless an epigastric hernia occurs in association with the diastasis recti. Frequently, patients or their families need to be counseled about the innocuous nature of the abnormality.

Omphalocele may be seen in the neonate and represents a defect in the closure of the umbilical ring. The herniated viscera are usually covered with a sac composed of amnion. *Gastroschisis* is a defect of the abdominal wall that is located lateral to the umbilicus. It is caused by a failure of closure of the body wall in which abdominal viscera protrude through the defect. No sac is present to cover the herniated intestine. Omphalocele and gastroschisis are discussed in Chapter 38.

Omphalomesenteric Duct Remnants. Remnants of the omphalomesenteric (vitelline) duct may present as abnormalities related to the abdominal wall. In the fetus, the omphalomesenteric duct connects the fetal midgut to the yolk sac. This normally obliterates and disappears completely. However, any or all of the fetal duct may persist and give rise to symptoms (Fig. 28–8).

An umbilical *polyp* is a small excrescence of omphalomesenteric duct mucosa that is retained in the umbilicus. Such polyps resemble umbilical granulomas except that they do not disappear after silver nitrate cauterization. They may be associated with a persistent vitelline duct or umbilical sinus. Appropriate treatment is excision of the mucosal remnant.

Umbilical *sinuses* result from the continued presence of the umbilical end of the omphalomesenteric duct. These resemble umbilical polyps, but close inspection reveals the presence of a sinus tract deep to the umbilicus. The morphology of the sinus tract can be readily delineated with a sinogram. Treatment is excision of the sinus.[30]

Persistence of the entire omphalomesenteric duct is heralded by the passage of enteric contents from the umbilicus. This is seen in the early neonatal period and should be treated promptly with laparotomy and excision of the duct to avoid intussusception or volvulus.

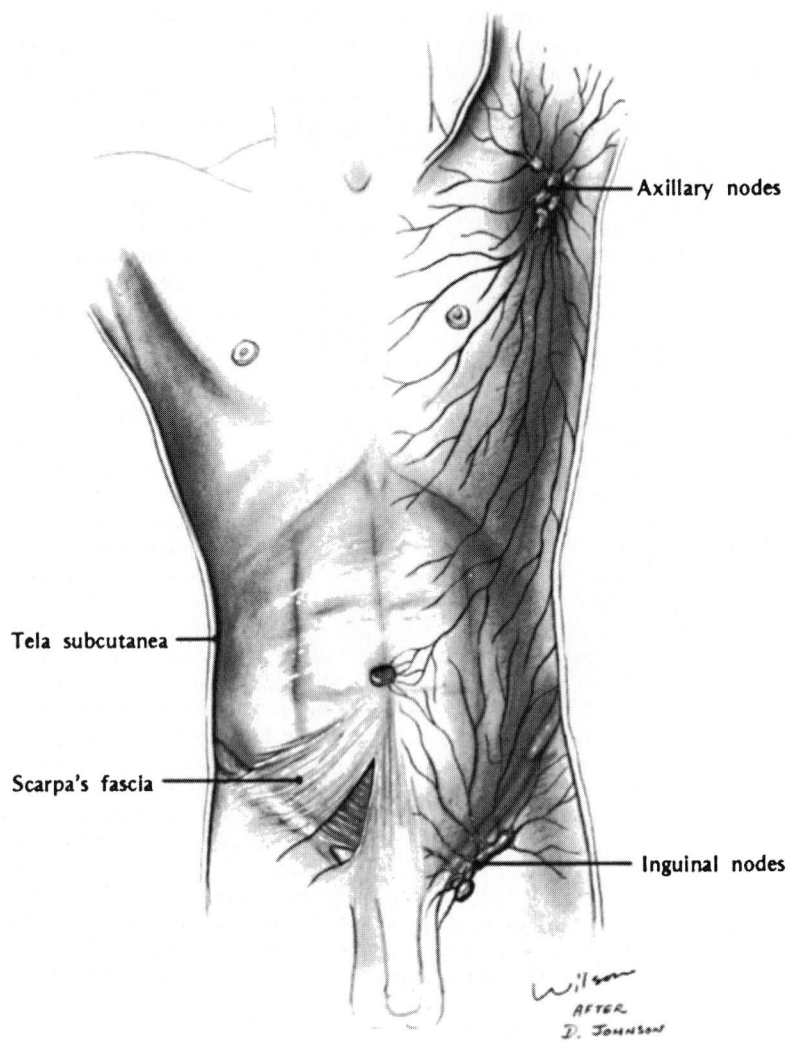

Figure 28–7. Schematic drawing of the lymphatic drainage of the abdominal wall, revealing drainage of the supraumbilical region to the axillary lymph nodes and drainage of the infraumbilical region to the inguinal lymph nodes. On the left, the tela subcutanea and Scarpa's fascia are depicted. (Modified from Healey, J. E., Jr.: A Synopsis of Clinical Anatomy. Philadelphia, W. B. Saunders, 1969.)

Cystic remnants of the omphalomesenteric duct may persist and be asymptomatic for long periods of time. The cysts may be connected to the ileum with a fibrous band that is a remnant of the obliterated omphalomesenteric duct. Patients may present with acute volvulus and intestinal obstruction or with acute abdomen because of cyst infection. The cysts usually remain undiagnosed until operation, at which time they should be excised.

Meckel's diverticulum results when the intestinal end of the omphalomesenteric duct persists. This is a true diverticulum of the intestine with all layers of the intestinal wall represented. It is discussed in detail in Chapter 38.

Urachal Anomalies. The urachus is a fetal structure that connects the developing bladder to the umbilicus. The urachus normally is obliterated by the time of birth. It may persist *in toto*, resulting in a vesicoumbilical fistula manifested by the drainage of urine from the umbilicus (Fig. 28–9). Proper treatment is excision of the fistula after distal urinary obstruction has been excluded.

Persistent *urachal sinus* results when the umbilical end of the urachus does not obliterate normally. Such sinuses present as the chronic drainage of small amounts of material from the umbilicus. They may become infected and should be totally excised. Cystic remnants of the urachus may persist between the bladder and umbilicus when urachal obliteration is incomplete. These cysts may become symptomatic at any time and present as lower abdominal masses or, occasionally, abscesses. They should be excised completely.

True *diverticula* of the urinary bladder result from incomplete obliteration of the distal end of the fetal urachus. They may result in recurrent urinary tract infections and are definitively diagnosed by cystography. Appropriate treatment is excision of the diverticulum and closure of the bladder.

Infections. The abdominal wall is occasionally the site of dermatoses and subcutaneous infections. Appropriate treatment is directed to the specific cause of the abnormality. The abdominal wall occasionally may be the site of severe bacterial gangrene and necrotizing fasciitis. The most serious form of this infection is seen in elderly patients with necrotizing fasciitis caused by mixed infections of aerobic and anaerobic bacteria. These infections are frequently associated with urinary extravasation or perirectal abscess, but they may present without obvious causes. Necrotizing fasciitis of the abdominal wall is a life-threatening infection that results in necrosis of the skin, subcutaneous tissue, and musculoaponeurotic abdominal wall. The only appropriate treatment is early wide débridement, with exteriorization of all infected planes. Appropriate antibiotic therapy is mandatory. Similar infections occasionally complicate wound healing after intestinal operations.

Omphalitis. Infection of the umbilicus may occur in infants and adults. It is generally an innocuous disease that results from poor hygiene and is treated with appropriate cleansing and local care to the umbilicus. However, in the neonatal period, omphalitis may result from bacterial infection and may potentially be associated with serious sequelae,

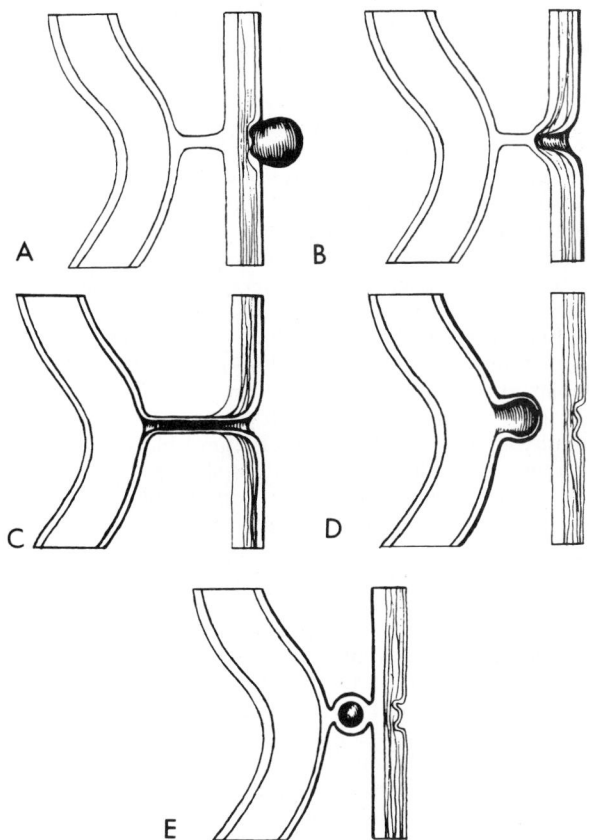

Figure 28–8. Vestiges of vitelline (omphalomesenteric) duct. *A*, Mucosal polyp (with band from bowel to umbilicus). *B*, Sinus in the umbilicus. *C*, Enteroumbilical fistula (patent omphalomesenteric duct). *D*, Meckel's diverticulum. *E*, Cyst between bowel and abdominal wall, which may communicate with the skin surface. (From Ravitch, M. M., et al.: Pediatric Surgery, 3rd ed. Chicago, Year Book Medical Publishers, 1979.)

such as portal vein thrombosis. In neonates, treatment includes systemic antibiotics.

Rectus Sheath Hematoma. Extravasation of blood into the rectus sheath resulting in a hematoma is rarely a life-threatening illness. However, it may mimic other abdominal diseases and must be considered in the differential diagnosis to avoid unnecessary laparotomy. Rectus sheath hematoma is usually the result of trauma, which may be as trivial as a paroxysm of coughing. Patients with rectus sheath hematomas most often give a history of receiving anticoagulant drugs for various conditions. When the hematoma develops, it ordinarily occurs at the level of the semicircular line of Douglas, where the inferior epigastric artery enters the rectus sheath. Patients may complain of an acute illness, with abdominal pain over the hematoma, nausea, and vomiting. Frequently, a tender mass is palpable. Operation is indicated only if more serious conditions cannot otherwise be excluded.

Abdominal Wall Tumors. Benign tumors of the abdominal wall may arise from any of the elements contained within the abdominal wall itself. Lipomas of the abdominal wall are common and are treated by excision. Benign fibromas, hemangiomas, and neurofibromas may be seen. The principles of their treatment are no different from those for similar tumors in other locations.

Desmoid tumors of the abdominal wall are benign fibrous tumors that arise from the musculoaponeurotic abdominal wall. These tumors are histologically benign but frequently are locally invasive and are prone to recurrence after local excision. They present as firm, subcutaneous masses that

grow slowly. They should be widely excised to prevent local recurrence. They do not have a propensity toward metastasis.

Primary malignancies of the abdominal wall are uncommon. Any of the cutaneous neoplasms may affect the abdominal wall and are treated like skin cancers elsewhere. Sarcomas arising from the abdominal wall are uncommon and are best treated by surgical excision.

The abdominal wall is occasionally the site of metastasis from primary malignancies located elsewhere. In particular, tumors of the ovary and prostate may metastasize to the lower abdominal wall. Tumors of the stomach, uterus, lung, kidney, breast, and colon occasionally give rise to metastases located within the abdominal wall.

Referred Pain. A consideration of the innervation of both the abdominal wall and the abdominal viscera is appropriate to understand the phenomenon of referred pain. Referred pain is pain of visceral origin (mediated through sympathetic nervous system pathways) that is perceived as somatic or cutaneous pain. None of the abdominal viscera are innervated by somatic afferent fibers, which are traditionally described as pain fibers. However, the abdominal viscera are innervated by afferent sympathetic nervous system fibers. These afferent sympathetic fibers join the central nervous system in a segmental manner, as do the somatic afferent fibers arising from the abdominal wall and skin. When a viscus becomes diseased or distended, the afferent sympathetic nervous system fibers are stimulated. These impulses are transmitted to the central nervous system and are perceived as somatic or cutaneous pain in segments of the body that are innervated from the same central nervous system segment that receives the afferent sympathetic impulses.

An example of referred pain is pain from distention of the vermiform appendix. The vermiform appendix, like all the gastrointestinal tract, has no somatic innervations. However, it has a rich sympathetic innervation. When the appendix becomes distended from obstruction, the resulting pain may be referred to the skin and abdominal wall around the umbilicus. This phenomenon is explained on an anatomic basis by the fact that the region of the umbilicus is innervated by the tenth thoracic spinal cord segment, which is the segment from which the sympathetic innervation of the vermiform appendix is derived. Numerous other examples of referred pain are well documented. These include pain from irritation of the diaphragmatic peritoneum, commonly referred to the

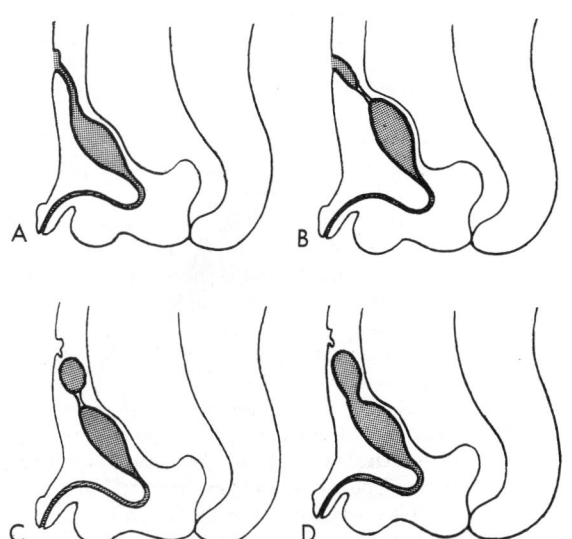

Figure 28–9. Vestiges of urachus. *A*, Urinary fistula. *B*, Sinus. *C*, Cyst. *D*, Bladder diverticulum. (From Ravitch, M. M., et al.: Pediatric Surgery, 3rd ed. Chicago, Year Book Medical Publishers, 1979.)

shoulder. Referred pain from an obstructed gallbladder is commonly perceived in the region of the scapula. Referred pain from renal colic is frequently perceived in the groin or scrotum.

General Diagnostic Signs. Many examples exist of diagnostic signs of abdominal and systemic disease that may be manifested in or on the abdominal wall. These include, among others, the Sister Mary Joseph nodule, which occasionally presents within the substance of the umbilicus. This lymph node, which was first appreciated by an observant operating room nun, is a manifestation of intra-abdominal malignancy.[24] It has the same diagnostic significance as Virchow's node in the neck. Grey Turner's sign of retroperitoneal hemorrhage, which was originally described in hemorrhagic pancreatitis, is well known. Grey Turner's sign also may be visible in patients with ruptured abdominal aortic aneurysm, retroperitoneal hemorrhage from trauma, and retroperitoneal hemorrhage that occurs as a complication of anticoagulation therapy. The caput medusa is a collection of distended veins around the umbilicus that results from portal venous hypertension. The caput medusa sign becomes apparent when there is shunting of blood from the portal venous circulation to the systemic venous system through the abdominal wall. Spider angiomas associated with chronic liver disease may be seen on the abdominal wall. Additionally, petechiae from thrombocytopenia or from fat embolus may present as abdominal wall findings. The striae of Cushing's disease are usually found on the abdominal wall. Distention of the abdomen is most readily appreciated by inspecting the abdominal wall, and the detection of ascitic fluid in the peritoneal cavity is easily appreciated after careful examination.

PERITONEUM

Embryology. The peritoneal cavity is a potential space containing the abdominal viscera. It develops from the primitive coelom, which is formed by a splitting of the lateral mesoderm into somatic and splanchnic layers. Originally there are two bilateral cavities separated by the developing gastrointestinal tract. The somatic mesoderm lines the body wall portion of the coelom, and the splanchnic mesoderm covers the intestine (Fig. 28–10). As the embryonic body wall closes ventrally, the two coelomic cavities fuse together in the midline. In between, the developing gut is covered on both sides by splanchnic mesoderm. That portion of this double layer of mesoderm from which the gut is suspended

is called the mesentery. As the ventral mesentery of the intestine is resorbed, the two coelomic cavities join to become one.

Physiology. The primary functions of the peritoneum have been derived by teleologic reasoning. The peritoneum does provide a frictionless surface over which the abdominal viscera can freely move, and the mesothelial lining secretes fluid that serves to lubricate the peritoneal surfaces. Normally, about 100 ml. of clear, straw-colored fluid is present in the peritoneal cavity of the adult. The quality and quantity of this fluid may change with various pathologic conditions.

When required to do so, the peritoneum serves as a bidirectional dialysis membrane through which water and solutes may move. Such movement is controlled largely by the osmolar gradient. This ability of the peritoneum to absorb substances is the basis for both experimental and clinical administration of fluid, electrolytes, and blood. Isotonic saline administered intraperitoneally is absorbed at a rate of 30 to 35 ml. per hour after an initial equilibration phase. However, if a hypertonic fluid is used, there is a large shift of water (up to 300 to 500 ml. per hour) from the intravascular space into the peritoneal cavity, which can result in hypotension and shock.[29] Studies in humans and animals show that intraperitoneal blood is absorbed at a slower rate, but approximately 70% eventually enters the bloodstream. This absorption occurs primarily through fenestrated lymphatic channels on the undersurface of the diaphragm. Such red blood cells have a normal survival time in the circulation.[28] Air and gases are also similarly absorbed. Air that enters the peritoneal cavity during laparotomy is present in diminishing amounts for 4 to 5 days.

Peritoneal dialysis is possible because of bidirectional transport across the peritoneal membrane. By adjusting that composition of the dialysate, excess water, sodium, potassium, and products of metabolism can be removed from the bloodstream. In addition, a variety of drugs can be removed with peritoneal dialysis (Table 28–1). Medications that are not dialyzable are shown in Table 28–2.

Intraperitoneal Fluid Collection

Ascites. Normally, there is a balance between fluid secretion and absorption in the peritoneal cavity. Ascites occurs when either the secretion rate increases or the absorption rate decreases disproportionate to the other. This fluid may be a transudate or exudate, and its composition is determined by the etiology of the ascites.

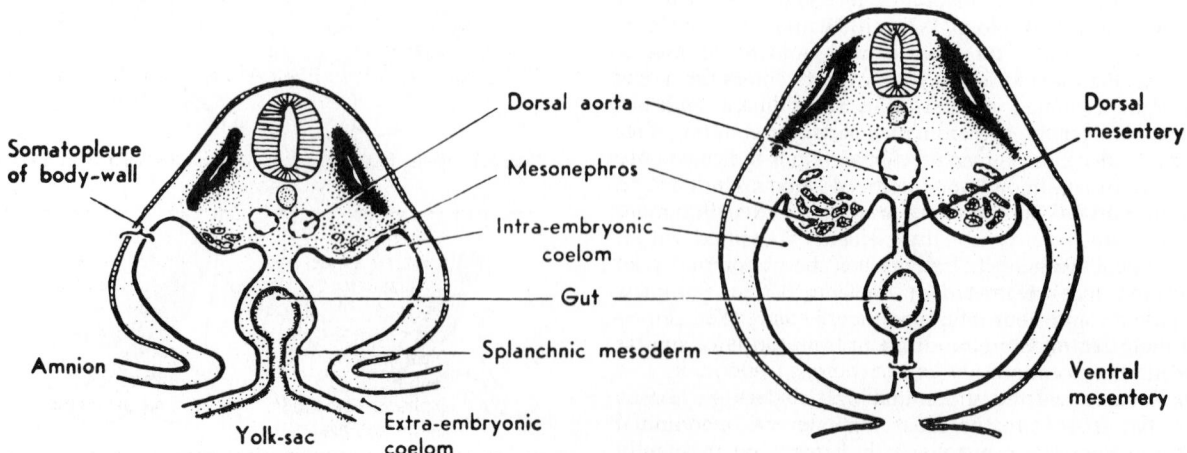

Figure 28–10. Diagram illustrating early stages in the development of the coelom and mesenteries. (From Patten, B. M.: Human Embryology, 3rd ed. New York, McGraw-Hill Book Company, 1969. Reproduced with permission of The McGraw-Hill Companies.)

TABLE 28–1. Substances That Can Be Removed by Peritoneal Dialysis

Ammonia	Chlorates
Amphetamines	Ergotamine
Aniline	Ethchlorvynol
Antibiotics	Fluorides
Carbenicillin	Iodides
Gentamicin	Iron (after deferoxamine)
Isoniazid	Lead (after edetate)
Kanamycin	Lithium
Neomycin	Magnesium
Nitrofurantoin	Meprobamate
Sulfonamides	Mercury (after dimercaprol)
Arsenic (after dimercaprol)	Methrobenzine
Aspirin	Mushrooms
Barbiturates	Paraldehyde
Boric acid	Phenacetin
Bromides	Phenytoin
Calcium	Potassium
Carbon tetrachloride	Quinidine
Chloral hydrate	

From Schuberth, K. C., and Zitelli, B. J.: The Harriet Lane Handbook, 8th ed. Chicago, Year Book Medical Publishers, 1979.

Chyle. Accumulation of lymph within the peritoneal cavity usually results from trauma or tumor involving lymphatic structures, abdominal surgical procedures, spontaneous bacterial peritonitis, cirrhosis, tuberculosis, congenital defects, or peritoneal dialysis. Proposed treatment regimens range from salt restrictions and diuretics to surgical ligation or peritoneovenous shunting.[4] Chyle differs from other fluid accumulations in the peritoneal cavity in that it has bacteriostatic properties, making infection less likely. In the laboratory, chyle layers out into an upper milky layer, a middle watery layer, and a lower opaque layer.

Bile. Uninfected bile is a mild irritant to the peritoneal cavity. It causes an increased production of peritoneal fluid, resulting in bile ascites or choleperitoneum. Patients with this condition may be relatively well as long as the fluid remains sterile, exhibiting only a mild jaundice from absorption of bile pigments. Infected bile, however, causes a severe peritonitis and necessitates urgent surgical therapy. Most cases of choleperitoneum follow biliary tract operations, but cases of spontaneous perforation of the bile duct have been reported in infants and some adults. This is reported to be the second most common cause of surgical jaundice in infancy.

Blood. The most common cause of hemoperitoneum is trauma to the liver or spleen. Less common causes include ruptured ectopic pregnancy, ruptured aortic aneurysm, and other intra-abdominal injuries. As mentioned earlier, approximately two thirds of the red blood cells in the peritoneal cavity are absorbed intact into the bloodstream. However, leaving blood in the peritoneal cavity after operative procedures is not recommended, because it may potentiate infection. It has been shown experimentally that intraperitoneal hemoglobin interferes with the immune response to peritonitis by interfering with clearance of bacteria from the peritoneal cavity.[33]

Urine. Urine collections within the peritoneal cavity are almost always due to trauma to the urinary tract. Urinomas may present as asymptomatic abdominal enlargement if sterile, but more often they are infected from associated injuries or underlying disease. Such injuries demand operation.

Air. Pneumoperitoneum is usually secondary to perforation of the gastrointestinal tract or to recent operation. It may result from alveolar rupture in patients on mechanical ventilators. Treatment is directed to the underlying cause of the pneumoperitoneum.

Meconium. The neonatal intestine contains sterile meconium.[9] Occasionally, perforation of the intestine occurs *in utero,* and meconium may leak into the peritoneal cavity. This can occur as early as the second trimester of pregnancy, and it results in a sterile inflammatory reaction, fluid accumulation, and eventual calcification of the peritoneal cavity. Depending on the time of the perforation, the newborn may present in one of several ways. Remote perforation is shown as fibrous adhesions and calcifications on roentgenograms. The infants may be asymptomatic and may develop problems from obstruction only later. More recent perforation may be walled off, forming a meconium pseudocyst, and infants with this present with an abdominal mass. Alternatively, the infant may be born with ascites from recent perforation and require urgent surgical therapy. In many cases, the cause of the perforation is obstruction of the intestine, with proximal distention and perforation. Some of these infants have meconium ileus and underlying cystic fibrosis.

Peritonitis

Peritonitis is inflammation of the peritoneum. It can be septic or aseptic, bacterial or viral, primary or secondary, and acute or chronic. Most surgical peritonitis is secondary to bacterial contamination from the gastrointestinal tract. Usually there is an underlying pathologic process or injury to the gut, and this form of peritonitis is discussed elsewhere. Other less common forms of peritonitis are discussed here.

Primary Peritonitis. Primary peritonitis refers to inflammation of the peritoneal cavity without a documented source of contamination. It occurs more commonly in children than in adults and in women more than in men. This latter distribution is thought to be explained by entry of organisms into the peritoneal cavity through the fallopian tubes. In children, incidence peaks in the neonatal period and again, at age 4 to 5 years. The patients present with an acutely tender abdomen, fever, and leukocytosis. There may be a history of antecedent ear or upper respiratory tract infection. It is often difficult in this situation to differentiate between primary and secondary peritonitis, and the diagnosis ultimately may be made at laparotomy. However, children with nephrotic syndrome and, less commonly, systemic lupus erythematosus are particularly susceptible to primary peritonitis. The bacteria in these cases are usually either hemolytic streptococci or pneumococci. A diagnosis can be made by peritoneal aspiration and Gram stain after excluding pneumonia and urinary tract infection. Adults with ascites from liver disease have an increased incidence of primary peritonitis.[14] In recent years, the bacterial flora has changed from gram-positive to gram-negative organisms. Thus, the distinction between primary and secondary peritonitis is more difficult to make by peritoneal aspirate alone.

Tuberculous Peritonitis. Tuberculous peritonitis has de-

TABLE 28–2. Substances Not Removed by Peritoneal Dialysis

Amitriptyline	Hallucinogens
Antidepressives	Imipramine
Antihistamines	Methaqualone
Atropine	Methyprylon
Chlordiazepoxide	Nortriptyline
Diazepam	Opiates
Digitalis	Oxazepam
Diphenhydramine	Propoxyphene
Diphenoxylate	

From Schuberth, K. C., and Zitelli, B. J.: The Harriet Lane Handbook, 8th ed. Chicago, Year Book Medical Publishers, 1979.

creased in frequency, as have other forms of tuberculosis.[34, 35, 39] In the past, it was seen commonly and carried a significant mortality. Presently the mortality rate is less than 5%. The tubercle bacillus presumably gains entry to the peritoneal cavity by one of three mechanisms: (1) transmurally from diseased bowel, (2) from tuberculous salpingitis, or (3) from the bloodstream. The majority of patients do not have radiographic evidence of pulmonary or gastrointestinal tuberculosis, but nearly all have such a focus identified at autopsy. All have positive tuberculin skin tests even if the tuberculosis is confined to the peritoneum.

The clinical manifestations of tuberculous peritonitis are of two types. The moist form consists of fever, ascites, abdominal pain, and weakness. The ascites is progressive and may become massive. The dry form presents in a similar manner but without ascites. Extensive adhesions within the peritoneal cavity result in a *matted* feeling on physical examination. In both forms, tuberculous implants (tubercles) are present on the peritoneal surfaces. Diagnosis may be made most reliably by open or closed peritoneal biopsy and culture. Barium studies are rarely helpful. Recently, laparoscopy has been employed to obtain peritoneal biopsies, which increases the yield over closed biopsy. The ascitic fluid in the moist form is an exudate. On smear examination, lymphocytes are mainly present and rarely acid-fast bacilli are seen. Cultures of the fluid are positive in fewer than half the cases. Treatment is generally nonoperative and includes appropriate antibiotics. Operation should be reserved for diagnosis if needle biopsy fails or for complications such as fecal fistula.

Aseptic Peritonitis. Aseptic peritonitis is generally due to chemical or foreign body irritants. It may be followed by secondary bacterial peritonitis. Most chemical peritonitis is due to various irritative body fluids (bile, meconium, gastric contents). Foreign bodies may result from external trauma or may be acquired at the time of operation in the form of sutures, sponges, or starch granules. There has been recent interest in starch peritonitis secondary to a reaction to glove powder. It is not clear whether this reaction is allergic or dose related, but the incidence of this complication can be reduced easily by careful glove washing before abdominal exploration. Pathologically, a granulomatous reaction occurs with giant cell formation. When this is examined under polarized light, the characteristic birefringent Maltese crosses can be seen in the granulomas.

Abscesses and Adhesions

Many forms of peritonitis lead to abscess and/or adhesion formation. Intraperitoneal abscess develops two basic patterns. Generalized peritonitis tends to result in abscess formation in anatomically dependent positions, such as the pelvis and paracolic gutters.[5] Localized peritoneal inflammation caused by contiguous disease or injury may result in localized abscesses rather than peritonitis. The common sites of intraperitoneal abscess formation are shown in Figure 28–11. Adhesions commonly form after peritonitis. Occasionally, adhesions develop to such an extent that the peritoneal cavity is nearly obliterated. This is compatible with life, although intestinal obstruction may occur. Partial obliteration of the peritoneal cavity with bandlike adhesions may also occur. Adhesions form from fibrin produced by the peritoneal surfaces. Most of this fibrin is lysed and absorbed, but some may remain and be invaded with fibroblasts, resulting in dense adhesions. Experimentally, adhesion formation is associated with a reduction in fibrinolysins and may be reduced using steroids, but this has not been validated clinically.[27] Because adhesion formation is a response to peritoneal irritation, meticulous surgical technique is probably the most important factor in prevention.

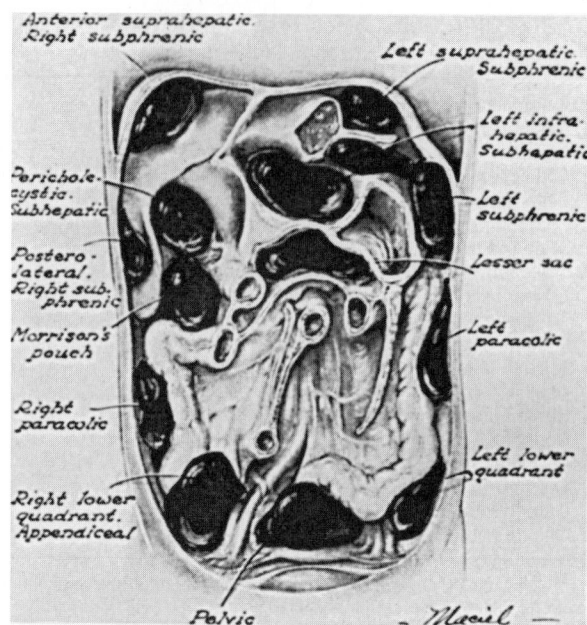

Figure 28–11. Anterior view of abdominal cavity illustrating the types, locations, and anatomic relationship of the various intraperitoneal abscesses. (From Altemeier, W. A., Culbertson, W. R., Fullen, W. D., and Shook, C. D.: Intra-abdominal abscesses. Am. J. Surg., *125*:71, 1973.)

MESENTERY AND OMENTUM

Embryology. As the peritoneal cavity develops, the splanchnic mesoderm covers the developing gut. Eventually, most of the ventral mesentery is resorbed except for that portion between the liver and the stomach that persists as the gastrohepatic (lesser) omentum. The dorsal mesentery remains intact but changes markedly in size and position as the gastrointestinal tract elongates and rotates. In the gastric region, the cardia of the stomach rotates to the left and the pylorus moves to the right. The dorsal mesogastrium grows with these changes but does so more than is necessary to accommodate the positional changes in the stomach. The mesogastrium elongates and forms a sac, the omental bursa, which eventually extends caudad over the transverse colon. The omentum fuses with the transverse mesocolon, and the two layers of the omental bursa fuse to become one layer. This apron of dorsal mesogastrium is called the greater omentum.

The intestine begins to elongate during the fifth week of development and forms a loop that extends into the umbilical cord, with the superior mesenteric artery extending from the apex to the loop. This is Stage I of midgut development. Stage II involves return of the duodenum to the abdominal cavity with its 270-degree counterclockwise rotation around the superior mesenteric artery. In Stage III, the right half of the colon returns to the abdomen and rotates 270 degrees in a counterclockwise direction to lie on the right side anterior to the superior mesenteric artery. This stage is completed with fixation of the intestine and its mesenteries. By the twelfth week of development, rotation is finished but fixation may not be completed until birth. With fusion of the mesentery of the ascending colon to the posterior abdominal wall, the root of the small intestine to extend from the transverse mesocolon to the ileocecal junction. This broad-based mesentery prevents volvulus. Malrotation and volvulus are discussed in Chapter 38.

Physiology. The greater and lesser omenta and the intestinal mesentery are rich in lymphatics and blood vessels.[18] Sequestration or obstruction of lymphatic vessels leads to

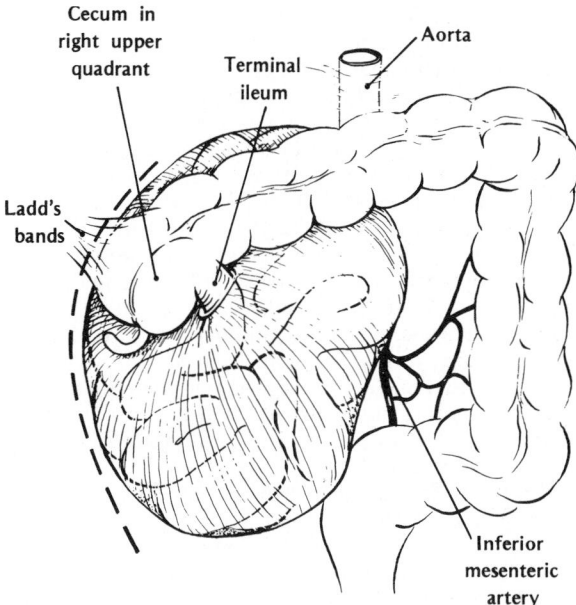

Figure 28–12. Right mesocolic hernia. The prearterial segment did not rotate during the second stage. The postarterial segment did rotate and has trapped most of the small bowel behind the ascending mesocolon containing the ileocolic, right colic, and middle colic vessels. The dashed line shows the incision for release of the hernia. (From Willwerth, B. M., Zollinger, R. M., Jr., and Izant, R. J., Jr.: Congenital mesocolic [paraduodenal] hernia. Am. J. Surg., *128*:358, 1974.)

various clinical entities, depending on anatomic location. Mesenteric, omental, and retroperitoneal cysts should be grouped together because mesenteric and omental structures are anterior extensions of what was originally retroperitoneal. In response to intraperitoneal inflammation, the omentum provides the major source of peritoneal macrophages and aids in removal of foreign material and bacteria.[18] It was previously thought that the omentum, the *policeman of the abdomen,* was capable of moving to sites of inflammation, but it has been demonstrated that omental movement is dependent on intestinal peristalsis and gravity. When in contact with a foreign body or inflamed area, the omentum can adhere firmly. In response to intestinal inflammation, the lymph nodes of the mesentery enlarge and may become symptomatic. The cause of this disorder is presumed to be viral, and it occurs primarily in children.

Congenital Intraperitoneal Hernias. Most intraperitoneal hernias result from anatomic variants present at birth. They can be divided into two types, based on etiology and the presence or absence of a hernia sac. Hernias that occur through defects in the peritoneum or mesentery do not have sacs, and those that occur secondary to variants in intestinal rotation do have sacs. The first type includes herniation through the epiploic foramen and through congenital defects in the mesentery of the small or large intestine or, less commonly, the broad ligament of the uterus. Some of the mesenteric defects occur secondary to trauma or operation, but most are congenital. Patients with transmesenteric hernia may present with a history of chronic incomplete obstruction or with an acute closed-loop obstruction. In many of these hernias, part of the constricting ring contains major vessels, and care must be taken not to injure these at operation.

The secondary type of intraperitoneal hernia includes the paraduodenal or mesocolic hernias.[40] These occur secondary to abnormal rotation of the intestine. The sac consists of intestinal mesentery, hence the name *mesocolic hernia.* They present more often in adults than in children, in contradis-

tinction to transmesenteric hernias. The right mesocolic hernia occurs secondary to incomplete rotation of the duodenum in Stage II. The duodenum rotates only 90 degrees and remains on the right side of the abdomen, during which time the large intestine rotates normally over it. The proximal small intestine then becomes trapped in the mesentery of the right colon. Operative correction of the right mesocolic hernia is most safely performed by dividing the peritoneal attachments of the right colon, thus moving the colon to the left and leaving the small bowel on the right (Fig. 28–12). The resulting configuration of intestine is then similar to that of an arrest at Stage I of rotation (nonrotation).

It was formerly thought that left mesocolic hernias occurred as a result of herniation of the small bowel through the paraduodenal fossa near the fourth portion of the duodenum. It is more likely that during Stage II of rotation the small bowel moves to the left and under the descending colon. With fixation of the colon, the intestine becomes trapped behind the left mesocolon. The inferior mesenteric vein often lies along the anterior rim of the neck of the sac. Reduction of this hernia, as with the right side, involves recognizing the anatomic abnormalities and correcting these according to embryogenesis. An incision is made along the border of the inferior mesenteric vein, which is the line of fusion of the left mesocolon, thus releasing the entrapped bowel (Fig. 28–13).

The mesocolic hernias may present with either vague abdominal symptoms or with acute intestinal obstruction. Abdominal films show the small intestine to be confined in one area of the abdomen, but often the diagnosis is not made until laparotomy.

Mesenteric Cysts. Mesenteric cysts are most often due to congenital lymphatic spaces that gradually enlarge as they fill with lymph.[22] According to Beahrs[8] and others, they may be divided into four groups based on their etiology:

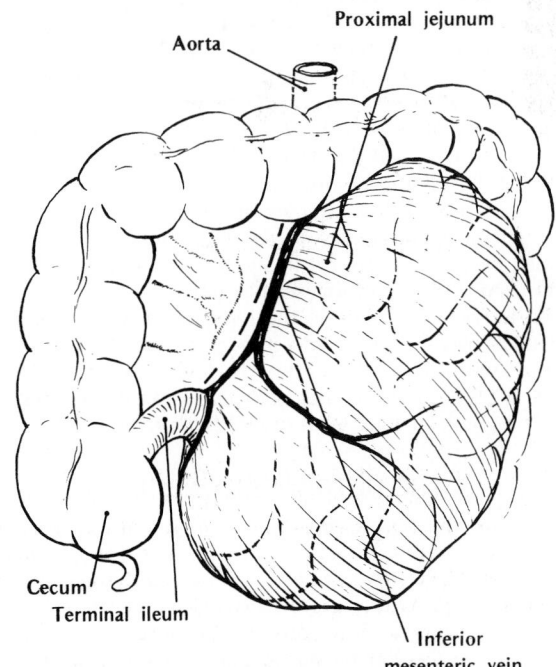

Figure 28–13. Left mesocolic hernia. A more extensive herniation has occurred, and the sac opening has fused along the dashed line. This line to the right of the inferior mesenteric vein also indicates the area for operative incision. After reduction of the small bowel to the right through this newly created neck, the inferior mesenteric vein, or right lateral margin of the sac, is secured to the retroperitoneum along the left side or root of the small-bowel mesentery. (From Willwerth, B. M., Zollinger, R. M., Jr., and Izant, R. J., Jr.: Congenital mesocolic [paraduodenal] hernia. Am. J. Surg., *128*:358, 1974.)

(1) embryonic and developmental cysts, (2) traumatic or acquired cysts, (3) neoplastic cysts, or (4) infective and degenerative cysts.

Mesenteric cysts usually present as abdominal masses accompanied by pain, nausea, and vomiting. These masses can generally be diagnosed on physical examination. They may display a characteristic lateral mobility and are treated most appropriately by surgical excision. Because of their intimate association with the bowel mesentery, intestinal resection may be required for their complete removal. At operation, they may be confused with duplication cysts of the intestine.[22]

Omental Cysts. Omental cysts are frequently asymptomatic but may present with vague discomfort or as a mobile abdominal mass that can cause torsion of the omentum. Diagnosis is sometimes difficult, but ultrasound examination may be helpful. On plain films, omental cysts characteristically lie anterior to the intestine. They are best seen in a lateral view. Treatment of omental cysts is by simple excision.

Omental Torsion and Infarction. Torsion of the omentum may be primary or secondary.[3] Primary torsion is rare, and the cause is unknown. Secondary torsion may be due to adhesions, omental cyst, or tumor. The right side of the omentum is involved more than the left, and the torsion generally occurs around two fixed points. Patients often present with signs and symptoms compatible with appendicitis, acute cholecystitis, or a twisted ovarian cyst. Diagnosis is usually not made before laparotomy.

Omental infarction may occur secondary to torsion, but it is usually unrelated to torsion. Omental infarction is a rare entity and may follow trauma or may be associated with collagen vascular disease. Treatment for both torsion and infarction entails local resection.

Uses of Omentum. The capability of the omentum to wall off infection and its rich vascular and lymphatic supply have led to many uses of omentum in a wide variety of disorders. Free omental grafts generally fibrose and do not function; but with construction of a vascular pedicle, the omentum can reach to the neck or the knee. Omentum has been used as a protective wrapping for intestinal anastomoses to prevent anastomotic leak and promote healing. Enthusiasm for the use of omentum in the treatment of lymphedema of the extremities has waxed and waned. This is discussed in Chapter 47 on lymphatic disorders. However, omental patches have been successfully employed in the closure of perforated duodenal ulcer and for esophageal perforations. Omentum has also been found useful in operative procedures on the genitourinary tract and in vascular reconstruction. After hepatic resection or trauma to the liver or spleen, an omental patch aids in hemostasis and in sealing of biliary leaks. In addition, with the advent of microvascular surgery, there are reports of the use of omental transplants to improve cerebral vascularity and in chest wall reconstruction.[29]

THE RETROPERITONEUM

Anatomy. The retroperitoneum is an actual space located between the peritoneal cavity and the posterior body wall (Fig. 28–14).[20] The diaphragm serves as the superior boundary, whereas the levator muscles of the pelvis delineate the inferior boundary of the retroperitoneal space. Anteriorly, this space is bounded by the posterior parietal peritoneum and the spaces between the leaves of the small and large bowel mesenteries. Posteriorly, it is bounded by the vertebral column and the psoas and quadratus lumborum and tendinous portions of the transversus abdominis muscles. Embryologically, ectoderm, mesoderm, and embryonal remnants constitute the contents of the retroperitoneum. It is, therefore, only natural that the majority of abnormalities in the retroperitoneum arise from the aforementioned cell lines. (Table 28–3 lists the contents of the retroperitoneum.)

Several disorders that lend themselves to surgical treatment can be approached by an extraperitoneal or retroperitoneal exposure. This approach has many advantages over the more commonly used transabdominal approach. When entrance through the peritoneal cavity is avoided, postoperative ileus is brief, if present at all. This allows the continued use of the alimentary tract to deliver nutritional support to the hypermetabolic postoperative patient. Retroperitoneal exposure avoids manipulation of the intestines and the subsequent development of adhesions. Intraoperative fluid and heat loss are markedly lessened, and postoperative atelectasis and pneumonia are seldom seen. If an abscess develops, it will be interstitial and not intraperitoneal. These advantages support the sound judgment to choose retroperitoneal or extraperitoneal exposure over transabdominal exposure when technically feasible.

Surgical Anatomy. The peritoneal *bag* can be dissected easily from the parietes throughout the bulk of its surface area. For practical purposes, dissection is limited in the posterior midline by the major visceral branches of the aorta. Superiorly, dissection is limited by fusion of the peritoneum to the undersurface of the diaphragm, although it can be free from the more caudal aspects of the diaphragm. It becomes progressively more difficult as the ligaments of the liver are approached. It is also easier to dissect the peritoneum from the posterior undersurface of the diaphragm than from the anterior undersurface. Inferiorly, dissection is limited in the depth of the pelvis only by the reflection of peritoneum onto the colon. Anteriorly, the peritoneum is densely fused to the posterior rectus sheath above the semicircular line. Below the semicircular line, dissection can cross the midline readily. Above the semicircular line, it is possible to extend dissection to the midline by dividing the lateral border of the rectus sheath in the semilunar line. This allows the posterior rectus sheath to come away from the rectus muscle while remaining attached to the peritoneum.

The areas where the parietal and visceral peritoneum form a juncture are shown in Figure 28–14. If the surgeon approaches these areas in the extraperitoneal plane laterally, it is possible to carry the dissection to the midline without entering the peritoneal cavity; however, if operating transperitoneally, it is not possible to reflect the right or left colon without entering the retroperitoneal space.

Retroperitoneal Infection. Many intra-abdominal abscesses are localized in such a way that a part of the limiting wall is the parietal peritoneum. Such abscesses, when recognized, are best evacuated through this portion of the abscess, because contamination of the general peritoneal cavity is thereby avoided. The common sites of abscesses, some of which may be drained by this approach, are shown in Figure 28–11. An abscess can be located by ultrasound studies, computed tomography, or more conventional means such as palpation or fluoroscopy. When operating on a patient with an abscess, the incision should be carefully planned to allow approach of the abscess without transgression of the free peritoneal cavity. Exploratory needle aspiration may be useful. If purulent material is located, the needle may be left in place and the incision extended into the abscess beside the needle. Some abscesses may present in the retroperitoneal space. This is more common with pancreatic abscesses. Because the pancreas is a retroperitoneal organ, an abscess or a pseudocyst that subsequently becomes infected may dissect behind the pancreas and down either or both sides of the abdomen. It is necessary to recognize the extent of these abscesses to obtain adequate drainage. Appendiceal abscesses secondary to perforated retrocecal appendix may also be retroperitoneal. Both computed tomography and ultraso-

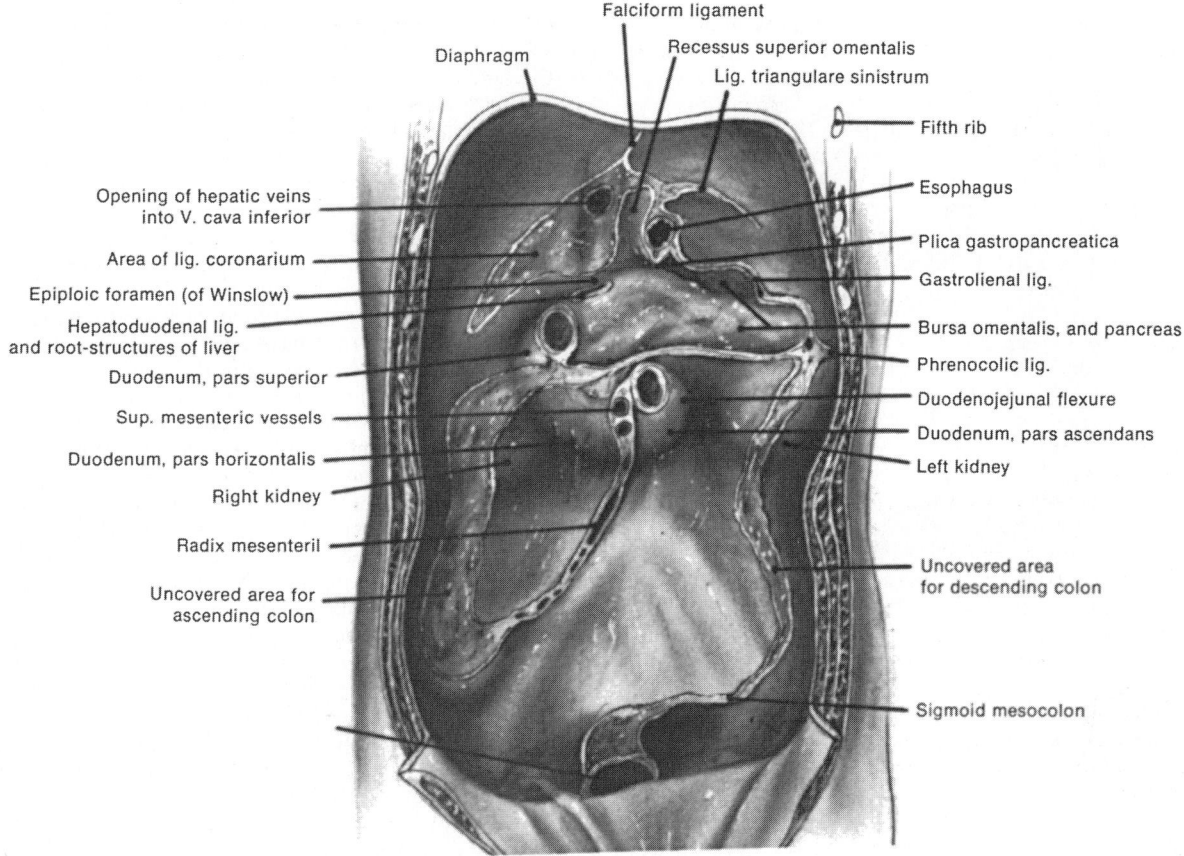

Figure 28–14. Reflection of the peritoneum on the posterior abdominal wall. (From Schaefer, G. P. [Ed.]: Morris' Human Anatomy, 10th ed. Philadelphia, Blakiston, 1951. Reproduced with permission of The McGraw-Hill Companies.)

nography may be used to localize abscesses and allow for percutaneous needle or catheter drainage. The choice depends on individual circumstances such as body habitus, patient stability, and mobility.[2]

Reflections of the peritoneum over intra-abdominal organs may influence the localization of intra-abdominal abscesses. From Figure 28–11, it can be seen that abscesses that arise from sources above the transverse mesocolon usually localize above the mesocolon. If the abscess extends, it likely extends either up into the subphrenic areas or down lateral to the ascending or descending colon. Abscesses that originate from sources below the mesocolon usually localize within the frame of the colon or extend into the pelvis. Occasionally,

TABLE 28–3. Structures That Can Be Approached Surgically Through the Retroperitoneum

Adrenal glands
Kidneys
Ureters
Bladder
Lumbar sympathetic chain
Splenic artery and vein
Renal artery and vein
Distal abdominal aorta
Inferior vena cava
Common iliac artery and vein
Internal iliac artery and vein
External iliac artery and vein
Distal pancreas
Groin hernias

giant abscesses encircle the abdomen, going around the colon through the pelvis and into either or both subphrenic spaces (Fig. 28–15).

Retroperitoneal Fibrosis. This unusual disease, which has some similarities to hypersensitivity or autoimmune disease, is relatively rare.[26, 38] The etiology is unknown, although a correlation between the ingestion of methysergide and the disease has been reported. About two thirds of all cases are considered idiopathic in that no specific cause can be proved. These are often called Ormond's disease.[7]

The most important clinical aspect of retroperitoneal fibrosis is that the fibrotic process frequently entraps and constricts the ureters, thereby causing obstructive uropathy. Patients' signs and symptoms depend on the presence or absence of ureteral stenosis, its severity, and the presence or absence of urinary infection. Presentation may vary from mild and nondescript back pain to uremia or sepsis.

The diagnosis of retroperitoneal fibrosis usually can be made accurately by intravenous pyelography if uremia is not present. The characteristic findings are hydronephrosis and hydroureter proximal to the site of extrinsic compression of the ureters. The ureters may be encased over a substantial distance, starting inferiorly and progressing superiorly. The ureters are deviated medially toward the midline. The disease is usually bilateral and symmetric but sometimes may involve only one ureter. When stenosis is severe and/or infection is present, nephrostomy may be urgently required. When the obstruction is minimal, a trial of nonoperative management may be indicated. Such management includes cessation of any drug therapy the patient is receiving, particularly methysergide. Corticosteroid therapy should be instituted. If a response does not occur within a matter of a few

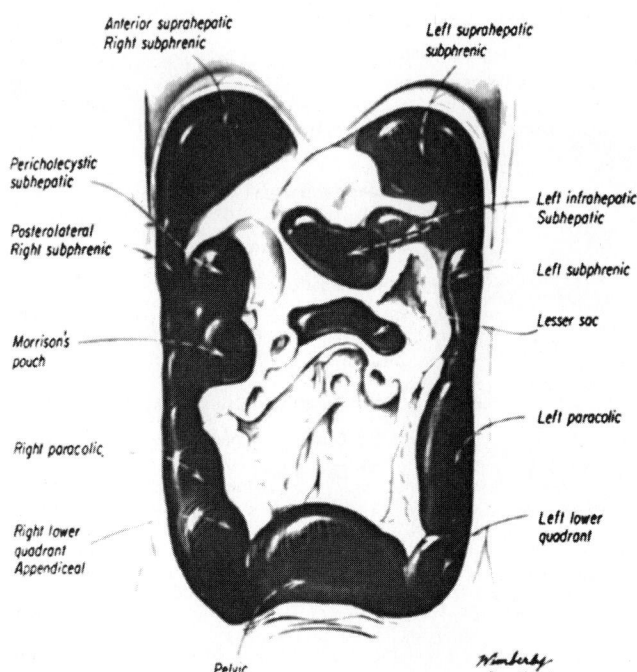

Figure 28–15. Anterior view of the abdominal and pelvic cavity illustrating size, component parts, location, and extent of giant horseshoe intra-abdominal abscess. (From Altemeier, W. A., Culbertson, W. R., and Fidler, J. P.: Giant horseshoe intraabdominal abscess. Trans. South Surg. Assoc., *86*:230, 1974.)

resonance imaging has assumed an increasingly important role in the evaluation of the primary tumor. Prospective studies comparing these modalities have shown that the two techniques complement one another, with magnetic resonance imaging often providing a greater degree of definition of muscle groups and vascular structures. Angiography continues to play an important role in the evaluation of retroperitoneal tumors.[36]

Successful treatment of these tumors remains primarily surgical. An *en bloc* resection of these malignancies provides the most favorable 5-year survival of 67%.[31] Although partial resection has a 0% 5-year survival, many patients symptomatically improve and may have a better response to radiation therapy and chemotherapy after the tumor has been debulked.

Retroperitoneal Vascular Procedures. Elective surgical procedures on the aorta and its branches are more commonly being approached from an extraperitoneal route today. Many advantages have already been mentioned, but others warrant discussion. The extraperitoneally exposed visceral aorta and its branches can be easily controlled for bypass, endarterectomy, splenorenal shunting, renal autotransplantation, and correction of aneurysmal disease. By avoiding the peritoneal cavity, the possibility of iatrogenic intestinal enterotomy and resultant graft contamination is removed. Operative time is also saved by removing the time-consuming and sometimes difficult step of reperitonealizing the aortic graft to prevent graft-enteric fistula formation. The retroperitoneal exposure of an aortic aneurysm does not disturb the periaortic tissue anterior to the proximal anastomosis.[23]

weeks, operative treatment should be advised. When renal function has been compromised, nonoperative treatment is not warranted.

Surgical treatment of retroperitoneal fibrosis centers on freeing the encased ureters from their fibrous encapsulation. Once freed, the ureters must be protected from recurrent fibrotic encasement. This has been successfully prevented by converting the ureters into intra-abdominal organs or wrapping them with omentum.[13] Renal autotransplantation also has been used as a means to treat retroperitoneal fibrosis surgically. With vascular and ureteral complications occurring in less than 5% of patients, it is a feasible surgical approach.[15] Nonspecific fibrosis can involve mediastinal structures (nonspecific mediastinal fibrosis), the thyroid gland (Reidel's struma), or the biliary tract (sclerosing cholangitis). These processes are similar and may or may not represent the same disease process involving different anatomic sites.

Retroperitoneal Tumors. At the time of presentation, the majority of retroperitoneal tumors have invaded adjacent organs and have reached considerable size. The relative inaccessibility of the retroperitoneum and the nonspecific symptoms associated with retroperitoneal tumors explain the delay in diagnosis.[12]

Primary retroperitoneal tumors are rare, with a reported incidence of 0.3% to 3%. Ackerman classified these tumors based on their histologic findings: tumors of nerve origin and tumors arising from embryonic origin.[19] The majority of these tumors (60% to 85%) are malignant; 75% are of mesodermal origin and 24% of nerve origin. Included in the mesodermally derived tumors are those arising from adipose tissue, smooth and striated muscles, connective tissues, blood vessels, and lymphatic structures.[12] These tumors are locally aggressive but rarely metastasize.

Computed tomography remains the most effective means of delineating abnormalities of the retroperitoneum. It provides evidence of local extension and resectability. Magnetic

SELECTED REFERENCES

Fry, D. E., and Osler, T.: Abdominal wall considerations and complications in reoperative surgery. Surg. Clin. North Am., 71:1, 1991.
This review article provides a clear description of the anatomy of the abdominal wall in association with reoperative abdominal surgery. It gives guidelines for placement of surgical incisions to prevent and treat abdominal wall complications.

Glenn, J., Sindelar, W. F., Kinsella, T., Glatstein, E., Tepper, J., Costa, J., Baker, A., Sugarbaker, P., Brennan, M. F., Seipp, C., Wesley, R., Young, R. C., and Rosenberg, S. A.: Results of multimodality therapy of resectable soft tissue sarcomas of the retroperitoneum. Surgery, 97:316, 1985.
This article from the National Cancer Institute reviews the use of adjuvant chemotherapy and radiation therapy in patients with resectable retroperitoneal sarcomas. The chemotherapy arm of the study was prospective and randomized and revealed that the chemotherapy regimen administered did not improve survival and was associated with major morbidity.

Hallak, A.: Spontaneous bacterial peritonitis. Am. J. Gastroenterol., 84:345, 1989.
This article clearly defines spontaneous bacterial peritonitis. It discusses the pathogenesis, clinical presentation, laboratory findings, therapy, and prognosis of this syndrome.

McGrath, P. C., Neifeld, J. P., Lawrence, W., Jr., DeMay, R. M., Kay, S., Horsley, J. S., III, and Parker, G. A.: Improved survival following complete excision of retroperitoneal sarcomas. Ann. Surg., 200:200, 1984.
This article concisely discusses the importance of aggressive surgical management of retroperitoneal sarcomas. It clearly illustrates that the improved 5-year survival rates achieved were the result of extensive surgical resections with microscopic clear margins.

REFERENCES

1. Ackerman, L. V.: Tumours of the retroperitoneum and peritoneum. *In* Atlas of Tumor Pathology, Section II, fascicle 23–24, p. 136. Washington, D.C., Armed Forces Institute of Pathology, National Research Council, 1954.
2. Adam, E. J., Page, J. E.: Intra-abdominal sepsis: The role of radiology. Baillieres Clin. Gastroenterol., 5:587, 1991.
3. Adams, J. T.: Primary torsion of the omentum. Am. J. Surg., 126:102, 1973.
4. Alban, J. C., Litooy, F. N., and Freeark, R. J.: Postoperative chylous ascites: Diagnosis and treatment. Arch. Surg., 125:270, 1990.
5. Altemeier, W. A., Culbertson, W. R., Fullen, W. D., and Shook, C. D.: Intra-abdominal abscesses. Am. J. Surg., 125:70, 1973.
6. Altemeier, W. A., Culbertson, W. R., and Fidler, J. P.: Giant horseshoe intra-abdominal abscess. Am. Surg., 181:716, 1975.

7. Amis, E. S., Jr.: Retroperitoneal fibrosis. AJR, *157*:321, 1991.

8. Beahrs, O. H., Judd, E. S., Jr., and Dockerty, M. B.: Chylous cysts of the abdomen. Surg. Clin. North Am., *30*:1081, 1950.

9. Birtch, A. G., Coran, A. G., and Gross, R. E.: Neonatal peritonitis. Surgery, *61*:305, 1967.

10. Blichert-Toft, M., Koch, F., and Neilson, O. V.: Anatomic variants of the urachus relating to clinical appearance and surgical treatment of urachal lesions. Surg. Gynecol. Obstet., *137*:51, 1973.

11. Brasfield, R. D., and Das Gupta, T. K.: Desmoid tumors of the anterior abdominal wall. Surgery, *65*:241, 1969.

12. Bryant, R. L., Stevenson, D. R., Hunton, D. W., Westbrook, K. C., and Casall, R. E.: Primary malignant retroperitoneal tumors: Current Management. Am. J. Surg., *144*:646, 1982.

13. Carini, M., Selli, C., Rizzo, M., Durval, A., and Costantini, A.: Surgical treatment of retroperitoneal fibrosis with omentoplasty. Surgery, *91*:137, 1982.

14. Conn, H., and Fessel, M.: Spontaneous bacterial peritonitis in cirrhosis: Variation on a theme. Medicine, *50*:161, 1971.

15. Deane, A. M., Gingell, J. C., and Pentlow, B. D.: Idiopathic retroperitoneal fibrosis: The role of autotransplantation. Br. J. Urol., *55*:254, 1983.

16. Duckett, J. W., Jr.: The prune belly syndrome. *In* Kelalis, P. P., and King, L. R. (Eds.): Clinical Pediatric Urology. Philadelphia, W. B. Saunders, 1976.

17. Goodman, P., Balachandran, S.: CT evaluation of the abdominal wall. Crit. Rev. Diagn. Imaging, *33*:461, 1992.

18. Hebra, A., Brown, M. F., McGeehin, K. M., and Ross, A. J.: Mesenteric, omental, and retroperitoneal cysts in children: A clinical study of 22 cases. South Med. J., *86*:173, 1993.

19. Kairaluoma, M. I., Krause-Makitalo, B., Pokela, R., Stahlberg, M., Laitinen, S., and Mokka, R. E. M.: Primary retroperitoneal tumours in adults. Ann. Chir. Gynaecol., *73*:313, 1984.

20. Klein, E. A., Streem, S. B., and Novick, A. C.: Intraoperative consultation for the retroperitoneum and adrenal glands. Urol. Clin. North Am., *12*:411, 1985.

21. Kling, S.: Patent omphalomesenteric duct: A surgical emergency. Arch. Surg., *96*:545, 1968.

22. Kurzweg, F. T., Daron, P. B., Williamson, J. W., Danna, S. J., and Johnson, J. F.: Mesenteric cysts. Am. J. Surg., *40*:462, 1974.

23. Leather, R. P., Shah, D. M., Kaufman, J. L., Fitzgerald, K. M., Chang, B. B., and Feustel, P. J.: Comparative analysis of retroperitoneal and transperitoneal aortic replacement for aneurysm. Surg. Gynecol. Obstet., *168*:387, 1989.

24. Majmudar, B., Wiskind, A. K., Croft, B. N., and Dudley, A. G.: The Sister (Mary) Joseph Nodule: Its significance in gynecology. Gynecol. Oncol., *40*:152, 1991.

25. Marschall, M. A., and Cohen, M.: The use of greater omentum in reconstructive surgery. Surg. Annu., *26*:251, 1994.

26. Ormond, J. K.: Bilateral ureteral obstruction due to envelopment and compression by an inflammatory retroperitoneal process. J. Urol., *59*:1072, 1948.

27. Replogle, R. L., Johnson, R., and Gross, R. E.: Prevention of postoperative adhesions with combined promethazine and dexamethasone therapy: Experimental and clinical studies. Ann. Surg., *163*:580, 1966.

28. Rochlin, D. B., Zill, H., and Blakemore, W. S.: Studies of resorption of chromium-51 tagged erythrocytes from the peritoneal cavity: The absorption of fluids and particulate matter from the peritoneal cavity. Surg. Gynecol. Obstet., *107*:1, 1958.

29. Samson, R., and Pasternak, B. M.: Current status of surgery of the omentum. Surg. Gynecol. Obstet., *149*:437, 1979.

30. Scherer, L. R., III, and Grossfield, J. L.: Inguinal hernia and umbilical anomalies. Pediatr. Clin. North Am., *40*:1121, 1993.

31. Serio, G., Tenchini, P., Nifosi, F., and Iacono, C.: Surgical strategy in primary retroperitoneal tumours. Br. J. Surg., *76*:385, 1989.

32. Shear, L., Swartz, C, Shinaberger, J. A., and Barry, K. G.: Kinetics of peritoneal fluid absorption in adult man. N. Engl. J. Med., *272*:123, 1965.

33. Simmons, R. L., Diggs, J. W., and Sleeman, H. K.: Pathogenesis of peritonitis: III. Local adjuvant action of hemoglobin in experimental *E. coli* peritonitis. Surgery, *63*:810, 1968.

34. Singh, M. M., Bhargava, A. N., and Jain, K. P.: Tuberculous peritonitis: An evaluation of pathogenic mechanisms, diagnostic procedures, and therapeutic measures. N. Engl. J. Med., *281*:1092, 1969.

35. Sochocky, S.: Tuberculous peritonitis: A review of 100 cases. Am. Rev. Respir. Dis., *95*:398, 1967.

36. Sondak, V. K., Economou, J. S., and Eilber, F. R.: Soft tissue sarcomas of the extremity and retroperitoneum: Advances in management. Adv. Surg., *24*:333, 1991.

37. Stiles, Q. R., Raskowski, H. J., and Henry, W.: Rectus sheath hematoma. Surg. Gynecol. Obstet., *12*:331, 1965.

38. Suby, H. I., Kerr, W. S., Graham, J. R., and Fraley, E.: Retroperitoneal fibrosis: A missing link in the chain. J. Urol., *93*:144, 1965.

39. Viranuvatti, V., Hitanat, S., Boonyapaknavig, V., Plengvanit, V., Kalayasiri, C., and Chearani, O.: Peritoneal biopsy: Experience with blind and direct vision biopsy. Am. J. Proctol., *17*:489, 1966.

40. Willwert, B. M., Zollinger, R. M., Jr., and Izant, R. J., Jr.: Congenital mesocolic (paraduodenal) hernia. Am. J. Surg., *128*:358, 1974.

THE ACUTE ABDOMEN

Arnold G. Diethelm, M.D., Robert J. Stanley, M.D., and
Michelle L. Robbin, M.D.

The diagnosis and treatment of acute abdominal pain remains one of the most important aspects of patient care, and the resolution of the problem usually resides with the surgeon. An accurate diagnosis is essential for the correct treatment, which in many cases will prevent the death of the patient. The natural history of abdominal pain depends on the pathologic process involved, which in some instances may resolve spontaneously with little or no treatment (e.g., gastroenteritis) and at other times may progress to generalized peritonitis and death (e.g., perforated viscus). The complexity of the entity known as the acute abdomen is such that a careful, methodical diagnostic approach is necessary to arrive at a correct diagnosis. Rapid or quick decisions are rarely necessary and if carried out may be incorrect or misleading. The history and physical examination remain the cornerstones of the diagnosis, which is confirmed by laboratory data and, when necessary, by radiographic studies. If this information is inadequate to establish a diagnosis and urgent or immediate operation is unnecessary, then periodic re-examination helps document the progression of the illness and often avoids surgical intervention. A thorough knowledge of the etiology of abdominal pain and its natural history is essential in the proper management of these patients. In addition, understanding the anatomy and physiology of the peritoneal cavity as well as the pathologic processes that occur within the abdomen is essential for an accurate diagnosis and treatment plan.

Perhaps no discovery had greater impact on intra-abdominal operations than the use of antibiotics in combination with operative treatment of intestinal disorders. In the past 10 years, the ability to accurately determine intra-abdominal pathology by radiologic imaging has allowed earlier and more accurate diagnosis. Today the combination of improved diagnostic procedures, antibiotics, and better anesthesia and preoperative and postoperative patient care has led to a decrease in morbidity and mortality of patients with acute septic and nonseptic conditions of the abdomen.

ANATOMY AND PHYSIOLOGY OF VISCERAL PAIN

The neurophysiology and anatomy of pain from viscera of the gastrointestinal tract, hepatobiliary tract, pancreas, kidneys, ureters, bladder, ovaries, fallopian tubes, and uterus are important to the understanding of the patient's complaint during an episode of acute abdominal pain. The lower esophagus receives its sensory innervation through rami from the splanchnic nerves and paravertebral ganglia, whereas pain from the cervical and thoracic esophagus is transmitted by sensory fibers in the vagi (Fig. 29–1). The sensation of pain from the stomach and duodenum travels by means of the splanchnic afferent fibers that enter the spinal cord at the seventh and eighth dorsal segments. Distention of the small intestine by a balloon causes discomfort that can be ablated by thoracolumbar ganglionectomy and splanchnicectomy;

however, in the presence of colon distention, the sensation of discomfort persists. Thus, colonic afferent axons travel in the sacral nerves. The primary cause of pain from the biliary tract is from distention of the common duct, cystic duct, gallbladder, and liver capsule. Pain from these structures travels though the major splanchnic nerve to the spinal cord through the seventh through ninth spinal roots. Pancreatic sensory fibers pass in the right and left splanchnic nerves from the celiac plexus. Sensation from the head of the pancreas is through the right splanchnic trunk and from the tail of the pancreas in the left splanchnic trunk. Renal pain and that from the cephalad portion of the ureter is transmitted through fibers in the vascular pedicle to the aorticorenal and celiac ganglia. From here, pain sensory fibers travel to the least splanchnic trunks and to the lowest thoracic ganglion. Thus, the main level of spinal innervation for the kidney and proximal ureter is through the tenth thoracic to the first lumbar segment. The sensory innervation of the bladder, vesical neck, and prostate is provided by the second, third, and fourth sacral nerves. Uterine pain travels through the superior hypogastric plexus and the preaortic nerves, with afferent fibers passing through the paravertebral ganglia to the twelfth thoracic and first lumbar sympa-

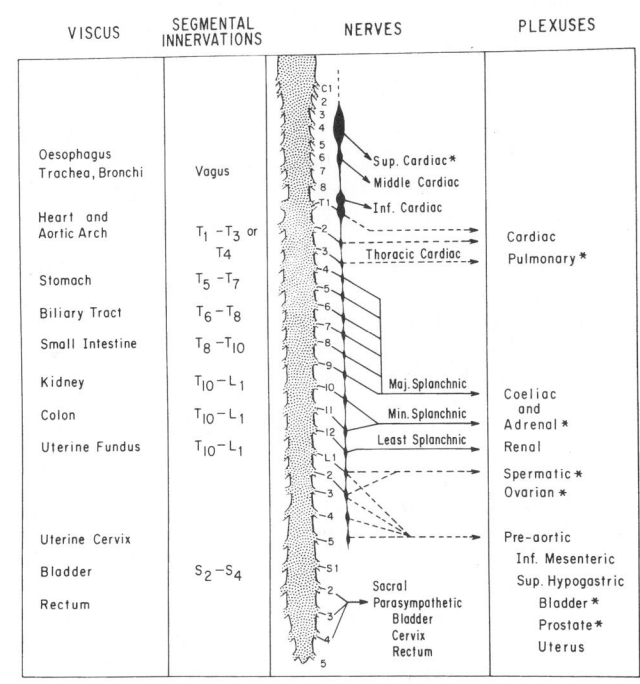

VISCUS	SEGMENTAL INNERVATIONS	NERVES	PLEXUSES
Oesophagus Trachea, Bronchi	Vagus	Sup. Cardiac* Middle Cardiac Inf. Cardiac	
Heart and Aortic Arch	$T_1 - T_3$ or T_4	Thoracic Cardiac	Cardiac Pulmonary*
Stomach	$T_5 - T_7$		
Biliary Tract	$T_6 - T_8$		
Small Intestine	$T_8 - T_{10}$		
Kidney	$T_{10} - L_1$	Maj. Splanchnic	Coeliac and Adrenal*
Colon	$T_{10} - L_1$	Min. Splanchnic	Renal
Uterine Fundus	$T_{10} - L_1$	Least Splanchnic	Spermatic* Ovarian*
Uterine Cervix			Pre-aortic Inf. Mesenteric Sup. Hypogastric
Bladder	$S_2 - S_4$		Bladder*
Rectum		Sacral Parasympathetic Bladder Cervix Rectum	Prostate* Uterus

* No known sensory fibers in sympathetic rami.

Figure 29–1. Sensory innervation of the viscera. (From White, J. C., and Sweet, W. H.: Pain and the Neurosurgeon. Springfield, IL, Charles C Thomas, 1969, p. 526.)

thetic rami and posterior spinal roots. Sensation of the cervix is transmitted by the sacral parasympathetics to the second, third, and fourth sacral segments. Ovarian pain is mediated through the sympathetic nerves passing along the ovarian arteries.

The multiple causes of abdominal pain require a thorough understanding of the anatomy and physiology of visceral pain and the patient's subjective interpretation of the pain. Pain can be characterized as sharp, stabbing, or burning or as heavy, diffuse, or dull. The autonomic response to visceral pain, often described as deep pain, is poorly localized; it includes sweating, nausea, and a decrease in blood pressure and differs from the sharp pricking pain originating from the skin. Visceral pain, which is pain arising from the abdominal and thoracic cavities, reaches the central nervous system by three routes: (1) the parasympathetic nerves, (2) the sympathetic nerves, or (3) the somatic nerves innervating the body wall and the diaphragm. It has long been recognized that visceral organs can be cut, crushed, or burned with little sensation. However, traction of the mesentery and stimulation of the parietal peritoneum cause pain. Stimulation of the visceral afferent fibers produces pain and includes (1) strong contractions or spasm, (2) sudden distention against resistance, and (3) chemical irritation and mechanical stimulation. Visceral reflexes and organic sensation travel by parasympathetic afferent nerves, whereas the sympathetic nerves conduct visceral pain. The exceptions are the pelvis, the esophagus, and trachea, where pain can be transmitted by the pelvic and vagus nerves.

Pain from visceral structures may occur at a considerable distance from the organ involved, such as shoulder pain with acute cholecystitis, and is called referred pain. This important observation has obvious clinical relevance. Visceral pain can be divided into two types: pain caused by stimulation of the parietal peritoneum and pain from the viscera itself. Both types of pain may be referred or nonreferred. The pain caused by inflammation from a perforated duodenal ulcer travels by somatic nerves. Referred parietal pain, such as diaphragmatic irritation, travels to the shoulder and neck, with the impulse ascending the phrenic nerve and entering the spinal cord at C3 and C4. Pain is then referred to these dermatome segments. The discrepancy between the point of origin of pain and its final point of referral can be explained by the caudal migration of the diaphragm during embryologic development. Referred visceral pain occurs from impulses initiated in the viscera traveling over visceral (usually sympathetic) nerves. Nonreferred visceral pain (splanchnic pain), such as pain from the gastrointestinal tract, is poorly localized and may be interpreted as being elsewhere than the site of stimulation. Visceral pain is usually described as a deep pain or ache. Rigidity and abdominal tenderness are common physical findings representing inflammation of the parietal peritoneum. In this circumstance, pain may be interpreted as regional rather than segmental.

This abbreviated description of abdominal pain is quite obviously, in clinical situations, dependent on the subjective interpretation by the patient. Careful questioning of the patient by the surgeon may provide additional information, such as whether the attention of the patient can be deflected during the examination and thus lessen the severity of the pain. An inappropriate response may suggest that the subjective expression of pain is less severe than that described by the patient. It is equally important to note the stoic patient, who has a high tolerance for pain and may express less discomfort than expected. All complaints of abdominal pain must be considered serious until all reasonable diagnostic efforts prove otherwise.

The assessment of abdominal pain in the patient who is acutely ill requires a complete knowledge of the anatomic relationship of the intraperitoneal organs, their innervation, and the location of referred pain. Generally, intra-abdominal pain is interpreted by the patient as being localized in various anatomic sites, which may be helpful to the surgeon in analyzing the potential pathologic cause. For example, biliary tract disease is localized more precisely than disease of the small and large intestines (Fig. 29–2). Acute cholecystitis presents with right upper quadrant pain and may extend to the epigastric region if pancreatitis or common duct stones are present. Thus, under such circumstances, the location of pain would overlap from the right upper quadrant to the epigastric region. The referral of pain to the right shoulder and scapula is frequently noted in patients with acute cholecystitis and is rarely seen with other causes of abdominal pain. Pain from acute duodenal ulcer disease, nonperforated, is noted in the epigastric region and is often highly circumscribed. If the ulcer is in the posterior wall of the duodenum and erodes into the pancreas, pain is referred directly to the back. This type of pain is often dull and constant and may be impossible to separate from carcinoma of the pancreas. Pain from the small intestine occurs in the periumbilical area and rarely radiates to the back or other intra-abdominal locations. Pain from the colon is more apparent in the suprapubic location and is ill defined in terms of character and radiation. Renal pain is not usually abdominal in location and only radiates when the ureter is involved. When a calculus is in the ureter, pain radiates to the groin, which is helpful in establishing an accurate diagnosis.

Although localization of pain in the four quadrants of the abdomen has some value to the examiner, it may not be relevant to the etiology of the pain. Knowledge of the embryologic development of the gastrointestinal tract is pertinent to the radiation of pain. The different innervations of the foregut, midgut, and hindgut are important in the assessment of the patient and in understanding that pain from visceral fibers is less well localized than pain from somatic nerves. This observation is due to a smaller number of sensory fibers that are unmyelinated.

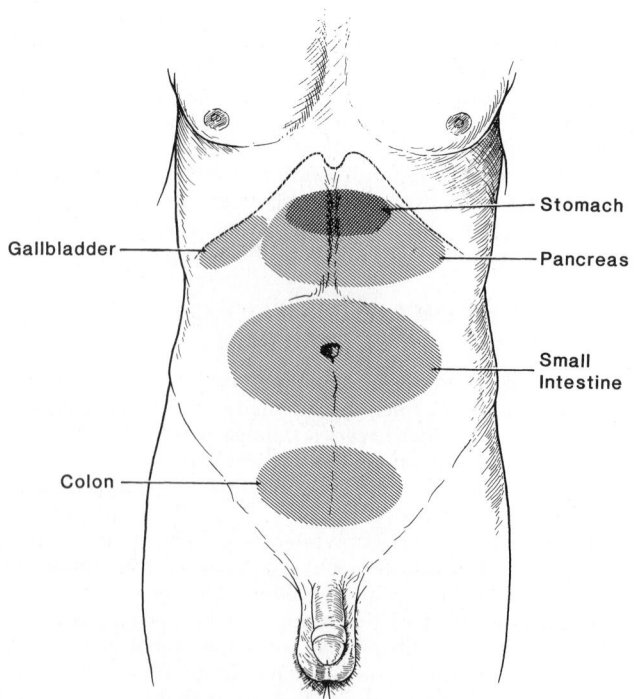

Figure 29–2. Pain from intra-abdominal viscera.

CLINICAL CONSIDERATIONS

The patient with acute abdominal pain requires a thorough clinical history and physical examination by an unhurried physician willing to take the necessary time to establish a correct diagnosis. It is important to assess the clinical situation in detail and obtain appropriate laboratory studies to avoid a superficial conclusion. Although most causes of abdominal pain are related to diseases of the gastrointestinal tract and the gynecologic subsystem, all potential causes must be considered in the overall analysis (Fig. 29–3).[38, 39]

History

Present Illness

Pain. Abdominal pain, either sudden or gradual in onset, frequently progresses in severity so that it becomes the dominant feature of the patient's illness. A careful and detailed history will define the time of onset of pain, its location, and whether a change in character occurs with various positions. Pain that persists for 6 hours or more and is of severe intensity usually requires operative intervention for treatment of the underlying process. The converse is true in those patients with pain of sudden onset who may experience complete resolution in 4 to 6 hours. The exact situation in which the onset of pain occurs may be important in establishing the diagnosis. Pain that is sharp, severe, and sudden in onset—awakening the patient from sleep or incapacitating the patient at work—often suggests a perforated viscus. Pain located in the upper abdomen favors peptic ulcer disease, acute cholecystitis, or pancreatitis, compared to ruptured ovarian cyst, perforated diverticulitis, or ruptured tubo-ovarian abscess, when pain is located in the lower abdomen. The character of the pain initially and later is important in the differentiation of pain from small bowel obstruction or strangulation of the intestine. The former pain is a cramping, intermittent type of pain, whereas the latter causes a dull, constant pain. The original location of the pain and its shifting or changing of position may provide a clue to the diagnosis, as is commonly seen with acute appendicitis. The character of the pain and the patient's description are of major importance. A sudden burning pain in the epigastric region suggests a perforated viscus; severe intermittent cramping pain with short pain-free intervals favors small bowel obstruction. Sudden excruciating tearing pain may be associated with a ruptured aneurysm. Radiation of the pain may be helpful in the diagnosis. Pain of acute cholecystitis frequently radiates around the right costal margin to the right scapula and to the shoulder. Pain in acute pancreatitis is usually epigastric in origin, with subsequent radiation along both costal margins to the back. Ureteral calculi causes pain radiating to the groin when the stone is in the cephalad portion of the ureter and produces perineal pain when the stone is near the ureterovesical junction. This type of pain is frequently excruciating. A sudden severe shearing or tearing pain of the chest or intracapsular region extending to the abdomen and occasionally into the upper or lower extremities suggests a dissection of the thoracic aorta.

Vomiting. Vomiting may result from the severity of the pain, but more often the cause is related to the gastrointestinal tract. Vomiting occurs uncommonly in the presence of a perforated ulcer but is frequently noted in patients with acute cholecystitis. Vomiting always occurs with obstruction of the small intestine and provides temporary relief from the cramping abdominal pain. The temporal relationship of abdominal pain to vomiting is important and may provide important diagnostic clues to the underlying etiology. Pain almost always precedes vomiting by 3 or 4 hours in patients with appendicitis. The converse is true in gastroenteritis. The frequency of vomiting may be significant in that one or two episodes may occur with gastroenteritis and then subside. Emesis occurs early and repeatedly in patients with small intestinal obstruction but presents late or not at all in the course of colon obstruction. The character of the emesis, including the volume, color, and content, is pertinent in regard to the site of obstruction. Clear vomitus suggests an obstructed pylorus, whereas bile-stained emesis indicates that the obstruction is distal to the entrance of the common bile duct into the duodenum. As the site of obstruction moves distally in the small intestine, the vomitus becomes brown and feculent. Cramping abdominal pain that is relieved by vomiting favors small bowel obstruction.

Anorexia. It is uncommon for patients with acute abdominal pain to desire food. Anorexia is usually associated with acute abdominal pain and, in patients with acute appendicitis, it may precede the onset of pain. This observation becomes especially important in children, in whom anorexia followed by vague periumbilical abdominal pain is suggestive of acute appendicitis.

Bowels. Constipation, diarrhea, and a recent change in bowel habits are important factors in the diagnosis of patients with abdominal pain. Profuse watery diarrhea for 12 or more hours with cramping abdominal pain is suggestive of gastroenteritis. In patients with acquired immunodeficiency syndrome (AIDS), profuse diarrhea is suggestive of cytomegalovirus infection as well as salmonellosis or cryptosporidiosis. The failure to pass flatus associated with cramping pain and vomiting strongly supports mechanical obstruction of the gastrointestinal tract. A description of subtle changes in bowel habits, although important, may be difficult to obtain from patients with extreme discomfort during abdominal pain.

Menstruation. An accurate menstrual history is especially valuable in the assessment of abdominal pain in the female, including frequency of the cycle and the duration of the menstrual period. The exact dates of the beginning and end of the period are important. Any change in volume of menstrual flow is pertinent, because an ectopic pregnancy may rupture at any time during the cycle as well as simultaneously with the menstrual period. The type of contraception and its duration of use is also important historical information.

Past Illnesses. The patient's history before the present illness is of special value, particularly in regard to previous operations (e.g., appendectomy, cholecystectomy, gastric, and intestinal procedures). The previous diagnosis of an abdomi-

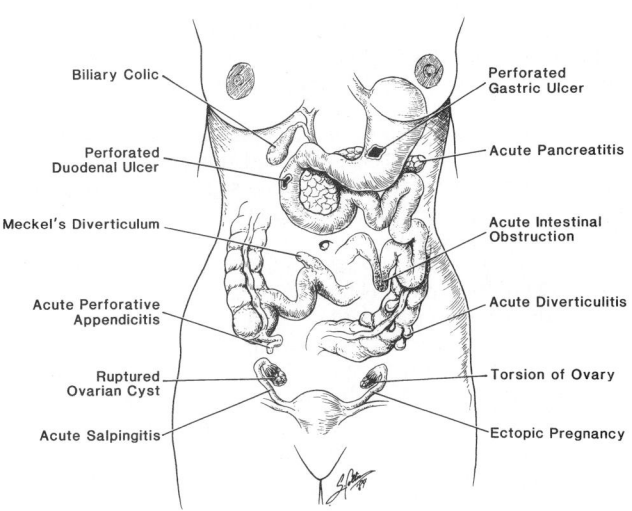

Figure 29–3. Common causes of abdominal pain.

nal or inguinal hernia may contribute to the diagnosis of the present illness. A history of similar pain is especially valuable, suggesting a recurrent problem such as a previous passage of a kidney stone or pelvic inflammatory disease. The natural history of a previous attack occasionally predicts the outcome of the current attack. It is important to record medications that may alter the severity of pain such as corticosteroids.

Family History. The probability of acute abdominal pain relating to a familial disease is unlikely but does occur in some circumstances. Familial Mediterranean fever (familial recurring polyserositis) occurs in persons of Armenian or Sephardic Jewish background as an inherited autosomal recessive trait with spontaneous attacks of abdominal pain. Sickle cell anemia in black patients is another example of hereditary influence on the etiology of abdominal pain. In such instances the patient is able to state with reasonable accuracy that the current pain is identical to that noted previously.

Organ System Review. A careful organ system review is essential to the patient's history and should be obtained in detail to avoid overlooking an extra-abdominal cause of pain, such as a pulmonary embolus to the lower lobe with diaphragmatic irritation or an acute myocardial infarction. Patients with a systemic illness, such as lupus erythematosus, nephrotic syndrome, porphyria, and sickle cell crisis, may also develop abdominal pain as a manifestation of their underlying illness and do not require surgical intervention.

Physical Examination

The physical examination coupled with a careful and accurate history, in most instances, provides or at least suggests an accurate diagnosis that may then be confirmed by the appropriately selected laboratory tests and radiologic imaging studies.

The physical examination includes a brief but complete assessment of the patient's appearance, ability to answer questions, position in bed, and degree of obvious pain or discomfort. The general appearance should be noted immediately on meeting the patient and the taking of the history. An anxious, pale, sweating patient who is either restless or lies quietly in a supine position in bed and complains of abdominal pain has a high probability of intra-abdominal disease or serious extra-abdominal disease with pain referred to the abdomen. The position in bed is important regarding whether the patient lies in a supine position or on his or her side with the knees and hips flexed. The presence of obvious dehydration with dry mucous membranes, sunken hollow eyes, and rapid shallow respiration all suggest generalized peritonitis. A rapid heart rate with hypotension occurs with hypovolemia and usually is caused by peritonitis and large plasma volume fluid shifts from the intravascular space to the extravascular space within the peritoneal cavity.

Examination of the abdomen always begins with a visual inspection of the chest and abdomen for previous scars, hernia, obvious masses, or abdominal wall defects. The inspection should include the size, shape, and contour of the abdomen and the respiratory rate of the patient. Rapid shallow breaths occur with peritoneal irritation. Auscultation of the abdomen includes all four quadrants, with special attention given to the frequency and pitch of bowel sounds and rushes of gas audible to the examiner that correlate to the facial expression of pain by the patient. Percussion of the abdomen should begin in the quadrant free of pain and be performed lightly so as to avoid eliciting pain at the onset of the examination. This is especially important in children with abdominal tenderness, in whom percussion may increase tenderness and cause them to lose confidence in the examining physi-

cian. The location of maximal tenderness should be confirmed in relation to the area of the abdomen and correlated with the history. Thus, maximal tenderness in the right lower quadrant over McBurney's point is suggestive of appendicitis if there is a history compatible with the disease. The abdomen should be palpated gently and begin in the quadrant away from that in which pain is described in the history.

A pelvic and rectal examination must be performed, preferably by the surgeon or physician responsible for the complete assessment of the patient. An umbilical or inguinal hernia should always be sought to document the presence of incarceration. The presence of peritoneal irritation can be assessed either by abdominal palpation with a quick release of the examining hand (rebound tenderness) or by gently rolling the patient from side to side with the examiner's hands placed on the patient's pelvis. Rigidity of the rectus muscles may be especially obvious in patients with generalized peritonitis due to a perforated viscus. Examination of the abdomen in such instances may be difficult. Flexion of the lower extremities at the knee and hip helps the patient relax the abdominal wall and allows a more complete examination. The lateral abdominal muscles are less rigid in acute peritonitis than the rectus muscles, and tenderness is less apparent in the older or obese patient with weak abdominal muscles. The abdomen should always be examined for free fluid, liver dullness, and iliopsoas rigidity due to inflammation of the psoas muscle. The pelvic examination may reveal the presence of cervical discharge or vaginal bleeding, and bimanual examination either confirms or excludes tenderness on uterine and adnexal palpation. A rectal examination should note the existence of a pelvic mass and the presence of a perirectal mass or abscess.

Diagnostic Imaging

The role of the radiologist in the evaluation of the patient with an acute abdomen has evolved greatly in the past decade. The plain supine and erect radiograph of the abdomen remains the most common first step in the diagnostic imaging evaluation of patients with abdominal pain, although more sensitive and more specific imaging methods, such as computed tomography (CT) and ultrasonography, play an increasing role in the evaluation of this complex, emergent clinical problem. Early enthusiasm for more sophisticated imaging technology was tempered by considerations of limited access, high cost, and delay of time required for the imaging procedure. CT and ultrasonography are now widely available methods, and techniques of examination have been streamlined. Although the cost of the more sophisticated examinations remains a factor, CT and ultrasonography often obviate organ-specific imaging studies such as excretory urograms, radionuclide examinations, and diagnostic arteriograms.

As greater experience in the use of CT and ultrasonography has been gained, it is recognized that there is a demonstrable morphologic correlate to almost all of the conditions associated with the clinical presentation of an acute abdomen. Although the plain abdominal film may provide specific, diagnostic findings, valuable in making correct therapeutic decisions, more often than not the findings are nonspecific or indeterminate. Whether one is dealing with acute, severe inflammatory disease affecting the gastrointestinal or genitourinary tract, complications of blunt abdominal trauma or acute vascular crises (e.g., acute mesenteric venous thrombosis or rupture of a visceral artery aneurysm), the plain film radiographic findings most often are not revealing and are substantially less informative than a carefully obtained history and physical examination. In contrast, CT and ultrasonography often provide differential morphologic information not obtainable by any other means short of exploratory operations, allowing the precise diagnosis of most of the entities associated with the acute abdomen.[36]

In this section, the appropriate role of the plain film, organ-specific contrast studies of the gastrointestinal and genitourinary tract, radionuclide imaging, CT, ultrasonography, and arteriography, as it applies to the evaluation of the acute abdomen, is presented.

Initial radiologic evaluation of the patient with an acute abdomen most often consists of the plain film of the abdomen obtained in the supine and erect position. The standard erect film of the abdomen, however, is not the most appropriate radiograph for the detection of free intraperitoneal air. This erect radiograph should be obtained with the central ray positioned at the level of the diaphragm to optimize the chances of detecting small quantities of free air trapped in subdiaphragmatic locations. If the patient is unable to assume the erect position, a lateral decubitus radiograph with the patient's left side down should be requested. In this instance the x-ray beam is in a horizontal cross-table orientation and the central ray should be positioned closer to the right lateral abdominal wall rather than toward the midline of the abdomen. Quantities of free air as small as 5 to 10 ml. can be detected in the space between the lateral aspect of the right lobe of the liver and the lateral abdominal wall.

Free intraperitoneal air can be the result of perforation of a gastric or duodenal peptic ulcer, perforation of the cecum due to obstruction and/or ischemia and necrosis, or perforation associated with colonic diverticulitis. Although the quantity of free air associated with a perforated duodenal ulcer is usually relatively small in volume, perforations of the stomach or colon may be associated with much larger quantities of free intraperitoneal air, a distinction of some differential diagnostic value. If the quantity of free air is great enough, its presence can be appreciated on the supine radiograph of the abdomen, when the inner and outer surface of the wall of a gas-filled loop of bowel can be clearly defined because of the presence of gas on either side of the soft tissue structure. In a similar fashion, the falciform ligament is occasionally visible as an obliquely oriented soft tissue structure extending from the right upper quadrant toward the umbilicus, when sufficiently large quantities of gas are present on either side of it. A sizeable hydropneumoperitoneum or pyopneumoperitoneum is easily recognized in the erect radiograph of the abdomen by the presence of an air-fluid level, which is too great in length for even an obstructed segment of colon (Fig. 29–4A). This same condition can be recognized on the supine radiograph of the abdomen by the detection of an oval- or football-shaped collection of gas beneath the anterior abdominal wall that does not conform to any recognizable loop of bowel (see Fig. 29–4B).

Abnormal calcific densities detectable on a plain radiograph of the abdomen and sometimes associated with the clinical presentation of an acute abdomen include gallstones, renal and ureteral calculi, appendicoliths, intrapancreatic calculi (most often associated with chronic pancreatitis), and curvilinear calcification located in the wall of an abdominal aortic or visceral artery aneurysm. Such plain radiographic information is only of value when correlated with the clinical presentation, because many of these findings occur in asymptomatic patients.

Plain radiographs of the abdomen play their greatest role in the evaluation of the question of mechanical obstruction of the gastrointestinal tract.[10] Supine and erect radiographs of the abdomen should allow the distinction between gastric outlet obstructions; proximal, mid, and distal small bowel obstructions; and colonic obstructive processes. If the plain films suggest a mid to distal small bowel obstruction, based on numerous air-fluid levels within loops of dilated small

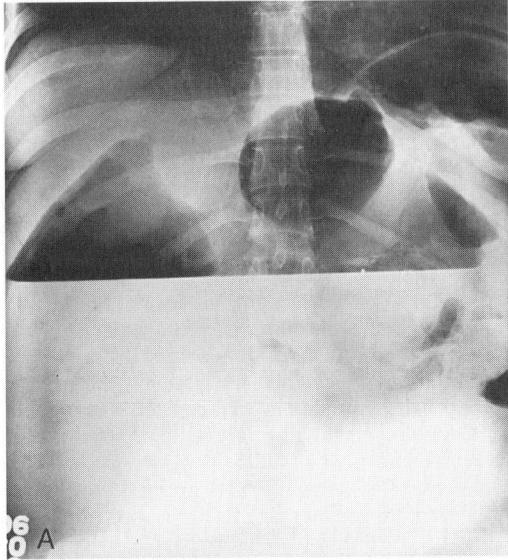
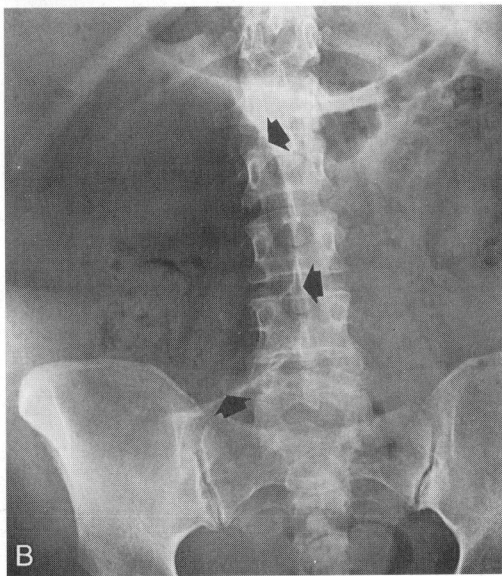

Figure 29–4. Plain film findings in hydropneumoperitoneum. *A*, Upright view shows fluid level too long to be within a loop of bowel. *B*, In the supine position, the free air is well defined by the interface with the fluid in the peritoneal cavity (arrows).

bowel, in association with partial or complete absence of gas within the colon, an immediate full-column barium enema clarifies the absence of colonic obstruction. If the ileocecal valve is sufficiently incompetent, the barium permits opacification of collapsed terminal ileum and possibly identifies the point of obstruction. High-grade obstructions of the right colon, such as those caused by a constricting neoplasm, may mimic a distal small bowel obstruction. It is in such cases that an immediate barium enema has its greatest value. Carcinomas of the cecum and ileocecal valve can also produce high-grade obstructions of the small bowel and are readily detected with a barium enema.

In contrast to the high diagnostic yield of a promptly performed barium enema in the presence of mid to distal small bowel obstruction, contrast studies from above, whether with barium or water-soluble contrast medium, frequently have little diagnostic value beyond reinforcing the impression of small bowel mechanical obstruction and often lead to delays in diagnosis and treatment. On the other hand, if the clinical presentation as well as the plain radiographs suggest obstruction of the gastric outlet or duodenum, an upper gastrointestinal examination is of considerable value, not only in confirming the presence of mechanical obstruction but also in suggesting the precise cause. Therefore, consultation with the radiologist can be of considerable value when assessing the plain film findings in the patient with an acute abdomen and planning further diagnostic imaging studies.

At times the patient with an acute abdomen presents with a radiographic bowel gas pattern suggestive of mechanical obstruction when, in fact, no mechanically obstructing process is present. Such varied entities as pneumonia, pulmonary infarction, diffuse peritonitis, acute severe pyelonephritis, vascular compromise of the small or large bowel, a variety of inflammatory processes affecting the gastrointestinal tract, as well as metabolic or drug-related effects on the motility of the bowel can all produce an abnormal bowel gas pattern. A decrease in peristalsis or its cessation is referred to as an *ileus*. This term can be applied to any type of intestinal obstruction, whether mechanical or not. Those conditions that produce diminished or absent bowel motility not due to a mechanical process are said to have caused an adynamic or paralytic ileus. It is, of course, crucial in the evaluation of the patient with an acute abdomen to make the important distinction between an adynamic ileus and a mechanical ileus. Plain film findings in a patient with an adynamic ileus include the presence of gas, both within the small intestine and colon. There is moderate distention of the caliber of the bowel throughout, rather than significant disproportions suggesting a point of transition. Air-fluid levels are at essentially the same level in the same loop of small bowel and on the erect radiograph (consistent with complete lack of motility) with a nonchanging appearance to the bowel gas pattern over a period of several hours. When it is difficult to differentiate an adynamic ileus pattern from a pattern suggestive of distal colonic obstruction, a carefully performed full-column barium enema will again provide rapid resolution of this diagnostic problem.

If the patient's clinical presentation suggests a free perforation of the bowel into the peritoneal cavity, and a contrast study of the gastrointestinal tract is still indicated, water-soluble contrast medium is appropriate to use to avoid the complications of a barium peritonitis.

Other plain film findings of diagnostic value include the detection of gas within the portal and mesenteric venous systems, intramural gas anywhere in the gastrointestinal tract, gas within the biliary tree in the absence of known, surgically created biliary enteric anastomoses, as well as abnormal gas collections associated with the gallbladder, the urinary tract, or retroperitoneal spaces in general. In patients with adequate perivisceral and retroperitoneal fat, obscuration of portions or all of the outlines of those organs and structures normally surrounded by fat may be an important clue to an associated or contiguous inflammatory or hemorrhagic process. The inflammation and abscess formation associated with appendicitis, for example, can obliterate the right psoas margin as well as the properitoneal fat flank stripe in the right lower quadrant. Whereas it is important to recognize these findings, they are still nonspecific and should lead to more definitive studies, such as CT.

When gas is detected within the portal or mesenteric venous systems on a plain radiograph of the abdomen, the inflammatory or ischemic process producing the release of gas into the venous system is generally far advanced and the finding is associated with a high mortality. In contrast, CT can detect minute quantities of gas within the portal and mesenteric venous systems and is often capable of demonstrating the causative condition at a far earlier stage of development. In general, by the time intra-abdominal pathologic

processes are detectable on a plain roentgenogram, they are usually far advanced. With the early use of CT, plain films of the abdomen that appear unremarkable or indeterminate have been shown to be insensitive to the readily recognizable morphologic changes on the CT examination associated with the conditions producing an acute abdomen (Fig. 29–5).

When the signs and symptoms of a patient with an acute abdomen suggest renal colic due to the passage of a renal calculus into the pelvis or ureter, an excretory urogram will often be diagnostic. The pain of renal colic can be simulated by other conditions, including a renal tumor, acute renal

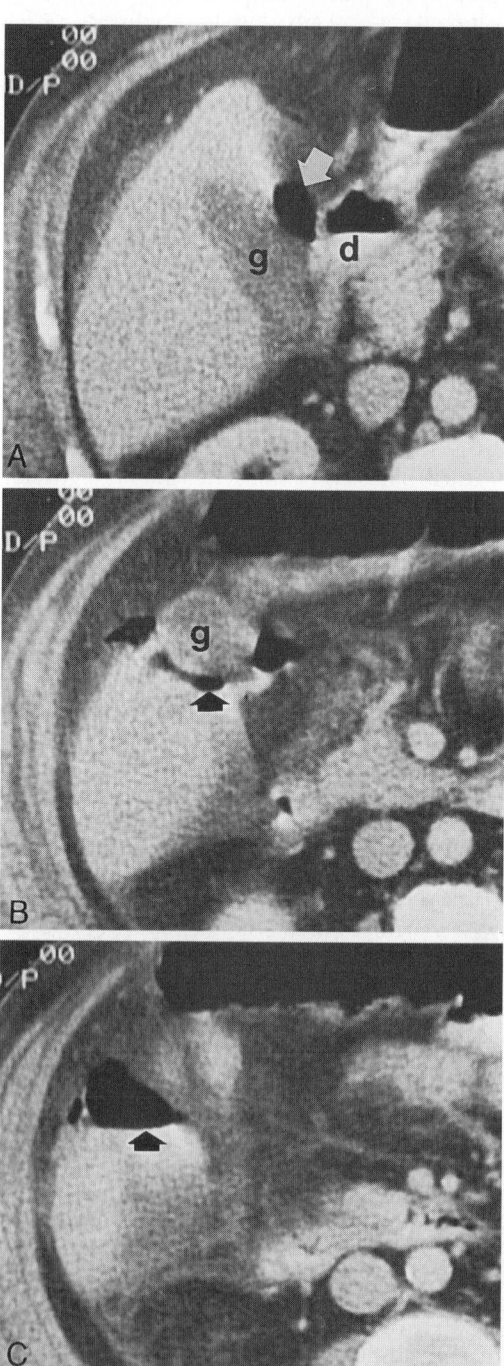

Figure 29–5. Unsuspected perforated duodenal ulcer. *A,* Small amount of extraluminal gas (arrow) lies lateral to duodenal bulb (d). g, gallbladder. *B,* At 3 cm. caudad, gas (arrow) tracks behind the gallbladder laterally. *C,* The air-fluid level (arrow) identifies the loculated extravasated duodenal contents. Inflammatory changes are present in the surrounding mesenteric fat.

inflammatory disease, or disease processes affecting the renal vascular pedicle, and often the excretory urogram establishes the correct diagnosis.

There are few indications for radionuclide imaging procedures in the evaluation of the acute abdomen. The role of biliary radiopharmaceuticals such as hepatoiminodiacetic acid (HIDA), in the evaluation of patients with suspected acute cholecystitis remains incompletely defined. Strong proponents of their use emphasize the diagnostic importance of the finding of nonfilling of the gallbladder by the radionuclide imaging agent in the presence of good excretion in the remainder of the biliary tree. However, a minimum of 4 hours must elapse before delayed filling of the gallbladder with a patent cystic duct can be excluded. Additionally, chronic cholecystitis has occasionally produced false-positive studies. Real-time ultrasonography is the more commonly used imaging study in the assessment of the patient with suspected acute cholecystitis. In a matter of minutes, the caliber of the biliary tree, the presence and location of biliary calculi, the morphology of the gallbladder wall, and the presence or absence of tenderness due to the pressure of the transducer directly over the gallbladder can be assessed (Fig. 29–6).

When acute abdominal pain develops after blunt trauma, radionuclide imaging studies of the liver and spleen are generally less informative than a properly performed CT examination of the abdomen. The radionuclide study is organ limited and, although it is sensitive to traumatic injuries of the liver and spleen, it is nevertheless insensitive to associated perisplenic or perihepatic processes. A radionuclide study may be indicated in the hemodynamically stable patient in whom the CT findings, for any one of a variety of technical problems, are indeterminate.

The indications for the use of CT and ultrasonography in the evaluation of the acute abdomen have increased dramatically in the past decade.[19–21] Ultrasonography can provide rapid evaluation of liver, spleen, pancreas, renal morphology, kidneys, ovaries, adnexa, and uterus. With the advent of color Doppler ultrasonography, the blood vessels of the abdomen can be studied with remarkable precision in a manner

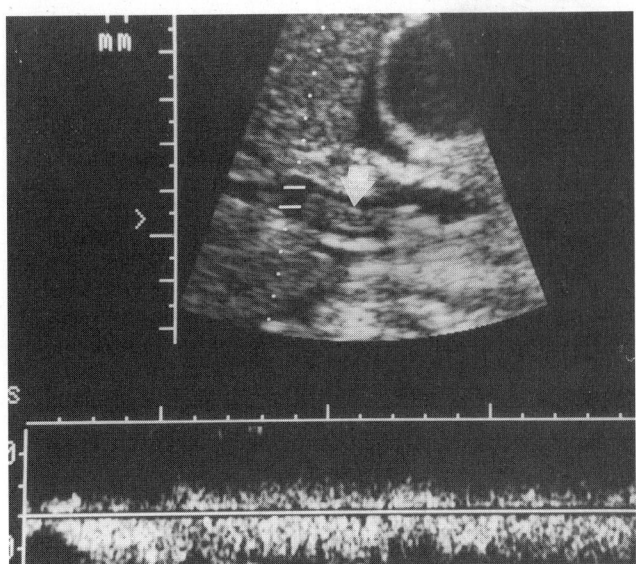

Figure 29–7. Thrombus in portal vein evident on pulsed Doppler ultrasonography. An echogenic thrombus (arrow) is within the lumen of the portal vein. Doppler tracing indicates flow within portal vein.

not possible as recently as the mid 1980s. Aortic and visceral artery aneurysms, thrombi within veins, arteriovenous fistulas, and vascular anomalies all are amenable to evaluation with modern ultrasound equipment (Fig. 29–7).

Because of the frequently occurring adynamic ileus in patients with an acute abdomen, large areas of the abdomen will be inaccessible for ultrasound evaluation due to the interposed gas, which poorly transmits a sound wave. CT is not hampered by overlying gas, bone, or adipose tissue, all of which present relative obstacles to the transmission of a sound wave. Additionally, whereas an experienced ultrasonographer can complete a general survey of the abdomen and pelvis in a relatively short period of time, a complete CT examination of the abdomen and pelvis can be performed in the same amount of time or less with a degree of thoroughness not achievable with ultrasonography. Therefore, CT plays a more useful role in the early evaluation of the patient with an acute abdomen, unless the signs and symptoms are highly indicative of a disease process in a specific organ system, such as acute cholecystitis or renal colic.

Considering one of the more common causes of the acute abdomen, namely appendicitis, plain films of the abdomen are occasionally helpful, and barium enemas have also been shown to clarify some cases with ambiguous findings. However, in the patient with uncomplicated appendicitis, ultrasonography has been found to be more sensitive for the detection of appendicoliths as well as in the demonstration of the abnormally distended and thick-walled appendix itself (Fig. 29–8). Periappendiceal and pericecal inflammatory changes are manifested as hyperechoic fat adjacent to the inflamed appendix, adding support to the diagnosis.[20]

CT is better in defining the changes associated with complicated appendicitis (Fig. 29–9). It is generally possible to differentiate a periappendiceal phlegmon from an abscess as well as differentiating a well-defined, well-localized abscess from a poorly localized, extensive abscess, all of which have therapeutic implications.

The differential diagnosis of appendicitis is extensive and includes acute cholecystitis, perinephric abscess, pyonephrosis, Crohn's disease, cecal or ileocecal carcinoma, psoas abscess, typhlitis (neutropenic enterocolitis), rectus hematoma, intestinal obstruction or infarction, diverticulitis with abscess, and salpingitis, possibly with rupture of the

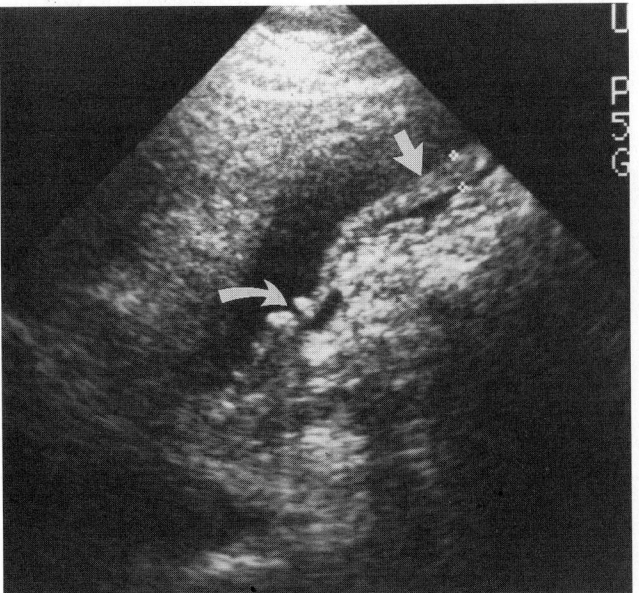

Figure 29–6. Acute cholecystitis. Ultrasound evaluation shows two small stones (curved arrow) present in the neck of the gallbladder. The wall of the gallbladder in the fundus (straight arrow) is thickened, and pericholecystic fluid is present.

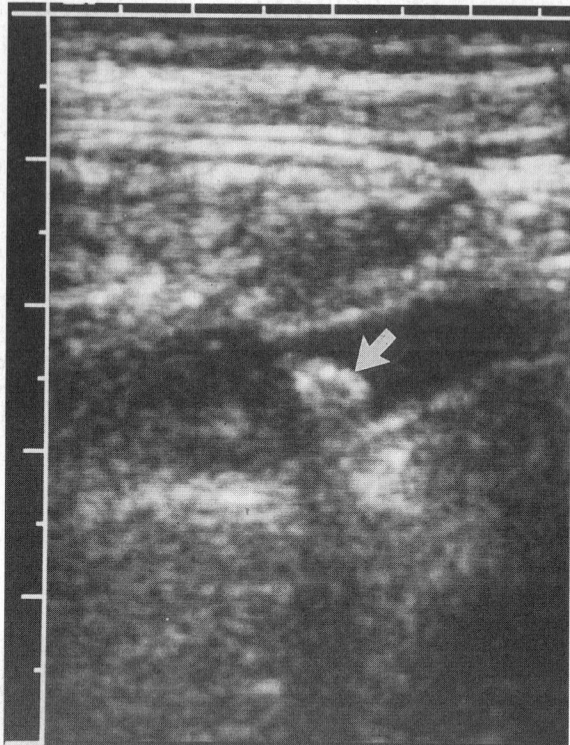

Figure 29–8. Acute appendicitis. On ultrasonography a radiographically nonopaque appendicolith (arrow) is evident within a thick-walled, distended appendix (longitudinal view).

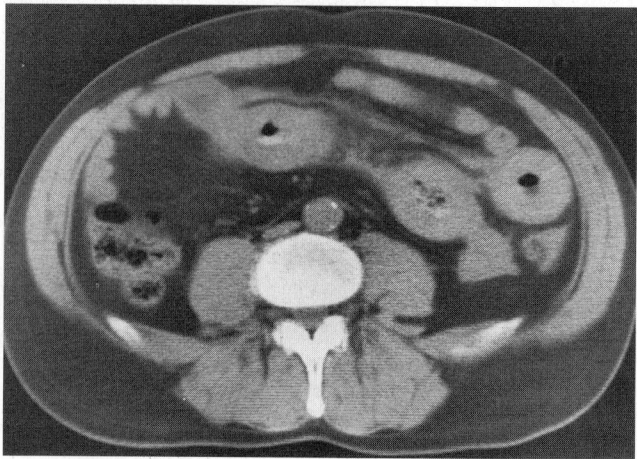

Figure 29–10. Intramural hematoma of small bowel. Uniform, concentric, high-density thickening of the wall of jejunal loops is characteristic.

pyosalpinx, as well as other causes of intraperitoneal pathology. CT allows differentiation of many, if not all, of these entities quickly.

Spontaneous as well as posttraumatic intra-abdominal hemorrhage is readily and accurately diagnosable with CT. Intramural intestinal hemorrhage from whatever cause may also cause acute abdominal pain and produce a characteristic appearance on CT (Fig. 29–10). Occasionally it is possible to identify the associated disease processes, such as pancreatitis, lymphoma, hepatic cirrhosis, and other diseases, that produce clotting disorders or vascular fragility. A rare cause of an acute abdomen related to hemorrhage is sudden, spontaneous adrenal hemorrhage, which can also result in an addisonian crisis. The findings on CT are pathognomonic.

The CT findings in bowel ischemia and infarction include wall thickening (a common but nonspecific feature) and, more specifically, intramural gas, venous gas, and vascular occlusion (Fig. 29–11). Pylephlebitis, a septic thrombophlebitis of the portal and mesenteric venous systems, usually caused by a suppurative intra-abdominal process, most often appendicitis, is a diagnosis that is rarely established on clinical grounds alone and is recognized only late in its course with plain film radiography. However, CT can image the causative inflammatory process, the thrombosed and inflamed vein, and even minute quantities of gas within the mesenteric venous system and the intrahepatic portions of the portal vein (Fig. 29–12). A similar condition seen in the postpartum patient in which endometritis was a complication is septic thrombosis of the ovarian vein. The CT findings in this entity are characteristic and include an enlarged, thrombosed, thick-walled ovarian vein surrounded by inflammatory changes in the retroperitoneal fat.[3]

Acute pancreatitis frequently presents as an acute abdomen. Since the advent of CT and ultrasonography, the understanding of the various inflammatory diseases affecting the pancreas has increased by a level of magnitude unsurpassed by that for any of the other disease processes within the abdomen. Before the era of CT and ultrasonography only the gross changes associated with complicated pancreatitis were

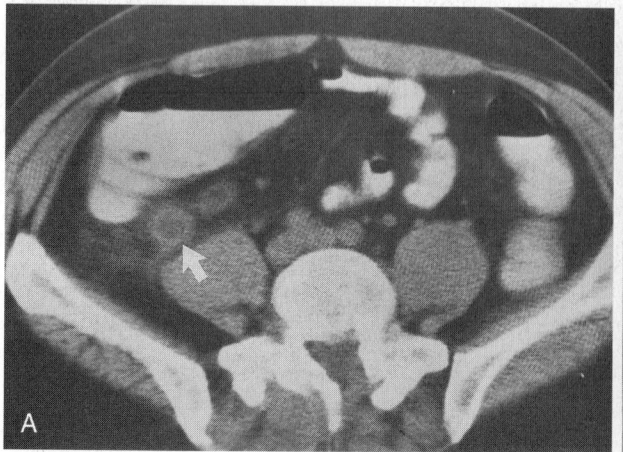

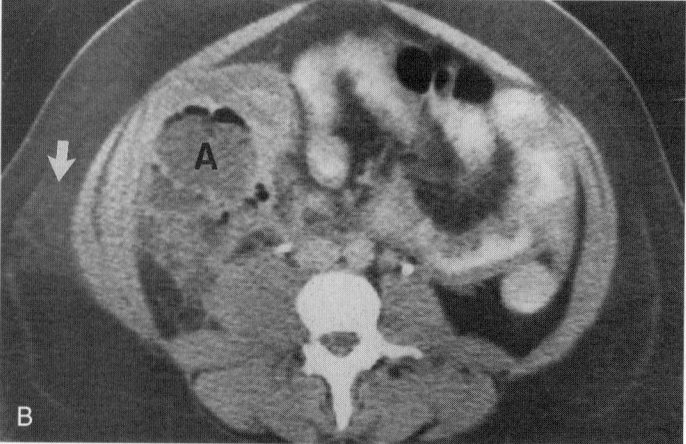

Figure 29–9. Appendicitis. *A*, CT scan of uncomplicated appendicitis. A thick-walled, distended, retrocecal appendix (arrow) is seen with inflammatory change in the surrounding fat. *B*, CT scan of complicated appendicitis. Retrocecal appendiceal abscess (A) with associated phlegmon posteriorly was found in a 3-week-postpartum, obese female patient. Inflammatory change extends through the flank musculature into the subcutaneous fat (arrow).

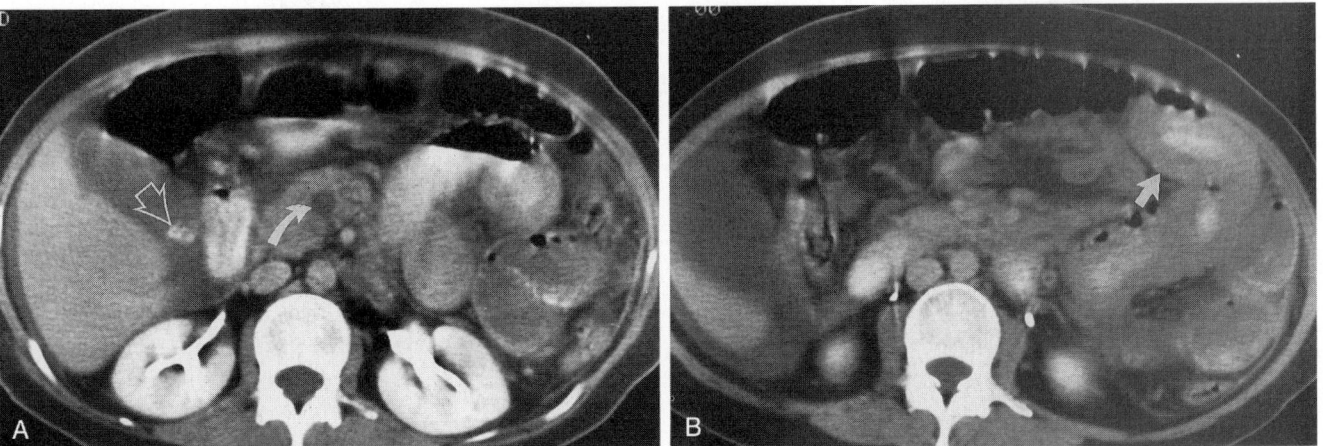

Figure 29–11. Small bowel infarction associated with mesenteric venous thrombosis. *A*, Note low-density thrombosed superior mesenteric vein (solid arrow) and incidental gallstones (open arrow). *B*, Thickening of proximal small bowel wall (arrow) coincided with several feet of infarcting small bowel at time of surgery.

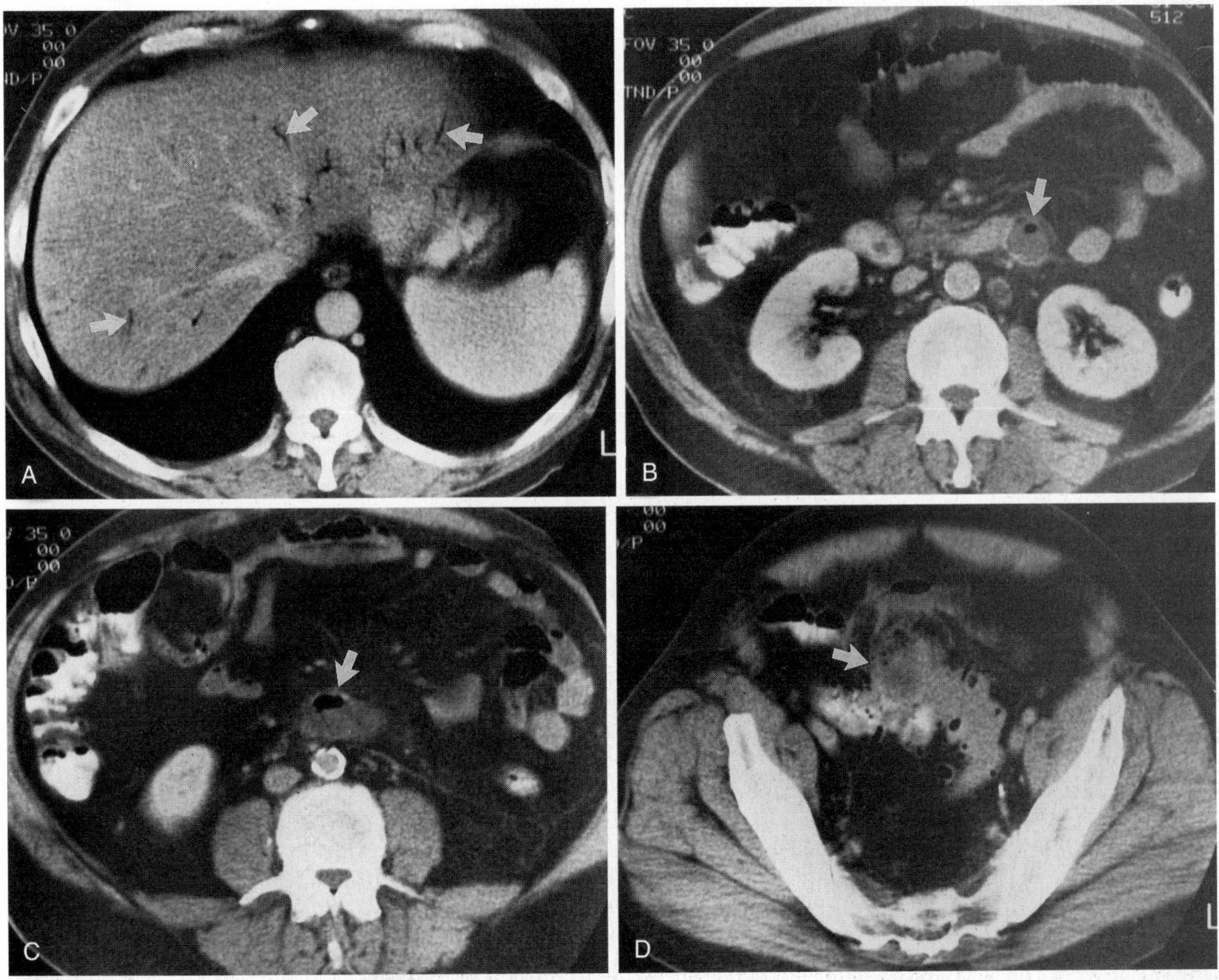

Figure 29–12. Acute pylephlebitis due to diverticulitis with abscess. *A*, Minute quantities of gas (arrows) within peripheral branches of the portal venous system were not visible on a plain radiograph. *B*, A gas-containing thrombus (arrow) is visible in the inferior mesenteric vein at its junction with the splenic vein. *C*, A chain of abscesses (arrow) extended along the course of the thrombosed inferior mesenteric vein. *D*, The septic thrombus led directly to a pericolonic abscess (arrow) caused by diverticulitis of the sigmoid colon.

recognizable with radiologic techniques. With regard to acute pancreatitis, it is now possible to show the morphologic changes in this disease, ranging from a minimal edema of the pancreatic parenchyma in interstitial inflammation to the extensive phlegmon, fluid collections, hemorrhage, and necrosis that develop in fulminant necrotizing hemorrhagic pancreatitis. The diagnosis of uncomplicated acute pancreatitis is generally established by the clinical presentation and biochemical tests without the need for diagnostic imaging. Although CT is not necessary in all cases of acute pancreatitis, it is valuable when the diagnosis has not been firmly established clinically or when complications are suspected.[2] Ultrasonography is generally more useful in assessing the pancreas and peripancreatic area in the subacute phase of pancreatitis after the associated ileus has resolved.

The radiographic assessment of pelvic pain in the female is a frequent necessity in the diagnostic evaluation of pathologic processes involving the ovary, fallopian tube, and uterus. The diseases may be of benign or malignant origin, an infection, or an ectopic pregnancy. The clinical impression can be best confirmed by ultrasonography.

Diagnostic arteriography serves a tertiary role in the evaluation of patients with an acute abdomen and should only be considered when the clinical presentation, supported by highly suggestive findings on CT or ultrasonography, indicate a vascular lesion amenable to diagnostic as well as potentially therapeutic angiographic techniques (Fig. 29–13). For example, spontaneous hemorrhage from an intrahepatic arterial aneurysm, diagnosed on a CT examination, can be confirmed by selective hepatic arteriography and therapeutically managed by selective embolization technique.

In summary, the diagnostic imaging evaluation of the patient with an acute abdomen has undergone significant change in the past decade. Technologically sophisticated imaging methods, primarily involving CT and ultrasonography, provide a more rapid and accurate diagnosis. One should now consider CT and ultrasonography early in the evaluation of the patient with an acute abdomen, when the diagnosis is not obvious based on the history and physical examination or apparent on the plain radiographs of the abdomen.

Clinicopathologic Diagnostic Studies

Patients evaluated for acute abdominal pain require certain basic laboratory studies that in most instances can be per-

formed rapidly on an emergency basis. The results are important in establishing a prompt and accurate diagnosis. Fortunately, those tests requiring a prolonged period of time for completion are rarely critical for the diagnosis and treatment of patients with acute abdominal pain. In some instances, the laboratory information may only confirm the clinical diagnosis and in the presence of generalized peritonitis play little or no role in the decision for operation. However, patients with mild to moderate abdominal pain with an uncertain diagnosis require frequent examinations of the abdomen before a decision for operation can be achieved. In such circumstances, a repeat complete blood cell count or other laboratory studies can be helpful in determining the progress of an acute intra-abdominal inflammatory process.

A complete blood cell count and urinalysis is essential in all patients evaluated for acute abdominal pain. The results need to be reviewed before a final decision is made regarding surgical intervention unless the urgency is such that immediate operation is required; laboratory tests that are especially helpful include a determination of the serum amylase level for patients with acute pancreatitis, a serum aspartate aminotransferase value to confirm the presence of acute hepatitis, and the human chorionic gonadotropin level to confirm the presence of an ectopic pregnancy. Liver function studies may be helpful in those patients with right upper quadrant pain, jaundice, and the possibility of hepatitis. Serum electrolytes obtained on an emergency basis are largely for the therapeutic management of the patient in preparation for admission and observation or in planning for operation.

A peritoneal diagnostic tap may be useful in determining the presence of intraperitoneal blood, fluid, and pus. Peritoneal lavage is more valuable in the presence of blunt abdominal trauma. The presence of blood, purulent material, or bacteria on Gram stain suggests the need for early exploration (Table 29–1).

PERITONITIS AND THE PERITONEAL CAVITY

The Peritoneal Cavity

The peritoneal cavity is covered by a single layer of mesothelial cells on connective tissue, including collagen, elastic fibers, macrophages, and fat cells. The parietal peritoneum, which covers the abdominal cavity, including the anterior

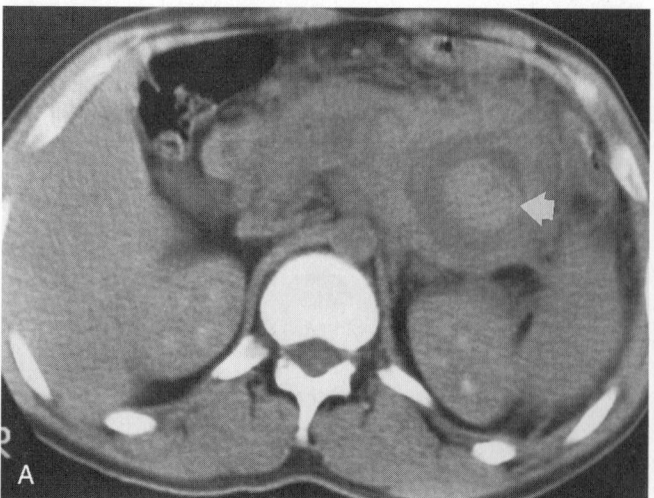
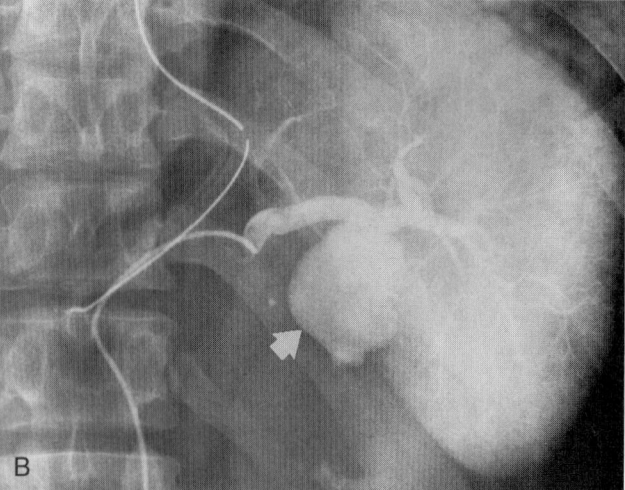

Figure 29–13. Hemorrhage and false aneurysm complicating pancreatitis. *A*, Intraparenchymal hemorrhage enlarges the body and tail of the pancreas. The lumen of the false aneurysm (arrow) is shown as an area of increased density due to the enhancement of the flowing blood. *B*, Selective splenic arteriogram. A false aneurysm (arrow) arises from a branch of the splenic artery and was successfully treated with transcatheter embolization.

TABLE 29–1. Causes of Hemoperitoneum

Gastrointestinal
   Traumatic laceration of liver, spleen, pancreas, mesentery,
      bowel
Gynecologic
   Ruptured ectopic pregnancy
   Ruptured graafian follicle
   Ruptured uterus
Vascular
   Ruptured aneurysm—aortoiliac, hepatic, renal, and splenic
      artery
Urologic
   Ruptured bladder
Hematologic
   Ruptured spleen

abdominal wall, diaphragm, and pelvis, is immediately adjacent to and reinforced by the transversalis fascia. The visceral peritoneum covers all the intraperitoneal viscera, creating a completely enclosed cavity except for the open ends of the fallopian tubes. The parietal peritoneum is innervated by both somatic and visceral afferent nerves. The peritoneum of the anterior abdominal wall is the area most sensitive to stimuli, and the pelvic peritoneum is the area least sensitive. Patients with abdominal pain may show tenderness to palpation of the abdomen; and if peritoneal irritation exists, they have rebound tenderness. Localized inflammation of the anterior parietal peritoneum may lead to voluntary muscle guarding. The visceral peritoneum is relatively insensitive and receives afferent innervation only from the autonomic nervous system. Stimuli from the visceral peritoneum are often poorly localized and are perceived as dull or intermittent cramping. The visceral afferent nerves have no receptors to mediate pain and temperature but do respond to distention, traction, and pressure. The biliary tract and mesentery of the small bowel have greater innervation than the small intestine. Thus, pain from the gallbladder and common duct is more accurately localized than that from the small intestine.

Peritonitis

The inflammatory response of the peritoneum to bacteria, endotoxin, or bile and gastric juice may involve the entire intra-abdominal cavity or only a portion of either the visceral or parietal peritoneum. The peritoneum responds to the trauma of inflammation, resulting in peritonitis with a transudation of fluid, edema formation, and vascular congestion of the tissue layer immediately adjacent to the single layer of mesothelium. The normal volume of 100 ml. of peritoneal fluid increases rapidly with the passage of a transudate of fluid from the extracellular compartment. This transudate, rich in protein content, is accompanied by a diapedesis of polymorphonuclear leukocytes, both of which play an important role in conjunction with fibrin in the containment of intraperitoneal infection. The peritoneal response to bacterial contact is first lymphatic absorption followed by phagocytosis. The activation of macrophages and complement play an important role in the cellular and humoral control of infection.

Peritonitis, classified as primary or spontaneous peritonitis, is a diffuse bacterial infection without an apparent intra-abdominal source of infection. The organisms are most commonly those of pneumococcus and hemolytic *Streptococcus* and occur more commonly in children than in adults. However, in adults with ascites and cirrhosis, spontaneous peritonitis may occur due to *Escherichia coli* and *Klebsiella*. Second-

ary peritonitis implies that the cause is the result of bacterial contamination from a known source, usually from within the abdomen and often from a perforation of the gastrointestinal tract. Occasionally, the source of infection may result from penetrating trauma or as an extension of a suppurative process from an intra-abdominal organ, such as a liver abscess or pyosalpinx. Secondary peritonitis is the most common form of peritoneal infection encountered by the surgeon; and because it is almost always of a suppurative origin, surgical intervention is required.

Chemical peritonitis refers to peritoneal inflammation from substances other than bacteria, and although this occurs initially, bacterial contamination soon follows. The substances commonly associated with chemical peritonitis include gastric contents, pancreatic exocrine fluid, bile, blood, urine, meconium, chyle, and barium. The most severe and common form of chemical peritonitis is that of a perforated peptic ulcer, causing a sudden outpouring of gastric juice and producing an acute inflammatory response in both the visceral and parietal peritoneum.

Bile peritonitis may occur as a result of perforation of the gallbladder with acute gangrenous cholecystitis. Hemoperitoneum, the result of a ruptured abdominal aneurysm, occurs so quickly that an inflammatory response is minor compared with the catastrophic event itself. However, slow bleeding into the abdomen from a ruptured graafian follicle or splenic injury from trauma produces surprisingly few signs of inflammation. If bacteria are also present, the hemoglobin and ferrous iron act to enhance the inflammatory response to the bacteria in producing suppurative peritonitis. Barium contamination of the peritoneal cavity secondary to spillage during a radiologic contrast examination causes severe peritoneal irritation. The outcome of gastrointestinal perforation is less favorable when both barium and bacteria are combined, producing an increased incidence of sepsis.

The cause of granulomatous peritonitis includes tuberculosis and iatrogenic causes, such as surgical glove powder (talc), which in some circumstances may lead to severe inflammation, exudation, and granuloma formation. Tuberculous peritonitis, now much less common than previously, still occurs in the chronically ill or malnourished patient. Although the primary focus of tuberculosis is usually the lung, the source may not be apparent clinically. The disease is, however, almost always due to the reactivation of pulmonary tuberculosis, with hematogenous spread to the peritoneum. The degree of peritoneal irritation varies from a dull generalized abdominal pain with minimal tenderness to a more severe form of abdominal peritonitis.

Osler[29] succinctly described the gross findings of peritonitis at the time of operation:

On opening the abdomen the intestinal coils are distended and glued together by lymph, and the peritoneum presents a patchy, sometimes a uniform injection. The exudation may be: (a) Fibrinous, with little or no fluid, except a few pockets of clear serum between the coils. (b) Serofibrinous. The coils are covered with lymph, and there is in addition a large amount of a yellowish, serofibrinous fluid. In instances in which the stomach or intestine is perforated this may be missed with food or faeces. (c) Purulent, in which the exudate is either thin and greenish yellow in color, or opaque white and creamy. (d) Putrid. Occasionally in puerperal and perforative peritonitis, particularly when the latter has been caused by cancer, the exudate is thin, grayish green in color, and has a gangrenous odor. (e) Haemorrhagic. This is sometimes found as an admixture in cases of acute peritonitis following wounds, and occurs in the cancerous and tuberculous forms.

This description more than 100 years ago is still accurate.

Signs and Symptoms. Peritonitis is usually associated with the abrupt onset of abdominal pain, often localized at first and then spreading throughout the abdomen. In some circumstances such as perforated diverticulitis, the pain may remain in one quadrant of the abdomen. A careful history often suggests the source of the problem, which is subsequently confirmed by the physical examination and radiographic studies. Perforated peptic ulcer presents suddenly as acute epigastric pain, often radiating to the right lower quadrant as the gastric juice drains caudad along the right gutter. The presence of bilateral shoulder pain suggests that peritonitis involves the parietal peritoneum of the diaphragm. Absent or hypoactive bowel sounds indicate generalized peritonitis with an adynamic ileus. Acute appendicitis with sudden perforation occurs rarely and is usually associated with an illness of several or more hours. The pain is eventually localized to the right lower quadrant unless the disease process has progressed to generalized peritonitis. Acute cholecystitis also has a several-hour history of right upper quadrant pain referred to the right scapula or shoulder. Perforation usually occurs after the disease has been in progress for hours or days, and free bile peritonitis develops only after gangrene and perforation of the gallbladder. Peritonitis due to acute ulcerative colitis is usually identified by the history of the primary disease. The peritoneal signs may be severe and generalized if perforation has occurred or diffuse and mild if only colonic inflammation exists without perforation. Crohn's disease may present as acute, severe, localized right lower quadrant pain and may be indistinguishable from acute appendicitis. Free perforation of the distal ileum with generalized peritonitis rarely occurs with Crohn's disease; however, formation of fistula tracts are common. Abdominal pain from obstruction and perforation of the small and large intestine is usually not of sudden onset except for cases of acute volvulus. Free perforation of a colonic neoplasm with generalized peritonitis is less common than a walled-off perforation with abscess formation.

The physical findings of patients with peritonitis depend on the etiology and duration and whether the process is diffuse or localized. In the early stages, the patient appears acutely ill and febrile with tachycardia. The blood pressure is normotensive or slightly hypotensive. As the disease progresses and the inflammatory process increases, the patient becomes severely ill with obvious signs of a decrease in circulating plasma volume. Hypotension and tachycardia are common. The patient may appear anxious and dehydrated with rapid respiration. Fever is always noted in the early hours after onset of peritoneal irritation but may disappear or the patient's temperature may even become subnormal with progression. The abdomen is distended with hypoactive or absent bowel sounds. Tenderness to percussion and palpation is present in all quadrants of the abdomen. Abdominal masses are rarely palpable in the presence of severe distention and tenderness or rectus muscle rigidity. Rectal and pelvic examination may or may not identify a pelvic mass but confirms peritoneal irritation.

Early recognition of peritoneal irritation is important, and proper preoperative management is critical if the patient is to survive. This management includes the insertion of a nasogastric tube, restoration of intravascular volume deficit, and improvement in the performance of the cardiovascular and renal subsystem. A Foley catheter should be placed as soon as possible to assess the hourly urine volume which, in turn, provides some indication of intravascular volume replacement. Immediate administration of intravenous antibiotics for broad coverage is essential to control sepsis. Hemodynamic monitoring using a central venous pressure or a Swan-Ganz line may be necessary in patients with hemodynamic instability.

Imaging experience has shown that many of the morphologic changes of peritonitis, such as thickening of the parietal and visceral peritoneum, inflammatory changes in the omen-

tum and mesentery, and free or loculated fluid collections, often with higher density than bland ascites, are well shown with CT (Fig. 29–14). The source of the peritonitis, such as a perforation of bowel, is often apparent as well (Fig. 29–15).

ORGAN SUBSYSTEM ANALYSIS

The etiology of acute abdominal pain can be separated according to the organ subsystem involved. Those body subsystems that contribute to abdominal pain include the gastrointestinal, renal, gynecologic, vascular, cardiac, pulmonary, neurologic, hematologic, metabolic, and musculoskeletal. If one considers the body as a whole to be composed of various organ subsystems, the examination of a patient with abdominal pain can be based on the analysis of those subsystems that may cause or contribute to the abdominal pain.

Gastrointestinal Subsystem

The most common cause of acute abdominal pain in the gastrointestinal subsystem relates to an inflammatory or mechanical process of the stomach, small and large intestine, gallbladder, common bile duct, liver, or pancreas (Table 29–2). The symptoms are often nonspecific and affected by the age of the patient, medication, and coexisting disease. For example, older patients, especially those with diabetes, may demonstrate fewer symptoms than younger patients. Corticosteroids and other immunosuppressive drugs may mask intraperitoneal inflammatory conditions, and patients receiving such medication are likely to minimize their symptoms. Nausea, vomiting, constipation, and abdominal pain are all common findings and often occur concomitantly.[41]

Perforated Peptic Ulcer. Free perforation of peptic ulcer disease, more often resulting from duodenal ulcer than from gastric ulcer, is usually found in male patients between the third and fourth decades. Perforation may occur in patients in good health without previous symptoms or in patients with a previous history of peptic ulcer disease that had worsened several days before the episode of pain. Perforation may occur nocturnally and awaken the patient from sleep. The pain is sudden, sharp, severe, and located first in the epigastrium and later over the entire abdomen. Shoulder pain is common and reflects referred pain from the diaphrag-

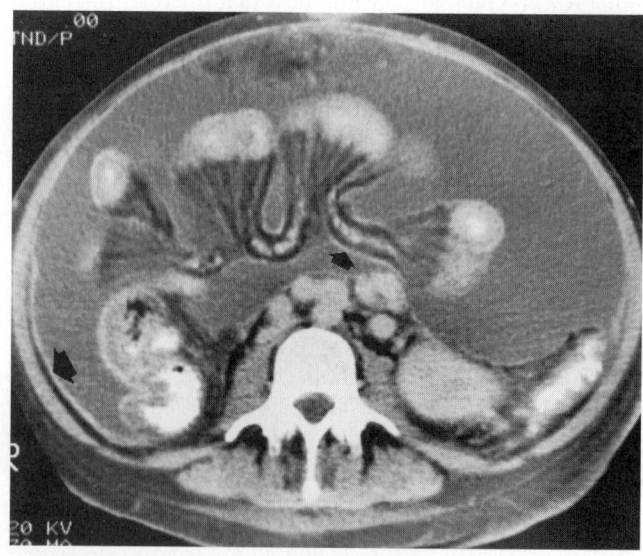

Figure 29–14. Peritonitis. CT scan shows inflammatory thickening of the parietal (large arrow) and visceral (small arrow) peritoneum. The ascitic fluid is of high density characteristic of peritonitis.

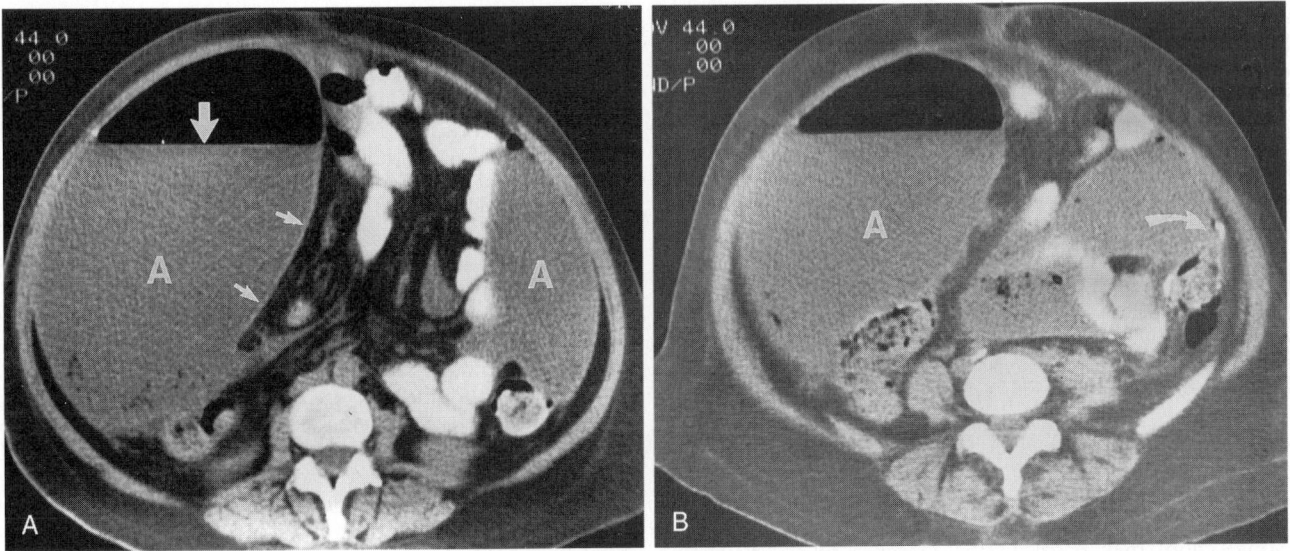

Figure 29–15. Pyopneumoperitoneum secondary to a perforated descending colon. *A*, Pyopneumo interface (large arrow). Inflammatory thickening of visceral peritoneum (small arrows). Seven liters of grossly infected ascitic fluid (A) were drained percutaneously. *B*, A trail of small gas bubbles in the left flank led to a point of discrete perforation of the descending colon (arrow), which was confirmed by contrast enema and surgically repaired.

matic irritation. Occasionally, the gastric contents will drain to the right lower quadrant, producing right lower quadrant pain and tenderness, suggesting acute appendicitis. Nausea is frequent; and although vomiting may occur, it is unusual. Hematemesis is also unusual. The patient with generalized peritonitis from a perforated ulcer usually lies in the supine position, avoiding any undue motion that might increase the abdominal pain.

During the examination, the patient lies quietly, often appearing acutely ill with tachypnea and tachycardia. Hypotension may be present if the process has existed for more than 4 to 6 hours because of plasma volume depletion. Respirations are shallow, and deep breathing or coughing produces severe abdominal pain. The patient may be afebrile soon after perforation but develops fever 6 to 8 hours later. In the first few hours, the abdomen may appear normal or scaphoid but will gradually progress to abdominal distention during the next 12 hours. Percussion reveals the abdomen to be extremely tender, especially in the epigastric region. Palpation of the abdomen reveals a firm *boardlike* appearance, with rigidity of the rectus muscles. Rebound tenderness is the rule, present in all four quadrants, and is worse in the epigastric region. Auscultation of the abdomen soon after perforation reveals hypoactive bowel sounds that progress to absent bowel sounds as the process of generalized peritonitis becomes worse. These findings confirm generalized peritonitis. Rectal examination is unremarkable unless there is pelvic peritonitis, in which case tenderness is present anterior to the examining finger.

Routine laboratory data usually include an elevated white blood cell count between 12,000 and 20,000 cells per cu. mm. with immature forms. The intravascular fluid shifts in the first 6 to 12 hours confirms the plasma volume loss resulting from peritonitis, and is reflected in the elevated hematocrit. The urinalysis shows a concentrated urine specific gravity, and there is little or no change in liver or renal function if there has been no pre-existing disease.

The plain radiograph of the abdomen or chest demonstrates free intraperitoneal air, present in approximately 75% of patients with a perforated ulcer. In patients in whom the clinical presentation is atypical and suggests a right mid or lower abdominal inflammatory process such as cholecystitis or appendicitis, a CT examination may show evidence of localized perforation of the duodenum with leakage in the area of the gallbladder and right flank, without gross free air being apparent (see Fig. 29–5).

Acute Cholecystitis. This disease most commonly occurs in women between the ages of 30 and 60 years who have had a previous history of pregnancy. The younger patients often have a family history of biliary tract disease. Although the episode of acute cholecystitis may begin several hours after a large meal and often occurs late at night or in the early morning hours, the disease may develop without a prior history of food intake. The attack is characterized by the onset of a constant dull right upper quadrant pain. Some patients move about, attempting to relieve the pain, whereas others lie restlessly in bed. Nausea and vomiting are common, with temporary improvement in the severity of pain after an episode of emesis. The emesis is of moderate quantity and green. The pain may subside after several hours; if so, the episode is considered to be biliary colic. The disease process may progress to acute cholecystitis, in which case there is steady severe right upper quadrant pain radiating to the right scapula or shoulder. If there is an associated common duct stone or acute pancreatitis, the pain may also be located in the midline of the epigastrium and may radiate along the right and left costal margins to the back. The temperature ranges from 37° C. to 39° C. (99° F. to 102° F.). A

TABLE 29–2. Abdominal Pain Secondary to Inflammatory Lesions of the Gastrointestinal Subsystem

Stomach
  Gastric ulcer
  Duodenal ulcer
Biliary tract
  Acute cholecystitis with or without choledocholithiasis
Pancreas
  Acute, recurrent, or chronic pancreatitis
Small intestine
  Crohn's disease
  Meckel's diverticulum
Large intestine
  Appendicitis
  Diverticulitis

high temperature and chills are not usually common unless the patient has cholangitis. This is rarely noted in the early stages of the disease and becomes apparent after 12 to 24 hours. Blood pressure is usually not altered, and the heart rate is seldom greater than 100 to 110 beats per minute.[14]

Examination of the abdomen reveals mild to moderate distention; and on inspection from the patient's feet, the abdomen may show asymmetry in the right upper quadrant with a mass that distends on deep inspiration. Bowel sounds are hypoactive to auscultation. Tenderness is maximal in the right upper quadrant. In the absence of perforation and generalized peritonitis, tenderness to palpation confirms the right upper quadrant tenderness to be worse with deep inspiration. Frequently, a mass can be palpated along the right costal margin, representing a distended tense gallbladder that descends with deep inspiration. Percussion tenderness over the right rib cage is the rule. The rectal examination rarely adds important information to the diagnosis.

Laboratory data reveal the white blood cell count to be often elevated (10,000 to 13,000 per cu. mm.); however, a normal count may occur in the presence of severe acute cholecystitis. This is especially true when the patient is over the age of 70 years, with or without diabetes, and in those patients receiving corticosteroid therapy. The urinalysis does not usually contribute to the diagnosis. An electrocardiogram is important to exclude the possibility of an acute myocardial infarction.

An elevated serum bilirubin to 2.0 or 2.5 mg. per 100 ml. may exist with uncomplicated acute cholecystitis. If, however, the bilirubin exceeds 3.0 mg. per 100 ml., common duct calculi should be considered. The significance of an increase in the serum amylase level is difficult to assess because acute cholecystitis may be associated with a mild amylase elevation and may reflect a chemical abnormality with little clinical evidence of pancreatitis.

The radiologic evaluation of acute cholecystitis has changed significantly in the past decade. Studies that once played a role—the oral cholecystogram and intravenous cholangiogram—have been essentially abandoned. Ultrasonography, the current most commonly used imaging method, can rapidly assess the caliber of the biliary tree, the presence or absence of biliary calculi, and the appearance of the gallbladder wall and contents as well as the surrounding structures (see Fig. 29–6). Further support for the diagnosis is provided by showing that pressure from the transducer directly onto the gallbladder elicits the patient's pain pattern.[5]

Radionuclide studies, employing agents such as HIDA, play a supportive role in cases where the diagnosis is not readily confirmed with ultrasound. If the gallbladder fails to show uptake of the agent within 4 hours in the presence of radionuclide activity in the bile duct and small bowel, cystic duct obstruction may be present. CT plays a limited role and is usually reserved for evaluating late complications of initially unrecognized acute cholecystitis.

Acute Pancreatitis. Pancreatitis may present with sudden onset characterized by severe epigastric pain radiating directly through to the back and around both costal margins with or without shoulder pain. The similarity of the description of the pain to acute perforation of peptic ulcer is obvious and may also simulate acute cholecystitis. The disease, however, most commonly is associated with biliary tract disease or chronic alcohol intake. Acute pancreatitis usually presents in patients between the ages of 30 and 50 years and has frequently been preceded by a similar episode with a previous diagnosis. The disease is uncommon in children and adolescents and in patients older than 70 years of age. The onset may be rapid, with the pain becoming intolerable in 3 to 4 hours. Anorexia, nausea, and vomiting are common, and emesis rarely provides significant relief. Examination reveals

an acutely ill patient with obvious severe abdominal pain, tachycardia, and tachypnea. Hypotension, rarely present in the early stages of the disease process, may develop after 4 to 6 hours if retroperitoneal hemorrhage occurs with intravascular volume extravasation. Abdominal tenderness is most evident in the epigastric region and is present with both percussion and palpation. Bowel sounds are usually hypoactive and may be absent. The classic Grey Turner's sign, with flank ecchymosis, and Cullen's sign, with discoloration of the skin around the umbilicus, are uncommon findings in the early phase of the disease.

Routine laboratory tests show a leukocytosis ranging from 12,000 to 22,000 cells per cu. mm. The hematocrit is normal in the early phase of the disease but becomes increased if retroperitoneal fluid loss is excessive. The key diagnostic test, the serum amylase value, is elevated within a few hours in most patients who have the acute form of the disease. If the attack is mild, the amylase elevation may be slight and transient, often returning to normal in 24 hours. Urinary amylase levels may be diagnostic in such patients when the serum amylase level has returned to normal. All patients suspected of having acute pancreatitis should have an immediate serum amylase determination; urinary amylase studies should be reserved for those patients with normal serum levels. Serum bilirubin levels may be elevated and, when combined with an increase in serum amylase, present a complex situation in differentiating primary biliary tract disease from pancreatitis. In general, the serum amylase level is not as high in patients with acute cholecystitis, and this elevation seldom persists for more than 2 or 3 days. If the attack of pancreatitis is severe, hypocalcemia may develop from calcium deposition in the pancreas and peripancreatic tissue.

Plain radiographs of the abdomen are often nondiagnostic in patients with acute pancreatitis. CT and ultrasonography are the next studies to confirm the clinical diagnosis or to assess suspected complications. Because of the frequent accompanying adynamic ileus, CT is better able to provide images of the entire pancreas and peripancreatic area. Pancreatic edema, intrapancreatic or peripancreatic fluid collections, inflammatory or phlegmonous changes in the surrounding anterior pararenal space, changes secondary to pancreatic hemorrhage (see Fig. 29–13), or necrosis and extension of the inflammatory process into distant intraperitoneal and retroperitoneal spaces can all be quickly defined.[2]

Acute Relapsing Pancreatitis. Acute relapsing pancreatitis differs from acute pancreatitis in that in the former the pain is recurrent with each exacerbation of pancreatitis and is associated with an increase in serum amylase level. The patient's previous history of pancreatitis usually confirms the diagnosis. The physical findings are identical to those noted with acute pancreatitis. However, the possibility of a pancreatic pseudocyst must always be considered. This diagnosis can be established by ultrasonography or a CT scan of the pancreas.

Chronic Pancreatitis. Patients with chronic pancreatitis differ from those with recurrent episodes of acute pancreatitis (acute relapsing pancreatitis) in that in the former the pain becomes constant. The history identifies the diagnosis from the patient's previous attacks, and radiographs of the abdomen often reveal calcification in the pancreas. The serum amylase level will be elevated if the pancreatic tissue has not been replaced by fibrous tissue.

Acute Appendicitis. Acute appendicitis, a common cause of abdominal pain, is especially difficult to diagnose in patients younger than age 3 and older than age 70. Although certain findings by history and physical examination are highly suggestive, establishing the correct diagnosis may be difficult. The symptoms relate to the anatomic position of the appendix and vary according to the age and coexistent disease of the patient. In patients with early acute appendicitis, there may be typical findings and an excellent surgical outcome, whereas in those patients with perforation and peritonitis, there may be a different clinical picture with a more complex recovery.[34]

A careful history is essential in making both an accurate and an early diagnosis. Abdominal pain typically begins in the epigastrium, then gradually migrates to the periumbilical region, and finally to the right lower quadrant. Anorexia, nausea, and vomiting are common. The prodromal symptoms of indigestion, irregularity of the bowels, nausea, and vomiting are all common findings. There is localization of the pain to the right lower quadrant after 6 to 8 hours of onset with tenderness to palpation and rebound tenderness. Guarding to palpation occurs when the process has progressed to localized peritonitis. Local hyperesthesia of the skin is a common finding. Rigidity is frequently present, although a flaccid abdomen does not preclude acute appendicitis. Abdominal distention is rarely present in the early stages of the disease but increases with time. It is especially important to remember that a retrocecal appendix may cause only mild abdominal tenderness. Regardless of all the possible findings, the most common complaint is right lower quadrant pain, and the most frequent physical finding is right lower quadrant tenderness to palpation. Rectal examination is especially important, and the findings may vary according to the appendiceal location. Abdominal tenderness is less severe when the appendix is in the retrocecal position. However, patients with the appendix lying free in the peritoneal cavity may elicit extreme tenderness on rectal examination, more so on the right side.

Laboratory data are nondiagnostic and often normal. The white blood cell count may be elevated, but this will depend on the duration of the illness. Those patients with symptoms for more than 24 hours with marked abdominal tenderness are more likely to have an elevated white blood cell count than those patients with symptoms of 6 hours or less. Most patients have a shift to the left in the differential count. The urinalysis is rarely helpful, although occasionally the appendix may lie in contact with the ureter or bladder and cause microscopic hematuria.

The plain film findings are not often helpful, although a fecalith is an exception to this observation. A dilated fluid-filled cecum may be present but is nondiagnostic. A free perforation of the appendix rarely has diagnostic findings, and intraperitoneal air is unusual. Scoliosis of the lumbar spine may occur with psoas spasm and the convex curvature to the right. Experience with ultrasonography and CT has shown both imaging methods helpful in defining the pathologic changes characteristic of appendicitis as well as its associated complications (see Figs. 29–8 and 29–9).[35]

Other diagnostic considerations in patients with appendicitis include perforated duodenal ulcer with spillage of gastric contents into the right lower quadrant (see Fig. 29–5). This produces right lower quadrant pain and tenderness. However, the symptoms relating to the peptic ulcer can usually be differentiated from appendicitis. Acute diverticulitis is a common intra-abdominal inflammatory process usually involving the sigmoid colon, especially in patients older than 60 years of age and when perforated may be difficult to differentiate from appendicitis if the sigmoid colon lies near the midline in the suprapubic area. The occurrence of marked left lower quadrant tenderness in the patient undergoing evaluation for acute appendicitis suggests either perforation with generalized peritonitis or acute diverticulitis. Ruptured graafian follicle is a common cause for right lower quadrant or left lower quadrant pain as a result of bleeding into the peritoneal cavity. The relationship to the menstrual cycle is of obvious importance, and the patient will often recollect

one or more previous similar episodes. Mittelschmerz pain is usually sudden in onset, sharp, often located in the pelvis, and not preceded by anorexia, nausea, or vomiting. If the left ovary is involved, the diagnostic considerations are less complicated. The process gradually subsides over a few hours, and most patients are well in a short period of time. Ectopic pregnancy in women of the childbearing years is an important consideration and must be considered in all women with abdominal pain, a history of missed menstrual periods, and an adnexal mass. Perforated typhoid enteritis is an uncommon entity in the United States but occurs elsewhere and therefore is an important diagnostic consideration.[24]

Pelvic inflammatory disease with acute salpingitis is a frequently encountered process causing acute pelvic pain originating in both lower quadrants. The prime consideration should be to differentiate the disease from acute appendicitis. Acute pelvic inflammatory disease often becomes symptomatic at the completion of or just after a menstrual period. The pain is not related to the gastrointestinal tract and is rarely associated with anorexia, nausea, or vomiting. Pain and tenderness are usually bilateral and are associated with a temperature of 38° C. to 39° C. (100° F. to 102° F.). If the patient has had previous symptoms of a similar nature, it is likely that chronic or recurrent pelvic inflammatory disease is the correct diagnosis. Inspection of the abdomen reveals mild to moderate distention in the suprapubic region. Bowel sounds are hypoactive. Abdominal tenderness to palpation usually exists in both lower quadrants, with marked tenderness on palpation of the cervix. Adnexal masses are common findings and often present as thickened areas bilaterally. A vaginal discharge is a frequent sequela. The diagnosis is confirmed by cervical smear and culture, with gonococcus being the most frequently found organism. It must be emphasized that salpingitis is primarily a disease of young women and rarely occurs after menopause. Septic thrombosis of the ovarian vein associated with endometritis in the immediate postpartum period can also simulate appendicitis if the right side is involved.[4]

Renal or ureteral calculi may cause abdominal pain; however, once the calculus begins to descend in the ureter, the pain pattern varies with radiation to the groin and perineum. The pain is sudden, is severe, and may subside in a few minutes. Hydronephrosis on the right side, a right pelvic kidney with pyelonephritis, or a polycystic kidney in a young person may all cause abdominal pain similar to that of acute appendicitis. Radiographs of the abdomen in a supine position, an intravenous pyelogram, and urinalysis can usually differentiate renal pain from that of nonrenal origin. Acute granulomatous ileocolitis (Crohn's disease) may present in an identical manner to that of acute appendicitis.[16] However, the CT demonstration of significant thickening of the wall of the terminal ileum with a surrounding sleeve of inflamed mesenteric fat serves to differentiate the two diseases.

Meckel's Diverticulitis. This condition, which involves the persistence of a portion of the vitelline duct on the antimesenteric border of the distal ileum, may produce bleeding, intestinal obstruction, and, less often, acute abdominal pain from diverticulitis. The disease, although uncommon, should always be considered in patients with an acute abdomen and with findings suggestive of acute appendicitis. The signs and symptoms of Meckel's diverticulitis are those of acute appendicitis, and only rarely will the true diagnosis be established preoperatively. The usual films of the abdomen in both supine and upright positions are unremarkable. The white blood cell count may be increased if surgical exploration is warranted on the basis of the acute abdominal findings; further diagnostic evaluation is not indicated. Whereas a focal inflammatory process in the area of the distal ileum is apparent on CT, the precise radiographic diagnosis of Meckel's diverticulitis is usually not possible. Other causes such as perforation by a foreign body (chicken bone) or granulomatous ileitis would also be considered. In the presence of an acute abdomen, barium contrast studies of the intestinal tract would not be indicated. The definitive diagnosis should be confirmed at the time of surgery.[9, 23]

Acute Diverticulitis. Acute diverticulitis may occur as a result of congenital or acquired diverticula. However, in most instances the disease is almost always a result of the acquired form of the disease in which the incidence increases with age. Diverticulitis, the result of inflammation of diverticula, is but one of several complications of diverticulosis. The process may involve the entire colon, but more commonly it occurs in the left colon, particularly in the sigmoid colon. The disease presents as left lower quadrant pain, chills, and fever. There is almost always a history of constipation, but vomiting and anorexia are uncommon. The patient is frequently febrile, with a temperature of 38° C. to 40° C. (101° F. to 104° F.).

Abdominal examination reveals the abdomen to be slightly distended, with tenderness in the left lower quadrant. A mass is often palpable just medial to the anterior-superior iliac spine. Bowel sounds are hypoactive and, if absent, the possibility of peritonitis must be considered. The rectal examination is rarely of diagnostic value unless a pelvic mass can be palpated. Sigmoidoscopy is performed with difficulty because of pain. The lumen is occluded owing to mucosal edema, but no intraluminal masses are noted.

Laboratory data reveal the white blood cell count to be increased to between 10,000 and 20,000 cells per cu. mm. The urinalysis may contain multiple white blood cells. Plain radiographs of the abdomen are most often indeterminate unless colonic obstruction or a gas-containing abscess is also present. If the diagnosis of diverticulitis is uncertain or complications are suspected, CT is the most definitive imaging method (see Fig. 29–12). Inflammatory changes in the pericolonic soft tissues and focal abscesses due to diverticulitis are apparent on CT but can be mimicked by a perforated colonic carcinoma. If the patient improves on medical therapy and operation is not necessary, a barium enema should be performed in 4 to 6 weeks when the patient is asymptomatic to exclude an occult colonic cancer with a focal perforation as the cause of the acute episode.[31, 32]

Acute Obstruction of the Small Intestine. Few conditions are more treacherous and demand a more accurate early diagnosis than obstruction of the small bowel. Obstruction from congenital disorders occurs most commonly in children and adolescents and includes intestinal atresia, meconium ileus, and intussusception (Table 29–3).

TABLE 29–3. Abdominal Pain Secondary to Obstructing Lesions of the Gastrointestinal Tract

Jejunum
  Malignancy
  Volvulus
  Adhesions
  Intussusception
Ileum
  Malignancy
  Volvulus
  Adhesions
  Intussusception
Colon
  Malignancy
  Volvulus—cecal or sigmoid
  Diverticulitis

The first symptom of acute obstruction of the small intestine is sudden, sharp, colicky abdominal pain, often periumbilical and cramping. Between episodes of colic, the patient is free of pain and may feel quite well. Nausea and vomiting occur soon after the onset of pain, and emesis may relieve the pain. The color of the vomitus is green at first and contains bile. The vomitus then changes to a yellow-brown color with a feculent odor. Frequent vomiting with epigastric pain is indicative of high small bowel obstruction, whereas cramping lower abdominal pain is noted with more distal abdominal obstruction. Inspection of the abdomen provides important diagnostic clues, such as previous incisions, ventral or inguinal hernia, or peristaltic waves. Abdominal distention does not occur with obstruction of the proximal jejunum (high small bowel obstruction) but is common when the site of obstruction occurs in the distal jejunum or ileum. Auscultation of the abdomen reveals hyperactive bowel sounds of increased pitch and intensity with audible rushes as the intestinal cramps increase in frequency. The increased activity in bowel sounds correlates with the visible peristaltic waves. Tenderness to percussion and palpation is minimal in the early stages but more apparent with the duration of time from the onset of symptoms. Patients with obstruction in the distal jejunum and ileum often have visible peristaltic waves that can be correlated with the patient's symptoms.

Patients with acute obstruction of the small intestine appear seriously ill with anxious facial expressions. Tachycardia is common; and as the disease process continues, hypotension may occur from fluid loss. Temperature is elevated from 37° C. to 40° C. (99° F. to 104° F.). During episodes of pain, the patient becomes restless and frequently draws the knees to the chest for relief. Rectal examination is seldom of diagnostic value.

Laboratory data reveal an increase in hematocrit caused by dehydration and fluid loss from the intravascular space into the intestinal lumen. If the obstruction has existed for several hours or more, the white blood cell count is increased from 12,000 to 20,000 per cu. mm. with an increase in immature forms. The serum amylase level may be normal or slightly elevated and may be misleading regarding an accurate diagnosis concerning acute pancreatitis.

Supine and erect radiographs of the abdomen are most helpful in the evaluation of patients with acute small bowel obstruction. If the level of obstruction is in the mid or distal small bowel, dilated loops of fluid and gas-filled small bowel are apparent, whereas the nonobstructed colon appears devoid of gas or feces. A high small bowel obstruction has less impressive plain film findings, especially if the patient has been vomiting. If high obstruction is clinically suspected and the plain film findings are consistent, an oral barium contrast study is valuable in confirming the diagnosis as to the level, as well as in some cases the cause, of obstruction, for example, obstructing carcinoma of the duodenum.

If the initial obstructive series indicates a mid to distal small bowel obstruction, the contrast study of choice to clarify the level and nature of obstruction is a barium enema, not an antegrade small bowel series. This quickly accomplished procedure can confirm that the colon is not involved in the obstructing process. If reflux through an incompetent ileocecal valve can be achieved, the study can also show the collapsed terminal ileum and may define the actual point of obstruction. Further imaging studies are usually not indicated and may only delay needed therapeutic intervention. However, when acute, severe abdominal pain is present and plain radiographs are nonrevealing, ultrasonography and CT may show clinically unsuspected small bowel obstruction, such as acute intussusception in an adult due to a small bowel tumor (Fig. 29–16). Ultrasonography for bowel ob-

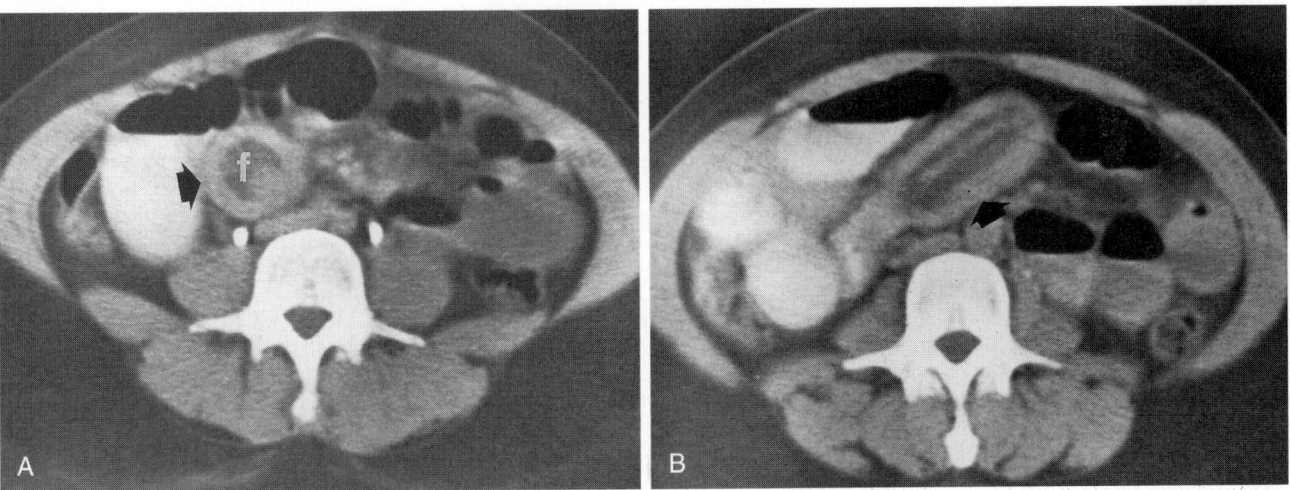

Figure 29–16. Acute small bowel intussusception. The patient had a sudden onset of severe mid-abdominal pain with nonspecific plain film findings. Cross-sectional *(A)* and longitudinal *(B)* CT scans of a small bowel intussusception (arrows). Mesenteric fat (f) accompanies the intussusceptum. A benign spindle cell tumor was the cause.

struction is a rapid, sensitive, and accurate method of diagnosis.[27]

A paralytic ileus can be differentiated from mechanical obstruction of the small intestine by the presence or absence of bowel sounds. However, the progression of cramping abdominal pain and hyperactive bowel sounds to a silent distended abdomen with signs of peritoneal irritation is a most dangerous sign, suggesting intestinal gangrene with necrosis, perforation of the bowel, and generalized peritonitis. Acute venous mesenteric thrombosis is difficult to differentiate from other causes of intestinal obstruction on clinical grounds alone. However, pulsed Doppler ultrasound and CT are capable of showing thrombosis of the portal and mesenteric venous systems as well as the associated bowel wall thickening (see Figs. 29–7 and 29–11). Acute occlusion of the superior mesenteric artery or its branches causes severe acute abdominal pain and is usually seen in older patients, particularly in those with atrial fibrillation or those with a low cardiac output after operation. The rapid progression of severe generalized abdominal pain, associated with clinical findings of generalized peritonitis and marked acidosis, suggests mesenteric arterial occlusion and gangrene of the small intestine. In the late stages of this disease, gas may be visible in the portal vein on a plain radiograph of the abdomen. In earlier stages, CT is capable of showing minute quantities of gas in the wall of the affected bowel and in the portal venous system, not detectable on a plain film of the abdomen (see Fig. 29–12).

Acute Obstruction of the Large Intestine. Obstruction of the large intestine occurs more often in patients older than the age of 40 years, is gradual in onset, and presents as constipation and abdominal distention. Contrary to obstruction of the small intestine, pain is minimal or absent unless peritonitis occurs. The most common causes of large bowel obstruction include carcinoma of the colon, acute diverticulitis, and volvulus. In many instances, carcinoma of the colon can be diagnosed by a careful history. Progressive constipation over a several month period, with or without thin pencil-sized stools streaked with blood, is frequently noted by patients with obstructing carcinoma of the sigmoid or rectosigmoid colon. Nausea and vomiting do not usually occur until the late stage of the disease. The patient may or may not be acutely ill, depending on the duration of the obstruction. The temperature, heart, and respiratory rates are often normal. The abdomen appears distended and tympanitic to percussion. Unless peritonitis or peritoneal irritation exists, there is

minimal abdominal tenderness to percussion and palpation. The distention may prevent the palpation of abdominal masses, and results of a rectal examination are negative unless the obstructing lesion is within reach of the examining finger.

Laboratory data reveal a normal or near-normal hematocrit and white blood cell count. The diagnosis can be suggested in most instances by a supine and an upright plain film of the abdomen. The descending and sigmoid colon are dilated to the point of the obstruction and extend cephalad to the cecum if the ileocecal valve is competent. If the ileocecal valve is not competent, the intraluminal air extends retrograde into the ileum. A sigmoidoscopy is necessary to assess the rectum and rectosigmoid, with a biopsy of the obstructing tumor if possible. If the obstructing lesion is cephalad to the sigmoidoscope and flexible sigmoidoscopy is not feasible, a barium enema should be obtained to confirm the presence, level, and nature of the obstructing lesion.

Acute diverticulitis with large bowel obstruction occurs most frequently in patients older than 45 years and in many instances has been preceded by other attacks. The location is almost always in the distal descending and sigmoid colon. There is frequently a recent increase in the severity of constipation with pain on defecation. The presenting signs and symptoms include left lower quadrant pain, chills, and fever. The patient usually appears ill with a distended, tympanitic, tender abdomen, especially marked in the left lower quadrant. A tender mass may be palpable just medial to the left anterior-superior iliac spine. Bowel sounds are hypoactive but are rarely absent unless generalized peritonitis has occurred. Rectal examination is usually unrevealing.

Laboratory data reveal a normal hematocrit with a normal or elevated white blood cell count. Supine and upright film views of the abdomen have similar findings to those seen in patients with carcinoma of the sigmoid colon. Sigmoidoscopy to examine the rectosigmoid colon is essential but usually does not reveal any obvious intrinsic lesions of the lumen. The sigmoidoscope, when passed to the point of inflammation, produces severe pain in contrast to the minimal discomfort observed in patients with carcinoma. When obstructive diverticulitis is acute, CT is a preferable imaging method to a contrast study of the colon and can demonstrate the presence of an abscess or an inflammatory mass associated with the obstruction (see Fig. 29–12).

Volvulus of the large intestine may cause acute intestinal obstruction and can occur in the cecum or sigmoid portion of the colon. Sigmoid volvulus is more common than cecal volvulus and occurs more often in patients older than the age of 65 years and in patients residing in nursing homes and psychiatric hospitals, in whom chronic constipation is a serious long-standing problem. Patients with a sigmoid volvulus present with large bowel obstruction of acute onset with little prior history. The patient is usually ill but with normal or near-normal temperature. Examination of the abdomen reveals findings similar to those noted in patients with large bowel obstruction due to carcinoma or diverticulitis. Rectal examination is generally noncontributory to the diagnosis. The diagnosis is established by the supine and upright radiographs of the abdomen, with a contrast enema revealing the characteristic point of torsion and nonfilling of the obstructed loop of sigmoid colon. When a sigmoid or cecal volvulus is strongly suspected, a water-soluble contrast enema is preferable to a barium enema. Sigmoidoscopy can be both diagnostic and therapeutic in that the sigmoidoscope, if passed into the obstructed colon, becomes quickly filled with liquid feces and a release of air. If the sigmoidoscope cannot be passed into the obstructed lumen, a catheter may be passed through the scope into the sigmoid colon and through the obstructed lumen with the same result. Cecal volvulus usually occurs in patients of the middle and older age group with sudden onset of cramping right lower quadrant and epigastric pain associated with nausea and vomiting. The diagnosis is best established by supine and upright radiographs of the abdomen demonstrating a dilated cecum and ascending colon, often with the gas distended cecum in the left upper quadrant. If the diagnosis is uncertain, sigmoidoscopy and a contrast enema examination may be required.

An expanding or ruptured abdominal aortic aneurysm almost always presents as abdominal pain. If the aneurysm is expanding, a previous history of back pain of several days' duration may be obtained. At physical examination, the aneurysm is palpable, is usually tender, and may be visible if the patient is thin without abdominal obesity. A plain film of the abdomen may demonstrate a calcified border of the aortic aneurysm that is also present in a two-dimensional view obtained with a cross-table lateral film. Ultrasonography is a rapid and simple diagnostic examination that can confirm the presence and size of an abdominal aortic aneurysm. CT examination is best for the diagnosis in the obese patient and can determine an early contained rupture in the retroperitoneal area.[17] An operation should be performed as soon as possible in patients with symptomatic aneurysms. If the aneurysm has ruptured, immediate exploration is indicated.[8]

Fecal impaction is a common cause of intestinal obstruction in elderly patients who are bedridden with long-standing constipation. Because of the patient's mental status, an accurate history may be impossible to obtain; and although the abdominal findings do not indicate an acute process, the possibility of the presence of obstructing colon carcinoma or diverticulitis cannot be excluded. Abdominal distention may exist, and although peritoneal signs are uncommon, the colon containing feces is often palpable. Sigmoidoscopy may be limited by the fecal content in the lumen, and multiple enema treatments may be required over a period of several days. After the colon has been emptied of fecal material, colonoscopy and a barium contrast study may be necessary to exclude other causes of intestinal obstruction.

Nonobstructive colonic dilatation, also described as pseudo-obstruction of the colon (Ogilvie's syndrome), refers to a clinical entity in which there are signs and symptoms of colonic obstruction but without mechanical obstruction.[28] This process, which is poorly understood in regard to etiology, may involve the entire colon or a segment of it and creates the risk of bowel rupture. The disease develops more commonly after previous operations and is often associated with other serious medical illnesses. Not infrequently, patients develop pseudo-obstruction while receiving narcotics or psychotropic drugs. Abdominal pain is a frequent complaint and is usually generalized. Vomiting is rare, and the patient may have constipation or frequent watery diarrhea. Abdominal distention is always present, developing over a period of 3 to 4 days with mild tenderness. Bowel sounds range from normal to hypoactive or hyperactive. The white blood cell count usually exceeds 12,000 per cu. mm. Supine radiographs of the abdomen may reveal generalized colon dilatation or cecal dilatation. When the transverse diameter of the colon exceeds 10 cm., impending rupture of the bowel may exist and surgical or endoscopic intervention is indicated.

Metastatic carcinoma with pelvic implantation may cause extrinsic compression on the sigmoid colon with obstruction. This rarely presents as a primary illness and usually occurs secondary to other malignant diseases. The patient's history includes progressive constipation over a period of several weeks, and the pelvic and rectal examinations may confirm a pelvic mass. Sigmoidoscopy excludes intrinsic colonic lesions involving the mucosa. A barium enema confirms the site of extrinsic compression, and a CT scan may provide additional information regarding the extent of the disease.[40]

Acute fulminating ulcerative colitis may present as abdominal distention and tenderness to percussion and palpation with hypoactive bowel sounds. The patient's history of chronic ulcerative colitis usually suggests the diagnosis, and the supine and upright abdominal radiographs document dilatation of the entire colon, often with pseudopolyps noted as outlined by the intraluminal air. A sigmoidoscopy should confirm the diagnosis by documenting the shaggy, friable bleeding appearance of the mucosa. A barium enema examination should not be performed in these circumstances to avoid colon perforation.

Acute Abdominal Pain After Blunt Trauma

Blunt trauma to the abdomen is a frequent cause of intra-abdominal injury, producing signs and symptoms of the acute abdomen. The injury itself is the inciting event, and the onset of abdominal pain may be immediate or delayed over a period of hours or even days. A careful history is especially important if the patient is alert and able to respond. If the injury is due to a motor vehicle accident in which the patient was a passenger or driver, certain information is particularly important. The speed of the vehicle, whether or not a seat belt was used, and the location of the passenger in the vehicle (i.e., driver, back-seat or front-seat passenger) are all important factors in the history taking.

If the patient is injured in an altercation with another person, the type of trauma is also pertinent to the diagnosis. Examination of the abdomen often reveals a distended tender abdomen with hypoactive bowel sounds with no visible skin marks or abrasions. The supine and upright plain films of the abdomen may reveal free air with rupture of an intraperitoneal viscus or a ruptured diaphragm with intra-abdominal contents in the pleural cavity. Free blood within the peritoneal cavity may have a *ground glass* appearance in the abdomen, and if the bleeding is retroperitoneal, the radiographic appearance of the psoas margins may be altered.[11] Occasionally, if the duodenum is ruptured, a small amount of air in the retroperitoneal tissues around the duodenum may be visualized. A single film intravenous pyelogram documents important information regarding the function of both kidneys and the position of the ureter. A cystogram is particularly valuable to exclude rupture of the bladder. Both anteroposterior and oblique views of the bladder during the cystogram are necessary if a small posterior retroperitoneal tear is to be excluded. All patients must have a complete blood cell count; urinalysis; determination of blood urea nitrogen, creatinine, serum electrolytes, and serum amylase; and a liver profile. Immediate peritoneal lavage is the definitive diagnostic test to confirm the presence of intraperitoneal hemorrhage. Free blood in the peritoneal cavity may result from a rupture of the spleen, liver, mesentery, and, occasionally, the pancreas and the bowel. Immediate laparotomy is indicated in these circumstances. A rupture of the pancreas may occur where the body of the organ overlies the vertebral column. This situation is especially common with automobile drivers who have blunt abdominal injury due to compression from the steering wheel. The clinical findings of an acute abdomen after blunt trauma usually require prompt surgical intervention. Patients who develop signs and symptoms of an acute abdomen several days after the trauma occurred present a more complex situation and require a careful assessment in which many or all of the original diagnostic procedures are repeated to confirm or exclude a perforated viscus, pancreatic injury, or a delayed rupture of the spleen or liver. For this reason, consideration for admission and careful observation is indicated for those who sustain severe blunt abdominal trauma. Serial CT examinations may be useful in establishing the presence of important visceral injury during the period of observation. The use of CT is only advised if the patient can tolerate the procedure based on his or her general medical condition.[25, 43]

Trauma to the kidney is less common than that to the liver and spleen because of its anatomic location. However, with violent trauma sustained in automobile accidents or in contact sports, the kidney may be ruptured with severe retroperitoneal bleeding. Because of its location, bleeding may be considerable before it is detected. Ureters are rarely injured in blunt abdominal trauma.

Injury to the large and small intestine and their mesenteric attachments may occur after blunt trauma. Laceration of the mesentery may cause arterial or venous bleeding with hemoperitoneum. Laceration of the bowel wall with a tear in the lumen causing bacterial peritonitis is less common and, when present, suggests generalized peritonitis. The omentum is rarely injured, partly because of its mobility, but it may bleed if the trauma initiates a laceration.

Growing experience with the use of CT in the evaluation of the severely traumatized patient, especially in situations where the patient has sustained closed-head trauma in addition to suspected chest and abdominal trauma, has shown it to be especially valuable. In a single CT survey of the abdomen and pelvis with intravenous contrast medium, complete assessment of the solid viscera, mesentery, retroperitoneum, gastrointestinal tract, abdominal wall, and skeletal structures can be accurately accomplished. The use of CT is only advised if the patient's general medical condition indicates that he or she can tolerate the procedure. Ultrasonography in this setting has little value.

Acute Abdominal Pain After Spinal Cord Injury

The progressive improvement in care after spinal cord injuries has allowed a substantial increase in the survival of patients during the past 30 years. However, conditions requiring consideration for abdominal surgical procedures occur in patients with spinal cord injuries and involve the entire gastrointestinal tract. Approximately 10% of all fatalities among patients with spinal cord injuries are the result of a perforated viscus and peritonitis.[6, 15, 18] The ability of a patient to describe the symptoms of acute abdominal pain depends on the location of the spinal cord injury. Conduction of pain to the spinal cord from abdominal viscera may occur

by the thoracic, sympathetic, splanchnic, hypogastric, or pelvic nerves and then proceeds to the dorsal root ganglion. Patients with cervical cord injuries are less able to document the site of abdominal discomfort, even though most of these patients experience some type of abdominal pain with a perforated viscus.[37] Patients with lower thoracic and lumbar cord injuries are able to more accurately describe the location and type of pain.

The most frequent signs of such injury are an increase in heart rate and occasionally an increase in blood pressure. Sudden high fever may accompany a perforate viscus. Sweating is frequent, and anorexia or a feeling of *something not right* is a common complaint. Abdominal examination is complicated by the neurologic injury. Distention is a frequent occurrence in patients with spinal cord injury, but tenderness is uncommon. When tenderness does exist, it suggests a perforated viscus or bladder. Palpation of the abdomen may not document rigidity of the rectus muscles because of spasticity or flaccidity. However, a generalized resistance may be present. Shoulder pain is common in patients with a perforated viscus and diaphragmatic irritation. If the spinal cord lesion is at T12 or below and there is normal bowel and bladder function, the sensation to the abdominal viscera will be intact.

The incidence of gastrointestinal hemorrhage in these patients is between 1% and 3%, and the diagnostic evaluation and treatment should be the same as that in patients without neurologic injury. The causes of the acute abdomen are the same in patients with spinal cord injury as in those without neurologic injury. Chronic urinary tract infections, acute pyelonephritis, and fecal impaction are common nonoperative problems that occur in these patients. Complications in the first 30 to 60 days after injury are different from those that occur at a later time. Gastric dilatation, ileus, peptic ulcer disease, and pancreatitis may occur in the early period after injury. In a chronic setting, fecal impaction, peptic ulcer disease, hepatitis, diverticulosis, and renal or ureteral calculus may occur. The possibility of appendicitis must be considered at all times and, frequently, it has perforated by the time that the patient presents. In such circumstances, a right lower quadrant mass is a common finding on examination.

Acute Gynecologic Disease

Acute abdominal pain caused by disorders of the gynecologic subsystem is a common and serious problem encountered by surgeons. A thorough history and complete pelvic and rectal examinations are essential for an accurate diagnosis (Table 29–4). Plain radiographs of the abdomen do not usually provide important information. Therefore, pelvic ultrasound is the diagnostic examination of choice.

Acute Salpingitis. This disease, most commonly due to gonococcal infection, has an index of highest frequency in patients between the ages of 15 to 35 years and is rarely seen

TABLE 29–4. Abdominal Pain Secondary to Lesions of the Gynecologic Subsystem

Ovary
Ruptured graafian follicle
Torsion of ovary
Fallopian tube
Ectopic pregnancy
Acute salpingitis
Pyosalpinx
Uterus
Uterine rupture
Endometritis

after menopause. The pain begins cephalad to the symphysis in the midline and radiates to the right and left lower quadrants. Occasionally, gonococcal hepatitis may occur and is difficult to differentiate from other forms of hepatitis. The pain of acute salpingitis develops over a period of hours, and the patient usually has few gastrointestinal complaints. Examination of the abdomen reveals right and left lower quadrant tenderness to percussion and palpation. Bowel sounds are hypoactive. There is severe cervical tenderness on palpation during pelvic examination. A vaginal discharge is frequent, and a positive diagnosis can be established with a cervical smear and culture. The diagnostic radiographic procedure of choice is ultrasonography to evaluate the presence of hydrosalpinx and/or tubo-ovarian abscess.

Ovarian Tumors. Ovarian neoplasms may present in an acute manner when torsion or rupture occurs. Pain is sudden, located in the lower abdomen, and is most severe in either the right or left lower quadrant, depending on the ovary involved. Anorexia is rare, but nausea and vomiting may occur in the presence of severe pain. If rupture occurs, generalized peritonitis with free intraperitoneal bleeding results. Pelvic examination is the key diagnostic maneuver, and a palpable mass may confirm the suspicion. The diagnosis of a ruptured ovarian cyst or ovarian torsion can be established by pelvic ultrasonography.

Ectopic Pregnancy. Tubal pregnancy may present as an acute intra-abdominal condition with sudden lower abdominal pain that is sharp and persistent, with or without nausea and vomiting. These symptoms indicate rupture of the fallopian tube and occur in the first trimester of pregnancy. The patient's history is the most important factor in the diagnosis. A missed menstrual period or an abnormally short scanty period precedes the abdominal pain. However, it may be difficult to obtain an accurate history at the time of the acute illness, contributing to the obscurity of the diagnosis.

The patient presents with acute abdominal pain in the lower abdomen that, with rupture, proceeds to generalized peritonitis, occasional diaphragmatic irritation, and referred pain to the shoulder. The pain worsens with time and, if blood loss is significant, hypotension and tachycardia occur. Examination of the patient reveals moderate distention of the lower abdomen and hypoactive or absent bowel sounds with marked tenderness to percussion or palpation. Pelvic examination may demonstrate blood in the vagina or cervical os. Motion of the cervix is painful, and an adnexal mass is often palpable. A hematoma may be present in the cul-de-sac. The cervix is frequently blue, and the uterus is slightly enlarged.

Laboratory data reveal a decrease in hematocrit to 30% or less with a leukocytosis of 15,000 per cu. mm. The human chorionic gonadotropin test result is positive. The simplest and most accurate radiographic study confirming intrauterine or ectopic pregnancy is ultrasonography.[33] However, a negative result on a study does not exclude the presence of an ectopic pregnancy. Peritoneoscopy may be of diagnostic value if the patient's condition is stable. Culdocentesis, paracentesis, or peritoneal lavage may demonstrate bloody peritoneal fluid. Because other conditions that cause acute abdominal pain, such as ruptured ovarian cyst, acute appendicitis, and perforated ulcer, may be difficult to differentiate from a ruptured ectopic pregnancy, surgical intervention is required for diagnosis and treatment.

Septic thrombosis of the left or right ovarian vein in the immediate postpartum period associated with endometritis is an uncommon and somewhat confusing clinical syndrome that is often misdiagnosed as acute appendicitis, peritonitis, or intra-abdominal abscess. Treatment is nonsurgical and involves measures directed toward the bacterial infection. The role of anticoagulation is uncertain. The appearance of this entity on CT is characteristic.[3]

Acute Abdominal Pain During Pregnancy

The presence of acute abdominal pain during pregnancy is complicated by the duration of the pregnancy, the enlarged uterus, and the difficulty in accurately examining the abdomen. Appendicitis, a common clinical problem of pregnant patients, has many clinical features similar to appendicitis in nonpregnant patients. Acute cholecystitis, another cause of abdominal pain during pregnancy, also presents in a manner similar to that in nonpregnant patients. Acute pancreatitis, perforated ulcer and acute diverticulitis are seen less frequently, probably because of the age of the patient and her general state of good health. Rupture of a splenic artery aneurysm in pregnant patients has been reported with an increased frequency over that expected in this age group. In this situation, the patient presents with severe epigastric pain, hypotension, and shock. Immediate surgical exploration is indicated for obvious reasons, and the diagnosis is usually established at that time. Rupture of the liver capsule after subcapsular hematoma in the pregnant patient is also an uncommon event, presenting as an urgent problem in diagnosis and management. Associated conditions that predispose to this entity include preeclamptic toxemia and disseminated intravascular coagulation. This illness most often occurs in women in their late 20s or 30s, of whom 80% are multipara. Fifty percent of women who experience rupture of the liver capsule do so in the third trimester of pregnancy, and 25% do so at term. Right upper quadrant and epigastric pain radiating to the back and associated with hypotension, shock, and hemoperitoneum are the usual sequence of events, often followed by death of the fetus. Other causes of abdominal pain during pregnancy include placental abruption, ruptured uterus, torsion of the ovary, pyelonephritis, and pulmonary embolus. The diagnostic imaging procedure of choice is ultrasonography in that it avoids ionizing radiation. However, the accurate diagnosis of appendicitis after the third or fourth month of gestation can be difficult because of uterine size.

Abdominal Pain with Acquired Immunodeficiency Syndrome and Organ Transplantation

During the past 15 years the increased incidence of AIDS has required frequent surgical consultation regarding the diagnosis and treatment of those patients with acute abdominal pain. The history of sexual preference and intravenous drug use are critical pieces of information in the work-up, as is the established diagnosis of AIDS. Causes of abdominal pain in this group of patients involves gastrointestinal infection, ileus, and/or hepatosplenomegaly and miscellaneous entities.[1, 30, 44] Patients with gastrointestinal infection have diffuse abdominal pain with watery diarrhea and occasionally hematochezia. Abdominal tenderness is usually generalized with few signs of peritoneal irritation. Rebound tenderness is uncommon. Although appendicitis is a consideration, the usual features of this disease are absent. Cytomegalovirus infection is a high probability and may be the cause of multiple mucosal ulcerations with or without bleeding. The ulcerations may occur throughout the gastrointestinal tract from the esophagus to the anus. Endoscopy is the diagnostic procedure of choice. Patients with ileus and/or hepatosplenomegaly and nonlocalized abdominal pain can be followed conservatively, and the abdominal pain usually resolves without surgical intervention in 24 hours. Patients with AIDS may also have the same causes of acute abdominal problems that confront those without the disease and include perforated ulcer, small bowel perforation, and diverticulitis. Radiographic diagnosis in this group of patients can be best established by ultrasonography if the pain is localized to the right upper quadrant or pelvis. Otherwise, CT is the examination of choice. As a general rule, laparotomy in patients with AIDS is infrequent for purposes of diagnosis and is usually reserved for acute abdominal conditions not related to AIDS.[26]

Patients who undergo organ transplantation followed by chronic immunosuppression may develop abdominal pain from causes similar to both the nonimmunosuppressed patient and to the patient with AIDS. The role of cytomegalovirus as a cause of colon perforation and gastrointestinal bleeding is well recognized. In some instances the lesions may appear to be identical, with lymphomas of the bowel requiring resection and the final diagnosis established by pathology. In the immunosuppressed posttransplant patient with cytomegalovirus infection, the systemic aspects of the disease, including fever, leukopenia, chills, and anorexia, assist in establishing the diagnosis.

Acute Abdomen in the Postoperative Patient

Acute postoperative pain in the first 10 to 14 days presents a problem of special concern because the primary decision is to separate a new condition from a complication of a just-completed operation. Postoperative complications include infection or technical problems involving the incision, peritonitis and abscess formation, intestinal obstruction, acute cholecystitis, and pancreatitis. These problems must be separated from a new and independent illness and require special attention to establish a prompt and accurate diagnosis.[12]

Nonsurgical Causes of the Acute Abdomen

There are a number of nonsurgical causes of acute abdominal pain that are important for the surgeon to consider to avoid operating in those circumstances in which a surgical procedure is not indicated (Table 29–5).[42]

Spontaneous bacterial peritonitis is defined as bacterial peritonitis that occurs without gastrointestinal perforation or intra-abdominal abscess.[7, 13] It occurs in patients with ascites and especially in those individuals with cirrhosis and poor

hepatic function. This disease process rarely occurs in patients with viral hepatitis. *Escherichia coli* organisms are responsible for more than half of the cases, with *Klebsiella* and other gram-negative bacteria in the other cases. The clinical features include ascites, fever, abdominal pain, and encephalopathy. Rebound tenderness occurs in half of the patients. The diagnosis can be best established by peritoneal fluid aspiration with Gram stain and assessment of polymorphonuclear leukocytes.

Sickle cell anemia, a hereditary hemolytic disturbance, is seen in patients of the black race. The disease presents early in life and is characterized by attacks of bone and joint pain as well as abdominal pain. The diagnosis can be established by a careful history, because patients usually have had previous episodes of a similar type. Cholelithiasis is common in this group of patients and may present acutely.

Gastroenteritis, if severe, may cause abdominal pain preceded by nausea and vomiting. Diarrhea is common and almost always occurs after the onset of abdominal pain. The illness may be related to specific food intake, and other family members may be affected. Fortunately, the process is self-limited and resolves in 6 to 10 hours.

Unrecognized, severe pseudomembranous colitis may present as an acute abdomen, suggesting the need for surgical intervention. Plain abdominal radiographs and sigmoidoscopy often establish the correct diagnosis and obviate operative intervention.

Lead poisoning is associated with colicky abdominal pain, often in the right lower quadrant, and may cause suspicion of acute appendicitis. The history is one of recurrent attacks and, in spite of the severity of pain, the clinical examination reveals minimal findings of abdominal tenderness.

Acute porphyria occurs with recurrent attacks of abdominal pain. The disease is rarely noted before puberty, is most common in women, and occurs in the third and fourth decades of life. The abdominal pain is moderate to severe in intensity, may be generalized or localized, and radiates to the back. The abdominal examination reveals minimal tenderness, much less than is expected with the severity of the pain. Fever and leukocytosis may exist, and abdominal radiographs show distended loops of bowel. This diagnosis is suggested by a history of previous similar attacks and is confirmed by the excessive porphobilinogen in the urine.

Familial Mediterranean fever, a disorder of persons of Jewish (Sephardic) or Armenian background, is inherited as an autosomal recessive trait. The paroxysms of abdominal pain are severe, may be associated with chest pain, and precede the fever. Fever may be as high as 40° C. (103° F.), and tachycardia, tachypnea, and abdominal tenderness, especially in the epigastric region, are noted. Because of the recurrent nature of the abdominal findings, a previous surgical exploration has been often performed.

Right- or left-lower-lobe pneumonia with involvement of the diaphragmatic pleura may present as right or left upper quadrant pain with symptoms of pulmonary infection. The leukocytosis and rapid respiratory rate combined with the radiographic findings of pneumonia suggest a supradiaphragmatic cause for the abdominal pain.

Acute myocardial infarction may produce epigastric pain and may mimic acute pancreatitis or perforated duodenal ulcer. The pain is of sudden onset and combined with dyspnea and cyanosis. The electrocardiogram provides the correct diagnosis.

Rectus sheath hematoma may cause acute abdominal pain and is frequently preceded by a paroxysm of coughing or straining after heavy exertion. The pain is localized to the rectus sheath, and the abdominal tenderness markedly decreases with tension of the rectus sheath. A tender mass is occasionally palpable. The process is self-limited and is of

TABLE 29–5. Nonsurgical Causes of Abdominal Pain

Cardia
    Myocardial infarction
    Acute pericarditis
Pulmonary
    Pneumonia
    Pulmonary infarction
Gastrointestinal
    Acute pancreatitis
    Gastroenteritis
    Acute hepatitis
Endocrine
    Diabetic ketoacidosis
    Acute adrenal insufficiency
Metabolic
    Acute porphyria
    Familial Mediterranean fever
    Hyperlipidemia
Musculoskeletal
    Rectus muscle hematoma
Central and peripheral nervous system
    Tabes dorsalis
    Nerve root compression
Genitourinary
    Pyelonephritis
    Acute salpingitis
Hematologic
    Sickle cell crisis

primary concern only in that it may suggest an acute intra-abdominal condition such as appendicitis. The presence and exact location of an acute hematoma in the abdomen can be accurately determined with CT.

Acute adrenal insufficiency may occur in the immediate postoperative period, precipitating acute abdominal pain. The diagnosis is straightforward in patients with Addison's disease or in those requiring corticosteroid replacement therapy who are on a subtherapeutic postoperative dosage. On the other hand, some patients may develop adrenal hemorrhage after operation, producing adrenal insufficiency characterized by fever, nausea, vomiting, abdominal pain, diarrhea, hypotension, and an apathetic affect. Failure to recognize the entity may result in death. The CT findings in this acute hemorrhagic process are diagnostic.

Hyperlipidemia may occur in patients with acute pancreatitis as well as in those patients with recurrent episodes of abdominal pain occurring in the absence of pancreatitis. The history of hyperlipidemia is the key factor in the diagnosis. The abdominal examination reveals generalized tenderness with occasional hepatomegaly and splenomegaly.

All patients with nonsurgical causes of abdominal pain must be evaluated carefully on each recurrence of pain to prevent a superficial and erroneous conclusion from being reached on the basis that the primary disease is of nonsurgical origin.

SELECTED REFERENCES

Jeffrey, R. B., Jr.: CT and Sonography of the Acute Abdomen. New York, Raven Press, 1989.
This excellent and comprehensive textbook covers the use of imaging techniques for the acute abdomen.

Lee, J. K. T., Sagel, S. S., and Stanley, R. J.: Computed Body Tomography with MRI Correlation, 2nd ed. New York, Raven Press, 1989.
This is a superb textbook that includes a complete study of CT and MRI of acute and chronic conditions of the abdomen.

Sawyers, J. L., and Williams, L. F.: The acute abdomen. Surg. Clin. North Am., 68:233, 1988.
A complete review of the diagnosis of the acute abdomen is provided.

Silen, W.: Cope's Early Diagnosis of the Acute Abdomen, 19th ed. New York, Oxford University Press, 1995.
The revised edition of this classic monograph is a discussion of patients with acute abdominal pain.

REFERENCES

1. Barone, J. E., Gingold, B. S., Arvanitis, M. L., and Nealon, J. F.: Abdominal pain in patients with acquired immune deficiency syndrome. Ann. Surg., 204:619, 1986.
2. Bradley, E. L., Murphy, F., and Ferguson, C.: Prediction of pancreatic necrosis by dynamic pancreatography. Ann. Surg., 210:495, 1989.
3. Brown, C. E. L., Lowe, T. W., Cunningham, F. G., and Weinreb, J. C.: Puerperal pelvic thrombophlebitis: Impact on diagnosis and treatment using x-ray computed tomography and magnetic resonance imaging. Obstet. Gynecol., 68:789, 1986.
4. Burnett, L. S.: Gynecologic causes of the acute abdomen. Surg. Clin. North Am., 68:385, 1988.
5. Carroll, B. A.: Preferred imaging techniques for the diagnosis of cholecystitis and cholelithiasis. Ann. Surg., 210:1, 1989.
6. Charney, K. J., Juler, G. L., and Comarr, A. E.: General surgery problems in patients with spinal cord injuries. Arch. Surg., 110:1083, 1975.
7. Conn, H. O., and Fessel, J. M.: Spontaneous bacterial peritonitis in cirrhosis: Variations on a theme. Medicine, 50:161, 1971.
8. DeBakey, M. E., Crawford, E. S., Cooley, D. A., Morris, G. C., Royster, T. S., and Abbott, W. P.: Aneurysm of the abdominal aorta: Analysis of results of graft replacement therapy 1 to 11 years after operation. Ann. Surg., 160:622, 1964.
9. DeBartolo, H. M., and Van Heerden, J. A.: Meckel's diverticulum. Ann. Surg., 183:30, 1976.
10. Eisenberg, R. L., Heineken, P., Hedgcock, M. W., Federle, M., and Gold-berg, H. T.: Evaluation of plain abdominal radiographs in the diagnosis of abdominal pain. Ann. Intern. Med., 97:257, 1982.
11. Feliciano, D.: Management of traumatic retroperitoneal hematoma. Ann. Surg., 211:109, 1990.
12. Flint, L. M.: Early postoperative acute abdominal complications. Surg. Clin. North Am., 68:445, 1988.
13. Gilbert, J. A., and Kamath, P. S.: Spontaneous bacterial peritonitis: An update. Mayo Clin. Proc., 70:365, 1995.
14. Glenn, F.: Pain in biliary tract disease. Surg. Gynecol. Obstet., 122:495, 1966.
15. Gore, R. M., Mintzer, R. A., and Calenoff, L.: Gastrointestinal complications of spinal cord injury. Spine, 6:538, 1981.
16. Greenstein, A. J., Sachae, D. B., Mann, D., Lachman, P., Heimann, T., and Aufses, A. H.: Spontaneous free perforation and perforated abscess in 30 patients with Crohn's disease. Ann. Surg., 205:72, 1987.
17. Hattery, R. R., Williamson, B., and Wallace, R. B.: Ultrasonic and computed tomographic imaging of the abdominal aorta. World J. Surg., 4:511, 1980.
18. Hoen, T. I., and Cooper, I. S.: Acute abdominal emergencies in paraplegics. Am. J. Surg., 75:19, 1948.
19. Jeffrey, R. B., Jr.: Abdominal imaging in the immunocompromised patient. Radiol. Clin. North Am., 30:579, 1992.
20. Jeffrey, R. B., Jr., Laing, F. C., and Townsend, R. R.: Acute appendicitis: Sonographic criteria based on 250 cases. Radiology, 167:327, 1988.
21. Jeffrey, R. B.: CT and Sonography of the Acute Abdomen. New York, Raven Press, 1989.
22. Lewis, F. R., Holcroft, J. W., Beoy, J., and Dunphy, J. E.: Appendicitis: A critical review of diagnosis and treatment in 1000 cases. Arch. Surg., 110:677, 1975.
23. Ludtke, F. E., Mende, V., Kobles, H., and Lepsien, G.: Incidence and frequency of complications and management of Meckel's diverticulum. Surg. Gynecol. Obstet., 169:537, 1989.
24. Meier, E. E., Imediegwu, O. O., and Tarpley, J. L.: Perforated typhoid enteritis: Operative experience with 108 cases. Am. J. Surg., 157:423, 1989.
25. Meredith, J. W., and Trunkey, D. D.: CT scanning in acute abdominal injuries. Surg. Clin. North Am., 68:255, 1988.
26. Nylander, W. A.: The acute abdomen in the immunocompromised host. Surg. Clin. North Am., 68:457, 1988.
27. Ogata, M., Mateer, J. R., and Condon, R. E.: Prospective evaluation of abdominal sonography for the diagnosis of bowel obstruction. Ann. Surg., 223:237, 1996.
28. Ogilvie, H.: Large intestine colic due to sympathetic deprivation: A new clinical syndrome. BMJ, 2:671, 1948.
29. Osler, W. M.: The Principles and Practice of Medicine. New York, D. Appleton, 1892, p. 462.
30. Parente, F., Cernuschi, M., Antinori, A., Moroni, M., Fasan, M., Rizzardini, G., Rovati, V., Morandi, E., Molteni, P., and Porro, G. B.: Severe abdominal pain in patients with AIDS: Frequency, clinical aspects, causes and outcome. Scand. J. Gastroenterol., 6:511, 1994.
31. Roberts, P. L., and Veidenheimer, M. C.: Current management of diverticulitis. Adv. Surg., 27:189, 1994.
32. Rodkey, G. V., and Welch, C. E.: Colonic diverticular disease with surgical treatment: A study of 338 cases. Surg. Clin. North Am., 54:655, 1974.
33. Russell, S. A., Filly, R. A., and Damato, N.: Sonographic diagnosis of ectopic pregnancy with endovaginal probes: What really has changed? J. Ultrasound Med., 3:145, 1993.
34. Schwartz, M. Z., Tapper, D., and Solenberger, R. I.: Management of perforated appendicitis in children. Ann. Surg., 197:407, 1983.
35. Schwerk, W. B., Wichtrup, B., Ruschoff, J., and Rothmund, M.: Acute and perforated appendicitis: Current experience with ultrasound-aided diagnosis. World J. Surg., 14:271, 1990.
36. Shaff, M. I., Tarr, R. W., Partain, C. L., and James, A. E.: Computed tomography and magnetic resonance imaging of the acute abdomen. Surg. Clin. North Am., 68:233, 1988.
37. Soderstrom, C. A., McArdle, D. Q., Ducker, T. B., and Militello, P. R.: The diagnosis of intra-abdominal injury in patients with cervical cord trauma. J. Trauma, 23:1061, 1983.
38. Staniland, J. R., Ditchburn, J., and DeDombal, F. T.: Clinical presentation of acute abdomen: Study of 600 patients. BMJ, 3:393, 1972.
39. Steinheber, F. U.: Medical conditions mimicking the acute surgical abdomen. Med. Clin. North Am., 57:1559, 1973.
40. Strodel, W. E., Nostrant, T. T., Eckhauser, F. E., and Dent, T. L.: Therapeutic and diagnostic colonoscopy in nonobstructive colonic dilatation. Ann. Surg., 197:416, 1983.
41. Svanes, C., Salvesen, H., Espehaug, B., Soreide, O., and Svanes, K.: A multifactorial analysis of factors related to lethality after treatment of perforated duodenal ulcer. Ann. Surg., 209:418, 1989.
42. Tedesco, F. J., Anderson, C. B., and Ballinger, W. F.: Drug induced colitis mimicking an acute surgical condition of the abdomen. Arch. Surg, 110:481, 1975.
43. Thal, E. R., and Meyer, D. M.: The evaluation of blunt abdominal trauma: Computerized tomography scan, lavage or sonography. Adv. Surg., 24:201, 1991.
44. Thuluvath, P. J., Connolly, G. M., Forbes, A., and Gazzard, B. G.: Abdominal pain in HIV infection. Q. J. Med., 78:275, 1991.

CHAPTER 30

THE STOMACH AND DUODENUM

I

HISTORICAL ASPECTS, ANATOMY, PATHOLOGY, PHYSIOLOGY, AND PEPTIC ULCER DISEASE

Theodore N. Pappas, M.D.

GASTRIC ANATOMY AND PHYSIOLOGY

The stomach resides in the upper abdomen and is dorsally bounded by the pancreas and retroperitoneum; the ventral border of the stomach is the anterior abdominal wall and left lobe of the liver. The stomach is anatomically defined at its superior margin by the gastroesophageal junction, which is normally found at the esophageal hiatus of the diaphragm, and inferiorly by the pylorus. It is bounded on the left by the spleen and on the right by the liver (Fig. 30–1). The blood supply to the stomach is extensive, with branches coming off the celiac axis in the form of the left gastric artery, which supplies the upper lesser curvature of the stomach. The right gastric artery branches off the hepatic artery, which originates from the celiac axis; it supplies blood to the distal lesser curvature. The left gastroepiploic artery is a branch off the short gastric vessels; it comes from the splenic and therefore originally from the celiac axis. The right gastroepiploic artery branches off the gastroduodenal artery, which comes originally from the hepatic artery and therefore from the celiac axis. The extensive blood supply to the stomach explains why it is possible to surgically remove a portion of the stomach involving three of the four major arterial supplies and still maintain blood supply to the gastric remnant (Fig. 30–2). The venous drainage of the stomach empties in a variety of directions, including venous tributaries along the esophagus, veins that flow with the short gastrics to the splenic vein, and venous drainage that is carried toward the duodenum and toward the portal vein in the coronary vein. Many of these veins become clinically important in conditions of portal venous hypertension or splenic vein thrombosis, because they may form varices.

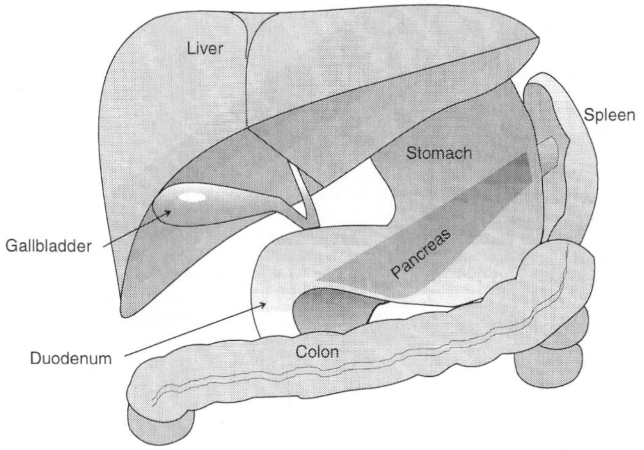

Neural input to the stomach is supplied predominantly by the vagus. An anterior (left) and posterior (right) vagus nerve courses with the esophagus until the gastroesophageal junction. At this point, they proceed along the lesser curvature of the stomach, sending nerve branches with the lesser curvature blood supply. The "criminal" nerve of Grassi is the first branch of the posterior vagal nerve innervating the greater curvature fundus. At the junction of the fundus and the antrum of the stomach, the vagal nerves branch and innervate the antrum. This vagal branch point is called the *crow's foot.* The hepatic branches of the vagus nerve that split from vagal trunks, noted in Figure 30–2, are preserved in a selective vagotomy but not in a truncal vagotomy. Highly selective vagotomy divides only the vagal branches to the parietal cell mass. Sympathetic innervation of the stomach occurs through the celiac ganglion, and postganglionic fibers run with the vascular supply to the stomach.

The stomach is divided into two major functional areas: the fundus and the antrum. The fundus is the acid-secretory storage site of the stomach. The antrum functions as a motility center and as an endocrine organ, in that it secretes gastrin. Further anatomic subdivisions of the stomach include the cardia, which is the most proximal portion of the stomach, and the body, which is the middle portion of the stomach (Fig. 30–3). The areas of the greater and lesser curvature on the left and right of the stomach indicate the long and short margins of the stomach, respectively.

The lesser sac is bounded ventrally by the stomach and is an important location during operation, in that it is a frequent space for fluid collection and is an important plane for the exposure of gastric anatomy. The greater and lesser omenta also have important surgical implications. The lesser omentum is a mesothelial structure lying between the lesser curvature and the liver. This represents the superior border of the lesser sac and contains the blood supply to the lesser curvature of the stomach. The greater omentum has a blood supply formed by the gastroepiploic vessels. The greater omentum emanates from the greater curvature of the stomach and is draped over the colon and attached only by adhesions, not by blood supply to the colon. The greater omentum is usually extensive and covers most of the abdominal organs. It is a favorite site of metastasis of gastric carcinoma and is rich in lymphatic support.

Figure 30–1. The anatomic relationships in the upper abdomen. The stomach is bounded on its left by the spleen, posteriorly (dorsally) by the pancreas, inferiorly (caudally) by the colon, and to its right by the duodenum along the liver's edge.

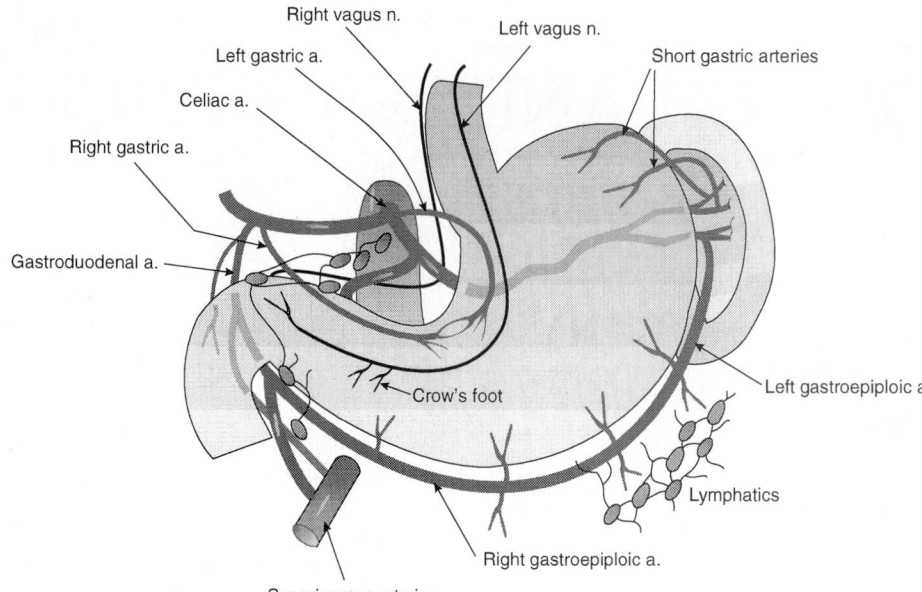

Figure 30–2. The anatomic location of arterial, venous, lymphatic, and neural supply of the stomach. The arterial supply comes mostly from the celiac system. The celiac artery sends branches to the lesser curve (left gastric and right gastric arteries) and to the greater curve (splenic, short gastric, left gastroepiploic, gastroduodenal, and right gastroepiploic arteries). The venous and lymphatic systems largely parallel the arterial system. The predominant cholinergic nerve input is through the vagal system, which sends branches to the liver near the hiatus. The gastric vagal input for antropyloric innervation is called the "crow's foot."

HISTOLOGY OF THE STOMACH

The gastric histology divides the stomach into three major parts: the cardia, fundus, and antrum, which are macroscopically similar but histologically distinct. The macroscopic view of the stomach demonstrates rugae, which are large folds of stomach protruding into the lumen. Microscopically, these rugae are covered with gastric glands and microvilli (Fig. 30–4). The gastric fundus is the acid-producing portion of the stomach, which contains five distinct cell types. The parietal cell is the major cellular component of the fundus and produces acid. Between the parietal cells are mucus-secreting cells. Zymogen-secreting cells, or chief cells, are also present; they produce pepsinogen, the precursor of the digestive enzyme pepsin. Endocrine cells (also called argentaffin cells) are scattered throughout the gastric glands. Undifferentiated cells are also found in the gastric glands. Gastric glands occur throughout the stomach; they contain parietal cells in the fundus, which are largely replaced by an overabundance of mucous cells in the cardia and gastrin-producing endocrine cells in the antrum (see Fig. 30–4).

The stomach wall is composed of circular and longitudinal muscles. The outer histologic margin of the stomach has a serosal lining. The intrinsic nerve fibers in the gastric wall include postganglionic nerve fibers that run with the longitudinal muscle. The pylorus muscle, which makes up the terminal part of the stomach, is a circular smooth muscle that can be hypertrophied in a variety of pathologic conditions; under normal conditions, it opens and closes as dictated by antral vagal innervation.

GASTRIC PHYSIOLOGY AND ACID SECRETION

Acid is secreted by the stomach through many avenues of stimulation. Vagal stimulation during cephalic-phase secretion is the trigger mechanism that initiates most forms of gastric acid stimulation. The vagal innervation of the stomach produces acid by two separate mechanisms: direct cholinergic innervation of the parietal cell, and indirect stimulation of the parietal cell via the hormonal mediator gastrin. The direct method is a vagal cholinergic innervation to an interneuron, which has a second cholinergic nerve ending on

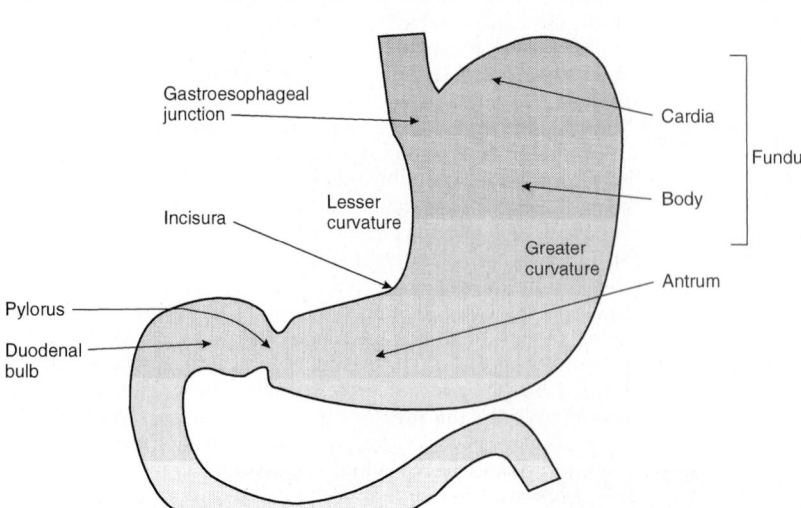

Figure 30–3. Anatomically, the stomach is divided into several segments. Functionally, the cardia and the antrum differ from the body in that they contain no acid secretory properties. The incisura is an area on the lesser curvature, which marks the antrum-body junction and is often easily seen on barium upper intestinal series.

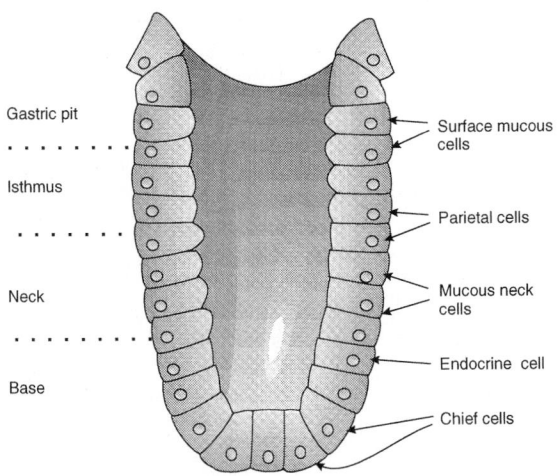

Figure 30–4. A stylized image of a human gastric gland from the body of the stomach. The gland contains parietal cells for acid production; mucous cells for the production of mucus and bicarbonate; endocrine (or argentaffin) cells, which produce a variety of paracrine; and hormonal agents and chief (or zymogenic) cells, which produce pepsinogen.

the parietal cell. In this way, cholinergic stimulation causes a direct increase in acid secretion via cholinergic receptors on parietal cells. The cholinergic receptor is one of three surface receptors on parietal cells. Vagal cholinergic stimulation also acts via an interneuron to stimulate the antral G cell to release gastrin. The neurotransmitter that causes gastrin release from the G cell is called gastrin-releasing peptide (GRP), or bombesin.[27] Gastrin acts as a true hormone through the bloodstream at gastrin receptors on parietal cells, the second surface receptor. The third parietal cell surface receptor responds to histamine (Fig. 30–5). Gastric mast cells release histamine, which can act locally to stimulate histamine receptors on parietal cells.[14] Gastrin and acetylcholine appear to assist in the mobilization of histamine stores and thereby indirectly stimulate the parietal cell via the histamine receptor.

Stimulation of the gastrin and acetylcholine receptors occurs through an intracellular calcium-dependent pathway to activate phosphorylase kinase, which leads to protein phosphorylation. The adenosine triphosphate (ATP) product drives the hydrogen-potassium ATPase that produces hydrogen ion (acid). Stimulation of the histamine receptor activates adenylate cyclase, producing adenosine monophosphate (AMP), which works through protein kinase to phosphorylate ATP to drive the hydrogen-potassium ATPase. In this way, parietal cell surface receptors can act through differing second-messenger systems to produce acid via a final common pathway. The site of final acid production is where the drug omeprazole works, explaining its ability to produce achlorhydria by inactivation of ATPase.[38, 51, 55]

Acid produced by the parietal cell is secreted through the mucous gel layer (Fig. 30–6) and resides in the stomach lumen to lower the intragastric pH. The back diffusion of acid is prevented by the mucous gel layer, which maintains a microenvironment of bicarbonate trapped near the surface of the parietal cell. In this way, the microenvironment of the cell maintains a pH of 7 while the lumen maintains a purely acid pH. Gastric bicarbonate is created by the mucous cell in very small quantities but can maintain a neutral pH in the mucous gel layer as long as the gel continues to be supported on the surface of the mucosa. The breakdown of the production of mucus or its position at the mucosal interface can lead to ulceration. Drugs that support the mucous gel layer or bicarbonate secretion are termed *cytoprotective*, since they treat ulcer disease without treating acid.[12, 43]

Downregulation of acid is controlled by a variety of inhibitors, including somatostatin. Somatostatin acts locally at the parietal cell and in the antrum to decrease both acid and gastrin release. The somatostatin cell (D cell) in the gastric fundus is innervated by the vagus and is released in response to vagal stimulation. This is a cholinergic-mediated response and allows somatostatin to act as an inhibitor of acid secretion. In a similar fashion, cholinergic innervation via a vagal interneuron acts at the somatostatin cell in the antrum to release somatostatin for downregulation of gastrin release. There is also a luminal control of acid secretion, which is pH

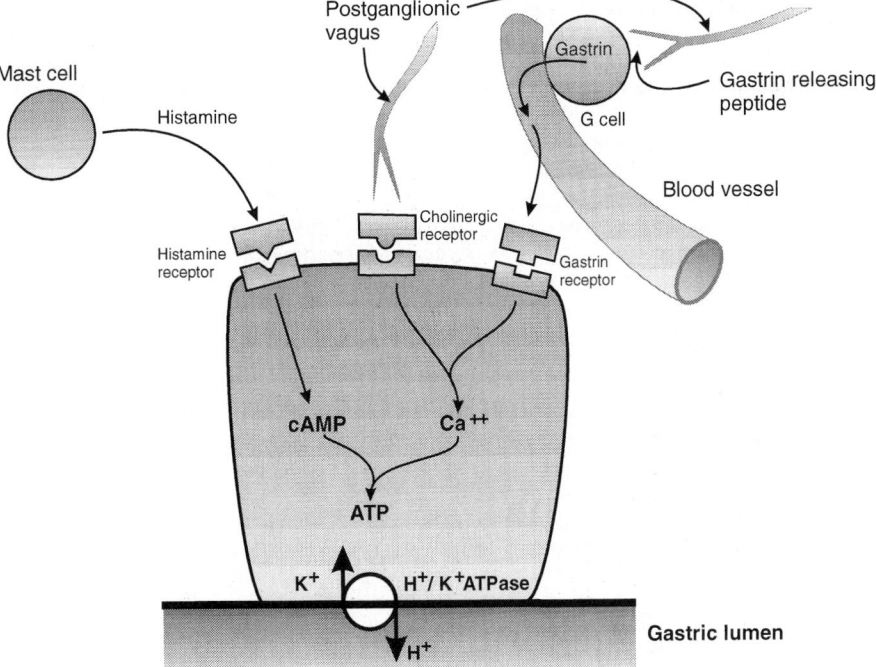

Figure 30–5. A parietal cell and the mechanisms that produce acid. The parietal cell has three stimulatory receptors: histamine, acetylcholine, and gastrin. Cholinergic stimulation and gastrin stimulation function synergistically, probably because they act through the same Ca^{++}-dependent second-messenger system. Histamine stimulation acts through a cAMP-dependent intracellular mechanism to stimulate the production of adenosine triphosphate (ATP) to drive the hydrogen-potassium ATPase (final common pathway of acid production).

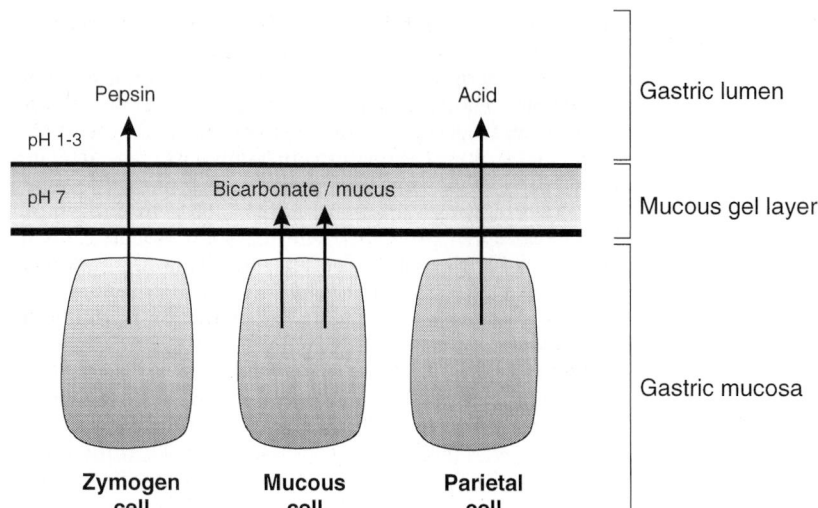

Figure 30–6. The importance of gastric mucus and bicarbonate to the production of the mucous gel layer is illustrated. Bicarbonate produced by the mucous cell is trapped in the gel layer that adheres to the gastric mucosa. This pH-neutral layer protects the mucosa from back diffusion of acid. Blocking the mucous cell function, such as occurs with nonsteroidal anti-inflammatory drugs, leads to back diffusion of acid and ulceration.

dependent. Alkaline pH (>3) releases gastrin from the antrum, producing acid. When the pH of the luminal antrum falls below 3, somatostatin is released, which closes the feedback loop and inhibits gastrin release.

PHYSIOLOGY OF GASTRIC EMPTYING

Functional aspects of gastric emptying depend on complete coordination of the anteropyloroduodenal complex. The anatomy of gastric emptying is divided into three parts: the fundus, which functions as a storage area of the particles that are being processed for emptying; the antrum, which functions as a grinder and sorter of particle size; and the pylorus, which functions with the antrum and duodenum to form a pressure gradient for the emptying of solids and liquids. The duodenum tends to act as a recipient and a regulator of the emptying process.

The process of gastric emptying starts with the acceptance of food in the stomach. Swallowed food enters the fundus, and the stomach accommodates this food bolus. The purpose of accommodation is to allow for an increase in gastric volume without an increase in gastric pressure. This is a vagal, cholinergic mechanism. In this way, the fundus responds to food by gradually dilating to meet the need of the approaching bolus. Vagotomy ablates the gastric accommodation and is thought to be associated with the dumping syndrome, allowing liquids to rapidly empty if the stomach outlet has been surgically altered.

Antral function is driven largely by vagal innervation. Vagal stimulation causes active contraction of the antrum, resulting in high pressure. This sends particles of 0.5 mm. or less through the pylorus to the duodenum. Particles greater than 1 mm. are processed back to the fundus for further digestion or trituration (particle size reduction). Ninety-nine percent of particles that leave the stomach are less than 1 mm., and 95% are less than 0.5 mm.[34]

The pylorus itself has little or no independent effect on gastric emptying. Large pyloroplasties probably alter gastric emptying when the pyloroplasty is extended well into the antrum, causing antral dysfunction.

The regulators of gastric emptying include a central mechanism, which probably acts largely through the vagus nerve. Neuropeptide Y and other brain neuropeptides may be responsible for triggering vagal mechanisms that affect gastric emptying.[45] There is also evidence that cholecystokinin in the brain influences gastric emptying, and the interplay between them may regulate the relationship between eating behavior

and gastric emptying after a meal.[44] The local phenomena that regulate gastric emptying include stretch receptors in the stomach, which feed back centrally to cause a slowing of gastric emptying. Although gastrin was previously thought to represent a regulator of gastric emptying, it probably works through the cholecystokinin receptors. Cholecystokinin is a physiologic inhibitor of gastric emptying and is released from the duodenum when food, particularly fats and amino acids, enter the duodenum.[10] This explains the delay in gastric emptying that occurs after a fatty meal. Duodenal acidification is also responsible for a delay in gastric emptying, mediated through secretin release. Finally, the distal gut has some impact on gastric emptying, in that distal gut stimulation slows gastric emptying. The ileum or colonic brake is a phenomenon that has been described by many investigators and is probably related to a hypothetical peptide *enterogastrone*. An enterogastrone-like substance, such as peptide YY, can be released from the distal gut and act in a hormonal fashion to decrease gastric emptying.[40] The current hypothesis suggests that peptide YY acts to decrease gut motility by blocking the release of acetylcholine on short postganglionic vagal fibers in the stomach wall.[42]

Gastric emptying of solids and liquids occurs at different rates. Gastric emptying of liquids occurs passively along the anteropyloroduodenal pressure gradient and therefore occurs in an exponential fashion. There is an early rapid phase of emptying for liquids, followed by a prolonged tail of the emptying curve.[9] The emptying of liquids is thought to result from contraction of the fundus, forcing fluid down the pressure gradient. The emptying of solids occurs after a lag phase, during which there is little emptying. Most solid particles are initially too large to pass the pylorus, so they are ground between the antrum and the fundus. Once the particles are sufficiently reduced in size, solid-phase gastric emptying becomes linear until the stomach is emptied.

The gastric pacemaker is found at the greater curvature in the upper third of the fundus and is responsible for initiating contractile waves in the upper gut. The gastric pacemaker produces cyclic electrical activity, which can produce a wave of up to three contractions per minute. In the fasting state, four phases of activity occur and are associated with varying rates of pacemaker propagation. These four phases of activity are termed the *migrating motor complex* (MMC). In phase I and II of the MMC, there is a pacemaker potential with intermittent wave propagation. The pacemaker electrical impulses are uniformly translated into contractile waves only during phase III of the MMC, when these contractions sweep the upper gut to carry large particles through the gut that did not pass previously. In phase IV, just prior to the fed state, the motor waves tend to decrease in frequency. In the fed state, contraction occurs frequently but is unrelated to the pacemaker.

DUODENUM

Anatomy and Physiology

The duodenum extends from the pylorus about 20 to 30 cm. and ends at the ligament of Treitz, which is where the jejunum begins. This is marked by adhesive bands between the duodenal-jejunal junction and the retroperitoneum on the left side of the abdomen. The duodenum is divided into four anatomic regions: the first portion, or the cap or bulb; the second portion, or the descending duodenum; the third, or transverse, portion; and the fourth, or ascending, portion (Fig. 30–7).

The duodenal cap lies just beyond the pylorus. Externally, the cap has attachments to the hepatoduodenal ligament in the pancreatic head. The cap is approximately 5 cm. long and directly overlies the passage of the common bile duct. Ninety percent of ulcers occur in the duodenal cap region. The gastroduodenal artery lies directly behind the duodenal cap, and penetrating ulcers into the pancreas initially erode through the gastroduodenal artery, accounting for the massive bleeding that occurs with these ulcers.

The second (descending) portion of the duodenum turns posteriorly and courses around the pancreatic head from the duodenal cap to the level of the first lumbar vertebra, where it turns into the third portion of the duodenum. This area of the duodenum is intricately attached to the pancreas, and these two organs share a blood supply. This portion overlies the vena cava and Gerota's fascia; mobilization of this portion has been termed a Kocher maneuver. Just superior to the junction between the duodenal cap and the second portion of the duodenum is the foramen of Winslow, which is bounded anteriorly by the hepatoduodenal ligament. *In situ*, the second portion is directly covered by the hepatic flexure, and mobilization of the hepatic flexure during a right colectomy requires careful preservation of this portion of the duodenum. The ampulla of Vater and the minor papilla both enter into the duodenum in this portion. The second portion of the duodenum is approximately 10 cm. in length.

The third and fourth portions of the duodenum (transverse and ascending portions) are mostly retroperitoneal. The third portion is attached to the uncinate process and crosses the abdomen and over the aorta. The third portion is trapped between the superior mesenteric artery (SMA) and the aorta. Compression of the junction of the third and fourth portions of the duodenum by the angle of the SMA and the aorta is called the SMA syndrome. The fourth portion of the duodenum blends into the jejunum at the ligament of Treitz, which attaches this junction to the retroperitoneum. Mobilization of the ligament of Treitz is necessary in duodenal resections. The ligament is often composed of small strands of striated muscle that eventually extend to the crus of the diaphragm. A fibromuscular band passing from the duodenum to the celiac axis is often present, and overaccentuated structures in this area can lead to compression of the celiac axis, presenting in a fashion similar to chronic upper gut ischemia.

The endoscopic view of the duodenal cap usually reveals a relatively small lumen, which includes fornices of the duodenal cap that require retroflexion to view. Occasionally, duodenal ulcers can be hidden in these fornices. Kerckring's folds of the duodenum begin just beyond the cap and continue throughout the duodenum. The concentric folds of Kerckring are approximately 1 to 2 mm. thick and 2 to 4 mm. high. They are usually separated by 2 to 4 mm. of flat duodenum. The major papilla enters the second portion of the duodenum and can be easily seen endoscopically, representing the ampulla of Vater. This usually appears as a hooded fold and is the site of the confluence of the common bile duct and main pancreatic duct (the duct of Wirsung). The duct of Santorini, or the accessory pancreatic duct, is present in most cases and is usually a little superior to the main papilla. The endoscopic appearance of the minor papilla is usually that of a small, 2-mm. polypoid structure. The endoscopic appearance of the third and fourth portions of the duodenum is unremarkable except for the presence of Kerckring's folds.

The blood supply of the duodenum is varied. The superior blood supply comes off the hepatic artery as the gastroduodenal artery, which splits into anterior and posterior pancreaticoduodenal arteries. These represent the superior seg-

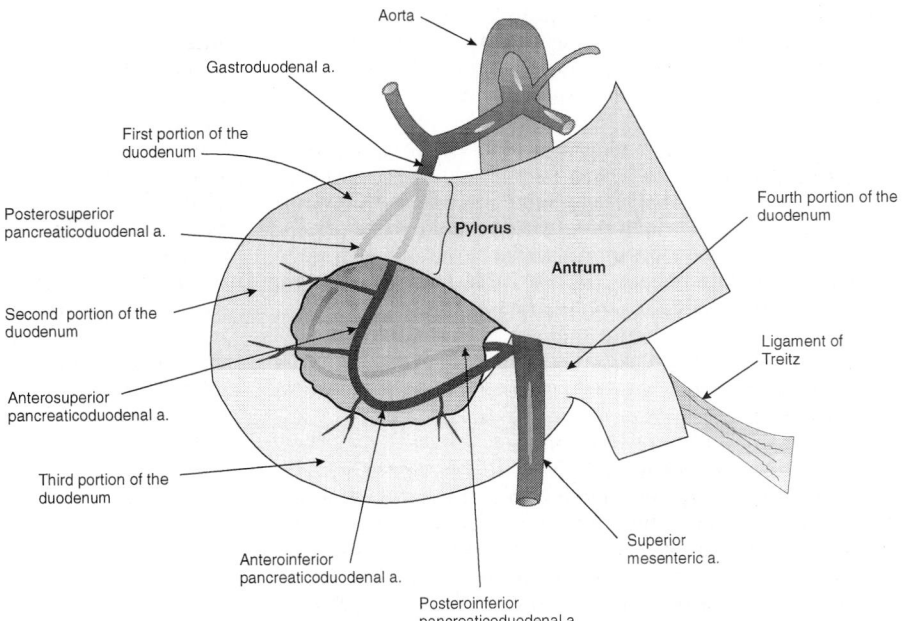

Figure 30–7. Gross anatomy of the duodenum. The arterial supply is passed off the celiac and gastroduodenal arteries, with anastomosis to the superior mesenteric artery. The first portion of the duodenum is where most duodenal ulcers occur. The second portion of the duodenum supports the ampulla of Vater (not shown). The ligament of Treitz divides the fourth portion of the duodenum from the jejunum.

Aorta

Gastroduodenal a.

First portion of the duodenum

Posterosuperior pancreaticoduodenal a.

Pylorus

Antrum

Fourth portion of the duodenum

Second portion of the duodenum

Ligament of Treitz

Anterosuperior pancreaticoduodenal a.

Third portion of the duodenum

Anteroinferior pancreaticoduodenal a.

Posteroinferior pancreaticoduodenal a.

Superior mesenteric a.

ments of an anastomosing group of vessels that eventually connect to the inferior pancreaticoduodenal arteries. There are anterior and posterior versions of these arteries. They join the superior mesenteric artery near its takeoff from the aorta. The vascular supply of this area generally courses through the pancreas itself, sending communicating vessels into the duodenum for its blood supply. The first portion of the jejunum is supplied by short branches of the superior mesenteric artery that also feed the terminal portion of the duodenum near the ligament of Treitz (see Fig. 30–7).

Histology of the Duodenum

The wall of the duodenum is made up of mucosa and muscle. The mucosa of the duodenum is predominantly secretory, with a small absorptive capacity. The mucosal thickness varies from 500 to 900 μm. and has an extensive surface area due to villi. The duodenal mucosa is rich with secretory capability and also has a predominant endocrine function.

Microscopically, the villi represent finger-like projections into the lumen of the bowel that contain mucus-secreting goblet cells and absorptive cells. The typical absorptive cell has microvilli at the lumen, and the base of the cell sits directly adjacent to capillaries. These cells are interspersed with goblet cells on most of the surface of the villi. A variety of cells exist in the crypts or valley areas of the multiple villi, including endocrine cells. The purpose of the goblet cells is to secrete mucigen. These goblet cells are narrow at the base and wide at the head, where the mucigen droplets are stored. The mucigen, which is secreted on the surface, acts as a lubricant. The crypt cells are predominantly endocrine or Paneth cells interspersed with other undifferentiated cells. The undifferentiated cells probably migrate to the tip of the villus as it becomes functional. Endocrine cells have an orientation somewhat different from that of absorptive cells. Absorptive cells tend to have nuclei that are basely located, in contrast to endocrine cells, in which the nuclei are positioned toward the lumen in the widest part of the cell and adjacent to the capillaries. The presumption is that this is in response to the endocrine function, with secretion of their product into the bloodstream as opposed to into the lumen. The function of the Paneth cells is unclear. The amine precursor uptake and decarboxylation (APUD) system represents cells that are endocrine in function and produce hormones, neuropeptides, and paracrine agents. Enterochromaffin cells represent APUD cells that secrete 5-hydroxytryptamine.

There are a variety of peptides that have biologic action and serve as the product of the endocrine portion of the duodenum (Fig. 30–8). Cholecystokinin (CCK) is a peptide that serves as a neurotransmitter in some areas and as a hormone in others. It is biologically available in a variety of molecular forms, although it is thought that the functional forms in the periphery are probably CCK 33 and 39. They are located in the duodenum and the first portion of the jejunum. CCK is released from the duodenum and jejunum in response to luminal fats and protein. There are several biologic actions of CCK that are thought to be physiologic, including gallbladder contraction, sphincter of Oddi relaxation, secretion of pancreatic protein, and delaying of gastric emptying; CCK may also have a role in the regulation of food intake.[5]

Secretin is a 27–amino acid peptide that is in the same family as glucagon, vasoactive intestinal peptide (VIP), and gastric inhibitory peptide (GIP). Secretin is found in the S cells, which are located predominantly in the duodenum and jejunum. It functions as a hormone by acting in the pancreas to increase the secretion of water and bicarbonate from the pancreas. Secretin works synergistically with CCK to produce pancreatic secretion. It is released from the duodenal mucosa in response to acid in the duodenum, particularly when the luminal pH of the duodenum falls below 4.5. The regulation of its secretion is pH dependent, in that pancreatic bicarbonate neutralizes acidic pH, thereby causing feedback inhibition of secretion.[6]

Somatostatin is a neuropeptide that works as a paracrine agent in the upper gut. It is biologically available as 14 and 28 amino acids and is produced by D cells in the gut. It appears to act as a paracrine agent in the pancreatic islets and also in the stomach, where it downregulates the production of acid and gastrin. The regulatory role of somatostatin in the control of pancreatic exocrine secretion is less well defined.[64]

GIP is a 42–amino acid peptide that belongs to the glucagon family. It functions as a hormone and is found in the mucosa of the duodenum and jejunum.[65] It is thought to augment the insulin response to an oral meal. Motilin, a 22–amino acid peptide found in the enterochromaffin cells in the mucosa of the upper gut, has been associated with the regulation of MMC. The timing of the MMC is coincident with the release of motilin in the bloodstream.[47]

Neurotensin is a 13–amino acid neurotransmitter produced by the N cells of the upper gut. It is found throughout most of the upper gut and in the colon, with its maximal concentration in the ileum and smaller concentrations in the duodenum. It is released in response to a mixed meal and fats, with smaller quantities released in response to carbohydrates and proteins. It is thought to have a physiologic role in gastric secretion, gastric emptying, pancreatic secretion, and motility.[62] Pancreatic glucagon and enteroglucagon belong to the secretin, VIP, and GIP family. Glucagon has 29 amino acids, in contrast to enteroglucagon, which has 37 amino acids. The pro-hormone for both of these peptides is glycinin. Enteroglucagon resides in the distal gut, whereas glucagon tends to reside more prominently in the upper gut. Glucagon has a physiologic role in the regulation of glucose homeostasis.[16]

PEPTIC ULCER DISEASE

Historical Perspective of Treatment

The history of the management of peptic ulcer disease has paralleled the understanding of the physiology and pathophysiology of acid secretion and gastric emptying in peptic ulceration. Initial management for complications of peptic ulcer disease was surgical in the nineteenth century, when Woefler, Billroth, and Von Rydigier described early gastric resections and gastroenterostomies. The modern management of peptic ulcer disease, based on the understanding of the vagal drive for acid secretion, was begun by Dragstedt, with his description of vagotomy and its use in peptic ulcer disease.[11] This led to the heyday of peptic ulcer surgical procedures in the 1940s and 1950s, when gastric operations for peptic ulcer disease rivaled cholecystectomy as the most common operation performed by general surgeons. During this period, extensive evaluations of the outcome of peptic ulcer operations, including long-term complications such as diarrhea and dumping, were performed. Several things have contributed to the fact that fewer peptic ulcer operations are being done, including a decreasing incidence of the disease and a general understanding of its pathophysiology, which led to improved medical therapy. In the late 1960s and early 1970s, Morton I. Grossman and Charles Code at the Center for Ulcer Research and Education (CURE) in Los Angeles established a large research group whose combined efforts paved the way for most of the physiologic knowledge about gastric function that was gained in the 1960s, 1970s, and 1980s. Medical and surgical scientists, including Andrew H.

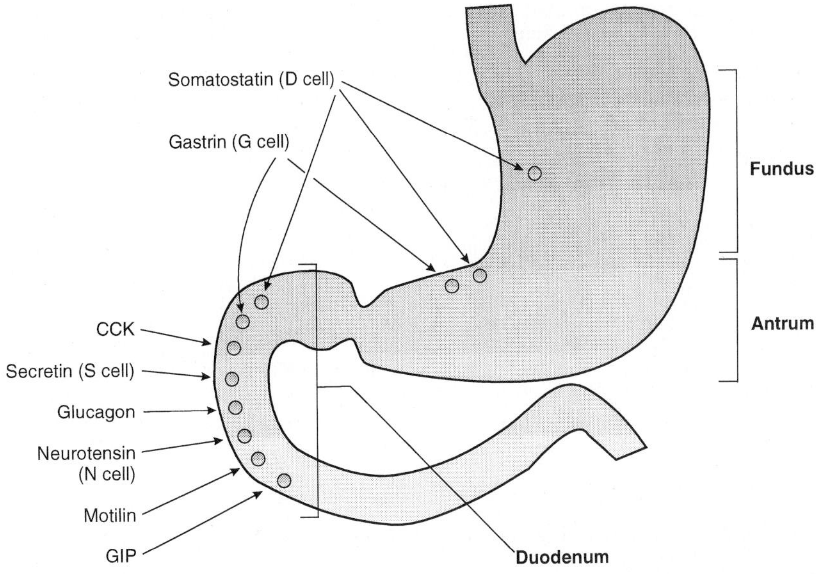

Figure 30–8. The upper gut has many endocrine functions, and some of the cells of origin are shown. The somatostatin cell is found over most of the gut and acts as a neurotransmitter or paracrine. The G cell is found mostly in the antrum, although smaller quantities of gastrin-producing cells are located in the duodenum. Cholecystokinin (CCK) cells are found in both duodenum and jejunum, as are secretin cells, gastric inhibitory polypeptide (GIP) cells, and motilin cells. Neurotensin- and glucagon-producing cells can be found well down into the colon.

Soll, Tadataka Yamada, John H. Walsh, Haile T. Debas, Edward J. Passaro Jr., John S. Fordtram, George Sachs, Leonard R. Johnson, and Ian L. Taylor, are only a small part of the large contingent of investigators that was spawned by CURE. This understanding of upper gut physiology led to the production and wide use of various antiulcer treatments, such as antacids, H$_2$ antagonists, omeprazole, and misoprostol.[54] These innovations in the pharmacologic management of this disease have vastly overshadowed surgical treatment in the 1980s and 1990s. Highly selected vagotomy is currently the only operation that has been perfected since World War II and is the operation of choice for the elective surgical management of peptic ulcer disease.[18]

Incidence

The incidence of peptic ulcer disease has been decreasing in the United States over the past 40 years. This decreased incidence has been documented by fewer physician visits and decreases in mortality, hospitalization, and operations for peptic ulcer disease.[2] The segment of the population in which peptic ulcer disease is increasing is the elderly, whose mortality and hospitalization are increasing, particularly among women. A decrease in peptic ulcer disease has also been documented in a variety of other countries including Europe, Asia, and North America.

Some of the specific complications of peptic ulcer disease continue to persist despite the decrease in overall incidence. Remarkably, the death rates for both duodenal and gastric ulcers have not changed since 1979. Again, this is largely due to the rising incidence in the elderly.[30] Currently, the vast majority of operations for peptic ulcer disease are performed for urgent and emergent complications of the disease, including hemorrhage, perforation, and obstruction.

The introduction of H$_2$ antagonists, such as cimetidine in 1977, had a dramatic effect on the treatment of peptic ulcer disease, but the falling incidence occurred much earlier. Although it is clear that these H$_2$ antagonists and now omeprazole have had a large impact on the modern-day management of this disease, it is not likely that the change in incidence is a result of this new medical management.

Etiology

The pathogenesis of peptic ulceration in the upper gut continues to be debated, but the central issue that links all theories is acid. All other hypotheses aside, acid must be present for nonmalignant ulceration of the upper gut to occur. The degree of acid secretion varies with the disease state, ranging from the extreme hyperacidity of Zollinger-Ellison syndrome to the hypoacidity present with Type I and IV gastric ulcers (Fig. 30–9). Still, the cornerstone of therapy for most routine duodenal ulcers is the diminution of acid, which appears to adequately treat 80% to 90% of patients. It is equally clear that acid hypersecretion is not necessary to create ulcers, in that only 40% of patients with duodenal ulcer disease can be described as hypersecretors. The total amount of acid secreted may not be as important as the time that the acid is secreted, particularly when patients have high secretory volumes in a basal state. Basal secretion in ulcer patients is usually high, and eradication of basal secretion, particularly nighttime secretion, can be sufficient to treat most peptic ulcers.[7, 15]

Gastric stasis can lead to peptic ulceration by inadequate clearance of normal amounts of acid. This can occur in patients who have delayed gastric emptying secondary to motility abnormalities or structural problems. Peptic ulcer disease often perpetuates itself by causing duodenal scarring, thereby delaying gastric emptying and leading to further ulceration.

A variety of environmental factors have been implicated in peptic ulceration. Medications, such as nonsteroidal anti-inflammatory drugs (NSAIDs), have been directly linked to gastric ulceration, particularly in elderly rheumatoid arthritis patients who require long-term therapy with NSAIDs (Table 30–1). NSAIDs appear to disrupt the prostaglandin-driven support of the mucosal barrier, as shown in Figure 30–6. Prostaglandins are directly related to the production of the mucous gel layer in the stomach.[24] This mucous gel layer protects the gastric and duodenal lining by trapping a neutral (pH 7) microenvironment at the cell surface. This allows the gastric lumen to have a very low pH while maintaining a protective barrier to the mucosa. Disruption of the mucous gel layer by NSAIDs often allows minimal amounts of acid to cause maximal ulceration in the upper gut.

Helicobacter pylori has recently become an important etiologic factor in peptic ulcer disease. This association was originally described in 1984 in mucosal samples of patients with peptic ulcers.[32] Recently, a large volume of work has demonstrated that many normal volunteers harbor *H. pylori* in their upper gut (up to 20%), whereas 100% of duodenal ulcer

A. Ulcers associated with relatively high acid

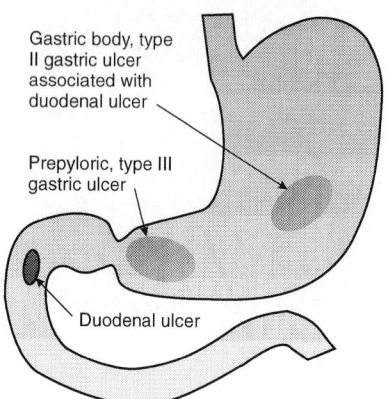

Gastric body, type II gastric ulcer associated with duodenal ulcer

Prepyloric, type III gastric ulcer

Duodenal ulcer

B. Ulcers associated with relatively low acid

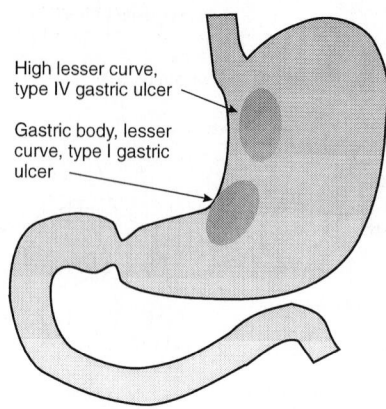

High lesser curve, type IV gastric ulcer

Gastric body, lesser curve, type I gastric ulcer

Figure 30–9. The four types of gastric ulcers. *A,* Ulcers related to high acid output include Type II (combination duodenal and gastric ulcer) and Type III ulcers (prepyloric). *B,* Ulcers associated with low acid output include Type IV (those located high on the lesser curve) and Type I (gastric body lesser curve) ulcers.

patients have demonstrable *H. pylori.* Current evidence suggests that eradication of the bacteria has led to a decreased recurrence rate and greatly supports the hypothesis that *H. pylori* is an etiologic factor. The presence of *H. pylori* and acid clearly predisposes to peptic ulceration, and eradication of both acid and *H. pylori* leads to high initial cure rates and marked decreases in recurrence rates.[13, 31, 46]

Cigarette smoking is another factor that appears to be related to peptic ulceration.[53, 56] The exact cause has not been clearly defined, although it has been suggested that cigarette smoking diminishes mucosal defense, similar to NSAIDs.

A decrease in bicarbonate production by the stomach and, more specifically, by the duodenum has been linked to peptic ulceration. Studies suggest that patients with duodenal ulcer disease have a reduced production of bicarbonate.[22] It has been proposed that patients with decreased bicarbonate production cannot maintain a pH-neutral microlayer above the mucosal lining and beneath the mucous gel layer. Drugs that increase bicarbonate production are being investigated for use in the treatment of peptic ulcer disease.[10]

Diagnosis and Management

The medical management of peptic ulcer disease has markedly changed over the past 30 years. There are now a host of

TABLE 30–1. Ulcerogenic Agents

Nonsteroidal anti-inflammatory drugs (NSAIDs)
  Aspirin
    Buffered
    Enteric coated
    Combination drugs
  Ibuprofen
  Ketorolac
  Naproxen
  Nabumetone
  Mefenamic acid
  Fenoprofen
  Meclofenamate
  Indomethacin
  Diclofenac
  Tolmetin
  Ketoprofen
  Etodolac
  Piroxicam
  Flurbiprofen
  Sulindac
  Diflunisal
Steroids, when used with NSAIDs
Cigarettes

medications with proven efficacy in the management of peptic ulcer disease (Table 30–2). All these treatments have evolved as the understanding of the physiology of acid secretion has matured. With improving medical management, intractability as an indication for surgical intervention has markedly diminished and now accounts for less than 5% of patients who undergo all types of ulcer operations (Table 30–3).

The medical management of upper gut ulceration varies for duodenal and gastric ulcers (Figs. 30–10 and 30–11). Duodenal ulcer disease is commonly treated after diagnosis is confirmed by either x-ray or endoscopy. First-line therapy includes an H_2 antagonist for 8 weeks and evaluation and treatment of *H. pylori,* whereas recurrent or persistent disease can be treated with omeprazole (Prilosec) and repeat investigation for *H. pylori.* Care should be taken to ascertain that these patients are not on ulcerogenic drugs. Rarely, patients fail to respond to these treatment courses and are referred for surgical therapy.

In contrast, gastric ulcer patients must be evaluated to rule out gastric cancer and are usually taking ulcerogenic medications, most commonly NSAIDs. All gastric ulcer patients should undergo initial endoscopy and biopsy to rule out malignancy. Prior recommendations for a repeat biopsy to guarantee healing and a follow-up endoscopy may not be necessary due to the accuracy of endoscopy and biopsy and the diminishing incidence of gastric adenocarcinoma. Current recommendations include initial therapy with an H_2 antagonist after tumor is excluded. Patients with the classic appearance of benign ulceration associated with NSAIDs who completely respond to therapy may avoid repeat biopsy. If any concern about malignancy remains, however, repeat biopsy is mandatory. Screening and treatment for *H. pylori* should be done for all recurrent or persistent gastric ulcers (see Fig. 30–11). Intractable gastric ulcers occasionally require surgical therapy, but most surgical evaluations are made when a suspicion of malignancy persists. Surgical intervention for peptic ulcer is most common for complications of the disease (Table 30–4).

Perforation

Perforation can be described as either free or contained. Free perforation occurs when duodenal gastric contents spill freely into the abdominal cavity, causing diffuse peritonitis. Contained perforation occurs when a full-thickness hole is created by an ulcer but free spillage is prevented by contiguous organs' creation of a *walled off* area. The term *penetrating ulcer* has been used to describe ulceration from the duode-

TABLE 30–2. Medical Therapy for Peptic Ulcer Disease

Drug	Site of Action	Advantages	Disadvantages
Antacids	Neutralizes gastric acid	Cost	Poor compliance
H_2 antagonists	Blocks histamine receptor on parietal cell	Efficacy	Cost
Omeprazole	Blocks H^+-K^+ ATPase (final common pathway of acid)	Efficacy, compliance (q.d. dosing)	Cost (treatment course restricted)
Misoprostol	Prostaglandin E analog inhibits acid, increases gastric bicarbonate and mucus	Cytoprotectron: ulcer prophylaxis in patients on NSAIDs	Cost, diarrhea, poor compliance (q.i.d. dosing)
Antibiotics and bismuth	Treats *H. pylori*	Decrease in recurrence rate	Should be used with antacid therapy and requires testing for *H. pylori*

NSAIDs, nonsteroidal anti-inflammatory drugs.

num into the pancreas, thereby being contained by the pancreatic tissue. Ninety per cent of perforated duodenal ulcers occur in the anterior duodenal bulb. Sixty per cent of gastric ulcers are located in the lesser curvature, and the other 40% are distributed throughout the stomach. Most perforations occur between meals on an empty stomach. NSAIDs have been implicated in perforated peptic ulcer disease in the elderly population.[1] Up to 20% of patients over the age of 60 who experience a perforated ulcer are on NSAIDs at the time of their perforation. A recent retrospective review showed that up to 52% of patients with perforations were taking ulcerogenic drugs.[58]

Presentation. Patients present with acute abdominal pain, whether they have perforated duodenal or gastric ulcers. The classic presentation is usually associated with a prodrome of gnawing abdominal pain for hours to months prior to perforation. The perforation generally occurs as a sudden, relatively catastrophic event associated with tachycardia, tachypnea, and hypotension. Occasionally, patients develop gastrointestinal bleeding at the time of perforation. The epigastric pain usually spreads, becoming a diffuse abdominal pain on acute perforation. On physical examination, the patient may be febrile and lies immobile, occasionally with the knees flexed. Bowel sounds are usually absent, and the abdomen shows evidence of acute diffuse tenderness and is often described as boardlike. On rare occasions, the predominant pain may be located in the right lower quadrant as enteral contents pool in the right gutter.

Laboratory tests show elevated white blood count, and some patients develop elevations in serum amylase, although large increases are unusual. Upright abdominal x-ray shows free abdominal air in approximately 70% of cases. Free abdominal air on computed tomography (CT) is much more common and is the most sensitive test for perforation. Because of the classic presentation in most patients, CT scanning is rarely required for diagnosis, however. Patients with perforated duodenal ulcers who are on steroid therapy or who are hospitalized for other abnormalities may develop occult causes of abdominal pain and sepsis. Gastrografin swallow and/or CT scanning may be required to determine the cause of occult abdominal sepsis.

Medical Therapy. Most patients with perforation of a peptic ulcer require operative therapy. On rare occasions, medical management of perforation is beneficial. Patients who may be managed medically include those with a long-standing perforation (greater than 24 hours) whose ulcer has been shown by Gastrografin radiograph to be sealed. If medical therapy is chosen, close surveillance is necessary, because the patient may deteriorate clinically, requiring invasive therapy. Patients who do poorly on medical therapy include those who have perforated gastric ulcers. They almost always require surgical therapy because (1) they fail to heal spontaneously with nonoperative therapy, (2) they occasionally have associated adenocarcinoma, and (3) the hypoacidity that occurs in the setting of gastric ulcer disease often leads to colonization of the upper gut, resulting in multiple abdominal abscesses after perforation. Other contraindications to medical therapy for perforation include the presence of steroids, which would diminish the patient's ability to seal the ulcer spontaneously. Additionally, patients who have continued leakage on a Gastrografin radiograph must proceed immediately to operation. Finally, patients who perforate while on active antacid therapy should undergo immediate surgical treatment, because they require a definitive ulcer operation (Table 30–5).

Published results of nonoperative therapy for peptic ulcer perforation are encouraging in selected patients.[8] A widely quoted randomized trial comparing surgical and nonsurgical therapy for perforated peptic ulcers showed similar mortality in each group (5%) and no difference in morbidity. The hospital stay was longer in the nonsurgical group, and patients over age 70 responded less well to nonoperative management.[59] Since the publication of that study, the authors have abandoned this technique, largely due to the extraordinary

TABLE 30–3. Operations Performed for Peptic Ulcer Disease

Vagotomy and pyloroplasty
  Finney pyloroplasty
  Heineke-Mikulicz pyloroplasty
  Jaboulay gastrojejunostomy
  Gastrojejunostomy
Vagotomy and antrectomy
  Billroth I
  Billroth II
  Roux-en-Y
Parietal cell vagotomy
Subtotal gastrectomy
Total gastrectomy

TABLE 30–4. Indications for Peptic Ulcer Surgery

Intractability
Perforation
Bleeding
Obstruction

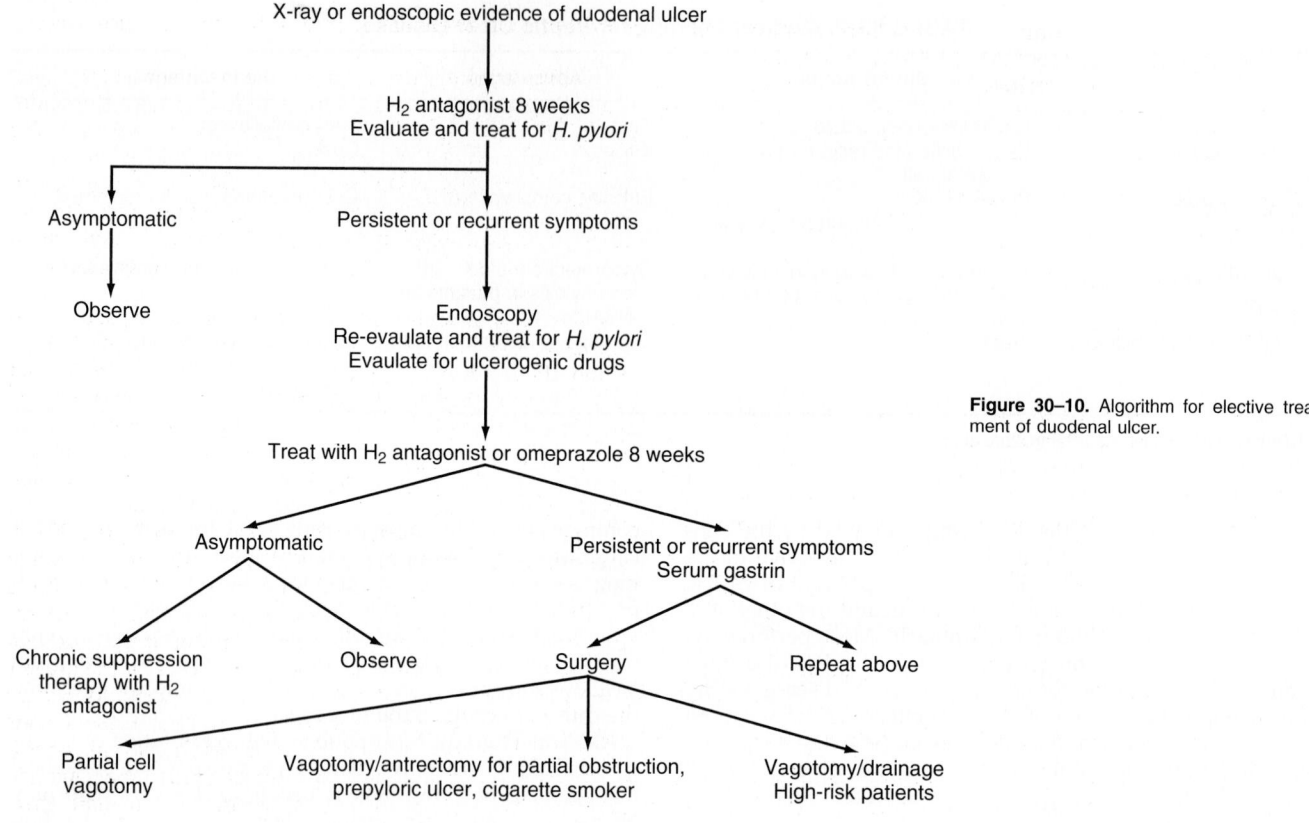

X-ray or endoscopic evidence of duodenal ulcer

H$_2$ antagonist 8 weeks
Evaluate and treat for *H. pylori*

Asymptomatic

Persistent or recurrent symptoms

Observe

Endoscopy
Re-evaulate and treat for *H. pylori*
Evaluate for ulcerogenic drugs

Figure 30–10. Algorithm for elective treatment of duodenal ulcer.

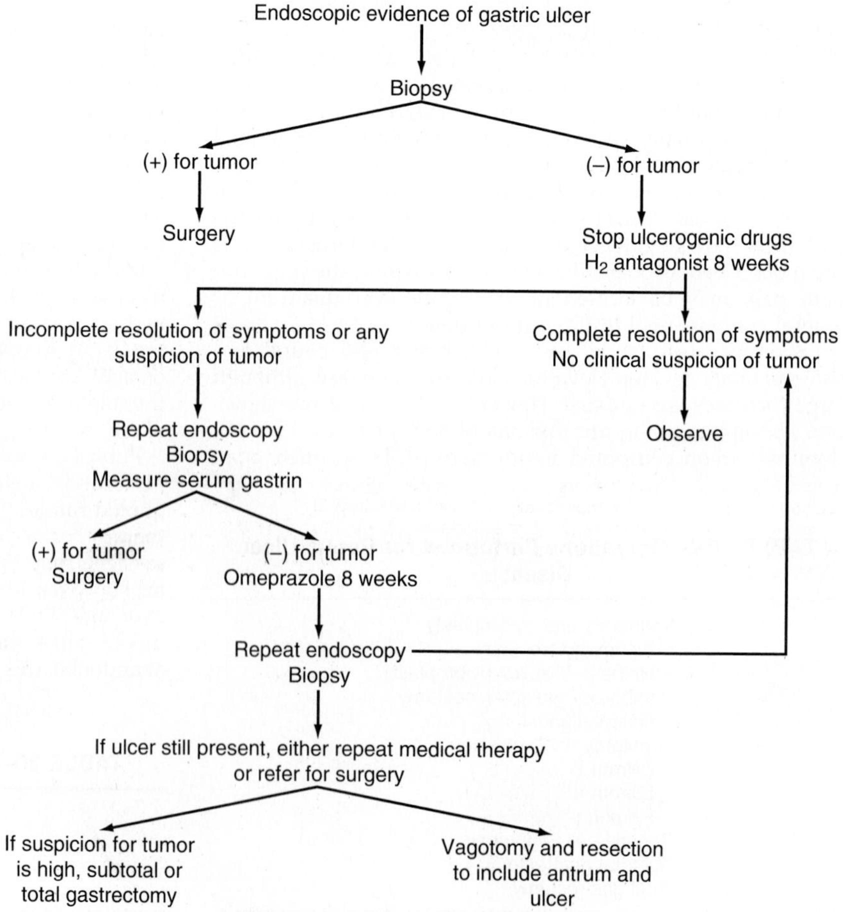

Treat with H$_2$ antagonist or omeprazole 8 weeks

Asymptomatic

Persistent or recurrent symptoms
Serum gastrin

Chronic suppression therapy with H$_2$ antagonist

Observe

Surgery

Repeat above

Partial cell vagotomy

Vagotomy/antrectomy for partial obstruction, prepyloric ulcer, cigarette smoker

Vagotomy/drainage
High-risk patients

Endoscopic evidence of gastric ulcer

Biopsy

(+) for tumor

(−) for tumor

Surgery

Stop ulcerogenic drugs
H$_2$ antagonist 8 weeks

Incomplete resolution of symptoms or any suspicion of tumor

Complete resolution of symptoms
No clinical suspicion of tumor

Figure 30–11. Algorithm for elective treatment of gastric ulcer.

Repeat endoscopy
Biopsy
Measure serum gastrin

Observe

(+) for tumor
Surgery

(−) for tumor
Omeprazole 8 weeks

Repeat endoscopy
Biopsy

If ulcer still present, either repeat medical therapy or refer for surgery

If suspicion for tumor is high, subtotal or total gastrectomy

Vagotomy and resection to include antrum and ulcer

TABLE 30–5. Relative Indications and Contraindications for Nonoperative Management of Peptic Ulcer Disease Perforation

Indications	Contraindications
Duodenal ulcer	Steroid use
Minimal peritonitis	Gastric ulcer
>24 hr. since perforation	Active medical treatment for ulcer disease prior to perforation
"Sealed" ulcer by Gastrografin swallow	Diagnostic uncertainty

amount of time required to observe the nonsurgical patients. Other studies have shown nonoperative therapy to be equally effective, documenting that as many as 81% of patients can be successfully treated nonoperatively. Unfortunately, up to 43% of these patients ultimately require surgery for complications of peptic ulcer disease.[26] On balance, the vast majority of patients who have perforated peptic ulcers require operative intervention to control ulcer diathesis and evacuate the abdomen of the enteral contents causing peritonitis.

Operative Management. More than 95% of patients with perforated peptic ulcers require emergent operative intervention. The complete surgical therapy includes preoperative management, closure of the ulcer, the addition of a definitive ulcer operation, and appropriate postoperative management. Preoperative therapy is important to ensure that the patients are adequately hydrated. The addition of broad-spectrum antibiotics is controversial but is usually advocated. The administration of intravenous H_2 antagonist is probably routine but has little or no benefit in patients who receive definitive ulcer operation. In patients who undergo simple closure of the perforation, use of H_2 antagonists, probably by continuous infusion, is necessary to control the virulent ulcer diathesis.[41]

The three missions during operative intervention for peptic ulcer disease are to close the perforation, irrigate the abdomen, and add a definitive ulcer operation as necessary. The majority of patients have culture-positive fluid in the abdomen that responds to generous irrigation. These patients do not usually require long-term antibiotic therapy. The management of the perforated ulcer is directly linked to the type of ulcer, its location, and whether a definitive ulcer operation will be undertaken.

Operative Strategies. Duodenal ulcers are grouped with peptic ulcers of the stomach, as shown in Figure 30–9. Type II and III ulcers share a common pathophysiology, in that most occur in patients who are relatively hypersecretory. The specific locations for peptic ulceration in the stomach include the prepyloric region and the lesser curvature. The management of duodenal and peptic gastric ulcers should be similar.

The closure of an anterior duodenal perforated ulcer can be done by simple omental patch, as shown in Figure 30–12. This suffices in controlling the ulcer perforation if a definitive ulcer operation is not required. In contrast, all gastric ulcers should be biopsied; if they clearly represent benign perforation, they can be patched in a similar fashion if they are in a peptic area, such as a prepyloric region. Ulcers on the greater curvature or high in the fundus are often managed by wedge resection of the stomach in an effort to biopsy these lesions and at the same time close the perforation. In extreme conditions when wedge resection cannot be undertaken, biopsy associated with patch closure is considered adequate therapy.[59]

The addition of a definitive ulcer operation comes into play in patients who have had a perforation for less than 24 hours, are hemodynamically stable, and have no obvious comorbidities that will limit the safety of an extended operation.[3] Patients who have a history of peptic ulcer disease,

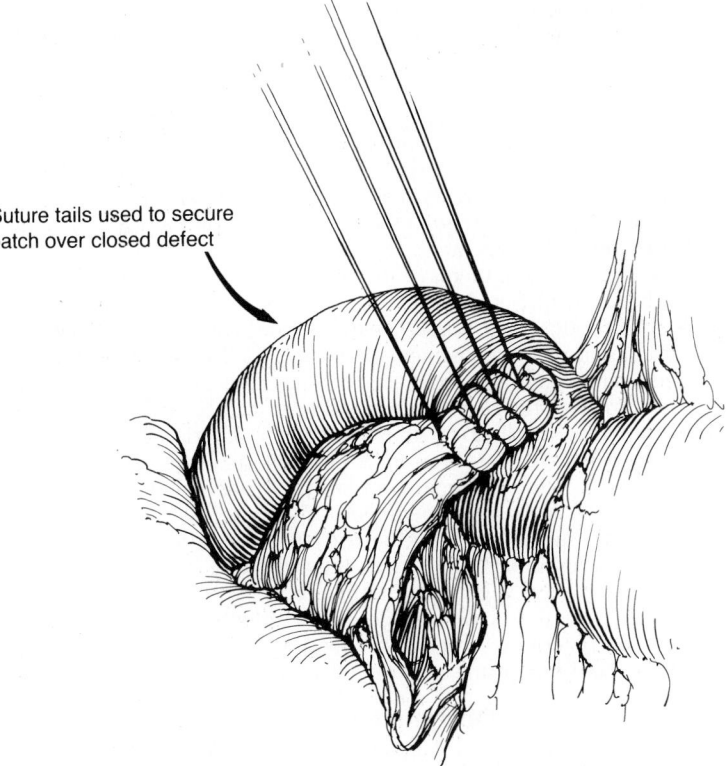

Suture tails used to secure patch over closed defect

Figure 30–12. The technique for patching a perforated ulcer. Sutures are placed across the perforation and the omental fat is sewn into the defect as a patch. (From Sabiston, D. C., Jr.: Atlas of General Surgery. Philadelphia, W. B. Saunders Company, 1994, p. 327.)

who have previously been treated for peptic ulcer disease, or who are on medications that predispose them to peptic ulcer disease should undergo definitive ulcer operation when it is medically feasible, as noted above. The type of definitive ulcer operation depends on the presentation of the ulcer and the expertise of the surgeon.

The time-honored operation for the treatment of perforated duodenal ulcer is a truncal vagotomy and pyloroplasty. The pyloroplasty often incorporates the perforation into the pyloroplasty closure. The advantage of vagotomy and pyloroplasty is the short operative time required and the short learning curve for this operation. An alternative technique, a highly selective vagotomy, has the advantage of adding a definitive ulcer operation without the side effects of a vagotomy and pyloroplasty. Disadvantages are that the operative time is somewhat longer and the operation requires greater surgical expertise. In the ideal patient, highly selective vagotomy is the recommended treatment for perforation.[52] Resection therapy, such as subtotal gastrectomy or vagotomy and antrectomy for perforated duodenal or prepyloric ulcer disease, is usually not indicated as first-line therapy in the urgent and emergent setting.

In all patients with perforated gastric ulcers, the exclusion of gastric carcinoma must be part of the treatment plan. Since gastric carcinoma can masquerade as benign disease, all gastric perforations should be biopsied and/or resected to be certain that treatment for malignancy is not required. Therefore, wedge resection and diagnostic biopsy are often the best choices for perforated gastric ulcers. The addition of an ulcer operation to the treatment for perforated gastric ulcers is controversial. Perforations in peptic areas of the stomach clearly are more likely to be considered for peptic ulcer operations. Some perforations may be caused by environmental factors and can be treated with simple biopsy and closure of the ulcer if the environmental factor can be eliminated (e.g., stopping NSAIDs). Resection therapy, such as antrectomy for perforated ulcers, is occasionally necessary in antral perforations. In these cases, antrectomy serves as part of the ulcer operation, removal of the perforation, and biopsy of the lesion.

Results of Operative Therapy. The mortality rate for perforated peptic ulcer disease can be as high as 23%, particularly if the patient population has a large proportion of elderly. The mortality rates for perforated gastric ulcers tend to be high, from 10% to 40%, and location is the most important determinant of overall mortality. Gastric ulcers occur more commonly in the elderly, are associated with ulcerogenic drugs, and are more common in the intensive care setting.[19, 28]

Laparoscopic Management. Recently, laparoscopy has been used to explore patients with viscus perforation. Many reports have documented the efficacy of laparoscopic management of peptic ulcer disease. Clearly, abdominal irrigation and evacuation of enteric contents that have spilled into the abdomen can be most easily done with the laparoscope. In addition, closure of a perforated peptic ulcer can be accomplished laparoscopically, particularly when the anterior duodenum is perforated, as it is in a majority of cases. The addition of a peptic ulcer operation is clearly dependent on the skill of the laparoscopic surgeon. Therefore, decisions about whether laparoscopy can be used to treat perforated ulcer disease continue to rest with the operating surgeon. Laparoscopic truncal vagotomy and pyloroplasty can also be accomplished in the acute setting, as can highly selective laparoscopic vagotomy, although the long operative time required for these procedures may be a clinical detractor.[25]

Obstruction

Peptic ulcer disease is a common cause of gastric outlet obstruction. Literature previous to 1975 suggested that the majority of patients with obstruction had benign disease. A current review showed that 37% of patients with gastric outlet obstruction have benign disease, with an increasing number of obstructions caused by gastric cancer.[49] Obstruction from peptic ulcer disease is invariably caused by a combination of acute and chronic disease. All these patients have chronic scarring of the pylorus and duodenum, with acute exacerbation resulting in obstruction. On rare occasions, an acute ulcer in the pyloric channel itself causes partial obstruction without concomitant fibrotic changes in the duodenum. These cases usually resolve with conservative management, whereas almost all other cases of chronic and acute ulceration require intervention. The classic presentation of obstruction from peptic ulcer disease includes nausea and vomiting in a majority of patients. These patients usually have early satiety and epigastric fullness, and many have weight loss. When vomiting occurs, the vomit commonly contains poorly digested food from previous meals. Longstanding gastric outlet obstruction often presents with very little pain and episodes of vomiting that are separated by long intervals. At this point, weight loss becomes pronounced and eventually culminates in an acute presentation, with dehydration and electrolyte imbalance.

Both barium swallow and upper endoscopy are useful in evaluating patients with gastric outlet obstruction. Barium swallow often shows a dilated stomach, with distortion of the pylorus and bulb. Estimates of gastric emptying based on a barium meal are often inadequate and should not be used to judge the functional significance of the gastric outlet obstruction. Upper endoscopy usually confirms the narrow, scarred duodenum and often visualizes acute ulceration in a field of chronic scarring. Sometimes the endoscope cannot be passed through the area of scarring. The importance of endoscopy is to rule out a malignant cause of the obstruction.

Medical management of gastric outlet obstruction includes nasogastric suction and repletion of electrolyte and volume abnormalities. Nutritional supplementation may be necessary in the face of long-standing obstruction associated with severe weight loss. Most patients with chronic and acute disease in the duodenum and pylorus respond to aggressive medical therapy, and their gastric emptying initially improves, most likely due to treatment of the acute ulceration. Unfortunately, these patients are usually left with chronic scarring of the duodenum, which continues to worsen with time. The vast majority of these patients develop a recurrent gastric outlet obstruction and therefore require some intervention. Patients who are poor operative candidates require medical management with an H_2 antagonist or omeprazole to control the large volume of acid retained in the stomach. Antacids are often unable to neutralize such large volumes of acid. Endoscopic dilatation of the strictured pylorus and duodenum has been shown to be successful in the short-term management of these patients.[29] There are no long-term data showing the efficacy of dilatation of scar in the duodenum. Still, in patients who are poor operative risks, medical management with endoscopic dilatation can be useful.

Over 75% of patients who present with outlet obstruction eventually require operative management.[23] Operative management involves relief of the obstruction with the addition of an antiulcer operation. The decision as to the type of operative intervention depends on the site and extent of the scarring. Vagotomy-antrectomy combined with Billroth II anastomosis is often the operation of choice if the duodenal stump can be closed. Unfortunately, in many of these patients, the duodenal stump is difficult or impossible to close, and a tube duodenostomy must be placed to control secretions until the stump can be closed by secondary intention. Vagotomy and pyloroplasty through the strictured duodenum is often not possible if the fibrosis in the duodenum is extensive. In many cases, vagotomy and Finney pyloroplasty or vagotomy and Jaboulay gastroduodenostomy are necessary to bypass the obstructed segment. In the same way, vagotomy and gastrojejunostomy can be useful in adding an ulcer operation to an outlet procedure. Highly selective vagotomy with dilatation of the duodenal scar has been reported but is associated with a high recurrence rate due to gastric stasis. As mentioned above, use of a laparoscopic approach to treat complications of peptic ulcer disease has been reported. The simplest operation for obstruction that can be accomplished laparoscopically is truncal vagotomy and gastrojejunostomy. The approach involves a hiatal dissection and sectioning of the vagal trunks under direct vision. The gastrojejunostomy can be accomplished with an endoscopic stapling device or by laparoscopic suturing techniques. Although other operations, such as vagotomy and antrectomy or vagotomy and gastroduodenostomy, are possible, they tend to be more technically challenging, requiring long laparoscopic operative time.

Bleeding

Bleeding from peptic ulcer disease often presents as a life-threatening complication, requiring a combination of skilled medical and surgical management. These patients often have a history of peptic ulceration, with an exacerbation presenting as hematemesis, hypotension, or anemia, and black tarry stools. The predictors of outcome in patients with upper gastrointestinal bleeding have been well described by a National Institutes of Health (NIH) consensus conference documenting clinical and endoscopic signs that predict rebleeding.[39] Patients who present with hypotension, multiple medical illnesses, hematemesis, a hematocrit under 30, and an inability to clear the stomach with aggressive gastric lavage often have a very high incidence of rebleeding in the hospital. These patients should be urgently evaluated and treated.

Aggressive medical management includes large-bore intravenous catheters, with adequate hydration and blood replacement as necessary. Patients with the aforementioned risk factors should be examined with upper endoscopy as early as possible for diagnostic purposes, due to the large variety of lesions that can cause upper tract bleeding (Table 30–6). Endoscopic therapy can be added to help control the bleeding diathesis. Patients who undergo endoscopy can also be evaluated for possible rebleeding, based on the ulcer appearance. Patients at highest risk for continued bleeding or rebleeding in the hospital are those who have active bleeding on endoscopy. These patients should be treated endoscopically in an effort to control the bleeding diathesis immediately. Endoscopic treatment for duodenal ulcer disease usually includes injection of epinephrine, heater probe coagulation, or laser coagulation. Most endoscopists now use either heater probe or epinephrine for immediate control of bleeding.[21] Patients with a visible vessel in the ulcer bed have at least a 50% chance of rebleeding during the current

hospitalization. These patients should also undergo endoscopic therapy to decrease the rate of rebleeding. Again, heater probe is the most common modality for the ablation of a visible vessel. Patients with overlying clot in an ulcer bed, cherry red spots, or a clean ulcer bed have a small incidence of rebleeding and are probably best followed with observation.[63] Patients who bleed after endoscopic therapy should be considered for operation after resuscitation with 6 units of blood. This is an arbitrary cutoff but is a useful marker for severity of bleeding. Arteriography with embolization should be reserved for the unusual patient who has either a difficult location of the upper gastrointestinal bleeding or comorbidities that prohibit operation.

The surgical management of upper gastrointestinal bleeding depends on the location of the bleeding ulcer. Patients with duodenal ulcers and *peptic ulceration* of the stomach (Type II, III) should have control of the ulcer bed with an ulcer operation added. Duodenal ulcers should be approached through a pyloroplasty incision, with the ulcer bed oversewn. Complete plication of the ulcer bed is often necessary to control hemostasis. Aggressive bleeding is often encountered because the ulcer has eroded into the gastroduodenal artery. After the ulcer is controlled, the pyloroplasty can be closed in the usual fashion, and the vagotomy is added to the ulcer operation. This approach is also useful for pyloric lesions and gastric lesions within 1 to 2 cm. of the pylorus in the stomach. In contrast, bleeding gastric ulcers are often managed in a different fashion. They usually require excision and biopsy to rule out malignancy. Operations should be designed as described previously for perforation. Greater curvature lesions can be wedged without difficulty, and an ulcer operation can be added as necessary if the patient requires antacid therapy.

On rare occasions, a patient's ulcer diathesis is directly related to pharmacologic agents, and the cessation of these drugs is the predominant factor in treatment. These patients need control of their ulcer diathesis without the addition of an ulcer operation.

As previously mentioned for perforation, resection therapy such as vagotomy and antrectomy is rarely indicated for the routine management of bleeding peptic ulcer disease. Most patients can be managed with nonresectional therapy. Unfortunately, severely ill patients with large bleeding lesions in the stomach, lesser curvature lesions, and bleeding ulcers associated with gastritis may require subtotal or near-total gastrectomy for control of hemorrhage.[48] Hemorrhagic gastritis is a rare disease that is occurring even less frequently. It is usually associated with multisystem organ failure and presents with massive upper gastrointestinal bleeding. The endoscopic appearance is classic, with diffuse hemorrhagic mucosa. The treatment of this disease is total gastrectomy, but it is often contraindicated because of the patient's overall condition. These patients are very difficult to manage by nonoperative means unless the source of their multisystem organ failure can be controlled. Occasionally, patients who undergo total gastrectomy survive if they resolve their multisystem failure.

TABLE 30–6. Causes of Upper Gastrointestinal Bleeding

Gastric ulcer
Duodenal ulcer
Esophagitis, esophageal ulcer
Gastritis
Gastric neoplasm
Dieulafoy
Mallory-Weiss syndrome
Varices

OPERATIONS FOR ULCER DISEASE

Parietal Cell Vagotomy. Parietal cell vagotomy, or highly selective vagotomy, is an operation that evolved from physiologic studies showing that preservation of antral innervation would provide the benefits of vagotomy without the side effects. The operation relies on selective sectioning of the vagal fibers of the fundus and the parietal cell mass while maintaining innervation to the antrum and the distal gut (Fig. 30–13). Technically, it is accomplished by devascularizing the lesser curvature of the stomach by dividing the ante-

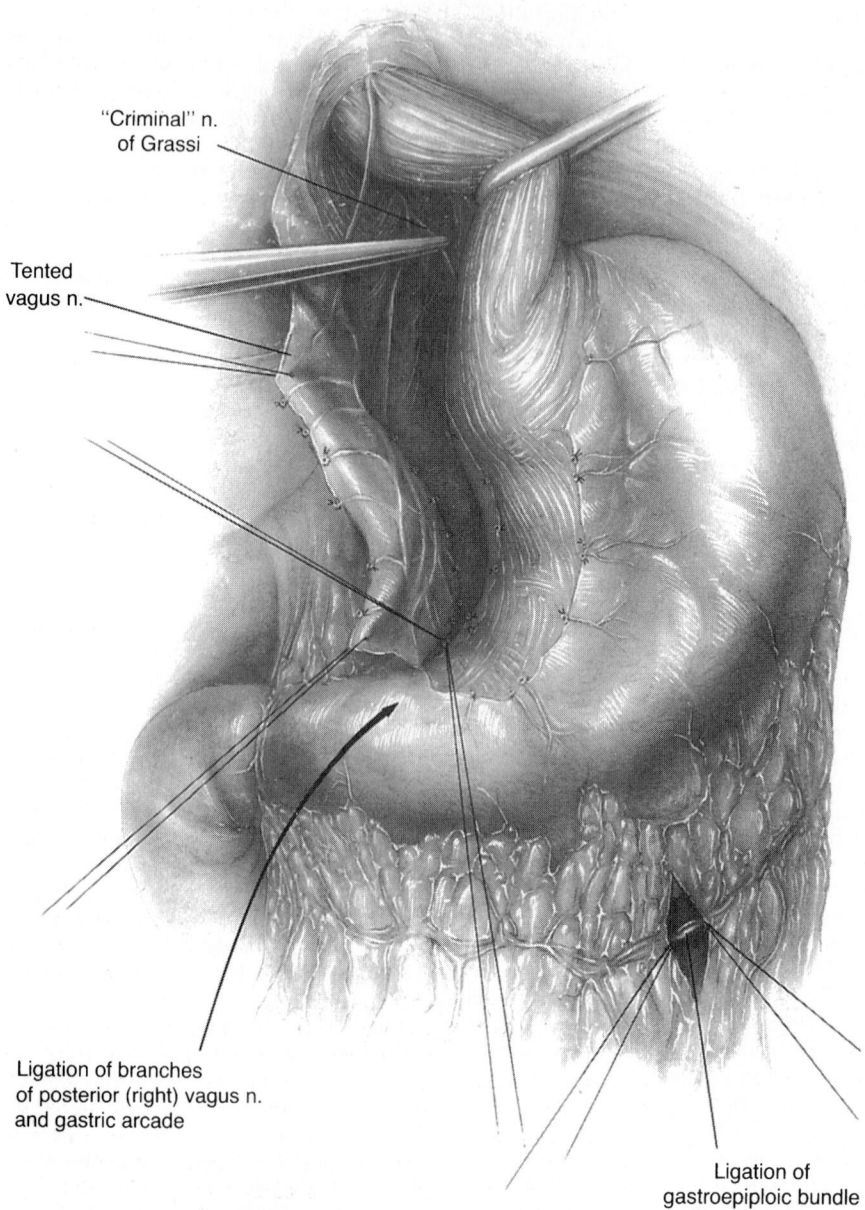

"Criminal" n. of Grassi

Tented vagus n.

Ligation of branches of posterior (right) vagus n. and gastric arcade

Ligation of gastroepiploic bundle

Figure 30–13. Parietal cell vagotomy (highly selective vagotomy) maintains vagal innervation to the antrum while denervating the parietal cell mass. The branches for both the anterior and the posterior vagus that innervate the parietal cells of the fundus are divided. (From Sabiston, D. C., Jr.: Atlas of General Surgery. Philadelphia, W. B. Saunders Company, 1994, p. 343.)

rior and posterior leaves of the lesser omentum proximal to the stomach. This begins approximately 7 cm. from the pylorus and progresses to the gastroesophageal junction. Most surgeons suggest skeletization of approximately 6 to 8 cm. of esophagus to ensure that the nerve of Grassi is sectioned. Parietal cell vagotomy is indicated for intractable duodenal ulcer disease. The relative contraindications to parietal cell vagotomy include prepyloric ulcers, gastric outlet obstruction, gastric ulcers, and patients who are likely to have high recurrence rates, such as cigarette smokers (Table 30–7). The incidence of dumping and diarrhea is extremely low with this operation, and measured gastric emptying rates 6 months after surgery are in the normal range.[36] This operation also decreases basal acid secretion.

The results of highly selective vagotomy are dependent on the overall operative experience of the surgeon. Centers with extensive experience with this operation report recurrence rates in the range of 5%. Other centers report high recurrence rates, with the highest being about 30%.[20] Factors that increase the rate of recurrence are gastric outlet obstruction and ulcers in the prepyloric region. It is thought that these

patients have delayed gastric emptying after this operation, resulting in perpetuation of their ulcer disease. Although recurrent ulceration rates are high after parietal cell vagotomy, management is relatively routine and rarely requires more extensive operations. Many recurrent ulcerations are

TABLE 30–7. Relative Indications and Contraindications for Parietal Cell Vagotomy

Indications	Contraindications
Elective treatment of intractable duodenal ulcer disease	Prepyloric or gastric ulcer
Emergent treatment of bleeding duodenal ulcer in a stable patient	Outlet obstruction
Emergent treatment of perforated duodenal ulcer in a stable patient (minimal soilage, few comorbidities)	Patient requiring ulcerogenic medications after diagnosis Cigarette smoker

asymptomatic, and those that are not can be easily managed with H_2 antagonists.

Vagotomy and Antrectomy. Given the fact that cholinergic- and gastrin-stimulated acid works synergistically, the elimination of both gastrin and cholinergic innervation leads to maximal reduction in acid secretion. For this reason, a combination vagotomy and antrectomy is the operation providing the lowest recurrence rate, short of total gastrectomy. The published recurrence rate is 2% or less, and this has held up over long-term follow-up. Vagotomy and antrectomy are associated with a mortality of approximately 1% and a morbidity of up to 20%. The most significant long-term complication is dumping, which occurs in up to 25% of patients. An additional 25% may experience some postvagotomy diarrhea. Of these patients, long-term morbidity is found in only 2% to 5% with refractory dumping or diarrhea. Although this percentage of patients is small, these complications are difficult to manage.

Technical considerations during vagotomy and antrectomy include the reconstruction, which can be accomplished in the Billroth I or Billroth II fashion (Fig. 30–14). Billroth I involves reanastomosis of the stomach to the duodenum, whereas Billroth II involves duodenal closure and a loop jejunostomy to the gastric remnant. This decision is often based on the degree of duodenal scarring from the peptic ulcer disease. An extremely scarred duodenum is often inadequate for reanastomosis. In these cases, a decision must be made whether to close the duodenal stump. A Billroth II is then accomplished or a duodenal catheter is placed in the duodenum to avoid duodenal *blowout.*

Laparoscopic vagotomy and antrectomy have been described anecdotally in the literature, but because of the technical difficulty of this operation, no large series has been undertaken. This undertaking should be left to extremely skilled laparoscopic surgeons.[57]

Vagotomy and Drainage. Truncal vagotomy was originally defined by Dragstedt[11] and was originally done without an outlet procedure. It was then realized that a drainage procedure was necessary to avoid gastric stasis. The simplest drainage procedure is the pyloroplasty. It alters the pylorus to avoid gastric stasis, as shown in Figure 30–14. Other alterations in the outlet can also be accomplished, including gastrojejunostomy, the Finney pyloroplasty, and the Jaboulay gastroduodenostomy (Fig. 30–15). The advantage of vagotomy and pyloroplasty is a relatively low recurrence rate (approximately 10%). It is a technically simple operation and has a very short learning curve. It can be accomplished in the emergency setting with a relatively low morbidity and mortality. Unfortunately, these patients have a high incidence of postvagotomy diarrhea and dumping syndrome. For this reason, vagotomy and pyloroplasty are usually reserved for emergency conditions. In patients who present electively, the preferred operation is highly selective vagotomy, which has few side effects; in patients who are unable to undergo highly selective vagotomy, a vagotomy and antrectomy provides the lowest recurrence rate.

SHORT-TERM COMPLICATIONS OF PEPTIC ULCER OPERATIONS

Rebleeding. Early recurrence of bleeding peptic ulcer disease after operation most commonly occurs in patients with multiple comorbidities who have a simple oversewing of an ulcer without an associated ulcer operation. Even patients who have vagotomy and pyloroplasty associated with oversewing have a recurrent bleeding rate that ranges from 0% to 17%.[35, 48] Although it is clear that resectional therapy such as vagotomy and antrectomy decreases the rebleeding rate, these patients are often extremely sick and benefit from shorter, less morbid operations. Therefore, intraoperative decisions must be made to limit the size and scope of the operation in favor of a short, safe operation. If recurrent bleeding occurs after a *lesser operation,* vagotomy plus resection should be done to diminish the possibility of further bleeding.

Gastroparesis. Gastroparesis occurs postoperatively in patients who originally present with gastric outlet obstruction and are operated on for this abnormality. These patients require vagotomy in addition to an outlet operation and frequently require long-term nasogastric suction or G-tube drainage until their gastric function returns. Prolonged, conservative management is wise, in that early operative intervention does not aid the gastroparesis. Barium and endoscopic evaluations usually reveal a clearly open gastrojejunostomy or outlet procedure, with little or no flow of barium in a static stomach. Simple observation is all that is necessary for management. Medical therapy can include erythromycin, metoclopramide, or cisipride as prokinetic agents. These medications appear to be most helpful in patients with diabetes but are occasionally effective in cases of idiopathic postoperative ileus. Repeat operative intervention should be reserved for patients with early marginal ulcers that are unresponsive to medical therapy, those with anatomic abnormalities of the gastric outlet, and patients without anatomic abnormalities who fail to empty at 1 month after the operation.

Duodenal Stump Disruption "Blowout." Vagotomy, antrectomy, and Billroth II operations are occasionally complicated by a duodenal stump blowout. This occurs when the closure of the duodenal stump breaks down, allowing bile, pancreatic juice, and duodenal contents to spill into the preperitoneal space. These patients present with severe abdominal sepsis, often requiring reoperation. Chronic scarring in the duodenum usually leads to a difficult to manage problem, in that simple closure of the duodenum can be impossible. A number of advanced techniques have been recommended for closure, but tube duodenostomy is often the best solution for control of secretions. A tube plus an external drain around the tube is often necessary to control secretion from a difficult duodenal stump. Once the diagnosis of duodenal stump blowout is considered in a postoperative patient, immediate attempts should be made to confirm this diagnosis by noninvasive means or by operative exploration, if necessary. Occasionally, this complication presents as a low-grade right upper quadrant sepsis that appears on CT as an abscess cavity. These patients respond to percutaneous drainage. The more common presentation is that of sepsis and an acute abdomen, resulting from free perforation of the duodenal stump into the peritoneal cavity. Such patients require exploration and wide drainage of the right upper quadrant, plus reclosure of the duodenal stump over a tube. This complication was once thought to be lethal in most cases, but currently the mortality is approximately 10%.[4]

Leaks or Fistulas. The perforation of a pyloroplasty or a duodenotomy after an ulcer operation is uncommon and occurs in approximately 5% of patients. These are often contained leaks, but they can present as lateral duodenal fistulas to the skin. Management of high-output lateral duodenal fistulas is formidable and requires parenteral nutrition, wide local drainage of the fistula site, and often broad-spectrum antibiotics to control local sepsis. Attempts to reoperate on the fistula for duodenal closure are rarely met with success.

Gastric Perforation. Gastric perforation after highly selective vagotomy is rare. This results from devascularization of the lesser curvature, resulting in an ischemic perforation. These patients develop sepsis approximately 5 to 7 days postoperatively and require exploration, débridement, and

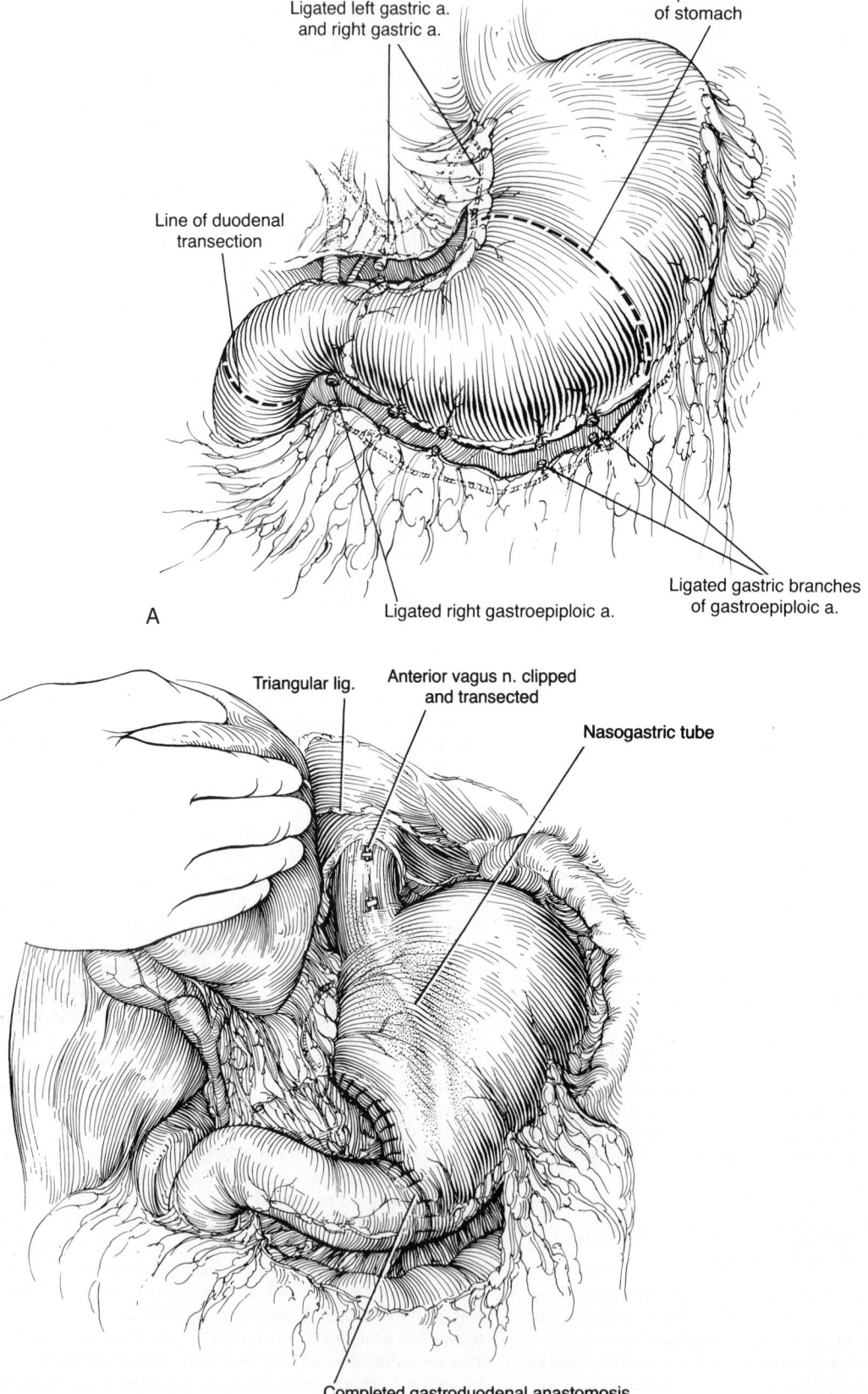

Ligated left gastric a. and right gastric a.

Line of stapled transection of stomach

Line of duodenal transection

Ligated right gastroepiploic a.

Ligated gastric branches of gastroepiploic a.

A

Triangular lig.

Anterior vagus n. clipped and transected

Nasogastric tube

Completed gastroduodenal anastomosis

B

Figure 30–14. The resection lines for antrectomy, plus two types of reconstruction. *A,* Lines of division over the duodenum and body during early stages of a vagotomy and antrectomy. *B,* Billroth I reconstruction, reanastomosing the stomach remnant to the duodenum.

Illustration continued on opposite page

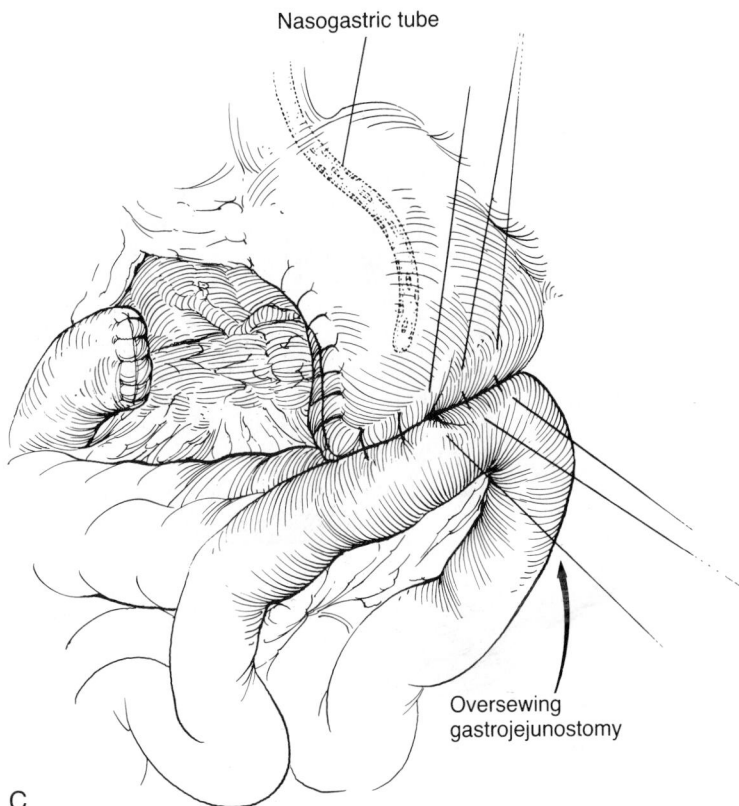

Nasogastric tube

Oversewing gastrojejunostomy

C

Figure 30–14 *Continued C,* Billroth II reconstruction, showing the closed duodenal stump with a gastrojejunostomy for reconstruction. (From Sabiston, D. C., Jr.: Atlas of General Surgery. Philadelphia, W. B. Saunders Company, 1994, pp. 271, 272, 285.)

plication of the perforation. On rare occasions, they require gastric resection to obtain adequate closure of the stomach.[61]

LONG-TERM COMPLICATIONS AFTER PEPTIC ULCER OPERATIONS

Patients who are stable after peptic ulcer operation can develop unique complications, discussed below. Most commonly, they are evaluated by the Visick criteria (Table 30–8). Visick Grade I or II is considered an adequate result after most peptic ulcer surgery. Most bad outcomes after peptic ulcer procedures fall in Grade III, and it is rare that patients end up as Visick Grade IV unless they have recurrent ulcers (Table 30–9).

Recurrent Peptic Ulceration. Recurrent peptic ulcer disease is a common complication after peptic ulcer procedures. The incidence ranges from 2% after vagotomy and antrectomy up to 15% to 29% after parietal cell vagotomy in some series.[33] Most recurrent ulcerations are managed medically with reasonable success. H₂ antagonists or omeprazole can be used to treat recurrent ulceration, or eradication of *H. pylori* may be necessary. Patients with marginal ulceration, which includes ulceration at a gastrojejunostomy site, often do not respond to medical therapy and may require reoperation. In cases of marginal ulcer after vagotomy and gastrojejunostomy, resectional therapy, including antrectomy, is often required. In patients who require operation after parietal

cell vagotomy, truncal vagotomy plus antrectomy is often necessary to control ulcer diathesis. If it is proved that the cause of ulceration after parietal cell vagotomy is delayed gastric emptying, then conversion to truncal vagotomy and pyloroplasty may be adequate treatment. Undiagnosed gastrinoma is a rare cause of recurrent ulceration but can easily be screened for with a fasting serum gastrin.

Dumping Syndrome. Dumping syndrome occurs after ulcer operations such as vagotomy. This syndrome, appearing after meals, is characterized by tachycardia, diaphoresis, hypotension, and abdominal pain. Dumping does not include diarrhea. Although this complication can occur in up to 25% of patients after truncal vagotomy, most of these patients have short-term dumping. Long-term morbidity from dumping occurs in less than 5% of patients with truncal vagotomy. Most patients with dumping have obvious symptoms immediately following surgical treatment that improve spontaneously with time. Symptoms can also be improved by separating the patient's solids and liquids at meals. Occasionally, conversion of a Billroth II to a Billroth I adequately manages dumping, as does conversion of a Billroth operation to a Roux-en-Y operation (Fig. 30–16). The latter is usually the greatest extent to which operative intervention should be undertaken. A variety of operations have been defined in the past, using an interposing reverse loop of ileum or jejunum to slow emptying. These operations are of historic interest only and have no foundation for use today.

It is likely that the cause of dumping is loss of receptive relaxation. Vagotomy eliminates the ability of the fundus to relax in response to a gastric load. In this way, gastric pressure increases during a meal and then decompresses through the gastric outlet procedure, such as the pyloroplasty. The rapid emptying of gastric contents is associated with the dumping syndrome. High-carbohydrate meals tend to worsen the symptoms.

Octreotide is a synthetic analog of somatostatin that can

TABLE 30–8. Visick Criteria

I.	No symptoms
II.	Symptoms that are mild and do not affect daily life
III.	Symptoms that are moderate, do not affect daily life, require treatment, but are not disabling
IV.	Recurrent ulceration or disabling symptoms

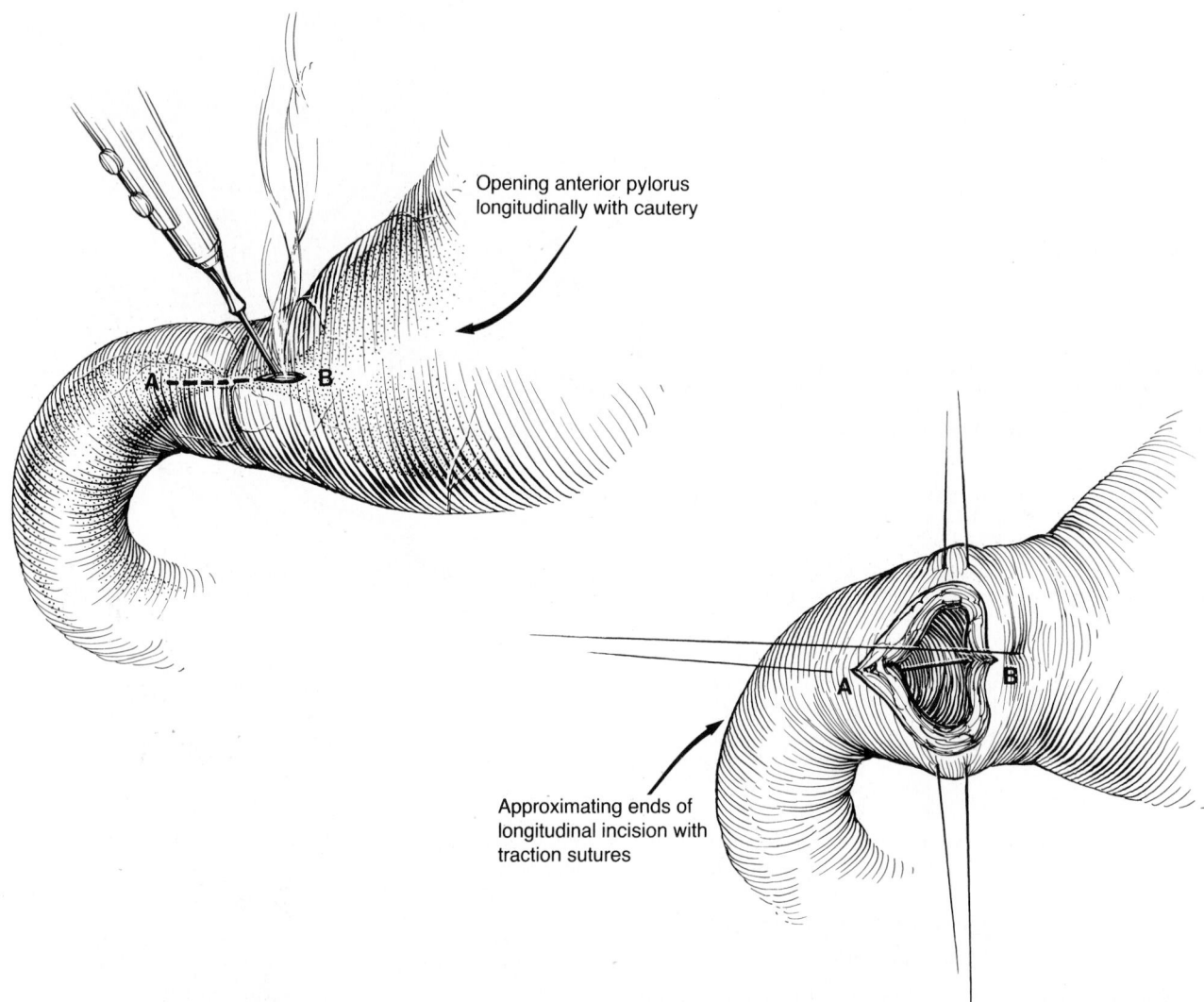

Figure 30–15. Vagotomy and pyloroplasty involve sectioning the trunk of both the anterior and the posterior vagus plus the addition of an outlet procedure, or "drainage." A simple Heineke-Mikulicz or Finney pyloroplasty is chosen, depending on the amount of scarring in the duodenum. With extensive scarring, the lengthening of the pyloroplasty past the scar (Finney) allows the creation of a wide gastroduodenal opening and avoids further obstruction. (From Sabiston, D. C., Jr.: Atlas of General Surgery. Philadelphia, W. B. Saunders Company, 1994, pp. 254, 260, 346.)

be given subcutaneously to treat the dumping syndrome.[17] A prospective randomized trial has shown that subcutaneous injection 30 minutes prior to a meal alleviates dumping syndrome. Twenty-five micrograms subcutaneously is below the therapeutic dose for antisecretory properties, but it appears to alleviate symptoms sufficiently to allow most patients to function normally.

Postvagotomy Diarrhea. Postvagotomy diarrhea should be

TABLE 30–9. Peptic Ulcer Surgery Outcome

	Parietal Cell Vagotomy*	Vagotomy and Antrectomy	Vagotomy and Drainage†
Morbidity	5–10%	15–20%	5–10%
Mortality	0–1%	0–2%	0–3%
Ulcer recurrence	1–25%	0–2%	5–10%
Dumping‡	0–6%	1–25%	1–12%
Diarrhea‡	0–5%	1–22%	2–20%
Advantage	Safe	Low recurrence rate	Safe for high-risk patients
Disadvantage	Recurrence rate is operator dependent	Early and late complications	Similar long-term morbidity as vagotomy and antrectomy, a higher recurrence rate

*Data for parietal cell vagotomy represent shorter follow-up, possibly explaining the 1% recurrence rate in some studies.
†Drainage implies pyloroplasty, gastrojejunostomy, or gastroduodenostomy.
‡Dumping and diarrhea data after vagotomy and antrectomy and vagotomy and drainage are expressed over a wide range due to varying definitions and the complications' mild to severe nature.

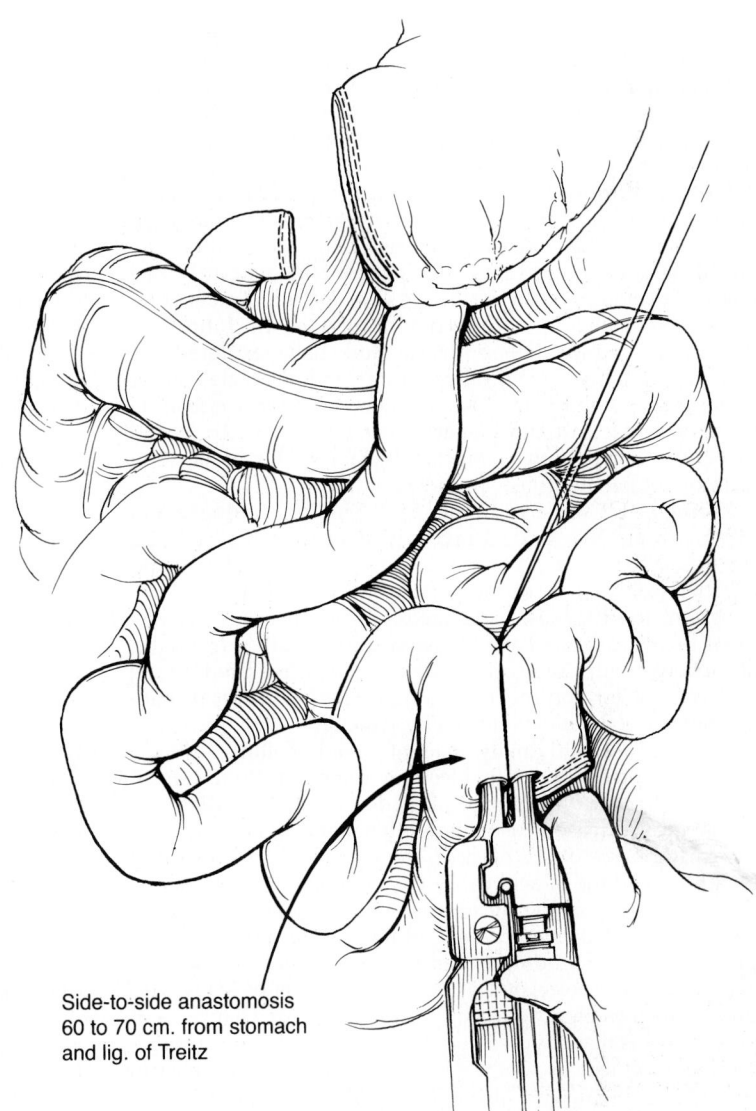

Figure 30–16. A Roux-en-Y reconstruction for the dumping syndrome occasionally alters postprandial symptoms. The Roux limb often leads to delayed gastric emptying, presumably changing the emptying pattern that was causing symptoms. (From Sabiston, D. C., Jr.: Atlas of General Surgery. Philadelphia, W. B. Saunders Company, 1994, p. 371.)

Side-to-side anastomosis
60 to 70 cm. from stomach
and lig. of Treitz

differentiated from the dumping syndrome, although both can occasionally be seen in the same patient. This diarrhea usually occurs 30 minutes after a meal and is watery in nature. Again, this complication tends to be worse immediately after the operation and improves with time. Aggressive management with antidiarrheal preparations tends to lessen the symptoms. Treatment with octreotide has been noted to benefit some patients, although not to the same degree as it benefits those with the dumping syndrome. Many operations have been described to reverse postvagotomy diarrhea but have no proven efficacy.

Malabsorption. Peptic ulcer and gastric operations are associated with malnutrition syndromes, the best documented of which is B_{12} deficiency. Operations that remove the parietal cell mass result in a B_{12} deficiency state, requiring exogenous B_{12}. This usually occurs after total gastrectomy, although B_{12} deficiencies have been described with lesser operations. The B_{12} deficiency results from loss of intrinsic factor, which is usually secreted by the parietal cell. Intrinsic factor is essential for the binding of B_{12} in the ileum for absorption. Total gastrectomy has been associated with poor nutritional outcome in many patients. This is largely due to a behavioral phenomenon. Patients are required to eat several small meals a day to attain adequate caloric intake, but many patients

insist on eating three large meals a day that provide insufficient calories due to their early satiety. There are no specific physiologic abnormalities resulting from subtotal or total gastrectomy that should limit patients' ability to maintain their weight.

Bile Reflux Gastritis. Bile reflux gastritis can occur when pylorus ablation is associated with bile stasis in the stomach. This can also occur with gastrojejunostomy, when bile is continually poured into the gastric remnant after vagotomy and antrectomy. The diagnosis of bile reflux gastritis can be made only when the patient has bile gastritis documented on biopsy, associated with bilious vomiting and abdominal pain.[50] The simple observation of bile-stained mucosa in a gastric remnant is not sufficient to make the diagnosis of bile reflux gastritis.

Careful distinction needs to be made between delayed gastric emptying and bile reflux gastritis. Both present as bile-stained gastric mucosa and persistent dyspeptic symptoms. These conditions require different management, so the distinction must be clear prior to therapy. The presence of biopsy-proven gastritis is essential for making the differentiation, as is the documentation of delayed gastric emptying. The treatment of bile reflux gastritis requires revising the patient's Billroth anatomy to a Roux-en-Y gastrojejunostomy (see Fig. 30–16). This diverts the bile away from the gastric remnant and completely cures this condition. In contrast, a Roux-en-Y reconstruction makes gastrostasis worse and precipitates a complete inability to eat. Gastroparesis after partial gastrectomy may eventually require completion gastrectomy.

Postgastrectomy Cancer. The incidence of gastric cancer in patients who have undergone partial gastrectomy has been extensively studied. Recent analysis of the world literature on this subject showed that such patients have an increased risk of developing gastric cancer.[58] The operation most commonly associated with this complication is the Billroth II surgical procedure. Other investigators have explored the relationship between truncal vagotomy and colorectal cancer in long-term follow-up. This relationship was ascribed to changes in bile salt and bile acid metabolism, which is said to be associated with colonic malignancy. This association has not yet been verified by corroborating studies.[37]

Zollinger-Ellison Syndrome. In 1955, Drs. Zollinger and Ellison from Ohio State University defined a new disease process in two patients with bleeding ulcer diathesis and non-beta-cell tumors of the pancreas.[67] Since that initial description, the diagnosis and medical and surgical management of this disease have changed dramatically. Originally, all patients with Zollinger-Ellison syndrome required a total gastrectomy for control of bleeding, whereas medical management is now suitable for many patients.

Presentation. Originally, patients with Zollinger-Ellison syndrome presented with bleeding diathesis. Today, most patients present with peptic ulcer disease and/or diarrhea. Peptic ulcer disease is usually duodenal and rarely jejunal in the early phases of the disease. The diarrhea is often caused by a high volume of acid as well as neutralization of pancreatic enzymes, causing steatorrhea-type diarrhea. Additionally, these patients may present with multiple endocrine neoplasm (MEN) syndrome, and their initial signs and symptoms may be related to the other aspects of MEN syndrome, such as parathyroid or pituitary disease. Diagnosis of gastrinoma is made with a high level of suspicion, prompting the measurement of serum gastrin. Screening serum gastrin should be obtained in all patients undergoing peptic ulcer surgery. Maximal elevations in serum gastrin in the 1000 to 2000 pg. per ml. range do not require secretin test confirmation. A simple gastric pH analysis to prove that the patient makes acid is enough to rule in gastrinoma. Minor elevations in serum gastrin should be evaluated by a gastric pH analysis followed by a secretin test. This test is accomplished by measuring basal serum gastrin and then injecting two clinical units of secretin per kilogram of body weight and repeating the serum gastrin measurements at various periods up to an hour. An abnormal secretin test result is an elevation in serum gastrin, occurring in patients with gastrinoma. Normal patients should have no change or a reduction in serum gastrin with intravenous secretin. Once gastrinoma has been proved, the patient must be evaluated further to determine whether operative intervention is necessary. Operative intervention is indicated for those who have sporadic gastrinoma that is not metastatic and for those who have gastrinoma and cannot tolerate or are resistant to medical management. Medical therapy alone is indicated for patients who have gastrinoma associated with MEN syndrome and patients who have metastatic gastrinoma.

Medical Management. Patients who have MEN syndrome usually have recurrence of elevated serum gastrin after surgical resection of tumors. Therefore, they are rarely cured surgically, and medical management is all that is necessary. They have a long survival, approaching 50% at 10 years.[66] Therefore, patients who have a family history of MEN syndrome, elevated calcium (a marker for hyperparathyroidism), or vi-

sual symptoms as a presentation for pituitary lesions should be considered for medical management. This medical management should consist of high-dose H_2 antagonists or omeprazole to control the ulcer disease. Controlling these patients' acid secretion controls the diarrhea.

Surgical Management. Evaluation of patients who are being considered for surgical management should include CT scanning to rule out metastatic disease. If the patient does not have MEN syndrome and does not have evidence of metastatic disease, further localization should continue. Occasionally, magnetic resonance imaging is more sensitive to determine whether the patient has metastatic disease to the liver. Although partial venous sampling for gastrin has occasionally been successful, intraoperative localization of gastrinoma is now considered the standard. The majority of patients have disease in the gastrinoma triangle, as shown in Figure 30–17.[60] This triangle has its apex at the cystic duct–common duct junction, and the base of the triangle is marked by the third portion of the duodenum. Between 60% and 75% of gastrinomas occur in this area.

If patients have no evidence of an obvious lesion on preoperative CT scanning, intraoperative exploration includes complete mobilization of the transverse colon to expose the entire surface of the pancreas. A generous Kocher maneuver is done for complete palpation of the pancreas. Ultrasonography is then used to assist in localizing the lesion, with a concentrated effort in the area of the duodenal sweep and the head of the pancreas. Lymph nodes should be biopsied frequently, because solitary gastrinomas in lymph nodes have been found. If ultrasonography of the entire pancreas, with concentration in the duodenal sweep, does not reveal the gastrinoma, a pyloroplasty is made, and palpation of the duodenal wall with an index finger in the lumen may be necessary to localize isolated duodenal gastrinomas. Resection of a duodenal gastrinoma often results in long-term cure of this disease; therefore, careful evaluation for small duodenal lesions should be undertaken. Gastrinomas in the duodenal wall or in the pancreas can usually be *shelled out* without major resection. Solitary lesions in the tail can be treated by tail resection. Rarely is a Whipple resection necessary or indicated for this disease.

In patients in whom no lesion is found, or in whom the

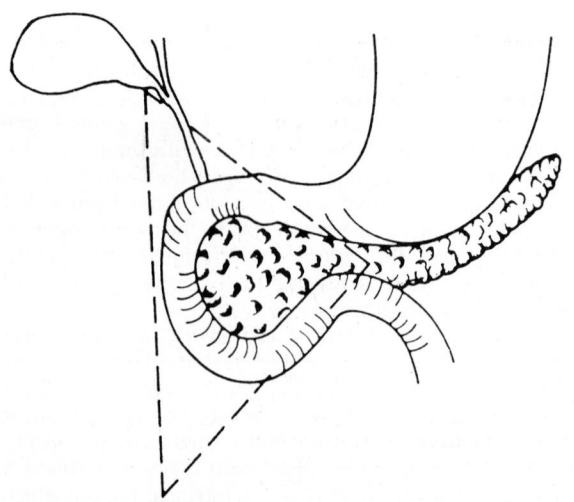

Figure 30–17. Gastrinoma triangle. Most gastrinomas are found in this triangle, with the apex near the cystic duct–common duct junction and the base of the triangle along the third portion of the duodenum. Gastrinomas found in this triangle include those in the head of the pancreas, duodenal gastrinoma, rare isolated nodal gastrinoma, and equally rare antral tumors. (From Tzu-Ming, C., Stabile, B. E., and Passaro, E., Jr.: Gastrinoma: Current medical and surgical therapy. Contemp. Surg., *29*:34, 1986.)

disease is multicentric or metastatic, a palliative ulcer operation can be added. If pyloroplasty has been done, a truncal vagotomy can be added. This operation decreases acid output by eliminating synergism between the gastrin and cholinergic innervation in the stomach. The addition of a vagotomy may allow a reduction in the dose of medication needed to control acid. An alternative to adding an ulcer operation is maintaining the patient on omeprazole. Highly selective vagotomy has been used in this setting, but the scarring that occurs after highly selective vagotomy at the lesser curvature makes later completion gastrectomy difficult. On rare occasions, total gastrectomy is required to control acid in patients who either do not respond to medical therapy or cannot tolerate the cost or side effects of medical therapy.

REFERENCES

1. Bliss, D. W., and Stabile, B. E.: The impact of ulcerogenic drugs on surgery for the treatment of peptic ulcer disease. Arch. Surg., 126:609, 1991.
2. Bloom, B., and Kroch, E.: Time trends in peptic ulcer disease and in gastritis and duodenitis: Morbidity, utilization, and disability in the United States. J. Clin. Gastroenterol., 17:333, 1993.
3. Boey, J., Choi, S. K. Y., Alagaratnam, T. T., and Poon, A.: Risk stratification in perforated duodenal ulcers: A prospective validation of predictive factors. Ann. Surg., 205:22, 1987.
4. Burch, J. M., Cox, C. L., Feliciano, D. V., Richardson, R. J., and Martin, R. R.: Management of the difficult duodenal stump. Am. J. Surg., 162:522, 1991.
5. Cheng, C. A., Geoghegan, J. G., Lawson, D. C., Berlangieri, S. U., Akwari, O., and Pappas, T. N.: Central and peripheral effects of CCK receptor antagonists L-365, 260 and MK-329 on satiety in dogs. Am. J. Physiol., 246:219, 1993.
6. Chey, W. Y., Kim, M. S., Lee, K. Y., and Chang, T. M.: Secretin is an enterogastrone in the dog. Am. J. Physiol., 240:G239, 1981.
7. Colin-Jones, D. G., Ireland, A., and Gear, P.: Reducing overnight secretion of acid to heal duodenal ulcers: Comparison of standard divided dose of ranitidine with a single dose administered at night. Am. J. Med., 77:116, 1984.
8. Crofts, T. J., Park, K. G. M., Steele, R. J. C., Chung, S. S. C., and Li, A. K. C.: A randomized trial of nonoperative treatment for perforated peptic ulcer. N. Engl. J. Med., 320:970, 1989.
9. Cullen, J. J., and Kelly, K. A.: Gastric motor physiology and pathophysiology. Surg. Clin. North Am., 73:1145, 1993.
10. Debas, H. T., Farooq, O., and Grossman, M. I.: Inhibition of gastric emptying is a physiological action of cholecystokinin. Gastroenterology, 68:1211, 1975.
11. Dragstedt, L. R.: Vagotomy for gastroduodenal ulcer. Ann. Surg., 122:973, 1949.
12. Feldman, M.: Gastric bicarbonate secretion in humans: Effect of pentagastrin, bethanechol, and 11,16,16-trimethyl prostagladin E_2. J. Clin. Invest., 72:295, 1983.
13. Fennerty, M.: Helicobacter pylori. Arch. Intern. Med., 154:721, 1994.
14. Gantz, I., Schaffer, M., DelValle, J., Logsdon, C., Campbell, V., Uhler, M., and Yamada, T.: Molecular cloning of a gene encoding the histamine H_2 receptor. Proc. Natl. Acad. Sci., 88:429, 1991.
15. Gitlin, N., McCullough, A. J., Smith, J. L., Mantell, G., and Berman, R.: A multicenter, double-blind, randomized, placebo-controlled comparison of nocturnal and twice-a-day famotidine in the treatment of active duodenal ulcer disease. Gastroenterology, 92:48, 1987.
16. Göke, R., Fehmann, H.-C., and Göke, B.: Glucagon-like peptide-1(7-36) amide is a new incretin/enterogastrone candidate. Curr. J. Clin. Invest., 21:135, 1991.
17. Gray, J. L., Debas, H. T., and Mulvihill, S. J.: Control of dumping syndromes by somatostatin analogue in patients after gastric surgery. Arch. Sachs., 126:1231, 1991.
18. Griffith, C. A., and Harkins, H. N.: Partial gastric vagotomy: An experimental study. Gastroenterology, 32:96, 1957.
19. Hamby, L. S., Zweng, T. N., and Strodel, W. E.: Perforated gastric and duodenal ulcer: An analysis of prognostic factors. Am. Surg., 59:319, 1993.
20. Hoffman, J., Olesen, A., and Jensen, H. E.: Prospective 14- to 18-year follow-up study after parietal cell vagotomy. Br. J. Surg., 74:1056, 1987.
21. Hui, W. M., Ng, M. M. T., Lok, A. S. F., Lai, C. L., Lau, Y. N., and Lam, S. K.: A randomized comparative study of laser photocoagulation, heater probe, and bipolar electrocoagulation in the treatment of actively bleeding ulcers. Gastrointest. Endosc., 37:299, 1991.
22. Isenberg, J. I., Selling, J. A., Hogan, D. L., and Koss, M. A.: Impaired proximal duodenal mucosal bicarbonate secretion in patients with duodenal ulcer. N. Engl. J. Med., 316:374, 1987.
23. Jaffin, B. W., and Kaye, M. D.: The prognosis of gastric outlet obstruction. Ann. Surg., 201:176, 1985.
24. Johansson, C., and Kollberg, B.: Stimulation by intragastrically administered E_2 prostaglandins of human gastric mucus output. Eur. J. Clin. Invest., 9:229, 1979.
25. Katkhouda, N., and Mouiel, J.: Laparoscopic treatment of peptic ulcer disease. In Hunter, J., and Sackier, J. (Eds.): Minimally Invasive Surgery. New York, McGraw-Hill, 1993, p. 123.
26. Keane, T. E., Dillon, B., Afdhal, N. H., and McCormack, C. J.: Conservative management of perforated duodenal ulcer. Br. J. Surg., 75:583, 1988.
27. Knuhtsen, S., Holst, J. J., Knigge, U., Olesen, M., and Nielsen, O. V.: Radioimmunoassay, pharmacokinetics, and neuronal release of gastrin-releasing peptide in anesthetized pigs. Gastroenterology, 87:372, 1984.
28. Koness, R. J., Cutitar, M., and Burchard, K. W.: Perforated peptic ulcer: Determinants of morbidity and mortality. Ann. Surg., 56:280, 1990.
29. Kozarek, R. A., Botoman, V. A., and Patterson, D. J.: Long-term follow-up in patients who have undergone balloon dilatation for gastric outlet obstruction. Gastrointest. Endosc., 36:558, 1990.
30. Kulber, D., Hartunian, S., Schiller, D., and Morgenstern, L.: The current spectrum of peptic ulcer disease in the older age groups. Am. Surg., 56:737, 1990.
31. Marshall, B.: Unidentified curved bacilli in gastric epithelium in active chronic gastritis. Lancet, 1:1273, 1983.
32. Marshall, B., and Warren, J.: Unidentified curved bacilli in the stomach of patients with gastritis and peptic ulceration. Lancet, 1:1311, 1984.
33. Meisner, S., Jorgensen, L. N., and Jensen, H.: The Kaplan and Meier and the Nelson estimate for probability of ulcer recurrence 10 and 15 years after parietal cell vagotomy. Ann. Surg., 207:1, 1988.
34. Meyer, J. H., Elashoff, J., Porter-Fink, V., Dressman, J., and Amidon, G. L.: Human postprandial gastric emptying of 1–3-millimeter spheres. Gastroenterology, 94:1315, 1988.
35. Millat, B., Hay, J., Valleur, P., Fingerhut, A., Fagniez, P., and the French Associations for Surgical Research: Emergency surgical treatment for bleeding duodenal ulcer: Oversewing plus vagotomy versus gastric resection, a controlled randomized trial. World J. Surg., 17:468, 1993.
36. Mistiaen, W., Van Hee, R., Blockx, P., and Hubens, A.: Gastric emptying for solids in patients with duodenal ulcer before and after highly selective vagotomy. Dig. Dis. Sci., 35:310, 1990.
37. Mullan, F. J., Wilson, H. K., Majury, C. W., Mills, J. O. M., Cromie, A. J., Campbell, G. R., and McKelvey, S. T. D.: Bile acids and the increased risk of colorectal tumours after truncal vagotomy. Br. J. Surg., 77:1085, 1990.
38. Negulescu, P. A., Reenstra, W. W., and Machen, T. E.: Intracellular Ca requirement for stimula-secretion coupling in parietal cell. Am. J. Physiol., 256:C241, 1989.
39. NIH Consensus Conference: Therapeutic endoscopy and bleeding ulcers. JAMA, 262:1369, 1989.
40. Pappas, T. N., Chang, A. M., Debas, H. T., and Taylor, I. L.: Peptide YY release by fatty acids insufficient to inhibit gastric emptying in dogs. Gastroenterology, 91:1386, 1986.
41. Pappas, T. N., and Debas, H. T.: Complications of peptic ulcer disease: Perforation and obstruction. In Taylor, M. B. (Ed.): Gastrointestinal Emergencies. Baltimore, Williams & Wilkins, 1992, p. 83.
42. Pappas, T. N., Debas, H. T., and Taylor, I. L.: Entergastrone-like effect of peptide YY is vagally mediated in the dog. J. Clin. Invest., 77:49, 1986.
43. Pappas, T. N., Mulvihill, S. J., Goto, Y., and Debas, H. T.: Advances in drug therapy for peptic ulcer disease. Arch. Surg., 122:447, 1987.
44. Pappas, T. N., Tache, Y., and Debas, H. T.: Opposing central and peripheral actions of brain-gut peptides: A basis for regulation of gastric function. Surgery, 98:183, 1985.
45. Pappas, T. N., Taylor, I. L., and Debas, H. T.: Postprandial neurohormonal control of gastric emptying. Am. J. Surg., 155:98, 1988.
46. Peterson, W. L.: Helicobacter pylori and peptic ulcer disease. N. Engl. J. Med., 324:1043, 1991.
47. Poitras, P.: Motilin is a digestive hormone in the dog. Gastroenterology, 87:909, 1984.
48. Poxon, V. A., Keighley, M. R. B., Dykes, P. W., Heppinstall, K., and Jaderberg, M.: Comparison of minimal and conventional surgery in patients with bleeding peptic ulcer: A multicentre trial. Br. J. Surg., 78:1344, 1991.
49. Quigley, R. L., Pruitt, S. K., Pappas, T. N., and Akwari, O.: Primary hypertrophic pyloric stenosis in the adult. Arch. Surg., 125:1219, 1990.
50. Ritchie, W. P.: Alkaline reflux gastritis: Late results on a controlled trial of diagnosis and treatment. Ann. Surg., 203:537, 1986.
51. Sachs, G., and Wallmark, B.: The gastric H^+, K^+-ATPase: The site of action of omeprazole. Scand. J. Gastroenterol., 24(suppl. 166):3, 1989.
52. Schirmer, B. D.: Current status of proximal gastric vagotomy. Ann. Surg., 209:131, 1989.
53. Schoon, I., Mellstrom, D., Oden, A., and Bengt-Olof, Y.: Peptic ulcer disease in older age groups in Gothenburg in 1985: The association with smoking. Age Ageing, 20:371, 1991.
54. Soll, A. H.: Pathogenesis of peptic ulcer and implications for therapy. N. Engl. J. Med., 322:909, 1990.
55. Soll, A. H., and Wollin, A.: Histamine and cyclic AMP in isolated canine parietal cells. Am. J. Physiol., 237:E444, 1979.
56. Sontag, S., Graham, D. Y., Belsito, A., et al.: Cimetidine, cigarette smoking, and recurrence of duodenal ulcer. N. Engl. J. Med., 311:689, 1984.
57. Taylor, T., and Bhandarkar, D.: Laparoscopic vagotomy: An operation for the 1990s? Ann. R. Coll. Surg. Engl., 75:385, 1993.
58. Toftgaard, C.: Gastric cancer after peptic ulcer surgery: A historic prospective cohort investigation. Ann. Surg., 210:159, 1989.
59. Turner, W. W., Thompson, W. M., and Thal, E. R.: Perforated gastric ulcers. Arch. Surg., 123:960, 1988.

60. Tzu-Ming, C., Stabile, B. E., and Passaro, E., Jr.: Gastrinoma: Current medical and surgical therapy. Contemp. Surg., 29:32, 1986.
61. Valen, B., Dregelid, E., Tonder, B., and Svanes, K.: Proximal gastric vagotomy for peptic ulcer disease: Follow-up of 483 patients for 3 to 14 years. Surgery, 110:824, 1991.
62. Walsh, J. H., and Mayer, E. A.: Gastrointestinal hormones. In Sleisenger, M. H., and Fordtran, J. S. (Eds.): Gastrointestinal Diseases, 5th ed. Philadelphia, W.B. Saunders, 1993, p. 18.
63. Wara, P.: Endoscopic prediction of major rebleeding—a prospective study of stigmata of hemorrhage in bleeding ulcer. Gastroenterology, 88:1209, 1985.
64. Yamada, T.: Local regulatory actions of gastrointestinal peptides. In Johnson, L. R., Christensen, J., Jacobson, M. J., and Walsh, J. H. (Eds.): Physiology of the Gastrointestinal Tract. New York, Raven Press, 1987, p. 131.
65. Yovos, J. G., O'Dorisio, T. M., Pappas, T. N., et al.: Effects of amino acids and gastric inhibitory polypeptide on insulin release in dogs. Am. J. Physiol., 242:E53, 1982.
66. Zollinger, R. M.: Gastrinoma: The Zollinger-Ellison syndrome. Semin. Oncol., 14:247, 1987.
67. Zollinger, R. M., and Ellison, E. H.: Primary peptic ulcerations of the jejunum associated with islet cell tumors of the pancreas. Ann. Surg., 142:709, 1955.

II

BENIGN TUMORS OF THE STOMACH

Mark W. Sebastian, M.D.

INCIDENCE

Approximately 7% of premortem gastric tumors are benign, including true neoplasms and other lesions that may be confused with neoplastic growths.[29] The reported incidence varies with the method of detection. A recent series of 5554 patients undergoing upper gastrointestinal endoscopy suggested an incidence of 0.8% of the total population screened. The mean age of the patient was 56 years, with a five-fold greater incidence in females. The polyps averaged 2.3 mm. in size, with an average of four polyps per patient.[24] Benign tumors constitute less than 2% of true gastric neoplasms, approximately 0.5% of neoplasms found at the time of autopsy, and approximately 3% of those discovered at the time of endoscopy in symptomatic patients. A classification of benign tumors of the stomach is presented in Table 30–10. Approximately 40% of these tumors are mucosal epithelial polyps, another 40% are leiomyomas, and all the remaining types are rare.[29]

CLINICAL PRESENTATION AND DIAGNOSIS

Benign gastric tumors occur predominantly in the middle decades of life and are most commonly located in the gastric antrum or corpus. Tumors of the cardia and pylorus proper are rare.

Because of the propensity of these tumors to ulcerate the associated mucosal epithelium, the resultant occult blood loss can cause iron-deficiency anemia. Deep ulcerations that overlie intramural tumors are notorious for their association with overt hemorrhage. Ulceration may cause a pain syndrome indistinguishable from that caused by peptic ulcer disease. Patients may therefore have an ill-defined sense of epigastric discomfort and an associated sense of fullness that is often caused by the large size of the tumor or by episodic obstruction of the digestive tract. Leiomyoma and the other mesenchymal tumors can reach a size that is palpable on abdominal examination. Tumors of the cardia and pylorus may cause partial obstruction early, which progresses to complete obstruction as the tumor grows larger. If it is pedunculated, the tumor, usually pyloric, can create intermittent obstruction as a result of a ball-valve effect. Frank gastroduodenal intussusception secondary to prolapsing gastric tumors may occur.[17]

The current widespread use of upper gastrointestinal endoscopy has undoubtedly greatly increased the rate of detection of benign gastric tumors. Still others are discovered by barium meal radiographs of patients with ill-defined abdominal complaints of pain, indigestion, nausea, weight loss, or unexplained anemia. In many instances, the diagnosis is serendipitous, there being no causal relationship between the lesion discovered on the radiograph and the nonspecific symptoms that prompted the investigation. These lesions cause concern not only because they simulate their malignant counterparts but also because of the potential for malignant transformation. Neither the radiologist nor the endoscopist can resolve these concerns. Increasing numbers of papers in the endoscopic literature continue to describe endoscopic appearance and to define the populations at risk for the development of polyps. It is uniformly agreed that histologic confirmation by endoscopic polypectomy or surgical excision for complete histologic diagnosis is mandatory.[42, 43]

Radiology is fairly sensitive in detecting gastric mucosal polyps, especially with the addition of air contrast techniques to procure good mucosal detail. Small size and the presence of a stalk support a benign diagnosis. Sessile polyps larger than 2 cm. in size with thickening of the surrounding gastric wall are more likely to be malignant. Benign tumors are more often associated with fluoroscopic pliability of the gastric wall. A properly performed and interpreted exfoliative cytologic examination is a sensitive diagnostic technique for mucosal lesions but is unreliable for submucosal lesions. Gastroscopy and biopsy through the fiberoptic gastroscope are not uniformly diagnostic of a specific type of polyp or of hyperplastic gastropathy.[24]

Biopsy material from a patient with intramural tumors is usually inadequate, because the biopsy forceps is unable to penetrate deeply enough for the surgeon to obtain a representative sample of the tumor for histologic examination. This is especially true with leiomyomas and other mesenchymal tumors with firm, rubbery consistencies.

Recent reports have described the utilization of sonography for examination of the gastric wall. Sonography shows five layers of the stomach: an inner hyperechoic layer, a second hypoechoic layer, a middle hyperechoic layer, a fourth hypoechoic layer, and a fifth outer hyperechoic area. The middle hyperechoic layer represents the submucosa, and the fourth hypoechoic layer represents the muscularis propria. The inner hyperechoic layer is the echo produced by acoustic mismatch between fluid in the gastric lumen and the mucosal surface. The second hypoechoic layer represents the mucosa; this has been verified in a study of pathologic specimens. Echocardiographic determination of obliteration of the second hypoechoic layer suggests mucosal erosion. This finding is believed to be a sensitive and specific tool in the detection

TABLE 30–10. Benign Tumors of the Stomach

Polyps

Hyperplastic polyp (Types I and II in Japanese literature)
Neoplastic or adenomatous polyps (Types III and IV in Japanese literature)
Mixed polyps (hyperplastic and neoplastic)
Fundic gland polyp
Familial polyposis and other polyposis syndromes
Peutz-Jeghers (hamartomatous) polyp
Inflammatory fibroid polyp
Retention (juvenile) polyp

Benign Hyperplastic Gastropathy

Ménétrier's disease *(polyadenomes en nappe)*
Associated with Zollinger-Ellison syndrome
Glandular type, without hypergastrinemia
Pseudolymphoma

Intramural Tumors

Leiomyoma
Other mesenchymal tumors (lipoma, neurogenic tumors, fibroma, vascular tumors)
Osteoma and osteochondroma
Heterotopic pancreas
Brunner's gland adenoma
Adenomyoma
Xanthoma (xanthelasma)

Inflammatory Tumors

Eosinophilic gastritis
  Diffuse
  Localized (inflammatory fibroid polyp)
Benign histiocytosis X
Granulomatous lesion (sarcoid, Crohn's disease)
Syphilis
Tuberculosis

Cysts

Intramucosal cyst (mucocele)
Submucosal cyst (gastritis cystica profunda)
Duplication cyst

Miscellaneous Conditions

Gastric varices
Aneurysm of gastric vessels (Dieulafoy's disease)
Antral vascular ectasia (watermelon stomach)

of mucosal erosion for the diagnosis of polyps and polypoid degeneration into cancer.[20]

The indications for extirpation of the tumor are elimination of any clinical symptoms and the necessity to exclude a diagnosis of malignancy. Ultimately, the tumor must be excised and recovered *in toto* either by endoscopic techniques or by surgical excision before a final disposition can be made. A recent review in the endoscopic literature suggests that Type I and II polyps removed and found to have well or moderately differentiated carcinoma limited to the mucosa need only be followed by regular endoscopy.[42] Specific aspects of the pathologic features and the management of the more frequently encountered benign tumors are considered individually below. There is relative consistency in the literature that the incidence of adenomas developing into carcinoma depends on histologic type and diameter of the adenoma. Red color of the polyp on endoscopy, lack of pedunculation, and surface erosion are associated with a higher incidence of carcinoma. Eleven percent of patients with biopsy-documented stomach adenoma were found to have synchronous or metachronous carcinoma.[42]

POLYPS

The word *polyp* is derived from the Greek *polypus,* which means "many footed," and is generically used to describe

any growth that protrudes into the gastric lumen. Almost all gastric polyps arise from the mucosal epithelium.[30] The nomenclature of gastric polyps is confusing largely because of early attempts to present them as being analogous to colorectal polyps in microscopic appearance and natural history. This is unfortunate, because most types of gastric polyps do not have an exact counterpart in the large bowel.[35] Unlike colonic polyps, gastric epithelial polyps are uncommon tumors, with an incidence of 0.4% to 0.8%. Early reports suggested that there was no distinction among the three histologic types of epithelial polyps (hyperplastic, adenomatous, fundic gland) by age, sex, location, symptoms, or endoscopic appearance.[5] The median age for gastric polyps is approximately 65 years, with a gender distribution that is equal or includes slightly more females. Recent reports and reviews suggest that glandular cyst and carcinoid tumors are small and located mostly in the corpus of the stomach. Pancreatic heterotopic growths, Brunner's gland heterotopias, and inflammatory fibroid polyps are approximately 1 cm. in diameter and located in the antrum. Other polyps vary between 1 and 2 cm. in diameter and have no predictable location within the stomach. However, multiple polyps in the same patient are almost always of the same histologic type.[5, 40]

Hyperplastic Polyps. Hyperplastic polyps (also known as regenerative, inflammatory, hyperplasiogenic, or hamartomatous polyps; or Type I and II polyps in the Japanese literature) constitute approximately 75% of all gastric epithelial polyps.[5] The polyps may be solitary or multiple and sessile or pedunculated. They are the result of glandular proliferation, since they are regenerative rather than neoplastic. They may vary in size from a few millimeters to several centimeters, although most are less than 2 cm. in diameter. Pedunculation usually occurs in larger polyps. Histologically, they show elongation, tortuosity, and dilatation (often cystic) of the gastric foveolae, with a component of pyloric or, less commonly, fundic-type glands in the deeper portion. The stroma is characterized by edema, patchy fibrosis, inflammatory cells, and scattered smooth muscle bundles from the muscularis (Fig. 30–18).

The gastric lesion termed *polyadenomes polypeux* by Ménétrier probably corresponds to multiple hyperplastic polyps (see Fig. 30–18).[24] The polypoid lesion that sometimes develops on the gastric side of gastroenterostomy stomas can also have a microscopic appearance similar to that of a hyperplastic polyp, except for its more diffuse nature and more prominent cystic component referred to as *gastritis polyposis cystica.*[29]

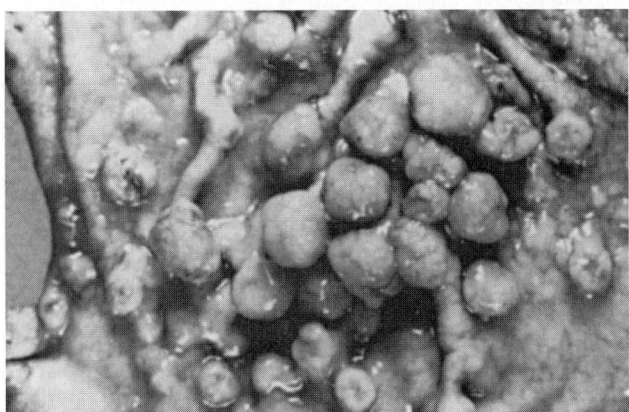

Figure 30–18. Multiple gastric polyps of the hyperplastic type occurring in a 65-year-old woman. Large sessile polyps of firm consistency occupied a large portion of the gastric mucosa. (From Rosai, J.: Gastrointestinal tract/stomach. *In* Rosai, J.: Ackerman's Surgical Pathology, 7th ed. St. Louis, C. V. Mosby, 1989, p. 496.)

Studies have demonstrated a modest association between hyperplastic polyps and adenocarcinoma arising in the non-polyp gastric mucosa.[5, 38] A coincident gastric carcinoma was present in 1 of 26 patients with hyperplastic polyps in the series by Deppisch and Rona.[5] The risk, if any, appears to be associated with the atrophic gastritis that frequently accompanies hyperplastic polyps rather than with the polyps themselves.[30] Patients with atrophic gastritis may be predisposed to both polyps and adenocarcinoma. Atrophic gastritis has been reported in 79% of patients with hyperplastic polyps,[46] and Neimark and Rogers[33] demonstrated that 5% of patients with atrophic gastritis develop hyperplastic polyps.

Neoplastic Polyps or Adenomas. Also known as Type III and IV polyps in the Japanese literature, these polyps are usually antral in location, are usually single and large, and may be sessile or pedunculated. Microscopically, they are composed of atypical glands with pseudostratified epithelium that has nuclear abnormalities and a high mitotic count. Like their large-bowel counterparts, they can be divided into adenomatous polyps (tubular adenomas) and villous adenomas.[28] Scattered endocrine cells that test positive for serotonin and a variety of peptide hormones have been identified in them. Carcinoembryonic antigen reactivity is usually found in the most cytologically atypical areas.[35]

Adenomatous polyps have long been associated with gastric adenocarcinoma.[46] This association is directly related to the size of the adenomatous polyp: up to 24% of polyps 2 cm. or greater in diameter were associated with adenocarcinoma, but only 4% of polyps with a diameter less than 2 cm. were associated with adenocarcinoma.[46] In an analogy to neoplastic polyps of the colorectum, the incidence of dysplasia, carcinoma in situ, and invasive adenocarcinoma appears to increase with gastric polyp size. The exact incidence of malignant transformation of these polyps is not known, but it appears to be relatively low, approximately 3.4%.[38] The presence of adenomatous polyps increases the risk of synchronous or metachronous carcinoma.

Fundic Gland Polyps. Fundic gland polyps (fundic gland hyperplasia, hamartomatous cystic polyps, polyps with fundic glandular cysts) present as multiple small polypoid projections in the gastric fundus or body. Their distinguishing microscopic feature is the presence of microcysts lined by fundic epithelium that includes oxyphilic cells; the overlying foveolae are usually shortened.[35] Fundic gland polyps, although particularly common in patients with familial polyposis syndromes, are not specific for that disorder, as previously claimed.[48] However, Nishiura and others believe that patients with familial polyposis may be identified by the histochemical findings of their gastric mucus.[34] The presence of O-acylated sialic acid may indicate the necessity of colorectal examination for polyposis in such patients.

Inflammatory Fibroid Polyps. Helwig and Rainer[14] named this lesion, also known as eosinophilic granuloma, granuloblastoma, neurofibroma, and hemangiopericytoma. Frequently associated with hypochlorhydria or achlorhydria, the lesion is probably not a true neoplasm. It is usually located in the antrum and may occur as single or multiple polyps. The gross appearance is similar to that of a pyogenic granuloma.

On microscopic examination, the lesion is shown to be centered in the submucosa and is characterized by fibroblastic proliferation in a whorl-like arrangement that simulates peripheral nerve tumors. There are abundant thin-walled blood vessels and a dense infiltrate of eosinophils, lymphocytes, histiocytes, and plasma cells. Ultrastructurally, many of the proliferating cells have a myofibroblastic appearance, which is in keeping with the presumed reactive nature of the process. An allergic cause has not been established, and peripheral eosinophilia is not associated with these polyps.

Thus, this condition should be distinguished from diffuse eosinophilic gastritis, in which peripheral eosinophilia is usually present and which probably has an allergic basis. The most intensive work continues in myofibroblast histochemistry and immunophenotypic differentiation within inflammatory fibroid polyps of the stomach.[18, 20]

Treatment

Symptomatic Polyps. Polyps that cause pain, bleeding, or gastric outlet obstruction should be removed. Total endoscopic excision of pedunculated lesions is advocated so that the nature of the polyp can be firmly established. Open surgical excision is indicated when the benignity of a pedunculated polyp greater than 2 cm. in diameter has not been firmly established, a safe total excision by endoscopic snare and cautery is not feasible, examination of the tissue removed endoscopically is consistent with invasive malignancy,[25] or a sessile polyp is present that exceeds 2 cm. in diameter.[4]

The role of individual surgical judgment regarding a specific polypoid lesion cannot be overemphasized. The guiding principle is to perform the least radical operation that allows complete removal.

A solitary sessile lesion is best excised with a margin of surrounding gastric wall and submitted for frozen section examination. Any further surgical procedure is dictated by the histologic diagnosis. Multiple polyps involving the distal stomach should be treated by subtotal gastrectomy. If a few polyps remain in the proximal pouch, they are removed by endogastric amputation and submitted for frozen section examination. When four to six polyps are randomly located in the stomach, a gastrotomy is indicated; endogastric excision, frozen section, and further treatment are dictated by the pathologic findings. A group of closely aligned polyps in the gastric corpus can be removed by wide local excision or sleeve resection of the involved segment of gastric corpus. In diffuse polyposis, a large portion of the gastric mucosal surface is involved with innumerable polypoid tumors. Here the decision must also take into account the fact that although these polyps are benign, they may be associated with coexisting adenocarcinoma elsewhere in the stomach. An especially difficult circumstance arises when diffuse polyposis involves the fundus of the stomach, where a coexisting adenocarcinoma may be masked and difficult to identify. A total gastrectomy may be indicated in these cases. Local wedge excision is adequate treatment for polyps that appear with focal atypia or carcinoma in situ.

Asymptomatic Polyps. The availability of endoscopic snare biopsy specimens and the insights provided by recent histologic and statistical studies have helped resolve much of the controversy surrounding these polyps. Biopsy specimens of asymptomatic polyps should be taken by endoscopic snare–cautery excision. Hyperplastic polyps can be safely observed, with annual endoscopic follow-up examinations to re-examine the polyps as well as to monitor the entire intervening gastric mucosa. If adenomatous epithelium is discovered, total endoscopic or open-wedge excision should be undertaken for lesions greater than 2 cm. in diameter. If reliable histologic diagnosis is unavailable, lesions 2 cm. or greater in diameter, especially if they are broad based and antral in location, should be surgically excised because of the risk of malignant transformation.

GASTRIC POLYPS IN POLYPOSIS SYNDROMES

Gastric involvement occurs in over 50% of patients with familial polyposis coli and the related Gardner's syndrome. These patients may also harbor polyps in the duodenum.

The gastric polyps can be adenomatous or hyperplastic or of the fundic gland hyperplasia type.[15] Other gastric tumors described in association with familial polyposis coli are adenocarcinoma and carcinoid tumors.

All patients confirmed as having familial adenomatous polyposis should have gastroduodenoscopy. Any polyps observed should be recorded, and representative biopsy specimens should be taken. If adenomas are found, they should be eradicated by endoscopic destruction. Since the adenomas are frequently multiple, they often require multiple treatments. Repeat examination should then be undertaken at 6- to 12-week intervals until no polyps remain. The examination is then carried out every 6 months as long as no new polyps are observed. When the initial examination is normal or when only fundic gland polyps are noted, endoscopy is repeated in 3 years.[36]

In Peutz-Jeghers syndrome, hamartomatous gastric polyps have been found in approximately 20% of patients, with an occasional coexisting adenocarcinoma.[12] These patients require endoscopic surveillance, especially when upper tract symptoms have been reported.

In generalized juvenile polyposis and the related Cronkhite-Canada syndrome, the incidence of gastric retention (juvenile) polyps is very high.[21]

Cowden's syndrome (Cowden is the family name of the index patient) was first described in 1963 by Lloyd and Dennis.[22] The patient presented with multiple orocutaneous hamartomas, a nontoxic goiter, fibrocystic disease of the breasts, and thyroid and breast cancer. This complex can also be accompanied by small sessile gastric polyps, most of which are of the hyperplastic type.[40] The feature of disseminated polyposis in the autosomal dominant disease has recently been emphasized. Gorensek and colleagues[11] have suggested that the term *disseminated hereditary gastrointestinal polyposis with orocutaneous hamartomatosis* is more descriptive; all four of their patients had hamartomas extending from the oral mucosa to the anus.

INTRAMURAL TUMORS

Smooth Muscle Neoplasm

Incidence. Leiomyomas are the most common benign tumor of the stomach reported at autopsy. Meissner[26] found a smooth muscle neoplasm in the gastric wall in 45% of his patients, and most of these neoplasms were less than 1 cm. in diameter. Among benign gastric neoplasms of mesodermal origin, those derived from smooth muscle constitute over 90% and demonstrate no strong sex predilection. Because it is rare for gastric leiomyomas less than 3 cm. in diameter to be symptomatic, considerably less than 2% of gastric neoplasms that are resected surgically are of smooth muscle origin.

Pathology. Leiomyomas may arise from the muscularis propria, the muscularis mucosae, or the smooth muscle present in the blood vessel wall. They are usually located antrally (25%) or corporally (40%). At an early stage of growth, the leiomyoma is intramural. With expansion, the tumor may protrude into the gastric lumen as a submucosal (endogastric) mass or develop as an exogastric (exophytic) mass. These types of presentation were described by Virchow[47] as *inneren* (submucosal) or *ausseren* (subserosal). Submucosal expansion is by far the more common mode of growth, occurring in about 60% of cases. Rarely, a dumbbell tumor occurs with both submucosal and subserosal components. The tumors may be smooth or lobulated. In time, a central ulceration occurs in the overlying mucosa of the tumor in approximately 50% of submucosal leiomyomas. Necrotic cavitation can occur in large tumors. Central cavities may communicate with the gastric lumen through one or more sinuses, or they may rupture into the peritoneal cavity. The gross appearance of an ulcerated leiomyoma and the radiologic image of such a lesion are demonstrated in Figure 30–19.

Gastric leiomyomas are not encapsulated, even though in tissue-section examinations they appear well circumscribed. In the absence of necrosis, they have a smooth, lobulated, or whorled-silk appearance. Microscopically, the tumor cells at the margin may intermingle with cells of the surrounding gastric wall. This is one factor that has led to confusion in distinguishing benign from malignant leiomyoma. Most smooth muscle tumors demonstrate well-differentiated smooth muscle cells with a variable degree of hyalinized connective tissue.[9] However, a relatively large number demonstrate a wide variation from this classic pattern. Peculiar features include extreme cellularity, presence of occasional large cells with bizarre hyperchromatic nuclei, marked dif-

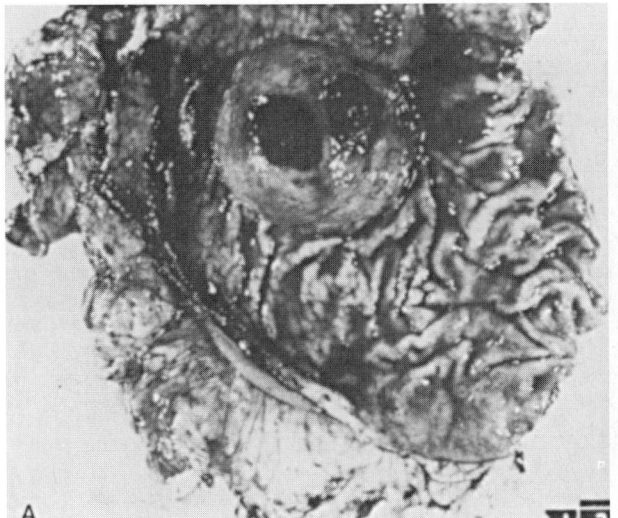
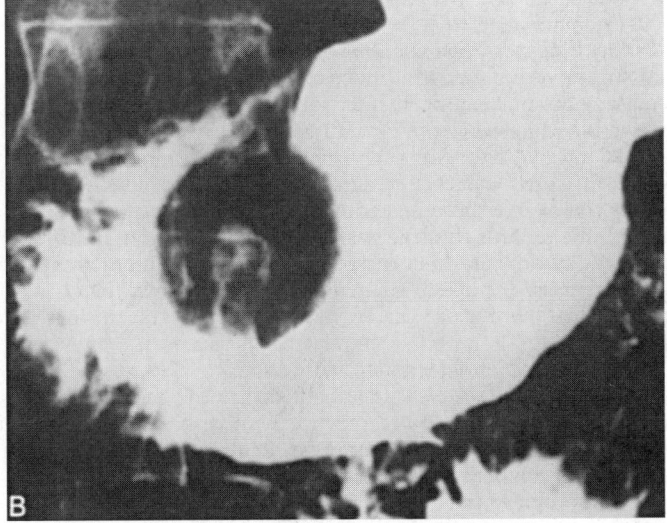

Figure 30–19. *A,* Leiomyoma of the stomach with two large necrotic ulcers on the surface of the lesion, which produced massive bleeding (specimen of case in *B*). The tumor has been removed by distal antrectomy. *B,* Barium meal examination of the stomach demonstrates a well-circumscribed mass-pedunculated leiomyoma of the proximal gastric antrum. Note the central ulcer with early cavitation of the stomach. (From Stavorovsky, M., Mora, G. B., Stavorovsky, H., and Papo, J.: Smooth muscle tumors of the alimentary tract. J. Surg. Oncol., *22*:109, 1983. Copyright © 1983. Reprinted by permission of John Wiley & Sons, Inc.)

fuse vascularity, regimentation of nuclei (palisading), and cells with a round shape and clear cytoplasm. Palisading leads to confusion between leiomyoma and neurilemoma. The neurilemoma is always encapsulated.

Stout[44] described a reasonably distinct variety of gastric smooth muscle tumor that he called *leiomyoblastoma* (bizarre smooth muscle tumor). The 69 cases he reported were characterized histologically by polyhedral smooth cells with central nuclei and abundant cytoplasm rather than by elongated cells. A clear zone that surrounds the central nucleus is probably an artifact of fixation. Appleman and Helwig[1] more recently suggested the designations *epithelial leiomyoma* or *leiomyosarcoma* for these tumors, depending on whether they have a benign or malignant pattern on histologic examination. Carney[3] described a syndrome characterized by the triad of multiple malignant leiomyoblastoma, pulmonary chondroma, and functioning extra-adrenal paraganglioma.

The criteria for distinguishing benign from malignant smooth muscle tumors are the same for the spindle cell and leiomyoblastoma cell types.[1] The most important criterion for distinguishing a leiomyoma from a leiomyosarcoma is the number of mitotic figures present. Golden and Stout[9] stated that "if two or more mitoses per high power field are present, one can feel fairly secure in predicting malignancy." However, correlation between mitotic activity and the clinical behavior of the tumor is not nearly as good for gastrointestinal smooth muscle tumors as it is for uterine smooth muscle tumors. Unfortunately, metastasis can occur in a smooth muscle tumor that is by all criteria histologically benign. Thus, the proposal has been made to designate as *smooth muscle tumors of indeterminate malignant potential* (STUMP) those neoplasms that are suspected of being malignant because of high cellularity, atypia, large size, and/or tumor cell necrosis but that have more than 5 mitoses per 10 high-power fields. In the final analysis, the only unchallengeable evidence of malignancy of a smooth muscle tumor is metastasis or invasive intragastric or extragastric growth noted either during a surgical procedure or following surgical resection. All smooth muscle tumors of the stomach should be suspected of being malignant until time and the demonstrable behavior of the tumor provide proof to the contrary. The malignant variant of leiomyoma can invade adjacent organs, but rarely involves lymph nodes except by direct extension; it can be seeded in the peritoneal cavity and can metastasize by hematogenous spread to the liver or lung.[39] In children and adolescents, gastric smooth muscle tumors are very rare; most are malignant.[49]

Clinical Aspects and Treatment. Smooth muscle tumors can cause overlying central mucosal ulceration, resulting in hematemesis, melena, or anemia caused by occult gastrointestinal blood loss. Bleeding from the tumor may be massive and/or intermittent. Although 20% of such tumors occur near the pylorus, obstruction is rare.[32] An occasional smooth muscle tumor may become pedunculated and then prolapse through the pylorus, causing gastric outlet obstruction. Huge exogastric tumors are frequently detected by the patient as a palpable mass. Incidental discovery at the time of laparotomy, during the course of a barium meal study, or during gastroscopy for a probably unrelated disease is the most common method of detection.

The principle of surgical treatment of smooth muscle tumors is local excision with a 2- to 3-cm. margin of surrounding gastric wall. In view of the difficulty in distinguishing between the benign and malignant variants, enucleation is an inappropriate method of treatment. The excised specimen should be submitted for pathologic examination. If a histologic diagnosis of malignancy is made on the basis of frozen section examination, an additional margin of gastric wall may be excised.

In the case of a very large tumor or a prepyloric tumor, a standard gastric resection may be the most expeditious form of excision. With tumors in the body of the stomach, local excision or sleeve resection is feasible. A more difficult decision is required when the tumor encroaches on the esophagogastric junction. Resection of the esophagogastric junction for a benign leiomyoma is not indicated.

Regional lymphadenectomy is not of proven value, and its practice is not consistent with the known biologic behavior of the tumor.

HETEROTOPIC PANCREAS

An aberrant rest of pancreatic tissue located in the wall of the stomach presents clinically as a tumor and must be considered in the differential diagnosis of benign gastric neoplasms. Although the tumor may project into the lumen of the stomach and may occasionally cause pyloric obstruction or hemorrhage, it is usually found incidentally at autopsy or laparotomy.[34]

The typical pancreatic rest is a hemispheric mass, a symmetrical cone, or a short cylindrical nipple-like projection measuring 0.5 to 3 cm. in diameter located in the antrum (61%) or the immediate prepyloric area (24%) of the stomach. The most characteristic gross feature is a central ductal orifice that may be identified by filling during a barium meal or gastroscopic examination. The orifice usually communicates with a filiform ductal system draining the mass of tightly packed pancreatic acini that form the tumor nodule. Approximately 85% of these lesions are in the submucosa, and most of the others are in the muscular layer.

Technically considered a hamartoma, the mass of heterotopic pancreas is composed of glands and intervening connective tissue. Islets of Langerhans are observed in only one third of the cases, and if they are present, their number is generally less than in the normal pancreas (Fig. 30–20). These lesions may be involved in the same types of pathologic processes that affect the pancreas proper. Debilitating pain is associated with inflammation occurring in these lesions; ductal dilatation and cyst formation can also occur. Some cases of intramural gastric carcinoma arising in these heterotopic tissues have been reported.[10]

Indeterminate or apparently symptomatic lesions should be excised, but if an accurate radiologic diagnosis can be made and the lesion is asymptomatic, expectant management

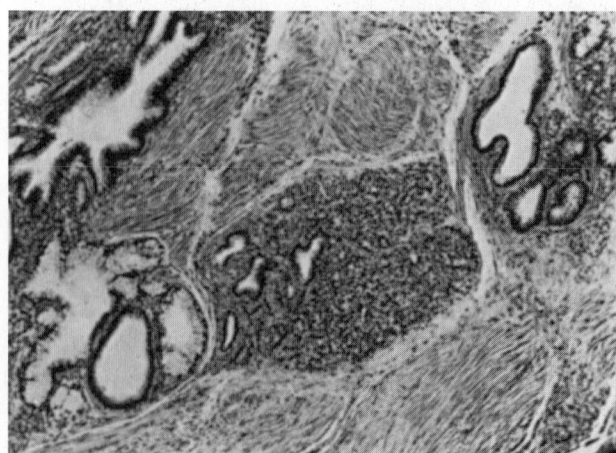

Figure 30–20. Microscopic appearance of pancreatic rest demonstrating ducts and acini. An islet is present in the middle of the photograph. Magnification, ×90. (From Edis, A. J.: Benign tumors of the stomach. *In* Schwartz, S. I., Ellis, H., and Husser, W. [Eds.]: Maingot's Abdominal Operations, 8th ed. New York, Appleton-Century-Crofts, 1985, p. 953.)

may be justified. From a practical point of view, however, most patients and physicians prefer surgical excision to avoid the uncertainty and the cost of frequent follow-up examinations.

BRUNNER'S GLAND ADENOMA

Brunner's gland adenoma can occur in the antrum or juxtapyloric region, representing heterotopic locations of a hamartomatous lesion that is usually found in the duodenum. This lesion is composed of intermingled glands and bands of smooth muscle fibers. Islands of pancreatic tissue may be present. Certain of these lesions may be referred to as *gastric adenomyomas.*[8]

HYPERPLASTIC GASTROPATHY

The general term *hyperplastic gastropathy* refers to a rare condition in which there is enlargement of the rugal folds in the stomach. The etiologic features of the hyperplastic process vary.

Of the two processes that Ménétrier described in 1888 under the common term *polyadenomes, polyadenomes polypeux* is probably equivalent to *multiple hyperplastic polyps,* whereas *polyadenomes en nappe* refers to *Ménétrier's disease.*

Ménétrier's Disease. Ménétrier's disease is characterized by gastric mucosal hypertrophy that may be so extensive that the rugae assume the appearance of convolutions of the brain (Fig. 30–21). Although this gross appearance is common to all cases of Ménétrier's disease, in individual cases, either the gastric glandular elements or the superficial epithelial elements of the gastric mucosa may predominate. Thus, acid secretion may be high, normal, or low; hypoproteinemia, formerly considered an essential component of the disease,

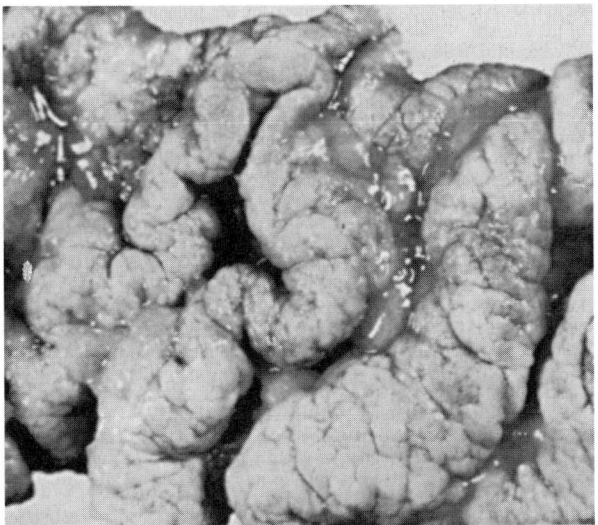

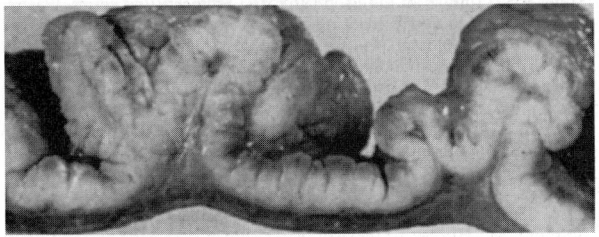

Figure 30–21. Ménétrier's disease in a 65-year-old woman. The gross pattern of the thickened rugae is reminiscent of convolutions of the brain. (From Rosai, J.: Gastrointestinal tract/stomach. *In* Rosai, J.: Ackerman's Surgical Pathology, 7th ed. St. Louis, C. V. Mosby, 1989, p. 499.)

may not be present. Sundt and associates[45] reported the lack of consensus in the literature regarding which features define the disease. Because the mucosal histologic character, level of acid secretion, and serum albumin levels are semiquantifiable along three graphic axes, Sundt and colleagues suggested describing the three cardinal abnormalities of Ménétrier's disease as *trivalent gastropathy.*

The cardia, fundus, and body of the stomach are usually diffusely thrown into folds and nodular areas that may resemble sessile polyps. The transition between normal and diseased mucosa is always abrupt. A lack of antral involvement is characteristic of the disease.

Microscopically, there is a striking foveolar hyperplasia that is accompanied by tortuosity, some degree of cystic dilatation, and extension into the base of the glands. The stroma is edematous and inflamed. Hyperrugosity may regress, atrophic gastritis may develop, and carcinoma of the stomach may ensue.

Abdominal distress or pain is present in over 80% of patients, blood loss is present in 34%, and symptoms of hypoproteinemia are present in 40%. Weight loss, edema, and malnutrition are common. It should be noted that only one patient described by Ménétrier exhibited the entire clinical syndrome.[27]

Ménétrier's disease can be diagnosed at any age.[19] The etiologic factors are unknown. Treatment is directed toward the debilitating effects of the protein-losing gastropathy; in view of reports of spontaneous resolution, nutritional support and a period of observation are justified when the precise diagnosis has been established.[6] Anticholinergics are sometimes prescribed because they diminish acid secretion and tighten gastric cell junctions, which limits protein losses by this route. H_2-blockers, which have many of the same effects, can be tried if the response to anticholinergics is suboptimal or the side effects become troublesome. Combination therapy with H_2-blockers and anticholinergics or administration of omeprazole may be useful in conjunction with parenteral nutrition.

If pharmacologic therapy fails, total gastrectomy and reconstruction with a long Roux-en-Y jejunal limb is the best therapy. The operation using a jejunal limb of adequate length obviates reflux esophagitis, eliminates the risk of gastric malignancy, and allows improved nutrition. Also, technical problems posed by the risk of anastomotic leakage and obstruction, which are common when distal gastrectomy is used for Ménétrier's disease, are avoided. The significant incidence of subsequent carcinoma of the stomach in even a small remaining portion of gastric mucosa should discourage the temptation to leave a small rim of stomach below the gastroesophageal junction.

An interesting aspect of the management of patients with Ménétrier's disease is their propensity to be in a hypercoagulable state, sometimes due to an occult gastric malignancy.[45] Hypercoagulability is a well-known complication of mucin-producing gastrointestinal adenocarcinomas. Gastric carcinoma occurs in approximately 1% to 15% of all cases of Ménétrier's disease.[37]

Roentgenographically and grossly, Ménétrier's disease can be confused with malignant lymphoma.

Pseudolymphoma. Extensive lymphocytic infiltration of a portion of the stomach can occur, predominantly in association with a benign gastric ulcer. A large portion of the stomach may be involved, and submucosal nodules, diffuse thickening, or enlarged rugal folds may be present. The infiltrate has a follicular pattern, leading to confusion with follicular lymphoma. Microscopically, the features favoring the diagnosis of pseudolymphoma are the presence of clearly reactive germinal centers throughout the lesions, a mixed population of inflammatory cells (including mature lymphocytes and

trasonography defined the layers of the stomach in normal regions in contrast to the infiltrative nature of gastric lymphoma.[10] This technique has a sensitivity of 83% and a positive predictive value of 87% for upper gut malignancy. It can also define metastatic perigastric lymph nodes in a large proportion of patients with very high sensitivity and specificity.[9] Because it is operator dependent, it has not gained wide acceptance.

Computed Tomography (CT). Most CT findings in gastric lymphoma are similar to those in adenocarcinoma of the stomach. Some of the unique characteristics of gastric lymphoma include diffuse involvement and lesions in more than one region of the stomach with widespread abdominal adenopathy.[7]

Gastrointestinal Endoscopy. Visual inspection of gastric lesions in these patients usually suggests gastric malignancy. Unfortunately, the visual diagnosis is correct in only half of patients.[42] The lesions appear as superficial stellate ulcers involving large areas of the stomach. The margin between the normal mucosa and the lesion is often very sharp, in contrast to adenocarcinomas, which have a dominant ulceration with an ill-defined margin between normal and abnormal tissue.[20] Biopsies and cytologic examination of these gastric lesions in patients with lymphoma make an accurate diagnosis in 36% to 96% of patients.[16, 23, 36, 37, 42, 43]

Immunophenotyping can be very effective in distinguishing malignant from benign disease.[50] Relatively large biopsies are required for immunophenotyping, but it is often impossible to obtain adequate quantities of tumor by endoscopic technique. Many patients therefore require exploratory laparotomy for definitive pathologic determination.

PATHOLOGY

Although primary gastric lymphoma usually occupies the distal part of the stomach, it can extend through the entire surface of the stomach. The five classifications of the gross morphology of these tumors are infiltrative, ulcerative, nodular, polypoid, and combined (any combination of the other four).

Histologic sections of primary lymphoma of the stomach are characterized by mucosal or submucosal lymphoid tissue. Infiltration of the gastric glands by follicle center cells forming characteristic lymphoid epithelial lesions is pathognomonic.[38] Primary gastric lymphoma is not associated with bone marrow or peripheral node involvement; it metastasizes to local nodes by contiguous spread and to the lymphoid tissue in the chest. The prognosis can be determined on the basis of histologic findings, including size, invasion, and nodal status.[5, 41]

Cytologic examination aids in the diagnosis of primary gastric lymphoma, with an accuracy varying from 35 to more than 80%, depending on the techniques used.[8, 37, 49] In one series, cytologic examination by abrasion plus endoscopic biopsy yielded a correct diagnosis in 14 of 15 patients.[8] In other series, cytologic diagnosis of gastric lymphoma has not been as encouraging.[45]

Pseudolymphoma represents 10% of all gastric lymphomas. Pseudolymphoma is benign gastric lymphomatosis, characterized by lymphoid infiltration of the gastric wall, predominantly in the mucosa, without evidence of nodal disease. Ulceration and extensive fibrosis are present, commonly with chronic peptic ulcer disease.[3, 25] The *sine qua non* for the diagnosis is germinal centers present within the gastric lesion.[6] Pseudolymphoma may represent a premalignant lesion that can convert to malignant lymphoma, as suggested by the occurrence of both pseudolymphoma and malignant lymphoma in specimens.[31] The recommended management for pseudolymphoma is conservative surgical resection,[7] with

nonoperative observation reserved for patients at high risk for operation. Complete resection offers cure and avoids malignant conversion. Adjuvant therapy is unnecessary.

Mucosa-associated lymphoid tissue (MALT) tumors are low-grade B-cell tumors that demonstrate mucosally based lymphoid tissue. They have growth characteristics that are less malignant than those of lymphomas. MALT tumors are associated with *Helicobacter pylori,* and recent reports suggest that eradication of the *H. pylori* leads to regression of the tumor. Clearly MALT tumors can progress to high-grade lymphomas, since they frequently coexist. Current management of MALT tumors is the same as for high-grade lymphomas until noninvasive techniques for management have proved their efficacy in long-term studies.[11, 12, 17, 27, 40]

TREATMENT

Many patients with primary gastric lymphoma present with a gastric mass and insufficient tissue to make a definitive diagnosis after endoscopic biopsy. At exploration, half the patients have Stage I or II disease.[36] The treatment of these tumors should be attempted cure with surgical resection.[5] This may include total gastrectomy in patients who are medically suitable. The reported mortality of resection ranges from 0% to 10%.[34, 37, 39, 47, 48] Intraoperative staging requires adequate sampling of regional lymph nodes and complete physical examination, including size of the spleen and the appearance of distant intra-abdominal nodes.

Surgical resection affords the greatest likelihood of long-term survival. Although all series are retrospective and therefore biased, most studies continue to demonstrate that surgically resected patients do better than those treated with only radiation therapy and chemotherapy. Approximately 75% of patients have resectable disease.[16, 26, 29, 47, 48] For all stages, curative resection should yield a 5-year survival in the range of 34% to 50%.[15, 26, 48] Those who undergo only palliative resections have a 5-year survival ranging from 25% to 35%,[41] and the stage of the tumor correlates well with survival. A 4-year survival of 90% of patients with Stage I and II disease has been reported,[36] contrasted with a 4-year survival of 25% of patients with Stage III and IV disease. Another series reported 95% Stage I survival, 78% Stage II survival, and 25% Stage IV survival at 5 years.[22]

Surgical resection improves not only survival but also postoperative palliative care. There are reports of bleeding and perforation in patients receiving adjuvant radiation therapy or chemotherapy before resection. Liang and colleagues reviewed 85 patients with primary abdominal lymphoma, 45 of whom had primary gastric lymphoma.[33] They found that 38% of patients who underwent chemotherapy before resection had complications of bleeding or perforation. Fleming and colleagues reported that preoperative treatment with combination chemotherapy led to upper gastrointestinal bleeding requiring emergency surgical therapy in four of five patients.[19] In contrast, Mittal and associates reviewed a series of 37 patients in whom radiation therapy did not lead to perforation or bleeding in any patient before resection.[37]

Adjuvant therapy for resected or unresected patients has been recommended for all stages of primary gastric lymphoma. Shimm and colleagues demonstrated that radiation therapy given postoperatively to patients with positive surgical margins improved survival.[46] Shiu and co-workers reviewed a series of 51 patients in whom resection alone yielded a 5-year survival of 33%, a 5-year survival of 67% was achieved if radiation was added to surgical resection.[47] Similarly, Hockey and associates showed that 5-year survival improved from 45% to 73% when radiation therapy was added to curative surgical resection for patients with Stage I disease.[26] In its aggressive form, this adjuvant therapy can include whole abdominal radiation, with an increase to the stomach bed totaling 3700 cGy.[48, 49] Chemotherapy usually includes either cyclophosphamide, vincristine, nitrogen mustard, procarbazine, and prednisone (CMOPP) or cyclophosphamide, doxorubicin, vincristine, and prednisone (CHOP).[16, 19, 36, 48]

Recent studies have shown that aggressive nonoperative management of gastric lymphoma with radiation therapy and chemotherapy yields results that are comparable to surgical therapy alone and are most impressive with early-stage tumors. These early results have not been substantiated by long-term follow-up, so aggressive nonoperative management for early-stage lymphomas must be evaluated in controlled studies before its acceptance as first-line therapy.[22]

In summary, all Stage I and II patients (disease confined to stomach and regional nodes) should undergo attempted curative resection followed by adjuvant chemotherapy, radiation therapy, or both. Stage III and IV patients who present with complications of bleeding, obstruction, or perforation should also undergo attempted primary resection followed by adjuvant therapy. Patients without complications presenting with preoperative documentation of Stage III or IV disease should be treated with radiation therapy and chemotherapy initially, and surgical resection should be reserved for persistent local disease of the stomach or for complications. If preoperative diagnosis and staging are not possible and exploration is undertaken for diagnosis, resection should be attempted unless precluded by the extent of the tumor.

SELECTED REFERENCES

Brooks, J. J., and Enterline, H. T.: Gastric pseudolymphoma: Its three subtypes and relation to lymphoma. Cancer, 51:476, 1983.
A complete review of pseudolymphoma of the stomach, with histologic findings.

Mentzer, S. J., Osteen, R. T., Pappas, T. N., Rosenthal, D. S., Canellos, G. P., and Wilson, R. E.: Surgical therapy of localized abdominal non-Hodgkin's lymphomas. Surgery, 103:609, 1988.
A series on abdominal lymphoma, with emphasis on presentation and management, reporting an excellent survival rate with surgical resection for Stages I and II.

Rosen, C. B., VanHeerden, J. A., Martin, J. K., Wold, L. E., and Ilstrup, D. M.: Is an aggressive surgical approach to the patient with gastric lymphoma warranted? Ann. Surg., 205:634, 1987.
A review of 84 patients, all with greater than 5-year follow-up, with emphasis on the necessity of attempted surgical cure and prognosis.

Shiu, M. H., Nisce, L., Pinna, A., Straus, D. J., Tome, M., Fillippa, D. A., and Lee, B. J.: Recent results of multimodal therapy of gastric lymphoma. Cancer, 58:1389, 1986.
A review of multimodal therapy for gastric lymphoma showing that surgical and adjuvant chemotherapy prolongs survival, these authors report the best survival data in the literature.

REFERENCES

1. Al-Bahrani, A., Al-Mondhiry, H., Bakir, F., Al-Saleem, T., and Al-Eshaiker, M.: Primary gastric lymphoma: Review of 32 cases from Iraq. Ann. R. Coll. Surg. Engl., 64:234, 1982.
2. Allison, J. E.: Gastrocolic fistula as a complication of gastric lymphoma. Am. J. Gastroenterol., 59:499, 1973.
3. Anderson, J. R., Lee, D., Naysmith, A., and Busuttil, A.: Gastric pseudolymphoma. Br. J. Surg., 67:672, 1980.
4. Aozasa, K., Ueda, T., Kurata, A., et al.: Prognostic value of histologic and clinical factors in 56 patients with gastrointestinal lymphoma. Cancer, 601:309, 1988.
5. Brooks, J. J., and Enterline, H. T.: Primary gastric lymphoma: A clinicopathologic study of 58 cases with long-term follow-up and literature review. Cancer, 51:701, 1983.
6. Brooks, J. J., and Enterline, H. T.: Gastric pseudolymphoma: Its three subtypes and relation to lymphoma. Cancer, 51:476, 1983.
7. Buy, J. N., and Moss, A. A.: Computed tomography of gastric lymphoma. A. J. R. Am. J. Roentgenol., 138:859, 1982.
8. Cabre-Fiol, V., and Vilardell, F.: Progress in the cytological diagnosis of gastric lymphoma: A report of 32 cases. Cancer, 41:1456, 1978.
9. Caletti, G. C., Ferrari, A., Brocchi, E., and Barbara, L.: Accuracy of endoscopic ultrasonography in the diagnosis and staging of gastric cancer and lymphoma. Surgery, 113:14, 1993.
10. Caletti, G. C., Zani, L., Bolondi, L., Guizzardi, G., Brocchi, E., and Barbara,
11. Castrillo, J. M., Montalban, C., Obeso, G., Piris, M. A., and Rivas, M. C.: Gastric B-cell mucosa associated lymphoid tissue lymphoma: A clinicopathologic study in 56 patients. Gut, 33:1307, 1992.
12. Chan, J. K. C., Ng, C. S., and Isaacson, P. G.: Relationship between high-grade lymphoma and low-grade B-cell mucosa-associated lymphoid tissue lymphoma (MALToma) of the stomach. Am. J. Pathol., 136:1153, 1990.
13. Dajani, Y. F., and Al-Jitawi, S.: Primary gastrointestinal lymphoma. Trop. Geogr. Med., 35:375, 1983.
14. Derchi, L. E., Banderali, A., Bossi, C., et al.: The sonographic appearance of gastric lymphoma. J. Ultrasound Med., 3:251, 1984.
15. Dworkin, B., Lightdale, C. J., Weingrad, N., et al.: Primary gastric lymphoma: A review of 50 cases. Dig. Dis. Sci., 27:986, 1982.
16. Economopoulos, T., Alexopoulos, C., Stathakis, N., et al.: Primary gastric lymphoma—the experience of a general hospital. Br. J. Cancer, 52:391, 1985.
17. Eidt, S., Stolte, M., Fischer, R.: Helicobacter pylori gastritis and primary gastric non-Hodgkin's lymphomas. J. Clin. Pathol., 47:436, 1994.
18. Eridani, S., and Singh, A. K.: Gastric non-Hodgkin's lymphoma after successful treatment of Hodgkin's disease. Oncology, 43:107, 1986.
19. Fleming, I. D., Mitchell, S., and Dilawari, R. A.: The role of surgery in the management of gastric lymphoma. Cancer, 49:1135, 1982.
20. Fork, F. T., Haglund, U., Hogstrom, H., and Wehlin, L.: Primary gastric lymphoma versus gastric cancer. Endoscopy, 17:5, 1985.
21. Ghahremani, G. G., and Fisher, M. R.: Lymphoma of the stomach following gastric surgery for benign peptic ulcers. Gastrointest. Radiol., 8:213, 1983.
22. Gobbi, P. G., Dionigi, P., Barbieri, F., Corbella, F., Bertoloni, D., Grignani, G., Jemos, V., Pieresca, C., and Ascari, E.: The role of surgery in the multimodal treatment of primary gastric non-Hodgkin's lymphomas: A report of 76 cases and review of the literature. Cancer, 65:2528, 1990.
23. Green, J. A., Dawson, A. A., Jones, P. F., and Brunt, P. W.: The presentation of gastrointestinal lymphoma: Study of a population. Br. J. Surg., 66:798, 1979.
24. Hayes, J., and Dunn, E.: Has the incidence of primary gastric lymphoma increased? Cancer, 63:2073, 1989.
25. Highman, L. M., Fantelli, F. J., and Hermann, R. E.: Pseudolymphoma of the stomach. Arch. Surg., 116:227, 1981.
26. Hockey, M. S., Powell, J., Crocker, J., and Fielding, J. W. L.: Primary gastric lymphoma. Br. J. Surg., 74:483, 1987.
27. Hussell, T., Isaacson, P. G., Crabtree, J. E., and Spencer, J.: The response of cells from low-grade B-cell gastric lymphomas of mucosa-associated lymphoid tissue to Helicobacter pylori. Lancet, 342:571, 1993.
28. Jamieson, N. V., Thiru, S., Calne, R. Y., and Evans, D. B.: Gastric lymphomas arising in two patients with renal allografts. Transplantation, 31:224, 1981.
29. Jones, R. E., Willis, S., Innes, D. J., and Wanebo, H. J.: Primary gastric lymphoma: Problems in staging and management. Am. J. Surg., 155:118, 1988.
30. Jones, T. E., and Carmody, M. G.: Lymphosarcoma of the stomach: Report of a case with a 19-year surgical cure. Ann. Surg., 101:1136, 1935.
31. Jung, S. S., Wieman, T. J., and Lindberg, R. D.: Primary gastric lymphoma and pseudolymphoma. Am. Surg., 54:594, 1988.
32. Kini, S. U., Pai, P. K., Rao, P. K., and Kini, A. J.: Primary gastric lymphoma associated with Crohn's disease of the stomach. Am. J. Gastroenterol., 81:23, 1986.
33. Liang, R., Todd, D., Chan, T. K., Ng, R. P., and Ho, F. C. S.: Gastrointestinal lymphoma in Chinese: A retrospective analysis. Hematol. Oncol., 5:115, 1987.
34. Lim, F. E., Hartman, A. S., Tan, E. G. T., Cady, B., and Meissner, W. A.: Factors in the prognosis of gastric lymphoma. Cancer, 39:1715, 1977.
35. McTamaney, J. P., Neifeld, J. P., Mendez-Picon, G., and Lee, H. M.: Primary gastric lymphoma following renal transplantation. J. Surg. Oncol., 18:275, 1981.
36. Mentzer, S. J., Osteen, R. T., Pappas, T. N., Rosenthal, D. S., Canellos, G. P., and Wilson, R. E.: Surgical therapy of localized abdominal non-Hodgkin's lymphomas. Surgery, 103:609, 1988.
37. Mittal, B., Wasserman, T. H., and Griffith, R. C.: Non-Hodgkin's lymphoma of the stomach. Am. J. Gastroenterol., 78:780, 1983.
38. Moore, I., and Wright, D. H.: Primary gastric lymphoma—a tumor of mucosa-associated lymphoid tissue: A histologic and immunohistologic study of 36 cases. Histopathology, 8:1025, 1984.
39. Orlando, R., Pastuszak, W., Preissler, P. L., and Welch, J. P.: Gastric lymphoma: A clinicopathologic reappraisal. Am. J. Surg., 143:450, 1982.
40. Parsonnet, J., Hansen, S., Rodriguez, L., Gelb, A. B., Warnke, R. A., Jellum, E., Orentreich, N., Vogelman, J. H., and Friedman, G. D.: Helicobacter pylori infection and gastric lymphoma. N. Engl. J. Med., 330:1267, 1994.
41. Rosen, C. B., VanHeerden, J. A., Martin, J. K., Wold, L. E., and Ilstrup, D. M.: Is an aggressive surgical approach to the patient with gastric lymphoma warranted? Ann. Surg., 205:634, 1987.
42. Russo, A., Grasso, G., Sanfillipo, G., Giannone, G., and Guerrera, G.: Gastroscopy and directed biopsy in the diagnosis of primary gastric lymphomas: Report of 16 personal cases. Tumor, 64:419, 1978.
43. Sandler, R. S.: Has primary gastric lymphoma become more common? J. Clin. Gastroenterol., 6:101, 1984.
44. Sato, T., Sakai, Y., Ishiguro, S., and Furukawa, H.: Radiologic manifestations of early gastric lymphoma. A. J. R. Am. J. Roentgenol., 146:513, 1986.

45. Seybolt, J. F., and Papanicolaou, G. N.: The value of cytology in the diagnosis of gastric cancer. Gastroenterology, 33:368, 1957.
46. Shimm, D. S., Dosoretz, D. E., Anderson, T., Linggood, R. M., Harris, N. L., and Wang, C. C.: Primary gastric lymphoma: An analysis with emphasis on prognostic factors and radiation therapy. Cancer, 52:2044, 1983.
47. Shiu, M. H., Karas, M., Nisce, L., Lee, B. J., Fillippa, D. A., and Lieberman, P. H.: Management of primary gastric lymphoma. Ann. Surg., 195:196, 1982.

48. Shiu, M. H., Nisce, L., Pinna, A., Straus, D. J., Tome, M., Fillippa, D. A., and Lee, B. J.: Recent results of multimodal therapy of gastric lymphoma. Cancer, 58:1389, 1986.
49. Spinelli, P., Gullo, C. L., and Pizzetti, P.: Endoscopic diagnosis of gastric lymphomas. Endoscopy, 12:211, 1980.
50. Villar, H. V., Wong, R., Paz, B., Bull, D., Neumayer, L., Grogan, T., and Spier, C.: Immunophenotyping in the management of gastric lymphoma. Am. J. Surg., 161:171, 1991.

IV ————————————————————————————

THE PATHOGENESIS, PROPHYLAXIS, AND TREATMENT OF STRESS GASTRITIS

Laurence Y. Cheung, M.D.

Stress gastritis occurs primarily in patients following severe burn, trauma, hemorrhagic shock, respiratory failure, or sepsis.[10, 17, 22, 23] These multiple, superficial erosions occur primarily in the fundus of the stomach and are clearly different from Cushing's ulcer, ulcer induced by drugs, and reactivation of a pre-existing chronic ulcer.[12, 25] A brief description of these other acute lesions should help distinguish them from stress gastritis.

Cushing's ulcer, which occurs with intracranial tumor, following head injury, or after a cranial operation, may involve the esophagus, stomach, and duodenum. Morphologically, Cushing's ulcer tends to be a single, deep ulcer. Therefore, perforation is a common complication of Cushing's ulcer but is rarely encountered in the more superficial stress gastritis. Hypersecretion of gastric acid and pepsin is common among patients with Cushing's ulcer but unusual in individuals with stress gastritis. Drug-induced ulcers are often indistinguishable from stress gastritis in their gross and microscopic appearance and distribution. Although both drug-induced and stress-induced ulcers share the same ultimate pathogenetic events at the cellular level, the initial factors that cause cellular damage may be different.[12] Occasionally, upper gastrointestinal bleeding in critically ill patients is caused by a pre-existing chronic duodenal or gastric ulcer. Also, during the course of another acute illness, a chronic ulcer diathesis could become activated. Reactivation of a previous chronic ulcer usually occurs at a single site with endoscopic evidence suggesting chronicity, whereas acute stress erosions are usually multiple with no evidence of chronicity. The distinction between these conditions and stress gastritis is important because the prognostic and therapeutic considerations are different.

INCIDENCE

Clinical studies that do not employ endoscopy underestimate the incidence of stress gastritis, because most of these erosions do not bleed. Gastroscopy showed the incidence of such gastric erosions to be 100% in 40 severely injured patients. In a similar study at the Brooke Army Surgical Research Institute, gastric erosions were found by sequential endoscopic examinations in 27 of 29 patients with major burns.[10] Acute gastric erosions were also found in most patients in the medical intensive care unit.[19] Recent endoscopic studies also reported a high incidence of stress gastritis in patients following cardiac procedures and head injury.[4] Most patients developed these lesions within 72 hours of admission to the intensive care unit. Fortunately, only a small number of these patients had significant gastrointestinal hemorrhage.

PATHOGENESIS

Although the precise mechanisms involved in the development of stress gastritis are still unknown, current evidence supports a multifactorial etiology.[17, 25] Most of the factors contribute to the development of stress gastritis by reducing the stomach's ability to protect itself against acid injury rather than by increasing the amount of acid secretion. This section focuses on some of these factors in patients at high risk for stress gastritis (Fig. 30–22).

Presence of Luminal Acid. There is no evidence that an increased quantity of secreted acid causes stress gastritis. Although hypersecretion is an unlikely cause, most experimental studies have shown that some hydrogen ions are necessary for the development of stress gastritis. Almost all experimentally induced stress gastritis, under conditions resembling clinical settings, require low gastric luminal pH.

Ischemia. Clinically, most patients who develop stress gastritis have experienced an episode of shock from hemorrhage, sepsis, or cardiac dysfunction. Diminished gastric mucosal blood flow is a common denominator in animal experiments that employ restraint, hemorrhage, or endotoxemia to produce acute ulceration. Virtually all investigators agree that one basic pathogenetic feature of stress gastritis is mucosal ischemia.[5]

Mucosal ischemia not only is caused by a reduction in blood flow secondary to episodes of shock from hemorrhage or sepsis, but more importantly is the result of gastric microcirculatory changes. Recent studies have provided evidence that microcirculatory dysfunction significantly contributes to prolonged mucosal ischemia following systemic insults such as hemorrhagic shock or sepsis.[15] Until recently, endothelial cells were presumed to play only a passive role, acting simply as a barrier between blood and vascular smooth muscle cells. However, accumulated evidence shows that these cells are actively involved in the control of microcirculatory function. Endothelial cells produce several vasoactive substances called endothelial-derived factors, including nitric oxide, prostacyclin, and endothelin-1, which have been shown to affect vascular tone, microvascular permeability, and leukocyte adherence to the microvasculature. These factors have a significant role in the regulation of tissue blood flow under normal conditions. Changes in the formation of these factors may initiate microcirculatory dysfunction and may represent an underlying cause of gastric mucosal ischemia in a variety of clinical settings, including shock and sepsis.[15, 29]

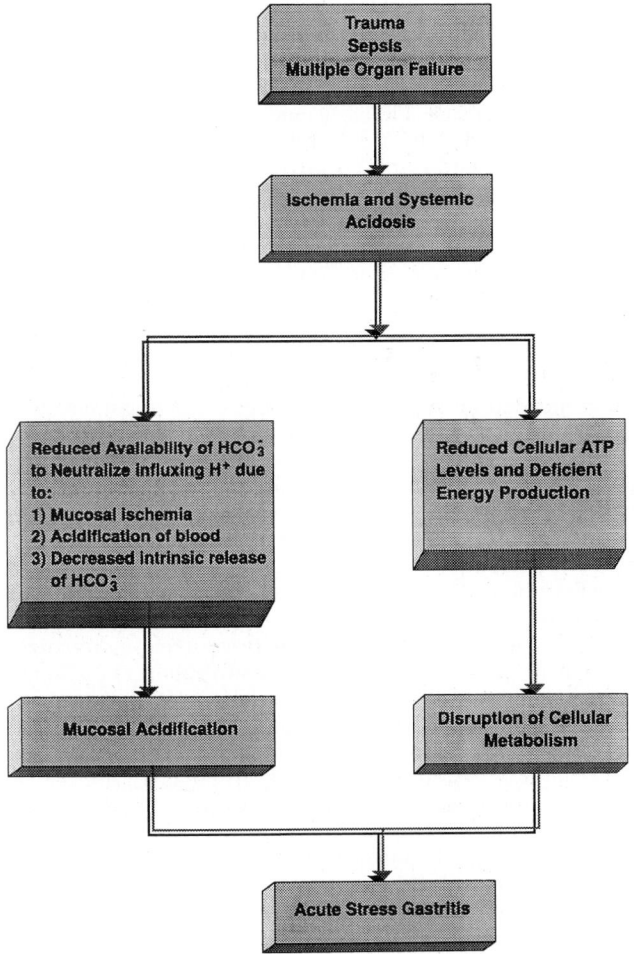

Figure 30–22. Proposed pathophysiologic mechanism for the development of acute stress gastritis.

One explanation for the cause-effect relationship between ischemia and stress erosions is the theory of energy deficit of the gastric mucosa. Ischemia may adversely affect gastric energy metabolism, an important factor in mucosal defense against injury. Menguy and associates have shown in a series of animal experiments that hemorrhagic shock produces a differential energy deficit (decreased levels of adenosine triphosphate and high-energy phosphate in the gastric mucosa).[14] This deficit is much greater in the fundic mucosa than in the antrum or other tissues such as the liver and muscle. Feeding before hemorrhage also causes a lesser degree of injury than fasting, presumably because of greater availability of energy sources. These data support the contention that a differential energy deficit exists between fundus and antrum and provide a possible explanation for the propensity of the fundus rather than the antrum to develop stress ulcers.

The other leading hypothesis to account for the association between ischemia and stress erosions is that gastric mucosal blood flow plays an important role in the disposal or buffering of the H^+ entering the tissue.[5, 25] Under normal conditions, a small amount of H^+ diffuses into the mucosa and may be rapidly cleared or neutralized by adequate mucosal blood flow. Ischemia reduces the capacity of the gastric mucosa to neutralize acid that enters the tissue, which in turns leads to accumulation of H^+ within the tissue, mucosal acidification, and ulceration. Recent studies measuring the mucosal pH with an electrode have supported this hypothesis.[1]

Furthermore, experimentally induced increases in mucosal blood flow by intra-arterial infusion of isoproterenol prevented ulcerations in dogs subjected to hemorrhagic shock.

Systemic Acid-Base Balance. Recent studies have suggested that the ability of the gastric mucosa to maintain its neutral pH depends not only on the rate of mucosal blood flow but also on the pH of the arterial blood perfusing the stomach.[6] This concept was first introduced by Cummins, Grossman, and Ivy in 1948. They demonstrated that if systemic acidosis induced by the constant intragastric infusion of acid was prevented by intravenous administration of sodium bicarbonate, the typical gastric and duodenal ulcers could be prevented. The author has also shown that mucosal injury produced by the combination of hemorrhagic shock and topical bile salts can be partially prevented by intravenous infusion of sodium bicarbonate.[6]

Secretory State of the Gastric Mucosa. It is well known that bicarbonate is released intrinsically within the mucosa during the active secretion of acid. However, the importance of this intramural release of bicarbonate in mucosal protection against luminal acid has only recently been recognized by Silen and associates.[25] They have clearly shown that an actively secreting stomach of a rabbit is much more resistant to ulceration than a metiamide-inhibited rabbit stomach, affirming that the alkaline tide is important in protecting the tissue against ulceration. Acid secretion requires a high consumption of energy and is usually reduced during mucosal ischemia. Therefore, the reduced acid secretion decreases the intrinsic release of bicarbonate, which renders the gastric mucosa more susceptible to acid injury.

Reflux of Bile and Disruption of Gastric Mucosal Permeability Barrier. Gastric mucosa has a unique ability to contain acid in the lumen and prevent excessive influx of acid into the tissue. This functional capability is defined as the gastric mucosal permeability barrier to acid. A significant amount of research has been done to evaluate the relationship between ischemia and the integrity of the gastric mucosal barrier. Most studies have failed to demonstrate disruption of the gastric permeability barrier during hemorrhagic shock. However, it is conceivable that reflux of duodenal contents and bile salts occurs in seriously ill patients, and bile salts are known to disrupt the barrier.[22] Bile salts not only increase mucosal permeability to acid but also produce direct injury to the surface cells of the stomach and render the gastric mucosa more susceptible to acid injury.

PREVENTION

Based on the various factors identified experimentally as being responsible for the pathogenesis of stress gastritis, a variety of prophylactic measures can be instituted in patients at high risk for its development. Since mucosal ischemia can alter a number of mechanisms by which the stomach normally protects itself against injury, vigorous efforts should be made to correct any shocklike state resulting from blood loss and/or sepsis. In addition, efforts should be made to improve ventilatory support, to correct any systemic acid-base abnormality, and to maintain adequate nutrition in these critically ill patients. Despite the lack of documentation, a strong impression exists among clinicians that the incidence and prevalence of stress gastritis have decreased significantly over the past decade, perhaps as a result of improved general care given to critically ill patients.

The "no acid, no ulcer" dictum has led to the concept that maintaining the gastric contents at a neutral pH may prevent the development of stress gastritis in critically ill patients. In fact, titration of gastric pH with antacid has effectively prevented gastrointestinal bleeding in such patients in several controlled prospective trials.[9, 13, 20, 30]

Several studies have reported that H_2-receptor antagonists are also useful in the prophylaxis of stress ulceration.[11, 18, 19] In a randomized, double-blinded, placebo-controlled study, Peura and Johnson showed that cimetidine can alleviate established lesions, prevent bleeding, and diminish the requirement for blood transfusion in patients admitted to a medical intensive care unit.[19] In a retrospective analysis of the combined data from 16 prospective trials, Shuman and associates concluded that acid reduction by either cimetidine or antacid, when compared with placebo, significantly reduces the risk of upper gastrointestinal bleeding in critically ill patients (Fig. 30–23). This finding is also confirmed by a recent study reported by Cook and colleagues.[9] They noted that H_2-receptor antagonists are even more effective than antacid at decreasing overt bleeding in critically ill patients. However, mortality rates in the intensive care unit are not decreased by stress ulcer prophylaxis. This is somewhat expected, because most such patients die from their underlying diseases rather than gastrointestinal bleeding.

The practice of prophylaxis of stress gastritis in critically ill patients with either antacids or H_2-receptor antagonists has been questioned for the potential serious side effect of neutralizing gastric content. Normal gastric acidity is an important component of the antibacterial defense of the upper gastrointestinal tract. Some reports indicate that neutralization of gastric acid or inhibition of acid secretion may increase the risk of nosocomial pneumonia by favoring gastric colonization with gram-negative bacilli.[11, 28] However, the results of other studies have not confirmed this finding. In fact,

a recent review of published studies indicates that stress ulcer prophylaxis with drugs that raise gastric pH does not increase the incidence of pneumonia in comparison with placebo or no therapy.[8] Given these findings, a strong argument can be made for early and aggressive reduction of intragastric acidity by intravenous administration of H_2-receptor antagonist or antacid in patients at risk for bleeding from stress gastritis.

A recent study showed that the enteral form of ranitidine given every 12 hours effectively provides a moderate to high serum ranitidine concentration.[18] The study also demonstrated a significant reduction (75%) in stimulated gastric acid secretion. Cost comparisons showed a significant reduction when using the enteral compound versus the parenteral route. Therefore, oral administration of ranitidine can be recommended for stress gastritis prophylaxis in patients who can tolerate oral intake of medications.

Sucralfate is a weak buffer that probably acts through pepsin absorption, mucosal protein binding, and cytoprotection. Several studies have shown that sucralfate provides adequate protection against stress bleeding without significantly increasing the intragastric pH.[3, 11, 28] Some studies suggest that the use of sucralfate may be preferable to using an antacid or H_2-blocker. However, these studies are preliminary and not yet conclusive. A large prospective randomized study is necessary to confirm whether sucralfate is preferable to an H_2-receptor antagonist.[8]

The efficacy of prophylaxis against stress gastritis in preventing gastrointestinal bleeding in critically ill patients has led to its widespread use. However, prophylaxis with an H_2-receptor antagonist, sucralfate, or antacid is expensive and may have adverse effects. A recent prospective multicenter study evaluated the potential risk factors for stress gastritis bleeding in patients admitted to intensive care units.[7] Of the 10 risk factors that were included in the study, respiratory failure and coagulopathy were shown to be two strong, independent risk factors for bleeding. The authors concluded from this study that it is safe to withhold prophylaxis against stress gastritis from intensive care patients who do not have coagulopathy or require mechanical ventilation for more than 48 hours.

TREATMENT

All patients with established stress gastritis with hemorrhage should be given adequate supportive care for shock and sepsis, with careful monitoring of the extent of hemorrhage. A patient with bleeding must be checked for coagulation defects, and any specific clotting abnormalities should be corrected. Initial management to control gastrointestinal hemorrhage should consist of gastric lavage with chilled solutions through a large-bore nasogastric tube. Lavage of the stomach aids in the fragmentation of clots and avoids gastric distention. Another benefit of gastric lavage is removal of duodenal contents that may have refluxed into the stomach as a result of adynamic ileus, since bile salts and pancreatic juice are injurious to gastric mucosa. Fortunately, most patients appear to stop bleeding following this general management. Occasionally, specific nonoperative or operative treatment is required.[4]

Endoscopic Therapy. Techniques for the treatment of stress gastritis via endoscopy include either electrocoagulation or laser photocoagulation.[4] Initial clinical experience with endoscopic therapy reports over 90% permanent hemostasis. However, only a small percentage of patients in these studies had bleeding from stress gastritis. Since upper gastrointestinal hemorrhage, whether from stress gastritis or other causes, stopped spontaneously in most patients, an evaluation of any new method requires a very large patient population in a

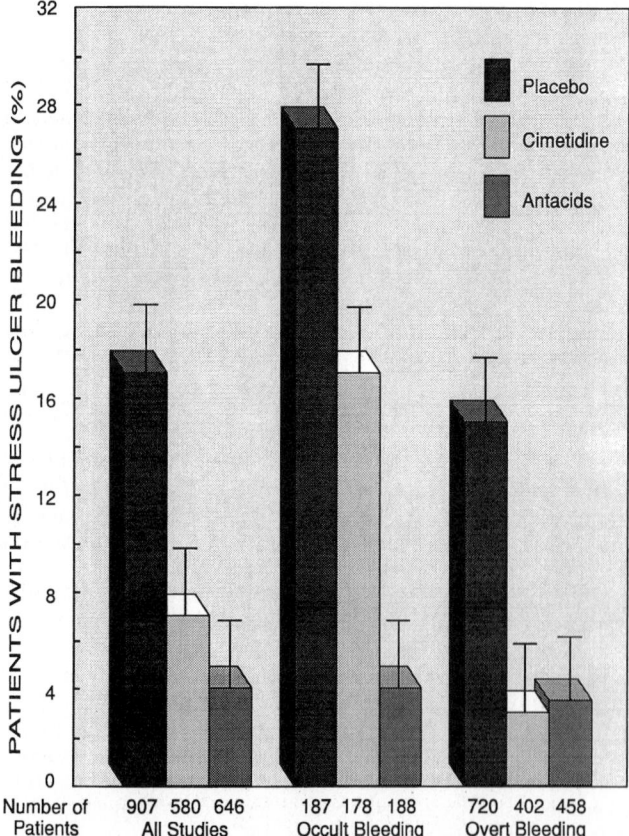

Figure 30–23. Incidence of stress ulcer bleeding in critically ill patients receiving placebo, cimetidine, or antacids for prophylaxis. Results are shown as percentages (means ± SD). All comparisons between treatment regimens within each group were statistically significant, except between antacid and cimetidine treatment in studies requiring overt bleeding. (Adapted from Shuman, R. B., Schuster, D. P., and Zuckerman, G. R.: Prophylactic therapy for stress ulcer bleeding: A reappraisal. Ann. Intern. Med., 106:562, 1987.)

controlled study to prove its efficacy. At present, endoscopic therapy provides an opportunity for direct control of bleeding from stress gastritis at institutions where this technique is available.

Angiographic Pharmacotherapy. The ability to selectively catheterize various branches of the splanchnic arterial circulation using angiographic methods represents an additional therapy. Several initial studies have reported a high success rate with this technique in the treatment of bleeding from stress gastritis. However, control of massive bleeding by selective intra-arterial infusion of vasopressin was not associated with an improved survival rate. Vasopressin helps decrease the amount of blood transfusion required during episodes of hemorrhage, and it provides the interval of time needed for a planned surgical approach to the problem. On the basis of these studies, the author recommends that this technique be attempted before surgical therapy is considered if facilities and trained personnel are available.

Somatostatin and Prostaglandins. Somatostatin is an endogenous gastrointestinal peptide. Exogenous administration of somatostatin inhibits acid secretion, reduces mucosal blood flow, and protects the gastric mucosa against stress-induced injury in experimental animals. These data suggest that somatostatin may be a clinically effective peptide in the treatment of stress-induced hemorrhagic gastritis. Several reports indicate that somatostatin is more effective than H_2-receptor antagonists in the control of upper gastrointestinal bleeding.[27] Unfortunately, only a small number of the patients in these studies were bleeding from stress gastritis. Therefore, somatostatin has not yet been used in a sufficient number of patients to determine its efficacy and long-term sequelae.

Prostaglandins are a group of long-chained, saturated fatty acids widely distributed throughout the body. The concentrations of various prostaglandins in the stomach are high relative to other tissue, and prostaglandins of the E, F, and I types have been detected in both gastric juice and mucosa. Exogenous prostaglandins have many effects on gastric function, including inhibition of basal and stimulated acid secretion, and changes in ion transport.[16] These actions appear to be involved in the ability of prostaglandins to reduce the severity of mucosal injury in a wide variety of experimental ulcer models. The mechanism of this property of prostaglandins is still not completely defined. The antisecretory and other protective effects of some prostaglandins may be useful in the treatment of stress ulceration.

Surgical Therapy. Persistent or recurring bleeding that does not respond to nonsurgical measures is an indication for operative intervention. The operative procedures used to control bleeding stress ulcers range from total gastrectomy to procedures of a smaller magnitude, such as pyloroplasty and vagotomy and the oversewing of bleeders.[26] No prospective clinical trials have substantiated the superiority of one form of therapy over another.[2] The ideal operation would be one that controls bleeding and has the lowest possible mortality and recurrent hemorrhage rates. In general, lesser procedures are associated with lower mortality rates but a higher incidence of rebleeding. Many surgeons advocate distal gastrectomy combined with bilateral truncal vagotomy.[2] Total gastrectomy is associated with high mortality and is reserved for patients who continue to bleed after the initial operation or who have diffuse bleeding lesions.

An alternative approach of gastric devascularization has been advocated by Richardson and Aust.[21] In this procedure, both the right and left gastric arteries and gastroepiploic arteries are ligated near their origins, with the entire gastric blood supply thereafter derived from the short gastric vessels. The rate of rebleeding following gastric devascularization is low, and no instances of gastric necrosis have been reported. However, mortality is high. The theoretical advantage of this approach is that serious postgastrectomy sequelae are avoided in patients who survive the underlying insult.

SELECTED REFERENCES

Cook, D. J., Fuller, H. D., Guyatt, G. H., Marshall, J. C., Leasa, D., Hall, R., et al.: Risk factors for gastrointestinal bleeding in critically ill patients. N. Engl. J. Med., 330:377, 1994.
In this report from a prospective multicenter cooperative study, the authors evaluate potential risk factors for stress ulcer bleeding in patients in intensive care units. Respiratory failure and coagulopathy were two strong independent risk factors for bleeding. Prophylaxis against stress ulcers should be strongly recommended for such patients with these two risk factors.

Michida, T., Kawano, S., Masuda, E., Kobayashi, I., Nishimura, Y., Tsujii, M., et al.: Role of endothelin 1 in hemorrhagic shock–induced gastric mucosal injury in rats. Gastroenterology, 106:988, 1994.
This is an excellent experimental study on the role of endogenous endothelin 1 in gastric microcirculatory disturbance during hemorrhagic shock. The results suggest that endogenous endothelin 1 has an important role in the pathogenesis of hemorrhagic shock–induced gastric mucosal damage. In addition, endothelin receptor antagonist BQ-123 has been demonstrated to improve gastric microcirculation during hemorrhagic shock and to reduce gastric mucosal damage.

Pemberton, L. B., Schaefer, N., Goehring, L., Gaddis, M., and Arrighi, D. A.: Oral ranitidine as prophylaxis for gastric stress ulcers in intensive care unit patients: Serum concentrations and cost comparisons. Crit. Care Med., 21:339, 1992.
The authors evaluate the efficacy of enteral ranitidine in reducing basal and stimulated acid secretion in surgical ICU patients. The results of this prospective study demonstrate that the serum concentration of ranitidine for both 150-mg. and 300-mg. enteral doses remains within or exceeds the therapeutic range in over 90% of acutely ill patients. This high serum concentration of ranitidine was associated with significant reduction (>50%) in stimulated acid secretion. Cost comparisons showed a significant saving when enteral ranitidine was compared with the parenteral route.

REFERENCES

1. Ashley, S. W., Soybel, D. I., Moore, C. D., and Cheung, L. Y.: Intracellular pH (pH_i) in gastric surface epithelium is more susceptible to serosal than mucosal acidification. Surgery, 102:371, 1987.
2. Bowen, J. C.: Surgical therapy in stress ulcerations. Scand. J. Gastroenterol., 19(suppl. 105):97, 1984.
3. Bresalier, R. S., Grendell, J. H., Cello, J. P., and Meyer, A. A.: Sucralfate suspension versus titrated antacid for the prevention of acute stress-related gastrointestinal hemorrhage in critically ill patients. Am. J. Med., 83:110, 1987.
4. Chamberlain, C. E.: Acute hemorrhagic gastritis. Gastroenterol. Clin. North Am., 22:843, 1993.
5. Cheung, L. Y., and Ashley, S. W.: Gastric blood flow and mucosal defense mechanisms. Clin. Invest. Med., 10:201, 1987.
6. Cheung, L. Y., and Porterfield, G.: Protection of gastric mucosa against acute ulceration by intravenous infusion of sodium bicarbonate. Am. J. Surg., 137:106, 1979.
7. Cook, D. J., Fuller, H. D., Guyatt, G. H., Marshall, J. C., Leasa, D., Hall, R., et al.: Risk factors for gastrointestinal bleeding in critically ill patients. N. Engl. J. Med., 330:377, 1994.
8. Cook, D. J., Laine, L. A., Guyatt, G. H., and Raffin, T. A.: Nosocomial pneumonia and the role of gastric pH: A meta-analysis. Chest, 100:7, 1991.
9. Cook, D. J., Witt, L. G., Cook, R. J., and Guyatt, G. H.: Stress ulcer prophylaxis in the critically ill: A meta-analysis. Am. J. Med., 91:519, 1991.
10. Czaja, A. F., McAlhand, J. C., and Pruitt, B. A., Jr.: Acute gastroduodenal disease after thermal injury. N. Engl. J. Med., 291:925, 1974.
11. Driks, M. R., Craven, D. E., Celli, B. R., Manning, M., Burke, R. A., Garvin, G. M., et al.: Nosocomial pneumonia in intubated patients given sucralfate as compared with antacids or histamine type 2 blockers: The role of gastric colonization. N. Engl. J. Med., 317:1376, 1987.
12. Fromm, D.: Drug-induced gastric mucosal injury. World J. Surg., 5:199, 1981.
13. Hastings, P. R., Skillman, J. J., Bushnell, L. S., and Silen, W.: Antacid titration in the prevention of acute gastrointestinal bleeding: A controlled, randomized trial in 100 critically ill patients. N. Engl. J. Med., 298:1041, 1978.
14. Menguy, R.: Role of gastric mucosal energy metabolism in the etiology of stress ulceration. World J. Surg., 5:175, 1981.
15. Michida, T., Kawano, S., Masuda, E., Kobayashi, I., Nishimura, Y., Tsujii, M., et al.: Role of endothelin 1 in hemorrhagic shock–induced gastric mucosal injury in rats. Gastroenterology, 106:988, 1994.
16. Miller, T. A.: Protective effects of prostaglandins against gastric mucosal damage: Current knowledge and proposed mechanisms. Am. J. Physiol., 245:G601, 1983.
17. Miller, T. A.: Stress erosive gastritis. *In* Moody, F. G., Carey, L. C., Jones, R. S., Kelly, K. A., Nahrwold, D. L., and Skinner, D. B. (Eds.): Surgical

similar symptoms and is discussed elsewhere. Carcinomas of the small intestine may be associated with Crohn's disease and are discussed in the next section. Connective tissue disorders such as scleroderma are known for their association with esophageal thickening and loss of motility; however, such findings may also be present in the small intestine. Rarely, endometriosis presents with obstructive symptoms or bleeding. Historically, the relationship can be established with menstrual periods. In the recent past, ulcers and strictures of the small intestine were associated with enteric-coated medications such as potassium chloride. Because such products are no longer commercially available, these lesions appear to be less common; however, a careful medication history should be elicited in all patients.

Radiation Damage. Radiation damage to the intestine after therapy for malignancy can cause endarteritis, with subsequent tissue anoxia and fibrosis. This can cause malabsorption, blood loss, and protein loss, as well as scarring and stenosis that may be mistaken for recurrent malignancy.[26]

MALIGNANT TUMORS OF THE SMALL INTESTINE

Adenocarcinoma. Adenocarcinoma of the small intestine is said to account for less than 1% of all intestinal carcinomas, but it is the most common small intestinal malignancy. In a Mayo Clinic series, 55 patients with small intestinal cancers were found, in contrast to 4597 with colon carcinomas and 4315 with gastric carcinomas in the same series.[29] The duodenum was the most common site for primary carcinoma in Rochlin and Longmire's review, with numbers decreasing distally.[32] Within the duodenum, the most common site is the periampullary region, with otherwise even distribution. Villous tumors of the duodenum are also most common in or near the ampulla of Vater, with an approximately 50% incidence of malignancy.[8] This malignancy is not necessarily associated with the size of the lesion, as is the case with villous adenomas of the colon. Within the area of the ampulla of Vater, carcinomas may arise from the mucosa of the wall of the duodenum or from the pancreatic ducts or the biliary ducts. Dawson and Connolly[12] emphasize that an analysis of mucin production from these tumors indicates the tissue of origin. Sialomucins arise from true ampullary tumors as a characteristic of biliary ductal epithelium and duodenal surface mucosa. Brunner's glands secrete neutral mucins, and the pancreatic duct produces predominantly sulfated mucins.[12] This study may be useful prognostically, because pancreatic neoplasms have a much lower cure rate than others in this area.

As noted above, there is an apparent increased incidence of adenocarcinoma of the small intestine associated with Crohn's disease. The incidence of cancer in patients with Crohn's disease has been estimated to be from 43 to over 100 times greater than that in the population at large. The average age at the time of diagnosis is the late forties, which is somewhat younger than the average age of all patients with adenocarcinoma of the small bowel in the absence of Crohn's disease. These patients with Crohn's disease and small intestinal cancer have had the disease for approximately 16 years. The mortality is expected to be 80% in 2 years, contrasted with a 50% 2-year mortality from cancer associated with ulcerative colitis. As is true with ulcerative colitis, these cancers are multicentric in 20% of patients. Screening for dysplasia in patients with Crohn's disease may be helpful in their management. There is also an apparent increase in bladder cancer in patients with Crohn's disease.[28] Adenocarcinomas of the small intestine develop in ileostomy stomata and in ileal conduits as a time-related phenomenon or as a manifestation of recurrence of urethral carcinoma.[6]

Sarcoma. Lymphomas are the most common small intestinal sarcoma (see Table 30–12). These may be primary or part of a more general disease pattern. Dawson and co-workers suggested four criteria for the diagnosis of primary bowel lymphoma: no generalized, superficial, or mediastinal lymphadenopathy is found; white blood cell (total and differential) count is normal; at laparotomy or autopsy, the bowel lesion drainage nodes are the only ones obviously affected; and the liver and spleen are free of tumor.[11]

The various manifestations of lymphoma, reticulum cell sarcoma, and Hodgkin's disease can all be primary in the intestine. Patterns of association exist with gluten-sensitive enteropathy and idiopathic steatorrhea. A specific pattern of duodenal lymphoma has been reported among young individuals in the Middle East. Leiomyosarcoma may be difficult to differentiate from leiomyoma because of a wide variety of histologic characteristics relating to cellularity, nuclear patterns, and so on. In many cases, the malignant nature of the tumor is established by the presence of metastatic disease.[37] There is not always a clear diagnosis of malignancy with solitary lesions. Other relatively rare sarcomas are fibromyxosarcomas and liposarcomas. Kaposi's sarcoma is a primary intestinal malignancy in AIDS.

Secondary Malignancies. Rarely, the small intestine is a site for metastases from the lung, stomach, colon, adrenal gland, kidney, ovary, uterine corpus, and cervix and from malignant melanoma, plasmacytomas, and leukemia.

Carcinoid and APUD Tumors. Carcinoid tumors are most common in the more distal intestine, particularly the appendix, but are found wherever argentaffin cells are located. APUDomas are most common in the stomach and rectum but are also found in the small intestine, most commonly the duodenum. Both of these tumors are well differentiated and slow growing. Criteria of malignancy are invasion of lymph nodes, blood vessels, and nerve sheath or the presence of distant (hepatic) metastasis. Initially, their ill effects are primarily endocrine.

RELATIONSHIP OF SMALL INTESTINAL TUMORS TO OTHER NEOPLASTIC GROWTH

Alexander and Altemeir reported that 83 of 112 patients with primary neoplasms of the small intestine had other independent neoplasms at death. Of those with benign intestinal neoplasms, 57% had benign neoplasms elsewhere in the small intestine, and 23% had secondary primary malignancies elsewhere.[1]

SYNDROMES ASSOCIATED WITH SMALL INTESTINAL NEOPLASMS

Bessauds-Hillmand-Augier Syndrome. Sexual infantilism is associated with intestinal polyposis.[30]

Carter-Horsley-Hughes Syndrome. Diffuse polyposis of the small and large intestine was noted in one family.[5]

Cowden's Disease or Multiple Hamartoma Syndrome. Hamartomatous, juvenile, lipomatous, or inflammatory polyps are present mainly in the stomach and colon but are also present in the small intestine. Benign and malignant breast and thyroid disease are also found in these patients, as well as mucocutaneous lesions, tricholemmas, acral keratoses, and oral papillomas.[16]

Cronkhite-Canada Syndrome. This syndrome is characterized by generalized gastrointestinal polyposis and ectodermal defects, such as alopecia, excessive skin pigmentations, and nail atrophy. In the intestinal polyps, dilated cystic glands are found in an edematous lamina propria. Loss of protein from the gut, along with calcium, magnesium, and potassium deficiencies, may occur.[10]

Familial Polyposis of the Colon. This syndrome is customarily associated with polyps of the colon, but cases of generalized polyposis have been recorded, with associated malignancy.[33]

Gardner's Syndrome. This syndrome is generally characterized by rectal and colonic polyposis, but generalized polyposis has been recorded. These polyps are involved in the development of adenocarcinoma. The syndrome also includes cysts of the skin, osteomas, fibrous and fatty tumors of the skin and mesentery, follicular odontomas, and dentigerous cysts and changes in the bony structures of the jaws. This syndrome is familial and is transmitted as an autosomal dominant trait.[13]

Gordon's Disease. This is a protein-losing gastroenteropathy, usually manifested as Ménétrier's disease, which involves mucosal hypertrophy, hyperplasia of the superficial epithelium, degeneration in the glandular layer, and hypoproteinemia due to leakage of proteins through the mucous membranes. A diffuse gastrointestinal polyposis associated with protein loss has also been reported.[15]

Juvenile Polyposis. Juvenile polyposis is most commonly found in the colon and rectum, but isolated examples of generalized gastrointestinal polyposis have been reported with and without family history or other congenital abnormalities. The polyps have normal propria.[34] There is no known relationship to malignancy, although the polyps may cause bleeding, obstruction, or intussusception.

Muir-Torre Syndrome. This syndrome was described by Muir and co-workers in 1967 and Torre in 1968 to include sebaceous adenomas, epidermoid cysts, fibromas, desmoids, lipomas, fibrosarcomas, and leiomyomas with visceral cancers.[9]

Peutz-Jeghers Syndrome. This syndrome is characterized by hamartomatous polyps of the gastrointestinal tract (stomach, small bowel, colon) that are associated with mucocutaneous pigmentation (lips, oral mucosa, fingers, forearm, toes, umbilical area). The skin pigmentation may fade after puberty, but that of the mucous membrane is retained.[20] Although there is said to be no relation between this syndrome and the development of cancer, River and associates reported that in 10 of 51 cases (19.6%), carcinomatous changes were observed in the polyps. The syndrome is probably transmitted as a dominant trait. The age of peak presentation in River's series was in the 10- to 29-year-old group.[31] The polyps usually develop later than the pigmentation.

Pseudoxanthoma Elasticum. Benign vascular lesions of the intestinal tract have been reported in association with this disease.[25]

Rendu-Osler-Weber Disease. This disease is described as telangiectasia of the nasopharynx or gastrointestinal tract. It is characterized by a familial incidence and also by lesions of the palmar surface of the hands and the nail beds.[25]

Turcot's Syndrome. Malignant brain tumors are associated with inherited intestinal adenomatous polyposis.[4]

Turner's Syndrome. Intestinal telangiectasia was noted in 4 of 55 patients in one series.[18]

von Recklinghausen's Disease. Generalized neurofibromatosis with café au lait skin pigmentation may also include neurofibromas of the gastrointestinal tract.[14]

SYMPTOMS AND COMPLICATIONS

The number and variety of small bowel tumors found at autopsy suggest that many such tumors are asymptomatic. When symptoms do arise, they are usually related to either obstructive phenomena or bleeding. Because the content of the small intestine is largely liquid, the degree of obstruction

must be almost complete before symptoms are noted. Epigastric discomfort or cramping pain associated with nausea and vomiting slowly increases in severity as the lesion occludes the intestinal lumen. Obstruction is the most common complication (50%) of benign tumors, and intussusception is the most common presentation. Bleeding is associated with angiomatous lesions and also with myomas, fibromas, fibromyomas, fibroadenomas, and metastatic tumors. The rate of bleeding is quite variable, from occult blood loss causing marginal anemia to exsanguinating hemorrhage.

Complications such as volvulus, necrosis, and peritonitis are less common. Malignant lesions more commonly present with symptoms of pain, anorexia, weight loss, and occult bleeding, whereas benign lesions may bleed more briskly, and the patient may have less anorexia and weight loss. Periampullary duodenal tumors are distinguished by association with painless jaundice, which varies as the tumor undergoes central necrosis and sloughs, with free passage of bile. The presence of a palpable gallbladder further supports the diagnosis of a neoplasm (Courvoisier's law).

DIAGNOSIS

The specific diagnosis of small intestinal neoplasms is possible by direct visualization and biopsy through various fiberoptic endoscopes that can traverse the entire small bowel from either end. Radiologic contrast studies using various forms of barium are the best technique for discovering lesions in the midrange of the small intestine (Figs. 30–24 and

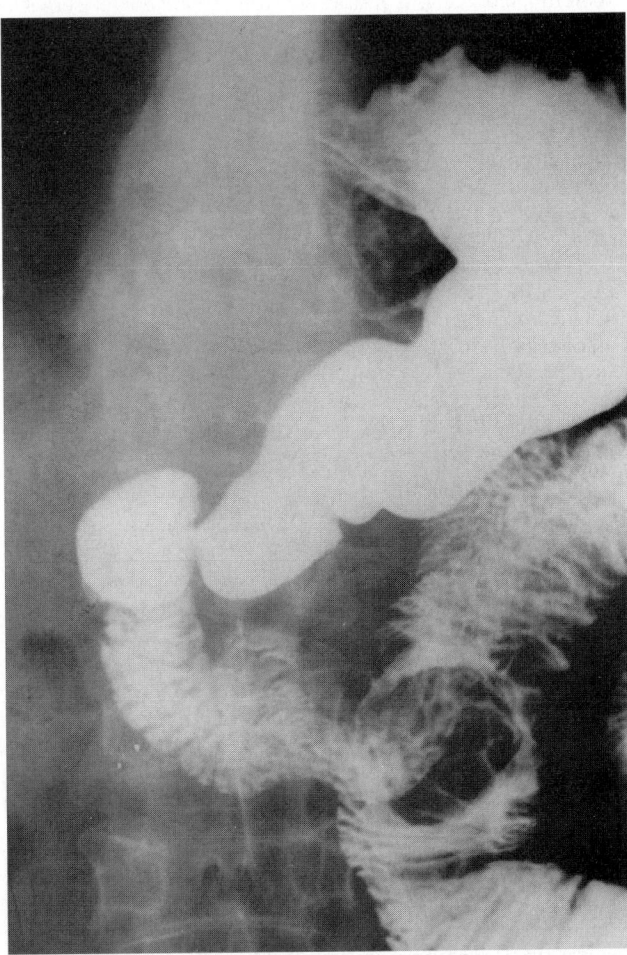

Figure 30–24. Upper gastrointestinal contrast study showing intraluminal mass (carcinoid tumor).

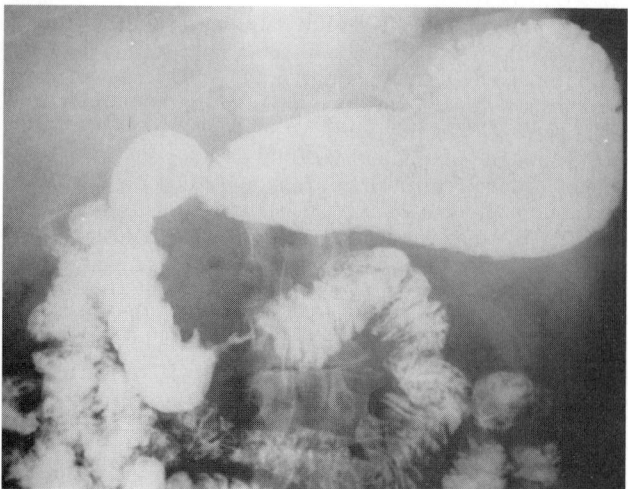

Figure 30–25. Upper gastrointestinal contrast study showing "apple-core" lesion of the jejunum (primary adenocarcinoma of the small intestine).

30–25). Sonography may be useful for large masses, such as leiomyosarcomas. Hypotonic duodenography involves the use of drugs such as glucagon to render the duodenum flaccid and relatively immobile, allowing more accurate delineation of mucosal abnormalities. The radiologic technique of enteroclysis may provide better diagnostic results than standard techniques, and computed tomographic scans with contrast may also be helpful (Fig. 30–26).

Overall, however, a routine barium small bowel series is probably as effective as other radiologic techniques.[35] Lesions bleeding at the time of investigation can be identified by arteriography if blood loss is greater than 1 to 2 ml. per minute. Laparotomy is often the diagnostic technique of choice, particularly for bleeding lesions, and it may be combined with intraoperative endoscopy. However, few experiences are more frustrating for the surgeon than the search for a poorly localized bleeding point that ceases to bleed actively when anesthesia is induced.

MANAGEMENT

Most small intestinal lesions can be treated successfully by resection and by end-to-end anastomosis of the residual bowel. Villous adenomas have a high incidence of malignancy (50%), but the diagnosis may not be evident on random biopsy or frozen section. Some investigators recommend

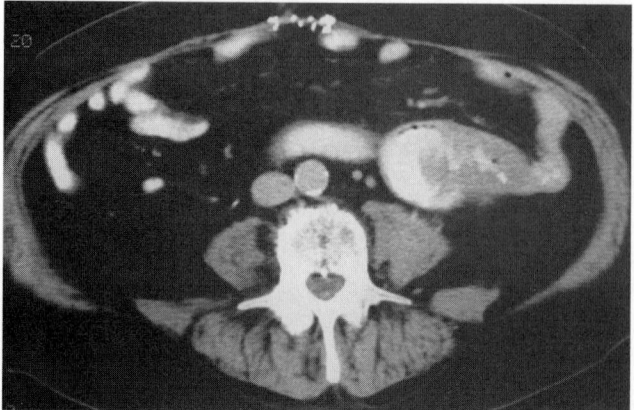

Figure 30–26. Computed axial tomography scan of the abdomen showing an intestinal mass (adenocarcinoma of the small intestine) partially obstructing contrast flow.

local excision, particularly in patients thought to be at greater risk of death from pancreatoduodenectomy. The degree of differentiation of the tumor is related to the prognosis and to the procedure recommended; local resections carry less likelihood of cure in undifferentiated tumors. The surgical treatment of duodenal carcinoma is essentially that of carcinoma of the head of the pancreas (see Chapter 35).

RESULTS

The results of therapy for carcinoma of the duodenum depend on the type of tumor, particularly at the ampulla of Vater. Here, duodenal mucosa and the mucosa of the ducts of Wirsung and Santorini and the common bile duct merge in or near the head of the pancreas. Characteristics of pancreatic tumors include perineural invasion, multicentricity, and local nodal metastases. Ampullary and duodenal lesions are more often of lower-grade malignancy, spread more locally, and do not invade bile duct perineural lymphatics or local nodes as frequently. Small bowel tumors are relatively rare, and malignant tumors are even less common. Because of the liquid content of the small intestine, symptoms are often a late manifestation of adenocarcinoma of the small intestine. The tumor has frequently spread through the wall and into regional lymph nodes and mesentery by the time laparotomy is performed. A 5-year survival rate with *en bloc* resection has been reported by various authors as ranging from 14% to 38%.[2]

Patients with localized lymphomas of the gastrointestinal tract treated by curative resection and 3000 to 4000 cGy have a 5-year survival as high as 85% (11 of 13).[23] For more advanced disease, combination chemotherapy of doxorubicin, prednisone, cyclophosphamide, and vincristine gains remission in up to 71% of patients.[27]

Leiomyosarcomas and fibrosarcoma are the most common lesions in the sarcoma group. Starr and Dockerty reported that 38% of patients with these lesions treated by resection were well 5 years later.[37] More advanced disease may show some response to a combination of doxorubicin and actinomycin D.[7]

Carcinoid tumors are extremely slow-growing, well-differentiated lesions. Some believe that all these lesions are malignant. MacDonald collected 356 gastrointestinal carcinoid tumors, 11% with hepatic metastases at operation.[24] In symptomatic patients, as many as 90% have metastases. Because of the slow rate of growth of carcinoid tumors, a 5-year span is probably inadequate to predict cure. Carcinoid tumors synthesize 5-hydroxytryptamine (serotonin), as well as kallikrein, bradykinin, and tachykinins.[24] Metastatic carcinoid tumors in the liver may release these and perhaps other substances into the blood to produce episodic symptoms of cutaneous flushing, diarrhea, asthma, and right-sided valvular heart disease (carcinoid syndrome). Management of this syndrome includes resection of hepatic masses and oral administration of methysergide and antihistamines. More recently, benefits have been reported with the use of somatostatin analogs.[39] Strodel and colleagues reported a 5-year survival of 35% and a 10-year survival of 15% for patients with hepatic metastases, compared with 72% and 59%, respectively, for patients without hepatic metastases.[38]

REFERENCES

1. Alexander, J. W., and Altemeir, W. A.: Association of primary neoplasms of the small intestine with other neoplastic growths. Ann. Surg., *167*:958, 1968.
2. Awrich, A. E., Irish, C. E., and Vetto, R. M.: A twenty-five year experience with primary malignant tumors of the small intestine. Surg. Gynecol. Obstet., *151*:9, 1980.
3. Bastlein, C., Decking, R., Voeth, C., and Ottenjann, R.: Giant brunneroma of the duodenum. Endoscopy, *20*:154, 1988.

4. Baughman, F. A., Jr., List, C. F., Williams, J. R., Muldom, J. P., Segarra, J. M., and Volkel, J. J.: The glioma-polyposis syndrome. N. Engl. J. Med., 281:1345, 1969.
5. Carter, B. N., Horsley, G. W., Horsley, J. J., and Hughes, R. D.: A new form of diffuse familial polyposis: A probable genetic explanation. Ann. Surg., 167:942, 1968.
6. Carter, D., Choi, H., Otterson, M., and Telford, G. L.: Primary adenocarcinoma of the ileostomy after colectomy for ulcerative colitis. Dig. Dis. Sci., 33:509, 1988.
7. Chang, P., Brenner, C. D., and Wiernik, P. H.: Adriamycin/actinomycin D therapy of advanced sarcomas—increasing response and toxicity. Proc. Am. Soc. Clin. Oncol., 17:422, 1979.
8. Chappuis, C. W., Divincenti, F. C., and Cohn, I., Jr.: Villous tumors of the duodenum. Ann. Surg., 209:593, 1989.
9. Cohen, P. R., Kohn, S. R., and Kurzrock, R.: Association of sebaceous gland tumors and internal malignancy: The Muir-Torre syndrome. Am. J. Med., 90:606, 1991.
10. Cronkhite, L. W., and Canada, W. J.: Generalized gastrointestinal polyposis: An unusual syndrome of polyposis, pigmentation, alopecia, and onychotrophia. N. Engl. J. Med., 252:1011, 1955.
11. Dawson, I. M. P., Coirnes, I. J., and Morson, B. D.: Primary malignant lymphoid tumors of the intestinal tract. Report of 37 cases with a study of factors influencing prognosis. Br. J. Surg., 49:30, 1961.
12. Dawson, P. J., and Connolly, M. M.: Influence of site of origin and mucin production on survival in ampullary carcinoma. Ann. Surg., 210:173, 1989.
13. Gardner, E. J.: Genetic and clinical study of intestinal polyposis: Predisposing factor for carcinoma of colon and rectum. Am. J. Hum. Genet., 3:167, 1951.
14. Ghrist, T. D.: Gastrointestinal involvement in neurofibromatosis. Arch. Intern. Med., 112:357, 1963.
15. Gill, W. J., and Wilken, B. J.: Diffuse gastrointestinal polyposis associated with hypoproteinemia. J. R. Coll. Surg. Edinb., 12:149, 1967.
16. Gold, B. M., Bagla, S., and Zarrabi, M. H.: Radiologic manifestations of Cowden disease. A. J. R. Am. J. Roentgenol., 135:385, 1980.
17. Griffen, W. O., Jr., Schaefer, J. W., Schindler, S., Hyde, G., and Bryant, L. R.: Ampullary obstruction by benign duodenal polyps. Arch. Surg., 97:444, 1968.
18. Haddad, H. M., and Wilkins, L.: Congenital anomalies associated with gonadal aplasia: Review of 55 cases. Pediatrics, 23:885, 1958.
19. Higgins, G. A., Lamm, E. W., and Yutzy, C. V.: Eosinophilic gastroenteritis. Arch. Surg., 92:476, 1966.
20. Jegher, H., McKusick, V. A., and Katz, K. H.: Generalized intestinal polyposis and melanin spots of oral mucosa, lips and digits. N. Engl. J. Med., 241:993, 1949.
21. Kepes, J. J., and Zacharias, D. L.: Gangliocytic paragangliomas of the duodenum. Cancer, 27:61, 1971.
22. Laarman, G. J., van der Wall, E. E., Muller, J. W., Eggink, H. D., and Hoekstra, J. B.: Extreme adenomatous hyperplasia of Brunner's glands in the proximal jejunum. Neth. J. Med., 32:20, 1988.
23. Loehr, W. J., Mujahed, Z., Zahn, F. D., Gray, G. F., and Thorbjarnarson, B.: Primary lymphoma of the gastrointestinal tract: A review of 100 cases. Ann. Surg., 170:232, 1969.
24. MacDonald, R. A.: Study of 356 carcinoids of gastrointestinal tract: Report of four new cases of carcinoid syndrome. Am. J. Med., 21:867, 1956.
25. Manley, K. A., and Skyring, A. P.: Some heritable causes of gastrointestinal disease. Arch. Intern. Med., 107:182, 1961.
26. Mason, G. R., Guernsey, J. M., Hanks, G. E., and Nelson, T. S.: Surgical therapy for radiation enteritis. Oncology, 22:251, 1968.
27. McKelvey, E. M., Gottlieb, J. A., Wilson, H. E., et al.: Hydroxyldaunomycin (Adriamycin) combination chemotherapy in malignant lymphoma. Cancer, 38:1484, 1976.
28. Persson, P., Karlen P., Bernell, O., Leijonmarck, C., Brostrom, O., Ahlborn, A., and Hellers, G.: Crohn's disease and cancer: A population based cohort study. Gastroenterology, 107:1675, 1994.
29. Raiford, T. S.: Tumors of small intestine. Arch. Surg., 25:112, 1932.
30. Ravitch, M. M.: Discussion of "a new form of diffuse familial polyposis" by Carter, B. N., Horsley, G. W., Horsley, J. J., and Hughes, R. D. Ann. Surg., 167:942, 1968.
31. River, L., Silverstein, J., and Tope, J. W.: Benign neoplasms of the small intestine: A critical comprehensive review with reports of 20 new cases. Int. Abstr. Surg., 102:1, 1956.
32. Rochlin, D. B., and Longmire, W. P., Jr.: Primary tumors of the small intestine. Surgery, 50:586, 1961.
33. Ross, J. R. E., and Mara, J. E.: Small bowel polyps and carcinoma in multiple intestinal polyposis. Arch. Surg., 108:736, 1974.
34. Sachatello, C. R., Pickren, J. W., and Grace, J. T., Jr.: Generalized juvenile gastrointestinal polyposis: A hereditary syndrome. Gastroenterology, 58:699, 1970.
35. Schwartz, S. S.: Book review of "Clinical Radiology of the Small Intestine" by Herlinger, H., and Maglinre, D. Gastroenterology, 97:1347, 1989.
36. Skaane, P., Eide, T. J., Westgaard, T., and Guaperaa, T.: Lipomatosis and true lipomas of the ileocecal valve. Fortschr. Rontgenstr., 135:663, 1989.
37. Starr, G. F., and Dockerty, M. B.: Leiomyomas and leiomyosarcomas of the small intestine. Cancer, 8:101, 1955.
38. Strodel, W. E., Talpos, G., Eckhauser, F., and Thompson, N.: Surgical therapy for small-bowel carcinoid tumors. Arch. Surg., 118:39, 1988.
39. Vinik, A., and Moattari, A. R.: Use of somatostatin analog in management of carcinoid syndrome. Dig. Dis. Sci., 34:14S, 1989.
40. Wattenberg, L. W.: Studies of polycyclic hydrocarbon hydroxylases of the intestine possibly related to cancer. Cancer, 28:99, 1971.

VI

VASCULAR COMPRESSION OF THE DUODENUM

Bruce D. Schirmer, M.D.

HISTORICAL ASPECTS

Vascular compression of the duodenum has had varying amounts of attention in the medical literature since its initial description by von Rokitansky[37] in 1842. In the late nineteenth century, Kundrat attributed incomplete duodenal obstruction to compression by the root of the mesentery.[1] In 1907, Bloodgood[6] reported three cases of fatal gastromesenteric ileus and suggested that an operative approach, creating a duodenojejunostomy, might prove helpful in such patients. This operation was successfully performed one year later by Stavely.[34]

By the 1920s, duodenojejunostomy to treat both duodenal obstruction and duodenal stasis was employed frequently relative to today's standards. In 1927, Wilkie[40] reported a series of 64 such operations with a 6% mortality rate. In 1933, Pool and colleagues[28] emphasized the then-current opinion that chronic duodenal stasis could benefit from timely operation under certain circumstances. This report marked the

height of the syndrome's popularity in the literature at that time. Since the differentiation between duodenal stasis and obstruction was never clearly defined in many of the early reports, results of treatment for the condition were variable, and popularity for surgical treatment markedly declined during the next two decades.

Attention to the problem increased in the 1960s,[5] including articles that suggested that the syndrome did not exist.[9] By the early 1970s, there was further interest in the subject and support for the syndrome's existence, as demonstrated by reports that more clearly defined the anatomic and clinical characteristics of patients with the condition,[22] as well as other reports of various clinical settings in which the condition occurred.[7, 11, 29, 38, 39]

During the twentieth century, this syndrome has been given various names in the literature. *Vascular compression of the duodenum* most accurately reflects the anatomic situation that is believed to produce this constellation of symptoms. It is also commonly known as *superior mesenteric artery syn-*

drome.[38] Other terms include Wilkie's syndrome,[40] cast syndrome,[10] chronic intermittent arteriomesenteric occlusion of the duodenum,[13] and arteriomesenteric duodenal obstruction.[35]

CLINICAL PICTURE

The symptoms that typically characterize vascular compression of the duodenum arise from obstruction of the third portion of the duodenum as it crosses under the superior mesenteric artery (Fig. 30–27). These include profound nausea and vomiting, abdominal distention, postprandial epigastric pain, and weight loss. Acute symptoms are classically relieved when the patient adopts the knee-chest, the left lateral, or occasionally the prone position. Symptoms vary from intermittent to constant, depending on the severity of the duodenal obstruction. If nausea and vomiting become protracted, dehydration can follow. Profound dehydration, cachexia, and aspiration as a result of vomiting have all caused death in patients with this problem.

Weight loss usually occurs before the onset of symptoms and contributes to the syndrome. The syndrome is most commonly seen in young asthenic individuals, with women being more commonly affected than men.

ANATOMY

The superior mesenteric artery originates behind the neck of the pancreas at the level of the first lumbar vertebra. Its origin is about 1.25 cm. below the celiac axis, and it exits the aorta at an acute angle through which passes the left renal vein and the uncinate process of the pancreas (Fig. 30–28). The duodenum crosses the lumbar spine from right to left, and there is a distinct ascendancy of the fourth portion of the duodenum relative to the third, which lies more posterior and to the right of the spine (see Fig. 30–27). It is at this

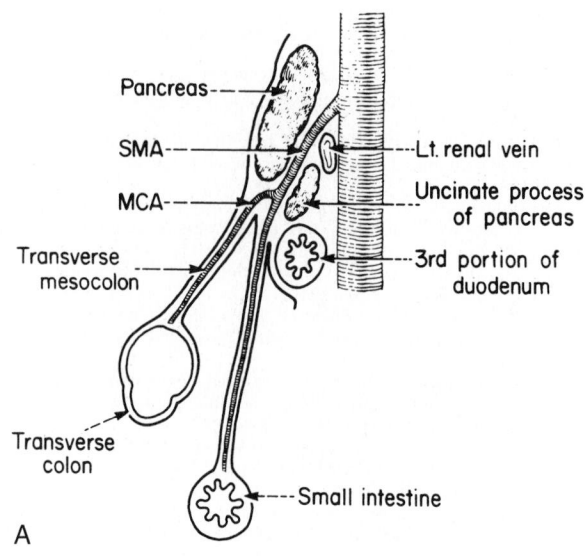

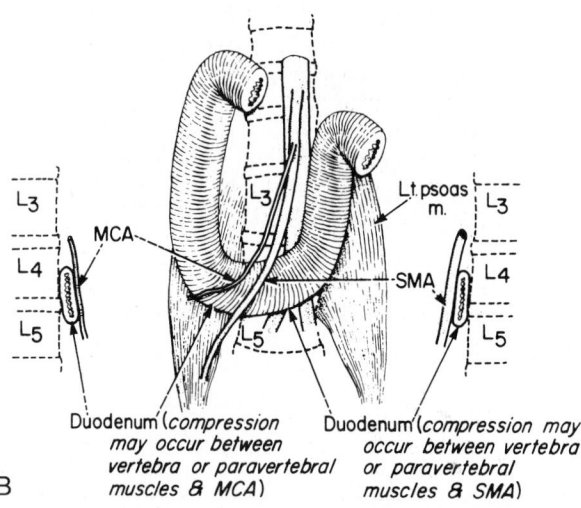

Figure 30–28. *A,* Diagrammatic sagittal section through the neck of the pancreas showing the relation of the third portion of the duodenum to the superior mesenteric artery (SMA), the middle colic artery (MCA), the aorta, and the mesentery. *B,* Anterior view of the duodenum, the SMA, the MCA, and the vertebral column. (From Akin, J. T., Gray, S. W., and Skandalakis, J. E.: Vascular compression of the duodenum: Presentation of ten cases and review of the literature. Surgery, *79:*515, 1976.)

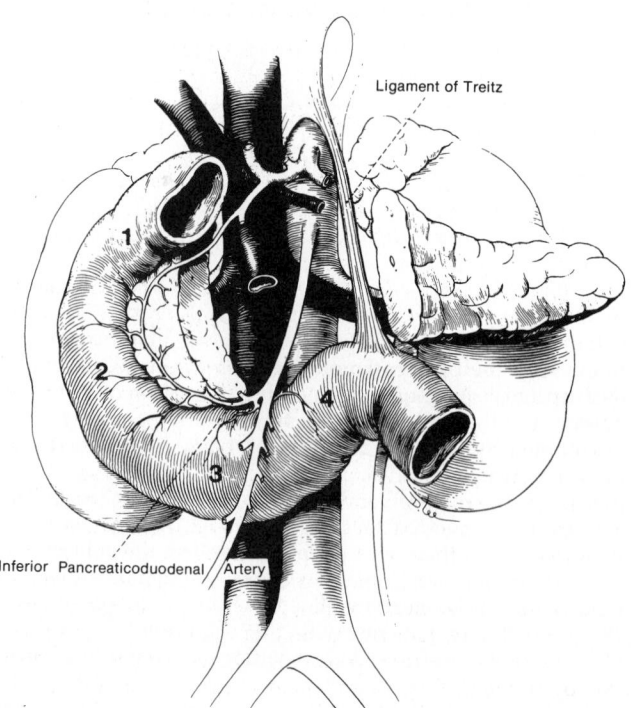

Figure 30–27. Anatomic structures involved in vascular compression of the duodenum. The numbers refer to the four portions of the duodenum. (From Thompson, N. W., and Stanley, J. C.: Vascular compression of the duodenum and peptic ulcer disease. Arch. Surg., *108:*674, 1974. Copyright 1974, American Medical Association.)

point, where the duodenum passes both upward and over the spine, that the bowel is most susceptible to anterior compression causing obstruction (see Fig. 30–28B). Lumbar lordosis is maximal at about the level of the fourth lumbar vertebra, accounting for occasional duodenal compression at this level.

The angle of the origin of the superior mesenteric artery from the aorta ranges from 30 to 41 degrees.[22] The distance from the angle of origin of the vessel to the duodenal midpoint (aortomesenteric distance) averages 10 cm. Studies of *in vivo* subjects by both Mansberger and co-workers[22] and Hearn[15] obtained measurements using simultaneous barium contrast studies and arteriography to define shortened mesenteric distances and markedly narrowed aortomesenteric angles in patients diagnosed with the syndrome (Fig. 30–29). Lukes and colleagues[21] reported an average aortomesenteric angle of only 8 degrees in three patients with vascular compression of the duodenum, as opposed to 37 degrees in

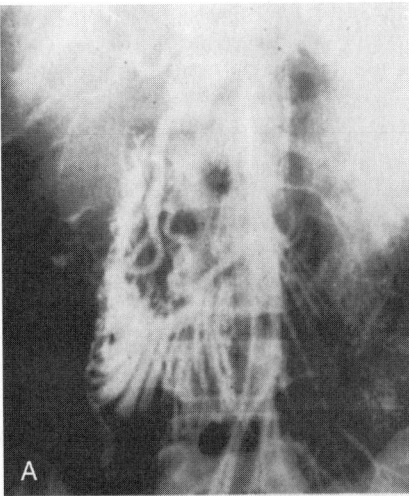
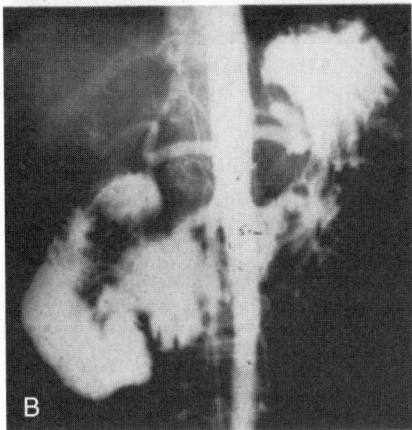

Figure 30–29. Combined gastrointestinal barium and aortography study revealing the point of compression and abnormal course of the superior mesenteric artery.

controls; the average aorta-to-mesentery distance was 3.3 mm. versus 18 mm. in controls (Fig. 30–30).

Factors that cause these anatomic differences include weight loss, with concomitant loss of fat normally located within the aortomesenteric angle; excessive lumbar lordosis; high fixation of the ligament of Treitz; the supine position; and a low origin of the superior mesenteric artery.[22]

DIAGNOSIS

Vascular compression of the duodenum is diagnosed radiologically, in the presence of the appropriate clinical findings. The most characteristic diagnostic criterion is the abrupt or near-total cessation of flow of barium from the duodenum to the jejunum during an upper gastrointestinal series (Fig. 30–31). Fluoroscopy helps confirm the diagnosis by allowing observation of what is usually described as a *to-and-fro peristalsis* of the barium in the proximal duodenum that is usually associated with significant pathologic change.[2] The termination is usually the distal third portion of the duodenum, where the anatomic course of the bowel is anterior and upward across the spine. Further confirmation is obtained by the abrupt relief of symptoms when barium passes the obstruction point as the patient assumes a position, such as the knee-chest position, that facilitates the relief of the obstruction. Hypotonic duodenography is actually the most accurate contrast study for making the diagnosis. It proved accurate when conventional barium studies were not diagnostic in several studies.[14, 21]

Computed tomography (CT) has been helpful in making the diagnosis radiologically, since this single study can demonstrate both duodenal distention and the close proximity of the superior mesenteric vessels. In one report, the symptoms resolved after improved nutrition but without a significant amount of new adipose tissue being deposited in the retroperitoneal area.[32]

Intraoperative confirmation of the diagnosis can be achieved by gastroduodenal insufflation with 150 to 300 ml. of air through a nasogastric tube.[17, 36] This maneuver, when followed by duodenal diameter dilatation of more than 3 to 4 cm., confirms distal duodenal obstruction.

The differential diagnosis of symptoms typical for vascular compression of the duodenum includes peptic ulcer disease, biliary tract disease, pancreatitis, and duodenitis. Obstruction of the duodenum or proximal jejunum from metastatic or primary tumors or metastatic involvement of the adjacent periaortic lymph nodes also produces similar symptoms.[2] Less common disorders such as visceral neuropathy, collagen vascular diseases, neuromuscular disorders, vitamin B deficiency, porphyria, postvagotomy syndrome, and surgical adhesions can also mimic vascular compression of the duodenum. Occlusion of the third portion of the duodenum by a phytobezoar can present with symptoms of vascular compression of the duodenum.[8]

INCIDENCE

The actual incidence of vascular compression of the duodenum is unknown, but it probably rarely occurs in its significantly symptomatic form. The combined incidence of the syndrome, as reported by several reviews, is shown in Table 30–13. Data have been obtained by reviewing either a hospital's experience of upper gastrointestinal series or overall hospital records. The syndrome may be more common in chronic care hospitals.[20]

ASSOCIATED CLINICAL SETTINGS

Associated clinical conditions that are predisposing factors for vascular compression of the duodenum, aside from weight loss, include supine immobilization, scoliosis, and the placement of a body cast. Akin and associates[1] found that approximately 25% of patients with vascular compression of the duodenum have one of these etiologic factors, whereas another 25% have weight loss as an aggravating factor, leaving 50% of the patients diagnosed with this condition as *idiopathic*.

Prolonged nausea and vomiting with gastric and duodenal dilatation after placement of a body cast was first referred to as the *cast syndrome* by Dorph.[10] Most cases of the cast syndrome have been reported in young patients, many of whom were treated for scoliosis, but the number of reported cases is low.[11, 16]

Two reviews of large series of patients treated in burn units reported the incidence of vascular compression of the duodenum to be 0.8%[38] and 1.12%[29] in this population. The syndrome occurred exclusively in patients with burns over more than 30% of the total body surface, and almost all had experienced significant weight loss (average 25.3% of initial body mass). Most patients developed the syndrome soon after injury. Gastroduodenal ulceration, aspiration, and sepsis were frequent concurrent problems. The syndrome may also develop with acute traumatic quadriplegia, where immobilization is a contributing factor.[31]

An association between vascular compression of the duodenum and peptic ulcer disease has been observed. One review showed that 32% of 291 patients described since 1960 had associated peptic ulcer disease.[36] Peptic ulcer disease was

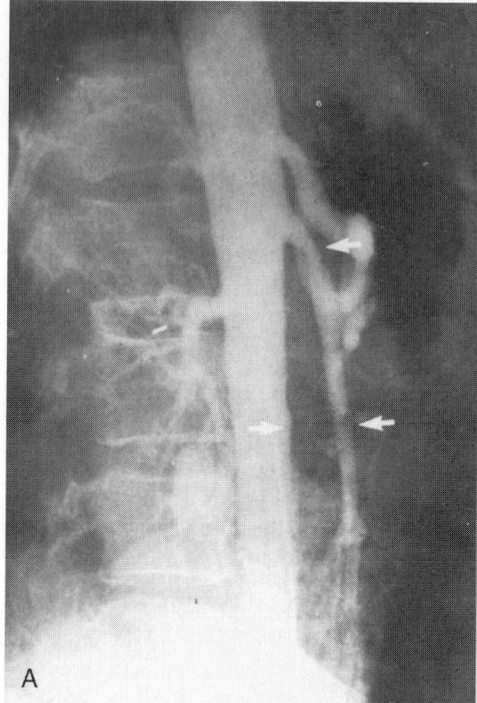
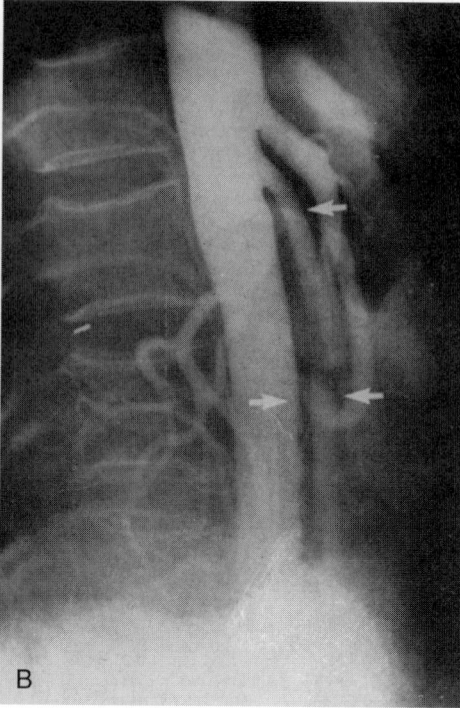

Figure 30–30. *A,* Abdominal aortography, lateral projection, normal case. *B,* Narrowed aortomesenteric angle and decreased aortomesenteric distance. (From Lukes, P. J., Rolny, P., Nilson, A. E., et al.: Diagnostic value of hypotonic duodenography in superior mesenteric artery syndrome. Acta Chir. Scand., *144:*39, 1978.)

most commonly associated with the chronic form of vascular compression of the duodenum, typically in men of normal body habitus.

Vascular compression of the duodenum has been reported in association with anorexia nervosa.[27] It has occurred following total proctocolectomy and J-pouch anal anastomosis;[3] reports implicate the process of placing the terminal ileum into the anal canal as possibly putting traction on the mesentery and contributing to duodenal compression. The syndrome has also been reported following resection of an arteriovenous malformation of the cervical cord.[4]

Traumatic mesenteric arteriovenous fistula causing compression of the duodenum from a false aneurysm has presented as the syndrome.[30] It has also been reported following repair of an abdominal aortic aneurysm.[19]

Marchant and colleagues[23] described the syndrome in 13 pediatric patients seen from 1974 to 1986. Of interest is the fact that 7 of the 13 were within the normal height and weight ranges for their age group, indicating that the syndrome need not be preceded by significant weight loss in children. A large series of pediatric patients with vascular compression of the duodenum has been described,[7] but most of these patients had either rapid growth or weight loss as part of the clinical picture. It has also been reported following orthopedic procedures, usually spinal operations, in patients whose average percentile for weight was only 18%.[16] Pediatric patients with this syndrome appear to be relatively free of the associated peptic ulcer disease seen in adults. One report in the literature describes vascular compression of the duodenum occurring in a familial cluster, with five of eight family members having the problem.[26]

TREATMENT

Treatment for the syndrome of vascular compression of the duodenum varies. Generally, conservative measures are

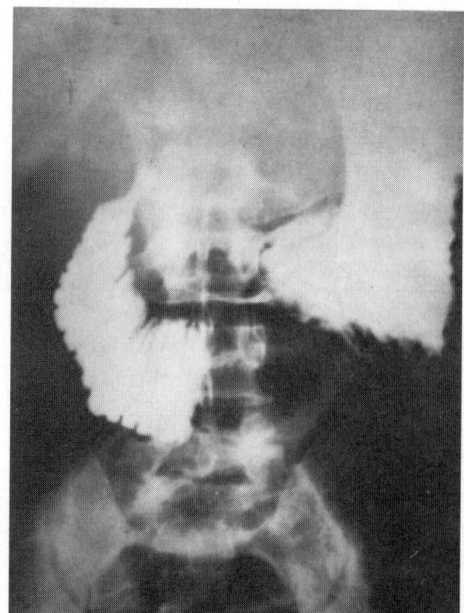

Figure 30–31. Radiograph from upper gastrointestinal series, supine position, showing complete obstruction of the duodenum. (From Reckler, J. M., Bruch, E. M., Munster, A. M., et al.: Superior mesenteric artery syndrome as a consequence of burn injury. J. Trauma, *12*(Nov):979–985, 1972.)

TABLE 30–13. Incidence of Vascular Compression of the Duodenum

Authors	No. of Cases Reviewed	No. Discovered	%
Goin and Wilk[13]	2080 (UGI series)	7	0.34
Anderson et al.[2]	6000 (UGI series)	12	0.20
Lee and Mangla[20]	3108 (chronic care hospital records)	3	0.0965
Lee and Mangla[20]	577,773 (acute care hospital records)	14	0.0024

UGI, upper gastrointestinal.

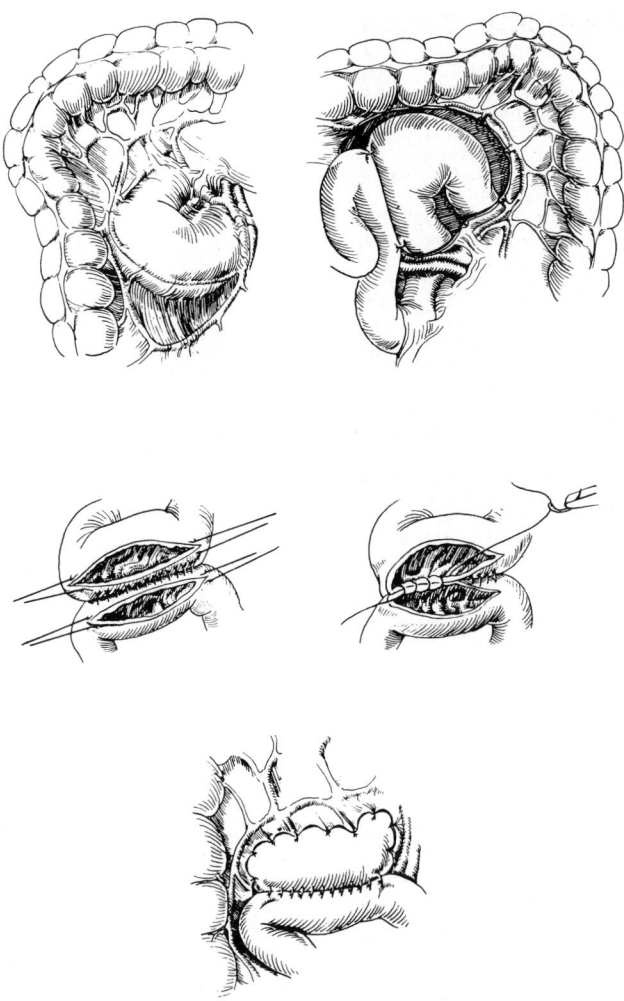

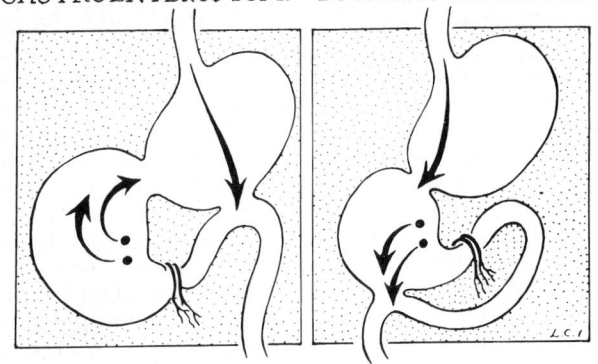

Figure 30–33. Gastroenterostomy necessitates a regurgitation of bile and pancreatic juice into the stomach, which is eliminated by a duodenojejunostomy. (From Jones, A. S., Carter, R., Smith, L. L., and Jorgensen, E. J.: Arteriomesenteric duodenal compression. Am. J. Surg., *100*:262, 1960.)

Figure 30–32. Duodenojejunostomy for vascular compression of the duodenum.

begun initially.[2] In recent years, such measures have been increasingly successful as definitive treatment.[12, 16, 19, 24, 33] Most patients reported in the literature, however, have been successfully treated surgically. There are two surgical approaches. The more common approach is a diverting bypass, with a duodenojejunostomy being the most frequently reported. The other includes performing some detachment of

the bowel from the ligament of Treitz, with or without additional derotation and resuspension of the parts of the bowel.

In 1958, Strong[35] advocated dividing the ligament of Treitz with downward displacement of the duodenum as definitive treatment. The derotation operation, developed more recently,[7] involves dividing not only the retroperitoneal attachments of the duodenum but also those of the right colon. The derotated small bowel is placed in the right abdominal gutter, and the colon is placed to the left. This operation has most commonly been performed by pediatric surgeons, based on their experience in treating Ladd's bands in congenital malrotation. This approach in the pediatric population has been about 90% successful.[7, 23]

Duodenojejunostomy is the operative treatment of choice for vascular compression of the duodenum and is illustrated in Figure 30–32. In one early review,[28] the authors dismissed all other operative treatments as ineffective. Another report concluded that Strong's operation failed to resolve the problem and that duodenojejunostomy was later required.[18] The disadvantage of using a gastroenterostomy for this problem is shown in Figure 30–33. The collective major reviews of this subject and the success of operative treatment are shown in Table 30–14. Medical treatment before surgical intervention is generally recommended.[13, 17]

Patients with the syndrome after placement of a body cast or a spinal procedure can be successfully treated conservatively with cast removal, nasogastric decompression, and intravenous fluid replacement.[16] Operative treatment has

TABLE 30–14. Results of Surgical Treatment of Vascular Compression of the Duodenum

Authors	No. of Operations Performed (% Successful)		
	Duodenojejunostomy	**Lysis of Ligament of Treitz**	**Gastrojejunostomy**
Barner and Sherman[5]	161 (95%)	6 (?)	31 (71%)
Pool et al.[28]	11 (82%)	—	—
Marchant et al.[23]		9 (89%)	1 (100%)
Burrington and Wayne[7]	2 (100%)	11 (100%)	—
Goin and Wilk[13]	2 (100%)	—	—
Reckler et al.[29]	5 (80%)	—	2 (100%)
Gustafsson et al.[14]	10 (100%)	—	1 (100%)
Jones et al.[17]	12 (100%)	—	5 (40%)
Lee and Mangla[20]			
Own series	8 (87.5%)	5 (80%)	2 (0%)
Reviewed	50 (92%)	24 (87.5%)	11 (63.6%)
Total	261 (94%)	55 (90%)	53 (66%)

been necessary less often in recent years, probably because supportive care has improved. Occasionally, those with the cast syndrome can be successfully treated with total parenteral nutrition.[25]

Often appropriate patient positioning and supportive care are all that is needed to relieve the symptoms of vascular compression of the duodenum. The Stryker frame can be used to position patients in the facedown position and relieve duodenal compression.[39]

Past studies suggested that nonoperative treatment should be used initially for severely burned patients only when suitable positioning to relieve the obstructive symptoms can be achieved. Otherwise, initial operative treatment produces better survival.[29, 38] However, in those early years, by the time the diagnosis was confirmed, patients were in an advanced state of malnutrition, weight loss, and deterioration, with a high failure rate for conservative measures.

SELECTED REFERENCES

Gustafsson, L., Falk, A., Lukes, P. J., and Gamklou, R.: Diagnosis and treatment of superior mesenteric artery syndrome. Br. J. Surg., 71:499, 1984.
This review summarizes the critical aspects of confirming the diagnosis of this syndrome and the treatment options available. It is one of the best articles on the subject.

Jones, A. S., Carter, R., Smith, L. L., and Jorgensen, E. J.: Arteriomesenteric duodenal compression. Am. J. Surg., 100:262, 1960.
This article covers experience with the syndrome up to 1960, emphasizing anatomic and diagnostic criteria. Preoperative and intraoperative confirmation of the diagnosis is detailed.

Mansberger, A. R., Hearn, J. B., Byers, R. M., et al.: Vascular compression of the duodenum. Am. J. Surg., 115:89, 1968.
This article documents the anatomic basis for the syndrome, providing data from gastrointestinal and arteriographic radiographs as well as autopsy studies.

Marchant, E. A., Alvear, D. T., and Fagelman, K. M.: True clinical entity of vascular compression of the duodenum in adolescence. Surgery, 168:381, 1963.
This well-written article details the diagnosis and treatment of this condition in the adolescent population. The efficacy of the derotation operation is described.

Milner, E. A., Cioffi, W. G., McManus, W. F., and Pruitt, B. A., Jr.: Superior mesenteric artery syndrome in a burn patient. Nutr. Clin. Practice, 8:264, 1993.
This review emphasizes current thinking regarding the benefits of providing appropriate nutritional support, preferably via the enteral route, to patients with this condition and thereby increasing the chances of successful nonoperative management.

REFERENCES

1. Akin, J. T., Gray, S. W., and Skandalakis, J. E.: Vascular compression of the duodenum: Presentation of ten cases and review of the literature. Surgery, 79:515, 1976.
2. Anderson, J. R., Earnshaw, P. M., and Fraser, G. M.: Extrinsic compression of the third part of the duodenum. Clin. Radiol., 33:75, 1982.
3. Ballantyne, G. H., Graham, S. M., Hammers, L., and Modlin, I. M.: Superior mesenteric artery syndrome following ileal J-pouch anal anastomosis: An iatrogenic cause of early postoperative obstruction. Dis. Colon Rectum, 30:472, 1987.
4. Balmaseda, M. T., Jr., Gordon, C., Cunningham, M. L., and Clairmone, A. C.: Superior mesenteric artery syndrome after resection of an arteriovenous malformation in the cervical cord. Am. J. Gastroenterol., 82:896, 1987.
5. Barner, H. B., and Sherman, C. D.: Vascular compression of the duodenum. Int. Abstr. Surg., 117:103, 1963.
6. Bloodgood, J. C.: Acute dilatation of the stomach, gastromesenteric ileus. Ann. Surg., 46:736, 1907.
7. Burrington, J. D., and Wayne, E. R.: Obstruction of the duodenum by the superior mesenteric artery—does it exist in children? J. Pediatr. Surg., 9:733, 1974.
8. Chung, S. C., Leung, J. W., and Li, A. K.: Phytobezoar masquerading as

9. Cohen, L. B., Field, S. P., and Sachar, D. B.: The superior mesenteric artery syndrome: The disease that isn't, or is it? J. Clin. Gastroenterol., 7:113, 1985.
10. Dorph, M. H.: The cast syndrome: Review of the literature and report of a case. N. Engl. J. Med., 243:440, 1950.
11. Evarts, C. M., Winter, R. B., and Hall, J. E.: Vascular compression of the duodenum associated with the treatment of scoliosis. J. Bone Joint Surg. [Am.], 53:431, 1971.
12. Fromm, S., and Cash, J. M.: Superior mesenteric artery syndrome: An approach to the diagnosis and management of upper gastrointestinal obstruction of unclear etiology. S. D. J. Med., 43:5, 1990.
13. Goin, L. S., and Wilk, S. P.: Intermittent arteriomesenteric occlusion of the duodenum. Radiology, 67:729, 1958.
14. Gustafsson, L., Falk, A., Lukes, P. J., and Gamklou, R.: Diagnosis and treatment of superior mesenteric artery syndrome. Br. J. Surg., 71:499, 1984.
15. Hearn, J. B.: Duodenal ileus with special reference to superior mesenteric artery compression. Radiology, 86:305, 1966.
16. Hutchinson, D. T., and Bassett, G. S.: Superior mesenteric artery syndrome in pediatric orthopedic patients. Clin. Orthop. Rel. Res., 250:250, 1990.
17. Jones, A. S., Carter, R., Smith, L. L., and Jorgensen, E. J.: Arteriomesenteric duodenal compression. Am. J. Surg., 100:262, 1960.
18. Kalouche, I., Leturgie, C., Tronc, F., Bokobza, B., Michot, F., Pons, P., and Menard, G.: The superior mesenteric artery syndrome: Apropos of a case and review of the literature. Ann. Chir., 45:609, 1991.
19. Lamont, P. M., Clarke, P. J., and Collin, J.: Duodenal obstruction after abdominal aortic aneurysm repair. Eur. J. Vasc. Surg., 6:107, 1992.
20. Lee, C. S., and Mangla, J. C.: Superior mesenteric artery compression syndrome. Am. J. Gastroenterol., 70:141, 1978.
21. Lukes, P. J., Rolny, P., Nilson, A. E., et al.: Diagnostic value of hypotonic duodenography in superior mesenteric artery syndrome. Acta Chir. Scand., 144:39, 1978.
22. Mansberger, A. R., Hearn, J. B., Byers, R. M., et al.: Vascular compression of the duodenum. Am. J. Surg., 115:89, 1968.
23. Marchant, E. A., Alvear, D. T., and Fagelman, K. M.: True clinical entity of vascular compression of the duodenum in adolescence. Surgery, 168:381, 1963.
24. Milner, E. A., Cioffi, W. G., McManus, W. F., and Pruitt, B. A., Jr.: Superior mesenteric artery syndrome in a burn patient. Nutr. Clin. Practice, 8:264, 1993.
25. Munns, S. W., Morrissy, R. T., Golladay, E. S., and McKenzie, C. N.: Hyperalimentation for superior mesenteric artery (cast) syndrome following correction of spinal deformity. J. Bone Joint Surg. [Am.], 66:1175, 1984.
26. Ortiz, C., Cleveland, R. H., Blickman, J. G., Jaramillo, D., and Kim, S. H.: Familial superior mesenteric artery syndrome. Pediatr. Radiol., 20:588, 1990.
27. Pentlow, B. D., and Dent, R. G.: Acute vascular compression of the duodenum in anorexia nervosa. Br. J. Surg., 68:665, 1981.
28. Pool, E. H., Niles, W. L., and Martin, K. A.: Duodenal statis: Duodenojejunostomy. Ann. Surg., 98:587, 1933.
29. Reckler, J. M., Bruch, E. M., Munster, A. M., et al.: Superior mesenteric artery syndrome as a consequence of burn injury. J. Trauma, 12:979, 1972.
30. Reed, J. K., McGiin, R. F., Gorman, J. F., and Thomford, N. R.: Traumatic mesenteric arteriovenous fistula presenting as the superior mesenteric artery syndrome. Arch. Surg., 121:1209, 1986.
31. Roth, E. J., Fenton, L. L., Gaebler-Spira, D. J., et al.: Superior mesenteric artery syndrome in acute traumatic quadriplegia: Case reports and literature review. Arch. Phys. Med. Rehabil., 72:417, 1991.
32. Santer, R., Young, C., Rossi, T., and Riddlesberger, M. M.: Computed tomography in superior mesenteric artery syndrome. Pediatr. Radiol. 21:154, 1991.
33. Smith, J. S., Jr., and Cooney, R. N.: Superior mesenteric artery syndrome in a tube-fed patient. Nutr. Clin. Practice, 9:151, 1994.
34. Stavely, A. L.: Acute and chronic gastromesenteric ileus with cure in a chronic case by duodenojejunostomy. Bull. Johns Hopkins Hosp., 19:252, 1908.
35. Strong, E. K.: Mechanics of arteriomesenteric duodenal obstruction and direct surgical attack upon etiology. Ann. Surg., 148:725, 1958.
36. Thompson, N. W., and Stanley, J. C.: Vascular compression of the duodenum and peptic ulcer disease. Arch. Surg., 108:674, 1974.
37. von Rokitansky, C. A.: Handbuch der pathologischen anatomic, 1st ed. Vol. 3. Wien, Braumuller and Seidel, 1842.
38. Wallace, R. G., and Howard, W. B.: Acute superior mesenteric artery syndrome in the severely burned patient. Radiology, 94:307, 1970.
39. Wayne, E., Miller, R. E., and Eisenman, B.: Duodenal obstruction by the superior mesenteric artery in bedridden combat casualties. Ann. Surg., 174:339, 1971.
40. Wilkie, D. P. D.: Chronic duodenal ileus. Am. J. Med. Sci., 173:643, 1927.

VII

ADENOCARCINOMA OF THE STOMACH

Gene D. Branum, M.D., and Aaron S. Fink, M.D.

EPIDEMIOLOGY

Fifty years ago, 20% to 30% of all cancer deaths in the United States could be attributed to gastric cancer. Today, only 3% of cancer deaths in men and even fewer in women are due to this disease (Fig. 30–34).[7] Despite intense scrutiny over the past quarter century, the reasons for this dramatic decline remain unclear.

The 5-year survival rate for all patients with adenocarcinoma of the stomach diagnosed between 1983 and 1987 was 17%.[7, 8] Moreover, tumors thought to be localized at the time of attempted curative resection carried survival rates of around 50%. These statistics demonstrate the insidious nature of gastric cancer, which has remained unchanged despite diagnostic advances such as dual-contrast radiography and endoscopy.

It is estimated that 24,000 new cases of gastric cancer were diagnosed in 1994, with 15,000 in men and 9,000 in women. With an estimated 14,000 deaths in 1994, the death rate in the United States is approximately 7.5 per 100,000. From 1988 to 1991, Costa Rica had an incidence of 77.5 deaths per 100,000; Russia, Japan, and Chile all had rates near 50 per 100,000 (Table 30–15).[8] A significant percentage of cases in Japan are discovered *early*. This is most likely due to the aggressive mass screening program instituted within the last quarter century.

The etiology and risk factors for gastric cancer have been intensely studied. It is known that gastric cancer occurs more frequently in males than in females and that the incidence and mortality increase with age. Higher rates of gastric cancer are associated with lower socioeconomic status, partially explaining the epidemiology of the disease. Although no single etiologic factor has been proved as a direct cause of gastric carcinogenesis, some associations are strong enough to attempt studies in prevention.

Environmental Factors. The incidence of gastric cancer varies from country to country as well as regionally within countries. In the United States, the incidence of gastric cancer among African Americans, Asian Americans, and Hispanics is almost double that among whites. Studies of migrants from Japan to the United States indicate only a moderate decrease in their risk, even if they migrate at an early age.[28] Second-generation Japanese in the United States have gastric cancer risk rates much closer to those of the general U.S. population.[20] This suggests that environmental factors that are important early in life.

Diet. Dietary factors have received significant attention as potential factors in the development of gastric cancer.

Epidemiologic data support the fact that the decline in gastric cancer in the United States has paralleled significant improvements in food, hygiene, and sanitation as well as general dietary improvements, including year-round availability of fresh fruits and vegetables. Gastric cancer appears to be correlated with a high intake of preserved foods (e.g., foods containing high levels of salt, nitrates, and nitrites), pickled vegetables, and salt—all of which can act as gastric irritants.[11, 12, 18, 38] Nitrates and nitrites can clearly be converted to active carcinogens, the n-nitrosamines. Certainly, free radical–induced injury by nitrosamines and bacterial by-products of *Helicobacter pylori* are potentially damaging. Both ascorbic acid and beta-carotene found in fresh fruits and vegetables act as antioxidants; further, ascorbic acid can prevent the conversion of nitrites to nitrosamines.[38, 46]

***Helicobacter Pylori* and Chronic Gastritis.** There is growing evidence that *H. pylori* infection plays a role in the development of gastric cancer. Striking parallels exist between regional rates of gastric cancer and *H. pylori* infection.[38] For example, in Central American regions, where virtually all adults are infected, gastric cancer rates are among the highest in the world. Interestingly, despite high *H. pylori* infection rates, many of these populations have low duodenal ulcer rates.[38] Based on examinations of banked sera, it appears that the *H. pylori* infection rate is decreasing over time in the United States, in parallel with the decrease in gastric cancer.[39] The bacterium seems to be associated more with intestinal-type cancer than with the diffuse type.[39] Tumors of the antrum, fundus, and body seem to be associated with the infection, whereas tumors of the cardia are not.[39]

Three important case-controlled studies in Great Britain, California, and Hawaii showed increased risk of gastric cancer in individuals with positive *H. pylori* antibody titers.[38, 39] Patients in these studies were followed from 6 to 25 years, and their estimated increases in relative risk were from 2.9- to 6-fold.

Although *H. pylori* is not known to produce carcinogens that directly damage gastric epithelia, several toxins such as ammonia and acetaldehyde are produced, which could lead to chronic inflammation and epithelial damage.[51] The link between *H. pylori* and gastric cancer is strengthened by the fact that *H. pylori* infection causes more than 80% of chronic gastritis cases.[47, 51] In addition, chronic *H. pylori* infection, if untreated, usually leads to chronic atrophic gastritis with metaplasia, with an associated high risk of gastric cancer.[51]

Experimental evidence demonstrates that *H. pylori* causes epithelial cell proliferation and production of growth regulatory peptides.[38] In addition, ammonia production and the recruitment of inflammatory cells (neutrophils) are augmented. These neutrophils generate free radicals and chloramine, both of which cause direct DNA damage.[38] Human mucosal tissue infected with *H. pylori* has been demonstrated to produce excessive reactive oxygen species by chemiluminescense.[38] A model for gastric carcinogenesis involving *H. pylori* has been proposed (Fig. 30–35).[38]

Trials aimed at gastric cancer prevention by the treatment of *H. pylori* infection are currently under way. Should the link be proved and prevention become feasible, it is estimated that from 35% to 89% of gastric cancer cases could be prevented by eradication of *H. pylori*.[38]

Adenomatous Polyps. Adenomatous gastric polyps are

TABLE 30–15. Deaths from Gastric Cancer per 100,000 Population, 1988–91

Country	Number
Costa Rica	77.5
Russia	52.8
Japan	50.5
Chile	48.8
England/Wales	17.6
Canada	11.4
United States	7.5

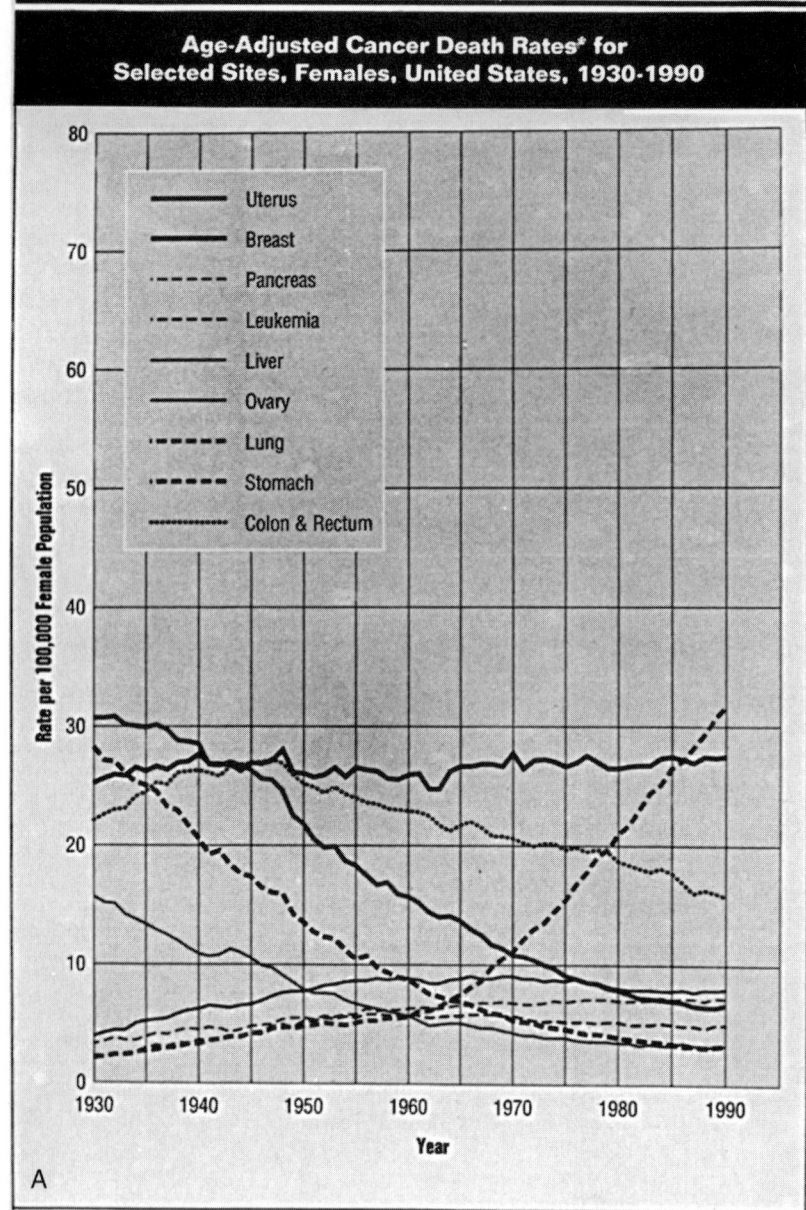

Figure 30–34. Cancer death rates for women *(A)* and men *(B)* in the United States, 1930 to 1990. (From Boring, C. C., Squires, T. S., Tong, T., and Montgomery, S.: Cancer statistics 1994. CA Cancer J. Clin., *44*:16, 1994.)

rare but carry a distinct potential for the development of malignancy. They occur most frequently between the fifth and seventh decades of life and have few symptoms or physical findings. The diagnosis is usually made on barium meal testing or as a coincidental finding during flexible fiberoptic endoscopy. The risk of developing cancer in adenomatous polyps is thought to be between 10% and 20% and is greatest for polyps 2 cm. or greater in diameter. The presence of an adenomatous polyp is a marker for increased risk of carcinogenesis in the remaining gastric mucosa. Pedunculated polyps should be removed endoscopically for pathologic examination. Wedge resection with a margin of normal mucosa is recommended for sessile polyps greater than 2 cm. in size. Patients with multiple polyposis or multiple recurrent adenomas should be considered for subtotal or total gastrectomy. Patients with frank malignancy and multiple polyps should undergo total gastrectomy.

Previous Gastric Operation. There is considerable evidence that gastric surgery for benign conditions increases the risk of gastric cancer by twofold to sixfold.[16, 36] Since the

increased incidence of malignancy occurs even though the most common site of gastric cancer (the antrum) has been resected, the risk may actually be greater. Most cases have occurred after Billroth II anastomosis, 15 to 20 years after the original surgical procedure.[36]

A sequence of events analogous to *H. pylori* infection with chronic atrophic gastritis is present after partial gastrectomy and vagotomy. The procedure causes hypo- or achlorhydria, allowing bacterial overgrowth. This bacterial overgrowth can lead to increased conversion of nitrites to nitrosamines, which, after a period of time, can cause metaplasia, dysplasia, and ultimately cancer. Cancers in the gastric remnant seem to have an especially poor prognosis. The lesions tend to present at a more advanced stage and in older patients, although the lesions themselves are no more aggressive than cancer arising in the intact stomach.[27] Routine radiologic endoscopic examinations in postgastrectomy patients beginning 15 years after their initial surgical procedures may improve treatment and survival in these patients due to earlier detection.

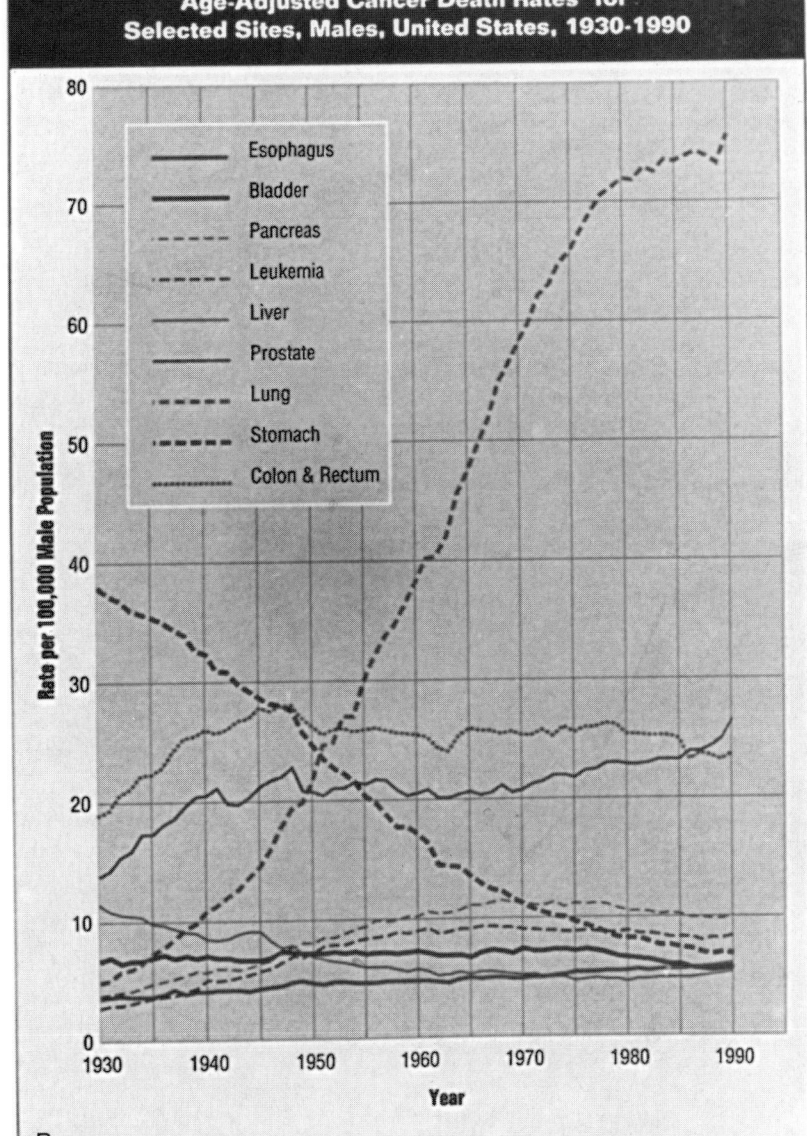

Figure 30–34 *Continued*

Other. Pernicious anemia and Ménétrier's disease have both been associated with gastric cancer. Based on the autopsy series by Zamcheck and associates in 1955, it was concluded that approximately 10% of patients with pernicious anemia might develop malignancy.[61] Hoffman later questioned the relationship between the two diseases after following 138 patients for 11 years, with no patient developing gastric cancer.[22]

Ménétrier's disease has clinical and roentgenologic findings that closely resemble multiple gastric polyps, and gastric cancer has been reported to occur in approximately 10% of cases. Interestingly, the majority of patients with Ménétrier's disease are hypochlorhydric, predisposing to the aforementioned mucosal injury sequence.

PATHOLOGY

Gastric adenocarcinoma can arise from gastric mucosal cells anywhere within the stomach. Tumors formerly arose with much greater frequency in the antral and pyloric re-

gions. However, most recent series indicate a much higher rate of involvement of the cardia and gastroesophageal junction than in the past.[10, 33, 44] This is an important observation, since the prognosis of proximal gastric tumors is worse than that for distal tumors. Approximately 10% to 15% of tumors are diffuse in character (linitis plastica), and the lesser curve is more commonly involved than the greater curve. It is unclear as yet whether the more proximal redistribution of tumors is a relative or absolute change. There is a much higher incidence of tumors of the cardia in smokers than of tumors elsewhere in the stomach.

In 1965, Lauren divided gastric cancers into intestinal and diffuse subtypes.[29] This classification is still used internationally and has prognostic importance. *Intestinal-type* tumors have a glandular structure resembling colonic carcinoma, with diffuse inflammatory cell infiltration and frequent intestinal metaplasia. The intestinal-type carcinomas are apparently preceded by a prolonged precancerous process and tend to predominate in geographic regions with a high incidence of gastric cancer. As regional gastric cancer risk is

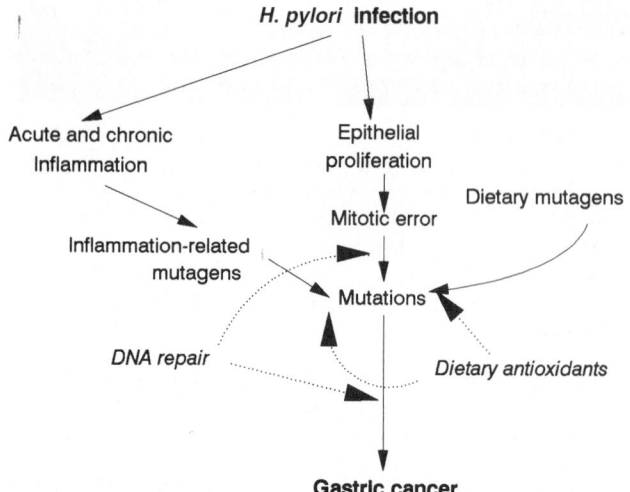

Figure 30–35. A model for gastric carcinogenesis incorporating *Helicobacter pylori* infection. Solid arrows indicate detrimental factors, and broken arrows indicate protective factors. *H. pylori*, by causing both proliferation and inflammation, increases the risk for mutation and eventual malignant transformation. (From Parsonnet, J.: *Helicobacter pylori* and gastric cancer. Gastroenterol. Clin. North Am., *22*:89, 1993.)

is seen with increasing frequency. Moreover, in the diffuse form of gastric cancer, lymphatic invasion and intraperitoneal metastases are frequently encountered. The diffuse subtype is seen more often in women, in younger patients, and in geographic regions where gastric cancer is less common.

Broeder's histologic grading system correlates well with survival in gastric cancer. The system classifies tumors as Grade I to IV, with Grade IV tumors representing the most anaplastic. Grade I patients have a 66% 5-year survival rate, whereas those with Grade IV tumors have an 11% 5-year survival rate.[8]

Ming's classification separates gastric tumors primarily by their biologic behavior, as evidenced by their growth pattern, rather than by their architectural structures. Gastric cancers are divided into *expanding-type* tumors, which form discrete tumor nodules that displace normal structures, and *infiltrative* tumors, in which the cells penetrate individually and widely, eventually causing diffuse gastric involvement. Expanding tumors tend to be fungating, whereas infiltrative tumors tend to be diffuse. Although both types of neoplasms are composed of mucin-producing cells, intestinal metaplasia occurs extensively only in expanding tumors, suggesting that the two types of cancers have a different histogenesis.[37] This scheme is similar to Lauren's classification but can be applied to unclassified tumors in Lauren's system.

Borrman proposed a gross classification of gastric cancer in 1926 (Fig. 30–36). The system is still used descriptively in the United States and is a more formal component of tumor staging in Japan. Borrman's four types supposedly have varying degrees of malignancy. Listed in ascending order of degree of malignancy, they are Group I—circumscribed, solitary, polypoid carcinomas without ulceration; Group II—ulcerated carcinomas with wall-like marginal elevation and sharply defined borders; Group III—partially ulcerated carci-

reduced, the intestinal-type tumors experience most of the reduction. *Diffuse-type* tumors are composed of tiny clusters of small uniform cells. In contrast to intestinal-type neoplasms, diffuse carcinomas are more widespread through the mucosa, have less inflammatory infiltration, and have a poorer prognosis. As the incidence of gastric cancer in the cardia becomes more predominant, the diffuse classification

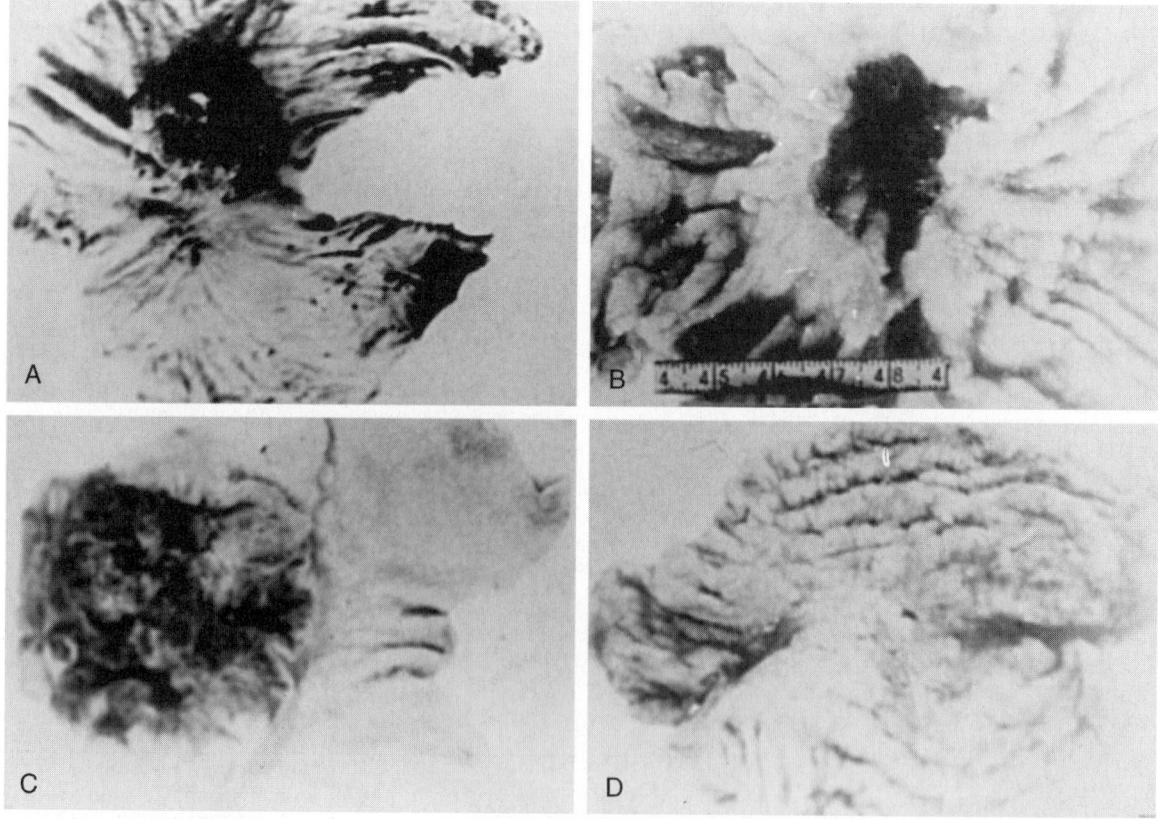

Figure 30–36. Illustrations of Borrman's classification of advanced gastric cancer. *A*, Type 1, polypoid. *B*, Type 2, ulcerating circumscribed. *C*, Type 3, ulcerating infiltrative. *D*, Type 4, diffusely infiltrative. (From Mori, M., and Sugimachi, K.: Clinicopathologic studies of gastric carcinoma. Semin. Surg. Oncol., *6*:19, 1990. Copyright © 1990. Reprinted by permission of John Wiley & Sons, Inc.)

TABLE 30–16. Genetic Alterations in Differentiated and Undifferentiated Gastric Cancer

Genetic Alteration	Differentiated Type, % (No.)	Undifferentiated Type, % (No.)
Amplification		
K-*sam*	0 (0/17)	21 (6/29)
c-*erb*B2	38 (5/13)	0 (0/27)
c-*met*	19 (5/26)	26 (10/38)
Point mutation		
c-Ki-*ras*	18 (3/17)	0 (0/18)
p53	42 (5/12)	33 (4/12)

From Katoh, M., and Terada, M.: Oncogenes and tumor suppressor genes. *In* Nishi, M., Schikawa, H., Nokajima, T., Maruyama, K., and Tahara, E. (Eds.): Gastric Cancer. Tokyo, Springer-Verlag, 1993.

nomas with marginal elevation and partial diffuse spread; Group IV—diffuse carcinomas.

Gastric cancers have several methods of extension, including spread within the gastric wall and into the regional lymphatics, as well as direct invasion of adjacent organs such as the liver, pancreas, transverse colon, or mesocolon. In addition, hematogenous spread via the portal vein to the liver or via the systemic circulation to the lungs, bones, and elsewhere produces distant metastases. Finally, involved gastric serosa can seed metastases throughout the peritoneum. The parietal peritoneum, ovary (Krukenberg's tumor), and other sites, including the pelvic cul-de-sac, may be involved. The latter may be palpated as a firm metastatic mass on rectal examination (Bloomer's shelf). Other named metastatic deposits include umbilical adenopathy (Sister Mary Joseph's node) and supraclavicular adenopathy, especially on the left (Virchow's node).

Molecular Genetics. The molecular and chromosomal alterations leading to the development of gastric adenocarcinoma of the stomach are under intense study (Tables 30–16 and 30–17). Investigation into the relationship between environmental factors and alteration in tumor suppressor genes and growth factors is in its infancy.

The relationship of the tumor suppressor gene p53 with the development and progression of gastric carcinoma has been evaluated.[30, 42] The p53 gene is located on chromosome 17p[13] and has 11 exons. The deletion of p53 or expression of aberrant p53 protein after missense mutation is regularly associated with transformation. Sano and co-workers found loss of heterozygosity at the p53 locus in 68% of gastric tumors.[45] More recently, Rhyu and colleagues found a 64% loss of heterozygosity in the malignant tissue, whereas no p53 alterations were found in the dysplastic gastric tissue surrounding the tumors. Moreover, analysis of the association of p53 abnormalities with the mutated in colon cancer (MCC) and the closely linked adenomatous polyposis coli (APC) genes (chromosome 5q) suggests that genetic alterations of all three genes may be related in gastric carcinogenesis.[9, 42, 57]

Allele loss has also been reported at the site of the deleted in colon cancer (DCC) gene on chromosome 18q.[59] As opposed to the p53 gene alterations, the 18q allele loss was identified in 60% of early intramucosal cases. Therefore, in gastric cancer, allele loss can occur on chromosomes 5q, 17p, and 18q.[59]

Alterations in epidermal growth factor (EGF) and its receptor (EGFR), as well as transforming growth factor alpha (TGFa), have been found in gastric cancer, Barrett's esophagus, and gastric metaplasia.[17, 55, 59] TGFa and EGFR are overexpressed in both esophageal and gastric cancer. Expression of the two is higher in the intestinal type (93%) than the diffuse type (30%). These early studies suggest that the increased expression and coexpression of EGFR and TGFa in precancer stages may represent an aberrant autocrine loop, which may play a role in malignant transformation.

The C-*erb*B-2 oncogene has also been demonstrated in gastric adenocarcinoma; malignant transformation may involve the loss of negative feedback control of the oncogene. C-*erb*B-2 overexpression was detected in 53% of intestinal-type tumors but only 8% of diffuse cancers, with gene amplifica-

TABLE 30–17. Genetic Alterations in Poorly and Well-Differentiated Stomach Cancer

Genetic Alteration	Frequency of Occurrence (%)	
	Poorly Differentiated Cancer Type	*Well-Differentiated Cancer Type*
Mutation		
K-*ras*	—	9
p53	66	50
APC	30*	40
Deletion		
p53	76	60
Chromosome 5q (APC locus)	—	60
Rb	7	5
bcl-2	—	43
Chromosome 18q (DCC locus)	—	50
Chromosome 1q	—	44
Chromosome 1p	38	25
Chromosome 7q (c-*met* locus)	—	50
Amplification		
c-*met*	39†	19
K-*sam*	33†	—
c-*erb*B2	—	18
Abnormal expression		
c-*met* 6.0 kb	73†	50

*Signet ring cell carcinoma.
†Scirrhous carcinoma.
From Tahara, E., Yokozaki, H., and Yasui, W.: Growth factors in gastric cancer. *In* Nishi, M., Schikawa, H., Nokajima, T., Maruyama, K., and Tahara, E. (Eds.): Gastric Cancer. Tokyo, Springer-Verlag, 1993.

tion detectable in 30% of cases.[60] It has been speculated that overexpression of EGFR and C-erbB-2 may be required in the early stages of carcinogenesis, with additional changes required for malignant development and progression. Since p53 alterations are rarely seen in metaplastic gastric epithelia and only rarely in dysplasia, it can be inferred that overexpression of EGFR and C-erbB-2 are early events, whereas p53 mutation is a late event in gastric carcinogenesis.

The K-sam oncogene is a rearranged fibroblast growth factor receptor gene whose amplification has been seen in higher percentages of undifferentiated compared with well-differentiated carcinomas.[59] Basic fibroblast growth factor 2 overexpression has been observed in gastric cancer.[59] The complexities of the interaction between fibroblast growth factor and EGF and their interactions with environmental or inflammatory (H. pylori) factors remain to be elucidated.

Staging. Staging of gastric cancer has evolved significantly over the past two decades. The Union Internacionale Contra la Cancrum (UICC) was the first to publish a classification system for stomach cancer in 1966, and this was updated in 1968. The American Joint Committee on Cancer (AJCC) established a task force on stomach cancer in 1969 to develop a classification system, the basis of which was published in 1970. The Japanese Cancer Committee (JCC), the AJCC, and the UICC independently met and updated their systems over the next 15 years. The surveillance, epidemiology, and end results (SEER) population-based study added more information, agreeing with the previous Japanese and American studies concerning the prognostic significance of depth of tumor invasion and regional lymphadenopathy. At international meetings held in 1983 and 1984, representatives of the UICC, AJCC, and JCC met to unify the classification system.[26] A unified staging system gradually evolved; in 1988, the publications of the UICC and AJCC contained the identical staging classification for gastric cancer. The current basis for gastric cancer staging in the United States is the AJCC staging classification, as published in the manual for staging of cancer.[4]

TNM Classification. Gastric cancer is staged according to the characteristics of the primary tumor (T), nodal metastases (N), and presence of metastatic disease (M). The most important prognostic indicators remain the depth of penetration by the primary tumor, the presence of cancer in local regional lymph nodes, and involvement of adjacent organs. Clinical classification of gastric cancer is based on diagnostic and pathologic data obtained prior to any surgical resection. Information may be gained from physical examination, imaging studies, endoscopy, and tissue obtained from primary or metastatic tumor.

Pathologic staging is based on the combination of clinical staging and analysis of resected specimens. Characteristics of the TNM assessments are presented in Table 30–18. Staging based on combinations of involvement is presented in Table 30–19.

Tumors are also grouped according to histopathologic type. Adenocarcinoma is the most common histopathologic type of gastric carcinoma. It may be further subdivided into intestinal, diffuse, and mixed histology, based on the Lauren classification. Other histopathologic types include papillary, tubular, or mucinous adenocarcinoma; signet ring cell carcinoma; squamous cell carcinoma; small cell carcinoma; and undifferentiated carcinoma. A grading system categorizes tumors as GX if grade cannot be assessed and G1 through G4 for well, moderately, poorly, and undifferentiated tumors. If controversy exists regarding staging of a tumor, the lower stage of those proposed should be assigned.

Early Gastric Cancer. With the frequent use of endoscopy in Japan, visualization and recognition of a superficial type of gastric cancer became possible. This entity was classified as early gastric cancer in 1962. The recognition of this tumor led to a mass screening program in Japan that, in 1988, led to the examination of approximately 5.2 million people over age 40. Of those screened, 6414 were discovered to have cancer, and most of these patients (98.7%) had operations. These patients represented 54% of detected cases, 62% of which were early gastric cancer.

Early gastric cancer is defined as disease involving the mucosa or submucosa, and as such may be fairly large. It may be associated with vague abdominal symptoms and positive lymph nodes at the time of resection (Fig. 30–37).[6] Early gastric cancer occurs predominantly in the distal stomach. Three types of macroscopic lesions are described: protruded (Type I), superficial (Type II), and excavated (Type

TABLE 30–19. American Joint Committee on Cancer's Stage Grouping of Gastric Cancer

Stage	TNM Classification		
0	Tis	N_0	M_0
IA	T_1	N_0	M_0
IB*	T_1	N_1	M_0
	T_2	N_0	M_0
II	T_1	N_2	M_0
	T_2	N_1	M_0
	T_3	N_0	M_0
IIIA	T_2	N_2	M_0
	T_3	N_1	M_0
	T_4	N_0	M_0
IIIB	T_3	N_2	M_0
	T_4	N_1	M_0
IV	T_4	N_2	M_0
	Any T	Any N	M_1

*Includes node-positive disease.

TABLE 30–18. TNM Classification

Primary Tumor (T)

T_1 Tumor limited to mucosa and submucosa regardless of its extent or location

T_2 Tumor involves the mucosa and the submucosa (including the muscularis propria) and extends to or into the serosa but does not penetrate through the serosa

T_3 Tumor prenetrates through the serosa without invading contiguous structures

T_4 Tumor penetrates through the serosa and invades the contiguous structures

Nodal Involvement (N)

N_0 No metastases to regional lymph nodes

N_1 Involvement of perigastric lymph nodes within 3 cm. of the primary tumor along the lesser or greater curvature

N_2 Involvement of the regional lymph nodes, more than 3 cm. from the primary tumor, which are removable at operation, including those located along the left gastric, splenic, celiac, and common hepatic arteries

N_3 Involvement of other intra-abdominal lymph nodes that are not removable at operation, such as the para-aortic, hepatoduodenal, retropancreatic, and mesenteric nodes

Distant Metastasis (M)

M_0 No (known) distant metastasis

M_1 Distant metastasis present

Surgical Results (R)

R_0 No residual tumor

R_1 Microscopic residual tumor

R_2 Macroscopic residual tumor

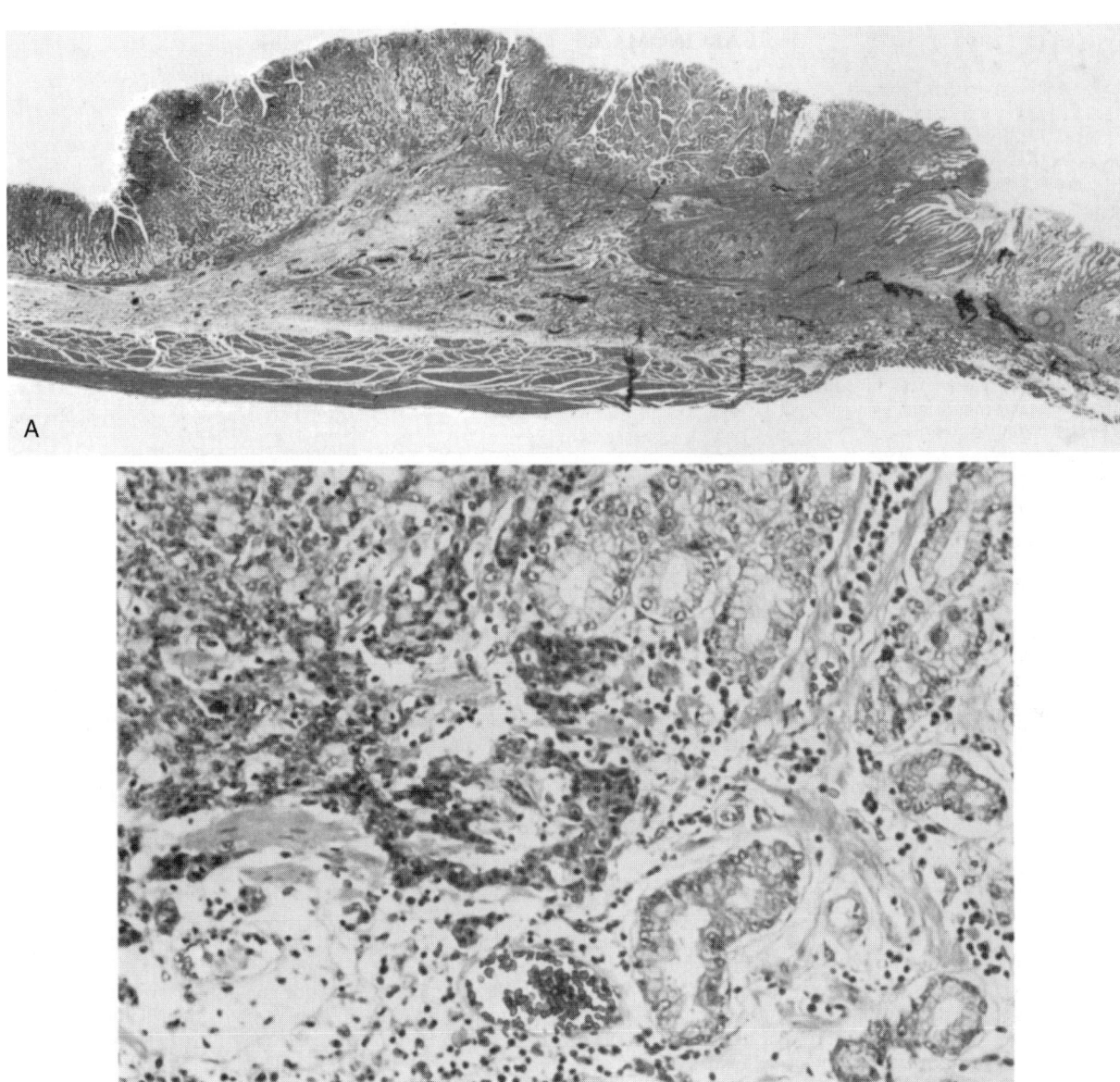

Figure 30–37. *A*, Photomicrograph of early gastric adenocarcinoma, Type IIa (superficial elevated type). *B*, Higher magnification of section from the same lesion, showing the junction of normal and neoplastic mucosa. (Courtesy of Professor Walter F. Coulson, Department of Pathology, UCLA School of Medicine.)

III) (Fig. 30–38). Type II is further divided into three subgroups, of which Type IIC is the most common. Although there have been objections that such a classification offers no special advantage over the TNM classification and that the TNM system provides greater prognostic significance, the Japanese classification appears to have stimulated recognition of this type of carcinoma by both endoscopists and radiologists. The Japanese and the TNM staging systems were reunified in 1993, and prognosis correlated well with stage. Unfortunately, early gastric cancer represents only 10% to 15% of diagnosed cases in Europe and North America.[58] Five-year survival after resection of early gastric cancer ranges from 70% to 95%, depending on the presence of nodal involvement.

Advanced Gastric Cancer. Advanced gastric cancer suggests invasion of the muscularis or beyond (Table 30–20). These lesions are frequently associated with distant or contiguous spread, have a higher stage, and are less often cured. Whereas advanced gastric cancer represents less than 50% of cases in Japan today, a recent survey by the American College

of Surgeons indicates that over 80% of cases in the United States were advanced gastric carcinomas at the time of diagnosis.

SYMPTOMS AND DIAGNOSIS

Regrettably, symptoms of early gastric cancer are vague and unspecific. They may mimic symptoms of benign gastric ulcer disease and may either be ignored by the patient or treated medically without further evaluation. Symptoms may not be evident until a tumor is of sufficient size to interfere significantly with gastric motor activity, decrease the size of the intraluminal passageway, or cause gross or occult bleeding from an ulcerated tumor mass.

Studies cite highly variable rates of symptoms in newly diagnosed patients.[33] Weight loss is clearly a symptom common to the series, occurring in from 20% to 60% of patients. The percentage of patients who present with abdominal pain is even more variable, ranging from 20% to 95%. A recent study of 18,000 patients in the United States revealed weight

CARCINOMA OF THE STOMACH

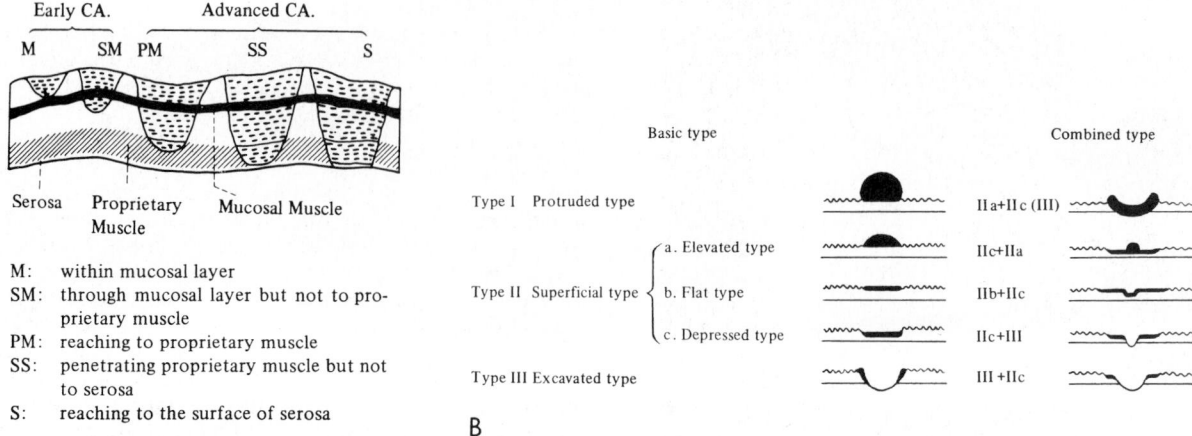

Figure 30–38. *A,* Schematic drawing of classification of carcinoma of the stomach based on depth of gastric wall penetration. *B,* Further detailed classification of early gastric cancer based on gross and microscopic presentation of the tumor in relation to the surrounding gastric wall. Classification proposed by Japanese Gastroenterological Endoscopic Society. (From Sakita, T., Oguro, Y., Takasu, S., Fukutomi, H., and Miwa, T.: The development of endoscopic diagnosis of early carcinoma of the stomach. Jpn. J. Clin. Oncol., *1*:118, 1971.)

loss in 62% and abdominal pain in 52%.[58] Nausea and anorexia were present in approximately 30%, dysphasia in 25%, and early satiety and ulcer-type pain in approximately 20%. Most studies cite weight loss and abdominal pain as the most common symptoms once symptoms occur.[58] Continuous abdominal pain generally suggests tumor extension beyond the stomach wall. Substernal or precordial pain may be associated with tumors of the cardia or gastroesophageal junction. Approximately 10% of patients present with signs or symptoms of disseminated disease, including supraclavicular or pelvic adenopathy, ascites, jaundice, or hepatomegaly.

Routine laboratory tests should include hematocrit, erythrocyte evaluation, liver function tests, and stool guaiac. In most cases of advanced disease, laboratory evidence of anemia develops; liver function tests are usually abnormal with hepatic metastasis. Currently, no serologic or gastric fluid tumor marker aids in the early diagnosis of gastric cancer.

Roentgenographic Studies

The double-contrast barium meal is a sensitive and cost-effective test for the detection of even small gastric cancers (Fig. 30–39). The technique was perfected in the 1950s by Shirakabe and colleagues.[48] In Japan, the technique of mass screening for gastric cancer involves the ingestion of 2 oz. of barium solution followed by six or seven radiographs from various angles, requiring only 3 to 4 minutes to perform.

Using this technique, approximately 87% of initial subjects are cleared, and 13% are subjected to further examinations.

A discussion of the nuances of the appearances of early gastric cancer on dual-contrast barium study is beyond the scope of this chapter, and the reader is referred to more detailed reports.[24] Advanced gastric cancer usually presents as a polypoid mass protruding into the gastric lumen, an ulcer crater, or a nondistensible stomach due to diffusely infiltrating carcinoma.

A polypoid mass leaves little doubt as to the presence of carcinoma. Demonstration of an ulcer crater, however, may present a difficult diagnostic problem. As seen radiographically, the character of a malignant ulcer crater lies in a mass and does not extend outside the boundary of the gastric wall. The mucosal folds do not radiate toward the center of the crater, maintaining their usual contour to and beyond the ulcer. Malignant ulcers are usually larger than 1 cm. and are surrounded by rigid gastric wall on fluoroscopy.

The techniques of double-contrast barium study and endoscopy are additive in certain situations. X-ray is better at detecting small lesions in certain sections of the posterior wall of the gastric body, whereas small lesions on the anterior wall are more easily diagnosed with endoscopy.[24]

As experience has increased, computed tomography (CT) scanning has been used with increased frequency to evaluate gastric cancer. Wanebo and co-workers reported that the use of CT scans in the United States to evaluate gastric cancer

TABLE 30–20. Lymph Node Involvement Versus Depth of Invasion of Primary Tumor

Level of Invasion	Number of Patients	Lymph Node Metastases (%)			
		None N_0	*Primary* N_1	*Secondary* N_2	*Tertiary* N_3
Intramucosal	34	88.2	8.8	2.9	—
Submucosal	46	78.3	17.4	4.3	—
Intermediate	94	48.9	30.9	18.1	2.1
Transmural	339	24.8	31.9	33.3	4.7
To neighboring organs	17	23.5	17.6	58.8	—
Total	530	37.7	28.5	30.3	3.4

From Yamada, E., et al: The surgical treatment of cancer of the stomach. Int. Surg., *65*:387, 1980.

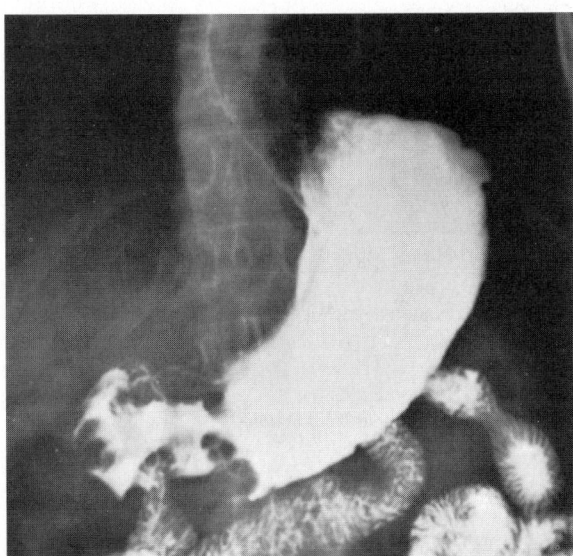

Figure 30–39. Barium upper gastrointestinal examination revealing classic example of distal polypoid gastric carcinoma. (Courtesy of Drs. Barbara Kadel and Marvin Weiner, Department of Radiology, UCLA School of Medicine.)

increased from 28% of patients in 1982 to 64% in 1987.[58] Two thirds of the scans in both groups were suggestive of cancer.

On CT scan, gastric cancer appears most often as gastric wall thickening. The CT appearance correlates with the histopathologic findings, with the tumor appearing localized, circumferential, or diffuse. Wall thickness ranges from 0.5 to 4 cm. and correlates with tumor penetration. Hada and associates suggest that when wall thickness is 2 cm. or greater, transmural extension is assured.[19] Scans may also suggest gastric ulceration, and the lesions can be characterized as polypoid or sessile. With improved sensitivity, CT scanning may suggest invasion of the gastrohepatic ligament, spleen, or diaphragm.[46] The extension of distal tumors into the pancreas, hepatoduodenal ligament, or peripancreatic lymph nodes can be suggested. Metastatic involvement of the liver, spleen, pancreas, and adrenal glands can be readily seen.

The use of CT for staging gastric cancer remains controversial. CT is clearly less accurate than exploration and may overstage or understage patients. Sussman and associates reported a comparison of 75 patients staged with CT scan and subsequent operative staging.[54] In this study, 31% of patients were understaged and 16% were overstaged by CT scan. Regional lymph node involvement was assessed with a sensitivity of 67% and a specificity of 61%. CT was only 27% sensitive in predicting pancreatic invasion and failed to detect peritoneal carcinomatosis in 6 of 20 patients. Andaker and colleagues likewise reported a 37% false-negative rate in the detection of cancer in regional or distant lymph nodes.[5] Cook and co-workers understaged 19 of 31 patients because of missed metastases to the liver, regional nodes, and omentum.[14] Three of six patients deemed unresectable by CT were resectable. Patients with CT findings of obvious metastatic disease, including liver and widespread intraperitoneal metastases, can be spared exploratory operations, except for palliation. Patients with limited or questionable CT findings, however, should undergo exploration for accurate staging and resection.

Flexible fiberoptic endoscopy is the most accurate method of diagnosing gastric cancer currently available. Use of the technique has evolved to the point that in experienced hands, detection of nonulcerative and even gastritis-like malignant lesions is not uncommon. In the American College of Surgeons study, the use of endoscopy increased from 88% to 93% from 1982 to 1987, with a diagnostic accuracy of 87%.[58] If biopsies were obtained, accuracy increased to 94%, and cytologic accuracy was 75%.

Studies concentrating on cytology obtained by multiple methods (fine-needle aspiration, lavage cytology, gastric aspirate, and brush cytology) yield a near 100% positivity.[35] The accuracy of endoscopic biopsy depends on the total number of specimens obtained. Ulcerated lesions should be biopsied at least twice in each quarter at the leading or rolled edge of the ulcer and not at the base, where necrotic tissue is common. Any polypoid or ulcerated lesion should be biopsied, since there is little correlation between the appearance of a lesion and its histopathology.

The endoscopic appearance of gastric cancer ranges from small, plaquelike lesions to polyps or small ulcers. Advanced lesions are typically ulcerated and have elevated margins with shaggy necrotic centers. Advanced diffuse cancers are easily recognized by an extensive tumor plaque or large polypoid mass. Linitis plastica is typified by a nondistensible stomach.

Endoscopic ultrasonography has proved to be the most accurate method of staging rectal and pancreatic head tumors in centers with extensive experience. The application of this technique to gastric cancer is proving highly accurate as well.[1] In six recent series reporting on over 700 patients, tumor stage was accurately predicted and confirmed pathologically in 81% to 92% of patients. Overestimation of stage recurred in 2% to 9% of patients, and underestimation occurred in 4% to 12%. Limitations of the technique lie in its insensitivity to microinvasion and the difficulty of evaluating anterior wall lesions. The technique's major drawback remains the insufficient prediction of lymph node status, with a diagnostic accuracy of less than 70%.[13]

Other Diagnostic Modalities

As previously mentioned, hypo- and achlorhydria are associated with increased risk for gastric cancer. Although not an effective screening or diagnostic tool itself, gastric acid analysis can diagnose patients with these conditions, who should be screened for gastric cancer. The use of molecular biologic techniques—such as cytologic evaluation for p53 or p21 protein, or the detection of alterations in *ras* or *c-myc* oncogenes—has not yet been developed to a clinically applicable stage. Important work in such diagnostic applications is ongoing.

TREATMENT

Patients with gastric cancer must be evaluated for comorbid conditions such as cardiovascular, pulmonary, or renal disorders. Patients with profound weight loss and metabolic complications of their cancer may be at higher surgical risk. Although these are not contraindications to exploration, they warn the surgeon of potential postoperative problems. Patients without obstruction or bleeding but who have been demonstrated to have Virchow's node, inguinal lymph nodes, obvious liver metastases, Sister Mary Joseph's node, or Bloomer's shelf should not be explored. Patients who are obstructed or bleeding should still be considered for exploration, as palliative resection may significantly improve their quality of life. If, at exploration, resection of an obstructing lesion is not possible, gastrojejunostomy can be performed, although results are better following palliative resection. In patients with metastatic obstructing proximal gastric tumors, satisfactory palliation is achieved less frequently. Prosthetic endoesophageal tubes or endoscopic laser therapy can be used in these situations.

When laparotomy is performed, the initial exploration must be thorough, with careful examination and biopsy of any suspicious areas of the pelvis, lower abdomen, and right upper quadrant, in addition to evaluating fixation and local extent of the primary tumor. If the lesion appears to be confined to the stomach except for possible regional lymphatic spread or direct extension, curative resection should be undertaken.

Clearly, surgical resection remains the only potentially curative therapy in gastric cancer. Nevertheless, much controversy persists regarding the extent of gastric resection, the necessity for lymphadenectomy, and the role of adjuvant chemoradiotherapy. At present, the answers to these questions vary not only among countries but also from center to center within countries.

Before an analysis of the current data can be undertaken, a means of comparison must be defined. The location of primary tumors can be defined as distal, middle, or proximal one third. Under the AJCC staging system, N_0 is defined as no regional lymph node metastasis.[4] N_1 lymph nodes lie within 3 cm. of the edge of the primary tumor. N_2 metastases lie more than 3 cm. from the edge of the primary tumor or in nodes along the left gastric, common hepatic, splenic, or celiac arteries. N_3 nodes are retropancreatic, para-aortic, or along the middle colic artery and are considered distant metastases. M_0 represents no distant metastasis, and M_1 is defined by the presence of distant metastases. The Japanese system defines 16 named sites corresponding with N_{1-3} (Fig. 30–40).

Surgical resection of the stomach and accompanying lymph nodes can be described using the terms R0 through

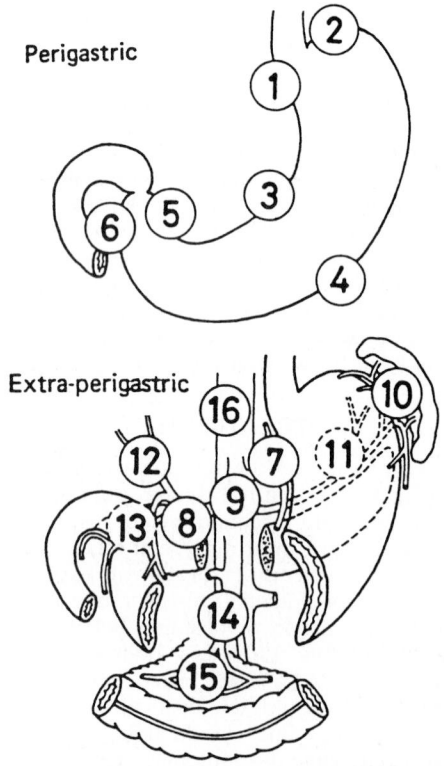

Figure 30–40. The Japanese Research Society for Gastric Cancer classification of regional lymph nodes of the stomach. The American Joint Committee on Cancer uses the same numerical system, classifying nodes in groups 12 through 16 as distant metastases. Perigastric lymph nodes: 1, right pericardial; 2, left pericardial; 3, lesser curvature; 4, greater curvature; 5, suprapyloric; 6, infrapyloric. Extra-perigastric lymph nodes: 7, left gastric artery; 8, common hepatic artery; 9, celiac artery; 10, splenic hilus; 11, splenic artery; 12, hepatic pedicle; 13, retropancreatic; 14, mesenteric root; 15, middle colic artery; 16, para-aortic. (From Mori, M., and Sugimachi, K.: Clinicopathologic studies of gastric carcinoma. Semin. Surg. Oncol., 6:19, 1990. Copyright © 1990. Reprinted by permission of John Wiley & Sons, Inc.)

Lower Third Lesions

R1

3 Lesser Curvature
4 Greater Curvature
5 Suprapyloric
6 Infrapyloric

R2

1 R Cardiac
7 L Gastric Artery
8 Hepatic
9 Celiac

Middle Third Lesions

R1

1 R Cardiac
3 Lesser Curvature
4 Greater Curvature
5 Suprapyloric
6 Infrapyloric

R2

2 L Cardiac*
7 L Gastric Artery
8 Hepatic Artery
9 Celiac
10 Splenic Hilar*
11 Splenic Artery

Upper Third Lesions (Includes Cardia)

R1

1 R Cardiac
2 L Cardiac
3 Lesser Curvature
4 Greater Curvature
and Short Gastric

R2

5 Suprapyloric*
6 Infrapyloric*
7 L Gastric Artery
8 Hepatic Artery
9 Celiac
10 Splenic Hilar
11 Splenic Artery
110 Paraesophageal
(Cardia Lesions)

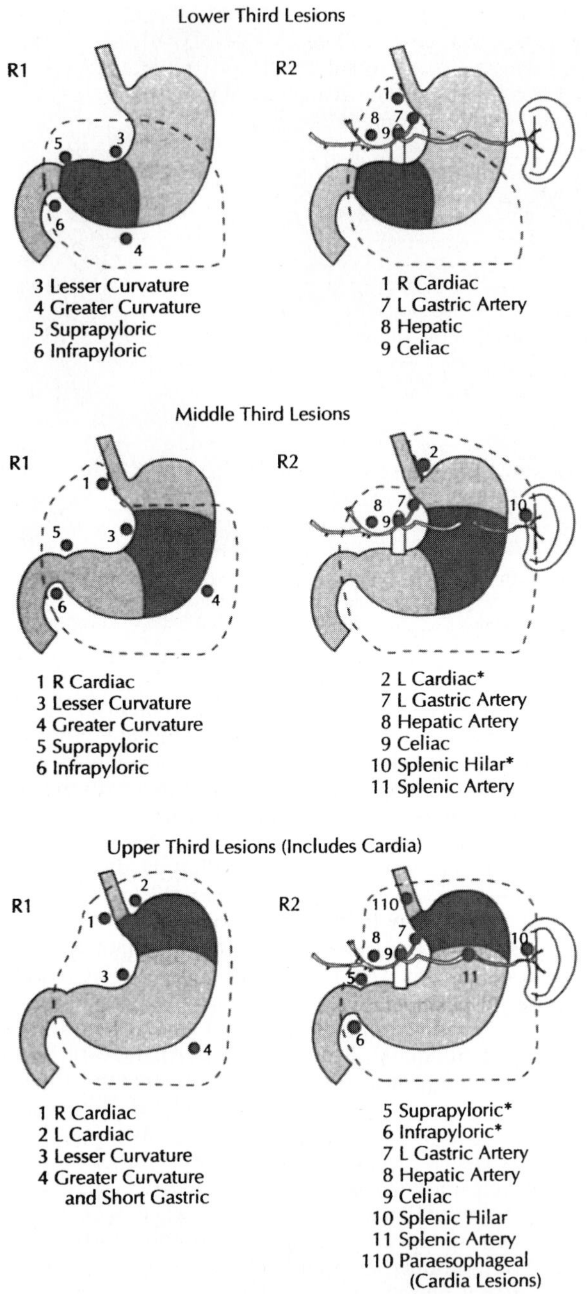

Figure 30–41. The extent of lymphadenectomy is shown by the broken line. R2 resection requires that all R1 and most R2 designated nodes in each category be removed. R indicates right, L left, and asterisks optional. (From Smith, J. W., Shiu, M. H., Kelsey, L., and Brennan, M. F.: Morbidity of radical lymphadenectomy in curative resection of gastric carcinoma. Arch. Surg., 126:1469, 1991.)

R4 (Fig. 30–41). R0 resection must be defined as palliative and implies incomplete removal of perigastric lymph nodes. R1 resection includes complete removal of perigastric nodes. R2 resection includes resection of the stomach, perigastric nodes, and lymph nodes along the named arteries of the stomach. R3 resection is R2 plus removal of the nodes of the celiac axis, and R4 resection includes R3 plus para-aortic nodes. Rn resection implies varying sites of nodal dissection depending on the location of the primary tumor.

An adequate proximal and distal surgical margin should be 4 to 6 cm. from the edge of the primary tumor. This should be confirmed with frozen section analysis at the time of surgery. This necessitates different resections in distal, middle, and proximal lesions. Moreover, in diffuse tumors with extensive submucosal involvement, total gastrectomy may be the only option available to achieve adequate margins, and even then it may be inadequate.

Early Gastric Cancer

R1 resection of early gastric carcinoma is usually curative. Survival rates of 95% or greater are regularly reported in Japanese series reviewing large numbers of early gastric cancer patients. For these lesions, resection typically includes the lesion with an adequate margin, as described earlier, and perigastric lymph nodes within 3 cm. of the lesion. Attempts should be made to preserve vagal branches if resection of the lesser curvature is not necessary.[31] Proximal- and middle-third lesions, especially along the greater curvature, allow for preservation of pyloric function. Distal-third lesions may require antrectomy with R1 reconstruction. Five to 6% of mucosal and 15 to 20% of submucosal early gastric cancers are accompanied by positive lymph nodes.[6]

Provocative reports have described endoscopic treatment of early gastric cancer using cauterization, local injection of drugs, and laser therapy. At present, lesions that appear to be amenable to endoscopic surgery include 1 cm. or smaller protruding-type lesions and 1 cm. or smaller depressed lesions with no ulcer or ulcer scar. Currently, these techniques should be reserved for patients at high risk for conventional operations due to age or concomitant medical problems. Patients must be informed that the results of endoscopic treatment are unknown, whereas surgical therapy typically yields high cure rates.

Advanced Gastric Cancer

During the first half of this century, the suggested extent of resection for gastric cancer became more and more radical. By the 1950s, total gastrectomy was routinely advocated and was accompanied by a high morbidity and mortality. Because of the high complication rate without demonstrable survival advantage, the recommended operation became somewhat less radical.[41] As currently practiced in the United States, a typical gastric resection for cancer includes subtotal gastrectomy for antral or pyloric lesions, subtotal or total gastrectomy for middle-third lesions (depending on the size and proximal extent of the tumor), and total gastrectomy with esophagojejunostomy for proximal-third, gastroesophageal junction, or extensive middle-third lesions (see Fig. 30–41). In addition, the perigastric lymph nodes along the lesser and greater curvatures and the lymph nodes along the left gastric artery are typically removed. The lesser and greater omenta are resected. Typically, however, celiac, hepatic, peripancrea-

tic, and splenic lymph nodes are left undissected. The American College of Surgeons study revealed that less than half of resected specimens were accompanied by gastric and perigastric lymph nodes.[58] Common hepatic, celiac, and splenic lymph nodes were included in only 6, 14, and 8% of specimens, respectively. Only 5% of patients having gastrectomy with clear margins had an R2 dissection as previously defined. The overall survival rate after resection was 19%, and the overall survival rate reflecting only deaths from cancer was 26%.

The Japanese experience with surgical resection for advanced gastric cancer is markedly different. Using a systematic approach, the standard operation in Japan for advanced gastric cancer is the R2 dissection with removal of N_1 and N_2 lymph node groups. Using this standard operation, Maruyama and colleagues from the National Cancer Center Hospital in Tokyo reported a postoperative mortality rate of 0.4% for R2 and R3 resections.[32] Moreover, the survival rates over the past 30 years have risen from 71% to 76% in Stage II, from 39% to 63% in Stage IIIA, from 28% to 39% in Stage IIIB, and from 2% to 10% in Stage IV disease (Table 30–21). Analysis of survival in the Japanese literature is largely retrospective. There are no prospective randomized trials of R1 versus R2, or R1 versus R2 and R3, resections for gastric cancer based on tumor stage. These are unlikely to be forthcoming, because the results of R2 resection for gastric cancer in Japan are so impressive and unmatched by any in the world. Factors possibly contributing to this success include the vast Japanese experience with the operation, the average younger age (10 years) and leaner body habitus of the Japanese patients compared with their Western counterparts, and the frequent underestimation of tumor stage in Western series due to incomplete removal of the lymph nodes necessary for accurate staging.

Prospective if not randomized results are beginning to appear in the literature.[7, 15, 25, 50] Siewert and colleagues assessed the value of systematic lymphadenectomy in a German series of gastric carcinoma patients (Table 30–22).[50] This prospective study of 2394 patients included 1654 curative resections; 1096 were considered radical, and 558 were considered standard, based on whether more or fewer than 26 lymph nodes were resected. This number was chosen because 26 lymph nodes corresponds to R1 resection; more than 26 corresponds to R2 resection when correlated with pathologic anatomic study. A multivariate analysis of the results indicates that there was no significant difference in the morbidity (29 versus 31%) or mortality (5.2 versus 5%) for standard versus radical surgical procedures. Radical resection was a positive independent prognostic variable for increased survival at 5 years in Stage II and IIIA disease (55 versus 27%, and 38 versus 25%, respectively). There was no advantage in either procedure for pathologic N_2 positive tumors. The

---

TABLE 30–21. Five-Year Survival Rates by Stage in Japanese Patients with Gastric Cancer

Stage	Percent Surviving 5 Yrs. (No.)			
	1963–1966 *Nationwide*	*1969–1973* *Nationwide*	*1974–1978* *Nationwide*	*1979–1990* *NCC*
I	94.4 (1016)	96.4 (3489)	96.6 (6952)	101.8 (1398)
II	56.1 (1070)	71.8 (1435)	72.0 (2179)	81.2 (303)
III	30.1 (910)	43.8 (3039)	44.8 (5292)	61.0 (565)
IV	9.3 (1523)	13.1 (2977)	7.7 (5487)	14.0 (558)
Unknown	40.2 (956)	58.1 (632)	58.8 (1614)	— (0)

NCC, National Cancer Center, Tokyo.
From Kinoshita, T., Maruyama, K., Sasako, M., and Okajima, K.: Treatment results of gastric cancer patients: Japanese experience. *In* Nishi, M., Schikawa, H., Nokajima, T., Marugama, K., and Tahara, E. (Eds.): Gastric Cancer. Tokyo, Springer-Verlag, 1993.

TABLE 30–22. Prospective Evaluation of Survival Based on Union Internacional Contra la Cancrum (UICC) Stage in Patients Undergoing Radical or Standard Resection

UICC Stage	Type of Lymph Node Dissection	Median (95% c.i.) Survival (mo.)	5-Yr Survival Rate, % (S.D.)	p*
IA	Radical (n = 130)	—	85.7 (3.1)	
	Standard (n = 96)	—	86.5 (3.7)	0.18
IB	Radical (n = 133)	—	68.7 (5.1)	
	Standard (n = 77)	—	72.4 (5.7)	0.2
II	Radical (n = 129)	—	55.2 (5.1)	
	Standard (n = 76)	25.6 (19.8–31.9)	26.8 (6.0)	<0.001
IIIA	Radical (n = 145)	28.9 (22.8–40.1)	38.4 (4.3)	
	Standard (n = 66)	14.3 (10.1–29.0)	25.3 (7.5)	0.03
IIIB	Radical (n = 130)	15.5 (12.4–19.7)	17.5 (4.0)	
	Standard (n = 30)	12.2 (9.9–17.4)	27.5 (8.7)	0.36
IV	Radical (n = 136)	12.5 (9.8–15.3)	16.1 (3.5)	
	Standard (n = 34)	16.1 (10.0–24.4)	28.2 (7.5)	0.13

*Log rank test.
c.i., confidence interval.
From Siewert, J. R., Böttcher, K., Roder, J. D., Busch, R., Hermanek, P., Meyer, H. J., and the German Gastric Carcinoma Study Group: Prognostic relevance of systematic lymph node dissection in gastric carcinoma. Br. J. Surg., *80:*1015, 1993.

study's final recommendation was that R2 resection be applied for at least Stage II and IIIA lesions.

These results are mirrored by those of the Memorial-Sloan Kettering group in the United States (Karpeh, personal communication). Their preliminary data are summarized in Table 30–23. This group previously suggested that, in experienced hands, R2 and R3 resections are as safe as R1 resection.[52] In their hands, R1 resection was accompanied by an 18% general medical and 16% surgical complication rate (34% total); patients undergoing R2 and R3 resections developed general medical and surgical complications 20 and 23% of the time, respectively (43% total). There were no deaths in 61 patients undergoing R0 or R1 resection, and 2 of 123 patients undergoing R2 or R3 resection died.

A recent prospective, randomized trial from Hong Kong compared R1 versus R3 resection for antral cancers.[43] Although only 55 patients were randomized in this study, the two groups were comparable for age, sex, tumor size, TNM stage, and length of follow-up. This study concluded that although both procedures could be performed with a low mortality rate, R3 resection had a much higher rate of intra-abdominal complications, but the overall survival rate, including all cases, was higher in the R3 group. However, based on their experience, radical resection was not recommended for the subgroup with antral cancers.

There are conflicting data in the literature concerning whether radical resection can be performed safely.[52, 53] It should be emphasized, however, that in experienced hands, a preponderance of data suggests that R2 resection can be performed as safely as R0 and R1 resection. Unfortunately, the vast majority of patients seen in the West present with advanced gastric cancer. In over 50% of patients, the tumor

TABLE 30–23. Data from Memorial Sloan-Kettering Cancer Center Comparing Survival Following R1 and R2 Resection of Gastric Cancer by Stage

Stage	Percent (No.) Surviving	
	R1	R2
IA	88 (16)	91 (43)
IB	56 (14)	85 (41)
II	39 (15)	58 (88)
IIIA	7 (22)	30 (163)
IIIB	0 (4)	12 (82)

is no longer localized when first identified, and the outcome is generally disappointing.

Adenocarcinoma of the cardia and gastroesophageal junction is becoming more prevalent, roughly doubling in incidence over the last 20 years.[58] The management of these tumors is controversial. The extent of gastric resection (total versus subtotal) must be decided, and it also must be determined whether a thoracotomy is necessary (versus blunt esophagectomy) and where the anastomosis will be sited (abdomen, chest, or neck).[23] The disease clearly occurs in an older patient population with a high percentage of advanced tumors (50 to 74%). Complete resection often requires thoracotomy or esophagectomy with anastomosis in the neck; mortality rates range from 11% to 16%, with leakage of the esophageal anastomosis being the most devastating complication. Regardless of which procedure is chosen, most recommend a radical operation, usually through a thoracoabdominal approach.[3] It is imperative to obtain frozen section analysis of the proximal and distal resection margins prior to restoring gastrointestinal continuity.

The issue of total versus subtotal gastrectomy for the treatment of gastric cancer has been addressed in multiple studies. The consensus is that a total gastrectomy that is unnecessary for adequate gastric wall margins does not improve survival and may increase postoperative morbidity.[40, 49] The issue of total gastrectomy for palliation has also been addressed in multiple studies and has recently been revisited. Monson and colleagues performed the procedure in 53 consecutive patients with a median survival rate of 19 months; 13 patients lived more than 2 years.[34] The quality of life was graded as good in 59% and poor in only 13%. There is little to be gained from performing the procedure in patients with bilobar liver involvement or if a safe proximal anastomosis cannot be easily performed. However, most do not believe that this procedure is an appropriate palliative intervention.

In summary, the surgical treatment for gastric cancer is still controversial (Table 30–24). For the purposes of staging and for the best chance at cure, extended resection (R2) should be performed when there is gastric serosal involvement or when local regional lymph nodes are involved. There is no proven survival advantage to routine R3 or combined resection at present. The extent of gastric resection should be tailored to the proximal extent of the primary lesion and geared toward obtaining negative proximal and distal margins. Total gastrectomy should be performed only for diffuse or large tumors of the middle or proximal third. Palliative

TABLE 30–24. Comparison of Published Japanese and Non-Japanese Series on Gastric Cancer Patients, 1970–1990

Factor	Japanese	Non-Japanese	Total
No. of series	15	85	100
No. of patients	19,048	80,738	99,786
Operation (%)	99.8	74.1	79.0
Resection (%)	93.1	35.2	46.3
Curative or radical resection (%)	58.6	17.8	25.6
Mean 5-yr. survival after curative or radical resection (%)	60.5 (6736 of 11,139)	39.4 (2836 of 7205)	52.2 (9572 of 18,344)

From Akoh, J. A., and Macintyre, I. M. C.: Improving survival in gastric cancer: Review of 5-year survival rates in English language publications from 1970. Br. J. Surg., *79*:293, 1992.

resection should be performed rather than palliative bypass, but both must be approached with caution.

Data from prospective randomized trials will be forthcoming from the Dutch trial, with the British Medical Research Council (MRC) trial to follow.[7] It is clear that a completely unified staging system, adherence to defined surgical terminology, and more broadly based randomized prospective trials are needed to answer the numerous uncertainties remaining in the treatment of gastric cancer.[56]

Adjuvant Therapy

The use of adjuvant chemotherapy, radiotherapy, and chemoimmunotherapy has recently been summarized by Agboola.[2] Reports of adjuvant chemotherapy in the treatment of adenocarcinoma of the stomach are generally pessimistic, although some trials have indicated success in selected subgroups of patients. A group of 134 patients underwent curative resection, and patients with T_1 to T_3 lesions and N_2 nodes were given mitomycin C (20 mg. per sq. m. intravenously once every 6 weeks for four courses). The treatment group had a survival advantage at 5 and 9 years (41 versus 26% 5-year survival). Of note was that there was a marked decrease in metastatic liver lesions in the treated patients but no difference in peritoneal recurrence.

Multiple prospective randomized trials of multiagent chemotherapy have been undertaken. Data from an early randomized trial of 5-fluorouracil, adriamycin, and mitomycin C (FAM) were confirmed in a randomized trial by the Eastern Cooperative Oncology Group (ECOG), demonstrating a survival advantage in advanced gastric cancer patients. The Southwestern Oncology Group (SWOG) and the International Collaborative Group (ICG) treated 536 patients with FAM. No survival advantage was noted in these patients, except for a small subset with T_3 and T_4 tumors and positive nodes. A significant problem with the trials mentioned is that, due to side effects of the regimen, fewer than 50% of patients enrolled in the trials received more than 75% of planned doses.

Five randomized trials between 1977 and 1985 were performed using 5-fluorouracil (5-FU) and nitrosourea. Only one of the groups, the Gastrointestinal Tumor Study Group (GITSG), reported a survival advantage at 4- and 11-year follow-ups. There are significant differences in the trials, however, both in the percentage of patients who received curative resection and in the number of patients who completed therapy. The regimen was toxic, with 45% of patients in the GITSG trial suffering from severe toxicities, and one therapy-related death. It was clear from other trials that patients who failed to complete planned chemotherapy had higher rates of recurrence.

Five randomized trials of mitomycin C alone or in combination with other agents have been published. Imanaga reported a trial of 2636 patients on four different regimens.[2] Only

one regimen showed a survival advantage of 13.5%. Mitomycin C was believed to decrease liver metastases but did not alter the incidence of serosal metastasis. Three trials of mitomycin C alone or combined with 5-FU-arabinoside or futrafur were completed.[2] One of the three showed a survival advantage in treated patients. In the two negative trials, there was a mild treatment advantage for Stage II and III cases, but not for Stage I and IV. Stage I patients given mitomycin C had a decreased survival rate compared with untreated controls. Mitomycin C demonstrated the greatest advantage in patients with serosal involvement and poorly differentiated tumors.

Overall results are mixed but generally disappointing. Only 2 of 16 randomized adjuvant chemotherapy trials showed a survival benefit for the treatment group. Neither of the positive trials has been confirmed by a follow-up trial in Europe or North America. Three Japanese trials, however, have confirmed a survival benefit for mitomycin C alone or futrafur (a derivative of 5-FU) and mitomycin C.

Results of combination chemotherapy and radiation therapy are mixed as well. An early report by Moertel indicated a significant advantage to patients given combination treatment.[2] This generated four other trials using radiation and either 5-FU or 5-FU plus methyl-CCNU or thiotepa. None of these trials reported a survival benefit; indeed, survival was generally better in patients with minimal residual disease regardless of the therapy given. The GITSG trial reported higher mortality rates in treated patients.

Two further studies by the British Stomach Cancer Group (1989) and the European Organization for Research and Treatment of Cancer (1989) using radiation alone or radiation combined with doxorubicin (Adriamycin), mitomycin C, or 5-FU showed no survival difference between treated and untreated control groups.[2]

It is well known that surgical exploration and/or resection along with blood transfusion compromises immunity in many patients. It is speculated that this immune depression encourages the growth of tumor cells in certain subsets of patients. Numerous immunomodulators have been found to enhance T-cell function and stimulate natural killer cells. However, immunotherapy alone has rarely been shown to be effective against residual tumors in patients with clinically measurable disease.

Thirteen prospective randomized trials of chemoimmunotherapy have been reported. Seven studies compared chemotherapy to chemoimmunotherapy, and four were three-arm studies of chemoimmunotherapy with chemotherapy or surgery alone as controls. The advantages were greatest in patients with Stage III and IV disease or patients who underwent R0 resection. Four trials reported no survival advantage, including two using levamisole and two using *Streptococcus pyogenes* antigens. In the studies indicating a survival advantage, the increased survival ranged from 13% to 29%, the highest being in a study of 216 patients curatively resected in which one treatment arm received 5-FU and adriamycin alone, in contrast to the second treatment arm, which included 5-FU, adriamycin, and polyadenylic polyuridylic acid.

In summary, a meta-analysis of prospective randomized trials in Europe and North America failed to show that the use of adjuvant chemotherapy in advanced gastric cancer is beneficial.[21] However, the use of mitomycin C and 5-FU or its derivative, futrafur, in Japanese trials is supported by several nonrandomized and two randomized trials.

Results of the use of chemoimmunotherapy in Eastern trials have been more encouraging. Several trials have shown positive results in patients who began therapy early in the postoperative period. This indicates that reversal of postoperative immunosuppression by immune stimulants may be beneficial. Experimentally, there is correlation between the degree of immune stimulation in postsurgical patients and their survival, independent of the stage of the disease.

The optimal postoperative adjuvant therapy for gastric cancer has not been developed. Needed are less toxic chemotherapeutic regimens, further evaluation of preoperative radiation and chemotherapy, and the development of regimens that are effective against peritoneal as well as visceral metastasis. The use of intraoperative radiation is undergoing evaluation, and its place in therapy has yet to be defined.

SUMMARY

Gastric cancer remains a devastating disease. With the exception of early gastric cancer, which is usually (>90%) cured with surgery alone, survival at 5 years remains 20% to 30% *at best*, especially in Western series, where early lesions make up only 8% to 10% of the total. Recent data from the United States indicate that less than 80% of patients are explored and less than 80% of those have a resection performed. The 5-year survival in patients with resection of all gross disease and clear margins ranged from 20% to 38%, indicating microscopic spread in a majority of apparently good candidates.

Although a preponderance of data indicates that extended resection (R2) can be performed safely, is useful in certain stages, and is the curative procedure of choice when there is serosal or locoregional lymph node involvement, it is doubtful that more radical operations (R3, combined resection) add any survival benefit. Current radiochemotherapy regimens are of marginal benefit, and more effective agents or combinations are needed.

The effectiveness of mass screening in high-risk populations has been demonstrated by the impressive Japanese results. Clearly, if an impact is to be made in the treatment of gastric cancer in the West, early detection and prevention are areas in which advances are needed. Investigations into the pathogenesis and molecular genetics of the disease are ongoing and may yield clinically applicable strategies in the near future.

SELECTED REFERENCES

Agboola, O.: Adjuvant treatment in gastric cancer. Cancer Treat. Rev., 20:217, 1994.
This article reviews the results of published randomized trials of adjuvant therapy for gastric cancer from 1967 to 1993. Forty-six trials comprising over 12,000 patients are reviewed, and it is concluded that comprehensive strategies remain to be developed that address local recurrence, peritoneal recurrence, and bloodborne metastasis. The potential for molecular strategies of diagnosis and therapy is emphasized.

Nishi, M., Schikawa, H., Nokajima, T., Maruyama, K., and Tahara, E.: Gastric Cancer. Tokyo, Springer-Verlag, 1993.
This treatise on gastric cancer contains chapters on all aspects of the epidemiology, pathology, molecular biology, diagnosis, staging, and treatment of the disease. Japanese, Korean, European, and American authors present treatment results and discuss future strategies.

Parsonnet, J., Friedman, G. D., Vandersteen, D. P., Chang, Y., Vogelman, J. H., Orentreich, N., and Sibley, R. K.: *Helicobacter pylori* infection and the risk of gastric cancer. N. Engl. J. Med., 325:1127, 1991.
This is a report of a cohort study of 186 patients with gastric cancer and matched controls taken from a group of 129,992 followed since the 1960s. Eighty-four percent of patients with gastric cancer had been infected with H. pylori, and 61% of controls had evidence of infection. Tumors of the gastroesophageal junction were not associated with an increased rate of infection, but H. pylori infection was a strong risk factor in women and blacks. A history of peptic ulcer disease was negatively correlated with cancer. It was concluded that H. pylori infection is associated with gastric cancer and may be a cofactor in its development.

Sawyers, J. L.: Gastric carcinoma. Curr. Probl. Surg., 32:101, 1995.
This excellent monograph by one of the giants of gastric surgery summarizes current diagnostic and therapeutic strategies. The status of basic research and adjuvant therapy is discussed.

Smith, J. W., Shiu, M. H., Kelsey, L., and Brennan, M. F.: Morbidity of radical lymphadenectomy in curative resection of gastric carcinoma. Arch. Surg., 126:1469, 1991.
Results from the Memorial Sloan-Kettering Cancer Center show no significant difference in operative time, time to resumption of diet, length of hospitalization, morbidity, or morality for <R2 versus ≥R2 resections. These results are in line with those of Japanese series and indicate that radical resection for gastric carcinoma may be undertaken without undue risk.

Wanabo, H. J., Kennedy, B. J., Chmiel, J., Steele, G., Jr., Winchester, D., and Osteen, R.: Cancer of the stomach: A patient care study by the American College of Surgeons. Ann. Surg., 218:583, 1993.
This important and enlightening study evaluated the status of gastric cancer treatment in the United States from 1982 to 1987. The treatment of 18,365 patients was analyzed, and the results are dismal. The need for greater uniformity in staging and reporting was emphasized. It was concluded that there is the potential for increasing survival through earlier diagnosis and the use of more adequate surgical techniques.

REFERENCES

1. Abe, S., Lightdale, C. J., and Brennan, M. F.: The Japanese experience with endoscopic ultrasonography in the staging of gastric cancer. Gastrointest. Endosc., 39:586, 1993.
2. Agboola, O.: Tumour review: Adjuvant treatment in gastric cancer. Cancer Treat. Rev., 20:217, 1994.
3. Akiyama, H., Miyazono, H., Tsurumaru, M., Hashimota, C., and Kawamura, T.: Thoracoabdominal approach for carcinoma of the cardia of the stomach. Am. J. Surg., 137:345, 1979.
4. American Joint Committee on Cancer: Stomach cancer. In Beahrs, O. H., Henson, D. E., Hutter, R. V. P., and Kennedy, B. T. (Eds.): Manual for Staging Cancer, 4th ed. Philadelphia, J. B. Lippincott, 1992, p. 63.
5. Andaker, L., Morales, O., and Hoger, H.: Evaluation of preoperative computed tomography in gastric malignancy. Surgery, 109:132, 1991.
6. Bogomoletz, W. V.: Early gastric cancer. Am. J. Pathol., 8:381, 1984.
7. Bonenkamp, J. J., Bunt, A. M. G., van de Velde, C. G. H., et al.: Radical lymphadenectomy for gastric cancer: A prospective randomized trial in the Netherlands. Surg. Oncol. Clin. North Am., 7:433, 1993.
8. Boring, C. C., Squires, T. S., Tong, T., and Montgomery S.: Cancer statistics 1994. Cancer J. Clin., 44:16, 1994.
9. Boynton, R. F., Blount, P. L., Yin, J., Brown, V. L., Huang, Y., Tong, Y., McDaniel, T., Newkirk, C., Resau, J. H., Haggitt, R. C., Raskind, W. H., Reid, B. J., and Meltzer, S. J.: Loss of heterozygosity involving the APC and MCC genetic loci occurs in the majority of human esophageal cancer. Proc. Natl. Acad. Sci. USA, 89:3385, 1992.
10. Cady, B., Choe, D. S.: Changing patterns of gastric cancer. In Neiburgs, H. E. (Ed.): Prevention and Detection of Cancer. New York, Marcel Dekker, 1981, p. 2041.
11. Chen, V. W., Abu-Elyazeed, R. R., Zavala, D. E., et al.: Risk factors of gastric precancerous lesions in a high-risk Colombian population. I. Salt. Nutr. Cancer, 13:59, 1990.
12. Chen, V. W., Abu-Elyazeed, R. R., Zavala, D. E., et al.: Risk factors of gastric precancerous lesions in a high-risk Colombian population. II. Nitrate and nitrite. Nutr. Cancer, 13:67, 1990.
13. Coletti, G., Ferrari, A., Brocchi, E., and Barbara, L.: Accuracy of endoscopic ultrasonography in the diagnosis and staging of gastric cancer and lymphoma. Surgery, 113:14, 1993.
14. Cook, A. O., Levine, B. A., Sirinek, K. R., and Gaskill, H. V.: Evaluation of gastric adenocarcinoma: Abdominal computed tomography does not replace celiotomy. Arch. Surg., 121:603, 1986.
15. Dent, D. M., Madden, M. V., and Price, S. K.: Randomized comparison of R1 and R2 gastrectomy for gastric carcinoma. Br. J. Surg., 75:110, 1988.
16. Domellof, L., Eriksson, S., and Janunger, K.-G.: Carcinoma and possible precancerous changes of the gastric stump after Billroth II resection. Gastroenterology, 73:462, 1977.
17. Filipe, M. I., and Jankowski, J.: Growth factors and oncogenes in Barrett's oesophagus and gastric metaplasia. Endoscopy, 25(suppl.):637, 1993.
18. Forman, D.: The etiology of gastric cancer. In O'Neill, J. K., Chen, J., and Bartsch, H. (Eds.): Relevance to Human Cancer of N-Nitroso Compounds,

Tobacco, Smoke, and Mycotoxins. Lyon (France), International Agency for Research on Cancer, 1991, p. 22.

19. Hada, M., Hihara, T., and Kakishita, M.: Computed tomography in gastric carcinoma: Thickness of gastric wall and infiltration to serosa surface. Radiat. Med., 2:27, 1984.

20. Haenszel, W., Kurihara, M., Segi, M., and Lee, R. K. C.: Stomach cancer among Japanese in Hawaii. J. Natl. Cancer Inst., 49:969, 1972.

21. Hermans, J., Bonenkamp, J. J., Boon, M. C., Bunt, A. M. G., Oyama, S., Sasako, M., and van de Velde, C. J. H.: Adjuvant therapy after curative resection for gastric cancer: Meta-analysis of randomized trials. J. Clin. Oncol., 11:1441, 1993.

22. Hoffman, N. R.: The relationship between pernicious anemia and the cancer of the stomach. Geriatrics, 25:90, 1970.

23. Hölscher, A. H., Siewert, J. R., Böttcher, K., et al.: Surgical classification for adenocarcinoma of the gastroesophageal junction. In Siewert, J. R., and Hölcher, A. H. (Eds.): Diseases of the Esophagus. Berlin, Springer-Verlag, 1988, p. 571.

24. Ichikawa, H.: X-ray diagnosis of early gastric cancer. In Nishi, M., Schikawa, H., Nokajima, T., Maruyama, K., and Tahara, E. (Eds.): Gastric Cancer. Tokyo, Springer-Verlag, 1993, p. 232.

25. Jaehne, J., Meyer, H.-J., Maschek, H., et al.: Lymphadenectomy in gastric cancer: A prospective and prognostic study. Arch. Surg., 127:290, 1992.

26. Kennedy, B. J.: The unified international gastric cancer staging classification system. Scand. J. Gastroenterol., 22:11, 1987.

27. Kidokoro, T., Hayashida, Y., and Urabe, M.: Long-term surgical results of carcinoma of the gastric remnant: A statistical analysis of 613 patients from 98 institutions. World J. Surg., 9:966, 1985.

28. Kmet, J.: The role of malignant population in studies of selected cancer sites: A review. J. Chronic Dis., 23:305, 1970.

29. Lauren, P.: The two histological main types of gastric carcinoma: Diffuse and so-called intestinal type carcinoma. An attempt at a histoclinical classification. Acta Pathol. Microbiol. Scand., 64:31, 1965.

30. Martin, H. M., Filipe, M. I., Morris, R. W., et al.: p53 expression and prognosis in gastric carcinoma. Int. J. Cancer, 50:859, 1992.

31. Maruyama, K., Sasako, M., and Kinoshita, T.: Preservation of sympathetic and vagal nerve system at gastric cancer surgery [in Japanese]. Igaku-no Ayumi, 159:898, 1991.

32. Maruyama, K., Sasako, M., and Kinoshita, T.: Role of systematic extended lymph node dissection, Japanese experience. In Nishi, M., Schikawa, H., Nokajima, T., Maruyama, K., and Tahara, E. (Eds.): Gastric Cancer. Tokyo, Springer-Verlag, 1993.

33. Meyers, W. S., Damiano, R. J., Postlehwait, R. W., and Rotolo, F. S.: Adenocarcinoma of the stomach: Changing patterns over the last decades. Ann. Surg., 205:1, 1987.

34. Monson, J. R. T., Donohue, J. H., McIlrath, D. C., Farnell, M. B., and Ilstrup, D. M.: Total gastrectomy for advanced cancer: A worthwhile palliative procedure. Cancer, 68:1863, 1991.

35. Mori, M., and Sugimachi, K.: Clinicopathologic studies of gastric carcinoma. Semin. Surg. Oncol., 6:19, 1990.

36. Nicholls, J. C.: Stump cancer following gastric surgery. World J. Surg., 3:731, 1979.

37. Oota, K., and Sobin, L. H.: Histological typing of gastric and oesophageal tumours. In International Histological Classification of Tumors, No. 18. Geneva, World Health Organization, 1977, p. 55.

38. Parsonnet, J.: Helicobacter pylori and gastric cancer. Gastroenterol. Clin. North Am., 22:89, 1993.

39. Parsonnet, J., Friedman, G. D., Vandersteen, D. P., Chang, Y., Vogelman, J. H., Orentreich, N., and Sibley, R. K.: Helicobacter pylori infection and the risk of gastric carcinoma. N. Engl. J. Med., 325:1127, 1991.

40. Pichlmayr, R., and Meyer, H.-J.: Patterns of recurrence in relation to therapeutic strategy. In Fielding, J. W. L., Newman, C. E., Ford, C. H. J., and Jones, B. G. (Eds.): Gastric Cancer. Oxford, Pergamon Press, 1981, p. 171.

41. Remine, W.: Indications and contraindications for surgery in gastric carcinoma. World J. Surg., 3:709, 1979.

42. Rhyu, M.-G., Park, W.-S., Jung, Y.-J., Choi, S.-W., and Meltzer, S. J.: Allelic deletions of MCC/APC and p53 are frequent late events in human gastric carcinogenesis. Gastroenterology, 106:1584, 1994.

43. Robertson, C. S., Chung, S. C. S., Woods, S. D. S., Griffin, S. M., Raimes, S. A., Lau, J. T. F., and Li, A. K. C.: A prospective randomized trial comparing R1 subtotal gastrectomy with R3 total gastrectomy for antral cancer. Ann. Surg., 220:176, 1994.

44. Rohde, H., Bauer, P., Stützer, H., Heitmann, K., Gebbensleben, B., and the German Gastric Cancer TNM Study Group: Proximal compared with distal adenocarcinoma of the stomach: Differences and consequences. Br. J. Surg., 78:1242, 1991.

45. Sano, T., Tsujino, T., Yoshida, K., Nakayama, H., Haruma, K., Ito, H., Nakamura, Y., Kajiyama, G., and Tahara, E.: Frequent loss of heterozygosity on chromosomes 1q, 5q, and 17p in human gastric carcinoma. Cancer Res., 51:2926, 1991.

46. Scatarige, J. C., and DiSantis, D. J.: CT of the stomach and duodenum. Radiol. Clin. North Am., 27:687, 1989.

47. Scott, N., Diament, R., Murday, V., et al.: Helicobacter gastritis and intestinal metaplasia in a gastric cancer family. Lancet, 1:728, 1990.

48. Shirakabe, H., Ichikawa, H., Kumakura, K., Nishizawa, M., Higurashi, K., Hayakawa, H., and Murakami, T.: Atlas of X-ray Diagnosis of Early Gastric Cancer. Philadelphia, J. B. Lippincott, 1966.

49. Shiu, M. H., Moore, E., Sanders, M., Huvos, A., Freedman, B., Goodbold, J., Chaiyaphruk, S., Wesdorp, R., and Brennan, M. F.: Influence of the extent of resection on survival after curative treatment of gastric carcinoma: A retrospective multivariate analysis. Arch. Surg., 122:1347, 1987.

50. Siewert, J. R., Böttcher, K., Roder, J. D., Busch, R., Hermanek, P., Meyer, H. J., and the German Gastric Carcinoma Study Group: Prognostic relevance of systematic lymph node dissection in gastric carcinoma. Br. J. Surg., 80:1015, 1993.

51. Sipponen, P.: Gastric cancer—a long-term consequence of Helicobacter pylori infection? Scand. J. Gastroenterol., 29(suppl. 201):24, 1994.

52. Smith, J. W., Shiu, M. H., Kelsey, L., and Brennan, M. F.: Morbidity of radical lymphadenectomy in curative resection of gastric carcinoma. Arch. Surg., 126:1469, 1991.

53. Sue-Ling, H. M.: Radical surgery is essential for treating gastric cancer. Eur. J. Surg. Oncol., 20:179, 1994.

54. Sussman, S. K., Halvorsen, R. A., Illescas, F. F., et al.: Gastric adenocarcinoma: CT versus surgical staging. Radiology, 167:335, 1988.

55. Tahara, E., Yokozaki, H., and Yasui, W.: Growth factors in gastric cancer. In Nishi, M., Schikawa, H., Nokajima, T., Maruyama, K., and Tahara, E. (Eds.): Gastric Cancer. Tokyo, Springer-Verlag, 1993, p. 213.

56. Thompson, G. B., van Heerden, J. A., and Sarr, M. G.: Adenocarcinoma of the stomach: Are we making progress? Lancet, 342:713, 1993.

57. Uchino, S., Tsuda, H., Noguchi, M., et al.: The APC gene responsible for familial adenomatous polyposis is mutated in human gastric cancer. Cancer Res., 51:2926, 1991.

58. Wanebo, H. J., Kennedy, B. J., Chmiel, J., Steele, G., Jr., Winchester, D., and Osleen, R.: Cancer of the stomach: A patient care study by the American College of Surgeons. Ann. Surg., 218:583, 1993.

59. Wright, P. A., and Williams, G. T.: Molecular biology and gastric carcinoma. Gut, 34:145, 1993.

60. Yokata, J., Yamamoto, T., Migajima, N., Toyoshima, K., Nomura, N., Soycamoto, H., Yoshida, T., Tenada, M., and Sugimura, T.: Genetic alterations of c-erbB-2 oncogene occur frequently in tubular adenocarcinoma of the stomach and are often accompanied by the amplification of the v-erbA homologue. Oncogene, 2:283, 1988.

61. Zamcheck, N., Grable, E., Ley, A., and Norman, L.: Occurrence of gastric cancer among patients with pernicious anemia at the Boston City Hospital. N. Engl. J. Med., 252:1103, 1955.

CHAPTER 31

THE SMALL INTESTINE

I

ANATOMY

R. Scott Jones, M.D.

The small intestine extends from the pylorus to the cecum. Its major function—absorption—depends on the complex integration of structural, physiologic, and chemical factors. The neurohormonal regulation of gastric, biliary, pancreatic, and intestinal secretion and of motor function enables complete digestion of foodstuffs and presentation of the digested products to the specialized intestinal epithelium for absorption. This section describes the structure and functions of this segment of the gut.

An essential anatomic characteristic of the small intestine, its large surface area, promotes absorption. The gross, microscopic, and ultrastructural features of the small intestine that account for this efficient function are intestinal length, mucosal folds, villi, and microvilli. Various types of intestinal movements also enhance the effectiveness of digestion and absorption.

GROSS ANATOMY

General Description. The length of the alimentary tract in normal humans averages about 453 cm. from the nose to the anus. The duodenum is approximately 21 cm. long, and the colon is approximately 109 cm. long. The combined length of the jejunum and ileum is 261 cm., or about three fifths of the entire canal.[16] Chapter 30 describes the duodenum. The jejunum begins at the duodenojejunal angle, supported by the ligament of Treitz. The jejunum constitutes the proximal two fifths of the small intestine, and the ileum makes up the distal three fifths; however, there is no clear demarcation between jejunum and ileum. The small intestine, which decreases in luminal diameter as it proceeds distally, is convoluted or folded upon itself to occupy the central and lower part of the abdominal cavity; it is enclosed laterally and superiorly by the colon.[13]

Mesentery. The mesentery, a large fold of peritoneum, suspends the small intestine from the posterior abdominal wall. The base of the mesentery attaches to the posterior abdominal wall to the left of the second lumbar vertebra and passes obliquely to the right and inferiorly to the right sacroiliac joint. The mesentery contains blood vessels, nerves, lymphatics, and lymph nodes, as well as considerable fat. It attaches to the small intestine along the length of one side, the mesenteric border, leaving the remainder of the surface of the bowel covered by its visceral peritoneum, the serosa. The broad-based attachment of the mesenteric base stabilizes the small bowel and prevents it from twisting upon its blood supply.

Blood Supply. The small intestine receives its blood supply from the superior mesenteric artery, the second large branch of the abdominal aorta. The superior mesenteric artery courses anterior to the uncinate process of the pancreas and

the third portion of the duodenum, where it divides to supply the pancreas, duodenum, and entire small intestine, as well as the ascending and transverse colon. The intestinal arteries branch within the mesentery to unite with adjacent arteries to form a series of arterial arcades before sending small straight arteries to the small intestine. The intestinal arteries contact the small intestine on the mesenteric border, where they pass toward the antimesenteric border, sending small branches into the layers of the intestine. The veins of the small intestine drain into the superior mesenteric vein, a major tributary to the portal vein.

Lymphatics. Peyer's patches are lymph nodules aggregated in the submucosa of the small intestine. These lymphatic nodules are most abundant in the ileum, but the jejunum also contains them. The lymphatic drainage from the small intestine passes into three sets of mesenteric nodes: a first set close to the wall of the small intestine, a second set adjacent to the mesenteric arcades, and a third set along the trunk of the superior mesenteric artery. The superior mesenteric preaortic group drains into the intestinal trunk, which drains into the cisterna chyli. The lymphatic drainage of the small intestine constitutes a major route for transport of absorbed lipid into the circulation.

Mucosa. The mucosal surface of the small intestine contains numerous circular mucosal folds called the *plicae circulares* (*valvulae conniventes*, or valves of Kerckring). These folds are 3 to 10 mm. in height; they are taller and more numerous in the distal duodenum and proximal jejunum, becoming shorter and fewer distally. Intestinal villi barely visible to the naked eye resemble tiny finger-like processes projecting into the intestinal lumen.

Innervation. The parasympathetic and sympathetic divisions of the autonomic nervous system provide the efferent nerves to the small intestine. The parasympathetic preganglionic fibers pass through the vagus nerves to synapse with neurons of the intrinsic plexuses of the intestine. The sympathetic preganglionic fibers arise from the ninth and tenth thoracic segments of the spinal cord and synapse in the superior mesenteric ganglion. The postganglionic sympathetic fibers pass along the branches of the superior mesenteric artery to the intestine. Pain from the intestine is mediated through thoracic visceral afferents, not vagal afferents. Although the vagus contains large numbers of afferent fibers, thoracic visceral afferents, not vagal afferents, mediate pain from the intestine.[6]

MICROSCOPIC ANATOMY

The small intestine consists of four layers. From the lumen outward, they are the mucosa, the submucosa, the muscularis, and the adventitia or serosa.

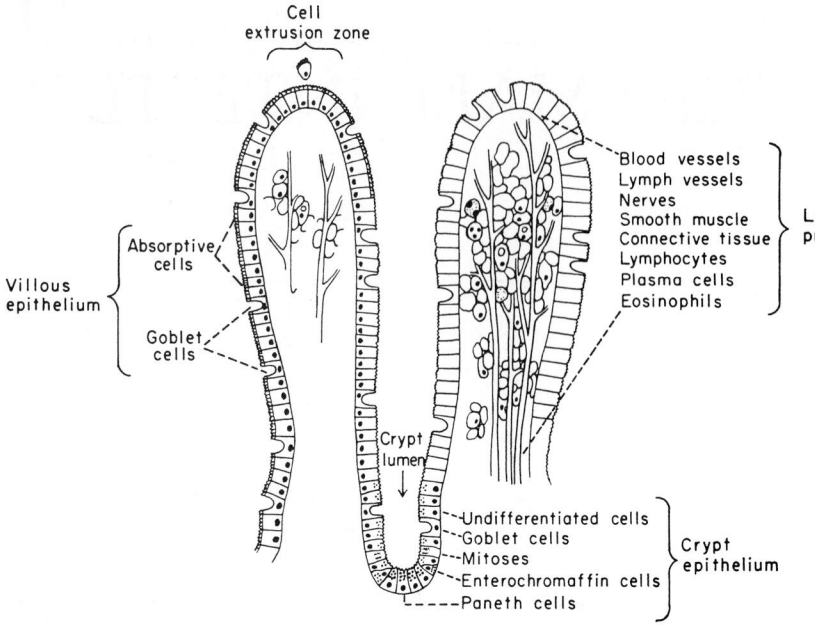

Figure 31–1. Schematic diagram of two sectioned villi and a crypt to illustrate the histologic organization of the small intestinal mucosa. (From Trier, J. S.: Morphology of epithelium of small intestine. *In* Code, C. F. (Ed.): American Physiological Society: Handbook of Physiology, Section 6, Alimentary Canal. Baltimore, Williams & Wilkins, 1968.)

Mucosa

The mucosa of the small intestine encompasses the epithelium, the lamina propria, and the muscularis mucosae. The mucosal surface has two important structural features: the villi and the crypts of Lieberkühn (Fig. 31–1). The villi have a columnar epithelial surface and a cellular connective tissue core of lamina propria. Each villus contains a central lymphatic vessel called a lacteal, a small artery, a vein, and a capillary network. Human jejunal villi measure 0.5 to 1.0 mm. high and number 10 to 40 villi per square millimeter of mucosal surface. In addition to the vessels, the villi contain smooth muscle fibers extending from the muscularis mucosae, providing contractility to each villus. The crypts of Lieberkühn, or intestinal glands, reside adjacent to the bases of the villi and extend down to, but not through, the muscularis mucosae. The lamina propria between the intestinal epithelium and the muscularis mucosae contains blood and lymph vessels, nerve fibers, smooth muscle fibers, fibroblasts, macrophages, plasma cells, lymphocytes, eosinophils, and mast cells, as well as elements of connective tissue.[3]

Scanning electron micrographs provide an in-depth perspective of the mucosa with excellent resolution (Fig. 31–2). The villi vary in shape from circular to flattened or finger-shaped. The finger-shaped villi are 0.1 to 0.25 mm. in diameter, are corrugated by deep horizontal clefts, and have holes 3 to 8 μ. across on the surface, representing the openings of the goblet cells.[23] The muscularis mucosa is a thin layer of smooth muscle separating the mucosa from the submucosa.

Cells of the Epithelium

Cells of the Villi. The columnar epithelial cells are responsible for absorption. These cells, 22 to 26μ. tall, exhibit a striated luminal border (brush border) and a basally placed nucleus (Fig. 31–3). The microvilli, which are projections 1 μ. tall and 0.1 μ. wide and are produced by numerous folds in the apical plasma membrane, account for the brush border appearance. The microvilli greatly increase the absorptive surface of the epithelial cell. The plasma membranes of the epithelial cells have a three-layered or trilamellar appearance and appear somewhat thicker over the microvilli than in the lateral and basal portion of the cell. The membrane of the microvillus is continuous, without fenestrations discernible by electron microscopic techniques, and it separates the lumen of the gut from the interior of the epithelial cell. A coat of fine filaments called the "fuzz" or glycocalyx, characterizes the luminal surface of the microvillus membrane (Fig. 31–4). The brush border contains high concentrations of digestive enzymes, particularly disaccharidases. The plasma membrane contains 80% to 90% of the disaccharidase activity of the intestinal cell. These findings indicate that the microvilli, besides increasing absorptive surface, perform an important digestive function.[6]

Three specialized areas of the lateral plasma membrane deserve comment. The *tight junctions* are fusions of the lateral plasma membranes between the terminal web and the intestinal lumen. This tight junction is present about the circumference of the cell. Immediately below the tight junction is an intermediate junction that has an intracellular space of

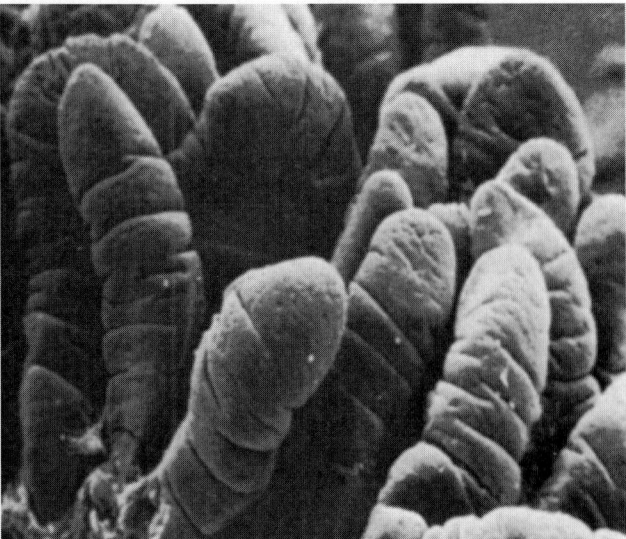

Figure 31–2. A scanning electron micrograph of human jejunal mucosa (× 42). The villi are finger shaped and are indented with numerous transverse grooves. The pitlike impressions on the villi are the openings of goblet cells. (Courtesy of A. L. Jones, M.D., University of California, San Francisco.)

approximately 200 Å. Occurring at intervals along the lateral plasma membranes are very close attachments of adjacent membranes called *desmosomes*. The intermediate junction and desmosomes bind adjacent cells together.[6]

The absorptive cells contain granular and agranular endoplasmic reticulum, which has an important synthetic function in the cell. The endoplasmic reticulum synthesizes the protein component of the chylomicron during fat absorption. This organelle also synthesizes triglyceride for an important step in fat absorption. The endoplasmic reticulum may synthesize the cytoplasmic enzymes of the absorptive cell.

The Golgi material probably stores or modifies substances absorbed or synthesized by the cell. Lysosomes contain lytic enzymes and eliminate waste materials by either lysing them or segregating the noxious substance for extrusion.

Goblet Cells. Goblet cells are present in both the villi and the crypts. These cells have cytoplasm filled with mucous granules between the nucleus and the apical brush border. Electron microscopic studies suggest that intestinal goblet cells secrete their mucus by merocrine secretion.[6]

Cells of the Crypts

Enterochromaffin Cells. Enterochromaffin cells reside in the crypts of the small intestine and in other parts of the gastrointestinal system as well, including the esophagus, stomach, colon, gallbladder, and pancreas. These cells do not contact the intestinal lumen, and their secretory granules are usually below the nuclei away from the lumen, suggesting secretion into the blood rather than the lumen. The enterochromaffin cells have an endocrine function.

Paneth Cells. Paneth cells occur in the base of the crypts and are structurally similar to cells known to secrete large amounts of protein, such as pancreatic or parotid acinar cells. The function of Paneth cells is unknown.

Undifferentiated Cells. Undifferentiated cells, the most frequent cell in the base of the crypts, multiply and differentiate to replace lost absorptive cells.

Epithelial Renewal. The epithelium of the small intestine is a dynamic, rapidly proliferating tissue in which old dying cells are constantly replaced by newly formed cells, thus maintaining the structural integrity of the mucosa. Mitotic division of undifferentiated cells occurs in the crypts. An undifferentiated cell may do one of three things: differentiate into an absorptive cell and migrate into the villus, remain in the crypt and continue mitotic activity, or remain in the crypt in a resting stage. The cells entering the villi migrate to the villus tips, where they are shed into the lumen. New growth replaces the population of intestinal epithelial cells every 3 to 7 days.[6]

Submucosa

The submucosa is a strong fibroelastic and areolar connective tissue layer containing vessels, nerves, and lymph nodules.

Muscular Layer and Intramural Neural Structures

Two distinct layers of smooth or nonstriated muscle, an outer longitudinal coat and an inner circular coat, form the muscular portion of the small intestine. Intestinal smooth muscle fibers are spindle-shaped structures about 250 μ long. Electron microscopic studies show intestinal smooth muscle cells as discrete structures. The plasma membrane of

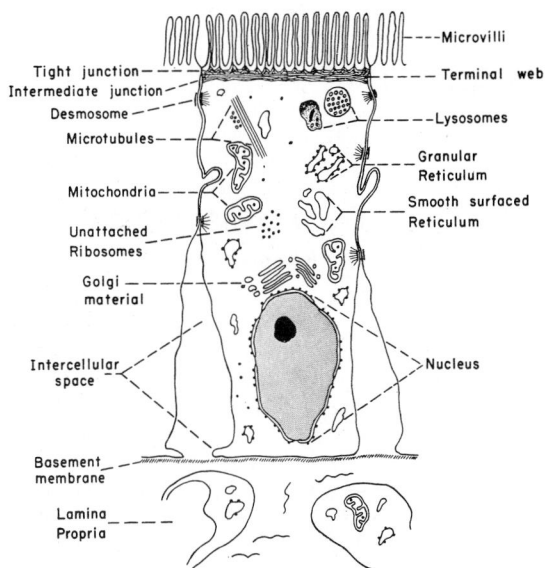

Figure 31–3. Schematic diagram of an intestinal absorptive cell. (From Trier, J. S., and Rubin, C. E.: Electron microscopy of the small intestine: A review. Gastroenterology, *49*:574, 1965.)

adjacent cells approximate at points, forming structures called nexuses. The nexuses allow electrical continuity between smooth muscle cells and permit conduction through the muscle layer.

The small intestine has four identifiable neural plexuses: (1) The subserous plexus, noticeable on the mesenteric attachment, forms the transition between the mesenteric nerve fibers and the myenteric plexus. Ganglia occur in the subserous plexus. (2) The myenteric plexus is located between the longitudinal and circular muscle layers and consists of three networks linking various ganglia and ramifying within the muscle layers. (3) The submucosal plexus is a network of nerve fibers and ganglia in the submucosa. (4) The mucous plexus consists of fibers from the submucosal plexus extending into the mucosa. This plexus does not contain nerve cell bodies.[3, 6, 20]

For references, see page 922.

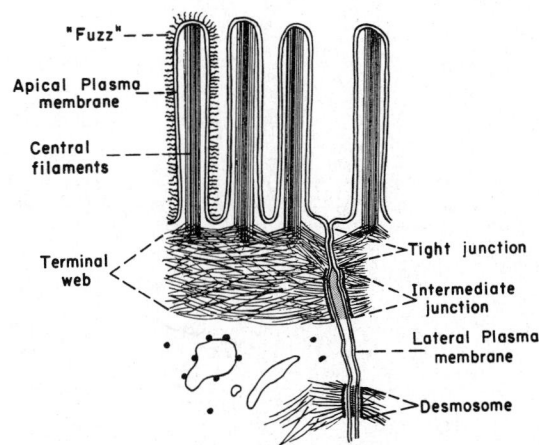

Figure 31–4. Schematic illustration of the specialization of the apical cytoplasm of the plasma membrane of intestinal absorption cells. (From Trier, J. S., and Rubin, C. E.: Electron microscopy of the small intestine: A review. Gastroenterology, *49*:574, 1965.)

II _____

PHYSIOLOGY

R. Scott Jones, M.D.

DIGESTION AND ABSORPTION

Carbohydrate

An adult may ingest about 350 gm. of carbohydrate daily, consisting of starch, sucrose, and lactose (Fig. 31–5). Dietary starch contains two glucose polymers, amylopectin and amylose. Amylopectin, the most abundant constituent of starch (80%) is a 1–4 linked straight chain of glucose molecules. Amylopectin also possesses a 1–6 branching side chain at approximately every 25 glucose units along the straight chain. Amylose has only 1–4 linkages of glucose molecules in a straight chain. Pancreatic and salivary amylases break the interior 1–4 glucose linkages, so the end product of amylose digestion by amylase is maltose (glucose-glucose) and maltotriose (glucose-glucose-glucose), which amylase cannot digest further because the only linkages present between glucose molecules in this circumstance are terminal bonds.

The 1–6 glucose linkages in amylopectin produce the end products of amylase digestion: maltose, maltotriose, and the residual branched saccharides, the dextrins. The digestion of starch by amylase probably occurs predominantly in the lumen of the alimentary tract. The high concentrations of digestive enzymes in isolated brush border preparations suggest that maltose, maltotriose, and dextrin, as well as the dietary disaccharides lactose (glucose-galactose) and sucrose (glucose-fructose), are completely broken down to the constituent monosaccharides by the microvilli, probably at the level of the glycocalyx (fuzz coat).

The intestinal cells actively transport glucose and galactose against a concentration gradient. Glucose and galactose compete for transport in a manner similar to competitive inhibition in other enzyme substrate systems. The active transport of sugars requires metabolic energy as well as oxygen. Sodium ion is important in the transport of glucose and galactose; however, only very small concentrations are required. Glucose and galactose are absorbed by carrier-mediated active transport. The absorption of glucose and galactose depends on Na^+ movement into the cell produced by the Na^+K^+

ATPase, located on the basolateral cell membrane. Fructose, the other significant monosaccharide, is not absorbed by active transport but probably enters the intestinal cells by *facilitated diffusion*.[6, 20]

Protein

The stomach initiates the digestion of protein in two ways: the acidic gastric environment favors denaturation of protein, and pepsin hydrolyzes protein to polypeptides. Digestion of protein is far from complete when gastric chyme enters the duodenum, where the higher pH inactivates pepsin. The pancreas secretes proteolytic enzyme precursors into the duodenum. The intestinal enzyme enterokinase converts trypsinogen to trypsin. The activation of trypsinogen is autocatalytic; that is, trypsin also activates trypsinogen. Trypsin likewise activates the other pancreatic proteolytic enzyme precursors. Trypsin, chymotrypsin, and elastase—pancreatic endopeptidases—split peptide bonds in the central portion of protein molecules, whereas carboxypeptidases—pancreatic exopeptidases—remove amino acids from the C-terminal position of protein molecules. Aminopeptidases are intestinal exopeptidases that split amino acids from the N-terminal position of protein molecules. Amino acids are the final product of protein digestion. However, some dipeptides are also absorbed.

Amino acids are absorbed from the intestinal lumen by carrier-mediated active transport.[6] The transport of amino acids requires oxygen and sodium. The sodium pump on the basolateral cell membrane of the intestinal epithelial cells maintains an electrical potential across the brush border. Transport of Na^+ into the cell is linked to the movement of amino acids and oligopeptides into the cell. Carrier-mediated active transport is supported by evidence that suggests that certain amino acids exhibit mutual competitive inhibition. Experiments on competitive inhibition of various L-amino acids have suggested several distinct pathways for absorption of amino acids, determined by their chemical structure. The brush border has three Na^+-dependent active transport systems for amino acids. The neutral brush border (NBB) system transports neutral amino acids, the PHE system transports phenylalanine and methionine, and the IMINO system transports proline and hydroxyproline. The L and y$^+$ transport systems on the brush border do not require Na^+. The L system transports neutral amino acids, and the y$^+$ system transports basic amino acids such as lysine and arginine.

Two Na^+-independent systems actively transport neutral amino acids across the basolateral plasma membrane: the A system and the ASC system. The Na^+-independent L system transports neutral amino acids across the basolateral membranes. In normal humans, digestion and absorption of protein are usually 80 to 90% completed in the jejunum.

Fat

Although emulsification of fat occurs in the stomach, little digestion of fat occurs except in the small intestine. The entry of gastric chyme into the duodenum is regulated in part by a negative feedback system in which fat in the duodenum inhibits gastric emptying. In the duodenum, dietary fat in

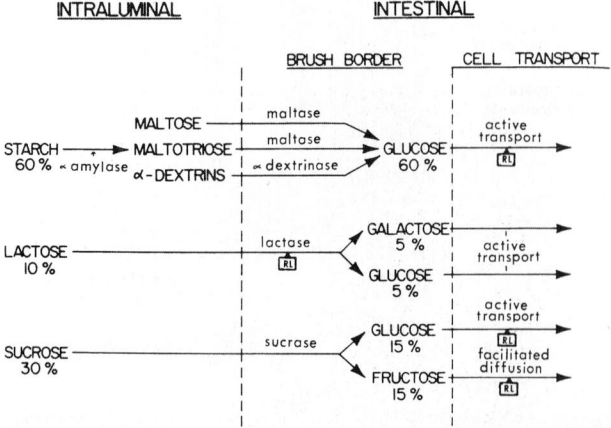

Figure 31–5. Outline of carbohydrate digestion and absorption in humans. Percentages refer to proportion of total carbohydrate in diet; RL locates the rate-limiting step in the overall digestion-absorption process for each carbohydrate ingested. (From Gray, G. M.: Carbohydrate digestion and absorption. Gastroenterology, *58*:96, 1970.)

the form of triglycerides mixes with biliary and pancreatic secretions, the important constituents of which are bile salts, lecithin, pancreatic lipase, and bicarbonate ion.[17]

The bile salts that occur in humans—glycine or taurine conjugates of cholic acid, deoxycholic acid, or chenodeoxycholic acid—are detergents; they are water-soluble at one portion of the molecule and fat-soluble at the other. In solution, substances produce polymolecular aggregates called *micelles*, which can dissolve fat. Lecithin, a phospholipid, greatly enhances the capacity of bile salts to form micelles and dissolve fat. Bile salt and lecithin solubilize lipid in an aqueous environment to produce a micellar solution. This provides an optimal physicochemical environment for the action of pancreatic lipase (Fig. 31–6). Pro-colipase is an intraluminal enzyme converted to colipase by the action of trypsin. Colipase binds to triglyceride; then lipase complexes with colipase, and triglyceride hydrolysis occurs.[20]

Pancreatic lipase catalyzes the hydrolysis of dietary triglyceride into 2-monoglyceride and fatty acids. The 2-monoglyceride and fatty acids then enter the micelles and are held in micellar solution. The bile salt–monoglyceride fatty acid micelle can also solubilize other lipids such as cholesterol, phospholipid, and fat-soluble vitamins. Pancreatic bicarbonate regulates the pH of the intestinal lumen to allow lipase to function optimally. An alkaline pH favors ionization of fatty acids and bile salts, which increases their solubility in micelles.[18] An alkaline pH also increases the solubility of bile salts. Three conditions impede the movement of lipids from the intestinal lumen into the absorptive cell: an unstirred water layer, a mucous coat on the brush border, and the lipid bilayer of the brush border membrane. When the micelles encounter the microvilli of the intestinal epithelial cells, the fatty acids and 2-monoglyceride pass into the epithelial cells by diffusion.

After entering the epithelial cell, 2-monoglyceride and fatty acids are synthesized into triglyceride in the endoplasmic reticulum. Fatty acid–binding protein participates in the movement of lipid from the brush border to the endoplasmic reticulum. The biosynthesis of triglyceride in the gut may occur by two pathways: the α-glycerophosphate pathway, in which the triglyceride is synthesized from glycerol and fatty acids, and the monoglyceride pathway, in which the triglyceride is formed by the addition of fatty acids to the 1 position of the 2-monoglyceride. The monoglyceride pathway is probably more important in humans (Fig. 31–7).

After triglyceride synthesis, triglycerides, phospholipid,

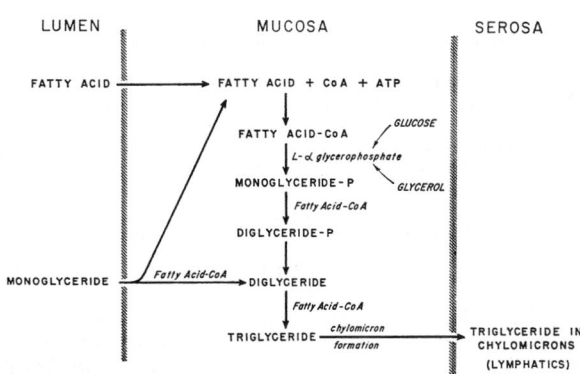

Figure 31–7. Major biochemical reactions in the transport of long-chain fatty acids and monoglycerides. (From Isselbacher, K. J.: Biochemical aspects of lipid malabsorption. Fed. Proc., *26*:1420, 1967.)

cholesterol, cholesterol esters, and protein form chylomicrons. The formation of chylomicrons requires the synthesis of lipoprotein. Although the lipoprotein content of the chylomicron is relatively small, the various apoproteins are important in determining subsequent chylomicron metabolism. Chylomicrons pass from the epithelial cells into the lacteals, where they pass through the lymphatics into the venous system (Fig. 31–8). All long-chain fat is absorbed in the manner just described; however, medium-chain triglyceride (C_8 to C_{10}) may be absorbed without hydrolysis and pass into portal blood rather than into lymph via the formation of chylomicrons.[6, 20]

The jejunum absorbs most dietary fat. Although unconjugated bile acids are absorbed in the jejunum by passive diffusion, the conjugated bile acids that form micelles are absorbed in the ileum by active transport. There they are almost completely absorbed and pass via the portal venous blood to the liver, for resecretion as bile. Only a small fraction of the pool of total bile salts, about 500 to 600 mg., escapes the enterohepatic circulation daily, and this small loss is replaced by hepatic synthesis of bile salts from cholesterol. In a normal adult, the bile acid pool of about 4 to 5 gm. circulates six to eight times daily. Normally, all dietary fat is absorbed, and the 5 gm. of fat excreted in the feces daily comes from desquamated cells and bacteria.[17]

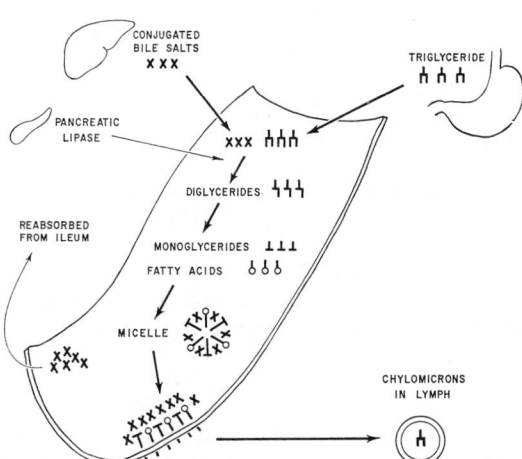

Figure 31–6. Diagram depicting the intraluminal events in fat absorption. (From Isselbacher, K. J.: Biochemical aspects of lipid malabsorption. Fed. Proc., *26*:1420, 1967.)

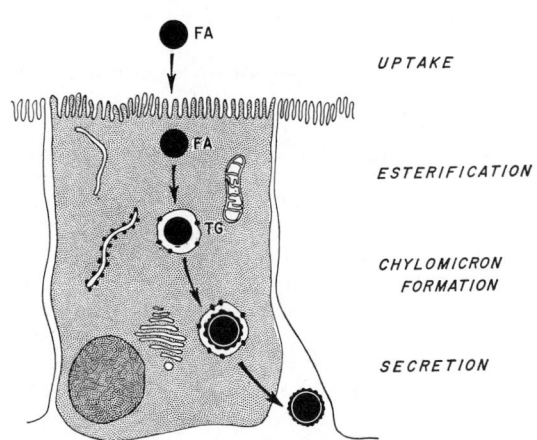

Figure 31–8. The major steps in the absorption of fat. This diagram depicts the role of the smooth endoplasmic reticulum in esterification and of the rough endoplasmic reticulum in protein synthesis, which is necessary for chylomicron formation. (From Isselbacher, K. J.: Biochemical aspects of lipid malabsorption. Fed. Proc., *26*:1420, 1967.)

Water and Electrolytes

Large quantities of water enter the small intestine. Some water is ingested, but the digestive glands secrete a larger amount to provide the luminal environment for optimal digestion and absorption. Five to 10 liters of water enters the small bowel daily, whereas only about 500 ml. or less leaves the ileum and enters the colon. The small intestine, therefore, absorbs large quantities of water. Experiments with isotopes reveal simultaneous movements of large quantities of water from intestinal lumen to blood and from blood to intestinal lumen. Intestinal absorption results from two large oppositely directed fluxes.[38] The net lumen-to-blood flux of water from an isotonic sodium chloride solution containing glucose in the human small intestine is an estimated 12.7 and 12.1 ml. per hour per cm. in jejunum and ileum, respectively.[36, 37]

The important factors in the movement of water across the intestinal mucosa are diffusion and osmotic filtration caused by osmotic or hydrostatic pressure differences across the membrane. In other words, water is absorbed as osmotic gradients are established by the active transport of solutes such as sodium ion, glucose, or amino acids into the cells. The intestinal mucosa behaves as if the absorptive cell plasma membrane were penetrated by aqueous channels called *pores*.[36, 37] These pores allow the transfer of water and water-soluble substances across the lipoidal cell membrane by a process of simple diffusion. The effective pore radii of the jejunum and ileum are 7.5 and 3.4 Å, respectively. The small size of these hypothetical pores prevents their identification by electron microscopy. Intestinal cells have a sodium pump (Na$^+$K$^+$ ATPase) on the basolateral cell membrane that moves Na$^+$ out of the cell into the basolateral intercellular space. Movement of K$^+$ into the cell accompanies the Na$^+$ movement. The sodium pump produces a concentration gradient that moves Na$^+$ into the cell from the lumen. This movement of Na$^+$ by the sodium pump also transports glucose, amino acids, and oligopeptide into the intestinal epithelial cells.[20]

In the human jejunum, absorption of sodium ions (net transfer from lumen to blood) occurs against a modest concentration gradient, is dramatically influenced by the rate and direction of water flux, and is stimulated by glucose, galactose, and bicarbonate ions. In the jejunum, a small portion of sodium absorption is mediated by active transport, but most of jejunal sodium absorption occurs by bulk flow along osmotic gradients. The jejunum effectively absorbs bicarbonate against steep electrochemical gradients. One explanation is that absorption of bicarbonate is mediated by H$^+$ secretion, and the relationship between Na$^+$ and HCO$_3$ is explained by an Na$^+$-H$^+$ exchange.[36]

The human ileum also absorbs Na$^+$ against steep electrochemical gradients; this absorption is unaffected by water flow and is not stimulated by glucose, galactose, or HCO$_3^-$. The observations suggest a very efficient Na$^+$ transport in the ileum. The human ileum also absorbs Cl$^-$ against steep electrochemical gradients. When net ileal Na$^+$ movement is zero, there is an equimolar exchange of Cl$^-$ and HCO$_3^-$ secretion.[36] Potassium is passively absorbed from the intestine according to its electrochemical gradients.

Calcium is absorbed, particularly in the proximal small intestine (duodenum and jejunum), by a process of active transport. This ion is absorbed better from an acid than from an alkaline environment, which may explain the better absorption in the proximal intestine. Vitamin D and parathyroid hormone enhance calcium absorption.[6, 20]

An important electrolyte absorbed by the small intestine is iron. One of the important functions of the small intestine is to regulate the body pool of iron. In a person with normal iron stores, there is only a slight transfer of iron from the intestinal absorptive cell to plasma, and only a small amount of iron enters the mucosal cell from the lumen. In a person with iron deficiency, there is no effective block to the transfer of iron from absorptive cell to plasma and no block to the entry of luminal iron into the mucosal cell.[1, 20]

MOTILITY

There are several types of visible small intestinal muscular activity. The *segmenting contraction* is a localized circumferential contraction of the circular muscle over a length of about 1 cm. of the small intestine. Segmenting contractions divide the luminal content within the area of contraction. Their rhythmic segmenting activity occurs in the proximal small intestine at about nine contractions per minute. Segmenting contractions occurring regularly and rhythmically in adjacent portions of the small intestine divide and subdivide the intestinal content, mixing it and exposing it to larger areas of mucosa, which facilitates digestion and absorption. *Peristalsis* consists of intestinal contractions passing aborally at a rate of 1 to 2 cm. per second through several centimeters of intestine. Peristalsis is somewhat slower in the distal than in the proximal small bowel. The major function of peristalsis is the distal movement of intestinal chyme. Under abnormal circumstances *peristaltic rushes* may occur. Peristaltic rushes usually begin in the proximal small bowel or duodenum and rapidly traverse the entire length of the small intestine. When the peristaltic rush ends, there may be a quiescent period of no motor activity.[6, 20]

The Migrating Myoelectrical Complex (MMC)

During the interdigestive period, there are cyclically occurring contractions that move aborally along the intestine every 75 to 90 minutes during fasting. Most of these fronts of activity begin in the stomach or duodenum, last about 4½ minutes, and pass along the gut at about 6.8 cm. per minute. The MMC is thought to sweep or cleanse the intestine during the interdigestive period. Motilin may regulate the MMC.[20, 29]

Regulation of Small Intestinal Motility

Myogenic Factors. Two types of electrical activity can be recorded from the small intestine. Slow-wave electrical activity begins in the longitudinal muscle layer of the duodenum and is propagated distally. In human adults, this activity occurs at 11.7 ± 0.5 (SEM) cycles per minute. This phenomenon, called the *basic electrical rhythm* (BER), is independent of the intrinsic neural plexuses, and is unrelated to motor activity. Intestinal *spike potential* may occur spontaneously during depolarization or from stretching of the bowel, and it is associated with motor activity.

Neurogenic Factors. Intrinsic neural regulation is initiated by stimulation of the mucosa, particularly by distention, which causes contraction of longitudinal and circular muscle, propelling luminal content distally. The intrinsic nerve supply regulates rather than initiates motor action. In general, sympathetic activity inhibits motor function, whereas parasympathetic activity stimulates it. Epinephrine inhibits small intestinal motor activity, whereas acetylcholine stimulates it. Distention of the small intestine can inhibit small intestinal motility by the intestinointestinal inhibitory reflex. Distention of the ureter, renal pelvis, or biliary system or peritoneal irritation may inhibit intestinal movements.[6]

Hormonal Factors. Gastrointestinal hormones may be important in regulating intestinal motility. Gastrin stimulates gastric and intestinal motility and relaxes the ileocecal sphincter. Cholecystokinin-pancreozymin (CCK-PZ) also stimulates intestinal motility and may decrease intestinal transit time. Secretin and chemically similar glucagon inhibit intestinal motility. The role of hormones in regulating intestinal motility is poorly understood.

ENDOCRINE FUNCTION

The mucosa of the small intestine is an important source of peptide hormones, whose main function is to regulate the gastrointestinal tract.[14]

Secretin

Secretin was the first gastrointestinal hormone described. This hormone, a helical polypeptide with 27 amino acid residues, is released from duodenal mucosal S cells in response to intraluminal H^+. Secretin promotes digestion by stimulating copious secretion of water and bicarbonate from the pancreas. This action facilitates entry of pancreatic enzymes into the intestinal lumen and provides a pH favoring digestion of fat. Secretin is also a choleretic and inhibits gastric acid secretion and gastrointestinal motility.

CCK-PZ

Cholecystokinin and pancreozymin are the same substance and are released from intestinal mucosal I cells bathed by amino acids or fatty acids. CCK-PZ facilitates digestion and absorption by stimulating emptying of the gallbladder as well as by increasing bile flow and relaxing the sphincter of Oddi. Another important action of CCK-PZ is stimulation of pancreatic enzyme secretion. CCK-PZ is a linear polypeptide having 33 residues. The C-terminal tetrapeptide of CCK-PZ is identical to that of another gastrointestinal hormone, gastrin, and this fragment possesses the action of both hormones. In general, CCK-PZ and gastrin share actions and differ mainly in potency for a given action.

Other Gut Hormones

During the past several years, the intestinal mucosa has been recognized as a source of several biologically active peptides. Not all these substances satisfy rigid physiologic criteria for hormone status, but they should be described briefly here. *Enteroglucagon* is released from the EG cells, which occur predominantly in the distal small intestine. This peptide occurs in two forms: one has a molecular weight of about 3500, and the other is a larger molecule. Enteroglucagon is released by carbohydrate and long-chain fatty acid and inhibits intestinal motility. *Vasoactive intestinal peptide* (VIP) is a member of the secretin-glucagon family of peptides and is found in high concentrations in bowel, brain, and peripheral nerve tissue. VIP shares some actions with secretin and glucagon. Blood levels of VIP do not change following meals, so VIP may act as a neurotransmitter or paracrine substance rather than as a hormone. *Gastric inhibitory polypeptide* (GIP) is also a secretin-glucagon–like peptide with 43 amino acids and a molecular weight of about 51,000. GIP is released from K cells, predominantly in the jejunum, on stimulation by carbohydrate or fat. The concentration of serum GIP increases after meals, and it is believed that its most significant action is to stimulate insulin secretion. *Motilin* is a 22-residue peptide with a molecular weight of about 2700; it is released from the EC cells of the intestine, predominantly the jejunum. Motilin inhibits gastric emptying in humans and may also alter the interdigestive myoelectrical complex and cause changes in the lower esophageal sphincter. *Somatostatin*, a tetradecapeptide, was recognized for its growth hormone release–inhibiting characteristics and has subsequently been shown to inhibit release of many hormones. Somatostatin is found in the brain, stomach, gut, and pancreas and is probably a paracrine substance. *Bombesin* may be secreted from the small bowel mucosa, and although it possesses several actions, its most important function seems to be to stimulate the secretion of gastric acid and the release of antral gastrin.

IMMUNOLOGIC FUNCTION OF THE INTESTINE

The intestine is a source of immunoglobulin, particularly IgA.[35] It is believed that this immunoglobulin arises from plasma cells in the lamina propria, and after linkage with a protein synthesized by epithelial cells, it is secreted into the lumen. Secretory IgA contains antibody activities, the exact roles of which are not yet known.

For references, see page 922.

III _____

INTESTINAL OBSTRUCTION

R. Scott Jones, M.D.

HISTORICAL ASPECTS

Hippocrates observed and treated intestinal obstruction. Praxagoras (350 B.C.), who created an enterocutaneous fistula to relieve an obstruction, performed the earliest known operation for intestinal obstruction. Nonoperative treatment remained the general rule, however, and included reduction of hernias, opium for pain, orally administered mercury or lead shot to open the occluded bowel, electrical stimulation, and gastric lavage.

In the nineteenth century, amid considerable debate, surgical procedures became more frequent for intestinal obstruction. Most of the significant advances in the management of this disorder occurred after the turn of the twentieth century. Hartwell and Hoguet[15] observed in 1912 that parenteral administration of saline solution prolonged the lives of dogs with intestinal obstruction. Administration of intravenous fluid has become a cardinal principle in the management of intestinal obstruction today. The second decade of the twentieth century saw the development of radiographic techniques for the diagnosis of intestinal obstruction. In the 1930s, nasogastric or intestinal tubes were employed to prevent or relieve intestinal distention in patients with intestinal obstruction. Antibiotics were added to the therapy of bowel obstruction in the 1940s and 1950s. Replacement fluids, intestinal decompression, antibiotics, and improvements in surgical and anesthetic techniques have reduced the mortality in simple intestinal obstruction; however, the recognition and treatment of strangulating intestinal obstruction remain important problems for surgeons today.[29]

ETIOLOGY

When gastrointestinal luminal content is pathologically prevented from passing distally, intestinal obstruction exists. Mechanical occlusion of the bowel into its lumen or paralysis of the intestinal muscle, called *paralytic ileus,* may cause intestinal obstruction.

Mechanical Obstruction

Three types of abnormalities may produce mechanical obstruction.[1, 2, 4, 7, 22, 25–27, 30, 32–34]

1. *Obstruction of the intestinal lumen* may be caused by several kinds of disease, such as polypoid tumors of the bowel. Intussusception is an invagination of the bowel lumen, with the invaginated portion (the intussusceptum) passing distally into the ensheathing outer portion (the intussuscipiens) by peristalsis. Unrelieved intussusception can occlude the blood supply of the intussusceptum. In adults, intussusception is usually caused by an abnormality of the bowel wall, such as a tumor or Meckel's diverticulum; in infants and children, intussusception may occur without apparent anatomic cause. Large gallstones, which can enter the intestinal lumen via a cholecystoenteric fistula, can cause obturation to produce a rare condition called *gallstone ileus.*

Feces, meconium, or bezoars may obstruct the intestine. Bezoars occur more frequently in children, the mentally retarded, and the toothless, and in patients after gastrectomy.

2. *Intrinsic bowel lesions* producing intestinal obstruction are often congenital (atresia, stenosis, duplication); they occur most commonly in infants and small children and are described in Chapter 38. Strictures of the intestine may result from neoplasm, as in carcinoma of the sigmoid colon, or from inflammation, as in Crohn's disease. Rarely, one encounters iatrogenic strictures following intestinal anastomosis or radiation therapy.

3. *Lesions extrinsic to the bowel* cause intestinal obstruction. Occlusion of the intestine by adhesions from previous operations or inflammation is the leading cause of small intestinal obstruction. Adhesions may obstruct by kinking or angulation or by creating bands of tissue that compress the bowel. External hernias are the second most common cause of mechanical small intestinal obstruction. Inguinal, femoral, umbilical, and incisional hernias are important causes of bowel obstruction. The risk of intestinal obstruction is the principal reason for the elective repair of hernias. Internal hernias due to congenital abnormalities of the mesentery or to surgical defects in the mesentery occasionally cause bowel obstruction. Extrinsic masses such as neoplasms and abscesses may cause mechanical bowel obstruction. A volvulus is an extrinsic abnormality in which a portion of the alimentary canal rotates or twists about itself; the twist usually involves the blood supply of the twisted portion of the bowel. This abnormality can kink the gut and produce mechanical obstruction, frequently occluding the blood supply to the bowel. A volvulus usually accompanies an underlying abnormality; for example, midgut volvulus is caused by the mesenteric abnormality of malrotation. Cecal volvulus occurs when the cecum or right colon is on a mesentery rather than being retroperitoneal. Sigmoid volvulus develops when the sigmoid colon is abnormally long or redundant. Another type of volvulus occurs when adhesions fix the intestine to a point that acts as a pivot for the volvulus. The most common causes of intestinal obstruction in adults are adhesions, usually from previous operations, hernias, and neoplasms. Neoplasms are the most common cause of colon obstruction.

Paralytic Ileus

Paralytic ileus, a common disorder, occurs to some extent in most patients undergoing abdominal operations. Several neural, humoral, and metabolic factors cause this abnormality. Reflexes that inhibit intestinal motility, such as the intestinointestinal reflex, result from prolonged intestinal distention. Distention of other organs, such as the ureter, can inhibit intestinal motility. Spine fracture, retroperitoneal hemorrhage, or trauma can also produce paralytic ileus. A humoral factor in paralytic ileus is suggested by experiments in dogs, in which motility of transplanted (denervated) intestinal loops was inhibited during experimental peritonitis.[21] The substances responsible for this phenomenon are unknown. Clinically, peritonitis causes paralytic ileus. Electrolyte imbalances, particularly hypokalemia, contribute to paralytic ileus by interfering with the normal ionic movements during smooth muscle contraction. Finally, ischemia of the intestine rapidly inhibits motility.

Idiopathic Intestinal Pseudo-Obstruction

Most patients with gaseous distention of the intestine have either mechanical intestinal obstruction or paralytic ileus. In most patients with ileus, the disorder can be readily ascribed to peritonitis, metabolic disturbances, or drugs. Idiopathic intestinal pseudo-obstruction is a chronic illness characterized by symptoms of recurrent intestinal obstruction without demonstrable mechanical occlusion of the bowel. Patients with this disease have impaired motor response to intestinal distention, but the duodenal and colonic slow waves may be normal. Some patients have aperistalsis of the esophagus, with failure of the lower esophageal sphincter to relax. Heredity plays a role in this disorder. The symptoms of intestinal pseudo-obstruction include cramping abdominal pain, vomiting, distention, diarrhea, and sometimes steatorrhea. Physical examination reveals abdominal distention. Intestinal pseudo-obstruction is distinguished from mechanical intestinal obstruction by the absence of the radiographic findings of mechanical obstruction. Surgical treatment for this condition should be avoided. Intravenous hyperalimentation may help manage these patients.[9]

PATHOGENESIS

Simple Mechanical Small Intestinal Obstruction

Mechanical obstruction of the small intestine causes accumulation of fluid and gas proximal to the obstruction, producing distention of the intestine. Ingested fluid, digestive secretions, and intestinal gas initiate the distention. As mentioned earlier, large volumes of saliva, gastric secretion, bile, and pancreatic juice enter the gut daily. The stomach has a very small capacity for absorbing fluid, so most alimentary fluid is absorbed by the small intestine.[38]

Peristalsis normally propels intestinal gas aborally for expulsion from the rectum as flatus. Gas accumulating in the intestine proximal to an obstruction originates from swallowed air, carbon dioxide from neutralization of bicarbonate, and organic gases from bacterial fermentation. Swallowed air is the most important source of gas in intestinal obstruction because its nitrogen content is very high, and the intestinal mucosa cannot absorb nitrogen. As a result, intestinal gas is predominantly (70%) nitrogen. The large amount of carbon dioxide produced in the lumen of the gut is readily absorbed and therefore contributes little to the distention.

One of the most important events during simple mechanical small bowel obstruction is loss of water and electrolytes from the body, caused mainly by intestinal distention. First, reflex vomiting may result from intestinal distention. In addition, intestinal distention is self-perpetuating in the obstructed small bowel, because distention increases intestinal secretion. Experiments on dogs show that intestinal distention initially causes decreased absorption (decreased lumen-to-blood flux of water) in the obstructed segment, but not in the intestine distal to the obstruction.[31] This phenomenon increases the accumulation of fluid in the bowel proximal to the obstruction, perhaps further accentuating dehydration and causing further intestinal distention, which proceeds proximally. Increased secretion in the obstructed bowel occurs in humans.[40]

The metabolic effects of fluid loss in simple mechanical obstruction of the small bowel depend on the site and the duration of the obstruction. Proximal obstruction of the small bowel causes relatively greater vomiting and less intestinal distention than distal obstruction. Proximal obstruction causes losses of water, Na^+, Cl^-, H^+, and K^+, producing dehydration with hypochloremia, hypokalemia, and metabolic alkalosis. Distal obstruction of the small bowel may entail loss of large quantities of fluid into the bowel; however, the abnormalities of serum electrolyte values are usually less dramatic, probably because less hydrochloric acid is lost.[22]

Oliguria, azotemia, and hemoconcentration can accompany dehydration. If dehydration persists, circulatory changes such as tachycardia, low central venous pressure, and reduced cardiac output may cause hypotension and hypovolemic shock. Other sequelae of intestinal distention include increased intra-abdominal pressure, decreased venous return from the legs, and elevation of the diaphragm sufficient to impair ventilation.

Rapid proliferation of intestinal bacteria occurs during intestinal obstruction. Normally the small intestine contains few bacteria and may be almost sterile. There may be several causes for the sparse bacterial population of the small intestine, but normal peristalsis and the interdigestive migrating myoelectrical complex (MMC), with continued aboral progression of luminal content, minimize the small intestinal flora. During small intestinal stasis, whatever the cause, intraluminal bacteria proliferate rapidly, especially in intestinal obstruction. The small intestinal contents thus become *feculent* during obstruction because of large quantities of bacteria. Normally the colon, an organ that functions as a reservoir, contains large numbers of bacteria.

The bacteria in the small intestine probably contribute little to the ill effects of simple mechanical small intestinal obstruction, although recent studies show that bacterial translocation may occur in the distended viable small intestine.[8]

Strangulation Obstruction

Strangulation occurs when the circulation to the obstructed intestine becomes impaired. Substantial increased intraluminal pressure impairs the bowel's circulation. Occlusion of the bowel lumen at two points along its length produces closed-loop obstruction. This type of obstruction may proceed more rapidly to strangulation than simple obstruction. Pressure necrosis can develop if the obstructed distending bowel is held by unyielding adhesive bands or hernial rings. The deformity or twisting of the mesentery, as in volvulus or intussusception, can occlude the mesenteric vessels. In strangulation obstruction, the patient may suffer all the ill effects of simple obstruction in addition to the effects of strangulation. Strangulation causes loss of blood and plasma into the strangulated segment. Predominant venous vascular obstruction may produce greater loss of blood or plasma than predominant arterial vascular obstruction. This loss of blood and plasma causes shock, particularly if the patient is already dehydrated. If strangulation produces gangrene, peritonitis and its sequelae occur. Rupture or perforation of a strangulated segment is possible and is a devastating complication.

In addition to the loss of blood and plasma, another important factor in strangulation obstruction is the toxic material from the strangulated loop. The luminal fluid from a strangulated intestinal loop and the bloody, malodorous peritoneal fluid are lethal when administered to normal animals. Bacteria and necrotic tissue appear to be necessary for the development of the toxic fluid. Apparently, this lethal fluid forms in the lumen of the strangulated intestine and passes through the injured intestinal wall. The peritoneum absorbs the toxic material, producing systemic effects.[21]

Colon Obstruction

In general, obstruction of the colon produces less fluid and electrolyte disturbance than mechanical obstruction of the small bowel. If the patient has a *competent* ileocecal valve, there may be little or no small bowel distention, but in this instance, the colon behaves like a closed loop. The massively distended colon may perforate. Because of its spherical shape and large diameter, the cecum is a likely site for perforation. However, the most common cause of colon obstruction is cancer, and the usual site of perforation is adjacent to the cancer. In patients with *incompetent* ileocecal valves, signs of small bowel distention may accompany colon obstruction. The colon is also subject to strangulation when obstruction compromises the blood supply.

DIAGNOSIS OF INTESTINAL OBSTRUCTION

The questions to ask in evaluating a patient suspected of having intestinal obstruction are: (1) Does the patient have bowel obstruction? (2) If so, where is it? (3) What is the anatomic and pathologic nature of the obstructing lesions? (4) Has strangulation occurred? (5) What is the general condition of the patient (fluid-electrolyte balance and other systemic disease)?

Abdominal pain, vomiting, obstipation, abdominal distention, and failure to pass flatus characterize intestinal obstruction. The typical crampy pain in intestinal obstruction occurs in paroxysms at 4- to 5-minute intervals in proximal obstruction and less frequently in distal obstruction. After a long period of mechanical obstruction, the crampy pain may subside because bowel distention inhibits motility. One should suspect strangulation with peritonitis when continuous severe abdominal pain replaces crampy abdominal pain.

Proximal intestinal obstruction can produce profuse vomiting and little abdominal distention. In distal obstruction, the vomiting is less frequent but is *feculent* because of the large bacterial population of intestinal contents. Obstipation and failure to pass gas from the rectum characterize complete obstruction, after the bowel distal to the obstruction empties. Increase in abdominal girth because of fluid and gas accumulating in the intestine accompanies distal obstruction of the small bowel, obstruction of the colon, or paralytic ileus.

Physical Examination

The physical examination should note certain points. Tachycardia and hypotension may indicate severe dehydration, peritonitis, or both. Fever suggests the possibility of strangulation. Poor skin turgor and dry mucous membranes may reflect dehydration. The abdomen is usually distended. Occasionally the examiner must distinguish bowel distention from ascites. A fluid wave, shifting dullness, and fullness in

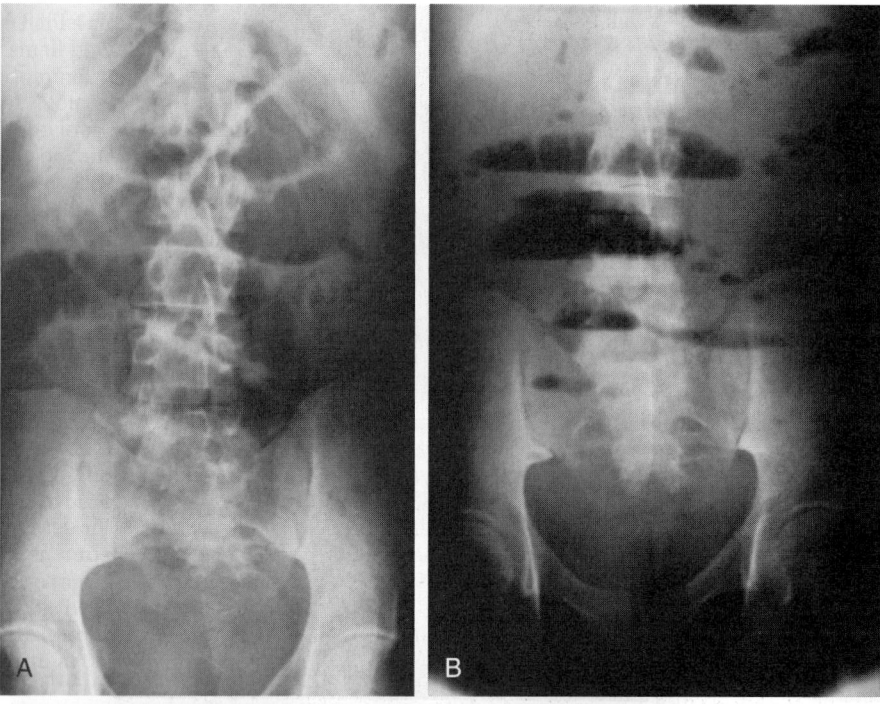

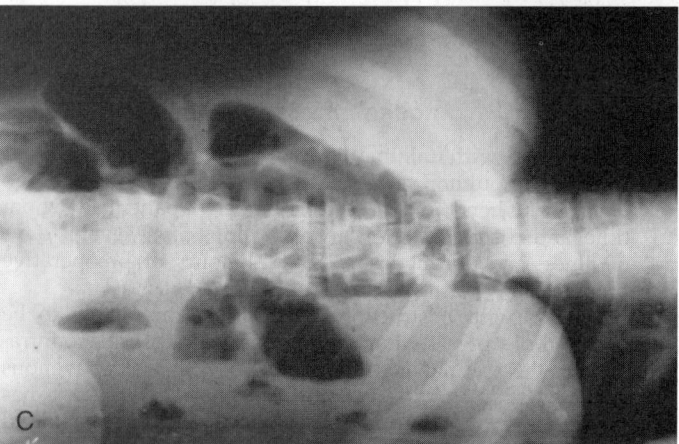

Figure 31–11. Supine *(A)*, upright *(B)*, and occasionally lateral decubitus *(C)* films usually confirm the diagnosis of acute complete mechanical obstruction of the small bowel by revealing distended small bowel loops, gas-fluid levels, inverted U-shaped loops, and the absence of gas in the colon or rectum.

do not respond well to conservative treatment, but malignant obstruction can frequently be relieved surgically. Judgment is required, however, in managing malignant intestinal obstruction in a terminally ill patient.[2] Certain patients with obstruction of the small bowel should undergo operation within several hours of admission to the hospital, including those with no history of previous abdominal surgery, those with incarcerated external hernias, those with signs of peritonitis, and any patient suspected of having strangulated bowel.[1]

Operation may be delayed under certain circumstances. In patients with pyloric obstruction, operation can safely be postponed to correct the fluid and electrolyte imbalance. A patient in whom intestinal obstruction develops immediately following an abdominal operation should initially be treated nonoperatively.[27] Overlooked strangulation is a risk in this instance, however. In one report of 41 patients with early postoperative obstruction of the bowel, the obstruction resolved in 30 patients without operation; however, two of those patients later required operation for bowel obstruction.[29] Infants with ileocecal intussusception respond to hydrostatic reduction of the intussusception, which avoids operation entirely. Adults with intussusception (Fig. 31–13)

should undergo operation because of the high frequency of bowel abnormalities causing the intussusception. In patients with sigmoid volvulus, sigmoidoscopy or colonoscopy can achieve decompression. In patients with intestinal obstruction due to an acute exacerbation of Crohn's disease, a period of conservative treatment may resolve the obstruction. Patients with chronic partial obstruction may be managed by less urgent operative treatment than patients with acute complete obstruction.

Operative Treatment for Intestinal Obstruction

In general, the nature of the problem determines the approach to management of intestinal obstruction. In simple obstruction, such as an incarcerated inguinal hernia, operative reduction and repair of the hernia suffice. Obstruction caused by peritoneal adhesions can be relieved by division of the adhesions. A second approach to obstructing lesions is to create an intestinal bypass. An example of this therapy is the treatment of radiation stricture of the ileum by ileotransverse colon anastomosis. The placement of a cutaneous fistula, such as a colostomy, proximal to the obstruction is

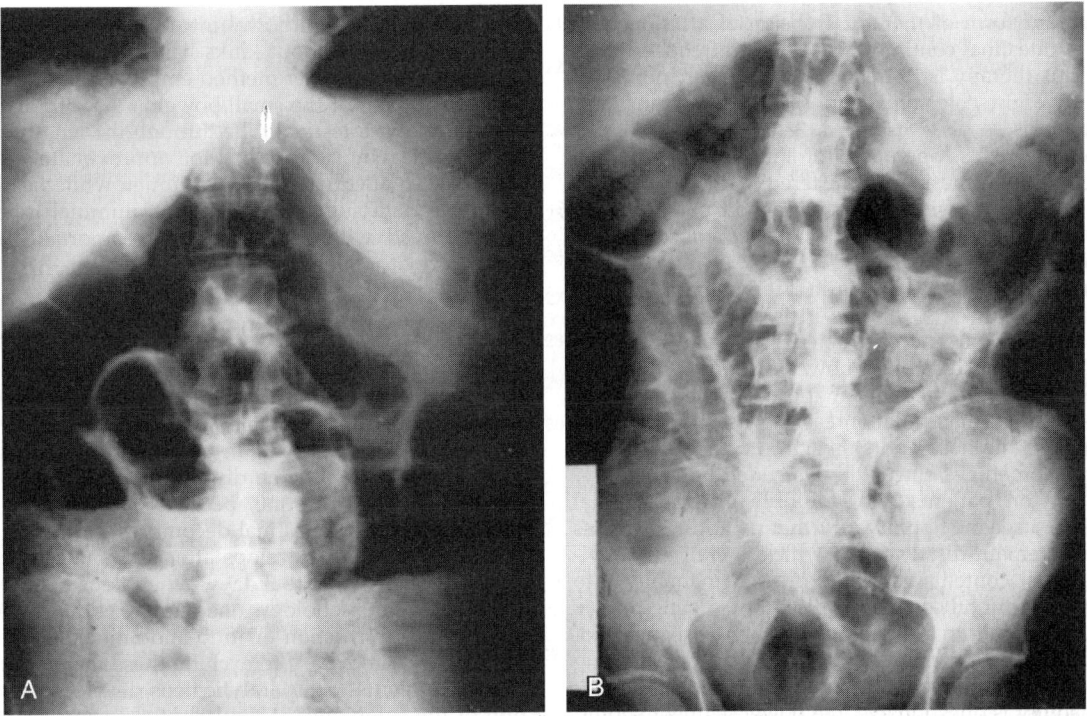

Figure 31–12. Paralytic ileus is usually difficult to distinguish from mechanical obstruction. The presence of gas in the stomach, small bowel, and colon suggests ileus, as shown in these films.

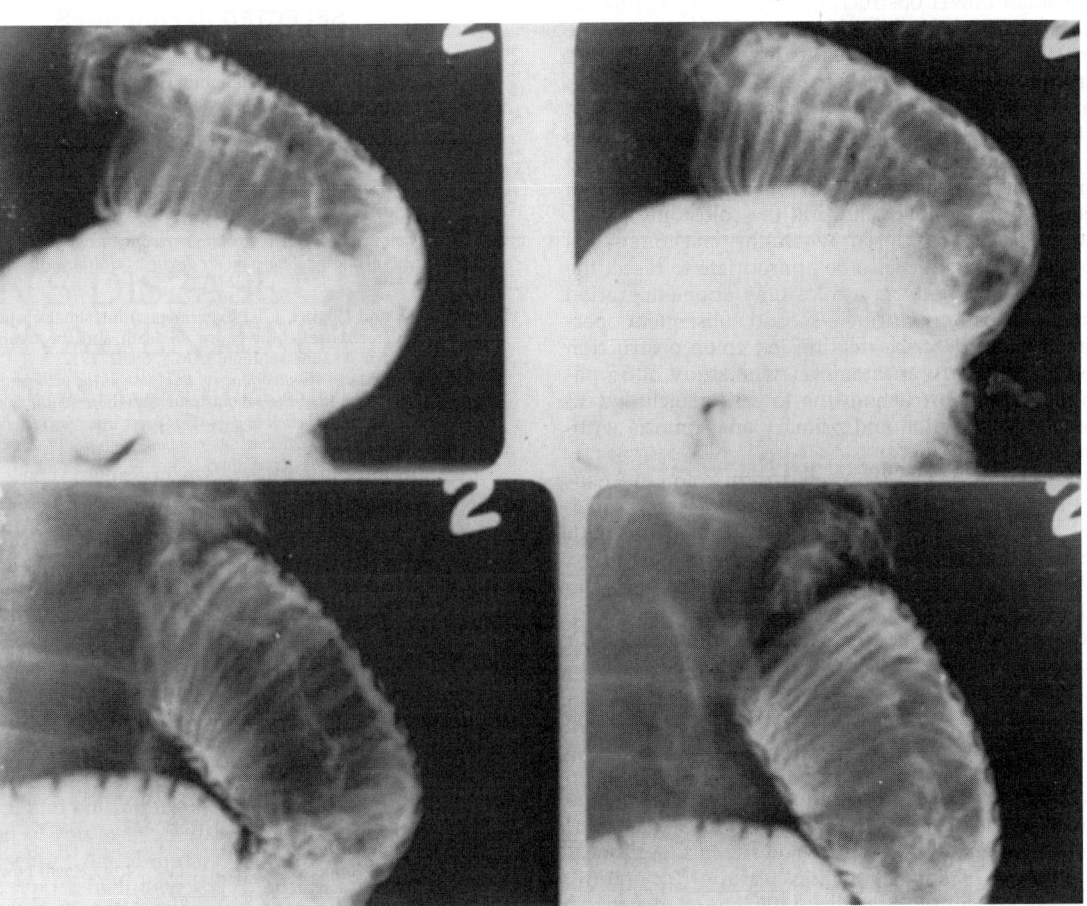

Figure 31–13. This series of spot films reveals an ileoileal intussusception in an adult.

a specific micro-organism that might be the cause of the disease; however, none has yet been identified. Recent reports of the isolation of *Mycobacterium paratuberculosis* from segments of bowel affected with Crohn's disease excited interest, but this organism as a specific etiology for the disease has yet to be proved. Also, no virus has been identified as an etiologic agent.

An immunologic origin of the disease has also been sought. No doubt an immunologic response to the condition does exist. Some have postulated that a childhood sensitization to milk impairs mucosal integrity and allows bacteria or bacteriologic products to enter the body. A cellular and humoral immune response to these products then ensues. The ileocolic epithelium, in particular, may be the target of a necrotizing immune response, with ensuing ulceration, tissue destruction, and the clinical appearance of the disease. Although an immunologic response certainly plays a role in the pathogenesis of the condition, its role as an etiologic agent is still unclear.

Other data suggest that environmental factors have an etiologic role in the disease. The disease is more common among persons living in temperate climates than among those living in tropical climates. Smoking may exert a stimulating effect on the disease; many patients with Crohn's disease are heavy smokers. Spouses of persons with Crohn's disease have a higher incidence of the disease than persons in the general population. Although these data suggest that environmental factors have a role, no specific environmental factor has been identified.

PATHOLOGY

Location of Lesions

Crohn's disease is a generalized inflammatory disorder of the alimentary tract that can involve any area from the mouth to the anus. The disease, however, is discontinuous and segmental. The small intestine and the large intestine are the most frequent sites of gross, macroscopic involvement. In one large series, 55% of patients had involvement of both small and large intestine, 30% of small intestine alone, and 15% of large intestine alone.[20] Of those with involvement of only the large intestine, one third (5% of the total patients) had anorectal involvement only. In contrast, anorectal involvement accompanied more proximal involvement in 48% of patients with Crohn's disease of the large intestine, in 41% of those with small and large intestinal Crohn's, and in 23% of those with small intestinal Crohn's.

Gross Pathologic Features

Aphthous Ulcers. One of the earliest macroscopic signs of Crohn's disease is the appearance of aphthous ulcers in the mucosa of the gastrointestinal tract. These small, flat, soft ulcers have a whitish center and a red border. They are scattered in the mucosa, with normal areas of mucosa in between. As the disease progresses, the aphthous ulcers deepen and coalesce, penetrating through the entire mucosa and forming longer ulcers that may reach 1 cm. or larger. The ulcers remain discontinuous and asymmetrical. They often appear first on the mesenteric border of the bowel and have a linear pattern along the wall of the intestine. Because of this, they are sometimes called *rake* ulcers, suggesting that a rake had been pulled across the mucosa in a longitudinal direction to create the pattern. Islands of normal mucosa can remain in between the ulcers to give the surface of the bowel a cobblestone appearance (Fig. 31–14).

Transmural Inflammation. As the ulcers grow and the inflammation spreads, the lesions extend deep into the wall

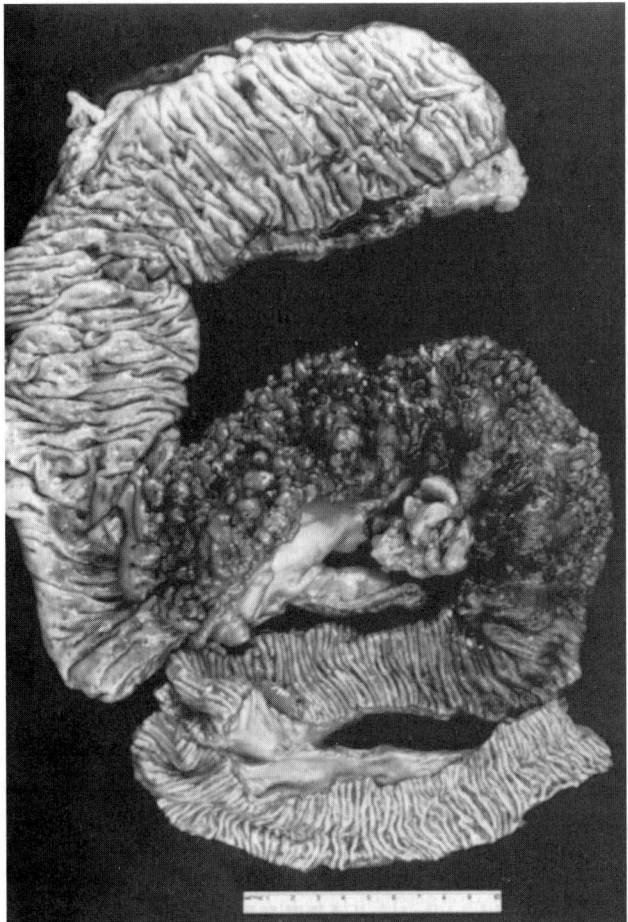

Figure 31–14. Photograph of ileum, cecum, and ascending colon resected for Crohn's disease of the terminal ileum, which demonstrates ulcerated ileal mucosa with a cobblestone appearance, thickened bowel wall, and enlarged adjacent ileal lymph nodes.

of the bowel through the mucosa and muscularis, out to the serosa, to form transmural fissures and thornlike defects. The inflammatory response creates a thickening of the bowel wall and a narrowing of its lumen, the so-called rubber-hose intestine. The inflammatory response on the serosa and adjacent mesentery also thickens these structures, and the fat of the mesentery creeps around the side of the bowel to add to the thickening. The intestinal lymphatic vessels are engorged, and the lymph nodes in the adjacent mesentery are enlarged.

Microscopic Features

Focal Chronic Inflammation. A chronic inflammatory infiltrate appears in the mucosa and submucosa and extends transmurally through the bowel wall (Fig. 31–15). The areas of inflammation are focal and scattered in between areas of uninvolved bowel. Distortion of the normal architecture of the intestinal crypts accompanies the inflammation.

Granulomas. A characteristic microscopic lesion of Crohn's disease is the granuloma, which appears in the mucosa, submucosa, or elsewhere in the wall of the bowel or its adjacent lymph nodes, in association with the chronic inflammatory response (see Fig. 31–15). The granulomas are nonspecific and contain chronic inflammatory cells and giant cells. They appear in 50% to 75% of patients.

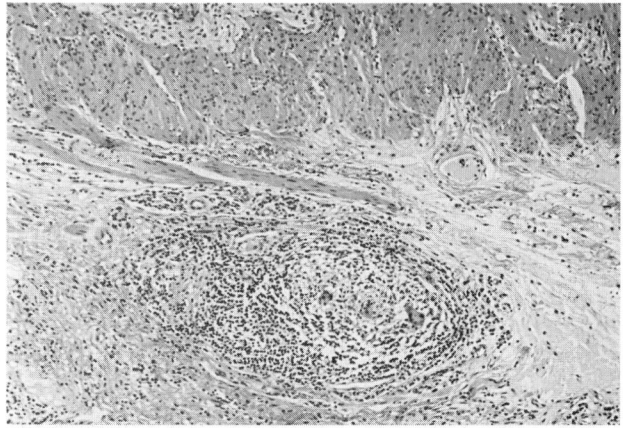

Figure 31–15. Photomicrograph of ileum with Crohn's disease, showing transmural inflammation and a subserosal, noncaseating granuloma.

Intestinal Complications

Two main intestinal complications develop from these lesions: obstruction and perforation. The chronic, fibrosing lesions of Crohn's disease may narrow the lumen of the bowel, producing partial or near-complete obstruction, with dilatation of the bowel proximal to the lesions and collapse of the bowel distal to the lesions. In contrast, lesions that penetrate into and perforate through the bowel wall result in localized abscesses near the sites of perforation and often fistulas between the sites of perforation and adjacent organs, such as loops of small and large intestine, the urinary bladder, the vagina (Fig. 31–16), the stomach, and sometimes the skin at sites of previous celiotomy. The perienteric fibrous response sometimes results in ureteral obstruction. Free perforations can occur directly into the generalized peritoneal cavity, but these are rare. The ulcerating mucosal lesions can also bleed, but this is also unusual. Patients with Crohn's disease of the large intestine may develop toxic megacolon, a condition of marked dilation of the colon, abdominal tenderness, ileus, and systemic signs such as fever, leukocytosis, tachycardia, and severe debility.

Long-standing lesions of the small and large intestine are premalignant. The incidence of carcinoma of the small bowel is six times greater in patients with Crohn's disease than in the general population; the incidence of carcinoma of the large bowel is four to six times greater. The cancers that appear in the small intestine of Crohn's patients have a different pattern than those that occur in the small intestine of patients without Crohn's. The Crohn's cancers are more likely to occur in males, in young patients, and in the ileum, and they have a worse prognosis. Large intestinal cancers associated with Crohn's are also usually more advanced when discovered and, therefore, have a worse prognosis than cancers arising in a colon without Crohn's. Cancers usually arise in segments of intestine that have been afflicted with Crohn's disease for 10 years or more.[27] Thus, patients with long-standing Crohn's disease should be examined annually or biannually using endoscopy and biopsy, looking for cancers or for premalignant changes, such as epithelial dysplasia.

Extraintestinal Manifestations

Extraintestinal manifestations are present in about 30% of patients with Crohn's disease. The most common are skin lesions, including erythema nodosum and pyoderma gangrenosum, iritis, uveitis, arthritis, spondylitis, pericholangitis, hepatitis, sclerosing cholangitis, and aphthous stomatitis (Table 31–1).

SYMPTOMS

The most common symptoms of Crohn's disease are those from the intestinal lesions, with abdominal pain, especially of a cramping nature, topping the list. Diarrhea is frequent. The stools may contain blood, although they often do not. Patients experience abdominal distention or flatulence and sometimes nausea and vomiting. Eating becomes difficult, because it induces symptoms. Patients therefore decrease their food intake and lose weight. Should fistulas develop, the pain and discharge of intestinal content at the site of the fistulas to the skin or in the perianal area produce localized symptoms in these areas. Systemic responses include fever and malaise; localized pain and discomfort are related to the sites of extraintestinal involvement in the skin, eyes, and joints.

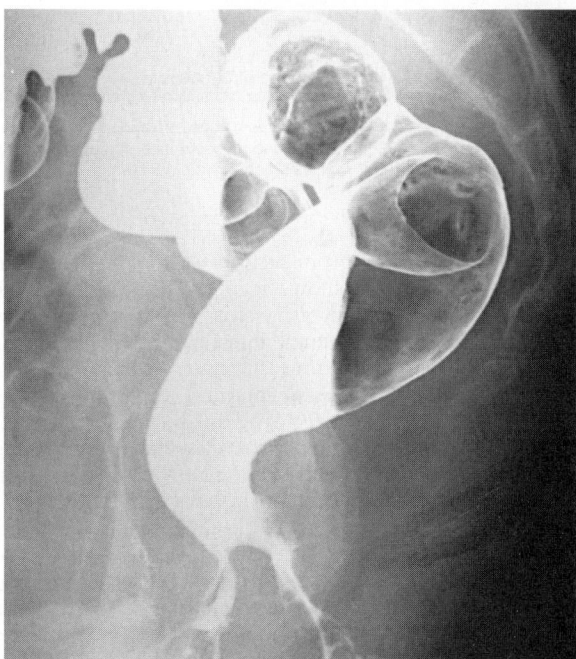

Figure 31–16. Radiograph demonstrating rectovaginal fistula secondary to Crohn's disease.

TABLE 31–1. Extraintestinal Manifestations of Crohn's Disease

Skin	**Liver**
Erythema multiforme	Nonspecific triaditis
Erythema nodosum	Sclerosing cholangitis
Pyoderma gangrenosum	**Kidney**
Eyes	Nephrotic syndrome
Iritis	Amyloidosis
Uveitis	**Pancreas**
Conjunctivitis	Pancreatitis
Joints	**General**
Peripheral arthritis	Amyloidosis
Ankylosing spondylitis	
Blood	
Anemia	
Thrombocytosis	
Phlebothrombosis	
Arterial thrombosis	

The course of the disease is one of exacerbations and remissions, but as the lesions mature and complications develop, the symptoms continue unabated and the disease becomes relentlessly progressive. About 70% of patients eventually come to operation, in spite of spontaneous remissions and medical or dietary therapy.

DIAGNOSIS

Diagnosis is based on the history, physical findings, and appropriate laboratory tests. The physical findings include the palpation of the thickened bowel wall or adjacent inflammatory response or abscesses in the abdomen. Hyperactive bowel tones are heard using auscultation, and peristaltic rushes in the small intestine may even be seen through a thin abdominal wall. Abdominal distention occurs. Fistulas are apparent, and probes and catheters can be passed through the cutaneous openings and into the lumen of the bowel through the tracts. On inspection, the perianal skin appears bluish, and perianal fissures, abscesses, and fistulas can be identified.

Proctoscopy often reveals the characteristic rectal aphthous ulcer with surrounding normal-appearing mucosa. With progressive and extensive involvement, the ulcerations involve more and more of the lumen of the bowel, with diminishing isolated segments of normal mucosa remaining. Anoscopy can show perianal abscesses, perianal fistulas, and even rectovaginal fistulas. Colonoscopy delineates the extent of the lesions in the large intestine. Sometimes the colonoscope can be passed through the colon and into the ileum to identify the ileal lesions of the disease. The hallmarks of Crohn's disease are the discontinuous and asymmetrical nature of the endoscopic findings. Biopsies taken during endoscopy show chronic inflammation and sometimes granulomas.

Roentgenographic examination of the gastrointestinal tract using $BaSO_4$ reveals the ulcerating lesions scattered in a segmental, irregular pattern along the wall of the involved intestine, producing irregular areas of ulceration, luminal narrowing, and thickened bowel wall (Fig. 31–17). Proximal dilatation of the bowel accompanies obstructing lesions. Long lengths of narrowed terminal ileum may reduce the caliber of the lumen to the size of a string (the string sign; Fig. 31–18). Areas of dilatation may alternate with areas of constriction (Fig. 31–19). The cobblestone appearance of the mucosa may be apparent, as may the rake ulcers. Fissures, fistulas, and perienteric abscesses may be found. Computed axial tomography may help delineate thickened bowel, perienteric abscesses, and perforations. In toxic megacolon, the transverse colon is greatly dilated and the bowel wall is thickened (Fig. 31–20). A mass accompanying a narrowed or ulcerated area suggests cancer. Free air in the abdomen is present with free perforation.

The differential diagnosis includes both specific and nonspecific causes of intestinal inflammation. Specific microbiologic diseases that may be confused with Crohn's disease include bacterial inflammations such as those caused by salmonella and shigella, typhoid fever, intestinal tuberculosis, and protozoan infections such as amebiasis. Appropriate cultures and biopsies reveal the causative organisms in these conditions and rule them out. In regard to nonspecific intestinal inflammation, chronic ulcerative colitis can usually be differentiated from Crohn's disease (Table 31–2). Although ulcerative colitis involves the mucosa of the large intestine, it does not extend deep into the wall of the bowel, as does Crohn's disease. Ulcerative colitis nearly always involves the rectum most severely, with lessening inflammation from the rectum to the ileocolic area. In contrast, Crohn's disease may be worse on the right side of the colon than on the left side, sometimes sparing the rectum. Ulcerative colitis also shows

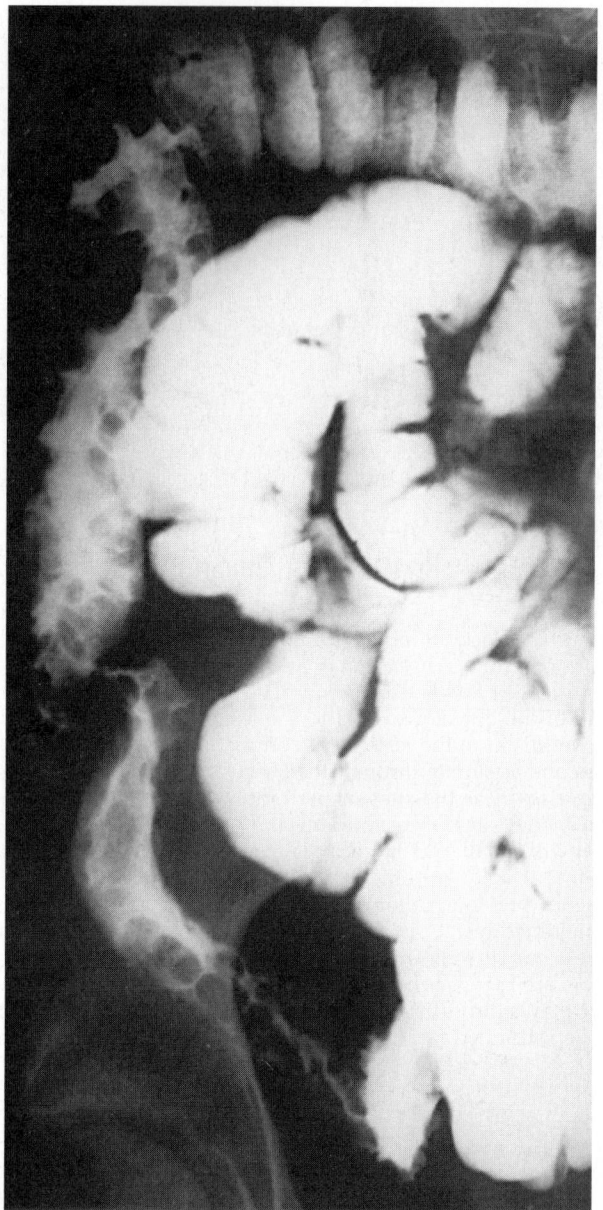

Figure 31–17. Radiograph of terminal ileum, cecum, and ascending colon involved by Crohn's disease, demonstrating mucosal ulceration with a cobblestone appearance, thickened bowel wall, and luminal narrowing.

continuous involvement from rectum to proximal segments, whereas Crohn's disease shows segmental lesions. Although nonspecific, so-called backwash ileitis may be present in ulcerative colitis, ileal and small intestinal involvement suggests Crohn's disease. Bleeding is a more common symptom in ulcerative colitis and is less common in Crohn's disease. Perianal involvement and rectovaginal fistulas are unusual in ulcerative colitis but are more common in Crohn's disease. In most instances, the two diseases can be clearly separated, but a subgroup of 5% to 10% of all patients with chronic nonspecific inflammatory bowel disease cannot be clearly classified as having ulcerative colitis or Crohn's disease. These patients are usually given a diagnosis of "indeterminate" colitis. The true diagnosis often becomes apparent as the patients are followed through the years.

Acute distal ileitis may be a manifestation of early Crohn's disease, but it also may be unrelated, such as when it is caused by a bacteriologic agent such as *Campylobacter* or

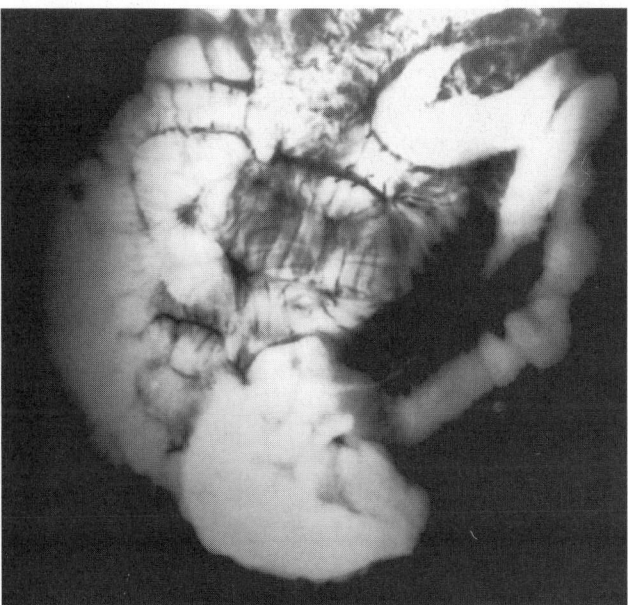

Figure 31–18. Radiograph of Crohn's disease of the small intestine, demonstrating marked narrowing (string sign) of the distal ileum.

Yersinia. Patients usually present in a manner similar to patients with acute appendicitis. They have a sudden onset of right lower quadrant pain, nausea, vomiting, and fever, with tenderness over the area of involvement. The diagnosis is made at operation by identifying an acutely inflamed segment of terminal ileum. No biopsy or resection should be

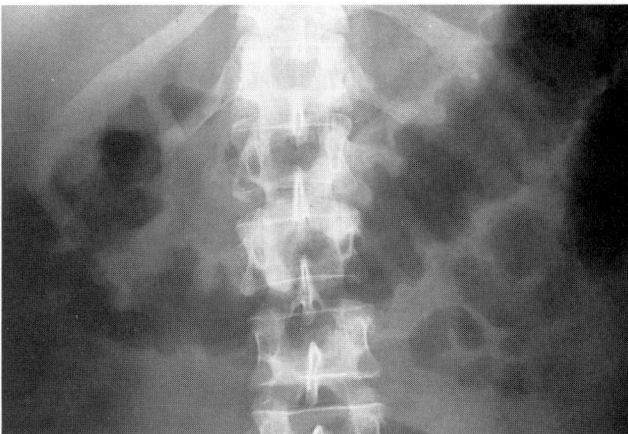

Figure 31–20. Radiograph of the abdomen in a patient with toxic megacolon secondary to Crohn's disease, demonstrating dilatation of the transverse colon, thickening of the bowel wall, and edematous haustral folds.

done. The condition almost always subsides spontaneously, and the segment should not be excised. If the cecum is not involved, the appendix should be removed to prevent subsequent bouts of right lower quadrant inflammation from being confused with appendicitis.

THERAPY

Medical and Dietary Therapy

Medical therapy consists of sulfasalazine, 5-aminosalicylic acid, corticosteroids, antibiotics such as metronidazole and ampicillin, and immunosuppressive agents such as azathioprine and cyclosporine. Because no specific etiology has been identified for Crohn's disease, the treatments are also nonspecific. They suppress inflammation and improve symptoms but are not curative.

Manipulations of the diet ordinarily have little effect on the progress of Crohn's disease. However, complete abstinence of oral intake with total parenteral nutrition may lead to temporary remission of symptoms in some patients with Crohn's disease. Sometimes enteroenteric or enterocutaneous fistulas close. Few long-term benefits of total parenteral nutrition have been achieved, however. When oral intake is resumed, the patients usually have recurring difficulty, and the symptoms of the disease return.

Surgical Therapy

Indications for Operation. Patients with Crohn's disease are usually operated on because an intestinal complication of Crohn's disease mandates the operation. All in all, about 70% of patients with Crohn's disease will come to operation. The most common complications leading to operation are recurrent intestinal obstruction, intestinal perforation with fistula formation and abscess, or a gastrointestinal bleeding.[2] Obstruction is usually partial and is seldom complete. With nasogastric suction and intravenous nutrition, the distended bowel usually decompresses, and bowel movements resume. Failure to achieve complete resolution or recurrence of obstructive symptoms with the resumption of oral feedings usually leads to operation. Perforation with fistula formation and resultant abdominal mass usually causes continuing pain, fever, malaise, and weight loss until operation can be accomplished. Perianal complications, such as abscess and fistula, commonly lead to operation. Bleeding, a less frequent cause of operation, is usually not massive, but it may be persistent and contribute to chronic anemia until the of-

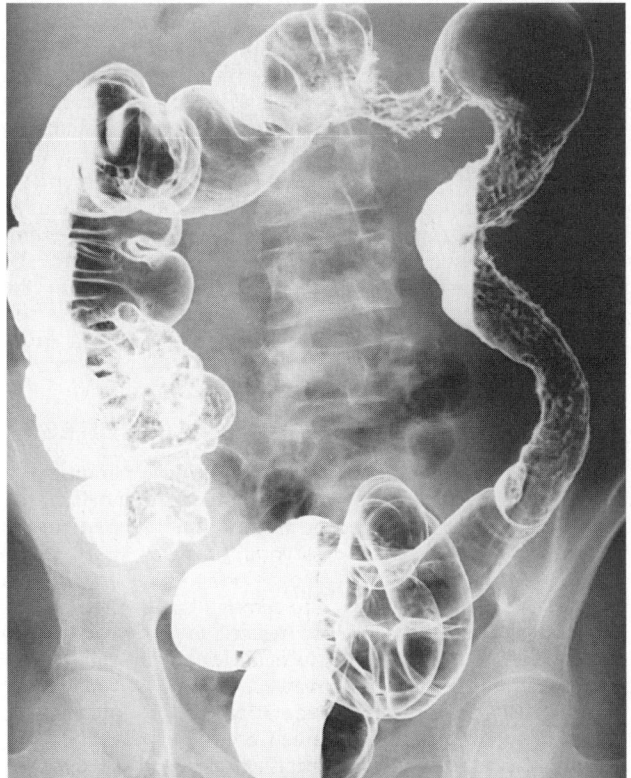

Figure 31–19. Radiograph of large intestine with Crohn's disease. Note the areas of narrowing with mucosal ulceration in the transverse colon, descending colon, and sigmoid colon, with spared, dilated segments of healthy colon and rectum in between.

TABLE 31–2. Diagnosis of Crohn's Colitis vs. Ulcerative Colitis

Observation	Crohn's Colitis	Ulcerative Colitis
Symptoms and signs		
Diarrhea	Common	Common
Rectal bleeding	Less common	Almost always
Abdominal pain (cramps)	Moderate to severe	Mild to moderate
Palpable mass	At times	No (unless large cancer)
Anal complaints	Frequent (>50%)	Infrequent (<20%)
Radiologic findings		
Ileal disease	Common	Rare (backwash ileitis)
Nodularity, fuzziness	No	Yes
Distribution	Skip areas	Rectum extending upward and continuously
Ulcers	Linear, cobblestone, fissures	Collar-button
Toxic dilatation	Rare	Uncommon
Proctoscopic findings		
Anal fissure, fistula, abscess	Common	Rare
Rectal sparing	Common (50%)	Rare (5%)
Granular mucosa	No	Yes
Ulceration	Linear, deep, scattered	Superficial, universal

fending lesion or lesions can be resected. Patients with small intestinal Crohn's disease usually require operation for obstruction or perforation, whereas those with large intestinal Crohn's are usually operated on for chronic debility and failure to respond to medical therapy.

Severe systemic symptoms, intractable medical therapy, and weight loss, especially with growth failure in children, can also lead to operation. Prepubertal and early pubertal patients experiencing growth failure from Crohn's can be expected to sustain *catch-up* and accelerated growth after resection.[16] Toxic megacolon and cancer of the small or large intestine are less common intestinal complications requiring operation. Extraintestinal complications (see Table 31–1) in and of themselves seldom require intestinal operation, but they often contribute to the decision to operate. Most of the extraintestinal complications, with the exception of ankylosing spondylitis and the hepatic complications, subside with the excision of intestine grossly involved with Crohn's disease.

Preoperative Preparation. The nutritional status of the patient is optimized before operation. This sometimes, but not often, requires parenteral caloric supplementation. Anemia is treated by blood transfusion. For patients currently on or recently receiving corticoid therapy, additional steroids—usually 100 mg. of hydrocortisone intravenously every 8 hours—are given to ensure an adequate supply during the operative stress. The bowels are cleansed with laxatives and enemas the day prior to operation. Alternatively, 4 liters of an electrolyte solution (GoLYTELY) can be given by mouth the night before operation.[36] Diet is restricted to clear liquids the day before operation.

The growth of enteric bacteria in patients having the laxative-enema preparation is suppressed by giving oral neomycin 0.5 gm. every 4 hours, and tetracycline, erythromycin, or metronidazole 250 mg. every 4 hours, for 18 hours prior to operation. When the GoLYTELY preparation is used, 2 gm. neomycin and 2 gm. metronidazole are given by mouth 12 hours and 8 hours before operation. With both preparations, cefazolin 0.5 gm. is given intravenously just prior to operation and is continued every 8 hours for two more doses.

General Principles of Operation. Because Crohn's disease involves nearly the entire gastrointestinal tract in most patients, total excision of the disease is not possible. Thus, surgical treatment is directed at the most severe areas of involvement, including those that account for the complications of obstruction, bleeding, or perforation.

The two main operative approaches are to excise the lesions or to bypass them. Currently, most surgeons advise excision rather than bypass. Bypass allows the diseased intestine to remain in place, where it can cause continuing symptoms, require treatment, and perhaps even develop malignancy. The risk of cancer in bypassed small and large intestine with Crohn's disease is greater than the risk in healthy bowel. Excision is done with 3-cm. "disease-free" margins on both sides of the area of involvement. The disease-free margins are established by gross inspection. Most surgeons do not use microscopic confirmation of healthy borders. Although the authors have found that when borders are free of microscopic involvement there are fewer recurrences over the long term than when the border is involved,[37] others have not found a higher recurrence rate when histologic findings of Crohn's are present in the margins.[14, 24] Certainly, demanding microscopic borders that are free of disease may lead to excessively large resections and result in the short bowel syndrome. Patients with this syndrome do not have enough intestine remaining to digest and absorb their food properly.

After resection and anastomosis of the index segment (or segments) of intestine that has led to the operation, fistulas from the index segment to adjacent organs, such as the stomach, colon, duodenum, bladder, or vagina, can usually be closed by suture of the entrance of the fistula into the adjacent segment. Resection of the adjacent segment is seldom required, unless it is primarily involved with gross Crohn's disease.

SURGICAL TREATMENT OF SPECIFIC SITES

The three most common sites requiring operation for Crohn's disease are the ileum, the colorectum, and the anorectum, with other sites needing surgical treatment less often.

Ileum

A vertical midline abdominal incision is made, skirting to the left of the umbilicus. This incision leaves the right lower quadrant of the abdomen unscarred and useful for the site of an ileostomy, should one be required at the initial operation or sometime in the future. Careful inspection of the abdominal content confirms the diagnosis and assesses the extent of the disease. Ileal Crohn's almost always involves the most distal terminal ileum, but "skip areas" can be found more proximally. Mucosal and submucosal lesions may not be apparent unless careful inspection of the small bowel from the stomach to the ileocolic valve is done. Subtle strictures can also be identified by passing a Foley catheter or a Baker tube into the lumen of the intestine through an enterotomy, threading the bowel onto the catheter, inflating the balloon of the catheter, and drawing the catheter back along the bowel. Areas of narrowing impede the withdrawal of the catheter. The diameter of the narrowed lumen can be assessed by noting the diameter of the balloon that can be pulled through the stricture. Strictures detected in this way may not be apparent on external inspection or palpation of the bowel. The length of healthy intestine from the ligament of Treitz to the first area of involvement should be carefully measured and recorded. The length of intestine grossly involved with Crohn's disease should also be measured.

Crohn's disease of the ileum should be excised with 3-cm. grossly disease-free margins on the proximal and distal ends. This usually means resecting the adjacent ileocolic valve, the cecum, and a small portion of ascending colon (Fig. 31–21). Obtaining microscopically disease-free margins at each end of the resected specimen may prolong the disease-free interval after operation,[37] but controversy exists about this point. Most surgeons do not demand histologic evidence of lack of disease at the margins during operation. No attempt should be made to resect the entire thickened adjacent mesentery; only enough mesentery to facilitate the removal of the diseased bowel and the anastomosis should be resected. Intestinal continuity is then restored with an end-to-end ileal-ascending colostomy. The anastomosis can be made with sutures or staples. The authors prefer to use a two-layer suture technique, using continuous 3-0 absorbable suture on the mucosal-submucosal layer to provide a water-tight closure and to control bleeding. Interrupted 3-0 or 4-0 absorbable or nonabsorbable (Dacron) sutures are used on the seromuscular layer to complete the anastomosis. The defect in the mesentery is closed by approximating the cut mesenteric edges with continuous 3-0 absorbable sutures. Necrotic debris, bowel content, blood, and bacteria are removed by irrigation of the site of excision with isotonic NaCl and aspiration of the irrigant. The abdomen is closed with interrupted or continuous no. 0 or no. 1 absorbable sutures.

Crohn's disease of the small bowel may involve segments not only of terminal ileum but also of more proximal ileum and even portions of jejunum. Areas of severe involvement

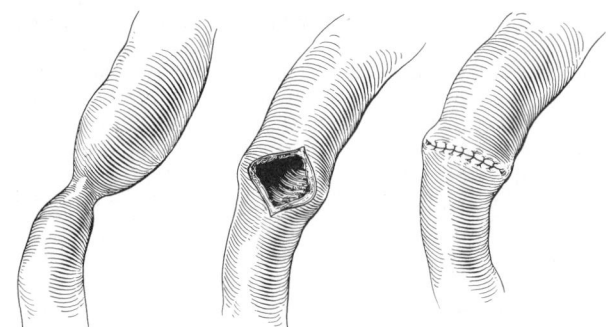

Figure 31–22. Diagram of "stricturoplasty" for localized segment of Crohn's disease of the small bowel. A longitudinal incision through the strictured segment is made, followed by a subsequent transverse closure with sutures. The procedure widens the lumen at the site of stricture yet resects no bowel.

(skip lesions) may be interspersed between areas of fairly normal bowel. Skip lesions close to the major area of involvement in the terminal ileum can be resected in continuity with the terminal ileum. However, when the area of small intestine involved in skip lesions or continuous lesions is great, the surgeon is faced with an operative dilemma. Total excision of all gross disease would involve such an extensive resection that the short bowel syndrome would result. Partial excision, however, would leave active, symptom-producing disease behind.

Two options are currently available to deal with this dilemma. The first, used more in the past than today, is to bypass the involved segments with a side-to-side anastomosis between the uninvolved proximal small intestine and the adjacent large intestine. This preserves small intestine and bypasses symptom-producing lesions, but it leaves diseased and often partially obstructed bowel in place. A second and better option is to excise only the most severe areas of involvement and to perform *stricturoplasties* on segments of remaining small bowel to relieve obstruction but to avoid excision.[1, 15] The stricturoplasties are performed by making a longitudinal incision through the narrowed areas and closing these incisions in a transverse direction using the two-layered technique described above (Fig. 31–22). This effectively widens the lumen at the sites of the narrowing yet does not remove any intestine. Stricturoplasty has the most application in those patients in whom multiple short areas of narrowing are present over long segments of intestine, in those patients who have already had several previous resections of the small intestine, and when the areas of narrowing are due to fibrous obstruction rather than acute inflammation.

Experience with stricturoplasty has been excellent. In one series, among 24 patients who underwent stricturoplasty for 86 strictures, obstruction was relieved and healing obtained without fistula in all patients.[4] Only one recurrent stricture appeared during a mean follow-up of 40 months. In another series involving 35 patients and 71 stricturoplasties, no perioperative complications occurred, and only 22% of patients had recurrent symptoms after operation.[30] In still another series, 54 patients underwent 215 stricturoplasties, with relief of obstructive symptoms in all but two patients and no deaths.[31]

Ileocolon

Another common distribution of Crohn's disease involves the ileum, cecum, and ascending colon. Under these circumstances, the diseased bowel is removed, again with 3-cm. gross disease-free margins, and an anastomosis is made between the ileum and the transverse colon in an end-to-end fashion.

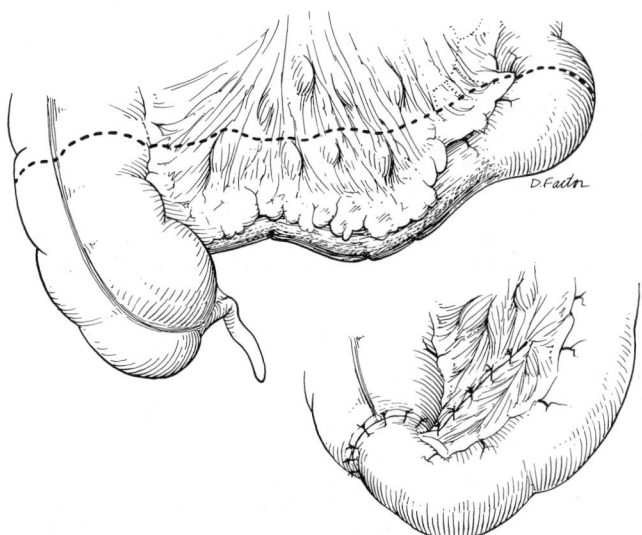

Figure 31–21. Diagram of resection of the ileum, ileocolic valve, cecum, and ascending colon for Crohn's disease of the ileum. Intestinal continuity is restored by end-to-end ileal-ascending colostomy.

Colorectum

The operative approach to Crohn's disease of the colo-rectum varies, depending on the sites of colorectal involvement and their severity. Patients with severe disease of the colon but mild or minimal rectal disease should have the cecum and colon removed and an ileorectostomy performed. Among 42 patients who had this operation at the Mayo Clinic, 91% had improved health and quality of life after operation, and 66% maintained an acceptable, functioning ileorectal anastomosis for at least 10 years. Older patients and male patients did better than younger patients and females. Patients with severe colonic disease and mild rectal disease, but with an anorectal complication such as an anorectal abscess or fistula, should have a colectomy, an end Brooke ileostomy, and a closure of the proximal rectum, leaving the rectum and the anal canal in place but excluded from the fecal stream. The plan is for a subsidence of the anorectal Crohn's disease with the intestinal bypass created by the ileostomy and with further medical and surgical treatment. Subsequent reanastomosis might be possible at a later date when the anorectal disease becomes quiescent or subsides, although it is unlikely.[9] Patients with toxic megacolon from Crohn's disease should also undergo colectomy, closure of the proximal rectum, and end ileostomy. This operation can be done expeditiously and leaves no anastomosis in the abdomen. Patients with toxic megacolon are extremely ill and heal anastomoses poorly. When both the colon and the rectum are severely involved, proctocolectomy with permanent end ileostomy (Brooke ileostomy) is usually required.[28]

The perineal wound may heal slowly after a complete proctectomy for Crohn's disease. In a past series from the Mayo Clinic, among 32 patients with Crohn's disease treated by complete proctectomy and primary closure, only 50% had healed *per primam* by 1 month after operation and only 90% by 1 year.[33] Persistent nonhealing of perineal wounds requires excision of the wound surface and secondary closure, skin grafts, a musculocutaneous flap, or some combination thereof.[25] To avoid the problem of the nonhealing wound, the authors employ endorectal and sphincter-saving excisions rather than wide excisions of the entire anorectum. In these current operations, the diseased mucosa and adjacent underlying and adherent submucosa and muscularis are excised, but most of the muscular complex of the anal sphincter and any associated sinuses or fistulous tracts are left in place. The remaining sphincteric muscle is approximated, and the anal canal is left open. With these techniques, healing is faster, and large, persistent draining wounds are avoided.

Several other options are available for patients with colorectal Crohn's. Localized segments of large intestinal inflammation can sometimes be handled by segmental resection with end-to-end anastomosis of the colon, recognizing that recurrence of Crohn's disease in the remaining colon is common. Another seldom-practiced operation is a diverting ileostomy, leaving the entire large intestine in place. The operation may have a role in patients who are severely ill with Crohn's colitis. Proponents state that a rapid improvement results from the fecal diversion.[10, 35] Continued activity of the colorectal disease, producing symptoms and requiring treatment, usually follows this operation, however. Patients with diverting ileostomies may eventually have their stomas closed, but after stomal closure, the colonic disease often flares again. Most eventually undergo proctocolectomy and have permanent ileostomies. Stricturoplasty has not been used for colorectal Crohn's; resection of strictured areas is preferred.

Sphincter-saving operations such as the continent ileostomy (Kock pouch) or the ileal pouch–anal canal anastomosis, both of which are commonly used in ulcerative colitis, are not often used for Crohn's disease. Kock and his colleagues performed the continent ileostomy in a series of patients with Crohn's disease. In this operation, after excision of the large intestine, a pouch is made from 30 cm. of the terminal ileum. A valve that prevents distal outflow from the pouch is created by intussuscepting the terminal ileum backward into the pouch and anchoring the intussusceptum in place with stainless-steel staples. The end of the terminal ileum is brought to the skin surface as a stoma. Once healed, the patient empties the pouch intermittently by passing a catheter through the stoma and valve into the pouch, draining the contents of the pouch directly into the toilet through the tube. In between intubations, the pouch is continent for both gas and stool. Kock and colleagues report that approximately 30% of their patients have had satisfactory long-term results with the operation. The risk of recurrence of Crohn's disease in the pouch, however, mandates against the use of the continent ileostomy in most patients with Crohn's disease.[8] Also, the ileal pouch–anal anastomosis is not recommended for Crohn's disease of the large intestine. This operation in patients with Crohn's usually results in recurrence of inflammation in the pouch, fistulas at the anastomosis, and peripouch abscesses.[13]

Anorectum

Conservative operations directed at relieving symptoms from anorectal Crohn's disease have been done with increasing frequency in recent years.[7] Abscesses have been drained, fissures excised, and anal fistulas opened and débrided, sometimes aided by the use of a *seton,* when the fistula goes through the anal sphincter. A seton is a suture of nonabsorbable material or a 1/4-inch Penrose drain passed through the cutaneous opening of the fistula, into the lumen of the anal canal, and then back out to the skin surface, where it is tied to itself. The intervening skin and mucosa are trimmed away under the seton. The seton is slowly tightened over a 2- to 3-week period. Peritract fibrosis occurs. The seton gradually cuts through to the luminal surface. If the seton does not cut through after 3 weeks, the fistula can be incised. The incision may divide some fibers of the anal sphincter, but the sphincter will not retract because it is now fixed by the peritract fibrosis. Anal sphincteric competence is maintained. Rectovaginal fistulas have been closed by débridement and direct suture of the opening of the fistula, followed by advancement of a rectal mucosal flap from the upper rectum over the opening of the fistula and down to the dentate line.

The emphasis when using anorectal operations for Crohn's disease is to be conservative. Wide excisions of large amounts of tissue should not be performed. Metronidazole 250 mg. given four times a day, used alone or in combination with operation, aids the healing of anorectal Crohn's. With conservative medical and surgical therapy, symptoms are often improved, and abscesses, fistulas, and fissures may be healed, especially when Crohn's does not involve the colon.[22]

Some have postulated that anorectal Crohn's disease will subside if more proximal areas of involvement in the small intestine or large intestine are excised. Little evidence exists, however, to support this hypothesis. Removal of a segment of severe ileal Crohn's disease, for example, is unlikely to alter the course of an associated anorectal complication of the disease.[38]

Duodenum

Duodenal Crohn's disease is almost always associated with ileal Crohn's disease. It most commonly results in duodenal obstruction, but duodenal perforation with fistulas into the pancreas and peripancreatic areas may also occur. When operation is required, gastrojejunostomy rather than duodenal resection is almost always performed, although duodenal stricturoplasty has been done in selected patients. Vagotomy to prevent marginal ulcer should not be done. The incidence of marginal ulcer is low (<5%), and such ulcers can usually be managed satisfactorily with medical therapy.

Stomach and Esophagus

Gastroesophageal Crohn's disease usually does not require surgical treatment and is almost always managed medically. When localized perforations, bleeding, or fistulas occur, however, local excisions of the grossly diseased areas are required, with closure or anastomosis at sites of excision.

POSTOPERATIVE MANAGEMENT

Postoperatively, patients take nothing by mouth, with nourishment being given by intravenous caloric and electrolyte solutions. The stomach and intestines should be decompressed by a nasogastric tube when patients have had extensive adhesiolysis, relief of intestinal obstruction, peritonitis, or abscess. Elastic stockings, sequentially inflating pneumatic cuffs placed on the legs, and early ambulation the day after operation are used to prevent phlebothrombosis and pulmonary embolism. A urinary bladder catheter is often required for the first 3 to 5 days after a pelvic procedure.

Instillation of a dilute solution of antibiotics into Type IV wounds via a 5-mm. polyethylene catheter placed in the subcutaneous space prior to skin closure and brought to the surface through a puncture site lateral to the wound is commenced the day of operation and continued for 4 more days. The catheter is connected to suction in between the instillations. This technique has decreased the incidence of wound infection.[6, 18]

Passage of flatus or bowel content per rectum or per stoma usually begins on or about the third postoperative day, at which time the nasogastric tube can be removed and oral feedings commenced. The authors begin with a pure liquid diet and gradually progress to solid content, so that patients are taking a soft general diet by about the sixth postoperative day. Once oral intake is adequate to support caloric, fluid, and electrolyte needs, intravenous feeding can be stopped. Antiembolism efforts are usually discontinued on about the fifth postoperative day. Parenteral hydrocortisone can be switched to oral prednisone once oral intake has resumed. For patients who have been on long-term steroids, the prednisone is gradually tapered and then discontinued over a 6-week period.

After discharge from the hospital, continued medical management directed at the prevention of recurrence of Crohn's disease may be of benefit. A recent preliminary report has shown that the administration of 5-aminosalicylic acid released in the small intestine reduces or delays recurrence after operation by 50% among patients with Crohn's disease of the distal ileum or colon.[19]

COMPLICATIONS OF OPERATION

Early Complications

The main complications of operation in the early postoperative period are intestinal obstruction from adhesions, intra-abdominal abscess, wound infection, anastomotic leaks, bleeding from areas of operation, phlebothrombosis and pulmonary embolism, atelectasis and pulmonary infections, urinary retention, and enterocutaneous fistulas. Most of these complications can be managed nonoperatively; reoperation should be required in less than 10% of patients. Operative mortality is unusual and should be less than 2% of patients at risk.

Late Complications

Resection of the ileum can result in malabsorption of vitamin B_{12}. The ileum is the sole site of absorption of this vitamin. Patients undergoing extensive resections of the ileum should receive 1 mg. of vitamin B_{12} parenterally each month on a long-term basis.

The ileum is also the area of intestine where bile salts are actively absorbed. Extensive ileal resections can result in depletion of the bile salt pool, resulting in steatorrhea from lack of sufficient bile salts in the enteric lumen for the formation of bile salt micelles. Micelles are needed for solubilization of fatty acids and their subsequent absorption. Steatorrhea may cause binding of calcium ion by fatty acids, making calcium unavailable in the enteric lumen for binding to oxalates. The unbound oxalate then passes into the large intestine, where it is absorbed. The absorbed oxalate is excreted in the urine, where it may precipitate to form oxalate urinary stones. Uric acid stones may also form in subjects with postresection diarrhea, with its resultant sodium, potassium, and water loss. The urine output decreases, the urine becomes more acidic, and uric acid urinary stones can form.

Steatorrhea can be treated by decreasing the intake of fatty food in the diet and ingesting medium-chain triglycerides. Hyperoxaluria can be improved by avoiding food with a high oxalate content, such as spinach, beets, rhubarb, and cocoa. A low-volume acidic urine output can be combatted by vigorous oral fluid intake, with increased ingestion of sodium ions.

The loss of bile salts may also lead to the formation of gallstones. The bile salt pool becomes depleted, and the concentration of bile salts in the bile becomes insufficient to solubilize the cholesterol in bile. Cholesterol gallstones then develop. Cholecystectomy may be required if symptoms develop from the gallstones.

Failure to absorb bile salts with extensive ileal resection allows unabsorbed bile salts to enter the colon, where they irritate the mucosa and stimulate the outpouring of water and electrolytes into the lumen. So-called choleraic diarrhea results. Cholestyramine 4 gm. per day, taken orally, binds bile salts and ameliorates choleraic diarrhea.

Extensive resections may leave insufficient small intestinal mucosa for the digestion and absorption of foodstuffs, vitamins, water, and electrolytes. The short bowel syndrome then develops. This condition is characterized by crampy abdominal pain, diarrhea, borborygmi, abdominal distention, and weight loss. The condition often results when less than 100 cm. of jejunoileum remain, although more extensive resections may be tolerated when the ileocolic valve and large intestine remain. Jejunal losses are tolerated better than ileal losses. The loss of intestine results in fecal outputs that exceed 1500 ml. per day. Malnutrition, dehydration, vitamin deficiencies, and deficiencies of electrolytes can occur. Loss of calcium, for example, may result in osteoporosis.

The short bowel syndrome often requires intravenous administration of nutrients, vitamins, minerals, and water. Elemental diets and liquids are tolerated better by mouth than are more complex foods and solids. Gastric hypersecretion of hydrochloric acid occurs and should be managed with histamine H_2-receptor blockers. Diarrhea can be decreased with antidiarrheal agents such as loperamide hydrochloride. Most patients with the short bowel syndrome improve over time, and after 6 months they may be able to stop intravenous supplementation. Reoperation, other than to drain pus, restore intestinal continuity, close fistulas, and relieve obstruction, usually has little benefit.

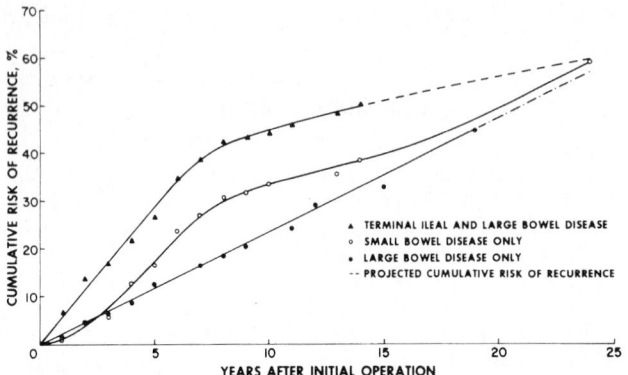

Figure 31–23. Cumulative rates of recurrence after resection for Crohn's disease of small intestine only, small intestine and large intestine, and large intestine only. (Reprinted by permission of *The New England Journal of Medicine* from Lock, M. R., Farmer, R. G., Fazio, V. W., et al.: Recurrence and reoperation for Crohn's disease. N. Engl. J. Med., *304*:1586, 1981, Copyright 1981, Massachusetts Medical Society.)

OUTCOME

Operations directed at Crohn's disease are palliative. They provide patients with symptomatic relief, but not cure. Reported rates of asymptomatic recurrence have been as high as 93% of patients at risk 1 year after operation.[23] Rates of symptomatic recurrence, however, are about 6% of patients at risk per year, or 30% at 5 years and 60% at 10 years. The 6% recurrence rate applies to patients after resection and anastomosis for ileal or ileocolic disease. In contrast, the rates of symptomatic recurrence after proctocolectomy and permanent ileostomy may be somewhat less. One paper reported that only 2.5% of patients at risk per year had a recurrence over 10 years after proctocolectomy and ileostomy, regardless of whether ileal disease was present at the time of operation.[28] Another paper also reported low early recurrence rates when ileostomy was done.[11] Regardless of the type of operation performed, however, rates of recurrence in patients with colonic Crohn's disease usually approach those of patients with ileal or ileocolic Crohn's disease, if the patients are followed long enough (25 years) after operation[17] (Fig. 31–23).The rates of recurrence are not affected or only minimally affected by age, sex, length of intestine involved in disease, interval between onset of disease and operation, and type and duration of medical treatment.[5] Recurrence rates are greater, however, when multiple sites of Crohn's disease are present and require treatment.[11, 21]

Recurrences usually occur at or just proximal to an anastomosis or stoma. They are diagnosed by symptoms, physical examination, endoscopy, and x-ray, and at reoperation with excision. Following a second operation for Crohn's disease, the rates of recurrence are similar to those following an initial operation. Thus, the results of reoperation, as with initial operation, are usually satisfactory and justify a continued operative approach to the disease. Some patients may require three or more operations. Nonetheless, the mortality rate from Crohn's disease rises slowly with time and is about two times that of a matched control group of healthy subjects drawn from the general population.[26] Deaths are caused directly by Crohn's disease, its digestive complications, or the complications arising from operation for the condition.

In spite of the risks of recurrence and the morbidity and possible mortality from operation, many patients who have had operation for Crohn's disease wish that they had had their operations sooner. Reasons given are that operation relieves symptoms, restores a feeling of well-being and the ability to eat normally, and abolishes the need for drugs.[29]

SELECTED REFERENCES

Fazio, V. W., Galandiuk, S., Fogelman, D. R., et al.: Strictureplasty in Crohn's disease. Ann. Surg., *210*:621, 1989.
  The authors report that stricturoplasty relieves obstruction in Crohn's disease without resection of bowel, with preservation of intestinal function, and with minimal anastomotic complications.

Lock, M. R., Farmer, R. G., Fazio, V. W., et al.: Recurrence and reoperation for Crohn's disease. N. Engl. J. Med., *304*:1586, 1981.
  The authors report that recurrence after operation for Crohn's disease occurs soonest with ileocolic disease, later with ileal disease, and latest with colonic disease, but provided the patients are followed long enough (25 years), the eventual rates of recurrence in all three cases are similar.

Mekhjian, H. S., Switz, D. M., Melnyk, C. S., et al.: Clinical features and natural history of Crohn's disease. Gastroenterology, *77*:898, 1979.
  A careful review of the clinical features and natural history of Crohn's disease in a large series of patients.

Van Patter, W. N., Bargen, J. A., Dockerty, M. D., et al.: Regional enteritis. Gastroenterology, *26*:347, 1954.
  An extensive review and description of Crohn's disease, its pathology, its sites of occurrence, and its clinical course.

Wolff, B. G., Beart, R. W., Jr., Frydenberg, H. B., et al.: The importance of disease-free margins in resections for Crohn's disease. Dis. Colon Rectum, *26*:239, 1983.
  An analysis of the continuing controversy regarding the extent of resection in Crohn's disease, favoring the position that achieving a disease-free margin at the time of resection lessens the likelihood of subsequent recurrence of the disease.

REFERENCES

1. Alexander-Williams, J., and Haynes, I. G.: Conservative operations for Crohn's disease of the small bowel. World J. Surg., *9*:945, 1985.
2. Andrews, H. A., Keighley, M. R., Alexander-Williams, J., and Allan, R. N.: Strategy for management of distal ileal Crohn's disease. Br. J. Surg., *78*:679, 1991.
3. Crohn, B. B., Ginzburg, L., and Oppenheimer, G. D.: Regional enteritis: A pathologic and clinical study. JAMA, *99*:1323, 1932.
4. Dehn, T. C. B., Kettlewell, M. G. W., and Mortensen, N. J. M.: Ten-year experience of strictureplasty for obstructive Crohn's disease. Br. J. Surg., *76*:339, 1989.
5. Farmer, R. G., Whelan, G., and Fazio, V. W.: Long-term follow-up of patients with Crohn's disease. Gastroenterology, *88*:1818, 1985.
6. Farnell, M. B., Worthington-Self, S., Mucha, P., Jr., Ilstrup, D. M., and McIlrath, D. C.: Closure of abdominal incisions with subcutaneous catheters: A prospective randomized trial. Arch. Surg., *121*:641, 1986.
7. Fry, R. D., Shemesh, E. I., and Kodner, I. J.: The management of anal and perineal Crohn's disease: Techniques and results. Surg. Gynecol. Obstet., *168*:42, 1989.
8. Handelsman, J. C., Gottlieb, L. M., and Hamilton, S. R.: Crohn's disease as a contraindication to Kock pouch (continent ileostomy). Dis. Colon Rectum, *36*:840, 1993.
9. Harling, H., Hegnhoj, J., Rasmussen, T. N., and Jarnum, S.: Fate of the rectum after colectomy and ileostomy for Crohn's colitis. Dis. Colon Rectum, *34*:931, 1991.
10. Harper, P. H., Truelove, S. C., Lee, E. C., Kettlewell, M. G., and Jewell, D. P.: Split ileostomy and ileocolostomy for Crohn's disease of the colon and ulcerative colitis: A 20 year survey. Gut, *24*:106, 1983.
11. Heimann, T. M., Greenstein, A. J., Lewis, B., Kaufman, D., Heimann, D. M., and Aufses, A. H., Jr.: Prediction of early symptomatic recurrence after intestinal resection in Crohn's disease. Ann. Surg., *218*:294, 1993.
12. Hellers, G.: Crohn's disease in Stockholm County, 1955–1974: A study of epidemiology, results of surgical treatment and long-term prognosis. Acta Chir. Scand. (Suppl.), *490*:1, 1979.
13. Hyman, N. H., Fazio, V. W., and Tuckson, W. B.: Consequences of ileal pouch–anal anastomosis for Crohn's colitis. Dis. Colon Rectum, *34*:653, 1991.
14. Kotanagi, H., Kramer, K., Fazio, V. W., and Petras, R. E.: Do microscopic abnormalities at resection margins correlate with increased anastomotic recurrence in Crohn's disease? Retrospective analysis of 100 cases. Dis. Colon Rectum, *34*:909, 1991.
15. Lee, E. C. G., and Papaionnou, N.: Minimal surgery for chronic obstruction in patients with extensive or universal Crohn's disease. Ann. Roy. Coll. Surg. Engl., *64*:229, 1982.
16. Lipson, A. B., Savage, M. O., Davies, P. S., Bassett, K., Shand, W. S., and Walker-Smith, J. A.: Acceleration of linear growth following intestinal resection for Crohn's disease. Eur. J. Pediatr., *149*:687, 1990.
17. Lock, M. R., Farmer, R. G., Fazio, V. W., Jagelman, D. G., Lavery, I. C., and Weakley, F. L.: Recurrence and reoperation for Crohn's disease: The role of disease location in prognosis. N. Engl. J. Med., *304*:1586, 1981.
18. McIlrath, D. C., van Heerden, J. A., Edis, A. J., and Dozois, R. R.: Closure of abdominal incisions with subcutaneous catheters. Surgery, *80*:411, 1976.
19. McLeod, R. S., Wolff, B. G., Steinhart, A. H., Carryer, P. W., O'Rourke, K., Andrews, D., Blair, J. E., Cangemi, J. B., Cohen, Z., Cullen, J. B., Chaytor,

R. G., Greenberg, G. R., Jaffer, N. M., Jeejeebjoy, K. N., MacCarty, R. L., Ready, R. L., and Weiland, L. H.: Delayed recurrence following surgery for Crohn's disease. Gastroenterology, *106*:A1733, 1994.

20. Mekhjian, H. S., Switz, D. M., Melnyk, C. S., Rankin, G. B., and Brooks, R. K.: Clinical features and natural history of Crohn's disease. Gastroenterology, *77*:898, 1979.

21. Michelassi, F., Balestracci, T., Chappell, R., and Block, G. E.: Primary and recurrent Crohn's disease: Experience with 1379 patients. Ann. Surg., *214*:230, 1991.

22. Nordgren, S., Fasth, S., and Hulten, L.: Anal fistulas in Crohn's disease: Incidence and outcome of surgical treatment. Int. J. Colorectal Dis., *7*:214, 1992.

23. Olaison, G., Smedh, K., and Sjodahl, R.: Natural course of Crohn's disease after ileocolic resection: Endoscopically visualised ileal ulcers preceding symptoms. Gut, *33*:331, 1992.

24. Pennington, L., Hamilton, S. R., Bayless, T. M., and Cameron, J. L.: Surgical management of Crohn's disease: Influence of disease at margin of resection. Ann. Surg., *192*:311, 1980.

25. Pezim, M. E., Wolff, B. G., Woods, J. E., Beart, R. W., Jr., and Ilstrup, D. M.: Closure of postproctectomy perineal sinus with gracilis muscle flaps. Can. J. Surg., *30*:212, 1987.

26. Prior, P., Gyde, S., and Allan, R. N.: Mortality in ulcerative colitis: Methods of analysis. Gastroenterology, *83*:524, 1982.

27. Ribeiro, M. B., Greenstein, A. J., Heimann, T. M., Yamazaki, Y., and Aufses, A. H., Jr.: Adenocarcinoma of the small intestine in Crohn's disease. Surg. Gynecol. Obstet., *173*:343, 1991.

28. Scammell, B. E., Andrews, H., Allan, R. N., Alexander-Williams, J., and Keighley, M. R.: Results of proctocolectomy for Crohn's disease. Br. J. Surg., *74*:671, 1987.

29. Scott, N. A., and Hughes, L. E.: Timing of ileocolonic resection for symptomatic Crohn's disease—the patient's view. Gut, *35*:656, 1994.

30. Spencer, M. P., Nelson, H., Wolff, B. G., and Dozois, R. R.: Strictureplasty for obstructive Crohn's disease: The Mayo experience. Mayo Clin. Proc., *69*:33, 1994.

31. Tjandra, J. J., and Fazio, V. W.: Strictureplasty without concomitant resection for small bowel obstruction in Crohn's disease. Br. J. Surg., *81*:561, 1994.

32. Van Patter, W. N., Bargen, J. A., Dockerty, M. G., Feldman, W. N., Mayo, C. W., and Waugh, J. M.: Regional enteritis. Gastroenterology, *26*:347, 1954.

33. Waits, J. O., Dozois, R. R., and Kelly, K. A.: Primary closure and continuous irrigation of the perineal wound after proctectomy. Mayo Clin. Proc., *57*:185, 1982.

34. Winship, D. H., Summers, R. W., Singleton, J. W., Best, W. R., Becktel, J. M., Lenk, L. F., and Kern, F., Jr.: National cooperative Crohn's disease study: Study design and conduct of the study. Gastroenterology, *77*:829, 1979.

35. Winslet, M. C., and Keighley, M. R.: Fecal diversion for Crohn disease of the colon. Surg. Ann., *23*(Pt. 2):99, 1991.

36. Wolff, B. G., Beart, R. W., Jr., Dozois, R. R., Pemberton, J. H., Zinsmeister, A. R., Ready, R. L., Farnell, M. B., Washington, J. A., and Heppell, J.: A new bowel preparation for elective colon and rectal surgery: A prospective, randomized clinical trial. Arch. Surg., *123*:895, 1988.

37. Wolff, B. G., Beart, R. W., Jr., Frydenberg, H. B., Weiland, L. H., Agrez, M. V., and Ilstrup, D. M.: The importance of disease-free margins in resections for Crohn's disease. Dis. Colon Rectum, *26*:239, 1983.

38. Wolff, B. G., Culp, C. E., Beart, R. W., Jr., Ilstrup, D. M., and Ready, R. L.: Anorectal Crohn's disease: A long-term perspective. Dis. Colon Rectum, *28*:709, 1985.

V

THE SURGICAL APPROACH TO MORBID OBESITY

Walter J. Pories, M.D.

Obesity is an increasingly serious health problem in the United States. About 50 million Americans, over one third of the adult population, are obese, exceeding their ideal body weight by more than 20%. Of these, at least 12 million are *morbidly* obese; that is, they exceed their ideal body weight by more than 100 pounds.[36, 51] Minority populations are affected out of proportion; nearly 50% of African American, Mexican American, and Native American women are overweight.

There is a direct relationship between the amount of excess weight and the incidence of morbidity and mortality from cardiovascular disease, diabetes, stroke, certain types of cancer, osteoarthritis, sleep apnea, and biliary disease. Mortality accelerates rapidly when an individual becomes 50% overweight; morbidly obese young males have a 12-fold increase in mortality. In females the picture is equally bleak. Sudden, unexplained deaths are common.[61] In addition to these health consequences, massive obesity also imposes severe limitations in function. Kral[33] summarized it well when he concluded that the morbidly obese are severely handicapped by every measure: physically, emotionally, economically, and socially. Morbid obesity is indeed a serious disease.

DEFINITIONS AND DIAGNOSIS

A number of indices have been developed for the quantification of obesity. Height and weight standards, shown in Table 31–3, have the virtue of clinical simplicity and continue to be widely used. The ideal body weights (IBWs) are derived from the midpoints for the average frame as listed in the 1983 Metropolitan Life Insurance Company tables. These standards, however, have been criticized for their skewed sampling, with underrepresentation of lower socioeconomic levels, minorities, and the elderly, as well as the arbitrary definition of body frame sizes. For example, African American girls have been reported to be heavier than Caucasian girls as early as age 9.[49]

The body mass index (BMI), defined as weight in kilograms divided by height in meters squared ($kg./m.^2$), although based on the same measurements as the height and weight insurance tables, has proved to be a better indicator of obesity. The formula emphasizes the relative fatness of individuals and minimizes the effects of height. The optimal value for the BMI lies between 20 and 27, according to the Ministry of National Health and Welfare of Canada. The National Academy of Sciences, however, emphasizes that the BMI rises with age; it subdivides optimal BMIs according to age, recommending values of 19 to 24 for young adults and 24 to 29 for those 65 and older.[37] In epidemiologic studies, the BMI correlates remarkably well with mortality, nullifies the gender differentiation required by the insurance tables, and serves as a reasonable surrogate for assessing body fat. Obesity is considered *morbid obesity* when the BMI exceeds 35, a value usually equivalent to the individual's exceeding the IBW by 100 pounds or more. Some use the term *superobese* to refer to the morbidly obese who exceed their IBW by more than 200 pounds. Table 31–3 also provides a comparison of weights in terms of BMI values. The IBW values of 1983 are significantly lower than the weights currently considered optimal in the United States.

Even though the BMI is a clinically useful index of "fatness," the formula can be misleading in muscular individuals. For example, an All-American running back on the

TABLE 31–3. Ideal Body Weights (IBWs) for Men and Women, with Comparisons to Weights for Body Mass Indexes (BMIs) of 24, 35,* and 40†

Ft.	Cm.	Lb.	Kg.	BMI = IBW	Lb. if BMI = 24	Lb. if BMI = 35	Lb. if BMI = 40
Women							
4'10"	147	115	52.2	24	114	166	190
4'11"	150	117	53.1	24	119	173	198
5'0"	152	120	54.2	23	122	178	203
5'1"	155	122	55.3	23	127	185	211
5'2"	158	125	56.7	23	132	192	220
5'3"	160	128	58.1	23	135	197	225
5'4"	163	131	59.4	22	140	205	234
5'5"	165	134	60.8	22	144	210	240
5'6"	168	137	62.1	22	149	217	248
5'7"	170	140	63.5	22	153	223	254
5'8"	173	143	64.9	22	158	230	263
5'9"	175	146	66.2	22	162	236	270
5'10"	178	149	67.6	21	167	244	279
5'11"	180	152	68.9	21	171	249	285
6'0"	183	155	70.3	21	177	258	295
Men							
5'2"	158	136	61.7	25	132	192	220
5'3"	160	138	62.6	24	135	197	225
5'4"	163	140	63.5	24	140	205	234
5'5"	165	143	64.6	24	144	210	240
5'6"	168	145	65.8	23	149	217	248
5'7"	170	149	67.6	23	153	223	254
5'8"	172	151	68.5	23	156	228	260
5'9"	175	154	69.8	23	162	236	270
5'10"	178	157	71.2	22	167	244	279
5'11"	180	160	72.6	22	171	249	285
6'0"	183	164	74.2	22	177	258	295
6'1"	185	167	75.7	22	181	264	301
6'2"	188	171	77.6	22	187	272	311
6'3"	191	175	79.2	22	193	281	321
6'4"	193	179	81.2	22	197	287	328

*Surgery is the therapy of choice for weight control when the BMI >35 in a patient with comorbidities such as diabetes and hypertension.
†Surgery is the therapy of choice for weight control when the BMI >40.
Data from the 1983 tables from the Metropolitan Life Insurance Company, New York, New York.

East Carolina University football team who was capable of running the 100-yard dash in less than 10 seconds had a BMI of 47 based on his height of 5'8" and his weight of 308 pounds. He was not obese, just very muscular. Hydroimmersion studies revealed his body composition included only 7% fat.

The failure of the height and weight measurements or the BMI to differentiate between the muscular and the fat has serious implications for those professions, such as the police and the military, in which failure to meet weight standards may lead to dismissal. In such cases, hydrodensitometry, or underwater weighing, is strongly recommended before proceeding with termination.

Measures of abdominal circumference, e.g., waist to hip ratios (WHRs), offer economical and readily available measures of obesity, with an emphasis on the distribution of fat. Although a good measure for the overweight, the ratios become increasingly inexact with increasing degrees of morbid obesity owing to the difficulties of locating the waists and hips for valid measures.

The most accurate (but clinically difficult) measure of obesity is probably provided by hydrodensitometry. Evans and colleagues[20] developed a head-above-water approach, which measures body composition in a clinically acceptable fashion. They showed that there is a significant inverse correlation (r = −0.21) between percent fat and relative fat-free weight (rel FFW = actual FFW/ideal FFW). As individuals increase body fat, they also add FFW to support the increased load during ambulation; however, at some critical point (fatness, total weight, cardiorespiratory impairment, orthopedic complications, etc.), mobility of the morbidly obese becomes restricted so that they *lose* or *atrophy* in the fat-free muscle compartment. The initial data suggest that this pathologic threshold for adiposity is 45% fat.

Other indices of relative adiposity include skinfold thickness, total body potassium, total body water, uptake of fat-soluble inert gases, energy balance, nitrogen balance, and various combinations of height versus weight calculations. Except for special research protocols, no clinical advantage is evident for any of these approaches.

Obesity is more complex than just "fat = intake > energy requirements." Obesity is still a poorly understood syndrome. Morbid obesity, especially, is not simply a matter of excessive food intake compared with *normal* food requirements; it may also be caused by unusually inefficient utilization of food, decreased energy expenditure from lessened activity, and/or altered metabolism, such as a reduced thermogenic response to food or attenuated loss of heat through the thickened subcutaneous fat. The examinations by Ravussin and colleagues[55] of the energy expenditure in Pima Indians suggest that some persons with similar physical characteristics are more *energy efficient* and thus more capable of weight gain than others.

Others continue to explore the set-point theory, which is based on the observation that the body weight of animals is remarkably constant. The theory states that body weight is set at a certain point, perhaps controlled at the hypothalamic level, and is defended at that level even when circumstances change in the environment. DuBois[18] suggested that the set point is based on a gene that allows the storage of energy in the form of fat during periods of plenty, favoring the survival of such fat individuals during times of famine. For such a gene to be fully expressed, one has to be in a situation of having unlimited amounts of food available continuously. The best example is that of the desert rat, which gorges after each rain and starves during dry spells. If placed in a cage with food available at all times, the rat becomes so fat that it is eventually unable to move. The Pima Indians, with their high prevalence of obesity, may have such a thrifty genotype developed through centuries of desert existence.

In the Minnesota starvation study,[30] volunteers lost 25% of their body weight, whereas in the Vermont prison overfeeding study,[60] men gained 50 or more pounds. In each study, when subjects were allowed to control their own food intake, body weight rapidly returned to normal. The pursuit of an appetite control center, perhaps in the ventromedial hypothalamus, is another fertile area for investigation. Studies of parabiotic rats (surgically produced Siamese twins) showed that when hypothalamic lesions cause obesity in one twin, the other twin decreases its food intake and may even die of starvation.[27] The body weight of the artificial twins seems to be regulated as a unit. Studies of lipectomy[21] support theories of the regulation of body weight; removing fat from one adipose depot is followed by a compensatory increase in fat in other depots.

ETIOLOGY OF HUMAN OBESITY: GENETIC OR ENVIRONMENTAL?

Although there is wide acceptance of the observation that obesity runs in families, the cause of that obesity, whether genetic or environmental, continues to be disputed. In a superb summary of the various studies noted below, Stunkard, in his classic Salmon lecture, concluded that both etiologies play a role.[62] The genetic argument rests on several findings: that most of the offspring of thin parents are thin, and most of the children of fat parents are fat; and that the strong inverse relationship between current socioeconomic status and obesity in women holds just as strongly when analyzed for socioeconomic status of origin. In addition, analysis of the Twin Register of the National Academy of Sciences/National Research Council showed that the concordance rates for obesity in monozygotic twins were approximately twice those at lesser degrees of overweight and even higher at greater degrees of overweight. Finally, the BMI of adoptees is strongly related to the BMI of the biologic parents and not of the adoptive parents. The recent cloning of the mouse satiety gene adds additional strong evidence for a genetic etiology for obesity.[67]

Similarly, there is evidence that environmental factors are also strong. For example, adoptees who are raised in a rural environment are more overweight than those who are raised in an urban setting. Studies of Danish draftees showed no change in the average weight of these men from 1943 to 1960, but in the following 12 years, there was an eightfold increase in the number with severe obesity, certainly too short a time for a change in the gene pool. It has been observed that attendance at "smorgasbord restaurants" by the obese was higher on the nights that buffets were featured. Currently, most authorities concur that both genetic and environmental factors play a role and that the genetic influences appear to be stronger.

COMPLICATIONS OF MORBID OBESITY

In addition to the physical and social handicaps from their massive bulk, many of the morbidly obese also suffer from serious health problems. Hypertension is the most common complication associated with morbid obesity, occurring in 59% of patients. As might be expected, the principal cause of death in the morbidly obese is directly related to hypertension-induced cardiovascular disease, usually in the form of stroke, acute coronary thrombosis, or arrhythmias. The role of the obesity is underscored by the observation that weight reduction alone lowers blood pressure in over half of hypertensive obese patients.

One third of the morbidly obese have fully developed adult-onset, Type II, diabetes (non-insulin-dependent diabetes mellitus, or NIDDM), another third demonstrate the glucose-impaired, prediabetic state defined by the World Health Organization. The diabetes seen in the morbidly obese seems to be identical to that seen in the general population, with equivalent abnormal metabolic disorders, morbidities, and mortality rates. In these patients, NIDDM is not caused by a lack of insulin; in fact, they generally exhibit significant hyperinsulinemia. Further, the insulin resistance in these obese individuals is caused not by alterations in the structure of the insulin receptors but by complex defects in the metabolism of the cell membrane, the cytoplasm, and the nucleus. Recent studies in human liver, muscle, and several types of fat continue to suggest a complex disorder with decreased availability of insulin receptors on the cell membrane, decreased insulin receptor kinase activity, inadequate generation of second messengers, and diminished activity of specific glucose transport proteins.[19] When diabetes complicates morbid obesity, mortality increases 40%.[17]

Pulmonary insufficiency develops in almost all the morbidly obese to some degree as the expiratory reserve volume falls with the continuing gain in weight. In those who develop the full-blown Pickwickian hypoventilation syndrome, the mortality exceeds 30%. Cholelithiasis is increased threefold. The morbidly obese often have difficulty conceiving; their infertility and the frequently seen amenorrhea generally reverse after surgically induced weight loss. Pregnancy, when it does occur, is associated with an increased risk of preeclampsia, hypertension, poor fetal weight gain, diabetes mellitus, and wound infections. The debilitating symptoms of degenerative arthritis are compounded by the severe stress placed on articulating joint surfaces by the patient's excessive weight. Other complications of obesity include gout, skin diseases, proteinuria, increased hemoglobin concentration, and immunologic impairment. In fact, morbid obesity probably affects every organ system.

The heart is especially burdened.[2] Obese patients have an increased cardiac output, stroke volume, central blood volume, plasma volume, and total blood volume; they also have decreased peripheral resistance.[2] If they are also hypertensive, the peripheral resistance is elevated as well. As the left ventricular volume is augmented in response to the high stroke volume, afterload is correspondingly increased. Not surprisingly, left ventricular function becomes impaired early in morbidly overweight patients, regardless of arterial pressure. The skeleton, stressed by the massive and poorly distributed weight, undergoes early joint and bone deterioration. The lungs expand poorly, because the weight of the chest wall, breasts, and abdominal organs limits the function of the intercostal and diaphragmatic muscles. Accordingly, the morbidly obese show significant decreases in their vital capacities, expired respiratory volume, and ventilatory ventilation, along with sharp increases in their carbon monoxide diffusing capacity.

Morbid obesity also exerts profound hormonal effects as a result of the excessive production of estrogen by the large volume of fat cells. In morbidly obese women, this hormonal change results in dysfunctional uterine bleeding, amenorrhea, and an inadequate luteal phase. In men, the high estrogen blood concentrations are associated with low serum testosterone and low testosterone-estradiol-binding globulin levels. In both sexes, the hypothalamic-pituitary-gonadal axis remains normal. The increased incidence of breast cancer in obese women may well be due to these high levels of estrogen.

WHO LIVES LONGER, APPLES OR PEARS?

Fat is not symmetrically distributed throughout the body but is more likely to be concentrated in the abdomen in the male and on the hips in the female. Five prospective studies examined this relation of fat distribution to morbidity and mortality.[3] Whether the abdominal to gluteal circumference ratio (WHR), the subscapular skinfold, or a combination of skinfolds was used as the indicator of abdominal fat, all five studies found a clear-cut and highly significant increase in the risk of death and/or an increased risk of diabetes, hypertension, or stroke in those individuals with large bellies and narrow hips (apples) versus those with a more gynecoid distribution (pears).[40] Fat distribution was a more important risk factor for morbidity and mortality than overweight or obesity per se and had a relative risk ratio of two or more. The data for WHR, divided into fifths for a cohort of residents of Gothenburg, Sweden,[41] showed that the quintile with the lowest WHR had a much greater chance of remaining free of myocardial infarction and of long-term survival compared with the quintile with the highest WHR. This effect was independent of total fatness. Before fully accepting the concept that "pears outlive apples," however, we need to heed Juczmarski's[28] warning that the definitions of waist and hip measures are inexact and vary throughout the literature. Future studies with computed tomography (CT) scans, ultrasonography, magnetic resonance imaging (MRI), and more accurately defined circumference measurements are badly needed to clarify this important question.

PSYCHOSOCIAL CONSEQUENCES OF MORBID OBESITY

Of greater immediate concern to patients than the physical consequences, however, and the major reason for seeking surgical treatment, are the psychologic and socioeconomic consequences of morbid obesity. Fat people are frequently objects of public scorn and malicious ridicule. They are viewed as lacking self-esteem and being slovenly by nature, with insufficient willpower to curtail excessive eating. Their obese physiques are the antithesis of the lean, trim, and muscular body habitus so highly prized in today's exercise-conscious Western society. Obese patients are often unable to fit into armchairs, find suitable clothing, obtain access to public toilets, and enter public conveyances. If they can enter an automobile, they may be unable to get out. Employers usually consider the morbidly obese poor candidates because of their unfavorable appearance, their inability to fit into office furniture or into factory environments, and their high absenteeism due to illness. In relationships with their peers, the severely obese make few friends and seldom find satisfactory marital or sexual partners, although the libidos of these obese individuals are often as great as their size. Obese women, particularly, tend to marry inadequate spouses who are afraid to accept the challenge of more desirable women. Frequently the object of jokes, the morbidly obese play the role of the jolly fat person, hiding their misery in public and soothing it by eating even more. Obesity limits the availability of educational opportunities and the opportunities for finding a mate. Finally, our patients frequently mention their inability to meet their parental and other social roles: their children and other family members are ashamed to be seen with them at school, at athletic events, and in social situations. The environment of the morbidly obese is neither happy nor filled with opportunities.

OBESITY: A COSTLY DISEASE

The arguments about the control of obesity are not merely academic. Obesity is the most common form of malnutrition in the United States today. According to Marketdata Enterprises, in 1993, nearly $33 billion was spent in the United States in the pursuit of diets, slimming programs, and the management of obesity. Additional billions are spent by pharmaceutical companies pursuing research to formulate various dietary supplements and to find the compounds that could safely alter metabolic rate, to introduce dietary fats that cannot be digested, or to change the appetite control center. Even the smallest towns have stores that specialize in clothing for the "stout or larger woman." Control of obesity, if achieved, would probably have an effect at least equal to that of controlling smoking in terms of the nation's health.

Further, the cost of diabetes cannot be overestimated. Health care for diabetes in 1992 was estimated to be $105 billion, with each diabetic spending an average of $9,493, compared with $2,604 spent by a nondiabetic individual (*American Medical News*, May 9, 1994). Most of these expenditures are for the 95% of diabetics who have the adult-onset form of the disease, an illness almost always associated with obesity.

The largest price is paid by the morbidly obese: not only do they have high health care costs; they often cannot meet their costs of daily living because they are unemployed and indigent. It is time to recognize, as the National Institutes of Health (NIH) Consensus Conference on Obesity[50] concluded, that morbid obesity is a serious, disabling, and common disease and that morbid obesity, like other diseases, deserves treatment and insurance coverage for therapy.

NONOPERATIVE TREATMENT OF MORBID OBESITY

Dieting

Although dieting remains the most useful method of weight control for individuals who are mildly or moderately overweight, it is generally ineffective for the morbidly obese. In most cases, even when massively obese patients are aided by groups such as Weight Watchers, by psychotherapy, by diuretics, by thyroid preparations, or by anorectic agents such as amphetamines, the lost pounds are usually regained along with a few extra ones as soon as the intense weight-reducing regimen has ceased. In fact, weight loss is usually disappointingly low. In a classic study of 100 patients subjected to an intensive weight-reducing regimen by four dietitians, 77% lost less than 10 pounds, and only one patient lost more than 20 pounds.[57] Stunkard and McLaren[63] reported similarly disappointing results. In their classic review of the literature on the failure rate of nonsurgical management of the grossly obese, they found that only 25% of the patients lost as much as 20 pounds, and only 5% lost 40 pounds or more. In their series of 100 consecutive patients, only 12% lost 20 pounds, 1% (one patient) lost 40 pounds, and 28% failed to return after the first visit. After pooling the data from several studies, Bray[3] found that the overall success rate over 1 year with diet alone is about 25%, with diet and medication it is about 40%, and with behavior modification it is nearly 50%. For individuals losing 40 pounds but still weighing 250 or 300 pounds, such losses are not adequate. Bray concluded that the long-term success rate by any of the nonoperative methods is not much more than 10 to 15%. The

1992 NIH Technology Assessment Conference on Methods for Voluntary Weight Control came to the same conclusion when it noted that in the morbidly obese, nonsurgical methods were not effective long-term; within 5 years of commencing any medical regimen, almost all participants gained back at least the weight lost.[12]

Although the use of drugs for the treatment of obesity has been disappointing in the past, advances are being made in the development of new agents and in the application of multiagent protocols. Appetite-suppressant drugs (amphetamines) have been in clinical use for over 50 years, but they have a long history of abuse. Safer new agents are now being introduced, including fenfluramine, phenylpropanolamine, and mazindol.[10] It is hoped that these new drugs will also prove useful in the morbidly obese. Until they are, operation remains the therapy of choice.

Wiring the Teeth

Wiring the teeth deserves mention as another unsuccessful approach to morbid obesity. Patients with fractured and immobilized jaws almost always lose weight, even though such loss could be prevented by the use of appropriate liquid nutrient formulas. Similarly, the morbidly obese lose weight if the jaws are wired shut. The approach has fallen into disuse for three reasons: (1) many morbidly obese patients are edentulous and therefore are not suitable candidates, (2) they tolerate wiring poorly because of their personality patterns and generally demand removal of the wires within a few days, and (3) most important, as soon as the wires are removed, even if a major change in appearance is apparent, they resume previous eating habits and quickly return to their original weight.[29] There may still be limited indications for wiring the teeth in poor-risk obese patients who are in cardiac or pulmonary failure and are being prepared for surgery. However, if this is done, it must be remembered that many morbidly obese patients are severely malnourished in spite of their size and that their liquid diets require considerable nutritional enrichment in order to minimize postoperative complications.

SURGICAL TREATMENT FOR MORBID OBESITY

Because diets are ineffective in the management of morbid and malignant obesity, most authorities now agree with the recommendation of the National Consensus Conference on Surgery for Obesity that operation is the treatment of choice for that small percentage of persons who suffer from severe obesity.[23] The evidence for that supremacy, however, has accumulated slowly. The history of bariatric operations is a story of procedures that were developed, enthusiastically adopted, and rapidly dropped without further follow-up as soon as the next operation or modification was described.

Historical Aspects

The progress of obesity operations is interesting not only because of its historical value but also because it represents a remarkable and useful record of physiologic and metabolic studies of the gut in man.

Intestinal Bypass. Kremen and associates[35] first reported the idea of reducing the length of functional intestine for therapeutic reasons. In 1954, after careful study in dogs, they reported a patient in whom an end-to-end jejunoileostomy was performed for weight reduction. In the discussion of that paper, Sandblom mentioned that Henrikson of Gothenburg, Sweden, had resected "an appropriate amount of small intestine" because of obesity and had induced weight loss

but had encountered difficulty in achieving nutritional balance. In 1956, Payne and DeWind[53] initiated the first clinical program of operations for obesity. Their initial procedure was designed to bypass most of the small intestine and half of the colon by an end-to-side anastomosis of the proximal 36 cm. of jejunum to the mid-transverse colon. When Payne and associates reported their series of patients in 1963, it was evident that the procedure produced dramatic weight loss but that liver failure was prohibitive. One patient died, and each of the remaining nine required reoperation. In six of these individuals, the original intestinal continuity was restored. In three patients, however, in recognition of the essentiality of the terminal ileum, end-to-side jejunoileostomies were performed with good results, except that these patients regained weight.

Because the end-to-side jejunoileostomy permits considerable reflux up the bypassed ileum and thus extends the absorptive surface area in an unpredictable fashion, other groups, notably Scott's[58] and Buchwald's[9] developed the end-to-end jejunoileostomy, draining the bypassed loop into the colon. Scott joined 30 cm. of proximal jejunum to 20 cm. of terminal ileum; Buchwald utilized corresponding 40-cm. and 4-cm. segments. In the massively obese who weigh over 158.9 kg. or 350 pounds, Scott employed 30-cm. and 15-cm. segments. Payne's original intestinal bypass and the later variations are shown in Figure 31–24.

Good results, in terms of weight loss, were reported in about 80% of the patients who underwent the intestinal bypass, with an average weight loss of 45 kg. or 100 pounds. Massively obese individuals lost more than the less obese; younger patients lost more than those in middle age. By the

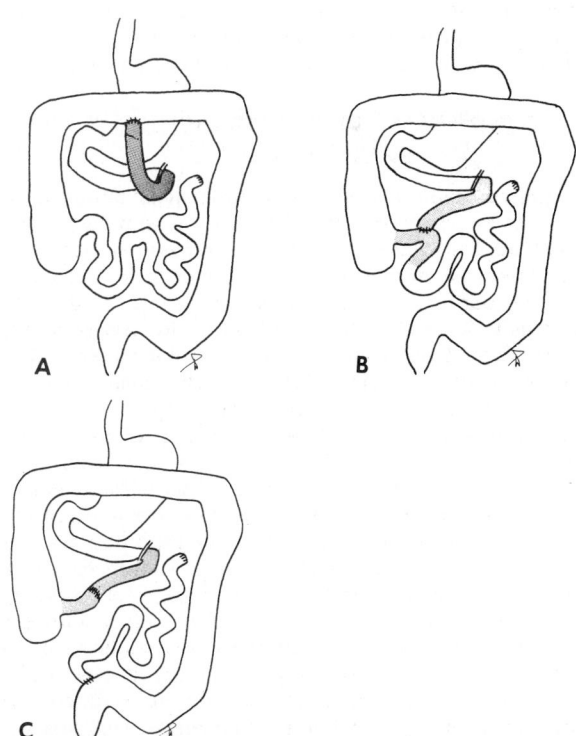

Figure 31–24. Various types of intestinal bypass. The functional areas of the gut are shaded. The early Payne jejunotransverse colostomy (A) bypassed the terminal ileum, with prohibitive metabolic consequences. The end-to-side jejunoileostomy (B) corrected that problem by providing a larger absorptive surface but produced unpredictable results because of the backwash of chyme into the bypassed segment. The end-to-end version (C) by Scott with 35 cm. of jejunum and 10 cm. of ileum was generally effective in producing weight loss but was associated with unacceptable metabolic complications due to malabsorption and overgrowth of bacteria in the excluded loop.

second or third year, almost all patients reached a plateau, and many regained their weight as adaptations for better absorption occurred in their intestines. Operations with more than 64 cm. (25 inches) of intestine in continuity produced unsatisfactory weight loss.

Jejunoileal bypass was associated with a high complication rate. The early in-hospital mortality and complication rates in six series of intestinal bypass operations demonstrated that the operative mortality varied from 1% to 8%, and the major complications included wound problems (10% to 20%), pulmonary emboli (1% to 4%), and hepatic failure (1% to 2%). Brolin et al.[5] reviewed 989 patients collected in the literature and reported the following causes for the 29 deaths (3%) during the first postoperative month: liver failure (five deaths); pulmonary embolism (eight deaths); cardiac failure (two deaths); surgical technique, including anastomotic leaks and sepsis (seven deaths); and other complications (seven deaths). They also reported a long-term follow-up on 1500 patients and found serious metabolic problems. Some resulted from the severe loss of minerals associated with diarrhea, including hypocalcemia, hypokalemia, hypomagnesemia, and iron and zinc deficiency. Hypoproteinemia and anemia were common. The diarrhea usually began about the fifth postoperative day and soon reached 12 to 20 liquid movements per day, gradually subsiding to 6 to 10 semiformed movements per day. Serum electrolyte, mineral, and vitamin levels had to be carefully monitored and corrected in order to avoid serious and occasionally uncontrollable symptoms. Vitamin B_{12} and folic acid deficiencies were common.

Gastrointestinal complications included intractable diarrhea, with associated rectal problems, hemorrhage, and *bypass enteritis*. The last is a syndrome that is probably caused by pathologic bacterial colonization of the bypassed bowel from the colon and is characterized by diarrhea, abdominal pain, fever of up to 39°C., and occasionally even pneumatosis intestinalis.

Biliary or urinary calculi developed in 8% of patients following intestinal bypass, possibly as a result of increased bile salt and glycine synthesis, hyperoxaluria, liver failure, and dehydration. Some patients developed renal failure severe enough to require surgical restoration of bowel continuity. The enhanced oxalate absorption is probably caused by increased fecal fat excretion. In the normal gut, fecal oxalate combines with calcium to form complexes that are poorly absorbed. Following intestinal bypass, however, fatty acids are present in large amounts. These combine with calcium even more readily than they combine with oxalate, effectively increasing the amount of soluble oxalate for absorption.

Liver disease was the most feared complication of intestinal bypass, and a number of fatalities were reported. Abnormalities in liver function occurred in about 40% of patients with an intestinal bypass. These changes were unpredictable and dangerous, appearing as early as 3 weeks or as late as 2 years after operation. Nausea, vomiting, jaundice, and enlargement of the liver were reported frequently; ascites and anasarca were rare. Hepatic coma and death occurred in 1% of all bypass patients. Although many patients showed improvement 6 to 12 months after operation, in 3% to 5% the changes were progressive and associated with marked fibrosis. In severe cases, the terminal changes were histologically indistinguishable from alcoholic cirrhosis. Many morbidly obese patients are particularly vulnerable, because fatty metamorphosis is common among the morbidly obese even prior to surgery; their fatty livers resemble those of force-fed geese.

Hepatic deterioration progressed in some patients in spite of restoration of good nutrition by hyperalimentation. O'Leary et al.[52] demonstrated that liver failure following in-

testinal bypass can be caused by an overgrowth of bacteroides, an organism that produces a hepatotoxic endotoxin, in the excluded intestinal limb. Antibiotics specific for bacteroides prevented liver damage in animal models.

In addition to hepatic dysfunction and urinary and biliary calculi, a large number of case reports cited a variety of problems, including unmanageable diarrhea, polyarthrosis, fatigue, lethargy, muscle cramps, uncontrollable nausea and bloating, tuberculosis, and nontuberculous granulomas. Besides the various metabolic problems, patients developed mechanical complications, including obstruction of the bypassed small intestine and intussusception of the blind loop into the colon. These two problems can be particularly puzzling and dangerous; roentgenographic findings may not be helpful, since the characteristic small bowel loops with airfluid levels may not be present.

Perhaps the most disappointing aspect of the intestinal bypass was that long-term weight control was poor. Twenty percent of the patients failed to lose weight satisfactorily, and some lost no weight at all. A significant number regained some of the lost weight during the second and third years after operation, and some of these patients required another procedure in which an additional segment of the now adapted small bowel was removed.

In summary, following intestinal bypass, most patients lost one third of their total body weight, with some improvement of insulin resistance, hypertension, cardiac failure, pulmo-

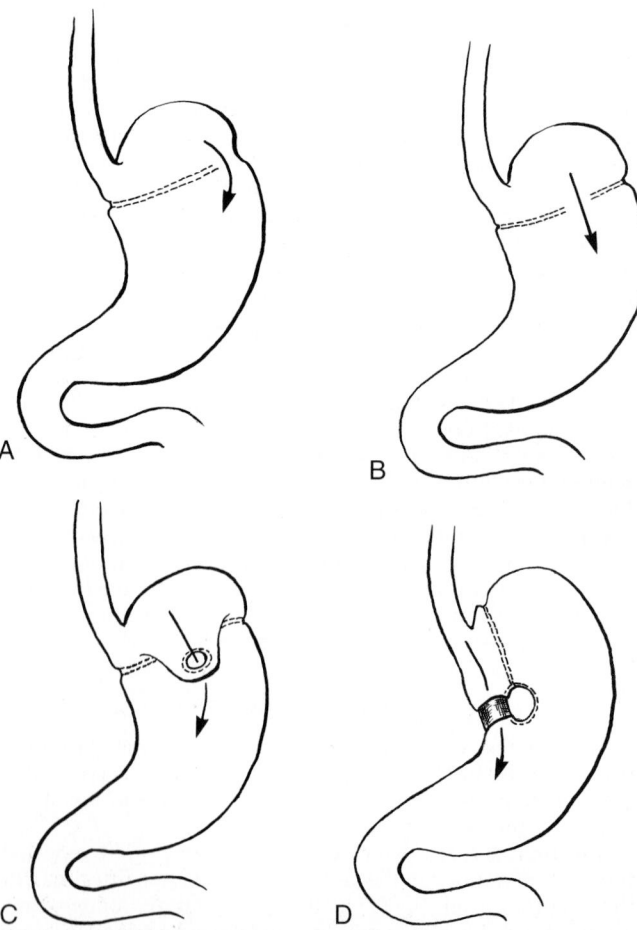

Figure 31–25. Various types of gastroplasty. The initial models (A, B, and C) failed because the pouches were too large, the staple lines disrupted, and the gastric pouch outlet stretched. Mason's vertical banded gastroplasty (D) improved outcomes by the use of a small measured collar, a double staple line, and a measured gastric outlet reinforced with a plastic mesh collar.

Figure 31–26. Various types of gastric bypass. The initial models *(A)* failed because pouches were too large, outlets were too wide, intestinal loops were of inadequate length, and staple lines were not durable. The current version of the gastric bypass *(B)* produces a gastric pouch of 15 to 30 ml., 8- to 15-mm. gastroenterostomies, more secure partitions prepared by division of the stomach or triple stapling techniques, and alimentary and afferent loops of 40 to 60 cm. and 40 to 200 cm., sized to the patient's needs. Scopinaro's biliopancreatic bypass *(C)* is the most radical approach. It may be useful for the superobese, with its gastrectomy, cholecystectomy, and a much shorter common small bowel channel.

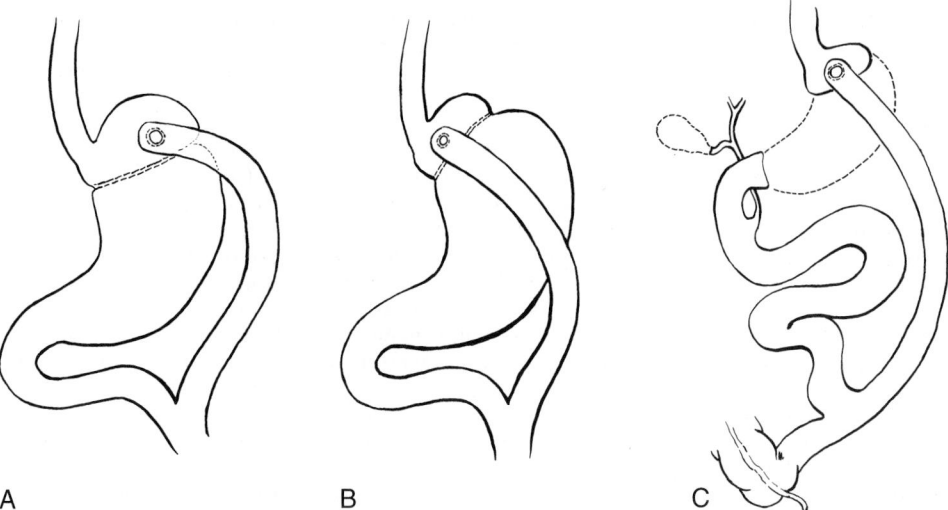

A　　　　　B　　　　　C

nary function, and hyperlipidemia. Unfortunately, the long-term complications were serious: persistent diarrhea, hypokalemia, profound hypomagnesemia and hypocalcemia, arthralgias, neurologic signs, enteropathies, intussusceptions, avitaminoses, trace element deficits, cholelithiasis, renal disease, and liver failure. Thousands of operations were done, and although there were a few long-term successes, over half of the patients required rehospitalization, and many had to have the bypasses reversed to prevent death from hepatic failure. Equally sad, most patients adapted their intestinal function and began to regain their weight in the second year. Griffen et al.[25] finally laid the procedure to rest after a review of the results: "Jejunoileal bypass is not an appropriate operation for morbidly obese patients and should be abandoned."

Gastric Operations. The most important advance in bariatric surgery occurred in 1966, when Mason and Ito,[46] concerned by the frequency and seriousness of the complications from intestinal bypass, devised the gastric bypass, which was designed to interfere with food intake rather than with digestion and absorption. The procedure and various modifications were rapidly adopted when others confirmed that the gastric bypass was not only safer but also as effective as the intestinal bypass in producing weight loss in the morbidly obese.

In the intervening decades, there have been a host of new gastric procedures, which can be divided into four types: gastroplasties, gastric bypasses, external constricting prostheses, and artificial bezoars or gastric balloons. All four procedures reduce the gastric reservoir and therefore limit intake. The gastroplasties, gastric bypasses, and banding procedures also delay gastric emptying with a small gastric outlet. The gastric bypasses also add variable degrees of malabsorption by excluding the chyme from the antrum, duodenum, and variable lengths of proximal jejunum. These four types of gastric bariatric procedures are shown in Figures 31–25, 31–26, and 31–27.

Although bariatric surgical procedures are still developing, they are no longer experimental approaches. Two operations are now well-established and recognized bariatric procedures: the vertical banded gastroplasty (VBG) and the gastric bypass (GB) operation. Two additional operations, Silastic gastric banding (SGB) and the biliopancreatic bypass (BPB), are increasingly used. There is a strong advantage in having several operations available, because morbidly obese patients differ, and "one size does not fit all." For example, patients who are addicted to sweets will lose more weight following gastric bypass than gastroplasty, because the bypass procedures cause dumping and the gastric restrictive procedures do not. Further, there are some early indications that results of the gastric bypass in the superobese can be improved by lengthening the biliopancreatic afferent limb of the Roux-en-Y and shortening the common channel.[59] Finally, bariatric operations may require a staged approach, as recommended by Kral,[34] in which simpler and less-demanding procedures are done first, with the understanding that if these prove to be inadequate, additional operations will be needed.

Figure 31–27. Gastroplasties and artificial bezoars. The total gastric wrap *(A)*, although successful in controlling weight, is no longer used because of problems with the large and occasionally eroding foreign body. The Garren gastric balloon *(B)* was an attempt to decrease weight with an artificial bezoar. It proved to be dangerous, caused little weight loss, and is no longer approved for use. The Kuzmak adjustable Silastic band *(C)* appears to offer a simple, safe approach with few complications. It produces less weight loss than the gastric bypass but does so without the danger of malnutrition due to malabsorption.

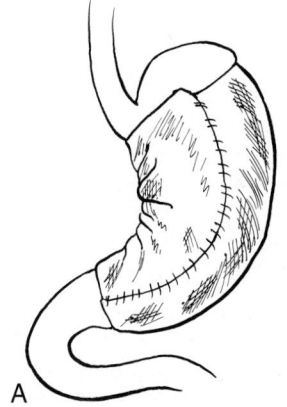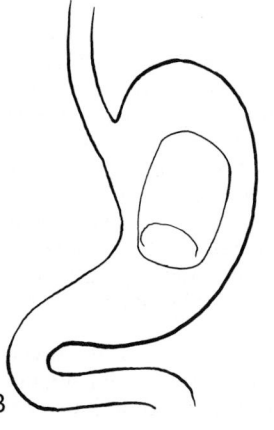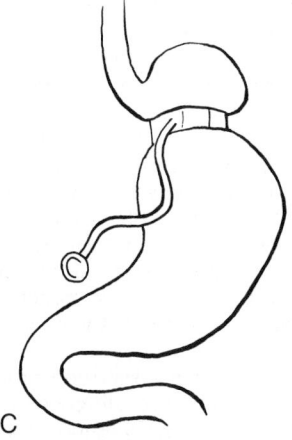

A　　　　　B　　　　　C

Restrictive Procedures: Gastroplasties and Banding Operations

Because Mason's first gastric bypass was a major technical challenge, other alternatives were developed that could also provide a small gastric pouch and a limited outlet without requiring gastric division or an intestinal anastomosis. These gastroplasties evolved around the same principle: the partition of the stomach with a stapler, leaving a small passage, about 1 cm. in diameter, in the center of the staple line or at the greater or lesser curvature. Others solved the problem with a gastro-gastroplasty, forming a small anastomosis between the two separated gastric pouches. All these eventually failed due to stretching of the opening or breakdown of the staple line.

Vertical Banded Gastroplasty. Mason, the real pioneer in bariatric operations, persevered through a number of model procedures and, in 1980, developed the VBG, which until recently was the most commonly performed bariatric operation in the United States. One area of concern in bariatric operations has been the fear that the small gastric reservoirs would produce reflux. That fear proved to be unfounded; reflux is rare and, in fact, the VBG, with its isolated gastric achlorhydric proximal tube, has been recommended as an antireflux procedure.[14]

Although the reader is advised to refer to Mason's detailed description,[45] the procedure is summarized below.

Description of the Operation. The abdomen is entered through a midline incision and carefully explored. If no contraindications are found, a 32-French Ewald tube is passed into the stomach and positioned against the lesser curvature; a Penrose drain is then passed around the esophagus just above the cardia, and the thin gastrohepatic ligament is entered. The fingers of the left hand are inserted into the lesser sac. A passage is made between the gastric neurovascular bundle and the gastric wall for the future collar. The Penrose drain is brought through, closely encompassing only esophageal and gastric tissue, excluding the vessels and branches of the vagus nerves. A 25-mm.-diameter end-to-end (EEA) stapler is used to create a window adjacent to the Ewald tube, which is positioned against the lesser curvature. The window may require reinforcement with absorbable sutures, especially if there is any doubt about the doughnut specimens excised by the stapler. The linear four-row stapler is then applied through the gastric window parallel to the Ewald tube to produce the pouch. The final pouch volume is adjusted to values of 9 to 25 ml., with an average of 15 ml., as measured through the tube. The collar is created with a 1.5- by 7-cm. strip of Marlex mesh marked and sewn to produce a 5-cm. opening. At the end of the procedure, the integrity of the pouch is tested with the insufflation of air with the abdomen filled with saline. The mesh is then covered with omentum. The abdomen is closed with absorbable suture, and the skin is reapproximated with staples.

Outcomes. Mason reported a combined series of 1000 patients from the University of Iowa Hospitals and Clinics in Iowa City and the St. Francis Memorial Hospital in San Francisco. The operative mortality was 0.33%. Three-year results showed sustained weight control, with a loss of 35 kg. (54% excess weight loss) in 45 patients whose initial weight was greater than 225% of ideal. The report suffers somewhat in that the size of the collar—the gastric pouch outlet—was changed during the series, and no data were provided regarding the intensity of the follow-up. Deitel and his associates[15] reported a series of 233 patients and confirmed Mason's excellent results with a follow-up of 94%, but for only 3 years. More recent studies,[43] but with division of the stomach rather than staple partition and a follow-up of at least 4 years, revealed a substantial failure rate, with

36% of patients requiring reoperation for stenosis or failure to lose weight.

Concerns. Surgeons are no longer as enthusiastic about the VBG as they were in previous years, for several reasons. First, weight loss is about 10% to 15% less than that attained with the GB operation. Second, on longer follow-up, a significant number of patients require reoperation with revision to a GB because of erosion of the Marlex band into the gastric lumen, stenosis of the outlet due to fibrosis and rotation of the band, or rupture of the pouch due to failure of the staple line. Finally, the VBG, in contrast to the GB, allows the intake of soft, sweet, high-calorie foods.[6] Even so, the VBG continues to be an acceptable and safe bariatric operation that deserves rigorous study to improve its long-term effectiveness and its late complication rate.

Willbanks's[66] silicone elastomere ring offers a simpler alternative for the reinforcement of the stoma in VBGs. The approach is technically easier than the VBG, since it avoids the need for the through-and-through EEA hole in the stomach and uses an easily placed 8-French radiopaque silicone ring. Although his follow-up is limited, he was able to report an operative mortality of 0.04% (1 of 2147) and only a 15% to 25% failure rate to maintain weight loss at 46 to 55 months.

Gastric Banding. The application of external prostheses to the stomach offers another way to limit the size of the reservoir. The concept of using gastric banding for the treatment of obesity originated in 1976 when Wilkinson[65] performed the first such operation, using a strip of Marlex mesh to pull the stomach into an hourglass configuration. When this approach failed to produce adequate weight loss, Wilkinson went on to wrap the entire stomach, but this operation failed as well. Molina[47] continued to explore banding with nylon and later with Dacron bands, placing these primarily by palpation through a small skin incision in an attempt to reduce the trauma of the operation. The most successful approach appears to be Kuzmak's[38] stoma adjustable silicone gastric banding (SASGB), in which a 1-cm.-wide soft, radiopaque, partly inflatable silicone band with a subcutaneous reservoir is used to develop a pouch, which is measured with an inflatable balloon. The stoma is precisely sized to a diameter of 12 to 13 cm. with a banding instrument equipped with an electronic sensor.

The procedure has become increasingly popular throughout the world since the introduction of the adjustable band and the demonstration that the operation can be performed with laparoscopy.[11]

Description of the Operation. An upper midline incision is made into the subcutaneous tissue. At about 10 cm. below the rib cage, subcutaneous fat is dissected from the right rectus sheath. The sheath is cut transversely, and part of the rectus muscle is transected to prepare the space for the reservoir. The abdomen is then entered through the midline. The avascular part of the hepatogastric ligament is opened, and blunt dissection is used to form a tunnel under the stomach and through the avascular suspensory ligament of the fundus. A Penrose drain is placed around the stomach for traction, and the fundus is further mobilized to obtain the correct size of the pouch. A small opening is then made next to the lesser curvature, 3 cm. below the gastroesophageal junction and medial to the gastric vessels and branches of the vagus nerve. A 1-cm.-wide soft band of silicone, reinforced with two layers of Dacron mesh and fitted with a 4-cm. inflatable segment connected to the reservoir, is threaded through the opening and around the stomach. When the band is placed around the stomach, the anesthesiologist inserts the calibrating tube, and the pouch is calibrated by inflating the balloon with 20 ml. of saline solution. The silicone band is then tightened with a buckle; an electronic sensor is used to determine the desired diameter of the stoma. When the correct tightness is reached, the band is sutured, and the buckle and the redundant part of the band are excised. The previously mobilized greater curvature is then sutured with three or four 3-0 silk sutures over the band to the pouch. As in all bariatric operations, attention to detail is essential, and reference to the author's original description and use of his materials is strongly advised.

Outcomes. Kuzmak's 7-year experience in 311 patients combines two groups: an initial cohort of 173 treated with a nonadjustable band, and the remainder treated with the adjustable modification. With an undefined level of follow-up, both groups demonstrated satisfactory weight loss. At 60 months, the nonadjustable group averaged a 47% excess weight loss, but at 36 months, the adjustable group had already demonstrated the advantage of the new modification, with 64.3% excess weight loss versus 49.4% in the nonadjustable group after the same time interval. With an average preoperative weight of 293 pounds, the average excess weight lost by those in the adjustable group who were followed was 42.1% ± 25.5% 1 year postoperatively; at 2 years, 60.1% ± 27.3%; at 3 years, 72.0% ± 26.5%; and at 4 years, 76.0% ± 22.8%. Slightly more than 28% of the patients reached a weight that was less than 30% above their estimated ideal weight. Operative mortality was 0.6% for the first group and 0.7% for the second group. Stoma complications occurred in about 8%: eight stomas required revision, and two bands eroded and required replacement. Kuzmak reported no wound infections, intra-abdominal infections, or dehiscences.

Concerns. Similar results were reported by Lise et al.[42] Others, however, report less satisfactory results. Granstrom and Backman,[24] in 72 patients followed for 12 to 54 months after gastric banding, had two operative deaths, and 22 of their patients required 33 reoperations. The difference may well be due to technique. Kuzmak is a meticulous surgeon who insists on precise placement and adjustment of the band.

The operation also has the limitations of the other gastroplasties, in that it can be defeated by those addicted to sweets. Also, weight loss is about 10% to 15% less than that following operations that include a malabsorptive component. Nevertheless, gastric banding offers a simple, safe, and reversible procedure that is adjustable to the patient's needs. Wider application of this procedure is likely.

Malabsorption Procedures

Gastric Bypass. The GB has undergone continuous modification since the initial description by Mason in 1963. The critical areas of the procedure have proved to be the volume of the proximal gastric pouch, partitioning of the stomach, the diameter of the gastrojejunostomy, and the length of the jejunal limbs.

The proximal gastric pouch has been reduced over the years to the currently accepted 30 ml. Some stretching can be expected with time so that, after about a year, most patients can eat about half a hamburger.

Partitioning of the stomach continues to be a troublesome challenge, because failure of the staple lines, with consequent transit of food into the distal gastric pouch, is responsible for the majority of bariatric operative failures. A number of approaches have been tried to divide the stomach securely: single staple lines, close and separated double staple lines, triple superimposed staple lines, and division of the stomach. Single staple lines—a double row of staples placed with one application of a TA90 instrument—were abandoned early because of their almost universal failure rate. Double staple lines—four rows of staples placed with a wider TA90—have a failure rate of almost 20% in our long-term follow-up, with some ruptures occurring as late as 10 years after the original

surgery. The ruptures may be caused by the isolation of a strip of stomach between the two staple lines, an exclusion that may act like a closed loop, with rupture into one of the gastric pouches. Two methods of partitioning seem to produce reliable results: the triple superimposed application of the single TA90 stapling device developed by Sugerman (personal communication, 1993), with a failure rate of less than 1%; and the division of the stomach, a far more challenging technique with a significant danger of a leak or fistula formation.[13]

The delay in gastric emptying by the gastrojejunostomy is most effective when the diameter of that anastomosis measures 8 to 10 mm. Smaller stomata frequently become occluded and require repeated dilatations; larger stomata are followed by inadequate weight loss. Dilatation of the anastomosis can be minimized with a double-layered continuous suturing technique with 3-0 polypropylene suture.

The length of the alimentary and the biliopancreatic jejunal limbs can also play a significant role in the success of the operation. Most bariatric surgeons now use a length of 40 to 75 cm. for the alimentary limb; longer segments, as long as 150 cm., are used for the superobese.[5] Scruggs and coworkers,[59] for example, recently reported satisfactory results with two modifications—a regular gastric bypass (R-GBP) with an alimentary limb of 90 cm. and an afferent limb of 60 cm., and an extended gastric bypass (X-GBP) with a similar alimentary proximal limb of 90 cm. but a much longer afferent limb that leaves only 180 to 240 cm. of common channel. (It is of interest that the weight loss did not differ substantially between the two groups.) The longer loops produce greater weight loss but do so with the increased danger of serious malnutrition.

Description of the Operation. The abdomen is entered through a midline incision, and exposure is provided by a mechanical retractor. If the exploration demonstrates no contraindications, the upper stomach is isolated by inserting the index finger gently into the angle at the cardia to the left of the esophagus. At this point there is a weak, thin area of the posterior peritoneum, which is easily entered by the dissecting finger. The dissection is gently continued behind the esophagus and cardia, and the finger is brought out not at the right side of the esophagus but between the ascending branches of the left gastric artery, 2.5 to 3.0 cm. below the esophagogastric junction. A no. 36 Malecot catheter, from which the bulbous end has been cut, is used to pull a TA90 stapling instrument through the passage. A proximal pouch measuring 4 cm. in width and 1.5 cm. in height, approximately the size of a thumb, is then prepared by firing the staples. Two additional layers of similar TA90 staples are superimposed and fired over the first set. A figure-of-eight suture is placed at each end of the staple line to close the ends securely and to serve as guy sutures. To prepare the Roux-en-Y, the jejunum is divided 40 to 60 cm. from the ligament of Treitz with the GIA stapling instrument and threaded through the mesocolon, the lesser sac, and back out by the bare area of the greater curvature. The proximal end of the distal jejunum is then sutured to the gastric pouch. The anastomosis is sewn to fit loosely around a 0.8-cm. Salem sump tube in two layers with continuous polypropylene. The Roux-en-Y enteroenterostomy is then completed by joining the proximal jejunum end-to-side to the distal jejunum 60 cm. below the gastroenterostomy with a GIA and TA55 stapling devices. It is important that the intestine is not constricted in its passage through the lesser sac. It is also important to fasten the Roux loop to the mesocolon to prevent an internal hernia and to oversew any bleeders in the enteroenterostomy before closing it. The abdomen is closed with a running double-stranded 0 monofilament absorbable suture. The skin is stapled. The operation can usually be performed in 60 to 75 minutes; blood loss rarely exceeds 300 ml.

Outcomes. Published reports of the GB demonstrate similar statistics in most series. The results described here in detail are included because the series offers the longest and most rigorous follow-up in the literature. In the 14-year study, personal contact was maintained with all but 9 of 608 patients, for a follow-up rate of 98%. The 608 morbidly obese patients were all treated with the Greenville modification of Mason's GB operation: a proximal gastric pouch of approximately 20 to 30 ml., an 8- to 10-mm. gastroenterostomy, and Roux-en-Y limbs varying from 40 to 60 cm. (These measurements are critical but are presented as honest ranges, given the limitations of working with tissues.) The first 519 gastric partitions were done with a four-row TA90 stapling device. Subsequently, to avoid further staple line failures, either the stomach is divided or triple superimposed layers of double-row TA90 staples are used. Except for the different approaches for partitioning, the operations were identical and can therefore be evaluated as one cohort. The operations were performed on 404 white and 102 black women and 87 white and 15 black men. The average age at the time of operation was 37.3 (range 14 to 64) years.

The operation produced significant and durable weight loss. An average maximum weight loss of 70% of excess body weight occurred approximately 2 years after operation. At the end of 5 years, mean weight loss was 58% of excess body weight; after 10 years, it was 55%; and after 14 years, 49% (Table 31–4).

Even more striking is the control of adult-onset diabetes. Before operation, 164 of the 608 (27%) had NIDDM, and another 166 (27.3%) proved to have impaired glucose tolerance (IGT). The normalization of glucose metabolism occurs with surprising speed, even before there is significant weight loss. After 10 days, there is no further evidence of NIDDM in most patients, even in those who required over 100 units of insulin preoperatively. Following operation, only 26 of those with NIDDM and 2 with IGT still had diabetic blood values. Seven died during follow-up, yielding a denominator of 323 patients. Thus 295 of 323 (91%) continue to be restored to euglycemia by the GB. No other therapy for diabetes, medical or surgical, has ever reported such a high rate of success in controlling the hyperglycemia and hyperinsulinemia associated with that disease.

Before operation, 353 (58.1%) of the patients had hypertension. After operation, this rate was reduced to 14%. The GB effectively reduced the proportion of body fat. Measurements of body composition with hydrodensitometry (underwater immersion weighing) in 220 of the patients demonstrated that the females fell from a preoperative mean of 50.92% fat to 38.46% fat, and males fell from 46.70% to 31.93% fat.[32] In addition to these improvements, patients generally demonstrated improvement in cardiopulmonary function, in their disabilities from arthritis, and in fertility.

The GB produced long-term improvement in the health and physical functioning of the morbidly obese, but the positive emotional and social changes proved to be temporary.

As reflected by the RAND scale measures, the emotional improvement seen in the patients returned to preoperative levels by 3 years after operation; only general health and vitality, both measures of physical performance, remained improved. The patients felt better and looked better, but those with inadequate preoperative personalities seemed to return to that state in spite of physical improvements. Whether counseling or other psychiatric intervention can alter this regression bears investigation. Relevant to these findings is the report by Ryden et al.,[56] who found depression to be more common in those patients who had excellent results after bariatric operations and concluded that "the marked weight loss leads to problems of adaptation, which in turn may trigger depressive reactions." Kopec et al.[31] reported that in a series of 45 patients who had undergone the VBG, 44% reported an improved social life after operation, 46% stated that it remained the same, and 9% thought that their social lives had deteriorated.

Improvement in daily function following bariatric operations was also documented by Deitel et al.,[16] who studied 44 morbidly obese patients who met the 17 Canadian criteria for severe disability before their operations. In these individuals, the disabilities disappeared in 22, became mild in 17, and became moderate in 3. Two were lost to follow-up.

Complications diminished with increasing experience. For the whole series, however, perioperative mortality was 9 of 608 (1.5%), with 6 dying of sepsis and 3 from pulmonary embolism. Perioperative morbidity during the first 30 days included the following complications: minor wound infections, 8.7%; wound seromas, 5.8%; severe wound infections, 3.0%; anastomotic stenosis, 3.0%; splenic tears, 2.5%; and subphrenic abscesses, 2.5%. Hospital readmissions were required in 8.2%, and 2.8% of the patients needed reoperations during the early postoperative period. The total mortality over the 14 years was 35 of 608, with the 26 late deaths divided into two groups: 12 from emotionally related causes, and 14 from more natural etiologies. The emotionally related deaths included three suicides, three cases of cirrhosis due to a return to drinking, one from bulimia, one from pernicious anemia due to a refusal to take vitamin B_{12}, and four, perhaps more questionable, from auto accidents. (We have had no such deaths in the last 3 years since we started a regular support group.) The other late deaths included four from cardiac causes, three from cancer, and one each from atherosclerosis, pneumonia, AIDS, peritonitis, pulmonary embolus, and two from unknown causes, presumably arrhythmias.

The most frequent late complications included vitamin B_{12} deficiency (40%), anemia (39%), hospital readmission (38.1%), incisional hernia (23.9%), depression (23.4%), staple line failure (15.1%), gastritis (13.2%), cholelithiasis (11.4%), and bile reflux (8.7%). Dumping developed in 70.6% of the patients, but although the syndrome is sometimes listed as a complication, it is actually a desired side effect, because it prevents these patients from gorging on sweets after operation. The mortality of a matched group of morbidly obese who did not undergo bariatric operation remains unknown. Although early data suggest that the surgical group does better in terms of function, disease, and mortality, a rigorous comparison is badly needed.

In spite of the complications and the limitation in food intake, only two of these patients have requested and undergone reversal of the GB. In those patients in whom the operation failed due to pouch dilatation, anastomotic widening, and staple failure, all but one requested that the defect be corrected as quickly as possible before they regained their previous weight. Few operations are performed that have such a high level of patient satisfaction.

Concerns. The GB is becoming the procedure of choice among bariatric surgeons because it produces durable weight

TABLE 31–4. Weight Loss in 608 Morbidly Obese Patients After Gastric Bypass over 14 Years

Time	Mean Weight (lb.)	Ranges (lb.)
Preoperative	304.4	198–615
1 yr.	192.0	104–466
5 yr.	205.4	107–512
10 yr.	206.5	130–388
14 yr.	204.7	158–270

loss, can be performed with a remarkably low mortality and complication rate in a very difficult group of patients, and provides excellent control of comorbidities such as diabetes and hypertension. However, two concerns remain: the rupture of the staple lines, and the stabilization of weight before reaching ideal levels, especially in the superobese. The failure of staple lines, a concern in all the bariatric procedures that require gastric partition, will probably be resolved by division of the stomach or a new stapling technique that produces scarring at the partition.

The attainment of normal weights by the superobese may not be a feasible goal, even with staged procedures. Recent attempts at improving weight loss by increasing the length of the limbs skirt close to the hazards of the intestinal bypass. The follow-up of these trials is still short; time will tell if the degree of malnutrition in these patients becomes a serious problem. A return to the ideal body weight may not, in fact, be appropriate, because correction of diabetes, hypertension, and other comorbidities occurs even with losses of 10% to 20% of body weight.[8]

Biliopancreatic Bypass. The biliopancreatic bypass represents a combination of the gastric bypass and the intestinal bypass, devised to produce even greater weight loss than is achievable with gastric bypass alone.[1] The operation, shown in Figure 31–26, includes a gastric resection, a cholecystectomy, and diversion of the biliopancreatic stream into a short common channel to inhibit digestion and absorption. Because of the gastrectomy, the operation is not reversible. The procedure has fewer complications than the intestinal bypass, perhaps because it avoids the bacterial overgrowth seen with totally excluded loops of small bowel. Weight loss is excellent, but recent reports of hepatic failure after the biliopancreatic bypass[26, 39] suggest that the operation should be used sparingly, perhaps being saved for those patients who have failed less demanding procedures.

Gastric Balloon

The gastric balloon is included in this chapter for completeness, so that others will not have to re-explore this idea. The balloon was introduced by Garren[22] on the premise that this artificial bezoar would produce early satiety and thus diminish intake. The device enjoyed rapid acceptance and widespread application through massive publicity and the scheduling of multiple well-attended national courses. Within a few years, thousands had been implanted. The Food and Drug Administration finally took the device off the market because of its lack of long-term effectiveness, the unjustifiable cost ($7,000 a year), and the high complication rates (including obstruction, ulceration, and perforation).

COMPARISON OF GASTRIC BYPASS, INCLUDING GASTROPLASTIES, AND GASTRIC BANDING

Several prospective studies compared the old gastroplasties—those performed prior to the VBG—with gastric bypasses; in each, the GB proved to be the better procedure. Whether the stoma was on the lesser or the greater curvature or in the middle of the staple line, the gastric pouches enlarged and the stomas stretched so that, within 1 or 2 years, the 20% mean weight loss was soon regained. Naslund and co-workers,[48] in a series of 57 patients followed for 2 years, found that weight loss at 1 year was significantly greater and failures significantly fewer in the 29 who underwent the GB. In a prospective and randomized series of 87 patients,[54] comparing the GB with gastric partition (gastric pouch stapling with a gastrogastrostomy) demonstrated that the GB patients lost 15% more of their original weight at 12 months

and 21% at 18 months, with fewer failures and a similar complication rate.

Zimmerman et al.[68] compared the results after GB and the Silastic-ring vertical gastroplasty in a small series of 35 patients with only a 1-year retrospective study. They concluded that the weight loss was roughly comparable but that the Silastic-ring series had a much greater problem with vomiting and food intolerance (76% versus 7%).

Only one well-controlled series comparing the GB with the true Mason's VBG has been published. Sugerman et al.[64] stopped the randomization at 9 months after 20 patients had undergone each procedure, because greater weight loss (p <0.05) was noted after the GB. The difference increased (p <0.01) with each 3-month interval through 3 years. In a later study, the same authors obtained their best results by assigning sweets eaters to the GB and recommended that VBG not be performed in patients who are addicted to sweets.

MacLean and his co-workers,[44] in a prospective randomized trial between the VBG and a vertical gastric bypass in 106 patients, reported a success rate of 39% with the gastroplasty and 58% for the bypass, due to failure of the staple lines. Their success rate, defined as a return of the patient to 150% of ideal body weight, rose to 83% when the gastric partition was performed with division rather than staples.

In summary, all three procedures—GB, Mason's VBG, and gastric banding—have been shown to be effective therapies for morbid obesity. Each has been reported to produce effective weight loss, to reverse hyperglycemia and hypertension, and to provide significant rehabilitation. All can be done with surprisingly low operative mortalities (<1% in good-risk patients, and <2% in those with severe comorbidities) and acceptable morbidity rates. Willbanks (personal communication, 1994) summarized the comparison nicely: "When statistically valid data become available, these will show the vertical gastroplasties to have a slightly lower complication rate and the gastric bypass to be slightly more effective and consistent." Perhaps the most important conclusion is that bariatric operations, like other operative therapies, need to be individualized to fit different patients, and in some, several staged operations will be necessary, as first recommended by Kral.[32]

MANAGEMENT OF THE MORBIDLY OBESE PATIENT

Patient Selection. Most groups operating for morbid obesity use similar criteria for the selection of their patients and, in general, manage their patients in the same way. Patients are considered to be candidates if their BMI is 40 and they have no comorbidities such as arthritis, diabetes, hypertension, the Pickwickian syndrome, sleep apnea, or other obesity-related disabling conditions; if their BMI is 35 and their obesity is complicated by these diseases; if they have realistic expectations of the outcomes after the procedure; and if they can tolerate the operation. The requirement by many insurance companies that patients provide evidence of physician-supervised diets is silly; virtually all morbidly obese have dieted all their lives and repeatedly failed. Bariatric operations are generally denied or delayed if the patient is physically unable to tolerate the procedure owing to causes such as irreversible cardiac disease; there is a history of alcohol or substance abuse within the preceding 5 years; the patient has inadequate intelligence to understand the procedure and its consequences; there is a previous pattern of severe depression or suicide attempts; the patient has unrealistic expectations and does not agree to long-term follow-up; and, occasionally, if there is an irreconcilably hostile and unsupportive family.

Preoperative Evaluation. The preoperative evaluation process proceeds slowly in order to ensure that the patient is well-educated about the procedure and to emphasize that the operation is a serious undertaking. The protocol begins with initial interviews, which include the family, if possible. Usually two visits suffice to determine whether the patient is an appropriate candidate, and if so, the preoperative work-up is begun. That evaluation includes a complete medical and dietary history, physical examination, complete blood count, urinalysis, SMA-12, electrolytes, a glucose tolerance test if the patient is not a known diabetic, electrocardiogram, posteroanterior and lateral chest roentgenograms, and pulmonary function tests with arterial blood gases. All patients are screened for psychopathology by the project psychologist or psychiatrist. Members of the family, if available, are counseled regarding the procedure. For the ongoing studies, a series of psychometric tests, special tests for glucose metabolism, and immersion hydrostatic weighing are performed. If indicated by the results of the work-up, patients may undergo more sophisticated studies, such as upper gastrointestinal series, fiberoptic endoscopy, echocardiography, stress testing, and cardiac angiography. Bariatric operations are a major undertaking; it is important that the patients be well prepared.

Preoperative Preparation. Patients are generally admitted on the morning of the procedure. Complicated cases, however, such as patients with cardiorespiratory failure, may require several days of preparation in the hospital to bring them to an optimal preoperative status. A cephalosporin is given intravenously for prophylaxis the morning of the procedure and for 2 days thereafter. Serious health problems need to be stabilized before surgery. Skin lesions need to clear as much as possible, and chronic problems such as asthma, chronic pulmonary infections, diabetes, and hypertension need to be stabilized; if the patient is on medications, these need to be reviewed and adjusted to appropriate levels.

Postoperative Care. In general, the postoperative care of bariatric patients resembles that following standard abdominal procedures and is therefore not described in detail, except to emphasize the need for prophylactic antibiotics; careful monitoring of vital signs, fluid balance, and glucose metabolism; and appropriate furniture and equipment to manage these massive individuals.

The first 24 hours are particularly critical because of the great seriousness of a leak or intra-abdominal infection in these individuals. If the pulse remains over 120, if there is a rise in temperature over 102° F., or if the patient looks ill in spite of normal vital signs, emergency exploration and the addition of other antibiotics may be needed. Barium swallows may be helpful but are not always reliable; several patients with anastomotic leaks demonstrated normal passage of barium without extravasation. Neglect of a perforation or intra-abdominal infection is associated with a high mortality rate. If there is doubt, it is best to proceed with the operation; an unnecessary exploration is a lot safer than a missed perforation.

Patients usually spend the first night on an intermediate unit with nurses who are familiar with bariatric care. Patients eat nothing by mouth until they pass flatus, usually on the third day; they are begun on half-strength Ensure Plus (30 ml. q.i.d.) with water (30 ml. q.h.) on the fourth day, and full-strength Ensure Plus with water, in the same doses, on the fifth and usually last day. After discharge, the patients are maintained on full fluids for 2 weeks and then cautiously progress to a full diet by the end of 6 weeks. Most patients gradually return to their previous diet in terms of variety, but with a marked reduction in quantity because they fill up quickly and the gastric pouch empties slowly. Most patients do not tolerate carbohydrates well because of the induced dumping. Meats may present difficulties; patients start slowly with fish, then progress to chicken, and finally, after some months, to red meat. By the end of 3 months, most patients eat a small but well-balanced diet.

The most common early complications seen in the clinic are wound abscesses, and as might be expected, these occur most commonly in diabetic patients. The wound infections generally present as red bulges that drain spontaneously or that can be drained through a small 1- to 2-cm. opening of the incision. It is not necessary to open the whole wound or significant lengths of the incision; such interventions may lead to long-term wound care and delays in healing. Late subphrenic abscesses can usually be drained percutaneously with interventional radiologic techniques.

Long-Term Follow-up. Patients generally do remarkably well and are a delight to follow with their new body images, their freedom from diabetes, and their new lives. Daily long-term intake of liquid or chewable total mineral and vitamin products is essential; 600 mg. per day of B_{12} is the recommended minimum dose. Omission of these supplements may lead to severe anemias, Wernicke-Korsakoff syndrome, or other neuropathies. Weight gain exceeding 12% above the lowest postoperative weight is generally the result of staple line breakdown, pouch or anastomotic dilatation, or compulsive snacking. Abdominal pain is most commonly due to cholecystitis, although some patients may develop marginal ulcers, which fortunately clear quickly with H_2 blockers. Recurrent vomiting usually signals overeating but may be due to stenosis of the gastrojejunostomy. Such strictures can almost always be relieved with one or two dilatations of the anastomosis. Finally, these patients require considerable emotional support from their referring physician, the surgical staff, and their own families. Monthly support groups are useful.

Revision of Failed Bariatric Procedures. All bariatric procedures have a failure rate, ranging from 80% or more for horizontal gastroplasties to about 5% to 10% for VBGs and GBs. Most of the failures are due to failed staple lines, stenosis of the gastric outlets, distended gastric pouches, or dilated gastrojejunostomies. Revision of these failures is technically challenging and is associated with a high complication and second failure rate.[8] The most useful approach has been to

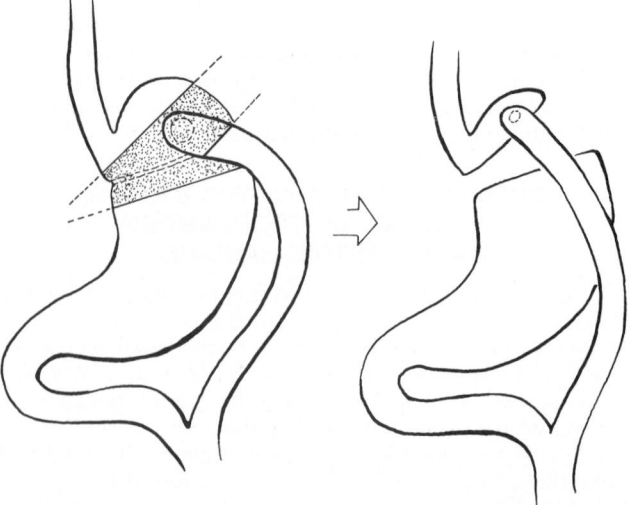

Figure 31–28. Revision of the failed bariatric procedure. Bariatric operations have failure rates of about 15%, usually from expansion of the gastric reservoir, dilatation of the gastric outlet, or disruption of the staple line and, occasionally, from the patient's continuous snacking on high-fat foods. The most effective approach for structural failures, although often complex and technically challenging, is to convert these to a divided gastric bypass.

define the stomach and the alimentary limb, expose the pouch and previous anastomosis, resect the old staple line and the gastroenterostomy, and reanastomose the jejunal limb to the now-divided gastric pouch (Fig. 31–28).

CONCLUSION

Morbid obesity is a serious and increasingly common disease that represents a severe handicap and is associated with major health problems, including diabetes, hypertension, biliary disease, arthritis, and a number of other disorders. Because diets rarely produce sustained weight loss in these patients, operation has become the treatment of choice. Three operations, the gastric bypass, the vertical banded gastroplasty, and Kuzmak's Silastic banding, have produced the best results to date. Scopinaro's biliopancreatic bypass operation has a limited role, perhaps in the rescue of patients who have failed with other procedures. These operations are no longer experimental but are effective procedures that can sharply ameliorate or reverse not only the excessive weight but also the complications. The operations are difficult, and the management of these patients is challenging but rewarding. Long-term follow-up is essential for the proper management of such late complications as nutritional deficiencies and psychologic problems. Failures due to pouch distention, anastomotic dilatation, and staple line breakdown are unusual, but revisions, though technically challenging, can be done with acceptable results.

SELECTED REFERENCES

Bray, G. A.: The inheritance of corpulence. Obes. Res., 2:601, 1994.
For those who would enjoy a historic review of the genetics of obesity.

Brownell, K. D., and Rodin, J.: The dieting maelstrom: Is it possible and advisable to lose weight? Am. Psychol., 49:781, 1994.
A thorough and recent review of the virtues and dangers of dieting.

Buchwald, H., and Campos, C. T.: Remedial operations following surgery for morbid obesity. Obes. Surg., 1:337, 1991.
An excellent review of bariatric surgery, with emphasis on treatment of surgical failures.

Esell, C.: Getting the skinny on obesity. J. NIH Res., 6:71, 1994.
An intriguing and unusually lucid summary of the molecular basis of obesity.

Mayer, J. M., and Stunkard, A. J.: Genetics and human obesity. In Stunkard, A. J., and Waddem, T. A. (Eds.): Obesity: Theory and Therapy, 2nd ed. New York, Raven Press, 1993.
An excellent and comprehensive review.

REFERENCES

1. Adami, G., Gianetta, E., Barreca, A., et al.: Body composition after "very-little-stomach" bilio-pancreatic bypass. Eur. Surg. Res., 19:91, 1987.
2. Benotti, P. N., Bistrian, B., Benotti, J. R., et al.: Heart disease and hypertension in severe obesity: The benefits of weight reduction. Am. J. Clin. Nutr., 55:586S, 1992.
3. Bray, G. A.: Surgical treatment of morbid obesity. Trans. Assoc. Life Insur. Med. Directors, 62:107, 1979.
4. Bray, G. A.: Management options in obesity. Hosp. Pract., April 1982.
5. Brolin, R. E., Kenler, H. A., Gorman, J. H., et al.: Long-limb gastric bypass in the superobese: A prospective randomized study. Ann. Surg., 215:387, 1992.
6. Brolin, R. E., Robertson, L. B., Kenler, H. A., et al.: Weight loss and dietary intake after vertical banded gastroplasty and Roux-en-Y gastric bypass. Ann. Surg., 220:782, 1994.
7. Brownell, K. D., and Rodin, J.: The dieting maelstrom: Is it possible and advisable to lose weight? Am. Psychol., 49:781, 1994.
8. Buchwald, H., and Campos, C. T.: Remedial operations following surgery for morbid obesity. Obes. Surg., 1:337, 1991.
9. Buchwald, H., Varco, R. L., Moore, R. B., et al.: Intestinal bypass procedures. Curr. Prob. Surg., Apr:1, 1975.
10. Bunker, A.: The use of drug therapy in the treatment of obesity: A status report. Parts I and II. The Bariatrician, Fall 1993 and Winter 1994.
11. Catona, A., Gossenberg, M., La Manna, A., et al.: Laparoscopic gastric banding: Preliminary series. Obes. Surg., 3:207, 1993.
12. Cowan, G. S.: The non-surgical treatment of serious obesity. Obes. Surg., 2:216, 1992.
13. Cucchi, B. S., Pories, W. J., and MacDonald, K. G.: Gastro-gastric fistulas, a complication of divided gastric bypass surgery. Ann. Surg., 1995 (in press).
14. Deitel, M., and Ilves, R.: Mechanism of antireflux in vertical banded gastroplasty. Problems Gen. Surg., 9:390, 1992.
15. Deitel, M., Jones, B. A., Petrov, I., et al.: Vertical banded gastroplasty: Results in 233 patients. Can. J. Surg., 29:322, 1986.
16. Deitel, M., Shahi, B., and Deitel, F. H.: Effect of weight loss in the morbidly obese patient with severe disability. Obes. Surg., 1:419, 1991.
17. Dublin, L. I., and Marks, H. H.: Mortality among Insured Overweights in Recent Years. New York, Recording and Statistical Recording Press, 1952.
18. Dubois, A.: Obesity and gastric emptying. Gastroenterology, 84:875, 1983.
19. Elton, C. W., Tapscott, E. B., Pories, W. J., and Dohm, G. L.: Effect of moderate obesity on glucose transport in human muscle. Horm. Metab. Res., 26:181, 1993.
20. Evans, P. E., Israel, R. G., Flickinger, E. G., O'Brien, K. F., and Donnely, J. E.: Hydrostatic weighing without head submersion in morbidly obese females. Am. J. Clin. Nutr., 50:400, 1989.
21. Faust, I. M., Johnson, P. R., and Hirsch, J.: Surgical removal of adipose tissue alters feeding behavior and the development of obesity in rats. Science, 197:393, 1977.
22. Garren, L. W.: Intragastric balloon in the treatment of morbid obesity. Presented at Symposium on Surgical Treatment of Obesity. Los Angeles, 1984.
23. Gastrointestinal surgery for severe obesity: NIH consensus development conference program and abstracts. Bethesda, Md., March 25–27, 1991.
24. Granstrom, L., and Backman, L.: Technical complications and related reoperations after gastric banding. Acta Chir. Scand., 153:215, 1987.
25. Griffen, W. O., Jr., Blivins, F. A., and Bell, R. M.: The decline and fall of the jejunoileal bypass. Surg. Gynecol. Obstet., 157:301, 1983.
26. Grimm, I. S., Schindler, W., and Haluszka, O.: Steatohepatitis and fatal hepatic failure after biliopancreatic diversion. Am. J. Gastroenterol., 88:321, 1993.
27. Hervey, G. R.: The effects of lesions in the hypothalamus in parabiotic rats. J. Physiol., 154:336, 1959.
28. Juczmarski, R. J.: The assessment of body fat distribution in population based surveys. In Workshop on Basic and Clinical Aspects of Regional Fat Distribution. Washington, D.C., National Institutes of Health, 1989, p. 47.
29. Kark, A. E.: Jaw wiring. Am. J. Clin. Nutr., 33:420, 1980.
30. Keys, A., Borzek, J., Henschel, A., et al.: The Biology of Human Starvation. Minneapolis, University of Minnesota Press, 1950.
31. Kopek, E., Gertler, R., Ramsey-Stewart, G., and Beaumont, P. J. V.: Psychosocial outcome and long-term weight loss after gastric restrictive for morbid obesity. Obes. Surg., 4:336, 1994.
32. Kral, J. G.: Surgical treatment of obesity. Med. Clin. North Am., 73:251, 1989.
33. Kral, J. G.: Overview of surgical techniques for treating obesity. Am. J. Clin. Nutr., 55:552S, 1992.
34. Kral, J. G., Strauss, R. J., and Wise, L.: Perioperative risk management in obese patients. In Deitel, M. (Ed.): Surgery for the Morbidly Obese Patient. Philadelphia, Lea & Febiger, 1989.
35. Kremen, A. J., Linner, J. H., and Nelson, C. H.: An experimental evaluation of the nutritional importance of the proximal and distal small intestine. Ann. Surg., 140:439, 1954.
36. Kuczmarski, R. J., Flegal, K. M., and Campbell, S. M.: Increasing prevalence of overweight among adults: The national health and nutrition examination surveys, 1960 to 1991. JAMA, 272:205, 1994.
37. Kushner, R. F.: Body weight and mortality. Nutr. Rev., 51:127, 1993.
38. Kuzmak, L. I.: A review of seven years' experience with silicone gastric banding. Obes. Surg., 1:403, 1991.
39. Langdon, D. E., Leffingell, T., and Rank, D.: Hepatic failure after biliopancreatic diversion. Am. J. Gastroenterol., 87:775, 1992.
40. Lapidus, L., Bengtsson, C., and Björntorp, P.: The quantitative relationship between "the metabolic syndrome" and abdominal obesity in women. Obes. Res., 2:372, 1994.
41. Lapidus, L., Bengtsson, C., Larsson, B., et al.: Distribution of adipose tissue and risk of cardiovascular disease and death: Twelve-year follow-up of participants in the population study of women in Gothenburg, Sweden. Br. Med. J., 289:1257, 1984.
42. Lise, M., Favretti, F., Belluco, C., et al.: Stoma adjustable silicone gastric banding: Results in 111 consecutive patients. Obes. Surg., 4:274, 1994.
43. MacLean, L. D., Rhode, B. M., and Forse, R. A.: A gastroplasty that avoids stapling in continuity. Surgery, 113:380, 1993.
44. MacLean, L. D., Rhode, B. M., Sampalis, J., et al.: Results of the surgical treatment of obesity. Am. J. Surg., 165:155, 1993.
45. Mason, E. E.: Gastric surgery for morbid obesity. Surg. Clin. North Am., 72:501, 1992.
46. Mason, E. E., and Ito, C.: Gastric bypass. Ann. Surg., 170:329, 1969.
47. Molina, M.: Gastric banding, an experience with more than 500 cases. Presented at Symposium on Surgical Treatment of Obesity, Los Angeles, 1984.
48. Naslund, I., Wickbom, G., Christorffersson, E., et al.: A prospective randomized comparison of gastric bypass and gastroplasty. Acta Chir. Scand., 152:681, 1986.
49. National Heart, Lung, and Blood Institute Growth and Health Study Research Group: Obesity and cardiovascular disease risk factors in black and white girls: The NHLBI growth and health study. Am. J. Public Health, 82:1613, 1992.

50. National Institutes of Health: Consensus development statement. Health implications of obesity. Washington, D.C., 1986.
51. National Task Force on Prevention and Treatment of Obesity: Towards prevention of obesity: Research directions. Obes. Res., 2:571, 1994.
52. O'Leary, J. P., Maher, J. W., Hollenbeck, J. I., et al.: Pathogenesis of hepatic failure after obesity bypass. Surg. Forum, 25:356, 1974.
53. Payne, J. H., and De Wind, L. T.: Surgical treatment of obesity. Am. J. Surg., 118:141, 1969.
54. Pories, W. J., Flickinger, E. G., Meelheim, H. D., et al.: The effectiveness of gastric bypass over gastric partition in morbid obesity. Ann. Surg., 196:389, 1982.
55. Ravussin, E., Llloja, S., Knowler, W. C., et al.: Reduced rate of energy expenditure as a risk factor for body weight gain. N. Engl. J. Med., 318:467, 1988.
56. Ryden, O., Olsson, W. A., and Danielsson, B. A.: Weight loss after gastroplasty: Psychologic sequelae in relation to clinical and metabolic observations. J. Am. Coll. Nutr., 8:15, 1989.
57. Schumacher, N., Groth, B., Kleinseck, J., et al.: Successful weight control for employees. J. Am. Diet. Assoc., 74:466, 1979.
58. Scott, H. W., Jr., Dean, R. H., Shull, H. J., et al.: Results of jejunoileal bypass in two hundred patients with morbid obesity. Surg. Gynecol. Obstet., 145:661, 1977.
59. Scruggs, D. M., Cowan, S. M., Jr., and Klesges, L.: Weight loss and caloric intake after regular and extended gastric bypass. Obes. Surg., 3:233, 1993.
60. Sims, E. A. H., and Horton, E. W.: Endocrine and metabolic adaptation to obesity and starvation. Am. J. Clin. Nutr., 21:1455, 1986.
61. Sjöström, L. V.: Mortality of severely obese subjects. Am. J. Clin. Rev., 55:516S, 1992.
62. Stunkard, A. J.: The Salmon lecture: Some perspectives on human obesity: Its causes. Some perspectives on human obesity: Treatment. Bull. N. Y. Acad. Med., 64:902, 1988.
63. Stunkard, A., and McLaren, H.: The results of treatment for obesity. Arch. Intern. Med., 103:79, 1979.
64. Sugerman, H. J., Londrey, G. L., and Kellum, J. M.: Weight loss with vertical banded gastroplasty and Roux-en-Y gastric bypass for morbid obesity with selective versus random assignment. Am. J. Surg., 157:93, 1989.
65. Wilkinson, L. H., and Peloso, O. A.: Gastric (reservoir) reduction for morbid obesity. Arch. Surg., 116:602, 1981.
66. Willbanks, O.: Silicone elastomere ring vertical gastroplasty: Extended follow-up. Obes. Surg., 1:369, 1991.
67. Zhang, Y., Proenca, R., Maffei, M., et al.: Positional cloning of the mouse obese gene and its human homologue. Nature, 372:425, 1994.
68. Zimmerman, V., Campos, C. T., and Buchwald, H.: Weight loss comparison of gastric bypass and Silastic ring vertical gastroplasty. Obes. Surg., 2:47, 1992.

VI

MECKEL'S DIVERTICULUM

Bryan M. Clary, M.D., and H. Kim Lyerly, M.D.

Meckel's diverticulum is the most commonly encountered congenital anomaly of the small intestine. Reported initially in 1598 by Hildanus, this abnormality was described in detail by Johann Meckel in 1809.[10] Autopsy studies have estimated the incidence of Meckel's diverticulum to be 1% to 2%, with men being more commonly affected than women by a ratio of 2:1.[3, 7] Although most commonly presenting as an incidental finding on laparotomy (and now laparoscopy), this entity can be associated with several life-threatening disease states.

EMBRYOLOGY

Meckel's diverticulum is an embryologic derivative of the vitelline duct. During the first few weeks of gestation, the primitive gut forms as the head, tail, and lateral folds incorporate the dorsal part of the yolk sac into the embryo. The midgut loop remains in open connection with the yolk sac by way of the vitelline duct (omphalomesenteric duct) until the 8th to 10th week of gestation, at which time the vitelline duct becomes obliterated (Fig. 31–29). Developmental anomalies related to persistence of the vitelline duct are among the most common abnormalities of digestive tract development (Fig. 31–30). Persistence of the vitelline duct may lead to (1) a fistula between the umbilicus and the ileum when the entire duct remains patent; (2) Meckel's diverticulum due to failure of closure of the intestinal end of the duct; (3) an umbilical sinus when the umbilical side of the duct is not obliterated; (4) a fibrous cord between the umbilicus and the ileum representing an obliterated duct and its vessels; or (5) any combination of these four entities, the most common being Meckel's diverticulum. As many as 25% of Meckel's diverticula are connected to the umbilicus by a fibrous strand. Meckel's diverticulum is a true diverticulum containing all layers of the intestinal wall, usually arising from the antimesenteric border of the ileum 45 to 90 cm proximal to the ileocecal valve (Fig. 31–31). As illustrated in Figure 31–31, the blood supply to a Meckel's diverticulum is provided by persistent vitelline vessels present within a distinct mesentery. It varies in length and diameter, ranging from 1 to 12 cm. As the cells lining the vitelline duct are pluripotent, it is not uncommon to find heterotopic tissue within a Meckel's diverticulum. Gastric mucosa is present in 50% of all Meckel's diverticula, but in more than 75% of symptomatic patients. Pancreatic mucosa is encountered in approximately 5% of diverticula. Less commonly, these diverticula may harbor colonic mucosa. Tumors are an uncommon find-

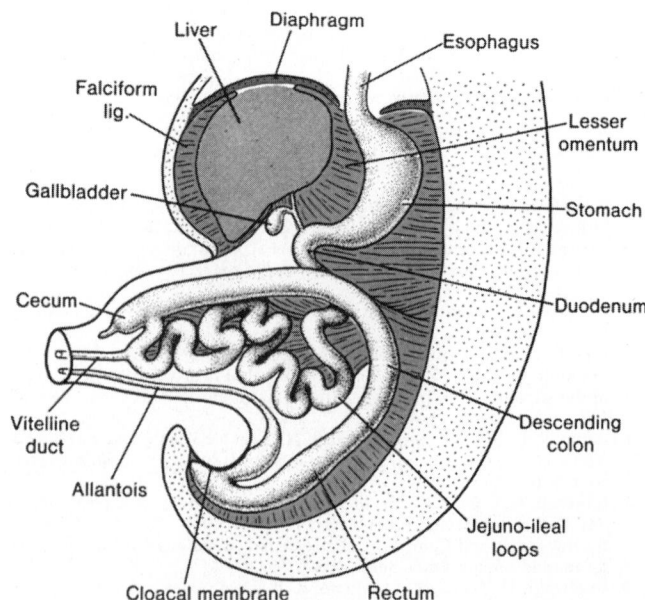

Figure 31–29. Embryo at approximately 8 weeks' gestation demonstrating the open communication of the midgut loop with the yolk sac via the vitelline duct. The midgut proximal to the vitelline duct rapidly elongates to become the coiled loops of small intestine, while distal to the duct, the loop becomes the distal ileum and the right and proximal transverse colon. (From Sadler, T. W.: Langman's Medical Embryology, 5th ed. Baltimore, Williams & Wilkins, 1985.)

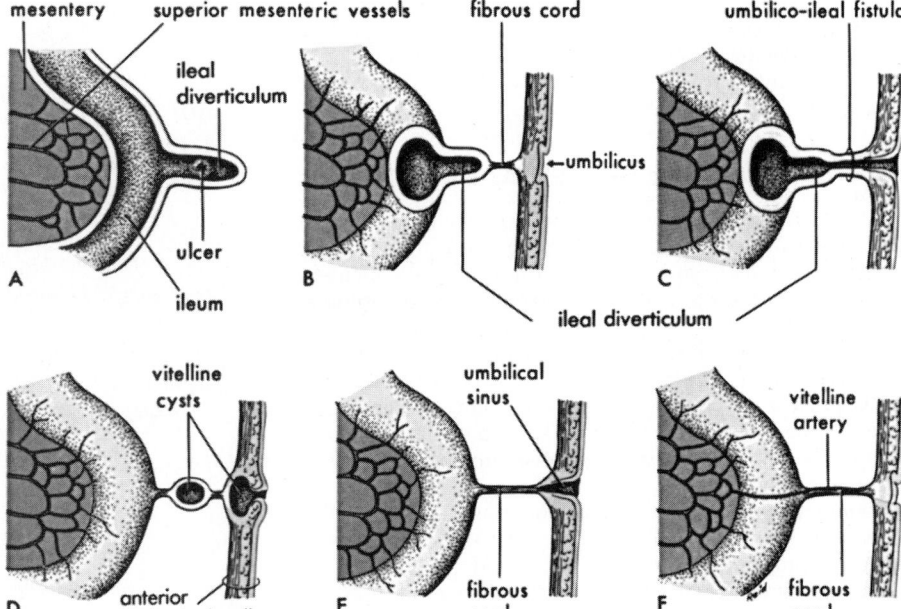

Figure 31–30. Anomalies of the vitelline duct. *A,* Meckel's (ileal) diverticulum secondary to persistence of the proximal aspect of the vitelline duct. *B,* Ileal diverticulum and fibrous cord. *C,* Umbilicoileal fistula secondary to persistence of the entire intra-abdominal portion of the vitelline duct. *D,* Vitelline cysts. *E,* Umbilical sinus resulting from persistence of the vitelline duct near the umbilicus. *F,* Persistence of the vitelline duct as a fibrous cord. (From Moore, K. L., and Persaud, T. V. N.: The Developing Human, 5th ed. Philadelphia, W.B. Saunders, 1993.)

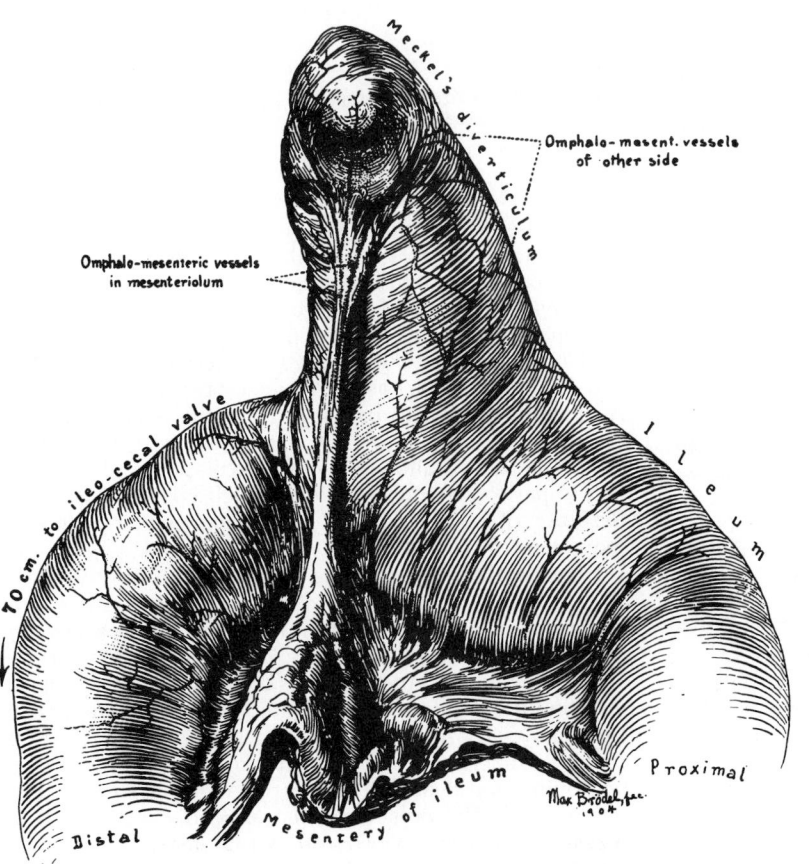

Figure 31–31. Meckel's diverticulum. Typical anatomic example of a Meckel's diverticulum. (From Kelly, H. A., and Hurdon, E.: The Vermiform Appendix and Its Diseases. Philadelphia, W. B. Saunders, 1905.)

ing in a Meckel's diverticulum and include the benign entities lipoma, leiomyoma, neurofibroma, and angioma. Malignant lesions, including leiomyosarcoma, carcinoid, and, less commonly, adenocarcinoma, have also been reported and probably arise from heterotopic gastric mucosa in most cases. Aside from the potential oncologic issues, these tumors serve as lead points for intussusception.

CLINICAL PRESENTATIONS

It is estimated that only 4% of patients who possess a Meckel's diverticulum become symptomatic during their lifetimes.[14] The most common clinical presentation is incidental identification during abdominal exploration. Symptomatic presentations are secondary to hemorrhage, small bowel obstruction, diverticulitis, perforation, associated umbilical abnormalities, and tumors (Table 31–5). More than half of patients presenting with symptoms are younger than 2 years of age. The average mortality rate in patients developing symptoms is 6%, with an excessive proportion of deaths occurring in the elderly.

Hemorrhage. One of the most common clinical problems associated with Meckel's diverticulum is gastrointestinal bleeding presenting as bright red blood per rectum. The usual source of the bleeding is a chronic acid-induced ileal ulcer in the ileum adjacent to a Meckel's diverticulum that contains gastric mucosa. Abdominal pain is rare; pallor and lethargy can be seen. Without treatment, intermittent episodes of bleeding recur. Hemorrhage is the most common symptomatic presentation for children aged 2 years or younger. Diagnosis of a Meckel's diverticulum possessing gastric mucosa can be made using ^{99m}Tc-pertechnetate radioisotope scanning. This isotopic compound is readily taken up by gastric mucosa. (Fig. 31–32). Pharmacologic intervention with pentagastrin or a histamine H_2 receptor blocker can significantly enhance the detection of a Meckel's diverticulum by enhancing uptake and inhibiting intraluminal release, respectively, minimizing false negative results.[6] Angiography, ultrasonography, and intestinal contrast studies have also been reported as means of preoperatively diagnosing a Meckel's diverticulum, but their use is not routine in these patients. False-negative results may be minimized by pentagastrin stimulation before the scan. Because of the high index of suspicion in young children with painless rectal bleeding, the diagnostic accuracy of this test is higher than 90%.

Intestinal Obstruction. Another common symptom associated with a Meckel's diverticulum is intestinal obstruction. The cause of this obstruction may be volvulus of the small bowel around a diverticulum associated with a fibrotic band attached to the abdominal wall, intussusception, or, rarely, incarceration of the diverticulum in an inguinal hernia

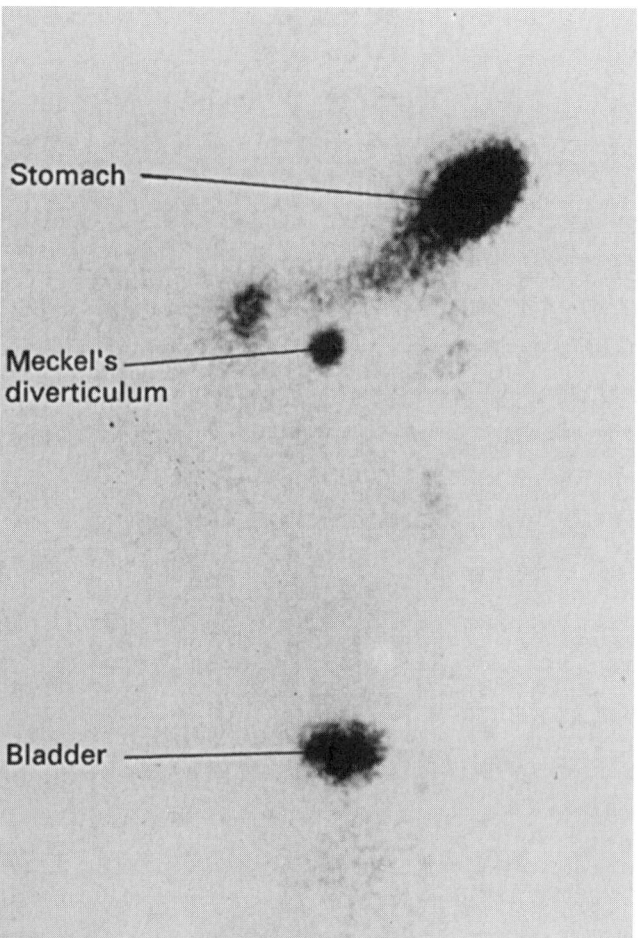

Figure 31–32. Radioisotopic scanning for Meckel's diverticulum shown as visualization of Meckel's diverticulum with ^{99m}Tc-pertechnetate.

(Littre's hernia). Volvulus is usually an acute event, and if allowed to progress, may result in strangulation of the involved bowel. In intussusception, a broad-based diverticulum invaginates and then is carried forward by peristalsis. This may be ileoileal or ileocolic and presents as acute obstruction associated with an urge to defecate, early vomiting, and occasionally, the passage of the classic *currant-jelly* stool. A palpable mass may be present. Barium enema reduction of an intussusception secondary to a Meckel's diverticulum can be performed although with a decreased level of success in comparison to non–Meckel's-associated intussusception. Resection of the diverticulum is indicated even if hydrostatic reduction is successful.

Diverticulitis. Diverticulitis accounts for approximately 10% to 20% of symptomatic presentations. In contrast with hemorrhage and obstruction, this complication is more common in older patients than in children younger than 2 years of age. Diverticulitis of a Meckel's diverticulum often appears indistinguishable from appendicitis, although the peritoneal signs may vary in location. As with appendicitis, failure to promptly diagnose the diverticulitis may lead to perforation, peritonitis, and death. During exploration for suspected appendicitis in instances when the appendix is found to be normal, it is critical to inspect the distal ileum for a Meckel's diverticulum. The indications for resection of the diverticulum in this clinical setting parallel that of appendectomy. Inflamed diverticula and diverticula incidentally found when other causes of the acute abdomen are not evident and that

---

TABLE 31–5. Clinical Presentations in Meckel's Diverticula*

Clinical Presentation	Frequency (%)
Hemorrhage	23
Ileus	31
Intussusception	14
Diverticulitis	14
Perforation	10
Miscellaneous (e.g., fistula and tumor)	8

*Occurrence in 1044 cases of Meckel's diverticula compiled from previously published reports.

Adapted from Schärli, A. F.: Vitello-intestinal disorders. *In* Freeman, N. V., Burge, D. M., Griffiths, D. M., and Malone, P. S. J. (Eds.): Surgery of the Newborn. Edinburgh, Churchill Livingstone, 1994.

do not preclude safe diverticulectomy should undergo resection.

Umbilical Anomalies. Umbilical abnormalities occur in approximately 8% to 10% of patients with a Meckel's diverticulum. These include fistulas, cysts, sinuses, and fibrous bands between the diverticulum and the umbilicus (filum enterale). A fibrous band, if found on laparotomy, should be removed because of the risk of internal herniation and volvulus. It is generally recommended to resect the diverticulum when a fibrous band is found, although in situations where this is not safe, simple resection of the fibrous band is sufficient. The identification of external umbilical abnormalities is usually not a difficult endeavor. The presence of intestinal mucosa at the skin level or persistent drainage from the umbilicus are the most common forms of presentation. To delineate the nature of the enterocutaneous fistula draining at the umbilicus, cannulation and dye injection are useful. Elective surgical exploration of the umbilicus is indicated in the management of these external umbilical abnormalities. Laparotomy may be necessary if fistulas are present, requiring closure of the small intestine.

SURGICAL MANAGEMENT OF ASYMPTOMATIC AND SYMPTOMATIC MECKEL'S DIVERTICULUM

The management of a Meckel's diverticulum found incidentally on laparotomy is controversial. It is clear that diverticulectomy under these circumstances has extremely low rates of morbidity and mortality. There is general agreement that diverticula that appear to have heterotopic mucosa on physical inspection should be resected, given their higher risk of subsequent complication.[2, 8] Age less than 40 years, diverticula longer than 2 cm.[8], and fibrous bands to the umbilicus or mesentery[15] are also risk factors for the development of complications and thus relative indications for resection. Resection of asymptomatic diverticula in children discovered on laparotomy is also generally recommended.

Because of the decreasing likelihood of complications associated with a Meckel's diverticulum with increasing age, the management of incidentally discovered diverticula in adults that are not found to have fibrous bands or believed to possess heterotopic mucosa is the subject of much controversy. In 1976 Soltero and Bill[14] estimated a 4.2% lifetime risk of developing complications from a Meckel's diverticulum using population-based life-table analysis. Using previously published mortality rates following resection of symptomatic (6%[12]) and asymptomatic (0%[13]) Meckel's diverticulum, they estimated that to save the life of one patient with an asymptomatic diverticulum, 800 asymptomatic diverticula would need to be resected. Assuming a morbidity rate of 9% following removal of an incidentally found Meckel's diverticulum (from Von Hedenberg[16]), Sortelo and Bill[14] opposed routine prophylactic diverticulectomy. Critics of this landmark article, which has greatly influenced surgical practice, cite the lower rates of morbidity associated with diverticulectomy and the fact that Sortelo and Bill's study was not truly population based. In an elegant epidemiologic, population-based study of 145 patients who underwent resection of a Meckel's diverticulum (87 incidental) in Olmsted County, Minnesota, Cullen and associates[4] demonstrated a 6.4% lifetime risk of developing a complication from a Meckel's diverticulum (assuming an incidence of 2%). In contrast with Sortelo and Bill[14] and other authors[2, 15] who have shown that complications from a Meckel's diverticulum occur more commonly in patients of younger ages, this study exhibited no trend consistent with age. Cullen and colleagues[4] reported an operative morbidity rate of 2% following resection of incidentally discovered diverticula. The risk of long-term complications

consisting mainly of adhesive small bowel disease was also 2%, compared with 7% of patients undergoing resection of complicated diverticular disease. Given the significant lifetime risk of developing complications from the Meckel's diverticulum and the low rate of short- and long-term postoperative complications following prophylactic removal, the authors of this study concluded that incidentally discovered diverticula should be resected in the absence of peritonitis or other conditions precluding the safe performance of this procedure. In addition, the ability to predict which patients are at risk for complication has been called into question by other studies thus further arguing for prophylactic resection.[1, 9] In summary, although the standard of care in recent decades has been the selective resection of incidentally discovered diverticula based on estimated risks of future complication, recent studies have demonstrated that the performance of prophylactic diverticulectomy under appropriate operative conditions is safe and may be beneficial.

Symptomatic Meckel's diverticula should undergo resection. Resection in this setting is associated with a 5% to 10% mortality rate. Controversy exists over whether diverticulectomy or segmental resection should be performed. In patients with hemorrhage from adjacent ileal ulcers, simple diverticulectomy does not remove the ulcer, and postoperative bleeding may recur. Segmental resection is also advocated in small children with broad-based diverticula for whom the risk of ileal stenosis is greater if diverticulectomy is performed. In other clinical scenarios, segmental resection of the diverticulum with careful attention to divide the associated blood supply is sufficient. This can be performed either by a hand-sewn technique or by stapling across the base of the diverticulum in a diagonal or transverse line so as to minimize the risk of subsequent ileal stenosis. Recent reports have demonstrated the feasibility of laparoscopic techniques in the performance of diverticulectomy.[5, 11] Although long-term results from these newer techniques are unavailable, the increasing frequency with which Meckel's diverticula are diagnosed via laparoscopic examination will lead to further controversy in the management of patients with asymptomatic diverticula.

SELECTED READINGS

Mackey, W., and Dineen, P.: A fifty-year experience with Meckel's diverticulum. Surg. Gynecol. Obstet., 156:56, 1983.
The authors report a 50-year experience with Meckel's diverticulum at the New York-Cornell Medical Center. Four hundred and two patients were involved in the study. Emphasis was placed on the fact that symptoms referable to the diverticulum occurred in 68 patients. Risk factors for complications of Meckel's diverticulum were identified.

Moses, W. R.: Meckel's diverticulum: A report of two unusual cases. N. Engl. J. Med., 237:118, 1947.
The largest collected series of Meckel's diverticulum, with 1605 cases. Also reported was the presence of leiomyosarcoma in 24 of the 1605 cases reviewed.

Soltero, M., and Bill, A.: The natural history of Meckel's diverticulum and its relation to incidental removal. Am. J. Surg., 132:168, 1976.
An excellent report on the natural history of Meckel's diverticulum using lifetime risk tables for a defined regional population. This landmark study helped define the selective resection of incidentally discovered diverticulum as the current standard of care.

Cullen, J. J., Kelly, K. A., Moir C. R., Hodge, D. O., Zinsmeister, A. R., and Melton, J.: Surgical management of Meckel's diverticulum. Ann. Surg., 220:564, 1994.
This recent study is one of the few to include long-term postoperative complications in the analysis of whether prophylactic resection of incidentally discovered diverticula is indicated. The authors concluded that incidentally discovered diverticula should be resected in most patients.

REFERENCES

1. Aubrey, A.: Meckel's diverticulum. Arch. Surg., 100:144, 1970.
2. Bemelman, W., Hugenholtz, E., Heij, H., and Wiersma, P.: Meckel's diver-

ticulum in Amsterdam: Experience in 136 patients. World J. Surg., *19*:734, 1995.
3. Christie, A.: Meckel's diverticulum: A pathological study of 63 cases. Am. J. Dis. Child., *42*:544, 1931.
4. Cullen, J. J., Kelly, K. A., Moir, C. R., Hodge, D. O., Zinsmeister, A. R., and Melton, J.: Surgical management of Meckel's diverticulum. Ann. Surg., *220*:564, 1994.
5. Echenique, M., Dominguez, A., Echenique, I., and Rivera, V.: Laparoscopic diagnosis and treatment of Meckel's diverticulum complicated by gastrointestinal bleeding. J. Lap. Surg., *3*:145, 1993.
6. Heyman, S.: Meckel's diverticulum: Possible detection by combining pentagastrin with histamine H_2 receptor blocker. J. Nucl. Med., *35*:1656, 1994.
7. Jay, G., Margulis, R., McGraw, A., and Northrup, R.: Meckel's diverticulum: A survey of 109 cases. Arch. Surg., *61*:158, 1950.
8. Mackey, W., and Dineen, P.: A fifty-year experience with Meckel's diverticulum. Surg. Gynecol. Obstet., *156*:56, 1983.
9. Matsagas, M., Fatouros, M., Koulouras, B., and Giannoukas, A.: Incidence,

complications, and management of Meckel's diverticulum. Arch. Surg. *130*:143, 1995.
10. Meckel, J.: Ueber die Divertikel am Darmkanal. Arch. die Physiol., *9*:421, 1809.
11. Sanders, L.: Laparoscopic treatment of Meckel's diverticulum. Surg. Endosc., *9*:724, 1995.
12. Schlicke, C., and Johnston, E.: Experiences with Meckel's diverticulum. Surg. Gynecol. Obstet., *126*:91, 1968.
13. Soderlund, S.: Meckel's diverticulum: A clinical and histologic study. Acta Chir. Scand., Suppl., *248*:13, 1959.
14. Soltero, M., and Bill, A.: The natural history of Meckel's diverticulum and its relation to incidental removal. Am. J. Surg., *132*:168, 1976.
15. St-Vil, D., Brandt, M., Panic, S., Bensoussan, A., and Blanchard, H.: Meckel's diverticulum in children: A 20-year review. J. Pediatr. Surg., *26*:1289, 1991.
16. von Hedenberg, C.: Surgical indications in Meckel's diverticulectomy. Acta Chir. Scand., *135*:530, 1969.

VII

CARCINOID TUMORS AND THE CARCINOID SYNDROME

Haile T. Debas, M.D., and Susan L. Orloff, M.D.

Although Merling described the gross pathology of a carcinoid tumor of the appendix in 1838, it was Oberndorfer in 1907 who coined the term *Karzinoide.*[29] In 1930, Kramer described similar tumors that arose from the Kulchitsky cells of the bronchial mucosa.[15] In 1934, Cassidy described malignant carcinoid syndrome.[6] That these tumors secreted humoral substances was suspected for a long time, but it was only after the discovery of serotonin by Rappaport and colleagues[34] in 1948, and the extraction of serotonin from a carcinoid tumor by Erspamer and Asero in 1952,[10] that the endocrine potential of the carcinoid tumor was recognized. Secretion of large quantities of 5-hydroxyindoleacetic acid (5-HIAA), the metabolite of serotonin, in the urine of patients with carcinoid tumors was recognized by Page and associates[31] in 1955. The carcinoid syndrome consisting of watery diarrhea, facial flushing, and right-sided cardiac valvular lesions was described by Pernow and Waldenstrom in 1954.[33]

CARCINOID TUMORS

Incidence

Carcinoid tumors are the most common gut endocrine tumors. They constitute 55% of all the gut endocrine tumors and 13% to 34% of all tumors of the small bowel. The incidence is 1.5 per 100,000 of the general population.[5]

The APUD Concept

In 1968, Pearse reported that certain cells in the gut and elsewhere share common histochemical characteristics. They have high *a*mine content in their cytoplasm, are capable of amine *p*recursor *u*ptake, and are able to *d*ecarboxylate these to produce amines and/or peptides. From this description, he coined the acronym APUD and suggested that all APUD cells derive from the embryonic neural crest.[32] In addition, these cells commonly produce neuron-specific enolase and chromogranins, both of which may be used as tumor markers.

This section describes carcinoid tumors that arise from the different portions of the gut itself: the foregut, the midgut, and the hindgut. Foregut carcinoid tumors arise mainly in

the stomach[45] and other embryologic derivatives of the foregut, of which the pancreas and lungs are important sites. Carcinoids of the midgut arise from the distal duodenum, jejunum, ileum, appendix, and ascending and right transverse colon. Of these, the appendix and terminal ileum are the most frequent sites. Carcinoids of the hindgut develop mostly in the rectum. The differential characteristics of carcinoid tumors from the different portions of the gut are listed in Figure 31–33.

Secretory Products

Carcinoid tumors secrete a wide variety of products, including amines, tachykinins (substance P, neurokinin A, neuropeptide K), and other peptides. The secretory products vary from tumor to tumor. The most common secretory products are listed in Table 31–6.

Pathology

Classically, carcinoid tumors are formed by solid nests of small monotonous cells with exceedingly rare mitoses and an occasional acinar or rosette formation. However, there is variability in histology, and five histologic types can be identified[38]:

Type A: tumors with nodular solid nests and peripheral invading cords
Type B: tumors with a trabecular or ribbon-like structure forming a frequent anastomosing pattern
Type C: tumors with a tubular, acinar, or rosette-like structure
Type D: tumors with structures of lower or atypical differentiations
Mixed type: tumors with mixed structures of any combination of the above four types

The mixed tumors that show an acinar and a glandular pattern have the best median survival time (4.4 years), whereas the undifferentiated pattern is associated with the poorest median survival (0.5 year).[14]

The benign or malignant nature of carcinoid tumors cannot be determined histologically; only the presence of metastases

CARCINOID TUMORS

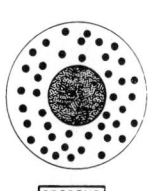 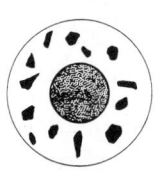 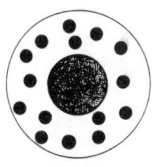

	FOREGUT	MIDGUT	HINDGUT
SITE	Bronchus, Stomach, Pancreas	Jejunoileum, Appendix	Colon, Rectum
HISTOLOGY	Trabecular	Nodular, Solid Nests of Cells	Trabecular Tendency
CELL TYPE			
Argentaffin	6%	65%	0%
Argyrophil	35%	20%	0%
SECRETION			
Tumor 5HT	Low	High	None
Urinary 5HIAA	High	High	Normal
5HTP	Frequent	Rare	None
CARCINOID SYNDROME	Frequent	Frequent	None
OTHER ENDOCRINE SECRETIONS	Frequent	Frequent	None
FUNCTIONAL MANIFESTATIONS	Atypical carcinoid, ZES, Acromegaly, Cushing's, Other	Carcinoid Syndrome	Silent
BONE METASTASES	Common	Unusual	Common

Figure 31–33. Cytologic, histochemical, biochemical, and clinical characteristics of carcinoid tumors arising in structures derived from the foregut, midgut, and hindgut. (Modified from Orloff, M. J.: Carcinoid tumors of the rectum. Cancer, *28*:175, 1971.)

TABLE 31–7. Site of Origin of Carcinoid Tumors and Metastases

Tumor Site	Cases (%)	Metastases (Average %)
Stomach	2.8	23
Duodenum	2.9	20
Jejunoileum	25.5	34
Appendix	36.2	2
Colon	6.0	60
Rectum	16.4	18
Bronchus	9.9	—
Ovary	0.5	6
Miscellaneous	0.2	—
Unknown primary	3.3	—

Data distilled from a study of 3718 cases[47] and 6965 cases.[45]

as young as 10 years and those in their ninth decade, with a peak incidence in the sixth and seventh decades.

Clinical Manifestations

Carcinoid tumors differ in their presentation, depending on their location. The most common carcinoid tumors of the foregut are those that occur in the stomach and bronchus. Gastric carcinoid tumors may be silent. When symptomatic, however, they may cause either upper abdominal pain or bleeding. Bronchial carcinoid tumors present with hemoptysis, with pneumonitis occurring behind the bronchus occluded by the tumor, or with localized wheezing. Midgut carcinoid tumors frequently occur in the appendix and small intestine. The tumors may be silent at both locations and found incidentally at operation for another condition. Appendiceal carcinoid tumors, however, may cause acute obstructive appendicitis. Carcinoid tumors of the small intestine are slow-growing and may be present for years without overt symptoms, and thus escape attention. A third of the patients with carcinoid tumors present with years of intermittent abdominal pain often ascribed to the irritable bowel syndrome. Malignant carcinoid tumors generally induce advanced fibrosis, which, by kinking of the intestine and by fibrous adhesions, may cause mechanical obstruction even when the primary tumor is small. Other symptoms include diarrhea, upper intestinal bleeding, weight loss, intussusception, and a palpable abdominal mass. The most frequent site of hindgut carcinoid tumors is the rectum. These rectal tumors may cause bleeding, and are frequently detected by digital or endoscopic examination. When carcinoid tumors of the hindgut occur in the colon, they may cause abdominal pain, a palpable mass, and rectal bleeding.

Diagnosis

Biochemical

The biochemical steps in the production of 5-hydroxytryptamine (5-HT) and 5-HIAA are as follows:

or invasion of adjacent structures is a true indicator of malignancy. Even when carcinoid tumors are malignant, however, they may be compatible with long survival. The overall 5-year survival rate can be as high as 62% for ileal carcinoid,[45] with the 5-year survival for malignant carcinoids being 20% to 40%.[43] The average time from the onset of symptoms to death from the disease is 8 years.[47]

Site of Origin

Carcinoid tumors may originate from neuroendocrine cells all along the gastrointestinal tract. About 85% of the tumors are located in the intestine, but they can also occur in the lungs or occasionally in the pancreas, biliary tract, or thymus.[12] The most common location of carcinoid tumors in the gastrointestinal tract is the appendix. Appendiceal carcinoids rarely metastasize. Ileal carcinoids have the highest propensity to metastasize. The site of origin and rate of metastases from data on carcinoid tumors distilled from two large clinical series are listed in Table 31–7.[45, 47]

The age distribution for carcinoid tumors includes patients

TABLE 31–6. Secretory Products of Carcinoid Tumors

Amines	Tachykinins	Peptides	Other
5-HT	Kallikrein	Pancreatic polypeptide (40%)	Prostaglandins
5-HIAA (88%)	Substance P (32%)	Chromogranins (100%)	
5-HTP	Neuropeptide K (67%)	Neurotensin (19%)	
Histamine		HCG$_\alpha$ (28%)	
Dopamine		HCG$_\beta$	
		Motilin (14%)	

5-HT, 5-hydroxytryptamine; 5-HIAA, 5-hydroxyindoleacetic acid; 5-HTP, 5-hydroxytryptophan.
Figures in parentheses represent percentage frequency. Data obtained from reference 41.

Tryptophan 5-hydroxylase
1. Tryptophan → 5-hydroxytryptophan (5-HTP)

Dopa-decarboxylase
2. 5-hydroxytryptophan → 5-hydroxytryptamine (5-HT)

Monoamine oxidase
3. 5-hydroxytryptamine → 5-hydroxyindoleacetaldehyde

Aldehyde dehydrogenase
4. 5-hydroxyindoleacetaldehyde → 5-hydroxyindoleacetic acid (5-HIAA)

In patients with typical carcinoid tumors, the rate-limiting step in the synthesis of serotonin is the conversion of tryptophan into 5-HTP by the enzyme tryptophan 5-hydroxylase. Once formed, 5-HTP is rapidly converted to 5-HT in the tumor. Most of the secreted 5-HT is taken up by platelets and stored in their secretory granules. The rest remains free in the plasma and is then largely converted into the urinary metabolite 5-HIAA by the ubiquitous enzyme monoamine oxidase (MAO) and by aldehyde dehydrogenase (AD). These enzymes are abundant in the kidney, and the urine typically contains large amounts of 5-HIAA. The normal range for 5-HIAA secretion is 2 to 8 mg. per 24 hours. Typical tumors are usually both argentaffin- and argyrophil-positive.

In patients with tumors of the foregut (atypical carcinoid tumors), the urine contains relatively little (but above-normal) 5-HIAA but large amounts of 5-HTP and 5-HT. These tumors are thought to be deficient in dopa-decarboxylase and have impaired conversion of 5-HTP into 5-HT, leading to 5-HTP secretion into the vascular compartment. Some 5-HTP is converted into 5-HT and 5-HIAA in extrarenal sites. Some of the 5-HTP is decarboxylated in the kidney and excreted into the urine as 5-HT, but some of the 5-HTP is excreted directly into the urine. Atypical carcinoid tumors are usually argentaffin-negative and argyrophil-positive. Serotonin-rich foods, such as bananas, plantains, pineapples, kiwi fruits, walnuts, hickory nuts, pecans, and avocados, and the analgesic acetaminophen may artificially increase 5-HIAA. False-negative results may be obtained in patients taking salicylates or L-dopa. Approximately half of patients with carcinoid tumors of gastrointestinal origin have evidence of serotonin production (manifested by elevated urinary 5-HIAA) whether or not an associated carcinoid syndrome is present.[11] Therefore, urinary 5-HIAA should be determined in patients with carcinoid tumors even in the absence of carcinoid syndrome. In patients with carcinoid tumors, neurotensin is elevated in 43%, substance P in 32%, motilin in 14%, somatostatin in 5%, and vasoactive intestinal polypeptide (VIP) rarely.[45]

Localization

Numerous techniques can identify the primary site of the tumor and evaluate the extent of the disease and the presence of metastases. A chest film or computed tomography (CT) is sufficient to detect a bronchial carcinoid tumor. Carcinoid tumors of the colon and rectum are usually demonstrable by barium enema examination or by colonoscopy. Routine barium studies often fail to demonstrate carcinoid tumors of the small intestine. Enteroclysis is more likely to give positive results. Ultrasonography, abdominal CT, and even magnetic resonance imaging (MRI) are usually not helpful because the tumors are too small for detection. Advanced intestinal carcinoid tumors may be visualized on barium examination when mesenteric fibrosis produces foreshortening, rigidity, fixation, and kinking of the bowel loops.[25, 40] CT is valuable for demonstrating the mesenteric fibrosis and can evaluate tumor extension in the mesentery, the retroperitoneal space, and the liver.[24] Superior mesenteric angiography in advanced

tumors may show segmental caliber changes or occlusions of branches of the superior mesenteric artery, which, together with the mesenteric veins, may be trapped by tumor or fibrosis. Angiography is the superior method for demonstrating hepatic metastases from carcinoid tumors. The most promising localizing techniques take advantage of the presence of somatostatin receptors in most carcinoid tumors. *In vivo* receptor scintigraphy can be performed using either [123]I- or [111]indium-labeled octreotide, the eight–amino acid analog of somatostatin. Kwekkeboom and colleagues[19] used both labels in 52 patients with or suspected of having carcinoid tumors. The tumor was visualized in 32 of 37 (86%) patients with known carcinoid lesions. However, the test identified hepatic metastases in only half of patients with known liver metastases. Sites previously not recognized with other imaging techniques were found in 20 of 37 patients.

The presence of a carcinoid tumor should be established by biopsy whenever this is clinically feasible. Positive argentaffin and argyrophil stains suggest the carcinoid nature of the tumor. However, electron microscopic demonstration of neurosecretory granules is probably the most specific test available. Endoscopy and biopsy are valuable for diagnosing primary gastric and rectal carcinoid tumors.[42]

Patients with ileal carcinoid tumors tend to develop a second neoplasm elsewhere, especially in the colon. The incidence of a second tumor was 36% in one series and 40% in another.[42] Thus, a search for synchronous, metachronous, and metastatic neoplasms should be undertaken.

Treatment

Early resection, while the tumor is small, offers the patient the best chance for cure. Carcinoid tumors should be treated by resection regardless of the presence of metastases, because growth of the primary neoplasm is slow and local complications, such as obstruction and intussusception, are frequent. The incidence of metastases depends on the size and location of the primary tumor.[3] Appendiceal carcinoid tumors are rarely malignant, and lesions smaller than 1.5 cm. can be safely treated by routine appendectomy. If the tumor is at the base of the appendix, a cecectomy may be necessary. For the rare appendiceal tumor larger than 1.5 cm., ileocolectomy is recommended. This procedure is also justified when local invasion or lymph node metastases are present. Gastroduodenal carcinoid tumors smaller than 1 cm. can be excised endoscopically.[3] For larger, invasive tumors, appropriate wide resection, which may include subtotal gastrectomy and omentectomy, is recommended.[46] Rectal carcinoid tumors smaller than 1 cm. can be treated by endoscopic excision. Tumors measuring 1 to 2 cm. should be excised operatively with margins, and those larger than 2 cm. may require anterior resection. When local excision has been performed, the depth of invasion should be investigated histologically. If there is invasion of the muscularis propria, wider excision or anterior resection is necessary.[42] Resection of carcinoid tumors of the midgut,[6] originating from the ileum and jejunum, sometimes presents a technical problem because of the fibrosis and foreshortening of the mesentery. Appreciation of this difficulty obviates more extensive resection than is necessary, and thus avoids creation of short gut syndrome. At clinical discovery, a large percentage (up to 70%) of the small intestinal tumors are metastatic to lymph nodes and/or liver.[40] Tumors with distant metastases should be managed by wide *en bloc* resection regardless of the size of the primary tumor. This may include ileocolectomy for lesions located in the distal ileum.[40]

Outcome

The published rates of survival vary. In general, the larger the primary tumor (>2 cm.), the worse the prognosis. Patients with noninvasive appendiceal and rectal tumors smaller than 2 cm. have 5-year survival approaching 100%.[35, 42] Survival declines to 40% when the tumor diameter is larger than 2 cm. Invasion of the muscle wall or the presence of lymph node metastases is a poor prognostic sign. In the presence of liver metastases, the 5-year survival has ranged from 21 to 42%.[22, 25, 40]

CARCINOID SYNDROME

Causes

Carcinoid syndrome occurs in less than 10% of patients with carcinoid tumors. The carcinoid syndrome is encountered when venous drainage from the tumor gains access to the systemic circulation so that vasoactive secretory substances escape hepatic degradation. This situation obtains in three circumstances: when hepatic metastases are present, when venous blood from extensive retroperitoneal metastases drains into paravertebral veins, and when the primary carcinoid tumor is outside the gastrointestinal tract, e.g., a bronchial, ovarian, or testicular tumor.

Clinical Manifestations

The principal features of carcinoid syndrome include flushing, sweating, wheezing, diarrhea, abdominal pain, cardiac valvular fibrosis, and pellagra dermatosis. Diarrhea is found in 83% of patients, flushing in 49%, dyspnea in 20%, and bronchospasm in 6%.[44] Two types of carcinoid flush are described.[45] With midgut carcinoid tumors, the flush is usually transient, is faint pink to red, and involves the face and the upper trunk. It may be provoked by alcohol, blue cheese, chocolate, and red wines. In contrast, the flush in foregut tumors is often more intense, is more protracted, is purplish in hue, involves the upper trunk and limbs, and leads to telangiectasias.

Many patients develop right-sided cardiac valvular disease with congestive heart failure. Serotonin and possibly other neurohumors produced by the tumor cause fibrosis, as well as eventual incompetence of the tricuspid and pulmonic valves. The lungs metabolize serotonin and the other mediators and protect the left heart from fibrosis. If one can establish that the tumor is slow growing, patients with carcinoid-induced cardiac lesions are candidates for valve replacement.

Biochemical Mediators

The specific etiologic agents for each of the protean manifestations of carcinoid tumors are not known. Serotonin, prostaglandins, 5-hydroxytryptophan, substance P, kallikrein, histamine, dopamine, and neuropeptide K are thought to be involved in the clinical manifestations of carcinoid tumors (see Table 31–6). Pancreatic polypeptide and motilin levels are often raised[44] and may serve as markers of tumor activity and provide a means of monitoring tumor growth and response to therapy.

Serotonin is thought to be largely responsible for both the diarrhea and the fibrosis. The cardiac lesions and tricuspid and pulmonic insufficiency are components of this fibrosing phenomenon. The vasomotor changes, however, are mediated by kinins and such vasoactive peptides as substance P, neuropeptide K, neurokinin A, and neurotensin. Other substances, such as histamine, VIP, and prostaglandins, may also contribute to the systemic manifestations in the carcinoid syndrome.

Diagnosis

Urinary 5-HIAA or whole blood and platelet-poor plasma 5-HT is the most reliable test to confirm the diagnosis of carcinoid syndrome. Occasionally, measurement of plasma levels of substance P and neurotensin by radioimmunoassay may also be helpful. Measurements of neuron-specific enolase and chromogranins, when available, provide nonspecific evidence of the presence of a neuroendocrine tumor.

A useful diagnostic aid is the pentagastrin provocative test, which induces facial flushing, gastrointestinal symptoms, elevation in circulating 5-HT, and release of the peptides substance P, neurokinin A, and neuropeptide K.[1, 27, 39]

Treatment

Surgical

Surgical cure of patients with the carcinoid syndrome is almost impossible in the presence of intra-abdominal and hepatic metastases. In rare instances in which the syndrome is secondary to bulky carcinoid tumors originating in teratomas or in the lung, all neoplastic tissue can be excised, with cure of both the malignant neoplasm and the clinical syndrome.[3] Surgical attempts at palliation should be considered, because the slow progression of this neoplasm often allows the patient many months or years of comfortable life if immediately life-threatening complications can be controlled.[13] Thus, metastatic tumors in the abdomen should be treated with *en bloc* resection, regardless of the size of the primary lesion.[40] Hepatic metastases can be treated by lobectomy, local resection, or enucleation.[2, 8] Debulking procedures have significantly relieved flushing and diarrhea with decreased levels of urinary 5-HIAA.[2] Another palliative approach involves ischemic treatment of the liver, which can be achieved by temporary surgical dearterialization of the liver[26] or by hepatic arterial embolization.[2, 26] A more recent and effective treatment of liver metastases and carcinoid syndrome involves embolization of the hepatic artery with chemotherapy (doxorubicin, 5-fluorouracil, cisplatin).[8, 36] In a prospective trial, Ruszniewski and associates[36] found that hepatic arterial chemoembolization with doxorubicin led to control of symptoms and regression or stabilization of liver metastases in 80% of 24 patients.

Liver Transplantation

Orthotopic liver transplantation has been used to treat patients with unresectable hepatic metastases from carcinoid tumors.[20, 37] Two patients with malignant carcinoid syndrome who received orthotopic liver transplants were free of associated symptoms and tumor at 26 and 34 months after operation.[37] Because of the very slow growth of carcinoid tumors, liver transplantation may be a potential therapeutic approach for some highly selected patients with unresectable hepatic metastases from carcinoid tumors. The effects of immunosuppressive therapy on the natural history of carcinoid tumor remain unknown.

Pharmacologic

Four types of pharmacologic agents are available for symptomatic control: serotonin antagonists (cryproheptadine, methotrimeprazine, and methysergide maleate), interferon, chemotherapeutic agents, and somatostatin and its analogs. The response to serotonin antagonists has largely been poor. Interferon, which acts by stimulating macrophages and T lymphocytes, has shown promising results in the control of flushing, diarrhea and 5-HIAA excretion, and stabilization of disease.[9] Interferon may directly inhibit hormone synthesis and tumor cell proliferation. No combination chemotherapy trial has generated any significant beneficial effect in patients with malignant carcinoid tumors and the carcinoid syndrome.[28] The response ranges from 9% to 30% with no prolongation of survival. The chemotherapeutic agents with the best response rates include streptozotocin and 5-fluorouracil with or without cisplatin or VP-16.

Somatostatin-14 and its long-acting analog octreotide successfully control symptoms of diarrhea and flushing.[7, 17, 23, 45] The single largest series is from the Mayo Clinic, where 66 patients with hepatic metastases and carcinoid syndrome were treated with octreotide. Flushing was abolished or significantly reduced in 87%, and diarrhea in over 75%. A fall of 50% or more in urinary 5-HIAA was observed. More important, the median survival of patients was increased by 3 years.[16] No major clinical side effects have been observed. Somatostatin analog therapy may also have direct antitumor activity.[4] The responsiveness of carcinoid tumors to somatostatin analog therapy may be predicted by the demonstration of somatostatin receptors in biopsies from tumors.[18] Octreotide can also rapidly reverse life-threatening hypotension during induction of anesthesia[21] and can successfully treat and prevent life-threatening carcinoid crisis.

SELECTED REFERENCES

Marshall, J. B., and Bodnarchuk, G.: Carcinoid tumors of the gut. J. Clin. Gastroenterol., 16:123, 1993.
A succinct and well-organized presentation of 55 cases of gastrointestinal carcinoid tumors as well as a review of the literature of carcinoid tumors and the carcinoid syndrome. A review of agents used to control symptoms of carcinoid syndrome and nonsurgical modalities to treat metastatic carcinoid tumors is presented.

Pearse, A. G. E., and Takor, T. T.: Neuroendocrine embryology and the APUD concept. Clin. Endocrinol., 5(suppl.):229s, 1976.
This classic paper formulates the amine precursor uptake and decarboxylation (APUD) concept and discusses the fate of cells originating from the embryonic neural crest. It provides a unified view of the diffuse neuroendocrine system, of which the gastrointestinal cells that give rise to carcinoid tumors are a part.

Thompson, G. B., van Heerden, J. A., Martin, J. K., Jr., Schutt, A. J., Ilstrup, D. M., and Carney, J. A.: Carcinoid tumors of the gastrointestinal tract: Presentation, management, and prognosis. Surgery, 98:1054, 1985.
An excellent discussion of the clinical presentation, pathology, and operative management of 154 surgically treated carcinoid tumors at the Mayo Clinic.

REFERENCES

1. Ahlman, H., Dahlstrom, A., Gronstad, K., Tisell, L. E., Oberg, K., Zinner, M. J., and Jaffe, B. M.: The pentagastrin test in the diagnosis of the carcinoid syndrome: Blockade of gastrointestinal symptoms by Ketanserin. Ann. Surg., 201:81, 1985.
2. Ahlman, H., Schersten, T., and Tisell, L. E.: Surgical treatment of patients with the carcinoid syndrome. Acta Oncol., 28:403, 1989.
3. Akerstrom, G.: Surgical treatment of carcinoids and endocrine pancreatic tumours. Acta Oncol., 28:409, 1989.
4. Anthony, L., Johnson, D., Hande, K., Shaff, M., Winn, S., Krozely, M., and Oates, J.: Somatostatin analogue phase I trials in neuroendocrine neoplasms. Acta Oncol., 32:217, 1993.
5. Buchanan, K. D., Johnston, C. F., O'Hare, M. M. T., et al.: Neuroendocrine tumors: A European view. Am. J. Med., 81(suppl. 66):14, 1986.
6. Cassidy, M. A.: Abdominal carcinomatosis associated with vasomotor disturbances. Proc. R. Soc. Med., 27:220, 1934.
7. Debas, H. T., and Gittis, G.: Somatostatin analogue therapy in functioning neuroendocrine gut tumors. Digestion, 54(suppl. 1):68, 1993.
8. Debas, H. T., and Mulvihill, S. J.: Neuroendocrine gut neoplasms: Important lessons from uncommon tumors. Arch. Surg., 129:965, 1994.
9. Di Bartolomeo, M., Bajetta, E., Zilembo, N., de Braud, F., Di Leo, A., Verusio, C., D'Aprile, M., Scanni, A., Iirillo, A., Barduagni, A., and Epifani, C.: Treatment of carcinoid syndrome with recombinant interferon alpha-2a. Acta Oncol., 32:235, 1993.
10. Erspamer, V., and Asero, B.: Identification of enteramine, the specific hormone of the enterochromaffin cell system, as 5-hydroxytryptamine. Nature, 169:800, 1952.
11. Feldman, J. M., and Jones, R. S.: Carcinoid syndrome from gastrointestinal carcinoids without liver metastasis. Ann. Surg., 196:33, 1982.
12. Godwin, J. D., II: Carcinoid tumors: An analysis of 2837 cases. Cancer, 36:560, 1975.
13. Gronbech, J. E., Soreide, O., and Bergan, A.: The role of resective surgery
14. Johnson, L. A., Lavin, P., Moertel, C. G., et al.: Carcinoids: The association of histologic growth pattern and survival. Cancer, 51:882, 1983.
15. Kramer, R.: Adenoma of bronchus. Ann. Otol. Rhinol. Laryngol., 39:689, 1930.
16. Kvols, L. K., et al.: Treatment of malignant carcinoid syndrome with long acting somatostatin analogue. Metabolism, 39:suppl. 2, 1990.
17. Kvols, L. K., and Reubi, J. C.: Metastatic carcinoid tumors and the malignant carcinoid syndrome. Acta Oncol., 32:197, 1993.
18. Kvols, L. K., Reubi, J. C., Horisberger, U., Moertel, C. G., Rubin, J., and Charboneau, J. W.: The presence of somatostatin receptors in malignant neuroendocrine tumor tissue predicts responsiveness to octreotide. Yale J. Biol. Med., 65:505, 1992.
19. Kwekkeboom, D. J., Krenning, E. P., Bakker, W. H., Oei, H. Y., Kooij, P. P. M., and Lamberts, S. W. J.: Somatostatin analogue scintigraphy in carcinoid tumors. Eur. J. Nucl. Med., 20:283, 1993.
20. Makowka, L., Tzakis, A. G., Mazzaferro, V., Teperman, L., Demetris, A. J., Iwatsuki, S., and Starzl, T.: Transplantation of the liver for metastatic endocrine tumors of the intestine and pancreas. Surg. Gynecol. Obstet., 168:107, 1989.
21. Marsh, H. M., Martin, J. K., Jr., Kvols, L. K., et al.: Carcinoid crisis during anesthesia: Successful treatment with a somatostatin analogue. Anesthesiology, 66:89, 1987.
22. Marshall, J. B., and Bodnarchuk, G.: Cardinoid tumors of the gut. J. Clin. Gastroenterol., 16:123, 1993.
23. Maton, P. N.: Use of octreotide acetate for control of symptoms in patients with islet cell tumors. World J. Surg., 17:504, 1993.
24. McCarthy, S. M., et al.: Computed tomography of malignant carcinoid disease. J. Comput. Assist. Tomogr., 8:846, 1984.
25. Moertel, C. G., Sauer, W. G., Dockerty, M. B., and Baggenstoss, A. H.: Life history of the carcinoid tumor of the small intestine. Cancer, 14:901, 1961.
26. Nobin, A., Mansson, B., and Lunderquist, A.: Evaluation of temporary liver dearterialization and embolization in patients with metastatic carcinoid tumour. Acta Oncol., 28:419, 1989.
27. Norheim, I., Theodorsson-Norheim, E., Brodein, E., and Oberg, K.: Tachykinins in carcinoid tumors: Their use as a tumor marker and possible role in the carcinoid flush. J. Clin. Endocrinol. Metab., 63:605, 1988.
28. Oberg, K.: The use of chemotherapy in the management of neuroendocrine tumors. Endocrinol. Metab. Clin. North Am., 22:941, 1993.
29. Oberndorfer, S.: Karzinoide Tumoren des Dunndarms. Z. Pathol., 1:426, 1907.
30. Orloff, M. J.: Carcinoid tumors of the rectum. Cancer, 28:175, 1971.
31. Page, I. H., Corcoran, A. C., Udenfriend, S., Sjoerdsma, A., and Weissbach, H.: Argentaffinoma as an endocrine tumor. Lancet, 1:198, 1955.
32. Pearse, A. G. E., and Takor, T. T.: Neuroendocrine embryology and the APUD concept. Clin. Endocrinol., 5(suppl.):229s, 1976.
33. Pernow, B., and Waldenstrom, J.: Paroxysmal flushing and other symptoms caused by 5-hydroxytryptamine and histamine in patients with malignant tumors. Lancet, 2:951, 1954.
34. Rapport, M. M., Green, A. A., and Page, I. H.: Partial purification of the vasoconstrictor in beef serum. J. Biol. Chem., 174:735, 1948.
35. Roggo, A., Wood, W. C., and Ottinger, L. W.: Carcinoid tumors of the appendix. Ann. Surg., 217:385, 1993.
36. Ruszniewski, P., Rougier, P., Roche, A., Legmann, P., Sibert, A., Hochlaf, S., Ychou, M., and Mignon, M.: Hepatic arterial chemoembolization in patients with liver metastases of endocrine tumors. Cancer, 71:2624, 1993.
37. Schweizer, R. T., Alsina, A. E., Rosson, R., and Bartus, S. A.: Liver transplantation for metastatic neuroendocrine tumors. Transpl. Proc., 25:1973, 1993.
38. Soga, J., and Tazawa, K.: Pathologic analysis of carcinoids: Histologic reevaluation of 62 cases. Cancer, 28:990, 1971.
39. Strodel, W. E., Vinik, A. I., Jaffe, B. M., Eckhauzir, F., and Thompson, N. W.: Substance P in the localization of a carcinoid tumor. J. Surg. Oncol., 27:106, 1984.
40. Strodel, W. E., Vinik, A. I., Thompson, N. W., Eckhauser, F. E., and Talpas, G. B.: Small bowel carcinoid tumors and the carcinoid syndrome. *In* Thompson, N. W., and Vinik, A. I. (Eds.): Endocrine Surgery Update. New York, Grune & Stratton, 1983, p. 277.
41. Theodorsson, E.: Regulatory peptides as tumour markers. Acta Oncol., 28:319, 1989.
42. Thompson, G. B., van Heerden, J. A., Martin, J. K., Jr., Schutt, A. J., Ilstrup, D. M., and Carney, J. A.: Carcinoid tumors of the gastrointestinal tract: Presentation, management, and prognosis. Surgery, 98:1054, 1985.
43. Tilson, M. D.: Carcinoid syndrome. Surg. Clin. North Am., 54:409, 1974.
44. Vinik, A. I., Strodel, W. E., Lloyd, R. V., and Thompson, N. W.: Unusual gastroenteropancreatic (GEP) tumors and their hormones. *In* Thompson, N. W., and Vinik, A. I. (Eds.): Endocrine Surgery Update. New York, Grune & Stratton, 1983, p. 293.
45. Vinik, A. I., Thompson, N., Eckhauser, F., and Moattari, A. R.: Clinical features of carcinoid syndrome and the use of somatostatin analogue in its management. Acta Oncol., 28:389, 1989.
46. Welch, J. P., and Malt, R. A.: Management of carcinoid tumors of the gastrointestinal tract. Surg. Gynecol. Obstet., 145:223, 1977.
47. Wilson, H., Cheek, R. C., Sherman, R. T., and Storer, E. H.: Carcinoid tumors. Curr. Probl. Surg., Nov:34, 1970.

in the treatment of the carcinoid syndrome. Scand. J. Gastroenterol., 27:433, 1992.

VIII

MALABSORPTION SYNDROMES

John P. Grant, M.D.

Knowledge of malabsorption began in antiquity, being mentioned in the Ebers Papyrus. The term *steatorrhea* apparently was first used in 1824 by Kunzmann. Modern understanding of malabsorption follows advances in knowledge of the physicochemical and biochemical processes involved in absorption and transport, the advent of electron microscopy, the use of radioisotopes, and peroral intestinal biopsy procedures.

DEFINITION OF MALABSORPTION

Malabsorption can be defined as impaired absorption of fat, carbohydrate, protein, vitamins, electrolytes, minerals, or water. Clinical manifestations include unexplained weight loss, steatorrhea and diarrhea, anemia, tetany, bone pain and pathologic fractures, bleeding, dermatitis, neuropathy, glossitis, and edema.

TESTS FOR MALABSORPTION

Screening Tests

Screening tests detect only the more clinically significant degrees of malabsorption.

Gross Inspection of Stool. With steatorrhea, the stool is bulky, sticky, foul smelling, and tends to float.

Microscopic Examination of Stool. Increased fat by Sudan II staining suggests impaired fat absorption. Increased numbers of striated muscle fibers suggest impaired protein digestion.

Fat Content of Random Stool Sample. With steatorrhea, the fat content of a random 24-hour stool sample may be 25 gm. or more.

Protein Content of Random Stool Sample. More than 3 gm. of protein per day in a random 24-hour stool sample is abnormal.

Serum Carotene Concentration. Carotene is poorly absorbed in the presence of steatorrhea. If dietary intake is adequate, low serum carotene concentrations strongly suggest fat malabsorption.

D-xylose Absorption. D-xylose is not metabolized, being excreted unaltered in the urine. This property makes it useful as a test for carbohydrate absorption. Normally, 5 gm. or more of D-xylose are excreted in the urine within the first 5 hours after oral ingestion of 25 gm. Improved sensitivity has been reported when only 5 gm. of D-xylose is given orally and blood xylose concentrations at 1 hour are corrected to a constant body surface area.[23]

Radiologic Examination. Radiologic examination is useful in evaluating intestinal transit time and motility. In addition, careful studies can identify abnormalities such as fistulas, strictures, mucosal diseases such as Crohn's disease, diverticula, and cancer.[26]

Intake-Output Balance Tests

Balance tests are more sensitive than screening tests and can identify milder degrees of malabsorption.

Fat Balance. A quantitative measurement of fat in a timed 3- to 5-day stool collection can be compared with measured fat intake (usually 100 gm. of fat per day). With malabsorption, more than 6 gm. of fat per 24 hours (or more than 5% of the measured ingested fat) passes unabsorbed in the stool.

Radioactive Tracer Tests. A ^{14}C-triolein breath test can evaluate intestinal absorption of neutral fats.[8] ^{13}C-trioctanion, a stable nonradioactive isotope, has also been used to quantitate fat malabsorption through measurement of 2-hour $^{13}CO_2$ respiratory excretion in a breath test.[59] These tests depend not only on normal absorption but also on normal fat metabolism. Measurement of the stool content of intravenously administered ^{131}I-albumin, ^{51}Cr-albumin, and ^{67}Cu-ceruloplasmin can identify patients with protein-losing enteropathies.

Tests for Malabsorption of Specific Nutrients

Lactose Tolerance Test. Abnormal absorption of lactose occurs with deficiency of the brush-border enzyme lactase as well as in many disorders of the small intestine. Of the various tests, the most common is the hydrogen breath test. Improved accuracy can be obtained by prolonging the test to 4 hours with simultaneous measurement of the orocecal transit time.[7]

Schilling Test. Abnormal absorption of vitamin B_{12} occurs in the absence of intrinsic factor and in dysfunction of the terminal ileum.

Other Radioactive Compounds. Radioisotopic methodologies are available to identify iron, calcium, various amino acids, folic acid, pyridoxine, and vitamin D malabsorption, as well as nearly any other compound that can be labeled with a radioisotope. Bile salt malabsorption can be estimated accurately by administration of ^{75}SeHCAT, a taurine conjugate of selenahomocholic acid.[46]

Small Intestinal Biopsy

Peroral small intestinal biopsy has been helpful in diagnosing various mucosal diseases, such as celiac disease, tropical sprue, and Whipple's disease.

CONDITIONS ASSOCIATED WITH MALABSORPTION

A useful classification system for malabsorption syndromes is that of Johnson (Table 31–8).[28] A significant number of malabsorption syndromes occur in the surgeon's domain; some are cured by operation, and others are the sequelae of removing or rearranging parts of the gastrointestinal tract.

Following Esophagectomy and Esophagogastrectomy

In two independent studies of absorption following esophagogastrectomy in 30 patients, only a moderate degree of fat malabsorption was identified.[45, 51] The amount of nitrogen excreted in the stool was only slightly abnormal. D-xylose and vitamin B_{12} absorption and small intestinal biopsies were normal. The malabsorption of fat following esophagectomy and esophagogastrectomy was most likely related to the vagotomy that was performed.

Following Total Gastrectomy

Total gastrectomy commonly causes nutritional abnormalities due to anorexia, loss of gastric storage capacity, inade-

TABLE 31–8. Classification of Malabsorption Syndromes

Intraluminal Factors

Decrease in effective length
  Resection of stomach or small bowel
  Intestinal fistulization
  Hypermotility (hyperthyroidism)
Decreased digestive activity
  Pancreatic juice
    Pancreatitis
    Carcinoma of pancreas
    Pancreatectomy
    Cystic fibrosis
    Pancreatic duct lithiasis with obstruction
    Pancreaticocutaneous fistula
  Bile
    Hepatitis
    Cirrhosis
    T-tube drainage
    Biliary obstruction
    Inadequate resorption of bile salts
    Congenital absence of bile salts
Changes in microorganism population
  Blind loop
  Small intestinal diverticula
  Intestinal stasis
    Visceral neuropathy (diabetes mellitus)
    Primary neurologic diseases
    Scleroderma
    Partial obstruction
  Oral antibiotics (neomycin)
  Giardiasis (also hookworm, whipworm)
  Acute infectious diarrhea
  Gastric achlorhydria

Changes in Intestinal Wall

Mucosal epithelial cell
  Celiac disease of childhood
  Gluten-induced enteropathy

Tropical sprue
  Disaccharidase deficiency
  Radiation enteritis
  Drug-induced (neomycin, etc.)
  Triglyceride enzyme deficiency
Ground substance
  Lymphoma, leukemia
  Whipple's disease
  Regional enteritis
  Systemic mast cell disease
  Amyloidosis
  Tuberculosis
  Carcinoma, sarcoma

Abnormalities in Blood or Lymphatic Channels

Blood
  Arterial or venous insufficiency
  Congestive heart failure
  Vasculitis
Lymphatics
  Intestinal lymphangiectasis
  Lymphatic obstruction

Indeterminate

Zollinger-Ellison syndrome
Malignant carcinoid
Abetalipoproteinemia
Protein-losing enteropathy
Pernicious anemia
Hyperthyroidism
Hypoparathyroidism
Pneumatosis cystoides intestinalis
Hemochromatosis
Kwashiorkor
Hypogammaglobulinemia
Adrenal-pituitary insufficiency
Tabes mesenterica

From Johnson, C. F.: Malabsorption syndromes: Clinical and theoretical consideration. Postgrad. Med. J., *37*:667, 1965.

quate mixing of food with digestive enzymes, and loss of intrinsic factor. Anorexia has been attributed to pain associated with reflux alkaline esophagitis and distention and dysmotility of the proximal segment of small intestine. Reflux esophagitis occurs with variable severity following different reconstructive procedures (Fig. 31–34). Scott and Weidner[50] suggested that a 16- to 18-inch Roux-en-Y esophagojejunostomy would eliminate reflux biliary esophagitis. This is the most common reconstruction used today. Longmire and Beal[3, 38] found that interposition of an isoperistaltic segment of jejunum or colon between the esophagus and the duodenum accomplished a similar result but significantly complicated the operation. The alternative of an end-to-side esophagojejunostomy with an enteroenterostomy between the ascending and descending jejunal limbs has not been as effective in reducing reflux. The most commonly used technique for construction of a reservoir pouch is that of a double loop of jejunum anastomosed side-to-side just below the esophagojejunostomy (Fig. 31–35).[42, 49] An alternative using a colonic segment has also been described.[43, 54] Scott and colleagues[48] studied the nutritional status of eight patients in whom a jejunal pouch was created. All eight patients were in a good state of nutrition 10 months to 3 years postoperatively.

Everson[15] collected results of all reported metabolic studies on patients who had undergone total gastric resection from 1897 to 1952. He found strong evidence for defective fat and protein absorption. Bradley and associates[5] evaluated 10 patients following total gastrectomy, combining their data with those of 12 similar patients reported in the literature. Sixty-nine percent of 22 patients showed fat malabsorption (more than 10% of ingested fat), and 42% demonstrated protein malabsorption. No significant difference appeared between patients who had jejunal pouches and those who did not. A major factor contributing to weight loss and failure to gain weight in their study was inadequate caloric intake. Armbrecht and co-workers[1] studied intestinal absorption in 11 patients after Roux-en-Y esophagojejunostomy reconstruction. A loss of 0 to 8 kg. was observed over an average of 19 months. D-xylose and lactose absorption was normal. All 11 had signs of steatorrhea, and the median transit time to the cecum was only 110 minutes. They attributed weight loss to a combination of rapid transit, bacterial overgrowth of the small intestine, and pancreatic understimulation. In a Swedish study of 10 patients following total gastrectomy, there was no decrease in dietary intake compared with healthy

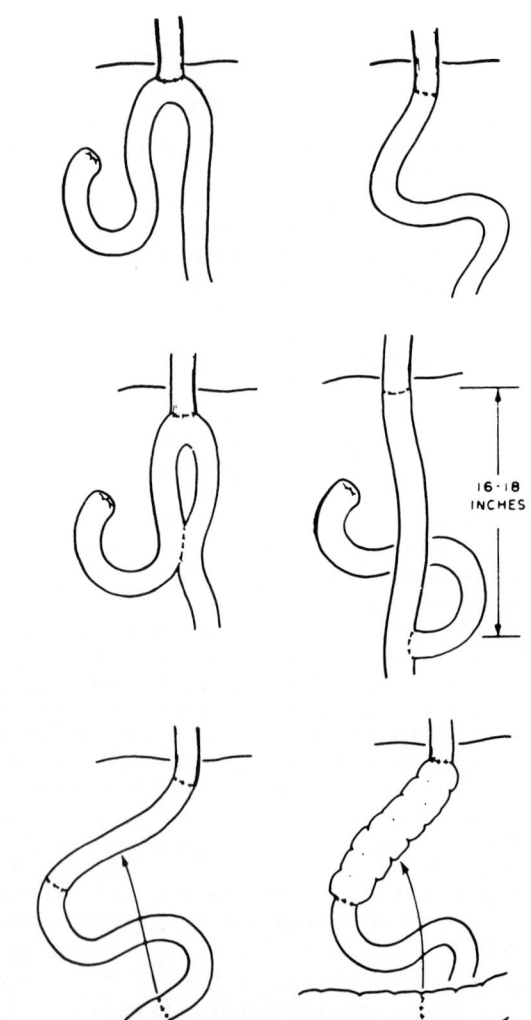

Figure 31–34. Methods of alimentary tract reconstruction most frequently used after total gastrectomy. (From Scott, H. W., Jr., and Law, D. H., IV: Malabsorption syndromes. Surg. Gynecol. Obstet., *121*:1231, 1965. By permission of Surgery, Gynecology and Obstetrics, now known as the JOURNAL OF THE AMERICAN COLLEGE OF SURGEONS.)

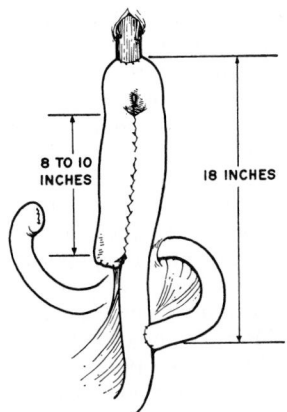

Figure 31–35. Alimentary reconstruction after total gastrectomy by Hunt-Lawrence jejunal pouch and Roux-en-Y esophagojejunostomy. (From Scott, H. W., Jr., Law, D. H., IV, Gobbel, W. G., Jr., and Sawyers, J. L.: Clinical and metabolic studies after total gastrectomy with a Hunt-Lawrence jejunal pouch. Am. J. Surg., 15:148, 1968.)

subjects.[53] Fat malabsorption was suggested, however, by depressed serum alpha-tocopherol and carotene concentrations. There was only mild weight loss.

The incidence of pernicious anemia following total gastrectomy is considerably lower than expected. One explanation is the normally large hepatic reserve of intrinsic factor. Another might be the poor survival of patients undergoing gastrectomy for gastric cancer. Still another explanation might be retention of as little as 1 to 2 cm. of normal fundic mucosa, which can provide sufficient intrinsic factor to prevent pernicious anemia. Hypochromic anemia has been observed in both humans and dogs after total gastrectomy. Such anemia usually responds favorably to oral iron.

Following Partial Gastrectomy

Partial gastrectomy is associated with less severe nutritional problems than is total gastrectomy. Intestinal continuity after subtotal gastrectomy can be restored by anastomosis of the stomach to the duodenum (Billroth I) or to a loop of jejunum (Billroth II), or by a Roux-en-Y gastrojejunostomy. Studies agree that the most common nutritional impairment following all types of anastomoses is loss of weight. In 1954, Zollinger and Ellison[64] reported that 127 of 203 patients were underweight after partial gastrectomy. Two thirds of the Billroth II patients were underweight, compared with one third of the Billroth I patients. Harkins and Nyhus[24] reported that 74% of patients with Billroth II anastomoses lost significant weight, compared with 42% of patients with Billroth I anastomoses. However, Fischer[16] reported minimal nutritional problems following Billroth II anastomoses in a 25-year follow-up study. Finally, Leth and associates[37] found little difference in weight loss among 18 patients randomized to either a Billroth I or Roux-en-Y reconstruction 2 years or more following operation.

Several factors appear to be significant in the development of malabsorption following subtotal gastrectomy. With all reconstructive procedures, there is decreased gastric digestion, more rapid and less regulated gastric emptying, and decreased intestinal transit time. When clinically severe, the early emptying and rapid transit are characterized by weakness, faintness, tachycardia, hemoconcentration, profuse perspiration, abdominal cramping and bloating, and urgent diarrhea. This is called the dumping syndrome. Weight loss due to reduced dietary intake, malabsorption, and dehydration from diarrhea can be dramatic. The dumping syndrome is

difficult to manage, and progressive malnutrition often ensues. The somatostatin analog octreotide has been of value in some but not all patients with severe dumping.[33, 40, 57]

Additional factors leading to malabsorption following a Billroth II or Roux-en-Y anastomosis include defective stimulation of biliary and pancreatic secretions due to bypass of the duodenum; possible inadequate mixing of pancreatic enzymes and bile salts with the gastric contents[41]; possible stasis in the afferent loop, leading to bacterial overgrowth and abnormalities of bile salt metabolism; and loss of the duodenum as the principal absorptive surface for iron, calcium, fat, and carotene. Small intestinal biopsies have shown inconsistent and nonspecific histologic changes in the mucosa that are not adequate to explain the changes in function. Metabolic balance studies have shown variable degrees of both fat and protein malabsorption.[4, 63] Malabsorption of fat is generally greater in patients who have had a Billroth II or Roux-en-Y compared with a Billroth I procedure. Approximately 50% demonstrate steatorrhea greater than 8 gm. in 24 hours. Nonetheless, less than 20% of patients develop clinically significant malabsorption. In contrast, only 25% of patients who have undergone a Billroth I procedure demonstrate steatorrhea, and less than 10% show clinically significant malabsorption.[14, 60] Leth and colleagues[37] reported a significantly greater fecal excretion of fat following Roux-en-Y reconstruction compared with Billroth I reconstruction. Because orocecal transit times and breath excretion of hydrogen after standardized test meals were similar, the increased excretion of fat was due to duodenal diversion, with poor mixing of pancreatic and biliary secretions with ingested food.

A common metabolic complication of subtotal gastrectomy is anemia, occurring in up to 30% of patients within 15 years. Causes include malabsorption of iron, folate, and, rarely, vitamin B_{12}. Oral administration of iron is usually helpful, although refractory cases may require intramuscular or intravenous administration of iron or blood transfusions. A metabolic bone disease similar to osteomalacia occurs in up to 33% of patients after 10 to 20 years, because of malabsorption of vitamin D and calcium.[36]

Following Vagotomy

Experimental studies have indicated that vagal denervation alters function of the stomach, pancreas, biliary system, and small intestine.[41] Malabsorption following truncal vagotomy may be due in part to diarrhea, poor mixing of pancreatic secretions and bile salts with food, and diminished release of cholecystokinin and secretin. The incidence of diarrhea following truncal vagotomy varies from 25% to 68%, but it is troublesome in only 1% to 5%.[32] The diarrhea is often intermittent, with 10 to 25 explosive, watery stools per day. The diarrhea may result from stasis of food in the stomach and small intestine, causing bacterial overgrowth; uncontrolled gastric emptying with dumping, supported by the lower incidence following selective vagotomy (less than 10%); and/or rapid small intestinal transit due to vagal denervation.[27]

Steatorrhea is common after vagal denervation. After truncal vagotomy without a drainage procedure, eight of nine patients showed excess excretion of fat.[19] Vagotomy and antrectomy in dogs interfered with absorption of solid but not liquid dietary fat.[12] There appears to be no difference between fecal fat levels after truncal vagotomy and those after selective vagotomy.[39] Abnormalities of gastric grinding and sieving of food particles were implicated, with larger fat particles being malabsorbed.

Absorption and metabolism of glucose are altered by vagotomy and pyloroplasty.[47] The malabsorption is attributed to rapid gastric emptying and decreased small intestinal transit time, overloading the limited glucose-absorbing capacity of the gut. Plasma glucose and insulin peaks are two to four times higher than normal, reflecting the rapid gastric emptying and initial absorption of glucose. Clearance of glucose from the blood is unaltered. The relatively short absorption period with normal clearance of glucose leads to the typically observed "reactive" hypoglycemia. The overall response to glucose intake is an early postprandial hyperglycemia followed by a reactive hypoglycemia.

Gastrointestinal Fistulas

Gastrocolic Fistula. A communication between the stomach and transverse colon is a result of a penetrating marginal ulcer at gastrojejunostomy, direct erosion of a large gastric ulcer or gastric or colonic carcinoma, or Crohn's disease. Either dumping of undigested food into the colon or severe bacterial gastritis with reflux of colonic bacteria into the stomach can cause malabsorption.

Enterocutaneous Fistula. If the enteric fistula is located distally in the intestine, fluid losses may be high, but malabsorption of nutrients is usually minimal, and nutritional depletion is uncommon. If the fistula is proximal, however, significant loss of ingested food may occur. Low-output fistulas (less than 200 ml. per day) seldom cause significant malnutrition. High-output fistulas (more than 800 ml. per day) are associated with marked malnutrition as well as formidable skin problems. Biliary and pancreatic fistulas may lead to malabsorption of fat, protein, and starch, depending on the amount of daily losses.

Pancreatic Insufficiency

Malabsorption may not be present despite significant pancreatic disease due to the organ's large functional reserve. When pancreatic insufficiency develops from chronic infection, tumor, or resection, however, malabsorption is common.

The diagnosis of exocrine pancreatic insufficiency is suggested by pancreatic calcification with normal D-xylose absorption in the presence of steatorrhea and/or increased losses of protein in the stool, and it can be confirmed by the secretin test. Treatment of malabsorption due to pancreatic insufficiency depends on the disease. Patients with chronic relapsing pancreatitis may benefit from pancreatic enzyme preparations. Patients with chronic relapsing pancreatitis with a dilated partially or completely obstructed pancreatic duct may benefit from anastomosis of the dilated duct to the gastrointestinal tract to restore intestinal flow of pancreatic enzymes. Patients with external pancreatic fistulas benefit temporarily from replacement of the fistula drainage via intestinal feeding tubes and benefit long term from implantation of the fistula tract into a segment of the intestine. Patients with pancreatic tumors and occlusion of the pancreatic duct should undergo resection, if possible, with implantation of the residual pancreas into the small intestine.

Total pancreatectomy produces both diabetes and malabsorption. Although insulin requirements are not as high as might be expected, control of the diabetes may be difficult. Loss of the counterregulatory hormones insulin and glucagon is associated with glucose instability, with frequent hypoglycemia.[13] Studies by Braga and colleagues[6] in patients after subtotal pancreatectomy and acinar destruction with polychloroprene injection of the pancreatic duct confirm that enterocyte function is normal in the absence of exocrine function, with no evidence of bacterial overgrowth or rapid transit. All observed malabsorption stemmed from the lack of lipase and protease, and oral pancreatic enzymes corrected the malabsorption. Dresler and associates[13] reported loss of

up to 16% of ingested fat in the stool following pancreatectomy, with accelerated fatty infiltration of the liver and marked osteopenia 5 years after operation.

Gastrin-secreting tumors of the pancreas cause marked gastric hypersecretion and hyperacidity. With an increased volume of gastric secretions, increased secretory response of the duodenal mucosa due to irritation from excess acid, and inactivation of pancreatic exocrine enzymes by duodenal acidity, malabsorption and diarrhea can be severe. Total gastrectomy as treatment of gastric hypersecretion can lead to malabsorption, as described above. H_2-receptor antagonists have fewer side effects than total gastrectomy, so they are frequently used. More recently, somatostatin, which suppresses gastrin production, has been quite effective. The long-term metabolic effects of global hormonal suppression by somatostatin are unknown.

Vasoactive intestinal peptide, when released in large amounts from pancreatic tumors, leads to a massive secretory response of the small intestine and severe diarrhea, with potential dramatic losses of electrolytes. Malabsorption varies, depending on the severity of diarrhea.

Biliary Tract Disease

Hepatobiliary disease can cause malabsorption through two mechanisms: inadequate amounts of bile in the intestinal tract, and the hepatic disease itself. Steatorrhea can occur with acute viral hepatitis, chronic intrahepatic cholestasis, chronic extrahepatic obstructive jaundice, and cirrhosis of the liver. The frequency of bone disease in patients with chronic intrahepatic cholestasis indicates a disturbance of calcium metabolism as well.[55] Bony changes may be those of both osteoporosis and osteomalacia.[2] It is presumed that the clinical abnormalities follow both malabsorption of vitamin D and calcium loss in the stool.

Treatment of patients with chronic cholestasis or obstructive jaundice, whether caused by obstruction of the bile duct or acute cholestasis, must include administration of fat-soluble vitamins A, D, E, and K and calcium salts. Diarrhea may be partially decreased by reducing fat intake, which may also reduce losses of fat-soluble vitamins and calcium in the stool. If obstructive jaundice is present, surgical intervention is indicated to re-establish bile flow into the intestinal tract. In patients with biliary fistulas, bile collected from the fistula can be returned to the gastrointestinal tract through an enteric tube as a temporary measure until the fistula closes spontaneously or is closed surgically.

Following Resection of the Small Intestine

Generally, resection of a short segment of small intestine is well tolerated with few, if any, signs of malabsorption. Yet even with removal of only a short segment, malabsorption of vitamin D and calcium can cause osteomalacia over time.[10] The incidence of malabsorption increases as more intestine is removed. With resection of more than 50% of the small intestine, malabsorption can be a significant clinical problem. Resection of all but 40 cm. or less usually leads to progressive weight loss, sepsis, and death unless intravenous nutritional support is given, both in the hospital and at home. Given time and adequate nutrition, the small intestine undergoes adaptive hyperplasia, increasing its absorptive surface and assuming absorptive functions normally performed by the resected segment.[62] Patients in whom the duodenum and 40 cm. or more of small intestine distal to the ligament of Treitz are preserved, along with part of the large intestine, may eventually tolerate an oral diet well enough to maintain body weight within 70% to 80% of their usual weight, allowing withdrawal of intravenous feeding.

Malabsorption following resection of the small intestine is due to several factors. Intestinal transit time is decreased, especially with resection of the distal small intestine and ileocecal valve, which affects absorption of all foodstuffs.[52] Resection of the terminal ileum may lead to vitamin B_{12} deficiency and malabsorption of bile salt. Depletion of the pool of bile salts causes steatorrhea. The increased fat in the stool binds intraluminal calcium, increasing absorption of oxalate salts (instead of excreting them as insoluble calcium). Oxaluria may lead to renal stone formation. Resection of the proximal small intestine may lead to malabsorption of calcium and iron. Gastric hypersecretion and hyperacidity occurs in direct proportion to the amount of small intestine removed.[20] The resultant high-solute load can contribute to diarrhea, along with increased duodenal secretions due to injury from hyperacidity. The hyperacidity may also inactivate the digestive enzymes lipase and trypsin. Finally, sugar intolerance—especially lactose, with loss of the brush-border enzyme lactase—may become clinically evident.

Patients with extensive resection of the small intestine require careful observation and management. Frequent feedings of low-fat, low-oxalate, high-protein dry diets are preferred. With extensive resections, total parenteral nutrition should be initiated within the first week and continued until intestinal adaptation permits an oral diet. Home intravenous nutrition may be necessary to allow for full adaptation. Addition of bile salts to treat steatorrhea or cholestyramine to treat bile salt diarrhea has been attempted but is of little benefit. Oral calcium carbonate may reduce steatorrhea and decrease oxalate absorption. Gastric hypersecretion should be treated aggressively with frequent antacids (calcium carbonate or aluminum hydroxide) and an H_2-receptor antagonist for up to 6 months to prevent peptic ulcer disease as well as to minimize diarrhea and malabsorption. The hypergastrinemia and need for H_2-receptor antagonists diminish over 6 to 12 months.

Blind Loop Syndrome

The term *blind loop syndrome* was originally used to describe complications of blind loops of the small intestine following operation. It is now applied whenever conditions give rise to intestinal stasis, such as with intestinal strictures, Crohn's disease, intestinal pseudo-obstruction, postvagotomy syndromes, scleroderma, and small intestinal diverticula. The syndrome is characterized by diarrhea, steatorrhea, anemia, weight loss, abdominal pain, and multiple vitamin deficiencies.

Hematologically, blind loop syndrome involves mainly vitamin B_{12} deficiency, although there may also be a deficiency in folic acid. The diagnosis of blind loop syndrome can be confirmed by the Schilling test, demonstrating intrinsic factor–resistant vitamin B_{12} malabsorption. There are two main hypotheses for the development of vitamin B_{12} deficiency: bacteria in the stagnant area use vitamin B_{12}, leaving an inadequate amount for absorption, or the bacteria produce a toxin that inhibits absorption of vitamin B_{12}. Steatorrhea most likely occurs when the bacteria present in the blind loop structurally alter bile salts, interfering with absorption of fat.[29]

Treatment of the blind loop syndrome should include surgical correction of the underlying cause of intestinal stasis, if feasible. If operation cannot be undertaken, antibiotics can improve symptoms. Useful drugs include chlortetracycline, clindamycin, and metronidazole. Neomycin is ineffective against anaerobes. With effective antibiotic therapy, the Schilling test should return to near normal and the diarrhea and steatorrhea should subside within a week. After treatment for 2 to 3 weeks, the antibiotics can be given intermittently

(1 to 2 weeks out of each month) to continue suppression of clinical symptoms.

SELECTED REFERENCES

Baron, J. H., Alexander-William, J., Allgower, M., Muller, C., and Spencer, J. (Eds.): Vagotomy in Modern Surgical Practice. London, Butterworths, 1982.
This comprehensive review of normal vagal function gives special attention to consequences of vagotomy in surgical practice. The series of articles was presented at the international symposium in Basel in 1981.

Koo, J., Lam, S. K., Chan, P., Lee, N. W., Lam, P., Wong, J., and Ong, G. B.: Proximal gastric vagotomy, truncal vagotomy with drainage, and truncal vagotomy with antrectomy for chronic duodenal ulcer: A prospective, randomized controlled trial. Ann. Surg., 197:265, 1983.
The metabolic side effects of three current operative procedures for peptic ulcer disease were compared in 152 patients—the largest of recent studies. Proximal gastric vagotomy had the fewest side effects of dumping, epigastric fullness, and diarrhea.

Thirlby, R. C.: Postsurgical syndromes. Gastroenterol. Clin. North Am., 23:2, 1994.
This is an excellent review of the current understanding of postsurgical syndromes following operations on the stomach and small bowel. There are separate chapters on postsurgical motility, absorption, and complications.

REFERENCES

1. Armbrecht, U., Lundell, L., Lindstedt, G., and Stockbruegger, R. W.: Causes of malabsorption after total gastrectomy with Roux-en-Y reconstruction. Acta Chir. Scand., 154:37, 1988.
2. Atkinson, M., Nordin, B. E. C., and Sherlock, S.: Malabsorption and bone disease in prolonged obstructive jaundice. Q. J. Med., 25:299, 1956.
3. Beal, J. M., Briggs, J. D., and Longmire, W. P., Jr.: Use of a jejunal segment to replace the stomach following total gastrectomy. Am. J. Surg., 88:194, 1954.
4. Bohmansson, G.: Studien uber die chiurgische Behandling von Gastroduodenalgeschwuren mit besonderer Berucksichtigung der Operationsanatomie und der postoperativen Digestionsphysiologie nebst einem Beitrag zur Frage der chirugischen Behandlung akuter Ulkusblutungen. Acta Chir. Scand., suppl. 7, 1926.
5. Bradley, E. L., 3rd, Isaacs, J., Hersh, T., Davidson, E. D., and Millikan, W.: Nutritional consequences of total gastrectomy. Ann. Surg., 182:415, 1975.
6. Braga, M., Cristallo, M., DeFranchis, R., Mangiagalli, A., Agape, D., Primignani, M., and DiCarlo, V.: Correction of malnutrition and maldigestion with enzyme supplementation in patients with surgical suppression of exocrine pancreatic function. Surg. Gynecol. Obstet., 167:485, 1988.
7. Brummer, R. J., Karibe, M., and Stockbruegger, R. W.: Lactose malabsorption: Optimalization of investigational methods. Scand. J. Gastroenterol. Suppl., 200:65, 1993.
8. Butler, R. N., Gehling, N. J., Lawson, M. J., and Grant, A. K.: Clinical evaluation of the 14C triolein breath test: A critical analysis. Aust. N. Z. J. Med., 14:111, 1984.
9. Cattel, R. B.: Massive resection of the small intestine. Lahey Clin. Bull., 4:167, 1945.
10. Compston, J. E., Ayers, A. B., Horton, L. W., Tighe, J. R., and Creamer, B.: Osteomalacia after small-intestine resection. Lancet, 1:9, 1978.
11. Doig, A., and Girdwood, R. H.: The absorption of folic acid and labeled cyanocobalamin in intestinal malabsorption. Q. J. Med., 29:333, 1960.
12. Doty, J. E., and Meyer, J. H.: Vagotomy and antrectomy impairs canine fat absorption from solid but not liquid dietary sources. Gastroenterology, 94:50, 1988.
13. Dresler, C. M., Fortner, J. G., McDermott, K., and Bajorunas, D. R.: Metabolic consequences of (regional) total pancreatectomy. Ann. Surg., 214:131, 1991.
14. Edwards, J. P., Lyndon, P. J., Smith, R. B., and Johnston, D.: Faecal fat excretion after truncal, selective, and highly selective vagotomy for duodenal ulcer. Gut, 15:521, 1974.
15. Everson, T. C.: Nutrition following total gastrectomy, with particular reference to fat and protein assimilation: Collective review. Surg. Gynecol. Obstet., 95:209, 1952.
16. Fischer, A. B.: The long-term results following Billroth II resection for duodenal ulcer. Dan. Med. Bull., 33:319, 1986.
17. Fletcher, R. F., Henly, A. A., Sammons, H. G., and Squire, J. R.: Case of magnesium deficiency following massive intestinal resection. Lancet, 1:522, 1960.
18. Floch, M. H.: Recent contributions in intestinal absorption and malabsorption: A review. Am. J. Clin. Nutr., 22:327, 1969.
19. Fox, H. J., and Grimson, K. S.: Defective fat absorption following vagotomy. J. Lab. Clin. Med., 35:362, 1950.
20. Frederick, P. L., Sizer, J. S., and Osborne, M. P.: Relation of massive bowel resection to gastric secretion. N. Engl. J. Med., 272:509, 1965.
21. Goulston, K., Bhanthumnavin, K., and Harrison, D.: Investigation of steatorrhea. Med. J. Aust., 2:462, 1968.

22. Grant, J. P.: Handbook of Total Parenteral Nutrition, 2nd ed. Philadelphia, W. B. Saunders, 1992.
23. Haeney, M. R., Culank, L. S., Montgomery, R. D., and Sammons, H. G.: Evaluation of xylose absorption as measured in blood and urine: A one-hour blood xylose screening test in malabsorption. Gastroenterology, 75:393, 1978.
24. Harkins, H. N., and Nyhus, L. M.: A comparison of the Billroth I and Billroth II procedures: Clinical and experimental studies. Bull. Soc. Int. Chir., 15:111, 1956.
25. Haymond, H. E.: Massive resection of the small intestine: An analysis of 257 collected cases. Surg. Gynecol. Obstet., 61:693, 1935.
26. Herlinger, H.: Enteroclysis in malabsorption: Can it influence diagnosis and management? Radiologe, 33:335, 1993.
27. Hobsley, M.: Dumping and diarrhoea. Br. J. Surg., 68:681, 1981.
28. Johnson, C. F.: Malabsorption syndromes: Clinical and theoretical considerations. Postgrad. Med. J., 37:667, 1965.
29. Kim, Y. S., Spritz, N., Blum, M., Terz, J., and Sherlock, P.: The role of altered bile acid metabolism in the steatorrhea of experimental blind loop. J. Clin. Invest., 45:956, 1966.
30. Kirsner, J. B.: Clinical observations on malabsorption. Med. Clin. North Am., 53:1169, 1969.
31. Knight, C. D., Jr., Van Heerden, J. A., and Kelly, K. A.: Proximal gastric vagotomy: Update. Ann. Surg., 197:22, 1983.
32. Koo, J., Lam, S. K., Chan, P., Lee, N. W., Lam, P., Wong, J., and Ong, G. B.: Proximal gastric vagotomy, truncal vagotomy with drainage, and truncal vagotomy with antrectomy for chronic duodenal ulcer: A prospective, randomized controlled trial. Ann. Surg., 197:265, 1983.
33. Lamers, C. B., Bijlstra, A. M., and Harris, A. G.: Octreotide, a long-acting somatostatin analog, in the management of postoperative dumping syndrome: An update. Dig. Dis. Sci., 38:359, 1993.
34. Law, D. H.: Medium chain triglyceride therapy of malabsorption. Clin. Res., 14:48, 1966.
35. Laws, J. W., Shawdon, H., Booth, C. C., and Stewart, J. S.: Correlation of radiological and histological findings in idiopathic steatorrhea. Br. Med. J., 1:1311, 1963.
36. Leading article: Osteomalacia after gastrectomy. Lancet, 1:77, 1986.
37. Leth, R. D., Abrahamsson, H., Kilander, A., and Lundell, L. R.: Malabsorption of fat after partial gastric resection: A study of pathophysiologic mechanisms. Eur. J. Surg., 157:205, 1991.
38. Longmire, W. P., Jr., and Beal, J. M.: Construction of a substitute gastric reservoir following total gastrectomy. Ann. Surg., 135:637, 1952.
39. Losowsky, M. S., Walker, B. E., and Kelleher, J.: Malabsorption in Clinical Practice. London, Churchill Livingstone, 1974.
40. Mackie, C. R., Jenkins, S. A., and Hartley, M. N.: Treatment of severe postvagotomy/postgastrectomy symptoms with the somatostatin analogue octreotide. Br. J. Surg., 78:1338, 1991.
41. Mayer, E. A., Thomson, J. B., Jehn, D., Reedy, T., Elashoff, J., Deveny, C., and Meyer, J. H.: Gastric emptying and sieving of solid food and pancreatic and biliary secretions after solid meals in patients with nonresective ulcer surgery. Gastroenterology, 87:1264, 1984.
42. McCorkle, H. J., and Harper, H. A.: The problem of nutrition following complete gastrectomy. Ann. Surg., 140:467, 1954.
43. Moroney, J.: Colonic replacement and restoration of the human stomach. Ann. R. Coll. Surg. Engl., 12:328, 1953.
44. Newcomer, A. D., Hofmann, A. F., DiMagno, E. P., Thomas, P. J., and Carlson, G. L.: Triolein breath test: A sensitive and specific test for fat malabsorption. Gastroenterology, 76:6, 1979.
45. Phillips, D. F., Wollaeger, E. E., Ellis, F. H., Jr., and Power, M. H.: Fecal excretion of fat and nitrogen after esophagogastrectomy in man. Surgery, 49:433, 1961.
46. Preece, J. D., Davies, I. H., and Wilkinson, S. P.: Use of the SeHCAT test in the investigation of diarrhoea. Postgrad. Med. J., 68:272, 1992.
47. Radziuk, J., and Bondy, D. C.: Abnormal oral glucose tolerance and glucose malabsorption after vagotomy and pyloroplasty: A tracer method for measuring glucose absorption rates. Gastroenterology, 83:1017, 1982.
48. Scott, H. W., Jr., Herrington, J. L., Jr., Edwards, L. W., Shull, H. J., Stephenson, S. E., Jr., Sawyers, J. L., and Classen, K. L.: Results of vagotomy and antral resection in surgical treatment of duodenal ulcer. Gastroenterology, 39:590, 1960.
49. Scott, H. W., Jr., Law, D. H., 4th, Gobbel, W. G., Jr., and Sawyers, J. L.: Clinical and metabolic studies after total gastrectomy with a Hunt-Lawrence jejunal food pouch. Am. J. Surg., 115:148, 1968.
50. Scott, H. W., Jr., and Weidner, M. G.: Total gastrectomy with Roux-en-Y esophagojejunostomy in treatment of gastric cancer. Ann. Surg., 143:682, 1956.
51. Shils, M. E., and Gilat, T.: The effect of esophagectomy on absorption in man: Clinical and metabolic observations. Gastroenterology, 50:347, 1966.
52. Singleton, A. O., Redmond, D. C., and McMurray, J. E.: Ileocecal resection and small bowel transit and absorption. Ann. Surg., 159:690, 1964.
53. Stael von Holstein, C., Ibrahimbegovic, E., Walther, B., and Akesson, B.: Nutrient intake and biochemical markers of nutritional status during long-term follow-up after total and partial gastrectomy. Eur. J. Clin. Nutr., 46:265, 1992.
54. State, D., Barclay, T., and Kelly, W. D.: Total gastrectomy with utilization of a segment of transverse colon to replace the excised stomach. Ann. Surg., 134:1035, 1951.
55. Summerskill, W. H. J., and Moertel, C. G.: Malabsorption syndrome associated with anicteric liver disease. Gastroenterology, 42:380, 1962.
56. Tovey, F. I., and Clark, C. G.: Anaemia after partial gastrectomy: A neglected curable condition. Lancet, 1:956, 1980.
57. Tulassay, Z., Tulassay, T., Gupta, R., and Tamas, G.: The effect of somatostatin in dumping syndrome after gastric surgery. Acta Gastroenterol. Belg., 56:219, 1993.
58. Tuna, N., Mangold, H. K., and Mosser, D. G.: Re-evaluation of the I-131-triolein absorption test. J. Lab. Clin. Med., 61:620, 1963.
59. Watkins, J. B., Schoeller, D. A., Klein, P. D., Ott, D. G., Newcomer, A. D., and Hofmann, A. F.: 13C-trioctanoin: A nonradioactive breath test to detect fat malabsorption. J. Lab. Clin. Med., 90:422, 1977.
60. Wheldon, E. J., Vanables, C. W., and Johnston, I. D. A.: Late metabolic sequelae of vagotomy and gastrojejunostomy. Lancet, 1:437, 1970.
61. Wilkins, R., Garvey, C., and DeLacey, G.: Radiological examination. In Booth, C. C., and Neale, G. (Eds.): Disorders of the Small Intestine. Oxford, Blackwell Scientific Publications, 1985, p. 5.
62. Williamson, R. C. N., and Chir, M.: Intestinal adaptation. N. Engl. J. Med., 298:1393, 1978.
63. Wilson, T. H.: Intestinal Absorption. Philadelphia, W. B. Saunders, 1962.
64. Zollinger, R. M., and Ellison, E. H.: Nutrition after gastric operations. JAMA, 154:811, 1954.

IX

RADIATION INJURY TO THE INTESTINE

Jerome J. DeCosse, M.D., Ph.D.

Radiation therapy is the primary method of management in some forms of curable cancer, such as squamous cell carcinoma of the cervix, carcinoma of the intrinsic larynx, and seminoma of the testis. Radiation therapy complements surgical therapy or is an alternative form of therapy for curable tumors at other sites, such as squamous cell carcinoma of the oral cavity, adenocarcinoma of the endometrium, and carcinoma of the breast, rectum, and prostate. Both radiation therapy and chemotherapy are applied in the curative treatment of lymphoma and pediatric tumors, such as Ewing's sarcoma and Wilms' tumor, and in bone marrow transplantation. Radiation therapy is also used frequently in the palliative management of incurable cancer. More than half of all patients with cancer receive curative or palliative radiation therapy.[5] The widespread application of megavoltage and technical advances in irradiation have improved safety and reduced skin damage even though more patients are receiving adjuvant or primary therapy. In effect, more patients are at less risk for visceral injury.[1, 11]

Roentgen, a physicist, discovered x-rays in 1895. The diagnostic potential of this discovery became apparent when he radiographed a colleague's hand for demonstration purposes. During the ensuing decade, the therapeutic potential and the hazards of irradiation were recognized in Europe. In the United States, advances have occurred rapidly since World War II.

The goal of radiation therapy is local control of tumor with minimal damage to normal tissue. To achieve this goal, the therapist must consider the total duration of a course of radiation therapy, the total dose, the number and size of fractions (small daily doses), the extent of the portal (area of the body to be exposed to irradiation), and the organ system or systems being irradiated. It is almost impossible to expose a tumor to irradiation without also exposing normal tissue. Both tumors and normal tissue vary in sensitivity to irradiation. The amount of irradiation that tissues can receive and still remain functional defines radiation tolerance. Elderly, thin women who have a deep cul-de-sac in which the small intestine resides are at increased risk for injury compared with young, obese men. Beyond these measurable factors, there is an important, variable individual sensitivity.

The energy absorbed in a biologic system is measured by the rad, which is defined as 100 ergs or 10^{12} primary ionizations per gram of tissue. One rad equals 0.01 Gy. The curative dose for cervical cancer is 70 to 75 Gy, whereas the maximal tolerance dose for intestine is 55 to 65 Gy. About 5% of patients who receive radiation therapy for abdominal or pelvic tumors experience late radiation injury requiring hospitalization.[29]

THE BIOLOGIC BASIS OF RADIATION INJURY

Therapeutic irradiation may be administered by a variety of external sources; by direct application to the tumor, as with radium; and by intravenous, intracavitary, or interstitial insertion with radioisotopes. Different forms of irradiation vary in linear energy transfer (LET), which is the amount of energy lost during the traversing of a given tissue. Gamma rays have high penetration and relatively low LET; that is, they dissipate energy evenly over a long distance. Alpha particles have low penetration and higher LET; they travel a shorter distance, and the energy concentration is higher at the end of their path. The penetration and LET of x-rays fall between these extremes (Table 31–9). Differences in LET cause similar doses of different types of ionizing radiation to vary in their biologic effects on a specific organ or site.

Within irradiated tissue, energy transferred by ionizing radiation generates a series of biochemical events. Ionized radicals injure DNA, RNA, intracellular fibers, and membranes. DNA appears to be the critical target associated with radiation-induced cell death. Mucosal injury leads to impaired absorption of metabolites. Carbohydrate malabsorption, which results from a decrease of disaccharidase located on the brush border of the intestinal wall, produces marked changes in the intestinal microflora, leading to excessive production of organic acids, carbon dioxide, and hydrogen ions;

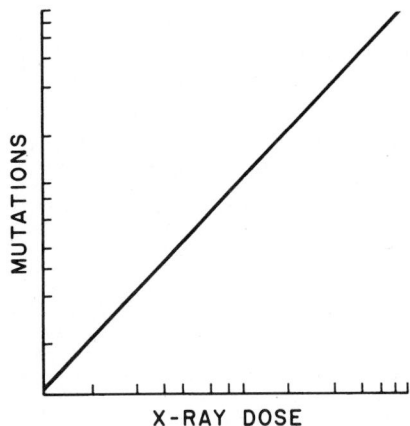

Figure 31–36. The frequency of mutations in *Drosophila* spermatozoa relates directly to the intensity of radiation administered.

impaired transport of water and electrolytes; and malabsorption of vitamin B_{12}. Decreased reabsorption of bile salts in the terminal ileum results in increased synthesis of unconjugated bile salts and an ensuing steatorrhea.

In addition to causing cell death, any type of ionizing radiation can induce true point mutations, with breakage and rearrangement of chromosomes (Fig. 31–36).[24] These effects of radiation, a linear function of dose, are persistent and cumulative over long periods of time.

Different types of cells vary considerably in their sensitivity to ionizing radiation. In general, the more frequently cells divide, the greater their sensitivity to irradiation. Hematopoietic cells, reproductive cells, and stem cells in the intestinal crypts proliferate rapidly and are at the greatest risk of radiation injury.[26] Static cell populations, such as nerve cells, are relatively resistant to radiation injury. Tissue and whole organ effects depend on age, sex, temperature, oxygenation, metabolic activity, weight, stress, species variation, and other variables.

In addition to injuring cells, irradiation causes progressive changes in fine vasculature and interstitial connective tissue. Subendothelial proliferation and medial thickening may progressively deplete the blood supply to irradiated tissue (Fig. 31–37). Interstitial collagen deposition also may cause severe scarring and further obliterate blood flow, causing tissue hypoxia and eventual necrosis, while fibrotic barriers inhibit revascularization and repair.

Systemic and topical agents have been applied before, during, and after irradiation to prevent injury to the host. Radioprotectants include elemental diets, glutamine supplements, vitamin A, nonsteroidal anti-inflammatory agents, the thiophosphate WR-2721, and several antioxidants.[10, 16, 33] To date, clinical benefit has been modest and confined to the acute phase of injury.

Prior surgical therapy or prior intra-abdominal infection may increase the risk of injury, because the serosal surface of the small or large intestine may adhere to tissue being irradiated.[8] Surgeons performing procedures to be followed by radiation therapy can reduce the risk of intestinal injury by accurately outlining the area to be treated with radiopaque markers, by reperitonealization, by excluding small bowel from the pelvis through omental transposition or other measures, and by scrupulous cleansing of the peritoneal cavity before closure.[3, 5, 20, 22]

ACUTE INTESTINAL INJURY

The acute effects of a given dose of ionizing radiation are inversely proportional to field size; that is, with small portals,

TABLE 31–9. Some Types of Ionizing Radiation and Their LET Values

Particle	Charge	Energy (MeV)	Description	LET (keV/μ)
Alpha	+2	5	Helium nucleus	100.0
Proton	+1	2	Hydrogen nucleus	16.0
		5		8.0
		10		4.0
Neutron	0	2.5	Neutron	20.0
		14.1		7.0
Electron	−1	0.001	Electron	12.3
		0.010		2.3
		0.100		0.42
		1.000		0.25
X-ray		3.000	Electromagnetic radiation	0.3
Gamma ray			Cobalt 60	0.3

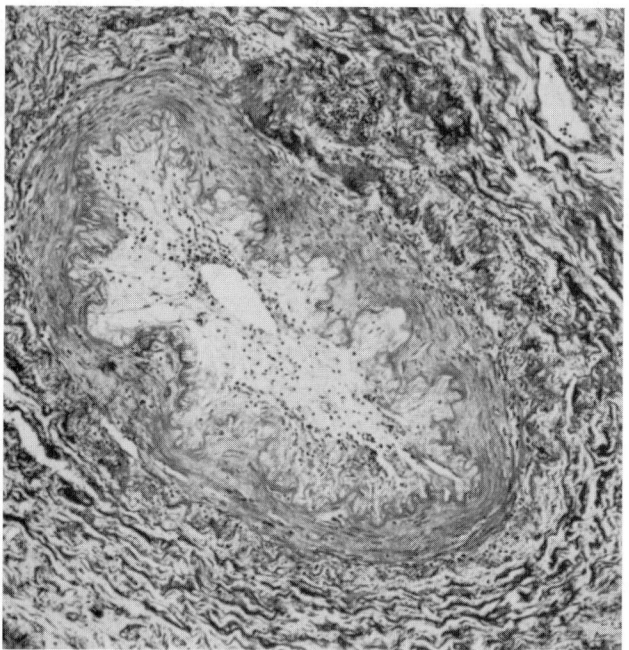

Figure 31–37. Photomicrograph (×80) of an ileal arteriole demonstrating occlusive radiation vasculitis and surrounding perivascular fibrosis, findings characteristic of chronic radiation injury.

and other physical factors being equal, large amounts of radiation can be given safely, whereas with total-body radiation, approximately 400 cGy constitute the median lethal dose (LD$_{50}$) in man. Radiation injuries have followed nuclear disasters and accidental radiation exposures, such as the nuclear accident at Chernobyl in 1986. Radiation at this level affects the proliferating cells in the crypts of Lieberkühn, which are no longer able to replete cells in the intestinal villi. The villi become flattened, and intestinal barrier function fails. Leakage of fluids into the intestinal lumen causes the patient to become dehydrated, and bacteria that normally live within the gastrointestinal tract enter the bloodstream, causing systemic toxemia. In a context of total-body radiation, damage to the bone marrow compounds the effect; pancytopenia due to hematopoietic depression may lead inexorably to the patient's death. At lower levels of total-body irradiation, prolonged and vigorous water and electrolyte replacement, antibiotic protection, and, in some cases, bone marrow transplantation—used with some success among Chernobyl victims—may enable patients to survive acute injury.[7]

Intestinal alterations that follow therapeutic irradiation are less devastating. Ordinarily, basic pathophysiologic mechanisms of mucosal damage are transient, self-limited, and localized and subside soon after completion of radiation therapy. Pelvic radiation therapy may place the patient at risk for acute radiation-induced (factitious) proctitis and for damage to other intestinal segments, especially a terminal ileum and cecum fixed by anatomy or by adhesions within the pelvis. Therapeutic irradiation to the periaortic area for lymphoma or testis cancer, or to the retroperitoneum for soft tissue sarcoma, can be associated with injury to the small intestine, the pancreas, and other viscera.

Patients with proctitis usually present with diarrhea, tenesmus, and rectal bleeding. Diarrhea also may follow impaired bile salt reabsorption in the injured terminal ileum. Nausea is common, and crampy abdominal pain may be present. Ordinarily, these symptoms subside shortly after completion of radiation therapy, and patients require only supportive

therapy with antidiarrheal, anticholinergic, and antispasmodic medication.

LATE INTESTINAL INJURY

Gastrointestinal symptoms may persist after radiation therapy and, in some patients, can progress over weeks, months, or even years to chronic injury. Late radiation injury is caused by progressive vasculitis, diffuse collagen deposition, and fibrosis rather than altered epithelial proliferative kinetics. The vasculitis causes tissue hypoxia, which may progress to necrosis, ulceration, chronic rectal bleeding, perforation, abscess formation, and fistulization.[4, 30]

In addition to general supportive therapy, gastrointestinal symptoms may be controlled by a low-fiber diet, stool softeners, opiates, hydrophilic colloids, acetylsalicylic acid, and, for anal pruritus, topical anesthetic agents and warm sitz baths. Clinical improvement has been shown with oral and rectal sucralfate and with oral sulfasalazine and rectal steroids.[13, 17]

Other patients experience a long symptom-free period before chronic radiation injury becomes evident. Subclinical injury may become overt when low-flow states, such as congestive heart failure or vascular narrowing from hypertension and arteriosclerosis, increase the hypoxia from radiation vasculitis until, finally, cellular oxygenation and nutrition are reduced below critical levels (Fig. 31–38).[9]

Some chemotherapeutic drugs, such as dactinomycin, doxorubicin, and 5-fluorouracil, enhance the effect of irradiation. Both treatments need not be administered at the same time; if they are applied sequentially, the subsequent effect is called a *recall phenomenon*. Although linked, the specific cellular damage caused by chemotherapy is probably different from that caused by radiation; in the gut, chemotherapy accelerates the depletion of crypt stem cells in zones of focal radiation ischemia.[27]

Chronic radiation injury of the intestine is frequently associated with injury to cutaneous, bony, and other visceral structures encompassed by the radiation portals. The radiation portal may be demarcated by a chronic dermatitis with capillary telangiectasia, epidermal atrophy, hyperkeratosis, and indolent ulceration. Sterility in men and amenorrhea in women may be evident. Genitourinary injury may be more life threatening than injury to the intestines.[29] Investigation of intestinal injury should include assessment by intravenous pyelography, cystoscopy, and computed tomography (CT) scanning for cystitis or urethral injury, as well as for radiation nephritis.

Short of biopsy, there is no specific test to distinguish

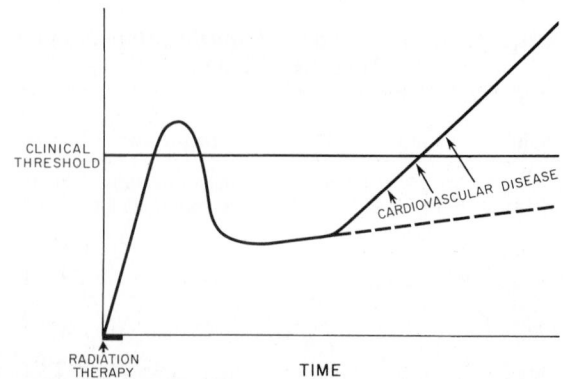

Figure 31–38. A model suggesting a pattern for radiation injury: early transient symptoms, a latent period of subclinical activity, and precipitation of clinical symptoms, often by onset of cardiovascular disease. (After Rubin, P., and Casarett, G. W.: Clinical Radiation Pathology. Philadelphia, W. B. Saunders, 1968.)

radiation damage from recurrent tumor, Crohn's disease, or ischemic colitis. Imaging may help identify recurrent tumor, and a CT-guided needle biopsy can be performed. A patient who appears well and maintains body weight but continues to have crampy abdominal pain often has a radiation injury rather than residual or recurrent cancer. Conditions associated with malabsorption, such as steatorrhea and hypocalcemia, point to a diagnosis of radiation injury to the small intestine.

Symptoms of partial intestinal obstruction may be insidious: limited nausea, no vomiting, only slight late postprandial crampy pain, and modest distention. In the presence of such symptoms, endoscopy and a small intestinal barium study should be conducted. Constricted, narrow loops of intestine or puddling of barium is indicative of partial obstruction (Fig. 31–39).[21] However, results may be difficult to interpret; the film may appear negative even when considerable pathologic change has occurred.

It is important not only to determine whether the obstruction is partial or complete but also to establish whether it involves vascular compromise. Patients with vascular compromise may have continuous abdominal pain between cramps, back pain suggesting torsion in the mesentery, involuntary guarding, localized and persistent tenderness to percussion or palpation, reduced or absent peristaltic sounds, a rectal temperature above 38° C., and a white blood count in excess of 12,000 cells per cu. mm.

Both vascular compromise and complete obstruction require surgical exploration. In the former case, exploration is urgent; in the latter, it should be preceded by nasogastric intubation and drainage, as well as volume repletion. At laparotomy, radiation-injured bowel is stenotic and thick-walled. The serosal surface is gray and opaque from serositis. Loose fibrinous adhesions congeal loops of small intestine to one another and to adjacent surfaces. Wide resection of the diseased bowel is the treatment of choice. Occasionally a bypass is necessary.[22, 31] Normal, unirradiated intestine should be used for the enteroenterostomy.

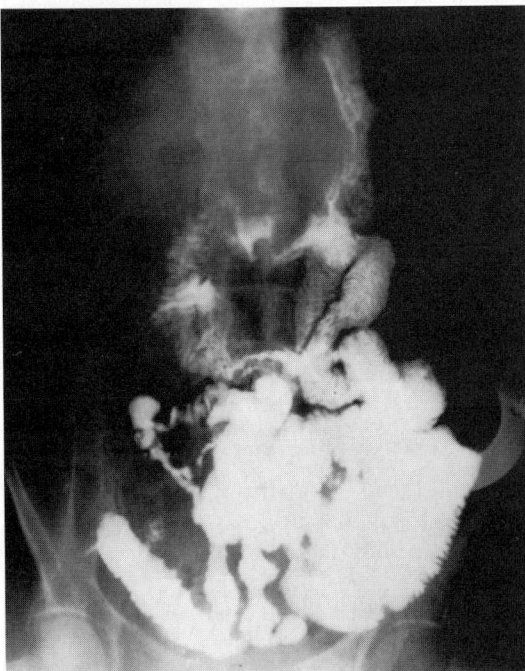

Figure 31–39. The relatively normal feathery appearance of the upper jejunum can be contrasted with stenosis, loss of valvular markings, and puddling evident in the distal radiation-injured small intestine.

Partial obstruction from radiation-induced stenosis of the small intestine may not require resection and should be managed initially by conservative intestinal decompression and fluid replacement. Oral steroids, sulfasalazine, and a low-residue diet may reduce symptoms to a tolerable level.

Obstruction and vascular occlusion can lead to hypoxia, necrosis, and perforation of the intestine. Perforation can cause (1) a diffuse peritonitis if the perforated loop has free access to the peritoneal cavity; (2) a localized abscess if matted loops of intestine and adjacent structures obstruct access to the free peritoneal cavity; or (3) fistulization if the perforation occurs into the bladder, ureter, vagina, intestine, or an operative wound agglutinated to the injured intestine. Operative management requires exteriorization of the perforated bowel, drainage, and proximal defunctionalization.[11, 20]

Fistulization between loops of bowel may exclude a segment of intestine and cause diarrhea or a blind loop syndrome with vitamin B_{12} deficiency. Urinary tract infections and pneumaturia (passage of air in the urine) may herald fistulization into the bladder. It is important to localize the site of the injury as accurately as possible by endoscopy, oral and rectal contrast studies, CT scanning, and fistulograms (instillation of iodinated water-soluble dyes) and to exclude recurrent cancer.

Patients with intestinal fistulas are usually severely ill—wasted, dehydrated, and toxic from chronic infection. A radiation-induced intestinal fistula rarely heals spontaneously; excision is almost always necessary.[2] However, a preliminary program of gastrointestinal decompression, resolution of pelvic sepsis, and nutritional replacement by total parenteral nutrition reduces operative risk and improves the likelihood of healing.

Some patients have persistent proctitis with severe pelvic pain, pain on defecation, and rectal bleeding. Persistence of these symptoms after radiation therapy merits assessment by endoscopy and barium enema examination. Some patients with severe rectal bleeding or intractable pain may require a proximal colostomy, but this procedure is not always successful.

Proctitis may progress to ulceration. At proctoscopy, the ulcer is located anteriorly at the level of the cervix or uterus and has a gray, shaggy, friable base but without the elevated perimeter suggestive of carcinoma. Rectal ulcers that do not heal may progress to perforation or formation of a rectovaginal fistula. Rectovaginal fistulas are often associated with recurrent carcinoma and therefore require biopsy.

Rectovaginal fistulas from radiation injury are rarely self-healing; they usually require defunctionalization of the rectum by a colostomy, which should be placed in the right transverse colon if a subsequent corrective operation is planned.[15] If pelvic fibrosis is extensive and the fistula involves a strictured distal rectum, the colostomy may be permanent. In recent years, some patients have had intestinal continuity restored by a low anterior resection, by a coloanal "sleeve" anastomosis,[12, 14, 25] or by interposition of a rotated flap of sigmoid colon.[6] Postoperative fecal incontinence may result from decreased rectal capacity and compliance, consequent to pelvic irradiation, particularly when combined with adjuvant chemotherapy.[19, 32] Another sequela of continued proctitis is rectal stenosis, which can usually be managed by conservative measures, including instrumental or digital dilations, but sometimes requires a colostomy.

Another long-term risk from radiation therapy is the development of neoplasia. The initial point of action of ionizing radiation in the induction of cancer may involve chromosomal damage. Low to moderate doses of radiation may be more carcinogenic than intensive therapeutic doses. In the latter, fibrosis and vasculitis may impair subsequent cellular proliferation.[18]

SELECTED REFERENCES

Kohn, H. I., and Fry, R. J. M.: Radiation carcinogenesis. N. Engl. J. Med., 310:304, 1984.
A review of the epidemiology of radiation carcinogenesis and the relation of epidemiologic observation to experimental radiation biology.

Muller, H. J.: Radiation damage to genetic material. Am. Sci., 38:33, 1950.
The author reviews his Nobel Prize–winning work on mutation frequency. His publications about this subject began in 1927, and this report summarizes his many important contributions.

Quastler, H.: The nature of intestinal radiation death. Radiat. Res., 4:303, 1956.
The cell kinetic evidence for radiation injury to the proliferative epithelium of the intestine is developed by an outstanding contributor in the field of cell cycle studies.

Rubin, P.: The Franz Bushke lecture: Late effects of chemotherapy and radiation therapy: A new hypothesis. Int. J. Radiat. Oncol. Biol. Phys., 10:5, 1984.
The author reviews previously published work about the pathophysiology of radiation effects and draws on documented histopathologic changes in clinical situations and in vivo and in vitro laboratory modeling to suggest a basis for differences between the late effects of chemotherapy and those of radiation therapy.

Warren, S. L., and Whipple, G. H.: Roentgen ray intoxication. I. Unit dose over thorax negative—over abdomen lethal. Epithelium of small intestine—sensitive to x-rays. J. Exp. Med., 35:187, 1922.
Two distinguished investigators and leaders of American medicine describe intestinal epithelial necrosis after radiation. This pioneering work is the first of a series by these authors on the pathology of acute and chronic radiation injury.

REFERENCES

1. Allan-Mersh, T. G., Wilson, E. J., Hope-Stone, H. F., and Mann, C. V.: Has the incidence of radiation-induced bowel damage following treatment of uterine carcinoma changed in the last 20 years? J. R. Soc. Med., 79:387, 1986.
2. Allen-Mersh, T. G., Wilson, E. J., Hope-Stone, H. F., and Mann, C. V.: The management of late radiation-induced rectal injury after treatment of carcinoma of the uterus. Surg. Gynecol. Obstet., 164:521, 1987.
3. Bakare, S. C., Shafir, M., and McElhinney, A. J.: Exclusion of small bowel from pelvis for postoperative radiotherapy for rectal cancer. J. Surg. Oncol., 35:55, 1987.
4. Berthrong, M.: Pathologic changes secondary to radiation. World J. Surg., 10:155, 1986.
5. Brady, L. W., Markioe, A. M., Sheline, G. E., Suntharalingam, N., and Sutherland, R. M.: Radiation oncology: Programs for the present and future. Cancer, 55:2037, 1985.
6. Bricker, E. M., Kraybill, W. G., and Lopez, M. J.: Functional results after postirradiation rectal reconstruction. World J. Surg., 10:249, 1986.
7. Champlin, R.: The role of bone marrow transplantation for nuclear accidents: Implications of the Chernobyl disaster. Semin. Hematol., 24:1, 1987.
8. Cox, J. D., Byhardt, R. W., Wilson, J. F., Haas, J. S., Komaki, R., and Olson, L. E.: Complications of radiation therapy and factors in their prevention. World J. Surg., 10:171, 1986.
9. DeCosse, J. J., Rhodes, R. S., Wentz, W. B., Regan, J. W., Dworken, H. J., and Holden, W. D.: The natural history and management of radiation-induced injury of the gastrointestinal tract. Ann. Surg., 170:369, 1970.
10. Delaney, J. P., Bonsack, M., and Hall, P.: Intestinal radioprotection by two new agents applied topically. Ann. Surg., 216:417, 1992.
11. Galland, R. B., and Spencer, J.: Surgical management of radiation enteritis. Surgery, 99:133, 1986.
12. Gazet, J. C.: Parks' coloanal pull-through anastomosis for severe, complicated radiation proctitis. Dis. Colon Rectum, 28:110, 1985.
13. Henriksson, R., Franzen, L., and Littbrand, B.: Prevention of irradiation-induced bowel discomfort by sucralfate. Am. J. Med., 91(suppl. 2A):151, 1991.
14. Kavanah, M. T., Feldman, M. I., Devereux, D. F., and Kondi, E. S.: New surgical approach to minimize radiation-associated small bowel injury in patients with pelvic malignancies requiring surgery and high-dose irradiation. Cancer, 56:1300, 1985.
15. Kimose, H. H., Fischer, L., Spjelldnaes, N., and Wara, P.: Late radiation injury of the colon and rectum: Surgical management and outcome. Dis. Colon Rectum, 32:684, 1989.
16. Klimber, V. S., Souba, W. W., Dolson, D. J., Salloum, R. M., Hautamaki, R. D., Plumley, D. A., Mendenhall, W. R., Bova, F. C., Bland, K. I., and Copeland, E. M.: Prophylactic glutamine protects the intestinal mucosa from radiation injury. Cancer, 66:62, 1990.
17. Kochhar, R., Patel, F., Dhar, A., Sharma, S. C., Ayyagari, S., Aggarwal, R., Goenka, M. K., Gupta, B. D., and Mehta, S. K.: Radiation-induced proctosigmoiditis: Prospective randomized, double-blind controlled trial of oral sulfasalazine plus rectal steroids versus rectal sucralfate. Dig. Dis. Sci., 36:103, 1991.
18. Kohn, H. I., and Fry, R. J. M.: Radiation carcinogenesis. N. Engl. J. Med., 310:304, 1984.
19. Kollmorgen, C. F., Meagher, A. P., Wolff, B. G., Pemberton, S. H., Martenson, J. A., and Ilstrup, D. M.: The long-term effect of adjuvant postoperative chemoradiotherapy for rectal carcinoma on bowel function. Ann. Surg., 220:676, 1994.
20. Makela, J., Nevasaari, K., and Kairaluomo, M. I.: Surgical treatment of intestinal radiation injury. J. Surg. Oncol., 36:93, 1987.
21. Mason, G. R., Dietrich, P., Friedland, G. W., and Hanks, G. E.: The radiological findings in radiation-induced enteritis and colitis. Clin. Radiol., 21:232, 1970.
22. Miholic, J., Schwarz, C., and Moeschl, P.: Surgical therapy of radiation-induced lesions of the colon and rectum. Am. J. Surg., 155:761, 1988.
23. Morganstern, L., Hart, M., Lugo, D., and Friedman, N.: Changing aspects of radiation enteropathy. Arch. Surg., 120:1225, 1985.
24. Muller, H. J.: Radiation damage to genetic material. Am. Sci., 38:33, 1950.
25. Parks, A. G., Allen, C. L. O., Frank, J. D., and McPartlin, J. F.: A method of treating post-irradiation rectovaginal fistulas. Br. J. Surg., 65:417, 1978.
26. Quastler, H.: The nature of intestinal radiation death. Radiat. Res., 4:303, 1956.
27. Rubin, P.: The Franz Bushke lecture: Late effects of chemotherapy and radiation therapy: A new hypothesis. Int. J. Radiat. Oncol. Biol. Phys., 10:5, 1984.
28. Russell, J. C., and Welch, J. P.: Operative management of radiation injuries to the intestinal tract. Am. J. Surg., 137:433, 1979.
29. Schellhammer, P. F., Jordan, G. H., and El-Mahdi, A. M.: Pelvic complications after interstitial and external beam irradiation of urologic and gynecologic malignancy. World J. Surg., 10:259, 1986.
30. Schofield, P. F., Carr, N. D., and Holden, D.: Pathogenesis and treatment of radiation bowel disease: Discussion paper. J. R. Soc. Med., 79:3030, 1986.
31. Smith, D. H., and DeCosse, J. J.: Radiation damage to the small intestine. World J. Surg., 10:189, 1986.
32. Varma, J. S., and Smith, A. N.: Anorectal function following coloanal sleeve anastomosis for chronic radiation injury to the rectum. Br. J. Surg., 73:285, 1986.
33. Wiseman, J. S., Senagore, A. J., and Chaudry, I. H.: Methods to prevent colonic injury in pelvic radiation. Dis. Colon Rectum, 37:1090, 1994.

X

APPENDICITIS

David C. Sabiston, Jr., M.D.

All physicians should have a thorough knowledge of appendicitis. Although most patients with acute appendicitis can be easily diagnosed, there are many in whom the signs and symptoms are quite variable, and a firm clinical diagnosis may be difficult to establish. It is for this reason that the diagnosis is made rather *liberally*, with the full expectation that some patients will be operated on and found to have a normal appendix. It is preferable to maintain broad indications, as this tends to include the group of patients with indefinite signs and symptoms who actually have the disease but do not fulfill the classic criteria for the diagnosis. Following this course, patients who might proceed to perforation of the appendix, with a host of possible secondary complications, are spared that fate. Therefore, it is generally agreed that 10% to 15% of patients having a diagnosis of acute appendicitis by acceptable standards in most hospitals will actually be found at operation to have a normal appendix.[8]

HISTORIC ASPECTS

There are a number of early reports of inflammation in and around the appendix that have been carefully summarized in a scholarly review by Williams.[12] Much credit is due Reginald Fitz for the first accurate description of acute appendicitis in 1886.[4] He clearly described the clinical history, physical findings, and pathologic aspects of acute appendicitis and advocated appendectomy as the appropriate treatment. Following this report, others rapidly accepted his concepts and urged that appendectomy be done prior to rupture of the appendix. Although appendicitis was formerly associated with a relatively high morbidity and mortality, today the vast majority of patients with acute appendicitis are diagnosed early in the course of the disease and undergo appendectomy with excellent results.

ANATOMY

The vermiform appendix is located in the right lower quadrant, arises from the cecum, and is generally 6 to 10 cm. in length. It has a separate mesoappendix with an appendicular artery and vein that are branches of the ileocolic vessels. The appendix is lined with colonic epithelium characterized by many lymph follicles numbering approximately 200, with the highest number occurring in the 10- to 20-year-old age group. After the age of 30, the number of lymph follicles is reduced to a trace, with total absence of lymphoid tissue occurring after the age of 60. The appendix may lie in a number of locations, essentially at any position on a clockwise rotation from the base of the cecum. It is important to emphasize that the *anatomic* position of the appendix determines the symptoms and the site of the muscular spasm and tenderness when the appendix becomes inflamed (Fig. 31–40).

PATHOPHYSIOLOGY

The pathogenesis of acute appendicitis is dependent primarily on obstruction of the appendiceal lumen. The most common pathologic cause of obstruction is marked hyperplasia of the lymphoid follicles, which obstruct the lumen. This occurs in approximately 60% of patients, most of whom are in the younger age groups. The presence of a fecalith may also be a cause of obstruction and occurs in some 35% of patients. In the remainder, foreign bodies, inflammatory strictures, and other rare causes are responsible. At times, no specific inciting cause can be found, and in some of these patients, it is probable that a fecalith initiated the inflammation and peristalsis propelled it into the lumen of the cecum.

Mucus continues to be secreted into the lumen following obstruction of the appendiceal lumen. Stasis is created by the obstruction, and bacteria multiply and secrete exotoxins and endotoxins, which damage the epithelium and ulcerate the mucosa. Bacteria can then penetrate through the ulcerated mucosa into the muscular layers of the appendix and establish an inflammatory process. The increased pressure within the lumen also elevates the interstitial pressure in the wall of the appendix, impeding arterial blood flow and creating a state of ischemia, with ultimate infarction and gangrene of the appendix. As the muscular layers become necrotic, perforation of the appendix occurs. Depending on the duration of the inflammatory process, either a walled-off abscess occurs at the site or, if the pathologic process has advanced rapidly, the perforation occurs free into the peritoneal cavity and causes generalized peritonitis. If the latter occurs, a very serious clinical situation ensues, and multiple intraperitoneal abscesses may follow at various sites in the pelvis and subhepatic and subdiaphragmatic spaces.

CLINICAL DIAGNOSIS

The diagnosis of acute appendicitis is made primarily on the basis of the history and the physical findings, with additional assistance from laboratory examinations. The *typical* history is one of onset of generalized abdominal pain followed by anorexia and nausea. The pain then becomes most prominent in the epigastrium and gradually moves toward the umbilicus, finally localizing in the right lower quadrant. Vomiting may occur during this time. Examination of the abdomen usually shows diminished bowel sounds, with direct tenderness and spasm in the right lower quadrant. As the process continues, the amount of spasm increases, with the appearance of rebound tenderness. The temperature is usually mildly elevated (approximately 38° C.) and usually rises to higher levels in the event of perforation. Direct tenderness is usually present in the right lower quadrant and may involve other parts of the abdomen, particularly if perforation has occurred. The appendix is usually situated at or around McBurney's point (a point one third of the way on a line drawn from the anterior superior spine to the umbilicus). However, it must be emphasized that the exact *anatomic location* of the appendix can be at any point on a 360-degree circle surrounding the base of the cecum, as shown in Figure 31–40. This is the site where the pain and tenderness are usually maximal, and the exact site may vary from patient to patient.

Rovsing's sign, elicited when pressure applied in the left lower quadrant reflects pain to the right lower quadrant, is often present. The *psoas* sign may be positive and is elicited by extension of the right thigh with the patient lying on the left side. As the examiner extends the right thigh with stretching of the muscle, pain suggests the presence of an inflamed appendix overlying the psoas muscle. The *obturator* sign can be elicited with the patient in the supine position with passive rotation of the flexed right thigh. Pain with this maneuver indicates a positive sign. Rectal examination generally elicits tenderness at the site of the inflamed appendix in the right lower quadrant. If the appendix ruptures, abdominal pain becomes intense and more diffuse, the muscular spasm increases, and there is a simultaneous increase

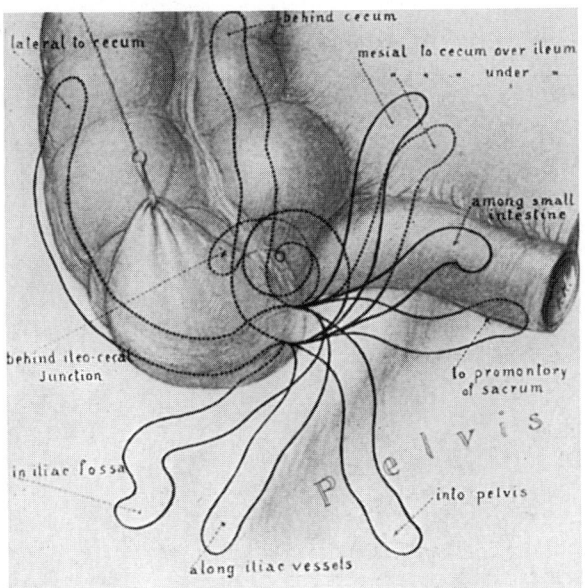

Figure 31–40. Diagram showing the various directions in which the appendix may be located. (From Kelly, H. A., and Hurdon, E.: The Vermiform Appendix and Its Diseases. Philadelphia, W. B. Saunders, 1905.)

in the heart rate above 100, with a rise in temperature to 39° or 40° C. At this time, the patient appears toxic, and it becomes obvious that the clinical situation has deteriorated.

LABORATORY DATA

The clinical history and physical examination are most important in establishing a diagnosis of acute appendicitis, but laboratory findings may be helpful. The majority of patients with acute appendicitis have an elevated leukocyte count of 10,000 to 20,000. For those in whom the level is normal, there is generally a shift to the left in the differential leukocyte count, indicating acute inflammation. However, it should be emphasized that a number of patients have a *normal* leukocyte count, especially the elderly. Urinary analysis may show a few red cells, indicating some inflammatory contact with the ureter or urinary bladder; a significant number of erythrocytes in the urine indicates a primary disorder of the urinary tract.

Radiographic studies are not indicated in classic cases of acute appendicitis but may be useful when the diagnosis is in doubt. Plain films of the abdomen may show a dilated cecum and fluid level and occasionally a calcified fecalith or foreign body. Barium enema may show an absence of filling of the appendix, which is suggestive of acute appendicitis. If the lumen of the appendix fills with barium, acute appendicitis is quite unlikely. *Ultrasonography* examination is sometimes helpful and may show signs indicating an enlarged appendix or an abscess. Similarly, a computed tomography (CT) scan of the abdomen may be helpful, particularly in establishing the presence of an abscess. However, it should be emphasized that in the vast majority of patients, these special studies are unnecessary and delay surgical therapy. It should also be mentioned that laparoscopic examination may be used to establish the diagnosis and, in appropriate instances, for appendectomy.

DIFFERENTIAL DIAGNOSIS

There are a number of acute abdominal disorders producing signs and symptoms similar to those of acute appendicitis.[9] These include acute gastroenteritis, cholecystitis, pyelitis, salpingitis, tubo-ovarian abscess, and ruptured ovarian cyst. Although diarrhea may occur with acute appendicitis, it is much more common with gastroenteritis. In young children, intussusception enters the differential diagnosis. Other less common differential disorders include ureteral stones, cystitis, perforated peptic ulcer, ectopic pregnancy, acute regional enteritis (particularly the first attack), epididymitis, and testicular torsion. If a patient persists in having pain in the right lower quadrant that cannot be explained by some other definitive diagnosis, the patient should be considered to have acute appendicitis and should be operated on or at least carefully observed.

TREATMENT

For the vast majority of patients with a diagnosis of acute appendicitis, the appropriate management is appendectomy. For patients with simple acute appendicitis, intravenous fluids should be initiated as well as an antibiotic agent effective against both aerobic and anaerobic organisms.[3] All patients are begun on antibiotics preoperatively and maintained postoperatively as needed. If the appendix is unruptured and not gangrenous, antibiotics can be discontinued after 24 hours. Although many agents are effective, cefoxitin is often the agent of choice on the basis of a multicenter randomized trial of 1735 patients. Half received 2 gm. of cefoxitin preoperatively. Three groups were evaluated: patients with a normal

appendix, those with an acutely inflamed appendix, and those with a gangrenous appendix. The incidence of wound infection was significantly lower in all three groups. However, the formation of intra-abdominal abscess was not influenced by preoperative antibiotics.[3] In a recent double-blind controlled study, prophylactic cefotetan was compared with prophylactic cefoxitin in the development of postoperative wound infections in patients with acute nonperforated appendicitis.[10] The results showed that single-dose cefotetan and multiple-dose cefoxitin are equally effective. However, because of the greater convenience and decreased cost, single-dose cefotetan was considered the prophylaxis of choice in appendectomy for nonperforated appendicitis.[10] Clindamycin with an aminoglycoside is indicated when *Bacteroides fragilis* is present; metronidazole can also be used for this organism.

Surgical Management

After appropriate preoperative preparation, a decision is made whether the appendix is to be removed by the *open* or the *laparoscopic* approach. If the open operation is done, anesthesia is administered, and a transverse incision is made in the skin lines in the right lower quadrant. The appendix is exposed through a gridiron, muscle-splitting incision (Fig. 31–41). If peritoneal fluid or exudate is present upon opening the peritoneum, the fluid should be cultured and the appendix exposed. Careful observation is made of the pathologic state and especially of the site of perforation or abscess formation. The appendix is then removed, as illustrated in Figures 31–42 through 31–44. If an abscess is present, it may be drained, but if *generalized* peritonitis is present, this is usually unnecessary.

If a normal appendix is found, additional exploration should follow to eliminate other possible causes, including inspection of the cecum and colon for inflammatory or neoplastic lesions, the terminal ileum for a Meckel's diverticulum, and the gallbladder and duodenum for primary disease. If further evidence of intra-abdominal disease is present, it

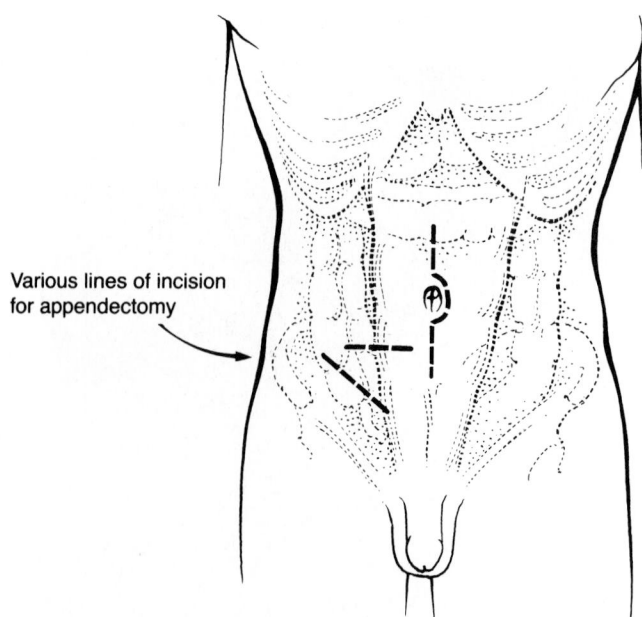

Various lines of incision for appendectomy

Figure 31–41. The incision for appendectomy can be a midline incision; a right lower quadrant transverse incision overlying the rectus muscle, with reflection of the muscle medially; or a gridiron, muscle-splitting incision. (From Sabiston, D. C., Jr. [Ed.]: Atlas of General Surgery. Philadelphia, W. B. Saunders, 1994.)

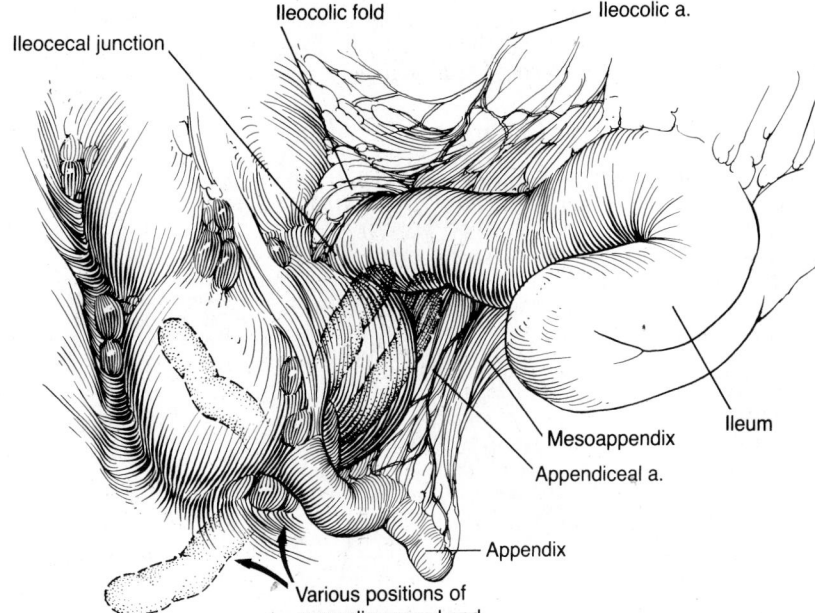

Figure 31–42. The appendix is located at the junction of the taeniae of the colonic wall at the tip of the cecum. It is supplied by the appendiceal artery, which must be ligated during removal of the appendix. It may be located in nearly any position, including retrocecal and extending upward toward the hepatic flexure of the colon. (From Sabiston, D. C., Jr. [Ed.]: Atlas of General Surgery. Philadelphia, W. B. Saunders, 1994.)

Ileocecal junction
Ileocolic fold
Ileocolic a.
Mesoappendix
Appendiceal a.
Ileum
Appendix
Various positions of appendix around and behind cecum

Ligature being placed
Ligature tied and base of appendix being transected
Pursestring suture
Base of appendix crushed

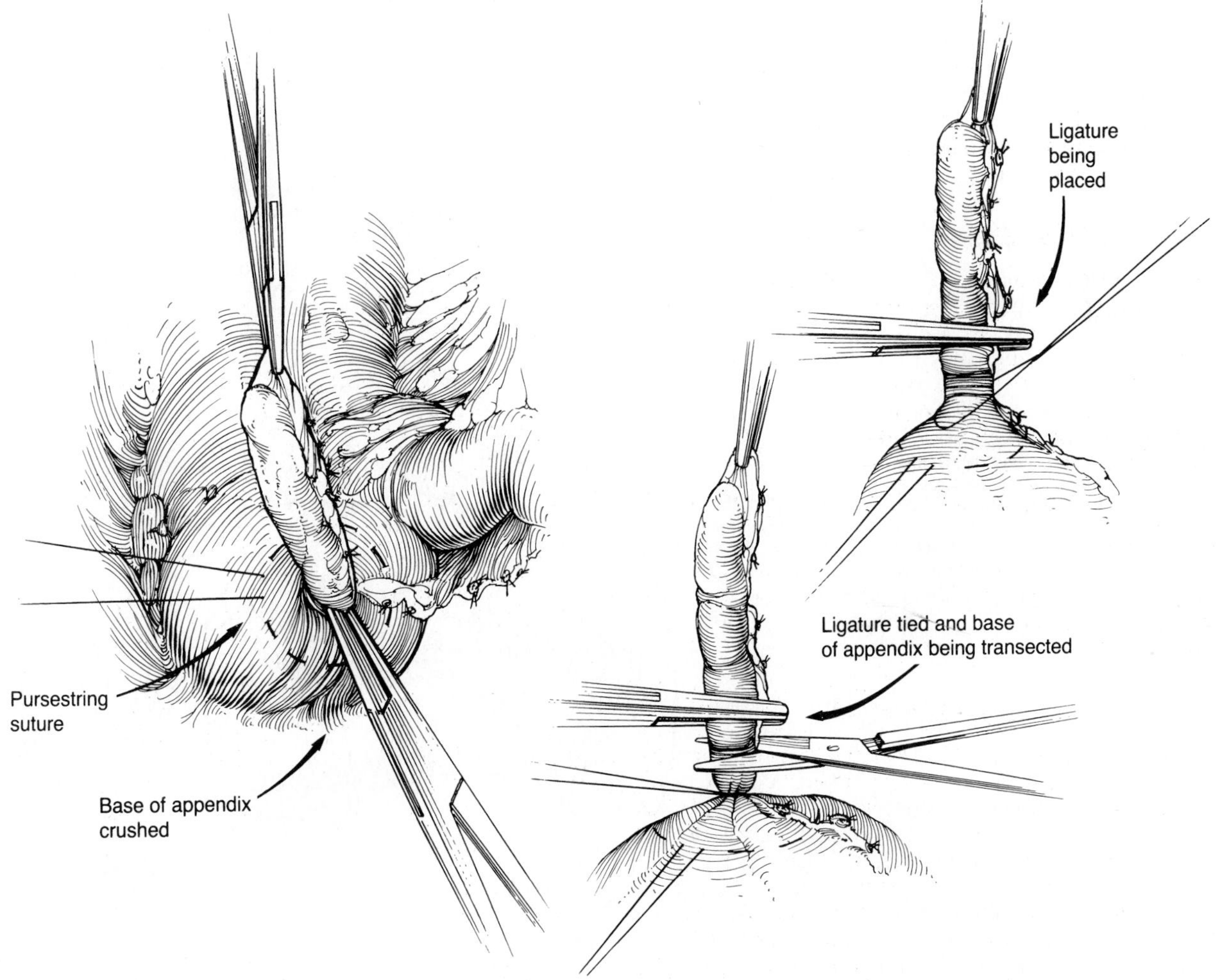

Figure 31–43. A pursestring suture is placed at the base of the appendix to crush the tissue. The lower hemostat is removed, and a 1-0 chromic catgut ligature is placed. (From Sabiston, D. C., Jr. [Ed.]: Atlas of General Surgery. Philadelphia, W. B. Saunders, 1994.)

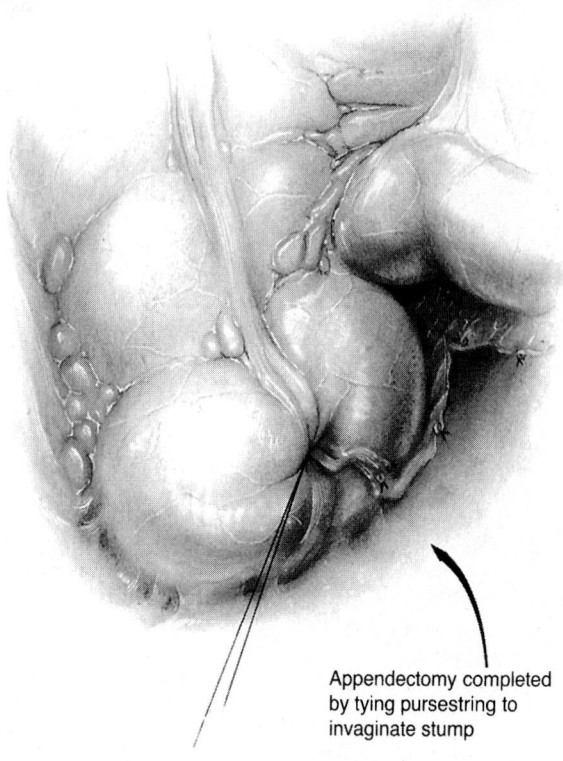

Figure 31–44. The appendix is divided, and the stump is invaginated by tying the pursestring suture. (From Sabiston, D. C., Jr. [Ed.]: Atlas of General Surgery. Philadelphia, W. B. Saunders, 1994.)

Appendectomy completed
by tying pursestring to
invaginate stump

Figure 31–45. A 10-mm. trocar is placed in the left lower quadrant in a tangential manner, obviating the need for closure of the fascia at the completion of the procedure. The abdomen is visually explored, and appendicitis is confirmed. An Endoloop is placed through a 5-mm. trocar, and the end of the appendix is snared for retraction. The mesoappendix is then easily visualized. (From Sabiston, D. C., Jr. [Ed.]: Atlas of General Surgery. Philadelphia, W. B. Saunders, 1994.)

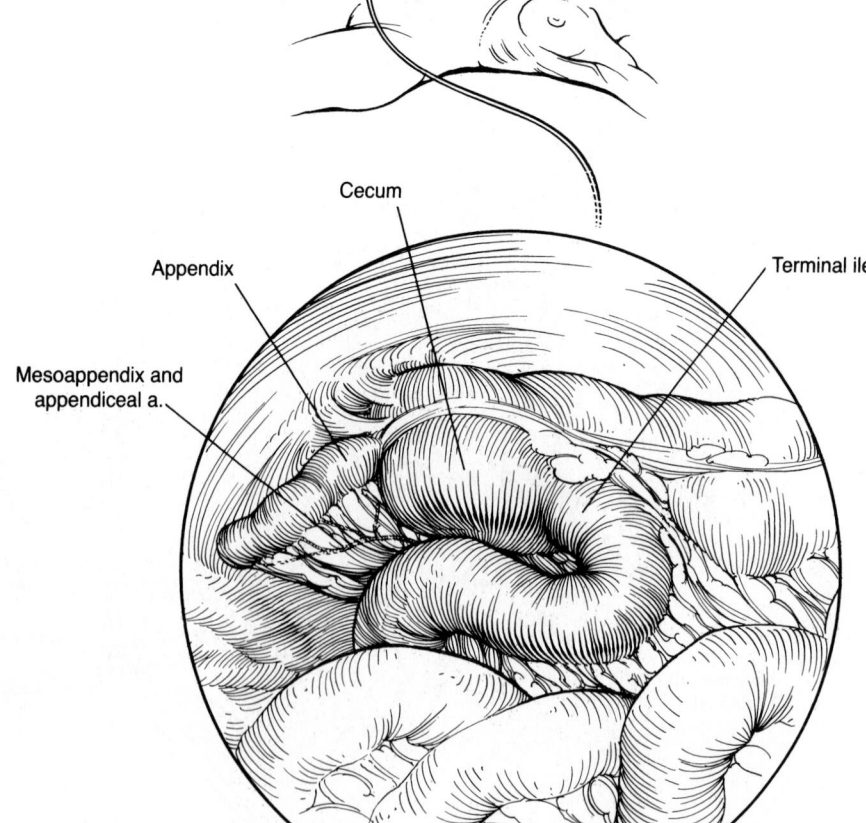

Cecum

Appendix

Terminal ileum

Mesoappendix and
appendiceal a.

may be necessary to enlarge the incision or perform a midline incision for more adequate exposure.

The laparoscopic approach may be chosen for selected patients. When the diagnosis is uncertain, this approach is helpful in achieving a more thorough examination of the abdominal contents. This procedure is shown in Figures 31–45 and 31–46. In a prospective, randomized trial comparing open versus laparoscopic appendectomy, 37 patients were assigned to the open appendectomy group and 38 patients to the laparoscopic group. It was concluded that patients who underwent laparoscopic appendectomy had a shorter duration of pain and returned to full activities sooner postoperatively than those undergoing open appendectomy. It was concluded that laparoscopic appendectomy is the procedure of choice in patients with acute appendicitis.[5]

Nonsurgical Management of Appendiceal Abscess

At times, a patient with an appendiceal perforation is seen late in the course of the disease and has a walled-off abscess in the right lower quadrant.[2] At this point, the process may be subsiding, with minimal systemic findings. In this situation, it may be appropriate to treat the patient with antibiotics and intravenous fluids and careful observation. When the process resolves, usually requiring 6 weeks to 3 months, an interval appendectomy should be performed, because the likelihood of recurrent appendicitis is quite high. Under these circumstances, it is preferable to remove the appendix electively rather than as an emergency.

Incidental appendectomy during the course of other abdominal operations has been raised, and opinion is divided. Elective appendectomy is probably performed most often in conjunction with gynecologic procedures. Removal of the appendix in these circumstances eliminates the possibility of postoperative acute appendicitis in patients who may later develop problems in the right lower quadrant. However, most surgeons do not electively remove a normal appendix during the course of general surgical procedures. There is also the likelihood that the rate of wound infection would be increased.[7]

SPECIAL FEATURES OF ACUTE APPENDICITIS

Appendicitis in infants and young children is difficult to diagnose preoperatively, since these patients cannot provide a history. Therefore, it is unusual to make a firm diagnosis in a patient under the age of 1 year unless perforation has occurred.

Acute appendicitis during pregnancy also presents diagnostic problems, because during the third trimester, the uterus is rapidly enlarging and causes displacement of the cecum and appendix into the right upper abdomen. Thus, acute appendicitis in these patients causes symptoms and signs higher and more lateral during the third trimester.[6]

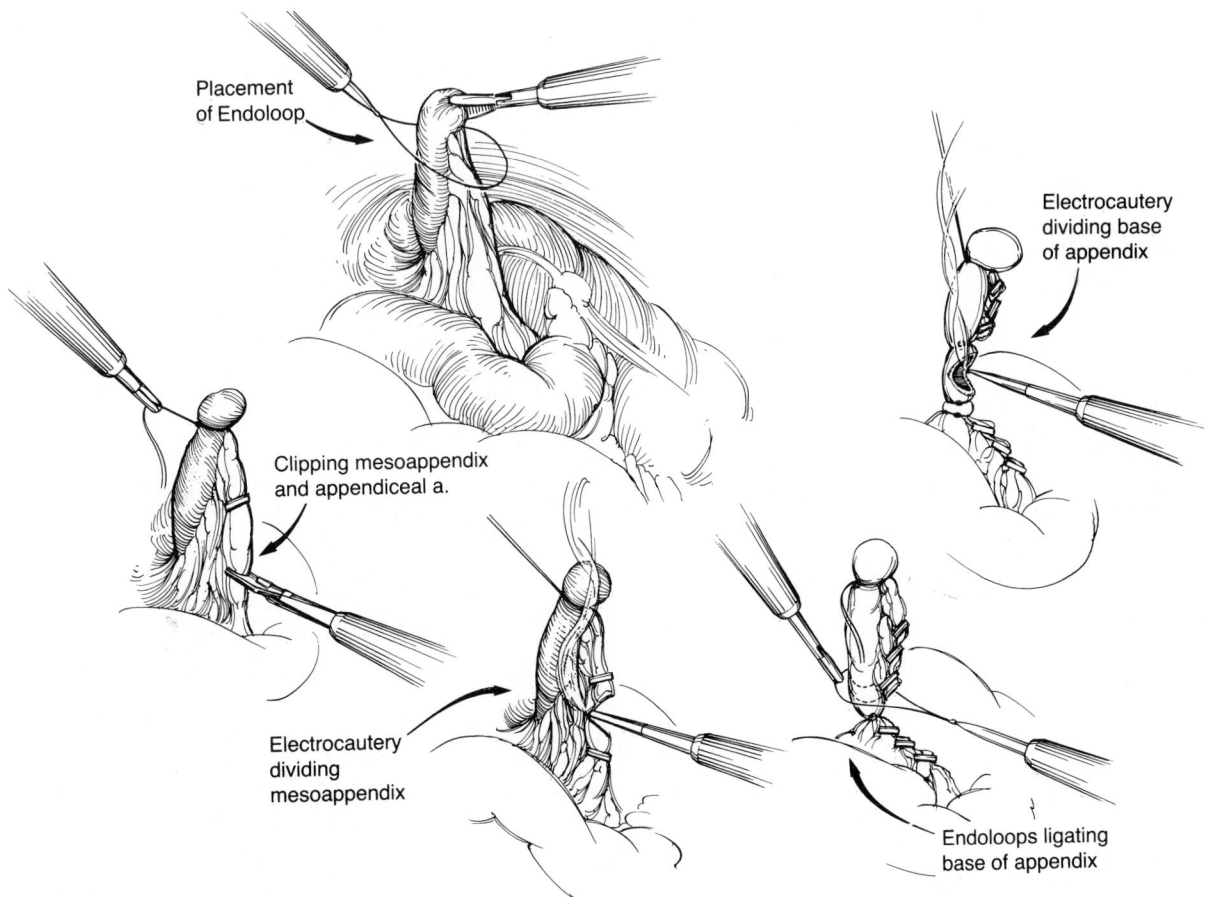

Placement of Endoloop

Clipping mesoappendix and appendiceal a.

Electrocautery dividing mesoappendix

Electrocautery dividing base of appendix

Endoloops ligating base of appendix

Figure 31–46. The mesoappendix is dissected via the 10-mm. port. The appendiceal artery and associated fat are controlled with electrocautery and clips. When the base of the appendix is easily seen, three additional Endoloops are placed sequentially on the appendix. Two are placed on the cecal side, and one is placed on the side of the specimen. The specimen is transected. Alternatively, an endoscopic linear stapler can be used through a 12-mm. port in the left lower quadrant to control both the appendiceal stump and the appendiceal artery. The electrocautery is used to cauterize the mucosa on the appendiceal stump. (From Sabiston, D. C., Jr. [Ed.]: Atlas of General Surgery. Philadelphia, W. B. Saunders, 1994.)

Appendicitis in young women also introduces a number of specific differential diagnoses, particularly those involving tubo-ovarian disorders. For these, *culdoscopy* or *laparoscopy* may be helpful in revealing the problem.

In the elderly, appendicitis may present with different clinical manifestations than in younger patients. The general tendency is for the *inflammatory* components to be less pronounced. The temperature is usually lower, as is the leukocyte count, and there is frequently less pain and tenderness. At times, the appendix in this age group may perforate with an abscess without causing the patient a significant earlier problem.

CARCINOMA OF THE APPENDIX

In one series of 5000 appendices, 41 cases of adenocarcinoma were found. Therefore, carcinoma of the appendix is an unusual neoplasm. The most common lesion is a carcinoid and accounts for some 90% of all primary tumors of the appendix. Malignant mucoceles are regarded as being well-differentiated adenocarcinomas. The clinical presentation of most patients with appendiceal carcinoma is typical of that for acute appendicitis. In many instances, the appendix is perforated, with a localized appendiceal abscess that requires drainage. In a study from the Mayo Clinic, 94 consecutive patients with adenocarcinoma of the appendix were evaluated (excluding patients with carcinoid). Of the group, 52 patients (55%) had mucinous tumors, of which 22 had pseudomyxoma peritonei. The most common presentation was that of acute appendicitis. The 5-year cure rate was 55% and varied with the stage: A, 100%; B, 67%; C, 50%; and D, 6%. Right hemicolectomy produced a higher survival (68%) than appendectomy alone (20%). For this reason, it was concluded that right hemicolectomy is indicated in treating carcinoma of the appendix.[11]

SELECTED REFERENCES

Bauer, T.: Antibiotic prophylaxis in acute nonperforated appendicitis: The Danish Multicenter Study Group III. Ann. Surg., *209*:307, 1989.
This multicenter study concerns the appropriate prophylactic regimen for the management of patients with acute nonperforated appendicitis. Definitive conclusions are drawn from the study, and it can be recommended as a reference for the role of antibiotics and prophylactic prevention of wound infection following appendectomy for acute appendicitis.

Frazee, R. C., Roberts, J. W., Symmonds, R. E., Snyder, S. K., Hendricks, J. C., Smith, R. W., Custer, M. D., 3rd, and Harrison, J. B.: A prospective randomized trial comparing open versus laparoscopic appendectomy. Ann. Surg., *219*:725, 1994.
In this study, a number of variables were considered, and it was concluded that patients undergoing laparoscopic appendectomy had a shorter duration of pain and returned to full activity sooner postoperatively than did patients with open appendectomy.

Liberman, M. A., Greason, K. L., Frame, S., and Ragland, J. J.: Single-dose cefotetan or cefoxitin versus multiple-dose cefoxitin as prophylaxis in patients undergoing appendectomy for acute nonperforated appendicitis. J. Am. Coll. Surg., *180*:77, 1995.
The authors report a double-blind controlled study of the use of cefotetan and cefoxitin to prevent postoperative wound infections in patients with acute nonperforated appendicitis. It was concluded that single-dose cefotetan is preferable.

Nitecki, S. S., Wolff, B. G., Schlinkert, R., and Sarr, M. G.: The natural history of surgically treated primary adenocarcinoma of the appendix. Ann. Surg., *219*:51, 1994.
The authors evaluate the natural history of surgically treated primary adenocarcinoma of the appendix in 94 consecutive patients. It was concluded that long-term survival is much improved by right hemicolectomy as compared with appendectomy alone.

REFERENCES

1. Anderson, A., Bergdahl, L., and Boquist, L.: Primary carcinoma of the appendix. Ann. Surg., *183*:53, 1976.
2. Arnbjornsson, E.: Management of appendiceal abscess. Curr. Surg., *41*:4, 1984.
3. Bauer, T.: Antibiotic prophylaxis in acute nonperforated appendicitis: The Danish Multicenter Study Group III. Ann. Surg., *209*:307, 1989.
4. Fitz, R. H.: Perforating inflammation of the vermiform appendix, with special reference to its early diagnosis and treatment. Trans. Assoc. Am. Physicians, *1*:107, 1886.
5. Frazee, R. C., Roberts, J. W., Symmonds, R. E., Snyder, S. K., Hendricks, J. C., Smith, R. W., Custer, M. D., 3rd, and Harrison, J. B.: A prospective randomized trial comparing open versus laparoscopic appendectomy. Ann. Surg., *219*:725, 1994.
6. Gomez, A., and Wood, M.: Acute appendicitis during pregnancy. Am. J. Surg., *137*:180, 1979.
7. Hayes, R. J.: Incidental appendectomies: Current teaching. JAMA, *238*:31, 1977.
8. Hobson, T., and Rosenman, L. D.: Acute appendicitis—when is it right to be wrong? Am. J. Surg., *108*:306, 1964.
9. Lewis, F. R., Holcroft, J. W., Boey, J., and Dunphy, J. E.: Appendicitis: A critical review of diagnosis and treatment in 1000 cases. Arch. Surg., *110*:677, 1975.
10. Liberman, M. A., Greason, K. L., Frame, S., and Ragland, J. J.: Single-dose cefotetan or cefoxitin versus multiple-dose cefoxitin as prophylaxis in patients undergoing appendectomy for acute nonperforated appendicitis. J. Am. Coll. Surg., *180*:77, 1995.
11. Nitecki, S. S., Wolff, B. G., Schlinkert, R., and Sarr, M. G.: The natural history of surgically treated primary adenocarcinoma of the appendix. Ann. Surg., *219*:51, 1994.
12. Williams, G. R.: A history of appendicitis with anecdotes illustrating its importance. Ann. Surg., *197*:495, 1983.

CHAPTER 32

THE COLON AND RECTUM

I —————————————————————————————————————

SURGICAL ANATOMY AND OPERATIVE PROCEDURES

Rolando Rolandelli, M.D., and Joel J. Roslyn, M.D.

The large intestine, or colon, extends from the ileocecal valve to the anus and is divided into the cecum, ascending and transverse colon, splenic flexure, descending and sigmoid colon, rectosigmoid, rectum, and anus. Although the average length of the large intestine is 135 to 150 cm., the location of the various anatomic divisions varies from person to person. The function of the colon, water absorption and evacuation of fecal waste, has been known for many years, but the mechanisms by which these specific activities are accomplished continue to be investigated. Surgical procedures are frequently performed in the management of patients with colonic diseases. A successful outcome depends largely on each surgeon's understanding and appreciation of anatomy, physiology, pathology, and microbiology of the colon.

SURGICAL ANATOMY

The colon originates in the right lower quadrant and courses in a horseshoe manner around the upper abdomen and down to the left lower quadrant and into the pelvis. Its anatomic relationships to both peritoneal and retroperitoneal organs are important for the surgeon when managing patients with colonic diseases. Although the colon is generally considered to be an intraperitoneal organ, the ascending and descending segments are frequently fixed by retroperitoneal attachments that give a portion of its circumference a retroperitoneal location. Developmental anomalies may affect the location of the ascending or sigmoid colon. The transverse colon is supported by a mesentery and found in a horizontal position or in a more dependent position traversing freely into the lower abdomen. The propensity to develop a cecal or sigmoid volvulus (i.e., a twist of the colon around its mesentery) is due to lax fixation of these organs to the retroperitoneum. Embryologically, the large intestine rotates in a counterclockwise manner around the axis of the superior mesenteric artery. The cecum rotates from the left side of the abdomen and comes to lie, in most individuals, in the right lower quadrant. Anomalies can occur in which the cecum arrests its development, causing malrotation. The cecum can, therefore, be found in the left or right upper quadrants of the abdomen. Although this change in location may not directly influence normal function, it may obscure the diagnosis of an otherwise straightforward condition such as appendicitis.

The colon contains the same inner circular muscular layer below the serosa as does the small bowel, but its outer longitudinal muscle layer is quite distinct. This outer longitudinal muscular coat is concentrated into three separate longitudinal strips, known as taeniae coli, which give the colon a characteristic appearance. At the level of the rectosigmoid junction, the taeniae generally coalesce and provide a complete longitudinal muscular coat for the rectum. The configuration of the taeniae coli and their state of contraction are responsible for the formation of haustra, which are sacculations or protrusions of the bowel wall between the taeniae. Unlike the valvulae conniventes of the small intestine, the haustra of the colon only partially encircle the large intestine. Their appearance on simple radiographs of the abdomen is characteristic and often allows distinction of the colon from the small intestine. The third gross characteristic unique to the colon is the appendices epiploicae, which are extensions of peritoneal fat.

The Ileocecal Valve and Cecum. The ileocecal valve is a sphincter located at the junction of the terminal ileum and the cecum. The fusion of an upper and lower lip, the muscular nature of which is not unlike the cecum itself, serves to function as a sphincter that prevents the reflux of material from the cecum back into the terminal ileum. The internal diameter of the colon is largest at the cecum, measuring 7 to 9 cm. The cecum is enveloped by peritoneum and free in the abdomen in most individuals. Therefore, the cecum usually has a certain degree of mobility that makes possible the development of cecal volvulus. As a result of the large diameter of the cecum, lesions such as tumors in this area rarely cause early obstructive symptoms but instead present in a more indolent course, frequently with anemia and generalized fatigue or other constitutional symptoms. Because of the characteristics of the cecum and Laplace's law, the cecum is usually the site of bursting when a lesion produces distal colonic obstruction and the ileocecal valve is continent.

The vermiform appendix generally projects from the inferior aspect of the medial portion of the cecum. Its length is variable, and it may ultimately come to lie in a pelvic or retrocecal position.

Ascending Colon and Hepatic Flexure. Coursing upward from the cecum to the transverse colon is the ascending colon and the hepatic flexure, which is the portion of the colon that turns medially and joins the transverse colon. During mobilization of the ascending colon and hepatic flexure, care must be exercised by the surgeon not to injure the right ureter or the duodenum. Occasionally, tumors involving the hepatic flexure can erode into the duodenum.

Transverse Colon. The transverse colon generally measures 35 to 50 cm. in length and lies between the hepatic flexure in the right upper quadrant and the splenic flexure in the left upper quadrant. It is the most mobile portion of the colon and may be found in the upper abdomen or as far down as the pelvis. With the exception of its most proximal and distal connections with the hepatic and splenic flexures, respectively, the transverse colon is generally considered to be completely intraperitoneal. It is suspended by the transverse mesocolon and is frequently enveloped anteriorly by the junction of the greater omentum and mesocolon. This area is frequently the site of either primary colonic tumors or neoplastic involvement from contiguous spread from gastric or pancreatic malignancies.

Splenic Flexure. The angle between the distal transverse colon and the descending colon is designated the splenic flexure and is frequently more angulated and in a more cephalad position than the hepatic flexure. The phrenocolic and splenocolic attachments should be carefully considered during mobilization of the splenic flexure to avoid injury to the spleen.

Descending Colon. The descending colon courses from the splenic flexure down into the sigmoid colon at the level of the pelvic brim and measures 20 to 25 cm. It is only partially peritonealized, is frequently in intimate association with the left ureter, and rarely has a free mesentery.

Sigmoid Colon. The sigmoid colon is the S-shaped segment of the colon that extends from the pelvic brim to the peritoneal reflection, where it joins the rectum. The sigmoid colon is frequently redundant, and its length varies between 10 and 30 cm. In some individuals the mesentery may become elongated and produce a sigmoid volvulus. Regardless of the extent and length of sigmoid colon, a constant finding is that it is situated 15 to 18 cm. from the anus. Therefore, tumors of the sigmoid colon can be visualized with a rigid sigmoidoscope.

Rectum. The junction between the sigmoid colon and the rectum is frequently marked by a flexure, with the rectum being directed posteriorly and downward to conform to the curve of the sacrum. As the rectum proceeds distally, the lumen enlarges. The most distal fusiform segment is frequently known as the rectal ampulla. There is considerable mobility in the rectum, and it is generally not fixed to the sacrum. As the rectum descends into the pelvis, the peritoneal investment becomes less apparent, such that the distal portion of the rectum has essentially no peritoneal covering. Therefore, much of the rectum can be considered extraperitoneal. The mobility of the rectum is responsible for the variability, and apparent change in location of rectal tumors, as when comparing preoperative assessment with intraoperative findings. The better understanding of the relationship of the rectum to the surrounding sphincteric mechanism has provided the rationale for sphincter-saving operations, such as those that are being performed for patients with ulcerative colitis and familial polyposis.[8]

Blood Supply of the Colon. A comprehensive understanding of the vascular supply to the colon (Fig. 32–1) is essential for all surgeons performing primary colonic procedures, as well as procedures in which the colon is used as a conduit, such as in esophageal replacements and urologic reconstructions. The cecum, ascending colon, hepatic flexure, and proximal portion of the transverse colon derive arterial blood supply from the ileocolic, right colic, and middle colic branches of the superior mesenteric artery. The inferior mesenteric artery supplies blood to the distal transverse colon, splenic flexure, descending colon, and sigmoid by means of the left colic artery and branches of the sigmoid and superior hemorrhoidal vessels. The rectum is supplied by a rich network of vessels from the middle hemorrhoidal and inferior hemorrhoidal arteries. As the main vessels course through the mesentery toward the bowel wall, they bifurcate and form arcades at 1 to 2 cm. from the mesenteric border and define a continuous chain of communicating vessels. This vascular structure is called the marginal artery

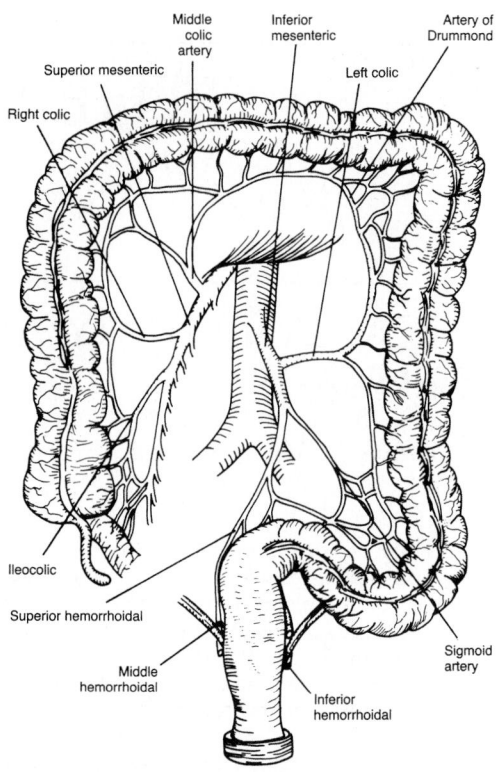

Figure 32–1. Anatomy and blood supply of the large intestine (From Beart, R. W., Jr., Nivatvongs, S., and Wolff, B.: The colon, rectum, and anus. *In* Nora, P. F. [Ed.]: Operative Surgery: Principles and Techniques, 3rd ed. Philadelphia, W. B. Saunders, 1990.)

of Drummond. The anastomosis or linking of arcades between the superior and inferior mesenteric vessels is known as the long anastomosis of Riolan. The colon is drained by a rich and vast network of lymphatics that frequently follow the course of the major vessels. The nodes may be involved with inflammatory or neoplastic diseases, and knowledge of their location is critical to curative cancer resections.

SURGICAL PROCEDURES

Surgical procedures for diseases of the colon continue to be among the most common operative procedures performed by surgeons (Fig. 32–2). When planning resections of the colon, it is essential to ensure adequate vascularity to all colonic anastomoses. The blood supply to the colon can be variable, specifically in segments that depend on marginal arcades. Ideally, one should be able to palpate pulsating vessels in the colonic mesentery and visualize active bleeding from the cut edges of the colon. This is particularly important with resections of the splenic flexure, because this area, known as a *watershed*, may be susceptible to ischemia. Adequate mobilization of the colon is necessary to minimize tension on an anastomosis. Attention to these details allows adequate healing of colonic anastomosis, whether by means of the traditional hand-sewn technique or with the use of stapling devices.

The basic principles of surgical oncology apply to tumors involving the colon. The surgeon should attempt to remove all of the malignant tissue from both the primary organ and any other structures locally involved, as well as the lymphatic channels and tissue through which the primary tumor is likely to spread. In the context of tumors involving the large intestine, adherence to these principles requires ligation of the appropriate vessels at their origin. In general, in benign

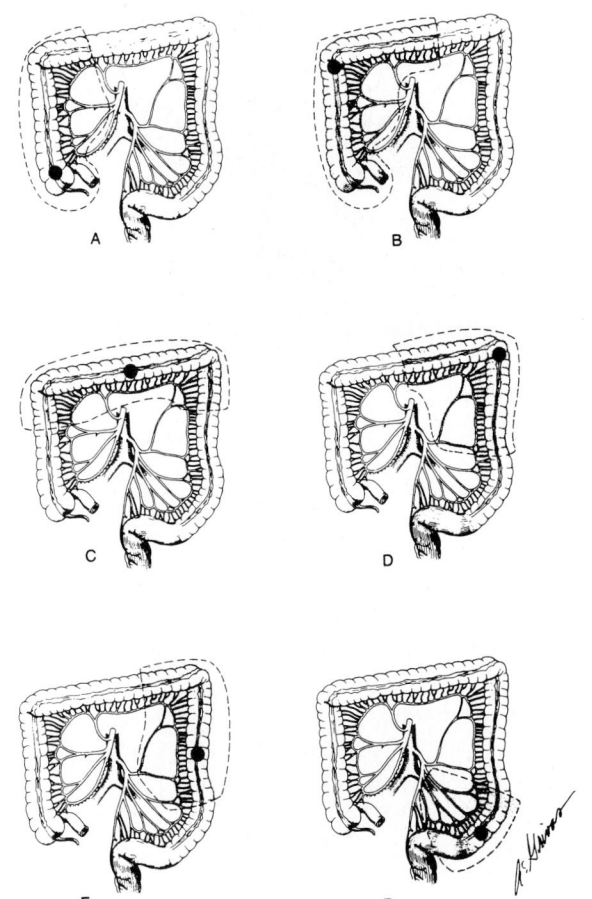

Figure 32–2. Extent of resection recommended for malignant lesions of colon. (From Beart, R. W., Jr., Nivatvongs, S., and Wolff, B.: The colon, rectum and anus. *In* Nora, P. F. [Ed.]: Operative Surgery: Principles and Techniques. Philadelphia, W. B. Saunders, 1990.)

tion of gastrointestinal continuity are best managed by a combined excision of the distal rectum and anus with anterior resection and abdominoperineal resection.

Total proctocolectomy—complete resection of the colon, rectum, and anus—has been the standard of care for patients with severe ulcerative colitis. In recent years, newer procedures have been developed to preserve transanal fecal flow, such as the ileal pouch–anal anastomosis or pull-through procedure.[8, 9, 31, 57]

Colostomy

Colostomy refers to the opening of the colon onto the surface of the abdomen. Colostomies may be necessary (1) to function as the outlet of feces when the distal colon or rectum has been removed; (2) to divert the fecal stream and protect a distal anastomosis; (3) to decompress a more distal colonic obstruction and serve as a *vent*; and (4) to temporarily divert the fecal stream from a pathologic process.[1] Depending on the specific indication and individual setting, the surgeon may choose to perform either a temporary or a permanent colostomy. The ideal temporary colostomy should provide adequate fecal diversion and be safe and easy to anastomose when one is restoring gastrointestinal continuity. A loop, or *double-barreled* colostomy, is typically performed when diversion is temporary. This is generally achieved by exteriorizing a segment of the colon and then making an opening in the loop of bowel through the taeniae. The question has arisen whether this procedure is completely diverting in nature.[78] To address this concern, many surgeons have developed the practice of stapling the distal segment and thereby creating, in essence, an end-colostomy. Although a transverse colostomy is a satisfactory temporary stoma, in general, it should not be performed in clinical settings in which permanent diversion is anticipated. Several problems can occur with this type of stoma, which although not life threatening can cause considerable nuisance and discomfort for the patient. The material discharged from a transverse colostomy is frequently semiliquid, and achieving a satisfactory seal with an appliance may therefore be difficult. In addition, the size of the stoma is often bulky, and this complicates the management of the appliance. Moreover, there appears to be a predisposition for prolapse and peristomal hernias with this type of colostomy. In general, permanent fecal diversion from this portion of the gastrointestinal tract can best be achieved by creation of an ileostomy rather than a proximal transverse loop colostomy.

When distal resection of the colon is needed but primary anastomosis is ill advised because of associated inflammation and/or intra-abdominal sepsis, a Hartmann procedure is often performed. This involves sigmoid resection with oversewing or closure of the distal rectal pouch and creation of an end-descending colostomy. This type of stoma, although generally temporary, should be created following the same principles and techniques of a more permanent stoma. A permanent colostomy is generally performed after abdominoperineal resection in patients with rectal tumors. Because of the position of the stoma in the distal colon, many of these patients are able to eliminate feces on a schedule and may not require an appliance. The ideal stoma should be situated in the left iliac fossa and pierce the abdominal wall through the rectus sheath. Positioning of the stoma in this location reduces the likelihood of peristomal herniation. Internal hernias around the colostomy can be avoided by securing the mesentery to the left paracolic gutter and closing this defect with a series of interrupted sutures. The key to providing an adequate cutaneous stoma for application of an appliance is

conditions of the colon, it is not necessary to remove the mesentery, and the mesentery can be divided close to the bowel wall.

Tumors of the cecum and ascending colon are generally managed by a right hemicolectomy with resection of the ileocecal valve, entire ascending colon, and proximal transverse colon to the level of, but not including, the middle colic vessels. If the concepts that have previously been stated are followed, malignant lesions in this area necessitate ligation of the ileocolic and right colic vessels at their origin from the superior mesenteric artery. Reconstruction is generally accomplished by an ileotransverse colostomy. Lesions involving the hepatic flexure are managed by a similar operative approach with resection of the transverse colon beyond the middle colic vessels. Lesions involving the midtransverse colon are managed by transverse colectomy. For lesions involving the descending colon, the splenic flexure and descending colon are generally removed. Sigmoid resections are frequently performed for malignant disease as well as benign conditions such as complications from diverticulitis. Anastomoses occurring after resection of lesions from the rectosigmoid can be safely performed either with a hand-sewn technique or with stapling devices. In fact, the advent of stapling devices and the continuing refinement in their development have allowed surgeons to perform low anastomoses (low anterior resection) that previously would not have been technically possible (Fig. 32–3). Tumors involving the rectum that preclude low anterior resection and restora-

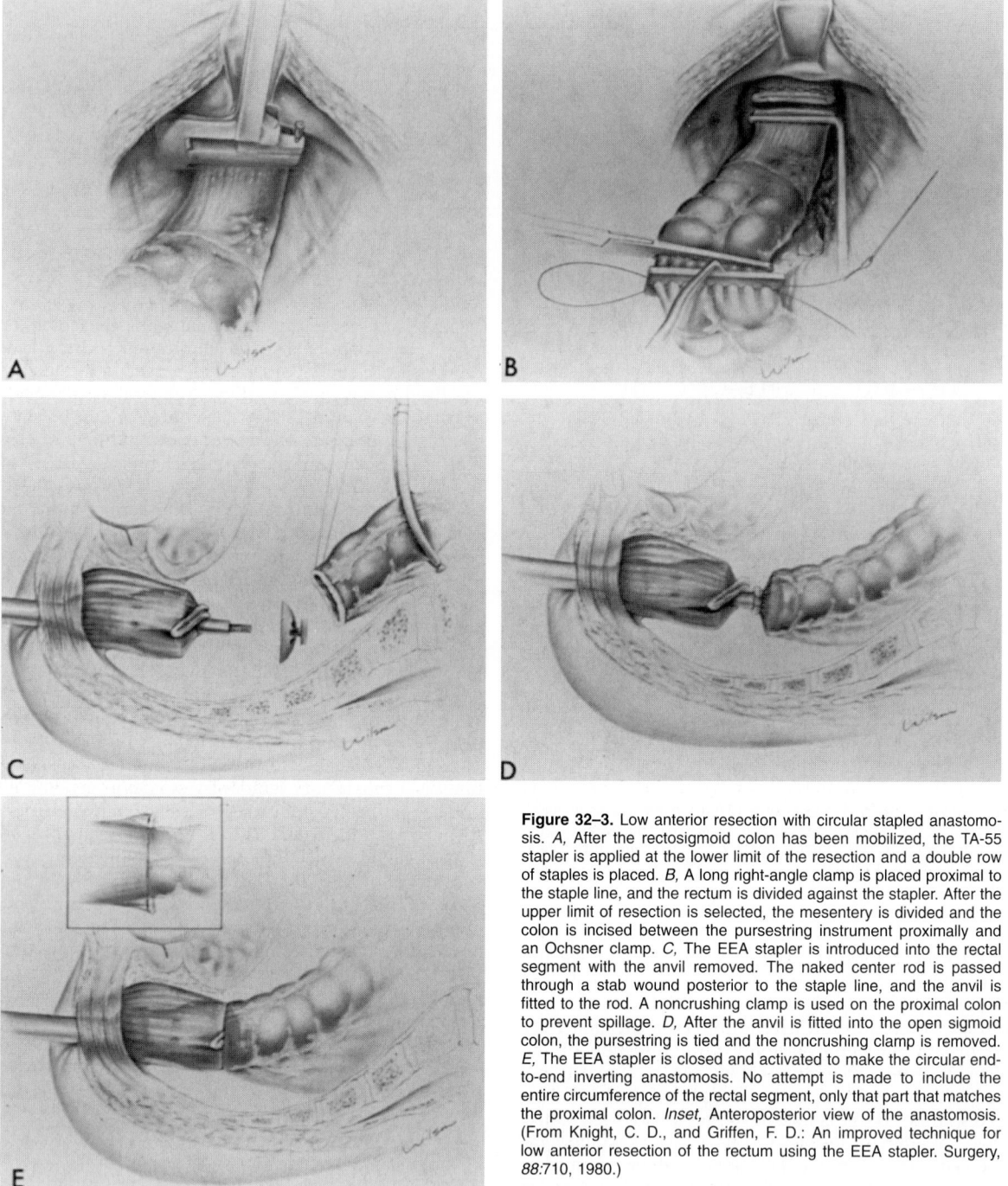

Figure 32–3. Low anterior resection with circular stapled anastomosis. *A*, After the rectosigmoid colon has been mobilized, the TA-55 stapler is applied at the lower limit of the resection and a double row of staples is placed. *B*, A long right-angle clamp is placed proximal to the staple line, and the rectum is divided against the stapler. After the upper limit of resection is selected, the mesentery is divided and the colon is incised between the pursestring instrument proximally and an Ochsner clamp. *C*, The EEA stapler is introduced into the rectal segment with the anvil removed. The naked center rod is passed through a stab wound posterior to the staple line, and the anvil is fitted to the rod. A noncrushing clamp is used on the proximal colon to prevent spillage. *D*, After the anvil is fitted into the open sigmoid colon, the pursestring is tied and the noncrushing clamp is removed. *E*, The EEA stapler is closed and activated to make the circular end-to-end inverting anastomosis. No attempt is made to include the entire circumference of the rectal segment, only that part that matches the proximal colon. *Inset*, Anteroposterior view of the anastomosis. (From Knight, C. D., and Griffen, F. D.: An improved technique for low anterior resection of the rectum using the EEA stapler. Surgery, 88:710, 1980.)

having the mesentery elevated through the stomal site and on minimal tension. One should strive to have a stoma that although not as high as an ileostomy is nevertheless a fourth to a half inch above the skin to permit application and good fitting of an appliance. The frequency with which patients eliminate feces through a colostomy varies from patient to patient. In some cases, frequency of evacuation can be regulated by diet. Potential complications associated with colostomies include stomal stenosis and necrosis secondary to ischemia, prolapse and peristomal hernias, internal hernias, and

more life-threatening complications such as bleeding and perforation.[69]

Colostomy takedown and restoration of gastrointestinal continuity is not an innocuous procedure and has been associated with significant morbidity.[42, 52, 60] The takedown of an end-colostomy has significantly more morbidity than takedown of a simple loop colostomy. Before colostomy closure, patients should undergo radiographic or endoscopic evaluation and bowel preparation.

For references, see page 980.

II _____

PHYSIOLOGY

Rolando Rolandelli, M.D., and Joel J. Roslyn, M.D.

Although the colon may not be essential for life, any alteration in its function may have profound effects on the quality of life and daily activities. Great efforts have been spent in recent years to develop new operative approaches to colonic and rectal disease so as to preserve relatively normal defecatory function. Although it has been known that the primary functions of the colon are to serve as an organ for storage and elimination of intestinal contents, only in recent years have we come to appreciate the complicated interaction and interdependence between physicochemical factors, central and enteric nervous system, and gut peptides that serve to coordinate and facilitate colonic absorptive activity and colonic motility.[22, 83] Progress in the area of colonic physiology has been facilitated by the similarities between human colonic physiologic processes and those that take place in the stomach of ruminants. Because ruminants have enormous economic implications for the food supply and can be readily accessed by investigators, the physiology of the rumen has been well studied.

The functions of the colon can be classified in two categories: (1) recycling of nutrients and (2) formation of stool and its elimination. The recycling of nutrients involves the metabolic activity of the colonic flora and active absorption. Stool formation also involves absorption of solutes and water and depends on dehydration of colonic contents. Elimination of intestinal waste through defecation is an elaborate process that intertwines reservoir, motor, continence, and evacuatory activities. The rectum is the site where complex mechanisms function to provide maintenance of continence and, ultimately, evacuation.[19] Interested readers should see the references on page 980 for several excellent reviews on this subject.

RECYCLING OF NUTRIENTS

During the digestive process, food is diluted within the gut lumen by mixing with bile salts and enzymes and by the secretion of gastrointestinal and hepatobiliary-pancreatic secretions. The small intestine absorbs the great majority of nutrients consumed and some of the fluid secreted into the lumen. Through an efficient enterohepatic circulation process, approximately 95% of bile salts are reabsorbed by the small intestine. The ileal effluent is rich in water, electrolytes, and some nutrients such as proteins (enzymes) and resistant carbohydrates. Colonic bacteria play a critical role in the process of nutrient recycling, conservation, and metabolism.

Metabolic Activity of the Colon

Fermentation. Dietary fiber is the main substrate for bacterial fermentation in the colon,[60] but not all dietary fibers are equally fermented.[65] Lignin is not fermented and produces bulk in the stool. Celluloses are only partially fermented whereas pectins are completely fermented in the normal colon. Colonic transit time and bulking of stool depend on the fermentability of the various fibers ingested. Poorly fermented fibers increase luminal bulk and accelerate transit time. Highly fermentable fibers provide minimal bulk and slow transit time. Consequently, the type of fiber ingested has a substantial impact on the evacuation of stool. Moreover, the amount and type of dietary fiber may predispose to

specific disease conditions. Constipation, diverticulosis, and colon cancer are all uncommon in populations with a high intake of roughage (i.e., water-insoluble fibers).[18] Water-insoluble fibers may be therapeutic for patients with constipation by the creation of bulk, whereas soluble fibers can be therapeutic for patients with diarrhea, by the generation of short-chain fatty acids (SCFA). In addition to dietary fiber, colonic bacteria ferment malabsorbed starches and proteins. In this manner, the caloric content of malabsorbed carbohydrates is transferred to SCFA and then recovered by the body. It is estimated that approximately 10% of the daily energy expenditure of a normal subject is obtained from the absorption of SCFA by the colon.

Urea Recycling. For many years, urea was thought to be the end product of nitrogen metabolism in humans.[89] This concept is only partially accurate; since humans do not produce urease, colonic bacteria are rich in this enzyme. Tracer studies have demonstrated that 10% of urea being synthesized is split by bacterial ureases in normal individuals. Urease-producing bacteria are firmly adherent to the colonic epithelium. Urea recycling is potentiated by a low protein and high fiber diet.[86] This phenomenon can be favorable in patients with renal failure.[42, 43] The exclusion of nonessential amino acids from the diet coupled with increased urea recycling, based in a larger pool of circulating urea, can either avoid or reduce the need for dialysis. Urea recycling is associated with adverse consequences in patients with hepatic insufficiency. Failure of the liver to reutilize urea nitrogen normally absorbed by the colon leads to increased amounts of ammonia passing across the blood-brain barrier that are responsible for hepatic encephalopathy.

FORMATION AND ELIMINATION OF STOOL

The formation of stool is a complex phenomenon that depends on the passage of nondigested material through the gastrointestinal tract (dietary fiber), absorption of water and solvents, bacterial metabolism of specific substrates, and secretion of fluid and electrolytes.

Absorption

Although the small intestine is responsible for the absorption of most nutrients entering the gastrointestinal tract, the colon is responsible for absorption of water from the ileal effluent. Although the entire length of the colon (approximately 135 cm.) has the capacity to absorb water and specific electrolytes, most of this absorptive activity occurs in the ascending colon. The total absorptive area of the large bowel is estimated to be approximately 900 sq. cm. Its capacity to absorb water and electrolytes is reflected by the 10-fold reduction in water volume that occurs there regularly. Numerous studies have suggested that 1000 to 1500 ml. of water is delivered from the ileum into the cecum during a 24-hour period. This effluent has a sodium concentration of approximately 200 mEq. per liter. The total volume of stool water is estimated to be only 100 to 150 ml. per day, with a sodium concentration of 25 to 50 mEq. per liter.[68] Therefore, despite the significant concentration effect and absorption of water, the sodium concentration is paradoxically low in the stool effluent. Based on *in vivo* and *in vitro* electrophysiologic experiments, various investigators have demonstrated that the mechanism (Fig. 32–4) of sodium absorption by the colonic epithelium is an active transport process directed against a combined transepithelial chemical, concentration, and electropotential difference.[14, 32, 39] Numerous factors have been identified that influence water and electrolyte movement by the colon. These include the mucosal cyclic adenosine monophosphate level,[13] pH, osmolarity, and ions such as fatty acids[15] and bile acids.[58] More recent information suggests that water and electrolyte movement is also controlled to some extent by the hormonal milieu.[12, 32, 39] The net effect of active sodium transport is the return of water from the lumen, and therefore absorption of water is a passive process.

In addition to recovering sodium and water, the colon also has an important role in the recovery of bile acids through the enterohepatic circulation. Bile acids are transported by nonionic or passive diffusion across the colonic epithelium.[59] This activity assumes even greater significance in patients in whom the terminal ileum is either diseased or surgically absent. In addition, the colon is the site of bile acid dehydroxylation, the process by which primary bile acids are converted to secondary bile acids. Bile acids affect colon transport of water and electrolytes. In the setting of ileal disease or after resection, conjugated bile acids that are normally absorbed in the distal small bowel are hydrolyzed by colonic bacteria and may induce a form of secretory diarrhea.

Absorption by the colonic mucosa depends on the availability of an energy source for epithelial cells. The colonic epithelium can utilize various fuels; however, *n*-butyrate is oxidized in preference to glutamine, glucose, or ketone bodies.[74] Because *n*-butyrate cannot be produced by mammalian cells, the colonic epithelium relies on luminal bacteria to produce it by fermentation of dietary fiber. The lack of *n*-butyrate, such as that produced by inhibition of fermentation by broad-spectrum antibiotics, leads to less sodium and water absorption and, thus, diarrhea.[73] Conversely, the perfusion of the colonic lumen with *n*-butyrate stimulates sodium and water absorption.[75] Acetate, *n*-butyrate, and propionate are SCFA produced by bacterial fermentation and constitute the main anions in stool.[76] Other physiologic effects of SCFA on the colon include stimulation of blood flow, mucosal cell renewal, and regulation of intraluminal pH with homeostasis of the bacterial flora.

Secretion

Studies in both animals[30] and humans[41] would suggest that potassium is actively secreted by colonic epithelium. This

activity is stimulated by exogenous or endogenous mineralocorticoids. There is also evidence that bicarbonate is secreted by the human colon as an active process directed against a difference in both chemical concentration and electrical potential.[29] Alterations in net fluid and electrolyte movement in the colon have been documented after administration of laxatives[11, 77] as well as in disease states, such as ulcerative colitis, granulomatous colitis, congenital chloridorrhea, and watery diarrhea syndrome.[71]

During the past 25 years, investigative efforts have focused on the hormonal regulation of ion transport in the small and large intestine in both health and disease. Several studies suggest that cyclic adenosine monophosphate,[13] prostaglandins,[70] and gut peptides, including vasoactive intestinal polypeptide,[12, 71] influence colonic ion transport. The true physiologic role of these substances on colonic absorptive and secretory function remains to be defined.[80]

MOTILITY

Fermentation of the colonic contents is the first step in the formation of stool. The process of fermentation is made possible by the distinct morphology of the colon.[28] Based on function, the colon can be divided into three anatomic segments. The right colon is the *fermentation chamber* of the human gastrointestinal tract because the bacteria in the cecum and ascending colon are the most active metabolically. The left colon is the site of storage and dehydration of stool. The rectum is the reservoir through which defecation is controlled. The storage and excretory functions of the colon are closely intertwined and regulated by the autonomic nervous system. A series of neural-mediated reflexes and smooth muscle contractions, characterized by reproducible myoelectrical activity, lead to propulsive activity through the colon. Parasympathetic nervous fibers supply the colon through the vagi and the pelvic nerves and are arranged in either the subserosal myenteric (Auerbach), submucosal (Meissner), or mucosal plexuses. The neurons of the myenteric plexus are concentrated along the taeniae coli and are more sparse between taeniae where the longitudinal muscle layer is thin. Sympathetic nerve fibers originate in the superior and inferior mesenteric ganglia and reach the colon through perivascular pathways. In general, the parasympathetic fibers are excitatory for the colon and inhibitory for the rectum, while the sympathetic fibers provide the opposite innervation.

The motility pattern is different in the three functional segments of the colon. In the right colon, there is evidence of *antiperistalsis* waves that generate retrograde flow of colonic contents back toward the cecum. In the left colon, contents are propelled caudad by tonic contractions, separating them into a series of globular masses. A third type of contraction, referred to as *mass peristalsis*, is interspersed with the propulsive and retropulsive contractions, occurring at varying intervals but typically more frequently after meals. Each mass peristaltic contraction is able to advance a column of colonic contents through one third of the colonic length. Finally, the rectum undergoes receptive relaxation to accommodate stool until defecation takes place.

Fecal continence and painless evacuation of stool are crucial to enjoy the normal activities of daily living. Fecal continence implies deferment of stool elimination; discrimination between gas, liquid, and solid stool; and selective elimination of gas without stool. Fecal continence is dependent on the presence of reservoir capacity within the rectum; a stiff, nondistensible rectum, such as in radiation proctitis, may produce incontinence even when the sphincter muscles are competent. The sphincteric mechanism surrounding the anorectum is composed of an internal and external anal sphincter.[22] The internal sphincter consists of circular smooth mus-

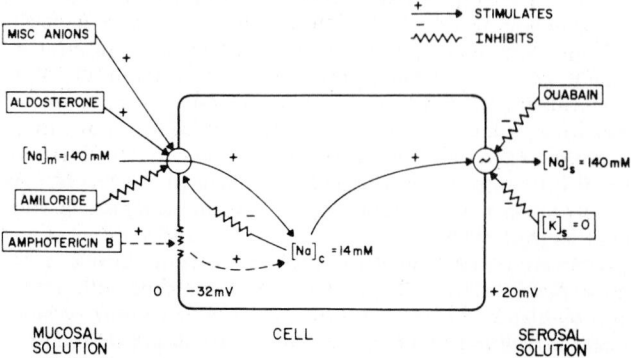

Figure 32–4. A cellular model for active sodium transport by mammalian colon. (From Schultz, E. G.: Ion transport by mammalian large intestine. *In* Johnson, L. R. [Ed.]: Physiology of the Gastrointestinal Tract. New York, Raven Press, 1981.)

cle, and it is tonically contracted to prevent passage of stool. Whereas the integrity of the internal and external sphincter muscles is believed to be essential for continence, partial disruption of the external sphincter during fistulotomy, for example, does not necessarily result in incontinence. As the rectum becomes distended, the internal sphincter is stimulated; and its activity in conjunction with the levator muscle groups serves to facilitate defecation and passage of stool.[19, 35]

The anorectum is richly innervated, and these sensory and motor pathways are essential to empty the rectum and ensure continence.[53] Increased understanding of the processes and anatomic structures responsible for defecation and incontinence has greatly facilitated the development of new and innovative procedures for sphincter preservation in patients with such diseases as ulcerative colitis and familial polyposis.

For references, see page 980.

III

DIAGNOSTIC STUDIES

Rolando Rolandelli, M.D., and Joel J. Roslyn, M.D.

The astute physician is directed toward the colon as the site of a pathologic process on the basis of the patient's complaints and history. Given the critical nature that the colon has in storage and evacuation of feces, diseases of the colon, whether inflammatory or neoplastic, often lead to alteration of gastrointestinal function. This is frequently reflected by change in the caliber of the stool, diarrhea, constipation or obstipation, hematochezia, melena, or rectal tenesmus or urgency. Because many systemic diseases and/or medications can affect colonic activity, it is essential that a complete history be obtained from all patients presenting for evaluation of a gastrointestinal disorder that may involve the colon or rectum. Many patients seek medical attention with a chief complaint of *diarrhea*. This term is often used indiscriminately, and careful questioning is essential to elucidate and define possible causes. In this setting, for example, patients need to be asked about frequency, consistency, color, and character of the stool so that the clinician can begin to distinguish between motility or mechanical disturbances and secretory disorders. It is not uncommon for patients with carcinoma of the ascending colon or cecum to have no disturbance of their gastrointestinal function but present with general fatigue, evidence of hypochromic, microcytic anemia, or heme-positive stools. In contrast, those individuals with malignant processes involving the sigmoid colon frequently present with obstructive symptoms. All patients in whom a diagnosis of colonic disease is being considered should undergo a complete physical examination, including pelvic and rectal examinations. Considerable information can often be gained from visualization and palpation, with specific attention given to systemic disease processes that may affect the colon, such as the presence of stigmata of portal hypertension, malnutrition, or the palpation of masses that may be inflammatory or neoplastic. Examination of the stool for blood either directly or by guaiac testing is an essential part of all physical examinations, especially in the setting in which carcinoma of the colon is being considered.[3] The efficacy of mass screening, however, remains to be defined.[82, 91]

Other diagnostic studies should be considered based on the individual clinical setting. Ordering tests for the sake of completeness should be avoided, and attention is focused on the specific problem with diagnostic tests ordered only as necessary. Urinalysis for laxatives (bisacodyl, phenolphthalein) may unmask surreptitious laxative abuse in patients who present with chronic diarrhea. Blood assays for gastrin, vasoactive intestinal peptide, and other enterohormones should be obtained when the history and stool analysis suggest secretory diarrhea of endocrine origin. Varying degrees of malnutrition may be present in individuals with either long-standing inflammatory bowel disease or with malignancies involving the colon. Baseline biochemical assessment of the patient's nutritional status provides important information concerning the problem and may assist in planning the timing of definitive therapy. Liver function tests are particularly helpful in the clinical evaluation of systemic processes or when liver metastases are suspected. The usefulness of carcinoembryonic antigen continues to be a source of considerable controversy.[16, 62] Most agree that a carcinoembryonic antigen level is appropriate for monitoring patients after resection for colon carcinomas.

In addition to the history, physical examination, and laboratory evaluation, a number of other diagnostic modalities should be considered in specific clinical settings.

RADIOGRAPHIC EVALUATION

Plain abdominal radiographs and contrast studies of the large intestine continue to be invaluable diagnostic methods in the assessment of patients with suspected colonic disease. These tests are quick, easy to perform, noninvasive, and associated with essentially no morbidity. They can be very helpful in directing the endoscopist and/or surgeon to the site of pathology. Today, contrast studies of the colon and colonoscopy should be viewed as complementary procedures. Although barium studies fail to detect small polyps and/or carcinomas, they continue to be an important screening test in patients with colon lesions. It is essential when ordering a barium enema examination that the clinician inform the radiologist of the presumptive diagnosis and, in addition, provide as much clinical information as possible. This dialogue facilitates the interpretation of the radiograph and enhances the ability to make an accurate diagnosis.

A colonic transit time test is mandatory for definitive confirmation of the diagnosis of constipation; it also assesses severity and locates segmental defects versus a global defect in colonic transit.[47] Plain films of the abdomen are obtained 4 and 6 days after the ingestion of radiopaque markers. A normal colonic transit should carry the markers throughout the colon in 5 days.

Cinedefecography involves instilling contrast media into the rectum and recording the act of defecation with static radiographs and video fluoroscopy.[55, 56] The static radiographs allow measurement of the anorectal angle and the relationship between the anus and the coccyx/pubis plane, both under resting conditions and when straining. Videofluoroscopy is used to detect *hidden* prolapse or rectal intussusception, which can be missed on static radiographs. Videofluoroscopy also demonstrates the coordinated function of the muscles involved in defecation.

ENDOSCOPY

With improving optics in a higher-quality instrument, diagnostic and therapeutic colonoscopy has become routine and has, in effect, revolutionized diagnostic capabilities in the management of patients with colonic disorders. Although colonoscopy should be performed only by trained surgical and gastrointestinal endoscopists, the introduction of a 60-cm. flexible sigmoidoscope has allowed the nonspecialist to participate in diagnostic evaluation of the colon. Nevertheless, expertise is required to manipulate the flexible sigmoidoscope, and all individuals practicing this technique should have basic training. Endoscopic evaluation of the colon remains the most important technique in the accurate diagnosis of colonic disease, especially carcinoma.[63] A variety of endoscopic instruments are available, depending on the expertise of the endoscopist and the presumed site of the lesion. The anoscope or proctoscope is invaluable for the assessment of internal hemorrhoids and rectal tumors that are within 8 to 10 cm. of the anal verge. Anoscopy is usually painless unless the patient has an anal fissure or thrombosed external hemorrhoids or unless the anoscope is introduced forcefully. Rigid sigmoidoscopy allows visualization of the distal 20 to 25 cm. of the colon. Physicians performing rigid sigmoidoscopy should be aware of the anatomic features of the rectum and sigmoid, including the posterior orientation and angulation, which usually occurs at the junction of the rectosigmoid and sigmoid colon. This examination can be performed with the patient in the knee-chest, jackknife, or lateral position. A flexible sigmoidoscope has the same capabilities as a colonoscope, including channels for biopsy, polypectomy, and electrocautery, but it is only 60 cm. long.

Colonoscopy is the most accurate method of assessing colonic disease. A skilled endoscopist can maneuver the scope to visualize the entire colon from the anus to the cecum. General indications for flexible sigmoidoscopy or for colonoscopy include (1) diagnosis, (2) biopsy to confirm or establish the nature of a disease process or malignant lesion, (3) therapeutic removal of polyps,[37] (4) management of bleeding lesions,[79] (5) surveillance and follow-up of lesions previously removed endoscopically or surgically, (6) detection and removal of foreign bodies, and (7) early cancer detection or another screening process. In addition, colonoscopy has also been used to facilitate endoscopic dilatation of anastomotic strictures.[10] Although vast experience throughout the world has suggested that colonoscopy is a safe procedure that can be performed with minimal morbidity and essentially no mortality,[40, 64] a number of potential contraindications should be considered. These include (1) suspected colonic perforation, (2) acute fulminating inflammatory bowel disease, (3) peritonitis with secondary paralytic ileus, and (4) acute inflammatory disease of the anus. Unlike rigid or flexible sigmoidoscopy, satisfactory performance of colonoscopy generally requires varying degrees of intravenous sedation. Therefore, the general medical condition of the patient and specifically the patient's cardiopulmonary status should be carefully considered before proceeding with a colonoscopic procedure. A number of medications are employed by endoscopists; some of the more popular ones are meperidine and the benzodiazepines, alone or in combination. In addition, glucagon administered intravenously is frequently used as an adjunct to facilitate smooth muscle relaxation. General anesthesia is generally not required for colonoscopy.

The efficacy and safety of diagnostic and/or therapeutic colonoscopy depend on the presence of a well-cleansed bowel. A satisfactory bowel preparation can be achieved by means of a number of techniques, including mechanical preparation with enemas and simple irrigation of the gastrointestinal tract with saline, mannitol preparation, or commercially available physiologic preparations.[24, 38, 61] The commercially available preparations, including solutions containing polyethylene glycol (PEG), are easy and safe and can be completed in a matter of hours. In the authors' experience, these latter preparations have largely replaced the more traditional regimens that required that the patient be maintained on clear liquids for 24 to 48 hours before the procedure as well as the administration of citrate of magnesia, castor oil, and tap water enemas. The specific regimen to be employed for bowel preparation should be carefully considered in patients with advanced diverticular disease, inflammatory bowel disease, or severe constipation. In those individuals in whom partial or total colonic obstruction is suspected, the use of tap water enemas is recommended rather than irrigating solutions.

The role of endoscopy has been well documented in intraluminal diseases and in the evaluation of diarrhea, constipation, and/or bleeding. Over the past several years, it has become increasingly apparent that endoscopy plays a vital role in the evaluation of patients with suspected motor abnormalities of defecation. For example, a rectal biopsy should be obtained in all patients with suspected aganglionosis.[2] The histologic specimens are examined for ganglion cells. A more reliable method for diagnosis of Hirschsprung's disease is the staining of biopsy specimens for acetylcholinesterase.[21] Acetylcholinesterase is significantly increased in Hirschsprung's disease. This method has a 99% accuracy in differentiating Hirschsprung's disease from idiopathic constipation. Routine hematoxylin/eosin staining fails to demonstrate ganglion cells in 39% of patients without Hirschsprung's disease.

Anorectal Laboratory Studies

Functional studies of the physiologic processes involved in defecation are essential in deciding whether a surgical procedure is indicated in a patient with chronic constipation.[6, 36] These studies include anorectal manometry, electromyography, sensory thresholds measurement, and colonic myoelectrical activity. Anorectal manometry is most commonly performed through open-tipped multilumen catheters perfused with fluid. These catheters are connected to a transducer and register the pressures of internal and external sphincter pressures and presence of the anorectal inhibitory reflex.[26] In patients with Hirschsprung's disease, the anorectal inhibitory reflex is abolished.[50] The results of anorectal manometry are less consistent in patients with idiopathic constipation. In these patients, some authors have reported elevated resting anal pressures[87] while others have found reduced resting pressures.[72] Electromyography records the action potential derived from the different muscles involved in defecation through endoscopically placed mucosal electrodes along the colon.[84] In patients with paradoxic pelvic floor contraction, the puborectalis muscle remains contracted during defecation. In patients with long-standing constipation, the nerves supplying the external sphincter and the puborectalis muscles can be damaged owing to perineal descent.[85] The pattern of myoelectrical activity in response to medications can differentiate between neurogenic and myogenic disorders and indicate the appropriate therapy. Sensory threshold measurements may disclose a high rectal threshold (insensitivity) in patients with idiopathic constipation, the extent of denervation, or myopathy in the colonic wall.

STOOL ANALYSIS

In all patients with diarrhea, a stool sample should be sent to the microbiology laboratory for isolation of enteropathogens and assay of *Clostridium difficile* toxin. In some patients with diarrhea it may be necessary to differentiate between malabsorptive and secretory diarrhea, which can be done by measurement of electrolytes and osmolality in stool. The osmotic gap is calculated by subtracting twice the amount of sodium plus potassium from the measured osmolality.[81] A negative osmotic gap indicates secretory diarrhea, while a positive osmotic gap indicates malabsorptive diarrhea. The diagnosis of malabsorptive diarrhea can be further investigated by measurement of fecal fat. An excretion of more than 7 gm. of fat per day is diagnostic of steatorrhea.

OTHER DIAGNOSTIC TESTS

The use of intravenous pyelography and ureteral stents in the management of patients undergoing laparotomy for colonic disease continues to be controversial. The ureters, either right or left, may be primarily or secondarily involved with inflammatory or malignant processes of the colon. Moreover, in patients who have already undergone previous laparotomy for gastrointestinal or vascular disease, the normal anatomic position of the ureters may be altered. Although it has not been the authors' practice routinely to obtain these studies or place stents preoperatively in all patients undergoing

colonic or pelvic operation, these measures are helpful in individuals with large malignant lesions, those with complex inflammatory processes, those undergoing reoperation, or those having had prior pelvic radiation. Computed tomographic scans and, more recently, magnetic resonance imaging have been particularly helpful in the assessment of patients with rectal tumors with regard to resectability. The evolving management of these patients, including the neoadjuvant use of radiation therapy, has heightened awareness of the utility of these studies. In addition, these scans may be helpful in the assessment of other malignant processes that may involve the gastrointestinal tract, contiguous organs, or the liver. The decision to proceed with one of these studies again should be individualized on the basis of the clinical setting. Other serum and radiologic examinations may be indicated, depending on the specific colonic disorder. A precise anatomic and pathologic diagnosis is now feasible in most patients with colonic disorders. The recognition of a number of motor disturbances involving primarily the anorectum has provided impetus for the development of several new diagnostic modalities that attempt to quantify motor activity in this region.[50, 51, 55, 56, 87, 92] The ultimate role of these tests remains to be defined.

For references, see page 980.

IV

INTESTINAL ANTISEPSIS

Rolando Rolandelli, M.D., and Joel J. Roslyn, M.D.

The microflora and microbiology of the colon are important to the activity of this organ in both health and disease. Maintenance of the normal ecologic relationships is responsible for the physiologic role that the colon has in the enterohepatic circulation of bile acids. Alterations in the microflora may be observed in clinically significant syndromes. Perhaps more important to the surgeon, however, is the effect that the qualitative and quantitative characteristics of the microbiologic environment in the colon have on the outcome of colonic surgery. Through the years, investigative efforts have focused on understanding this interaction, and attempts have been directed to control the microbiologic environment to facilitate safe surgical therapy. The methods employed in preparing the bowel for both endoscopic and surgical procedures have evolved over the past 30 to 40 years. Understanding the scientific basis for this evolution is critical for the surgeon involved in planning treatment and management of patients with colonic disease.

MICROBIOLOGY OF THE COLON

The human colon is the site of more than 400 bacterial species. Unlike the stomach and proximal small bowel, both of which have a bacterial count generally considered no greater than 10^5 organisms, the colon has a bacterial concentration that approaches 10^{12} colony-forming units per ml. The organisms found in the colon vary widely, depending on the clinical situation, but, in general, include large numbers of both aerobic and anaerobic bacteria (Table 32–1). Nearly one third of the fecal dry weight consists of bacteria. The predominant bacteria are anaerobic and include *Bacteroides, Bifidobacterium,* and *Eubacterium.* There are a number of host and microbial factors that interact to maintain a relatively stable

microfloral population within the colon. When these factors are altered, groups of bacteria may proliferate and normal physiologic function may be impaired, or the patient may be at increased risk for development of subsequent infection. A series of epidemiologic studies has attempted to demonstrate a link between colon cancer and intestinal microflora.[4, 17] The exact mechanism responsible for this link remains to be identified. Perhaps the most important clinical manifestation of colonic microflora concerns the risk of infection following colonic surgical procedures. Analysis of the available literature suggests that the rate of wound infection in patients undergoing colonic procedures who have not received prophylactic antibiotics may be as high as 75%.[20, 46, 90] This concept has been largely responsible for the development of approaches for intestinal antisepsis.

TABLE 32–1. Concentration of Bacteria Present in Normal Human Small and Large Intestine

Bacteria	Ileum	Colon
Total bacterial count	10^3–10^9	10^8–10^{12}
Anaerobes		
Bacteroides sp.	10^3–10^7	10^9–10^{12}
Lactobacillus	10^2–10^5	10^6–10^{12}
Clostridium sp.	10^2–10^4	10^3–10^{10}
Aerobes		
Coliforms	10^2–10^7	10^5–10^8
Streptococcus sp.	10^2–10^6	10^4–10^7
Lactobacillus	10^2–10^5	10^3–10^7
Staphylococcus sp.	10^2–10^4	10^2–10^4

MECHANICAL PREPARATION

As previously stated, much of the dry weight of feces is bacteria. To reduce the bulk of feces and bacteria within the colon, mechanical cleansing of the colon has long been an integral feature of intestinal antisepsis and colon preparation. However, it appears that mechanical cleansing alone does not produce a significant reduction in the colony count of bacteria within the colon. For many years, mechanical preparation of the bowel consisted of a 3-day period during which the patient was maintained on clear liquids and received a variety of purgatives and laxatives. Whereas the details of the specific regimens may have varied from institution to institution, they all shared certain potential problems. They were time consuming, frequently requiring several days of hospitalization preoperatively, and were associated with varying degrees of physical exhaustion, patient compliance, and dissatisfaction. During the past 10 years, colonic lavage with a variety of solutions has been introduced as a viable alternative to the 3-day mechanical preparation component of the intestinal antisepsis program. The earliest attempts at colonic lavage with saline were associated with problems and potential risks, especially in elderly patients, owing to sodium and water retention.[24] This system was modified to include the use of oral mannitol.[63] During the past several years, a commercially available electrolyte–polyethylene glycol solution has been introduced and widely tested.[34] Clinical trials have examined the efficacy of this solution as compared with more conventional mechanical preparations for colonoscopy and have clearly determined the newer solution to be safe, well tolerated, and cost effective. This type of solution administered orally in 4 liters the day before operation generally provides excellent mechanical preparation of the bowel. Use of this solution has become the standard regimen for mechanical bowel preparation for an elective colonic procedure. Currently, many patients undergoing an elective colonic surgical procedure are asked to go through this process on an outpatient basis the day before operation.

ORAL VERSUS PARENTERAL ANTIBIOTICS FOR COLONIC SURGERY

The rationale for the use of antibiotics preoperatively for patients undergoing a colonic operation is to reduce the number of bacteria within the colon. This concept is well accepted. However, there continues to be controversy concerning the most efficacious way of achieving this goal.[7] The role of oral antibiotics rather than parenteral agents, together with the selection of specific agents, continues to be debated and studied. In 1973, Nichols and associates[64] demonstrated the benefit of orally administered, nonabsorbable antibiotics in combination with mechanical cleansing, contrasted to only the latter. The findings of this limited study were confirmed several years later in a prospective, randomized, multi-institutional trial. This study of over 1000 patients undergoing colonic surgery suggested that there was no significant benefit from the addition of parenteral antibiotic prophylaxis to an appropriate mechanical preparation with oral nonabsorbed antimicrobial agents.[5] A large number of studies have subsequently attempted to identify the ideal agents for either oral antimicrobial therapy or parenteral administration.[25, 27, 33, 44–46, 48, 88] There are certain characteristics that any ideal prophylactic antibiotic regimen, whether oral or parenteral, should include. The regimen selected should provide broad suppression of fecal flora with high activity against aerobic and anaerobic organisms. Toxicity should be minimal, and there should be no emergence of resistant organisms. Additionally, a single agent is preferable to multiple drugs, there should be a short term of administration, and the drugs should be

TABLE 32–2. Common Regimens for Oral Antibiotic Bowel Preparation

Drugs	Regimen
I. Neomycin	1 gm. orally at 1 P.M., 2 P.M., and 11 P.M. the day before surgery
Erythromycin base	1 gm. orally at 1 P.M., 2 P.M., and 11 P.M. the day before surgery
II. Metronidazole	750 mg. every 8 hours for 72 hours

cost effective. Orally administered neomycin and erythromycin base or metronidazole have become the most common agents used for oral antibiotic preparation (Table 32–2). These agents are generally administered at 1 P.M., 2 P.M., and 11 P.M. the day before operation. It was initially thought that absorption of these drugs was not desirable. It is now thought that increased tissue levels of the drug at sites distant from the colon aid the normal host resistance mechanisms when contamination of the wound occurs.

Appropriate regimens for parenteral antibiotics should include agents that have considerable activity against aerobes and anaerobes. Several investigators have reviewed multiple-drug regimens, including aminoglycosides and metronidazole or clindamycin, rather than single-agent regimens. In recent years, the second-generation cephalosporins have gained considerable popularity as useful agents for antimicrobial prophylaxis. However, these combinations or single agents are not effective against group D streptococci (enterococci). More recent studies have compared the third-generation cephalosporins used as a single dose compared with multiple-dose administration of the second-generation cephalosporins.[44, 67] These types of studies may ultimately help define the nuances of antibiotic utilization in patients undergoing colonic operation. In the future, continuation of the evolution in management of patients undergoing elective and emergent colonic surgery will ensue. Undoubtedly, new antibiotics will be described, and perhaps understanding of the host factors that dictate the response to clinical infection will be such that whole new techniques will be described for colon and intestinal antisepsis.

SELECTED REFERENCES

Corman, M. D.: Colon and Rectal Surgery. Philadelphia, J. B. Lippincott, 1989.
   A very thorough and up-to-date discussion of all facets of colon and rectal surgery, this text contains excellent reviews of technical considerations.

DeCosse, J. J., and Todd, I. P.: Anorectal Surgery. Edinburgh, Churchill Livingstone, 1988.
   In addition to an excellent overview of surgical principles pertinent to anus and rectum, this volume contains an outstanding discussion and review of anorectal physiology.

Goligher, J., Duthrie, H., and Nixon, H.: Surgery of the Anus, Rectum, and Colon, 5th ed. London, Bailliere-Tindall, 1983.
   This work continues to be the classic text and provides an authoritative and thorough review of all clinical problems involving the large intestine, rectum, and anus.

Kelvin, F. M., and Gardiner, R.: Clinical Imaging of the Colon and Rectum. New York, Raven Press, 1987.
   This is a radiology text that is beautifully written and provides an excellent reference book for all clinicians involved in the care of patients with colorectal disease.

Shinya, H.: Colonoscopy: Diagnosis and Treatment of Colonic Diseases. New York, Igaku-Shoin, 1982.
   This work is a simple, well-written text covering the fundamentals of colonoscopy. The book is written by a surgical endoscopist and provides basic information.

REFERENCES

1. Abrams, J. S.: Abdominal Stomas: Indications, Operative Techniques, and Patient Care. Boston, John Wright. PSG, 1984.

2. Aldridge, R. T., and Campbell, P. E.: Ganglion cell distribution in the normal rectum and anal canal: A basis for the diagnosis of Hirschsprung's disease by anorectal biopsy. J Pediatr. Surg., 3:475, 1968.

3. American Cancer Society: Guidelines for the cancer-related checkup. CA, 30:208, 1980.

4. Aries, V., Crowther, J. S., Drassar, B. S., Hill, M. J., and Williams, R. E. O.: Bacteria and the etiology of cancer of the large bowel. Gut, 10:334, 1969.

5. Bartlett, J. G., Condon, R. E., Gorbach, S. L., et al.: Veterans Administration's cooperative study on bowel preparation for elective colorectal operations. Ann. Surg., 188:249, 1978.

6. Bassotti, G., Betti, C., Pelli, M. A., and Morelli, A.: Extensive investigation on colonic motility with pharmacological testing is useful for selecting surgical options in patients with inertia colica. Am. J. Gastroenterol., 87:143, 1992.

7. Baum, M. L., Anish, D. S., Chalmers, T. C., et al.: A survey of trials of antibiotic prophylaxis in colon surgery: Evidence against further use of no-treatment controls. N. Engl. J. Med., 305:795, 1981.

8. Becker, J. M.: Anal sphincter function after colectomy, mucosal proctectomy, and endorectal ileoanal pull-through. Arch. Surg., 119:526, 1984.

9. Becker, J. M., and Raymond, J. L.: Ileal pouch-anal anastomosis: A single surgeon's experience with 100 consecutive cases. Ann. Surg., 204:375, 1986.

10. Bedogni, G., Rica, E., Pedrazzoli, C., et al.: Endoscopic dilatation of anastomotic colonic stenosis by different techniques: An alternative to surgery? Gastrointest. Endosc., 33:21, 1987.

11. Binder, H. J.: Pharmacology of laxatives. Annu. Rev. Pharmacol. Toxicol., 17:355, 1977.

12. Binder, H. J.: New modes for regulating intestinal ion transport. Gastroenterology, 78:642, 1980.

13. Binder, H. J., Felburn, C., and Volpe, B. T.: Bile salt alteration of colonic electrolyte transport: Role of cyclic adenosine monophosphate. Gastroenterology, 68:503, 1975.

14. Binder, H. J., Foster, E. S., Budinger, M. E., and Hayslett, J. P.: Mechanism of electroneutral sodium chloride absorption in distal colon of the rat. Gastroenterology, 93:449, 1987.

15. Binder, H. J., and Mehtan, P.: Short-chain fatty acids stimulate active sodium chloride absorption in vitro in the rat distal colon. Gastroenterology, 96:989, 1989.

16. Bland, K. I., and Polk, H. C., Jr.: Therapeutic measures applied for the curative and palliative control of colorectal carcinoma. Surg. Annu., 15:123, 1983.

17. Burkitt, D. P.: Epidemiology of cancer of the colon and rectum. Cancer, 28:3, 1971.

18. Burkitt, D. P., Walker, A. R. P., and Painter, N. S.: Effect of dietary fibre on stools and transit-times and its role in the causation of disease. Lancet, 2:1408, 1972.

19. Burleigh, D. E., and D'Mello, A.: Physiology and pharmacology of the internal anal sphincter. In Henry, M. M., and Swash, M. (Eds.): Coloproctology and the Pelvic Floor: Pathophysiology and Management. London, Butterworths, 1985.

20. Burton, R. C.: Postoperative wound infection in colonic and rectal surgery. Br. J. Surg., 60:363, 1973.

21. Causse, E., Vaysse, P., Fabre, J., Valdiquie, P., and Thouvenot, J. P.: The diagnostic value of acetylcholinesterase/butyl-cholinesterase ratio in Hirschsprung's disease. Am. J. Clin. Pathol., 88:477, 1987.

22. Christensen, J.: Motility of the colon. In Johnson, L. R. (Ed.): Physiology of the Gastrointestinal Tract. New York, Raven Press, 1990.

23. Christensen, J.: Intestinal pseudo-obstruction and paralytic ileus. In Moody, F. G., et al. (Eds.): Surgical Treatment of Digestive Disease. Chicago, Year Book Medical, 1990.

24. Chung, R. S., Gurll, N. J., and Berglund, E. M.: A controlled clinical trial of whole gut lavage as a method of bowel preparation for colonic operations. Am. J. Surg., 137:75, 1979.

25. Clarke, J. S., Condon, R. E., Bartlett, J. G., et al.: Preoperative oral antibiotics reduce septic complications of colon operations: Results of a randomized double-blind clinical trial. Ann. Surg., 186:251, 1977.

26. Coller, J. A.: Clinical application of anorectal manometry. Gastroenterol. Clin. North Am., 16:17, 1987.

27. Condon, R. E., et al.: Efficacy of oral and systemic antibiotic prophylaxis in colorectal operations. Arch. Surg., 118:496, 1983.

28. Cummings, J. H., and Branch, W. J.: Fermentation and the production of short chain fatty acids in the human large intestine. In Vahouny, G. B., and Kritchevsky, D. (Eds.): Dietary Fiber: Basic and Clinical Aspects: New York, Plenum Press, 1986, p. 131.

29. Donowitz, M., Asarkof, N., and Pike, G.: Calcium dependence of serotonin-induced changes in rabbit ileal electrolyte transport. J. Clin. Invest., 66:341, 1980.

30. Donowitz, M., and Binder, H. J.: Mechanism of fluid and electrolyte secretion in the germ-free rat cecum. Dig. Dis. Sci., 24:551, 1979.

31. Dozois, R. R., Kelly, K. A., Welling, D. R., et al.: Ileal pouch-anal anastomosis: Comparison of results in familial adenomatous polyposis and chronic ulcerative colitis. Ann. Surg., 210:268, 1989.

32. Edmonds, C. J., and Marriott, J.: Electrical potential and short-circuit current in rat colon in vivo and the effect of aldosterone. J. Physiol., 210:1021, 1970.

33. Edmondson, H. T., and Rissing, J. P.: Prophylactic antibiotics in colon surgery: Cephaloridine vs. erythromycin and neomycin. Arch. Surg., 118:227, 1983.

34. Ernstoff, J. J., Howard, D. A., Marshall, J. B., Jumshyd, A., and McCullough, A. J.: A randomized, blinded clinical trial of a rapid colonic lavage solution (Golytely) compared with standard preparation for colonoscopy and barium enema. Gastroenterology, 84:1512, 1983.

35. Felt-Bersma, R. J. F., Strijars, R. L. M., Janssen, J. J. W. M., et al.: The external anal sphincter: Relationship between anal manometry and anal electromyography and its clinical relevance. Dis. Colon Rectum, 32:112, 1989.

36. Fleshman, J. W., Fry, R. D., and Kodner, I. J.: The surgical management of constipation. Baillieres Clin. Gastroenterol., 6:145, 1992.

37. Forde, K. A.: Colonoscopic management of polypoid lesions. Surg. Clin. North Am., 69:1287, 1989.

38. Fordtran J. S., Santa Ana, C. A., and Cleveland, MvB.: A low-sodium solution for gastrointestinal lavage. Gastroenterology, 98:11, 1990.

39. Foster, E. S., Zimmerman, T. W., Hayslett, J. P., and Binder, H. J.: Corticosteroid alteration of active electrolyte transport in rat distal colon. Am. J. Physiol., 245:G668, 1983.

40. Ghazi, A., and Grossman, M.: Complications of colonoscopy and polypectomy. Surg. Clin. North Am., 62:889, 1982.

41. Gingell, J. C., Davies, M. W., and Shields, R.: Effect of a synthetic gastrin-like pentapeptide upon the intestinal transport of sodium, potassium, and water. Gut, 9:111, 1968.

42. Giordano, C., De Pascali, C., Balestrieri, C., Cittadine, D., and Crescenzi, A.: The incorporation of urea N into serum proteins of uremic patients on low-nitrogen diets. J. Clin. Invest., 45:1013, 1966.

43. Giovanetti, S., and Meggiore, Q.: Low nitrogen diets with proteins of high biological value for severe chronic uraemia. Lancet, 1:1000, 1964.

44. Goransson, G., Nilsson-Ehle, I., Olsson, S., et al.: Single- versus multiple-dose doxycycline prophylaxis in elective colorectal surgery. Acta Chir. Scand., 150:245, 1984.

45. Groner, J. I., Edmiston, C. E. Jr., Krepel, C. J., et al.: The efficacy of oral antimicrobials in reducing aerobic and anaerobic colonic mucosal flora. Arch. Surg., 124:281, 1989.

46. Guglielmo, B. J., Hohn, D. C., Koo, P. J., et al.: Antibiotic prophylaxis in surgical procedure: A critical analysis of the literature. Arch. Surg., 118:943, 1983.

47. Hinton, J. M., Lennard-Jones, J. E., and Young, A. C.: A new method for studying gut transit time using radio-opaque markers. Gut, 10:842, 1969.

48. Khubchandani, I. T., Karamchandani, M. D., Sheeb, J. A., et al.: Metronidazole vs. erythromycin, neomycin, and cefazolin in prophylaxis for colonic surgery. Dis. Colon Rectum, 32:17, 1989.

49. Knox, A. J., Birkett, F. D. H., and Collins, C. D.: Closure of colostomy. Br. J. Surg., 58:669, 1971.

50. Lawson, J. O. N., and Nixon, H. H.: Anal canal pressures in the diagnosis of Hirschsprung's disease. J. Pediatr. Surg., 2:544, 1967.

51. Lestar, B., Penninckx, F. M., and Kerremaus, R. P.: Defecometry: A new method for determining the parameters of rectal evacuation. Dis. Colon Rectum, 32:197, 1989.

52. Livingston, D. H., Miller, F. B., and Richardson, J. D.: Are the risks after colostomy closure exaggerated? Am. J. Surg., 158:17, 1989.

53. Lubowski, D. Z., Nicholls, R. J., Swash, M., and Jordan, M. J.: Neural control of internal anal sphincter function. Br. J. Surg., 74:668, 1987.

54. Macrae, F. A., Tank, G., and Williams, C. B.: Toward safer polypectomy: A report on the complications of 5000 diagnostic or therapeutic colonoscopies. Gut, 24:376, 1983.

55. Mahieu, P., Pringot, J., and Bodart, P.: Defaecography. I: Description of a new procedure and results in normal patients. Gastrointest. Radiol., 9:247, 1984.

56. Mahieu, P., Pringot, J., and Bodart, P.: Defecography. II: Contribution to the diagnosis of defecation disorders. Gastrointest. Radiol., 9:253, 1984.

57. Martin, L. W., Lecoultre, C., and Schubert, W. K.: Total colectomy and mucosal protectomy with preservation of continence in ulcerative colitis. Ann. Surg., 186:477, 1977.

58. Mekhjian, H. S., and Phillips, S. F.: Perfusion of the canine colon with unconjugated bile acids: Effect of water and electrolyte transport, morphology, and bile acid absorption. Gastroenterology, 59:120, 1970.

59. Mekhjian, H. S., Phillips, S. F., and Hofmann, A. F.: Colonic absorption of unconjugated bile acids: Perfusion studies in man. Dig. Dis. Sci., 24:545, 1979.

60. Miller, T. L., and Wolin, M. J.: Fermentations by saccharolytic intestinal bacteria. Am. J. Clin. Nutr., 32:164, 1976.

61. Minervini, S., Alexander-Williams, J. I. A., Bentley, S., and Keighley, M. R. B.: Comparison of three methods of whole bowel irrigation. Am. J. Surg., 140:400, 1980.

62. Moertel, C. G., Schutt, A. J., and Go, V. L. W.: Carcinoembryonic antigen test for recurrent colorectal carcinoma: Inadequacy for early detection. JAMA, 239:1065, 1978.

63. Neugut, A. I., and Pita, S.: Role of sigmoidoscopy in screening for colorectal cancer: A critical review. Gastroenterology, 95:492, 1988.

64. Nichols, R. L., Broido, P., Condon, R. E., et al.: Effect of preoperative neomycin-erythromycin intestinal preparation on the incidence of infectious complications following colon surgery. Ann. Surg., 178:453, 1973.

65. Nyman, M., and Asp, N. G.: Fermentation of dietary fiber components in rat intestinal tract. Br. J. Nutr., 47:357, 1982.

66. Parks, S. E., and Hastings, P. R.: Complications of colostomy closure. Am. J. Surg., 149:672, 1985.

67. Periti, P., Mazzei, T., and Tonelli, F.: Single-dose cefotetan vs. multiple-dose cefoxitin-antimicrobial prophylaxis in colorectal surgery: Results of a prospective, multicenter, randomized study. Dis. Colon Rectum, 32:121, 1989.

68. Phillips, S. F., and Giller, J.: The contribution of colon to water and electrolyte conservation in man. J. Lab. Clin. Med., 81:733, 1973.

69. Porter, J. A., Salvati, E. P., Rubin, R. J., and Eisenstat, T. E.: Complications of colostomies. Dis. Colon Rectum, 32:299, 1989.

70. Racusen, L. D., and Binder, H. J.: Effect of prostaglandin on ion transport across isolated colonic mucosa. Dig. Dis. Sci., 25:900, 1980.

71. Rambaud, J. C., Modigliani, R., Matuchansky, C., et al.: Pancreatic cholera studies on tumoral secretions and pathophysiology of diarrhea. Gastroenterology, 69:110, 1975.

72. Read, N. W., Timms, J. M., Barfield, L. J., Donnelly, T. C., and Bannister, J. J.: Impairment of defecation in young women with severe constipation. Gastroenterology, 90:53, 1986.

73. Roediger, W. E. W.: Role of anaerobic bacteria in the metabolic welfare of the colonic mucosa in man. Gut, 21:793, 1980.

74. Roediger, W. E. W.: Utilization of nutrients by isolated epithelial cells of the rat colon. Gastroenterology, 83:424, 1982.

75. Roediger, W. E. W., and Moore, A.: Effect of short chain fatty acids on sodium absorption in isolated human colon perfused through the vascular bed. Dig. Dis. Sci., 26:100, 1981.

76. Roediger, W. E. W., and Rae, D. A.: Trophic effects of short chain fatty acids on mucosal handling of ions by the defunctionalized colon. Br. J. Surg., 69:23, 1982.

77. Saunders, D. R., Sillery, J., and Rachmilewitz, D.: Effect of dioctyl sodium sulfosuccinate on structure and function of rodent and human intestine. Gastroenterology, 69:380, 1975.

78. Schofield, P. F., Cade, D., and Lambert, M.: Dependent proximal loop colostomy: Does it defunction the distal colon? Br. J. Surg., 67:201, 1980.

79. Schrock, T. R.: Colonoscopic diagnosis and treatment of lower gastrointestinal bleeding. Surg. Clin. North Am., 69:1309, 1989.

80. Schultz, S. G.: Ion transport by mammalian large intestine. In Johnson, L.

R. (Ed.): Physiology of the Gastrointestinal Tract, Vol. 2. New York, Raven Press, 1983.

81. Shiau, Y. F., Feldman, G. M., Resnick, M. A., and Coff, P. M.: Stool electrolyte and osmolality measurements in the evaluation of diarrheal disorders. Ann. Intern. Med., 102:773, 1985.

82. Simon, J. B.: Occult blood screening for colorectal carcinoma: A critical review. Gastroenterology, 88:820, 1985.

83. Smith, F. W., and Sleisenger, M. H.: Physiology of the colon. In Sleisenger, M. H., and Fordtran, J. S. (Eds.): Gastrointestinal Disease: Pathophysiology, Diagnosis, Management. Philadelphia, W. B. Saunders, 1989.

84. Snooks, S. J., and Swash, M.: Electromyography and nerve latency studies. In Gooszen, H. G., Cate Hoedemaker, H. O., Weterman, I. T., and Keighley, M. R. B. (Eds.): Disordered Defecation. The Netherlands, Nijhoff, Dordrecht, 1987.

85. Snooks, S. J., Barnes, P. R. H., Swash, M., and Henry, M. M.: Damage to the innervation of the pelvic floor musculature in chronic constipation. Gastroenterology, 89:977, 1985.

86. Tanaka, N., Kubo, K., Shirakik, Koishi H., and Voshimura, H.: A pilot study on protein metabolism in the Papua New Guinea highlanders. J. Nutr. Sci. Vitaminol, 26:247, 1980.

87. Taylor, I., Hammond, P., and Darby, C.: An assessment of anorectal motility in the management of adult megacolon. Br. J. Surg. 67:754, 1980.

88. Tonelli, F., Ficari, F., DeFarra, F., et al.: Short or long-term prophylaxis with cefoxitin in elective colonic surgery. Coloproctology, 7:84, 1985.

89. Walser, M., and Bodenlos, L.: Urea metabolism in man. J. Clin. Invest., 38:1617, 1959.

90. Washington, J. A., Dearing, W. H., Judd, E. S., and Elveback, L. R.: Effect of postoperative antibiotic regimen on development of infection after intestinal surgery: A prospective randomized, double-blind study. Ann. Surg., 180:567, 1974.

91. Winawer, S. J.: Detection and diagnosis of colorectal cancer. Cancer, 51:2519, 1983.

92. Womack, N. R., Williams, N. S., Holmfield, J. H., Morrison, J. F., and Simpkins, K. C.: New method for the dynamic assessment of anorectal function in constipation. Br. J. Surg., 72:994, 1985.

V

DIVERTICULAR DISEASE OF THE COLON

Anthony L. Imbembo, M.D.

HISTORICAL ASPECTS

Until the early 1900s, diverticular disease of the colon was only of occasional interest, being described in sporadic case reports. In 1904, its anatomic basis was defined, and it was suggested that diverticular inflammation was due to impaction of a fecalith. The latter observation was also correlated with the pathologic findings of perforation, abscess formation, and fistulization. In 1907, the first report advocating surgical resection for complicated diverticulitis was presented by Dr. William J. Mayo at the American Surgical Association. Even in this early report, the advantages of creating a diverting colostomy ("temporary anus") or of performing a primary resection, when technically feasible, were expressed. Since these initial accounts, the incidence at autopsy of diverticular disease in Western civilizations seemingly has increased from an estimated 5% in 1910 to more than 40% in 1970.[13] This dramatic increase has been attributed both to increased recognition of diverticular disease and to changing environmental conditions.

DEFINITION

Diverticula are saclike protrusions of the colonic wall, varying in size from a few millimeters to several centimeters. True diverticula contain all layers of the colon wall and are believed to be congenital. They are very uncommon in the colon. False or *pseudodiverticula* represent herniations of the mucosa and submucosa through the circular muscle of the bowel wall. Unless otherwise stated in the text, the term *diverticula* refers to the predominant lesion, namely, colonic pseudodiverticula. The term *diverticulosis* simply indicates the presence of multiple diverticula of the colon.

PREVALENCE, PATHOGENESIS, AND PATHOLOGIC ANATOMY

The prevalence of diverticular disease in the general population ranges between 35% and 50%, as estimated by several large autopsy and radiographic series.[13] Prevalence directly correlates with age, estimated to be less than 5% at age 40, increasing to 30% by age 60, and as high as 65% by age 85.[25] Males and females appear to be affected equally. Geographically, diverticular disease is much more common in the United States and Western Europe than in other less industrialized regions such as Africa, South America, and Asia. Although diet is thought by many to contribute significantly to the development of diverticular disease, the complete etiology is likely to involve other, as yet unrecognized, factors. For example, diverticular disease in Asian populations is localized predominantly to the right colon, in distinct contrast to the left-sided predilection observed in Western civilizations. Such variations in the anatomic distribution of diverticula among civilizations might suggest that factors other than diet alone exert a substantial influence on the character of this disease worldwide.

Mechanical Factors. Clinical studies within the past 30 years have implicated low fiber diets as a prominent etiologic factor in the development of diverticular disease.[24, 25] Diets lacking vegetable fiber are presumed to predispose to the development of diverticula by altering colonic motility. Colonic motility is a complex process serving to transport feces distally while also permitting storage, thereby facilitating fluid and electrolyte absorption. Colonic motility is modulated by myogenic, hormonal, and neural influences.[14] There is evidence that patients with diverticular disease manifest exaggerated contractile responses to feeding and hormonal stimuli.[14, 27] Resting pressures are usually normal, however. These abnormal muscular contractions are believed to cause colonic smooth muscle hypertrophy, a characteristic of diverticular disease.

Some patients with diverticulosis also exhibit various types of colonic dysmotility that are thought to contribute to formation of diverticula. Normal fecal transport is modulated by coordinated, segmental muscular contractions that serve to separate the colonic lumen into a series of chambers [24, 26] (Fig. 32–5). Contraction of any one chamber tends to increase intraluminal pressure within that segment. Under normal circumstances, the chamber is open at one end, thereby allowing passage of feces, which results in lowering of intraluminal pressure. Patients with diverticulitis exhibit such segmentation, but individual chambers tend to become occluded at both ends during muscular contraction. When outflow from a particular segment is obstructed both proximally and distally, massive increases in intraluminal pressures, as high as 90 mm. Hg, have been noted.[26] Such isolated increases of intraluminal pressure are thought to predispose to herniation of mucosa through the bowel wall and, thus, to the development of diverticula (see Fig. 32–5).

The possible role of dietary fiber in the development of diverticula is best explained by effects on colonic diameter and stool consistency. It has been postulated that colonic segments with bulky fecal contents and large luminal diameters are less likely to exhibit exaggerated segmentation. Low-fiber diets are associated with a narrowed colon filled with small, hardened feces; segmentation is enhanced, and high luminal pressures tend to develop. Although this concept has been widely disseminated, definitive evidence for a causal relationship between low dietary fiber and the development of diverticular disease does not exist.[31, 39] Nonetheless, high-residue diets are in widespread use in the management of diverticular disease. Whether such therapy has a significant influence on the natural history of diverticular disease is unclear.

A possible increase in colonic wall strength in patients with diverticulosis is supported by the finding of elevated intraluminal pressures and colonic wall hypertrophy in these patients. Others, however, measuring the response of the sigmoid colon to intraluminal balloon distention suggest that the colon in diverticulosis may be weakened.[36] The presence of a structural defect in the colonic wall is suggested by the progressive decrease in tensile strength associated with aging. This decrease is associated with a progressive increase in the amounts of collagen, elastin, and reticular tissue in the colon wall.[6] Presently, it is generally accepted that diverticula are caused by various factors that intermittently increase colonic intraluminal pressure coupled with progressive decrease in colonic wall strength. The mechanisms responsible have not been defined precisely.

Anatomic Features. Diverticula tend to develop at specific points in the circumference of the colon. This localization is determined, in part, by the anatomic relationship between the colonic musculature and its nutrient blood supply (Fig. 32–6). Diverticula form at so-called weak points where the nutrient blood vessels (vasa recta) penetrate the circular muscle layer en route to the mucosa. These *perforating* vessels tend to penetrate the colonic wall along the mesenteric border of the two antimesenteric taeniae. The gaps in the circular muscle layer where the vasa recta penetrate constitute points of potential weakness through which the mucosa and submucosa can herniate, forming diverticula. Diverticula, therefore, are usually located between the single mesenteric taenia and either of the two antimesenteric taeniae (Fig. 32–7). Less commonly, diverticula form in the area between the antimesenteric taeniae. Although also consisting of mucosal herniation through the muscular layers of the colonic wall, these diverticula tend to be less prominent. In many instances the mucosal herniation does not quite extend to the serosa, causing these to be referred to as intramural diverticula.[20]

The distribution of diverticula throughout the colon also tends to follow a pattern, but with considerable individual variation (Fig. 32–8). The overwhelming majority of diverticula occur in the descending and sigmoid colon. It is estimated that 90% to 95% of patients with diverticulosis will have involvement of the sigmoid colon.[13, 31, 32] Approximately 65% of patients will have disease limited to the sigmoid colon alone.[28, 31] Conversely, only a small number of patients

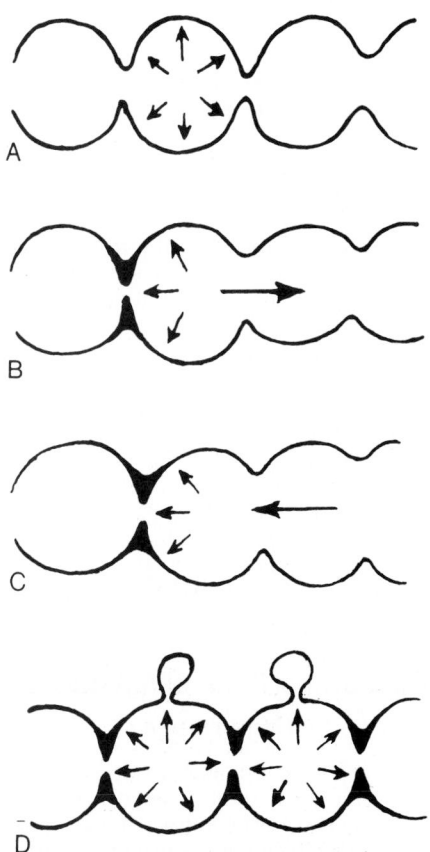

Figure 32–5. Schema demonstrating the process of segmentation. *A,* Contraction of a single chamber results in increased intraluminal pressure. Under normal circumstances the chamber is not completely isolated, thereby preventing dramatic increases in pressure. *B,* Relaxation at one end of a chamber during contraction allows fecal matter to be transported distally along the lumen. *C,* Failure to relax at one end of a chamber can slow or even halt transit of intestinal contents along the lumen. *D,* Complete isolation of one or more chambers during contraction results in diverticular formation. (From Painter, N. S.: The aetiology of diverticulosis of the colon with special reference to the action of certain drugs on the behavior of the colon. Ann. R. Coll. Surg. Engl., *34:*111, 1964.)

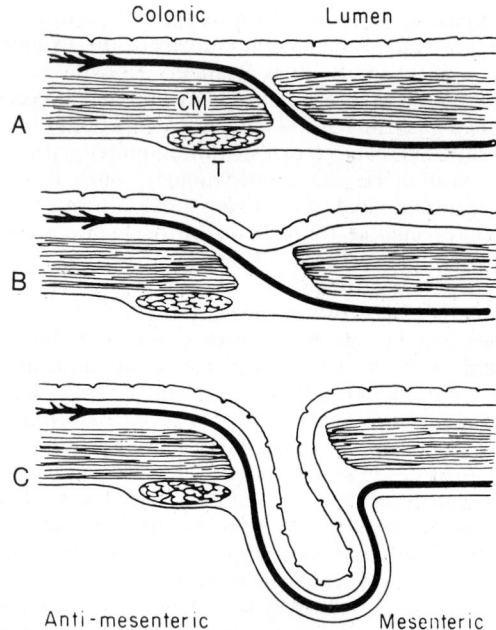

Figure 32–6. Drawing demonstrating the relation of a diverticulum to mural vasculature. *A*, The vasa recta penetrate the colonic wall obliquely at specific sites in the circular muscle (CM), usually along the mesenteric side of the taeniae (T). *B*, As a diverticulum begins to herniate through the colonic wall the blood vessels are drawn along. *C*, The vasa recta eventually become draped over the dome of the diverticulum and are prone to rupture after injury arising from within the lumen of the colon. (From Meyers, M. A., et al.: Pathogenesis of bleeding colonic diverticulosis. Gastroenterology, *71*:577, 1976.)

(2% to 10%) will have disease confined to the right colon.[31] Solitary diverticula occur most commonly in the cecum.

NATURAL HISTORY

Most patients with diverticulosis remain asymptomatic throughout their lifetime. It is estimated that between 10% and 25% of patients eventually develop signs and symptoms of diverticulitis.[28] Another 15% present with diverticular hemorrhage. As in most conditions, the prognosis of any one

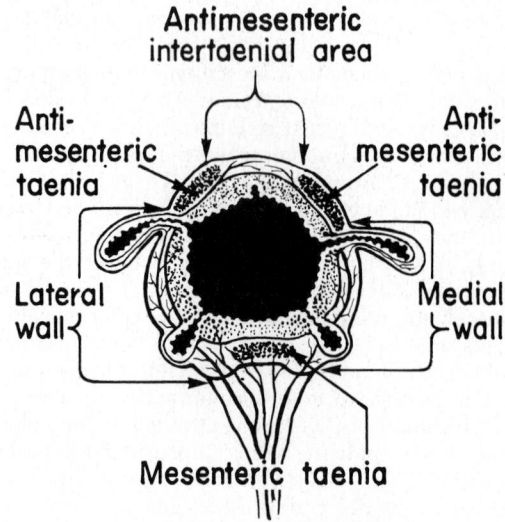

Figure 32–7. Transverse section of the colon demonstrating the relationship of diverticula to colonic taeniae and vasculature. (From Goligher, J.: Diverticulosis and diverticulitis of the colon. *In* Duthie, H., and Nixon, H. [Eds.]: Surgery of the Anus, Rectum, and Colon. London, Bailliere, 1984, p. 1083.)

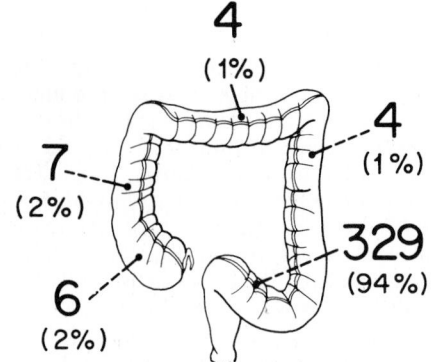

Figure 32–8. Diagram illustrating the prevalence of diverticular disease by location within the colon. (From Rodkey, G. V., and Welch, C. E.: Changing patterns in the surgical treatment of diverticular disease. Ann. Surg., *200*:466, 1984.)

episode of bleeding or inflammation varies according to the patient's general health and the severity of the underlying disease process. Patients with mild diverticulitis can be treated conservatively with excellent results, while patients with free intra-abdominal perforation of a diverticulum require emergent operation and can be expected to incur a 20% mortality.[32] An overall mortality of less than 5% can be expected in association with an initial attack of diverticulitis.[28]

After the first episode of diverticulitis, approximately one third of patients will sustain a second attack, usually within 3 to 5 years.[28] Another 30% to 40% will suffer from intermittent symptoms of discomfort and crampy abdominal pain, without requiring hospitalization. The remainder can be expected to remain symptom free. The prognosis is worse after a second attack, with only 10% of patients remaining symptom free. The morbidity and the mortality from recurrent attacks are also higher than that associated with an initial episode. Complications such as abscess formation or fistulization develop in approximately 20% of patients after a single attack of diverticulitis, while the complication rate approaches 60% in patients who have had previous episodes.[28]

Because diverticulosis is an acquired disease, the incidence of which clearly increases with age, it would seem logical that the number and size of diverticula would also increase with time. However, only 30% of patients demonstrate radiologic evidence of progression of their disease, either in the form of an increased number of diverticula or involvement of other segments of the colon. Progression of disease after resection of involved colon is also unusual, occurring in less than 10% to 15% of patients.[1]

COMPLICATIONS OF DIVERTICULOSIS

Hemorrhage

Diverticular disease is the most common cause of massive lower gastrointestinal bleeding in adults. Although, overall, colon carcinoma is the most common source of gastrointestinal blood loss, such bleeding is usually small in volume, often being detected only as occult blood on chemical testing.

Incidence and Etiology. Bleeding can be expected to develop in 15% of patients with diverticulosis, and before the use of angiography and emergent colonoscopy, diverticula were thought to account for up to 90% of significant lower intestinal hemorrhage. Actual localization of bleeding to a diverticulum was uncommon, however, because the diagnosis was often established primarily by excluding other potential sources of hemorrhage, such as carcinoma. With the ad-

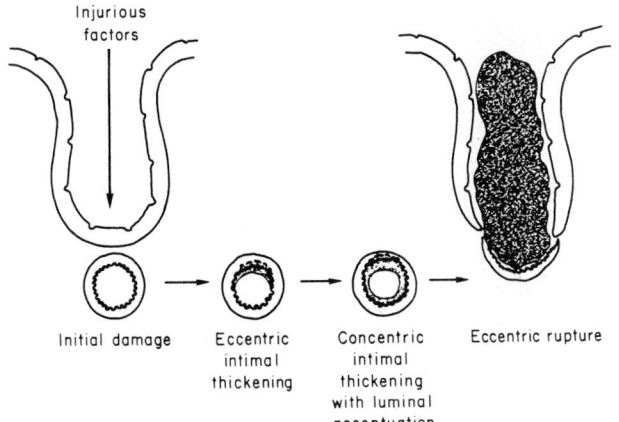

Figure 32–9. Drawing demonstrating proposed mechanism of diverticular hemorrhage. Arterial branches of the vasa recta lie in close proximity to the dome of the diverticulum. Over time, the artery is subjected to injury, but only along the side of the vessel facing the diverticular lumen. Eccentric (toward the colonic lumen) intimal thickening develops with eventual rupture into the colon. (From Meyers, M. A., et al.: Pathogenesis of bleeding colonic diverticulosis. Gastroenterology, *71*:577, 1976.)

vent of improved localization techniques, angiodysplastic lesions, also known as arteriovenous malformations, have been implicated with increasing frequency as a cause of colonic bleeding. It is estimated that 30% to 50% of massive colonic bleeding is due to diverticulosis while angiodysplasia is responsible for another 20% to 30%.[40] Remaining causes include colonic neoplasms, inflammatory bowel disease, ischemic colitis, and rare congenital lesions. Because as many as 30% to 40% of patients with lower intestinal hemorrhage never have the site of bleeding accurately determined, there is significant variation in the reported incidence of diverticular bleeding.[40]

Diverticular hemorrhage arises from the right colon in 70% to 90% of patients.[3] The explanation for this right-sided predilection is not entirely clear but may be related to the thinner wall of the right colon. Approximately 70% of patients with diverticular hemorrhage will stop bleeding spontaneously, often before presentation at the hospital. The risk of rebleeding is only 30%, but it increases to 50% after a second episode of hemorrhage.

Diverticular hemorrhage is thought to result from injury and subsequent rupture of blood vessels lying adjacent to a diverticulum (Fig. 32–9). Diverticula develop at potential weak points in the colonic wall where the nutrient blood vessels penetrate the circular muscle layer, en route to the mucosa. As a diverticulum begins to herniate, it tends to carry one of the penetrating vessels with it. Eventually, the vessel becomes draped over the dome of the diverticulum, separated from the colonic lumen only by the thin mucosal layer. This anatomic relationship predisposes to injury with subsequent rupture. Characteristic pathologic changes in the vasa recta of bleeding diverticula have been observed. These consist of eccentric thickening of the intima and thinning of the underlying media.[22] In all cases, rupture occurs eccentrically into the lumen of the diverticulum. Diverticular hemorrhage usually occurs in the absence of acute or chronic inflammation.[22]

Clinical Features. Many patients with diverticular hemorrhage present with self-limited or minor episodes of bleeding. Patients often describe intermittent, sporadic passage of bright red or maroon blood per rectum. Fifty percent of patients will give a history of a previous episode of colonic hemorrhage.[3] Usually, abdominal pain or discomfort is absent and physical examination is unremarkable.

One third of patients with diverticular hemorrhage (or about 5% of all patients with diverticulosis) present with massive, exsanguinating hemorrhage. Such patients demand immediate resuscitation and therapeutic intervention. The overwhelming majority of these patients are elderly, usually in their seventh or eighth decade. Consequently, 70% of these patients have serious comorbid diseases. These associations undoubtedly contribute to the high morbidity and mortality (10% to 20%) associated with diverticular hemorrhage.[40]

Diagnosis. The first step in the management of any patient with massive gastrointestinal hemorrhage is resuscitation. Monitoring should be instituted rapidly, as for any patient with the potential for hypovolemic shock. The passage of a nasogastric tube helps exclude an upper gastrointestinal source of bleeding. Resuscitative measures should commence before any further diagnostic maneuvers are undertaken.

All patients with massive lower gastrointestinal hemorrhage should undergo proctoscopy as soon as possible. The main purpose of this examination is to exclude the rectum as the bleeding source. Although difficult in the face of active hemorrhage, identification of bleeding from hemorrhoids or other rectal lesions is extremely important. Emergency subtotal colectomy for exsanguinating colonic hemorrhage should not be performed until every effort has been made to exclude the rectum as the site of bleeding. Failure to do so results occasionally in a patient who continues to bleed postoperatively from a previously unidentified rectal source.

Seventy to 80% of patients will stop bleeding spontaneously; such patients should undergo elective evaluation. Continued massive bleeding in a hemodynamically unstable patient is an indication for emergent operation.[5] However, in actively bleeding patients who maintain relative hemodynamic stability, attempts at localization of the bleeding site should be made. Emergent selective mesenteric arteriography will successfully identify the site of hemorrhage in 40% to 60% of patients.[3, 40] (Fig. 32–10). The high rate of spontaneous cessation of bleeding after initial resuscitative management

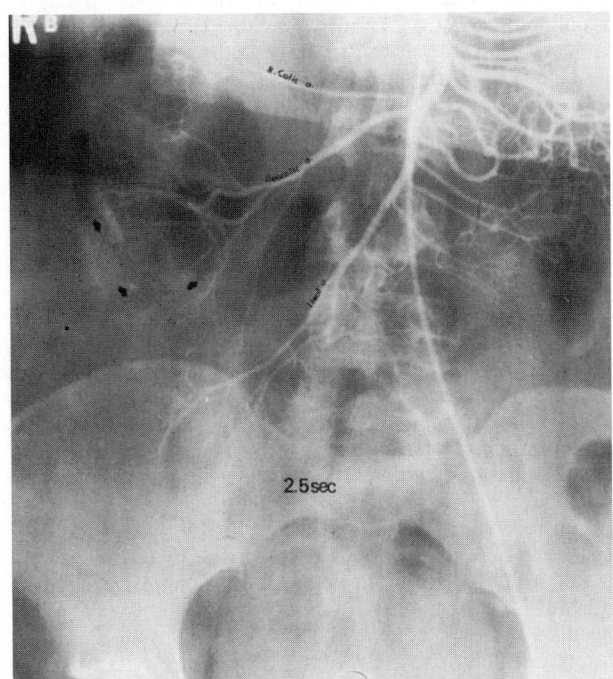

Figure 32–10. Selective mesenteric radiograph demonstrating extravasation of contrast (arrows) from diverticular hemorrhage. This specific case represents an unusual situation in which multiple, simultaneous bleeding sites were detected.

probably contributes to a relatively high rate of nondiagnostic arteriograms.[40] For arteriography to be diagnostic, bleeding must be taking place at a minimal rate of 0.5 ml. per minute and both the superior mesenteric and inferior mesenteric vessels must be studied. Therefore, performing selective mesenteric arteriography in all patients with lower gastrointestinal hemorrhage, regardless of the rate of bleeding, results in lower diagnostic yields. Limiting arteriography to those patients with ongoing hemorrhage results in a diagnostic yield of 70% to 100%.

Another alternative, even in the actively bleeding patient, is to perform diagnostic colonoscopy. Jensen and Machicado have demonstrated that combined colonoscopy and esophagogastroduodenoscopy is extremely effective in localizing the site of bleeding, provided that the colon has been rapidly and adequately purged with large amounts of a nonabsorbable, polyethylene-glycol solution (GoLytely).[15] In a group of 80 patients with lower gastrointestinal hemorrhage, they reported an 86% diagnostic accuracy rate. They either detected lesions in the colon (74%) or noted the absence of such lesions in patients with bleeding emanating from above the ileocecal valve (20%). Emergent colonoscopy was not associated with an increased technically related complication rate. However, congestive heart failure, secondary to the voluminous (3 to 7 liters) purge of the gastrointestinal tract, occurred in 4% of patients.

Radioisotope scans are of two basic types: technetium-99m–labeled sulfur colloid or red blood cells. ^{99m}Tc-sulfur colloid, once injected intravenously, is cleared from the circulation by the liver, spleen, and bone marrow within several minutes. However, any labeled colloid that extravasates into the intestinal lumen is not cleared and remains, it is hoped, near the site of bleeding. Abnormal radioactive pooling can be detected on scanning. The study is completed within a short time, and bleeding rates as low as 0.1 ml. per minute can be detected (Fig. 32–11). Labeled erythrocytes, on the other hand, have a relatively long half-life within the circulation. Scanning can be repeated at 24 or 36 hours after injection. Therefore, the tagged red blood cell scan may be useful in detection of chronic or intermittent bleeding.[11] Tagged red blood cell studies are also capable of detecting extremely slow rates of bleeding, as little as 0.1 ml. per minute.

Radioisotope scans are variably successful in actually localizing the site of hemorrhage. In one series of 59 patients, the site of bleeding was suggested in 36 (61%), but in only 25 patients (42%) did the activity on scintigraphy correlate with an actual pathologic lesion demonstrated by other means (endoscopy, angiography, or surgery).[11] Others have reported localization accuracy rates ranging from 24% to 91%.[41] One reason for the relatively poor localization rates is that blood within the intestinal lumen does not remain stationary. For example, blood originally extravasated into the cecum may pass rapidly into the distal colon after only a few peristaltic waves. Similarly, with an incompetent ileocecal valve, blood may reflux proximally into the small intestine. In either case, subsequent scanning might lead to inaccurate localization. Normal anatomic relationships also may account for diagnostic errors. Bleeding lesions in the upper gastrointestinal tract may superimpose on adjacent colon, thereby resulting in an incorrect diagnosis of colonic hemorrhage. Similarly, lesions in the transverse colon, although an unusual site for hemorrhage, may be interpreted as an upper intestinal bleeding source. Bleeding from a redundant loop of sigmoid colon, which drapes toward the patient's right lower quadrant, may be falsely identified as bleeding from the right colon. For all these reasons, segmental colon resection based solely on the results of a positive bleeding scan should be undertaken with extreme caution.

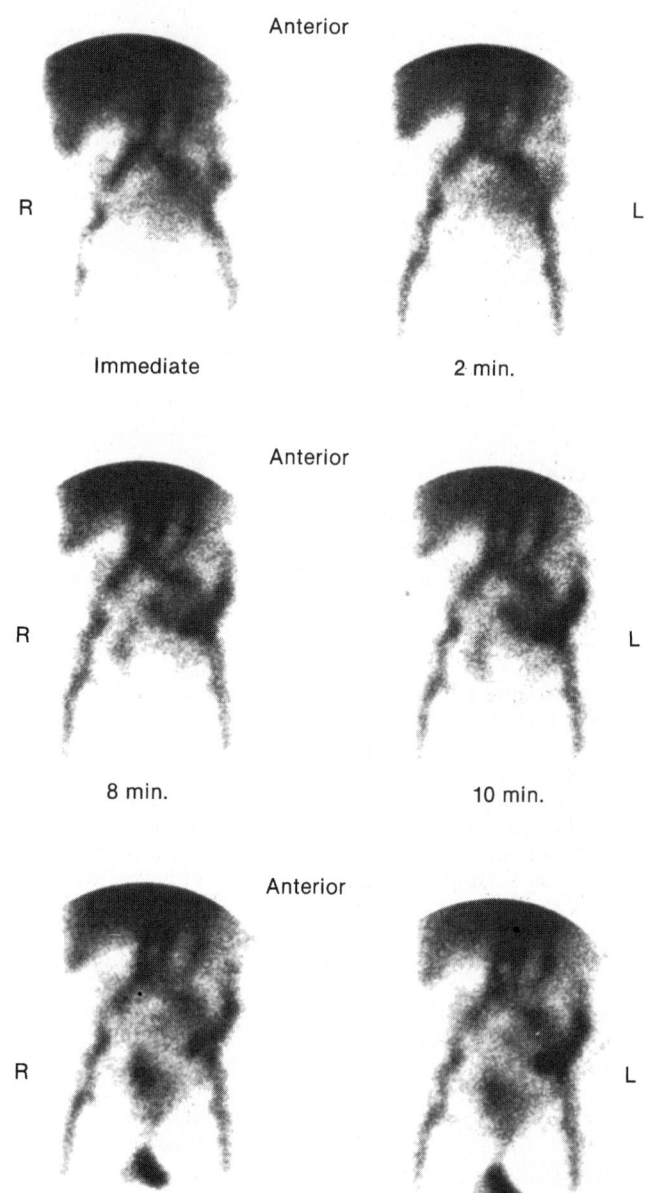

Figure 32–11. Radionuclide scan with technetium-99m demonstrates rapid extravasation of tracer into the left colon of a patient with bleeding diverticular disease. The tracer can be seen almost immediately in the left colon. At 8 to 10 minutes tracer is clearly present within the sigmoid colon and by 16 to 18 minutes tracer has already passed distally into the rectum.

Despite the wide variations noted, such scans are frequently obtained as the initial diagnostic study in patients with intestinal hemorrhage. Currently, several centers use nuclear scanning as a screening test to determine the need for subsequent arteriography.[38] Patients with positive bleeding scans proceed to selective arteriography, while those with no evidence of active bleeding are observed for signs of further hemorrhage. Bleeding scans are extremely sensitive in detecting active bleeding, with false-negative and false-positive rates of less than 10%.[41] By reserving arteriography for the patient with a positive scan, the diagnostic accuracy of this study can be substantially improved, often to greater than 90%.

In patients who have ceased bleeding, diagnostic studies can be performed on a more elective basis. The colon can be adequately prepared and colonoscopy performed with outstanding diagnostic accuracy. Elective colonoscopy should have a diagnostic sensitivity of 90% in detecting nonbleeding lesions of the colon. The double-contrast barium enema is still a useful test, but it may have a sensitivity of only 70% in this situation. A barium enema evaluation should never be performed in the actively bleeding patient. Once barium contrast has been introduced into the colon, it obscures any subsequent attempts at visualization by arteriography or colonoscopy.[38]

Treatment. Initial resuscitative measures, as for any patient with gastrointestinal hemorrhage and hypovolemia, should be begun promptly. With adequate fluid resuscitation, blood transfusion, and correction of coagulation abnormalities, 70% to 80% of patients cease bleeding spontaneously. However, approximately 15% of all patients presenting with massive diverticular hemorrhage will require emergent operation before further diagnostic information can be obtained. The mortality in this group is high, often approaching 30% to 50%.[40]

If a bleeding source can be localized at arteriography, selective intra-arterial infusion of vasopressin (0.1 to 0.4 units per minute) or embolization with thrombotic agents, such as absorbable gelatin or autologous clot, have been used with success. In patients with an identifiable site of bleeding, selective intra-arterial infusion of vasopressin (a potent vasoconstrictor) can be expected to control hemorrhage in over 90% of cases.[2] The infusion should be started at a rate of 0.2 unit per minute. If the bleeding is not controlled promptly, the rate can be increased to a maximum of 0.4 unit per minute. Continued bleeding despite vasopressin infusion is an indication for other therapeutic measures, usually a surgical procedure. If, however, bleeding stops with the administration of vasopressin, the infusion should be maintained for another 24 hours. If bleeding does not recur, the infusion should be tapered gradually and discontinued over the subsequent 12 hours. The catheter should be left in place for an additional 8 to 12 hours for use if bleeding recurs. Selective vasopressin infusion, however, is not without problems. Its vasoconstrictive effects are often only temporary, with up to 50% of patients rebleeding after the infusion has been stopped.[2] Vasopressin is also associated with infrequent but potentially serious side effects. Major complications can include myocardial, mesenteric, and cerebral ischemia; arrhythmias; hypertension; hyponatremia; and fluid overload. Embolic, thrombotic, and septic complications due to the indwelling arterial catheter also contribute to an overall complication rate of 4% to 6%. Still, selective arterial infusion of vasopressin may convert an emergent situation to an elective or semi-elective one, thereby decreasing the operative mortality in this elderly, high-risk patient population.

Transcatheter embolization might be an alternative to vasopressin, especially in situations where vasopressin has not been effective or is contraindicated. However, use of embolization for the treatment of lower intestinal hemorrhage is controversial. Due to a postembolic colon infarction rate of 13%, transcatheter embolization has been used more often for control of upper intestinal hemorrhage.[33] On rare occasions, colonoscopy may reveal an actively bleeding lesion at the base of a diverticulum, thereby permitting attempts at electrocoagulation or laser photoablation. Diverticular hemorrhage, however, is usually not amenable to endoscopic therapy.[15] Although the barium enema has been used in the past in an attempt to tamponade diverticular hemorrhage, the validity of this approach is questionable.[38]

Emergent operation should be performed in any patient who continues to bleed despite resuscitative and therapeutic maneuvers. Indications for surgery include persistent hemodynamic instability, a transfusion requirement of greater than 2000 ml. over a 24-hour period, and recurrent hemorrhage. Emergent operation can be either *directed* or *nondirected*, de-

pending on the success or failure of preoperative localization. If a bleeding site has been identified by colonoscopy or arteriography, a segmental resection can be performed with the expectation that bleeding will be controlled in over 90% of patients. A primary anastomosis is usually possible because fecal matter has usually been removed secondary to passage of large amounts of blood.

If the source of bleeding has not been identified, total abdominal colectomy with ileoproctostomy should be performed. This procedure will cure the patient with colonic bleeding but is associated with high mortality rates (30% to 50%).[2] However, even with angiographic localization and a limited segmental resection, an operative mortality rate of 20% to 30% can be expected in emergent circumstances. Segmental resection should not be performed when the site of colonic hemorrhage has not been identified. Blind segmental resection is associated with an extremely high rate of rebleeding (35% to 50%). Attempts at intraoperative localization of previously unidentified bleeding sites, either by multiple enterotomies or divided colostomies, are usually unsuccessful. Other maneuvers that have been used sporadically to localize bleeding intraoperatively include Doppler scanning, transillumination of the bowel lumen, intra-arterial injection of methylene blue dye, and intraoperative colonoscopy, all with very limited success. Total abdominal colectomy with ileoproctostomy should be selected in the absence of localization because this obviates the even higher morbidity and mortality associated with inability to control hemorrhage at the initial operation. Elective colon resection is recommended in any patient with a history of previous diverticular bleeding who presents with a second episode of hemorrhage.

DIVERTICULITIS

The term *diverticulitis* simply refers to inflammation of one or more diverticula. It comprises a spectrum of disease ranging from mild, well-localized inflammation to a fulminant process resulting in free perforation and generalized peritonitis. It is thought that diverticulitis represents, at an anatomic level, perforation of a diverticulum into the pericolic, or *peridiverticular*, space. However, as many as one third of patients undergoing colon resection for symptomatic diverticulitis will not have pathologic evidence of inflammation on subsequent histologic examination. Because many patients may have abdominal symptoms in the absence of active inflammation, a clear distinction between diverticulitis and painful colonic spasm is often difficult. Patients with diverticulosis may also have coexistent irritable bowel syndrome. Thus, a patient's symptoms may be totally unrelated to his or her diverticular disease.

The inflammatory process may be classified as either simple or complicated. Simple diverticulitis can be expected to resolve, in most cases, with medical therapy. Patients with complicated diverticulitis manifest one or more of the serious sequelae of the disease, such as abscess formation, obstruction, free perforation, or fistulization. Such patients generally require surgical intervention.

Incidence and Pathogenesis. Diverticulitis will develop in 15% to 20% of patients with diverticulosis sometime during their lifetime. Although 65% of diverticula are confined solely to the sigmoid colon, inflammation will be limited to this segment in over 90% of cases.[32] Right-sided diverticular inflammation occurs in only 5% of patients with diverticulitis.[9, 10, 34] Approximately three fourths of cases with right-sided diverticulitis are not diagnosed until laparotomy for presumptive acute appendicitis.[10]

The pathogenesis of diverticulitis is usually believed to be secondary to perforation, either microscopic or macroscopic, of a diverticulum. The perforation is preceded by chronic effacement and erosion of the diverticular wall caused by increased intraluminal pressure or inspissated food particles trapped within the diverticular lumen. Eventually, sufficient inflammation and focal necrosis ensues, leading to perforation. In most settings, the inflammatory process is relatively mild and of sufficient duration so that the entire perforation is confined by the pericolic fat and surrounding mesentery. Involvement of other abdominal organs in this walling-off process occasionally leads to small bowel obstruction or fistulization. If the inflammatory process does not resolve despite containment, a localized abscess may develop. If the perforation is not well contained, free perforation with generalized peritonitis may supervene. The pathogenesis of diverticulitis previously was thought to be quite similar to that of appendicitis. However, luminal obstruction of a diverticular neck by a fecalith or inspissated food particles is believed to be an extremely rare event.[31]

Clinical Features. The presenting clinical features of diverticulitis vary according to the location and severity of the underlying inflammatory process. Patients with painful colonic spasm or irritable bowel syndrome may present with abdominal complaints similar to those associated with mild, acute diverticulitis. Patients with true acute diverticulitis, however, usually manifest signs and symptoms of ongoing inflammation, such as progressive localized pain, anorexia, fever, leukocytosis, and the physical findings consistent with local peritonitis.

Left lower quadrant pain is the most common complaint of patients with diverticulitis. It is present in over 70% of patients and is the most common reason for hospitalization.[29, 31] The pain is usually present for several days before hospitalization, thus helping to differentiate the condition from other acute surgical problems, such as appendicitis or perforated peptic ulcer. Only 17% of patients present with symptoms of less than 24 hours' duration.[32] A history of previous episodes of pain is given by one half of patients.[19] Nausea and vomiting occur in only 20% of patients.[29] Diarrhea is present in one third, and constipation occurs in almost one half of cases. Urinary tract symptoms such as dysuria, urgency, and increased frequency are present in only 10% to 15% of patients.[19, 29] The presence of symptoms in addition to pain is associated with an overall worsened prognosis.[28, 29]

Physical examination usually reveals direct abdominal tenderness, characteristically localized to the left lower quadrant. A tender abdominal mass is found in 20% of cases, and its presence portends a worse prognosis.[29] Occasionally, tenderness may be manifest in the right lower quadrant. This may be due to either right-sided diverticulitis or inflammation of a redundant loop of sigmoid colon. Such cases are often initially confused with acute appendicitis and usually are not diagnosed until laparotomy. Overall, abdominal distention is reported in up to two thirds of patients. Low-grade fever and mild leukocytosis are common.[19] Patients with white blood cell counts greater than 15,000 per cu. mm. are more likely to have an intra-abdominal abscess. Urinalysis may demonstrate an increased number of white blood cells if the inflammatory process is adjacent to ureter or bladder. The presence of bacteria, especially colonic flora, in the urine is a strong indication that a fistula exists between the inflamed colon and the urinary tract.

Diagnosis. Most patients can be diagnosed on the basis of their clinical presentation. However, because other acute surgical conditions such as appendicitis, perforated colon cancer, or perforated duodenal ulcer can present with a similar clinical picture, confirmation of the diagnosis is of considerable importance.

Routine abdominal and chest radiographs are usually unremarkable. Only one third of such films demonstrates any abnormality.[23] Despite this, they are helpful in excluding other acute surgical problems such as intestinal obstruction or a perforated viscus. Free air beneath the diaphragm is an unusual finding with diverticulitis. Occasionally, plain films may demonstrate retroperitoneal air or a mass effect secondary to a large paracolic abscess.

Contrast radiography or colonoscopy should be undertaken with caution in patients with suspected acute diverticulitis. The increased luminal pressure from the injected contrast material or from insufflation of air may lead to free rupture of a previously well-localized peridiverticular abscess or phlegmon.[31] The fear of extravasation of barium and/or feces into the peritoneal cavity causes most clinicians to delay contrast studies until signs of active inflammation have subsided. Although studies have suggested that both contrast enema and colonoscopy, when performed by experienced personnel, can be done safely with a high diagnostic yield, the introduction of computed tomographic (CT) scanning has substantially reduced their use.

CT scanning has been shown to be as accurate as barium enema evaluation in diagnosing diverticulitis (Fig. 32–12). Evidence of pericolic inflammation, bowel wall edema, abscess formation, and even fistulization is present in 63% to 95% of patients.[23] CT scanning has the advantages of being noninvasive, avoiding increased intraluminal pressure, and being able to detect extraluminal disease (i.e., the presence of ureteral obstruction or distant abscess formation). It is especially useful in identifying and localizing abscess or phlegmon formation, and it is also an objective way to follow resolution of the inflammatory process.

In contrast, elective evaluation of a patient after complete resolution of an episode of diverticulitis should include colonoscopy, barium enema, or both. Contrast studies of the colon may reveal coexistent lesions such as polyps or colon cancer. It is imperative that the entire colon be evaluated in any patient with suspected diverticulitis to establish the extent of the underlying disease (Fig. 32–13). Even if a patient has an otherwise normal-appearing colon by barium study, colonoscopy can add important information. For example, diverticular inflammation can lead to severe stricture formation that mimics colon cancer (Fig. 32–14). Colonoscopy with multiple biopsies should be undertaken in such a situation.

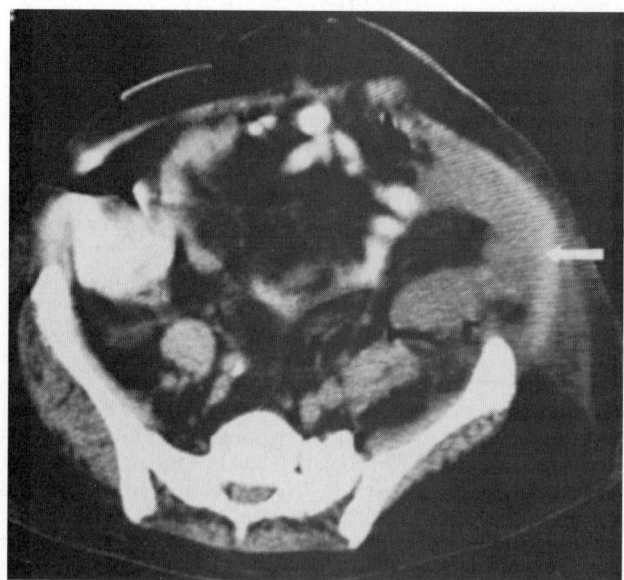

Figure 32–12. CT scan of the abdomen demonstrating severe diverticulitis. A pericolic abscess (arrow) is present in the left lower quadrant and significant signs of inflammation (bowel wall edema, "dirty fat" appearance to mesentery) are present through the lower abdomen.

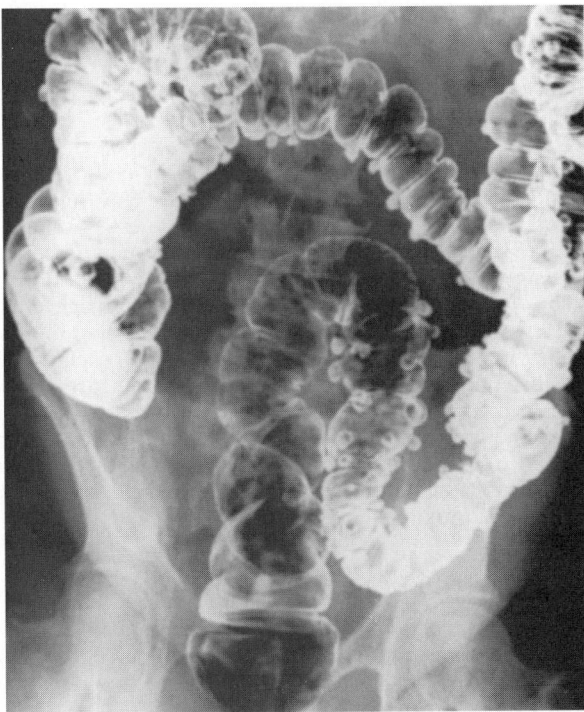

Figure 32–13. Barium enema demonstrating a typical case of severe diverticulosis. This patient has pancolonic disease, but the highest concentration is in the left and sigmoid colon.

Even with multiple negative biopsies, the gross appearance of the lesion may resemble carcinoma so closely that urgent resection is recommended.

Treatment. A few patients with minor episodes of diverticulitis can be treated on an outpatient basis with oral antibiotics and a clear liquid diet. Patients who do not improve with such treatment require hospitalization. Except for the most minor of attacks, however, a patient with acute diverticulitis

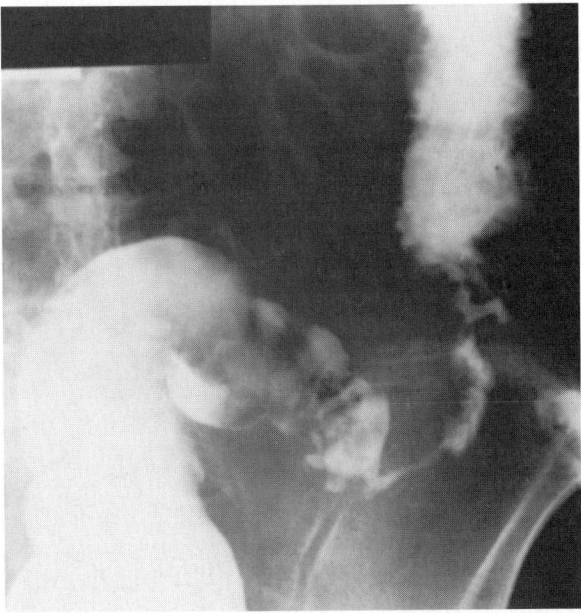

Figure 32–14. Barium enema demonstrating a severe stricture in the sigmoid colon secondary to diverticular disease. Severe disease such as shown here is often difficult to differentiate from colon carcinoma; therefore, colonoscopy is often necessary to exclude malignancy.

should be hospitalized for treatment and close observation. Therapy consists of bowel rest (including use of nasogastric suction if nausea, vomiting, or abdominal distention are present), intravenous antibiotics, and intravenous fluids. Antispasmodics and analgesia are often added to improve patient comfort. The antibiotic regimen should provide coverage of normal colonic flora. Common regimens include cefoxitin or, in more severe cases, an aminoglycoside in combination with either clindamycin or metronidazole for anaerobic coverage. With resolution of clinical evidence of inflammation, oral intake can be instituted. Before discharge the patient should be placed on a high-fiber diet. Psyllium seed preparations may be prescribed to add bulk to the stool with the aim of minimizing segmentation. Barium enema and/or colonoscopy should be performed within several weeks of the acute episode.

Patients who fail to respond or deteriorate within the first 24 to 48 hours usually require urgent surgical intervention. Occasionally, patients who are known to have a diverticular abscess can be stabilized temporarily by percutaneous, CT-guided drainage. Studies have suggested that this maneuver may provide valuable time for adequate resuscitation of a critically ill patient before further management.[37] However, such drainage should never be construed as definitive treatment.

Approximately 20% of patients who develop acute diverticulitis eventually require operation.[12, 32] After a second attack, the incidence of complications approaches 50% to 60%, with a mortality rate that is twice that associated with an initial attack.[28] Most clinicians agree that recurrence of acute diverticulitis warrants surgical resection once active inflammation has subsided.[31] Indications for operation are listed in Table 32–3. Septic complications such as abscess formation and free perforation are the most common indications for surgical intervention. Other less common indications include intestinal obstruction, fistulization, intractable abdominal pain, the presence of a persistent abdominal mass, and the inability to exclude the presence of a colon carcinoma. In several distinct subgroups, surgical treatment is also recommended; patients younger than the age of 40, those with suspected right-sided diverticulitis, and those who are immunocompromised usually do not respond to medical treatment.

Surgical Options. The type of surgical treatment depends largely on the severity and extent of the underlying inflammatory process. Patients undergoing an elective surgical procedure for recurrent attacks, the presence of a persistent abdominal mass, or intractable symptoms are usually best served by resection of the involved segment and primary anastomosis. Adequate bowel preparation is usually possible,

TABLE 32–3. Indications for Surgical Treatment

Absolute

Complications of the disease
    Intractable or recurrent hemorrhage
    Sepsis (abscess, peritonitis)
    Fistula
    Obstruction
Recurrent episodes of inflammation
Intractable symptoms or signs (persistent pain or mass)
Clinical deterioration
Inability to exclude carcinoma

Relative

Chronic stricture
Young patient
Corticosteroid use
Right-sided diverticulitis

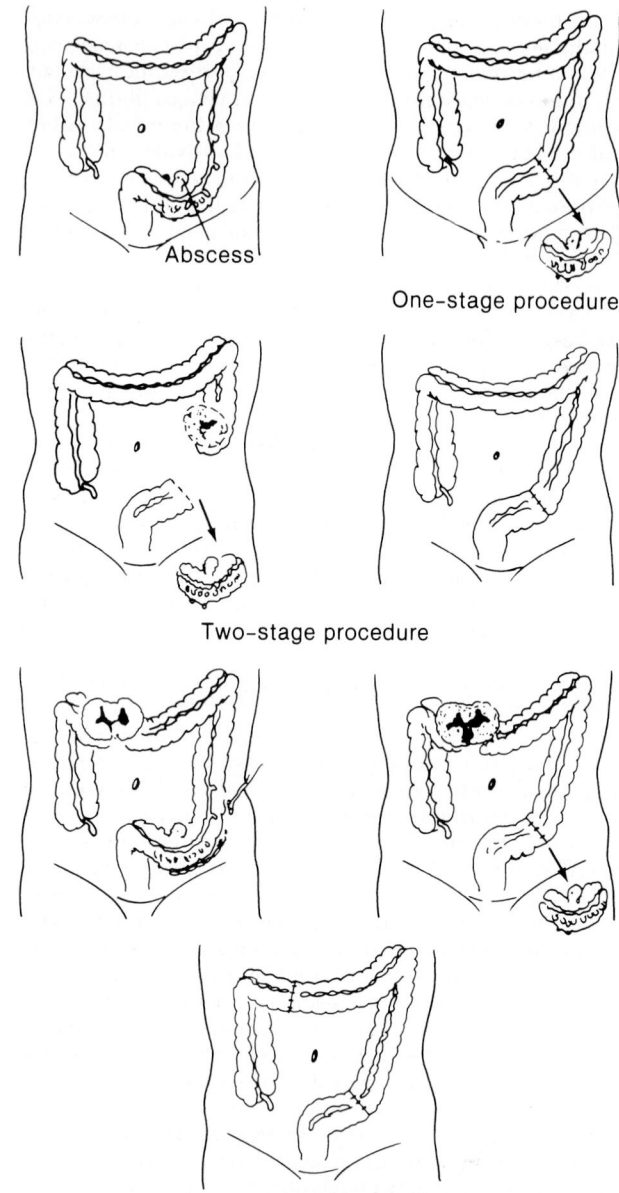

Abscess

One-stage procedure

Two-stage procedure

Three-stage procedure

Figure 32–15. Drawing illustrating the options in the surgical treatment of diverticular disease. One-stage procedure: (1) Resection of the diseased segment of colon with primary anastomosis. Two-stage procedure: (1) Resection of the diseased segment with formation of a temporary end-colostomy. (2) Closure of colostomy. Three-stage procedure: (1) Simple drainage of the diseased region with formation of a proximal, diverting colostomy. (2) Resection of the diseased segment with primary anastomosis. The colostomy is left intact. (3) Closure of colostomy. (Redrawn from Rege, R. V., and Nahrwold, D. L.: Diverticular disease. Curr. Probl. Surg., *26:*136, 1989.)

and both oral and systemic antibiotics can be administered safely and easily. The mortality for elective colon resection after the resolution of inflammatory diverticular disease should be less than 2%.[32]

Patients presenting with progressive or fulminant disease usually require emergent intervention. Because bowel preparation is not usually possible, two- and three-stage procedures have been advocated (Fig. 32–15). The two-stage procedure entails resection of the involved colon with creation of an end-colostomy initially. The colostomy is then closed as a subsequent procedure, which is often deferred for 8 to 12 weeks. The three-stage procedure consists of drainage of the

involved segment along with creation of a proximal diverting colostomy. This is followed 3 to 6 months later by resection of the diseased segment with primary anastomosis. The third operation consists of closure of the proximal colostomy 1 to 3 months later. If the inflammatory process is well localized and if the colon can be safely mobilized, resection is strongly recommended, usually with creation of an end-colostomy and mucous fistula or Hartmann's pouch. The three-stage approach is now largely of historical interest. Numerous studies have documented that primary resection is associated with a significantly lower mortality (0% to 10%) and morbidity (25% to 30%) as compared with simple drainage of the abscess with proximal colostomy. The mortality and morbidity following the latter approach 30% and 50%, respectively.[7, 19, 32] Most failures of the three-stage approach are due to failure to control sepsis after the initial procedure. Only in the extremely rare circumstance where the diseased segment is densely adherent to adjacent structures, such as the ureter or iliac vessels, should resection be abandoned in favor of drainage and proximal colostomy.

SEQUELAE OF DIVERTICULITIS

Common sequelae of diverticulitis include abscess formation, free intraperitoneal perforation, intestinal obstruction, and fistulization (Fig. 32–16). Each of these conditions may coexist in any given patient. Complications develop in up to 25% of patients with active diverticulitis, and surgical intervention is necessary in almost all such instances.[12, 32] Of patients requiring operation, the distribution of the various complications is abscess formation (40% to 50%), intestinal obstruction (10% to 30%), free perforation (10% to 15%), and fistulization (4% to 10%).[19, 29, 32]

Abscess Formation. Diverticular abscesses are extremely common and are characterized, according to their location, as either peridiverticular, retroperitoneal, mesenteric, or pelvic. Occasionally, such collections spread to adjacent structures and present as a hip, thigh, or anterior abdominal wall abscess. Hepatic abscess may develop as a secondary complication on occasion. Primary resection of the involved segment with colostomy and adequate local drainage is the most appropriate treatment. Successful preoperative percutaneous drainage of diverticular abscesses has been reported. Such measures may help to stabilize critically ill patients. It is

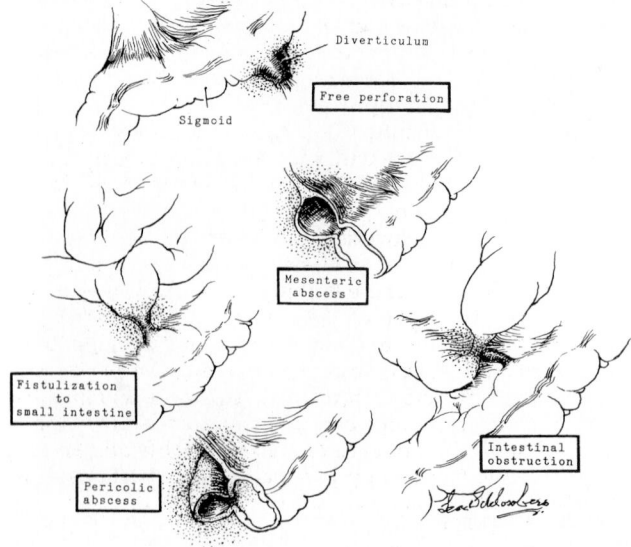

Figure 32–16. Complications of diverticulitis.

argued that these patients are then able to undergo elective, one-stage resection of the diseased colon at a later date. However, since the underlying focus of infection is not removed, caution should be exercised in choosing this approach. Advocates suggest that sepsis can be controlled in up to 80% of patients. The presence of a fecal fistula after percutaneous drainage usually means that sepsis may not be adequately controlled.[37]

Obstruction. Chronic diverticulitis may cause progressive large bowel obstruction due to stricture formation. Such obstruction is rarely complete. Occasionally, a loop of small intestine may become densely adherent to the inflammatory process in the colon, resulting in partial or complete small bowel obstruction. Resection of the involved segment with either primary anastomosis or colostomy is the treatment of choice, depending on the adequacy of bowel preparation proximal to the diseased segment.

Free Perforation. Although most episodes of perforated diverticulitis are confined to the peridiverticular region or pelvis, an occasional patient presents with signs of generalized peritonitis. Free intraperitoneal contamination may develop secondary to rupture of an inflamed diverticulum or of an established diverticular abscess. These patients require emergent surgical intervention. The overall mortality is high (20% to 40%), largely due to complications such as septic shock and multiple organ failure.[12] Resection of the perforated segment with end-colostomy, followed by copious irrigation of the peritoneal cavity is the appropriate treatment.

Fistulization. Although less common than abscess formation or intestinal obstruction, colonic fistulas may develop secondary to diverticulitis. Over 90% of cases of acute diverticulitis are localized to the sigmoid colon and, therefore, fistulization most commonly involves this segment. The most common type is the colovesical fistula, accounting for up to two thirds of all internal diverticular fistulas.[42] Colocutaneous fistulas are the second most common type of diverticular fistula, followed by colovaginal and coloenteric fistulas, in decreasing order of frequency. Other fistulas such as colouterine, colouteric, and colosalpingian are extremely rare.

The most common diverticular fistula, the colovesical fistula, serves as an excellent example of the clinical features, diagnostic evaluation, and therapeutic options in management of this complication. Colovesical fistula is three to five times more common in men than in women. This discrepancy has been attributed to the presence of an intervening uterus in females, which serves as a protective anatomic barrier between the inflamed colon and the bladder. This is supported by the fact that 61% of women who develop a colovesical fistula have had a previous hysterectomy. Patients with colovesical fistulas present with dysuria (29% to 94%), fecaluria (48% to 75%), and pneumaturia (41% to 75%) as the most frequent complaints.[16] Only 25% to 30% of patients will present with abdominal pain or evidence of systemic infection. The occurrence of recurrent urinary tract infections is a common presentation.

The diagnosis of a colovesical fistula can often be made on the basis of a history of pneumaturia and the finding of fecaluria on urinalysis. These findings do not, however, identify the underlying cause of the fistula. Colovesical fistulas may develop secondary to either diverticulitis (52%), granulomatous colitis (18%), or carcinoma (11%) or other pelvic malignancies.[16] Therefore, further diagnostic evaluation is necessary. Cystoscopy and barium enema are studies most likely to confirm the presence of a colovesical fistula and to define its cause. Cystoscopy is usually the most helpful in confirmation, with diagnostic accuracy of 80% to 95%. The most common finding on cystoscopy is localized inflammation and bullous edema of the bladder mucosa, with actual demonstration of the fistula occurring in only 20% of patients. Barium enema demonstrates nonspecific colonic abnormalities in almost all cases; however, actual visualization of the fistula tract can be expected in only 30%. Other diagnostic options include cystography, colonoscopy, and CT scanning. Of these, CT scanning with rectal contrast is probably the most helpful.[18] CT scanning has the advantage of being able to evaluate the extent of disease outside the colon or bladder. The low diagnostic yield (20%) of cystography and colonoscopy in detecting colovesical fistula has limited their use for this purpose.

Operative procedures should be performed in all patients with the diagnosis of colovesical fistula. Most patients with a colovesical fistula present with long-standing disease and, therefore, usually can be prepared for operation on an elective basis. After antibiotic administration (oral and systemic) and mechanical preparation, segmental colon resection, primary bladder repair, and primary colon anastomosis can usually be performed. A one-stage repair can be performed safely in 90% of patients with colovesical fistula of diverticular origin.[16] The mortality associated with a colovesical fistula is 4% to 5%.[42] The surgical treatment of diverticular fistula involves organs other than the bladder and usually consists of segmental colon resection and primary anastomosis with repair or resection of the involved organ.

SPECIAL CONSIDERATIONS

Diverticular Disease in the Immunocompromised Patient. Immunosuppression is associated with an increased incidence of colon perforation in patients with diverticular disease. The most common form of immunosuppression is long-term corticosteroid therapy. Immunocompromised patients with diverticulitis tend to present with minimal or no symptoms or suggestive physical findings. The masking of the clinical features of colon perforation is an important reason for delayed diagnosis in this group. Medical treatment of acute diverticulosis is successful in 75% of nonimmunocompromised patients, but operation may be required in almost all patients who are immunocompromised.[30] Patients with impaired immune response are more likely to present with a free intraperitoneal perforation because of the inability of the immunocompromised patient to adequately wall-off an inflammatory process. Early operative intervention should be considered in any immunocompromised patient with acute diverticulitis. Some surgeons even advocate elective colon resection in patients with diverticular disease who are about to undergo kidney transplantation.

Diverticular Disease in Young Patients. Symptomatic diverticular disease in patients younger than age 40 comprises only 2% to 4% of all patients with diverticulosis.[8] Although diverticular disease is unusual in younger patients, several important distinctions from the usual situation exist. Of patients younger than 40 years of age with diverticulitis, 90% are men.[17] The reason for this predominance is unclear, although obesity may be a predisposing factor.[35] The correct admitting diagnosis of acute diverticulitis is made in only 15% to 35% of these patients.[8] Because of the uncommon occurrence of diverticula in this age group, the diagnosis of acute diverticulitis is often not even considered in the evaluation of abdominal pain. Despite the fact that the inflammatory process originates in the sigmoid colon in 70% to 85% of cases, a preoperative diagnosis of acute appendicitis is made in one third of patients.[8] The disease also tends to follow a more fulminant course and is associated, therefore, with a higher incidence of complications. Up to 70% of patients with diverticulitis in this age group may eventually require operative intervention.[8] Therefore, symptomatic diverticular disease in patients younger than 40 is a strong indication for surgical resection.

Right-Sided Diverticulitis. Isolated diverticula of the right colon occur in 1% to 3% of all patients with diverticular disease; however, right-sided diverticulitis accounts for 4% to 9% of all operations for inflammatory complications.[9]

Two types of diverticula are generally recognized. Acquired right-sided diverticula are false diverticula, their walls consisting only of mucosa, submucosa, and serosa. They develop secondary to the same pathologic process that leads to formation of diverticula concentrated in the sigmoid colon. The incidence of these acquired lesions also increases with age. Congenital diverticula are usually solitary lesions and are most commonly found in the right colon, with 88% located in the cecum. Their incidence does not increase with age. Congenital diverticula often contain fecaliths, which may lead to inflammation and perforation.

The average age of patients with right-sided diverticula (i.e., 44 years) is less than that of patients with sigmoid diverticula. Patients usually present with right lower quadrant pain, thereby leading to a diagnosis of acute appendicitis. Appendicitis is the preoperative diagnosis in 60% of patients with right-sided diverticulitis.[9, 34] Several clinical features, however, may help to differentiate diverticulitis from appendicitis. Patients with diverticulitis are usually older. Symptoms are often of a longer duration (average, 3.3 days) as opposed to less than 24 hours in patients with appendicitis.[9, 10] The pain begins in the right lower quadrant and remains there, unlike the migrating history typical of appendicitis. Episodes of nausea and vomiting are less common (about 20% of patients) than with appendicitis (about 80% of patients).[10] Right-sided diverticulitis is diagnosed correctly in only 5% to 7% of cases, with the diagnosis frequently being made at laparotomy.[9, 34] Physical examination is usually not helpful in making the correct diagnosis. Barium enema and, more recently, CT scanning occasionally provide diagnostic assistance.[4] In patients with an atypical clinical presentation for acute appendicitis, consideration should be given to obtaining one of these studies. At exploration, two thirds of patients will have an isolated, inflamed diverticulum that can be treated by local resection. One third of patients will have developed a large, inflammatory mass that is extremely difficult to distinguish from a neoplasm. Right partial colectomy or hemicolectomy is then indicated.

Giant Diverticula. Giant colonic diverticula are extremely uncommon.[21] Giant diverticula, otherwise known as *giant air cysts*, most commonly present with vague abdominal pain and an enlarging abdominal mass that is mobile and tympanitic on physical examination. Plain abdominal radiographs reveal a large, usually solitary, air-filled cystic cavity. Although, on rare occasions, the gallbladder, urinary bladder, small intestinal diverticula, and intra-abdominal abscesses can present as large, air-filled cavities, volvulus of the colon is the major differential diagnosis. Three distinct pathologic forms of giant colonic diverticula have been identified.[21] One variant represents an unusual enlargement of the commonly recognized *false* colonic diverticula and occurs in the absence of perforation or active inflammation. The second variant develops after perforation of a diverticulum with subsequent formation of an abscess cavity. The abscess cavity remains in communication with the colonic lumen, with enlargement of the cavity occurring secondary to either a continued air leak or the presence of gas-forming organisms within it. The third variant contains all three layers of the colonic wall, representing, therefore, a true congenital lesion. Giant diverticula usually arise from the sigmoid colon and are treated by resection of the involved bowel segment.

SELECTED REFERENCES

Meyers, M. A., Alonso, D. R., Gray, G. F., and Baer, J. W.: Pathogenesis of bleeding colonic diverticulosis. Gastroenterology, 71:577, 1976.

The authors describe the presumed pathogenesis of diverticular hemorrhage. Precise anatomic localization of the sites of diverticular hemorrhage was performed using arteriographic and microangiographic techniques. Consistent changes in the microvasculature of the colon were identified on histologic section. Excellent diagrams are provided describing the development of bleeding colonic diverticula.

Painter, N. S.: The cause of diverticular disease of the colon, its symptoms and its complications: Review and hypothesis. J. R. Coll. Surg. Edinb., 30:118, 1985.

The author provides an in-depth summary of the roles of segmentation and dietary factors in the development of diverticular disease. The discussion is also related to the development of symptoms and the proposed etiology of complications secondary to diverticulitis.

Parks, T. G.: Natural history of diverticular disease of the colon. Clin. Gastroenterol., 4:53, 1975.

The author provides an excellent and detailed review of the natural history of diverticular disease. The discussion is broken down into clear, concise subgroups that relate prognosis to factors such as age, sex, number of diverticula, extent of disease, nature of the symptomatology, and numerous other aspects that are not readily discussed in most texts.

Rege, R. V., and Nahrwold, D. L.: Diverticular disease. Curr. Probl. Surg., 26:133, 1989.

An in-depth and clear discussion of the pathogenesis, clinical manifestations, complications, and management of diverticular disease is provided. This extensive review of the currently available data on important and controversial aspects of diverticular disease is superbly rendered. Readers interested in a more detailed analysis of diverticular disease are referred to this monograph.

Rodkey, G. V., and Welch, C. E.: Changing patterns in the surgical treatment of diverticular disease. Ann. Surg., 200:466, 1984.

This well-recognized work summarizes a 70-year surgical experience with diverticular disease at the Massachusetts General Hospital. Clinical features, complications, and management are expertly reviewed.

REFERENCES

1. Benn, P. L., Wolff, B. G., and Ilstrup, D. M.: Level of anastomosis and recurrent colonic diverticulitis. Am. J. Surg., 151:269, 1986.
2. Browder, W., Cerise, E. J., and Litwin, M. S.: Impact of emergency angiography in massive lower gastrointestinal bleeding. Ann. Surg., 204:530, 1986.
3. Casarella, W. J., Kanter, I. E., and Seaman, W. B.: Right-sided colonic diverticula as a cause of acute rectal hemorrhage. N. Engl. J. Med., 286:450, 1972.
4. Crist, D. W., Fishman, E. K., Scatarige, J. C., and Cameron, J. L.: Acute diverticulitis of the cecum and ascending colon diagnosed by computed tomography. Surg. Gynecol. Obstet., 166:99, 1988.
5. Drapanas, T., Pennington, D. G., Kappelman, M., and Lindsey, E. S.: Emergency subtotal colectomy: Preferred approach to management of massively bleeding diverticular disease. Ann. Surg., 177:519, 1973.
6. Eastwood, M. A., Watters, D. A. K., and Smith, A. N.: Diverticular disease: Is it a motility disorder? Clin. Gastroenterol., 11:545, 1982.
7. Eng, K., Ranson, J. H. C., and Localio, S. A.: Resection of the perforated segment: A significant advance in treatment of diverticulitis with free perforation or abscess. Am. J. Surg., 133:67, 1977.
8. Eusebio, E. B., and Eisenberg, M. M.: Natural history of diverticular disease of the colon in young patients. Am. J. Surg., 125:308, 1973.
9. Gouge, T. H., Coppa, G. F., Eng, K., Ranson, J. H. C., and Localio, S. R.: Management of diverticulitis of the ascending colon: 10 years' experience. Am. J. Surg., 145:387, 1983.
10. Graham, S. M., and Ballantyne, G. H.: Cecal diverticulitis: A review of the American experience. Dis. Colon Rectum, 30:821, 1987.
11. Gupta, S., Luna, E., Kingsley, S., Prince, M., and Herrera, N.: Detection of gastrointestinal bleeding by radionuclide scintigraphy. Am. J. Gastroenterol., 79:26, 1984.
12. Haglund, U., Hellberg, R., Johnsen, C., and Hulten, L.: Complicated diverticular disease of the sigmoid colon: An analysis of short and long term outcome in 392 patients. Ann. Chir. Gynecol., 68:41, 1979.
13. Hughes, L. E.: Postmortem survey of diverticular disease of the colon: I. Diverticulosis and diverticulitis. Gut, 10:336, 1969.
14. Huizinga, J. D.: Electrophysiology of human colon motility in health and disease. Clin. Gastroenterol., 15:879, 1986.
15. Jensen, D. M., and Machicado, G. A.: Diagnosis and treatment of severe hematochezia: The role of urgent colonoscopy after purge. Gastroenterology, 95:1569, 1988.
16. Kirsch, G. M., Hampel, N., Shuck, J. M., and Resnick, M. I.: Diagnosis and management of vesicoenteric fistulas. Surg. Gynecol. Obstet., 173:91, 1991.
17. Konvolinka, C. W.: Acute diverticulitis under age forty. Am. J. Surg., 167:562, 1993.
18. Labs, J. D., Sarr, M. G., Fishman, E. K., Siegelman, S. S., and Cameron, J. L.: Complications of acute diverticulitis of the colon: Improved early diagnosis with computerized tomography. Am. J. Surg., 155:331, 1988.
19. Letwin, E. R.: Diverticulitis of the colon: Clinical review of acute presentations and management. Am. J. Surg., 143:579, 1982.
20. Marcus, R., and Watt, J.: The "pre-diverticular state": Its relationship to diverticula in the antimesenteric intertaenia areas of the pelvic colon. Br. J. Surg., 51:676, 1976.

21. McNutt, R., Schmitt, D., and Schulte, W.: Giant colonic diverticula: Three distinct entities: Report of a case. Dis. Colon Rectum, 31:624, 1988.
22. Meyers, M. A., Alonso, D. R., Gray, G. F., and Baer, J. W.: Pathogenesis of bleeding colonic diverticulosis. Gastroenterology, 71:577, 1976.
23. Morris, J., Stellato, T. A., Haaga, J. R., and Lieberman, J.: The Utility of Computed Tomography in Colonic Diverticulitis. Ann. Surg., 204:128, 1986.
24. Painter, N. S.: The cause of diverticular disease of the colon, its symptoms and its complications: Review and hypothesis. J. R. Coll. Surg. Edinb., 30:118, 1985.
25. Painter, N. S., and Burkitt, D. P.: Diverticular disease of the colon, a 20th century problem. Clin. Gastroenterol., 4:3, 1975.
26. Painter, N. S., Truelove, S. C., Ardran, G. M., and Tuckey, M.: Segmentation and the localization of intraluminal pressures in the human colon, with special reference to the pathogenesis of colonic diverticula. Gastroenterology, 49:169, 1965.
27. Parks, T. G., and Connell, A. M.: Motility studies in diverticular disease of the colon: I. Basal activity and response to food assessed by open-ended tube and miniature balloon techniques. Gut, 10:534, 1969.
28. Parks, T. G.: Natural history of diverticular disease of the colon. Clin. Gastroenterol., 4:53, 1975.
29. Parks, T. G.: Reappraisal of clinical features of diverticular disease of the colon. Br. Med. J., 4:642, 1969.
30. Perkins, J. D., Shield, C. F., III., Chang, F. C., and Farha, G. J.: Acute diverticulitis: Comparison of treatment in immunocompromised and non-immunocompromised patients. Am. J. Surg., 148:745, 1984.
31. Rege, R. V., and Nahrwold, D. L.: Diverticular disease. Curr. Probl. Surg., 26:136, 1989.
32. Rodkey, G. V., and Welch, C. E.: Changing patterns in the surgical treatment of diverticular disease. Ann. Surg., 200:466, 1984.
33. Rosenkrantz, H., Bookstein, J. J., Rosen, R. J., Goff, W. B., II, and Healy, J. F.: Postembolic colonic infarction. Radiology, 142:47, 1982.
34. Sardi, A., Gokli, A., and Singer, J. A.: Diverticular disease of the cecum and ascending colon: A review of 881 cases. Am. Surg., 53:41, 1987.
35. Schauer, P. R., Ramos, R., Ghiatas, A. A., and Sirinek, K. R.: Virulent diverticular disease in young obese men. Am J. Surg., 164:443, 1992.
36. Smith, A. N., Sheppard, J., and Eastwood, M. A.: Pressure changes after balloon distension of the colon wall in diverticular diseases. Gut, 22:841, 1981.
37. Stabile, B. E., Puccio, E., van Sonnenberg, E., and Neff, C.: Preoperative percutaneous drainage of diverticular abscesses. Am. J. Surg., 159:99, 1990.
38. Steer, M. L., and Silen, W.: Diagnostic procedures in gastrointestinal hemorrhage. N. Engl. J. Med., 309:646, 1983.
39. Talbot, J. M.: Role of dietary fiber in diverticular disease and colon cancer. Fed. Proc., 40:2337, 1981.
40. Uden, P., Jiborn, H., and Jonsson, K.: Influence of selective mesenteric arteriography on the outcome of emergency surgery for massive, lower gastrointestinal hemorrhage: A 15-year experience. Dis. Colon Rectum, 29:561, 1986.
41. Winzelberg, G. G., Froelich, J. W., McKusick, K. A., Waltman, A. C., Greenfield, A. J., Athanasoulis, C. A., and Strauss, H. W.: Radionuclide localization of lower gastrointestinal hemorrhage. Radiology, 139:465, 1981.
42. Woods, R. J., Lavery, I. C., Fazio, V. W., Jagelman, D. G., and Weakley, F. L.: Internal fistulas in diverticular disease. Dis. Colon Rectum, 31:591, 1988.

VI

BENIGN NEOPLASMS OF THE COLON, INCLUDING VASCULAR MALFORMATIONS

Anthony L. Imbembo, M.D., and Alan T. Lefor, M.D.

Benign lesions of the colon are being identified with increasing frequency, owing largely to the use of colonoscopy in the evaluation and follow-up of patients with a variety of disorders. Many benign lesions remain asymptomatic. The most frequent clinical presentation is occult bleeding. Occasionally, vague abdominal pain or a change in character or frequency of stools may develop. Most discussions of benign neoplasms and polyps of the colon have been hampered by variable terminology. The classification outlined in Table 32–4 provides a useful basis for discussion.

COLORECTAL POLYPS

Submucosal Lesions

Submucosal lesions may cause elevation of the overlying epithelium, thereby appearing polypoid (Fig. 32–17). Endoscopic biopsy of these areas frequently demonstrates normal mucosa only. Lymphoma, lipomas, and fibromas may arise in any part of the large intestine but are extremely uncommon. Occasionally, hypertrophied lymph follicles may mimic a submucosal mass or polyp.

Gastrointestinal carcinoid tumors arise most commonly in the appendix (35% to 40%), but they may also arise in the rectum (15%) or the remainder of the colon (10%). Rectal carcinoids may have a more benign course than do those arising in the small bowel or proximal colon. Rectal carcinoids measuring less than 2 cm. in diameter are excised locally by the transanal route, including part of the underlying muscularis with the lesion. However, the risk of malignancy is estimated to be about 20% for tumors of greater diameter. A more aggressive approach, such as low anterior resection, may be warranted for these large lesions, although it is unclear whether a more extensive resection provides any survival benefit. Carcinoids of the intraperitoneal colon tend to be malignant, so that segmental resection encompassing the lymphatic drainage is standard treatment.

Air-filled cysts in the submucosa of the colon may take the appearance of polyps. Full-thickness biopsy establishes the diagnosis of pneumatosis cystoides intestinalis. The condition may develop secondary to a fulminant colitis, with invasion of the bowel wall by gas-forming bacteria. Pneumatosis may also occur in association with conditions such as chronic obstructive pulmonary disease or scleroderma. The pathophysiology of these associations is not understood; but an infectious etiology is doubtful, and resection is not required.

Nonneoplastic Mucosal Lesions

Hyperplastic (Metaplastic) Polyps. Hyperplastic polyps are the most common nonneoplastic polyps found in the colon and rectum. They are generally multiple, sessile, and less than 5 mm. in size; it is extremely uncommon to find a hyperplastic polyp larger than 10 mm. During colonoscopic examination of asymptomatic patients, hyperplastic polyps are identified in approximately 10%. These lesions generally remain small and asymptomatic. However, because they are grossly indistinguishable from neoplastic polyps, they are commonly removed.

Histologically, hyperplastic polyps demonstrate an orderly papillary configuration of the mucosa with elongated crypts. There is no cellular atypia. The crypts show orderly maturation with mitoses at the bases. The genesis of these lesions is unclear, but they may result from the failure of normal cells

TABLE 32–4. Classification of Polyps of the Colon and Rectum

Submucosal Lesions

Carcinoid tumors
Pneumatosis cystoides intestinalis
Lymphoid polyps
Lipomas
Metastatic neoplasms
Others

Mucosal Lesions

Nonneoplastic
    Hyperplastic polyps
    Juvenile polyps
    Inflammatory polyps (pseudopolyps)
Neoplastic
    Benign
        Tubular adenomas
        Tubulovillous adenomas
        Villous adenomas
    Malignant
        Carcinomas *in situ*
        Invasive carcinomas

Adapted from Itzkowitz, S. H., and Kim, Y. S.: Gastrointestinal polyposis syndromes. *In* Sleisenger, M. H., and Fordtran, J. [Eds.]: Gastrointestinal Disease, 5th ed. Philadelphia, W. B. Saunders, 1993.)

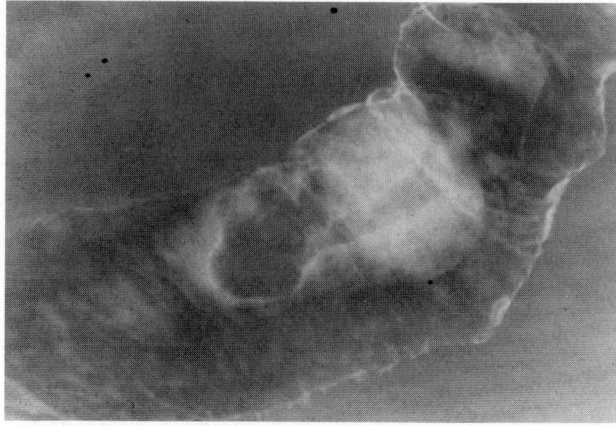

Figure 32–18. Appearance of a pedunculated polyp on barium enema showing the stalk.

to detach during the maturation process, resulting in a large proliferative zone.[25] There is no specific therapy required for these lesions. Follow-up colonoscopy is not mandated merely by the presence of hyperplastic polyps.

Juvenile Polyps. Because juvenile polyps are rarely found in patients younger than 1 year of age, they are considered to be acquired lesions. They are almost always found in children younger than the age of 10. The prevalence is unknown because screening endoscopy is not performed in this age group. Juvenile polyps are hamartomas, with up to 25% of patients having multiple lesions. They are most commonly found in the distal colon, with over three fourths occurring in the rectum. Grossly, they appear cherry-red and pedunculated, with a smooth surface contour. Size varies from a few millimeters to 2 cm. Microscopically, the abundant glands are elongated and dilated, with areas of mucus-filled cystic dilatation, hence the alternative name *retention polyp*. An intense inflammatory infiltrate and excessive lamina propria are usually present. Both the columnar and numerous goblet cells show little atypia. The stroma is usually edematous and markedly vascular. Abundant lymphoid tissue and hamartomatous elements such as bone may also be present. Areas of necrosis and ulceration are often seen.

Although massive hemorrhage is rare, nearly all patients with juvenile polyps have hematochezia due to the rich vascularity of the stroma. Because most of these polyps are pedunculated, torsion can lead to infarction and resultant sloughing. Prolapse occurs in about one third of patients, with the child presenting with a cherry-red or *beefy* protrusion from the anus. Propulsion of the polyp and its stalk by peristalsis creates traction, which may cause crampy abdominal pain. Intussusception is rare.

Juvenile polyps have no malignant potential. They should be removed for histologic confirmation and relief of symptoms. Most can be removed endoscopically, with care being taken to control completely the highly vascular pedicle. Lesions low in the rectum or those that have prolapsed can be removed transanally. Recurrence is very rare after excision.

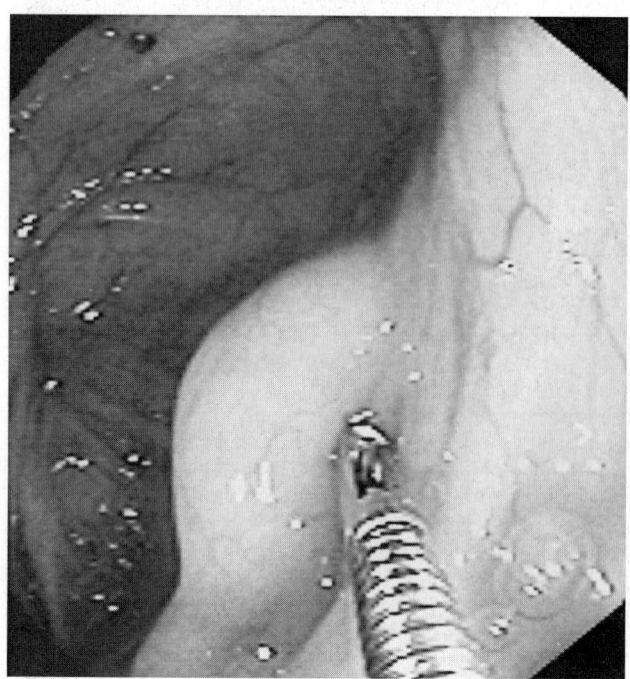

Figure 32–17. Endoscopic view of a submucosal polyp in the cecum.

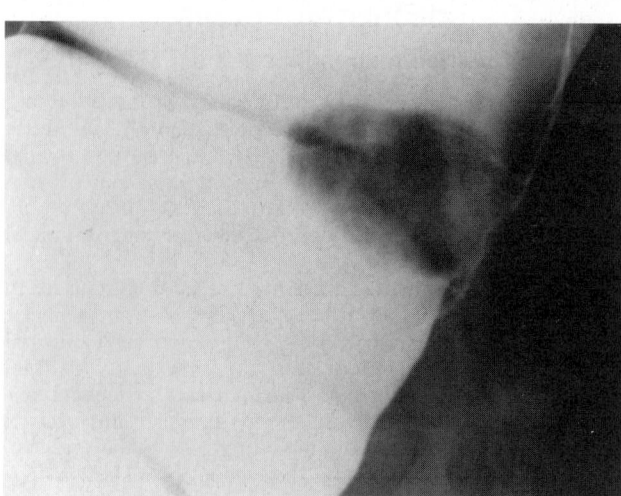

Figure 32–19. Appearance of a sessile polyp on barium enema.

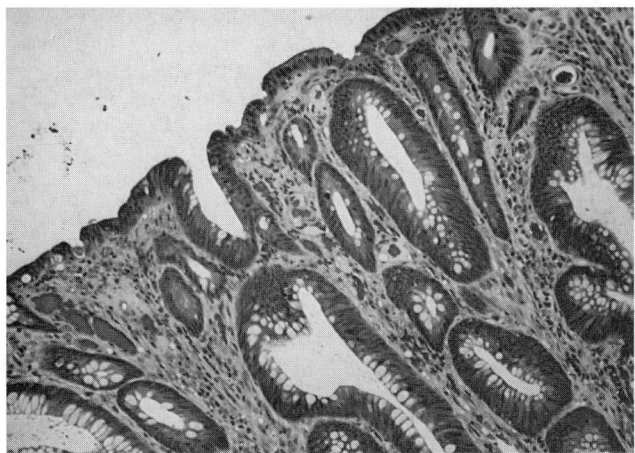

Figure 32–20. Microscopic appearance of a tubular adenoma (adenomatous polyp) showing a network of glandular structures.

Inflammatory Polyps (Pseudopolyps). Inflammatory polyps consist of regenerating epithelium in response to inflammation. They may arise secondary to any inflammatory process but are most commonly associated with idiopathic ulcerative colitis. They can also develop secondary to infectious processes, such as amebic colitis, chronic schistosomiasis, or bacterial dysentery. Inflammatory polyps have no malignant potential, but in ulcerative colitis they may coexist with areas of dysplasia or malignancy.

Neoplastic Mucosal Lesions

The most common polypoid lesions of the colon and rectum are neoplasms, both benign and malignant (see Table 32–4). Neoplastic polyps are assigned a histologic type based on the predominant pattern seen on microscopic examination. Each type of neoplastic polyp can be either pedunculated or sessile (Figs. 32–18 and 32–19).

Tubular Adenoma. Tubular adenomas are the most common histologic type, accounting for 60% to 80% of neoplastic mucosal polypoid lesions. The incidence increases with age, being extremely rare in individuals younger than 20 years old. On endoscopic examination they may appear as pedunculated lesions with a stalk or as sessile lesions with a broad base. Histologically, tubular adenomas have complex branching glands (Fig. 32–20). As shown in Table 32–5, most small (<10 mm.) neoplastic polyps are tubular adenomas. The likelihood of a polyp being malignant is directly related to its size (Table 32–6). Most tubular adenomas feature only mild dysplasia. However, as many as 20% will demonstrate severe atypia, carcinoma *in situ*, or invasive carcinoma.[36] Overall, only 5% of tubular adenomas are malignant.

Tubulovillous Adenoma. These polyps contain the histologic features of both tubular adenomas and villous adeno-

TABLE 32–5. Relation of Adenoma Size to Histologic Type (2489 lesions)

Type	Size (%)		
	<10 mm.	*10–20 mm.*	*>20 mm.*
Tubular	77	20	4
Tubulovillous	25	47	28
Villous	14	26	60

Adapted from Muto, T., Bussey, J. H. R., and Morson, B. C.: The evolution of cancer of the colon and rectum. Cancer, *36*:2251, 1975.

TABLE 32–6. Relation of Adenoma Size to Percentage Containing Carcinoma

Type	<10 mm.	10–20 mm.	>20 mm.	% Total
Tubular	1	10	35	5
Tubulovillous	4	7	46	23
Villous	10	10	53	41

Adapted from Muto, T., Bussey, H. J. R., and Morson, B. C.: The evolution of cancer of the colon and rectum. Cancer, *36*:2251, 1975.

mas (Fig. 32–21). There are both branching glandular patterns, as well as glands arranged in long fingerlike projections. The tubulovillous pattern is the most common one seen in polyps, measuring 10 to 20 mm. (see Table 32–5). Tubulovillous adenomas have an intermediate likelihood of being malignant (see Table 32–6).

Villous Adenoma. These polyps have glands arranged in elongated, fingerlike patterns (Fig. 32–22). Most villous adenomas contain some tubular elements. The villous pattern is the one most commonly seen in polyps greater than 20 mm. (see Table 32–5) and overall is most likely to contain malignant foci (see Table 32–6).

Adenoma-Carcinoma Sequence. The major clinical concern regarding colorectal neoplastic polyps, other than symptoms such as bleeding or obstruction, is their relationship to carcinoma. Although a direct causal relationship may not be provable, evidence strongly supports the concept that nearly

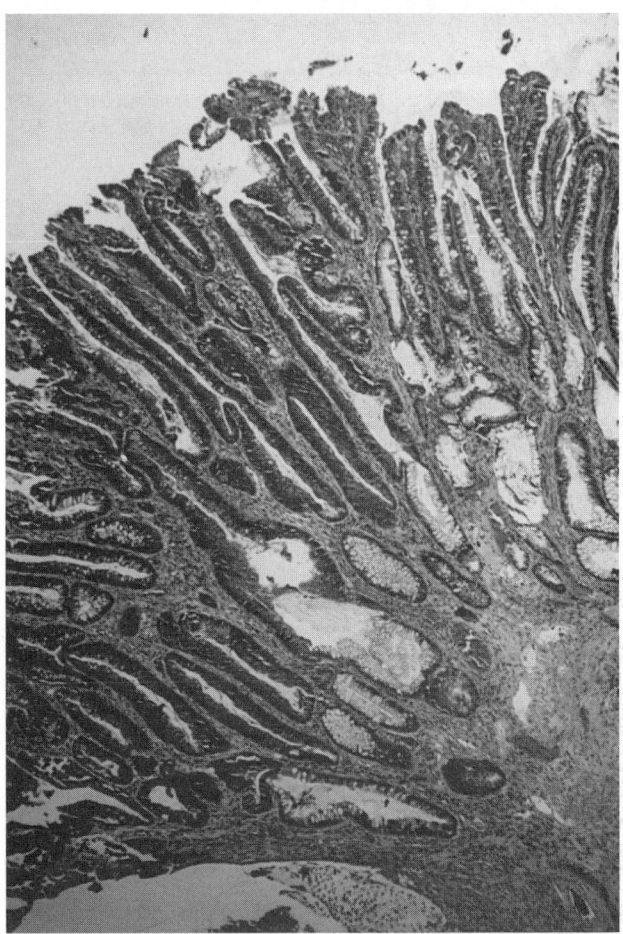

Figure 32–21. Microscopic appearance of a tubulovillous adenoma (H&E, ×40), demonstrating both tubular and villous elements.

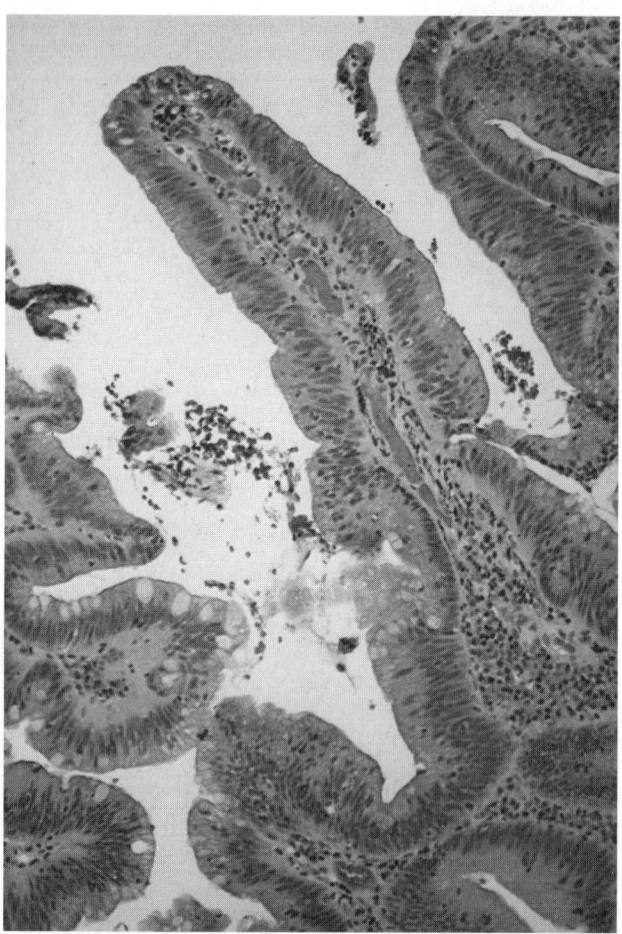

Figure 32–22. Microscopic appearance of a villous adenoma (H&E, ×40), demonstrating long villi.

all carcinomas of the colon develop in previously benign polyps. The prevalence of adenomas and carcinomas is parallel. As a group, patients with adenomas are generally 5 to 7 years younger than those with carcinomas.[4] It has also been observed that larger adenomas are more likely to demonstrate cellular atypia and abnormal chromosome patterns,[38] suggesting that adenomas are precursors to carcinomas. Furthermore, the anatomic distribution of adenomas and carcinomas is similar.[4] Histologic studies have shown that the three types of neoplastic polyps occur with equal frequency contiguous to carcinomas, which suggests a progressive increase in malignant potential from adenomatous polyp to villous adenoma.[38] Some have suggested that there are two carcinogenesis pathways: the adenoma-carcinoma sequence and *de novo* carcinogenesis.[3] These two pathways may be associated with different etiologic factors, and one or the other may predominate in different parts of the large intestine.

Molecular Biology of Malignant Transformation. The molecular genetics of cancer has been the subject of an intense investigative effort, which has provided important information about the process of carcinogenesis. Colorectal cancer is the prototypical disease in these investigations for a number of reasons, including the fact that specimens of tumors and tumor precursors (polyps) are easily available owing to the high prevalence of the disease, and familial adenomatous polyposis and hereditary nonpolyposis colorectal cancer are heritable diseases, making it possible to search for specific genetic errors.

No single genetic defect has yet been identified that is common to all cancers. Instead, the process of carcinogenesis is believed to be due to a sequence of genetic alterations, which ultimately result in both the activation of oncogenes and the inactivation of tumor suppressor genes. A possible sequence of events in the multistep process of carcinogenesis is shown in Figure 32–23.

The loss of tumor suppressor gene function serves to promote carcinogenesis. Two such genes have been described at the FAP locus on chromosome 5q, including the *MCC* (mutated in colon cancer) and the *APC* (adenomatous polyposis coli) genes. Because mutations at the *APC* site have been seen in very small polyps (60% of those less than 5 mm.) and are preserved in carcinomas, it has been suggested that this is a very early event, possibly responsible for the development of hyperproliferative epithelium.[29]

The K-*ras* oncogene, located on chromosome 12p, has been extensively investigated in colorectal malignancies. In an early study of the genetic alterations in colorectal cancer development, Vogelstein and colleagues found that while *ras* mutations were found in only 9% of adenomas under 1 cm., this gene was mutated in 58% of adenomas greater than 1 cm. and in 47% of carcinomas.[39] This suggests that mutation of the K-*ras* oncogene plays an intermediate role in the development of colorectal cancer.

The *DCC* (deleted in colon cancer) tumor suppressor gene has also been implicated in the multistep process of carcinogenesis. This gene is located on chromosome 18q, with mutations occurring in approximately 75% of colorectal carcinomas and 47% of large adenomas.[7] These data suggest that loss of this locus occurs before *p53* alterations during carcinogenesis.

The *p53* tumor suppressor gene has been suggested to play a role in the later stages of tumorigenesis. It is located on chromosome 17p, and its loss is associated with a wide variety of malignancies. Genetic alterations of *p53* are associated with the transformation from adenoma to focal carcinoma,[26] because changes are very uncommon in adenomas but are found in more than 75% of colorectal cancers.

Therapy for Neoplastic Polyps. Because most colonic malignancies begin as polyps, it seems intuitive that removal of the polyps should decrease the incidence of malignancy. However, until recently there were no data to support this contention. A report from the National Polyp Study Workgroup has shown that colonoscopic polypectomy results in a lower-than-expected incidence of colorectal cancer.[42] This study evaluated 1418 patients who underwent colonoscopic removal of one or more adenomas with periodic follow-up colonoscopy. The incidence of colorectal cancer was compared with that in three reference groups, including two groups in which colonic polyps were not removed and one general population registry matched for age, sex, and polyp size. The reductions in the incidence of colorectal cancer were 90%, 88%, and 76%, respectively. None of the patients developing cancer was symptomatic. This study is the first to demonstrate that colonoscopic polypectomy reduces the incidence of colorectal cancers, supporting a program of population surveillance. It seems that an interval of at least 3 years is appropriate before follow-up examination after complete colonoscopic removal of newly diagnosed adenomatous polyps.[43]

Fiberoptic colonoscopy permits the identification and resection of approximately 70% of colorectal polyps. The histologic identification of invasive carcinoma in a polyp resected endoscopically presents a therapeutic problem, because complete staging of the disease cannot occur without evaluating especially the status of regional lymph nodes. It has been argued that failure to identify positive lymph nodes could result in a poorer outcome. Therefore, it has been advocated by some that all patients with invasive cancer in a polyp

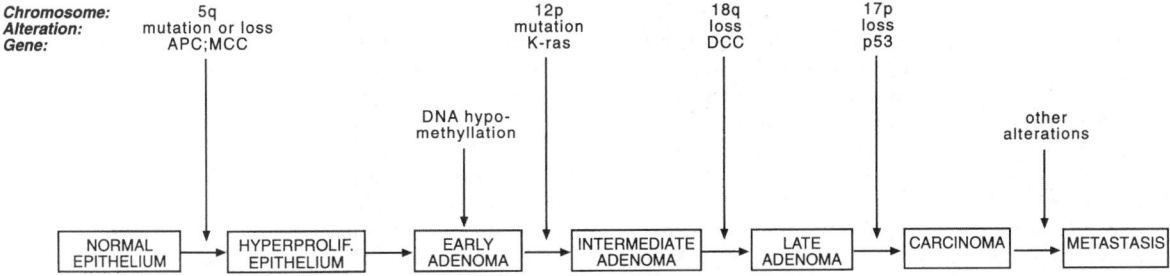

Figure 32–23. Molecular genetic alterations in the adenoma-carcinoma sequence. (Adapted from Vogelstein, B., et al.: Genetic alterations during colorectal tumor development. N. Engl. J. Med.; reprinted, by permission of the New England Journal of Medicine, 319:525, 1988.)

undergo colon resection.[8] However, using a numerical system to grade the level of invasion into the stalk, it has been shown that rectal location and invasion into the submucosa were the only significant adverse prognostic factors in 64 patients with carcinoma in a polyp.[16] Histologic characteristics of the polyps have also been used to determine optimal resective management.[9] In general, when a pedunculated polyp contains moderate to well-differentiated carcinoma invading into the submucosa but without extension to the base of the polyp, and without lymphatic or vascular invasion, polypectomy is adequate therapy. Although the risk of residual tumor after resection of a pedunculated polyp is 0.3%, patients with sessile lesions have an approximately 1.5% risk of harboring residual tumor in the base of an endoscopically resected polyp. This risk must be weighed against the operative risk of formal bowel resection. In general, patients older than 50 years of age should not undergo bowel resection for a favorable sessile polyp, while resection should be considered for younger patients because operative mortality generally is less than the risk of residual malignancy.[41]

It has been shown that adenomatous polyps have increased colonic mucosal prostaglandin E_2 levels, and this has been suggested as an explanation for the beneficial effects of nonsteroidal anti-inflammatory drugs in suppressing colonic tumorigenesis.[31] However, in a trial of sulindac or piroxicam in patients with unresected adenomatous polyps, no significant regression of polyps was seen.[17]

Endoscopic Surveillance. The follow-up of patients having undergone colonoscopic resection of adenomas should be individualized. It is recommended that patients with polyps detected by barium enema undergo complete colonoscopy to permit biopsy as well as to search for other lesions.[4] It has been observed that after endoscopic resection of neoplastic polyps nearly one half of older men will have new lesions at 2 years.[18] Patients with hyperplastic polyps found on flexible sigmoidoscopic examination do not necessarily require colonoscopy.[30] Endoscopic resection of a large sessile polyp necessitates follow-up colonoscopy within 3 to 6 months to ensure complete excision. Any residual polyp should be resected, and the patient is reassessed in another 3 to 6 months. Failure to completely excise the lesion in two or three attempts necessitates surgical resection in most cases.[4] After complete excision, repeat colonoscopy is performed at 3 years for most patients. With a negative follow-up examination, patients are thereafter examined every 5 years.[4]

MULTIPLE POLYPOSIS SYNDROMES

Inherited Adenomatous Polyposis Syndromes

The understanding of this group of diseases has been markedly enhanced by the identification of the familial adenomatous polyposis (FAP) locus on the long arm of chromosome 5. The actual familial polyposis gene was identified in 1991 and called *APC,* for adenomatous polyposis coli.[24]

Familial Adenomatous Polyposis. This is a rare condition that occurs in 1:10,000 to 1:30,000 births.[5] The genetic defect has a high penetrance, with nearly all persons carrying the mutated gene developing hundreds to thousands of colonic adenomas, most of which are small (<5 mm.) (Fig. 32–24). Histologic examination shows these lesions to be indistinguishable from sporadically occurring adenomatous polyps. The biologic potential of the adenomas in these patients, however, is significantly different; patients who are untreated will inevitably develop colorectal cancer.[5] Upper gastrointestinal polyps occur in 40% to 90% of patients with familial adenomatous polyposis. These sites include the gastric antrum, duodenum, periampullary area, and terminal ileum. Because the risk of duodenal and periampullary cancer is increased, endoscopic surveillance of the upper gastrointestinal tract is probably indicated.

The clinical manifestations of the disease are undoubtedly related to the specific mutation in the *APC* gene but show great variability even in patients with the identical point mutation.[14] The phenotypic variations concern such factors as age at onset, size and density of polyps, as well as the presence of extracolonic manifestations. The variability suggests that environmental or other genetic factors play a role in the phenotypic expression of the *APC* gene mutation. It has also been shown that familial adenomatous polyposis has an impact on tumorigenesis at other sites, including thyroid, stomach, and the periampullary region, suggesting the need for intensive follow-up in these patients.[20]

The average age of patients at the onset of polyposis is 25 years. Even in the presence of hundreds of polyps, patients may be asymptomatic. The average age at onset of symptoms is 33 years, with complaints consisting of crampy abdominal pain, diarrhea, hematochezia, or iron-deficiency anemia.[6] The

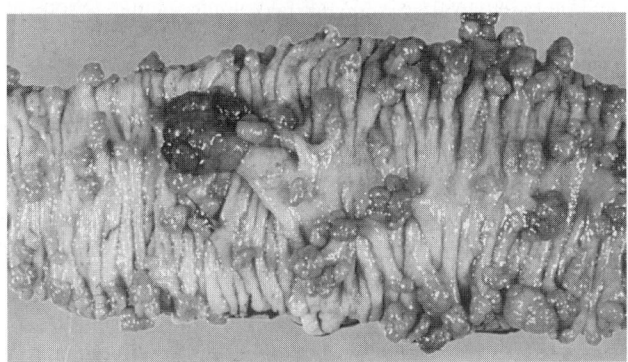

Figure 32–24. Surgical specimen demonstrating densely arranged polyps in a patient with familial adenomatous polyposis. (Courtesy of Dr. Francis Giardiello.)

average age at diagnosis of colon cancer is 42 years. As many as 20% of patients do not have a family history of familial adenomatous polyposis, suggesting spontaneous mutation of the *APC* gene. The disease is associated with extracolonic manifestations. For example, mandibular osteomas, occasionally multiple, and other sclerotic bony lesions are sometimes found.

In view of the inevitable progression to malignancy, colonic resection is indicated. The optimal timing and extent of surgery must be individualized for each patient. Surveillance colonoscopy is not sufficiently reliable for detection of malignancy at an early stage. There are a number of surgical options. Whereas total proctocolectomy with ileostomy completely eliminates the risk of developing colonic carcinoma, the permanent stoma is not generally well accepted by patients. Total abdominal colectomy with ileorectal anastomosis has been recommended by some. However, carcinoma may develop in the retained rectum, with a risk as high as 37% at 20 years.[20] The development of rectal cancer is the principal cause for decreased survival in patients undergoing ileorectal anastomosis. Thus, this procedure is best suited to the older patient and mandates intensive endoscopic follow-up.[37] More recently, total abdominal colectomy and rectal mucosectomy with an ileoanal pull-through procedure has been used, usually with creation of a small bowel reservoir to reduce the frequency of bowel movements. Although pharmacologic treatment of these patients with sulindac has been reported, a controlled trial demonstrated that the number and size of adenomas is reduced but the effect is incomplete.[13]

Gardner's Syndrome. Gardner's syndrome is a familial disease consisting of gastrointestinal adenomatous polyposis; osteomas of the mandible, skull, and long bones; and a variety of soft tissue lesions, including sebaceous cysts, fibromas, lipomas, and desmoid tumors.[12] The colon is the most common site for polyposis, but the stomach, duodenum, small bowel, and periampullary area may also be involved. The diagnostic evaluation, malignant potential, and management is identical to that for familial adenomatous polyposis.

The extracolonic manifestations of Gardner's syndrome are frequent and varied. The small intestine, particularly the duodenum and periampullary area, is subject to neoplastic development, with an overall incidence of malignant degeneration as high as 12% in these locations. In the stomach, multiple adenomas, microcarcinoids, hyperplastic polyps, and/or lymphoid polyps can develop. Generally, the gastric lesions can be followed by surveillance, because gastric carcinoma is rare in association with Gardner's syndrome. Bony abnormalities, consisting of osteomas, exostoses, and cortical thickening, can occur in the skull, mandible, and facial and long bones. Associated dental anomalies include odontomas, dentigerous cysts, supernumerary teeth, or unerupted teeth. The bony changes may predate the colonic manifestations of the disease.

It is the presence of cutaneous and subcutaneous lesions that most often serves to differentiate Gardner's syndrome from familial adenomatous polyposis. Epidermal cysts, fibromas, and lipomas can occur on the face, neck, trunk, and scalp. Desmoid tumors are rare in the general population (0.03%) but are seen in up to 4% of patients with neoplastic polyposis.[22] These locally aggressive tumors in the abdominal wall usually arise from a surgical scar or are secondary to trauma; however, spontaneous occurrence is also seen. Histologically, desmoid tumors vary from well-differentiated fibromas to borderline fibrosarcomas. Cultured fibroblasts from patients with polyposis have exhibited an enhanced tritiated thymidine incorporation and increased tetraploidy. These findings suggest that impaired control of fibroblast proliferation constitutes a significant defect. An enlarging

desmoid tumor may extend intra-abdominally, usually when the tumor has arisen in a pre-existent scar. Diffuse mesenteric or retroperitoneal fibrosis may result, causing gastrointestinal, vascular, or ureteral obstruction. Desmoid tumors occur in 8% to 13% of patients with Gardner's syndrome and constitute the second leading cause of death. Due to encasement of vital structures, they are usually not completely resectable. Indeed, mesenteric fibrosis may be further stimulated after laparotomy. Occasional responses to radiation have been reported.[23] There are also reports of partial regression of desmoid tumors with sulindac, tamoxifen, and progesterone, but the mechanisms of action, if any, are unclear.

Familial adenomatous polyposis and Gardner's syndrome are inherited as autosomal dominant traits. As in familial adenomatous polyposis, the *APC* germ-line mutations lead to colonic polyposis in Gardner's syndrome. No differences have yet been detected in the spectrum of mutations in patients with familial adenomatous polyposis and Gardner's syndrome to account for the variation in expression of the extracolonic manifestations in these disorders. The biologic basis of the varied expression remains to be identified.

Turcot's Syndrome. Also known as glioma-polyposis, Turcot's syndrome is characterized by familial colonic polyposis and malignant brain tumors.[2] Although the mode of inheritance is not definite, it is believed to be autosomal recessive, because parents may not have the features of the disease. The diagnosis should be suspected in a young individual with colonic polyposis and a high-grade malignant brain tumor. Some studies have found no linkage to the *APC* gene in kindreds with Turcot's syndrome.[33]

Noninherited Hamartomatous Polyposis Syndromes

The most important disease among these rare conditions is the Cronkhite-Canada syndrome. This was first described in 1955 and is characterized by the presence of diffuse gastrointestinal polyps, hyperpigmentation, alopecia, a progressive protein-losing enteropathy with diarrhea and weight loss, and dystrophy of the fingernails. The polyps associated with the Cronkhite-Canada syndrome are hamartomas, are similar to juvenile polyps, and occur in 52% to 96% of patients.[10]

This condition usually presents as malabsorption, which progresses in an unrelenting manner, often resulting in death within 18 to 24 months. It is usually identified in adults, who are often older than the age of 50. There is no specific therapy. Fluid and electrolyte deficiencies are coupled with large protein losses. Surgical intervention is limited to complications of the polyps such as bleeding, gastric outlet obstruction, intussusception, or rectal prolapse. Aggressive nutritional support has been reported to result in symptomatic remissions.[10] Antibiotics may be of benefit in patients with bacterial superinfections.

Inherited Hamartomatous Polyposis Syndromes

These uncommon diseases are inherited in an autosomal dominant fashion. They include five syndromes: Cowden's disease, basal cell nevus syndrome, neurofibromatosis, Peutz-Jeghers syndrome, and juvenile polyposis.

Cowden's Disease. Also called multiple hamartoma syndrome, this disease is characterized by multiple hamartomas of ectodermal, mesodermal, and endodermal origin.[35] Mucocutaneous lesions include verrucous papules, acral keratoses, and oral papillomas. Breast lesions ranging from fibrocystic disease to carcinoma are found in as many as one half of patients. Other extracolonic manifestations include multinodular goiter, thyroid cancer, cutaneous lipomas, and ovarian cysts. Polyps can occur anywhere in the gastrointestinal tract. The polyps are usually small and are typically hamartomas. Lipomatous and inflammatory polyps also occur. There is no known risk of cancer associated with the gastrointestinal polyps.

Basal Cell Nevus Syndrome. This syndrome is characterized by colonic hamartomas associated with multiple basal cell carcinomas.

Neurofibromatosis Type I. Also known as von Recklinghausen's disease, this condition is characterized by multiple submucosal neurofibromas of the gastrointestinal tract as well as café-au-lait pigmentation, bony abnormalities, and neurofibromas of both central and peripheral nerves. Gastrointestinal involvement occurs in up to 25% of cases.[19] Neurofibromas occur most frequently in the stomach and jejunum, but the colon may also be involved. The lesions consist of an overgrowth of neural tissue along with other mesenchymal elements. Gastrointestinal neurofibromas may cause occult bleeding, luminal obstruction, or intussusception. Therapy is directed to symptomatic lesions only. Malignant transformation of submucosal neurofibromas into neurofibrosarcomas has been reported.

Peutz-Jeghers Syndrome. This syndrome is characterized by mucocutaneous pigmentation and gastrointestinal polyposis. It appears to be inherited as an autosomal dominant trait. Melanin deposits may appear in infancy or early childhood and tend to occur on or around the lips, buccal linings, nostrils, hands, feet, or perianal area. The melanin deposits, other than the buccal pigmentation, may fade at puberty. The gastrointestinal polyps are unique hamartomas with a very prominent smooth muscle component, deriving from the muscularis mucosa, surrounded by glandular epithelium. They are usually multiple and, though they may occur anywhere within the gastrointestinal tract, are most frequently found in the small bowel.[21] The most common complications are intussusception, obstruction, and bleeding. Cancers of the duodenum, small bowel, and colon have been reported in patients with Peutz-Jeghers syndrome. The tumors may arise from adenomatous elements within the hamartomas or from synchronous adenomatous polyps. It has been estimated that as many as 50% of patients will develop either intestinal or extraintestinal cancers. Ovarian cysts and unique sex cord tumors occur in 5% to 12% of female patients. The counterpart in young boys is Sertoli cell testicular tumors with feminizing features. Other neoplasms include breast cancer, pancreatic cancer, cancer of the gallbladder, and cholangiocarcinoma.[15]

Juvenile Polyposis Syndromes. There are at least three distinct familial syndromes, all autosomal dominant, defined according to whether the polyps are located in the stomach, colon, or diffusely throughout the gastrointestinal tract.[34] Unlike the familial adenomatous polyposis syndromes, juvenile polyposis produces symptoms in childhood. Typical manifestations include obstruction, bleeding, and intussusception. Although the juvenile polyps are hamartomas, and as such do not carry malignant potential, it appears that the risk of developing colon cancer is increased. Colon cancer arises either in mixed adenomatous-juvenile polyps or synchronous adenomatous polyps.[27] This premalignant condition is not associated with mutations of the *APC* gene.

VASCULAR MALFORMATIONS OF THE COLON AND RECTUM

Angiodysplasia

Also known as arteriovenous malformations, angiodysplasia may occur anywhere in the gastrointestinal tract and is responsible for about 6% of all cases of lower gastrointestinal tract bleeding.[11] The large intestine is most commonly involved, usually on the right side. Malformations, most often seen in the older population, are believed to be due to a nonspecific degenerative process. Venules within the colonic wall become progressively dilated with disruption of capillaries and formation of small arteriovenous shunts.[11] The process may be due to increased intraluminal pressure or partial obstruction of draining veins.

Most of these lesions remain asymptomatic. When symptomatic, the clinical presentation is that of gross lower gastrointestinal hemorrhage, although chronic blood with anemia also occurs. Angiodysplasia may be diagnosed endoscopically, but this may be difficult in the setting of active hemorrhage. The best diagnostic tool remains selective visceral angiography. A tortuous knot of blood vessels is usually seen, sometimes with early filling of a large vein (Fig. 32–25). Therapy usually consists of colonoscopic electrocoagulation and/or laser photoablation. Those lesions that do not respond may require surgical resection, but preoperative localization is imperative because these lesions are impossible to identify by palpation or external inspection of the bowel. Estrogen therapy has been attempted, but prospective randomized trials have failed to conclusively demonstrate any benefit.[11]

A number of conditions, including von Willebrand's disease, aortic stenosis, cirrhosis, and pulmonary disease, have been reported to be associated with a higher incidence of angiodysplasia of the gastrointestinal tract. However, the data are not at all conclusive. Patients with chronic renal failure may have an increased likelihood of bleeding from angiodysplastic lesions, which, in this case, occur throughout the gastrointestinal tract.

Hemangiomas

Hemangiomas of the colon are much less common than angiodysplasia and are composed of large blood-filled sinuses within a connective tissue framework. Gastrointestinal hemangiomas are classified as capillary, cavernous, or mixed

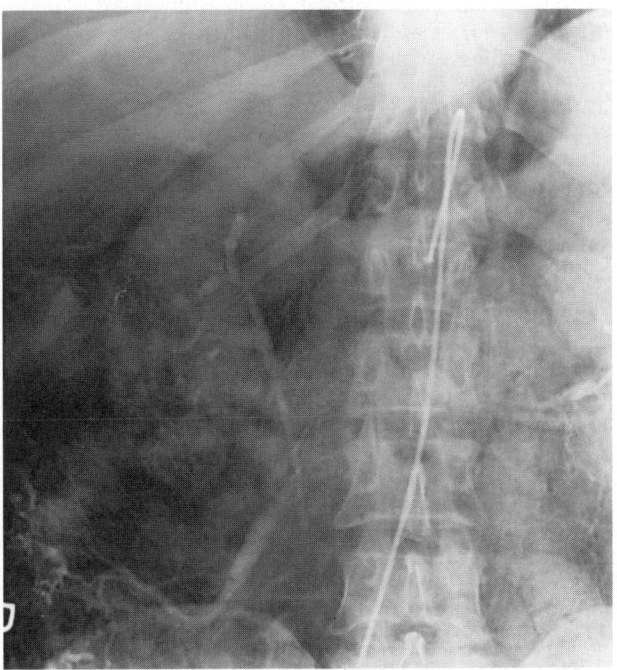

Figure 32–25. Angiographic appearance of angiodysplasia of the colon. Note the early filling of the large vein due to arteriovenous shunts.

and probably arise from the rich submucosal vascular plexus. Most often they are solitary and of the cavernous type.[1] Overall, the rectum is the most common location.

Kaposi's sarcoma, a common manifestation of the acquired immunodeficiency syndrome, is a neoplastic vascular malformation that is considered a variety of hemangioma.[40] Half of Kaposi's sarcomas are found in the gastrointestinal tract, with the duodenum being the most common location. The colon and rectum may also be involved.

Hemangiomas present with occult blood loss or gross hemorrhage, even in childhood. Endoscopy is often an effective diagnostic modality. On angiography, hemangiomas show a characteristic tumor blush and abnormal vessels. Contrast radiographs are usually not diagnostic. Thirty percent of hemangiomas contain phleboliths visible on plain radiographs.

Hemangiomas are treated either by local excision or segmental resection of the involved segment of bowel. Because of their vascularity and the potential for serious hemorrhage, endoscopic coagulation should not be attempted. Kaposi's sarcoma is considered for resection only in the presence of obstruction or intractable bleeding.

Mesenteric Varices

Varices in the colon may develop from portal hypertension. Localized mesenteric venous outflow obstruction due to tumor, lymphadenopathy, or adhesions may also be responsible on occasion. Both endoscopy and mesenteric angiography with attention to the late venous phase are effective diagnostic studies. Asymptomatic varices require no treatment. Bleeding varices are addressed according to their cause. Bleeding varices at the site of a colostomy may be difficult to control because of repeated trauma to the area from stoma appliances. Diffuse intestinal varices may require a procedure for portal decompression. Isolated varices are best treated by segmental resection, if possible.

Telangiectasias

Telangiectasias of the colon usually occur as part of the hereditary hemorrhagic telangiectasias syndrome (Osler-Weber-Rendu syndrome). Gastrointestinal bleeding occurs in up to 40% of patients with this condition, often not until middle age. Frequently, there is a family history for the disease. Telangiectasias are usually small and do not produce a mass effect. The diagnosis is best made by endoscopy or angiography.

Management is complicated by the multiplicity of these lesions. Endoscopic photoablation or electrocoagulation has been used. Unfortunately, other lesions may subsequently become symptomatic.[32] Extensive surgical resection is not indicated for episodic bleeding but may be for massive hemorrhage. Some have suggested that oral estrogens may decrease the tendency for these lesions to bleed.

SELECTED REFERENCES

Bond, J. H.: Polyp guideline: Diagnosis, treatment and surveillance for patients with nonfamilial colorectal polyps. Ann. Int. Med., *119*:836, 1993.
This article provides a set of practical guidelines for the management of patients with nonfamilial colorectal polyps. The guidelines were derived from multiple clinical trials and serve as an excellent practical guide.

Haggitt, R. C., Glotzbach, R. E., Soffer, E. E., and Wruble, L. D.: Prognostic factors in colorectal carcinomas arising in adenomas: Implications for lesions removed by endoscopic polypectomy. Gastroenterology, *89*:328, 1985.
The treatment of patients with carcinomas arising in adenomas is discussed, with the level of invasion being identified as the major factor in determining prognosis and therapy.

Peltomaki, P., Aaltonen, L. A., Sistonen, P., Pylkkanen, L., et al.: Genetic

mapping of a locus predisposing to human colorectal cancer. Science, *260*:810, 1993.
This important work serves as a landmark in the molecular genetics of colon cancer because it reports the identification of the gene involved in hereditary nonpolyposis colorectal cancer.

Tierney, R. P., Ballantyne, G. H., and Modlin, I. M.: The adenoma to carcinoma sequence. Surg. Gynecol. Obstet., *171*:81, 1990.
This serves as a good review of the adenoma-carcinoma sequence.

Winawer, S. J., Zauber, A. G., Ho, M. H., O'Brien, M. J., et al.: Prevention of colorectal cancer by colonoscopic polypectomy. N. Engl. J. Med., *329*:1977, 1993.
This important paper demonstrates that colonoscopic polypectomy resulted in a lower-than-expected incidence of colorectal cancer, validating the aggressive approach taken by colonoscopists and demonstrating a definite impact on the incidence of this disease.

REFERENCES

1. Abrahamson, J., and Shandling, B.: Intestinal hemangiomata in childhood and a syndrome for diagnosis: A collective review. J. Pediatr. Surg., *8*:487, 1973.
2. Baughman, F. A., Jr., List, C. F., Williams, J. R., Muldoon, J. P., Segarra, J. M., and Volkel, J. S.: The glioma polyposis syndrome. N. Engl. J. Med., *281*:1345, 1969.
3. Bedenne, L., Faivre, J., Boutron, M. C., Piard F., Cauvin, J. M., and Hillon, P.: Adenoma-carcinoma sequence or "de novo" carcinogenesis?" Cancer, *69*:883, 1992.
4. Bond, J. H.: Polyp guideline: Diagnosis, treatment and surveillance for patients with nonfamilial colorectal polyps. Ann. Intern. Med., *119*:836, 1993.
5. Burt, R. W.: Hereditary aspects of the polyposis syndromes. Hematol. Oncol. Ann., *2*:163, 1994.
6. Bussey, H. J. R.: Familial Polyposis Coli. Baltimore, Johns Hopkins University Press, 1975.
7. Cho, K. R., and Vogelstein, B.: Genetic alterations in the adenoma-carcinoma sequence. Cancer, *70*:1727, 1992.
8. Colacchio, T. A., Forde, K. A., and Scantlebury, V. P.: Endoscopic polypectomy: Inadequate treatment for invasive colorectal carcinoma. Ann. Surg., *194*:704, 1981.
9. Cranley, J. P., Petras, R. E., Carey, W. D., Paradis, K., and Sivak, M. V.: When is endoscopic polypectomy adequate therapy for colonic polyps containing invasive carcinoma? Gastroenterology, *91*:419, 1985.
10. Daniel, E. S., Ludwig, S. L., Lewin, K. J., Ruprecht, R. M., Rajacich, G. M., and Schwabe, A. D.: The Cronkhite-Canada syndrome: An analysis of the pathologic features and therapy in 55 patients. Medicine, *61*:293, 1982.
11. Foutch, P. G.: Angiodysplasia of the gastrointestinal tract. Am. J. Gastroenterol., *88*:807, 1993.
12. Gardner, E. J.: A genetic and clinical study of intestinal polyposis, a predisposing factor for carcinoma of the colon and rectum. Am. J. Hum. Genet., *3*:167, 1951.
13. Giardiello, F. M., Hamilton, S. R., Krush, A. L., Piantadosi, S., et al.: Treatment of colorectal adenomas with sulindac in familial adenomatous polyposis. N. Engl. J. Med., *328*:1313, 1993.
14. Giardiello, F. M., Krush, A. J., Petersen, G. M., Booker, S. V., et al.: Phenotypic variability of familial adenomatous polyposis in 11 unrelated families with identical APC gene mutations. Gastroenterology, *106*:1542, 1994.
15. Giardiello, F. M., Welsh, S. B., Hamilton, S. R., et al.: Increased risk of cancer in the Peutz-Jeghers syndrome. N. Engl. J. Med., *316*:1511, 1987.
16. Haggitt, R. C., Glotzbach, R. E., Soffer, E. E., and Wruble, L. D.: Prognostic factors in colorectal carcinomas arising in adenomas: Implications for lesions removed by endoscopic polypectomy. Gastroenterology, *89*:328, 1985.
17. Hixson, L. J., Earnest, D. L., Fennerty, M. B., and Sampliner, R. E.: NSAID effect on sporadic colon polyps. Am. J. Gastroenterol., *88*:1652, 1993.
18. Hixson, L. J., Fennerty, M. B., Sampliner, R. E., McGee, D. L., and Garewal, H.: Two-year incidence of colon adenomas developing after tandem colonoscopy. Am. J. Gastroenterol., *89*:687, 1994.
19. Hochberg, F. H., Dasilva, A. B., Galdabini, J., Richardson, E. P., Jr.: Gastrointestinal involvement in von Recklinghausen's neurofibromatosis. Neurology, *24*:1144, 1974.
20. Iwama, T., Mishima, Y., and Utsunomiya, J.: The impact of familial adenomatous polyposis on the tumorigenesis and mortality at the several organs. Its rational treatment. Ann. Surg., *217*:101, 1993.
21. Jeghers, H., McKusick, V. A., and Katz, K. H.: Generalized intestinal polyposis and melanin spots of the oral mucosa, lips and digits. N. Engl. J. Med., *241*:993, 1031, 1949.
22. Jones, I. T., Jagelman, D. G., Fazio, V. W., Lavery, I. C., Weakley, F. L., and McGannon, E.: Desmoid tumors in familial polyposis coli. Ann. Surg., *204*:94, 1986.
23. Kiel, K. D., and Suit, H. D.: Radiation therapy in the treatment of aggressive fibromatoses (desmoid tumors). Cancer, *54*:2051, 1984.
24. Kinzler, K. W., Nilbert, M. C., Su, L. K., Vogelstein, B., et al.: Identification of FAP locus genes from chromosome 5q21. Science, *253*:661, 1991.
25. Lane, N., Kaplan, H., and Pascal, R. R.: Minute adenomatous and hyperplastic polyps of the colon: Divergent patterns of epithelial growth with specific associated mesenchymal changes. Gastroenterology, *60*:537, 1971.

26. Ohue, M., Tomita, N., Monden, T., Fujita, M., et al.: A frequent alteration of *p53* gene in carcinoma in adenoma of colon. Cancer Res., *54*:4798, 1994.

27. O'Riordain, D. S., O'Dwyer, P. J., Cullen, A. F., McDermott, E. W., and Murphy, J. J.: Familial juvenile polyposis coli and colorectal cancer. Cancer, *68*:889, 1991.

28. Peltomaki, P., Aaltonen, L. A., Sistonen, P., Pylkkanen, L., et al.: Genetic mapping of a locus predisposing to human colorectal cancer. Science, *260*:810, 1993.

29. Powell, S. M., Zilz, N., Beaser-Barclay, Y., Bryan, T. M., et al.: APC mutations occur early during colorectal tumorigenesis. Nature, *359*:235, 1992.

30. Provenzale, D., Garrett, J. W., Condon, S. E., and Sandler, R. S.: Risk for colon adenomas in patients with rectosigmoid hyperplastic polyps. Ann. Intern. Med., *113*:760, 1990.

31. Pugh, S., and Thomas, G. A. O.: Patients with adenomatous polyps and carcinomas have increased colonic mucosal prostaglandin E_2. Gut, *35*:675, 1994.

32. Reilly, P. J., and Nostrant, T. T.: Clinical manifestations of hereditary hemorrhagic telangiectasia. Am. J. Gastroenterol., *79*:363, 1984.

33. Rustgi, A. K.: Hereditary gastrointestinal polyposis and nonpolyposis syndromes. N. Engl. J. Med., *331*:1694, 1994.

34. Sachatello, C. R., Pickren, J. W., and Grace, J. T.: Generalized juvenile gastrointestinal polyposis: A hereditary syndrome. Gastroenterology, *58*:699, 1970.

35. Salem, O. S., and Steck, W. D.: Cowden's disease (multiple hamartomas and neoplasia syndrome): A case report and review of the English literature. J. Am. Acad. Dermatol., *8*:686, 1983.

36. Shinya, H., and Wolff, W. I.: Morphology, anatomic distribution and cancer potential of colonic polyps. Ann. Surg., *190*:679, 1979.

37. Skinner, M. A., Tyler, D., Branum, G. D., Cucchiaro, G., et al.: Subtotal colectomy for familial polyposis: A clinical series and review of the literature. Arch. Surg., *125*:621, 1990.

38. Tierney, R. P., Ballantyne, G. H., and Modlin, I. M.: The adenoma to carcinoma sequence. Surg. Gynecol. Obstet., *171*:81, 1990.

39. Vogelstein, B., et al.: Genetic alterations during colorectal tumor development. N. Engl. J. Med., *319*:525, 1988.

40. Wall, S. D., Friedman, S. L., Margulis, A. R.: Gastrointestinal Kaposi's sarcoma in AIDS: Radiographic manifestations. J. Clin. Gastroenterol., *6*:165, 1984.

41. Waye, J. D., and Haggit, R. C.: Controversies, dilemmas, and dialogues: When is colonoscopic resection of an adenomatous polyp containing a "malignancy" sufficient? Am. J. Gastroenterol., *85*:1564, 1990.

42. Winawer, S. J., Zauber, A. G., Ho, M. H., O'Brien, M. J., et al.: Prevention of colorectal cancer by colonoscopic polypectomy. N. Engl. J. Med., *329*:1977, 1993.

43. Winawer, S. J., Zauber, A. G., O'Brien, M. J., et al.: Randomized comparison of surveillance intervals after colonoscopic removal of newly diagnosed adenomatous polyps. N. Engl. J. Med., *328*:901, 1993.

VII

ULCERATIVE COLITIS

James M. Becker, M.D., and Frank G. Moody, M.D.

Ulcerative colitis, a diffuse inflammatory disease of the mucosal lining of the colon and rectum, is characterized by bloody diarrhea that exacerbates and abates without apparent cause. It is difficult to realize that a disease so devastating remains without an identified etiology or specific medical therapy. Total removal of the affected organs—the colon and rectum—provides a complete cure, but at a sacrifice, since patients so treated must learn to live with an external abdominal stoma (an ileostomy) for the remainder of their lives. Since the disease has its peak onset in early and middle adulthood, this represents a long time span for most patients. Fortunately, new surgical alternatives have eliminated the need for a permanent ileostomy without sacrificing definitive treatment of the disease.

ETIOLOGY

The etiology of ulcerative colitis remains unknown despite intensive work by many investigators. The examination of bacterial and viral agents continues to be an area of great activity. Whether the infectious agents are more likely to be triggers of disease or perpetuators of disease is of great controversy. To be a trigger, an infectious agent would have to act by initiation or reactivation. Agents could initiate an autoimmune response by altering antigens, affecting molecular immunity, or increasing immune responsiveness. The microbial agent might also trigger the pathologic response by increasing mucosal permeability or stimulating epithelial injury or localized ischemia. The microbial agent could reactivate the inflammatory process directly, by secondary infection, or by the release of toxins. Evidence for microbial agents as triggers in inflammatory bowel disease is only indirect.

Other investigators have suggested that infectious agents may perpetuate the disease. The full clinical expression of ulcerative colitis requires an intact mucosal immune system and depends on normal intestinal flora and their products. Thus, alterations in the disease may result from changes in intestinal flora. In addition, treatment interventions may af-

fect disease activity by altering the flora and therefore the energetic or immunologic environment. As discussed later in this chapter, short-chain fatty acids are effective in treating diversion colitis and are natural products of the intestinal flora. Metronidazole may have an effect on ulcerative colitis by altering the flora. Finally, remissions of inflammatory bowel disease have been anecdotally observed in patients with acquired immunodeficiency syndrome. Despite scattered reports suggesting that *Chlamydia*, cytomegalovirus, or *Yersinia* is involved in the pathogenesis of ulcerative colitis, these reports have not been substantiated by further work. *Clostridium difficile* toxin activity has been associated with relapses of ulcerative colitis but appears to be better correlated with prior antibiotic administration than with disease activity. Ljungh and Wadstrom[60] have isolated *Escherichia coli* with unique binding characteristics from patients with ulcerative colitis. The immune response to this strain is being investigated, in an effort to examine factors that might lead to chronic infections with a resultant chronic autoimmune inflammatory disease of the colon. A viral cause also appears unlikely, since the disease cannot be transmitted and viral particles have not been identified. Specifically, rotavirus and Norwalk agents cannot be identified serologically as important factors in recurrences. A cytopathic agent with physical and chemical characteristics suggestive of a 16-nm. RNA virus has been identified in patients with ulcerative colitis, but this finding has not been duplicated. Although serum lysozymes are elevated in patients with Crohn's disease, they are normal in those with ulcerative colitis.[28, 115]

Genetic factors may have a role, since most studies have suggested that ulcerative colitis is two to four times more common in Jewish than in non-Jewish white populations and is probably about 50% less frequent in nonwhite than in white populations.[2, 55] Gilat and colleagues,[35] however, in a study of Jews in Tel Aviv, reported a remarkably decreased incidence of ulcerative colitis in that city (3.7 per 100,000 population), compared with the incidences reported from Copenhagen (7.3 per 100,000), Oxford, England (7.3 per

100,000), and Rochester, Minnesota (7.2 per 100,000). In addition, the female to male ratio was only 0.8, as compared with 1.3 for the other studies. A greater frequency (10% to 15%) of ulcerative colitis has been identified in family members of patients with confirmed ulcerative colitis. Some families have reportedly had up to six members affected. The disease occurs with greater frequency in monozygotic twins. Finally, HLA phenotypes AW24 and BW35 are associated with ulcerative colitis in those Israeli Jews of European origin mentioned previously. The AW24 phenotype also occurs with increased frequency in patients with an early onset of chronic ulcerative colitis and moderate to severe disease. The genetic mechanisms involved are not known, although multiple gene alterations are likely. Genetic possibilities in ulcerative colitis include a polygenetic mode of inheritance, a specific form of somatic gene mutation in mesenchymal stem cells, the growth of a forbidden clone of cells whose mutant humoral products attack the colonic mucosa, and a rare additive major gene.[53] The identification of specific biologic markers of chronic ulcerative colitis would greatly facilitate genetic epidemiologic studies and further clarify the nature of the disorder. It is hoped that the study of the genetically modified transgenic rat model and the genetic "knockout" animal model will provide important clues to the genetic nature of ulcerative colitis. Obviously, geographic as well as racial differences influence the occurrence of the disease. The incidence of ulcerative colitis is highest in developed or urban regions of the world and lowest in developing regions, although there are recent signs that the incidence rates of inflammatory bowel disease may be leveling off in the developed countries and starting to increase in the developing world. Ulcerative colitis is being reported with increasing frequency in Japan, India, Thailand, and other countries in Asia.

Psychologic factors have long been thought to have a critical role in exacerbations of the disease.[27] It is now clear that patients with ulcerative colitis have no unusual predisposing factors when compared with matched controls.[69] Moreover, colectomy is usually followed by a marked improvement in pre-existing morbid psychologic states such as depression or social estrangement. Psychosomatic factors most likely only facilitate the colonic mucosal reaction to another as yet unidentified causative agent.

There has been considerable speculation that ulcerative colitis is an autoimmune disease.[27] For example, many patients have circulating antibodies to normal colonic epithelium that cross-react with specific enterobacterial lipopolysaccharide antigens.[70] In addition, lymphocytes may be rendered cytotoxic to colonic epithelium by incubation with serum from patients with ulcerative colitis. These patients have also been found to have alterations of their T- and B-cell lymphocyte activation and homing properties. Whereas total lymphocyte and T-cell lymphocyte counts are normal in patients with ulcerative colitis, thymosine-dependent T-lymphocyte response may be abnormal, suggesting an immune-deficient state.[11] These interesting aberrations have been reviewed by members of Work Group VIII on Progress in Digestive Disease, who point out that these changes may not necessarily contribute to the pathogenesis of the disease but may indeed be a consequence of its activity.[15] In fact, Brandtzaeg and colleagues[8] demonstrated quite clearly that rather than a defect occurring in immunoglobulin activity at the tissue level in the remaining glands of patients with ulcerative colitis, IgA transport is normal, whereas IgG immunocyte response is five times that of control patients. It is possible, therefore, that IgG antibodies have a role in the chronicity of the disease but may not be involved in its onset.

Another area of great interest has been that of cytokines and immunoregulatory molecules involved in the control of the immune response.[61] The production of interferon during inflammation could have a significant role in the differentiation of mature memory and effector cells within the intestine. Specific activities of interleukins that are potentially relevant to inflammatory bowel disease have been identified. Most important of these may be interleukin-1 (IL-1), which activates T and B lymphocytes as well as macrophages and neutrophils. IL-1 stimulates production of eicosanoids, cytokines, growth factors, and destructive enzymes; increases adhesion of neutrophils and monocytes to endothelial cells; induces acute-phase response as well as fever, anorexia, and sleep; and stimulates collagen production and thus fibrosis. IL-1 has been shown to be elevated in ulcerative colitis as well as in experimental models of colitis. The increase in IL-1 levels seems to correlate with severity of disease. Alterations in IL-2, IL-6, IL-8, and interferon-gamma have been identified in tissues from patients with ulcerative colitis. The production of interferon during inflammation could play a significant role in the differentiation of mature memory and effector cells within the intestine. Tumor necrosis factor may also be particularly important in the activation of mesenchymal cells but has not been fully evaluated in ulcerative colitis. Thus, it appears that cytokines are integrally involved in the pathogenesis of inflammatory bowel disease with both immunoregulatory and proinflammatory properties.

Abnormalities in complement function or metabolism have also been reported. The finding of deficient activity of IL-2 in patients with ulcerative colitis suggests abnormal T-cell proliferation and clonal expansion response, leading to a chronic inflammatory reaction. Low levels of IL-2, however, have not correlated with duration, activity, or anatomic location of disease or response to corticosteroid therapy.[32, 98, 102] Other investigators have explored the role of helper T cells in controlling intestinal immune responses. In conclusion, although abnormalities in immune regulation have been implicated in ulcerative colitis, definitive proof of basic immunologic defects or autoimmune phenomena in this disorder is still lacking.

Several exciting alternative approaches to the pathogenesis of ulcerative colitis have been taken. Roediger[85] suggested that ulcerative colitis represents an energy-deficient disease of the colonic epithelium. Colonocytes from patients with ulcerative colitis demonstrated lower oxidation of butyrate to carbon dioxide and decreased free coenzyme A (CoA). In pigs, it was found that the induction of low colonic mucosal CoA content produced a colitis that resembled human ulcerative colitis. In this model, resolution of the colitis occurred when CoA deficiency was corrected with pantothenic acid. The precise cause of the decreased fatty acid oxidation was not speculated on, but this failure of fatty acid oxidation was thought to represent a state of energy deficiency of the colonic mucosal cells.

A further clue comes from the work of Harig and associates.[44] Patients with diversion colitis were found to have reduced short-chain fatty acid (SCFA) levels within the bypassed segments. Treatment with intraluminal instillation of an isotonic SCFA solution caused complete endoscopic healing in all patients and recurrence when saline was substituted for the SCFA solution. Luminal SCFAs have also been shown to accelerate healing of surgical anastomoses,[86] increase regional blood flow and oxygen intake,[58] and have contrasting effects on epithelial proliferation *in vitro* as compared with *in vivo*.[91, 114] Thus, whereas short-chain fatty acids may have a role in the pathogenesis and treatment of inflammatory bowel disease, this requires further study in patients with ulcerative colitis.

Podolsky and Isselbacher[79] suggested that there might be alterations in colonic mucosal glycoprotein composition in patients with ulcerative colitis. Mucin profiles were performed on mucosa from patients with ulcerative colitis, and a selective decrease in mucin species IV was identified. Normal mucin profiles were found in patients with Crohn's disease, ischemic colitis, infectious colitis, and radiation colitis. Patients with ulcerative colitis were found to have this abnormality even in the absence of active disease. It was thought, therefore, that this alteration might be *permissive* for injury by an additional factor or factors. It is unclear, however, whether this defect is a cause or an effect of the disease.

A relationship between cigarette smoking and ulcerative colitis has been suggested. Several studies have found that current and former smoking has opposite effects on the risks of this disease. Boyko[7] critically reviewed the available literature on this topic and found that current smokers had a 60% reduction in risk of ulcerative colitis compared with those who never smoked, whereas former smokers had a twofold increase in risk compared with those who never smoked. Plausible biologic mechanisms for these relationships have yet to be defined.

Further experimental and clinical work is necessary to evaluate the etiologic possibilities in ulcerative colitis. Over the last decade, animal models of intestinal inflammation have substantially augmented our understanding of the pathogenesis of ulcerative colitis, particularly in the areas of inflammatory mediators and cytokine regulation, genetic susceptibility, and the influence of ubiquitous luminal bacterial constituents.[93–95, 105] Inducible models, such as administration of acetic acid, trinitrobenzene sulfonic acid–ethanol, and indomethacin to rats and feeding dextran sodium sulfate to mice, are cheap, easily accomplished, and reproducible, making these models the preferred routes for testing novel pharmaceutical agents. Submucosal injection of the bacterial cell wall polymer peptidoglycan-polysaccharide[64] and intravenous administration of preformed immune complexes after rectal installation of formalin[16] elicit more immunologically and environmentally relevant inflammatory responses than the toxin-induced models, permitting more in-depth dissection of immunoregulatory mechanisms of acute and chronic intestinal inflammation. The cotton-top tamarin monkey is unique in that it exhibits spontaneous colitis with associated adenocarcinoma of the colon.

Unprecedented advances in molecular biology now provide techniques to routinely overexpress or delete selected genes in rodents. *In vivo* overexpression (transgenic) or deletion (knockout) of genes encoding targeted cytokines, T-cell receptors, HLA molecules, and intracellular messengers by basic scientists outside of the inflammatory bowel disease field have unexpectedly created a whole new class of animal models. Spontaneous intestinal inflammation in these genetically engineered rodents, in addition to colitis that follows a spontaneous genetic mutation in C3H/HeJ mice and restoration of T-lymphocyte subsets in immunocompromised hosts, now permits exciting new approaches to explore mechanisms of chronic, spontaneous gastrointestinal inflammation.

PATHOLOGY

Ulcerative colitis is, for the most part, a disease confined to the mucosal and submucosal layers of the colonic wall, progressing from mucosal edema and lipemia to vascular congestion, superficial ulcers, increased cellular infiltration of the lamina propria, and cyst abscesses beginning in the rectum and advancing proximally to involve the entire colon. In 10% of patients, the terminal ileum may show mild inflammation and dilation, a process that has been called *backwash ileitis*. On gross inspection, the colonic mucosa demonstrates healed granular superficial ulcers superimposed on a friable and thickened mucosa with increased vascularity. Patients may also demonstrate superficial fissures and small

and regular pseudopolyps. This is in contradistinction to the transmural inflammatory changes found in Crohn's disease of the colon, in which all layers may be involved in a granulomatous inflammatory process. The pathologic changes observed in ulcerative colitis, however, are nonspecific and can be seen in shigellosis, amebiasis, and gonorrheal colitis.

In its earliest stage, the typical lesion consists of infiltration of round cells and polymorphonuclear leukocytes into the crypt abscesses Light microscopy reveals poor staining and vacuolization of overlying epithelial cells. There is swelling of mitochondria, widening of intercellular spaces, and broadening of the endoplasmic reticulum observed by transmission electron microscopy. As the lesions progress, there is a coalescence of crypt abscesses and desquamation of overlying cells to form an ulcer. This is associated with undermining of adjacent, relatively normal mucosa, which becomes edematous and assumes a polypoid configuration as it becomes isolated between adjacent ulcers. Collagen and a luxurious growth of granulation tissue occupy the areas of ulceration, which extend down to, but rarely through, the muscularis. The histologic features of a typical ulcer and pseudopolyp are shown in Figure 32–26. In fulminating ulcerative colitis and toxic megacolon, such lesions may penetrate through the full thickness of the bowel wall and lead to perforation into the peritoneal cavity. Fortunately, these forms of the disease are infrequent (15% and 3%, respectively). The pathologic changes described offer a clear explanation of the clinical manifestations of the disease. It is little wonder that a colon as shown in Figure 32–27 allows almost constant passage of 20 or more bloody bowel movements per day. The denuded, remarkably distorted mucosal lining provides little opportunity for absorption of sodium or water. Each bowel action milks large volumes of blood from the exposed hillocks of granulation tissue. Loss of haustral markings, an early roentgenographic finding, is thought to be due to paralysis of the muscularis mucosa. The foreshortening of the colon and its rigid *stovepipe* appearance on barium roentgenograms are consequences of repeated injury and the scar that forms with repair of these injuries (Fig. 32–28).

Little is known about why some patients have involvement of only the rectum and others develop changes throughout the colon. Moreover, the factors determining the severity and time course of the disease are poorly understood. Possibly these factors relate to the extent of immunologic disturbance engendered by the initial attack. There is also some evidence that prostaglandins may have a role in acute episodes of the disease.[99] Unfortunately, a positive response to prostaglandin synthetase inhibitors, such as indomethacin, has not yet been reported. More recent evidence suggest that acute episodes of colitis may in fact be associated with prostaglandin deficiencies.[82]

CLINICAL MANIFESTATIONS

The initial presentation of ulcerative colitis can take many forms. Bloody diarrhea is the most common early symptom. Occasionally, extraintestinal manifestations, including arthritis, iritis, hepatic dysfunction, and skin lesions, may be paramount. The most common clinical manifestations are enumerated in Table 32–7. The disease presents as a chronic, relatively low-grade illness in most patients. In a small number of patients (15%), it has an acute and catastrophic fulminating course. Such patients present with frequent bloody bowel movements (up to 30 per day), high fever, and abdominal pain. The disease therefore has a wide spectrum of clinical manifestations, ranging from a mild diarrheal illness to an overwhelming life-threatening event of short duration that demands immediate medical attention.

Onset of the disease occurs in patients less than 15 years

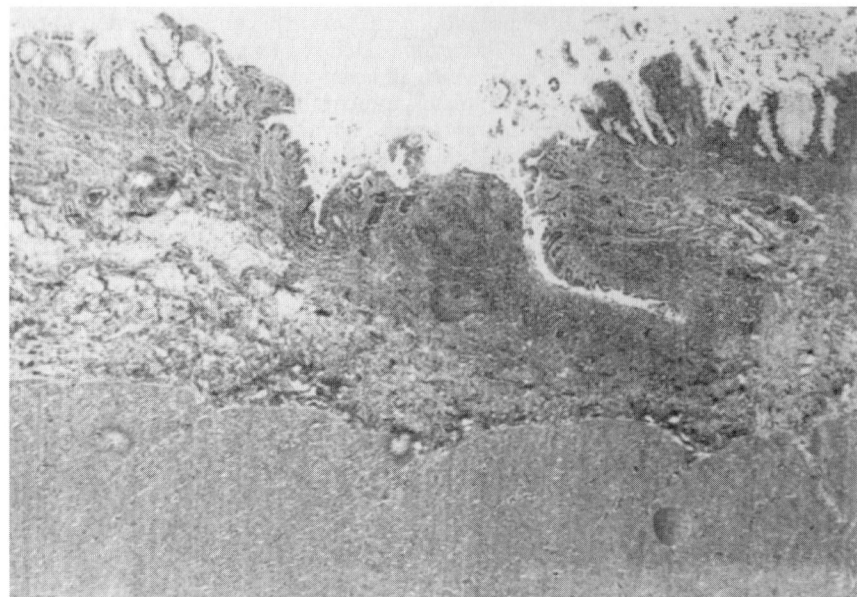

Figure 32–26. This low-power photomicrograph reveals the details of a chronic mucosal ulceration of the colon in ulcerative colitis. Note the round cell infiltration and granulation tissue at its base. The mucosa at its margins is edematous and hypertrophic, providing a pseudopolypoid appearance. The poor staining of the mucosal cells is a characteristic finding. (From Goligher, J. C., de Dombal, F. T., Watts, J. M., and Watkinson, G.: Ulcerative Colitis. Baltimore, Williams & Wilkins, 1968.)

of age in approximately 15% of cases, and presentation in patients over 40 years of age is not uncommon. The incidence of ulcerative colitis is 3.5 to 6.5 per 100,000 population, and the prevalence is 60 per 100,000. A slight female predominance has been reported.[11]

Physical findings are directly related to the duration and presentation of the disease. Weight loss and pallor are usually present. In the active phase, the abdomen, in the region of the colon, is usually tender to palpation. There may be signs of an acute abdomen accompanied by fever and decreased bowel sounds. This is especially true during acute attacks or in the fulminating form of the disease. Abdominal distention is unusual, except in patients who have toxic megacolon, in which case the patient is usually febrile and has signs of an acute abdomen. The perianal area may be excoriated from the numerous wipings associated with bowel movements. There may be evidence of perianal inflammation in the form of a fissure, abscess, or fistula in ano, although the last is more common in Crohn's disease. Rectal examination is almost always painful and, in the presence of perianal inflammation, should be done with gentle care. Examination of the integument, tongue, joints, and eyes is important, since

the presence of disease in these areas suggests ulcerative colitis as a likely cause of the diarrheal illness.

Proctosigmoidoscopy is a helpful and specific diagnostic aid, since ulcerative colitis involves the distal colon and rectum in 90% to 95% of cases. In fact, the mucosa of both the rectum and the sigmoid colon is usually erythematous and granular and bleeds easily when touched by the endoscope or rubbed with a cotton swab. Normal colonic vascular markings may be absent, or the mucosa may be hyperemic; in the disease-bearing mucosa, superficial (less than 2 mm.) mucosal alterations are seen. The intercolonic haustra are thick and blunted. Cobblestoning and deep linear ulceration, which are common endoscopic findings in Crohn's disease,

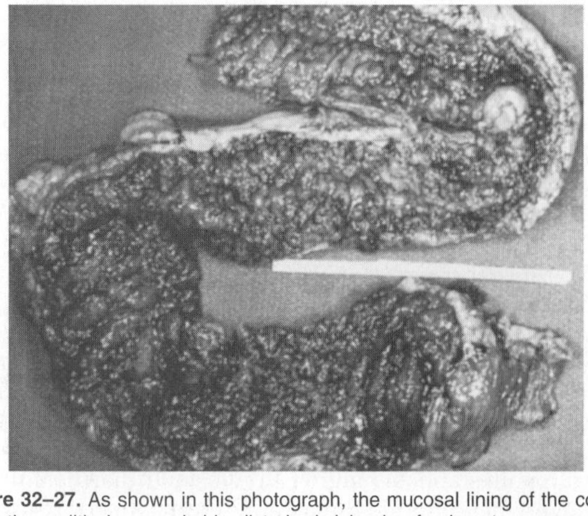

Figure 32–27. As shown in this photograph, the mucosal lining of the colon in ulcerative colitis is remarkably disturbed. Islands of edematous mucosa are isolated by ulcerations that are contiguous throughout the entire colon in this case. Note that the process stops abruptly at the ileocecal valve.

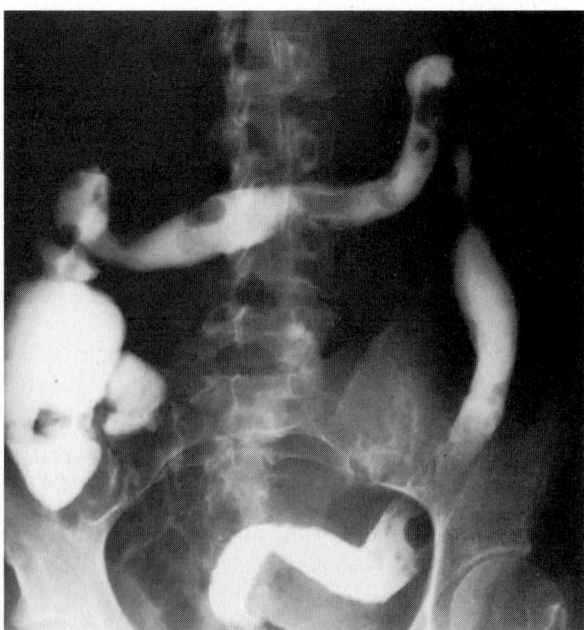

Figure 32–28. The contracted, *stovepipe* appearance of this colon, as viewed by barium roentgenogram, is typical of advanced ulcerative colitis in its chronic phase. The large lucent areas in the barium column probably represent fecal matter, whereas the smaller, more subtle shadows along the left colon are most likely pseudopolyps.

TABLE 32–7. Principal Symptoms of Ulcerative Colitis (525 Cases)

Diarrhea	79%
Abdominal pain	71%
Rectal bleeding	55%
Weight loss	18%
Tenesmus	16%
Vomiting	14%
Fever	11%
Constipation	5%
Arthralgia	2%

From Peete, W. P. J., and Sabiston, D. C., Jr.: Ulcerative colitis. *In* Sabiston, D. C., Jr. (Ed.): Davis-Christopher Textbook of Surgery, 10th ed. Philadelphia, W. B. Saunders, 1972.

are unusual in ulcerative colitis. In advanced disease, ulcers may be present, surrounded by hyperplastic areas of granulation tissue and edematous mucosa, which may assume a polypoid appearance (pseudopolyps). Mucosal bridging is also commonly found. In chronic advanced disease, the lumen of the rectosigmoid may be remarkably contracted. The use of flexible sigmoidoscopy has improved diagnostic accuracy and patient acceptance. Colonoscopic examination is of value in determining the extent and activity of the disease. Unless a distinct granuloma is identified, endoscopic biopsies are of little value in differentiating ulcerative colitis from Crohn's colitis.

Although recent studies suggest that previous reports may have overestimated the risk of cancer in the adult population with ulcerative colitis, patients with this disease still appear to be confronted with at least a 10% to 20% likelihood of developing carcinoma within 20 years of the diagnosis of ulcerative colitis.[100] Adenocarcinoma in association with ulcerative colitis is multicentric in 15% of patients. In addition, the cancers tend to be flatter and perhaps more infiltrating. These tumors are more evenly distributed throughout the colon, with approximately 50% being found proximal to the splenic flexure. Carcinoma in association with ulcerative colitis is more difficult to diagnose by history and physical examination, stool guaiac testing, and radiographic studies. The likelihood of carcinoma in patients with ulcerative colitis appears to relate to both the extent of colonic involvement and the duration of disease. Although it is generally accepted that patients with extensive total ulcerative colitis are at increased risk of developing carcinoma, the question of what constitutes extensive colitis is still not fully resolved. In addition, the assessment is variable if judged radiographically or colonoscopically. The evidence that patients with left-sided ulcerative colitis, by any criteria, are at increased risk when compared with the general population—which carries a 4% to 6% likelihood of developing colorectal carcinoma, with three fourths of these cancers occurring on the left side—is far from overwhelming. The likelihood of cancer may be related to duration of activity and age of onset, although this has not been clearly established. Although it was held for some time that the carcinoma associated with ulcerative colitis was more aggressive than that in the general population, recent studies have demonstrated that the natural evolution of the cancer is likely the same in both groups.

Rectal biopsies have also been advocated to assess the presence or absence of dysplasia. Morson and Pang[71] advocate a surveillance program of rectal biopsy to assess the point at which a patient becomes at high risk for colonic cancer. When dysplasia of the rectal mucosa is identified, colectomy has been advocated. Other investigators in this field have found the test less useful, with false-negative results of 20% to 40% and false-positive results of 30% to 40%.[90]

Colonoscopy may improve the accuracy of surveillance; however, random biopsies have a very low yield because of the immense sampling problem. Between 20 and 25 equally spaced biopsies are required on a 10-cm. length of colon to reasonably detect a patch of dysplasia 2 cm. in diameter. Moreover, the endoscopic appearances of both dysplasia and carcinoma in ulcerative colitis remain nearly undocumented. The biopsy of target lesions, that is, any lesion that cannot be reasonably accepted as part of the chronic disease state, is recommended. In addition, the end-point of surveillance remains controversial. Many gastroenterologists recommend colectomy only in the presence of high-grade dysplasia, a dysplasia-associated mass lesion, or a frank carcinoma. Unfortunately, the presence of dysplasia, whether low-grade or high-grade, can give rise directly to an invasive carcinoma, and all large centers have had patients under surveillance who developed and died of colorectal carcinoma. Some evidence suggests that even low-grade dysplasia unassociated with severe inflammation, if it is unequivocal, should prompt colectomy. To date, no prospective study has clearly demonstrated that surveillance lowers the mortality from colorectal cancer in association with ulcerative colitis,[14] although a large review from St. Marks suggested an overall 5-year survival of 87% in those patients who underwent surveillance and 55% in those who did not.[17]

A plain abdominal film may reveal a variant of the disease called *toxic megacolon,* in which there may be free air within the peritoneal cavity from perforation of the colon. A more common sign is a remarkable dilation of the transverse colon (Fig. 32–29).

Barium enema examination, usually with air contrast, can be performed safely in most patients and is extremely helpful in identifying the extent and severity of the disease. Barium roentgenographic signs include loss of haustral markings and irregularities of the colon wall, which represent small ulcerations. These are well demonstrated in Figure 32–30,

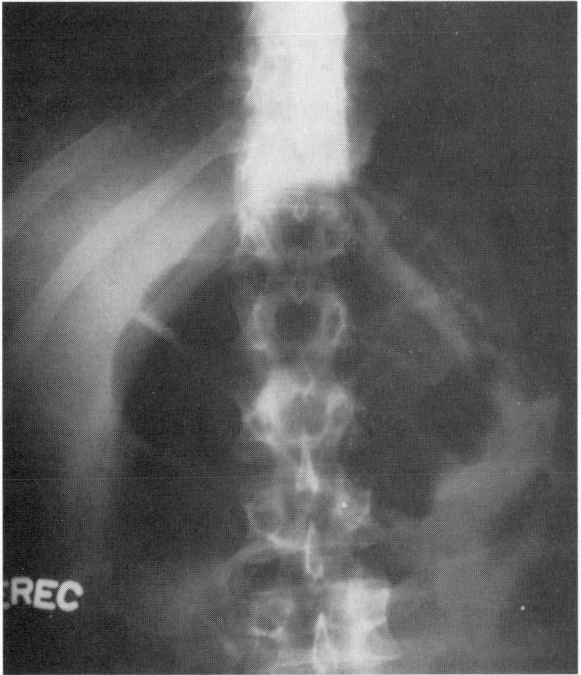

Figure 32–29. Toxic megacolon is characterized by massive distention of the right colon by air as shown in this upright roentgenogram of the abdomen. Distention of the cecum in excess of 12 to 14 cm. is believed to represent a sign of impending perforation. The irregularities in the air column represent pseudopolyps within the lumen of the colon.

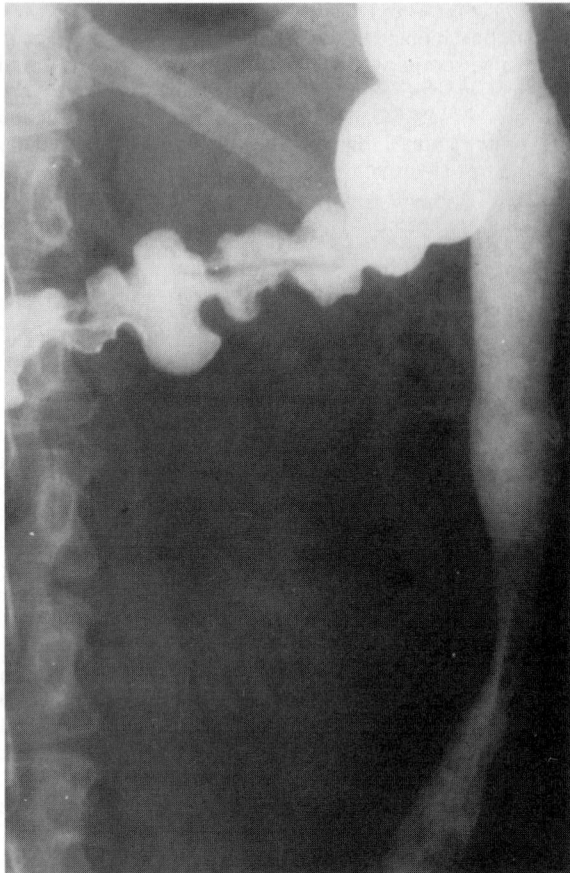

Figure 32–30. This barium roentgenogram of the splenic flexure of the colon reveals loss of haustral markings in the descending colon, in contrast with their presence in the transverse colon. The irregular appearance of the barium column in the descending colon is indicative of the inflammation and ulceration of its mucosal lining.

which contrasts the appearance of the left side of the splenic flexure and that of the right. As the disease progresses, pseudopolyps become a prominent roentgenographic sign (Fig. 32–31). In advanced disease, the colon assumes the appearance of a rigid contracted tube (see Fig. 32–28). The barium roentgenogram, although useful, should be avoided in the presence of toxic megacolon, since it may exacerbate the colitis. When diarrhea is not present, a liquid diet for 3 days prior to examination is recommended. Barium roentgenogram should be omitted when the clinical signs of toxic megacolon are present. Upper gastrointestinal contrast studies are also indicated in most patients to exclude Crohn's disease.

The aforementioned clinical manifestations and simple diagnostic tests usually help identify the presence of ulcerative colitis. It is necessary, however, to obtain stool smears and cultures to exclude colitis due to viruses, *Chlamydia,* bacterial pathogens, and parasites. Particularly important and difficult to exclude are pseudomembranous colitis, the proctocolitis seen increasingly in homosexual males, and traveler's diarrhea. Cello and Meyer[12] provided a useful schema for distinguishing ulcerative colitis from granulomatous colitis (Table 32–8). Note, however, the low frequency of discriminating clinical characteristics, except for associated small bowel disease or skip areas within the colon, when the etiology is Crohn's disease.

The strong association of cancer of the colon with ulcerative colitis bears further emphasis.[115] For example, 40% of patients with total colonic involvement may die of cancer if

they survive their disease and the colon is left in place.[62] Three percent of children with ulcerative colitis have cancer of the colon at 10 years; 20% develop cancer during each ensuing decade.[20] With the availability of far more acceptable surgical alternatives to proctocolectomy and ileostomy, it is hoped that patients will obtain definitive treatment for the disease well before they enter the phase of accelerating cancer risk. These data support close medical management for such patients and surgical intervention, on this basis alone, when chronicity is well established.

The extracolonic manifestations of ulcerative colitis can be categorized as the colitis group, the pathophysiologic group, and the miscellaneous group of disorders. The colitis group of extracolonic manifestations generally parallels the activity of the underlying bowel disease, being present and most active when the colitis is active and usually subsiding when the colitis goes into remission induced by medical therapy, by surgical intervention, or spontaneously. It appears most likely that these extracolonic disorders represent antigen-antibody immune complex disorders. Ocular manifestations are common in ulcerative colitis and include conjunctivitis, iritis, and choroiditis. These are closely related to disease activity and respond to steroid therapy. More severe and rare eye diseases, including ulcerative panophthalmitis, are more difficult to treat, even with high-dose steroid suppression. Articular disorders, including peripheral joint disease, arthralgias, swelling, pain, and redness with migratory involvement, usually parallel the intensity of the colitis and respond to medical or surgical treatment. The joints of the lower extremities are most frequently involved. Fortunately, permanent deformity of these joints is very uncommon. A certain percentage of patients go on to develop clear evidence of rheumatoid arthritis even after colectomy. Ankylosing spondylitis and sacroiliitis, in contrast, can cause permanent fixa-

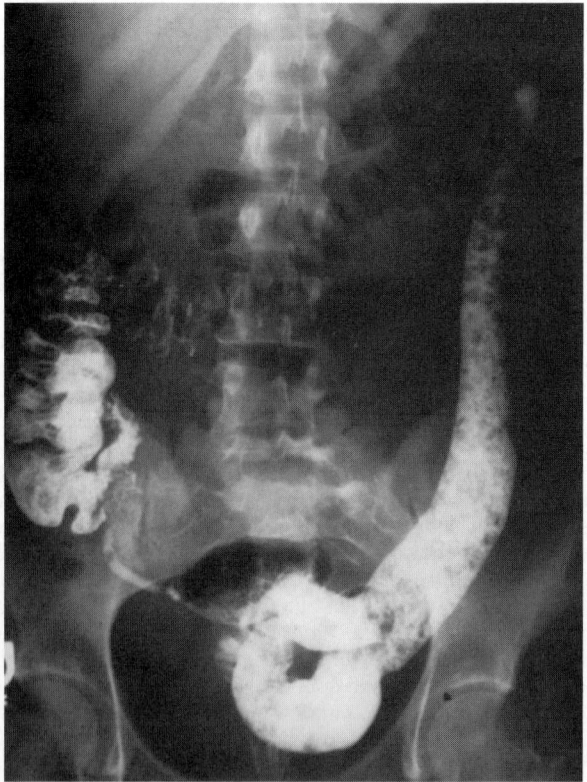

Figure 32–31. Mucosal pseudopolyp formation is well demonstrated in the descending colon in this barium roentgenogram. The right colon appears relatively spared.

TABLE 32–8. Pathologic Features Distinguishing Crohn's Colitis from Ulcerative Colitis

Pathologic Finding	Percentage of Cases with Finding	
	Crohn's Colitis	Ulcerative Colitis
Macroscopic		
Bowel wall thickened	74	17
Superficial discrete ulcers	53	13
Confluent linear ulcers	37	0
Deep fissures	37	0
Skip lesions	21	0
Bowel lumen narrowing	68	35
Cobblestoning of mucosa	21	0
Microscopic		
Transmural inflammation	95	17
Submucosal thickening	79	4
Fissures	95	35
Increased submucosal cellularity	100	30
Granulomas	100	0
Submucosal fibrosis	63	4
Full mucosal thickness ulceration	79	43

From Cello, J. P., and Meyer, J. H.: Crohn's disease of the colon. In Sleisenger, M. H., and Fordtran, J. S. (Eds.): Gastrointestinal Disease. Philadelphia, W. B. Saunders, 1978, p. 1660.

tion of the spine and need to be treated aggressively. Bone involvement specific to the axial skeleton is less closely related to the severity of the inflammatory state of the colon and, in fact, may precede frank evidence of ulcerative colitis. Patients with ulcerative colitis frequently experience dermatologic disorders, including erythema nodosum and pyoderma gangrenosum. Although these difficult problems resolve after colectomy in most patients, in others, they may precede the colonic disease or may not become manifest until after proctocolectomy has been performed.

Pathophysiologic disorders are more often seen in Crohn's disease than in ulcerative colitis, since in ulcerative colitis, the normal physiology of the terminal ileum is not disturbed. Liver disease is common in patients with both ulcerative colitis and Crohn's disease. Nonspecific inflammation and fatty metamorphosis manifested by mild increases in the serum transaminase values are common in ulcerative colitis. Pruritus and elevation of the alkaline phosphatase are commonly associated with the pericholangitis that occasionally accompanies ulcerative colitis. The most dreaded complication, sclerosing cholangitis, presents with pruritus, alkaline phosphatase elevation, right upper quadrant pain and tenderness, and jaundice. The diagnosis is most often made by endoscopic retrograde cholangiopancreatography or transhepatic cholangiography. It has been estimated that 50% of patients who present with sclerosing cholangitis already have or will develop frank ulcerative colitis. Controversy surrounds the treatment of this disorder. Whereas some patients respond to colectomy, many others show progression of their disease even after colon resection. Surgical drainage, internal stent placement, antibiotics, and ultimately liver transplantation have all been reported to be of value in the treatment of symptomatic sclerosing cholangitis. Cholangiocarcinomas have also been reported in patients with ulcerative colitis, usually after many years of sclerosing cholangitis.[41, 53]

MEDICAL MANAGEMENT

The outcome of an acute episode of ulcerative colitis relates to the severity of the disease as manifested by systemic symptoms. Duration of the disease and extent of involvement of the colon do not appear to be determinants of survival if ulcerative proctitis is excluded from consideration. Those who present with advanced signs of acute illness require hospitalization and supportive, as well as specific, therapy for associated metabolic and hematologic derangements. Because of the massive fluid and electrolyte loss per rectum, such patients often present with metabolic acidosis, contracted extravascular volume, and prerenal azotemia. The serum potassium level is usually low because of excessive loss in stool and urine. Intravenous administration of balanced salt solutions in amounts sufficient to replace these losses is an initial step in management. Patients with longstanding disease may have lost considerable protein and probably are in a depleted nutritional state. The precise role of specialized nutritional support in ulcerative colitis and, in particular, of total parenteral nutrition is unclear. Despite early enthusiasm, total parenteral nutrition does not appear to have a specialized therapeutic role in this disease. Total parenteral nutrition improves the overall nutritional state of patients with ulcerative colitis and may reverse growth retardation in children, but it certainly does not replace conventional medical treatment or prevent or delay colectomy. In fact, in patients with severe acute colitis, it may be impossible to attain a positive nitrogen balance while the colon is still in place.[22, 26, 66, 84]

Corticosteroids and immunosuppressive agents have both been demonstrated to be effective in the management of ulcerative colitis. Both agents, however, are capable of producing significant side effects. In general, corticosteroids have been more readily accepted by the medical community as therapeutic agents and remain the mainstay of therapy in acute attacks. Between 40 and 60 mg. of prednisone in a single daily dose is effective in inducing remission.[110] Rectal steroids have been shown to be effective in left colon disease or proctitis and may have therapeutic efficacy in universal colitis as well, perhaps because approximately 30% of the steroid given rectally is absorbed into the systemic circulation. In an attempt to avoid systemic effects of steroid enemas, tixocortol pivalate was synthesized by adding a thiol ester group at position 21 on the hydrocortisone molecule. In trials, this agent has been useful for treating patients with left-sided colitis and has resulted in a reduction in systemic steroid side effects. The controversy over intravenous steroids versus intravenous adrenocorticotropic hormone (ACTH) has now been resolved by a randomized trial that revealed a similar response to equipotent doses of either hormone.[49] A recent study suggests that ACTH may be more effective in patients not previously treated with corticosteroids, whereas corticosteroids appear to be preferable for patients already receiving steroid therapy.[68] A steroid-induced remission is not more likely to exacerbate than a spontaneous remission, and an ACTH-induced remission is not more likely to exacerbate than a corticosteroid-induced remission. The usual recommended doses are 300 mg. of hydrocortisone or 40 units of ACTH per day. Occasionally, massive doses of steroids (over 1 gm. per day) are required. The usual response is rapid, and acute signs of inflammation subside within a few days. The optimal duration of intravenous steroid therapy is 5 to 7 days, although this may be extended in patients supported nutritionally with total parenteral nutrition. Proctoscopic examination is useful in following response to therapy. There is still controversy as to whether maintenance steroid thereby reduces recurrence of the disease. Although maintenance steroids may be useful in controlling symptoms of patients with continuing activity, maintenance therapy with low-dose corticosteroids for patients with inactive disease has not been demonstrated to prevent relapse.[59] Patients must be monitored carefully for the long-term adverse sequelae of corticosteroid use, including hypertension, hyperglycemia, cataracts, osteoporosis, and osteomalacia.

Sulfasalazine has enjoyed widespread use in the chronic phases of ulcerative colitis. Its mode of action is unknown. Sulfasalazine may exert this prophylactic effect by inhibiting mucosal prostaglandin synthesis,[49] although not all studies have supported this mechanism.[81] Whatever the mechanism of action, sulfasalazine appears to be associated with fewer exacerbations as assessed by controlled randomized trials.[21, 108] The drug appears to be of lesser value in severe ulcerative colitis. Sulfasalazine is metabolized by bacteria to 5-aminosalicylic acid (5-ASA) and sulfapyridine. Dose-related side effects of sulfasalazine include nausea, vomiting, headache, and abdominal discomfort. Reversible hypospermia and infertility are observed in males. Hypersensitivity effects include fever, skin rash, agranulocytosis, and hemolytic anemia. Studies have indicated that the sulfapyridine produced by bacterial degradation of sulfasalazine is responsible for the majority of the side effects, whereas the 5-ASA component appears to be the effective moiety of the drug. Five-aminosalicylic acid is now available in this country for clinical use. In all studies to date, these compounds have been shown to be as efficacious as sulfasalazine in treating acute ulcerative colitis as well as in preventing relapse.

A third approach has been the use of immunosuppressive agents. Rosenberg and colleagues[88] concluded, based on a well-controlled study, that azathioprine allows reduction of the use of steroids in chronic cases but does not, in itself, control exacerbation of the disease. In a more recent controlled trial, however, Kirk and Lennard-Jones[54] demonstrated that clinical improvement may occur in about 25% of patients treated with a dose of azathioprine at 2 to 2.5 mg. per kg. Uncontrolled trials have demonstrated a favorable response to 6-mercaptopurine (6-MP) in 64% to 70% of patients with refractory ulcerative colitis.[81] Because these drugs do not produce a clinical response for several months, they have no role in the treatment of acute flares of ulcerative colitis. Cyclosporine (CS), which has a more rapid onset of action, has been advocated for the treatment of severe, refractory acute ulcerative colitis. Both uncontrolled trials and one controlled study suggest that high-dose CS is efficacious for severe ulcerative colitis. There is, however, significant theoretical risk of irreversible CS-associated nephropathy following treatment with high-dose CS. Severe infectious complications may also occur.[92] A trial of 6-MP or CS may be warranted when steroids and sulfasalazine have failed, when the disease is confined to the left side of the colon or rectum, when the patient is compliant, and when there is no absolute indication for immediate surgical therapy.[80] However, before prescribing these immunosuppressive agents, one must be fully familiar with the dosing, monitoring, toxicity, and possible induction of lymphoma or other malignancies associated with these drugs.

Although widely prescribed for both ulcerative colitis and Crohn's disease, metronidazole and other antibiotics have no proven value in the treatment of inflammatory bowel disease.

The major therapeutic problem between acute episodes is control of diarrhea and maintenance of nutrition. Diet therapy is no longer recommended, and patients are encouraged to eat a substantial diet of their choice. Milk products are to be avoided only if they cause problems such as increasing diarrhea or cramps (as they may in about half of patients with ulcerative colitis). The reason for this is not clear but relates to something specific in cow's milk rather than to the lactase deficiency that exists in many patients with ulcerative colitis. Opiates such as codeine or paregoric should be avoided. Nocturnal diarrhea can be controlled by anticholinergics or diphenoxylate with atropine. The synthetic peripheral-acting opioid loperamide may be more effective than

diphenoxylate in this situation and avoids the atropine side effect associated with this drug.[74] Stool bulk formers, such as psyllium, are also helpful. Finally, the importance of rest and peace of mind cannot be overemphasized. Patients are advised to remain at rest during episodes of exacerbation.

INDICATIONS FOR SURGICAL TREATMENT

Since total removal of the colon and rectum (proctocolectomy) cures ulcerative colitis, one might reasonably ask why all patients with established chronicity are not so treated. The incidence of surgical intervention appears to be related to the availability of skilled and knowledgeable gastrointestinal surgeons and enlightened physicians. For example, the clinic at Leeds offers surgical care to approximately half of its patient population,[38] whereas in another center the reported operative rate is below 10%.[35] There are several well-identified complications that require urgent operation for survival.[36] These include massive, unrelenting hemorrhage; toxic megacolon with impending or frank perforation; fulminating acute ulcerative colitis that is unresponsive to steroid therapy; obstruction from stricture; and suspicion or demonstration of colonic cancer. Surgical therapy is also recommended in children who fail to mature at an acceptable rate. The largest number of colectomies for ulcerative colitis are performed for less dramatic indications, as the disease enters an intractable chronic phase and becomes both a physical and a social burden to the patient.

Acute perforation occurs infrequently, with the incidence directly related to both the severity of the initial episode and the extent of the disease in the bowel. Although the overall incidence of perforation during a first attack is less than 4%, if it is severe, the incidence rises to 9.7%. If the total colon is involved, the perforation rate is 14.6%, and if the attack is both severe and involves the total colon, it increases to 19.2%.[37]

Obstruction caused by benign stricture formation occurs in 11% of patients, 34% of these occurring in the rectum.[19] They usually follow submucosal fibrosis and occasionally mucosal hyperplasia. Although they do not usually cause acute obstruction, the lesions must be differentiated from carcinoma by biopsy or excision, and particular attention should be given to excluding Crohn's disease. Strictures caused by carcinoma are less common than those caused by benign disease and are more prone to perforate.

Massive hemorrhage secondary to ulcerative colitis is rare, occurring in less than 1% of patients.[37] Prompt surgical intervention is indicated after hemodynamic stabilization. More than 50% of patients with acute colonic bleeding have toxic megacolon, so one should be suspicious of the coexistence of the two complications. Uncontrollable hemorrhage from the entire colorectal mucosa may be the one clear indication for emergency proctocolectomy. If possible, the rectum should be spared for later mucosal proctectomy with ileoanal anastomosis.

Acute toxic megacolon can occur in both ulcerative colitis and Crohn's disease. Its incidence is between 6% and 13% in patients with ulcerative colitis.[30] Patients usually present clinically with the onset of abdominal pain and severe diarrhea (greater than 10 stools per day), followed by abdominal distention and generalized tenderness. Once megacolon and toxicity develop, fever, leukocytosis, tachycardia, pallor, lethargy, and shock ensue. It is important to note that any of these manifestations can be masked by chronic steroid use and the generally poor nutritional condition of the patient. An abdominal radiograph usually shows dilation of the transverse and occasionally the sigmoid colon that is greater than 5 cm. and averages 9.2 cm. (see Fig. 32–29).[30] Thickening and nodularity of the bowel wall due to mucosal inflammation are also noted. Caprilli and colleagues[10] reported abnormal gaseous distention of the small bowel in association with toxic megacolon; thus, this finding may be a useful predictor of its development in patients with severe colitis.

The morbidity and mortality for acute toxic megacolon remain high. Soyer and Aldrete[103] reported a series of 12 patients in which the incidence of postoperative sepsis was 50%, wound infection 58%, abscess of fistula 33%, and delayed wound healing 25%. Postoperative mortality ranges from 11% to 16%; for the subset of patients with perforation, mortality is 27% to 44%.[42, 47] These data support the use of combined aggressive medical and surgical treatment of this disease.

Initial treatment for toxic megacolon includes intravenous fluid and electrolyte resuscitation, nasogastric suction, broad-spectrum antibiotics to include anaerobic and aerobic gram-negative coverage, and total parenteral nutrition to improve nutritional status. Proctoscopy may be helpful in determining the etiology of the attack, as may culture of the stool. Although the efficacy of steroids is still in question,[67] most patients presenting with toxic megacolon are already on steroid therapy and thus need stress doses of corticosteroids to prevent adrenal crisis. Most clinicians think that steroids help reduce the inflammation and may *cool down* an acute toxic episode in up to 50% of patients, although long-term remissions are not achieved.[40] Moreover, the short-term use of corticosteroids does not appear to increase surgical morbidity. Long-term use of larger doses, however, does increase the incidence of wound and septic complications. The authors agree with Fazio[30] that, provided the patient is stable, initial medical trial is warranted in order to make the operation elective rather than urgent. If no clear response is obtained within 24 to 48 hours, surgical therapy is warranted. Larger doses of steroids after initial medical failure probably will not benefit the patient and, as noted, may be deleterious. During medical therapy, serial blood counts, serum electrolyte levels, and abdominal roentgenograms should be closely monitored.

In the presence of acute toxic megacolon caused by ulcerative colitis, surgical therapy can be associated with a high operative morbidity and mortality. Block and colleagues[6] noted an overall mortality following emergency operation of 8.7%; 6.1% after total abdominal colectomy, and 14.7% after proctocolectomy. This suggests that more conservative surgical intervention is appropriate in the acute setting. Also, with the recent popularity of anal sphincter–sparing procedures, when operating for acute ulcerative colitis, one should weigh the possibility of subsequent surgical correction for continence. Specifically, leaving the rectum intact allows its use for subsequent surgical mucosal proctectomy and ileoanal anastomosis. When urgent colectomy is required, total abdominal colectomy, Brooke ileostomy, and Hartmann's pouch are appropriate.[39, 97] Although ileostomy alone for acute complications has been abandoned, it has been used in the recent past with good success by Turnbull and co-workers,[111] in combination with skin-level transverse and sigmoid colostomies, for toxic megacolon. This is a relatively simple procedure that spares such desperately ill patients a major operative intervention until their acute illness has subsided. Because the procedure involves only decompression of the colon and does not remove the acutely inflamed tissue, most surgeons prefer colon resection.

SURGICAL MANAGEMENT

Total proctocolectomy with permanent Brooke ileostomy offers definitive treatment for ulcerative colitis by eliminating diseased mucosa and the risk of malignant transformation. Nevertheless, it remains controversial and is poorly accepted by patients and their physicians. Patients with a permanent ileostomy are incontinent of gas and stool and must wear a collecting bag day and night. As many as 40% to 50% of patients with Brooke ileostomies have appliance-related problems, and the psychologic and social implications, particularly for young patients, are tremendous.[78, 89] Therefore, the search has continued for adequate alternatives to proctocolectomy and ileostomy.

Until recently, single-stage total proctocolectomy was the procedure of choice when complications of the disease were treated electively. This procedure is performed through a midline incision. The rectum is excised from the abdomen after mobilization and circumferential incision from the perineum. When cancer is not suspected, excision is performed rapidly, with division of the mesentery close to the bowel wall. This principle is especially important in the pelvic colon and rectum, where injury to the sacral parasympathetic nerves may lead to bladder and sexual dysfunction. Endorectal mucosal resection, as described later, appears to offer the best way to avoid such serious complications.[34] After standard proctocolectomy, management of the perineal wound is a problem, since chronic infection and poor healing may cause a lingering sinus tract between the buttocks. The authors' preference is to apply active closed drainage to this area for 3 to 5 days following operation. Gauze packing of the perineum should be reserved for pelvic hemorrhage that cannot otherwise be controlled. Perineal wound problems may be reduced by performing an intersphincteric proctectomy, which entails dissecting between the internal and external anal sphincter when removing the rectum, thus preserving the levator ani and external anal sphincter muscles. These muscles can then be included in the closure of the perineum. Using this technique, complete healing of the perineum approaches 95% at 6 months.[113]

The importance of providing patients with a well-functioning, trouble-free ileostomy cannot be overemphasized. Most surgeons have accepted the technique of Brooke (Fig. 32–32). The principles include passing the end of the ileum through an opening in the midaspect of the right rectus muscle at a point below the umbilicus that allows convenient placement of the forepiece of an ileostomy bag. Placement that is too low or too lateral may lead to serious problems in ileostomy care and function. The length of the stoma is important. Approximately 5 cm. should be withdrawn above the skin so that when the tip is folded back upon itself, 2 to 3 cm. protrude from the surface. The folding back or *maturing* prevents the development of an inflammatory response in the serosa and provides more substance to the protruding ileal nipple. Easily applied receptacles are now available. In the final analysis, it is the need for an external stoma that limits the more general use of colectomy for patients with established ulcerative colitis. Proctocolectomy and ileostomy continue to have a role in the surgical management of ulcerative colitis, being used most commonly in elderly patients, those with poor sphincter function, or those with carcinomas in the lower rectum.

At present, there are several alternatives to proctocolectomy and Brooke ileostomy (Table 32–9). Subtotal colectomy with ileorectal anastomosis has been employed as a compromise operation for ulcerative colitis for decades (Fig. 32–33). One advantage of the operation is that it eliminates an abdominal ileostomy and can be offered to patients who adamantly refuse ileostomy. In addition, since the pelvic autonomic nerves are not disturbed, impotence or bladder dysfunction is not encountered. The disadvantages of ileorectal anastomosis, however, are considerable, and with the availability of newer alternatives, these disadvantages may outweigh any advantages. The operation does not eliminate the proctitis. At least 10% of patients require proctectomy

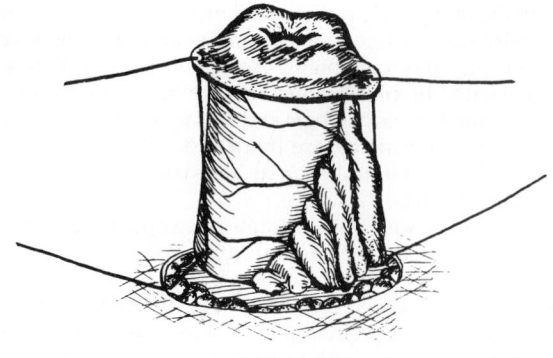

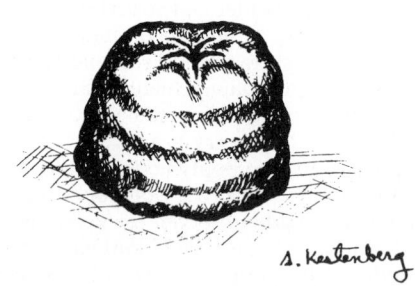

Figure 32–32. Technique of construction of an end-ileostomy as described by Brooke. The ileum is brought 5 cm. through an abdominal defect and then everted and sutured to the dermis to "mature" the ileostomy.

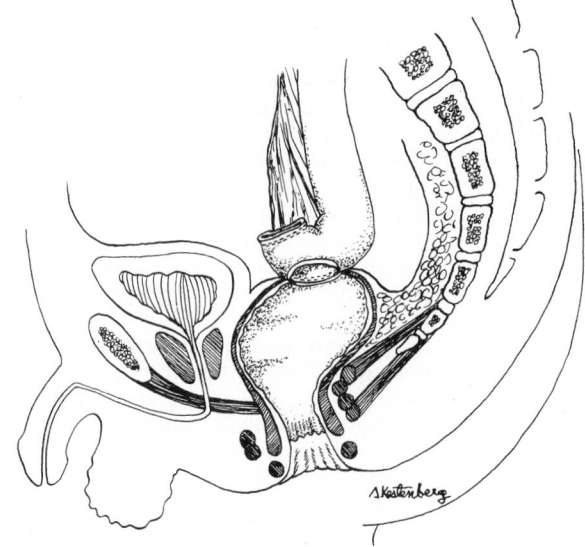

Figure 32–33. Ileorectal anastomosis following subtotal colectomy. This operation eliminates proctectomy with its attendant complications but does not provide definitive treatment for ulcerative colitis.

for control of the inflammatory disease alone. Patients with ileorectal anastomosis have a considerable risk of developing carcinoma in the rectal remnant: 15% at 30 years in the series of Johnson and colleagues.[50] Functional results also vary, with a high stool frequency necessitating subsequent proctectomy in another 10% of patients.[29] The authors therefore believe that subtotal colectomy with ileorectal anastomosis should be considered only in patients who are not candidates for ileoanal anastomosis and who refuse proctectomy.

In 1969, Kock described a new type of ileostomy, a continent ileostomy, made entirely of terminal ileum and consisting of a pouch that would hold intestinal contents and an ileal conduit that led from the pouch to a cutaneous stoma. This was modified in 1973 to include an intestinal valve between the pouch and the stoma, the valve being constructed by intussuscepting the terminal ileum in a retrograde manner into the pouch for 3 to 4 cm. (Fig. 32–34). Patients would then empty the pouch via the stoma. This technique offered the patient a new lifestyle by making the ileostomy continent, thereby avoiding the need for an external appliance.[56] Although results with the Kock pouch have

improved, technical and anatomic complications still necessitate reoperation in up to 40% to 50% of patients. The majority of the problems revolve around the nipple valve, including valve disintussusception and stenosis.[24] Currently, there are few indications for the continent ileostomy. It is an option for patients who have undergone proctocolectomy or who present with carcinoma in the lower rectum. Patients who have a poor anal sphincter mechanism and those who have a failed ileoanal anastomosis are also potential candidates for a continent ileostomy. The latter is currently the most frequent indication for a continent ileostomy. Crohn's disease is an absolute contraindication to the continent ileostomy.

In 1947, Ravitch and Sabiston proposed an anal sphincter–sparing operation that consisted of abdominal colectomy, mucosal proctectomy, and endorectal ileoanal pull-through and anastomosis (Fig. 32–35).[76, 84] As initially proposed, the operation was performed by first resecting the colon in the standard manner. Rather than removing the entire rectum and anus, the disease-bearing mucosa of the rectum was dissected free and resected, preserving an intact rectal muscular cuff and anal sphincter mechanism. Continuity of the intestinal tract was re-established by extending the terminal ileum into the pelvis within the muscular tube and circumferentially suturing it to the anus. The potential advantages of this approach are elimination of all diseased mucosa; preservation of parasympathetic innervation to the bladder and genitalia, and thus avoidance of impotence; avoidance of a permanent abdominal ileostomy; and preservation of the

TABLE 32–9. Outcome of Operations for Ulcerative Colitis

Procedure	Fecal Continence Preserved	Stoma Present	Intubations Required	Disadvantages
Brooke ileostomy	No	Yes	No	Ileostomy bag required
Ileal pouch–anal anastomosis	Yes	No	No	Frequent stooling, occasional fecal leakage, pouchitis may appear
Kock pouch	Yes	Yes	Yes	Valve malfunction, pouchitis may appear
Ileorectostomy	Yes	No	No	Rectal mucosa may cause symptoms, may develop cancer

From Kelly, K. A.: Ileoanal anastomosis. *In* Bayless, T. M. (Ed.): Current Management of Inflammatory Bowel Disease. Philadelphia, B. C. Decker, 1989, p. 129.

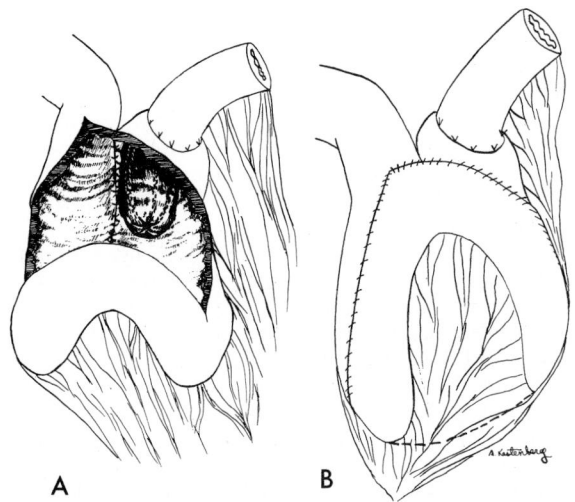

Figure 32–34. *A* and *B*, The Kock continent ileostomy consists of an intestinal reservoir and nipple valve constructed by intussuscepting the efferent limb of ileum and tacking it in place with sutures or staples. This provides a continent internal reservoir that the patient can drain by intubating the pouch several times throughout the day.

anorectal sphincter apparatus, which is responsible for fecal continence. Despite these theoretical advantages, the operation was associated initially with a high complication rate and an unpredictable functional result, and enthusiasm for ileoanal anastomosis among surgeons declined. During the late 1970s, there was a resurgence of interest in the ileoanal pull-through operation, in part because of disillusionment with the Kock pouch, but mainly because of the improved success of the operation. This improvement was in part a result of the generalized advancement in perioperative and intraoperative surgical care, but specifically, it was the result of several technical alterations in the operation.

Perhaps the most important modification of the operation was the creation of an ileal pouch or reservoir proximal to the ileoanal anastomosis. This addition was partially prompted by the physiologic studies of Heppel and co-workers,[48] which showed an inverse correlation between ileal compliance or capacity and stool frequencies in patients following straight ileoanal pull-through. Several pouch configurations exist: J, S, and W (in increasing size) (Fig. 32–36). Studies comparing the functional result following ileoanal anastomosis with and without an ileal reservoir found that 24-hour stool frequency was significantly reduced in patients with ileal pouches, particularly in the early postoperative period.[45, 63, 73]

For most patients, the operation is performed in two stages. The first stage consists of abdominal colectomy, mucosal proctectomy, endorectal ileal pouch–anal anastomosis, and diverting loop ileostomy. During the second stage, performed at least 8 weeks after the initial operation, the loop ileostomy is closed. In patients in whom an emergency colectomy was required, the operation is staged. The first stage consists of abdominal colectomy, ileostomy, and Hartmann closure of the rectum. During the second stage, the rectal mucosa is dissected free and the ileoanal anastomosis is performed with loop ileostomy. Finally, the loop ileostomy is closed. Patients who required prior abdominal colectomy followed by a staged mucosal proctectomy with ileal pouch–anal anastomosis were compared with matched patients who had undergone colectomy with ileoanal anastomosis at a single operation.[31, 117] Previous abdominal colectomy was associated with a higher cumulative operative morbidity, prolonged hospital stay, increased costs, and a less optimal functional result. Aggressive and overly extended medical therapy, including cyclosporine, has been associated with an increased incidence of patients requiring staged subtotal colectomy with delayed ileoanal anastomosis. Therefore, patients with acute ulcerative colitis should be managed initially with a clearly defined course of medical therapy. However, if they have not responded within a reasonable period (i.e., 7 to 10 days), they should undergo prompt surgical intervention, preferably to include single-stage colectomy and ileal pouch–anal anastomosis.

The postoperative morbidity and functional results in most large series after ileoanal pull-through have been encouraging. Eighty-two percent of the patients in a series were operated on for ulcerative colitis and 18% for familial polyposis coli.[5] The mean age was 35 years, with a range of 11 to 67

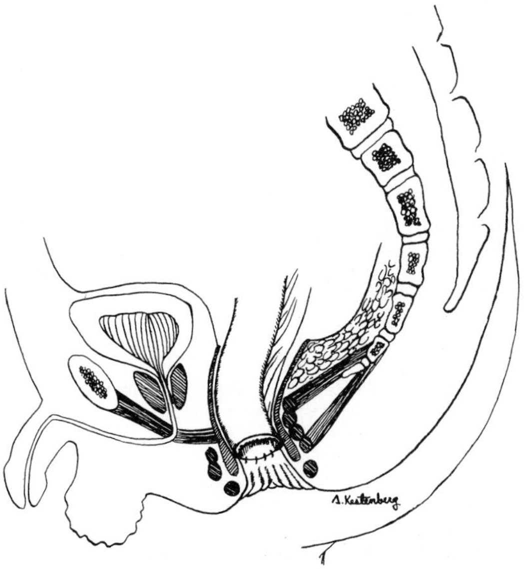

Figure 32–35. End-to-end ileoanal anastomosis following colectomy, mucosal proctectomy, and endorectal ileoanal pull-through. After abdominal colectomy, the rectal mucosa is circumferentially dissected from the rectal muscle and anal sphincter. The ileum is then extended down into the pelvis endorectally and anastomosed to the dentate line of the anus.

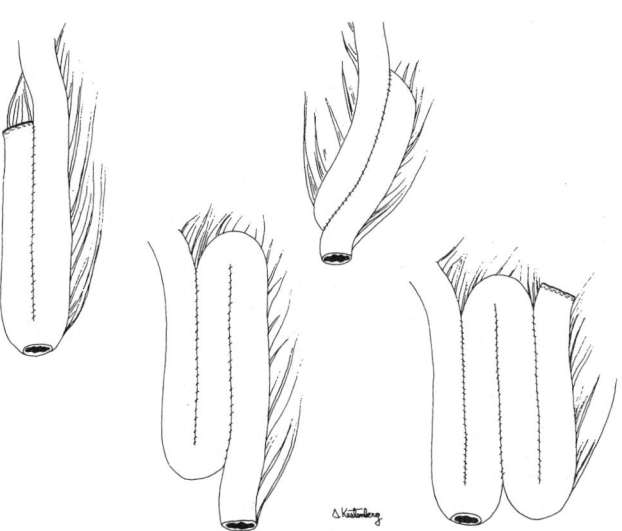

Figure 32–36. Ileal pouch configurations in patients undergoing endorectal ileoanal anastomosis. (From Becker, J. M., and Parodi, J. E.: Total colectomy with preservation of the anal sphincter. Surg. Annu., *21*:263, 1989. Used with permission.)

years. Sixty-two percent of the patients were male. Experience with ileal pouch–anal anastomosis supports the absence of mortality and low morbidity that can be achieved with this operation if it is performed frequently, carefully, and with a standard operative technique. No operative deaths occurred in the series, and the overall operative morbidity after the ileal pouch–anal anastomosis portion of the operation was about 10%. The major operative morbidity was bowel obstruction, both after the initial operation and after loop ileostomy closure. The bowel obstruction rate requiring reoperation compares favorably with the 7% to 13% incidence of reoperation reported after proctocolectomy and ileostomy. An obstruction rate of 10% to 25% is reported in most series of patients undergoing ileal pouch–anal anastomosis. Pelvic and wound infections have been reported to occur in 10% to 20% of patients undergoing ileoanal anastomosis, although the overall infection rate was reduced to about 5% in several more recent large series. A 5% to 10% failure rate necessitating conversion to permanent ileostomy has been reported in several series.

The functional results of ileoanal anastomosis in the largest series with adequate late follow-up data are summarized in Table 32–10. These studies demonstrated that the number of bowel movements during the day is in the range of 1.5 to 6.2, with an average of 5. Nocturnal bowel movements occur 0.2 to 1.8 times nightly, with a mean of slightly more than 1. Of greater importance were control and urgency of bowel movements, which were variable, depending on the time after the operation. Daytime incontinence was extremely uncommon, although nocturnal seepage occurred in 0.6% to 52% of patients. Improvement in these functions continued for more than 2 years postoperatively.

Although results with mucosal proctectomy and ileal pouch–anal anastomosis have been excellent, divergent points of view have arisen regarding the operative technique and its effect on anal physiology and functional result. In recent years, a number of surgeons have advocated an alternative approach to conventional endoanal rectal mucosal resection that eliminates distal mucosal proctectomy altogether.[40, 77, 107] Instead, the distal rectum is divided near the pelvic floor, leaving the anal canal largely intact. The ileal pouch is then stapled to the top of the anal canal. The rationale for this approach is that, by preserving the mucosa of the anal transition zone, the anatomic integrity of the anal canal is preserved and the rate of fecal incontinence improved. Although several studies have suggested that patients have improved sensation and better functional results following preservation of the anal transition zone, this has

not been documented by prospective study. The obvious concern is that, by leaving disease-bearing mucosa in the anal canal, the patients are exposed to a lifelong risk of persistent or recurrent inflammatory disease as well as the potential for malignant transformation. Until this technique is further evaluated, patients require careful lifetime surveillance. Mucosectomy must be recommended in patients with rectal dysplasia, proximal rectal cancer, diffuse colonic dysplasia, and familial polyposis.[77]

Several recent reports have questioned the need for a proximal diverting ileostomy at the time of ileal pouch–anal anastomosis for ulcerative colitis.[112] The avoidance of a diverting loop ileostomy has several theoretical advantages: it eliminates the additional surgery needed to close the ileostomy, it eliminates the complications of ileostomy and ileostomy closure, and it may reduce diversion enteritis. A diverting ileostomy, however, reduces the risk of leakage from the ileal pouch or ileoanal anastomosis, a serious complication associated with significant morbidity and the potential for total loss of the ileal pouch. Only prospective, randomized, controlled trials will answer the question.

The most frequent late complication in patients undergoing ileoanal anastomosis is ileal pouch dysfunction or pouchitis, which has been reported to occur in 10% to 50% of patients undergoing this procedure for ulcerative colitis. Pouchitis is an incompletely defined and poorly understood clinical syndrome consisting of increased stool frequency, watery stools, cramping, urgency, nocturnal leakage of stool, arthralgias, malaise, and fever. The syndrome is similar to that found in patients with Kock continent ileostomy pouches. The etiology of this condition is unknown; speculations have included early Crohn's disease, bacterial overgrowth or bacterial dysbiosis, either primary or secondary malabsorption, stasis, ischemia, and nutritional or immune deficiencies.[75]

Fortunately, a short course of metronidazole is successful in treating approximately two thirds of patients with pouchitis. The remaining patients have recurrent pouchitis, which responds to repeat metronidazole therapy, or a chronic unresponsive form. It has been argued that, with the high incidence of pouchitis observed in some patients following ileoanal anastomosis, one disease (chronic ulcerative colitis) is simply being replaced by another (pouchitis). Analysis of data from the major large clinical series, however, suggests an overall incidence of pouchitis of approximately 15%.[84] Of these patients, only 10% appear to develop a recurrent or unresponsive variant of pouchitis.

Mortality for elective surgical therapy is in the range of 0% to 2%; for emergency operation, it is about 4% to 5%; and

TABLE 32–10. Functional Results of Ileoanal Reservoirs

Series	No. of Patients	Frequency of Bowel Movements (No. of Times)		Leakage (%)			Soiling (%)		
		Day	Night	Day	Night	24-Hour	Day	Night	24-Hour
Becker & Parodi[4]	250	5.4	0.7	0	22	—	0	0	—
Fleshman et al.[32a]	102	6.2	—	18	23	—	1	7	—
Fonkalsrud & Ament[34]	138	4.8	—	—	—	—	—	—	—
Kelly[52a]	1193	4.5	0.5	—	—	25	—	—	—
Pemberton et al.[77]	389	6	1	22	52	—	—	—	—
Reissman et al.*,[84a]	140	5.4	1.2	0	0.6	—	5.4	8.1	—
Schoetz et al.[95a]	86	4.9	0.2	—	—	12	—	—	1
Sugarman & Newsome*,[106a]	75	5.1	1.8	4	4	—	8	17	—
Wexner et al.[113a]	114	1.5	—	12	29	—	2	1	—

*Double-stapled.

TABLE 32–11. Performance Status After Proctocolectomy

Type of Operation	No. of Patients	% Wanting Change	Activities					
			Sex		Social		Sports	
			% Improved	% Restricted	% Improved	% Restricted	% Improved	% Restricted
Brooke	675	40	15	29	28	21	15	43
Kock pouch	330	11	31*	29	38*	17	26*	21*
Ileoanal	50	6	34†	8‡	52†	12†	40†	8‡

*Differs from Brooke, p <0.05.
†Ileoanal > Brooke, p <0.02.
‡Ileoanal < Brooke, p <0.002.
Modified with permission from Dozois, R. R., and Kelly, K. A.: Newer operations for ulcerative colitis and Crohn's disease. *In* Kirsner, J. B., and Shorter, R. G. (Eds.): Inflammatory Bowel Disease, 3rd ed. Philadelphia, Lea & Febiger, 1988, p. 661.

for toxic megacolon, it rises to 17%.[5] These are remarkable statistics when one considers the debilitating nature of the disease and the fact that many patients have had long-term steroid therapy. The major complication in all reported series is sepsis, either in the wound or in the intra-abdominal cavity. There is little evidence that the development of more potent and specific antibiotics has significantly reduced the incidence of this complication; attention to the details of operative management continues to be the best way to ensure a smooth postoperative course. The most common late complication of resectional therapy with ileostomy or ileoanal anastomosis is intestinal obstruction, which occurs in about 10% of patients. Other bothersome but nonlethal complications following proctocolectomy include delay in perineal closure (25%), sexual dysfunction (5% to 10%), and renal stones (10%). Ileostomy dysfunction as a consequence of stenosis has been reduced to 2% by the Brooke-Turnbull ileostomy. Additional uncommon complications include prolapse, herniation, and ulceration of the stoma, which is usually a sign of the development of Crohn's disease within the ileal stoma. Whether the outcome following surgical therapy for Crohn's disease of the colon is as favorable as for ulcerative colitis continues to be a source of controversy.[104]

Results with ileoanal anastomosis in patients with ulcerative colitis are such that this operation is preferable in most patients. The authors[4] and others[23, 65] have found that more than 90% of patients are satisfied with their results, would not consider another alternative, and have fewer restrictions in their daily activities than do patients with Brooke ileostomies or Kock pouches (Table 32–11).

The formation of social groups (ileostomy clubs) has provided an important mechanism for the education of patients by those who have already mastered the technique of ileostomy management. Some hospitals have enterostomal therapists. These professionals are highly skilled in dealing with the physical and emotional problems of stomal management. In institutions that perform a large number of ileal pouch operations, specialized patient-oriented support groups are essential.[25]

These are extraordinary advances for patients who suffer from this poorly understood disease. New advances in surgical therapy have made the operative approach even more attractive to patients with ulcerative colitis. The cumulative mortality, as reported by Goligher and associates in their excellent monograph on the subject,[38] suggests that operative therapy should be administered quite liberally in the chronic or acutely fatal forms of the disease. In most patients, fortunately, ulcerative colitis is episodic and mild. Unfortunately, the high incidence of cancer in the presence of persistent disease (especially after 10 years' duration) does not allow these patients a life free of concern.

SELECTED REFERENCES

Becker, J. M.: Ileal pouch–anal anastomosis: Current status and controversies. Surgery, 113:599, 1993.
This article reviews the controversies surrounding technical aspects of ileal pouch–anal anastomosis.

Becker, J. M., and Parodi, J. E.: Total colectomy with preservation of the anal sphincter. Surg. Annu., 263:302, 1989.
This article analyzes the results in patients following ileoanal anastomosis.

Burakoff, R., and MacDermott, R. P.: Inflammatory Bowel Diseases. Philadelphia, Lippincott-Raven.
A new journal devoted to the science and medicine of inflammatory bowel diseases.

Lukash, W. M., and Johnston, R. B. (Eds.): The Systemic Manifestations of Inflammatory Bowel Disease. Springfield, Ill., Charles C. Thomas, 1975.
This monograph describes in detail the various colonic and extracolonic manifestations of ulcerative colitis. Associated liver, eye, skin, joint, blood, metabolic, and endocrine problems are covered in detail.

MacDermott, R. P., and Stenson, W. F. (Eds.): Inflammatory Bowel Disease. New York, Elsevier, 1992.
A concise review of the current diagnosis and treatment of inflammatory bowel disease.

Peppercorn, M. A. (Ed.): Inflammatory bowel disease. Gastroenterol. Clin. North Am. 24:1, 1995.
An excellent, concise review of inflammatory bowel disease, including current medical and surgical therapy of chronic ulcerative colitis.

Targan, S. R., and Shanahan, F.: Inflammatory Bowel Disease: From Bench to Bedside. Baltimore, Williams & Wilkins, 1994.
The authors provide a readable, authoritative text on the various facets of ulcerative colitis that relate to diagnosis, medical management, and natural history of the disease. The discussion of newer concepts of etiology places the numerous variables in a contemporary perspective.

Turnbull, R. B., Jr., and Weakley, F. L.: Atlas of Intestinal Stomas. St. Louis, C. V. Mosby, 1967.
The authors provide a stepwise, reliable method of constructing an ileostomy, The technical features offered cannot be overemphasized and, if adhered to, minimize ileostomy problems.

REFERENCES

1. Adams, F.: The Genuine Works of Hippocrates. Baltimore, Williams & Wilkins, 1939.
2. Almy, T. P., and Sherlock, P.: Genetic aspects of ulcerative colitis and regional enteritis. Gastroenterology, 51:757, 1966.
3. Baker, W. N. W., Glass, R. E., Ritchie, J. K., and Aylett, J. S. O.: Cancer of the rectum following colectomy and ileorectal anastomosis for ulcerative colitis. Br. J. Surg., 5:862, 1978.
4. Becker, J. M., and Parodi, J. E.: Total colectomy with preservation of the anal sphincter. Surg. Annu., 21:263, 1989.
5. Becker, J. M., and Raymond, J. L.: Ileal pouch–anal anastomosis: A single surgeon's experience with 100 consecutive cases. Ann. Surg., 204:375, 1986.
6. Block, G. E., Moosa, A. R., Siminowitz, D., et al.: Emergency colectomy for inflammatory bowel disease. Surgery, 82:531, 1977.
7. Boyko, E. J.: A critical review of the association between cigarette smoking and risk of ulcerative colitis. *In* MacDermott, R. P. (Ed.): Inflammatory Bowel Disease: Current Status and Future Approach. Amsterdam, Excerpta Medica, 1988, p. 671.
8. Brandtzaeg, P., Baklien, K., Fausa, O., and Hoel, P. S.: Immuno-histochem-

ical characterization of local immunoglobulin formation in ulcerative colitis. Gastroenterology, 66:1123, 1974.

9. Bubrick, M. P., Jacobs, D. M., and Levy, M.: Experience with the endorectal pull-through and S pouch for ulcerative colitis and familial polyposis in adults. Surgery, 98:689, 1985.

10. Caprilli, R., Verrua, P., Catella, G., et al.: Early recognition of toxic megacolon, J. Clin. Gastroenterol., 9:160, 1987.

11. Cello, J. P.: Ulcerative colitis. In Sleisenger, M. H., and Fordtran, J. S. (Eds.): Gastrointestinal Disease. Philadelphia, W. B. Saunders, 1983, p. 1122.

12. Cello, J. P., and Meyer, J. H.: Crohn's disease of the colon. In Sleisenger, M. H., and Fordtran, J. S. (Eds.): Gastrointestinal Disease. Philadelphia, W. B. Saunders, 1978, p. 1660.

13. Cohen, Z., McLeod, R. S., Stern, H., et al.: The pelvic pouch results. Am. J. Surg., 105:601, 1985.

14. Collins, R. H., Feldman, M., and Fordtran, J. S.: Colonic cancer, dysplasia, and surveillance in patients with ulcerative colitis: A critical review. N. Engl. J. Med., 316:1654, 1987.

15. Colonic and inflammatory bowel disease. Work Group VIII. Gastroenterology, 69:1140, 1975.

16. Cominelli, F., Nast, C. C., Clark, B. D., et al.: Interleukin-1 (IL-1) gene expression, synthesis, and effect on specific IL-1 receptor blockade in rabbit immune complex colitis. J. Clin. Invest., 86:972, 1990.

17. Connell, W. R., Talbot, I. C., Harpaz, N., Britto, N., Wilkinson, K. H., Kamm, M. A., and Lennard-Jones, J. E.: Clinicopathological characteristics of colorectal carcinoma complicating ulcerative colitis. Gut, 35:1419, 1994.

18. Crohn, B. B.: An historic note on ulcerative colitis (Letter). Gastroenterology, 42:366, 1962.

19. deDombal, F. T., Watts, J., Watkinson, G., and Goligher, J. C.: Local complications of ulcerative colitis: Stricture, pseudopolyposis and carcinoma of the colon and rectum. Br. Med. J., 1:1142, 1966.

20. Devroede, G. H., Taylor, W. F., Sauer, W. G., et al.: Cancer risk and life expectancy of children with ulcerative colitis. N. Engl. J. Med., 285:17, 1971.

21. Dick, A. P., Grayson, M. J., Carpenter, R. G., and Petrie, A.: Controlled trial of sulphasalazine in the treatment of ulcerative colitis. Gut, 5:437, 1964.

22. Dickinson, R. J., Ashton, M. G., Axon, A. T. R., et al.: Controlled trial of intravenous hyperalimentation and total bowel rest as an adjunct to the routine therapy of acute colitis. Gastroenterology, 79:1199, 1980.

23. Dozois, R. R.: Ileal pouch–anal anastomosis, Surg. Rounds, 10:34, 1987.

24. Dozois, R. R., Kelly, K. A., Bert, R. W., and Beahrs, O. H.: Improved results with continent ileostomy. Ann. Surg., 1923:19, 1980.

25. Dunnegan, D., and Becker, J. M.: Support groups for ileal pouch patients. In Bayless, T. M. (Ed.): Current Management of Inflammatory Bowel Disease. Philadelphia, B. C. Decker, 1989.

26. Elson, C. O., Layden, T. J., Nemchausky, B. A., et al.: An evaluation of total parenteral nutrition in the management of inflammatory bowel disease. Dig. Dis. Sci., 25:41, 1980.

27. Engle, G. L.: Studies of ulcerative colitis. III. The nature of the physiological process. Am. J. Med., 19:231, 1955.

28. Falchuk, K. R., Perotto, J. L., and Isselbacher, K. J.: Serum lysozyme in Crohn's disease and ulcerative colitis. N. Engl. J. Med., 292:395, 1975.

29. Farnelli, M. B., Van Heerden, J. A., Bert, R. W., Jr., et al.: Rectal preservation in non-specific inflammatory diseases of the colon. Ann. Surg., 192:249, 1980.

30. Fazio, V. W.: Toxic megacolon: Natural history and management. In Jagelman, D. G. (Ed.): Mucosal Ulcerative Colitis. New York, Futura, 1986, p. 159.

31. Ferzoco, S. J., and Becker, J. M.: Does aggressive medical therapy for acute ulcerative colitis result in a higher incidence of staged colectomy? Arch. Surg., 129:420, 1993.

32. Fiocchi, C., Hilfiker, M. L., Youngman, K. R., Doerder, N. C., and Finke, J. H.: Interleukin-2 activity of human intestinal mucosa mononuclear cells: Decreased levels in inflammatory bowel disease. Gastroenterology, 86:734, 1984.

32a. Fleshman, J. W., Cohen, Z., Mcleod, R. S., et al.: The ileal reservoir and ileoanal anastomosis procedure: Factors affecting technical and functional outcome. Dis. Colon Rectum, 31:10, 1988.

33. Fonkalsrud, E. W.: Endorectal ileal pull-through with isoperistaltic ileal reservoir for colitis and polyposis. Ann. Surg., 202:145, 1985.

34. Fonkalsrud, E. W., and Ament, M. E.: Endorectal mucosal resection without proctectomy as an adjunct to abdominoperineal resection for nonmalignant conditions. Ann. Surg., 188:245, 1978.

35. Gilat, T., Ribak, J., Benaroya, Y., Zemishlany, Z., and Weissman, I.: Ulcerative colitis in the Jewish population of Tel-Aviv Yafo. Gastroenterology, 66:335, 1974.

36. Goligher, J. C.: Surgical aspects of ulcerative colitis and Crohn's disease of the large bowel. Adv. Surg., 11:71, 1977.

37. Goligher, J. C.: Ulcerative colitis. In Goligher, J. C. (Ed.): Surgery of the Anus, Rectum and Colon. New York, Macmillan, 1980, p. 689.

38. Goligher, J. C., deDombal, F. T., Watts, J. M., and Watkinson, G.: Ulcerative Colitis. Baltimore, Williams & Wilkins, 1968.

39. Goligher, J. C., Hoffman, D. C., and deDombal, F. T.: Surgical treatment of severe attacks of ulcerative colitis with special reference to the advantages of early operation. Br. Med. J., 4:703, 1970.

40. Grant, C., and Dozois, R. R.: Toxic megacolon and ultimate fate of patients after successful medical management. Am. J. Surg., 147:106, 1984.

41. Greenstein, A. J., Janowitz, H. D., and Sachar, D. B.: The extra-intestinal complications of Crohn's disease and ulcerative colitis: A study of 700 patients. Medicine, 55:401, 1976.

42. Greensten, A. J., Sachar, D. B., Gibas, A., et al.: Outcome of toxic dilatation in ulcerative and Crohn's colitis. J. Clin. Gastroenterol., 7:137, 1985.

43. Gyde, S. N., Prior, P., Thompson, H., et al.: Survival of patients with colorectal cancer complicating ulcerative colitis. Gut, 25:228, 1984.

44. Harig, H. M., Soergel, K. H., Komorowski, R. A., and Wood, C. M.: Treatment of diversion colitis with short-chain-fatty-acid irrigation. N. Engl. J. Med., 230:23, 1989.

45. Harms, B. A., Pellet, J. R., and Starling, J. R.: Modified quadruple-loop (W) ileal reservoir for restorative proctocolectomy. Surgery, 101:234, 1987.

46. Heimann, T., Gelernt, I., Bauer, J., et al.: Mucosal proctectomy without reservoir. Am. J. Surg., 145:674, 1983.

47. Heppel, J., Farkouh, E., Dube, S., et al.: Toxic megacolon, an analysis of 70 cases. Dis. Colon Rectum, 29:789, 1986.

48. Heppel, J., Kelly, K. A., Phillips, S. F., et al.: Physiologic aspects of continence after colectomy, mucosal proctectomy and endorectal ileoanal anastomosis. Ann. Surg., 195:435, 1982.

49. Hoult, J. R. S., and Moore, P. K.: Sulphasalazine is a potent inhibitor of prostaglandin 15-hydroxydehydrogenase: Possible basis for therapeutic action in ulcerative colitis. Br. J. Pharmacol., 64:6, 1978.

50. Johnson, W. R., McDermott, F. T., Pihl, E., and Hughes, E. S. R.: Mucosal dysplasia, a major predictor of cancer following ileorectal anastomosis. Dis. Colon Rectum, 26:697, 1983.

51. Kaplan, H. P., Portnoy, B., Binder, H. J., et al.: A controlled evaluation of intravenous adrenocorticotropic hormone and hydrocortisone in the treatment of acute colitis. Gastroenterology, 69:91, 1975.

52. Keighley, M. R. B.: Abdominal mucosectomy reduces the incidence of soiling and sphincter damage after restorative proctocolectomy and J pouch. Dis. Colon Rectum, 30:386, 1987.

52a. Kelly, K. A.: Anal sphincter–saving operations for chronic ulcerative colitis. Am. J. Surg., 163:5, 1992.

53. Kern, F.: Extra-intestinal complications of chronic ulcerative colitis and Crohn's disease of the colon. In Kirsner, J. B., and Shorter, R. G. (Eds.): Inflammatory Bowel Disease. Philadelphia, Lea & Febiger, 1980, p. 217.

54. Kirk, A. P., and Lennard-Jones, J. E.: Controlled trial of azathioprine in chronic ulcerative colitis. Br. Med. J., 284:1291, 1982.

55. Kirsner, J. B.: Genetic aspects of inflammatory bowel disease. Clin. Gastroenterol., 21:557, 1973.

56. Kock, N. G.: Continent ileostomy. Prog. Surg., 12:180, 1973.

57. Kraft, S. C., and Kirsner, J. B.: Present status of immunological mechanisms in ulcerative colitis. Gastroenterology, 51:788, 1966.

58. Kvietys, P. R., and Granter, D. N.: The effect of volatile fatty acids on blood flow and oxygen uptake by the dog colon. Gastroenterology, 80:962, 1981.

59. Lennard-Jones, J. E., Misiewica, J. J., Connell, A. M., et al.: Prednisone as maintenance treatment for ulcerative colitis in remission. Lancet, 1:188, 1965.

60. Ljungh, A., and Wadstrom, T.: Subepithelial connective tissue protein binding of Escherichia coli isolated from patients with ulcerative colitis. In MacDermott, R. P. (Ed.): Inflammatory Bowel Disease: Current Status and Future Approach. Amsterdam, Excerpta Medica, 1988, p. 571.

61. MacDermott, R. P.: Overview of current and future approaches to research in the inflammatory bowel diseases. In MacDermott, R. P. (Ed.): Inflammatory Bowel Disease: Current Status and Future Approach. Amsterdam, Excerpta Medica, 1988, p. v.

62. MacDougall, I. P. M.: The cancer risk in ulcerative colitis. Lancet, 2:655, 1964.

63. Martin, L. W., Sayers, H. S., Alexander, F., et al.: Anal continence following Soave procedure. Ann. Surg., 203:525, 1986.

64. McCall, R. D., Haskill, S., Zimmerman, E., et al.: Tissue IL-1 and IL-1 receptor antagonist expression in enterocolitis in resistant and susceptible rats. Gastroenterology, 106:960, 1994.

65. McHugh, S. M., Diamont, N. E., McLeod, R., and Cohen, Z.: S-pouches versus "J" pouches colon: A comparison of functional outcomes. Dis. Colon Rectum, 30:671, 1987.

66. McIntyre, P. B., Powell-Tuck, J., Wood, S. R., Lennard-Jones, J. E., Lerebours, E., Hecketsweiler, P., Galamiche, J.-P., and Colin, R.: Controlled trial of bowel rest in the treatment of severe acute colitis. Gut, 276:481, 1986.

67. Meyers, S., and Janowitz, H. D.: The place of steroids in the therapy of toxic megacolon. Gastroenterology, 75:729, 1978.

68. Meyers, S., Sachar, D. B., Goldberg, J. D., and Janowitz, H. D.: Corticotrophin versus hydrocortisone in the intravenous treatment of ulcerative colitis: A prospective, randomized, double-blind clinical trial. Gastroenterology, 85:351, 1983.

69. Monk, M., Mendeloff, A. I., Siegel, C. I., and Lilienfeld, A.: An epidemiological study of ulcerative colitis and regional enteritis among adults in Baltimore. III. J. Chron. Dis., 22:565, 1970.

70. Montiero, E., Fossey, J., Shiner, J. M., Drasser, B., and Allison, A.: Antibacterial antibodies in rectal and colonic mucosa in ulcerative colitis. Lancet, 1:249, 1971.

71. Morson, B. C., and Pang, L. S.: Rectal biopsy as an aid to cancer control in ulcerative colitis. Gut, 8:423, 1967.

72. Nasmyth, D. G., Williams, N. S., and Johnston, D.: Comparison of the function of triplicated and duplicated pelvic ileal reservoir after mucosal proctectomy and ileoanal anastomosis for ulcerative colitis and adenomatous polyposis. Br. J. Surg., 73:361, 1986.

73. Nicholls, R. J., and Pezim, M. E.: Restorative proctocolectomy with ileal reservoir for ulcerative colitis and familial adenomatous polyposis: A comparison of three reservoir designs. Br. J. Surg., 72:470, 1985.

74. Palmer, K. R., Corbett, C. L., and Holdsworth, C. D.: Double-blind cross-over study comparing loperamide, codeine, and diphenoxylate in the treatment of chronic diarrhea. Gastroenterology, 79:1272, 1980.

75. Pemberton, J. H.: The problem with pouchitis. Gastroenterology, 104:1209, 1993.

76. Pemberton, J. H., Heppel, J., Bert, R. W., et al.: Endorectal ileoanal anastomosis. Surg. Gynecol. Obstet., 155:417, 1982.

77. Pemberton, J. H., Kelly, K. A., Beart, R. W., Jr., et al.: Ileal pouch–anal anastomosis for chronic ulcerative colitis. Ann. Surg., 206:504, 1987.

78. Pemberton, J. H., Phillips, S. F., Dozois, R. R., et al.: Current clinical results of conventional ileostomy. In Dozois, R. R. (Ed.): Alternatives to Conventional Ileostomy. Chicago, Year Book Medical Publisher, 1985, p. 40.

79. Podolsky, D. K., and Isselbacher, K. J.: Glycoprotein composition of colonic mucosa: Specific alterations in ulcerative colitis. Gastroenterology, 87:991, 1984.

80. Present, D. H.: Mercaptopurine and other immunosuppressive agents in the treatment of Crohn's disease and ulcerative colitis. Gastroenterol. Clin. North Am., 18:57, 1989.

81. Present, D. H., Chapman, M. G., and Rubin, R. H.: Efficacy of 6-mercaptopurine in refractory ulcerative colitis (Abstract). Gastroenterology, 94:A359, 1988.

82. Rampton, D. S., McNeil, N. I., and Sarner, M.: Analgesic ingestion and other factors preceding relapse in ulcerative colitis. Gut, 24:187, 1983.

83. Rampton, S. S., Sladen, G. E., and Youlten, L. J. F.: Rectal mucosal prostaglandin E$_2$ release and its relation to disease activity, electrical potential difference, and treatment in ulcerative colitis. Gut, 21:591, 1980.

84. Ravitch, M. M., and Sabiston, D. L., Jr.: Anal ileostomy with preservation of the sphincter: A proposed operation in patients requiring total colectomy for benign lesions. Surg. Gynecol. Obstet., 84:1095, 1947.

84a. Reissman, P., Piccirillo, M. F., Ulrich, A., et al.: Long-term outcome of the double-stapled ileoanal reservoir [abstract]. Dis. Colon Rectum, 37:(4):3, 1994.

85. Roediger, W. E. W.: The colonic epithelium in ulcerative colitis: An energy deficiency disease? Lancet, 2:712, 1980.

86. Rolandelli, R. H., Koruda, M. J., Settle, R. G., et al.: The effect of enteral feedings supplemented with pectin on the healing of colonic anastomoses in the rat. Surgery, 99:703, 1986.

87. Rombeau, J. L., Barot, L. R., Williamson, C. E., et al.: Preoperative total parenteral nutrition and surgical outcome in patients with inflammatory bowel disease. Am. J. Surg., 143:139, 1982.

88. Rosenberg, J. L., Wall, A. J., et al.: A controlled trial of azathioprine in the management of chronic ulcerative colitis. Gastroenterology, 69:96, 1975.

89. Roy, P. H., Sauer, W. G., Beahrs, O. H., et al.: Experiences with ileostomies: Evaluation of long-term rehabilitation in 497 patients. Am. J. Surg., 119:77, 1970.

90. Rubio, C. A., Johansson, C., Slezak, P., Ohman, V., and Hammarberg, C.: Villous dysplasia: An ominous histologic sign in colitic patients. Dis. Colon Rectum, 27:283, 1984.

91. Sakata, T.: Stimulatory effect of short-chain fatty acids on epithelial cell proliferation in rat intestine: A possible explanation for trophic effects of fermentable fibre, gut microbes and luminal trophic factors. Br. J. Nutr., 58:95, 1987.

92. Sandborn, W. J.: A critical review of cyclosporine therapy in inflammatory bowel disease. Ann. Intern. Med., 1:48, 1995.

93. Sartor, R. B.: Insights into the pathogenesis of inflammatory bowel diseases provided by new rodent models of spontaneous colitis. Inflam. Bowel Dis., 1:64, 1995.

94. Sartor, R. B.: Animal models of intestinal inflammation: Relevance to IBD. In MacDermott, R. P., Stenson, W. (Eds.): Inflammatory Bowel Disease. New York: Elsevier, 1991, p. 337.

95. Sartor, R. B.: Current concepts of the etiology and pathogenesis of ulcerative colitis and Crohn's disease. Gastroenterol. Clin. North Am. (in press).

95a. Schoetz, D. J., Coller, J. A., and Veidenheimer, M. C.: Can the pouch be saved? Dis. Colon Rectum, 31:671, 1988.

96. Schoetz, D. J., Jr., Coller, J. A., and Veidenheimer, M. C.: Ileoanal resevoir for ulcerative colitis and familial polyposis. Arch. Surg., 121:404, 1986.

97. Scott, H. W., Jr., Sawyers, J. L., Gobbel, W. G., Jr., et al.: Surgical management of toxic dilatation of the colon in ulcerative colitis. Ann. Surg., 179:647, 1974.

98. Sharon, P., and Stenson, W. F.: Enhanced synthesis of leukotriene B$_4$ by colonic mucosa in inflammatory bowel disease. Gastroenterology, 86:453, 1984.

99. Sharon, P., Lingmsky, M., Rachmilewitz, D., and Zor, V.: Role of prostaglandins in ulcerative colitis. Gastroenterology, 75:638, 1978.

100. Sinclair, T. S., Brunt, P. W., and Mowat, N. A. G.: Nonspecific proctocolitis in northeastern Scotland: A community study. Gastroenterology, 85:1, 1983.

101. Smith, L. E.: A review of twenty-one rectal mucosectomy and ileal pouch pull-through procedures. Am. Surg., 52:182, 1986.

102. Smolen, J. S., Gangl, A., Polterauer, P., Manzel, E. J., and Mayr, W. R.: HLA antigens in inflammatory bowel disease. Gastroenterology, 82:34, 1982.

103. Soyer, M. T., and Aldrete, J. S.: Surgical treatment of toxic megacolon and proposal for a program of therapy. Am. J. Surg., 140:421, 1980.

104. Steinberg, D. M., Allan, R. D., Brooke, B. N., et al.: Sequelae of colectomy and ileostomy: Comparison between Crohn's colitis and ulcerative colitis. Gastroenterology, 68:33, 1975.

105. Stenson, W. F.: Animal models of inflammatory bowel disease. In Targan, S. R. (Ed.): Inflammatory Bowel Disease: From Bench to Bedside. Baltimore, Williams & Wilkins, 1994, p. 180.

106. Stout, C., and Snyder, R. L.: Ulcerative colitis–like lesion in saimang gibbons. Gastroenterology, 57:256, 1969.

106a. Sugarman, J. H., and Newsome, H. H.: Stapled ileoanal anastomosis without a temporary ileostomy. Am. J. Surg., 167:58, 1994.

107. Sugarman, H. J., Newsome, H. H., DeCosta, G., and Zfass, A. M.: Stapled ileoanal anastomosis for ulcerative colitis and familial polyposis without a temporary diverting ileostomy. Ann. Surg., 213:606, 1991.

108. Taffet, S. L., and Das, K. M.: Sulfasalazine: Adverse effects and desensitization. Dig. Dis. Sci., 28:833, 1983.

109. Trickson, W., Tavery, I., Fazio, V., Oakley, J., Church, J., and Nilson, J.: Manometric and functional comparison of ileal pouch anastomosis with and without anal manipulation. Am. J. Surg., 161:90, 1991.

110. Truelove, S. C., et al.: Cortisone in ulcerative colitis: Final report on a therapeutic trial. Br. Med. J., 2:1041, 1955.

111. Turnbull, R. B., Jr., Hawk, W. A., and Weakley, F. L.: Surgical treatment of toxic megacolon, ileostomy and colostomy to prepare patient for colectomy. Am. J. Surg., 122:325, 1971.

112. Utsunomiya, J., Iwama, T., Imajo, M., et al.: Total colectomy, mucosal proctectomy and ileoanal pull-through. Dis. Colon Rectum, 23:459, 1980.

113. Weiss, E. G., and Wexner, S. D.: Surgical therapy for ulcerative colitis, Gastroenterol. Clin. North Am., 24:559, 1995.

113a. Wexner, S. D., Jensen, L., Rothenberger, D. A., et al.: Long-term functional analysis of ileoanal reservoir. Dis. Colon Rectum, 32:275, 1989.

114. Whitehead, R. H., Young, G. P., and Bhathal, P. S.: Effects of short-chain fatty acids on a new human colon carcinoma cell line (LIM1215). Gut, 27:1457, 1986.

115. Yardley, J. H., Bayless, T. H., and Diamond, M. P.: Cancer in ulcerative colitis. Gastroenterology, 76:221, 1979.

116. Yoshimura, H. H., Estes, M. K., and Graham, D. Y.: Search for evidence of a viral etiology for inflammatory bowel disease. Gut, 25:347, 1984.

117. Zenilman, M. E., Soper, N. J., Dunnegan, D., and Becker, J. N.: Previous abdominal colectomy affects functional results after ileal pouch–anal anastomosis. World J. Surg., 14:594, 1990.

VIII

VOLVULUS OF THE COLON

Anthony L. Imbembo, M.D., and Karl A. Zucker, M.D.

Volvulus is the abnormal twisting or rotation of a portion of the bowel about its mesentery. This may cause occlusion of the lumen at each end of the segment, with resultant obstruction and/or vascular compromise. Colonic volvulus has been recognized since antiquity. Descriptions of this disease, as well as its natural history, were detailed in the Egyptian Papyrus Ebers.[8] Colonic volvulus was also described in the writings of ancient Greek and Roman physicians, who administered purgatives as the preferred treatment. Hippocrates is credited with the use of a 12-inch-long suppository and of anal insufflation with air to untwist the bowel, methods somewhat similar to those currently used to treat sigmoid volvulus.[1] Today, volvulus is an uncommon cause of obstruction in the developed countries of Western Europe and North America, accounting for approximately 1% to 3% of all admissions for bowel obstruction.[6] It remains a major health problem in parts of Africa, Iran, India, Pakistan, Turkey, Eastern Europe, and South America, however, where volvulus is one of the most common causes of intestinal obstruction.[10]

The various forms of colonic volvulus were described by Von Rokitansky in the mid-nineteenth century. The sigmoid colon, cecum or right colon, transverse colon, or splenic flexure may be involved.[16] Colonic volvulus generally occurs in the setting of a dilated redundant colonic segment that has a narrow mesenteric base. The redundant segment is freely mobile within the peritoneal cavity, and the points of fixation are quite close, serving as a fulcrum for the development of volvulus. These features may be acquired, as in sigmoid volvulus, or congenital in origin, as is likely with cecal volvulus. Left untreated, volvulus generally progresses rapidly from colonic obstruction to strangulation and gangrene.

SIGMOID VOLVULUS

The sigmoid colon is the most common site for colonic volvulus, accounting overall for about three quarters of cases. In Olmstead County, Minnesota, where comprehensive medical records are available for all residents, there was an incidence of 1.47 episodes of sigmoid volvulus per 100,000 population per year. Sigmoid volvulus was also found to be 20 times more common in individuals above age 60 than in those who were younger.[6]

Much of the international literature has ascribed the pathogenesis of sigmoid volvulus to an acquired redundancy of sigmoid colon secondary to the ingestion of high-residue diets.[4, 5] In the United States, the most prominent association appears to be chronic constipation. Almost all patients have a long-standing history of disordered bowel habits, with excessive reliance on laxatives or enemas. Other contributing factors may include underlying neurologic or psychiatric disorders such as Parkinson's disease, Alzheimer's disease, multiple sclerosis, traumatic paralysis, chronic schizophrenia, pseudobulbar palsy, and senility. These associations have generally been attributed to the frequent bedridden state of these patients and/or the use of various neuropsychotropic drugs, which are both known to alter bowel motility. Thus, in the United States, up to 50% of patients admitted with sigmoid volvulus are referred from chronic care facilities.[4, 5] Adhesions from prior abdominal procedures have also been implicated as a causative factor in some patients, with the scar tissue serving as a pivot point around which the bowel can twist. In one study, 53% of 59 patients with sigmoid volvulus gave a history of prior abdominal operations,[6] but others have failed to confirm this association.[10] Although, overall, sigmoid volvulus is an uncommon complication in pregnant women, it appears to be the most frequently encountered cause of intestinal obstruction during pregnancy.[4, 5, 10]

The age and sex distributions of patients with sigmoid volvulus have been detailed in a number of international reports, with two distinct patterns emerging. Patients in Iran, Africa, India, and Eastern Europe are predominantly middle-aged males (mean age 40 to 50 years), whereas in the United States, Australia, the United Kingdom, and Canada, volvulus occurs in elderly patients (mean age 60 to 70 years) of either sex. In a large collected series from the United States, approximately two thirds of the patients were black; racial differences have not been noted in reports from other countries, however.[4, 5] Marked tribal differences have been noted in Africa and Pakistan.[10]

The diagnosis of sigmoid volvulus is usually straightforward and is based on the patient's history, physical examination, and plain abdominal radiographs. Acute sigmoid volvulus generally presents with the sudden onset of severe, colicky abdominal pain, obstipation, and abdominal distention. Distention is usually rapidly progressive as the twisted sigmoid continues to fill with gas and feces without the possibility of egress. The development of generalized abdominal pain, tenderness, fever, and hypovolemia suggests that strangulation has occurred. Occasionally, patients present with a history of intermittent abdominal pain and distention consistent with chronic intermittent volvulus.

Plain abdominal radiographs often reveal a dilated colon forming the so-called bent inner tube or omega loop sign. The convexity of the loop points toward the right upper quadrant, or away from the point of obstruction (Fig. 32–37). Two air-fluid levels, commonly at different levels, are frequently seen within the sigmoid loop. If the appearance of the plain radiograph is equivocal, a limited barium enema usually establishes the diagnosis. The column of barium tapers to a narrow point, the appearance having been described as a "bird's beak" pointing toward the site of obstruction. Barium enema is contraindicated whenever strangulation is suspected.

The treatment for acute sigmoid volvulus has evolved from attempts to untwist the bowel nonoperatively, as advocated by Hippocrates and his successors, to primary operative detorsion, to a combination of early nonoperative reduction followed by definitive surgical therapy. Operative detorsion of sigmoid volvulus was popularized in the late nineteenth century, with Atherton reporting the first successful experience in the United States in 1883.[3] However, operative mortality was high, especially since surgical intervention generally occurred very late in the course of the disease. Nonoperative reduction of sigmoid volvulus was rapidly

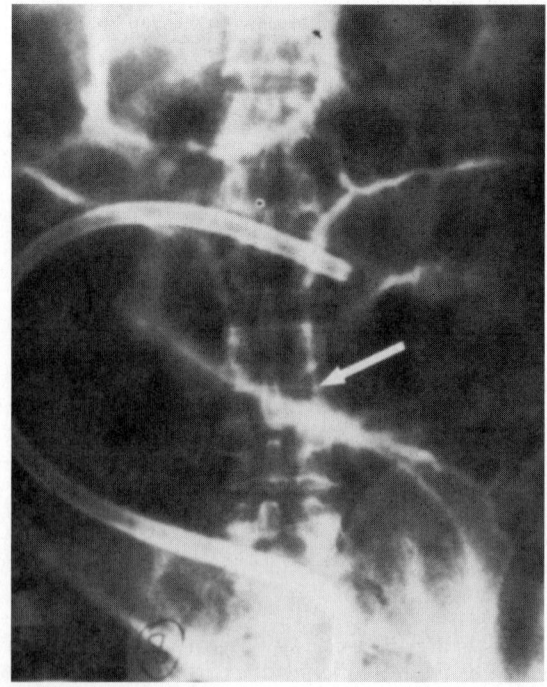

Figure 32–37. Sigmoid volvulus with rectal tube placement for decompression. The convexity of the loops (arrow) points toward the right upper quadrant. (Courtesy of G. H. Ballantyne, M.D.)

adopted following the report of Bruusgaard in 1947.[9] He found that in 82% of 148 patients, sigmoid volvulus was successfully reduced by a combination of rigid proctoscopy and rectal tube insertion. With this approach, overall mortality was only 14.2%.

In the United States, initial treatment of sigmoid volvulus consists of an attempt at nonoperative reduction, which can be expected to be successful in approximately 70% to 80% of patients.[4, 5] Successful detorsion of a sigmoid volvulus permits deferral of a surgical procedure in an acutely ill patient with an unprepared colon. Techniques that have been successful in reducing sigmoid colon volvulus include proctoscopy alone, enemas alone, proctoscopy and placement of a rectal tube, and barium–water-soluble contrast enemas. The latter modality is occasionally employed as part of the radiologic evaluation if there is some question about the diagnosis after plain films and may itself untwist the volvulus. Flexible fiberoptic colonoscopy has been advocated in those patients who fail rigid proctoscopy. In a report from the University of Ife in Nigeria, colonoscopic decompression was successful in 83 of 92 patients (90.2%) with sigmoid volvulus.[2] The fiberoptic colonoscope is especially useful when the sigmoidoscope fails to reach the point of obstruction. Some now advocate its use as the primary modality for detorsion. Flexible endoscopy has been shown to be a safe and effective diagnostic and therapeutic tool in patients with suspected colonic volvulus.[7]

The most widely used nonoperative procedure for reduction of sigmoid volvulus is the combination of proctoscopy and rectal tube placement. With the patient in the lateral knee-chest position, a rigid proctoscope is carefully advanced through the rectum into the distal sigmoid colon. The advancing proctoscope, along with the gentle insufflation of air to distend the bowel, often untwists the colon. A well-lubricated rectal tube is then passed through the proctoscope and eased past the point of torsion. With reduction of the volvulus, there is usually explosive decompression, with passage of gas and liquid feces. The return of bloody intraluminal contents or the presence of discolored colonic mucosa is a reliable sign of colonic ischemia. Such evidence of vascular compromise on proctoscopy necessitates immediate surgical intervention.

When the flexible fiberoptic endoscope is used successfully for detorsion, the maintenance of decompression is somewhat more complicated. Once the endoscope has been positioned within the sigmoid colon, a blunt guide wire is passed through the biopsy channel into the intestinal lumen. The length of endoscope within the bowel is noted, and then it is withdrawn, with the guide wire left in position. A well-lubricated, large-bore rectal tube is passed over the guide wire to the identical distance as that of the endoscope. The guide wire is withdrawn, and the tube is secured to the thigh or buttock. A plain abdominal radiograph confirms the proper position of the tube in the sigmoid loop.

If there is no evidence of bowel wall ischemia and nonoperative reduction is successful, delayed sigmoid colon resection is recommended for most patients. This procedure should be performed after the patient has been adequately resuscitated and nutritionally repleted and has undergone appropriate bowel preparation. With a delayed, elective resection, primary anastomosis can be performed safely in most patients. In those patients who fail nonoperative reduction, however, the appropriate surgical approach can be much less clear. Colostomy alone, proximal to the site of volvulus, is contraindicated, as this procedure will not prevent strangulation of the segment or recurrent volvulus. Operative detorsion alone carries a recurrence rate of up to 40% and, by itself, is not an acceptable procedure in most cases.[14] Other procedures that have been used in conjunction with operative detorsion include tube sigmoidostomy, extraperitonealization of the sigmoid colon, sigmoidopexy to the transverse colon, sigmoidopexy to the peritoneum, fixation of the sigmoid mesentery, and resection with end-colostomy (with or without mucous fistula).[4, 5] Unfortunately, there is insufficient experience reported to evaluate the efficacy of these procedures. Presently, the most common recommendation is initial operative reduction followed by delayed resection and primary anastomosis. If gangrene is present at the time of laparotomy, immediate resection is indicated, with creation of an end-colostomy and mucous fistula or Hartmann's pouch.

There is little information regarding the recurrence rate following operation for sigmoid volvulus. In a study of 29 patients undergoing a variety of operative procedures for sigmoid volvulus, the overall recurrence rate was 36%.[12] Although the rate varied slightly according to the procedure, the most significant factor correlating with recurrence was the extent of colonic disease at the time of the procedure. The recurrence rate was 6% when disease was limited to the sigmoid, but 82% for those with associated diffuse megacolon. Thus, subtotal colectomy may be appropriate in selected patients.[12]

The main determinant of patient mortality from acute sigmoid volvulus is viability of the sigmoid colon. In the United States, patients undergoing successful nonoperative reduction followed by elective resection have an expected mortality of 6% to 10%. Patients with gangrenous colon have a mortality of 50% to 70%.[4, 5] Prompt nonoperative or operative intervention in the hope of preventing strangulation of sigmoid volvulus appears to be the most important principle of treatment. Recurrence of volvulus after nonoperative reduction ranges from 55% to 90%. The mortality rate relative to recurrent volvulus or its treatment can be as high as 20% to 30%.[4, 5] Therefore, maximal survival is achieved by early elective resection, even in an elderly population.

CECAL VOLVULUS

Cecal volvulus accounts for 20% to 40% of all cases of colonic volvulus. In 502 patients with volvulus of the colon collected from 16 series, 34% were found to have cecal volvulus.[6] Approximately 90% of patients with cecal volvulus have an axial twist of a segment of the proximal colon (Fig. 32–38; see also Fig. 32–40B) or even of the entire right colon; in the remainder, there is a cephalad fold of the cecum across the ascending colon (cecal bascule) (Figs. 32–39 and 32–40A). A mobile cecum is a prerequisite for development of cecal volvulus. Various anomalous patterns of cecal attachment allow for such mobility. A detailed study of 125 cadavers at Northwestern University revealed that over one third of cecums examined were mobile enough to allow a volvulus to occur.[17] Poor fixation usually results from malrotation of the colon, setting the stage for torsion, often around the pedicle of the ileocolic artery.

Various risk factors have been associated with the development of cecal volvulus. As with sigmoid volvulus, high-fiber diets among developing populations and the use of various neuropsychotropic drugs in Western populations have been implicated. In the United States, as many as one half to two thirds of these patients have undergone previous abdominal surgical procedures; in one series, 68% of these operations were appendectomies.[13] Colonic distention resulting from distal obstruction has also been implicated in the development of cecal volvulus and should be ruled out in each instance.

Cecal volvulus generally presents with the acute onset of severe, colicky pain, nausea, vomiting, and obstipation. Often, abdominal distention develops along with a compressible mass extending from the right lower quadrant to the

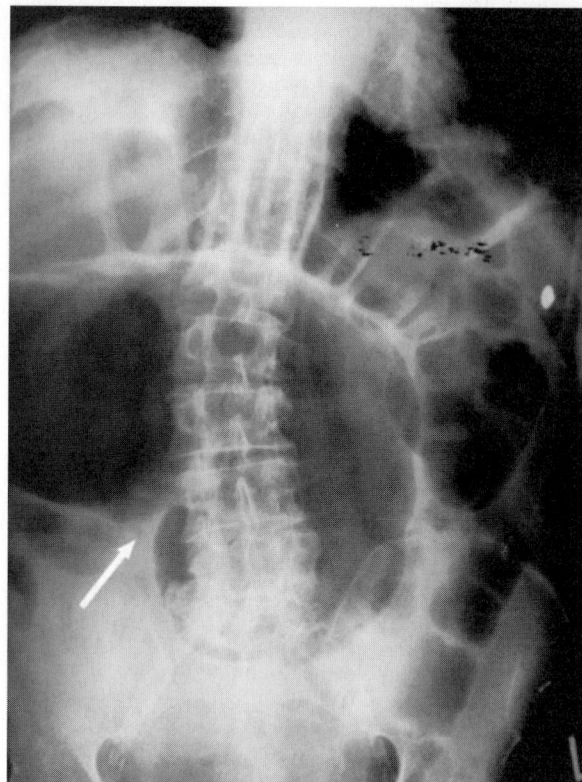

Figure 32–38. Cecal volvulus with an axial twist at the level of the mid-ascending colon. In contrast to sigmoid volvulus, the convexity of the loops (arrow) points toward the left upper quadrant. (Courtesy of G. H. Ballantyne, M.D.)

Figure 32–39. Cecal bascule with a cephalad fold of the cecum across the ascending colon (arrow). The ileocecal valve and terminal ileum are visible over the L2–3 interspace. (Courtesy of G. H. Ballantyne, M.D.)

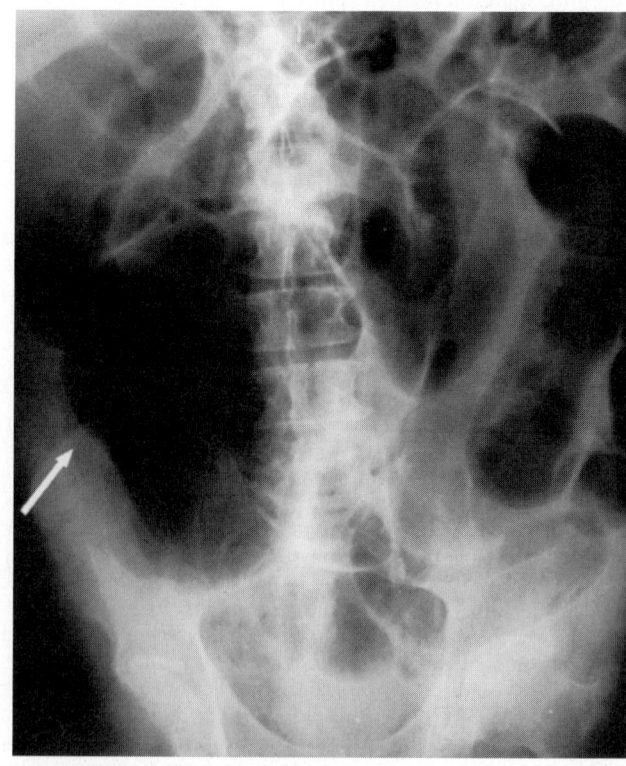

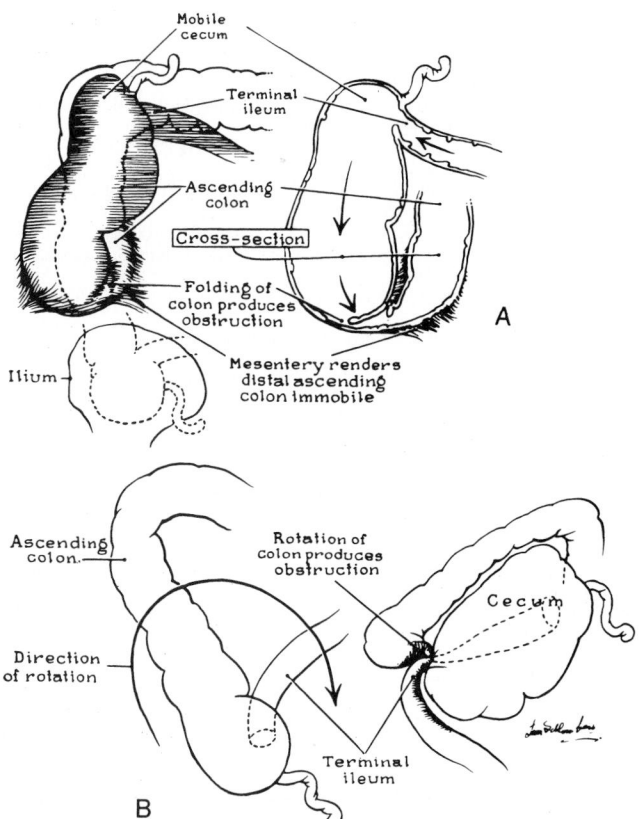

Figure 32–40. Diagrammatic representation of cecal volvulus caused by an anterior cephalad displacement of the cecum, resulting in obstruction at the site of transverse folding. Dotted lines show usual position of the cecum in relation to the ilium. B, Demonstration of cecal volvulus produced by a clockwise rotation of the terminal ileum, cecum, and ascending colon. (From O'Mara, C. S., Wilson, T. M., Jr., Stonesifer, G. L. and Cameron, J. L.: Cecal volvulus. Ann. Surg., 189:724, 1979.)

midabdominal region. Chronic abdominal symptoms occur in many patients because of the tendency for cecal volvulus to resolve spontaneously, only to recur. These patients often obtain relief by the self-administration of enemas or by assumption of the knee-chest position. Plain abdominal roentgenograms may reveal marked distention of the cecum as well as small bowel dilatation. Barium enema classically reveals the narrowing accompanying the twisting of the colon (so-called bird's neck deformity); however, such studies may be misinterpreted as showing obstruction secondary to neoplasm. The filling of the entire left colon on barium enema can differentiate cecal from sigmoid volvulus.

Nonoperative techniques for the reduction of cecal volvulus have been much less successful than for sigmoid volvulus. Reduction of the volvulus by barium enema may occur in a small number of patients, but early recurrence is the rule.[11] Colonoscopic reduction has been reported in a small number of patients but is accompanied by a high failure rate; it often delays necessary operative reduction and is unwise in the setting of ischemic bowel.[7]

The physical examination, as well as the presence of fever and leukocytosis, correlates poorly with the presence or absence of gangrenous bowel in patients with cecal volvulus.[13] Approximately 25% of patients are found to have gangrenous changes at the time of laparotomy. Mortality in the setting of gangrenous bowel approaches 40%; in patients with viable bowel, it is generally less than 10%.[15] Therefore, once the diagnosis of cecal volvulus has been made, prompt surgical intervention is advised. When the cecum is gangrenous, re-

section is mandatory, usually with ileotransverse colostomy. However, in the setting of viable bowel, the procedure of choice is less clear. The available options include detorsion alone, cecopexy, cecostomy, and colonic resection. Operative detorsion alone without fixation is associated with a high recurrence rate and consequent mortality.[6, 15] Cecopexy performed by suturing the colon to the parietal peritoneum eliminates hypermobility, with quite satisfactory overall results. Cecostomy accomplishes both fixation and venting of the obstructed colon, but this procedure inevitably results in spillage of colonic contents, increasing the risk of intraabdominal sepsis or wound complications. Right hemicolectomy for nongangrenous cecal volvulus is the procedure of choice in a number of institutions.[15] In this way, the possibility of recurrent volvulus is eliminated. However, results from 15 reports of patients with cecal volvulus comparing the various treatment options revealed no significant difference in overall mortality.[15] Controlled trials are necessary to determine whether there is an optimal procedure.

VOLVULUS OF THE TRANSVERSE COLON

Fewer than 100 cases of transverse colon volvulus have been reported. In a collected series of international reports, these patients were found to be middle-aged, with females outnumbering males by two to one.[6] Patients present with the typical signs and symptoms of colonic obstruction. Diagnosis of transverse colon volvulus is difficult on plain abdominal x-rays and, in most series, was not suspected preoperatively. Contrast radiologic studies may be more specific. Reported attempts at nonoperative reduction of transverse colon volvulus have been few and generally unsuccessful. Urgent surgical intervention is recommended in all cases, and the principles of treatment are similar to those for cecal volvulus. If gangrenous bowel is encountered, resection is mandatory. In patients with viable colon, detorsion alone appears to be associated with a high rate of recurrence and mortality.[6] Transverse colectomy, colopexy, and transverse tube colostomy have all been used successfully. The procedure of choice is unknown at this time.

VOLVULUS OF THE SPLENIC FLEXURE

The splenic flexure is the least common site for colonic volvulus, with fewer than 50 cases reported. The splenic flexure is fixed in position by the gastrocolic, splenocolic, and phrenocolic ligaments. Congenital absence or iatrogenic division of one or more of these attachments may predispose to splenic flexure volvulus. Approximately two thirds of reported patients with splenic flexure volvulus have undergone previous abdominal operation.[6] Urgent surgical intervention is recommended. Resection is mandated in cases of ischemic bowel. The majority of patients with nongangrenous bowel have also been treated by resection, although there have been reports of patients treated successfully by colopexy or splenic flexure colostomy.

SELECTED REFERENCES

Ballantyne, G. H.: Review of sigmoid volvulus: history and results of treatment. Dis. Colon Rectum, 25:494, 1982.
A lucid summary of the history of sigmoid volvulus, along with a summary of various forms of therapy from the international literature. Results of the various surgical options in the treatment of nongangrenous sigmoid volvulus are presented.

Ballantyne, G. H., Brandner, M. D., Beart, R. W., and Ilstrup, D. M.: Volvulus of the colon: Incidence and mortality. Ann. Surg., 202:83, 1985.
This is an excellent review of colonic volvulus. It describes 137 patients from the Mayo Clinic with sigmoid, cecal, transverse, and splenic volvulus from 1960 to 1980. Methods of diagnosis, treatment, and outcome are discussed in these patients and compared with the experience in the literature.

Gibney, E. J.: Volvulus of the sigmoid colon. Surg. Gynecol. Obstet., *173*:243, 1991.
An outstanding collective review of the international literature on sigmoid volvulus.

O'Mara, C. S., Wilson, T. H., Stonesifer, G. L., and Cameron, J. L.: Cecal volvulus: Analysis of 50 patients with long-term follow-up. Ann. Surg., *189*:724, 1979.
The authors report the diagnosis, management, and outcome of 50 patients with cecal volvulus from the Johns Hopkins University. The diagnosis of cecal volvulus was made preoperatively in less than half of the patients. Thirty-eight percent had undergone one or more previous abdominal operations, the majority being appendectomies. When gangrene of the cecum was present, resection was performed. Otherwise the authors recommend cecopexy because of the low mortality and recurrence rates.

Tejler, G., and Jiborn, H.: Volvulus of the cecum: Report of 26 cases and review of the literature. Dis. Colon Rectum, *31*:445, 1988.
The management of 26 patients with cecal volvulus treated at the Malmo General Hospital is described, along with a review of 350 patients in the literature. The pathogenesis of cecal volvulus as a result of colonic malrotation with a common ileocolic mesentery is discussed. The authors recommend resection as the treatment of choice when there is no gangrene present.

REFERENCES

1. Adams, F. (Trans. and Ed.): The Genuine Works of Hippocrates. London, Sydenham Society, 1849.
2. Arigbabu, A. O., Badejo, O. A., and Akinola, D. O.: Colonoscopy in the emergency treatment of colonic volvulus in Nigeria. Dis. Colon Rectum, *28*:795, 1985.
3. Atherton, A. B.: Cases of internal strangulation of the bowels: Laparotomy. Boston Med. Surg. J., *108*:531, 1883.
4. Ballantyne, G. H.: Review of sigmoid volvulus: Clinical patterns and pathogenesis. Dis. Colon Rectum, *25*:823, 1982.
5. Ballantyne, G. H.: Review of sigmoid volvulus: History and results of treatment. Dis. Colon Rectum, *25*:494, 1982.
6. Ballantyne, G. H., Brandner, M. D., Beart, R. W., and Ilstrup, D. M.: Volvulus of the colon. Ann. Surg., *205*:83, 1985.
7. Brothers, T. E., Strodel, W. E., and Eckhauser, F. E.: Endoscopy in colonic volvulus. Ann. Surg., *206*:1, 1987.
8. Brothwell, D., and Sandison, A. T. (Eds.): Diseases in Antiquity, A Survey of the Diseases, Injuries, and Surgery of Early Populations. Springfield, Ill., Charles C. Thomas, 1967.
9. Bruusgaard, C.: Volvulus of the sigmoid colon and its treatment. Surgery, *22*:466, 1947.
10. Gibney, E. J.: Volvulus of the sigmoid colon. Surg. Gynecol. Obstet., *173*:243, 1991.
11. Hjelmstedt, A.: Volvulus of the right colon. Acta Chir. Scand., *118*:455, 1960.
12. Morrissey, T., and Deitch, E.: Recurrence of sigmoid volvulus after surgical intervention. Am. Surg., *60*:329, 1994.
13. O'Mara, C. S., Wilson, T. H., Stonesifer, G. L., and Cameron, J. L.: Cecal volvulus. Ann. Surg., *189*:724, 1979.
14. String, S. T., and DeCosse, J. J.: Sigmoid volvulus: An examination of the mortality. Am. J. Surg., *121*:293, 1971.
15. Tejler, G., and Jiborn, H.: Volvulus of the cecum: Report of 26 cases and review of the literature. Dis. Colon Rectum, *31*:445, 1988.
16. Von Rokitansky: A Manual of Pathologic Anatomy. London, Sydenham Society, 1849.
17. Wolfer, J. A., Beaton, L. E., and Anson, B. J.: Volvulus of the cecum: Anatomical factors in its etiology. Surg. Gynecol. Obstet., *74*:882, 1942.

IX

CARCINOMA OF THE COLON, RECTUM, AND ANUS

H. Kim Lyerly, M.D.

Carcinoma of the colon and rectum is one of the most common malignancies in the United States and one of the most lethal. An understanding of the biology of colorectal cancer and improvements in surgical techniques have led to significant improvements in the management of early or preneoplastic lesions, as well as reduction in the morbidity associated with colorectal carcinoma.

Advances in our understanding of the cellular and molecular events that lead to the development of colon and rectal cancer have proceeded in two overlapping areas: (1) the examination of the molecular events that occur in the pathogenesis of adenoma formation and progression to colonic malignancy, and (2) the study of inherited syndromes and familial clustering of colorectal carcinoma.[5, 20, 42, 54] These advances have led to the widely accepted paradigm that cancer appears to develop by an orderly progression. Rather than a random event that can attack at any point within the intestinal mucosa, cancer is a process that develops in a sequential fashion, arising from normal colonic epithelium and progressing through premalignant adenomatous polyps prior to developing into frankly invasive carcinoma. This orderly progression from adenomatous polyps to invasive carcinoma forms the theoretic basis for the modern management of colon and rectal cancer. An appreciation that adenomatous polyps can be identified and treated prior to the development of invasive and metastatic cancer provides the rationale and justification for screening populations for preinvasive disease as well as cancer and the use of therapeutic procedures to remove precursor lesions. Ultimately, the identification of mucosa at risk for the development of invasive carcinoma provides the background for trials of agents to prevent progression of premalignant lesions. Therefore, this chapter provides an overview of the molecular biology of colonic and rectal neoplasia, a discussion of the impact of inheritance on the risk of colon cancer, and the biologic basis for the current management of the common sporadic forms of colon and rectal cancer.

Because adenomatous polyps have a central role in the progression from normal colonic epithelium to invasive carcinoma, and their management plays a critical role in colorectal malignancies, they are specifically reviewed.

INTESTINAL POLYPS

An intestinal polyp is grossly defined as an elevation of the mucosal surface. Estimates of the prevalence of asymptomatic polyps in the general population range from 1.6% to 12%; however, in the population older than 70 years of age, it may be as high as 40%.[18] Polyps are therefore relatively common, and an understanding of their biology and natural history is critical for appropriate management. The biologic and clinical ramifications of intestinal polyps vary substantially with the microscopic appearance and are due in large part to their potential to degenerate from a benign condition to an invasive carcinoma. Polyps are therefore classified as neoplastic or nonneoplastic, as shown in Table 32–12, with neoplastic being premalignant and requiring management with the potential clearly in mind.

Although most polyps are asymptomatic, they may be continuously growing, requiring as long as 10 years to double their diameter. Polyps may grow sufficiently to cause symptoms, that is, by becoming the lead point of intussuscep-

TABLE 32–12. Intestinal Polyps

Nonneoplastic	Neoplastic
Hamartomatous polyps	Adenomatous polyps
Cowden's disease	Tubular
Cronkhite-Canada syndrome	Tubulovillous
Peutz-Jeghers syndrome	Villous
Juvenile (retention) polyps	
Inflammatory polyps	
Benign lymphoid polyps	
Inflammatory polyps (pseudopolyps)	
Metaplastic or hyperplastic polyps	

tion or by ulcerating and causing bleeding. Polyps may also achieve sufficient size to prolapse through the rectum, and rarely, may be of sufficient size or number to lead to obstruction. Less commonly, large polyps may secrete sufficient mucus to cause diarrhea or protein-losing enteropathy.

Symptomatic polyps are usually treated by endoscopic removal or local resection; however, asymptomatic polyps may also require intervention. Although the gross appearance of asymptomatic neoplastic and nonneoplastic polyps may be similar, it is critical to determine the *histologic* appearance of polyps to classify them as neoplastic or nonneoplastic. Neoplastic polyps have the potential for progression to invasive carcinoma and must be removed appropriately to eliminate this risk. A review of the histologic subtypes of polyps with associated symptoms and natural history follows.

Nonneoplastic Polyps

An *intestinal hamartoma* is a localized overgrowth of normal mature intestinal epithelial cells that is usually pedunculated, with the stalk lined with normal mucosa. Intestinal hamartomas can cause intussusception but are more often asymptomatic. The malignant potential of hamartomas appears to be small, and prophylactic resection of a known hamartoma is not warranted. Multiple intestinal hamartomas are found in Peutz-Jeghers syndrome and Cowden's disease.

Peutz-Jeghers syndrome is an autosomal dominant condition in which numerous hamartomatous polyps are present throughout the gastrointestinal tract, including the small intestine, large intestine, and stomach.[12] More than 95% of patients with this syndrome also have a brownish pigmentation of their lips, buccal surfaces, periocular skin, and perianal regions. Conversely, less than 5% of patients with these characteristic mucocutaneous melanotic macules do not have this syndrome. Rarely, exostoses, ovarian tumors, and polyps of the bladder occur. The hamartomatous polyps associated with Peutz-Jeghers syndrome may grow to sufficient size to cause bleeding, obstruction, or intussusception but are not considered premalignant. Removal of gastric and small intestinal polyps is performed to manage complications.

An increased risk of cancer in patients with Peutz-Jeghers syndrome appears to be linked with adenomatous elements that may be found in association with the hamartomas.[22] Therefore, although patients with this syndrome are at an increased risk for the development of colon cancer, it is not sufficiently high enough to justify prophylactic colectomy. Nonetheless, colonic polyps should be aggressively managed and endoscopically removed, even if asymptomatic. Children with this syndrome are also at increased risk for the development of unusual tumors of the reproductive system and bladder and should be screened.

Cowden's disease is an autosomal dominant condition consisting of multiple intestinal hamartomas.[56] Associated lesions include hyperkeratotic cutaneous and gingival lesions, such as trichilemmomas, acral keratoses, and oral mucosal papillomas. These associated findings are important for the diagnosis of Cowden's disease. Patients with Cowden's disease are at increased risk for cancers of the breast, thyroid, and skin.

Juvenile or *retention polyps* occur mainly in children and are hamartomatous epithelial retentions, composed of cystically dilated glands filled with mucus and inflammatory debris. Most juvenile polyps are pedunculated, although some are small and sessile. The peak ages for patients to experience symptoms are 5 and 6 years, when these polyps may cause rectal bleeding, mucous discharge, and diarrhea and abdominal pain, or, less frequently, intussusception or rectal prolapse. Hamartomatous polyps do not appear to be premalignant; however, patients with multiple retention polyps or the juvenile polyposis syndrome, inherited as an autosomal dominant trait, have an increased incidence of adenomatous polyps as well as having the juvenile polyps. Therefore, in some patients with juvenile polyposis syndrome, there is an increased incidence of adenocarcinoma of the colon and rectum (arising from coexistent adenomatous polyps).[46] Operation is indicated to obtain biopsy specimens of polyps to confirm their histologic diagnosis and to treat symptoms. Prophylactic colectomy to reduce the risk of development of invasive colon carcinoma is not indicated.

Inflammatory polyps are usually multiple and are associated with ulcerative colitis and Crohn's disease. Most are small and sessile, but they can rarely become large or numerous enough to obstruct the colon. They may bleed, leading to anemia. Treatment consists of attention to the underlying inflammatory bowel disease.

Cronkhite-Canada syndrome is a nonfamilial condition characterized by diffuse juvenile-type hamartomatous polyps throughout the gastrointestinal tract. It is characterized by accompanying dystrophy of the nails, alopecia, and cutaneous hyperpigmentation. Weight loss, diarrhea, and malnutrition may occur, and therapy is supportive and directed toward nutritional replacement. The polyps associated with Cronkhite-Canada syndrome are not reported to have malignant potential.

Hyperplastic polyps are the most common small benign tumors of the colon and are the product of excessive replication of the mucosal epithelium, causing small sessile mucosal elevations. These are usually asymtomatic but may be associated with rectal bleeding or diarrhea if numerous enough. They are not premalignant, but a small number of polyps cannot be strictly classified as hyperplastic or adenomatous, and up to one third of hyperplastic polyps have been found to contain adenomatous elements. Therefore, these polyps are treated by removal, and patients are followed as if the polyps were adenomatous.

Neoplastic Polyps

Neoplastic or *adenomatous polyps* are relatively common in patients in the United States and may be either sporadic or associated with an inherited polyposis syndrome. Although the inherited forms of polyps occur in young patients, there is an increased incidence of the sporadic type with advancing age, with adenomatous polyps being most common in patients older than 60 years of age. These polyps may be histologically classified as tubular or villous, depending on the glandular pattern. Patients with the inherited forms of adenomatous polyps or polyposis have an extremely high incidence of colorectal carcinoma, suggesting that with genetically inherited colorectal carcinoma, there is a link between adenomas and carcinomas. However, even in spontaneous colorectal carcinomas, a number of epidemiologic, clinical, and histologic, and genetic observations provide evidence about the validity of the adenoma-carcinoma sequence. Adenomatous polyps are therefore considered premalignant, and most, if not all, colorectal carcinomas are believed to arise from these polyps in a succession of events termed the *adenoma-carcinoma sequence.*

Evidence to support the adenoma-carcinoma sequence includes the fact that, except for the inherited polyposis syndromes, polyps are most commonly found in patients older than 60 years of age, which is similar to the age distribution of colorectal cancer. There is a geographic variation in the frequency of polyps that parallels that of colorectal carcinoma, which suggests that environmental or dietary factors may have a role in adenoma formation and carcinogenesis.

If the adenoma-carcinoma sequence is valid, one would expect to see further associations of adenomas with invasive carcinomas. Indeed, there is a high incidence of associated polyps in patients with colorectal carcinomas, since about one third of resected colorectal carcinomas have one or more associated adenomas. In addition, there is evidence that the presence of these additional adenomas reflects an intestinal mucosa that is at high risk for the development of subsequent carcinomas. In fact, these additional adenomas double the risk of a metachronous colorectal carcinoma. Finally, about 75% of patients with synchronous colorectal carcinomas also have adenomas.

In addition to the epidemiologic and clinical association of adenomas and carcinomas is the physical association of adenomas and carcinomas in operative specimens. This association appears to be consistent with a continuum of histologic appearances from adenoma to carcinoma, with an intermediate, mixed histologic appearance in between. For example, the frequency of cancer in adenomas less than 1 cm. in diameter is less than 1%, but this frequency increases with the size of the adenoma. In adenomas larger than 1 cm. but less than 2 cm. in diameter, the frequency of cancer is 10%, whereas in adenomas larger than 2 cm. it may be as high as 50%. A corollary to this observation is that well-differentiated carcinomas are likely to contain some adenomatous elements, whereas advanced or poorly differentiated carcinomas rarely contain adenomatous components.

This evidence has led to the current management of adenomatous polyps as premalignant lesions, which should theoretically lead to a reduction in incidence of invasive colorectal carcinomas. As a justification of these presumptions, recent large clinical trials have indeed demonstrated a reduction in incidence and mortality due to colorectal carcinoma in patients with adenomatous polyps treated by polypectomy and surveillance.[43, 69]

Therefore, the progressive and orderly histologic and clinical development of colorectal neoplasms constitutes an ideal system for studying the genetic alterations responsible for tumor initiation and progression. Genetic studies of tumors of various histologic sizes and stages have revealed several basic principles underlying colorectal tumorigenesis, most notably the accumulation of somatically acquired mutations in colorectal adenomas and carcinomas that parallels the histologic progression of tumorigenesis. A description of the progressive molecular changes in the pathologic sequence from adenoma to carcinoma is described in detail in the following section.

MOLECULAR CARCINOGENESIS

The pathologic development of human colon cancer is a complex, multistep process. The series of progressive changes in the colonic epithelial cells appears to correlate with a series of progressive genetic changes that involves multiple but specific events culminating in deregulation of cell proliferation and progression from adenomas to carcinoma. Several

genetic abnormalities commonly occur during the genesis of colorectal carcinoma, and the cumulative total of genetic abnormalities appears to be more important than their order of appearance (see Chapter 2).[20]

Molecular studies have provided a theoretic framework for understanding the nature of colorectal neoplasia. Each adenoma appears to arise from a single epithelial cell of a mucosal crypt, and tumor progression represents the selection for a clonal predominance of those cells that have acquired certain additional mutations. The acquisition of multiple changes in an adenoma increases the likelihood of its progression to the carcinoma, whereas in a carcinoma, the more advanced degrees of genetic change are associated with metastatic behavior.[70]

CLINICAL FEATURES OF INHERITED SYNDROMES AND FAMILIAL CLUSTERING OF COLORECTAL CANCER

Relatives of patients with colon cancer are known to have an increased risk for this malignancy. Well-characterized inherited syndromes account for some of this risk, but in most instances the risk is less well defined. Some familial syndromes characterized by multiple neoplastic colonic polyps may account for less than 1% of colon cancer cases. Hereditary nonpolyposis colorectal carcinoma (HNPCC) may occur in up to 5% of cases. Most familial cases of colon cancer, however, cannot be classified as well-defined syndromes. These poorly defined familial cases may represent a large fraction of colon cancers and may result from partially penetrant inherited susceptibility.[50]

Familial Adenomatous Polyposis. Familial adenomatous polyposis (FAP) has four variants: typical FAP, Gardner's syndrome, Turcot's syndrome, and attenuated polyposis coli (AAPC).[7, 11]

FAP has an approximate prevalence of 1 in 10,000 births and is characterized by the presence of hundreds to thousands of colonic adenomatous polyps. Polyps occur at an average age of 15 years, and all affected persons exhibit polyps by 35 years of age. Colon cancer occurs at an average age of 39. Seven per cent of untreated patients develop cancer by age 21 and 90% by age 45. The disease is inherited in an autosomal dominant fashion, and nearly all persons who carry the gene develop polyposis.

Upper gastrointestinal polyps are also common in patients with FAP.[31] Gastric polyps occur in 50% and duodenal polyps in at least 90% of affected persons. Gastric polyps are fundic gland polyps histologically with no malignant potential. Duodenal polyps are adenomas. There is some malignant potential, with persons with FAP having a 10% lifetime risk of duodenal cancer. Small bowel cancer distal to the duodenum is rare.

FAP is classified as *Gardner's syndrome* when the intestinal findings are accompanied by certain benign extraintestinal growths, including osteomas (particularly of the mandible or long bones), epidermoid cysts, desmoid tumors, and congenital hypertrophy of the retinal pigment epithelium. These growths may precede the development of polyposis and are generally cosmetic in nature. Desmoid tumors, however, may sometimes compress and invade intra-abdominal vessels and other structures and are a cause of significant morbidity and sometimes mortality.[53]

Turcot's syndrome refers to intestinal polyposis in combination with brain tumors.[4] Some families with Turcot's syndrome exhibit colonic polyposis typical of FAP, whereas others have fewer, larger polyps. Autosomal dominant transmission is apparent in most kindreds, although recessive inheritance is suggested in some. The brain tumors of

Turcot's syndrome are mostly gliomas and normally occur in the first or second decade of life.

AAPC is an attenuated form of FAP that has been recognized in a number of families.[17] Affected patients have a high risk of colon cancer but have fewer colonic polyps. These polyps are distributed more proximally in the colon than they are in typical FAP. The average age of cancer diagnosis is 54 years.

Eighty per cent of FAP families have a different and distinct mutation of the APC gene, usually causing a truncation in the protein. Although Gardner's syndrome also arises from mutation in the APC gene, it is not clear how such mutations cause the particular phenotype exhibited by patients with this variant syndrome. Some relationship between the location of mutations in the APC gene and phenotype has been observed. One study suggested that a higher density of colonic polyps follows from mutations near the center portion of the APC gene. AAPC arises from mutations in the extreme proximal end of the APC gene. Families with congenital hypertrophy of the retinal pigment epithelium consistently have mutations distant to exon 9 of the gene.

Genetic testing can now be used to diagnose FAP and its variants.[54] DNA markers are sufficiently accurate to diagnosis more than 95% of people at risk for FAP, usually with greater than 99% accuracy. The problem with this method, called *linkage testing,* is that at least two people in a family must already have a firm clinical diagnosis of FAP for additional members to be tested. A newly developed genetic method identifies truncated APC protein fragments and successfully detects 87% of people with APC mutations. This method is advantageous in that it can be applied to those without knowledge of whether other family members have the disease.

Present screening recommendations for FAP include flexible sigmoidoscopy every 1 to 2 years, beginning at 10 to 12 years of age in those at risk for the disease. Genetic testing should be performed at the same age. Those who have negative results by genetic testing should probably undergo occasional sigmoidoscopy until more longitudinal experience is gained. Those who test positive should have periodic sigmoid screening until adenomas enlarge and an appropriately timed colectomy is planned. Upper gastrointestinal screening with endoscopy should be performed every 1 to 3 years once colonic polyposis develops.

The management of the polyposis syndromes is different than the management of sporadic polyps because the familial syndromes may be associated with hundreds or thousands of colonic polyps that are premalignant. Total colectomy with ileostomy eliminates the risk of malignancy, but a consequent creation of a permanent abdominal stoma and loss of rectal continence make this procedure unacceptable to many patients. Total abdominal colectomy leaving the rectal mucosa at risk for polyps and malignant degeneration mandates continued endoscopic surveillance of the retained rectum. Unfortunately, even though residual rectal polyps may regress transiently, the risk of malignancy is not eliminated. In the management of premalignant polyposis syndromes and ulcerative colitis, resection of the rectal mucosa is required if the procedure is to be considered curative.

Until recently, total proctocolectomy with Brooke ileostomy was the procedure of choice, but there are several alternatives, including abdominal colectomy with ileorectal anastomosis. Because a segment of rectum with its mucosa is retained, the risk for carcinoma of the colon remains, and the patient must be followed closely by proctoscopy and digital examination. Another alternative is proctocolectomy with creation of a continent ileostomy. The continent ileostomy or Kock pouch involves creation of an intestinal reservoir composed of ileum with an ileal conduit leading to a cutaneous stoma. Intussusception of the terminal ileum into the pouch for 3 to 4 cm. further improves continence. Drainage of these pouches is accomplished by passing a tube through the valve into the pouch via the stoma.

In 1947 Ravitch and Sabiston described abdominal colectomy, mucosal proctectomy, and ileoanal pull-through and anastomosis, which in a modified form has become a commonly used procedure.[52] After abdominal colectomy, the rectal mucosa is circumferentially dissected from the rectal muscle and anal sphincter. An ileal reservoir is then created by folding the ileum on itself and, with a stapling device, eliminating the common wall of the folded segments. The terminal ileum is then anastomosed to the dentate line of the anus.

The use of nonsteroidal anti-inflammatory drugs (NSAIDs) such as sulindac has been advocated to reduce the risk of polyps in patients with FAP.[64] Sulindac may cause regression of rectal and colonic polyps and related symptoms, but it is not clear that it reduces the risk of colorectal carcinoma in patients with FAP.[64]

Hereditary Nonpolyposis Colorectal Cancer. HNPCC includes site-specific colorectal cancer and cancer family syndrome, which are synonymous with Lynch syndrome I and II, respectively.[36] Autosomal dominant inheritance of colorectal cancer is observed in both syndromes; the average patient age at cancer diagnosis is 45 years. People with HNPCC have a high occurrence of synchronous and proximal colonic malignancies. Those affected usually show one or several adenomatous polyps. The polyps on average are larger, have more villous histology, and occur at a younger age than adenomas in the general population. Cancer family syndrome also includes other malignancies, especially endometrial, but also ovarian, gastric, small intestinal, or renal cancer.

In most of the HNPCC families studied genetically, the disease results from inherited mutations of *mismatch repair genes* (also called *mutator genes*).[21, 33, 34, 45, 48] It was known that a gene responsible for HNPCC lay on chromosome 2 (from genetic mapping studies with chromosome 2 DNA markers) and that the DNA in tumors from these patients had widespread alterations in short tandem repeats (STRs). This finding suggested that a candidate gene for this disorder might be involved in DNA mismatch repair, or *genetic proofreading,* because a similar instability of STRs was observed in mismatch repair-defective bacteria and yeast mutants.

The clinical criteria for HNPCC are the following: (1) three family members should have colon cancer, two of whom should be first-degree relatives of the other; (2) at least two successive generations should be affected; and (3) one relative should have a diagnosis of colon cancer when younger than 50 years of age. Genetic testing for HNPCC currently includes analysis of hMSH2, hMLH1, hPMS1, and hPMH2 genes in peripheral blood leukocytes. Clinical screening of affected family members includes full colonoscopy every 2 to 3 years, beginning either at age 25 or when the family member in question is 5 years younger than the person with the earliest colonic cancer diagnosis in the family. Periodic screening for other cancers, especially uterine by endometrial biopsy and pelvic ultrasonography, should also be performed.

In patients with previous colorectal cancer, the probability of developing a second or metachronous lesion is approximately three times higher than that in the general population. When colonic polyps are found in a specimen resected for primary colorectal cancer, the risk may be as high as six times the expected development. If the initial tumor was in the cecum, the likelihood of developing a second primary colon cancer is greatest. Metachronous lesions vary in incidence from 1.9% in patients with colonic cancer to a high of

5% after 25 years. The average elapsed time for development of a metachronous lesion is approximately 13.5 years.[26]

Adenomatous Polyps

Colorectal adenomas tend to grow slowly and continuously, and a polyp may take 10 years to double in size. Adenomas may be sessile (flat) or pedunculated (long stalked). Although polyps may cause symptoms related to blood loss from an ulcerated surface, they are most frequently occult and are detected by barium enema, proctosigmoidoscopy, or colonoscopy. Adenomas may rarely cause hemorrhage or diarrhea, although villous adenomas may sometimes produce a mucoid diarrhea with resultant hypokalemic alkalosis. Villous adenomas may also produce an excessive secretion of mucus with loss of protein, which rarely causes hypoalbuminemia. Very large polyps may cause abdominal pain from partial intestinal obstruction or may be the lead point in colonic intussusception in an adult.

Treatment. It is essential that the entire colon be examined because adenomas are often multiple. Removal of all colorectal polyps is recommended.[9] Pedunculated polyps may be excised by endoscopic snare cautery. Fractionated excision of sessile adenomas is discouraged because the removed fragments are difficult for the pathologist to orient properly.

Careful histopathologic assessment of all excised adenomas is mandatory for proper management of patients. It is necessary to resect and retrieve all polyps and to submit the tissue for examination promptly. Carcinomas occurring in adenomas are usually well differentiated and occur most commonly at the tip of the adenoma. If there is no invasion, these represent *in situ* carcinomas that rarely metastasize and are adequately treated by polypectomy. In some cases, cancers in adenomas may invade the muscularis mucosa and potentially invade lymphatics and metastasize. Therefore, if the lesion has penetrated the muscularis mucosa and invaded lymphatics, if the cancer is poorly differentiated, or if it extends to the margin of the excision, then segmental resection as used routinely for the treatment of adenocarcinoma of the colon is indicated.

With large polyps that have a high risk of malignant change, such as a large villous adenoma, a segmental colectomy is often indicated. Villous adenomas have a marked predilection for malignant degeneration, and complete excision is required.

Follow-up. Following endoscopic polypectomy, the patient should have routine colonoscopic surveillance to detect new or additional lesions, since about 40% of patients will have another adenoma at follow-up. Many endoscopists perform a follow-up colonoscopy 6 months to 1 year after polypectomy.[9]

Other Colonic Neoplasms

A variety of submucosal lesions that occur throughout the colon and rectum includes lipomas, fibromas, leiomyomas, and carcinoids. Many are asymptomatic, but problems do occur, including blood loss secondary to ulceration and intestinal obstruction. Angiodysplasia or arteriovenous malformations may occur anywhere in the gastrointestinal tract. The most frequently encountered subset is an acquired lesion that tends to localize in the right colon. These malformations are believed to develop secondary to altered vascular dynamics in the bowel wall. They occur primarily in older patients, and there may also be an increased incidence in patients with aortic valvular disease and chronic renal failure. Angiodysplasias may cause chronic blood loss with anemia or acute hemorrhage; they are the second leading cause of lower gastrointestinal hemorrhage in adults. Diagnosis of these le-

sions may be difficult, with angiography or endoscopy being most useful. When identified, endoscopic coagulation or laser photoablation may be effective. Segmental resection is reserved for failure of endoscopic therapy, particularly in the presence of ongoing hemorrhage when definitive localization has been accomplished.

Gastrointestinal hemangiomas are less common than angiodysplasia and are most often of the cavernous type. They may be associated with similar lesions in the central nervous system or other organs. Because of their vascularity, endoscopic coagulation should not be attempted. Segmental resection is the definitive treatment.

Kaposi's sarcoma is a neoplastic lesion associated with acquired immunodeficiency syndrome. Half of these lesions occur in the gastrointestinal tract, with most in the duodenum. Treatment is resection for symptomatic relief.

COLORECTAL MALIGNANCIES

Although much has been learned about colorectal malignancies at the molecular level, the management of patients continues to rely on surgical principles of *en bloc* resection of malignant lesions, although advances in surgical technique and in multimodality therapy provide promise for improving the morbidity of therapy and perhaps the outcome.[8, 37, 57]

Incidence

More than 152,000 new cases of colon or rectal cancer occur annually in the United States, making it the second most frequent cancer in men and women, and more than 57,000 patients die each year from colorectal cancer. Carcinoma of the colon and rectum is generally a disease of older people, with equal incidence in males and females. In the general population, the incidence of colon cancer begins to rise significantly after the age of 40 to 45 years and increases each decade thereafter until it peaks at age 75. The probability of developing colorectal cancer from birth to age 70 is 4%.

Twice as many cancers arise in the colon than in the rectum. The incidence of colon cancer has risen among blacks, with the black and white male adjusted incidence being equal. Among white and black females, age-adjusted incidence rates are approximately equal. Mortality rates parallel the incidence rates. Mortality from colon cancer has decreased slightly among white females but has risen among other population groups. Mortality from rectal cancer has declined slightly in all groups.

Cancer Prevention

As discussed previously, several genetic factors are associated with an increase in the incidence of colorectal malignancies, including inherited polyposis and nonpolyposis syndromes,[19] but there are other conditions that predispose to colorectal carcinoma such as ulcerative colitis. The incidence of colon cancer is 5 to 10 times higher in patients with colitis than in the general population, increasing about 10 years after the onset of the disease, and is estimated to be about 20% to 30% at 20 years. High-risk groups include those with the onset of disease before 25 years of age and those with pancolitis and unremitting disease. Since all available screening tests are problematic, most patients with this unusually high risk of colon cancer probably benefit at some point from prophylactic colectomy. When ileoproctectomy is performed preserving the distal rectum and anus, a worrisome incidence of carcinoma is still observed. Proctocolectomy with a Brooke ileostomy or abdominal colectomy with mucosal proctectomy and ileoanal reconnection with a reservoir procedure is useful. Granulomatous colitis is also generally associated with a higher risk of colon cancer, especially if onset is before 21 years of age.

Other well-known conditions that predispose to colon and rectal cancer include the formation of a ureterosigmoidostomy. A 5% to 10% incidence of colon cancer has been found as long as 15 to 20 years after this procedure is performed to correct congenital exstrophy of the bladder. Tumors characteristically develop distal to the ureteral implant at the site at which the mucosa is exposed to urine and feces. Recognition of this complication has led to the use of alternative urinary conduits in the modern management of urologic reconstruction.

Although much has been learned about the development of colon cancer from inherited forms of cancer, most colon cancer cases are considered sporadic. Nonetheless, population studies have consistently demonstrated a twofold to threefold increased risk of colorectal cancer in first-degree relatives of persons with so-called sporadic colon cancer. The number of colon cancer cases in a family and the age at cancer diagnosis can be used clinically to stratify the severity of familial risk in common or sporadic cases of large bowel cancer. Those with two first-degree relatives with colorectal cancer have at least twice the risk of developing large bowel cancer compared with people with a single affected first-degree relative. The risk of colorectal cancer for first-degree relatives is twice that of the general population if the index case has large bowel cancer diagnosed at 55 years of age or older. The risk is triple that of the general population if the cancer is diagnosed between the ages of 45 and 55 and quadruple that of the general population if the diagnosis is made before the age of 45. Other clinical features that confer familial risk to a lesser degree include adenomatous polyps in first-degree relatives and colorectal cancer in more distant relatives. All colonic sites of tumors are associated with familial risk, although the rectum is implicated to a lesser degree.

All first-degree relatives of those with colorectal cancer should undergo standard large bowel cancer screening. This includes yearly fecal occult blood testing and sigmoidoscopy every 3 to 5 years. Both tests should be initiated between the ages of 35 and 40 because of the higher risk and thus improved predictive value in this setting. Colonoscopy is an alternative approach that is indicated especially if the index case was diagnosed at younger than 55 years of age or if two first-degree relatives have colon cancer. If three or more relatives have been diagnosed with colorectal cancer, HNPCC and FAP should be excluded. Adenomas in first-degree relatives and colorectal cancer in second- and third-degree relatives would indicate that standard screening should also be encouraged.

Population Screening

Because the morbidity and mortality associated with colorectal cancer are so significant in the United States, strategies for early diagnosis of polyps or cancer in the general population are considered attractive cancer prevention measures.[68] Screening tests of asymptomatic patients include digital rectal examination, routine stool guaiac testing, proctosigmoidoscopy, or pancolonoscopy and barium enema with air contrast studies. Rules for screening are empiric or dependent on data derived from statistical models. Major studies attempting to determine the benefit of screening large populations for occult blood in the stool have led to mixed results. Application of statistical methods to non-high-risk people has shown that the most cost-effective application of occult blood testing and either colonoscopy or air contrast barium enema begins at age 40, and, if nothing is found, should be repeated every 5 years.

At present serum carcinoembryonic antigen (CEA) as well as other experimental serologic tumor markers is ineffective for cancer screening since no marker is tumor specific. The detection of neoplastic cells or of DNA encoding for activated oncogenes in the stool of patients is theoretically possible, and the feasibility of these approaches has been demonstrated. Unfortunately, the practical application of these strategies remains unproven.

Prevention

Recent data regarding the pathogenesis of colorectal cancer at the molecular level have provided a greater understanding of the biology of these neoplasms. They provide possible explanations of the influence of diet and changes in the bowel microenvironment that lead to genetic changes required for malignant transformation.

A number of environmental risk factors have been suggested to be related to the development of colorectal carcinoma. This is inferred from studies of those who emigrate from an area of low incidence, such as Japan, to an area of higher incidence, such as the United States. These groups have a likelihood of developing colorectal cancer similar to that of the population of the new country, suggesting environmental and dietary influences. Dietary factors associated with a higher incidence of colorectal carcinoma include those with low dietary fiber and high dietary fat and sugar intake. In industrialized countries, including the United States and those of Western Europe, large amounts of animal fat, protein, and refined carbohydrates are consumed. In these geographic areas the incidence of colorectal cancer is much higher than in the developing countries of Africa, South America (excluding Argentina and Uruguay, where meat consumption is high), and Japan, where considerably less meat is consumed and the diet is significantly higher in vegetable fiber. Specifically, the death rate from colon carcinoma in the United States is approximately 17 per 100,000 population but is as high as 24 per 100,000 in New Zealand and as low as 3 per 100,000 in Mexico. These variations are not believed to be due to genetic differences, primarily because certain immigrant groups tend to assume the colon cancer incidence rates of their adopted countries. For example, in a study comparing Japanese immigrants to Hawaii with second-generation Japanese immigrants already resident, a higher incidence of large bowel cancer was found in those who discontinued the practice of eating at least one Japanese-style meal daily. The increased consumption of meat is the major dietary difference between residents of Japan and Hawaii, and such an increase in beef consumption paralleled the higher risk of bowel cancer among Japanese immigrants. A correlation between the daily consumption of meat and the incidence of large bowel cancer also has been noted in people from many countries, suggesting an etiologic role.

A recent study of the association between dietary factors and the incidence and recurrence of colorectal adenomatous polyps demonstrated the expected relationship between dietary fat intake and recurrent adenoma.[44] Among women, recurrent polyps showed an association with total dietary fat (odds ratio 3.8) and total fiber (odds ratio 0.2). No consistent relationship was observed with men, although an increase in caloric intake increased the risk for incidence and recurrence in both men and women.

In patients who have developed polyps, endoscopic polypectomy has been believed to prevent the development of colorectal carcinoma. This assumption is supported by recent results reported from the National Polyp Study. The National Polyp Study Workgroup studied 1418 patients who had a complete colonoscopy, during which one or more adenomas of the colon or rectum was removed. The patients subsequently underwent periodic colonoscopy during an average follow-up of 5.9 years. Five asymptomatic early-stage cancers were detected by colonoscopy, and no symptomatic cancers were detected. The numbers of colorectal cancers expected in this age group were then compared, and it was noted that colonoscopic polypectomy had led to a reduction in the incidence of colorectal carcinoma of between 76% and 90%. These results have supported the view that adenomas progress to adenocarcinomas, as well as the current practice of searching for and removing adenomatous polyps to prevent colorectal carcinoma.[43, 69]

In addition to colonoscopy and polypectomy, other strategies have been advocated for the prevention of colorectal carcinoma. Obviously, prophylactic colectomy has a role in patients with some of the polyposis syndromes and in some cases of ulcerative colitis; however, other nonsurgical forms of cancer prevention should also be considered. Since investigators showed that the sulindac could decrease adenomas in colon polyposis syndromes, there have been a series of reports showing that NSAIDs, including aspirin, reduce all forms of neoplasms of the colon and rectum. In a study of aspirin use to evaluate the risk of colorectal carcinoma and adenoma in male health professionals,[51] 529 male health professionals between 40 and 75 years of age were enrolled in a study comparing the use of aspirin with other variables, including smoking, weight, and family history.[23] There was a steady decrease in the relative risk of developing a malignancy among the patients who took aspirin at least twice a week. When this level of intake was maintained over the 6-year period of the study, the relative risk of developing a malignancy decreased to 0.38. During the final 2 years of the study, 42 new cases of colorectal carcinoma were found among the nonaspirin users, compared with 20 from the aspirin group.

Clinical Features

The clinical features of colorectal carcinomas are related to the tumor size and location. Seventy to 80% of these lesions are located below the mid-descending colon. Tumors in this location are often infiltrating or annular and may cause obstructive symptoms, changes in bowel habits, or bleeding. Because of the semisolid or solid contents and the small diameter in this location, gas pains, a decrease in caliber of the stool, and the use of laxatives are common symptoms. In the right colon, large bulky tumors are more common, owing perhaps to the wide diameter of the colon and its liquid contents, which allow growth into the lumen without symptoms of obstruction. Patients may complain of abdominal pain that may be confused with gallbladder or peptic ulcer disease or may have bleeding, weight loss, or anemia.

Diagnosis

The diagnosis of colorectal carcinomas requires a high index of suspicion and evaluation of all symptoms, especially in high-risk patients. Tests for fecal blood are usually accomplished using Hemoccult guaiac-impregnated paper. Proctosigmoidoscopy is an important diagnostic test in the symptomatic patient, and flexible instruments have much better patient tolerance and a marked increase in diagnostic accuracy. Colonoscopy is frequently used to evaluate all patients with symptoms or occult fecal blood, since lesions can be detected and excised and biopsy specimens can be obtained. Limitations include failure to evaluate the splenic or hepatic flexure or cecum. However, these technical considerations depend on having a well-trained endoscopist perform the procedure. Barium enema with air contrast is complementary to colonoscopy and usually detects all colonic lesions at least

5 mm. in diameter. Contraindications include acute, severe inflammatory bowel disease, suspected perforation, and recent injury to the bowel wall. The entire colon must be evaluated for synchronous lesions when a tumor is found. Complete blood count, blood chemistries, chest films, liver function studies, urinalysis, and CEA titer are routinely obtained preoperatively. If symptoms are present or if results of the blood tests suggest further studies, they should be obtained, including abdominal computed tomographic scan, magnetic resonance imaging, or intravenous pyelogram.

The diagnostic value of conventional transabdominal ultrasonograpy is limited because of the numerous artifacts caused by gas-filled bowel; however, some trials with hydrocolonic sonography have shown accuracy rates as high as 97% in the detection of colorectal carcinomas.[13] A recent possibility of preoperative staging of colonic tumors is endoscopic ultrasonography of the large bowel, which provides an intraluminal ultrasonographic evaluation of the colorectal diseases. This method may be important in the future for the planning of minimal invasive surgical procedures since it may provide better staging criteria to select cases of colonic carcinoma suitable for laparoscopic resection.[29, 63]

Treatment

The true pathologic extent of disease can be determined only after resection and examination of the specimen with staging. Carcinoma of the colon and rectum extends by six routes: intramucosal extension, direct invasion of adjacent structures, lymphatic spread, hematogenous spread, intraperitoneal spread, and anastomotic implantation. The modes and routes of spread must be considered in deciding on the appropriate surgical extirpation to provide the highest cure rate and to appropriately stage the patient.

Therefore, any modern surgical approach to colorectal cancer must consider margins of resection and the *en bloc* resection of the draining lymphatic tissue. In addition, alternative routes of tumor spread must be considered, including neural, venous, peritoneal implantation, and direct extension. Consequently, resection of the primary tumor must include adequate margins of normal tissue, the adherent lymph node compartment, and delimiting fascia, notably Waldeyer's fascia in the presacral space or the plane behind the seminal vesicles, but it can also include Gerota's fascia of the kidney.

Almost 90% of patients have tumors that can be resected completely, and the mortality rate ranges from 2% to 10%. The critical determinant of success is the degree to which the tumor has spread at the time of operation. Inadequate resection close to the macroscopic tumor border, tumor inoculation into the anastomotic region, and spread of tumor cells within the operative field are examples of common technical maneuvers that produce suboptimal outcomes. In addition to adequate margins and *en bloc* resection of draining lymphatics, important principles of surgical resection include restoration of continuity of the intestine and maintenance of function, whenever possible, with minimal morbidity and mortality.

The exact surgical procedure for a particular carcinoma is therefore dependent on the location of the tumor. Selection for the appropriate surgical procedure is influenced by the degree of local tumor invasion, tumor mobility, accessibility, size, and presence of involved lymph nodes, particularly the mesorectal lymph nodes associated with rectal carcinomas. Although colonoscopy or barium enema may be sufficient localizing procedures for colon cancer, careful digital examination and sigmoidoscopy are critical in the evaluation of rectal tumors to determine tumor level, mobility, size, and intraluminal appearance. Unfortunately, the depth of invasion and lymph node involvement cannot be accurately assessed.[16]

Endorectal ultrasound (EUS) can be used to correctly assess the depth of invasion in about 90% of rectal tumors.[24] The accuracy of EUS for the detection of large stage T3 and T4 tumors is very high, making the correct identification of these patients likely. This assessment may be necessary to allow some patients to be treated preoperatively with neoadjuvant forms of therapy. Reports on the effectiveness of EUS in the detection of perirectal lymph nodes show accuracy rates of 73% to 80%. The main difficulty in staging lymph nodes by EUS is the existence of so-called transitional forms in which the echo structure cannot clearly be assessed as hypoechoic or hyperechoic. Advances in image analysis and computer-based systems to aid in the evaluation of these transitional forms are needed.

Preoperatively, patients should undergo bowel preparation and be psychologically prepared if either a temporary or permanent colostomy is anticipated. They also should be counseled about postoperative sexual dysfunction if extensive pelvic dissection is anticipated. Wide margins surrounding the primary tumor must be removed with an *en bloc* resection of the draining lymphatics. The necessity to remove the draining lymphatics requires interruption of the blood supply to a region of the colon as the lymphatic drainage parallels the blood supply.

Employing the principles just described, the standard treatment of neoplasms of the cecum and ascending colon is right colectomy, which includes a segment of the terminal ileum, the cecum, and the right half of the transverse colon and removal of the corresponding mesocolon and a space around the superior mesenteric artery at the origin of the middle colic vessels. Carcinomas of the splenic flexure or descending colon are treated by excision of the distal transverse, descending, and sigmoid colon, together with the associated mesocolon excised to the aorta. For tumors of the sigmoid colon, the proximal resection can be limited, and the transverse colon need not necessarily be removed. For carcinomas in the upper rectum, an anterior resection and reanastomosis can be performed; however, preservation of the distal rectum to provide continence is extremely important.

For tumors involving the upper rectum, a low anterior colon resection may be performed with a distal margin of 2 inches or 5 cm. as shown in Figure 32–41. Distal intramural spread of cancer is usually restricted, and a 5-cm. segment

of normal colon or rectum is adequate as a resection margin. Although lymphatic spread may occur downward, it has been shown that upward and lateral displacement through superior hemorrhoidal and inferior mesenteric lymphatics is by far the most important type of spread. Therefore, the decision to perform an *abdominoperineal resection* (APR) or a *low anterior resection* (LAR) is determined primarily by the distance of the lower border of the cancer from the anus. The lateral pelvic extension of the two operations, both of which remove the upper lymphatic drainage areas, is essentially the same.

In general, tumors within 7 to 8 cm. of the anal verge are treated by APR, whereas those more than 12 cm. from the anal verge are adequately managed by LAR. Lesions lying between 7 and 11 cm. from the anal verge may be managed by either procedure, depending on the size of the lesion, the size of the pelvis, and the differentiation of the tumor.[50] In general, a lesion that is easily palpated with the examining finger is often removed by APR. However, if the neoplasm can be delivered to the level of the abdominal incision following mobilization of the rectum, an adequate resection may be performed. The use of circumferential stapling devices greatly facilitates the construction of the LAR.

In many series, there is no difference in operative mortality between the two approaches, with a slightly superior survival rate in patients having anterior resections, although it is probably related to the smaller tumor size in those having anterior resections. Local recurrence rates have ranged from 7% to 20% for patients with LAR and APR.[71]

New combined-treatment modalities have made it possible to perform sphincter-sparing operations for rectal carcinomas that would have previously been managed by APR. These modalities include preoperative radiation therapy combined with chemotherapy. The response of the tumor mass may allow previously unresectable lesions to be removed and may permit LAR rather than an APR to be performed. Long-term follow-up studies demonstrating an improvement in survival have not yet been performed, but short-term results suggest that a decrease in the local recurrence rate may be achieved by neoadjuvant therapy in selected patients.

As an alternative to both LAR or APR, local excision has been advocated by some in patients with small, well-differentiated lesions limited to the mucosa (T1 lesions).[3, 25] In patients with compromised cardiovascular status or other comorbid conditions, selective local therapy may be considered in lesions with favorable characteristics. Although a number of techniques have been described for improving the results of surgical excision and preserving the sphincter in these patients, data are sparse concerning their true efficacy. Neoadjuvant therapy, including preoperative chemotherapy and preoperative radiation therapy, is being evaluated to determine its role in carcinoma of the rectum.[25, 38]

Laparoscopically Assisted Procedures for Colon Cancer. The rapid acceptance of laparoscopic cholecystectomy began a new era in abdominal surgery, as minimally invasive techniques were rapidly applied to benign disorders such as hernia, appendicitis, and reflux esophagitis.[58] Not surprisingly, the success of laparoscopic procedures for many benign abdominal disorders led to the application of laparoscopic or laparoscopically assisted procedures for malignant diseases of the intestinal tract, specifically palliative and curative operations on the colon.

Laparoscopic colectomy is usually performed by using the laparoscopic instruments to mobilize the colon and prepare the mesentery for resection. Since an incision is necessary to remove the specimen, and it must be large enough to extract the colon and mesentery, most surgeons perform the anastomosis used for specimen retrieval through the incision. The actual resection of the colon can often be performed extracor-

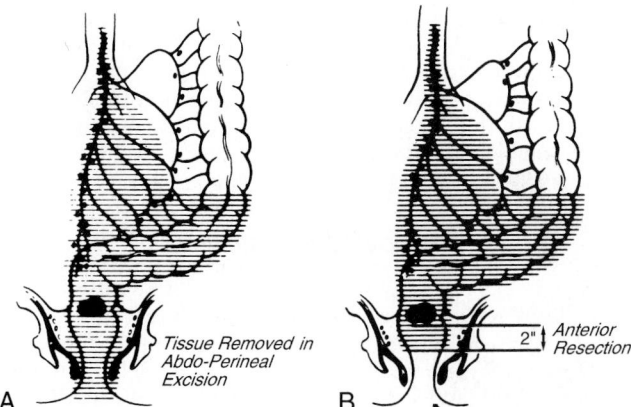

Figure 32–41. The shaded area shows the extent of removal for carcinoma of the upper rectum by abdominal perineal resection *(A)* and by anterior resection *(B)*. Note the necessity for a 2-inch or 5-cm. margin to the lesion in an anterior resection. If this cannot be accomplished, an abdominoperineal resection of the rectum should be performed. (From Butcher, H. R., Jr.: Carcinoma of the rectum: Choice between anterior resection and abdominoperineal resection of the rectum. CANCER, Vol. 28, Jul, 1971, pp. 204–207. Copyright ©1971 American Cancer Society. Reprinted by permission of Wiley-Liss, Inc., a subsidiary of John Wiley & Sons, Inc.)

poreally as well. The colon can be resected and an anastomosis performed using staplers or by resecting and hand sewing an anastomosis as one would an open anastomosis—either an ileocolostomy or a colocolostomy. The anastomosed bowel is then returned into the abdominal cavity and inspected laparoscopically. Mesenteric defects are usually closed laparoscopically.

Several recent reports about the feasibility and safety of laparoscopic and laparoscopically assisted colectomy for malignant disease have emerged. However, issues such as compromised cancer control and complications appeared in discussions of the role of laparoscopic surgery in curative resections. Cancer control issues include the extent of lymphadenectomy, the implantation of malignant cells in the wound, the adequacy of intraperitoneal staging, and the no-touch technique.[47] A limitation of laparoscopic colectomy is the inability to palpate the liver. There is a lack of tactile sensation during a laparoscopic procedure that may limit the surgeon's ability to stage the disease adequately. However, it is not known whether such a discovery of extensive metastatic disease has a significant impact on cancer control and patient survival.

Another major concern of laparoscopic colectomy is whether the lymphadenectomy is equivalent to that achieved by open colectomy.[30] Investigators have found that an equal number of lymph nodes are harvested via both laparoscopic and open colectomies. Furthermore, node sampling and mesenteric resection may be related but may not have a major impact on survival. In a randomized study of segmental colectomy versus radical colectomy for descending colon cancer, no difference in survival was noted. For colon tumors, lymph node metastasis may not be governors but rather indicators of survival.

Another concern is tumor implantation either at the port site or specimen retrieval wound site. Implantation of carcinoma after laparoscopic colectomy has been noted in the literature. The true incidence of this complication is unknown, since the total number of laparoscopic colectomies performed without implantation is unknown. Nonetheless, techniques to reduce this occurrence have been promoted, including avoidance of grasping the colonic wall with an instrument near the tumor to avoid shedding tumor cells, using a specimen extraction site large enough to avoid squeezing the specimen through a small opening, and using a plastic protective shield at the site of wound extraction.

The potential of laparoscopic colectomy to reduce the morbidity of operations for colon cancer may be great, if reduced postoperative pain and ileus result. Many questions regarding the potential benefits and pitfalls of this technique await the results of large multi-institutional studies that randomize patients between open and laparoscopic colectomy. Current procedures for staging and palliation appear warranted.[35]

Complicated Colon Cancers

Complete intestinal obstruction occurs in 8% to 23% of patients with colorectal cancer and usually presents with abdominal pain.[55] Patients with obstructing cancers have a generally poor prognosis, with an overall mortality rate of 15% and a higher postoperative complication rate. The high perioperative mortality rate is probably because of the inability to perform an adequate bowel preparation, as the patients who survive operation compare with patient survival following elective colon resection. The most critical determinant of long-term survival after a successful emergency operation is the pathologic stage of the lesion.

Colonic perforation tends to increase operative and perioperative morbidity and mortality and decrease long-term survival. Operative mortality rates of higher than 30% with 5-year survival rates of less than 10% have been reported. This may be related to peritoneal seeding of colon cancer cells following perforation. Surgical management of acute obstruction or perforation due to carcinoma of the colon depends on the judgment and experience of the surgeon, who must consider the dilation and viability of the bowel, the physical status of the patient with associated comorbidities, and the degree of contamination. Usually a resection of the primary carcinoma can be accomplished with a proximal diverting colostomy. Resection is preferable if more than minimal survival is expected, because a large fungating cancer may bleed and possibly require more invasive intervention.

Direct extension of colon and rectal cancer to adjacent organs necessitates *en bloc* resection of these organs, because the adhesions usually contain tumor cells. Although the number of patients with extended surgical procedures for colon cancer is relatively small, several features should be considered when extensive lesions are encountered. It has been established that the size of the primary lesion is not a determinant of regional metastases. Thus, finding a direct extension of a cancer into an adjacent organ statistically is not a more adverse prognostic sign than regional lymph node metastasis. In fact, advanced colorectal tumors that have invaded other organs but have not metastasized to the lymph nodes may have favorable biologic characteristics. A series of patients with extended resections that usually include colectomy and partial or total excision of an invaded organ has been reported, thus favoring an aggressive approach to locally advanced disease. The response of the tumor to preoperative radiation therapy may allow tumors fixed to adjacent bony structures to be resected.

Bilateral oophorectomy is recommended in all postmenopausal women with carcinoma of the colon to decrease the morbidity of neoplastic change. The procedure should be considered in all premenopausal women with ovarian abnormalities at operation or in the presence of peritoneal implants.

Pathologic Staging and Survival

The original pathologic staging system was developed by Dukes and was further modified by Astler and Collier in 1954. Most recently the TNM system has been recommended by the American Joint Committee on Cancer (Table 32–13). A number of new techniques are being applied to these tumors in the hope of obtaining better prognostic information.[1, 66]

Another method of viewing prognosis is by examining the patterns of failure of patients with colorectal carcinoma. August and coworkers have reviewed in detail the outcome of 100 patients with large bowel cancer seen at the National Cancer Institute.[2] Figure 32–42 summarizes the results of that analysis, which illustrates the fact that recurrent disease does not necessarily portend death from cancer.

Postoperative Follow-up

Colonoscopy or barium enema for imaging the entire colon is recommended in the postoperative period, usually within 2 to 3 months. Colonoscopy should be repeated annually for at least the first 4 years following the resection. Routine physical examination with complete blood count and liver function tests should be obtained every 3 months for 2 years, then every 6 months for 2 years, then annually.[62] A chest film should be obtained every 6 months for 3 years, then annually.

Recommendations for CEA level monitoring had generally been assessment every 3 months for 2 years, then every 4 months for 2 years, then annually. A recent analysis of CEA monitoring for detecting surgically curable recurrence of co-

TABLE 32–13. TNM Cancer Classification System

Primary Tumor (T)

Tx   Primary tumor cannot be assessed
T0   No evidence of primary tumor
Tis Carcinoma *in situ*
T1   Tumor invades submucosa
T2   Tumor invades muscularis propria
T3   Tumor invades through the muscularis propria into the subserosa or into nonperitonealized percolic or perirectal tissue
T4   Tumor perforates the visceral peritoneum or directly invades other organs or structures (including invasion of other segments of the colon across serosa)

Regional Lymph Node (N)

NX   Regional lymph nodes cannot be assessed
N0   No regional lymph node metastasis
N1   Metastasis to 1 to 3 pericolic or perirectal lymph nodes
N2   Metastasis to 4 or more pericolic or perirectal lymph nodes
N3   Metastasis to any lymph node along the course of a named vascular trunk

Distant Metastases (M)

MX   Presence of distant metastasis cannot be assessed
M0   No distant metastasis
M1   Distant metastasis

From Sabiston, D. C., Jr., and Lyerly, H. K.: Essentials of Surgery, 2nd ed. Philadelphia, W. B. Saunders, 1994, p. 355.

lon cancer was performed by collecting clinical data from a national surgical adjuvant trial in which CEA monitoring was elective.[40] Eighty-four per cent of 1216 patients had CEA monitoring, and 417 had recurrence, with 59% of patients having a preceding CEA level elevation. Sixteen of 600 patients without recurrence had a false-positive test result. Surgical exploration was performed in 115 patients with CEA elevations, and 47 recurrences, usually hepatic, were resected with curative intent. Thirty-eight patients with normal CEA concentrations and 23 patients not monitored also underwent such resections, usually for pulmonary or local recurrence. Of all CEA-monitored patients 2.3% are alive and disease free more than 1 year after salvage surgery. Of patients with

no CEA monitoring, 2% are alive and disease free more than 1 year after salvage surgery.

A recent analysis of the cost of patient follow-up after potentially curative colorectal cancer treatment analyzed the costs associated with 11 separate surveillance strategies.[67] Medicare-allowed charges varied widely for the 5 years of posttreatment follow-up, with variations of 28-fold among strategies. There was no indication that higher cost strategies increased survival or quality of life.

Operations for Metastatic Disease

Despite complete preoperative evaluation, the identification of metastatic disease at the time of laparotomy is not uncommon. Excision of the primary lesion is desirable, if only for prevention of obstruction in the future, even in the presence of widespread metastatic disease. If resection is not possible, proximal diverting colostomy is indicated. In patients with rectal lesions and tenesmus or bleeding, APR can be used as a palliative procedure.[65]

A single small hepatic metastatic lesion can be considered for resection at the time of treatment of the primary tumor. This can be accomplished with a wedge resection with minimal morbidity. The performance of a hepatic lobectomy concurrently with colon resection is not indicated. Identification of a single large hepatic metastasis should prompt a curative colon procedure to be followed by complete imaging studies and possible hepatic resection later. Although it seems likely that operative resection of metastatic disease would have minimal impact on long-term survival, many authors have demonstrated that the judicious application of resection for metastatic colon cancer can prolong life. In general, the metastases must be confined to one organ, and single lesions are associated with a better prognosis than multiple ones.

It is usually not necessary to perform formal anatomic liver resections to remove metastatic liver disease; however, a margin of uninvolved liver should be excised with the tumor. Patients with unresectable hepatic metastases have been treated with a number of modalities, including hepatic intra-arterial chemotherapy. However, because of toxicity and the inability to demonstrate a clear survival advantage from intra-arterial 5-fluorouracil (5-FU), this approach remains in-

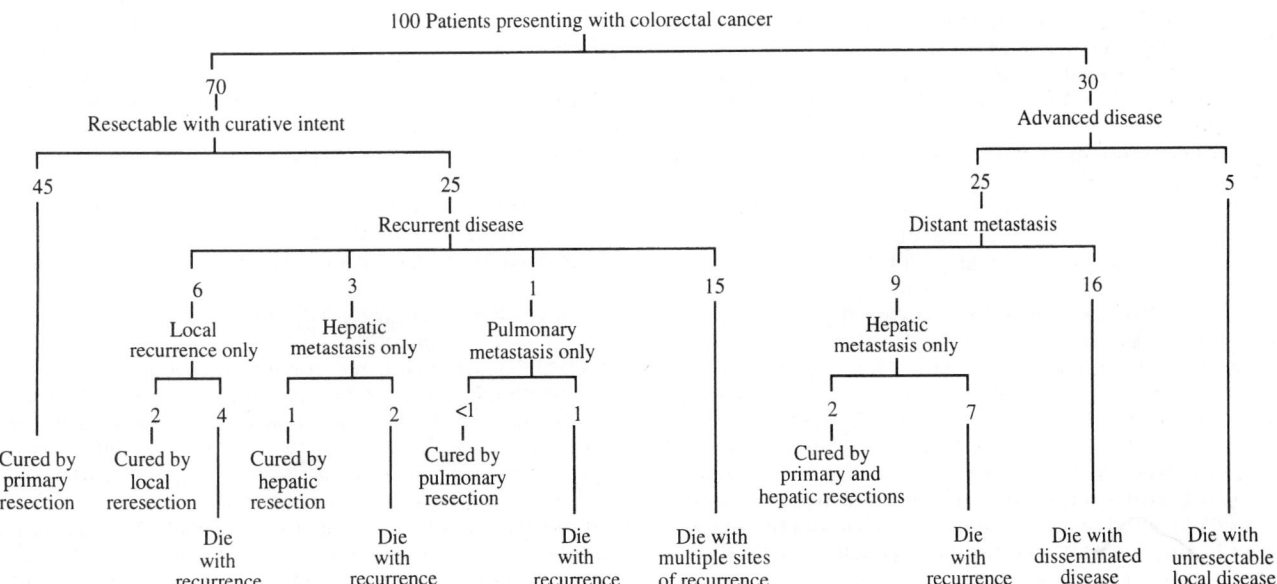

Figure 32–42. Outcomes of treated patients with colorectal cancer. The algorithm depicts the natural spectrum of treatment outcomes in 100 patients with colorectal carcinoma. Of 100 patients clinically presenting with colorectal cancer, 70 will have local disease, while 30 will have advanced disease. Of the 30 patients with advanced disease, 25 will have distant metastasis, and so forth.

vestigational. Other forms of therapy for hepatic metastases include cryotherapy for nonresectable lesions.

Isolated pulmonary metastases occur in less than 10% of patients with metastases, but 5-year relapse-free survivals have been reported following pulmonary resection confined to the lungs. Patients considered for these procedures must have no evidence of hepatic metastases, and often a laparoscopy is advocated prior to thoracotomy to examine the liver. If enteroabdominal disease is not present, a thoracotomy is indicated.

In the presence of multiple unresectable metastases, the management of the primary colon cancer consists of resection of the primary lesion. Although the survival is determined by the metastases, it has been demonstrated that those with primary resection have a more favorable course owing to the prevention of anemia, protein loss, obstruction, and pain. Anastomotic recurrences represent a major form of treatment failure and occur in 2% to 15% of all curative resections. Reexploration is necessary to determine resectability. Patients who develop local recurrence after LAR may need to undergo APR for local control.

Adjuvant Therapy

Both radiation therapy and chemotherapy have been used as adjuvant therapy following resection of colon cancer with a high risk of recurrence. The application of combination therapy seems appropriate both in patients with stage III colon cancer receiving surgical therapy plus chemotherapy and in patients with stage II and III rectal cancer most often receiving surgical treatment chemotherapy, and radiation therapy.[51, 60]

Adjuvant Systemic Therapy. Fifty to 60% of patients with colorectal cancer have tumors that penetrate the serosa or involve the regional lymph nodes. Most tumors in this category eventually recur and end fatally. Therefore, adjuvant therapy to improve the mortality was sought for this group of patients. The most active drug used against colon cancer is 5-FU, but it achieves only a 10% to 20% response in patients with advanced disease.[39, 41] *Levamisole* is believed to be an immunomodulating agent in advanced colorectal carcinoma. Randomized, controlled trials of 5-FU with levamisole, levamisole alone, and surgical resection in patients with Dukes B2 or C colon cancer were performed and demonstrated that levamisole plus 5-FU and levamisole alone improve disease-free survival for patients with Dukes B and C lesions. Subsequent analysis demonstrated that Dukes C patients receiving levamisole and 5-FU also had slightly prolonged survival.

A larger, confirmatory intergroup trial was launched demonstrating that in patients with Dukes C carcinomas of the colon, adjuvant treatment for 1 year with levamisole combined with 5-FU reduced the risk of cancer recurrence by 41%, with overall mortality reduced by 33%, but the results in patients with Dukes B2 disease were equivocal.

Current recommendations for adjuvant therapy are based on the efficacy of adjuvant therapy and the risk of treatment failure. Patients with stage I or Dukes A and B1 disease are at low risk of recurrence and should not receive adjuvant treatment. Optional adjuvant therapy for stage II and III colon cancer has been advised owing to the higher risk of recurrence. Based on the current clinical trial data, stage III or Dukes C patients unable to enter clinical trials should be offered adjuvant 5-FU and levamisole, as it was administered by the intergroup trial. The survival benefit is considered to be at least 25% to 30% compared with surgery alone. Specific adjuvant therapy for Dukes 2 or B2 patients has not been recommended by the National Institutes of Health outside clinical trials. However, ongoing and further trials are apt to modify these recommendations.

Adjuvant Liver Infusion Therapy. Since the liver is the predominant site of distal failure in colon cancer, eradication of micrometastases in the liver in the perioperative period is believed to be a reasonable approach to the treatment of colon cancer.[61] Studies have shown improved survival and decreased liver recurrence following portal vein infusion of 5-FU beginning within 5 days of operation. Other confirmatory trials have revealed a uniform lack of benefit in reducing liver recurrence. Adjuvant portal vein and hepatic artery infusion may be a complex way to deliver systemic therapy and is not recommended outside a clinical trial at this time.

Preoperative Radiation Therapy for Rectal Cancer. Because neither APR nor LAR resection eliminates local recurrence in the pelvis, especially in patients with stage III or Dukes C disease, investigators have attempted to add other treatments to improve local control of rectal cancer.[14] In theory, administration of preoperative radiation therapy has the advantage that undisturbed oxygenated tissues are more susceptible to ionizing irradiation than the vascular planes created by operation and treated with postoperative irradiation. Furthermore, more than two thirds of nodal metastases are smaller than 4 mm. in diameter and may be controlled by radiation therapy.

The results of preoperative radiation therapy include significant downstaging of regional disease. However, there has been no significant improvement in local control or survival in randomized trials of preoperative radiation therapy using relatively low doses to the tumor and pelvis. Therefore, higher doses of radiation therapy have been applied (40 to 50 Gy) with the performance of sphincter-saving operations for low and midrectal carcinomas with good results. Relatively few patients have undergone local excision after preoperative radiation therapy, possibly because healing in the irradiated field is poor.

Preoperative radiation therapy may decrease local recurrence; however, some authors believe that it may downstage the disease and hinder healing. Further clinical trials may resolve the usefulness of preoperative radiation therapy, and clinical trials are in progress to evaluate the role of radiation therapy combined with chemotherapy in the treatment of rectal carcinoma.

Postoperative Radiation Therapy for Rectal Cancer. Although the role of neoadjuvant therapy for rectal carcinoma is being investigated, radiation therapy should be part of the postoperative adjuvant therapy for rectal cancer that has penetrated the rectal wall or metastasized to regional nodes (stage II or III).[15] Postoperative radiation therapy combined with chemotherapy using 5-FU and methyl CCNU significantly decreases local recurrence in patients with stage II and III or Dukes B2 and C lesions in the rectum. This approach has produced a significant improvement in survival. Thus, the standard of practice for adenocarcinomas of the rectum that penetrate the rectal wall or involve regional lymph nodes is radical resection followed by chemotherapy and radiation therapy.

Limited Resection of Rectal Carcinoma. Although the role of combined therapy has been directed toward prolonging survival and reducing recurrences, preservation of organs and function is also considered a goal of cancer therapy. With this perspective, limited resection to preserve the anus and continence has been advocated. In the narrow confines of the pelvis, a local excision of a primary carcinoma with *en bloc* removal of mesorectal fat may have a lateral margin that is comparable with that of a standard radical resection. In patients who are carefully selected to minimize the chance of lymph node metastasis, it may be possible to locally excise rectal carcinomas and achieve cure rates similar to those of radical resection. With this policy, T1 and T2 low rectal cancers have been locally excised, with survival rates at 2 years comparable with those achieved with radical resection. Excision is usually performed by the transanal approach. However, other sphincter-preserving approaches may be used, including transsacral resection. Low resections with coloanal anastomosis are also used to preserve continence.[8]

An alternative to transanal approaches to rectal tumor is transanal endoscopic microsurgery, which was introduced in 1989. The procedure is performed through the rectoscope with a diameter of 4 cm. and length of 12 to 20 cm. The rectoscope is closed and equipped with an enlarging optic, which allows video imaging. The rectal cavity is visualized by carbon dioxide insufflation, and instrument channels allow for manipulation of the tumor. In carefully selected patients with low-risk T1 lesions, local excision consisting of full-thickness excision with partial removal of the perirectal fat can be performed.

Long-term follow-up to determine the role of these lesions is required. The roles of adjuvant chemotherapy and radiation therapy, along with local excision and sphincter-sparing operations, are being studied.

Squamous Cell Carcinoma of the Anus. Anal carcinoma is relatively uncommon, but squamous cell carcinoma comprises about 70% of all anal cancers. The most common treatment for these lesions has been surgical excision by APR, but the results have been disappointing, with 5-year survival rates of 24% to 62%. Combination therapy using radiation therapy and chemotherapy has improved the survival to as much as 83% and is now the treatment of choice for this tumor. Biopsy specimens of the area of the primary lesion are obtained, and the patient begins radiation therapy to the pelvis. If inguinal lymph nodes are enlarged, biopsy specimens of that tissue are also obtained, usually by fine-needle aspiration, and, if the findings are positive, the lymph nodes are included in the field of radiation.

Following radiation therapy, the patients receive intravenous 5-FU and mitomycin C. After treatment, a biopsy specimen of the lesion is obtained. If residual tumor is present, salvage radiation therapy and chemotherapy are given. A biopsy of the tumor site is again performed, and if the results are negative, no further treatment is given. If residual tumor is present, an APR is performed. If enlarged lymph nodes remain after treatment, a node dissection on the involved side is indicated.

Patients who fail therapy have limited options, including additional chemotherapy or radiation therapy. Salvage therapy may also include APR, lymphadenectomy, or a diverting colostomy, depending on the nature of the recurrence.

SELECTED REFERENCES

Bleday, R., and Wong, R. D.: Recent advances in surgery for colon and rectal cancer. Curr. Probl. Cancer, 17:1, 1993.
A comprehensive review of major surgical advances in the modern management of colorectal cancer. This volume is written by an authoritative group and is well illustrated and referenced.

Burt, R. W., DiSario, J. A., and Cannon-Albright, L.: Genetics of colon cancer: Impact of inheritance on colon cancer risk. Annu. Rev. Med., 46:371, 1995.
A brief, definitive, state-of-the-art review of the modern concepts of colon cancer genetics.

Moertel, C. G., Fleming, T. R., et al.: Fluorouracil plus levamisole as effective adjuvant therapy after resection of stage III colon cancer: A final report. Ann. Intern. Med., 122:321, 1995.
A landmark paper regarding the role of adjuvant chemotherapy for advanced colon cancer.

Muller, A. D., and Sonnenberg, A.: Prevention of colorectal cancer by flexible endoscopy and polypectomy. Ann. Intern. Med., 123:904, 1995.
A landmark paper describing results from the National Polyp Study Workgroup, in which the incidence of colon and rectal cancer is reduced by therapeutic polypectomy.

Rustgi, A. K.: Hereditary gastrointestinal polyposis and nonpolyposis syndromes. N. Engl. J. Med., 331:1694, 1994.
A comprehensive review of polyposis and nonpolyposis syndromes. This review also provides specific guidelines regarding the clinical management of suspected inherited syndromes, with an overview of available clinical and genetic testing.

Moerel, C. G., et al.: An evaluation of the carcinoembryonic antigen (CEA) test for monitoring patients with resected colon cancer. JAMA, 270:943, 1993.
A provocative paper regarding the role of surveillance CEA monitoring in patients who have been treated for colorectal cancer.

Giovanniuccie, E., et al.: Aspirin use and risk for colorectal cancer and adenomas in male health professionals. Ann. Intern. Med., 121:241, 1994.
A provocative paper regarding the role of routine aspirin use in preventing adenomatous polyps and colorectal cancer.

REFERENCES

1. American Joint Committee on Cancer. Beahrs, O. H., Henson, D. E., Hutter, D. E., et al. (Eds): Manual for Staging of Cancer, 3rd edition. Philadelphia, J. B. Lippincott, 1988.
2. August, D.A., et al.: Clinical perspective of human colorectal cancer metastasis. Cancer Metastasis Rev., 3:303, 1984.
3. Baron, P. L., and Sigurdson, E. R.: Local surgical treatment of rectal cancer. Cancer Invest., 13(5):612, 1995.
4. Baughman, F. A., Jr., List, C. F., Williams, J. R., Muldoon, J. P., Segarra, J. M., and Volkel, J. S.: The glioma-polyposis syndrome. N. Engl. J. Med., 281:1345, 1969.
5. Burt, R. W., DiSario, J. A., and Cannon-Albright, L.: Genetics of colon cancer: Impact of inheritance on colon cancer risk. Annu. Rev. Med., 46:371, 1995.
6. Burt, R. W., and Groden, J.: The genetic and molecular diagnosis of adenomatous polyposis coli. Gastroenterology, 104:1211, 1993.
7. Burt, R. W., and Samowtiz, W. S.: The adenomatous polyp and the hereditary polyposis syndromes. Gastroenterol. Clin. North Am., 17:657, 1988.
8. Bleday, R., and Wong, R. D.: Recent advances in surgery for colon and rectal cancer. Curr. Probl. Cancer, 17:1, 1993.
9. Bond, J. H.: Polyp guideline: Diagnosis, treatment, and surveillance for patients with nonfamilial colorectal polyps. The Practice Parameters Committee of the American College of Gastroenterology. Ann. Intern. Med., 119:836, 1993.
10. Bosman, F. T.: Prognostic value of pathological characteristics of colorectal cancer. Eur. J. Cancer, 31A(7–8):1216, 1995.
11. Bussey, H. J. R., Veale, A. M. O., and Morson, B. C.: Genetics of gastrointestinal polyposis. Gastroenterology, 74:1325, 1978.
12. Burdick, D., and Prior, J. T.: Peutz-Jeghers syndrome: A clinicopathologic study of a large family with 27-year follow-up. Cancer, 50:2139, 1982.
13. Chui, D. W., Gooding, G. A. W., McQuaid, K. R., Griswold, V., and Grendell, J. H.: Hydrocolonic ultrasonography in the detection of colonic polyps and tumors. N. Engl. J. Med., 331(25):1685, 1994.
14. Cummings, B. J.: Adjuvant radiation for rectal cancer: When and with what? Curr. Opin. Gen. Surg., 1:85, 1994.
15. Cummings, B. J.: Radiation treatment for rectal cancer. World J. Surg., 19(2):275, 1995.
16. Durdey, P., and Williams, N. S.: Preoperative evaluation of patients with low rectal carcinoma. World J. Surg., 16(3):430, 1992.
17. Leppert, M., Burt, R., Hughes, J. P., et al.: Genetic analysis of an inherited predisposition to colon cancer in a family with a variable number of adenomatous polyps. N. Engl. J Med., 322:905, 1990.
18. Eide, T. J.: Risk of colorectal cancer in adenoma-bearing individuals within a defined population. Int. J. Cancer, 38:173, 1986.
19. Fath, R. B., Jr., and Winawer, S. J.: Early diagnosis of colorectal cancer. Annu. Rev. Med., 34:501, 1983.
20. Fearon, E. R., and Vogelstein, B.: A genetic model for colorectal tumorigenesis. Cell, 61:759, 1990.
21. Fishel, R., Lescoe, M. K., Rao, M. R. S., et al.: The human mutator gene homolog MSH2 and its association with hereditary nonpolyposis colon cancer. Cell, 75:1037, 1993. [Erratum, Cell, 77:167, 1994.]
22. Giardello, F. M., Welsh, S. B., Hamilton, S. R., et al.: Increased risk of cancer in the Peutz-Jegher syndrome. N. Engl. J. Med., 316:1511, 1987.
23. Giovanniuccie, E., et al.: Aspirin use and risk for colorectal cancer and adenoma in male health professionals. Ann. Intern. Med., 121:241, 1994.
24. Glaser, F., Schlag, P., Herfarth, C.: Endorectal ultrasonography for the assessment of invasion of rectal tumours and lymph node involvement. Br. J. Surg., 77:883, 1990.
25. Graham, R. A., Garnsey, L., and Jessup, J. M.: Local excision of rectal carcinoma. Am. J. Surg., 160:306, 1990.
26. Groden, J., Thliveris, A., Samowitz, W., et al.: Identification and characterization of the familial adenomatous polyposis coli gene. Cell, 66:589, 1991.
27. Hall, A.: A biochemical function for Ras—at last. Science 264:1413, 1994.
28. Harris, C. C., and Hollstein, M.: Clinical implications of the p53 tumor-suppressor gene. N. Engl. J. Med., 329:1318, 1993.
29. Hölscher, A. H., Siewert, R., and Fink, U.: Endoscopic ultrasonography: I. Staging concepts of gastrointestinal malignancies: The importance of preoperative locoregional T- and N-staging. Gastrointest. Endosc. Clin. North Am. 5(3):529, 1995.
30. Hohenberger, P., Schlag, P., Kretzschmar, U., Herfarth, C.: Regional mesenteric recurrence of colorectal cancer after anterior resection or left hemicolectomy: Inadequate primary resection demonstrated by angiography of the remaining arterial supply. Int. J. Colorect. Dis., 6:17, 1991.
31. Jarvinen, H., Nyberg, M., and Peltokallio, P.: Upper gastrointestinal tract polyps in familial adenomatosis coli. Gut, 24:333, 1983.

32. Kinzler, K. W., Nilbert, M. C., Su, L. K., et al.: Identification of FAP locus genes from chromosome 5q21. Science 253:661, 1991.

33. Leach, F. S., Nicolaides, N. C., Papdopoulos, N., et al.: Mutations of mutS homolog in hereditary nonpolyposis colerectal cancer. Cell, 75:1215, 1993.

34. Liu, B., Parsons, R. E., Hamilton, S. R., et al.: hMSH2 mutations in hereditary nonpolyposis colorectal cancer kindreds. Cancer Res, 54:4590, 1994.

35. Lyerly, H. K., and Mault, J.: Laparoscopic ileostomy and colostomy. Ann. Surg., 219:317, 1994.

36. Lynch, H. T., Kimberling, W., Albano, W. A., et al.: Hereditary nonpolyposis colorectal cancer (Lynch syndromes I and II): Clinical description of resource. Cancer, 56:934, 1985.

37. McGinnis, L. S.: Surgical treatment options for colorectal cancer. Cancer, 74(7 Suppl):2147, 1994.

38. Minsky, B. D.: Conservative treatment of rectal cancer with local excision and postoperative radiation therapy. Eur. J. Cancer, 31A(7/8):1343, 1995.

39. Moertel, C. G., Fleming, R. R., MacDonald, J. S., Haller, D. G., Laurie, J. A., Tangen, C. M., Ungerleider, J. S., Emerson, W. A., Tormey, D. C., Glick, J. H., Veeder, M. H., and Mailliard, J. A.: Fluorouracil plus levamisole as effective adjuvant therapy after resection of stage III colon carcinoma: A final report. Ann. Intern. Med. 122(5):321, 1995.

40. Moertel, C. G., Fleming, T. R., MacDonald, J. S., Haller, D. G., Laurie, J. A., and Tangen, C.: An evaluation of the carcinoembryonic antigen (CEA) test for monitoring patients with resected colon cancer. JAMA, 270(8):943, 1993.

41. Moertel, C. G.: Chemotherapy for colorectal cancer. N. Engl. J. Med., 330:1136, 1994.

42. Muto, J. L., Busset, H. J., and Morson, B. C.: The evolution of cancer of the colon and rectum. Cancer, 36:2251, 1975.

43. Muller, A. D., and Sonnenberg, A.: Prevention of colorectal cancer by flexible endoscopy and polypectomy. Ann. Intern. Med., 123:904, 1995.

44. Neuget, A. I., Garbowski, G. C., Lee, W. C., Murray, T., Nieves, J. W., Forde, K. A., Treat, M. R., Waye, J. D., and Fenoglio-Preiser, C.: Dietary risk factors for the incidence and recurrence of colorectal adenomatous polyps: A case-control study. Ann. Intern. Med., 118(2):91, 1993.

45. Nicolaides, N. C., Papadopoulos, N., Liu, B., Wei, Y. F., Carter, K. C., Ruben, S. M., Rosen, C. A., Haseltine, W. A., Fleischmann, R. D., Fraser, C. M., et al.: Mutations of two PMS homologues in hereditary nonpolyposis colon cancer. Nature, 371(6492):75, 1994.

46. O'Riordain, D. S., O'Dwyer, P. J., Cullen, A. F., McDermott, E. W., and Murphy, J. J.: Familial juvenile polyposis coli and colorectal cancer. Cancer, 68:889, 1991.

47. Ota, D. M., Nelson, J., and Weeks, J. C.: Controversies regarding laparoscopic colectomy for malignant diseases. Curr. Opin. Gen. Surg., 1:208, 1994.

48. Papadopoulos, N., Nicolaides, N. C., Wei, Y. F., Ruben, S. M., Carter, K. C., Rosen, C. A., Haseltine, W. A., Fleischmann, R. D., Fraser, C. M., Adams, M. D., et al.: Mutation of a mutL homolog in hereditary colon cancer Science, 263(5153):1625, 1994.

49. Papillon, J., and Berard, P.: Endocavitary irradiation in the conservative treatment of adenocarcinoma of the low rectum. World J. Surg., 16(3):451, 1992.

50. Phillips, R. K.: Adequate distal margin of resection for adenocarcinoma of the rectum. World J. Surg., 16(3):463, 1992.

51. Posner, M. R., Bleday, R., Huberman, M., et al.: Impact of combined modality therapy on the treatment of adenocarcinoma of the colon. Semin. Surg. Oncol., 9(1):33, 1993.

52. Ravitch, M. M., and Sabiston, D. C., Jr.: Anal ileostomy with preservation of sphincter: A proposed operation in patients requiring total colectomy for benign lesions. Surg. Gynecol. Obstet., 84:1095, 1947.

53. Ricards, R. C., Rogers, S. W., and Gardner, E. J.: Spontaneous mesenteric fibromatosis in Gardner's syndrome. Cancer, 47:597, 1981.

54. Rustgi, A. K.: Hereditary gastrointestinal polyposis and nonpolyposis syndromes. N. Engl. J. Med., 331(25):1694, 1994.

55. Runkel, N. S., Schlag, P., Schwarz, V., and Herfarth, C.: Outcome after emergency surgery for cancer of the large intestine. Br. J. Surg., 78:183, 1991.

56. Salem, O. S., and Steck, W. D.: Cowden's disease (multiple hamartoma and neoplasia syndrome): A case report and review of the English literature. J. Am. Acad. Dermatol., 8:686, 1983.

57. Shirasawa, S., Furuse, M., Yokoyama, N., and Sasazuki, T.: Altered growth of human colon cancer cell lines disrupted at activated Ki-ras. Science, 260(5104):85, 1993.

58. Soper, N. J., Brunt, L. M., and Kerbl, K.: Laparscopic general surgery. N. Engl. J. Med., 330:409, 1994.

59. Steele, G.: Advances in the treatment of early- to late-stage colorectal cancer: 20 years of progress. Ann. Surg. Oncol., 2(1):77, 1995.

60. Steele, G., Jr.: Accomplishment and promise in the understanding and treatment of colorectal carcinoma. Lancet, 324:1092, 1993.

61. Swiss Group for Clinical Cancer Research (SAKK): Long-term results of single course of adjuvant intraportal chemotherapy for colorectal cancer. Lancet, 345:349, 1995.

62. Sugarbaker, P. H.: Follow-up of colorectal cancer. Tumori, 81(3 Suppl):126, 1995.

63. Tio, T. L., Coene, P. P., van Delden, O. M., and Tytgat, G. N. J.: Colorectal carcinoma: Preoperative TNM classification with endosonography. Radiology, 179:165, 1991.

64. Tonelli, F., Valanzano, R., and Dolara, P.: Sulindac therapy of colorectal polyps in familial adenomatous polyposis. Dig. Dis., 12:259, 1994.

65. Turk, P. S., and Wanebo, H. J.: Results of surgical treatment of nonhepatic recurrence of colorectal carcinoma. Cancer, 71(12 Suppl):4267, 1993.

66. Hermanek, P., and Sobin, L. H. (Eds.): UICC: TNM Classification of Malignant Tumours, 4th edition. Berlin, Springer, 1987.

67. Virgo, K. S., Vernava, A. M., Longo, W. E., et al.: Cost of patient follow-up after potentially curative colorectal cancer treatment. JAMA, 273(23):1837, 1995.

68. Wanebo, H. J., Fang, W. L., Mills, A. S., and Zfass, A. M.: Colorectal cancer: A blueprint for disease control through screening by primary care physicians. Arch. Surg., 121:1347, 1986.

69. Winawer, S. J., et al.: Prevention of colorectal cancer by colonoscopic polypectomy. N. Engl. J. Med., 329:1978, 1993.

70. Yaremko, M. L., Wasylyshyn, M. L., Westbrook, C. A., and Michelassi, F.: Oncogenes, suppressor genes, and allele losses in colon cancer. Adv. Surg., 26:323, 1993.

71. Yeatman, T. J., and Bland, K.: Sphincter-saving procedures for distal carcinoma of the rectum. Ann. Surg., 201:11, 1989.

X

DISORDERS OF THE ANAL CANAL

Roger R. Dozois, M.D.

The region of the anal canal can be the site of many lesions. Most conditions arising in this area are common and benign but may be incapacitating and interfere with the daily quality of life. Moreover, these disorders are often misdiagnosed and/or maltreated, sometimes leading to disastrous consequences. A better knowledge of the functional anatomy of this most distal portion of the gastrointestinal tract as well as recent changes in our understanding of its physiology and that of the pelvic floor should facilitate the diagnosis and management of these ailments and result in more favorable outcome.

ANATOMY

The anal canal, which extends for a distance of about 4 cm. from the anorectal ring to the hairy skin of the anal verge, is the most distal portion of the alimentary canal. Its lining and its musculature have important features that, together with the structures of the pelvic floor, contribute significantly to the regulation of defecation and continence. Its borders include the coccyx posteriorly, the ischiorectal fossa and its contents bilaterally, and, anteriorly, the perineal body and vagina in women and the urethra in men.

Anal Canal Lining

The epithelium that lines the anal canal differs at various levels. The characteristically serrated dentate (pectinate) line made up of anal valves anatomically demarcates the cephalad, pleated mucosa from the caudad, smooth, anoderm mucosa. The proximal mucosa is corrugated into a series of 12 to 14 columns of Morgagni, with corresponding crypts between each fold. Opening into these crypts are a variable number of anal glands that traverse the submucosa to enter the internal sphincter and terminate in the intersphincteric plane.[11] Thus, infection of these cryptoglandular structures may cause fistulas that can be expected to communicate with the dentate line area.

The mucosa of the upper anal canal, like that of the rectum, is pinkish in color and is lined by columnar epithelium. The mucosa distal to the dentate line is paler and lined by squamous epithelium devoid of hair and glands.[26] The change between the two types of epithelium is not abrupt, however, and the mucosa of the so-called transitional zone that lies immediately proximal to the dentate line consists of layers of cuboid cells interspersed with tongues of columnar epithelium that is purplish in color. Thus, diseases affecting the rectal mucosa, such as ulcerative colitis, can extend to the transitional zone area.[3] At the anal verge, the lining acquires the characters of normal skin with its apocrine glands.

Anal Canal Musculature

The musculature of the anal canal and its sphincteric apparatus constitute the terminal muscular channel of the gastrointestinal tract and can be conceptualized as two tubular structures overlying each other.[37] The inner component is a continuation of the smooth circular layer of the rectum and forms the thickened, rounded internal sphincter, which ends 1.5 cm. below the dentate line slightly cephalad to the external sphincter (intersphincteric groove). The outer component is a continuous sheet of striated muscle constituting the pelvic floor, which comprises the levator ani muscle, the puborectalis muscle, and the external sphincter (Fig. 32–43). The latter is elliptical and engulfs the anal canal and the internal sphincter, beyond which it terminates in a subcutaneous portion. The other two portions—the superficial and deep divisions—constitute a single muscular unit that is continuous superiorly with the puborectalis and levator ani muscles.[11] The external sphincter, bulbospongiosus, and transverse perineal muscles meet centrally on the perineum to constitute the perineal body. The funnel-shaped configuration of the paired levator ani muscles forms the major part of the pelvic floor, and their fibers decussate medially with the contralateral side to fuse with the perineal body around the prostate or vagina.

TABLE 32–14. Fecal Continence: Controlling Factors

Anorectal
    Sphincters
    Angulation
    Sensory and reflex mechanisms
    Motility
Rectal
    Compliance
    Tone
    Evacuability
Pelvic floor
    Coordinated muscular activity
Colon
    Transit
    Stool volume and consistency

The internal sphincter is innervated by the autonomic nervous system and is independent of voluntary control. The external sphincter, which is supplied by the inferior rectal branch of the internal pudendal nerve and the perineal branch of the fourth sacral nerve, is under voluntary control.[26]

PHYSIOLOGY

The physiology of the anal canal and pelvic floor is complex, but the advent of sophisticated means of evaluating their functions, such as manometry, defecography, evacuability testing, and electromyography, has improved our understanding. The principal function of the anal canal is the regulation of defecation and the maintenance of continence, which depend on intricate and interrelated factors (Table 32–14). Conditions such as constipation, incontinence, solitary rectal ulcer, rectal intussusception, and prolapse are likely caused by disordered motor function in this area.

The anal canal, which has a mean length of 4 cm., lengthens with squeezing of the external sphincter and shortens with straining.[19] *Resting pressure* or tone, which depends largely on the internal sphincter, averages 90 cm. H_2O and is lower in women and older patients than in men and younger patients.[22] This high-pressure zone increases resistance to the passage of stool. *Squeeze pressure*, generated by contraction of the external anal sphincter and puborectalis muscle, more

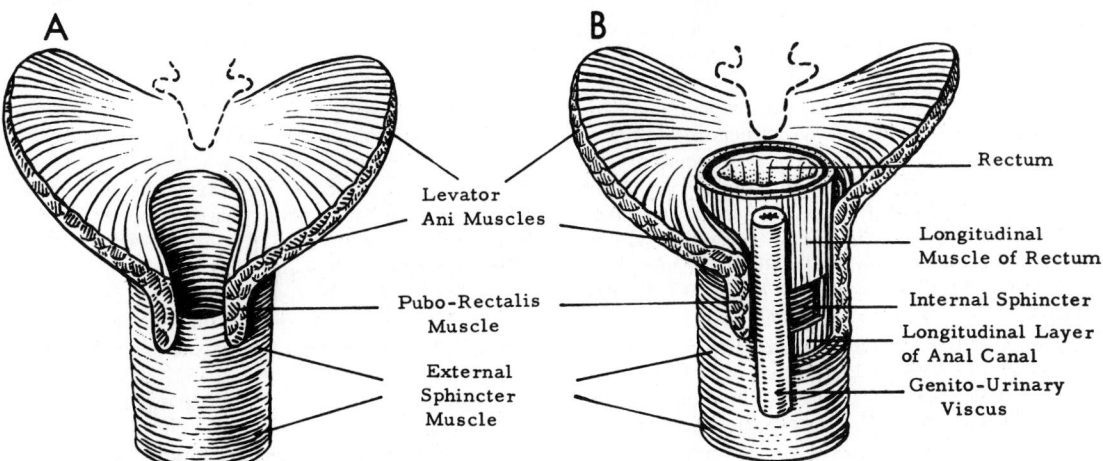

Figure 32–43. The anal canal mechanism comprises two components, visceral and somatic, each of which is tubular. The visceral tube is enclosed by a skeletal muscle tube by means of which continence is maintained. *A*, Diagrammatic representation of the skeletal muscle component. *B*, Composite arrangement after insertion of a simple visceral component. (From Parks, A. G.: Hemorrhoidectomy. *In* Welch, C. E. [Ed.]: Advances in Surgery. Copyright © 1971, Year Book Medical Publishers. Used by permission.)

than doubles intra-anal canal resting pressure. This maximal increase lasts for only a minute at most; consequently, squeeze pressure serves only to prevent leakage when the rectal content is presented to the proximal anal canal at inappropriate times. The principal mechanism that provides continence is the pressure differential between the rectum (6 cm. H_2O) and the anal canal (90 cm. H_2O).[10] The anorectal angle produced by the anterior pull of the puborectalis muscle as it encircles the rectum at the anorectal ring also contributes to fecal continence. This angle may act as a flap valve[27] or have a sphincter-like function.[4] Maneuvers that sharpen this angle augment continence, whereas those that straighten it favor defecation. *Anorectal sensation* allows discrimination of the character of the enteric content (gas, liquid, or solid) and detection of the need to pass that content through sensory receptors located in either the rectal muscular wall or the pelvic floor musculature.[22] The fact that such sensation persists after proctectomy and ileoanal anastomosis suggests that the receptors are situated in the pelvic floor.[5] In order for the enteric content to reach the anal canal for discrimination, the internal sphincter must relax while the rectum distends and contracts (rectal anal inhibitory reflex). The reflex involves inhibitory neurons of the myenteric plexus, which innervates the internal sphincter and involves intramural nerves and neurotransmitters.[22] Transient relaxation of the internal anal sphincter brings the rectal content into contact with the sensory mucosa of the proximal anal canal so that it can be recognized. Other factors important to continence include rectal compliance, tone, and capacity; the characteristics of rectal filling and emptying; and the stool volume and consistency.[22]

DIAGNOSIS

Systematic evaluation of anorectal disorders includes a careful history and physical examination of the anal canal area prior to laboratory testing.

History

Important symptoms include bleeding, pain, discharge (mucoid, purulent, or fecal), and change in bowel habits. It is also paramount to know about associated illnesses, medication, family history, bleeding tendency, and exposure through travel or sexual contacts.

Bleeding per anus helps differentiate between anorectal conditions and bowel diseases above the level of the anorectum. Inquiry into the type of bleeding should include whether the blood is dark or bright red or associated with clots, whether it is mixed with the stool or separate, and whether it drips into the toilet bowl or only appears on the toilet paper. Blood that drips, is separate from stools, and is bright red is most commonly seen with bleeding internal hemorrhoids. Blood on toilet tissue may be associated with minor hemorrhoidal disease but also with anal fissure. Clots or melena indicate colonic or more proximal bleeding, respectively. Anorectal pain occurring during or immediately after stooling that is described as severe is usually associated with anal fissure. Pain that may or may not be related to stooling and is throbbing in nature most often is seen with an abscess or a poorly draining fistula. Pain totally unrelated to stooling is likely to be associated with proctalgia fugax or levator ani syndrome, a condition characterized by painful episodes of short duration (less than 20 to 30 minutes) often occurring at night and relieved by walking, warm baths, or other maneuvers. To ascertain a change in bowel habits, it is necessary to establish by careful inquiry the previous pattern. Indeed, constipation may mean different conditions to different patients, and it is important to know whether the condition is of

recent onset or chronic in order to determine the appropriate course of investigation.

Physical Examination

The left lateral position with the buttocks projecting slightly beyond the edge of the table is most suitable for patient and surgeon alike. Inspection with good lighting should precede any other types of examination. Skin tags, excoriations, scars, and any changes in the color or appearance of perianal skin are easily recognized. A patulous anus may indicate incontinence and possibly prolapse. Inspection while the patient is straining may help determine the presence of hemorrhoidal or rectal prolapse, and in multiparous women, a protruding anus may be an indication of descending perineum syndrome. A careful and systematic digital examination with a well-lubricated index finger gradually inserted into the anal canal helps appreciate any mass, induration, or stricturing, as well as the pelvic floor muscles. In men, the prostate should be palpated; in women, the posterior vaginal wall should be pushed forward to detect rectocele.

After the preliminary evaluation has been completed, proctosigmoidoscopy following enema preparation enables satisfactory visualization of the anorectum. Early signs of mucosal inflammation include the loss of the vascular pattern with erythema, granularity, friability, and even ulcerations. Gross lesions such as polyps or carcinoma should be readily identifiable. Any suspicious area or mass should be biopsied, with the patient's permission, so that a precise histopathologic diagnosis can be established. On retrieving the scope, the anorectal area can be assessed for mucosal prolapse, hemorrhoids, fissure, polyps, and so forth. The anoscope can be used for the same purpose.

Other investigations include barium enema, flexible sigmoidoscopy or colonoscopy, and stool examination, especially if one is suspicious of infectious diarrhea or sexually transmitted diseases. Special studies such as manometry, defecography, and electromyography may help in the assessment of anorectal incontinence, constipation, or other pelvic floor disorders. More recently, ultrasonography and magnetic resonance imaging (MRI) have shown promise in the evaluation of anorectal suppurative processes. The indications for and usefulness of these tests are discussed under the specific disorders.

PELVIC FLOOR DISORDERS

Incontinence

Voluntary control of defecation is obviously desirable. A distinction must be made between minor incontinence, such as occasional staining of undergarments and/or loss of gas, and true incontinence (complete loss of solid stools). Careful questioning is important, because many incontinent patients who seek surgical assistance have either a history of previous trauma to the anal canal region or rectal prolapse.

Trauma may follow previous surgical procedures for hemorrhoids, fissures, or fistulas; forceful dilatation of the anal canal; or obstetric injuries—either directly because of a tear or breakdown of episiotomy repair or indirectly from stretching of the pudendal nerve during labor.[21] It is important to remember that the latter may develop decades later. Other factors include aging, trauma such as impalement, primary disease of the anal canal, irradiation, and neurogenic processes. A careful history pertaining to possible etiologic factors and a simple physical examination are useful. A patulous anus, which may indicate procidentia; scars and deformities, such as a keyhole-shaped one in the posterior midline; or large, protruding hemorrhoids may all lead to at least partial incontinence or soiling. The integrity of the anal sphincters can be assessed by manometry. Electromyography with pudendal nerve terminal motor latency helps locate the severed ends of the sphincter muscle and establish the integrity of sphincter innervation. The assessment is critical, since the therapeutic approach depends on the underlying cause.

Treatment may be nonoperative, including medications to slow transit or increase stool consistency or diet and sphincter exercises, but in general, these approaches have been disappointing. More recently, biofeedback training has been used, but results have been variable, depending on the compliance of the patient and the underlying cause of incontinence. Operation, primarily an overlapping sphincteroplasty consisting of approximating and suturing the severed ends,[12] has provided very good to excellent results in the majority of well-selected patients. When no anatomic disruption of the sphincter mechanism can be demonstrated, some authors have advocated a posterior sphincteroplasty with suturing of the puborectalis, or a so-called postanal repair.[27] The results have been quite variable,[12] and some authors believe that the procedure restores the anatomy but not the function.[32] More aggressive approaches such as transposition of gracilis or gluteal muscles, free muscle grafts, neosphincter construction, and artificial sphincter implantation are either complex or experimental or both and should be reserved for the ultraspecialist. In some instances, a colostomy is the last recourse but may prove to be quite beneficial. Whether proctectomy should also be included depends on the patient and the underlying cause of incontinence. In most cases, the morbidity of proctectomy should be balanced against that of a defunctionalized rectum.

Prolapse of the Rectum

Prolapse of the rectum, or procidentia, is an uncommon problem of obscure etiology characterized by full-thickness eversion of the rectal wall through the anus and its external protrusion as a series of concentric rings (Fig. 32–44). The exact cause is unclear, but the disorder tends to predominate in women, in those who strain excessively, and in those with chronic mental disorders.[9] Pregnancy and delivery cannot be the cause, as the condition can occur in men and in nulliparous women. Studies strongly support the concept that rectal prolapse is the result of intussusception or infolding of the rectum or rectosigmoid.[35] As the intussusception progresses caudally, the intussusceptum gradually pulls the upper rectal wall away from its sacral and lateral moorings. With continued straining, the bowel continues to roll inside out until initially the mucocutaneous junction and eventually the rectal wall itself evert completely.[9] This progressive phenomenon may explain why some patients have occult or hidden prolapse and why the sigmoid mesentery may elongate, the cul-de-sac deepen, and the pelvic floor musculature increasingly weaken.[9] Such findings have been implicated as causative, but it is more likely that they are the result of the prolonged process of gradual prolapsing of the rectum.

The symptoms of early prolapse may be vague, including discomfort or a sensation of incomplete evacuation during defecation. A long history of constipation and excessive straining is common. When prolapse is complete, protrusion of the rectum is noted as a mass during and after defecation. By the time the diagnosis is secured, half of the patients have fecal incontinence. In patients with occult prolapse, a feeling of pressure and a sensation of incomplete evacuation may be the only symptoms. On endoscopy, these patients may have redness of the anterior rectal mucosa or a solitary ulcer anteriorly, 6 to 8 cm. from the anal verge.[9] Defecography may show intussusception of the distal sigmoid and proximal rectum into the distal rectum. Anal manometry can help document the degree of anal sphincter damage and aid in planning the surgical procedure.

Surgical correction of complete prolapse of the rectum is imperfect, as can be surmised from the large number of

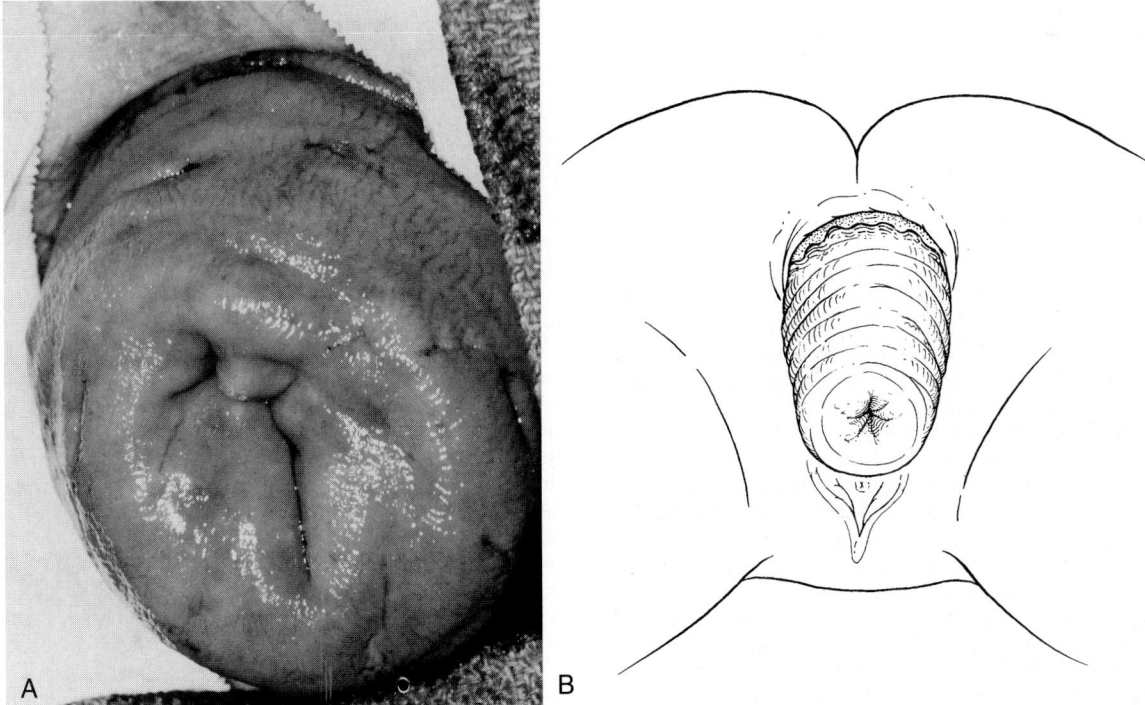

A   B

Figure 32–44. Complete rectal prolapse. *A,* The everted rectal wall appears as a tubular mass made up of several concentric mucosal folds. *B,* Schematic representation of complete rectal prolapse. (From Dozois, R. R., and Nivatvongs, S.: Prolapse of the rectum. *In* Block, G. E., and Moossa, A. R. [Eds.]: Operative Colorectal Surgery. Philadelphia, W. B. Saunders, 1994.)

TABLE 32–15. Hemorrhoids: Classification and Management

Condition	Symptoms and Signs	Management
First degree	Painless bleeding	Exclusion of other causes of bleeding Diet, psyllium or bran Rubber-band ligation Infrared coagulation Bipolar electrocoagulation
Second degree	Protrusion with defecation with spontaneous reduction Bleeding	Rubber-band ligation Infrared coagulation Bipolar electrocoagulation
Third degree	Protrusion, spontaneous or with bowel movement, requiring manual reduction Bleeding	Rubber-band ligation Infrared coagulation Bipolar electrocoagulation Closed hemorrhoidectomy
Fourth degree	Permanently prolapsed Irreducible Bleeding	Closed hemorrhoidectomy
Prolapsed strangulated hemorrhoids	Painful, edematous, tender unreducible hemorrhoids	Emergency closed hemorrhoidectomy
Thrombosed external hemorrhoids	If painful	Excision under local anesthesia

Modified from Nivatvongs, S.: Hemorrhoids. *In* Gordon, P. H., and Nivatvongs, S. (Eds.): Principles and Practice of Surgery for the Colon, Rectum, and Anus. St. Louis, Quality Medical Publishing, Inc., 1992.

operations that have been proposed over the years. In most instances, the preferred operation is anterior resection with rectal fixation.[9] This operation provides excellent long-term results, is safe if done at a level above the promontory after mobilizing the rectum and resecting the redundant sigmoid, and can be done by most surgeons. Simple fixation of the stalks to the presacral fascia with sutures is technically easy to perform and avoids complications resulting from foreign materials such as obstruction and perforation with Marlex mesh.[17] Transperineal repairs may provide less satisfactory results over the long term but are safer. They are usually reserved for elderly and/or debilitated patients. If the prolapsing rectal segment is shorter than 3 to 4 cm., a modification of the Delorme procedure consisting of anorectal mucosectomy with plication of the muscular coat of the rectum can be used.[9] If the prolapsed segment is longer than 3 to 4 cm., a transperineal rectal amputation of the Altemeier type is preferred.[9] It is now widely held that the incontinence that follows prolapse may be due to chronic stretching and ensuing damage of the pudendal innervation of the anal sphinc-

ter.[30] This belief would explain why all incontinence is not reversible after correction of procidentia. Since as many as 50% to 75% of incontinent patients with a prolapsed rectum improve over 6 to 12 months after surgical repair,[27] direct repair of the continence mechanism is not attempted at the time of the abdominal repair. In incapacitated patients, a postanal repair can be performed at a later date with some degree of success.[18, 27]

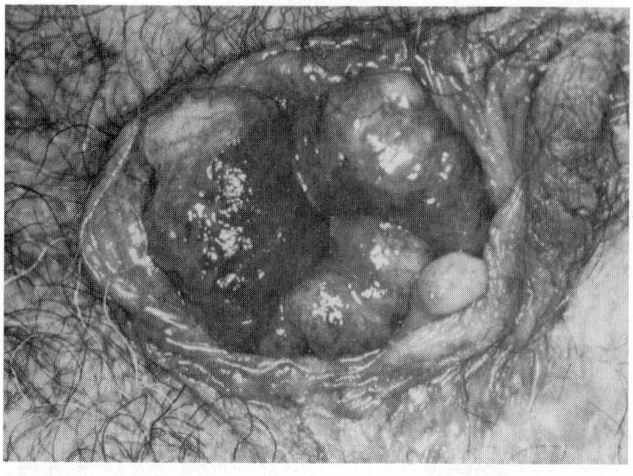

COMMON ANAL CANAL DISORDERS

Hemorrhoids

Within the anal canal there are specialized, highly vascularized *cushions* forming discrete masses of thick submucosa containing blood vessels, smooth muscle, and elastic and connective tissue.[36] They are located in the left lateral, right anterior, and right posterior quadrants of the canal to aid in anal continence. By definition, the term *hemorrhoids* should be restricted to clinical situations in which these cushions are abnormal and cause symptoms. The cause of hemorrhoids remains unknown. They may be no more than the downward sliding of anal cushions associated with straining and irregular bowel habits.[37] Hemorrhoids have been classified by degree of symptoms, which in turn influences treatment (Table 32–15). The diagnosis is based on the history, physical examination, and endoscopy. External hemorrhoids are covered with anoderm and are distal to the dentate line; they may swell, causing discomfort and difficult hygiene, but cause severe pain only if actually thrombosed. Internal hemorrhoids cause painless, bright red bleeding associated with defecation. The patient may report dripping or even squirting of blood in the toilet bowl. Chronic occult bleeding leading to anemia is rare, and other causes of anemia must be excluded. Prolapse below the dentate line area occurs with straining and may lead to mucus and fecal leakage and pruritus. Pain is not usually associated with uncomplicated hemorrhoids but more often with fissure, abscess, or external hemorrhoidal thrombosis. Inspection with or without straining may reveal signs of late hemorrhoidal disease (Fig. 32–45) and help exclude other anal pathology. Digital examination enables assessment of hemorrhoidal disease and anal canal tone

Figure 32–45. Third-degree hemorrhoids. Note the squamous epithelial change and the darkened mucosa.

and the exclusion of other lesions, especially low rectal or anal canal neoplasms. Anoscopy is the definitive examination, but a flexible proctosigmoidoscopy should always be added to exclude proximal inflammation or neoplasia. Colonoscopy or barium enema should be added if the hemorrhoidal disease is unimpressive, the history is somewhat uncharacteristic, and the patient is over 45 years of age or has risk factors for colon cancer, such as a family history.

Depending on the degree of disease, treatment falls into two main categories: nonsurgical and hemorrhoidectomy. In many patients, hemorrhoidal symptoms can be ameliorated or relieved by simple measures such as better local hygiene, avoidance of excessive straining, and better dietary habits supplemented by medication to keep stools formed but soft (see Table 32–15). Of the various nonsurgical therapies, rubber-band ligation is probably the most widely used, the simplest, and the least expensive. It can be performed in the office without sedation through an anoscope using a ligator. Two rubber bands are applied on each hemorrhoidal bundle. The bands should be placed on the rectal mucosa just proximal to the enlarged hemorrhoid. Preferably, only one site should be banded each time. Patients should be instructed to go immediately to the emergency room if delayed or undue pain, inability to void, or fever develops.[33] The procedure should be avoided in immune-deficient patients, especially those who are HIV-positive. Infrared coagulation is a controlled burn produced at the junction of the rectal and anal canal mucosa that causes mucosal fixation. The equipment required is expensive, and there is a risk of secondary hemorrhage. Anal stretch can be associated with incontinence and is not advocated. Cryotherapy should no longer be used.

Hemorrhoidectomy is the best means of curing hemorrhoidal disease and should be considered whenever patients fail to respond satisfactorily to repeated attempts at conservative measures, hemorrhoids are severely prolapsed and require manual reduction, or they are complicated by strangulation or associated pathology such as ulceration, fissure, fistula, or very large anal tags.[25] The choice of anesthesia should be individualized, based on the patient's preference, the patient's build and medical status, and the individual surgeon. In most instances, local anesthesia with mild sedation can be used safely. Closed hemorrhoidectomy is preferred and may be performed in the ambulatory setting (Fig. 32–46). Other types of hemorrhoidectomy include the excision and ligation technique, which leaves the wound open,[37] and the rarely used modified Whitehead procedure.[40] Laser hemorrhoidectomy offers no definite advantage over conventional techniques. For thrombosed external hemorrhoid, excision is the therapy of choice (Fig. 32–47).

Fissure in Ano

Fissure in ano is a linear ulcer of the lower half of the anal canal usually located in the posterior commissure in the midline (Fig. 32–48). Location may vary, and an anterior midline fissure is seen more often in women, although most fissures in women occur in the posterior midline. Characteristically associated findings include a sentinel pile or tag externally and an enlarged anal papilla internally. Fissures away from these two locations should raise the possibility of associated diseases, especially Crohn's disease, hidradenitis suppurativa, or sexually transmitted diseases. Because it involves the highly sensitive squamous epithelium, it is often a very painful condition. With defecation, the ulcer is stretched, causing pain that may last for some time thereafter and mild bleeding. The pain may be such that patients avoid defecation, resulting in hard stools, which compounds the problem. The exact cause is unknown, but many factors appear likely, such as the passage of large, hard stools, which may be the initiating factor; inappropriate diet; previous anal procedure; childbirth; and laxative abuse. Numerous authors have documented a higher-than-normal resting anal canal pressure, which explains why internal sphincterotomy relieves symptoms and heals the ulceration.[20] The diagnosis is secured by the typical history of pain with defecation, especially if associated with prior constipation and confirmed by inspection after gently parting the posterior anus. Digital and proctoscopic examination may trigger severe pain, interfering with the ability to visualize the ulcer. An examination under anesthesia may then be necessary. Treatment is usually quite satisfactory. In some patients, the fissure heals with the use of conservative measures to avoid constipation and decrease pain. The remainder require minor surgical procedures in the form of lateral internal sphincterotomy (Fig. 32–49). Any fissure that fails to heal should be biopsied. Conservative measures include emollient suppositories, psyllium seeds,

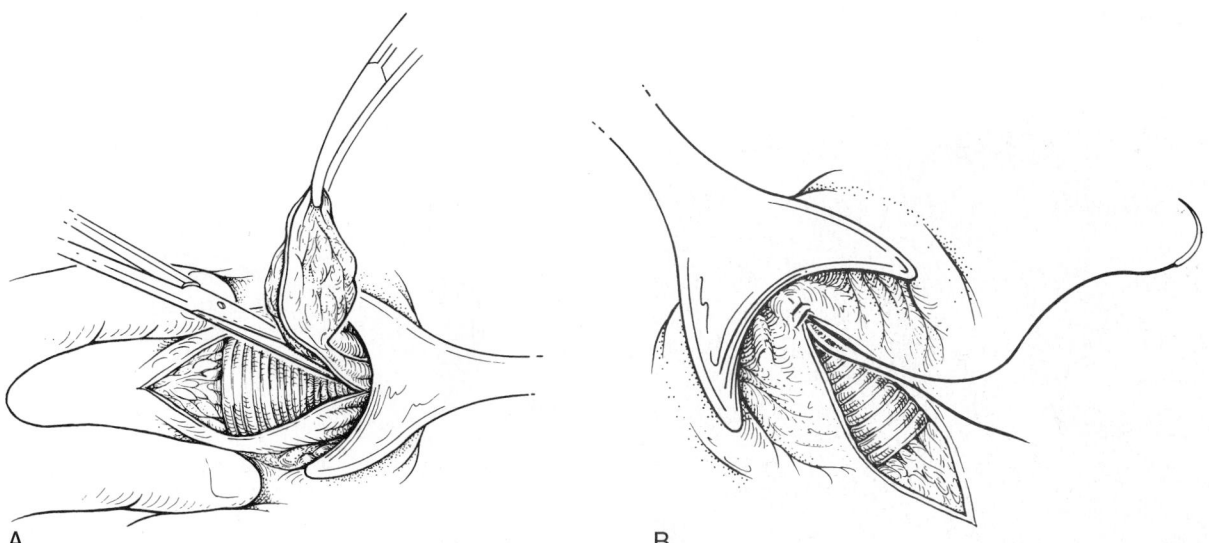

A   B

Figure 32–46. Closed hemorrhoidectomy. *A,* The operation involves dissecting hemorrhoidal tissues superficial to the internal sphincter muscle. *B,* After transfixing the vascular pedicle, the defect is closed with a running absorbable suture. (From Prager, E.: Common ailments of the anorectal region. *In* Block, G. E., and Moossa, A. R. [Eds.]: Operative Colorectal Surgery. Philadelphia, W. B. Saunders, 1994.)

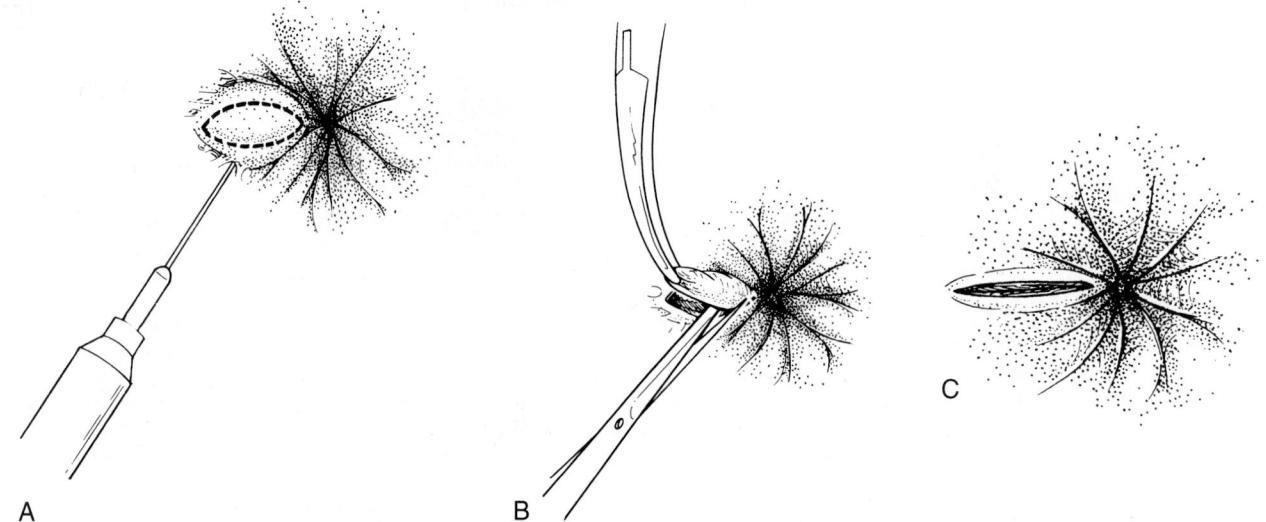

Figure 32–47. Excision of thrombosed external hemorrhoid. The area is infiltrated with local anesthetic, and the future elliptical incision is outlined *(A)*. The thrombosed hemorrhoid is excised sharply with scissors *(B)*, and the edges of the wound are left open after ensuring hemostasis *(C)*. (From Prager, E.: Common ailments of the anorectal region. *In* Block, G. E., and Moossa, A. R. [Eds.]: Operative Colorectal Surgery. Philadelphia, W. B. Saunders, 1994.)

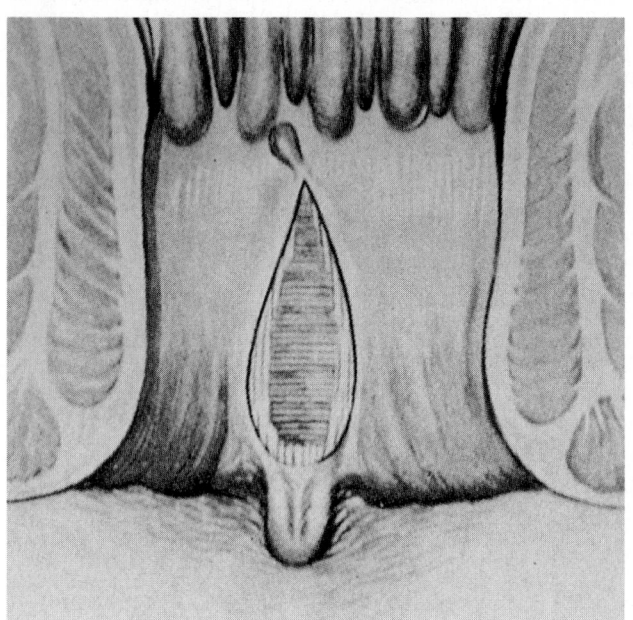

Figure 32–48. Typical appearance of a posterior anal fissure showing the sentinel pile, the circular muscle fibers at the base of the ulcer, and the enlarged anal papilla. (From Morgan, C. N., and Thompson, H. R.: Surgical anatomy of the anal canal with special reference to the surgical importance of the internal sphincter and conjoint longitudinal muscle. Ann. R. Coll. Surg. Engl., *19*:88, 1956.)

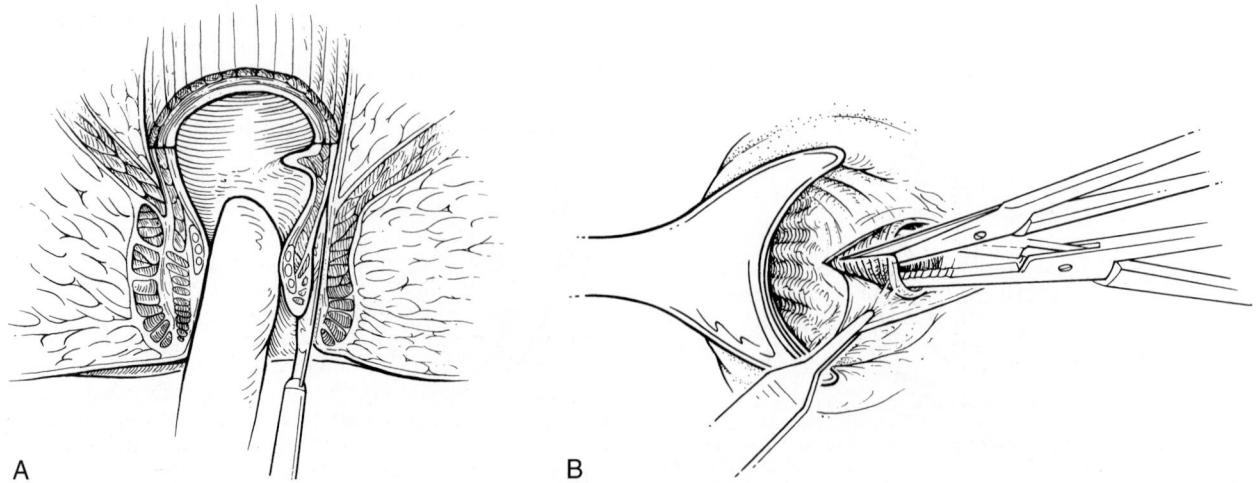

Figure 32–49. Lateral internal sphincterotomy: closed technique *(A)* and open technique *(B)*. (From Prager, E.: Common ailments of the anorectal region. In Block, G. E., and Moossa, A. R. [Eds.]: Operative Colorectal Surgery. Philadelphia, W. B. Saunders, 1994.)

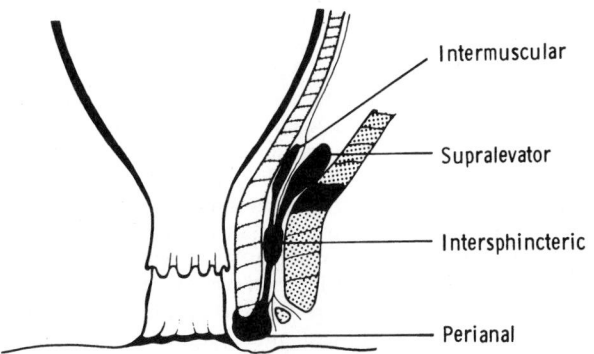

Figure 32–50. Upward and downward vertical spread of infection from an intersphincteric abscess. (From Parks, A. G., and Thomson, J. P. S.: Abscess and fistula. *In* Thomson, J. P. S., Nichols, R. J., and Williams, C. R. [Eds.]: Colorectal Disease. Copyright © 1981. London, William Heissemann Medical Books, and New York, Appleton-Century-Crofts. Used by permission.)

and sitz baths.[37] In the only reported prospective trial, a combination of sitz baths and sufficient amounts of bran (5 gm. per day) appeared to be effective.[16] If the fissure persists or recurs, one should treat the patient with conservative measures before proceeding with another sphincterotomy. In general, the results are excellent with minimal complications.

Anorectal Suppuration

Although there may be several causes of anorectal suppuration, by far the most common is a nonspecific infection of cryptoglandular origin. Other causes are quite rare, except for Crohn's disease and hydradenitis suppurativa. The pathogenesis of both abscesses and fistulas is usually the same, with the abscess representing the acute phase and the fistula the chronic sequela.[28]

Abscess

Infection originates in the intersphincteric plane, most likely in one of the anal glands. This may cause a simple intersphincteric abscess, or it may extend vertically either upward or downward (Fig. 32–50), horizontally (Fig. 32–51), or circumferentially (Fig. 32–52), resulting in a number of clinical presentations.[37]

An *intersphincteric abscess* is limited to the primary site of origin; it may be asymptomatic or cause severe, throbbing

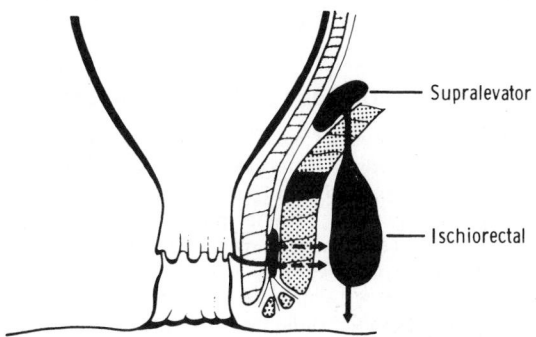

Figure 32–51. Horizontal spread of infection medially into the anal canal and laterally into the ischiorectal fossa. The level at which the primary tract crosses the external sphincter may not be the same as the level of the internal opening. Vertical spread of infection may then occur across the levator ani muscle. (From Parks, A. G., and Thomson, J. P. S.: Abscess and fistula. *In* Thomson, J. P. S., Nichols, R. J., and Williams, C. R. [Eds.]: Colorectal Disease. Copyright © 1981. London, William Heissemann Medical Books, and New York, Appleton-Century-Crofts. Used by permission.)

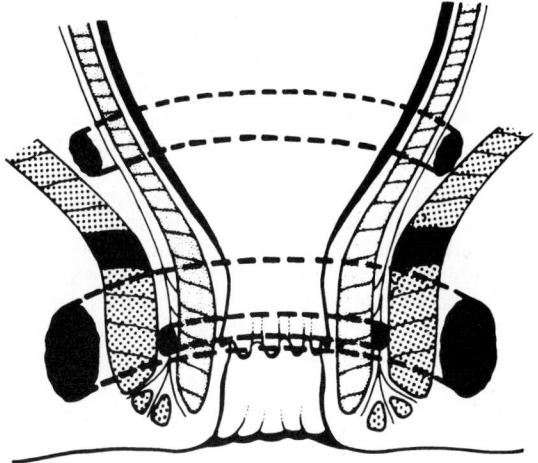

Figure 32–52. Circumferential spread of infection can occur in the intersphincteric and supralevator spaces and the ischiorectal fossa. (From Parks, A. G., and Thomson, J. P. S.: Abscess and fistula. *In* Thomson, J. P. S., Nichols, R. J., and Williams, C. R. [Eds.]: Colorectal Disease. Copyright © 1981. London, William Heissemann Medical Books, and New York, Appleton-Century-Crofts. Used by permission.)

pain that resembles the pain of a fissure.[37] Pain persisting after adequate treatment of a coexisting fissure should raise suspicion of an underlying, unrecognized intersphincteric abscess. A *perianal abscess* follows the vertical downward spread of an intersphincteric infection to the anal margin and presents as a tender swelling that can be misinterpreted as a thrombosed external hemorrhoid.[37]

If the infection spreads vertically upward, an *intermuscular abscess* within the rectal wall itself or a *supralevator abscess* may develop, depending on which side of the longitudinal muscle the infection has tracked.[37] These abscesses are difficult to diagnose, because the patient may complain of vague discomfort, external manifestations are absent, and the presence of rectal induration and swelling may be clearly established only with the aid of an examination under anesthesia.

Horizontal spread of infection may track across the internal sphincter into the anal canal or in the opposite direction across the external sphincter into the ischiorectal fossa to form an *ischiorectal abscess*. The abscess may be quite large, especially if it is neglected or treated only with antibiotics. It may expand to the roof of the fossa or even through it into the supralevator space after traversing the levator ani muscle and downward to the perianal skin.[37] The patient may complain of pain and fever before an erythematous mass is detectable. Ultimately, an obvious red, fluctuant mass is visible. The infectious process may spread circumferentially from one side to the other of the intersphincteric space, the supralevator space, or the ischiorectal fossa, producing a complex horseshoe abscess.

Abscesses should be drained when diagnosed. An intersphincteric abscess is drained by dividing the internal sphincter to the level of the abscess. For a perianal abscess, a simple skin incision is all that is necessary. Both an intermuscular abscess and a supralevator abscess, as long as it is not an ischiorectal abscess extension, need to be drained into the lower rectum and upper anal canal.[37] An ischiorectal abscess requires immediate wide, local drainage after excision through an appropriate cruciform incision through the skin and subcutaneous tissue overlying the infected space. The cavity should be gently digitalized to break down loculations, and the pus should be cultured. Neglected abscesses can lead to devastating, necrotizing infections of the perineum that can spread with dramatic rapidity and be lethal.

Failure of response to local treatment or recurrent abscesses may suggest inadequate drainage with residual pus, the presence of a fistula, or immunoincompetence. Under these circumstances, antibiotics may be useful, together with examination under anesthesia after preliminary evaluation by computed tomography (CT) of the pelvis and perineum. For a horseshoe abscess, the deep postanal space should be drained through a posterior midline incision extending from the subcutaneous portion of the external sphincter over the abscess to the tip of the coccyx, separating the superficial external sphincter and thus unroofing the postnatal space and its ischioanal extension. Para-anal incisions are made to drain the anterior extensions of the abscess. A rubber seton is placed through the fistulous tract posteriorly around the internal sphincter and the lower portion of the external sphincter.[14]

Fistula in Ano

Anorectal sepsis can be complicated by a fistula in ano in about 25% of patients during the acute phase of sepsis or within 6 months thereafter.[15] Most fistulas derive from sepsis originating in the glands of the anal canal at the dentate line, and the path of the fistula is determined by the local anatomy. Most commonly, they track in the fascial or fatty planes, especially the intersphincteric space between the internal and external sphincters into the ischiorectal fascia. In such instances, the track passes directly to the perineal skin. In some instances, circumferential spread may occur in the ischiorectal fossa, with the track passing from one fossa to the contralateral one via the posterior rectum (a horseshoe fistula). Fistulas usually fall under four main anatomic categories as described by Parks and associates (Table 32–16).[29]

Intersphincteric fistulas constitute 70% of all fistulas in ano. In most cases, the infectious process passes directly downward to the anal margin, but there are some variants that are less common and more complex to treat. For instance, the track may travel upward in the rectal wall (higher track), with or without a perineal opening. Rarely, an intersphincteric fistula originates in the pelvis from the colon.[29] In *transsphincteric fistulas* (25%), the track traverses the external sphincter, passes through the ischiorectal fossa, and ends at the perineal skin. If it passes through the muscle at a low level, it is uncomplicated and readily treatable; if it penetrates the upper portion of the sphincter (high blind track), it presents a more difficult therapeutic dilemma. It may be felt digitally through the wall of the rectum and may lead the surgeon to create an artificial connection with the rectum by forceful probing, which can have disastrous consequences. *Suprasphincteric fistulas* are rare (4%) and difficult to treat and should not be dealt with by inexperienced surgeons. The track may first course upward in the intersphincteric plane before taking a lateral direction over the top of the puborectalis and finally downward through the ischiorectal fossa to the perineal skin. Since its trajectory is above all the muscles that are important to continence, division of all external muscles causes incontinence. Moreover, the fistula may have an additional extension into the pelvis that runs parallel to the rectum (high blind track). In this instance, an indurated area can be palpated through the rectal wall. Finally, *extrasphincteric fistulas* are fortunately very rare (1%), as their treatment is hazardous. The fistula travels from the perineal skin to the rectal wall above the levator ani that it pierces, and the track is completely outside the sphincteric apparatus. Causes include external or internal trauma (for instance, fish bone piercing one wall of rectum), carcinoma, and Crohn's disease. Treatment is difficult and lengthy and usually involves colostomy.

The fistula may first present as an acute abscess or simply as a draining sinus that irritates the perineal skin. On examination, subcutaneous induration may be traced from the external opening to the anal margin. Digital examination may reveal a palpable nodule in the wall of the anal canal, an indication of the primary source of infection. A probe can be eased gently (not forcefully) from the external skin opening to the internal anal canal opening.

Management of fistula in ano includes the following steps:

1. Accurate definition of the abnormal anatomy by palpation for induration, gentle probing, and partially laying open the defect to curet the excess granulation tissue.

2. Drainage of primary intersphincteric infection in all types of fistulas, as well as the primary track across the external sphincter and secondary tracks within the anorectal fossa. Suprasphincteric and extrasphincteric fistulas should be referred to specialists.[37]

3. Close follow-up and careful nursing of the wound by a doctor-nurse team. Sitz baths and wound irrigation and packing ensure healing from the depth of the wound to the surface. A seton of monofilament nylon tied loosely around the fistulous track may be used to drain the transsphincteric track traveling above the anal valves for suprasphincteric fistula.[13] It can be removed 2 to 3 months later, at which time the track may heal spontaneously. If not, the track may be divided, since fibrosis can cause minimal separation of the cut ends. Failure of the track to heal may be due to residual infection, which may require examination under anesthesia; excess granulation tissue, which may need to be cauterized with silver nitrate or cureted; or ingrowth of hair due to lack of shaving.[37] Crohn's disease should also be excluded. A difficult and persistent high fistula can be treated by a sliding flap advancement made of mucosa, submucosa, and circular muscle to cover the internal opening.[13] Goodsall's rule is often helpful but is of little help in defining the anatomy of complex fistulas (Fig. 32–53).

Crohn's Disease of the Anorectum

Anal manifestations of Crohn's disease can be devastating because of their painful nature and their threat to the patient's continence.[1] They may occur in nearly 20% of patients with this disease. Patients may suffer from fissures, fistulas, and abscesses. Symptoms and signs of anal Crohn's disease include pain, swelling, bleeding, soilage or frank incontinence, and fever. Pain may be due to skin excoriation and maceration, hemorrhoids, fissures, or abscess-fistula disease.[1] Edematous purplish tags are characteristic of the disease. Bleeding may be from distal proctitis, fissures, hemorrhoids, or granulating fistulas. Soilage may follow prolapsing rectal mucosa, seepage of liquid stool, drainage from abscess, or poor continence. The latter may result from sphincter damage caused by the disease or an aggressive procedure, anoperineal fistulas, rectovaginal fistulas, or loss of rectal

---

TABLE 32–16. Classification of the Anorectal Fistulas

Intersphincteric (the most common): the fistula track is confined to the intersphincteric plane

Transsphinteric: the fistula connects the intersphincteric plane with the ischiorectal fossa by perforating the external sphincter

Suprasphincteric: similar to transsphincteric, but the track loops over the external sphincter and perforates the levator ani

Extrasphincteric: the track passes from the rectum to perineal skin, completely external to the sphincteric complex

Based on the classification by Parks, A. G., Gordon, P. H., and Hardcastle, J. E.: A classification of fistula-in-ano. Br. J. Surg., *63*:1, 1976; with permission of Blackwell Science Ltd.

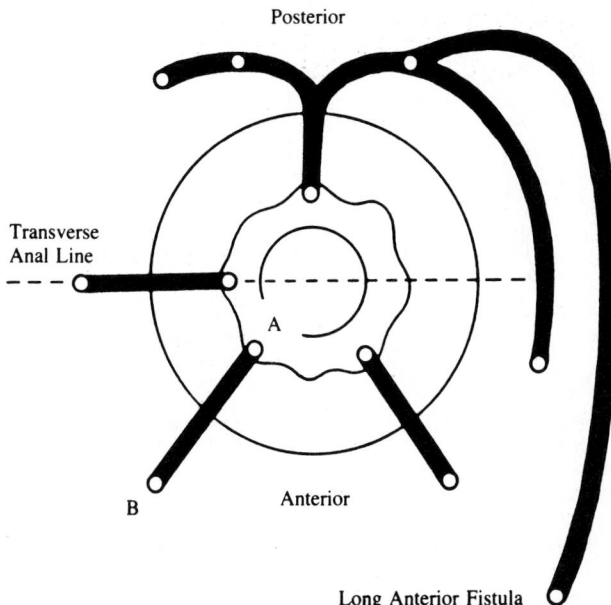

Figure 32–53. Goodsall's rule. The usual relationship of primary and secondary fistula orifices is diagrammed. The internal (primary) orifice is marked A. The rule predicts that if a line is drawn transversely across the anus, an external opening (B) anterior to this line will lead to a straight radial tract, whereas an external opening that lies posterior to the line will lead to a curved tract and an internal opening in the posterior commissure. The long anterior fistula is an exception to the rule. (From Schrock, T. R.: Benign and malignant disease of the anorectum. *In* Fromm, O. [Eds.]: Gastrointestinal Surgery. New York, Churchill Livingstone, 1985.)

compliance.[1] Anorectal examination should include inspection, digital examination, anoscopy, and proctosigmoidoscopy. If the examination cannot be performed satisfactorily due to pain, the patient should be evaluated under anesthesia. The remainder of the gastrointestinal tract should also be assessed. Although conservatism is paramount, patients should not be undertreated if treatment is indicated. Surgical therapy is usually warranted for pain due to a poorly draining or undrained abscess. Fissures are often located atypically off the midline and usually respond to conservative measures such as sitz baths, stool softeners, and oral analgesics. Occasionally, excision of skin tags surrounding deep ulcers to favor better drainage and gentle stretch may be sufficient. Sphincterotomy and fissurectomy should be avoided. Metronidazole and immunosuppressive drugs such as steroids, 6-mercaptopurine, azathioprine, and cyclosporine have produced mixed results.[1] In some patients, a proctectomy may ultimately be required. The dissection should be done in the intersphincteric plane to favor better perineal healing and help reduce the risk of sexual dysfunction.

Neoplastic Disorders

Neoplasms of the anal area are rare and represent a wide spectrum of benign and malignant tumors. Benign lesions range from innocuous *in situ* Bowen's disease to clinically aggressive verrucous lesions. Malignant lesions range from favorable early-stage squamous cell cancers of the anal margin to anal canal adenocarcinoma and melanoma.[23] In all instances, it is essential for clinicians to consider the location of the tumor with reference to clear landmarks such as anal verge, dentate line, and anorectal ring.

Preoperative assessment should include a complete history and physical examination. The nature and duration of local anal symptoms such as a mass, bleeding, and pruritus and distant manifestations such as weight loss should be docu-

mented. The perianal area should be closely inspected for skin alterations. Digital examination helps establish the location, mobility, or fixity of the tumor, as well as the integrity of the sphincter mechanism. Anoscopy or rigid proctosigmoidoscopy verifies the size and location of the tumor in relationship to the dentate line, anal verge, or anorectal ring. A systemic search for organomegaly and groin adenopathy, as well as CT, is important when evaluating a malignant lesion.

Anal Margin Tumors

Bowen's disease is an *in situ* intraepithelial squamous cell carcinoma that rarely (5%) invades or metastasizes.[23] Most patients are asymptomatic or have minor complaints such as burning or pruritus. The perianal skin may be erythematous and thickened, with fissuring, brown-red plaques, or nodules, or it may appear normal. Multiple punch biopsies can establish the diagnosis. Women should be evaluated for concomitant genital disorders. Wide local excision with clear surgical margins confirmed by frozen sections, with either primary closure or V-Y advancement flaps, is the treatment of choice. Patients who have invasion of the sphincter should be considered for abdominoperineal resection. Postoperative follow-up is imperative to detect recurrent disease or development of invasive disease.

Paget's Disease

Extramammary Paget's disease of the anus is a rare intraepithelial adenocarcinoma. Unlike Bowen's disease, it is more common in older patients, is associated with an underlying carcinoma in 50% to 86%, and has a poor prognosis.[23] The typical appearance of Paget's disease is that of well-demarcated eczematoid plaques with whitish-gray ulcerations or papillary lesions.[23] The diagnosis is confirmed by microscopy. Treatment is based on the local extent of the disease and on the presence or absence of underlying malignancies. Limited Paget's disease can be widely excised and the defect closed primarily or with V-Y advancement flaps. Biopsies of the proximal anal canal and distal anal skin margins help map the extent of resection.[23] Patients with underlying rectal adenocarcinoma should undergo abdominoperineal resection, and those with epidermoid anal canal cancer can be treated with combined radiation and chemotherapy.[24] Following the procedure, patients should be monitored closely for recurrence.

Basal Cell Carcinoma

This type of anal canal tumor is very rare. Macroscopically, these lesions have the same pearly borders with a central depression that other basal cell cancers of the skin have. On occasion, it may be difficult to differentiate a cloacogenic (or basaloid) carcinoma arising in the transitional zone from a basal cell cancer arising in the anal skin. The distinction is critical because of the dramatic behavioral difference and is based on location as well as histologic features.[23] Most often, these tumors can be treated adequately by wide local excision, reserving abdominoperineal resection for extensive lesions.[23]

Squamous Cell Carcinoma

Although their oncologic behavior resembles that of skin tumors elsewhere, their location causes site-specific symptoms such as a mass, chronic pruritus, bleeding, pain, and associated fistulas and condylomata.[23] Wide local excision is recommended for early anal margin squamous cell carcinoma, with excellent results.[6] Recurrences can be managed

Operative view

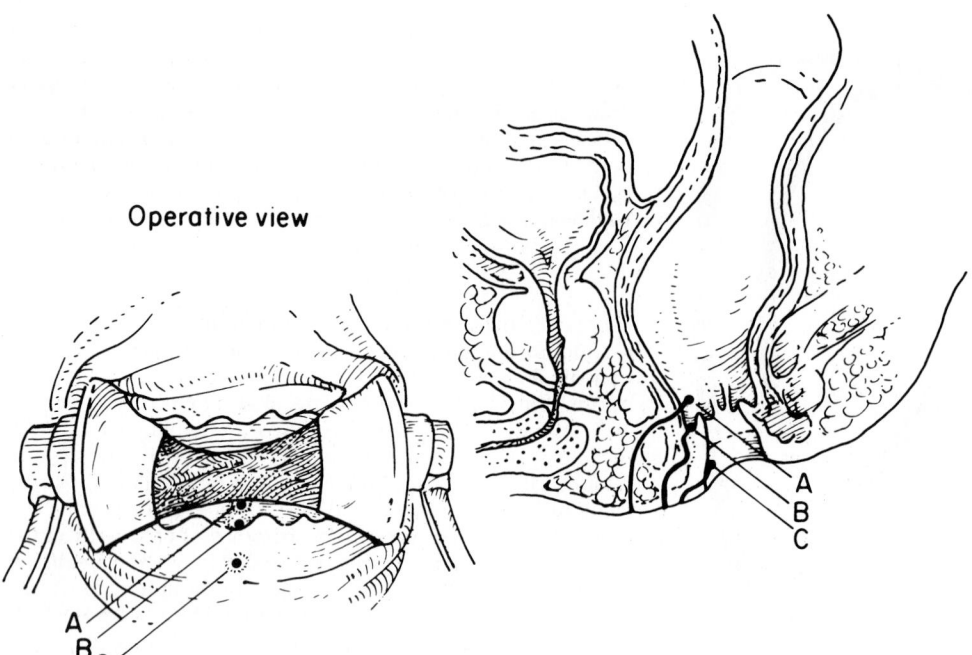

Figure 32–54. Relationship of fistulous tracts in Crohn's disease above the dentate line (A); cryptoglandular abscess-fistula disease at the dentate line (B); and hidradenitis suppurativa distal to the dentate line (C). (From Culp, C. E.: Chronic hidradenitis suppurativa of the anal canal: A surgical skin disease. Dis. Colon Rectum, *26*:669–676, 1983. By permission of Mayo Foundation.)

by re-excision or preferably by abdominoperineal resection, especially if locally advanced.

Verrucous Carcinoma

Verrucous carcinoma, also referred to as giant condyloma acuminatum or Buschke-Löwenstein tumor, is poorly defined and is best considered an intermediate lesion between condyloma acuminatum and invasive squamous cell carcinoma, based on their common human papillomavirus etiology.[23] The large, wartlike lesions are soft and slow growing. They may fistulize, become infected, and undergo malignant transformation.[23] Radical wide local excision or abdominoperineal resection is recommended. A poor prognosis can be expected for tumors progressing to invasive squamous cell carcinoma, although some respond favorably to combined radiation and chemotherapy.

Anal Canal Neoplasms

Tumors arising in the anal canal or in the transitional zone that have a squamous, basaloid, cloacogenic, or mucoepidermoid epithelium share a similar clinical presentation, response to treatment, and prognosis[23] and are considered collectively. They typically present as a mass, sometimes with bleeding and pruritus. At the time of diagnosis, 50% are less than 3 cm. in size, and the rest are larger.[23] Nearly a quarter are superficial or *in situ*.[23] In the past, treatment modalities included either surgery alone or radiation alone. Patients with tumors confined to epithelial or subepithelial tissue have been treated by local excision, and patients with more advanced lesions by abdominoperineal resection.[7] The introduction of multimodality therapy, combining radiation and chemotherapy, promised to preserve continence, avoid colostomy, and offer similar survival advantages. In keeping with this concept, local excision alone remains a good option for superficial, early-stage lesions, which have been associated with survivorship ranging from 61% to 87% and, in at least one study, 100% if the lesion was less than 2 cm.[7] Variations in survival and rate of recurrence may be related at least in part to bias in patient selection. Patients with lesions greater

than 2 cm. with any suggestion of fixation or sphincter involvement on digital examination or anal ultrasonography should not be treated by local excision. Thus, the majority of patients who are not candidates for local excision are best treated by combined chemotherapy and radiation therapy (Table 32–17).

Combined modality therapy has evolved as the preferred alternative to radical surgical procedures, since, in theory, surgical mortality and morbidity are largely avoided and survival rates compare favorably with those for operation. Several questions remain unanswered, however, including whether radiation alone could be as effective as radiation plus chemotherapy; whether lesions greater than 5 cm. are better treated by primary abdominoperineal resection; what the long-term morbidity of combined chemoradiation is, including the need for later colostomy; and whether mitomycin C is necessary, considering its toxic effects, including death.[23] Refinements in multimodality therapy for anal canal cancers no doubt will be the focus of future studies.

Melanoma

Melanomas involving the anal canal can produce a mass, pain, or bleeding and are not infrequently lacking pigmentation. Overall, the outlook for patients with such tumors is quite poor, with 5-year survival hovering around 10% or less.[23] Survival depends on the stage of the disease. In gen-

TABLE 32–17. Chemoradiation Therapy for Anal Cancer

External irradiation: 3000 cGy. to primary tumor and pelvic and inguinal nodes. Start day 1 (200 cGy./day)
Systemic chemotherapy:
1. 5-fluorouracil: 1000 mg./sq. m. for 24 hours as a continuous infusion for 4 days. Start day 1.
2. Mitomycin C: 15 mg./sq. m. intravenous bolus. Day 1 only.
3. 5-fluorouracil: Repeat 4-day infusion. Start day 28.

From Nigro, N. D., Vaitkevicius, V. K., and Considine, B., Jr.: Dynamic management of squamous cell cancer of the anal canal. Invest. New Drugs, 7:83, 1989.

eral, survival is poor whether the surgical procedure is conservative or radical. Abdominoperineal resection seems reasonable for advanced lesions if complete resection and palliation are to be achieved. It should also be noted that the only 5-year survivors have been patients who have undergone abdominoperineal resection for early lesions.[38] Prophylactic inguinal node dissection offers no benefit.

Adenocarcinoma

Adenocarcinoma of the anal canal is rare. Such tumors originate from anal ducts and are often extramucosal in location. Because of their rarity, their diagnosis is frequently delayed. Like melanoma, the tumor is occasionally found incidentally during hemorrhoidectomy. Whether the tumor is locally excised or widely removed by abdominoperineal resection, the prognosis is poor.[23]

Other Tumors

Connective tissue sarcomas such as leiomyosarcoma, rhabdomyosarcoma, and myoblastoma are rare.[31] Lymphoma of the anus is quite unusual. Carcinoid tumors occasionally originate from anal canal endocrine cells, and abdominoperineal resection may be required, especially for those exceeding 2 cm.[37]

Other Disorders

Hidradenitis suppurativa is an inflammatory process affecting the apocrine glands of the region, characterized by abscesses and sinus formation. Affected individuals frequently have seborrheic skin and may have involvement of other areas where apocrine sweat glands are present, such as the axillary, mammary, inguinal, and genital regions. Patients complain of burning, itching, and hyperhidrosis. The affected areas have a purplish appearance, with drainage of watery pus. The condition must be differentiated from cryptoglandular fistulas, which communicate with the dentate line, and Crohn's disease, which may track to the anorectum proximal to the dentate line (Fig. 32–54). Treatment consists of unroofing of sinuses in limited disease and wide local excision in more advanced disease.[8]

Condyloma acuminatum, or perianal warts, is characterized by multiple papillary acanthotic and parakeratotic growths involving the perianal region, the external genitals, and, at times, the anal canal itself. The causative agent is believed to be an autoinoculable and transmissible papillomavirus.[37] The prevalence in the anorectal and urogenital regions points toward a sexual mode of transmission, and the lesions occur with greatest frequency in male homosexuals. Thus, other focuses of sexually transmitted diseases (STDs) should be excluded. If few lesions are present, local applications of podophyllin are sufficient; when the condition is extensive, electrocoagulation or laser therapy of small lesions is effective, but larger lesions or massive involvement may require surgical excision under general anesthesia. Immunotherapy has produced an impressive cure rate of greater than 90%.[2]

A history of sexual preference and promiscuity provides clues to several STDs and HIV infection.[34] Gastrointestinal manifestations of STDs may be found from the mouth to the anus, and HIV-infected patients can be expected to acquire other opportunistic infections. Patients, especially homosexual men, may have colitis, proctitis, or proctocolitis. Amebiasis, giardiasis, and shigellosis are common causes of enteritis. Smears should be obtained as part of the endoscopic evaluation for Gram's stain and culture, looking for *Neisseria gonorrhoeae*, *Chlamydia trachomatis*, *Treponema pallidum*, and herpesvirus Type 2.[34] A discrete ulcer on the genitals, the perianal

skin, or the anorectum should alert the examiner to consider syphilis, chancroid, herpes, and lymphogranuloma venereum. A mass should suggest possibilities such as abscess, lymphoma, Kaposi's sarcoma, and anal carcinoma.

Disorders of the anorectum are frequent in those with AIDS,[39] including abscess or fistula and, less often, neoplasia such as Kaposi's sarcoma, lymphoma, Bowen's disease, and epidermoid carcinoma. The main focus of treatment includes drainage, biopsy, fistulotomy, and local excision.[39]

SELECTED REFERENCES

Block, G. E., and Moossa, A. R. (Eds.): Operative Colorectal Surgery. Philadelphia, W. B. Saunders, 1994.
Well-illustrated compendium of the various surgical procedures commonly used in colon and rectal surgery, including the anorectal area, by well-known surgeons. Each chapter is supplemented by the editors' views.

Gordon, P. H.: Anorectal abscesses and fistula-in-ano. *In* Gordon, P. H., and Nivatvongs, S. (Eds.): Principles and Practice of Surgery for the Colon, Rectum and Anus. St. Louis, Quality Medical Publishers, 1992.
Comprehensive and detailed review of this complex subject by an expert in the field. The illustrations are particularly useful for understanding the various types of abscesses and fistulas and their trajectories.

Nelson, H., and Dozois, R. R.: Anal neoplasms. Perspect. Colon Rectal Surg., 7:16, 1994.
The most recent review of these rare tumors, focusing on the debated aspects of treatment. The review is supplemented by expert commentary by Stuart Quan, an authority in the field.

REFERENCES

1. Abcarian, H.: Perianal Crohn's disease. Semin. Colon Rectal Surg., 5:210, 1994.
2. Abcarian, H., and Sharon, N.: The effectiveness of immunotherapy in the treatment of anal condyloma acuminatum. J. Surg. Res., 22:231, 1977.
3. Ambroze, W. L., Pemberton, J. H., Dozois, R. R., and Carpenter, H. A.: Does retaining the anal transition zone (ATZ) fail to extirpate chronic ulcerative colitis (CUC) after ileal-pouch anal anastomosis (IPAA)? Dis. Colon Rectum, 34:P20, 1991.
4. Bartolo, D. C. C., Roe, A. M., Lock-Edmunds, J. C., Virjee, J., and Mortensen, M. J.: Flap-valve theory of anorectal continence. Br. J. Surg., 73:1012, 1986.
5. Beart, R. W., Dozois, R. R., Wolff, B. G., and Pemberton, J. H.: Mechanisms of rectal continence: Lessons from the ileoanal procedure. Am. J. Surg., 149:31, 1985.
6. Beahrs, O. H., and Wilson, S. M.: Carcinoma of the anus. Ann. Surg., 184:422, 1976.
7. Boman, B. M., Moertel, C. G., O'Connell, M. J., Scott, M., Weiland, L. H., Beart, R. W., Gunderson, L. L., and Spencer, R. J.: Carcinoma of the anal canal: A clinical and pathologic study of 188 cases. Cancer, 54:114, 1984.
8. Culp, C. E.: Chronic hidradenitis suppurativa of the anal canal: A surgical skin disease. Dis. Colon Rectum, 26:669, 1983.
9. Dozois, R. R., and Nivatvongs, S.: Prolapse of the rectum. *In* Block, G. E., and Moossa, A. R. (Eds.): Operative Colorectal Surgery. Philadelphia, W. B. Saunders, 1994.
10. Ferrara, A., Pemberton, J. H., Levin, K. E., and Hanson, R. B.: Relationship between anal canal tone and rectal motor activity. Dis. Colon Rectum, 36:337, 1993.
11. Fozard, J. B. J., and Pemberton, J. H.: Applied surgical anatomy: Pelvic contents. *In* Fielding, L. P., and Goldberg, S. M. (Eds.): Rob and Smith's Operative Surgery: Surgery of the Colon, Rectum and Anus, 5th ed. London, Chapman and Hall Medical, 1994.
12. Gordon, P. H.: Anal incontinence. *In* Gordon, P. H., and Nivatvongs, S. (Eds.): Principles and Practice of Surgery for the Colon, Rectum and Anus. St. Louis, Quality Medical Publishers, 1992.
13. Gordon, P. H.: Anorectal abscesses and fistula-in-ano. *In* Gordon, P. H., and Nivatvongs, S. (Eds.): Principles and Practice of Surgery for the Colon, Rectum and Anus. St. Louis, Quality Medical Publishers, 1992.
14. Hanley, P. H., Ray, J. E., Pennington, E. E., and Grablowsky, O. M. Fistula-in-ano: A ten-year follow-up study of horseshoe-abscess fistula-in-ano. Dis. Colon Rectum, 19:507, 1976.
15. Henrichsen, S., and Christiansen, J.: Incidence of fistula-in-ano complicating anorectal sepsis: A prospective study. Br. J. Surg., 73:371, 1986.
16. Jensen, S. L.: Treatment of first episodes of acute anal fissure: Prospective randomized study of lignocaine ointment versus hydrocortisone ointment or warm sitz baths plus bran. Br. Med. J., 292:1167, 1986.
17. Keighley, M. R. B., Fielding, J. W., and Alexander-Williams, J.: Results of Marlex mesh abdominal rectopexy for rectal prolapse in 100 consecutive patients. Br. J. Surg., 70:229, 1983.
18. Keighley, M. R. B., and Matheson, D. M.: Results of treatment for rectal prolapse and fecal incontinence. Dis. Colon Rectum, 24:449, 1981.

19. Kerremans, R.: Morphological and Physiological Aspects of Anal Continence and Defecation. Brussels, Arscia, Ultgavon, 1969.

20. Kuijpers, H. C.: Is there really sphincter spasm in anal fissure? Dis. Colon Rectum, 26:493, 1983.

21. Laurberg, S., Swash, M., and Henry, M. M.: Delayed external sphincter repair for obstetric tear. Br. J. Surg., 75:786, 1988.

22. Lee, S. J., Meagher, A., and Pemberton, J. H.: Structure and function of the lower gastrointestinal tract. In Saclarides, T., and Brubaker, L. (Eds.): The Female Pelvic Floor—Disorders of Function and Support. In press.

23. Nelson, H., and Dozois, R. R.: Anal neoplasms. Perspect. Colon Rectal Surg., 7:16, 1994.

24. Nigro, N. D., Vaitkevicius, V. K., and Considine, B., Jr.: Dynamic management of squamous cell cancer of the anal canal. Invest. New Drugs, 7:83, 1989.

25. Nivatvongs, S.: Hemorrhoids. In Gordon, P. H., and Nivatvongs, S. (Eds.): Principles and Practice of Surgery for the Colon, Rectum and Anus. St. Louis, Quality Medical Publishers, 1992.

26. Nivatvongs, S., and Gordon, P. H.: Surgical anatomy. In Gordon, P. H., and Nivatvongs, S. (Eds.): Principles and Practice of Surgery for the Colon, Rectum and Anus. St. Louis, Quality Medical Publishers, 1992.

27. Parks, A. G.: Anorectal incontinence. Proc. R. Soc. Med., 68:681, 1975.

28. Parks, A. G.: Pathogenesis of fistula-in-ano. Br. Med. J., 1:463, 1961.

29. Parks, A. G., Gordon, P. H., and Hardcastle, J. D.: A classification of fistula-in-ano. Br. J. Surg., 63:1, 1976.

30. Parks, A. G., Swash, M., and Urich, H.: Sphincter denervation in anorectal incontinence and rectal prolapse. Gut, 18:656, 1977.

31. Randleman, C. D., Jr., Wolff, B. G., Dozois, R. R., Spencer, R. J., Weiland, L. H., and Ilstrup, D. M.: Leiomyosarcoma of the rectum and anus: A series of 22 cases. Int. J. Colorectal Dis., 4:91, 1989.

32. Scheuer, M., Kuijpers, H. C., and Jacobs, P. P.: Postanal repair restores anatomy rather than function. Dis. Colon Rectum, 32:960, 1989.

33. Shemesh, E. I., Kodner, I. J., Fry, R. D., et al.: Severe complication of rubber band ligation of internal hemorrhoids. Dis. Colon Rectum, 30:199, 1987.

34. Smith, L. E.: Sexually transmitted diseases. In Gordon, P. H., and Nivatvongs, S. (Eds.): Principles and Practice of Surgery for the Colon, Rectum and Anus. St. Louis, Quality Medical Publishers, 1992.

35. Theuerkauf, F. J., Jr., Beahrs, O. H., and Hill, J. R.: Rectal prolapse: Causation and surgical treatment. Ann. Surg., 171:819, 1970.

36. Thompson, W. H. F.: The nature of hemorrhoids. Br. J. Surg., 62:542, 1975.

37. Thomson, J. P. S., and Akwari, O. E.: Disorders of the anal canal. In Sabiston, D. S. (Ed.): Textbook of Surgery: The Biological Basis of Modern Surgical Practice, 14th ed. Philadelphia, W. B. Saunders, 1991.

38. Wanebo, H., Woodruff, J. M., Farr, G. H., and Quan, S. H.: Anorectal melanoma. Cancer, 47:1891, 1981.

39. Wexner, S. D., Smithy, W. B., Milson, J. W., and Dailey, T. H.: The surgical management of anorectal diseases in AIDS and pre-AIDS patients. Dis. Colon Rectum, 29:719, 1986.

40. Wolff, B. G., and Culp, C. E.: The Whitehead hemorrhoidectomy: An unjustly maligned procedure. Dis. Colon Rectum, 31:587, 1988.

CHAPTER 33

THE LIVER

William C. Meyers, M.D.

DEVELOPMENT OF HEPATOBILIARY SURGERY

Surgeons have learned to operate successfully on the liver primarily during the past three decades. For centuries, the liver was a mysterious organ with complex anatomy, an overwhelming number of functions, and an extraordinary capability to regenerate. The organ's large size and abundant blood supply contributed to the respect paid to this organ in most civilizations and operating theaters. Improved understanding of anatomy and physiology, combined with a number of recently developed surgical techniques, led from myth and mystery to the emergence of the specialty of hepatobiliary surgery.

Laparoscopic cholecystectomy rivals Langenbuch's contribution of the open technique (he performed the first successful cholecystectomy in 1882) with respect to surgical importance. Not only has laparoscopic cholecystectomy opened the field to other new procedures, laparoscopic surgery has contributed greatly to present interest in shortened hospital stays, lessened costs, and the rethinking of surgical dogma such as wide exposure.

The development of hepatobiliary surgery culminates in the rise and increased safety of hepatic resections and liver transplantation. A large number of hepatic resections are performed by specialized surgeons in major centers. The mortality of elective resection has decreased from 20% two decades ago to less than 1%. This increased safety follows improved technology and understanding of the anatomy and physiology of the liver. With improved safety has come an increased confidence in liver surgery, a wide expansion of the indications for resection, and development of other aggressive procedures such as cryoablation and chemoembolization. The most common indication for partial liver resection in most centers remains neoplasia.

A spectacular advance in hepatic surgery and hepatic therapy in general has been the success of liver transplantation. Welch performed the first experimental liver transplant in 1955 using a heterotopic technique in dogs, but the procedure was abandoned because of difficulties in maintaining vascular inflow and adequate biliary drainage. In 1959, Moore and Starzl independently achieved successful orthotopic liver transplantation in dogs, the same year that Kasai and Suzuki reported the first hepatoportoenterostomy for biliary atresia. The first human liver transplant was performed by Starzl in 1963. Subsequently, Starzl and Calne developed large series of liver transplants. Other important advances in transplantation include identification of the immunosuppression characteristics of cyclosporine by Borel in 1972 and the clinical trials of newer agents such as tacrolimus (FK506) in the 1990s. An important achievement, which combined the advances in hepatic resection and transplantation, was the successful transplantation of the left lateral segment from a live parent to a child, performed in 1989 at the University of Chicago by Broelsch and Emond. Success with monitoring human life using a pig liver suggests there is great promise for xenotransplantation, perhaps with transgenic livers.

It is interesting to note the exchange of roles surgery and medicine have had in the treatment of hepatobiliary disorders over the past two decades. The development of endoscopic and endosurgical approaches has radically changed the treatment of gallstones. Many of the traditional medical disorders such as cirrhosis and metabolic deficiencies are being treated by liver transplantation. The development of minimally invasive techniques for hepatobiliary diseases raises important new questions with respect to the definition of surgery. It is likely the next decade will see consolidated educational programs for the training of physicians and surgeons in this field. A unified International Hepato-Pancreato-Biliary Association has led to the development of the American Hepato-Pancreato-Biliary Association (AHPBA), which promotes a union of surgeons, gastroenterologists, radiologists, and other specialists who work within this dynamic field.

SELECTED REFERENCES

Beal, J. M.: Historical perspective of gallstone disease. Surg. Gynecol. Obstet., *158*:181, 1984.
The surgical aspects of gallstone disease are detailed.

Chen, T. S., and Chen, P. S.: Understanding the Liver, a History. Westport, CT, Greenwood Press, 1984.
This remarkable book on the development of hepatology examines in detail the historical aspects of the understanding of anatomy, physiology, and diseases pertinent to hepatobiliary surgery.

Meyers, W. C., and Jones, R. S.: Development of liver and biliary surgery. In Meyers, W. C., and Jones, R. S. (Eds.): Textbook of Liver and Biliary Surgery. Philadelphia, J. B. Lippincott, 1990.
Details on many of the historical aspects of hepatobiliary surgery are included.

Robinson, J. O.: Silvergirl's Surgery: Biliary Tract. Austin, TX, Silvergirl, 1985.
Some of the key historical, original articles in hepatobiliary surgery are reproduced in this work.

Starzl, T. E., Iwatsuki, S., Van Thiel, D. H., et al.: Evolution of liver transplantation. Hepatology, 2:614, 1982.
A historical review of liver transplantation is presented by the surgeon and his colleagues who have contributed the most.

REFERENCES

1. Admirand, W. H., and Small, D. M.: The physiochemical basis of cholesterol gallstone formation in man. J. Clin. Invest., *47*:1043, 1968.
2. Beck, J.: Surgery of the liver. JAMA, *78*:1063, 1902.
3. Bengmark, S.: Progress in Surgery of the Liver, Pancreas and Biliary System. Dordrecht, Martinus Nijhoff, 1988.
4. Bernard, C.: Sur le mécanisme de la formation du sucre dans le foie. Compt. Rend., *41*:461, 1855.
5. Budd, G.: Diseases of the Liver. Philadelphia, Blanchard & Lea, 1853.
6. Cahill, K. M.: Platonic concepts of hepatology. Arch. Intern. Med., *111*:819, 1963.
7. Calne, R. Y., and Williams, R.: Survival after orthotopic liver transplantation: A follow-up report of two patients. Br. Med. J., *3*:436, 1970.
8. Cantlie, J.: On a new arrangement of the right and left lobes of the liver. J. Anat. Physiol. (Lond.), *32*:iv, 1877.
9. Celsus, A.: De Medicina, Books I, II, IV, and VII. Spencer, W. G. (Trans.). Cambridge, MA, Loeb Classical Library, Harvard University Press, 1935.
10. Chakravorty, R. C., and Wanebo, H. J.: Historic preamble: Liver and biliary cancer. In Wanebo, H. J. (Ed.): Hepatic and Biliary Cancer. New York, Marcel Dekker, 1987.
11. Charcot, J. M.: Leçons sur les Maladies du Foie, des Voies Biliaires, et des Reins. Paris, Progress Medical, 1877.

12. Chari, R. S., Collins, B. H., Magee, J. C., et al.: Brief report: Treatment of hepatic failure with *ex vivo* pig-liver perfusion followed by liver transplantation. N. Engl. J. Med., *331*:234, 1994.
13. Couinaud, C.: Bases anatomiques des hepatectomies gauche et droite réglées, techniques que en deroulent. J. Chir. Paris, *70*:933, 1954.
14. Disse, J.: Über die Lymphbahnen der Saugetierleber. Arch. Mikr. Anat., *36*:203, 1890.
15. Donovan, A. J., and Covey, P. C.: Early history of the portacaval shunt in humans. Surg. Gynecol. Obstet., *147*:423, 1978.
16. Eck, N. V.: The question of ligature of the portal vein. Voen. Med. Zh. (St. Petersburg), 130:1877. Translated into English in Child, C. G.: Eck's fistula. Surg. Gynecol. Obstet., *96*:375, 1953.
17. Frerichs, F. T.: A Clinical Treatise on Diseases of the Liver, Vols. I and II. Murchinson, C. (Trans). London, New Sydenham Society, 1860–1861.
18. Glenn, F.: Biliary tract disease since antiquity. Acad. Med. Bull. N. Y., *47*:329, 1971.
19. Glenn, F., and Grafe, W. R., Jr.: Historical events in biliary tract surgery. Arch. Surg., *93*:848, 1966.
20. Glisson, F.: Anatomie Hepatis. Amsterdam, Ravesteyn, 1659. Cited in Heaton, K. W. (Ed.): Bile Salts in Health and Disease. Edinburgh, Churchill Livingstone, 1972.
21. Goldsmith, N. A., and Woodburne, R. T.: The surgical anatomy pertaining to liver resections. Surg. Gynecol. Obstet., *105*:310, 1957.
22. Healey, J. E., Jr., and Schroy, P. C.: Anatomy of the biliary ducts within the human liver. Arch. Surg., *66*:599, 1953.
23. Hjortsjo, C. H.: The topography of the intrahepatic duct systems. Acta Anat. (Basel), *11*:599, 1951.
24. Jastrow, M.: The Liver in Antiquity and the Beginnings of Anatomy. Philadelphia, Transactions of the College of Physicians, 1907.
25. Keen, W. W.: On resection of the liver. Boston Med. Surg. J., *126*:405, 1892.
26. Kiernan, F.: The Anatomy and Physiology of the Liver. Phil. Trans., 1833.
27. Kupffer, C. von: Über Sternzellen der Leber. Arch. Mikr. Anat., *12*:353, 1876.
28. Langenbuch, C.: Ein Fall von Extirpation der Gallenblase wegen chronischer Cholelithiasis. Berlin Clin. Wochenschr., *48*:725, 1882.
29. Mall, F. P.: A study of the structural unit of the liver. Am. J. Anat., *5*:2270, 1906.
30. Moore, F. D., et al.: One-stage homotransplantation of the liver following total hepatectomy in dogs. Transplant. Bull., *6*:103, 1959.
31. Rappaport, A. M.: The structural and functional units in the human liver (liver acinus). Anat. Rec., *130*:673, 1958.
32. Rex, H.: Beitrage zur Morphologie der Saugerleber. Morphol. Jahrb. (Leipzig), *14*:517, 1888.
33. Rokitansky, C.: A Manual of Pathological Anatomy. Sieveking, E. (Trans.). Philadelphia, Blanchard & Lea, 1855.
34. Singer, C.: A Short History of Anatomy and Physiology from the Greeks to Harvey. New York, Dover, 1975.
35. Starzl, T. E., et al.: Homotransplantation of the liver in humans. Surg. Gynecol. Obstet., *117*:659, 1963.
36. The Southern Surgeons Club: A prospective analysis of 1518 laparoscopic cholecystectomies. N. Engl. J. Med., *324*:1073, 1991.
37. Trendelenburg, F.: Die ersten 25 Jahre der deutschen Gesellschaft für Chirurgie. Berlin, Springer, 1923.
38. Warren, W. D., et al.: Selective trans-splenic decompression of gastroesophageal varices by distal splenorenal shunt. Ann. Surg., *166*:437, 1967.
39. Young, F. G.: Claude Bernard and the discovery of glycogen: A century of retrospect. BMJ, *1*:1431, 1957.
40. Young, J.: Malpighi. N. Z. Med. J., *20*:1, 1921.

I

ANATOMY AND PHYSIOLOGY

William C. Meyers, M.D., and Ravi S. Chari, M.D.

ANATOMY

Modern concepts of gross hepatobiliary anatomy differ considerably from the anatomy suggested by the ligamentous reflections of the peritoneum, particularly the falciform ligament. For centuries the *right* lobe of the liver was defined as all the hepatic parenchyma to the right of the falciform ligament and the *left* lobe as only the substance to the left of the ligament. There are now two new classifications of the gross anatomy that have much more applicability to surgery. The first is the lobar system used most frequently in the United States and often called the American System. The second is the French segmental system, which has the most applicability.

Anatomic features that enable the liver to be an important integrator between the digestive system and the rest of the body include (1) a dual blood supply, with portal blood from the splanchnic system and the hepatic artery; (2) a specific architectural arrangement of single cells and cell masses that facilitates exchange between blood and hepatocytes; (3) a specific orientation of the hepatocytes that compartmentalizes biliary versus blood pathways; and (4) an organized biliary excretory system that regulates the enterohepatic circulation. In this section aspects of the anatomic organization of the liver are considered that are important for both hepatic physiology and surgery.

Gross Anatomy

General Description

The liver lies in the right upper quadrant of the abdomen, beneath the diaphragm and connected to the digestive tract by means of the portal vein and the biliary drainage system.

The largest gland in the body, it weighs approximately 1500 gm. in the adult (Fig. 33–1). The liver accounts for 2% of the body weight of the adult and about 5% of the body weight of a newborn. Hepatic extramedullary hematopoiesis produces the relatively larger liver size in newborns. The normal adult liver resides under the protective rib cage. It extends in the midclavicular line from as high as the fourth intercostal space down to slightly below the costal margin. The gallblad-

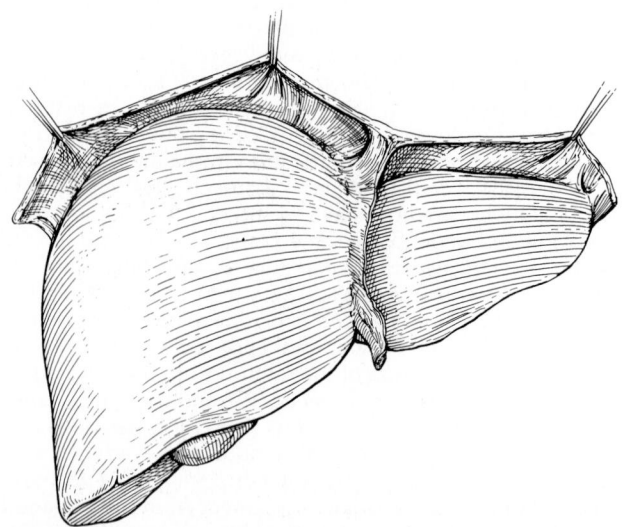

Figure 33–1. The anterior surface of the liver as viewed in the peritoneal cavity. Whereas the falciform ligament is the primary topographic landmark, the true anatomic left and right lobes are approximately determined by an anteroposterior plane through the gallbladder and vena cava.

der lies on the dorsal surface of the liver in a transpyloric plane. A peritoneal membrane (Glisson's capsule) covers the liver and extends as fibrous septa into the parenchyma with blood vessels and bile ducts. The superior surface of the liver conforms to the undersurface of the right diaphragm. Only the liver to the left of the falciform ligament contacts the left diaphragm. The inferior surface of the liver touches the duodenum, colon, kidney, adrenal gland, esophagus, and stomach. Peritoneum invests the entire liver except for a *bare* area under the diaphragm on the posterosuperior surface adjacent to the inferior vena cava and hepatic vein.

Normal Development

The liver primordium appears at about the third week as a ventral thickening of the entoderm at the distal end of the foregut (future duodenum). The major portion of this primordium produces hepatic parenchyma and the main bile duct. A secondary caudal proliferation will become the gallbladder and cystic duct. The hepatic primordium is formed of cellular cords, which colonize the ventral mesogastrium (septum transversum). The vitelline (omphalomesenteric) veins connected to the digestive tube consist of an anastomotic network around the duodenum and then cross the septum transversum. Proliferation of the entodermal cords forming the hepatic primordium fragments the vitelline veins into a vascular labyrinth: the hepatic sinusoids. The hepatocytes arrange themselves into cords surrounding the sinusoidal capillaries.

When the yolk sac disappears, the vitelline veins regress almost totally and persist only in their mesenteric branches. Caudad to the liver, the anastomotic network of vitelline veins fuse into a single trunk, the portal vein. In a cranial direction the vitelline veins open into the sinus venosus. When the left horn of the sinus venosus disappears, the right vitelline trunk receives the anastomosis of the inferior vena cava and becomes the terminal segment. Extension and proliferation of hepatocytes into the entire septum transversum result in concurrent fragmentation of the umbilicoallantoic

veins (more lateral to the vitelline veins). The right umbilicoallantoic vein regresses in the sixth week, leaving the left one to drain blood coming from the placenta to the liver. The left umbilical vein drains into the left portal vein and passes through a temporary, short circuit (ductus venosus) directly into the inferior vena cava (Fig. 33–2). The ductus venosus and left umbilical vein are obliterated after birth to form the ligamentum venosum and the ligamentum teres.

The hepatocytes proliferate, and the liver protrudes from the transverse septum into the abdomen, with the bare area a reminder of its origin. Bile ducts differentiate from hepatic cells and join the extrahepatic biliary system, appearing first in the hilum and then spreading peripherally. Bile formation may be evident as early as the third month.

Topographic Anatomy

The reflections of peritoneum that attach the liver to the abdominal wall, diaphragm, and abdominal viscera determine the topographic anatomy of the liver. Three sets of ligaments include the following:

1. The *falciform ligament,* which attaches the liver to the anterior abdominal wall from the diaphragm to umbilicus and incorporates the ligamentum teres hepaticus in its dorsal border. In persons with portal hypertension, the umbilical vein recanalizes and connects the periumbilical superficial venous system with the portal system.

2. The anterior and posterior right and left *coronary ligaments,* which in continuity with the falciform ligament connect the diaphragm to the liver. The lateral aspects of the anterior and posterior leaves of the coronary ligaments fuse to form the right and left triangular ligaments. The area encompassed by the falciform, coronary, and triangular ligaments over the inferior vena cava and under the diaphragm is the *bare* area of the liver.

3. The *gastrohepatic* and *hepatoduodenal ligaments,* which consist of the anterior layer of lesser omentum and are continuous with the left triangular ligament. The hepatoduodenal ligament contains the hepatic arteries, portal vein, and

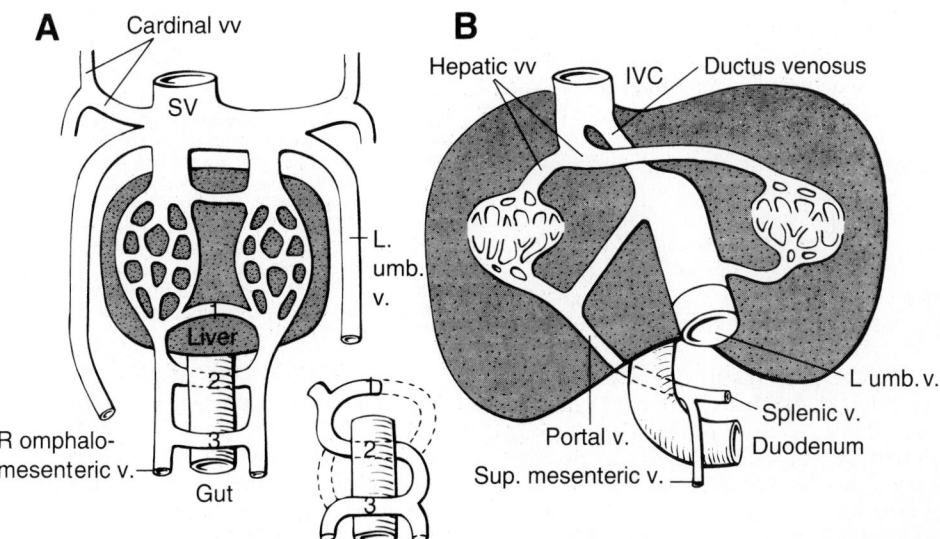

Figure 33–2. The changes undergone by the vitelline (omphalomesenteric) and umbilical veins in the region of the developing liver. *A,* Ventral view of the liver at about 4 weeks' gestation. The omphalomesenteric veins drain into the hepatic sinusoids and thence into the sinus venosus. Three cross-anastomoses between the omphalomesenteric veins encircle the gut. Anastomosis 2 (the future portal vein) passes dorsal to the duodenum (inset). The umbilical veins also drain into the sinus venosus but will soon be tapped by the hepatic sinusoids. *B,* Ventral view of the liver at approximately 6 weeks' gestation. Basically, the right omphalomesenteric vein has become the portal vein caudally and hepatic veins cranially. The right umbilical vein has disappeared, whereas the left umbilical vein has enlarged and carries oxygenated blood in a new, diagonal route (the ductus venosus) through the sinusoids and on to the inferior vena cava. 1, 2, 3, cross anastomoses; IVC, inferior vena cava; SV, sinus venosus. (From O'Rahilly, S., and Muller, B.: Human Embryology and Teratology. New York, Wiley-Liss, 1992. Copyright © 1992. Reprinted by permission of John Wiley & Sons, Inc.)

extrahepatic bile ducts. It forms the anterior boundary of the epiploic foramen of Winslow and the communication between the greater and lesser peritoneal cavities.

Four lobes of the liver are commonly described: right, left, quadrate, and caudate. The topographic right lobe includes a portion of the liver to the right of the falciform ligament and the topographic left lobe portion to the left. The quadrate lobe is a rectangular junction on the inferior surface bounded by the umbilical fissure on the left, the gallbladder fossa on the right, and the portal triad posteriorly. The posterior (transverse) extension of the falciform ligament (ligamentum venosum) on the left and the impression of the inferior vena cava on the right delineate the caudate (spigelian) lobe.

Lobar Anatomy (The American System)

The distribution of the major branches of the veins, arteries, or bile ducts of the liver does not conform precisely with the topographic anatomy (Fig. 33–3). The general relationships between the hepatic veins and portal vein branches determine the lobar anatomy of the liver, which is best demonstrated by direct injection of its blood supply with substances such as methylene blue or colored celloidin. A plane called the *portal fissure* (Cantlie's line) passes from the left side of the gallbladder fossa to the left side of the inferior vena cava to divide the liver into right and left lobes. The left lobe consists of a medial segment, which lies to the right of the falciform ligament and umbilical fissure, and a lateral segment, which lies to the left of the falciform ligament. The right lobe consists of an anterior and a posterior segment. No visible surface marking delineates the lobar segmental anatomy. Conventionally, most of the topographic caudate lobe is in the medial segment of the left lobe, but it extends over the plane between the gallbladder and the inferior vena cava into the anatomic right lobe. The conceptual division of the liver into lobes and segments forms the basis for the four classic types of major hepatic resection (Fig. 33–4). The lobes may be further divided into subsegments that correspond to segments in the French system, described next.

French Segmental System

Another nomenclatural system for hepatic anatomy was developed by Soupault and Couinaud. This system shows more consideration for the hepatic venous drainage and cau-

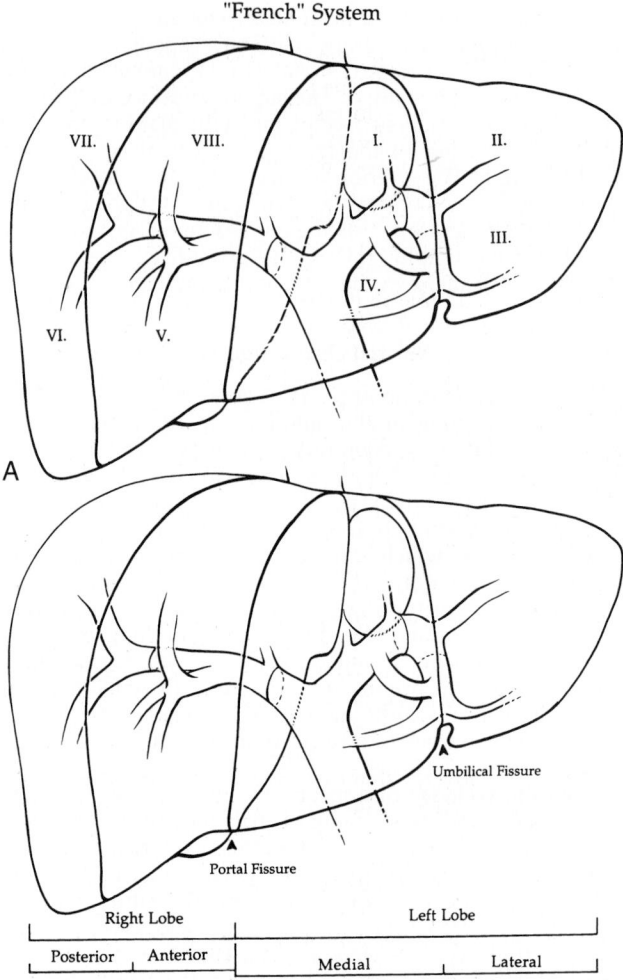

Figure 33–4. *A,* Segmental anatomy as defined by Couinaud (the "French" system). According to Couinaud's description, the three main hepatic veins divide the liver into four sectors. He terms the planes through which the veins course the *portal scissurae.* The right, main, and left portal scissurae define the four sectors, each of which receives a portal pedicle. The main portal scissura divides the liver into right and left sectors. The right portal scissura divides the right and left livers into sectors. It also divides the right liver into anterior and posterior sectors, each of which sectors contains two segments: the anterior sector has segment V inferiorly and segment VIII superiorly, and the posterior sector has segment VI inferiorly and segment VII superiorly. The left portal scissura divides the left liver into superior and inferior sectors. The umbilical fissure divides the anterior sector into two segments: segment IV medially and segment III laterally. The posterior sector has only one segment, segment II, which forms the posterior part of the left lobe. The caudate lobe comprises segment I. The portal veins and hepatic arteriole branches correspond to the segmental anatomy. Likewise, the bile ducts provide segmental drainage. *B,* The "American" system. (From Jones, R. S.: Atlas of Liver and Biliary Surgery. Chicago, Year Book Medical Publishers, 1990; with permission of Mosby-Year Book.)

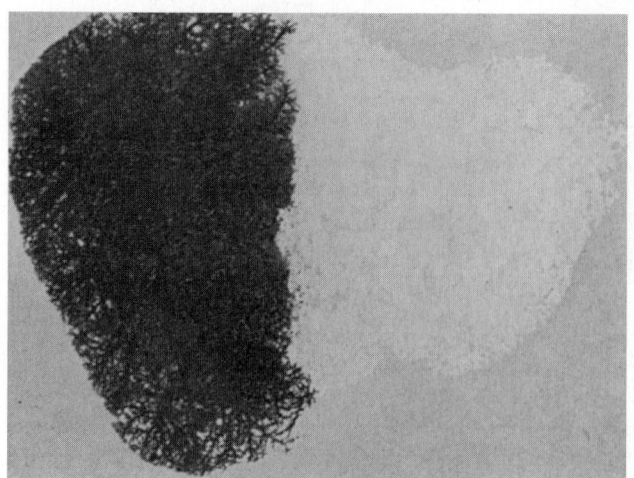

Figure 33–3. A corrosion case with the right and left portal veins injected with vinyl acetate of different colors demonstrates the true lobar anatomy of the liver. (From Mays, E. T.: Anatomy of the liver. *In* Calne, R. Y., and Della Rovere, G. Q. [Eds.]: Liver Surgery. Philadelphia, W. B. Saunders, 1982.)

date lobe but also applies to the portal, biliary, and arterial anatomy. Instead of four, there are eight segments: four on the right, three on the left, and one corresponding to the topographic caudate lobe. Segment I corresponds to the caudate lobe; segments II to IV constitute the left lobe; and segments V to VIII the right lobe. The three main hepatic veins divide the liver into four *sectors.* The planes containing the right, middle, and left hepatic veins are called portal scissurae, while the planes containing portal pedicles are called hepatic scissurae. The caudate lobe is its own autonomous segment in the French system. In general, the segments described in the French classification correspond to the subsegments described in the lobar anatomic classification.

Portal Vein

The portal vein provides about three fourths of the liver's blood supply (Fig. 33–5). The junction of the superior mesenteric and splenic veins forms the portal vein, dorsal to the neck of the pancreas. The portal vein then passes superiorly, posterior to the first part of the duodenum at the level of the second lumbar vertebra. This vein varies from 1 to 3 cm. in diameter and 5 to 8 cm. in length before dividing into right and left branches at the porta hepatis. In about 10% of persons there appear to be three main trunks of the portal vein, with two going to the right lobe and one to the left lobe. The extra trunk represents the right branch of the portal vein dividing into segmental (sectoral) branches before entering the liver. The portal vein usually passes behind the bile duct and hepatic artery in the hepatoduodenal ligament. The portal vein rarely varies. Although the portal vein neatly divides into right and left branches, it does not distribute splanchnic blood equally to the hepatic lobes. Radioactive phosphorus injected into the superior mesenteric vein preferentially flows into the right lobe, whereas splenoportography demonstrates the two lobes nonselectively. Despite the preferential flow, the two lobes function similarly. However, the preferential flow has pathologic significance; for example, amebic abscesses appear predominantly in the right lobe.

The portal trunk divides into left and right hepatic branches in the portal fissure. The left branch of the portal vein is longer and consists of two portions: (1) the pars transversus, which traverses the base of segment IV, and (2) the pars umbilicus, which turns into the umbilical fissure. Two branches to the lateral segment of the left lobe (segments II and III) usually arise from the pars umbilicus near the plane of the falciform ligament. Branches from both the pars transversus and umbilicus supply the medial segment of the left lobe (segment IV). The right branch of the portal vein divides into anterior and posterior segments approximately at the point of entry into liver parenchyma. The portal vein divides into small veins and venules, which finally enter hepatic sinusoids. Abundant vascular intercommunications exist at the sinusoidal level.

The absence of portal vein valves has several important implications: (1) pressures observed in portal vein tributaries reflect portal vein pressure, and therefore, during surgery for portal hypertension, portal pressure is conveniently measured in a small mesenteric or omental vein; (2) the intrahepatic portal vein's low resistance sustains a large amount of flow despite loss of much kinetic energy to the capillary network of the digestive system; and (3) the specialized intrahepatic architecture accommodates both the high-pressure hepatic arteries and the portal veins.

Numerous tributaries of the portal vein connect outside the liver with the systemic venous system. Under normal circumstances these communications have little physiologic significance. However, if portal hypertension develops, these rudimentary portosystemic communications develop into large channels with increased collateral flow. The most important natural portosystemic anastomoses include (1) the submucosal veins of the proximal stomach and distal esophagus, which can receive blood from the coronary and short gastric veins to drain into the azygous veins (high blood flow through this pathway produces gastric varices, esophageal varices, or both); (2) umbilical and periumbilical veins, recanalized from the obliterated umbilical vein in the ligamentum teres hepaticus, and which may cause spectacular physical findings such as caput medusae or the loud Cruveilhier-Baumgarten bruit; (3) tributaries of the inferior mesenteric vein, which include the superior hemorrhoidal veins that communicate with the middle and inferior hemorrhoidal veins of the systemic circulation and may cause large hemorrhoids; and (4) other retroperitoneal communications, including connections to the renal and adrenal veins.

Hepatic Artery

The extrahepatic arterial system does not parallel the portal channels, although the intrahepatic system does (Fig. 33–6). Over 50% of the population have the same anatomic pattern. The hepatic artery arises from the celiac axis and passes along the upper part of the pancreas toward the liver. Poste-

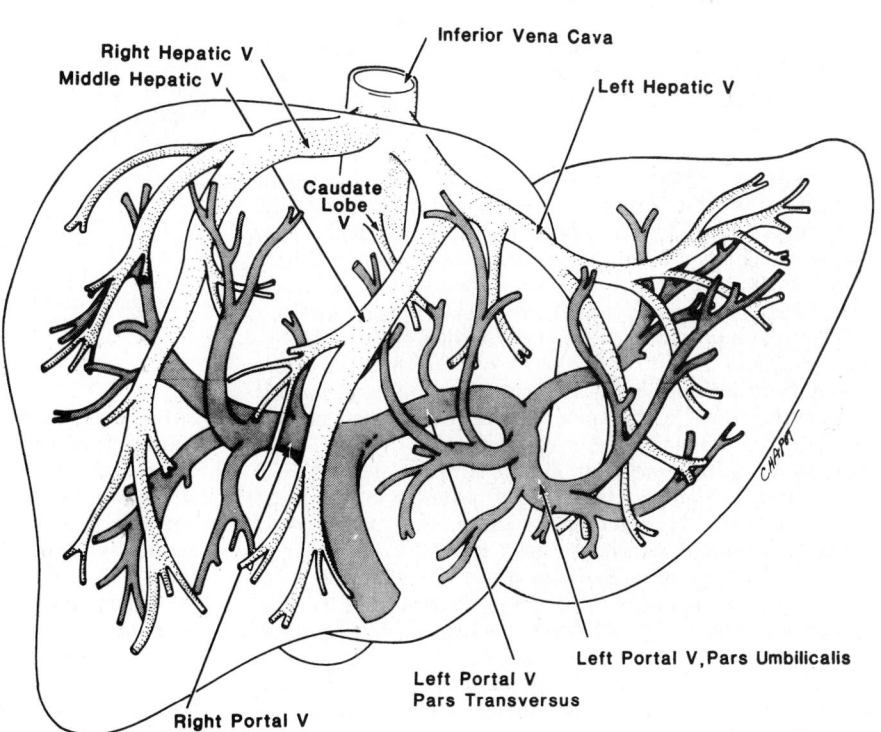

Figure 33–5. Hepatic veins and portal vein. There are three major hepatic veins: right, middle, and left. The portal vein divides into a right and left trunk, with the left curving in the falciform ligament as the pars umbilicus (where the umbilical vein joined it). (From Campra, J. L., and Reynolds, T. B.: The hepatic circulation. *In* Arias, I., et al. [Eds.]: The Liver: Biology and Pathobiology. New York, Raven Press, 1982.)

Right Hepatic V
Middle Hepatic V
Inferior Vena Cava
Left Hepatic V
Caudate Lobe V
Left Portal V, Pars Umbilicalis
Left Portal V Pars Transversus
Right Portal V

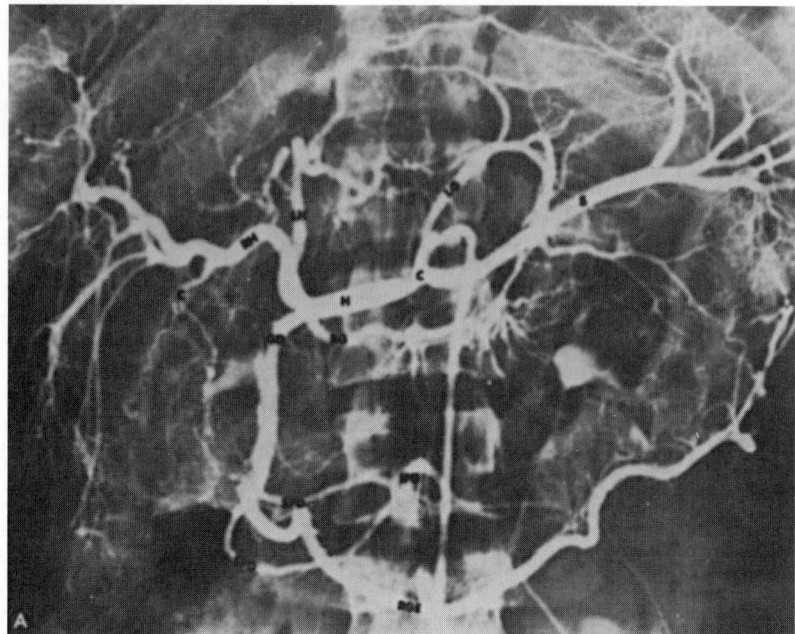
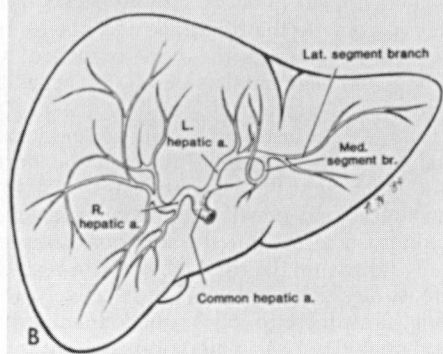

Figure 33–6. *A,* Celiac axis with usual branching pattern. The angiographic catheter is located at the origin of the celiac axis (C), and the following arteries are demonstrated: splenic (S), left gastric (LG), hepatic (H), right gastric (RG), gastroduodenal (GD), superior and inferior pancreatoduodenal (SPD and IPD), and right gastroepiploic (RGE). The left and right hepatic arteries (LH and RH) are also visualized. (From Campra, J. L., and Reynolds, T. B.: The hepatic circulation. *In* Arias, I., et al. [Eds.]: The Liver: Biology and Pathobiology, 2nd ed. New York, Raven Press, 1988.) *B,* Diagram of the branches of the common hepatic artery.

rior and superior to the duodenum it gives off the gastroduodenal artery. The terms *proper* or *common* hepatic arteries refer to the segment proximal or distal to the origin of the gastroduodenal artery. Note that some anatomic textbooks denote those terms in reverse (proper: distal; common: proximal to the gastroduodenal artery). Therefore, using the entire phrase "hepatic artery *proximal* or *distal* to the gastroduodenal artery" is suggested. Within the hepatoduodenal ligament the hepatic artery divides into right and left branches and subsequently into smaller branches corresponding to the portal venous system, segmental, or subsegmental anatomy. Because of abundant collaterals, ligation of the hepatic artery proximal to the gastroduodenal artery fails to damage the liver. Ligation of the hepatic artery distal to the gastroduodenal artery can produce hepatic necrosis and death but also may not result in serious consequences because of development of a rich collateral extrinsic blood supply from the celiac axis, superior mesenteric, and inferior phrenic arteries. Ligation of the right or left hepatic artery usually results in elevated enzyme levels but often without severe clinical manifestations. A diffuse subcapsular arterial plexus may contribute significantly to the hepatic arterial collateral circulation. One angiographic study has shown that rich collaterals can also develop in the liver's suspensory ligaments.

The most important variations of the hepatic arterial system are a right hepatic artery and a common hepatic artery arising from a superior mesenteric trunk (*replaced* hepatic arteries) (Fig. 33–7). Other anomalies include the left hepatic artery arising from the left gastric artery, the right hepatic artery traveling anterior rather than posterior to the bile duct, and the right hepatic artery traveling posterior to the portal vein. In addition, the right hepatic artery often has a curved extrahepatic course, which may lead to inadvertent ligation during cholecystectomy. The cystic artery usually arises from the right hepatic artery but occasionally arises from the gastroduodenal artery, the left hepatic artery, or the common hepatic artery. Double cystic arteries occasionally occur. When significant hepatic arterial branches arise from the superior mesenteric artery, they usually pass to the right side of and posterior to the portal vein.

Hepatic Veins

Most of the hepatic venous effluent drains into the three major hepatic veins—*right, middle,* and *left.* Each has only a short extrahepatic segment before draining into the inferior vena cava. In general, the short extrahepatic segment makes surgical accessibility difficult, particularly for control of traumatic bleeding. The right hepatic vein, the largest of the three, provides the principal drainage for the right lobe of the liver. The main trunk of the right hepatic vein follows an intersegmental plane between the French segments or the anterior and posterior segments (American system). Several small veins also normally drain directly from the right lobe into the vena cava. The middle hepatic vein lies in the lobar (portal) fissure draining the medial segment of the left lobe and a portion of the anterior segment of the right lobe. The middle hepatic vein joins the left hepatic vein in 80% of dissections. The exact site of juncture varies considerably. The left hepatic vein provides the principal venous drainage of the left lateral segment. In addition, several small veins from the caudate lobe drain posteriorly directly into the vena cava. After thrombosis of the major hepatic veins (Budd-Chiari syndrome), these small posterior caudate veins become particularly important.

Biliary System

The biliary drainage system begins at the hepatocyte level, where portions of the hepatocyte membrane form small channels called canaliculi. Bile drains from the canaliculi into intrahepatic ducts that follow the segmental anatomy determined primarily by the vascular supply. The convergence of canaliculi and proximal ductal systems is called the canal of Hering. The ductal pattern becomes more variable distally. The left lobar duct forms in the umbilical fissure from the union of ducts from segments II, III, and IV, then passes to the right across the base of segment IV (medial segment of the left lobe, topographic quadrate lobe), and unites with the right lobar duct to form the common hepatic duct. The right hepatic duct drains segments V and VIII and arises usually

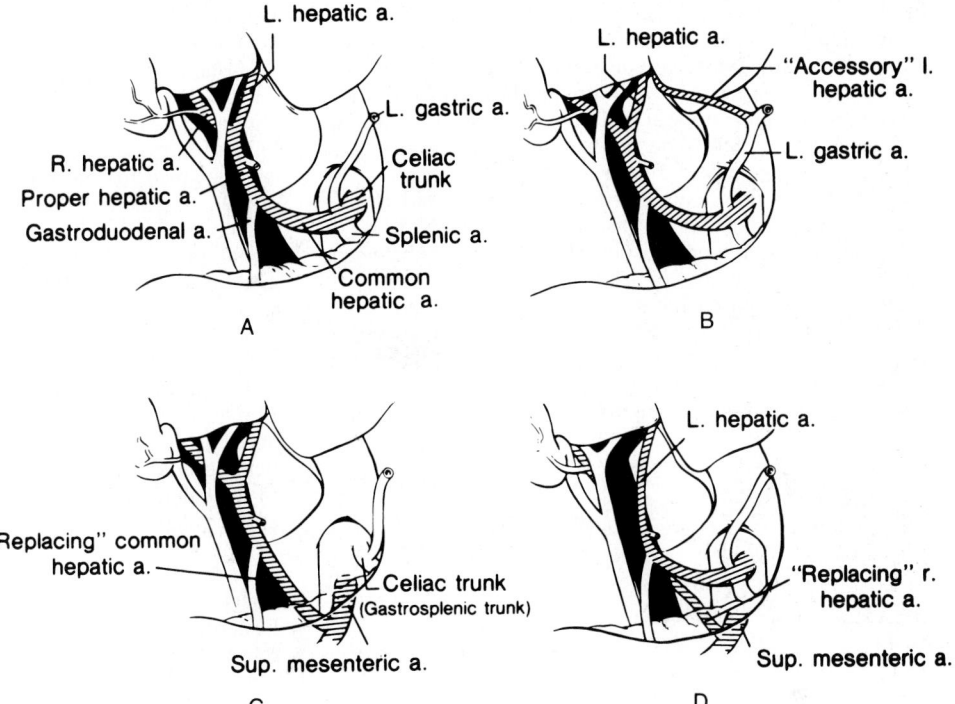

Figure 33–7. *A–D,* The four most common variations of the hepatic arterial system. (From Skandalakis, L. J., Gray, S. W., Colburn, G. L., and Skandalakis, J. E.: Surgical anatomy of the liver and associated extrahepatic structures. *In* Contemporary Surgery. Glenview, IL, Bobbit Publishing Company, 1987.)

from the junction of the anterior and posterior segmental (sectoral) ducts. The right posterior duct usually follows almost a horizontal course before joining with the anterior duct, where it descends more vertically. The junction of the two main right biliary channels is usually found above the right branch of the portal vein.

The shorter extrahepatic right lobar duct joins the longer left duct at the base of the right lobe. The extrahepatic portion of the left lobar duct characteristically is about 2 cm. long. The right and left lobar ducts join outside the liver to become the common hepatic duct, which passes anterior to the portal vein in most persons. The left hepatic duct joins the right hepatic duct at a much more anterior and acute angle, which is an anatomic consistency of importance during exploration of the common duct or cholangiography. The length of the common hepatic duct varies according to the location of its junction with the cystic duct, where it becomes the common bile duct. The hepatic duct confluence varies considerably with respect to the union of the right and left main hepatic ducts. The biliary drainage of the topographic caudate lobe (segment I) varies considerably but enters both the right and left hepatic duct systems in about 80% of persons. In about 15% of cases, the caudate lobe drains only into the left hepatic duct system, and in about 5% it drains only into the right hepatic duct.

The upper limit of normal for the diameter of the common bile duct is controversial. Most references give the upper limit as 6 to 8 mm. except after cholecystectomy, when the common bile duct may dilate to 10 to 12 mm. Intrahepatic and extrahepatic ducts usually lie anterior to the corresponding portal branches. The extrahepatic bile ducts lie within the hepatoduodenal ligament. The common hepatic artery ascending to the left of the common bile duct gives off the right hepatic artery, which usually courses dorsal to the bile duct. Like the common hepatic duct, the common bile duct varies in length. It passes posterior to the first part of the duodenum and then courses through the pancreas and the wall of the duodenum to form the papilla of Vater on the medial duodenal wall. The major pancreatic duct (duct of Wirsung) joins the common duct in about 90% of cases, forming the ampulla of Vater.

Sphincter of Oddi. The circular smooth muscle fibers in the ampulla of Vater area constitute the sphincter of Oddi, which regulates the flow of bile from the liver into the duodenum. The three principal parts of the sphincter of Oddi are the sphincter of the choledochus (i.e., the circular muscle fibers surrounding the intramural and submucosal bile duct); the pancreatic sphincter, which consists of the amuscular septum between the bile and pancreatic ducts; and an ampullary sphincter. The ampullary sphincter, the most important component of the sphincter of Oddi, includes a layer of longitudinal muscle fibers that help prevent reflux of intestinal contents into the ampulla. Relaxation of the ampullary sphincter may promote reflux into the pancreatic duct. About 10% of papillas have clearly distinct, separate openings of the common bile duct and pancreatic duct. The blood supply of the common bile duct arises from the gastroduodenal, common hepatic, and right hepatic arteries. A plexus formed on the duct provides two axial vessels, the 3 o'clock and 9 o'clock arteries, named for their positions relative to a cross-section of the duct.

Gallbladder. The gallbladder, a pear-shaped, distensible appendage of the extrahepatic biliary system, usually holds 30 to 50 ml. of bile. It has a fundus, body, and neck. The gallbladder fills and empties through the cystic duct, which varies in length and usually contains spiral valves of Heister that regulate bile flow. The valves may be extremely tortuous, complicating cannulation during intraoperative cholangiography. Enlargement of the neck of the gallbladder such as from a stone may form a pouch (Hartmann's pouch). The triangle bounded by the cystic duct, common hepatic duct, and inferior border of the liver is the triangle of Calot. The gallbladder receives its blood supply from the cystic artery, which originates from the right hepatic artery, usually after the latter passes beneath the common hepatic duct. Venous drainage of the gallbladder enters principally into the portal vein. The lymphatics drain into cystic duct nodes near the superior aspect of the cystic duct. Venous and lymphatic channels also enter into the liver parenchyma.

Biliary System Variants. Variations in the gallbladder and related anatomy are important during surgery, because failure to recognize variants can produce iatrogenic injury (Fig. 33–8). Small accessory ducts (ducts of Luschka) between the liver and gallbladder easily escape detection. Low extrahepatic right segmental duct insertions (most notably VII–VIII or VI) can also join the cystic duct. The latter injury has been recognized since the use of laparoscopic cholecystectomy. Occasionally, liver parenchyma is partially embedded in the gallbladder, and rarely one may encounter a completely intrahepatic gallbladder. The length of the cystic duct varies, and it occasionally passes for several centimeters ensheathed with the common hepatic duct. Passage of the cystic duct

posterior and around the common hepatic duct to form a left-sided junction (spiral union) occurs in less than 5% of persons. The cystic duct may also join the right or left hepatic duct or be absent. Rarely, major hepatic ducts drain separately into the gallbladder.

Common variations in the anatomy of the hepatic artery of relevance to this biliary anatomy include a bend in the course of the hepatic artery, which can mimic the cystic artery origin, a short cystic artery takeoff from the right hepatic artery, dual cystic arteries, or an artery that courses anterior to the hepatic ductal system.

Nerves

The portal and pericapsular regions harbor a distinct, complex system of nerves of unknown clinical importance. An anterior neural plexus consists primarily of sympathetic fibers derived bilaterally from ganglia T7 to T10 and synapsing in the celiac plexus or of fibers from the right and left vagus and right phrenic nerves. The anterior plexus surrounds the hepatic arteries. A posterior plexus that intercommunicates with the anterior plexus lies around the portal vein and bile ducts. The sympathetic nerves innervate the hepatic arteries. Distention of the liver capsule or gallbladder causes pain referred to the right shoulder or scapula by means of the third and fourth cervical nerves. Interruption of the anterior neural plexus may have various physiologic effects, such as on the composition of secreted bile and the accumulation of fat in the liver. The significance of these findings is not known.

Lymphatics

Hepatic lymph forms in the perisinusoidal spaces of Disse and in the clefts of Mall to drain into larger lymphatics in the porta hepatis, subsequently into the cisterna chyli, and eventually into the thoracic duct. Lymphatic vessels also lie near the hepatic vein in Glisson's capsule and around the bile ducts. Lymphatics also pass through the diaphragm into the thoracic duct. Hepatic lymph nodes are found in the porta hepatis, celiac region, and near the inferior vena cava. Cirrhosis, veno-occlusive disease, and glycogenosis produce lymph vessel dilation. Alterations in the permeability of sinusoidal epithelial cells can alter lymph flow and protein content, an observation important in the pathogenesis of ascites. Injection of dye into the bile duct under supraphysiologic pressure reveals communication with the hepatic lymph vessels, but the importance of these communications under physiologic conditions is unknown.

Anomalous Development of the Liver

Incomplete or maldevelopment of the hepatobiliary system can cause a number of anomalies that are encountered clinically. Complete absence of the liver is rare and not reported after birth. Absence of the left lobe has been seen. Hepatic transposition has been reported with *situs inversus*. Occasionally, a tongue of liver tissue extends inferiorly from the right lobe (Riedel's lobe); more frequently encountered in the female, this condition usually causes no symptoms, although it may be associated with colonic or pyloric obstruction. Heterotopic liver tissue has been seen in the gallbladder, pancreas, adrenals, spleen, or within an omphalocele. Four cases of supradiaphragmatic liver have been reported in the absence of a hernia sac.

Although biliary variants are extremely common, true anomalies are not. Biliary atresia and choledochocele are the most common serious biliary problems seen after birth. Other abnormalities include congenital absence of gallbladder, in-

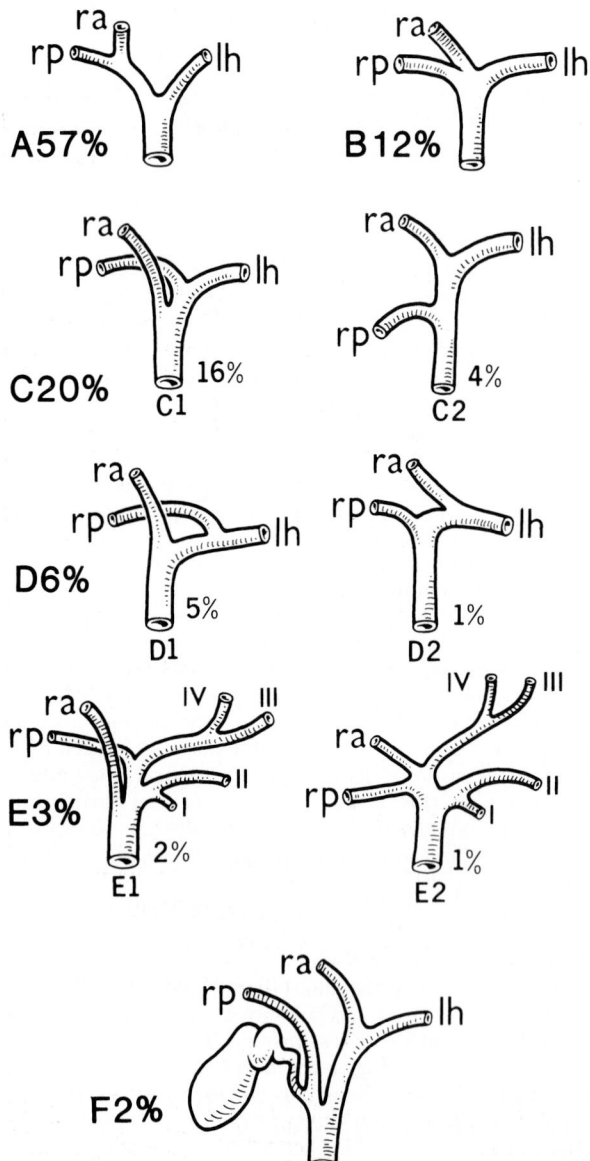

Figure 33–8. Anatomy of the hepatic duct confluence. *A*, Most common anatomy. *B*, Triple confluence. *C*, Drainage of right anterior or right posterior segment into common hepatic duct. *D*, Drainage of right anterior or right posterior segment into left hepatic duct. *E*, Absence of a well-defined confluence. (From Smadja, C.: The anatomy of the biliary tract and biliary exposure. *In* Blumgart, L. H. [Ed.]: Surgery of the Liver and Biliary Tract. Edinburgh, Churchill Livingstone, 1988.)

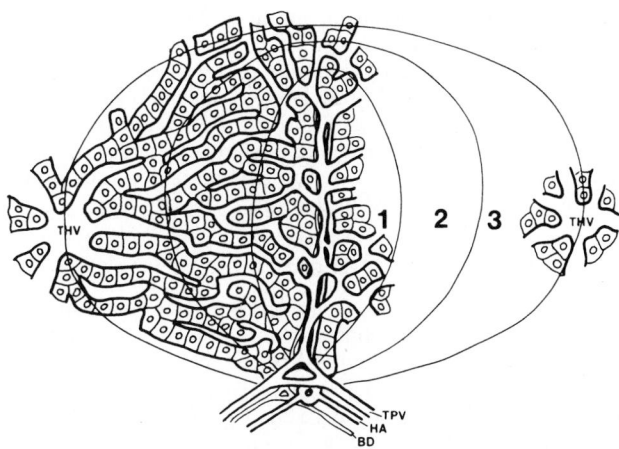

Figure 33–9. Diagram of liver acinar unit as described by Rappaport. Terminal extensions of a terminal portal venule (TPV), hepatic arteriole (HA), and bile ductule (BD) are labeled. Zone 1 represents the area nearest to the sinusoidal axis. Blood flows sequentially through zones 1, 2, and 3 into terminal hepatic venules (THV). (From Gumucio, J. J., and Miller, D. L.: Liver cell heterogeneity. *In* Arias, I., et al. [Eds.]: The Liver: Biology and Pathobiology. New York, Raven Press, 1982.)

trahepatic or left-sided gallbladder, multiple gallbladders, and abnormalities in the shape of the gallbladder. The definition of multiple gallbladders is determined by the presence of more than one cystic duct. Other gallbladder anomalies include septation, bilobation, and duplication of the cystic duct. Occasionally the gallbladder has a long mesentery predisposing to torsion. Portal vascular abnormalities include portal agenesis, congenital portocaval shunt, a preduodenal portal vein, and anomalous pulmonary veins that traverse the diaphragm and enter the portal system.

Microscopic Anatomy

The Acinar Unit

The smallest functional unit of the liver is the acinus, a structure first named by Rappaport (Fig. 33–9). In an acinar unit, the portal venule is accompanied by a hepatic arteriole, a bile ductule, lymphatics, and nerves. Blood flows from the terminal portal venules into the sinusoids and comes in contact with hepatocytes in the unit. The blood drains into the terminal hepatic venule. The solutes are removed by the hepatocytes, and their concentration decreases as the blood flows toward the terminal hepatic venule. The hepatocytes around the portal venule axis are divided arbitrarily into three zones. In zone 1, the area immediately adjacent to the portal venule, the sinusoids are smaller in diameter and more anastomotic than in zones 2 and 3, which are farther away from the portal venule. This concept explains centrilobular necrosis that occurs with hypotension; zone 1 cells are the first to receive blood and oxygen and the last to experience hypoxia.

Microcirculation

The terminal branches of the major inflow system (the portal vein) and the major outflow system (the hepatic vein) do not meet but are regularly interspersed with space between them filled with hepatic cell plates and sinusoids. The portal veins and their branches become progressively smaller as they penetrate the liver substance, while the terminal hepatic veins connect with the sinusoidal bed, piercing through closely applied cell plates. This anatomy is clearly a result of the embryologic development of the liver. Flow of

portal blood in the sinusoids is partially regulated via the periphery of the cell plates.

The branches of the hepatic artery similarly decrease in caliber as they penetrate the parenchyma, and their size and composition change accordingly. In the terminal branches, they form a general plexus, which eventually terminates in the sinusoids. A special capillary plexus encompasses the bile ducts; this network also terminates in the sinusoids. The peribiliary plexus appears to play an important role in ductular bile secretion and absorption. Cuffs of smooth muscle surrounding the terminal arterioles help regulate the flow into the sinusoids (see Blood Flow).

The hepatic sinusoids are 7 to 15 μm. wide, but the width may increase to 180 μm. under physiologic conditions. Pressure within the sinusoids is only 2 to 3 mm. Hg, making this an extremely low resistance system (Fig. 33–10). Three anatomic features characterize this low resistance system:

1. The sinusoids are lined by Kupffer's and endothelial cells, which overlap loosely and are not attached to one

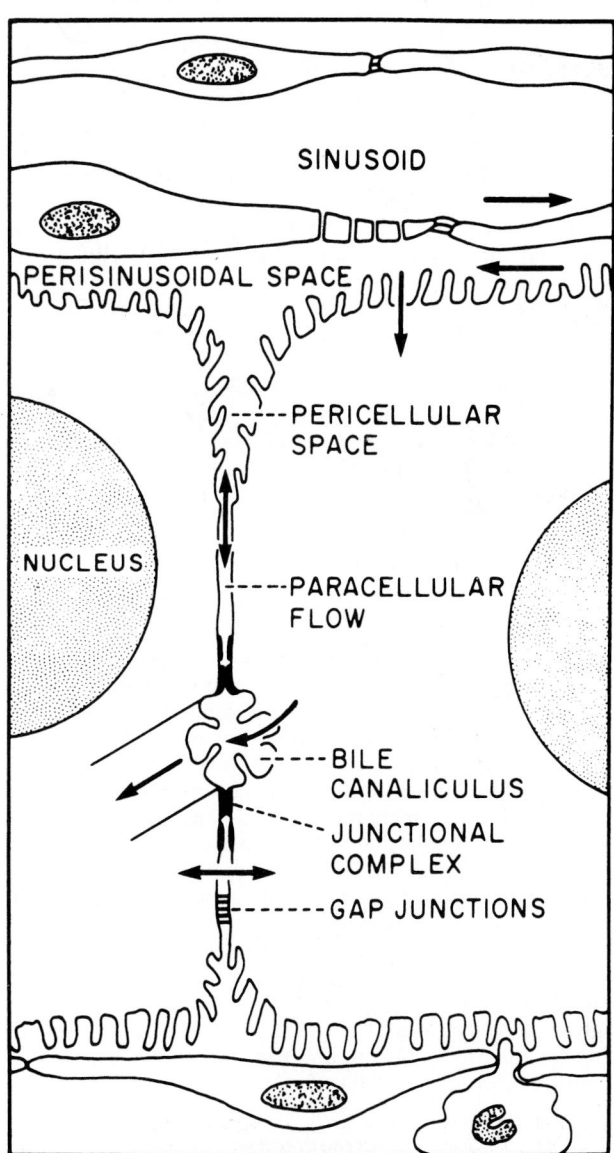

Figure 33–10. Diagram of hepatic sinusoids, perisinusoidal space of Disse, and principal hepatocyte surfaces. Arrows show the direction of fluid flow. (From Arias, I., et al. [Eds.]: The Liver: Biology and Pathobiology. New York, Raven Press, 1982.)

another. The stellate Kupffer's cell cannot be distinguished from endothelial cells by light microscopy. However, the former are much larger, and have irregular surfaces with folds and microvilli.

2. The endothelial cells are flat and fenestrated, with openings varying from 0.1 to 2 μm. in diameter.

3. Hepatocyte and membrane microvilli project through the fenestrations of the endothelial cells and therefore facilitate and maximize hepatocyte exposure to sinusoidal contents.

The space between the endothelial lining of the sinusoid and the hepatocyte is the perisinusoidal *space of Disse.* Important cells located in the perisinusoidal space of Disse include fibroblasts, Ito cells (lipocytes), and neurons. Sinusoids are freely permeable to low- and high-molecular-weight substances in solution. The sinusoids empty into terminal hepatic venules, which in turn empty into hepatic veins of increasing caliber. The space of Disse is the primary site for the formation of hepatic lymph.

Hepatocytes and Sites of Bile Formation

Hepatocytes represent approximately 60% of the cells of the adult human liver and 80% of the cytoplasmic mass. These diameters vary between 13 and 30 μm. The cells have both a microvillar and smooth surface, with the microvillar surface lining the perisinusoidal space. The smooth surface is capable of forming microvilli, particularly during regeneration and cholestasis. The microvilli of the hepatocytes are not as extensive as the microvilli of the intestinal epithelial lining, increasing the surface area 1.6-fold compared with 24-fold for the latter. Approximately 15% of the plasma membrane encompasses bile canaliculi that remain separated from the pericellular space by tight junctions and desmosomes. The main source of canalicular bile is across the canalicular membrane, although some paracellular flow of small solutes also occurs. The canaliculi measure approximately 1 μm. in diameter. The epithelial ductular or ductular lining cells measure 10 μm. in diameter and have a distinct basement membrane, in contrast to hepatocytes.

Hepatocyte Ultrastructure

The organization and structure of the hepatocyte organelles permit the liver to carry out its metabolic functions. Mitochondria occupy approximately 18% of the liver cell by volume and participate in oxidative phosphorylation and the oxidation of fatty acids. Lysosomes catabolize endogenous substances as well as some exogenous wastes. Multivesicular bodies contain large amounts of protein derived from plasma. Microtubules and associated mechanotransducers may regulate the direction of vesicular transport in the cell. The liver is unique in that both the smooth and rough endoplasmic reticulum are well developed. As many as 50 Golgi complexes occupy a hepatocyte. The smooth and rough endoplasmic reticulum and Golgi complexes are collectively known as the liver microsomal fraction. The liver microsomes are known to participate in glycogenolysis; synthesis of cholesterol and bile salts; esterification of free fatty acids to triglycerides; synthesis of albumin, fibrinogen, and other proteins destined for export to the plasma; and glucuronidation of bilirubin, drugs, and bile salts.

FUNCTION

The liver has an extraordinary spectrum of functions. The organ regulates a massive amount of energy; stores, distributes, and disposes of various nutrients; and synthesizes, transforms, and metabolizes many endogenous substrates and pollutants. Over the past 5 years, major advances have occurred in molecular and cellular biology and immunobiology, including increased knowledge of mechanisms of signal transduction, growth control and cell death, and membrane physiology. This section capsulizes some of this fundamental biology and practical knowledge that influences our understanding of liver function and surgical disease.

Energy

Most of the body's metabolic needs are regulated in some way by the liver. To accomplish this, the liver expends approximately 20% of the body's energy and consumes 20% to 25% of the total utilized oxygen, despite constituting only 4% to 5% of the total body weight. The liver architecture seems specific for these demands. The blood supply includes the portal system between the intestinal and hepatic capillary bed, which helps establish a remarkably efficient extrahepatic circulation. The acinar unit permits each cell to be bathed by sinusoidal blood and at the same time separates a biliary compartment within a portion of its membrane to ensure an excretory pathway. The hepatocellular organelles in plasma membranes permit specific functions and, at the same time, interrelate with an extracellular matrix, which facilitates metabolic exchange between blood and hepatocytes.

The liver not only conducts a large number of functions but also manufactures a large number of substances, such as plasma proteins, carnitine, and creatine, which service solely other organs or tissues. The liver collects and transforms such substrates to meet the fuel requirements of other tissues in response to various metabolic signals. It is the only organ that produces acetoacetate for use by muscle, brain, and kidney but not itself. The liver also uses little glucose for its own requirements and expends little of the energy generated by degradation of glycogen. It uses fatty acids that originate from the diet and fat, but also easily makes fatty acids as triacylglycerols and phospholipids, which are exported. The liver has a special capacity for gluconeogenesis from alanine arising in muscle but has little capacity for transamination of leucine, isoleucine, and valine.

The energy-related functions of the liver are remarkably regulated by hormones, other agonists, and substrates coming to and from the liver. No doubt there are many other signals that regulate these exchanges. The contribution of this energy metabolism to the body's overall acid-base balance must be great, but surprisingly undiscovered are the signaling responses so important in this regulation.

Functional Heterogeneity and Sinusoidal Membrane Traffic

Under light microscopy, liver cells look basically the same. However, the cells from different acinar zones behave differently. In fact, many of the markers on the cell surfaces are different depending on the zone, or even depth within a segment. Krebs cycle enzymes (i.e., urea synthesis enzymes and glutaminase) are found highest in concentration in zone 1, whereas glutamine synthetase is highest in zone 3. The drug-metabolizing P-450 enzymes are concentrated in zone 3, particularly after enzyme induction by phenobarbital. The hepatocytes in zone 1, as expected, are more important for bile salt–dependent bile formation, because they are the first to come into contact with and readily absorb the detergents. In contrast, the hepatocytes in zone 3 are more important to bile salt–independent bile formation. The differences relate not only to blood flow but also to gene transcription rates.

Receptor-mediated endocytosis is responsible for the transfer of large molecules, such as growth factors and carrier proteins. When they become occupied, the receptors on the sinusoidal membrane cluster into a pit when endocytosis begins. Sinusoidal plasma membrane is particularly receptor rich and metabolically important. A lateral domain, important in cell-cell interaction, separates it from the bile canaliculus. Endothelial cells and perisinusoidal cells patrol the sinusoids and have an increasingly recognized diverse set of functions, including protection, immune surveillance, and regulation of some major hepatic processes, including regeneration. Perisinusoidal cells consist of the Kupffer's cells so important in phagocytosis and antigen presentation, the fat-storing cells, or Ito cells, important in collagen metabolism and storage of vitamin A, and the rare pit cells that have natural killer cell and neuroendocrine activities. The sinusoidal cells also appear to be important in the production of growth-regulating molecules.

Blood Flow

The liver receives blood from the arterial and portal circulation; processes nutrients and metabolizes toxins and wastes; and stores, transforms, and distributes them to the vascular, biliary, or lymphatic circulations. Mean total hepatic blood flow has been estimated to be 100 to 130 ml. per kg. per minute. Seventy per cent to 75% of total hepatic blood flow comes from the portal vein, while the remainder comes from the hepatic artery. There is a reciprocal increase in hepatic arterial flow in response to a reduction in the portal flow, but the converse does not occur; portocaval shunt or ligation of the superior mesenteric artery results in an almost 100% increase in hepatic arterial flow. The compensation is not complete, however, so total hepatic flow does not return to normal. Reflex neural control and autoregulation appears to be an important regulatory factor for hepatic arterial flow but not for portal venous flow. To a large extent, portal venous flow into the liver is regulated by extrahepatic factors such as the rate of flow from the intestines and spleen. Food, bile salts, secretin, cholecystokinin, pentagastrin, epinephrine, vasoactive intestinal peptide, glucagon, and isoproterenol all increase portal blood flow. Although it is conceivable that flow would increase based on nutritional status, because of hepatic arterial flow regulation the total flow does not vary with metabolic state of the organism.

Both intrinsic and extrinsic factors appear to be important in controlling the variable arterial blood flow. Intrinsic flow regulation occurs through arterial autoregulation based on the local concentration of adenosine surrounding the hepatic arteriole and portal venule. Adenosine is a potent arteriolar dilator; an increase in portal flow washes out perivascular adenosine and results in constriction of the hepatic arteriole, thereby maintaining a constant level of hepatic blood flow. Less is known about the extrinsic control mechanisms. Possible humoral regulators of extrinsic regulation include gastrin, glucagon, secretin, and bile salts. The hepatic artery is also densely innervated by sympathetic nerves and constricts in response to alpha-adrenergic receptor stimulation. Hepatic arterial flow and pressures reflect the systemic system.

Portal blood flow appears to be controlled by resistance across a distinct hepatic venous–like zone. In normal liver there is no resistance attributable to either the portal venule or sinusoid. In experimental models, hepatic venous sphincters appear to contract in response to histamine, norepinephrine, and angiotensin. Portal venous pressures range from 7 to 10 mm. Hg, while sinusoidal pressures are 2 to 4 mm. Hg above the pressure in the inferior vena cava.

Intrinsic liver flow is to a degree comparable to a sponge, but with various methods of regulation. The microvasculature is regulated by a series of sinusoidal inlet and outlet sphincters. Hepatic inflow increases with expiration and de-

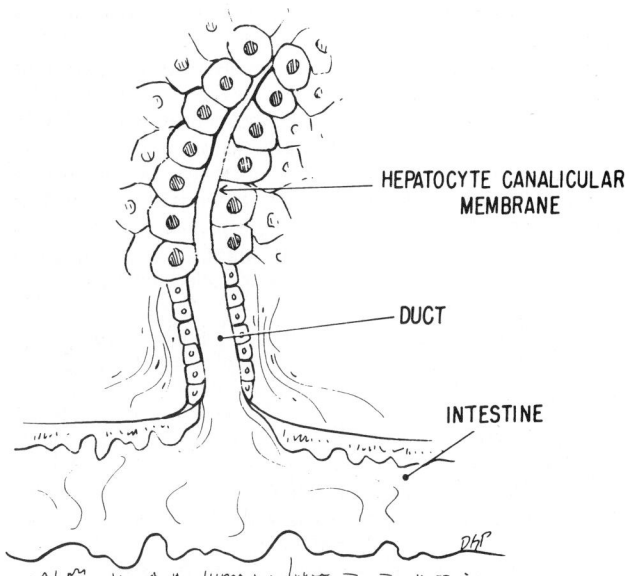

Figure 33–11. Schematic diagram demonstrating the two principal cellular sites of bile production: (1) the canalicular membranes of the hepatocyte and (2) epithelial cells of the bile ductules or ducts distally. In addition to these sites, a paracellular route is also operative (see Fig. 33–13).

creases with inspiration, which is opposite to the phasic flow in the vena cava. During vigorous exercise, total hepatic blood flow is decreased because of shunting of blood to muscle and the brain. The liver serves as a physiologic reservoir of blood: 25% to 30% of its volume is composed of blood, and during acute blood losses, 300 ml. or more can be released into the systemic circulation without adverse effects on liver function. Conversely, in the face of right-sided heart failure, up to 1000 ml. of blood can be stored in the liver without affecting liver function.

Bile Formation

Bile secretion is an active process, relatively independent of total liver blood flow, except in conditions of shock. Bile is formed at two sites: (1) the canalicular membrane of the hepatocyte and (2) the bile ductules or ducts (Fig. 33–11). Total unstimulated bile flow in a 70-kg. man has been estimated to be 0.41 to 0.43 ml. per minute. Eighty percent of the total daily production of bile (1500 ml.) is secreted by hepatocytes and 20% is secreted by the bile duct epithelial cells. The principal organic compounds in bile are the conjugated bile acids, cholesterol, phospholipids, and protein (Table 33–1). Because of the excellent correlation between bile acid output and bile flow, the term *bile acid–dependent flow* is used to describe this fraction of bile formation: bile flow is linearly related to bile acid output. Secretion of cholesterol and phospholipid is closely linked to the output of bile acids,

TABLE 33–1. Composition of Hepatic Bile

Inorganic Ions (mEq./L.)		Organic Solutes	
Na$^+$	(140–165)	Bile acids	(5–50 mmol./L.)
K$^+$	(3.8–5.8)	Cholesterol	(100–340 mg./100 ml.)
Cl$^-$	(93–123)	Phospholipids	(150–800 mg./100 ml.)
HCO$_3^-$	(15–55)	Proteins	(25–500 mg./100 ml.)
CA^{2+}	(1.4–5.0)		
Mg^{2+}	(1.5–3.0)		

except under certain conditions such as insulin or glucagon stimulation.

The bile canaliculus is a long narrow channel that begins as a space of approximately 1 μm. in diameter, bounded by two or three hepatocyte canalicular membranes. It has no wall of its own, but the membrane has numerous microvilli. Canalicular flow may be generated in near absence of bile acids or during stabilized bile acid–dependent flow, and this is termed the *bile acid–independent canalicular fraction.* Abundant evidence exists now, suggesting that this *independent* fraction of bile may actually be controlled by hepatic bile production.

As bile passes through the biliary ductules or ducts it is modified by secretion or absorption of epithelial cells. The highest cells in the biliary ductules have functions and architecture in common with both hepatocytes and ductular cells and so are called cholangiocytes. Secretion from biliary epithelial cells (canalicular bile) appears to be dependent on chloride channel stimulation. The best characterized hormone stimulator is secretin. Extracellular signaling molecules may control ion channels on the apical surface of the bile duct epithelial cells. The presence of such signals suggests an origin upstream of the canalicular membrane. These molecules may provide alternate methods to stimulate canalicular bile flow in conditions such as bile stasis or secretin-associated chloride channel defects (such as cystic fibrosis). Cholangiocytes contain receptors for epidermal growth factor, secretin, and somatostatin.

The only known function of the gallbladder is to concentrate and store bile during fasting. Approximately 90% of the water in gallbladder bile is absorbed in 4 hours. Bile acids within the gallbladder may reach 50 times their concentration in hepatic bile. Cholecystokinin appears to be the principal physiologic stimulator of gallbladder concentration. It is released from the mucosa of the proximal intestine in response to food and simultaneously relaxes the sphincter of Oddi. Other peptides, such as vasoactive intestinal peptide, neuropeptide Y, motilin, histamine, prostaglandins, pancreatic polypeptide, and somatostatin, may be involved in control of gallbladder storage and emptying. Cholinergic stimulation causes contraction of the gallbladder and relaxation of the sphincter of Oddi. Bile acids in the intestine appear to have a negative feedback effect on release of cholecystokinin from the intestine. The importance of gallbladder function is debatable because humans have no nutritional consequences after cholecystectomy.

Bile is a micellar solution (see Table 33–1). Sodium is the most important cation involved in canalicular secretion, while chloride plays an important role at the ductular level. Osmolality is approximately 300 mOsm per kg., which is isosmotic with plasma. The low osmolality reflects in part the aggregation of bile acids in micelles and consequent reduction of osmotic activity. The concentrations of the major electrolytes resemble those of lactated Ringer's solution (see Table 33–1); thus, lactated Ringer's solution is the fluid of choice for replacement of fluid lost through a biliary fistula. A prolonged biliary fistula results in impaired lipid and lipid-soluble vitamin absorption. These effects, for the most part, are reversed by replacement of bile into the upper gastrointestinal tract. Surprisingly, most patients are able to drink their own bile when it is mixed with orange juice or other drinks. Bile secretory pressure is usually 10 to 20 cm. of saline. Maximal secretory pressure is 30 to 35 cm., even in the presence of complete biliary obstruction. Numerous proteins are present in physiologic bile; the most abundant is IgA. The presence of IgA depends on an active secretory process, whereas that of albumin does not. It is likely that IgA is important to the immunocompetence of the gastrointestinal tract.

Enterohepatic Circulation

Bile salts secreted into the biliary system empty into the intestine, where they are efficiently absorbed into the enterohepatic circulation (Fig. 33–12). The liver extracts the bile acids and transports them back to the canalicular membrane where they are resecreted back into the biliary system. This process is referred to as the enterohepatic circulation (see Fig. 33–8). Total bile pool size in humans is 2 to 5 gm. and undergoes this circulation 2 to 3 times per meal and 6 to 10 times a day, depending on dietary habits. In addition, 0.2 to 0.6 gm. is lost in the stool per day, and this quantity is replaced with newly synthesized bile acids. Therefore, 20 to 40 times more bile acid than is normally synthesized is delivered into the intestine, underscoring the importance of this circulation. Under normal circumstances, serum bile acid levels are low (~5 μmol.) because of the 95% extraction efficiency of the liver: the liver can remove 80% of the bile acids delivered to it in a single pass. Serum bile acid levels are frequently increased in a patient with liver failure.

The active secretion of bile acids across the canalicular membrane is the primary metabolic pump of the enterohepatic circulation. In discussing the enterohepatic circulation, it is useful to distinguish between primary and secondary bile acids. Primary bile acids are synthesized from cholesterol by the liver and consist of cholic acid and chenodeoxycholic acid in humans. Secondary bile acids are formed in the intestinal lumen by bacterial dehydroxylation and consist of deoxycholic and lithocholic acid from cholic acid and chenodeoxycholic acid, respectively. Essentially all primary and secondary bile acids are conjugated with the amino acids glycine and taurine. Amino acid conjugation lowers the pKa of bile acids so they remain ionized in the intestinal lumen and are not passively absorbed through nonionic diffusion.

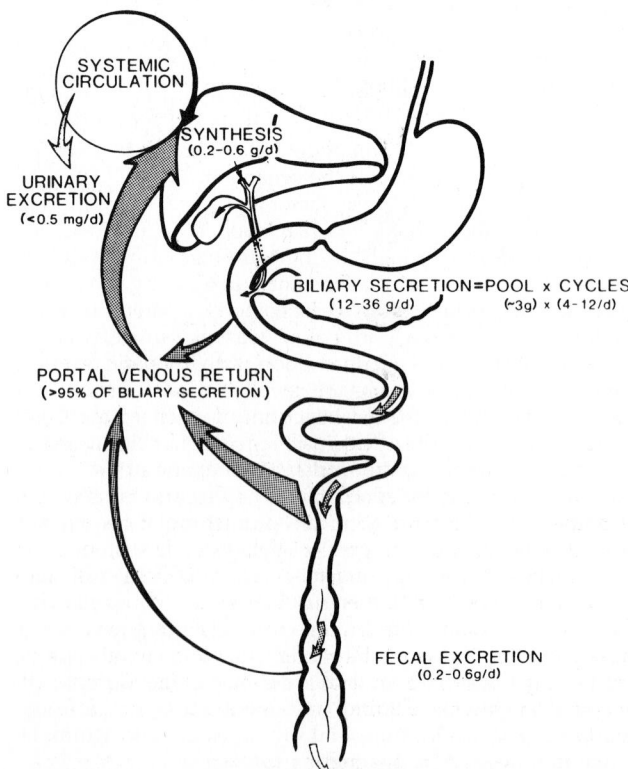

Figure 33–12. The enterohepatic circulation of bile salts with some general kinetic values for man. (From Carey, M. C.: The enterohepatic circulation. *In* Arias, I., et al. [Eds.]: The Liver: Biology and Pathobiology. New York, Raven Press, 1982.)

Conjugated bile acids also form micelles, which more effectively facilitate lipid digestion and absorption from the small intestine. Various intestinal problems such as regional enteritis, ileal resection, Zollinger-Ellison syndrome, radiation enteritis, and blind loop syndrome may be associated with deficient bile acid absorption, which leads to diarrhea, steatorrhea, or vitamin B_{12} deficiency. A decreased bile acid pool may also predispose to the formation of gallstones. In blood, bile salts are tightly bound to both serum albumin and lipoproteins, particularly high-density lipoprotein. Hepatic uptake is carrier mediated and follows Michaelis-Menten kinetics.

Bilirubin Metabolism

Bilirubin, a breakdown product of heme, is excreted almost entirely in the bile. With hepatocellular disease or extrahepatic biliary obstruction, free bilirubin may accumulate in blood and tissues. Approximately 75% of bilirubin is derived from senescent red blood cells. Bilirubin circulates bound to albumin, which protects tissue from its toxicity. It is rapidly removed from the plasma by the liver through a carrier-mediated transport system. In the hepatocyte, bilirubin is bound to other proteins (Y and Z), which probably have a role in transport. It is conjugated with glucuronide and secreted in bile. Conjugated bilirubin may form a covalent bond with albumin; this is called delta bilirubin. The implications of delta bilirubin are still being investigated.

Disorders of bilirubin metabolism leading to predominantly unconjugated hyperbilirubinemia include neonatal hyperbilirubinemia, Crigler-Najjar Type I (which usually leads to kernicterus and death), the more benign Crigler-Najjar Type II, and Gilbert's syndrome. Disorders characterized by predominantly conjugated hyperbilirubinemia include Dubin-Johnson syndrome, Rotor's syndrome, and recurrent intrahepatic cholestasis; patients with these disorders usually have a benign course.

In the intestine, bilirubin is reduced by bacteria to mesobilirubinogen and stercobilinogen, collectively termed *urobilinogen.* These are both excreted in the stool. A fraction of urobilinogen is oxidized to urobilin, which is brown pigment and gives stool its normal color. Part of urobilinogen is resorbed in the intestine and excreted in the urine. With complete biliary obstruction, urobilinogen cannot form and, therefore, will not appear in the urine.

Carbohydrate Metabolism

The liver has a central role in energy metabolism: it helps provide a continuous source of glucose for the central nervous system and red blood cells. During the fed state, results of intestinal carbohydrate digestion (glucose: 80%; and galactose and fructose: 20%) are delivered to the liver. The latter two are rapidly converted to glucose. Glucose absorbed by the hepatocyte is converted directly to glycogen for storage up to a maximum of 65 gm. of glycogen per kg. of liver mass. Excess glucose is converted to fat. Glycogen is also produced by muscle, but this is not available for use by any other tissues. During the fasting state, this glycogen is the primary source of glucose. However, after 48 hours of fasting, liver glycogen is exhausted, and proteins mobilized primarily from muscle, mainly alanine, are converted by the liver to glucose.

Lactate produced by anaerobic metabolism is metabolized only in the liver. Ordinarily it is converted to pyruvate and subsequently back to glucose. This shuttling of glucose and lactate between liver and peripheral tissue is carried out in the Cori cycle. The brain does not participate in this cycle, and a continuous source of glucose for the brain must come at the expense of muscle proteins.

In liver disease, the metabolism of glucose is often deranged. Frequently, in patients with cirrhosis, the portosystemic shunting causes decreased exposure of portal blood to the hepatocytes, producing an abnormal result of the oral glucose tolerance test. Hypoglycemia is rare in chronic liver disease, since the synthetic capacity of hepatocytes is preserved until late in the disorder. In fulminant hepatic failure, however, there is extensive loss of hepatocyte mass and function, and hypoglycemia supervenes as gluconeogenesis fails.

Lipid Metabolism

There are three sources of free fatty acid available to the liver: fats absorbed from the gut, fat liberated from adipocytes in response to lipolysis, and fatty acids synthesized from carbohydrates and amino acids. These fatty acids are esterified with glycerol to form triglyceride. The export of triglycerides is dependent on the synthesis of very low density lipoproteins. In cases of excess supply of fatty acid, there is lipid accumulation in the liver because there is an imbalance of triglyceride relative to very low density lipoproteins. This is seen in obesity, corticosteroid use, pregnancy, diabetes, and total parenteral nutrition. Simple protein malnutrition or protein-calorie imbalance may also result in fatty change of liver, based on decreased export of triglycerides, because of limited supply of precursors for hepatic synthesis of lipoproteins.

The fatty infiltration of alcohol abuse is the result of several abnormalities: (1) alcohol is a source of calories, which are converted to acetyl-coenzyme A, which is a substrate for fat synthesis; (2) the reduced form of nicotinamide-adenine dinucleotide produced in the metabolism of alcohol inhibits fatty acid oxidation and shifts metabolism toward triglyceride synthesis and esterification; and (3) chronic alcoholism may, because of malnutrition, inhibit synthesis of very low density lipoproteins.

The liver also has a central role in cholesterol metabolism. It is the most active site of cholesterol and bile salt synthesis. In mammals, 90% of cholesterol is synthesized *de novo* from its precursor acetyl-coenzyme A. Hydroxymethylglutaryl coenzyme A reductase is the rate-limiting enzyme of cholesterol metabolism. A competitive antagonist, mevinolin, can block this enzyme and effectively lower plasma cholesterol. Cholesterol can enter the liver cell with four different species of lipoprotein: chylomicrons, very low density lipoproteins, low density lipoproteins, and high density lipoproteins. The major carriers of cholesterol are low density lipoproteins. Bile salt synthesis is the major catabolic pathway of cholesterol in liver, and 7-alpha-hydroxylase is the rate-limiting enzyme for the conversion of cholesterol to bile acids. The other important route of cholesterol elimination is direct secretion into the bile.

Protein Metabolism

Hepatic protein synthesis and catabolism are vitally important. At least 17 of the major human plasma proteins are synthesized and secreted by the liver. The liver is the only organ that produces serum albumin and alpha-globulin, and it synthesizes most of the urea in the body. Production of various serum proteins is an important index of liver function. Albumin is the most abundant serum protein, its synthesis accounting for 11% to 15% of total hepatic synthesis. Synthesis of albumin is influenced by nutritional status, thyroxine, insulin, glucagon, cortisol, and cytokines produced in the systemic inflammatory response.

Dramatic changes in both type and amount of plasma

protein produced by the liver take place in systemic inflammatory states. The *acute-phase reactants* produced by the liver in response to interleukin-6 increase in a sudden transient rise in production of several proteins. These include C-reactive protein, serum amyloid A, and fibrinogen. Albumin synthesis decreases. The acute-phase proteins have a wide range of biologic activities, including inhibition of proteases, blood clotting, opsonization of bacteria and debris, modulation of the immune response, and binding of heavy metals. In general, it is thought that the acute-phase reactants localize and limit the tissue damage while enhancing microbial clearance.

Vitamin Metabolism

The liver has many important roles in the uptake, storage, and mobilization of vitamins. Most important are the fat-soluble vitamins A, D, E, and K. The absorption of these is dependent on bile salts. The vitamins appear in the thoracic duct 2 to 6 hours after oral administration. Vitamin A is exclusively stored in the liver, and excessive ingestion of vitamin A may be associated with significant liver injury. A role for the storage of vitamin A in Ito cells has been suggested. The initial step in vitamin D activation occurs in the liver, where vitamin D_3 is converted to 25-hydroxycholecalciferol.

Of particular surgical significance was the discovery of vitamin K. This vitamin is essential for the gamma-carboxylation of the vitamin K–dependent coagulation factors II, VII, IX, and X. These factors are inactive without gamma carboxylation. In 1929, Dam observed that chicks developed hemorrhages when fed fat-free diets. He designated the active ingredient in normal feed as vitamin K, after the German word *Koagulation*. The veterinary hematologic disorder called sweet clover disease, first reported in 1922 in cattle that developed fatal hemorrhages, was later found to be caused by *bis*-hydroxycoumarin, a vitamin K antagonist. The minimal daily requirement of vitamin K is small, less than 0.1 µg. per kg. of body mass.

Coagulation

The liver synthesizes 11 proteins critical for hemostasis; all the procoagulant factors except von Willebrand's factor are produced by the liver. Factors I, VII, IX, and X share the unique characteristic of having gamma carboxyl glutamic acid in their amino acid sequence and are dependent on vitamin K for activation; without vitamin K, they do not undergo gamma-carboxylation and are inactive. Warfarin (Coumadin) impairs the formation of vitamin K–dependent factors by reducing the amount of vitamin K available to participate in gamma carboxylation of these factors. Clinically, warfarin is followed by observing the prothrombin time. Reversal of the effect of warfarin occurs by parenteral administration of vitamin K or coagulation factors.

Classically, there are two pathways for fibrin formation (*intrinsic* and *extrinsic*); physiologically, it is more likely that the two act in concert. The extrinsic pathway causes large amounts of clot to be formed in seconds and is limited only by the amount of tissue thromboplastin released. The intrinsic pathway requires several minutes to form a clot and can be blocked by a number of inhibitors. In clinical practice, the extrinsic pathway is monitored by measuring the prothrombin time, whereas the intrinsic pathway is monitored by measuring the partial thromboplastin time or accelerated partial thromboplastin time. Factor VII has the shortest half-life (5 to 7 hours), and in patients with hepatic dysfunction the synthetic ability of the liver may be assessed by monitoring the prothrombin time, because this test is dependent on adequate amounts of functional factor VII.

Metabolism of Drugs and Toxins

Drug and toxin metabolism is primarily a hepatic function. The range of metabolic transformations that foreign compounds undergo is conveniently categorized into two broad headings: (1) the phase I reactions of oxidation, reduction, and hydrolysis and (2) the phase II reactions, in which a compound is combined with an endogenous molecule to form a conjugate. Oxidative reactions represent most of the phase I biotransformations in what has come to be known as the cytochrome P-450 system.

Regeneration

Clinically, the regenerative capacity of the liver is well known and typically triggered by partial hepatectomy. During the midlife of humans, the liver will regenerate to a volume of 25 ± 1.2 ml. per kg. However, the exact time course for the regenerative phase in humans is lacking. Van Thiel and associates have previously presented clinical data on two patients receiving livers from donors an average of 10 kg. smaller than the recipients, which resulted in livers 29% and 59% smaller than expected had the donor liver and recipient been ideally matched. Serial computed tomographic scans after transplantation revealed an average increase of 70 ml. per day of liver volume, until achievement of a liver volume consistent with that expected for the recipient's size, age, or sex was achieved.

Interestingly, whereas plasma levels of amino acids, glucagon, and insulin and standard liver injury tests have been monitored, none has correlated with changes in graft size. Most of these are generally believed to be poor indices of the hepatocyte proliferation, and there is still no specific clinical marker for hepatocyte proliferation. Timetables of test results during regeneration suggest that bilirubin levels return to normal at 3 weeks and albumin levels normalize after 5 weeks.

Potential growth promoters include prostaglandins, platelet-derived growth factor, epidermal growth factor, hepatocyte growth factor (released from platelets by thrombin), and epinephrine. To date, the most important negative growth factors are tumor growth factor-beta and age. The regenerative capacity of the hepatocytes may be determined by factors other than the hepatocytes themselves. This inference comes from studies of reduced-size liver grafts from related donors, in which the transplanted livers regenerated faster than the residual liver in the donor. These observations substantiate previous findings that regeneration is determined by an intrinsic liver/host body:volume ratio, independent of functional liver mass. Further investigations are necessary to characterize more fully the regenerative response of the liver.

Future Developments

A number of areas of active research are likely to develop new concepts with respect to disease and therapy. Advances are likely in the following fields: (1) characterization of liver stem cells, (2) methods of molecular modification of the genome, (3) hepatocyte transplantation or replacement, and (4) apoptosis. Studies of liver development have shown that committed endodermal cells form hepatoblasts that have dual lineage progenitor capacity and give rise to mature hepatocytes, intrahepatic bile ducts, and portions of the extrahepatic ducts. Certain chemicals induce the proliferation of *oval cells*, which may play some role in carcinogenesis. Considerable research is ongoing with respect to permissive conditions for hepatocyte engraftment and survival. Transplantation of hepatocytes in ectopic sites has led to some enthusiasm with respect to their use in acute liver failure and also in methods of altering the genes of cells for better integration into the host. Gene therapy seems to have a great deal of potential applicability to the liver. This research is divided into two general strategies, somatic cell and germ cell therapy (i.e., introduction of foreign genes into nongerm cell versus germ cell lines). The strategies can be further subdivided into gene replacement or augmentation strategies, *ex vivo* and *in vivo*. Some progress has been reported by using viral vectors or other carriers, and by targeted delivery of polynucleotides to inhibit gene expression. Apoptosis, or DNA-encoded cell death, appears to play an important role in the cessation of liver regeneration. Early validation of this concept in the liver has led to a great flurry of research relating apoptosis to benign or malignant conditions.

Assessment of Liver Function

Although there is no magic test, a number of methods are useful in the diagnostic evaluation of the patient with potential liver disease. In this section are mentioned only some routine tests of liver function and several quantitative estimates of liver function (Table 33–2).

Routine Tests

Routine tests of liver function (see Table 33–2) include the liver transaminases, which are named either by the products of the reaction (i.e., serum glutamic oxaloacetic transaminase [SGOT] and serum glutamic pyruvic transaminase [SGPT]) or by the amino group donor (i.e., aspartate transaminase [AST] or alanine transaminase [ALT]); alkaline phosphatase (ALP); gamma-glutamyl transpeptidase (GGT); leucine aminopeptidase (LAP); 5'-nucleotidase; serum albumin and transferrin; and serum lipids and lipoproteins.

Liver Transaminases. Increased liver transaminase levels in liver disease reflect leakage from injured liver cells. The degree of elevation of the transaminases generally reflects the severity of hepatic necrosis, except in the important setting of alcoholic hepatitis, when levels seldom exceed 200 to 300 I.U. per liter.

Alkaline Phosphatase Activity. Activity of ALP is detected in many tissues, including the liver, bile ducts, intestines, bone, kidneys, placenta, or white blood cells. The serum ALP level is also elevated in a number of conditions not associated with hepatobiliary disease, such as pregnancy, normal growth, bone tumors, and liver tumors (the Regan isoenzyme). The reason for ALP elevation is apparent in most cases. When the reason is not apparent, several methods, such as electrophoresis and relative heat stability, differentiate the hepatobiliary enzyme from other isoenzymes. The most available solution in the clinical setting is to order a 5'-nucleotidase, LAP, or GGT activity measurement. These generally parallel ALP levels in hepatobiliary disease. Increased serum hepatobiliary ALP activity indicates bile duct obstruction, parenchymal disease, infiltrative lesions of the liver, or repair after hepatocyte injury. Increased ALP activity reflects both increased enzyme synthesis and altered biliary excretion or leakage from damaged cells. The highest levels of ALP occur, in general, with extrahepatic bile duct obstruction, followed by intrahepatic cholestasis and then neoplasms of the liver. The degree of ALP elevation is a predictor of the degree of liver involvement or metastatic disease.

Other Enzymes. LAP is a ubiquitous cellular peptidase, and 5'-nucleotidase is a plasma membrane enzyme. GGT is present in many tissues, and its elevation suggests hepatobiliary disease, myocardial infarction, or pancreatic or neuromuscular disease. GGT also monitors the degree of ingestion of alcohol.

Albumin. Albumin is a useful clinical marker of synthetic function in chronic hepatic insufficiency. It is synthesized only in the liver, and its level in the blood is determined by liver function, nutritional state, thyroid hormone, or adrenal corticosteroids. The normal rate of albumin synthesis is 110 to 200 mg. per kg. per day. The exact mechanisms involved in albumin metabolism in the healthy state are not clear. Albumin loss is augmented in certain disease states, such as burns, sepsis, nephrotic syndrome, and protein-losing enteropathies. When other mechanisms of albumin loss are excluded, the serum albumin level is an accurate marker of liver failure or altered hepatic function. Unfortunately, because of its long half-life, albumin measures just chronic and not acute liver failure.

TABLE 33–2. Laboratory Tests in Liver Disease

Laboratory Test	Change in Liver Disease	Significance of Change in Liver Disease
Alanine aminotransferase	Increase	Correlates with hepatic cell death
Aspartate aminotransferase	Increase	Correlates with hepatic cell death
Alkaline phosphatase	Increase	Biliary duct obstruction Liver tumor, metastatic liver tumor *Note:* normally increased during growth and pregnancy; increased in bone tumors; heat stability/electrophoresis can distinguish isoenzyme; increased 5'-nucleotidase, leucine aminopeptidase, gamma-glutamyl transferase with alkaline phosphatase suggestive of biliary disease
Gamma-glutamyl transferase	Increase	Extrahepatic biliary obstruction *Note:* increased in chronic alcoholics; increased in myocardial infarction and neuromuscular disease; useful in following alcohol consumption
Leucine aminopeptidase	Increase	Cholestasis *Note:* increased in pregnancy; ubiquitous enzyme
5'-Nucleotidase	Increase	Cholestasis
Albumin	Decrease	Chronically impaired liver function *Note:* dependent on nutritional status of patient; decreased in conditions associated with loss/consumption (nephrotic syndrome, protein-losing enteropathy, sepsis, burns); need adequate thyroid and adrenal function
Transferrin	Decrease	Reflects more acute changes in liver function and nutritional status

Transferrin. Also synthesized in the liver, transferrin has a much shorter half-life than albumin. Changes in transferrin levels reflect more acute changes in liver function than do changes in albumin levels. Lipid and lipoprotein electrophoreses also change in acute or chronic liver disease, owing to abnormal or altered synthesis. Much work has gone into investigating these patterns, but their measurement has not yet proved particularly useful clinically.

Specific Tests. Specific tests of liver disease include screening tests for hepatitis and for other benign chronic liver disease. Such tests include antimitochondrial (primary biliary cirrhosis), smooth muscle (sclerosing cholangitis), antinuclear antibody, alpha$_1$-antitrypsin (antitrypsin deficiency), blood alcohol, plasma ceruloplasmin, or amylase levels. Specific markers for neoplasms include alpha-fetoprotein and carcinoembryonic antigen levels. Infectious serologic markers include cytomegalovirus, Epstein-Barr virus antibodies, leptospiral agglutination, fasciola, ameba, hydatid complement fixation tests, and the Wasserman reaction.

Quantitative Assessment

Bromsulphalein and Indocyanine Green. These dyes are removed from the circulation by the liver. Such intravenous tests have been used to assess liver dysfunction in the absence of jaundice. Each is a measure of biliary excretion and is a more specific quantitative test than any of the routine tests of liver function or cholestasis. However, neither has particular clinical utility, and bromsulphalein has a long history of being put on and taken off the commercial market.

Galactose Elimination Capacity. This test reflects hepatocellular function but requires multiple determinations over a 2-hour period. Galactose is safe and injected intravenously at a dose that saturates the enzyme system responsible for its elimination. The preliminary step is the initial phosphorylation by galactokinase.

Aminopyrine Breath Test. Aminopyrine as well as caffeine have been used as breath test substances that measure the efficiency of the cytochrome P-450 (microsomal) system where they are metabolized. Aminopyrine is labeled with carbon-14 and given by mouth. Carbon dioxide samples labeled with carbon-14 are collected at intervals over 2 hours. This test reflects the residual functional microsomal mass and, thus, viable hepatic tissue. It has more value in assessing prognosis than for screening. Serial salivary caffeine clearance is a similar measure. Antipyrine clearance can also be measured, but the test requires over 30 hours.

Lidocaine Metabolite Formation (MEGX Test). Lidocaine similarly is metabolized by oxidative *N*-demethylation by the cytochrome P-450 system. Monoethylglycinexylidide (MEGX) is formed correlating with lidocaine clearance. Clearance 15 minutes after injection gives a quantitative assessment of liver function, which may correlate with graft survival before liver transplantation.

Tests of Coagulation. The prothrombin time is in general a sensitive marker of the severity of liver failure. Prolongation indicates deficiency not only of the thrombin complex but also of factors XI and XII. Estimation of individual clotting factors is rarely required. However, some evidence suggests that a factor V concentration of less than 10% on admission in acetaminophen-induced acute liver failure predicts a poor outcome. The ratio of factor VIII to factor V may also be valuable. Prognostic significance of several other clotting factors relating to various kinds of fulminant failure is receiving intensive scrutiny.

SELECTED REFERENCES

Bismuth, H.: Surgical anatomy and anatomical surgery of the liver. *In* Blumgart, L. H. (Ed.): Surgery of the Liver and Biliary Tract. Edinburgh, Churchill Livingstone, 1992.
This is an excellent review of the French segmental system of liver anatomy.

Lautt, W. W., and Greenway, C. V.: Conceptual review of the hepatic vascular bed. Hepatology, 7:952, 1987.
This overview details some of the current understanding of hepatic microvascular circulation.

Rappaport, A. M.: The microcirculatory hepatic unit. Microvasc. Res., 6:212, 1973.
The work of this investigator permits the understanding of the functional unit of the liver and the heterogeneity of hepatocyte function.

Tavaloni, N., and Berk, P. D. (Eds.): Hepatic Transport and Bile Secretion. New York, Raven Press, 1993.
This text is a detailed outline of the current understanding of the liver and biliary physiology at the molecular level.

Zucker, S. D., and Gollan, J. L.: Physiology of the liver. *In* Haubrich W. S., and Schaffner, F. (Eds.): Gastroenterology, 5th ed. Philadelphia, W. B. Saunders, 1995.
This recent edition includes basic physiologic principles and detailed discussions of the current concepts of hepatic physiology.

REFERENCES

1. Adson, M. A., and Beart, R. W.: Elective hepatic resections. Surg. Clin. North Am., 57:339, 1977.
2. Amenta, F., Cavalotti, C., Ferrant, F., and Tonelli, F.: Cholinergic nerves in the human liver. Histochem. J., 13:419, 1981.
3. Arias, I. M.: Multidrug resistance genes, P-glycoproteins and the liver. Hepatology, 12:159, 1990.
4. Arias, I. M.: The biology of the bile canaliculus. Hepatology, 17:318, 1993.
5. Berk, P. D., Howe, R. B., Bloomer, J. R., and Berlin, N. I.: Studies of bilirubin kinetics in normal adults. J. Clin. Invest., 48:2176, 1969.
6. Boyer, J. L., and Bloomer, J. R.: Canalicular bile secretion in man: Studies utilizing the biliary clearance of ¹⁴C mannitol. J. Clin. Invest., 54:773, 1974.
7. Campbell, H. A., and Link, K. P.: Studies on the hemorrhagic sweet clover disease: IV. The isolation and crystalization of the hemorrhagic agent. J. Biol. Chem., 138:21, 1941.
8. Campra, J. L., and Reynolds, T. B.: The hepatic circulation. *In* Arias, I. M., Popper, H., Schacter, D., and Shafritz, D. A. (Eds.): Pathobiology of the Liver. New York, Raven Press, 1982, pp. 627–645.
9. Cantlie, J.: On a new arrangement of the right and left lobes of the liver. J. Anat. Physiol. (Lond.), 32:iv, 1898.
10. Chiandusi, L., Greco, F., Stardi, G., Vaccarino, A., Ferraris, C. M., and Curti, B.: Estimation of hepatic arterial and portal venous blood flow by direct catheterization of the vena porta through the umbilical vein in man. Acta Hepatosplenol. (Stuttg.), 15:166, 1968.
11. Corless, J. K., Middleton, H. M.: Normal liver function—a basis for understanding hepatic disease. Arch. Intern. Med., 143:2291, 1983.
12. Couinaud, C.: Les envelopes vasculobiliares de foie ou capsule de Glisson: Leur intérêt dans la chirurgie vesiculaire, les resections hepatique et l'abord du hile du foie. Lyon Chir., 49:589, 1954.
13. Disse, J.: Über die Lymphbahnen der Saugetierleber. Arch. Mikr. Anat., 36:203, 1890.
14. Elias, H.: Appositional growth of the embryonic liver. Rev. Int. Hepatic, 14:317, 1964.
15. Elias, H., and Petty, D.: Gross anatomy of blood vessels and ducts within the liver. Am. J. Anat., 90:59, 1952.
16. Emond, J. C., and Renz, J. F.: Surgical anatomy of the liver and its applications to hepatobiliary surgery and transplantation. Semin. Liver Dis., 14:158, 1994.
17. Fitz, J. G., Basavappa, S., McGill, J., Milhas, O., and Cohn, J. A.: Regulation of membrane chloride currents in rat bile duct epithelial cells. J. Clin. Invest., 91:319, 1993.
18. Gebhardt, R.: Metabolic zonation of the liver: Regulation and implications for liver function. Pharmacol. Ther., 53:275, 1992.
19. Geuze, H. J., Van der Donk, H. A., Simmons, C. F., et al.: Receptor-mediated endocytosis in liver parenchymal cells. Int. Rev. Exp. Pathol., 29:113, 1986.
20. Gilfillan, R. S.: Anatomic study of the portal vein and its branches. Arch. Surg., 61:449, 1950.
21. Hahn, P. F., et al.: Physiologic bilaterality of portal circulation: Streamline blood flow into liver as shown by radioactive phosphorus. Am. J. Physiol., 143:105, 1945.
22. Havel, R. J., and Hamilton, R. L.: Hepatocytic lipoprotein receptor and intracellular lipoprotein catabolism. Hepatology, 8:1689, 1988.
23. Hoffman, A. F.: Chemistry and enterohepatic circulation of bile acids. Hepatology, 4(suppl. 5):4, 1984.
24. Hoffman, A. F.: Bile acid secretion, bile flow and biliary lipid secretion in humans. Hepatology, 12:17S, 1990.
25. Jones, A. L.: Anatomy of the normal liver. *In* Zakim, D., and Boyer, T. D. (Eds.): Hepatology. Philadelphia, W. B. Saunders, 1982, pp. 3–31.
26. Jones, A. L., Schmucker, D. L., Renston, R. H., et al.: The architecture of bile secretion: A morphological perspective of physiology. Dig. Dis. Sci., 25:609, 1980.
27. Jones, R. S., and Meyers, W. C.: Regulation of hepatic biliary secretion. Ann. Rev. Physiol., 141:67, 1970.

28. LaRusso, N. F.: Proteins in bile: How they get there and what they do. Am. J. Physiol., 247:G199, 1984.
29. Lautt, W. W., and Greenway, C. V.: Conceptual review of the hepatic vascular bed. Hepatology, 7:952, 1987.
30. Lautt, W. W., Legare, D. J., and Ezzat, W. R.: Quantitation of the hepatic arterial buffer response to graded changes in portal blood flow. Gastroenterology, 98:1024, 1990.
31. Longmire, W. P. J., and Tompkins, R. K.: Anatomy. *In* Longmire, W. P. J., and Tompkins, R. K. (Eds.): Manual of Liver Surgery. New York, Springer-Verlag, 1981, pp. 13–25.
32. Mall, F. P.: A study of the structural unit of the liver. Am. J. Anat., 5:227, 1906.
33. Marzolo, M. P., Rigotti, A., and Nervi, F.: Secretion of biliary lipids from the hepatocytes. Hepatology, 12:134S, 1990.
34. McGill, J. M., Basavappa, S., Gettys, T. W., and Fitz, J. G.: Secretin activates Cl⁻ channels in bile duct epithelial cells through a cAMP-dependent mechanism. Am. J. Physiol., 266:G731, 1994.
35. Meyers, W. C., and Jones, R. S.: Glucagon or insulin suppressed biliary lipid excretion in dogs and man. Ann. Surg., 190:709, 1979.
36. Michalopoulos, G. K.: Liver regeneration: Molecular mechanisms of growth control. FASEB J., 4:176, 1990.
37. Michalopoulos, G. K.: Liver regeneration and growth factors: Old puzzles and new perspectives. Lab. Invest., 67:413, 1992.
38. Michel, N. A.: Newer anatomy of the liver and its variant blood supply and collateral circulation. Am. J. Surg., 112:337, 1966.
39. Molino, G.: The functioning liver mass. Ric. Clin. Lab., 21:9, 1991.
40. Mosely, R. H.: Hepatic uptake of amino acids. *In* Tavaloni, N., and Berk,

P. D. (Eds.): Hepatic Transport and Bile Secretion. New York, Raven Press, 1993, pp. 337–349.
41. Nakamura, S., and Tsuzuki, T.: Surgical anatomy of the hepatic veins and the inferior vena cava. Surg. Gynecol. Obstet., 152:43, 1981.
42. Rappaport, A. M.: The microcirculatory hepatic unit. Microvasc. Res., 6:212, 1973.
43. Rappaport, A. M.: Physioanatomic considerations. *In* Schiff, L., and Schiff, E. R. (Eds.): Diseases of the Liver. Philadelphia, J. B. Lippincott, 1982, pp. 1–57.
44. Rappaport, A. M., and Schniederman, J. H.: The function of the hepatic artery. Rev. Physiol. Biochem. Pharmacol., 76:129, 1976.
45. Scharschmidt, B. F., and Van Dyke, R. W.: Mechanism of hepatic electrolyte transport. Gastroenterology, 85:1199, 1983.
46. Schenk, W. G. J., McDonald, J. C., McDonal, K., and Drapanas, T.: Direct measurement of hepatic blood flow in surgical patients: With related observations on hepatic flow dynamic in experimental animals. Ann. Surg., 156:463, 1962.
47. Stark, M. E., and Szurszewski, J. H.: Role of nitric oxide in gastrointestinal and hepatic function and disease. Gastroenterology, 103:1928, 1992.
48. Truttmann, M., and Sasse, D.: The lymphatics of the liver. Anat. Embryol., 190:201, 1994.
49. Zakim, D.: Metabolism of glucose and fatty acids by the liver. *In* Zakim, D., and Boyer, T. D. (Eds.): Hepatology. Philadelphia, W. B. Saunders, 1990, pp. 65–96.
50. Zucker, S. D., and Gollan, J. L.: Physiology of the liver. *In* Haubrich, W. S., and Schaffner, F. (Eds.): Gastroenterology. Philadelphia, W. B. Saunders, 1995, pp. 1858–1905.

II

PYOGENIC AND AMEBIC LIVER ABSCESS

Gene D. Branum, M.D., and William C. Meyers, M.D.

Liver abscess remains a formidable diagnostic and therapeutic problem, but significant strides in management have occurred over the past two decades. Changing etiologies of liver abscess reflect both improvements in health care and increased recognition of the condition in sicker, often immunocompromised patients. Pyogenic (bacterial) and amebic abscesses share many clinical features and are therefore discussed together. The pyogenic type is much more common in most sections of the United States; yet amebic abscess is endemic in many areas of the world and requires clinical suspicion for correct diagnosis. Fungi, cytomegaloviruses, and other organisms also cause liver abscess, predominantly in the immunocompromised host, but are less common and usually cause more diffuse hepatic disease. Echinococcosis generally has a different clinical presentation from pyogenic or amebic abscess, unless there is secondary bacterial involvement.

Liver abscess has been recognized since Hippocrates (circa 400 B.C.), who speculated that prognosis is related to the type of fluid within the lesion.[21] In the early nineteenth century, Bright[6] suggested that amebae might contribute to the formation of hepatic abscess, and Koch, in 1883, described amebae in the wall of a hepatic abscess. Fitz[10] and Dieulafoy[9] both emphasized the importance of intra-abdominal (bacterial) sources of infection in the pathogenesis of the disease. Dieulafoy[9] coined the term *la foie appendiculaire* in describing multiple hepatic abscesses subsequent to perforated appendicitis with pyelophlebitis (Fig. 33–13). Ochsner and DeBakey provided classic treatises on pyogenic and amebic hepatic abscess in 1938 and 1943. The latter authors reviewed a large personal experience and the world literature and emphasized the similarity in clinical presentation between the two types

of abscesses. Although clinical signs have remained the same, radiologic methods of diagnosis have greatly improved, and it is rare that a lesion is overlooked when ultrasonography or computed tomography (CT) is used. Antibiotic therapy has also improved, but the principal advance in the management of hepatic abscess has been the application of percutaneous aspiration or of laparoscopic techniques for diagnosis or treatment.

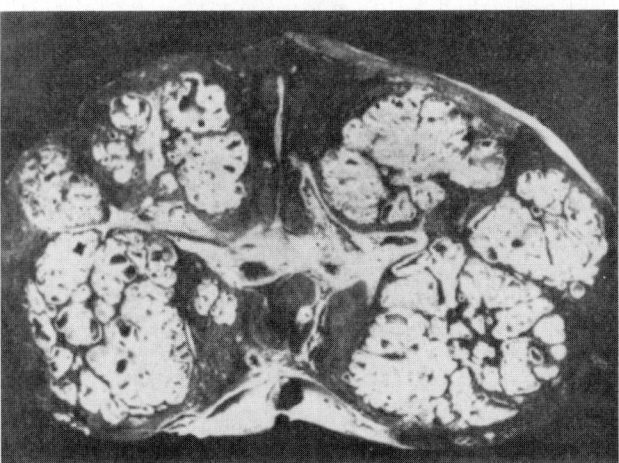

Figure 33–13. "Foie appendiculaire." Liver with multiple pyogenic abscesses. The patient died 3 weeks after operation for suppurative appendicitis. (From Bras, G., and Brandt, K. H.: Vascular disorders. *In* MacSween, R. N. M., Anthony, P. P., and Scheuer, P. J. [Eds.]: Pathology of the Liver. Edinburgh, Churchill Livingstone, 1987, p. 481.)

INCIDENCE

The overall incidence of liver abscess remains relatively stable, although the distribution of causes is changing. Pyogenic abscess represents approximately 80% of the cases in the United States, and superinfection represents another 10%. Amebae are the primary cause of 10%, and fungi and other organisms cause less than 10%. The overall rate of pyogenic abscess in the United States is estimated to be between 8 and 15 per 100,000 population. The incidence of both pyogenic and amebic abscess is higher in nations where medical care is not immediately available. For example, in Malaysia, pyogenic abscess constitutes 0.85% of total hospital admissions.

Amebic infestation is higher in countries in tropical or subtropical zones, locations with poor sanitation, and mental institutions. In the United States in 1975, the Center for Disease Control (CDC) noted 1.3 cases of amebiasis reported per 100,000 population. The CDC recorded 3500 cases of amebiasis per year, data that probably underestimate the actual number of cases. Immigrants and tourists from developing countries have a higher incidence, and American tourists to tropical areas are more likely to develop invasive amebiasis than permanent residents. Amebae are estimated to infest 15% to 30% of the population of Mexico, Africa, Southeast Asia, and South America. Local inhabitants are less likely than visitors to manifest symptoms, presumably due to partial immunity.

Hepatic abscess is the most common extraintestinal manifestation of amebiasis. Hepatic amebiasis is reported in 3% to 10% of afflicted patients. DeBakey and Ochsner found an average incidence of hepatic involvement associated with intestinal disease to be 13.2%. In certain severely infested locations up to a 40% incidence of hepatic involvement is reported. Liver abscess of both types affects both sexes and all age groups. In recent years, pyogenic abscess affected slightly more males than females, which is consistent with earlier series. The 40- to 60-year-old age group is the most commonly afflicted, and children represent a distinct group because of a higher rate of immunosuppression in hospitalized youth. In a series from Duke University Medical Center all six patients with pyogenic abscess who were younger than 15 years of age were male. Over the past several years in Los Angeles, the male-to-female ratio has been nearly 2:1 in young patients. This changing sex distribution in younger patients probably reflects the impact of the acquired immunodeficiency syndrome (AIDS). Amebic abscess affects males more than females in as much as a 9 to 10:1 ratio. In general the patients are younger, with the highest incidence in the 20- to 50-year-old age group. Several recent reports indicate a marked increase in the incidence of amebic liver abscess in children younger than the age of 3. There does not appear to be any particular racial susceptibility except for that related to living conditions. Examples include Mexican-Americans in the American Southwest and the predisposition of South African blacks compared with South African whites.

PATHOGENESIS

The pathophysiology of liver abscess in general or pyogenic abscess in particular involves two basic elements: the presence of the organism and the vulnerability of the liver. The spread of bacterial or other organisms to the hepatic parenchyma may occur through (1) the portal system; (2) ascension from the biliary tree; (3) the hepatic artery during generalized septicemia; (4) direct extension from subhepatic or subdiaphragmatic infection; or (5) a direct route following trauma (Fig. 33–14).

Most organisms enter the liver through the portal route. Hepatic clearance of portal bacteria is probably a very common event in healthy persons. The human liver remains

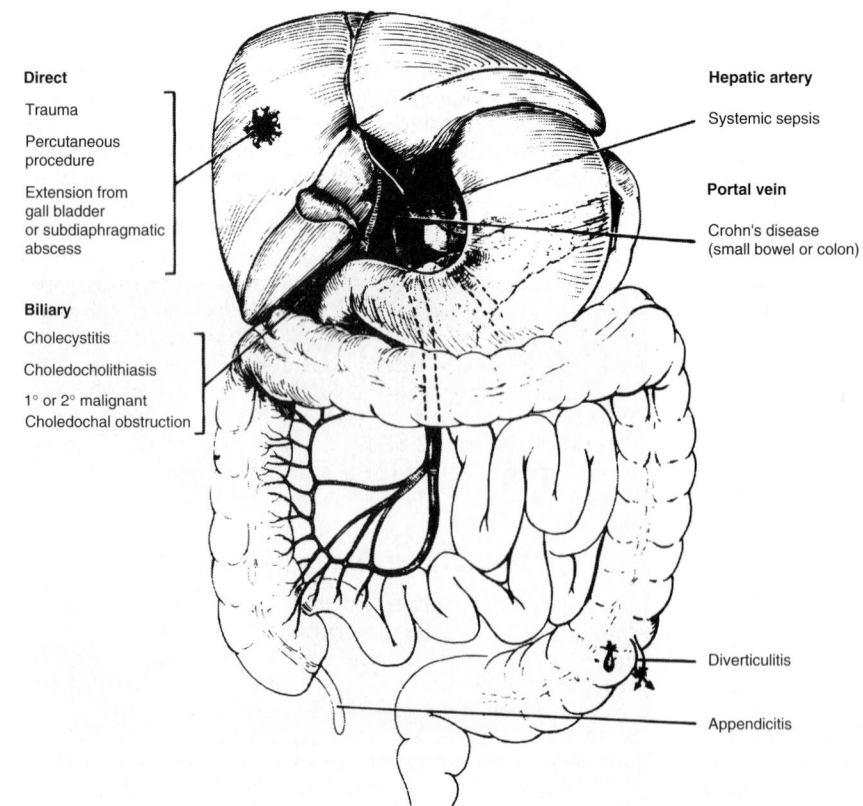

Direct

Trauma

Percutaneous procedure

Extension from gall bladder or subdiaphragmatic abscess

Biliary

Cholecystitis

Choledocholithiasis

1° or 2° malignant Choledochal obstruction

Hepatic artery

Systemic sepsis

Portal vein

Crohn's disease (small bowel or colon)

Diverticulitis

Appendicitis

Figure 33–14. Sources of organisms invading the liver in pyogenic hepatic abscesses.

sterile in most circumstances because of an efficient clearance mechanism that prevents colonization of hepatic sinusoids or parenchyma. Multiplication, tissue invasion, and abscess formation occur secondary to the introduction of other factors such as necrotic tissue, hepatic injury, malignant tumors, microemboli, poor perfusion, or congenital or acquired biliary or vascular obstruction. Pyogenic hepatic abscess usually represents an infective process in another organ. The process is usually within the abdomen. Appendicitis was by far the common source in most earlier series, representing 35% of the total group in Ochsner's patients. Appendicitis is involved in only approximately 10% of cases in more recent series (Table 33–3).[5a]

The other most common sources are cholecystitis, biliary or pancreatic cancer with obstruction, diverticulitis, regional enteritis, trauma, generalized sepsis, and pelvic inflammatory disease. Patients receiving chemotherapy for hematologic or solid malignancies are at increased risk. Other important associations with hepatic abscess in adults include colon cancer, diabetes, and cardiopulmonary disease. Associated conditions in children are malignancy, non-AIDS immunodeficiency states, AIDS, polycystic disease, cholecystitis, necrotizing enterocolitis, and congenital hepatic fibrosis. The most common non-AIDS immunodeficiency states occur after transplantation, as a result of liver failure, after treatment of malignancy, or with chronic granulomatous disease of childhood.

Despite advances in diagnostic techniques and an aggressive search for a source, no probable cause of hepatic abscess has been identified in 13% to 35% of cases since 1984. Cryptogenic abscesses constituted 22% of Ochsner's collected series in 1938. This incidence may increase further with more use of percutaneous drainage techniques because of fewer opportunities for abdominal exploration. In most previous series, cryptogenic abscesses were usually solitary, and the associated mortality was low. It is also possible that mortality associated with cryptogenic abscess could increase because of more undetected problems, such as underlying malignancy.

Portal pyelophlebitis is an infection of the portal vein, usually manifested radiographically by air in the portal vein. Although portal venous infection undoubtedly occurs more frequently than the demonstration of portal venous air, the latter complication is usually lethal. Pyelophlebitis is a likely cause of hepatic abscess. In this condition, mesenteric veins at the site of an inflammatory process thrombose and subsequently extend into the portal system and embolize to the liver. The septic emboli block venous radicles, giving rise to polymorphonuclear leukocyte, lymphocyte, and macrophage migration to the region and an intense inflammatory reaction.

Foci are usually multiple, but multiple sites may coalesce into a "solitary" abscess, with or without septation. Multiple, microscopic hepatic abscesses are often found at autopsy in patients dying of sepsis with portal pyelophlebitis. More abscesses occur in the right than in the left lobe. This is probably secondary to preferential laminar drainage of the superior mesenteric vein to the right lobe, although some controversy exists concerning this explanation.

Abscess formation secondary to biliary obstruction follows a slightly different pattern, with similar results. After obstruction of bile ducts, bacteria multiply and ascend into intrahepatic biliary radicles and canaliculosinusoidal channels, producing cholangitis. Bacterial proliferation causes further biliary distention with lymphatic and portal invasion and formation of a pyelophlebitic abscess. Further coalescence allows escape of pus into surrounding hepatic tissue with formation of multiple pockets and subsequent septations of a predominant cavity.

Biliary tract disease has supplanted appendicitis as the most common gastrointestinal problem associated with liver abscess. Bile ducts, biliary lymphatics, and periductal vascular channels are the primary routes by which abscesses develop in association with biliary infection. Liver abscess occurs most commonly with cholecystitis, choledocholithiasis, and malignant or benign biliary stricture. Malignant obstruction or metastatic adenocarcinoma causes more cases of liver abscess than observed previously because of improved palliative treatments, such as percutaneous or endoscopic biliary drainage techniques. Patients undergoing biliary-enteric bypass are at increased risk of abscess formation, even when there is no demonstrable stricture. Several studies suggest that choledochoduodenal anastomoses are associated with a high incidence of bacteremia or abscess than Roux-en-Y hepaticojejunostomy or choledochojejunostomy. A greater potential for reflux of foodstuffs in the former drainage procedure supports the latter observation. The incidence of a potential biliary source in association with liver abscess is estimated at 30% to 50%.

Trauma predisposes hepatic parenchyma to abscess formation by several mechanisms: bile leakage, decreased perfusion, foci of hepatic necrosis, direct introduction of bacteria through penetrating high- or low-velocity missiles, and hematoma formation. The combination of bile leakage, hematoma, and necrotic tissue provides a rich culture medium for bacteria introduced by the trauma itself or entrapment of bacteria borne in blood or bile. Modern therapy for various tumors has introduced an important new etiology for pyogenic abscess—iatrogenic cell death. Specific therapies relatively commonly associated with hepatic abscess include chemoembolization, alcohol injection, or cryoablation of hepatic tumors. In one report from the National Cancer Institute, bacterial abscesses were more common in older patients with solid tumors and invasive procedures; in contrast, fungal abscesses occurred more in younger patients with leukemia or lymphoma after chemotherapy and resultant neutropenia.

PATHOLOGY AND MICROBIOLOGY

Pyogenic hepatic abscesses have some characteristic gross and microscopic pathologic features. In most series, right hepatic abscesses predominate by a nearly 3:1 ratio. The presumed explanation for this is streaming of the superior mesenteric vein fraction of portal flow to the right lobe of the liver as well as its relatively greater volume. Bilobar metastases occur in 1% of patients. Most series indicate a nearly equal distribution between solitary and multiple liver abscesses. Abscesses vary from less than a millimeter to several centimeters. They may appear honeycombed with

TABLE 33–3. Source of Pyogenic Abscess in Four Series[5a] of Patients Since 1985*

	No.	Percentage
Cryptogenic	32	18.7
Biliary		
Benign	41	23.9
Malignant	17	9.9
Colonic		
Benign	29	16.9
Malignant	2	1.2
Hematogenous (arterial)	14	8.2
Other portal	12	7.0
Trauma	10	5.8
Other (chronic granulomatous disease, local extension, abdominal surgery)	9	5.3

*n = 171.

multiple lesions, although this appearance is unusual except with fungal organisms. Interestingly, the size of solitary abscesses nearly tripled in one study between 1945 to 1957 and 1971 to 1983. Grossly, hepatic abscesses appear yellow, compared with the normal, deep maroon hepatic parenchyma that surrounds them. The organ is usually subtly enlarged, and palpation may reveal fluctuant areas corresponding to the pus-filled cavity. The liver is often adherent to surrounding organs or the diaphragm because of associated capsular inflammation. Small abscesses deep within the parenchyma rarely exhibit these findings. Most traumatic abscesses are solitary and localized near the site of injury. Microscopically, acute inflammatory reaction is observed with necrosis and hepatocyte cords in the portal triad regions, and cholestasis may be evident in adjacent tissue.

Organisms recovered from liver abscesses vary greatly but generally reflect bile or enteric flora (Table 33–4). Reasons for the variability include differences in antibiotics before culture, culture techniques, or patient populations. In most recent series, most patients have a positive culture, and over half harbor more than one organism. Solitary abscesses are more likely than multiple ones to grow multiple organisms. The high frequency of "sterile" abscesses found in earlier studies was probably due primarily to an inability to isolate anaerobic or microaerophilic organisms. At present, the most likely reason for a sterile culture is effective antibiotic therapy. The most common aerobic organisms in most series are *Escherichia coli, Klebsiella,* and *Enterococcus.* The most common anaerobes are *Bacteroides,* anaerobic streptococci, and *Fusobacterium* species. Streptococcal species (aerobic, anaerobic, or microaerophilic) are found in 25% to 30% of cultured abscesses and are believed to be of increasing importance in the pathogenesis of pyogenic abscess. The presence of isolated colonies of *E. coli* or *Klebsiella* should raise the suspicion of a biliary source, while the presence of anaerobes suggests a colonic source. One interesting observation is the more common appearance of staphylococcal abscesses in young males, compared with other patient groups. More than half of patients not receiving antibiotics may have microorganisms cultured from the peripheral blood.

Amebic liver abscess follows intestinal infestation by *Entamoeba histolytica.* The most common mode of transmission of *E. histolytica* is by individual contact rather than contaminated drinking water or food. Venereal transmission usually causes genital, gut, or visceral disease. Two forms of the protozoan may be found in stool specimens: trophozoites and cysts. Trophozoites are the invasive form and are derived from cysts. The factors that determine clinically significant disease are poorly understood. The simple finding of trophozoites or cysts in the stool is so common that this alone is not evidence of active disease.

The incidence of liver disease in patients with intestinal amebiasis is reported to be between 3% and 25%. There is a latency period of several weeks between intestinal infection and observable hepatic involvement. The amebae reach the

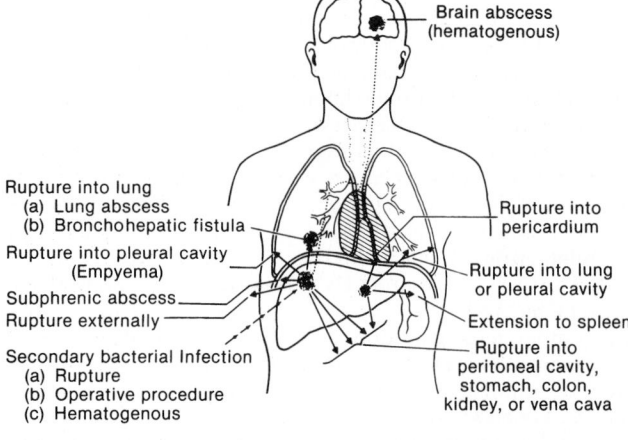

Figure 33–15. Sites of rupture or extension of amebic abscess. A slight but real possibility of hematogenous spread exists, as illustrated by the development of a brain abscess.

liver through the portal vein. The trophozoites either degenerate in the portal venous radicles or migrate to an adjacent area, causing necrosis and liquefaction. The areas of destruction coalesce to form most commonly a single large cavity in the right lobe. The abscess may vary from less than 1 cm. to 25 cm. in diameter. The contents are a mixture of necrotic hepatic parenchyma and blood that yields a classic "anchovy paste" appearance. This is usually sterile and odorless. Secondary bacterial infection occurs in approximately 10% of cases and may change the color and odor of the contents. Protozoa are usually found only in a rim of necrotic tissue and are therefore unlikely to be aspirated.

Seventy-five per cent to 90% of abscesses are found in the right lobe. Left lobe or bilobar involvement usually indicates more advanced disease. Right lobe lesions are more likely to rupture intraperitoneally, whereas left lobe lesions rupture into the pericardium or pleural space (Fig. 33–15). As with pyogenic abscess, the liver is usually enlarged. Capsular adhesions to the diaphragm or adjacent tissue are generally not as numerous. Early or acute lesions have thin walls with little fibrosis, whereas older abscesses have a more well-formed fibrous capsule, sharply demarcating them from normal liver parenchyma. There is usually marked necrosis of hepatic parenchyma within the lesions, with little polymorphonuclear cell infiltration. As the abscess matures, it becomes spherical, and more eosinophilic staining debris develops. Calcification is unusual except in chronic abscesses.

Like pyogenic hepatic abscess, the amebic variety may be associated with depressed immunologic states. Experimental infection is easier to induce after splenectomy, probably because of decreased macrophage clearance of the parasite. Antimacrophage serum exacerbates and bacille Calmette-Guérin improves host defenses against amebae. Cell-mediated immunity is impaired during the first 2 weeks of infection in normal patients without treatment. Therefore, suppression of immune response during systemic infection may have a role in amebic liver abscess.

DIAGNOSIS

The diagnosis of hepatic abscess is challenging because clinical signs are usually not specific. Early differentiation between pyogenic and amebic liver abscess may be even more difficult because of the similarity in signs, symptoms, and radiologic features. Both pyogenic and amebic abscess should be considered lethal unless detected early. For pyogenic abscess, two diagnoses are necessary for optimal man-

TABLE 33–4. Most Common Organisms Isolated in Five Series[3a, 5, 5a, 16a, 22a] of Pyogenic Abscess Reported Since 1985*

	No.	Percentage
Escherichia coli	72	33
Klebsiella pneumoniae	39	18
Bacteroides species	53	24
Streptococcal species	80	37
Microaerophilic streptococci	26	12

*n = 219.

agement: the abscess condition itself and the underlying source. Neither diagnosis may be apparent initially, but both can usually be discovered with appropriate evaluation. The diagnosis of hepatic abscess is apparent at the time of admission in a minority of patients but, if suspected, is readily diagnosed by ultrasonography or CT in over 95% of patients.

The majority of patients with hepatic abscess have symptoms of less than 2 weeks' duration, although one third have been affected a month or longer. The primary symptoms are fever, malaise, chills, anorexia, weight loss, abdominal pain, and nausea. With amebic abscess, a recent diarrheal syndrome can be documented in only a minority of patients. An occasional historical feature is a long-standing respiratory infection occurring before the development of abdominal symptoms. Fever of unknown origin is the presentation in a significant number of patients. Rarely, patients with either amebic or pyogenic abscess are admitted with diffuse peritonitis, shock, or hepatic failure. Possible physical findings include right upper quadrant tenderness, pleural dullness to percussion, fever, hepatomegaly, and jaundice. Tenderness may be elicited by either direct palpation or percussion of the right rib cage. Most patients have leukocytosis and some liver enzyme abnormality. The most common findings on plain abdominal or chest radiographs are right-sided atelectasis, an elevated hemidiaphragm, pleural effusion, or pneumonia. Occasionally, a subdiaphragmatic air-fluid collection is observed with pyogenic abscess or a superinfected amebic abscess (Fig. 33–16). In addition to ultrasonography or liver CT, a liver scan usually accurately localizes the abscess. CT should routinely be enhanced with intravenous injection of contrast medium to demonstrate the relative hypovascularity of the abscess.

Specific Imaging Tests

Ultrasonography. Ultrasonography is the most useful screening test when the suspicion of hepatic abscess arises (Fig. 33–17*A* and *B*). The test is highly sensitive (85% to 95%), is more accurate than CT in imaging the biliary tree, and allows diagnostic or therapeutic drainage or biopsy at the time of performance. Limitations of ultrasonography arise in nonhomogeneous livers, in those situated high beneath the

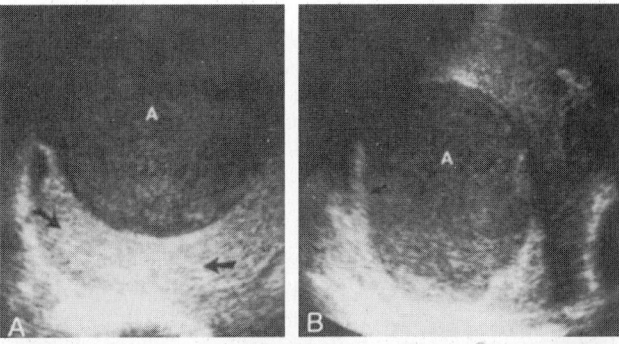
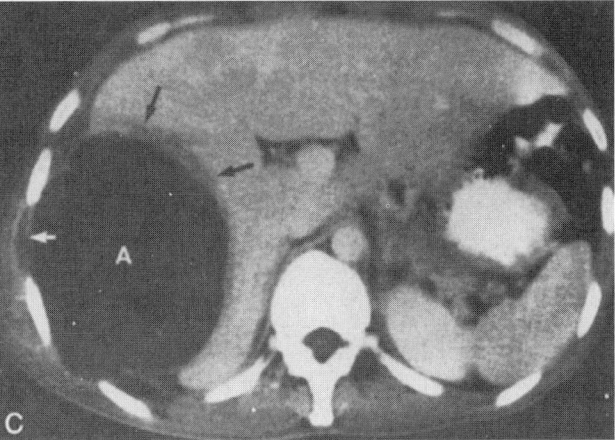

Figure 33–17. Ultrasonographic and computed tomographic (CT) appearance of an amebic abscess. *A*, Large, rounded abscess (A) in the right lobe with slight distal acoustic enhancement (arrows). *B*, Location of the abscess (A) immediately adjacent to the diaphragm (arrow). *C*, CT scan revealing abscess (A) with surrounding low-density peripheral zone of edema (black arrows) and extrahepatic extension of abscess into intercostal space (white arrow). (From Jeffrey, R. B., Jr.: CT and Sonography of the Acute Abdomen. New York, Raven Press, 1989, p. 25.)

thoracic cage, and in extremely obese or uncooperative patients.

Computed Tomography. CT is the most sensitive of the imaging procedures (95% to 100%) and allows diagnostic or therapeutic intervention to be performed (see Fig. 33–17*C*). The appearance of an abscess on a CT scan is variable, and lesions may appear cystic or isodense, with solid metastatic lesions. A minority of hepatic lesions contain gas, making this criterion generally of little use but diagnostic if present. The phenomenon of an enhancing rim surrounding an abscess is apparent in a small percentage of cases.

Radionuclide Scans. Technetium-99m sulfur colloid scanning has been useful in the diagnosis of abscesses for four decades. The labeled colloid is engulfed by hepatic Kupffer's cells, in which the technetium is reduced to a lower energy state, and the radiation emitted is measured by a photon-sensitive crystal. The ability of the test to demonstrate an abscess lies in the difference of Kupffer cell activity within and surrounding the abscess. The test is very sensitive but has the significant limitations of being unable to detect lesions smaller than 2 cm. as well as to discriminate between solid and cystic structures. The liver scan is an adequate screening test but is not useful in planning treatment strategies. Newer radionuclide scans with gallium and indium have been reported but add nothing to the standard technetium scan and are not as useful as ultrasonography or CT.

Other Techniques. Hepatic arteriography has been used in the past in diagnosing pyogenic abscesses, but this invasive technique offers no benefit over CT scan with percutaneous aspiration for diagnosis. At present, magnetic resonance im-

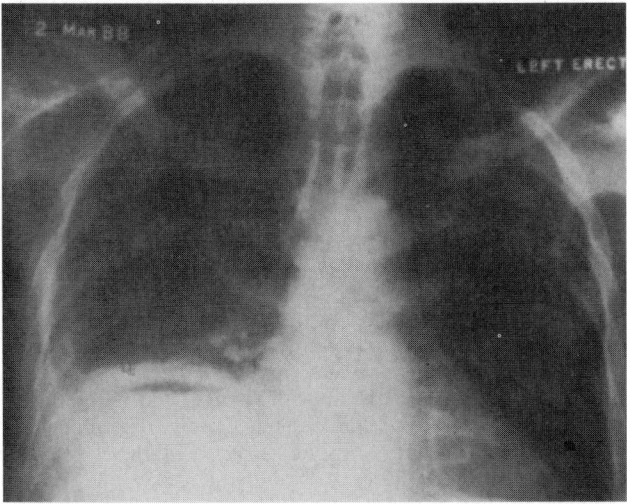

Figure 33–16. Typical appearance of a pyogenic abscess on a plain chest roentgenogram. Note the elevated right hemidiaphragm, blunted right costophrenic angle, and intrahepatic air-fluid level. (From Meyers, W. C., and Jones, R. S.: Textbook of Liver and Biliary Surgery. Philadelphia, J. B. Lippincott, 1990, p. 133.)

aging offers no advantage over CT and cannot be used for percutaneous procedures. The diagnosis of the underlying source may be apparent from the history, physical examination, or initial laboratory tests. If ultrasonography and CT do not reveal the underlying source, barium studies, colonoscopy, endoscopic retrograde cholangiopancreatography, or other tests may be indicated.

DIFFERENTIAL DIAGNOSIS

Correct and expedient diagnosis of pyogenic versus amebic abscess is important because the treatments are radically different (Table 33–5). The standard treatment of pyogenic abscess remains external drainage with an appropriate course of antibiotics. Management also includes consideration of the underlying cause of the abscess. Treatment of uncomplicated amebic abscess is primarily nonsurgical.

When an abscess has been demonstrated, the distinction must be made between pyogenic and more unusual types. *Echinococcus* can usually be excluded by history. Serum antibody titer for *E. histolytica* and counterimmunoelectrophoresis are highly specific and of great benefit when positive. Major centers should have results available in 24 to 36 hours. Percutaneous aspiration may help in the identification of a bacterial organism. However, such aspiration is not usually helpful in the diagnosis of amebae, and in only 10% to 20% of cases can amebae be found on microscopic analysis of rectal mucosa secretions. If the latter results are positive, the finding still may be coincidental with a pyogenic abscess. If amebic serologic testing is not available or the results delayed, the best method of early distinction between pyogenic and amebic abscess is a trial of an amebicidal agent. Metronidazole is usually selected because it is also effective against many organisms causing pyogenic abscess. If the patient has not responded clinically in a 24- to 36-hour trial, pyogenic abscess should be the primary diagnosis. Clinical response is determined by relief of pain, fever, and leukocytosis.

The radiologic and chemical features of amebic abscess are nearly indistinguishable from those of a solitary pyogenic abscess. Leukocytosis is characteristic, although a white blood cell count in excess of 20,000 per cu. mm. suggests secondary bacterial infection. Symptoms are also similar, except that rigors are rare in amebic abscess.

MANAGEMENT
Pyogenic Abscess

Untreated pyogenic abscesses are 95% to 100% fatal. Death follows rupture, sepsis, or both. Spontaneous drainage is most often directly into the peritoneal or pleural cavity, usually causing septic shock and death. Rarely an abscess can resolve by spontaneous drainage externally or into the intestine. The likelihood of rupture is related to size and location. The larger the size, the more prone the abscess is to rupture, and left lateral segment lesions are more likely to rupture than right lobe lesions. Prognostic factors include the patient's age, multiplicity of abscesses, multiplicity of organisms, and the presence of associated malignant or other immunosuppressive disease. Survival from pyogenic abscess has improved in recent years with earlier diagnosis and treatment. Mortality was 80% in 1938 and over the past decade has decreased to less than 20%.

Effective management of pyogenic abscess involves elimination of both the abscess and the underlying source. At the time of diagnosis of the abscess the underlying problem has usually been present for a variable period and the concern is usually focused on treatment of the abscess. The treatment of pyogenic abscess usually includes both intravenous antibiotics and effective drainage. A 1- or 2-day period of intravenous antibiotics may be reasonable before drainage. During this time, the patient's clinical response is closely observed and possible sources are evaluated. Effective drainage is accomplished by percutaneous or open surgical methods. Factors that should be considered in the selection of method include available expertise, the accessibility of the abscess, the number and size of the abscesses, and treatment of the underlying condition.

The course of management must be individualized. For example, the combination of appendiceal and hepatic abscess is usually best treated by open drainage of both. However, percutaneous drainage may be useful as definitive therapy in many patients, in the preoperative period in a septic patient not adequately treated by antibiotics or in a patient for whom a search for a primary source continues. An example of an abscess particularly accessible to percutaneous drainage is a solitary one in the peripheral posterior aspect of the right lobe. In contrast, a large left lateral segment lesion may be more prone to spillage into the peritoneal cavity and the controlled exposure of laparotomy may be of benefit. Numerous small abscesses cannot usually be effectively drained and should be treated initially by antibiotics alone, although percutaneous aspiration for culture may aid in the choice of antibiotics. Drainage and antibiotics are unlikely to be curative in two exceptional situations: secondary infection of a hepatic malignancy and hepatic abscess associated with chronic granulomatous disease of childhood. In both instances the best treatment is hepatic resection if safely achievable. Interferon gamma has been reported to be effective in the treatment of chronic granulomatous disease of childhood. The drug has been given alone or after operation. Prophylactic interferon gamma (0.05 mg./sq. m.) three times weekly in these children may help prevent hepatic abscesses.

Recent series have documented the ease, effectiveness, and safety of percutaneous drainage of most hepatic abscesses. Percutaneous drainage has the disadvantages of an increased likelihood of secondary procedures and the possibility of an underlying source remaining unknown. Some surgeons have reported a high incidence of sepsis in association with the procedures. Fortunately, repeated percutaneous drainage attempts are associated with little increase in mortality. Multiple abscesses remain difficult management problems by either percutaneous, open, or even a combination of the two approaches. The variability in patients precludes a good prospective study of percutaneous versus open surgical drainage. Most studies report a higher rate of complications and mortality with open drainage but include patients who required open drainage after percutaneous methods had failed. Any comparative analysis must closely consider the underly-

TABLE 33–5. Comparison of Characteristics in Amebic Versus Pyogenic Abscess in the United States

	Amebic	Pyogenic
Demographics		
Age (yr)	Mean <40	Mean >50
Sex	Males 9–10:1	Approximately equal
Race	>90% Hispanic origin	No predisposition
Symptoms		
Right upper quadrant pain	60–65%	30–40%
Fever	95–100%	95–100%
Chills	<30%	75–80%
Laboratory		
Serologic tests positive for *Entamoeba histolytica*	98–100%	<5%
Mortality	<5%	10–15%

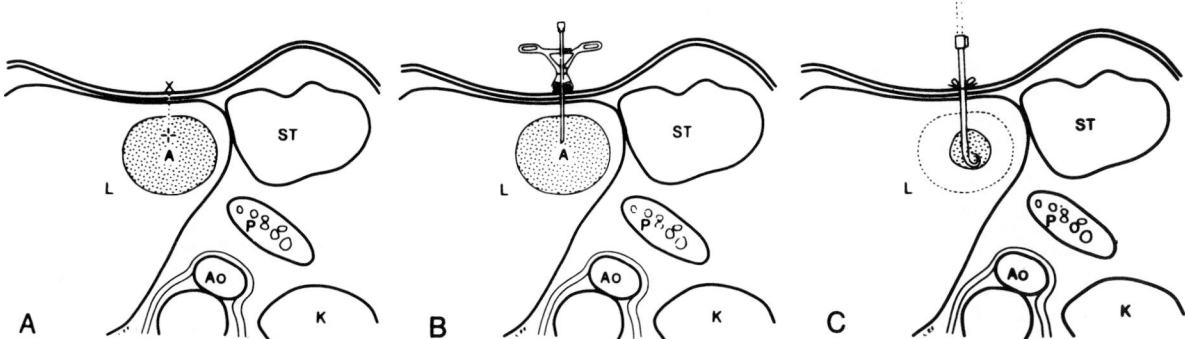

Figure 33–18. The modified Seldinger technique for the percutaneous drainage of a hepatic abscess. *A,* A transverse diagram shows a 5-cm. abscess (A) in the left lobe of the liver (L). The cursor (×—+) marks the entry site and depth. *B,* A 20-gauge Teflon sleeve with a needle stop is inserted over the route shown in A. *C,* After the insertion of a J-wire, a No. 8- to 14-French dilator and then pigtail catheters are advanced over the wire. The abscess is evacuated by manual syringe suction, and the catheter is secured to the skin. P, pancreas; K, kidney; ST, stomach; Ao, aorta. (From Gerzof, S. G.: Percutaneous drainage technique. *In* Doudelinger, R. F., Rossi, P., Kurdziel, J. C., and Wallace, S. [Eds.]: Interventional Radiology. New York, Thieme Medical Publishers, 1990, p. 353.)

ing conditions involved in the abscesses because these are changing (e.g., the increased incidence of abscess as a complication in immunosuppressed patients). Continuing studies are evaluating intravenous antibiotics as primary therapy for hepatic abscess. However, nondrainage therapy must presently be considered still experimental, considering the high risk of this treatment in many previous retrospective analyses.

Adjunctive antibiotic therapy is critical to effective treatment of hepatic abscesses. Directed therapy may be based on results of Gram's stain or culture of diagnostic abscess aspirates. The most common isolates are gram-negative aerobes, colonic anaerobes, and microaerophilic streptococcal species. Anaerobes are rarely isolated singly and therefore necessitate broad coverage if discovered. An appropriate regimen might include an aminoglycoside; an antibiotic directed primarily against anaerobes, such as clindamycin or metronidazole; and a penicillin. This regimen is adjusted appropriately after definitive culture results become known. The appropriate length of antibiotic therapy is unknown, but recommendations include 3 to 12 weeks. The duration of drainage, of course, depends on the method and effectiveness of external drainage.

The choice among several surgical approaches for open drainage of hepatic abscesses has been a controversial subject for many years. Three approaches are available: transpleural, extraperitoneal, and transperitoneal. Percutaneous drainage has eliminated much of this controversy. Most surgeons prefer the transperitoneal route if the abscess requires open surgical therapy. This approach allows inspection of the entire abdominal cavity for an underlying source as well as the best mobilization for appropriate drainage. Intraoperative ultrasound has added to the surgeon's ability to detect multiple hepatic or extrahepatic sites. The transpleural route is occasionally useful for high posterior lesions. The extraperitoneal route is usually through the twelfth rib (posterior) approach or an anterior retroperitoneal dissection. Recent reports also demonstrate three distinct advantages of laparoscopic drainage of pyogenic abscesses. These are the potential use of larger drains, avoidance of transthoracic drainage, and the search for a primary source of infection.

Percutaneous drainage is accomplished by localization of the abscess with ultrasound or CT guidance (Fig. 33–18). A Chiba needle is introduced through the safest anatomic route possible; and when the cavity is located, a trocar or an 18-gauge sheathed needle is passed with progressive dilatation of the tract using a guide wire and sheath. An 11- to 14-French pigtail catheter is subsequently left within the cavity, and it is irrigated with sterile saline and attached to gravity

drainage, with the catheter being irrigated two or three times daily. The sterile pleural space is usually avoided in this technique.

Amebic Abscess

Except when there is rupture or secondary infection, amebicidal agents are the treatment of choice for hepatic amebiasis. The best drug is usually metronidazole or a related agent. Alternative drugs include emetine, dehydroemetine, and chloroquine. The usual dosage of metronidazole is 750 mg. orally three times a day for 7 to 14 days. If the patient is too ill to receive oral agents, intravenous administration is effective. For acute intestinal amebiasis, the recommended dosage is similar. The dosage for amebic hepatic abscess in children is 35 to 50 mg. per kg. every 24 hours in divided doses for 10 days. Emetine and dehydroemetine may cause cardiotoxicity but may be useful if metronidazole is not curative.

If clinical symptoms do not resolve within 48 hours after treatment, an incorrect diagnosis or secondary bacterial infection should be suspected. Peritoneal aspiration or surgical drainage may then be considered. Surgical therapy also has a role in suspected rupture, erosion, or perforation of an adjacent viscus and extrahepatic problems such as colonic obstruction and toxic megacolon. Such colonic problems are extremely rare; and when they occur, they usually involve the right colon. Mortality from amebic liver abscess should be less than 5% in the absence of secondary bacterial infection.

SELECTED REFERENCES

Balasegaram, M.: Management of hepatic abscess. Curr. Probl. Surg., 18:218, 1981.
This excellent review of one surgeon's extensive experience with both pyogenic and amebic abscesses was done over a 15-year period.

Barnes, P. F., DeCock, K. M., Reynolds, T. N., and Ralls, P. W.: A comparison of amebic and pyogenic abscess of the liver. Medicine, 66:472, 1987.
The differentiation of amebic and pyogenic abscess is often difficult. The details of epidemiology, diagnosis, and therapy in a large series of patients with both entities are reviewed.

Branum, G. D., Tyson, G. S., Branum, M. A., and Meyers, W. C.: Hepatic abscess: Changes in etiology, diagnosis, and management. Ann. Surg., 212:655, 1990.
This report chronicles some important changes in the presentation of hepatic abscesses during the past decade.

DeBakey, M. E., and Ochsner, A.: Hepatic amebiasis: A 20-year experience and analysis of 263 cases. Int. Abstr. Surg., 92:209, 1951.
A review of 263 cases of amebic abscess in the era before liver scans, ultrasonography, and CT scans emphasizes the prevalence of amebic infestation.

Ochsner, A., DeBakey, M., and Murray, S.: Pyogenic abscess of the liver: II.

An analysis of forty-seven cases with review of the literature. Am. J. Surg., 40:292, 1938.

This is the classic early reference on the diagnosis, treatment, and outcome of pyogenic abscess. Timeless principles of therapy are discussed, and the world literature to date is reviewed.

REFERENCES

1. Adams, E. B., and MacLeod, I. N.: Invasive amebiasis: II. Amebic liver abscess and its complications. Medicine, 56:325, 1977.
2. Altemeier, W. A., Schowengerdt, C. G., and Whiteley, D. H.: Abscesses of the liver: Surgical considerations. Arch. Surg., 101:258, 1970.
3. Barbour, G. L., and Juniper, K., Jr.: A clinical comparison of amebic and pyogenic abscess of the liver in sixty-six patients. Am. J. Med., 53:323, 1972.
3a. Barnes, P. F., DeCock, K. M., Reynolds, T. N., and Ralls, P. W.: A comparison of amebic and pyogenic abscess of the liver. Medicine, 66:472, 1987.
4. Bernardino, M. E., Berkman, W. A., Plemmons, M., Sones, P. J., Jr., Price, R. B., and Casarella, W.: Percutaneous drainage of multiseptated hepatic abscess. J. Comput. Assist. Tomogr., 8:38, 1984.
5. Bertel, C. K., van Heerden, J. A., and Sheedy, P. F.: Treatment of pyogenic hepatic abscesses: Surgical vs. percutaneous drainage. Arch. Surg., 121:554, 1986.
5a. Branum, G. D., Tyson, G. S., Branum, M. A., and Meyers, W. C.: Hepatic abscess: Changes in etiology, diagnosis, and management. Ann. Surg. 212:655, 1990.
6. Bright, R.: Observations on jaundice. Guys Hosp. Rep., 1:630, 1836.
7. Cappuccino, H., Campanile, F., and Knecht, J.: Brief clinical report: Laparoscopy-guided drainage of hepatic abscess. Surg. Laparosc. Endosc., 4:234, 1994.
8. Chou, F. F., Sheen-Chen, S. M., Chen, Y. S., Chen, M. C., Chen, F. C., and Tai, D. I.: Prognostic factors for pyogenic abscess of the liver. J. Am. Coll. Surg., 179:727, 1994.
9. Dieulafoy: Le foie appendiculaire: Abcès du foie consecutifs à l'appendicite. Sem. Med. (Paris), 18:449, 1898.
10. Fitz, H. R.: Perforating inflammation of the vermiform appendix. Am. J. Med. Sci., 92:321, 1886.
11. Gallin, J. I., Malech, H. L., Weening, R. S., Curnutte, J. T., Quic, P. G., Jaffe, H. S., and Ezekowitz, R. A. B. (The Internal Chronic Granulomatous Disease Cooperative Study Group): A controlled trial of interferon gamma to prevent infection in chronic granulomatous disease. N. Engl. J. Med., 324:509, 1991.
12. Gerzof, S. G., Johnson, W. C., Robbins, A. H., and Nabseth, D. C.: Intrahepatic pyogenic abscesses: Treatment by percutaneous drainage. Am. J. Surg., 149:487, 1985.
13. Gerzof, S. G., Robbins, A. H., Johnson, W. C., Birkett, D. H., and Nabseth, D. C.: Percutaneous catheter drainage of abdominal abscesses: A five year experience. N. Engl. J. Med., 305:653, 1981.
14. Goldenring, J. M., and Flores, M.: Primary liver abscesses in children and adolescents. Clin. Pediatr., 25:153, 1986.
15. Greenwood, L. H., Collins, T. L., and Trizarry, J. M.: Percutaneous management of multiple liver abscesses. AJR, 139:390, 1982.
16. Griffin, F. M., Jr.: Failure of metronidazole to cure hepatic amebic abscess. N. Engl. J. Med., 288:1397, 1973.
16a. Gyorffy, E. J., Frey, C. F., Silva, J., Jr., and McGahan, J.: Pyogenic liver abscess. Ann. Surg., 206:699, 1987.
17. Hague, R. A., Eastham, E. J., Lee, R. E. J., and Cant, A. J.: Resolution of hepatic abscess after interferon gamma in chronic granulomatous disease. Arch. Dis. Child., 69:443, 1993.
18. Halvorsen, R. A., Korobkin, J., Foster, W. L., Silverman, P. M., and Thompson, W. M.: The variable CT appearance of hepatic abscesses. AJR, 142:941, 1984.
19. Hanazaki, K., Kajikawa, S., Horigome, N., Shiohara, E., Haba, Y., Kuroda, T., and Iida, F.: Gas-forming liver abscess after transcatheter arterial embolization for hepatocellular carcinoma: Report of a case. Surg. Today Jpn. J. Surg., 23:747, 1993.
20. Hashimoto, T., Mitani, T., Nakamura, H., Hori, S., Kozuka, T., Kobayashi, S., Nakata, A., and Tsujimura, T.: Fatal septic complication of transcatheter chemoembolization for hepatocellular carcinoma. Cardiovasc. Intervent. Radiol., 16:325, 1993.
21. Hippocrates. *In* The Genuine Works of Hippocrates. Translated from the Greek with a preliminary discourse and annotations by Adams, F. Vols. I and II. New York, William Wood & Co., 1886, pp. 57–58, 266–267.
22. Ibarra-Perez, C.: Thoracic complications of amebic abscess of the liver: Report of 501 cases. Chest, 79:672, 1981.
22a. Klatchko, B. A., and Schwartz, S. I.: Diagnostic and therapeutic approaches to pyogenic abscess of the liver. Surg. Gynecol. Obstet., 168:332, 1989.
23. Lambiase, R. E., Deyoe, B. C., Cronan, J. J., and Dorfman, G. S.: Percutaneous drainage of 335 consecutive abscesses: Results of primary drainage with 1 year follow-up. Interven. Radiol., 184:167, 1992.
24. Malmvall, B. E., and Follin, P.: Successful interferon-γ therapy in a chronic granulomatous disease (CGD) patient suffering from *Staphylococcus aureus* hepatic abscess and invasive *Candida albicans* infection. Scand. J. Infect. Dis., 25:61, 1993.
25. Marcus, S. G., Walsh, T. J., Pizzo, P. A., and Danforth, D. N., Jr.: Hepatic abscess in cancer patients: Characterization and management. Arch. Surg., 128:1258, 1993.
26. McCorkell, S. J., and Niles, N. L.: Pyogenic liver abscesses: Another look at medical management. Lancet, 1:803, 1985.
27. McDonald, M. I., Corey, G. R., Gallis, H. A., and Durack, D. R.: Single and multiple pyogenic liver abscesses: Natural history, diagnosis and treatment, with emphasis on percutaneous drainage. Medicine, 63:291, 1984.
28. Okada, S., Aoki, K., Okazaki, N., Nose, H., Yoshimori, M., et al.: Liver abscess after percutaneous ethanol injection (PEI) therapy for hepatocellular carcinoma: A case report. Hepatogastroenterology, 40:496, 1993.
29. Pitt, H. A.: Surgical management of hepatic abscesses (Review). World J. Surg., 14:498, 1990.
30. Reed, R. A., Teitelbaum, G. P., Daniels, J. R., Pentecost, M. J., and Katz, M. D.: Prevalence of infection following hepatic chemoembolization with cross-linked collagen with administration of prophylactic antibiotics. JVIR 5:367, 1994.
31. vanSonnenberg, E., Ferrucci, J. T., Jr., Mueller, P. R., Wittenberg, J., and Simeone, J. F.: Percutaneous drainage of abscesses and fluid collections: Technique, results, and applications. Radiology, 142:1, 1982.
32. Wallace, R. J., Jr., Greenberg, S. B., Lau, J. M., Kalchoff, W. P., Mangold, D. E., and Martin, R. R.: Amebic peritonitis following rupture of an amebic liver abscess. Arch. Surg., 113:322, 1978.
33. Yanaga, K., Kitano, S., Hashizumf, M., Ohta, M., Matsumata, T., and Sugimachi, K.: Laparoscopic drainage of pyogenic liver abscess. Br. J. Surg., 81:1022, 1994.

III

NEOPLASMS OF THE LIVER

William C. Meyers, M.D.

The development of hepatobiliary surgery as a distinct specialty reflects the increasing sophistication in the management of liver tumors. Health care economists have identified specialty care such as this as costly. However, the benefits of these operations are great, and the costs are minimized by early detection of liver neoplasms and appropriate and skillful treatment. During the past decade surgeons have encountered more liver tumors. This increase is due to four principal factors: (1) an apparent increase in incidence of tumors; (2) improved detection; (3) continued enthusiasm about the success of surgical treatment; and (4) combined, aggressive approaches to reduce tumor volume even in apparently incurable situations. In addition, over the past 30 years several

new categories of tumors have been recognized. New etiologic factors have been identified, such as the hepatitis B and C viruses, hemochromatosis, exposure to vinyl chloride, oral contraceptive use, Thorotrast injection, liver adenoma, and chronic liver disease of almost any etiology. Other factors have been implicated, such as agent orange (dioxin), and there is renewed interest in other types of environmental induction. In contrast to other oncologic diseases, primary liver cancer seems much more a disease of acquisition than of genetic predisposition.

The challenges of cost effectiveness in this dynamic specialty are considerable. For example, computed tomographic (CT) portography, magnetic resonance imaging (MRI), and positron emission tomography have greatly increased the sensitivity and specificity of preoperative imaging. These tests are also, to a certain degree, complementary. Therefore, thoughtful algorithms concerning their use are important, as is early operation in appropriate cases.

It is also interesting to reflect over the past 5 or so years and note the development of the surgeon as a diagnostician in addition to a therapist. This development closely parallels the increased use of laparoscopy. Laparoscopic cryoablation of liver tumors may be a culmination of modern technology with respect to both diagnosis and therapy.

THE SURGEON'S DEVELOPING ROLE

The traditional role of the hepatic surgeon has been to safely control the liver's blood supply during surgery. The earliest hepatic surgery was performed almost exclusively for trauma. The earliest resection for tumor was by Langenbuch in 1888. In 1889, Keen reviewed the liver resections performed to that time. In 1911, Wendel performed the first successful major hepatic resection using selective hilar ligation of the vessels. With improved understanding of the anatomy and physiology of the liver has come increased confidence in surgical treatment, a significant increase in the number of resections performed, a wide expansion of the indications for resection, and a reduction in the mortality for elective hepatic resection in selected major liver centers to less than 1%.

Much of modern medicine seems to be focusing on cost issues and the streamlining of health care delivery. In deference to the modern focus on cost issues, this chapter is reorganized slightly to conform to recent algorithms (Fig. 33–19). The surgeon approaches hepatobiliary disease in the modern era in terms of two basic categories: operable and inoperable. *Operable* can be variably defined to include or exclude intervention such as endoscopic retrograde cholangiopancreatography (ERCP), percutaneous transhepatic cholangiography (PTC), or the new transjugular intrahepatic portosystemic shunt (TIPS) procedure. Treatment of many problems is changing. For example, operable diseases of 10 to 20 years ago are now treated by ERCP, and *nonoperable* diseases from that era are now treated by transplantation. The current classifications (Table 33–6) are meant to allow a

TABLE 33–6. Categorization of Operable and Nonoperable Liver Diseases

Resectable Liver Disease	Disorders Involving Other Surgical Options
Cystic disease	Polycystic disease
Neoplastic disease	Nonresectable tumors
Liver abscess, unusual types	Liver abscess
Hydatid disease	Portal hypertension
Large hemangiomas	Hemobilia
Infarctions	Variceal bleeding
Caroli's disease	Infections and infestations of the liver
Pseudotumors	Ascites
Hepatic stone disease	Ruptured hepatocellular carcinoma
Transplantable Liver Disease	**Nonoperable Liver Disease**
Chronic advanced liver disease	Disease considered inappropriate for operation
Unresectable hepatic cancer (selected cases)	Operable disease but patient inappropriate for operation
Fulminant hepatic failure	Overriding factors
Inborn errors of metabolism	
Budd-Chiari syndrome	

From Chari, R. S., and Meyers, W. C.: The liver. *In* Levine, B. A., et al. (Eds.): Current Practice of Surgery. New York, Churchill Livingstone, 1994, p. 18.

general approach to the management of the various hepatobiliary problems, not definitive categorization. Operable liver disease in its new classification means hepatobiliary disease treated by open or laparoscopic operation. The three main categories are hepatic resection, transplantation, and other surgical options. Considerable overlap occurs, of course, among the various options. In this discussion the focus is on resectable liver disease, specifically neoplastic disease, cystic and parasitic disease, and several other specific lesions. This subject is discussed elsewhere in this text in the discussions of liver transplantation and portal hypertension.

PRIMARY MALIGNANT TUMORS

Familiarity with the types and relative incidences of primary or secondary liver tumors is important for both the surgeon and primary care physician. Take, for example, the workup of a young woman with right upper quadrant pain. One could perform ultrasonography as the initial diagnostic test and then order a battery of more expensive imaging tests, blood chemistries, hepatology or general surgery consultations, ERCP, PTC, and biopsies. An alternative scenario might be early laparoscopy with definitive diagnosis and surgical treatment at the same operative sitting.

Hepatocellular Carcinoma

Hepatocellular carcinoma (HCC) is the most prevalent malignant disease in the world, killing up to 1.25 million persons annually. It constitutes 90% to 95% of primary liver cancers. HCC is the most common primary malignant liver tumor in adults. Hepatoblastoma is the most common primary hepatic cancer of young children. The variability and prevalence of HCC remain dramatic. This malignancy has nearly doubled in the United States over the past 20 years. Hepatoma is much more common in sub-Saharan Africa, Southeast Asia, Japan, the Pacific islands, Greece, and Italy than it is in North and Central America, Great Britain, most parts of Europe, the Middle East, the former Soviet Union, and Australia. In Africa, the incidence of HCC varies from 13.5 per 100,000 annually in Swaziland to 143.8 per 100,000 individuals in Mozambique. In contrast, North Africa has an incidence that varies from 0.8 per 100,000 to 9.0 per 100,000 in Sudan.

Five different studies demonstrate HCC to have doubled

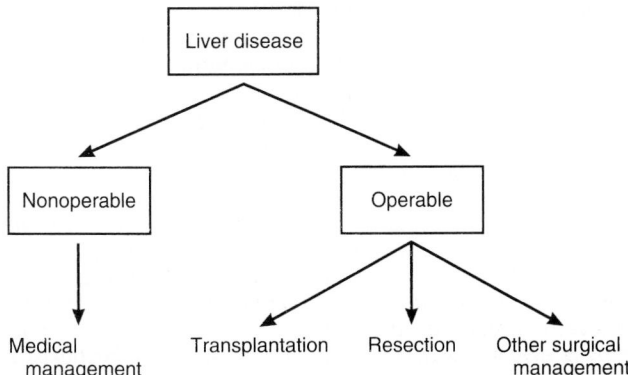

Figure 33–19. The surgeon approaches hepatobiliary disease in terms of two basic categories: operable and inoperable. "Operable" can be variably defined to include or exclude interventions, such as endoscopic retrograde cholangiopancreatography, percutaneous transhepatic cholangiography, or the new transjugular intrahepatic portocaval shunt procedure. Operable liver disease by this new classification means hepatobiliary disease treatable by open or laparoscopic operation. The three main categories are hepatic resection, transplantation, and "other" surgical options. Considerable overlap occurs, of course, among the various options. (From Chari, R. S., and Meyers, W. C.: The liver. *In* Levine, B. A., et al. [Eds.]: Current Practice of Surgery. New York, Churchill Livingstone, 1994, p. 19.)

over the past 30 years in the United States. HCC occurs four to nine times more frequently in males than in females, except in the group without pre-existent liver disease, in whom the ratio is 1:1. Asians in the United States are approximately eight times at risk for developing the tumor compared with white populations. HCC makes up a relatively small proportion of the total primary cancers diagnosed on a yearly basis in the United States. It has an annual incidence in the United States of 1 to 7 per 100,000 population and is the twenty-second most common type of cancer.

Studies of histocompatibility antigens in southern African blacks do not support a genetic basis for the increased susceptibility to HCC. The higher risk of men in certain populations probably reflects a greater exposure to environmental carcinogens. The differences include not only a higher hepatitis B carrier rate in males but also dietary carcinogens and varying rates of metabolism within the sexes. Chinese patients with HCC are usually considerably older than their black counterparts. There are rural-born blacks in South Africa who migrate as young adults to cities and are at lower risk from the disease. HCC occurs about two decades later in blacks who remain in the rural setting. The carcinogen aflatoxin is increasingly implicated. In populations with low incidences of HCC, the elderly are the predominant group affected. In the Far East, HCC develops predominantly in the fifth and sixth decades. In sub-Saharan Africa, the tumor develops at a younger age, with a peak incidence in the third through fifth decades. In high-incidence locations, the tumor more often occurs in patients treated for cirrhosis for a long period of time.

Etiology. Chronic liver disease of any cause probably plays an important role in development of HCC in any part of the world. Epidemiologic and laboratory studies have firmly established a strong and specific association between hepatitis B virus (HBV) and HCC. Other well-documented risk factors include alcoholic cirrhosis, blood group B, hepatic adenoma, repeated ingestion of aflatoxin, other types of cirrhosis or chronic active hepatitis, and persistent hepatitis C viral infection. Implicated risk factors for HCC include other various mycotoxins, plant alkaloids, oral contraceptives, androgens, vinyl chloride, Thorotrast, parasites, porphyria, organochloride pesticides, membranous obstruction of the inferior vena cava, hemochromatosis, alpha$_1$-antitrypsin deficiency, and even cigarette smoking. The relative risk of each factor also appears to vary by geography, although the reason for this difficulty may be both incomplete reporting and the presence of more than one major risk factor.

Hepatitis B Virus. The evidence for the causal relationship between chronic infection with HBV and the disease is compelling and has accumulated over the past two decades. As many as 98% of indigenous persons are infected with the virus at some time in their lives, and approximately 10% are persistently infected. Studies from both Asia and Africa suggest that HBV is present in as many as 70% to 80% of patients with HCC. In 97 consecutive autopsies of patients with HCC in Los Angeles, 21% had HBV infection. In addition, 40% of 55 patients dying of HBV cirrhosis had HCC at autopsy. One third of the patients with HCC studied at autopsy had a cryptogenic cirrhosis. Whether HCC occurs as a consequence of chronic HBV infection or as a result of chronic liver disease is not certain. Since HBV vaccine has been available for only a short period of time, it is not known if this will have a significant impact on the incidence of the disease in endemic areas. HBV does not contain an oncogene, but insertional mutagenesis is a potential mechanism. Overexpression of c-*myc*, c-*phos*, and c-*erb*-A oncogenes has been demonstrated in tumors from African blacks, but the relationship may be coincidental. A number of other studies in individual patients or cell lines has suggested lost tumor suppressor genes.

The relative risk of developing HCC among HBV carriers is 9.7. Observations that strongly implicate HBV are as follows: (1) the HBV carrier state exists in the same geographic distribution as HCC; (2) HCC patients have a 100-fold greater sensitivity to hepatitis B surface antigen (HBsAg) than do population-matched controls; (3) HBV infections precede the development of HCC; (4) in a 5-year study, HBsAg-positive patients had a 1000-fold increased risk of developing HCC; (5) progression from chronic active HBV to cirrhosis and subsequently HCC is well documented; and (6) HBV DNA resides in the HCC cell genome.

Hepatitis C. In contrast to HBV infection, most of the information showing an association between chronic hepatitis C virus (HCV) infection and HCC has been accumulated in Western civilizations, where there is relatively little overlap with HBV. HBV and HCV do act as independent risk factors, plus the two viruses may have a synergistic effect. HCV is a single-stranded RNA that does not become integrated host to DNA. Therefore, it is not certain whether the virus is directly carcinogenic or its marked propensity to cause chronic necroinflammatory disease is the real culprit. Interaction of either HBV or HCV with the p53 protein might also provide a growth advantage to cells harboring a mutation. Studies in Japan have also implicated HCV as the predominant cause of cirrhosis and HCC. HCV infection is present in 51% of the patients with HCC in Japan, as opposed to 26% with HBV infection.

Other Risk Factors. Alcoholic cirrhosis is certainly a major predisposing factor for HCC in the United States; 8% to 10% of patients dying of alcoholic cirrhosis have HCC. In one study, 55% of patients with alcoholic cirrhosis who have stopped drinking had HCC at autopsy, leading to the suggestion that abstinence from alcohol use allows the alcoholic patient to live long enough to develop a tumor. Aflatoxins are important carcinogens in experimental animals. They are products of the fungus *Aspergillus flavus,* which is found in wheat, soybeans, corn, rice, oats, bread, milk, cheese, and peanuts. The United States Food and Drug Administration limits the amount of aflatoxins allowed in peanut butter to 20 parts per billion. Ingestion of raw materials is another likely reason for the geographic variability of HCC. In Taiwan, the risk may be regulated through a guanine to thymine mutation in the *p53* suppressor gene.

The exact risk of HCC developing with the use of oral contraceptives is not clear, although a number of carcinomas have been reported arising within benign adenomas in oral contraceptive users. A type of carcinoma termed *fibrolamellar carcinoma* characteristically develops in persons younger than the age of 35, and it is possible that some of these tumors are also linked etiologically to oral contraceptives. A number of cases of hepatoma have been reported in males after administration of antigenic or other anabolic steroids for the treatment of aplastic anemia, although it is also possible that multiple transfusions contributed to anemia in these patients. There does appear to be a greater hormone responsiveness in these androgen-related HCCs.

Most of the research relating to coexistence of cirrhosis in HCC has focused on the high turnover rates of those cells. Interestingly, primary biliary cirrhosis did not appear to be associated with HCC. On the other hand, the reported association of HCC with hemochromatosis-related cirrhosis is between 10% and 30%.

Symptoms and Signs. The most common symptoms of HCC relate to its late discovery. They include weakness, malaise, anorexia, upper abdominal pain, and weight loss. In one series in the United States, an abdominal mass was the main complaint in 19 of 140 of patients (14%) with primary hepatic malignant tumors and jaundice was present in 34 patients (24%). Obstructive jaundice is the initial problem in 1% to 10% of patients. The biliary obstruction is caused by necrotic tumor embolism or extrinsic compression of the biliary system. Approximately two thirds of the patients are hospitalized with an obvious cancer in the liver with symptoms or signs including abdominal pain and tenderness, dyspnea, asthenia, weight loss, hepatomegaly, jaundice, ascites, peripheral edema, or evidence of portal hypertension. Approximately 5% of the patients present with a manifestation of metastatic lesions, of which pulmonary metastases are the most common.

A minority of patients initially experience an acute abdominal event, such as rupture of the tumor or hemorrhage, or fever of unknown origin. More often, the tumor represents an occult process. In endemic areas, HCC is the most common cause of nontraumatic acute hemoperitoneum in males. In general, the duration of symptoms of patients with HCC is often surprisingly short. In one series, over 75% of patients had symptoms of less than 6 weeks' duration.

Physical findings depend on the stage of the disease. Hepatomegaly is the most common sign found in patients. Interestingly, an arterial bruit can be heard in 15% to 20% of patients, which may be diagnostically valuable. Two thirds of the patients admitted with an obvious cancer exhibit many signs of liver disease (e.g., abdominal pain and tenderness, dyspnea, asthenia, hepatomegaly, splenomegaly, jaundice, ascites, peripheral edema, weight loss, spider angiomas, or evidence of portal hypertension). The few patients who initially have an acute abdominal event representing rupture or hemorrhage into the liver (6.9%) or peritoneal cavity generally have a poor prognosis. Ninety percent of the patients have metastatic disease at initial presentation.

Many paraneoplastic manifestations are associated with HCC. The most common of these manifestations is probably hypoglycemia. Other manifestations include serum protein abnormalities of alpha-fetoprotein, globulins, haptoglobin, ceruloplasmin, alpha$_1$-antitrypsin, choriogonadotropins and choriosomatotropins, alkaline phosphatase, and isoferritins. Associated hematologic abnormalities include erythrocytosis, hemolysis, plasmacytosis, and dysfibrinogenemias. Other abnormalities include hypercholesterolemia, hypertriglyceridemia, porphyria, cystathioninuria, ethanolaminuria, pseudohyperparathyroidism, sexual changes, hypertrophic pulmonary osteoarthropathy (hepatopulmonary syndrome), increased thyroxine-binding globulin, and carcinoid syndrome. Increased carcinoembryonic antigen (CEA) occurs in 8% of cases. Other hormonal syndromes include hypertension secondary to the overproduction of angiotensin, a sensorimotor polyneuropathy that affects all four limbs, and hyperthyroidism caused by increased circulatory thyroid-stimulating hormone, thyroxine, triiodothyronine, and free triiodothyronine.

Diagnosis. The oncofetoprotein alpha-fetoprotein (AFP) deserves special mention because of its diagnostic value. This protein has a molecular weight of 64,000 to 74,000 daltons. It is present in large quantities during fetal development but decreases rapidly after birth and thereafter remains at the normal adult level of 10 ng. per ml. or less. When a relatively insensitive immunodiffusion method is used, 28% to 87% of patients with HCC are shown to have significant elevations of AFP in their sera. Radioimmunoassay for AFP increased positivity for tumor detection in Chinese patients to 69% to 93%. In the United States, 75% of patients with HCC arising in association with HBV cirrhosis had AFP levels above 400 ng. per ml. Sixty-five percent of patients with HCC secondary to alcoholic cirrhosis had positive results, whereas only 33% of patients with carcinoma arising in a noncirrhotic liver had positive assays. In one study, 14 of 16 patients who under-

went laparotomy for a positive AFP level found on screening tests had resectable cancers. AFP may return to normal after successful surgical resection and is a useful level to follow. Mild elevations of AFP may be found in acute viral hepatitis, chronic liver disease, and some cases of metastatic cancer. Higher levels may be found in adult patients with fulminant type HBV infection. Markedly elevated levels may also be found in patients with teratocarcinomas, yolk sac tumors, and, rarely, hepatic metastatic carcinomas from the stomach or pancreas.

Recently the value of real-time ultrasonography has been realized in both Japan and Taiwan as a screening test for HCC in high-risk populations. One study in Japan disclosed that ultrasonography detected 72.5% of tumors that developed in a group of patients with chronic liver disease undergoing routine follow-up evaluation. In another study, ultrasonography detected 92% of HCCs less than 5 cm. in diameter, compared with scintigraphy, which demonstrated only 50%. Arteriography confirmed the majority of lesions. It was also learned that ultrasonography performed at 4- to 5-month intervals theoretically detects all tumors less than 3 cm. in diameter. The time interval was determined by calculation of estimated tumor growth rate. In one study, 4.6 months ensued for a rapidly growing 1-cm. HCC to reach the size of 3 cm. In one prospective study of 115 patients with cirrhosis in Japan, HCC developed in 12 (10.4%): the tumor developed in 7 of 30 (23%) HBsAg-positive patients and 5 of 85 (6%) seronegative patients. A more recent development is the use of intraoperative ultrasonography for the detection of occult tumors. Several reports now document the usefulness of this technique in combination with preoperative AFP determinations.

In the United States, three fourths of patients with an HCC greater than 5 cm. in diameter have AFPs greater than 100 μg. per liter (normal, 0 to 20 μg/L). A level greater than 4 μg. per liter is generally diagnostic for HCC. Acute hepatitis usually produces only transient rises in AFP, whereas chronic hepatitis generally produces a low level AFP elevation, which correlates with the degree of transaminase elevations. Therefore, minor elevations in the AFP level in such patients prompt re-evaluation in 3 months. From 10% to 15% of liver tumors do not produce AFP; therefore, ultrasonography is a better screening study in general for HCC. A National Institutes of Health Consensus Panel recommends the use of both ultrasonography and AFP to detect HCC in high-risk populations.

A number of radiologic investigations may be helpful in the diagnosis of HCC (Fig. 33–20). Plain radiographs are nonspecific and may show an enlarged liver, elevated hemidiaphragm, and, rarely, calcification of the tumor. Ultrasonography is generally noninvasive and expensive. Radionuclide scans are relatively sensitive but have more false-positive results than ultrasonography or CT. Lesions less than 1 to 2 cm. in diameter are often not detected by ultrasonography or radionuclide scans. CT, with and without enhancement with intravenously injected contrast material, has emerged as the procedure of choice in most cases to define the HCC. CT may detect lesions as small as 1 cm. in diameter, and it may also differentiate among fatty, cystic, and solid lesions. However, MRI has probably overtaken conventional CT with respect to sensitivity and characterization of the tumors.

Hepatic arteriography is occasionally helpful in determining the extent of the disease and, in particular, portal or arterial involvement. It can also predict the usefulness of direct arterial infusion or chemoembolization for HCC, which may be either hypervascular or hypovascular. A preoperative arteriogram may also be helpful in determining anatomic variability. A distinct disadvantage of arteriography is the

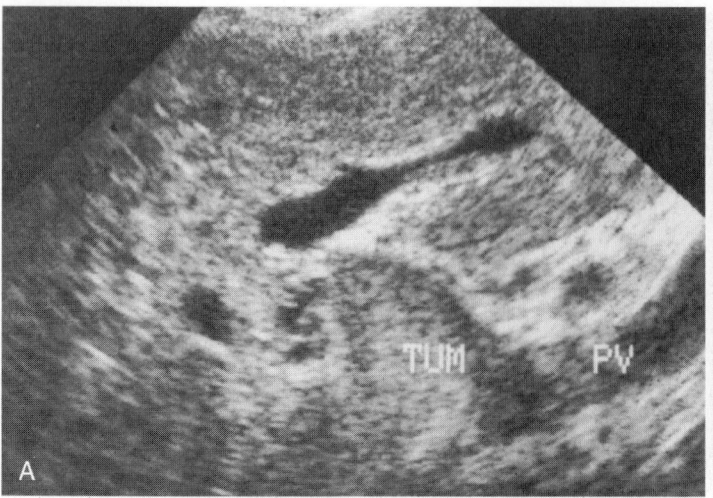
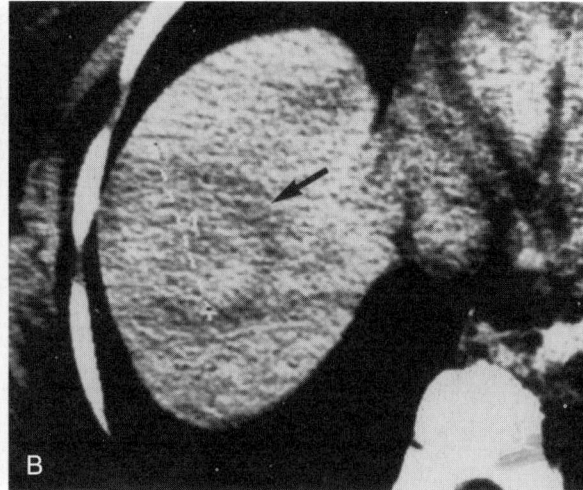
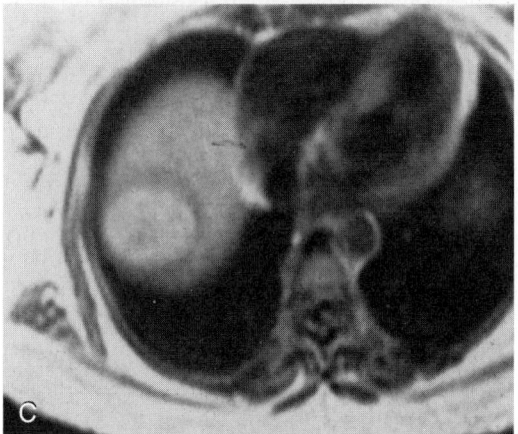

Figure 33–20. Imaging studies of HCC. *A,* Ultrasound image of tumor (TUM) invading main portal vein (PV), making this lesion unresectable. *B,* Computed tomography of HCC showing pseudocapsule or edema (arrow). *C,* magnetic resonance imaging of similar lesion as in *B.* (From Terblanche, J. [Ed.]: Hepatobiliary Malignancy: Its Multidisciplinary Management. Boston, Little, Brown & Co., 1994, pp. 69, 80.)

possibility of thrombosing an artery to the remaining lobe when major hepatic resection is anticipated. Splenoportography may demonstrate the intrahepatic spread of tumor and invasion of the portal vein, but the procedure is not widely used because invasion may also be seen during the venous stage of arteriography. Percutaneous or retrograde cholangiography may be helpful in selected patients.

Laparoscopy is emerging as a procedure of choice in the diagnosis of HCC or other suspected liver tumors. Five separate studies demonstrate its usefulness before anticipated resection, particularly in the detection of occult metastases not demonstrated by other modalities. Laparoscopy also offers an opportunity for limited treatment. An unpublished Duke University series included 22 patients who underwent laparoscopic cryoablation, alcohol injection, minor resection, or a combination of therapies. Percutaneous needle biopsy or fine-needle aspiration for cytodiagnosis generally adds little to the evaluation of potentially resectable, indeterminant liver masses, plus needle biopsy or aspiration has some hazard for hypervascular masses. These techniques are reported to diagnose two thirds of HCCs, and an indeterminant or negative biopsy aspirate adds little to the decision-making process, except perhaps to establish cirrhosis.

Pathology. Various classifications confuse the understanding of the pathology of HCC. The traditional classification of Eggel divides the tumors into massive, nodular, or diffuse. The more recent classification of Nakashima has four groups: infiltrative, expansive, mixed infiltrative and expansive, and diffuse. The latter classification also recognizes two special gross types of HCC: small (less than 2 cm. in diameter) and pedunculated. The classifications are further divided

by histopathology. The most common histologic pattern is trabecular, which encompasses the pseudoglandular, pseudofollicular, and mixed trabecular-acinar types. Other histologic adjectives often used with HCC include pseudoglandular, solid, compact, scirrous, clear cell (replacing), giant cell, pseudocapsular, and sarcomatous. More important than these classifications are the recognition of distinctive variants of HCC and the presence or absence of cirrhosis.

The gross pathologic appearance of HCC varies considerably, depending on the presence or absence of pre-existing cirrhosis. In the cirrhotic liver, it is most often multinodular, whereas in the noncirrhotic liver, it is usually a single mass. The tumor probably begins in an otherwise normal liver as a fairly homogeneous mass and then develops satellite lesions. Most satellite lesions occur within the same segment. The more diffuse multifocal disease in the cirrhotic liver is probably a function of the end-stage disease of the liver.

Distinctive HCC Variants

Fibrolamellar HCC. During the past two decades, the fibrolamellar variant of HCC has emerged as a distinct clinical and pathologic entity. The tumor occurs primarily in young patients with noncirrhotic livers and has a more favorable prognosis than does standard HCC. The distinguishing histologic features are sheets of well-differentiated hepatocytes sandwiched between lamellae of collagen and fibroblasts (Fig. 33–21). The neoplasm accounts for only 1% to 2% of all HCCs, but as many as 40% of such tumors in patients younger than 35 years old. A female sex predilection is debated. Two thirds of such tumors occur in the left lobe. Table 33–7 is a summary of the available comparative data between HCC and fibrolamellar carcinoma. Characteristic

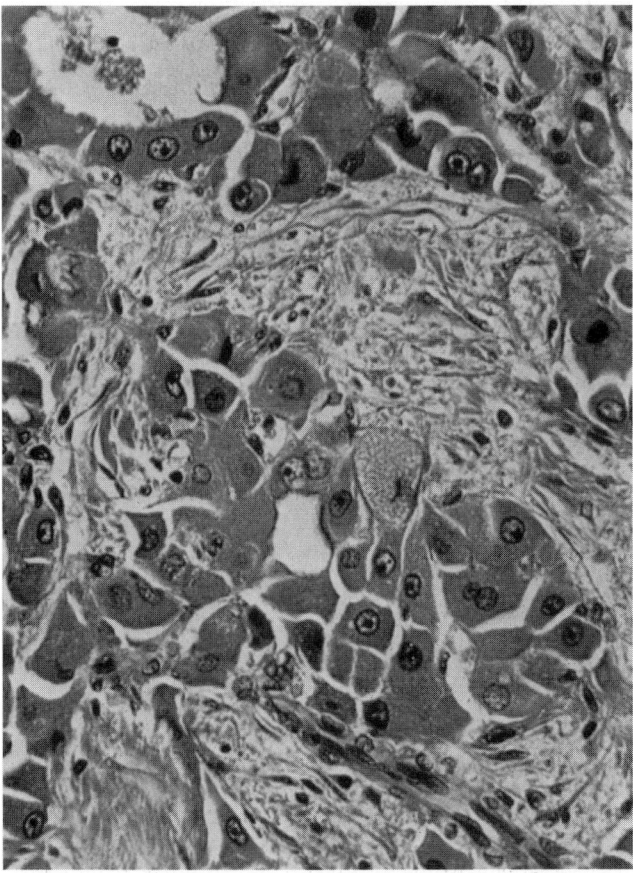

Figure 33–21. Fibrolamellar HCC. Abundant collagen is evident interconnecting clusters of cells. The cells are often in single-layer sheets. An acinus is present in the left upper field. (From Edmondson, H. A.: Differential diagnosis of tumors and tumor-like lesions in infancy and childhood. Am. J. Dis. Child., *91*:168–186, 1956. Copyright 1956, American Medical Association. Pediatrics Tumor Registry, NY, courtesy of Dr. Alexander Brunschwig.)

gross features include a sharply circumscribed solitary mass with scalloped borders, often with adjacent small satellite nodules, fibrous septa within the tumor that mimic the central scars of focal nodular hyperplasia, and a distinct vascular supply. The resemblance of fibrolamellar carcinoma to focal nodular hyperplasia suggests malignant transformation, but this remains unlikely. The cause of the tumor remains uncertain. The location and distribution of metastases are similar

TABLE 33–7. Hepatocellular Carcinoma Compared with Fibrolamellar Carcinoma

Characteristic	Hepatocellular Carcinoma	Fibrolamellar Carcinoma
Male to female ratio	4:1–8:1	1:1–1:2
Tumor	Multiple nodules; large, invasive tumors	Well localized at time of diagnosis
Resectability	Less than 50%	50–75%
Mean survival	3–4 months	32–68 months
Cirrhosis	77%	4%
Increased α-fetoprotein	83%	7%
Hepatitis B positive	65%	6%

From Levine, B. A., et al. (Eds.): Current Practice of Surgery. New York, Churchill Livingstone, 1994, p. 27.

to those in HCC, except in association with a more prolonged course.

Fibrolamellar carcinoma usually remains well localized at the time of diagnosis, yielding a 50% to 75% resectability rate. Mean survival from the time of diagnosis is 32 to 68 months. An aggressive operative approach to this disease is obviously warranted.

Childhood HCC. The underlying hepatic disorders that lead to HCC in childhood distinguish this category of HCC. Those disorders include biliary atresia, glycogen storage disease Type I, hereditary tyrosinemia, hyperalimentation, and HBV infection. In most cases, the gross features of childhood HCC include multifocality and bilaterality. The histologic features may resemble the underlying problem such as glycogen storage disease. It is not clear whether these patients have a different prognosis.

Spindle Cell HCC and Carcinosarcoma. An increasing number of tumors show features of both HCC and spindle cell carcinoma. For this reason, the term *carcinosarcoma* is usually reserved for similar tumors but with the sarcoma being a non–spindle cell variety. Pedunculated HCCs represent an unusually large number of these tumors. Although metastases may be more common in these tumors, these patients may actually live longer than those with the more common HCC.

Clear Cell Carcinoma. This tumor represents a significant problem distinguishing it from metastatic renal cell carcinoma. In fact, the two tumors have been found to coexist in the same patients. The Hong Kong experience suggests that this cell type has a better prognosis, but all patients in that series had a generally short survival. A better prognosis has not been reproduced in other series.

Giant Cell Carcinoma. This tumor refers to carcinomas in which more than 50% of the primary tumor is composed of either multinucleated or pleomorphic large cells. The exact cell of origin is not apparent but certainly may be hepatocellular. These tumors apparently have a similar prognosis to standard HCCs.

Combined HCC (Hepatocellular-Cholangiocellular). Ductal transformation of HCCs actually occurs in 5% to 10% of tumors. The term *mixed hepatic tumor* refers to a distinct tumor type in which both hepatocellular and mesenchymal components are present. A number of patients have also been reported with both entities as separate tumors. Histologic evidence suggests that these tumors are similar to the spindle cell carcinoma/HCC variant, but the prognosis with this tumor is not clearly different from that of standard HCC.

Other Primary Malignant Tumors

Epithelial Tumors

Hepatoblastoma. Hepatoblastoma is a malignant tumor of embryonic or fetal hepatocytes that often has mesenchymal elements and occurs in children younger than 3 years of age. The tumors are generally divided into epithelial or mixed epithelial and mesenchymal types, depending on the number of mesenchymal cells seen. Other terms employed for some tumors are teratoid and anaplastic. These tumors are responsible for 50% of all primary hepatic tumors requiring surgery in a 10-year survey of pediatric surgeons in the United States. These tumors are about one tenth as frequent as Wilms' tumors. There is a white male predominance, and metabolic effects include osteopenia, hypoglycemia, isosexual precocity, and hemihypertrophy. Possible striking effects include marked elevations of beta-human chorionic gonadotropin, thrombocytosis, serum alpha-fetoprotein elevation, cystathioninuria, virilization, and radiographic calcification. Cirrhosis is usually absent. The tumor is often solitary but multinodular with a variegated appearance. Over 50% long-term survival in patients who undergo resection of the tumor is expected. Recurrence can occur in up to half the patients. Several recent studies suggest that prognosis is predicted by histologic grading and ploidy analysis. Large-scale studies of therapy for this tumor have not been reported.

Bile Duct Cancer (Cholangiocarcinoma). Several authors suggest using the term *bile duct cancer* for central lesions and *cholangiocarcinoma* for tumors in more peripheral ducts. The terms are nonetheless interchanged in the literature. Bile duct cancers represent 5% to 20% of primary carcinoma of the liver. They may occur within the liver parenchyma and small ducts or ductules or arise from major hepatic ducts outside the liver substance. The intrahepatic type of cholangiocarcinoma is associated with chronic cholestasis, cirrhosis, hemochromatosis, and congenital cystic disease of the liver. *Clonorchis sinensis* infestation is associated with more than 90% of cholangiocarcinomas in Hong Kong. However, one third of patients without bile duct carcinoma also have infestation with this fluke. Extrahepatic bile duct cancers arise anywhere along the hepatic ducts or bile duct and represent 10% of primary hepatic malignancies. There is a 3:2 male-to-female predominance. Pruritus, vague abdominal pain, mild cholangitis, and jaundice are the usual initial symptoms. Physical examination may reveal slight hepatomegaly or jaundice but usually no other findings except a large gallbladder when the lesion is distal. Both intrahepatic and extrahepatic bile duct cancers have been associated with ulcerative colitis and may also be confused with sclerosing cholangitis. There is a clear association with biliary cystic disease as well as with gallstones.

On pathologic examination the lesion is generally a markedly sclerosing adenocarcinoma. This tumor may extend into the parenchyma along the biliary ducts. Twenty per cent to 25% of the tumors are found to be resectable even when the lesion involves the bifurcation of the hepatic ducts (Klatskin tumors). The treatment of choice probably remains surgical resection, which provides longest survival (Fig. 33–22). The average survival in one series after surgical resection was approximately 2 years. There is a 15% to 20% 5-year survival rate after resection. Most cures occur after resection of distal-third lesions; cure is unusual for proximal bile duct cancers. If the tumor cannot be resected, a bypass or intubation procedure may provide excellent palliation. Before these palliative procedures were used, survival was usually only several months. With more aggressive palliation, average survival has been extended to 1 or 2 years. Adjunctive iridium seed implantation through a biliary drainage tube is often employed, with or without external beam iridium, but whether this leads to significant improvement in survival remains unclear. Percutaneous or endoscopic biliary drainage is offered as a primary treatment for poor-risk surgical patients or those with obviously unresectable tumors. The long-term results of percutaneous or endoscopic drainage compared with open dilation and intubation have not been fully evaluated. Intrahepatic ductal enteric anastomoses, such as the Longmire or falciform ligament approaches, have had mixed success in the treatment of unresectable cholangiocarcinoma.

One might expect that patients with bile duct cancer would be a particularly favorable group for hepatic transplantation because of the slow-growing and localized nature of the tumor. However, results of transplantation have generally been disappointing, primarily because of tumor recurrence. This has, in part, been the stimulus for *cluster* operations being performed by several transplant groups in which most of the upper abdominal viscera are transplanted *en bloc.* Results of this aggressive surgical procedure are disappointing. At present, chemotherapy is considered an ineffective primary treatment modality.

Other primary predisposing factors for cholangiocarci-

noma are primary sclerosing cholangitis, inflammatory bowel disease, intrahepatic calculi, and possibly certain environmental toxins. The Mayo Clinic series of primary sclerosing cholangitis patients suggested a 17% incidence of carcinoma development during a period of observation before transplantation. A review from Johns Hopkins Hospital suggests that early resection of the extrahepatic ductal system for primary sclerosing cholangitis reduces the incidence of carcinoma development.

Hepatic Cystadenocarcinoma. Most hepatobiliary cystadenocarcinomas probably arise from hepatobiliary cystadenomas. A predisposing condition (i.e., pre-existent cyst) has been traced to about half of those tumors in one series. However, in general, the prognosis of patients with these tumors is poor in contrast to that of patients with pancreatic cystadenocarcinoma. The poor prognosis may be related to the relatively low number of resections performed for this disease. Resection does offer a chance for cure.

Squamous Cell Carcinoma. The primary consideration with this disease is the possibility of a metastatic lesion. Primary squamous cell carcinoma of the liver has occurred with long-standing biliary or hepatic cystic disease and has been cured by resection. However, the tumor is rare.

Primary Malignant Mesenchymal Tumors. Primary hepatic sarcomas have received much attention because of their association with vinyl chloride or Thorotrast. Angiosarcoma is the principal tumor associated with this agent. It usually occurs as multiple nodules of variable size that rapidly disseminate intravascularly. No single incidence of cure for angiosarcoma has been reported. The longest reported survivor (5 years) received radiation therapy. Other tumors such as leiomyosarcoma, fibrosarcoma, rhabdomyosarcoma, and mesenchymal sarcoma also rarely appear in the liver. Undifferentiated sarcoma is also generally associated with an extremely poor prognosis, although the authors had a patient who had undergone tumor resection who was a 5-year survivor.

Epithelioid hemangioendotheliomas are considered malignant because of their characteristically diffuse involvement within the liver and ability to metastasize. Their clinical presentation and course are extremely variable, with most patients dying of liver failure 1 to 10 years after diagnosis. Other malignant tumors reported rarely as primary lesions in the liver include malignant fibrous histiocytoma, familial erythrophagocytic lymphohistiocytosis, lymphoma, teratoma, yolk sac tumor, schwannoma, osteosarcoma, and carcinoid.

Treatment of Primary Malignant Liver Tumors

Two common misconceptions about HCC are that it grows rapidly and that it is universally fatal (Fig. 33–23). HCC is actually slower growing, in general, than other neoplasms, such as colon cancer and bronchogenic carcinoma. Resection has often resulted in cure, particularly in the absence of cirrhosis. Most carcinomas resected in the presence of underlying cirrhosis or chronic hepatitis recur in the liver, although this may not happen for several years. Whether the recurrences are actually new lesions arising in the presence of cirrhosis is not known.

When one considers all persons within an endemic population such as Africa, the overall survival of patients with untreated HCC is only 3 to 4 months after symptoms appear. In the United States, the course seems more benign. Average survival after resection is reported to be approximately 3 years. Five-year survival rates after resection (including liver transplantation) in several large series varied from 11% to 46%. At present, resection is the only therapy that substan-

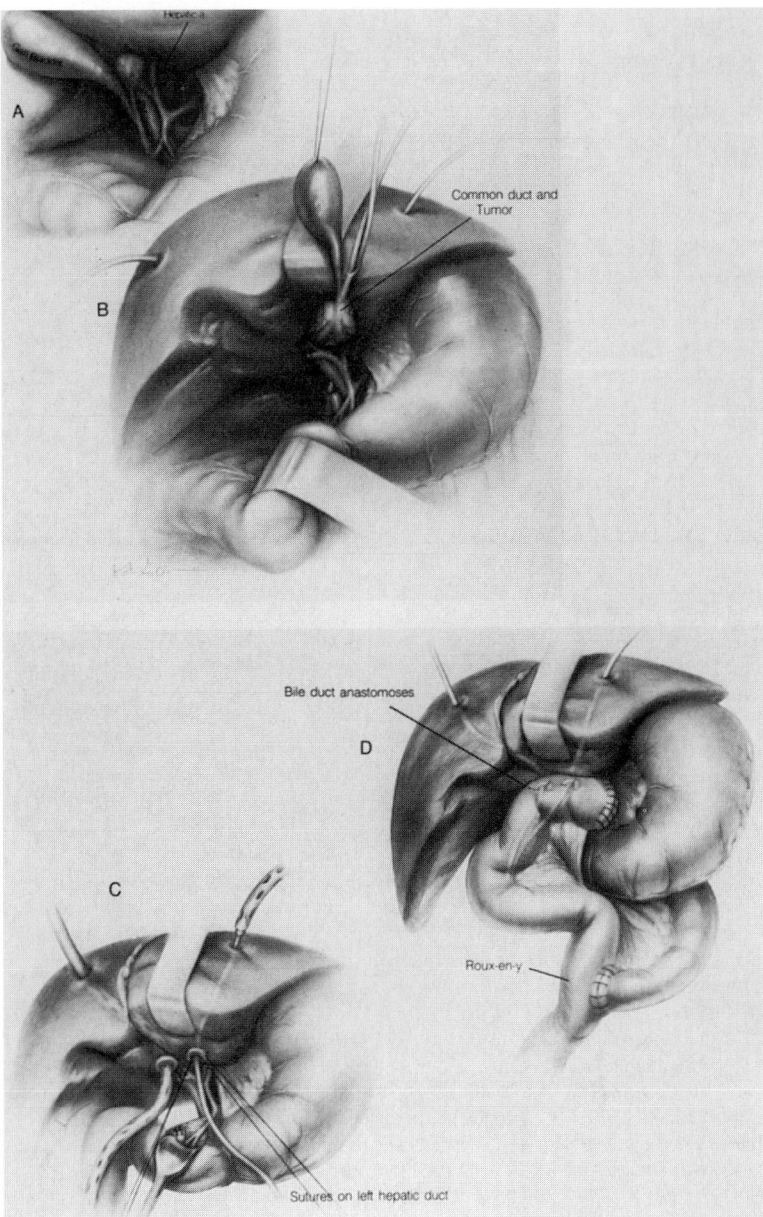

Figure 33–22. Illustration of proximal bile duct tumor resection. *A,* Intact anatomy with tumor. *B,* The distal common duct has been divided, and the proximal system with gallbladder, radiologic tubes, and tumor has been lifted up to complete the dissection. *C,* The tumor has been resected, and percutaneous tubes are being replaced with larger ones. The left tube is in the process of being exchanged. The multiple side holes in the tubes permit internal biliary drainage. The proximal ends of the tubes exit percutaneously. The biliary reconstruction depicted in *D* is with a Roux-en-Y jejunal limb. The posterior biliary-jejunal anastomosis can be seen ghosted near the closed end of the jejunum. (From Meyers, W. C., and Jones, R. S. [Eds.]: Textbook of Liver and Biliary Surgery. Philadelphia, J. B. Lippincott, 1990.)

tially prolongs survival. Exploration is indicated unless there is an obviously unresectable tumor or distant metastases or end-stage cirrhosis. Operative mortality from major hepatic resection has decreased from nearly 20% before 1950 to approximately 1% currently. The mortality still relates primarily to postoperative liver failure from accompanying cirrhosis. Prognostic indices have developed to calculate the risk of hepatectomy in HCC and cirrhosis. Most are based on the modifications of Child's classification, percentage of remaining liver tissue, and patient age. In cirrhosis, wedge resection is as effective as more radical procedures in many patients. In addition to detection of occult lesions, intraoperative ultrasonography helps to determine the extent of resection and identification of the precise segment of liver to be removed, which can be done after injection of stain into the portal vein to that segment.

The impact of early discovery and treatment of subclinical HCC is best depicted in studies from Shanghai. The overall 5-year survival from that disease increased dramatically from 1.7% in the period from 1950 to 1966 to 7.1% in the period

from 1967 to 1975 and 19.5% in the period from 1976 to 1984. This dramatic increase was clearly the result of improved detection and resective treatment of subclinical HCC. No 5-year survivor was reported in the absence of resection. Most patients underwent limited resection, which usually consisted of a 1- to 2-cm. margin around the tumor.

In the 1980s, liver transplantation was performed only for otherwise unresectable tumors, with only a 20% 2-year survival. In contrast, there was an 80% to 90% cure rate, with coincidental cancers found at pathologic examinations of the cirrhosis after transplantation. Fibrolamellar HCC had a better prognosis with transplantation, that is, 30% to 40% 1-year tumor-free survival, compared with 10% survival of patients with nonfibrolamellar tumors. Most deaths after transplantation for tumor are attributable to tumor recurrence.

Nonprospective studies suggest a doubling of the chance for survival with transplantation compared with resection, when resection is an option. This outcome is most evident in patients with cirrhosis and with solitary lesions less than 5 cm in diameter. These data may also support an aggressive,

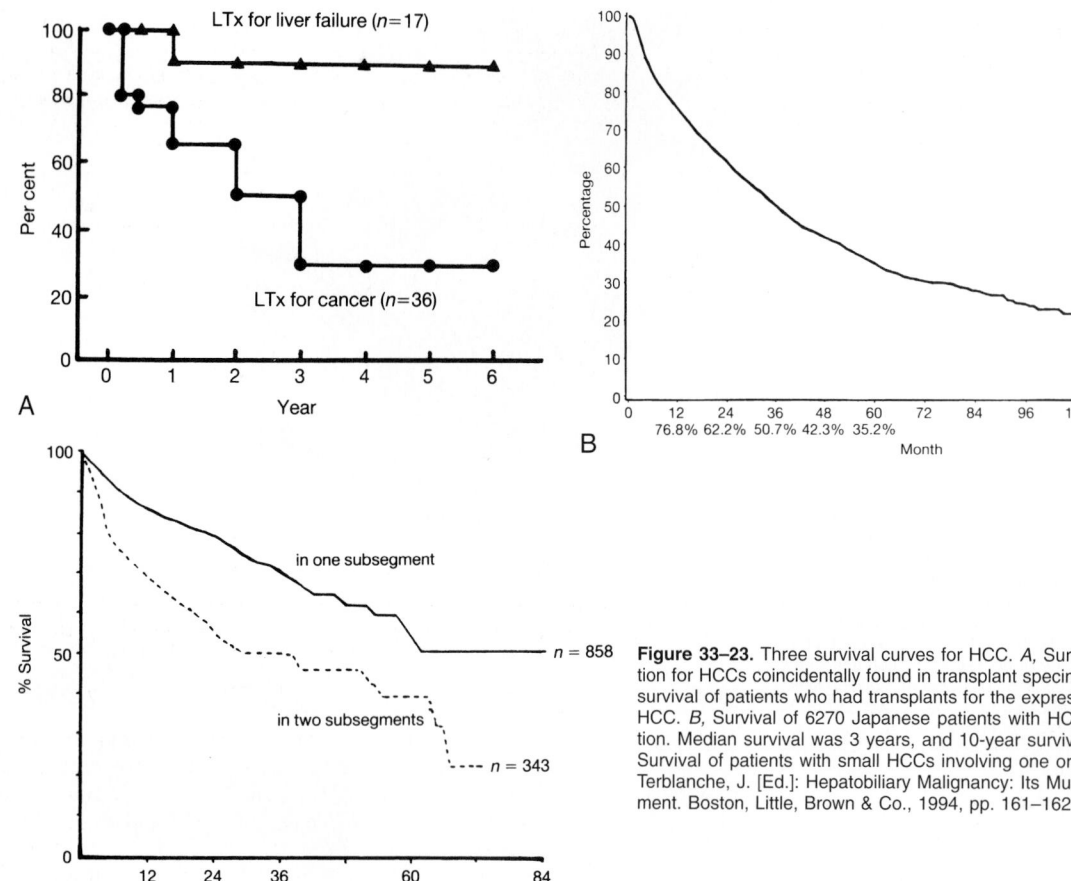

Figure 33–23. Three survival curves for HCC. *A,* Survival after transplantation for HCCs coincidentally found in transplant specimens is compared with survival of patients who had transplants for the expressed purpose of curing HCC. *B,* Survival of 6270 Japanese patients with HCC after hepatic resection. Median survival was 3 years, and 10-year survival was about 20%. *C,* Survival of patients with small HCCs involving one or two segments. (From Terblanche, J. [Ed.]: Hepatobiliary Malignancy: Its Multidisciplinary Management. Boston, Little, Brown & Co., 1994, pp. 161–162.)

combined approach to HCC, to include resection or transplantation plus another modality such as chemotherapy, chemoembolization, or cryoablation. Because of the shortage of donor livers, some authorities argue that transplantation for HCC, with its best long-term survival of only 20% to 30%, is not acceptable. This argument has led to proposals in certain donor regions to stratify the donor pool according to disease, with the less favorable organ going to the patient with carcinoma.

Cryoablation. Cryoablation has emerged as a potentially useful surgical technique in the treatment of HCC and certain other malignancies. The technique is effective in local kill of tumor, particularly after a double-freeze technique. The overall operative morbidity and mortality of cryoablation may be less compared with resection. Therefore the number of nodules that can be treated may increase or the margin of resection may widen. Preliminary analyses from Boston, Pittsburgh, and New Haven in the United States and from Australia all suggest a slight prolongation of survival for patients with malignancies that were otherwise unresectable. Long-term data on cryoablation of primary or secondary liver malignancies are not available. Nonetheless, the technique raises a number of interesting possibilities in terms of combined therapy.

Nonsurgical Treatment. Nonsurgical treatment of HCC includes hepatic artery ligation, arterial embolization, intra-arterial chemotherapy, targeting irradiation or chemotherapy, direct tumor injection, or combination of methods. Iodine-121 antiferritin therapy combined with external radiation and/or chemotherapy has not achieved satisfactory results. Mean survivals were 5 and 10 months in AFP-negative and AFP-positive patients, respectively, in one carefully designed

study. Interestingly, arterial embolization has yielded the best results in unresected patients. However, the improvement in survival is still less than 6 months by that approach. In some studies investigators have suggested improved survival with the combination of an external-beam linear accelerator and direct percutaneous ultrasound-guided alcohol injection.

Because HBV infection is now unequivocally linked to development of HCC, it would appear that HBV vaccine would reduce the incidence of this disease in endemic populations. However, economic factors have thus far prohibited wide distribution of this vaccine in endemic parts of the world. The most consistent response rates (~25%) with respect to systemic chemotherapy have been reported with doxorubicin (Adriamycin). The best results have occurred in black South African patients.

METASTATIC TUMORS

Metastatic cancer comprises the largest group of malignant tumors in the liver. Most metastatic lesions likely arise in the liver as a result of primary shedding into the vascular system. According to a large autopsy study in the United States, bronchogenic carcinoma is the most common primary lesion causing hepatic metastases (Table 33–8). Next in order of frequency are primary tumors in the prostate, colon, breast, pancreas, stomach, kidney, and cervix. The liver is involved in 60% to 66% of small cell carcinomas of the lung, 40% of lung adenocarcinomas, and 22% of squamous cell carcinomas. Some reports indicate that over 40% of patients with breast cancer develop liver metastases before death. In total, about 40% of patients dying with a solid tumor develop liver metastases. The tumor that most concerns liver surgeons in

TABLE 33–8. Most Common Nonlymphoma Malignant Tumors Metastatic to the Liver

Tumor	Number of Primary Tumors	Number with Hepatic Metastases	Percentage with Hepatic Metastases	Percentage of Patients with Hepatic Metastases Who Were Icteric
Bronchogenic	682	285	41.8	9
Colon	323	181	56.0	34
Pancreas	179	126	70.4	51
Breast	218	116	53.2	30
Stomach	159	70	44.0	60
Unknown primary	102	59	57.0	35
Ovary	97	47	48.0	0
Prostate	333	42	12.6	0
Gallbladder	49	38	77.6	60
Cervix	107	34	31.7	10
Kidney	142	34	23.9	15
Melanoma	50	25	50.0	13
Urinary bladder and ureter	66	25	37.9	11
Esophagus	66	20	30.3	29
Testis	45	20	44.4	14
Endometrial	54	17	31.5	<20
Thyroid	70	12	17.1	14

Data obtained at Los Angeles County University of Southern California Medical Center and John Wesley County Hospital. From Edmondson, H. A., and Peters, R. L.: Neoplasms of the liver. *In* Schiff, L., and Schiff, E. R. (Eds.): Diseases of the Liver, 5th ed. Philadelphia, J. B. Lippincott Company, 1982, pp. 1101–1157.

the United States is metastatic colorectal cancer. At least 20,000 patients with colorectal cancer develop hepatic metastases annually. Liver metastases are detected in 30% of these patients at the time of primary anastomosis. Between 10% and 20% of patients discovered with liver metastases from colorectal cancer have potentially resectable disease.

Pathogenesis

Primary tumors that drain into the portal system contribute seven times as many hepatic metastases as tumors arising outside the portal drainage system. Only 2% to 3% of patients with hepatic metastases have no detectable extrahepatic disease. The factors governing the distribution of hepatic metastases within the liver are not well understood. Unanswered questions include (1) why some patients have only one or several tumors confined to one lobe and others exhibit multiple tumors throughout the liver; (2) when hematogenous spread occurs; and (3) what other factors, such as age or sex, influence the natural history of hepatic metastases. Some factors governing number in distribution of hepatic metastases undoubtedly include the number and viability of tumor emboli, hemodynamic factors related to distribution of liver blood flow, *receptiveness* of the liver tissue to implantation and growth, and the tumor's inherent aggressiveness.

Detection

The most common symptoms of hepatic metastatic disease are pain, ascites, jaundice, palpable mass, weight loss, anorexia, fever, and vague gastrointestinal complaints. Most of these symptoms generally indicate advanced disease. Therefore, one cannot rely on development of symptoms for early detection of metastases to the liver. A correlative observation is that most resectable lesions are found by early laboratory detection before symptoms or signs develop. For this reason, close follow-up of patients with colorectal cancer is required. Liver enzyme and CEA determinations in combination with appropriately timed imaging studies are recommended in the routine follow-up of patients with colorectal cancer.

CEA is a 200,000-dalton glycoprotein secreted into the glycocalyceal surface of intestinal cells. The human digestive organs elaborate CEA between the second and sixth months *in utero*. Human colorectal cancer often secretes sufficient amounts of CEA to permit its use as a tumor marker. An elevated CEA level was formerly believed to be specific for colorectal malignancy. Unfortunately, this is not the case, because increased CEA concentrations occur in other malignancies and in benign conditions such as alcoholic cirrhosis, pancreatitis, inflammatory bowel disease, rectal polyps, and diabetes mellitus. CEA is usually elevated only mildly in most of these benign conditions. Therefore, serial CEA determinations after surgical removal of colorectal cancer are still an important test for recurrent disease. Marked elevation of CEA reliably indicates recurrent or persistent cancer in most cases but does not provide anatomic localization of the tumor. Elevated CEA levels in a patient with colon cancer indicate a search for a site of recurrent disease. A serum CEA concentration greater than 9 ng. per ml. combined with a positive result of a liver imaging test predicts metastases with 98% accuracy. Conversely, a normal CEA value combined with a negative hepatic imaging test result is about 95% accurate in excluding hepatic metastases from colorectal cancer. An elevated serum alkaline phosphatase concentration is reported to have a 75% sensitivity in the detection of hepatic metastases, and the combination of alkaline phosphatase and CEA has a sensitivity of nearly 90%, with a false-positive rate of about 10%.

Other blood tests that can reflect the presence of hepatic metastases include determination of levels of gamma-glutamyl transpeptidase, 5'-nucleotidase, alanine transaminase, and lactate dehydrogenase. The lactate dehydrogenase study is reported to have the highest sensitivity (85%) of all standard liver function tests but also the highest false-positive rate (about 50%). The latter observation illustrates the difficulty in using routine liver function tests alone in surveillance for recurrent disease. A prospective study by the National Institutes of Health concluded that laboratory tests alone were inadequate for detecting liver metastases. The consensus group recommended a single liver imaging study plus selected blood tests as a screening protocol for liver metastases for colorectal cancer. The imaging studies most commonly used for this purpose are ultrasonography, CT, and MRI.

Each imaging test has its advantages and disadvantages. Ultrasonography is relatively inexpensive but operator dependent. It is highly accurate in the characterization of certain liver masses such as cysts and permits easily guided liver biopsies. The CT scan is generally considered the most favored test because of its availability and overall accuracy in the detection of liver metastases. The sensitivity of CT varies widely according to the technique, the experience of the radiologist, and the generation of equipment used. The two most common techniques involving CT are bolus-dynamic CT and CT portography. In one study of bolus-dynamic CT, liver metastases were found in 93% (26 of 28) of patients with metastatic disease and 92% (86 of 93) of tumor nodules were detected. CT portography uses knowledge on the differences in blood supply between normal liver parenchyma and liver metastases. Whereas liver parenchyma normally receives 75% of its blood supply from the portal inflow, liver metastases derive nearly all their vascular inflow from branches of the hepatic artery. The same is true of most primary tumors of the liver. The procedure is done in two phases—a conventional arteriogram and then a CT scan performed during the portal venous phase of a superior mesenteric arterial or splenic arterial injection. Therefore, lesions show up as dark spaces.

CT portography is by far the most sensitive available imaging test but also one of the least specific and most expensive (Fig. 33–24). The sensitivity in detecting lesions as small as 5 mm. in diameter is about 97%. However, many of the lesions need correlation with ultrasonography, MRI, or open surgical techniques. The technique also requires a large volume of injected contrast material and therefore considerable periprocedural patient hydration. A distinct alternative for potentially resectable lesions is to bypass CT portography and go directly to laparoscopic exploration with ultrasonography before a traditional incision. The latter approach is less expensive and possibly more efficient.

A variety of techniques are being developed that use MRI. T1-weighted images are used primarily for determination of anatomy. T2-weighted sequences remain the most useful, plus there are some developments that show great promise for detection of pathologic processes. Gadolinium-enhanced techniques are probably useful for both detection and characterization of liver lesions. Fast spin-echo and gradient refocusing are reducing scan times and expense. MR cholangiography and various arterial and portal flow techniques are also showing great promise. In contrast, nuclear scans have lost most of their practicality because of improvement in the sensitivity and accuracy of other tests. Various antibody tests to CEA and other tumor markers have developed but not achieved great reliability. The latter test may have limited usefulness for the patient with a markedly elevated serum CEA value but no metastasis detectable by other modalities.

Treatment

Resection, if possible, is the treatment of choice for metastatic colorectal cancer to the liver. Liver lesions detected on careful follow-up will often be resectable, and several studies have documented the unfavorable prognosis of untreated hepatic metastases from colorectal cancer. Without treatment, 60% to 70% of patients die within 1 year and close to 100% have died within 3 years. Although earlier reports suggested

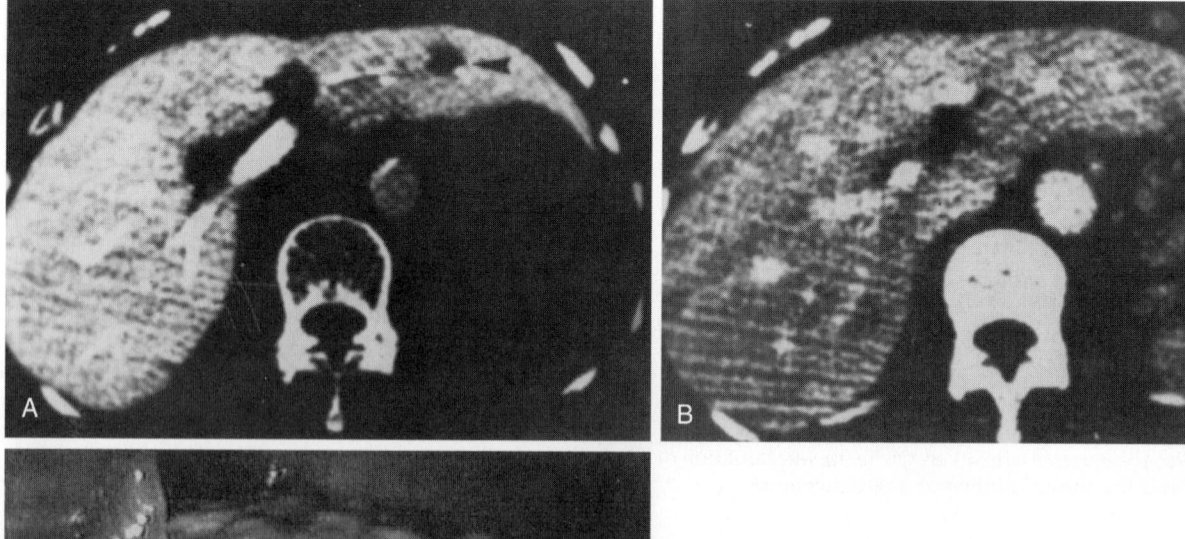

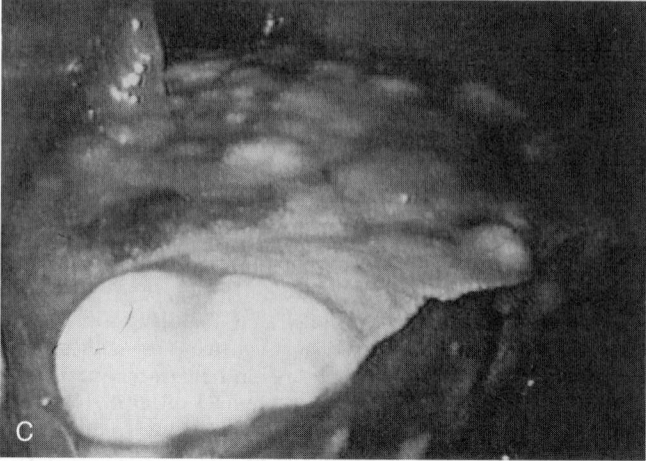

Figure 33–24. Two main choices for preoperative work-up of a patient with potentially resectable metastatic colon cancer. *A,* CT portography. *B,* Note lesion that is not seen on conventional CT. *C,* Example of a lesion found in a cirrhotic patient during laparoscopy. (*A* and *B* from Meyers, W. C., and Jones, R. S. [Eds.]: Textbook of Liver and Biliary Surgery. Philadelphia, J. B. Lippincott, 1990; and *C* from Chari, R. S., and Meyers, W. C.: The liver. *In* Levine, B. A., et al. [Eds.]: Current Practice of Surgery. New York, Churchill Livingstone, 1994, p. 15.)

that patients with untreated solitary liver metastases did not live much longer than those with multiple tumors, some critical analyses have demonstrated small but significant differences in survival among patients based on the number of metastases. No doubt the natural history of patients with hepatic metastases is variable. However, rarely does an individual with unresected disease live more than 3 years with the diagnosis of metastatic liver cancer. Resection of a solitary metastatic lesion from a colorectal primary tumor can have as much as a 40% 5-year survival rate.

When a synchronous hepatic metastasis is found during operation with a primary tumor in colorectal malignancy, the hepatic lesion may be removed simultaneously or at a second procedure. The decision is based on the adequacy of colon preparation, magnitude of the principal procedure, anticipated extent of hepatic resection, general status of the patient, and experience of the surgeon. Because no randomized prospective studies have been performed, it has not been proved whether the prolongation of survival after resection of hepatic metastases is a function of the resection or the natural biology of the tumor.

With the improved safety of hepatic resection, the indications for hepatic resection of metastases have expanded. Examples include resection of large symptomatic lesions in the presence of extrahepatic disease and resection of residual hepatic disease in combination with aggressive chemotherapy.

In general, contraindications to major hepatic resection for metastatic disease include total hepatic involvement, advanced cirrhosis, jaundice (except from extrinsic hepatic ductal obstruction), vena cava or main portal vein invasion, and extrahepatic tumor involvement. Transplantation of the liver for metastatic disease has generally been unsuccessful except for select tumors such as carcinoid.

A review of 345 patients who underwent surgery for hepatic metastases revealed that 70% had primary colorectal lesions. Wilms' tumor, melanoma, and leiomyosarcoma represented another 10%, and a variety of other tumors made up the remaining 20%. The cumulative 5-year survival rate after hepatic resection of colorectal metastases was 22%. Patients with tumors more than 5 cm. in diameter had a poorer outcome. Survival did not correlate with the time interval between resection of the primary tumor and resection of the metastatic tumor, nor with the extent of liver resection. No difference in survival was found between patients with synchronous and those with metachronous lesions or between patients with solitary lesions and patients with multiple lesions in the same lobe. In addition, the status of colonic lymph node involvement in the resected primary tumor had no effect on survival. Data are beginning to indicate that a number of factors are predictors of survival after resection of colorectal hepatic metastases. These include size, number of metastases, and presence of residual local disease. Logic, but little data, suggests that the colonic lymph node status should be another predictor. Interestingly, several studies suggest that females have a better survival after hepatic resection of colorectal hepatic metastases.

Other Treatment Modalities. A variety of other treatment modalities have been advocated for treatment of metastatic colorectal cancer to the liver. The chemotherapeutic agent 5-fluorouracil has about a 20% reported response rate when given systemically for treatment of tumors of the gastrointestinal tract. However, the response appears to be even less in the presence of hepatic metastases. Leucovorin or levamisole appears to add to this rate.

A hepatic artery infusion pump (Infusaid) is used in several centers. Failure to accrue enough patients for large studies of the pump in the mid 1980s led to general pessimism about the use of the pump for treatment of colorectal metastases. Seven randomized trials now have demonstrated higher partial and complete response rates of intrahepatic versus systemic infusion in the treatment of hepatic metastases from colorectal carcinoma. The toxicity of direct hepatic arterial therapy is surprisingly low. A rare and irreversible problem is severe biliary sclerosis, which is related to biliary ischemia.

Cryoablation, hyperthermia, and various chemoembolic hepatic artery occlusion techniques continue to be investigated in several centers. Chemoembolization has had its best success with metastatic leiomyosarcoma. Radiation therapy has had no real success in the treatment of hepatic metastases.

Resection of Noncolorectal Metastases. Neuroendocrine malignancies, including metastatic carcinoid, represent the second most common indication for resection of secondary liver tumors. About 80% of patients who undergo resection with metastatic neuroendocrine tumors are symptomatic. Ninety percent of such patients with carcinoids have an endocrine syndrome. The primary indication for resection in most cases is palliation. The chance of cure with resection is small. Reduction of tumor volume by resection or cryoablation results predictably in elimination or amelioration of symptoms, often for years. There has usually already been a failure of medical management of the syndrome, such as after octreotide (Sandostatin) therapy or chemotherapy.

Hepatic metastases from primary malignancies other than colorectal and neuroendocrine (including lung, breast, stomach, pancreas, melanoma, and the rest of the gastrointestinal tract) connote dismal outcomes. Solitary metastases from these lesions are rare, probably related to the natural biology of these tumors. However, data on aggressive, combined medical/surgical treatment are sparse. Rare favorable results with liver resection have also been reported with Wilms' tumor, renal cell carcinoma, gallbladder cancer, bile duct cancer, and even adrenal cancer. Long-term survival has not been reported after resection of melanoma nor pancreatic cancer. The authors have treated 20 patients with residual liver deposits of breast cancer after bone marrow transplantation chemotherapy, and more than half the patients have survived well over a year, suggesting a benefit.

BENIGN HEPATIC NEOPLASMS

Benign tumors of the liver are relatively common, occurring in about 1% of autopsies. CT and MRI are considerably more sensitive than autopsy and find some kind of liver lesion in about 5% of patients. Benign tumors may be classified into true neoplasms, hamartomas, and pseudotumors. The nonbiliary neoplasms of the liver can also be classified as hepatocellular, vascular, and other nonvascular lesions. This section discusses the most common benign lesions with their characteristic features.

Adenomas and Focal Nodular Hyperplasia

Liver cell adenoma and focal nodular hyperplasia are frequently difficult to differentiate, although each has its own distinct pathologic and clinical features. The striking similarities are that both occur primarily in young women and are associated with the use of oral contraceptives and that pathologically both are composed of hepatocytes. Hepatic adenomas are usually solitary and may vary in size up to 38 cm. in diameter. Occasionally they may be multiple and cluster within families. They are prone to hemorrhage and necrosis, and tumor rupture or dramatic bleeding occurs in approximately one third of patients. Malignant change is possible. The remaining patients present because of pain or a palpable mass. The patient with an unresected adenoma who discontinues using oral contraceptives and becomes pregnant is at considerable risk for tumor rupture and hemorrhage. Microscopically, the adenomas are closely approximated cords of hepatocytes that have vacuolated sinusoidal borders (Fig. 33–25). Centers of the adenomas may undergo degenerative changes. Adenomas have an abundant blood supply; the benign tumor appears separate from adjacent normal hepatic tissue. In contrast, focal nodular hyperplasia does not produce symptoms; and hemorrhage, rupture, or other problems, such as malignant change, are exceedingly rare. Histologically, this lesion has a central stellate scar and no true encapsulation, and the cells, which are slightly different in color, usually blend with the normal hepatic parenchyma. The ultrastructure of the hepatocytes in nodular hyperplasia is similar to that of normal hepatocytes. The blood supply to areas of focal nodular hyperplasia is quite different from that to hepatic adenomas, with most of the supply arising centrally rather than peripherally.

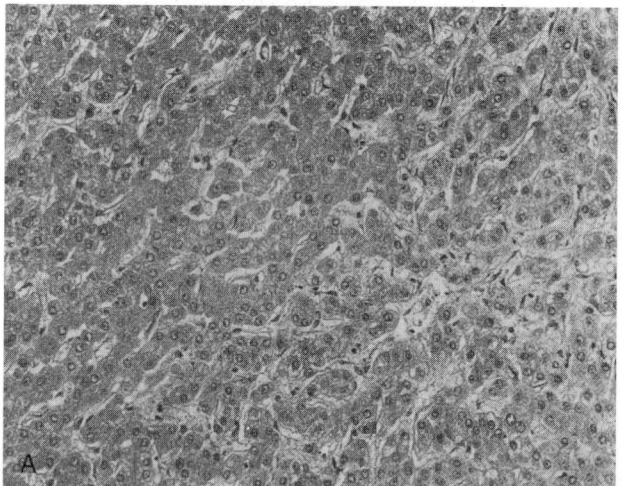

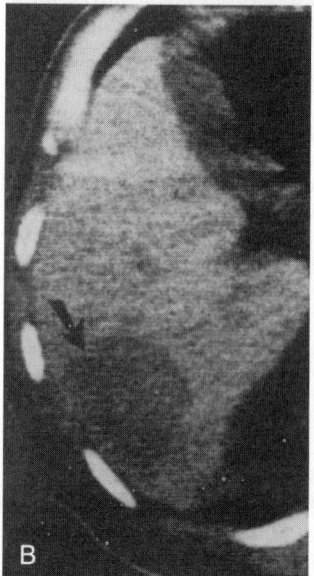
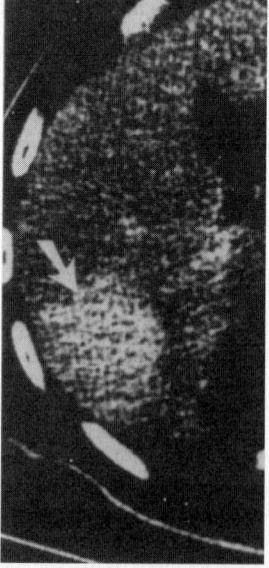

Figure 33–25. Benign lesions of liver. *A,* Histology of a hepatic adenoma. Note the bland pattern of cells resembling hepatocytes and the absence of portal triads. Focal nodular hyperplasia would have portal triads. (From Chari, R. S., and Meyers, W. C.: The liver. *In* Levine, B. A., et al. [Eds.]: Current Practice of Surgery. New York, Churchill Livingstone, 1994, p. 22.) *B,* CT scan of a hemangioma *(arrows)* demonstrating nearly complete filling of the lesion with intravenous contrast medium. A particularly hypervascular hepatoma or metastasis must still be considered. (From Cronon, J. J., Esparza, A. A., and Dorfman, G. S.: Management of cavernous hemangioma of liver: Role of percutaneous biopsy. *Radiology, 166:*136, 1988.)

Nodular Regenerative Hyperplasia

Nodular regenerative hyperplasia is, by definition, a noncirrhotic diffuse hepatocellular process characterized by multiple nodules in intervening areas of hepatic atrophy. It is similar to focal nodular hyperplasia in that both are not true neoplasms. Nodular regenerative hyperplasia is more frequently confused with cirrhosis. Both are frequently associated with portal hypertension, but the former is distinguished by the absence of severe fibrosis. Although this condition is generally considered rare, because of the understandable confusion between this entity and cirrhosis the incidence is reported quite variably.

Cavernous Hemangiomas

Cavernous hemangiomas occur in all age groups, often grow during pregnancy, and are usually successfully diagnosed by ultrasonography, CT, MRI, radionuclide scan, or arteriography (see Fig. 33–25). Approximately 2% of livers at autopsy contain cavernous hemangiomas, making this the most common liver tumor encountered coincidentally at laparotomy. Most hemangiomas are small and do not cause symptoms. However, they may be large and when associated with diffuse hemangiomatosis can nearly replace the liver. Spontaneous rupture is unusual but can be dramatic. Rare complications include congestive heart failure due to arteriovenous shunts and consumptive coagulopathy. Biopsy of a cavernous hemangioma may lead to severe, uncontrollable hemorrhage. Indications for resection are usually determined by the presence of symptoms, the danger of rupture, and the amount of liver tissue involved. Symptoms usually indicate enlargement and are associated with increased incidence of rupture. The occupation of the patient and size of the lesion influence the decision to resect. For example, a large lesion in a professional football player should be removed. On the other hand, most hemangiomas do not have to be treated.

Other Benign Solid Tumors

Other benign solid tumors that may appear in the liver include lipomas, fibromas, leiomyomas, myxomas, teratomas, carcinoid tumor, and mesenchymal hamartomas. Carcinoid is an exceedingly rare primary liver tumor and is associated with the carcinoid syndrome. Mesenchymal hamartomas are rare but important to recognize because they grow to an extremely large size in an infant or young child and require surgical resection. Biliary cystadenomas and bile duct adenomas are exceedingly rare and may cause pain or extrahepatic biliary obstruction. Other even rarer benign biliary tumors include meningioma, fibroma, granular cell myoblastoma, and carcinoid. Tiny biliary hamartomas, or tufts of biliary hyperplasia, are extremely common. Another lesion usually of little pathologic significance but relatively common is focal fatty change.

Some benign conditions that can be confused with hepatic neoplasms include hereditary hemorrhagic telangiectasia, peliosis hepatis, and hepatic pseudotumor. Hereditary hemorrhagic telangiectasia is a diffuse telangiectatic process in the liver with numerous arteriovenous fistulas; it is rare, associated with fibrosis, and considered by some authorities to be a form of cirrhosis. Peliosis hepatis is also a rare lesion characterized by variably sized blood lakes and the most common association is with anabolic steroid therapy. Rarely is the condition clinically important. Over 50 cases of inflammatory *pseudotumor* have been reported, most probably resulting from healed abscesses.

NONPARASITIC CYSTS

Cysts of the liver are generally benign. They may be solitary or multiple and may or may not communicate with the hepatic ductal system. Large solitary parenchymal cysts appear to be very rare; only 48 have been observed by investigators at a major medical center in the past 30 years. Most cysts are lined by biliary epithelium but may also have a mesothelial cell lining or rarely other types of lining. They are more common in the right lobe of the liver. It has been presumed that most of these cysts are congenital. They occur four times as frequently in females as in males. Although most cysts are small and asymptomatic, they may be quite large; in fact, one reported cyst contained 17,000 ml. of fluid. The most common presenting symptoms of large cysts are increased abdominal girth, vague pain, occasional bleeding or infection, and rarely evidence of significant hepatocyte compromise such as obstructive jaundice. Small cysts require no treatment, although if they are discovered incidentally at the time of operation they may simply be aspirated. For large cysts from which clear fluid is aspirated, the preferred treatment is excision. However, major vascular and ductal structures may be proximal to the wall, in which case unroofing and external drainage is the treatment of choice. Many of these excisions have been performed laparoscopically at several centers. An infected cyst should be treated like an abscess, that is, with open drainage. If the cyst contains biliary contents, a communication to the bile duct system should be presumed and excision or Roux-en-Y cystojejunostomy is the treatment of choice.

Polycystic liver disease often accompanies polycystic kidneys. The number of cysts varies, but most do not cause liver function compromise; and rupture, hemorrhage, and infection are rare. When indicated, they may be treated in a manner similar to solitary cysts. Injection of sclerosing solutions such as tetracycline and formalin has been performed with only limited success. Simple aspiration is a temporizing maneuver. The surgical procedure of choice for a symptomatic dominant cyst in polycystic disease is the fenestration operation, in which the symptomatic cyst is made to communicate with the peritoneal cavity.

Cysts may also form as a consequence of trauma or inflammation; however, these are not true cysts, because they have a fibrous rather than an epithelial lining. There are no special aspects of treatment of these cysts. Cystadenomas, cystadenocarcinomas, and other neoplasms with necrotic centers obviously may present as cysts and should be treated by excision. Cystadenoma is thought to be a precursor of cystadenocarcinoma. Despite the rarity of cystadenoma, there have been several large series of resection of cystadenomas. This disparity suggests there may be some confusion in the diagnosis of this lesion. Other unusual cysts include teratomas, necrotic cysts secondary to infarction, intrahepatic duodenal duplications, and cysts associated with congenital hepatic fibrosis. Peliosis hepatis is a dilation of the hepatic sinusoids often associated with steroids, chemotherapy, and tuberculosis.

Choledochal or other solitary ductal cysts are more common in Asia than in the United States. They occur more commonly in females than in males, but the pathogenesis is unknown. Sixty percent are diagnosed before the age of 10. Associated intrahepatic ductal dilation is frequent. The most common type of choledochal cyst is one that involves the common bile duct and cystic duct but does not involve the junction of the common hepatic duct. A number of other types may occur, including a diverticulum, diffuse biliary ductal involvement, and segmental dilation. Treatment of choledochal or hepatic ductal cysts or dilation is surgical and is supplemented by antibiotics to control infection. Because of the significant likelihood of biliary obstruction, cholangitis, calculi, and carcinoma, the procedure of choice is excision whenever possible. However, this may not be practical anatomically. In addition, the drainage procedures such as hepaticoenterostomy or cystoenterostomy are preferred. The incidence of carcinoma in congenital biliary duct cysts appears to be 5% to 8%. Occasionally this occurs after cyst excision. The incidence of stricture after cystoenterostomy has been reported to be as high as 40% to 50%.

Multiple cystic dilations of the intrahepatic ducts (Caroli's disease) are a congenital malformation often associated with congenital hepatic fibrosis. It may be confined to one segment or lobe but is usually diffuse. This problem also appears to be more common in Asia. Symptoms of biliary tract disease, such as colic or cholangitis, may be associated with Caroli's disease. Treatment depends on the location and extent of the intrahepatic ductal dilation. Both drainage and resection in selected patients have been reported to provide good results.

ECHINOCOCCAL CYSTS

Echinococcosis, or hydatidosis, is the most frequent cause of liver cysts in the world. The problem is endemic in Greece, other parts of Eastern Europe, South America, Australia, and South Africa. Echinococcosis is rare in the United States, although it is prevalent enough to be seen by most general surgeons during their careers. The most common form is due to *Echinococcus granulosus*, although occasionally *E. multilocularis* is the infective agent. The adult *E. granulosus* is a tapeworm that resides in the jejunum of dogs. Eggs are passed in the stool and ingested by cows, sheep, moose, caribou, or humans. Embryos pass through the intestinal mucosa into the portal circulation and are filtered by the liver and occasionally by the lungs. They then develop into cysts that have two layers, an outer fibrous layer and an inner parasite-derived layer. The inner layer is the germinal membrane that contains the scolices and daughter cysts and may float freely in the clear cyst fluid.

Approximately 80% of hydatid cysts are initially single and in the right lobe. The most common presenting symptoms or signs are abdominal pain and palpation of a mass in the right upper quadrant. The cysts are usually greater than 5 cm. in diameter when they cause symptoms. The complications of echinococcal cysts include infection, rupture, anaphylaxis, biliary obstruction, and liver replacement. The patient may have eosinophilia and mildly elevated results of liver function tests. Of the serologic tests, the indirect hemagglutination test and the Casoni skin test have approximately an 85% sensitivity. Problems with the Casoni skin test are that the test itself may sensitize the host, which may cause false-positive serologic tests or even anaphylaxis, and there is a high frequency of false-positive tests due to poor standardization of the nitrogen content in the antigen. The complement fixation test has approximately a 70% sensitivity. Calcification of the cystic wall is present in over half the patients. Liver scan, ultrasonography, CT, and arteriography all can have nearly 100% sensitivity (Fig. 33–26). Endoscopic retrograde cholangiopancreatography and cholangiography have been reported to be helpful occasionally. The finding of daughter cysts or hydatid *sand* on ultrasonography and CT helps differentiate this cyst from pyogenic or amebic liver abscess. This entity must be suspected to avoid percutaneous needle aspiration, which may cause spillage and spread of the cysts. Communication of the cyst with the biliary tract may be seen on the preoperative cholangiogram or intraoperatively in approximately one fourth of patients. Treatment is primarily surgical.

At exploration, the abdomen is carefully packed with pads around the cysts to reduce the risk of peritoneal soilage. The

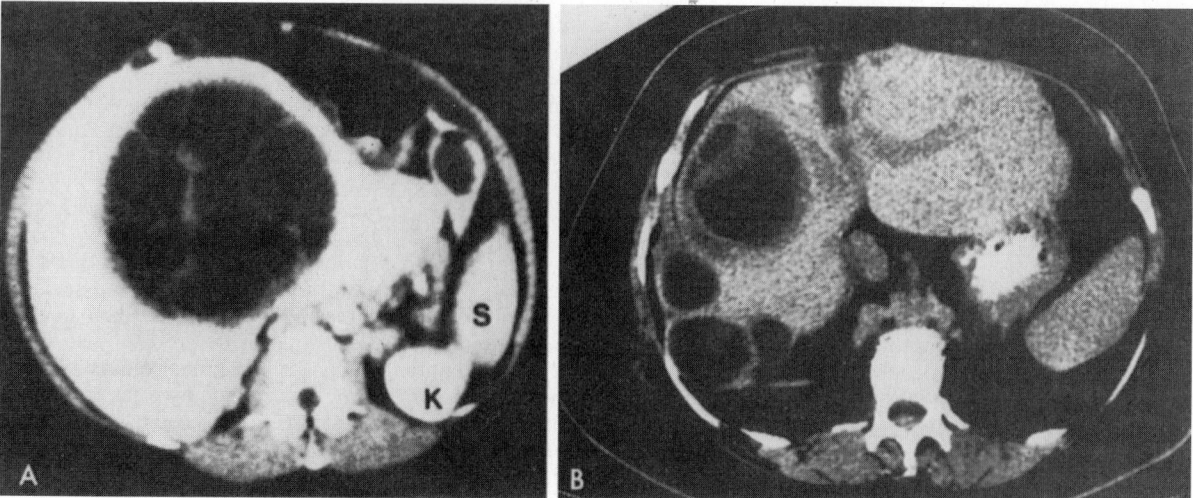

Figure 33–26. Solitary *(A)* and multiple *(B)* recurrent echinococcal cysts with septa seen on computed tomography (K, kidney; S, spleen). (*A* reprinted with permission from Gutierrez, O. H., and Schwartz, S. I. [Eds.]: Atlas of Hepatic Tumors and Focal Lesions. New York, McGraw-Hill Book Company, 1984.)

cyst may then be aspirated as completely as possible with a closed system. If the fluid color suggests biliary communication, a sclerosing solution should not be used. Hypertonic saline, chlorhexidine, 80% alcohol, and 0.5% cetrimide are all useful as scolecidal agents and may be instilled into the cyst cavity. Formalin is no longer used because of the risk of systemic toxicity. After 5 minutes, the procedure is repeated and then the cyst cavity is unroofed. The fluid in the echinococcal cyst cavity is highly antigenic and therefore anaphylaxis as well as spread is a risk of cyst rupture. Instillation of scolecidal agents is effective in destroying 80% to 90% of scoleces. There are two alternatives in the management of the cyst cavity: drainage and obliteration without drainage. Except in cases with biliary communication, drainage is accompanied by greater postoperative morbidity and prolonged hospitalization. Therefore, most surgeons prefer not to drain the cyst cavities. Small intrahepatic or extrahepatic cysts may be excised. Recently, mebendazole has been found to be an effective agent in some cases of echinococcal cysts, and this drug may be used for cases not amenable to surgical therapy.

The treatment of the more aggressive *E. multilocularis,* or alveolar hydatid disease, is excision whenever possible. However, this is rarely possible. This disease is limited geographically to the Northern Hemisphere, being endemic in Alaska and Canada. Natural hosts include the fox, coyote, and small rodents.

MAJOR HEPATIC RESECTION

With reduction of elective operative mortality to less than 1%, major hepatic resection has gained wide acceptance as the primary therapy for many primary and metastatic tumors to the liver and other selected benign conditions. Those conditions include segmental Caroli's disease or hepatolithiasis, echinococcosis, or solitary hepatic abscesses in chronic granulomatous disease of childhood. Formerly, only four types of major hepatic resection were employed, based on the lobar (American) system of anatomy: (A) right hepatic lobectomy, (B) left hepatic lobectomy, (C) right trisegmentectomy, and (D) left lateral segmentectomy (Fig. 33–27). Now, a number of new resections have become commonplace in major centers. Most are based on the French segmental system (Fig. 33–28).

Basically, there are three types of hepatic resection: (1)

anatomic resection, (2) enucleation operation, and (3) nonanatomic resection. The primary concept behind anatomic resection according to the segmental anatomy is that malignant cells distribute along the portal venous segmental supply. Enucleation operations are used for specific benign lesions with limited chance of local invasion (e.g., hemangioma, developmental cysts, focal nodular hyperplasia, or even hepatic adenoma). Nonanatomic resections are appropriate for pathologic processes in which a limited margin is appropriate (e.g., echinococcal cysts and abscess excision in chronic granulomatous disease).

The techniques of resection are distinguished by the presence or absence of partial or complete vascular occlusion. Vascular occlusion has the advantage of reduction of blood loss and the disadvantage of ischemic injury relating to the duration of occlusion. Most experienced surgeons use vascular occlusion selectively, depending on the individual cases. At Duke University Medical Center, a selective approach with respect to occlusion is used and about half the patients require blood transfusion. The techniques of parenchymal dissection have been greatly facilitated by the development

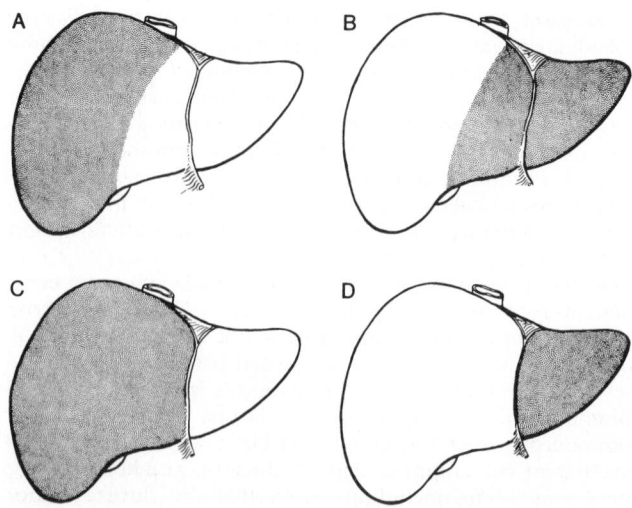

Figure 33–27. Four classic major hepatic resections: *A,* right hepatic lobectomy; *B,* left hepatic lobectomy; *C,* right trisegmentectomy; and *D,* left lateral segmentectomy.

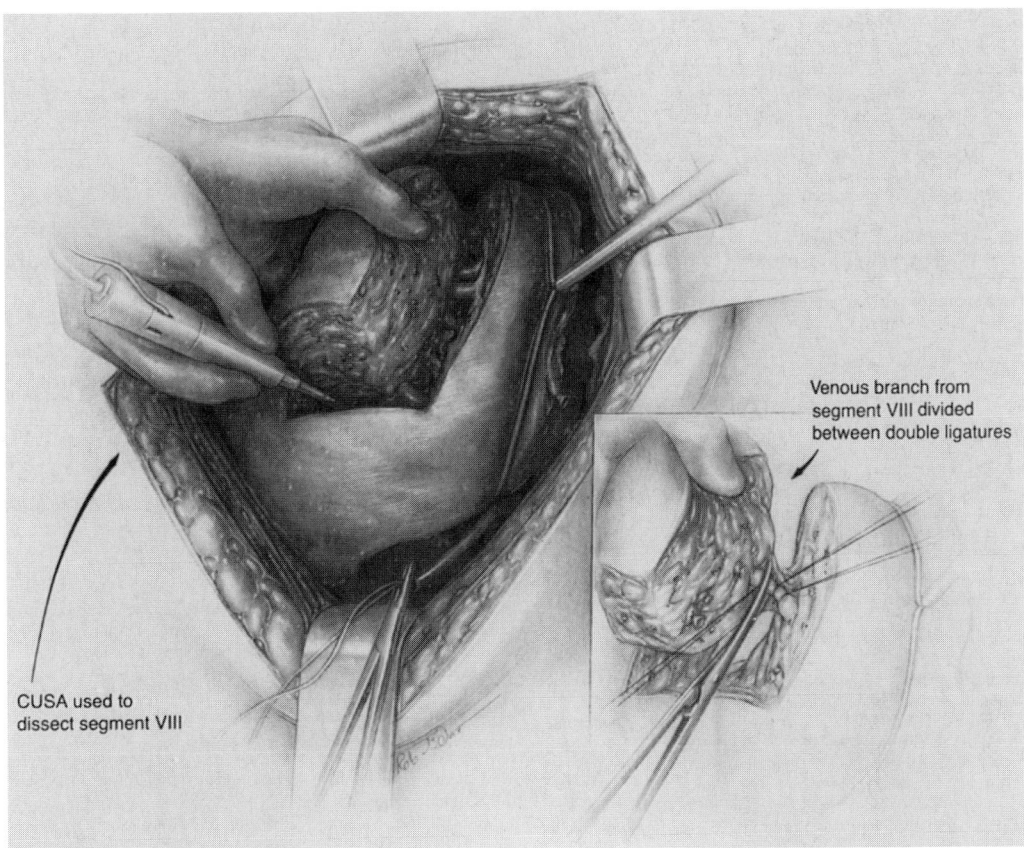

CUSA used to
dissect segment VIII

Venous branch from
segment VIII divided
between double ligatures

Figure 33–28. Any of the French segments can now be resected with safety, either alone or in combination with other segments. Depicted here is a method of resecting segment VIII using the Cavitron ultrasonic aspirator and temporary portal occlusion if necessary. (From Meyers, W. C.: Segmental hepatic resection. *In* Sabiston, D. C. [Ed.]: Atlas of General Surgery. Philadelphia, W. B. Saunders, 1994, p. 543.)

of various instruments, such as the argon beam coagulator and the Cavitron ultrasonic aspirator. The latter instrument has a metal tip that vibrates at an ultrasonic frequency that fragments and detaches parenchymal cells. An irrigation port lifts the cells so that a suction port can remove them. Major biliary or vascular structures remain intact, permitting their isolation and ligation, even without hilar dissection. Through the use of these and other techniques, many more lesions can be safely resected than was formerly believed and partial hepatic transplantation has become possible.

A variety of incisions may be used for hepatic resection. Most surgeons stay below the diaphragm with a right subcostal incision and a left subcostal extension if necessary. The incision can be extended as a median sternotomy or right thoracotomy. A paramedian incision is preferred by many surgeons in Asia. Lobectomy and trisegmentectomy usually require hilar dissection, whereas segmental resections generally do not. Branches of the portal vein, hepatic artery, and bile duct of the lobe to be removed are ligated and divided. The hepatic veins may be ligated extrahepatically or during the parenchymal dissection. Parenchymal dissection is performed with a small clamp, handle of the knife, or finger fracture. A variety of noncrushing liver clamps may be applied to control parenchymal bleeding, and surgical staplers are useful during the latter stages of the parenchymal dissection.

Compulsive preoperative hydration is key to a benign postoperative course. Dehydration leads to rapid intraoperative volume resuscitation, which leads to hepatic venous congestion, the chief cause of morbidity and mortality.

Hypoglycemia and hypoproteinemia frequently occur in the postoperative period after major hepatic resection. These should be treated supportively and usually resolve within 1 week after the operation. Alkaline phosphatase and transaminase elevations frequently occur, and transient hyperbilirubinemia is not uncommon. Up to 80% or 90% of the liver may be removed without serious consequence if the remaining liver is normal. Patients with pre-existing diffuse liver disease are at greatly increased risk for liver failure after resection. Regeneration is nearly complete by 3 weeks postoperatively, except in elderly patients, whose livers grow back more slowly.

SELECTED REFERENCES

Chari, R. S., and Meyers, W. C.: The liver. In Levine, B. A., et al. (Eds.): Current Practice of Surgery. New York, Churchill Livingstone, 1994.
An algorithmic approach to the care of patients with potentially surgical liver disease is presented.

Craig, J. R., Peters, R. L., and Edmondson, H. A.: Atlas of Tumor Pathology. Washington, D.C., Armed Forces Institute of Pathology, 1988.
This is one of the classic references for the pathology of liver and biliary neoplasms.

Foster, J. H., and Berman, M. M.: Solid Liver Tumors. Philadelphia, W. B. Saunders, 1977.
This remains a landmark monograph on the subject.

Meyers, W. C., and Jones, R. S. (Eds.): Textbook of Liver and Biliary Surgery. Philadelphia, J. B. Lippincott, 1990.
This relatively recent comprehensive textbook covers hepatobiliary surgery with emphasis on the pathobiology and historical perspectives that guide current therapy.

Terblanche, J. (Ed.): Hepatobiliary Malignancy: Its Multidisciplinary Management. London, Edward Arnold, 1994.
This recent monograph on hepatobiliary malignancy provides views on the subject from surgeons, pathologists, radiologists, gastroenterologists, and other specialists.

REFERENCES

1. Adson, M. A.: The resection of hepatic metastases: Another view. Arch. Surg., 124:1023, 1989.

2. Aoki, K.: Cancer of the liver: International mortality trends. World Health Stat. Rep., *31*:28, 1978.
3. Belmaric, J.: Malignant tumors in Chinese. Int. J. Cancer, *4*:560, 1979.
4. Bismuth, H., and Chiche, L.: Surgery of hepatic tumors. Prog. Liver Dis., *11*:269, 1993.
5. Bismuth, H., Castaing, D., and Garden, O. J.: The use of operative ultrasound in surgery of primary liver tumors. World J. Surg., *11*:610, 1987.
6. Blumgart, L. H., Benjamin, I. S., Hadis, N. S., and Beazler, R.: Surgical approaches to cholangiocarcinoma at confluence of hepatic ducts. Lancet, *1*:66, 1984.
7. Bonfanti, G., Bombelli, L., Bozzetti, F., et al.: The role of CEA and liver function tests in the detection of hepatic metastases from colorectal cancer. HPB Surg., *3*:29, 1990.
8. Brown, H. W.: Basic Clinical Parasitology, 3rd ed. New York, Appleton-Century-Crofts, 1969, chaps 10 to 13.
9. Castaing, D., Garden, O. J., and Bismuth, H.: Segmental liver resection using ultrasound-guided selective portal venous occlusion. Ann. Surg., *210*:20, 1989.
10. Chitwood, W. R., Meyers, W. C., Heaston, D. K., et al.: Diagnosis and treatment of primary extrahepatic bile duct tumors. Am. J. Surg., *143*:99, 1982.
11. Colombo, M.: Hepatocellular carcinoma in cirrhotics. Semin. Liver Dis., *13*:374, 1993.
12. Couinaud, C.: Bases anatomiques des hepatectomies gauche et droite reglées: Techniques qui en deroulent. J. Chir., *70*:933, 1954.
13. Cuschieri, A., Crosthwaite, G., Shimi, S., Pietrabissa, A., Joypaul, V., Tair, I., and Naziri, W.: Hepatic cryotherapy for liver tumors: Development and clinical evaluation of a high-efficiency insulated multineedle probe system for open and laparoscopic use. Surg. Endosc., *9*:483, 1995.
14. Dalton, R. R., and Eisenberg, B. L.: Surgical management of recurrent liver tumors. Semin. Oncol., *20*:493, 1993.
15. Dunham, L. J., and Bailar, J. C.: World maps of cancer mortality rates and frequency rates. J. Natl. Cancer Inst., *41*:155, 1968.
16. Dusheiko, G. M., Hobbs, K. E., Dick, R., and Burroughs, A. K.: Treatment of small hepatocellular carcinomas. Lancet, *340*:285, 1992.
17. Ezaki, T., Stansby, G. P., and Hobbs, K. E.: Intraoperative ultrasonographic imaging in liver surgery: A review. HPB Surg., *3*:1, 1990.
18. Farmer, D. G., Rosove, M. H., Shaked, A., and Busuttil, R. W.: Current treatment modalities for hepatocellular carcinoma. Ann. Surg., *219*:236, 1994.
19. Fausto, N., and Webber, E. M.: Mechanisms of growth regulation in liver regeneration and hepatic carcinogenesis. Prog. Liver Dis., *11*:115, 1993.
20. Ferrucci, J. T.: Liver tumor imaging: Current concepts (see comments). AJR, *155*:473, 1990.
21. Foster, J. H., and Berman, M. M.: The malignant transformation of liver cell adenomas. Arch. Surg., *129*:712, 1994.
22. Herndier, B. G., and Friedman, S. L.: Neoplasms of the gastrointestinal tract and hepatobiliary system in acquired immunodeficiency syndrome. Semin. Liver Dis., *12*:128, 1993.
23. Hughes, K., Scheele, J., and Sugarbaker, P. H.: Surgery for colorectal cancer metastatic to the liver: Optimizing the results of treatment. Surg. Clin. North Am., *69*:339, 1989.
24. Iwatsuki, S., Gordon, R. D., Shaw, B. W., and Starzl, T. E.: Role of liver transplantation in cancer therapy. Ann. Surg., *202*:401, 1985.
25. Jaffe, B. M., Donegan, W. L., Watson, F., and Spratt, J. S., Jr.: Factors influencing survival in patients with untreated hepatic metastases. Surg. Gynecol. Obstet., *127*:1, 1968.
26. Jenkins, R. L., Johnson, L. B., and Lewis, W. D.: Surgical approach to benign liver tumors. Semin. Liver Dis., *14*:178, 1994.
27. John, T. G., and Garden, O. J.: Needle track seeding of primary and secondary liver carcinoma after percutaneous liver biopsy. HPB Surg., *6*:199, 1993.
28. Keen, W. W.: Report of a case of resection of the liver for the removal of a neoplasm, with a table of 76 cases of resection of the liver for hepatic tumors. Ann. Surg., *30*:267, 1899.
29. Kemeny, M. M.: Chemotherapy after hepatic resection of colorectal metastases. Cancer Treat. Res., *69*:121, 1994.
30. Kemeny, N.: Review of regional therapy of liver metastases in colorectal cancer. Semin. Oncol., *19*:155, 1992.
31. Kemeny, N. E.: Is hepatic infusion of chemotherapy effective treatment for liver metastases? Yes. Important Adv. Oncol., 207, 1992.
32. Kortz, W. J., Meyers, W. C., Hanks, J. B., et al.: Hepatic resection for metastatic cancer. Ann. Surg., *199*:182, 1984.
33. Langenbuch, C.: Ein Fall von Resektion eines linksseitigen Schnurlappens der Leber, Heilung. Berl. Klin. Wochenschr., *25*:37, 1888.
34. Langer, J. C., Rose, D. B., Keystone, J. S., et al.: Diagnosis and management of hydatid disease of the liver: A 15-year North American experience. Ann. Surg., *199*:412, 1984.
35. Lygidakis, N. J., and Tytgat, G. N. J. (Eds.): Hepatobiliary and Pancreatic Malignancies: Diagnosis, Medical and Surgical Management. New York, Thieme Medical Publishers, 1989.
36. Pichlmayr, R., Weimann, A., and Ringe, B.: Indications for liver transplantation in hepatobiliary malignancy. Hepatology, *20*:33S, 1994.
37. Reddy, K. R., and Schiff, E. R.: Approach to a liver mass. Semin. Liver Dis., *13*:423, 1993.
38. Robinson, W. S.: The role of hepatitis B virus in the development of primary hepatocellular carcinoma: II. J. Gastroenterol. Hepatol., *8*:95, 1993.
39. Robinson, W. S.: The role of hepatitis B virus in the development of primary hepatocellular carcinoma: I. J. Gastroenterol. Hepatol., *7*:622, 1992.
40. Sanfilippo, P. M., Behars, O. H., and Weiland, L. H.: Cystic disease of the liver. Ann. Surg., *179*:922, 1974.
41. Schwartz, M. E.: Primary hepatocellular carcinoma: Transplant versus resection. Semin. Liver Dis., *14*:135, 1994.
42. Schwartz, S. I.: Hepatic resection. Ann. Surg., *211*:1, 1990.
43. Soulen, M. C.: Chemoembolization of hepatic malignancies. Oncology, *8*:77, 1994.
44. Steele, G., Jr.: Cryoablation in hepatic surgery. Semin. Liver Dis., *14*:120, 1994.
45. Todani, T., Tabuchi, K., Watanabe, Y., and Kobayashi, T.: Carcinoma arising in the wall of congenital bile duct cysts. Cancer, *44*:1134, 1979.
46. Wendel, W.: Beitrage zur Chirurgie der Leber. Arch. Klin. Chir., *95*:887, 1911.
47. Wilson, J. F., and Rausch, R. L.: Alveolar hydatid disease: A review of clinical features of 33 indigenous cases of *Echinococcus multilocularis* infection in Alaskan Eskimos. Am. J. Trop. Med. Hyg., *29*:1340, 1980.
48. Wu, A. H., and Sell, S.: Markers for hepatocellular carcinoma. Immunol. Ser., *53*:403, 1990.

IV

HEMOBILIA

Ravi S. Chari, M.D., and William C. Meyers, M.D.

Hemobilia, a term introduced by Sandblom in 1948, refers to a relatively common and occasionally severe clinical problem. A severe case should engender in the clinician certain reflex responses with respect to diagnosis and treatment.

Glisson provided the first modern description of bleeding within the biliary tract in 1654, recognizing that it was probably a relatively common consequence of trauma. Rupture of a hepatic artery aneurysm into the biliary tract was first reported by Jackson in 1921. In 1948, Sandblom recognized the classic triad of pain, jaundice, and hematemesis. With severe bleeding, blood usually moves in both directions in the gastrointestinal tract, causing both hematemesis and melena. Recently, the more common causes of identifiable hemobilia reflect advances in hepatobiliary diagnostic and therapeutic techniques. These include percutaneous liver biopsy, transhepatic or endoscopic cholangiography, extracorporeal lithotripsy, transjugular intrahepatic portosystemic shunt, and laparoscopic cholecystectomy.

ETIOLOGY

Bleeding may arise anywhere within the biliary system, that is, from liver parenchyma, intrahepatic or extrahepatic bile ducts, gallbladder, pancreas, or the ampullary region. The communication between the vascular and biliary systems may be caused by laceration, pressure necrosis, tumor, or infection. In addition, thrombolysis in bile may contribute to continued bleeding. Because of its higher pressure, the arterial system is more often involved than the venous system.

In earlier reviews, operative trauma represented approximately 15% of cases of hemobilia. Other causes include major procedures on or near the liver that may produce minor or major bleeding, such as liver, stomach, or colon resections; cholecystectomy; or extraction of intrahepatic calculi (Fig. 33–29). The procedure most likely to cause bleeding within the biliary system is common bile duct exploration. The peribiliary arterial plexus is often involved in the bleeding. Hepatic artery false aneurysms may follow unsuspected injury and later erode into the bile duct. Postoperative dislodgment of a T-tube may also produce the problem. The diagnosis of thrombus within the biliary tree is easily made by cholangiography if a catheter such as a T-tube is within the common bile duct. Thus, thrombus may occasionally be confused with a retained stone. Recently, percutaneous cholangiography has become an important cause of bleeding into the biliary system. Hemobilia occurs after 4% of percutaneous transhepatic cholangiograms and 9% of percutaneously placed biliary drainage catheters. Some degree of hemobilia occurs in 5% to 10% of therapeutic endoscopic procedures. In these patients, thrombus in the biliary tree usually evolves from the sphincterotomy site. Some degree of hemobilia occurs in 8% to 14% of extracorporeal hepatic biliary lithotripsy and 4% to 8% of extracorporeal gallstone lithotripsy. In nearly all of the latter cases the reported bleeding has been minor and inconsequential.

In a review of 545 patients in 1972, trauma was the most important causative factor in 48% of cases, followed by infection in 28%, gallstones in 10%, aneurysms in 7%, and tumor in 5%. Trauma included both blunt and penetrating injuries, with that resulting from vehicular accidents leading the list. Blunt trauma may cause deep liver injury with or without disruption of Glisson's capsule. Probably the most frequent reason for hemobilia occurring after liver injury is bleeding deep within the substance of the liver when the capsule remains intact, is sutured closed, or heals superficially. If the resultant hematoma expands, it may rupture into the biliary

system; or a false aneurysm may occur and lead to the same problem in a delayed manner. These are the principal reasons that suture closure of a liver laceration is generally not recommended. Penetration may cause hemobilia by a similar mechanism or by creating a direct communication of a vascular structure with the biliary system.

Infection may also be an important factor in the development of hemobilia. In the Far East, the parasites *Clonorchis sinensis* and *Ascaris* may cause cholangitis or pericholangitic abscesses, which may cause hemobilia. Less commonly, amebic abscess, tuberculosis, and *Echinococcus* infestation are implicated. Biliary tract infection in North America is more often caused by calculi, which may also cause hemobilia by direct trauma to the ampulla or other sites within the duodenal ductal system. Before the development of oral cholecystography, the coexistence of biliary colic with blood in the stool was considered a reliable sign of gallstones. The term *hemocholecyst* refers to bleeding within the gallbladder, which rarely may be the cause of biliary colic. Pyogenic liver abscess may lead to hemobilia by direct erosion into a vessel, by formation of a pseudoaneurysm, or as a complication of treatment. Hemobilia may also follow a mycotic aneurysm complicating subacute bacterial endocarditis or another disease process. Pancreatitis may cause hemobilia by erosion of a large vessel such as the splenic or gastroduodenal artery and communication with the pancreatic duct; the outcome is usually fatal. Hemobilia due to pancreatic disease is unusual except when cancer has, by erosion, entered the biliary system. Hemobilia can also occur as a manifestation of rupture of an echinococcal or amebic abscess.

Various aneurysms may cause hemobilia by pressure necrosis. Arteriosclerotic, congenital, false, or mycotic aneurysms of the hepatic or gastroduodenal artery have all been reported to cause this problem. In one series, 43 of 103 ruptured hepatic artery aneurysms (42%) led to hemobilia. Hepatoma secondary to cirrhosis is the most common tumor causing hemobilia. Other tumors that have been reported to induce hemobilia include gallbladder cancer, cholangiocarcinoma, hemangioma, angiosarcoma, adenomas, cystadeno-

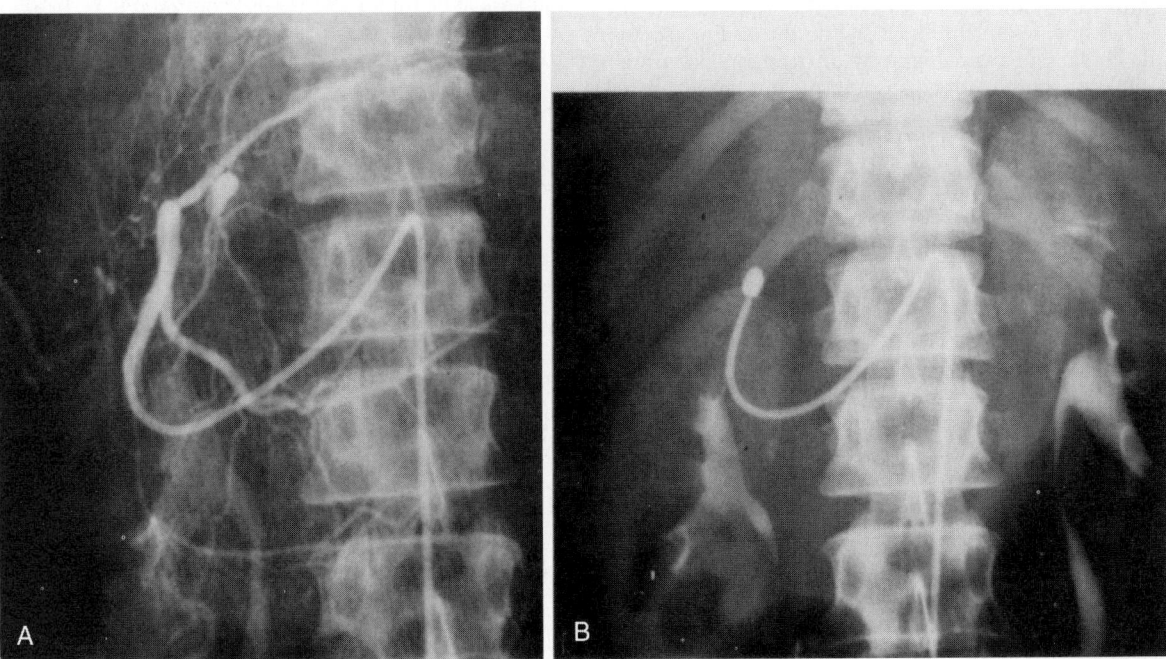

Figure 33–29. *A,* Intraparenchymal hepatic artery aneurysm causing hemobilia after percutaneous liver biopsy. *B,* Arteriographic balloon used to occlude and thrombose artery and aneurysm. (Radiographic films selected with the assistance of N. Reed Dunnick, M.D., from a case reported by Dunnick, N. R., Doppman, I. L., and Brereton, H. D.: Balloon occlusion of segmental hepatic arteries: Control of biopsy-induced hemobilia. JAMA, *238:*2524, 1977. Copyright 1977, American Medical Association.)

mas, cystadenocarcinomas, and metastatic lesions of the liver parenchyma, gallbladder, and bile ducts. Hemobilia may also occur in association with choledochal cyst or may appear spontaneously in association with vasculitis, heterotopic gastric mucosa, or hemolytic disease such as sickle cell anemia.

In the authors' unpublished review of hemobilia during the past 3 years, 24 of 43 cases were the direct result of iatrogenic trauma, 12 were postsurgical, 6 followed laparoscopic cholecystectomy, and 2 were complications of cryoablation of liver masses. Others were caused by complications of transcatheter arterial embolization, alcohol injection of liver lesions, transjugular intrahepatic portosystemic shunt, percutaneous liver biopsy, lithotripsy, endoscopic sphincterotomy, percutaneous abscess drainage, and transhepatic cholangiography. Twelve patients had hemobilia as the initial presentation of a hepatobiliary tumor and 8 of the 12 tumors were resected.

SYMPTOMS AND SIGNS

The classic triad of hemobilia comprises gastrointestinal bleeding, right upper quadrant pain, and jaundice. These features may also suggest other diseases, including terminal cancer. In the setting of trauma, general good health, or any type of hepatobiliary manipulation, this triad should suggest the possibility of hemobilia. All three symptoms are not necessarily present. Acute bleeding usually first causes pain, followed by hematemesis or melena. Hemobilia may occur days, weeks, or months after trauma. A palpable mass representing the liver or gallbladder may accompany these symptoms. When a right upper quadrant bruit is heard with the classic triad, a visceral artery aneurysm causing hemobilia should be considered.

DIAGNOSIS

Early diagnosis may be lifesaving with severe hemobilia. A pseudoaneurysm should immediately be suspected, and arteriography remains the single most accurate and helpful diagnostic test. Liver or biliary scans, ultrasonography, computed tomography, or magnetic resonance imaging may provide helpful information such as evidence of anatomic defects or abnormalities in the liver or bile ducts. Endoscopic retrograde cholangiopancreatography or percutaneous transhepatic cholangiography may be helpful, but these procedures, particularly the last one, may confuse the diagnosis because this manipulation may also create a new source of bleeding. Ultrasonography may yield an erroneous impression of normal duct size in the presence of fresh blood or clot because of its variable echogenicity. Technetium-labeled or another red blood cell scan may occasionally be an efficient way of establishing a diagnosis, particularly in stable patients, but may also delay definitive diagnosis and treatment in severely bleeding patients. An external biliary drainage catheter may demonstrate the bleeding, or injection of the catheter with contrast material may document thrombus within the biliary system (Fig. 33–30). Immediate surgical therapy is rarely required to establish the diagnosis of severe hemobilia, although it may occasionally be indicated. If the operation is performed before diagnosis, a cause such as hepatic artery aneurysm, calculi, or tumor may be evident, or the biliary system may be the site of a collection of blood.

MANAGEMENT

The conditions associated with hemobilia can cause severe blood loss and, in some cases, hemorrhagic shock. Initial management of the patient should be general evaluation and resuscitation, with blood transfusions as needed (Fig. 33–31).

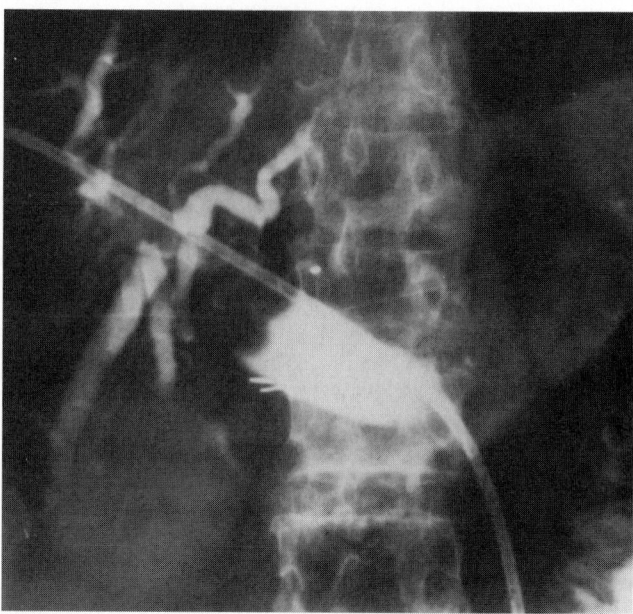

Figure 33–30. Large amount of thrombus within a markedly dilated common duct in a patient with obstructing carcinoma of the head of the pancreas. Thrombus prevented effective drainage of the catheter, and significant intraperitoneal hemorrhage at the hepatic entrance site occurred.

Careful monitoring with blood replacement is important in the care of these patients. If anticipated, coagulopathy may be prevented or managed by administration of blood components such as fresh frozen plasma or platelets. After the diagnosis of hemobilia is established, there are several options for treatment. The majority of cases of hemobilia, particularly those involving intrahepatic false aneurysms, may be effectively treated with arteriographic techniques such as embolization with clot, steel coils, or other emboli.

Selection of operative versus nonoperative treatment is based on the severity of bleeding, the underlying cause, and the age and general state of the patient. If the bleeding appears to be minor and easily monitored (e.g., in a postoperative situation), it is best managed expectantly. With acute trauma and hemoperitoneum, management of the acute

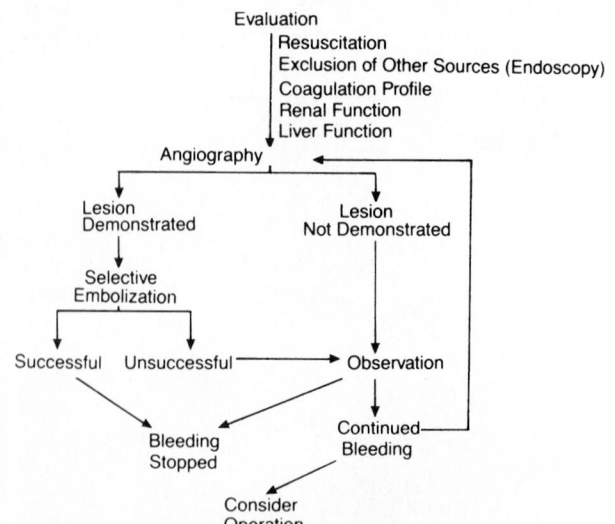

Figure 33–31. Management scheme for patients with suspected hemobilia. (From Czerniak, A., et al.: Hemobilia—a disease in evolution. Arch. Surg., *123*:718, 1988. Copyright 1988, American Medical Association.)

bleeding is a primary concern. Hepatic parenchymal bleeding may be controlled by a variety of methods, including direct ligation of the bleeding vessel and resection, packing, or ligation of the proper, common, right, or left hepatic artery. Ligation of the proper hepatic artery rarely causes any clinical problem because of abundant collateral vessels. Ligation of the common, right, or left hepatic artery more often causes enzyme abnormalities but is usually tolerated by the patient, particularly if it is a lifesaving maneuver. Cholecystectomy is curative with bleeding into the gallbladder. A false aneurysm within the parenchyma of the liver is best treated nonoperatively by embolization of the involved arterial branch or balloon tamponade with arteriographic control. Underlying processes, such as biliary calculi, infection, or tumor are usually best managed simultaneously with control of hemobilia. If a common bile duct exploration is performed, selective occlusion of the right or left hepatic artery may indicate which system is involved in the bleeding. In addition, selective occlusion of the right and left hepatic ducts may determine which duct is bleeding after extraction of multiple intrahepatic calculi. In selected cases, moderate to severe bleeding in children has been treated by vigorous supportive therapy, including blood replacement and serial angiography to monitor progressive healing. Visceral artery aneurysms may be treated operatively by ligation and usually with arterial repair.

Hemobilia after percutaneous transhepatic cholangiography is usually minor and ceases spontaneously. However, it may cause several problems, including ineffective biliary drainage, difficulty in determining the diagnosis of the primary problem, or continued bleeding from the catheter into the biliary system or into the peritoneal cavity. If these problems do not resolve, operation may be indicated. All reported cases after gallstone lithotripsy have been minor; but with increased use of this technique, severe bleeding is likely to occur occasionally. The overall mortality from severe hemobilia is estimated to be between 10% and 20%, depending on the age of the patient and the underlying etiology, but mortality decreases with increased awareness of the condition and prompt, appropriate therapy. Treatment of hemobilia due to other iatrogenic causes depends on the severity of the bleeding and type of manipulation. Most bleeding of this type can be controlled with arteriography.

SELECTED REFERENCES

Czerniak, A., Thompson, J. N., Hemmingway, A. P., et al.: Hemobilia—a disease in evolution. Arch. Surg., 123:718, 1988.
  This is a review that provides a sound approach to diagnosis and management.

Fagan, E. A., Allison, D. J., Chadwick, V. S., et al.: Treatment of hemobilia by selective arterial embolization. Gut, 21:541, 1980.
  Arterial embolization is an important therapeutic modality in the management of hemobilia.

Merrell, S. W.: Hemobilia—evolution of current diagnosis and treatment. West. J. Med., 155:621, 1991.
  This is a review and update on the diagnosis and management of hemobilia.

Pinheiro, E. A.: Hemobilia as a complication of laparoscopic cholecystectomy. Surg. Laparosc. Endosc., 4:301, 1994.
  This article describes the complication of laparoscopic cholecystectomy and reviews the incidence and management of hemobilia in this setting.

Sandblom, P.: Hemobilia (Biliary Tract Hemorrhage). Springfield, Ill., Charles C Thomas, 1972.
  This is a classic monograph on the subject. Sandblom reviews the cases of hemobilia in the world literature up to 1972.

REFERENCES

1. Barba, C. A., Bret, P. M., and Hinchey, E. J.: Pseudoaneurysm of the cystic artery: A rare cause of hemobilia. Can. J. Surg., 37:64, 1994.
2. Bloechle, C., Izbicki, J. R., Rashed, M. Y., et al.: Hemobilia: Presentation, diagnosis, and management. Am. J. Gastroenterol., 89:1537, 1994.
3. Boyer, J.: Endoscopic sphincterotomy and lithiasis of the common bile duct: Reality and perspectives (editorial). Gastroenterol. Clin. Biol., 17:241, 1993. In French.
4. Cappell, M. S., Marks, M., and Kirschenbaum, H.: Massive hemobilia and acalculous cholecystitis due to benign gallbladder polyp. Dig. Dis. Sci., 38:1156, 1993.
5. de Sio, I., Castellano, L., and Calandra, M.: Hemobilia following percutaneous ethanol injection for hepatocellular carcinoma in a cirrhotic patient. J. Clin. Ultrasound, 20:621, 1992.
6. Genyk, Y. S., Keller, F. S., and Halpern, N. B.: Hepatic artery pseudoaneurysm and hemobilia following laser laparoscopic cholecystectomy: A case report. Surg. Endosc. 8:201, 1994.
7. Grisendi, A., Lonardo, A., and Della Casa, G.: Hemoductal pancreatitis secondary to gastroduodenal artery–ruptured pseudoaneurysm: A rare cause of hematemesis. Am. J. Gastroenterol., 86:1654, 1991.
8. Katz, P. O., and Salas, L.: Less frequent causes of upper gastrointestinal bleeding. Gastroenterol. Clin. North Am., 22:875, 1993.
9. Kotoh, K., Satoh, M., Kyoda, S., et al.: Successful control of hemobilia secondary to metastatic liver cancer with transcatheter arterial embolization. Am. J. Gastroenterol., 86:1642, 1991.
10. Kuipers, E. J., van Leeuwen, M. A., Nikkels, P. G., et al.: Hemobilia due to vasculitis of the gallbladder in a patient with mixed connective tissue disease. J. Rheumatol., 18:617, 1991.
11. Lygidakis, N. J., Okazaki, M., and Damtsios, G.: Iatrogenic hemobilia: How to approach it. Hepatogastroenterology, 38:454, 1991.
12. Monroe, P. S., Deeter, W. T., and Rizk, P.: Delayed hemobilia secondary to expandable metal stent. Gastrointest. Endosc., 39:190, 1993.
13. Muller, M. F., Siewert, B., Stokes, K. R., et al.: MR angiographic guidance for transjugular intrahepatic portosystemic shunt procedures. J. MRI, 4:145, 1994.
14. Okazaki, M., Ono, H., Higashihara, H., et al.: Angiographic management of massive hemobilia due to iatrogenic trauma. Gastrointest. Radiol., 16:205, 1991.
15. Rosch, J., Petersen, B. D., Hall, L. D., and Ivancev, K.: Interventional treatment of hepatic arterial and venous pathology: A commentary. Cardiovasc. Intervent. Radiol., 13:183, 1990.
16. Shapiro, M. J.: The role of the radiologist in the management of gastrointestinal bleeding. Gastroenterol. Clin. North Am., 23:123, 1994.
17. Tanaka, J., Fujimoto, K., Iwakiri, R., et al.: Hemobilia in a case of Bernard-Soulier syndrome (Letter). Am. J. Gastroenterol., 88:2142, 1993.

V

SURGICAL COMPLICATIONS OF CIRRHOSIS AND PORTAL HYPERTENSION

Layton F. Rikkers, M.D.

HISTORICAL REVIEW

Cirrhosis was first described in a fourth century B.C. Hippocratic aphorism: "In cases of jaundice it is a bad sign when the liver becomes hard."[4] Although the deleterious effect of alcohol on the liver was appreciated by Galen and his contemporaries in the second century A.D., alcoholic liver disease as an entity was first recognized by Baillie and other English writers after the "gin plague" in the eighteenth century. Shortly thereafter, Laënnec introduced the term *cirrhosis*, which was derived from the Greek word *kirrhos*, meaning "orange-yellow." Nineteenth-century European and English pathologists, including Carswell and Rokitansky, described the gross and histopathologic characteristics of the disease. Although alcoholic cirrhosis was thought to be due to toxins other than alcohol or to malnutrition during much of the twentieth century, recent investigations have established alcohol itself as a hepatotoxin.

Cirrhosis is the end result of a variety of mechanisms causing hepatocellular injury, including toxins (alcohol), viruses (hepatitis B and hepatitis C), prolonged cholestasis (extrahepatic and intrahepatic), autoimmunity (lupoid hepatitis), and metabolic disorders (hemochromatosis, Wilson's disease, alpha$_1$-antitrypsin deficiency). Although the mechanisms are diverse, the pathologic response is uniform: hepatocellular necrosis followed by fibrosis and nodular regeneration. Each of these elements may exist alone (necrosis, uncomplicated hepatitis; fibrosis, congenital hepatic fibrosis; nodular regeneration, partial nodular transformation), but all three are required for the development of cirrhosis. Cirrhosis is always a diffuse process and may be classified either morphologically or by etiology. Alcoholic cirrhosis, which is usually micronodular, and posthepatitic cirrhosis, which is generally macronodular, are the two most common varieties in the United States. Because the pathologic response to various mechanisms of hepatocellular injury is so similar, occasionally the cause cannot be ascertained (cryptogenic cirrhosis).

Cirrhosis causes two major phenomena: hepatocellular failure and portal hypertension. Even after the noxious agent is removed (e.g., abstinence from alcohol), the disease may progress. Although the mechanism is not clear, both ischemia, secondary to extensive fibrosis and intrahepatic and extrahepatic shunts, and autoimmune factors may play roles. The altered hepatic architecture and perisinusoidal fibrosis cause increased hepatic vascular resistance, resulting in portal hypertension and its associated complications of variceal hemorrhage, encephalopathy, ascites, and hypersplenism.

Autopsy studies suggest an incidence of cirrhosis of between 3.5% and 5.0%. Only 15% of heavy drinkers develop alcoholic cirrhosis. However, because of the large number of alcoholics in the United States, as well as a significant percentage of patients with nonalcoholic causes of chronic liver disease, cirrhosis presently ranks as the sixth leading cause of death between the ages of 35 and 54 for both males and females. Hepatic failure and variceal hemorrhage are the first and second most common causes of death, respectively, in patients with cirrhosis.

Historically the treatment of cirrhosis has been the treatment of the complications of portal hypertension. Presently, medical treatment of cirrhosis with antifibrogenesis drugs such as colchicine and penicillamine is experimental. In contrast, since 1980 the surgical management of chronic liver disease with hepatic transplantation has been highly successful with long-term survival rates generally above 70%. A major challenge to the physician or surgeon managing patients with cirrhosis is to determine when definitive treatment (transplantation) rather than palliative treatment (e.g., operations to prevent recurrent variceal hemorrhage) should be applied.

ANATOMY, PHYSIOLOGY, AND PATHOPHYSIOLOGY OF PORTAL HYPERTENSION

The liver is a unique organ in that it has a dual blood supply: portal venous and hepatic arterial. The portal vein is formed from the confluence of the superior mesenteric and splenic veins (Fig. 33–32). The left gastric or coronary vein drains the distal esophagus and lesser curvature of the stomach, generally entering the portal vein near its origin. The splenic vein lies beneath the pancreas and is usually joined by the inferior mesenteric vein just before its confluence with the superior mesenteric vein.

The hepatic artery, one of three major branches of the celiac axis, lies medial to the common bile duct and portal vein in the hepatoduodenal ligament. Common variations include origins of the right and left hepatic arteries from the superior mesenteric artery and of the left gastric artery, respectively, both of which occur in nearly 20% of the population.

Hepatic blood flow averages 1500 ml. per minute, which represents approximately 25% of the cardiac output. The portal vein contributes two thirds of the total hepatic blood

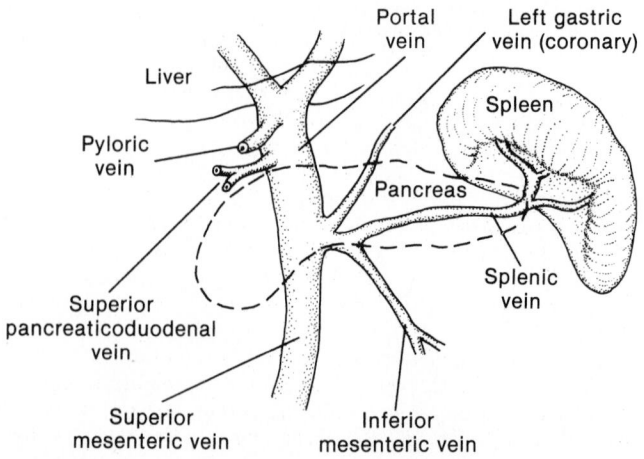

Figure 33–32. The extrahepatic portal venous circulation. (From Rikkers, L. F.: Portal hypertension. *In* Goldsmith, H. [Ed.]: Practice of Surgery. Philadelphia, Harper & Row, 1981, pp. 1–37.)

flow, while hepatic arterial perfusion accounts for over one half of the liver's oxygen supply. The volume of portal venous flow is indirectly regulated by vasoconstriction and vasodilation of the splanchnic arterial bed. In contrast, hepatic arterioles respond to circulating catecholamines and sympathetic nervous stimulation; thus, hepatic arterial flow is directly regulated. However, even intense vasoconstrictive influences can be overcome by a hepatic arterial autoregulatory or *buffer* response, which maintains total hepatic blood flow as near to normal as possible when portal perfusion is decreased in patients with shock or in those with either disease-induced or surgically created portosystemic shunts.[23]

Many splanchnic hormones are important regulators of hepatic metabolism. Insulin is particularly important because it is a hepatotrophic hormone and is essential for maintenance of liver structure and function. Thus, even if the quantity of hepatic blood flow is maintained in the normal range by hepatic arterial compensation for decreased portal flow, hepatic physiology may be impaired.

Because increased portal venous resistance is usually the initiator of portal hypertension, classifications of this disorder are generally based on the site of elevated resistance. However, increased portal venous inflow secondary to a hyperdynamic systemic circulation and splanchnic hyperemia is often a major contributor to the maintenance of portal hypertension. The cause of the elevated cardiac output and splanchnic hyperemia is not known, but splanchnic hormones, such as glucagon, and decreased sensitivity of the splanchnic vasculature to catecholamines probably play a role.[2]

The most common cause of prehepatic portal hypertension is portal vein thrombosis, which accounts for approximately 50% of cases of portal hypertension in the pediatric age group. When the portal vein is thrombosed in the absence of liver disease, hepatopetal (to the liver) portal collateral vessels develop to restore portal perfusion. This combination is termed *cavernomatous transformation of the portal vein*. Isolated splenic vein thrombosis (left-sided portal hypertension) is usually secondary to pancreatic inflammation or neoplasm. The result is gastrosplenic venous hypertension, while superior mesenteric and portal venous pressures remain normal. The left gastroepiploic vein becomes a major collateral vessel, and gastric varices are generally more prominent than esophageal varices. This variant of portal hypertension is important to recognize because it is easily reversed by splenectomy alone.

The site of increased resistance in intrahepatic portal hypertension may be at the presinusoidal, sinusoidal, or postsinusoidal level. Frequently, more than one level is involved. The most common cause of intrahepatic, presinusoidal hypertension is schistosomiasis. In addition, many causes of nonalcoholic cirrhosis also result in presinusoidal portal hypertension, especially early in their course. Alcoholic cirrhosis, the most common cause of portal hypertension in the United States, usually causes increased resistance to portal flow at the sinusoidal (secondary to deposition of collagen in Disse's space) and postsinusoidal levels (secondary to regenerating nodules distorting small hepatic veins). Postsinusoidal causes of portal hypertension are rare and include the Budd-Chiari syndrome (hepatic vein thrombosis), constrictive pericarditis, and heart failure. Rarely, increased portal venous flow alone, secondary either to massive splenomegaly (idiopathic portal hypertension) or a splanchnic arteriovenous fistula, causes portal hypertension.

A portal pressure above the normal level of 5 to 10 mm. Hg stimulates portosystemic collateralization. Collateral vessels usually develop where the portal and systemic venous circulations are in close proximity (Fig. 33–33). Although the collateral network through the coronary and short gastric veins to the azygos vein is the most important one clinically, be-

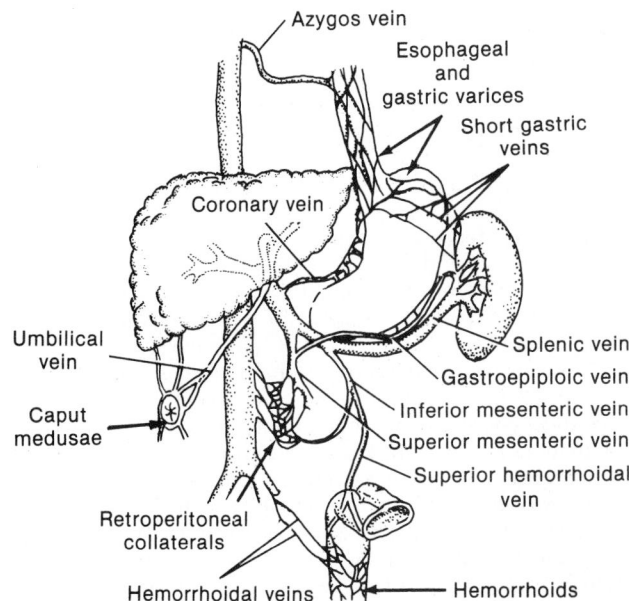

Figure 33–33. Portosystemic collateral pathways develop where the portal venous and systemic venous systems are in close apposition (large arrows). (From Rikkers, L. F.: Portal hypertension. *In* Miller, T. A. [Ed.]: Physiologic Basis of Modern Surgical Care. St. Louis, C. V. Mosby, 1988, pp. 417–428.)

cause it results in formation of esophagogastric varices, other sites include a recanalized umbilical vein from the left portal vein to the epigastric venous system, retroperitoneal collateral vessels, and the hemorrhoidal venous plexus. In addition to extrahepatic collateral vessels, a significant fraction of portal venous flow passes through both anatomic and physiologic (capillarization of hepatic sinusoids) intrahepatic shunts. As hepatic portal perfusion decreases, hepatic arterial flow generally increases (buffer response).[23]

EVALUATION OF THE PATIENT WITH CIRRHOSIS

Key aspects of the assessment of an individual with suspected chronic liver disease or one of the complications of portal hypertension are the following: (1) diagnosis of the underlying liver disease, (2) estimation of functional hepatic reserve, (3) definition of portal venous anatomy and hepatic hemodynamic evaluation, and (4) identification of the site of upper gastrointestinal hemorrhage if present. These diagnostic categories take on varying levels of importance depending on the clinical situation. For example, estimation of functional hepatic reserve is useful in determining the risk of therapeutic intervention and whether definitive (hepatic transplantation) or palliative treatment (e.g., endoscopic sclerotherapy or shunt procedure) is indicated. Knowledge of portal anatomy and physiology guides the surgeon in selecting an appropriate operation for control of variceal bleeding. Precise identification of the site of bleeding is essential because hemorrhage secondary to portal hypertension may be from esophageal varices, gastric varices, or portal hypertensive gastropathy and because a significant fraction of patients with portal hypertension bleed from other lesions.

History and Physical Examination. In a patient with nonspecific constitutional complaints such as weight loss, malaise, and weakness, a past history of chronic alcoholism, hepatitis, complicated biliary disease, or exposure to hepatotoxins should lead one to include cirrhosis in the differential diagnosis. Subtle clues to the presence of underlying chronic liver disease on physical examination are spider angiomas, palmar erythema, testicular atrophy, and gynecomastia. A palpable spleen in association with these signs suggests portal hypertension. Confirmatory evidence of cirrhosis is provided by signs of hepatic functional decompensation or advanced portal hypertension such as jaundice, ascites, palpation of a firm irregular liver edge, dilated abdominal wall veins, and impairment of mental status or the presence of asterixis (liver flap).

Laboratory Tests. Cirrhosis is often accompanied by anemia, leukopenia, and thrombocytopenia. Anemia may be secondary to bleeding, nutritional deficiencies, hemolysis, or bone marrow depression secondary to alcoholism. Although many patients with portal hypertension have some degree of hypersplenism, it is unusual to find a platelet count of less than 50,000 per cu. mm. or a white blood cell count less than 2000 per cu. mm. In addition to thrombocytopenia, coagulation may be impaired by a prolonged prothrombin time because many of the coagulation factors are synthesized by the liver and by primary fibrinolysis, which is present in many patients with chronic liver disease.

A chemistry profile is helpful in both the diagnosis and assessment of severity of cirrhosis. Hypoalbuminemia is usually a reliable index of chronic rather than acute liver disease. Elevation of the hepatocellular enzymes, aspartate aminotransferase and alanine aminotransferase, to more than three times their normal level is indicative of significant, ongoing hepatocellular necrosis, which is often present in patients with alcoholic hepatitis and chronic active hepatitis due to a variety of causes. Increased disease activity may be an important risk factor in patients who undergo surgery. A ratio of alanine aminotransferase to aspartate aminotransferase of greater than 2 is highly suggestive of alcohol as the cause of liver disease. Although mild elevations of the enzymes alkaline phosphatase and gamma glutamyl transpeptidase are nonspecific, marked increases in these enzymes are indicative of either intrahepatic or extrahepatic cholestasis (primary or secondary biliary cirrhosis). In the absence of prior blood transfusions, a total bilirubin level of greater than 3 mg. per 100 ml. is indicative of severe hepatic decompensation and a high operative risk status.

Hepatitic serology should be obtained in most patients with cirrhosis. A significant fraction of patients with hepatitis B and hepatitis C develop cirrhosis, whereas hepatitis A generally causes only acute liver disease. The most common internal malignancy worldwide is hepatocellular carcinoma, which is frequently secondary to hepatitis B infestation. However, this malignancy frequently develops in patients with other causes of cirrhosis and occasionally in patients without chronic liver disease. Unexpected hepatic functional deterioration is sometimes due to the development of hepatocellular carcinoma, which can be diagnosed in approximately 60% of patients by an elevated alpha-fetoprotein level.

Common serum electrolyte abnormalities in cirrhosis are hyponatremia, hypokalemia, and metabolic alkalosis. These metabolic disorders are secondary to hyperaldosteronism, diarrhea, and recurrent emesis, which frequently accompany cirrhosis. Deleterious consequences of metabolic alkalosis are shift of the oxyhemoglobin dissociation curve to the left, which impairs tissue oxygen delivery, and conversion of ammonium chloride to ammonia, which facilitates transport of this purported cerebral toxin across the blood-brain barrier.

Liver Biopsy. Percutaneous liver biopsy is a useful technique for establishing the cause of cirrhosis and for assessing activity of the liver disease. When the diagnosis is known and the chemistry profile suggests quiescent disease, liver biopsy is probably not necessary before surgical intervention for variceal hemorrhage. Percutaneous liver biopsy should not be done when either coagulopathy or moderate ascites is present.

Measurement of Hepatic Functional Reserve. The time-honored method of assessing hepatic functional reserve is Child's classification (Table 33–9). Although this classification scheme includes three clinical variables in addition to two biochemical indices and, therefore, is not a direct measure of hepatic functional reserve, no other test has surpassed it with respect to predicting operative outcome or assessing long-term prognosis in the unoperated patient. In most clinical series, operative mortality rates for Child's Class A, B, and C patients are in the range of 0% to 5%, 10% to 15%, and greater than 25%, respectively. Because many patients with acute variceal hemorrhage present with decompensated hepatic function as reflected by their Child's class, an interval of medical management to improve the patient from Child's Class C to Class A or B is worthwhile before surgical intervention.[16]

True quantitative measures of hepatocellular function, such as galactose elimination capacity, aminopyrine breath test, and hepatic clearance of amino acids, are not available in most institutions. However, these tests may be valuable indicators of limited hepatic reserve in some patients with nearly normal conventional measures of liver function. Now that hepatic transplantation has become a realistic option for many patients with cirrhosis, accurate quantitation of hepatocellular function to determine which patients are transplant candidates has become even more important.

Hepatic Hemodynamic Assessment. In patients with alcoholic cirrhosis and many varieties of nonalcoholic cirrhosis, portal pressure can be indirectly estimated by measurement of hepatic venous wedge pressure. Because hepatic venous wedge pressure is normal in patients with presinusoidal portal hypertension, portal pressure in these individuals can be measured only directly by transhepatic or umbilical venous cannulation of the portal venous system or by percutaneous puncture of the spleen. However, because magnitude of portal venous pressure predicts neither likelihood of bleeding nor ultimate prognosis, the only useful application of these techniques is in differentiating between presinusoidal and sinusoidal/postsinusoidal causes of portal hypertension.

Because splanchnic venous thrombosis may be the cause of portal hypertension or develop secondary to cirrhosis, portal venous anatomy should be defined before performing a portosystemic shunt operation. Selective visceral angiography has been the most frequently used method for visualization of the portal venous system and for qualitative estimation of hepatic portal perfusion.[28] A complete angiographic study generally consists of selective injections of radiographic contrast medium into the superior mesenteric and splenic arteries followed by late venous phase films to define splenic, superior mesenteric, and portal veins. If the renal vein is to be used in shunt construction, this vessel should also be cannulated and opacified. Hepatic portal perfusion can be estimated from the venous phase of the superior mesenteric angiogram and graded as follows: Grade 1, normal perfusion; Grade 2, visualization of intrahepatic portal venous radicles; Grade 3, opacification of portal vein only; Grade 4, nonvisualization of portal vein (Fig. 33–34).[28] This grading system is particularly valuable for assessment of portal blood flow before and after a selective shunt, because one of the objectives of such a procedure is preservation of hepatic portal perfusion. Postoperative venography, either indirectly after arterial injection or directly by means of venous shunt cannulation, is the most accurate method of determining shunt patency.

Duplex ultrasonography is a noninvasive alternative to angiography for assessment of portal venous patency, direction of portal flow, and shunt patency status.[29] This technique

TABLE 33–9. Child's Criteria for Hepatic Functional Reserve

	A Minimal	B Moderate	C Advanced
Serum bilirubin (mg./100 ml.)	<2.0	2.0–3.0	>3.0
Serum albumin (gm./100 ml.)	>3.5	3.0–3.5	<3.0
Ascites	None	Easily controlled	Poorly controlled
Neurologic disorder	None	Minimal	Advanced, "coma"
Nutrition	Excellent	Good	Poor, "wasting"

From Boyer, T. D.: Portal hypertension and its complications: Bleeding esophageal varices, ascites, and spontaneous bacterial peritonitis. *In* Zakim, D., and Boyer, T. D. (Eds.): Hepatology: A Textbook of Liver Disease. Philadelphia, W. B. Saunders, 1982, pp. 464–499.

is less accurate in assessing superior mesenteric and splenic vein anatomy and flow characteristics. Likewise, duplex ultrasonography usually accurately assesses patency status of central shunts (e.g., portacaval) but is of less value for evaluating more peripheral shunts (e.g., distal splenorenal).

Diagnosis of Bleeding. In the absence of hematemesis, a nasogastric tube should be inserted to determine whether bleeding is from the upper gastrointestinal tract. The key procedure for diagnosing the site of upper gastrointestinal hemorrhage in a patient with portal hypertension is endoscopy. Before endoscopy the patient should be hemodynamically stabilized and the stomach evacuated of blood clots with a large-bore lavage tube.

Upper gastrointestinal tract bleeding in patients with portal hypertension is secondary to portal hypertension in approximately 90% of instances. The remaining 10% of patients bleed from Mallory-Weiss tears, gastric ulcers, and duodenal ulcers, all of which are more common in patients with alcoholic cirrhosis than in the general population. Portal hypertensive bleeding is most commonly from esophagogastric varices (esophageal varices = 90%; gastric varices = 10%). The endoscopic diagnosis of variceal hemorrhage can be established by either observing a bleeding varix (approximately 25% of patients) or by observation of moderate- to large-sized varices and no other lesions in a patient who has recently experienced a major upper gastrointestinal tract hemorrhage (>2 units of blood).

The only nonvariceal cause of portal hypertensive bleeding is portal hypertensive gastropathy.[27] The frequency of this lesion is unknown, but it is probably more common after eradication of varices by endoscopic sclerotherapy. Portal hypertensive gastropathy mainly involves the fundus and body of the stomach and has an endoscopic appearance of a white reticular network with enclosed erythematous areas. Because varices and portal hypertensive gastropathy often coexist, it may be difficult to determine which lesion is responsible for any given episode of bleeding. Occasionally, massive bleeding in a patient with cirrhosis makes an endoscopic diagnosis initially impossible, in which case endoscopy should be repeated after bleeding is controlled.

VARICEAL HEMORRHAGE

Bleeding from esophagogastric varices is the single most life-threatening complication of portal hypertension, responsible for approximately one third of all deaths in patients with cirrhosis. The risk of death from bleeding in any individual patient is mainly related to the underlying hepatic functional reserve. Patients with extrahepatic portal venous obstruction and normal hepatic function rarely die of bleeding varices, whereas individuals with decompensated cirrhosis (Child's Class C) face a mortality rate in excess of 25%. The greatest risk of death from variceal bleeding is within the first few days after the onset of hemorrhage and declines rapidly between then and 6 weeks, when it returns to the prehemorrhage risk level.[40]

Pathogenesis

Varices in the distal esophagus and proximal stomach are a component of the collateral network that diverts high pres-

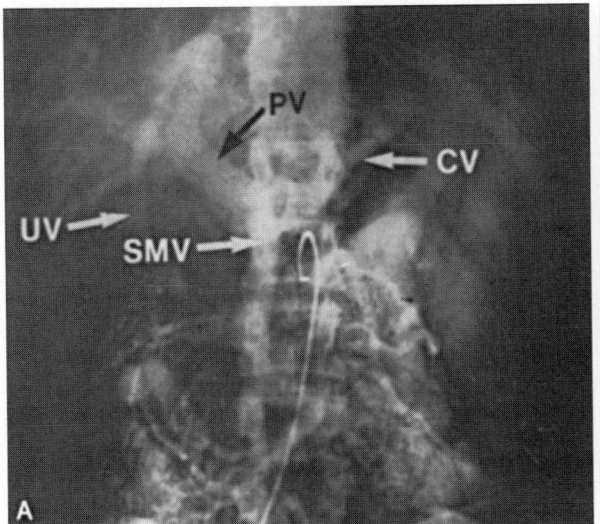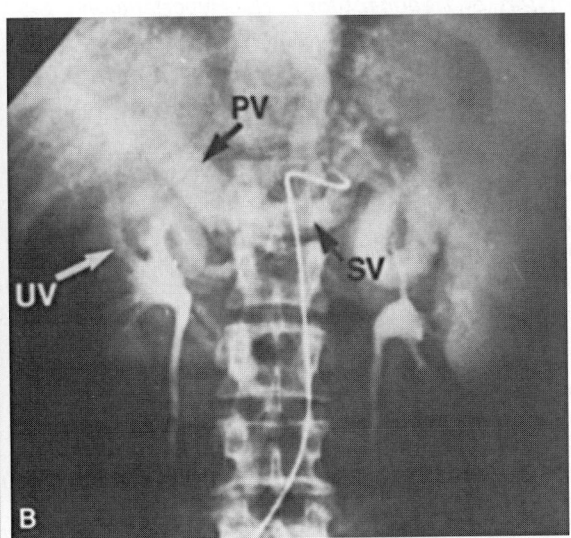

Figure 33–34. Venous phase films following superior mesenteric (A) and splenic (B) angiograms in a patient with portal hypertension secondary to alcoholic cirrhosis. The portal perfusion grade is 2. PV, portal vein; SMV, superior mesenteric vein; UV, umbilical vein; CV, coronary vein; SV, splenic vein. (From Rikkers, L. F.: Portal hypertension. *In* Goldsmith, H. [Ed.]: Practice of Surgery. Philadelphia, Harper & Row, 1981, pp. 1–37.)

sure portal venous flow through the left and right gastric veins and the short gastric veins to the azygous system. Less commonly, varices develop at other sites in the gastrointestinal tract but are less prone to rupture in those locations. Esophagogastric varices do not develop until portal pressure exceeds 12 mm. Hg and, once present, bleed in only one third to one half of patients. The pathogenesis of variceal rupture is incompletely understood but is most likely multifactorial. Polio and Groszmann[31] have put forth a unifying hypothesis of variceal rupture based on LaPlace's law. Although it has been observed that variceal size, magnitude of portal pressure, and thickness of the epithelium overlying the varix all significantly separate bleeders from nonbleeders, the overlap between groups is large when any one of these variables is considered independently. LaPlace's law states that variceal wall tension is directly related to transmural pressure and varix radius and inversely related to variceal wall thickness, thus combining all three of these variables. Because all of these parameters cannot be measured clinically, there are inherent inaccuracies in predicting which patients with varices may bleed. However, endoscopic classification schemes that consider size of varices and characteristics such as cherry-red spots and red wale markings, which are related to the thickness of the overlying epithelium, have improved the predictability of variceal hemorrhage. These prognostic indices are especially important when considering prophylactic therapy (treatment of varices that have not previously bled).

Treatment

Therapy for portal hypertension and variceal bleeding has evolved over the past 100 years. The many treatment modalities available suggest that no single therapy is entirely satisfactory for all patients or for all clinical situations. Nonoperative treatments are generally preferred for acutely bleeding patients since they are often high operative risks because of decompensated hepatic function. Therapies that are effective (a low rebleeding rate) and minimally alter hepatic physiology are optimal for long-term prevention of recurrent bleeding. Only treatments associated with minimal morbidity and mortality can be considered for prophylaxis, because many patients will be treated unnecessarily (only one third to one half of patients with varices eventually bleed).

History of Treatment for Portal Hypertension

Table 33–10 presents a chronology of the treatment of portal hypertension, which began with the description of the Eck fistula (end-to-side portacaval shunt) in 1877.[4] Eck's main concerns were to determine if survival was possible after complete portal flow diversion and to develop a treatment for ascites. Probably the most important contribution to this field was made by Pavlov's group in 1893. These investigators perfected the technique of portacaval shunting and, after carefully observing 20 surviving dogs, described in detail the syndrome of "meat intoxication" or portosystemic encephalopathy, which they believed was due to intestinally absorbed cerebral toxins bypassing their site of metabolism in the liver. They also found from autopsy studies that dogs with encephalopathy had patent portacaval shunts and atrophic livers whereas animals with normal cerebral function and preserved hepatic structure had thrombosed shunts and maintenance of hepatic portal perfusion through collateral vessels.

The modern era of treatment for variceal hemorrhage can be dated from 1945, when Blakemore, Lord, and Whipple introduced the portacaval and conventional splenorenal shunts into clinical practice. Although balloon tamponade

and endoscopic sclerosis of varices were initially described in the 1930s, these were found to be only temporizing measures. During the ensuing 20 years, several varieties of nonselective shunts (complete portal decompression and portal flow diversion) were described and the portacaval shunt was evaluated in randomized, controlled trials. Motivated by the discouraging results of these trials, Warren, Zeppa, and Fomon introduced the concept of selective variceal decompression (distal splenorenal shunt) in 1967.[46] An initial wave of enthusiasm for the distal splenorenal shunt (partial portal flow diversion) was followed by several randomized trials, which produced inconsistent results. A report from Johnston and Rodgers in 1973 of a large series of patients successfully treated by endoscopic sclerotherapy led to a resurgence of interest in this treatment, which has now become the most widely applied therapy for bleeding varices.[20] Although pharmacotherapy was first used for acute hemorrhage in 1956, drug treatment for long-term prevention of initial or recurrent hemorrhage is a phenomenon of the 1980s. Improved immunosuppression (cyclosporine) and surgical techniques have led to the recent widespread application of hepatic transplantation for patients with end-stage liver disease. Finally, a nonoperative means of portal decompression (transjugular intrahepatic portosystemic shunt [TIPS]), first described by Rosch in animals in 1969, has been widely applied to the problem of variceal bleeding.

Treatment of the Acute Bleeding Episode

Because many patients with acute variceal bleeding have decompensated hepatic function secondary to either recent alcoholism or hypotension, they are high risks for emergency surgical intervention.[26] In addition, these individuals often have other complications of chronic liver disease such as encephalopathy, ascites, coagulopathy, and malnutrition. Therefore, emergency treatment should be nonoperative whenever possible. Endoscopic treatment (sclerosis or ligation), which has become the mainstay of nonoperative treatment of acute hemorrhage in most centers, controls bleeding in over 85% of patients, allowing an interval of medical management for improvement of hepatic function, resolution of ascites and encephalopathy, and enhancement of nutrition before definitive treatment for prevention of recurrent bleeding. Although pharmacotherapy and balloon tamponade still play an important role in emergency management in some patients (e.g., endoscopic treatment failures and those bleeding from gastric varices), these modalities are used less frequently than in the past. The place of the TIPS in managing acute variceal bleeding is evolving. Emergency surgical intervention may be the preferred approach in selected patients, especially those in whom less invasive methods fail to control bleeding or are not indicated. A management scheme for acute variceal hemorrhage is outlined in Figure 33–35.

Resuscitation and Diagnosis. The highest priority in emergency management is restoration of circulating blood volume, which should be accomplished before upper gastrointestinal endoscopy. Although initial resuscitation is usually with isotonic crystalloid solutions, a minimum of six units of blood should be typed and crossmatched for most patients with variceal bleeding. Volume status is assessed by central venous pressure measurements, urinary output measured with a Foley catheter, and a Swan-Ganz pulmonary artery catheter if necessary. If the prothrombin time is prolonged more than 3 seconds, fresh frozen plasma should be a component of the resuscitation volume. Although moderate hypersplenism is a common accompaniment of portal hypertension, platelet transfusions are necessary only when the platelet count is less than 50,000 per cu. mm.

Endoscopy to determine the cause of bleeding should be

TABLE 33–10. History of Treatment of Portal Hypertension

Year	Author	Contribution
1877	Eck	Portacaval shunt (dog)
1893	Pavlov	Encephalopathy (dog)
1903	Vidal	Clinical portacaval shunt (ascites)
1930	Westphal	Balloon tamponade
1939	Crafoord, Frenckner	Endoscopic sclerotherapy
1945	Blakemore, Lord, Whipple	Clinical portacaval and splenorenal shunts (bleeding)
1950	Sengstaken, Blakemore	Balloon tamponade
1956	Kehne	Vasopressin
1967	Warren, Zeppa, Fomon	Distal splenorenal shunt
1967	Starzl	First successful liver transplant
1968	Inokuchi	Left gastric–vena caval shunt
1969	Rosch	Transjugular intrahepatic portosystemic shunt (TIPS) in animals
1973	Johnston, Rodgers	Reintroduction of endoscopic sclerotherapy
1973	Sugiura, Futagawa	Extensive esophagogastric devascularization
1980	Calne	Cyclosporine for transplantation
1981	Lebrec	Propranolol for bleeding
1983	Colapinto	TIPS in humans

Data from Chen, T. S., and Chen, P. S.: Understanding the Liver. Westport, Conn., Greenwood Press, 1984.

performed as soon as the patient is stabilized. If a bleeding esophageal varix is observed or suspected because of an overlying clot, sclerotherapy should be performed during the initial endoscopy if the expertise is available. Bleeding from gastric varices or from portal hypertensive gastropathy should be initially treated with pharmacotherapy. Because these lesions are often incompletely controlled by nonoperative means, such patients frequently require either insertion of a TIPS or early surgical intervention.

Pharmacotherapy. Vasopressin, which is a potent splanchnic vasoconstrictor, has been the most commonly used drug in the acute setting and controls hemorrhage in approximately 50% of patients. Vasopressin is usually administered intravenously as a bolus dose of 20 units over 20 minutes and then as a continuous infusion of 0.4 units per minute. Because vasopressin also constricts systemic arterioles, it frequently causes hypertension, bradycardia, decreased cardiac output, and coronary vasoconstriction. Therefore, the use of this drug should be confined to the intensive care unit where the patient can be appropriately monitored. The adverse systemic effects of vasopressin can be effectively counteracted by simultaneous infusion of nitroglycerin or nitroprusside. The combination of vasopressin and nitroglycerin may also be more effective in controlling variceal hemorrhage than vasopressin alone.[8]

Recent randomized trials have shown that somatostatin

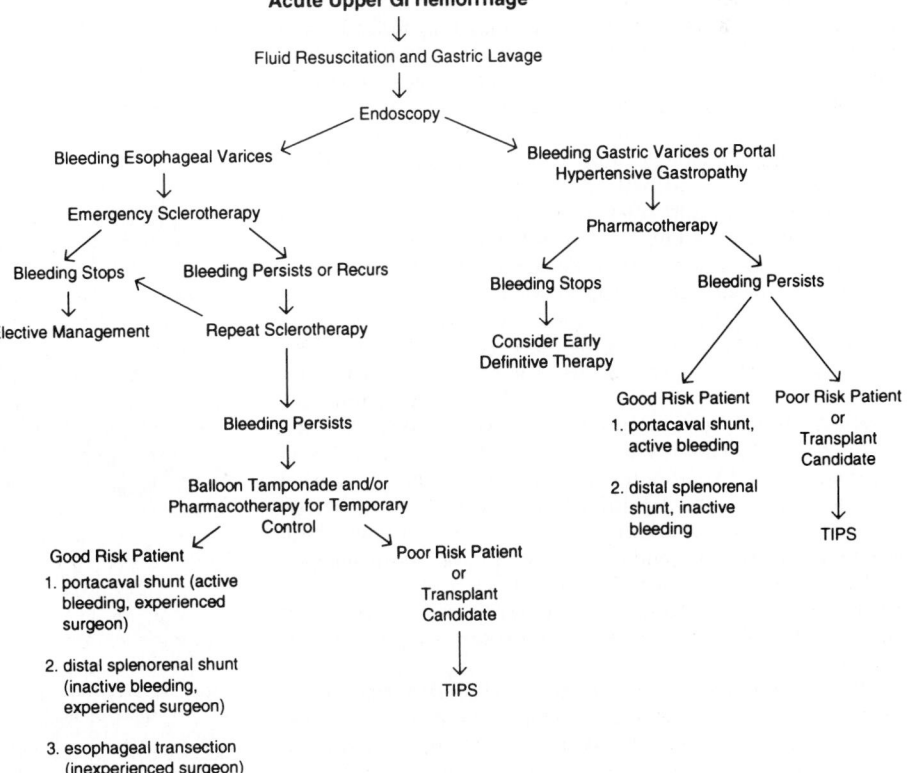

Figure 33–35. Algorithm for management of acute variceal hemorrhage (see text). (From Rikkers, L. F.: Portal hypertension. In Levine, B. A., et al. [Ed.]: Current Practice of Surgery, vol. 3. New York, Churchill Livingstone, 1995.)

and its analog octreotide are as efficacious as endoscopic treatment for control of acute variceal bleeding.[30] These agents are also associated with fewer adverse side effects than vasopressin. Because of their ease of administration and effectiveness, these newer drugs may return pharmacotherapy to a more central role in the treatment of acute portal hypertensive bleeding, especially when endoscopic treatment is unlikely to be effective (failed chronic sclerotherapy, gastric varices, and portal hypertensive gastropathy). Somatostatin is administered as a 250-μg. intravenous bolus, followed by a continuous infusion of 250 μg. per hour for 2 to 4 days. Octreotide is given as an intravenous infusion of 25 to 50 μg. per hour for a similar length of time.

Balloon Tamponade. The major advantages of variceal tamponade with the Sengstaken-Blakemore tube are immediate cessation of bleeding in more than 85% of patients and widespread availability of this device, including small community hospitals. Significant disadvantages of balloon tamponade are frequent recurrent hemorrhage after balloon deflation, considerable discomfort for the patient, and a high incidence of serious complications when the device is used by inexperienced personnel. The potentially lethal complications of esophageal perforation secondary to intraesophageal inflation of the gastric balloon, ischemic necrosis of the esophagus secondary to overinflation of the esophageal balloon, and aspiration can be avoided by using balloon tamponade only in an intensive care unit and adhering to a strict protocol.

Because of the effectiveness of endoscopic treatment and pharmacotherapy for acute variceal bleeding, balloon tamponade is infrequently required. However, it may be lifesaving when exsanguinating hemorrhage prevents acute endoscopic treatment and in patients in whom sclerotherapy has failed and who do not respond to pharmacotherapy. Because balloon deflation is followed by a high rebleeding rate, definitive treatment such as endoscopic therapy, TIPS, or operation should be planned for most patients in whom the Sengstaken-Blakemore tube is used.

Endoscopic Treatment. Endoscopic treatment (variceal sclerosis or ligation) is the most commonly used therapy for both management of the acute bleeding episode and prevention of recurrent hemorrhage. In early trials, variceal sclerosis was performed through a rigid esophagoscope with the patient under general anesthesia. However, most sclerotherapists now prefer to use a flexible endoscope because complications are fewer and general anesthesia can be avoided. Both intravariceal and paravariceal techniques of injection are used, and often these two techniques are purposefully or inadvertently combined (Fig. 33–36). The most commonly used sclerosants in the United States are sodium morrhuate and sodium tetradecyl sulfate.

When experienced personnel are available, the initial sclerotherapy injections can often be done during the endoscopy at which diagnosis of variceal bleeding is made. Each varix is usually injected with 1 to 2 ml. of sclerosant just above the esophagogastric junction and 5 cm. proximal to it. Alternatively, each varix can be ligated with a rubber band as shown in Figure 33–37. A subsequent treatment session is planned for 4 to 6 days later. Additional endoscopic treatments depend on the effectiveness of the initial ones in controlling bleeding and whether endoscopic therapy has been selected as definitive treatment for that patient.

Emergency sclerotherapy of esophageal varices has been highly effective with control of hemorrhage in over 85% of patients. However, this technique has been generally unsuccessful for bleeding gastric varices. Controlled trials have confirmed the effectiveness of endoscopic treatment in acutely bleeding patients.[26] Recent investigations have suggested that rubber band ligation of varices may be more

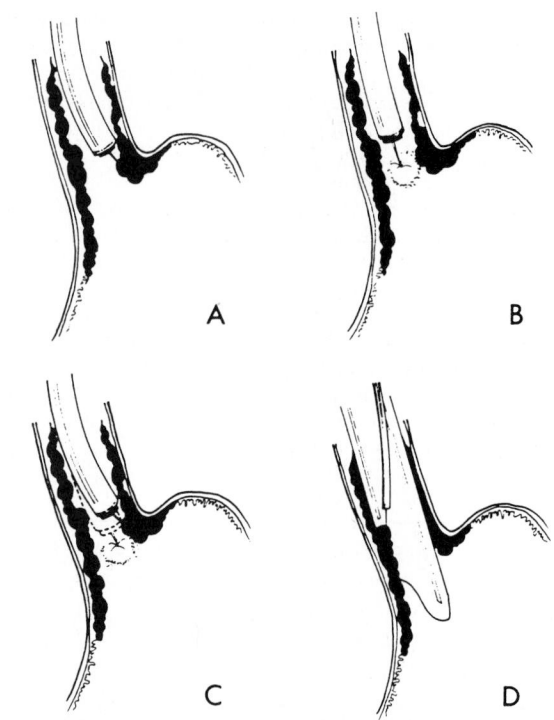

Figure 33–36. Techniques of endoscopic sclerotherapy. A flexible endoscope is used for intravariceal injection *(A)*, paravariceal (submucosal) injection *(B)*, and combined paravariceal and intravariceal injection *(C)*. Less commonly a rigid esophagoscope with a slot is used for intravariceal injection *(D)*. This latter technique requires general anesthesia. (From Terblanche, J., Burroughs, A. K., and Hobbs, E. F.: Controversies in the management of bleeding esophageal varices. N. Engl. J. Med., *320*:1393–1398, 1989. Reprinted by permission of *The New England Journal of Medicine.* Copyright 1989, Massachusetts Medical Society.)

effective and associated with fewer complications than sclerosis.[43]

Minor complications of sclerotherapy, including retrosternal chest pain, esophageal ulceration, and fever, occur commonly. More serious complications, which account for the

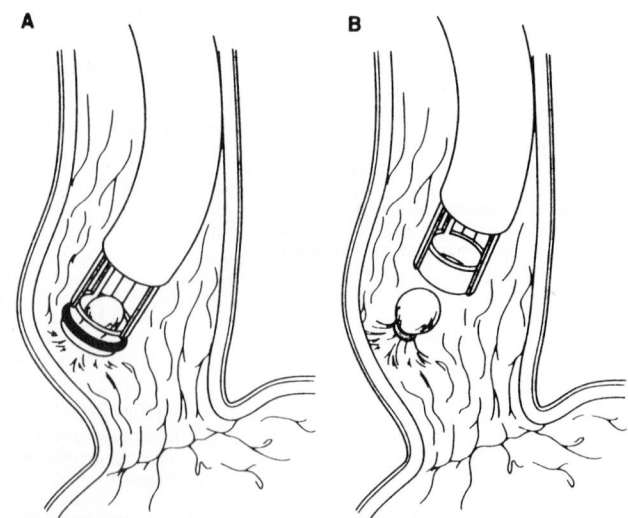

Figure 33–37. Endoscopic ligation of esophageal varices. *A,* The varix is drawn into the ligator by suction. *B,* An "O" ring is applied. (From Turcotte, J. G., Roger, S. E., and Eckhauser, F. E.: Portal hypertension. *In* Greenfield, L. J., Mulholland, M. W., and Oldham, K. T. [Eds.]: Surgery: Scientific Principles and Practice. Philadelphia, J. B. Lippincott, 1993, p. 899.)

1% to 3% mortality rate of this procedure, are esophageal perforation, worsening of variceal hemorrhage, and aspiration pneumonitis. Failure of sclerotherapy should be declared when two sessions fail to control hemorrhage. Unless urgent surgery is performed in such patients, mortality exceeds 60%.

Transjugular Intrahepatic Portosystemic Shunt. TIPS is a technique that accomplishes portal decompression without an operation.[21, 37] Because of the complexity of the procedure, an experienced interventional radiologist is required. Access is gained to a major intrahepatic portal venous branch through puncture through a hepatic vein. A parenchymal tract between hepatic and portal veins is then created with a balloon catheter and a 10-mm. expandable metal stent is inserted, thereby creating the shunt (Fig. 33–38).

In large series, the success rate of TIPS has been over 90%, but experience with this technique is limited in acutely bleeding patients, who generally make up only a small fraction of patients receiving TIPS. One evaluation of TIPS in the emergency setting revealed an in-hospital mortality of 56% and incomplete control of bleeding in 26% of patients.[11] At the present time, TIPS should not be recommended as initial therapy for acute variceal hemorrhage but should be used only after less invasive treatments such as endoscopic therapy and pharmacotherapy have failed to control bleeding.

One clear indication for TIPS is as a short-term bridge to liver transplantation for patients in whom endoscopic treatment has failed. In addition to controlling bleeding, advantages in this situation are that the lower portal pressure may make the transplant operation easier and that the shunt is removed when the recipient liver is excised. Patients with advanced hepatic functional decompensation (Child's Class C), even when they are not transplant candidates, may be better served by TIPS than by an emergency operation when less invasive approaches fail to control bleeding.

Hemodynamic studies suggest that TIPS is a nonselective shunt and several investigations have demonstrated a similar frequency of encephalopathy after TIPS· as has been previously reported after nonselective shunts. Another disadvantage of the procedure is that shunt stenosis or occlusion develops in as many as 50% of patients within 1 year of TIPS insertion.[6] This situation can often be remedied by repeated angiographic intervention, however.

Emergency Surgery. Although nonoperative therapies are effective for the majority of patients with acute variceal bleeding, emergency operation should be promptly done when less invasive measures fail to control hemorrhage or are not indicated.[34] The most common situations requiring either urgent or emergency surgery are failure of acute endoscopic treatment, failure of long-term endoscopic therapy, and hemorrhage from gastric varices or portal hypertensive gastropathy. Selection of the appropriate emergency operation should mainly be guided by the experience of the surgeon. Esophageal transection with a stapling device is rapid and relatively simple, but rebleeding rates after this procedure are high and there is little evidence that operative mortality rates are less than after surgical portal decompression. The most commonly performed shunt operation in the emergency setting is the portacaval shunt because it rapidly and effectively decompresses the portal venous circulation. However, when the patient is not actively bleeding at the time of surgery and in those individuals in whom bleeding is temporarily controlled by pharmacotherapy or balloon tam-

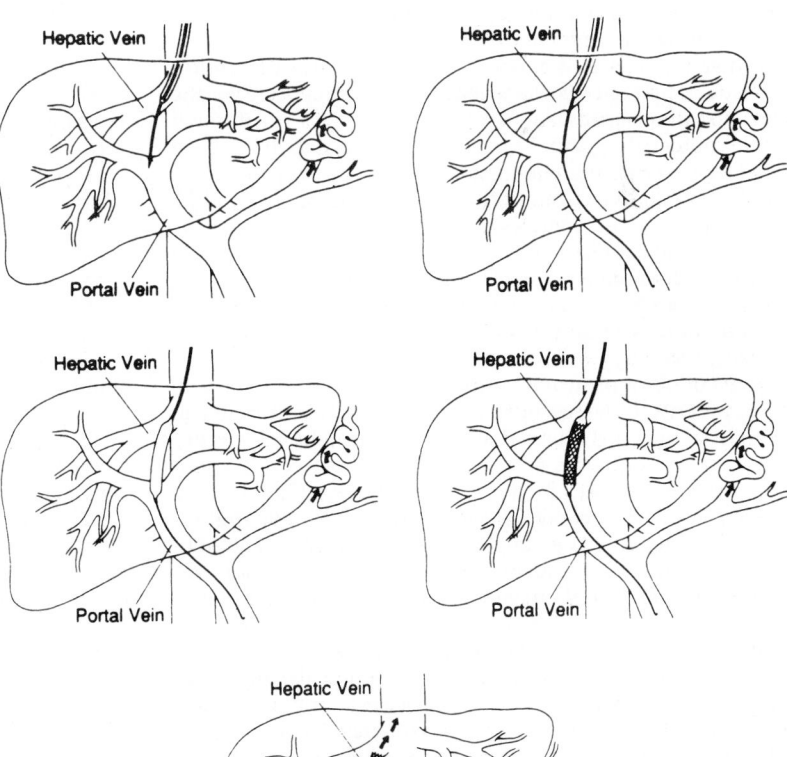

Figure 33–38. Transjugular intrahepatic portosystemic shunt (TIPS). A needle is advanced from a hepatic vein to a major portal vein branch *(top left)* and a guide wire is placed *(top right).* A hepatic parenchymal tract is created by balloon dilation *(middle left)* and an expandable metal stent is placed *(middle right),* thereby creating the shunt *(bottom).* (From Zemel, G., Katzen, B. T., Becker, G. J., et al.: Percutaneous transjugular portosystemic shunt. JAMA, *266*:390, 1991. Copyright 1991, American Medical Association.)

ponade, a more complex operation such as the distal spleno-renal shunt may be appropriate. The major disadvantage of emergency surgery is that operative mortality rates exceed 25% in most reported series. Early postoperative mortality is usually related to the status of hepatic functional reserve rather than to the type of emergency operation selected.

Prevention of Recurrent Hemorrhage

Once a patient has bled from varices, the likelihood of a repeat episode exceeds 70%. Because most persons with variceal hemorrhage have chronic liver disease, the challenge of long-term management is both prevention of recurrent bleeding and maintenance of satisfactory hepatic function. Options available for definitive treatment include pharmacotherapy, chronic sclerotherapy, TIPS, three hemodynamic types of shunt operations (nonselective, selective, and partial), a variety of nonshunt procedures, and hepatic transplantation.

Pharmacotherapy. Pharmacotherapy for the prevention of recurrent variceal bleeding was introduced in 1984 by Lebrec and co-workers, who reported that a dose of propranolol sufficient to decrease the heart rate by 25% resulted in a decreased frequency of recurrent hemorrhage and prolongation of survival in good-risk patients with alcoholic cirrhosis.[25] Multiple subsequent investigations have shown inconsistent results.[24] Invasive hemodynamic monitoring of patients on propranolol has demonstrated minimal or no reduction of portal pressure in many individuals and no correlation between decrease in portal pressure and reduction in pulse rate, which has been the parameter used in most studies to assess therapeutic effect. Thus, two obstacles to effective treatment with propranolol are variability of response to the drug and the lack of an easily measured hemodynamic index to monitor therapy.

A meta-analysis of the many controlled trials of nonselective beta-adrenergic blockade has shown it to decrease the likelihood of recurrent hemorrhage by about 20%.[24] Although multiple other drugs and combinations of agents have been tested, none has been demonstrated to be superior to nonselective beta-blockers. Long-term pharmacotherapy should be limited for use in compliant patients who are observed closely by their physicians. Although an attractive approach because of its noninvasiveness, pharmacotherapy is not yet a practical option for most patients who bleed from varices.

Endoscopic Therapy. During the past 15 years, chronic endoscopic therapy has become the most common treatment for prevention of recurrent variceal hemorrhage. The increasing popularity of endoscopic treatment can be attributed to several factors: (1) disenchantment with shunt surgery among several gastroenterologists and surgeons; (2) endoscopic therapy is less invasive than surgery; (3) there are no adverse hemodynamic effects of endoscopic therapy; (4) endoscopic treatment can be administered by gastroenterologists to whom most patients are initially referred; and (5) several controlled trials have confirmed its therapeutic efficacy.[3]

The objective of chronic endoscopic therapy is to eradicate esophageal varices (see Fig. 33–36). Although the timing of repeat sessions varies from series to series, variceal eradication is usually successful in approximately two thirds of patients. Fewer treatment sessions are required to eradicate varices when variceal ligation rather than sclerosis is used (see Fig. 33–37). After eradication is achieved, diagnostic endoscopy should be performed at 6-month to 1-year intervals, because varices do recur and recurrent varices can bleed. Some investigators have noted an increased frequency of bleeding from gastric varices and portal hypertensive gastropathy after eradication of esophageal varices.

Several controlled trials comparing chronic endoscopic therapy to conventional medical management have been completed.[3] Although fewer patients receiving endoscopic treatment rebled than medically treated patients in all of the investigations, recurrent bleeding still occurred in approximately 50% of endoscopic therapy patients. Rebleeding is most frequent during the initial year and the rate decreases to approximately 15% per year thereafter. Although a single episode of recurrent hemorrhage does not signify failure of therapy, uncontrolled hemorrhage, multiple major episodes of rebleeding, and hemorrhage from gastric varices and portal hypertensive gastropathy all require that endoscopic therapy be abandoned and another treatment modality substituted. Endoscopic treatment failure secondary to rebleeding occurs in as many as one third of patients.[13, 35] Thus, chronic endoscopic therapy is a rational, initial treatment for many patients who bleed from esophageal varices, but subsequent treatment with TIPS, a shunt procedure, nonshunt operation, or hepatic transplantation should be anticipated for a significant percentage of patients. Because of its relatively high failure rate, a course of chronic endoscopic therapy should not be undertaken for noncompliant patients and those living a long distance from advanced medical care.[35]

Transjugular Intrahepatic Portosystemic Shunt. TIPS is being increasingly used as a definitive treatment for patients who bleed from portal hypertension (see Fig. 33–38).[21, 37] However, a major limitation of TIPS is a high incidence (up to 50%) of shunt stenosis or shunt thrombosis within the first year.[6] Shunt stenosis, which is usually secondary to neointimal hyperplasia, is more common than thrombosis and can often be resolved by balloon dilation of the TIPS or, in some cases, by placement of a second shunt. Total shunt occlusion occurs in 10% to 15% of patients. Both shunt stenosis and shunt thrombosis are often followed by recurrent portal hypertensive bleeding. Except for prosthetic interposition shunts, a surgically created shunt rarely fails in the late postoperative interval. Until TIPS technology improves, an operative shunt is preferable for patients who require long-term portal decompression.

Angiographic and duplex ultrasound studies suggest that TIPS, when it effectively decompresses varices, is a nonselective shunt and completely diverts portal flow. Clinical evidence of the nonselectivity of TIPS is its effectiveness in resolving medically intractable ascites and a fairly high frequency of post-TIPS encephalopathy in some of the reported series. Thus far, all clinical studies regarding TIPS are compromised by a relatively brief period of follow-up. It is likely that the frequency of encephalopathy increases as the interval of follow-up lengthens.

The major advantage of TIPS is that it is nonoperative. Because of this, it would appear to be the ideal therapy when only short-term portal decompression is required. Thus, liver transplant candidates who fail sclerotherapy are well suited for TIPS followed by a transplant when a donor organ becomes available. Not only is the patient protected from bleeding in the interim, but the transplant procedure itself may be facilitated by the lower portal pressure. Another group of patients in whom TIPS may be advantageous are those with advanced hepatic functional decompensation who are unlikely to survive long enough for the TIPS to malfunction.

Although TIPS, because it functions as a side-to-side portosystemic shunt, is effective in the treatment of ascites, it is questionable whether ascites alone is a reasonable indication for its use. The adverse side effects of TIPS, such as total portal diversion and encephalopathy, may be more serious problems than ascites.

Portosystemic Shunts. Portosystemic shunts are clearly the most effective means of preventing recurrent hemorrhage in patients with portal hypertension. These procedures are effective because they all, to some degree, decompress the portal venous system by shunting portal flow into the low-pressure systemic venous system. However, diversion of portal blood, which contains hepatotrophic hormones, nutrients, and cerebral toxins, is also responsible for the adverse consequences of shunt operations, namely, portosystemic encephalopathy and accelerated hepatic failure. Depending on whether they completely decompress, compartmentalize, or partially decompress the portal venous circulation, portosystemic shunts can be classified as nonselective, selective, or partial. In addition to variceal decompression, the goal of selective and partial portosystemic shunts is preservation of hepatic portal perfusion, thereby preventing or minimizing the adverse consequences of these procedures.

Nonselective Shunts. Commonly used varieties of nonselective shunts, all of which completely divert portal flow, include the end-to-side portacaval shunt (Eck fistula), the side-to-side portacaval shunt, large-diameter interposition shunts, and the conventional splenorenal shunt (Fig. 33–39). The end-to-side portacaval shunt is the prototype of nonselective shunts and is the only shunt procedure that has been compared with conventional medical management in randomized, controlled trials.[36] Figure 33–40 combines survival data from the four controlled investigations of the therapeutic portacaval shunt (performed in patients with prior variceal hemorrhage). The most common causes of death in medically treated and shunted patients were rebleeding and accelerated hepatic failure, respectively. Although no survival advantage could be demonstrated for shunt patients, all of these studies had a crossover bias in favor of medically treated patients, several of whom received a shunt when they developed intractable recurrent variceal hemorrhage. In addition, nearly all of the trial patients were alcoholic cirrhotics, so these results do not necessarily apply to other causes of portal hypertension. Other important findings of these randomized trials include reliable control of bleeding in shunted patients, variceal rebleeding in over 70% of medi-

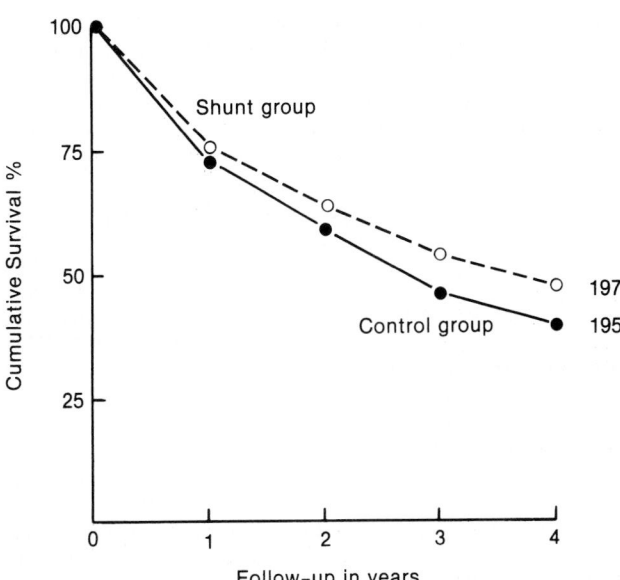

Figure 33–40. Cumulative survival data from four controlled trials of the portacaval shunt versus conventional medical management. (From Boyer, T. D.: Portal hypertension and its complications: Bleeding esophageal varices, ascites, and spontaneous bacterial peritonitis. *In* Zakim, D., and Boyer, T. D. [Eds.]: Hepatology: A Textbook of Liver Disease. Philadelphia, W. B. Saunders, 1982, pp. 464–499.)

cally treated patients, and spontaneous, often severe, encephalopathy in 20% to 40% of shunted patients.

All of the other nonselective shunts in Figure 33–39 maintain continuity of the portal vein, thereby connecting the portal and systemic venous systems in a side-to-side fashion. Therefore, these procedures decompress both the splanchnic venous circulation and the intrahepatic sinusoidal network. Because the liver and intestines are both important contributors to ascites formation, side-to-side portosystemic shunts are the most effective shunt procedures for relieving ascites as well as preventing recurrent variceal bleeding. However, because they completely divert portal flow like the end-to-side portacaval shunt, side-to-side shunts also accelerate hepatic failure and lead to frequent postshunt encephalopathy. One controlled investigation of the end-to-side versus the side-to-side portacaval shunt showed no significant clinical differences between these procedures.[32]

Synthetic grafts or autogenous vein may be interposed between the portal and systemic venous circulations at a variety of locations (see Fig. 33–39). The interposition mesocaval shunt in particular became popular during the 1970s after an initial report showed a lower frequency of encephalopathy after this procedure than after other nonselective shunts. However, subsequent data, including a randomized trial of the interposition mesocaval shunt versus the direct side-to-side portacaval shunt, has documented that there are no clinical or hemodynamic differences between these two operations.[44] A major disadvantage of prosthetic interposition shunts is a high graft thrombosis rate that approaches 35% during the late postoperative interval.[41] On the other hand, advantages of these procedures are that they are relatively easy to construct; the hepatic hilum is avoided, thereby making subsequent liver transplantation less complicated; and they can be easily occluded if intractable postshunt encephalopathy develops.

The conventional splenorenal shunt consists of anastomosis of the proximal splenic vein to the renal vein. Splenectomy is also done. Because the smaller proximal rather than the larger distal end of the splenic vein is used, shunt throm-

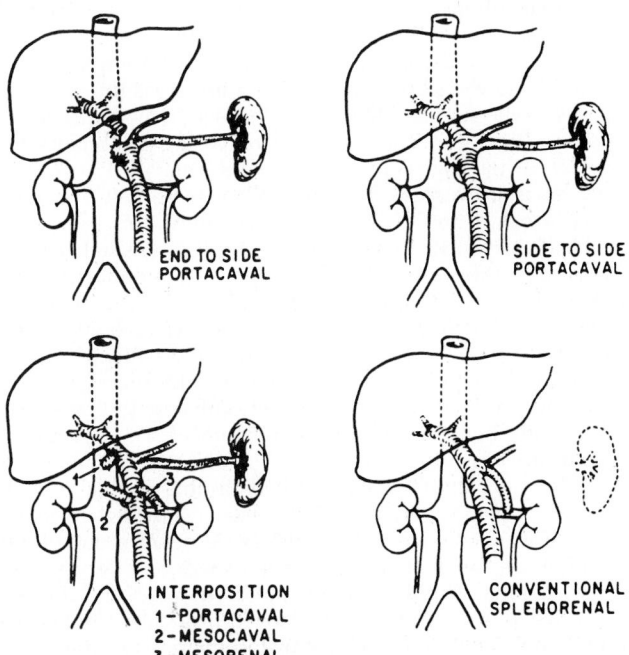

Figure 33–39. Nonselective shunts completely divert portal blood flow away from the liver. (From Rikkers, L. F.: Portal hypertension. *In* Moody, F. G., et al. [Eds.]: Surgical Treatment of Digestive Disease. Chicago, Year Book Medical Publishers, 1986, pp. 409–424.)

bosis is more frequent after this procedure than after the distal splenorenal shunt. Although early series noted that postshunt encephalopathy was less common after the conventional splenorenal shunt than after the portacaval shunt, subsequent analyses have suggested that this low frequency of encephalopathy was probably due to restoration of hepatic portal perfusion after shunt thrombosis developed in many patients. A conventional splenorenal shunt that is of sufficient caliber to remain patent gradually dilates and eventually causes complete portal decompression and portal flow diversion. A purported advantage of the procedure is that hypersplenism is eliminated by splenectomy. However, the thrombocytopenia and leukopenia that accompany portal hypertension are rarely of clinical significance, making splenectomy an unnecessary procedure in most patients.

In summary, nonselective shunts effectively decompress varices. However, because of complete portal flow diversion, they are complicated by frequent postoperative encephalopathy and accelerated hepatic failure. Side-to-side nonselective shunts effectively relieve ascites as well as prevent variceal hemorrhage. Presently, the only indications for nonselective shunts are in the emergency setting, in patients with both variceal hemorrhage and medically intractable ascites, and as a bridge to hepatic transplantation in patients in whom bleeding is not controlled by sclerotherapy.

Selective Shunts. The hemodynamic and clinical shortcomings of nonselective shunts stimulated development of the concept of selective variceal decompression. In 1967, Warren and colleagues[46] introduced the distal splenorenal shunt; and in the following year Inokuchi and associates[18] reported their initial results with the left gastric vena caval shunt. The latter procedure consists of interposition of a vein graft between the left gastric (coronary) vein and the inferior vena cava and, thus, directly and selectively decompresses esophagogastric varices. However, only a minority of patients with portal hypertension have appropriate anatomy for this operation; experience with it has been limited to Japan, and no controlled trials have been conducted.

The distal splenorenal shunt consists of anastomosis of the distal end of the splenic vein to the left renal vein and interruption of all collateral vessels, such as the coronary and gastroepiploic veins, connecting the superior mesenteric and gastrosplenic components of the splanchnic venous circulation (Fig. 33–41). This results in separation of the portal venous circulation into a decompressed gastrosplenic venous circuit and a high pressure superior mesenteric venous system that continues to perfuse the liver. Although the procedure is technically demanding, it can be mastered by most well-trained surgeons who are knowledgeable in the principles of vascular surgery.

Not all patients are candidates for the distal splenorenal shunt. Because sinusoidal and mesenteric hypertension is maintained and important lymphatic pathways are transected during dissection of the left renal vein, the distal splenorenal shunt tends to aggravate rather than relieve ascites. Thus, patients with medically intractable ascites should not undergo this procedure. However, the larger population of patients who develop transient ascites after resuscitation from a variceal hemorrhage are candidates for a selective shunt. Other contraindications to a distal splenorenal shunt are prior splenectomy and a splenic vein diameter less than 7 mm.

Although selective variceal decompression is a sound physiologic concept, the distal splenorenal shunt remains controversial after an extensive clinical experience spanning more than 25 years.[19] The key questions regarding this procedure are how effective is it in preserving hepatic portal perfusion and is it superior to nonselective shunts with respect to duration or quality of survival?

Although the distal splenorenal shunt results in portal flow preservation in over 85% of patients during the early postoperative interval (Fig. 33–42), the high pressure mesenteric venous system gradually collateralizes to the low pressure shunt, resulting in loss of portal flow in approximately 50% of patients by 1 year. The degree and duration of portal flow preservation depends on both the cause of portal hypertension and on technical details of the operation (extent to which mesenteric and gastrosplenic venous circulations are separated). Henderson and coworkers[14] have shown that portal flow is maintained in the majority of patients with nonalcoholic cirrhosis and noncirrhotic portal hypertension (e.g., portal vein thrombosis). In contrast, portal flow rapidly collateralizes to the shunt in individuals with alcoholic cirrhosis.

Modification of the distal splenorenal shunt by purposeful or inadvertent omission of coronary vein ligation results in early loss of portal flow. Even when all major collateral vessels are interrupted, portal flow may be gradually diverted through a pancreatic collateral network (pancreatic siphon). This pathway can be discouraged by dissecting the full length of the splenic vein from the pancreas (splenopancreatic disconnection). In an uncontrolled series, the Emory group has shown that portal flow can be preserved into the late postoperative interval in the majority of patients with alcoholic cirrhosis when splenopancreatic disconnection is done.[15] However, this extension of the procedure makes it technically more challenging, which may be a significant disadvantage in an era when fewer shunts are being done because of increasing utilization of endoscopic therapy, TIPS, and hepatic transplantation.

Six of the seven controlled comparisons of the distal splenorenal shunt to nonselective shunts have included predominantly alcoholic cirrhotic patients.[19] None of these trials has demonstrated an advantage to either procedure with respect to long-term survival. Three of the studies have found a lower frequency of encephalopathy after the distal splenorenal shunt, whereas the other trials have shown no difference in the incidence of this postoperative complication. In contrast to survival, encephalopathy is a subjective end-point that was assessed with a variety of methods in the different trials. One of the more objective investigations quantified encephalopathy by the number of postoperative hospital admissions required for the treatment of this complication.[22] This trial showed significantly fewer admissions for encephalopathy in the selective than in the nonselective shunt group. Another important end-point in comparing treatments for variceal hemorrhage is the effectiveness with which recurrent bleeding is prevented. In nearly all uncontrolled and controlled series of the distal splenorenal shunt, this procedure has been equivalent to nonselective shunts.[19] A single exception is one of the controlled trials that was complicated by a high rebleeding rate in the distal splenorenal shunt group (30%).[10] Mainly because of these inconsistent results of the controlled trials, there is no consensus as to which shunting procedure is superior in patients with alcoholic cirrhosis. However, since the quality of life (encephalopathy rate) was significantly better in the distal splenorenal shunt group in three of the trials, there would appear to be an advantage to selective variceal decompression even in this population.[33]

There are considerably fewer data regarding selective shunting in nonalcoholic cirrhosis and in noncirrhotic portal hypertension. Because hepatic portal perfusion after the distal splenorenal shunt is better preserved in these disease categories, one might expect improved results. A single controlled trial in patients with schistosomiasis (presinusoidal portal hypertension) demonstrated a lower frequency of encephalopathy after the distal splenorenal shunt than after a conventional splenorenal shunt (nonselective).[5] There were few deaths in either limb of this trial. Two large uncontrolled

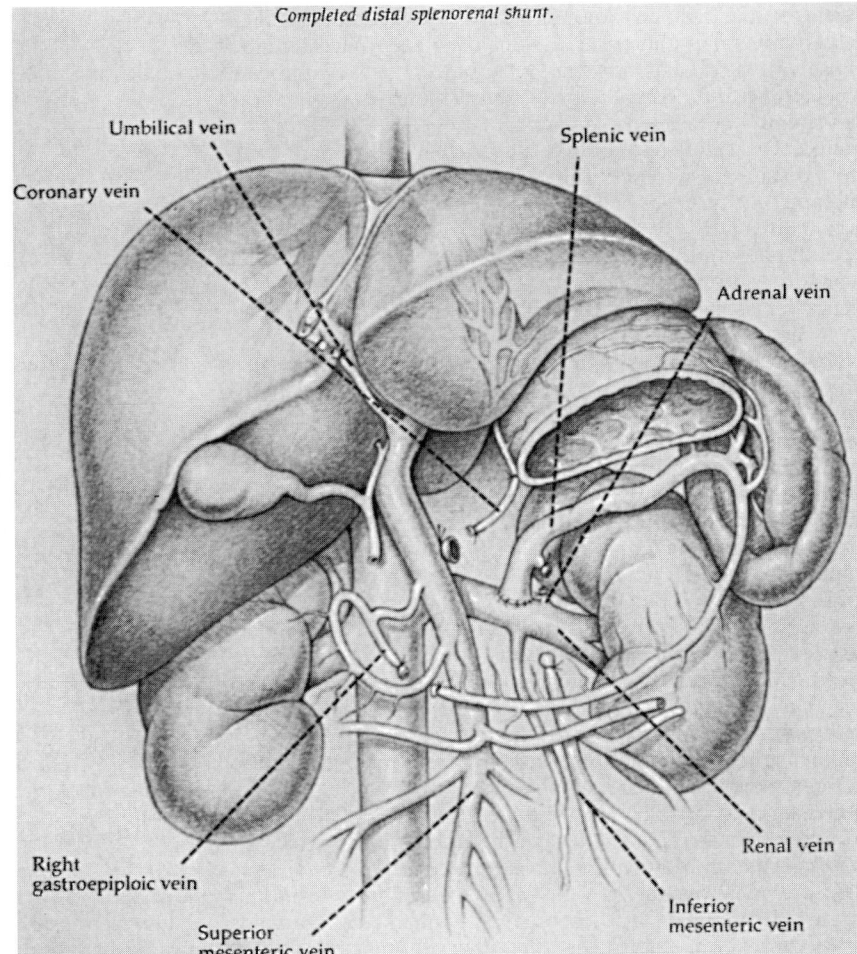

Figure 33–41. The distal splenorenal shunt provides selective variceal decompression through the short gastric veins, spleen, and splenic vein to the left renal vein. Hepatic portal perfusion is maintained by interrupting the umbilical vein, coronary vein, gastroepiploic vein, and any other prominent collaterals. (From Rikkers, L. F.: Distal splenorenal shunt for portal hypertension. Surgery Illustrated. 1988. Drawing by William B. Westwood. Courtesy of LTI Medica and the Upjohn Company. Copyright 1988 by Learning Technology Incorporated.)

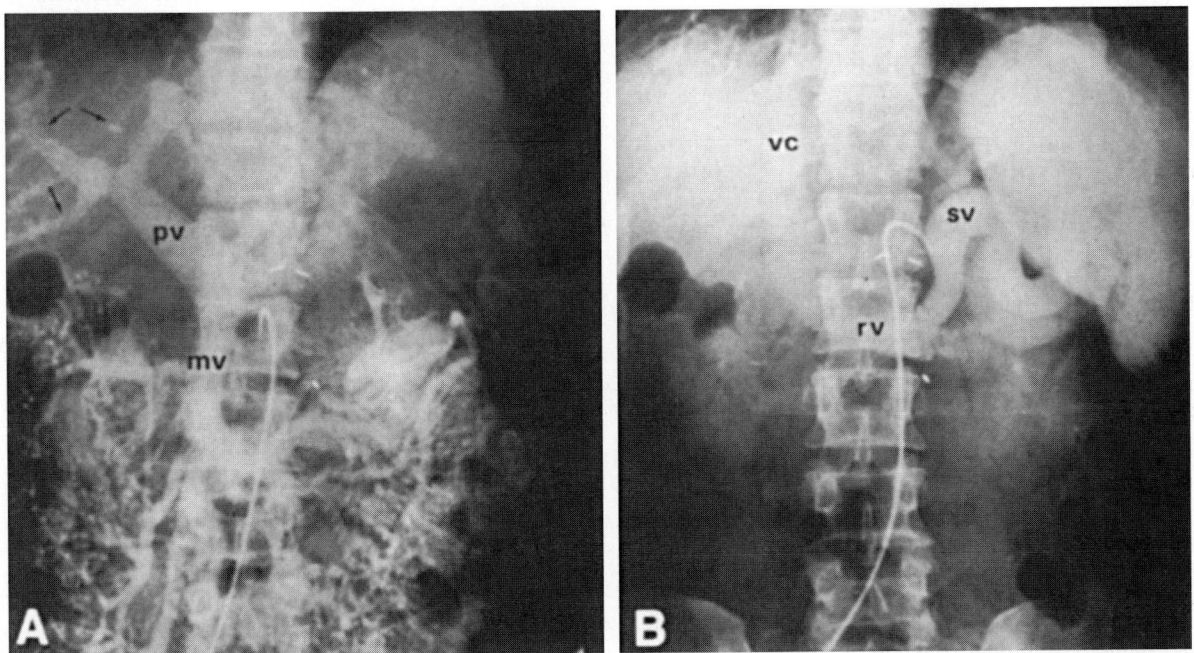

Figure 33–42. Selective superior mesenteric (A) and splenic (B) angiograms after a distal splenorenal shunt. The venous phase of the superior mesenteric angiogram visualizes the superior mesenteric vein (MV), portal vein (PV), and intrahepatic portal vein branches (arrows). The venous phase of the splenic angiogram opacifies the splenic vein (SV), left renal vein (RV), and inferior vena cava (VC). (From Rikkers, L. F., Rudman, D., Galambos, J. T., et al.: A randomized, controlled trial of the distal splenorenal shunt. Ann. Surg., *188*:271, 1978.)

series of the distal splenorenal shunt have demonstrated better survival in patients with nonalcoholic cirrhosis than in those with alcoholic cirrhosis.[45, 47] However, this has not been a consistent finding in all centers in which the distal splenorenal shunt is performed.

Recently completed controlled trials have also compared the distal splenorenal shunt with chronic endoscopic therapy.[13, 35] In these investigations, recurrent hemorrhage was more effectively prevented by selective shunting than by sclerotherapy, but hepatic portal perfusion was maintained in a significantly higher fraction of patients undergoing sclerotherapy. Despite this hemodynamic advantage, encephalopathy rates have been similar after both therapies. The two North American trials were dissimilar with respect to the effect of these treatments on long-term survival. Sclerotherapy with surgical rescue for the one third of sclerotherapy failures resulted in significantly better survival than selective shunt alone in one study.[13] In this investigation, 85% of sclerotherapy failures could be salvaged by surgery. In contrast, a similar investigation conducted in a sparsely populated area (Intermountain West and Plains) showed superior survival after the distal splenorenal shunt.[35] Only 31% of sclerotherapy failures could be salvaged by surgery in this trial. The survival results of these two studies suggest that endoscopic therapy is a rational, initial treatment for patients who bleed from varices if sclerotherapy failure is recognized and such patients promptly undergo surgery. However, patients living in remote areas are less likely to be salvaged by shunt surgery when sclerotherapy fails, and a selective shunt may be preferable initial treatment for such patients.

Partial Shunts. The objectives of partial and selective shunts are the same: (1) effective decompression of varices, (2) preservation of hepatic portal perfusion, and (3) maintenance of some residual portal hypertension. Initial attempts at partial shunting consisted of small-diameter vein-to-vein anastomoses, but these generally either thrombosed or dilated with time, thereby becoming nonselective shunts.

More recently, a small-diameter interposition portacaval shunt using a polytetrafluoroethylene graft, combined with ligation of the coronary vein and other collateral vessels, has been described (Fig. 33–43). When the prosthetic graft is 10 mm. or less in diameter, hepatic portal perfusion is preserved in the majority of patients, at least during the early postoperative interval.[39] Early experience with this small-diameter, prosthetic shunt is that despite the small diameter, fewer than 15% of shunts have thrombosed and most of these have been successfully opened by interventional radiologic techniques. A recent prospective, randomized trial of partial (8-mm. diameter) and nonselective (16-mm. diameter) interposition portacaval shunts has shown a lower frequency of encephalopathy after the partial shunt but similar survival after both types of shunts.[38] However, the number of patients included in this investigation was small and further trials need to be done to confirm this finding.

Nonshunt Operations. The objectives of these procedures are either ablation of varices or, more commonly, extensive interruption of collateral vessels connecting the high-pressure portal venous system with the varices. One exception is splenectomy, which is effective in left-sided portal hypertension caused by splenic vein thrombosis.

The simplest nonshunt operation is transection and reanastomosis of the distal esophagus with a stapling device. This operation, which has generally been used in the emergency setting, is frequently followed by recurrent hemorrhage.[34] The most effective nonshunt operation is extensive esophagogastric devascularization combined with esophageal transection and splenectomy (Fig. 33–44). The Sugiura procedure preserves the coronary and paraesophageal veins to maintain a portosystemic collateral pathway and thus discourage re-

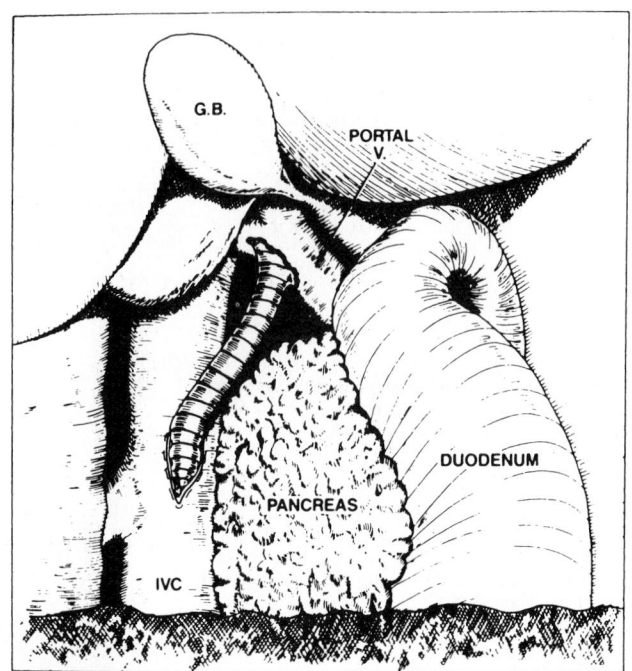

Figure 33–43. A small-diameter (8 to 10 mm.) interposition portacaval shunt partially decompresses the portal venous system and may preserve hepatic portal perfusion. G.B., gallbladder; IVC, inferior vena cava. (From Sarfeh, I. J., Rypins, E. B., and Mason, G. R.: A systematic appraisal of portacaval H-graft diameters: Clinical and hemodynamic perspectives. Ann. Surg., *204*:356, 1986.)

formation of varices. In Japan, the results with this operation have been excellent.[17] However, extensive devascularization procedures have generally been less successful in North American patients with alcoholic cirrhosis. Long-term follow-up in American series has revealed rebleeding rates of 35% to 55%, which are similar to the endoscopic sclerotherapy experience. In many centers, esophagogastric devascularization procedures are mainly used for unshuntable patients

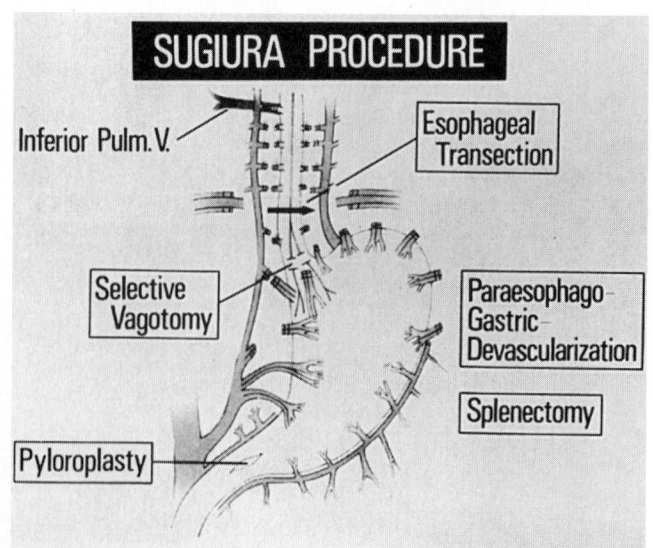

Figure 33–44. The Sugiura procedure combines esophageal transection, extensive esophagogastric devascularization, and splenectomy. The paraesophageal collateral vessels are preserved to discourage re-formation of varices. (From Sugiura, M., and Futagawa, S.: Further evaluation of the Sugiura procedure in the treatment of esophageal varices. Arch. Surg., *112*:1317, 1977. Copyright 1977, American Medical Association.)

with diffuse splanchnic venous thrombosis and for individuals with distal splenorenal shunt thrombosis.

Hepatic Transplantation. Of the numerous therapeutic options for prevention of recurrent variceal hemorrhage, hepatic transplantation is the only one that addresses the underlying liver disease in addition to providing reliable portal decompression.[12] However, because of economic factors and a limited supply of donor organs, hepatic transplantation is not available to all patients. In addition, transplantation is not indicated for some of the more common causes of variceal bleeding, such as schistosomiasis (normal liver function) and active alcoholism (noncompliant).

Patients with variceal bleeding who are transplant candidates include nonalcoholic cirrhotics and abstinent alcoholic cirrhotics with either limited hepatic functional reserve (Child's Class C) or a poor quality of life secondary to their disease (e.g., encephalopathy, fatigue, or bone pain). In such individuals, the acute hemorrhage should be treated with endoscopic therapy and the patient's transplant candidacy immediately activated. If sclerotherapy is ineffective, a TIPS should be inserted as a short-term bridge to transplantation.

There are few data presently as to the best therapy for eventual transplant candidates who have well-compensated liver disease (Child's Class A and B) when they bleed from varices. Although the majority of these individuals should initially be treated with chronic endoscopic therapy, it is unclear whether hepatic transplantation or a nontransplant operation is preferable for sclerotherapy failures and for patients who bleed from gastric varices or portal hypertensive gastropathy. The issue is not whether these patients should undergo transplantation but when this formidable procedure should be undertaken. If a nontransplant operation (e.g., selective shunt or devascularization procedure) is performed initially, these patients should be carefully assessed at 6-month to 1-year intervals and hepatic transplantation considered when other complications of cirrhosis develop or hepatic functional decompensation is evident either clinically or by careful assessment with quantitative tests of liver function.

Overall Treatment Plan. An algorithm for definitive management of variceal hemorrhage is shown in Figure 33–45. Patients are first grouped according to their transplant candidacy. This decision is based on multiple factors: etiology of portal hypertension, abstinence for alcoholic cirrhotic patients, the presence or absence of other diseases, and physiologic rather than chronologic age. Transplant candidates with either decompensated hepatic function or a poor quality of life secondary to their liver disease should be transplanted as soon as possible. Most future transplant and nontransplant candidates should undergo initial endoscopic therapy unless they bleed from gastric varices or portal hypertensive gastropathy or live in remote geographic locations and have limited access to emergency tertiary care. These latter individuals and those who fail sclerotherapy should receive a selective shunt if they meet the criteria for this operation. Patients with medically intractable ascites and those with diffuse splanchnic venous thrombosis are best treated with a side-to-side portosystemic shunt and a devascularization procedure, respectively. TIPS is indicated for patients with endoscopic treatment failure who may require transplantation in the near future and for nontransplant candidates with advanced hepatic functional deterioration. Future transplant candidates should be carefully monitored so they undergo transplantation at the appropriate time before they become poor operative risks.

Prevention of Initial Variceal Hemorrhage (Prophylactic Therapy)

The rationale for treating patients with varices before they bleed is the high mortality rate associated with the initial hemorrhage. However, because only a third of patients with varices eventually bleed, unless potential bleeders are more reliably identified, approximately two thirds of patients undergoing prophylactic therapy would be treated unnecessarily.

The first trials of prophylaxis for variceal hemorrhage compared the portacaval shunt to conventional medical therapy. In these investigations, survival of shunted patients was actually less than that of medically treated patients, because of accelerated hepatic failure secondary to complete portal diversion.[9] In addition, a significant fraction of shunted patients developed postshunt encephalopathy.

The major impetus to reconsideration of prophylactic therapy was the development of relatively noninvasive treatments (endoscopic therapy and pharmacotherapy), which

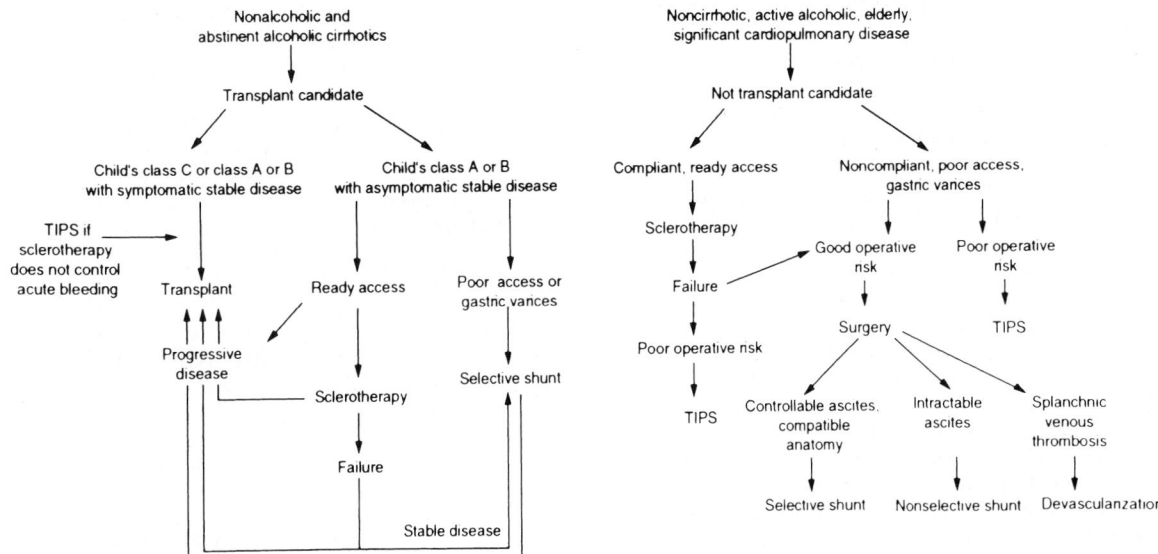

Figure 33–45. Algorithm for definitive therapy of variceal hemorrhage (see text). (From Rikkers, L. F.: Portal hypertension. *In* Levine, B. A., et al. [Eds.]: Current Practice of Surgery, vol. 3, New York, Churchill Livingstone, 1995.)

should be associated with less morbidity than major operative procedures. However, endoscopic treatment cannot be presently advocated for prophylaxis because controlled trials have shown no consistent benefit and some have demonstrated a higher rebleeding rate and a lower survival rate in the sclerotherapy group than in medically treated controls.[9] In contrast, all trials of beta blockade as prophylactic therapy have found a reduced incidence of initial variceal hemorrhage in treated patients.[9, 24] In several of these studies, the decreased bleeding rate in the treatment group was statistically significant and in one study survival was prolonged in patients receiving beta blockade. Because beta blockade has been associated with few adverse side effects, it can be recommended for reliable patients with varices that have never bled.

PORTOSYSTEMIC ENCEPHALOPATHY

Portosystemic encephalopathy is a psychoneurologic syndrome that may have a variety of manifestations, including alterations in the level of consciousness, intellectual deterioration, personality changes, and neurologic findings such as the flapping tremor, asterixis.[7] Although encephalopathy may sometimes develop spontaneously in patients with chronic liver disease, it more often occurs after portosystemic shunt procedures. It is particularly common (20% to 40% of patients) in individuals who undergo nonselective shunts.

Although the pathogenesis of encephalopathy is uncertain, most theories are based on circulating cerebral toxins that are intestinally absorbed and bypass the liver by means of shunts or fail to be inactivated by the liver's decreased metabolic capacity. Purported cerebral toxins include ammonia, mercaptans, and gamma-aminobutyric acid. The false neurotransmitter hypothesis, based on the high ratio of aromatic to branched-chain amino acids present in the blood of patients with chronic liver disease, has also been proposed to explain the psychoneurologic disturbances observed.

Encephalopathy develops spontaneously in less than 10% of patients. More commonly, one or more of the following precipitating factors induce the syndrome: gastrointestinal hemorrhage, excessive diuresis, azotemia, constipation, sedatives, infection, and excess dietary protein.

Most episodes of encephalopathy can be successfully treated by identifying and then eliminating the precipitating factors responsible. Dietary protein should be restricted, infections should be treated, all sedatives should be discontinued, and intestinal catharsis to remove blood within the gastrointestinal tract should be accomplished. Stool softeners and dietary protein restriction should be prescribed for patients who have chronic encephalopathy.

Pharmacologic treatment of encephalopathy is indicated for individuals with chronic, intermittent symptoms and for those with persistent, acute psychoneurologic disturbances despite elimination of precipitating factors. The only drugs with proven effectiveness are neomycin, a poorly absorbed antibiotic that suppresses urease-containing bacteria, and lactulose, a nonabsorbable disaccharide that acidifies colonic contents and also has a cathartic effect. Acute episodes of encephalopathy can be treated equally effectively by neomycin and lactulose. Neomycin is orally administered in a dose of 1.5 gm. every 6 hours, whereas in the acute setting lactulose should be given in a dose of 30 gm. every 1 or 2 hours until a cathartic effect is noted. The patient should then be maintained with 20 to 30 gm. of lactulose two to four times a day or as needed to result in two soft bowel movements daily. Neomycin should not be used for treatment of chronic encephalopathy because nephrotoxicity or ototoxicity may develop. Lactulose combined with mild protein restriction (60 to 80 gm. per day) is the preferred treatment for chronic, intermittent encephalopathy.

Enteral or parenteral administration of nutritional formulas enriched in branched-chain amino acids has been suggested as the treatment of both acute and chronic encephalopathy. These solutions have improved mental status in patients in some controlled trials.

Surgery plays a minor role in the management of encephalopathy. Cerebral function has been improved in some patients with chronic encephalopathy after interruption of a completely diverting portosystemic shunt (nonselective shunt). Likewise, in isolated cases, occlusion of a major portosystemic collateral vessel such as the coronary vein has reversed encephalopathy after the distal splenorenal shunt. Although both total colectomy and colonic exclusion have resolved encephalopathy in some patients, the significant morbidity and mortality rates after these operations in patients with decompensated hepatic disease have prevented their widespread use.

ASCITES

Ascites is another complication of portal hypertension that rarely requires surgical treatment.[1] Portal hypertensive ascites is initiated by altered hepatic and splanchnic hemodynamics, which cause transudation of fluid into the interstitial space. When the rate of interstitial fluid formation exceeds lymph drainage capacity, ascites accumulates. This pathophysiologic process results in an intravascular volume deficit, which initiates compensatory mechanisms such as aldosterone secretion to restore plasma volume. Both the liver and intestines are important sites of ascites formation, and clinically detectable ascites is rare in patients with extrahepatic portal hypertension.

Medical management resolves ascites in approximately 95% of patients.[1] Dietary salt restriction and diuretic therapy are the mainstays of medical treatment. A rational first-line diuretic is spironolactone because secondary hyperaldosteronism is present in most patients. A combination of salt restriction (20 to 30 mEq. per day) and spironolactone in a dose of 100 to 400 mg. per day results in effective diuresis in approximately two thirds of patients.[1] If this regimen fails to mobilize ascites, a more potent diuretic such as hydrochlorothiazide or furosemide should be added. Recent studies have shown that intermittent, large-volume paracentesis either with or without intravenous infusion of colloid is also effective.[1] Contrary to earlier beliefs, large-volume paracentesis in a stable patient does not markedly alter systemic hemodynamics or renal function.

Surgical therapy should be reserved for the unusual patient with medically intractable ascites. The safest and most effective surgical procedure is the peritoneovenous shunt. However, controlled trials have shown that this relatively simple operation is followed by significant morbidity and that survival is not prolonged when compared with medical management.[42] Although side-to-side portosystemic shunts are also effective in relieving ascites, these operations should not be used for ascitic patients unless they have bled from esophagogastric varices. TIPS, a nonoperative side-to-side portosystemic shunt, has also been effectively used to relieve medically intractable ascites.[21, 37] However, because of the high long-term failure rate of TIPS and the adverse consequences of total portal diversion secondary to this procedure (i.e., encephalopathy and accelerated hepatic failure), its use should be limited to highly selected patients.

SELECTED REFERENCES

Groszmann, R. J., and Grace, N. D. (Eds.): Complications of portal hypertension: Esophagogastric varices and ascites. Gastroenterol. Clin. North Am., 21(no. 1), 1992.

This is a monograph of 11 chapters on treatment of esophagogastric variceal hemorrhage and 3 chapters devoted to management of cirrhotic ascites, all by authorities in these fields.

Langer, B. (Ed.): World progress in surgery—treatment of portal hypertension 1994: State of the art. World J. Surg., *18*(no. 2), 1994.
Included in this issue is a compendium of 14 articles on the state of the art treatment of the complications of portal hypertension. Eight articles are devoted to surgical treatment (shunts, nonshunt operations, and liver transplantation) of variceal bleeding. Other entries deal with endoscopic treatment, pharmacotherapy, portal hypertension in children, surgical treatment of ascites, and prophylactic therapy for varices that have not bled.

W. Dean Warren Memorial Issue: Am. J. Surg., *160*(no. 1), 1990.
This issue was published in memory of Dr. W. Dean Warren, who died in 1989. It contains 22 articles on the treatment of variceal bleeding. Several entries deal with the selective distal splenorenal shunt, which was originated by Dr. Warren.

Rikkers, L. F. (Ed.): Management of variceal hemorrhage. Surg. Clin. North Am., *70*:2, 1990.
This series of 14 articles by recognized authorities deals with all aspects of acute and definitive treatment of variceal hemorrhage. Individual articles are devoted to pharmacotherapy, endoscopic sclerotherapy, each of the major types of portosystemic shunts, nonshunting operations, and hepatic transplantation. Additional articles consider pathophysiology of portal hypertension, nonoperative emergency treatment, emergency surgery, diagnosis and hemodynamic evaluation, prophylactic therapy, and management of children with variceal bleeding.

Terblanche, J., Burroughs, A. K., and Hobbs, K. E. F.: Controversies in the management of bleeding esophageal varices (two parts). N. Engl. J. Med., *320*:1393–1398 and 1469–1475, 1989.
This excellent review consists of three parts: emergency management, long-term management, and prophylactic management of esophageal varices. The many controlled trials of pharmacotherapy, endoscopic sclerotherapy, and surgery are summarized. The several remaining controversies concerning the treatment of variceal hemorrhage are discussed and, where appropriate, the authors' conclusions are presented. The bibliography is comprehensive and current.

REFERENCES

1. Arroyo, V., Gines, P., and Planas, R.: Treatment of ascites in cirrhosis: Diuretics, peritoneovenous shunt, and large-volume paracentesis. Gastroenterol. Clin. North Am., *21*:237, 1992.
2. Benoit, J. N., and Granger, D. N.: Splanchnic hemodynamics in chronic portal hypertension. Semin. Liver Dis., *6*:287, 1986.
3. Burroughs, A. K., and McCormick, P. A.: Prevention of variceal rebleeding. Gastroenterol. Clin. North Am., *21*:119, 1992.
4. Chen, T. S., and Chen, P. S.: Understanding the Liver. Westport, Conn., Greenwood Press, 1984.
5. da Silva, L. C., Strauss, E., Gayotto, L. C. C., et al.: A randomized trial for the study of the elective surgical treatment of portal hypertension in Mansonic schistosomiasis. Ann. Surg., *204*:148, 1986.
6. Dohrenwend, M., Saddekni, S., Memel, D. S., et al.: Clinical outcome, shunt patency, and survival after transjugular intrahepatic portosystemic shunt. Gastroenterology, *106*:A885, 1994.
7. Fraser, C. L., and Arieff, A. I.: Hepatic encephalopathy. N. Engl. J. Med., *313*:865, 1985.
8. Gimson, A. E., Westaby, D., Hegarty, J., et al.: A randomized trial of vasopressin and vasopressin plus nitroglycerin in the control of acute variceal hemorrhage. Hepatology, *6*:410, 1986.
9. Grace, N. D.: Prevention of initial variceal hemorrhage. Gastroenterol. Clin. North Am., *21*:149, 1992.
10. Harley, H. A., Morgan, T., Redeker, A. G., et al.: Results of a randomized trial of end-to-side portacaval shunt and distal splenorenal shunt in alcoholic liver disease and variceal bleeding. Gastroenterology, *91*:802, 1986.
11. Helton, W. S., Belshaw, A., Althaus, S., et al.: Critical appraisal of the angiographic portacaval shunt (TIPS). Am. J. Surg., *165*:566, 1993.
12. Henderson, J. M.: Liver transplantation for portal hypertension. Gastroenterol. Clin. North Am., *21*:197, 1992.
13. Henderson, J. M., Kutner, M. H., Millikan, W. J., Jr., et al.: Endoscopic variceal sclerosis compared with distal splenorenal shunt to prevent recurrent variceal bleeding in cirrhosis: A prospective, randomized trial. Ann. Intern. Med., *112*:262, 1990.
14. Henderson, J. M., Millikan, W. J., Jr., Wright-Bacon, L., et al.: Hemodynamic differences between alcoholic and nonalcoholic cirrhotics following distal splenorenal shunt: Effect on survival. Ann. Surg., *198*:325, 1983.
15. Henderson, J. M., Warren, W. D., Millikan, W. J., et al.: Distal splenorenal shunt with splenopancreatic disconnection: A 4-year assessment. Ann. Surg., *210*:332, 1989.
16. Holman, J. M., and Rikkers, L. F.: Success of medical and surgical management of acute variceal hemorrhage. Am. J. Surg., *140*:816, 1980.
17. Idezuki, Y., Kokudo, N., Sanjo, K., and Bandai, Y.: Sugiura procedure for management of variceal bleeding in Japan. World J. Surg., *18*:216, 1994.
18. Inokuchi, K., Beppu, K., Koyanagi, N., et al.: Fifteen years' experience with left gastric venous caval shunt for esophageal varices. World J. Surg., *8*:716, 1984.
19. Jin, G., and Rikkers, L. F.: Selective variceal decompression: Current status. HPB Surg., *5*:1, 1991.
20. Johnston, G. W., and Rodgers, H. W.: A review of 15 years' experience in the use of sclerotherapy in the control of acute haemorrhage from oesophageal varices. Br. J. Surg., *60*:797, 1973.
21. LaBerge, J. M., Ring, E. J., Gordon, R. L., et al.: Creation of transjugular intrahepatic portosystemic shunts with the Wallstent endoprosthesis: Results in 100 patients. Radiology, *187*:413, 1993.
22. Langer, B., Taylor, B. R., Mackenzie, D. R., et al.: Further report of a prospective randomized trial comparing distal splenorenal shunt with end-to-side portacaval shunt. Gastroenterology, *88*:424, 1985.
23. Lautt, W. W., and Greenway, C. V.: Conceptual review of the hepatic vascular bed. Hepatology, *7*:952, 1987.
24. Lebrec, D.: Long-term management of variceal bleeding: The place of pharmacotherapy. World J. Surg., *18*:229, 1994.
25. Lebrec, D., Poynard, T., Bernau, J., et al.: A randomized controlled study of propranolol for prevention of recurrent gastrointestinal bleeding in patients with cirrhosis: A final report. Hepatology, *4*:355, 1984.
26. Matloff, D. S.: Treatment of acute variceal bleeding. Gastroenterol. Clin. North Am., *21*:103, 1992.
27. McCormack, T. T., Sims, J., Eyre-Brook, I., et al.: Gastric lesions in portal hypertension: Inflammatory gastritis or congestive gastropathy? Gut, *26*:1226, 1985.
28. Nordlinger, B. M., Nordlinger, D. F., Fulenwider, J. T., et al.: Angiography in portal hypertension: Clinical significance in surgery. Am. J. Surg., *139*:132, 1980.
29. Ozaki, C. F., Anderson, J. C., Lieberman, R. P., and Rikkers, L. F.: Duplex ultrasound as a noninvasive technique of assessing portal hemodynamics. Am. J. Surg., *155*:70, 1988.
30. Planas, R., Quer, J. C., Boix, J., et al.: A prospective randomized trial comparing somatostatin and sclerotherapy in the treatment of acute variceal bleeding. Hepatology, *20*:370, 1994.
31. Polio, J., and Groszmann, R. J.: Hemodynamic factors involved in the development and rupture of esophageal varices: A pathophysiologic approach to treatment. Semin. Liver Dis., *6*:218, 1986.
32. Resnick, R. H., Iber, F. L., Ishihara, A. M., et al.: A controlled study of the therapeutic portacaval shunt. Gastroenterology, *67*:843, 1974.
33. Rikkers, L. F.: Is the distal splenorenal shunt better? Hepatology, *8*:1705, 1988.
34. Rikkers, L. F., and Jin, G.: Surgical management of acute variceal hemorrhage. World J. Surg., *18*:193, 1994.
35. Rikkers, L. F., Jin, G., Burnett, D. A., et al.: Shunt surgery versus endoscopic sclerotherapy for variceal hemorrhage: Late results of a randomized trial. Am. J. Surg., *165*:27, 1993.
36. Rikkers, L. F., Sorrell, W. T., and Jin, G.: Which portosystemic shunt is best? Gastroenterol. Clin. North Am., *21*:179, 1992.
37. Rossle, M., Haag, K., Ochs, A., et al.: The transjugular intrahepatic portosystemic stent shunt procedure for variceal bleeding. N. Engl. J. Med., *330*:165, 1994.
38. Sarfeh, I. J., and Rypins, E. B.: Partial versus total portacaval shunt in alcoholic cirrhosis. Ann. Surg., *219*:353, 1994.
39. Sarfeh, I. J., Rypins, E. B., and Mason, G. R.: A systematic appraisal of portacaval H-graft diameters: Clinical and hemodynamic perspectives. Ann. Surg., *204*:356, 1986.
40. Smith, J. L., and Graham, D. Y.: Variceal hemorrhage: A critical evaluation of survival analysis. Gastroenterology, *82*:968, 1982.
41. Smith, R. B., III, Warren, W. D., Salam, A. A., et al.: Dacron interposition shunts for portal hypertension: An analysis of morbidity correlates. Ann. Surg., *192*:9, 1980.
42. Stanley, M. M., Ochi, S., Lee, K. K., et al.: Peritoneovenous shunting as compared with medical treatment in patients with alcoholic cirrhosis and massive ascites. N. Engl. J. Med., *321*:1632, 1989.
43. Stiegman, G. V., Goff, J. S., Mihaletz-Onody, P. A., et al.: Endoscopic sclerotherapy as compared with endoscopic ligation for bleeding esophageal varices. N. Engl. J. Med., *326*:1527, 1992.
44. Stipa, S., Ziparo, V., Anza, M., et al.: A randomized controlled trial of mesentericocaval shunt with autologous jugular vein. Surg. Gynecol. Obstet., *153*:353, 1981.
45. Warren, W. D., Millikan, W. J., Jr., Henderson, J. M., et al.: Ten years' portal hypertensive surgery at Emory. Ann. Surg., *195*:530, 1982.
46. Warren, W. D., Zeppa, R., and Fomon, J. J.: Selective transsplenic decompression of gastroesophageal varices by distal splenorenal shunt. Ann. Surg., *166*:437, 1967.
47. Zeppa, R., Hutson, D. G., Levi, J. U., and Livingstone, A. S.: Factors influencing survival after distal splenorenal shunt. World J. Surg., *8*:733, 1984.

VI _____

PERITONEOVENOUS SHUNTS FOR INTRACTABLE ASCITES

Paul D. Greig, M.D., and Bernard Langer, M.D.

Ascites is the pathologic accumulation of fluid in the peritoneal cavity. It may be part of a generalized third-space fluid loss in conditions such as chronic renal disease, congestive heart failure, or massive fluid overload, but it is more often related to intra-abdominal factors that cause formation of peritoneal fluid at a more rapid rate than it can be absorbed (Table 33–11). Of these conditions, chronic liver disease is by far the most common.

PATHOPHYSIOLOGY OF ASCITES FORMATION IN CIRRHOSIS

In cirrhosis with portal hypertension, the accumulation of ascites is caused by abnormal renal function that is characterized by sodium and water retention.[1] The degree of renal dysfunction ranges from minimal in compensated cirrhosis without ascites with only a mild abnormality of sodium homeostasis (e.g., inability to excrete a sodium load) to advanced dysfunction in decompensated cirrhosis with marked sodium retention and progressive ascites. These patients have a reduction in renal blood flow with decreased glomerular filtration rate from intrarenal shunting of blood to medullary nephrons in spite of normal or increased circulating blood volume and cardiac output. Associated with these renal and hemodynamic changes are increases in plasma renin, angiotensin, and aldosterone levels. These factors contribute to sodium and water retention with low urinary volume and sodium concentration. The end stage of this spectrum is a functional form of renal failure with progressive oliguria, rising creatinine, and intense sodium retention, termed *hepatorenal syndrome.*[2] Studies of the mechanism of ascites formation have enhanced understanding of many aspects of this functional renal disorder that accompanies postsinusoidal portal hypertension; however, there is no single theory that unifies the many pathophysiologic disturbances that have been identified.

The classic *underfill theory* focuses on portal hypertension

TABLE 33–11. Causes of Ascites

General extravascular fluid accumulation
  Chronic renal failure
    Nephrotic syndrome
  Chronic right-sided heart failure
    Constrictive pericarditis, cardiac tamponade, tricuspid
      stenosis or insufficiency
  Malnutrition
  Marked fluid overload
Intra-abdominal causes
  Acute liver disease
    Viral hepatitis
    Acute hepatic necrosis
  Chronic liver disease
    Cirrhosis
    Budd-Chiari syndrome
  Pancreatic ascites
  Chylous ascites
  Malignancy, especially ovary, colon, metastatic breast
  Tuberculosis

and hypoalbuminemia as the initiating factors in ascites formation. The fibrosis and nodular regeneration that occur in the cirrhotic liver increase the resistance to portal blood flow, which increases the pressure in the portal and splanchnic veins. This increased hydrostatic pressure promotes the movement of fluid from the intravascular to the extravascular compartment. Although some of this increased interstitial fluid can be taken up by mesenteric lymphatics (producing increased flow in the thoracic duct), fluid production exceeds the capacity of lymphatic absorption and ascites is produced off the surfaces of the liver, bowel, and mesentery. The hypoalbuminemia associated with liver disease may contribute to the formation of ascites through a decrease in oncotic pressure in the postcapillary venule.

The underfill theory postulates that portal hypertension and hypoalbuminemia produce an imbalance of Starling forces across the portal vasculature with the loss of intravascular volume as ascites. Together with sequestration of blood in the splanchnic bed (caused by portal hypertension), this third-space loss of ascitic fluid produces a decrease in the effective circulating volume. This accounts for the secondary decreases in renal blood flow and glomerular filtration rate and stimulation of the renin-angiotensin-aldosterone system, which all contribute to sodium and water retention. This retention of sodium and water further aggravates the ascites, and the process becomes cyclical. The underfill theory, however, which focuses on portal hypertension as the primary etiologic factor, does not explain why in conditions of presinusoidal portal hypertension, including schistosomiasis and portal vein thrombosis, ascites was uncommon whereas in postsinusoidal obstruction, including acute right-sided heart failure and Budd-Chiari syndrome, ascites was characteristic.

It has now become clear that renal sodium and water retention with plasma volume expansion occurs before the development of ascites in man. This is the basis of the *overflow theory* originally proposed by Lieberman and associates in 1970,[3] which postulates a primary abnormality of renal function with progressive sodium and water retention in patients who have postsinusoidal portal hypertension. The cause of this lesion has yet to be defined.[4] It may be initiated by intrahepatic pressure receptors and may be neural or hormonally mediated. Abnormalities of atrial natriuretic factor responsiveness, impaired intrarenal prostaglandin production, sympathetic nervous system overactivity and unresponsiveness, and increased production of nitric oxide[5] may contribute to the progressive renal sodium retention. Sodium and water retention lead to expansion of the plasma volume. The alteration in Starling forces identified in the underfill theory account for the subsequent accumulation of the retained sodium and water as ascites in the abdominal cavity. The response to peritoneovenous shunting has been used to study the pathogenesis of ascites. Acutely, it decompresses the peritoneal cavity and, by establishing a sustained volume expansion, it has identified the role of hemodynamics,[6, 7] renin and aldosterone,[6, 7] vasopressin,[8] prostaglandins,[9] catecholamines,[10] and atrial natriuretic factor[4] in the etiology of sodium and water retention.

Although the overflow theory explains many of the observations early in the pathogenesis of ascites, it appears insufficient to explain the spectrum of renal dysfunction, particularly in decompensated cirrhosis, where the increased sympathetic nervous system activity, relative arterial hypotension, and elevated renin-angiotensin-aldosterone activity are more consistent with circulatory underfilling than volume expansion.

The most recent theory—the peripheral arterial vasodilatation hypothesis proposed by Schrier and colleagues[11] in 1988—suggests that the integrity of the arterial circulation, not the total plasma volume, is the major determinant of renal sodium and water handling. It proposes that the progressive arterial vasodilatation accompanies the stages of cirrhosis (from compensated to decompensated to hepatorenal syndrome). The major site of this vasodilatation may be the splanchnic arteries; however, the etiology of this vasodilatation remains unclear. Many factors, including opening of pre-existing shunts, increased nitric synthase activity, vasodilating prostaglandins, and others have been proposed. Arterial vasodilatation is accompanied by activation of the neurohumoral responses to arterial underfilling, which causes sodium and water retention and leads to plasma volume expansion. It is postulated that much of this expansion occurs in the venous compartment, which is estimated to comprise over 85% of the circulating volume, and that arterial refilling is not achieved. Sodium and water retention therefore persists. Whether this hypothesis can account for the events that initiate sodium retention or whether the primary hepatorenal dysfunction postulated by the overflow hypothesis can induce the onset of ascites without arterial vasodilatation remains to be determined.

CLINICAL MANIFESTATIONS OF ASCITES IN CHRONIC LIVER DISEASE

Although the development of ascites is usually chronic, ascitic fluid may accumulate rapidly in the presence of a hepatoma, hepatic vein thrombosis, or acute hepatitis superimposed on chronic cirrhosis. Transient ascites may develop after a laparotomy or from aggressive resuscitation of patients with variceal bleeding with large volumes of fluid. The presence of ascites in the patient with chronic liver disease usually indicates an advanced degree of liver dysfunction and is associated with a poor prognosis. One-year survival figures of less than 50% have been reported for patients with resistant ascites,[12] a prognosis that is similar to that of patients who have bled from esophageal varices.

In well-compensated cirrhotic patients, a small amount of ascites may go unnoticed, other than for a slight increase in abdominal girth, and requires no treatment. Severe ascites, however, may become disabling, with significant interference in activities of daily living. There may be pleural effusions and atelectasis with shortness of breath, swelling of the legs, and the development of umbilical and inguinal hernias. Patients with ascites are at risk for developing spontaneous bacterial peritonitis, which carries a 70% mortality rate. Abdominal distention may produce anorexia, which when combined with dietary restrictions for encephalopathy causes protein-calorie malnutrition with progressive muscle wasting.

MEDICAL TREATMENT OF ASCITES

When ascites becomes symptomatic, treatment is directed toward the reduction, but not necessarily the complete elimination of ascites. Some patients can be managed with dietary restriction of 1 gm. sodium and 1 liter of fluid per day. If the ascites is more resistant, diuretics may be added, beginning with an aldosterone antagonist such as spironolactone or amiloride. If this is insufficient, a loop diuretic, such as furosemide or a thiazide, should be added. In general, loop diuretics should not be the sole therapeutic agents. Diuretics should be added cautiously, and renal function must be closely monitored. In general, any peripheral edema responds to diuretics before ascites. Once dependent edema has resolved, diuretic therapy should aim to mobilize no more than 1 liter of fluid or 1 kg. of body weight per day.

Serious complications can result from the chronic and overly aggressive use of diuretics in cirrhotic patients, particularly when combined with intermittent therapeutic paracentesis. These include hyponatremia, hypokalemia, metabolic alkalosis, hypocalcemia, and hypomagnesemia. When these diuretics are used, muscle cramps, particularly in the calves, are common and difficult to manage. Excessive diuresis can aggravate hypovolemia and produce prerenal failure with oliguria and acute tubular necrosis or may precipitate the hepatorenal syndrome.

Therapeutic paracentesis can be effective in removing all ascites and may be necessary in patients with tense ascites with shortness of breath from the increased intra-abdominal pressure and elevated diaphragm. Despite previous concerns that after large-volume paracentesis (more than 5 liters) the reaccumulation of ascites might reduce intravascular volume and precipitate hypotension and/or renal failure, a number of carefully designed trials have demonstrated the safety of carefully supervised, repeated paracenteses with 5% albumin infusion[13] or single total paracentesis with albumin infusion.[14] These studies demonstrated that, compared with diuretic therapy alone, paracentesis with albumin infusion is more effective in eliminating ascites, does not cause significant changes in hemodynamics or hepatic or renal function, was associated with a lower incidence of electrolyte abnormalities, and had a shorter hospitalization with similar rates of readmission and survival. A subsequent trial of large-volume paracentesis without albumin infusion, however, was associated with significant impairment of renal function,[15] emphasizing the importance of colloid infusion after large volume paracentesis and close monitoring of the patient. Smaller, repeated paracenteses without colloid infusion appear to be safe.[13] In a randomized trial comparing paracentesis and albumin infusion against the LeVeen shunt, peritoneovenous shunting controlled the ascites better in the long term; however, total hospitalization and overall survival were the same.[16] Intermittent large-volume paracentesis with albumin replacement (performed on an outpatient basis) with judicious use of sodium restriction and diuretics and close monitoring of renal function has become a common strategy for the long-term management of diuretic-resistant ascites. This technique is also valuable in the cirrhotic patient who develops acute ascites after portosystemic shunt to avoid an ascitic leak through the wound.

SURGICAL TREATMENT OF ASCITES

The majority of patients with ascites respond to diet and diuretic therapy. In those with persistent ascites and adequate hepatic function, surgical intervention may be an alternative to long-term, repeated large-volume paracentesis. Surgical procedures for intractable ascites have been directed toward either decreasing production of ascites or increasing its resorption (Table 33–12).

Portosystemic Shunting. Physiologic side-to-side portosystemic shunts (side-to-side portacaval, mesocaval, or proximal splenorenal anastomoses) lower pressure in both the splanchnic veins and the intrahepatic portal system, which theoretically should decrease the rate of ascites formation. There is substantial evidence from animal models and in patients with the Budd-Chiari syndrome to support the use of side-to-side shunting when both bleeding and uncontrolled ascites require surgical treatment.[17] In a study of pa-

TABLE 33–12. Surgical Management of Intractable Ascites

Decreases production
    Lymphovenous anastomosis
    Side-to-side portosystemic shunting
    Omentopexy
Increases removal or resorption
    Paracentesis
    Paracentesis with reinfusion
    Peritoneovenous anastomosis
    Peritoneovenous shunting

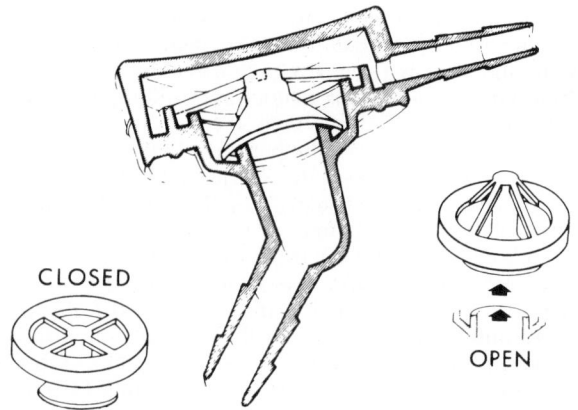

Figure 33–46. A cross section of the LeVeen valve. Note that the silicone rubber struts are attached to a ring that attaches to the valve casing. The valve is in the normally closed position and opens with 3 cm. of water pressure. (From LeVeen, H. H., et al.: Further experience with peritoneovenous shunt for ascites. Ann. Surg., *184*:574, 1976.)

tients undergoing a portosystemic shunt procedure for bleeding esophageal varices, compared with patients managed with injection sclerotherapy or esophageal transection, the probability of developing ascites was lower (15% vs. 73%) and the incidence of both spontaneous bacterial peritonitis and hepatorenal syndrome was lower (2% to 4% vs. 21% for each) in the shunted group.[18]

Side-to-side shunting has been used for intractable ascites alone, but because of the mortality and the incidence of postshunt encephalopathy, the risk of portosystemic shunting for ascites alone has been considered prohibitive. More recent experience with portosystemic shunting for ascites alone in carefully selected patients has confirmed its effectiveness in controlling ascites, but the 50% incidence of encephalopathy is a strong argument against its general acceptance.[19]

Transjugular Intrahepatic Portosystemic Shunt. The transjugular intrahepatic portosystemic shunt was first described in man in 1982 as therapy for bleeding varices.[20] With the addition of an expandable stent to maintain patency, its ability to significantly reduce portal pressure has been applied more widely.[21] It has become attractive as a *bridge* to liver transplantation in patients whose bleeding varices have not been well controlled with sclerotherapy.[22] Hemodynamically, it functions as a type of side-to-side portacaval shunt. It may be expected therefore that this shunt should be effective in controlling ascites. Preliminary reports of small numbers of patients who had ascites at the time of the shunt procedure have suggested a response rate of 50% to 67%.[20, 24] The complications of shunt occlusion (over 30%) and hepatic encephalopathy (over 20%) may limit the usefulness of this new technology as primary therapy for ascites.

Peritoneovenous Shunting. Peritoneovenous shunting is based on an extension of the principles of paracentesis with reinfusion studies and involves the implantation of a prosthetic conduit with a one-way valve between the peritoneal cavity and the intrathoracic vascular compartment. The shunt receiving the widest use and most careful study is that devised by LeVeen and first reported in 1974 (Fig. 33–46).[25] It consists of a pressure-activated one-way valve with peritoneal and venous Silastic catheters. The pressure gradient between positive intraperitoneal and negative intrathoracic pressures promotes fluid flow from the abdomen to the intrathoracic vascular space.

Other valves, such as the Denver shunt (Fig. 33–47),[26] have been developed as alternatives to the LeVeen valve and incorporate features that allow active pumping of fluid from the peritoneal cavity to the venous compartment. One randomized trial in 21 cirrhotic patients has suggested that the LeVeen valve has a superior patency rate of 40% at 2 years compared with the Denver shunt; however, the survival was similar in the two groups.[27]

Indications. The most common indication for a peritoneovenous shunt is chronic intractable ascites due to cirrhosis. Up to 10% of patients with significant ascites become refractory to management with diet and diuretics with or

without repeated large-volume paracentesis and colloid reinfusion. Intractable ascites has been associated with progressive muscle loss, and repeated paracentesis may be complicated by intra-abdominal bleeding, bacterial infection, and loculation of ascites. In some patients, a strategy of repeated paracentesis may not be logistically possible and others may require repeated hospital admissions for their ascites. The peritoneovenous shunt may be effective in achieving better long-term control.[16] The results of peritoneovenous shunting vary depending on the severity of the renal and hepatocellular dysfunction of the patient being shunted. The shunt should not be used in patients who can be managed with diet and diuretics but should be reserved for those who fail closely supervised medical management.

The peritoneovenous shunt has been used in the treatment of the hepatorenal syndrome. This form of functional renal failure must be distinguished from prerenal failure produced by diuretic- or paracentesis-induced central blood volume constriction with acute tubular necrosis. The peritoneovenous shunt has been reported to reverse the hepatorenal syn-

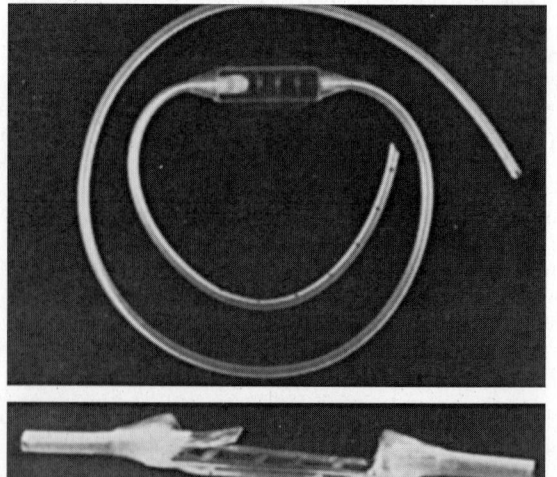

Figure 33–47. Denver peritoneovenous shunt. The shunt is made of silicone rubber and consists of a fenestrated peritoneal catheter, a pump chamber with a one-way valve, and a venous catheter. The valve is shown magnified with the pump chamber partly removed. (Reprinted with permission from Turner, W. W., Jr., and Pate, R. M.: The Denver peritoneovenous shunt: Relationship between hepatic reserve and successful treatment of ascites. Am. J. Surg., *144*:619, 1982. Copyright 1982 by Excerpta Medica Inc.)

drome, but because of advanced liver disease, these patients are a very high risk for the procedure and postoperative complications.[28] Postoperative ascites may develop in the cirrhotic patient after any abdominal operation, but especially after portosystemic shunting procedures. This may be secondary to aggressive intravenous therapy in the perioperative period combined with the division of periportal or retroperitoneal lymphatics at the time of the procedure. Repeated large-volume paracentesis with colloid infusion is successful in most patients. If the postoperative ascites is severe and reaccumulates rapidly, an early peritoneovenous shunt is usually effective.

Contraindications. Peritoneovenous shunting is contraindicated in any patient with infected peritoneal fluid or other source of sepsis, acute viral or alcoholic hepatitis, end-stage liver disease, or uncorrectable coagulopathy. A serum bilirubin value of more than three times the upper limit of normal has generally been considered a contraindication.[29, 30] The presence of any one of the following risk factors has been reported to be associated with a 50% mortality within the first postoperative month and should be considered a relative contraindication[31]: (1) an episode of gastrointestinal bleeding or peritonitis within the previous month; (2) hepatic encephalopathy greater than Grade 1; (3) complications of alcoholism such as pancreatitis, cardiomyopathy, or neuropathy; (4) an uncomplicated hernia; (5) severe malnutrition; (6) a prothrombin time prolonged more than 4 seconds; or (7) a serum creatinine value more than 2.3 times the upper limit of normal. Patients who have had a previous variceal hemorrhage remain at risk for rebleeding after shunting because of the transient increase in portal pressure and the coagulopathy that accompanies the procedure. If the esophageal varices have not been obliterated by repeated injection sclerotherapy, or there has been recent bleeding, patients may be better treated by a side-to-side portosystemic shunt.

Procedure. A diagnostic paracentesis is performed to exclude infection (negative culture and a cell count less than $250 \times 10^6/L.$) or malignancy. Liver biopsy (transjugular) and detailed liver tests including coagulation studies are performed. Perioperatively, prophylactic antibiotics, such as a cephalosporin and an aminoglycoside, should be administered to cover both skin and gastrointestinal tract organisms.

The shunt may be inserted with the patient under local or general anesthesia (Fig. 33–48). The LeVeen valve is placed in the abdominal wall deep to the rectus muscle. A pumpable valve (e.g., Denver shunt) is placed over the chest wall or lower end of the sternum. The peritoneal end lies freely in the ascites. The venous limb is tunneled subcutaneously and may be inserted into the superior vena cava through either the internal jugular or the subclavian vein. During the operation, the tip is directed under radiologic control to lie just below the junction of the superior vena cava and the right atrium. A tip that is left too high in the superior vena cava or innominate vein will predispose to catheter blockage and venous thrombosis. Meticulous hemostasis is important to prevent the occurrence of hematoma and ecchymosis. The incidence of postoperative coagulopathy may be reduced by draining all of the ascitic fluid and replacing it with body-temperature Ringer's lactate.[25, 26] Some surgeons discard most of the ascitic fluid at surgery to reduce the incidence of pulmonary edema.[23]

Prophylactic antibiotics are continued for up to 48 hours. Inspiratory exercises are used to decrease intrathoracic pressure and increase the gradient across the valve and promote ascites flow. Small doses of intravenous furosemide may be necessary to maintain the urine output at greater than 60 ml. per minute. Body weight, abdominal girth, and the hematocrit, serum electrolytes, and coagulation status are monitored closely.

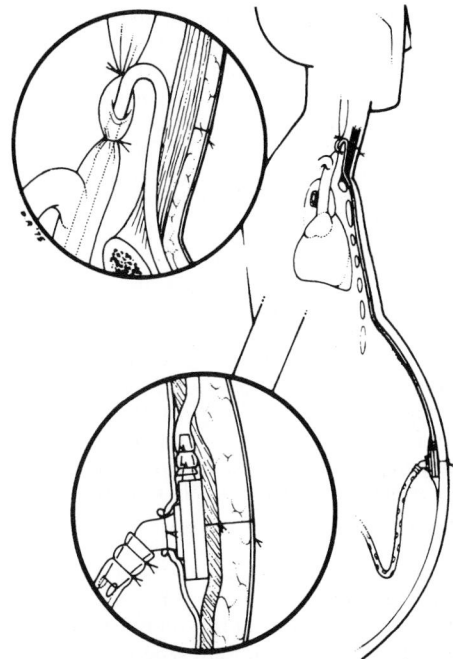

Figure 33–48. The valve lies outside the peritoneum and deep to the abdominal muscles. The venous collecting tube traverses the subcutaneous tissue of the chest wall into the neck, where it enters the internal jugular vein. The top of the tubing is pushed into the superior vena cava (7.5 cm.). (From LeVeen, H. H., et al.: Further experience with peritoneovenous shunt for ascites. Ann. Surg., *184*:574, 1976.)

Results. With reinfusion of the ascitic fluid there is an increase in the total circulating blood volume, a hemodilutional fall in hematocrit, an increase in the cardiac output, and a decrease in the systemic vascular resistance. There is an early rise in renal blood flow and glomerular filtration rate and an associated decrease in renin and aldosterone levels. In some patients, spontaneous natriuresis and diuresis occur; however, most patients require small doses of furosemide to produce and maintain the diuresis and natriuresis that are characteristic of a functioning shunt and that lead to progressive loss of ascites, abdominal girth, and weight.[6]

Early postoperative complications occur in up to 80% of patients[33, 34] and include infection, leak of ascitic fluid, variceal hemorrhage, pulmonary edema, coagulation disorders, shunt migration or blockage, and cardiac arrhythmias. All patients develop a degree of coagulopathy with prolongation of the prothrombin and partial thromboplastin times and a fall in platelet count, and up to 20% may develop clinical manifestations of disseminated intravascular coagulation.[35] The degree of coagulopathy and the incidence of disseminated intravascular coagulation have been reduced by discarding most of the ascites intraoperatively, with or without replacement with saline or Ringer's lactate.[30, 32] Clinical disseminated intravascular coagulation is treated by temporarily ligating the shunt and providing fresh frozen plasma, cryoprecipitate, and platelets. Epsilon-aminocaproic acid may also be useful in this setting.[35] The coagulation defect is usually self-limited, resolving after a few days.

Patients undergoing peritoneovenous shunting are a high risk group for infectious complications from malnutrition and reduced cell-mediated immunity.[36] Previous episodes of spontaneous bacterial peritonitis increase the risk of postoperative shunt infection. When it occurs, shunt infection is a serious complication that always requires shunt removal and systemic antibiotic therapy.

Blockage of the shunt may occur by omentum migration

into the tubing, kinking, thrombus formation at the tip of the venous limb, or the collection of fibrin and other peritoneal debris within the valve. The diagnosis of shunt occlusion can be made with either an intraperitoneal injection of technetium-99m sulfur colloid and scanning of the chest[37] or a direct percutaneous injection of radiopaque contrast medium into the venous limb.[38] With the latter technique, a more precise identification of point of occlusion (valve, venous tubing, or thrombus) can be made. In the event of a blocked valve with a patent venous limb, it is usually possible to replace only the valve and peritoneal limb.

The operative mortality ranges up to 30%.[33] The major causes of early death are infection and complications of the underlying liver disease, including hepatic failure and variceal hemorrhage. Variations in operative mortality and survival reported reflect the severity of the liver disease and renal dysfunction in the groups of patients being selected for shunting procedures. With careful patient selection and improved perioperative care, operative mortality may be less than 5%.[30]

The renal and hemodynamic changes persist in the late postoperative period. Most patients have normal levels of renin and aldosterone and persistent improvements in creatinine clearance and sodium and water excretion. However, many continue to retain sodium when challenged with a high-sodium diet, and most require small doses of diuretics even with a functioning shunt.[39] Others become free of ascites without diet or diuretic therapy.[36] In some patients, ascites remains under control with diuretics, even if the shunt becomes blocked.[40, 41]

With the control of ascites, many patients demonstrate an improvement in nutritional status with an increase in serum albumin and transferrin levels, an improvement in cell-mediated immunity,[36] and an increase in lean body mass[36, 42] with an obvious gain in muscle bulk. These improvements likely result from an improved well-being and increase in appetite and dietary intake.[42]

Late complications occur in a significant proportion of surviving patients and include shunt blockage, infection, superior vena caval thrombosis, and obstruction of the small bowel. The shunt patency rate of 5-year survivors has been reported to be as low as 40%, and the incidence of thrombosis of the superior vena cava has been over 25%.[40] With improved patient selection and perioperative technique, the shunt occlusion rate may be reduced to 12% at 2 years.[30] Most of the late postoperative deaths are due to bleeding esophageal varices and hepatic failure.

Peritoneovenous shunting does not prolong life. One study comparing the peritoneovenous shunt with diuretic therapy in 28 patients refractory to sodium restriction alone suggested improved survival with the shunt.[43] However, two subsequent multicenter, randomized studies of 57 patients in France[34] and 299 men in the United States[31] showed no difference between diet and diuretic therapy and peritoneovenous shunting. In both groups, the early mortality (30 days) ranged from 20% to 50%, depending on the severity of the liver disease, and the 1-year survival ranged from 25% to 79%. These authors identified a modest benefit in favor of the shunt, which was limited to control of ascites predominantly in the first month. A subsequent prospective, randomized trial of LeVeen shunting versus repeated paracentesis with albumin infusion in 89 patients in Spain demonstrated equivalence between the two therapies.[16] The ascites response rate was the same. Although the initial hospitalization was longer for the shunted patients, and the readmission rate was higher with paracentesis, total hospitalization was the same. The 3-year survival was the same (approximately 33%). In other uncontrolled series, the survival curves after insertion of the peritoneovenous shunt have been similar to older studies of patients who developed ascites before the introduction of the LeVeen valve, with a 50% to 75% 1-year survival and 30% to 40% survival at 2 years.[16, 27, 29] A more recent report has suggested that with careful patient selection and improved perioperative technique, the 2-year survival after shunting may be improved to 55%.[30]

In cirrhotic patients with intractable ascites, peritoneovenous shunting should be considered to be only a palliative procedure. Although the operation is appealing because of its apparent technical simplicity and the early postoperative diuresis, the postoperative complication rate is high. Long-term survival appears to be determined mainly by the natural history of the liver disease. A review in 1990 concluded that the patient undergoing peritoneovenous shunting may be expected to have an 18% perioperative mortality, a 46% survival rate at 21 months, and control of ascites in 59% of those who survive more than 18 months.[41] The equivalent efficacy of either diuretic therapy or repeated paracentesis compared with shunting has led to a significant reduction in the use of the peritoneovenous shunt.

Patients must be selected carefully. In a patient who is or may be a candidate for liver transplantation, peritoneovenous shunting should be avoided—it does not alter the course of the underlying liver disease, the procedure has a significant morbidity and mortality, and the occurrence of thrombosis of the superior vena cava poses a significant relative contraindication to the transplant operation. Two groups of patients appear to be the best candidates for peritoneovenous shunting: (1) those in whom uncontrollable ascites develops immediately after abdominal operations and (2) those whose chronic, intractable ascites is out of keeping with the other complications of portal hypertension and hepatocellular dysfunction.

PERITONEOVENOUS SHUNT FOR MALIGNANT ASCITES

Malignant ascites occurs most commonly with intraperitoneal spread of ovarian, colonic, or breast cancer caused by increased fluid production (from the tumor or peritoneal surface inflammation) and reduced reabsorption (from lymphatic obstruction).[44] The majority of patients obtain palliation from a combination of paracentesis and chemotherapy and/or radiation therapy. In selected patients who are unresponsive to this treatment and who do not have loculated fluid, peritoneovenous shunting may be indicated and the ascites may be controlled in approximately two thirds of patients.[45]

In a series of 42 patients with malignant ascites treated with a peritoneovenous shunt, compared with 43 treated with paracentesis followed by intraperitoneal doxorubicin, the ascites was controlled by the shunt in 64%. The median survival from the time of diagnosis of ascites was 137 days in the shunted group and 91 days in those not shunted. Survival was best for those with breast cancer. There was no difference in total hospitalization or measurements of quality of life between the two groups.[45] The equivalence of paracentesis with peritoneovenous shunting suggests a limited role for surgery in these patients with limited life expectancy.

Complications are similar to those in the cirrhotic population,[46] and the operative mortality is similar.[40] Shunt occlusion is more frequent, especially in patients with bloody or viscid ascitic fluid, high protein content (greater than 4.5 gm. per liter), or positive cytology. These factors are therefore relative contraindications to its use. Tumor embolism occurs in approximately 5% of patients and occasionally produces acute respiratory failure and death.[47] In spite of these complications, 60% to 75% of patients obtain useful palliation, with the best results occurring in patients with carcinoma of the ovary or breast.[46] In general, the median reported survival, however, is only 3 months.[46, 47]

SELECTED REFERENCES

LeVeen, H. H., Christoudias, G., Ip, M., Luft, R., Falk, G., and Grosberg, S.: Peritoneovenous shunting for ascites. Ann. Surg., 180:580, 1974.
This is the first report of the clinical use of the LeVeen valve. It outlines the principle of the pressure-activated valve and the experimental data behind the first clinical application of the device.

Blendis, L. M., Greig, P. D., Langer, B., Baigrie, R. S., Ruse, J., and Taylor, B. R.: The renal and hemodynamic effects of the peritoneovenous shunt for intractable hepatic ascites. Gastroenterology, 77:250, 1979.
This is a report of the clinical, hemodynamic, and metabolic changes in 15 patients with chronic liver disease having peritoneovenous shunts. This study also documents the significant complication rate associated with this procedure in poor-risk patients with advanced liver disease.

Stanley, M. M., Ochi, S., Lee, K. K., Nemchausky, B. A., Greenlee, H. B., Allen, J. I., et al.: Peritoneovenous shunting as compared with medical treatment in patients with alcoholic cirrhosis and massive ascites. N. Engl. J. Med., 321:1632, 1989.
This prospective study randomized 299 men with alcoholic cirrhosis and ascites resistant to a standard medical regimen to receive a LeVeen shunt or intensive diet and diuretic therapy. Patients were grouped into four risk categories on the basis of the severity of liver dysfunction, previous complications, and renal dysfunction. The authors conclude that peritoneovenous shunting alleviates disabling ascites more rapidly than medical management and delays its recurrence; however, the duration of survival was more closely related to the severity of the illness and was not altered by shunting. This is an important study that has identified a number of risk factors that constitute contraindications to LeVeen shunting.

Wong, F., and Blendis, L. M. (Eds.): Hepatorenal Disorders. Semin. Liver Dis., 14:1, 1994.
This is a collection of manuscripts by many of the basic and clinical investigators of the pathogenesis of ascites formation in cirrhotic patients with portal hypertension. The current knowledge regarding the pathophysiology that has been identified in the progressive phases of ascites and the current, somewhat conflicting, theories which may explain the initiation and ongoing formation of ascites are presented.

Hillaire, S., Labianca, M., Borgonovo, G., Smadja, C., Grange, D., and Franco, D.: Peritoneovenous shunting of intractable ascites in patients with cirrhosis: Improving results and predictors of failure. Surgery, 113:373, 1993.
This report of the results of peritoneovenous shunting in 56 cirrhotic patients with intractable ascites demonstrates how careful patient selection and improved perioperative management can combine to improve the morbidity and mortality of the procedure. The long-term outcome was dictated by the development of complications of the underlying liver disease with most deaths attributable to bleeding esophageal varices and spontaneous bacterial peritonitis. The authors suggest that the peritoneovenous shunt may be beneficial only in selected patients who would not be candidates for liver transplantation.

REFERENCES

1. Epstein, M.: Renal sodium handling in cirrhosis. *In* Epstein, M. (Ed.): The Kidney in Liver Disease, 3rd ed. Baltimore, Williams & Wilkins, 1988, pp. 3–30.
2. Levy, M.: Pathophysiology of the hepatorenal syndrome and potential for therapy. Am. J. Cardiol., 60:661, 1987.
3. Lieberman, F. L., Denison, E. K., and Reynolds, T. B.: The relationship of plasma volume portal hypertension, ascites, and renal sodium retention in cirrhosis: The overflow theory of ascites formation. Ann. N.Y. Acad. Sci., 170:202, 1970.
4. Wong, F., and Blendis, L.: Pathophysiology of sodium retention and ascites formation in cirrhosis: Role of atrial natriuretic factor. Semin. Liver Dis., 14:59, 1994.
5. Michielsen, P. P., and Pelckmans, P. A.: Hemodynamic changes in portal hypertension: New insights in the pathogenesis and clinical implications. Acta Gastroenterol. Belg., 57:194, 1994.
6. Blendis, L. M., Greig, P. D., Langer, B., Baigrie, R. S., Ruse, J., and Taylor, B. R.: The renal and hemodynamic effects of the peritoneovenous shunt for intractable hepatic ascites. Gastroenterology, 77:250, 1979.
7. Greig, P. D., Blendis, L. M., Langer, B., Ruse, J., and Taylor, B. R.: The acute effects of sustained volume expansion on the renin-aldosterone system and renal function in human hepatic ascites. J. Lab. Clin. Med., 98:127, 1981.
8. Reznick, R. K., Langer, B., Taylor, B. R., Seif, S., and Blendis, L. M.: Hyponatraemia and arginine vasopressin secretion in patients with refractory hepatic ascites undergoing peritoneovenous shunting. Gastroenterology, 84:713, 1983.
9. Shaw-Stiffel, T., Campbell, P. J., Sole, M. J., Greig, P. D., Wong, P. Y., and Blendis, L. M.: Renal prostaglandin E_2 and other vasoactive modulators in refractory hepatic ascites: Response to peritoneovenous shunting. Gastroenterology, 95:1332, 1988.
10. Blendis, L. M., Sole, M. J., Campbell, P., Lossing, A. G., Greig, P. D.,
11. Schrier, R. W.: Pathogenesis of sodium and water retention in high-output and low-output cardiac failure, nephrotic syndrome, cirrhosis and pregnancy. N. Engl. J. Med., 319:1065, 1988.
12. Capone, R. R., Buhac, I., Kohberger, R. C., et al.: Resistant ascites in alcoholic liver disease: Course and prognosis. Dig. Dis. Sci., 23:867, 1979.
13. Gines, P., Arroyo, V., Quintero, E., Planas, R., Bory, F., Cabrera, J., Rimola, A., Viver, J., Camps, J., Jimenez, W., Mastai, R., Gaya, J., and Rodes, J.: Comparison of paracentesis and diuretics in the treatment of cirrhotics with tense ascites. Gastroenterology, 93:234, 1987.
14. Tito, L. I., Gines, P., Arroyo, V., and Rodes, J.: Total paracentesis associated with intravenous albumin in the management of patients with cirrhosis and ascites. Gastroenterology, 98:146, 1990.
15. Gines, P., Tito, L. I., Arroyo, V., and Rodes, J.: Randomized comparative study of therapeutic paracentesis with and without intravenous albumin in cirrhosis. Gastroenterology, 94:1493, 1988.
16. Gines, P., Arroyo, V., Vargas, V., Planas, R., Casafont, F., Panes, J., Hoyos, M., Viladomiu, L., Rimola, A., Morillas, R., Salmeron, J. M., Gines, A., Esteban, R., and Rodes, J.: Paracentesis with intravenous infusion of albumin as compared with peritoneovenous shunting in cirrhosis with refractory ascites. N. Engl. J. Med., 325:829, 1991.
17. Orloff, M. J.: Pathogenesis and surgical treatment of intractable ascites associated with alcoholic cirrhosis. Ann. N.Y. Acad. Sci., 170:202, 1970.
18. Castells, A., Salo, J., Planas, R., Quer, J. C., Gines, A., Boix, J., Gines, P., Gassull, M. A., Teres, J., Arroyo, V., and Rodes, J.: Impact of shunt surgery for variceal bleeding in the natural history of ascites in cirrhosis: A retrospective study. Hepatology, 20:584, 1994.
19. Elcheroth, J., Vons, C., and Franco, D.: Role of surgical therapy in management of intractable ascites. World J. Surg., 18:240, 1994.
20. Colapinto, R. F., Stronell, R. D., Birch, S. J., Greig, P. D., Taylor, B. R., and Langer, B.: Creation of an intrahepatic portosystemic shunt with a Gruntzig balloon catheter. Can. Med. Assoc. J., 26:267, 1982.
21. Richter, G. M., Noeldge, G., Roessle, M., et al.: Transjugular intrahepatic portosystemic stent shunt (TIPSS). Radiology, 174:1027, 1990.
22. Freeman, R. B., Jr., FitzMaurice, S. E., Greenfield, A. E., Halin, N., Haug, C. E., and Rohrer, R. J.: Is the transjugular intrahepatic portacaval shunt beneficial for liver transplant patients? Transplantation, 58:297, 1994.
23. Rousseau, H., Vinel, J. P., Bilbao, J. I., Longo, J. M., Maquin, P., Zozaya, J. M., Garcia-Villareal, L., Coustet, B., Railhac, N., and Railhac, J. J.: Transjugular intrahepatic portosystemic shunts using the Wallstent prosthesis: A follow-up study. Cardiovasc. Intervent. Radiol., 17:7, 1994.
24. Ferral, H., Bjarnason, H., Wegryn, S. A., Rengel, G. J., Nazarian, G. K., Rank, J. M., Tadavarthy, S. M., Hunter, D. W., and Castaneda-Zuniga, W. R.: Refractory ascites: Early experience in treatment with transjugular intrahepatic portosystemic shunt. Radiology, 189:795, 1993.
25. LeVeen, H. H., Christoudias, G., Ip, M., Luft, R., Falk, G., and Grosberg, S.: Peritoneovenous shunting for ascites. Ann. Surg., 180:580, 1974.
26. Turner, W. W., Jr., Pate, R. M.: The Denver peritoneovenous shunt: Relationship between hepatic reserve and successful treatment of ascites. Am. J. Surg., 144:619, 1982.
27. Fulenwider, J. T., Galambos, J. D., Smith, R. B., III, Henderson, J. M., and Warren, W. D.: LeVeen vs Denver peritoneovenous shunts for intractable ascites of cirrhosis: A randomized, prospective trial. Arch. Surg., 121:351, 1986.
28. Epstein, M.: Peritoneovenous shunt in the management of ascites and the hepatorenal syndrome. Gastroenterology, 82:790, 1982.
29. Fulenwider, J. T., Smith, R. B., III, Redd, S. C., Ansley, J. D., Henderson, J. M., Millikan, W. F., Galambos, J. T., and Warren, W. D.: Peritoneovenous shunts: Lessons learned from an eight-year experience with 70 patients. Arch. Surg., 119:1133, 1984.
30. Hillaire, S., Labianca, M., Borgonovo, G., Smadja, C., Grange, D., and Franco, D.: Peritoneovenous shunting of intractable ascites in patients with cirrhosis: Improving results and predictors of failure. Surgery, 113:373, 1993.
31. Stanley, M. M., Ochi, S., Lee, K. K., Nemchausky, B. A., Greenlee, H. B., Allen, J. I., et al.: Peritoneovenous shunting as compared with medical treatment in patients with alcoholic cirrhosis and massive ascites. N. Engl. J. Med., 321:1632, 1989.
32. Biagini, J. R., Belghiti, J., and Fekete, F.: Prevention of coagulopathy after placement of peritoneovenous shunt with replacement of ascitic fluid by normal saline solution. Surg. Gynecol. Obstet., 163:315, 1986.
33. Greig, P. D., Langer, B., Blendis, L. M., Taylor, B. R., and Glynn, M. F. X.: Complications after peritoneovenous shunting for ascites. Am. J. Surg., 139:125, 1980.
34. Bories, P., Compean, D. G., Michel, H., Bourel, M., Capron, J. P., Gauthier, A., Lafon, J., Levy, V. G., Pascal, J. P., Quinton, A., Tournieux, B., and Weill, J. P.: The treatment of refractory ascites by the LeVeen shunt: A multi-centre controlled trial (57 patients). J. Hepatol., 3:212, 1986.
35. LeVeen, H. H., Ahmed, N., Hutto, R. B., Ip, M., and LeVeen, E. G.: Coagulopathy post peritoneovenous shunt. Ann. Surg., 205:305, 1987.
36. Franco, D., Charra, M., Jeambrun, P., Belghiti, J., Cortesse, A., Sossler, C., and Bismuth, H.: Nutrition and immunity after peritoneovenous drainage of intractable ascites in cirrhotic patients. Am. J. Surg., 146:652, 1983.
37. Kirchmer, N., and Hart, U.: Radionuclide assessment of LeVeen shunt patency. Ann. Surg., 185:145, 1977.
38. Taylor, B. R., and Langer, B.: The effect of peritoneovenous shunting on catecholamine metabolism in patients with hepatic ascites. Hepatology, 7:143, 1987.

38. Schwartz, M. L., and Miller, R. P.: Angiographic assessment of peritoneovenous shunt malfunction. Arch. Surg., *116*:435, 1981.
39. Greig, P. D., Blendis, L. M., Langer, B., Taylor, B. R., and Colapinto, R. F.: Renal and hemodynamic effects of the peritoneovenous shunt: II. Long-term effects. Gastroenterology, *80*:119, 1981.
40. Franco, D., Meakins, J. L., Wu, A., Smadja, C., Bonnet, P., Gouffier, E., and Campillo, B.: Long-term results (>5 years) in patients with peritoneovenous shunting for intractable ascites: Liver function and cancer mortality. HPB Surg., *1*:185, 1989.
41. Moskovitz, M.: The peritoneovenous shunt: Expectations and reality. Am. J. Gastroenterol., *85*:917, 1990.
42. Blendis, L. M., Harrison, J. E., Russell, D. M., Miller, C., Taylor, B. R., Greig, P. D., and Langer, B.: Effects of peritoneovenous shunting on body composition. Gastroenterology, *90*:127, 1986.

43. Wapnick, S., Grosberg, S. J., and Evans, M. I.: Randomized prospective matched pair study comparing peritoneovenous shunt and conventional therapy in massive ascites. Br. J. Surg., *66*:667, 1979.
44. Nagy, J. A., Hertzberg, K. T., Dvorak, J. M., and Dvorak, H. F.: Pathogenesis of malignant ascites formation: Initiating events that lead to fluid accumulation. Cancer Res., *53*:2631, 1993.
45. Gough, I. R., and Balderson, G. A.: Malignant ascites: A comparison of peritoneovenous shunting and nonoperative management. Cancer, *71*:2377, 1993.
46. Edney, J. A., Hill, A., and Armstrong, D.: Peritoneovenous shunts palliate malignant ascites. Am. J. Surg., *158*:598, 1989.
47. Cheung, D. K., and Raaf, J. H.: Selection of patients with malignant ascites for a peritoneovenous shunt. Cancer, *50*:1204, 1982.

VII

VIRAL HEPATITIS AND THE SURGEON

John D. Hamilton, M.D.

Blumberg's discovery of the Australia antigen in 1965 and the technological advances of the past three decades have led to a virtual explosion of new information about viral hepatitis. Although itself not a surgical disease, viral hepatitis is an important concern to both the surgical patient and the surgeon. In this section the basic concepts about the viral hepatitides are summarized, focusing particularly on those viruses most relevant to the practicing surgeon. Excellent texts, reviews, monographs, and papers are available and should be consulted for more detailed information.[6, 13, 26, 33, 37]

HISTORY

The landmarks in the evolution of knowledge about viral hepatitis are shown in Table 33–13. It is noteworthy how rapidly understanding of this disorder has accelerated.

DEFINITION

Viral hepatitis is an infection of the liver caused by one of at least six groups of viruses: hepatitis A virus (HAV) (known formerly as causing infectious hepatitis); hepatitis B virus (HBV) (known formerly as causing serum hepatitis); hepatitis C virus (HCV), the recently recognized virus that is associated with parenterally transmitted non-A, non-B hepatitis (PT-NANB); hepatitis D virus (HDV), known also as the agent that causes delta-associated hepatitis; hepatitis E virus (HEV), the virus responsible for enterically transmitted non-

A, non-B hepatitis (ET-NANB); and two new viruses, designated hepatitis F and G (HFV and HGV), that cause clinical disease but are distinct from each other and from hepatitis A–E.[14, 34]

ETIOLOGY

Virus Characterization. Selected features of each viral agent are listed in Table 33–14. Until recently, the causes of viral hepatitis were not distinguished other than by certain epidemiologic criteria. It is now evident that the viral causes are very different.

Nomenclature. Familiarity with the terms that describe the hepatitis virus antigens and antibodies is essential to the understanding of this group of diseases. The currently recommended terms and the available tests and their interpretation are shown in Table 33–15. The sequence of development of the various hepatitis markers is presented in Figure 33–49.

No antigens common to two or more viral agents have been identified. Within each class of virus, no differences in the virulence or the nature of the ultimate disease have been found between subtypes or strains, although there is now a description of viral variants that seem to modify the immune response and therefore, potentially, the clinical consequences.[16]

PATHOGENESIS

The pathogenesis of viral hepatitis is incompletely understood, but two theories have been proposed. One theory

TABLE 33–13. Chronology of the History of Hepatitis

Period/Date	Event	Source
Early civilizations	Recognition of jaundice as a disease	Talmud/Hippocrates
1885	"Hepatitis" determined to be parenterally transmitted	Lurman
1942	28,000 cases of epidemic hepatitis in U.S. military	Seeff
1947	Epidemiology distinguished bloodborne (hepatitis B) and enteric hepatitis (hepatitis A)	MacCallum
1965	Australia antigen (hepatitis B surface antigen) discovered	Blumberg
1966	Non-A, non-B hepatitis (NANB) proposed	Mosley
1970	Complete hepatitis B virion visualized	Dane
1973	Hepatitis A visualized by electron microscopy	Feinstone
1977	Hepatitis D antigen detected and found dependent on hepatitis B	Rizzetto
1987	Hepatitis E discovered to be one form of enterically transmitted NANB	Balayan
1989	Parenterally transmitted NANB found to be hepatitis C	Choo
1994	Non A–E hepatitis virus suggested	Bradley

TABLE 33–14. Characteristics of the Hepatitis Viruses

Virus	Virus Family/ Genus	Size	Nucleic Acid	Sequenced and/or Cloned	Grown in Tissue Culture	Identified by Electron Microscopy	Specific Serologic Tests	Infectious for Animals	Special Characteristics
HAV	Picornaviridae/ hepatovirus 72	27 nm.	Single-stranded positive-sense RNA; 7.5 kb.	Yes	Yes	Yes	Yes	Yes	
HBV	Hepadnaviridae/ hepadnavirus type 1	42-nm. Dane particle 22-nm. surface antigen	Primarily circular, double-stranded DNA; 3.2 kb.	Yes	Yes*	Yes	Yes	Yes	
HCV	Togavirus-like	36–62 nm.	Positive-stranded RNA	Yes	No	No	Yes	Yes	
HDV	Defective virus	35–37 nm.	Negative-stranded RNA 1.7 kb.	Yes	No	Yes	Yes	Yes	Requires HBV for replication
HEV	Calicivirus-like	32–34 nm.	RNA† Positive-stranded; 7.6 kb.	Yes	No	Yes	Yes‡	Yes	Recognized only in developing countries
HFV	Unknown	Unknown	Unknown	No	No	No	No	No	Recognized only by the exclusion of hepatitis A–E

*Reported.
†Provisional.
‡Immune electron microscopy.

suggests direct cytopathogenicity of liver cells by virus, and the other proposes humoral and cell-mediated immunopathogenetic mechanisms for all types of viral hepatitis. It is possible that both mechanisms occur. The extrahepatic manifestations of HBV, HCV, and HDV infections are thought to be due to the localization of antigen-antibody complexes in the affected tissue (synovium, arteries, kidneys, and skin).[21]

EPIDEMIOLOGY

To understand viral hepatitis, it is important to consider the trends in occurrence, risk factors, and modes of transmission. In 1993, the Centers for Disease Control and Prevention (CDC) received reports of 24,238 cases of infection with HAV, 13,361 cases of infection with HBV, and 4786 cases of NANB infection. From these figures they project that in the United States 300,000 cases of HBV and 5000 deaths yearly are due

to viral-induced cirrhosis and hepatocellular carcinoma. HAV infection increased in the late 1980s but is now on the decline. It still, however, accounts for 56% of all reported cases of hepatitis. HBV infection cases increased progressively through the mid 1980s and then steadily decreased, now accounting for 30% of the total. Although the number of reported cases of HCV infection is relatively low, it is the most common cause of posttransfusion hepatitis. The other hepatitis viruses are either rarely recognized or rarely reported in the United States.

VIRAL TRANSMISSION

Some of the epidemiologic characteristics associated with disease transmission are shown in Table 33–16. HBV, HCV, and HDV are typically transmitted by parenteral routes, although not always.[6, 32, 37] Transmission of HBV and HCV

TABLE 33–15. Nomenclature of the Hepatitis Virus Antigens and Antibodies and Their General Interpretation

Virus	Antigens		Antibodies	
	Name	*Interpretation*	*Name*	*Interpretation*
Hepatitis A virus (HAV)	HA Ag (major antigen of HAV)*	Acute infection	Anti-HA IgG IgM	Immune to HAV Recurrent or current acute infection
Hepatitis B virus (HBV)	HBsAg (surface antigen of HBV) Subtypes ayw, ayw₂, ayw₃, ayw₄, ayr, adw₂, adw₄, and adr	Prior exposure to HBV Distinctive strains of HBV	Anti-HBs	Immune to HBV
	HBcAg (core antigen of HBV)*	Infectivity—acute or chronic	Anti-HBc	Early or late convalescence or chronic hepatitis
	HBeAg (core-related antigen)	Infectivity—acute or chronic	Anti-HBe	Late convalescence
Posttransfusion non-A, non-B hepatitis virus (HCV)	Not available	Not available	Anti-HBc	Late convalescence or chronic hepatitis
Delta-associated agent (HDV)	Delta antigen*	Acute delta-associated hepatitis	Anti-delta	Immune to delta-associated hepatitis (low titer) or chronic HDV
Enterically transmitted non-A, non-B hepatitis virus (HEV)	Viruslike particles by immune electron microscopy*	Acute infection	Anti-HEV*	Immune to HEV

*Research tools only.

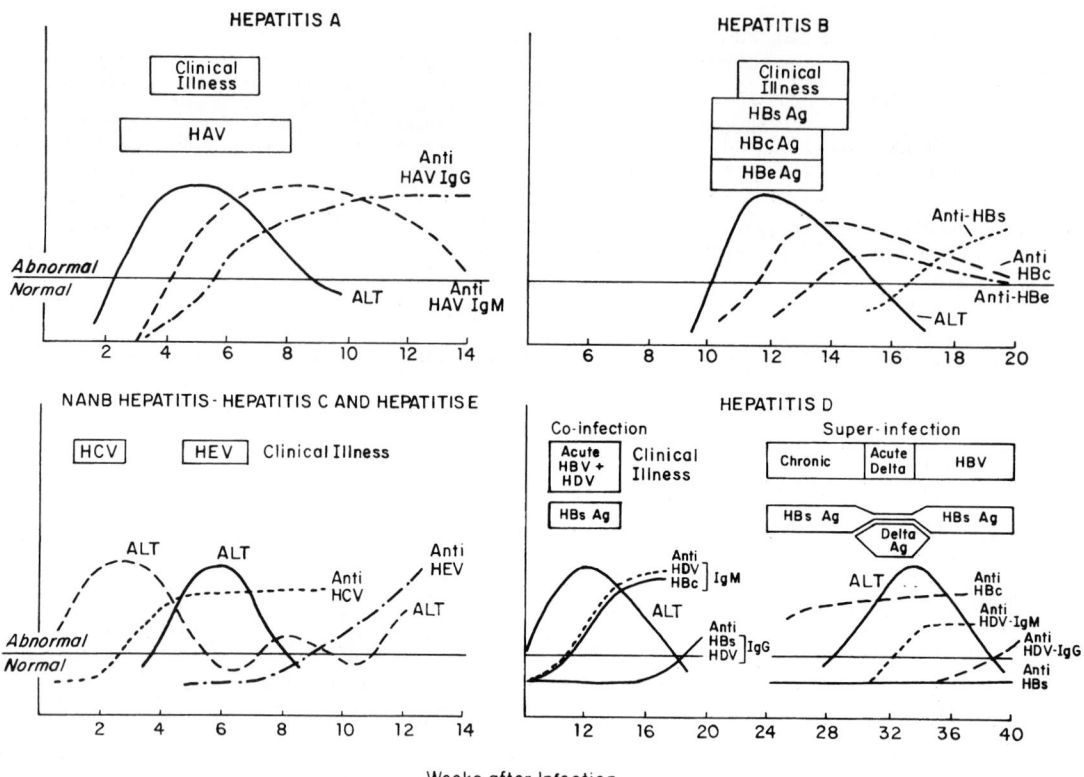

Figure 33–49. Sequence of development of the various hepatitis markers.

through transfused blood is facilitated by the ability of these viruses to exist in an infectious form in the serum of otherwise normal blood donors, making the period of infectivity potentially very long. HDV, a defective virus that requires HBV for replication, may also persist chronically in asymptomatic individuals, although this has been more difficult to establish. Certainly HAV and HEV, and likely the two new agents as well, do not seem to constitute any special risk for the surgeon and will not be discussed further here in any detail.

Blood and blood products from different sources have a greater or lesser risk of possessing infectious virus. Most whole blood and its derivatives that are not prepared by pooling of units have a relatively smaller risk of inducing infection with HBV. This is largely due to the infrequency of viral carriage in the normal adult population, the exclusion of potentially infected donors defined by questionnaire, and, perhaps most important, the routine testing of donor blood for hepatitis B surface antigen (HBsAg), hepatitis B core antigen (HBcAg), HCV antibody, and serum alanine amino-

transferase, positive results for which eliminate these units for use. Such procedures are especially important when the donor pool may include individuals at risk for HBV, HCV, and HDV infections, such as intravenous drug users and those who engage in high-risk sexual practices. The prevalence of one or another form of hepatitis in these groups approaches 100%. Preparations generally considered to be safe include serum albumin, thrombin, profibrinolysin, fibrinolysin, immune serum globulin, and all hyperimmune globulins, although one report identified contaminated intravenous immune globulin as the source of a sizable epidemic of HCV infection in Scandinavia.[11] The blood and blood products that pose a higher risk are those from commercial as opposed to volunteer donors and from pools of plasma and clotting factors.[11, 44] Washed and frozen human blood cells are not reliably virus free.[7]

Other predictable means of parenteral exposure include accidental needlestick or accidental injury, such as might occur during a surgical procedure. It is this occupational risk

TABLE 33–16. Epidemiology of Viral Hepatitis Transmission

Virus	No. of Cases 1990*	Major Infectious Body Fluid	Route†				
			Transfusion/ Intravenous Drug Use	Fecal-Oral	Sexual	Vertical	Occupational
HAV	29,000	Feces	−/−	4+	1+	−	+/−
HBV	20,000	Blood and other body fluids	−/4+	+/−	3+	3+	3+
HCV	3,000	Blood	2+/4+	+/−	1+	+/−	2+
HDV	NR	Blood	−/4+	1+	3+	3+	+/−
HEV	NR	Feces	−/−	4+	Unk	Unk	Unk

*Approximate number.
†Estimates of the relative frequency and/or efficiency.
NR, not reported; Unk, unknown.

that represents a continuous threat over the period of a surgical career and constitutes the basis for individual protection, including scrupulous surgical technique and HBV vaccine.

There is strong evidence that certainly HAV and HEV—and probably also HBV and HCV—may be transmitted by close, personal contact. Sexual transmission is one such route for HAV and HBV and possibly for HCV.[3–5, 19, 42] It is currently not possible to quantify the frequency of nonparenteral transmission in nonepidemic circumstances, but cases of hepatitis B and C occur without a prior known opportunity for parenteral exposure. It seems likely that the efficiency of disease transmission is much lower in these cases. There has been no documentation of a nonparenteral transmission of HDV.

Vertical transmission *in utero* and perinatal transmission occur with HBV, HCV, and HDV.

CLASSIFICATION AND CLINICAL DISEASE

All hepatitis viruses cause a wide spectrum of clinical disease, and in the majority of instances the resultant syndromes are indistinguishable. Some of the characteristic clinical events are summarized in Table 33–17. Typically, three types of infection occur most often: (1) inapparent and asymptomatic, (2) anicteric but symptomatic, and (3) icteric and symptomatic. The precise incidence of these alternatives is unknown, but inapparent disease appears to occur several to many times more frequently than symptomatic clinical disease, especially in children with HAV infection. The clinical illness typically found in about 90% of symptomatic patients may comprise lassitude, anorexia, weakness, nausea, dark urine, fever, vomiting, headache, chills, and abdominal discomfort, with other miscellaneous symptoms occurring somewhat less commonly. Laboratory abnormalities reflect liver cell necrosis and include primarily an elevation of alanine aminotransferase and, less commonly, elevations of levels of alkaline phosphatase and bilirubin.[12] In most typical cases of viral hepatitis, the pathologic findings in the liver consist of combinations of portal, periportal, and lobular hepatitis. There is an accumulation of inflammatory cells and parenchymal cell necrosis throughout the liver.[29, 46] Differences in histopathology generally correlate with the clinical severity and resolve completely with recovery from the illness. Recovery is complete in about 85% to 90% of patients 2 to 6 weeks after the onset of illness.[38] The course of HFV infection has been incompletely defined; it appears to be a milder acute disease than HCV infection, for example, but to have a frequency of chronicity of 10% to 29%.[14]

HBV and HCV infections, however, have variants of typical disease, representing 10% and 30%, respectively, of the clinically detectable cases. In HBV infection, manifestations may be atypical by virtue of the type of abnormalities or the severity or duration of the abnormality. As to the first

possibility, extrahepatic manifestations of hepatitis B most frequently occur in the form of arthralgias, predominantly involving the small joints.[40] Other reported *immune phenomena* include arteritis, nephritis, and dermatitis.[20] Extrahepatic manifestations occur with HCV and HDV infections as well. Viral hepatitis, particularly that caused by HCV, may also present atypically with a primarily cholestatic profile of liver function abnormalities.[41] Patients with this profile may have profound jaundice and pruritus but no anatomic obstruction of the biliary system.

Atypical viral hepatitis manifestations that differ in duration or severity are described as follows by the expert panel contributing to *The Hepatitis Knowledge Base*.[10] *Prolonged viral hepatitis* is defined simply as typical acute disease lasting 4 to 12 months. It differs from *relapsing viral hepatitis* in that the latter resolves within several months but only after an unsettling relapse or two of typical disease. Prolonged viral hepatitis is not easily distinguished from *chronic persistent hepatitis*, which seems to share most of its features. All three entities share the features of an ultimately self-limited disease, no demonstrated effective therapy, and no sequelae. After typical acute viral hepatitis, *post-hepatitis hyperbilirubinemia* (with normal liver histology) may persist as the sole abnormality, only to resolve spontaneously.

Carriers of HBsAg, about whom most is known, are asymptomatic and represent less than 1% of the normal population in this country, although the estimate worldwide is over 200 million carriers.[26] Acute HBV infections result in long-term carriage of HBsAg and sometimes other markers of HBV in approximately 5% of clinically identified cases. It is not unusual to lack a history of prior infection, and the carrier may or may not be infectious. Currently available tests do not make that distinction, but several guidelines may be useful. The carrier is more likely to be infectious: the closer he or she is to the acute infection, the higher the titer of anti-HBcAg, the higher the titer of hepatitis B e antigen (HBeAg), and the more immunocompromised the carrier is. In contrast, the presence of antibodies to HBsAg or HBeAg makes the individual less likely to be infectious. From a practical point of view, all carriers should be considered potentially infectious, particularly when an invasive procedure is contemplated. Judgments about the timing for a surgical procedure are dictated primarily by the indications for operation. In elective procedures, however, when it is not possible to distinguish the true chronic carrier from an individual with incubating acute viral hepatitis, a period of observation is a worthwhile precaution to allow the circumstances to clarify. Because it has not been possible to detect HCV or its antigens conclusively and because the development of antibody seems to occur later and perhaps less reliably than with HBV, it has not been possible to ascertain the frequency of the infectious carrier of HCV or to determine the consequences of exposure. That transmission from asymptomatic carriers occurs and that disease ensues in the

TABLE 33–17. Clinical Characteristics and Consequences of Viral Hepatitis

Virus	Asymptomatic (%)	Incubation Period (days)	Acute	Extrahepatic Manifestations	Fulminant/ Mortality	Chronic Hepatitis			Associated with Cirrhosis/Hepatocellular Carcinoma
						Persistent	*Aggressive*	*Carrier*	
HAV	Children >80% Adults <20%	25	+	–	+/1–4%	–	–	–	–/–
HBV	>50%	75	+	+	+/1–4%	2–4%	2–4%	5%	+/+
HCV	75%	14–28	+	+	+/0.1	15%	30%	+	+/+
HDV	Unknown	28–90	+	+	+/+	2–4%	2–4%	5%	+/–
HEV	Unknown*	22–60	+	–	+/†	–	–	–	–

*Usually recognized as part of epidemic.
†Pregnant women.

TABLE 33–18. Recommendations for Use of Immune Globulins

Virus Exposure	Time of Evaluation	Nature of Exposure	Immune Globulin Recommended	
			ISG*	HBIG†
HAV	Pre-exposure	Travel to endemic area, primate animal handlers	+	NA
	Postexposure	Household/day-care center	+	NA
		School or work	−	NA
		Institution	+/−	NA
		Primate handler	+	NA
		Medical and paramedical personnel	−	NA
		Common-source epidemic	+	NA
HBV	Pre-exposure	Personnel or family members attending an infected patient	−	+
	Postexposure	Parenteral transfusion of HBsAg-positive blood	−	+
		Accidental needlestick or surgical injury or blood on open wound or mucous membrane	−	+
		Nonparenteral		
		Intimate contact	+	+ (optional)
		Postnatal	−	+
HCV	Postexposure	Parenteral		
		Transfusion	+	NA
		Accidental	+	NA
HDV			−	NA
HEV			−	NA

*ISG dose, 0.02 ml./kg. of body weight before or within 14 days of exposure if possible; 0.06 ml./kg. every 5 months for prolonged travel.
†HBIG dose, 0.05 to 0.07 ml./kg. within 7 days of exposure and repeated 1 month later.

recipient is certain, however, in view of the frequency of posttransfusion hepatitis[2] and the frequency of the documented instances of HCV infection after an accidental needlestick. Screening procedures on patients who serve as the source of a potentially infected needlestick, for example, are controversial. Neither normal results of liver function tests nor absence of HCV antibody preclude the possibility that the individual is infectious, although the risks should be substantially reduced.

Of some concern to the surgeon is the possibility that he or she may become infected and subsequently be a carrier of HBV or HCV.[22, 25] Although the level of risk to patients has not been conclusively defined, most authorities agree that HBV transmission from physician to patients, although documented, is a very unusual event and that common hygienic measures, not to mention scrupulous surgical technique, reduce that risk perhaps to the vanishing point.[31, 36] Because of a single instance in which another bloodborne virus, human immunodeficiency virus (HIV), was transmitted from a health care provider (a dentist) to six patients, the CDC formulated a policy, now in effect in all states, that requires self-notification of all health care providers known to be positive for HBV or HIV to the state health department.[18] Routine testing of health care providers has not been mandated, and most authorities do not recommend such a practice.

Of the serious sequelae, acute fulminant viral hepatitis, chronic aggressive hepatitis, and viral hepatitis with confluent hepatic necrosis (subacute hepatic necrosis) appear to represent points on a spectrum from more to less advanced.[46] Any of these sequelae may progress to cirrhosis with its complications. Finally, there is an association between hepatoma (hepatocellular carcinoma) and HBV and possibly HCV infection, suggesting the oncogenic potential of these viruses. For HBV infection, considerable epidemiologic, molecular, and animal evidence exists; and current thinking about the most likely mechanism is that integration of the viral DNA is subjected to mutagenic stimuli over a prolonged period, resulting in hepatocellular carcinoma.[8, 39] No association with carcinoma has been identified with other classes of hepatitis virus.

HCV infection appears to result in chronic hepatitis even more frequently than HBV infection does. Initially, chronic hepatitis caused by HCV was considered to be more benign than that associated with HBV.[9] Subsequently, however, follow-up biopsy studies found that in as many as 30% of the originally detected cases of chronic aggressive hepatitis the patients developed cirrhosis.[27]

Because HDV does not cause disease in the absence of HBV, its contribution to chronicity is somewhat complicated. Available evidence suggests that co-infection with HBV and HDV results in a long-term course indistinguishable from that with infection with HBV alone, whereas superimposed infection of HBV with HDV results in chronic HDV infection. A worsened histopathologic picture and accelerated liver disease appear to accompany the latter scenario.[23, 37]

PREVENTION

The mainstays of viral hepatitis prevention are the correct diagnosis and reporting of new cases, the attention to standard principles of cleanliness and hygiene, and specific measures to eliminate the sources of infection. Because these methods are only partially successful, additional measures have been used. Passive immunity through the use of immune globulin is one such approach. The current recommendations for the use of immune serum globulin or hyperimmune hepatitis B immune globulin are summarized in Table 33–18.[17] There is general, but not complete, agreement on these recommendations among authorities.

Active immunization is the most reliable option for the prevention of HBV infection. The first licensed vaccine (Heptavax-B) is a preparation of purified HBsAg from the plasma of known chronic carriers of HBV.[24, 43] In addition, there are now effective vaccines prepared by recombinant DNA technology (Recombivax HB and Engerix-B), and they also consist of purified HBsAg. The recommendations of the United States Public Health Service for recipients of HBV vaccine are shown in Table 33–19. Special recommendations exist for immune-compromised patients because of their reduced ability to respond to standard regimens, and there is

TABLE 33–19. Hepatitis B Vaccine Recommendations

	Vaccine
Pre-exposure	
Health care workers	+
Institutions for mentally retarded	
Staff	+
Clients	+
Hemodialysis patients	+
Homosexually active males	+
Illicit injectable drug users	+
Recipients of certain blood products	+
Household and sexual contacts of HBV carriers	+
Postexposure	
Perinatal	+
Percutaneous	+
Sexual	+
HAV*	
Travelers to developing countries	+
Children and staff in day-care centers	+
Homosexually active men	+
Intravenous drug users	+
Penal and institutions for the mentally retarded	+
Food handlers	+
Household contacts of acute cases	+

*Proposed target groups when licensed.

now a mandate for universal immunization of all young children.[1, 28]

In addition, vaccines have been developed for HAV. Approaches include vaccines made from live, attenuated, or inactivated virus, as well as recombinant viral vaccines. Vaccine efficacy has been demonstrated using either inactivated or attenuated vaccines,[35, 45] and the former may be licensed in the United States in the near future.

TREATMENT

No specific form of therapy other than supportive care is available for acute hepatitis. A variety of forms of treatment have been used in the treatment of chronic hepatitis, with some being more effective than others in selected patient subsets with HBV, HCV, and HDV infections. In a review of studies before 1986, no conclusively beneficial therapeutic regimen was found.[15] Subsequently, trials of interferon with or without a prior tapered course of prednisone have demonstrated reduced liver function abnormalities and viral replication for up to 9 to 12 months in as many as 50% to 60% of patients with chronic hepatitis.[46] The addition of the prednisone taper appears beneficial. Although less well studied, benefits of these or similar regimens have been detected for chronic HCV[30] and HDV infections.[23] It is not yet clear, however, that these courses of therapy for any chronic form of hepatitis will be durably effective or practical in all patients.

ADDENDUM

Subsequent to the preparation of this chapter, an RNA virus, designated as *hepatitis G virus* (HGV), was identified. It is associated with acute and chronic hepatitis and persistent viremia for up to 9 years. It is transfusion transmissible, global in distribution, and present in the blood donor population in the United States. The virus is closely related to the GBV-A and GBV-B viruses recently isolated from tamarins and distantly related to hepatitis C virus.[34]

SELECTED REFERENCES

Alter, M. J., Margolis, H. S., Krawczynski, K., et al.: The natural history of community acquired hepatitis C in the United States. N. Engl. J. Med., 327:1899, 1992.
This paper, written by the group from the CDC, is a current synthesis of the clinical and epidemiologic facts about this relatively newly defined viral cause of non-A, non-B hepatitis.

Bradley, D. W.: Hepatitis E: Epidemiology, aetiology and molecular biology. Rev. Med. Virol., 2:19, 1992.
In 1993 new serologic techniques were used to document hepatitis E in six U.S. travelers. This earlier paper summarizes the current state of knowledge about this new cause of enterically transmitted non-A, non-B hepatitis.

Hollinger, F. B.: Hepatitis B virus. *In* Fields, B. N., and Knipe, D. M. (Eds.): Fields' Virology, New York, Raven Press, 1990, p. 2171.
Detailed information concerning all aspects of hepatitis B is contained in this exhaustive review of the literature by one of the authorities in the field. The depth of information is exceptional.

Lemon, S. M., Ping, P.-H., Day, S., et al.: Immunobiology of hepatitis A virus. *In* Hollinger, F. B., Lemon, S. M., and Margolis, H. S. (Eds.): Viral Hepatitis and Liver Disease. Baltimore, Williams & Wilkins, 1991, p. 20.
Although HAV has long been recognized as a cause of hepatitis, an understanding of its immunobiology has advanced dramatically only in recent years. This reference represents an excellent review of this subject.

Purcell, R. H., and Gerin, J. L.: Hepatitis delta virus. *In* Fields, B. N., and Knipe, D. M. (Eds.): Fields' Virology, 2nd ed., vol. 1. New York, Raven Press, 1990, p. 2275.
For the reader interested in the latest information on HDV, or "delta" hepatitis, this chapter is ideal. The author is a leading authority in the field of viral hepatitis.

REFERENCES

1. AAP Committee on Infectious Diseases: Universal hepatitis B immunization. Pediatrics, 89:795, 1992.
2. Alter, M. J.: Non-A, non-B hepatitis: Sorting through a diagnosis of exclusion. Ann. Intern. Med., 110:583, 1989.
3. Alter, M. J.: Transmission of hepatitis C virus: Route, dose, and titer. N. Engl. J. Med., 330:784, 1994.
4. Alter, M. J., Ahtone, J., Weisfuse, I., Starko, K., Vacalis, T. D., and Maynard, J. E.: Hepatitis B virus transmission between heterosexuals. JAMA, 256:1307, 1986.
5. Alter, M. J., Coleman, P. J., Alexander, W. J., Kramer, E., Miller, J. K., Mandel, E., Hadler, S. C., and Margolis, H. S.: Importance of heterosexual activity in the transmission of hepatitis B and non-A, non-B hepatitis. JAMA, 262:1201, 1989.
6. Alter, M. J., Margolis, H. S., Krawczynski, K., et al.: The natural history of community acquired hepatitis C in the United States. N. Engl. J. Med., 327:1899, 1992.
7. Alter, M. J., Tabor, E., Meryman, H. T., Hoofnagle, J. H., Kahn, R. A., Holland, P. V., Gerety, R. J., and Barker, L. F.: Transmission of hepatitis B virus infection by transfusion of frozen deglycerolized red blood cells. N. Engl. J. Med., 298:637, 1978.
8. Beasley, R. P.: Hepatitis B virus: The major etiology of hepatocellular carcinoma. Cancer, 61:1942, 1988.
9. Berman, M., Alter, H. J., Ishak, K. G., Purcell, R. H., and Jones, E. A.: The chronic sequelae of non-A, non-B hepatitis. Ann. Intern. Med., 91:1, 1979.
10. Bernstein, L. H., Koff, R. S., Siegel, E. R., Merritt, A. D., Goldstein, C. M., and Panel, E.: The hepatitis knowledge base: A prototype information transfer system. Ann. Intern. Med., 93:169, 1980.
11. Bjøro, K., Frøland, S. S., Yun, Z., Sarndal, H. H., and Hasland, T.: Hepatitis C infection in patients with primary hypogammaglobulinemia after treatment with contaminated immune globulin. N. Engl. J. Med., 331:1607, 1994. (See also the accompanying editorial: Schiff, R. I.: Transmission of viral infection through intravenous immune globulin, p. 1649.)
12. Boggs, J. D., Melnick, J. L., Conrad, M. E., and Felsher, B. F.: Viral hepatitis: Clinical and tissue culture studies. JAMA, 214:1041, 1970.
13. Bradley, D. W.: Hepatitis E: Epidemiology, aetiology, and molecular biology. Rev. Med. Virol., 2:19, 1992.
14. Bradley, D. W.: New hepatitis virus in the alphabet soup of viral hepatitis. Presented before the Interscience Conference on Antimicrobial Agents and Chemotherapy, Orlando, Fla., October 7, 1994.
15. Burke, C. A.: A statistical view of clinical trials in chronic hepatitis B. J. Hepatol., 3:S261, 1986.
16. Carman, W. F., Thomas, H. C., Zuckerman, A. J., et al.: Molecular variants. *In* Zuckerman, A. J., and Thomas, H. C. (Eds.): Viral Hepatitis: Scientific Basis and Clinical Management. London, Churchill Livingstone, 1993, p. 115.
17. Centers for Disease Control: Protection against viral hepatitis. MMWR, 39:1, 1990.
18. Ciesielski, C., Marianos, D. W., Schochetman, G., Witte, J. J., and Jaffe, H. W.: The 1990 Florida dental investigation. Ann. Intern. Med., 121:886, 1994.
19. Corey, L., and Holmes, K. K.: Sexual transmission of hepatitis A in homosexual men: Incidence and mechanism. N. Engl. J. Med., 302:435, 1980.

20. Dienstag, J. L.: Immunopathogenesis of the extrahepatic manifestations of hepatitis B virus infection. Springer Semin. Immunopathol., 3:461, 1981.

21. Dienstag, J., Bhan, A., Klingenstein, R., and Savarese, A.: Immunopathogenesis of liver disease associated with hepatitis B. *In* Szmuness, W., Alter, H., and Maynard, J. E. (Eds.): Viral Hepatitis. Philadelphia, Franklin Institute Press, 1982, p. 221.

22. Dienstag, J. L., and Ryan, D. M.: Occupational exposure to hepatitis B virus in hospital personnel: Infection or immunization. Am. J. Epidemiol., 115:26, 1982.

23. Farci, P.: Hepatitis D virus in the alphabet soup of viral hepatitis. Presented before the Interscience Conference on Antimicrobial Agents and Chemotherapy, Orlando, Fla., October 7, 1994.

24. Francis, D., Hadler, S., Thompson, S., Maynard, J., Ostrow, D., Altman, N., Braff, E., O'Malley, P., Hawkins, D., Judson, F., Denley, K., Nylund, T., Christie, G., Meyers, F., Moore, Y., Gardner, A., Doto, I., Miller, J., Reynolds, G., Murphy, B., Schable, C., Clark, B., Curran, J., and Redeker, A.: The prevention of hepatitis B with vaccine: Report of the Centers for Disease Control multicenter efficacy trial among homosexual men. Ann. Intern. Med., 97:362, 1982.

25. Grady, G. F.: Hepatitis B from the medical professions: How rare? How preventable? N. Engl. J. Med., 296:995, 1977.

26. Hollinger, F. B.: Hepatitis B virus. *In* Fields, B. W., and Knipe, D. M. (Eds.): Fields' Virology. New York, Raven Press, 1990, p. 2171.

27. Hollinger, F. B.: Non-A, non-B hepatitis virus. *In* Fields, B. W., and Knipe, D. M. (Eds.): Fields' Virology. New York, Raven Press, 1990, p. 2239.

28. Immunization Practices Advisory Committee. Hepatitis B virus: A comprehensive strategy for eliminating transmission in the U.S. through universal childhood immunization. MMWR, 4:RR-13, 1991.

29. Ishak, K.: Light microscopic morphology of viral hepatitis. Am. J. Clin. Pathol., 65:787, 1976.

30. Jacyna, M. R., Brooks, M. G., Loke, R. H., Main, J., Murray-Lyon, I. M., and Thomas, H. C.: Randomised controlled trial of interferon alfa (lymphoblastoid interferon) in chronic non-A, non-B hepatitis. Br. Med. J., 298:80, 1989.

31. Kiernan, T. W., and Powers, R. J.: Hepatitis B virus: Inappropriate reactions to transmission risks. JAMA, 241:585, 1979.

32. Krugman, S., and Giles, J.: Viral hepatitis, type B (MS-2 strain): Further observations on natural history and prevention. N. Engl. J. Med., 288:755, 1973.

33. Lemon, S. M., Ping, P.-H., Day, S., et al.: Immunobiology of hepatitis A virus. *In* Hollinger, F. B., Lemon, S. M., and Margolis, H. S. (Eds.): Viral Hepatitis and Liver Disease. Baltimore, Williams & Wilkins, 1991, p. 20.

34. Linnen, J., Wages, J., Jr., Zhang-keck, Z.-Y., et al.: Molecular cloning and disease association of hepatitis G virus: A transfusion-transmissible agent. Science, 271:505, 1996.

35. Mao, J. A., Dong, D. X., and Zhang, S. Y.: Further studies of attenuated live hepatitis A vaccine (H2 strain) in humans. *In* Hollinger, F. B., Lemon, S. M., and Margolis, H. S. (Eds.): Viral Hepatitis and Liver Disease. Baltimore, Williams & Wilkins, 1991, p. 110.

36. Occupational exposure to bloodborne pathogens: Final rule. Fed. Register, 56:64175, 1991.

37. Purcell, R. H., and Gerin, J. L.: Hepatitis delta virus. *In* Fields, B. N., and Knipe, D. M. (Eds.): Fields' Virology, 2nd ed., vol. 2. New York, Raven Press, 1990, p. 2275.

38. Redeker, A. G.: Viral hepatitis: Clinical aspects. Am. J. Med. Sci., 270:9, 1975.

39. Robinson, W. S.: Hepadnaviridae and their replication. *In* Fields, B. N., and Knipe, D. M. (Eds.): Fields' Virology. New York, Raven Press, 1990, p. 2137.

40. Schumacher, H. R., and Gall, E. P.: Arthritis in acute hepatitis and chronic active hepatitis. Am. J. Med., 57:655, 1974.

41. Shouval, D., Levij, I. S., and Eliakim, M.: Chronic active hepatitis with cholestatic features: I. A clinical and immunologic study; II. A histopathological study. Am. J. Gastroenterol., 72:542, 1979.

42. Szmuness, W., Much, M. I., Prince, A. M., Hoofnagle, J. H., Cherubin, C. E., Harley, E. J., and Black, G. H.: On the role of sexual behavior in the spread of hepatitis B infection. Ann. Intern. Med., 83:489, 1975.

43. Szmuness, W., Stevens, C. E., Harley, E. J., Zang, E. A., Olesko, W. R., William, D. C., Sadovsky, R., Morrison, J. M., and Kellner, A.: Hepatitis B vaccine: Demonstration of efficacy in a controlled clinical trial in a high-risk population in the United States. N. Engl. J. Med., 303:833, 1980.

44. Trepo, C., Hantz, D., Jacquier, M. F., Nemoz, G., Cappel, R., and Trepo, D.: Different fates of hepatitis B markers during plasma fractionation: A clue to the infectivity of blood derivatives. Vox Sang., 35:143, 1978.

45. Werzberger, A., Mensch, B., Kuter, B., et al.: A controlled trial of a formalin-inactivated hepatitis A vaccine in healthy children. N. Engl. J. Med., 327:453, 1992.

46. Zuckerman, A. J., and Thomas, H. C. (Eds.): Viral Hepatitis: Scientific Basis and Clinical Management. London, Churchill Livingstone, 1993.

CHAPTER 34

THE BILIARY SYSTEM

David L. Nahrwold, M.D.

HISTORICAL OVERVIEW

Most of the progress in the diagnosis and treatment of biliary tract disease has been made in the last 150 years, but gallstones and their sequelae, which cause most of the clinical problems, are not a malady of just modern times. The earliest known gallstone dates back to the twenty-first Egyptian dynasty (1085–945 B.C.), having been discovered in the mummy of a priestess of Amen. Ironically, this ancient specimen was destroyed in the bombing of England during World War II. Much later, during the time of the Roman Empire, Pliny described the rare anomaly of double gallbladder,[45] and the well-known physician Soranus of Ephesus described jaundice and the associated signs of extrahepatic obstruction, including acholic stools, dark urine, and itching.[4] Gallstones were first described in the fifth century by a Greek physician, Alexander Trallianus, who wrote about calculi within the bile ducts.

The surgical relevance of biliary tract disease was first made obvious by the Islamic physician Ibn Sina (980–1037), who stated that a biliary-cutaneous fistula could follow drainage of an abdominal wall abscess. Perforation of an acutely inflamed gallbladder into the abdominal wall with abscess formation may have been the underlying problem. Joenisius first extracted gallstones through a biliary fistula that had formed from spontaneous drainage of an abdominal wall abscess. According to Power,[48] Jean Louis Petit (1674–1760) noted that a gallbladder could become adherent to the abdominal wall and proposed that it be punctured through the wall of the abdomen by a trocar. He believed that the wound should be enlarged with a knife if stones could be felt with a sound passed through the trocar. It is not clear that he actually performed the procedure, however.

The first cholecystotomy was performed by John Stough Bobbs in Indianapolis on June 15, 1867.[9] His patient, a 32-year-old woman, had a large abdominal mass, which proved to be the gallbladder filled with clear serous fluid and gallstones. Obviously, she had hydrops of the gallbladder. He opened the gallbladder, removed the stones, and closed it by suture. His patient survived until the age of 77, when she died of arteriosclerosis.

Carl Langenbuch of Berlin performed the first cholecystectomy in June of 1882, using the aseptic technique that Joseph Lister had initiated in 1868 (the year in which Bobbs reported the first cholecystotomy). The patient was a 43-year-old man who had suffered from biliary colic for 16 years. He was released from the hospital 8 weeks after operation. Four years later, in 1886, the first cholecystectomy in the United States was performed by Justus Ohage of St. Paul, Minnesota. The basic technique remained unchanged until 1986, when Mühe performed the first cholecystectomy laparoscopically.[36] Ludwig Courvoisier of Basel performed the first successful choledocholithotomy in 1890 and made several contributions to the understanding of bile duct obstruction at the turn of the century.

Important advances in diagnostic testing have been made in the twentieth century. This field was opened by the development of cholecystography by Graham and Cole, culminating in the first cholecystogram in man in 1924.[15] Cholescintigraphy was first reported in 1953.[63] Improved imaging techniques and better contrast agents and nuclides led to the present high-resolution oral cholecystography and cholescintigraphy. Operative cholangiography was described in 1932; cholangiography by the percutaneous transhepatic and the endoscopic retrograde routes has been developed since 1950. The application of ultrasonography, computed tomography, choledochoscopy, and interventional radiologic techniques to the diagnosis and management of biliary tract disease has occurred in the past 2 decades.

ANATOMY

The gallbladder and extrahepatic bile ducts are derived from the primitive foregut and are formed in conjunction with the liver. The shape of the gallbladder is approximately that of a pear, with a bulbous fundus at the distal end, a middle corpus that tapers to a neck, and a proximal cystic duct that enters the common bile duct (Fig. 34–1). The organ is about 7 cm. long and holds 30 to 50 ml. of bile. The corpus nestles into the substance of the liver for a variable distance, and the entire organ is held to the liver by a peritoneal covering, which is a reflection of the visceral peritoneum covering the liver. The fundus protrudes slightly beyond the edge of the liver and lies anteriorly in the region of the costal arch at the lateral border of the rectus muscle. The cystic duct lies posteriorly on a plane with the duodenum, but superiorly to it at the level of the first lumbar vertebra. The neck of the gallbladder is lax, because it is not bound to the liver by peritoneum. The distal portion of the gallbladder has the appearance of a diverticulum, which is called *Hartmann's pouch.* The cystic duct is 2 to 4 cm. long and contains the spiral valves of Heister, which allow easy entry of bile into the gallbladder but offer resistance to its outflow.

The extrahepatic bile ducts lie within the hepatoduodenal ligament. Normally, the right anterior and posterior segmental bile ducts join to form the right hepatic duct, a confluence that is usually just within the substance of the liver. The left lateral and left medial segmental ducts form the left hepatic duct, which joins the right hepatic duct to form the common hepatic duct. The right and left hepatic ducts are 1 to 4 cm. long, with the left more accessible because it has a more transverse course before entering the liver. The length of the common hepatic duct is extremely variable because it is determined by the point at which the cystic duct joins it. The common bile duct courses through the pancreas and the wall of the duodenum to form the papilla of Vater on the medial wall of the duodenum (Fig. 34–2). Its distal end is enveloped by the sphincter of Oddi, which regulates the flow of bile from the liver into the duodenum. The pancreatic duct may share a common orifice on the papilla of Vater with the common bile duct, it may join the common duct proximal to its entrance into the duodenum, or the two ducts may open

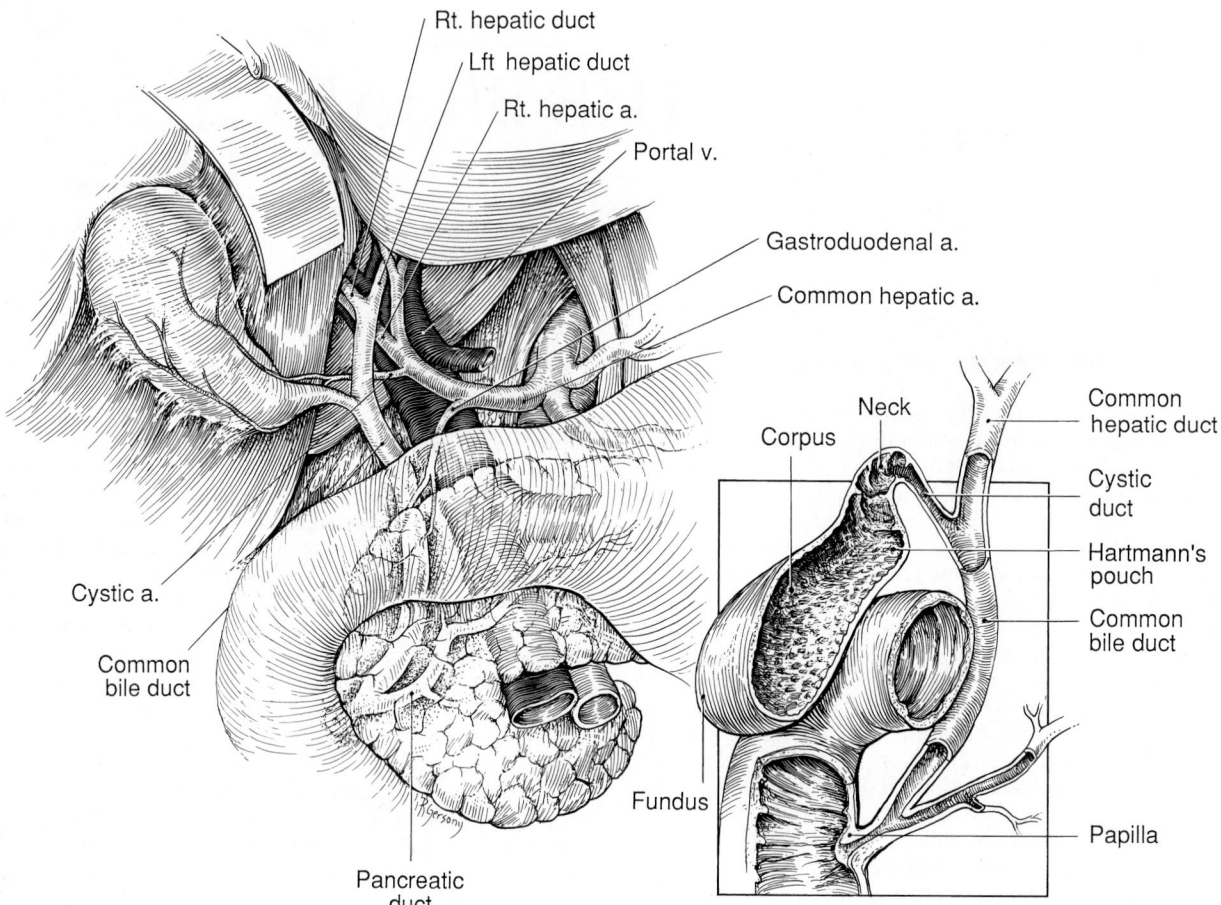

Figure 34–1. Anatomy of the biliary system and its relationship to surrounding structures.

separately on the papilla (Fig. 34–2). A common channel, ranging from 1 mm. to several centimeters in length, is present in about 75% of individuals, and in about 25% the common bile duct and pancreatic duct open separately on the papilla.

The common bile duct receives its blood supply from the retroduodenal, the common hepatic, and the right hepatic arteries. Their branches form a plexus on the duct that is joined together by two axial vessels, the 3 o'clock and 9 o'clock arteries, named for their positions in reference to a cross section of the duct. The gallbladder is supplied by branches of the cystic artery, which normally originates from the right hepatic artery. The venous drainage of the gallbladder and extrahepatic ducts is into the portal vein. Lymphatics from the gallbladder drain into the cystic duct lymph node, located near the superior aspect of the junction of the infundibulum of the gallbladder and the cystic duct. Lymph nodes along the posterior aspect of the common bile duct and the common hepatic duct drain these structures.

The triangle of Calot, a surgical landmark used to identify important structures during cholecystectomy, is bounded by the cystic duct, the common hepatic duct, and the inferior border of the liver. The right hepatic and cystic arteries are located within it, and anomalous structures often pass through it.

Significance of Variations in Anatomy. Variations in the anatomy of the gallbladder, the bile ducts, and the arteries that supply them and the liver are important to the surgeon, because failure to recognize them can cause iatrogenic injury to the biliary tract. The significant variations in ductal anatomy are shown in Figure 34–3. The cystic duct may be long,

illustrating the need for its complete dissection. The duct may pass behind the common hepatic duct to enter on its posterior wall or on its left lateral aspect. In chronic cholecystitis, the gallbladder may be small and shrunken, and the cystic duct may be absent or extremely short; in this circumstance, the common bile duct may easily be mistaken for the cystic duct as dissection proceeds from the gallbladder fundus toward the cystic duct. A very long cystic duct may enter the common bile duct a variable distance from the sphincter of Oddi and may be fused with the common duct, in which case the two ducts should not be separated because they share a common wall. Finally, an *accessory* duct from the liver may enter the cystic duct or the common hepatic duct. Actually, this is not an accessory duct but an anomalous entry and course of either the right anterior or right posterior segmental duct from the liver.

Variations in the anatomy of the hepatic and cystic arteries that are of surgical significance are shown in Figure 34–4. A bend in the course of the right hepatic artery, throwing it into the configuration of a *caterpillar hump,* invites injury unless it is carefully dissected free. A very short cystic artery also puts the hepatic artery at risk. Occasionally, the right hepatic artery courses anterior to the common bile duct.

CONGENITAL ANOMALIES OF THE GALLBLADDER

Absence of the gallbladder is rare and apparently has a genetic predisposition, because several family members may be affected.[62] Patients with gallbladder agenesis fall into three categories.[5] Some are born with other congenital anomalies,

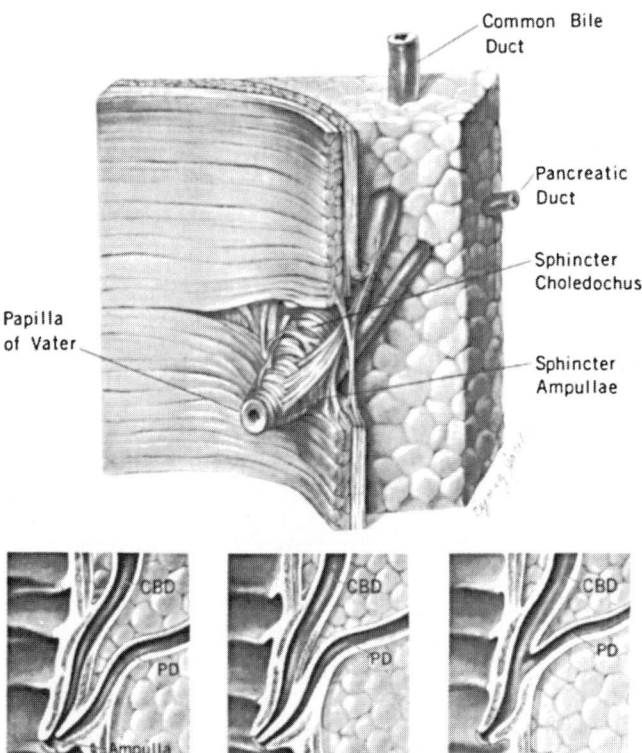

Figure 34-2. The choledochoduodenal junction and variations in the entrances of the common bile duct and the pancreatic duct.

including biliary atresia and cardiovascular or other gastrointestinal malformations. They often die in infancy. Others are asymptomatic throughout life. Slightly more than half have symptoms suggestive of biliary tract disease; in these patients, dilatation of the bile duct system or choledocholithiasis is a frequent finding.

Agenesis of the gallbladder is rarely diagnosed preoperatively in patients with symptoms of biliary tract disease, because the sonogram is interpreted as showing a small, contracted gallbladder, and oral cholecystography and scintigraphy show nonvisualization of the gallbladder, all of which suggest the presence of gallbladder disease. A thorough search for the gallbladder in possible ectopic locations should be made during operation. If none is found, an operative cholangiogram is indicated.

An ectopic location of the gallbladder is also rare. An intrahepatic location on the right side makes cholecystectomy hazardous, and a cholecystostomy with removal of the stones is the preferred treatment of cholelithiasis in patients with this anomaly. A left-sided gallbladder is located to the left of the falciform ligament and is usually partially embedded in the substance of the left lobe of the liver. The cystic duct may drain into the left hepatic duct or the common hepatic duct. In retrodisplacement of the gallbladder, the organ is located beneath the posterior and inferior surfaces of the liver. Torsion may occur in a *floating* gallbladder, in which the organ is completely peritonealized and free from the liver or attached to the liver by a long mesentery.

Double and triple gallbladders have been reported, the latter being extremely rare. Double gallbladders may share a common cystic duct and be completely separated, or they may be divided by a septum. When they do not share a common outlet, the cystic ducts of double or triple gallbladders open separately into the common bile duct or, less commonly, into the right hepatic duct.[26]

Choledochal Cysts

Cysts of the biliary duct system are uncommon, and the understanding of them is incomplete. About 80% are diagnosed during childhood, and the remainder become apparent in adulthood. Originally, they were described as cystic dilatations of the extrahepatic duct system, which Alonso-Lej and colleagues classified with regard to their location and their fusiform or diverticular configuration.[2] Subsequently, Todani extended this classification to include the frequent association with cystic dilatation of the duct system within the liver, a condition described in 1958 and now known as *Caroli's disease*.[13, 57, 58] The basic types are shown in Figure 34-5, but variations are frequent. For example, the fusiform dilatation may extend proximally to involve the entire common hepatic duct, there may be multiple extrahepatic cysts, and intrahepatic cysts may occur alone or be unilateral, bilateral, cystic, or fusiform. The solitary fusiform type accounts for approximately 80% of cases. The etiology is uncertain, but some evidence suggests that fusiform dilatation results from distal obstruction and destruction of the proximal bile duct epithelium by pancreatic juice, because the pancreatic duct enters proximal to the ampulla in most of these patients, and distal obstruction and damage to the epithelium cause cysts in puppies.[41, 57]

The classic symptoms are abdominal pain, jaundice, and an abdominal mass, but not all children have a mass. In both children and adults, cholangitis is frequent, probably because of bile stasis and colonization with bacteria. Most cysts can be detected by ultrasonography or by radionuclide scanning, but the definitive diagnosis requires cholangiography.

Choledochal cysts should be treated by complete excision and Roux-en-Y hepaticojejunostomy whenever possible. The results are excellent.[25, 42] The long-term results of procedures in which the cyst remains *in situ* are not good because of recurrent pancreatitis in about one third of patients and the development of carcinoma in the cyst in about one fourth of them.[37] Recent evidence suggests that excision of the extrahepatic portion of the cyst alone eliminates the risk of subsequent cholangiocarcinoma in patients who have both intrahepatic and extrahepatic cystic disease, perhaps because the reflux of pancreatic juice is prevented.[14]

CHOLEDOCHOLITHIASIS

Common duct stones are found in 8% to 16% of patients who have cholelithiasis. The incidence increases with age. In most instances, bile duct stones migrate from the gallbladder; the fact that they often are larger than the cystic duct suggests that they are able to grow within the bile duct system. Most are cholesterol stones, in keeping with their high incidence in the gallbladder.

Stones may form *de novo* within the bile ducts. These calculi, called *primary common duct stones*, are usually composed of calcium bilirubinate. They are ovoid, brown stones that crumble easily and are always associated with bile duct obstruction. Frequently, infection or bacterbilia is present. Arbitrarily, those stones discovered more than 2 years after cholecystectomy are designated primary common duct stones. The etiology of calcium bilirubinate stones is thought to be precipitation of unconjugated bilirubin as its calcium salt. Normally, bilirubin is conjugated as glucuronide. Stone formation begins when the soluble bilirubin diglucuronide is deconjugated by beta glucuronidase, an enzyme produced by bacteria such as *Escherichia coli* and by the epithelium of the biliary tract, leaving insoluble, unconjugated bilirubin to precipitate with calcium.[43] Bacteria also release phospholipases, which hydrolyze lecithin in bile to lysolecithin, stearate, and palmitate. The binding of biliary calcium forms

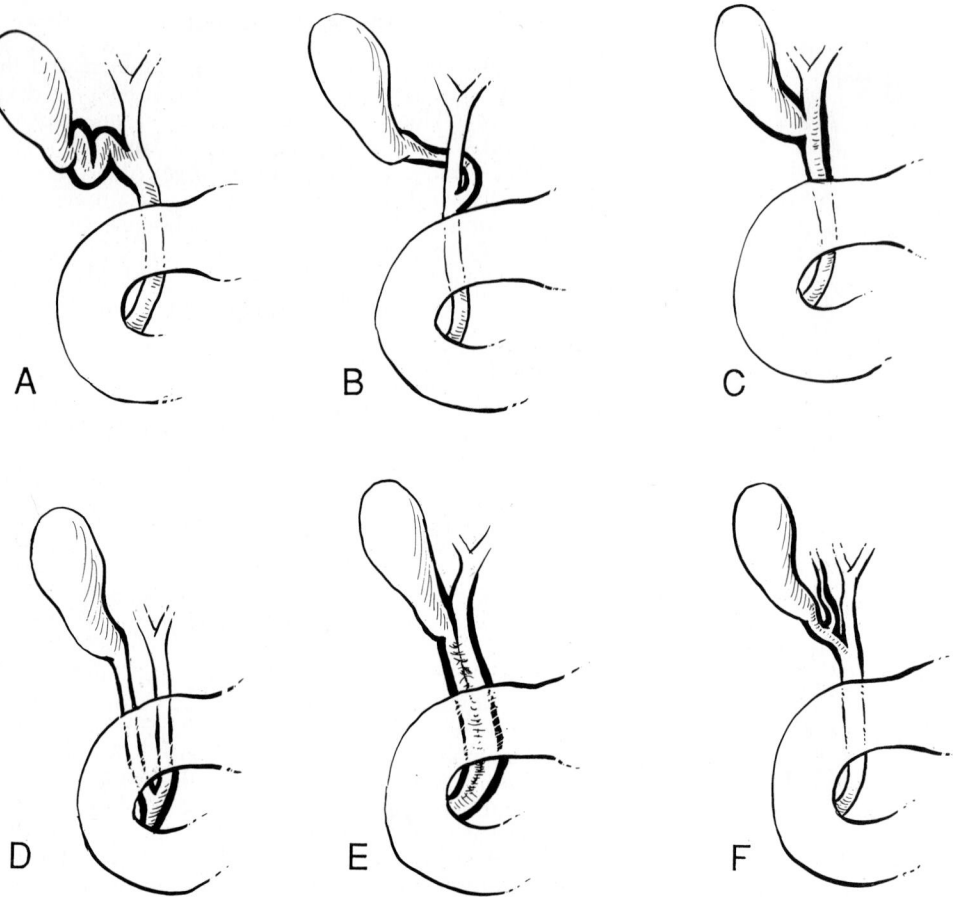

Figure 34–3. Surgically significant variations in ductal anatomy. *A,* Long, tortuous cystic duct. *B,* Cystic duct crosses common hepatic duct posteriorly and joins common duct on left side. This junction is posterior in some patients. *C,* Very short or absent cystic duct, usually seen in severe, chronic inflammation. *D,* Long cystic duct with low insertion into common duct. *E,* Long cystic duct fused to common hepatic duct. *F,* Anomalous entry of right anterior or posterior segmental duct into cystic duct; it may also enter the common hepatic duct.

calcium stearate and palmitate, which form layers in calcium bilirubinate stones.[50] The clinical settings in which this occurs include posttraumatic biliary stricture, a narrowed biliary-enteric anastomosis, stenosis of the sphincter of Oddi, sclerosing cholangitis, and Asian cholangiohepatitis. A suspected but unproved cause of primary common duct stones is dysfunction of the choledochal sphincter mechanism, with bile stasis and marked dilatation of the bile duct system.

Clinical Manifestations and Diagnosis. Common duct calculi may be asymptomatic or cause biliary colic, bile duct obstruction, cholangitis, or pancreatitis. The pain may be mild or severe and cannot be differentiated from pain arising

in the gallbladder. Jaundice will be intermittent if the obstruction is partial and intermittent, or it may be progressive if a stone becomes impacted in the distal duct. Chills and fever are usually associated with slight abdominal discomfort and a mild elevation of serum bilirubin, but any of these signs of cholangitis may be absent. Occasionally, symptoms of cholangitis are accompanied by shock and confusion, coma, or other central nervous symptoms, which signal the presence of acute toxic cholangitis, a condition in which infected bile or pus is under pressure within the duct system. Immediate resuscitation and emergency decompression of the duct system are necessary to prevent death. In routine cases of

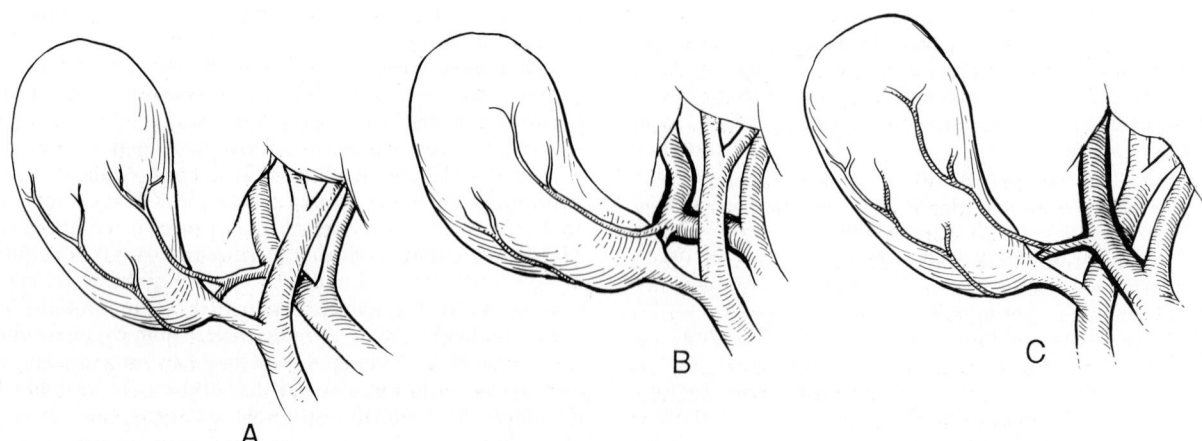

Figure 34–4. Important variations in the anatomy of the cystic and right hepatic arteries. *A,* Normal. *B,* "Caterpillar hump" right hepatic artery, which is amenable to injury. *C,* Right hepatic artery passing anterior to common hepatic duct, where it could be mistaken for cystic duct or cystic artery.

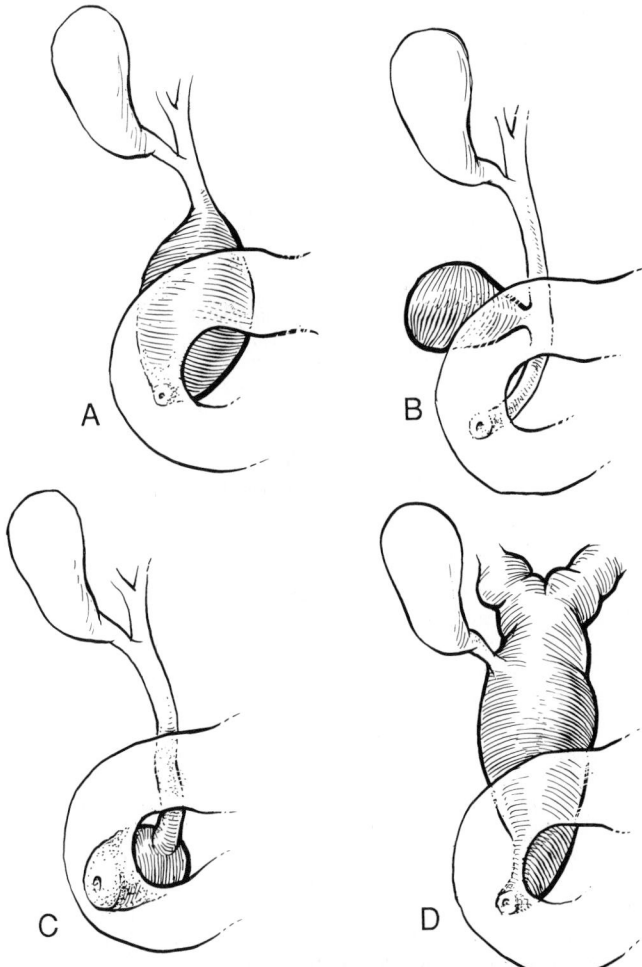

Figure 34–5. Cysts of the extrahepatic bile ducts. *A*, Classic fusiform choledochal cyst. *B*, Extrahepatic supraduodenal diverticulum. *C*, Choledochocele. *D*, Fusiform extrahepatic and intrahepatic cysts. (*A* to *D* from Alonso-Lej, F., Rever, W. B., Jr., and Pessagno, D. J.: Congenital choledochal cyst, with a report of 2, and an analysis of 94 cases. Surg. Gynecol. Obstet., *108*:1, 1959. By permission of SURGERY, Gynecology & Obstetrics, now known as the JOURNAL OF THE AMERICAN COLLEGE OF SURGEONS.)

Treatment. Cholangitis should be treated with antibiotics. Defervescence usually occurs rapidly. If it does not, acute toxic cholangitis may be present, and decompression of the duct system must be carried out immediately. This can be done by establishing percutaneous, transhepatic biliary drainage or by endoscopic sphincterotomy, but immediate laparotomy and insertion of a T-tube should be done if these simpler procedures fail or are not available.

Prior to the development of laparoscopic cholecystectomy, bile duct stones were suspected preoperatively on the basis of certain risk factors and identified by palpation or operative cholangiography during open cholecystectomy. Stones were then removed through a choledochotomy. Not all bile duct stones can be removed by laparoscopic cholecystectomy using the imperfect techniques currently available, and not all surgeons are expert in their use. Therefore, preoperative clearance of stones from the duct system by endoscopic sphincterotomy and stone extraction is preferred. Risk factors are used to make the diagnosis of choledocholithiasis prior to laparoscopic cholecystectomy. They include gallstone pancreatitis, cholangitis, clinical jaundice, dilatation of the common bile duct on ultrasonography (>8 mm.), elevated serum bilirubin and/or alkaline phosphatase, and identification of a bile duct stone on ultrasonography. Only identification of the stone on ultrasonography is always accurate; none of the other risk factors are more than approximately 50% reliable unless various combinations of them are used.[33, 47] Unfortunately, these risk factors falsely predict choledocholithiasis in up to three fourths of patients.[3] Patients thought to have choledocholithiasis preoperatively undergo ERCP. When stones are identified, endoscopic sphincterotomy and stone extraction is performed, a procedure that is successful in 90% of patients.[16, 38, 52] Success rate is low in patients who have more than five stones or any one stone larger than 1 cm. Open choledocholithotomy and cholecystectomy are performed if the duct system cannot be cleared of stones.

When risk factors are used to screen patients for bile duct stones and preoperative endoscopic stone removal is carried out, less than 5% of patients have stones identified on operative cholangiography at the time of laparoscopic cholecystectomy.[33, 44] In such patients, the stones must be removed by laparoscopic techniques, open choledocholithotomy, or postoperative endoscopic sphincterotomy and extraction.

Laparoscopic Choledocholithotomy. Common bile duct stones are managed laparoscopically by inserting a choledochoscope through a longitudinal incision in the cystic duct. In most instances, the cystic duct requires dilatation by graduated dilators or a pneumatic device to accommodate the scope. Guide wires and stone baskets can be passed directly into the duct or through a working channel in the scope to facilitate retrieval of stones.[28] Disadvantages are that stones larger than approximately 8 mm. in diameter cannot be retrieved, and bile duct stones located proximal to the entrance of the cystic duct are inaccessible because the choledochoscope cannot be directed proximally. Some advocate balloon dilatation of the sphincter of Oddi to facilitate flushing or pushing the stones into the duodenum,[46] but others believe that this is unwise. Successful clearance of stones from the bile duct system in selected patients ranges from 57% to 96%.[46]

Laparoscopic techniques in which stones are removed through a longitudinal choledochotomy in the common bile duct have been developed, but they require advanced skills and are not uniformly successful.[22, 56] A technique has been developed to perform antegrade sphincterotomy through a choledochoscope inserted into the duct system via the cystic duct. A duodenoscope is used to guide the operator in performing the sphincterotomy.[19] Further development of instrumentation and skills is needed.

choledocholithiasis, the physical examination may be normal. Jaundice and mild tenderness in the epigastrium and right upper quadrant may be present.

The white blood cell count is usually elevated when cholangitis is present, but in the absence of active infection, it is normal. Elevations of the serum bilirubin and alkaline phosphatase levels are characteristic. The mean serum bilirubin level in choledocholithiasis is about 9 mg. per deciliter, and values above 15 are rare.[61] Serum amylase measurement should always be done; when elevated, gallstone pancreatitis must be considered.

The early symptoms of choledocholithiasis cannot be easily distinguished from gallbladder colic or acute cholecystitis. Ultrasonography should be done to detect the presence or absence of gallstones and dilatation of the bile ducts. Ultrasonography is not reliable in the detection of common duct stones. Endoscopic retrograde cholangiopancreatography (ERCP) is indicated for most patients who have bile duct obstruction, as manifested by persistent jaundice or bile duct dilatation on ultrasonography or abnormal liver function tests. Percutaneous transhepatic cholangiography (PTC) is an alternative, but ERCP permits visualization of other portions of the gastrointestinal tract and allows for the performance of pancreatography and endoscopic sphincterotomy with stone extraction, when indicated.

Open Choledocholithotomy. Patients who are not candidates for laparoscopic procedures and those in whom endoscopic cholangiography and stone extraction are not possible may require open choledocholithotomy. Operative cholangiography should be performed routinely. The common duct should be opened longitudinally, examined with the choledochoscope, and explored carefully with stone forceps, scoops, and balloon catheters. Choledochoscopy is especially valuable to rule out intraductal papillary tumors and occult cancers. Stones impacted in the distal duct may be impossible to remove from above, and a duodenotomy and sphincterotomy may be necessary. After the stones have been removed, the duct should be closed around a Moss-Whelan T-tube, which has a large side arm, allowing percutaneous stone removal later, if necessary. A T-tube cholangiogram should be done before the abdomen is closed to check the position of the tube and to make certain that no stones remain.

Consideration must be given to a common duct drainage procedure in certain circumstances. These include the presence of more than five stones, marked dilatation of the duct, the inability to remove all the stones, and a previous choledocholithotomy. The author's preference is a large side-to-side choledochoduodenostomy, but division of the common duct and an end-to-side anastomosis are preferred by some. In some situations, sphincteroplasty is more efficacious than choledochoduodenostomy, especially when a stone is impacted in the distal duct, ampullary stenosis is present, or the duct is small in diameter.

In choledocholithotomy patients, the T-tube should not be removed prior to a postoperative cholangiogram, nor should it be removed earlier than 10 days postoperatively. When stones are present, the tube should be left in place for about 6 weeks, at which time percutaneous extraction of the calculi can be carried out through the mature, fibrous tract created by the tube (Fig. 34–6).

Choledocholithiasis in a patient who has had previous cholecystectomy is best treated by endoscopic sphincterotomy.[27] The success rate for endoscopic sphincterotomy and extraction of stones is about 90%,[16, 52] and the mortality rate is 1.0 to 1.5%,[23] which compares favorably with the mortality

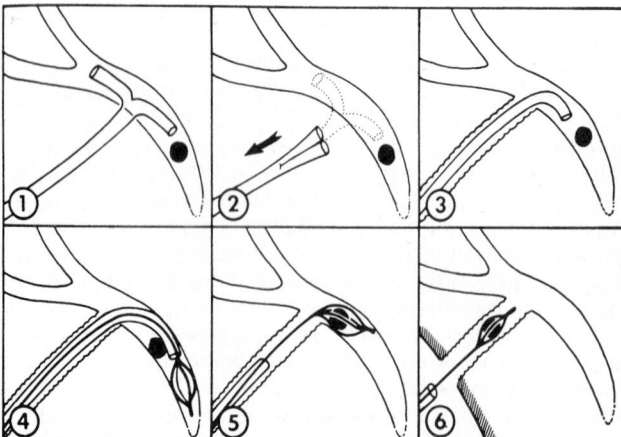

Figure 34–6. Steps in instrument extraction of retained common duct stone. (1) Repeat T-tube cholangiogram is obtained on the day of stone extraction 4 to 5 weeks after choledochotomy. (2) After the location of the retained stone has been ascertained, the T-tube is withdrawn. (3) Using the sinus tract of the T-tube, the steerable catheter is guided into the bile duct, and its movable tip is advanced beyond the retained stone. (4) The basket is inserted through the steerable catheter, the catheter is withdrawn, and the basket is opened. (5) The open basket is withdrawn in order to engage the stone. The basket is only retracted, never advanced outside the enclosure of the steerable catheter. (6) The stone is extracted through the drain tract. (From Burhenne, H. J.: Nonoperative retained biliary tract stone extraction: A new roentgenologic technique. A. J. R. Am. J. Roentgenol., *117*:388, 1973.)

associated with surgical choledocholithotomy. Extraction of stones larger than 1.5 cm. in diameter is often not possible, and the success rate for clearance of the duct when numerous stones are present is low. In such instances, surgical choledocholithotomy may be necessary. The endoscopic approach cannot be used in patients who have had a Billroth II reconstruction, and it should also be avoided when a distal common duct stricture is present. Other contraindications include the presence of duodenal diverticula in certain locations, coagulation disorders, and recent pancreatitis.

BILE DUCT INJURIES

More than 90% of bile duct leaks and strictures are due to inadvertent injury during cholecystectomy, bile duct surgery, or hepatic transplantation. Strictures also result from abdominal trauma, chronic pancreatitis, impaction of a calculus within the duct system, or chemical injury. Over 80% follow cholecystectomy and are due to inadvertent injury to the common hepatic or common bile duct. Knowledge of anatomic variants, routine operative cholangiography, and meticulous care in dissection are the keys to preventing injury. Iatrogenic strictures of the distal common bile duct usually result from injury by probes, forceps, or dilators during common duct exploration. The healing of bile duct injuries is characterized by extensive scarring and fibrosis, probably because of damage to the blood supply of the duct system and the fibrosing effect of bile on injured tissue.[39] More than 70% of injuries involve the common hepatic duct or the confluence of the right and left hepatic ducts.[60]

Early Management of Bile Duct Injuries. Leakage of bile into the peritoneal cavity or through an abdominal wound during the first postoperative week is often the first manifestation of bile duct injury. Patients may have fever, jaundice, increasing abdominal girth, and a failure to improve. Liver function tests are usually abnormal. Suspected leaks should be confirmed by a [99m]technetium-iminodiacetic acid scan. ERCP is performed to identify the site of bile leakage and to determine whether the duct has been transected or partially excised. When the duct system is intact, placement of a stent endoscopically produces excellent results,[10, 54] although long-term follow-up for possible stricture development has not been possible. Stents are removed after approximately 60 days.

Leakage of bile from the cystic duct stump or a minor injury immediately after cholecystectomy may be complicated by a distal bile duct calculus. The leak will not close unless the obstruction is relieved. This usually requires endoscopic sphincterotomy and extraction of the offending stone, followed by placement of a stent through the site of the leak.

When the ERCP shows that the duct system is not intact, PTC with placement of stents is essential. Cholangiography must demonstrate both right and left duct systems, and each of them must be cannulated with a stent. In this manner, the complete extent of the injury is delineated, and any anomalous ductal anatomy is clearly identified in preparation for the most efficacious reconstructive procedure. Computed tomography (CT) of the abdomen is performed to identify and drain fluid collections.

Reconstruction is performed as soon as the patient's condition is stable. End-to-side Roux-en-Y hepaticojejunostomy is usually possible when the confluence of the right and left hepatic ducts is intact. Higher injuries require anastomosis of each duct to the side of the Roux-en-Y limb. Sometimes the adjoining walls of the two hepatic ducts can be sewn together and the resulting complex anastomosed to the Roux-en-Y limb of jejunum. The previously placed transhepatic stents are placed across the biliary enteric anastomoses.

Late Strictures. Strictures due to bile duct injury can present in the immediate postoperative period or many years later. Recurrent cholangitis is the most common manifestation of a stricture that develops months or years after operation. Stricture is a rare cause of acute suppurative cholangitis, in which the biliary duct system contains pus under pressure. In long-standing strictures, jaundice may be the only manifestation; sometimes this is due to the formation of stones proximal to the site of narrowing. Life-threatening conditions caused by a stricture include sepsis from cholangitis and the development of cirrhosis, portal hypertension, and hemorrhage from esophageal varices. Therefore, symptoms of biliary tract obstruction following cholecystectomy or other biliary tract operations should always be investigated. The development of jaundice or symptoms of cholangitis is an indication for liver function tests. Elevated serum bilirubin and alkaline phosphatase are indicative of obstruction. Cholangiography is essential. The common practice is to perform ERCP, but PTC may be necessary to define precisely the extent of stricturing and to insert Ring catheters.

Management of Late Strictures. Surgical reconstruction of the duct system has been the traditional treatment of late strictures. The goal is to construct a wide, tension-free anastomosis, with mucosa-to-mucosa apposition, between normal bile duct and the intestine. This is best accomplished by an end-to-side choledochoduodenostomy or a Roux-en-Y hepaticojejunostomy (Fig. 34–7). The former is applicable to distal bile duct strictures, such as those caused by chronic pancreatitis. Most iatrogenic strictures are in the proximal portion of the extrahepatic duct system and cannot be treated by choledochoduodenostomy, because a tension-free anastomosis is not possible. The Roux-en-Y limb permits a tension-free anastomosis that can be sized according to the diameter of the bile duct. A stent is left in place only when the anastomosis is narrow; it is removed after 2 or 3 months. Excellent results are obtained after surgical treatment in over 75% of patients.[20, 34] Serum bilirubin and alkaline phosphatase should be monitored, and if either is elevated persistently, cholangiography is indicated. A stricture may recur as long as 20 years after repair.

Growing experience in the treatment of biliary strictures by the placement of stents suggests that good results can be obtained in selected patients. Removable plastic stents, placed endoscopically, are changed every 3 months and removed from 6 to 18 months after the initial procedure. Tight strictures may require catheter or balloon dilatation to facilitate placement of the stent. The results are good to excellent in approximately 80% of patients, but follow-up is short.[6, 20, 24, 34] The most frequent complication is recurrent cholangitis.

The role of percutaneous transhepatic balloon dilatation of benign strictures is not clear.[35] The proximal ducts are not dilated in some patients, and hemobilia is a risk of the

transhepatic approach. However, balloon dilatation was successful in up to 76% of patients after 2 years.[44]

BILE DUCT CANCER

Carcinomas of the extrahepatic bile ducts are rare and are often recognized late in their course. Because of their location in close proximity to the liver, hepatic artery, and portal vein, they may not be resectable. Nevertheless, these tumors do not have a high propensity to metastasize, so palliation for significant periods of time may be possible.

The average age of onset is about 60 years. Males and females are equally affected. Bile duct cancer has been categorized according to anatomic location.[10, 31, 54] Cancers in the upper third occur between the undersurface of the liver and the cystic duct; 50% to 75% are located in this area. Mid-third lesions are between the cystic duct and the superior border of the duodenum; 10% to 25% are found here. Lower-third lesions are located between the superior border of the pancreas and the ampulla, accounting for 10% to 20% of lesions, but carcinomas of the ampulla itself are not included in this category.

Associations. Approximately 30% of patients with cholangiocarcinoma have gallstones, but this is no different from the incidence of gallstones in a population matched for age and sex.[29] Cholangiocarcinoma is associated with primary sclerosing cholangitis,[51] infestation with *Clonorchis sinensis*,[53] exposure to certain chemicals, and congenital cystic disease of the biliary tract, including choledochal cyst and Caroli's disease.[7] Patients with ulcerative colitis are predisposed to the development of primary sclerosing cholangitis. However, cholangiocarcinoma is associated with primary sclerosing cholangitis, not ulcerative colitis.[51]

Clinical Manifestations and Diagnosis. About 90% of patients present with jaundice.[1, 59] Weight loss and pain occur in about half, but the pain is not severe. Pruritus is frequent. Sometimes the disease presents with cholangitis—chills, fever, abdominal pain, and jaundice. Physical examination reveals an enlarged, tender liver. The gallbladder may be palpable when lesions are distal to the entrance of the cystic duct and obstruction is complete. The presence of ascites and splenomegaly signifies portal vein invasion and implies a grave prognosis. Laboratory tests show elevation of bilirubin and alkaline phosphatase.

As in all cases of extrahepatic bile duct obstruction, cholangiography is necessary to determine the location of the tumor and its resectability. The author prefers PTC, because the proximal extent of the lesion can be visualized. However, brushings can be obtained if ERCP is performed. CT may be helpful in determining the extent of the lesion in the radial direction, and angiography may delineate growth into a major vessel, usually the portal vein.[8] In distal lesions, endoscopy may be helpful to rule out carcinoma of the ampulla of Vater. Cytologic diagnosis is possible by percutaneous, directed fine-needle aspiration of the tumor or by brushings obtained via the endoscope.

Treatment. Surgical resection of the tumor is the only chance for cure. Proximal- and middle-third lesions require removal of the common bile duct and surrounding tissue, with dissection at least 1 cm. proximal to the most proximal extent of the tumor. This often requires resection of portions of both hepatic ducts and sometimes hepatic lobectomy. Reconstruction should be by Roux-en-Y hepaticojejunostomy, splinted by catheters brought out through the liver and skin proximally. The ability to change catheters under fluoroscopic guidance has obviated the need to bring the distal end out through the Roux-en-Y limb and the skin as U-tubes.

Although an indwelling catheter may not be necessary to protect the anastomosis, especially if it is large, one should

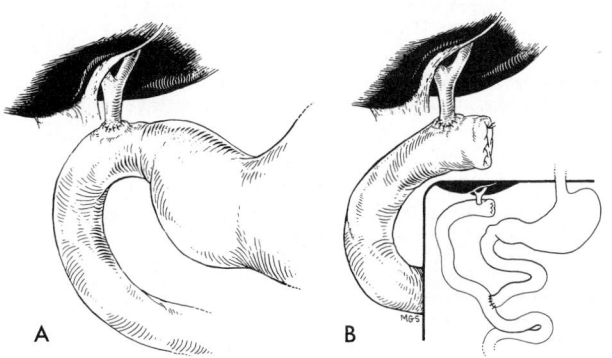

Figure 34–7. Choledochoduodenostomy *(A)* and anastomosis to a Roux-en-Y limb *(B)*. Note that the end of the jejunum is closed so that a precise, appropriately sized mucosa-to-mucosa anastomosis can be done to the jejunum.

be used if radiation therapy is contemplated, because bile duct epithelium is easily damaged by radiation.[55]

Carcinomas in the distal third of the bile duct are, by definition, in the intrapancreatic portion of the duct and must be treated by the Whipple procedure. Often, it is not possible to differentiate them from pancreatic cancers preoperatively.

Patients who have disseminated cancer or involvement of the hepatic artery, the portal vein, or their branches can be treated by palliative stenting.[18] Frequent catheter changes under fluoroscopic guidance are necessary because of the problem of recurrent cholangitis (Fig. 34–8).

The prognosis is poor. Taken as a group, about 10% of patients who have bile duct cancer are cured.[12, 49] Cure is rare for proximal-third lesions, approximately 10% for middle-third cancers, and about 25% for those in the lower third. The role of radiation therapy and chemotherapy in enhancing survival is not clear.

SCLEROSING CHOLANGITIS

Sclerosing cholangitis is an inflammatory disease of the bile ducts that causes fibrosis and thickening of their walls and multiple short, concentric strictures. Both the intrahepatic and extrahepatic portions of the duct system, as well as the gallbladder, may be involved. The disease is progressive and gradually causes cirrhosis, portal hypertension, and death from hepatic failure. Patients with sclerosing cholangitis have an increased incidence of cholangiocarcinoma, which may have a similar cholangiographic appearance.

Many cases of sclerosing cholangitis occur primarily, but some are associated with inflammatory bowel disease, most notably ulcerative colitis, which is associated with about 70% of cases.[21] Retroperitoneal and mediastinal fibrosis, pancreatitis, pancreatic fibrosis, orbital pseudotumors, and Peyronie's disease have also been reported in association with sclerosing cholangitis.[30] The etiology has been linked to altered immunity, toxins, and infectious agents, and there is indirect evidence to support each of these theories.

About two thirds of cases occur in persons younger than 45 years of age, and the male-to-female ratio is 3:2. Fatigue, anorexia, weight loss, and the insidious development of jaundice and pruritus are the usual findings. Vague upper abdominal pain is sometimes present. Cholangitis may develop and may become a vexing problem after surgical

intervention or the placement of indwelling tubes or stents percutaneously. The diagnosis is made by the typical cholangiographic appearance, usually obtained by ERCP, the clinical findings, and liver biopsy.

Medical therapy consists of corticosteroids and long-term antibiotic administration when cholangitis is a recurrent problem. Immunosuppressants, bile acid–binding agents, colchicine, and penicillamine have been used. There is no solid evidence that these agents alter the slow, progressive course of the disease. Ursodeoxycholic acid improves the associated biochemical abnormalities and is currently being evaluated.[40]

Surgical intervention in the form of extrahepatic bile duct and liver biopsies may be necessary, especially when cholangiocarcinoma cannot be ruled out. More often, consideration of percutaneous balloon dilatation or stenting arises when the patient is jaundiced and clearly has one or more points of obstruction within the biliary tree. Some patients are improved by these procedures.[17, 32] The treatment of each patient must be individualized.

In the very rare patient who has an isolated obstruction within the extrahepatic duct system, a Roux-en-Y choledochojejunostomy proximal to the obstruction may be indicated. When the extrahepatic duct system is severely involved, the most severe constriction may be at or near the bifurcation of the common hepatic duct. In this situation, Cameron and associates[11] recommend excision of the extrahepatic duct system distal to the bifurcation and individual anastomoses of the right and left hepatic ducts to a Roux-en-Y limb of jejunum. Each of the anastomoses is then splinted with a transhepatic U-tube stent. The short-term results have been good.

The definitive management of patients with sclerosing cholangitis is hepatic transplantation. At present, the 5-year survival rates are approximately 60%—about the same as those for other types of chronic liver disease.

SELECTED REFERENCES

Cotton, P. B.: Endoscopic management of bile duct stones (apples and oranges). Gut, 25:587, 1984.
This classic article describes problems in and results of the endoscopic management of choledocholithiasis.

Glenn, F., and Grafe, W. R., Jr.: Historical events in biliary tract surgery. Arch. Surg., 93:848, 1966.
The authors review the significant events in biliary tract surgery and provide excellent references for those who wish to study the subject.

Petelin, J. B.: Laparoscopic approach to common duct pathology. Am. J. Surg., 165:487, 1993.
Extensive experience with the laparoscopic management of bile duct stones is detailed by a leader in the field.

Strasberg, S. M., Hertl, M., and Soper, N. J.: An analysis of the problem of biliary injury during laparoscopic cholecystectomy. J. Am. Coll. Surg., 180:101, 1995.
The causes, classification, diagnosis, and management of biliary injuries are set forth in this comprehensive review of the literature.

Tompkins, R. K.: Treatment and prognosis in bile duct cancer. World J. Surg., 12:109, 1988.
An experienced surgeon reviews a large series of cases and suggests the best procedures, based on outcome and the extensive experience at his institution.

REFERENCES

1. Alexander, F., Rossi, R. L., O'Bryan, M., Khettry, U., Braasch, J. W., and Walkins, E., Jr.: Biliary carcinoma: A review of 109 cases. Am. J. Surg., 147:503, 1984.
2. Alonso-Lej, F., Rever, W. B., Jr., and Pessagno, D. J.: Congenital choledochal cyst, with a report of 2, and an analysis of 94 cases. Surg. Gynecol. Obstet., 108:1, 1959.
3. Arregui, M. E., Davis, C. J., Arkush, A. M., and Nagan, R. F.: Laparoscopic cholecystectomy combined with endoscopic sphincterotomy and stone extraction or laparoscopic choledochoscopy and electrohydraulic lithotripsy for management of cholelithiasis with choledocholithiasis. Surg. Endosc., 6:10, 1992.

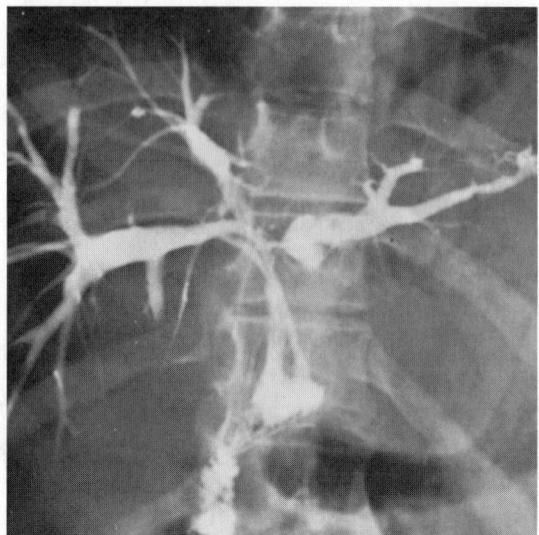

Figure 34–8. Carcinoma involving the common hepatic duct and both hepatic ducts through which a tube has been passed for palliation.

4. Beal, J. M.: Historical perspective of gallstone disease. Surg. Gynecol. Obstet., *158*:181, 1984.
5. Bennion, R. S., Thompson, J. E., Jr., and Tompkins, R. K.: Agenesis of the gallbladder without extrahepatic biliary atresia. Arch. Surg., *123*:1257, 1988.
6. Berkelhammer, C., Kortan, P., and Haber, G. B.: Endoscopic biliary prosthesis as treatment for benign postoperative bile duct strictures. Gastrointest. Endosc., *35*:98, 1989.
7. Bloustein, P. A.: Association of carcinoma with congenital cystic conditions of the liver and bile ducts. Am. J. Gastroenterol., *67*:40, 1977.
8. Blumgart, L. H., Hadjis, N. S., Benjamin, I. S., and Beazley, R.: Surgical approaches to cholangiocarcinoma at confluence of hepatic ducts. Lancet, *1*:66, 1984.
9. Bobbs, J. S.: Case of lithotomy of the gallbladder. Trans. Ind. State Med. Soc., *18*:68, 1868.
10. Branum, G., Schmitt, C., Baillie, J., Suhocki, P., Baker, M., Davidoff, A., Branch, S., Chari, R., Cucchiaro, G., Murray, E., Pappas, T., Cotton, P., and Meyers, W. C.: Management of major biliary complications after laparoscopic cholecystectomy. Ann. Surg., *217*:532, 1993.
11. Cameron, J. L., Pitt, H. A., Zimmer, M. J., Herlong, H. F., Kaufman, S. L., Boitnott, J. K., and Coleman, J.: Resection of hepatic duct bifurcation and transhepatic stenting for sclerosing cholangitis. Ann. Surg., *207*:614, 1988.
12. Cameron, J. L., Pitt, H. A., Zimmer, M. A., Kaufman, S. L., and Coleman, J.: Management of proximal cholangiocarcinomas by surgical resection and radiotherapy. Am. J. Surg., *159*:91, 1990.
13. Caroli, J., Soupalt, R., Kossakowski, J., Plocker, L., and Paradowska, M.: La dilatation polikistique congenitale des voies biliares intrahepatiques: Essai de classification. Sem. Hop. Paris, *34*:488, 1958.
14. Chijüwa, K., Komura, M., and Kameoka, N.: Postoperative follow-up of patients with type IVA choledochal cysts after excision of extrahepatic cyst. J. Am. Coll. Surg., *179*:641, 1994.
15. Cole, W. H.: The development of cholecystography: The first fifty years. Am. J. Surg., *136*:541, 1978.
16. Cotton, P. B.: Endoscopic management of bile duct stones (apples and oranges). Gut, *25*:587, 1984.
17. Cotton, P. B., and Nickl, N.: Endoscopic and radiologic approaches to therapy in primary sclerosing cholangitis. Semin. Liver Dis., *11*:40, 1991.
18. Crist, D. W., Kadir, S., and Cameron, J. L.: Proximal biliary tract reconstruction: The value of preoperatively placed percutaneous biliary catheters. Surg. Gynecol. Obstet., *175*:579, 1987.
19. Curet, M. J., Pitcher, D. E., Martin, D. T., and Zucker, K. A.: Laparoscopic antegrade sphincterotomy: A new technique for the management of complex choledocholithiasis. Ann. Surg., *221*:149, 1995.
20. Davids, P. H. P., Tanka, A. K. F., Ramros, E. A. J., van Gulik, T. M., van Leeuwen, D. J., de Wit, L. T., Verbeek, P. C. M., Huibregtse, K., van der Heyde, M. N., and Tytgat, G. N. J.: Benign biliary strictures: Surgery or endoscopy? Ann. Surg., *217*:237, 1993.
21. Farrant, J. M., Hayllar, K. M., Wilkinson, M. L., Karani, J., Portmann, B. C., Westaby, D., and Williams, R.: Natural history and prognostic variables in primary sclerosing cholangitis. Gastroenterology, *100*:1710, 1991.
22. Ferzli, G. S., Massaad, A., Ozuner, G., and Worth, M. H., Jr.: Laparoscopic exploration of the common bile duct. Surg. Gynecol. Obstet., *174*:419, 1992.
23. Frost, R. A.: Prospective multi-center study of British sphincterotomy: Initial results and complications. Gut, *25*:549, 1984.
24. Geenen, D. J., Geenen, J. E., Hogan, W. J., Schenck, J., Venu, R. P., Johnson, G. K., and Jackson, A., Jr.: Endoscopic therapy for benign bile duct strictures. Gastrointest. Endosc., *35*:367, 1989.
25. Grosfeld, J. L., Rescorla, F. J., Skinner, M. A., West, K. W., and Scherer, L. R., III: The spectrum of biliary tract disorders in infants and children: Experience with 300 cases. Arch. Surg., *129*:513, 1994.
26. Harlaftis, N., Gray, S. W., and Skandalakis, J. E.: Multiple gallbladders. Surg. Gynecol. Obstet., *145*:928, 1977.
27. Hawes, R., Cotton, P. B., and Vallon, A.: Follow-up 6 to 11 years after duodenoscopic sphincterotomy for stones in patients with prior cholecystectomy. Gastroenterology, *98*:1008, 1990.
28. Hunter, J. G.: Laparoscopic transcystic common bile duct exploration. Am. J. Surg., *163*:53, 1992.
29. Koga, A., Ichimiya, H., Yamaguchi, K., Miyazaki, K., and Nakayama, F.: Hepatolithiasis associated with cholangiocarcinoma: Possible etiologic significance. Cancer, *55*:2828, 1985.
30. LaRusso, N. F., Wiesner, R. H., Ludwig, J., and MacCarty, R. L.: Primary sclerosing cholangitis. N. Engl. J. Med., *310*:899, 1984.
31. Longmire, W. P., Jr.: Tumors of the extrahepatic biliary radicles. Curr. Probl. Cancer, *1*:1, 1976.
32. May, G. R., Bender, C. E., La Russo, N. F., and Wiesner, R. H.: Nonoperative dilatation of dominant strictures in primary sclerosing cholangitis. A.J.R. Am. J. Roentgenol., *145*:1061, 1985.
33. Miller, R. E., Kimmelstiel, F. M., and Winkler, W. P.: Management of common bile duct stones in the era of laparoscopic cholecystectomy. Am. J. Surg., *169*:273, 1995.
34. Millis, J. M., Tompkins, R. K., Zinner, M. J., Longmire, W. P., Jr., and Roslyn, J. J.: Management of bile duct strictures: An evolving strategy. Arch. Surg., *127*:1077, 1992.
35. Mueller, P. R., vanSonnenberg, E., Ferrucci, J. T., Jr., Weyman, P. J., Butch, R. J., Malt, R. A., and Burhenne, H. J.: Biliary stricture dilatation: Multicenter review of clinical management in 73 patients. Radiology, *160*:17, 1986.
36. Mühe, E.: Die erste cholecystektomie durch des laparoskop. Langenbecks Arch. Chir., *369*:804, 1986.
37. Nagorney, D. M., McIlrath, D. C., and Adson, M. A.: Choledochal cysts in adults: Clinical management. Surgery, *96*:656, 1984.
38. Neoptolemos, J. P., Carr-Locke, D. L., and Fossard, D. P.: Prospective randomised study of preoperative endoscopic sphincterotomy versus surgery alone for common bile duct stones. Br. Med. J., *294*:470, 1987.
39. Northover, J. M. A., and Terblanche, J.: A new look at the arterial supply of the bile duct in man and its surgical implications. Br. J. Surg., *66*:379, 1979.
40. O'Brien, C. B., Senior, J. R., Arora-Mirchandani, R., Batta, A. K., and Salen, G.: Ursodeoxycholic acid for the treatment of primary sclerosing cholangitis: A 30-month pilot study. Hepatology, *14*:838, 1991.
41. Okada, A., Oguchi, Y., Kamata, S., Ikeda, Y., Kawashima, Y., and Saito, R.: Common channel syndrome—diagnosis with endoscopic retrograde cholangiopancreatectography and surgical management. Surgery, *93*:634, 1983.
42. O'Neill, J. A., Templeton, J. M., Schnaufer, L., Bishop, H. C., Ziegler, M. M., and Ross, A. J., III: Recent experience with choledochal cyst. Ann. Surg., *205*:533, 1987.
43. Ostrow, J. D.: The etiology of pigment gallstones. Hepatology, *4*:2155, 1984.
44. Pace, B. W., Cosgrove, J., Breuer, B., and Margolis, I. B.: Intraoperative cholangiography revisited. Arch. Surg., *127*:448, 1992.
45. Palmisano, D. J.: Double gallbladder. Am. J. Surg., *118*:463, 1969.
46. Petelin, J. B.: Laparoscopic approach to common duct pathology. Am. J. Surg., *165*:487, 1993.
47. Phillips, E. H., Carroll, B. J., Pearlstein, A. R., Daykovsky, L., and Fallas, M. J.: Laparoscopic choledochoscopy and extraction of common bile duct stones. World J. Surg., *17*:22, 1992.
48. Power, D.: Gallstones: A plea for earlier operation. Br. J. Surg., *1*:12, 1913.
49. Reding, R., Buard, J.-L., Lebeau, G., and Launois, B.: Surgical management of 552 carcinomas of the extrahepatic bile ducts (gallbladder and periampullary tumors excluded): Results of the French Surgical Association survey. Ann. Surg., *213*:236, 1991.
50. Robins, S., Fasulo, J., and Patton, G.: Lipids of pigment gallstones. Biochim. Biophys. Acta, *712*:21, 1987.
51. Rosen, C. B., Nagorney, D. M., Wiesner, R. H., Coffey, R. J., and La Russo, N. F.: Cholangiocarcinoma complicating primary sclerosing cholangitis. Ann. Surg., *213*:21, 1990.
52. Safrany, L.: Endoscopic treatment of biliary tract disease. Lancet, *2*:983, 1978.
53. Sher, L., Iwatsuki, S., Lebeau, G., and Zajko, A. B.: Hilar cholangiocarcinoma associated with clonorchiasis. Dig. Dis. Sci., *34*:1121, 1989.
54. Sherman, S., Shaked, A., Cryer, H. M., Goldstein, L. I., and Busuttil, R. W.: Endoscopic management of biliary fistulas complicating liver transplantation and other hepatobiliary operations. Ann. Surg., *218*:167, 1993.
55. Sindelar, W. F., Tepper, J., and Travis, E. L.: Tolerance of bile duct to intraoperative radiation. Surgery, *92*:533, 1982.
56. Stoker, M. E., Leveillee, R. J., McCann, J. C., Jr., and Maini, B. S.: Laparoscopic common bile duct exploration. J. Laparoendosc. Surg., *1*:287, 1991.
57. Todani, T., Watanabe, Y., Fujii, T., and Uemura, S.: Anomalous arrangement of the pancreatobiliary ductal system in patients with choledochal cyst. Am. J. Surg., *147*:672, 1984.
58. Todani, T., Watanabe, Y., Narusue, M., Tabuchi, K., and Okajima, K.: Congenital bile duct cysts: Classification, operative procedures, and review of thirty-seven cases including cancer arising from choledochal cyst. Am. J. Surg., *134*:263, 1977.
59. Tompkins, R. K., Thomas, D., Wile, A., and Longmire, W. P., Jr.: Prognostic factors in bile duct carcinoma: Analysis of 96 cases. Ann. Surg., *194*:447, 1981.
60. Warren, K. W., Mountain, J. C., and Midell, A. I.: Management of strictures of the biliary tract. Surg. Clin. North Am., *51*:711, 1971.
61. Way, L. W., Admirand, W. H., and Dunphy, J. E.: Management of choledocholithiasis. Ann. Surg., *176*:347, 1972.
62. Wilson, J. E., and Dietrick, J. E.: Agenesis of the gallbladder: Case report and familial investigation. Surgery, *99*:106, 1986.
63. Yuhl, E. T., Stirrett, L., Hill, M. R., Jr., and Beal, J. M.: The cholescintigram: A preliminary report. Surgery, *34*:724, 1953.

I

ACUTE CHOLECYSTITIS

David L. Nahrwold, M.D.

Acute cholecystitis is a chemical or bacterial inflammation of the gallbladder that may cause severe peritonitis and death unless proper treatment is instituted. In about 95% of cases, gallstones are present in the gallbladder (calculous cholecystitis), and in about 5% they are not (acalculous cholecystitis).

ACUTE CALCULOUS CHOLECYSTITIS

The incidence of acute calculous cholecystitis is higher in females, with a female-to-male ratio of 3:1 up to about the age of 50 and a ratio of approximately 1.5:1 thereafter.

The exact incidence of acute cholecystitis among patients who harbor gallstones is not known, but about 20% of patients who enter a hospital for biliary tract disease have acute cholecystitis. The percentage of cholecystectomies done for acute cholecystitis has increased, especially in the elderly.[8] Patients who have symptoms from gallstones should be advised to have elective cholecystectomy to avoid the mortality and morbidity of acute cholecystitis and its complications.

Pathogenesis. Acute calculous cholecystitis appears to be caused by obstruction of the cystic duct or the junction of the gallbladder and the cystic duct by a stone or by edema formed as the result of local mucosal erosion and inflammation caused by a stone. The obstruction causes gallbladder distention, followed by subserosal edema, venous and lymphatic obstruction, cellular infiltration, and localized areas of ischemia. Perforation at the site of ischemic gangrene may cause bile peritonitis or, if confined by omentum, a localized pericholecystic abscess. Rarely, a gangrenous area may perforate into the wall of the duodenum or small intestine, causing a cholecystoenteric fistula. Gallstones then may be discharged into the small intestine, and if one is sufficiently large, the rare syndrome of mechanical obstruction of the distal ileum, gallstone ileus, may result.

The role of bacteria in the pathogenesis of acute cholecystitis is not clear; positive cultures of bile or gallbladder wall are found in 50% to 75% of cases.[17, 25] Nevertheless, deaths and complications from untreated cholecystitis are almost always related to septic complications of the disease, and the organisms involved are those that most often colonize the stone-containing gallbladder. An important feature of the pathogenesis may be erosion of the mucosa by a stone, giving highly concentrated bile salts access to tissue planes. Bile salts are toxic to cells because they have detergent properties that allow them to solubilize the lipids in cell membranes. This causes destruction of cells, necrosis, and, eventually, perforation of the gallbladder.

Although obstruction by a stone is essential for the development of acute calculous cholecystitis, other factors appear to be involved, because acute cholecystitis is not the inevitable consequence of obstruction. Hydrops of the gallbladder, in which the outlet is obstructed by a stone, produces marked distention, but acute inflammation does not follow. In animals, ligation of the cystic duct alone does not produce acute cholecystitis. Thus, it appears that outlet obstruction plus another factor are essential for the development of acute cholecystitis. In animal experiments, the presence of pancreatic juice, gastric juice, or concentrated bile in the lumen of the obstructed gallbladder causes acute cholecystitis.[33, 39]

Pathology. The inflamed gallbladder is enlarged, and the serosal surface is congested and may have areas of gangrene or necrosis. The wall is edematous and thickened. The obstructing stone is usually impacted in the infundibulum or the cystic duct. Pus or bloody bile may be found within the lumen. Mucosal sloughing is usually present, although this may be apparent only on microscopic examination. Neutrophils are found within 24 hours and become more prominent as time progresses; the neutrophilic response is more prominent in gangrene, perforation, and empyema. *Empyema* is the term used to denote an acutely inflamed gallbladder that contains pus. Empyema of the gallbladder is the equivalent of an intra-abdominal abscess and may be associated with severe sepsis. Cystic duct obstruction is the *sine qua non* for its development. In neglected cases, the empyema may drain spontaneously through the abdominal wall.

About 65% of gallbladders involved with acute cholecystitis also have the manifestations of chronic cholecystitis: fibrosis of the wall, chronic inflammatory cell infiltrate, Rokitansky-Aschoff sinuses, and mucosal flattening.[18] This is evidence that recurrent attacks of acute cholecystitis occur. As the acute process resolves, fibrosis of the wall and a chronic inflammatory infiltrate become prominent features.

Symptoms. Most patients have symptoms referable to the gallbladder prior to the development of acute cholecystitis, but 20% to 40% are asymptomatic. Persistent pain in the area of the gallbladder is present in almost every case. The absence of pain essentially rules out the diagnosis. Frequently, the pain develops after ingestion of a meal and probably results from forceful contraction of the gallbladder against a fixed obstruction, usually a stone impacted in the infundibulum or the cystic duct. As the development of acute cholecystitis progresses through the sequence of distention, edema, venous and lymphatic obstruction, and ischemia, the pain is probably caused by gallbladder distention and, later, by inflammation of the gallbladder and adjacent peritoneal surfaces. Depending on the build of the patient and the precise location of the organ, the pain may be in the right upper quadrant, the epigastrium, or both. Radiation of the pain is around the right side toward the tip of the scapula. Pain in the right shoulder is present when the diaphragm is irritated by the inflammatory process. The persistence and severity of pain serve to distinguish the development of acute cholecystitis from an attack of gallbladder colic. The former may last for several days, but the latter rarely lasts for more than a few hours.

Nausea and vomiting, which occur in 60% to 70% of patients, are the only other significant symptoms. This appears to be a reflex phenomenon, associated with a rapid rise in gallbladder pressure. Frequently, patients attempt to induce vomiting, having the sensation that they will feel better afterward.

Physical Findings. The inflammatory nature of acute cholecystitis results in an elevated temperature in about 80% of patients. Fever may be absent in elderly or immunocompromised patients and in those who take steroids or nonsteroidal anti-inflammatory drugs. The most common and reliable finding on physical examination is tenderness in the right upper quadrant, the epigastrium, or both. Subjective tenderness is so common that its absence should raise serious questions about the diagnosis. About half of all patients have muscle rigidity in the right upper quadrant, and about one fourth have rebound tenderness. The frequency of these findings, which are indicative of peritonitis, increases as the disease progresses. Murphy's sign, consisting of inspiratory arrest during deep palpation of the right upper quadrant, is not a consistent finding but is almost pathognomonic when present. Unless generalized peritonitis has developed, acute cholecystitis usually does not cause paralytic ileus distal to the duodenum; therefore, bowel sounds are absent in only about 10% of patients. A mass in the region of the gallbladder is palpable in about 40%. This may be the distended gallbladder or the omentum attached to the gallbladder, in response to the inflammation. Late in the course of the disease, a mass may signify the development of a pericholecystic abscess.

Jaundice occurs in approximately 10% of patients, possibly due to entry of bile pigments into the circulation through the damaged gallbladder mucosa, or to physiologic obstruction of the bile duct system from choledochal sphincter spasm induced by the adjacent inflammatory process.[28] The presence of jaundice should suggest the possibility of concomitant choledocholithiasis, which occurs in 10% to 15% of cases.

Laboratory Findings. The white blood cell count is elevated in 85% of cases, but it may not be increased in those who take anti-inflammatory drugs or in the elderly. One half have elevation of the serum bilirubin, and the serum amylase is increased in one third.

Imaging Studies. The specific test for acute cholecystitis is cholescintigraphy with a derivative of ^{99m}technetium-iminodiacetic acid (technetium-IDA scan). Normally, the scan outlines the liver and the extrahepatic biliary tract, including the gallbladder, and shows the nuclide flowing into the upper small intestine as well (Fig. 34–9). In acute cholecystitis, the gallbladder is not seen on the scan, presumably because the gallbladder outlet or the cystic duct is obstructed (Fig. 34–10).

In acute calculous cholecystitis, cholescintigraphy has a sensitivity of almost 100%, meaning that the test will be positive in almost all patients who actually have acute cholecystitis; it has a specificity of 95%, meaning that the scan is negative in 95% of individuals who do not have the disease.[37] Complete obstruction of the common bile duct or the common hepatic duct is detectable on the technetium-IDA scan, but the degree of resolution is not sufficient to diagnose stones or other lesions.

Calculi within the gallbladder can be accurately detected by ultrasonography, but this test is not specific for acute calculous cholecystitis. A thickened gallbladder wall and pericholecystic fluid are sometimes present. Ultrasonography can detect right upper quadrant masses and enlargement of the bile ducts and pancreas, so it may be useful in complicated cases or when the diagnosis is obscure.[5] Although some have advocated routine ultrasonography in suspected acute cholecystitis to confirm the presence of gallstones, the technetium-IDA scan is more specific and is the indicated test in patients who present with the classic clinical manifestations.

Differential Diagnosis. Acute cholecystitis must be differentiated from other acute abdominal conditions, including acute appendicitis, perforated or penetrating duodenal ulcer, acute or perforated gastric ulcer, and acute pancreatitis. Most cases of acute appendicitis can be differentiated easily, but those in which the tip of a long, retrocecal appendix lies near the gallbladder can be vexing. Cholescintigraphy is helpful in this situation.

In approximately 15% of cases of acute cholecystitis, the serum amylase is elevated, suggesting the possibility of acute pancreatitis. The cause of hyperamylasemia in uncomplicated acute cholecystitis is unknown; hyperamylasemia does not

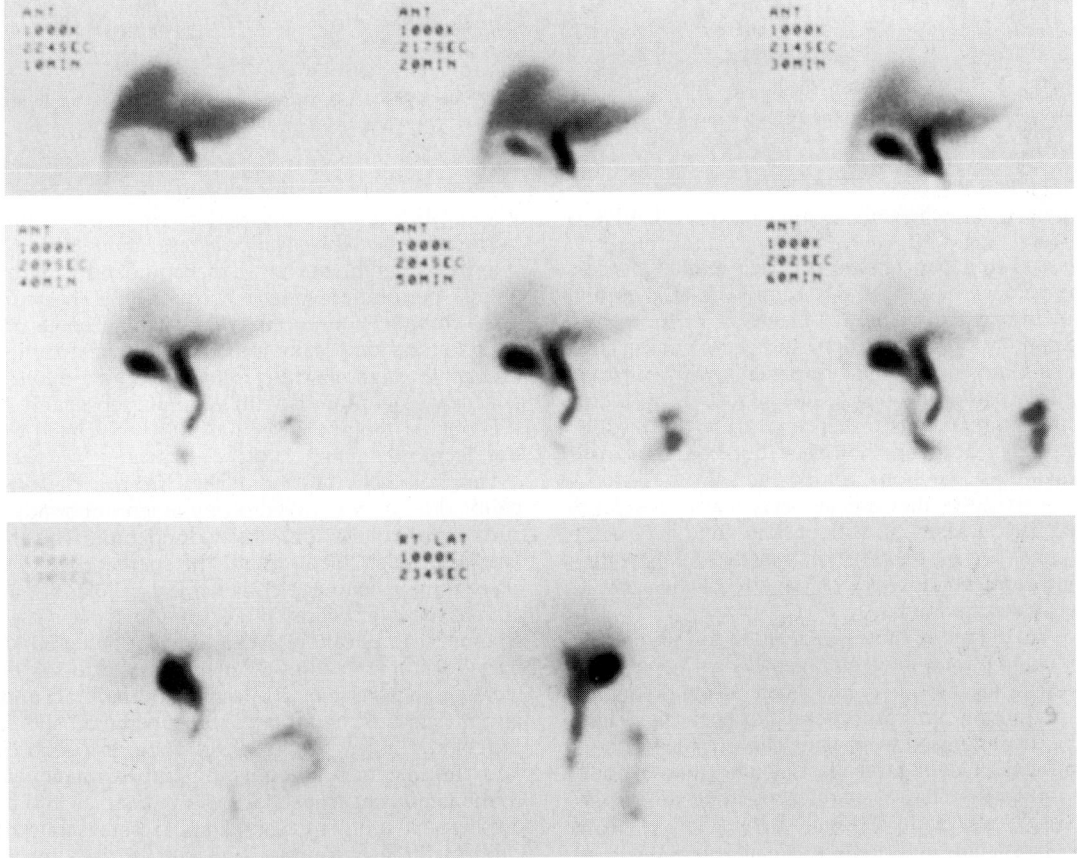

Figure 34–9. Normal cholescintigram showing liver, bile duct, gallbladder, and small intestine. Reading from left to right, scans were done every 10 minutes in the anterior view. The two bottom scans are the right anterior oblique view (left) and the right lateral view (right).

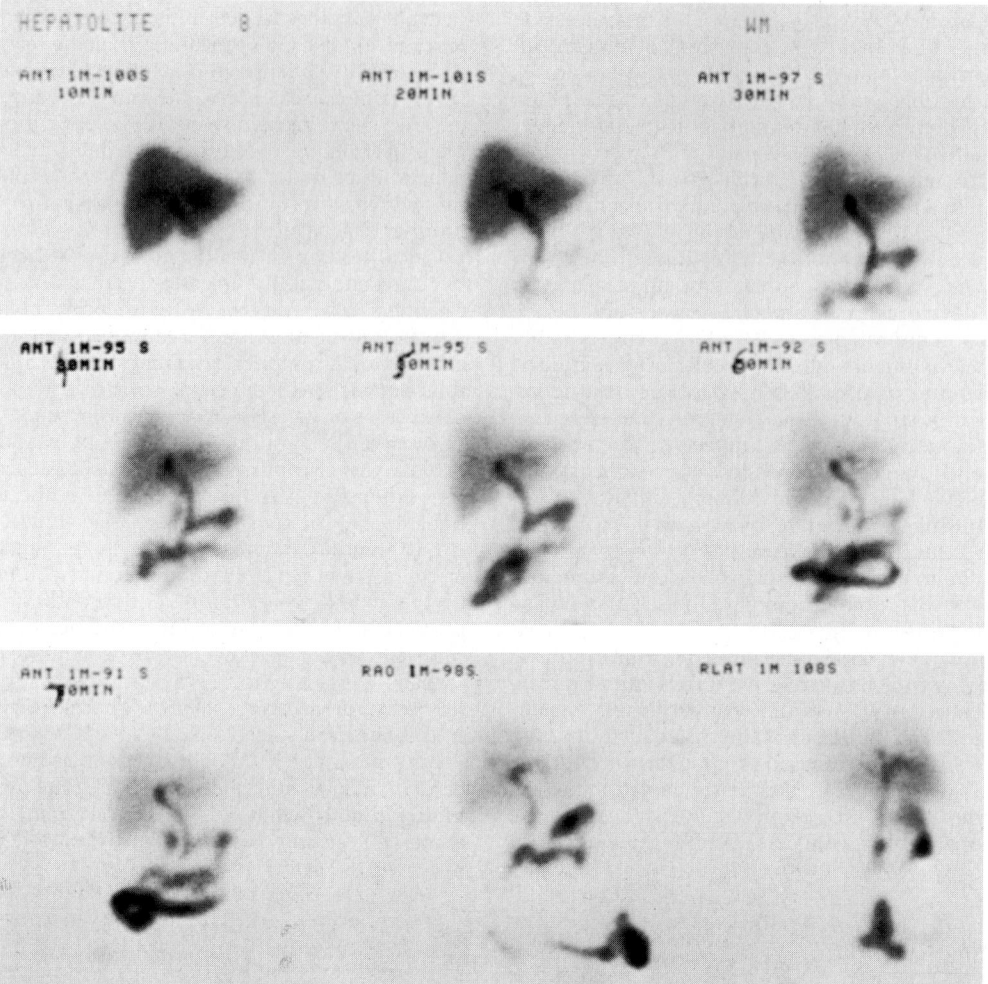

Figure 34–10. Abnormal cholescintigram in a patient with acute calculous cholecystitis. The gallbladder is not visualized. Reading from left to right, scans were done every 10 minutes in the anterior view. The last two scans are the right anterior oblique view and the right lateral view, respectively.

necessarily mean that clinically significant pancreatitis is present.

Gallstone-associated pancreatitis is a self-limited process related to the passage of a stone through the distal common bile duct and into the duodenum.[1] Elevation of the serum amylase is common in this situation, and acute cholecystitis is present in as many as one third of patients with gallstone pancreatitis. The pathophysiology and sequence of events that lead to the simultaneous presence of acute cholecystitis and gallstone pancreatitis are not clear, but both processes seem to resolve once the stone has passed into the duodenum. The importance of the association is that acute cholecystitis should be considered in patients known to have acute pancreatitis, and the possibility of gallstone pancreatitis should be considered in patients who have acute cholecystitis and elevation of serum amylase.

The differential diagnosis must also include conditions that cause pain due to rapid liver enlargement or hepatic inflammation, including viral hepatitis, acute alcoholic hepatitis, right heart failure, and gonococcal perihepatitis. These can usually be distinguished from acute cholecystitis without difficulty. Gallbladder colic rarely lasts longer than 3 hours and does not have the clinical manifestations of an inflammatory process. Other acute abdominal conditions such as small bowel obstruction and acute regional enteritis can be differentiated easily by a carefully taken history and a thorough physical examination.

Complications. Complications of acute cholecystitis are perforation, pericholecystic abscess, and fistula. All are consequences of gallbladder wall ischemia and gangrene.

Free perforation, which accounts for about one third of these complications, occurs when a gangrenous area becomes necrotic and bile leaks into the peritoneal cavity. Diffusion of bile throughout the peritoneal cavity frequently causes generalized peritonitis with systemic sepsis and death unless it is treated promptly. The mortality associated with perforation is approximately 20%.[20, 36]

Pericholecystic abscess results from a perforation of the gallbladder that is walled off by omentum or adjacent organs such as the colon, stomach, or duodenum. The abscess forms between the gallbladder and the surrounding structures. An abscess may also form between the gallbladder and the bare area of the liver behind it. Pericholecystic abscess is the most common complication, accounting for about 50% of cases.

Fistulization occurs when the gallbladder becomes attached to a portion of the gastrointestinal tract and perforates into it. The duodenum is the most common site, followed by the colon. Cholecystojejunal and cholecystogastric fistulas are rare. Fistulization accounts for approximately 15% of the complications of acute cholecystitis. Fistulas into the gallbladder may have other causes, such as penetrating peptic ulcer, Crohn's disease, trauma, tuberculosis, and intra-abdominal abscess. When a stone is discharged from the gallbladder into the small intestine and is sufficiently large to obstruct the narrow terminal ileum, the resulting gallstone ileus creates an additional hazard for a patient with a cholecystoenteric fistula.

The symptoms of these complications are generally indistinguishable from those of acute cholecystitis. In one report, only 59% of patients had signs of peritoneal irritation, and less than half had diffuse abdominal tenderness or absent bowel sounds.[20] Furthermore, none of the three types of complications is consistently manifested by a specific symptom complex.

Complications may develop as early as 2 days after the onset of the symptoms of acute cholecystitis, and as late as several weeks. The average is approximately a week, but this information is not helpful in managing an individual case. The overall mortality from complications is about 20%.[9, 13, 20, 36]

Treatment. Patients suspected of having acute cholecystitis should be hospitalized. Preoperative management should include administration of an antibiotic that is effective against the enteric organisms found in the bile of approximately 80% of patients with gallstones and acute cholecystitis. These organisms include both gram-positive and -negative aerobes and anaerobes. Those present most frequently are *Escherichia coli, Klebsiella* species, *Streptococcus faecalis, Clostridium welchii, Proteus* species, *Enterobacter* species, and anaerobic *Streptococcus* species. A single organism is found in about 40% of cases, two species in about 30%, three in 20%, and four or more in the remainder.[22] Obviously, no single antibiotic is effective against all these organisms. The broadest coverage can be achieved by a combination of ampicillin or ampicillin-sulbactam plus gentamycin, but the toxicity of the latter is of concern. Therefore, the author favors administration of a second-generation cephalosporin for most cases of acute cholecystitis and reservation of the triple drug combination for patients who are seriously ill with sepsis. The incidence of postoperative septic complications is markedly reduced by prophylactic antibiotic administration.[3, 34] The incidence of wound infection, for example, is reduced to such an extent that it is difficult to demonstrate that one antibiotic provides better protection against wound infection than another. Antibiotic therapy should be initiated as soon as the diagnosis is made and should be continued for 24 hours postoperatively, unless the degree of peritonitis in surrounding tissues is severe, in which case it should continue for 7 days. Changes in the regimen may be indicated by the response of the patient and the results of the cultures of bile and gallbladder wall taken at operation.

The definitive treatment of acute cholecystitis is cholecystectomy. The timing of operation was debated until data from several prospective trials showed that the mortality rates for early and delayed surgical procedures are equal and that there are no significant differences in the frequency or severity of postoperative complications.[21, 27] These and other studies have also shown that length of hospital stay is shorter, and return to productivity is sooner, when early cholecystectomy is done.

Laparoscopic cholecystectomy is the preferred operation (see Part II in this chapter for details). Usually, the tense, distended gallbladder must be aspirated of its contents to facilitate grasping the organ and dissecting structures in the triangle of Calot. The infundibulum and cystic duct, which may be very friable, must be dissected with care to avoid injury to the extrahepatic bile ducts. The author prefers to perform operative cholangiography routinely unless the extent of inflammation makes it unsafe. The management of choledocholithiasis is discussed in Chapter 34.

Conversion to open cholecystectomy is indicated when the laparoscopic procedure cannot be completed safely or when bleeding or a bile leak cannot be stopped without risking injury to important structures. Conversion is also required in

the rare patient who has a fistula from the gallbladder into the bile duct or intestine and in some patients who have perforation and an abscess in the right upper quadrant.

Although acute cholecystitis has been cited as a risk factor for bile duct injury during laparoscopic cholecystectomy,[2] there is no solid evidence that the incidence of bile duct injury is higher in this patient population.[35] The need to convert to an open procedure is no greater in patients with acute cholecystitis than in those without inflammation. A patient who is too ill from a concomitant condition to withstand general anesthesia can be treated by percutaneous cholecystostomy. Resolution of the inflammation usually follows decompression of the gallbladder, although gangrenous areas may perforate subsequently. Careful observation is essential after percutaneous cholecystostomy.

Cholecystectomy for acute cholecystitis is performed with a mortality rate of less than 0.2% and a major morbidity rate of less than 5%. The incidence of bile duct injury is approximately 0.4%.[7]

ACUTE ACALCULOUS CHOLECYSTITIS

Acute acalculous cholecystitis is acute inflammation of the gallbladder in the absence of gallstones. It accounts for approximately 4% to 8% of all cases of acute cholecystitis. In contrast to calculous cholecystitis, which is more common in females, the male-to-female ratio is approximately 1.5:1.[19]

The disease has a tendency to occur after, or in association with, other conditions, especially major trauma, burns, or operations. Other conditions known to be precedents include multiple transfusions, childbirth, bacterial sepsis, and debilitating diseases such as sarcoidosis, polyarteritis nodosa, and lupus erythematosus. These patients are often critically ill, requiring extensive monitoring and life-support procedures. Cases associated with the administration of total parenteral nutrition have been reported.[30] No apparent precipitating factor is present in up to 50% of cases.

Acute postoperative cholecystitis and *acute posttraumatic cholecystitis* are terms used to describe the most frequently associated conditions. Not all such cases of cholecystitis are of the acalculous variety, however.[11] About two thirds of those that occur postoperatively, and about 15% of posttraumatic cases, are associated with gallstones.[19, 29]

The pathology of acute acalculous cholecystitis does not differ from that of the calculous type, except that the incidence of gangrene and perforation is higher. Whether this is an inherent feature of the disease or the result of delayed diagnosis and treatment is conjectural. The masking of symptoms and findings by the effects of recent trauma, operation, or other illness frequently leads to a delay in recognizing the condition. This could be partially responsible for the higher mortality seen in acalculous cholecystitis, although coexisting disease may add to the usual risk factors as well.[1] Thus, the association with other conditions does not denote the presence or absence of gallstones.[19, 29]

Etiology. The etiology of acute acalculous cholecystitis is uncertain and may be multifactorial. Stasis of gallbladder bile occurs in the absence of regular contraction, stimulated by cholecystokinin, which is released by the presence of certain products of digestion in the upper small intestine. Maximal concentration and extraction of water from gallbladder bile reduce it to a viscid material known as *sludge*, which may even contain soft concretions. Possibly, viscid bile and sludge may lead to the release of inflammatory mediators such as prostaglandins and interleukins from the gallbladder epithelium, producing inflammation, venous and lymphatic obstruction, ischemia, and necrosis. Stasis of gallbladder bile may also render it more susceptible to colonization with bacteria and the possibility of bacterial invasion of the gallbladder wall. Lack of oral intake frequently accompanies several of the conditions with which acalculous cholecystitis is associated, including trauma, major operative procedures, and serious debilitating disease. Administration of narcotics may be a contributing factor. Thus, stasis may be an important mechanism in some patients with these conditions, as well as in long-term total parenteral nutrition patients. However, the disease does occur in patients who have eaten normally, and other factors must be involved.

Ischemia has been implicated because of the high incidence of gangrene and necrosis of the gallbladder wall. Brief or prolonged periods of hypotension or low blood flow are not uncommon during operations, following trauma and burns, or in association with sepsis. Decreased blood flow to the gallbladder epithelium could cause it to slough, and concentrated bile acids, which are toxic to tissues, would then have access to the gallbladder wall.

Diagnosis. Recognition of the disease may be delayed when a patient cannot communicate well because of concomitant disease or his or her postoperative or posttraumatic state. The symptoms are identical to those of acute calculous cholecystitis, except that they may be absent or masked by symptoms of an underlying or precedent condition. Pain in the right upper quadrant, the epigastrium, or both occurs in about 70% of patients, and vomiting in about 35%. Whereas pain is almost always present in acute calculous cholecystitis, it may be absent or masked in the acalculous variant because of narcotic administration, decreased level of consciousness, or abdominal pain from an incision or other disease process.

The most significant physical findings include tenderness in the right upper quadrant and fever, which occur in about 75% of cases. Abdominal distention and absent or hypoactive bowel sounds are present in about 25%, and a right upper quadrant mass and jaundice are even less frequent.[30] Usually, the diagnosis can be made from the physical examination, but only about half the cases are correctly diagnosed preoperatively when abdominal surgery or trauma has been antecedent.

The inflammation is reflected in an elevated white blood cell count in 70% of patients, and the alkaline phosphatase or aspartate aminotransferase (AST) is elevated in over 50%.

Cholescintigraphy should be done when acute acalculous cholecystitis is suspected,[14] but the accuracy, about 88%, is not as high as in calculous cholecystitis.[16] The problem is a higher incidence of false-positive scans.[12] Patients at risk for acute acalculous cholecystitis may have inadequate oral intake, and their gallbladders may contain viscid bile from lack of contraction. Therefore, the radionuclide may not be able to enter the otherwise normal gallbladder. Ultrasonography may be helpful by showing distention and thickening of the wall. However, these signs are not always present, and when they are, they may be nonspecific. For example, thickening of the gallbladder wall occurs in ascites, congestive heart failure, and hypoalbuminemia. Percutaneous aspiration of bile from the gallbladder and establishment of a percutaneous tube cholecystostomy are being used more often as a combined diagnostic and therapeutic maneuver. The bile is examined for the presence of bacteria and leukocytes.

Treatment. The standard treatment has been emergency cholecystectomy. In contrast to the calculous form, for which some have advocated delaying operation, the high risk of gangrene and perforation mandates early treatment. Unless the inflammation is so severe as to make it dangerous, operative cholangiography should be done to rule out the possibility of passage of a single gallstone into the common bile duct. The mortality rate of acute acalculous cholecystitis is higher than that of the calculous variety because the antecedent or concomitant condition usually increases the risk and because the diagnosis is often delayed. Some have advocated

the periodic ingestion of fat or cholecystokinin administration in total parenteral nutrition patients to empty the gallbladder and prevent stasis and, presumably, the development of acute cholecystitis.[24, 30]

Percutaneous cholecystostomy is performed to treat acute cholecystitis in high-risk patients. A summary of reported cases revealed a success rate of 99% and morbidity and mortality rates of 25% and 10%, respectively.[38]

UNUSUAL TYPES OF ACUTE CHOLECYSTITIS

Acute Emphysematous Cholecystitis

Acute emphysematous cholecystitis accounts for only about 1% of all cases and is characterized by the presence of gas in the wall and lumen of the gallbladder.

Emphysematous cholecystitis is more common in diabetics; about 40% of the reported cases have this association.[26] Approximately 75% of cases occur in males, and the average age of afflicted patients is about 60 years. The onset of emphysematous cholecystitis is abrupt, and, in addition to right upper quadrant pain, nausea, and vomiting, patients rapidly become toxic.

The pathognomonic diagnostic sign is the presence of gas within the lumen and wall of the gallbladder on a plain radiograph of the abdomen (Fig. 34–11). The gas is produced by bacteria; *Clostridium perfringens*, *E. coli*, *Klebsiella*, or a mixture of organisms is usually found. *C. perfringens* has been cultured in about half the reported cases.[26] Gangrene of the gallbladder is usually present. Stones are absent in about 30% of cases. Emergency cholecystectomy is the appropriate treatment. The high incidence of gangrene invites perforation and sepsis unless the gallbladder is removed.

Typhoid Cholecystitis

Acute cholecystitis occurs rarely in patients who have typhoid fever, usually during the third week of the illness or later. Gallstones are not present, and the offending organism, *Salmonella typhi*, is found in the bile. Perforation of the gallbladder is a frequent occurrence.

A more common problem is colonization of the gallbladder bile with *S. typhi* in patients who have had typhoid fever, which may or may not have been clinically apparent. These individuals become typhoid carriers and excrete the organism in their feces. Gallstones and chronic cholecystitis may develop. The quinolone antibiotics are effective in eradicating

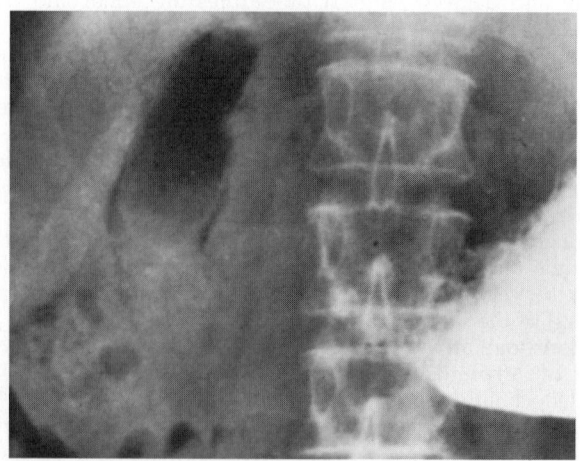

Figure 34–11. Radiograph showing air in the wall and lumen of the gallbladder in acute emphysematous cholecystitis.

the carrier state in a majority of patients,[31] but when gallstones are present, they serve as a continuing nidus for infection, and cholecystectomy may be necessary.[10, 15]

Torsion of the Gallbladder

Hemorrhagic infarction of the gallbladder occurs when the organ twists 180 degrees or more. Two anatomic anomalies permit torsion. In the rarest type, the gallbladder has no mesentery or attachment to the liver and is completely peritonealized. It lies free in the peritoneal cavity, suspended only by the cystic duct and cystic artery, both of which may have a short mesentery. The propensity for infarction is obvious and it usually occurs in childhood.[4] More commonly, the gallbladder is suspended from its usual position on the liver by a mesentery that is sufficiently long to allow torsion in either direction. Gallstones are present in a significant percentage of cases,[23] and it has been suggested that the weight of the stones contributes to the torsion. However, the weight of gallstones is not much different from the weight of the bile they displace.

Acute torsion causes abdominal pain on the right side, and the twisted, infarcted gallbladder may be palpable as a mass in the right lower quadrant. The correct diagnosis is often missed preoperatively, frequently being mistaken for acute appendicitis. Some patients have periodic episodes of abdominal pain that are presumed to be caused by incomplete volvulus and spontaneous reduction. The treatment of torsion of the gallbladder is cholecystectomy.

Tumors

Carcinoma of the gallbladder occasionally presents as acute cholecystitis. This is not surprising, given its frequent association with gallstones and the possibility that the cancer itself may obstruct the gallbladder outlet.

Granular cell myoblastomas—firm yellow nodules that are thought to be of neuroectodermal origin—are found in the wall of the cystic duct, the common bile duct, or the gallbladder.[6] They are benign tumors that tend to occur in young black females. Gallstones may be present. Those tumors that obstruct the cystic duct may cause acute cholecystitis, empyema, or hydrops of the gallbladder.[32] The treatment is cholecystectomy, with excision of the portion of the cystic duct that bears the tumor.

Tumors of the gallbladder are often incidental findings, even though they may cause acute cholecystitis. This reinforces the dictum that excised gallbladders should always be opened in the operating room and inspected for neoplasm, so that gallbladder cancer can be treated properly.

SELECTED REFERENCES

Glenn, F.: Acute cholecystitis. Surg. Gynecol. Obstet., 143:56, 1976.
This is a classic review of over 2000 cases by the late master biliary tract surgeon. He emphasizes the serious risk factors and the increased mortality in elderly patients. An aggressive approach to patients with acute cholecystitis is described.

Glenn, F.: Acute acalculous cholecystitis. Ann. Surg., 189:458, 1979.
Experience with 139 cases is described, and the associated illnesses are emphasized. The author's management resulted in a mortality of 6.5%, one of the lowest reported in the literature.

Norrby, S., Herlin, P., Holmin, T., Sjodahl, R., and Tagesson, C.: Early or delayed cholecystectomy in acute cholecystitis? A clinical trial. Br. J. Surg., 70:163, 1983.
This article reports on a trial to determine the best management method for patients with acute cholecystitis. The results show that mortality and morbidity are the same with early and delayed surgery, but that length of hospital stay is reduced and patients return to productivity sooner with early surgery.

Weedon, D.: Pathology of the Gallbladder. New York, Masson, 1984.
This book describes the pathogenesis, clinical findings, and pathology for all known conditions that affect the gallbladder, as well as their complications. The illustrations are excellent, and the references are complete. Anyone who wishes to gain comprehensive knowledge of acute cholecystitis or study the nuances of individual cases will find this monograph helpful.

Werbel, G. B., Nahrwold, D. L., Joehl, R. J., Vogelzang, R. L., and Rege, R. V.: Percutaneous cholecystostomy in the diagnosis and treatment of acute cholecystitis and the high-risk patient. Arch. Surg., 124:782, 1989.
An experience with percutaneous cholecystostomy in critically ill patients who have acute acalculous or calculous cholecystitis is presented. The role of this technique in diagnosis is emphasized. The results of other reports are summarized.

REFERENCES

1. Acosta, J. M., Pelligrini, C. A., and Skinner, D. B.: Etiology and pathogenesis of acute biliary pancreatitis. Surgery, 88:118, 1980.
2. Asbun, H. J., Rossi, R. L., Lowell, J. A., and Munson, J. L.: Bile duct injury during laparoscopic cholecystectomy: Mechanism of injury, prevention, and management. World J. Surg., 17:547, 1993.
3. Chetlin, S. H., and Elliott, D. W.: Preoperative antibiotics in biliary surgery. Arch. Surg., 107:319, 1973.
4. Chilton, C. P., and Mann, C. V.: Torsion of the gallbladder in a 9-year-old boy. J. R. Soc. Med., 73:141, 1980.
5. Deitch, E. A., and Engle, J. M.: Acute acalculous cholecystitis: Ultrasonic diagnosis. Am. J. Surg., 142:290, 1981.
6. Dewar, J., Dooley, J. S., Lindsay, I., George, P., and Sherlock, S.: Granular cell myoblastoma of the common bile duct treated by biliary drainage and surgery. Gut, 22:70, 1981.
7. Deziel, D. J., Millikan, K. W., Economou, S. G., Doolas, A., Ko, S. T., and Airan, M. C.: Complications of laparoscopic cholecystectomy: A national survey of 4292 hospitals and an analysis of 77,604 cases. Am. J. Surg., 165:9, 1993.
8. Diettrick, N. A., Cacioppo, J. C., and Davis, R. P.: The vanishing elective cholecystectomy. Arch. Surg., 123:810, 1988.
9. Diffenbaugh, W. G., Sarver, F. E., and Strohl, E. L.: Gangrenous perforation of the gallbladder: Analysis of 19 cases. Arch. Surg., 59:742, 1949.
10. Dinbar, A., Altmann, G., and Tulcinsky, D. B.: The treatment of chronic biliary salmonella carriers. Am. J. Med., 47:236, 1969.
11. DuPriest, R. W., Jr., Khaneja, S. C., and Cowley, R. A.: Acute cholecystitis complicating trauma. Ann. Surg., 189:84, 1979.
12. Echevarria, R. A., and Gleason, J. L.: False-negative gallbladder scintigram in acute cholecystitis. J. Nucl. Med., 21:841, 1980.
13. Essenhigh, D. M.: Perforation of the gallbladder. Br. J. Surg., 55:175, 1968.
14. Fox, M. S., Wilk, D. J., Weissmann, H. S., Freeman, L. M., and Gliedman, M. L.: Acute acalculous cholecystitis. Surg. Gynecol. Obstet., 159:13, 1984.
15. Freitag, J. L.: Treatment of chronic typhoid carriers by cholecystectomy. Public Health Rep., 79:567, 1964.
16. Freitas, J. E.: Cholescintigraphy in acute and chronic cholecystitis. Semin. Nucl. Med., 12:18, 1982.
17. Fukunaga, F. H.: Gallbladder bacteriology, histology and gallstones: Study of unselected cholecystectomy specimens in Honolulu. Arch. Surg., 106:169, 1973.
18. Gunn, A. A.: A surgeon's appraisal of cholecystitis. J. R. Coll. Surg. Edinb., 20:180, 1975.
19. Howard, R. J.: Acute acalculous cholecystitis. Am. J. Surg., 141:194, 1981.
20. Isch, J. H., Finneran, J. C., and Nahrwold, D. L.: Perforation of the gallbladder. Am. J. Gastroenterol., 55:451, 1971.
21. Jarvinen, H. J., and Hastabacka, J.: Early cholecystectomy for acute cholecystitis, a prospective randomized study. Ann. Surg., 191:501, 1980.
22. Keighley, M. R. B.: Microorganisms in the bile. Ann. R. Coll. Surg. Engl., 59:329, 1977.
23. Levene, A.: Acute torsion of the gallbladder: Postmortem finding in two cases. Br. J. Surg., 45:338, 1958.
24. Long, T. N., Heimbach, D. M., and Carrico, C. J.: Acalculous cholecystitis in critically ill patients. Am. J. Surg., 136:31, 1978.
25. Lou, M. A., Mandal, A. K., Alexander, J. L., and Thadepalli, H.: Bacteriology of the human biliary tract and the duodenum. Arch. Surg., 112:965, 1977.
26. Mentzer, R. M., Jr., Golden, G. T., Chandler, J. G., and Horsley, J. S., III: A comparative appraisal of emphysematous cholecystitis. Am. J. Surg., 129:10, 1975.
27. Norrby, S., Herlin, P., Holmin, T., Sjodahl, R., and Tagesson, C.: Early or delayed cholecystectomy in acute cholecystitis? A clinical trial. Br. J. Surg., 70:163, 1983.
28. Ostrow, J. D.: Absorption of bile pigments by the gallbladder. J. Clin. Invest., 46:2035, 1967.
29. Ottinger, L. W.: Acute cholecystitis as a postoperative complication. Ann. Surg., 184:162, 1976.
30. Petersen, S. R., and Sheldon, G. F.: Acute acalculous cholecystitis: A complication of hyperalimentation. Am. J. Surg., 138:814, 1979.
31. Rodriguez-Noriega, E., Andrade-Villanueva, J., and Amaya-Tapia, G.: Quinolones in the treatment of Salmonella carriers. Rev. Infect. Dis., 11:S1179, 1989.
32. Serpe, S. J., Todd, D., and Baruch, H.: Cholecystitis due to granular cell myoblastoma of the cystic duct. Am. J. Dig. Dis., 5:824, 1960.
33. Stephenson, S. E., Jr., and Nagel, C. B.: Acute cholecystitis: An experimental study. Ann. Surg., 157:687, 1963.
34. Stone, H. H., Hooper, C. A., Kolb, L. D., Geheber, C. E., and Dawkins, E.

J.: Antibiotic prophylaxis in gastric, biliary and colonic surgery. Ann. Surg., *184*:443, 1976.

35. Strasberg, S. M., Hertl, M., and Soper, N. J.: An analysis of the problem of biliary injury during laparoscopic surgery. J. Am. Coll. Surg., *180*:101, 1995.

36. Strohl, E. L., Diffenbaugh, W. G., Baker, J. H., and Cheema, M. H.: Gangrene and perforation of the gallbladder (Int. Abstr. Surg.). Surg. Gynecol. Obstet., *114*:1, 1962.

37. Weissmann, H. S., Badia, J., Sugarman, L. A., Kluger, L., Rosenblatt, R., and Freeman, L. M.: Spectrum of 99m-Tc-IDA cholescintigraphic patterns in acute cholecystitis. Radiology, *138*:167, 1981.

38. Werbel, G. B., Nahrwold, D. L., Joehl, R. J., Vogelzang, R. L., and Rege, R. V.: Percutaneous cholecystostomy in the diagnosis and treatment of acute cholecystitis in the high-risk patient. Arch. Surg., *124*:782, 1989.

39. Womack, N. A., and Bricker, E. M.: Pathogenesis of acute cholecystitis. Arch. Surg., *44*:658, 1942.

II

CHRONIC CHOLECYSTITIS AND CHOLELITHIASIS

David L. Nahrwold, M.D.

The term *chronic cholecystitis with cholelithiasis* is often used to connote symptomatic gallbladder disease. Chronic inflammatory changes are found in the gallbladders of many symptomatic patients with gallstones, but gallstones may also be present in otherwise normal gallbladders, and gallbladder symptoms may occur in the absence of inflammation.[19] Approximately 98% of patients with symptomatic gallbladder disease have gallstones. The understanding of the pathogenesis of gallstones and their relationship to gallbladder disease is central to the management of patients with chronic cholecystitis.

PATHOGENESIS OF GALLSTONES

An estimated 20 million people in the United States harbor gallstones. Approximately 500,000 cholecystectomies are done annually. The prevalence increases with increasing age. Women of childbearing age have a higher incidence than men of the same age; in an autopsy series, gallstones were found in about 17% of women and 8% of men over age 20.[15] Much of the present knowledge of cholesterol gallstones comes from a study of Pima Indian women in the southwestern United States, who have an incidence of about 75% between the ages of 25 and 34 years.[22] In the Far East, pigment gallstones predominate, and their incidence in blacks is higher than in whites. Gallstones are classified as cholesterol, pigment, and mixed types, but most stones do not fit into this rigid classification system. Pure cholesterol stones, having the appearance of white pearls, are rare. Most cholesterol stones contain significant amounts of pigment and are more aptly called predominantly cholesterol stones. Pigment calculi are divided into black pigment stones, which are associated with hemolysis and cirrhosis, and the earthy calcium bilirubinate type, which is associated with infection in the biliary system.

Predominantly Cholesterol Stones

The primary constituents of bile are water, electrolytes, pigments, cholesterol, phospholipids (mostly lecithin), and bile salts. Cholesterol, insoluble in water, is soluble in bile because it is associated with phospholipids and bile salts through the formation of mixed micelles and vesicles. Lecithin is incorporated into the bile salt micelle. Mixed bile salt–lecithin micelles become swollen because water penetrates them, allowing cholesterol to be *packaged* within them and, therefore, solubilized in bile. Because cholesterol, phospholipids, and bile salts form micelles and vesicles, the total amount of any one of these substances relative to the total

amounts of the other two determines the maximum amount of cholesterol, for example, that can be solubilized. When the relative amounts of the three substances are insufficient to *package* all the cholesterol in micelles and vesicles and therefore solubilize it, cholesterol crystals form on the surfaces of vesicles, making possible the formation of a cholesterol gallstone. Bile is said to be lithogenic when the solubility of cholesterol is exceeded. The relationships among the three substances were first expressed by Admirand and Small[1] by a triangular coordinate graph and were later modified by Holzbach and co-workers[13] (Fig. 34–12). Increased output

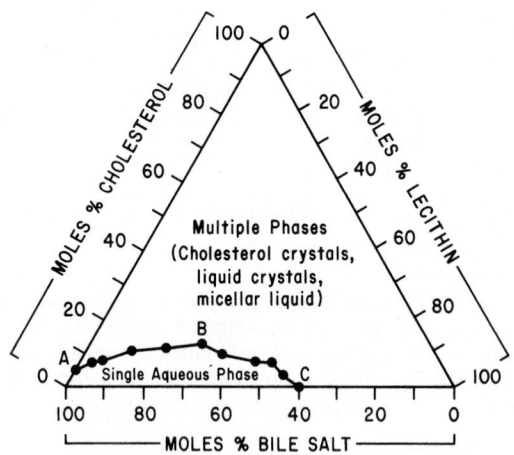

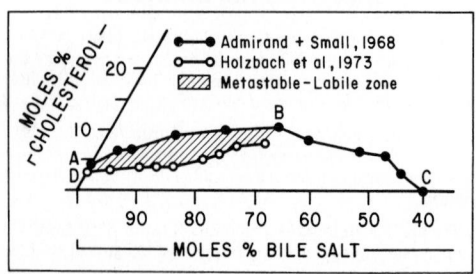

Figure 34–12. Triangular diagram in which the amounts of lecithin, bile salt, and cholesterol are used to express the lithogenicity of bile. Lines are drawn into the triangle perpendicular from the appropriate point on each side of the triangle. If the point at which they intersect is above line ABC, cholesterol is completely soluble; if beneath, the bile is supersaturated. Between lines ABC and DBC is a metastable-labile zone in which stone formation could occur if specific nucleating factors are present.

of cholesterol in bile occurs with obesity, estrogen therapy, and age.[9, 10]

Bile salts are secreted by the liver, concentrated and stored in the gallbladder, and released into the intestine during a meal. About 95% are reabsorbed in the intestine, mainly in the ileum. About 5% are excreted in the feces, and this amount is replaced by hepatic synthesis. In healthy people, the size of the bile salt pool remains fairly constant, and the pool circulates 6 to 10 times each day. The primary bile acids, cholic and chenodeoxycholic, are conjugated with taurine or glycine in the liver. Bacteria in the distal ileum and colon may deconjugate and dehydroxylate them, forming the secondary bile acids, deoxycholic and lithocholic, which are absorbed by passive diffusion in the colon. The constant recycling of bile acids is known as the enterohepatic circulation, and the size of the pool and its frequency of cycling may be important in the formation of predominantly cholesterol stones. Bile acids are synthesized in the liver from cholesterol, a process that is influenced by a negative feedback system. Sequestration of bile acids in the gallbladder during fasting contracts the pool and initially causes a decrease in bile acid secretion relative to cholesterol secretion, with formation of lithogenic bile. But after eating, bile acid secretion increases, and the bile is no longer saturated. Prolonged fasting produces lithogenic bile.[3] Cholecystectomy causes redistribution of the bile acid pool in the enterohepatic circulation and increases the frequency of cycling. This exerts negative feedback on bile acid synthesis and causes a reduction in the pool size. These changes favor formation of a nonlithogenic bile in many patients after cholecystectomy.

Stone formation is initiated by nucleation, a complex process that requires more than saturation with cholesterol alone. Bile proteins and pigments, bacteria, cellular debris, gallbladder mucus, calcium salts, and other substances have been implicated as nucleating agents. When gallbladder emptying is impaired, bile containing mucoprotein and cholesterol crystals forms gallbladder sludge, which is associated with the development of gallstones. Sludge forms during pregnancy, prolonged fasting, and parenteral nutrition administration. Growth of a stone is also a complicated process that is not understood very well. The mixed nature of predominantly cholesterol stones gives rise to many unanswered questions about how pigment and other bile constituents are incorporated into a stone as it becomes larger.

The precise cause of predominantly cholesterol gallstones is not yet known, and current evidence suggests that it is multifactorial. Cholesterol saturation of bile, stasis of bile within the gallbladder, and nucleating factors appear to be important. The incidence of predominantly cholesterol gallstones increases with age and is higher in females. Obesity, exogenous estrogen administration, truncal vagotomy, and pregnancy are other predisposing factors. Gallstones are also the consequence of caloric restriction in individuals on certain diets.[4] Genetic factors, as exemplified by the high incidence in the Pima and Chippewa Indians, may also play a role.

Pigment Stones

About 30% of patients with cholelithiasis in the United States have pigment stones. They are of two types: black pigment stones and earthy calcium bilirubinate stones. Pigment stones are much more common in Asian than in Western countries, but the extent to which they are found in the United States has not been appreciated until recently. Stones associated with ileal resection or disease and total parenteral nutrition are the pigment type.[7, 20]

Black pigment stones are black or dark brown in color and are found almost exclusively in the gallbladder. They are associated with cirrhosis and conditions that cause hemolysis, including sickle cell disease, thalassemia, hereditary spherocytosis, and artificial cardiac valves. They consist of an insoluble black pigment polymer, some calcium bilirubinate, calcium carbonate, and calcium phosphate. From 10% to 60% of the weight is residue, probably a mucin glycoprotein. Typically, the bile of patients with black stones is sterile. The black pigment is a polyvinyl network polymer of bilirubinate.

Earthy calcium bilirubinate stones are earthy brown to orange in color and soft in consistency and are found almost exclusively in the bile ducts. They form in circumstances that predispose to bacterbilia and infection, such as in the bile ducts of patients who have had a previous biliary-enteric anastomosis and in patients with strictures or Caroli's disease. Earthy calcium bilirubinate stones are found within the ducts of the liver and extrahepatic ducts in recurrent pyogenic cholangitis or Asian cholangiohepatitis, a common disease in Southeast Asia in which the bile duct system is infected with parasites and/or enteric organisms, usually E. coli. These stones consist mainly of calcium bilirubinate, calcium soaps of fatty acids derived from lecithin, and cholesterol. The mucin glycoprotein residue found in black pigment stones is also present in calcium bilirubinate stones.

The etiology of the two types of pigment stones is not completely clear, but the bile of patients with pigment stones contains an excess of unconjugated bilirubin, compared with the bile of patients with cholesterol stones or no stones. Many also have abnormally high activity of beta glucuronidase, an enzyme produced by bacteria, especially E. coli, which is also found in the epithelium of the biliary tract. Presumably, beta glucuronidase hydrolyzes soluble bilirubin glucuronide to insoluble unconjugated bilirubin and glucuronic acid. The unconjugated bilirubin may then form insoluble calcium bilirubinate.[17] Unconjugated bilirubin may be secreted into bile and become at least partially solubilized by bile salts in the presence of calcium. Theoretically, a decrease in the amount of bile salts present could cause precipitation of calcium bilirubinate. The mechanisms by which calcium bilirubinate precipitates and forms a calcium bilirubinate stone, or polymerizes and forms a black pigment stone, are not known. The presence of ova or other foreign bodies at the center of calcium bilirubinate stones suggests that a nucleating factor may be necessary. Precipitates of calcium phosphate or carbonate could serve this function in the formation of black pigment stones. Stasis of bile in the gallbladder may be a factor, as it appears to be in cholesterol stone formation. Sludge, a soft, black, amorphous substance, is found in gallbladders that have not contracted normally and has been identified as calcium bilirubinate. Sludge is often present in the gallbladders of patients on long-term total parenteral nutrition therapy. These patients have an increased incidence of pigment gallstones.[20]

PATHOLOGY

The pathologic findings in chronic cholecystitis are best interpreted in light of the clinical manifestations of the disease. Two types of chronic cholecystitis exist: that which follows an episode of acute cholecystitis, and that which occurs primarily without antecedent acute cholecystitis. The former is called secondary chronic cholecystitis, and the latter primary chronic cholecystitis.[8]

Acute cholecystitis is caused by gallbladder outlet obstruction, almost always by a stone. Marked thickening of the gallbladder wall from edema is characteristic, and there is subserosal hemorrhage, a marked inflammatory infiltrate, and mucosal necrosis. In cases that do not progress to perforation, these abnormalities gradually resolve over 3 to 4

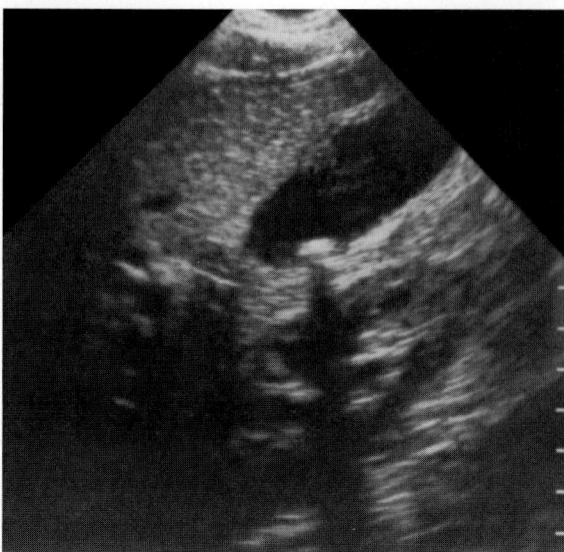

Figure 34–13. Ultrasonogram of the gallbladder showing a large stone with acoustic shadowing.

weeks. Simultaneously, granuloma formation begins at the end of the first week, and after 2 or 3 weeks, fibroblast proliferation and collagen formation commence. These features, typical of chronic cholecystitis, become the dominant findings by 5 weeks. The granulomas frequently contain cholesterol clefts; Rokitansky-Aschoff sinuses, outpouchings of the mucosa, are present. The mucosa itself becomes thin and loses its villous appearance. Fibrosis occurs in the muscular coat.

In contrast, primary chronic cholecystitis is characterized by a thin-walled gallbladder, with an intact mucosa that retains its villous configuration. Sometimes the muscular coat is hypertrophic, and in these cases, crypt formation is frequent. The inflammatory cell infiltrate is primarily lymphocytes. Stones are almost always present in both forms of chronic cholecystitis. Primary chronic cholecystitis lacks an initial acute inflammatory phase, and the exact pathophysiologic events that lead to its development are not known.

DIAGNOSIS

Chronic cholecystitis is characterized by recurrent attacks of right upper quadrant or epigastric pain or discomfort, usually following meals. Nausea and vomiting may occur during the attack, and self-induced vomiting frequently makes the patient feel better. The discomfort may persist for several days or only a few hours. Intervals between attacks are variable; they may be almost continuous or separated by several years. Patients often complain of the sensation of right upper quadrant fullness or of bloating between attacks. These symptoms may follow an episode of acute cholecystitis or they may begin insidiously. No fever or other signs of inflammation are present.

It is unlikely that the pain in primary chronic cholecystitis, and in most patients with secondary chronic cholecystitis, is related to inflammation of the gallbladder. Rather, the pain is gallbladder colic, which results from the temporary obstruction of the gallbladder outlet by a stone in the cystic duct or the infundibulum. The frequent occurrence after a large meal is explained by gallbladder contraction, induced by cholecystokinin, against the fixed obstruction. The pain persists for the duration of the contraction and is relieved as the gallbladder relaxes, a process that may be hastened by opiates. Gallbladder pain characteristically radiates around

the side toward the tip of the right scapula. However, some patients complain of radiation straight through to the back or radiation into the substernal area. Approximately 10% of patients with cholelithiasis have choledocholithiasis, and their gallstones sometimes first become manifest by the symptoms of cholangitis.

Patients with gallstones may complain of intolerance to fatty foods, flatulence, bloating, belching, pyrosis, and vague upper abdominal sensations. The best evidence suggests that these symptoms alone probably are not due to chronic cholecystitis or cholelithiasis.[21] The cardinal symptom of chronic cholecystitis and cholelithiasis is pain.

Physical findings are present only during an attack. They include right upper quadrant or epigastric tenderness to palpation and voluntary muscle guarding, but signs of peritonitis are absent. The gallbladder is not palpable. The temperature is normal. Jaundice is not a feature of cholelithiasis or chronic cholecystitis unless common duct obstruction is also present. The blood tests are unremarkable; specifically, the white blood cell count and the differential counts are normal.

Imaging Studies

The diagnosis is confirmed by ultrasonography of the gallbladder, which is a highly sensitive and accurate test for the diagnosis of gallstones, with a sensitivity and specificity of 98%.[6] The important criteria include demonstration that the stones move to the dependent portion of the gallbladder when the position of the patient is changed and that the stone produces acoustic shadowing (Fig. 34–13). Reverberations at the edges of small stones are also a helpful sign. The advantages of ultrasonography are that it is accurate and safe, does not use radiation, and can be performed rapidly without preparation. For these reasons, it has replaced oral cholecystography, in which oral administration of iopanoic acid is followed by x-ray examination of the right upper quadrant 12 to 24 hours later. The dye enters the gallbladder and outlines the stones (Fig. 34–14). Nonvisualization of the gallbladder indicates obstruction of the cystic duct, presumably by a stone, and therefore also confirms the diagnosis of cholelithiasis. However, this finding may be falsely positive if the patient did not ingest the dye tablets, if the tablets were not absorbed, or if liver function is compromised, as indicated by a serum bilirubin value above approximately 3 mg. per 100 ml. Although ultrasonography should be the initial diagnostic test, oral cholecystography should be done when the symptoms are suggestive and ultrasonography is negative or nondiagnostic.

TREATMENT

The initial treatment of biliary colic, after the diagnosis has been made, is parenteral administration of a narcotic to re-

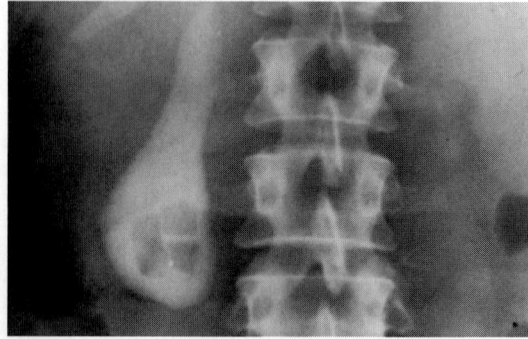

Figure 34–14. Oral cholecystogram showing faceted gallstones outlined by the contrast material.

lieve pain. This may help induce relaxation of the gallbladder as well. Nasogastric suction probably is of no benefit. Hospitalization is not necessary, unless the diagnosis is obscure. Many patients believe that a low-fat diet is helpful, but this has not been proved scientifically.

Preoperative Preparation

The most frequent cause of death after elective cholecystectomy is cardiovascular disease. This emphasizes the importance of taking a good history to detect angina pectoris and carefully examining the electrocardiogram for ischemia or evidence of previous myocardial infarction. Symptoms of cerebrovascular disease, especially transient ischemic attacks, should also be sought, and a noninvasive carotid artery flow study should be done if the history is positive or questionable. Elective cholecystectomy should be delayed until after coronary artery bypass or carotid artery revascularization, if either is indicated. Diseases of the liver and biliary tract, principally cirrhosis, are second to cardiovascular disease as a cause of death after elective cholecystectomy. Intraoperative hemorrhage is the primary problem, but hepatic failure and sepsis also occur.[24]

Septic complications after elective cholecystectomy have been reduced markedly since the introduction of prophylaxis in selected patients. In 10% to 15% of patients with chronic cholecystitis, the bile is colonized with bacteria; this climbs to about 50% in patients with resolving acute cholecystitis. The organisms are enteric, most commonly *E. coli, K. aerogenes,* and *Streptococcus faecalis. Clostridium, Bacteroides,* and *Proteus* species are also found frequently. The incidence of bacterbilia increases significantly with age. In patients with cholelithiasis and chronic cholecystitis, antibiotic prophylaxis should be given to those older than 60 years of age, those recovering from an episode of acute cholecystitis, and those known to have concomitant common duct stones. The author prefers a second-generation cephalosporin administered 1 hour before operation. Some surgeons give antibiotic prophylaxis to all patients.

Technical Considerations

The definitive treatment for symptomatic gallstones is laparoscopic cholecystectomy. Although this procedure has been performed on a regular basis for less than a decade, the results are outstanding, and open cholecystectomy is indicated only in patients in whom the laparoscopic technique is impossible or unsafe. The latter patients include those in whom it is impossible to establish safe access to the peritoneal cavity for the induction of pneumoperitoneum or those in whom adhesions or other anatomic abnormalities prevent safe access to the gallbladder. The surgeon should have a low threshold for converting to the open technique if the gallbladder and bile duct anatomy is unclear and when bleeding or leakage of bile cannot be controlled satisfactorily. Currently, conversion to the open technique is necessary in less than 5% of patients.

Pneumoperitoneum is established by many surgeons by blindly puncturing the peritoneal cavity with a Verres needle and insufflating carbon dioxide to a pressure of 10 to 15 mm. Hg. To further reduce the already low incidence of bowel, bladder, and vascular injury, the author prefers the Hasson open method, in which a small incision is made inferior to the umbilicus and a trocar is introduced into the peritoneal cavity under direct vision, through which carbon dioxide is insufflated. Thereafter, the laparoscope is introduced into the umbilical port, and three other ports are established, as shown in Figure 34–15. The gallbladder is grasped through the lateral port and retracted anteriorly and superiorly, after which adhesions to the gallbladder are lysed.

A grasper inserted through the subcostal port in the midclavicular line is used to pull the infundibulum of the gallbladder inferiorly and to the right, exposing the structures within the triangle of Calot (Fig. 34–16). The cystic duct is completely dissected free from its junction with the gallbladder to its junction with the common bile duct and divided between clips. Prior to dividing the cystic duct, some perform operative cholangiography,[14] but other surgeons employ this procedure only in selected cases.[16] Finally, the cystic artery or its branches are dissected free and divided between clips as close to the gallbladder as possible (Fig. 34–17).

The gallbladder is excised by placing traction on the distal end and incising the peritoneal and hepatic attachment with cautery (Fig. 34–18). Usually, the laparoscope is placed in the superior midline port, and the gallbladder is removed through the umbilical port, which is easier to enlarge, when necessary (Fig. 34–19). The organ should always be opened and inspected for the unsuspected, though rare, carcinoma.

Results

The mortality of laparoscopic cholecystectomy is as low as that previously reported for open cholecystectomy and ranges from 0% to 0.3%.[11] Most experienced surgeons successfully complete the procedure laparoscopically in more than 95% of patients. The general complication rate in a group of reports ranged from 1.3% to 11.2%, which is well within the complication rates previously reported for open cholecystectomy.[11]

The major advantages of the laparoscopic procedure are that patients have less pain and a shorter hospitalization and are able to return to their normal activities sooner than after open cholecystectomy.[2] Data on cost effectiveness vary and are not sufficiently refined to draw definitive conclusions.

The higher incidence of major bile duct injury after laparoscopic as compared with open cholecystectomy is disconcerting. Reconstructive procedures, although successful in approximately 80% of patients, are difficult and costly. Liver transplantation may be the last resort for some. During the introduction of laparoscopic cholecystectomy, the bile duct injury rate was approximately 0.5%, whereas the rate for open cholecystectomy was probably no higher than 0.1% to 0.2%.[25] Subsequent reports are not all easy to interpret, but an ongoing rate of major bile duct injury is estimated at 0.4%.[26] The hope is that with improved training, more experience, identification of the risk factors, and improved instrumentation, this problem will decrease.

Other Treatments

Although laparoscopic cholecystectomy is the standard method for treating patients with symptomatic cholelithiasis or those with complications of cholelithiasis, other treatments may be useful in selected patients.

Oral Dissolution Therapy. The oral administration of the bile acids chenodeoxycholic acid (CDCA) or ursodeoxycholic acid (UDCA) dissolves predominantly cholesterol gallstones in selected patients. At therapeutic dosages, CDCA causes diarrhea, induces transient abnormalities in liver function tests, and increases the concentration of serum low-density lipoprotein cholesterol in some patients, whereas UDCA is free of side effects and has therefore become the preferred oral agent. The stones must be radiolucent in a gallbladder that functions on oral cholecystography. The results are related to the initial size of the stones. Radiolucent gallstones less than 15 mm. in diameter will dissolve in up to 40% of patients within 2 years; longer therapy does not increase

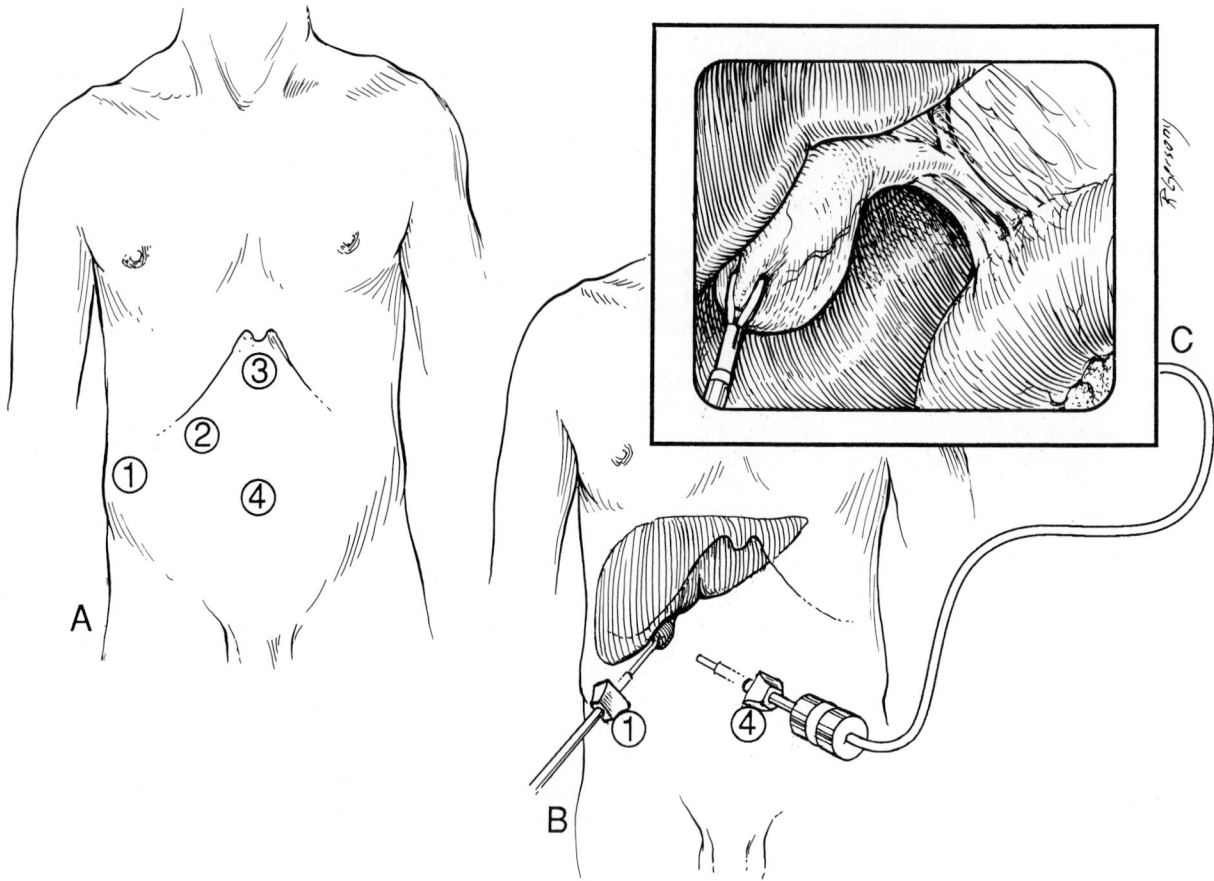

Figure 34–15. *A*, The standard sites of the four ports used in laparoscopic cholecystectomy. *B*, The gallbladder is retracted through the lateral port, and the laparoscope is inserted through the umbilical port.

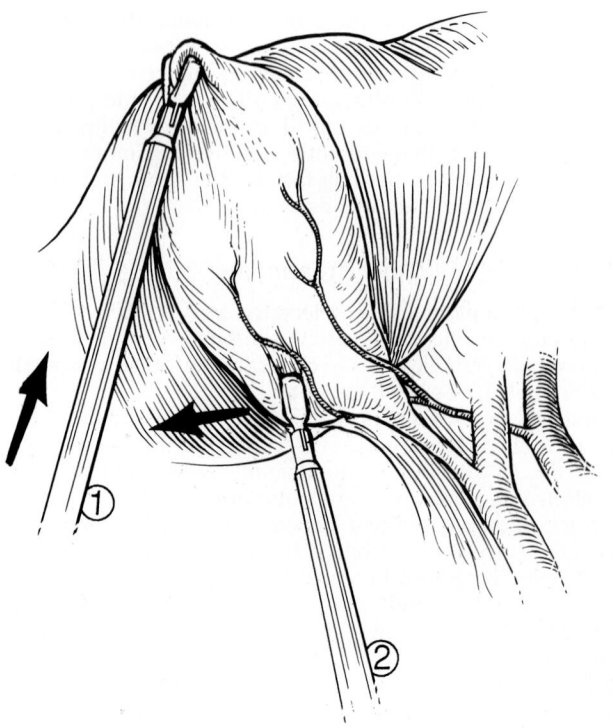

Figure 34–16. Traction superiorly and anteriorly via the grasper in port 1, and traction inferiorly and to the right via the grasper in port 2, facilitate exposure of Calot's triangle and the important structures within it.

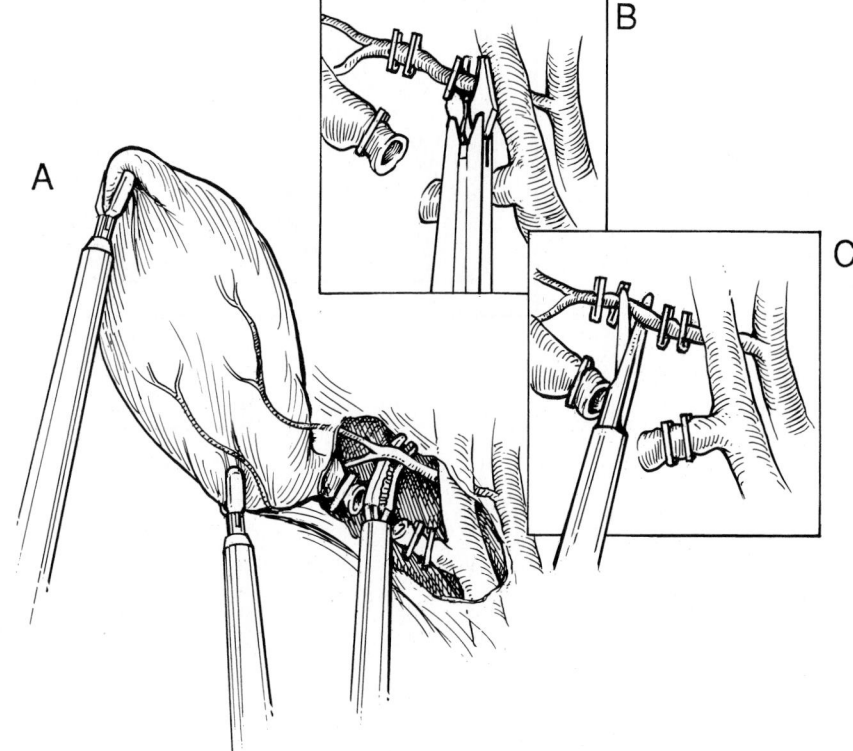

Figure 34–17. *A–C,* The entire cystic duct and the cystic artery are completely dissected free prior to the application of clips and transection.

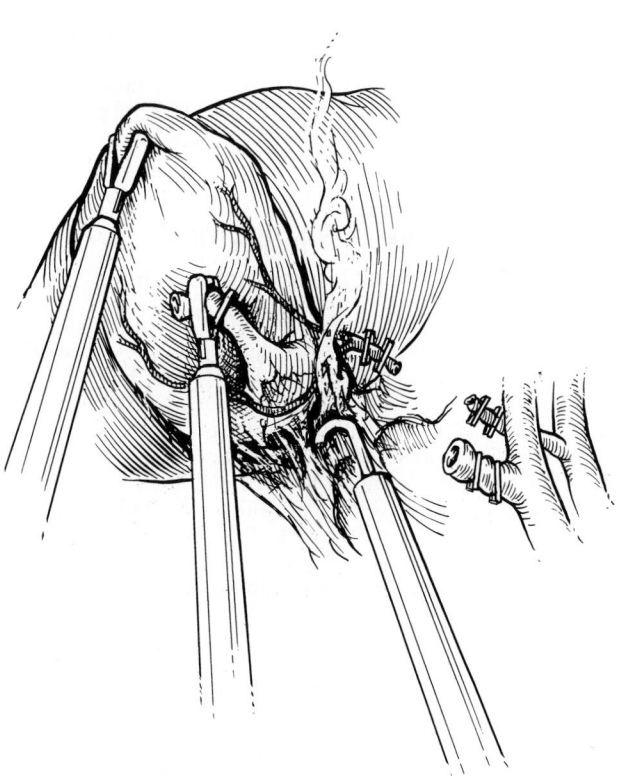

Figure 34–18. After the gallbladder is grasped near the infundibulum, traction in an anterior and superior direction exposes the lateral peritoneal reflections over the gallbladder, as well as its bed within the liver, making removal with complete hemostasis possible.

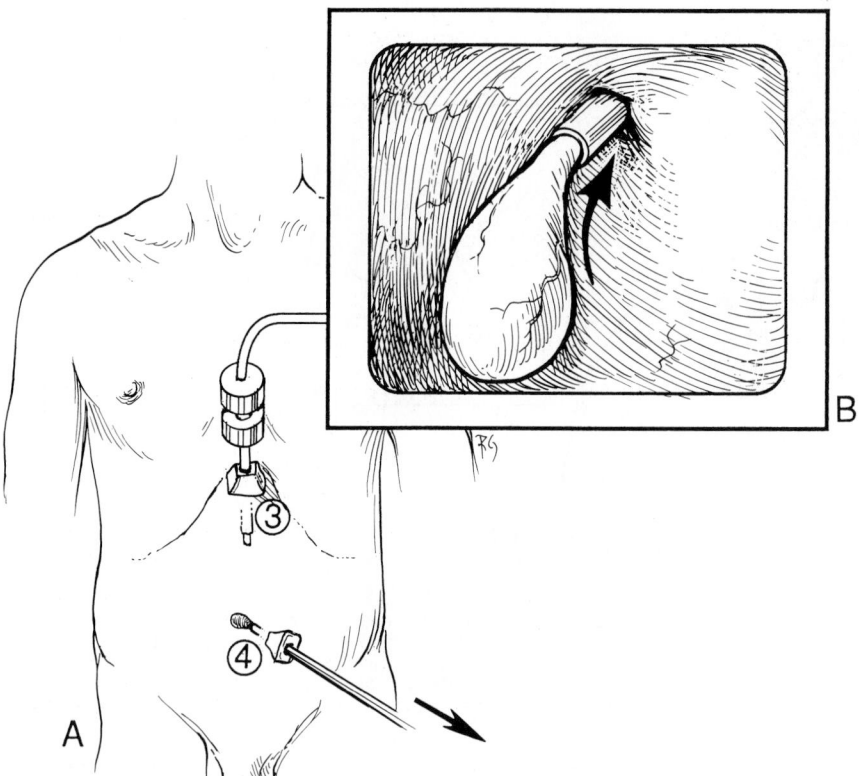

Figure 34–19. When the gallbladder is completely free of its attachments, the laparoscope is placed in the superior midline port and the gallbladder is removed through the umbilical port, which is easy to enlarge, if necessary. Some surgeons prefer to remove it through the superior midline port, and some place the gallbladder in a protective bag prior to removal to avoid spillage of bile and stones into the peritoneal cavity during the extraction process.

efficacy. Approximately 15% of patients will require cholecystectomy during therapy, and gallstones recur in approximately 50% of patients within 5 years without prophylaxis. The ideal candidate for oral dissolution is a thin, young female who has a small number of small, floating stones. Oral dissolution therapy may be useful in selected symptomatic patients who are unwilling to undergo laparoscopic cholecystectomy or who have precluding risk factors.[23]

Contact Dissolution Therapy. Methyl tert-butyl ether is a potent lipid solvent that dissolves gallstones within hours when introduced into the gallbladder through a pigtail catheter appropriately positioned under local anesthesia by an experienced radiologist. An automatic infusion-withdrawal device prevents overflow into the duodenum and washes the gallbladder free of debris as the stones disintegrate. In carefully selected patients, this investigational technique dissolved approximately 95% of the stone mass within about 12.5 hours.[27]

Extracorporeal Shock Wave Lithotripsy. Treatment of selected symptomatic gallstone patients by lithotripsy under protocols approved by the Food and Drug Administration showed that approximately 75% of patients with a single stone 20 mm. or less in diameter were stone free 6 months after treatment. The procedure was less efficacious in patients who had larger or multiple stones.[18] Accordingly, the procedure was not approved for treatment of gallstones.

Asymptomatic Stones

The indications for treatment of patients with cholelithiasis include symptoms that can reasonably be attributed to the presence of gallstones. Asymptomatic stones may be discovered at operation for other illnesses or on routine testing for unrelated abdominal complaints. The question is whether cholecystectomy should be done in healthy asymptomatic patients to prevent the development of acute cholecystitis and its complications. The best evidence suggests that the rate of development of symptoms is about 2% per year in patients with truly asymptomatic stones, and that mortality and morbidity in this group are approximately equal to those associated with cholecystectomy.[12] Some do not believe that truly asymptomatic patients should have cholecystectomy, unless it can be done safely during an operation for another condition. Cholecystectomy is recommended by some in asymptomatic patients who are candidates for heart or renal transplantation, in patients who must receive total parenteral nutrition indefinitely, and during bariatric surgery for morbid obesity.

SPECIAL CONSIDERATIONS

Chronic Acalculous Cholecystitis

Acute inflammation of the gallbladder without stones is a recognized entity that requires cholecystectomy. Occasionally, patients have signs and symptoms of gallbladder disease, but stones cannot be demonstrated by repeated ultrasonography or oral cholecystography. The criteria for cholecystectomy in this situation are not clearly defined, but a significant number of patients are found to have gallbladder pathology and are subsequently free of symptoms. How many patients have relief because of the placebo effect of surgical procedures is unknown, however. The presence of cholesterol crystals in bile has been taken to mean that small gallstones may be forming and causing symptoms as they pass through the biliary tract. Recently, duodenal drainage during administration of cholecystokinin has been used to obtain samples of bile from the gallbladder for examination for crystals. Prior to the test, iopanoic acid is administered to opacify the gallbladder and to monitor its contraction fluoroscopically. Criteria for a positive test include the presence of crystals, reproduction of pain, and either hypocontraction or hypercontraction of the gallbladder. Positive responders have a high incidence of chronic acalculous cholecystitis, cholelithia-

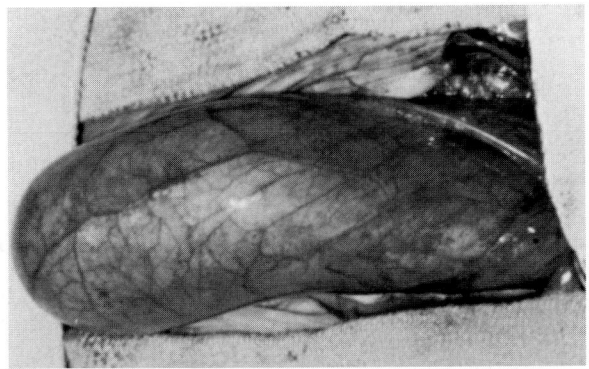

Figure 34–20. Hydrops of the gallbladder. Elongated, tense gallbladder filled with clear, mucoid material protrudes through the wound.

sis, cholesterolosis, and adenomyomatosis, and about three fourths of the cholecystectomized patients become asymptomatic.[5] More experience is needed with this diagnostic test.

Hydrops of the Gallbladder

Hydrops of the gallbladder is caused by obstruction of the outlet, usually by an impacted stone, but occasionally by a tumor or fibrosis. The organ becomes filled with mucoid material and distends to an extremely large size (Fig. 34–20). There is little evidence of inflammation. The mucoid material undoubtedly comes from the gallbladder epithelium, but the pathophysiology is not known. Although most cases occur in adults, children develop hydrops in association with a wide range of infectious diseases and as the result of a congenitally narrow cystic duct. The average age is about 5 years.

Hydrops causes pain in the area of the gallbladder, which may be located as far inferiorly as the pelvis, depending on its size. The gallbladder is usually palpable and may be tender. Some patients are asymptomatic. The gallbladder does not visualize on oral cholecystography because of the cystic duct obstruction, but it may be identified easily by ultrasonography. In children, the process usually resolves without treatment; in adults, cholecystectomy is indicated.

SELECTED REFERENCES

Fromm, H.: Gallstone dissolution therapy: Current status and future prospects. Gastroenterology, 91:1560, 1986.
> *The epidemiology and natural history of gallstones are set forth, and a comprehensive discussion of the mechanisms by which bile acids and solvents dissolve gallstones is presented. The indications, treatment regimens, and complications of bile acid therapy are described.*

Gadacz, T. R.: U.S. experience with laparoscopic cholecystectomy. Am. J. Surg., 162:71, 1991.
> *An excellent compilation of results, morbidity, mortality, and problems taken from a large number of reports.*

Gallstones and laparoscopic cholecystectomy. NIH Consensus Statement, 10:1, 1992.
> *This monograph represents the consensus of experts and should be required reading by all who care for gallstone patients.*

Johnston, D. E., and Kaplan, M. M.: Pathogenesis and treatment of gallstones. N. Engl. J. Med., 328:412, 1993.
> *A well-referenced overview of all the current issues and problems pertaining to all aspects of gallstones, their clinical manifestations, diagnosis, and treatment.*

McSherry, C. K., and Glenn, F.: The incidence and causes of death following surgery for nonmalignant biliary tract disease. Ann. Surg., 191:271, 1980.
> *This classic paper details the causes of death following 11,808 biliary tract operations. Detailed information about mortality rates for subgroups is presented. This experience provides a standard with which the results in other hospitals or individual practices can be compared. High-risk groups are identified.*

REFERENCES

1. Admirand, W. H., and Small, D. M.: The physiochemical basis of cholesterol gallstone formation in man. J. Clin. Invest., 47:1043, 1968.
2. Barkun, J. S., Barkun, A. N., Meakins, J. L., and the McGill Gallstone Treatment Group: Laparoscopic versus open cholecystectomy: The Canadian experience. Am. J. Surg., 165:455, 1993.
3. Bolondi, L., Gaiani, S., Testa, S., and Labo, G.: Gallbladder sludge formation during prolonged fasting after gastrointestinal tract surgery. Gut, 26:734, 1985.
4. Broomfield, P. H., Chopra, R., Sheinbaum, R. C., Bonorris, G. G., Silverman, A., Schoenfield, L. J., and Marks, J. W.: Effects of ursodeoxycholic acid and aspirin on the formation of lithogenic bile and gallstones during loss of weight. N. Engl. J. Med., 319:1567, 1988.
5. Burnstein, M. J., Vassal, K. P., and Strasberg, S. M.: Results of combined biliary drainage and cholecystokinin cholecystography in 81 patients with normal oral cholecystograms. Ann. Surg., 196:627, 1982.
6. Cooperberg, P. L., and Burhenne, H. J.: Real-time ultrasonography: Diagnostic treatment of choice in calculous gallbladder disease. N. Engl. J. Med., 302:1277, 1980.
7. Coyle, J. J., Hoyt, D. B., and Sedaghat, A.: Relationship of intestinal bypass operations and cholelithiasis. Surg. Forum, 31:139, 1980.
8. Edlung, Y., and Zettergren, L.: Histopathology of the gallbladder in gallstone disease related to clinical data. Acta. Chir. Scand., 116:460, 1958.
9. Einarsson, K., Nilsell, K., Leijd, B., and Angelin, B.: Influence of age on secretion of cholesterol and synthesis of bile acids by the liver. N. Engl. J. Med., 313:277, 1985.
10. Everson, G. T., McKinley, C., and Kern, F., Jr.: Mechanisms of gallstone formation in women: Effects of exogenous estrogen (Premarin) and dietary cholesterol on hepatic lipid metabolism. J. Clin. Invest., 87:237, 1991.
11. Gadacz, T. R.: U.S. experience with laparoscopic cholecystectomy. Am. J. Surg., 165:450, 1993.
12. Gracie, W. A., and Ransohoff, D. F.: The natural history of silent gallstones. Gastroenterology, 80:1161, 1981.
13. Holzbach, R. T., March, M., Olszewski, M., and Holan, K.: Cholesterol solubility in bile with evidence that supersaturated bile is frequent in healthy man. J. Clin. Invest., 52:1467, 1973.
14. Hunter, J. G.: Avoidance of bile duct injury during laparoscopic cholecystectomy. Am. J. Surg., 162:71, 1991.
15. Lieber, M. M.: The incidence of gallstones and their correlation with other diseases. Ann. Surg., 135:394, 1952.
16. Lorimer, J. W., and Fairfull-Smith, R. J.: Intraoperative cholangiography is not essential to avoid duct injuries during laparoscopic cholecystectomy. Am. J. Surg., 169:344, 1995.
17. Maki, T.: Pathogenesis of calcium bilirubinate gallstones: Role of E. coli, β-glucuronidase, and coagulation by inorganic ions, polyelectrolytes, and agitation. Ann. Surg., 165:90, 1966.
18. Nahrwold, D. L.: Gallstone lithotripsy. Am. J. Surg., 165:431, 1993.
19. Nahrwold, D. L., Rose, R. C., and Ward, S. P.: Abnormalities in gallbladder morphology and function in patients with cholelithiasis. Ann. Surg., 184:415, 1976.
20. Pitt, H. A., Berquist, W. E., Mann, L. L., Porter-Fink, V., Fonkalsrud, E. W., and Ament, M. E.: Parenteral nutrition induces calcium bilirubinate gallstones. Gastroenterology, 84:1274, 1983.
21. Price, W. H.: Gallbladder dyspepsia. Br. Med. J., 2:138, 1963.
22. Sampliner, R. E., Bennett, P. H., Comess, L. J., Rose, F. A., and Burch, T. A.: Gallbladder disease in Pima Indians: Demonstration of high prevalence and early onset by cholecystography. N. Engl. J. Med., 283:1358, 1970.
23. Schoenfield, L. J., and Marks, J. W.: Oral and contact dissolution of gallstones. Am. J. Surg., 165:427, 1993.
24. Schwartz, S. I.: Biliary tract surgery and cirrhosis: A critical combination. Surgery, 90:577, 1981.
25. Southern Surgeons Club: A prospective analysis of 1518 laparoscopic cholecystectomies. N. Engl. J. Med., 324:1073, 1991.
26. Strasberg, S. M., Hertl, M., and Soper, N. J.: An analysis of the problem of biliary injury during laparoscopic cholecystectomy. J. Am. Coll. Surg., 180:101, 1995.
27. Thistle, J. L., May, G. R., Bender, C. E., Williams, H. J., LeRoy, A. J., Nelson, P. E., Peine, C. J., Petersen, B. T., and McCullough, J. E.: Dissolution of cholesterol gallbladder stones by methyl tert-butyl ether administered by percutaneous transhepatic catheter. N. Engl. J. Med., 320:633, 1989.

III

CHOLANGITIS

David L. Nahrwold, M.D.

Cholangitis, originally described by Charcot in 1877,[3] is a bacterial, parasitic, or chemical inflammation of the bile duct system. How bacteria, parasites, and other foreign material enter the bile duct system is not entirely clear, but several routes are possible. Normally, small numbers of bacteria pass into the portal venous system from the intestine, enter the liver, and are phagocytosed by the reticuloendothelial system of the liver. Occasionally, the normal defense mechanisms are unable to prevent the entry of bacteria into bile. In normal individuals with intact bile duct systems, the flow of bile is sufficient to clear the bile of bacteria, whereas in patients who have obstructing lesions of the duct system, colonization and, eventually, symptoms of cholangitis might supervene.

Bacteria could also ascend from the duodenum through the sphincter of Oddi. This is an obvious possibility after a sphincterotomy or other biliary surgery in which the normal, periodic occlusive action of the sphincter of Oddi is absent, such as in a patient who had a choledochoduodenostomy.[24]

Finally, organisms can be introduced into a normal or abnormal bile duct system by the tubes, catheters, scopes, guide wires, and other instruments used for the diagnosis and treatment of biliary tract disorders.[13, 23]

Experimental evidence in animals and clinical observations in humans suggest a relationship between the entry of bacteria into the circulation and the pressure within the bile duct system. Early observations that T-tube cholangiography caused cholangitis led to the demonstration that small particles appeared in the bloodstream after cholangiography and that pressures of about 20 cm. H_2O are necessary for cholangiovenous reflux to occur.[15] Bile canaliculi—the terminal tributaries of the bile duct system that are lined by hepatocytes—communicate directly with hepatic sinusoids at their terminal ends, so the anatomic arrangement within the liver permits reflux of bacteria from canaliculi directly into the venous circulation.[4, 5] Small particles about the size of a virus can pass into the circulation at pressures less than the secretory pressure of the liver,[7] and radioactively labeled bacteria enter the circulation at pressures slightly higher than the secretory pressure of the liver.[8]

Cholangitis often occurs in patients who have only partial bile duct obstruction, and it is logical to assume that intraductal pressure could be normal in the absence of complete obstruction. This question has been addressed experimentally, and higher than normal pressures have been found in patients and animals with partial obstruction, although they are not as high as when complete obstruction is present.[25]

The exact circumstances under which cholangiovenous reflux occurs in patients with partial obstruction are not known, but high intraductal pressure for varying lengths of time could be caused by temporary impaction of an otherwise freely movable stone. Short-lived increases in intra-abdominal pressure caused by movement, coughing, or other maneuvers could also produce cholangiovenous reflux when the choledochal sphincter mechanism is closed.

ASSOCIATED PATHOLOGY

The conditions that affect the biliary tract and are associated with cholangitis are listed in Table 34–1. The most common cause of acute cholangitis is choledocholithiasis, which accounts for approximately 60% of the cases.[22] Common duct stones usually occur in association with cholelithiasis but may also be found in patients who have had cholecystectomy (Fig. 34–21). Common duct stones may migrate from the gallbladder and grow within the common duct. They may be undetected at the time of cholecystectomy (retained stones). Stones may also form *de novo* within the common duct. Arbitrarily, stones discovered 2 years after cholecystectomy are designated primary common duct stones (see Fig. 34–21). They are linked to bacterial colonization of bile, in that their primary constituent is calcium bilirubinate. Normally, insoluble bilirubin is conjugated to its soluble form, bilirubin diglucuronide, and excreted in bile. When beta glucuronidase, an enzyme produced by bacteria, including *E. coli*, is present in bile, bilirubin diglucuronide is deconjugated, leaving bilirubin to precipitate as calcium bilirubinate, the principal constituent of primary common duct stones. This theory is supported by the fact that common duct stones made of calcium bilirubinate are found in association with bacterbilia and in conditions that lend themselves to bacterbilia, such as biliary-enteric anastomoses, benign strictures, and the presence of foreign bodies. The signs and symptoms of acute cholangitis are the most frequent manifestations of both primary and secondary common duct stones, and the diagnosis of acute cholangitis usually prompts the studies that lead to their discovery.

Malignant tumors that cause bile duct obstruction are carcinoma of the head of the pancreas, the bile ducts, and the ampulla of Vater. Strictures associated with these tumors are an infrequent cause of cholangitis,[2, 22] so studies leading to their detection are usually prompted by the occurrence of jaundice rather than signs and symptoms of infection. Malig-

---

TABLE 34–1. Biliary Tract Conditions Associated with Cholangitis

Choledocholithiasis	Cholangiography
Malignant strictures	T-tube
Cholangiocarcinoma	Percutaneous transhepatic
Pancreatic cancer	Endoscopic retrograde
Ampullary cancer	Parasitic infestations
Gallbladder cancer	*Clonorchis sinensis*
Benign strictures	*Ascaris lumbricoides*
Anastomotic stenosis	Ischemia
Impacted stone	Chemical irritation
Ampullary stenosis	Carbamazepine
Indwelling tubes or stents	Clinoril

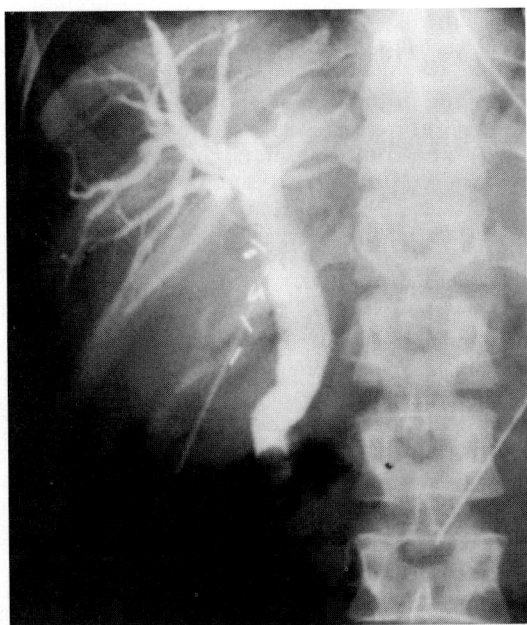

Figure 34–21. Cholangiogram in a patient who had cholecystectomy 3 years previously and presented with cholangitis. A stone was impacted in the distal common bile duct.

nant strictures are associated with bacterbilia in one fourth to one third of cases—less frequently than other lesions that predispose to cholangitis. However, cases of cholangitis associated with malignancies are much more likely to be severe and life-threatening than those associated with other obstructive lesions. About half the cases reported by Boey and Way[2] had acute suppurative cholangitis, the most severe form of the disease. This high incidence is probably due to the completeness of obstruction in malignant disease.

Benign strictures of the duct system are often heralded by an episode of cholangitis. Most of them are due to primary sclerosing cholangitis, but a few result from operative trauma during cholecystectomy.

Almost all patients with stricture have bacterbilia. As mentioned previously, calcium bilirubinate stones are prone to form proximal to a stricture, so the development of cholangitis may be the result of both stricture and stone. Another cause of bile duct stricture, seen with increasing frequency, is chronic pancreatitis. This stricture, located in the intrapancreatic portion of the common bile duct, may first become manifest through the development of acute cholangitis.

Patients who have biliary-enteric anastomoses are prone to bacterbilia because of reflux of chyme into the biliary tract, even though some protection may be afforded by a Roux-en-Y anatomic arrangement. There is no solid evidence that bacterbilia in such patients is harmful, or that such patients are predisposed to cholangitis. However, when the anastomosis is too narrow, cholangitis does occur (Fig. 34–22). Acute suppurative cholangitis is rare in patients with a biliary stricture or a biliary-enteric anastomosis in the absence of an accompanying stone that produces complete obstruction, but benign strictures are second only to choledocholithiasis as a cause of acute cholangitis.

At some institutions, invasive procedures may be the most common cause of acute cholangitis. The frequency of chills and fever after T-tube cholangiography has led to various regimens to prevent it, including drainage of bile for 24 hours after the procedure and antibiotic coverage. This complication, which results from cholangiovenous reflux and bacteremia, can be avoided by careful attention to sterile technique

and slow injection of the contrast material. The T-tube should not be removed or clamped for about 24 hours after cholangiography, but antibiotic coverage is unnecessary. Acute cholangitis may follow percutaneous transhepatic cholangiography (PTC), endoscopic retrograde cholangiopancreatography (ERCP), or cholangiography done by injection of contrast through other indwelling biliary drainage tubes, such as the U-tubes sometimes used to splint biliary-enteric anastomoses. Other biliary tract procedures that may be complicated by cholangitis include percutaneous transhepatic biliary drainage, endoscopic sphincterotomy, percutaneous extraction of calculi, and insertion of an endoprosthesis. Obviously, contamination of bile may occur during these procedures, and they are almost always carried out for conditions that are associated with bacterbilia. Temporary increases in biliary tract pressure are frequent during these procedures, and concomitant cholangiography is frequently necessary, so the high incidence of cholangitis is not surprising.

The presence of a T-tube or stent within the bile duct system results in bacterial colonization of the bile within a week in more than 90% of cases.[19] This accounts for the high frequency of cholangitis in these patients, especially when obstruction and increased pressure occur after indwelling tubes are clamped or become occluded with the *sludge* that typically forms on foreign bodies in the biliary tract. This problem has led to the recommendation that tubes and catheters expected to be indwelling on a long-term basis be irrigated daily, when possible.

Parasites are a cause of cholangitis and biliary strictures in Asia. They include *Clonorchis sinensis*, *Trichuris trichiura*, and *Ascaris lumbricoides*, which obstruct the bile duct system and are associated with bacterbilia. These problems are rare in the United States.

Bacteriology

The organisms found in the bile of patients with gallstones and other diseases of the biliary tract are those that are cultured from the blood and the biliary tract during episodes of acute cholangitis or acute toxic cholangitis. Most are aerobic bacteria, including the gram-negative organisms *E. coli*; species of *Klebsiella*, *Proteus*, and *Pseudomonas*; and the gram-positive organisms *Streptococcus faecalis* and *Enterococcus* species. But the anaerobic bacterial species *Bacteroides*, *Clostridium*, and even *Candida* have been isolated. A single species is

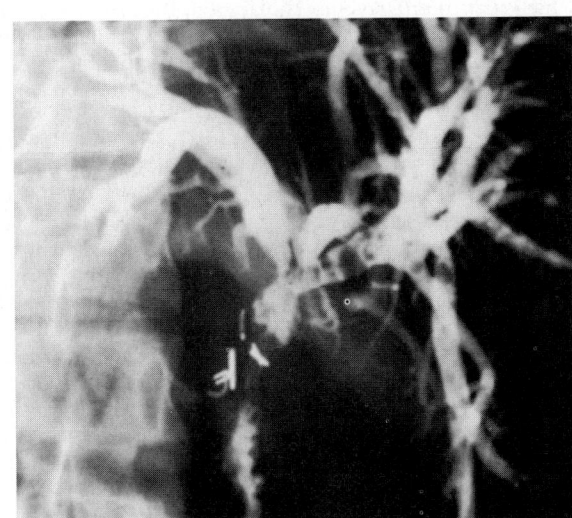

Figure 34–22. Cholangiogram in a patient who had a bile duct injury at cholecystectomy, followed by a Roux-en-Y choledochojejunostomy, which is now strictured. Note the many calculi within the intrahepatic ducts.

isolated in about 40% of patients; two or more are found in a similar percentage, and as many as three species are found in approximately 20% of patients.[9]

CLINICAL MANIFESTATIONS

The original description of cholangitis by Charcot consisted of intermittent chills and fever, jaundice, and abdominal pain. *Charcot's triad*, as this combination is now known, remains the hallmark of acute cholangitis, by definition. His original description referred to the presence of pus or purulent mucus mixed in stagnant bile. Reynolds and Dargan described patients who had shock and central nervous system (CNS) depression in addition to Charcot's triad and noted that this lethal combination of symptoms, now known as Reynolds' pentad, occurred in the presence of complete obstruction of a bile duct system that contained pus under pressure.[21] It is now known that pus may be present in partially obstructed as well as completely obstructed ducts, and that some patients with cholangitis may develop shock and coma without having frank pus within the duct system. The significance of Reynolds' pentad (intermittent chills and fever, abdominal pain, jaundice, shock, and CNS depression) is that this condition is rapidly lethal without emergency intervention, whereas Charcot's triad is an acute but less toxic condition for which immediate intervention is usually not necessary.

Accordingly, degrees of severity of inflammation of the biliary tract have become apparent, ranging from clinically inapparent bacterbilia, to an episode of cholangitis manifested by mild, short-lived fever and abdominal pain, to a lethal form of the disease—acute toxic cholangitis—in which complete bile duct obstruction converts the bile duct system into an abscess cavity that contains pus under pressure. The concept of this spectrum of cholangitis is important, because the severity of clinical signs and symptoms determines the appropriate therapy and its timing. Because cholangitis does not occur in the absence of other biliary tract pathology, the treatment varies according to the type of obstructing lesion present. When the diagnosis of cholangitis is made, appropriate tests must be done to find the associated lesion.

An accurate history is essential in making the diagnosis. The details of previous biliary tract problems or operations should be obtained, keeping in mind the possibilities of retained or primary common duct stones, operative injury to the bile ducts, or a previous biliary-enteric anastomosis, all of which may predispose to cholangitis. Recurrent episodes of pancreatitis may suggest a distal common duct stricture. Similarly, the possibility of malignant stricture should be explored by questioning the patient about anorexia, pain, and weight loss.

The complete symptom triad of chills and fever, abdominal pain, and jaundice occurs in only 50% to 70% of patients who have cholangitis.[2, 13, 17] The most frequent symptom is fever, which is present in over 90%, but a history of chills is not as frequent. Abdominal pain, usually in the right upper quadrant, occurs in about 80% and is characteristically mild. Severe abdominal pain is very unusual. Clinically apparent jaundice is present in about 80%. Nausea and vomiting, not part of Charcot's triad, are the only other frequent symptoms.

Other than elevated temperature and jaundice, the positive physical findings are limited to the abdomen. Sixty per cent to 80% of patients have abdominal tenderness, which is almost always in the right upper quadrant or epigastrium. Signs of peritoneal irritation are not commonly found. In general, the abdominal tenderness is mild to moderate. Bowel sounds are usually normal. Occasionally, a mass may be present in the right upper quadrant due to an enlarged gallbladder, a tumor, or an abscess. In patients with biliary stricture and biliary cirrhosis, the liver may be enlarged. They may have other stigmata of biliary cirrhosis as well.

The laboratory findings in acute cholangitis reflect the infectious nature of the disease and the fact that biliary tract obstruction is a prerequisite for its development. The white blood cell count is elevated in approximately 75% of cases. In some instances, a shift to the left is the only abnormality. The presence or absence of an abnormal white blood cell count depends on the interval between symptoms and the time of measurement. Obviously, a patient who had an episode of chills and fever a week prior to examination is unlikely to have an abnormal count, whereas the opposite is true for a patient who has bacteremia at the time of testing. More than 90% of patients with acute cholangitis have hyperbilirubinemia. The degree of hyperbilirubinemia varies according to the underlying biliary tract problem, but 20% of patients have a serum value of 2.0 mg. per deciliter or less.[2, 14] As mentioned previously, 70% to 80% have jaundice detectable on physical examination, so measurement of serum bilirubin is essential to detect the remaining 20% to 30% of cases. Serum alkaline phosphatase values are elevated in over 90%, and the same is true of aspartate aminotransferase (AST) and alanine aminotransferase (ALT) levels. Serum amylase is frequently increased, but this is probably a nonspecific finding, except in patients with concomitant pancreatitis, in whom the values are elevated to at least twice normal. The importance of measuring serum bilirubin, alkaline phosphatase, and transaminases in patients who are not jaundiced cannot be overemphasized, because this directs attention to the biliary tract in the face of nonspecific symptoms such as nausea and vomiting, chills, fever, and abdominal pain. The possibility of cholangitis must be raised in any patient who has intermittent fever without other symptoms. This aspect of the diagnostic process in patients with fever of undetermined origin is often overlooked.

In many cases, the clinical picture of cholangitis suggests bacteremia, especially when chills and fever are present. Patients suspected of having acute cholangitis should have cultures of their blood drawn during a chill, when possible, because of the importance of determining the organism's sensitivity to specific antibiotics in case the initial antibiotic treatment fails. Slightly less than half of patients with acute cholangitis have positive blood cultures.[2, 14, 22] Most patients who have chills and fever would probably have positive cultures if it were possible to obtain blood samples more frequently and at the most appropriate times. Not surprisingly, the type of organisms cultured and the frequency with which each is found in the blood correlate very well with the types found later, at operation, in the bile of the same patients. The organisms most frequently cultured from the blood of patients with acute cholangitis are, in decreasing order, *E. coli*, *Klebsiella pneumoniae*, and *S. faecalis*. These organisms are the ones most commonly found in bile, in the same order of frequency. About two thirds of patients have multiple organisms present in their bile. Anaerobic organisms, usually *Bacteroides fragilis*, are found rarely in both bile and blood, but anaerobic cultures of blood should be made.

About 15% of all patients with cholangitis have symptoms that include shock and CNS depression. The latter may take the form of coma, disorientation, drowsiness, confusion, or inappropriate behavior—the same CNS symptoms seen in patients with severe, persistent sepsis from other causes. In general, the symptoms of acute toxic cholangitis are more severe, but the characteristic features are the persistent and progressive nature of the symptoms and the patient's failure to respond rapidly to conventional therapy for sepsis. This, of course, is the signal for emergency measures to find the septic focus and drain it immediately. In acute toxic cholangitis, this means emergency decompression of the bile duct system.

DIAGNOSIS OF THE UNDERLYING CONDITION

The underlying biliary tract disease must be delineated when the diagnosis of acute cholangitis is made. Cholangiography is the definitive test and is necessary for planning definitive therapy, but it should not be done until the acute process is under control. Injection of contrast material under pressure into the biliary tract may produce cholangiovenous reflux and exacerbate the sepsis unless appropriate antibiotic therapy has controlled the infection. Patients with acute cholangitis should have an ultrasound examination, with special emphasis on the presence or absence of cholelithiasis, bile duct dilatation, masses in the head of the pancreas or within the hepatic portal, and choledocholithiasis. Ultrasonography is highly accurate in the detection of gallbladder calculi and bile duct enlargement, but less so in the delineation of common duct calculi.

Once the cholangitis is under control, further testing may proceed, using the ultrasound examination as a guide. If a mass in the pancreas or the hepatic portal is suspected, computerized axial tomography should be done to delineate its extent, as well as to assess the liver for hepatic metastases. Cholescintigraphy is helpful in differentiating between acute cholecystitis and acute cholangitis, but its role in the diagnosis of conditions that underlie cholangitis is limited. Complete bile duct obstruction can be diagnosed by cholescintigraphy, but delineation of lesions causing incomplete obstruction is not possible (Fig. 34–23).

The essential procedure is cholangiography, which can be obtained by the percutaneous transhepatic or endoscopic retrograde technique. PTC should be done when ultrasonography shows a dilated proximal duct system, and ERCP is indicated when the duct system is normal. The endoscopic technique should be considered when concomitant upper gastrointestinal endoscopy is indicated, such as in a suspected carcinoma of the ampulla of Vater, or when pancreatography is necessary, such as in chronic pancreatitis. Certain aspects of PTC and ERCP that have a bearing on the therapy of acute cholangitis and acute toxic cholangitis are discussed below.

TREATMENT

The principles of therapy for acute cholangitis are, first, to achieve complete control of the septic process and, second, to correct the underlying cause. All patients with significant symptoms of acute cholangitis or acute toxic cholangitis should receive antibiotic therapy. An occasional patient may have a history of mild, short-lived symptoms suggestive of acute cholangitis but be asymptomatic at the time of examination. Under these circumstances, clinical investigation for the underlying cause may proceed without antibiotic coverage, except when indicated for invasive procedures. To date, there is no ideal antibiotic regimen. The choice should be based on the organisms most often cultured from the blood, which are *E. coli*, *K. pneumoniae*, and *S. faecalis*. The first two organisms are best treated by an aminoglycoside such as gentamycin or tobramycin, but these agents are not effective against *S. faecalis* or other enterococci. Enterococci are best managed by a combination of a penicillin and an aminoglycoside. To further complicate the situation, anaerobes, most commonly *B. fragilis*, are cultured from bile in one fourth to one third of cases. This organism is best treated by clindamycin or metronidazole. Therefore, patients with severe acute cholangitis are treated with a combination that includes a penicillin such as ampicillin, an aminoglycoside, and either clindamycin or metronidazole. Some might dispute the need for gram-negative anaerobe coverage because of the rela-

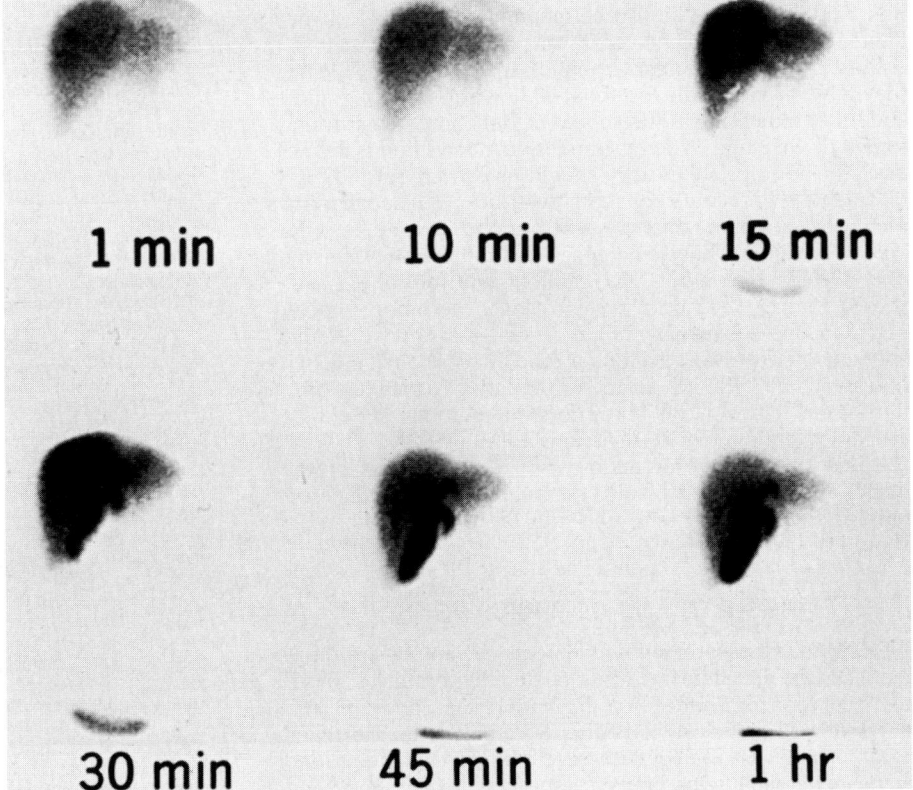

Figure 34–23. Hepatobiliary scan showing complete obstruction of the distal common bile duct.

1 min   10 min   15 min

30 min   45 min   1 hr

tively low frequency with which these organisms are actually cultured from the blood in cholangitis patients. The major disadvantage of this regimen is the nephrotoxicity of the aminoglycosides, which is made even more likely because of the septic shock and hyperbilirubinemia seen in some cholangitis patients. Serum levels of aminoglycosides and creatinine should be monitored to minimize this problem.

In patients with mild cholangitis and no evidence of continuing, severe sepsis, antibiotic therapy with a second- or third-generation cephalosporin is adequate. These agents are effective against *E. coli, K. pneumoniae*, and other gram-negative aerobic organisms but not against the more rarely cultured *S. faecalis* and other enterococci.

The newer penicillins, such as piperacillin, mezlocillin, and imipenem, appear to be effective against gram-negative aerobes and enterococci and may prove to be the safest and most effective agents for acute cholangitis. The results of blood cultures and sensitivities should be used to adjust antibiotic therapy and to discontinue nephrotoxic agents when less toxic agents can be substituted.[16] The emphasis on the concentration of antibiotics in bile may be less important than originally thought. Although there are theoretical advantages to high bile concentrations, such as the elimination of organisms from bile, tissue and serum concentrations may be more important. In acute toxic cholangitis with complete bile duct obstruction, for example, high concentrations might not be achieved because of failure of the liver to secrete the antibiotic into bile.

Elderly and debilitated patients who have acute cholangitis, and all patients with acute toxic cholangitis, require careful monitoring of hemodynamic parameters, urine output, and blood gases. Direct arterial blood pressure monitoring should be instituted if the blood pressure is unstable or urine output is abnormal. In such cases, measurements of central venous and pulmonary wedge pressures are necessary, and frequent determinations of cardiac output and systemic vascular resistance should be made so that decisions about volume replacement, inotropic agents, and vasoactive drugs can be made on the basis of the data at hand. Coagulation parameters should also be monitored, especially in patients who have chronic liver disease.

Most cholangitis patients respond rapidly to therapy. After they have been afebrile for about 48 hours, cholangiography and other indicated studies should be done under continuing antibiotic coverage. When the underlying condition is delineated, the appropriate therapy should be carried out.

Patients with acute cholangitis who do not respond completely to antibiotic therapy and supportive care or who deteriorate should have emergency decompression of the bile duct system. Numerous trials, although uncontrolled, have shown that the bile duct system can be decompressed by percutaneous transhepatic biliary drainage or by endoscopic sphincterotomy and concomitant nasobiliary drainage, when necessary.[6, 10, 12] The advantage of the latter is that concomitant stone removal can be performed, but this should be attempted only under ideal circumstances.

When transhepatic or endoscopic decompression of the biliary system is not available or possible, immediate laparotomy and insertion of a T-tube into the common bile duct should be carried out.

RESULTS AND COMPLICATIONS

The results of treatment of mild acute cholangitis are excellent. Deaths are almost always related to complications of the operation performed for the underlying condition and are unrelated to the original episode of cholangitis. However, the mortality associated with severe acute cholangitis and acute toxic cholangitis is high, especially when shock and CNS symptoms are present. In one review of 86 patients, the mortality rate was 100% in untreated patients and 50% in those who had bile duct decompression.[1] The high mortality of nonoperative therapy has been confirmed in other reviews.[17, 18] More recent data suggest that the mortality of properly treated acute toxic cholangitis is 20% to 25%.[11, 17]

The most serious complication of acute cholangitis and acute toxic cholangitis is hepatic abscess. Biliary tract disease, including cholangitis, accounts for about half of all cases of hepatic abscess.[20] Because they occur in association with cholangitis, hepatic abscesses are often overlooked. They should be suspected in all patients who fail to respond to treatment of cholangitis. Antibiotic treatment should include coverage for anaerobic organisms, because they are frequently cultured from hepatic abscesses. They are successfully treated by surgical or percutaneous drainage, but the mortality rate approaches 100% when multiple abscesses are present. The best approach to this problem is to prevent them by prompt attention to biliary tract obstruction and cholangitis.

SELECTED REFERENCES

Csendes, A., Diaz, J. C., Burdiles, P., Maluenda, F., and Morales, E.: Risk factors and classification of acute suppurative cholangitis. Br. J. Surg., 79:655, 1992. *This large prospective study of patients was designed to determine the clinical and laboratory values that predict the severity of cholangitis. Operative mortality for each group is provided.*

Lai, E. C. S., Mok, F. P. T., Tan, E. S. Y., Chung-Mau, L., Sheung-Tat, F., Kok-Tjang, Y., and Wong, J.: Endoscopic biliary drainage for severe acute cholangitis. N. Engl. J. Med., 326:1582, 1992. *The authors showed a remarkable reduction in mortality by employing emergency endoscopic biliary drainage as opposed to definitive surgery.*

Nahrwold, D. L.: Acute cholangitis. Surgery, 112:487, 1992. *The rationale for a specific regimen of antibiotic therapy for acute cholangitis is presented.*

REFERENCES

1. Andrew, D. J., and Johnson, S. E.: Acute suppurative cholangitis, a medical and surgical emergency. Am. J. Gastroenterol., 54:141, 1970.
2. Boey, J. H., and Way, L. W.: Acute cholangitis. Ann. Surg., 191:264, 1980.
3. Charcot, J. M.: Lecons sur les maladies du foie des voies filiares et des reins. Paris, Faculte' de Medecine de Paris, 1877.
4. Edlund, Y., and Hanzon, V.: Demonstration of the close relationship between bile capillaries and sinusoid walls. Acta Anat., 17:105, 1953.
5. Hampton, J. C.: An electron microscope study of the hepatic uptake and excretion of microscopic particles injected into the blood stream and into the bile duct. Acta Anat., 32:262, 1958.
6. Huang, M., and Ker, C.: Ultrasonic guided percutaneous transhepatic bile drainage for cholangitis due to intrahepatic stones. Arch. Surg., 123:106, 1988.
7. Hultborn, A., Jacobsson, B., and Rosengren, B.: Cholangiovenous reflux during cholangiography. Acta Chir. Scand., 123:111, 1962.
8. Jacobsson, B., Kjellander, J., and Rosengren, B.: Cholangiovenous reflux. Acta Chir. Scand., 123:316, 1962.
9. Keighley, M. R. B., and Blenkharn, F. I.: Infection and the Biliary Tree: Surgery of the Liver and Biliary Tract. New York, Churchill Livingstone, 1988.
10. Lai, E. C. S., Paterson, I. A., Tam, P. C., Choi, T. K., Fan, S. T., and Wong, J.: Severe acute cholangitis: The role of emergency nasobiliary drainage. Surgery, 107:268, 1990.
11. Lai, E. C. S., Tam, P., Paterson, I. A., Ng, M. M. T., Fan, S., Choi, T., and Wong, J.: Emergency surgery for severe acute cholangitis. Ann. Surg., 211:55, 1990.
12. Leese, T., Neoptolemos, J. P., Baker, A. R., and Carr-Locke, D. L.: Management of acute cholangitis and the impact of endoscopic sphincterotomy. Br. J. Surg., 73:988, 1986.
13. Lipsett, P. A., and Pitt, H. A.: Acute cholangitis. Surg. Clin. North Am., 70:1297, 1990.
14. Longmire, W. P., Jr.: Suppurative cholangitis. In Hardy, J. M. (Ed.): Critical Surgical Illness. Philadelphia, W. B. Saunders, 1971, p. 397.
15. Mixer, H. W., Rigler, L. G., and Gonzales-Oddone, M. V.: Experimental studies on biliary regurgitation during cholangiography. Gastroenterology, 9:64, 1947.
16. Nahrwold, D. L.: Acute cholangitis. Surgery, 112:487, 1992.
17. O'Connor, M. J., Schwartz, M. L., McQuarrie, D. G., and Sumner, H. W.: Acute bacterial cholangitis. Arch. Surg., 117:437, 1982.

18. Pitt, H. A., and Longmire, W. P., Jr.: Suppurative cholangitis. *In* Hardy, J. M. (Ed.): Critical Surgical Illness, 2nd ed. Philadelphia, W. B. Saunders, 1980, p. 380.
19. Pitt, H. A., Postier, R. G., and Cameron, J. L.: Bacteremia after tube cholangiography. Ann. Surg., *191*:30, 1980.
20. Pitt, H. A., and Zuidema, G. D.: Factors influencing mortality in the treatment of pyogenic hepatic abscess. Surg. Gynecol. Obstet., *140*:228, 1975.
21. Reynolds, B. M., and Dargan, E. L.: Acute obstructive cholangitis: A distinct clinical syndrome. Ann. Surg., *150*:299, 1959.
22. Saharia, P. C., and Cameron, J. L.: Clinical management of cholangitis. Surg. Gynecol. Obstet., *142*:369, 1976.
23. Sinanan, M. N.: Acute cholangitis. Infect. Dis. Clin. North Am., *6*:571, 1992.
24. Sun, J. Y., Leung, J. W. C., Shaffer, E. A., Lam, K., Olson, M. E., and Costerton, J. W.: Ascending infection of the biliary tract after surgical sphincterotomy and biliary stenting. J. Gastroenterol. Hepatol., *7*:240, 1992.
25. Williams, R. D., Fish, J. C., and Williams, D. D.: The significance of biliary pressure. Arch. Surg., *95*:374, 1974.

IV

GALLSTONE ILEUS AND FISTULA

Francis E. Rosato, M.D.

BILIARY FISTULAS

A biliary fistula is an established and abnormal connection between any portion of the biliary tree and some other area. If this abnormal connection is between the biliary tree and the exterior, it is termed an *external fistula*; a connection between the biliary tree and an internal structure constitutes an *internal fistula*. Gallstones, peptic ulcer, trauma, and neoplasia are common causes of such fistulas. In general, external fistulas are most likely caused by trauma, particularly operative trauma; internal fistulas most often follow peptic ulcer, gallstone disease, and cancer.

The mode of presentation varies, depending on the cause and the type of fistula. Most external fistulas occur in a postoperative setting, usually after the formation of an extrabiliary accumulation of bile. Internal biliary fistulas are more insidious in their presentation, since the antecedent neoplastic or inflammatory adherence to another body structure occurs over a protracted period of time. The most common biliary fistulas and their symptom complexes are listed in Table 34–2. Cholangitis is likely to be associated with any biliary fistula. In addition, biliary tract connections have been made into the kidney, urinary bladder, uterus, vagina, portal vein, inferior vena cava, and pericardial sac.

External Biliary Fistula

The most common setting for external biliary fistula is after operation on the biliary tree, particularly when exploration or reconstruction of the common bile duct is included. If bile leakage occurs, it results in a walled-off collection of bile, producing a chemical peritonitis. This is usually accompanied by a characteristic rise in conjugated serum bilirubin due to absorption from the peritoneal cavity, followed several days later by an elevation of serum alkaline phosphatase, probably due to pericholangitis.[10] Rarely, bile peritonitis may pursue a more indolent course, producing a mild jaundice and abdominal distention termed *bile ascites*.[17] However, a walled-off bile collection usually occurs, typically producing fever and abdominal tenderness that persist until the bile is removed either operatively by the placement of drains (or

the reopening of drain tracts) or spontaneously. Occasionally, in the absence of any bile duct obstruction, such external fistulas may rapidly close. With sonographic or computed tomographic imaging, percutaneous catheter placement successfully resolves 80% of fistulas.[14] Even with distal common duct obstruction, endoscopic papillotomy allows improved bile flow and passage of common duct stones, permitting nonoperative closure.[6, 13]

Internal Biliary Fistula

Ninety per cent of internal biliary fistulas are caused by gallstone disease, and 5% are secondary to peptic ulcer.[19] Ulcers on the posterior duodenum invade the common duct;[2, 11] those on the anterior and lateral wall attach and erode into the gallbladder. Gastric ulcers typically erode into the gallbladder, where they also produce fistulas. Tumors of the stomach, gallbladder, pancreas, and common duct erode into contiguous structures, producing different types of fistulas.[9] After the connection between the biliary tree and the adjacent structure has been established, the symptom complex of cholangitis ensues. At times, an internal biliary fistula may begin as a localized bile collection; for example, a choledochobronchial fistula usually follows a bile collection that leads to an inflammatory process, producing a connection between these two physically disparate structures.[8]

Complications of Fistula

There are four important complications of biliary fistula, regardless of the type of fistula or the particular structures involved (Fig. 34–24).[12]

Hyponatremia. The sodium content of bile is approximately 150 mEq. per liter, and the loss of such bile can produce severe hyponatremia.

Inanition and Weight Loss. The critical role of bile as an emulsifying agent facilitating the absorption of fats and fat-soluble vitamins is well established. The external loss of bile produces a malabsorption problem, and the resultant diarrhea may additionally jeopardize protein and carbohydrate absorption. When internal biliary fistulas form, particularly between the biliary system and the upper reaches of the intestinal tract, this complication is minimized.

Infection. There are two principal modes by which infection ensues in the presence of biliary fistula. The first is from a transient leakage of bile, with resultant contamination of the peritoneal space. Bile is not sterile and, especially in fistulas, contains coliform organisms and occasionally anaerobic clostridia. Bile leakage into body cavities produces tran-

TABLE 34–2. Symptoms of Biliary Fistulas

Fistula Type	Symptom Complex
Biliary-cutaneous	Bile peritonitis and/or external bile leakage
Biliary-intestinal	Gallstone ileus
Biliary-pleurobronchial	Bile-tinged sputum (biloptysis)

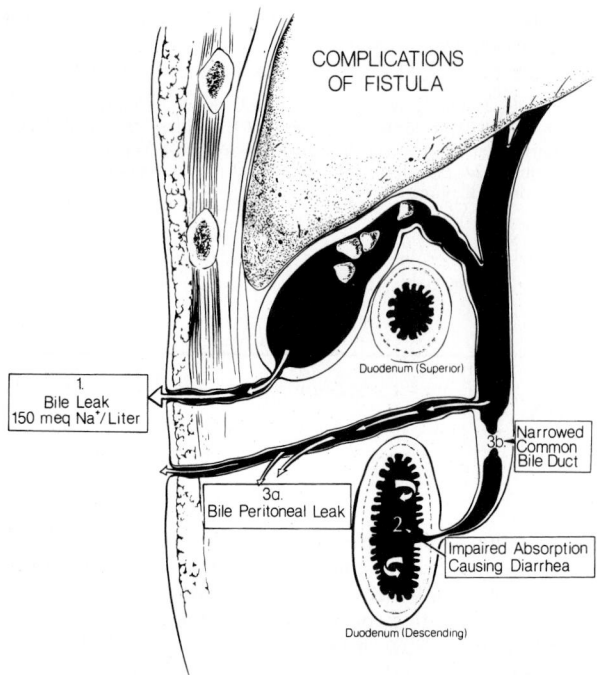

Figure 34–24. Diagrammatic representation of major biliary fistula complications.

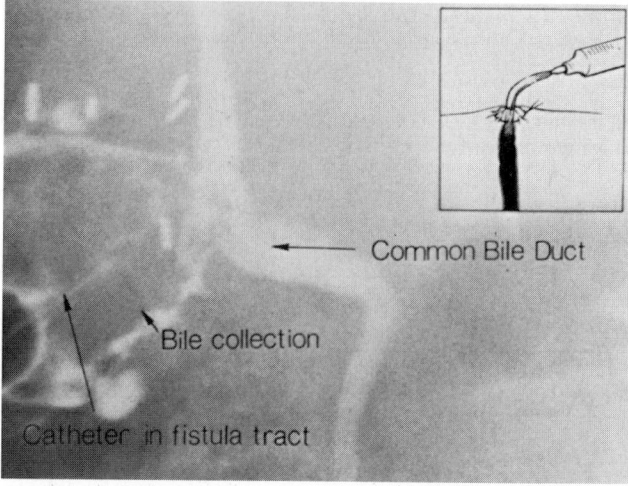

Figure 34–25. Catheter (inset) introduced into fistula tract, and resultant fistulogram demonstrating a choledochocutaneous fistula. The tortuosity of the common bile duct resulted from bile-induced inflammation.

sient episodes of bacterial infection, in addition to the anticipated chemical inflammation. The second factor in infection is cholangitis, which occurs in about 10% to 15% of cholecystoenteric fistulas. The exact mechanism is not clearly understood, since the pressure gradients generally favor the distal flow of bile; in addition, cholangitis does not ensue even when reflux has been demonstrated in surgically created biliary-enteric fistulas. Some degree of bile stasis and obstruction appears to be essential in the production of cholangitis. Cholangitis is ushered in with the classic Charcot's triad of jaundice, fever, and chills.

Gallstone Ileus. Gallstone ileus is considered separately, later in this section.

Therapy

The management of a biliary fistula should be considered in sequential steps.

1. Establish the Anatomy of the Fistula. When the fistula is external, an 8- or 10-French red rubber tube can be inserted in the external orifice and held in place with a pursestring suture of 2-0 silk. Injection of contrast material serves to delineate the site of origin and the fistula tract (Fig. 34–25). When an internal fistula is present, attempts are made through upper gastrointestinal series, barium enema, cholangiography, bronchoscopy, or cystography to delineate the anatomic extent of the fistula (Fig. 34–26).[1] Endoscopic retrograde cholangiopancreatography allows visualization of the distal biliary tree; transhepatic cholangiography demonstrates the intrahepatic biliary system and the extrahepatic ductal system, often pinpointing the biliary origins of the fistula.

2. Attempt to Establish the Cause of the Fistula. In attempting to localize the fistula, one can often obtain additional information on the underlying cause. Studies such as gastroduodenoscopy, radioactive scanning of the liver, sonography (particularly to detect nonopacified gallstones), and cytologic evaluation of a number of aspirated specimens

may be required. The value of surgical exploration for final determination of the cause cannot be overemphasized; very often, initial studies localize the fistula, and surgical therapy delineates its cause. Historically, those 5% of fistulas caused by peptic ulcer disease can be suspected when ulcer symptoms subside with the appearance of the fistula, presumably due to alkaline bathing of the ulcer through the choledochoduodenal fistula.

3. Control Infection. Since infection is one of the major complications of fistula, appropriate antibiotics must be chosen to combat infection. In the case of external fistulas, cultured bile is often helpful in making the correct choice of antibiotics. In general, drugs with a high degree of enterohepatic recirculation and that are effective against gram-negative bacilli, including those that are effective against anaerobes, are ideal for such patients. Ampicillin or cefoxitin (Mefoxin) is an ideal initial agent.

4. Correct Electrolyte Abnormalities. Particular attention should be paid to possible sodium depletion. With the advent

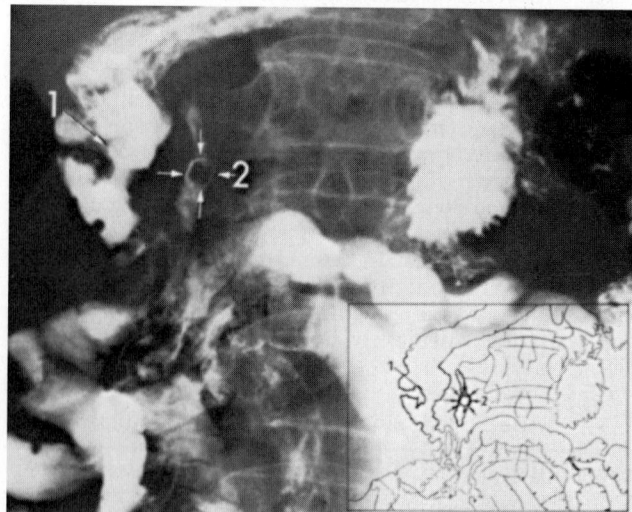

Figure 34–26. Upper gastrointestinal series showing duodenum (1) and shortly thereafter opacification of common bile duct. This sequence is pathognomonic of choledochoduodenal fistula. Note stone in common bile duct (2).

of intravenous hyperalimentation, nutritional problems can be corrected while studying the type and cause of the fistula.

5. Undertake Surgical Therapy. As mentioned, the initial approach to both internal and external biliary fistulas is to establish drainage (usually by computed tomographic or ultrasound guidance) and to relieve obstruction, where it exists, by endoscopic papillotomy. Thus, most fistulas can *dry out* without surgical intervention.[4] However, continuing jaundice, sepsis, or electrolyte disturbances may force a surgical approach.

When inflammation is the cause of the fistula, surgical separation of the adjacent structures is usually done, with surgical closure of each. When neoplasia is the underlying problem, separation may not be possible, although it is obviously preferred. Often the relief of distal obstruction to bile flow may be sufficient to cause complete resolution of the fistula without direct operative intervention. In general, operative cholangiography may be of help in deciding the appropriate surgical therapy. Inflammatory fistulas are usually *taken down* and attention given to the relief of any attendant biliary obstruction.

Neoplastic fistulas often cannot be closed, and in this situation, relief of any obstruction to the bile flow is recommended. For example, cholangitis in cholecystogastric fistulas due to prepyloric tumors can often be controlled by gastrojejunostomy alone.

GALLSTONE ILEUS

This particular complication follows internal fistulas in which a gallstone or common duct stone gains entrance into the intestinal tract through an internal biliary fistula. The usual potential complications of any internal biliary fistula are possible, particularly ascending cholangitis. In addition, with gallstone ileus, the presence of a large stone in the intestinal tract produces an obstruction at the point where its diameter exceeds that of the intestinal lumen. A typical presentation of gallstone ileus is a history of frequent previous episodes of partial bowel obstruction that exacerbate and abate as the stone negotiates its way into a narrower region of the intestinal tract. This phenomenon is called a *tumbling obstruction*.

Three fourths of the spontaneous fistulas underlying gallstone ileus occur between the gallbladder and the duodenum. Most gallstones that enter the gastrointestinal tract are either passed or vomited, but 10% to 15% may lead to the condition described above. This disorder represents only 1% of all cases of intestinal obstruction but 25% of simple obstruction in those over age 70.[7] The common site of obstruction, found in two thirds of patients, is the ileum.

The diagnosis is easily made if a large mass lesion is found at the site of bowel obstruction; this *mass* is readily identified if the gallstone is opaque. Sometimes, even if it is nonopaque, it can be observed because of surrounding intestinal air. In addition, the finding of air in the biliary tree makes the diagnosis almost certain. Ultrasonography has been helpful in identifying this condition.[16]

Treatment

The proper treatment of gallstone ileus is relief of the intestinal obstruction, usually by the performance of an enterotomy and removal of the stone. Concomitant definitive correction of the internal fistula is advocated if the patient is in good condition and has sustained no prolonged preoperative losses or intraoperative complications and there is no significant inflammatory reaction at the fistula site.[5] There is a 10% recurrence of gallstone ileus after enterotomy alone. In addition, recurrent cholecystitis, recurrent cholangitis, and

a reportedly higher incidence of gallbladder carcinoma in association with biliary-enteric fistula all reinforce the recommendation of complete correction after enterotomy. This may be delayed and performed as a separate procedure if the patient is judged too ill to withstand a prolonged single operation.[3] In the largest single published review of this condition, 80% of the 1001 patients were treated by enterotomy and stone extraction only, and the recurrence rate of gallstone ileus was noted to be 4% to 7%.[15] Most recently, the obstruction has been successfully overcome by shock wave lithotripsy without surgical intervention.[18]

SELECTED REFERENCES

Deitz, D. M.: Improving the outcome in gallstone ileus. Am. J. Surg., *151*:572, 1986.
The author presents a retrospective 32-year experience covering 24 patients with gallstone ileus. The article emphasizes the preponderance of females over 70 years of age who have this condition, the small percentage with the correct preoperative diagnosis, and the significant mortality of 13%.

Fox, P. F.: Planning the operation for cholecystoenteric fistula with gallstone ileus. Surg. Clin. North Am., *50*:93, 1970.
This article reviews 13 patients with gallstone ileus, including technical details of the surgical intervention.

Papanicolaou, N.: Abscess-fistula association: Radiologic recognition and percutaneous management. A.J.R. Am. J. Roentgenol., *143*:811, 1984.
This is one of the larger earlier series detailing the new and important contribution of percutaneous catheter drainage to successful resolution of biliary fistulas, even when such fistulas are associated with abscesses.

Reisner, R. M.: Gallstone ileus: A review of 1001 reported cases. Am. Surg., *60*:441, 1994.
This review is an exhaustive consolidation of all reported cases from 1953 through 1993 in the English-language literature. It covers all aspects of epidemiology, diagnosis, therapy, and complications and emphasizes the adequacy of enterolithotomy alone in the majority of cases.

Safaie-Shirazi, S.: Spontaneous enterobiliary fistulas. Surg. Gynecol. Obstet., *137*:769, 1973.
This is one of the larger case review series presenting data on 92 patients with spontaneous enterobiliary fistula. It emphasizes clinical presentation, diagnosis, and long-term results of management.

REFERENCES

1. Calonje, M. A., Ozenstark, J. L., and Nice, C. M., Jr.: Internal biliary fistulas. JAMA, *179*:112, 1962.
2. Constant, E., and Turcotte, J. C.: Choledochoduodenal fistula: The natural history and management of an unusual complication of peptic ulcer disease. Ann. Surg., *167*:220, 1968.
3. Cooperman, A. M., Dickson, E. R., and ReMine, W. H.: Changing concepts in the surgical treatment of gallstone ileus: A review of 15 cases with emphasis on diagnosis and treatment. Ann. Surg., *167*:377, 1968.
4. Czerniak, A., Thompson, J. N., Soreido, O., et al.: The management of fistulas of the biliary tract after injury to the bile duct during cholecystectomy. Surg. Gynecol. Obstet., *167*:33, 1988.
5. Day, E. A., and Marks, C.: Gallstone ileus: Review of the literature and presentation of thirty-four new cases. Am. J. Surg., *129*:552, 1975.
6. Del Olmo, L., Meroño, E., Moreira, V. F., et al.: Successful treatment of postoperative external biliary fistulas by endoscopic sphincterotomy. Gastrointest. Endosc., *34*:307, 1988.
7. Dietz, D. M., Standage, B. A., Pinson, C. W., et al.: Improving the outcome in gallstone ileus. Am. J. Surg., *151*:572, 1986.
8. Gugenheim, J., Ciardullo, M., Traynor, O., and Bismuth, H.: Bronchobiliary fistulas in adults. Ann. Surg., *207*:90, 1988.
9. Hicken, N. F., and Coray, Q. B.: Spontaneous gastrointestinal biliary fistulas. Surg. Gynecol. Obstet., *82*:723, 1946.
10. McCarthy, J. D., and Picazo, J. G.: Bile peritonitis—diagnosis and course. Am. J. Surg., *116*:664, 1968.
11. Misra, M. C., Grewal, H., and Kapur, B. M.: Spontaneous choledochoduodenal fistula complicating peptic ulcer disease—a case report. Jpn. J. Surg., *19*:367, 1989.
12. Norcross, J. W., and Dadey, J. L.: Medical complications of operative bile duct injuries. N. Engl. J. Med., *257*:1216, 1957.
13. O'Rahilly, S., Duignan, J. P., Lennon, J. R., and O'Malley, E.: Successful treatment of a postoperative external biliary fistula by endoscopic papillotomy. Endocrinology, *15*:68, 1983.
14. Papanicolaou, N., Mueller, P. R., Ferrucci, J. R., Jr., et al.: Abscess-fistula association: Radiologic recognition and percutaneous management. A.J.R. Am. J. Roentgenol., *143*:811, 1984.
15. Reisner, R. M., and Cohen, J. R.: Gallstone ileus: A review of 1001 reported cases. Am. Surg., *60*:441, 1994.

16. Renner, W., Went, J., McLean, J., and Plattner, G.: Ultrasound demonstration of a non-calcified gallstone in the distal ileum causing small bowel obstruction. Radiology, *144*:884, 1982.

17. Rosato, E. F., Berkowitz, H. D., and Roberts, B.: Bile ascites. Surg. Gynecol. Obstet., *130*:494, 1970.

18. Sackman, M., Holl, J., Haerlin, M., Sauerbruch, R., et al.: Gallstone ileus successfully treated by shock-wave lithotripsy. Dig. Dis. Sci., *36(12)*:1794, 1991.

19. Safaie-Shirazi, S., Zike, W. L., and Printen, K. J.: Spontaneous enterobiliary fistulas. Surg. Gynecol. Obstet., *137*:769, 1973.

V

CARCINOMA OF THE GALLBLADDER

David Fromm, M.D.

Carcinoma of the gallbladder is the most common malignant lesion of the biliary tract and accounts for 5% of all cancers found at autopsy.[1] Ninety-one per cent of patients who develop this malignancy are 50 years of age or older (Fig. 34–27).[18] The incidence of the cancer in females is three to four times that in males and is in contrast to the predominance of cancer of the bile ducts in males.

INCIDENCE AND ASSOCIATIONS

Cancer of the gallbladder has its highest incidence in American Indians, Americans of Mexican origin, Alaskan natives, northeastern Europeans, Israelis, and Japanese who have immigrated to the United States. The frequency of this cancer in Alaskan natives is approximately the same as that in the Indians of New Mexico,[3] which has been estimated to be more than six times greater than the frequency in the non-Indian population. American Indian females are twice as likely to develop cancer of the gallbladder as Spanish American females, who in turn are almost 10 times as likely to develop the cancer as non-Spanish American whites.[4] The lowest rates are reported for black Americans, black Rhodesians, Indians in India, and Spaniards in Spain.

The association between cancer of the gallbladder and gallstones is well established and is present in at least 70% of patients, a figure far greater than that found in the age-matched general population. A parallel exists between the epidemiology of cancer of the gallbladder and that of gallstones. In both conditions there is a higher incidence in females, an increasing incidence with age, and variation among ethnic groups. Cancer of the gallbladder associated with cholelithiasis is found in about 0.5% of autopsies, whereas it is present in about 1% to 2% of patients undergoing cholecystectomy. There is no predilection for the development of carcinoma in a gallbladder containing single or multiple stones. It has been suggested that there may be some relationship between carcinoma and the size of a stone. A patient with a 3-cm. gallstone is reportedly 10 times more likely to develop carcinoma than someone with a stone less than 1 cm.,[5] but more precise data indicate no relationship to size.[14]

There are several other pathologic conditions of the gallbladder in addition to gallstones that are associated with the development of carcinoma. There is believed to be a 15% incidence of carcinoma of the gallbladder in patients who have or have had a cholecystoenteric fistula,[2] and the tumor may develop as much as 16 years later. The incidence of carcinoma in a calcified, or porcelain, gallbladder is reported to range from 12.5% to 61%. It is now generally accepted that adenoma of the gallbladder is a precancerous lesion. Adenomas present as polypoid lesions, which are best detected by ultrasonography. Surgical treatment of a polypoid lesion is recommended if the lesion exceeds 1 cm. in diameter, the lesion is single, the polyp is associated with stones, or the patient is older than 50 years.[27] These features are more often associated with a malignant polyp. It has been suggested that xanthogranulomatous cholecystitis, a rare form of chronic cholecystitis that may grossly mimic cancer of the gallbladder, is also associated with a higher than expected incidence of carcinoma.[19] Cancer of the gallbladder is more frequent in the presence of congenital biliary dilatation, in which case there appears to be a lower incidence of associated gallstones. However, congenital bile duct dilatation is frequently related to a long common channel, distal to the entry of the pancreatic duct. A long common channel alone (that is, even without ductal dilatation) is believed to be associated with a higher incidence of gallbladder carcinoma.[24] Ulcerative colitis has a well-known association with biliary tract malignancy. Although the majority of such malignancies involve the bile ducts, as many as 13% originate in the gallbladder. Adenomyomatosis is believed by some to be associated with cancer, but it is not clear whether this is coincidental.

PATHOGENESIS

Although the etiology of carcinoma of the gallbladder is unknown, there are several experimental studies suggesting that malignant transformation may be caused by foreign bodies. These data are controversial and do not explain instances in which gallstones are not found. Other experimental data suggest that stones alone do not cause carcinoma but, in the presence of a carcinogen, may facilitate the devel-

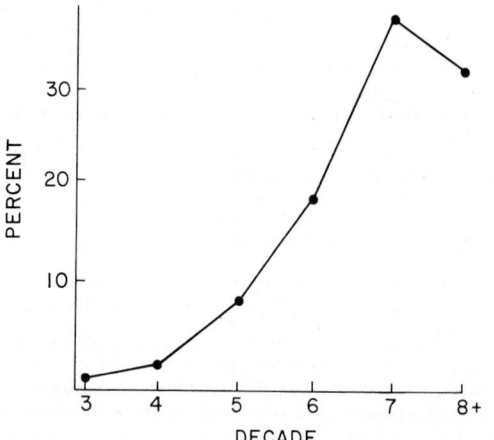

Figure 34–27. Frequency of carcinoma of the gallbladder relative to age. Note the increase with each decade. Data were compiled from 1728 patients in 29 reports. (From Piehler, J. M., and Crichlow, R. W.: Primary carcinoma of the gallbladder. Surg. Gynecol. Obstet., *147*:929, 1978.)

opment of a tumor. It is possible that bacteria associated with gallstones produce a carcinogen, but this has not yet been identified in man.

TYPE

Adenocarcinoma constitutes 82% of gallbladder carcinomas and may be scirrhous, papillary, or mucin producing. Undifferentiated carcinoma accounts for 7%, and squamous cell for 3%. The latter is believed to arise from pluripotential cells in the basal layers of the epithelium. Mixed carcinoma, or adenoacanthoma, occurs in 1% of cases. Unusual tumors include lymphosarcoma, rhabdomyosarcoma, reticulum cell sarcoma, fibrosarcoma, melanoma, carcinoid,[23] and carcinosarcoma.

ROUTES OF METASTASIS

The spread of carcinoma of the gallbladder can take several routes: lymphatic, vascular, intraperitoneal seeding, neural, intraductal, and direct extension.[8] All four major types of tumor (adenocarcinoma, undifferentiated, squamous, and mixed) seem to spread in a similar manner. Although metastases to practically every organ can occur, this is a late phenomenon, probably occurring through venous routes. Spread to adjacent organs occurs with some frequency and usually involves the liver, stomach, duodenum, hepatic flexure of the colon, abdominal wall at the site of a previous cholecystectomy, omentum, or a combination of these. Lymphatic metastases involve the pericholedochal nodes in the lesser omentum and those behind the first portion of the duodenum (Fig. 34–28). Most of the lymphatic trunks draining the left side of the gallbladder terminate in the cystic lymph node. The lymphatic trunks on the right side pass into the pericholedochal nodes, lying to the right of the common duct. Vital staining shows progression from the latter nodes to those

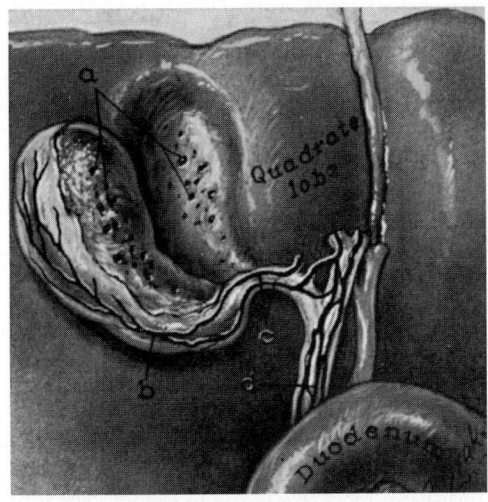

Figure 34–29. Venous drainage of the gallbladder. a, Cholecystic veins entering the gallbladder bed and draining into the quadrate lobe. b, Subserosal cholecystic veins communicating with veins of the gallbladder neck. c, Veins of the neck drain into the quadrate lobe or venous plexus around the bile ducts. d, The latter also drain into the quadrate lobe. The venous drainage from the gallbladder emptying into the quadrate lobe ultimately communicates with the hepatic veins. (From Fahim, R. B., McDonald, J. R., Richards, J. C., and Ferris, D. O.: Carcinoma of the gallbladder: A study of its modes of spread. Ann. Surg., *156*:114, 1962.)

posterior to the head and neck of the pancreas and finally to the interaortocaval nodes adjacent to the left renal vein.[20] Unless there is blockage of the lymphatics, lymph flow from the gallbladder does not ascend toward the hepatic hilum. There are extensive connections between the various sets of lymph vessels, but the lymphatics along the hepatic artery do not connect with those from the gallbladder.

Involvement of the liver usually occurs early and can result from spread along the bile ductules, veins, and lymphatics or by direct extension. Direct extension and spread through lymphatic vessels are the most common. The disseminated multinodular form of liver involvement is probably due to retrograde lymphatic spread or can be the first manifestation of widespread vascular metastases. The lymphatic drainage of the liver on the right side empties for the most part into the pericholedochal nodes (see Fig. 34–28). Involvement of the liver can occur in the absence of lymph node metastases.

Spread of metastases by the venous route most often involves cholecystic veins draining into the gallbladder bed, terminating in the quadrate lobe (segment IV). The venous system along the peritoneal side of the gallbladder also drains into the quadrate lobe (Fig. 34–29). The tumor may also extend along the cystic duct into the common duct. This is more typical for papillary adenocarcinoma but does not occur in all cases of this tumor. Intraductal spread may represent instances of multifocal cancer.

DIAGNOSIS

The symptoms of carcinoma of the gallbladder are not specific. Pain occurs in 66% of patients, weight loss in 59%, jaundice in 51%, anorexia in 40%, and right upper quadrant mass in 40%.[22, 25] The clinical presentation differs, depending on the stage of the disease, but there is no distinct picture because the presenting symptoms and their duration are dependent on the site of the lesion, its extent, and the presence or absence of pre-existing biliary symptoms. Malignancy in patients with pre-existing biliary symptoms generally produces a noticeable change in symptoms.

A right upper quadrant mass may be apparent and is

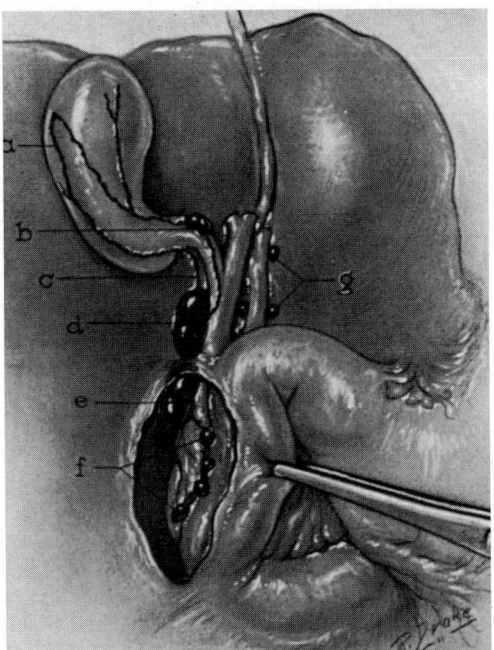

Figure 34–28. Lymphatic drainage of the gallbladder. a, Subserosal lymphatics. b, Cystic node. c, Lymph vessels ending in lower lymph nodes. d, Node of hiatus. e, Superior pancreatoduodenal node. f, Posterior pancreatoduodenal nodes. g, Nodes along the hepatic artery do not connect with those draining the gallbladder. (From Fahim, R. B., McDonald, J. R., Richards, J. C., and Ferris, D. O.: Carcinoma of the gallbladder: A study of its modes of spread. Ann. Surg., *156*:114, 1962.)

usually tender. The presence of a palpable gallbladder represents advanced disease. Jaundice most often is due to invasion of the common duct or compression from involved pericholedochal lymph nodes or, less frequently, involvement of the liver; rarely, it is due to concurrent stones in the biliary tract.[25] Jaundice is accompanied by pain in the majority of patients, which may be of use in distinguishing this disease from periampullary carcinoma. A cancerous gallbladder can perforate into adjacent organs or into the free peritoneal cavity. The latter has been reported in as many as 5% of patients.[1]

Symptomatic invasion or development of a fistula to an adjacent organ frequently leads to the diagnosis of carcinoma originating in the symptomatic organ. Invasion of the upper gastrointestinal tract can lead to obstruction or bleeding, mimicking peptic ulcer disease. Hemorrhage may follow invasion of adjacent organs, hematobilia, or liver failure. Patients presenting with acute cholecystitis tend to have less advanced disease, most likely due to the incidental presence of tumor.

With the deceptive nature of the disease's presentation and its relative rarity, the correct preoperative diagnosis is seldom made. However, certain combinations of signs and symptoms should arouse suspicion. These include an elderly female with biliary complaints presenting with a change in frequency or severity of pain, right upper quadrant mass or hepatomegaly, and constitutional symptoms of malignant disease. By the time these factors are noted, however, the disease is rarely (if ever) curable. Those with early, resectable lesions tend to have symptoms of benign biliary disease.

The diagnosis is infrequently made by radiographic studies. A nonfunctioning gallbladder is apparent on the majority of oral cholecystograms. The rare occurrence of visualization (1% to 2%) is usually of poor quality, and the diagnosis is not evident. An upper gastrointestinal barium study may show compression of the antroduodenal area, but this can also be found in benign, acute inflammatory gallbladder disease. Patients with an abnormal upper gastrointestinal series from carcinoma of the gallbladder have been found to have extensive disease. Nearly two thirds of cases may be correctly diagnosed by computed tomographic scans.[12] Diagnostic accuracy of ultrasonography and computed tomography are reported to be 36% and 70%, respectively.[17] Angiography provides a high degree of diagnostic accuracy, but the majority of tumors diagnosed in this fashion are unresectable.

PROGNOSIS

Carcinoma of the gallbladder is usually associated with a dismal prognosis, with some 88% of patients dead within a year of diagnosis and only about 4% alive after 5 years in a review of nearly 6000 patients.[18] Most of the long-term survivors are those in whom the surgeon was unaware of the presence of the tumor at the time of cholecystectomy (approximately 12% of cases), with the diagnosis being made by the pathologist. It is an unusual patient who is symptomatic from the tumor and enjoys prolonged survival following operative treatment.

Those neoplasms that are localized are generally associated with a longer survival. The depth of invasion and surgical margin are independent variables.[26] Spread that is limited to the muscle coat is usually associated with 100% 5-year survival, but there are a few exceptions. Extension to the subserosa with negative resection margins is associated with a 95% 1-year survival and a 65% 3- and 5-year survival. However, extension to the subserosa with a positive resection margin is associated with a 43% 1-year survival and no survival at 3 years.

Regional lymph nodes are often involved, and invasion of the liver occurs in the majority of patients by the time they undergo operation. Patients with papillary adenocarcinoma, which tends to be localized, have a median survival of almost 6 months after diagnosis, with 24% of patients alive at the end of 1 year.[10] In contrast, patients with other types of adenocarcinoma have a median survival of 2 months after diagnosis, with 10% of patients alive after 1 year. Those with anaplastic carcinoma have a median survival of less than 1 month, with only 4% of patients alive after 1 year. Squamous cell tumors of the gallbladder tend to behave like anaplastic carcinomas. For those with localized disease, knowledge of the depth of invasion is important prognostically. Practically all patients with invasion confined to the mucosa and muscularis and who survive operation are alive at 5 years, whereas only about 7% with serosal (or adventitial) involvement are alive at 5 years.[15]

TREATMENT

Increasing concern has been raised about tumor seeding of laparoscopic port sites and intraperitoneal dissemination that becomes evident within a few months after cholecystectomy when the cancer was not recognized at the time of operation.[9] Thus, it is recommended that a biopsy not be done in the presence of resectable disease. If there is suspicion of (resectable) cancer at laparoscopy, it should be converted to an open procedure.

The routes of spread suggest that the extent of the tumor can be excised in some patients with tumor invasion beyond the confines of the gallbladder wall. However, debate continues over the utility of radical resection of the tumor. Proponents of a radical approach optimistically maintain that up to 30% of patients present with tumors that could be encompassed by radical cholecystectomy, which includes in-continuity resection of its hepatic bed, right hepatic lobectomy, or even trisegmentectomy, as well as regional lymph node dissection. Yet only a handful of long-term survivors has been reported following radical surgery. Furthermore, the operative morbidity and mortality of radical resection remain high for a disease associated with an extremely poor prognosis. Radical excision may be followed by death from disseminated metastases as soon as 2 months later,[22] in spite of what appeared to be adequate resection at operation.

It is generally held that radical resection does not significantly influence prognosis, but a recent series from Japan suggests that radical excision with intent to cure may indeed improve survival.[16] The number of confounding variables makes the data difficult to place in perspective. Furthermore, data from a number of series imply that the intrinsic nature of the tumor rather than the extent of treatment accounts for survival.[7] Although it has been concluded that patients who undergo hepatopancreatoduodenectomy (to encompass lymph nodes posterior to the pancreatic head and neck) have a significantly lower survival than other surgical patients, some continue to advocate this approach in selected patients.[16] There are insufficient conclusive data to support the proposition that a patient with unexpected carcinoma found histologically should undergo reoperation for radical excision. The controversy about the efficacy of resection beyond cholecystectomy continues. There are indirect suggestions that the prognosis of gallbladder carcinoma may be improving, but it is not clear whether this is spontaneous or due to either earlier diagnosis or surgical management.[17]

Moderate palliation can occasionally be achieved by operation, even though its benefits are usually of short duration. Palliation is directed chiefly at relieving common duct obstruction or bypassing an obstructed portion of the gastrointestinal tract. Some palliation may also be achieved by removing the gallbladder, when feasible, in the hope of delaying obstruction of surrounding structures. Reports dealing with chemotherapy[13] and/or radiation therapy suggest that the benefit of these modalities is questionable.

Obstructive jaundice occurring sometime after cholecystectomy can be difficult to treat by operation because of tumor encroachment in the porta hepatis. Endoscopic sphincterotomy followed by placement of a prosthesis retrogradely through a malignant stricture in the common duct or at the hepatic bifurcation can reduce symptoms relating to biliary obstruction. However, long-term palliation appears to be more related to tumor extent than to resolution of jaundice.[11] Percutaneous insertion of a biliary prosthesis can also be used to decompress the biliary tree, but such catheters tend to be painful, and their use is occasionally complicated by the appearance of painful malignant deposits along the catheter site.[21]

Since the prognosis of carcinoma of the gallbladder is so poor, some maintain that nearly all patients with asymptomatic gallstones should undergo cholecystectomy. For every 100 cholecystectomies done during a year, one fewer death from cancer of the gallbladder probably occurs.[6] However, given the incidence of gallstones, this proposition would place an inordinate drain on surgical resources to prevent a generally fatal condition of relatively low incidence in the general population. In fact, the chances of developing other complications from cholelithiasis are much greater than the chance of eventually developing a malignancy. Yet there appears to be an association between the increasing rate of cholecystectomy and a decreasing mortality from cancer of the gallbladder. This may be fortuitous, since the incidence of carcinoma of the stomach has also been declining, but not due to prophylactic gastrectomy.[4]

SELECTED REFERENCES

Diehl, A. K.: Epidemiology of gallbladder cancer: A synthesis of recent data. J. Natl. Cancer Inst., 65:1209, 1980.
One of the better summaries of the epidemiology of gallbladder cancer.

Fahim, R. B., McDonald, J. R., Richards, J. C., and Ferris, D. O.: Carcinoma of the gallbladder: A study of its modes of spread. Ann. Surg., 156:114, 1962.
A classic study of the routes of metastases, providing the anatomic basis for radical excision.

Ogura, Y., Mizumoto, R., Isaji, S., Kususa, T., Matsuda, S., and Tabata, M.: Radical operations for carcinoma of the gallbladder: Present status in Japan. World J. Surg., 15:337, 1991.
Analyzes the surgical outcome of 1686 cases, making it one of the largest collections of radical operative results. The authors' advocacy of radical resection is controversial.

Piehler, J. M., and Crichlow, R. W.: Primary carcinoma of the gallbladder. Surg. Gynecol. Obstet., 147:929, 1978.
A thorough review of the literature, extending that of Arminski to 1976.

Yang, H. L., Sun, Y. G., and Wang, Z.: Polypoid lesions of the gallbladder: Diagnosis and indications for surgery. Br. J. Surg., 79:227, 1992.
An analysis of 172 cases of polypoid lesions—one of the largest analyses of such lesions.

REFERENCES

1. Arminski, T. C.: Primary carcinoma of the gallbladder: A collective review with the addition of twenty-five cases from the Grace Hospital, Detroit, Michigan. Cancer, 2:379, 1949.
2. Berliner, S. D., and Burson, L. C.: One-stage repair of cholecyst-duodenal fistula and gallstone ileus. Arch. Surg., 90:313, 1965.
3. Boss, L. P., Lanier, A. P., Dohan, P. H., and Bender, T. R.: Cancers of the gallbladder and biliary tract in Alaskan natives: 1970–79. J. Natl. Cancer Inst., 69:1005, 1982.
4. Diehl, A. K.: Epidemiology of gallbladder cancer: A synthesis of recent data. J. Natl. Cancer Inst., 65:1209, 1980.
5. Diehl, A. K.: Gallstone size and the risk of gallbladder cancer. JAMA, 250:2323, 1983.
6. Diehl, A. K., and Beral, V.: Cholecystectomy and changing mortality from gallbladder cancer. Lancet, 1:187, 1981.
7. Donohue, J. H., Nagorney, D. M., Grant, C. S., Tsushima, K., Ilstrup, D. M., and Adson, M. A.: Carcinoma of the gallbladder: Does radical resection improve outcome? Arch. Surg., 125:237, 1990.
8. Fahim, R. B., McDonald, J. R., Richards, J. C., and Ferris, D. O.: Carcinoma of the gallbladder: A study of its modes of spread. Ann. Surg., 156:114, 1962.
9. Fong, Y., Brennan, M. F., Turnbull, A., Colt, D. G., and Blumgart, L. H.: Gallbladder cancer discovered during laparoscopic surgery. Arch. Surg., 128:1054, 1993.
10. Hart, J., and Modan, B.: Factors affecting survival of patients with gallbladder neoplasms. Arch. Intern. Med., 129:931, 1972.
11. Huibregtse, K., Schneider, B., Coene, P. P., and Tytgat, G. N. J.: Endoscopic palliation of jaundice in gall bladder cancer. Surg. Endosc., 1:143, 1987.
12. Itai, Y., Araki, T., Yoshikawa, K., Furui, S. H., Yashiro, N., and Tasaka, A.: Computed tomography of gallbladder carcinoma. Radiology, 137:713, 1980.
13. Makela, J. T., and Kairaluoma, M. I.: Superselective intra-arterial chemotherapy with mitomycin for gallbladder cancer. Br. J. Surg., 80:912, 1993.
14. Moerman, C. J., Lagerwaard, F. J., Bueno De Mesquita, H. B., Van Dalen, A. V., Van Leeuwen, M. S., and Schrover, P.: Gallstone size and the risk of gallbladder cancer. Scand. J. Gastroenterol., 28:482, 1993.
15. Nevin, J. E., Moran, T. J., Kay, S., and King, R.: Carcinoma of the gallbladder: Staging, treatment, and prognosis. Cancer, 37:141, 1976.
16. Ogura, Y., Mizumoto, R., Isaji, S., Kususa, T., Matsuda, S., and Tabata, M.: Radical operations for carcinoma of the gallbladder: Present status in Japan. World J. Surg., 15:337, 1991.
17. Ouchi, K., Suzuki, M., Saijo, S., Ito, K., and Matsuno, S.: Do recent advances in diagnosis and operative management improve the outcome of gallbladder carcinoma? Surgery, 113:324, 1993.
18. Piehler, J. M., and Crichlow, R. W.: Primary carcinoma of the gallbladder. Surg. Gynecol. Obstet., 147:929, 1978.
19. Reed, A., Ryan, C., and Schwartz, S. I.: Xanthogranulomatous cholecystitis. J. Am. Coll. Surg., 179:249, 1994.
20. Shirai, Y., Yoshida, K., Tsukada, K., Ohtani, T., and Muto, T.: Identification of the region lymphatic system of the gall bladder by vital staining. Br. J. Surg., 79:659, 1992.
21. Shorvon, P. J., Leung, J. W. C., Corcoran, M., Mason, R. R., and Cotton, P. B.: Cutaneous seeding of malignant tumors after insertion of percutaneous prosthesis for obstructive jaundice. Br. J. Surg., 71:694, 1984.
22. Solan, M. J., and Jackson, B. T.: Carcinoma of the gall-bladder: A clinical appraisal and review of 57 cases. Br. J. Surg., 58:593, 1971.
23. Strauch, G. O.: Primary carcinoma of the gallbladder: Presentation of seventy cases from the Rhode Island Hospital and a cumulative review of the last ten years of the American literature. Surgery, 47:368, 1960.
24. Tanaka, K., Nishimura, A., Yamada, K., Ishibe, R., Ishizaki, N., Yoshimine, M., Hamada, N., and Taira, A.: Cancer of the gallbladder associated with anomalous junction of the pancreatobiliary duct system without bile duct dilatation. Br. J. Surg., 80:622, 1993.
25. Tanga, M. B., and Ewing, J. B.: Primary malignant tumors of the gallbladder: Report of 43 cases. Surgery, 67:418, 1970.
26. Yamaguchi, K., and Tsuneyoshi, M.: Subclinical gallbladder carcinoma. Am. J. Surg., 163:382, 1992.
27. Yang, H. L., Sun, Y. G., and Wang, Z.: Polypoid lesions of the gallbladder: Diagnosis and indications for surgery. Br. J. Surg., 79:227, 1992.

CHAPTER 35

THE PANCREAS

Charles J. Yeo, M.D., and John L. Cameron, M.D.

Historically, the first description of the pancreas is credited to Herophilus of Chalkaidon around the year 300 B.C. Four centuries later, in approximately A.D. 100, this abdominal organ was named the pancreas by Rufus of Ephesus. The first operative intervention on the pancreas has been attributed to LeDentu in the year 1862, involving percutaneous aspiration of a pancreatic mass with an unfavorable outcome. Much evidence has accumulated during the years, adding to knowledge of the basic anatomy and physiology of the pancreas and to the pathophysiology of pancreatic disease.

EMBRYOLOGY

The pancreas begins development during the fourth week of gestation, when the embryo is 3 to 4 mm. in size. Pancreatic tissue originates from the endodermal lining of the duodenum, from which form two pouches that develop into a large dorsal and a smaller ventral pancreas (Fig. 35–1). The dorsal pouch arises first, directly from the duodenal endoderm, and normally forms the bulk of adult pancreatic tissue. The ventral pouch forms from the endoderm of the hepatic diverticulum, and it maintains a close association with the common bile duct throughout development. As the duodenum rotates to assume a C configuration, the ventral pancreatic pouch migrates dorsally in a clockwise direction to assume a position adjacent to the posterior inferior surface of the more rapidly expanding dorsal pancreatic primordium (Fig. 35–2). At approximately the eighth week of gestation, the parenchyma of the dorsal and ventral primordia fuse, as do their respective ductal systems. The ventral primordium forms the uncinate process and the inferior aspect of the head of the adult gland. The dorsal primordium becomes the superior aspect of the head as well as the entirety of the neck, body, and tail of the gland.

The fusion of the pancreatic ductal systems during fetal development produces the most typical anatomic arrangement of the pancreatic ductular structures. More than 85% of the time, the ventral pancreatic duct fuses with the more distal dorsal pancreatic duct to create the duct of Wirsung, also known as the main pancreatic duct. This duct joins with the common bile duct in an intrapancreatic location and empties pancreatic exocrine secretions through the ampulla of Vater at the major duodenal papilla. The proximal aspect of the dorsal pancreatic duct (duct of Santorini) often remains in communication with the duct of Wirsung and may empty small amounts of exocrine pancreatic secretions through a separate minor duodenal papilla located on the medial aspect of the duodenum proximal to the major papilla.

Clinically recognized malformations of pancreatic embryology include heterotopic pancreas, pancreas divisum, and annular pancreas. The development of pancreatic tissue outside the confines of the main gland is a congenital abnormality referred to as heterotopic pancreas. Most commonly, heterotopic pancreatic tissue is found in the stomach, duodenum, small bowel, or Meckel's diverticulum. In most locations, heterotopic pancreatic tissue resides in a submucosal location, presenting as firm, yellow, irregular nodules that vary in size from millimeters to several centimeters. The mucosa overlying typical heterotopic pancreatic tissue commonly has a central umbilication. There may be a duct draining exocrine pancreatic secretions from the aberrant tissue into the intestinal lumen. Histologically, heterotopic pancreatic tissue can vary from entirely normal architecture, including ductular structures, acini, and islets of Langerhans, to rudimentary pancreatic structures with markedly aberrant histology. The clinical significance of heterotopic pancreas is dependent on resultant complications. Intestinal obstruction may ensue, rarely as a result of the size of the mass, and more commonly following intussusception, with the ectopic pancreatic tissue serving as the intussusceptum. Other complications of heterotopic pancreas include ulceration and hemorrhage. Appropriate treatment is indicated for the complications of heterotopic pancreas, usually involving local excision of the heterotopic tissue, with histologic examination to exclude the presence of malignancy.

Pancreas divisum is an anatomic variant that follows failure of fusion of the two primordial ductal systems. This anomaly has been recognized in up to 10% of patients undergoing endoscopic retrograde pancreatography for presumed pancreatic disease. In this entity, the major portion of the pancreas is drained via the duct of Santorini via the minor duodenal papilla. The major duodenal papilla usually communicates with a small duct of Wirsung, which drains the ventral pancreas, consisting of the inferior head and uncinate process. The significance of pancreas divisum remains controversial. In selected series of patients undergoing endoscopic pancreatography for *idiopathic pancreatitis*, the incidence of pancreas divisum approaches 25%. In these cases, it is unknown whether the ductal anomaly has any causal relationship to the pancreatitis. Some have speculated that pancreas divisum, when associated with relative stenosis of the minor duodenal papilla, can cause pancreatitis. Patients with this abnormality have been treated with endoscopic stenting of

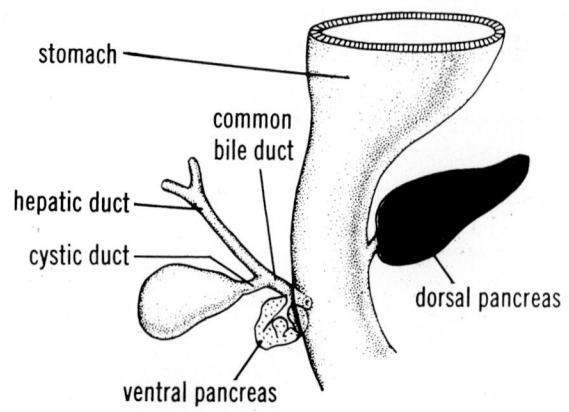

Figure 35–1. The smaller ventral pancreas initially develops as an outpouching from the hepatic diverticulum. The larger dorsal pancreas originates directly from the endodermal epithelium of the duodenum. (From Langman, J.: Medical Embryology, 3rd ed. Baltimore, Williams & Wilkins, 1975, p. 287.)

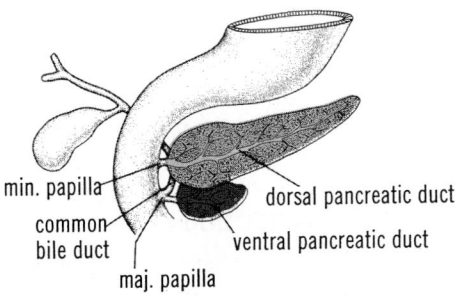

Figure 35–2. After clockwise rotation in a dorsal direction, the ventral pancreas comes to lie adjacent to the dorsal pancreas, as shown here. The dorsal pancreatic duct enters the duodenum at the minor papilla and the ventral pancreatic duct at the major papilla. (From Langman, J.: Medical Embryology, 3rd ed. Baltimore, Williams & Wilkins, 1975, p. 288.)

pancreas to form a complete ring or may remain as an incomplete ring. Varying degrees of duodenal obstructive symptoms may be observed in this condition. In children, there is a common association with other serious congenital anomalies such as intracardiac defects, Down's syndrome, and intestinal malrotation. For an unexplained reason, some children have no symptoms from this anomaly, and instead they may present as adults, commonly in the fourth decade of life. In adults, symptoms may appear to be those of upper gastrointestinal obstruction, chronic pancreatitis, or peptic ulcer. Obstructive symptoms are an indication for operation. Resection or division of the normal pancreatic tissue constituting the annulus is not recommended, because of the high incidence of duodenal or pancreatic fistula. Instead, a bypass procedure in the form of duodenojejunostomy is indicated.

the minor papilla or transduodenal sphincteroplasty of the minor papilla, with mixed results. Pancreas divisum associated with extensive dorsal pancreatic parenchymal injury or multiple ductular stenoses is not optimally treated with stenting or transduodenal minor papillary sphincteroplasty and instead may require pancreatic resection or pancreatic ductular drainage via longitudinal pancreaticojejunostomy.

Annular pancreas is a rare condition that results when histologically normal pancreatic tissue completely or partially encircles the second portion of the duodenum. Annular pancreas is thought to arise from failure of normal clockwise rotation of the ventral pancreatic primordia, possibly related to abnormal fixation at the free end. With annular pancreas, the tissue originating from the ventral primordium lies anterior to the duodenum, where it can fuse with the dorsal

ANATOMY

The pancreas occupies a retroperitoneal position in the abdomen, lying posterior to the stomach and lesser omentum. It extends obliquely from the duodenal C loop to a more cephalad position in the hilum of the spleen (Fig. 35–3). The normal adult pancreas varies in weight from 75 to 125 gm., in length from 10 to 20 cm., and in cephalad to caudad width from 3 to 5 cm. In the anteroposterior axis, the pancreas is thickest at the head, varying from 1.5 to 3.5 cm., and thinnest at the tail, 0.8 to 2.5 cm. The gland has a distinctive yellow/tan/pink color and is multilobulated. The pancreas is covered by peritoneum anteriorly, and posteriorly it lies in proximity to the inferior vena cava, right renal vein, aorta at the level of the first lumbar vertebra, superior mesenteric vessels, and splenic vein.

The gland is divided into four portions: the head (which

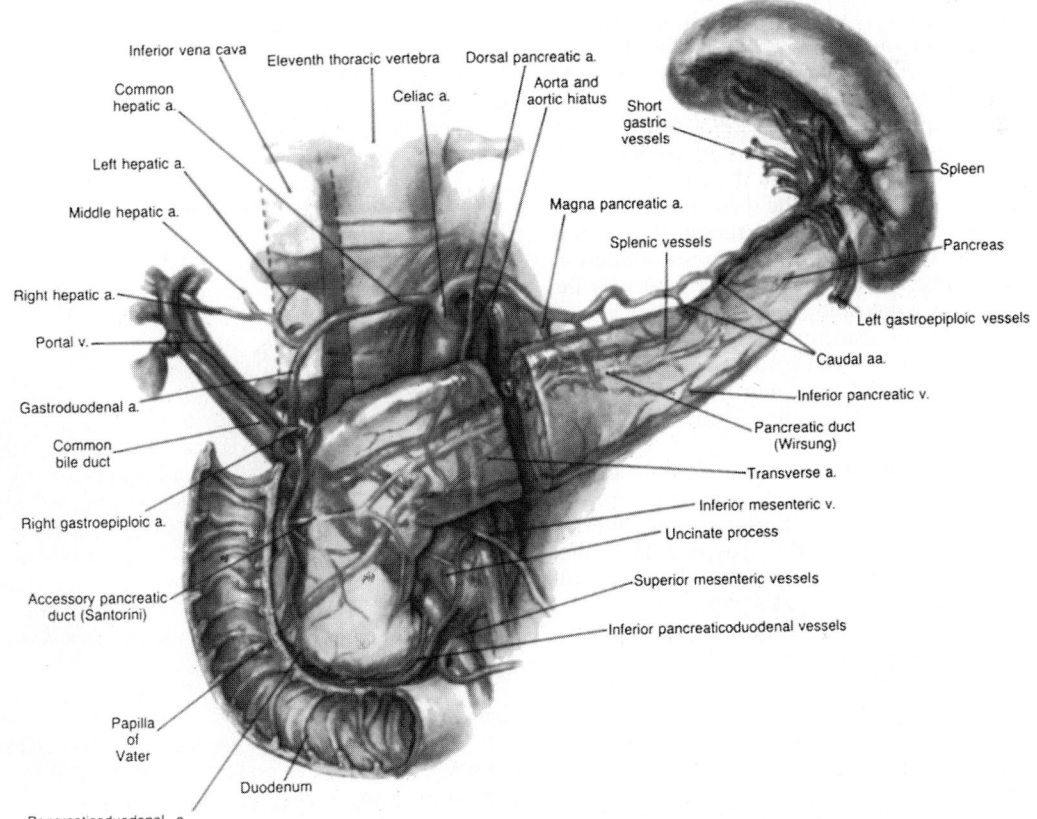

Figure 35–3. Anatomic relationships of the pancreas, including the adjacent viscera, arterial and venous systems, and pancreatic ducts. (From Schlossberg, L., and Zuidema, G. D.: The Johns Hopkins Atlas of Human Functional Anatomy, 3rd ed. Baltimore, The Johns Hopkins University Press, 1986, Plate 48.)

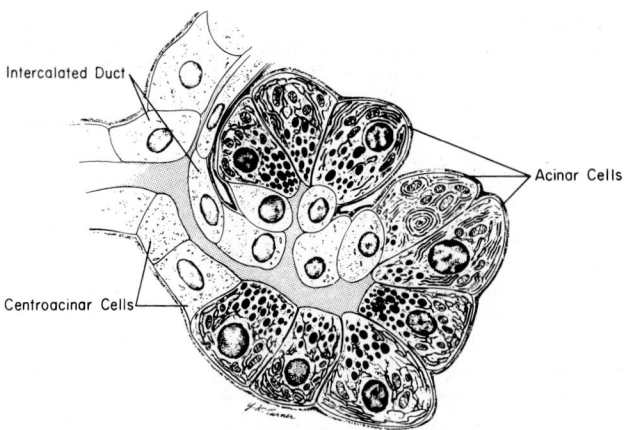

Figure 35–4. Illustration demonstrating the relationships of a terminal branch of the pancreatic ductal system to the centroacinar cells and acinar cells. (From Bloom, W., and Fawcett, D. W.: A Textbook of Histology, 10th ed. Philadelphia, W. B. Saunders, 1975, p. 738.)

includes the uncinate process), the neck, the body, and the tail. That portion of the pancreas anterior to the superior mesenteric vein is designated the neck of the gland. The head of the gland extends to the right of the neck, lying within the confines of the duodenal C loop; it includes the posteroinferior extension arising from the ventral primordium, designated the uncinate process. The uncinate process extends posterior to the superior mesenteric vein, ending at the right margin of the superior mesenteric artery. The body of the pancreas lies immediately to the left of the neck; the tail of the pancreas extends to the left of the body into the splenic hilum.

An extensive arterial system originating from multiple sources supplies the pancreas. The head of the pancreas is intimately associated with the second portion of the duodenum, and these two structures are jointly supplied by two arterial arcades known as the anterior and posterior pancreaticoduodenal arteries. These arteries originate from the superior and inferior pancreaticoduodenal vessels as branches of the celiac axis and superior mesenteric artery, respectively. The blood supply to the body and tail of the pancreas is via a more variable complex of arteries. The distal body and tail of the pancreas are supplied by short branches of the splenic and left gastroepiploic arteries. Within the posterosuperior and posteroinferior aspects of the body of the pancreas lie the superior and inferior pancreatic arteries, respectively.

The venous drainage of the pancreas corresponds with the arterial anatomy. Veins draining the pancreatic parenchyma eventually terminate in the portal vein, which arises posterior to the neck of the pancreas at the junction of the splenic and superior mesenteric veins.

Multiple lymph node groups drain the pancreas. From the head of the gland, nodes in the pancreaticoduodenal groove communicate with subpyloric, portal, mesocolic, mesenteric, and aortocaval nodes. Lymphatics in the body and tail of the pancreas drain to retroperitoneal nodes in the splenic hilum or to celiac, aortocaval, mesocolic, or mesenteric nodes.

A dual sympathetic and parasympathetic innervation subserves the pancreas. Preganglionic sympathetic axons arise from cell bodies within the thoracic sympathetic ganglia and travel as the greater, lesser, and lowest splanchnic nerves to terminate within the celiac ganglia. From these, postganglionic sympathetic fibers traverse retroperitoneal tissue to innervate the pancreas, serving as the principal pathways for pain of pancreatic origin. This sympathetic pathway is the target during splanchnicectomy for the relief of pain of pancreatic origin. The parasympathetic innervation of the pan-

creas commences with preganglionic fiber cell bodies that reside within the vagal nuclei, the axons of which terminate in parasympathetic ganglia within the pancreatic parenchyma. Postganglionic parasympathetic fibers then traverse a short course to innervate the pancreatic islets, acini, and ducts, serving an exclusively efferent function.

HISTOLOGY

Two distinct organ systems share residence within the human pancreas. The endocrine portion of pancreatic function is served by the structures termed the islets of Langerhans. The islets are nearly spherical collections of cells scattered throughout the pancreatic parenchyma. Up to a million islets per gland exist. Each islet has an extensive blood supply, marked by a network of intercommunicating sinusoids, and is composed of several distinctive cell types. The insulin-producing beta cells compose the majority of the islet population. The alpha cells produce glucagon and constitute approximately 20 to 25% of the total islet cell number. Scattered about the periphery of the islets, constituting approximately 5% of the islet cells, are the somatostatin-producing delta cells, which appear to function as paracrine modulators of islet cell function. Small minorities of islet cells have been shown by immunohistochemical techniques to contain pancreatic polypeptide (PP), gastrin, and vasoactive intestinal polypeptide (VIP).

The acini and ductal systems constitute the exocrine portion of the pancreas (Fig. 35–4). On a macroscopic level, the exocrine pancreas is analogous to clusters of grapes (representing individual acini) on a vine (representing minor ducts) and terminating in a major trunk (representing the major pancreatic duct). Each acinus has an approximately spheroid configuration and is composed of a single layer of acinar cells. Acinar cells contain zymogen granules (Fig. 35–5) in their narrow, centrally located apical portion and rest on a distinct basal lamina supported by delicate reticular fibers at the periphery. The pancreatic ductal system originates in the centroacinar cells of each individual acinus, includes intercalated duct cells along the ductal pathway, and terminates in the main excretory duct of the pancreas.

PHYSIOLOGY

Exocrine. Investigation of the physiology of exocrine pancreatic secretion has attracted much attention for more than

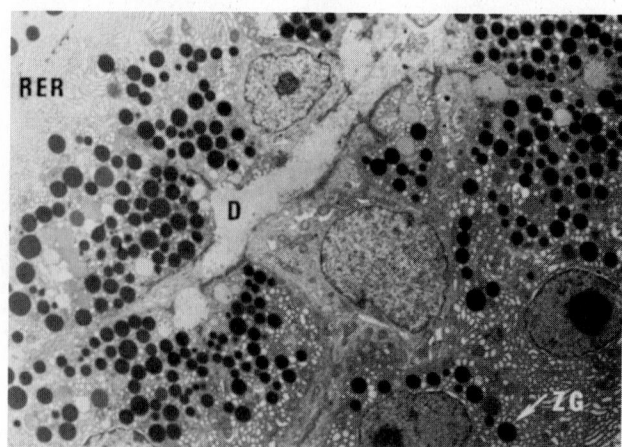

Figure 35–5. Electron micrograph of multiple acinar cells and a portion of a terminal duct (D). The acinar cells contain extensive rough endoplasmic reticulum (RER) and electron-dense zymogen granules (ZG). Uranyl acetate and lead citrate, ×2000.

a century. Heidenhain in 1875 first demonstrated the effect of vagal stimulation on pancreatic secretion. This work was extended by Pavlov and later by Babkin, who reported the cholinergic nature of the stimulus to pancreatic exocrine secretion. Bayliss and Starling first demonstrated the presence of a substance in duodenal mucosa—secretin—which stimulated pancreatic secretion.

The final products of pancreatic exocrine secretion derive from the interplay of an intricate system of acinar and ductal cell functions. The final secretory product of the human exocrine pancreas is a clear isotonic solution with a pH in the range of 8 and a specific gravity that varies between 1.007 and 1.035. There are two distinct components of pancreatic exocrine secretion: enzyme secretion originates from acinar cells, and water and electrolyte secretion originate from the centroacinar and intercalated duct cells. From endoscopic pancreatic cannulation studies, basal secretory rates of pancreatic exocrine products average 0.2 to 0.3 ml. per minute, with rates approaching 5.0 ml. per minute with maximal secretin stimulation.

The secretion of water and electrolytes is under both vagal and humoral control. The electrolyte composition of exocrine pancreatic juice varies with the rate of pancreatic secretion (Fig. 35–6). Over the entire spectrum of secretory rates, the composition of sodium and potassium in the pancreatic exocrine effluent remains constant, with the concentrations of these cations being approximately equivalent to plasma. In contrast, the anion concentration of pancreatic exocrine secretion is dependent on the secretory rate. At low secretory rates, the concentrations of chloride and bicarbonate ions are nearly equivalent to those of plasma, whereas with neurohumoral stimulation, the bicarbonate component increases in concentration and the chloride anion concentration decreases. Secretin is the most potent endogenous stimulant of pancreatic bicarbonate secretion. The term *hormone* was first used in reference to secretin, a 27–amino acid peptide. Secretin is synthesized in the mucosal S cells of the crypts of Lieberkühn of the proximal small intestine and is released in the presence of luminal acid and bile. Secretin circulates in the blood and binds to secretin receptors on pancreatic ductal cells, effecting signal transduction via the intracellular adenylate cyclase system, to yield an increase in intracellular cyclic adenosine monophosphate (cAMP).

An entirely distinct sequence of intracellular events mediates the synthesis and excretion of the digestive enzyme exocrine products from pancreatic acinar cells. Experiments using radioactive labeling techniques have delineated a sophisticated and stepwise sequence of intracellular events that produce the final exocrine digestive enzyme products. Messenger RNA is translated into proenzymes on the microsomes of the rough endoplasmic reticulum. These proenzymes subsequently pass to the Golgi apparatus, where they are packaged within a glycoprotein vesicular membrane. These zymogen granules formed at the level of the Golgi apparatus contain a full complement of digestive enzymes. Zymogen granules then migrate to the acinar cell apex, where zymogen granule membranes fuse with the acinar cell plasma membrane (exocytosis), yielding extrusion of the zymogen granule contents into the centroacinar luminal space. Specific enzymes synthesized and released include endopeptidases such as trypsin, chymotrypsin, elastase, and kallikrein, as well as exopeptidases such as carboxypeptidase A and B. Other synthesized enzymes include phospholipase, lipase, colipase, nonspecific carboxylesterase, amylase, ribonuclease, and deoxyribonuclease. The peptidases synthesized by acinar cells are released into the pancreatic ductal system in inactive forms. Peptide activation commences after the peptidase enters the duodenum, where mucosal enterokinase cleaves trypsinogen to trypsin, leaving trypsin to further activate the other peptidases. In contrast to the peptidases, ribonuclease, deoxyribonuclease, amylase, and lipase are released into the pancreatic ductal system in their active forms. The control of pancreatic acinar cell secretion is mediated by specific secretagogues acting on acinar cell receptors. Secretagogues such as cholecystokinin (CCK) and acetylcholine stimulate acinar cell enzyme secretion via a membrane transduction process involving the accumulation of intracellular cyclic guanosine monophosphate (cGMP) and the mobilization of intracellular calcium. CCK is the most potent endogenous hormone known to stimulate pancreatic enzyme secretion.

Three classic phases of digestion describe the response of the pancreas to a meal. During the cephalic phase of digestion, stimuli such as the smell, sight, and taste of food activate vagal efferent signals, which follow parasympathetic pathways to stimulate pancreatic enzyme release. In addition, cephalic phase stimulation of gastric acid secretion causes duodenal acidification, which stimulates secretin release and subsequent pancreatic bicarbonate secretion. In all, the net effect of cephalic phase stimulation is the secretion of an enzyme-rich bicarbonate-poor fluid. During the gastric phase of digestion, the gastric G cell product, gastrin, serves a major function. Antral distention and antral protein stimulate the release of gastrin, which promotes gastric acid secretion and also serves as a weak stimulator of pancreatic enzyme secretion. The ability of gastrin to serve as a weak stimulator of pancreatic enzyme secretion can be explained by the sequence homology between gastrin and the C terminal pentapeptide-amide sequence of CCK, yielding an affinity for the CCK receptor on pancreatic acinar cells that is 1/1000 times as strong as CCK. Gastrin-stimulated gastric acid secretion contributes to pancreatic bicarbonate secretion via duodenal acidification and subsequent secretin release. Stimulation of vagal afferents by antral distention also has a role in the gastric phase of pancreatic exocrine secretion, as is proved by the reduction in antral distention-induced pancreatic exocrine secretion following truncal vagotomy. During the intestinal phase of digestion, the hormones secretin and CCK serve a major function in mediating pancreatic exocrine secretion. Duodenal acid and bile stimulate secretin release, with resultant pancreatic bicarbonate secretion from duct cells. Duodenal fat and protein release CCK, with subsequent stimulation of pancreatic enzymes from acinar cells. In addition to these humorally mediated events, bile salts, fatty acids, and amino

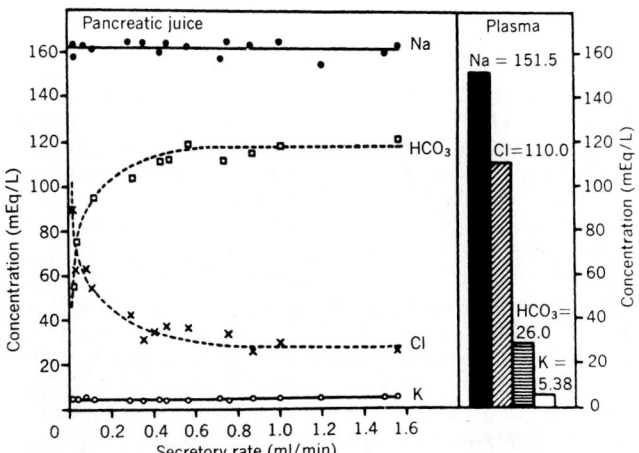

Figure 35–6. Relationship between the rate of secretion and the concentration of electrolytes in pancreatic juice, compared with the electrolyte composition of plasma. (From Bro-Rasmussen, F., Killmann, S. A., and Thaysen, J. H.: The composition of pancreatic juice as compared to sweat, parotid saliva and tears. Acta Physiol. Scand., *37*:97, 1956.)

acids in the duodenum can stimulate pancreatic exocrine secretion via neural pathways.

Endocrine. The best known endocrine function of the pancreas involves glucose homeostasis. The association between diabetes mellitus and the pancreas was established more than a century ago, in 1889, in a canine experiment in which glucose intolerance developed after removal of the pancreas. In the 1920s, Banting and Best isolated pancreatic extracts that were highly active against hyperglycemia. Later, insulin was crystallized and found to contain two polypeptide chains linked by a disulfide bridge. Insulin is the secretory product of the beta cell within the islets of Langerhans. The secretory granules of beta cells contain the storage form of insulin (Fig. 35–7). The release of insulin from the beta cell into the portal blood is controlled by multiple factors, including the level of glycemia, vagal interactions, and local concentrations of somatostatin, among others.

Glucagon is a single-chain 29–amino acid peptide synthesized and released from islet alpha cells. A major stimulus for glucagon release is a substantial drop in serum glucose. Glucagon causes hyperglycemia by promoting hepatic glycogenolysis and gluconeogenesis from proteins. Although the primary effect of glucagon appears to be on glucose homeostasis, other effects of glucagon have been described, including inhibition of gastric acid secretion, inhibition of gastrointestinal motility, and stimulation of choleresis and triglyceride lipolysis.

Pancreatic polypeptide (PP) is a 36–straight-chain amino acid peptide localized predominantly to non–beta islet cells of the head and uncinate process of the pancreas. PP is released into the blood in a biphasic manner following a meal, with both cholinergic and adrenergic modulation. At physiologic levels, PP has been reported to decrease pancreatic exocrine secretion and to alter biliary tract motility. It has also been implicated as a glucoregulatory hormone. In PP-deficient states such as postpancreatectomy or chronic pancreatitis, there has been demonstrable hepatic resistance to insulin, reversed by chronic, but not acute, administration of PP.

Somatostatin is a cyclic tetradecapeptide synthesized and released from islet delta cells as well as other brain-gut sources. The gastrointestinal tract contains 70% of the body's somatostatin. Stimulants of somatostatin release into the blood include a meal, vagal stimulation, bombesin, CCK, gastrin, and secretin. Somatostatin has a broad spectrum of gastrointestinal activity, including inhibition of hormone release (gastrin, secretin, VIP, PP, insulin, and glucagon), inhibition of gastric acid and pepsin secretion, inhibition of pancreatic exocrine secretion, and inhibition of gastrointestinal motor activity, as well as reduction of gastrointestinal blood flow.

ACUTE PANCREATITIS

Although the disease now classified as acute pancreatitis has been recognized since antiquity, it was not until the mid-nineteenth century that the importance of the pancreas and the severity of its inflammatory disorders became evident. Operative intervention for acute pancreatitis associated with pancreatic gangrene or abscess formation was suggested by Senn in 1886. In 1889, Fitz presented a succinct clinical and pathologic description of acute pancreatitis. In 1901, Opie, at the Johns Hopkins Hospital, documented a gallstone impacted in the ampulla of Vater during the postmortem examination of a patient, operated on by Halsted, who had died of gallstone pancreatitis, thereby first describing the pathogenetic mechanism of gallstone pancreatitis. Moynihan in 1925 described acute pancreatitis as "the most terrible of all the calamities that occur in connection with the abdominal viscera." This statement still underscores the importance of acute pancreatitis as a major cause of morbidity and mortality today.

Acute pancreatitis includes a broad spectrum of pancreatic disease, which varies from mild parenchymal edema to severe hemorrhagic pancreatitis associated with loss of parenchymal viability, with subsequent gangrene and necrosis. The clinical presentation of acute pancreatitis is quite variable, from episodes of mild abdominal discomfort alone to a severe illness associated with hypotension, metabolic derangements, sepsis, fluid sequestration, multiple organ failure, and death. Nine out of 10 patients experience the disease with mild to moderate symptoms and a self-limited course and improve with supportive care. In contrast, in 1 of 10 patients, a severe life-threatening form of acute pancreatitis evolves. Two recent autopsy studies reviewed the causes of death in patients with acute pancreatitis. In 126 patients with fatal acute pancreatitis, the late complications of multisystem organ failure and pancreatic abscess contributed to most of the deaths.[46] In a review of 405 postmortem examinations, the dominant pathologic finding in 95% of patients dying within 7 days of admission was pulmonary edema and congestion. In contrast, the dominant finding in 77% of patients expiring after day 7 was infection.[32]

Etiology

Many causes of acute pancreatitis exist (Table 35–1). In 90% of the cases, the cause is related to excessive alcohol intake or biliary tract disease. The relative frequency of these two principal causes of acute pancreatitis varies according to patient population.[40] In urban settings in the United States, alcohol abuse is the principal cause of acute pancreatitis. In other areas of the United States and in many regions of Asia and Europe, gallstone-associated pancreatitis predominates.

Alcohol is implicated as the etiologic agent in many patients with acute pancreatitis. Although the exact mechanism of alcohol-related injury is unknown, the association between alcohol abuse and acute pancreatitis is undeniable. Several theories exist to explain alcohol-related acute pancreatitis. First, alcohol-related pancreatitis may be the result of pancreatic exocrine hypersecretion in the presence of partial ampullary obstruction. Alcohol is a known stimulant of gastric acid secretion, and the resultant duodenal acidification is a stimulus for the release of secretin, which increases the exocrine secretion of pancreatic water and bicarbonate. Alcohol

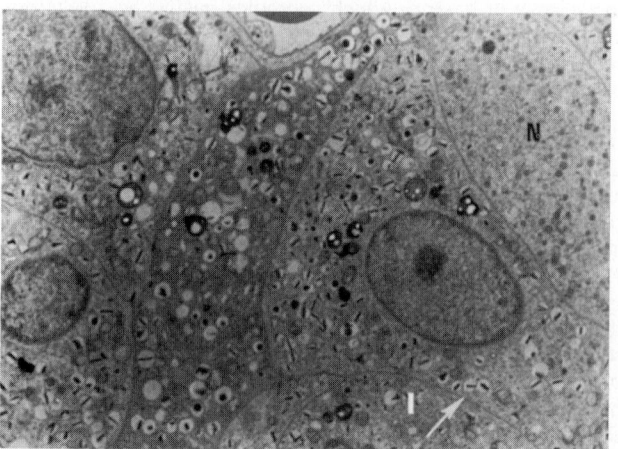

Figure 35–7. Electron micrograph of a portion of an islet of Langerhans. Most of the cells are beta cells, with characteristic insulin-containing granules (I) seen as tubular densities within clear vacuoles (arrow). A non-beta cell (N) is seen near the top right. Uranyl acetate and lead citrate, ×3000.

TABLE 35–1. Causes of Acute Pancreatitis

Alcohol
Biliary tract disease
Hyperlipidemia
Hypercalcemia
Familial
Trauma
    External
    Operative
    Retrograde pancreatography
Ischemia
    Hypotension
    Cardiopulmonary bypass
    Atheroembolism
    Vasculitis
Pancreas duct obstruction
    Tumor
    Pancreatic divisum
    Ampullary stenosis
    Ascaris infestation
Duodenal obstruction
Viral infection
Scorpion venom
Drugs
Idiopathic

is also known to increase the resistance of the sphincter of Oddi at the ampulla of Vater, thereby at least theoretically causing partial obstruction to the flow of pancreatic exocrine secretion. In a feline model, enterally administered alcohol was shown to increase pancreatic duct pressure and permeability to macromolecules. Thus, this first theory implicating alcohol in the etiology of acute pancreatitis suggests that the pancreatic parenchyma is injured by pancreatic enzyme extravasation, facilitated by an increase in pancreatic ductal permeability, and occurs in the presence of exocrine hypersecretion and partial ampullary obstruction. A second mechanism to explain the etiologic role of alcohol suggests that alcohol may initiate enzyme extravasation and cause pancreatic injury as a result of protein obstruction of the pancreatic duct. A third postulated mechanism to explain alcohol-induced pancreatitis involves the intermediate state of hypertriglyceridemia. Transient hypertriglyceridemia is known to occur after alcohol ingestion in some individuals. Clinical and laboratory studies suggest that toxic levels of free fatty acids, produced from the lipolysis of triglycerides, may induce pancreatic injury by causing acinar cell or capillary endothelial cell injury. A fourth mechanism to explain alcohol-induced pancreatitis involves injury generated by oxygen-derived free radicals, such as the superoxide radical and the hydroxyl radical. In experimental models, such injury can be ameliorated by free radical scavengers such as superoxide dismutase and catalase, and by a xanthine oxidase inhibitor such as allopurinol.[27]

The etiologic role of gallstones in the pathogenesis of acute pancreatitis first suggested by Opie now involves gallstone migration through the ampulla of Vater, causing diversion of bile into the pancreatic duct and subsequent bile-induced pancreatic parenchymal injury. Evidence supporting this mechanism is derived from clinical studies documenting the retrieval of gallstones in the stool of approximately 90% of patients with acute gallstone pancreatitis. These data suggest that it is the migration of a gallstone, and not necessarily its impaction, that initiates the pancreatic injury. Further evidence to support the gallstone migration theory evolves from cholangiographic studies that demonstrate a common channel between the common bile duct and the pancreatic duct in up to 90% of patients with a history of gallstone pancreatitis,

compared with only a 20 to 30% incidence of a common channel in patients with calculous biliary tract disease and no history of pancreatitis. Additional evidence is demonstrated on intraoperative cholangiograms performed at cholecystectomy, which show that pancreatic duct reflux is demonstrable in more than 60% of patients with a history of pancreatitis, a nearly fourfold increase, compared with those patients lacking a history of pancreatitis. Of note, recent experimental evidence suggests that biliary-pancreatic reflux is not essential in the initiation of gallstone-associated pancreatitis; obstruction of the pancreatic duct alone is sufficient to initiate pancreatic injury. Thus, gallstone-associated pancreatitis is associated with the anatomic existence of a common channel between the pancreatic and bile ducts, and it occurs in the setting of gallstone migration through the ampullary region.

Many other causes of acute pancreatitis exist. Hyperlipidemia alone, without excessive alcohol intake, is an etiologic agent. Hyperlipidemia may occur secondary to nephritis, castration, or exogenous estrogen administration, or it may occur as hereditary hyperlipidemia (Fredrickson Types 1 and 5), notable for hypertriglyceridemia and chylomicronemia.

Hypercalcemia is associated with acute pancreatitis, generally arising as a result of hyperparathyroidism. The mechanism of hypercalcemia-related pancreatitis may involve calcium-induced trypsinogen activation, with subsequent parenchymal autodestruction, calcium-associated stone precipitation in the pancreatic duct causing ductal obstruction, or calcium-stimulated pancreatic exocrine hypersecretion.

Familial cases of acute pancreatitis have been reported with no definite mechanism defined. Acute pancreatitis may also occur after pancreatic trauma, i.e., penetrating or blunt external trauma, intraoperative manipulation, or ampullary manipulation and pancreatic ductal overdistention during retrograde pancreatography.[37]

Pancreatic ischemia is also implicated in the etiology of acute pancreatitis. Ischemic episodes may occur during systemic hypotension or cardiopulmonary bypass or may be associated with visceral atheroembolism or vasculitis. Impairment of the pancreatic microcirculation has been correlated with the severity of experimental pancreatitis.[2] Ischemic pancreatitis has been produced with the use of an *ex vivo* isolated canine pancreatic preparation.[35] In this model, pancreatic ischemia has caused parenchymal edema, hyperamylasemia, and pathologic findings mimicking acute pancreatitis.

Recently it has been demonstrated that many patients with idiopathic pancreatitis harbor small biliary stones or sludge, termed *microlithiasis*, which appear to be the cause of their pancreatitis.[20] In these patients, cholecystectomy or endoscopic sphincterotomy prevented relapses of pancreatitis, providing evidence to support the theory that these occult small stones were the cause of the acute pancreatitis.

Numerous drugs (Table 35–2) have been linked to the initiation of acute pancreatitis. The most substantive evidence supports estrogens and azathioprine in the direct causation of pancreatitis. Direct causation has not been definitively proved for other substances.

The actual events on a cellular and molecular level responsible for the initiation of pancreatic parenchymal injury causing acute pancreatitis have not been fully elucidated. To assist in delineating the cellular and subcellular events that incite acute pancreatitis, a number of animal models have been developed. In 1975, Lombardi and co-workers reported that in young female mice fed a choline-deficient diet supplemented by 0.5% ethionine (the CDE diet), acute hemorrhagic pancreatitis developed with a reproducible mortality.[24] Lampel and Kern, in 1978, showed that the intravenous infusion of supramaximal doses of the cholecystokinin analog cerulein caused reproducible acute edematous pancreatitis in rats.[18]

TABLE 35–2. Drugs Implicated in the Initiation of Acute Pancreatitis

Definite Association	Probable Association
Azathioprine	Thiazide diuretics
Estrogens	Furosemide
	Ethacrynic acid
	Sulfonamides
	Tetracycline
	L-asparaginase
	Corticosteroids
	Phenformin
	Procainamide
	Valproic acid
	Clonidine
	Pentamidine
	Dideoxyinosine

Results of CDE diet and cerulein infusion experiments involving pulse labeling techniques and tritiated amino acid incorporation into zymogen granules, as well as cytochemical and immunohistochemical analyses, suggest that some pancreatitis-inducing stimuli prevent the extrusion of zymogen granules from individual acinar cells. This prevention of zymogen granule exocytosis causes fusion of the zymogen granules with intracellular lysosomes, activation of the zymogen proenzyme trypsinogen (Fig. 35–8), and generation of active intracellular trypsin, which is capable of cellular autodigestion.[38] Pathologic examination of human tissue examined by electron microscopy during acute pancreatitis confirms the findings of zymogen granule enlargement and formation of large autophagosomes. Although this mechanism is supported by several models of acute pancreatitis, it appears not to be applicable to all.

Clinical Presentation

In acute pancreatitis, a diverse spectrum of illness is seen, varying from a mild, short-lived, self-limited disease to a

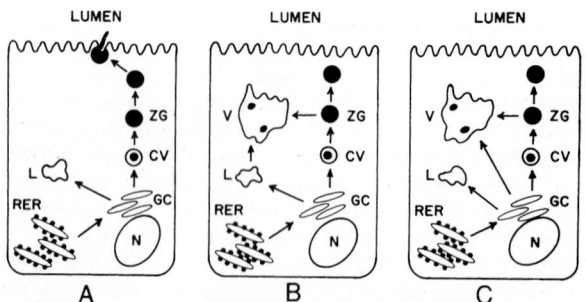

Figure 35–8. Intracellular transport of digestive enzymes and lysosomal hydrolases. *A,* Normal pattern, with synthesis of digestive enzymes and lysosomal hydrolases in the rough endoplasmic reticulum (RER), with subsequent transport to the Golgi complex (GC) adjacent to the nucleus (N). Lysosomal hydrolases are then transported to lysosomes (L), while digestive enzymes are concentrated in condensing vacuoles (CV) and zymogen granules (ZG). Zymogen granules fuse with the luminal plasma membrane and release their contents by exocytosis. *B,* Changes in mice fed the CDE diet, which blocks exocytosis and causes digestive enzymes and zymogen granules to accumulate. The zymogen granules fuse with lysosomes in a process termed crinophagy, causing the formation of large vacuoles (V). *C,* Changes in rats given supramaximal doses of cerulein. Here, transport to the Golgi complex is unaffected, but impaired separation of lysosomal hydrolases and digestive enzymes results in the formation of abnormal large vacuoles that contain both types of enzymes. Mature zymogen granules also fuse with these vacuoles, and exocytosis at the luminal plasma membrane is prevented. (From Steer, M. L., and Meldolesi, J.: The cell biology of experimental pancreatitis. N. Engl. J. Med., *316:*144, 1987. Copyright 1987, Massachusetts Medical Society.)

severe toxic condition associated with shock, hypovolemia, multiple metabolic derangements, and ultimate death. The clinical presentation alone may be quite suggestive of the diagnosis. The predominant clinical feature of acute pancreatitis is abdominal pain. Pain normally begins in the mid epigastrium, achieving maximal intensity several hours into the illness. Paroxysmal pain is uncommon. In most patients, the pain has a penetrating quality, radiating to the back. Although the pain is most commonly located in the mid epigastrium, it may predominate in the right or left upper quadrants. Generalized nonlocalized abdominal pain may also be observed. In patients with alcohol-associated pancreatitis, pain often commences between 12 and 48 hours after an episode of inebriation. In contrast, patients with gallstone-associated pancreatitis typically experience the onset of pain after a large meal. Nausea and vomiting frequently accompany the abdominal pain. The vomiting may be severe and protracted. Rare patients with acute pancreatitis may present without abdominal pain but with a severe systemic illness marked by hypotension, hypoperfusion, and depression of mental status. In these patients, the diagnosis of acute pancreatitis may be particularly difficult to establish.

Typical findings on physical examination in patients with acute pancreatitis include fever, tachycardia, epigastric tenderness, and abdominal distention. Abdominal distention may be the result of a paralytic ileus arising from retroperitoneal irritation or may occur secondary to a retroperitoneal phlegmon. Severe pancreatitis associated with hemorrhage into the retroperitoneum may produce two distinctive physical signs: Turner's sign (bluish discoloration in the left flank) and Cullen's sign (bluish discoloration of the periumbilical region). These physical signs, which occur in less than 3% of patients with pancreatitis, are the result of the tracking of blood-stained retroperitoneal fluid through the tissue planes of the abdominal wall to the flank or along the falciform ligament to the umbilical area. These signs signal the presence of a severe episode of acute hemorrhagic pancreatitis, with an overall mortality that may exceed 30%.

Jaundice is an uncommon finding at the initial presentation of acute pancreatitis. Jaundice may occasionally be seen in patients with gallstone-associated pancreatitis, where it represents distal common bile duct obstruction by gallstones. Jaundice may also follow compression of the distal common bile duct by edema of the pancreatic head.

Patients with severe pancreatitis may manifest major circulatory derangements such as hypotension, hypovolemia, hypoperfusion, and obtundation. Formerly, the etiology of this shock state was attributed to a putative circulating myocardial depressant factor thought to be elaborated during severe hemorrhagic pancreatitis. Recent investigations have shown that the detrimental effects of acute pancreatitis on cardiovascular function are related primarily to hypovolemia and decreased preload to the heart and are not related to a depressant factor released in response to the disease.

Extra-abdominal manifestations of acute pancreatitis may be found on careful physical examination in many patients. Up to one third of patients have evidence of a left pleural effusion or left hemidiaphragm elevation. Less frequently, patients manifest signs of acute pulmonary failure, marked by tachypnea, dyspnea, and cyanosis. The etiology of this respiratory dysfunction remains unclear, although it has been linked to abnormalities of circulating phospholipase A, circulating free fatty acids generated from triglyceride lipolysis, pulmonary surfactant, and volume overload in the setting of pulmonary capillary leakage. Nonpulmonary findings associated with acute pancreatitis include subcutaneous fat necrosis and cerebral abnormalities of a nonlateralizing nature, including belligerence, confusion, psychosis, and coma. It has been speculated that these cerebral abnormalities follow hyperosmolarity, hypoperfusion and hypoxia, cerebral fat embolism, or disseminated intravascular coagulopathy.

Diagnosis

Acute pancreatitis is often suspected on the basis of clinical presentation, with the diagnosis supported by appropriate laboratory determinations and radiographic findings (Table 35–3).

Laboratory Determinations. The determination of serum amylase is the most widely used laboratory test in the diagnosis of acute pancreatitis. In most cases, hyperamylasemia is observed within 24 hours of the onset of symptoms, with gradual return to normal values during the subsequent 7 days. Persistent hyperamylasemia beyond the initial week of the illness may indicate the development of complications such as pancreatic pseudocyst, phlegmon, or abscess or may indicate ongoing acute pancreatic inflammation. The degree of initial hyperamylasemia is not a reliable predictor of the severity of pancreatitis. However, the magnitude of hyperamylasemia is an independent predictor that differentiates gallstone-associated pancreatitis from alcohol-induced pancreatitis when examined by regression analysis in patient populations with diverse causes of pancreatitis.

Despite its widespread use, serum amylase is not an ideal marker for the diagnosis of acute pancreatitis. Serum amylase alone is limited as a predictor of acute pancreatitis because of high false-positive and high false-negative rates. In an acute hospital setting, nearly one third of the detected elevations of serum amylase are unrelated to acute pancreatitis (false-positive). A multitude of other causes of hyperamylasemia exists (Table 35–4). In addition, there is a false-negative rate of approximately 10%, indicating that hyperamylasemia is observed in only 90% of patients subsequently proved to have acute pancreatitis. Thus, the absence of hyperamylasemia does not exclude the diagnosis of acute pancreatitis. There are several possible explanations for the absence of hyperamylasemia in cases of acute pancreatitis. In some patients, only brief hyperamylasemia may occur prior to medical evaluation, normoamylasemia being observed at the initial presentation. The lack of hyperamylasemia may also reflect extensive pancreatic necrosis or failure of a chronically diseased gland to elaborate sufficient circulating amylase at the time of acute inflammation. Moreover, most patients with hyperlipidemia-induced acute pancreatitis present with normoamylasemia, possibly related to a circulating inhibitor of amylase activity in these hyperlipidemic patients.

The measurement of pancreatic isoenzyme components improves the accuracy of the diagnosis in acute pancreatitis. Normally, P type amylase isoenzyme arises from the pancreas, representing 40% of circulating amylase. The remaining 60% of total circulating amylase, designated S type isoamylase, derives from salivary glands, fallopian tubes, ovaries, endometrium, prostate, breast, lung, and possibly liver. Isoenzyme analyses have been shown to be of some benefit in

TABLE 35–3. Diagnosis of Acute Pancreatitis

Laboratory Tests	Radiographic Procedures
Serum amylase	Plain chest roentgenogram
Serum amylase isoenzymes	Plain abdominal roentgenogram
Urinary amylase	Upper gastrointestinal contrast series
Amylase-creatinine clearance ratio	Ultrasonography
	Computed tomography
Serum lipase	Magnetic resonance imaging
Serum methemalbumin	
Peritoneal fluid analysis	

TABLE 35–4. Disorders Associated with Hyperamylasemia

Intra-abdominal	Extra-abdominal
Pancreatic disorders	Salivary gland disorders
Acute pancreatitis	Mumps
Chronic pancreatitis	Parotitis
Trauma	Trauma
Carcinoma	Calculi
Pseudocyst	Irradiation sialadenitis
Pancreatic ascites	Impaired amylase excretion
Abscess	Renal failure
Nonpancreatic disorders	Macroamylasemia
Biliary tract disease	Miscellaneous
Intestinal obstruction	Pneumonia
Mesenteric infarction	Pancreatic pleural effusion
Perforated peptic ulcer	Mediastinal pseudocyst
Peritonitis	Cerebral trauma
Afferent loop syndrome	Severe burns
Acute appendicitis	Diabetic ketoacidosis
Ruptured ectopic pregnancy	Pregnancy
Salpingitis	Drugs
Ruptured aortic aneurysm	Bisalbuminemia

excluding the diagnosis of acute pancreatitis, particularly in patients with hyperamylasemia and an absence of P type isoenzyme elevation.

The measurement of urinary amylase excretion has also been proposed as a sensitive index of the disease. Urinary amylase elevations persist for a longer period of time than serum elevations, with the magnitude of urinary elevations frequently surpassing the magnitude of serum elevations. However, hyperamylasuria alone is not diagnostic of pancreatitis and may be observed in most other disorders associated with hyperamylasemia. In addition, a normal urinary amylase value does not preclude the diagnosis of acute pancreatitis.

The measurement of the renal clearance of amylase has been suggested as a means of improving the accuracy of the diagnosis of acute pancreatitis. The equation for the calculation is

$$\frac{\text{urine amylase}}{\text{serum amylase}} \times \frac{\text{serum creatinine}}{\text{urine creatinine}} \times 100$$

$$= \text{the amylase-creatinine clearance ratio}$$

Many authors have supported the use of the amylase-creatinine clearance ratio in the diagnosis of acute pancreatitis, noting that the renal glomerular permeability to amylase appears to be increased in the disease. Normally, this ratio varies from 1 to 4%. A ratio of greater than 6% is consistent with the diagnosis of acute pancreatitis; ratios up to three times this level are frequently observed in severe pancreatitis. Unfortunately, acute pancreatitis may occur with a normal amylase-creatinine clearance ratio. Additionally, false-positive elevated ratios may be seen in disease states such as renal insufficiency, perforated peptic ulcer, pancreatic carcinoma, burns, and diabetic ketoacidosis. Thus, the amylase-creatinine clearance ratio is not a totally specific or totally sensitive indicator of acute pancreatitis.

The elevation of serum lipase is a more accurate indicator of acute pancreatitis than is the elevation of serum amylase, because lipase is solely of pancreatic origin. In addition, the duration of hyperlipasemia often exceeds that of hyperamylasemia, making this test beneficial in patients with late clinical presentation. However, hyperlipasemia is not entirely specific for acute pancreatitis, being observed in other disease states such as perforated peptic ulcer, acute cholecystitis, and intestinal ischemia.

The finding of serum lactescence is one of the most specific indicators of acute pancreatitis. Lactescent serum occurs when circulating triglyceride values exceed 500 mg. per 100 ml. Serum lactescence may be seen in patients with hereditary hyperlipidemia-associated pancreatitis or in alcohol-associated pancreatitis. Patients with lactescent serum usually have falsely normal serum amylase levels, making the demonstration of serum lactescence a valuable diagnostic indicator supporting the diagnosis of acute pancreatitis.

Additional support for the diagnosis of acute pancreatitis can be derived from a number of standard laboratory tests. Although these tests are not specific for the diagnosis of acute pancreatitis, they may provide important information substantiating the diagnosis. Hematologic evaluation may reveal hemoconcentration from third-space fluid sequestration. An elevated white blood cell count above 10,000 cells per cu. mm. is typical. Serum chemistries often reveal hyperglycemia, mild azotemia, abnormalities of liver function tests, and hypocalcemia. Hyperglycemia appears to be the result of relative hypoinsulinemia and relative hyperglucagonemia, and it is associated with the degranulation of beta cells by electron microscopy.[48] Mild azotemia is related to fluid sequestration, resultant hypovolemia, and diminished cardiac output. Hypocalcemia is the consequence of dilutional hypoalbuminemia, calcium deposition in areas of fat necrosis, and resistance of skeletal bone to parathyroid hormone stimulation. Derangements of calcitonin and vitamin D do not appear to be acutely implicated in pancreatitis-induced hypocalcemia. Abnormalities of liver function tests are more commonly found in gallstone-associated pancreatitis, in which they reflect some obstruction to the free flow of bile through the ampulla of Vater. Using stepwise logistic regression analyses, a number of investigators have confirmed that elevated bilirubin, alkaline phosphatase, γ-glutamyl transferase, alanine aminotransferase, and aspartate amino transferase serve as independent predictors favoring a common bile duct stone as the initiator of the attack of pancreatitis.

In a minority of patients with pancreatitis, arterial blood gas abnormalities occur. However, in up to 10% of patients, generally those with severe attacks, severe progressive pulmonary dysfunction marked by dramatic hypoxemia and hyperventilation may occur. Severe pancreatitis may also cause dramatic coagulation abnormalities marked by hypercoagulability, disseminated intravascular coagulation, and hypofibrinogenemia.

Diagnostic paracentesis is occasionally utilized to confirm the diagnosis of acute pancreatitis. Elevations in peritoneal fluid amylase and lipase may be found in settings where their respective serum levels are normal. However, diagnostic paracentesis is not an ideal test for the confirmation of the diagnosis of acute pancreatitis due to its invasive nature, its potential for complications, and the lack of complete specificity of peritoneal fluid enzyme elevations for acute pancreatitis.

Radiographic Procedures. Clinical and laboratory evidence of acute pancreatitis can be supported by radiographic procedures such as plain chest and abdominal radiographs, gastrointestinal contrast studies, sonography, computed tomography (CT), and magnetic resonance imaging (MRI) studies.

Chest film findings supportive of the diagnosis of acute pancreatitis, but not specific for the disease, include left basal atelectasis, elevation of the left hemidiaphragm, and left pleural effusion. These findings reflect the presence of a significant peridiaphragmatic, retroperitoneal inflammatory process occurring in the region of the pancreas. Chest films are also useful in eliminating other diagnoses from the differential diagnosis in a patient with abdominal pain. For example, the findings of pneumoperitoneum or lobar pneumonia

on an upright chest film would lead the clinician away from the diagnosis of acute pancreatitis.

There are no specific indicators of acute pancreatitis on abdominal radiographs. However, they reveal nonspecific abnormalities in the majority of patients. Most frequently seen on the abdominal plain film is the presence of air in the duodenal loop, representing a local duodenal ileus secondary to the adjacent inflammatory reaction in the head of the gland. Also common is the abnormality referred to as the *sentinal loop sign*, representing a dilated proximal jejunal loop localized to the upper abdomen, adjacent to the pancreatic bed. The *colon cutoff sign* may also be observed, indicative of distention of the colon to the level of the transverse colon, with little to no air being present in the splenic flexure and more distal colon. Other possible findings on abdominal films include gallstones in the gallbladder, obliteration of the psoas margin secondary to retroperitoneal edema, or a nonspecific ileus pattern. One specific marker of pancreatic disease is the presence of pancreatic calcifications, although this is not an indicator of acute pancreatitis, but rather of chronic pancreatitis.

Upper gastrointestinal contrast studies were formerly used to assist in the diagnosis of acute pancreatitis. Typical findings included widening of the duodenal C loop, anterior displacement of the stomach by an inflamed retroperitoneal process, and subtle duodenal mucosal abnormalities reflecting duodenal wall inflammation. However, no findings on upper gastrointestinal series are specific for acute pancreatitis, and more sensitive and specific radiographic evaluations are now available.

Abdominal sonography may be used to assist in the diagnosis of acute pancreatitis. Unfortunately, the value of ultrasonography is often limited by the presence of air and fluid-filled loops of bowel overlying and obscuring the pancreas. In the absence of this limitation, ultrasound can be used to detect pancreatic edema and acute peripancreatic fluid collections. In addition, in patients with suspected gallstone-associated pancreatitis, the gallbladder can be assessed for gallstones, and the common bile duct can be evaluated for size and the presence of stones.

Currently, the most widely accepted and sensitive method used to confirm the diagnosis of acute pancreatitis is CT. The accuracy of CT scanning is improved with both oral and intravenous contrast enhancement. Nearly all patients with acute pancreatitis have some abnormalities on CT scan. Specific CT findings in acute pancreatitis can be categorized into pancreatic and peripancreatic changes (Table 35–5). Pancreatic changes include diffuse or focal parenchymal enlargement, edema, or necrosis with liquefaction. Peripancreatic changes include blurring or thickening of the surrounding

---

TABLE 35–5. Computed Tomographic Findings in Acute Pancreatitis

Pancreatic changes
  Parenchymal enlargement
    Diffuse
    Focal
  Parenchymal edema
  Necrosis
Peripancreatic changes
  Blurring of fat planes
  Thickening of fascial planes
  Presence of fluid collections
Nonspecific findings
  Bowel distention
  Pleural effusion
  Mesenteric edema

tissue planes and the presence of fluid collections. An approximate correlation exists between the degree of CT abnormality and the clinical course and severity of the acute pancreatitis. CT is additionally useful for the demonstration of structural complications that develop during the course of acute pancreatitis, such as pancreatic abscess, pseudocyst, or necrosis.

MRI holds promise for more sophisticated imaging and more accurate diagnosis of acute pancreatitis. Currently, MRI and CT appear to provide equivalent information regarding the presence and extent of fluid collections and parenchymal irregularity. High-resolution ^{31}P spectral analysis has been used in longitudinally evaluating the severity of acute pancreatitis in several experimental settings. The stepwise depletion of the high-energy compounds adenosine triphosphate and phosphocreatine was found to parallel the progression of the acute pancreatitis in one study and to be associated with the presence of ischemic pancreatitis in another. Active investigation is currently under way to elucidate the role of MRI and spectroscopy in the clinical assessment of pancreatitis.

Endoscopic retrograde pancreatography is an invasive procedure that has proven diagnostic utility in occasional patients with recurrent attacks of acute pancreatitis without obvious etiology. In these settings, endoscopic pancreatography has been useful in identifying potentially correctable abnormalities in up to 50% of patients. In such patients, the findings of pancreas divisum, stenosis of the ampulla of Vater, and focal pancreatic duct abnormalities may be demonstrated. However, endoscopic retrograde pancreatography has no role in the standard diagnostic evaluation of the majority of patients with acute pancreatitis.

Clinical Course

The clinical course in up to 90% of patients with acute pancreatitis follows a mild, self-limited pattern. However, in 10 to 15% of patients with acute pancreatitis, a severe form of illness develops that may be attended by lengthy hospitalization and specific complications, with significant associated morbidity and mortality. Patients with severe pancreatitis provide a major management challenge, often requiring intensive care support, invasive hemodynamic monitoring, frequent laboratory and radiographic evaluation, and experienced management.

It is possible to predict the severity of an attack of pancreatitis and the overall prognosis using routinely available clinical and laboratory determinations. The most widely used predictive criteria involve 11 prognostic signs identified by Ranson in 1974 and, which are most useful in patients with pancreatitis not related to gallstones.[30] A modification of this prognostic system has been verified for patients with gallstone-induced pancreatitis (Table 35–6). These prognostic signs are clinically valuable in guiding the therapy of each individual patient with acute pancreatitis. Patients who present with two or fewer prognostic signs have essentially no mortality, and generally simple supportive care suffices in their management. Patients with three or four prognostic signs have a mortality that approximates 15%, with nearly half the patients requiring intensive care unit support. If five or six prognostic signs are present, intensive care unit support is usually required, and mortality approaches 50%. Patients with seven or more prognostic signs have an even higher predicted mortality and represent a group of patients that tests the limits of modern medicine. The application of this prognostic scoring system allows early stratification of patients based on predicted outcome and allows the triaging of patients to appropriate treatment modalities. Patients assessed to have severe pancreatitis are at risk for the development of life-threatening complications, and they are optimally managed in the intensive care setting with hemodynamic monitoring, aggressive fluid resuscitation, and consideration of antibiotic administration as prophylaxis against infectious complications.

Although the Ranson prognostic scoring system has gained widespread use, many other predictive indicators have been proposed. Methemalbuminemia loosely correlates with the presence of severe hemorrhagic pancreatitis. Diagnostic peritoneal lavage can assess the severity of illness and serves as a predictor of prognosis. Serum ribonuclease activity has been suggested as a marker of severe parenchymal necrosis. Other scoring systems based on laboratory and radiographic evidence have also been proposed. These include the second version of the Acute Physiology and Chronic Health Enquiry (APACHE II), the Medical Research Council Sepsis (MRCS) score, and the Simplified Acute Physiology (SAP) score, among others.

Nonoperative Management

Following initial clinical assessment, confirmation of diagnosis by laboratory and radiographic study, and prediction of prognosis, the initial management of patients with acute pancreatitis is nonoperative (Table 35–7). Standard therapy in all patients includes intravenous fluid resuscitation, electrolyte replacement, and analgesics. Nasogastric decompression is reserved for patients with significant ileus, in whom it is used to prevent emesis and aspiration. Patients with severe pancreatitis often require nutritional support via parenteral alimentation, antibiotic administration for prevention or treatment of septic complications, or respiratory support for pulmonary dysfunction. In addition to these standard supportive measures, a number of specific therapies have undergone trial under experimental or clinical conditions to test their efficacy in reducing the degree of pancreatic

TABLE 35–6. Ranson's Early Prognostic Signs of Acute Pancreatitis

Criteria for Pancreatitis Not Due to Gallstones

At Admission	During Initial 48 Hours
Age over 55 yr.	Hematocrit fall >10 percentage points
WBC >16,000 cells/cu. mm.	
Blood glucose >200 mg./100 ml.	BUN elevation >5 mg./100 ml.
Serum lactate dehydrogenase >350 I.U./L.	Serum calcium fall to <8 mg./100 ml.
AST >250 U./100 ml.	Arterial P_{O_2} <60 torr
	Base deficit >4 mEq./L.
	Estimated fluid sequestration >6 L.

Criteria for Gallstone Pancreatitis

At Admission	During Initial 48 Hours
Age over 70 yr.	Hematocrit fall >10 percentage points
WBC >18,000 cells/cu. mm.	
Glucose >220 mg./100 ml.	BUN elevation >2 mg./100 ml.
Serum lactate dehydrogenase >400 I.U./L.	Serum calcium fall to <8 mg./100 ml.
AST >250 U./100 ml.	Base deficit >5 mEq./L.
	Estimated fluid sequestration >4 L.

WBC, white blood cell count; AST, aspartate aminotransferase; BUN, blood urea nitrogen.

Data from Ranson, J. H. C., Rifkind, K. M., Roses, D. F., et al.: Prognostic signs and the role of operative management in acute pancreatitis. Surg. Gynecol. Obstet., *139*:69, 1974; and Ranson J. H. C.: Etiological and prognostic factors in human acute pancreatitis: A review. Am. J. Gastroenterol., *77*:633, 1982.

TABLE 35–7. Proposed Nonoperative Therapies for Acute Pancreatitis

Supportive measures
    Intravenous fluid therapy
    Electrolyte replacement
    Analgesia
    Nutritional support
    Antibiotics
    Respiratory support
Pancreatic exocrine secretion suppression
    Nasogastric suction
    Histamine H_2-receptor antagonists
    Antacids
    Anticholinergics
    Glucagon
    Calcitonin
    Somatostatin
    Peptide YY
    Cholecystokinin-receptor antagonists
Pancreatic enzyme inhibition
    Protease inhibitors
        Aprotinin
        Gabexate
        Camostate
        Fresh frozen plasma
    Antifibrinolytics
    Chloroquine
    Phospholipase A inhibitors
Pancreatic protection from oxygen-derived free radicals
    Free radical scavengers
    Xanthine oxidase inhibitors
    Isovolemic hemodilution
Elimination of toxic intraperitoneal compounds
    Peritoneal dialysis

parenchymal injury, subsequent complications, and overall mortality.

Standard Supportive Measures. Acute pancreatitis is commonly associated with massive fluid sequestration. Fluid can accumulate within the bowel lumen secondary to paralytic ileus, or there can be marked edema in the peripancreatic region. External fluid losses may also occur in the form of emesis. An essential initial step in the management of acute pancreatitis involves generous fluid resuscitation directed at correcting hypovolemia and restoring circulating blood volume. The adequacy of volume replacement is assessed by the response of the heart rate, blood pressure, and urinary output. In patients with pre-existing cardiac, pulmonary, or renal disease, or in patients with severe pancreatitis, invasive monitoring, including urethral catheterization, central venous pressure measurement, or measurement of cardiac output and cardiac filling pressures via a Swan-Ganz catheter, is often indicated. In rare cases, shock may be intractable to fluid resuscitation alone, requiring the use of potent vasopressor agents during initial resuscitation. Crystalloid solutions are generally used for fluid resuscitation in acute pancreatitis. Severe hemorrhagic pancreatitis may require blood transfusion or the transfusion of clotting factors to correct a markedly abnormal coagulation status. However, clinical trials of colloid therapy have failed to delineate benefit from routinely administering fresh frozen plasma as a specific therapy in acute pancreatitis.

During the initial phase of resuscitation, a variety of electrolyte abnormalities may be encountered. A hypochloremic contraction alkalosis may follow persistent emesis and is treated with vigorous volume replacement with normal saline, supplemented with exogenous potassium chloride. Intravascular volume contraction may cause hypernatremia correctable by isotonic volume replacement. Serum calcium

is often depressed secondary to hypoalbuminemia; however, if the ionized calcium level is normal, the patient does not require exogenous calcium replacement. Patients with depressed ionized calcium levels should receive supplementation. Hypomagnesemia may also be observed and should be corrected, because this may hasten the normalization of serum ionized calcium. Mild hyperglycemia is a frequent finding that improves with volume resuscitation. Marked hyperglycemia or glycosuria mandates cautious insulin administration.

Abdominal pain is treated with careful administration of narcotic analgesics. Meperidine is the preferred drug, and it may be administered using patient-controlled analgesia (PCA) systems. Morphine is avoided because of its potential for causing sphincter of Oddi spasm, an entity that could theoretically potentiate ongoing pancreatic parenchymal injury. Infrequently used techniques to manage the abdominal pain of acute pancreatitis include percutaneous splanchnic nerve blocks and epidural anesthesia.

In patients with acute pancreatitis, oral intake is initially prohibited. Oral intake can generally be resumed during the first week of treatment when abdominal pain and tenderness have improved, ileus has resolved, and hyperamylasemia is normalizing. Premature return to oral intake has been associated with the formation of pancreatic abscess and reactivation of pancreatic inflammation. In a subgroup of patients, the return to eating is necessarily delayed as a result of persistent pain, ileus, or the occurrence of a complication such as pseudocyst, phlegmon, or abscess. Under these circumstances, standard parenteral nutrition using carbohydrate- and amino acid–based solutions is indicated. Intravenous lipids can also be used as a calorie source in most patients. Lipid administration should be restricted in patients with underlying hyperlipidemia and in those rare patients who demonstrate hypertriglyceridemia with exogenous intravenous lipid administration.

Antibiotics are not indicated in the routine treatment of mild to moderate pancreatitis. In severe pancreatitis—defined as greater than three Ranson prognostic signs associated with CT evidence of pancreatic or peripancreatic necrosis—a recent randomized multicenter trial showed that prophylactic imipenem administered intravenously every 8 hours for 2 weeks significantly reduced the incidence of pancreatic sepsis.[29] A further study showed a beneficial effect of selective decontamination of the intestinal tract (using norfloxacin, colistin, and amphotericin) in patients with severe acute pancreatitis.[25] Thus, accumulating data support the use of some form of prophylactic regimen in patients with severe pancreatitis. Respiratory complications of acute pancreatitis such as atelectasis, effusion, pneumonia, and mild respiratory insufficiency generally require supportive care with supplemental oxygen administration, physical therapy, and treatment of infection. Progressive respiratory failure that is unresponsive to lesser supportive modalities may require endotracheal intubation and positive pressure ventilation.

Pancreatic Exocrine Secretion Suppression. Therapeutic attempts to suppress pancreatic enzyme secretion have included nasogastric suction, histamine H_2-receptor antagonists, antacids, anticholinergics, glucagon, calcitonin, somatostatin, peptide YY and cholecystokinin-receptor antagonists such as proglumide. All these therapies have some theoretic potential to improve the outcome in patients with acute pancreatitis, based on the hypothesis that pancreatic exocrine hypersecretion in the presence of partial ampullary obstruction is important in the pathogenesis of the disease. In fact, currently, none of these therapies has proved effective in shortening the duration of the disease, reducing complications, or reducing mortality.

Treatment directed at the reduction of gastric acid delivery to the duodenum (such as nasogastric suction, histamine H$_2$-receptor antagonists, antacids, and anticholinergics) is designed to reduce duodenal acidification-induced secretin release from the duodenum, thereby reducing the volume of pancreatic exocrine secretion. However, no beneficial effect has been demonstrated. Nasogastric suction is, however, indicated in a subset of patients who present with gastric distention, persistent emesis, or altered mental status at risk for aspiration. Histamine H$_2$-receptor antagonists or antacids are indicated as prophylaxis against upper gastrointestinal tract hemorrhage in patients with severe pancreatitis. The adverse side effects of anticholinergics, such as urinary retention, tachycardia, and prolongation of ileus, make them unattractive for use in the treatment of acute pancreatitis.

Both glucagon and calcitonin, the hormonal product of the thyroid parafollicular C cell, suppress pancreatic exocrine and gastric acid secretion. Neither has documented efficacy in altering the outcome of acute pancreatitis.

Somatostatin is also a potent inhibitor of pancreatic exocrine secretion and gastric acid output. Native somatostatin has a circulating half-life in the blood of less than 3 minutes and thus must be delivered by continuous intravenous infusion. Octreotide is a long-acting octapeptide analog of the native tetradecapeptide that is now available for clinical use. In animal models of established experimental pancreatitis, somatostatin has been effective in reducing mortality from bile-induced pancreatitis and in hastening the return to normoamylasemia. However, multicenter clinical trials have failed to document a statistically significant reduction in overall mortality in patients with acute pancreatitis. Evaluation of octreotide therapy in acute pancreatitis is continuing.

The cholecystokinin-receptor antagonist proglumide has proved efficacious in models of experimental pancreatitis. In animal models using both cerulein-induced and CDE diet–induced pancreatitis, proglumide treatment has reduced mortality. Further investigations are needed to clarify the role of cholecystokinin-receptor antagonists in the management of clinical pancreatitis.

Pancreatic Enzyme Inhibition. The treatment of acute pancreatitis by inhibition of pancreatic enzyme activation has a sound theoretical basis. Protease inhibitors such as aprotinin, gabexate, camostate, and fresh frozen plasma have been studied. However, in clinical trials, none was of value in the treatment of acute pancreatitis.

Clinical studies have also failed to demonstrate a beneficial effect of antifibrinolytics such as ε-aminocaproic or ρ-aminomethylbenzoic acid. Phospholipase A inhibitors such as calcium disodium-EDTA also have not decreased morbidity or mortality in human pancreatitis.

Pancreatic Protection from Oxygen-Derived Free Radicals. Systemic hypotension, low flow states associated with cardiopulmonary bypass, emboli to mesenteric vessels, or obstruction to visceral flow from vasculitis can cause relative pancreatic ischemia with resultant acute pancreatitis. Attempts to improve pancreatic perfusion using isovolemic hemodilution with dextran have proved beneficial in experimental, but not clinical, pancreatitis. Experimental models of acute pancreatitis have been used to demonstrate that free radical scavengers such as superoxide dismutase and catalase or xanthine oxidase inhibitors such as allopurinol can prevent acute experimental pancreatitis when administered before initiation of the parenchymal injury. However, these treatments are not effective in arresting the progression of established experimental pancreatitis and are unlikely to be clinically beneficial in the treatment of established acute pancreatitis.

Elimination of Toxic Intraperitoneal Contents. Potentially toxic intraperitoneal compounds such as histamine, vasoactive kinins, elastase, prostaglandins, phospholipase A, trypsin, and chymotrypsin have been identified in the peritoneal exudate from acute pancreatitis. These compounds may mediate many adverse systemic effects such as hypotension, pulmonary failure, hepatic failure, and altered vascular permeability. Peritoneal dialysis appears theoretically attractive as a means of accelerating the removal of these activated toxic compounds. Studies in experimental pancreatitis have yielded favorable responses to peritoneal dialysis, with improvement in outcome. Prospective randomized trials using nonlavaged control groups compared with lavage treatment groups have failed to reveal any beneficial effect of peritoneal lavage on overall outcome. One prospective study[41] and other noncontrolled trials have suggested that peritoneal lavage may be of benefit in reducing the early systemic complications of severe pancreatitis. Further study is needed to clarify the role of peritoneal dialysis in patients with severe acute pancreatitis.

Operative Management

Operative intervention in patients with acute pancreatitis is indicated in four specific circumstances: (1) uncertainty of diagnosis, (2) treatment of secondary pancreatic infections, (3) correction of associated biliary tract disease, and (4) progressive clinical deterioration despite optimal supportive care.

Uncertainty of Clinical Diagnosis. Since there is no single test or combination of studies that is capable of diagnosing acute pancreatitis with 100% accuracy, it may occasionally be difficult to exclude other diagnoses that mimic acute pancreatitis and require operative intervention. Examples of such conditions include perforated viscus or acute mesenteric ischemia. In these situations, when the clinical diagnosis is not firm, exploratory laparotomy may be indicated to exclude a surgically correctable disease with a potentially fatal outcome in the unoperated state. With the widespread availability of abdominal CT scanning, these situations are becoming less frequent. At the time of exploration, any ascitic fluid present is sampled for amylase, lipase, aerobic and anaerobic culture, and cell counts. If no extrapancreatic disease is discovered, the gastrocolic omentum is opened to fully expose the body and tail of the pancreas. If uncomplicated acute pancreatitis is present, no manipulation is indicated, and the operation is terminated. In patients with systemic toxicity and gross evidence of severe pancreatitis associated with large amounts of peritoneal fluid exudate, the placement of a peritoneal dialysis catheter for postoperative lavage should be considered. In patients with cholelithiasis and presumed gallstone-associated pancreatitis, definitive biliary surgery, including cholecystectomy and intraoperative cholangiography, is favored if the clinical circumstances permit. In patients with severe hemorrhagic pancreatitis with necrosis but without frank infection, formal pancreatic resection is no longer favored. Instead, cautious débridement of necrotic tissue is performed, and wide retroperitoneal drainage is established.

Treatment of Secondary Pancreatic Infections. Pancreatic abscess, infected pancreatic pseudocyst, and infected pancreatic necrosis are three serious and life-threatening complications of acute pancreatitis, occurring in up to 5% of all patients. They occur with increasing frequency in direct proportion to the severity of acute pancreatitis. In patients with six or more of Ranson's prognostic signs, over 50% develop a pancreatic septic complication that typically occur as a result of a secondary infection of necrotic pancreatic and peripancreatic tissue. The organisms may arise from transmural migration of bacteria from adjacent inflamed bowel or from hematogenous seeding. Enteric organisms predominate. Polymicrobial infection is common, occurring in the majority of cases. Fungal infection is being recognized with increased frequency. The abscesses may be unilocular but are usually multilocular, and they may be located in any region adjacent to the pancreas. It is not uncommon to find large abscesses that extensively dissect retroperitoneal planes, residing behind the ascending or descending colon laterally or extending in the midline inferior to the base of the small bowel mesentery. Pancreatic abscess and infected pseudocysts are associated with little or no necrosis. Patients with diffuse or focal areas of nonviable pancreatic parenchyma, often associated with peripancreatic fat necrosis, are categorized as having infected or noninfected pancreatic necrosis.[4]

The development of pancreatic septic complications should be suspected in patients with severe pancreatitis, in patients with documented bacteremia, in patients with clinical deterioration after the first week, and in patients in whom pancreatitis fails to resolve within the first week to 10 days. Clinical manifestations include fever, abdominal pain, abdominal distention, and a palpable abdominal mass. Associated laboratory abnormalities include persistent hyperamylasemia, nonspecific elevations of liver function tests, and leukocytosis. The diagnosis of pancreatic septic complications is assisted by radiographic studies. Plain abdominal films may show extraluminal retroperitoneal air, described as the *soap bubble sign*, in 15% of patients. Abdominal ultrasonography and nuclear medicine scans using gallium and indium-labeled leukocytes may suggest a diagnosis but cannot accurately differentiate abscess from phlegmon. Currently, dynamic, contrast-enhanced CT scanning is the most widely used and accurate procedure for evaluating potential pancreatic septic complications. Findings on a CT scan such as air bubbles in the retroperitoneum are diagnostic of a pancreatic abscess, infected pseudocyst, or infected necrosis, but unfortunately, they are absent in many cases. The combination of abdominal CT scan and guided percutaneous needle aspiration has been demonstrated to be highly reliable in different- iating pancreatic abscess from sterile peripancreatic phlegmon. Fluid sampled at percutaneous needle aspiration is immediately Gram-stained and cultured. The aspiration is considered positive for pancreatic abscess if either Gram's stain or the culture reveals organisms.

Treatment of secondary pancreatic infections combines antibiotic therapy with prompt drainage. Occasional patients with solitary, well-defined abscesses or infected pseudocysts may be managed via percutaneous drainage techniques. Operative débridement is necessary to remove the thick, debris-filled, pastelike collections of infected necrotic material in patients with infected pancreatic necrosis. The two accepted alternatives for management of infected pancreatic necrosis and many pancreatic abscesses are (1) laparotomy with débridement and wide sump drainage and (2) laparotomy with débridement and open packing. In either case, the anterior transperitoneal approach to the abdomen is used to facilitate exposure. The gastrocolic omentum is divided, and the retroperitoneum is débrided of devitalized tissues. Anatomic resection is usually avoided. The peripancreatic region is copiously irrigated with saline and topical antibiotic solutions. Subsequently, wide sump drainage of the retroperitoneum or open packing is instituted. The wide sump drainage technique allows fascial closure of the abdomen and places multiple large-bore drains in dependent positions to drain the infected area. With this technique, 16% to 40% of patients require reoperation for persistent peripancreatic sepsis, and mortality varies from 5% to 50%, averaging 30%. The alternative to wide sump drainage involves open packing (marsupialization) of the pancreatic abscess cavity. With this technique, the abdominal fascia is not closed; multiple packing changes, initially in the operating room and subsequently in the intensive care unit, allow repetitive access to the abscess cavity. Retrospective studies have observed an improvement

in outcome with the open drainage technique, compared with the wide sump drainage technique. However, no randomized prospective trials have been reported.

Correction of Associated Biliary Tract Disease. Formerly, definitive biliary tract operations for gallstone-associated pancreatitis were often deferred up to 8 weeks after the acute episode of pancreatitis. This approach has gradually lost favor, primarily because the natural history of gallstone-associated pancreatitis without early surgical intervention is that of frequent recurrences. Up to 50% of patients awaiting deferred elective operation experience a recurrence of gallstone-associated pancreatitis. Since typical episodes of gallstone-associated pancreatitis follow a mild, short-lived clinical course, and since definitive biliary tract operations at the time of the index admission have proved safe and cost-effective, early biliary tract procedures are now favored in most patients. This approach eliminates the need for a second hospitalization and reduces the overall length of stay. At this time, most surgeons proceed with biliary tract operations, usually laparoscopic cholecystectomy, during the index admission but after clinical resolution of pancreatitis. The one exception to this treatment plan involves patients with severe gallstone pancreatitis who have a prolonged clinical course marked by ileus, abdominal distention, a CT scan showing multiple peripancreatic fluid collections, and slow resolution of hyperamylasemia. These patients appear to benefit from a delay in elective operation. In these cases, a nonoperative management course is followed as long as clinical improvement persists, thereby allowing resolution of pancreatic and peripancreatic inflammation. Two to 4 weeks are allowed to elapse between hospitalization for acute pancreatitis and readmission for definitive biliary tract surgery.

Another treatment option for operative intervention in patients with gallstone-associated pancreatitis involves early surgical intervention within the first 72 hours after the onset of the disease. The rationale for such early intervention is that early elimination of ampullary obstruction by a common duct calculus can theoretically reduce the severity of the episode of pancreatitis. In studies comparing historic controls managed by delayed operative intervention with a group undergoing immediate cholecystectomy and common bile duct exploration for calculus retrieval, mortality was 16% versus 2%. However, the mortality in this historic control group is inappropriately high by today's standards, and the conclusion that immediate surgical treatment is indicated in all patients with gallstone pancreatitis is unsupported. In a randomized study of patients with gallstone-associated pancreatitis, it was demonstrated that early operation within 72 hours of admission can be performed safely, with equivalent morbidity and mortality when compared with patients undergoing delayed procedures 3 months after the acute illness.[42] However, patients undergoing early operation required more complicated surgical procedures because the incidence of choledocholithiasis was 64%, versus 18% in the delayed operative group. Further data have failed to reveal any advantage to early operation in patients with gallstone pancreatitis. Early surgical therapy appears to offer no advantage in the majority of patients, often requires more complicated operative intervention, and appears to be overly aggressive, since most patients improve with standard supportive measures, passing their common bile duct calculi without further incident. Thus, the current recommendation for management of patients with gallstone-associated pancreatitis favors initial supportive care, followed by delayed biliary operation during the index admission.

In those patients with a prolonged deteriorating clinical course, the use of endoscopic retrograde cholangiopancreatography (ERCP) or percutaneous transhepatic cholangiography can document the presence of choledocholithiasis, and impacted ampullary stones may be retrieved nonoperatively. For those patients with severe gallstone-associated pancreatitis, recent data support the use of early ERCP and endoscopic sphicterotomy (ES).[26] In that study, 121 patients with acute gallstone pancreatitis were randomized to treatment with ERCP and ES versus conventional therapy. ERCP was performed within 72 hours of admission, and if common bile duct stones were identified, ES and stone extraction were performed. In the subgroup of 46 patients with severe pancreatitis, significantly fewer complications occurred with ERCP and ES (such as pseudocyst, pulmonary insufficiency, and death), and the patients had a shorter mean hospital stay compared with the group managed with supportive care alone. Therefore, in patients with severe attacks of gallstone pancreatitis, the use of early ERCP, combined with ES in the presence of common bile duct stones, appears appropriate.

Deterioration of Clinical Status. In patients with acute pancreatitis and a deteriorating clinical condition who fail to respond to nonoperative supportive care, operative intervention has been advocated. This issue remains the most controversial indication for surgical therapy in patients with acute pancreatitis. Among proponents of early operative intervention, recommended operative procedures range from local débridement of obviously necrotic tissue (necrosectomy) to formal total pancreatectomy. Beger and associates recently generated renewed interest in early necrosectomy in patients judged to have necrotizing pancreatitis by clinical and CT criteria. However, to date, no controlled randomized clinical trials allow realistic evaluation of the efficacy of such early resectional therapies. In a canine model, in a comparison with a nonoperated control group, resectional therapy increased mortality. Overall, there are few objective clinical or experimental data to support the use of routine early pancreatic resection in patients with severe pancreatitis. Nonetheless, operative intervention may still be indicated in selected patients with clinical deterioration and the presumed diagnosis of pancreatitis for the exclusion of another surgically correctable lesion or for the detection and treatment of early pancreatic abscess formation.

CHRONIC PANCREATITIS

Chronic pancreatitis is a clinical entity that includes recurrent or persistent abdominal pain and evidence of exocrine and endocrine pancreatic insufficiency.[39] It is marked pathologically by irreversible parenchymal destruction of pancreatic tissue. Pathologic findings in chronic pancreatitis in both humans and animal models[48] include evidence of acinar loss, glandular shrinkage, proliferative fibrosis, calcification, and ductal stricturing. Electron microscopic findings in chronic pancreatitis reveal evidence of dense collagen and fibroblastic proliferation in the parenchyma; this fibroproliferative response separates large clusters of islet cells with normal or nearly normal ultrastructural features.

Etiology

Chronic pancreatitis is associated with alcohol abuse, hyperparathyroidism, cystic fibrosis, congenital anomalies of the pancreatic duct such as pancreas divisum, and pancreatic trauma. The most common cause of chronic pancreatitis in industrialized countries is alcohol abuse. The exact mechanism whereby alcohol induces the disease is unknown. Dietary factors may have a permissive role in alcohol-related chronic pancreatitis, since the risk of chronic pancreatitis associated with alcohol intake increases in proportion to the protein intake and is maximized by ingestion of a high-fat diet. In underdeveloped or developing countries, chronic pancreatitis, termed tropical pancreatitis, appears to be re-

lated to nutritional deficiencies or toxin ingestion. In patients with hyperparathyroidism, the associated hypercalcemia is believed to be responsible for the chronic pancreatitis, possibly by overstimulating the exocrine secretions of the gland and by predisposing to precipitation of protein aggregates within the main pancreatic ductal system. In some patients with idiopathic chronic pancreatitis, the etiology of the disease is unknown. Various mechanisms may play a role in the pathogenesis of chronic pancreatitis. These include hypersecretion of protein from acinar cells, plugging of the pancreatic ducts with protein precipitates, and pancreatic ductal hypertension, among others.

Clinical Presentation

The incidence of chronic pancreatitis in the United States approximates 4 per 100,000 population. Typically, patients present with a history of alcohol abuse in the fourth or fifth decades of life. Abdominal pain is the feature that prompts consultation. The pain is commonly epigastric in location but may be localized to the right or left side of the midline. Radiation of the pain to the back is common. Some patients have continuous and unremitting pain, whereas others have recurrent episodes of pain that entirely resolve between attacks. Anorexia and weight loss may be present. Insulin-dependent diabetes mellitus occurs in up to one third of patients. Up to one quarter have steatorrhea, indicative of a major reduction in pancreatic exocrine function. Thus, the clinical tetrad of abdominal pain, weight loss, diabetes, and steatorrhea serves as a classic presentation in patients with chronic pancreatitis. Additionally, many patients present with a history of narcotic analgesic abuse in an effort to control their abdominal pain.

Diagnosis

Chronic pancreatitis is usually suspected on clinical findings. Routine laboratory tests are rarely helpful. Radiographic evaluation may reveal pancreatic calcifications on plain abdominal films, a finding at least 95% specific for chronic pancreatitis.

A CT scan of the abdomen is useful in the evaluation of both parenchymal and ductal disease. The size and texture of the gland are evaluated and inspected for pancreatic parenchymal calcifications, nodularity, and inhomogeneous densities, as well as pseudocyst formation or dilatation of the pancreatic ductal system. Important information is gained by the use of endoscopic retrograde pancreatography. Pancreatography can document ductal abnormalities not convincingly demonstrated by CT scan. Also, pancreatography has an essential role in guiding surgical therapy, by providing anatomic information that directs therapy to specific pathology (Fig. 35–9). Characteristic early changes in chronic pancreatitis observed via pancreatography include ductal dilatation and filling of secondary and tertiary branches, which ordinarily are not visualized. Patients with well-established chronic pancreatitis demonstrate ductal strictures and calculi and often show pseudocyst formation. The characteristic *chain of lakes* pancreatogram, representing ductal dilatation in concert with ductal stricturing, is a classic finding in chronic pancreatitis, but it is not observed as frequently as uniform ductal dilatation. An entirely normal pancreatogram in a patient with abdominal pain safely eliminates the diagnosis of chronic pancreatitis.

Pancreatic function tests are occasionally used in the workup of chronic pancreatitis. These tests are generally reserved for difficult diagnostic problems and clinical research and are not essential for preoperative evaluation. The purpose of these tests is to document exocrine pancreatic insufficiency

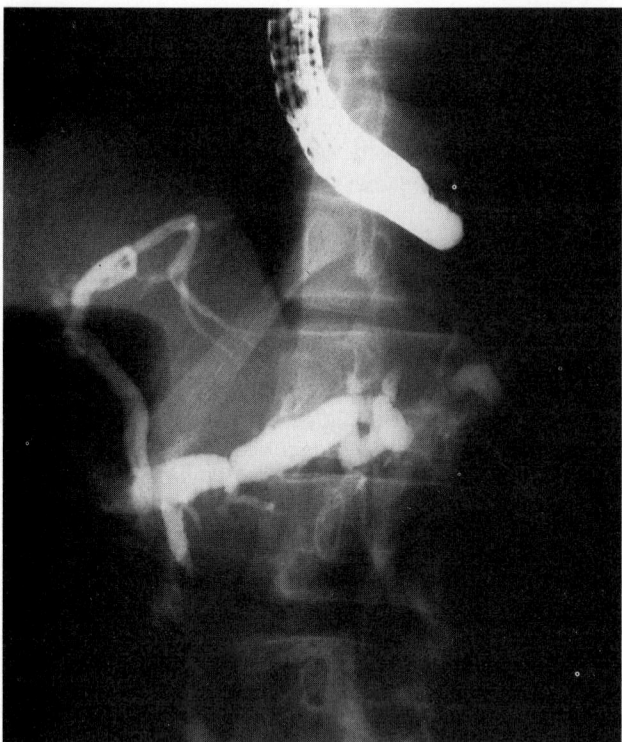

Figure 35–9. An endoscopic retrograde cholangiopancreatogram of a patient with chronic pancreatitis resulting from alcohol abuse. The bile duct appears normal, and the pancreatic duct is diffusely dilated with scattered strictures.

as a marker for parenchymal pathology. Tests such as the Lundh test meal, duodenal essential amino acid perfusion, and the intravenous secretin and cholecystokinin stimulation tests require gastroduodenal intubation with collection of the pancreatic effluent for assessment. Simpler approaches include the bentiromide or pancreolauryl tests, both of which involve the oral administration of test substances with measurement of digestion products in the urine. Another simple test is to examine the stool for increased fat with a 72-hour fecal fat measurement and the Sudan stain.

Pancreatic endocrine function is normally assessed by glucose tolerance testing. More than two thirds of all patients with chronic pancreatitis have abnormal studies. Fortunately, less than one third of patients are insulin-dependent. Chronic pancreatitis-associated diabetes is generally mild and is rarely associated with ketoacidosis or vascular complications. Peripheral neuropathy is a common finding and appears to be related to both the diabetes and the effects of alcohol. Experimental data in a canine model suggest that pancreatic parenchymal fibrosis associated with chronic pancreatitis is associated with abnormal islet responsiveness, causing a circulating insulin deficiency and glucose intolerance, in the presence of histologic and ultrastructural evidence of intact islets of Langerhans.[48] Endocrine function is generally unaffected by ductal drainage procedures but is reduced by resectional therapies.

Nonoperative Management

Three areas are encompassed in the nonoperative management of chronic pancreatitis: control of abdominal pain, treatment of endocrine insufficiency, and treatment of exocrine insufficiency.

The control of abdominal pain can be a major problem, and it is generally the sole indication for operative intervention. In the typical setting of alcohol-related chronic pancre-

atitis, total abstinence from alcohol is mandatory for nonoperative pain relief and is successful in some patients. In addition to abstinence, dietary manipulation, including small-volume, frequent, low-fat meals, is recommended, although controlled data proving efficacy are lacking. High-dosage regimens of exogenous pancreatic enzyme supplements, which theoretically decrease pancreatic secretion and thereby reduce pain, have had variable outcomes and are of limited efficacy. Octreotide has been studied in small numbers of patients, with modest improvements seen in a minority of those treated. Attempts to control pain often require early use of nonnarcotic analgesics, followed later by narcotic analgesics.

Exogenous insulin therapy in patients with chronic pancreatitis-associated diabetes must be used cautiously: one must attempt to control glycosuria and avoid hypoglycemia. In this group of patients, hypoglycemia following insulin administration can arise as the result of poor nutrient absorption secondary to malabsorption or the irregular caloric intake typical of alcoholics.

Digestive enzyme insufficiency with associated steatorrhea or malabsorption occurs in a minority of patients with chronic pancreatitis. When present, exocrine insufficiency is treated with a low-fat diet and with exogenous pancreatic enzyme supplementation. During a typical 4-hour postprandial period, adequate digestion requires the administration of approximately 30,000 I.U. of lipase and 10,000 I.U. of trypsin. Should malabsorption persist even with adequate exogenous pancreatic enzyme supplementation, the addition of histamine H_2-receptor antagonists may prove efficacious by diminishing the gastric acid–induced degradation of the exogenous enzyme preparations.

Operative Management

Surgical treatment of chronic pancreatitis can be broadly categorized into three groups: ampullary procedures, ductal drainage procedures, and ablative procedures. Ablative procedures are usually considered the last step in surgical treatment for patients with chronic pancreatitis because of the fear of producing insulin-dependent diabetes mellitus. The primary goal of operative management is relief of pain, the secondary consideration being to preserve maximal endocrine and exocrine function. Prior to consideration of surgical intervention, mandatory evaluation of pancreatic disease involves parenchymal imaging by CT scan as well as assessment of pancreatic ductal anatomy by endoscopic retrograde pancreatography. The role of therapeutic endoscopic interventions such as stenting of the major or minor pancreatic duct is currently being evaluated.

Ampullary Procedures. Favorable results following sphincteroplasty of the ampulla of Vater for chronic pancreatitis were reported by Doubilet and Mulholland in 1956. At that time, the procedure was designed to eliminate pancreatitis by preventing bile reflux into the pancreatic duct in the setting of a common channel between the distal common bile duct and the pancreatic duct. Results in the intervening years in patients treated by sphincteroplasty have not been favorable, and therefore enthusiasm for the procedure has diminished. Ampullary procedures currently have limited application. In patients with the rare finding of a focal obstruction at the ampullary orifice, transduodenal sphincteroplasty of the major pancreatic duct orifice may be helpful. Also, for patients with recurrent pancreatitis associated with pancreas divisum and relative stenosis of the minor pancreatic duct papilla, transduodenal minor papilloplasty may be successful in up to 85% of patients. However, the results are less favorable in patients with pancreas divisum and established chronic pancreatitis.

Ductal Drainage Procedures. A ductal drainage procedure intended to decompress the pancreatic duct in a retrograde manner was described by Duval in 1954. This procedure involved a limited distal pancreatectomy and an end-to-end pancreaticojejunostomy. It was used as treatment to relieve proximal pancreatic duct obstruction. Although this procedure was successful in selected patients, the enthusiasm for caudal pancreaticojejunostomy diminished as failures of the operation were reported and as knowledge of pancreatic ductal pathology revealed more widespread ductal disease.

In 1958, Peustow and Gillesby described the side-to-side pancreaticojejunostomy, a procedure subsequently modified by Partington and Rochelle. This procedure is now more widely used than the caudal pancreaticojejunostomy, and it has been evaluated in many large clinical series with success rates of 60% to 90%. It is theoretically more appealing than the caudal pancreaticojejunostomy because it decompresses nearly the entire pancreatic duct. Determinants of success for the side-to-side pancreaticojejunostomy include a pancreatic duct greater than 1 cm. in diameter, the presence of pancreatic calcifications, and a pancreatic-jejunal anastomosis longer than 6 cm. Currently, side-to-side pancreaticojejunostomy is the most commonly applied pancreatic ductal drainage procedure, and it is recommended in patients with a dilated pancreatic duct in need of operative therapy for chronic pancreatitis. Ductal drainage does not improve established pancreatic exocrine or endocrine dysfunction, although it may delay the rate of progressive functional impairment in patients with early disease.

Ablative Procedures. The operative treatment of chronic pancreatitis by surgical resection of the pancreas is associated with variable success and the potential for postoperative complications. In carefully selected patients with isolated parenchymal disease in the body and tail of the pancreas, often secondary to trauma, limited distal pancreatectomy (40% to 80% pancreatectomy) has documented success. Such a resection extends no further than to the neck of the pancreas, to the level of the superior mesenteric vein. Subtotal distal pancreatectomy (95% pancreatectomy) involves distal pancreatic resection extending beyond the pancreatic neck to the level of the intrapancreatic portion of the common bile duct (Fig. 35–10). It has been applied to patients with severe diffuse parenchymal disease. Subtotal distal pancreatectomy has a nearly universal risk of postoperative insulin-dependent diabetes mellitus. Sixty to 80% of patients treated by subtotal distal pancreatectomy obtain adequate pain relief. This operation should be reserved for patients who have diffuse parenchymal destruction without duct dilatation or in whom prior lesser procedures have failed.

Pylorus-preserving pancreaticoduodenectomy (modified Whipple operation) should be considered in cases of chronic pancreatitis without ductal dilatation when parenchymal disease affects primarily the head of the gland. In these circumstances, resection of the head of the pancreas and duodenum by pancreaticoduodenectomy provides relief of associated biliary or duodenal obstruction and preserves a substantial mass of islet cell tissue in the body and tail of the gland. Up to 80% of properly selected patients obtain satisfactory results after pancreaticoduodenectomy.

Total pancreatectomy for chronic pancreatitis, combined with the necessary duodenal resection, is usually utilized as a completion pancreatectomy in patients with refractory pain after lesser procedures. In such circumstances, over 60% of patients have been rendered pain-free. However, the significant problems associated with labile insulin sensitivity, steatorrhea, and weight loss dictate that total pancreatectomy be applied as a last resort in carefully selected patients.

Several newer surgical treatments have been reported for the management of patients with chronic pancreatitis. Warren and associates proposed a duodenum-preserving resection of the pancreatic head combined with denervation of the body and tail. Beger and associates reported a similar duodenum-preserving resection of the pancreatic head combined with Roux-en-Y drainage of the retained pancreatic duct.[3] A modified side-to-side pancreaticojejunostomy with an anterior central resection or *coring out* of the pancreatic head has been utilized by Frey and Smith.[12] Recent prospective comparisons between pylorus-preserving pancreaticoduodenectomy and the duodenum-sparing alternatives of Beger and Frey have shown roughly equivalent results.[6, 15]

Pancreatic autotransplantation remains an uncommonly used procedure in patients with chronic pancreatitis. Autotransplantation following resectional therapy, using either islet cell suspensions or segmental grafts, has theoretical value in preserving endocrine function but has had only limited success. Currently, pancreatic autotransplantation for chronic pancreatitis, intended to avert surgically induced diabetes mellitus, has limited indication and utility.

DISRUPTIONS OF THE PANCREATIC DUCT

In adults, disruptions of the main pancreatic duct are most commonly found in the setting of alcoholic pancreatitis, although they may occasionally occur following pancreatitis caused by other factors and as a result of pancreatic trauma or neoplasms. In children, trauma is the leading cause of pancreatic duct disruption. In pancreatic duct disruption, pancreatic exocrine secretions exit the duct at the site of the disruption. Disruptions of the main pancreatic duct cause external or internal pancreatic fistulas. If the pancreatic exocrine secretions drain externally through a drain site or a wound, an external pancreaticocutaneous fistula results. If the exocrine secretions extravasate into the peritoneal cavity but are walled off by adjacent tissues, a pancreatic pseudocyst may occur. Pancreatic ascites occurs when the exocrine secretions extravasate anteriorly from the pancreatic duct, are not walled off, but drain freely into the peritoneal cavity. Pancreatic pleural effusion can result if the secretions extravasate into the retroperitoneum and track cephalad through the diaphragm to enter the thorax, draining into one or both pleural spaces. Rarely, pancreatic secretions may extravasate into a hollow viscus, forming a pancreatic-enteric fistula.

External Pancreatic Fistula

Drainage of pancreatic fluid through an abdominal wound or drain tract that persists for greater than 7 days is, by

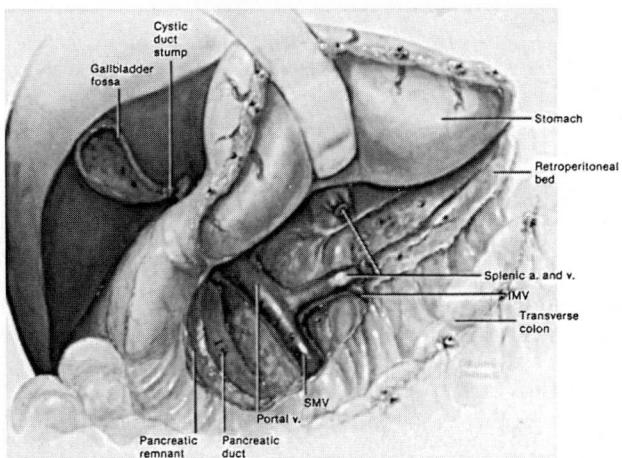

Figure 35–10. Illustration of a 95% pancreatectomy, performed for chronic pancreatitis. (From Cameron, J. L.: Atlas of Surgery. Vol. 1. Toronto, B. C. Decker, 1990, p. 365. Illustration by Corinne Sandone.)

definition, an external pancreatic fistula. Pancreaticocutaneous fistulas follow pancreatic operations in as many as 25% of patients. Fistulas that drain less than 200 ml. per day are classified as low-output fistulas, whereas those draining in excess of 200 ml. per day are high-output fistulas. Complications of pancreaticocutaneous fistulas include sepsis, fluid and electrolyte abnormalities, and skin excoriation. Sinography and CT are used to delineate the anatomy of the fistulous tract and to exclude the presence of undrained cavities. The skin surrounding the fistulous tract is protected by means of appropriate skin care products. Attention is paid to fluid and electrolyte status, with appropriate replacement. Total parenteral nutrition is often utilized to avoid pancreatic stimulation by oral intake and to maximize tissue anabolism. The long-acting somatostatin analog octreotide has been reported to be of benefit in expediting closure of external pancreatic fistulas that fail to close by standard treatment. The majority of external pancreatic fistulas close with nonoperative management. Refractory fistulas may require surgical management. Prior to operation, endoscopic retrograde pancreatography is essential in delineating the anatomy of the pancreatic duct. Fistulas originating from the tail of the pancreas in association with a normal proximal pancreatic duct may best be managed by distal pancreatectomy. Distal pancreatic fistulas associated with abnormalities of the proximal pancreatic duct may be managed by distal pancreatectomy and pancreaticojejunostomy or by pancreaticojejunostomy to the fistula site itself. Fistulas localized in the head, neck, or body of the gland are best managed by Roux-en-Y pancreaticojejunostomy to the fistula tract.

Internal Pancreatic Fistula

Pancreatic Pseudocyst. Pancreatic pseudocysts are localized collections of pancreatic secretions in a cystic structure that lack an epithelial lining and occur as a result of surrounding tissues walling off and containing a pancreatic duct disruption. Pancreatic pseudocysts may be located within the pancreatic parenchyma but more often are adjacent to or near the pancreas in one of the potential spaces that separate the pancreas from adjacent abdominal viscera. Pancreatic pseudocysts represent well over 75% of cystic lesions of the pancreas. Electrolyte concentrations in pseudocyst fluid are equivalent to those in plasma. Pseudocysts contain high concentrations of pancreatic enzymes, including amylase, lipase, and trypsin. Pseudocysts persist for as long as the cyst remains in continuity with the disrupted pancreatic duct. Should the communication between the pancreatic duct and the pseudocyst close secondary to cicatrization, the fluid contents of the cyst are absorbed, and the pseudocyst disappears. Pancreatic pseudocysts develop in up to 10% of patients after an attack of acute alcoholic pancreatitis. Pseudocysts are also associated with acute pancreatitis with other causes, as well as with chronic pancreatitis, pancreatic trauma, and pancreatic neoplasm. By convention, collections of fluid containing pancreatic enzymes that occur within the first 3 weeks after an episode of acute pancreatitis are termed *acute fluid collections* and are not considered pseudocysts.

Clinically, patients with pancreatic pseudocysts most often present with upper abdominal pain, which may be found in up to 90% of patients. Nonspecific symptoms at presentation include nausea and vomiting, as well as weight loss. Physical examination reveals abdominal tenderness in the majority of patients, and an abdominal mass is present in less than half. The most common clinical scenario of a patient with a pancreatic pseudocyst involves abdominal pain as well as early satiety, nausea, and vomiting secondary to gastroduodenal obstruction from the mass effect of the pseudocyst. More uncommon modes of clinical presentation include pru-

ritus and jaundice secondary to common bile duct obstruction, variceal bleeding secondary to either splenic vein or portal vein obstruction, evidence of sepsis secondary to pseudocyst infection, and evidence of intra-abdominal hemorrhage secondary to bleeding from a pseudoaneurysm in adjacent visceral vessels.

Laboratory findings in patients with pancreatic pseudocysts are nonspecific. Many have elevations of serum amylase, and a small percentage of patients have evidence of liver function test abnormalities. Although a pancreatic pseudocyst may be suspected by clinical and laboratory findings, radiographic studies are necessary for definitive diagnosis. A CT scan of the abdomen is the favored study in an initial assessment for determining the presence of a pancreatic pseudocyst (Fig. 35–11). Ultrasound evaluation is nearly as accurate as CT scanning and can be recommended in the follow-up of patients with known pseudocysts for assessment of interval size changes. Analysis of the fluid within a peripancreatic cystic structure may help distinguish between such entities as pseudocyst, mucinous cystic tumor, or serous cystic tumor.[21] However, in most patients, such invasive testing is not needed, as the diagnosis of a pseudocyst is supported by the clinical postpancreatitis setting.

The management of patients with pseudocysts is guided by the natural history. Previous reports suggested that spontaneous resolution of pseudocysts occurred in less than 25% of patients. The natural history of pseudocysts followed by ultrasound has been reported by Bradley and associates.[5] These data indicated that pseudocysts documented to be present for less than 6 weeks had a 40% spontaneous resolution rate and a 20% complication rate, whereas pseudocysts present for greater than 12 weeks never resolved and were associated with a complication rate of 67%. Pseudocyst size has also been considered to be a factor in determining the need for surgical therapy; most authors suggest operative therapy for pseudocysts greater than 5 to 6 cm. With these criteria for operation, the operative treatment of pancreatic pseudocysts has a mortality of 5 to 12% and morbidity of 21 to 53%. The advent of CT scanning for patients suspected of having pancreatic pseudocysts has allowed more precise documentation of the natural history. In a report of 75 patients followed at Johns Hopkins Hospital, patients with asymptomatic pseudocysts were preferentially managed nonoperatively, independent of pseudocyst size.[47] Operative management was performed only for persistent abdominal

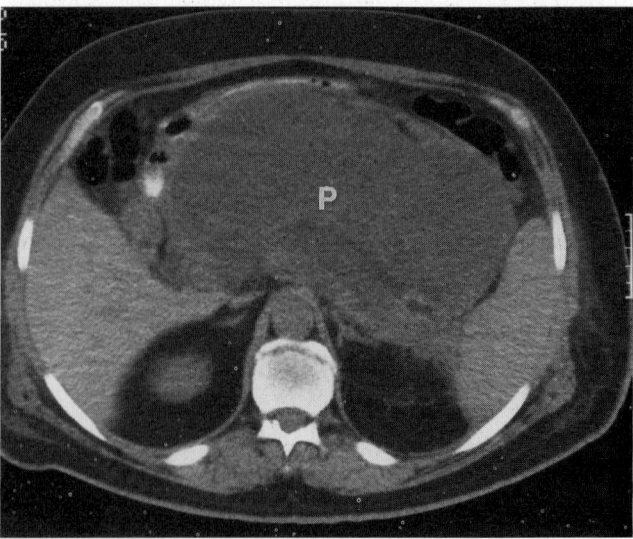

Figure 35–11. CT scan of a patient with a large retrogastric pancreatic pseudocyst (P), which developed after an attack of gallstone pancreatitis.

pain, pseudocyst enlargement, or pseudocyst complications. Forty-eight percent of the entire group was successfully managed nonoperatively, whereas 52% required surgical therapy. In the group managed without operation, with a mean follow-up of 1 year, 60% had complete pseudocyst resolution documented radiographically, and 40% had pseudocysts that remained stable or decreased in size. No pseudocyst-related mortality occurred in either group. Pseudocyst size correlated with eventual need for operation: 67% of patients with pseudocysts larger than 6 cm. required surgical therapy, and those with pseudocysts 6 cm. or less required operations significantly less frequently. Twenty-seven percent of pseudocysts greater than 10 cm. in size were successfully managed nonoperatively. Similar results have been reported from the Mayo Clinic by Vitas and Sarr.[45] These data suggest that strict size criteria alone are not sufficient to determine the need for operative versus nonoperative management.

Currently, treatment of patients with pancreatic pseudocysts is based on the clinical setting, the presence or absence of symptoms, the age and size of the pseudocyst, and the presence or absence of complications. In the most common clinical settings, a pseudocyst is discovered after an episode of acute alcoholic pancreatitis. With the resolution of pancreatitis, a patient who is free of complications and able to tolerate oral intake is discharged from the hospital, with follow-up CT or ultrasound studies obtained at monthly intervals to assess for pseudocyst enlargement, stability, or resolution. In contrast, if, after an episode of acute pancreatitis, a pseudocyst is associated with pain or early satiety precluding oral intake and hospital discharge, the patient remains hospitalized, supported with total parenteral nutrition, while pseudocyst size and clinical symptoms are assessed. Persistent symptoms, failure to tolerate oral intake, or pseudocyst-related complications require intervention. A 6-week period is generally allowed between the episode of pancreatitis and elective operative intervention, to allow satisfactory internal drainage.

Occasional patients are encountered without an obvious history of pancreatitis or trauma and with a pseudocyst of indeterminate age. If asymptomatic, these patients are followed with outpatient CT or ultrasound studies for several months, with observation of pseudocyst resolution or size diminution. However, if at the time of presentation significant symptoms exist, intervention is indicated, if one assumes that pseudocyst wall maturation has already occurred.

For pseudocysts that fail to resolve and require intervention, specialized preoperative studies other than abdominal ultrasound or CT scan are not mandatory. Endoscopic retrograde pancreatography is not essential prior to surgical therapy, although it may be useful in recurrent or multiple pseudocysts or to better define pancreatic duct anatomy prior to operative intervention. If endoscopic pancreatography is employed prior to surgical intervention, it is recommended that it be performed within 24 hours of operation to reduce the risk of pseudocyst infection. Options for the management of pseudocysts include internal drainage, pseudocyst excision, external drainage, and percutaneous or endoscopic techniques. When possible, treatment of pancreatic pseudocysts includes biopsy of the pseudocyst wall to exclude the possibility of a cystic neoplasm.

The preferred operative therapy in uncomplicated pseudocysts is internal drainage. The three options for operative internal drainage of pseudocysts are drainage to a defunctionalized Roux-en-Y jejunal limb (cystojejunostomy), drainage into the stomach (cystogastrostomy), and drainage into the duodenum (cystoduodenostomy). Cystojejunostomy is the most versatile and useful method of cyst drainage (Fig. 35–12), being particularly appropriate when the pseudocyst presents at the base of the transverse mesocolon or is not adher-

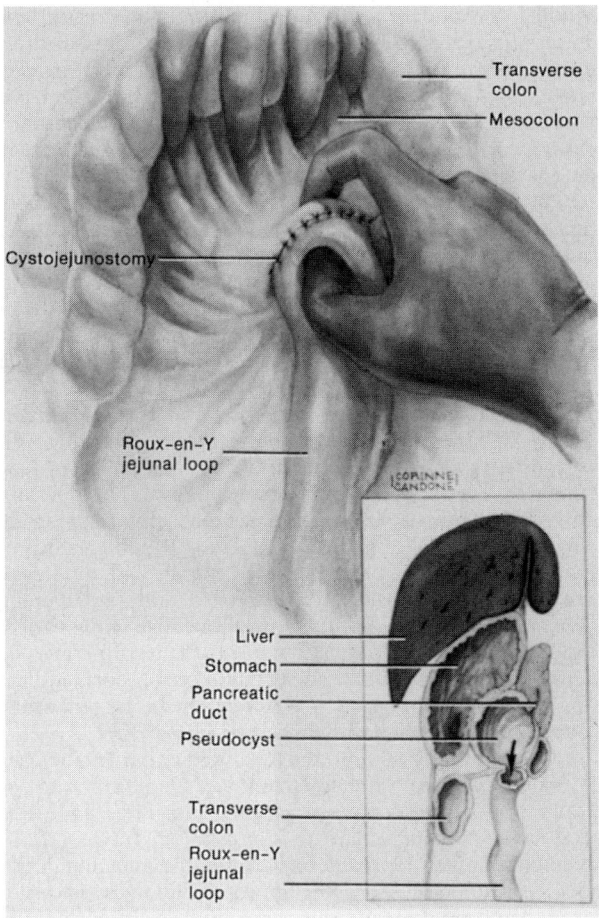

Figure 35–12. Illustration of internal drainage of a pancreatic pseudocyst by Roux-en-Y cystojejunostomy through the base of the transverse mesocolon. (From Cameron, J. L.: Atlas of Surgery. Vol. 1. Toronto, B. C. Decker, 1990, p. 379.)

ent to the posterior gastric wall. Cystogastrostomy can be used when the pseudocyst is adherent to the posterior wall of the stomach. When feasible, cystogastrostomy is a faster and less technically demanding procedure than Roux-en-Y cystojejunostomy. The final option for internal drainage involves cystoduodenostomy. This procedure has limited utility, being applicable to pseudocysts in the head of the pancreas within 1 cm. of the duodenal lumen. Cystoduodenostomy has the potential for the formation of a duodenal fistula. It is best performed similar to the way in which cystogastrostomy is performed, by opening the lateral duodenal wall and creating a connection between the pancreatic pseudocyst and the duodenum through a medial duodenotomy. The majority of pancreatic pseudocysts treated operatively are drained internally by means of cystojejunostomy or cystogastrostomy.

Excisional therapy of pancreatic pseudocysts is utilized in a minority of cases, usually limited to distal pancreatic resections for pseudocysts in the tail of the gland. Distal pancreatectomy with or without splenectomy in this setting may be a technically challenging procedure because of peripancreatic and pericystic inflammation. Following distal pancreatectomy, if an obstructed proximal pancreatic duct is present, drainage of the pancreatic remnant by means of a Roux-en-Y pancreaticojejunostomy is indicated.

External drainage of pancreatic pseudocysts via the operative route is indicated with gross infection, intraoperatively in an unstable patient in whom more complex surgical intervention is precluded, and with immature pseudocysts with thin, nonfibrous walls that do not allow safe internal drainage. A pancreaticocutaneous fistula occurs after external drainage, which often closes spontaneously. Persistent pancreaticocutaneous fistulas may require operative closure.

Nonoperative approaches to the drainage of pancreatic pseudocysts have gained popularity in recent years.[50] Both percutaneous and endoscopic techniques have been used. Currently, the most common technique is percutaneous catheter drainage. Typical methods use either a tandem trocar catheter insertion technique or the Seldinger technique. After the pseudocyst is entered, the fluid is aspirated, and catheters ranging from 7 to 16 French are placed into the pseudocyst cavity. The catheters are exteriorized and irrigated with small amounts of saline several times a day. The typical duration of catheter drainage ranges from several days to several months. It appears that pseudocysts communicating with the pancreatic duct on sinography require longer catheter drainage.[11] To date, the only study to evaluate operative versus percutaneous drainage in a prospective fashion has been reported by Lang and colleagues.[19] In this study of patients with severe pancreatitis as manifested by five or more Ranson prognostic signs, surgical and percutaneous drainage appeared to be equally efficacious. However, the long-term efficacy of percutaneous catheter drainage has been poorly documented, and several recent reports indicate that caution should be exercised to temper the current enthusiasm for percutaneous drainage approaches.

Endoscopic approaches to the treatment of pancreatic pseudocysts include two different techniques. One technique uses flexible upper endoscopy to localize, aspirate, and drain pseudocysts bulging into the stomach or duodenum via placement of an endoprosthesis between the intestinal lumen and the pseudocyst. A newer approach involves placement of transpapillary drainage catheters either to drain the pseudocyst directly or to stent (bridge) the pancreatic ductal disruption associated with the pseudocyst. Although reports of such therapies have been encouraging, further analysis of these techniques is ongoing.[8, 17]

Pancreatic Ascites and Pancreatic Pleural Effusion. Similar pathophysiology and etiology apply to the entities of pancreatic ascites and pancreatic pleural effusion. Both entities occur as a result of a pancreatic duct disruption secondary, in most cases, to alcohol abuse. Often these entities occur in the absence of a history of clinical pancreatitis. In pancreatic ascites, pancreatic exocrine secretions exiting a pancreatic duct disruption drain anteriorly into the peritoneal cavity. In pancreatic pleural effusion, the exocrine secretions drain from a duct disruption posteriorly into the retroperitoneum and then in a cephalad direction into the mediastinum and pleural space.

Patients with pancreatic ascites usually present with painless massive ascites and are often thought to have alcoholic cirrhosis with ascites.[23] The diagnosis of pancreatic ascites is best made by paracentesis, in which analysis of the ascitic fluid reveals it to be high in amylase (greater than 1000 units per liter) and high in albumin (greater than 3 gm. per 100 ml.). Patients with pancreatic pleural effusion generally present with primary pulmonary symptoms such as dyspnea, chest pain, and cough. Abdominal symptoms may be absent. Findings on physical examination are consistent with pleural effusion. The diagnosis of pancreatic pleural effusion is made by thoracentesis, again revealing a greatly elevated pleural fluid amylase and a high albumin content. Up to one quarter of patients may present with both pancreatic ascites and pancreatic pleural effusion. In both conditions the serum amylase is usually but not invariably elevated.

Nonoperative treatment is initially indicated in patients with pancreatic ascites and pancreatic pleural effusion (Table

TABLE 35–8. Management of Patients with Internal Pancreatic Fistula

Nonoperative treatment
  Prohibition of oral intake
  Nasogastric tube suction
  Paracentesis (for pancreatic ascites)
  Thoracentesis or chest tube (for pancreatic pleural effusion)
  Hyperalimentation
  Somatostatin (octreotide)
Operative treatment
  Direct duct leak
    Roux-en-Y drainage of duct leak
    Pancreatic resection for distal duct leak, with Roux-en-Y drainage of proximal pancreatic remnant if proximal duct disease present
Leaking pseudocyst
  Roux-en-Y drainage of pseudocyst to jejunum
  Small, distal pseudocyst—possible resection, with Roux-en-Y drainage of proximal pancreatic remnant if proximal duct disease present
External drainage

35–8). The rationale of treatment is to decrease pancreatic exocrine secretion, thereby encouraging the pancreatic duct disruption to seal. Management includes the prohibition of oral feeding, nasogastric suction, total parenteral nutrition, and the use of paracentesis or thoracentesis, as appropriate, to eliminate the ascites or pleural fluid and thereby encourage the apposition of serosal surfaces. The long-acting somatostatin analog octreotide may be of some benefit in selected cases.[28] Nonoperative management is recommended for a 2- to 3-week period and may resolve the clinical entity in 50% of patients. In patients not cured by nonoperative management, surgical therapy is indicated after delineation of pancreatic duct anatomy using endoscopic retrograde pancreatography (Fig. 35–13). Most patients with pancreatic ascites or pancreatic pleural effusion are leaking from an incompletely formed or ruptured pseudocyst, and a minority have

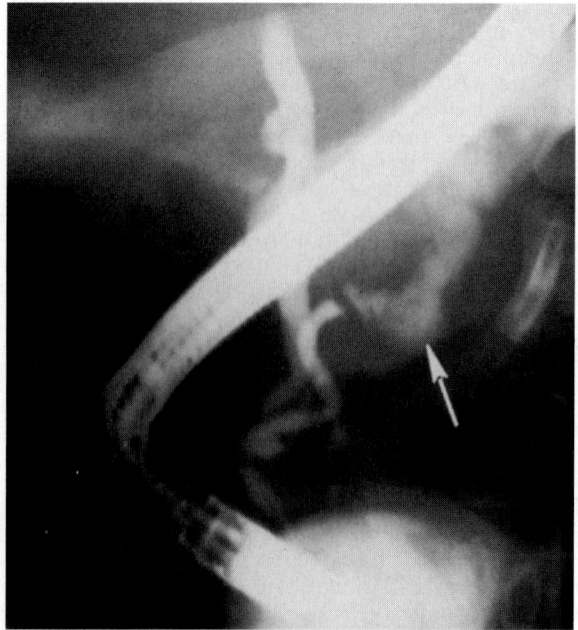

Figure 35–13. Endoscopic retrograde cholangiopancreatogram in a patient with pancreatic ascites. The pancreatic duct disruption is well visualized, demonstrating an abrupt cutoff with contrast extravasating into the lesser sac (arrow).

direct duct leaks. Surgical therapy is based on the findings of pancreatography. Distal pancreatic duct disruption or a leaking pseudocyst in the body or tail of the pancreas may be treated with distal pancreatectomy or with Roux-en-Y pancreaticojejunostomy. Pancreatic duct leaks in the more proximal aspects of the gland are treated with Roux-en-Y pancreaticojejunostomy to the site of pancreatic duct or pseudocyst disruption.

Pancreatic-Enteric Fistula. Spontaneous decompression of a pancreatic pseudocyst or abscess into an adjacent hollow viscus can produce the unusual finding of a pancreatic-enteric fistula. Most commonly, these fistulas occur between the pancreas and the splenic flexure or transverse colon. Less frequently involved organs include the stomach, duodenum, small bowel, and extrahepatic biliary tree. Symptomatic pancreatic pseudocysts have rarely been reported to be cured by spontaneous decompression into an enteric structure. In most cases, however, spontaneous rupture of a pseudocyst or abscess into a hollow viscus causes bleeding or sepsis, and appropriate operative intervention becomes necessary for correction of the disorder.

NEOPLASMS OF THE PANCREAS
Exocrine Tumors
Cancer of the Exocrine Pancreas

In the United States there are approximately 28,000 cases of cancer of the exocrine pancreas diagnosed each year. Cancer of the pancreas is the fifth most common cause of cancer death, exceeded only by lung, colorectal, breast, and prostate cancers. Ninety percent of patients die within the first year after diagnosis. In both men and women, pancreatic cancer represents 3% of all cancers and 5% of all cancer deaths. Since 1960, the relative 5-year survival rate for all cases of pancreatic cancer has increased from 1% to 3%. Considering only cancers of the digestive tract, cancer of the pancreas ranks second, behind colorectal cancer, in incidence and cancer death rates. Cancer of the pancreas is more common in blacks than in whites, more common in smokers than in nonsmokers, more common in males than in females, and appears to be linked to the presence of diabetes mellitus. Cancer of the pancreas is possibly linked to both a history of previous chronic pancreatitis and the ingestion of a high-fat diet. A small percentage of patients appear to have an inherited or familial form of pancreatic cancer.

Pathologically, over 90% of malignant pancreatic exocrine tumors are classified as duct cell adenocarcinomas. The most common site of origin of duct cell adenocarcinomas is the pancreatic head, where two thirds of the cases are localized. Subtypes of duct cell adenocarcinoma include mucinous and adenosquamous varieties. Less common types of pancreatic exocrine cancer include cystadenocarcinoma and acinar cell carcinoma.

Recent studies have identified recurrent chromosome abnormalities in pancreatic adenocarcinoma, which can provide clues to the specific genes involved in the pathogenesis of this tumor. Griffin and co-workers analyzed 62 primary pancreas cancers and found frequent loss of chromosomes 18, 13, 12, and 6, as well as gains of chromosomes 20 and 7.[14] Using a complementary approach, Seymour and colleagues constructed an allelotype (an extensive survey of the loss of alleles) in a series of pancreatic adenocarcinomas.[36] In these allelic loss studies, the most frequently lost chromosome arms were 17p and 18q, followed by 3p, 4q, 7p, 10p, 11q, 12q, and 16q. Since the loss of one allele at a tumor suppressor gene results in the loss of gene function if the second copy is mutated, these patterns of allelic loss suggest certain regions of the genome that may be tumor suppressor gene

loci. In fact, recent evidence indicates that at least three tumor suppressor genes are involved in pancreatic adenocarcinoma: *p53*, *DPC4*, and *MTS1*.[7, 14a, 31]

In addition to the presence of tumor suppressor genes, activating point mutations in k-*ras* have been found in over 80% of pancreatic cancers studied. Such activating mutations have been found to be more prevalent in cancers obtained from patients who had smoked cigarettes at some point during their lives than in nonsmokers. This association suggests that carcinogens in cigarette smoke are responsible for some of the mutations in k-*ras*, a premise that is supported by three additional lines of evidence. First, cigarette smoking is a major risk factor for the development of pancreatic cancer; second, nitrosamines contained in cigarette smoke are capable of inducing G-to-A transitions at the second nucleotide of a GG pair, a mutation that is the single most common alteration found in k-*ras* mutation-positive tumors; and third, the administration of nitrosamines found in cigarette smoke has been found to induce the development of pancreatic adenocarcinomas containing point mutations in codon 12 of k-*ras*. Thus, the identification of mutations in pancreatic cancers obtained from smokers has strengthened the epidemiologic link between pancreatic cancer and cigarette smoking.

Somewhat like the mutations in oncogenes and tumor suppressor genes found in colon cancer, an emerging pattern of acquired somatic mutations appears to be involved in the development of pancreatic adenocarcinoma. K-*ras*, p53, DPC4, and MTS1 all appear to be frequent targets of mutation or deletion. Cytogenetic studies and molecular studies assessing allelic loss suggest that several additional tumor suppressor genes involved in the pathogenesis of pancreatic carcinoma remain to be discovered.[9]

PERIAMPULLARY ADENOCARCINOMA

Diagnosis. Neoplasms originating in the region of the ampulla of Vater are categorized as periampullary tumors. Clinically, radiographically, intraoperatively, and pathologically, it is often difficult to accurately differentiate cancer of the head of the pancreas from three other malignant periampullary neoplasms: ampullary carcinoma, duodenal carcinoma, and carcinoma of the distal common bile duct. Approximately 85% of these tumors arise from the head of the pancreas; less than 10% represent ampullary carcinomas, and duodenal carcinomas and carcinomas of the distal common bile duct represent less than 5% each. The most common clinical features in patients with periampullary carcinoma are jaundice, weight loss, and abdominal pain. Approximately three quarters of patients present with jaundice, and it is this symptom that normally causes the patient to seek medical attention. Weight loss occurs in over 75% of patients. Abdominal pain is found in 70% of patients, generally reflected as a dull, aching pain in the mid epigastrium or the right upper quadrant, with possible radiation to the back. Anorexia, weakness, pruritus, and alteration of bowel habits may also be present. The most common physical finding at initial presentation is jaundice. Hepatomegaly and a palpable gallbladder may also be noted.

The majority of patients with periampullary carcinoma have laboratory abnormalities marked by elevated serum bilirubin and alkaline phosphatase, with mild elevations of hepatic transaminases. Serologic markers for pancreatic carcinoma have been evaluated, including carcinoembryonic antigen (CEA), DU-PAN-2, alpha-fetoprotein (AFP), pancreatic oncofetal antigen (POA), and carbohydrate antigen 19–9 (CA 19–9). No currently available serologic test is completely accurate for diagnosis; the tests are limited by cross-reactivity with other tumors and low sensitivity for small, potentially resectable lesions. At present, CA 19–9 is used most frequently to assist in diagnosis and follow-up.

In patients with suspected periampullary carcinoma, radiologic intervention is extremely important for diagnosis, staging, and management. Older techniques such as barium upper gastrointestinal series may be positive in patients with large tumors, showing widening of the duodenal sweep or the *inverted 3* sign. Sonography is a useful screening examination, particularly in patients less than 40 years old, who are more likely to have cholestatic jaundice. In older patients, CT scanning is an essential procedure for the evaluation of periampullary neoplasms. Dynamic, thin-section, contrast-enhanced CT scanning is superior to sonography, in that it allows visualization of the entire pancreas, without distortion from overlying bowel gas, and it provides better accuracy in detecting hepatic metastases, determining the size of the periampullary neoplasm, and locally staging the tumor. MRI appears to offer no advantage over CT.

After CT scanning, the site of biliary obstruction is defined by cholangiography. Cholangiography can suggest the site of tumor origin and is essential in planning successful resection and reconstruction (Fig. 35–14). Percutaneous transhepatic cholangiography (PTHC) has nearly a 100% success rate in visualizing the biliary tree in the setting of dilated intrahepatic ducts, with a 75% success rate in visualizing the biliary tree in settings of nondilated ducts. PTHC in the setting of an obstructing periampullary neoplasm is generally combined with catheter drainage of the biliary tree via the percutaneous transhepatic route. ERCP has a role in patients with periampullary neoplasms. ERCP is particularly valuable in the diagnosis of duodenal or ampullary carcinoma, where diagnostic tissue can be obtained by endoscopic biopsy. ERCP may also be useful in cases of partial biliary obstruction, where the endoscopically injected contrast can fill the proximal biliary tree above the tumor, thus defining the proximal biliary anatomy for subsequent biliary-enteric reconstruction. Biliary endoprostheses may be placed at the time of ERCP as a short- or long-term maneuver to palliate biliary obstruction and allow for reduction in the degree of jaundice.

Selective celiac and mesenteric angiography, combined with the evaluation of portal venous anatomy, can be used for delineation of major arterial and venous anatomy and for staging for resectability. In a review of the use of staging angiography for 90 patients with periampullary neoplasms at Johns Hopkins Hospital, the resectability rate was 77% in patients with normal studies, 35% in patients with encasement of the portal or superior mesenteric veins or the superior mesenteric or hepatic arteries, and 0% in patients with visceral vessel occlusion.[10] Laparoscopy has been advocated by some as a means of improving staging, particularly addressing the issue of small, unsuspected liver metastases or peritoneal implants. Recently, endoscopic ultrasound has been applied to the staging of periampullary neoplasms, with early results in skilled hands appearing to be comparable to those obtained with CT and angiography.[34]

Management. The majority of patients presenting with periampullary neoplasms are operative candidates and are treated surgically. In a minority of patients, nonoperative therapy may be appropriate.

Nonoperative Therapy. Nonoperative therapy is an option in patients with documented distant metastases, unresectable local disease, and acute or chronic debilitating illnesses. In patients treated nonoperatively, attempts are made to acquire a tissue diagnosis and to palliate features of the disease such as abdominal pain and biliary obstruction. Tissue diagnosis can be obtained via biopsy of distant metastases, biopsy of hepatic metastases, cytologic specimens acquired by ERCP or PTHC, or percutaneous needle biopsy of the primary pancreatic neoplasm. Percutaneous needle biopsy of the primary tumor is generally reserved for those patients who are to be treated nonoperatively and is not used preoperatively in patients with localized, apparently resectable tumors. Following tissue diagnosis, palliation of tumor-associated pain commences with oral analgesics. Poorly controlled pain may require percutaneous celiac ganglion blocks. Palliation of biliary obstruction can be achieved nonoperatively via a percutaneous transhepatic drainage catheter or by an endoprosthesis. Percutaneous transhepatic internal drainage allows constant access to the biliary tree but requires an external catheter. Endoprostheses have the advantage of avoiding external catheters, but their use is limited by prosthesis migration and side hole obstruction by biliary sludge, which mandate repeat endoscopy for manipulation or replacement. There appears to be some advantage to using the newer metallic endoprostheses as compared with the older plastic varieties. Nonoperative palliation of duodenal obstruction, which occurs in up to one third of patients, can be difficult, with very limited possibilities for success with the use of systemic chemotherapy or external beam radiotherapy. High-grade duodenal obstruction generally requires operative intervention for gastroenterostomy.

Operative Therapy. The majority of patients with periampullary carcinoma are managed operatively. Preoperative preparation includes (1) assessment and supplementation of nutritional status; (2) standard mechanical and oral antibiotic bowel preparation; (3) assessment of coagulation status, with correction of prolonged prothrombin time by exogenous vitamin K; (4) intravenous antibiotic prophylaxis administered perioperatively to reduce the possibility of a wound infection; and (5) consideration of placement of a percutaneous transhepatic catheter or endoscopic placement of an endoprosthesis. Drainage of the biliary tree is best applied in patients with biliary sepsis secondary to cholangitis or in patients with major nutritional deficiency states and high-grade biliary obstruction. Randomized, prospective studies have shown that routine percutaneous transhepatic biliary drainage does not reduce operative mortality and may prolong hospital stay.

RESECTIONAL THERAPY. At exploration, care is taken to assess distant intra-abdominal metastases. Hepatic metastases, serosal implants, and lymph node metastases outside of the resection area indicate unresectable disease. The duodenum and head of the pancreas are elevated from the retroperitoneum, lifting these structures off the inferior vena cava and the aorta (Kocher's maneuver). The superior mesenteric ar-

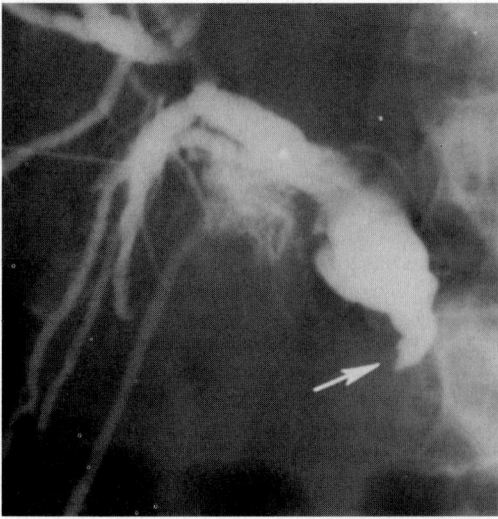

Figure 35–14. Percutaneous transhepatic cholangiogram of a patient with periampullary adenocarcinoma, showing a dilated intrahepatic and extrahepatic biliary tree with a typical *bird's beak* obstruction (arrow) at the level of the common bile duct.

tery is palpated for the purpose of ensuring that the vessel is not encased by tumor extending from the uncinate process. The common bile duct is isolated in the hepatic portal, as is the anterior surface of the portal vein and the hepatic artery. At the inferior aspect of the neck of the pancreas, the anterior surface of the superior mesenteric vein is identified. The plane between the neck of the pancreas and the anterior surface of the superior mesenteric vein is developed, fully elevating the pancreatic neck from the vein. If no tumor is encountered outside of the resection margin during these maneuvers, resection is performed. The role of intraoperative biopsy to obtain a tissue diagnosis prior to resection remains controversial. Benign periampullary lesions presenting as solid periampullary masses in patients in their sixth and seventh decades causing pain, weight loss, and jaundice are unusual; therefore, few resections are performed for benign disease in this setting. If resection is performed and the permanent pathology reveals chronic pancreatitis, resection remains appropriate and effective therapy. Currently, for all patients explored with curative intent for a preoperative diagnosis of periampullary carcinoma, the resectability rate approaches 35% to 40%. The resectability rate is lowest for adenocarcinoma of the head of the pancreas (15% to 20%), is approximately 80% for ampullary carcinoma, and averages 60% for duodenal and distal common bile duct tumors. Preoperative staging using MRI, visceral angiography, and/or preoperative laparoscopy can significantly improve these resectability rates.

The first successful resection of a periampullary carcinoma was performed by Halsted at Johns Hopkins Hospital in 1898. He performed a local resection of an ampullary tumor. Presently, standard resection for periampullary carcinoma involves a pancreaticoduodenectomy, first performed successfully by Kausch in 1909 and popularized by Whipple in 1935. The gallbladder, common bile duct, entire duodenum, head of the pancreas to the level of the superior mesenteric vein, pylorus, and distal stomach are resected (Fig. 35–15). Restoration of gastrointestinal tract continuity utilizes the proximal jejunum brought through the transverse mesocolon for pancreaticojejunostomy, hepaticojejunostomy, and gastro-

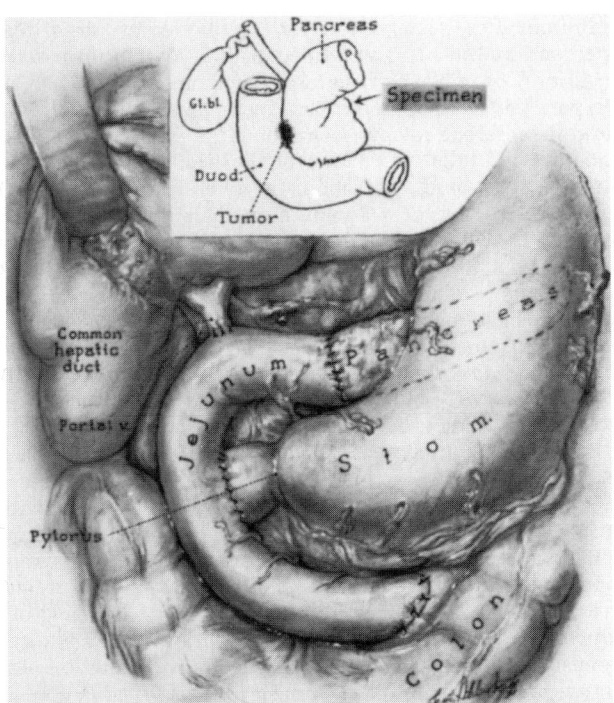

Figure 35–16. Illustration of a pylorus-preserving pancreaticoduodenectomy and the subsequent reconstruction. The inset at the top depicts the resected specimen. (From Cameron, J. L.: Current status of the Whipple operation for periampullary carcinoma. Surg. Rounds, September: 77, 1988.)

jejunostomy. The standard Whipple resection remains the classic therapy for periampullary carcinoma and can be successfully performed in experienced hands with a perioperative mortality of less than 5%. A modification of the standard Whipple resection, the pylorus-preserving pancreaticoduodenectomy (Fig. 35–16), has gained popularity in recent years. This modification eliminates gastric resection and leaves a 2-cm. cuff of duodenum for enteric reconstruction as a duodenojejunostomy. Operative time is shortened somewhat, and the incidence of postgastrectomy complications such as dumping and marginal ulceration, which are associated with the standard Whipple procedure, is reduced. A further theoretical advantage is that the postprandial release of gastrin and secretin are nearly normal in patients who undergo the pylorus-saving procedure, compared with patients who undergo a standard Whipple resection. Accumulated data to date indicate no compromise in survival in patients undergoing pylorus preservation.

Formerly, total pancreatectomy was proposed as a more appropriate operation for pancreatic carcinoma. Support was based on a reported 30% to 40% incidence of multifocality of pancreatic cancer, a concern about tumor cell implantation into the remnant pancreatic duct at Whipple resection, and the high mortality and morbidity associated with the pancreaticojejunostomy required in the Whipple reconstruction. It now appears that concerns about tumor seeding and multicentricity are not relevant, because the 5-year survival rate in patients who undergo the classic total pancreatectomy is equivalent to that in patients who undergo Whipple resection. Also, improved techniques and postoperative management have made pancreaticojejunostomy safer. Total pancreatectomy necessarily removes all exocrine and endocrine pancreatic function, requiring exogenous pancreatic enzyme and insulin administration.

At present, the overall 5-year survival rate for all patients with resected periampullary carcinoma approximates 15 to 25%. A major determinant of survival is the site of origin of

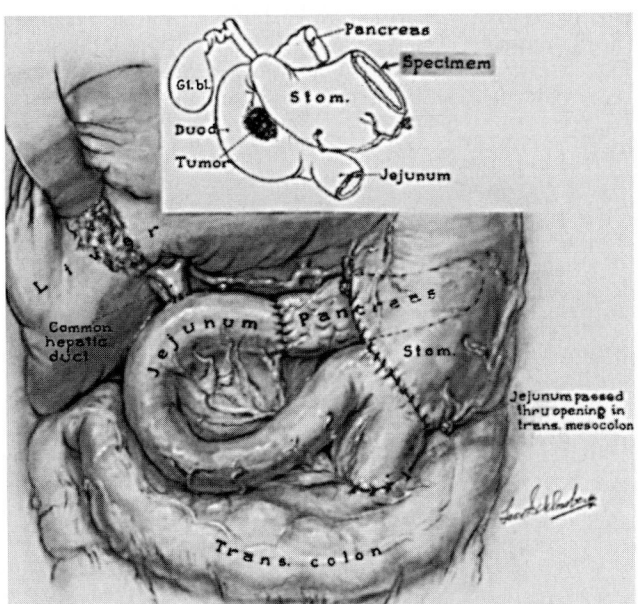

Figure 35–15. Illustration of a standard pancreaticoduodenectomy (Whipple procedure) and the subsequent reconstruction. The inset at the top depicts the resected specimen. (From Cameron, J. L.: Current status of the Whipple operation for periampullary carcinoma. Surg. Rounds, September: 77, 1988.)

the tumor. Resectable cancers of the duodenum, distal bile duct, and ampulla are associated with 5-year survival rates of 40 to 60%, whereas resectable carcinoma of the head of the pancreas is associated with a 5-year survival rate of 5 to 25%. In a recent review from Johns Hopkins Hospital of patients with adenocarcinoma of the head of the pancreas undergoing Whipple resection, the overall actuarial 5-year survival rate was 21%, with a median survival of 15.5 months.[49] Multivariate analysis indicated that the strongest predictors of long-term survival were diploid tumor DNA content, tumor diameter less than 3 cm., negative nodal status, and negative resection margins. Additionally, analysis of patient outcomes over time indicated a significant improvement in survival for patients resected from the 1970s to the 1990s, partially explained by the increased use of postoperative chemoradiation therapy.

PALLIATIVE SURGERY. Palliative surgery for periampullary carcinoma is performed in patients with unresectable disease discovered at the time of laparotomy or in patients with prohibitive risk for resectional therapy (advanced age, limited cardiopulmonary reserve, and so forth) whose symptoms are poorly alleviated nonoperatively. Palliative surgical treatment seeks to alleviate biliary obstruction, duodenal obstruction, and tumor-associated pain. Multiple authors have extensively reviewed the results of palliative operations for unresectable periampullary cancer. Biliary obstruction is treated with biliary-enteric bypass, by means of the gallbladder or the common hepatic duct. Although symptomatic gastroduodenal obstruction is uncommon at initial diagnosis of periampullary cancer, up to one third of patients with unresectable tumors develop obstructive symptoms prior to death. For this reason, gastrojejunostomy is usually performed at the time of biliary bypass. Prophylactic gastrojejunostomy does not add to the morbidity or mortality of palliative surgery for unresectable disease. Abdominal and back pain associated with unresectable periampullary tumors can be a major problem. Chemical splanchnicectomy using 50% alcohol can be performed intraoperatively in an effort to achieve pain control, with significant improvement in both subjective and objective measures of pain.[22]

Adjuvant Therapy. The bulk of available data indicates that chemotherapy alone has no role after curative resection or as palliative therapy of periampullary carcinoma. Single-agent therapy with 5-fluorouracil, mitomycin C, streptozotocin, or high-dose methotrexate yields partial response rates of 10 to 20%, but it does not prolong survival. Although combination drug therapy appears to improve response rates in carefully selected patients, there has been only limited improvement in survival demonstrated for any chemotherapeutic regimens.

The combination of radiation and chemotherapy has been shown to prolong survival following curative Whipple resection. In a controlled prospective trial reported by the Gastrointestinal Tumor Study Group (GITSG), patients receiving 40 Gy external beam radiation therapy (EBRT) and weekly intravenous 5-fluorouracil following curative resection demonstrated a significantly longer median survival (20 months), compared with the resected group receiving no adjuvant therapy (11 months).[16] In this study, the 2-year actuarial survival was 42% in the treated group versus 15% for the control group. A follow-up study by the GITSG confirmed improved survival with combination radiation and chemotherapy,[13] and recent results from Johns Hopkins Hospital also indicated a survival benefit in treated patients.[49]

Results of treatment of unresectable periampullary cancer are not as promising as those for resectable tumors. The median survival in patients with unresectable tumors is approximately 6 to 9 months. EBRT alone does not prolong survival, according to most reports. The combination of EBRT

and chemotherapy, usually 5-fluorouracil, has yielded mixed results on overall survival, with several reports suggesting improved outcome compared with EBRT alone, and others showing no advantage. In an effort to boost the irradiation dose delivered directly to unresectable tumors, several studies of intraoperative radiation therapy (IORT) have been undertaken. IORT alone does not improve survival and appears to increase perioperative complications. IORT in combination with EBRT with or without chemotherapy has had conflicting results, with most studies showing improved local control of the tumor but little improvement in long-term survival. Neoadjuvant therapy for periampullary tumors, typically involving preoperative EBRT and 5-fluorouracil-based chemotherapy, is currently being evaluated. Early results indicate no convincing survival benefits in patients who receive such preoperative neoadjuvant regimens.

CARCINOMA OF THE BODY AND TAIL OF THE PANCREAS

Adenocarcinomas of the body and tail of the pancreas represent up to 30% of all cases of pancreatic carcinoma. Tumors in this location generally grow to a large size prior to the development of symptoms. This silent course occurs as a result of the retroperitoneal location of the body and tail of the pancreas away from the common bile duct and duodenum. Thus, these tumors do not cause early obstructive jaundice or gastrointestinal obstructive symptoms.

The clinical presentation of patients with carcinoma of the body and tail of the pancreas generally involves weight loss and pain, which are present in up to 90% of patients. Weight loss may be significant, often involving up to 20% of the patient's body weight. Because of the distance between the primary tumor and the intrapancreatic portion of the common bile duct, less than 10% of patients present with jaundice. On physical examination, the findings are often nonspecific. Vague abdominal tenderness may be present, or an abdominal mass may be palpated. Evidence of metastatic dissemination may be found and can include hepatomegaly, ascites, a Blumer's shelf, or lymph node metastases to Virchow's nodes.

The diagnosis of carcinoma of the body and tail of the pancreas depends on radiographic assessment. Serum tests for tumor-associated antigens such as CEA and CA 19–9 are usually positive with large tumors, but they may be negative. The abdominal CT scan is the best initial radiographic study (Fig. 35–17). The CT scan can demonstrate the primary tumor in the pancreas, can be used for assessment of liver metasta-

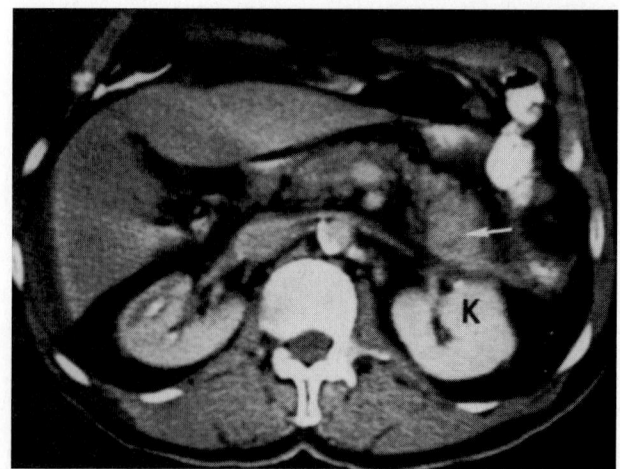

Figure 35–17. CT scan of a patient with adenocarcinoma of the body and tail of the pancreas. The tumor (arrow) is seen anterior and adjacent to the left kidney (K). At operation, the tumor was invading Gerota's fascia.

ses, and may give information regarding involvement of adjacent visceral and vascular structures or lymph node metastases. Endoscopic retrograde pancreatography usually documents a pancreatic duct abnormality. The most common abnormality on ERCP is a pancreatic duct cutoff, representing obstruction to the flow of contrast material by the neoplasm. The proximal pancreatic duct is generally normal. In the absence of prior abdominal trauma and an otherwise normal pancreatogram, a finding such as stenosis or obstruction of the pancreatic duct in the region of the body or tail of the pancreas is highly suggestive of a pancreatic neoplasm.

Following the radiographic identification of an abnormality in the body or tail of the pancreas, an attempt at obtaining a tissue diagnosis should be considered. Pathologic evaluation can differentiate pancreatic adenocarcinoma, which is rarely resectable in this region, from more favorable neoplasms such as pancreatic islet cell tumors or benign pancreatic neoplasms, which are often resectable. Tissue diagnosis may be obtained at laparotomy or via percutaneous needle aspiration of the primary mass. Prior to laparotomy, visceral arteriography may be helpful. Evaluation of the celiac axis, splenic artery and vein, and superior mesenteric artery and vein is performed. Splenic artery or vein involvement by tumor does not preclude curative resection. However, tumor involvement of the main trunk of the celiac axis, superior mesenteric artery, or superior mesenteric vein usually indicates unresectability. Good-risk patients without evidence of metastatic disease and with favorable CT or arteriographic findings are best served by abdominal exploration with the intent of tumor resection. In the unusual patient with a resectable adenocarcinoma, distal pancreatectomy and *en bloc* splenectomy provide an opportunity for cure and serve as good palliation of tumor-associated pain. In patients with unresectable disease diagnosed at laparotomy, intraoperative chemical splanchnicectomy should be used to palliate pain. In the majority of patients with carcinoma of the body and tail of the pancreas, biliary bypass and duodenal bypass are not indicated. However, a proportion of patients with carcinoma of the body and tail of the pancreas have tumor encroachment at the level of the duodenojejunal junction, and this small group of patients may be well served by a palliative gastroenterostomy. Poor-risk patients or those with evidence of metastatic or clearly unresectable tumors by CT scan or arteriography are not explored and instead undergo percutaneous biopsy for tissue diagnosis.

The resectability rate for carcinoma of the body and tail of the pancreas is low (less than 7%), and the prognosis is generally dismal (mean survival, 5 to 6 months). The few reported 5-year survivors following resection generally had their tumors discovered incidentally during evaluation of other intra-abdominal pathology. Patients undergoing resection of adenocarcinoma of the body and tail of the pancreas with curative intent may be benefited by adjuvant chemotherapy and postoperative EBRT, although confirmatory data are lacking. Unresectable tumors usually respond poorly to radiation or chemotherapy.

CYSTADENOCARCINOMA OF THE PANCREAS

Cystadenocarcinoma generally arises in females between the ages of 40 and 60, and it represents less than 2% of all pancreatic exocrine neoplasms. Cystadenocarcinomas often present as cystic masses in the body and tail of the pancreas, associated with abdominal and back pain. CT scan of the abdomen typically reveals a tumor mass with associated cysts, which may be misinterpreted as representing a pancreatic pseudocyst. Histologically, these cystic tumors are lined with an epithelium with disordered columnar cells associated with mucin production and papillary features. When this diagnosis is suspected, resectability is assessed by contrast-enhanced CT or arteriography. Tissue diagnosis in patients with metastatic or unresectable disease may be obtained by percutaneous biopsy. Patients without evidence of metastatic or unresectable disease are candidates for exploration. At the time of laparotomy, it may be impossible to distinguish between a malignant cystadenocarcinoma and a benign cystadenoma. Resectable lesions in the body and tail of the pancreas are treated by distal pancreatectomy and *en bloc* splenectomy. Resectable lesions in the head of the pancreas, which are less common, are treated by pancreaticoduodenectomy. The long-term survival rate for resected cystadenocarcinomas approaches 50%, greatly in excess of the rate for the more common pancreatic ductal adenocarcinoma.

ACINAR CELL CARCINOMA OF THE PANCREAS

This is a rare malignancy of the pancreas that has no sexual predominance. These tumors are usually discovered when they are already large in size and are associated with weight loss and pain. Histologically, they consist of epithelium with tall cylindric cells, containing an eosinophilic cytoplasm with periodic acid–Schiff (PAS) positivity in their apical regions. Electron microscopy reveals classic features of intracellular zymogen granules. Patients with these tumors are diagnosed, assessed for resectability, and managed in a similar fashion to patients with pancreatic ductal adenocarcinoma.

Benign Neoplasms of the Exocrine Pancreas

CYSTADENOMA

The majority of cystic lesions of the pancreas are pancreatic pseudocysts. Cystadenomas constitute less than 10% of cystic pancreatic lesions, with a predilection for middle-aged and older women. It is frequently difficult to differentiate between benign and malignant cystic neoplasms of the pancreas based on clinical, radiographic, or gross pathologic findings. Symptoms are often vague and may include abdominal pain, gastrointestinal obstructive symptoms, or, rarely, obstructive jaundice. Grossly, these tumors usually appear as large unilobulated or multilobulated cystic masses. The two most common forms of these cystic tumors are serous neoplasms and mucinous neoplasms. Serous tumors are almost always benign, typically fail to express CEA in the epithelial cells, and histologically are composed of a honeycomb of small-diameter cysts lined by a glycogen-rich low-cuboidal epithelium. Mucinous tumors represent a more heterogeneous group, with a variable potential for malignant degeneration. Histologically, mucinous cystic neoplasms contain a tall columnar epithelium and may stain positively for CEA. Resection is recommended for good-risk patients with suspected cystic neoplasms.

SOLID AND PAPILLARY NEOPLASMS OF THE PANCREAS

These unusual tumors have a notable female predominance and are usually found in patients between 10 and 35 years of age. Most occur in the body or tail of the gland. These tumors tend to grow to a large size, and evidence of local invasion is observed frequently. On gross examination, these neoplasms are large, rounded masses often containing hemorrhagic areas. Histologic findings reveal a mixture of solid, papillary, and microcystic changes with cystic degeneration. These tumors are potentially curable by resection, and most patients have long-term survival. Appropriate pancreatic resection involves distal pancreatectomy for lesions of the body and tail of the pancreas and pancreaticoduodenectomy for lesions of the head.

Endocrine Tumors

Endocrine tumors of the pancreas are rare, with an annual clinically recognized incidence of 5 per 1 million population.

TABLE 35–9. Classification of Functional Pancreatic Endocrine Tumors

Tumor Name	Major Hormone(s)	Cell Type	Syndrome	Malignancy Rate	Extrapancreatic Location
Insulinoma	Insulin	Beta cell	Hypoglycemia	<15%	Rare
Gastrinoma (Zollinger-Ellison syndrome)	Gastrin	Non-beta cell	Peptic ulcer Diarrhea	50%	Frequent
VIPoma (Verner-Morrison syndrome)	VIP Prostaglandins	Non-beta cell	Watery diarrhea Hypokalemia Achlorhydria	Majority	Occasional
Glucagonoma	Glucagon	Alpha cell	Hyperglycemia Dermatitis	Majority	Rare
Somatostatinoma	Somatostatin	Delta cell	Hyperglycemia Steatorrhea Gallstones	Majority	Rare

In contrast, the prevalence of these tumors in unselected autopsy material approximates 1 per 100, where they are usually noted as incidental findings. Pancreatic endocrine cells are presumed to originate from neural crest cells. Cells of this origin are termed APUD cells, indicating that they have a high content of *a*mine, have capacity for amine *p*recursor *u*ptake, and contain an amino acid *d*ecarboxylase. A generalized derangement of the APUD system may cause abnormalities of multiple endocrine cells, as is observed in the multiple endocrine neoplasia (MEN) syndromes. Recent genetic observations have added to our knowledge of pancreatic endocrine tumors. Up to 50% of malignant tumors have been found to have clonal chromosome abnormalities, with an absence of *ras* oncogene mutations. Both sporadic and MEN-associated tumors have been shown to harbor mutations on the long arm of chromosome 11 (11q) in many cases, indicating the presence of a tumor suppressor gene.

Functional endocrine tumors of the pancreas are conventionally named according to the major hormone produced by the tumor (Table 35–9). The majority (more than 75%) of tumors discovered *premortem* are functional and elaborate one or more hormonal products into the bloodstream. Patients with normal serum levels of hormones and no recognized clinical manifestations who have pancreatic endocrine tumors are considered to have nonfunctional islet cell tumors.

All endocrine tumors of the pancreas have a similar light-microscopic appearance. Routine histologic examination does not predict the biologic behavior or endocrine manifestations of these neoplasms. Immunofluorescence techniques and the peroxidase-antiperoxidase procedure allow demonstration of specific hormones within tumor cells. Malignancy is determined by the presence of local invasion, spread to regional lymph nodes, or existence of hepatic or distant metastases.

The general principles applicable to the management of patients with suspected functional pancreatic endocrine tumors involve, first, the recognition of the abnormal physiology or characteristic syndrome; second, the detection of hormone elevations in serum by radioimmunoassay; and third, the localization and staging of the tumor in preparation for operative therapy. Characteristic clinical syndromes have been well described for insulinoma, gastrinoma, VIPoma, and glucagonoma. Radioimmunoassay is widely available for measurement of serum insulin, gastrin, VIP, and glucagon. Less widely available are the assays for somatostatin, PP, prostaglandins, and other hormonal markers. The standard techniques used for pancreatic endocrine tumor localization include CT scanning with intravenous and oral contrast, visceral angiography, transhepatic portal venous sampling, and ultrasonography, either endoscopic or intraoperative. The

place of MRI in the evaluation of pancreatic islet cell tumors remains to be defined. The accuracy of the CT scan in detecting the primary tumor within the pancreas varies from 35 to 85% and is largely based on the size of the tumor. Larger lesions are more easily detectable (Fig. 35–18). The CT scan is also used in the evaluation for hepatic metastases. In a patient with biochemical documentation of hormone excess, particularly for insulinoma and gastrinoma, it is not uncommon for the CT scan to be normal. The next step in radiographic assessment may be visceral angiography. The angiogram is particularly useful in identifying an enhancing tumor blush in lesions less than 1 cm. in size not demonstrated by CT scan (Fig. 35–19). Two newer techniques that appear promising in tumor localization include endoscopic ultrasonography and somatostatin receptor imaging. Tumors not localized by CT, angiography, endoscopic ultrasound, or somatostatin receptor imaging may be localized by the invasive technique of transhepatic portal venous sampling. In experienced hands, this technique is safe and useful, based on the ability to demonstrate a step-up in hormone concentration at the portal venous drainage site of the primary tumor.

At exploration, a thorough evaluation of the pancreas and peripancreatic region is undertaken. The pancreatic head is assessed bimanually by means of Kocher's maneuver, and the body and tail are explored by dividing the gastrocolic

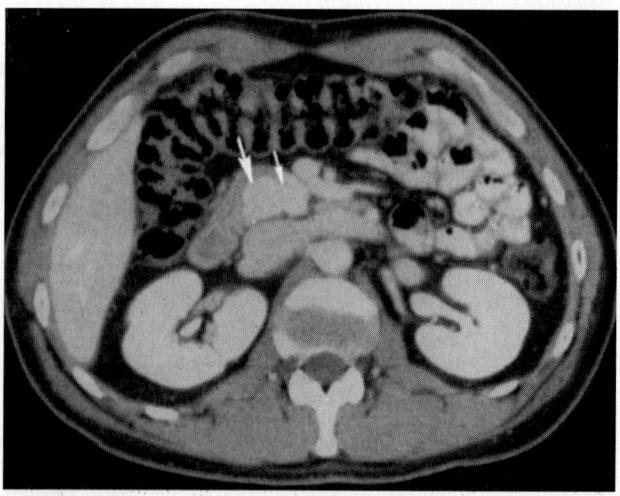

Figure 35–18. Contrast-enhanced CT scan of a patient with a malignant insulinoma of the head and uncinate process of the pancreas. The 3-cm. tumor (large arrow) lies adjacent to the superior mesenteric vein (small arrow). The tumor was resected by pylorus-preserving pancreaticoduodenectomy, and the hyperinsulinism was cured.

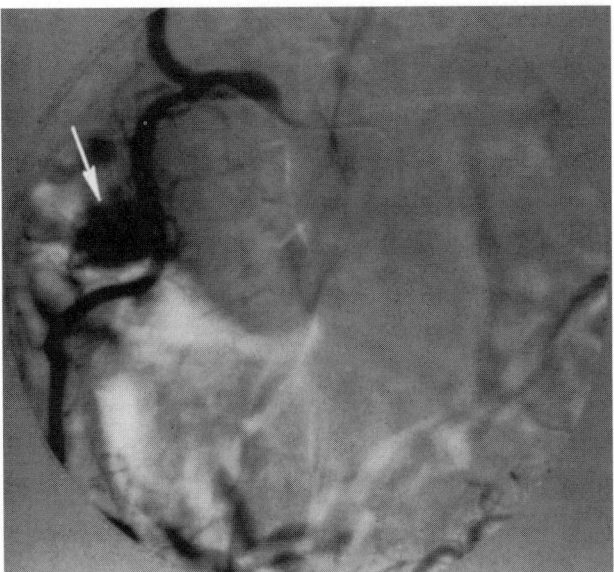

Figure 35–19. Selective celiac arteriogram in a patient with Zollinger-Ellison syndrome. The hepatic artery injection fills the gastroduodenal artery, which reveals a tumor blush (arrow) in the region of the duodenum or head of the pancreas. At exploration, a 2-cm. benign duodenal gastrinoma was identified and locally resected.

ligament and the peritoneum at the inferior pancreatic margin. The liver is carefully assessed for evidence of hepatic metastases. Tumors are sought at common extrapancreatic sites, such as the duodenum, small bowel mesentery, and lymph nodes. Small pancreatic lesions may be difficult to detect by bimanual palpation alone, and intraoperative real-time ultrasound may assist in their identification. The distribution of pancreatic endocrine tumors varies, with gastrinomas, somatostatinomas, and PPomas most commonly found in the head of the gland and insulinomas and glucagonomas tending to be evenly distributed throughout the pancreas. The goals of surgical therapy for pancreatic islet cell tumors include control of symptoms due to hormone excess, excision of maximal neoplastic tissue, and prevention of tumor recurrence. Operative strategies vary for the different tumors.

Insulinoma

The most common endocrine tumor of the pancreas is the insulinoma. The first recognition of the insulinoma syndrome is attributed to Whipple and associates. Insulinoma is associated with Whipple's triad, which consists of (1) symptoms of hypoglycemia at fasting, (2) documentation of blood glucose levels of less than 50 mg. per 100 ml., and (3) relief of symptoms following administration of glucose. Insulinomas synthesize and secrete insulin autonomously in the presence of low blood glucose levels, causing spontaneous hypoglycemia and characteristic clinical symptoms. These symptoms can be categorized into two groups: hypoglycemia-induced catecholamine-surge symptoms (tremor, irritability, weakness, diaphoresis, tachycardia, and hunger) and neuroglycopenic symptoms (personality change, confusion, obtundation, seizure, and coma). Typically, the relief of symptoms is achieved by the consumption of carbohydrate-rich foods.

In an adult population, the differential diagnosis of hypoglycemia includes functional hypoglycemia associated with gastrectomy or gastroenterostomy, chronic adrenal insufficiency, hypopituitarism, extensive hepatic insufficiency, surreptitious administration of insulin or ingestion of sulfonylureas, and reactive hypoglycemia. Of these diagnoses,

reactive hypoglycemia is the most common, normally causing symptoms 3 to 5 hours after meals and not associated with fasting hypoglycemia.

The most reliable method for diagnosing insulinomas involves a monitored 72-hour fast. Blood for glucose and insulin determinations is sampled every 4 to 6 hours during the fast and particularly when symptoms develop. Symptomatic hypoglycemia with fasting is usually associated with concurrent serum insulin levels greater than 25 μU. per ml. Additional support for the diagnosis of insulinoma is derived from the calculation of the insulin-to-glucose ratio. Normal values are less than 0.3, whereas nearly all patients with insulinomas demonstrate insulin to glucose ratios greater than 0.4 after an overnight fast. As C peptide and proinsulin are synthesized in excess along with insulin by insulinoma cells, C peptide and proinsulin levels are usually elevated in the presence of insulinoma. Further support for the diagnosis of insulinoma is obtained by screening for the possibility of surreptitious insulin or sulfonylurea administration. Sulfonylureas are a group of oral hypoglycemic agents that stimulate insulin secretion and are used for the treatment of noninsulin-dependent adult-onset diabetes. The presence of sulfonylureas can be assessed by serum screening.

Following biochemical diagnosis and appropriate localization studies, the treatment of insulinoma is surgical. Up to 90% of patients have benign solitary pancreatic adenomas amenable to surgical cure. Malignant insulinoma is present in 10 to 15% of cases.

At the time of exploration, insulinomas are found evenly distributed throughout the pancreas, with one third located in the head, one third in the body, and one third in the tail. Small benign adenomas not in proximity to the pancreatic duct, located anywhere in the gland, may be enucleated (Fig. 35–20). In the body and tail of the gland, larger benign lesions or those in proximity to the pancreatic duct are usually excised by distal pancreatectomy. Large benign lesions in the head of the pancreas, not amenable to local excision, may be resected by pancreaticoduodenectomy.[44] If at the time of exploration no tumor is identified, a blind distal pancreatic resection to the level of the superior mesenteric vein may be considered, in the hope of excising a previously unidentified adenoma. Another option is to close the patient without resection and perform a postoperative transhepatic portal venous insulin sampling, to allow definitive localization prior to resectional therapy.

In cases of malignant insulinoma, resection of the primary tumor and accessible metastases should be considered. Such resections may include distal pancreatectomy for lesions of the body and tail of the gland or pancreaticoduodenectomy for resectable lesions of the head of the gland. Tumor debulking may be helpful in reducing hypoglycemic symptoms in patients not well controlled by medical therapy preoperatively. Pharmacologic therapy may be useful in patients with residual tumor following resection when symptomatic hypoglycemia is not avoided by frequent feedings. Diazoxide, in doses of 600 or 1000 mg. per day, can improve hypoglycemic symptoms because of its ability to directly inhibit the release of insulin from beta cells. Salt and water retention following diazoxide therapy can be improved by the use of a thiazide diuretic, which also has a synergistic effect in improving hypoglycemia via inhibition of insulin secretion. As with other pancreatic islet cell tumors, there is evidence to support the use of adjuvant chemotherapy or hormonal therapy in patients with unresectable disease (e.g., streptozotocin, octreotide).

Gastrinoma (Zollinger-Ellison Syndrome)

Following the first report of an islet cell tumor of the pancreas associated with peptic ulcer disease by Sailer and

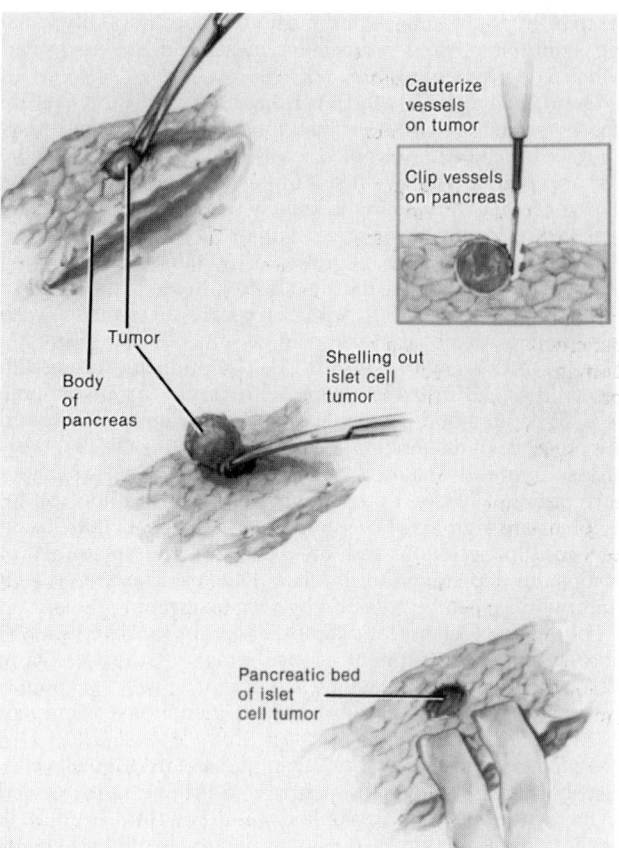

Figure 35–20. Technique used for enucleation of a benign insulinoma, using scissors (top left and center) or electrocautery (top right). After enucleation, the site of tumor excision is drained (bottom right). (From Cameron, J. L.: Atlas of Surgery. Vol. 1. Toronto, B. C. Decker, 1990, p. 441.)

Zinninger in 1946, Zollinger and Ellison in 1955 described two patients with florid peptic ulcer disease and pancreatic islet cell tumors. The diagnostic triad proposed for this syndrome at that time included (1) the presence of primary peptic ulcerations in unusual locations, (2) gastric hypersecretion of gigantic proportions that persists despite adequate therapy, and (3) the identification of an islet cell tumor of the pancreas. In the intervening decades, much information has accumulated regarding these gastrin-secreting tumors and the associated Zollinger-Ellison syndrome.[1] It is estimated that 0.1% of patients with primary duodenal ulcer disease and up to 2% of patients with recurrent ulcers following standard ulcer therapy harbor a gastrinoma. Seventy-five percent of gastrinomas occur sporadically, in the absence of other endocrinopathies, whereas 25% are associated with the MEN-I syndrome (hyperparathyroidism, pancreatic endocrine tumors, and pituitary tumors). Formerly, over 60% of gastrinomas were regarded as malignant on the basis of the findings of metastatic disease at the time of laparotomy. More recent information suggests that as screening for hypergastrinemia becomes more widespread, the diagnosis of gastrinoma is being made earlier, with discovery of a higher percentage of solitary, benign, curable tumors.

Clinical manifestations of gastrinoma are nearly exclusively related to hypergastrinemia. Peptic ulceration of the upper gastrointestinal tract and abdominal pain are the most common findings, occurring in 90% of patients. Although the finding of postbulbar duodenal ulcers is suggestive of Zollinger-Ellison syndrome, the most frequently found ulcer is in the duodenal bulb. Diarrhea occurs in up to 50% of patients, and 10% of patients present with diarrhea as the

TABLE 35–10. Diagnosis: Suspect and Screen for Gastrin

Initial diagnosis of peptic ulcer disease
Recurrent peptic ulcer
Failure of medical therapy for peptic ulcer
Postoperative peptic ulcer
Postbulbar peptic ulcer
Family history of peptic ulcer
Peptic ulcer and diarrhea
Prolonged undiagnosed diarrhea
MEN Type I kindred
Known nongastrinoma pancreatic endocrine tumor
Prominent gastric rugal folds on upper gastrointestinal series

sole manifestation of the syndrome. The diarrhea observed in patients with gastrinoma arises as a result of gastric hypersecretion, and it can be eliminated by nasogastric suction or adequate doses of gastric antisecretory medications. A history compatible with peptic esophageal injury can be obtained in up to 10% of patients, representing acid injury to the esophagus as a result of gastroesophageal reflux.

The diagnosis of gastrinoma requires a proper level of suspicion in several clinical settings (Table 35–10). When it is suspected, fasting serum gastrin levels should be obtained. In patients with gastrinoma, the fasting serum gastrin level is usually elevated above the normal range of 100 to 200 pg. per ml. A fasting gastrin over 1000 pg. per ml. is generally diagnostic of gastrinoma when accompanied by well-established acid peptic disease or hyperchlorhydria. Many patients with gastrinomas have fasting gastrin values in an intermediate range of 200 to 1000 pg. per ml. The documentation of fasting hypergastrinemia alone is not sufficient for diagnosis. Gastrin is the normal secretory product of antral G cells, and hypergastrinemia may exist in other pathophysiologic states, both ulcerogenic and nonulcerogenic (Table 35–11). Identification of the correct cause of hypergastrinemia utilizes knowledge of the clinical setting as well as two additional diagnostic modalities: gastric acid analysis and provocative testing.

Gastric acid analysis differentiates ulcerogenic from nonulcerogenic states. The analysis is performed after stopping antisecretory medications and allows the measurement of the basal acid output (BAO) and the maximal acid output (MAO). A BAO in excess of 15 mEq. per hour in nonoperated patients or in excess of 5 mEq. per hour in patients with previous acid-reducing operations supports the diagnosis of gastrinoma. A BAO/MAO ratio in excess of 0.6 provides additional support for the diagnosis.

Provocative testing should be employed when the diagnosis is considered, particularly in patients with fasting gastrin levels in the range of 200 to 1000 pg. per ml. Provocative testing can be helpful in differentiating between gastrinoma, antral G-cell hyperplasia/hyperfunction, and other causes

TABLE 35–11. Disease States Associated with Hypergastrinemia

Ulcerogenic (Hyperchlorhydric)	Nonulcerogenic (Nonhyperchlorhydric)
Zollinger-Ellison syndrome	Postvagotomy
Retained excluded antrum	Pernicious anemia
Gastric outlet obstruction	Atrophic gastritis
Antral G-cell hyperplasia/hyperfunction	Short gut syndrome
	Renal failure

of ulcerogenic hypergastrinemia. The intravenous secretin stimulation test is the provocative test of choice. The test is performed after an overnight fast, by administering 2 units of Kabi secretin per kg. of body weight as an intravenous bolus and obtaining serum samples for gastrin for up to 30 minutes. An absolute increase in the gastrin level of 200 pg. per ml. over the baseline level is diagnostic of gastrinoma. Patients with antral G-cell hyperplasia/hyperfunction have a flat gastrin response to secretin. The gastrin response to a test meal is also helpful in distinguishing the causes of ulcerogenic hypergastrinemia. In the fasting state, serum gastrin levels are measured before and at 15-minute intervals for 1 hour after a test meal. Patients with gastrinoma have little to no postprandial change in serum gastrin (a less than 50% increase over basal), whereas patients with antral G-cell hyperfunction have a greater than 100% increase in serum gastrin.

After the diagnosis of gastrinoma, patient management follows two distinct, yet interrelated, pathways: (1) control of gastrin acid hypersecretion, and (2) alteration of the natural history of the gastrinoma (i.e., tumor localization, assessment of metastatic disease, and resection of localized tumor for cure). Formerly, patients with gastrinoma died of complications from overwhelming gastric acid hypersecretion. At that time, total gastrectomy provided the most reliable means of controlling the ulcer diathesis without effect on the natural history of the gastrinoma. Since the advent of powerful antisecretory medications such as histamine H_2-receptor antagonists and substituted benzimidazoles, the pharmacologic control of gastric acid hypersecretion has improved, and total gastrectomy is rarely indicated. However, it is now recognized that tumor progression continues in the presence of antisecretory medications, and the majority of patients with unresected gastrinoma succumb to the neoplastic process. The current strategy for patients with gastrinoma, particularly those with *sporadic* gastrinomas not associated with the MEN Type I syndrome, involves careful evaluation at initial diagnosis for potential curative resection.

The substituted benzimidazoles (omeprazole and lansoprazole) have now replaced the histamine H_2-receptor antagonists as the drugs of choice for gastrinoma. Omeprazole and lansoprazole selectively inhibit the H^+-K^+-adenosine triphosphatase (proton pump) on the luminal surface of the gastric parietal cell. These drugs are effective in patients with gastrinoma, either as primary treatment before exploration or in patients with unresectable lesions who will require long-term therapy. Typical daily doses for gastrinoma patients vary from 40 to 160 mg. per day for omeprazole and from 30 to 90 mg. per day for lansoprazole. The doses should be adjusted to achieve a nonacidic gastric pH during the hour immediately prior to the next dose of the drug.

After the institution of appropriate pharmacologic therapy to control gastric hypersecretion, all patients undergo radiographic studies in an effort to localize the primary tumor and to assess metastatic disease. Patients with radiographically suspected unresectable metastatic disease to the liver should undergo percutaneous biopsy for histologic verification. If unresectable metastatic tumor is documented, the patient is not explored and is maintained on antisecretory medication. In the absence of documented unresectable disease, all patients should undergo exploration with curative intent.

At the time of exploration, the entire abdomen is carefully assessed, paying particular attention to the pancreas and to the known locations of extrapancreatic gastrinomas. Abnormal masses and peripancreatic lymph nodes are excised and submitted for frozen section. Intraoperative ultrasound may be valuable in identifying nonpalpable intrapancreatic disease. If no tumor is encountered, a longitudinal duodenotomy can be performed at the second portion of the duodenum (Fig. 35–21), and the duodenum can be bimanually palpated and carefully everted in a search for duodenal gastrinomas. Duodenal gastrinomas are typically submucosal in location, and they are resected with a small margin of normal duodenal tissue. Another method used to identify duodenal tumors is intraoperative transillumination, performed by passing a flexible upper endoscope into the duodenum via the oral route. Tumors within the pancreas are resected by enucleation or partial pancreatectomy. Tumors that are easily accessible to the pancreatic surface, small (less than 2 cm.), and well-encapsulated may be carefully enucleated. Larger tumors without defined capsules or situated deep in the pancreatic parenchyma usually require pancreatic resection. Tumors of the neck, body, and tail are treated by distal pancreatectomy; tumors in the pancreatic head or uncinate process are resected by pancreaticoduodenectomy.

Despite extensive preoperative localization studies and meticulous surgical exploration, some patients with gastrinoma have no tumor demonstrable at laparotomy. The proportion of such patients varies from 5 to 40%, depending on such factors as the security of the diagnosis, the availability of and experience with localization techniques, the experience of the surgeon, and the use of blind resection based solely on transhepatic portal venous sampling results. If exploration is negative, several alternatives are available to the surgeon, including closure without intervention, parietal cell vagotomy, and total gastrectomy. Closure without intervention appears to be appropriate in patients with controlled acid hypersecretion. Parietal cell vagotomy may be considered a means of reducing antisecretory drug requirements in patients on high-dose therapy without previous life-threatening complications. Total gastrectomy is best reserved for patients with past life-threatening complications of ulcer disease while under appropriate medical management.

Results of selected recent series of patients with gastrinoma treated surgically have revealed improving results. Up to 35% of patients explored for gastrinoma with curative intent have been rendered eugastrinemic at follow-up. Considering only those patients who underwent exploration and who were thought to have had successful resection, the cure rate was 60%. These results represent a major change in the management of these patients during the past several decades and support the practice of initial short-term pharmacologic control of gastric hypersecretion, followed by aggressive tumor localization and staging in anticipation of curative resection.

At present, the cause of death in the majority of gastrinoma

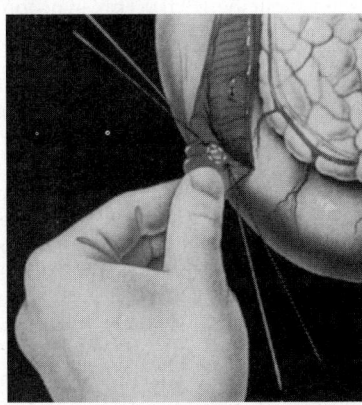

Figure 35–21. Illustration depicting a longitudinal duodenotomy used to identify a duodenal gastrinoma (indicated by dashed white circle) that is to be locally resected. (From Thompson, N. W., Vinik, A. I., and Eckhauser, F. E.: Microgastrinomas of the duodenum: A cause of failed operations for the Zollinger-Ellison syndrome. Ann. Surg., *209*:396, 1989.)

patients is tumor growth and dissemination. Chemotherapy, hormonal therapy with octreotide, hepatic transplantation, hepatic embolization, and interferon have all been used to treat patients with unresectable or metastatic gastrinoma. The overall response to chemotherapy is poor. A recent prospective study of monthly cycles of streptozotocin 3 gm. per sq. m., 5-fluorouracil 1.2 gm. per sq. m., and doxorubicin 40 mg. per sq. m. in patients with metastatic gastrinoma showed that 60% of the patients failed to respond. In the 40% of patients with a response, no complete responses occurred. Survival rates have not been significantly altered by the use of chemotherapy. Hormonal therapy with the long-acting somatostatin analog octreotide has been reported to ameliorate symptoms, reduce hypergastrinemia, and diminish hyperchlorhydria in patients with metastatic gastrinoma. However, the role of octreotide, which must be parenterally administered, will probably remain limited, because adequate doses of oral antisecretory medications can control hyperchlorhydria and acid peptic symptoms in most patients. Neither hepatic transplantation nor embolization therapy have proved to be of consistent benefit in the management of gastrinoma metastatic to the liver. Human leukocyte interferon has been used in small numbers of patients and has been reported to cause a 50% reduction in tumor size or serum gastrin levels. Overall, further trials are awaited in an effort to define the proper role of these adjuvant therapies either alone or in combination in the management of patients with unresectable metastatic gastrinoma.

Patients with gastrinoma and MEN Type I require cautious management. Omeprazole or lansoprazole should be used to control gastric acid hypersecretion. Surgical treatment of hyperparathyroidism should precede operative treatment of gastrinoma. MEN Type I gastrinoma typically involves multiple pancreatic and/or duodenal neoplasms, and localization techniques must be utilized to guide resection. In limited numbers of MEN Type I gastrinoma patients, hypergastrinemia has been corrected by surgical resection. The overall cure rates for MEN Type I gastrinoma are lower than those for sporadic gastrinoma.

VIPoma (Verner-Morrison Syndrome)

Verner and Morrison described two cases of islet cell tumor and diarrhea in 1958 and have been credited with the definition of the syndrome. Pancreatic islet cell tumors associated with watery diarrhea, hypokalemia, and either achlorhydria or hypochlorhydria (WDHA) can produce a variety of biologically active substances. The primary candidates for the active agent in this syndrome include VIP, prostaglandins, and peptide histidine-isoleucine (PHI). This syndrome has many names, including *Verner-Morrison syndrome, WDHA syndrome,* and *pancreatic cholera.*

Patients typically present with intermittent severe diarrhea, often of a watery nature. Unlike the diarrhea associated with Zollinger-Ellison syndrome, the diarrhea in WDHA syndrome is not relieved by nasogastric suction, since it represents a secretory diarrhea caused by elevated circulating hormones. Cutaneous flushing may be observed in some patients. Gastric analysis usually reveals hypochlorhydria, although patients usually respond to pentagastrin with an increase in acid production. The diagnosis is generally suspected on the basis of the clinical syndrome, and elevations in serum VIP or pancreatic polypeptide (a marker for islet cell tumors) may provide further support for the diagnosis. As VIP secretion may be episodic, several fasting serum VIP values should be measured.

Tumor localization and staging are performed by the standard tests used for endocrine tumors of the pancreas, as previously discussed. Preoperative preparation must include correction of fluid and electrolyte losses by volume and electrolyte replacement. The long-acting somatostatin analog octreotide has proved efficacious in reducing circulating VIP levels and controlling diarrhea in selected cases.

The definitive treatment of WDHA syndrome is surgical excision of the tumor. Over half of the reported cases have had evidence of malignancy, with documented tumor metastases outside of the confines of the pancreas. The majority of tumors have been found in the body or tail of the pancreas. In less than 20% of cases, diffuse islet cell hyperplasia has been found as the etiology of the syndrome. If no tumor is found in the pancreas, a careful exploration of the retroperitoneum, including both adrenals, is performed. If no tumor is identified, subtotal pancreatectomy to the level of the superior mesenteric vein can be considered. When the tumor is identified as incurable because of metastatic spread, palliative debulking of safely resectable tumor is indicated. In patients with symptomatic unresectable or recurrent tumor, indomethacin or octreotide therapy may be beneficial.

Glucagonoma

The hallmarks of the glucagonoma syndrome are mild diabetes and severe dermatitis. In addition, patients may demonstrate malnutrition, anemia, glossitis, hypocholesterolemia, hypoproteinemia, and venous thrombosis. The diabetes characteristic of this disorder is mild and is only rarely associated with ketoacidosis. The characteristic skin rash (necrolytic migratory erythema) usually exhibits cyclic migrations, with spreading margins and a healing point of resolution within its center. It is typically located on the lower abdomen, perineum, perioral area, or feet. In patients with the syndrome, glucagon determinations usually show values in excess of 500 pg. per ml., with normal levels being less than 120 pg. per ml. Elevated basal insulin levels are also characteristic, as is dramatic hypoaminoacidemia.

Preoperative management consists of treatment of the dermatitis and stabilization of the diabetes, with concurrent tumor localization and staging by means of standard tests. The dermatitis has been reported to improve with steroid and zinc therapy, as well as with the institution of total parenteral nutrition and octreotide therapy.

Exploration is recommended in essentially all patients suspected of having glucagonoma. The majority of glucagonomas are found in the body and tail of the pancreas and tend to be large at the time of exploration. Metastases are found in up to 80% of patients, and complete resection is possible in only 30%. Tumor debulking is performed when feasible and safe and has been associated with a return to euglycemia and complete resolution of the dermatitis. Patients with incurable or recurrent disease have been treated with the chemotherapeutic agents streptozotocin and dacarbazine (DTIC) with some success. Hormonal therapy with octreotide has also been reported to control the hyperglycemia and dermatitis.

Somatostatinoma

The somatostatinoma syndrome, encompassing the presence of gallstones, diabetes, and steatorrhea, was first described by Ganda and associates in 1977 and shortly thereafter by Kregs and co-workers. Many of the symptoms observed in this syndrome are related to the ability of somatostatin to inhibit the function of most of the digestive organs. Somatostatin has also been shown to reduce the circulating levels of a number of hormones. Somatostatinoma is a rare pancreatic endocrine tumor with an estimated annual incidence of 1 in 40 million people. Serum somatostatin levels, which are normally less than 100 pg. per ml., may be extremely elevated, often over 10 ng. per ml. The syndrome is difficult to diagnose because the early findings are nonspecific. In the small number of cases reported in the English literature, the primary tumor was located in the head of the pancreas in the majority of patients, often with liver metastases present at exploration. Management of patients with somatostatinoma encompasses preoperative treatment of hyperglycemia and malnutrition, combined with standard radiographic localization and staging studies. Gallbladder ultrasonography should be performed to determine the presence of gallstones. At exploration, resection for cure is uncommon, although safe resection and debulking are indicated. Cholecystectomy appears to be indicated because of the known increased incidence of cholelithiasis with persistent hypersomatostatinemia.

Nonfunctional Islet Cell Tumors

The majority of clinically detected islet cell tumors of the pancreas are associated with characteristic clinical syndromes caused by hypersecretion of hormonal products. Fifteen to 25% of pancreatic endocrine tumors are found to be nonfunctional, on the basis of the absence of a defined clinical syndrome and the lack of elevated serum hormone levels. The one hormone that may be elevated in the serum of patients with nonfunctional tumors is pancreatic polypeptide (PP). Nonfunctioning or clinically silent tumors are morphologically indistinguishable from their functional counterparts. These nonfunctioning islet cell tumors frequently have clinical manifestations similar to those of the more common exocrine malignancies. Thus, these patients frequently present with abdominal pain, weight loss, and jaundice, all related to the mass effect of the tumor. Nonfunctioning islet cell tumors are associated with a higher malignancy rate (90%) than their functioning counterparts, and they are most commonly located in the head of the pancreas. However, in contrast to the poor prognosis associated with ductal adenocarcinoma of the exocrine pancreas, these nonfunctional islet cell tumors are often indolent and slow-growing. Surgical exploration follows routine radiographic studies and staging efforts. At operation, localized tumors are resected by pancreaticoduodenectomy when lesions are located in the head and by distal pancreatectomy when they are in the distal gland. Patients with surgically incurable disease may benefit from primary tumor debulking or surgical palliation of jaundice and gastric outlet obstruction by biliary-enteric or gastroenteric bypass, respectively. Five-year survival for all patients averages 25 to 45%. Five-year survival without curative resection has been documented in several cases. Chemotherapy with 5-fluorouracil and streptozotocin or other combinations may be associated with a favorable objective response.

PANCREATIC LYMPHOMA

Primary involvement of the pancreas with non-Hodgkin's lymphoma occurs and represents an unusual neoplasm of the pancreas. Equal numbers of affected males and females have been reported. The clinical presentation commonly includes weight loss and abdominal pain and may include jaundice and symptoms of gastric outlet obstruction. The most common physical finding is a palpable abdominal mass. The abdominal CT scan may suggest the diagnosis by revealing a large soft-tissue mass in the vicinity of the pancreas with peripancreatic lymphadenopathy (Fig. 35–22). In suspected cases of pancreatic lymphoma, radiographically guided needle biopsy may establish the diagnosis. After the pathologic diagnosis of non-Hodgkin's lymphoma, further staging is performed via bone marrow biopsy and accurate review of the chest and abdominal CT scans. Staging laparot-

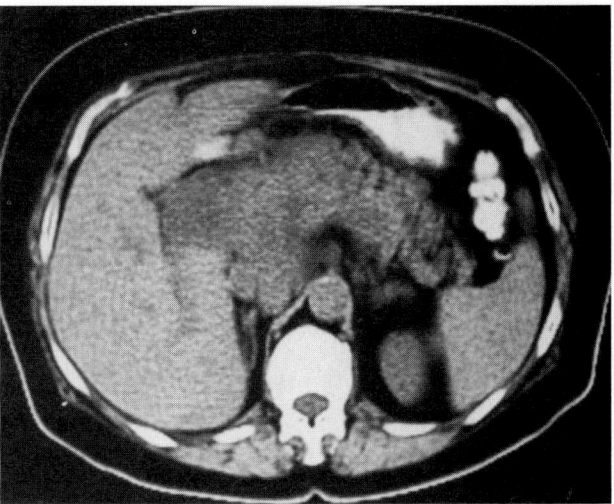

Figure 35–22. CT scan of a patient with pancreatic lymphoma demonstrating a large soft tissue mass in the region of the pancreas. (From Webb, T. H., Lillemoe, K. D., Pitt, H. A., et al.: Pancreatic lymphoma: Is surgery mandatory for diagnosis or treatment? Ann. Surg., 209:25, 1989.)

omy or laparoscopy is performed only if the percutaneous needle biopsy fails to be diagnostic. There is no role for extensive resection in the management of patients with pancreatic lymphoma. Nonjaundiced patients appear to be best treated by doxorubicin-based combination chemotherapy regimens. In patients with obstructive jaundice, temporary biliary decompression is performed with a percutaneous transhepatic catheter. Chemotherapy begins with nonhepatotoxic agents such as cyclophosphamide and prednisone until resolution of jaundice is achieved, and then doxorubicin-containing regimens are initiated. Long-term remission can be obtained with chemotherapy alone.

PANCREATIC TRAUMA

The pancreas is injured in less than 2% of patients with abdominal trauma. Two thirds of pancreatic injuries are associated with penetrating abdominal trauma, and one third are associated with blunt abdominal trauma. As a consequence of the retroperitoneal location of the pancreas, a significant proportion of patients with pancreatic trauma have injuries to adjacent organs and major vascular structures. In penetrating pancreatic injuries, the lowest mortality is associated with stab wounds (approximately 5 to 10%), with intermediate mortality associated with gunshot wounds, and the highest mortality (50%) observed with close-range shotgun wounds. Blunt pancreatic trauma is associated with mortality of 15 to 50%. In the majority of fatal cases, death is the result of hemorrhage from nearby vascular structures. The second most common cause of death involves delayed mortality from intra-abdominal sepsis.

In blunt abdominal trauma, the extent and location of pancreatic injury are determined by the mechanism of injury and the location of impact. Injuries occurring secondary to midline forces, such as classic steering wheel injuries, are associated with pancreatic neck transections, which occur when the vertebral column acts as a fulcrum over which the pancreas is sheared. Forces to the left of the vertebral column in the left upper quadrant are associated with distal pancreatic contusions or injuries of the spleen or left kidney. Forces confined to the right of the vertebral column may cause contusions to the pancreatic head, liver laceration, gallbladder injury, duodenal injury, avulsion of the common bile duct, or right renal injury.

Clinical Presentation

Pancreatic injury is associated with many clinical presentations. Patients with penetrating abdominal trauma generally present with obvious external injury and frequently show signs of ongoing hemorrhage, progressive peritonitis, and hypovolemia. The presentation of blunt abdominal trauma with pancreatic injury may be varied. Patients with pancreatic injury and solid organ injury to the liver or spleen may present with signs of obvious hypovolemia and peritonitis requiring exploration. In contrast, blunt abdominal trauma without other solid organ injury may produce subtle pancreatic injury that is difficult to diagnose. Such patients can present with mild epigastric pain and abdominal tenderness with otherwise unimpressive physical findings. In these patients, progressive clinical deterioration may herald the diagnosis of a pancreatic injury.

Diagnosis

No laboratory test is sufficiently accurate for the specific diagnosis of pancreatic injury. Hyperamylasemia is present in up to 90% of patients with blunt pancreatic injury but is present in only a minority of patients with penetrating pancreatic injury. Moreover, hyperamylasemia may occur in up to 50% of patients with blunt abdominal trauma without pancreatic injury. Thus, hyperamylasemia is an insensitive and nonspecific indicator of pancreatic injury. Nonspecific laboratory tests such as the hematocrit and the white blood cell count provide little assistance in the initial assessment of patients with suspected pancreatic injury, although they may be useful during serial observation of such patients. Peritoneal lavage, which has proved useful in the assessment of patients with blunt abdominal trauma, is inaccurate and unreliable for the diagnosis of pancreatic trauma. This is due to the retroperitoneal location of the pancreas and the existence of other sources for intraperitoneal amylase other than the pancreas, such as the bile duct, intestine, and fallopian tubes.

Chest and abdominal films are often not helpful in diagnosing pancreatic injury. Unusual and often late findings on abdominal films associated with pancreatic injury include obliteration of the psoas shadow, the presence of retroperitoneal air, and displacement of the stomach secondary to a retroperitoneal mass. Injury to the head of the pancreas with associated duodenal injury can be evaluated by means of an upper gastrointestinal series with water-soluble contrast. Extraluminal contrast extravasation indicates disruption of duodenal integrity and a major injury. A duodenal hematoma may be diagnosed by the typical *coiled spring* appearance of duodenal luminal narrowing.

In the setting of blunt abdominal trauma, the CT scan has gained importance in the serial evaluation of pancreatic injury. An abdominal CT scan obtained within hours of pancreatic trauma may reveal subtle abnormalities suggestive of pancreatic injury, such as hemorrhagic infiltration of the peripancreatic fat or peripancreatic thickening due to fluid sequestration. In the appropriate clinical setting, serial assessment by CT scan may be of benefit in following subtle peripancreatic abnormalities and documenting acute fluid collection, pancreatic pseudocyst, or pancreatic abscess.

Endoscopic retrograde pancreatography (ERP) is occasionally useful in the acute setting following abdominal trauma. In general, however, abnormalities found at the time of acute injury, such as minor pancreatic ductal extravasation or small pseudocyst formation, require only expectant observation. Thus, the information gained by acute ERP is of little benefit in the management of such patients. In contrast, the use of ERP in a delayed setting following blunt abdominal trauma is important in defining pancreatic ductal abnormalities associated with pancreatic pseudocysts or other pancreatic ductal disruptions. In this setting, the definition of duct anatomy and pathology may be of great importance in planning definitive operative management.

Management

Patients with pancreatic injury suggested by clinical and radiographic examination who have stable vital signs and lack a specific indication for exploration may initially be managed nonoperatively. In this setting, patients are observed clinically, with laboratory evaluation of the hematocrit, white blood cell count, and serum amylase and with abdominal CT scan. Such patients are followed for the development of complications such as pancreatic abscess, pseudocyst formation, or retroperitoneal phlegmon.

Patients who undergo laparotomy for abdominal trauma require complete assessment of the pancreas at the time of surgical exploration. Assessment involves performance of Kocher's maneuver for evaluation of the duodenum and the head of the pancreas and division of the gastrocolic ligament for entrance into the lesser sac for visualization of the neck, body, and tail of the pancreas. Bimanual palpation of the body and tail may be accomplished by opening the peritoneum inferior to the pancreas and by reflecting the spleen and distal pancreas from the retroperitoneum toward the midline. In the setting of blunt or penetrating trauma, all peripancreatic hematomas should be explored to exclude and repair any major vascular injury.

The goals of operative therapy for pancreatic injury include control of hemorrhage; débridement of nonviable tissue, with maximal preservation of viable pancreatic tissue; and adequate drainage of exocrine secretions. Operative therapy is dependent on the degree of pancreatic injury. Pancreatic injury can be categorized into four classes. In order of increasing severity, they are (1) pancreatic contusion without capsular rupture, (2) pancreatic capsular and parenchymal rupture without injury to the main pancreatic duct, (3) severe pancreatic parenchymal injury with rupture of the main pancreatic duct, and (4) combined severe pancreatic and duodenal injuries.

Class I Injury. Pancreatic contusion without capsular rupture is treated by external drainage alone. External drainage for Class I injuries is recommended because of the difficulty in assessing pancreatic capsular injury intraoperatively. By draining Class I injuries, occult capsular disruptions that could potentially cause accumulation of pancreatic secretions and subsequent pancreatic pseudocyst, abscess, or pancreatic ascites are prevented. Drains are usually left in place until oral intake is re-established.

Class II Injury. More severe pancreatic injuries that involve pancreatic capsular or parenchymal rupture but are not associated with injury to the main pancreatic duct constitute Class II injuries. These injuries are treated by cautious débridement of devitalized tissue, achievement of adequate hemostasis, careful suture closure of major capsular disruption, and external drainage of the injury site.

Class III Injury. Pancreatic parenchymal injuries associated with rupture or destruction of a major pancreatic duct constitute Class III injuries. These injuries require individualized treatment, based on injury location and associated injuries to adjacent structures. Class III injuries may be diagnosed preoperatively by ERP, or they may be discovered at the time of laparotomy via intraoperative pancreatography or operative findings. Class III injuries to the body and tail of the pancreas are best treated by distal pancreatectomy encompassing the site of the injury, with or without splenectomy. Following distal pancreatectomy, the transected surface of the pancreatic remnant is closed, and the closure is externally drained. Distal resection up to the level of the superior mesenteric vein can be performed with reasonable rapidity, rarely causes pancreatic endocrine insufficiency, and has a low incidence of persistent external pancreatic fistula. As an alternative to distal pancreatectomy, Class III injuries to the body of the pancreas may be treated with Roux-en-Y pancreaticojejunostomy to the distal pancreatic remnant, with oversewing of the proximal pancreas. This procedure requires the creation of a Roux-en-Y jejunal limb, but no distal pancreatic resection is performed. This procedure requires more time than distal pancreatic resection, requires two gastrointestinal anastomoses, and may be complicated by postoperative leak from the pancreatic-enteric anastomosis. Thus, it is not commonly chosen for Class III injuries to the body of the pancreas.

Class III injuries to the head of the pancreas not associated with duodenal injury are uncommon and usually follow penetrating trauma. Isolated injuries of the inferior head or uncinate process may be débrided and externally drained or drained via Roux-en-Y pancreaticojejunostomy. Injuries in the proximity of the pancreatic neck may be treated by distal pancreatectomy to the level of the injury. Injuries adjacent to the duodenal C loop in the central aspect of the pancreatic head are treated as Class IV injuries.

Class IV Injury. Combined severe injuries to the pancreas and duodenum represent a minority of cases of pancreatic trauma. These Class IV injuries are frequently associated with injuries to adjacent visceral or major vascular structures, and they are attended by mortality in up to 45% of cases. There are several different surgical options for the treatment of Class IV injuries. First, the serosal patch technique employs healthy small bowel serosa to patch defects in the duodenal wall that cannot be safely closed primarily. This technique has utility when discrete duodenal injuries occur in combination with injury to the head of the pancreas that does not require pancreatic resection. In such instances, a serosal patch may provide secure duodenal closure, whereas the pancreatic injury is managed with hemostasis, débridement, and external drainage.

More extensive injuries to the duodenum and head of the pancreas can be treated by a second approach: duodenal decompression with triple ostomy. This technique uses tube gastrostomy, retrograde tube jejunostomy for duodenal drainage, and antegrade tube jejunostomy for enteral feeding. These triple ostomies are combined with secure duodenorrhaphy and wide drainage of the duodenum and head of the pancreas.

Patients with more severe injuries to the duodenum and head of the pancreas may be managed by a third technique: the duodenal diverticularization procedure. This procedure, as initially described, involved closure of the duodenal defect, placement of a proximal tube duodenostomy, pyloroantrectomy with gastrojejunostomy, truncal vagotomy, T-tube placement, and wide drainage of the retroperitoneum (Fig. 35–23). The goal of this therapy is to achieve widespread drainage of the retroperitoneum and a reduction in the flow of luminal contents through the duodenum. The pyloric exclusion procedure is a more recent modification of the duodenal diverticularization technique. In the exclusion procedure, the pylorus is closed from within the gastric lumen with an absorbable suture. A gastrojejunostomy is performed, and the injury to the duodenum is repaired primarily. Vagotomy and antrectomy are not performed, thus avoiding their late complications and saving operative time. Marginal ulceration at the gastrojejunal anastomosis is prevented by postoperative histamine H_2-receptor antagonist therapy. Both the diverticularization and the exclusion procedures are applicable to pancreaticoduodenal injuries of intermediate severity.

Devitalizing injuries of the duodenum and head of the

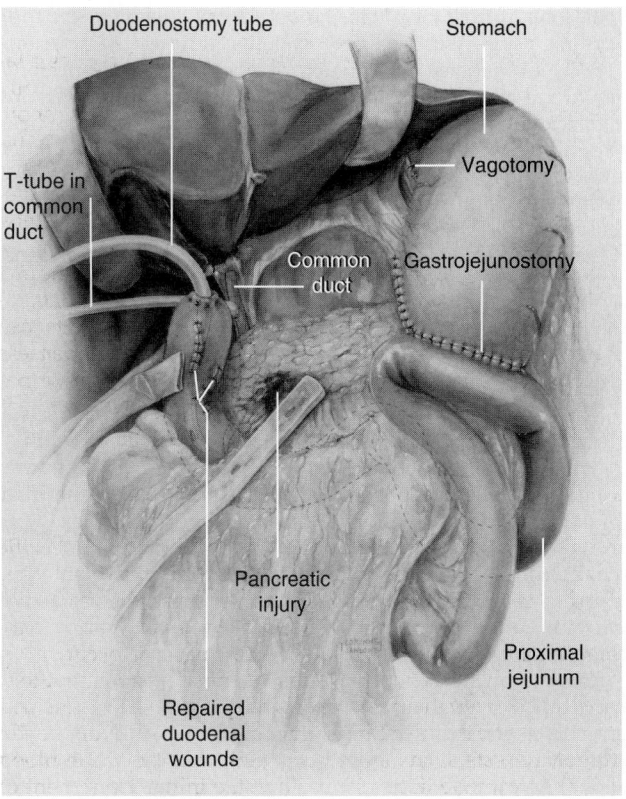

Figure 35–23. Illustration of the duodenal diverticularization procedure used for Class IV injuries to the duodenum and head of the pancreas. (From Cameron, J. L.: Atlas of Surgery. Vol. 1. Toronto, B. C. Decker, 1990, p. 461.)

pancreas that are not amenable to lesser procedures are treated by pancreaticoduodenectomy. Indications for pancreaticoduodenectomy in the setting of abdominal trauma include massive destruction of the duodenum and pancreatic head, avulsion of the bile duct and pancreatic duct at the ampulla of Vater, and, rarely, jeopardized vascularity of the pancreaticoduodenal region. Pylorus-preserving pancreaticoduodenectomy may be accomplished if the most proximal duodenum is free of injury. Mortality following pancreaticoduodenectomy in the setting of abdominal trauma varies from 0 to 60%. Mortality is related to many factors, including the magnitude of injury to associated structures, the condition of the patient prior to operation, the length of operation, the overall blood loss, and the experience of the surgeon.

PANCREATIC TRANSPLANTATION

In the United States there are approximately 1 million Type I diabetics. Half of these diabetics develop significant long-term metabolic complications such as nephropathy, neuropathy, vasculopathy, and retinopathy within 20 years of the onset of their disease. Well-controlled glucoregulation in these patients not only prevents ketoacidosis, hypercholesterolemia, and hyperlipidemia but also appears to reduce the long-term metabolic complications. Until recently, the primary therapy for insulin-dependent diabetes involved intermittent administration of subcutaneous insulin. Now, newer methods of treatment include (1) fine regulation of serum glucose by sophisticated insulin delivery systems, (2) pancreatic islet cell transplantation, and (3) vascularized pancreas (segmental or whole) transplantation.

A number of insulin delivery systems are currently available; others are undergoing testing. Delivery systems can involve external or internal (implantable) devices with an open-loop format or a closed-loop format using a glucose sensor. Results with delivery systems indicate that insulin-dependent diabetes can be successfully treated without daily parenteral injections, with doses of insulin that mimic physiologic secretion, and with satisfactory glycemic control as assessed by glycosylated hemoglobin. For the future, the most attractive system appears to be an implantable pump with a peritoneal insulin delivery arm combined with a glucose-sensing closed-loop system.

Pancreatic transplantation serves as an alternative method of treating insulin-dependent diabetes. The first human pancreas transplant was performed by Kelly and associates in 1966. In the ensuing years, multiple different techniques have evolved, and varied experiences have been gained in the field of experimental and human pancreatic transplantation.[33, 43]

Pancreas transplantation remains confined to a select group of patients with insulin-dependent diabetes mellitus. Pancreas transplantation can be performed (1) in a nonuremic patient, (2) simultaneously with a kidney transplant in a uremic patient with end-stage diabetic nephropathy, or (3) at an interval after successful kidney grafting in a patient with renal failure. Contraindications for pancreas transplantation vary but generally include the presence of malignancy, active infection, advanced cardiovascular disease, and major psychiatric illness.

Enthusiasm for pancreatic islet transplantation has waxed and waned over the past 3 decades. Theoretically, islet cell grafting is attractive because it avoids transplantation of the antigenic exocrine tissue and because it has the potential to allow harvesting of islets for multiple recipients from a single donor. The isolation, processing, and purification of islet tissues have been topics of renewed inquiry. Prevention of islet rejection in the allogeneic transplant setting has been studied with standard immunosuppressive regimens as well as immunoalteration and immunoisolation techniques. The best results with islet cell transplantation have been observed in patients undergoing autografting as part of resectional therapy for chronic pancreatitis.

Enthusiasm for segmental or whole pancreas transplantation has increased greatly since the late 1970s. Worldwide, a number of techniques for vascularized pancreatic allotransplantation are utilized (Fig. 35–24). In the United States, whole organ grafts are generally performed, providing venous drainage to the systemic circulation and exocrine drainage via a duodenal segment to the urinary bladder. In Europe, segmental pancreatic grafts have been preferred, with exocrine secretion managed by drainage into a Roux-en-Y jejunal limb or prevented by ductal polymer injection. Bladder-drained grafts appear to achieve significantly better 1-year function than enterically drained or duct-injected grafts. The improvement in function observed with bladder-drained grafts has been attributed largely to the ability to serially follow urinary amylase excretion as a measure of graft function. Immunosuppressive regimens for segmental or whole pancreas transplantation usually involve quadruple drug therapy with prednisone, azathioprine, cyclosporine, and polyclonal anti-T-lymphocyte antibody. Initial therapy for rejection episodes usually involves monoclonal antibody therapy with OKT-3.

Specific surgical complications are well recognized after vascularized pancreatic transplantation. These include posttransplant pancreatitis, transplant vascular thrombosis, peritransplant hemorrhage, and sepsis. Posttransplant pancreatitis may have several causes, including injury to the pancreas during the procurement procedure, preservation injury, rejection, and ductal obstruction. No specific treatment is available for the management of posttransplant pancreatitis. The incidence of graft thrombosis following transplantation has been reported to be as high as 20%. Graft thrombosis

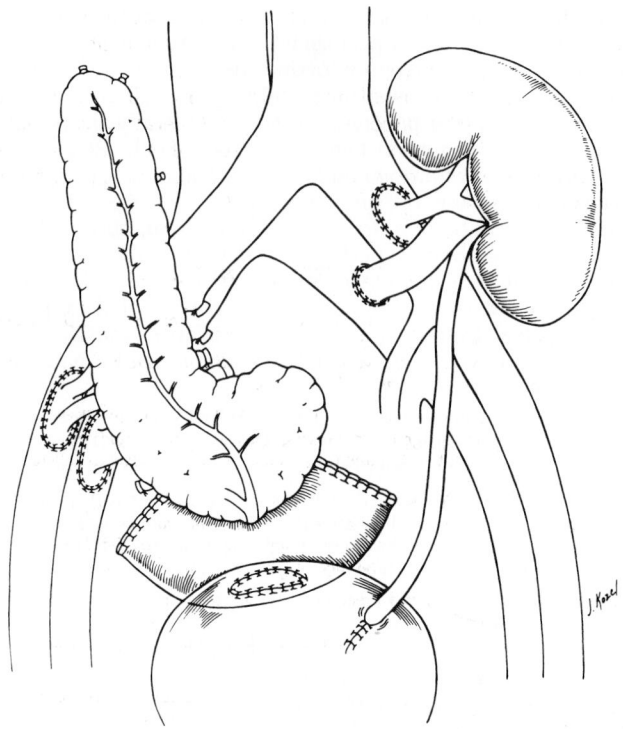

Figure 35–24. Illustration of combined pancreas and kidney transplantation. The pancreas graft is anastomosed to the right iliac vessels, with the pancreatic secretions drained via a duodenal segment to the urinary bladder. The renal graft is anastomosed to the left iliac vessels, with the graft ureter anastomosed to the bladder via neoureterocystostomy. (From Sollinger, H. W.: Pancreas transplantation in humans. *In* Moody, F. G. [Ed.]: Surgical Treatment of Digestive Disease, 2nd ed. Chicago, Year Book, 1990, p. 577.)

is more frequent after segmental pancreatic transplantation, partially because of the low flow through the graft and the large caliber of the draining splenic vein. Local sepsis after pancreatic transplantation is not uncommon, particularly after enteric drainage of the pancreatic graft. Infection may be the result of an anastomotic leak or may arise from small areas of necrotic transplanted pancreatic tissue.

The results of pancreatic allotransplantation using vascularized grafts have been steadily improving. The most recent data available indicate a 60 to 90% 1-year graft survival for synchronous pancreas and kidney transplants. The graft survival rates are lower for pancreas transplants performed alone or after renal transplantation. Although there appears to be no distinct advantage in pancreatic graft survival between segmental or whole organ grafts, bladder-drained grafts appear to be favored over enterically drained or polymer-injected grafts.

After successful pancreatic transplantation, carbohydrate metabolism reliably improves. Posttransplant patients with functioning grafts demonstrate nearly normal glucose tolerance testing, fasting euglycemia, and improved functional status. Although graft function eliminates the need for exogenous insulin therapy, standard immunosuppressive therapy is substituted. The ultimate purpose of pancreatic transplantation is to reverse or halt the secondary complications of diabetes. Patients receiving successful combined pancreatic and renal transplants have been noted to have an absence of electron microscopic evidence of diabetic nephropathy in the transplanted kidney, supporting a protective effect of pancreatic transplantation against diabetic nephropathy. Successful pancreatic transplantation has also been associated with a subjective improvement in peripheral neuropathy, as well as an objective improvement in motor nerve conduction velocities in the upper and lower extremities. The effects on diabetic retinopathy have not been as universally favorable, although subjective visual improvement or stabilization has been observed after successful grafting. Overall, accumulating evidence supports a beneficial effect of pancreas transplantation on the various end organs commonly injured by diabetes mellitus.

SELECTED REFERENCES

DiGiuseppe, J. A., and Hruban, R. H.: Pathobiology of cancer of the pancreas. Semin. Surg. Oncol., 11:87, 1995.
A review of the pathology and genetics of pancreatic adenocarcinoma, including recent findings in the field of molecular genetics.

Neoptolemos, J. P., Carr-Locke, D. L., London, N. J., et al.: Controlled trial of urgent endoscopic retrograde cholangiography and endoscopic sphincterotomy versus conservative treatment for acute pancreatitis due to gallstones. Lancet, 2:979, 1988.
The authors describe the results of ERCP plus sphincterotomy to retrieve common duct stones versus supportive care alone in patients with gallstone pancreatitis. In patients with severe pancreatitis, the endoscopic intervention reduced the complication rate and the length of hospital stay.

Steer, M. L., Waxman, I., and Freedman, S.: Chronic pancreatitis. N. Engl. J. Med., 332:1482, 1995.
A succinct review of chronic pancreatitis, including etiologic aspects and treatment options.

Steinberg, W., and Tenner, S.: Acute pancreatitis. N. Engl. J. Med., 330:1198, 1994.
A current review of acute pancreatitis, which includes a discussion of epidemiology, etiology, pathophysiology, and complications.

Yeo, C. J., Cameron, J. L., Lillemoe, K. D., et al.: Pancreaticoduodenectomy for cancer of the head of the pancreas: 201 patients. Ann. Surg., 221:721, 1995.
This paper describes a large, single-institution experience with the Whipple operation for pancreatic carcinoma, focusing on patient outcome and prognostic factors influencing survival. The most important prognostic factors favoring lengthy survival were small tumor size, absence of lymph node metastases, negative resection margins, and diploid tumor DNA content.

REFERENCES

1. Andersen, D. K.: Current diagnosis and management of Zollinger-Ellison syndrome. Ann. Surg., 210:685, 1989.
2. Bassi, D., Kollias, N., Fernandez-del Castillo, C., et al.: Impairment of pancreatic microcirculation correlates with the severity of acute experimental pancreatitis. J. Am. Coll. Surg., 179:257, 1994.
3. Beger, H. G., Buchler, M., Bittner, R. R., et al.: Duodenum-preserving resection of the head of the pancreas in severe chronic pancreatitis: Early and late results. Ann. Surg., 209:273, 1989.
4. Bradley, E. L., III: A clinically based classification system for acute pancreatitis. Arch. Surg., 128:586, 1993.
5. Bradley, E. L., III, Clements, J. L., Jr., and Gonzalez, A. C.: The natural history of pancreatic pseudocysts: A unified concept of management. Am. J. Surg., 137:135, 1979.
6. Buchler, M. W., Friess, H., Muller, M. W., et al.: Randomized trial of duodenum-preserving pancreatic head resection versus pylorus-preserving Whipple in chronic pancreatitis. Am. J. Surg., 169:65, 1995.
7. Caldas, C., Hahn, S. A., daCosta, L., et al.: Frequent somatic mutations and homozygous deletions of the MTS1 gene in pancreatic adenocarcinoma. Nature Genet., 8:27, 1994.
8. Cremer, M., Deviere, J., and Engelholm, L.: Endoscopic management of cysts and pseudocysts in chronic pancreatitis: Long-term followup after 7 years of experience. Gastrointest. Endosc., 35:1, 1989.
9. DiGiuseppe, J. A., and Hruban, R. H.: Pathobiology of cancer of the pancreas. Semin. Surg. Oncol., 11:87, 1995.
10. Dooley, W. C., Cameron, J. L., Pitt, H. A., et al.: Is preoperative angiography useful in patients with periampullary tumors? Ann. Surg., 211:649, 1990.
11. Freeny, P. C.: Percutaneous management of pancreatic fluid collections. Baillieres Clin. Gastroenterol., 6:259, 1992.
12. Frey, C. F., and Smith, G. J.: Description and rationale of a new operation for chronic pancreatitis. Pancreas, 2:701, 1987.
13. Gastrointestinal Tumor Study Group: Further evidence of effective adjuvant combined radiation and chemotherapy following curative resection of pancreatic cancer. Cancer, 59:2006, 1987.
14. Griffin, C. A., Hruban, R. H., Morsberger, L. A., et al.: Consistent chromosome abnormalities in adenocarcinoma of the pancreas. Cancer Res., 55:2394, 1995.
14a. Hahn, S. A., Schutte, M., Shamsul Hoque, A. T. M., et al.: *DPC4,* a

candidate tumor suppressor gene at human chromosome 18q21.1. Science, 271:350, 1996.
15. Izbicki, J. R., Bloechle, C., Knoefel, W. T., et al.: Duodenum-preserving resection of the head of the pancreas in chronic pancreatitis: A prospective, randomized trial. Ann. Surg., 221:3250, 1995.
16. Kalser, M. H., and Ellenberg, S. S.: Pancreatic cancer: Adjuvant combined radiation and chemotherapy following curative resection. Arch. Surg., 120:899, 1985.
17. Kozarek, R. A., Ball, T. J., Patterson, D. J., et al.: Endoscopic transpapillary therapy for disrupted pancreatic duct and peripancreatic fluid collections. Gastroenterology, 100:1362, 1991.
18. Lampel, M., and Kern, H. F.: Acute interstitial pancreatitis in the rat induced by excessive doses of a pancreatic secretagogue. Virchows Arch. [A], 373:97, 1977.
19. Lang, E. K., Paolini, R. M., and Pottmeyer, A.: The efficacy of palliative and definitive percutaneous versus surgical drainage of pancreatic abscesses and pseudocysts: A prospective study of 85 patients. South. Med. J., 84:55, 1991.
20. Lee, S. P., Nicholls, J. F., and Park, H. Z.: Biliary sludge as a cause of acute pancreatitis. N. Engl. J. Med., 326:589, 1992.
21. Lewandrowski, K. B., Southern, J. F., Pins, M. R., et al.: Cyst fluid analysis in the differential diagnosis of pancreatic cysts. Ann. Surg., 217:41, 1993.
22. Lillemoe, K. D., Cameron, J. L., Kaufman, H. S., et al.: Chemical splanchnicectomy in patients with unresectable pancreatic cancer: A prospective randomized trial. Ann. Surg., 217:447, 1993.
23. Lipsett, P. A., and Cameron, J. L.: Internal pancreatic fistula. Am. J. Surg., 163:216, 1992.
24. Lombardi, B., Estes, L. W., and Longnecker, D. S.: Acute hemorrhagic pancreatitis (massive necrosis) with fat necrosis induced in mice by DL-ethionine fed with a choline-1 deficient diet. Am. J. Pathol., 79:465, 1975.
25. Luiten, E. J. T., Hop, W. C. J., Lange, J. F., et al.: Controlled clinical trial of selective decontamination for the treatment of severe acute pancreatitis. Ann. Surg., 222:57, 1995.
26. Neoptolemos, J. P., Carr-Locke, D. L., London, N. J., et al.: Controlled trial of urgent endoscopic retrograde cholangiography and endoscopic sphinterotomy versus conservative treatment for acute pancreatitis due to gallstones. Lancet, 2:979, 1988.
27. Nordback, I. H., Olson, J. L., Chacko, V. P., et al.: Detailed characterization of experimental acute alcoholic pancreatitis. Surgery, 117:41, 1995.
28. Parekh, D., and Segal, I.: Pancreatic ascites and effusion: Risk factors for failure of conservative therapy and the role of octreotide. Arch. Surg., 127:707, 1992.
29. Pederzoli, P., Bassi, C., Vesentini, S., et al.: A randomized multicenter clinical trial of antibiotic prophylaxis of septic complications in acute necrotizing pancreatitis with imipenem. Surg. Gynecol. Obstet., 176:480, 1993.
30. Ranson, J. H. C., Rifkind, K. M., Roses, D. F., et al.: Prognostic signs and the role of operative management in acute pancreatitis. Surg. Gynecol. Obstet., 139:69, 1974.
31. Redston, M. S., Caldas, C., Seymour, A. B., et al.: p53 mutations in pancreatic carcinoma and evidence of common involvement of homocopolymer tracts in DNA microdeletions. Cancer Res., 54:3025, 1994.
32. Renner, I. G., Savage, W. T., III, Pantoja, J. L., et al.: Death due to acute pancreatitis: A retrospective analysis of 405 autopsy cases. Dig. Dis. Sci., 30:1005, 1985.
33. Robertson, R. P.: Pancreatic and islet transplantation for diabetes—cures or curiosities? N. Engl. J. Med., 327:1861, 1992.
34. Rosch, T., Braig, C., Gain, T., et al.: Staging of pancreatic and ampullary carcinoma by endoscopic ultrasonography: Comparison with conventional sonography, computed tomography, and angiography. Gastroenterology, 102:188, 1992.
35. Sanfey, H., Bulkley, G. B., and Cameron, J. L.: The role of oxygen-derived free radicals in the pathogenesis of acute pancreatitis. Ann. Surg., 200:405, 1984.
36. Seymour, A. B., Hruban, R. H., Redston, M., et al.: Allelotype of pancreatic carcinoma. Cancer Res., 54:2761, 1994.
37. Sherman, S., and Lehman, G. A.: ERCP- and endoscopic sphincterotomy-induced pancreatitis. Pancreas, 6:350, 1991.
38. Steer, M. L., and Meldolesi, J.: The cell biology of experimental pancreatitis. N. Engl. J. Med., 316:144, 1987.
39. Steer, M. L., Waxman, I., and Freedman, S.: Chronic pancreatitis. N. Engl. J. Med., 332:1482, 1995.
40. Steinberg, W., and Tenner, S.: Acute pancreatitis. N. Engl. J. Med., 330:1198, 1994.
41. Stone, H. H., and Fabian, T. C.: Peritoneal dialysis in the treatment of acute alcoholic pancreatitis. Surg. Gynecol. Obstet., 150:878, 1980.
42. Stone, H. H., Fabian, T. C., and Dunlop, W. E.: Gallstone pancreatitis: Biliary tract pathology in relation to time of operation. Ann. Surg., 194:305, 1981.
43. Sutherland, D. E. R., Gores, P. F., Farney, A. C., et al.: Evolution of kidney, pancreas, and islet transplantation for patients with diabetes at the University of Minnesota. Am. J. Surg., 166:456, 1993.
44. Udelsman, R., Yeo, C. J., Hruban, R. H., et al.: Pancreaticoduodenectomy for selected pancreatic endocrine tumors. Surg. Gynecol. Obstet., 177:269, 1993.

45. Vitas, G. J., and Sarr, M. G.: Selected management of pancreatic pseudocysts: Operative versus expectant management. Surgery, *111*:123, 1992.

46. Wilson, C., Imrie, C. W., and Carter, D. C.: Fatal acute pancreatitis. Gut, *29*:782, 1988.

47. Yeo, C. J., Bastidas, J. A., Lynch-Nyhan, A., et al.: The natural history of pancreatic pseudocysts documented by computed tomography. Surg. Gynecol. Obstet., *170*:411, 1990.

48. Yeo, C. J., Bastidas, J. A., Schmieg, R. E., Jr., et al.: Pancreatic structure and glucose tolerance in a longitudinal study of experimental pancreatitis-induced diabetes. Ann. Surg., *210*:150, 1989.

49. Yeo, C. J., Cameron, J. L., Lillemoe, K. D., et al.: Pancreaticoduodenectomy for cancer of the head of the pancreas: 201 patients. Ann. Surg., *221*:721, 1995.

50. Yeo, C. J., and Sarr, M. G.: Cystic and pseudocystic diseases of the pancreas. Curr. Probl. Surg., *31*:165, 1994.

CHAPTER 36

THE SPLEEN

*George F. Sheldon, M.D., Robert D. Croom III, M.D.,
and Anthony A. Meyer, M.D., Ph.D.*

ANATOMY

Embryonic development of the spleen begins in the fifth week of gestation as a small cluster of mesenchymal cells in the dorsal mesogastrium between the stomach and pancreas. Mesenchymal remnants that do not fuse with the main splenic mass account for the high incidence (15%–30%) of accessory spleens in adjacent tissues.

The spleen is the second largest organ of the reticuloendothelial system. It is located in the posterior left upper quadrant of the abdomen where its relationships to the diaphragm, stomach, pancreas, left kidney, and splenic flexure of the colon are maintained by suspensory ligaments. The splenophrenic, splenorenal, and splenocolic ligaments are usually relatively avascular, except in patients with portal hypertension, and their transection allows the spleen to be displaced medially and anteriorly. The gastrosplenic ligament, which extends from the greater curvature of the body and fundus of the stomach to the spleen, contains the short gastric arteries and veins. Located in the most medial aspect of the splenorenal ligament and attached to the spleen at the hilum, the splenic pedicle contains the splenic artery and vein, lymphatic structures, and often the tail of the pancreas (Fig. 36–1).

The arterial supply to the spleen is derived from the celiac artery from both the splenic artery and the short gastric arteries, which usually arise as branches of the gastroepiploic or the splenic arteries (Fig. 36–2). The splenic vein is formed by a coalescence of polar veins in the splenic hilum and courses with the splenic artery along the dorsal surface of the pancreas to enter the portal system.

The normal adult spleen is a slightly concave, solid, dark red organ that measures approximately $3 \times 8 \times 14$ cm., weighs between 100 and 175 gm., and frequently has fetal lobulations on its anterior edge. A thin peritoneal capsule encloses the deeper organ pulp and easily strips from it. In elderly individuals or in those with prior splenic injury, irradiation, or recurrent infarction, the splenic capsule may become firm and thickly scarred ("sugar coated") and adherent to the diaphragm.

A trabecular connective tissue framework extends into the splenic pulp from the internal capsular surface to subdivide the organ into small communicating compartments. After entering the spleen at the hilum, arterial vessels branch into the trabeculae to enter the pulp. Veins and lymphatics draining the pulp also pass in the trabeculae to leave the spleen at the hilum. The splenic pulp is conventionally divided into three areas: red pulp, white pulp, and an interfacing marginal zone. The red pulp, so designated due to its gross appearance from the presence of blood, is composed almost entirely of

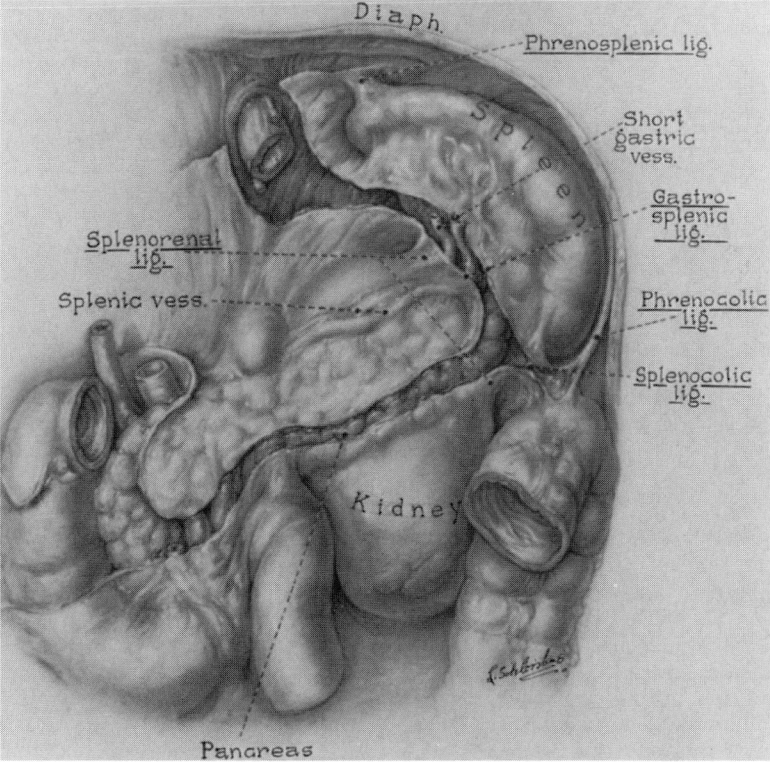

Figure 36–1. Suspensory ligaments of the spleen. (From Ballinger, W. F., and Erslev, A. J.: Splenectomy: Indications, technic and complications. Curr. Probl. Surg., 1–51, February 1965.)

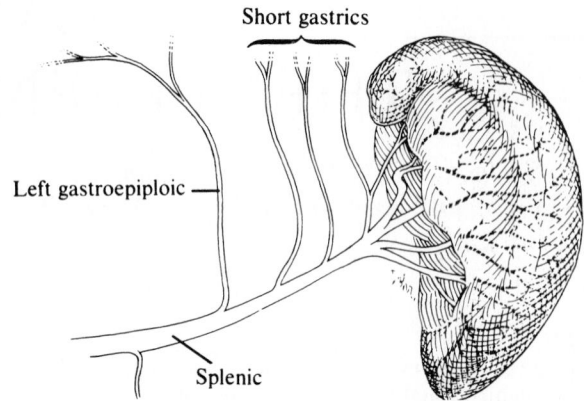

Figure 36–2. The arterial supply of the spleen is derived from the splenic artery through five or six branches that arise in or proximal to the hilus. The most proximal branch of the splenic artery is the left gastroepiploic artery. Four to six short gastric arteries are present in the gastrosplenic ligament between the proximal greater curvature of the stomach and the spleen. (From Blaisdell, F. W., and Trunkey, D. D.: Trauma Management. New York, Thieme-Stratton, 1982, p. 186.)

large, branching, thin-walled blood vessels, called splenic sinuses or sinusoids, and thin plates or cords of cellular tissue lying between the sinuses to form splenic cords. Within this cordal meshwork, erythrocytes, platelets, and some granulocytes are crowded with macrophages and plasma cells, with macrophages often being the predominant cells. Lying within and surrounded by the red pulp are small gray-white zones of lymphatic tissue consisting of lymphocytes, plasma cells, and macrophages, which constitute the white pulp. The white pulp forms periarterial lymphatic sheaths and lymphatic nodules, which, like those of lymph nodes, may contain germinal centers. The marginal zone constitutes the interface between the red and white pulp and is an ill-defined vascular space where many arterial vessels terminate.[49]

Controversy has surrounded the exact nature of the splenic microcirculation for 300 years. Billroth is credited with the *open circulation* theory, in which either arterioles empty blood directly into tissue spaces or arterial capillaries open into pulp cords, with blood cells then passing through pores in the walls of splenic sinusoids to enter the venous circulation. In the *closed circulation* theory, splenic blood follows an endothelialized pathway throughout to flow directly into sinusoids (Fig. 36–3). Studies in rabbits using plastic microspheres too large to pass through pores of the venous sinuses confirm the unique *open* splenic microcirculation. Ninety percent of splenic arterial flow enters the open circulation of the red pulp, with only 10% of the blood in arterial capillaries emptying directly into venous sinuses. Blood cells and particles such as particulate antigens must circulate through the meshwork of splenic cords before squeezing through 0.5 to 2.5 μm. pores between endothelial cells of the sinuses to enter the venous circulation.[8]

FUNCTION

During early fetal development, the spleen produces red and white blood cells. By the fifth month of gestation, the spleen and other extramedullary sites of blood cell production no longer have hematopoietic function but retain the capability throughout life. As a result of a singular microcirculation, the spleen is a sophisticated filter having both blood cell monitoring and management functions and important immune functions. When the spleen is removed, these functions are lost.

Normal red cells usually traverse the splenic circulation but may undergo *repair* by having surface abnormalities such as pits or spurs removed. Reticulocytes pass through the spleen more slowly than mature red cells and lose nuclear remnants and excess membrane before entering the circulation as mature cells. In reducing the membrane surface area, the spleen converts the red cell from a target appearance to a biconcave disc. The spleen also removes high-molecular-weight surface protein, Howell-Jolly bodies (nuclear remnant), Heinz bodies (denatured hemoglobin), Pappenheimer bodies (iron granules), and spur cells. These *cleaned* red cells, if they have the deformability to pass through the splenic circulation, re-enter the bloodstream. Aged red cells (120 days) that have lost enzymatic activity and membrane plasticity are trapped and destroyed in the spleen (Table 36–1).[8]

The normal filtering function of the spleen also enables it to remove abnormal blood cells. Morphologically abnormal erythrocytes, such as the spherocytes of hereditary spherocytosis, fixed sickled cells, and rigid hemoglobin C cells, are trapped by the splenic filter. Blood cells coated with IgG are destroyed by the splenic monocytes, which have surface receptors for the Fc fragment of the IgG coating the cells.[8] Because the spleen removes cells coated with IgG or IgM, it is the site of destruction in diseases such as autoimmune hemolytic anemia (AIHA), immune thrombocytopenic purpura, and probably Felty's syndrome. Parasites with intra-erythrocytic habitation, such as malaria, can be *pitted* from the red cell by the spleen.[8] Red cells that are unable to deform to pass into the splenic sinuses are eventually destroyed by the histiocytes/macrophages of the red pulp.

In addition to blood cell morphology and surface characteristics, rate of blood flow through the splenic microcirculation and alterations of splenic pulp pressure affect the filtering function of the spleen. For example, patients with splenic vein thrombosis have slow red cell passage through the splenic microcirculation due to elevated portal-splenic pulp pressure, with resultant increased red cell sequestration and destruction.[8, 40]

The spleen is involved in specific and nonspecific immune responses. Properdin and tuftsin, which are synthesized in the spleen, are opsonins. Tuftsin binds to granulocytes to promote phagocytosis, while properdin can initiate the alternative pathway of complement activation to produce destruction of bacteria as well as foreign and abnormal cells. Because these opsonic proteins are also produced in other organs, the loss of the splenic contribution to their synthesis is probably small. However, serum levels of both tuftsin and properdin are below normal after splenectomy and in some diseases associated with hyposplenism.[8]

The macrophages and histiocytes of the spleen remove bacteria and abnormal or foreign cells and are especially effective in removing bacteria coated with antibody or opsonic proteins. If bacteria for which the host lacks pre-existing antibody are present in the bloodstream, the spleen's unique circulation makes it the major site for clearance of these bacteria as well as the initial site for synthesis of IgM.[8] When radioactively labeled bacteria are administered to animals, the liver clears most of the well-opsonized microorganisms while the spleen removes those that are poorly opsonized.[8] When specific antibody is lacking to facilitate bacterial removal by the liver, the spleen becomes the primary site for clearance. Encapsulated bacteria, which resist antibody binding, are less effectively removed in an asplenic individual than in a normal host.[8]

The role of the spleen in removing malignant tumor cells is probably underestimated. Although large metastases to the spleen are uncommon, micrometastases occur frequently, with one study reporting 50% of spleens from patients with solid tumors containing neoplastic cells. Experimental evi-

THE SPLEEN

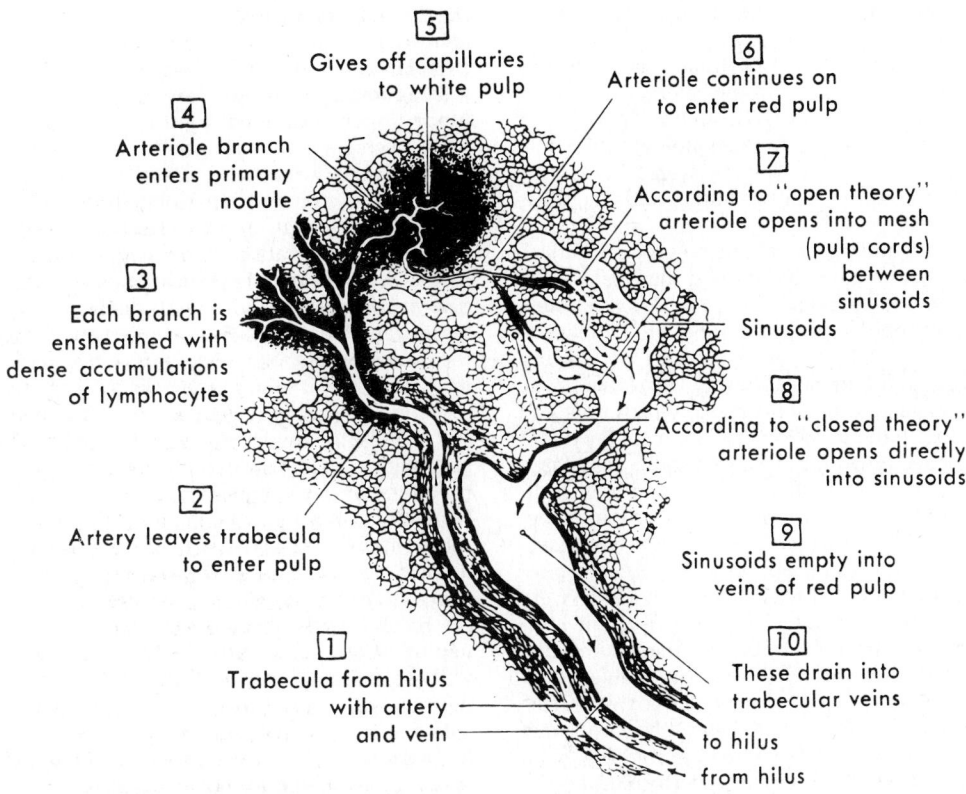

Figure 36–3. Diagram of the blood circulation through the spleen illustrating the *open* and *closed* theories of blood flow.

dence suggests that intense destruction of malignant cells in the spleen limits the incidence of clinically apparent metastases.[8]

A third important immune function of the spleen is the production of specific antibody, especially IgM. Particulate antigens, such as *Salmonella* flagella, lodge in the splenic red pulp and are transported by macrophages into the germinal centers where the IgM response is thought to occur.[8] In asplenic individuals, IgM levels fall and the antibody response to a blood-borne antigen diminishes.[8] Because of the

anatomy of the splenic microcirculation, humoral and cellular antigens remain in contact with macrophages and lymphocytes for longer periods than in other areas of the reticuloendothelial system. The importance of an adequate time period for interaction of these cells after antigen exposure is becoming apparent as lymphocyte and macrophage subpopulations responsible for humoral and cellular immunity are identified.

INDICATIONS FOR SPLENECTOMY

Two large series of studies illustrate the changing indications for splenectomy that have accompanied improved diagnosis and therapy of hematologic diseases.[46, 50] In one report of a 30-year experience, splenectomy was performed for primary and secondary hypersplenism (41%), incidental to other operations (30%), for trauma (10.5%), for diagnosis (9%), for Hodgkin's staging (8%), and for non-Hodgkin's lymphoma (NHL) (1.5%). The more recent 5-year experience, at the University of North Carolina, Chapel Hill, showed the indications for splenectomy in 473 cases to be Hodgkin's staging (27%), incidental to other operations (20%), hypersplenism (16%), trauma (14%), NHL (7%), and diagnosis (7%).[46]

In a comparison between two series of splenectomies performed for hematologic disorders between 1946 and 1962 and 1963 and 1982, 400 splenectomies (20 per year) were performed between 1963 and 1982, compared with 94 (5.5 per year) during the earlier interval.[50] A sharp decline occurred in the number of splenectomies performed each year between 1974 and 1982. The evolution of the staging laparotomy for lymphomas, particularly Hodgkin's disease, with the decline in the average annual incidence of staging laparotomies since 1974 was the major factor responsible. Contributing to the

TABLE 36–1. Biologic Substances Removed by the Spleen

In Normal Subjects
Red blood cell membrane
Red blood cell surface pits and craters
Howell-Jolly bodies
Heinz bodies
Pappenheimer bodies
Acanthocytes
Senescent red blood cells
Particulate antigen

In Patients with Disease
Spherocytes (hereditary spherocytosis)
Sickled cells, Hb C cells
Antibody-coated red blood cells
Antibody-coated platelets
Antibody-coated white blood cells

Modified from Eichner, E. R.: Splenic function: Normal, too much and too little. Am. J. Med., *66*:311, 1979.

differences was an increase in the total number of splenecto-mies for hereditary spherocytosis, idiopathic hypersplenism, and myeloproliferative disorders. The average number of splenectomies for immune thrombocytopenic purpura in-creased significantly between the two time periods. Hairy cell leukemia (HCL) and Felty's syndrome emerged as indica-tions for splenectomy during the second time period. Of the 400 splenectomies performed for hematologic disorders between 1963 and 1982, the indications were therapeutic splenectomy (57%), Hodgkin's staging (40%), and diagnosis (3%).[50]

An improved understanding of immune anemia, thrombo-cytopenia, and neutrocytopenia has clarified the role of sple-nectomy in many hematologic diseases. Some diseases, such as immune thrombocytopenic purpura, appear to be increas-ing in incidence. Splenectomy as a means of staging Hodgkin's disease is no longer such an important diagnostic test in the overall approach to that disease, which now can be controlled in most patients using radiation therapy and chemotherapy. Splenectomy for splenomegaly associated with selected leukemias and NHLs is less commonly indi-cated because chemotherapy and radiation therapy have be-come more effective. Hypersplenism, both primary and sec-ondary, is now diagnosed less commonly because of better definition and classification of diseases that previously were labeled as hypersplenic syndromes. The most frequent indi-cations for splenectomy are now traumatic injury, immune thrombocytopenic purpura, and hypersplenism (Table 36–2).

In another report of splenectomy for hematologic disease, 81% of the patients underwent splenectomy to control ane-mia, thrombocytopenia, neutropenia, or discomfort from splenomegaly.[36] In 19%, splenectomy was performed for di-agnostic purposes, most commonly Hodgkin's disease stag-ing. The morbidity rate of 25% accurately reflects the fre-quency of complications that are related primarily to bleeding and infection. Sepsis is the usual cause of death after splenectomy for hematologic disease, and the mortality rate ranges from 5% to 27% (Table 36–3).[36]

Splenic Trauma

The spleen is the most common intra-abdominal organ injured in blunt trauma and is frequently injured in penetrat-ing abdominal injury. Selected older reports reveal mortality rates for splenic injury as high as 20%. Although some recent series report no deaths from splenic trauma, others still show a mortality rate approaching 10% because of the frequent association of other major organ injuries.

Diagnosis. Injury to the spleen should be suspected in blunt upper abdominal injuries, which commonly occur in motor vehicle or bicycle accidents. Splenic injuries are often associated with fractured ribs of the left chest. The diagnosis and clinical course of an isolated splenic injury is variable. The spleen receives approximately 5% of the cardiac output, and a large laceration through the body of the spleen can extend into the splenic pedicle, causing extensive and contin-ued hemorrhage, abdominal distention with hemoperito-neum, and shock. More commonly, a laceration deep into the pulp occurs or an adhesion between the spleen and its ligaments or diaphragm causes capsular avulsion with cessation of hemorrhage after an initial blood loss of 500 to 750 ml. If the injury does not involve the major splenic vasculature and is limited to the pulp or capsule, the patient may remain hemodynamically stable. However, subcapsular hematomas can form, which have the potential to rupture at a time remote from the injury, accounting for the phenome-non of *delayed* rupture of the spleen. Alternatively, some subcapsular hematomas evolve into splenic cysts while oth-ers resolve with fibrosis and scarring (Fig. 36–4). Unfortu-nately, in the acute setting of evaluating the stable patient with splenic injury, it is difficult to identify which splenic injuries will resolve without operative management.

If a splenic injury is suspected, admission to the hospital for monitoring is mandatory. Although many useful mea-sures are available to aid in the diagnosis of splenic injury, their application requires a high index of clinical suspicion. A careful history should be obtained to include delineation of pain and a mechanism of injury consistent with splenic trauma. Usually injury to the left upper abdomen associated with fractured ribs of the left anterior chest alerts the clinician to proceed with evaluation by specific diagnostic tests. If the patient is in shock with hemoperitoneum, the diagnosis of splenic injury is established at laparotomy.

The signs and symptoms of splenic trauma are those of hemoperitoneum. Generalized and nonspecific abdominal pain in the left upper quadrant occurs in approximately one third of patients with splenic injury. Pain referred to the tip of the left shoulder (Kehr's sign) is inconstant, varying in incidence from 15% to 75%, and is unreliable for excluding splenic injury but is useful for enhancing the diagnostic probability if present. Kehr's sign is elicited by bimanual compression of the left upper quadrant after the patient has been in Trendelenburg's position for several minutes preceding the maneuver. On rare occasions, patients with splenic injury have a palpable tender mass in the left upper quadrant (Ballance's sign), caused by an extracapsular or subcapsular hematoma with omentum adherent to the injured spleen.

Patients with splenic trauma usually have hemoglobin/hematocrit values that are 10% to 30% below normal and a moderate leukocytosis. Diagnostic peritoneal lavage is a use-ful and inexpensive maneuver, which may reveal gross blood or an elevated red blood cell count diagnostic of intraperito-neal hemorrhage. When intraperitoneal hemorrhage is diag-nosed by peritoneal lavage, laparotomy is performed to diag-nose and treat all bleeding viscera, including the spleen.

A variety of imaging techniques are useful in the diagnosis of splenic injury. Standard abdominal or contrast radiogra-phy may reveal depression of the splenic flexure of the colon and medial displacement of the stomach in patients with an injured spleen but are less reliable in establishing the diagno-sis of splenic trauma than isotope or scanning techniques.

TABLE 36–2. Indications for Splenectomy

To Control or Stage Basic Disease

Hereditary spherocytosis
Autoimmune anemia
Hodgkin's disease
Ruptured spleen
Immune thrombocytopenic purpura
Thrombotic thrombocytopenic purpura
Primary cysts or tumors

For Chronic and Severe Hypersplenism

Hairy cell leukemia
Lymphoproliferative disorders (non-Hodgkin's lymphoma, chronic lymphocytic leukemia)
Felty's syndrome
Agnogenic myeloid metaplasia
Thalassemia major
Gaucher's disease
Hemodialysis splenomegaly
Splenic vein thrombosis
Sickle cell disease, HbS/C disease
Acquired immunodeficiency syndrome
Thrombocytopenia associated with drug abuse

Modified from Eichner, E. R.: Splenic function: Normal, too much and too little. Am. J. Med., 66:311, 1979.

TABLE 36–3. Characteristics of 306 Patients Who Underwent Splenectomy for Hematologic Disease

Diagnosis	Number of Patients	Mean Age (Range)	Sex (M:F)	Number with Complications (%)	Deaths (%)	Mean Spleen Weight (gm.) (Range)
Idiopathic thrombocytopenic purpura	65	35 (0.5–73)	0.3	14 (22)	1 (2)	171 (26–660)
Hodgkin's disease	40	26 (5–57)	1.5	4 (10)	2 (5)	349 (50–1698)
Hereditary spherocytosis	39	15 (4–44)	0.8	2 (5)	0	430 (57–1500)
Non-Hodgkin's lymphoma	25	49 (7–76)	0.9	9 (36)	1 (4)	573 (60–2050)
Idiopathic hypersplenism	21	48 (5–74)	2.0	9 (43)	5 (24)	798 (357–2050)
Myelofibrosis	17	55 (30–72)	2.4	8 (47)	3 (18)	1776 (205–5180)
Felty's syndrome	16	56 (20–80)	0.6	3 (19)	0	766 (225–1250)
Hairy cell leukemia	16	52 (32–68)	15.0	3 (19)	1 (6)	1904 (319–5400)
Autoimmune hemolytic anemia	14	44 (16–67)	0.6	3 (21)	0	762 (175–2800)
Chronic myelogenous leukemia	9	49 (21–87)	3.5	5 (56)	3 (33)	2981 (1102–6040)
Splenomegaly with portal hypertension	9	44 (21–62)	0.1	4 (44)	0	862 (500–1830)
Chronic lymphocytic leukemia	7	62 (49–71)	2.4	5 (71)	0	2113 (685–5500)
Other*	28	35 (1–77)	0.6	7 (25)	0	773 (120–3060)
Total	306			76 (25)	16 (5)	

*This category includes ill-defined myeloproliferative disorders (4), pure red cell aplasia (3), pyruvate kinase deficiency (2), thalassemia (2), aplastic anemia (2), splenomegaly without cytopenia (2), infectious mononucleosis (2), congenital nonspherocytic hemolytic anemia (1), systemic lupus erythematosus (1), amyloidosis (1), sickle cell anemia (1), Letterer-Siwe disease (1), Gaucher's disease (2), polycthemia vera (1), mast cell leukemia (1), and subacute monocytic leukemia (1).

From Musser, G., Lazar, G., Hocking, W., and Busuttil, R. W.: Splenectomy for hematologic disease: The UCLA experience with 306 patients. Ann. Surg., *200*:41, 1984.

Splenic angiography can demonstrate a variety of splenic injuries but is used infrequently because of the equal or greater accuracy of diagnostic peritoneal lavage and less invasive imaging techniques. Ultrasonography of the spleen can provide evidence of free blood and hematoma surrounding the splenic capsule with reasonable accuracy. Isotope scans (^{99m}Tc sulfur colloid) are popular in many centers for the acute diagnosis of splenic injury with a diagnostic accuracy rate exceeding 90%. However, computed tomography (CT) is probably the most accurate method available for diagnosing splenic injury (Fig. 36–5).

Reports of imaging techniques reveal a high sensitivity and specificity (>90%) for the diagnosis of splenic injury; however, considerable variation exists in the skill and enthusiasm of different radiologic units performing the tests for suspected splenic injury. Although CT and isotope imaging techniques are accurate methods for establishing the diagnosis of an injured spleen, the accuracy in individual instances is in large part dependent on the skill of the radiologist.

Changing Concepts in the Treatment of Ruptured Spleen. In recent years the spleen's important role in cellular and humoral immunity has been clarified and the danger of overwhelming bacterial infection in asplenic patients has been established.[8, 30, 42, 43] Consequently, operative techniques for splenic preservation have been developed, and a concept for nonoperative management of selected splenic injuries is evolving.[33, 34, 37, 42, 43] Although periodic reports of repairing injured spleens by use of suture or cauterization have been available for many years, interest in partial splenectomy has been rekindled since 1960. In animal and human studies, it has been shown that segmental resection of the spleen is practical and safe.[42, 43] In addition to partial splenectomy, splenorrhaphy, ligation of segmental vessels, and capsular repair are useful techniques for splenic salvage (Figs. 36–6

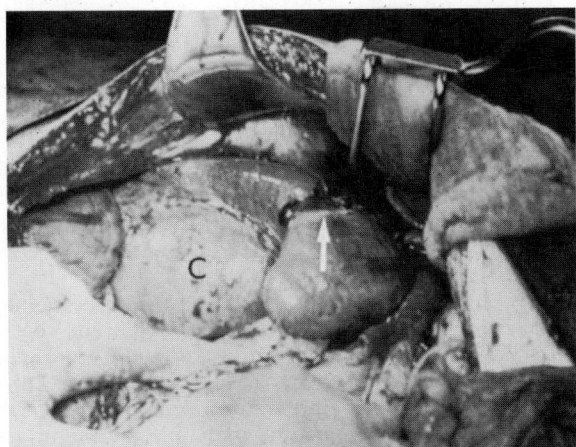

Figure 36–4. Operative photograph showing a traumatic laceration (arrow) producing avulsion of the lower pole of the spleen and a splenic cyst (C), an incidental finding produced by untreated injury 8 years previously. Splenic salvage was precluded by dense inflammatory adhesions between the spleen and the diaphragm.

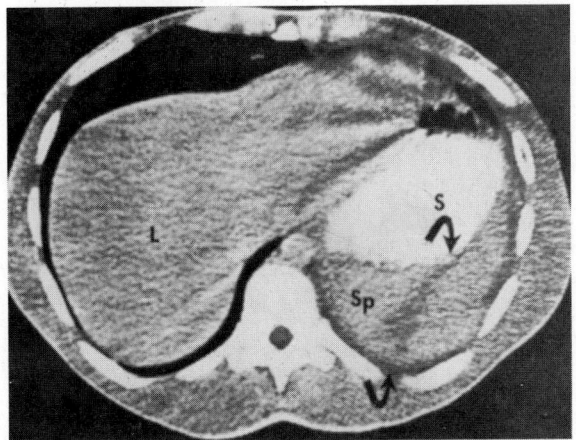

Figure 36–5. Computed tomogram revealing a laceration of the spleen (arrows). The liver (L) and stomach (S) were uninjured. (From Federle, M. P., Crass, R. A., Jeffrey, R. B., and Trunkey, D. D.: Computed tomography in blunt abdominal trauma. Arch. Surg., *117*:645, 1982. Copyright 1982, American Medical Asssociation.)

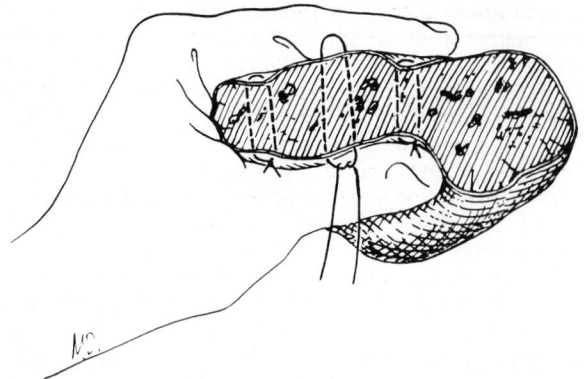

Figure 36–6. Technique of hemostasis after partial splenectomy. The spleen should be adequately mobilized to identify and control the injury. Compression facilitates identification of bleeding vessels, which are occluded by sutures or small metal clips, and placement of absorbable mattress sutures to control bleeding from the raw surface. (From Blaisdell, F. W., and Trunkey, D. D.: Trauma Management. New York, Thieme-Stratton, 1982, p. 194.)

and 36–7). Splenic salvage operations have been greatly aided by the development and use of topical hemostatic agents such as microfibrillar collagen (Avitene) and a variety of absorbable *envelopes* to aid in hemostasis from splenic injuries.[28] Although technically more difficult than splenectomy, splenic repair can be performed with comparable transfusion requirements, reoperation rates, and morbidity.

Conservatism in the management of splenic injury has extended beyond repairing and preserving an injured spleen when possible. Because bleeding from splenic trauma appears to be more self-limited in children than in adults, nonoperative therapy may prove to be safe in selected pediatric patients. Nonoperative therapy requires a stable patient who is found by diagnostic tests to have an isolated splenic injury. At The Hospital for Sick Children (Toronto), where nonoperative management of splenic injury has been pioneered, 75 children with splenic injury were treated between 1981 and 1986. Ten (13%) required splenectomy or splenorrhaphy, but the remaining 65 patients (87%) were successfully managed nonoperatively. Of those patients treated nonoperatively, only 23% required blood transfusions. In comparison to an earlier report, current guidelines for management have resulted in an increased number of patients managed nonop-

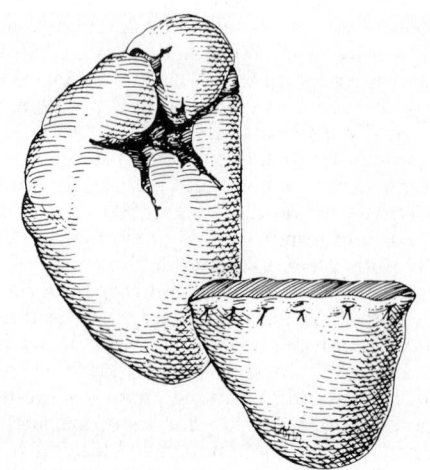

Figure 36–7. Technique of splenorrhaphy. Stellate lacerations that are deep or involve the hilus are best treated by resection of the injured segment. (From Blaisdell, F. W., and Trunkey, D. D.: Trauma Management. New York, Thieme-Stratton, 1982, p. 194.)

eratively, a reduction in the number of patients receiving blood transfusions, and a decrease in the length of both hospital stay and time spent in the intensive care unit.[37]

In one large series of injuries associated with splenic trauma an appropriate note of caution was suggested before nonoperative management of splenic trauma is adopted.[47] In 258 patients with splenic injury, concomitant injuries requiring operative therapy were present in 36.5% of those with blunt trauma and 94% of patients with penetrating injury. Children younger than the age of 16 had an incidence of intra-abdominal injuries in addition to the spleen of 32.6% for blunt trauma and 100% for penetrating trauma.[48]

One pitfall of nonoperative management of splenic trauma lies in the significant possibility of failing to diagnose and treat concomitant intra-abdominal injuries. An additional concern is that most reported series of nonoperative management of splenic injuries include patients with blood transfusion requirements substantial enough to expect an incidence of transfusion-related hepatitis greater than the statistical probability of postsplenectomy sepsis. In addition, hospital time is usually longer for nonoperative management (13–16 days) compared with operative management (7 days) with a longer period for convalescence.[47]

The recommended management in adults with hemoperitoneum and demonstrated splenic injury is laparotomy with the expectation that 30% to 50% of spleens may be salvaged with sufficient (>50%) splenic pulp retained to preserve immune function. In both children and adults with splenic injury secondary to penetrating wounds, laparotomy should be performed because of the risk of significant injury to other intra-abdominal organs. All patients in shock or with significant transfusion requirement should have exploratory laparotomy for control of hemorrhage from the spleen and management of any other injured structures.

Nonoperative treatment of splenic trauma in children is prudent only for the stable patient who is being followed in an appropriate hospital area by surgeons experienced in nonoperative management. There should be no hesitation to proceed with laparotomy and splenic repair. Operation is well tolerated, and splenic salvage techniques are probably more feasible in children than adults because of the higher ratio of splenic capsule to pulp. Any mortality from nonoperative management of splenic injury in children is unacceptable.

Delayed Rupture of the Spleen. As early as 1866, Evans suggested that the spleen might bleed catastrophically at a time remote from injury.[43] It was postulated that injury to the pulp of the spleen could not be contained indefinitely by the thin splenic capsule under continuous arterial pressure. The usual interval between injury and the onset of clinically apparent intra-abdominal hemorrhage (*period de latence,* Baudet, 1907) is within 2 weeks, although longer intervals have been reported.[43] Although the incidence of delayed rupture of the spleen has been reported to be 15% to 30%, the criteria for diagnosis are variable and unconvincing.[43] It is apparent from splenic injuries managed nonoperatively that many heal by fibrosis and without sequelae. The entity of delayed rupture of the spleen is more properly referred to as *delayed diagnosis* of splenic injury. As imaging techniques for follow-up of suspected or proved splenic trauma become commonplace, it is likely that delayed rupture of the spleen will cease to be an entity with clinical meaning or application.

Splenosis and Splenic Implants. Splenosis is the autotransplantation of splenic tissue after splenic trauma. Although fewer than 200 cases have been reported, the true incidence of splenosis undoubtedly is more common because of the high incidence of traumatic injury to the spleen. Appearing as sessile or pedunculated dark red nodules, splenic implants vary from a few millimeters to several centimeters in diameter. Splenic implants depend on a blood supply from small arteries penetrating the capsule and usually remain small or outgrow their blood supply and undergo infarction. Splenosis may occur anywhere in the peritoneal cavity and has been reported on the pericardium and the pleura as well as in the subcutaneous tissue of abdominal incisions.[10] Splenosis seldom causes symptoms and is usually discovered as an incidental finding at reoperation years after splenic trauma. Isolated reports have described splenosis producing intestinal obstruction from adhesions, stomach masses simulating carcinoma, and pain, presumably from torsion.[10]

Recent interest in the postsplenectomy sepsis syndrome has heightened interest in splenosis as potentially valuable for preservation of immune function by providing splenic implants at the time of removal of an injured spleen. Splenosis can be produced in a variety of animals by transplantation of splenic pulp.[10] Von Stubenrauch seeded crushed splenic pulp throughout the peritoneal cavity in dogs and believed that *splenoids* arose *de novo* from the peritoneum. Perla described the histologic sequence of splenic transplants in rats. After transplantation, splenic implants underwent degeneration with only the reticulum cells at the periphery remaining viable after 24 hours. Regeneration of splenic tissue appeared to originate from the reticulum cell precursor.[10] Recently, investigators interested in preserving the immune function of the spleen have injected splenic pulp into the liver to avoid mechanical problems from adhesions that sometimes develop in association with splenosis.

Splenosis, *the born-again spleen*, may provide the blood management functions of the spleen.[37] The absence of Howell-Jolly bodies, siderocytes, and other postsplenectomy blood changes as well as the recurrence of the hematologic disease for which splenectomy was performed should raise suspicion of splenosis or the presence of accessory splenic tissue.[23, 38, 40, 41, 51] Splenosis has been reported in conjunction with the expected postsplenectomy blood changes, suggesting a critical mass of splenic tissue is needed for recovery of splenic function. Residual splenic tissue can be detected by isotope scanning using ^{99m}Tc sulfur colloid (Fig. 36–8).

Splenic reticuloendothelial function has been investigated in a series of patients previously undergoing total splenectomy, partial splenectomy and splenic repair, and splenic autotransplantation.[48] Partial splenectomy and splenorrhaphy resulted in normal splenic reticuloendothelial function that was indistinguishable from a control group of patients sustaining trauma but who had intact spleens. Extraperitoneal

splenic autotransplantation resulted in the preservation of a small amount of reticuloendothelial function. The subnormal reticuloendothelial function achieved by splenic autotransplantation was clearly superior to that resulting from total splenectomy without deliberate splenic autotransplantation. Splenic autotransplantation, which in this study involved placing thin slices of spleen weighing a total of 25 to 30 gm. into an anterolateral extraperitoneal pocket, appeared to be safe and was not associated with increased postoperative complications.[48]

Although autotransplanted splenic tissue, accessory splenic tissue, and splenosis can restore some of the spleen's blood management functions and antibody synthesis, it is unclear how much splenic tissue is needed for protection against overwhelming postsplenectomy sepsis. Studies have failed to identify re-establishment of resistance to postsplenectomy sepsis after autotransplantation of splenic tissue. Death from postsplenectomy sepsis has occurred in children and adults having a total mass of residual splenic tissue weighing 3 to 92 gm.[48] Although residual splenic tissue can restore some of the spleen's functions, a critical amount of splenic tissue is required for full protection against postsplenectomy sepsis.[8, 30, 42]

Immune Thrombocytopenic Purpura

Immune thrombocytopenic purpura (ITP, previously called idiopathic thrombocytopenic purpura) is a syndrome characterized by a persistently low platelet count. The thrombocytopenia is caused by a circulating antiplatelet factor that causes platelet destruction by the reticuloendothelial system. In most patients, the antiplatelet factor is an immunoglobulin (IgG) antibody directed toward a platelet-associated antigen. Circulating immune complexes may have a causal role in some cases, but their precise role is unclear. Proof of autoimmunity is lacking.[31]

The majority of patients with ITP are young women. In Schwartz's series, the average age was 36 years and the duration of clinical symptoms before splenectomy was 24 weeks, with an average preoperative platelet count of 33,000 per cu. mm.[41] ITP is increasing in frequency, and the disease is being diagnosed more often now in men. This increase results in part from the association of immune thrombocytopenia with the acquired immunodeficiency syndrome (AIDS) and an increasing occurrence of ITP in three groups of patients at risk for developing AIDS—homosexual men positive for human immunodeficiency virus (HIV), parenteral drug abusers, and hemophiliacs receiving multiple transfusions.[21] The diagnosis of ITP is suggested by spontaneous and easy bruising, petechiae, and mucosal bleeding. Menorrhagia is common, and prolonged bleeding after shaving trauma may be an initial complaint in males. Intracranial hemorrhage is a rare and usually fatal complication.

The propensity for hemorrhage is reflected by the level of thrombocytopenia. A bleeding diathesis is unlikely with thrombocytopenia in the range of 50,000 to 100,000 per cu. mm. Bleeding with minor trauma or surgical procedure can be expected with platelet counts in the range of 20,000 to 100,000 per cu. mm. Spontaneous bleeding with purpura and petechiae, epistaxis, menorrhagia, gingival bleeding, and so on, occurs commonly with platelet counts below 20,000 per cu. mm. and especially below 5,000 per cu. mm.[26]

Crosby has suggested classifying patients with thrombocytopenia into those with *dry purpura* (petechiae and ecchymoses) and those with *wet purpura* (active bleeding from mucosal surfaces). This distinction postulates that patients with wet purpura are at increased risk for central nervous system bleeding and thus require aggressive treatment.[31]

Patients with easy bruisability or hemorrhage require a

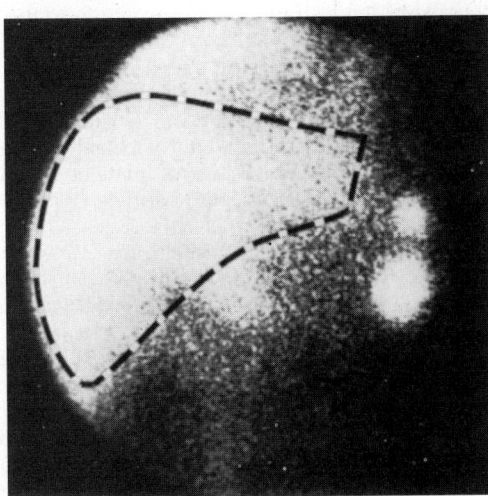

Figure 36–8. ^{99m}Tc sulfur colloid scan reveals two accessory spleens in the left upper quadrant. The liver is outlined.

careful history with special emphasis on recent exposure to quinine, quinidine, sulfonamides, and thiazides that may produce drug-dependent antibodies and immune thrombocytopenia. Isoantibodies against transfusion products can also cause thrombocytopenia. Collagen disease such as systemic lupus erythematosus may be indistinguishable in initial presentation from ITP.[26, 31] Pseudothrombocytopenia, a phenomenon in which the platelet count is spuriously low, results when antibodies in the patient's serum react with platelets in blood anticoagulated with ethylenediaminetetraacetic acid (EDTA), causing agglutination. Platelet clumping results in a falsely low platelet count that will be at variance with the estimated number of platelets present on a peripheral blood smear obtained by fingertip puncture. EDTA-dependent platelet antibodies have been detected in several patients erroneously diagnosed as having ITP.[23, 51] Diagnosis of immune thrombocytopenia requires the exclusion of drug-dependent antibodies, isoantibodies, collagen vascular disease, lymphoproliferative disorders, thyroid disease, recent viral illness, and spurious thrombocytopenia.[23, 26, 31, 51] Patients with *classic* ITP rarely have a palpable spleen (<2%), whereas a palpable spleen that reflects mild to moderate enlargement and an associated high incidence of generalized lymphadenopathy have been found in ITP associated with AIDS.[23, 51]

ITP is diagnosed definitively only after exclusion of other illnesses or conditions that cause or are associated with thrombocytopenia. Except for thrombocytopenia, patients with ITP usually have normal blood cell counts. Antinuclear antibodies are rarely present, but autoantibodies have been noted in some patients. A peripheral blood smear shows thrombocytopenia, occasionally with an increased number of large platelets. A bone marrow aspirate reveals normal granulocytic and erythrocytic elements with an increased megakaryocyte count.[23, 31, 51]

Platelet Kinetics and the Immune System in ITP. Platelet kinetics in patients with ITP are markedly altered with an increased platelet production (four to five times normal) and an increased megakaryocyte mass being present in association with a greatly shortened platelet survival.[31] In patients with ITP, body-surface counts show primarily splenic sequestration of platelets with significant liver sequestration occurring only in patients with severe disease. The amount of platelet-associated antibody reflects the severity of the clinical disease and is inversely correlated with the patient's platelet count and intravascular platelet life span. The antiplatelet factor probably is an IgG antibody directed against a platelet-associated antigen. In some patients, the IgG antibody functions in combination with IgM, IgA, or both.[31] Antiplatelet antibody assays are now routinely available, and the value for platelet-associated IgG normally is less than 1200 gamma-globulin molecules per platelet.

The spleen is an important site of antibody production, and splenic cells from patients with chronic ITP produce five to six times more IgG in culture than control splenic cells.[31] The initial immune response to the platelet antigen probably occurs in the spleen, or in the bone marrow where intramedullary platelets and megakaryocytes share antigenic determinants and may trigger a response. In its function as a monitor of the intravascular space, the spleen probably is more important in the early response. Less involved initially, the marrow assumes an important role as the immune response becomes generalized. With development and recirculation of memory cells (both B and T lymphocytes), the marrow becomes a major site of antibody production. The liver produces little or no antiplatelet antibody, and the lymph nodes are not deeply involved in the response to intravascular antigens.[31]

Platelet destruction in ITP requires sufficient quantities of antigen (platelets), antibody, and phagocytic cells in an environment that provides time for antibody binding and subsequent platelet phagocytosis.[31] The spleen is ideally suited for this function, and once platelet sensitization has occurred, phagocytosis is triggered by the Fc portion of the IgG molecule or by complement activation with C3b fixation to the platelet surface. The macrophage Fc receptor mechanism clearly is important as increased platelet-bound IgG is present in essentially all patients with ITP. Macrophage Fc and C3b receptors may act synergistically, resulting in a greatly enhanced phagocytic efficiency.[31]

Because 30% of the total circulating platelet mass is within the spleen at all times as an exchangeable platelet pool, the spleen is the most active site of platelet destruction.[31] The stagnant blood flow in the splenic microcirculation allows sensitized platelets to be readily removed by phagocytic cells lining the reticular network of the red pulp. Having no resident platelet pool and possessing a rapid microcirculation by contrast, the liver assumes a major role in platelet destruction when severe disease and high antibody titers result in heavily sensitized platelets. The bone marrow is the most likely source of antibody in patients who have undergone splenectomy.[31] Intramedullary platelet destruction and inhibition of thrombopoiesis may occur as a result of antiplatelet antibody binding to both platelets and megakaryocytes, although the efficiency of the marrow reticuloendothelial system is below that of the liver and the spleen.[31]

A study investigating the mechanisms of increase in the platelet count after treatment of ITP determined the survival time and localization of radiolabeled autologous platelets and measured platelet-associated immunoglobulin levels before and after prednisone therapy or splenectomy.[12] Prednisone therapy produced an increased platelet count from increased platelet production. The increased platelet count after splenectomy correlated with increased platelet survival. The degree of radiolabeled platelet localization in the liver was normal in patients in whom splenectomy was effective and was increased to above normal in patients in whom splenectomy was ineffective. The conclusion that prednisone improves platelet counts primarily by increasing platelet production requires modification of the pathophysiologic concept of ITP to incorporate the hypothesis that in some patients the predominant cause of thrombocytopenia is ineffective marrow production of platelets rather than accelerated platelet removal.[12]

In summary, thrombocytopenia in patients with ITP usually occurs from a combination of intramedullary platelet removal by reticuloendothelial cells, causing ineffective platelet production and decreased survival of circulating platelets due to peripheral sequestration and destruction in the spleen and liver. Successful therapy may produce an increase in the platelet count either by increasing the effective production of platelets or by decreasing peripheral platelet sequestration and destruction. Splenectomy appears to increase platelet survival by removing a major organ of peripheral destruction. If the liver is the major site of platelet destruction, splenectomy may not result in improvement in the platelet count.[12]

Treatment. The goal of therapy in chronic ITP is to obtain a complete and sustained remission of the disease and to remove the patient from the risks of hemorrhage.[30] This can be achieved in 80% to 90% of patients (Table 36–4).

When ITP is initially diagnosed, the patient should be hospitalized. A patient having active bleeding should remain at bed rest and have specific therapy instituted. Platelet transfusions provide immediate benefit and should be administered as needed to control bleeding. Although transfused platelets rapidly become coated with antibody and destroyed and provide only transient benefit, they afford protection against life-threatening bleeding.[26, 31] High-dose intravenous

TABLE 36–4. Results of Therapy in Immune Thrombocytopenic Purpura

Therapy	Number of Cases	Average Dose	Response Time (Days)	Response (%)*			
				Excellent	Good	Fair	Poor
Splenectomy	756		1–14	80	←———— 20 ————→		
Corticosteroids	253	60–100 mg./day	14	19	←——— 34 ———→		47
Cyclophosphamide	61	50–200 mg./day	14–56	42	14	12	32
Vinblastine	20	10 mg./wk.	10	5	←——— 56 ———→		39
Vincristine	21	2 mg./wk.	10	←——— 28 ———→		48	24
Azathioprine	92	100–250 mg./day	60–120	8	18	26	48

*Response definitions: excellent, normal platelet count after therapy; good, normal platelet count during therapy; fair, improved platelet count during therapy; poor, no response. In some cases, details of the reports did not permit accurate placement, and in those cases percentages may apply to more than one response category (arrows).

Adapted from McMillan, R.: Chronic idiopathic thrombocytopenic purpura. N. Engl. J. Med., 1981, *304*:1135. Copyright 1981. Massachusetts Medical Society. All rights reserved.

gamma-globulin is also useful but requires several days for a beneficial platelet increase to occur.

Corticosteroid therapy (prednisone, 1 mg. per kg. per day or the therapeutic equivalent) is instituted at the time of diagnosis. Most patients with ITP are improved with administration of corticosteroids, with an increase in the platelet count occurring within 3 to 7 days and reaching a maximum in several weeks.[31] Complete and sustained remission with corticosteroid therapy is rare, although rates as high as 25% have been reported.[31] In most cases, even if the platelet count becomes normal, the response is transient, and thrombocytopenia recurs as the corticosteroid dose is tapered.

Splenectomy should be performed in patients with ITP that is refractory to corticosteroid therapy. In the majority of patients, splenectomy is performed electively. Emergent splenectomy is necessary in patients with ITP who have evidence of central nervous system bleeding.

Complete remission after splenectomy is more likely in patients who have shown a response to corticosteroids. Additional clinical features indicating the likelihood of a favorable response to splenectomy include patients who are younger than 60 years old, who have disease of relatively short duration, and who exhibit a prompt thrombocytosis with platelet counts reaching 500,000 per cu. mm. or more after splenectomy.[26, 31] Most patients, however, are improved after splenectomy, even if their platelet counts were not significantly increased by corticosteroid therapy.

Eighty-eight percent of Schwartz's patients responded to splenectomy and developed normal platelet counts. Of those responding to splenectomy, 20% had platelet counts exceeding 100,000 per cu. mm. by the third postoperative day, and 90% of them had normal platelet counts after 1 week. The remaining responders developed normal platelet counts within 1 to 6 months postoperatively. In three patients, thrombocytopenia recurred after a long interval and was attributed in one patient to an accessory spleen.[41]

The level of platelet-associated IgG falls to normal after a response to splenectomy due to the removal of a large site of antiplatelet antibody production.[31] A corticosteroid response is also accompanied by a decrease in platelet-associated IgG. An increase in the platelet count often occurs before platelet-associated IgG falls because of the corticosteroid influence on the reticuloendothelial system. A response to immunosuppressants such as cyclophosphamide and vincristine is also associated with a decrease in platelet-associated IgG.[31]

ITP During Childhood. In children, particularly those younger than age 6, ITP often appears after a viral upper respiratory tract infection. In contrast to the adult form of the disease, childhood ITP usually undergoes spontaneous remission without specific therapy. A short course of prednisone therapy is usually prescribed; however, a clear benefit has not been demonstrated.[26]

Intracranial hemorrhage is a life-threatening complication of childhood ITP and occurs in 1% to 2% of cases. It is responsible for the majority of deaths from the disease in this age group. The risk of intracranial hemorrhage is greatest during the first month of the illness. Most reported cases appear to be spontaneous, but minor head trauma may result in intracranial hemorrhage in patients with platelet counts below 10,000 to 20,000 per cu. mm.[52] Development of intracranial hemorrhage in ITP is an indication for emergency splenectomy.

Spontaneous and complete remission occurs in approximately 85% of children with ITP. Those in whom spontaneous remission does not occur within 1 year are considered to have chronic ITP and usually undergo elective splenectomy to avoid the risks of chronic thrombocytopenia.

Splenectomy and Perioperative Therapy for ITP. Most patients are referred for splenectomy after corticosteroid therapy has failed to achieve a complete and sustained remission. A small group of patients have ITP diagnosed due to abnormal bleeding during surgical procedures or after injury. A third group of patients require emergent splenectomy for intracranial hemorrhage.

High-dose intravenous gamma-globulin is very effective in achieving an increase in the platelet count preoperatively in patients who do not respond to corticosteroids or are not candidates for corticosteroid therapy. It is postulated that intravenous gamma-globulin therapy promotes a rise in the platelet count due to temporarily reducing platelet destruction by saturating macrophage Fc receptors, thus producing a transient blockade of the reticuloendothelial system. A significantly improved platelet count (100,000–250,000/cu. mm.) occurs within 4 to 6 days and provides a *therapeutic window* for performance of splenectomy.[23, 51] In addition to affecting an increase in the platelet counts of patients failing to respond to corticosteroids or who are not candidates for corticosteroid therapy, high-dose gamma-globulin therapy is appropriate for the patient with ITP needing urgent splenectomy in whom a trial of corticosteroids is not warranted and in the pregnant patient with ITP late in the third trimester of pregnancy.

Immunizations with polyvalent pneumococcal vaccine (Pnu-Imune 23 or Pneumovax 23), *Haemophilus influenzae* vaccine, and *Neisseria meningitidis* vaccine should be administered as soon as it becomes likely that splenectomy will be performed. Ideally these immunizations should be carried out 10 to 14 days preoperatively. It is probable that patients receiving corticosteroids have a suboptimal early response to these vaccines but ultimately will develop protective antibody titers. The availability of blood and platelets for transfusion should be ensured, although the need for blood transfusion is rare. Intraoperative thrombocytopenic bleeding usually ceases after the splenic artery is ligated. In Schwartz's series, platelets were not used preoperatively and were administered intraoperatively or postoperatively in only 9 of 120 patients having splenectomy for ITP.[41] Although a nasogastric tube is advisable for postoperative gastric decompression in most patients undergoing splenectomy, some avoid use of a nasogastric tube in patients with ITP because of the potential risk of precipitating hemorrhage from the nose or nasopharynx.

Splenectomy can be performed through a variety of abdominal incisions. The midline incision is preferred in ITP because it allows entry into the peritoneal cavity without transection of abdominal muscles and thus reduces the potential for postoperative muscle hematoma. The spleen, usually of normal size, is assessed for adhesions and the nature of its ligamentous attachments. Splenic ligaments vary considerably in composition, being thin membranes affording easy dissection in some patients and being thick and tendinous in others. The technique for splenectomy is a matter of personal preference. The authors prefer the sequence of initially incising the posterior splenic ligaments followed by mobilizing the spleen and tail of the pancreas toward the midline for subsequent dissection of the splenic vessels in the hilus. Caution is taken to avoid excessive traction or trauma to the tail of the pancreas. Division of the gastrosplenic ligament is performed with suture ligation of the gastric ends of the short gastric arteries. After removal of the spleen, laparotomy pads are placed in the left upper quadrant while a search is made for accessory splenic tissue. Approximately 20% of patients have an accessory spleen, and common sites are the splenic hilus, adjacent to the splenic vessels and tail of the pancreas, greater omentum, and gastrosplenic and gastrocolic ligaments. Rarely has an accessory spleen been found in the intestinal mesentery, presacral, and gonadal regions.[9, 40] The left upper quadrant is not drained routinely. Indications for closed suction drainage are injury to the pancreas during hilar dissection and incomplete hemostasis.

During the immediate postoperative period, corticosteroid therapy is continued intravenously, and the platelet count is monitored. It usually is possible to begin tapering the corticosteroid dose immediately, and in patients demonstrating a satisfactory thrombocytosis, corticosteroids are gradually reduced over 4 to 6 weeks and discontinued.

The mortality rate for splenectomy in ITP is under 2% and occurs primarily in patients with intracranial hemorrhage. In approximately 80% of adult patients who have splenectomy for ITP, the platelet count returns to normal or above-normal levels within the first 6 weeks after operation.[31] In approximately 15% there is substantial improvement in the platelet count from preoperative levels, but it does not reach a normal level. Only about 5% of patients remain severely thrombocytopenic after splenectomy and require some form of chronic therapy. In these patients with refractory ITP, therapy having the least side effects is chosen to maintain the platelet count at a safe level (30,000 to 50,000/cu. mm.). Ingestion of antiplatelet drugs, trauma, azotemia, fever, and infection increases the bleeding tendency in thrombocytopenic patients.[31] Immunosuppressants such as cyclophosphamide, *Vinca* alkaloids (vincristine and vinblastine), azathioprine, and danazol, a modified androgen, have been used to treat patients with refractory ITP, with variable results (see Table 36–4).

Thrombotic Thrombocytopenic Purpura

Thrombotic thrombocytopenic purpura (TTP, Moschcowitz's syndrome) is a syndrome characterized by thrombocytopenia, microangiopathic hemolytic anemia, fluctuating neurologic abnormalities, progressive renal failure, and fever. TTP is produced by widespread deposition of platelet microthrombi, and the pentad of clinical manifestations results from occlusion of arterioles and capillaries by subendothelial and intraluminal deposits of *hyaline* material composed of aggregated platelets and fibrin. The etiology of TTP is unknown, and approximately 90% of the cases of TTP are idiopathic. The pathologic response in TTP may be initiated by various stimuli, including viral and bacterial infection, pregnancy, drugs (oral contraceptives, mitomycin, and cyclosporine), and nonspecified toxins. The syndrome has been associated with systemic lupus erythematosus and other connective tissue disorders, malignancies, and more recently with AIDS. TTP has a peak incidence in the third decade of life and occurs more frequently in females than in males.[23, 51]

The differential diagnosis includes hemolytic-uremic syndrome, disseminated intravascular coagulation, drug reaction, eclampsia, aplastic anemia, idiopathic AIHA, ITP, leukemia, paroxysmal nocturnal hemoglobinuria, periarteritis nodosa, infection, systemic lupus erythematosus, and exposure to toxins. The exact role of the spleen in TTP is unclear, but approximately 20% of patients will have splenomegaly.[23, 51]

Prognosis for untreated patients with TTP is very poor, with less than 10% surviving beyond 1 year.[23] The current therapeutic regimen of infusions of fresh-frozen plasma results in dramatic improvement for the majority of patients with TTP. A combined therapeutic approach using plasma therapy, antiplatelet agents (aspirin and dipyridamole) and high-dose corticosteroid therapy is instituted immediately after the diagnosis is established. Plasma infusion or plasma exchange using plasmapheresis and replacement with fresh-frozen plasma achieves response rates between 70% and 90%.[23] It is speculated that plasma infusion or plasma exchange replaces a deficient plasma component or removes some toxic substance.[23, 51] Immunosuppressive drugs (vincristine and azathioprine) are also beneficial adjunctive agents in the present combined therapeutic approach for TTP. If combined-modality therapy fails, splenectomy should be performed. Splenectomy occasionally results in spectacular improvement, particularly when combined with high-dose corticosteroid therapy and antiplatelet drugs.[23] Although a clear physiologic explanation is lacking for this occasional response to splenectomy, prior experience has documented that 70% of the long-term survivors with TTP were patients who had undergone splenectomy.[41]

Hypersplenism

Hypersplenism is a concept, probably first used by Chauffard in 1907, which refers to a variety of ill effects resulting from increased splenic function that may be improved by splenectomy.[23, 51] Criteria for diagnosis include: (1) anemia, leukopenia, thrombocytopenia, or combinations thereof; (2) compensatory bone marrow hyperplasia; (3) splenomegaly; and (4) improvement after splenectomy.[8, 23, 51] Hypersplenism is classified as primary when an underlying disease cannot be identified to account for the exaggerated splenic function. Secondary hypersplenism refers to those cases in which a specific or more-or-less well-defined disorder has been diagnosed. Because it now is possible to obtain more specific diagnoses for many patients who previously would have been thought to have primary hypersplenism, primary hypersplenism is now diagnosed much less frequently than secondary hypersplenism.

Primary hypersplenism was initially described in 1939 by Doan and Wiseman as an illness consisting of neutropenia and splenomegaly for which splenectomy was curative.[40] The definition of the syndrome subsequently was broadened to include patients with variable degrees of anemia, thrombocytopenia, or pancytopenia. Subclassification of primary hypersplenism is used to describe splenic hyperfunction producing depression of one or more of the formed elements of the blood (red cells, white cells, and platelets). Primary splenic panhematopenia (pancytopenia) refers to depression of all formed elements, whereas in primary splenic neutropenia, depression of the white blood cells is the prominent feature.

Most patients with primary hypersplenism are women. Clinical manifestations are dependent on the specific formed elements that are depressed and include pallor and other signs of anemia, fever, recurrent infections, oral ulcerations, ecchymoses, and petechiae. Splenomegaly is common. The peripheral blood smear shows leukopenia or varying degrees of pancytopenia without evidence of leukemia or myeloproliferative disorders. Pancellular hyperplasia is present in the bone marrow.

Primary hypersplenism is a diagnosis of exclusion and should be accepted only after an exhaustive search for a specific etiology of hypersplenism has been unrewarding. Corticosteroids are seldom of benefit in primary hypersplenism. Splenectomy is indicated when the diagnosis is established and usually results in marked hematologic improvement for virtually all patients. Occasional patients have subsequently developed reticulum cell sarcoma or histiocytic lymphoma.[40, 51]

Lymphoma having primary presentation in the spleen may present as asymptomatic splenomegaly with or without hypersplenism. Radionuclide studies, CT, and magnetic resonance imaging usually reveal nonspecific, featureless organ enlargement. If parenchymal expansion secondary to tumor infiltration and congestion becomes massive, splenic pooling and increased regional blood flow may result in hypersplenism. Lymphoma with primary presentation in the spleen may result in the diagnosis of *idiopathic splenomegaly* until splenectomy permits accurate histopathologic diagnosis.

Secondary hypersplenism classically refers to a syndrome of pancytopenia (anemia, thrombocytopenia, and leukopenia) associated with portal hypertension from intrahepatic or extrahepatic portal or splenic vein obstruction. Hypersplenism associated with portal hypertension secondary to cirrhosis seldom requires splenectomy. Cytopenias commonly are improved after a shunt between the portal and systemic circula-

tions, presumably caused by relief of congestive splenomegaly.[40] Splenic vein thrombosis with bleeding from gastric varices should be treated by splenectomy, which usually cures the gastric variceal bleeding and any existing hypersplenism.[6, 42]

Secondary hypersplenism includes a number of diseases sharing the common feature of splenomegaly. Rather than listing these, it is more appropriate to consider the mechanisms producing splenic enlargement (Table 36–5).[8] Work hypertrophy from immune response and/or red blood cell destruction, venous congestion, myeloproliferation, infiltration, and neoplastic proliferation within the spleen produce variable degrees of splenomegaly. Diverse pathophysiologic mechanisms are involved in the resulting hypersplenism (Table 36–6).[8] In both primary and secondary hypersplenism, the degree of splenomegaly does not correlate closely with the severity of clinical symptoms or the degree of depression of formed elements of the blood.

Hyposplenism

Hyposplenism is a potentially lethal syndrome characterized by diminished splenic function. Hyposplenism was first described by Dameshek in 1955 in a patient with sprue who had an asplenic peripheral blood picture with Howell-Jolly bodies and target cells.[8] As in the asplenic patient, other peripheral blood findings that suggest hyposplenism are the presence of acanthocytes and siderocytes, a long-term lymphocytosis and monocytosis, and a mild thrombocytosis.[8] Diagnosis of hyposplenism is confirmed by an isotope scan (^{99m}Tc sulfur colloid) revealing an atrophic spleen. Hyposplenism can occur in the presence of a normal sized or an enlarged spleen (Table 36–7).

The danger of hyposplenism is the risk of developing potentially lethal sepsis (see The Problem of Overwhelming Postsplenectomy Sepsis). Sickle cell anemia is the most common disease associated with hyposplenism. Children with sickle cell anemia are vulnerable to overwhelming pneumococcal infection similar to that seen in asplenic children. The child with sickle cell anemia is most vulnerable when the spleen is enlarged. By the time the spleen becomes atrophic from recurrent infarctions (*autosplenectomy*), the patient will have developed some immunity from exposure to different pneumococcal strains.[8]

The most common surgical disease associated with hyposplenism is chronic ulcerative colitis, in which 40% or more of patients develop hyposplenism as the pancolitis progresses. Other conditions associated with hyposplenism

TABLE 36–6. Etiology of Hypersplenism in Selected Diseases

Disease	Probable Mechanism
Hairy cell leukemia	Retention of hairy cells in splenic pulp
Portal hypertension (cirrhosis, splenic vein thrombosis)	Increased pooling of blood cells
Felty's syndrome	Immune system work hypertrophy
Thalassemia major	Reticuloendothelial system work hypertrophy
Hemodialysis splenomegaly	Immune and reticuloendothelial system work hypertrophy
Gaucher's disease	Increased pooling and flow-induced dilutional anemia
Agnogenic myeloid metaplasia	Extramedullary hematopoiesis

Modified from Eichner, E. R.: Splenic function: Normal, too much and too little. Am. J. Med., 66:311, 1979.

TABLE 36–5. Etiology of Splenomegaly

Mechanism	Example
Work hypertrophy: immune response	Subacute bacterial endocarditis Infectious mononucleosis Felty's syndrome
Work hypertrophy: red cell destruction	Spherocytosis Thalassemia major Pyruvate kinase deficiency
Congestive	Cirrhosis Splenic vein thrombosis
Myeloproliferative	Chronic myelocytic leukemia Myeloid metaplasia
Infiltrative	Sarcoidosis Amyloidosis Gaucher's disease
Neoplastic	Lymphoma Hairy cell leukemia Chronic lymphocytic leukemia Metastatic cancer

Modified from Eichner, E. R.: Splenic function: Normal, too much and too little. Am. J. Med., 66:311, 1979.

TABLE 36–7. Diseases Associated with Hyposplenism

Atrophic Spleen

Ulcerative colitis
Celiac disease
Dermatitis herpetiformis
Thyrotoxicosis (Graves' disease)
Hemorrhagic thrombocythemia
Thorotrast administration
Sickle cell anemia (chronic)

Normal-Sized or Enlarged Spleen

Sickle cell anemia, HbS/C disease
Sarcoidosis
Amyloidosis
Corticosteroid administration (?)

Modified from Eichner, E. R.: Splenic function: Normal, too much and too little. Am. J. Med., *66*:311, 1979.

in which the surgeon is commonly involved include thyrotoxicosis, corticosteroid administration, and patients who have received Thorotrast (thorium dioxide) as a radiocontrast agent.[8] If a patient is suspected or proved to have hyposplenism, the same precautions against sepsis recommended for asplenic patients should be instituted.

Hodgkin's Disease

Described by Thomas Hodgkin in 1832, Hodgkin's disease is a malignant lymphoma characterized by the presence of typical, multinucleate giant cells. The unique cell, described by Sternberg and later Reed around the turn of the century, is essential for diagnosis. Hodgkin's disease is relatively rare, with a bimodal age-incidence curve that peaks in the late 20s and declines to the mid 40s. After age 45, the incidence of Hodgkin's disease increases with age. The disease is slightly more common in men than women.[3, 23, 51]

Most patients with Hodgkin's disease have asymptomatic lymphadenopathy at the time of diagnosis. The site of initial nodal involvement is the cervical area in most patients (65%–80%), followed by the axillary (10%–15%) and inguinal (6%–12%) regions. Retroperitoneal lymph nodes may be involved but require lymphangiography or CT for diagnosis. Mediastinal involvement occurs in 6% to 11% of patients at the time of diagnosis.[3, 23, 51]

Constitutional symptoms (B symptoms) such as fever, night sweats, weight loss, and pruritus are usually indicative of widespread involvement and are unfavorable prognostic signs. They may appear simultaneously with lymph node enlargement or may precede development of lymphadenopathy. A typical fever pattern is a high temperature alternating for a few days with an afebrile period (Pel-Ebstein fever). Less specific constitutional symptoms include localized acute discomfort in areas of adenopathy after ingestion of alcoholic beverages, malaise, lethargy, easy fatigability, generalized weakness, and anorexia.[3, 23, 51]

Many patients have a mild normochromic normocytic anemia. One third have a leukocytosis due to a neutrophil increase, and eosinophilia is present frequently. Lymphopenia is common in the later stages of the disease. The platelet count is normal initially but is frequently depressed in advanced disease. There is a progressive loss of T-lymphocyte function with reduced cell-mediated immunity.

A classification of Hodgkin's disease was developed by the international symposium held in Rye, New York, in 1965, at which time the earlier classifications were simplified. In the Rye classification there are four histopathologic subtypes of Hodgkin's disease: lymphocyte predominance, nodular

sclerosis, mixed cellularity, and lymphocyte depletion. Lymphocyte predominance and nodular sclerosis subtypes have a more favorable prognosis than mixed cellularity and lymphocyte depletion subtypes. However, the prognostic implications of subtyping are becoming less useful because of the excellent results of current aggressive treatment.[3, 23, 51]

Hodgkin's disease metastasizes initially in a predictable, nonrandom pattern through lymphatic channels to contiguous lymph node groups and organs with a prominent lymphatic tissue component. The predictable mode of spread of Hodgkin's disease provides the basis for irradiation of adjacent lymph node areas in patients with apparently localized disease.[3] Treatment and ultimately survival of the patients with Hodgkin's disease depend on the anatomic distribution of the disease and the presence or absence of specific symptoms, the stage of the disease, and the histopathologic subtype.[3, 23, 51]

Histopathologic diagnosis is made by lymph node biopsy in which the largest and most centrally placed node should be selected for excision. In a matted group or cluster of nodes, a central node from the group should be excised or a generous incisional biopsy specimen obtained. Nodes from the lower cervical or axillary areas provide the most satisfactory tissue for histopathologic evaluation, because nodes from the parotid, submandibular, and inguinal regions often show changes due to previous inflammatory processes in their regions of drainage. When only mediastinal adenopathy is present, biopsy is performed through mediastinoscopy or thoracotomy, as indicated. Laparotomy is seldom required to obtain the initial diagnosis in Hodgkin's disease.[3]

Since the concept of staging was introduced approximately 30 years ago, the staging process has undergone continued modification with the intent of accurately defining the anatomic sites of involvement and thus improving patient selection for the most appropriate type and amount of therapy. Stage I disease indicates nodal involvement in only one lymph node region. Stage II disease is limited to two or more lymph node regions on the same side of the diaphragm. Stage III refers to disease involving lymph node regions on both sides of the diaphragm (the spleen is considered a lymph node). Stage IV disease encompasses diffuse or disseminated involvement of one or more distant extranodal organs with or without associated lymph node involvement. Stage IV is further classified as A (absence) or B (presence) with regard to fever, night sweats, weight loss, and pruritus. The subscript E is used to classify selected patients having localized extranodal disease in Stages I to III (e.g., lung, muscle, bone, skin) contiguous to involved nodes. In general, the E designation is reserved for patients having extralymphatic disease so limited in extent and/or location that it is amenable to definitive treatment by radiotherapy. The S subscript indicates splenic involvement.[3, 22, 23, 42, 51] Anatomic substages of Stage IIIA disease have been designated to differentiate between upper abdominal disease (III_1) and lower abdominal disease (III_2). A biologic difference or prognostic significance has not been clearly shown with respect to 5-year survival or disease-free survival between upper and lower abdominal involvement.[42] Both a clinical stage designation and a pathologic stage designation are implied by the Ann Arbor staging classification (Fig. 36–9).

Clinical stage is dependent on history and physical examination, the initial diagnostic biopsy, laboratory tests, and the results of radiographic and imaging studies. Pathologic stage is more accurate than the clinical stage because histopathologic data from the bone marrow, liver, spleen, intra-abdominal lymph nodes, and other involved tissues (e.g. bone, skin, lung) provide precise knowledge of the extent of the disease.[3, 23, 24, 51]

Lymphangiography and abdominal CT are reliable and

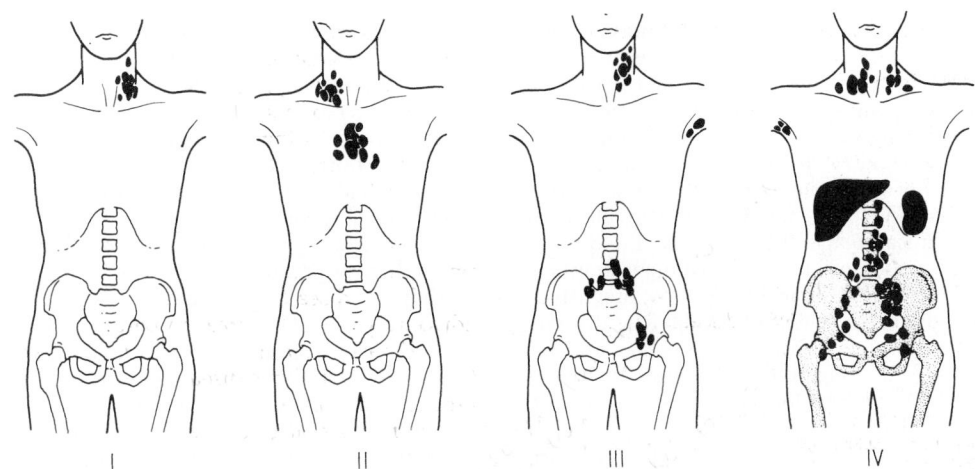

Figure 36–9. Ann Arbor Staging Classification for Hodgkin's Disease. (From Hoffbrand, A. V., and Pettit, J. E.: Essential Hematology. Oxford, England, Blackwell Scientific Publications, 1980, p. 141.)

complementary tests to evaluate retroperitoneal and abdominal nodal involvement. Lymphangiography has an overall accuracy of 80% to 90% with high sensitivity and specificity and can detect disease in nodes that are not significantly enlarged. Shortcomings include the need for bipedal incisions and a failure to adequately visualize the celiac, splenic hilar, and portal nodes. These and other enlarged lymph nodes can be detected by CT, which has lower overall accuracy, sensitivity, and specificity than lymphangiography.[42] CT is not helpful in detecting splenic involvement unless extensive splenic disease exists.[24, 25] When the lymphangiogram is positive, involvement of retroperitoneal nodes by Hodgkin's disease is confirmed by staging laparotomy in 80% to 90% of cases.[24, 42] Additionally, approximately 40% of patients with abnormal lymphangiograms have another site of Hodgkin's disease within the abdomen, most commonly the spleen.[24] A normal lymphangiogram usually indicates that the retroperitoneal lymph nodes are uninvolved (10%–15% incidence of false-negative results) but does not exclude other abdominal sites of occult disease. Approximately 20% of patients with negative lymphangiograms have intra-abdominal disease, usually in the spleen.[24]

Subdiaphragmatic Hodgkin's disease is frequently confined to the spleen and splenic hilar lymph nodes. The probability of subdiaphragmatic Hodgkin's disease is related closely to histopathologic subtype, with mixed cellularity and lymphocyte depletion subtypes having greater likelihood of subdiaphragmatic extension than lymphocyte predominance and nodular sclerosis subtypes. The probability of splenic involvement increases with increasing spleen size and is almost always present in spleens weighing more than 400 gm.[23, 24, 51] The absence of splenomegaly does not exclude splenic involvement. Hodgkin's disease involving the spleen is commonly apparent on gross examination as grayish white nodules ranging from several millimeters to several centimeters (Fig. 36–10). Liver involvement with Hodgkin's disease rarely occurs in the absence of splenic disease.[23–25, 42, 51] Hepatic disease, in contrast to splenic disease, may not be apparent from inspection and palpation.

In a report of the Stanford experience, the spleen was found to be involved with Hodgkin's disease in 39% of patients undergoing staging laparotomy.[42] In 50% of these, the spleen was the only site of intra-abdominal disease detected by staging laparotomy. Splenic involvement consisted of fewer than five nodules in 27%, with all of the nodules being too small to have been detected by CT or found on random biopsy. All positive liver and accessory spleen speci-

mens were associated with positive splenic involvement, suggesting that the spleen is the trigger for visceral dissemination.[42]

Staging laparotomy, which in the past was frequently employed for pathologic staging of Hodgkin's disease, is now being used less frequently. Its use as a diagnostic test has been based on the following:

1. Hodgkin's disease generally begins in a single area and spreads initially in a predictable and nonrandom manner through lymphatic channels to contiguous lymph node areas and organs having a prominent lymphatic tissue component.

2. Selection of therapy is dependent on pathologic stage.

3. Assignment of stage using clinical criteria alone is often inaccurate. Twenty-five to 30% of clinically staged patients will have their stage of disease increased (upstaged), and 10% to 15% will be downstaged after laparotomy for a total alteration in stage of approximately 40%.[24, 25, 42] (Patients with AIDS who develop Hodgkin's disease have great likelihood of being upstaged by laparotomy.)

4. Prognosis is related primarily to the pathologic stage of the disease.

The role of staging laparotomy continues to be re-evaluated as a routine staging procedure for Hodgkin's disease. Diagnostic advantages and contributions of staging laparotomy have helped to significantly change the understanding

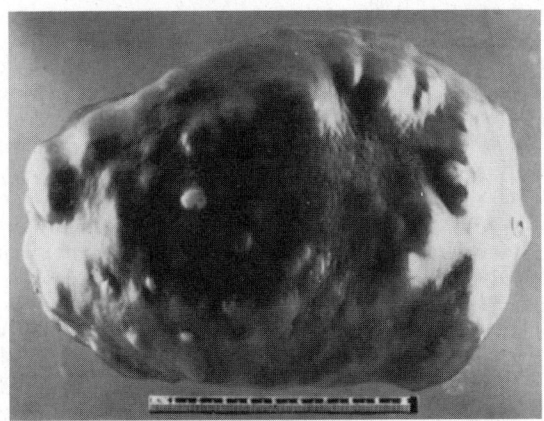

Figure 36–10. Spleen weighing 960 gm. exhibits typical gross nodules of Hodgkin's disease. The spleen, which was palpable preoperatively, was removed during staging laparotomy.

and therapeutic management of patients with Hodgkin's disease, and the current success and widespread use of combination chemotherapy has challenged the need to know the precise anatomic extent of the disease required for treatment by radiation therapy.[31] Staging laparotomy is not applicable to all patients with Hodgkin's disease and should be performed only in patients in whom the results may change management decisions and plans for therapy. Patients with advanced disease, clinical Stage IIIB or Stage IV, do not benefit from staging laparotomy because treatment employs combination chemotherapy. (If splenomegaly is present or develops in these advanced stages of Hodgkin's disease, splenectomy may be of value to control cytopenias and reduce tumor burden.) Staging laparotomy has been restricted by the recognition of the limitations of radiation therapy for patients with extensive mediastinal presentation or with multiple extranodal sites. The success of combination chemotherapy in treating minimal or occult disease and for controlling recurrent disease after radiation therapy is a major consideration in further restricting the use of staging laparotomy.[31] Splenectomy in Hodgkin's staging has been shown to be a predisposing risk factor for acute leukemia in patients older than 40 years of age who have received combination chemotherapy (MOPP—mechlorethamine, vincristine, procarbazine, and prednisone). This surprising association suggests that staging laparotomy with splenectomy should not be done in patients of this age group who may eventually require MOPP-like chemotherapy.[31]

Controversy continues regarding the role of staging laparotomy, and improved noninvasive diagnostic tests and the introduction of more effective and less toxic chemotherapy continue to reduce the indications for this procedure.[31] Currently, staging laparotomy is appropriate for selected patients with Hodgkin's disease of low clinical stage (Stage IA, IIA, and IIIA) in whom the results will have major influence on therapeutic management.

Staging laparotomy is based on a systematic abdominal exploration with an organized approach to tissue sampling and consists of splenectomy, liver biopsy, and selective excision of abdominal and retroperitoneal lymph nodes based on CT, lymphangiographic, and operative findings. The operation is performed through a midline incision. The liver is examined initially, and if no gross evidence of disease is identified, a 2-cm. wedge of tissue is excised from the left hepatic lobe, and deep biopsy samples are obtained from the right and left lobes with a Trucut needle. Splenectomy is then performed with biopsy of splenic hilar lymph nodes and placement of identifying metal clips on the splenic pedicle. Partial splenectomy does not provide an adequate degree of accuracy in staging to justify its use as an alternative to splenectomy.[25, 42, 44] The lesser omentum is incised, and a lymph node is removed from the celiac axis region. The hilum of the liver, cystic duct, and distal common duct areas are inspected, and representative lymph nodes are removed. Representative nodes are excised from the small intestinal mesentery and mesocolon. Exposure of the para-aortic, para-caval, and iliac lymph nodes is necessary to adequately examine these areas. If any abnormal or suspicious retroperitoneal nodes were demonstrated on the lymphangiogram, the nodes are excised and the sites are marked with metal clips. Confirmation that the specific node or nodes have been excised can be obtained by comparing an intraoperative abdominal radiograph with the lymphangiogram. Ten to 15% of patients with normal lymphangiograms will have involvement of the retroperitoneal lymph nodes by Hodgkin's disease (false-negative), and representative nodes should be excised even if the lymphangiogram is normal. A bone marrow biopsy should be obtained from the iliac crest to conclude the staging aspects of the operation. Preoperative bone marrow

biopsy has a false-negative rate of 2% to 3% and would constitute a significant treatment error if not corrected by staging laparotomy findings.[42]

Oophoropexy (ovarian translocation) is advisable in the premenopausal woman in whom radiation therapy using an inverted Y port is likely. Both ovaries should be moved from the potential field of radiation and identified with metal clips. Lead shielding is an important adjunct to the protective effects offered by oophoropexy, and menstrual function is retained in approximately 55% of women receiving pelvic irradiation for Hodgkin's disease after oophoropexy and lead shielding.[45] Ancillary procedures such as appendectomy or cholecystectomy add an unnecessary risk to the staging laparotomy and are not recommended.

Staging laparotomy has minimal morbidity, and the mortality rate is less than 0.5%. The risk of developing postsplenectomy sepsis in patients with Hodgkin's disease is 10% or higher.

Current treatment of Hodgkin's disease integrates radiation therapy and combination chemotherapy to achieve the maximum potential for cure. The success of combination chemotherapy in controlling and even curing Hodgkin's disease in patients demonstrating recurrence after radiation therapy has been a major therapeutic advance. In the Stanford experience from 1974 to 1980 for patients at all stages of Hodgkin's disease, survival was 86%, and freedom from progression (FFP) was 77% in surgically staged patients.[42] For patients with Stage IA and IIA disease being treated by irradiation only, survival and FFP were 91% and 82%, respectively, with no advantage being shown by adding chemotherapy (usually MOPP). Adding chemotherapy to radiation improved survival from 65% to 92% and FFP from 70% to 82% in patients with Stage IIIA disease. Patients with Stage IIIB disease had a generally poorer prognosis even with combination therapy, but alternating chemotherapy and radiation therapy has yielded significantly improved survival. Extensive extranodal disease (Stages IIE, IIIE, IV) has a poor survival (approximately 60% at 5 years), whether irradiation or combined therapy is used.[42]

Most patients with Hodgkin's disease present with Stage II or III disease. Ten to 15% present with Stage I or IV. Untreated Hodgkin's disease has a 5-year survival rate of 5%. Current survival rates for Hodgkin's disease, however, approximate 85% for all stages. The gold standard for the management of Stage I and IIA Hodgkin's disease is external-beam radiation. The potential contribution of adjuvant radiation therapy to the management of advanced-stage Hodgkin's disease remains controversial. The cornerstone of therapy for advanced Hodgkin's disease is combination chemotherapy. It is the staging between IIA and IIIA that might make some difference.

There are subsets of patients in whom the likelihood of any staging change that would alter therapy is remote. The risk of having abdominal involvement is less than 10% in women with clinical Stage I disease, in men with clinical Stage I disease with lymphocyte predominance, and in women with clinical Stage II disease who are younger than 27 years of age with three different sites of involvement. Alternatively, the patient with Stage I disease who has a large mediastinal mass now usually requires chemotherapy in addition to external-beam radiation, because of recurrence outside the radiation ports and the fact of cardiac, especially pericardial, complications from radiation. Patients with Stage IIIB disease require no staging, nor do ones with multiple E, IIA$_2$. Another contraindication or reason for the decline in staging has been the appearance in significant numbers of patients of acute myeloid leukemia in patients who have had MOPP therapy and have received staging laparotomy with splenectomy.

The approximate results of different stages of Hodgkin's disease, then, are as follows: Stages I and IIA treated by external-beam radiation alone have an 80% FFP (free from progression) and a 90% regression-free survival; Stage IIIA has a 94% relapse-free survival at 10 years with MOPP; and Stage IVA with alternating MOPP and ABD has an 80% remission. The potential of bone marrow transplantation adding to the treatment is an additional therapeutic maneuver.

The reason, then, that staging laparotomies are less frequently done currently is not entirely due to the ability to better stage the disease by noninvasive means (e.g., CT, laparoscopic surgery). It in part results from the effectiveness of the various therapeutic modalities available. Salvage after recurrence is quite possible with most patients with Hodgkin's disease, making it less important that the small differential that would be changed from a staging process at the present time would make much difference in overall survival.

Non-Hodgkin's Lymphomas

Non-Hodgkin's lymphomas constitute a diverse group of primary malignancies of lymphoreticular tissue. The clinical course and natural history of NHL are more variable than those of Hodgkin's disease, the pattern of spread is irregular, and more patients have leukemic features.[3, 22, 23, 51] Current histologic classifications incorporate the nomenclature based on light and electron microscopic morphology, histochemical studies, and selected cell-surface antigens.[3, 22, 23, 51] For prognostic and therapeutic purposes, NHL is classified according to nodular (favorable) and diffuse (unfavorable) types.

In contrast to Hodgkin's disease, only about two thirds of patients with NHL initially have asymptomatic lymphadenopathy. In 20% to 35% of patients, the onset of NHL occurs in an extranodal site.[3] In addition to peripheral and mediastinal lymphadenopathy, NHL is commonly found initially as an abdominal mass (retroperitoneal or mesenteric) or as hepatic and/or splenic enlargement. Constitutional symptoms such as fever, weight loss, and night sweats are frequently present. Occasionally the first manifestation of NHL is an oncologic emergency such as superior vena caval syndrome, spinal cord compression, or ureteral obstruction.

In NHL the mode of spread generally is unpredictable, and most patients have disseminated disease at the time of presentation.[3, 23, 51] In patients with initial nodal involvement, early spread may be limited to contiguous lymphatic sites or adjacent extranodal sites. More often, NHL spreads rapidly to distant nodal and extranodal sites through the bloodstream. Progression of NHL arising in extranodal areas may be through (1) local invasion of adjacent structures, (2) extension to regional lymph nodes, and/or (3) dissemination to noncontiguous lymph nodes and/or distant extranodal sites. The extranodal spread of NHL is comparable to the pattern of metastasis observed in carcinoma.[3]

The median age at the time of diagnosis is 50 years, without sex preference. Patients younger than age 35 and older than 65 are more likely to have diffuse histology. The majority of NHLs are monoclonal B-cell tumors that are sometimes associated with an IgM or IgG protein. In some patients, particularly children with a mediastinal mass, the disease is thymic.[22, 23, 51]

As with Hodgkin's disease, chemotherapy and/or radiation therapy are the primary forms of treatment. Therapeutic considerations are based on the histopathologic type of lymphoma and the stage (extent) of disease. Because the majority of patients with NHL have disseminated disease at the time of presentation, staging laparotomy is seldom required and is indicated only for the patient with limited disease in whom laparotomy findings may influence selection of therapy.

NHL having primary presentation in the spleen may present as asymptomatic splenomegaly, with or without hypersplenism. Radionuclide scanning, CT, and magnetic resonance imaging usually reveal nonspecific, featureless organ enlargement. If parenchymal expansion secondary to tumor infiltration and congestion becomes massive, splenic pooling and increased regional blood flow may result in hypersplenism. NHL with primary presentation in the spleen may result in the diagnosis of *idiopathic splenomegaly* until splenectomy permits accurate histopathologic diagnosis.

Splenectomy in NHL is also performed for hematologic depression secondary to hypersplenism or to relieve symptomatic splenomegaly or discomfort from recurrent splenic infarctions. Hypersplenism may produce symptomatic anemia requiring red blood cell transfusions, dangerous levels of thrombocytopenia, and leukopenia with recurrent infections. The severity of the cytopenia may require withholding of chemotherapy and radiation therapy.[1, 13, 23, 51] Immunohemolysis or AIHA occasionally contributes to the anemia in NHL and is diagnosed by a positive Coombs test.

The bone marrow typically has significant infiltration by neoplastic cells and additionally shows erythroid hypoplasia and decreased megakaryocytes. Because most patients with NHL have received chemotherapy or radiation therapy before becoming candidates for splenectomy, the splenic contribution to the pancytopenia can only be determined by the response to splenectomy.[13] Almost all patients with NHL undergoing splenectomy for hypersplenism require red cell and platelet transfusions preoperatively.

Significant therapeutic benefit can be achieved by splenectomy in 80% to 90% of patients with advanced lymphomas (including Hodgkin's disease).[1, 13] Although patients with both NHLs and Hodgkin's disease may develop remission with reinstituted chemotherapy after correction of cytopenias, the eventual outcome of the underlying disease is unchanged. Most patients with well-differentiated lymphocytic lymphoma survive for 5 years, and many live 10 years after the diagnosis is made. The prognosis is more favorable for the nodular than for the diffuse forms of NHL.[13, 23, 51]

Chronic Lymphocytic Leukemia

Chronic lymphocytic leukemia (CLL) is a lymphoproliferative abnormality that occurs primarily in the elderly (sixth decade of life or older), with a male predominance (2:1). Proliferation and accumulation of abnormal lymphocytes in lymphatic tissues result in the major signs of lymphadenopathy, splenomegaly, and lymphocytosis in the peripheral blood. The most constant abnormality on physical examination is lymph node enlargement, which frequently is found either by the patient or on routine physical examination. Splenomegaly is present in most patients and is progressive during the course of the disease. Hepatomegaly is a frequent finding, and lymphocytic infiltration of the skin and gastrointestinal and respiratory tracts occurs as the disease progresses. The diagnosis is based on the increase in the total leukocyte count due to a large number of abnormal, small, immature lymphocytes. Bone marrow examination demonstrates a variable and progressive degree of infiltration by abnormal lymphocytes.[23, 51]

Therapy for CLL incorporates the judicious use of chemotherapeutic agents, corticosteroids, irradiation, and splenectomy.[22, 23, 51] Although CLL is not cured by available therapeutic modalities, effective palliation is achieved in most patients, and many lead relatively normal lives. The disease progresses over 5 to 10 years with gradual increases in lymphadenopathy, splenomegaly, and hepatomegaly and development of weakness, weight loss, anemia, and thrombocytopenia. CLL is frequently complicated by development of immune hemolysis (AIHA), in which the hemolytic anemia is nearly always Coombs positive. If hemolysis becomes severe and cannot be controlled by medical therapy, splenectomy is useful to ameliorate the hemolytic process. As in NHL, splenectomy in chronic lymphocytic leukemia is performed primarily for hematologic depression secondary to hypersplenism and for palliation of symptomatic splenomegaly (Fig. 36–11). Significant hematologic improvement occurs after splenectomy in 80% to 90% of patients, but the natural course of CLL is unchanged.[1, 13, 23, 51] Unless another illness supervenes, death usually occurs from hemorrhage or infection.

Chronic Myeloid Leukemia

Chronic myeloid (granulocytic, myelocytic) leukemia (CML, CGL) is a myeloproliferative abnormality characterized by marked elevation of the leukocyte count from myeloid cells in all stages of maturation and by neoplastic overgrowth of granulocytes in the bone marrow. The incidence of CML increases with age and is more frequent in males than in females (ratio 3:2). Splenomegaly is the most common physical finding, and sternal tenderness, lymphadenopathy, and hepatomegaly are frequently present.[23, 51] A unique chromosomal abnormality designated the Philadelphia chromosome (Ph) occurs in 90% of patients with CML. Patients who are Ph-negative have an atypical course and a poorer prognosis than patients with CML who have the Ph chromosome.[23, 51] Chemotherapy (busulfan, hydroxyurea), irradiation, radioactive phosphorus, and extracorporeal irradiation of the blood can control symptoms and most physical and laboratory abnormalities of CML during the chronic or *treatable* phase, which lasts from 1 to 4 years.[23, 51] Development of *myeloblastic crisis* appears to be an intrinsic feature of CML and indicates an accelerated or acute stage of the disease, which results in death from infection or hemorrhage within 3 to 6 months.[23, 51]

Splenectomy may be of benefit in selected patients during the chronic stage of CML to palliate severe thrombocytopenia and/or anemia and to relieve pain from splenic infarctions or massive splenomegaly. Splenectomy offers no benefit in delaying the onset of blastic transformation, improving the quality of life after the development of blastic crisis, or in prolonging survival.[32]

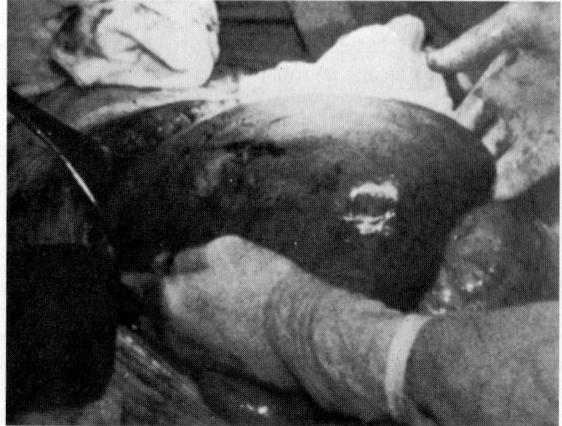

Figure 36–11. Operative photograph showing removal of a 5660-gm. spleen in a patient with chronic lymphocytic leukemia and hypersplenism.

Hairy Cell Leukemia

Hairy cell leukemia (leukemic reticuloendotheliosis) is an uncommon form of leukemia characterized by pancytopenia, splenomegaly without significant lymphadenopathy, and characteristic mononuclear cells in the blood and bone marrow. The disease is more common in males (ratio 4:1). The typical patient is a middle-aged man with moderate splenomegaly, absence of significant peripheral adenopathy, and variable hepatomegaly.[16]

Initial complaints among symptomatic patients are abdominal fullness or discomfort due to splenomegaly, nonspecific symptoms of fatigue, weakness, and weight loss, easy bruising from thrombocytopenia, or recurrent infections associated with leukopenia. In approximately 25% of patients, splenomegaly and cytopenias are detected during a routine examination or during evaluation for an unrelated illness.

HCL is characterized by the presence of malignant cells that have irregular, filamentous cytoplasmic projections on light microscopy that give the cells a hairy appearance. The surface projections are demonstrable by electron microscopy as broad-based, undulating ruffles and patches of short, blunt microvilli.

A pancytopenia of moderate severity is present in approximately two thirds of patients at the time of diagnosis. Hairy cells are frequently present in the peripheral blood and often account for a large proportion of the total white cell count. Demonstration in the hairy cells of tartrate-resistant acid phosphatase (TRAP) isoenzyme activity as a red reaction product is helpful supporting evidence for diagnosis. Although not required for diagnosis, the *TRAP positive* reaction product occurs in 90% to 95% of patients with HCL. Bone marrow biopsy permits definitive diagnosis of HCL from characteristic morphology.[16]

Ten to 15% of patients with HCL have an indolent course with a nearly normal life expectancy and require no specific therapy. These are usually elderly men who have minimal splenomegaly, relatively few hairy cells in the blood, and asymptomatic neutropenia. The remaining 85% to 90% require treatment because of one or more cytopenias resulting in symptomatic anemia requiring transfusions, thrombocytopenic bleeding, and repeated infections attributable to neutropenia. Pancytopenia develops from concurrent splenic pooling secondary to infiltrative splenomegaly and bone marrow replacement with hairy cells. Symptomatic splenomegaly and recurring splenic infarctions are other indications for therapy. For the majority of patients who require some form of therapy shortly after diagnosis, splenectomy continues to be an early consideration. Splenectomy is most appropriate for those patients with severe cytopenias, a large spleen, and patchy bone marrow infiltration. It results in rapid palliation, and almost all patients have hematologic improvement. Blood cell counts return to normal in 40% to 50% of patients, with the response lasting for many years and almost half the patients requiring no further therapy.[17, 18]

Patients with HCL having diffuse infiltration of the bone marrow, minimal splenomegaly, and severe cytopenias gain only minor or short-term benefit from splenectomy and require additional therapy. In the past 5 years interferon alfa and pentostatin have been found to be highly effective systemic therapy for HCL. Randomized trials of interferon alfa versus pentostatin are in progress, both for newly diagnosed HCL patients and those patients previously having had splenectomy. Presently, interferon alfa remains the systemic therapy of choice, with pentostatin being indicated for patients with HCL that is refractory to interferon alfa. Splenectomy likely will continue to have a place in the sequential treatment of those patients with HCL requiring therapy.[17, 18]

SPLENECTOMY FOR ANEMIA

Hemolytic anemia results from an increase in the rate of red blood cell destruction. The adult bone marrow can produce red cells at six to eight times the normal rate, and hemolysis must be reasonably severe before laboratory or clinical evidence of anemia occurs.[22, 23, 51] Diagnostic evaluation should include a detailed family history because many hemolytic anemias that improve after splenectomy have a hereditary basis. Congenital hemolytic anemias have a defect intrinsic to the red blood cell that may involve the cell membrane (hereditary spherocytosis), cellular metabolism (pyruvate kinase deficiency, glucose-6-phosphate dehydrogenase [G-6-PD] deficiency), hemoglobin structure (sickle cell anemia), or hemoglobin chain synthesis rates (thalassemia). Acquired hemolytic anemias have an extracorpuscular factor that affects normal red cells. Chromium-51–labeled red cell survival studies are sometimes useful to confirm hemolysis and a shortened red cell life span and to determine sites of red cell destruction.[22, 23, 51]

Clinical features include variable pallor related to the degree of anemia, mild, fluctuating jaundice, and splenomegaly. Pigment gallstones are common after childhood and may produce biliary tract symptoms. Valuable laboratory studies include serum direct and total bilirubin and haptoglobin levels. Jaundice associated with hyperbilirubinemia resulting from hemolysis is caused by an excess of unconjugated (free) bilirubin and is measured by an increase in the indirect reacting fraction of bilirubin. The unconjugated bilirubin that is bound to albumin does not enter the urine, and indirect hyperbilirubinemia thus is not associated with biliuria. Reticulocytosis and bone marrow erythroid hyperplasia reflect increased red cell production. Red cell morphology is often abnormal, as is osmotic fragility. Red cells tagged with chromium-51 demonstrate a shortened red cell survival.[22, 23, 51]

Hereditary Spherocytosis

Hereditary spherocytosis is a relatively common, genetically determined red blood cell membrane disorder that results in hemolytic anemia. The erythrocyte membrane defect results from a deficiency in spectrin, a major component of the membrane skeleton that is thought to be responsible for the shape, strength, and reversible deformability of the red blood cell.[2, 23, 51] The membrane abnormality leads to a gradual loss of red cell surface area, so that instead of remaining a flexible biconcave disc, the red cell becomes small and spherical. Lacking adequate deformability to traverse the splenic microcirculation, spherocytes are trapped in the splenic red pulp and are eventually destroyed by reticuloendothelial cells.

Hereditary spherocytosis occurs primarily by autosomal dominant inheritance with variable expression. Twenty to 25% of the cases appear sporadically.[2, 23, 51] The severity of the anemia and other clinical manifestations are variable. The disease may be so severe that repeated blood transfusions are required to maintain a functional hemoglobin level, or it may be so mild as to go unnoticed in childhood, becoming manifest in adult life with development of symptomatic cholelithiasis. Aplastic crisis, which usually is precipitated by a viral illness such as human parvovirus, may produce a rapidly worsening anemia that may be life threatening. Fluctuating jaundice due to hemolysis is common, and pigment gallstones are frequent, with the incidence being directly related to the severity of the hemolysis and patient age. Cholelithiasis develops in 20% to 55% of patients with hereditary spherocytosis but is uncommon before age 10. Moderate splenomegaly is a characteristic physical finding.[7]

Diagnosis is established by the presence of spherocytes in the peripheral blood, reticulocytosis (usually 5%–20%), an increased osmotic fragility, and a negative Coombs test.[22, 23, 51]

Splenectomy is indicated in virtually all patients. In children, splenectomy is usually performed after age 6 but can be done at a younger age if warranted by the severity of the anemia and the need for frequent transfusions. After splenectomy, hemolysis is alleviated, and clinical cure of the anemia is achieved in most patients. The intrinsic red cell membrane defect is unaltered by splenectomy, but red cell survival becomes normal. With resolution of hemolysis, jaundice disappears, and the increased risk of calculous biliary tract disease is removed. Gallbladder ultrasonography is advisable before splenectomy in anticipation of combining cholecystectomy with splenectomy if gallstones are demonstrated.[7]

Hereditary Elliptocytosis

Hereditary elliptocytosis is a relatively common heterogeneous red blood cell membrane disorder characterized by an abundance of elliptical red cells. The abnormality usually produces a mild anemia, and most patients remain asymptomatic throughout their lives.[5, 23, 51] Like hereditary spherocytosis, hereditary elliptocytosis is caused by an abnormal erythrocyte membrane skeleton. Several defects in the red cell membrane skeleton have been identified in hereditary elliptocytosis and include impaired association of spectrin chains and a quantitative deficiency of protein 4.1.[2, 23, 51] Symptomatic individuals have a mild hemolytic anemia with clinical and laboratory features similar to those of hereditary spherocytosis except for the elliptical appearance of the erythrocytes. Splenectomy is indicated in symptomatic patients, and results are uniformly good, although the abnormal erythrocyte morphology persists.[5, 23, 51]

Hereditary Pyropoikilocytosis

Hereditary pyropoikilocytosis (HPP) is a rare congenital hemolytic anemia that is catalogued along with hereditary elliptocytosis because of certain molecular and morphologic similarities. Distinguished from hereditary elliptocytosis (and hereditary spherocytosis) by marked alterations in red cell morphology and by the pattern of inheritance, this severe hemolytic disorder occurs most commonly in blacks. Erythrocytes in HPP are severely deformed, and virtually all red cells are poikilocytic, fragmented, spherocytic, or elliptocytic. Osmotic fragility is increased, and red cells in HPP exhibit increased susceptibility to thermal injury. The decision for splenectomy in HPP is deferred until the natural course of the disease has been established. In some newborns, HPP gradually evolves into a morphologic picture characteristic of hereditary elliptocytosis. *True* HPP persists as a severe hemolytic anemia that usually requires early splenectomy, which greatly reduces hemolysis.[23, 51]

Hereditary Nonspherocytic Hemolytic Anemia

A number of erythrocyte enzyme deficiencies associated with hemolytic syndromes constitute this group of hemolytic anemias. Pyruvate kinase (PK) deficiency is the prototype of the enzymopathies involving the Embden-Meyerhof pathway of anaerobic glycolysis in the red cell. PK deficiency is inherited as an autosomal recessive trait and affects both sexes equally. An unusually high incidence exists among the Pennsylvania Amish.[23, 51] A discrepancy between red cell energy needs and adenosine triphosphate–generating capacity produces irreversible membrane injury with cellular distortion, rigidity, dehydration, and premature destruction of the red cells by the spleen.[23, 51] The severity of the anemia is variable.

Splenectomy results in improvement, but hemolysis is not abolished, and mild anemia persists. After splenectomy, transfusion requirements are reduced, young children experience a period of rapid *catch-up* growth, and the danger from aplastic crises is reduced.[23, 51]

It is important to differentiate between pyruvate kinase deficiency and other erythrocyte enzymopathies that cause hemolytic anemia such as G-6-PD deficiency and its variants. Specific enzyme assays are employed for this purpose. In G-6-PD deficiency, hemolysis is precipitated by infection and other acute illness, certain drugs, and fava beans. Splenic enlargement is rare, in contrast to frequent splenomegaly with pyruvate kinase deficiency, and splenectomy is not indicated for patients with G-6-PD deficiency.[5, 23, 51] A role for splenectomy in other erythrocyte enzyme deficiency states has not been established.

Sickle Cell Anemia

Sickle cell anemia is a hereditary hemolytic anemia occurring in blacks who are homozygous for the sickle hemoglobin (HbS) gene. Sickle hemoglobin (HbS) differs from normal adult hemoglobin (HbA) only in the substitution of valine for glutamic acid in the sixth position of the beta chain. HbS, which results from this single amino acid substitution, imparts the sickle shape to deoxygenated red blood cells and is responsible for the wide spectrum of clinical features that characterize sickle cell anemia. The highest incidence of HbS occurs among black Africans and descendants of emigrants from equatorial Africa. Sickle cell anemia (homozygous state for HbS) occurs in approximately 0.5% of the black population, and sickle cell trait (heterozygous state for HbS) is present in approximately 8% of African Americans. In the homozygous state, HbA is totally lacking and the red cells contain predominantly HbS. The red cells of individuals with sickle cell trait contain both HbA and HbS, with the relative amount of HbS ranging between 35% and 45%. A combination of two variant hemoglobin genes or a combination of a variant hemoglobin and an interacting thalassemia gene results in doubly heterozygous states designated by both aberrant gene products (e.g., HbS/C, HbS/beta thalassemia).[23, 51]

Under conditions of reduced oxygen availability, red cells containing HbS acquire the sickle-shaped deformity due to the intracellular polymerization of the HbS molecules. Sickling of erythrocytes containing HbS occurs more readily with a reduced pH, higher intracellular concentration of HbS, low intracellular concentrations of HbF (fetal hemoglobin), and conditions favoring hemoglobin deoxygenation. Increased blood viscosity due to the sickled cells and an increased adhesion of sickled cells to vascular endothelium result in circulatory stasis and stagnation that leads to further reduction in oxygen tension, further sickling, and a *vicious cycle* of erythrostasis. The consequent thrombosis, ischemia, necrosis, and organ fibrosis result in the clinical features of sickle cell anemia.[23, 51]

Patients with sickle cell anemia characteristically are without symptoms until the second half of the first year of life due to an initial sufficiency of HbF that limits clinically significant sickling. Clinical features of sickle cell anemia, which are both acute and episodic *(crises)* and chronic and progressive, are more a consequence of the rheologic properties of the sickle cells than of the anemia itself. Patients with sickle cell crisis often have severe abdominal pain and signs of peritoneal irritation similar to those of acute surgical illnesses such as acute cholecystitis and appendicitis. Clinical features of abdominal crises in patients with sickle cell anemia tend to be similar for a given individual, and deviation from previous patterns may be an important differentiating feature of an acute surgical illness in patients with sickle

cell anemia.[27] Chronic features of sickle cell anemia include retarded growth and development after the first decade; bone and joint disease; cardiovascular, pulmonary, hepatobiliary, genitourinary, and neurologic manifestations; hematuria; priapism; and ulcerations over the malleoli and distal portions of the legs. The incidence of pigment gallstones in patients with sickle cell anemia increases with age. Calculi appear first in childhood (2–4 years of age) and are present in approximately 70% of adult patients.[23, 51]

Diagnosis is established by the presence of characteristic sickle cells on blood smear, hemoglobin electrophoresis demonstrating predominantly HbS, variable amounts of HbF (5%–15%) and no HbA, and the presence of the sickle cell trait in both parents. Treatment is palliative and is directed toward minimizing complications of the disease. Many patients die during childhood from infections, renal failure, and heart failure. Rarely will a patient with sickle cell anemia have a relatively normal life span.[23, 51]

The role of the spleen in sickle cell anemia is unclear. Sequestration crisis characterized by sudden trapping of blood in the spleen is a complication that occurs almost exclusively in infants and young children whose spleens are chronically enlarged. Further enlargement of the spleen occurs rapidly at the expense of the blood volume, and hypovolemic shock and death may occur within hours.[23, 51] Splenomegaly first becomes apparent after 6 months of age and characteristically persists throughout childhood. Despite splenomegaly, splenic hypofunction may be documented as early as 5 months of age, and the risk of overwhelming infection exists in a child with sickle cell anemia by age 1 year.[23, 51] By adolescence or early adult life, recurrent infarctions have resulted in splenic atrophy and functional asplenia (hyposplenism). (See Hyposplenism and The Problem of Overwhelming Postsplenectomy Sepsis.) Splenectomy may be beneficial to the occasional child with sickle cell anemia in whom excessive red cell sequestration occurs in an enlarged spleen. The beneficial effect of splenectomy clearly is related to spleen size and is most effective in children with large spleens.[23, 51]

Sickle cell trait is rarely associated with significant clinical or hematologic manifestations, although splenic infarction has occurred in patients flying at high altitudes in unpressurized aircraft.[23, 51]

Thalassemia (Thalassemia Syndromes)

These hereditary hemolytic anemias result from a defect in hemoglobin synthesis in which one of the hemoglobin polypeptide chains is synthesized at a markedly reduced rate. Specific pairs of genes are responsible for synthesis of the alpha, beta, gamma, and delta chains of the hemoglobin molecule, and a deficiency in synthesis of one of these subunits may lead to one of the thalassemia syndromes. Thalassemia is classified by the deficient peptide chain.[23, 51] Beta-thalassemia, in which there is a quantitative reduction in the rate of beta chain synthesis, is the most common type of thalassemia. When the abnormal gene is inherited from both parents (homozygous), severe anemia, termed *thalassemia major*, results. Heterozygous patients have a mild anemia termed *thalassemia minor*. The term *thalassemia intermedia* is used to describe some homozygous patients who have a milder than usual course and some heterozygous patients who have a more severe course than usual. In thalassemia major, the reduction in the rate of beta chain synthesis produces a marked decrease in the amount of normal adult hemoglobin (HbA) with a compensatory increase in fetal hemoglobin (HbF). Homozygous alpha-thalassemia is incompatible with life, and these infants are stillborn or die shortly after birth. Patients with heterozygous alpha-thalassemia have a mild form of anemia similar to that in heterozygous beta-thalassemia.[23, 51]

The pathogenesis of hemolysis in thalassemia lies in the unbalanced synthesis of the polypeptide chains. Because of the absence of the complementary polypeptide chain with which to bind, the overproduced normal chains form aggregates that precipitate within the red cell cytoplasm and lead to premature cell destruction. In homozygous beta-thalassemia (thalassemia major), the deficiency of beta chain synthesis causes a relative overproduction of alpha chains, which undergo aggregation to form insoluble inclusions in bone marrow erythroid precursors. Ineffective erythropoiesis occurs because of the death of many of these cells. Additionally, the inclusion-bearing red cells are detained in the spleen, where they sustain mechanical and metabolic injury that facilitates their ultimate destruction.[23, 51]

Thalassemia major results in a severe anemia and clinical manifestations, usually within the first year of life. Pallor, retarded growth, and enlargement of the head with *thalassemic facies* are present, along with splenomegaly and hepatomegaly. The intense erythroid hyperplasia in the bone marrow causes expansion of the medullary cavities and attenuation of the cortex, producing bony abnormalities and a predisposition to fractures. Iron overload due to defective iron utilization coupled with increased iron absorption and frequent blood transfusions is a common complication.

The peripheral blood smear in thalassemia major shows a microcytic hypochromic anemia with a severe degree of poikilocytosis, anisocytosis, and polychromatophilia. Nucleated red cells are invariably present and may outnumber the leukocytes. Reticulocytosis and leukocytosis are characteristic, but the platelet count is generally normal. Hemoglobin electrophoresis in thalassemia major reveals absence or almost complete absence of HbA with the presence of large amounts of HbF.

Treatment consists of transfusion therapy and iron chelation, and splenectomy is effective in selected patients. Although the basic hematologic disease is not influenced, splenectomy decreases blood transfusion requirements and relieves discomfort from splenomegaly. Most patients with thalassemia major die during the second decade of life from complications of iron excess with myocardial hemosiderosis. Patients with alpha-thalassemia minor and beta-thalassemia minor rarely need treatment, and an important therapeutic consideration for patients with thalassemia minor is avoidance of therapeutic iron to minimize the risk of iron overload.[22, 51]

Autoimmune Hemolytic Anemia

Autoimmune hemolytic anemia is an acquired hemolytic anemia resulting from antibodies that are produced by the body against its own red cells. Patients with AIHA have the usual manifestations of hemolysis with anemia, reticulocytosis, a shortened erythrocyte survival time, fluctuating jaundice, and splenomegaly. The blood smear in AIHA shows spherocytes and microspherocytes in numbers exceeded only in hereditary spherocytosis. The distinguishing feature of AIHA is a positive direct Coombs test, which identifies antibody on the red cell surface. The type of antibody attached to the red cell determines the mechanism of hemolysis as well as the site for primary destruction of the sensitized cells. Anti–red cell antibodies are classified as warm reactive or cold reactive, depending on whether they bind to red cells most avidly at 37° C or have progressively greater affinity for erythrocytes as the temperature approaches 0° C.[22, 51]

Warm-reactive antibodies usually are IgG (less commonly IgM, IgA, or a combination) and facilitate sequestration and destruction of sensitized erythrocytes in the spleen. When IgG-coated red cells become attached to splenic macrophages, which have receptors for the Fc portion of the IgG molecule, portions of the red cell membrane are removed, rendering the erythrocyte more spherical and more susceptible to sequestration and premature destruction. Red cells coated by both IgG and complement are destroyed by the reticuloendothelial system generally and not primarily by the spleen.[21, 22, 51] Cold-reactive antibodies usually are IgM (rarely IgG or IgA) and bind to red cells mainly in the peripheral circulation where the blood temperature is cooled. Cold-reactive antibodies may cause either immediate intravascular hemolysis by complement-mediated mechanisms or sequestration and destruction of sensitized red cells by the liver. These patients usually have chronic hemolysis that is acutely worsened by cold exposure and often demonstrate acrocyanosis (Raynaud's phenomenon) due to intracapillary red cell agglutination.[23, 51]

The designation *autoimmune* in AIHA must not obscure the fact that in many cases the hemolytic process is associated with or related to a drug or a reversible disease that can be eliminated. Drugs associated with AIHA include penicillin, cephalothin, streptomycin, methyldopa (Aldomet), quinidine, quinine, phenacetin, *p*-aminosalicylic acid, and several sulfonamides.[23, 51] AIHA may occur in association with another disease, such as mycoplasmal pneumonia, viral infections, chronic lymphocytic leukemia, lymphoma, Hodgkin's disease, systemic lupus erythematosus, infectious mononucleosis, and AIDS. When a drug exposure or an underlying disease is identified, AIHA is termed secondary. When no other etiologic association is demonstrable, AIHA is classified as primary or idiopathic. AIHA occurs at any age and in both sexes but is more common in women older than age 50. Pallor and splenomegaly are the main physical findings in idiopathic AIHA, whereas in secondary AIHA additional clinical features of the underlying disease are present. The severity and duration of the hemolytic anemia may vary, and in some patients the course is rapid and fulminating. Severe hemolysis may produce hemoglobinuria and acute tubular necrosis. When AIHA follows mycoplasmal pneumonia, the disease may be acute and self-limited over several weeks and require no therapy. More often the disease is chronic, with varying degrees of severity over months or years.[21, 23, 51]

Treatment is directed toward the hemolytic anemia and any underlying disease. Blood transfusions, corticosteroid therapy, and splenectomy are important aspects of treatment for the anemia. Splenectomy is usually performed in patients with AIHA in whom either corticosteroids are ineffective or an excessive corticosteroid dose is required, or when complications preclude corticosteroid use. Chromium-51–labeled red cell studies are useful to measure the degree of splenic sequestration and to serve as a guide for selecting patients who are most likely to respond to splenectomy.[23, 40, 51] Splenectomy results in a favorable response, with complete hematologic remission in approximately 80% of patients demonstrating significant splenic sequestration. Lack of significant red cell sequestration by the spleen does not preclude a good response to splenectomy. Splenectomy is more likely to induce a complete and sustained remission in primary (idiopathic) AIHA in which only IgG (warm-reactive) antibodies coat the red cells. In addition to removing the primary site for destruction of the sensitized red cells, splenectomy can be expected to significantly reduce production of anti-red cell antibody, because the spleen is a major site for IgG antibody production. The prognosis for patients with secondary AIHA depends mainly on the underlying disease and is generally favorable when the hemolytic anemia follows a viral illness or is related to a drug exposure. Prognosis is poor when

and the reticuloendothelial system. Splenic cysts and primary tumors are rare but must be considered in the differential diagnosis of a left upper quadrant mass.

Cystic lesions of the spleen comprise parasitic and nonparasitic cysts. Parasitic cysts are due almost exclusively to echinococcal disease and account for 60% to 70% of splenic cysts in countries where hydatid disease is endemic (South America, Australia, and Greece). Because echinococcal disease is rare in the United States, nonparasitic cysts are encountered much more frequently in this country. Nonparasitic cysts are classified as primary or true cysts, which have an epithelial lining, and pseudocysts. Pseudocysts are much more common and probably result from liquefaction of old hematomas or areas of infarction and inflammation. True cysts of the spleen are very rare and include epidermoid and dermoid cysts, cystic hemangiomas, and cystic lymphangiomas.

Symptoms of splenic cysts are vague and are caused primarily by mass effect, compression of adjacent viscera, and diaphragmatic irritation. Although selected nonparasitic cysts may be effectively managed by aspiration, splenectomy should be performed for all large cysts and those with uncertain diagnosis. In some patients a splenic cyst may be suitably located for excision by partial splenectomy. Intraoperative drainage may facilitate dissection and splenectomy for very large cysts. External drainage and marsupialization have an unacceptable incidence of infection, bleeding, and cyst reaccumulation and are inappropriate techniques for management of splenic cysts.

Malignant and benign primary tumors of the spleen are rare. Most primary malignant tumors are angiosarcomas, although primary splenic lymphoma may occur. Before primary parenchymal lymphoma is diagnosed in the spleen, the bone marrow, nodal regions, liver, and other areas must be evaluated and found to be free of disease. Benign splenic tumors include hamartomas, lymphangiomas, hemangiomas, and lipomas.[42]

Except for involvement with Hodgkin's disease and NHLs, metastatic disease to the spleen is diagnosed infrequently (Fig. 36–13). The spleen's effective filtering mechanism and high blood flow suggest that the spleen would develop metastatic lesions more often. Although spleens from patients dying of metastatic tumors frequently reveal malignant cells, metastatic deposits are rare. Studies in rodents have confirmed that metastatic tumors rarely develop in the spleen after injection of tumor cells into the splenic artery. It is probable that the splenic immune mechanisms that so efficiently destroy abnormal red cells also eliminate the majority of metastatic tumor cells that are trapped in the red pulp.[8]

Splenic Vein Thrombosis

Since the pathophysiology of splenic vein thrombosis was first elucidated 50 years ago, this uncommon cause of upper gastrointestinal variceal hemorrhage has been found to be eminently curable by splenectomy.[6] Pancreatitis is the cause of splenic vein thrombosis in more than half of the reported cases. Other causes include pancreatic carcinoma, pancreatic pseudocyst, penetrating gastric ulcer, retroperitoneal fibrosis, and myeloproliferative disorders.[6] The underlying disease produces thrombosis of the splenic vein with subsequent development of venous collateral channels. Because the collateral pathways are usually the short gastric veins to the submucosal venous plexus of the gastric cardia and fundus, gastric varices develop.

Splenic vein thrombosis should be suspected in a patient with upper gastrointestinal hemorrhage, isolated gastric varices on endoscopy, and a history of pancreatitis or pancreatic cancer. Splenomegaly is variable, and if present it is not

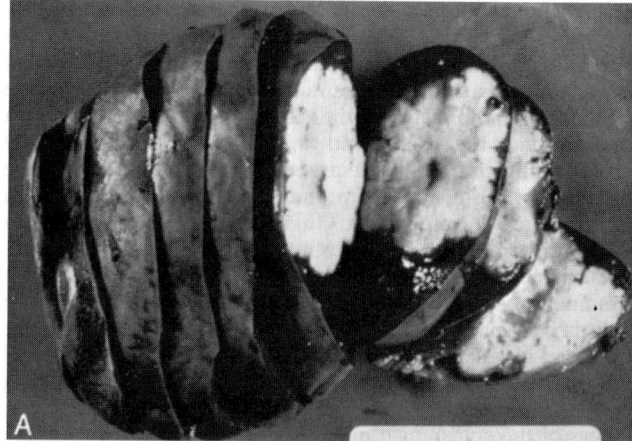
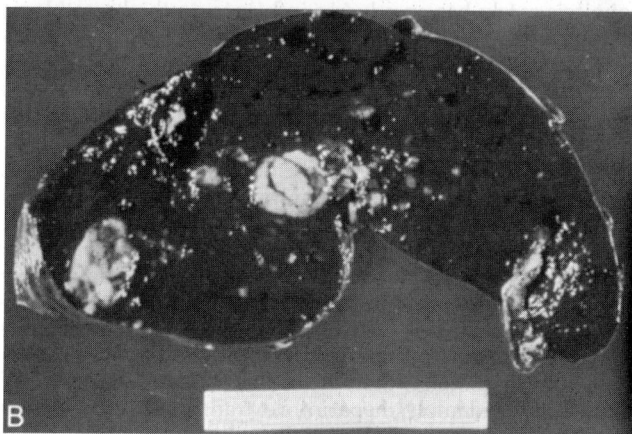

Figure 36–13. *A,* Large metastatic deposit in the spleen (480 gm.) from gastric adenocarcinoma. *B,* Metastatic plasmacytomas in the spleen (1000 gm.) of a patient with multiple myeloma who developed hypersplenism.

associated with other stigmata of cirrhosis. Anemia is usually present, but tests of liver function are normal. Definitive diagnosis is made by celiac angiography, which demonstrates absence of the splenic vein. Splenomegaly may be noted along with venous collaterals in the splenic hilus.[6, 42]

Splenectomy is curative and eliminates the increased blood flow through collaterals to the gastric venous plexuses. Although there are no studies that have followed the course of asymptomatic patients with splenic vein thrombosis, it seems prudent to consider splenectomy if this diagnosis is made.

Infectious Mononucleosis

Infectious mononucleosis is a disease characterized by fever, sore throat, lymphadenopathy, and atypical lymphocytes in the blood smear. The atypical lymphocytes are believed to be T cells reacting against B lymphocytes infected with Epstein-Barr virus. Most patients are young adults, but the disease also occurs in middle-aged individuals.[22, 23, 51] The diagnosis is made by finding a pleomorphic atypical lymphocytosis and heterophilic antibodies in the serum as demonstrated by a mono spot test.

Clinical symptomatology is akin to that of a severe upper respiratory tract infection. The spleen is enlarged and palpable in over 50% of young patients, in contrast to the 3% incidence of a palpable spleen found normally in this age group.[8, 23, 51] Hepatomegaly is present in 15% of patients.

Splenic rupture may occur, probably resulting from minor trauma to an enlarged and diseased spleen rather than from *spontaneous rupture.* There has been minimal experience with

TABLE 36–8. Morbidity and Mortality in Splenectomy, 1948 to 1978

Indication	Number of Patients	Per Cent	Morbidity (%)	Mortality (%)
Hypersplenism	999	41	15	7
Primary	557	23	10	2
Secondary	442	18	22	13
Incidental	659	27	36	13
Trauma	257	10.5	30	16
Hodgkin's staging	203	8	4	0
Other	299	12	—	—
Total	2417	100	34	9.25

Modified from Traetow, W. D., Fabri, P. J., and Carey, L. C.: Changing indications for splenectomy: 30 years' experience. Arch. Surg., 115:447, 1980. Copyright 1980, American Medical Association.

splenic preservation for rupture associated with infectious mononucleosis. Most series of splenectomy for bleeding in patients with infectious mononucleosis report a higher mortality than with splenectomy for trauma.

Incidental Splenectomy

The spleen is vulnerable to injury during operative procedures in the upper abdomen. Operations on the stomach, esophageal hiatus, vagus nerves, pancreas, left kidney and adrenal gland, and transverse and descending colon carry risk of splenic injury. When the splenic capsule is torn, splenectomy is frequently performed (Table 36–8).

In most series, morbidity and mortality are higher with iatrogenic injury requiring incidental splenectomy than with splenectomy for a specific disease. One large series reported an earlier (before 1974) morbidity rate of 44% and a mortality rate of 14%.[46] More recent experience from the same institution has revealed a pronounced decrease in the incidence of incidental splenectomy but a continued significant morbidity (26%) and mortality (12%). Awareness of the risk for overwhelming postsplenectomy sepsis and the high complication and death rates from incidental splenectomy indicate and emphasize the need for avoiding intraoperative splenic injury. Most iatrogenic injuries occur to the capsule, and techniques for splenic repair and preservation should be employed instead of splenectomy.

SPLENECTOMY

Operations for splenic injury or disease should be preceded by specific preoperative preparations. All patients should receive polyvalent pneumococcal vaccine (Pnu-Imune 23 or Pneumovax 23), polyvalent meningococcal vaccine, and *Haemophilus influenzae* type b conjugate vaccine as early as possible before operation. Blood and blood products should be sought sufficiently in advance to allow for crossmatching, which may be difficult in patients with acquired hemolytic anemia, thalassemia, or isoantibodies from previous transfusions. Platelet availability is advisable in severely thrombocytopenic patients for use after removal of the spleen if thrombocytopenic bleeding occurs. The operating room and blood and blood products should be warmed before use. This is especially important in patients with CLL or lymphoma who may have developed cold hemagglutinin disease and thus have an increased risk for hemolysis.

Splenectomy can be performed through several standard abdominal incisions. It is rarely necessary to use a thoracoabdominal incision, even to remove massively enlarged spleens. The midline incision is preferred, although a left subcostal incision is favored by some surgeons, especially in children. Palpation is carried out to detect any inflammatory adhesions to the spleen that might cause a capsular tear and troublesome bleeding if not carefully divided. The spleen is mobilized by dividing its posterior ligamentous attachments, which may contain blood vessels requiring control by electrocauterization or ligation. The short gastric vessels are divided and suture ligated, avoiding injury or ischemia to focal areas of the greater gastric curvature that might produce necrosis and gastric fistula formation. Some instances of postsplenectomy bleeding are due to inadequately secured short gastric vessels in patients who develop gastric distention postoperatively. A nasogastric tube is advisable for most patients undergoing splenectomy, although some do not use a nasogastric tube in patients with ITP because of the potential risk of causing bleeding from the nose or nasopharynx.

The spleen may be removed at laparotomy by either of two techniques. Splenic ligaments may be divided and the spleen mobilized toward the midline before securing the hilar vessels, a technique applicable for normal sized, slightly enlarged, and ruptured spleens (Fig. 36–14). Initial ligation of the splenic artery and vein along the upper edge of the pancreas before splenic mobilization is a very useful technique with massive splenomegaly, because it controls the major portion of the vascular supply and allows safer mobilization of the spleen and dissection of its hilar branches (Fig. 36–15).[15] Isolation and ligation of blood vessels in the hilus should be performed carefully to avoid injuring the tail of the pancreas. Accessory splenic tissue occurs in approximately 20% of patients, and a thorough search for an accessory spleen should be performed in all patients undergoing splenectomy for hematologic disease (Fig. 36–16). The left upper quadrant should not be drained routinely. When injury

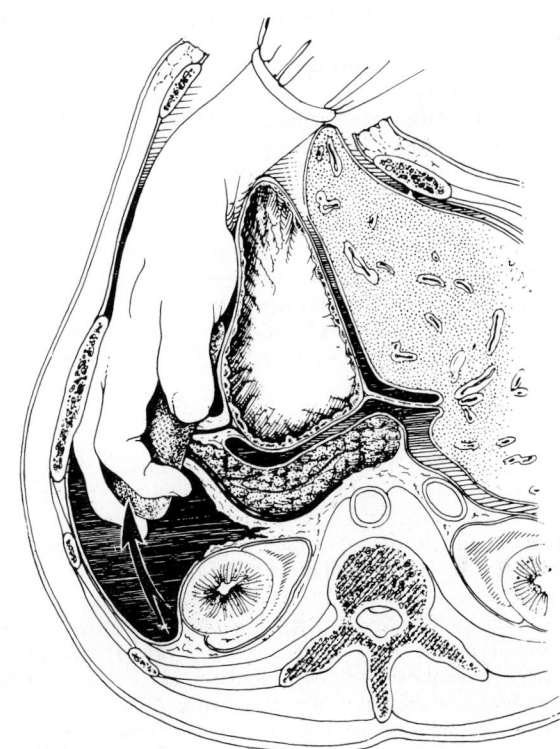

Figure 36–14. Technique of splenic mobilization for splenectomy or splenorrhaphy. The spleen is easily mobilized to the midline after dividing its posterior ligaments. The plane of dissection lies posterior to the body and tail of the pancreas and can be developed rapidly by blunt dissection. (From Blaisdell, F. W., and Trunkey, D. D.: Trauma Management. New York, Thieme-Stratton, 1982, p. 190.)

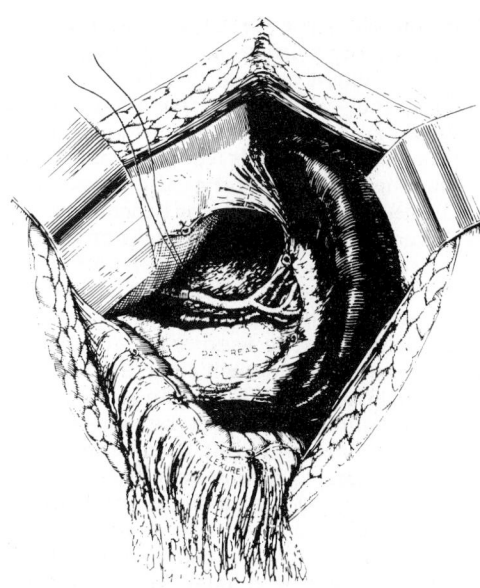

Figure 36–15. Technique of splenectomy showing in continuity ligation of the splenic artery and vein before mobilizing the spleen. The gastrosplenic ligament has been partially divided. Initial control of the splenic artery and vein in this manner minimizes the danger of major bleeding in performing splenectomy for very large spleens. (From Cooper, P.: The Craft of Surgery, 2nd ed. Boston, Little, Brown, and Co., 1971, p. 1314.)

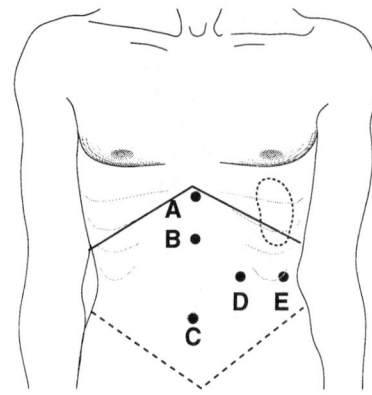

Figure 36–17. Position of operating ports for laparoscopic splenectomy. (From Flowers, J. L., Lefor, A. T., Steers, J., Heyman, M., Graham, S. M., and Imbembo, A. L.: Laparoscopic splenectomy in patients with hematologic diseases. Ann. Surg., *224*:19, 1996.)

BLOOD COMPOSITIONAL CHANGES IN THE ASPLENIC OR HYPOSPLENIC PATIENT

The absence of functional splenic tissue results in characteristic compositional changes in the circulating blood. Some of these are predictable and desirable results of splenectomy

to the tail of the pancreas or incomplete hemostasis indicate the advisability for left upper quadrant drainage, a system of closed suction drainage should be employed. Depending on the indication for splenectomy, most patients tolerate the operation well. The most common postoperative complication is left lower lobe atelectasis. Other more serious complications include postoperative hemorrhage, subphrenic abscess, pancreatitis, pneumonia, wound infection, and portal vein and mesenteric venous thrombosis.

In the recent past the *laparoscopic* approach to splenectomy has become increasingly important and is often used. It is now regarded by some as being preferable to open splenectomy for hematologic diseases in view of its efficacy and reduction in morbidity and mortality. Return of gastrointestinal function is prompt, there is less postoperative pain, and return to a normal status and work is more rapid. The patient benefits from use of this approach in removing the spleen are summarized in a report by Flowers and associates.[11] The technique is illustrated in Figures 36–17 and 36–18.

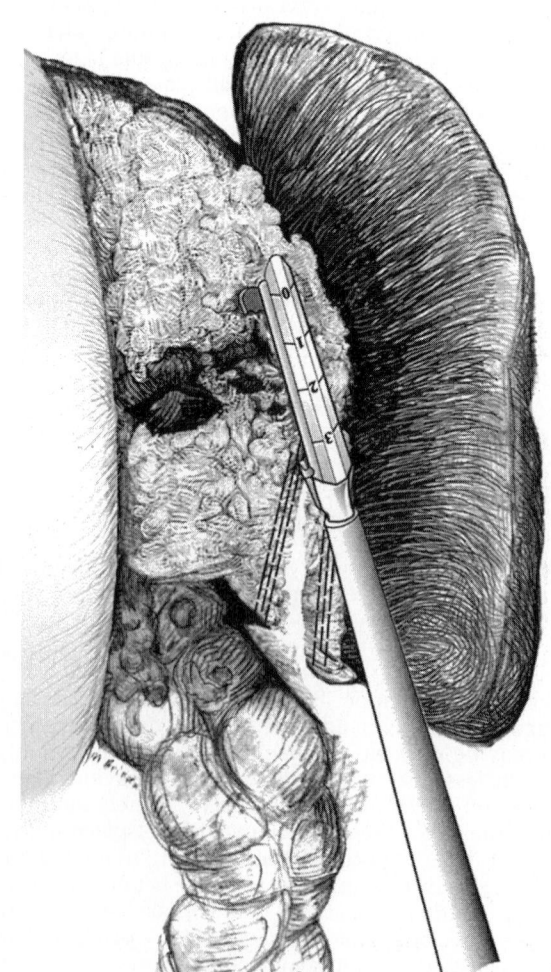

Figure 36–18. The hilar vessels are clamped with a 3-cm. linear laparoscopic stapler. (From Flowers, J. L., Lefor, A. T., Steers, J., Heyman, M., Graham, S. M., and Imbembo, A. L.: Laparoscopic splenectomy in patients with hematologic diseases. Ann Surg., *224*:19, 1996.)

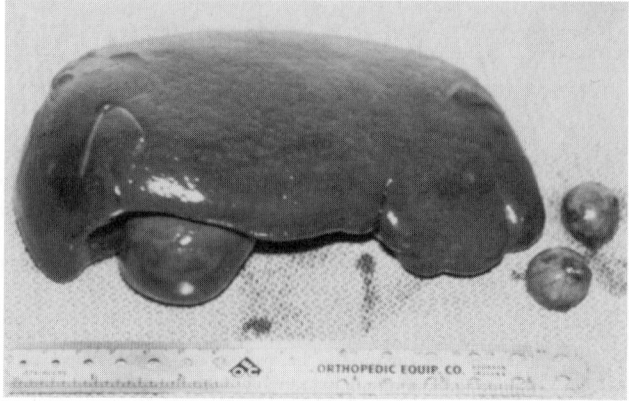

Figure 36–16. A spleen (440 gm.) demonstrating prominent fetal lobulations and two accessory spleens from a patient with hereditary elliptocytosis.

and are a measure of its success when splenectomy is performed for a hematologic disease.

In its normal filtering function, the spleen removes excess red cell membrane, surface abnormalities such as pits and spurs, and a variety of intracellular inclusions. Red cells that cannot be adequately molded and pitted are culled.[8] In the absence of the spleen, this function is lost, and several characteristic red cell changes can be identified in the peripheral blood. Howell-Jolly bodies (nuclear remnants) are typically present in asplenic patients, and absence of Howell-Jolly bodies after splenectomy suggests the presence of functional residual splenic tissue (accessory spleen or splenosis).[8, 38] Target cells, red cells with fine inclusions (stippled red cells), acanthocytes (spur cells), Heinz bodies (denatured hemoglobin), and Pappenheimer bodies (iron granules) are also predictable findings in asplenic patients. Granulocytosis, lymphocytosis, and monocytosis commonly occur after splenectomy but are variable in occurrence, magnitude, and duration.[8, 23, 51]

Thrombocytosis occurs immediately after splenectomy in most patients and is often the desired therapeutic result. Up to 75% of patients who have had splenectomy develop thrombocytosis (platelet count of greater than 400,000/cu. mm.), and platelet counts in excess of 1 million per cu. mm. develop in some patients. Generally this has not been associated with an increased risk of thromboembolism.[4] An exception to this is seen in patients with myeloproliferative disorders who clearly have an increased risk of thromboembolic complications after splenectomy.[19, 23, 51] In these patients, and especially in those with thrombocytosis preoperatively, specific antiplatelet therapy should be used. The spectrum of antiplatelet therapy includes administration of *p*-aminosalicylic acid, dipyridamole, heparin, dextran, hydroxyurea, and busulfan. Hydroxyurea is especially useful in controlling thrombocytosis. A rapid reduction of the thrombocytosis can be achieved by plateletpheresis (thrombocytopheresis) in patients with thrombohemorrhagic manifestations.[19, 23, 51]

After splenectomy, depression of serum levels of at least two important opsonins occurs. Diminution in these two opsonic proteins, tuftsin and properdin, is partially responsible for the increased susceptibility of asplenic patients to infection from encapsulated bacteria. The exact role of these opsonins is unclear. Children with sickle cell anemia have low levels of properdin and an impaired alternate pathway of complement activation, which decrease their ability to opsonize pneumococci. However, children with splenectomy for trauma have normal pneumococcal opsonizing activity in spite of subnormal levels of properdin and tuftsin.[8]

THE PROBLEM OF OVERWHELMING POSTSPLENECTOMY SEPSIS

Asplenic patients and those with deficient splenic function have an increased susceptibility to the development of overwhelming infection characterized by fulminant bacteremia, meningitis, or pneumonia. Although it was suggested as early as 1919 that removal of the spleen would increase susceptibility to infection (Morris and Bullock), the increased risk of fatal sepsis was first documented by King and Shumacker in 1952.[30, 42, 43] Singer's review of 2796 patients with splenectomy described a 4.2% incidence of sepsis and a 2.5% mortality rate (Table 36–9). The risk of overwhelming sepsis is approximately 60 times greater than normal after splenectomy and may be as high as 0.5% to 1.0% per year. Although a lifetime risk of fulminant sepsis is incurred with splenectomy, the risk is greatest in children younger than 4 years of age and within 2 years of splenectomy (80% of cases).[8] In one series of adults, the average time period between splenectomy and fulminant sepsis was 5.8 years, with a range of 7 months to 25 years.[30] A follow-up of 740 servicemen with splenectomy for trauma demonstrated an increased mortality rate from pneumonia and ischemic heart disease.[30, 42]

The risk for overwhelming postsplenectomy sepsis is highest in patients requiring splenectomy for thalassemia and reticuloendothelial system diseases such as Hodgkin's disease, histiocytosis X, or the Wiscott-Aldrich syndrome.[8, 30] It is lowest for patients with splenectomy for trauma, ITP, and hereditary spherocytosis (see Table 36–9).[8]

The postsplenectomy sepsis syndrome typically occurs in a previously healthy individual after a mild upper respiratory tract infection associated with fever. Within hours, nausea, vomiting, headache, confusion, shock, and coma occur; and death follows within 24 hours. Laboratory studies reveal hypoglycemia, acidosis, electrolyte abnormalities, and disseminated intravascular coagulation.[8, 30] Blood cultures reveal *Streptococcus pneumoniae, Neisseria meningitidis, Escherichia coli,* or *Haemophilus influenzae* in 75% of the cases, with *S. pneumoniae* accounting for 50%.[30] Patients with pneumococcal sepsis have no obvious site of primary infection, and the bacteremia, which may reach extraordinary proportions ($>10^6$ bacteria/ml.), is of cryptic origin. The peripheral blood smear shows vacuolated polymorphonuclear leukocytes, thrombocytopenia, and, occasionally, pneumococci.[8, 30] The fulminant nature of the syndrome makes it difficult to diagnosis early enough for therapy to be effective. Adrenal hemorrhage is a common autopsy finding.[30]

The spleen has both mechanical and humoral roles in pro-

TABLE 36–9. Incidence of Postsplenectomy Sepsis

Reason for Splenectomy	Number of Patients	Number of Patients with Sepsis (%)	Number of Fatalities from Sepsis (%)	Increased Risk of Death from Sepsis (×)
Trauma	688	10 (1.4)	4 (0.58)	58
Incidental to operation	233	5 (2.1)	2 (0.86)	86
Idiopathic thrombocytopenic purpura	489	10 (2.0)	7 (1.43)	140
Hereditary spherocytosis	850	30 (3.5)	19 (2.23)	220
Acquired hemolytic anemia	67	5 (7.5)	2 (2.90)	290
Portal hypertension	221	18 (8.2)	13 (5.90)	590
Primary anemia	70	6 (8.5)	5 (7.01)	700
Reticuloendothelial disease	69	8 (11.5)	7 (10.10)	1000
Thalassemia	109	27 (24.8)	12 (11.00)	1100
Total	2796	119 (4.2)	71 (2.50)	

Modified from Singer, R.: Postsplenectomy sepsis. Perspect. Pediatr. Pathol., *1:*285, 1973. Reprinted with permission of J. Karger Basel.

tecting against bacterial infection, and the exact mechanism whereby postsplenectomy sepsis develops is unclear. Among the immunologic defects that occur after splenectomy are decreased serum properdin and tuftsin levels, decreased serum IgM, an impaired alternate pathway of complement activation, and a reduced response to particulate antigens.[8, 30, 42] Opsonization is critically important in the phagocytosis of *S. pneumoniae*, but animal studies indicate an adequate splenic mass is also important in pneumococcal clearance.[30, 42] Evidence suggests that approximately 50% of the normal mass of splenic tissue is necessary to preserve protection against encapsulated bacteria.[30, 42] Because postsplenectomy sepsis and death have occurred in patients having a total mass of residual splenic tissue weighing 3 to 92 gm., preservation of a sufficient *critical* splenic mass appears necessary for the maintenance of normal host defenses.[8, 42] Antibiotic prophylaxis or early antibiotic therapy may be effective in reducing the incidence of postsplenectomy sepsis. Because half of the patients develop sepsis from *S. pneumoniae*, penicillin can be administered prophylactically or immediately with the onset of a febrile upper respiratory tract illness. In patients who have had splenectomy for Hodgkin's disease staging, the incidence of overwhelming sepsis has been reduced by penicillin prophylaxis.[30] The authors' practice is to administer penicillin prophylactically for an indefinite period after splenectomy in young children. If allergy to penicillin exists, erythromycin or trimethoprim-sulfamethoxazole is substituted. Each adult patient is instructed to obtain and wear a Medic Alert tag indicating their asplenic state and increased risk for infection. In addition, the danger of overwhelming postsplenectomy sepsis and the importance of seeking immediate medical attention with the onset of a febrile upper respiratory tract illness are stressed to adult patients and to the parents of children who have had splenectomy.

Considerable hope exists for preventing postsplenectomy sepsis by immunization using specific vaccines. Ideally, patients should be immunized well in advance of splenectomy (2 to 3 weeks preoperatively) to allow development of protective antibodies. Polyvalent vaccines against capsular polysaccharides from pneumococcal strains responsible for the majority of serious pneumococcal disease (Pnu-Imune 23 [23 strains] and Pneumovax 23 [23 strains]) are available. Polyvalent meningococcal vaccines are also available, and *H. influenzae* type b conjugate vaccines provide immunization against type b *Haemophilus*, a leading cause of serious systemic bacterial disease. Although the efficacy of vaccination to reduce the incidence of overwhelming infection is difficult to assess owing to the infrequent occurrence of postsplenectomy sepsis, polyvalent pneumococcal vaccine has provided significant protection from pneumococcemia in children with sickle cell anemia.[8, 30] Not all splenectomized patients are capable of developing protective antibody titers after vaccination. Children younger than 2 years of age and patients with Hodgkin's disease who are receiving chemotherapy and/or radiation therapy do not respond consistently to polyvalent pneumococcal vaccine. An additional shortcoming of immunization is that current vaccines do not immunize against all bacteria capable of producing overwhelming postsplenectomy sepsis. It is unclear if and how often patients should be reimmunized after splenectomy. As new vaccines become available and further studies are completed, a more definitive immunization program may become standard. Presently, repeat immunization every 5 years seems reasonable.

RARE SPLENIC DISORDERS

Wandering (Ectopic) Spleen. Congenital deficiency or acquired laxity of the suspensory ligaments of the spleen may cause extreme splenic mobility. This rare condition, which is termed *wandering* or *ectopic spleen*, permits a normal-sized spleen to be palpable in the lower abdomen or in the pelvis. The majority of cases of wandering spleen have occurred in young and middle-aged women in whom multiparity and laxity of the abdominal wall and splenic ligaments due to the hormonal effects of pregnancy have been cited as predisposing causes. A wandering spleen may be an incidental finding on physical or radiographic examination. An elongated splenic pedicle predisposes a wandering spleen to torsion, leading either to development of acute symptoms due to splenic volvulus and infarction or to chronic and intermittent abdominal discomfort due to spontaneous torsion and detorsion. Useful diagnostic tests in the patient who is asymptomatic or has chronic and recurring symptoms include abdominal CT or ultrasonography, a splenic radionuclide scan, and visceral arteriography. Splenic volvulus with infarction requires emergency splenectomy. Selected asymptomatic patients and those with chronic and recurring symptoms may sometimes be managed successfully by splenopexy, which preserves splenic function and avoids the potential danger of postsplenectomy sepsis.

Splenic Artery Aneurysm. Aneurysms of the splenic artery are rare and occur more frequently in females, in whom

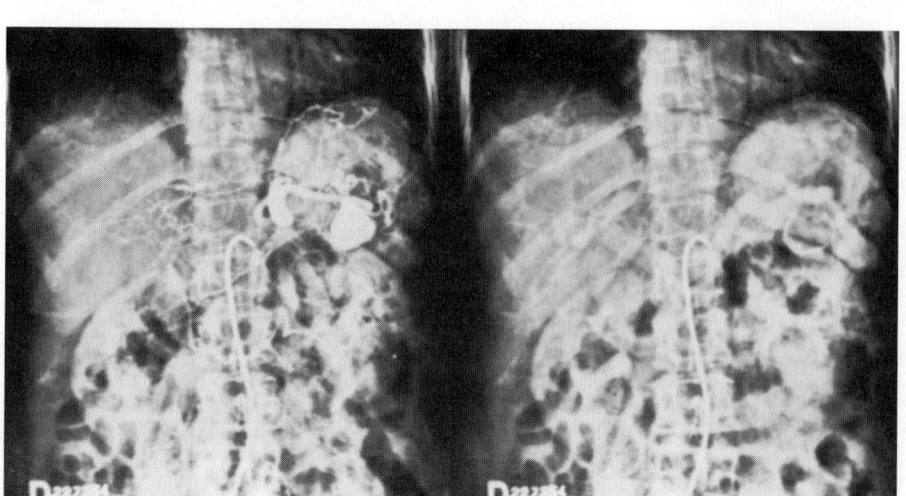

Figure 36–19. A splenic arteriogram disclosing an aneurysm of the distal splenic artery. *A*, The aneurysm is filled with contrast material. *B*, In a later radiograph the egg-shell calcification characteristic of an arteriosclerotic aneurysm is evident. Excision of the aneurysm was performed and required splenectomy.

A   B

the most common etiology is medial dysplasia of the arterial wall. Atherosclerosis accounts for the majority of splenic artery aneurysms in males. Additional causes include focal arterial injury due to pancreatitis, trauma or arteritis due to septic emboli, portal hypertension with splenomegaly, and an ill-defined pathogenesis associated with multiparity.[42] Most splenic artery aneurysms are asymptomatic, and characteristic eggshell calcification of an arteriosclerotic aneurysm may be an incidental finding on an abdominal radiograph (Fig. 36–19). When symptoms are present, they are variable and consist primarily of vague left upper quadrant discomfort. Aneurysmal rupture may occur, and the rupture initially may be contained within the lesser sac. Initial aneurysmal rupture into the peritoneal cavity or delayed rupture from the lesser sac are associated with findings of hemoperitoneum and exsanguinating hemorrhage. Rarely, a splenic artery aneurysm ruptures into the gastrointestinal tract, pancreatic duct, or splenic vein. The mortality with a ruptured splenic artery aneurysm remains high. Excision of the aneurysm is advisable for symptomatic aneurysms and for asymptomatic aneurysms in patients who are acceptable operative risks. This is especially important for women of childbearing age who have an increased propensity for aneurysmal rupture during pregnancy. Elective operation has a low risk of mortality and minimal morbidity. In the treatment of splenic artery aneurysm, the spleen should be preserved if possible.[42]

Splenic Abscess. Splenic abscess occurs rarely and usually results from (1) bacteremia associated with a primary septic focus such as bacterial endocarditis or lung abscess or (2) secondary infection in an area of the spleen damaged by infarction (sickle cell anemia or leukemia), trauma, or parasitic infestation. Clinical features of splenic abscess are those of left subphrenic suppuration and include fever, chills, left upper quadrant tenderness, and often splenomegaly. Imaging techniques (ultrasonography and radionuclide and CT scans) are useful in differentiating splenic abscess from left subphrenic abscess and in determining whether there is a single abscess or multiple abscesses within the spleen. CT is probably the most direct way of evaluating the spleen and establishing an early diagnosis.[42]

Splenectomy has been the preferred treatment for most patients in the past and remains a standard means of safe and rapid management. Splenotomy and abscess drainage may be advisable for selected patients with a single abscess and extensive adhesions between the spleen and adjacent structures. Image-guided percutaneous drainage may be appropriate in the management of some patients with splenic abscess. Percutaneous drainage is most likely to be successful, if the abscess is unilocular and if the abscess contents are amenable to complete evacuation by an in-dwelling suction catheter.[14]

SELECTED REFERENCES

Croom, R. D., McMillan, C. W., Sheldon, G. F., and Orringer, E. P.: Hereditary spherocytosis: Recent experience and current concepts of pathophysiology. Ann. Surg., 203:34, 1986.
A thorough review of this important hemolytic anemia is presented along with case reports that illustrate the recessively inherited form of hereditary spherocytosis. This article contains a concise description of the hypothesized erythrocyte membrane skeleton and the relationship to current concepts of pathophysiology of this disease.

Eichner, E. R.: Splenic function: Normal, too much and too little. Am. J. Med., 66:311, 1979.
This exceptionally thoughtful and complete review discusses splenic function in normal and pathologic conditions. The indications for splenectomy are presented from the viewpoint of a hematologist.

Leonard, A. S., Giebink, G. S., Baesl, T. J., and Krivit, W.: The overwhelming postsplenectomy sepsis problem. World J. Surg., 4:423, 1980.
This article contains a complete discussion of the postsplenectomy sepsis syndrome and the postulated immune defects. Invited commentary by Doctors Filler, Grosfeld, Lynn, and Singer is included along with their experiences with this problem and therapeutic recommendations.

McMillan, R.: Chronic idiopathic thrombocytopenic purpura. N. Engl. J. Med., 304:1135, 1981.
This article provides a complete discussion of this complex immune syndrome and reviews the mechanisms of pathogenesis and results of therapy.

Schwartz, S. I., Adams, J. T., and Bauman, A. W.: Splenectomy for Hematologic Disorders. Chicago, Year Book Medical Publishers, 1971.
Although published 19 years ago, this monograph by a premier surgical hematologist is a classic. The immunologic mechanisms have undergone some revision since publication, but the presentation of surgical concepts and the clear writing style are noteworthy.

Schwartz, S. I.: Progress symposium—Diseases affecting the spleen. World J. Surg., 9:377, 1985.
This symposium focuses on traumatic, infectious, vascular, neoplastic, and selected hematologic indications for operations on the spleen and its blood vessels. Indications, results, and complications of operation are reviewed, and a thorough overview of postsplenectomy sepsis is presented.

Sherman, R.: Perspectives in management of trauma to the spleen: 1979 Presidential Address, American Association for the Surgery of Trauma. J. Trauma., 20:1, 1980.
This article was the presidential address to the American Association for the Surgery of Trauma in 1979. It provides a comprehensive and scholarly review of the evolution of concepts and techniques for management of splenic trauma.

REFERENCES

1. Adler, S., Stutzman, L., Sokal, J. E., and Mittelman, A.: Splenectomy for hematologic depression in lymphocytic lymphoma and leukemia. Cancer, 35:521, 1975.
2. Agre, P., Orringer, E. P., and Bennett, V.: Deficient red-cell spectrin in severe, recessively inherited spherocytosis. N. Engl. J. Med., 306:1155, 1982.
3. Bonadonna, G., and Santoro, A.: Current Diagnosis and Treatment of Malignant Lymphomas. Evansville, IN, Mead Johnson & Company, 1983.
4. Boxer, M. A., Braun, J., and Ellman, L.: Thromboembolic risk of postsplenectomy thrombocytosis. Arch. Surg., 113:808, 1978.
5. Brain, M. C., and McCulloch, P. B.: Current Therapy in Hematology-Oncology: 1983–1984. Toronto, B. C. Decker, 1983.
6. Bunt, T. J., Hackler, M. T., and Greene, F. L.: Isolated splenic vein thrombosis: The curable variceal hemorrhage. South. Med. J., 76:936, 1983.
7. Croom, R. D., McMillan, C. W., Sheldon, G. F., and Orringer, E. P.: Hereditary spherocytosis: Recent experience and current concepts of pathophysiology. Ann. Surg., 203:34, 1986.
8. Eichner, E. R.: Splenic function: Normal, too much and too little. Am. J. Med., 66:311, 1979.
9. Eraklis, A. J., and Filler, R. M.: Splenectomy in childhood, a review of 1413 cases. J. Pediatr. Surg., 7:382, 1972.
10. Fleming, C. R., Dickson, E. R., and Harrison, E. G., Jr.: Splenosis: Autotransplantation of splenic tissue. Am. J. Med., 61:414, 1976.
11. Flowers, J. L., Lefor, A. T., Steers, J., Heyman, M., Graham, S. M., and Imbembo, A. L.: Laparoscopic splenectomy in patients with hematologic diseases. Ann. Surg., 224:19, 1996.
12. Gernsheimer, T., Stratton, J., Ballem, P. J., and Slichter, S. J.: Mechanisms of response to treatment in autoimmune thrombocytopenic purpura. N. Engl. J. Med., 320:974, 1989.
13. George, J. N., El-Harake, M. A., and Raskob, G. E.: Chronic idiopathic thrombocytopenic purpura. N. Engl. J. Med., 331:1207, 1994.
14. Gill, P. G., Souter, R. G., and Morris, P. J.: Splenectomy for hypersplenism in malignant lymphomas. Br. J. Surg., 68:29, 1981.
15. Gleich, S., Wolin, D. A., and Herbsman, H.: A review of percutaneous drainage in splenic abscess. Surg. Gynecol. Obstet., 167:211, 1988.
16. Goldstone, J.: Splenectomy for massive splenomegaly. Am. J. Surg., 135:385, 1978.
17. Golomb, H. M.: Hairy cell leukemia: Lessons learned in twenty-five years. J. Clin. Oncol., 1:652, 1983.
18. Golomb, H. M., and Ratain, M. J.: Recent advances in the treatment of hairy cell leukemia. N. Engl. J. Med., 316:870, 1987.
19. Golomb, H. M., and Ratain, M. J.: What is the choice of treatment for hairy cell leukemia? J. Clin. Oncol., 7:156, 1989.
20. Gordon, D. H., Schaffner, D., Bennett, J. M., and Schwartz, S. I.: Postsplenectomy thrombocytosis: Its association with mesenteric, portal, and/or renal vein thrombosis in patients with myeloproliferative disorders. Arch. Surg., 113:713, 1978.
21. Guzzetta, P. C., Connors, R. H., Fink, J., and Barranger, J. A.: Operative technique and results of subtotal splenectomy for Gaucher disease. Surg. Gynecol. Obstet., 164:359, 1987.
22. Hoballah, J. J., Kim, E. H., and Dumont, A. E.: Thrombocytopenic purpura in parenteral drug abusers. Surg. Gynecol. Obstet., 168:497, 1989.
23. Hoffbrand, A. V., and Pettit, J. E.: Essential Haematology. London, Blackwell Scientific Publications, 1980.
24. Jandl, J. H.: Blood: Textbook of Hematology. Boston, Little, Brown & Co., 1987.
25. Jones, S. E.: Importance of staging Hodgkin's disease. Semin. Oncol., 7:126, 1980.
26. Kinsella, T. J., and Glatstein, E.: Staging laparotomy and splenectomy for Hodgkin's disease: Current status. Cancer Invest., 1:87, 1983.

27. Koller, C. A.: Immune thrombocytopenic purpura. Med. Clin. North Am., *64*:761, 1980.
28. Kudsk, K. A., Tranbaugh, R. F., and Sheldon, G. F.: Acute surgical illness in patients with sickle cell anemia. Am. J. Surg., *142*:113, 1981.
29. Lange, D. A., Zaret, P., Merlotti, G. J., Robin, A. P., Sheaff, C., and Barrett, J. A.: The use of absorbable mesh in splenic trauma. J. Trauma., *28*:269, 1988.
30. Laszlo, J., Jones, R., Silberman, H. R., and Banks, P. M.: Splenectomy for Felty's syndrome: Clinicopathological study of 27 patients. Arch. Intern. Med., *138*:597, 1978.
31. Leonard, A. S., Giebink, G. S., Baesl, T. J., and Krivit, W.: The overwhelming postsplenectomy sepsis problem. World J. Surg., *4*:423, 1980.
32. McMillan, R.: Chronic idiopathic thrombocytopenic purpura. N. Engl. J. Med., *304*:1135, 1981.
33. Medical Research Council's Working Party for Therapeutic Trials in Leukaemia: Randomized trial of splenectomy in Ph1-positive chronic granulocytic leukaemia, including an analysis of prognostic features. Br. J. Haematol., *54*:415, 1983.
34. Morgenstern, L.: Salvaging the spleen. Contemp. Surg., *23*:27, 1983.
35. Morgenstern, L., and Uyeda, R. Y.: Nonoperative management of injuries of the spleen in adults. Surg. Gynecol. Obstet., *157*:513, 1983.
36. Morgenstern, L.: The surgical inviolability of the spleen: Historical evolution of a concept. London, Wellcome Institute of the History of Medicine, 1974, p. 62.
37. Musser, G., Lazar, G., Hocking, W., and Busuttil, R. W.: Splenectomy for hematologic disease: The UCLA experience with 306 patients. Ann. Surg., *200*:40, 1984.
38. Pearl, R. H., Wesson, D. E., Spence, L. J., Filler, R. M., Ein, S. H., Shandling, B., and Superina, R. A.: Splenic injury: A 5-year update with improved results and changing criteria for conservative management. J. Pediatr. Surg., *24*:428, 1989.
39. Pearson, H. A., Johnston, D., Smith, K. A., and Touloukian, R. J.: The born-again spleen: Return of splenic function after splenectomy for trauma. N. Engl. J. Med., *298*:1389, 1978.
40. Rosenberg, S. A.: Exploratory laparotomy and splenectomy for Hodgkin's disease: A commentary. J. Clin. Oncol., 6:574, 1988.
41. Salgia, R., Skarin, A. T., Kraus, M. D., and Osteen, R. T.: The Spleen: An Oncopathologic Approach. Contemp. Surg., *45*:197, 1994.
42. Schwartz, S. I., Adams, J. T., and Bauman, A. W.: Splenectomy for Hematologic Disorders. Chicago, Year Book Medical Publishers, 1971.
43. Schwartz, S. I., Hoepp, L. M., and Sachs, S.: Splenectomy for thrombocytopenia. Surgery, *88*:497, 1980.
44. Schwartz, S. I.: Progress Symposium—Diseases affecting the spleen. World J. Surg., *9*:377, 1985.
45. Sherman, R.: Perspectives in management of trauma to the spleen: 1979 Presidential Address, American Association for the Surgery of Trauma. J. Trauma., *20*:1, 1980.
46. Sterchi, J. M., Buss, D. H., and Beyer, F. C.: The risk of improperly staging Hodgkin's disease with partial splenectomy. Am. Surg., *50*:20, 1984.
47. Stillman, R. J., Schiff, I., and Schinfeld, J.: Reproductive and gonadal function in the female after therapy for childhood malignancy. Obstet. Gynecol. Survey, 37:385, 1982.
48. Traetow, W. D., Fabri, P. J., and Carey, L. C.: Changing indications for splenectomy. Arch. Surg., *115*:447, 1980.
49. Traub, A. C., and Perry, J. F., Jr.: Injuries associated with splenic trauma. J. Trauma., *21*:840, 1981.
50. Traub, A., Giebink, G. S., Smith, C., Kuni, C. C., Brekke, M. L., Edlund, D., and Perry, J. F.: Splenic reticuloendothelial function after splenectomy, spleen repair, and spleen autotransplantation. N. Engl. J. Med., *317*:1559, 1987.
51. Weiss, L.: Cell and Tissue Biology: A Textbook of Histology, 6th ed. Baltimore, Urban & Schwarzenberg, 1988.
52. Wilhelm, M. C., Jones, R. E., McGeheek, R., Mitchener, J. S., Sandusky, W. R., and Hess, C. E.: Splenectomy in hematologic disorders: The ever-changing indications. Ann. Surg., *207*:581, 1988.
53. Wintrobe, M. M.: Clinical Hematology, 9th Ed. Philadelphia, Lea & Febiger, 1990.
54. Woerner, S. J., Abildgaard, C. F., and French, B. N.: Intracranial hemorrhage in children with idiopathic thrombocytopenic purpura. Pediatrics, *67*:453, 1981.

CHAPTER 37

HERNIAS

Steve Eubanks, M.D.

The surgical management of the groin hernia has undergone extensive reevaluation with renewed emphasis during the past five years. The rejuvenation of the surgeon's interest related to herniorrhaphy is partially attributable to the controversy regarding the application of laparoscopic techniques to this disease entity. Alterations in health care economics have also contributed to the renewed scrutiny with which the surgical treatment of hernia is viewed. The introduction of new techniques for the repair of hernia has highlighted the necessity for the surgeon to obtain a thorough understanding of the anatomy and pathophysiology of the hernia regardless of the repair technique applied.

A hernia is the abnormal protrusion of a peritoneal-lined sac through the musculoaponeurotic covering of the abdomen. The word *hernia* is a Latin term that means rupture of a portion of a structure.[1] Weakness of the abdominal wall, congenital or acquired in origin, results in the inability to contain the visceral contents of the abdominal cavity within their normal confines.

ANATOMIC CONSIDERATIONS

No disease of the human body, belonging to the province of the surgeon, requires in its treatment, a better combination of accurate, anatomical knowledge with surgical skill than Hernia in all its varieties.

Sir Astley Paston Cooper, 1804

The complex anatomy of the inguinal region is often poorly understood by students of surgery. The anatomy of the groin is frequently taught by describing layers of the abdominal wall, as are other regions of the human anatomy (Table 37–1). However, the inguinal region must be understood with regard to its three-dimensional configuration and relations. A knowledge of the convergence of tissue planes is essential for the surgical cure of hernia.[1]

The option of repairing a groin hernia laparoscopically mandates a knowledge of the inguinal region from the peritoneal surface outward. The significant structures are consistently present and reliably arrayed. Variability in anatomy is found with regard to the size and location of the hernia, degree of adiposity, and distortion from previous operations. The laparoscopic approach uses the concept of a frame on which the reinforcing mesh is placed. The laparoscopic surgeon should be able to consistently locate and demonstrate Cooper's ligament, the transversus abdominis aponeurotic arch, and the iliopubic tract. These structures serve as the borders of the frame. The deep inguinal ring, ductus deferens, spermatic vessels, and external iliac vessels are important anatomic landmarks that are frequently seen through the peritoneum. Although they are rarely visualized, the surgeon must also be aware of the precise location of the femoral nerve, genitofemoral nerve, and lateral femoral cutaneous nerves to minimize the risk of nerve entrapment syndromes (Fig. 37–1).

The inguinofemoral region is lined by the peritoneum. The preperitoneal space is a potential optical cavity that can be easily established by balloon dissection. The preperitoneal tissues are bound by the peritoneum and the transversalis fascia. The preperitoneal space contains adipose tissue, blood vessels, the ductus deferens, and nerves. The major vessels in the inguinofemoral region are the external iliac artery and vein, which pass under the iliopubic tract through the femoral canal. The inferior epigastric artery and deep circumflex iliac artery are major branches of the external iliac artery. The external iliac vein lies medial and slightly posterior to the external iliac artery and receives branches that parallel the arterial vessels. The inferior epigastric veins are usually two in number, running on either side of the artery (Fig. 37–2).[2]

The pubic arterial branch of the external iliac artery courses medially from the femoral canal and then gives off an inferior-directed branch, the obturator artery, across Cooper's ligament and continues medially as the arteria corona mortis on the cephalad surface of Cooper's ligament.

Several structures in the inguinal region merit individual description and comment. These structures are discussed below.

Inguinal Canal

The adult inguinal canal is approximately 4 cm. in length and is located 2 to 4 cm. cephalad to the inguinal ligament. A canal extends between the internal (deep inguinal) ring and the external (superficial inguinal) ring opening. The inguinal canal contains either the spermatic cord or the round ligament of the uterus.[3] The inguinal canal must be understood in the context of its three-dimensional anatomy. The canal courses from lateral to medial, deep to superficial, and cephalad to caudad. The inguinal canal is bounded superficially by the external oblique aponeurosis. The cephalad wall is composed of internal oblique muscle, transversus abdominis muscle, and the aponeuroses of these muscles. The inferior wall of the inguinal canal is formed by the inguinal ligament and lacunar ligament. The posterior wall (floor) of the inguinal canal is formed by the transversalis fascia and the aponeurosis of the transversus abdominis muscle. The

TABLE 37–1. Layers of the Abdominal Wall at the Level of the Inguinal Canal

Skin
Subcutaneous tissue
  Camper's fascia
  Scarpa's fascia
External oblique fascia
Cremasteric muscle fibers
Spermatic cord structures
Cremasteric muscle fibers
Transversus abdominis aponeurosis
Transversalis fascia
Preperitoneal tissues (fat, vessels, nerves,
  lymphatics, ductus deferens)
Peritoneum

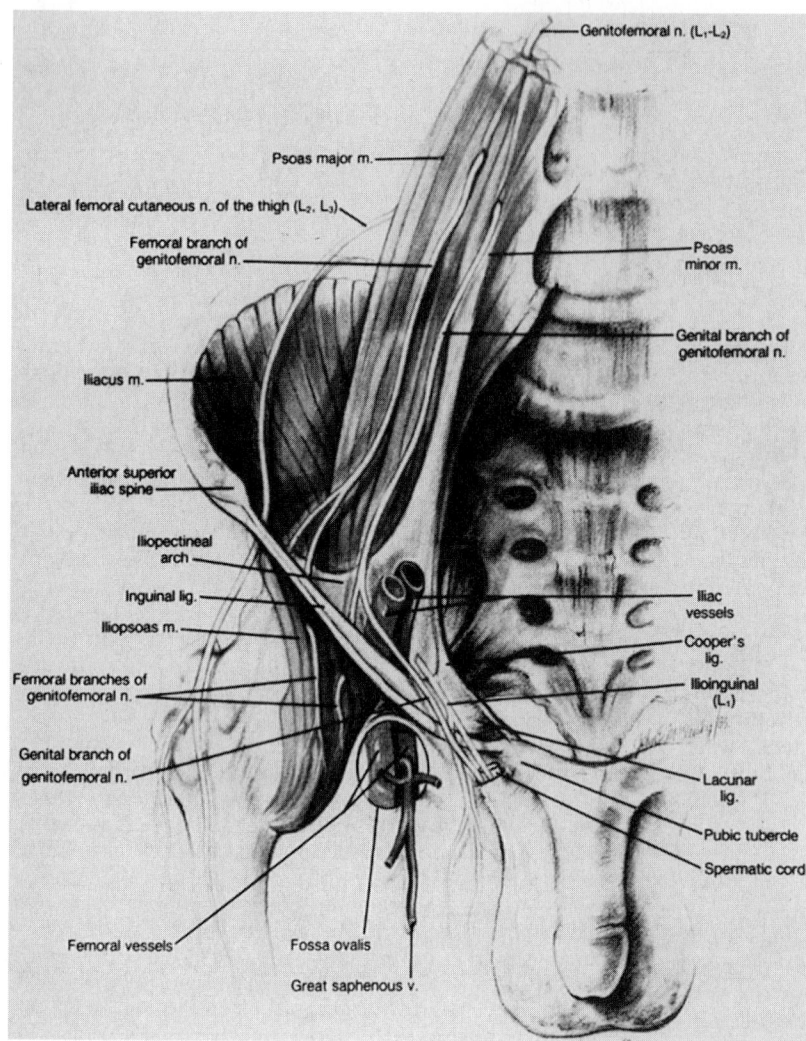

Figure 37–1. The neuroanatomy of the ilioinguinal region (the iliohypogastric nerve is not shown). (From Gray, S. W., Skandalakis, J. E., and McClusky, D. A.: Atlas of Surgical Anatomy for General Surgeons. Baltimore, Williams & Wilkins, 1985.)

floor of the inguinal canal is the most important structure of the inguinal canal from an anatomic and surgical standpoint.

The inferior epigastric vessels serve as the superolateral border of *Hesselbach's triangle*. The medial border of the triangle is formed by the rectus sheath, and the inguinal ligament serves as its inferior border. Hernias occurring within Hesselbach's triangle are considered direct hernias, whereas hernias occurring lateral to the triangle are indirect hernias. The original description of Hesselbach's triangle defined the inferior border as Cooper's ligament.[4] The borders were subsequently modified, substituting the inguinal ligament for Cooper's ligament, to allow an easier identification of the area by surgeons who use the traditional anterior approach for herniorrhaphy (Fig. 37–3).[5]

External Oblique Aponeurosis

The aponeurosis of the external oblique muscle is formed by two layers, a superficial and a deep layer. Together with the bilaminar aponeurosis[6] of the internal oblique and transversus abdominis, they form the rectus sheath and, finally, the linea alba by linear decussation.[3] The external oblique aponeurosis serves as the superficial border of the inguinal canal and reflects posteriorly in a curvilinear fashion to form the inguinal ligament. The inguinal ligament extends from the anterior superior iliac spine to the pubic tubercle.

Internal Oblique Muscle

The internal oblique muscle serves as the cephalad (or superior) border of the inguinal canal. The medial aspect of the internal oblique aponeurosis fuses with the fibers from the aponeurosis of the transversus abdominis near the pubic tubercle to form the conjoined tendon. The incidence of a true conjoined tendon has been debated but is thought by most surgeons to occur in less than 10% of patients.

Transversalis Fascia

The transversalis fascia is considered to be the downward continuation of the transversalis muscle and its aponeurosis. The transversalis fascia was described by Cooper[7] as having two layers: "The fascia transversalis may be divided into two portions, the one being placed a little before the other . . . the inner portion is thinner than the former; . . . it rises to the tendon of the transversalis muscle on the inner side of the spermatic cord and is firmly attached to the linea semilunaris. It appears that the internal ring is not a circumscribed aperture like the external abdominal ring but is formed by the separation of two portions."[8]

The transversus abdominis muscle arises from the lateral portion of the iliopubic tract, the iliac crest, the lumbodorsal fascia, and the inner surface of the cartilage of the lower six ribs. The lower free margin of this muscle arches with the

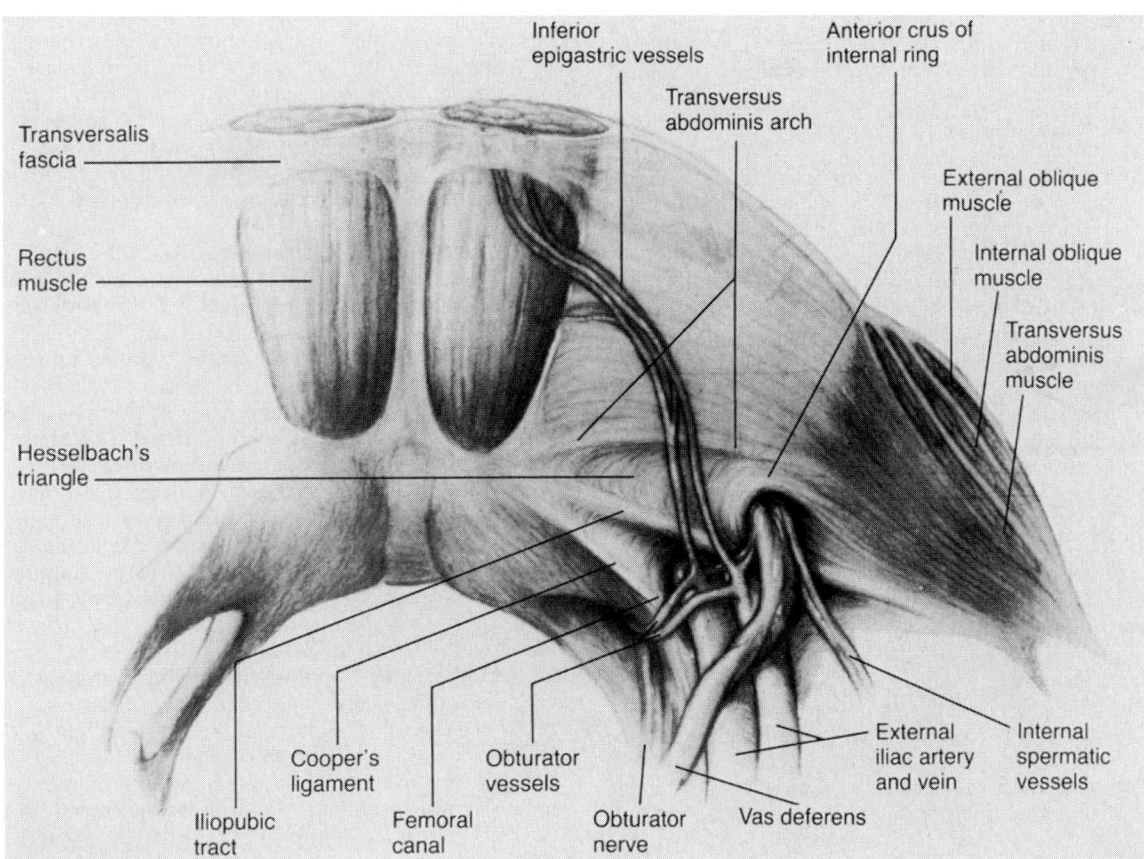

Figure 37–2. The preperitoneal inguinal anatomy (peritoneum and preperitoneal fat removed). (From Madden, J. L.: Abdominal Wall Hernias: An Atlas of Anatomy and Repair. Philadelphia, W. B. Saunders, 1989.)

Figure 37–3. Hesselbach's triangle as originally described (left) and as accepted today (right). (From Skandalakis, P. N., Skandalakis, L. J., Gray, S. W., and Skandalakis, J. E.: Supravesical hernia. In Nyhus, L. M., and Condon, R. E. [Eds.]: Hernia, 4th ed. Philadelphia, J. B. Lippincott, 1995.)

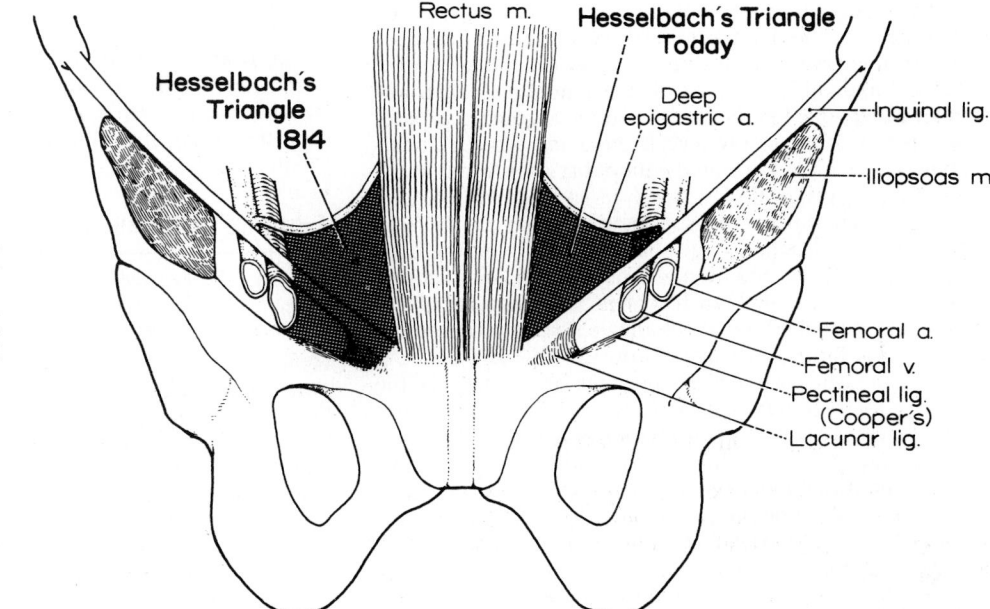

internal oblique muscle over the internal inguinal ring to form the *transversus abdominis aponeurotic arch.* The transversus aponeurosis usually joins the internal oblique at the rectus sheath. However, in approximately 5% to 10% of cases, the transversus abdominis aponeurotic arch fuses with the internal oblique aponeurosis to form the conjoined tendon.

Iliopubic Tract

The iliopubic tract is a fibrous condensation of endoabdominal fascia that arises from the iliopectineal arch and inserts on the anterior superior iliac spine and inner lip of the wing of the ilium. The iliopubic tract is located posterior to the inguinal ligament. This structure arches over the femoral vessels, composing a portion of the femoral sheath. The iliopubic tract is located at the inferior border of the internal (deep) inguinal ring. The medial insertion is along the superior border of the pubic ramus and pubic tubercle and Cooper's ligament.

The iliopubic tract is an extremely important structure in the repair of femoral hernias and in the preperitoneal repair (open and laparoscopic) of inguinal hernias. The lateral iliopubic tract (lateral to the internal inguinal ring) serves as the inferior border below which staples should not be placed during a laparoscopic inguinal hernia repair. The lateral femoral cutaneous and genitofemoral nerves are located inferior to the lateral iliopubic tract.

Cooper's Ligament

Cooper's ligament is located on the posterior aspect of the superior ramus of the pubis and is formed of periosteum and fascial condensations. Cooper's ligament is extremely important in laparoscopic hernia repair as well as McVay's repair.

Preperitoneal Space

The preperitoneal space contains adipose tissue, lymphatics, blood vessels, and nerves. The nerves of specific concern to the hernia surgeon include the lateral femoral cutaneous nerve and the genitofemoral nerve. The lateral femoral cutaneous nerve originates as a root of L2 and L3 and is occasionally a branch of the main femoral nerve. The nerve courses along the anterior surface of the iliac muscle and under the iliac fascia and under or through the lateral attachment of the inguinal ligament at the anterior superior spine. A laparoscopic view of the anatomy reveals the nerve passing underneath or occasionally through the iliopubic tract lateral to the internal inguinal ring.[9]

The genitofemoral nerve usually arises from L2, or from L1 and L2, or occasionally from L3. It descends on the front of the psoas muscle and divides into genital and femoral branches. The genital branch enters the inguinal canal through the deep ring, whereas the femoral branch enters the femoral sheath lateral to the artery.[10] Vessels traversing this preperitoneal space include the external iliac vessels, the inferior epigastric artery and veins, the obturator artery, and the arteria corona mortis. The inferior epigastric artery and veins are frequently seen through the peritoneum and serve as important landmarks for the laparoscopic surgeon.

The ductus deferens courses through the preperitoneal space from caudad to cephalad and medial to lateral to enter the deep inguinal ring.

Adipose tissue, containing lymphatics, is found in the preperitoneal space, and the quantity of adipose tissue is highly variable. Cloquet's lymph node is consistently present at the level of the abdominal wall along the medial aspect of the femoral canal.

DIAGNOSIS, CLASSIFICATION, AND INCIDENCE

A patient with a groin hernia usually presents with the complaint of a bulge in the inguinal region. The patient may describe minor pain or vague discomfort associated with the groin bulge. Extreme pain related to a hernia in the absence of incarceration and intestinal vascular compromise is unusual and should raise the surgeon's suspicion of another etiology of the pain. Occasionally, patients present with paresthesias related to irritation or compression of inguinal nerves by the hernia.

Masses other than hernias can occur in the inguinal region. The differentiation of the groin hernia from these other entities can usually be accomplished by the physical examination. Once hernia has been excluded, the determination of the nature of other groin masses may involve a more extensive evaluation (Table 37–2).

The inguinal area is examined with the patient standing and facing the physician, who is sitting on a chair or stool. Visual inspection of the groin frequently reveals a loss of symmetry in the inguinal area or a discrete bulge. Having the patient perform Valsalva's maneuver or cough may accentuate the bulge, making it clearly visible. Fingertips are then placed on the abdominal wall over the inguinal region, and the patient is asked to repeat Valsalva's maneuver. A fingertip is then placed in the inguinal canal, and Valsalva's maneuver is repeated. A bulge that progresses from a lateral to medial direction against the fingertip is most consistent with an indirect hernia. A bulge that progresses against the finger from deep to superficial through the floor of the canal is most consistent with a direct inguinal hernia. Differentiation between indirect and direct hernias at the time of examination is not essential, because both types can be repaired through the same approach. A bulge below the inguinal ligament is consistent with a femoral hernia and should be differentiated from an inguinal hernia at the time of examination. The patient is then examined in the supine position, repeating the steps used during the standing examination. A groin mass described by the patient but not demonstrated on examination may become palpable or visible after having the patient ambulate or stand for a period of time. Infrequently, it is necessary to have the patient return at a later time so that the groin can be re-examined.

An incarcerated hernia can be reduced manually in many instances. Gentle pressure on the hernial mass toward the inguinal ring, usually with the patient in the head-lowered (Trendelenburg's) position, is generally effective. If the mass

---

TABLE 37–2. Differential Diagnosis of Groin Masses

Inguinal hernia
Femoral hernia
Inguinal adenitis
Ectopic testes
Lipoma
Varicocele
Hematoma
Psoas abscess
Femoral adenitis
Hydrocele
Lymphoma
Tuberculosis
Metastatic neoplasm
Epididymitis
Testicular torsion
Femoral aneurysm or pseudoaneurysm
Sebaceous cyst
Hidradenitis of inguinal apocrine glands

is tender and the pressure causes pain, appropriate analgesic agents can be administered to relieve the discomfort while the procedure is repeated.[11] Gangrenous bowel can rarely be reduced by this method, and suspected patients should be followed for the development of peritoneal signs. Reduction *en masse*, or reduction of the entire hernia sac with the intestine remaining incarcerated within the sac, is also an unusual but reported occurrence. Any attempt to reduce an incarcerated hernia should be abandoned prior to traumatizing the incarcerated viscera. The inability to manually reduce an incarcerated hernia necessitates immediate operation.

Numerous classification systems for groin hernias exist. Their purpose is to provide a common language for physician communications and to allow appropriate comparisons of therapeutic options. A simple and widely used classification system of groin hernias is the Nyhus classification (Table 37–3). It allows consistent descriptions of groin hernias and can serve as a guide for the selection of technical approaches.

Approximately 700,000 inguinal herniorrhaphies are performed as outpatient procedures each year.[12] According to data from the National Center for Health Statistics, the five most common major surgical operations performed by general surgeons in 1991 were groin hernia (680,000), cholecystectomy (571,000), lysis of peritoneal adhesions (339,000), appendectomy (255,000), and partial excision of large intestine (220,000).[13]

Approximately 75% of all hernias occur in the inguinal region. Approximately 50% of hernias are indirect inguinal hernias, and 24% are direct inguinal hernias. Incisional and ventral hernias account for approximately 10% of all hernias, and femoral hernias for 3%; unusual hernias account for the remaining 5% to 10%. The vast majority of hernias occur in males. The most common hernia in males and females is the indirect inguinal hernia. Femoral hernias occur much more frequently in females than in males. Twenty-five percent of males and only 2% of females will develop inguinal hernias in their lifetimes. Hernias occur more commonly on the right side than the left.

CAUSES OF GROIN HERNIA

The factors leading to the development of a hernia are traditionally divided into two categories: congenital origins and acquired defects. Congenital factors are responsible for the majority of groin hernias.

The lack of obliteration of the processus vaginalis is the primary factor leading to the development of an indirect inguinal hernia. Prematurity and low birth weight are docu-

mented as significant risk factors. Congenital abnormalities, such as pelvic deformities or exstrophy of the urinary bladder, can cause abnormalities of the inguinal canal, leading to indirect inguinal hernia formation. In rare cases, congenital deformities or collagen deficiencies may cause the development of direct inguinal hernias.

Direct hernias are attributed to the wear-and-tear stresses of life. Straining to urinate or defecate, coughing, and heavy lifting have been implicated as causative factors, leading to trauma and weakening of the inguinal floor.

Several biologic and intracellular factors are closely associated with hernia formation. A decrease in the content of hydroxyproline, the major amino acid component of collagen, in the aponeurosis of patients with groin hernias has been demonstrated. Abnormal proliferation of fibroblasts cultured from the anterior rectus sheath of patients with groin hernias has also been shown. Additionally, the ultrastructure of rectus sheath collagen contains irregular microfibril in patients with direct hernias.[14] Read extracted rectus sheath collagen and demonstrated an altered capacity for precipitation and a reduced hydroxyproline ratio, suggesting impaired hydroxylation and lysyl oxidase activity. Synthesis of hydroxyproline, and therefore collagen, was shown to be inhibited.[15]

An association between cigarette smoking and groin hernias has been demonstrated.[15] Through the use of a fibrinopeptide cleavage product of fibrinogen, evidence of free, active, unbound neutrophil elastase activity has been detected in the plasma of cigarette smokers.[16] Levels of circulating serum elastolytic activity have been shown to be significantly greater than normal in patients with direct herniation who smoke.[17] Groin hernias have been demonstrated to occur more frequently in smokers than in nonsmokers, especially women.[18]

The multifactorial process of wound healing provides many clues to the etiology of groin hernia. It is suspected, but not proved, that malnutrition and vitamin deficiency lead to the weakening of strength layers and decreased collagen content, which may lead to hernia formation. Advanced age and chronic illness are risk factors associated with the development of hernias. Strenuous physical activity and athletics have also been proposed as chronic stresses that can lead to hernia formation. Herniography has been used to demonstrate clinically occult hernias in athletes who present with groin pain.[19]

SURGICAL MANAGEMENT OF INGUINAL HERNIAS

I know more than a hundred surgeons whom I would cheerfully allow to remove my gallbladder but only one to whom I should like to expose my inguinal canal.

Sir Henage Ogilvie

Surgical repair of a groin hernia can be simple, but in some cases, the distortion and attenuation of normal anatomy provide an extreme technical challenge. Approximately 100,000 recurrent hernias present each year, suggesting the need for technical precision, an awareness of the potential for progressive weakening of tissues, and the need for a broad individual experience by surgeons.

Inguinal hernias should be surgically repaired following diagnosis by physical examination. Rarely, extenuating circumstances cause a physician to advise against surgical repair. A terminally ill, immunosuppressed, or extremely old patient may fall into the category of those who should be followed without operative correction. The natural history of groin hernia is one of progressive enlargement and weaken-

---

TABLE 37–3. Nyhus Classification of Groin Hernia

Type I: Indirect inguinal hernia—internal inguinal ring normal (e.g., pediatric hernia)

Type II: Indirect inguinal hernia—internal inguinal ring dilated but posterior inguinal wall intact; inferior deep epigastric vessels not displaced

Type III: Posterior wall defect
  A. Direct inguinal hernia
  B. Indirect inguinal hernia—internal inguinal ring dilated, medially encroaching on or destroying the transversalis fascia of Hesselbach's triangle (e.g., massive scrotal, sliding, or pantaloon hernia)
  C. Femoral hernia

Type IV: Recurrent hernia
  A. Direct
  B. Indirect
  C. Femoral
  D. Combined

ing, with the potential for incarceration and obstruction of the intestine and subsequent compromise of the vascular supply to the bowel (strangulation), leading to intestinal infarction. Hernias do not resolve spontaneously or improve with time. Wearing a truss does not cure a hernia. Repair of a groin hernia can be planned electively unless incarceration or strangulation is present.

Open hernia repair is begun with a curvilinear incision approximately two finger breadths above the inguinal ligament. The curve of the incision should follow Langer's lines. Dissection is carried through the subcutaneous tissues, and the external oblique fascia is incised. Care should be taken to avoid injuring the ilioinguinal and iliohypogastric nerves, which provide cutaneous innervation of the skin of the lower abdomen, penis, and scrotum. The spermatic cord is mobilized by placing a finger around the cord structures at the level of the pubic tubercle. Mobilization of the spermatic cord lateral to the pubic tubercle can cause improper identification of tissue planes and result in disruption of the floor of the inguinal canal, with damage to the transversalis fascia.

The cremasteric muscle fibers of the mobilized cord are divided and separated from the underlying cord structures. The hernia sac is carefully dissected free from the adjacent cord structures and cleared to the level of the internal inguinal ring. The hernia sac is opened and examined for visceral contents. The neck of the sac is suture-ligated at the level of the internal ring, and excess sac is excised. The options for reconstruction of the inguinal floor are numerous, and several of the more popular approaches are described.

Bassini Repair

The Bassini procedure and its modifications are frequently used for indirect inguinal hernias and small direct hernias. The conjoined tendon of the transversus abdominis and the internal oblique muscles is sutured to the inguinal (Poupart's) ligament. The technique for this operation is demonstrated in Figure 37–4.

The classic Halsted-Ferguson operation differs little from the Bassini repair, with the exception of the management of

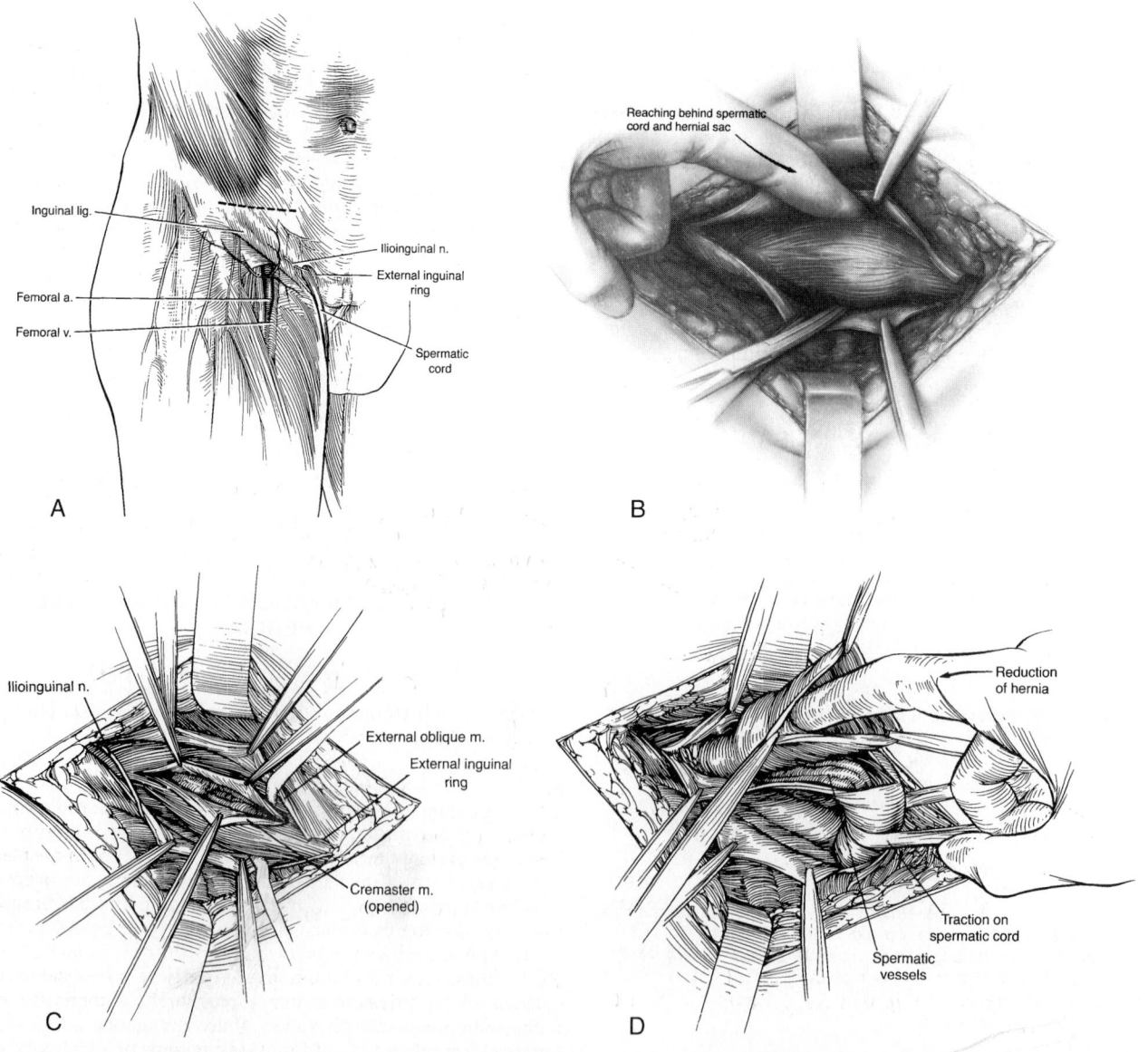

Figure 37–4. *A*, The Bassini repair is begun with an incision cephalad to the inguinal canal. *B*, The spermatic cord is mobilized at the level of the pubic tubercle after incising the skin, dermis, subcutaneous tissues, and external oblique fascia. *C*, The indirect hernia sac is identified by dissecting the cremaster muscle off the medial aspect of the spermatic cord structures. *D*, The hernia sac is carefully dissected free of the spermatic cord structures to the level of the abdominal wall. The sac is opened at its apex, and its contents are manually reduced.

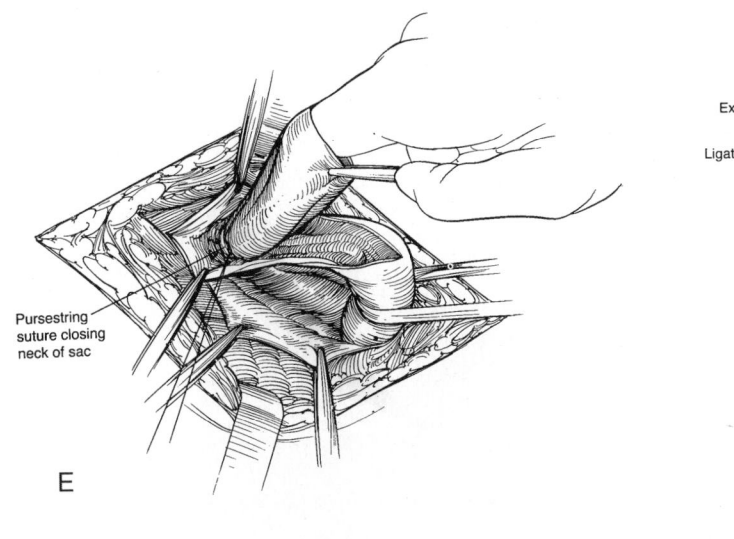

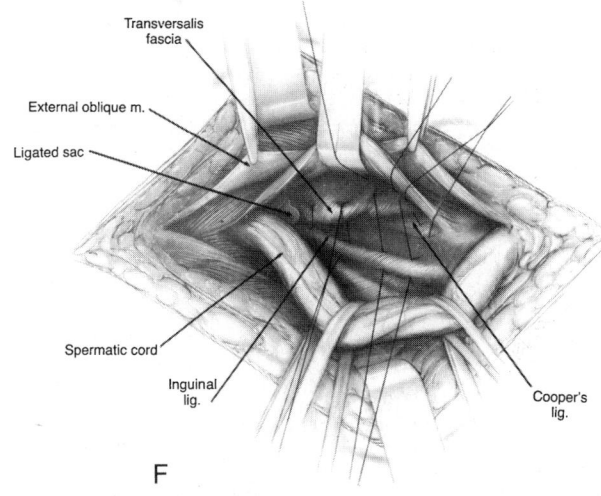

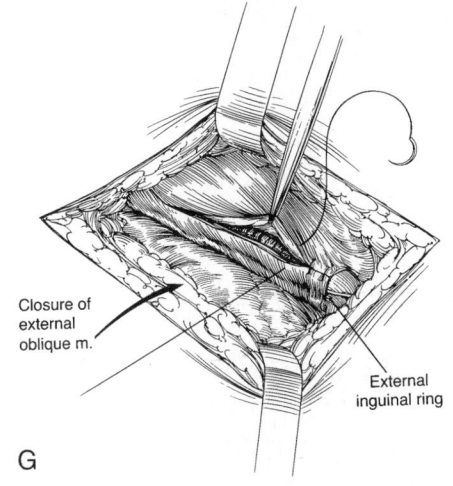

Figure 37–4 *Continued E,* The pursestring suture closure of the neck of the sac is performed at the level of the internal inguinal ring. The remaining distal sac is resected. *F,* Interrupted sutures are used to approximate the conjoined tendon and internal oblique muscular edge to the shelving edge of the inguinal ligament. The medial aspect of the floor is repaired by suturing the conjoined tendon or lateral edge of the rectus sheaths to Cooper's ligament. Following the repair of the floor of the inguinal canal, the spermatic cord is returned to its normal anatomic position and the external oblique fascia is approximated over the cord structures. *G,* Following the repair of the floor of the inguinal canal, the spermatic cord is returned to its normal anatomic position and the external oblique fascia is approximated over the cord structures. (From Moylan, J. A.: Inguinal herniorrhaphy: Bassini [inguinal ligament]. *In* Sabiston, D. C. [Ed.]: Atlas of General Surgery. Philadelphia, W. B. Saunders, 1994.)

the external oblique fascia. The aponeurosis of the external oblique is imbricated, with the medial flap overlapping the lateral flap. The Halsted I technique transplanted the spermatic cord external to the external oblique fascial closure. The Halsted II procedure returned the spermatic cord structures to their normal anatomic location.

McVay (Cooper's Ligament) Repair

The Cooper's ligament operation (McVay) is a popular repair for the correction of large inguinal hernias, direct inguinal hernias, recurrent hernias of the groin, and femoral hernias (Fig. 37–5). It is essential to clearly identify Cooper's ligament and the transversus abdominis aponeurotic arch. The conjoined tendon is sutured to Cooper's ligament from the pubic tubercle laterally to the femoral canal. The femoral canal must be narrowed when using this approach for the correction of a femoral hernia. The repair is continued at the level of the femoral canal by making a transition from Cooper's ligament anteriorly so that the conjoined tendon is sutured to the inguinal ligament beyond the femoral canal. The internal inguinal ring is recreated with adequate laxity to allow the passage of the tip of a Kelly clamp adjacent to the cord structures.

Shouldice (Canadian) Repair

The Shouldice (Canadian) repair emphasizes a multilayer, imbricated repair of the floor of the inguinal canal with running sutures (Fig. 37–6). The Shouldice approach encourages preoperative weight loss, the use of local anesthesia, and intraoperative testing of the repair by the patient's performance of Valsalva's maneuver. Shouldice repair proponents have reported very low recurrence rates with large series of patients.

Lichtenstein (Tension-Free) Repair

One of the most commonly performed open herniorrhaphy techniques is the tension-free (Lichtenstein) repair popularized by Irving L. Lichtenstein and colleagues (Fig. 37–7). Lichtenstein emphasized the lack of logic in repairing a hernia by placing together attenuated tissues under tension. Berliner proposed that "total absence of tension on the suture line is the *sine qua non* for the (hernia) repair."[20] Lichtenstein demonstrated that a tension-free hernioplasty performed with mesh reinforcement of the inguinal floor significantly decreases the recurrence rate.

The Lichtenstein repair is routinely performed in an outpatient setting with local anesthesia. A Marlex mesh patch is sutured to the aponeurotic tissue overlying the pubic bone, with continuation of this suture along the shelving edge of the inguinal (Poupart's) ligament to a point lateral to the internal inguinal ring. The lateral edge of the mesh is slit to allow passage of the spermatic cord between the split limbs of the mesh. The cephalad edge of the mesh is sutured to the

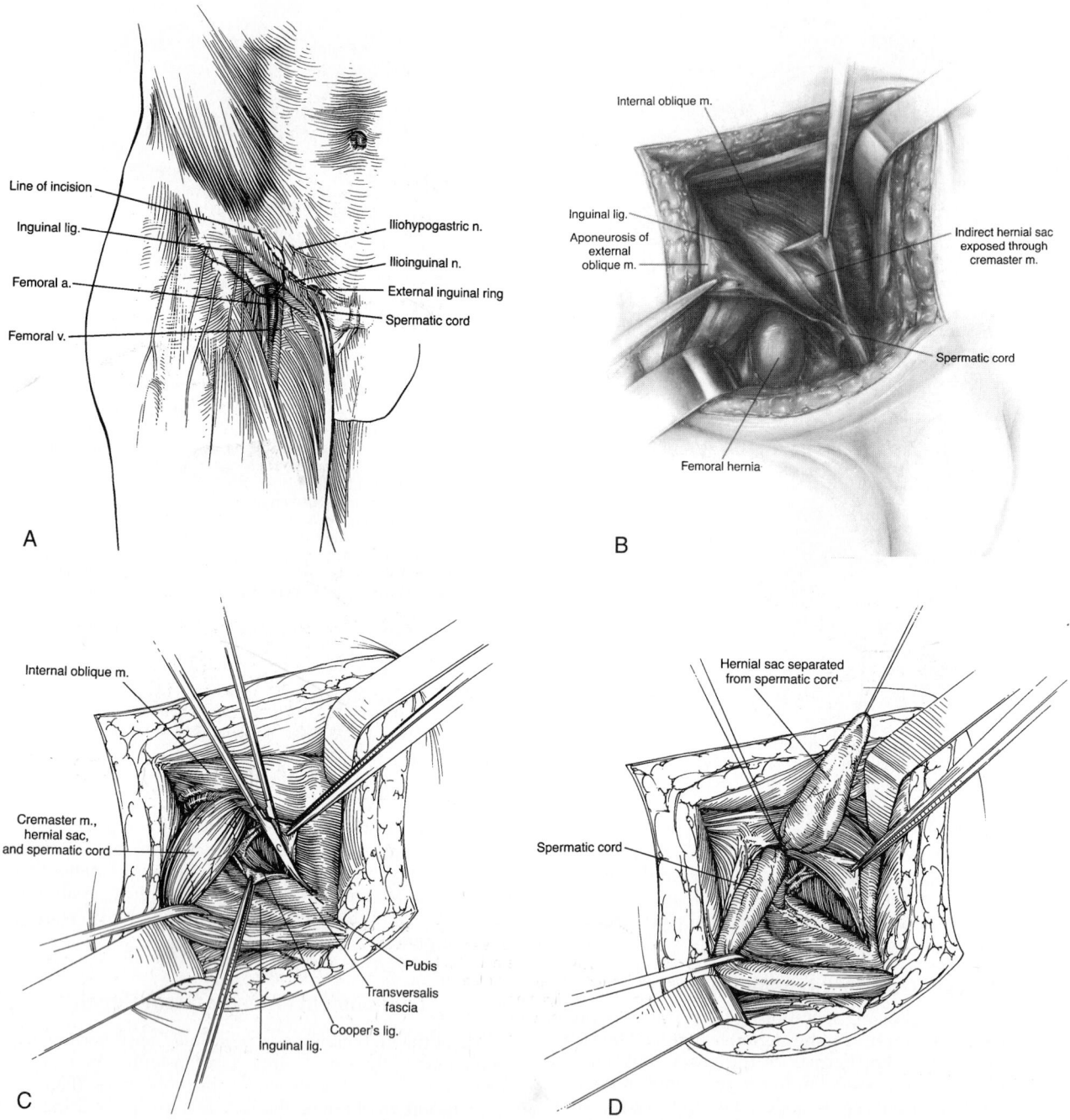

Figure 37–5. *A,* The McVay (Cooper's ligament) repair is initiated through a curvilinear incision placed cephalad to the inguinal ligament. *B,* The external oblique fascia is opened, exposing the cord structures covered with cremasteric muscle fibers. An incision in the cremasteric muscle on the medial surface demonstrates an underlying indirect inguinal hernia sac. A femoral hernia is demonstrated below the inguinal ligament. *C,* The posterior wall (transversalis fascia) of the inguinal canal is incised from the internal inguinal ring to the pubic tubercle. Cooper's ligament is dissected free of overlying tissue. *D,* The cremasteric muscle fibers overlying the spermatic cord are opened, and the indirect hernia sac is dissected to the level of the peritoneum. The sac is opened, its contents are reduced, and it is suture-ligated with a pursestring suture at the level of the peritoneum. The transversus abdominis aponeurotic arch is developed along the cephalad aspect of the wound, and the spermatic cord is retracted inferiorly.

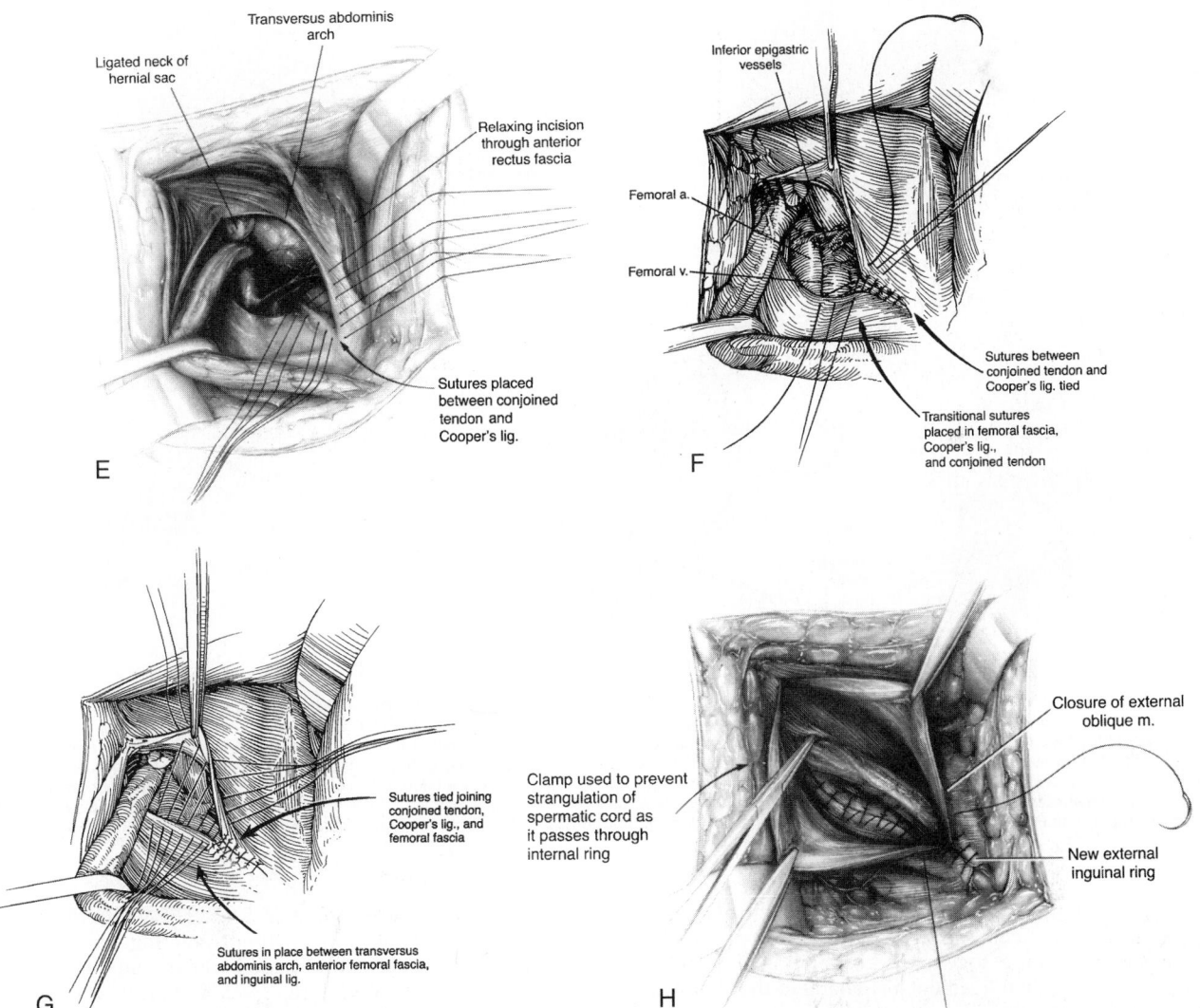

Figure 37–5 *Continued E,* The conjoined tendon and transversus abdominis aponeurotic arch are sutured to Cooper's ligament using interrupted permanent sutures. A relaxing incision through the anterior rectus fascia is made prior to tying the sutures. The sutures are carried laterally to the level of the medial aspect of the femoral vein. *F,* The femoral canal is reconstructed by placing interrupted sutures between the transversus abdominis aponeurotic arch and the anterior femoral fascia. The iliopubic tract may be incorporated into these sutures to provide strength for the closure. *G,* The repair is continued laterally by placing sutures between the transversus abdominis arch, the anterior femoral fascia, and the inguinal ligament, continuing laterally beyond any indirect sac so that the cord actually emerges obliquely laterally at the new inguinal ring. No sutures are placed lateral to the cord. *H,* The new inguinal ring admits only a Kelly clamp tip. Reinforcement with a layer of Marlex mesh may be necessary if the tissues are extremely weak or attenuated. The spermatic cord is returned to the inguinal canal and the external oblique aponeurosis is closed over the spermatic cord. (From Peete, W. P. J.: Inguinal herniorrhaphy: McVay [Cooper's ligament]. *In* Sabiston, D. C. [Ed.]: Atlas of General Surgery. Philadelphia, W. B. Saunders, 1994.)

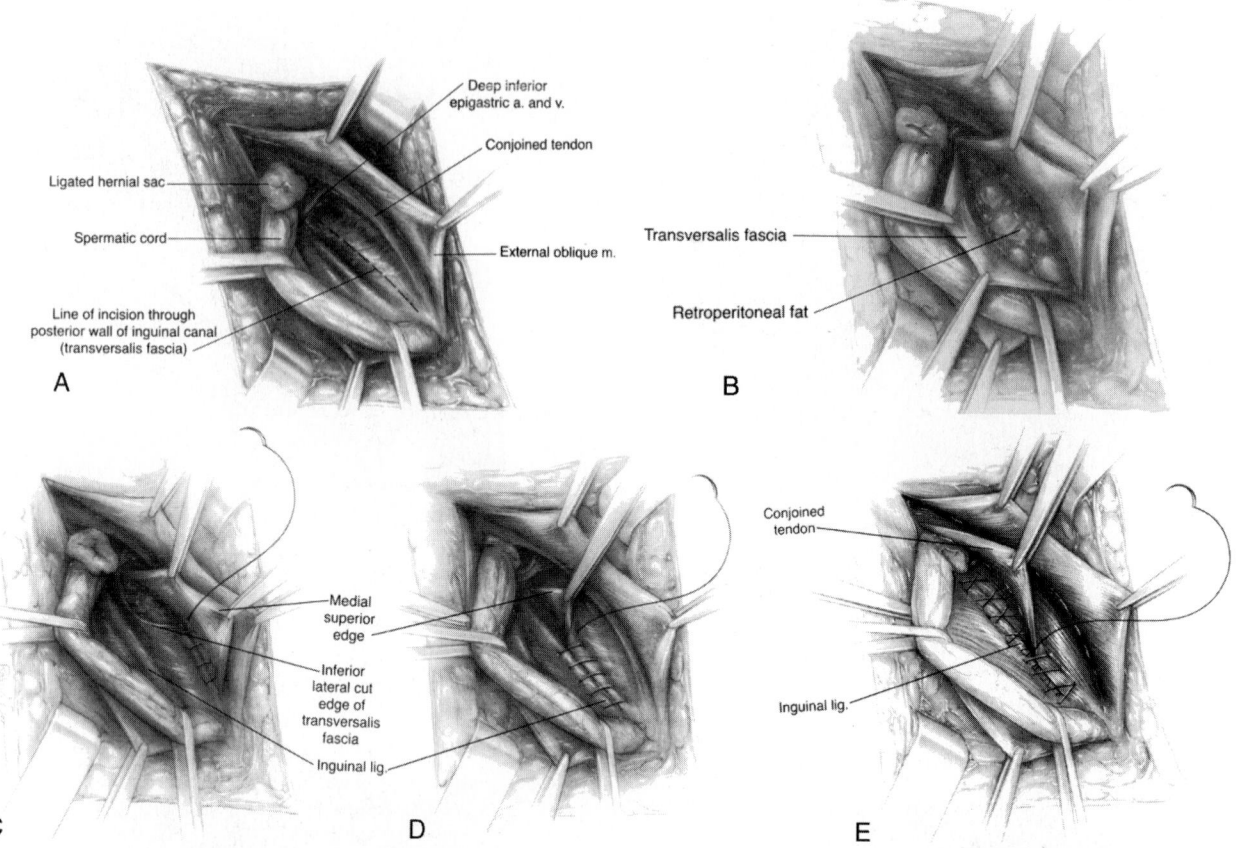

Figure 37–6. *A,* The Shouldice inguinal floor reconstruction is performed following spermatic cord dissection and high ligation of the indirect hernia sac. The transversalis fascia of the inguinal canal is incised from the internal inguinal ring to the level of the pubic tubercle. *B,* The inferior epigastric vessels may be divided if necessary to facilitate opening the internal inguinal ring. The preperitoneal fat is identified underneath the incised transversalis fascia. *C,* The lateral (or inferior) cut edge of the transversalis fascia is sutured medially to the undersurface of the internal oblique muscle. *D,* Imbrication of the tissue layers is continued by suturing the medial (or superior) cut edge of transversalis fascia to the inguinal ligament. *E,* The conjoined tendon is sutured to the inguinal ligament, thereby reinforcing the underlying imbricated tissue layers. The spermatic cord structures are returned to the inguinal canal, and the external oblique aponeurosis is closed over the spermatic cord. (From Peete, W. P. J.: Inguinal herniorrhaphy: Shouldice. *In* Sabiston, D. C. [Ed.]: Atlas of General Surgery. Philadelphia, W. B. Saunders, 1994.)

conjoined tendon, with the internal oblique edge overlapped by approximately 2 cm. The two tails of the lateral aspect of the mesh are sutured together, incorporating the shelving margin of the inguinal ligament just lateral to the completion knot of the lower suture.

Lichtenstein encouraged patients to resume activity rapidly. Excellent results have been achieved by those adopting Lichtenstein's technique. The Stoppa technique and the plug-and-patch technique are based on similar principles using prosthetic reinforcement without tension.

Laparoscopic Hernia Repair

The use of the laparoscope in the repair of groin hernias has added an exciting and highly controversial dimension to herniorrhaphy. The laparoscope allows the surgeon to visualize the hernia defect and surrounding anatomy with enhanced clarity and magnification. Early attempts at laparoscopic repair of inguinal hernias resulted in exceptionally high recurrence rates, but these early repairs were performed in a nonanatomic fashion.

The current popular techniques for laparoscopic hernia repair include the transabdominal preperitoneal (TAPP) repair and the totally extraperitoneal approach (TEPA). The actual hernia repair is similar in both these techniques. The main difference between TAPP and TEPA is the manner in which access to the preperitoneal space is achieved. TAPP uses intraperitoneal trocars and the creation of a peritoneal

flap over the posterior inguinal area. TEPA provides access to the preperitoneal space without entering the peritoneal cavity.[21] The skin incision is made in the periumbilical region, and dissection is carried to the level of the rectus sheath. The rectus sheath is entered, and a balloon dissector is placed along the anterior surface of the posterior rectus sheath and advanced to the level of the pubis. The balloon is then inflated, thereby creating an optical cavity in the preperitoneal space and allowing additional trocars to be placed in this cavity without traversing the peritoneum. The identical cavity may be created by blunt dissection, which is less costly but slower, more tedious, and less precise.

Laparoscopic hernia repair is based on the preperitoneal approach introduced by Cheatle,[22] Henry,[23] Nyhus,[24] Stoppa,[25] and Read.[26] The principles of the tension-free hernioplasty popularized by Lichtenstein are also incorporated into laparoscopic hernia repair. Publication of the results of cadaveric dissections enhanced the laparoscopic surgeon's understanding of the preperitoneal anatomy.[27] A prosthetic mesh is secured to the posterior inguinal wall to consistently present anatomic structures. Medial to the inferior epigastric vessels, the mesh is secured to Cooper's ligament, the lacunar ligament, the posterior rectus musculature, and the transversus abdominis aponeurotic arch. Laterally, the mesh is attached to the lateral extension of the transversus aponeurotic arch and the superior edge of the iliopubic tract.

Staples should not be placed below the lateral iliopubic tract because of potential injury to the genitofemoral nerve

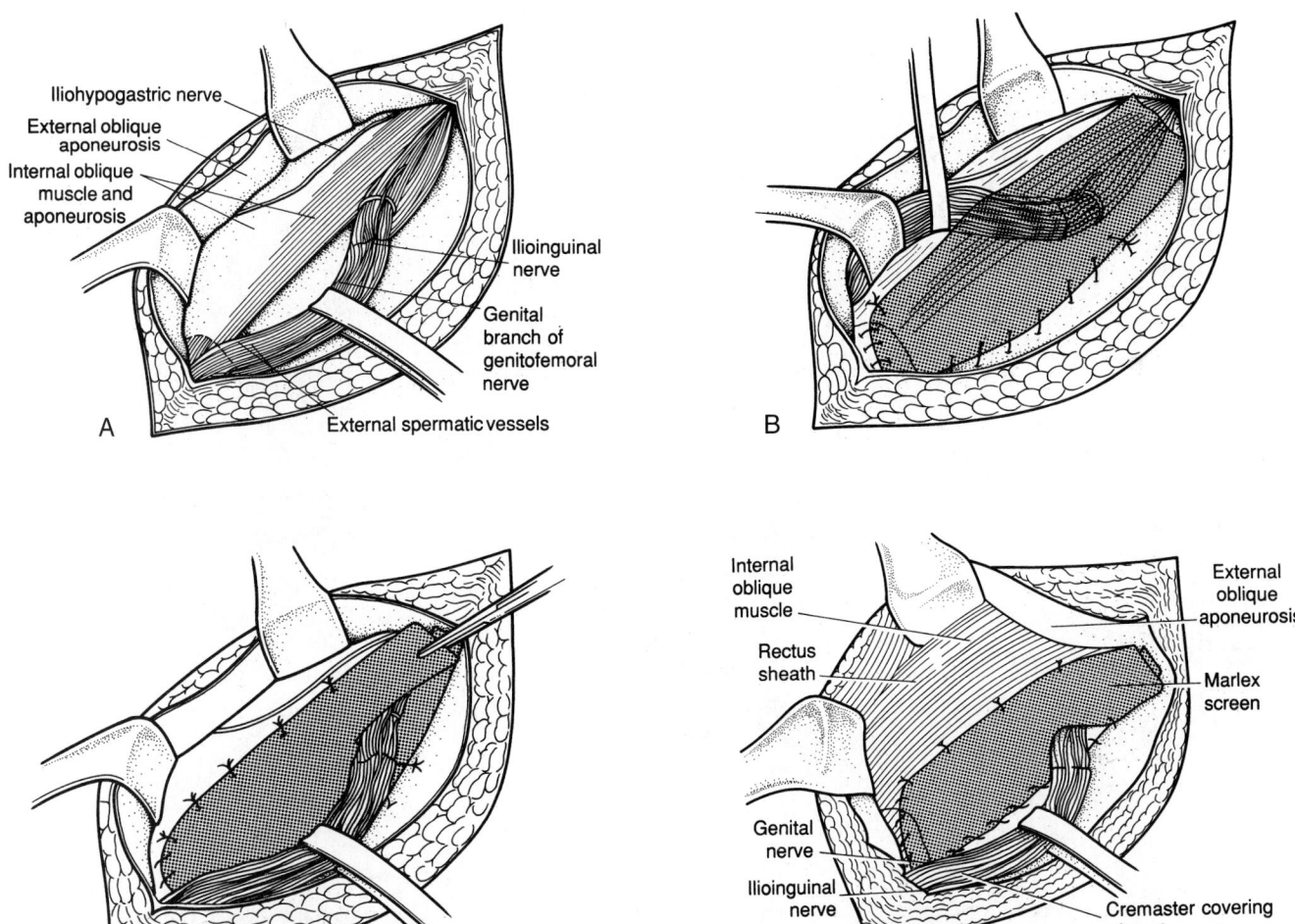

Figure 37–7. *A*, The Lichtenstein tension-free hernioplasty is performed by careful dissection of the inguinal canal. High ligation of an indirect hernia sac is performed, and the spermatic cord structures are retracted inferiorly. The external oblique aponeurosis is separated from the underlying internal oblique muscle high enough to accommodate a 6- to 8-cm.-wide mesh patch. Overlap of the internal oblique muscle edge by 2 to 3 cm. is necessary. An 8- by 16-cm. sheet of Marlex mesh is fashioned to fit the inguinal canal. A slit is made in the lateral aspect of the mesh, and the spermatic cord is placed between the two tails of the mesh. *B*, The spermatic cord is retracted in the cephalad direction. The medial aspect of the mesh overlaps the pubic bone by approximately 2 cm. The mesh is secured to the aponeurotic tissue overlying the pubic tubercle using a running suture of nonabsorbable monofilament material. The suture is continued laterally by suturing the inferior edge of the mesh to the shelving edge of the inguinal ligament to a point just lateral to the internal inguinal ring. *C*, A second monofilament suture is placed at the level of the pubic tubercle and continued laterally by suturing the mesh to the internal oblique aponeurosis or muscle approximately 2 cm. from the aponeurotic edge. *D*, The lower edges of the two tails are sutured to the shelving edge of the inguinal ligament to create a new internal ring made of mesh. The spermatic cord structures are placed within the inguinal canal overlying the mesh. The external oblique aponeurosis is closed over the spermatic cord. (Reproduced with permission from Arregui, M. E., and Nagan, R. F. [Eds.]: *Inguinal Hernia: Advances or Controversies?* Oxford, Radcliffe Medical Press, 1994.)

and the lateral femoral cutaneous nerve in this region. Stapling is also avoided in the triangular area inferior to the internal inguinal ring, called the *triangle of doom*. The triangle is bordered by the ductus deferens medially and the spermatic vessels laterally in the male. The apex of the triangle is at the level of the internal inguinal ring. Located between the ductus deferens and the spermatic vessel are the external iliac artery and vein and the femoral nerve. The obturator artery is located medial to the triangle of doom but should also be avoided when securing the mesh to Cooper's ligament. The techniques for the TAPP and TEPA repairs are illustrated in Figures 37–8 and 37–9.

Numerous modifications of the TAPP and TEPA techniques have been introduced. Most of these modifications are minor and relate primarily to the size or configuration of the mesh prosthesis. An innovative and increasingly popular modification that has been used primarily in recurrent hernias is the double-buttress laparoscopic herniorrhaphy.[28] The double-buttress technique is performed by placing in the groin a 10- by 6-cm. sheet of polypropylene mesh that has

been slit to surround the spermatic cord structures. After securing the initial piece of mesh with staples to the anatomic frame, a larger 15- by 15-cm. sheet of mesh is secured with staples overlying the initial prosthesis. This technique ensures adequate closure of the internal ring and complete coverage of the entire floor.[29]

The use of laparoscopic techniques for the repair of groin hernias has incited heated debate. Proponents of this technique emphasize the benefits of excellent visualization, minimal pain, rapid return to work and normal activities, small incisions that provide improved cosmesis and decreased wound infection complications, and potential cost savings secondary to decreased work loss. Payne and colleagues demonstrated, through a randomized prospective trial, the potential for laparoscopic herniorrhaphy patients to return to work and achieve baseline exercise capabilities more rapidly than patients undergoing conventional tension-free hernioplasties.[30] Numerous studies have demonstrated the benefits of laparoscopic herniorrhaphy over various conventional approaches in selected patients.[31–36]

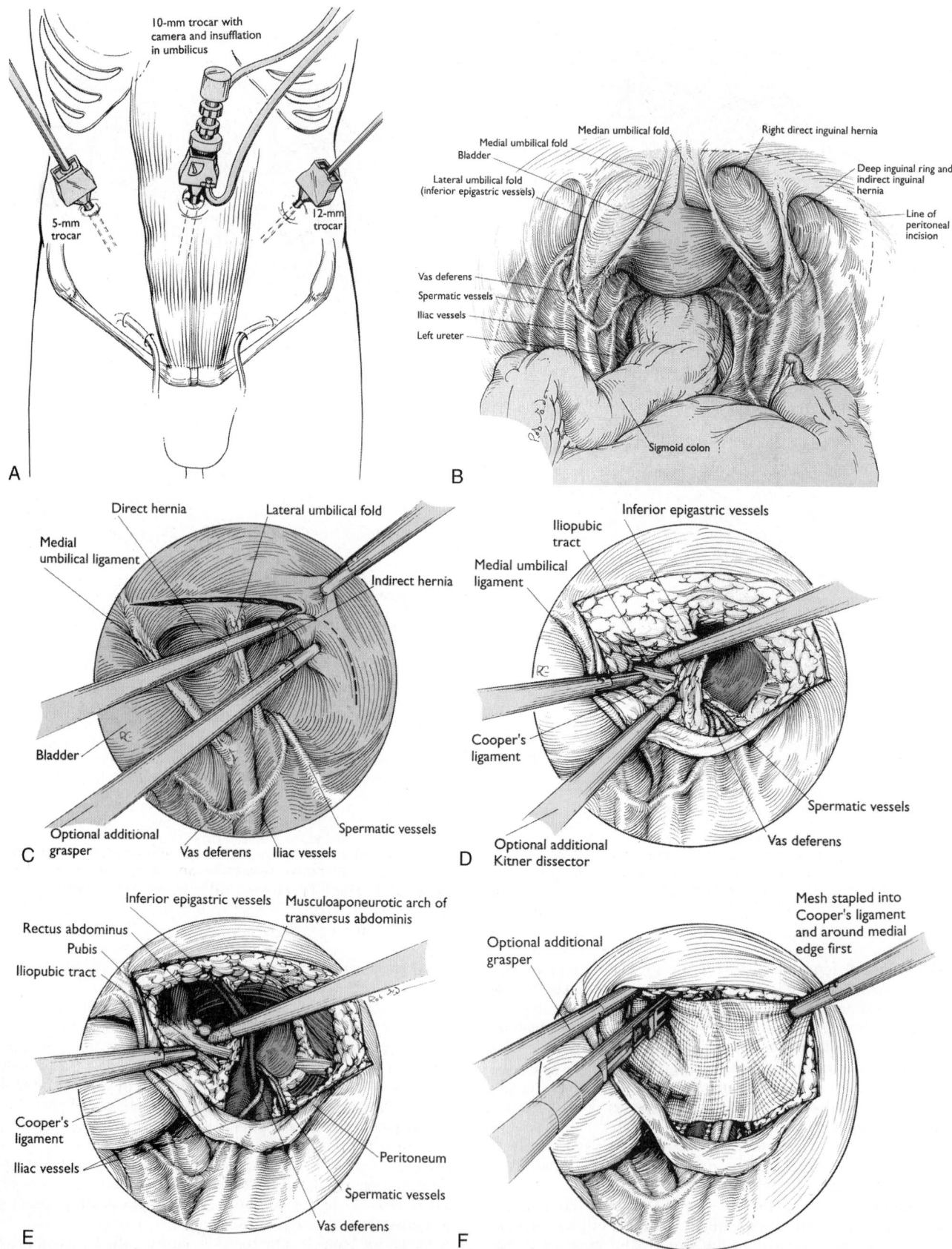

Figure 37–8. *A,* Trocar placement for the transabdominal preperitoneal (TAPP) laparoscopic hernia repair. *B,* Laparoscopic view of the groin anatomy prior to incision of the peritoneum. *C,* A transverse curvilinear peritoneal incision is made cephalad to the internal inguinal ring. The incision extends from the medial umbilical ligament to a point 2 to 3 cm. lateral to the internal inguinal ring. The incision may be made from medial to lateral or from lateral to medial. Countertraction on the peritoneum inferior to the line of incision facilitates dissection and reduces the risk of injury to underlying structures (e.g., inferior epigastric vessels). *D,* Blunt dissection of the inguinal floor. *E,* Completed dissection of the inguinal floor skeletonizes Cooper's ligament, the iliopubic tract, the lateral edge of the rectus abdominis, and the transversus abdominis aponeurotic arch. *F,* The mesh is secured to the anatomic frame with a hernia stapler.

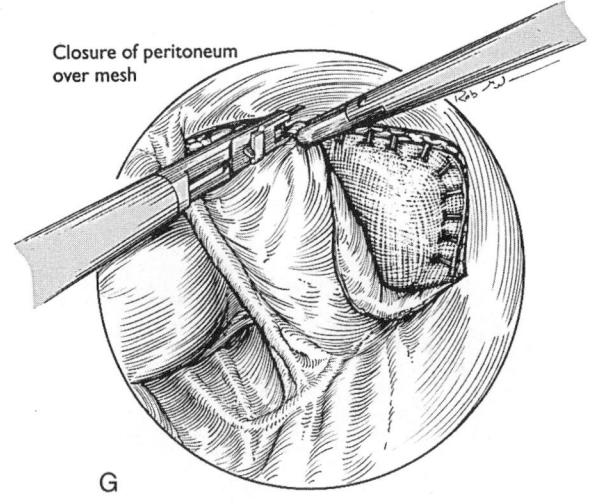

Closure of peritoneum over mesh

G

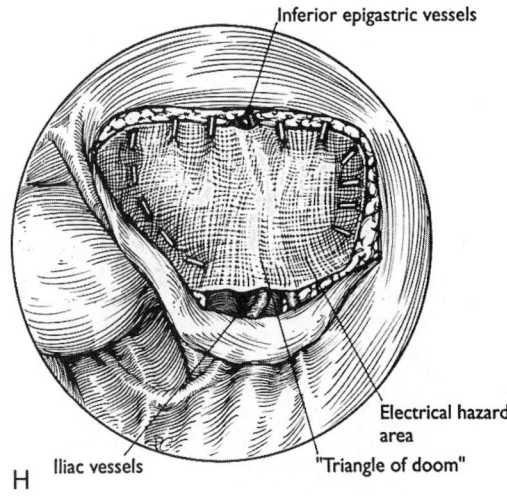

Inferior epigastric vessels

Electrical hazard area

Iliac vessels "Triangle of doom"

H

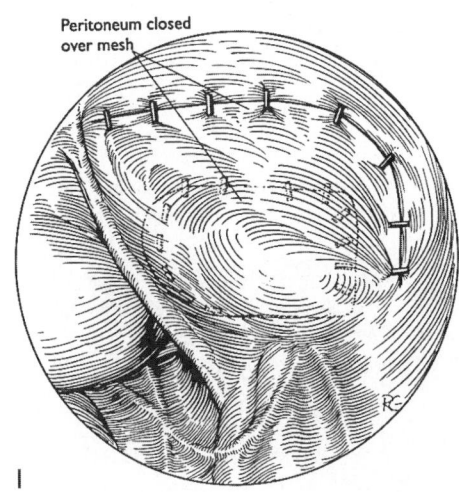

Peritoneum closed over mesh

I

Figure 37–8 *Continued G,* The mesh is stapled to Cooper's ligament, the posterior rectus abdominis, the transversus abdominis aponeurotic arch, and the lateral iliopubic tract. Staples are avoided in the region of the inferior epigastric vessels, the "triangle of doom," and below the lateral iliopubic tract. *H,* The peritoneum is closed over the mesh. *I,* A completed repair is demonstrated. (*A* to *I* from Shadduck, P. P., Schwartz, L. B., and Eubanks, W. S.: Laparoscopic inguinal herniorrhaphy. *In* Pappas, T. N., Schwartz, L. B., and Eubanks, W. S. [Eds.]: Atlas of Laparoscopic Surgery. Philadelphia, Current Medicine, 1996. Copyright © 1996 by Current Medicine. Reproduced by permission of the publisher.)

Critics of laparoscopic hernia repair emphasize the necessity for general anesthesia, the operative costs, the violation of the peritoneal cavity (with the TAPP repair), the necessity for advanced laparoscopic skills, and the lack of long-term follow-up to document recurrence rates. Most opponents of laparoscopic herniorrhaphy accept this approach as a viable alternative for the repair of recurrent inguinal hernias that have previously been repaired using a conventional anterior technique. Another widely accepted indication for laparoscopic hernia repair is the simultaneous repair of bilateral inguinal hernias.[37] The greatest threat to the broad application of laparoscopic techniques in the repair of inguinal hernias is the changing socioeconomic medical environment. Definitive outcome and cost-effectiveness studies are not available in sufficient quantity to determine the long-term role of laparoscopic hernia repair.

FEMORAL HERNIAS

A femoral hernia occurs through a space bounded superiorly by the iliopubic tract, inferiorly by Cooper's ligament, laterally by the femoral vein, and medially by the insertion of the iliopubic tract into Cooper's ligament. On examination, a femoral hernia produces a mass below the inguinal ligament. Femoral hernias are more common in females than males.

A femoral hernia can be repaired using a standard Cooper's ligament (McVay) repair. The preperitoneal approach and the laparoscopic approach also provide excellent visualization and access. The essential elements of femoral hernia repair include dissection and removal of the hernia sac and coverage of the femoral space with mesh or approximation of the iliopubic tract to Cooper's ligament. Viability of the intestine must be ensured when incarceration is detected at the time of hernia repair. The preperitoneal suture repair of a femoral hernia is illustrated in Figure 37–10.

UMBILICAL HERNIAS

The vast majority of umbilical hernias are congenital in origin. There is a strong predisposition toward the development of umbilical hernias in individuals of African descent. In the United States, the incidence of umbilical hernia is as much as eight times higher in black infants than in white infants.[38] The umbilical defect closes spontaneously by the age of 2 years in the vast majority of patients. Umbilical hernias that persist after the age of 5 years are frequently repaired surgically, although complications related to umbilical hernias are unusual in children.

Umbilical hernias presenting during adulthood are considered acquired hernias. Incarceration and strangulation are unusual; rupture can also occur. Patients with conditions that result in increased intra-abdominal pressure can develop umbilical hernias. Pregnancy, ascites, or acute abdominal distention (e.g., intestinal obstruction) may cause an umbilical hernia or bring an occult hernia to attention.

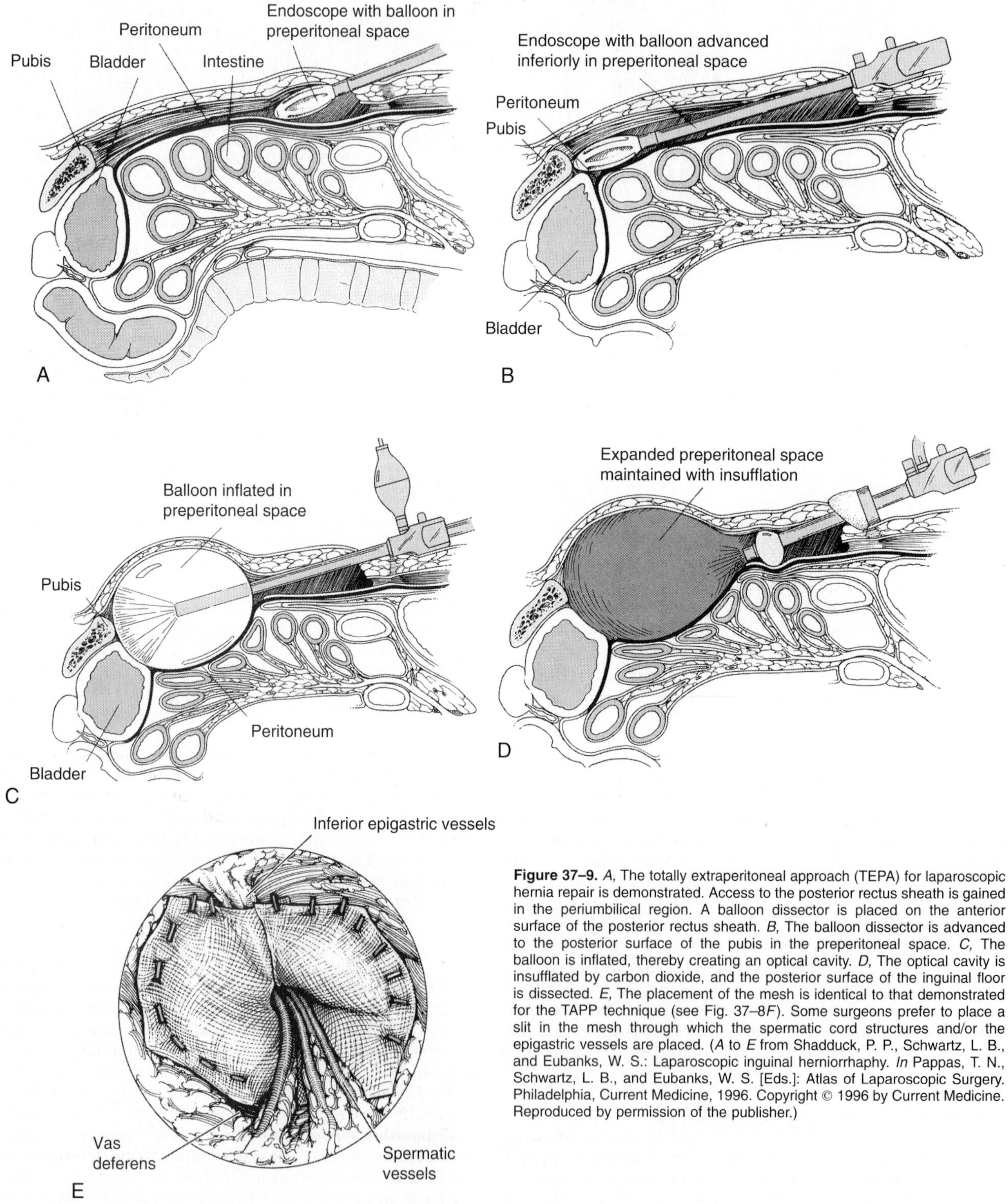

Pubis Bladder Peritoneum Intestine Endoscope with balloon in preperitoneal space

A

Endoscope with balloon advanced inferiorly in preperitoneal space

Peritoneum Pubis

Bladder

B

Balloon inflated in preperitoneal space

Pubis

Peritoneum

Bladder

C

Expanded preperitoneal space maintained with insufflation

D

Inferior epigastric vessels

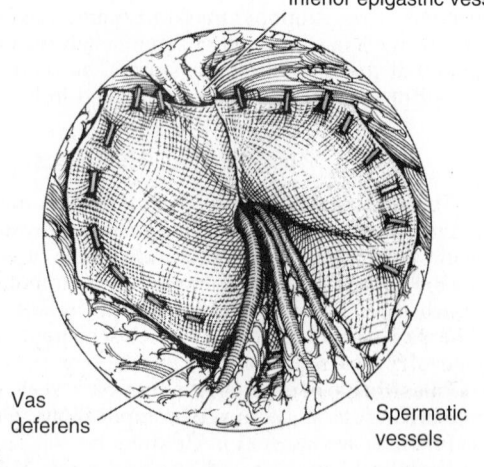

Vas deferens

Spermatic vessels

E

Figure 37–9. *A,* The totally extraperitoneal approach (TEPA) for laparoscopic hernia repair is demonstrated. Access to the posterior rectus sheath is gained in the periumbilical region. A balloon dissector is placed on the anterior surface of the posterior rectus sheath. *B,* The balloon dissector is advanced to the posterior surface of the pubis in the preperitoneal space. *C,* The balloon is inflated, thereby creating an optical cavity. *D,* The optical cavity is insufflated by carbon dioxide, and the posterior surface of the inguinal floor is dissected. *E,* The placement of the mesh is identical to that demonstrated for the TAPP technique (see Fig. 37–8*F*). Some surgeons prefer to place a slit in the mesh through which the spermatic cord structures and/or the epigastric vessels are placed. (*A* to *E* from Shadduck, P. P., Schwartz, L. B., and Eubanks, W. S.: Laparoscopic inguinal herniorrhaphy. *In* Pappas, T. N., Schwartz, L. B., and Eubanks, W. S. [Eds.]: Atlas of Laparoscopic Surgery. Philadelphia, Current Medicine, 1996. Copyright © 1996 by Current Medicine. Reproduced by permission of the publisher.)

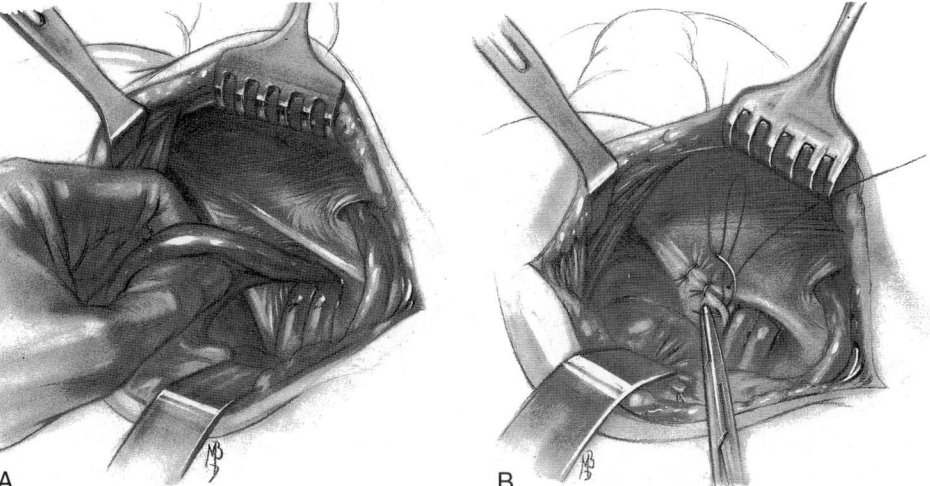

Figure 37–10. *A,* Femoral hernia. The peritoneal sac of the femoral hernia is reduced by traction and blunt dissection. *B,* The femoral canal is narrowed by sutures placed between the iliopubic tract above and Cooper's ligament below. (From Nyhus, L. M.: The preperitoneal approach and iliopubic tract repair of all groin hernias. *In* Nyhus, L. M., and Harkins, H. N. [Eds.]: Hernia. Philadelphia, J. B. Lippincott, 1964.)

Umbilical hernias can be repaired in a *pants over vest* manner, as proposed by Mayo in 1907.[39] A simple transverse closure of an adult umbilical hernia has been demonstrated to be highly effective.[40] Recurrence of umbilical hernias is extremely uncommon.

VENTRAL (INCISIONAL) HERNIA

Ventral hernias usually occur as a result of inadequate healing of a previous incision or excessive strain at the site of an abdominal wall scar. These hernias can be particularly bothersome due to their high recurrence and complication rates. Many of the factors that lead to the development of incisional hernias persist at the time of a second repair. Some of these factors can be altered during a phase of preoperative preparation, whereas others are lifelong or progressively worsening conditions.

Obesity is one of the leading causing of the development of incisional hernias. The bulk associated with a fatty omentum and excessive subcutaneous tissue provides increased strain on the operative wound during early healing. Many of these individuals have an associated loss of muscle mass and tone and therefore possess inadequate strength at the fascial level to compensate for the added strain. An attempt at weight reduction is often recommended prior to the repair of an incisional hernia, but few patients actually comply with this recommendation to a degree that lowers the risks associated with reoperation. Surgical repair in an obese patient is associated with an increased potential for pulmonary complications, wound infection, pulmonary embolus, and similar risks, and these should be discussed with the patient.[41]

Other factors that increase the risk of developing an incisional hernia include advanced age, malnutrition, ascites, postoperative hematoma, peritoneal dialysis, pregnancy, and other conditions causing increased strain on the abdominal wall. The most common causative factor in the development of incisional hernias is postoperative wound infection. Infection may lead to impaired wound healing and subsequent weakness of the incision. Postoperative pulmonary complications are an infrequent cause of incisional hernias.

Certain medications have been demonstrated to lead to poor wound healing. Steroids and chemotherapy are two of the more commonly used drug regimens that have been implicated in the development of incisional hernias. These drugs may blunt normal inflammatory responses and impair the usual healing process.

Timing of the surgical repair of an incisional hernia must be individualized. Whenever possible, the repair should occur when the patient's underlying medical conditions have been stabilized and nutritional status optimized. Weight loss, cessation of smoking, rigid control of diabetes, and avoidance of medications that may impair wound healing are ideal goals during the preoperative preparation. Most incisional hernias can be repaired on an elective basis. There should be no evidence of residual wound infection at the time of prosthetic mesh repair of an incisional hernia. The presence of pus or bacteria at the site of an incisional hernia makes recurrent wound infection likely if prosthetic material is placed prior to eradication of the infection.

Primary repair of an incisional hernia can occasionally be accomplished. A small incisional hernia with adequate surrounding tissues can be repaired with simple interrupted or mattress sutures. However, it is much more common to encounter an incisional hernia that requires prosthetic materials. Some small incisional hernias are repaired with the placement of an onlay prosthetic mesh, which overlaps each of the wound edges by several centimeters. More commonly, prosthetic mesh is used in place of approximating the wound edges. The second alternative provides the opportunity to repair the hernia in a tension-free manner. Polypropylene mesh and expanded polytetrafluoroethylene (e-PTFE) have been used successfully in the repair of incisional hernias. Autogenous tissues have also been used instead of prosthetic materials to repair incisional hernias.

SLIDING HERNIA

A sliding inguinal hernia is defined as one in which a viscus forms a portion of the wall of the hernia sac. Most commonly, the viscus involved is a segment of bowel or urinary bladder. The cecum is most commonly involved with a right inguinal hernia, whereas the sigmoid colon is the organ most frequently involved on the left side. Indirect inguinal hernias are the most common type of sliding hernias, although femoral and direct sliding hernias occur.

The primary danger associated with a sliding hernia is the failure to detect the visceral component of the hernia prior to injury to the bowel or bladder. The hernia sac should be opened on the anteromedial border, as the visceral component most commonly constitutes the posterolateral wall of the hernia sac. Essential to the repair of a sliding hernia is reduction of the viscera into the peritoneal cavity and ligation of the hernia sac. A standard floor reconstruction can be performed following reduction of the viscera and closure of the peritoneum. Ponka[42] described the repair of a sliding hernia by complete dissection of the hernia sac from the spermatic cord and subsequent medial and lateral sac incision to separate the bowel from the hernia sac. After reduction of the bowel into the abdominal cavity, the peritoneal ring was reconstructed with suture-ligation and a conventional inguinal floor repair was accomplished.

Another repair option is the placement of a series of pursestring sutures with progressive inversion of the sliding portion of the hernia sac. The key to successful repair of a sliding hernia is the recognition of the visceral component and the safe return of the viscera to the abdominal cavity, with a careful reconstruction of the inguinal canal.

UNUSUAL HERNIAS

Epigastric Hernia

Hernias of the linea alba occur more commonly above the umbilicus than below. These hernias are usually small and can be difficult to diagnose in obese patients. Patients complain of a painful, pulling sensation at the midline upon reclining. These hernias can usually be repaired with simple suture closure. The surgeon should be aware that these hernias are frequently multiple, and adequate exposure at the linea alba adjacent to the hernia may reveal additional occult hernias.

Richter's Hernia

For a hernia to be considered a Richter hernia, the antimesenteric border of the intestine must protrude into the hernia sac, but never to the point of involvement of the entire circumference of the intestine.[43] The symptoms and clinical course vary widely, depending on the degree of obstruction related to the amount of bowel circumference involved. Strangulation can occur, presenting with a painful mass, nausea, vomiting, and abdominal distention. Conversely, a small, asymptomatic Richter hernia may remain unrecognized until the time of operation. A Richter hernia can occur within any type of abdominal wall hernia, but the most common location is at the site of a femoral hernia.

Richter's hernias have received increased attention with the dramatic increase in the use of the laparoscope. Anecdotal reports have appeared describing Richter's hernias at trocar incisional hernias.[44]

Repair of a Richter hernia is based on the location of the hernia. Critical to the repair of a Richter hernia is an adequate evaluation of the intestine for viability. In some situations, it is impossible to adequately assess or treat the compromised bowel through the incision for hernia repair. In these cases, an additional midline incision may be indicated to perform an adequate exploratory laparotomy. Diagnostic laparoscopy can be used as an alternative to exploratory laparotomy to evaluate the intestine.

Littre's Hernia

The presence of a Meckel diverticulum as the sole component of the hernia sac defines a Littre hernia. This rare entity can be extremely difficult to diagnose due to the frequent lack of obstructive symptoms. Strangulation of the Meckel diverticulum can occur, resulting in abscess or fistulization as the presenting complaint. Surgical management includes repair of the hernia with or without resection of the Meckel diverticulum. A symptomatic or strangulated Meckel diverticulum should be resected. The elective resection of an asymptomatic Meckel diverticulum should be based on the patient's age and overall clinical condition.

Spigelian Hernia

A hernia through the fascia along the lateral edge of the rectus muscle at the space between the semilunar line and the lateral edge of the rectus muscle is a spigelian hernia. Most commonly, spigelian hernias occur inferior to the semicircular line of Douglas. The lack of posterior rectus fascia below the line of Douglas contributes to inherent weakness in this area. Many patients presenting with spigelian hernias are obese, and preoperative diagnosis is correct in only 50% of patients.[11] Spigelian hernias may be found incidentally by ultrasonography or computed tomography (CT).

Spigelian hernias are usually successfully repaired at the initial operation. Approximation of the tissues adjacent to the defect with interrupted sutures is adequate in most patients. However, if the defect is large or the tissues attenuated, prosthetic mesh reinforcement may be indicated.

Obturator Hernia

The obturator canal is covered by a membrane pierced by the obturator nerve and vessels. Weakening of the obturator membrane and enlargement of the canal may result in the formation of a hernia sac, which can lead to intestinal incarceration and obstruction. The obturator canal, which is 2 to 3 cm. long, may contain a fat pad, considered by many surgeons to be pathologic. The patient may present with evidence of compression of the obturator nerve, resulting in pain in the medial aspect of the thigh. This was described by John Howship[45] in 1840 and independently by Moritz Heinrich Romberg[46] in 1848.

Surgical repair of obturator hernias has been performed through various approaches. The abdominal approach, open or laparoscopic, is preferred when compromised bowel is suspected. The retropubic (preperitoneal) approach is preferred by many surgeons when there are no signs of obstruction or intestinal involvement. The obturator, inguinal, and combination approaches have been described. Regardless of the approach, reduction of the contents and inversion of the hernia sac are the initial steps in the surgical treatment of obturator hernias. Gentle manipulation of the obturator nerve with a blunt nerve hook may facilitate reduction of the fat pad from the canal into the pelvis. The fat pad can then be dissected free from the canal, thus relieving the pressure on the obturator nerve. The dilated obturator foramen is repaired with interrupted sutures.

Lumbar (Dorsal) Hernia

Lumbar or dorsal hernias can occur in the lumbar region through the posterior abdominal wall. Grynfeltt's hernia appears through the superior lumbar triangle, whereas Petit's hernia occurs through the inferior lumbar triangle. Diffuse lumbar hernias, a third type, are most often iatrogenic. Most diffuse lumbar hernias occur following flank incisions for kidney operations.

Lumbar hernias usually enlarge in size and become progressively and cosmetically troublesome. Simple suture repair of small hernias is feasible. With larger hernias, reconstruction is challenging. Overlapping and imbricating suture repairs are possible in some patients. However, patients with large hernias or those presenting with extremely attenuated tissues may require mesh reinforcement, pedicle flaps, or free flaps.

Sciatic Hernia

The greater sciatic foramen can be the size of hernia formation. These extremely unusual hernias are difficult to diag-

TABLE 37–4. Postoperative Complications in 548 Adult Patients with Indirect Inguinal Hernias

Complication	Number
Wound complications	
Early	**52**
Seroma	22
Hematoma	9
Minor wound infection	8
Wound abscess	6
Swelling and induration	2
Stitch abscess	1
Minor wound separation	4
Late	**4**
Numbness	3
Keloid	1
Skin reactions	**6**
Sensitivity to tape	5
Reaction to antiseptic	1
Testicular	**34**
Scrotal edema, swelling, induration, and ecchymosis	20
High-riding testicle	8
Impotency	3
Atrophic testicle	2
Bilaterally atrophic testes	1
Urinary tract	**11**
Urinary retention	9
Cystitis	2
Pulmonary	**11**
Bronchitis-pneumonitis	3
Atelectasis	3
Upper respiratory tract infection	2
Pulmonary infarcts (questionable)	3
Thrombophlebitis	**1**
Complications attributable to spinal anesthesia	**3**
Headache	1
Backache	2
Cardiovascular	**4**
Vasovaginal reaction	1
Congestive heart failure	1
Supraventricular tachycardia	1
Anginal attack	1
Total	**126**

From Ponka, J. L.: Hernias of the Abdominal Wall. Philadelphia, W.B. Saunders, 1980, p. 174.

nose, and the patient may be symptom free until intestinal obstruction occurs. Other patients present with a mass in the gluteal or infragluteal area, which causes discomfort when standing. Sciatic nerve pain is rarely caused by pressure from a sciatic hernia. These hernias can be surgically repaired transabdominally or through a transgluteal approach.

TABLE 37–5. Systemic Complications in Adults Following Inguinal Hernia Repair (961 Operations)

Complication	Number	Per Cent
Cardiovascular-pulmonary	39	4.1
Atelectasis, pneumonitis	(24)	(2.5)
Thrombophlebitis	(13)	(1.4)
Coronary occlusion	(2)	(0.2)
Urinary retention (requiring TUR)	10	1.0
Urinary infection	5	0.5
Miscellaneous	12	1.3
Total	66	6.9

TUR, transurethral resection.
From Rydell, W. B., Jr.: Inguinal and femoral hernias. Arch. Surg., 87:493, 1963. Copyright 1963, American Medical Association.

TABLE 37–6. Local Complications in Adults Following Repair of 1053 Hernias

Complication	Number	Per Cent
Wound	21	2.0
Major infection	(14)	(1.3)
Hematoma	(7)	(0.7)
Scrotal and cord (924 male hernias)	62	6.7
Marked swelling	(24)	(2.6)
Testicular atrophy	(16)	(1.8)
Postoperative hydrocele	(5)	(0.5)
Ilioinguinal neuritis	(14)	(1.5)
Cut vas deferens	(3)	(0.3)
Total	83	8.7

From Rydell, W. B., Jr.: Inguinal and femoral hernias. Arch. Surg., 87:493, 1963. Copyright 1963, American Medical Association.

Perineal Hernia

Perineal hernias caused by congenital or acquired defects are very uncommon. These hernias may occur following abdominoperineal resection, prostatectomy, or removal of the pelvic organs. A myocutaneous flap or mesh reinforcement is frequently required to repair a perineal hernia.

COMPLICATIONS

In adult patients, complication rates from open inguinal herniorrhaphy vary from 1% to 26%, with most reports ranging from 7% to 12%.[12] With approximately 700,000 inguinal herniorrhaphies performed each year, complications occurring in approximately 10% of these individuals poses a problem of significant magnitude. Local and systemic complications related to conventional (open) herniorrhaphy have been well documented for many years (Tables 37–4, 37–5, and 37–6). Other series from specialized hernia clinics have reported extremely low complication rates (Table 37–7).

The rate, magnitude, and nature of complications are similar whether the laparoscopic or open approach is used. Differences occur in the pattern of nerve injury, etiology of visceral injury, and risk of postoperative wound hernia.

Intraoperative complications include injury or transection of spermatic cord structures, vascular injury producing hemorrhage, severance or entrapment of nerves, visceral (usually bowel or bladder) injury, and systemic complications such as cardiac arrest or death. With the exception of an injury to a nerve, intraoperative complications are usually immediately recognized and repaired.

Postoperative wound complications include infection, hematoma, ecchymosis, and seroma. Complications related to the scrotum and testicles include hematoma, atrophy, sterility, swelling, ecchymosis, and hydrocele. Genitourinary post-

TABLE 37–7. Complications in 4114 Hernioplasties of the Groin

Complication	Number	Per Cent
Wound infection	24	0.58
Hematoma	18	0.43
Pulmonary embolus	3	0.07
Hemorrhage	1	0.02
Ischemic orchitis	25	0.61
Testicular atrophy	14	0.34

Wantz, G. E.: The Canadian repair of inguinal hernia. In Nyhus, L. M., and Condon, R. E. (Eds.): Hernia, 3rd edition. Philadelphia, J. B. Lippincott, 1989, pp. 236–248.

operative complications include urinary retention and urinary tract infection.

Numerous systemic postoperative complications have been described, which are related to the specific procedure performed. Pulmonary complications such as atelectasis, pneumonia, pneumonitis, and pulmonary embolus have been described following inguinal hernia repair. Deep venous thrombosis can occur following laparoscopic or open hernia repair. Cardiac arrhythmia and cardiac arrest have been reported following inguinal hernia repair, and intraoperative cardiac arrhythmias are frequently documented. Mortality related to the repair of a groin hernia is extremely unusual, but because of the advanced age and comorbid conditions of many patients, deaths have occurred.

Recurrence of a groin hernia is frequently excluded from lists of complications but is discussed here due to the morbidity associated with recurrence. Reported recurrence rates vary from less than 1% to 7% for indirect inguinal hernias, from 4% to 10% for direct inguinal hernias, from 1% to 7% for femoral hernias, and from 5% to 35% for recurrent hernia repair. Recurrence may result from technical failure, inadequate fascial strength, impaired wound healing, trauma, progressive weakening of surrounding tissues, or tissue approximated under excessive tension.

Nerve injuries are a well-documented complication of inguinal hernia repair.[47–50] The nerves most commonly affected during an open herniorrhaphy are the ilioinguinal and iliohypogastric nerves; during a laparoscopic hernia repair, the lateral femoral cutaneous nerve and the genitofemoral nerve are most often affected. Compression or entrapment of the lateral femoral cutaneous nerve results in *meralgia paresthetica*—pain and paresthesias in the anterolateral thigh.[9] Rarely, the main trunk of the femoral nerve is injured during an open or laparoscopic inguinal hernia repair.

Transection of a sensory nerve of the groin usually results in an area of cutaneous numbness corresponding to the dermatomal distribution of the involved nerve (Fig. 37–11). Transient neuralgias are frequently self-limited and resolve within days to weeks following the operation. Persistent neuralgias may be secondary to postoperative inflammatory changes or mild injury to the nerve and surrounding tissues. Occasionally, a nerve injury is the result of entrapment by a suture or staple and causes much more troublesome symptoms. A patient with nerve entrapment usually presents with pain and paresthesias in the groin and/or in the dermatomal distribution of the affected nerve. Similar symptoms may be produced as a nerve becomes encased in scar tissue or from compression secondary to a recurrent hernia. Patients presenting with nerve entrapment syndromes may require reoperation for removal of the offending agent or transection of the involved nerve. In the event that a postoperative neuralgia is diagnosed, a trial of conservative therapy is warranted, as many patients experience resolution of symptoms without repeat operation.

REFERENCES

1. Ger, R.: The laparoscopic management of groin hernias. Contemp. Surg., 39:15, 1991.
2. Condon, R. E., and Carilli, S.: The biology and anatomy of inguinofemoral hernia. Semin. Laparosc. Surg., 1:75, 1994.
3. Skandalakis, J. E., Colborn, G. L., Gray, S. W., et al.: Embryologic and anatomical basis of modern herniorrhaphy: Part II. Anatomy, physiology, and etiology of hernias. Em. Univ. J. Med., 6:177, 1992.
4. Nyhus, L. M., Klein, M. S., and Rogers, F. B.: Inguinal hernia. Curr. Probl. Surg., 6:401, 1991.
5. Annibali, R. G.: Surgical anatomy of the inguinal region and lower abdominal wall from the laparoscopic perspective. *In* Nyhus, L. M., and Condon, R. E. (Eds.): Hernia, 4th ed. Philadelphia, J. B. Lippincott, 1995.
6. Rizk, N. N.: A new description of the anterior abdominal wall in man and mammals. J. Anat., 131:373, 1990.

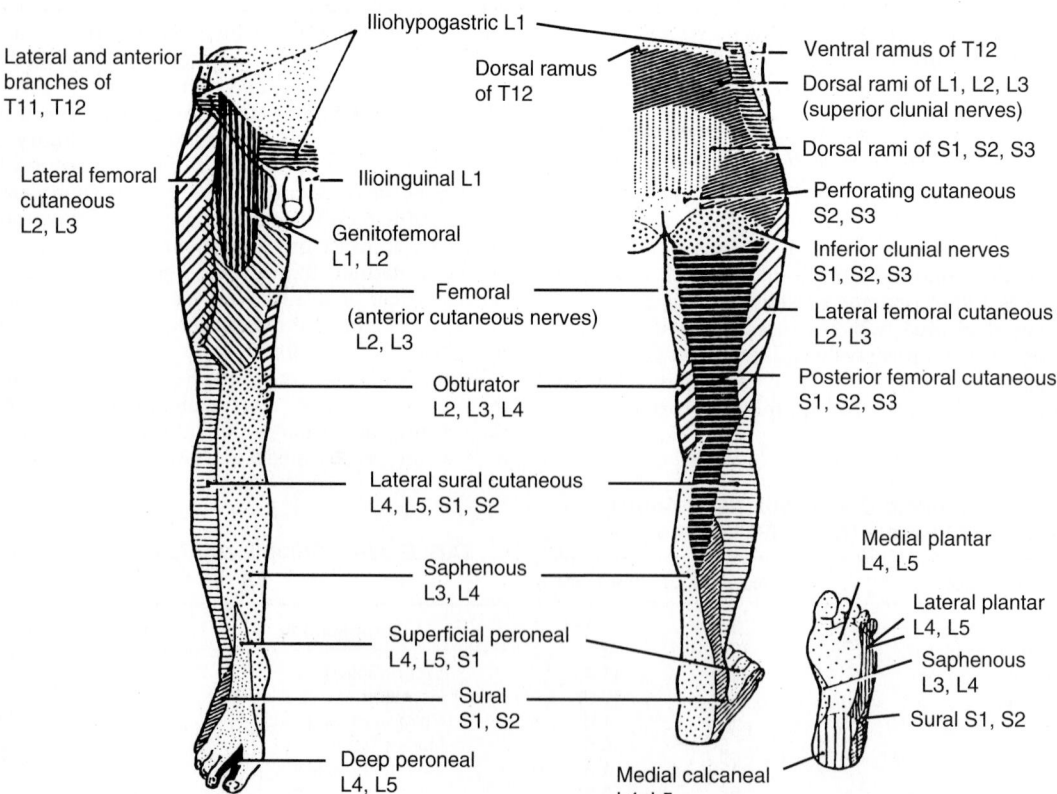

Figure 37–11. Sensory innovation of the lower extremity (From Omer, G. E., and Spinner, E.: Management of Peripheral Nerve Problems. Philadelphia, W. B. Saunders, 1980.)

7. Cooper, A. P.: The Anatomy and Surgical Treatment of Inguinal and Congenital Hernia. London, Longman, 1804.
8. Read, R. C.: The transversalis and peritoneal fasciae—a reevaluation. *In* Nyhus, L. M., and Condon, R. E. (Eds.): Hernia, 4th ed. Philadelphia, J. B. Lippincott, 1995.
9. Eubanks, S. E., Newman, L. N., et al.: Meralgia paresthetica: A complication of laparoscopic herniorrhaphy. Surg. Laparosc. Endosc., 3:381, 1993.
10. Gardner, E., Gray, D. J., and O'Rahilly, R.: Blood vessels, lymphatic drainage, and nerves. *In* Anatomy: A Regional Study of Human Structure, 4th ed. Philadelphia, W. B. Saunders, 1975.
11. Kortz, W. J., and Sabiston, D. C.: Hernias. *In* Sabiston, D. C. (Ed.): Sabiston's Essentials of Surgery. Philadelphia, W. B. Saunders, 1987.
12. MacFadyen, B. V., and Mathis, C. R.: Inguinal herniorrhaphy: Complications and recurrences. Semin. Laparosc. Surg., 1:128, 1994.
13. Rutkow, I. M.: Open versus laparoscopic groin herniorrhaphy: Economic realities. *In* Arregui, M. E., Nagan, R. F. (Eds.): Inguinal Hernia: Advances or Controversies? Oxford, Radcliff Medical Press, 1994.
14. Read, R. C.: Attenuation of rectus sheath in inguinal herniation. Am. J. Surg., 120:610, 1970.
15. Read, R. C.: Collagen synthesis and direct inguinal herniation. *In* Arregui, M. E., and Nagan, R. F. (Eds.): Inguinal Hernia: Advances or Controversies? Oxford, Radcliff Medical Press, 1994.
16. Weitz, J. I., Crowley, K. A., Landman, S. L., Lipman, B. I., and Yu, J.: Increased neutrophil elastase activity in cigarette smokers. Ann. Intern. Med., 107:686, 1987.
17. Read, R. C.: The role of protease-antiprotease in the pathogenesis of herniation and abdominal aortic aneurysm in certain smokers. Postgrad. Gen. Surg., 14:161, 1992.
18. Bielecki, K., and Puawski, R.: Is cigarette smoking a causative factor in the development of inguinal hernia? Pol. Tyg. Lek., 43:974, 1988.
19. Gullmo, A., Broome, A., and Smedberg, S.: Herniography. Surg. Clin. North Am., 64:229, 1984.
20. Berliner, S. D.: An approach to groin hernia. Surg. Clin. North Am., 64:197, 1984.
21. McKernan, J. B., and Laws, H. L.: Laparoscopic preperitoneal prosthetic repair of inguinal hernias. Surg. Rounds, 15:610, 1994.
22. Cheatle, G. L.: An operation for the radical cure of inguinal and femoral hernia. Br. Med. J., 2:68, 1920.
23. Henry, A. K.: Operation for femoral hernia by a midline extraperitoneal approach: With a preliminary note on the use of this route for reducible inguinal hernia. Lancet, 1:531, 1936.
24. Nyhus, L. M., Stevenson, J. K., Listerud, M. V., and Harkins, H. N.: Preperitoneal herniorrhaphy: A preliminary report in 50 patients. West. J. Surg. Obstet. Gynecol., 67:48, 1959.
25. Stoppa, R., Petit, J., Abourachid, H., et al.: Procède original de la plastique des hernies de l'aine: linterposition sans fixation d'une prothèse en tulle de dacron par voie médiane sous-péritonéale. Chirurgie, 99:119, 1973.
26. Read, R. C.: Preperitoneal exposure of inguinal herniation. Am. J. Surg., 116:653, 1968.
27. Spaw, A. T., Ennis, B. W., and Spaw, L. P.: Laparoscopic hernia repair: The anatomic basis. J. Laparoendosc. Surg., 1:269, 1991.
28. Felix, E., and Michas, C.: The double-buttress laparoscopic herniorrhaphy. J. Laparoendosc. Surg., 1:1, 1993.
29. Felix, E. L., Michas, C. A., and McKnight, R. L.: Laparoscopic repair of groin hernias. *In* Arregui, M. E., and Nagan, R. F. (Eds.): Inguinal Hernia: Advances or Controversies? Oxford, Radcliff Medical Press, 1994.
30. Payne, J. H., Grininger, L. M., Izawam, T., et al.: Laparoscopic or open inguinal herniorrhaphy? A randomized prospective trial. Arch. Surg., 129:973, 1994.
31. Newman, L., Eubanks, S., Mason, E., and Duncan, T. D.: Is laparoscopic herniorrhaphy an effective alternative to open hernia repair? J. Laparoendosc. Surg., 3:121, 1993.
32. Shultz, L., Graber, J., Pietrafitta, J., and Hickok, D.: Laser laparoscopic herniorrhaphy: A clinical trial preliminary results. J. Laparoendosc. Surg., 1:41, 1990.
33. Arregui, M. E., Davis, C. J., Yucel, O., and Nagan, R. F.: Laparoscopic mesh repair of inguinal hernia using a preperitoneal approach: A preliminary report. Surg. Laparosc. Endosc., 2:53, 1993.
34. Fitzgibbons, R. J., Camps, J., Cornet, D. A., et al.: Laparoscopic inguinal herniorrhaphy: Results of a multicenter trial. Ann. Surg., 221:3, 1995.
35. Stoker, D. L., Spiegelhalter, D. J., Singh, R., and Wellwood, J. M.: Laparoscopic versus open inginal hernia repair: Randomised prospective trial. Lancet, 343:1243, 1994.
36. Millikan, K. W., Kosik, M. L., and Doolas, A.: A prospective comparison of transabdominal preperitoneal laparoscopic hernia repair versus traditional open hernia repair in a university setting. Surg. Laparosc. Endosc., 4:247, 1994.
37. Brooks, D. C.: A prospective comparison of laparoscopic and tension-free open herniorrhaphy. Arch. Surg., 129:361, 1994.
38. Radhakris, H., and Nan, J.: Umbilical hernia. *In* Nyhus, L. M., and Condon, R. E. (Eds.): Hernia, 4th ed. Philadelphia, J. B. Lippincott, 1995.
39. Mayo, W. J.: Radical cure of umbilical hernia. JAMA, 48:1842, 1907.
40. Farris, J. M., Smith, G. K., and Beattie, A. S.: Umbilical hernia: An inquiry into the principle of imbrication and a note on the preservation of the umbilical dimple. Am. J. Surg., 98:236, 1956.
41. Condon, R. E.: Incisional hernia. *In* Nyhus, L. M., and Condon, R. E. (Eds.): Hernia, 4th ed. Philadelphia, J. B. Lippincott, 1995.
42. Ponka, J. L.: Surgical management of large bilateral indirect sliding inguinal hernias. Am. J. Surg., 112:52, 1966.
43. Tito, W. A., and Perez-Tamayo, A.: Richter and Littre's hernias. *In* Nyhus, L. M., and Condon, R. E. (Eds.): Hernia, 4th ed. Philadelphia, J. B. Lippincott, 1995.
44. Williams, M. D., Flowers, S. S., et al.: Richter hernia: A rare complication of laparoscopy. Surg. Laparosc. Endosc., 5:419, 1995.
45. Howship, J.: Practical Remarks on the Discrimination and Appearances of Surgical Disease. London, John Churchill, 1840.
46. Romberg, M. H.: Die Operation des singeklemmten Bruches des eirunden Loches: Operatio herniae foraminis ovalis incarceratae. *In* Dieffenbach, J. F. (Ed.): Die Operative Chirurgie, Vol. 2. Leipzig, F. A. Brockhaus, 1848.
47. Harms, B. A., DeHaas, D. R., and Starling, J. R.: Diagnosis and management of genitofemoral neuralgia. Arch. Surg., 119:339, 1984.
48. Starling, J. R., Harms, B. A., Schroeder, M. E., and Eichman, P. L.: Diagnosis and treatment of genitofemoral and ilioinguinal entrapment neuralgia. Surgery, 102:581, 1987.
49. Starling, J. R., and Harms, B. A.: Diagnosis and treatment of ilioinguinal genitofemoral neuralgia. World J. Surg., 13:586, 1989.
50. Laha, R. K., Rao, S., Pedgeon, C. N., and Dujovny, M.: Genitofemoral neuralgia. Surg. Neurol., 8:280, 1977.

CHAPTER 38

PEDIATRIC SURGERY

Jay L. Grosfeld, M.D.

HISTORICAL ASPECTS

The first text in pediatric surgery is credited to the Swiss surgeon Felix Wurtz in the year 1563.[172] Further development of the speciality followed the publication of a pediatric surgical text by Forster (England)[47] and published lectures on childhood surgical conditions by Guersant (France) in 1864.[70] In the late 1870s, the Hospital for Sick Children in London and the Hôpital des Enfants Malades in Paris developed separate surgical programs. The first textbook of pediatric surgery in the United States was published by Kelly in 1909.[89] By 1920, a number of surgeons began to devote much of their energies to the care of children. Following World War II, the growth of pediatric surgery flourished under the direction of Drs. William E. Ladd and Robert E. Gross at the Boston Children's Hospital, Dr. Willis Potts of Chicago, and Sir Dennis Browne in London.[69, 94, 129] Their special clinical and educational contributions to the field are well recognized.

More recently, the evolution of sophisticated neonatal intensive care, early detection of numerous anomalies by prenatal ultrasonography, development of high-risk obstetric centers, combined programs of cancer care, and emergence of other pediatric subspecialties in surgery (neurosurgery, orthopedics, urology, cardiology), pathology, anesthesia, and radiology have further enhanced the growth, importance, and popularity of pediatric surgery. In 1988, the specialty established its first independent surgical forum session at the annual meeting of the American College of Surgeons, indicative of efforts in the field to promote clinical excellence, quality education, and innovative scientific research.

SPECIAL CONSIDERATIONS
Newborn Physiology

A newborn infant is a unique surgical patient who is physically and physiologically different from an adult. A neonate presents a significant challenge in patient care management, involving both congenital and acquired conditions. Because of small size, limited volume capacities, and functional immaturity of organ systems, an infant's response to and ability to cope with the stress related to a serious illness and major operative procedure may be marginal.

Cardiovascular System

The cardiovascular system of a newborn must convert from a fetal circulation that bypasses the lungs to a postnatal state with both a systemic and a pulmonary circulation. In the absence of intracardiac defects or anomalies of the aortic arch, the newborn heart functions quite well. The elevated pulmonary artery pressure in a neonate, in association with a patent foramen ovale and ductus arteriosus, may result in right-to-left shunting. A neonate's cardiac output is rate dependent, and the infant heart has a limited ability to increase the stroke volume, so cardiac output decreases with

episodes of bradycardia. The pathophysiology of congenital heart defects is covered elsewhere in this text.

Thermoregulation

A newborn infant must be kept in a neutral thermal environment (73° F., 22.7° C.) to minimize caloric expenditure, reduce oxygen consumption, and diminish metabolic demands. A baby's temperature must be closely monitored by skin probes or axillary probes, as the rectal temperature is not an accurate measure of body temperature in a neonate, and insertion of a rectal thermometer may cause rectal perforation. The normal skin temperature is 36 to 36.5° C. An infant's relatively large body surface area, lack of hair and subcutaneous tissue, and increased insensible losses make it vulnerable to hypothermia. A neonate cannot shiver but responds to cold stress by increasing its metabolic rate and oxygen consumption by mobilizing brown fat deposits in the neck, axilla, mediastinum, and perirenal area (nonshivering thermogenesis).[95] Continued exposure to cold ultimately leads to decreased perfusion and metabolic acidosis. Heat loss can occur as a result of radiant and evaporative heat loss and by conduction and/or convection.[28] Overhead radiant heaters, warming lights, tin-foil caps, heat shields, extremity wraps, and warmed prep solutions are frequently used to reduce skin exposure and heat loss.

Pulmonary Function

The lungs are not fully mature at birth. There are 17 subdivisions of the tracheobronchial tree *in utero,* and the lungs continue to add new respiratory units (terminal bronchioles and alveoli) until 8 years of age. The more immature the patient, the fewer the number of pulmonary units present. A premature baby has fewer Type II pneumocytes and lower surfactant levels, making it susceptible to alveolar collapse, atelectasis, hyaline membrane formation, and barotrauma. A neonate is also at risk for the development of persistent pulmonary hypertension (formerly called persistent fetal circulation), a condition in which the pulmonary vascular resistance is equal to or greater than systemic vascular resistance, causing hypoxemia due to extrapulmonary right-to-left shunting. This may occur in a variety of conditions, including hyperviscosity, decreased lung mass (diaphragmatic hernia), or decreased vessel radius (reactive vasoconstriction, pulmonary venous obstruction, total anomalous venous drainage, or hypoplastic left heart). The tidal volume in a neonate is 6 to 10 ml. per kg. The airway diameter is quite small (trachea 2.5 to 4.0 mm.) and is easily plugged with secretions (Table 38–1). The respiratory rate may be as high as 60 per minute and still be normal. Respiratory distress is heralded by tachypnea, grunting, nasal flaring, intercostal and substernal retraction, and cyanosis. Infants are nasal and diaphragmatic breathers. A newborn infant does not mouth breathe. If a newborn baby needs gastric drainage, the tube should be inserted through the mouth rather than the nose. Any condition that obstructs the nasal passages (e.g., choanal atresia)

TABLE 38-1. Tracheal Tube Size in Infants and Children

Age of Patient	Internal Tracheal Tube Diameter
Premature	2.5 mm.
0–3 months	3.0 mm.
3–7 months	3.5 mm.
7–15 months	4.0 mm.
15–24 months	4.5 mm.
2–10 years	$\frac{16 + age (yr.)}{4} = mm.$
10–19 years	6.0–8.0 mm. (cuffed)

or interferes with diaphragmatic function (e.g., eventration, diaphragmatic hernia) may result in severe respiratory distress. Administration of maternal steroids 48 hours prior to the anticipated birth of a premature baby at risk for respiratory distress often results in early lung maturation. Use of exogenous surfactant and the administration of nitric oxide have ameliorated respiratory illness in neonates.

Normal blood gas tensions in a newborn are different from those in an adult because of shunting (foramen ovale, patent ductus) and a more rapid respiratory rate. The PaO_2 is usually 75 to 80 torr in a blood sample obtained from the right radial artery (above the ductus) and may be only 60 torr from a sample taken from the umbilical artery (below the ductus). The $PaCO_2$ is usually 30 to 35 torr because of the relatively rapid respiratory rate. The lower the $PaCO_2$, the less the risk of pulmonary vasoconstriction. The apH is usually normal (7.3 to 7.4). Pulse oximetry is a useful method of monitoring O_2 saturation.

Renal Function

Although the newborn kidney may not concentrate urine normally, it functions quite well otherwise and responds to a fluid load. This occurs despite a reduced glomerular filtration rate and immature tubular function. A urine osmolality of less than 150 mOsm. may indicate overhydration, whereas one greater than 400 mOsm. may reflect dehydration. A urinary output of 1 to 2 ml. per kg. per hour is considered normal in infants.

Immunologic Function

A neonate is relatively immunodeficient, as it has decreased levels of opsonins; IgA, IgG, and IgM; and the C3b component of complement. The more immature the infant, the poorer the ability of the polymorphonuclear leukocytes to phagocytize bacteria. A premature infant is therefore at an increased risk for severe infection.[28] Prolonged rupture of fetal membranes, perinatal asphyxia, and maternal peripartum infection increase the risk of neonatal infection. The evaluation of sepsis in a newborn requires an extensive workup, including blood, urine, and cerebrospinal fluid cultures; chest x-ray; urinalysis; complete blood count and differential smear; platelet count; culture of any eye drainage; ear examination (for otitis); evaluation of intravenous or arterial catheter sites, including the umbilicus; careful evaluation of the wound in a postoperative patient; and, in premature infants, evaluation for possible necrotizing enterocolitis. Combination antibiotic therapy is administered empirically after acquisition of cultures. Group B beta streptococcus (gram positive)

and *Escherichia coli* (gram negative) are the two most common serious infections. There has also been a resurgence of antibiotic-resistant *Staphylococcus albus*.

Metabolic and Endocrine Function

Liver function in a newborn is immature. Most infants have some deficiency in hepatic enzyme function, particularly those enzymes involved in the conjugation of indirect to direct bilirubin (glucuronyl transferase, Y and Z protein) and the detoxification of certain drugs (sulfonamides) and anesthetic agents. A premature infant is more prone to hyperbilirubinemia and kernicterus due to passage of indirect bilirubin across the blood-brain barrier. Most endocrine activity in a full-term neonate is at a near-normal level. Hypoglycemia is the major cause of seizures in newborns and is defined as a concentration of less than 20 mg. per 100 ml. in a premature infant and 30 mg. per 100 ml. in full-term infant.[14] Hypoglycemia is most commonly noted in babies that are small for their gestational age. These infants have intrauterine growth retardation and inadequate glycogen stores in the liver. Progeny of diabetic mothers may also have hypoglycemia as a result of temporary excess insulin production stimulated during intrauterine life by the mother's elevated glucose levels. Infants with pancreatic islet cell dysplasia (nesidioblastosis) have severe hypoglycemia that may be resistant to treatment with steroids and diazoxide and require a somatostatin analog or total parenteral nutrition to maintain the blood sugar level until a 95% pancreatectomy can be performed.

Hypocalcemia (<7.0 mg. per 100 ml.) can present with jitteriness, hypotonicity, or seizures and is most frequently observed in premature infants, infants of diabetic mothers, and asphyxiated infants. Hypomagnesemia and pyridoxine deficiency are more rare causes of seizures in newborns.

Fluid and Electrolyte Balance

In a full-term newborn, the total body water space is 80% of body weight.[28] The extracellular water space constitutes more than two thirds of the total body water space. A neonate has increased insensible water losses (30 to 35 ml. per kg. per day) when compared with an adult (15 ml. per kg. per day). In premature infants weighing less than 1500 gm., insensible losses are significantly higher (45 to 60 ml. per kg.). Radiant heat warmers, phototherapy for hyperbilirubinemia, fever, and respiratory distress increase the insensible losses. Water requirements for maintenance in a normal newborn vary from 100 to 125 ml. per kg. per day in a full-term infant up to 140 to 150 ml. per kg. per day in a premature infant (particularly very low birth weight babies less than 1.0 kg.) (Table 38–2). Ten per cent dextrose in 0.25% saline is used as

TABLE 38-2. Daily Fluid Requirements for Neonates and Infants

Weight	Volume
Premature <2.0 kg.	140–150 ml./kg./day
Neonates and infants (2–10 kg.)	100 ml./kg./day (for first 10 kg.)
Infants and children (10–20 kg.)	1000 ml. + 50 ml./kg./day >10 kg.
Children >20 kg.	1500 ml. + 20 ml./kg./day >20 kg.

a maintenance solution. Potassium and sodium requirements are 2 to 3 mEq. per kg. per day. Fluid losses related to gastric drainage are replaced in equal volumes with lactated Ringer's solution if the drainage is bilious and 5% dextrose in 0.45% normal saline if it is clear. A postoperative patient may need somewhat less fluid because of antidiuretic hormone secretion and cortisol release. Body weight, skin turgor, urine and serum osmolality, and urine specific gravity are reasonable means to assess fluid requirements. Normal serum osmolarity is 280 mOsm. Poor urine output and high urine specific gravity may reflect third-space interstitial fluid shifts requiring an additional intravenous bolus (10 ml. per kg. of lactated Ringer's solution over 30 minutes). Large volume losses from an enterostomy can be replaced with 0.5 ml. of lactated Ringer's solution per 1.0 ml. of stomal effluent.

The total blood volume in a newborn is approximately 8% of body weight and decreases to approximately 5% in older infants. This can be calculated as 80 ml. per kg. A safe transfusion for an infant is 10 ml. per kg. (packed red blood cells). In instances of thrombocytopenia, 10 ml. per kg. of platelets is an adequate transfusion volume. If an infant has hypotension, a rapid infusion of 20 ml. per kg. of lactated Ringer's solution reduces the pulse rate, increases the blood pressure, and often restores hemodynamic stability.

Nutrition

A neonate has a metabolic rate that is higher than that of an older child and 2.5 times that of an adult. A neonate requires 120 calories per kg. per day for growth. Most infant formulas contain 20 calories per ounce, so the caloric need can be determined by the following: weight (kg.) × 6 oz. = volume of formula necessary to deliver 120 calories per kg. Major illness (sepsis), trauma, or fever may increase the caloric requirements. Half of the calories provided are carbohydrates, 35% are fat, and 15% are protein. Infants require more protein, vitamins, and minerals than adult patients. Linoleic acid is an essential fatty acid, and histidine, tyrosine, and cystine are essential amino acids for infants, in addition to the eight other essential amino acids required by adults. Breast milk (296 mOsm.) is recommended for most infants when possible. In some instances, modification of the diet is necessary. Following gastrointestinal surgery, lactose-containing formulas (Enfamil, Similac) should be avoided, because flattening of the intestinal villi occurs in unfed neonates and is associated with decreased lactase levels, producing poor absorption and diarrhea. Lactose also produces a large curd, which may obstruct a small anastomosis. Low-osmolar nonlactose formulas, such as the soybean formulas Isomil or Prosobee (260 mOsm.) are useful in postoperative patients. Feedings are started when the gastric returns are clear and of low volume (2.0 ml. per hour). Initial feedings should be diluted (e.g., quarter strength, half strength) and gradually increased in volume and then density as tolerated. The swallowing mechanism in premature infants is immature, indicating that these babies should be given small, frequent gavage feedings containing specially designed formulas. In patients with short bowel syndrome, a more defined formula (pediatric elemental diet) given by a continuous drip technique may be necessary. Babies with obstructive jaundice thrive on Vital, a non-long-chain fat–containing diet that delievers 30 calories per ounce. If the infant cannot tolerate an enteral diet, intravenous nutrition may be needed.

Total Parenteral Nutrition (TPN)

The advent of parenteral nutrition was one of the most important developments in pediatric surgical care. This tech-

nique permits the delivery of adequate amounts of carbohydrates, fats, and amino acids to ensure appropriate caloric intake, supporting growth of an infant even in the absence of enteral intake. Patients most commonly managed with TPN therapy include those with short bowel syndrome, necrotizing enterocolitis, severe gastroenteritis due to nonspecific diarrhea syndromes, Crohn's disease with internal fistulas, gastroschisis, extensive thermal burns, cancer, corrected intestinal atresia, and many nonsurgical disorders leading to inadequate enteral intake.[28] The nonprotein calorie–gram of nitrogen ratio is maintained at greater than 150:1. A continuous drip of a solution containing 17% to 18% carbohydrate in newborns and 25% carbohydrate concentration in older children, 2.5 gm. per kg. of amino acids in newborns, and 3.5 gm. per kg. in older children, and no more than 4 gm. per kg. of fat emulsion administered as either a 10 or 20% solution of intralipid usually delivers 120 to 130 calories per kg. per day.[84] Venous access for TPN is most readily achieved by inserting a Silastic catheter (Broviac or Hickman) into the external jugular vein and, under fluoroscopic control, placing the end of the catheter in a central high-flow location in the superior vena cava at the entrance of the right atrium. The cephalic vein, subclavian vein, facial vein, internal jugular vein, and saphenofemoral entry can be used as alternative venotomy sites. The amount of fat must be reduced (0.5 gm. per kg. per day) if the patient is jaundiced or the triglyceride level is greater than 200 mg. per 100 ml. The amount of glucose may need to be lowered in patients with respiratory conditions associated with hypercarbia (PCO_2). Appropriate sodium (3 to 4 mEq. per kg. per day) and potassium (2 to 3 mEq. per kg. per day) are added to the infusion. Multivitamins, calcium, phosphorus, magnesium, zinc, copper, and folate are also added to the solution. A weight gain of 15 to 30 gm. per day is anticipated, barring untoward events (e.g., sepsis or other complications) that increase metabolic demand and require additional calories. Technical complications may be encountered at the time of central venous catheter insertion; they include bleeding, pneumothorax, and vein perforation. Late complications related to the presence of the catheter include catheter-related sepsis, vena caval thrombosis, and, rarely, pulmonary embolus due to mural thrombus. Myriad metabolic complications have been observed, including hyperglycemia, hyperosmolality, hypoglycemia, hypocalcemia, hypophosphatemia, fluid overload characterized by pulmonary and peripheral edema, fatty acid and mineral deficiencies, and cholestatic jaundice.[28] Most of the metabolic problems can be obviated by careful monitoring and the addition of fat infusions and trace element solutions. Cholestatic jaundice remains a problem and is most often observed in prematures with sepsis, including peritonitis. Premature infants' inability to tolerate the high amino acid load due to immature enzyme function is suspected. The amount of amino acids infused may need to be reduced to 1.0 gm. per kg. per day. Cholestasis is often improved by initiating enteral feedings or administering cholecystokinin. Chronic liver disease (cirrhosis) and a few instances of hepatoblastoma or hepatoma have been observed as late complications of prolonged TPN administration in the neonatal period.

ALIMENTARY TRACT OBSTRUCTION

Neonatal alimentary tract obstruction is often heralded by a number of signs, including maternal polyhydramnios, bilious vomiting, abdominal distention, and failure to pass normal amounts of meconium in the first 24 hours of life. Although none of these observations are pathognomonic of obstruction, all are consistent with an obstructive phenomenon and should be carefully evaluated.

Polyhydramnios refers to the presence of excess fluid in the amniotic sac (>2000 ml.). Twenty-five to 40% of the amniotic fluid is swallowed by the fetus and absorbed in the jejunum. Instances of high alimentary tract obstruction are associated with maternal polyhydramnios, including esophageal atresia without tracheoesophageal (TE) fistula, pyloric atresia, duodenal atresia, and high jejunal atresia. Other maternal causes are related to cardiac, renal, and hepatic disease and toxemia. Fetal causes include swallowing problems due to central nervous system disorders such as anencephaly, diaphragmatic hernia, and cystic adenomatoid malformations, which compress the esophagus and interfere with swallowing.[1, 2] In addition, some cases are idiopathic in nature. Any pregnant woman with abnormalities of amniotic fluid should have a prenatal ultrasonography examination. Many of the above-noted lesions are detected on the sonogram and can be anticipated at the time of delivery, allowing early treatment and improved results.

Bilious vomiting is always pathologic, whether occurring in a neonate or an octogenarian. The presence of bile in the stomach at birth should be carefully investigated. A newborn infant's stomach usually contains less than 15 ml. of clear gastric juice at birth. Greater than 20 to 25 ml. of clear gastric juice or any bile may signify the presence of alimentary tract obstruction.[57, 122] Bilious vomiting may also occur in cases of neonatal sepsis with adynamic ileus. The presence of bile indicates that the level of obstruction is distal to the ampulla of Vater.

Abdominal distention is a sign of distal intestinal obstruction. The normal contour of a newborn's abdomen is round, unlike the usual scaphoid appearance of an adult's. Physical findings associated with distention include visible veins on the abdominal wall due to attenuation, visible loops of intestine *(intestinal patterning)* with or without noticeable peristalsis, and occasionally respiratory distress caused by elevation of the diaphragm. A recumbent and erect abdominal radiograph is obtained to evaluate the nature of the distention. Distention may be related to free air (perforated viscus), fluid (hemoperitoneum from birth injury, chyloperitoneum), or distended bowel (intestinal obstruction or adynamic ileus).

Failure to pass normal amounts of meconium in the first 24 hours of life is another cardinal sign of potential bowel obstruction. Normal meconium is composed of amniotic fluid and debris (squames, lanugo hairs), succus entericus, and intestinal mucus. Meconium is dark green or black in color and sticky in consistency, and up to 250 gm. may be passed per rectum. Failure to pass this material in the first day of life may be pathologic. Infants with Hirschsprung's disease, meconium plug syndrome, small left colon syndrome, and colonic neuronal dysplasia may present with failure to pass meconium. There are other causes, however, including intestinal pseudo-obstruction, sepsis with adynamic ileus, hypothyroidism, and being born to a narcotics addict.

Esophageal Atresia and TE Fistula

Infants with esophageal atresia frequently present with severe respiratory distress and excessive salivation. Choking, coughing, and cyanosis are often encountered on the first attempted feeding. Infants with an associated TE fistula may also develop acute gastric dilatation due to air entering the distal esophagus and stomach with each inspired breath. As most neonates have an incompetent lower esophageal sphincter, this ultimately leads to reflux of gastric acid through the fistula into the tracheobronchial tree, producing aspiration and chemical pneumonitis. There are five recognized anatomic variants of esophageal atresia (Fig. 38–1): proximal esophageal atresia with a distal TE fistula (Gross Type C—the most common variant, occurring in 85% of patients), proximal esophageal atresia without a TE fistula (Type A—8%), an *H-type* TE fistula without esophageal atresia (Type E—4%), proximal esophageal atresia with a proximal TE fistula (Type B—1%), and proximal esophageal atresia with a double (proximal and distal) TE fistula (Type D—2%).[80, 120] The incidence of this anomaly is 1:1500–3000 live births, with both sexes equally affected. Infants with esophageal atresia without a TE fistula have mothers with polyhydramnios. Approximately 33% of these infants are low birth weight, and 60 to 70% have associated anomalies (gastrointestinal, cardiac, genitourinary, musculoskeletal, and central nervous system). Cases of esophageal atresia have been noted in infants with Down's syndrome and trisomy 18. In addition, 10% of patients have the VATER association, an acronym for a nonhereditary concurrence of anomalies including vertebral or vascular defects, anal anomalies, TE fistula, esophageal atresia, and radial limb or renal anomalies. An alternative acronym is VACTERL (vertebral, anal, cardiac, tracheal, esophogeal, renal, and limb).

The diagnosis of esophageal atresia is not difficult to confirm. Attempted passage of a firm red-rubber catheter through each naris (to rule out choanal atresia) demonstrates the level of esophageal atresia by coming up against an obstruction. A frontal and lateral chest x-ray confirms the location of the tube in the blind proximal pouch. If gas is present in the gastrointestinal tract below the diaphragm, an associated TE fistula must also be present.[80, 122, 148] If no gas is seen below the diaphragm, a distal fistula is highly un-

ESOPHAGEAL ATRESIA
TE FISTULA

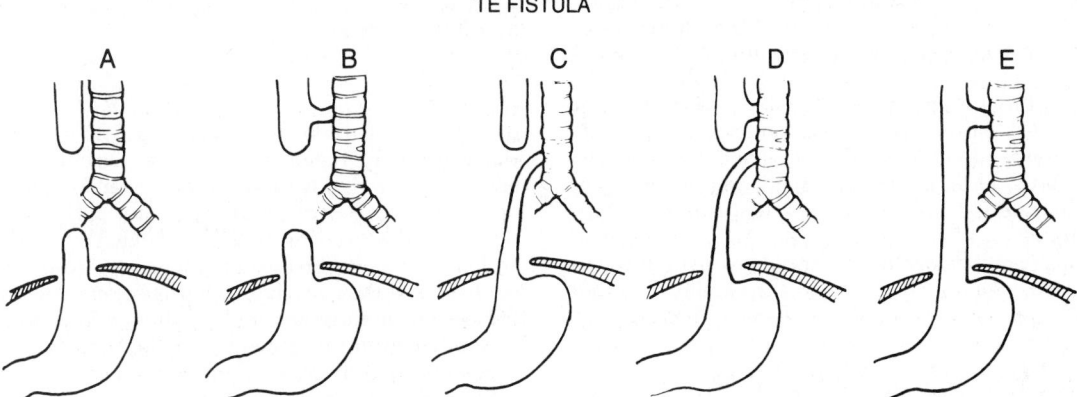

A   B   C   D   E

Figure 38–1. The five variants of esophageal atresia and tracheoesophageal (TE) fistula. Proximal atresia with a distal TE fistula (Type C) is the most common type observed.

likely.[37, 125] These simple observations yield a diagnosis in 95% of cases. Bronchoscopy usually demonstrates the fistula in cases of Type B, D, and E. Contrast studies with isosmolar sterile Omnipaque is an alternative but runs the risk of aspiration.

Emergency care of the infant includes insertion of a sump suction catheter in the proximal pouch, which is placed on constant suction to control oral secretions. The infant is evaluated for other associated anomalies by physical examination and ultrasonography studies of the heart, head, and kidneys. These studies should also note the location of the aortic arch (left or right). Parenteral antibiotics—ampicillin (100 to 200 mg. per kg. per day) and gentamycin (5 to 7 mg. per kg. per day)—are administered. Although the Waterston risk classification[165] was used for many years to determine the timing of operative therapy (immediate versus staged), more recent assessment of the physiologic status of neonates has refined these criteria; birth weight, gestational age, and pulmonary status—previously considered essential determinants—are now excluded.[40, 120, 143] Currently, therapy is more individualized. Infants with stable cardiac and respiratory status undergo immediate thoracotomy and repair.[40, 120] Anomalies that are not life-threatening and the presence of physiologic derangements that are easily correctable are included in the determination of stability. Intercostal retractions, oxygen requirements, endotracheal intubation, and minor pulmonary infiltrate are not considered absolute contraindications for immediate repair, as long as the infant is stable.[120]

The operation is performed through a right extrapleural thoracotomy in the fourth intercostal space. The procedure can be done through the left chest if there is a right aortic arch. The TE fistula is usually identified at the site where the azygous vein passes over the trachea to enter the superior vena cava. The azygous vein is divided between 4-0 silk ties, and the fistula is identified. The tracheal end is sutured with interrupted 5-0 silk or polypropylene suture. The tracheal suture line is covered with mediastinal pleura to reduce the risk of a recurrent TE fistula should an anastomotic leak occur. The proximal blind atretic esophageal pouch is identified and dissected superiorly into the neck (if possible) to attain adequate length. The dissection along the esophagotracheal plane must be done very cautiously to avoid entering the trachea and weakening the tracheal wall in an attempt to reduce the incidence of postoperative tracheomalacia. If there is an excessive gap between the two ends of the esophagus, a proximal circular myotomy (Livaditis technique) is performed 1 to 2 cm. above the blind end of the atresia, often resulting in a tension-free, end-to-end anastomosis accomplished with one layer of interrupted 4-0 absorbable Maxon or PDS suture with the knots on the outside (Fig. 38–2).[112, 140] In stable patients, a gastrostomy (which was once used in almost every patient with esophageal atresia and TE fistula) is avoided.[40, 120, 143] A high incidence of gastroesophageal reflux is noted in patients with esophageal atresia and may be enhanced by a Stamm gastrostomy.[19, 115] A small orogastric tube is passed through the anastomosis to drain the stomach postoperatively. A barium swallow is obtained on the sixth or seventh postoperative day to evaluate the anastomosis for a leak. If none is observed, oral feedings are initiated. The patient can usually be discharged in 7 to 10 days, barring complications.

Infants considered unstable are candidates for either delayed primary repair or staged repair. Instability is determined by the presence of significant cardiac defects with heart failure, sepsis, hyaline membrane disease, and pulmonary insufficiency due to aspiration pneumonia.[120] In these infants, the proximal atretic pouch is kept on suction and a temporary Stamm gastrostomy is inserted, often under local anesthesia, using 0.25% lidocaine without epinephrine. When

HAIGHT–TELESCOPIC ANASTOMOSIS

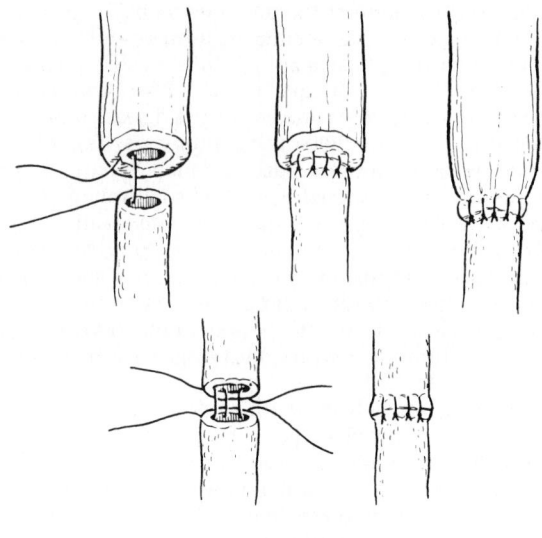

A   one-layer

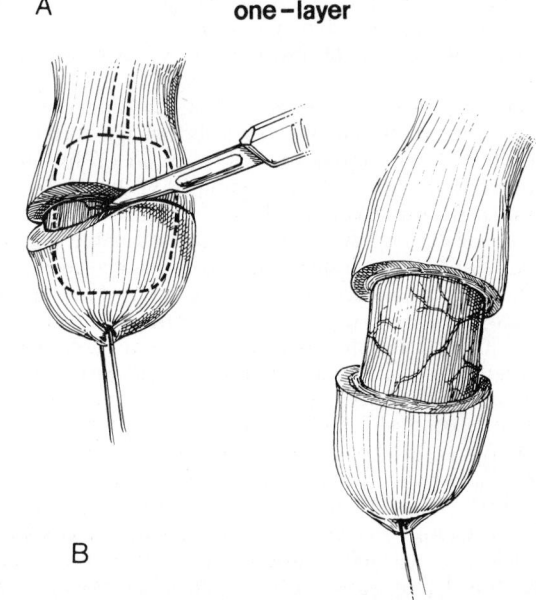

B

Figure 38–2. *A,* Primary anastomosis is accomplished using the telescopic technique described by Haight or a single-layer end-to-end anastomosis, which is favored by most surgeons in the current era. *B,* In instances of long gap atresia, a proximal esophagomyotomy may permit the safe performance of a primary anastomosis and avoid the need for esophageal replacement. (*B* from Ballantine, T. V. N.: Surgery of the esophagus. *In* Waldhausen, J. A., and Pierce, W. E. [Eds.]: Johnson's Surgery of the Chest, 5th ed. Chicago, Year Book Medical Publishers, 1985, p. 199.)

the underlying problems subside and the patient becomes stable, primary repair is performed as noted above. Some babies with severe cardiac anomalies and/or severe pulmonary compromise who need ventilator support may require staging and life-saving division of the TE fistula because of an inability to ventilate such infants due to air loss through the fistula. If they survive, they may eventually become candidates for thoracotomy and an attempted anastomosis.

Another group of patients that benefits from staging are those infants with Type A atresia without a TE fistula. These babies undergo a Stamm gastrostomy as newborns and daily dilatations of the atretic proximal pouch for 6 to 12 weeks. Some investigators suggest that the proximal segment will grow and extend further into the mediastinum without dilatations. Between dilatations, the proximal pouch is also kept on long-term suction. At thoracotomy, most of these infants require a single or double circular esophageal myotomy (or spiral myotomy) to achieve an end-to-end esophageal anastomosis.[100, 140, 143] This technique produces esophageal salvage and obviates the need for esophageal replacement procedures (gastric tube, colon interposition, or gastric pullup) in most patients. A few infants have an extra long gap between the two ends of the esophagus that cannot be brought together. Under these circumstances, the distal esophagus is at the level of the diaphragm. A proximal cervical esophagostomy is constructed between the heads of the sternocleidomastoid muscle on either the left side of the neck, if a gastric tube is contemplated, or the right side of the neck, if a substernal colon interposition is considered for later reconstruction.[37, 40, 126, 149]

In infants with an H-type TE fistula without atresia, the repair can often be performed through a cervical approach.[80] Division of the TE fistula is facilitated by endoscopic (bronchoscopic) passage of a small catheter through the fistula to aid in its intraoperative identification. Following division of the fistula, rotation of a strap muscle between the esophageal and tracheal suture lines promotes healing and avoids recurrence of the fistula.

Postoperative complications are common and include atelectasis, pneumonia, esophageal motility disorders, gastroesophageal reflux (25 to 50%), anastomotic stricture (15 to 30%), leak (10 to 20%), and tracheomalacia (8 to 15%).[40, 120] Due to the use of the extrapleural approach, a leak does not result in empyema, and spontaneous closure is the rule. Most strictures respond to esophageal dilatation, except if the anastomotic suture line is continually bathed with gastric acid due to significant gastroesophageal reflux. If the stricture is resistant to dilatation, an antireflux procedure should be performed. The most popular antireflux procedure is a loose, floppy Nissen fundoplication. Due to poor esophageal motility in instances of esophageal atresia, an antireflux operation occasionally results in a physiologic obstruction. In addition, the success rate of antireflux procedures is lower in infants with esophageal atresia. Survival is achieved in all good-risk patients who are considered stable at initial evaluation and in most patients (90 to 95%) who are staged. Deaths are attributed to severe cardiac defects, pulmonary insufficiency with end-stage bronchopulmonary dysplasia, and chromosomal disorders. Because of esophageal dysmotility, long-term follow-up is important.

Pyloric Atresia

Pyloric atresia accounts for 1% of all cases of alimentary tract obstruction. There may be a family occurrence, with cases observed in siblings and occasionally associated with epidermolysis bullosa. Maternal polyhydramnios is observed in more than 60% of cases.

These infants present with vomitus of clear gastric juice on any attempted feedings. Plain x-ray of the abdomen shows a single upper abdominal gas bubble, consistent with swallowed air in the stomach or a gastric air-fluid level. The infant may develop hypochloremic alkalosis from vomiting and loss of hydrochloric acid. An orogastric tube should be inserted to aspirate the stomach, prevent vomiting, and avoid the risk of aspiration. Intravenous fluids are administered to replete electrolytes and fluid losses from vomiting. When stable, the infant is taken to the operating room. The atretic lesion is most often a mucosal web. Excision of the prepyloric atretic web and a pyloroplasty is an efficacious procedure. Occasionally, the distal stomach and duodenum are separated, requiring a gastroduodenostomy. Postoperatively, an orogastric tube is left in place for gastric drainage until normal motility and appropriate gastric emptying are demonstrated.

Duodenal Obstruction

Duodenal atresia probably occurs during early intrauterine life. The most frequently encountered anomaly is an incontinuity mucosal atresia. Occasionally the two ends are separated by a small distance. In some cases, an intrinsic obstructive web has a *wind-sock* deformity. Obstruction may be complete (atresia) or incomplete (stenosis). In 85% of cases, the obstruction occurs just distal to the ampulla of Vater and presents with bilious vomiting.[122] In 15% of cases, however, the obstruction occurs proximal to the ampulla, and the infant may vomit clear gastric juice. Polyhydramnios is noted in 33 to 50% of cases, and the anomaly can be detected by prenatal ultrasonography examination. Infants with duodenal obstruction are often premature (40 to 50%), 33% have Down's syndrome, and 50 to 75% have associated anomalies, including cardiac, renal, and other gastrointestinal defects (esophageal atresia with TE fistula and imperforate anus).[60] At birth, the infant usually fails to tolerate attempted feeding. Bilious vomiting is observed and initiates a diagnostic evaluation. Plain x-ray of the abdomen demonstrates a *double-bubble*, with one air bubble in the stomach and the second in the duodenum proximal to the obstruction (Fig. 38–3). If atresia is present, no air is seen distal to the duodenum. However, if stenosis is present, some air is seen in the intestine beyond the duodenum. Contrast studies are usually not

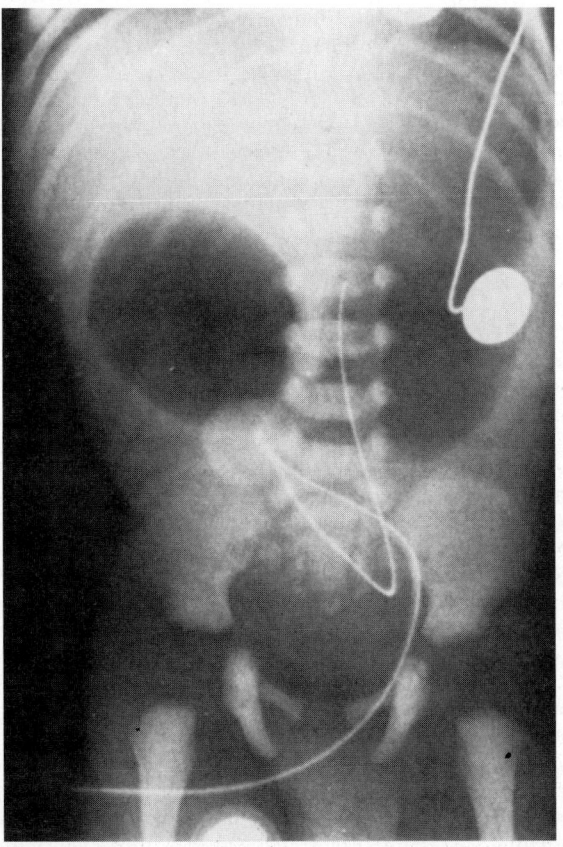

Figure 38–3. Plain roentgenogram of the abdomen demonstrates a *double-bubble* sign consistent with a diagnosis of duodenal obstruction. Air outlines the stomach and the first part of the duodenum. (From Rescorla, F. J., and Grosfeld, J. L.: Intestinal atresia and stenosis: Analysis of survival in 120 cases. Surgery, 98:668, 1985.)

necessary to confirm the diagnosis. An orogastric tube is passed into the stomach to decompress the area of obstruction and avoid aspiration. Fluid and electrolyte disturbances are corrected to replete any losses related to prior vomiting and dehydration. Antibiotics are administered, especially if the infant also has a cardiac anomaly. Ampicillin 100 mg. per kg. per day and gentamycin 5 to 7 mg. per kg. per day are given parenterally in divided doses. Peak and trough levels are obtained for the latter medication. During the preoperative preparation, a cardiac echogram and electrocardiogram are obtained and reviewed by a pediatric cardiologist.

When stable (usually within 24 to 48 hours), the infant undergoes laparotomy under general endotracheal anesthesia through a right upper quadrant transverse incision. The operation of choice is a duodenoduodenostomy to bypass the obstruction. In instances of wind-sock web, a duodenotomy and excision of the web at its takeoff is preferred. The ampulla should be identified in each case by gently compressing the gall bladder, which results in a jet of bile from the ampulla. The anastomosis is accomplished in either one or two layers of interrupted 5-0 silk sutures. An end-to-end or a diamond-shaped anastomosis is equally effective. At the time of the procedure, a small (8 to 10 French) red-rubber catheter should be passed distally to rule out a second mucosal web. Anular pancreas and/or malrotation are observed in 25 to 30% of cases. Although side-to-side duodenojejunostomy was a popular procedure in the past, this anastomosis is rarely indicated in the current era. When the proximal atretic duodenal pouch is grossly dilated, an antimesenteric tapering is a useful adjunct. Although gastrostomy was recommended in the past, a gastrostomy tube is now rarely used because of its potential role in causing gastroesophageal reflux and the risk of aspiration. An orogastric tube effectively decompresses the stomach until the anastomosis functions.

Postoperatively, the infant receives intravenous maintenance support with 100 ml. per kg. per day of 0.25% saline in 10% dextrose in water with 2 to 3 mg. per kg. per day of potassium chloride added. Antibiotics are given for 24 to 48 hours and then discontinued. Feedings are started when bowel movements are observed and the volume of gastric drainage is minimal. Half-strength, low-osmolar, small-curd formulas such as a soybean-based formula or quarter-strength Pregestamil are useful diets. When tolerated, the density and volume can be increased to full strength, 20 calories per ounce, in amounts adequate to deliver 120 calories per kg. per day. The current survival is 88 to 90%, with most deaths related to associated anomalies, particularly those affecting the cardiovascular system. There are some late complications, including gastroesophageal reflux and delayed gastric emptying. Duodenal stenosis presents with a partial obstruction and may not be detected until beyond the newborn period. Poor eating habits, bilious vomiting, and failure to thrive are often observed. Plain abdominal x-rays often show dilatation of the stomach and proximal duodenum, with some air noted distally. Duodenal stenosis may be due to anular pancreas, malrotation with Ladd's bands (incomplete rotation and fixation), an anterior portal vein, or a mucosal web with a small diaphragm. The preparation and operative treatment are similar to that noted above for duodenal atresia.

Jejunoileal Atresia and Stenosis

Small bowel atresia is related to a late mesenteric vascular accident, as a result of intrauterine volvulus, malrotation, internal hernia, intussusception, and strangulation in a tight abdominal wall defect (e.g. gastroschisis and omphalocele). Atresias occur slightly more commonly in the jejunum than in the ileum. Most are single, but in 10 to 15% of cases,

multiple atresias are observed. Ten to 12% of cases occur in infants with cystic fibrosis, which suggests that a sweat chloride determination should be obtained prior to hospital discharge. The pathologic findings are classified as Type I, a mucosal web or diaphragm (which may be due to epithelial plugging); Type II, in which an atretic cord exists between two blind ends of the bowel with an intact mesentery; Type IIIa, in which there is a complete separation of the blind ends of the bowel by a V-shaped mesenteric *gap* defect; Type IIIb, which represents an apple-peel or Christmas tree deformity in which the distal bowel receives a retrograde blood supply from the ileocolic or right colic artery; and Type IV or multiple atresias, which are often characterized by a *string-of-sausage* appearance (Fig. 38–4).[53]

Jejunal Atresia

High jejunal atresia usually presents with bilious vomiting and three to four loops of air- and fluid-filled bowel on plain abdominal x-ray. A history of polyhydramnios may be elicited in 35% of cases. These patients are often full-term infants and have fewer associated anomalies than babies with duodenal atresia. Jaundice is noted in as many as 40% of cases. An orogastric tube is inserted into the stomach, and fluid and electrolyte repletion is accomplished with administration of parenteral electrolyte solution. Fluid resuscitation is accomplished within a short time, and exploratory laparotomy should be carried out in an expeditious fashion. Operation is performed through a right upper quadrant transverse incision. The proximal dilated atretic segment is often atonic and should be resected back to the ligament of Treitz (in instances with near-normal bowel length), where an end-to-end anastomosis is performed. The distal bowel should be evaluated for additional atresias or stenosis by passage of a soft red-rubber catheter or by injection of saline. In patients with short bowel syndrome due to a volvulus, the proximal

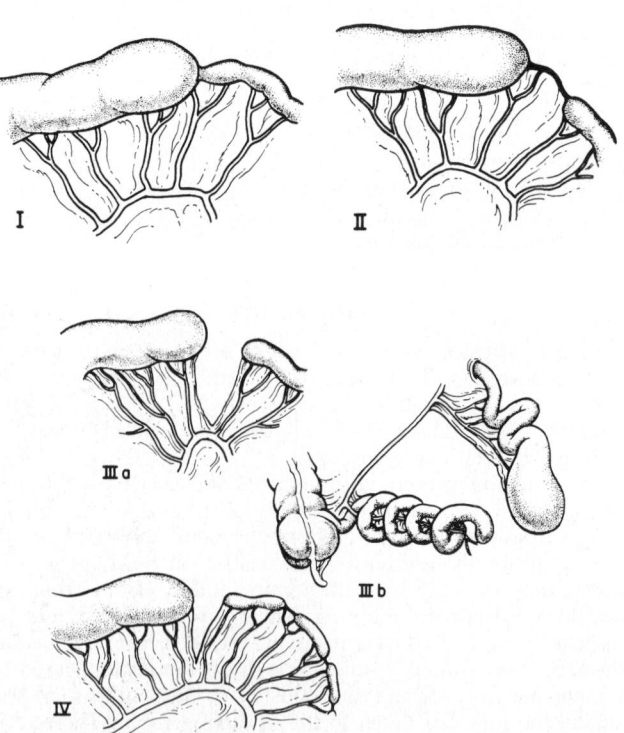

Figure 38–4. Classification of jejunoileal atresia. The most common type of atresia noted was Type IIIa gap defect. (From Grosfeld, J. L., et al.: Operative management of intestinal atresia based on pathologic findings. J. Pediatr. Surg., *14*:368, 1979.)

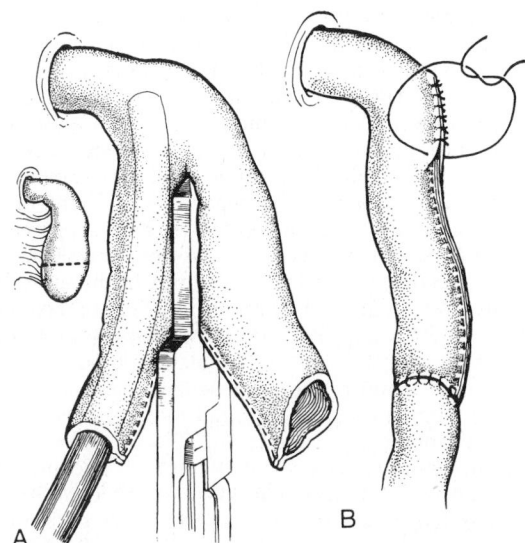

Figure 38–5. The technique employed in the performance of a tapering jejunostomy in cases of proximal jejunal atresia. (From Grosfeld, J. L., et al.: Operative management of intestinal atresia based on pathologic findings. J. Pediatr. Surg., *14*:368, 1979.)

atretic segment can be preserved by performing an antimesenteric tapering enteroplasty. Disparity in the size of the dilated proximal bowel and the smaller distal end may be alleviated by an end-to-oblique interrupted 5-0 silk anastomosis (Fig. 38–5). Anastomotic function may be delayed for 7 to 10 days. The stomach is kept decompressed by an orogastric tube. Nutritional support is accomplished with postoperative parenteral nutrition using glucose (17 to 18%), amino acids (2.5%), and intralipids (4 gm. per kg. per day) until bowel function is restored. When bowel motions occur and clear gastric juice with low volume is noted, the orogastric tube can be removed and diet instituted. A low-osmolar, small-curd, easily absorbed formula such as Pregestamil or a soybean-based formula can be used. Feedings are increased in both density and volume as tolerated. Most modern infant formulas contain adequate vitamin and iron supplements. For some formulas, that do not contain supplements, iron must be administered on a daily basis for the first year of life (0.6 ml. Fer-in-sol per day). In instances of short bowel syndrome, special formulas and drip feedings may be re-

quired in addition to long-term total parenteral nutrition to ensure adequate caloric intake for growth.

Ileal Atresia

Infants with ileal atresia frequently present with abdominal distention, bilious vomiting, and failure to pass meconium. Erect and recumbent abdominal radiographs demonstrate many dilated intestinal loops, often with air-fluid levels. The atretic loop may be much larger than the other loops of bowel. Since haustral markings are not present on the plain abdominal x-ray of a neonate, a barium enema must be performed in each case of low intestinal obstruction. The first enema the newborn baby receives is a barium enema. Preparation of the colon for this study is not necessary. The barium enema discerns between small intestine and colonic distention, determines if the colon is used or unused (microcolon), and therefore identifies the level of obstruction (e.g., small bowel or colon) and evaluates the position of the cecum in regard to possible anomalies of intestinal rotation and fixation.[122] Occasionally, areas of calcification are seen on the abdominal radiographs and signifies the presence of meconium peritonitis. This is a sign of intrauterine bowel perforation (12% of cases). The sterile fetal meconium results in an intense local inflammatory reaction and eventually becomes calcified. The two most common causes of low small bowel obstruction in newborns are ileal atresia and meconium ileus.

On plain abdominal x-ray, infants with ileal atresia have dilated intestine with air-fluid levels, and the atretic loop is often much larger than the other bowel. Barium enema usually shows a microcolon (unused), limiting the obstruction to the small bowel (Fig. 38–6A and B). The majority of patients have Type IIIa pathology, and when reasonably normal bowel length is preserved, operative management includes resection of the dilated atretic loop and an interrupted 5-0 silk end-to-oblique anastomosis (Fig. 38–6C). At the time of the procedure, the distal bowel should be checked for additional areas of atresia or stenosis. This can be demonstrated by injecting saline into the distal bowel. In cases associated with short bowel syndrome, a tapering ileostomy is performed to preserve an intestinal length compatible with survival. In the presence of severe peritonitis or when bowel viability is in question, a temporary enterostomy may be required. Infants with ileal atresia who have an intact ileocecal valve have better absorptive capability and survival than those in whom the ileocecal valve is resected. This is proba-

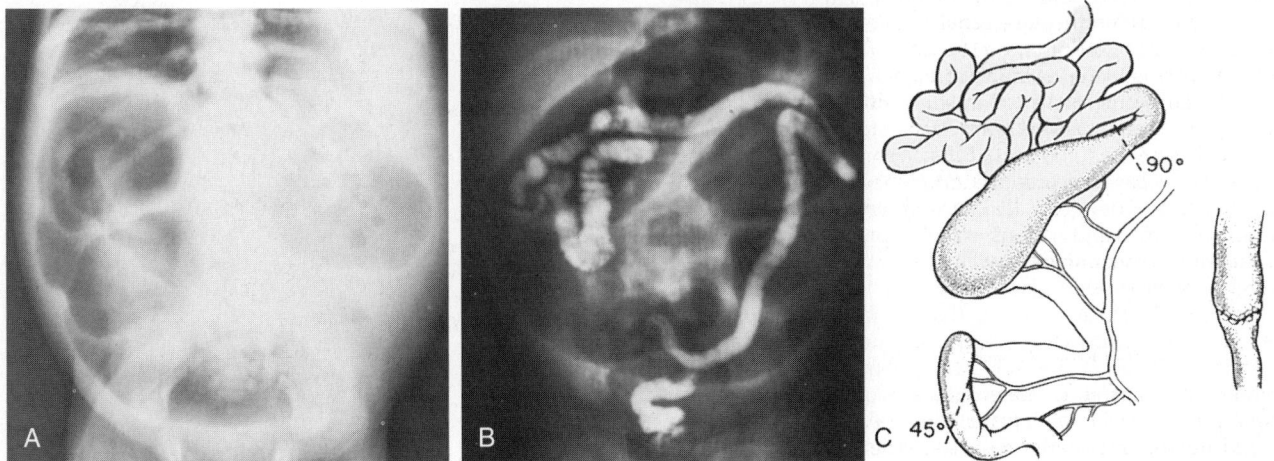

Figure 38–6. *A,* Flat plate of abdomen shows distended intestine. *B,* Barium enema demostrates a microcolon in an infant with ileal atresia. *C,* The technique for an end-to-oblique anastomosis of the ileum. (From Grosfeld, J. L., et al.: Operative management of intestinal atresia based on pathologic findings. J. Pediatr. Surg., *14*:368, 1979.)

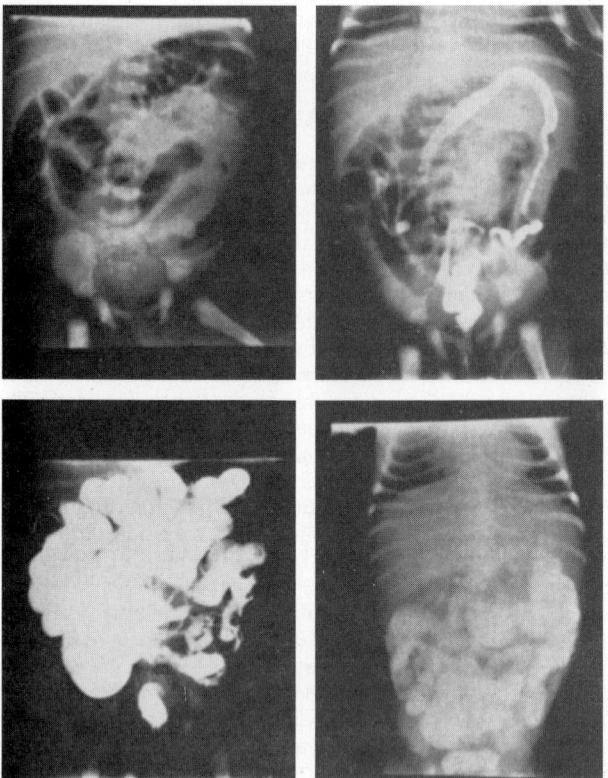

Figure 38–7. Composite of abdominal roentgenograms demonstrating the diagnosis and successful treatment of uncomplicated meconium ileus using a hypertonic Gastrografin enema. (From Rescorla, F. J., et al.: Changing patterns of treatment and survival in neonates with meconium ileus. Arch. Surg., *124*:837, 1989. Copyright 1989, American Medical Association.)

bly related to improved fat and vitamin B_{12} absorption and an improved enterohepatic circulation of bile from the distal ileum rather than to the valve itself.

Meconium Ileus

Meconium ileus is a unique form of congenital obstruction that occurs in 10 to 15% of infants born with cystic fibrosis.[106, 107, 111] A deficiency of pancreatic enzymes and an abnormality in the composition of the meconium are responsible for the presence of the solid meconium concretions that cause an obturator form of obstruction. A careful family history should be obtained at the time of birth. The cystic fibrosis transmembrane conductance regulator gene has been identified on the long arm of chromosome 7q, and the delta F508 mutation at this locus is responsible for 70% of the abnormal genes.[43] The occurrence of low small bowel obstruction in identical twins is almost always due to meconium ileus. Infants present with abdominal distention, bilious vomiting, and failure to pass meconium. Certain abdominal x-ray findings may help distinguish ileal atresia from meconium ileus. Babies with meconium ileus often demonstrate significant dilatation of similar-sized bowel loops, with few, if any, air-fluid levels. A ground-glass appearance in the right lower quadrant (Neuhauser's sign or the *soap-bubble* sign) may be observed and represents viscid meconium mixed with air.[107, 124] Although this is not pathognomonic of meconium ileus (it is also seen in some cases of colon atresia), it is a frequent finding. Barium enema commonly demonstrates an unused microcolon similar to cases of ileal atresia; however, reflux of contrast material into the distal ileum may identify the small obstructive intraluminal concretions characteristic of this hereditary disorder.

The treatment of meconium ileus depends on whether it is uncomplicated (simple obturator obstruction) or complicated by atresia, volvulus, perforation, or giant cystic meconium peritonitis.[20, 73, 124] The treatment of choice in cases of uncomplicated meconium ileus is nonoperative clearance of the obstructive intraluminal meconium pellets using a Gastrografin enema.[107, 124] This radiopaque substance allows direct visualization under fluoroscopic control while its hypertonicity draws fluid into the bowel lumen that separates the abnormal meconium pellets from the bowel wall, causing relief of obstruction (Fig. 38–7). This form of therapy causes significant fluid shifts and requires infusion of crystalloid and/or colloid during the procedure to prevent hypovolemia. Careful attention to fluid balance, blood pressure, pulse rate, and urine output is essential. Occasionally, the Gastrografin enema must be repeated to relieve the obstruction. This technique is successful in 50% of uncomplicated cases. Unsuccessful nonoperative attempts in uncomplicated cases and all cases of meconium ileus with complications require operative intervention. The procedure currently favored in uncomplicated cases is intraoperative irrigation of the viscid meconium and clearing of the obstructive pellets through an enterotomy.[73, 124] The bowel is irrigated with saline and dilute Hypaque or Gastrografin, which lowers the viscosity of the meconium, flushes the debris, and relieves the obstruction by washing the pellets into the colon, where evacuation follows (Fig. 38–8). This procedure obviates the need for enterotomy in most uncomplicated cases and avoids a second operation (e.g., enterostomy closure). The Bishop-Koop enterostomy or double-barrel enterostomy, which were popular methods of treatment in the past, are rarely necessary in the present era.[12] Avoidance of an enterostomy facilitates early discharge from the hospital and reduces the risk of hospital-acquired cross-infection. In instances of meconium ileus complicated by atresia, volvulus, perforation, or gangrenous bowel, bowel resection and anastomosis or temporary enterostomy is required. Gastrografin enema is contraindicated in these cases.

After correction of the obstruction, careful family counseling and parental instruction regarding diet, enzyme replacement, and pulmonary toilet using percussion and postural drainage are important components in the overall care of

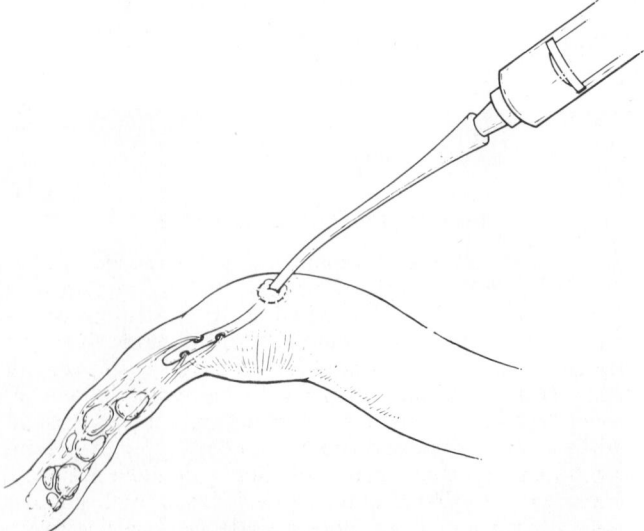

Figure 38–8. The technique of intraoperative enterotomy and catheter irrigation of the obstructing meconium pellets. (From Rescorla, F. J., et al.: Changing patterns of treatment and survival in neonates with meconium ileus. Arch. Surg., *124*:837, 1989. Copyright 1989, American Medical Association.)

these patients. The survival for this condition has improved dramatically in recent years, with more than 90% of patients currently surviving the neonatal period.

Long-term follow-up is essential. In addition to the occurrence of severe chronic pulmonary disease, these children are at risk of developing meconium ileus equivalent as a result of poor enzyme compliance and decreased fluid intake during episodes of infection. This results in severe intraluminal obstruction with inspissated fecal material that mimics the findings of meconium ileus in neonates. Recognition of this late complication of cystic fibrosis allows for nonoperative intervention with either a Gastrografin swallow or enema. Operation can be avoided in most cases. Recently, colonic strictures have been identified in children with cystic fibrosis, related to the use of high-density enteric-coated pancreatic replacement. These patients require colon resection.

COLONIC OBSTRUCTION

Causes of colon obstruction in neonates include meconium plug syndrome, aganglionic megacolon (Hirschsprung's disease), colon atresia, small left colon syndrome, neuronal colonic dysplasia, intestinal pseudo-obstruction, and the various presentations of imperforate anus.

Colon Atresia

Colon atresia as an isolated entity (unassociated with imperforate anus or cloacal exstrophy) is relatively uncommon. Failure to pass meconium in the first 24 hours of life, abdominal distention, and bilious vomiting are the usual clinical manifestations.[122] Infants with colon atresia are usually full term and rarely have associated anomalies. Erect and recumbent abdominal radiographs demonstrate dilated intestine with air-fluid levels. The atretic loop often has a soap-bubble appearance due to the admixture of meconium and air. Diagnosis is confirmed by barium enema, which demonstrates a blind-ending distal end of a microcolon and dilated air-filled loops of proximal intestine. Most cases occur in the transverse colon and are type IIIa atresias with a V-shaped gap between the atretic ends, probably caused by a vascular injury (volvulus) to the mesentery. The sigmoid colon is the second most common site of colon atresia. Type I mucosal atresia has also been noted in the colon. Colon atresia is treated with a preliminary colostomy in the newborn period and subsequent closure with anastomosis at age 3 to 6 months. All 12 infants with isolated colon atresia treated at the author's institution in this fashion have survived. Other reports concerning colon atresia recommend primary anastomosis for right-sided lesions and a temporary colostomy for atresia affecting the sigmoid colon.

Meconium Plug Syndrome

The meconium plug syndrome was first described in 1956. The exact etiology is unknown and is thought to be related to some factor or factors that dehydrate the meconium. Meconium plug syndrome is unrelated to meconium ileus and in the vast majority of cases is not a sequela of cystic fibrosis. Although an occasional infant with meconium plug syndrome has a positive sweat chloride determination consistent with cystic fibrosis, most do not.[111, 133] Infants typically present with significant abdominal distention and failure to pass meconium in the first 24 hours of life. Plain abdominal radiographs demonstrate many loops of distended bowel with air-fluid levels. Barium enema shows a microcolon extending up to the descending or transverse colon, at which point the colon becomes dilated and copious intraluminal material (thick meconium plug) is observed. The barium enema is often both diagnostic and therapeutic. Following instillation of the contrast material, large pieces of inspissated meconium plugs are passed and the obstruction is completely relieved. Occasionally, a second enema (usually using Gastrografin) is required to effect a complete evacuation of the thickened meconium. If any signs of obstruction recur, aganglionic megacolon must be considered as the cause of these symptoms. Five percent of cases of Hirschsprung's disease present with a clinical picture of meconium plug syndrome in the neonatal period. Under these circumstances, a screening submucosal suction biopsy should be performed, and the tissues should be examined for the presence or absence of ganglion cells. In premature infants, meconium plugging has been noted in the distal small bowel, producing bowel obstruction.

Aganglionic Megacolon (Hirschsprung's Disease)

Aganglionic megacolon is a neurogenic form of intestinal obstruction in which there is an absence of ganglion cells in the myenteric (Auerbach's) and submucosal (Meissner's) plexuses. Hypertrophic nerve fibers are often observed. The absence of parasympathetic innervation causes a failure of relaxation of the internal anal sphincter. Abnormalities in purinergic and peptidergic fibers and nitric oxide synthase deficiency have also been observed. Aganglionosis begins at the anorectal line and in 80% of cases involves the rectosigmoid area; it extends proximal to the splenic flexure in 10% of cases, and the entire colon and distal ileum or more proximal small bowel may be involved in 10% of cases.[125] Relatively rare cases of total aganglionosis of the entire gastrointestinal tract have also been reported. Three to 5% of patients have Down's syndrome. Hirschsprung's disease has a definite family history. If the first infant in a family had rectosigmoid involvement, the risk of a second child being born with Hirschsprung's disease is approximately 6%. The incidence of a second child having Hirschsprung's disease in cases in which the first infant had total colonic aganglionosis is 12%. An abnormal locus on the tenth chromosome has been identified in some families. Eighty percent of affected infants are boys; in cases of total colonic aganglionosis, 35% are girls. Occasionally, this condition occurs with other neurocristopathies, including Ondine's curse (sleep apnea), Von Waardenburg's syndrome, and neuroblastoma.[134]

Most infants with Hirschsprung's disease are symptomatic at birth. More than 95% present with delayed passage of meconium in the first 24 hours of life. Almost all babies with aganglionosis are full-term babies with an average birth weight greater than 3 kg. Abdominal distention and bilious vomiting are other presenting findings. Abdominal distention is often severe, with obvious dilated loops of bowel visible on the abdominal wall (intestinal patterning). In some instances (10 to 15% of cases), the infants may have severe diarrhea alternating with constipation. This diarrhea is known as the enterocolitis of Hirschsprung's disease and is associated with colonic ulceration and an increased morbidity and mortality. Erect and recumbent abdominal radiographs demonstrate many dilated loops of bowel. A barium enema is performed in each suspected case of aganglionic megacolon. This contrast study usually demonstrates that the colon is slightly dilated; however, in most newborns, there is no definitive cutoff point indicating the transition zone where the narrow distal aganglionic rectum or rectosigmoid meets the obstructed dilated normal proximal colon containing ganglion cells. It may take 3 to 6 weeks for the transition zone to become apparent in some cases. Unlike normal newborns who evacuate the contrast from a barium enema in 10 to 18 hours, infants with Hirschsprung's disease retain the barium for 24 to 48 hours. This observation emphasizes the importance of obtaining a delayed (>24 hours) follow-up abdominal x-ray.[125] A transition zone may be seen more clearly on the delayed x-ray. In older babies, the transition zone is usually appreciated on the initial barium study. The barium enema may look entirely normal in babies with short segment disease affecting only the rectum and demonstrates a comma-shaped rectosigmoid, flattened flexures, and occasionally a microcolon in instances of total colonic aganglionosis.

The differential diagnosis of Hirschsprung's disease includes hypothyroidism, meconium plug syndrome, colonic neuronal dysplasia, adynamic ileus associated with sepsis, intestinal pseudo-obstruction, and being born to a narcotics addict. These conditions are also associated with delayed passage of meconium at birth. The diagnosis of Hirschsprung's disease is confirmed by obtaining a rectal biopsy. A submucosal suction biopsy is adequate in more than 90% of cases. Ganglion cells are either identified or absent in the Meissner's submucosal plexus. This determination must be done with permanent stains and is usually not amenable to frozen-section techniques. In more emergent circumstances, a definitive diagnosis requires a full-thickness operative rectal biopsy that can be evaluated for the presence or absence of ganglion cells in Auerbach's myenteric plexus by frozen-section technique. If no ganglion cells are seen on at least 10 sections, the diagnosis of Hirschsprung's disease is confirmed. Acetylcholinesterase (Ach) staining is also a useful diagnostic tool. Increased Ach staining of neurofibrils is characteristic of Hirschsprung's disease. Anorectal manometry may be a useful diagnostic adjunct. This technique measures the anorectal intraluminal pressure with a balloon probe connected to a pressure transducer and polygraph recorder. In infants with Hirschsprung's disease, this study usually demonstrates an absent rectoanal inhibitory reflex, indicating a lack of relaxation of the internal sphincter, characteristic of aganglionosis.

Although some surgeons recommend a one-stage pull-through procedure in the first few weeks of life, most consider the treatment of choice in the neonatal period to be a temporary decompressing colostomy at least 10 cm. proximal to the transition zone. This site is evaluated at the time of operation for the presence of ganglion cells on frozen section to avoid placing the stoma in obstructed aganglionic bowel. If there are no ganglion cells present in the sigmoid colon, a biopsy is obtained in the transverse colon. If there are no ganglion cells noted there, the appendix should be removed. If no ganglion cells are noted in the appendix, the disease process extends into the small bowel and the biopsy process continues until ganglion cells are identified. At 6 months to 1 year of age, a definitive pull-through procedure using the Soave (endorectal), modified Duhamel (retrorectal), or Swenson (rectosigmoidectomy) procedure may be performed in infants with rectosigmoid disease. The choice of procedure is up to the pediatric surgeon in charge of the case. All these operations are acceptable procedures, with the Soave and Duhamel being the most popular currently. In cases of total colonic aganglionosis, the pull-through procedure may be delayed until 18 months of age. Many pediatric surgeons favor the modified Duhamel operation for total colonic aganglionosis. When the aganglionic process extends proximal to the mid–small bowel, a vascularized antimesenteric aganglionic patch of right colon has been a useful adjunct to aid fluid absorption and slow transit time.[90, 93] The extended side-to-side Martin modification of the *long* Duhamel procedure, which employed the entire aganglionic colon in a side-to-side anastomosis with the distal small bowel, has been abandoned because of a significant complication rate associated with this technique, particularly recurring enterocolitis. In rare cases of aganglionosis affecting the entire small bowel, an extensive

enteromyotomy and myectomy as advocated by Ziegler and associates may result in relief of obstruction.[173] Infants with extensive aganglionosis extending into the proximal small intestine almost always require total parenteral nutrition to achieve adequate caloric intake.

The survival of babies with Hirschsprung's disease has improved significantly in the past decade. Rare deaths occur in infancy due to delays in diagnosis complicated by enterocolitis and sepsis and in instances of total colonic aganglionosis with significant proximal extension into the small intestine. Many of the deaths have been observed in babies with Down's syndrome. Infants who present with enterocolitis preoperatively are more likely to have this complication postoperatively following both colostomy and pull-through procedures. Overall, survival is achieved in more than 90% of cases. Long-term follow-up is important. Most patients (more than 96%) are continent, but soiling is a problem in 2 to 3% of cases; rarely (in 1%), incontinence is observed. Some patients (10 to 20%) may have constipation, but this can usually be improved with a high-fiber diet and stool softeners. Most children with postoperative symptoms improve with age.[125]

ANORECTAL ANOMALIES

There is a wide spectrum of anorectal anomalies that fit under the general category of anal atresia, imperforate anus, and rectal atresia. In 1984, an important symposium was held that led to a unified international classification of these anomalies, called the Wingspread classification (Table 38–3).[145] Anal atresia refers to an inappropriate ascent of the proctodeum, resulting in a thin, veil-like membrane covering the normal anal canal and residing within the normal sphincter. This is treated simply by puncturing the skin membrane that is often seen bulging with meconium. Anal dilatations avoid the need for any extensive surgical procedures. Anorectal anomalies can be classified as low, intermediate, or high, according to whether the rectal atresia has descended below the puborectalis sling, is at the level of the puborectalis, or remains above that level.[34, 145, 158]

Eighty-five to 90% of infants with imperforate anus and rectal atresia have an associated fistulous tract originating from the rectal segment. In males, the fistulous tract is usually to the perineum (low lesion) or to the verumontanum of the urethra (intermediate or high). Anal atresia with a perineal fistula can be treated definitively in the neonatal period with a *cutback* perineal Y-V anoplasty. Infants with rectal atresia and a fistula to the urethra are best managed with a diverting sigmoid colostomy in the neonatal period with a subsequent posterior sagittal anorectoplasty (as advocated by Peña) performed between 6 and 12 months of age (Figs. 38–9 and 38–10).[34, 35, 117] In girls, a variety of anomalies are observed. Anal atresia with a rectoperineal fistula can be repaired in a neonate by performing a perineal Y-V anoplasty. Rectal atresia with a rectofourchette fistula (to the fourchette of the vagina), an intermediate-level lesion, can be treated by transplantation of the fistula to a site within the circular fibers of the external sphincter.[103, 158] The timing of the procedure varies according to the surgeon's choice. Although this could be accomplished in the neonatal period, the preferred method involves gently dilating the fistula on a daily basis to maintain evacuation of feces, and then performing a transplant anoplasty at age 3 to 6 months when the tissues are firmer. Transplantation of the fistula allows preservation of the perineal body and an improved perineal appearance. Separation of the rectal and vaginal openings by the perineal body reduces the risk of urinary tract infection and vaginal soiling. If the tissues seem fragile at the time of the repair, a backup colostomy to divert the fecal stream may facilitate

TABLE 38–3. Wingspread Classification of Anorectal Anomalies

Level	Female	Male
High	Anorectal agenesis with rectovaginal fistula	Anorectal agenesis with rectoprostatitis, urethral fistula
	Rectal atresia	Rectal atresia
Intermediate	Rectovestibular fistula	Rectobulbar urethral fistula
	Rectovaginal fistula	
	Anal agenesis without fistula	Anal agenesis without fistula
Low	Anovestibular fistula	Anocutaneous fistula
	Anocutaneous fistula	Anal stenosis*
	Anal stenosis*	
	Cloacal malformations	
	Rare malformations	Rare malformations

*Previously called "covered anus."
From Smith, E. D.: The bath water needs changing but don't throw out the baby: An overview of anorectal anomalies. J. Pediatr. Surg., *22*:335, 1988.

healing and avoid breakdown of the repair. Alternatively, a colostomy can be performed in the neonatal period, using the posterior sagittal technique of Peña to repair the fourchette fistula. Girls with intermediate or high rectal atresia and rectovaginal fistula or a cloaca require a colostomy in the neonatal period.[102, 103, 158] Subsequent division of the fistula and posterior sagittal anorectoplasty are performed at 6 to 12 months of age. The colostomy is left in place postoperatively in both boys and girls until adequate healing of the anoplasty has occurred and the anoplasty site is dilated to a 13 to 14 Hegar dilator size.[158] This is usually accomplished in 3 to 6 months.

The operations performed on children with imperforate anus should be carried out by pediatric surgeons with considerable expertise in the management of these cases. The first operation is the most important, and there is no room for error. Infants undergoing perineal anoplasty in the newborn period usually develop good external sphincter tone and have a bright outlook for developing continence. The higher the rectal atresia, the worse the potential outcome of the operation in terms of obtaining fecal continence. Long-term care and follow-up are required in such patients, and their families must be carefully counseled not to expect the normal progression of bowel training in these children. If the puborectalis sling and deep and superficial fibers of the external sphincter are preserved at the time of the pull-through procedure, many of these children have a reasonable chance of obtaining socially acceptable continence. This may not be achieved, however, until a stage of maturity is reached (6 to 9 years) that allows the child to voluntarily participate in his or her attempts to stay clean and avoid fecal odor at school or during play. Abnormal motility in the rectal segment, causing severe obstipation, may also be a late problem. Perfect continence may never be achieved due to the absence or

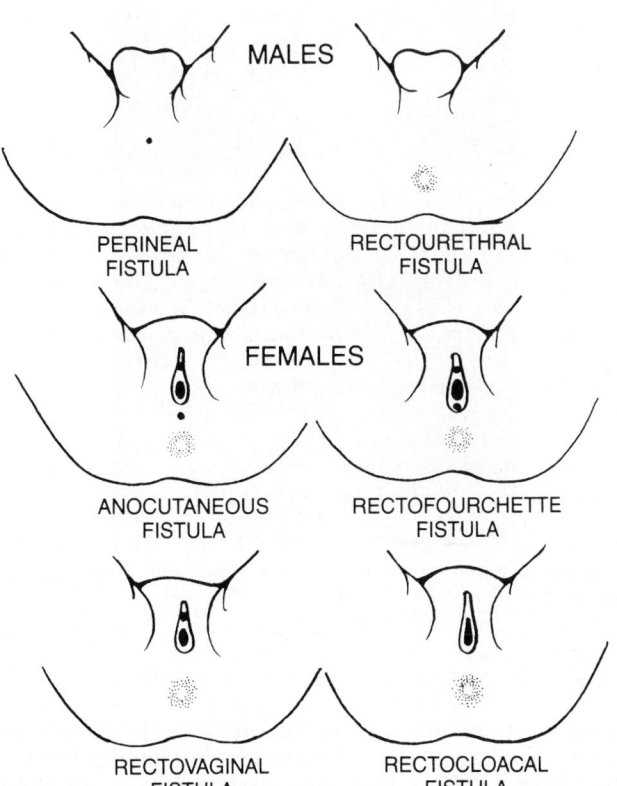

Figure 38–9. Perineal appearance of anorectal anomalies in boys and girls. (From Grosfeld, J. L.: Anorectal malformations. *In* Zuidema, G., and Condon, R. E. (Eds.): Surgery of the Alimentary Tract, 3rd ed. Vol. 4. Philadelphia, W. B. Saunders, 1990.)

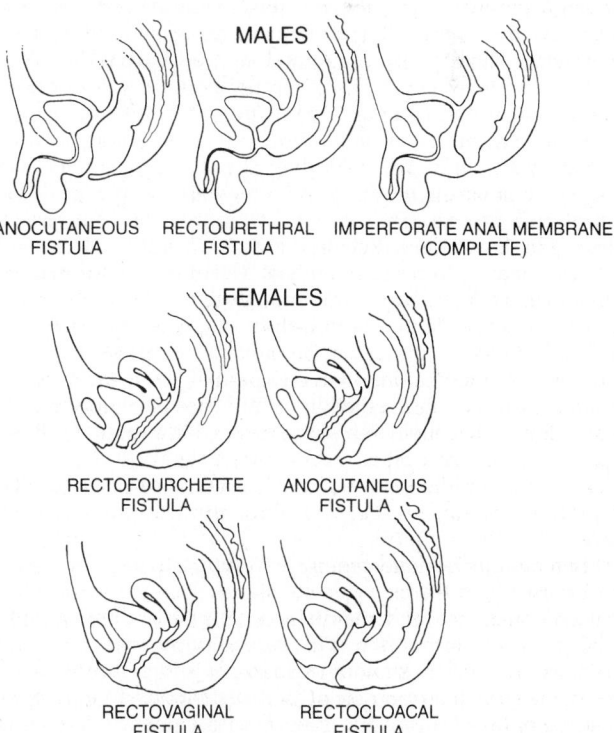

Figure 38–10. Lateral view of pelvis demonstrating the anorectal anomalies of boys and girls. (From Grosfeld, J. L.: Anorectal anomalies. *In* Zuidema, G., and Condon, R. E. (Eds.): Surgery of the Alimentary Tract, 3rd ed. Vol. 4. Philadelphia, W. B. Saunders, 1990.)

deficiency of a true internal sphincter component in many of these patients, and some require a system of morning enema washouts to stay clean.

Many children with imperforate anus have sacral vertebral anomalies and/or associated spinal dysraphic syndromes (30%) that may not be detected until they are older.[86, 160] These anomalies are best detected by magnetic resonance imaging (MRI) of the spinal canal and pelvic musculature. Neural contribution to continence is also quite important and must be thoroughly evaluated in problematic cases. Infants with imperforate anus have a high rate of associated anomalies in other systems. A careful system review involving other areas of the gastrointestinal tract (looking for esophageal atresia, duodenal atresia), cardiovascular system, musculoskeletal system, genitourinary tract, and central nervous system should be carried out early to delineate these problems and initiate treatment before they get out of hand and cause the unnecessary demise of the patient.

NECROTIZING ENTEROCOLITIS

Necrotizing enterocolitis (NEC) is a life-threatening intra-abdominal condition affecting 1 to 2% of patients admitted to most neonatal intensive care facilities. The vast majority of cases occur in premature and low-birth-weight infants. The exact etiology is unknown, but a number of conditions seem to predispose to the onset of this potentially catastrophic illness. These include shock, hypoxia, respiratory distress syndrome, apneic episodes, sepsis, polycythemia, hyperviscosity, exchange transfusions, patent ductus arteriosus, hyperosmolar feedings, and cyanotic heart disease.[24, 58] The common underlying pathophysiologic insult involves splanchnic vasoconstriction, diminished splanchnic perfusion, mucosal ischemic injury, gut immaturity, and probable bacterial translocation and invasion.[58] Symptoms and signs include increased gastric residuals with gavage feedings, abdominal distention, vomiting (often bilious), lethargy, occult or gross rectal bleeding, fever or in some instances hypothermia (<96.5° F. [35.8° C.]), abdominal mass, abdominal wall erythema, oliguria, jaundice, and apnea-bradycardia. Any evidence of these signs or symptoms should result in cessation of attempted feedings and a prompt evaluation. These observations can be accompanied by a variety of abdominal radiographic findings, including fixed dilated intestinal loops, pneumatosis intestinalis, portal vein air, free fluid (ascites), and free air (Fig. 38–11). Laboratory data frequently show a leukocytosis with a shift to the left on the differential smear, anemia, hypoalbuminemia, electrolyte disturbances, metabolic acidosis, hyper- or hypoglycemia, and a progressive decrease in the platelet count. In some instances, disseminated intravascular coagulation may also be present. Resuscitation of the patient involves cessation of feedings, insertion of an orogastric tube, repletion of intravascular volume with crystalloid and colloid infusions, ventilator support as indicated, acquisition of blood cultures, parenteral administration of systemic antibiotics (ampicillin, gentamycin, and clindamycin), blood transfusion, and platelet transfusion as necessary.

Some infants respond promptly to supportive therapy with an improvement in their general status. They are kept without enteral intake and maintained on gastric drainage and antibiotics and supported with parenteral nutrition for 7 to 10 days. If serial abdominal radiographs show improvement of the pneumatosis and decreased distention, nonoperative therapy is often successful. Infants with evidence of free air on abdominal radiographs, abdominal wall erythema (consistent with perforation and abscess), and/or the presence of an abdominal mass require operative intervention. In addition, infants started on nonoperative therapy who demonstrate

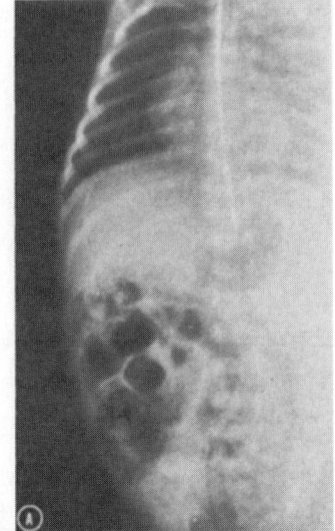

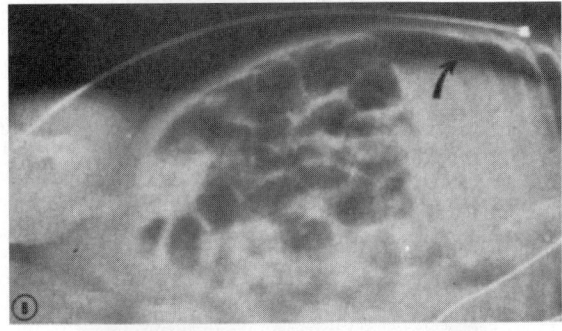

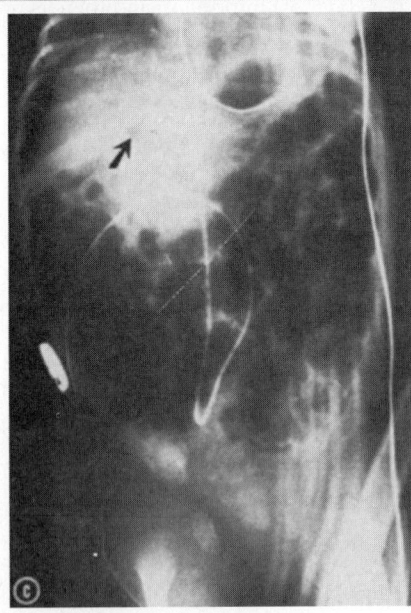

Figure 38–11. Abdominal roentgenogram demonstrates the presence of pneumatosis intestinalis, consistent with the diagnosis of necrotizing enterocolitis. (From Cikrit, D., et al.: Necrotizing enterocolitis. Surgery, *96*:648, 1984.)

progressive clinical deterioration characterized by shock, unstable vital signs, decreasing serial platelet counts, continued gross rectal bleeding, persistent acidosis, rising serum phosphorus levels, increasing abdominal distention, or the presence of turbid brown fluid containing bacteria on paracentesis (in those with ascites) require operation.[58] When an operation is necessary, these high-risk prematures require expert pediatric anesthesia support and the availability of blood, platelets, and fresh frozen plasma in the operating theater.

At laparotomy, the surgical treatment of the patient is individualized according to the pathologic findings in each case. Patients with ischemic necrosis and perforation require bowel resection; often, a temporary stoma is created to facilitate the procedure and control peritonitis. Extensive involvement from the duodenum to mid–transverse colon is seen in 15% of cases. Under these dire circumstances, no resection is performed, the abdomen is closed, and supportive care is continued for 24 to 48 hours. If the infant improves, a second-look laparotomy is performed to see whether any bowel is viable. This procedure has been successful in a few patients. The majority of infants with extensive NEC succumb. Under very unusual circumstances, when the ischemic involvement is limited to a short segment of bowel, a primary anastomosis may be considered.

Postoperative complications are common. These include further bowel necrosis, gram-negative sepsis, disseminated intravascular coagulation, wound infection and breakdown, stomal complications, cholestasis, short bowel syndrome, and severe malabsorption with dietary intolerance.[24, 58, 62] A stricture in the distal bowel (usually the colon) can follow either surgical or nonoperative management. The etiology of intestinal stricture following treatment of NEC is most likely related to mucosal destruction and healing by the formation of a circumferential cicatrix. Stenotic lesions are more common in the colon than in the small bowel. Recognition of this complication is important, especially when a proximal stoma is in place and closure of the enterostomy is being considered. These cases should be evaluated preoperatively by acquiring a barium enema.

Mortality rates vary according to treatment, severity and extent of disease, the presence of multiorgan failure, gestational age, birth weight, and the development of postoperative complications. Patients who respond to medical therapy are often less ill and have less disease. Surgically treated patients have already failed attempted medical therapy and have a more severe form of the disease. Survival after medical therapy is approximately 80% but is only 60 to 70% following surgical treatment.[58] An increased mortality is seen in infants with birth weight below 1000 gm. and gestational age less than 27 weeks. The presence of portal vein air is a sign of advanced disease and is often associated with rapid clinical deterioration.[24] Late complications are frequently noted, and an additional 20% of survivors of early therapy subsequently succumb to these problems. In addition to the sequelae of short bowel syndrome, long-term survivors have problems with both motor and intellectual developmental delays, cerebral palsy, failure to thrive, below-level school performance, attention deficits, and the like.

MALROTATION AND MIDGUT VOLVULUS

Anomalies of intestinal rotation result from a failure of normal bowel rotation from the fifth to twelfth weeks of fetal development. The small bowel lacks appropriate fixation to the posterior wall, the cecum fails to migrate to the right lower quadrant, and the colon fails to attach to the lateral abdominal wall. This results in a right upper abdominal position for the cecum, which may extend fixation bands across the duodenum and cause obstruction. The bowel hangs from a narrow pedicle based on the superior mesenteric artery and vein. Due to the presence of abnormal bands, the small bowel can twist in a clockwise direction, resulting in volvulus of the midgut. Congenital diaphragmatic hernia, abdominal wall defects, duodenal atresia, and prune belly

syndrome are conditions associated with anomalies of rotation and fixation.

Approximately one third of all cases of midgut volvulus occur in the first week of life, and 85% of cases are recognized by 1 year of age. Infants usually present with the sudden onset of bilious vomiting and become seriously ill. If the condition is not recognized promptly, midgut infarction may ensue, causing either death or the need for massive enterectomy. On physical examination, the abdomen may be tender and distended. Bilious material is usually observed when an orogastric tube is passed into the stomach. In some cases, bloody tissue can be passed per rectum. The plain abdominal radiograph may show an airless abdominal cavity beyond the level of the duodenum or many air-fluid levels. Both barium enema and upper gastrointestinal barium study may prove useful in achieving a diagnosis. The enema documents that the cecum is in an abnormal position in the upper abdomen. The upper gastrointestinal contrast study demonstrates obstruction at the level of the second to third portion of the duodenum at the point of volvulus around the superior mesenteric vessels (the corkscrew effect). The infant is given intravenous antibiotics and fluid resuscitation with crystalloid solutions (lactated Ringer's solution) and is taken to the operating room on an emergent basis.

At the time of laparotomy, the volvulus is identified and reduced counterclockwise. Although the bowel may look dusky, it often returns to a normal appearance. The use of a sterile intraoperative Doppler probe or fluorescein with a Wood's light may be useful in documenting the viability of the intestine. Obviously infarcted intestine is resected. Any fixation bands (Ladd's bands) from the abnormally located cecum across the duodenum or jejunum are divided, and the colon is moved to the left side of the abdomen, with the cecum placed next to the sigmoid colon. All the small bowel then drops straight down from the duodenum on the right side of the abdomen. An appendectomy is also performed because the cecum is then located in an atypical position, making the future diagnosis of possible appendiceal pathology difficult. If the viability of most of the bowel remains in question at the time of detorsion, the abdomen is closed and the patient is given supportive therapy. A second-look procedure is performed after 24 to 36 hours to evaluate whether the bowel is viable. The mortality for midgut volvulus remains high (18 to 25%). Even those infants who can be salvaged may have significant morbidity, since short bowel syndrome can be a consequence of extensive bowel resection.[46] Because midgut volvulus can occur at any time, when malrotation is identified either *de novo* or at the time of a laparotomy for another condition, a Ladd's procedure and an appendectomy should be performed.

ABDOMINAL WALL DEFECTS

Defects of the anterior abdominal wall (gastroschisis and omphalocele) represent a relatively common cause of admission to most major children's centers. Anterior abdominal wall defects can be identified on prenatal ultrasonography examination, and most of these births are anticipated and delivery is carried out at a high-risk tertiary obstetric center with the availability of neonatal intensive care and pediatric surgical specialists.

Omphalocele

An omphalocele is a covered defect of the umbilical ring into which abdominal contents herniate. The sac is composed of an outer layer of amnion and an inner layer of peritoneum. Omphalocele occurs in approximately 1 per 5000 births. There is a high incidence of associated anomalies. More than

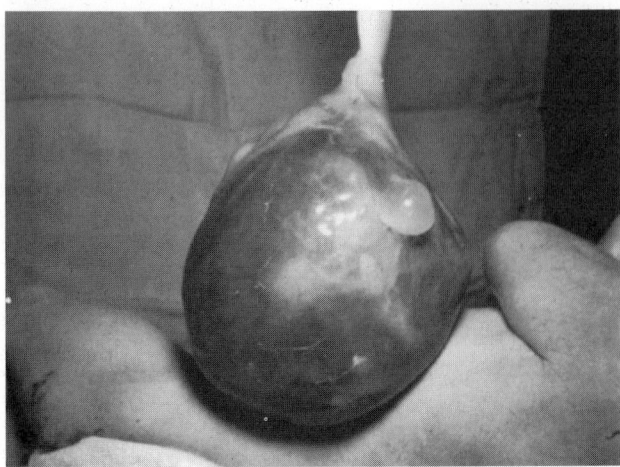

Figure 38–12. A large omphalocele containing the liver. (From Grosfeld, J. L., et al.: Contemporary management of abdominal wall defects. Surg. Clin. North Am., *61*:1037, 1981.)

50% of cases have other serious defects involving the alimentary tract and the cardiovascular, genitourinary, musculoskeletal, and central nervous systems. Many infants with omphalocele are premature. Others may be affected by a number of syndromes, including Beckwith-Wiedemann syndrome (gigantism, macroglossia, and an umbilical defect—umbilical hernia or omphalocele), chromosomal abnormalities (trisomy 13–15, 16–18), exstrophy of the bladder or cloaca, and the pentalogy of Cantrell (omphalocele, anterior diaphragmatic hernia, sternal cleft, ectopia cordis, and intracardiac defects, most commonly a ventricular septal defect and occasionally a diverticulum of the left ventricle). The size of the omphalocele defect may vary from 2 to 10 cm. (Fig. 38–12). The smaller the defect, the better the prognosis. The contents of the sac may include only bowel; frequently, however, the liver as well as the entire gastrointestinal tract is within the sac. The extra-abdominal location of the viscera *in utero* produces a small abdominal cavity, which may make attempts at primary repair difficult. In addition, malrotation is almost always present as a coexisting anomaly.

The emergency care of patients with omphalocele includes the insertion of an orogastric tube to decompress the stomach and prevent swallowed air from causing bowel distention, which may interfere with attempted reduction of the viscera at the time of repair. If the infant requires transfer to a tertiary high-risk pediatric center, transportation in a thermally neutral environment should be provided, and the intact omphalocele sac should be kept covered with a sterile dressing and protected from injury. Excessively wet dressings may macerate the sac and cause temperature decrease by cooling and evaporative loss. Intravenous fluids (10% dextrose in water with 0.25% normal saline) and parenteral antibiotics are administered (ampicillin 100 mg. per kg. per day and gentamycin 5 mg. per kg. per day). The patient's general condition should be carefully assessed in regard to cardiorespiratory status and the occurrence of additional anomalies. Since the viscera are covered by a physiologic sac, the surgeon has a number of treatment options. Operative management depends on the circumstances and the anatomy in each case. Small defects (2 cm.) can be managed by direct primary closure of the abdominal wall. Medium to large defects may require a staged closure, using a Dacron-reinforced Silastic silo as a temporary housing for the bowel. The prosthesis is sutured to the edge of the defect with continuous 3-0 Prolene suture. The silo can gradually be reduced over 3 to 7 days in

the neonatal intensive care unit and the baby returned to the operating room for a formal closure of the abdominal wall. On rare occasions, when the defect is very large (>10 cm.) or in cases of suspected chromosomal syndromes (trisomy 13, 18), conservative management using topical application of an escharotic agent is reasonable therapy. Topical therapy is also useful as a temporizing measure in a premature infant with an omphalocele and hyaline membrane disease or in heart failure. The definitive repair can be delayed until the infant's cardiopulmonary status is improved. Escharotic agents include 0.25% Mercurochrome, Silvadene, and 0.5% silver nitrate solution. Twice-daily applications allow the sac to thicken and epithelialize.

The overall survival for infants with omphalocele depends on the size of the defect, whether the infant is premature, whether the sac ruptures, and the number and severity of associated anomalies. Infants with chromosomal syndromes and those with the pentalogy of Cantrell have a significant mortality. The overall mortality at the author's institution is 37%.

Gastroschisis

Gastroschisis (Greek for *belly cleft*) is a defect of the anterior abdominal wall just lateral to the umbilicus. The defect is almost always to the right of an intact umbilical cord. This anomaly is probably the result of a defect that occurs at the site where the second umbilical vein involutes. Unlike instances of omphalocele, there is no peritoneal sac, so evisceration of the bowel occurs through the defect during intrauterine life. The irritating effect of amniotic fluid (pH 7.0) on the exposed bowel wall results in a chemical form of peritonitis characterized by a thick edematous membrane that is occasionally exudative. The exposed viscera may be congested, and the bowel appears foreshortened (Fig. 38–13). Nonrotation always accompanies this condition. In contrast to omphalocele, the incidence of associated anomalies in patients with gastroschisis is relatively infrequent. The exception to this general observation is the occurrence of intestinal atresia, which may complicate gastroschisis in 10 to 15% of

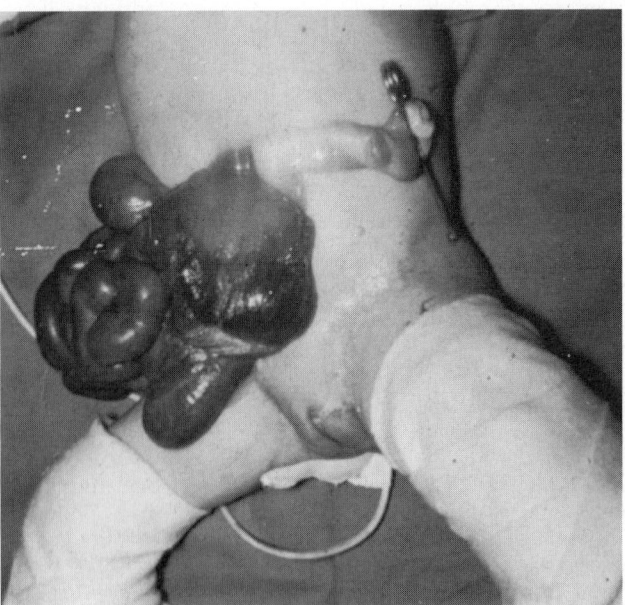

Figure 38–13. The typical appearance of an infant with gastroschisis. The viscera herniated *in utero* through a small defect in the abdominal wall just to the right of the umbilicus. (From Grosfeld, J. L., et al.: Contemporary management of abdominal wall defects. Surg. Clin. North Am., *61*:1037, 1981).

cases. Atresia of the bowel is often related to intrauterine volvulus or an interruption of the blood supply to a segment of exposed intestine by compression in a very tight defect in the abdominal wall. The liver is almost never eviscerated; however, the ovaries and fallopian tubes or abdominal testes are occasionally found outside the defect. The sexes are equally affected, and 40% of the patients are either premature or small for gestational age. Of interest is that 20 to 25% of the patients are born to unwed teenage mothers.

Despite the fact that gastroschisis can frequently be detected on a prenatal ultrasonography study, there is no evidence that early cesarean section improves the outcome. Spontaneous vaginal delivery is reasonable for these infants. Once delivered, an infant with gastroschisis is at risk for a variety of problems due to an increase in insensible losses related to exposure of the eviscerated bowel. Hypothermia, hypovolemia, and sepsis are the major problems to avoid. Significant third-space fluid deficits occur as a result of sequestration of interstitial fluid. The lower half of the baby (including the eviscerated bowel) is placed in a sterile bowel bag. Fluid requirements are 2.5 times that of a normal newborn in the first 24 hours of life. The infant is resuscitated with a bolus of 20 ml. per kg. of 10% dextrose in lactated Ringer's solution given over 30 minutes. Additional fluid is administered until urine output is established. Acid-base balance is closely monitored, as metabolic acidosis is commonly observed due to poor perfusion related to hypovolemia. An orogastric tube is placed in the stomach to prevent air swallowing and aspiration of intestinal contents, as an infant with gastroschisis has an associated adynamic ileus. The infant is given parenteral antibiotics (ampicillin and gentamycin).

At operation, the abdominal wall and exposed viscera are prepared with an iodophor solution. The defect is enlarged 1 to 2 cm. in both a cephalad and a caudad direction. The stomach contents are aspirated by the anesthesiologist, and meconium in the left colon is evacuated through the rectum by external compression of the viscera. The abdominal wall is manually stretched to enlarge the relatively small peritoneal cavity. Primary reduction of the viscera is attempted using a maximum ventilatory pressure of 35 cm. H_2O and PaO_2 as a guide and is successful in 70% of cases. The abdominal closure is accomplished using one layer of through-and-through interrupted 3-0 polypropylene sutures. The umbilicus can usually be preserved for cosmetic purposes. Some infants, however, require a staged closure using a Dacron-reinforced Silastic silo as a temporary extra-abdominal housing. The viscera can be gradually reduced by gentle pressure in the neonatal intensive care unit starting on the second to third postoperative day. The silo can usually be removed and closure of the abdominal wall completed in the operating room within a week in most cases. Antibiotics are discontinued when the silo is removed.

Due to a prolonged adynamic ileus, most infants with gastroschisis require 3 to 4 weeks of TPN for adequate caloric support. Most infants begin to tolerate oral intake by 2 to 3 weeks of age and can usually take all their calories enterally by 1 month. In infants with an associated intestinal atresia, a temporary enterostomy is constructed at the time of the initial abdominal wall repair. Closure can be accomplished at a later date. Although a primary anastomosis can be performed, due to inflammatory changes in the bowel wall at birth, stricture complicates a significant number of cases. Patients with atresia often have longer delays in gastrointestinal recovery and prolonged hospitalization. With appropriate neonatal resuscitation, surgical treatment, and nutritional support, the current survival rate in infants with gastroschisis is better than 90%.

SURGICALLY CORRECTABLE CAUSES OF RESPIRATORY DISTRESS

Congenital Diaphragmatic Hernia

Congenital posterolateral diaphragmatic hernia (foramen of Bochdalek) is a defect in the developing pleuroperitoneal fold through which the viscera ascend and enter the chest, usually in the eighth to tenth weeks of fetal life. The herniated bowel acts as a space-occupying lesion and prevents normal lung development.[2, 168] The risk of occurrence is 1 per 2200 live births; males are more commonly affected. The infants are often full term and weigh more than 3 kg. The defect is on the left side in 88% of cases, on the right side in 10%, and rarely bilateral (1 to 2%).[33] The defect can be detected *in utero* by prenatal ultrasonography. Polyhydramnios may be noted and is a poor prognostic sign.[2] High-risk mothers are brought to a tertiary care obstetric center with the immediate availability of neonatal intensive care, pediatric surgical expertise, and resources for extracorporeal membrane oxygenation (ECMO).[168] At birth, infants with diaphragmatic hernia develop symptoms of respiratory distress, either in the delivery room or shortly thereafter, as the bowel in the chest becomes distended with swallowed air. This further compresses the ipsilateral lung (which is often hypoplastic) and causes a mediastinal shift, interfering with ventilation of the contralateral lung. The infant appears dyspneic, tachypneic, and cyanotic and has severe retractions with an increased chest diameter and a relatively scaphoid abdomen. Bowel sounds may be heard on auscultation of the affected chest. An anteroposterior and lateral chest x-ray demonstrates air-filled viscera in the chest, confirming the diagnosis (Fig. 38–14). The infant may have severe hypoxia and respiratory acidosis. A combined metabolic acidosis may also be present when insufficient tissue perfusion coexists with pulmonary embarrassment.

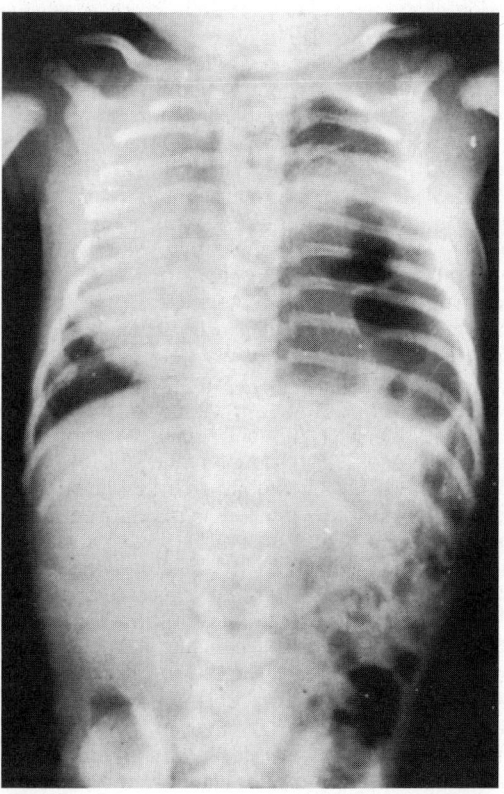

Figure 38–14. Chest x-ray demonstrates bowel gas in the left chest, consistent with the diagnosis of congenital diaphragmatic hernia.

Treatment can be conveniently divided into three main areas: (1) stabilization and preoperative preparation, (2) operative treatment, and (3) postoperative respiratory, circulatory, metabolic, and nutritional support. Infants with diaphragmatic hernia should have direct endotracheal intubation and ventilatory support with high oxygen flow (FiO_2 of 1.0). The respiratory rate is set intentionally rapid to induce respiratory alkalosis. Excessive ventilatory pressure should be avoided to reduce the risk of barotrauma and contralateral pneumothorax.[168] An arterial catheter should be inserted in the right wrist to serially monitor preductal PaO_2, pH, and $PaCO_2$. An umbilical artery catheter is a viable alternative to monitor postductal blood gas tensions. An orogastric tube is inserted to decompress the stomach and prevent further air from entering the gastrointestinal tract. If the infant becomes stabilized and demonstrates a PaO_2 greater than 100 torr and an arteriolar-alveolar gradient of less than 600, operative correction of the defect is attempted but can be safely delayed for 24 hours or longer. Repair is best accomplished by a transabdominal approach using a subcostal incision on the affected side.[33] The bowel is carefully reduced from the chest, avoiding injury to the spleen and left lobe of the liver on the left side and the right lobe of the liver on the right side. Infants with diaphragmatic hernia have malrotation, and if coloduodenal or duodenojejunal bands are noted, a Ladd's procedure should be performed. The hernia defect is evaluated; a sac is present in 10% of cases, and the distal rim can usually be identified above the renal fossa. A chest tube is inserted under direct vision. Primary diaphragmatic repair is accomplished, when feasible, using horizontal 3-0 or 2-0 nonabsorbable mattress sutures. If there is inadequate diaphragmatic tissue or an absent diaphragm, a synthetic patch is necessary to reconstruct the barrier between the abdominal and thoracic cavities. A Gore-Tex patch is often preferred. The abdomen is closed in layers if not excessively tight. In some instances, the abdominal cavity is extremely small, and either an intentional ventral hernia with skin closure or application of a temporary Dacron-reinforced Silastic housing may be necessary.

Postoperatively, the infant is monitored in the neonatal intensive care unit in a thermal neutral environment. The endotracheal tube is kept in place, and ventilation is supported using an FiO_2 of 1.0, maintaining the PaO_2 greater than 150 torr for a period of time. The infant is slowly weaned from high inspired oxygen requirements over a 48- to 72-hour period to avoid the honeymoon phenomenon characterized by an early smooth course followed by the sudden development of pulmonary vasoconstriction and potentially lethal persistent pulmonary hypertension.

Unfortunately, few neonates with congenital diaphragmatic hernia who present shortly after birth have a benign course. More often, the babies have severe hypoxemia and some degree of hypercarbia, which in the past did not respond to mechanical ventilation or the administration of pharmacologic agents such as prostaglandins, tolazoline, acetylcholine, and thorazine to induce pulmonary vasodilatation. The response to these agents was generally disappointing, and survival was less than 30%—lower if polyhydramnios was observed (15%).[2, 33, 74, 168] Mortality is directly related to the degree of pulmonary hypoplasia (especially if the contralateral lung is also hypoplastic) and the presence of associated congenital anomalies, including cardiac defects or chromosomal abnormalities. The advent of prenatal ultrasonography and early recognition of the defect *in utero* allowed for optimal prenatal and perinatal care but did not improve the overall survival of these patients with conventional therapy.[2, 33] In fact, the mortality actually increased in many centers. This observation was probably related to early identification (prenatal ultrasound), delivery at high-risk centers,

better neonatal transport, and improved techniques of resuscitation, permitting the treatment of babies with diaphragmatic hernia who previously never made it to tertiary neonatal intensive care centers prior to their demise. Currently, infants with congenital diaphragmatic hernia are intubated, stabilized, and observed on ventilator support (often using a high-frequency jet ventilator) for at least 24 hours. Only those infants who demonstrate adequate oxygenation (PaO_2 >100 on FiO_2 of 1.0) and the ability to ventilate at the alveolar level (PCO_2 < 60) are subjected to early operative repair. The rapid development of ECMO has led to a number of innovative clinical programs.[8, 9, 168] A baby who develops persistent pulmonary hypertension following an apparently successful repair of a diaphragmatic hernia (the honeymoon phenomenon) can almost always be salvaged by the use of ECMO (Fig. 38–15). However, infants with severe pulmonary hypoplasia do not reap the same postoperative benefits from ECMO and continue to have a high mortality.[2] Placing an unstable baby on ECMO preoperatively has also been employed.[8] When the baby's general condition improves (3 to 5 days), the infant can be weaned from the ECMO circuit, and the defect can be repaired. In some centers, repair of the diaphragmatic hernia is performed while the infant is still on the ECMO circuit and the baby is weaned from the circuit postoperatively. There have been some survivors in each clinical setting; however, not enough data are available for definitive recommendations at this time.[168]

There is no doubt that ECMO has a significant role in the management of certain patients with diaphragmatic hernia, but it is not a panacea for all cases.[8, 9] An oxygenation index (OI) greater than 40 has a mortality risk of 80% and is an indication for ECMO (OI = MAP [mean airway pressure] × FiO_2 × $100/PaO_2$), based on three of five postductal arterial blood gas determinations.[8] Gestational age less than 34 weeks, Grade III–IV intracranial hemorrhage, neurologic impairment, anomalies incompatible with a meaningful life expectancy, and irreversible lung disease are contraindications for ECMO. Although some patients with diaphragmatic hernia and presumed bilateral pulmonary hypoplasia (e.g., PaO_2 <50 without adequate oxygenation during a honeymoon pe-

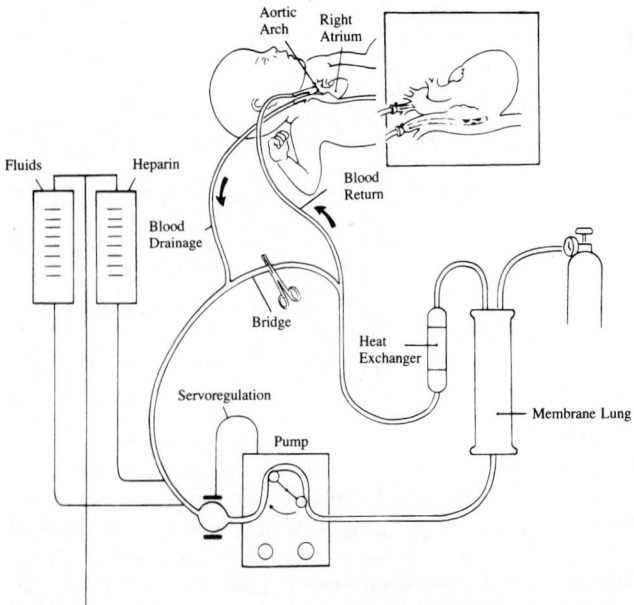

Figure 38–15. The extracorporeal membrane oxygenation (ECMO) circuit used for extracorporeal support in the neonatal unit. (From Bartlett, R. H.: Extracorporeal life support in neonatal respiratory failure. Surg. Rounds, *12*:41, 1989.)

riod) do not improve on ECMO, others have survived, indicating that the criteria are not absolute. Recent reports indicate survival rates of 70 to 90% using ECMO for all diaphragmatic hernia candidates who fail conventional treatment and have no other contraindications for life-support therapy. Recent data suggest that venovenous (V-V) perfusion during ECMO often obviates the need for arteriovenous (A-V) perfusion and avoids carotid artery ligation. V-V perfusion requires an adequate cardiac output. Conversion to A-V perfusion may be required in 10 to 15% of cases. The decision to employ ECMO must continue to be individualized until more definitive and absolute criteria become available.

The availability of nitric oxide (a potent pulmonary vasodilator) and surfacant in combination with the jet ventilator may reduce the need for ECMO in the future. Prenatal intrauterine surgical repair of congenital diaphragmatic hernia with subsequent live birth has been accomplished by Harrison and co-workers.[74] However, this approach must still be considered a courageous undertaking and remains an experimental program that has significant ethical overtones and cannot be routinely recommended.[74]

In a small percentage of cases, the diagnosis of diaphragmatic hernia is not achieved until after the infant is 24 hours old. All these patients should survive following successful repair, without the need for ventilator support. Rare instances of delayed presentation of right diaphragmatic hernia are noted in association with beta-hemolytic streptococcal infection.[5, 127] Some cases are not detected until later in infancy, presenting with failure to thrive, obstructive jaundice, and chronic recurring pulmonary symptoms.

There are other congenital abnormalities of the diaphragm that may also result in respiratory compromise. These include anterior parasternal diaphragmatic hernia into the space of Larrey, commonly referred to as Morgagni's hernia, and eventration of the diaphragm. Morgagni's hernia is relatively uncommon in infants and children and usually presents with respiratory distress or abdominal or substernal pain due to entrapment of the transverse colon in the defect. In rare instances, there may be bilateral defects on either side of the sternum. Diagnosis can be suspected on the lateral chest x-ray, demonstrating an air-filled structure in the anterior mediastinum. This can be confirmed by ultrasonography examination or a barium enema showing the colon in the chest. Repair is best accomplished through an abdominal approach. Eventration refers to a thin, floppy attenuation of the central portion of the diaphragm, allowing the intra-abdominal viscera to push the diaphragm upward and encroach on the lung. This condition may occur *de novo*, but it is more often a complication of phrenic nerve injury from a difficult breech delivery or inadvertent trauma during congenital heart surgery. Atelectasis, tachypnea, dyspnea, and cyanosis may be noted. The elevated diaphragm changes the esophagogastric angle and may produce gastroesophageal reflux, vomiting, and aspiration pneumonia. Severe hypoxia may require intubation and ventilator support. When the infant is stable, plication of the eventrated diaphragm can be more safely accomplished on an elective basis with a thoracotomy. The infant can almost always be extubated in the first 24 hours postoperatively.

Congenital Cystic Lung Disease

The lung is derived as an outpouching of the primitive foregut. A number of foregut-derived malformations may present with severe respiratory distress. These include instances of congenital and acquired lobar emphysema, pulmonary sequestration, congenital cystic adenomatoid malformation, bronchogenic cyst, and enteric duplication.[33] Lobar emphysema presents in the first 4 to 5 months of life with an overdistended, hyperaerated lobe (usually an upper or right middle lobe) that compresses the ipsilateral lung, causing atelectasis and resulting in a shift of the mediastinum to the contralateral side. The treatment of choice is thoracotomy and lobectomy. Sequestrations may be intralobar (in older children) or extralobar (in infants), and both have a systemic blood supply with direct arterial inflow from the aorta. Extralobar lesions drain into the azygous venous system and do not communicate with the lung, whereas intralobar lesions are within the lung tissue (lower lobes), drain through the pulmonary veins, and are frequently associated with pulmonary infection. The arterial supply can be detected by ultrasonography and may arise from the subdiaphragmatic aorta. The treatment of choice is resection, which includes a lobectomy for intralobar lesions. Congenital cystic adenomatoid malformations (CCAMs) have a *Swiss cheese* appearance on chest x-ray and disproportionate cartilagenous elements in relation to alveoli. Air is trapped in the lesion, causing overdistention and compression of normal tissues. One third of these patients are stillborn. Maternal polyhydramnios is often observed. Many of these lesions can be detected by prenatal ultrasonography and classified into three distinct types. Infants can develop severe respiratory compromise shortly after birth, with persistent pulmonary hypertension; in some instances, pulmonary hypoplasia coexists. A few babies have been salvaged with ECMO after lobectomy failed to alleviate the respiratory distress. Fetuses with Type III CCAM on ultrasound have been successfully resected *in utero*.[1] These observations indicate that if a CCAM is recognized on prenatal ultrasonography, the patient should be managed at a high-risk obstetric and neonatal intensive care center with immediate pediatric surgical expertise and ECMO resources available. Bronchogenic cysts are usually located near the bifurcation of the trachea and cause compression of the bronchus (most commonly on the left side), producing severe respiratory distress. Diagnosis is achieved by chest x-ray and ultrasonography. Treatment of choice is excision of the cyst. Enteric cysts of the esophagus can compress the trachea and in some instances may communicate with the tracheobronchial tree, the lung, or the spinal canal (neurenteric cyst). Rarely, hemorrhage into the tracheobronchial tree as a result of peptic ulceration from ectopic gastric mucosa in the cyst has been observed. Diagnosis is achieved with barium esophagram and ultrasonography. Extramucosal resection of the esophageal cyst is the operation of choice.

Other Causes

Respiratory distress can be caused by congenital abnormalities of the oropharynx, nasopharynx, jaw, tongue, and trachea, including micrognathia with Pierre-Robin and Stickler syndromes; choanal atresia or stenosis; hemangiomas; lymphangiomas; and teratomas of the pharynx or tongue, which can cause obstruction of the airway. Tracheomalacia, subglottic stenosis, laryngotracheal clefts, and congenital tracheal stenosis are other important conditions to consider. The appropriate diagnosis can usually be arrived at with a careful physical examination, laryngoscopy, and bronchoscopy.[33]

PYLORIC STENOSIS

Pyloric stenosis is a common condition in infancy of unknown etiology. It is hereditary and occurs in 1 per 750 births. It is far more common in boys and is often noted in the first-born son. Pyloric obstruction is the result of gradual hypertrophy of the circular smooth muscle of the pylorus. The condition presents with progressive, often projectile, nonbilious vomiting following attempted feeding. The onset of vomiting usually begins between the second and third weeks of life and increases in frequency and force. The infant fails to gain weight and may actually lose weight. The number of bowel movements and times of voiding diminish. Eight percent of cases may have bloody gastric vomitus related to gastritis or esophagitis. Five to 8% of patients are jaundiced; indirect bilirubin is elevated because of decreased glucuronyl transferase levels, which are caused by a lack of substrate delivered to the liver because of limited caloric intake. On physical examination, visible gastric waves may be observed progressing across the upper abdomen from left to right during feedings. Diagnosis can be established by palpation of a pyloric mass (olive shaped) in the midline, one third to one half the distance from the umbilicus to the xiphoid, when the stomach is empty. This is best accomplished while offering the infant an oral feeding of dextrose and water. Careful examination can identify the pyloric mass in 85% of cases.

If the *olive* cannot be palpated, ultrasonography may show an elongated pyloric channel (>17 mm.) and thickened muscle wall (>3.5 to 4.0 mm.). If the ultrasound study is not diagnostic, a barium contrast study is obtained to evaluate the pylorus as well as other possible causes of nonbilious vomiting. The gastrointestinal series may show an elongated pylorus with an antral shoulder and either a single string sign or a double railroad track sign, consistent with pyloric stenosis. The differential diagnosis includes pylorospasm, milk allergy, hiatal hernia, pyloric duplication, prepyloric antral web, gastroesophageal reflux, adrenogenital syndrome (salt-losing type), and certain aminoacidurias associated with electrolyte derangements and gastric waves. If the diagnosis is made early in the course of the illness (prior to the onset of dehydration), operative correction can be accomplished without excessive preparation. Infants with prolonged vomiting, however, may present with dehydration associated with hypochloremic alkalosis. Hypokalemia may coexist as a result of excessive urinary losses of K⁺. Serum pH, electrolytes, blood urea nitrogen, urine output and specific gravity, and the infant's weight should be carefully evaluated.

Pyloric stenosis is never a surgical emergency, but it may be a medical emergency requiring aggressive intravenous resuscitation in a dehydrated infant and the occasional patient with peripheral collapse and shock due to severe hypovolemia. Dehydration and metabolic derangements must be corrected prior to operation. Percutaneous insertion of a short Silastic (22- to 24-gauge) intravenous catheter is used to administer parenteral fluid therapy. Cutdown by venesection is almost never needed. The infant is kept without oral intake, and the stomach is emptied of old formula and retained secretions using a 10-French orogastric tube. In an infant with severe dehydration, an initial fluid infusion of 20 ml. per kg. of 5% dextrose in 0.9% (normal) saline or 5% Plasmanate (colloid) is rapidly administered over a 30-minute period. This volume load usually stabilizes the infant and improves renal plasma flow. The infusion is then continued with 5% dextrose in 0.45% saline at a rate of 200 ml. per kg. per day for an 8-hour period. Potassium (3 to 4 mEq. per kg. per day) is added when urine output is established. A safe rate of K⁺ infusion is 4 mEq. per 100 ml. of infusate (40 mEq. per liter). After the first 8 hours, the intravenous infusion rate is reduced slightly to 125 to 150 ml. per kg. per day for the next 16 hours. Patients with mild isotonic dehydration can be safely prepared with an infusion of 5% dextrose in 0.25% saline at a rate of 125 ml. per kg. per day and operated on promptly. All but the most severely depleted infants are usually ready for operation after 24 hours of fluid therapy. It is not necessary to use ammonium chloride to correct the alkalosis. Operation may be safely performed when the pH is less than 7.5, serum chloride greater than 88 mEq. per liter, serum CO₂ combining power less than 30 mEq. per liter, and

serum potassium greater than 3.2 mEq. per liter when urine output is satisfactory (1 to 2 ml. per kg. per hour) and the specific gravity is less than 1.020.

A 10- or 12-French orogastric catheter or sump drainage tube is inserted just prior to the anticipated operation to empty the stomach and diminish the risk of aspiration. The infant is similarly intubated while awake to prevent possible aspiration because of gastric outlet obstruction. General endotracheal anesthesia is employed. Operation is performed through a small transverse right upper abdominal incision made over the oblique muscles and the lateral border of the rectus muscle, which is retracted medially. The stomach is mobilized, and the pylorus is brought into the wound. Pyloromyotomy (Ramstedt-Fredet procedure) is accomplished by an incision on the relatively avascular anterior surface of the white glistening *pyloric tumor,* starting at the pyloric vein (pyloroduodenal line) distally and extending proximally onto the normal prepyloric antrum. Downward pressure over the incision site using the back of the scalpel handle cracks the muscle. Gentle spreading of the thick, hypertrophic circular muscle with a hemostat or pyloric spreader allows the submucosa and mucosa to bulge out and relieve the obstruction. Independent motion of the two sides of the divided pyloric muscle indicates an adequate pyloromyotomy. If the distal extent of the incision is kept at the pyloroduodenal line, entry into the duodenum is avoided. If entry does occur, the opening is sutured with 4-0 Vicryl and then covered with omentum. Closure of the abdomen is accomplished in layers of continuous 4-0 Vicryl. A 4-0 white Vicryl subcuticular suture is used to appose the skin edges, which may be sealed and supported with either collodion or Steri-Strips. Although successful laparoscopic pyloromyotomy has been reported, it offers little or no advantage to the open technique.

Postoperatively, the patient is placed in a crib with the head elevated at a 30-degree angle. The orogastric tube is maintained on suction for 6 hours and then removed and feeding is initiated. In cases of intraoperative duodenal entry, feedings are withheld for 24 hours. Feedings are started by offering 15 ml. (½ oz.) of Pedialyte every 2 hours for two feedings. If tolerated, feedings are advanced to 15 ml. of half-strength (10 calories per ounce) formula every 2 hours for two feedings. The volume of intake is increased to 30 ml. (1 oz.) of half-strength formula every 3 hours. On the following day, the concentration of the formula is increased to full strength (20 calories per ounce), which is offered every 3 hours. An intravenous infusion is kept in place, using 5% dextrose in 0.25% saline at a rate of 100 ml. per kg. per day for the first 24 hours to prevent hypoglycemia and dehydration if the early feedings are not well tolerated. Early postoperative vomiting is not uncommon but is usually self-limited. If repeated vomiting occurs, an orogastric tube is reinserted and the stomach is gently lavaged with normal saline or 5% sodium bicarbonate. Feedings are then resumed. If the infant was breast-fed prior to operation, nursing may be resumed late on the first postoperative day. If feedings are well tolerated, the volume of full-strength formula is advanced to 45 ml. (1.5 oz.) every 3 hours. This is further advanced to 60 ml. (2 oz.) and then 75 ml. (2½ oz.) later that day. The infant is usually discharged on the second postoperative day on 3 to 4 oz. every 3 to 4 hours. Pyloromyotomy is one of the most gratifying of all surgical procedures. The infant rapidly resumes an adequate caloric intake and gains weight, to the delight of both parents and physician. The expected morbidity is quite low (an occasional wound infection), and the mortality rate should be zero.

GASTROESOPHAGEAL REFLUX

In the past decade, gastroesophageal reflux (GER) has become one of the most common clinical conditions managed by pediatric surgeons. The largest group of patients with clinically symptomatic GER are infants and children with neurologic impairment. More than 70% of GER cases are reported in this impaired patient population. Infants with apnea and bradycardia and children with chronic pulmonary conditions due to asthma, bronchopulmonary dysplasia, and cystic fibrosis represent an additional group of patients with significant GER. Many of these children receive bronchodilator medications (e.g., aminophylline) that reduce the lower esophageal sphincter pressure and may result in active GER. Choking, asthma-like symptoms, coughing at night, and recurring episodes of pneumonia related to aspiration of gastric contents are being recognized with an increasing frequency. Dysfunction of the lower esophageal sphincter may also be observed in children with scleroderma, familial dysautonomia, Cornelia de Lange's syndrome, myotonic dystrophy, and nemaline myopathy of infancy.[6, 7, 21, 32] GER has also been implicated as an etiologic factor in the sudden infant death syndrome (SIDS).[6] Another group of infants at high risk of GER are those with congenital anomalies, including esophageal atresia with or without TE fistula, and those in whom tight closure of the abdominal wall following repair of omphalocele and gastroschisis is associated with increased abdominal pressure. GER is also common in disorders associated with diaphragmatic distortion, such as eventration, diaphragmatic hernia, and severe diaphragmatic elevation due to a large upper abdominal mass, which may alter the esophagogastric angle. Dysfunction of the lower esophageal sphincter, reduced length of the sphincter, disordered esophageal motility, poor esophageal clearance, and delayed gastric emptying all play a role in the severity of the symptoms.

The common presentation of symptomatic GER includes failure to thrive, vomiting, and repeated episodes of respiratory infection due to aspiration of gastric contents. Diagnosis can be achieved by a number of tests, including barium esophagram with fluoroscopic control, lower esophageal sphincter manometrics, gastric scintigraphy, 24-hour pH-probe measurements, and esophagoscopy. Delayed gastric emptying is observed in 25 to 50% of cases. This is documented with a quantitative gastric scintiscan using radiolabeled scrambled eggs in older children and thickened formula in infants. Medical therapy includes the administration of antacids, H_2-blockers and omeprazole, and parasympathomimetic and prokinetic agents (bethanechol, metoclopramide, and cisapride).[46] Keeping infants in a head-up position on an incline board reduces the risk of reflux. In infants, small frequent feedings and occasionally nasojejunal feedings are useful. Unfortunately, prospective randomized double-blind studies evaluating the effects of parasympathomimetic medications show little benefit of their administration.[113] Indications for operative intervention include continued failure to thrive, persistent vomiting, repeated episodes of respiratory infection, the presence of Barrett's esophagus, esophagitis (with blood-tinged or coffee-ground vomitus), and stricture.[45] Simultaneous demonstration of decreased esophageal pH (<4) associated with apnea and episodes of bradycardia is also an indication for fundoplication in these cases.

A number of antireflux operations are used to treat GER. These include the Nissen fundoplication procedure (360-degree wrap), Thal procedure, Dor modification of the Nissen (270-degree) procedure, Hill repair, Toupet procedure, and anterior plication of Boix-Ochoa.[6, 13, 32] The most popular antireflux operation is the Nissen fundoplication procedure. This is constructed using a short, floppy gastric wrap (no longer than 2.5 to 3.0 cm. in length) performed over the largest size esophageal dilator that will safely fit within the lumen of the intra-abdominal portion of the esophagus at the time the sutures are inserted. Suture placement is important and requires a healthy seromuscular bite of stomach (using 3-0 silk

in neonates, 2-0 silk in older infants and children), a bite of the anterior wall of the esophageal smooth muscle (avoiding esophageal lumen entry), and then another healthy bite on the wrapped portion of the gastric fundus. Heavy sutures are necessary to prevent wrap breakdown. In some cases, one or two short gastric vessels must be divided to acquire a tension-free wrap. The vagus nerves are carefully preserved to avoid postoperative gastric atony. If the crura of the hiatus were dissected to free the distal intra-abdominal esophagus, these should be carefully reapproximated with interrupted 2-0 silk sutures in infants and 0-silk in older children to prevent herniation of the fundic wrap into the mediastinum. If significant delayed gastric emptying (less than 35%) is identified preoperatively, a concomitant pyloroplasty is performed.[82, 83, 115] The authors prefer a one-layer technique, using a Gambee stitch of 4-0 interrupted silk in infants and 3-0 silk in older children. The sutures are left long, and a portion of omentum is placed over the pyloroplasty site and tied. In patients with severe neurologic impairment and swallowing disorders, a gastrostomy tube is inserted for feeding purposes. In otherwise normal children, the gastrostomy is omitted. Both clinical and laboratory evidence indicates that a Stamm gastrostomy placed along the anterior gastric wall near the greater curvature may result in GER.[19, 114] This has been documented in many patients in whom a gastrostomy was initially performed for feeding purposes, only to be followed by severe postoperative vomiting due to GER. The incidence of postgastrostomy GER is similar after percutaneous endoscopically placed gastrostomy tubes, indicating that fixation of the stomach to the anterior abdominal wall is responsible for this event. These observations strongly suggest that a complete work-up to evaluate both the esophagus and the stomach should be carried out prior to the performance of feeding gastrostomy. Recent information suggests that a gastrostomy placed along the lesser curvature may reduce the risk of GER postoperatively.

The success rate of antireflux procedures is in the 90th percentile. Recent reports suggest the similar success rates can be achieved with laparoscopic fundoplication. Complications are observed in 16% of cases. The complication rate is higher in infants and children with neurologic impairment and in patients with esophageal atresia.[32] The most frequent complications involve the wrap itself (8%), with wrap breakdown or herniation into the mediastinum being most common.[32] Postoperative small bowel obstruction occurs in 4% of cases. Of interest is that some of these events are related to postoperative small bowel intussusception rather than adhesions. Wound infection, dehiscence, inadvertent splenectomy, and pancreatitis have also been documented as complications of fundoplication. Gagging, gas-bloat syndrome, and early satiety are postprandial problems that may be related to disordered gastric motility. In some instances, significant delays in gastric emptying can be documented by gastric scintigraphy, and these postoperative symptoms have been ameliorated by performance of an emptying procedure (pyloroplasty).[83, 115] These latter observations further indicate the importance of a complete preoperative work-up of patients with feeding disorders and GER. In children with recurrent symptoms of GER due to wrap breakdown, a second Nissen fundoplication procedure has the same success rate as a primary procedure (greater than 90%).[32] It is therefore reasonable to recommend reoperation in these cases. Multiple failures (more than three) of a Nissen fundoplication procedure usually require resection of the lower esophagus and jejunal interposition.

INTUSSUSCEPTION

Intussusception is a relatively frequent cause of intestinal obstruction in infancy and early childhood. More than 50%

of cases are observed between the ages of 3 months and 1 year, and 80% occur by age 2 years. Intussusception is more common in boys, and most are well-nourished and otherwise healthy babies. The exception is a child with cystic fibrosis who may fail to thrive and intussusception as a sequela in children with Henoch-Schönlein purpura. Approximately 30% of cases follow a bout of viral gastroenteritis or an upper respiratory infection. The clinical presentation of intussusception typically includes the sudden onset of abdominal pain (85%) characterized by episodic screaming and drawing the legs up. This may be followed by vomiting (60%), which initially may be clear but eventually becomes bilious in nature as obstruction progresses. The appearance of blood in the stool is a common finding and may vary from occult blood to bright red bleeding; the classic description of currant-jelly stool, consisting of blood mixed with mucus, is the most common observation. On physical examination, the abdomen is often distended, the right lower quadrant may feel empty, and a sausage-shaped mass may be palpable in the upper right to midabdomen (65%). The intussusceptum can sometimes be palpated on rectal examination. The child may appear gravely ill if symptoms are present for more than 24 to 48 hours, sometimes mimicking meningitis. The child is often febrile, and the blood count may show a leukocytosis. Plain erect and recumbent radiographs of the abdomen may demonstrate dilated loops of small intestine, air-fluid levels, or a soft tissue mass effect in the right upper quadrant. A diagnostic barium enema may demonstrate the intussusceptum with a coil-spring sign at the point of bowel invagination (Fig. 38–16).

An infant with intussusception is managed by insertion of a nasogastric tube, intravenous fluid resuscitation, and antibiotics. After rehydration, the child is taken to the radiology suite for an attempted hydrostatic reduction of the intussusception. A sedative should be administered prior to the examination once hypovolemia has been corrected. The surgical staff should be in attendance for the attempted reduction, with the anesthesiologist and operating room staff alerted and standing by should reduction be unsuccessful.

Hydrostatic barium enema has been the mainstay of nonoperative treatment. The enema is performed with a 3-foot column and limitation of continuous hydrostatic pressure to

5-minute time frames. Reduction is considered satisfactory when the intussusceptum is reduced through the ileocecal valve and the contrast material refluxes into multiple small bowel loops.[170] Air reduction of intussusception was introduced in a large number of cases in China.[71] This technique is now commonly performed in the United States and Canada. Reports suggest that this technique is as effective as barium enema reduction. The air pressure must be monitored, with a maximum of 110 mm. Hg in children and 80 mm. Hg in infants. The procedure is performed under fluoroscopic control, and it is safe to make two to three attempts at reduction. The perforation rate is similar to that observed with hydrostatic barium enema. This almost always occurs in the uninvolved intussuscipiens. Perforation occurs more commonly in babies less than 6 months of age with symptoms present for more than 3 days.[36, 38]

The rate of successful reduction varies from center to center but is in the range of 50 to 75%. Some centers do not attempt reduction if the infant has had symptoms for longer than 72 hours and has a severe obstructive bowel pattern on plain abdominal x-ray. Unsuccessful reduction is followed by an immediate trip to the operating room suite.[170] Laparotomy is carried out through a right lower quadrant transverse abdominal incision. The intussusception is identified, and manual reduction is attempted using a milking technique to squeeze the mass retrograde through the ileocecal valve. Following reduction, an appendectomy is performed and, when present, Jackson's veil is divided. This band of tissue tends to draw the terminal ileum toward the cecum. Recurrence of intussusception after barium or air reduction is between 8 and 12%, and recurrence following surgical reduction is extremely rare. Failure of manual reduction is often a sign of bowel necrosis. Reduction attempts should cease when bowel wall muscle splitting is noted, to avoid intraoperative perforation and soiling. Bowel resection is required in 35 to 40% of cases. Although performance of a primary anastomosis in obstructed unprepared bowel is controversial, many such procedures have been successful. In the presence of bowel obstruction with severe distention or in those cases complicated by barium perforation and peritonitis, resection should be followed by formation of a temporary enterostomy. Intussusception in older children may be due to a pathologic lead point. These cases include instances of B-cell lymphoma, Peutz-Jeghers polyps, inversion of a Meckel's diverticulum, submucosal hemangioma, carcinoid tumor, juvenile polyposis coli, and *Ascaris lumbricoides* worm infestation.

Postoperative complications include prolonged adynamic ileus, fever, wound infection, pneumonitis, urinary tract infection, enterostomy stenosis, wound dehiscence, and subhepatic abscess. Despite considerable morbidity, in recent studies, the mortality rate has been zero. A high index of suspicion, early recognition, and diagnostic barium enema often allow a prompt diagnosis and nonoperative reduction. When symptoms have been present for more than 72 hours and a severe obstructive pattern is noted on the plain abdominal radiograph, a low success rate with hydrostatic reduction can be anticipated. In these cases, confirming the diagnosis with a gentle barium enema and operating promptly without attempted hydrostatic reduction are suggested.

MECKEL'S DIVERTICULUM

Meckel's diverticulum is the most common form of persistent vitelline duct remnant. The diverticulum occurs on the antimesenteric border of the ileum, usually within 60 cm. of the ileocecal valve, and contains all layers of the intestinal wall. Other vitelline duct anomalies include persistent vitelline duct (which presents at the umbilicus as a draining fistula), a fibrous band connecting the ileum to the undersur-

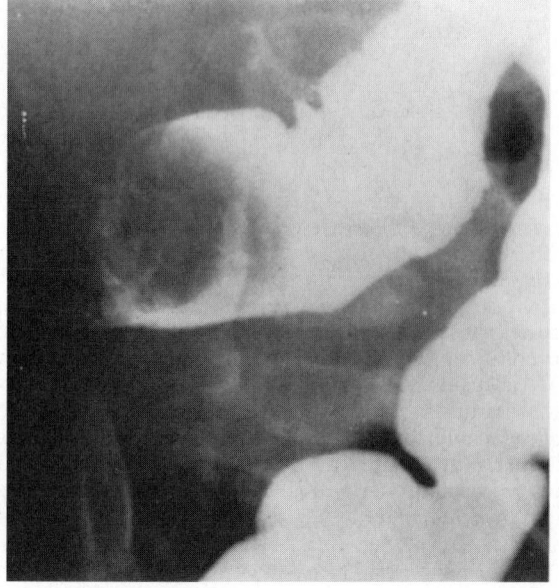

Figure 38–16. Barium enema in an infant with idiopathic ileocolic intussusception shows the intussusceptum in the right upper quadrant.

face of the umbilicus, a patent vitelline sinus beneath the umbilicus and an obliterated bowel portion, and a vitelline duct cyst (Fig. 38–17). Ectopic tissue of gastric or pancreatic origin is frequently noted in these lesions. Ectopic gastric mucosa is most common and is responsible for the most frequent complication of this anomaly—peptic ulceration with hemorrhage (22%). Other complications include inflammation (2%); bowel obstruction due to internal hernia around a vitelline duct band (13%); intussusception, with Meckel's diverticulum acting as a lead point (<1%); and a T-shaped prolapse of both efferent and afferent intestine through a persistent vitelline duct fistula at the umbilicus in a neonate (<1%).[162] Hemorrhage is related to peptic ulceration occurring at the margin between ectopic gastric mucosa and ileal mucosa. Hemorrhage from a Meckel's diverticulum presents as painless rectal bleeding, which is often significant. The hemoglobin is often less than 8 gm. per 100 ml., and the child may require blood transfusion. Spontaneous cessation of bleeding is the rule; however, life-threatening hemorrhage may occur.

Diagnostic evaluation of a patient with a suspected bleeding Meckel diverticulum should start with a 99mTc-pertechnetate scintiscan (Fig. 38–18). This isotope is picked up by gastric mucosa and may be enhanced by giving the infant cimetidine and pentagastrin before the test. Ectopic mucosa is also present in intestinal duplications—a lesion that must be included in the differential diagnosis. Barium studies are usually unre-

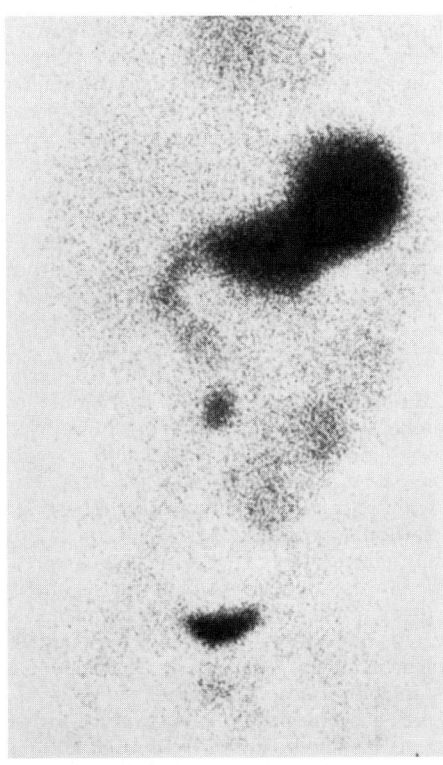

Figure 38–18. 99mTechnetium-pertechnetate scintiscan identifies an area of lower abdominal isotope pickup, consistent with ectopic gastric mucosa in a Meckel's diverticulum.

warding. A visceral angiogram is occasionally useful when the rate of bleeding is greater than 1 ml. per minute. The treatment of choice is resection of the Meckel's diverticulum. This can be accomplished by a wedge excision, bowel resection and anastomosis, or use of a stapling device.[116] Successful resection of a Meckel's diverticulum can also be accomplished with laparoscopy, using an endoscopically designed autostapling device. In some cases, a primitive persistent right vitelline artery originating from the mesentery supplies the diverticulum and must be identified and ligated. Instances of bowel obstruction may be related to a volvulus around a persistent vitelline band or under a persistent vitelline artery, causing bowel infarction. These cases often present with fever, leukocytosis, and sepsis. Cases of inflammation and perforation are treated with antibiotics (ampicillin, gentamycin, and clindamycin). All these latter complications of vitelline duct anomalies usually require resection and bowel anastomosis.

MESENTERIC AND OMENTAL CYSTS

Both mesenteric and omental cysts are probably the result of an abnormality of the lymphatic system. These cysts have a fibrous wall that is lined by a single layer of endothelial cells and have small lymphatic spaces. In most cases, omental cysts are detected in the first few years of life and present with an asymptomatic large abdominal mass. Omental cysts are often located anteriorly and displace the stomach posteriorly. Almost all omental cysts are serous and contain clear straw-colored fluid of low specific gravity. Mesenteric cysts may be single or multiple and can occur anywhere in the abdominal cavity. Mesenteric cysts frequently present with abdominal pain, vomiting, abdominal distention, and evidence of intestinal obstruction due to volvulus around the cysts. Sudden enlargement has been observed after relatively

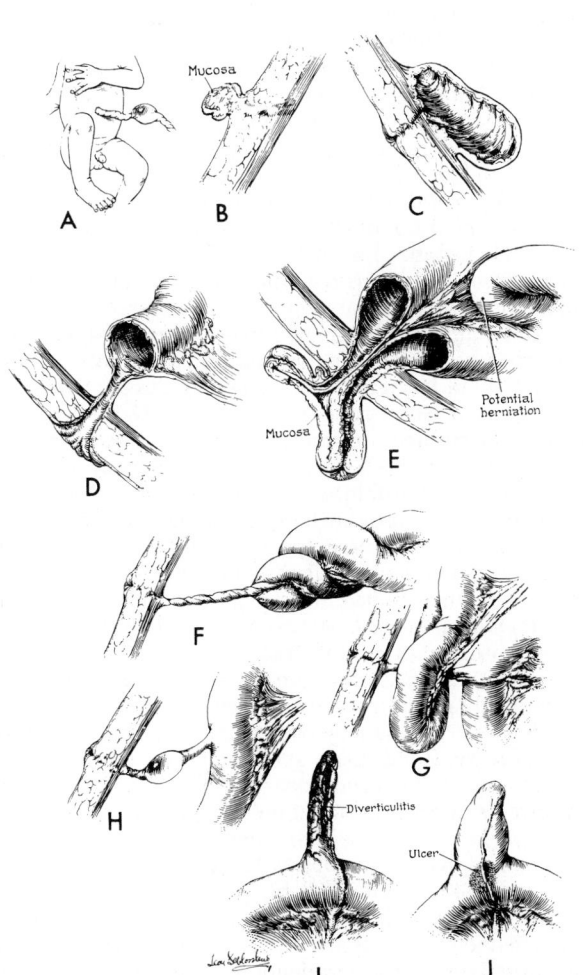

Figure 38–17. Variants of a persistent vitelline duct. The most common variant is a Meckel's diverticulum. (From Ravitch, M. M.: Meckel's diverticulum. *In* Rhoads, J. E., et al. (Eds.): Surgery: Principles and Practice, 4th ed. Philadelphia, J. B. Lippincott, 1970.)

minor episodes of blunt abdominal trauma, causing hemorrhage into the mesenteric cyst. The most common sites include the ileal mesentery, lesser sac, and jejunal mesentery. Those cysts affecting the small bowel may be chylous, whereas most mesenteric cysts involving the colon are serous. Diagnosis is easily achieved with abdominal ultrasonography, which demonstrate a large unilocular or septated nonspecific sonolucent cystic mass with a smooth wall. The treatment of choice is resection of the cyst. In some instances, this requires resection of the cyst with a segment of intestine due to adherence of the cyst wall and the adjacent bowel.

ENTERIC DUPLICATIONS

Enteric duplications are relatively rare anomalies that can occur anywhere in the alimentary tract, from the mouth to the anus. The most common site is the small intestine. Duplications share a common mesenteric blood supply and muscular wall with the normal intestine. These lesions may be cystic or tubular, and in 20% of cases they communicate with the normal intestine. The duplication may contain ectopic gastric mucosa and, in some instances, pancreatic tissue as well. Clinical presentation includes a shifting abdominal mass (due to its mesenteric attachment) that may be palpated in different areas of the abdomen at separate examinations. Symptoms include cramping abdominal pain or vomiting due to compression of the normal bowel by the duplication cyst. In some instances, the presenting finding is melena related to hemorrhage from peptic ulceration, caused by ectopic gastric mucosa in the duplication that communicates with the normal bowel. An ultrasound examination of the abdomen detects a cystic mass, and a ^{99m}Tc-pertechnetate scintiscan demonstrates the presence of ectopic gastric tissue. The therapy of choice is resection of the duplication cyst. This may require resection of the involved segment of normal intestine. In instances of long tubular duplications, the mucosal lining may be stripped to remove potential sites of ectopic mucosa, and the duplication is joined side to side with the normal bowel to obviate the need for extensive bowel resection. A similar technique can be used for duodenal duplications to avoid the necessity of a pancreatoduodenectomy. A blind-loop syndrome caused by bacterial overgrowth in a tubular duplication that communicates proximally but not distally may also occur. This unusual occurrence can be detected with the use of a diagnostic small bowel barium enteroclysis. This syndrome can be treated by resection or distal anastomosis of the blind end to the normal bowel and mucosal strapping.

INTESTINAL POLYPS

A number of polypoid conditions can affect the alimentary tract of children, including juvenile polyps of the colon, Peutz-Jeghers syndrome with hamartomatous polyps, Cronkhite-Canada syndrome, familial polyposis, Gardner's syndrome, Turcot's syndrome, and generalized juvenile polyposis coli.

Juvenile polyps are the most frequent polyps noted in children. These polyps present between the ages of 4 and 14 years, are inflammatory in nature, and may have a cystic component. The polyp may contain significant eosinophiles, implicating an allergenic cause. The most common symptom is rectal bleeding. In some cases, a polyp with a long stalk can prolapse out of the rectum with a bowel movement. The most accurate method of diagnosis is to perform proctosigmoidoscopy, which detects 85% of polyps. In more than 80% of cases, the polyp is solitary. Multiple polyps can occur, however, and an air-contrast barium enema and colonoscopy should be performed in these cases to determine the exact site of the polyps. The natural history of most juvenile polyps is autoamputation and spontaneous involution. Very few require treatment, except for those associated with significant bleeding, cramping abdominal pain from intussusception, and recurring prolapse. In most cases, polypectomy can be accomplished with the use of the sigmoidoscope or colonoscope without the need for laparotomy. Children with familial generalized juvenile polyposis coli have myriad polyps throughout the entire colon and can present with failure to thrive, anemia, hypoproteinemia, and hypokalemia from rectal bleeding and loss of mucus rich in protein and potassium. These patients require abdominal colectomy and ileorectal anastomosis. Proctoscopy is performed every 6 months to evaluate the rectal segment for polyps. Although juvenile polyposis is not a premalignant condition, recurring rectal polyps may require resection of the rectal mucosa and an ileoanal pull-through at a future time. Unlike in cases of solitary juvenile polyps, in generalized juvenile polyposis, the polyps persist into adult life and may involve the small intestine as well. The other polypoid conditions noted above are covered extensively elsewhere in this text.

BILIARY TRACT DISORDERS

Cholestasis in Infancy

Neonatal jaundice is a common occurrence and is considered a physiologic event produced by an immaturity of the enzyme glucuronyl transferase. Appropriate delivery of substrate (caloric intake) to drive the enzyme system usually resolves the jaundice in a week to 10 days. The elevation in serum bilirubin is almost entirely due to an increase in the indirect unconjugated fraction. Jaundice persisting more than 2 weeks following birth must be considered pathologic and is accompanied by an elevation of the direct fraction (conjugated) of bilirubin (greater than 1 mg. per 100 m.), indicating some form of cholestatic syndrome or obstruction. Babies with hepatic dysfunction are at risk for developing sequelae from cholestasis regardless of its etiology. A prompt evaluation of the cause of jaundice is in order.

The differential diagnosis of persistent jaundice includes a wide spectrum of disorders, including breast milk jaundice, Rh and ABO incompatibilities, hemolytic disease (hereditary spherocytosis), Gilbert's disease, and Crigler-Najjar syndrome, in which the indirect unconjugated bilirubin fraction is elevated (more than 80%). Those patients in whom more than 20% of the total bilirubin is direct have either cholestasis or obstruction; these cases include metabolic conditions (tyrosinemia, Gaucher's disease, galactosemia, cystic fibrosis, hypothyroidism, iron storage disease, infantile copper overload, fructosemia, and alpha$_1$-antitrypsin deficiency), infectious agents (cytomegalovirus, herpesvirus, rubella virus, hepatitis B virus, varicella, coxsackievirus, echovirus, toxoplasmosis, and syphilis), sepsis, total parenteral nutrition, intrahepatic disorders (idiopathic neonatal hepatitis, intrahepatic cholestasis due to arteriohepatic dysplasia [Alagille's syndrome], Byler's disease, Zellweger's syndrome, and absence of bile ductules), and those conditions that affect the extrahepatic biliary tree and cause obstruction (biliary atresia, biliary hypoplasia, bile duct stenosis, spontaneous perforation of the bile duct, and inspissated bile syndrome).

A number of tests are available to distinguish some of the causes of cholestasis from obstructive jaundice. The presence of bile in the duodenal aspirate, green- or brown-colored stool, sweat chloride determination, thyroxine and thyroid-stimulating hormone levels, cultures, TORCH screen and VDRL titers, metabolic screen for aminoacidurias, evaluation of urine-reducing substances, and an abnormal alpha$_1$-antitrypsin level eliminate most causes of cholestasis that do not require surgical intervention. Most babies with biliary atresia have persistent and progressive jaundice associated with elevation of the serum bilirubin and alkaline phosphatase levels. Hepatomagaly is the most common finding on physical examination. The liver is often quite firm on palpation. Splenomegaly is also noted, but in slightly older infants (older than 6 weeks). Ascites and the presence of prominent venous patterning on the abdominal wall above the level of the umbilicus are usually signs of more advanced liver disease (with portal hypertension) and are less common in infants evaluated in the first 6 weeks of life. The stools are acholic, and the urine may appear dark and contains bile but no urobilinogen.

None of the clinical findings and tests currently available for evaluation of infants with biliary atresia are pathognomonic but simply indicate instances of obstruction. Ultrasound examination of the biliary tree may demonstrate the presence of a gallbladder or, rarely, a choledochal cyst—neither of these findings, however, excludes biliary atresia. The intrahepatic bile ducts are never enlarged in cases of biliary atresia. In a jaundiced baby with elevated direct bilirubin fraction, acholic stools, and a negative duodenal aspirate, a ^{99m}technetium–diisopropyl iminodiacetic acid (^{99m}Tc-DISIDA) scintiscan should be performed. If the radioisotope appears in the intestine, obstruction can be ruled out, whereas failure of hepatic clearance indicates obstruction. Although many centers pretreat infants with a 5-day course of phenobarbital or ursodiol prior to the DISIDA scan, recent reports indicate that babies with obstructive jaundice who receive phenobarbital have a higher incidence of liver failure when given a halogenated general anesthetic at the time of definitive surgical correction of the biliary obstruction.[108] These latter observations suggest that phenobarbital administration be avoided or, if it is deemed vital for diagnosis, that a slight delay in proceeding with surgical correction is in order. In addition, a nonhalogenated anesthetic agent can be employed. Eighty to 85% of babies with an obstructive DISIDA-scan have biliary atresia. Although percutaneous needle biopsy may be helpful in distinguishing between biliary atresia (proliferating bile ducts) and idiopathic neonatal hepatitis (giant cells and focal areas of necrosis), there is a significant overlap, with atresia patients often demonstrating the presence of giant cells and the like. A minilaparotomy with operative cholangiography (when possible) should be performed. This culls the cases of neonatal hepatitis, biliary hypoplasia, and Alagille's syndrome by demonstrating an intact but small patent biliary tree with tiny intrahepatic branches and passage of contrast into the duodenum.[59] A confirmatory open liver biopsy should be obtained and the abdomen closed. If biliary atresia is documented, however, the incision can be enlarged and a formal exploration of the porta hepatis carried out under the same anesthetic.

Biliary Atresia

The etiology of biliary atresia is probably related to a dynamic intrauterine inflammatory process caused by fibrosis of both the intrahepatic and extrahepatic biliary tree. Although biliary atresia was once considered a postnatal condition, a number of cases with associated cystic dilatation of the atretic duct have been identified in utero by prenatal ultrasound examination or at laparotomy in the newborn for other congenital anomalies such as duodenal and jejunal atresia. Some reports suggest that the etiology of the inflammatory process responsible for fibrosis of the bile ducts may be the result of an REO-3 viral infection or rotavirus-C; however, solid scientific evidence is still needed to confirm these relationships. The incidence of biliary atresia is 1 per 15,000 live births. This condition is slightly more common in

females. Infants with biliary atresia have associated anomalies in 25 to 30% of cases, including duodenal atresia or stenosis, anular pancreas, malrotation, polysplenia syndrome, situs inversus, and anterior (preduodenal) portal vein. In addition, 15% of patients may have a congenital heart defect.

An important consideration in the management of babies with biliary atresia is to recognize the disadvantages of delayed diagnosis and treatment.[59, 98, 109] Laparotomy should be performed by 2 months of age. A number of recent reports clearly indicate that the success rate for surgical correction of biliary atresia is much improved when done in the first 2 months of life and that the operation is probably an unrewarding technical exercise after 4 months of age, because of progressive ductular fibrosis (extra- and intrahepatic). At operation, the pathologic variants of biliary atresia include fibrous obliteration of the gallbladder with a fibrous bile duct up to the level of the porta hepatis in the majority of cases (80%), a *correctable* form of atresia with a blind-ending cystic dilatation of the common hepatic duct in 5 to 6% of cases, and a patent gallbladder (containing white bile) and distal common bile duct with no evidence of proximal ducts in 15% of cases. The procedure of choice is a modification of the Kasai hepatoportoenterostomy.[88] The fibrous cord representing the bile duct is followed up to the porta hepatis, and a biopsy with frozen section of the thick fibrous structure above the bifurcation of the portal vein is obtained. Microscopic bile ductules are usually seen by the pathologist. A Roux-en-Y hepatoportoenterostomy is performed with one layer of interrupted 5-0 absorbable suture (Maxon or PDS). The bifurcation of the portal vein must be mobilized and retracted inferiorly to allow incorporation of the entire porta hepatis in the anastomosis (Fig. 38–19).[109] The Roux limb is brought out as a temporary biliostomy to evaluate bile flow and perhaps reduce the incidence and severity of postoperative cholangitis.[59, 163] Some pediatric surgeons do not use a cutaneous stoma but prefer establishing an antireflux intussuscepted valve between the distal end of the limb and the duodenum.[128] Others have used a vascularized pedicle of appendix in a hepatoportal-appendicoduodenostomy, with the distal appendix tunneled in the muscular wall of the duodenum to prevent reflux and cholangitis.[29] In cases in which the gallbladder and distal common duct are patent, a hepatoportocholecystostomy has been an alternative technique to restore bile flow.[59, 163]

Postoperatively, the infant is placed on trimethoprim-sulfamethoxazole as a prophylactic biliary antibiotic and is also given phenobarbital and ursodiol to stimulate bile flow. Fat-soluble vitamins (including A, D, E, and K) are administered daily.[109, 112] Postoperative complications include cholangitis, progressive cirrhosis manifested by portal hypertension with bleeding esophageal varices, ascites, hypoalbuminemia, hypoprothrombinemia, fat-soluble vitamin deficiencies, micronutrient deficiency (calcium, phosphorus, and zinc), and malabsorption of long-chain triglycerides. Cholangitis is characterized by a decrease in bile secretion, recurrence of jaundice, fever, and leukocytosis.[112] This event should be documented by a positive blood culture that identifies the offending organism. However, this is not always done, and the infant should be started on a third-generation cephalosporin or imipenem and cholerectics (phenobarbital, glucagon, and steroids), even in the absence of a positive blood culture. Intravenous aminoglycoside can be added if there is no response to the initial treatment. Some surgeons use steroids empirically to ameliorate the risk of recurring cholangitis and progressive disease.[87, 109, 112] Reoperation should be limited to patients with recurring episodes of cholangitis and to re-establish bile flow in those infants who drain adequate bile after the initial hepatoportoenterostomy, are anicteric, and then suddenly become jaundiced.[48, 59] In these latter

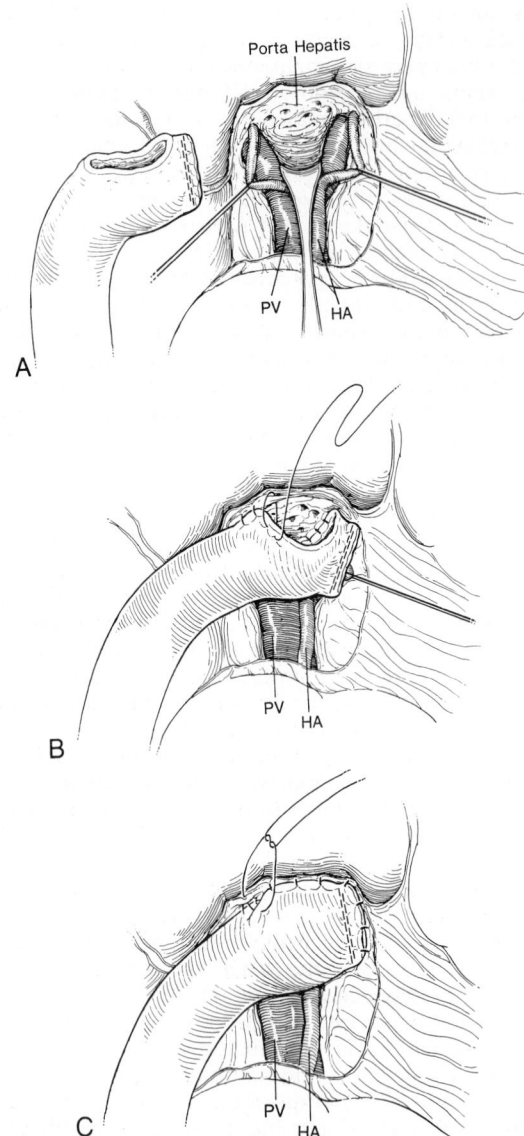

Figure 38–19. *A* to *C*, The bifurcation of the portal vein is the landmark for the dissection of the porta hepatis in infants with biliary atresia. The bifurcation is freed and retracted inferiorly so that the entire fibrous porta can be included in the hepatoportoenterostomy anastomosis (*B* and *C*). PV, portal vein; HA, hepatic artery. (From Grosfeld, J. L., et al.: The efficacy of hepatoportoenterostomy in biliary atresia. Surgery, *106*:692, 1989.)

cases, there may be an underlying mechanical cause for obstruction of the Roux loop.[59]

Successful outcome following hepatoportoenterostomy is related to proper performance of the procedure, the age of the patient (less than 3 months), the severity of liver disease at the time of the operation, the presence of microscopic ductules at the porta hepatis, and whether or not adequate bile flow is achieved.[59, 109, 163] Patients can be staged postoperatively and placed in prognostic groups by 4 to 6 weeks after the procedure.[59] Infants who produce adequate amounts of bile (more than 6 mg. per 100 ml. per day) from the biliostomy and are completely relieved of their jaundice fall into a successful category; they can expect long-term survival and normal or near-normal liver function, and they rarely require liver transplantation. If the bile flow is moderate but the infant remains mildly jaundiced and the liver disease is stabilized, extended survival can be expected; however, the infant will require liver transplantation in later years. In instances

in which little or no bile flow is achieved and the infant's liver disease is progressive, the procedure must be considered a failure, and the patient becomes a candidate for liver transplantation within months. Babies in whom the diagnosis was delayed and referral for surgical evaluation occurs after 4 months of age are candidates for liver transplantation as the primary procedure. Most infants with biliary atresia should undergo an attempt at hepatoportoenterostomy. Approximately 30 to 40% of those patients operated on early have a successful outcome and may not require liver transplantation. An additional group of patients are improved, have an extended survival, and can delay the liver transplant to a time when the donor organ pool size is larger. In the remaining infants who either fail to improve following hepatoportoenterostomy or are referred late, liver transplantation is a vital and life-saving complementary procedure. In these more urgent cases, the use of reduced-size orthotopic grafts has decreased the waiting period for donor organs and improved the overall survival of candidates for liver transplantation, particularly those who used to die while on the waiting list. Some of the best results of liver transplantation are achieved in patients with biliary atresia (85 to 93% survival).[61]

Choledochal Cyst

Cystic enlargement of the common bile duct is referred to as a choledochal cyst. The etiology of choledochal cyst is controversial and includes a common channel theory, with destructive effects of pancreatic enzymes causing damage in the wall of the common duct. These lesions are more common in females (4:1), and approximately half the patients present with jaundice, a right upper quadrant mass, and abdominal pain. Both the pain and jaundice may be intermittent. In some instances, the initial presentation is acute pancreatitis due to an abnormal insertion of the pancreatic duct. Cholelithiasis and cirrhosis may complicate cases of choledochal cyst that are not recognized early.[61]

There are five main variants of choledochal cyst (Fig. 38–20): (1) fusiform dilatation of the common hepatic and common bile duct, with the cystic duct entering the cyst (the distal common bile duct may be stenotic); (2) a lateral saccular cystic dilatation; (3) a choledochocele represented by an

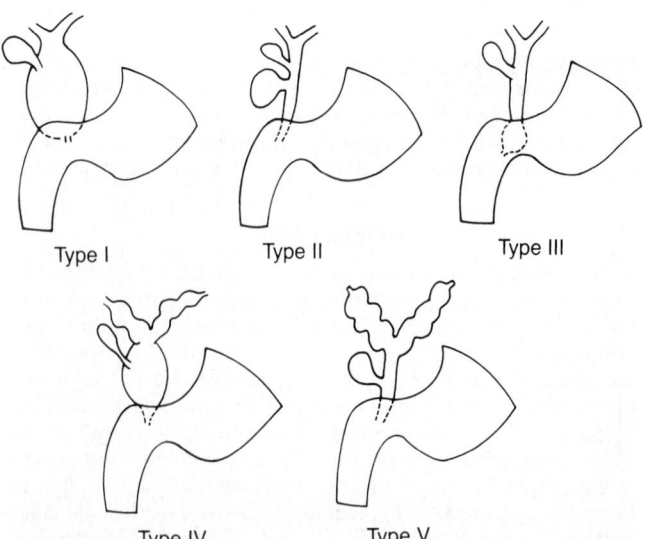

Figure 38–20. The five types of choledochal cyst. Type I is the most common form. (From O'Neill, J. A., et al.: Recent experience with choledochal cyst. Ann. Surg., *205*:533, 1985.)

intraduodenal cyst; (4) extrahepatic and intrahepatic ductal dilatation, and (5) intrahepatic cystic dilatation only. Diagnosis is achieved by ultrasound examination, which usually demonstrates the choledochal cyst and dilated intrahepatic ducts.[112] Although preoperative percutaneous transhepatic cholangiography and endoscopic retrograde cholangiopancreatography (ERCP) can demonstrate the cyst and the biliary system, these studies are probably unnecessary in most cases. Definitive operation is performed through a transverse or subcostal right upper quadrant incision. An operative cholangiogram is performed through the gallbladder or the cyst wall itself and clarifies the pathology, including the site of an abnormally inserted pancreatic duct (Fig. 38–21). Internal drainage procedures such as cystduodenostomy and cystjejunostomy, which were popular procedures in the past, are no longer recommended.[61, 112] The choledochal cyst is usually devoid of epithelium, and the wall is fibrous and fails to contract, resulting in poor emptying and significant bile stasis. These prior diversionary procedures were complicated by cholangitis, cholelithiasis, cirrhosis, and malignant degeneration in the cyst wall. The risk of subsequent malignancy is approximately 20% over 20 years. Currently, the operation of choice is complete resection of the cyst and a Roux-en-Y hepatojejunostomy[23] performed with interrupted 5-0 absorbable suture (Maxon or PDS). The cyst wall must be carefully dissected from the anterior surface of the portal vein, and an abnormally high insertion of the pancreatic duct must be identified to prevent injury. The distal end of the bile duct is oversewn at the duodenum. In cases of significant inflammation, the cyst can be resected, leaving the outer posterior layer of the cyst wall in place on the portal vein to decrease the risk of excessive hemorrhage. Postoperative complications are relatively few, and the operative mortality has been negligible. The risks of cholangitis, anastomotic stricture, progressive liver disease, and carcinoma are significantly reduced by resection of the choledochal cyst. The occurrence of a protein plug in the pancreatic duct and late intrahepatic cysts are relatively rare. Long-term follow-up is important.

Cholelithiasis

The etiology of gallstones in infants and children differs somewhat from the causes noted in adults. The most common cause of cholelithiasis in infants and young children is pigment stones due to congenital hemolytic disorders,

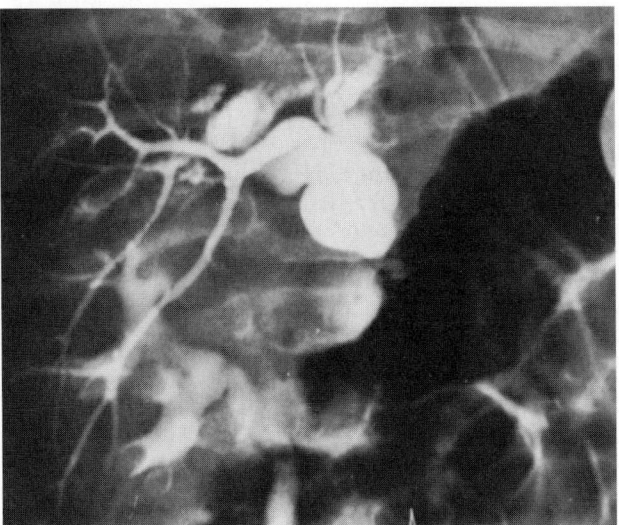

Figure 38–21. Intraoperative cholangiogram demonstrates a Type I choledochal cyst.

including hereditary spherocytosis, thallassemia, pyruvic-kinase deficiency, and sickle cell disease. Other causes include cholestasis following long-term treatment with total parenteral nutrition and cystic fibrosis.[61] Children with extensive bowel resection due to malrotation with midgut volvulus, necrotizing enterocolitis, or intestinal atresias who have distal ileum resection have an abnormal enterohepatic circulation of bile and secrete a more concentrated cholesterol in the bile, which increases the rate of gallstone formation.[61, 62] In older patients, especially adolescent females, use of birth control pills, obesity, a positive family history of gallstones, and teenage pregnancy are associated with an increased risk of cholesterol gallstone formation. Diagnosis is achieved in a manner similar to that in adult patients, relying heavily on the results of ultrasonographic studies and the occasional use of ERCP when indicated. The treatment of choice is laparoscopic cholecystectomy, which is an efficient procedure in both children and adults.

ACUTE APPENDICITIS

Acute appendicitis is one of the most common causes of acute abdomen in the childhood age group. A careful clinical history and thorough physical examination are paramount for arriving at an early, accurate diagnosis of appendicitis. The pathophysiology of appendicitis involves obstruction of the appendix by a fecalith, producing a *closed-loop* obstruction. The classic presentation of appendicitis includes the onset of epigastric or periumbilical pain followed by anorexia, nausea, and vomiting. The pain then radiates to the right lower quadrant. The pain is persistent and becomes more localized and intense than the earlier periumbilical pain.[75]

The appendix is a finger-like projection that may reside in a variety of locations, including the pelvis, right upper quadrant under the gallbladder, across the top of the bladder, and in a retrocecal site. Other unusual locations of the appendix are the left lower quadrant in cases of situs inversus and the upper midabdomen in instances of malrotation. Under these circumstances, the site of localized pain may occur at locations other than the classic presentation of pain in the right lower quadrant. When the appendix lies behind the cecum, irritation of the parietal peritoneum often does not occur, and the classic shift of pain to the right lower quadrant may be absent. Localized right lower quadrant pain indicates that the patient may have appendicitis, and in the absence of findings suggesting otherwise, prompt operation should be performed to prevent perforation. In young children, perforation occasionally occurs after 12 to 15 hours of documented pain[67]; it is present in 25% at 24 hours from the onset of symptoms, in 50% by 36 hours (half are gangrenous or perforated), and 80% at 48 hours.[75] Gangrenous or perforated appendicitis occurs in one third to one half of patients admitted to most children's hospitals.[67, 75, 125, 137] At least half of these patients have been seen in a physician's office or an emergency room and sent home with an incorrect diagnosis. This is especially true for infants less than 2 years of age, in whom appendicitis is relatively unusual.[67] A very young child with a ruptured appendix commonly has free perforation and peritonitis because of the inability of the short, flimsy omentum to wall off the process. Appendiceal perforation in the newborn period may be related to distal obstruction from Hirschsprung's disease, meconium plug syndrome, or a localized process due to necrotizing enterocolitis.[67]

A careful, detailed history is important to establish the exact time of the onset of pain and the sequence of events.[75] In appendicitis, vomiting follows periumbilical pain, but it often precedes abdominal pain in gastroenteritis. Documenting the character and frequency of diarrhea may prove useful. Mucoid, infrequent, small-volume episodes of diarrhea may be associated with pelvic irritation due to appendicitis and follows the onset of abdominal pain. High-volume, frequent, watery diarrhea that may or may not precede the onset of crampy abdominal pain may be indicative of gastroenteritis or inflammatory bowel disease. Careful documentation of symptoms in other systems is important, such as recent urinary tract infection. In adolescent female, information regarding the menstrual cycle, previous episodes of pelvic inflammatory disease, and mittelschmerz; an accurate sexual history; and a prompt urine test for pregnancy are important. The physical examination is the most important single determinant in a child with an acute abdomen and forms the basis for decisions regarding surgical intervention. In some cases, observation and periodic re-examination by the same physician may be necessary to confirm or exclude the diagnosis of appendicitis. Physical examination must include a careful and meaningful abdominal and rectal examination, with the patient cooperative enough to make the evaluation valid. The examination should document guarding, muscle spasm, and possible rebound tenderness consistent with peritoneal irritation. Evaluation of the obturator and psoas signs may be helpful. The rectal examination may detect a mass in the pelvis consistent with a pelvic abscess or elicit tenderness due to irritation of the pelvic peritoneum from exudate or fluid from pelvic appendicitis. In some cases, the rectal exam may detect a fecal impaction due to severe constipation, which can cause significant abdominal pain. If the child is not cooperative, a short-acting nonanalgesic medication (seconal 4 mg. per kg. given intramuscularly) is administered to relieve anxiety but not reduce the pain response. Most patients with appendicitis have a low-grade temperature (98.6 to 102° F. [37 to 38.8° C.]). Patients with pyelonephritis, pelvic inflammatory disease, and gastroenteritis from a variety of organisms (including *Salmonella, Shigella, Campylobacter,* and *Yersenia*) often have a higher temperature.

The laboratory evaluation includes a complete blood count with differential smear and urinalysis. Although the white blood cell count is greater than 10,000 per cu. mm. in more than 90% of cases, a normal count should not delay surgical exploration in a child with localized right lower quadrant tenderness or peritonitis. The urinalysis is important in differentiating between pyelonephritis or a renal calculus and acute appendicitis. The urine may contain a few red and white blood cells if an inflamed appendix lies near the ureter or bladder. An elevated urine specific gravity is consistent with hypovolemia and dehydration and is more common in cases of perforation. In teenage girls, an erythrocyte sedimentation rate should be obtained. This test is normal in appendicitis, but an elevation may reflect the presence of pelvic inflammatory disease. Other laboratory tests are unnecessary unless the patient is severely dehydrated and hypovolemic, in which case blood urea nitrogen and serum electrolytes are obtained. Radiologic evaluation should include a chest x-ray (to rule out right-middle or lower-lobe pneumonia) and flat and erect abdominal radiographs. Although the abdominal radiographs may be nonspecific, a calcified appendicolith is observed in 15% of cases and is consistent with a diagnosis of appendicitis. Although there has been recent enthusiasm for the use of a diagnostic barium enema to rule in or out acute appendicitis, the author has not found it particularly useful. Both false-negative and false-positive studies have been reported.[76] Ultrasound imaging may demonstrate an appendiceal abscess but is of no use in detecting early appendicitis.[75] In teenage girls, diagnostic laparoscopy may be helpful in distinguishing appendicitis from pelvic inflammatory disease.

In addition to the conditions previously mentioned, the differential diagnosis includes idiopathic intussusception, in-

testinal obstruction and volvulus, Meckel's diverticulum, Crohn's disease, ovarian torsion (cyst or tumor), perforated ulcer, pancreatitis, mittelschmerz, Henoch-Schönlein purpura, pelvic inflammatory disease, ruptured ectopic pregnancy, hemorrhage from a tumor (Wilms' tumor, neuroblastoma), and other pathology.

In instances of early acute appendicitis, the child is promptly prepared for operation with an intravenous infusion in the left upper extremity, and a preoperative dose of cefotetan or triple antibiotics (ampicillin, gentamycin, and clindamycin) is started at least 30 minutes before the incision, as gangrenous changes or perforation cannot always be excluded. In cases of a ruptured appendix, the child may be severely dehydrated and have a high temperature, rapid pulse, and adynamic ileus related to peritonitis. The patient must be carefully resuscitated with a rapid intravenous infusion of lactated Ringer's solution 20 ml. per kg. over 30 minutes, and then at a rate of 200 ml. per kg. per day until the pulse rate decreases and urine output is established. Triple antibiotics (as noted above) and pain medication are administered, and a nasogastric tube is inserted and placed on intermittent suction. It may take 2 to 4 hours to adequately prepare a patient with perforation for the operating room.

Appendectomy is accomplished through a right lower quadrant (Rockey-Davis) incision. Nonperforated cases are managed by appendectomy and closure of the wound in layers. Antibiotics are discontinued after two doses. Patients can usually resume oral intake after 24 hours, and in most cases, the child is discharged in 72 hours. In instances of perforation, however, all pus is drained, cultures are obtained, an appendectomy is performed, and the pelvis and right gutter are irrigated with saline or an antibiotic solution and aspirated dry. If there is a localized abscess, this may be drained through a separate stab wound below the main wound. In instances of generalized peritonitis, the peritoneal cavity is irrigated and aspirated dry, but drainage is not performed.[67, 75, 141] The muscular layers of the wound are closed in layers, but the skin is packed open. Antibiotics are continued for 5 to 7 days or at least until the temperature returns to normal and the white blood cell count diminishes. In some centers, the use of triple antibiotics has reduced the incidence of intra-abdominal abscess and postoperative wound infection, even when the wound is primarily closed and no intra-abdominal drains are employed.[141] The nasogastric tube remains in place until alimentary tract function returns. Diet is advanced, and the patient is discharged when afebrile and a postoperative rectal exam confirms no evidence of pelvic abscess. Children who present with a mass (abscess or phlegmon) may respond to antibiotic treatment without operation or by ultrasound-guided percutaneous drainage. These patients are treated by internal appendectomy 6 to 8 weeks later. The morbidity and mortality of appendicitis in children have gradually decreased over the past 2 decades, despite the fact that the incidence of ruptured appendix at diagnosis remains high. Most deaths are noted in the very young, when the diagnosis is not considered and long delays in treatment occur, and in those patients with ruptured appendix who are poorly prepared for operation and develop renal failure, hyperpyrexic events (including seizures), and gram-negative sepsis.

INFLAMMATORY BOWEL DISEASE

Crohn's disease can occur in childhood and adolescence and often presents with growth failure, cramping abdominal pain, diarrhea, perianal disease, and stricture resulting in bowel obstruction. This transmural condition most commonly affects the distal ileum and right colon. Multiple areas of small intestine may be involved, and in some cases, the only area of involvement is the colon. Rare cases of duodenal involvement have also been documented in children.[96] Diagnosis is usually achieved by barium enteroclysis of the small bowel, barium enema, and proctosigmoidoscopy and biopsy. Medical management includes the use of sulfadine and steroids.[96] In resistant cases, cyclophosphamide (Cytoxan), 6-mercaptopurine, and cyclosporin A have been used to induce a remission.[3, 17, 97] Indications for surgical intervention in children include growth failure, intestinal obstruction, perforation with internal fistulas, and the presence of a mass, indicating perforation into the mesentery. Patients are often anemic, hypoalbuminemic, and malnourished. Leukocytosis, an elevated erythrocyte sedimentation rate, and an elevated platelet count are frequently noted. A course of total parenteral nutrition and administration of metronidazole often result in significant improvement of the patient's nutrition and general status in preparation for surgery.[28] Limited resection of obstructive segments or sites of fistulas, with preservation of bowel length (occasionally resorting to stricturoplasty) when possible, is recommended. Occasionally, a total colectomy is required for granulomatous colitis. In cases of duodenal involvement, gastroenterostomy and vagotomy is a useful procedure. Recurrence following surgical intervention occurs in as many as 50% of cases, and symptoms extend into adult life. Long-term follow-up is essential. The best results are obtained in patients with an isolated short-segment distal ileal stricture. This condition and information concerning ulcerative colitis are presented in detail elsewhere in this text.

TRAUMA

Accidents are the leading cause of death in children between the ages of 1 and 15 years. Each year, approximately 15,000 children die as a result of traumatic events, which represents almost 50% of all deaths reported in the pediatric age group.[119] Motor vehicle accidents are responsible for the greatest number of deaths, followed by falls, bicycle injuries, drowning, burns, and the unique aspects of pediatric trauma, such as child abuse and birth trauma.[119, 139, 166] In recent years, an increasing number of deaths have been related to violence, including the use of firearms. In addition, more than 20 million children sustain some type of injury each year that requires treatment and causes more than 100,000 cases of permanent disability.[123]

Although there are many similarities in the management of adult and child trauma patients, there are several differences worthy of mention. These include response to stress; psychological trauma and communication difficulties; thermoregulation; a relatively small total blood volume; increased metabolic requirements related to growth and an increased metabolic rate; aerophagia with acute gastric dilatation and an increased risk of aspiration; smaller airway diameter, which can be more easily plugged by secretions and can make intubation difficult; a greater risk for postsplenectomy sepsis; and a different physiologic response to severe head injury (with incomplete sutures) than in an adult.[28, 119] In addition, the accident pattern is quite different, as most pediatric injuries are the result of blunt trauma, whereas injuries in adults are relatively evenly divided between blunt and penetrating trauma. Furthermore, the trauma scores used to evaluate injury severity in adult patients are inadequate for pediatric patients, leading to the development of a pediatric trauma score (Table 38–4).[28] A pediatric trauma score of less than 8 or 9 indicates an injury that places the child at risk for dying and suggests that the patient should be transported to a pediatric trauma facility. Although adult trauma centers have reduced the mortality for adult patients, this has not

TABLE 38–4. Pediatric Trauma Score

Parameter	Coded Value
Size	
>20 kg.	+2
10–20 kg.	+1
<10 kg.	−1
Airway	
Normal	+2
Maintainable	+1
Not maintainable	−1
Systolic blood pressure	
>90 mm. Hg	+2
50–90 mm. Hg	+1
<50 mm. Hg	−1
In the absence of a proper size BP cuff, assess BP by assigning these values:	
Pulse palpable at wrist	+2
Pulse palpable at groin	+1
Pulse not palpable	−
Central nervous system status	
Awake	+2
Partially conscious or unconscious	+1
Comatose or decerebrate	−1
Open wounds	
None	+2
Minor	+1
Major	−1
Skeletal injury	
None	+2
Closed fracture	+1
Open/multiple fractures	−1
Total score Range	−6 to +12

Scoring triage criterion for direct transport of the child to a level-1 trauma center = < 9.

From Coran, AG: The pediatric surgical patient. Scientific American Surgery, Wilmore, DW, Cheung, LY, Harken, AH, et al. (Eds.). Section VII, Subsection 14. © 1996 Scientific American, Inc. All rights reserved.

been the case for severely injured children. Pediatric trauma patients should have access to appropriate transport and receive care at a regional pediatric trauma center that is experienced in managing the complex treatment requirements of seriously injured children. This represents between 5 and 10% of the total number of children injured, as the majority of the cases (greater than 90%) can be managed at most local medical facilities; this emphasizes the importance of adequate trauma outreach programs designed to educate ambulance transport and emergency room personnel at the community level.

The pediatric trauma center includes a multidisciplinary group of pediatric surgical, anesthetic, and medical specialists in an integrated system of care. Multiple-injury patients are ideally admitted to the pediatric surgical trauma service for initial resuscitation and complete evaluation of their status. Other surgical specialists are available as necessary for the evaluation of injuries in their areas of expertise (e.g., neurosurgery, orthopedics) and play a vital role in the overall care of the patient. Head injuries are more common in children and represent the most frequent cause of death in the pediatric age group.[28] Early identification of severe head injury and aggressive management of increased intracranial pressure have significantly reduced the mortality of pediatric head injury in the last decade to less than 10%.

The resuscitation of a pediatric trauma victim follows the basic guidelines of adult trauma care by initiating the traditional ABCs—establishing an airway, stopping external sources of bleeding, and restoring the circulating volume. The cervical spine should be stabilized and the oropharynx cleared of blood and debris such as food and broken teeth. If necessary, intubation is accomplished with a noncuffed pediatric endotracheal tube, using the fifth fingernail as a guide for sizing. A large-bore intravenous catheter is inserted in either the upper or lower extremity, and if the blood pressure is low (less than 90 mm. Hg.), crystalloid (lactated Ringer's solution) is rapidly infused at a rate of 20 ml. per kg. to restore the circulating volume, reduce the rapid pulse rate, and increase blood pressure to greater than 90 mm. Hg. A nasogastric tube is inserted to decompress the distended stomach and prevent aspiration. A Foley catheter is inserted to monitor urine output. If the blood pressure drops again, an additional bolus of crystalloid is administered. Continued low blood pressure and rapid pulse rate are indicative of ongoing blood loss, and O-negative noncrossmatched blood is administered. The possibility of intrathoracic trauma and pneumothorax should be considered. If this is ruled out, an unstable patient who does not respond to fluid resuscitation most likely has a significant intra-abdominal injury with bleeding and needs to go directly to the operating room.[119] If an abdominal injury is considered after the patient has become hemodynamically stable, a more definitive evaluation can be accomplished by obtaining a computed tomography (CT) scan.[85, 110, 123] If the patient has an associated head injury, the CT scan of the head is followed by a study of the abdomen. The CT scan with both intravenous and oral contrast can document injury to the liver and spleen, evaluate for possible duodenal laceration or hematoma, image the pancreas, localize abnormal fluid collections, identify free air from bowel perforation, and adequately assess both kidneys with one examination. Although most adult trauma centers commonly use diagnostic peritoneal lavage as an important clinical maneuver to establish the presence of an intra-abdominal injury, bloody lavage fluid return in children does not necessarily indicate the need for laparotomy. Nonoperative management of the injured spleen and liver is a well-accepted method of therapy in the childhood age group.[85, 91, 110, 116, 123] As long as the child's vital signs remain stable and blood loss is minimal (less than 40 ml. per kg.), operation is unnecessary.[116] A child with a stable spleen or liver injury is transferred to the pediatric intensive care facility on the pediatric surgical service. The facility must have in-house surgical staff available around the clock. The patient may resume oral intake after 48 hours and is transferred from the intensive care unit to a regular pediatric floor. A 1-week hospitalization is usually all that is necessary for children with an isolated splenic injury. The child must refrain from any physical activity for a few weeks and avoid contact sports for 3 months.

Continued bleeding (more than one half of blood volume), multiple injuries, or the presence of free air is an indication for operative intervention. Following complete mobilization, the injured spleen can be salvaged by a number of techniques, including topical hemostatic agents, splenorrhaphy, partial splenectomy, and splenic artery ligation.[91, 116, 123] The fact that infants and children are more susceptible to overwhelming postsplenectomy infection due to encapsulated bacteria within a cell wall (pneumococcus, *Haemophilus influenzae*) makes conservative management and splenic salvage important considerations.[169] Complete splenectomy is rarely indicated. When the spleen is removed, the child should be immunized with Pneumovax vaccine (which contains 23 serotypes of pneumococcus) and placed on oral prophylactic penicillin. For children under 8 years of age, immunization with vaccines against *H. influenzae* and meningococcus should be considered. In children with liver injury, the major indication for surgical intervention is significant intra-abdominal bleeding (more than 40 ml. per kg.). These cases are usually identified early, with the patient's course unstable from the onset of care.[110, 123] Careful control of he-

mostasis (with the aid of the Pringle maneuver) and adequate débridement of devitalized liver tissue and drainage are the essential aspects of surgical care. The cell saver and rapid autotransfuser are helpful intraoperative adjuncts. Hepatic resection is rarely indicated. In some instances of coagulation defects due to excessive bleeding and multiple transfusions, the only way to control hemorrhage is by placing packs in the right upper quadrant.[123] The packs are removed in the operating room at a second-look procedure 24 to 48 hours later, when levels of coagulation factors return to normal. Compressing the liver with a Vicryl mesh wrap is occasionally useful in controlling bleeding as well.

Injuries to the small intestine are less common than those to the spleen and liver.[63] These injuries are related to blunt trauma that compresses the second and third portions of the duodenum against the spine.[166] Duodenal hematomas can be identified by contrast studies and can be treated conservatively in most cases with nasogastric drainage and total parenteral nutrition.[166, 171] Although duodenal laceration can be detected by the presence of free air or air bubbles in the retroperitoneum, the best method of diagnosis is administration of oral contrast material at the time of a CT scan of the abdomen. Surgical management includes primary suture of the duodenal laceration and drainage, jejunal serosal patch, and occasionally, in severe combined pancreatic-duodenal injuries, pyloric exclusion with temporary gastroenterostomy or duodenal diverticularization.[139, 164] The latter procedures are more commonly required with an associated injury to the head of the pancreas. Pancreatic injuries are also related to direct compression of the midportion of the gland against the vertebral column.[161] Although the CT scan is the most accurate diagnostic tool in instances of pancreatic injury, some cases of ductal injury can be missed.[152, 161] Most pancreatic injuries in children can be treated conservatively; however, if the pancreatic duct is transected, a distal pancreatectomy with splenic salvage (when possible) is advised. Serial ultrasound studies can follow the course of the injury and determine if a pseudocyst or abscess develops. Some pseudocysts resolve spontaneously, others that persist can be treated with ultrasound-guided percutaneous drainage. Failure of these techniques usually indicates a missed ductal injury that can be confirmed by ERCP and often requires either an internal drainage procedure or a distal pancreatectomy. Instances of pancreatic abscess are usually associated with a febrile course, often complicated by sepsis, and require operative débridement and drainage.[161]

Renal injuries require surgical intervention in less than 20% of cases. Significant leakage of pyelogram contrast material from the kidney, persistent hemorrhage, and failure to visualize the kidney, suggestive of a hilar vascular injury (confirmed by angiogram), are the major indications for operation. Bleeding from the urethra is a common finding in cases of pelvic fractures. Rectal exam may demonstrate a high-riding prostate gland. A urethrogram should be performed to detect a urethral rupture prior to attempted passage of an indwelling urinary catheter. A suprapubic cystostomy is necessary to establish urinary drainage.

Although the survival following severe blunt polytrauma has improved in recent years, the key to improvement rests with innovative prevention programs to reduce the number of victims. The topic of trauma is also covered elsewhere in this text, and the reader is encouraged to peruse this section for further information about other aspects of injury management.

NECK MASSES

The appearance of a neck mass is a common occurrence in infancy and childhood and is a source of parental alarm. The etiology of the neck mass may be congenital, infectious, or neoplastic.

Lymphadenitis

Lymphadenitis is characterized by the presence of enlarged, often tender lymph nodes. Most are the result of a local infection that is controlled by the natural barrier established in the lymphoid tissues. Most cases resolve with treatment of the primary source of infection (e.g., otitis media, tonsillitis). Cervical lymph gland enlargement is often the result of a suppurative bacterial infection due to *Staphylococcus* or *Streptococcus* infection. Acutely infected lymph nodes often enlarge quickly, are painful, and may show erythema (cellulitis) in the skin overlying the mass. Fever and leukocytosis are often present. Antibiotics are started, using a third-generation cephalosporin. The therapy of choice for suppurative lymphadenitis is incision and drainage of the infected lymph node when the mass becomes fluctuant. Appropriate cultures are obtained. Antibiotics are discontinued after 48 hours if the temperature returns to normal. Daily changes of the wound packing that was inserted at the time of drainage are performed by the parents at home. Recurring cases of suppurative lymphadenitis may be caused by an immunodeficiency syndrome (e.g., chronic granulomatous disease, AIDS, Bruton's syndrome).

Lymphadenitis can also be caused by a more indolent chronic inflammatory process, such as atypical mycobacterial infection, cat-scratch disease, or fungal infection (histoplasmosis).[4] Lymph node enlargement is of longer duration than in acute infectious cases, and multiple lymph nodes may be affected. The lymph nodes are also less tender and may be complicated by a draining sinus; there may be enlarged lymph nodes in the mediastinum as well. A chest x-ray should always be obtained when a chronic inflammatory process is suspected. The chest x-ray is usually normal in instances of atypical mycobacterial infection but may show enlarged mediastinal lymph nodes in cases of histoplasmosis. Skin tests should be planted using intermediate PPD (which is usually positive for atypical mycobacterium), and complement fixation titers for histoplasmosis should also be obtained.

The therapy of choice for chronic lymphadenitis due to mycobacteria and occasionally fungi is complete excision of the involved lymph nodes to eradicate the infection, which may be resistant to drug therapy. In some instances, a modified radical neck dissection is necessary to accomplish this goal. Cultures of the lymph node itself should be sent for evaluation of mycobacterium and fungi in addition to bacterial cultures.

Cervical Anomalies

The most common benign cervical anomalies include branchial cleft cysts and sinuses, thyroglossal duct cysts, cystic hygromas, dermoid cysts, hemangiomas, and torticollis.[42, 156]

Bronchial cleft anomalies are remnants of the four paired embryonic branchial arches, clefts, and pouches. These lesions may present as sinuses, fistulas, or cartilaginous rests in infants but more commonly present as cysts in older children, adolescents, and adults. The first branchial cleft sinus presents anterior to the ear and connects with the eustachian tube. The most frequently observed anomaly involves the second branchial cleft remnant, which may present clinically anywhere along the anterior border of the sternocleidomastoid muscle from the angle of the jaw (as a cystic mass) to the lower third of the neck (as a sinus tract). The sinus tract passes cephalad in a deeper path under the digas-

tric muscle, between the branches of the carotid artery, and under the hypoglossal nerve to end in the tonsillar fossa. The tract is excised using a stepladder technique (two incisions) with high ligation at the tonsillar fossa. The third and fourth branchial clefts develop into the lower and upper parathyroid glands, respectively. A deficiency in their development may be part of a pharyngeal pouch deficiency syndrome characterized by absent parathyroids and an absent or depleted thymus (DiGeorge's syndrome), producing an immunosuppressive syndrome (T-cell depletion), hypocalcemia, and seizures. Aortic arch vascular anomalies may also coexist. Therapy includes administration of vitamin D and calcium and fetal thymic tissue or bone marrow transplantation. The fifth embryonic branchial cleft involutes.

Thyroglossal duct anomalies are midline lesions that originate at the base of the tongue at the foramen caecum and pass through the central portion of the hyoid bone. The thyroglossal duct usually obliterates in the sixth intrauterine week. Persistence of this fetal structure postnatally results in a midline swelling over the hyoid bone that moves with deglutition. Infection is the most common complication. A sinus tract may develop as a result of infection. The differential diagnosis of upper midline neck masses includes inflamed submental lymph node, pretracheal dermoid cyst, or ectopic thyroid tissue. The lymph node usually responds to antibiotics, is movable, and is separate from the hyoid bone. Ectopic thyroid is rare, does not get infected, and always appears solid on ultrasonography. Dermoid cysts are usually small and spherical and contain keratin-like material. They do not go through the hyoid bone and shell out easily from the pretracheal fascia at operation. In older individuals, the thyroglossal duct may contain thyroid remnants, which occasionally become malignant. This is extremely rare in children. The treatment of choice is complete excision of the mass with the central portion of the hyoid bone and high suture ligation of the duct at the foramen caecum (Sistrunk's procedure). The recurrence rate is 6 to 9% and is more common following infection. Inadequate resection of the hyoid centrum and recurrence of duct patency at the base of the tongue are the most frequent findings at reoperation.

Cystic hygroma is another neck mass frequently encountered in children. This developmental lymphangioma is derived from the primitive embryonic jugular venolymphatic sacs. In some instances, the mass is detected by prenatal ultrasonography. More commonly, however, the mass is either noted at birth or presents when sudden enlargement of a neck hygroma occurs during an upper respiratory infection and causes severe tracheal compression and air hunger. In 10% of cases, the mass extends into the axilla or mediastinum. A chest x-ray or neck and chest ultrasonography usually identifies these cases. Complete excision is the therapy of choice; however, this is not always possible, as the mass may be more solid in nature and infiltrate structures such as the tongue or pharynx. The cystic form is frequently intimately adherent to vital structures (e.g., vagus nerve, phrenic nerve) that should not be sacrificed, since this lesion is benign. Sclerosing agents, steroid injection, and irradiation have been used but have not been effective. Recent reports indicate that injection of a bleomycin-fat emulsion or intralesional streptococcal lysin may eradicate the hygroma.

Torticollis refers to a hard, spindle-shaped, fibrous tumor within the sternocleidomastoid muscle. The mass is usually detected in the first 2 to 4 weeks of life. The incidence is 0.4% of live births. The most likely cause of this lesion is a birth injury. Torticollis occurs more commonly following breech delivery and may be associated with eventration of the diaphragm and Erb's palsy on the same side. The clinical presentation includes a hard mass within the sternocleidomastoid muscle, ipsilateral facial hemihypoplasia, plagiocephaly, head turned away from the side of the mass, and, occasionally, ipsilateral trapezius atrophy. An underlying cervical vertebral abnormality should be ruled out by obtaining an x-ray of the cervical spine. In older children, a spinal cord tumor at the cervical level should be suspected. In 80% of cases, the mass responds to conservative therapy, which includes ipsilateral stimulation to feeding, light, sound, and so on and range-of-motion exercises twice daily. Approximately 10 to 15% of patients require division of the affected sternocleidomastoid muscle below the level of the exit of the spinal accessory nerve. The two ends should be separated, and any adhesions to the cervical fascia divided.

Neck masses in children can also be caused by a benign or malignant tumor.[42] Primary tumors that arise in the neck in the pediatric age group include teratomas, neurofibromas, salivary gland tumors (submandibular and parotid), thyroid and parathyroid tumors, Hodgkin's disease, non-Hodgkin's lymphomas, cervical neuroblastoma, rhabdomyosarcoma, leukemia, histiocytosis-X, and others that are described in more detail elsewhere in this text.

INGUINAL HERNIA AND HYDROCELE

Inguinal hernia is a common finding in infants and children and represents the condition most frequently requiring surgical repair in the pediatric age group.[54] Persistence of all or part of the embryonic processus vaginalis (which follows the descent of the testis down to the scrotal sac) causes a variety of inguinal anomalies, including scrotal hernia, distal obliteration with proximal hernia sac, communicating hydrocele (which is a hernia with a small connection to the peritoneal cavity), hydrocele of the spermatic cord, and hydrocele of the tunica vaginalis (Fig. 38–22). The incidence of inguinal hernia varies with gestational age, ranging from 9 to 11% in preterm infants to 3.5 to 5% in full-term babies. Inguinal hernia is more common in males than females, has a definite familial tendency, and presents more frequently on the right side as a result of later descent of the right testis and delayed obliteration of the processus vaginalis. Clinical presentation is on the right side in 60% of cases, the left side in 30%, and bilateral in 10%. Bilateral inguinal hernias are more common in preterm infants.[121] The major risk factor in cases of inguinal hernia is the occurrence of bowel incarceration and possible strangulation. The rate of bowel incarceration is significantly higher in premature infants and babies in the first year of life (31%), compared with the general pediatric age group (12 to 15%).[55, 118, 121, 135] Bowel obstruction, gonadal infarction, and intestinal gangrene requiring resection occur more commonly in the first 6 months of life as a result of incarceration.[118, 121] It is often possible to safely reduce an incarcerated hernia in infants and convert an emergent problem that requires an immediate operation to an elective procedure.[54, 55] Sedation, positioning, and gentle taxis to reduce the hernia are successful in 70% of cases. The postoperative complication rate is more than 20% in incarcerated cases, as compared with 1 to 2% in elective procedures.[55, 135] These observations suggest that the best time to repair an inguinal hernia in infancy is shortly after making the diagnosis and before complications occur.

A number of recent trends have influenced the type of patients currently being referred for hernia repair. Advances in neonatal intensive care have resulted in the survival of many small premature infants who have a high incidence of inguinal hernia.[51, 121] A significant number of these babies have been hospitalized for birth asphyxia, respiratory distress syndrome, apnea, bradycardia, and so forth and develop a symptomatic hernia in the neonatal intensive care unit. These babies should have their hernias repaired just prior to hospital discharge.[51, 121] Recent information regarding the depletion of germ cells and volume loss in the first 6 months of life in boys with undescended testes has stimulated the performance of early orchiopexy at 1 year of age. More than 90% of these infants have associated inguinal hernias that require repair at the time of orchiopexy.[54] The use of the peritoneal

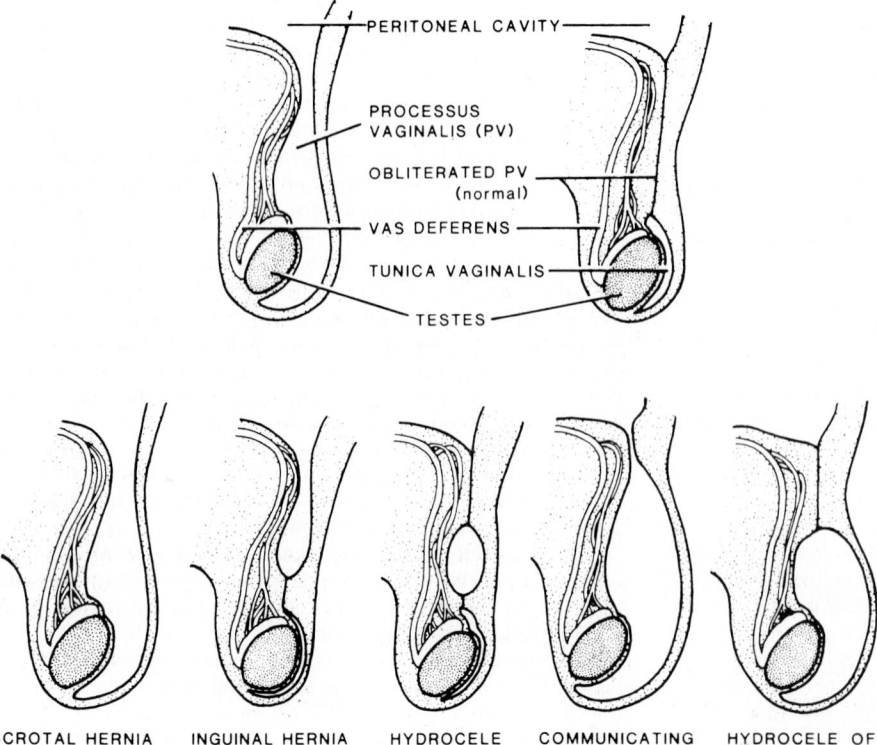

PERITONEAL CAVITY

PROCESSUS VAGINALIS (PV)

OBLITERATED PV (normal)

VAS DEFERENS

TUNICA VAGINALIS

TESTES

SCROTAL HERNIA   INGUINAL HERNIA   HYDROCELE OF THE CORD   COMMUNICATING HYDROCELE   HYDROCELE OF TUNICA VAGINALIS

Figure 38–22. The upper portion of this illustration shows the fetal development of the processus vaginalis and the normal full-term appearance following its obliteration. The lower set of illustrations indicates the common variants of inguinal canal anomalies in infants and children characterized by persistence of all or part of the processus. (From Grosfeld, J. L.: Current concepts in inguinal hernia in infants and children. World J. Surg., *13*:506, 1989.)

cavity for fluid absorptive purposes in infants with hydrocephalus treated by ventriculoperitoneal shunts and continuous ambulatory peritoneal dialysis for chronic renal failure or metabolic derangements (hyperammonemia, lactic acidosis) cause increased intra-abdominal pressure, leading to a high incidence of previously unrecognized inguinal hernia.[54, 151, 154] Recognition of these and other conditions associated with an increased incidence of inguinal hernia (Table 38–5) should allow early identification and treatment prior to the development of serious complications.

The technical details of inguinal hernia repair in children have been previously published.[55] Most infants can be successfully managed by high-suture ligation of the indirect hernia sac at the level of the internal ring with nonabsorbable suture. In some patients with a large internal ring, the transversalis fascia inferior to the internal ring is snugged to reduce the size of the excessively large opening without causing compression of the spermatic vessels. Contralateral exploration of the opposite groin is routinely performed in the first 2 years of life, in females less than 3 years old (who have a higher rate of bilaterality), in patients with ventriculoperitoneal shunts, and in babies less than 2 years old who present with a clinical hernia on the left side.[55, 136] Some suggest that insertion of a laparoscopy port through the clinical hernia sac allows detection of a contralateral hernia with an angled endoscope.

All full-term infants and older children without underlying illness can undergo hernia repair in an outpatient setting. Outpatient hernia repair in children is safe, effective, and well tolerated; it avoids the psychological trauma of hospitalization, reduces the cross-infection rate, and is cost-effective. Outpatient surgery centers for children must have skilled pediatric anesthesia and nursing staffs, a pleasant environment, appropriately sized pediatric equipment and monitoring capability, and the ability to admit a baby postoperatively to a pediatric inpatient facility if necessary. Some infants with symptomatic inguinal hernias need to be admitted to the hospital. Those with bronchopulmonary dysplasia, a history of prematurity (up to 6 months of age), a history of apnea or bradycardia, severe congenital heart disease, and seizure disorders should be admitted postoperatively (23-hour admission) for monitoring purposes.[99, 150]

In instances of communicating hydrocele, the child's parent often describes a changing size of the scrotal sac due to

exchange of fluid between a narrow connection of the hydrocele and the peritoneal cavity. Communicating hydrocele is a misnomer, as the pathology is that of a hernia that requires repair. A hydrocele of the spermatic cord often presents as a spherical mass in the inguinal canal. In most instances, the hydrocele has a small connection with the peritoneal cavity and should be treated by surgical excision and high ligation of the sac. In young females, this presents as a hydrocele in the canal of Nuck. Occasionally, females have sliding hernias containing the ovary and fallopian tube. These should be repaired promptly, as there is a risk of ovarian torsion in the inguinal canal. The hydrocele of the tunica vaginalis may spontaneously resolve in the first 6 months of life. If it persists beyond that time, there is probably a connection to the peritoneal cavity, indicating that surgical intervention is warranted. Acquired hydroceles can develop in older children as a result of tumor, trauma, or inflammation and may require hydrocelectomy.

UMBILICAL HERNIA

Umbilical hernia is a defect of the umbilical ring. The sac has an inner lining of peritoneum, which is adherent to the undersurface of the umbilical skin. Umbilical hernia is more common in females and black children. The natural history of umbilical hernia is spontaneous involution in 80% of cases. The defect in these cases is usually less than 2 cm. Hernia defects greater than 2.0 cm. often do not close. Unlike inguinal hernias, umbilical hernias are rarely associated with complications. As it is a low-risk lesion, it is reasonable to observe an umbilical hernia for 3 to 4 years in anticipation of its spontaneous closure. In cases that persist for more than 4 years, an umbilical hernia repair should be performed with suture inversion of the undersurface of the umbilical skin for cosmetic purposes. If the patient requires a general anesthetic for repair of an inguinal hernia, the umbilical hernia can be repaired at the same time before 3 to 4 years of age.

UNDESCENDED TESTES

Undescended testes are observed in 1 to 2% of full-term boys. The actual incidence varies considerably with gestational age. Up to 30% of preterm babies may have an undescended testis.[92] The cryptorchid testis is associated with both histologic and morphologic changes in the affected testis, characterized by loss of volume and progressive germ cell depletion starting at 6 months of age.[39] Other histologic changes occur, including atrophy of Leydig cells, decreased tubular diameter, and reduced number of spermatogonia by 2 years of age. Since some undescended testes noted in premature infants eventually descend by 1 year of age, the infant is usually observed until that time. The differential diagnosis includes *bashful* (retractile) testis, ectopic testis, and monorchism. A retractile testis can be brought into the scrotal sac on physical examination in a frogleg position and is managed nonoperatively. Ectopic testis is usually detected in an aberrant location after exiting from the external ring at the time of inguinal exploration. Although some clinicians advocate therapy with human chorionic gonadotropin (hCG), the results have been discouraging, and the response rate is worst between 1 and 2 years of age.[39] Early orchiopexy with dartos pouch fixation is recommended at 1 year of age. For nonpalpable intra-abdominal testis, retroperitoneal laparoscopy can identify the presence and location of the testis and facilitate a staged repair.

TABLE 38–5. Conditions Associated with an Increased Incidence of Inguinal Hernia

Prematurity
Positive family history
Hydrops
Meconium peritonitis
Chylous ascites
Liver disease with ascites
Abdominal wall defects
Ambiguous genitalia
Hypospadias, epispadias
Exstrophy of bladder, cloaca
Cryptorchid testes
Cystic fibrosis
Connective tissue disorders
Ventriculoperitoneal shunt
Continuous ambulatory peritoneal dialysis
Hunter-Hurler syndrome
Mucopolysaccharidosis

Patients seen at the J. W. Riley Hospital for Children, Indiana University Medical Center, Indianapolis, Ind.
From Grosfeld, J. L.: Current concepts in inguinal hernia in infants and children. World J. Surg., *13*:506, 1989.

TUMORS

Significant advances have been made in the management of infants and children with malignant solid tumors. Improved understanding of tumor behavior and response to combined modalities of treatment has resulted in improved survival in a number of neoplasms. Many of these advances have been made possible by the development of cooperative study groups and multidisciplinary care.

Wilms' Tumor

Wilms' tumor (nephroblastoma) is an embryonal tumor of renal origin. Approximately 500 new cases of this pediatric malignancy are seen in the United States annually.[49, 65] Most are managed according to protocols of the National Wilms' Tumor Study Group (NWTS).[15, 30] An abdominal mass is often detected by a parent while bathing the infant or child. Hematuria is noted in 10 to 15% of cases, often after relatively minimal trauma to an unsuspected renal tumor. Hypertension is present in 20% of cases and is related to compression of the juxtaglomerular apparatus by the tumor, causing a renin-angiotension release. The majority of patients are diagnosed between 1 and 4 years of age. However, Wilms' tumor occurs in older children and occasionally adolescents or young adults. Wilms' tumor is more commonly observed in infants with sporadic aniridia, hemihypertrophy, Beckwith-Wiedemann syndrome, neurofibromatosis, horseshoe kidney, and Pearlman's syndrome; in families with genitourinary anomalies; and as a hereditary factor associated with the eighth and eleventh chromosomes.[65] The WT-1 gene is located on the eleventh chromosome $(11p^{13})$.[18] The WT-2 gene has been identified on the $11p^{15}$ locus in children with Beckwith's syndrome. Some children with aggressive, unresponsive tumors have an abnormal locus on the sixteenth chromosome.

On physical examination, Wilms' tumor presents as a round, smooth, hard flank mass. The mass is usually nontender. Ultrasonography demonstrates a solid intrarenal lesion and also indicates whether the tumor has extended into the renal vein, inferior vena cava, or occasionally the right atrium. The next diagnostic test obtained is a CT study of the abdomen with intravenous contrast.[26, 31] This demonstrates a renal mass and a pyelogram effect showing intrinsic distortion of the collecting system with medial displacement of the kidney. The CT study usually separates the kidney from other organs (e.g., adrenal glands), indicates whether the tumor involves the liver on the right side or the diaphragm on either side by direct extension, identifies the presence of enlarged and suspicious perirenal and para-aortic lymph nodes, evaluates for a second tumor in the opposite kidney, and determines whether the patient has liver metastases.[25] A chest x-ray and chest CT scan are obtained to evaluate for lung metastases. Bone survey is obtained in children with clear-cell renal tumors who are at risk for bone metastasis, which is rare in patients with Wilms' tumor. Arteriograms and MRI are rarely helpful in the preoperative evaluation of Wilms' tumor, and for most patients, these tests are both unnecessary and unduly expensive. Special (helical) CT with three-dimensional reconstruction is useful in determining the resectability of tumors in close proximity to large vessels.

The treatment of Wilms' tumor depends on the staging of the specific case by preoperative and postoperative evaluation of the extent of disease based on preliminary studies as outlined above; the resectability of the primary tumor; the status of perirenal, capsular, and lymph node involvement; local invasion of nearby organs and structures (e.g., liver, diaphragm, mesentery); tumor histology; and the presence or absence of distant metastases or contralateral involvement (second Wilms' tumor). Operative management includes a carefully planned, well-monitored radical resection of the affected kidney through a long transverse transabdominal incision under general endotracheal anesthesia.[55, 65] The incision should be large enough to examine both sides and remove the tumor without spillage. The opposite kidney and the liver are first evaluated for possible tumor involvement. The colon attachment and mesentery are carefully separated from the tumor and moved medially. The duodenum and liver are carefully freed on the right side, and the splenic flexure of the colon is mobilized on the left. The spleen and pancreas are elevated and retracted anteriorly and superiorly on the left side, exposing the entire upper retroperitoneal space and diaphragm. When feasible, the hilum of the kidney is approached initially, and the renal artery and vein are identified, doubly ligated, and divided.[56] This controls blood loss during the resection and also theoretically reduces the risk of blood-borne and lymphatic metastases during the procedure. This may not always be possible, and mobilization of the tumor may be necessary in some instances to clearly identify the vascular pedicle without injuring other structures (e.g., superior mesenteric artery). The tumor is dissected free from the aorta, and the specimen includes lymph node–bearing tissues in the renal hilum and ipsilateral para-aortic region, which are excised for staging purposes. The retrorenal fossa is freed, and any attachments to the diaphragm may require *en bloc* excision with the tumor. On the right side, direct extension of tumor into the liver also requires *en bloc* resection in 1.5 to 7% of cases. The adrenal gland can be spared if the tumor is small or is located in the inferior pole; however, this organ must be excised if the primary lesion involves the superior pole of the kidney. In rare instances, the tumor may not be amenable to safe resection at the first procedure. Under these circumstances, a biopsy is obtained to confirm the histology (which is inadequate with a needle biopsy), and the patient is treated with two courses of chemotherapy to shrink the tumor. A successful second-look resection of the tumor is almost always possible.[68, 125, 132, 159] Postoperative complications are infrequent.[65, 123, 130]

The current staging system of the NWTS-4 is listed in Table 38–6. Following surgical excision, treatment depends on both stage and histology. The histologic evaluation of Wilms' tumor is accomplished in a central pathology center to confirm local impressions. Histology is divided into *favorable* (FH) and *unfavorable* (UH) types, which reflect invasiveness of the tumor and probable response to therapy. Favorable lesions represent 89% of cases, unfavorable 11%.[15, 49] The former are characterized by blastemal, epithelial, mixed, and even glomerular elements, and the latter are anaplastic. Anaplastic tumors are characterized by nuclear pleomorphism and extreme hyperdiploidy. Stage I and II cases with FH are treated with actinomycin-D and vincristine in pulse courses and have a 95% survival. Anaplastic tumors are rare under the age of 2 years. If an anaplastic tumor is completely resected and considered Stage I, the outcome is similar to Stage I infants with FH. In more advanced stages, however, anaplastic tumors have a 55% relapse rate and 45% mortality. The overall survival for FH tumors is 90% for all stages. The few patients with FH tumors who succumb are nonresponsive to

TABLE 38–6. Staging for Wilms' Tumor

Stage	Description
I	Tumor limited to the kidney and completely resected
II	Tumor extends beyond the kidney but is completely resected; capsule invasion, perirenal tissues may be involved
III	Residual nonhematogenous tumor confined to the abdomen, including tumor rupture (or biopsy) or peritoneal implants; lymph nodes involved
IV	Hematogenous metastases (lung, distant lymph nodes, brain)
V	Bilateral renal involvement

treatment and usually have primitive blastemal tumors, which are more invasive in nature.[116] In Stages I and II, these tumors are more adherent to surrounding structures, and there may be tumor in intrarenal vessels. Stage III patients have an 80% survival, and even in the presence of metastatic disease (Stage IV), 60% survive.[30, 65] These advanced cases are treated with three-drug chemotherapy, with the addition of adriamycin to the treatment protocol. Unresponsive cases are treated with second-phase drugs, including ifosfamide and cis-platinum.

The treatment of pulmonary metastases is still controversial. Treatment with chemotherapy and whole-lung irradiation (1800 cGy to each side) appears to be as effective alone as when combined with surgical excision of multiple metastases.[50] The incidence of pulmonary relapse is quite low (7%), but 13% of patients acquire radiation pneumonitis as a complication of therapy. Another special circumstance is management of intracaval involvement, which occurs in 4% of cases. Appropriate excision of the primary tumor and tumor thrombus is advised. The level of tumor thrombus is an important preoperative consideration (infrahepatic cava, 61%; intrahepatic cava, 14%; and suprahepatic inferior vena cava or right atrium, 21%). In the latter cases, cardiopulmonary bypass should be an available surgical adjunct. Cardiovascular bypass has been used successfully by a number of investigators to safely remove tumor thrombus from the right atrium and pulmonary artery.[65] The level of thrombus involvement does not affect outcome. Recent data suggest that intravascular tumor can be successfully managed with preoperative chemotherapy and delayed surgical intervention, if necessary.[126, 131]

The overall survival is 88%, 89%, and 62% for Stages II, III, and IV, respectively. The key indicator of survival is tumor histology. In cases of massive involvement, using preoperative chemotherapy to shrink the tumor may make the resection safer.[154] In Stage V disease (bilateral Wilms' tumor), a very conservative approach to therapy is recommended in an attempt to preserve renal parenchyma and to avoid bilateral nephrectomy, the need for dialysis, and renal transplantation. Treatment options include bilateral heminephrectomy if feasible, initial bilateral biopsy, chemotherapy, avoidance of irradiation therapy and second- or even third-look laparotomies to limit renal resection, and total nephrectomy on one side and partial nephrectomy on the other. In a relatively large group of NWTS patients, the 3-year survival was 76%, despite institutional variation in therapy. Currently, unless both tumors are small and allow bilateral partial nephrectomy, bilateral biopsy and chemotherapy at the onset of treatment are favored. Fortunately, most patients have favorable histology (86%). Ten percent have UF, and 4% have discordant pathology, with FH on one side and UH on the other. This latter observation indicates that both kidneys must always be biopsied. The best prognosis in Stage V disease is in patients less than 3 three years of age with FH, negative lymph node involvement, and lower staging of the more advanced of the two renal lesions.

Mesoblastic Nephroma

Mesoblastic nephroma (renal embryoma) is a renal tumor that usually presents in infants less than 3 to 4 months of age.[22] The tumor is embryonic in nature and has been detected on prenatal ultrasound examination. The mass appears as a solid lesion with a concentric ring pattern. An abdominal CT examination with contrast shows a solid neoplasm (which occassionally contains calcium) with intrarenal distortion of the collecting system. The treatment of choice is nephrectomy with lymph node sampling, since the tumor rarely behaves in a malignant fashion. More than 95% of mesonephric nephromas are benign and need no other treatment.

Nephroblastomatosis

Nephroblastomatosis (nodular renal blastema) is a benign condition characterized by subcapsular nests of primitive metanephric epithelial rests around the rim of the kidney. This condition may be multifocal and involve both kidneys. The nephrogenic rest may undergo sclerosis, involution, or hyperplastic overgrowth, with tumor induction to a neoplastic rest, which has the potential to progress to a Wilms' tumor (with mitosis) or an adenomatous rest (no mitosis). Nephroblastomatosis is therefore an accumulation of multiple nephrogenic rests. Ninety percent of cases of synchronous bilateral Wilms' tumor and 94% of metachronous bilateral tumors contain areas of intralobar nephrogenic rests. The risk of a nephrogenic rest becoming malignant is 1 to 3%.

Neuroblastoma

Neuroblastoma is an embryonal tumor of neural crest origin that may arise anywhere in the sympathetic nervous system, including the neck (3%), posterior mediastinum (20%), pelvis (3%), para-aortic paraspinal ganglia (24%), and adrenal medulla (50%).[52] This is the most common solid malignant tumor of infancy and occurs in 1 per 7000 to 10,000 live births. More than 50% of cases occur in the first 2 years of life and 90% by 8 years. The tumor may be observed in patients with Hirschsprung's disease, fetal alcohol syndrome, and Beckwith-Weidemann syndrome and in children born to mothers taking phenylhydantoin for seizures.[52, 134] The tumor could be classified as an APUD tumor, since it secretes a number of hormones and other substances, including vasoactive intestinal polypeptide (VIP), vasoactive substances such as catecholamines and their by-products (homovanillic acid [HVA], vanillylmondelic acid [VMA], 3-methyltyrosine [3-MT], metanephrines, and dopamine), ferritin, and rarely acetylcholine. Symptoms vary according to tumor location and whether metastases have occurred. An abdominal mass is palpable in 50% of cases and is firm, nodular, and somewhat tender. Respiratory distress (mediastinal tumor), Horner's syndrome (upper chest or neck lesion), proptosis or bilateral black eyes (so-called panda eyes) from orbital metastases, leg pain and refusal to walk from bone metastases, hepatomegaly, and subcutaneous tumor nodules are other findings. Systemic manifestations, such as anemia, failure to thrive, weight loss, and poor nutritional status, may be observed in cases with bone marrow metastases and advanced disease. Paraplegia or cauda equina syndrome is related to extradural extension of tumor. Hypokalemic watery diarrhea syndrome (due to VIP secretion) and opsomyoclonus and nystagmus (dancing-eye syndrome) may also be indicative of a neurogenic tumor.[157] Hypertension is noted in 20 to 35% of cases due to release of catecholamines. Neuroblastoma has been characterized cytogenetically with loss of heterozygosity (deletion at the 1p36 chromosomal position).[16, 44] Diagnosis is achieved with plain x-ray and a CT examination of the area involved. Stippled calcification within the mass and paraspinal widening may also be noted. CT scans usually discern between a renal tumor and neuroblastoma, which displaces the kidney either downward (adrenal tumor) or laterally (paraspinal lesion).[52] Spinal involvement is best detected with an MRI study. Bone survey and bone-seeking MIBG (I^{123} metaiodobenzylguanidine) or ^{99m}Tc scintiscan are useful in detecting bone metastases. These isotopes may also be picked up by the primary tumor. Bone marrow aspirate can demonstrate the presence of tumor rosettes. A 24-hour urinary collection to measure urinary VMA, HVA, and metanephrines confirms elevated levels in more than 85% of cases. Preoperative serum ferritin, neuron-specific enolase (NSE), coagulation profile, and complete blood count are obtained.

TABLE 38–7. Staging for Neuroblastoma (Evans)

Stage	Description
I	Tumor is confined to organ of origin (totally excised)
II	Tumor extends beyond organ of origin but does not cross the midline; regional lymph nodes may be involved
III	Tumor extends beyond the midline to encroach on tissues on opposite side (exclude overhanging tumor)
IV	Distant metastases (skeletal, other organs, soft tissues, distant lymph nodes)
IV-S	Localized primary tumor not crossing the midline with remote disease confined to liver, subcutaneous tissues, and bone marrow, but without evidence of bone cortex involvement

Therapy depends on the extent of disease as determined by preoperative clinical and operative staging. The most frequent staging system utilized has been the Evans system (Table 38–7).[41] A new international staging system has been developed to allow comparison of data among groups and countries (Table 38–8).[146] Very few patients are classified as Stage I (5%), and 25% are Stage II. The majority of patients have advanced disease, with Stage III affecting 20%; more than 50% have metastases at diagnosis (Stage IV or IV-S). Complete surgical excision is the only treatment required for Stage I disease. In patients with Stage II disease, surgical excision alone may also be reasonable therapy if the tumor histology is favorable (Shimada classification stoma-rich, low mitotic karyorrhectic index [MKI]), DNA-flow cytometry shows an aneuploid tumor, and there are fewer than three copies of the N-*myc* oncogene.[105, 143, 144, 155] Normal NSE levels, low serum ferritin, and low *trk* proto-oncogene levels are also useful determinants of a less aggressive tumor.[16, 101, 104] If some of these tests are unfavorable (especially diploidy, more than 10 copies of N-*myc*, and stroma-poor, high MKI, unfavorable Shimada histology), then aggressive chemotherapy programs are added.[16, 105] In Stage III, surgical therapy alone may be reasonable if total excision can be accomplished and all tumor markers are negative. However, at the initial opera-

TABLE 38–8. Proposed International Staging System for Neuroblastoma

Stage	Description
I	Localized tumor confined to the area of origin; complete gross excision, with or without microscopic residual disease; identifiable ipsilateral and contralateral lymph nodes negative microscopically
IIA	Unilateral tumor with incomplete gross excision; identifiable ipsilateral and contralateral lymph nodes negative microscopically
IIB	Unilateral tumor with complete or incomplete gross excision; with positive ipsilateral regional lymph nodes; identifiable contralateral lymph nodes negative microscopically
III	Tumor infiltrating across the midline with or without regional lymph node involvement; or unilateral tumor with contralateral regional lymph node involvement; or midline tumor with bilateral regional lymph node involvement
IV	Dissemination of tumor to distant lymph nodes, bone, bone marrow, liver and/or other organs (except as defined for Stage IV-S)
IV-S	Localized primary tumor as defined for Stage I or IIA, with dissemination limited to liver, skin, or bone marrow

From Smith, E. I., et al.: Surgical perspective on the current staging in neuroblastoma: The international neuroblastoma staging system proposal. J. Pediatr. Surg., 24:386, 1989.

tion, most Stage III cases consist of large, often unresectable neoplasms. Following a biopsy to evaluate histology, *trk*, N-*myc*, and DNA-flow cytometry, these patients are treated with aggressive programs of chemotherapy to shrink the tumor and, it is hoped, allow second-look resection prior to the development of metastases.[53, 58, 68, 72] Unfortunately, many Stage III patients develop metastases early and require the same type of aggressive treatment programs as infants and children with Stage IV (metastatic) disease. This includes multiple drug chemotherapy programs (*cis*-platinum, adriamycin, VP-16, and cyclophosphamide) combined with delayed primary tumor excision,[53, 58] regional radiation therapy for residual nonresectable retroperitoneal disease, total-body irradiation, or near-lethal melphalan therapy and rescue with an autologous bone marrow transplant in which the marrow has been purged of potential neuroblasts with monoclonal antibodies, as retinoic acid has been used as an agent that stimulates tumor maturation. Operation in Stage IV cases permits evaluation of lymph node involvement and resection of the primary tumor, converts cases from a partial response to a complete tumor response at the local site, and determines whether local irradiation is required for unresectable tumor. In some small series, the only survivors with metastatic disease had their primary tumors resected, and in cooperative group studies, surgical resection has also proved advantageous. Survival in Stage IV-S disease is controversial. Although the author usually resects the primary tumor, survival in these unusual cases with hepatic metastases, subcutaneous tumor nodules, and sometimes bone marrow metastases without bone cortex involvement has been achieved even without treatment. Stage IV-S patients with bone marrow metastases and those with more than 10 copies of the N-*myc* oncogene and low *trk* have a guarded outlook and should be treated with chemotherapy. Stage IV-S patients with significant hepatomegaly may develop respiratory distress due to diaphragmatic elevation, coagulopathy, and renal failure, which can be improved with radiation to the liver (600 to 1000 cGy) and/or low-dose cyclophosphamide. The creation of a temporary ventral hernia using Dacron-reinforced Silastic sheeting has been attempted in some cases; however, this is not routinely recommended.

The Japanese have initiated mass screening programs evaluating urinary levels of VMA and HVA in infants at 6 months of age. This has uncovered a large number of infants with neuroblastoma who have an exceptional survival compared with the survival of patients who present with clinical disease. One report of 170 patients detected by screening reported survival in 165 (97%). Screening programs have doubled the detected incidence of neuroblastomas in young infants but have not decreased the number of cases in older children.[11] Many of the cases detected by early screening probably represent tumors that spontaneously regress in patients who do not present with clinical disease.[11] The majority of tumors detected by screening do not have N-*myc* amplification. In addition, mass screening may be negative at 6 months in some children who later present with advanced disease. Ishimoto et al. reported six patients with false-negative urine tests at 6 months who later presented with advanced disease (one Stage III, five Stage IV) and recommended repeat screening at 18 months of age.[81]

The two key determinants of survival in neuroblastoma have been the age of the patient and the stage of disease at diagnosis. In 266 children with neuroblastoma at the author's institution, survival for children less than 1 year of age was 76%, versus 32% for those greater than 1 year of age. Survival for Stage I patients has been near 100%; Stage II, 80%; Stage III, 37%; Stage IV, 12%; and Stage IV-S, 81%. Survival for Stage IV patients less than 1 year of age is 50 to 75%, compared with less than 10% for those over 1 year.[6, 52] Survival by site was 100% for both pelvic and neck primary tumors, 81% for mediastinal lesions, and only 28% for retroperitoneal tumors. The overall survival was 44%. However, 87 of 119 survivors had Stage I, II, or IV-S disease, and 56 patients were less than 1 year of age. Children with VIP secretion and opsomyoclonus or nystagmus have an excellent prognosis, with more than 90% of these patients surviving following tumor resection.[157] These data indicate that an improved prognosis can be anticipated in infants less than 1 year old with Stage I, II, or IV-S; normal NSE and serum ferritin; favorable Shimada tumor histology[144]; aneuploid DNA-flow cytometry[155]; high trk[104]; fewer than three copies of N-myc; normal chromosomal analysis; primary tumors affecting the pelvis, neck, and mediastinum; and good nutrition. In contrast, a poor prognosis might be expected in children with Stage III or IV retroperitoneal tumors,[77] elevated HVA:VMA ratio, elevated NSE and serum ferritin levels, low trk,[104] more than 10 copies of N-myc,[105, 142] diploid DNA-flow cytometry, unfavorable Shimada tumor histology,[144] loss of heterozygosity at the 1p36 chromosomal locus,[44] and malnutrition at diagnosis. An improved understanding of the immune aspects of neuroblastoma, clarification of the role of screening programs for early detection of unsuspected disease in infancy,[11, 138] refinements in combined treatment programs (altering chemotherapy protocols and use of bone marrow transplant early in the treatment phase), and a more careful selection of patients for aggressive therapy based on age, stage, histology, tumor markers, and biologic characteristics such as DNA-flow cytometry, trk levels, and the number of copies of N-myc may prove useful in reducing the mortality of this unusual and highly lethal pediatric cancer.

Rhabdomyosarcoma

Rhabdomyosarcoma is a highly malignant soft tissue sarcoma of infancy and childhood, with an incidence of approximately 8 cases per 1 million children less than 15 years of age. Children with rhabdomyosarcoma have an increased incidence of genitourinary and central nervous system anomalies, including the Arnold-Chiari malformation. Rhabdomyosarcoma has also been observed in the fetal alcohol syndrome, Beckwith-Weidemann syndrome, and Li-Fraumeni syndrome, with familial instances of breast and lung cancer and glioblastoma, and is probably associated with a germ line mutant p53 suppressor gene. Rhabdomyosarcoma invades local structures early, and metastasis occurs via lymphatic and hematogenous spread. Rhabdomyosarcoma can occur in many areas of the body, including the head, neck, orbit, chest wall, mediastinum, respiratory tract, trunk, extremities, perianal region, retroperitoneum, bile duct, bladder, prostate, uterus, vagina, and paratesticular tissues.[66] The survival of infants and children with rhabdomyosarcoma depends on the site of occurrence, extent of disease (stage), and tumor histology.[66] The location of the primary tumor is often age dependent, with lower genitourinary, head, neck, perianal, and bile duct lesions more common in infancy and early childhood; trunk, extremity, and uterine lesions are more common in adolescents. Diagnostic work-up involves a CT scan of the involved region, which also assesses the extent of tissue involvement and local tumor spread. Ultrasonography is useful for a suspected bile duct lesion, and cystoscopy and vaginoscopy are important in staging and acquiring a biopsy in instances of bladder or vaginal tumors. MRI is useful in evaluating possible spinal canal encroachment by a paraspinal tumor or muscle planes in extremity lesions. Spiral CT (helical) with three-dimensional reconstruction is helpful in assessing resectability when the tumor involves large vessels and other vital structures. Since there

are no known tumor markers for rhabdomyosarcoma, an accurate diagnosis is dependent on a tissue biopsy.

Staging is carried out according to the Intergroup Rhabdomyosarcoma Staging (IRS) System (Table 38–9). Accurate staging requires preoperative radiologic assessment, bone marrow aspirate, and histologic evaluation of the surgical margins from resected specimens and lymph nodes, as well as the tumor type. In one survey of 146 patients, 21% had Stage I, 22% Stage II, 28% Stage III, and 29% Stage IV disease at the time of diagnosis.[66] The pathology of rhabdomyosarcoma has been in flux in the past few years. The commonly referred to cell lines are embryonal, alveolar, indeterminate, and unclassified. Botryoid tumor refers to a physical appearance of grapelike clusters of an embryonal tumor growing into a cavity from the wall of the bladder, vagina, and bile duct. The indeterminate and unclassified sarcomas account for 15 to 20% of cases. Embryonal tumors have a favorable prognosis, and alveolar tumors are considered an unfavorable histologic type. Alveolar tumors are more common in the trunk and extremities. The nuclear characteristics of the tumor cells and the predominance of tumor subtype within a specific neoplasm determine the prognosis. Disease-free survival for favorable tumors is 65 to 70% at 2 years but is less than 40% for unfavorable lesions.

The most important phase of therapy for rhabdomyosarcoma is resection of the primary tumor when possible. Patients with complete resection do significantly better than those with gross residual disease, particularly in trunk and extremity tumors. In early IRS group studies, vincristine, actinomycin-D, and cyclophosphamide (VAC) were the chemotherapy agents commonly employed. Stage I patients with favorable histology received adjunctive chemotherapy without radiation. Adriamycin was not additive when given with the VAC program in Stage III cases and could induce cardiotoxicity. Ifosfamide, cis-platinum, and VP-16 were employed for more advanced, recurrent, or unresponsive cases. Local radiotherapy (4000 cGy) to the tumor bed is required in Stage II, III and IV cases and in instances of tumor relapse and reduces the risk of local tumor recurrence. Some sites of primary tumor occurrence preclude a wide cancer resection (e.g., head and neck, pelvis) making adjunctive therapy (chemotherapy and radiation) the mainstay of treatment. For genitourinary tumors, initial biopsy is employed as primary treatment, with combination chemotherapy in attempts to avoid anterior pelvic exenteration.[78] Genitourinary lesions often have favorable histology and tend to stay localized for extended periods, making this approach reasonable. More localized resection of the primary tumor, including partial

TABLE 38–9. Staging for Rhabdomyosarcoma

Stage	Description
I	Localized disease, completely resected, no lymph node involvement
	a. Tumor confined to the muscle or organ of origin
	b. Tumor infiltration outside this structure
II	Localized or regional disease with total gross resection
	a. Primary tumor grossly resected, with "microscopic residual" disease, regional nodes negative
	b. Completely resected primary tumor, i.e., no "microscopic residual" disease in which there is extension into an adjacent organ
	c. Resected primary tumor, with evidence of "microscopic residual" disease and positive nodes (all resected)
III	Incomplete resection or biopsy, with residual unresected disease (either primary tumor or regional nodes)
IV	Distant metastatic disease present at diagnosis (regional nodes excluded)

cystectomy and partial vaginectomy, have been successfully accomplished in some cases. Salvage cystectomy may be possible when relapse occurs. The survival for patients with bladder and prostate tumors is 70%.[78, 101] These results, however, do not compare to the greater than 90% survival in cases of bladder or prostate tumors managed by anterior pelvic exenteration.[66] In addition, functional bladder salvage has been achieved in less than 50% of cases. Patients with vaginal lesions have a greater than 90% survival, but only 40 to 50% of those with uterine tumors survive.[79]

For patients with head and neck primary tumors, especially those with a parameningeal location (sinus, middle ear), craniospinal irradiation and intrathecal chemotherapy reduced the incidence of meningeal spread from 35 to 6% and increased survival. Unfortunately, this treatment caused late complications characterized by cognitive deficits. Craniospinal irradiation is now used only in cases of known intracerebral lesions. The overall survival for those with tumors of the head and neck is 60%. Orbital tumors have an excellent prognosis (greater than 90% survival) with either primary chemotherapy or extirpation of the globe.

Survival in patients with extremity lesions has been adversely affected by attempts to treat these patients with biopsy and primary chemotherapy (converting potential Stage I cases to Stage III) and the high incidence of alveolar histology (44%). Stage III patients have a 35% survival and high rate of local recurrence. Preoperative chemotherapy has been ineffective. Optimal treatment involves early wide local excision (when possible), paying careful attention to the involved muscle compartments during the resection. Limb salvage is usually possible, with survival greater than 70 to 75% in Stage I and II cases after appropriate chemotherapy (VAC) and radiation therapy in Stage II. If microscopic residual disease is noted on histologic evaluation of the initial specimen (Stage IIa), re-excision of the primary tumor site within 2 weeks of the previous surgery results in a statistically improved survival.

Excellent survival is achieved in instances of paratesticular rhabdomyosarcoma (greater than 90%). Most of these cases have favorable histology.[167] The treatment of choice is an orchiectomy with high ligation of the spermatic cord on the affected side through an inguinal incision. The spermatic cord is controlled at the level of the internal inguinal ring prior to mobilizing the tumor and testis. If a biopsy had been done elsewhere through the scrotal sac, a scrotectomy should also be done at the time of definitive resection. Retroperitoneal exploration to evaluate for lymph node involvement (45%) is performed selectively using CT guidance and/or laparoscopic biopsy for staging purposes.[167] The fact that chemotherapy (VAC) is so effective in these cases suggests that radiation therapy may not be necessary for most paratesticular tumors.

Although excellent results have been obtained for certain tumor sites, primary tumors affecting the chest wall, bile ducts, buttocks, and retroperitoneum continue to have a poor prognosis. Infants with tumors involving the perianal area have fared well following abdominoperineal resection, permanent colostomy, chemotherapy, and irradiation. Recently, the author treated two additional children with initial biopsy, chemotherapy, and limited local resection, with no evidence of tumor residual at 2 years.

A review of 3000 patients from IRS-III indicates that the overall 3-year survival rate is 70%. The 5-year survival for the IRS-I study was only 55% but increased to 63% in IRS-II. Stage, site, histology, and tumor size were the main predictors of outcome. Although significant advances have been achieved in certain tumor sites, other locations remain a problem, and Stage IV cases continue to have a dismal outcome (less than 20% survival over 10 years). Pilot studies using more aggressive chemotherapy programs, perhaps in conjunction with bone marrow transplantation (as currently employed in Stage IV neuroblastoma) and second-look procedures to accurately assess complete response to chemotherapy, are currently being considered for advanced cases of rhabdomyosarcoma in the future. The IRS-IV revised the current staging system to include a TNM (T, tumor; N, nodal staging; M, presence of metastases) component for randomization of chemotherapy and radiotherapy treatment areas (Table 38–10). Ifosfamide, cis-platinum, and VP-16 are included as initial agents in advanced stages (Stages III and IV). The efficacy of conventional and hyperfractionated radiotherapy will also be compared.

Hepatic Tumors

Liver tumors in children can be benign or malignant. Benign tumors include hemangioma, hemangioendothelioma, mesenchymal hamartoma, teratoma, and focal nodular hyperplasia. Hepatic adenoma is occasionally seen in teenage girls on birth control pills. Hemangioma is the most frequent benign liver tumor in infancy. These lesions can be solitary and involve a single segment or lobe or present as multiple hemangiomatosis involving the entire liver.[10, 27, 149] On rare occasions, a large vascular malformation ruptures and causes hemoperitoneum. A dynamic CT scan with intravenous bolus contrast is usually diagnostic and shows a characteristic pattern of heterogeneous areas within the liver, with increased filling and rapid emptying of the contrast. Liver hemangiomas follow the natural history of most hemangiomas—spontaneous involution. Unfortunately, some babies present with a syndrome of hepatomegaly, cutaneous hemangioma, and cardiac failure due to A-V shunting within the liver. Treatment includes corticosteroids, diuretics, and digoxin. Recent reports document the efficacy of alpha-interferon in causing involution. Occasionally, continued symptoms require more aggressive treatment. Hepatic resection may be possible for hemangiomas affecting a single liver segment or lobe. In some cases, hepatic artery embolization or ligation may be necessary. The mortality in these latter cases remains high (20 to 33%). Malignant tumors include hepatoblastoma, hepatoma, and rare sarcomas. Hepatoblastoma is seen in infants in the first 3 years of life, and hepatic carcinoma is observed in older children and adolescents.

Liver tumors may be associated with a loss of heterozygosity on the long arm of the fifth chromosome (5q). Liver tumors are more common in children with hemihypertrophy, Beckwith-Weidemann syndrome, Fanconi's disease, and cir-

TABLE 38–10. Staging for Rhabdomyosarcoma by Site and TNM Status

Stage	Site	TNM Status
I	Orbit, genitourinary (nonbladder, nonprostate), head, and neck (nonparameningeal)	T1 or T2, A or B, N0 or N1, M0
II	Genitourinary (bladder, prostate), extremity, parameningeal, other	T1 or T2, A, N0, M0
III	Genitourinary (bladder, prostate), extremity, parameningeal, other	T1 or T2, A or B, N0 or N1, M1
IV	Any site	T1 or T2, A or B, N0 or N1, M1

A, <5 cm.
B, >5 cm.
M0, no distant metastasis; M1, distant metastasis present.
N0, no nodal metastasis; N1, nodal metastasis present.
T1, confined to site of origin; T2, extension or fixation to surrounding tissue.

rhosis due to a variety of conditions, including biliary atresia, histocytosis, cholestasis from the use of total parenteral nutrition in infancy, Type 1 glycogen storage disease, and hereditary tyrosinemia. There is also a relationship between hepatic carcinoma and hepatitis B virus. The patient is usually not jaundiced. The main findings on physical examination are abdominal distention and a right upper quadrant mass that moves with respiration. Serum alpha-fetoprotein (AFP) and ferritin levels may be elevated and can be used as tumor markers. AFP is elevated in 90% of children with hepatoblastoma. Diagnosis can be achieved by observing a right upper quadrant mass (sometimes containing calcium) on a plain abdominal x-ray and CT scan of the abdomen with contrast. The CT scan usually outlines the site of the tumor, clarifies its relationship to the central structures, and evaluates for multicentricity (common in hepatoma patients) and involvement of the contralateral lobe. Spiral (helical) CT with contrast and three-dimensional reconstruction can often predict resectability. An ultrasound study determines if the tumor is solid and also detects tumor extension into the hepatic veins or vena cava. Although an arteriogram was routinely obtained in every prospective candidate for liver resection in the past, a greater appreciation of the segmental anatomy and vascular variations and other more effective diagnostic modalities have made this invasive test less necessary today.

The treatment of choice is complete resection of the tumor by lobectomy or trisegmentectomy. The availability of Cavitron ultrasonic surgical aspiration (CUSA) and rapid transfusers has made hepatic resection a much safer and well-controlled procedure. Recent data indicate that a biopsy and courses of preoperative chemotherapy (Cis-platinum, 5-fluorouracil, and vincristine) in cases of very large primary tumors or those initially considered unresectable result in significant reduction of tumor size and allow for subsequent second-look or delayed primary hepatic resection and long-term survival.[153] The biopsy may be performed with an open technique; however, when preoperative imaging indicates extension of tumor to the opposite lobe or evidence of multifocal disease, a percutaneous biopsy may be performed to confirm the diagnosis.

Malignant liver tumors are staged according to whether the tumor is completely resected (Stage I), resected with microscopic residual disease (Stage II), unresectable tumor or gross residual disease (Stage III), and the presence of metastases, usually to the lungs (Stage IV) (Table 38–11). The best survival (85 to 90%) is achieved in patients with Stage I disease with a complete resection who receive chemotherapy. A recent Intergroup Hepatoma Study showed that four short courses of adriamycin in completely resected Stage I hepatoblastoma with pure fetal histology resulted in a greater than 95% cure rate. The effects of cis-platinum and adriamycin versus cis-platinum, 5-fluorouracil, and vincristine on survival in cases of hepatoma and hepatoblastoma Stages I (90%), II (70%), III (48%), and IV (18%) were similar, but

adriamycin-treated patients had unacceptable toxicity (eight treatment-related deaths) and longer hospital stays. In addition to infants with fetal histology, children with a fibrolamellar hepatocellular histology also have an improved prognosis. The 3-year event-free survival for all cases of hepatoblastoma is 63% but is only 13% for hepatocarcinoma.

Teratomas

Teratomas are composed of tissues from all three germ layers (endoderm, ectoderm, and mesoderm). These lesions can be cystic or solid and occur along the para-axial tissues throughout the body, including the brain, tongue, neck, anterior mediastinum, retroperitoneum, liver, gonadal tissues, and sacrococcygeal regions. In neonates, the sacrococcygeal area is the most common site of tumor occurrence. These tumors are often detected by prenatal ultrasonography in both the cervical and the sacral areas. In the latter instances, delivery by cesarean section may be necessary. In some cases, A-V shunting through the tumor produces a shocklike syndrome associated with severe metabolic acidosis and requires emergency resection in an attempt to salvage the infant. Sacrococcygeal tumors are much more common in females (4:1 ratio). A family history of twinning is observed in 10% of cases. Plain x-ray may demonstrate calcium within the tumor. An ultrasound examination may demonstrate extension of the tumor into the pelvis or abdomen and may also show that the bladder and rectum are displaced anteriorly and the ureters are partially obstructed, causing hydroureter and hydronephrosis. Malignancy is rarely observed in neonates.

Elective resection should be performed in the first week of life. Long delays in recognition, diagnosis, and surgical excision may be associated with a higher rate of malignancy. Malignant teratomas are either endodermal sinus tumors (yolk sac tumors) or embryonal carcinomas. Serum AFP and human chorionic gonadotropin levels may be elevated in instances of yolk sac tumor and can be used as tumor markers. The treatment of choice for sacrococcygeal teratoma is complete excision through a chevron-shaped buttocks incision, with careful preservation of the rectal sphincter muscles. The coccyx should always be resected with the tumor. Failure to do so results in a 35 to 40% tumor recurrence rate. During the dissection, early control of the midsacral vessels that supply the tumor is important and prevents significant hemorrhage, which is the most common operative complication. In instances of malignancy, a careful search for metastatic disease in the liver, lungs, retroperitoneum, and bone marrow, along with chest x-ray, CT scan, and bone marrow aspirate, are in order. Malignant cases are treated with cis-platinum, vinblastine, and bleomycin. Radiation therapy is probably not indicated, since these agents result in an excellent tumor response. When a malignant tumor is not resectable, courses of chemotherapy may shrink the tumor, convert the tumor to a benign-appearing teratoma, and allow complete resection at a second-look procedure, with gratifying survival in some cases.

Teratoma is the most common ovarian tumor in children. The patient may present with a mass or abdominal pain due to torsion of the tumor. The diagnosis is suspected when a calcified mass is noted in the pelvis on plain x-ray of the abdomen. CT scan can confirm this impression and may detect liver and retroperitoneal lymph node involvement in malignant cases. Operative excision, lymph node biopsy (both pelvic and retroperitoneal), peritoneal washings and biopsy, and omentectomy followed by combination chemotherapy result in a favorable outcome in greater than 60% of cases.

TABLE 38–11. Staging for Hepatic Tumors

Stage	Description
I	Confined to the liver and completely removed by surgery
II	Confined to the liver and further subdivided into Stage IIA and IIB: Stage IIA is defined as microscopic residual disease at the margin of resection after surgery; Stage IIB is defined by the presence of regional disease
III	Macroscopic residual tumor remains after surgery; this stage includes tumors that have been ruptured or with nodal involvement
IV	Metastatic disease

SELECTED REFERENCES

Ashcraft, K. W., and Holder, T. M.: Pediatric Esophageal Surgery. Orlando, Grune & Stratton, 1986.
This is an excellent monograph covering disorders of the esophagus in children. The section on embryology is quite thorough. The book is nicely illustrated and is a useful resource for practicing surgeons.

Ashcraft, K. W., and Holder, T. M.: Pediatric Surgery, 3rd ed. Philadelphia, W. B. Saunders, 1993.
This is an updated edition of the standard textbook on pediatric surgery, with new chapters, a contemporary look at topics, and numerous authors.

Dehner, L.: Pediatric Surgical Pathology, 2nd ed. Baltimore, Williams & Wilkins, 1987.
This text is complete and well written, and the content allows the reader to correlate the clinical aspects of the various pediatric disease states with an in-depth review of the pathologic findings.

Gross, R. E.: The Surgery of Infancy and Childhood. Philadelphia, W. B. Saunders, 1953.
This was the most influential textbook on pediatric surgery for more than two decades. The content reflects the enormous personal experience of the late Dr. Robert E. Gross from Boston Children's Hospital. In addition to its historic significance as a reference source, the text is so well written that it is worthwhile reading.

Hays, D. M.: Pediatric Surgical Oncology. Orlando, Grune & Stratton, 1986.
This monograph is an important resource for surgeons interested in pediatric surgical oncology. Each chapter is written by a contributing author who is an expert in the field. Information based on data accrued from cooperative, multidisciplinary tumor study groups is carefully presented, highlighting the current management of solid pediatric malignancies.

Jones, K. L.: Smith's Recognizable Patterns of Human Malformations, 4th ed. Philadelphia, W. B. Saunders, 1986.
This superb textbook is a readable repository of human malformations, including developmental anomalies and intrauterine acquired conditions. The text is well written and beautifully illustrated and presents a concise review of the etiology, history, and prognosis for each syndrome.

Rogers, M. C.: Textbook of Pediatric Intensive Care, 2nd ed. Baltimore, Williams & Wilkins, 1987.
This two-volume text is the most comprehensive resource concerning the rapidly expanding field of pediatric intensive care and critical care. It exposes the reader to the mainstream concepts of intensive care practice in the pediatric setting.

Rowe, M. I., O'Neill, J. A., Jr., Grosfeld, J. L., Fonkalsrud, E. W., and Coran, A. G. (Eds.): Essentials of Pediatric Surgery. St. Louis, Mosby Year Book, 1995.
This concise, contemporary text has easily readable chapters, all of which were written by the five editors. It is excellent for students and residents, is well illustrated, and has good algorithms.

Stephens, F. D., Smith, E. D., and Paul, N. W.: Anorectal Malformations in Children: Update 1988 (Birth Defects Foundation). Vol. 24. New York, Alan R. Liss, 1988.
This leading text describes the various types of congenital anorectal anomalies. It includes the new Wingspread classification of these complex defects and a detailed clinical presentation of current methods of diagnosis and treatment. The recommended surgical techniques are well described and illustrated.

Welch, K. W., Randolph, J. G., Ravitch, M. M., O'Neill, J. A., and Rowe, M. I. (Eds.): Pediatric Surgery, 4th ed. Chicago, Year Book Medical Publishers, 1986.
This two-volume textbook of pediatric surgery is the best comprehensive resource for information about patient care management. The text covers all areas of pediatric surgical care and has numerous contributors who have written chapters in their areas of expertise.

REFERENCES

1. Adzick, N. S., and Harrison, M. R.: Fetal surgery for cystic adenomatoid malformation of the lung. J. Pediatr. Surg., 40:315, 1993.
2. Adzick, N. S., Vacanti, J. P., Lillihei, C. W., et al.: Fetal diaphragmatic hernia: Ultrasound diagnosis and clinical outcome in 38 cases. J. Pediatr. Surg., 24:654, 1989.
3. Allam, B. F., Tillman, J. E., Thomson, T. J., Crossling, F. T., and Gilbert, L. M.: Effective intravenous cyclosporine therapy in a patient with severe Crohn's disease on parenteral nutrition. Gut, 28:1166, 1987.
4. Altman, R. P., and Margileth, A. M.: Cervical lymphadenopathy from atypical mycobacteria: Diagnosis and surgical treatment. J. Pediatr. Surg., 10:419, 1975.
5. Ashcraft, K. W., Holder, T. M., Amoury, R. A., et al.: Diagnosis and treatment of right Bochdalek hernia associated with Group B-streptococcal septicemia. J. Pediatr. Surg., 18:480, 1983.
6. Ashcraft, K. W., Holder, T. M., and Amoury, R. A.: The Thal fundoplication for gastroesophageal reflux. J. Pediatr. Surg., 19:480, 1984.
7. Axelrod, F. B., and Abubbrage, J. J.: Familial dysautonomia: A prospective study of survival. J. Pediatr., 101:234, 1982.
8. Bartlett, R. H.: Extracorporeal life support in neonatal respiratory failure. Surg. Rounds, 12:41, 1989.
9. Bartlett, R. H., Gazzaniga, A. B., et al.: Extracorporeal membrane oxygenation (ECMO) in neonatal respiratory failure: 100 cases. Ann. Surg., 204:236, 1986.
10. Becker, J. M., and Heitler, M. S.: Hepatic hemangioendotheliomas in infancy. Surg. Gynecol. Obstet., 168:189, 1989.
11. Bessho, F., Hashizome, K., Nakajo, T., et al.: Mass screening in Japan increased the detection of infants with neuroblastoma without a decrease in cases in older children. J. Pediatr., 119:237, 1991.
12. Bishop, H. C., and Koop, C. E.: Management of meconium ileus: Resection, Roux-en-Y anastomosis and ileostomy irrigation with pancreatic enzymes. Ann. Surg., 145:410, 1957.
13. Boix-Ochoa, J.: The physiologic approach to the management of gastric esophageal reflux. J. Pediatr. Surg., 21:1032, 1986.
14. Bradburn, N. C., and Schreiner, R. L.: Neonatal seizures. In Schreiner, R. L., and Bradburn, N. C. (Eds.): Care of the Newborn, 2nd ed. New York, Raven Press, 1988, p. 153.
15. Breslow, N., Churchill, G., et al.: Prognosis for Wilms' tumor patients with nonmetastatic disease at diagnosis: Results of the 2nd national Wilms' tumor study. J. Clin. Oncol., 3:521, 1985.
16. Brodeur, G. M., and Fong, C. T.: Molecular biology and genetics of human neuroblastoma. Cancer Genet. Cytogenet., 41:153, 1989.
17. Brynskov, J., Freund, L., Rasmussen, S. N., Lauritzen, K., et al.: A placebo-controlled, double-blind, randomized trial of cyclosporine therapy in active Crohn's disease. N. Engl. J. Med., 321:845, 1989.
18. Call, C. M., Glaster, T., Ito, C. Y., et al.: Isolation and characterization of a zinc-finger polypeptide gene at the human chromosome 11 Wilms' tumor locus. Cell, 60:509, 1990.
19. Canal, D. F., Vane, D. W., Goto, S., and Grosfeld, J. L.: Reduction of lower esophageal sphincter pressure with Stamm gastrostomy. J. Pediatr. Surg., 22:54, 1987.
20. Caniano, D. A., and Beaver, B. L.: Meconium ileus: A 15 year experience with 42 neonates. Surgery, 102:699, 1987.
21. Cates, M., Billmire, D. F., Bull, M. J., and Grosfeld, J. L.: Gastroesophageal dysfunction in Cornelia deLange syndrome. J. Pediatr. Surg., 24:248, 1989.
22. Chan, H. S. L., Cheng, M. Y., Mancer, K., et al.: Congenital mesoblastic nephroma: A clinicoradiologic study of 17 cases representing the pathologic spectrum of disease. J. Pediatr., 111:64, 1987.
23. Cheney, M., Rustad, D. G., and Lilly, J. R.: Choledochal cyst. World J. Surg., 9:244, 1985.
24. Cikrit, D., Mandastrea, J., West, K. W., Schreiner, R. L., and Grosfeld, J. L.: Necrotizing enterocolitis: Factors affecting mortality in 101 surgical cases. Surgery, 96:648, 1984.
25. Cohen, M. D.: Current controversy: Is computed tomography scan of the chest needed in patients with Wilms' tumor? Am. J. Pediatr. Hematol. Oncol., 16:191, 1994.
26. Cohen, M. D., Siddiqui, A., and Weetman, R. M.: A rational approach to the radiologic evaluation of children with Wilms' tumor. Cancer, 50:887, 1982.
27. Cohen, R. C., and Myers, N. A.: Diagnosis and management of massive hepatic hemangiomas in childhood. J. Pediatr. Surg., 21:6, 1986.
28. Coran, A. G.: Perioperative care of the pediatric surgical patient. In Wilmore, D. W., Brennan, M. F., Harken, A. H., Holcroft, J. W., and Meakins, J. L. (Eds.): Care of the Surgical Patient. Vol. 1. New York, Scientific American, 1989, p. 1.
29. Crombleholme, T. M., Harrison, M. R., Langer, J. C., and Longaker, M. T.: Biliary appendicoduodenostomy: A nonrefluxing conduit for biliary reconstruction. J. Pediatr. Surg., 24:665, 1989.
30. D'Angio, G. J., Evans, A. E., et al.: Results of the 3rd national Wilms' tumor study (NWTS-3): A preliminary report. Proc. Am. Assoc. Cancer Res., 183:25, 1984.
31. D'Angioi, G. J., Rosenberg, H., Sharples, K., et al.: Position paper: Imaging methods for primary renal tumors of childhood: Costs vs. benefits. Med. Pediatr. Oncol., 21:205, 1993.
32. Dedinsky, G. K., Vane, D. W., Black, C. T., and Grosfeld, J. L.: Complications and reoperation after Nissen fundoplication in childhood. Am. J. Surg., 153:177, 1987.
33. deLorimier, A. A.: Congenital malformations and neonatal problems of the respiratory tract. In Welch, K. J., Randolph, J. G., Ravitch, M. M., O'Neill, J. A., and Rowe, M. I. (Eds.): Pediatric Surgery, 4th ed. Chicago, Year Book Medical Publishers, 1986, p. 639.
34. deVries, P. A., and Cox, K. L.: Surgery of anorectal anomalies. Surg. Clin. North Am., 65:1139, 1985.
35. deVries, P. A., and Pena, A.: Posterior sagittal anorectoplasty. J. Pediatr. Surg., 17:638, 1982.
36. Ein, S. H., Mercer, S., Humphrey, A., and MacDonald, P.: Colon perforation during attempted barium enema reduction of intussusception. J. Pediatr. Surg., 16:313, 1981.
37. Ein, S. H., Shandling, B., and Heiss, K.: Pure esophageal atresia: Outlook in the 1990's. J. Pediatr. Surg., 28:1147, 1993.
38. Ein, S. H., Shandling, B., Reilly, B. J., and Stringer, D. A.: Hydrostatic reduction of intussusception caused by lead points. J. Pediatr. Surg., 21:883, 1986.
39. Elder, J. S.: The undescended testis: Hormonal and surgical management. Surg. Clin. North Am., 68:983, 1988.

40. Engum, S. E., Grosfeld, J. L., West, K. W., et al.: Analysis of morbidity and mortality in 227 cases of esophageal atresia and/or tracheoesophageal fistula over two decades. Arch. Surg., in press.

41. Evans, A. E., D'Angio, G. J., and Randolph, J. G.: A proposed staging for children with neuroblastoma. Cancer, 27:374, 1971.

42. Filston, H. C.: Head and neck: Sinuses and masses. In Holder, T. M., and Ashcraft, K. W. (Eds.): Pediatric Surgery. Philadelphia, W. B. Saunders, 1981, p. 1062.

43. Fong, C. T.: Molecular diagnosis of genetic disease. Pediatr. Ann., 22:304, 1993.

44. Fong, C. T., Dracopoli, N. C., White, P. S., et al.: Loss of heterozygosity for the short arm of chromosome 1 in human neuroblastomas: Correlation with N-myc amplification. Proc. Natl. Acad. Sci., 86:3753, 1989.

45. Fonkalsrud, E. W., Berquist, W., Vargas, J., Turner, M. K., Ament, M. E., and Foglia, R. P.: Surgical treatment of gastroesophageal reflux syndrome in infants and children. Am. J. Surg., 154:11, 1987.

46. Forbes, D., Hodgson, M., and Hill, R.: The effects of gaviscon and metoclopramide in gastroesophageal reflux in children. J. Pediatr. Gastroenterol. Nutr., 5:549, 1986.

47. Forster, J. C.: The Surgical Diseases of Children. London, John W. Parker & Son, 1860.

48. Frietas, L., Gauthier, F., and Valayer, J.: Second operation for repair of biliary atresia. J. Pediatr. Surg., 22:857, 1987.

49. Green, D. M., Breslow, N. E., and D'Angio, G. J.: The treatment of children with unilateral Wilms' tumor. J. Clin. Oncol., 11:1009, 1993.

50. Green, D. M., Fernbach, D. J., Norhool, P., et al.: The treatment of Wilms' tumor in patients with pulmonary metastases detected only with computed tomography: A report from the National Wilms' Tumor Study. J. Clin. Oncol., 9:1776, 1991.

51. Groff, D., Nagaraj, H. S., and Pietsch, J. B.: Inguinal hernias in premature infants operated on before discharge from the neonatal intensive care unit. Arch. Surg., 120:962, 1985.

52. Grosfeld, J. L.: Neuroblastoma in infants and childhood. In Hays, D. M. (Ed.): Pediatric Surgical Oncology. Orlando, Grune & Stratton 1986, p. 63.

53. Grosfeld, J. L.: Operations for neuroblastoma. In Spitz, L., and Nixon, H. H. (Eds.): Operative Surgery (Pediatric Surgery), 4th ed. London, Butterworth, 1988, p. 478.

54. Grosfeld, J. L.: Current concepts in inguinal hernia in infants and children. World J. Surg., 13:506, 1989.

55. Grosfeld, J. L.: Groin hernia in infants and children. In Nyhus, L. M., and Condon, R. E. (Eds.): Hernia. Philadelphia, J. B. Lippincott, 1989, p. 81.

56. Grosfeld, J. L.: Resection of Wilms' tumor. Surg. Rounds, 12:17, 1989.

57. Grosfeld, J. L., Ballantine, T. V. N., and Shoemaker, R.: Operative management of intestinal atresia based on pathologic findings. J. Pediatr. Surg., 14:368, 1979.

58. Grosfeld, J. L., Cheu, H., Schlatter, M., et al.: Changing trends in necrotizing enterocolitis: Experience with 302 cases in two decades. Ann. Surg., 214:300, 1991.

59. Grosfeld, J. L., Fitzgerald, J. F., Predaina, R., West, K. W., and Vane, D. W.: The efficacy of hepatoportoenterostomy in biliary atresia. Surgery, 106:692, 1989.

60. Grosfeld, J. L., and Rescorla, F. J.: Duodenal atresia and stenosis: Reassessment of treatment and outcome based on antenatal diagnosis, pathologic variance and long-term follow-up. World J. Surg., 17:301, 1993.

61. Grosfeld, J. L., Rescorla, F. J., Skinner, M. A., et al.: The spectrum of biliary tract disorders in infants and children: Experience with 300 cases. Arch. Surg., 129:513, 1994.

62. Grosfeld, J. L., Rescorla, F. J., and West, K. W.: Short bowel syndrome in infants and children: Analysis of survival in 60 cases. Am. J. Surg., 151:41, 1986.

63. Grosfeld, J. L., Rescorla, F. J., West, K. W., and Vane, D. W.: Gastrointestinal injuries in childhood: Analysis of 53 cases. J. Pediatr. Surg., 24:580, 1989.

64. Grosfeld, J. L., Rescorla, R. J., West, K. W., et al.: Neuroblastoma in the first year of life: Clinical and biologic factors influencing outcome. Semin. Pediatr. Surg., 2:37, 1993.

65. Grosfeld, J. L., and Weber, T. R.: Surgical considerations in the treatment of Wilms' tumor. In Gonzales-Crussi, F. (Ed.): Wilms' Tumor (Nephroblastoma) and Related Neoplasms of Childhood. Boca Raton, CRC Press, 1984, p. 263.

66. Grosfeld, J. L., Weber, T. R., Weetman, R. M., and Baehner, R. L.: Rhabdomyosarcomas in childhood: Analysis of survival in 98 cases. J. Pediatr. Surg., 18:141, 1983.

67. Grosfeld, J. L., Weinberger, M., and Clatworthy, H. W., Jr.: Acute appendicitis in the first two years of life. J. Pediatr. Surg., 8:285, 1973.

68. Grosfeld, J. L., West, K. W., and Weber, T. R.: The role of second-look procedures in the management of retroperitoneal tumors in children. Am. J. Pediatr. Hematol. Oncol., 16:441, 1984.

69. Gross, R. E.: The Surgery of Infancy and Childhood. Philadelphia, W. B. Saunders, 1953.

70. Guersant, P. L. B.: Notices sur la Chirurgie des Infants. Paris, Asselin, 1864.

71. Guo, J. B., Ma, X., and Zhou, Q.: Results of air pressure enema reduction of intussusception: 6,396 cases in 13 years. J. Pediatr. Surg., 12:1201, 1986.

72. Haase, G. M., O'Leary, M. C., Ramsay, N. K. C., et al.: Aggressive surgery combined with intensive chemotherapy in proven survival in poor risk neuroblastoma. J. Pediatr. Surg., 26:1119, 1991.

73. Harberg, F. J., Senekjian, E. K., and Pokorny, W. J.: Treatment of uncomplicated meconium ileus via T-tube ileostomy. J. Pediatr. Surg., 16:61, 1981.

74. Harrison, M. R., Langer, J. C., Adzick, N. S., et al.: Correction of congenital diaphragmatic hernia in utero. V. Initial clinical experience. J. Pediatr. Surg., 25:47, 1990.

75. Hatch, E. I.: The acute abdomen in children. Pediatr. Clin. North Am., 32:1151, 1985.

76. Hatch, E. I., Naffis, D., and Chandler, N. W.: Pitfalls in the use of barium enema in appendicitis in children. J. Pediatr. Surg., 16:309, 1981.

77. Hayes, F. K., Green, A., et al.: Surgicopathologic staging of neuroblastoma: Prognostic significance of regional lymph node metastases. J. Pediatr., 102:59, 1983.

78. Hays, D. M., Raney, R. B., and Lawrence, W.: Primary chemotherapy in the treatment of children with bladder-prostate tumor in the intergroup rhabdomyosarcoma study (IRS II). J. Pediatr. Surg., 17:813, 1982.

79. Hays, D. M., Shimada, H., Raney, R. B., et al.: Clinical staging and treatment results in rhabdomyosarcoma of the female genital tract among children and adolescents. Cancer, 61:1893, 1988.

80. Holder, T. M., Ashcraft, K. W., Sharp, R. J., and Amoury, R. A.: Care of infants with esophageal atresia, tracheoesophageal fistula, and associated anomalies. J. Thorac. Cardiovasc. Surg., 94:828, 1987.

81. Ishimoto, K., Kiyokawa, N., Fujita, H., et al.: Problems of mass screening for neuroblastoma: Analysis of false negative cases. J. Pediatr. Surg., 25:398, 1990.

82. Jolley, S. G., Leonard, J. C., and Tunell, W. P.: Gastric emptying in children with gastroesophageal reflux. II. The relationship to retching symptoms following antireflux surgery. J. Pediatr. Surg., 22:929, 1987.

83. Jolley, S. G., Tunell, W. P., Leonard, J. C., Hoelzer, D. J., and Smith, E. I.: Gastric emptying in children with gastroesophageal reflux. I. An estimate of effective gastric emptying. J. Pediatr. Surg., 22:923, 1987.

84. Jones, M. O., Pierro, A., Lloyd, D. A., et al.: The metabolic response to operative stress in infants. J. Pediatr. Surg., 28:1258, 1993.

85. Karp, M. P., Cooney, D. R., Pros, G. A., Newman, B. M., and Jewett, T. C.: The nonoperative management of pediatric hepatic trauma. J. Pediatr. Surg., 18:512, 1983.

86. Karrer, F. M., Flannery, A. M., Nelson, M. D., McLone, D. G., and Raffensperger, J. G.: Anorectal malformations: Evaluation of associated spinal dysraphic syndrome. J. Pediatr. Surg., 23:45, 1988.

87. Karrer, F. M., and Lilly, J. R.: Corticosteroid therapy in biliary atresia. J. Pediatr. Surg., 20:593, 1985.

88. Kasai, M., Kimura, S., Asakura, Y., et al.: Surgical treatment of biliary atresia. J. Pediatr. Surg., 3:665, 1985.

89. Kelley, S. W.: Surgical Diseases of Children: A Modern Treatise on Pediatric Surgery. New York, E. B. Treat, 1909.

90. Kimura, K., Nishijima, E., Muraji, T., et al.: A new surgical approach to extensive aganglionosis. J. Pediatr. Surg., 16:840, 1981.

91. King, D. R., Lobe, T. E., Haase, G. M., et al.: Selective management of the injured spleen. Surgery, 90:677, 1981.

92. Kogan, S. J.: The case for early orchiopexy. In King, L. R. (Ed.): Urologic Surgery in Neonates and Infants. Philadelphia, W. B. Saunders, 1988, p. 396.

93. Kottmeier, P. K., Jongco, B., Velcek, F. T., and Klotz, D.: Absorptive function of the aganglionic ileum. J. Pediatr. Surg., 16:275, 1981.

94. Ladd, W. E., and Gross, R. E.: Abdominal Surgery of Infancy and Childhood. Philadelphia, W. B. Saunders, 1941.

95. Lemons, J. A., and Bradburn, N. C.: Temperature regulation. In Shreiner, R. L., and Bradbum, N. C. (Eds.): Care of the Newborn, 2nd ed. New York, Raven Press, 1988, p. 42.

96. Lenaerts, C., Roy, C. C., Vaillancourt, M., Weber, A. M., Morin, C. L., and Seidman, E.: High incidence of upper gastrointestinal tract involvement in children with Crohn's disease. Pediatrics, 83:777, 1989.

97. Lennard-Jones, J. E.: Azopriothine and 6-mercaptopurine have a role in the treatment of Crohn's disease. Dig. Dis. Sci., 26:364, 1981.

98. Lilly, J. R., Karrer, F. M., Hall, R. J., Stellin, G. P., Vasquez-Estevez, J. J., Greenholz, S. K., Wanek, E. A., and Schroter, G. P.: The surgery of biliary atresia. Ann. Surg., 210:289, 1989.

99. Liu, L. M. P., Cote, C. J., Goudsouzian, N. G., and Ryan, J. F.: Life-threatening apnea in infants recovering from anesthesia. Anesthesiology, 59:506, 1983.

100. Livaditis, A.: Esophageal atresia: A method of bridging large segmental gaps. Z. Kinderchir., 13:298, 1973.

101. Loughlin, K. R., Retik, A. B., Weinstien, J., et al.: Genitourinary rhabdomyosarcoma in children. Cancer, 63:1600, 1989.

102. Lund, D. P., and Hendren, W. H.: Cloacal exstrophy: Experience with 20 cases. J. Pediatr. Surg., 28:1360, 1993.

103. Mollard, P., Marechal, J. M., and Jaubert de Beaujen, J.: Surgical treatment of high imperforate anus with definition of the puborectalis sling by an anterior perineal approach. J. Pediatr. Surg., 13:499, 1978.

104. Nakagawara, A., Arima-Nakagawara, M., Scavarda, N. J., et al.: Association between high levels of expression of the trk gene and favorable outcome in human neuroblastoma. N. Engl. J. Med., 328:847, 1993.

105. Nakagawara, A., Ikeda, K., Yokoyama, T., et al.: Surgical aspects of N-myc oncogene amplification of neuroblastoma. Surgery, 104:34, 1988.

106. Neuhauser, E. D.: Roentgen changes associated with pancreatic insufficiency in early life. Radiology, 46:319, 1946.

107. Noblett, H.: Meconium ileus. In Ravitch, M. M., Welch, K., Benson, C. D.,

Aberdeen, E. I., and Randolph, J. G. (Eds.): Pediatric Surgery, 3rd ed. Chicago, Year Book Medical Publishers, 1979, p. 943.

108. Nomura, F., Hatano, H., Ohnishi, K., Akikusa, B., and Okuda, K.: Effects of anticonvulsant agents on halothane-induced liver injury in human subjects and experimental animals. Hepatology, 6:952, 1986.

109. Ohi, R., Hanamatsu, M., Modizuki, I., et al.: Progress in the treatment of biliary atresia. World J. Surg., 2:285, 1985.

110. Oldham, K. I., Guice, K. S., Kaufman, R. A., et al.: Blunt hepatic injury and elevated hepatic enzymes: A clinical correlation in children. J. Pediatr. Surg., 19:457, 1984.

111. Olsen, M. M., Luck, S. R., Lloyd-Still, J., and Raffensperger, J. G.: The spectrum of meconium disease in infancy. J. Pediatr. Surg., 17:479, 1982.

112. O'Neill, J. A., Templeton, J. M., Schnaufer, L., Bishop, H. C., Ziegler, M. M., and Ross, A. J.: Recent experience with choledochal cyst. Ann. Surg., 205:533, 1985.

113. Orenstien, S. R., Lofton, S. W., and Orenstien, D. M.: Bethanechol for pediatric gastroesophageal reflux: A prospective, blind, controlled study. J. Pediatr. Gastroenterol. Nutr., 5:556, 1986.

114. Papaila, J. G., Vane, D. W., Colville, C., Berend, M., Mallik, G., Canal, D., and Grosfeld, J. L.: The effect of various types of gastrostomy on the lower esophageal sphincter. J. Pediatr. Surg., 22:1198, 1987.

115. Papaila, J. G., Wilmot, D., Grosfeld, J. L., Rescorla, F. J., West, K. W., and Vane, D. W.: Increased incidence of delayed gastric emptying in children with gastroesophageal reflux. Arch. Surg., 124:933, 1989.

116. Pearl, R. H., Wesson, D. E., Spence, L. J., et al.: Splenic injury: A five year update with improved results and changing criteria for conservative management. J. Pediatr. Surg., 24:121, 1989.

117. Pena, A.: Atlas of Surgical Management of Anorectal Malformations. New York, Springer-Verlag, 1989.

118. Puri, P., Guiney, E. J., and O'Donnell, B.: Inguinal hernia in infants: The fate of the testis following incarceration. J. Pediatr. Surg., 19:44, 1984.

119. Ramenofsky, M. L.: Pediatric abdominal trauma. Pediatr. Ann., 16:318, 1987.

120. Randolph, J. G., Newman, K. D., and Anderson, K. D.: Current results in repair of esophageal atresia with tracheoesophageal fistula using physiologic status as a guide to therapy. Ann. Surg., 209:526, 1989.

121. Rescorla, F. J., and Grosfeld, J. L.: Inguinal hernia repair in the perinatal period and early infancy. J. Pediatr. Surg., 19:832, 1984.

122. Rescorla, F. J., and Grosfeld, J. L.: Intestinal atresia and stenosis: Analysis of survival in 120 cases. Surgery, 98:668, 1985.

123. Rescorla, F. J., and Grosfeld, J. L.: Splenic and liver trauma in children. Indiana Med., 82:516, 1989.

124. Rescorla, F. J., and Grosfeld, J. L.: Contemporary management of meconium ileus. World J. Surg., 17:318, 1993.

125. Rescorla, F. J., Morrison, A. M., Engles, D., et al.: Hirschsprung's disease: Evaluation of mortality and long-term function in 260 cases. Arch. Surg., 127:934, 1992.

126. Rescorla, F. J., West, K. W., Scherer, L. R., III, and Grosfeld, J. L.: The complex nature of Type A (long gap) esophageal atresia. Surgery, 116:658, 1994.

127. Rescorla, F. J., Yoder, M. C., West, K. W., and Grosfeld, J. L.: Delayed presentation of a right sided diaphragmatic hernia and Group B streptococcal sepsis. Arch. Surg., 124:1083, 1989.

128. Reynolds, M., Luck, S. R., and Raffensperger, J. G.: The valved conduit prevents ascending cholangitis: A follow-up. J. Pediatr. Surg., 20:696, 1985.

129. Rickham, P. P.: Denis Browne: Surgeon. In Rickham, P. P. (Ed.): Progress in Pediatric Surgery. Vol. 20. Berlin, Springer-Verlag, 1986, p. 69.

130. Ritchie, M. L., Kelalis, P. P., Breslow, N. B., et al.: Surgical complications following nephrectomy for Wilms' tumor—a report from NWTS-3. Surg. Gynecol. Obstet., 175:507, 1993.

131. Ritchie, M. L., Kelalis, P. P., Haase, G. M., et al.: Preoperative therapy for intracaval and atrial extension of Wilms' tumor. Cancer, 71:4104, 1993.

132. Ritchie, M. L., Pringle, K. C., and Breslow, N. E.: Management and outcome of inoperable Wilms' tumor. Ann. Surg., 220:683, 1994.

133. Rosenstien, B. J.: Cystic fibrosis presenting with the meconium plug syndrome. Am. J. Dis. Child., 132:167, 1978.

134. Roshkow, J. E., Haller, J. O., Berdon, W. E., and Sane, S. M.: Hirschsprung's disease, Ondine's curse, and neuroblastoma—manifestations of neurocristopathy. Pediatr. Radiol., 19:45, 1988.

135. Rowe, M. I., Clatworthy, H. W., Jr.: Incarcerated and strangulated hernias in children. Arch. Surg., 101:136, 1970.

136. Rowe, M. I., and Marchildon, M. G.: Inguinal hernia and hydrocele in infants and children. Surg. Clin. North Am., 61:1137, 1981.

137. Savin, R. A., Clatworthy, H. W., Jr.: Appendiceal rupture: A continuing problem. Pediatrics, 63:36, 1979.

138. Sawada, T., Kidowaki, T., Sakamoto, I., et al.: Neuroblastoma: Mass screening for early detection and its prognosis. Cancer, 53:2731, 1984.

139. Schorr, R. M., Greaney, G. C., and Donovan, A. J.: Injuries of the duodenum. Am. J. Surg., 154:938, 1987.

140. Schwartz, M. Z.: An improved technique for circular myotomy in long gap esophageal atresia. J. Pediatr. Surg., 18:833, 1983.

141. Schwartz, M. Z., Tapper, D. M., and Solenberger, R. I.: Management of perforated appendicitis in children. Ann. Surg., 197:407, 1983.

142. Seeger, R. C., Brodeur, G. M., Sather, H., et al.: Association of multiple copies of the N-myc oncogene with rapid progression of neuroblastoma. N. Engl. J. Med., 313:1111, 1985.

143. Shaul, D. B., Schwartz, M. Z., Marr, C., and Tyson, K. R.: Primary repair without routine gastrostomy is the treatment of choice for neonates with esophageal atresia and tracheoesophageal fistula. Arch. Surg., 124:1188, 1989.

144. Shimada, H., Chatten, J., and Newton, W. A.: Histopathologic prognostic factors in neuroblastic tumors. J. Natl. Cancer Inst., 73:409, 1984.

145. Smith, E. D.: The bath water needs changing but don't throw out the baby: An overview of anorectal anomalies. J. Pediatr. Surg., 22:335, 1988.

146. Smith, E. I., Haase, G. M., Seeger, R. C., and Brodeur, G. M.: A surgical perspective on the current staging in neuroblastoma: The international neuroblastoma staging system proposal. J. Pediatr. Surg., 24:386, 1989.

147. Spitz, L.: Gastric transposition for esophageal substitution in children. J. Pediatr. Surg., 27:252, 1992.

148. Spitz, L., Kiely, E., and Brerton, R. J.: Esophageal atresia: A five year experience with 148 cases. J. Pediatr. Surg., 22:103, 1987.

149. Stanley, P., Geer, G. D., Miller, J. H., Gilsanz, V., Landing, B. H., and Boechat, I. M.: Infantile hepatic hemangiomas—clinical features, radiologic investigations, and treatment in 20 patients. Cancer, 64:936, 1989.

150. Steward, D. J.: Preterm infants are more prone to complications following minor surgery than are fullterm infants. Anesthesiology, 59:304, 1982.

151. Stone, M. M., Fonkalsrud, E. W., Salusky, I. B., Takiff, H., Hall, T., and Fine, R. N.: Surgical management of peritoneal dialysis catheters in children: Five-year experience with 1,800 patient-month followup. J. Pediatr. Surg., 21:1177, 1986.

152. Synn, A. Y., Mulvihill, S. I., Fonkalsrud, E. W.: Surgical disorders of the pancreas in infancy and childhood. Am. J. Surg., 156:201, 1988.

153. Tagge, E. P., Tagge, D. V., Reyes, J., et al.: Resection, including transplantation for hepatoblastoma and hepatocellular carcinoma: Impact on survival. J. Pediatr. Surg., 27:292, 1992.

154. Tank, E. S., and Hatch, E. I.: Hernias complicating chronic ambulatory peritoneal dialysis in children. J. Pediatr. Surg., 21:41, 1986.

155. Taylor, S. R., Blatt, J., Costantino, J. P., et al.: Flow cytometric DNA analysis of neuroblastoma and ganglioneuroma: A 10 year retrospective study. Cancer, 62:749, 1988.

156. Telander, R. L., and Deane, S. A.: Thyroglossal duct and branchial cleft cysts and sinuses. Surg. Clin. North Am., 57:779, 1977.

157. Telander, R. L., Smithson, W. A., and Groover, R. V.: Clinical outcome in children with acute cerebellar encephalopathy and neuroblastoma. J. Pediatr. Surg., 24:11, 1989.

158. Templeton, J. M., and O'Neill, J. A.: Anorectal malformations. In Welch, K., Randolph, J. G., Ravitch, M. M., O'Neill, J. A., and Rowe, M. I. (Eds.): Pediatric Surgery, 4th ed. Chicago, Year Book Medical Publishers, 1986, p. 1022.

159. Tournade, M. F., Com-Nouge, C., Voute, P. A., et al.: Results of the 6th International Society of Pediatric Oncology Wilms' tumor trial study: A risk adopted therapeutic approach to Wilms' tumor. J. Clin. Oncol., 11:1014, 1993.

160. Tunell, W. D., Austin, J. C., Barnes, P. A., and Reynolds, A.: Neuroradiologic evaluation of sacral abnormalities in imperforate anus complex. J. Pediatr. Surg., 22:58, 1987.

161. Vane, D. W., Grosfeld, J. L., West, K. W., and Rescorla, F. J.: Pancreatic disorders in infancy and childhood: Experience with 92 cases. J. Pediatr. Surg., 24:771, 1989.

162. Vane, D. W., West, K. W., and Grosfeld, J. L.: Vitelline duct anomalies: Experience with 217 childhood cases. Arch. Surg., 122:542, 1987.

163. Vasquez-Estevez, J. J., Stewart, B. A., Shikes, R. A., et al.: Biliary atresia: Early determination of prognosis. J. Pediatr. Surg., 24:48, 1989.

164. Vaughn, G. D., III, Frazier, O. H., Graham, D. Y., et al.: The use of pyloric exclusion in the management of severe duodenal injury. Am. J. Surg., 134:785, 1977.

165. Waterston, D., Bonham-Carter, R., and Aberdeen, E.: Oesophageal atresia and tracheoesophageal fistula: A study of survival in 218 infants. Lancet, 1:819, 1962.

166. Weeks, D. A., Beckwith, J. B., and Luckey, D. W.: Relapse-associated variables in Stage I favorable histology Wilms' tumor. Cancer, 60:1204, 1987.

167. Weiner, E. S., Lawrence, W., Hays, D., et al.: Retroperitoneal node biopsy in paratesticular rhabdomyosarcoma. J. Pediatr. Surg., 29:171, 1994.

168. Weinstein, S., and Stolar, C. J.: Newborn surgical emergencies, congenital diaphragmatic hernia and ECMO. Pediatr. Clin. North Am., 40:1315, 1993.

169. West, K. W., and Grosfeld, J. L.: Postsplenectomy sepsis: Historical background and current concepts. World J. Surg., 9:477, 1985.

170. West, K. W., Stephens, B., Vane, D. W., and Grosfeld, J. L.: Intussusception: Current management in infants and children. Surgery, 102:704, 1987.

171. Winthrop, A. L., Wesson, D. E., and Filler, R. M.: Traumatic duodenal hematoma in the pediatric patient. J. Pediatr. Surg., 21:757, 1986.

172. Wurtz, F.: Practica der Wundartzney, Basel, 1563.

173. Ziegler, M. M., Ross, A. J., and Bishop, H. L.: Total intestinal aganglionosis: A new technique for prolonged survival. J. Pediatr. Surg., 22:82, 1987.

CHAPTER 39

SURGICAL DISORDERS OF THE EARS, NOSE, PARANASAL SINUSES, PHARYNX, AND LARYNX

James B. Snow, Jr., M.D.

THE EARS

Progress in surgical therapy of the ear began in 1853 when Sir William Wilde of Dublin, father of Oscar Wilde, advocated a postauricular incision for the drainage of subperiosteal abscesses in acute mastoiditis. The next major advance occurred with Herman Schwartze's introduction in 1873 of the complete mastoidectomy. This operation gained great popularity because of its effectiveness in resolving acute mastoiditis. Emanuel Zaufal recognized that the operation did not solve the problem in the presence of a cholesteatoma and in 1890 described the radical mastoidectomy, in which the disease process in the middle ear, antrum, and mastoid cell area is exteriorized by removal of the posterior and superior portion of the bony canal wall. Bondy observed that removal of the tympanic membrane remnants and auditory ossicles was not always necessary to exteriorize cholesteatomas and in 1910 introduced the modified radical mastoidectomy, in which a cholesteatoma lateral to the ossicles could be exteriorized and the hearing preserved. In the 1930s Lempert popularized endaural incisions. The development of the binocular surgical microscope by Holmgren and improved illumination was followed by the introduction of tympanoplasty by Wullstein and Zöllner in the 1950s.[45] The next major advance occurred in 1952 when Rosen mobilized the stapes in a patient with otosclerosis.[34] Shea introduced stapedectomy in 1958 and brought a century of surgical therapy for the middle ear to a dramatic climax.[36] House later developed endolymphatic subarachnoid shunt surgery for Meniere's disease and translabyrinthine and middle cranial fossa approaches to the internal auditory meatus for removal of acoustic neurinomas, vestibular neurectomy, and vascular decompression of the eighth nerve.[21–23] Over the last 30 years, sensory prostheses for individuals who are deaf have been developed. Since deafness from most causes produces loss of the hair cells with relative preservation of the eighth nerve fibers in the cochlea, introduction of electrodes into the scala tympani permits electrical stimulation of the remaining auditory nerve fibers. Single-electrode devices have given way to multichannel cochlear implants.[6] Early cochlear implants provided aid in speech reading, recognition of environmental sounds, and limited open-set speech understanding.[14, 33] Two current strategies of speech processing—compressed analog presentation of the continuous acoustic waveform of speech, and continuous interleaved sampling of speech designed to reduce channel interaction through nonsimultaneous pulses at a high rate of stimulation—promise to improve open-set speech understanding.[43] Cochlear implants have become appropriate therapy for adults who develop deafness postlingually and are habilitation and rehabilitation options for children with congenital or acquired hearing impairment so severe as to preclude benefit from a hearing aid. Auditory brain stem implants are being developed for individuals who have lost both eighth nerves from trauma or from bilateral acoustic neurinomas, as in neurofibromatosis Type 2.

Anatomy of the Ear

The external auditory canal makes a slightly S-shaped curve. The outer third has a cartilaginous skeleton, and the inner two thirds has a bony skeleton. Sebaceous glands and hair are borne in the outer third. The plane of the tympanic membrane makes an angle of 55 degrees with the long axis of the external auditory canal. The tympanic membrane is divided into the pars tensa and the pars flaccida. The pars tensa is composed of three layers: the outer stratified squamous epithelium, which is continuous with the skin of the canal; the fibrous layer; and the inner mucous membrane, which is continuous with the rest of the mucous membrane of the middle ear. The fibrous layer thickens toward the periphery of the tympanic membrane to form the anulus tympanicus, which rests in the sulcus tympanicus, a groove in the most medial aspect of the canal. The fibrous layer ends at the anterior and posterior malleolar folds. The pars flaccida has only two layers, the stratified squamous epithelium laterally and the mucous membrane medially (Fig. 39–1). The long process of the malleus is embedded in the fibrous layer of the tympanic membrane, and the short process projects laterally. The head of the malleus articulates with the body of the incus. The lenticular process of the incus articulates with the head of the stapes. The footplate of the stapes articulates with the oval window (Fig. 39–2).

The middle ear space is irregular and compressed laterally. The part superior to the level of the tympanic membrane is the epitympanum, or attic. The mesotympanum lies directly medial to the tympanic membrane. The hypotympanum is inferior to the level of the tympanic membrane. The basal turn of the cochlea makes an impression on the medial wall of the middle ear, termed the promontory. The tegmen, or roof, of the tympanum is opposite the middle cranial fossa. The tegmen tympani extends posteriorly to become the tegmen of the antrum and mastoid process. The middle ear communicates with the mastoid process through the antrum. All mastoid air cells communicate one through another with the antrum. Pneumatic cells also extend into the petrous pyramid from the antrum, attic, and hypotympanum. The floor of the middle ear is the roof of the jugular fossa.[2]

The cochlea makes two and three-quarter turns in the human. A cross section through the modiolus, or central bony framework, demonstrates in each turn the scala vestibuli, the scala media, and the scala tympani (Fig. 39–3). The scala vestibuli is separated from the scala media by

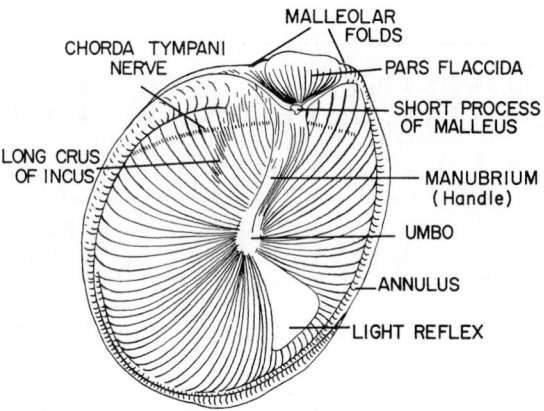

Figure 39–1. Landmarks of the right tympanic membrane. (From Saunders, W. H.: Ears, nose and throat. *In* Prior, J. H., and Silberstein, J. S.: Physical Diagnosis: The History and Examination of the Patient. St. Louis, C. V. Mosby Company, 1963.)

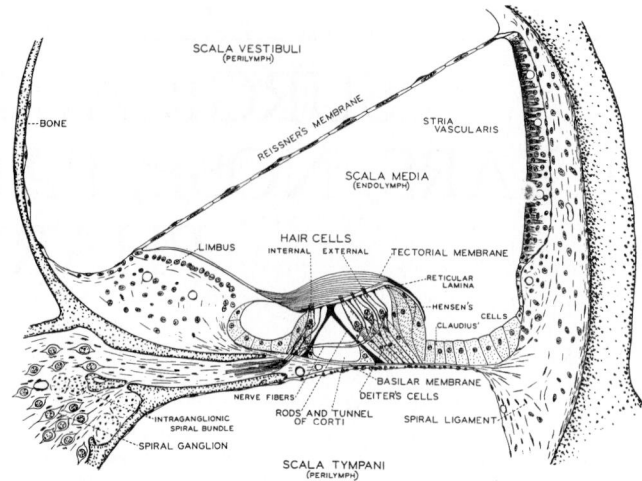

Figure 39–3. Cross section of a turn of the cochlea. (From Davis, H., et al.: Acoust. Soc. Am., *25*:1180, 1953.)

Reissner's membrane. The scala media is separated from the scala tympani by the basilar membrane. The organ of Corti, with its hair cells and their supporting cells, rests on the basilar membrane. The hairs of the hair cells are in contact with the tectorial membrane. Dendrites of the first-order neurons, of which the cell bodies are in the spiral canal of Rosenthal in the modiolus, arborize around the base of the hair cells.

The axons terminate in the dorsal and ventral cochlear nuclei in the medulla. The pathway to the auditory cortex consists of at least four orders of neurons and includes the superior olivary complexes, the lateral lemnisci, the inferior colliculi, and the medial geniculate bodies. Crossing of the midline occurs at the level of the brain stem nuclei and the inferior colliculi. In humans the auditory cortex lies in the posterior portion of the superior temporal gyrus in the sylvian fissure, which is termed Heschl's gyrus.

The saccule is spherical and is connected with the scala media through the canalis reuniens of Hensen (Fig. 39–4). The saccular duct joins the utricular duct to form the endo-

lymphatic duct. The utricle is larger than the saccule and is ovoid. The utricle has five openings for the three ampullated ends of the semicircular canals, the crus simplex of the horizontal semicircular canal, and the crus commune of the superior and posterior semicircular canals. The endolymphatic duct extends through the vestibular aqueduct to the endolymphatic sac, which is located between sheaves of dura on the posterior surface of the petrous pyramid.

The membranous labyrinth contains endolymph. The space between the bony labyrinth and the membranous labyrinth is filled with perilymph. The perilymphatic space communicates with the subarachnoid space through the cochlear aqueduct, which enters the scala tympani. The endolymph is chemically similar to intracellular fluid, with a high K^+ concentration and a low Na^+ concentration, whereas the perilymph resembles extracellular fluid, with a low K^+ and a high Na^+. There is a resting direct current potential difference of 80 millivolts between the endolymph in the scala media and the perilymph, and the endolymph is positively charged relative to the perilymph.

Physiology of the Ear

The external auditory canal maintains the temperature and humidity of the external environment of the tympanic membrane, and this environment varies very little regardless of

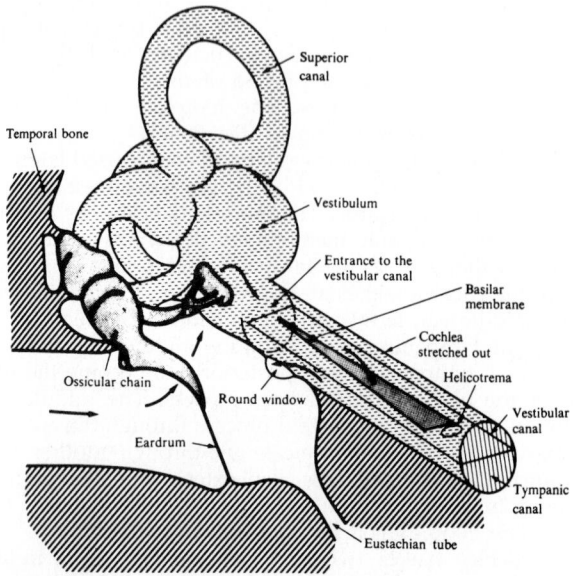

Figure 39–2. Functional diagram of the external, middle, and inner ear with the cochlea unrolled. (From von Békésy, G.: Cochlea mechanics. *In* Theoretical and Mathematical Biology, edited by Talbot H. Waterman and Harold J. Morowitz © 1965, Xerox.)

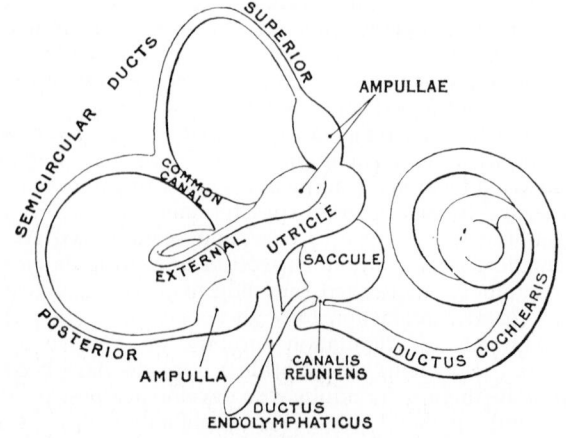

Figure 39–4. Membranous labyrinth. (After Goss, C. N. (Ed.): Gray's Anatomy of the Human Body, 27th ed. Philadelphia, Lea & Febiger, 1959.)

the ambient temperature or humidity. The canal is self-cleansing. Debris is carried by the migration of a sheet of desquamated epithelial cells from the center of the tympanic membrane to its periphery and from the medial portion of the canal to its lateral extent.

Sound waves impinging upon the tympanic membrane set the tympanic membrane in motion. Movement of the tympanic membrane then causes movement of the malleus, incus, and stapes. Movement of the stapes causes pressure changes in the fluid in the inner ear. These pressure changes cause deformation of the basilar membrane. A traveling wave is propagated in the basilar membrane from the base to the apex of the cochlea. Along the length of the basilar membrane, a point of maximal displacement occurs with each traveling wave. The location of the point of maximal displacement depends on the frequency of the stimulating tone. High-frequency tones cause maximal displacement near the base of the cochlea. As the frequency of the stimulating tone is decreased, the point of maximal displacement moves from the base to the apex.

Displacement of the basilar membrane causes movement of the organ of Corti and deformation of the hairs of the hair cells. As the hairs of the hair cells are bent away from the modiolus, a depolarization occurs within the hair cell. An alternating current potential known as the cochlear potential or cochlear microphonic occurs in response to stimulation of the hair cells. The cochlear potential faithfully reproduces the frequency and intensity of the acoustic stimulation through a wide intensity range. In response to mechanical stimulation, the outer hair cells undergo alternating contraction and elongation. Motility of the outer hair cells is thought to alter the physical properties of the organ of Corti and enhance the intensity sensitivity and frequency selectivity of the inner hair cells. A chemical transmitter is released in the region of the boutons terminaux of the afferent eighth nerve fibers. This chemical transmitter initiates depolarization of the dendritic terminals of the afferent nerve fibers.

Trauma and Foreign Bodies

Blunt trauma to the pinna causes a subperichondrial hematoma. When bleeding occurs between the cartilage and the perichondrium, the pinna becomes a reddish-purple shapeless mass. Because the perichondrium carries the blood supply to the cartilage, the cartilage undergoes avascular necrosis if the hematoma is present on both sides of the cartilage, and with time the pinna becomes shriveled. A hematoma may become organized and calcify, which produces the cauliflower ear characteristic of wrestlers and boxers. Treatment consists of incision for aspiration of the clot and approximation of the perichondrium to the cartilage by the use of closed suction drainage so that the cartilage and its blood supply are in contact.[11]

Lacerations of the pinna extending through skin, cartilage, and skin are repaired by suturing of the skin margins of the wound, external splinting of the cartilage of the pinna with a molded splint of cotton soaked in benzoin, and protective dressing. Sutures are not placed in the cartilage.

Perichondritis of the pinna causes accumulation of pus between the perichondrium and the cartilage and leads to avascular and septic necrosis of the cartilage. The infection persists for long periods. The treatment for perichondritis is wide incision for drainage and systemic antibiotic therapy. Often, perichondritis follows a gram-negative rod infection, and culture and sensitivities are of considerable importance. Incisions in the skin of the pinna on its lateral surface for drainage of hematomas and perichondritis should be made just anterior to the antihelix so that the scar is not visible on the lateral view of the ear.

Incision of superficial infections of the pinna is avoided for fear of initiating perichondritis.

Foreign bodies in the external auditory canal are a common problem. Beads, erasers, beans, and other objects may be inserted by children and their siblings into their ears. An insect may find its way into the ear canal and is particularly annoying to the patient until it is killed or removed. Foreign bodies are removed by passing a blunt hook deep to the foreign body for extraction (Fig. 39–5). A forceps is likely to push smooth foreign bodies ahead of it. If the foreign body is far medial, it is difficult to remove without injuring the tympanic membrane and ossicular chain. If a child is uncooperative or the mechanical problem is difficult, a general anesthetic is used for the removal of a foreign body. Metal and glass beads may be removed by irrigation, but care is used to be certain that the foreign body is not hygroscopic, like a bean, because swelling with the addition of water complicates removal. An insect is killed to give the patient immediate relief and facilitate its removal by filling the ear canal with mineral oil. The dead insect is removed with a forceps.

The force of blows to the mandible may be transmitted to the anterior wall of the external auditory canal, which is the posterior wall of the glenoid fossa. In fractures of the anterior wall of the canal, fragments may be displaced to such a degree that stenosis of the canal results. The displaced fragments are reduced or excised under general anesthesia.

The tympanic membrane may be perforated with twigs of a tree, cotton applicators, and other objects placed in the ear canal, missiles such as hot slag in welding, and a sudden overpressure in an explosion (acoustic trauma). Perforations of the tympanic membrane may be associated with dislocation of the ossicular chain. Vertigo or a sensorineural hearing loss suggests that a portion of an ossicle or a missile has been driven into the inner ear or that there is a fistula between the perilymphatic space of the vestibule and the middle ear.[37] These conditions require prompt exploration of the middle ear with an operative microscope and repair of the labyrinthine fistula. Most perforations of the tympanic membrane heal spontaneously in 6 weeks. Instrumentation to approximate the wound margins of the tympanic membrane should be performed under aseptic conditions and microscopic control. It is important to avoid infection during the healing period. The patient must be careful to avoid getting water in the ear. Topical applications have the risk of introducing microorganisms. Prophylactic antibiotic therapy in the form

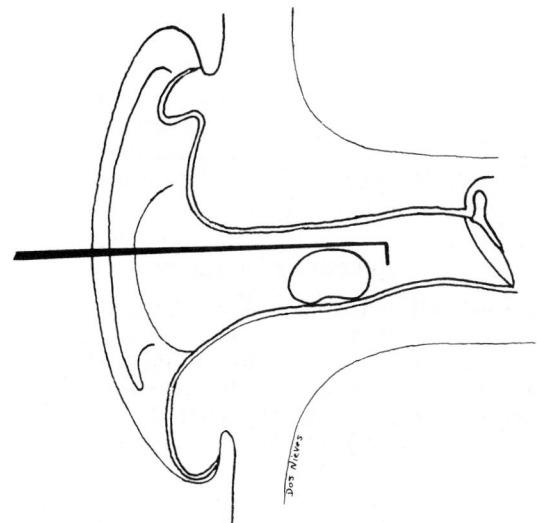

Figure 39–5. Technique for the removal of foreign bodies of the ear canal. The foreign body is raked out with a blunt Day hook.

of oral penicillin for the first 7 days is recommended. If the perforation fails to heal or if there is a persisting conductive hearing loss suggesting discontinuity of the ossicular chain, the middle ear is explored and repaired.

Fractures of the Temporal Bone. Basal skull fractures follow blunt trauma to the head, particularly to the occipital area. Basal skull fractures are, in essence, fractures of the temporal bone, and they are a frequent cause of profound sensorineural hearing loss. Bleeding from the ear following an injury to the skull is pathognomonic of a fracture of the temporal bone whether the bleeding is medial to an intact tympanic membrane, from the middle ear through a rupture of the tympanic membrane, or from a fracture line in the ear canal. Hemotympanum gives the tympanic membrane a blue-black color. Usually, there is a communication with the subarachnoid space through the fracture line. Often there is cerebrospinal fluid otorrhea. Cleaning of the ear canal should be avoided for fear of introducing microorganisms. The immediate danger to the patient is the development of meningitis. Therefore, prophylactic antibiotic therapy is initiated and continued for 7 to 10 days. More fractures of the temporal bone are longitudinal (80%) than are transverse (20%) to the long axis of the petrous pyramid. Longitudinal fractures extend through the middle ear into the ear canal and cause rupture of the tympanic membrane. Transverse fractures extend across the cochlea and fallopian canal to produce a profound, permanent sensorineural hearing loss and a facial paralysis.[39] These fractures are usually well demonstrated with computed tomography (CT). Approximately 35% of longitudinal fractures produce a sensorineural hearing loss, and approximately 15% produce facial paralysis. The fracture extending through the middle ear may cause a dislocation of the ossicular chain that requires subsequent repair. Persistence of a facial paralysis requires decompression of the facial nerve under certain circumstances.

Perilymphatic Fistulas. Strenuous physical exertion or abrupt changes in ambient atmospheric pressure, as occurs during flying or diving, may cause a communication between the perilymphatic space in the inner ear and the middle ear through the footplate of the stapes or the round window membrane. Perilymphatic fistulas also occur spontaneously. The patient may experience a popping sound or the feeling of an explosion in the ear at the onset. Tinnitus, a sensory hearing loss that may fluctuate, and persistent or intermittent vertigo may occur. Increasing and decreasing the pressure in the external auditory canal with a pneumatic otoscope may cause vertigo and nystagmus; this is known as a positive fistula test. The nystagmus can also be demonstrated with electronystagmography during tympanometry, in which the pressure in the ear canal is increased and decreased. The fistula may be found in an exploratory tympanotomy by observing the leak of perilymph through a defect in or around the footplate of the stapes or a laceration of the round window membrane. The fistula may be repaired with a graft of fibrous tissue.

Infectious Diseases

External Otitis. Infection of the ear canal occurs in a diffuse form involving the entire canal, termed otitis externa diffusa, and a localized form due to furunculosis, termed otitis externa circumscripta. The diffuse form may be caused by a gram-negative rod such as *Escherichia coli*, *Pseudomonas aeruginosa*, or *Proteus*, or by *Staphylococcus aureus*. Rarely a fungus may have a pathogenic role. Furunculosis is usually due to *S. aureus*.

Patients with diffuse external otitis complain of itching, pain, foul-smelling discharge, and loss of hearing if the canal becomes swollen or filled with purulent debris. Tenderness

on traction of the pinna and on pressure over the tragus tends to distinguish it from otitis media. The skin of the external auditory canal appears red, swollen, and littered with moist purulent debris.

Treatment with topical antibiotics and corticosteroids is efficacious. Systemic therapy is rarely necessary unless there is a spreading cellulitis around the ear. Furuncles of the canal should be allowed to resolve, because incision may cause perichondritis of the pinna.

Malignant External Otitis. An unusually virulent form of external otitis due to infection with *P. aeruginosa* occurs in diabetics, particularly elderly diabetics with poor metabolic control. It produces pain, purulent otorrhea, and hearing loss. Characteristically, the external auditory canal contains granulation tissue. There is destruction of the bone of the external auditory canal, and the osteomyelitis may spread along the base of the skull to the midline or even to the opposite side.[30] Facial paralysis often occurs owing to involvement of the fallopian canal. Its lethal potential follows the infection's ability to spread intracranially. Surgical intervention is of limited value. Therapy is based on the antibiotic sensitivities of the causative *Pseudomonas* organism and usually requires 6 weeks of oral ciprofloxacin or intravenous administration of an aminoglycoside antibiotic and a semisynthetic penicillin. Careful control of the diabetes is an essential part of the treatment.

Acute Otitis Media. Acute otitis media is an infectious inflammatory process in the middle ear, usually secondary to an upper respiratory tract infection. It is the most common localized infection in children. Most children between 1 and 5 years of age have two or three episodes of acute otitis media each winter. Acute otitis media may be viral or bacterial. Viral otitis media may resolve, or the middle ear may be secondarily invaded by bacteria. In neonates, otitis media is caused by gram-negative enteric bacilli, especially *E. coli*, and *S. aureus*. In older infants and children under 15 years of age, acute suppurative otitis media is caused by group A beta-hemolytic streptococci, *Streptococcus pneumoniae*, *S. aureus*, *Moraxella catarrhalis*, and *Haemophilus influenzae*. In adults, streptococcal, pneumococcal, and staphylococcal infections are most common. Rarely *E. coli*, *Klebsiella pneumoniae*, and *Bacteroides* may produce acute otitis media in children.

Penicillin is the drug of choice for acute otitis media in patients over 14 years of age and adults. In those under 15 years of age, amoxicillin is preferred because of the frequency of *H. influenzae* infections. The treatment is continued for 12 days to ensure resolution and prevention of the sequelae of streptococcal infections.

A myringotomy is indicated when bulging of the tympanic membrane persists despite antibiotic therapy or when the pain and systemic symptoms and signs such as fever, vomiting, and diarrhea are severe. A large curvilinear incision is made parallel to the anulus in the inferior quadrants midway between the umbo and the canal wall (Fig. 39–6). The appearance and movement of the tympanic membrane, tympanometry, and the patient's hearing are followed until there is complete resolution. The management of incomplete resolution is discussed later under *Serous and Secretory Otitis Media*.

The infectious complications of acute otitis media are acute mastoiditis, petrositis, labyrinthitis, facial paralysis, conductive and sensorineural hearing loss, epidural abscess, meningitis, brain abscess, lateral sinus thrombosis, subdural empyema, and otitic hydrocephalus. The most common intracranial complication of acute otitis media is meningitis.

Acute Mastoiditis. In acute otitis media, the infection almost invariably extends through the mastoid antrum into the mastoid cells. However, the term *acute mastoiditis* is not used clinically until destruction of the bony partitions between

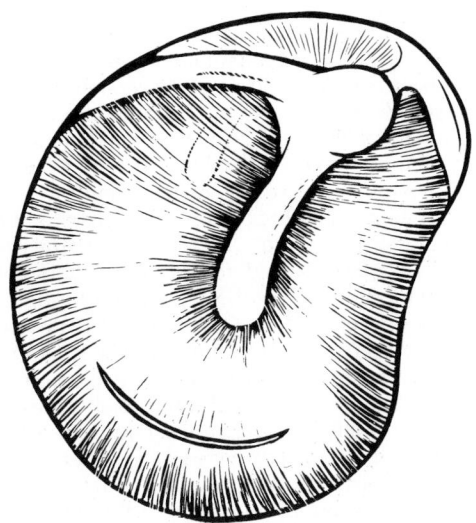

Figure 39–6. Myringotomy incision that occupies one fourth of the circumference of the tympanic membrane midway between the umbo and the annulus tympanicus.

the mastoid air cells has occurred. Progression of the acute infectious stages in the mastoid process is so regularly aborted by antibiotic therapy that clinically apparent acute mastoiditis has become a rare condition. The responsible bacteria are the same as those responsible for acute otitis media.

Acute mastoiditis becomes clinically apparent 14 days or more after the onset of acute otitis media as one of the cortices of the mastoid process is destroyed. Usually associated with this destruction of the mastoid cortex is an exacerbation of the aural pain, fever, and otorrhea. The pain tends to be persistent and throbbing, and the discharge is usually creamy and profuse. Increasing hearing loss is characteristic of acute mastoiditis.

The lateral mastoid cortex is most frequently the first to be destroyed, and a postauricular subperiosteal abscess develops. The first signs are thickening of the postauricular tissue, reduced mobility of the skin over the mastoid cortex, and blunting of the postauricular crease. As pus exudes from the mastoid cortex deep to the periosteum, an erythematous, warm, tender, fluctuant postauricular mass develops, displacing the pinna laterally and inferiorly.

In acute otitis media, there is increased density of the mastoid air cells due to swollen mucous membrane and purulent fluid in the air cells on CT scanning of the temporal bones. In coalescent mastoiditis, the partitions between the air cells become indistinct. The individual septa can no longer be seen as one air cell coalesces with another.

In early cases of acute mastoiditis in which there are postauricular signs of tenderness and edema but no fluctuant subperiosteal abscess, antibiotic therapy may effect complete resolution, with spontaneous healing of the tympanic membrane, reventilation of the middle ear, and return of hearing to the preinfection level.

In the presence of a subperiosteal abscess, complete exenteration of the mastoid air cells (Schwartze operation) should be performed. The operation should include inspection of a small area of the middle and posterior fossa dura to exclude an epidural abscess. The objective of the complete mastoidectomy is to drain the abscess in the mastoid air cells and antrum. Through-and-through drainage of the middle ear is provided by the myringotomy or by perforation of the tympanic membrane anteriorly and through the antrum posteriorly. The goals of this operation are resolution of the

infection, prevention of intracranial infectious complications, spontaneous healing of the perforation of the tympanic membrane, reventilation of the middle ear, and return of hearing to the preinfection level.

Serous and Secretory Otitis Media. Serous and secretory otitis media are manifested as effusions in the middle ear. Such effusions follow incomplete resolution of acute otitis media or eustachian tube obstruction due to inflammatory processes in the nasopharynx, allergic manifestations, hypertrophic adenoids, or benign or malignant nasopharyngeal neoplasms. Normally the middle ear is ventilated three to four times per minute as the eustachian tube opens during swallowing. If the patency of the eustachian tube is compromised, oxygen in the middle ear is absorbed by the blood in the vessels of the mucous membrane of the middle ear, and a relative negative pressure develops. At first there is mild retraction of the tympanic membrane. Soon a transudate of fluid occurs from the blood in the vessels in the mucous membrane of the middle ear. The presence of fluid in the middle ear may be recognized by an amber or dark gray color of the tympanic membrane, immobility of the tympanic membrane, a tympanogram indicating negative pressure in the middle ear, and conductive hearing loss. Rarely an air-fluid level or bubbles of air may be observed through the tympanic membrane. Although there is usually little evidence of acute inflammation, pathogenic bacteria may be cultured from the middle ear in approximately half of children with effusions.[17] In adults, the possibility of a malignant tumor of the nasopharynx must be excluded, requiring careful inspection and often biopsy of the nasopharynx.

Myringotomy for aspiration of the fluid and insertion of a tympanostomy tube for ventilation of the middle ear ameliorate the problem of eustachian tube obstruction regardless of the cause (Fig. 39–7). In children, thorough adenoidectomy is frequently a necessary part of the treatment. Allergic evaluation and management with either elimination of the allergen from the patient's environment or immunotherapy are helpful if there is an underlying allergic manifestation.

In children with middle-ear effusions, initial treatment consists of antibiotic therapy appropriate for acute otitis media for 6 weeks. The antibiotic therapy may sterilize the middle ear as well as ameliorate the eustachian tube obstruction secondary to purulent rhinitis, sinusitis, or adenoiditis. It results in resolution of the middle-ear effusion in one third to one half of patients. Immunologic investigation is occasionally helpful. The Valsalva maneuver and politzerization are employed in the absence of tympanostomy tubes.

Chronic Otitis Media. Chronic otitis media means a permanent perforation of the tympanic membrane. Perforations

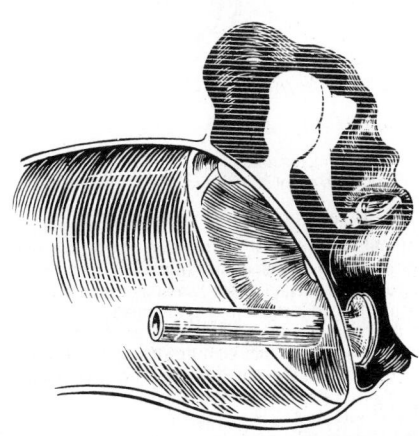

Figure 39–7. Tympanostomy tube placed through a myringotomy incision for ventilation of the middle ear in serous and secretory otitis media.

follow acute otitis media, mechanical trauma, thermal and chemical burns, and blast injuries. Chronic otitis media can be divided into two major categories, depending on the type of perforation present. There is a benign tubotympanic type, with a central perforation of the tympanic membrane, and a dangerous type, with a pars flaccida or marginal perforation.

A central perforation is one in which there is some substance of the tympanic membrane between the rim of the perforation and the bony sulcus tympanicus. These perforations follow commonly from acute otitis media produced by relatively virulent microorganisms. Exacerbations of the chronic otitis media cause painless, purulent otorrhea, which may be foul-smelling and occur secondary to upper respiratory infections and when water gains access to the middle ear in bathing and swimming.

The middle ear can generally be repaired in chronic otitis media with a central perforation. A tympanoplasty provides sound protection for the round window and restores sound-pressure transformation to the oval window.[45] Wullstein categorized tympanoplastic procedures into five types (Fig. 39–8). The Type I tympanoplasty is applicable to a patient with a perforation of the tympanic membrane in which the ossicular chain is intact and mobile. The Type I tympanoplasty, sometimes termed a myringoplasty, restores the tympanic mem-

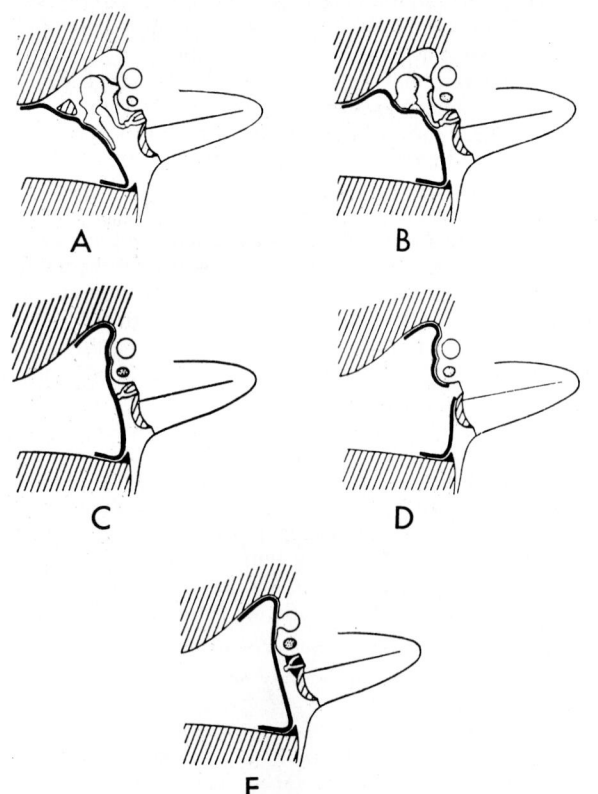

Figure 39–8. Five types of tympanoplasty: *A,* Type I: Perforation of the tympanic membrane repaired with soft tissue graft to the tympanic membrane remnants. *B,* Type II: Perforation of the tympanic membrane and discontinuity of the ossicular chain repaired by soft tissue graft to the tympanic membrane remnants and by rearrangement of the ossicles, bony graft, or prosthesis. *C,* Type III: Perforation of the tympanic membrane and destruction of the incus and malleus repaired by applying to the tympanic membrane remnants a soft tissue graft, which is placed in contact with the head of the stapes (columellar effect). *D,* Type IV: Perforation of the tympanic membrane with destruction of the superstructure (head, neck, and crura) of the stapes repaired by creating an air-filled space between the round window and the eustachian tube to provide sound protection for the round window. *E,* Type V: Perforation of the tympanic membrane with destruction of the stapedial superstructure and fixation of its footplate repaired by protecting the round window from sound and fenestrating the horizontal semicircular canal. (From Shambaugh, G. E., Jr.: Surgery of the Ear, 2nd ed. Philadelphia, W. B. Saunders Company, 1967.)

brane by the use of a graft of soft tissue such as temporalis muscle fascia.[20] A Type II tympanoplasty is required if there has been greater damage to the middle ear. Disruption of the ossicular chain, which often occurs as a result of necrosis of the long process of the incus, must be repaired in addition to grafting of the tympanic membrane.[20] Often the remnant of the incus or the head of the malleus can be remodeled and repositioned for the purpose of re-establishing the continuity of the ossicular chain. Alloplastic materials such as hydroxylapatite are also used for restoring the sound-conducting mechanism.[16] A Type III tympanoplasty is required for a still more severely damaged middle ear in which the malleus and incus are not usable and only the stapes remains. Under these circumstances, the graft is placed in contact with the head of the stapes for the purpose of producing a columellar effect similar to the single middle ear ossicle or columella found in birds. Tympanoplasty Types I, II, and III include sound protection for the round window as well as sound-pressure transformation for the oval window. In more severe degrees of damage to the middle ear in which the superstructure of the stapes has been destroyed, only sound protection of the round window can be achieved by grafting from the promontory to the inferior remnant of the tympanic membrane. This Type IV tympanoplasty creates a small closed space that communicates with the eustachian tube and provides an air-filled cushion over the round window. A Type V tympanoplasty is utilized when the footplate of the stapes is fixed. It provides sound protection for the round window as in a Type IV tympanoplasty and fenestration of the horizontal semicircular canal for the admission of acoustic energy into the inner ear. This type of tympanoplasty is rarely used.

The dangerous type of chronic otitis media occurs with pars flaccida and marginal perforations. Pars flaccida perforations lead into the epitympanum and are termed attic perforations. Marginal perforations usually occur in the posterosuperior portion of the pars tensa. There is no substance of tympanic membrane between the periphery of the perforation and the bony sulcus tympanicus. The anulus tympanicus has been destroyed.

Theories of the pathogenesis of perforations of the pars flaccida include progressive retraction of the pars flaccida secondary to eustachian tube obstruction, rupture during acute otitis media, and hyperactivity of the basal layer of the epidermis of the pars flaccida due to long-standing inflammation in the middle ear. Each of these mechanisms may cause an invasive cholesteatoma.

A cholesteatoma occurs when the middle ear is lined with stratified squamous epithelium. The stratified squamous epithelium desquamates in this closed space. The desquamated epithelial debris cannot be cleared and accumulates in ever enlarging concentric layers. This debris serves as a culture medium for microorganisms. Cholesteatomas have the ability to destroy bone, including the tympanic ossicles, probably because of the elaboration of collagenase.

Pars flaccida and marginal perforations are frequently associated with cholesteatomas. Those cholesteatomas arising in association with pars flaccida perforations are classified as primary acquired cholesteatomas and may develop as an integral part of the development of the perforation or from the migration of stratified squamous epithelium when perforation has occurred.

Marginal perforations are produced by acute otitis media with an especially virulent bacterium, particularly a group A beta-hemolytic streptococcus, or in association with other infectious diseases such as diphtheria, chickenpox, or measles. This necrotizing otitis media destroys large areas of the tympanic membrane, including the anulus tympanicus and the middle ear-mucous membrane, as well as the ossicles and their vascular and ligamentous support. During the healing process, the remaining epithelium of the mucous membrane of the middle ear migrates to cover the denuded areas. Likewise, the stratified squamous epithelium of the ear canal migrates into the middle ear to re-epithelialize the denuded areas. When stratified squamous epithelium is established in the middle ear, it begins to desquamate, and a cholesteatoma results. Cholesteatomas developing by this mechanism are classified as secondary acquired cholesteatomas.

The presence of a cholesteatoma greatly increases the probability of the development of a serious complication such as purulent labyrinthitis, facial paralysis, or intracranial suppurations. Intracranial infections include meningitis, brain abscess, lateral sinus thrombosis, subdural empyema, and epidural abscess. Magnetic resonance imaging (MRI) readily allows identification and differentiation of these entities. The propensity of cholesteatomas to produce these complications stems from their ability to destroy bone and the persistence of infection in the area bearing cholesteatoma.

Cholesteatomas are usually recognized by the small bits of white, amorphous debris in the middle ear and by the destruction of the external auditory canal bone superior to the pars flaccida or marginal perforation. Cholesteatomas are often associated with aural polyps, which may conceal the epithelial debris and bone destruction. CT of the temporal bone may demonstrate destruction of bone due to the cholesteatoma. Destruction of the scutum of Leidy (lateral wall of the epitympanum) and enlargement of the antrum greater than 1 cm. in diameter can be considered evidence of cholesteatoma.

Cholesteatomas require surgical treatment. The objective of surgical therapy is to exteriorize the cholesteatoma and, if possible, remove it. In a radical mastoidectomy, the middle ear, including the attic and the antrum, and the mastoid air cell area are converted into one cavity that communicates with the exterior through the ear canal. If the cholesteatoma lies superficial to the remnants of the tympanic membrane and ossicles, a modified radical mastoidectomy can be performed (Fig. 39–9). The modified radical mastoidectomy spares the tympanic membrane remnants and ossicles and preserves the remaining hearing. Under favorable circumstances, the cholesteatoma can be completely removed and the middle ear reconstructed. Exteriorization or removal of the cholesteatoma greatly reduces the possibility of intracranial complications. The primary goal of operation for cholesteatoma is to make the ear safe, and the secondary goal is to maintain or improve the hearing.

Congenital Malformations

The auricle may stand out too far from the skull and be termed an outstanding ear, lop ear, or protruding ear. The basic deformity is a lack of development of the antihelix. This deformity can be corrected surgically by weakening the spring of the cartilage of the pinna so that an antihelical fold can be created. This deformity is ideally corrected at age 5 to 6 years.

Preauricular cysts and sinuses are fairly common and may be unilateral or bilateral. They are usually asymptomatic but may become infected and require incision and drainage and later excision. Complete excision is difficult because the ramification of these sinuses may be in proximity to the branches of the facial nerve. Excision is recommended only if recurrent infection has become a problem.

Severe congenital deformities of the external ear are referred to as microtia, which describes a small and misshapen pinna. With absence of a major portion of the auricular cartilage, surgical reconstruction rarely produces a satisfactory cosmetic result. An artistic prosthesis is the best solution to

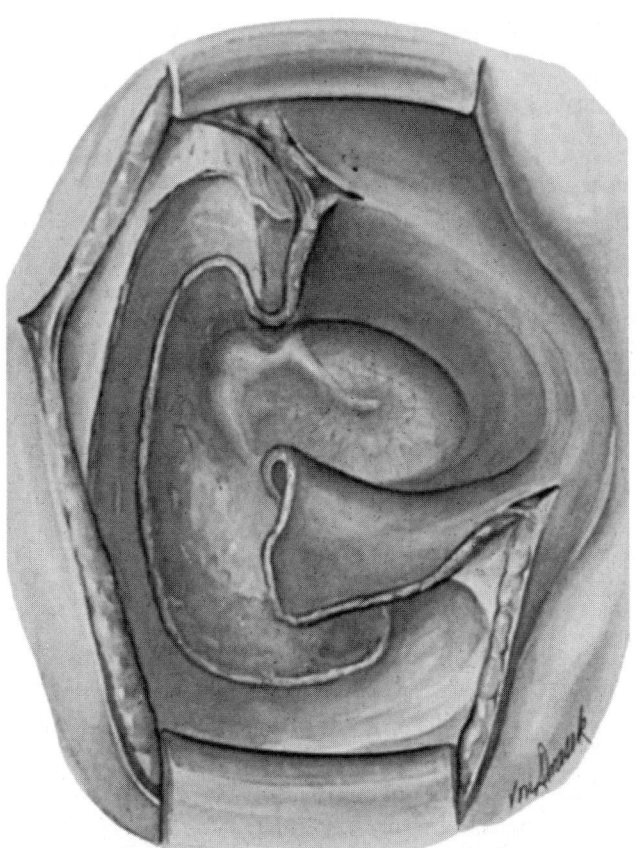

Figure 39–9. Modified radical mastoidectomy for exteriorizing a cholesteatoma that is superficial to the remnants of the tympanic membrane and ossicles. The remnants of the tympanic membrane and ossicles are preserved. (From Shambaugh, G. E., Jr.: Surgery of the Ear, 2nd ed. Philadelphia, W. B. Saunders, 1967.)

this cosmetic problem. Microtia is often associated with stenosis or atresia of the external auditory canal. These deformities are often associated with developmental abnormalities in the middle ear, causing profound conductive hearing losses. The course of the facial nerve in the temporal bone may also be abnormal, and surgical repair of the sound-pressure transformation apparatus of the middle ear is hazardous.[9] In unilateral defects with normal hearing in the other ear, middle-ear reconstruction is not recommended because of the danger of facial nerve injury. However, if there is a bilateral profound hearing loss, attempts at reconstruction should be made. A bone conduction hearing aid contributes to habilitation if surgical reconstruction is not feasible. Congenital malformations of the inner ear causing profound sensorineural hearing losses may or may not be associated with abnormalities of the external and middle ear. The evaluation of congenital malformation of the ear is facilitated by CT of the temporal bone.

Idiopathic Diseases

Otosclerosis. Otosclerosis is the most common cause of a progressive conductive hearing loss in an adult with a normal ear drum. Otosclerosis is a disease of the bone of the otic capsule, with a predilection for the anterior part of the oval window. Histologically, foci of otosclerosis demonstrate irregularly arranged, immature bone interspersed with numerous vascular channels. As the focus of the otosclerotic bone enlarges, it causes ankylosis of the footplate of the stapes and produces a conductive hearing loss. A second site of predilection is the posterior part of the oval window.

Otosclerosis tends to be familial. It is more common in women than in men. Approximately 10% of the adult white population have foci of otosclerosis. Only 1 in 10 of these, or approximately 1% of the white population, has clinical otosclerosis as evidenced by conductive hearing loss. Otosclerosis is rare in blacks, Native Americans, and Japanese. It is common in Asiatic Indians. Otosclerosis also produces a sensorineural hearing loss when the focus is adjacent to the scala media. The conductive hearing loss becomes clinically evident in the late teenage and early adult years. The fixation of the stapes may progress rapidly during pregnancy. The conductive hearing loss can be corrected surgically in most instances. With microsurgical techniques, the superstructure (head, neck, and crura) of the stapes is removed and replaced with a prosthesis. A widely used prosthesis is one composed of a stainless steel wire and a Teflon piston. The wire, which is shaped like a shepherd's crook, is crimped around the long process of the incus, and the piston is placed through a hole created in the footplate of the stapes (Fig. 39–10). The sound conduction characteristics of this arrangement are excellent. The complication of a profound sensorineural hearing loss occurs in 2 to 4% of patients. If a good initial hearing result is obtained, ordinarily a good result is maintained.

Meniere's Disease. Meniere's disease is characterized by hearing loss, tinnitus, and recurrent prostrating vertigo. The pathologic change in the inner ear is generalized dilation of the membranous labyrinth, or endolymphatic hydrops. Only one ear is involved in 85% of patients with Meniere's disease. The sensorineural hearing loss is initially more severe in the lower frequencies than in the higher frequencies. The hearing tends to fluctuate. It is depressed after an attack of vertigo. The tinnitus has a low-pitched, roaring quality and is worse just before, during, or after an attack of vertigo. The attacks of vertigo occur suddenly, last from a few to 24 hours, and subside gradually. The attacks are associated with nausea and vomiting. The patient often has a full feeling or a pressure sensation in the affected ear. Over the course of many years, hearing loss progressively worsens. Early in the course

of the disease, the ratio of the amplitudes of the summating potential and eighth nerve action potential is increased.[28]

Neither medical nor surgical therapy has been demonstrated to be effective in arresting the progression of the hearing disorder or preventing recurrent attacks of vertigo. There are a number of drugs that are effective in suppressing the vertigo and its side effects. Cholinolytic agents such as atropine and scopolamine reduce the autonomic side effects. Phenothiazines, antihistamines, and barbiturates are effective, and diphenhydramine is widely used. Perhaps the most effective agent in suppressing vertigo is diazepam.[29] A number of operations have been advocated for the treatment of patients who are disabled by the frequency of the recurrent attacks of vertigo. Fick introduced the sacculotomy, in which the saccule is ruptured with a pick placed through the footplate of the stapes.[12] Cody has advocated the placement of a stainless steel tack through the footplate of the stapes so that a sacculotomy is performed each time the membranous labyrinth begins to distend.[5] House has advocated the production of an artificial communication between the membranous labyrinth and subarachnoid space.[21] Transection of the vestibular division of the eighth nerve is a logical approach to the control of vertigo in Meniere's disease. A labyrinthectomy can be performed if the vertigo is sufficiently disabling and the hearing has degenerated to a useless level.

Benign Paroxysmal Positional Vertigo and Nystagmus. Vertigo that occurs with changes in position may follow lesions in the inner ear, eighth nerve, brain stem, or cerebellum. Positional vertigo and nystagmus arising from the inner ear is termed benign paroxysmal positional vertigo and nystagmus. The patient experiences vertigo when lying on or rolling over onto the affected ear or when tilting the head back to look up. There is a latency of a few seconds after assuming the provocative position before the vertigo and nystagmus begin. The vertigo is characterized by an intense sensation of spinning, and the nystagmus is rotary and counterclockwise when the affected right ear is placed under and clockwise when the affected left ear is placed under. The quick component of the nystagmus is always toward the affected ear. The vertigo and nystagmus last less than 20 seconds, and the response fatigues with repeated assumption of the provocative position. Peripheral (inner ear) positional vertigo and nystagmus are distinguishable from central (brain stem or cerebellum) positional vertigo and nystagmus. In the central form, there is no intense subjective sensation of spinning, latency of response, or fatigability on repeated testing, and the nystagmus persists as long as the provocative position is maintained. There are no auditory symptoms or signs in benign paroxysmal positional vertigo and nystagmus that differentiate it from Meniere's disease and acoustic neurinomas. The symptoms rarely last more than several weeks or months but may recur.

The finding of basophilic calcium-containing concretions in the ampulla of the posterior semicircular canal has led some to refer to this condition as cupulolithiasis.[35] Epley has designed a useful set of head maneuvers for displacing the cupulolith to an insensitive part of the semicircular canal, which provides immediate and usually prolonged relief of recurrent vertigo. If the condition persists for more than 1 year, the nerve to the posterior semicircular canal can be divided in the singular canal through the middle ear, providing relief of symptoms in 90% of patients.[13]

Bell's Palsy. Bell's palsy is a unilateral facial paralysis that develops suddenly and is accompanied by pain in the postauricular area. It is thought to be of viral etiology. All divisions of the nerve are paralyzed; this distinguishes the disease from a supranuclear lesion. The lesion is in the internal auditory meatus or the intratemporal course of the nerve. The initial pathologic changes are hyperemia and edema. The

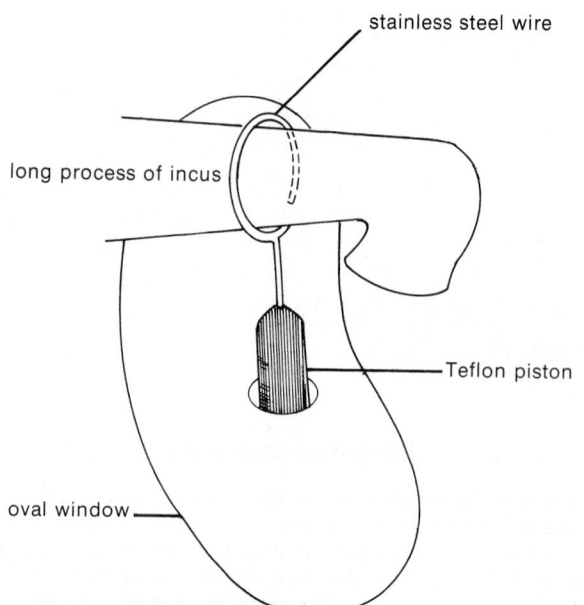

Figure 39–10. Stapedectomy with wire and Teflon piston prosthesis. The wire is crimped around the long process of the incus, and the Teflon piston is placed through a hole created in the fixed footplate of the stapes.

edema compresses the blood supply to the nerve because of the bony confines of the fallopian canal. A conduction block develops without death or degeneration of the axons. Release of the pressure on the nerve produces rapid recovery of function. This type of paralysis is termed neurapraxia. It should be differentiated from axonotmesis, in which the pressure on the nerve is sufficiently severe to cause death of the axons distal to the compression within a period of several days. Neurotmesis designates complete transection of the facial nerve. In neurapraxia, the flow of axoplasm has been interrupted; with resumption of the flow of axoplasm, the function of the distal axon recovers.

Corticosteroid therapy is initiated as soon as possible after the onset of the paralysis and is continued for 10 days to minimize the inflammatory reaction.

Nerve excitability testing or electroneurography is performed to determine whether neurapraxia or axonotmesis or neurotmesis exists. As long as muscular contraction can be induced at approximately the same direct current stimulus intensity on the affected side as on the normal side with nerve excitability testing, the paralysis is probably a neurapraxia, and complete recovery may be anticipated. Loss of nerve excitability or 90% or greater nerve degeneration found on electroneurography is an indication for decompression of the facial nerve by removing the bone of the fallopian canal. Approximately 85% of all patients with idiopathic facial nerve paralysis recover spontaneously. If recovery has not begun at 3 weeks after the onset of the facial paralysis, the possibility of spontaneous recovery is greatly reduced. Ordinarily, facial nerve decompression is performed 3 weeks after the onset if there has been no recovery, or at any time when the nerve excitability deteriorates.

Neoplasms

Squamous cell and basal cell carcinomas frequently develop on the pinna of those who are exposed to the sun. Early lesions can be successfully treated with irradiation or cautery and curettage. Surgical excision of a V-shaped wedge or larger amounts of the pinna is required in more advanced lesions. Invasion of cartilage usually dictates against radiation therapy and makes surgical therapy the treatment of choice. Squamous cell and basal cell carcinomas also arise in the external auditory canal and under these circumstances require extensive resection in order to offer the best likelihood of cure. *En bloc* resection of the external auditory canal with sparing of the facial nerve is performed for lesions that are limited to the ear canal and have not invaded the middle ear.[7] Squamous cell carcinoma may arise in the middle ear. Persistent otorrhea of chronic otitis media predisposes to squamous cell carcinomas arising in the middle ear and the external auditory canal. Squamous cell carcinoma involving the middle ear requires resection of the temporal bone to obtain an adequate margin around the tumor. Preoperative or postoperative radiation therapy increases the likelihood of cure.

Ceruminomas arise in the outer third of the external auditory canal. Although these neoplasms appear to be benign histologically, they behave in a malignant manner and should be widely excised.

Chemodectomas arise in the middle ear. These nonchromaffin paragangliomas are termed glomus jugulare or glomus tympanicus tumors, depending on their site of origin. The glomus tympanicus tumor arises from the area of Jacobson's nerve in the tympanic plexus on the promontory of the middle ear. The glomus jugulare tumor arises from the glomus jugulare body in the jugular bulb. Both tumors consist of rich networks of vascular spaces surrounded by epithelioid cells. Usually the neoplasms grow slowly, and symptoms may not be evident until the neoplasm is quite large. Pulsatile tinnitus, facial nerve paralysis, otorrhea, hemorrhage, vertigo, and paralysis of cranial nerves IX, X, XI, and XII are often the presenting symptoms and signs. Characteristically, a red mass that pulsates and blanches with compression with a pneumatic otoscope can be seen in the ear canal or middle ear. The pulsation can also be demonstrated with tympanometry. There may be evidence of bone erosion in the mastoid process, middle ear, or petrous pyramid on CT. The extent of the lesion is best demonstrated with MRI with enhancement with gadolinium. Angiography is a necessary part of the preoperative evaluation. Treatment consists of excision of the smaller neoplasms with or without a radical mastoidectomy. With large lesions, treatment choices are a skull-base approach, which is necessary to deal safely with the sigmoid sinus and jugular bulb and vein and the internal carotid artery, as well as the cranial nerves, or radiation therapy.

Acoustic neurinomas represent approximately 7% of all intracranial neoplasms. They arise twice as often from the vestibular division of the eighth nerve as from the auditory division. These neoplasms are derived from Schwann cells. Initially, they produce tinnitus and a neural hearing loss. The patient complains of unsteadiness or imbalance. True vertigo is not a common complaint. The hearing loss is predominantly a high-tone loss, with greater impairment of speech discrimination than would be expected with a cochlear lesion producing the same amount of pure-tone hearing loss. Loudness recruitment is absent. Tone decay is present. Decay of the acoustic reflex is pronounced. There is a decrement in speech discrimination with increasing intensity. The structure of the five waves in auditory brain stem responses is disrupted, the interwave latency is increased, and the interaural latency difference of the fifth peak is increased.[3] Hallpike caloric testing usually demonstrates canal paresis on the involved side. Initially, the tumor is confined to the internal auditory meatus. As it increases in size, it projects into the cerebellopontine angle and begins to compress the cerebellum and brain stem. With the passage of time, the fifth and ultimately the seventh cranial nerves become involved. Papilledema is a late sign of acoustic neurinomas. Early diagnosis is based on auditory findings suggesting a neural loss of hearing. Auditory brain stem responses have become the most effective means of differentiating sensory from neural hearing losses. Acoustic neurinomas as small as 6 mm. can be visualized with MRI with enhancement with gadolinium. For the removal of small tumors, microsurgical approaches have been developed that utilize a translabyrinthine route if no useful hearing remains and a middle cranial fossa route for the preservation of the remaining hearing.[22] Both routes allow preservation of the facial nerve. For very large neoplasms, the combined suboccipital and translabyrinthine approach offers the best likelihood of complete removal. New closed skull radiation therapy through 201 sharply focused cobalt 60 sources (gamma knife) offers an alternative form of treatment for the elderly, those with bilateral acoustic neurinoma, and those with tumors affecting the only hearing ear.[24]

THE NOSE AND THE PARANASAL SINUSES

In ancient India, adultery was punished by amputation of the nose. Suśruta (circa A.D. 1000) described the reconstruction of the nose with a pedicle flap from the cheek. Another ancient Indian method described the forehead flap. Tagliacozzi in Renaissance Italy developed the arm-to-nose pedicle graft. Sir William Ferguson in 1845 introduced an approach for tumors of the nose and paranasal sinuses. It included splitting of the lip in the midline as well as a horizontal incision along the inferior orbital rim to reflect the soft tissues of the face laterally. Ingals introduced nasal septal surgery by partial excision of the nasal septum for deviation of the septum in 1882. This operation was later improved by Krieg in 1899 and by Freer in 1902.

In 1903, Killian was the first to operate for an infection in the frontal sinus; in 1904, he refined the submucous resection of the nasal septum. At the same time, Caldwell in New York and Luc in Paris were describing a reliable procedure for dealing with infection in the maxillary sinus. Osteoplastic obliteration of the frontal sinus, popularized by Goodale and Montgomery, provided a definitive procedure for recalcitrant frontal sinusitis and mucoceles. Open procedures for the paranasal sinuses have been partially replaced by functional endoscopic sinus surgery. Joseph, at the turn of the century in Berlin, developed techniques and principles upon which modern rhinoplasty is based.

Anatomy of the Nose and Paranasal Sinuses

The skeleton of the nose consists of the nasal bones, the ascending processes of the maxilla, the upper lateral cartilages, the lower lateral cartilages, and the septal cartilage. The nasal septum is the medial wall of each nasal cavity. The lateral wall of each nasal cavity provides the attachment for the three turbinates. The inferior turbinate is the largest of the three. It extends from far anterior in the nasal cavity to the choana. The middle turbinate is somewhat smaller. Although it extends to the choana, its anterior tip is 2 cm. posterior to the anterior tip of the inferior turbinate. Its attachment to the lateral wall of the nasal cavity is oblique from superior anteriorly to inferior posteriorly. The superior turbinate arises from the far posterosuperior portion of the lateral wall of the nasal cavity. Inferior to the inferior turbinate is the inferior meatus. The nasolacrimal duct opens into the inferior meatus. The middle meatus lies between the middle turbinate and the inferior turbinate. The ostia of the maxillary and anterior ethmoid cells and the nasofrontal duct are in the middle meatus. The superior meatus lies between the superior turbinate and the middle turbinate. The ostia of the posterior ethmoid cells are in the superior meatus. The ostium of the sphenoid sinus is in the posterior part of the superior meatus, the sphenoethmoid recess.

Trauma and Foreign Bodies

Nasal Fracture. The nose is a vulnerable leading part. Fractures of the nasal bones are the most common fractures of the facial bones. Fractures of the nose may involve the ascending processes of the maxillae and the nasal processes of the frontal bones as well as the nasal bones. A fracture of the nose is usually an open fracture. The skin of the dorsum of the nose may be lacerated, and the mucous membrane in the nasal cavity is generally torn. The most common deformity is a deviation of the nasal bones to the right, with depression of the nasal bones on the left, characteristically occurring with a right hook. Fractures of the nose may be associated with septal fractures and hematomas.

Fractures of the nasal bones are generally associated with bleeding from the nose owing to the tear of the mucous membrane. A fracture should be suspected if blunt injury causes bleeding from the nose. Soft tissue swelling occurs fairly promptly and may tend to obscure the underlying bony deformity. Ecchymosis may spread into the upper and lower eyelids. The diagnosis can ordinarily be established by gentle palpation of the dorsum of the nose. Any deformity suggests a fracture. Radiographs of the nasal bones tend to confirm the diagnosis. Linear radiolucencies parallel to the long axis of the nasal bones are usually nutrient vessels.

Radiolucencies transverse to the long axis of the nasal bones are usually fractures. Displacement of the bony fragments may be demonstrated; however, the degree of displacement is more readily determined by physical examination.

Fractures of the nasal complex are often associated with fractures of other facial bones, and a CT scan of the paranasal sinuses should be obtained. Trauma to the facial bones is often associated with a cerebrospinal fluid rhinorrhea. After injury to the central portion of the face, the patient is specifically examined for cerebrospinal fluid rhinorrhea by tipping the head forward and collecting any drainage from the nose. Cerebrospinal rhinorrhea requires prophylactic antibiotic therapy to prevent meningitis. The patient is instructed to avoid blowing the nose. In most cases, cerebrospinal fluid rhinorrhea ceases spontaneously. The location of a cerebrospinal fluid leak may be determined with CT scanning with intrathecal iohexol. If the site of the suspected leak is not found in this manner, its presence or absence can be determined by the introduction of a radioactive isotope into the cerebrospinal fluid at lumbar puncture, and cotton pledgets placed in the nasal cavities are counted for radioactivity after several hours. If the rhinorrhea does not cease within 14 to 21 days, the dural leak is repaired through a frontal craniotomy or through a transethmoid approach to the roof of the nasal cavity.

Nasal fractures in adults may be reduced under local anesthesia. General anesthesia is necessary for the reduction of nasal fractures in children. The local anesthesia required is similar to that used for a rhinoplasty. Through anesthesia is necessary for a satisfactory reduction of the nasal bones. The fracture is manipulated into a good position by internal traction on the fracture fragments with a blunt periosteal elevator in association with external traction with the fingers. The need for internal and external splinting depends on the postreduction stability of the fracture.

If blunt trauma to the nose is neglected, it causes permanent deformity that ultimately requires septal surgery to improve the airway and rhinoplasty to improve the appearance of the nose.

Fractures of the nasal septum may be reduced at the same time as the reduction of the fracture of the nasal bones. Often these fractures are difficult to maintain in a position of good alignment and require a subsequent septoplasty or submucous resection of the nasal septum.

Septal hematomas lie between the quadrangular cartilage and the perichondrium. When the perichondrium has been elevated from both sides of the septal cartilage, the cartilage undergoes avascular necrosis. Septal hematomas frequently become infected, and abscess formation produces avascular and septic necrosis of the septal cartilage, which causes a saddle deformity of the nose. Septal hematomas are incised and drained as soon as the diagnosis is made. An incision in the mucoperichondrium over the anterior part of the hematoma allows access for aspiration. The perichondrium is placed in contact with the septal cartilage by packing the nasal cavity with petrolatum gauze.

Septal abscesses are located between the cartilage and the perichondrium. They may involve both sides of the cartilage. Septal abscesses are incised and drained under general anesthesia as soon as the diagnosis is established. Incisions are made bilaterally if there is pus on both sides of the septum. A small rubber drain is sutured to a lip of the wound until the drainage subsides. Vigorous systemic antibiotic therapy is employed.

Deviations of the Nasal Septum. Deviations of the nasal septum may be caused by trauma or may occur as developmental abnormalities, particularly in individuals with highly arched palates. The nasal bones and septum are frequently fractured at the time of birth. This injury is of the greenstick type, and it often corrects itself. However, correction is usually accomplished by moving the nose digitally back toward the midline. Slight anterior traction is applied to the tip of the nose during this maneuver. No internal or external splinting is required.

Deviations of the nasal septum produce varying degrees of nasal obstruction and predispose the patient to sinusitis, particularly if the deviation tends to obstruct one of the ostia of the paranasal sinuses during acute inflammatory processes, and to epistaxis as a result of drying air currents over the deflected septum. The caudal edge of the nasal septum may be dislocated and produce an external deformity of the columella.

Deviations of the septum are corrected by septoplasty or submucous resection of the nasal septum. In these procedures, the mucoperichondrium is elevated from the cartilage. The deviated cartilage and bone are resected or remodeled to straighten the septum.

Perforations of the nasal septum may be secondary to nasal surgery or repeated trauma, as in picking the nose. In the past, perforations due to syphilis and tuberculosis were common. Perforations of the septum produce crusting around their margins and repeated epistaxis. Small perforations whistle. The crusting and bleeding can be controlled with the use of a Silastic septal button, which is shaped like a collar button. The post extends through the perforation, and the two flanges cover the perforation on each side of the nasal septum. Septal perforations are closed by the development of opposing mucoperichondrial flaps.

Rhinoplasty is performed for physiologic as well as cosmetic purposes. A deformed nose is usually associated with airway obstruction. The aims of rhinoplasty are to eliminate the airway obstruction and to correct the external deformity of the nose. Usually rhinoplasty is performed under local anesthesia. The surgical procedure is directed toward the cartilaginous and bony framework of the nose. The soft tissue of the nose conforms postoperatively to the modification of the bony and cartilaginous framework. Generally, modification of each element of the nasal skeleton is necessary for aesthetically pleasing results. Saddle deformities of the nose may be corrected by augmentation with autogenous bone or silicone rubber implants.

Foreign Bodies. Children put all manner of objects in their noses. Erasers, beans, buttons, pebbles, wool nap, paper, and sponge rubber are common foreign bodies. A foreign body in the nasal cavity produces a severe inflammatory reaction and causes a foul-smelling, bloody, unilateral discharge. Removal of the foreign body is facilitated by producing vasoconstriction anterior to it with a topical sympathomimetic amine such as phenylephrine. The foreign body is removed by placing a blunt hook posterior to it and raking it anteriorly. Attempts at grasping smooth, firm foreign bodies with forceps tend to push them farther posteriorly. General anesthesia is used if good cooperation from a child cannot be obtained by gentle reassurance.

If a foreign body dwells long in the nose, mineral salts are deposited on it and produce a rhinolith. The rhinolith tends to conform to the contour of the nasal cavity, and its removal is usually difficult and requires general anesthesia.

Sinusitis

Acute rhinitis is the usual manifestation of a common cold. Acute sinusitis is usually initiated by an acute respiratory tract infection of viral etiology. Nearly all cases of acute sinusitis and most cases of chronic sinusitis respond well to antibiotic therapy. The complications of acute and chronic sinusitis often require surgical therapy, as does unresponsive chronic sinusitis. Complications of maxillary sinusitis are rare. Ethmoid sinusitis is frequently complicated in children by orbital cellulitis and abscess. Eighty percent of all cases of orbital cellulitis are secondary to ethmoid sinusitis. In a patient who presents with erythema and swelling of the eyelids, proptosis, and displacement of the globe laterally and inferiorly, the source of the infection is sought by inspection of the nose for mucopus in the middle meatus and by CT scanning of the paranasal sinuses for ethmoid sinusitis. CT scanning of the orbits may allow differentiation of orbital cellulitis from orbital abscess. Ethmoid sinusitis and orbital cellulitis respond well to systemic antibiotic therapy. If the proptosis fails to subside or progresses, incision and drainage of the abscess, which is between the lamina papyracea and the orbital periosteum, is performed through a Killian incision that extends from the lateral aspect of the nose to the eyebrow. The orbital periosteum is elevated from the medial wall of the orbit so that the abscess cavity can be reached. The optic nerve tolerates 11 to 14 mm. of proptosis. The point at which extraocular motion is lost is also the limit of stretch of the optic nerve. Therefore, incision and drainage of an orbital abscess are performed prior to complete loss of extraocular motion to prevent permanent blindness.

Frontal sinusitis may cause intracranial complications such as meningitis, epidural abscess, subdural empyema, and brain abscess. In severe acute frontal sinusitis that fails to respond promptly to systemic antibiotic therapy, the floor of the frontal sinus is trephined through an incision just inferior to the medial part of the eyebrow. An opening of approximately 7 to 8 mm. is made, and a catheter is placed in the sinus to maintain drainage. Trephination is performed in an attempt to prevent the intracranial complications of frontal sinusitis.

Fractures of the frontal sinus lead to the development of mucoceles. Mucoceles follow duplication of the mucous membrane. They gradually enlarge and destroy the floor of the frontal sinus; as they expand into the orbital cavity, they produce proptosis and inferior and lateral displacement of the eye. Mucoceles and other forms of chronic frontal sinusitis that do not respond to medical management or endoscopic sinus surgery can be managed surgically by an osteoplastic flap approach for obliteration of the frontal sinus (Fig. 39–11). The incision in the bone is made at the periphery of the frontal sinus, and the anterior wall is rotated inferiorly on the hinge of periosteum at the floor of the sinus. Infected mucous membrane is removed with a gas-driven burr under microscopic control, and the cavity of the frontal sinus is obliterated by the implantation of fat taken from the abdominal wall.

Approximately 25% of cases of chronic maxillary sinusitis are secondary to a dental infection. In chronic maxillary sinusitis, radiographs of the apices of the teeth should be obtained to exclude the possibility of a periapical abscess.

Infection and allergy can lead to hyperplastic tissue in the confluence of the ostia of the maxillary, anterior ethmoid, and frontal sinuses in the middle meatus, which produces obstruction of the ostia of these sinuses. Inflammation in the ostiomeatal complex is thought to account for a great deal of subacute and chronic maxillary, ethmoid, and frontal sinusitis. Endoscopic excision of inflammatory tissue in the ostiomeatal complex is credited with resolution of chronic sinusitis without open operative procedures.

Chronic maxillary sinusitis that does not respond to medical management or endoscopic sinus surgery may be controlled with the Caldwell-Luc operation, which is a maxillary sinusotomy performed through an incision in the canine fossa. The bone of the anterior wall of the maxillary sinus is resected to permit access to the interior of the sinus for removal of infected mucous membrane, cysts, and epithelial

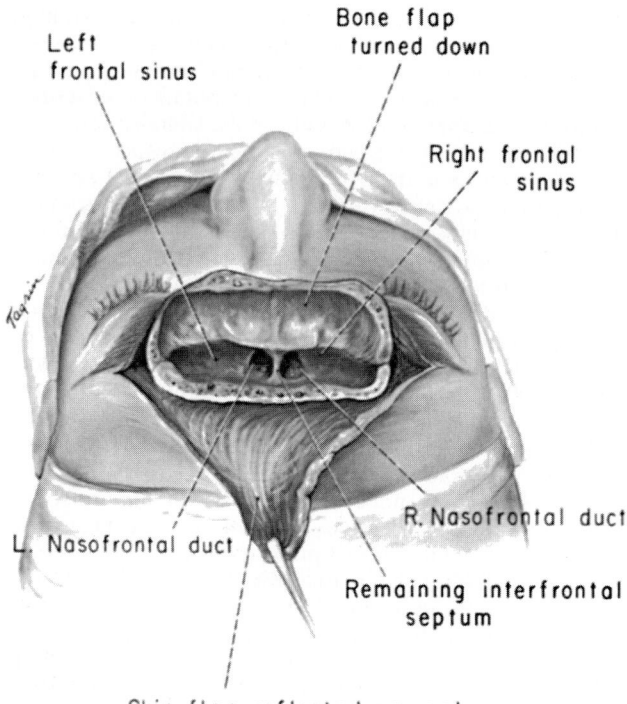

Figure 39–11. Approach to the frontal sinuses by the use of an osteoplastic flap for obliteration of the sinuses. (From Goodale, R. L., and Montgomery, W. W.: Technical advances in osteoplastic frontal sinusectomy. Arch. Otolaryngol., *79*:522, 1964. Copyright 1964, American Medical Association.)

debris. Drainage of the maxillary sinus is improved by creating a nasoantral window in the inferior meatus.

Chronic ethmoid sinusitis is often associated with allergic rhinitis and the formation of nasal polyps. In those individuals in whom the formation of nasal polyps and the symptoms of ethmoid sinusitis cannot be controlled adequately with medical management, including topical corticosteroid therapy and immunotherapy, an ethmoidectomy is indicated. Ethmoidectomy is performed intranasally with endoscopic guidance and through an external approach utilizing a Killian incision. In the external ethmoidectomy, the orbital periosteum is elevated, and the lamina papyracea is removed for the purpose of giving access to the ethmoid air cells. Infected mucous membrane, polypoid tissue, and epithelial debris are removed. The anterior half of the middle turbinate is excised for creation of a large opening between the ethmoid air cells and the nasal cavity. In essence, an ethmoidectomy incorporates the ethmoid air cell area into the nasal cavity.

Chronic sphenoid sinusitis that does not respond to medical management may be controlled by an operation in which the sphenoid sinus is approached with endoscopic guidance or through an external ethmoidectomy. After an ethmoidectomy has been accomplished, the anterior wall of the sphenoid sinus is resected to remove infected mucous membrane, polypoid tissue, and epithelial debris. The anterior and inferior walls of the sphenoid sinus are removed. In this way, the interior of the sphenoid sinus is incorporated in the posterior part of the nasal cavity and the nasopharynx, and, in essence, the sphenoid sinus is eliminated as a separate entity.

Epistaxis

Bleeding from the nose is a common clinical problem. Ninety per cent of the time, epistaxis occurs from a plexus of vessels in the anteroinferior part of the septum. In the other 10% of cases, nasal bleeding occurs from the posterior part of the nose, particularly from far posterior in the inferior meatus at the junction of the inferior meatus and the nasopharynx. It is from this area that individuals with arteriosclerosis and hypertension are likely to bleed. This type of bleeding may be difficult to control and is associated with a 4% to 5% mortality. Mild epistaxis from the anterior part of the nasal septum is usually effectively controlled by steady pressure applied by squeezing the mobile portion of the nose between the index finger and thumb for 5 to 10 minutes. Treatment for epistaxis that is not controlled by this simple measure requires visualization of the bleeding point. The bleeding point can be controlled temporarily and anesthesia achieved with pressure applied over a cotton pledget impregnated with a vasoconstrictor and a topically active local anesthetic such as lidocaine. The bleeding point can be cauterized chemically or with electrocautery. Silver nitrate is preferred as the cauterizing agent, since it produces satisfactory intravascular coagulation without a severe burn of the mucous membrane. If the bleeding cannot be easily controlled with cautery or if the bleeding point cannot be visualized, strips of ½-inch petrolatum gauze are used for applying pressure to the bleeding point. Pressure is applied as atraumatically as possible. This method is preferred in a patient with a bleeding tendency because the periphery of a cauterized area may begin to bleed.

In order to pack the posterior part of the nasal cavity, the choana is obstructed with the balloon of a Foley catheter (Fig. 39–12) or a postnasal pack (Fig. 39–13). Although the Foley catheter is easier to insert, the gauze postnasal pack is more secure. The postnasal pack is made by folding and rolling 4- by 4-inch gauze squares into a tight pack and tying the pack with two strands of no. 2 black silk. The ends of one tie are oriented inferiorly, and the ends of the other tie are oriented superiorly. After topical anesthesia of the nose, nasopharynx, and pharynx has been induced, a catheter is introduced through the nasal cavity on the side of the bleeding and brought out through the mouth. The superiorly oriented ends of the tie are tied to the catheter, and the catheter is withdrawn from the nose as the pack is placed posterior to the soft palate into the nasopharynx. The inferiorly oriented ends of the tie are trimmed below the level of the soft palate so that they can be utilized in removing the pack. The

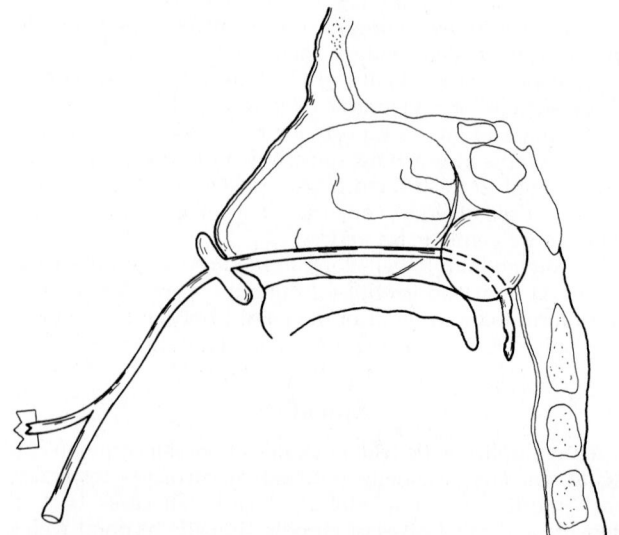

Figure 39–12. Use of a Foley catheter to obstruct the choana so that petrolatum gauze may be used to pack the nasal cavity tightly without prolapse of the packing in the nasopharynx.

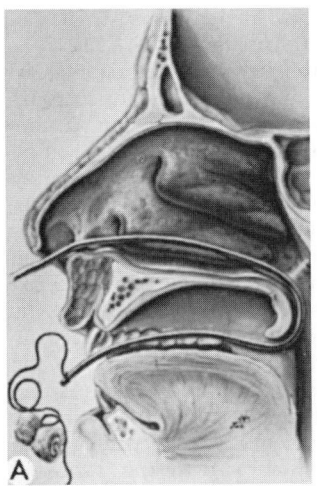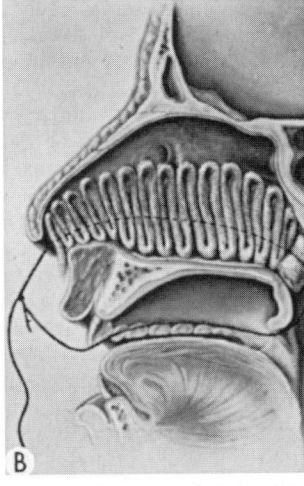

Figure 39–13. Packing of the nose for epistaxis with a postnasal pack and an anterior nose pack. (From Boles, L. R., et al.: Fundamentals of Otolaryngology: A Textbook of Ear, Nose, and Throat Diseases, 4th ed. Philadelphia, W. B. Saunders, 1964.)

superiorly oriented strands are held taut while the nasal cavity is firmly packed with petrolatum gauze. If the bleeding point is in the inferior meatus, this area is packed tightly. The superiorly oriented strands are tied over a roll of a 4- by 4-inch gauze square. The packing is left in place for 4 days. Prophylactic antibiotic therapy is indicated to prevent sinusitis and otitis media. Patients requiring postnasal packing generally have serious systemic vascular diseases. They have a low arterial PO_2 while the packing is in place and should be given supplemental humidified oxygen by mask.

An alternative treatment method for patients with severe bleeding from the posterior part of the nose is ligation of the internal maxillary artery (Fig. 39–14).[4] The artery is reached through the maxillary sinus. An incision is made in the canine fossa, and the anterior wall of the maxillary sinus is removed as in the Caldwell-Luc operation. The bone of the posterior wall of the sinus is removed, and the internal maxillary artery and its branches are gently dissected under microscopic control from the adipose tissue in the pterygomaxillary fossa. Metallic clips are placed on the internal maxillary artery as it enters the fossa and its major branches, the sphenopalatine and descending palatine arteries, as they leave the fossa. This method avoids nasal packing and the problems of hypoxemia associated with it, requires less hospitalization, and involves less discomfort for the patient.

Percutaneous transfemoral embolization of the internal maxillary artery with polyvinyl alcohol particles has a high success rate in controlling bleeding, but major neurologic complications remain relatively high, although often transient.[10]

Severe epistaxis is often associated with pre-existing liver disease. Large amounts of blood may have been swallowed prior to the nasal packing. Blood is eliminated from the gastrointestinal tract as promptly as possible by the use of cathartics and enemas. Sterilization of the gastrointestinal tract to prevent the breakdown of blood by microorganisms and the absorption of ammonia is indicated by the presence of liver disease.

Replacement of blood lost as a result of the epistaxis is carried out as indicated by the hemoglobin and hematocrit determinations, as well as by the patient's vital signs.

A particularly debilitating form of epistaxis occurs in hereditary hemorrhagic telangiectasia (Rendu-Osler-Weber disease). Patients with this disease have frequent bleeding from the nose and gastrointestinal tract. Often the bleeding from the nose is sufficient to cause a chronic anemia that cannot be overcome by iron supplementation. A septal dermoplasty, in which the mucous membrane of the anterior portions of the nasal cavity is replaced with a split-thickness skin graft, is very effective in reducing the severity and frequency of the epistaxis so that the hemoglobin concentration may be brought to the normal level.

Congenital Malformations

Choanal Atresia. Choanal atresia is a malformation in which the opening of the nasal cavity into the nasopharynx is obstructed by a partition of mucous membrane and bone. The malformation may occur unilaterally or bilaterally. If it occurs bilaterally, it produces respiratory distress in the neonate. Newborn infants are obligatory nasal breathers. If there is obstruction to the nasal airway, asphyxia occurs. The newborn presses his tongue against the roof of his mouth during the inspiratory effort. Fortunately, crying, with its attendant mouth breathing, often allows some ventilatory exchange. This diagnosis should be made in the delivery room. Choanal atresia should be considered in an infant who makes respiratory effort but fails to accomplish ventilatory exchange. The immediate solution to the problem is the insertion of an oral airway. The nursing care of the oral airway during the next 2 to 3 weeks must be extremely meticulous. After 2 to 3 weeks, the newborn learns to breathe through his mouth, and the danger abates. Most experts advocate perforation of the atretic area in the neonatal period for the insertion of polyethylene tubes. This operation often fails to provide permanent improvement, and a better repair can be performed when the child is 4 to 5 years of age through a transpalatal approach (Fig. 39–15). With careful nursing supervision of the oral airway, a tracheotomy can be avoided in the neonatal period. The diagnosis is made by attempting without success to pass a catheter through the nose into the pharynx. The diagnosis is confirmed by instilling radiopaque dye into the nasal cavity and taking a lateral radiograph of the nasophar-

Figure 39–14. Approach through the canine fossa as in the Caldwell-Luc operation to ligate the internal maxillary artery. The anterior and posterior walls of the maxillary sinus have been removed to expose the artery. (From Chandler, J. R., and Serrins, A. J.: Transantral ligation of the internal maxillary artery for epistaxis. Laryngoscope, 75:1151, 1965.)

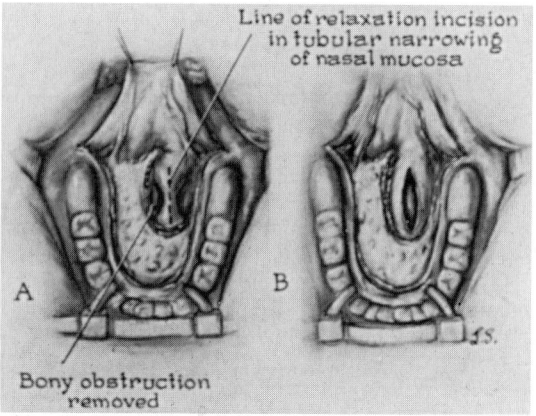

Figure 39–15. Transpalatal approach for repair of choanal atresia. (From Cherry, J., and Bordley, J. E.: Surgical correction of choanal atresia. Ann. Otol. Rhinol. Laryngol., 5:911, 1966.)

ynx in the supine position. If choanal atresia is present, the dye pools in the posterior part of the nasal cavity. The thickness, composition, and location of the atretic plate and the contour of the walls of the adjacent nasal cavities can be precisely determined with CT.

Nasal Gliomas, Dermoids, Encephaloceles, and Meningoceles. Nasal gliomas and dermoids may present as a malformation of the dorsum of the nose evident at birth or as a mass in the nasal cavity. Nasal gliomas and dermoids often have intracranial connections that can be demonstrated with CT. Under these circumstances, a frontal craniotomy is performed prior to the removal of the nasal glioma. Encephaloceles and meningoceles may present in the nasal cavity through defects in the cribriform plate. Clinically they have an appearance similar to that of a nasal polyp. Nasal polyps ordinarily arise from the middle meatus. If what appears to be a nasal polyp does not arise from the middle meatus, CT with iohexol introduced into the cerebrospinal fluid is performed to exclude an encephalocele or meningocele.

Neoplasms

Benign Neoplasms of the Nose and Paranasal Sinuses. Exophytic squamous cell papillomas occur in the nasal cavity and are thought to be caused by the human papillomavirus. Exophytic papillomas occasionally recur after excision but have a benign course. Inverted papillomas are invasive and behave in a locally malignant manner. They arise from the lateral wall of the nasal cavity and invade bone. Inverted papillomas require removal of a margin of normal tissue through a lateral rhinotomy. Fibromas, hemangiomas, and neurofibromas occur occasionally in the nasal cavity. Fibromas, neurolemmomas, and ossifying fibromas occur in the paranasal sinuses.

Malignant Neoplasms of the Nose and Paranasal Sinuses. The most common malignant neoplasm occurring in the nose and paranasal sinuses is squamous cell carcinoma. Adenoid cystic carcinomas, adenocarcinomas (particularly in the ethmoid sinuses), mucoepidermoid carcinomas, malignant mixed tumors, lymphomas, fibrosarcomas, osteosarcomas, chondrosarcomas, and melanomas also occur in the nose and paranasal sinuses. Metastatic tumors may involve the paranasal sinuses, and the most common neoplasm to metastasize to the paranasal sinuses is the hypernephroma.

Early squamous cell and basal cell carcinomas of the skin of the nose are treated with radiation therapy or cauterization and curettage. Larger carcinomas involving cartilage require

excision. Nasal septal carcinomas often require sacrifice of the columella as well as adjacent structures.

A combination of radiation therapy and radical resection provides the best survival rates in carcinomas and sarcomas of the nasal cavities and paranasal sinuses. Malignant neoplasms of the lateral wall of the nose require lateral rhinotomy. Malignant neoplasms of the maxillary sinus require partial or radical maxillectomy. A radical maxillectomy usually includes exenteration of the orbit. Malignant neoplasms of the ethmoid sinus require radical resection of the ethmoid complex, including exenteration of the orbit and partial maxillectomy. Malignant neoplasms of the frontal sinus and the sphenoid sinus are not satisfactorily resected and are usually treated with radiation therapy. Lymphomas limited to the nasal cavities or paranasal sinuses are treated with radiation therapy. Disseminated lymphomas require chemotherapy. Melanomas arising in mucous membrane are treated with surgical therapy and radiation therapy, with only rare success.

THE PHARYNX

Celsus is generally recognized as the first to describe tonsillectomy in his first-century *De medicina*. However, the Asiatic Indians frequently performed the operation 1000 years earlier.

Anatomy of the Pharynx

For descriptive purposes, the pharynx can be divided into the nasopharynx, oropharynx, and hypopharynx. However, from a functional point of view, the pharynx remains united by the constrictors of the pharynx. They have a common insertion in the median pharyngeal raphe and form a musculomembranous tubular passage from the base of the skull to the opening of the esophagus. The lymphoid structures of the pharynx include the pharyngeal tonsil or adenoid, the palatine tonsils, the lateral bands, and the lingual tonsils.

Foreign Bodies

Foreign bodies of the pharynx are likely to be found in four locations: the palatine tonsils, the lingual tonsils, the valleculae, and the pyriform sinuses. Sharp foreign bodies, such as fish bones, are particularly likely to lodge in the palatine tonsils and the lingual tonsils. Smooth, small, oval foreign bodies, such as capsules, are likely to come to rest in the valleculae. Irregular sharp foreign bodies are likely to be retained in the pyriform sinuses. Rarely, foreign bodies are coughed into the nasopharynx and become trapped there. Radiopaque foreign bodies may be located in a lateral neck film. Foreign bodies in the palatine tonsil are removed by grasping the foreign body with a hemostat. Foreign bodies in the nasopharynx require general anesthesia for their removal. Foreign bodies of the hypopharynx are removed during direct laryngoscopy under local anesthesia.

Nasopharynx

The Adenoids. Adenoid hypertrophy in childhood often leads to obstruction of the eustachian tubes and the choanae. This lymphoid hyperplasia may be physiologic or secondary to infectious and allergic manifestations. Obstruction of the eustachian tubes leads to serous or secretory otitis media, recurrent acute otitis media, and exacerbations of chronic otitis media. Obstruction of the choanae produces mouth breathing, a hyponasal voice, and rhinorrhea.

Recurrent serous or secretory otitis media is the most common indication for the removal of the adenoid tissue. An effusion in the middle ear in a child lasting 6 weeks or longer, occurring *de novo* or following acute otitis media, that does not respond to medical management responds regularly but not invariably to the use of myringotomies with the insertion of tympanostomy tubes. In patients with recurrent or persistent serous or secretory otitis media, adenoidectomy increases the likelihood of success.

Chronic otitis media in children is another indication for adenoidectomy. The procedure reduces the severity and frequency of exacerbations of chronic otitis media. It prepares the patient for subsequent mastoidectomy and tympanoplasty. Recurrent acute otitis media is a fairly frequent indication for these procedures. Many children between the ages of 1 and 6 years have two or three episodes of acute otitis media per year that completely resolve with antibiotic therapy. However, a child who is on antibiotic therapy for otitis media half of the time should be considered for this procedure. The duration of the pain, the presence of spontaneous perforation, the regularity with which myringotomy is required, and the associated systemic symptoms deserve consideration. Febrile convulsions with acute otitis media weigh heavily in favor of adenoidectomy, since antibiotic therapy ordinarily is not initiated prior to the convulsion.

Persistent nasal obstruction due to adenoid hypertrophy is a problem in which the age of the patient is considered as well as the severity, since lymphoid tissue reaches a relative and absolute maximum at puberty. Persistent and recurrent purulent rhinorrhea despite adequate antibiotic therapy is occasionally encountered in association with adenoid hypertrophy and chronic adenoiditis. Chronic sinusitis in children without an underlying immune or other defense mechanism defect such as agammaglobulinemia or hypogammaglobulinemia, cystic fibrosis, or Kartagener's syndrome is relatively rare but is rather regularly improved or eliminated by adenoidectomy.

An adenoidectomy is performed under general anesthesia. The adenoid tissue is sheared from the posterior nasopharyngeal wall with a guillotine-type adenotome placed posterior to the soft palate. The lymphoid tissue is removed superficial to the fascia of the superior constrictor of the pharynx without damaging the fascia or the underlying musculature.

Tornwaldt's Cyst. Cysts occasionally form in the region of the medial recess of the nasopharynx. These cysts become symptomatic when they become infected. There may be persistent purulent drainage that has a foul taste and odor. Symptoms of eustachian tube obstruction and sore throat may be prominent. Excision or marsupialization of the cyst with an adenotome is the treatment of choice.

Benign Neoplasms of the Nasopharynx. Juvenile angiofibromas are very vascular neoplasms that occur in pubescent males. They develop in the vault of the nasopharynx from the area of the basisphenoid and grow to a large size. Angiofibromas may extend into and obstruct the nasal cavity, and their extensions may develop parasitic attachments distant to their site of origin. They may encroach upon the paranasal sinuses, the orbit, and the intracranial cavity. Histologically, these neoplasms are composed of fibrous tissue and numerous thin-walled vessels without contractile elements. Angiofibromas tend to involute at maturity.

Epistaxis is the major problem with angiofibromas, and the magnitude of the bleeding can be great. The neoplasms are red and quite firm. Those portions of the neoplasm that project into the airway often become ulcerated during upper respiratory tract infections and bleed from the ulcerated surface. Their surgical removal is necessitated by recurrent massive bleeding. The extent of the neoplasm can be determined with CT and angiography. The pterygomaxillary fissure is often widened on the sagittal plane of the CT of the lateral part of the nasopharynx by the extension of the neoplasm

into the infratemporal fossa. These neoplasms have a characteristic vascular pattern on angiography. The main blood supply is usually from the branches of the internal maxillary artery, although the branches of the internal carotid artery and the middle meningeal artery also may contribute. Usually, they are removed through a transpalatal approach. Often a lateral rhinotomy offers important advantages. The blood loss during excision is often great, and rapid blood replacement is required. Treatment with estrogens and embolization of the internal maxillary artery at angiography have been used to reduce the operative blood loss. These neoplasms are responsive to radiation therapy. This is often the treatment of choice for a neoplasm that has invaded the orbit or the intracranial cavity or receives a large blood supply from intracranial vessels.

Malignant Neoplasms of the Nasopharynx. Malignant neoplasms of the nasopharynx include squamous cell carcinomas, adenocarcinomas, adenoid cystic carcinomas, mucoepidermoid carcinomas, malignant mixed tumors, melanomas, chordomas, sarcomas (including fibrosarcoma, rhabdomyosarcoma, liposarcoma, and myxosarcoma), plasmacytomas, and lymphomas. Among children, lymphomas are the most common malignant neoplasms arising from and secondarily involving the nasopharynx. Among the carcinomas, lymphoepithelioma or squamous cell carcinoma is the most common type.

Carcinoma of the nasopharynx occurs at relatively young ages, and there is an unusually high incidence among the Chinese. There are immunologic similarities among patients with Burkitt's lymphoma, carcinoma of the nasopharynx, and infectious mononucleosis. Elevated titers of anti–Epstein-Barr virus antibodies are present in 45% of patients with Stage I carcinoma of the nasopharynx and 100% of patients with Stage V lesions.[19] The majority of patients with carcinoma of the nasopharynx present with nasal or eustachian tube obstruction. Obstruction of the eustachian tube may cause a middle-ear effusion. The nasal obstruction may be associated with purulent, bloody rhinorrhea and frank epistaxis. The more dramatic symptoms caused by cranial nerve paralysis and cervical lymph node metastasis are, unfortunately, common presenting complaints. Metastasis tends to be limited to the neck until the late stages of the disease. A granular mass or ulcer may be seen in the nasopharynx. The palate may be deformed by the bulk of the nasopharyngeal mass, or its mobility may be limited by paralysis of the levator veli palatini. Not infrequently, the neoplasm extends deep to the mucous membrane, appears only as a slight fullness, and produces no abnormality of the mucous membrane. It is this feature of carcinoma of the nasopharynx that makes biopsy through apparently normal mucous membrane occasionally fruitful.

The diagnosis is made by biopsy of the primary tumor. Adequate access to the nasopharynx ordinarily requires general anesthesia. General anesthesia also allows the opportunity to judge the extent of the primary lesion by palpation. Biopsy of the metastasis in the neck should be avoided until the nasopharynx has been inspected and palpated and any suspicious lesion has been biopsied. Biopsy of the cervical metastasis violates the integrity of the block of tissue that is removed in a radical neck dissection. It may cause implantation of the neoplasm in the skin and subcutaneous tissue. The necessity of demonstrating the neoplasm in the nasopharynx prior to treatment remains, even if a histologic diagnosis is obtained from biopsy of the cervical metastasis.

The treatment of choice for carcinoma of the nasopharynx is irradiation with a supervoltage source. The radiation should be delivered to the primary tumor-bearing area of the nasopharynx and to both sides of the neck whether or not there is clinically demonstrated metastasis. Operations have no role in the initial therapy of carcinoma of the nasopharynx. Those cervical metastases that remain clinically palpable following radiation therapy or that subsequently become apparent should be eradicated by radical neck dissection. Generally, control of the metastatic lesions should be attempted only after there is evidence that the primary lesion has been controlled. The overall 5-year survival for carcinoma of the nasopharynx is approximately 35%.

Oropharynx

Peritonsillar Abscess. Peritonsillar cellulitis and abscess are complications of acute tonsillitis in which the infection has spread deep to the tonsillar capsule. Pus forms between the tonsillar capsule and the superior constrictor of the pharynx, and the tonsil is displaced medially. The uvula becomes tremendously edematous and is displaced to the opposite side. The soft palate is very red and displaced forward. There is marked trismus due to irritation of the pterygoid muscles, and the head is held tilted toward the side of the abscess. It is painful for the patient to talk and to swallow. Swallowing is so painful that the patient drools. The breath is foul-smelling. The temperature is usually 38 to 40° C. Peritonsillar cellulitis or abscess is rare in children under the age of 10 to 12 years and is usually caused by a group A beta-hemolytic streptococcus or anaerobe. If a cellulitis without pus formation exists, it responds in a matter of 24 to 48 hours to penicillin therapy. If pus is present, it may resolve or require incision and drainage. The pus may be difficult to locate. Incision is performed as the mucous membrane overlying the pus assumes a pale yellow color. The patient is placed in the sitting position to avoid aspiration of the pus. Under topical anesthesia, the incision is made in the anterior pillar parallel to its free edge. The incision need only split the mucous membrane, and the pus is obtained by spreading gently with a hemostat. No drain is required because the abscess cavity is emptied by each swallow.

These abscesses tend to recur and are an indication for tonsillectomy, which is usually performed 6 weeks after the acute infection. At the time of tonsillectomy, 1 to 2 ml. of pus is often encountered between the capsule and the tonsillar fossa. This persistent abscess is the apparent reason for the recurrence of these abscesses. Some advocate that the tonsillectomy be performed within a day or two after the antibiotic therapy is initiated.

Parapharyngeal Abscess. Parapharyngeal abscess may occur in infants and young children as well as in adults. The abscess is usually secondary to streptococcal pharyngitis or tonsillitis. Pus forms in the parapharyngeal space secondarily from the breakdown of lymphadenitis. The pus is located lateral to the superior constrictor of the pharynx and adjacent to the carotid sheath. The tonsil and soft palate may be displaced medially, but there may be no inflammatory reaction in the pharynx. There is marked swelling in the anterior cervical triangle. Penicillin is the antibiotic of choice. Pus formation can be demonstrated with CT or MRI before the abscess becomes fluctuant. When pus formation has been demonstrated, the abscess is incised and drained. The abscess is not drained through the lateral pharyngeal wall because of the proximity of the internal carotid artery and the internal jugular vein. An incision is made parallel to the skin folds over the anterior border of the sternocleidomastoid muscle. The anterior border of the muscle is identified, and blunt dissection is carried toward the carotid sheath, where the pus is encountered. A drain is sewn in place and removed when the drainage subsides.

Retropharyngeal Abscess. Retropharyngeal abscess occurs in infants and young children and is rare after the age of 10 years. These infections are located between the constrictors

of the pharynx and the prevertebral fascia. They are secondary to pharyngitis and are due to the breakdown of retropharyngeal lymphadenitis. Infants with retropharyngeal abscesses usually present with stridor and hyperextension of the neck. A lumbar puncture is the appropriate diagnostic procedure in a febrile infant who presents in opisthotonos. If the cerebrospinal fluid is normal, the possibility of a retropharyngeal abscess must be excluded. The diagnosis is made by palpating the posterior pharyngeal wall. The infant is held in the prone position for the examination so that if the abscess is ruptured during the examination, the pus flows out of the infant's mouth and is not aspirated. The abscess has a boggy fluctuant texture, and the bodies of the cervical vertebrae are not palpable. Inspection of the pharynx may not demonstrate the abscess, because the whole posterior pharyngeal wall may be displaced forward and there may be no inflammatory reaction in the mucous membrane. The abscess can also be demonstrated by a radiograph of the lateral neck in which the posterior pharyngeal wall is displaced anteriorly or by CT of the neck. To maintain the airway, the child should be allowed to hyperextend the neck. A tracheotomy is rarely necessary. In addition to penicillin therapy, the posterior pharyngeal wall should be incised under general endotracheal anesthesia with the patient in the Rose position. The mucous membrane at the posterior wall of the pharynx is incised vertically. The incision need only split the mucous membrane. The pus is obtained by gently spreading a hemostat in the wound toward the retropharyngeal space. No drain is necessary because the abscess cavity tends to be emptied on swallowing.

Tonsillectomy. Recurrent acute bacterial tonsillitis caused by a group A beta-hemolytic streptococcus occurring three to four times during the year in children from 2 to 7 years of age can be adequately managed with penicillin or other appropriate antibiotics administered for 12 days. The rationale for this length of treatment is that a shorter period may not eliminate a streptococcal infection. In addition to inappropriate selection of antibiotics and inadequate duration of therapy, passage of the streptococcus among family members is a cause of failure in the medical management of tonsillitis. This situation requires simultaneous cultures of the entire family and simultaneous treatment of all carriers. Despite these precautions, in some patients, tonsillitis repeatedly develops within a few days after the completion of adequate treatment. When this pattern cannot be altered by medical management, tonsillectomy is indicated.

Chronic tonsillitis with persistent sore throat, either briefly relieved or not at all relieved by antibiotic therapy, constitutes another indication for tonsillectomy. One peritonsillar abscess is an indication for tonsillectomy.

Tonsillar and adenoid hypertrophy frequently causes upper airway obstruction in children, causing sleep apnea. Tonsillectomy and adenoidectomy regularly solve this problem.

In adults, tonsillectomy is performed under local or general anesthesia. In children, general anesthesia is required. The technique involves an incision in the free edge of the tonsillar pillars. The dissection of the tonsil from the tonsillar fossa is performed in the plane between the tonsillar capsule and the superior constrictor muscle of the pharynx and is completed by closing a snare placed inferior to the lower pole of the tonsil. The objective is to remove the tonsil and its capsule intact and spare the musculature of the tonsillar fossa.

Uvulopalatopharyngoplasty. Snoring is usually due to the vibration of the soft palate during respiration. Relaxation of the soft palate can also contribute to the airway obstruction in obstructive sleep apnea. Other contributing factors include the posterior displacement of the base of the tongue and collapse of the hypopharyngeal airway, for which obesity is a predisposing condition. It is important to differentiate obstructive from central sleep apnea by overnight evaluation in a sleep laboratory. Uvulopalatopharyngoplasty (UPPP) involves removing the uvula, approximately 1 cm. of the free edge of the soft palate, and the palatine tonsils if they have not previously been removed. The resulting scarring tends to stiffen the soft palate and is fairly reliable in reducing snoring but is less efficacious in relieving obstructive sleep apnea. With life-threatening obstructive sleep apnea, a tracheotomy is indicated.

Carcinoma of the Tonsil. Carcinoma of the tonsil represents 1.5 to 3% of all cancers and is second in frequency only to carcinoma of the larynx among malignant neoplasms of the upper respiratory tract. It is predominantly a disease of males, and smoking cigarettes and consuming more than 100 ml. of ethanol per day are etiologic factors. Squamous cell carcinoma is the predominant histologic type. These carcinomas may be exophytic with superficial ulceration or deeply invasive. At times they present as lobulated submucosal masses. The neoplasm frequently extends into the base of the tongue. Carcinoma of the tonsil usually remains asymptomatic until it has reached considerable size. Sore throat is the most common presenting complaint, and pain often radiates to the ear on the same side. Not infrequently, the patient presents with a metastatic mass in the neck as the first symptom. The diagnosis is established by biopsy of the primary lesion. Treatment requires combined radiation therapy and operation. Radiation therapy may be given preoperatively or postoperatively. If preoperative irradiation is utilized, 5000 cGy are delivered to the primary lesion and both sides of the neck over a 5-week period. The patient is given a 6-week rest. The operation consists of radical resection of the tonsillar fossa, hemimandibulectomy, and radical neck dissection if there are palpable metastases. If postoperative irradiation is utilized, 6000 cGy are delivered to the primary site and 5000 cGy to both sides of the neck. The 2-year disease-free survival approximates 50%.

Hypopharynx

Diverticulum of the Hypopharynx. Pharyngoesophageal diverticula follow herniation of the mucous membrane of the hypopharynx through weak points in the inferior constrictor muscle; spasm of the cricopharyngeal muscle may have an etiologic role. They occur in older patients. These pulsion diverticula usually occur on the left side. The sac lies between the prevertebral fascia and the left posterolateral wall of the esophagus. Although the origin of the diverticulum is the hypopharynx, the esophagus is compressed by the diverticulum, and dysphagia and weight loss follow. During deglutition, the diverticulum fills with food and fluid. When the patient lies down, the diverticulum empties into the pharynx, and aspiration of food and fluid into the lower respiratory tract may occur and may cause recurrent and debilitating pneumonitis. The diverticulum is demonstrated with a barium swallow. Treatment consists of cricopharyngeal myotomy and excision of the diverticulum through a cervical incision or by endoscopic cautery of the party wall between the cervical esophagus and the diverticulum.

THE LARYNX

Caelius Aurelianus credits Asclepiades with having first employed tracheotomy in cynanche (probably diphtheria) in the century before the birth of Christ. In 1778, the French surgeon Pelletan performed a successful laryngofissure for the removal of a bolus of meat that had become entrapped between the vocal cords. In 1854, Manuel Garcia, a Spanish singing teacher, succeeded in observing his own larynx with

two mirrors and the sun as a light source. In 1856, Türck and Czermak independently developed the laryngoscope in Vienna. After the development of the laryngoscope, peroral endolaryngeal surgery flourished in many centers. It remains the principal approach to restoration of the voice. In the 1870s, Bergman performed laryngotomies for removal of parts of the larynx involved with carcinoma. Billroth performed the first successful laryngectomy in 1873. Laryngofissure for cordectomy was developed in the first half of this century, and hemilaryngectomy, partial supraglottic laryngotomy, and subtotal laryngectomy followed. After many attempts at rehabilitation of laryngectomy patients with tracheoesophageal communications, the Blum-Singer procedure proved to be a practical alternative to the development of esophageal speech. Augmentation of the paralyzed vocal cord with the injection of Teflon paste opened a new era of voice restoration.[27] Improvement of voice quality in several disease entities and rehabilitation for vocal cord paralysis have been achieved through modification of the laryngeal skeleton, known as thyroplasty.[25]

Anatomy of the Larynx

The skeleton of the larynx consists of the thyroid cartilage, the cricoid cartilage, the arytenoid cartilages with corniculate and cuneiform cartilages, and the epiglottis. Phylogenetically, the arytenoid cartilages are the oldest elements of the laryngeal skeleton. This fact emphasizes the primeval role of the larynx as a sphincter rather than a conduit for air. The cricoid cartilage completely encircles the airway and maintains its patency. The arytenoid cartilages articulate with the cricoid cartilage. The true vocal cords are attached to the vocal processes of the arytenoid cartilages and to the isthmus of the thyroid cartilage. The superior surfaces of the true vocal cords are flat, and the inferior surfaces are concave. The inferior surfaces of the false vocal cords are flat, and the superior surfaces of the false vocal cords are convex. The true vocal cords and the false vocal cords make a double-layered sphincter. The configuration of the true vocal cords makes them a good barrier to the ingress of air and a poor barrier to the egress of air. The configuration of the false vocal cords makes them a poor barrier to the ingress of air and a good barrier to the egress of air. The true vocal cords can be regarded as an inlet valve and the false vocal cords as an outlet valve.

Physiology of the Larynx

The primary function of the larynx is that of a sphincter. During deglutition, both the true vocal cord sphincter and the false vocal cord sphincter are closed, and the epiglottis is drawn posteriorly over the closed sphincter and serves as a watershed, deflecting food and fluid into the pyriform sinuses. The larynx also serves as a sphincter during parturition, coughing, and defecation. At these times, it serves primarily as an outlet valve. In lifting heavy objects and climbing hand over hand, such as climbing a tree, the pull of the shoulder girdles on the thorax tends to expand the thoracic cage. The larynx limits the ingress of air as an inlet valve and thereby stabilizes the thorax.

The larynx serves as the sounding source for speech. A fundamental tone is produced by the movement of the vocal cords, which is brought about by the flow of exhaled air past lightly approximated vocal cords. The fundamental tone and its overtones are modified into meaningful symbols or speech by articulators such as the pharynx, palate, tongue, teeth, and lips. Synchrony of the vibration of the two vocal cords exists normally at any given instant, but aperiodicity over time also occurs. The fundamental tone varies with the sex and age of the individual. Adult males produce a fundamental tone of 125 Hz., and adult females produce a fundamental tone of 250 Hz. In the healthy voice, the predominant overtones of these fundamental tones are partial and whole-number multiples of the fundamental tone. The predominance of harmonic overtones gives the voice a musical quality. The distribution of the harmonics gives the voice a timbre that is characteristic of that individual. In the healthy voice, there are frequent changes in the frequency of the fundamental tone that provide it with a melodious quality. The normal speaker usually uses changes in frequency rather than changes in intensity for emphasis.

Pathophysiology of the Larynx

Various pathologic changes in the vocal cords cause the prominence of nonharmonic noise components in the voice. In contrast to the healthy musical voice, overtones that are not partial or whole-number multiples of the fundamental tone produce a noisy voice or hoarseness. Structural changes in the vocal cords cause greater aperiodicity and asynchrony of the vibration of the vocal cords. Aperiodicity and asynchrony disrupt the harmonic relationships of the voice by limiting the possibility of the occurrence of overtones that are partial and whole-number multiples of the fundamental tone. Characteristically, the abnormal voice is monotonous. A monotone may occur because of loss of flexibility in the frequency range of the larynx due to a disease process, or it may be acquired as a habit, particularly in speakers who tend to use increases in intensity rather than changes in frequency for emphasis. Structural changes in the vocal cords often interfere with their approximation and result in air wastage, which gives the voice a breathy quality.

Structural Changes in the True Vocal Cords Secondary to Misuse and Abuse of the Voice

Abuse and misuse of the voice can cause structural changes in the true vocal cords. Using the voice too loudly and too long produces acute and chronic changes in the true vocal cords. Prolonged use of intensity rather than frequency for emphasis, the employment of a monotone, the affectation of a frequency that is too low, and an abrupt onset of high intensities (sharp glottal attack) produce structural changes in the true vocal cords.

Polyps of the Vocal Cords. Polyps of the true vocal cords develop in response to using the voice too loudly and too long, as in an individual who must speak over a great deal of background noise in a factory or who demonstrates wares in a department store or barks at a circus or carnival. Chronic subepithelial edema develops in the lamina propia of the true vocal cords. Similar pathologic changes follow chronic allergic reactions and the chronic inhalation of irritants such as tobacco smoke and industrial fumes. Such polypoid swellings of the free edge of the true vocal cord interfere with the approximation of the true vocal cords and with the maintenance of periodicity and synchrony of the vibration of the vocal cords. They produce hoarseness and give a breathy quality to the voice. To restore the voice, polyps are removed with the use of an operation microscope during direct laryngoscopy, with the patient under general anesthesia.

Vocal Nodules. Vocal nodules are caused by using a fundamental frequency that is unnaturally low and using the voice too loudly and too long. Vocal nodules occur in children as well as adults and are likely to occur in robust, athletic boys 8 to 12 years of age who yell frequently. Men affect an unnaturally low pitch to give an air of authority; women do it to give an impression of sexiness; and young boys probably do it to identify with older males in the family or community.

Vocal nodules are condensations of hyaline connective tissue in the lamina propria at the junction of the anterior one third and the posterior two thirds of the true vocal cord. These nodules produce hoarseness and give the voice a breathy quality. In adults, these lesions are removed during direct laryngoscopy to restore the voice. However, it is necessary to begin voice therapy prior to surgical therapy, because if the underlying misuse of the voice is not corrected, the nodules recur. In children, surgical removal is not usually necessary, because the vocal nodules regress with voice therapy, which consists of voice rest, reduction in intensity and duration of voice production, and elevation of the pitch.

Contact Ulcers. Contact ulcers of the larynx are thought to follow misuse and abuse of the voice, particularly in the form of a sharp glottal attack, and reflux of gastric contents. They occur unilaterally or bilaterally over the vocal process of the arytenoid. The presence of these lesions causes mild pain on phonation and swallowing and varying degrees of hoarseness. The ulcers have a shaggy or granular base. Gastroesophageal reflux should be identified and managed if found on esophageal intraluminal pH testing or barium esophagography. Biopsy of these ulcers to exclude the possibility of carcinoma is done during direct laryngoscopy. Voice therapy to correct the underlying misuse of the voice is important. However, prolonged voice rest is required for most contact ulcers to heal.

Trauma

Trauma has replaced infectious diseases such as diphtheria, streptococcal croup, syphilis, tuberculosis, rhinoscleroma, and typhoid fever as the most common cause of laryngeal stenosis. Automobile accidents in which the patient is thrown forward and the larynx is crushed between the cervical vertebrae and the object against which it decelerates are the single most important cause of laryngeal stenosis. Children may fracture the larynx by falling against the handlebars of a bicycle or riding a horse or bicycle under a taut line. Another cause of laryngeal stenosis is a high tracheostomy in which perichondritis of the cricoid cartilage follows pressure of the tube on the cartilage. Prolonged endotracheal intubation frequently causes subglottic stenosis, as do infectious processes. Subglottic stenosis is a frequent complication of neonatal intubation, particularly in low-birth-weight infants.

Fractures of the thyroid cartilage may cause supraglottic, glottic, or transglottic stenosis. Individuals with long, slender necks are more likely to sustain supraglottic injuries in which the hyoid bone is also fractured. The suprahyoid muscles are disrupted, and the thyrohyoid membrane is ruptured. Fracture of the cricoid cartilage causes subglottic stenosis. Fractures of the cricoid cartilage are more likely to occur in males with short, thick necks and are relatively rare in females. Often a blow to the neck spares the larynx but transects the trachea.

Patients with crush injuries of the larynx complain of pain on swallowing. Hoarseness may progress to aphonia. Hemoptysis is usually present. Progressive dyspnea due to upper respiratory obstruction is to be anticipated. Subcutaneous emphysema is usually present in fractures of the larynx or trachea. The laryngeal cartilages cannot be distinctly palpated, nor can the trachea, owing to soft tissue swelling. Lateral neck radiographs should be performed to exclude or demonstrate associated fractures or dislocations of the cervical vertebrae. On direct laryngoscopy, the laryngeal lumen appears disrupted or obliterated, and there may be exposed cartilage and lacerated mucous membrane. Vocal cord paralysis may be noted. A barium swallow is required to exclude a perforation of the hypopharynx or cervical esophagus if the patient's condition permits. CT scanning of the neck indicates the type and degree of injury.

In the initial management of a patient with a laryngeal fracture, a tracheostomy is performed and followed by direct laryngoscopy and tracheoscopy. Often, patients with multiple injuries are treated with a tracheostomy because of upper airway obstruction, and the reason for the tracheostomy is forgotten during the management of thoracic and abdominal or perhaps intracranial injuries. The laryngeal trauma is rediscovered 10 or so days later, when it appears that it would be appropriate to remove the tracheostomy tube. Evaluation of the larynx should be performed early to be certain that there has not been a fracture of the laryngeal cartilages that requires early repair.

The repair of the fracture is done through a transverse incision in the neck. To gain access to the interior of the larynx, a laryngofissure is performed by dividing the thyroid cartilage at its isthmus, or the fracture in the thyroid and cricoid cartilage is utilized. Mucous membrane lacerations are repaired, and the cartilages are returned to their normal alignment.[38] Internal splinting is maintained with a solid-core mold for as long as 6 weeks. Failure to reduce a dislocated or fractured cartilage causes laryngeal stenosis. Late repair of laryngeal stenosis can sometimes be accomplished by an arytenoidectomy. At other times, a supraglottic partial laryngectomy is required to restore the airway and the functional integrity of the laryngeal sphincter. A keel is often employed to repair the angle of the anterior commissure. Subglottic stenosis can be relieved in adults by laser therapy or repaired by excision of the stenotic area and internal splinting for a period of 6 weeks or more. Subglottic stenosis in infants is successfully repaired with an anterior or anterior and posterior cricoid cartilage split (vertical transection), with or without costal cartilage grafts.

In addition to external trauma, tracheal stenosis occurs secondary to pressure necrosis of the tracheal walls caused by the inflated cuff in prolonged endotracheal intubation. Tracheal stenosis also occurs secondary to tracheostomy, particularly when the wound becomes infected and there is cicatricial healing of large eroded tracheostomas. Tracheal stenosis may be managed by dilations, excision of the stenotic area with internal splinting for 6 weeks or more, or excision of the stenotic area with end-to-end anastomosis of the trachea. As much as 50% of the length of the trachea can be resected and end-to-end anastomosis performed.[15]

Vocal Cord Paralysis

Vocal cord paralysis follows traumatic, infectious, and neoplastic involvement of the vagus and recurrent laryngeal nerves and degenerative neurologic disorders. Unilateral vocal cord paralysis produces hoarseness and aspiration. Bilateral vocal cord paralysis causes upper airway obstruction with little adverse effect on the voice. In unilateral vocal paralysis, injection of Teflon paste during direct laryngoscopy lateral to the vocalis muscle causes medialization and augmentation of the paralyzed vocal cord so that the unaffected vocal cord can approximate with it. Teflon injection produces improvement of the voice and elimination of aspiration.[27] Similar results have been obtained with phonosurgical techniques in which the paralyzed vocal cord is moved toward the midline with the implantation of autografts lateral to the vocal cord.[25]

The upper airway obstruction caused by bilateral vocal cord paralysis usually requires a tracheostomy initially. Subsequent improvement in the airway can be obtained with an arytenoidectomy.

Foreign Bodies of the Larynx, Tracheobronchial Tree, and Esophagus

Foreign bodies are retained in the larynx because they are sharp and stick into the mucous membrane or are irregular and soft and are caught between the two vocal cords in laryngospasm. A frequently fatal laryngeal foreign body is a bolus of meat. The resulting laryngospasm completely occludes the larynx and makes a choking person mute. This *café coronary* may be distinguished from a myocardial infarct by the respiratory effort without exchange and the marked suprasternal, intercostal, and subxiphoid retraction. Death occurs rapidly unless an alternative airway is established or the foreign body is dislodged. As long as adequate respiratory exchange occurs, the choking individual should be allowed to employ protective reflexes to manage the problem. Maneuvers such as striking the choking individual on the back or turning a choking child upside down may make it more difficult for the choking individual to handle the problem successfully and may convert the situation into one that is less easily managed. If the choking individual is mute and makes no respiratory exchange, the Heimlich (abdominal thrust) maneuver should be attempted.[18] In this maneuver, the operator places his arms around the choking individual from behind, grasps the fist of one hand in the other hand, and brings both hands up in the subxiphoid area briskly to apply pressure to the diaphragm. The pressure increases the intrathoracic pressure and may expel the foreign body. Should this maneuver fail, an alternative airway must be established by the prompt performance of a tracheostomy. Even nonobstructing foreign bodies of the larynx induce a degree of laryngospasm that makes their removal difficult without general anesthesia, and a tracheostomy is often the first step in their removal, particularly subglottic foreign bodies such as sand or grass burrs. The site of the foreign body is exposed with a laryngoscope, and the foreign body is grasped, disengaged, and removed with alligator or other appropriate forceps.

Smooth objects such as nuts, kernels of corn, watermelon seeds, beans, peas, and plastic toys pass through the larynx into the tracheobronchial tree. At the onset, there is severe spasmodic coughing that continues for approximately 30 minutes. During this time, the foreign body migrates from one portion of the tracheobronchial tree to another. It more frequently comes to rest in the right bronchus because the right bronchus is larger than the left and makes less of an angle with the long axis of the trachea, and the carina is to the left of the midline of the tracheal lumen. As it finally comes to rest, the coughing subsides, and a latent period begins during which the patient is free of symptoms. The mistaken inference is often made by the family and the physician in attendance that the foreign body has been expelled. However, careful auscultation of the chest may demonstrate an expiratory wheeze and the signs of obstructive emphysema. The most common mechanism of the bronchial obstruction due to a foreign body is a one-way valve through which air may enter the bronchus distal to the foreign body during inspiration but that affords limited egress on expiration. This type of obstruction produces emphysema distal to the foreign body. The obstructive emphysema may become apparent radiographically only on expiration or by fluoroscopy. The mediastinum shifts away from the obstructed lung, and the obstructed portion of the lung becomes radiolucent, compared with the normal lung. This type of partial obstruction of the bronchus is likely to occur with the aspiration of nuts. In the evaluation of a patient with a suspected nonradiopaque foreign body of the bronchus, comparison of inspiratory and expiratory chest films and fluoroscopy of the chest may demonstrate obstructive emphysema that would not be apparent on inspiration radiographs.

A foreign body that completely obstructs the bronchus causes the rapid development of a more serious pathophysiologic state. Complete atelectasis of the obstructed lung occurs as a result of absorption of the remaining air in the lung. The mediastinum shifts toward the atelectatic lung, and the remaining lung undergoes compensatory emphysema (Fig. 39–16). The atelectatic lung is useless as far as ventilatory exchange is concerned, and the efficiency of the emphysematous lung is greatly reduced. Rapid cardiorespiratory failure occurs unless the foreign body is removed. This type of complete bronchial obstruction is likely to occur with smooth hygroscopic foreign bodies, such as beans, that swell in the bronchus.

Vegetable foreign bodies are very poorly tolerated. Metallic and plastic foreign bodies that cause partial obstruction of the bronchus may be tolerated for long periods. Nuts, particularly peanuts, produce a severe tracheobronchitis. After a latent period of 24 hours, the patient develops a cough productive of purulent sputum, and a febrile course begins. A long-indwelling foreign body of the bronchus may produce bronchiectasis, recurrent pneumonitis, lung abscess, and empyema. Tracheobronchial foreign bodies are removed with general anesthesia through an open bronchoscope with forceps designed specifically for each type of foreign body.

Foreign bodies of the esophagus are likely to lodge just below the cricopharyngeus muscle. Ninety-five percent of esophageal foreign bodies are found in this location. Other locations are the gastroesophageal junction and the indentations of the esophagus caused by the left bronchus and the arch of the aorta. The constrictors of the pharynx are very strong and can propel almost any irregular object through the cricopharyngeus muscle. When the foreign body has passed the cricopharyngeus, the muscular activity is very weak, and progress occurs mainly by gravity. Therefore, irregular objects are brought to an abrupt stop just below the cricopharyngeus muscle.

The symptoms of a foreign body of the esophagus are

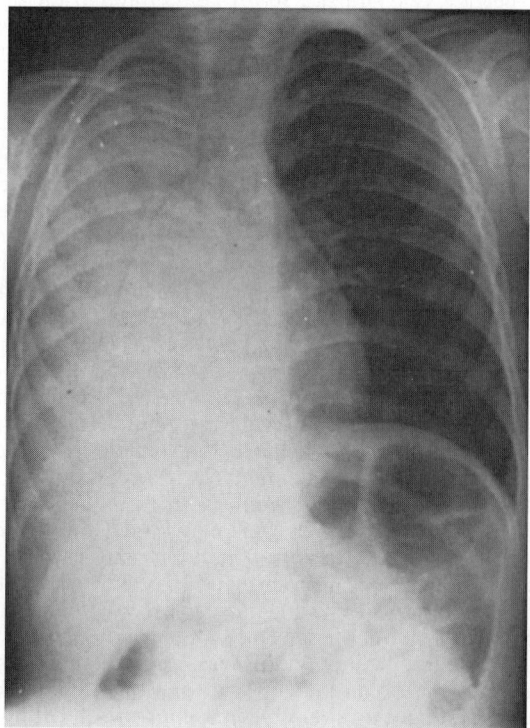

Figure 39–16. Posteroanterior radiograph of the chest of a child with a pinto bean in the right bronchus. There is atelectasis of the right lung and compensatory emphysema of the left lung.

dysphagia and pain in the suprasternal area on swallowing. Bulky foreign bodies in the cervical esophagus may produce upper airway obstruction by extrinsic pressure through the membranous posterior wall of the trachea. Foreign bodies can be identified on a lateral neck film if they are radiopaque. If they are radiolucent, evidence of a foreign body may still be obtained, because the foreign body tends to hold the esophageal walls apart and air may be observed in the cervical esophagus. If the foreign body cannot be located on a lateral neck radiograph, posteroanterior and lateral chest films are obtained. If the foreign body cannot be located in this manner, an esophagogram may demonstrate it. A small pledget of cotton saturated with a solution of barium sulfate may hang on a sharp foreign body. A foreign body of the esophagus is removed under general anesthesia through an open esophagoscope. The foreign body is grasped, disengaged, and removed as a trailing foreign body or through the esophagoscope with a foreign body forceps appropriate to the object. The longer a foreign body remains in the esophagus, the greater the risk of perforation of the esophagus. Perforation of the esophagus causes air and soft tissue swelling in the paraesophageal tissue that may be demonstrated on physical examination and radiographically.

Infectious Diseases

Croup. There are two forms of croup, epiglottitis and laryngotracheobronchitis. Croup occurs primarily in children over 1 year and under 5 years of age. It may be viral or bacterial. Parainfluenza Type I is the most frequently isolated agent in viral croup. *Haemophilus influenzae* is the most frequently isolated agent in bacterial croup, but *Staphylococcus* and *Streptococcus* may also cause croup.

H. influenzae Type b is the predominant microorganism in epiglottitis and frequently causes a bacteremia. Both epiglottitis and laryngotracheobronchitis may produce the rapid onset of upper respiratory obstruction with inspiratory stridor and suprasternal, supraclavicular, intercostal, and subxiphoid retractions. The voice may be hoarse, and the cough has a brassy quality with subglottic edema. The supraglottic swelling may be demonstrated on a lateral neck radiograph (Fig. 39–17). In laryngotracheobronchitis, the major problem is subglottic edema.

Epiglottitis or supraglottic laryngitis is more likely to cause abrupt and complete airway obstruction. When the diagnosis of epiglottitis is made, nasotracheal intubation is performed and maintained for 48 hours until the supraglottic swelling subsides.[42] Fortunately, the *H. influenzae* Type b (Hib) vaccine against meningitis also reduces the incidence of epiglottitis. In laryngotracheobronchitis, the airway obstruction results in part from edema, but there are also tenacious mucoid secretions. Humidification of the inspired atmosphere liquefies the material, and the patient may cough it out to reduce the degree of airway obstruction. Antibiotic therapy is initiated at the onset of both diseases; amoxicillin is the drug of choice (pending blood culture and sensitivities) because the infection is frequently caused by *H. influenzae*. There is usually bacteremia when it is the causative microorganism. Corticosteroid therapy is controversial, but it may be initiated in an attempt to reduce the inflammatory swelling. Oxygen saturation is continuously monitored transcutaneously. With evidence of desaturation or fatigue, endotracheal intubation is accomplished. Prolonged endotracheal intubation increases the risk of laryngeal and subglottic stenosis in laryngotracheobronchitis. If tracheostomy is elected, it can be performed under general anesthesia in a relaxed patient and under unhurried and ideal circumstances. This approach reduces the incidence of pneumothorax and other complications.

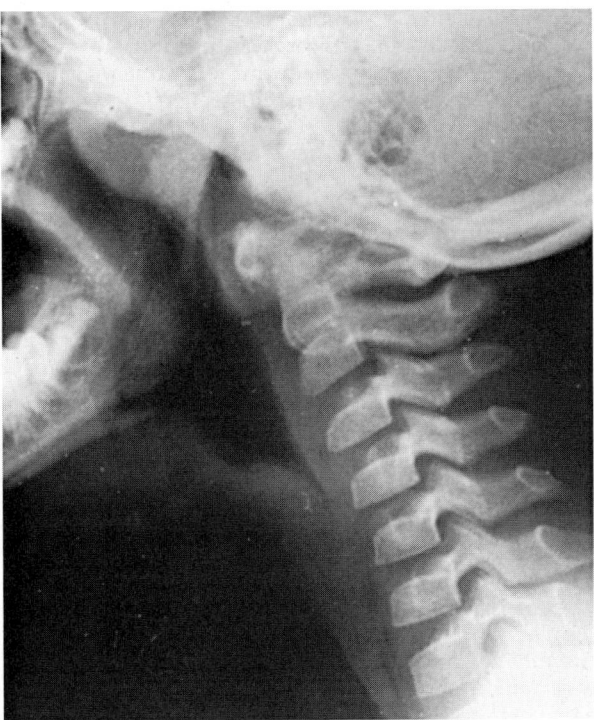

Figure 39–17. Lateral radiograph of the neck in a child with supraglottic laryngitis. Note the swelling of the epiglottis, aryepiglottic folds, and arytenoids.

Tracheostomy. The indications for tracheostomy form three broad categories: upper respiratory obstruction, inability to handle upper respiratory secretions, and inability to handle lower respiratory secretions. Among those causes of upper respiratory obstruction that frequently require tracheostomy are congenital malformations of the upper respiratory tract, laryngotracheobronchitis, diphtheria, foreign bodies, bilateral vocal cord paralysis, neoplasms of the larynx, postintubation edema, allergic reactions, and maxillofacial and laryngeal trauma. The importance of a tracheostomy in patients who are having difficulty managing upper respiratory secretions became well recognized during the polio epidemics. Neurologic problems other than infections, such as intracranial trauma and neoplasms, also lead to difficulty in managing upper respiratory secretions. Patients with ineffective respiratory effort on a neurologic or mechanical basis, chronic obstructive pulmonary disease, and parenchymal infections may have difficulty managing lower respiratory secretions. Many of these problems can be managed with endotracheal intubation on a short-term basis.

A tracheostomy has several advantages and disadvantages. It relieves upper respiratory obstruction and allows more effective access to the lower respiratory tract for suctioning the tracheobronchial tree. It decreases the dead space and reduces the work required for effective ventilation. A tracheostomy can readily be used as a route for the delivery of respiratory assistance. It eliminates the normal warming and humidification of the inspired air by bypassing the upper respiratory tract. A very serious disadvantage of tracheostomy is the loss of an effective cough. It opens the lower respiratory tract to environmental pathogens and increases the vulnerability to *Pseudomonas* infections.

Recurrent Respiratory Papillomatosis. Recurrent respiratory papillomatosis is a chronic infection caused by the human papillomavirus. Its most frequent manifestation is laryngeal papillomas. Although these lesions may occur as early as 1 year of age, they more commonly make their appearance

in the second or third year of life. Papillomas may recur promptly after excision. Exuberant growth from multiple sites in the larynx makes maintenance of an adequate airway difficult. Many children with laryngeal papillomas require a tracheostomy. The papillomas are periodically vaporized with a laser or removed gingerly during direct laryngoscopy under general anesthesia to maintain the voice and the airway.[41] Involution of the papillomas usually occurs at puberty.

Congenital Malformations

Congenital malformations of the larynx may produce varying degrees of airway obstruction. Among the well-recognized causes of laryngeal obstruction encountered in the immediate neonatal period are bilateral vocal cord paralysis and subluxation of the arytenoids secondary to traumatic delivery, laryngomalacia or the exaggerated infantile larynx, stenosis and atresia of the larynx, cysts, and subglottic hemangioma. Tracheal obstruction may be due to intrinsic tracheal lesions such as tracheomalacia, absence of tracheal rings, and tracheal stenosis or to extrinsic tracheal compression from neoplasms of the thyroid, thymus, esophagus, and mediastinum and vascular rings. Tetany of the newborn with laryngospasm is usually recognized by other characteristics of this condition. Newborns with tracheoesophageal fistulas have respiratory distress due to aspiration, but usually no true airway obstruction.

In the delivery room, exposure of the vocal cords with a laryngoscope relieves the obstruction of an exaggerated infantile larynx, in which the flexible epiglottis and arytenoids prolapse into the glottis with inspiration. Inserting a laryngoscope does not relieve obstruction from bilateral vocal cord paralysis, stenosis, or subglottic hemangiomas. Insertion of a 3.5-mm. bronchoscope improves ventilation in these laryngeal lesions but does not relieve tracheal obstruction until the bronchoscope is passed beyond it. These maneuvers are risky in a newborn and should not be undertaken unless the infant's exchange is inadequate for survival. In general, if the exchange is adequate, the infant should be managed expectantly in the neonatal period. Most forms of congenital stridor improve with time. Inappropriate instrumentation may convert a tolerable degree of airway obstruction into one requiring prolonged endotracheal intubation or a tracheostomy. A tracheostomy in a newborn is hazardous and difficult to manage.

Laryngoceles

Laryngoceles are epithelium-lined diverticula of the laryngeal ventricle and may be located internal or external to the laryngeal skeleton. An internal laryngocele may displace and enlarge the false vocal cord and may cause hoarseness and airway obstruction. External laryngoceles pass through the thyrohyoid membrane and present as a mass in the neck over the thyrohyoid membrane. The mass rises with the larynx on swallowing. Internal and external laryngoceles may coexist. Laryngoceles are more common in glassblowers, wind instrument musicians, and others who develop high intraluminal pressures. Initially, laryngoceles are filled with air and expand and collapse with changes in the intraluminal pressure. They are expanded during the Valsalva maneuver. They appear as smooth, ovoid, air-filled masses on CT scans of the neck. Laryngoceles may fill with mucoid fluid and become infected, under which circumstance the term *laryngopyocele* is appropriate. External laryngoceles are excised through a transverse cervical incision. The sac is dissected from surrounding tissue to its point of penetration of the thyrohyoid membrane. The sac is transected, and the mucous membrane of the ventricle is repaired. Internal laryngoceles are managed by the same approach but require extension of the dissection into the larynx through a thyrotomy.

Neoplasms

Benign neoplasms, including papillomas, fibromas, myxomas, chondromas, neurofibromas, hemangiomas, and so forth, may involve any part of the larynx, including the true vocal cords. Such lesions can ordinarily be removed during direct laryngoscopy, with restoration of the voice, the airway, and the functional integrity of the laryngeal sphincter.

Malignant Neoplasms of the Larynx. The majority of malignant neoplasms of the larynx are squamous cell carcinomas. Squamous cell carcinomas of the larynx cause approximately 2% of all cancer deaths. It is a disease mainly of males, with a sex ratio of 5:1.[8] The peak incidence of carcinoma of the larynx is in the fifth and sixth decades of life. Twelve thousand new cases are expected each year in the United States. Laryngeal carcinoma occurs more commonly in individuals with a large ethanol intake. It rarely develops in an individual who does not smoke. Dysplasia follows the inhalation of irritants such as tobacco smoke that contain known potent carcinogens, including 3,4-benzpyrene and other polycyclic aromatic hydrocarbons. It is a premalignant condition from which carcinoma may develop after a period of months or years.

Carcinoma may arise from the mucous membrane of any part of the larynx; however, there is a predilection for the true vocal cords, particularly the anterior portions of the true vocal cords. The epiglottis, pyriform sinus, and postcricoid area also are common sites of origin of carcinoma. For purposes of clinical staging and end result reporting, carcinomas of the larynx can be divided into supraglottic, glottic, subglottic, and hypopharyngeal lesions.[1] Supraglottic lesions involve the epiglottis, aryepiglottic fold, and false vocal cords. Glottic lesions are limited to the area of the true vocal cords. Subglottic lesions include the glottic area as well as the subglottic area. Hypopharyngeal lesions may be divided into lesions of the pyriform sinus, postcricoid area, and posterior pharyngeal wall.

The natural history of the carcinoma varies considerably from one location to another. The early symptom of carcinoma of the true vocal cords is hoarseness. In any patient with hoarseness lasting 2 weeks, indirect laryngoscopy should be done. Any discrete lesions of the mucous membrane of the larynx should be biopsied. Carcinomas of the true vocal cord limited to the middle third of the true vocal cord and not impairing the mobility of the cord are treated with radiation therapy or cordectomy, with an overall 5-year survival rate of 85% to 95%. Because cordectomy causes permanent hoarseness and irradiation usually returns the voice to normal, radiation therapy is the treatment of choice. Cordectomy is reserved for the 5% to 15% who have persistent carcinoma following radiation therapy. The likelihood of metastasis in early carcinoma of the true vocal cord is very slight.

The mobility of the vocal cord becomes impaired in more advanced carcinomas as a result of invasion of the intrinsic musculature and cartilage. With invasion of the intrinsic musculature, the rate of metastasis increases. With invasion of the thyroid cartilage, the rate of 5-year survival with radiation therapy decreases precipitously. Operation becomes the treatment of choice for lesions that involve the anterior commissure where cartilage is invaded early and for larger glottic lesions in which the mobility of the true vocal cord is impaired. Often a vertical hemilaryngectomy can be performed to preserve the phonatory and sphincteric functions of the larynx.[31] In more advanced cases, total laryngectomy is required, and the laryngectomy may be combined with a radi-

cal neck dissection if palpable metastases are present.[40] In view of the fact that only 15% to 20% of patients with glottic carcinomas have nonpalpable metastasis present at the time of initial treatment, a radical neck dissection is not performed electively.

Supraglottic carcinomas tend to be asymptomatic until they reach considerable size. They may produce hoarseness by secondary involvement of the vocal cords, or they may produce pain on swallowing as the first symptom. Often the pain radiates to the ears. Not infrequently, a patient with a supraglottic carcinoma presents with the chief complaint of a swelling in the neck that represents a metastasis. The chance of nonpalpable metastasis being present is 35%. Early supraglottic carcinoma is successfully treated with radiation therapy to the primary lesion and both sides of the neck, but in advanced lesions, better survival rates are obtained with a combination of radiation therapy and surgical therapy.[32] Better local and regional control is obtained with postoperative radiation therapy than with preoperative radiation therapy.[26] The 2-year disease-free survival approximates 70%. In many patients with supraglottic carcinomas, the neoplasm can be completely removed by supraglottic partial laryngectomy, with preservation of the phonatory and sphincteric functions of the larynx. If the glottis is involved, a total laryngectomy is usually required. These procedures are often combined with a radical neck dissection if there are palpable metastases.

Subglottic lesions represent more advanced glottic carcinomas in which the neoplasm has secondarily invaded the subglottic area as well as the supraglottic area. Metastasis to the same side is present in 50% of patients. Subglottic extension of the carcinoma requires a total laryngectomy and radical neck dissection with thyroid lobectomy on the same side. The overall 5-year survival rate for patients with glottic or subglottic carcinomas treated with total laryngectomy for all stages approximates 65%.

Pyriform sinus carcinomas tend to remain asymptomatic for long periods of time. Often the patient presents with dysphagia and pain on swallowing that may radiate to the ear on the same side. Often the presenting complaint is a mass in the neck that represents a metastasis. A combination of preoperative or postoperative radiation therapy and operation yields better survival rates than operation alone. The results of preoperative and postoperative radiation therapy are equivalent in this site.[26] Depending on the location of the lesion in the pyriform sinus, a partial laryngectomy can sometimes be accomplished, with preservation of the phonatory and sphincteric functions of the larynx. More often, a total laryngectomy is required. More extensive lesions require pharyngolaryngectomy, with replacement of the pharynx with a free jejunal graft with microvascular anastomosis. Either of these procedures is combined with a radical neck dissection if there are palpable metastases. The 5-year survival rate for all stages is 30%.

Postcricoid carcinoma has a female predominance of 10 to 1. Women with Plummer-Vinson syndrome have a predilection for the development of postcricoid carcinoma. The presenting complaint is usually pain on swallowing and dysphagia. Metastasis to both sides of the neck is common. A combination of preoperative or postoperative radiation and surgical therapy is usually employed, and the operation required is pharyngectomy, total laryngectomy, and, if there are palpable metastases, radical neck dissection on one side followed by radical neck dissection on the other side in approximately 6 weeks. The 5-year survival rate for all stages is 25%.

Combinations of induction (preoperative) chemotherapy and radiation therapy have allowed the use of conservation surgery (something less than total laryngectomy) in advanced laryngeal carcinoma.[44]

A total laryngectomy requires the formation of a permanent tracheostomy in which the trachea is transected and anastomosed to the skin of the lower part of the neck. Rehabilitation of the postlaryngectomy patient requires the development of alaryngeal or esophageal speech. In this technique, the patient draws air into the esophagus during inspiration and gradually eructs the air through the cricopharyngeus muscle. The opening of the esophagus vibrates and serves as the sounding source. The sound is articulated by the pharynx, palate, tongue, teeth, and lips into speech. For those individuals who, because of age or other physical or emotional reasons, cannot develop alaryngeal speech, an electrolarynx can serve as the sounding source for modification by the articulators. The oscillator of the electrolarynx is placed in the submandibular area, and the sound is articulated into speech. Alternatively, a communication between the trachea and cervical esophagus can be established and maintained with a prosthetic valve that provides a source of air to produce sound generation in the esophagus. The sound can be articulated into meaningful speech with the pharynx, palate, tongue, teeth, and lips. Most individuals who require a laryngectomy may return to their former occupation. With proper guidance in their rehabilitation, laryngectomy patients may resume all activities except swimming.

SELECTED REFERENCES

Alberti, P. W., and Ruben, R. J.: Otologic Medicine and Surgery. New York, Churchill Livingstone, 1988.
A complete encyclopedia of otology.

Ballenger, J. J., and Snow, J. B.: Otorhinolaryngology: Head and Neck Surgery, 15th ed. Baltimore, Williams & Wilkins, 1995.
An up-to-date and authoritative compendium of diseases and disorders of the ears, nose, and throat and head and neck in general, and their management.

Cummings, C. W., et al. (Eds.): Otolaryngology—Head and Neck Surgery, 2nd ed. St. Louis, C. V. Mosby, 1993.
Excellent presentation of major concerns in head and neck oncology.

Montgomery, W. W.: Surgery of the Upper Respiratory Tract, 2nd ed. Baltimore, Williams & Wilkins, 1995.

Schuknecht, H. F.: Pathology of the Ear. 2nd ed. Philadelphia, Lea & Febiger, 1993.
A comprehensive compendium of otopathology that incorporates much of the author's vast knowledge of otology.

REFERENCES

1. American Joint Committee on Cancer: Manual for Staging of Cancer, 4th ed. Philadelphia, J. B. Lippincott, 1992.
2. Anson, B. J., and Donaldson, J. A.: The Surgical Anatomy of the Temporal Bone and Ear. Philadelphia, W. B. Saunders, 1967.
3. Brackman, D. E.: Electric response audiometry in a clinical practice. Laryngoscope, 87(Suppl. 5):1, 1977.
4. Chandler, J. R., and Serrins, A. J.: Transantral ligation of the internal maxillary artery for epistaxis. Laryngoscope, 75:1151, 1965.
5. Cody, D. T. R., Simonton, K. M., and Hallberg, O. E.: Automatic repetitive decompression of the saccule in endolymphatic hydrops (Tack operation). Laryngoscope, 77:1480, 1967.
6. Cohen, N. L., Waltzman, S. B., and Fisher, S. G.: A prospective randomized study of cochlear implants. N. Engl. J. Med., 328:233, 1993.
7. Conley, J. J., and Novack, A. J.: The surgical treatment of malignant tumors of the ear and temporal bone. Arch. Otolaryngol., 71:635, 1960.
8. De Rienzo, D. P., et al.: Carcinoma of the larynx. Arch. Otolaryngol. Head Neck Surg., 117:681, 1991.
9. Eavey, R. D.: Microtia and significant auricular malformation. Arch. Otolaryngol. Head Neck Surg., 121:57, 1995.
10. Elahi, M. M., Parnes, L. S., Fox, A. J., Pelz, D. M., and Lee, D. H.: Therapeutic embolization in the treatment of intractable epistaxis. Arch. Otolaryngol. Head Neck Surg., 121:65, 1995.
11. Eliachar, I., Golz, A., Joachims, H. Z., and Goldsher, M.: Continuous portable vacuum drainage of auricular hematomas. Am. J. Otolaryngol., 4:141, 1983.
12. Fick, I. A. van N.: Decompression of the labyrinth. Arch. Otolaryngol., 79:447, 1964.
13. Gacek, R. R.: Singular neurectomy update. Ann. Otol. Rhinol. Laryngol., 91:469, 1982.
14. Gantz, B. J., et al.: Evaluation of five different cochlear implant designs: Audiologic assessment and predictors of performance. Laryngoscope, 98:1100, 1988.
15. Grillo, H. C.: Obstructive lesions of the trachea. Ann. Otol. Rhinol. Laryngol., 82:770, 1973.
16. Grote, J. J.: Reconstruction of the middle ear with hydroxylapatite implants: Long-term results. Ann. Otol. Rhinol. Laryngol., 99(Suppl. 144):12, 1990.
17. Healy, G. B., and Teele, D. W.: The microbiology of chronic middle ear effusions in children. Laryngoscope, 87:1472, 1977.
18. Heimlich, H. J.: A life-saving maneuver to prevent food-choking. JAMA, 234:398, 1975.
19. Henle, W.: Elevated antibody titers to Epstein-Barr virus in nasopharyngeal carcinoma, other head and neck neoplasms and control groups. J. Natl. Cancer Inst., 44:225, 1970.
20. Hough, J. V. D.: Tympanoplasty with the interior fascial graft technique and ossicular reconstruction. Laryngoscope, 80:1385, 1970.
21. House, W. F.: Subarachnoid shunt for drainage of hydrops. Arch. Otolaryngol., 79:328, 1964.
22. House, W. F.: Transtemporal bone microsurgical removal of acoustic neuromas. Arch. Otolaryngol., 80:601, 1964.
23. Jannetta, P. T., Moller, M. D., and Moller, A.: Disabling positional vertigo. N. Engl. J. Med., 310:1700, 1984.
24. Kamerer, D. B., Lunsford, L. D., and Moller, M.: Gamma knife: An alternative treatment for acoustic neurinomas. Ann. Otol. Rhinol. Laryngol., 97:631, 1988.
25. Koufman, J. A.: Laryngoplasty for vocal cord medialization: An alternative to Teflon. Laryngoscope, 96:726, 1986.
26. Kramer, S., Gelber, R. D., Snow, J. B., Marcial, V. A., Lowry, L. D., Davis, L. W., and Chandler, R.: Combined radiation therapy and surgery in the management of advanced head and neck cancer: Final report of study 73-03 of the Radiation Therapy Oncology Group. Head Neck Surg., 10:19, 1987.
27. Lewy, R. B.: Experience with vocal cord injection. Ann. Otol. Rhinol. Laryngol., 85:440, 1976.
28. Margolis, R. H., Rieks, D., Fournier, E. M., and Levine, S. E.: Tympanic electrocochleography for diagnosis of Meniere's disease. Arch. Otolaryngol. Head Neck Surg., 121:44, 1995.
29. McCabe, B. F.: Central aspects of drugs for motion sickness and vertigo. Adv. Otorhinolaryngol., 20:458, 1973.
30. Nadol, J. B.: Histopathology of *Pseudomonas* osteomyelitis of the temporal bone starting as malignant external otitis. Am. J. Otolaryngol., 1:359, 1980.
31. Ogura, J. H., and Biller, H. F.: Glottic reconstruction following extended frontolateral hemilaryngectomy. Laryngoscope, 75:2181, 1965.
32. Ogura, J. H., Sessions, D. G., and Spector, G. J.: Conservation surgery for epidermoid carcinoma of the supraglottic larynx. Laryngoscope, 85:1808, 1975.
33. Osberger, M. J., Maso, M., and Sam, L.: Speech intelligibility of children with cochlear implants, tactile aids and hearing aids. J. Speech Hear. Res. 36:186, 1993.
34. Rosen, S.: Mobilization of the stapes to restore hearing in otosclerosis. N. Y. J. Med., 53:2650, 1953.
35. Schuknecht, H. F.: Cupulolithiasis. Arch. Otolaryngol., 90:765, 1969.
36. Shea, J. J., Jr.: Fenestration of the oval window. Ann. Otol. Rhinol. Laryngol., 67:932, 1958.
37. Silverstein, H., Fabian, R. L., Stool, S. E., and Hong, S. W.: Penetrating wounds of the tympanic membrane and ossicular chain. Trans. Am. Acad. Ophthalmol. Otolaryngol., 77:125, 1973.
38. Snow, J. B.: Diagnosis and therapy for acute laryngeal and tracheal trauma. Otolaryngol. Clin. North Am., 17:101, 1984.
39. Snow, J. B.: Management and therapy of trauma to the external ear and auditory and vestibular systems. In Alberti, P. W., and Ruben, R. J. (Eds.): Otologic Medicine and Surgery. New York, Churchill Livingstone, 1988, p. 1561.
40. Snow, J. B.: Surgical management of head and neck cancer. Semin. Oncol., 15:20, 1988.
41. Strong, M. S., Vaughan, C. W., Healy, G. B., Cooperband, S. R., and Clemente, M. A. C. P.: Recurrent respiratory papillomatosis: Management with the CO$_2$ laser. Ann. Otol. Rhinol. Laryngol., 85:508, 1976.
42. Tos, M.: Nasotracheal intubation in acute epiglottitis. Arch. Otolaryngol., 97:373, 1973.
43. Wilson, B. S., Finley, C. C., Lawson, D. T., Wolford, R. D., et al.: Better speech recognition with cochlear implants. Nature, 352:236, 1991.
44. Wolf, G. T., et al.: Induction chemotherapy plus radiation compared with surgery plus radiation in patients with advanced laryngeal cancer. N. Engl. J. Med., 324:1685, 1991.
45. Wullstein, H.: The restoration of function of the middle ear in chronic otitis media. Ann. Otol. Rhinol. Laryngol., 65:1020, 1956.

CHAPTER 40

PLASTIC AND MAXILLOFACIAL SURGERY

Greg J. Mackay, M.D., Grant W. Carlson, M.D., Robert J. Wood, M.D., and John Bostwick III, M.D.

We bring back, refashion and restore to wholeness the features which nature gave but chance destroyed, not that they may charm the eye but that they may be an advantage to the living soul.[1]

G. TAGLIACOZZI

Plastic surgery is the branch of surgery that concentrates on restoring form and function to the human body. Plastic (Gr., *plastikos*, meaning "fit for molding") is the surgical technique of repair. It is a specialty that is not confined to one system or anatomic region but involves aesthetic and reconstructive problems throughout the body.

HISTORICAL ASPECTS

The history of plastic surgery dates to antiquity. The earliest recorded attempts at wound closure can be found in the *Edwin Smith Papyrus*, the oldest surgical medical record known to man, written in Egypt around 3000 to 2500 B.C. Early attempts at reconstruction of the nose and earlobes are described by the noted Indian practitioner Sushruta in 600 B.C.[2] Celsus, a Roman (25 B.C.–A.D. 50), described operations on the lip, nose, and ears and was the first to use an advancement flap for lip and cheek defects.

Between the Roman Empire and the Renaissance, little was recorded about plastic surgery. During the Renaissance (1400–1600) in Italy, crimes of violence related to political and religious feuds were common as assassinations and mutilations among the common people became a daily occurrence. Branca, of Sicily, in 1430 developed the Italian method of nasal reconstruction, being the first to use a flap from the arm to fashion a new nose. Tagliacozzi, of Bologna (1545–1599), the modern *father of plastic surgery*, also described the arm flap for nasal reconstruction (Fig. 40–1).

At the start of the twentieth century and during World War I plastic surgery became a subspecialty. Stimulated by the challenge to reconstruct facial injuries after gunshot wounds, integrated teams of dental, oral, and general surgeons were created. Gillies, an otolaryngologist, is credited for his pioneer work in setting up a treatment center for the wounded in Great Britain. He would later write *Plastic Surgery of the Face*, detailing his war experience. Kazanjian, of Boston, set up another allied war reconstructive center in France. Kazanjian was a dental surgeon and used his knowledge to reconstruct mandibular defects by fixation.

Davis is credited with advocating the establishment of the first division of plastic surgery at the Johns Hopkins Hospital in 1916. His book, *Plastic Surgery, Its Principles and Practice* was published in 1916 and was the first American text devoted solely to plastic surgery. The American Board of Plastic Surgery was established in 1937.

World War II casualties stimulated the principles of soft tissue reconstruction of the extremities and hand. Bunnell is

credited with developing many of the techniques used in hand surgery today, along with the postwar establishment of specialized centers for the treatment of hands and burns. Research in tissue transplantation began with Medawar's work in 1944; and in 1955, Murray, a plastic surgeon in

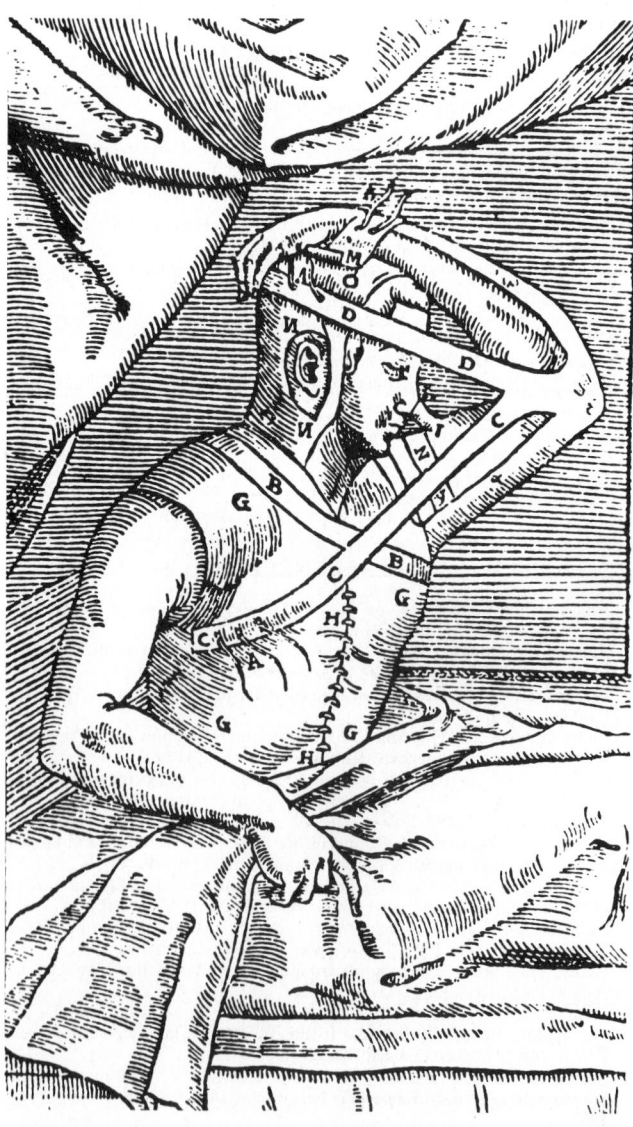

Figure 40–1. Plate VIII illustrating the arm flap to reconstruct a nose. (From Tagliacozzi, G.: De Curtorum Chirurgia per Insitionem. Venice, Gaspare Bindoni, 1597.)

Boston, performed the first successful renal allotransplantation in monozygotic twins.

In the early 1960s the deltopectoral flap was introduced by Bakamjian for head and neck reconstruction. McGregor and Jackson described the groin flap, an axial pattern flap, based on the blood supply of the superficial circumflex iliac artery in 1972. Ger (1971) introduced the local muscle flap for the treatment of lower-extremity wounds, and further pioneering work by Vasconez, Bostwick, and McCraw (1974) and by Mathes and Nahai (1979) established the musculocutaneous flap.[3, 4] Development of the operating microscope allowed for microvascular anastomosis between vessels of very small diameter (1.0–3.0 mm.), and successful free tissue transfers were reported by Daniel and Taylor (1972), McLean and Buncke (1972), and Harii and Ohmori (1973).

In 1967, Tessier introduced his concepts of craniofacial surgery techniques, which permitted correction of severe craniofacial deformities.[5] Multispecialty clinics composed of plastic surgeons, neurosurgeons, orthodontists, and speech pathologists have been established for the treatment of craniofacial disorders and cleft lip and palate deformities. Recent advances in craniofacial surgery include the application of endoscopic surgical techniques and osteodistraction of the facial skeleton.[5a]

BASIC PRINCIPLES

Wound Closure

Wound healing is a complex and dynamic process and can be influenced by surgical technique. Optimal wound healing, with a minimal scar that compromises neither appearance nor function, is the desired result. This process is affected by both local and systemic factors.[6] Many local conditions are readily controlled at the time of wound closure, and several fundamental principles of surgical wound closure exist that should be adhered to in the management of any skin wound to improve optimal healing (Table 40–1).[7]

Complex wounds can result from trauma, severe infections with widespread tissue necrosis, or a surgical procedure. To successfully manage a wound, both the type and anatomic location must be considered in determining the technique of wound closure. The *type* of injury can be clean or contaminated and may be an abrasion, contusion, puncture, laceration, or avulsion. Most traumatic civilian wounds can be closed primarily after adequate sharp débridement and copious pulsatile irrigation. Certain exceptions include human bites or wounds with heavy bacterial contamination. The key to the closure of any wound is adequate débridement to ensure that infection is minimized. Nonviable tissue acts as a nidus for infection. The viability of traumatized tissue can be assessed by seeking active circulation. Tissue blanching with pressure, the presence of dermal bleeding, and the contraction of underlying muscle indicate an intact active circulation.[8] Abrasions can be scrubbed or dermabraded if necessary to remove dirt or other foreign material buried in the dermis that otherwise may result in traumatic tattoos. Perma-

nent discoloration due to buried dirt can occur if the dirt is not removed within 24 to 48 hours. Lacerations and avulsion injuries require assessment for tissue viability to determine the extent of débridement. Avulsed tissue can be placed back into its anatomic position if it has been defatted and placed onto a well-vascularized bed, where it can survive as a free graft. Puncture wounds should be evaluated for underlying damage and may require formal wound exploration. Human bites and animal bites need to be managed with aggressive débridement and antibiotics to prevent the often-devastating infections that can follow these injuries.

The anatomic location of the injury significantly affects the approach to the initial closure of a wound. Injuries to the face, where cosmesis is of greatest concern, require a more conservative approach to débridement and closure to preserve key anatomic landmarks such as the eyelid, eyebrow, nostril, vermilion-cutaneous border, and helical rim. Generally, in managing more extensive facial wounds with loss of soft tissue, it is better to débride only the foreign and grossly nonviable tissues, leaving the questionable areas intact and replacing the tissue into its correct anatomic position. If a primary closure is not attainable, the defect can be closed with a split-thickness skin graft, which minimizes wound contracture and permits a more definitive closure at a later date. Injuries involving cartilaginous structures require special attention. Exposed cartilage, as might occur with ear injuries, should be covered with available soft tissue or topical antibiotic ointment to prevent the development of chondritis. Perichondral hematomas in the ear and nasal septal hematomas should be drained immediately to prevent permanent damage to the underlying cartilage.

Amputated body parts, if retrieved intact, should be replaced within 6 hours if possible. The amputated part should be covered with saline-moistened gauze, placed in a plastic bag, and then placed in ice for transport and preservation until replantation.[9]

Skin Incisions

In any plastic surgical procedure, skin incisions are placed to minimize the scar. Langer, in 1861, described the lines of minimal tension within the skin. These lines usually run perpendicular to the long axis of underlying muscles (Fig. 40–2). When an incision is placed within these lines of minimal tension, the resulting scar is not subjected to the transverse pull of underlying muscles, which could result in widening of the scar. These lines of minimal tension are easily recognized in the face, because they are produced by repeated contraction of the underlying muscles of facial expression (Fig. 40–3). If the wrinkle lines or lines of minimal tension are not readily apparent, they can often be identified by having the patient simulate a facial expression. In certain areas of the face the lines of minimal tension develop in relation to the eyes and mouth, such as the nasolabial fold, at the lateral canthus of the eye as crow's-feet, and as frown lines in the forehead. Incisions should be placed within or parallel to these wrinkle lines whenever possible. If this is not possible, then the incisions should be placed such as to distract the viewer's eye from the scar. This can be accomplished by hiding the scar in the junction lines of the face that exist around the base of the ala, the nostril rim, the preauricular region, and the lower eyelid just below the eyelashes in the subciliary region (Fig. 40–4).

Certain anatomic areas are particularly prone to forming large unsightly scars because of the associated skin tension in the region. For instance, incisions placed in and around the shoulders and sternal area tend to form hypertrophic scars, particularly in large muscular athletes and in women with large pendulous breasts.

TABLE 40–1. Fundamental Techniques of Wound Closure

1. Handle all tissues gently and débride only devitalized areas.
2. Eliminate tension at skin edges.
3. Evert wound edges.
4. Ensure complete hemostasis before wound closure.
5. Use fine sutures whenever possible and remove them early.
6. Place incisions in natural skin folds when possible.
7. Allow time for scar maturation before revision is undertaken.

Surgical Technique

The aim in surgical wound closure is to achieve precise approximation of skin edges with minimal or no tension. Wounds closed under tension tend to pull apart, resulting in large hypertrophic scars and suture marks, or "railroad tracks" form where the suture has cut through the underlying tissue owing to the tension and re-epithelialized suture holes. Inverted wound edges heal with a scar that is depressed and create a shadow, which draws attention to it. Inverted wound edges follow poorly coapted skin edges or tension on the skin closure (Fig. 40–8). To relieve tension at the skin closure site, the deeper layers of tissue should first be reapproximated with sutures. A simple interrupted suture or an everting vertical mattress suture may then be used to close the skin edges. The vertical mattress suture is often used in wounds where the skin edges are thin or slight tension exists and the wound edges are difficult to evert. This suture brings the wound edges close together with the outer bite and allows for eversion of the edges under less tension (Fig. 40–9). Occasionally it is necessary to undermine the skin edges by 3 to 6 mm. to achieve the correct amount of eversion for proper wound closure.

Wounds may be closed with either interrupted or continuous-running sutures. If cosmetic closure is the goal, then interrupted sutures should be placed, because the wound edges can be aligned to a more accurate degree. The continuous suture can be used in many areas where the wound edges are already well aligned and can save time in closure. The intradermal stitch is especially useful for reapproximating wound edges where there is concern about leaving suture marks (Fig. 40–10).

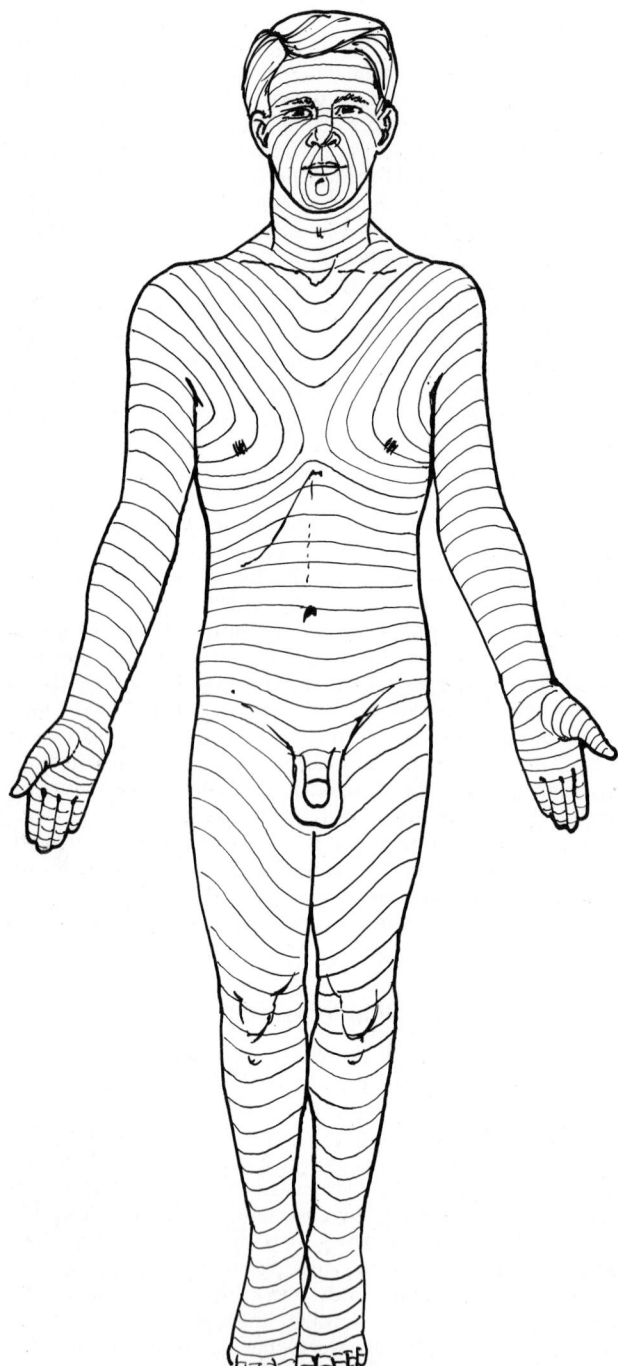

Figure 40–2. Langer's lines of minimal tension.

Incisions placed across joint surfaces should be oriented across the joint in an oblique or transverse manner so that as a scar forms it will not limit or restrict range of motion (Fig. 40–5). Incisions designed to remove skin lesions should be oriented along relaxed skin tension lines and made as a long ellipse approximately two and one-half to three times longer than they are wide (Fig. 40–6). If the ellipse is too short, excess tissue will form at the end and require excision.[10] If the orientation of the natural minimal tension skin lines is not evident, then the lesion can be excised circularly and the surrounding tissue undermined in all directions. The circular defect will reorient into an ellipse as a result of the natural skin tension (Fig. 40–7).

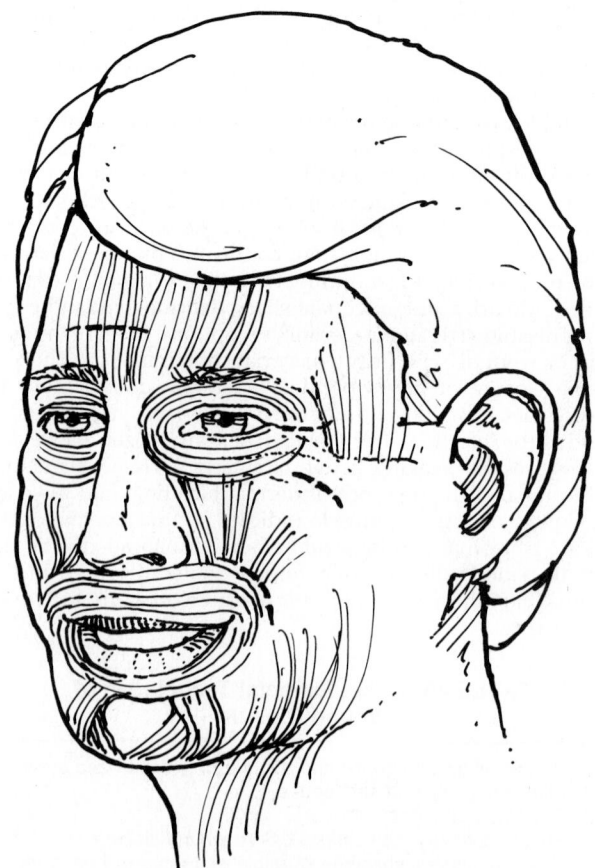

Figure 40–3. Muscles of facial expression and their relationship to lines of minimal tension in the face.

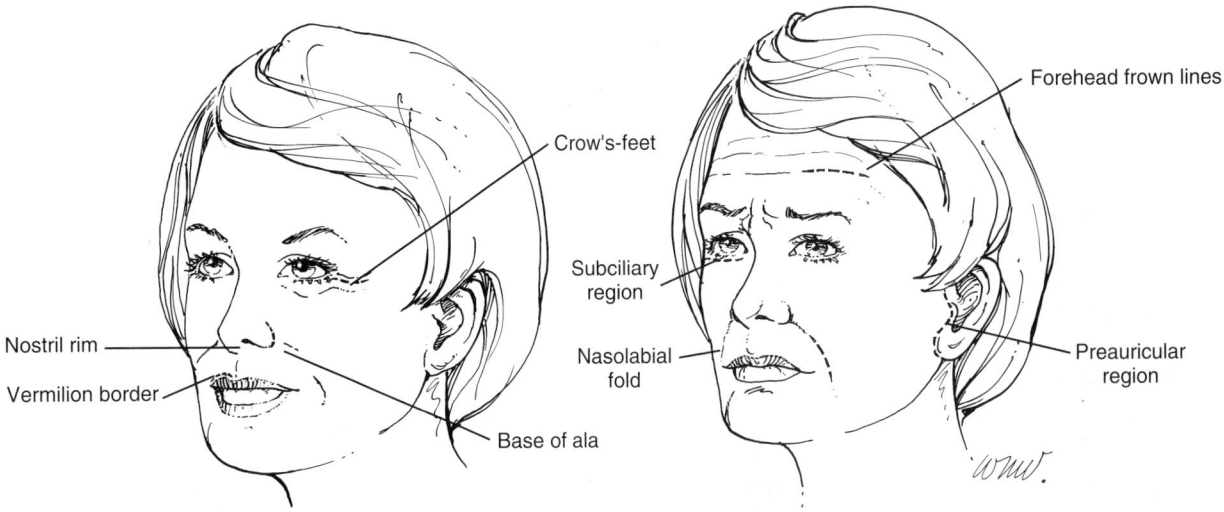

Figure 40–4. Proper placement of incisions to conceal scars in the face.

When an elliptical or oval defect is closed, there often is excess tissue at the end of the wound, known as a *dog ear.* To remove it, a hook is placed in the end of the wound and the excess tissue is elevated to define the exact amount of tissue for removal. The excess tissue is then incised at its base as an ellipse or a triangle. An alternative method is to extend the incision as an ellipse and then remove the excess tissue (Fig. 40–11).

A great variety of sutures as well as stapling devices are available for wound closure. Sutures can be absorbable or nonabsorbable. Absorbable sutures include plain or chromatized catgut, polyglactin-910 (Vicryl), polydioxanone (PDS),

and polyglycolic acid (Dexon). It generally takes 1 to 2 weeks for the body to break down the plain catgut, and approximately 3 to 4 weeks to break down chromatized gut. Fine plain gut is very useful in closing skin lacerations and incisions about the face, particularly in children in whom removing sutures may be as traumatic as placing them. Plain gut does elicit a significant inflammatory response, and in older children and adults a nonabsorbable suture may be indicated. The other absorbable sutures, polyglycolic acid and polyglactin-910, are produced by polymerization of glycolic acid. These are often used to close subcutaneous tissues or as intradermal sutures and are generally hydrolyzed by the

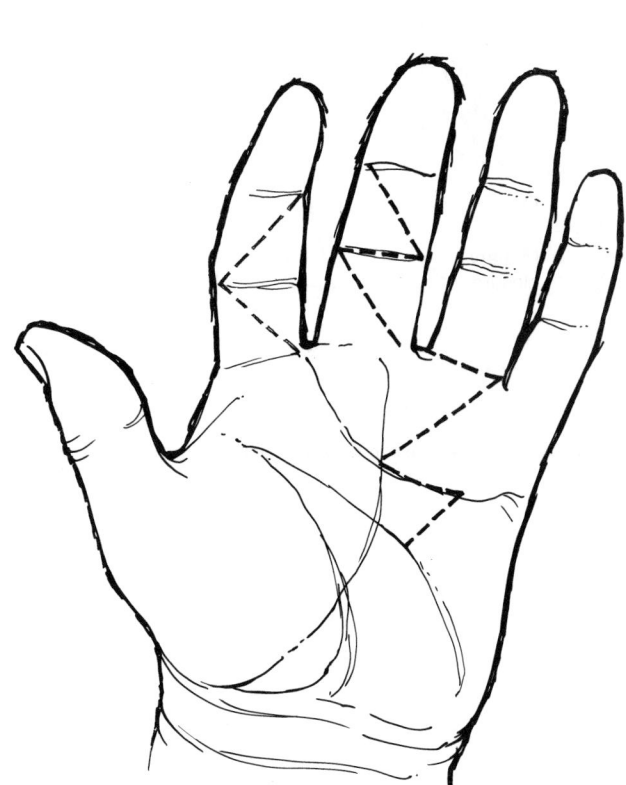

Figure 40–5. Proper placement of incisions across joint surfaces.

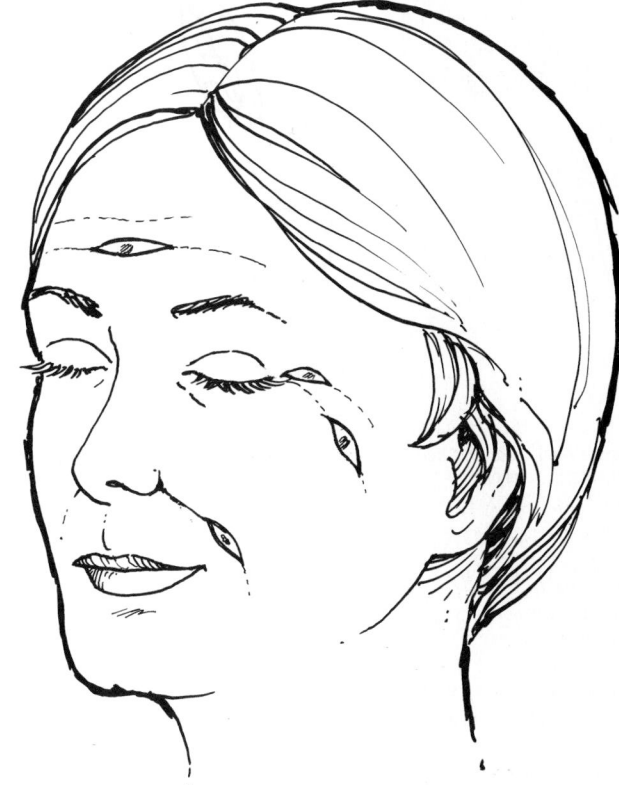

Figure 40–6. Elliptical incisions to remove lesions should follow the lines of facial expression.

the underlying dermis or split thickness when they include a portion of the underlying dermis.

Once harvested, skin grafts can be expanded or meshed in ratios of 1:1.5, 1:2, 1:3, or up to 1:9. Split-thickness grafts undergo less primary contraction than full-thickness grafts when harvested. Primary contraction is the amount a graft contracts immediately after being harvested and is related to recoil of the elastic fibers of the dermis. Full-thickness grafts contract about 40% of their original volume. Split-thickness skin grafts contract 10% to 20% of their original volume. Split-thickness skin grafts undergo greater secondary contraction than full-thickness grafts. Secondary contraction is the amount a graft shrinks after it has healed at the recipient site, and is related to contraction of the wound and dermal thickness of the graft.

Split-thickness skin grafts are not as durable as full-thickness grafts and may demonstrate abnormal pigmentation, but they have a better chance of survival.[11] Meshed split-thickness skin grafts are most useful for covering large areas of skin loss. Meshed grafts are not indicated for use in the face because of cosmetic reasons or over joints where they may contract.

Full-thickness skin grafts undergo less secondary contraction and maintain their normal pigment. They are especially useful in closing defects on the face, where color and texture match is important, and for closing finger defects to avoid contractures. The donor site of a full-thickness graft must be closed primarily, because the entire epidermis and underlying dermis has been removed.

Selection of the donor site depends on the anatomic site to be grafted and the type of graft to be harvested. In general,

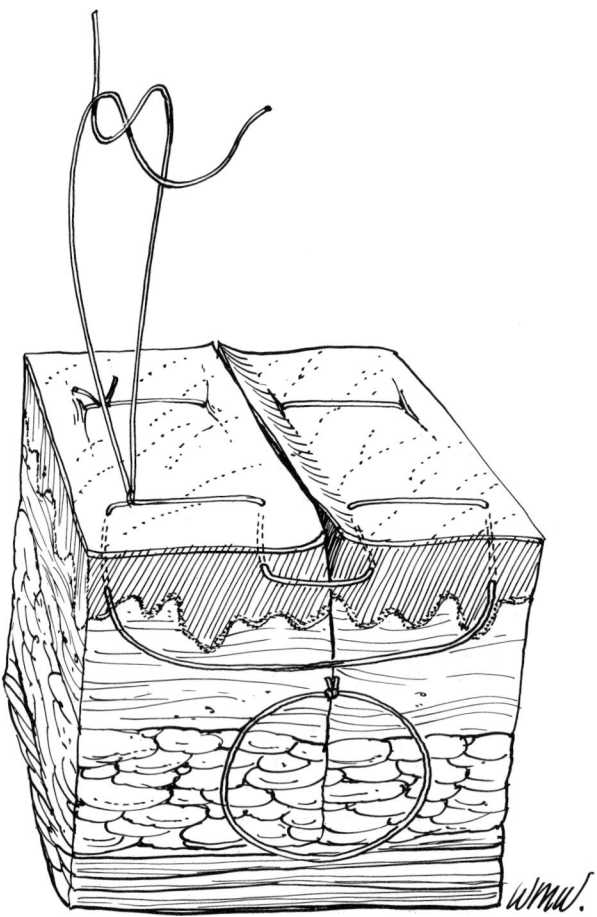

Figure 40–9. The vertical mattress suture everts the wound edges.

Tiss
be e:

body over a 1- to 3-month period. Polydioxanone loses most of its strength in 6 weeks.

The nonabsorbable sutures include silk, cotton, steel, nylon, polypropylene (Prolene), and Dacron. These sutures elicit a much weaker inflammatory response and have much greater tensile strength. They are excellent for closing skin incisions and subcutaneous lacerations, especially if cosmesis is a primary concern, and should be removed within 5 to 7 days to prevent the development of permanent suture marks.

Skin Grafts and Flaps

The technique used to close a wound is determined largely by the defect, its anatomic location, and the surgeon's preference. When minimal tissue loss is evident and the wound can be closed without undue tension, direct closure is indicated. When there has been significant tissue loss or when direct closure of a wound might result in compromise of function or form, a skin graft or flap may be indicated. The reconstructive ladder illustrates a logical approach to the closure of difficult wounds (Fig. 40–12).

Grafts

The technique of skin grafting permits the closure of large wounds by transplanting a sheet of epidermis with underlying dermis of variable thickness from one part of the body to another. The transplanted skin is completely detached from one area and attached to the recipient or host site. Skin grafts may be considered full thickness when they include all

Figure 40–7. A to D, Circula natural skin tension.

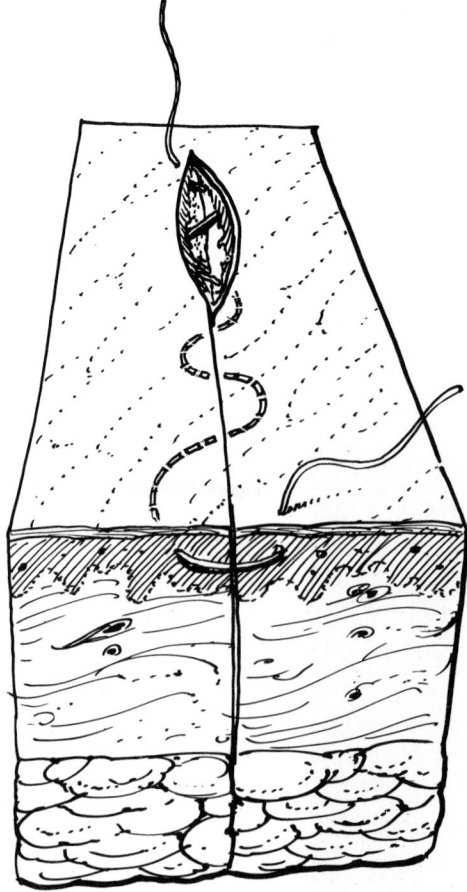

Figure 40–10. Intradermal suture placement for wound closure.

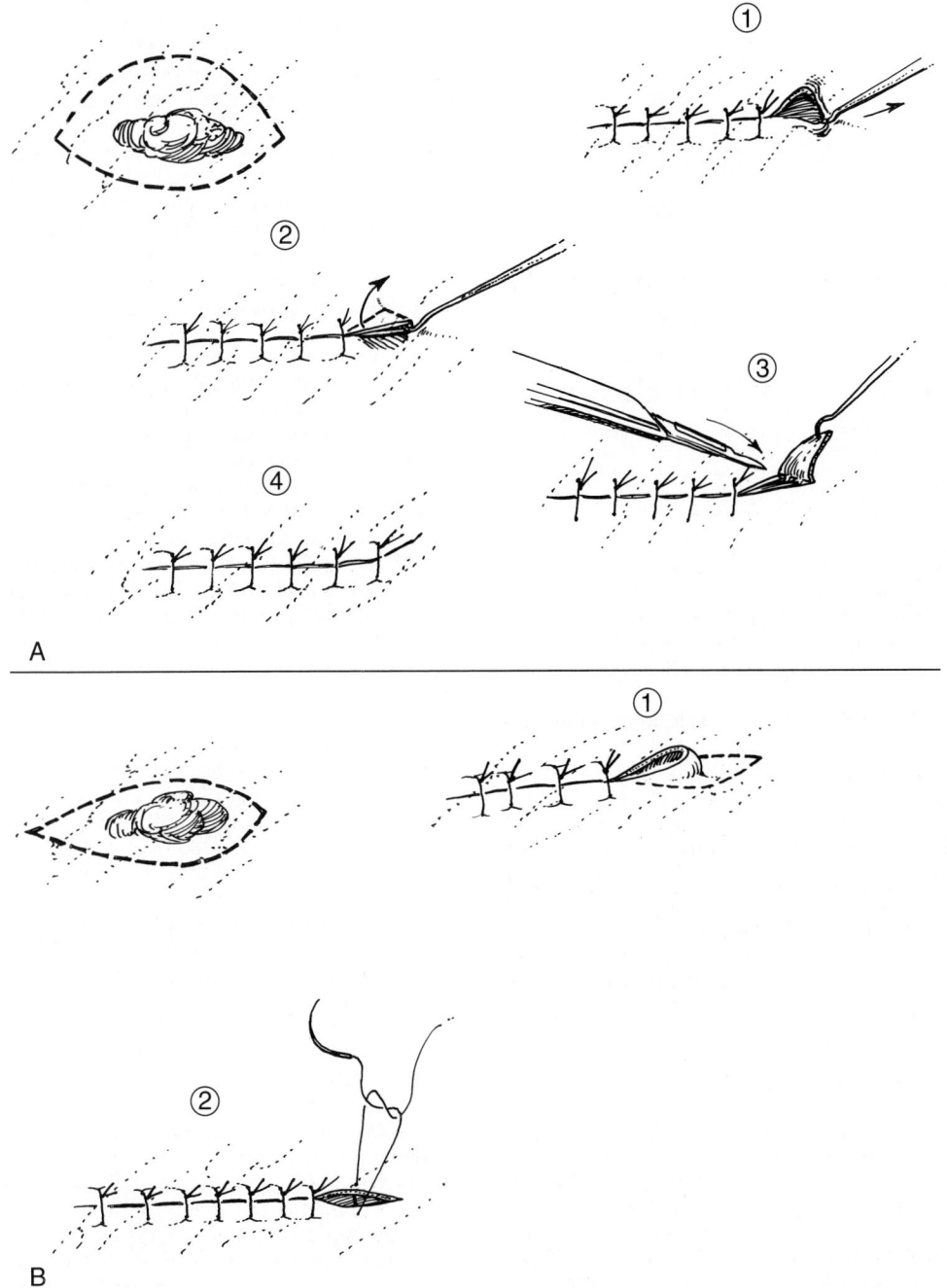

Figure 40–11. *A,* Removal of "dog ear" as a triangle of excess skin. *B,* Removal of dog ear by extending the incision as an ellipse.

Reconstructive ladder

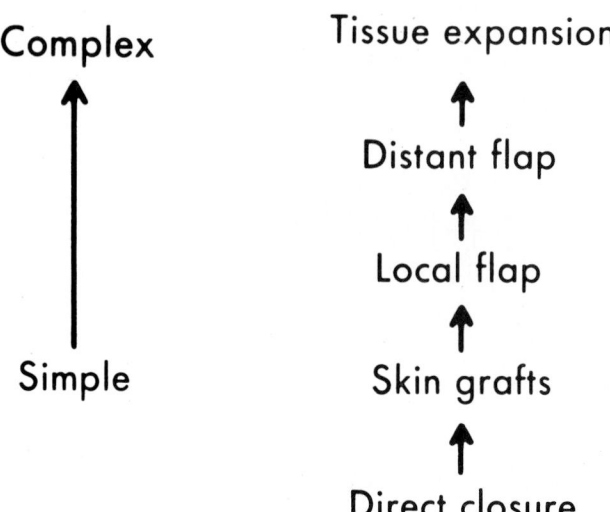

Figure 40–12. Techniques available for surgical wound management progressing from simple to complex. (Modified from Mathes, S. J., and Nahai, F.: Clinical Applications for Muscle and Musculocutaneous Flaps. St. Louis, C. V. Mosby, 1982.)

split-thickness skin grafts are harvested from the thighs, buttocks, or abdominal wall. When possible the skin is harvested from an area that is hidden by an undergarment. Full-thickness grafts for the face are taken from the postauricular area, the supraclavicular region, or the upper eyelid to achieve the best match in color and texture to that of the face. Additional donor sites for full-thickness skin grafts include the antecubital crease or groin crease.

Clean granulating wounds or surgically prepared wounds provide adequately vascularized beds for skin grafts to *take.* Fascia, well-vascularized fat, peritenon, perineurium, and periosteum all provide suitable beds. Grafts, however, do not survive on bare cortical bone, denuded tendon, nerve, or cartilage. Infected wounds with bacterial counts of more than 10^5 per gram of tissue or wounds that have been previously irradiated and may be poorly vascularized may not support a skin graft. Before the placement of any skin graft, meticulous hemostasis is absolutely necessary. Any underlying hematoma existing between a skin graft and the underlying host bed can result in failure of skin graft survival.

Adequate contact between the graft and host bed is imperative for a graft to survive. A secure dressing to immobilize the graft is important, and often a tie-over-bolster dressing is helpful. If a graft is placed in an area that is difficult to dress, it may be left open. Skin grafts develop some nerve reinnervation with time. They assume the sensory pattern of the area in which they are placed, as the surrounding regional nerves grow into the graft through the remaining neurilemmal sheaths. Sensory recovery begins at 1 to 5 months and is complete by 1 to 2 years. These grafts also develop limited sebaceous secretions and sweating, depending on the amount of glandular tissue left in the transplanted skin. Full-thickness grafts and thicker split-thickness grafts have more intact sweat and sebaceous glands, and often redevelop normal function.

Hyperpigmentation of skin grafts occurs, especially in the thinner split-thickness skin grafts in dark-skinned individuals. To minimize the amount of hyperpigmentation, patients should wear sunscreen for at least the first year after operation.

Flaps

In many instances, wound closure with a skin graft is not possible or is not the method of choice for reconstructing a defect. This situation occurs when there are greater functional or aesthetic needs that cannot be met with a skin graft (e.g., breast reconstruction, pressure sores, full-thickness face defects, or exposed tendon or bone) or when the vascularity of the wound defect is inadequate to support a skin graft. When these situations occur, it is often necessary to reconstruct the defect with a flap of tissue composed of either skin, subcutaneous tissue, fascia, muscle, bone, or any combination of these. Technically, a flap is tissue transferred from one site to another with its vascular supply intact. Knowledge of the blood supply to a flap is essential in determining how large a flap can be made, how far it can be moved, and what its pivotal point should be. Flaps are generally classified by their method of movement (i.e., local or distant), by their blood supply (i.e., random, axial, fasciocutaneous, or musculocutaneous), and by their composition.

Classification by Method of Flap Movement. Local skin flaps are in close proximity to the defect and are classified by their method of movement as either rotation, transposition, advancement, or interpolation (Fig. 40–13). These local cutaneous flaps are transferred into the defect and inset so as to reconstruct the deformity. The donor site is then closed primarily or skin grafted. A rotation or transposition flap is any flap of skin and subcutaneous tissue that rotates about a pivot point into the defect to be closed. There is little difference between the two flaps. An advancement flap is any flap that involves movement of skin and subcutaneous tissue in a forward direction for defect closure. An interpolation, or *island,* flap is one that rotates about a pivot point into a defect close to but not adjacent to the flap so that its pedicle must pass over or under the intervening tissue.

One major advantage of a local flap over a skin graft is that it is obtained from the surrounding area of the defect and therefore likely to be of similar color and texture to the skin at the site of the defect.[12] Local flaps tend to contract very little when compared with skin grafts, and they provide an additional source of blood supply. The main disadvantage of local skin flaps is that they require extensive planning and experience to prevent their failure, which can result in an even greater functional or cosmetic deformity.

Distant flaps (Fig. 40–14) are those attached directly to the defect either by bringing the defect to the flap (e.g., groin flap for hand wounds) or by raising a flap at a site remote from the defect, which can then be easily moved to fill the defect (e.g., transverse rectus abdominis musculocutaneous [TRAM] flap). Free-tissue transfers also fall under the category of distant flaps.

Classification by Blood Supply. As well as being classified as either local or distant, flaps are generally classified according to their blood supply. The blood supply to the skin and subcutaneous tissue is through musculocutaneous arteries or by direct septocutaneous vessels (Fig. 40–15). Segmental vessels that come directly off the aorta branch out to the various tissues. From the segmental vessels arise musculocutaneous perforating branches and direct cutaneous perforating branches (Fig. 40–16). The musculocutaneous perforators supply blood to the muscle as well as the fascia, skin, and subcutaneous tissue through the dermal-subdermal plexus. The direct cutaneous perforators supply blood to the fascia, skin, and subcutaneous tissue by directly feeding the dermal-subdermal plexus.

Random cutaneous flaps are perfused by the dermal-subdermal plexus of multiple vessels, but they do not incorporate a specific cutaneous perforator. They are therefore limited in their overall size and, in particular, their length-

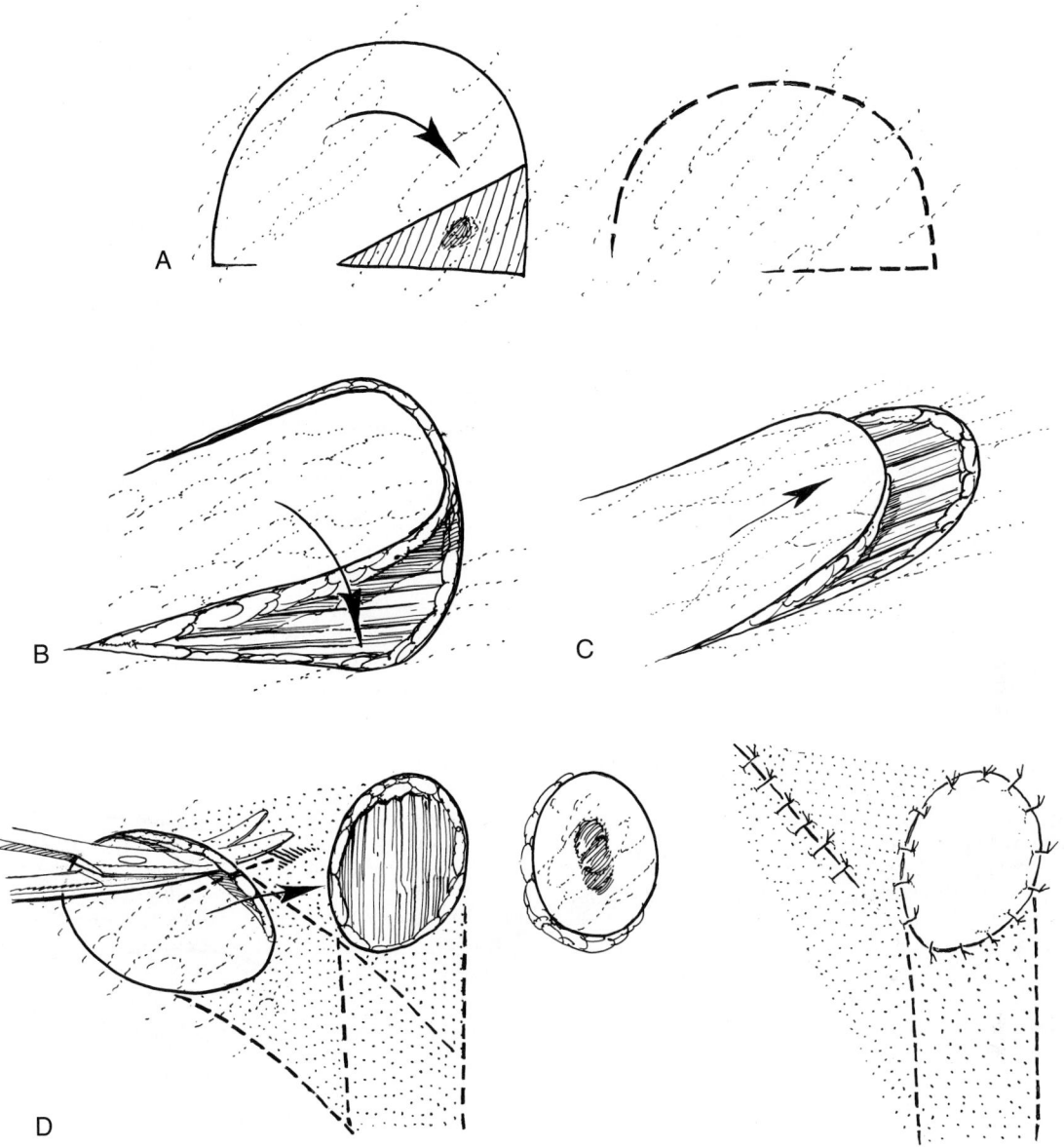

Figure 40–13. Various local skin flaps: *A*, Rotation flap; *B*, transposition flap; *C*, advancement flap; and *D*, interpolation, or island flap.

to-width dimensions. Axial/arterial flaps are based on blood supply to the skin and subcutaneous tissue by a specific cutaneous perforator. Examples of these flaps include the groin, scapular, or radial forearm flap. Their size and mobility are limited only by the length and territory supplied by the underlying vessel. Axial flaps can be used as free flaps if they are transferred to a distant site and their dominant vessel is reanastomosed using microsurgery. Fasciocutaneous flaps are composed of skin, subcutaneous tissue, and the underlying deep fascia of a muscle. The fascia has its own system of vessels that course throughout it and sends branches to the overlying subdermal-dermal plexus to supply the skin. If the underlying fascia is included in a random cutaneous flap, its vascularity is greatly improved. Musculocutaneous flaps are composed of skin, subcutaneous tissue, and the underlying muscle. The blood supply to the skin and subcutaneous tissue is dependent on the underlying muscle and the musculocutaneous perforators, which are supplied by large dominant segmental vessels. Often, more than one segmental vessel supplies a muscle. The muscle

without the overlying cutaneous paddle can be transferred alone, based solely on its segmental perforating vessel. These large robust flaps can supply well-vascularized tissue for covering exposed bone and filling in dead space, or they can be shaped for such purposes as reconstructing a breast (i.e., TRAM flap). Musculocutaneous flaps can be transferred locally to reconstruct a defect, depending on their type of vascular pedicle, the size of the muscle, and their arc of rotation; or they may be transferred as free flaps.

Free Tissue Transfer

The development of microsurgery has made it possible to transfer a composite of tissue or flap from one segment of the body to a distant recipient site. A single anastomosis between an artery and a vein in the flap, usually of 1.0 to 3.0 mm., to the recipient artery and vein allows for revascularization of the transferred tissue.

These microvascular tissue transfers or free flaps offer several immediate advantages to the previously pedicled local

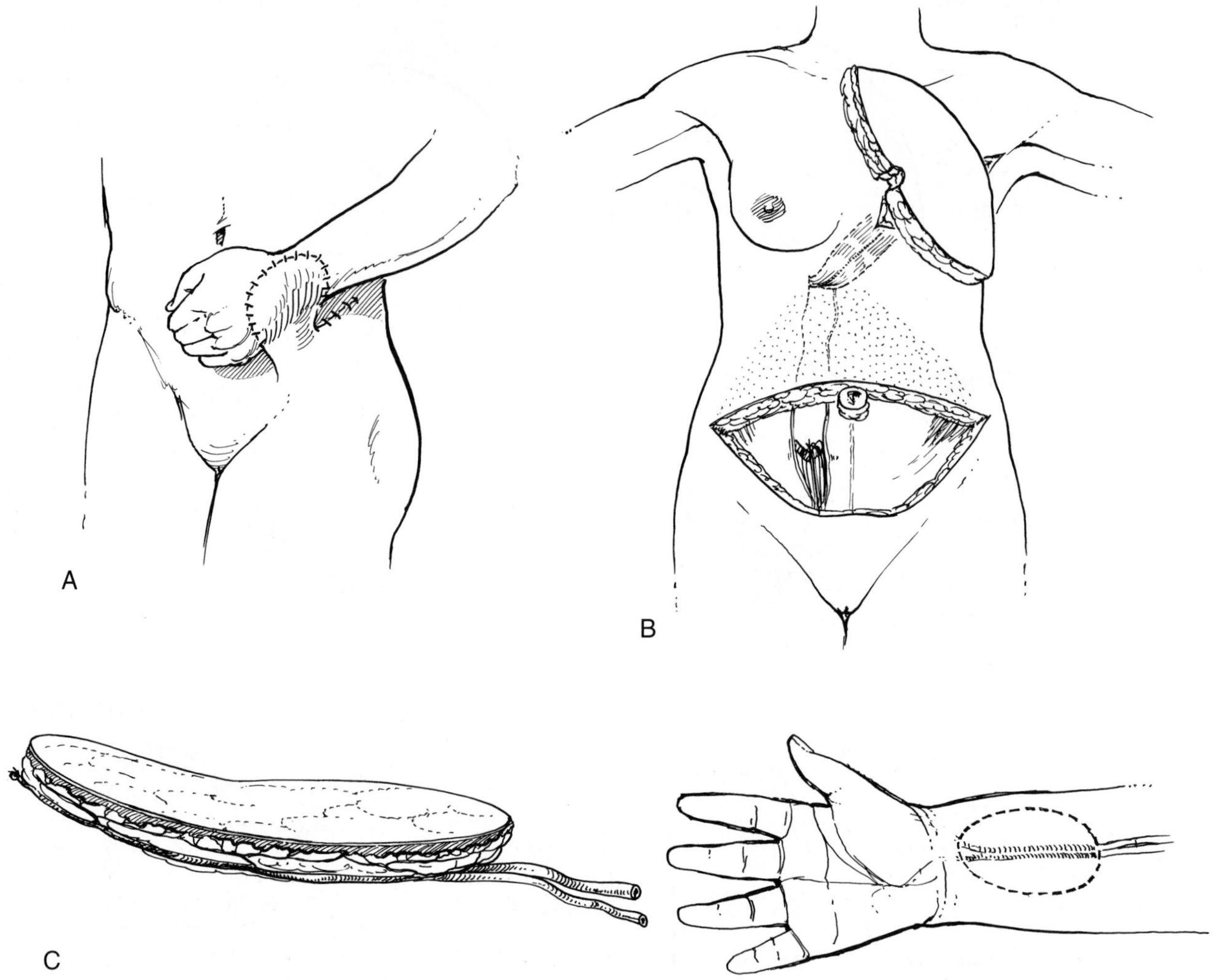

A

B

C

Figure 40–14. Distant flaps: *A*, Groin flap; *B*, transverse rectus-abdominis musculocutaneous (TRAM) flap; and *C*, radial forearm free flap.

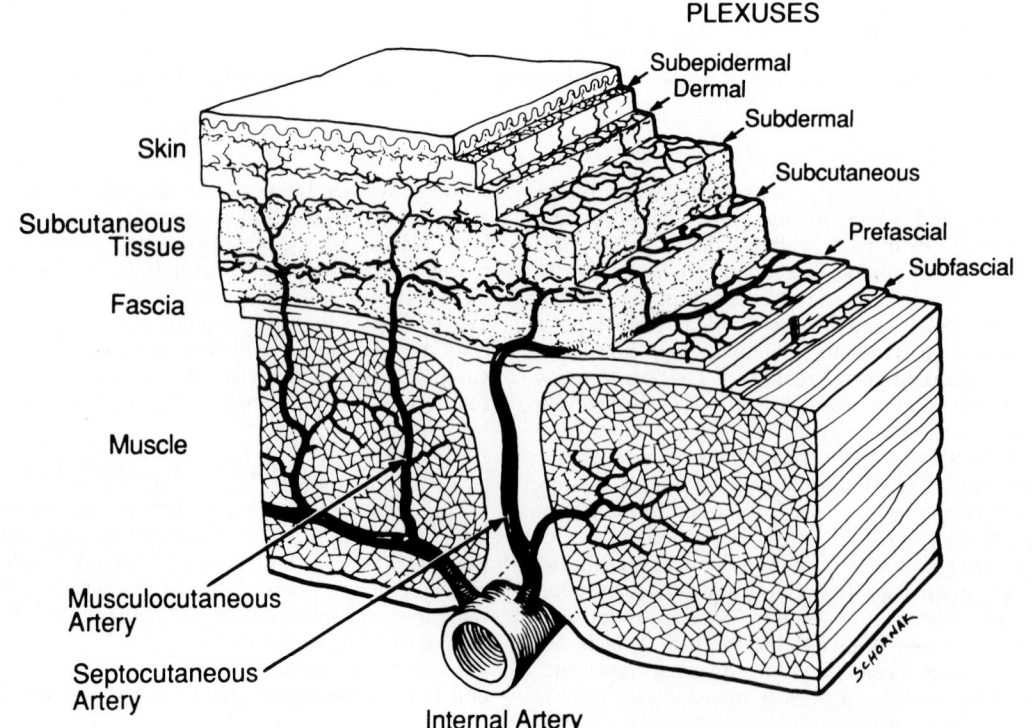

PLEXUSES

Figure 40–15. Blood supply to the skin and subcutaneous tissue. (From McCarthy, J. G. [Ed.]: Plastic Surgery. Philadelphia, W. B. Saunders, 1990.)

MUSCULOCUTANEOUS ARTERIES:

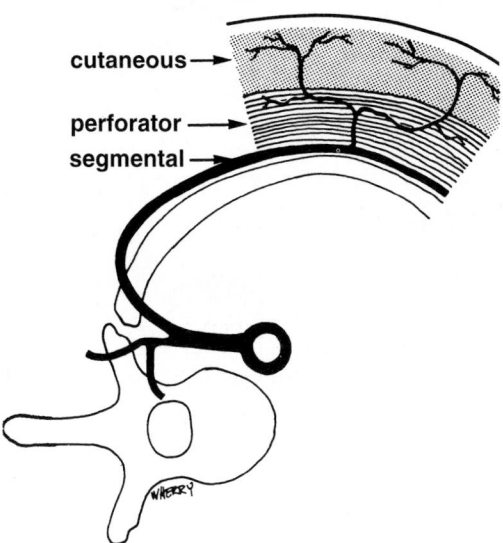

DIRECT CUTANEOUS ARTERIES:

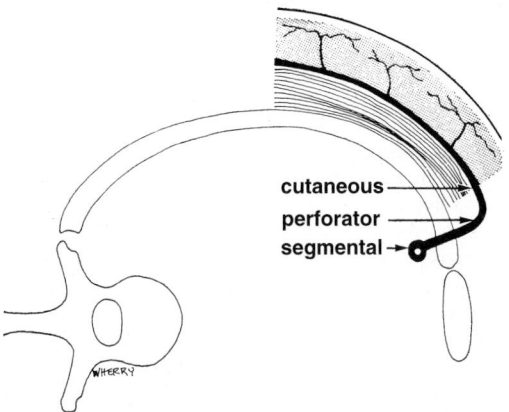

Figure 40–16. Schematic representation of musculocutaneous (upper) and direct cutaneous (lower) vascular system. (From Daniel, R. K., and Williams, H. B.: The free transfer of skin flaps by microvascular anastomosis: An experimental study and a reappraisal: V. The vascular supply of the skin. Plast. Reconstr. Surg., *52*:16, 1973.)

flaps. Free tissue transfer permits the movement of a wide variety of tissues, including bone, cartilage, muscle, skin, or any combination of the above for reconstruction of a defect (Table 40–2).[13] The tissue can be transferred in one stage, with immediate closure of the defect, contrasted to the multi-

TABLE 40–2. Tissues Available for Microsurgical Transfer

Axial skin flaps
Muscle and musculocutaneous flaps
Fascia and fasciocutaneous flaps
Omentum
Vascularized osseous transfers
Sensory transfers
Functional muscle transfers
Composite transfers: toe-to-hand, wrap-around flap, vascularized joint, free jejunum

From Jurkiewicz, M. J., et al.: Plastic Surgery: Principles and Practice. St. Louis, C. V. Mosby, 1990.

ple-stage repairs that often require local flaps or skin grafts. The tissue to be transferred can be designed specifically to reconstruct the defect and to provide its separate microcirculation, which greatly enhances the surrounding tissue's ability to heal infected or irradiated wounds.

The disadvantage of free tissue transfer is that it is a technically demanding procedure that often requires lengthy operating times, in the range of 3 to 8 hours. In addition, total flap failure can occur if there is a problem with the single-vessel anastomosis. To ensure flap survival and minimize the risk of vessel thrombosis, adequate recipient vessels must exist to which the flap can be anastomosed. If the only recipient vessels available are located within a large zone of injury, as may occur with lower extremity trauma or within a previously irradiated field as in many head and neck reconstructions, then suitable vessels away from the injury zone must be sought. Vein grafts are often needed to bridge the gap between the free flap vessels and the newly located recipient vessels.

The success rate for free flaps in most major microvascular centers is greater than 90%, but total flap failure can occur and inherent risks with microvascular surgery exist.[14] Appropriate postoperative monitoring of the free flap by a skilled member of the microvascular team is crucial to ensure that any potential problems with the flap are recognized early and corrected.

CONGENITAL CRANIOFACIAL DEFORMITIES

Cleft Lip

Cleft lip and palate are the most common of the major congenital craniofacial deformities. Few defects have the emotional impact of the facially disfigured child for the family. Those surgeons attempting a lip repair must be aware that this work will "face" the public for perhaps 100 years and may determine the outlook of the patient's life.

In the normal upper lip (Fig. 40–17), the central segment of the lip forms a vertical depression known as the philtrum. This is bounded by two mounds of tissue known as the philtral columns. The vermilion cutaneous junction, or mucocutaneous ridge, is marked by a fine white line known as the white roll. Any disruption in the white roll, either by operation or trauma, is usually obvious. The vermilion cutaneous

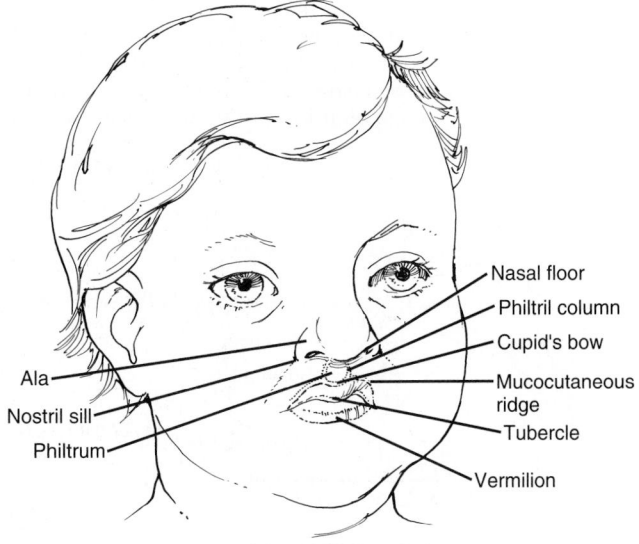

Figure 40–17. Anatomy of normal upper lip.

junction forms two gentle peaks at each philtral column. This forms the characteristic configuration of the vermilion cutaneous junction known as cupid's bow.

The primary and secondary palate are delineated by the embryology of the lip and palate (Fig. 40–18). The primary palate includes the lip, alveolus, and hard palate to the incisive foramen. The secondary palate begins at the incisive foramen and extends posteriorly to include the remainder of the hard palate and the entire soft palate. With this terminology a cleft palate is a cleft of the secondary palate and a cleft lip is a cleft of the primary palate.

The overall incidence of clefting is approximately 1 in 700 live births. The incidence appears to be slowly increasing, possibly due to improved neonatal care of the more severely affected syndromic children. Eighty-five per cent of cleft lips are nonsyndromal, meaning that they are unassociated with other congenital deformities or with known genetic aberrations. In these cases, the etiology is generally believed to be multifactorial.[15] Risk factors for clefting include systemic conditions such as maternal diabetes, increased parental age, drug use, and smoking during pregnancy. Approximately 15% of cleft lips are part of a syndrome. There are over 200 known syndromes associated with these clefts. One of the more important is Van der Woude's syndrome, which presents as a cleft lip with lip pits. Its importance lies in its mode of transmission. This syndrome exhibits autosomal dominant transmission, and offspring of the affected individual have a 50% chance of being affected.

Cleft lips present either as a unilateral or bilateral deformity in various degrees of severity. A complete cleft of the primary palate extends through the lip and nostril floor and across the alveolus to the incisor foramen (Fig. 40–19). Any lesser form, such as a cleft lip without cleft alveolus, is known as an incomplete cleft of the primary palate. A cleft lip is associated with a characteristic nasal deformity that also varies in severity according to the severity of the cleft. The typical nasal deformity in a unilateral cleft lip is posterior, with inferior displacement of the alar cartilage on the affected side.

Presurgical orthopedic devices are sometimes used to realign the cleft lip, alveolus, and nose before definitive lip repair.[16] When these devices are used, an impression is obtained of the child's cleft lip, alveolus, and palate soon after birth. A plaster mold is then made from this impression, and this plaster cast is used to fabricate the orthopedic appliance. The use of presurgical appliances is somewhat controversial, but advocates claim that presurgical realignment of the cleft segments facilitates a superior repair.

Lip repair is generally undertaken at between 3 and 4 months of age or according to the time-honored *rule of tens*. This means the lip repair should be undertaken when the child has attained an age of at least 10 weeks, a weight of at

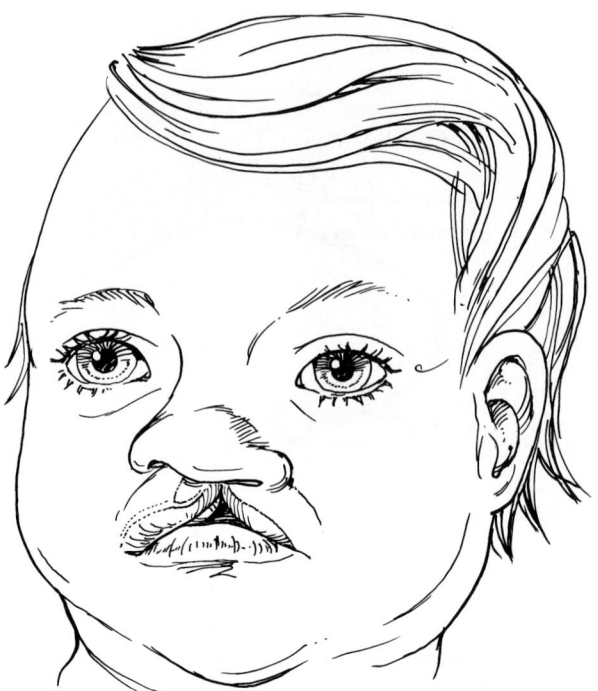

Figure 40–19. Unilateral cleft lip with associated cleft nasal deformity.

least 10 pounds, and a hemoglobin value of at least 10 gm. per 100 ml. The lip repair usually requires general anesthesia, and there are many techniques used for repair of the cleft lip. All repairs have as their goal reconstitution of the orbicularis muscle sling, reconstruction of a horizontal cupid's bow, and an inconspicuous scar. In the United States, the rotation advancement repair as described by Millard is the most popular repair for correction of the unilateral cleft lip (Fig. 40–20). This repair is based on a medial rotation flap that serves to lengthen the lip and create a horizontal cupid's bow. Some surgeons close the alveolar cleft at the time of lip repair. The goal in rehabilitating a child with a unilateral cleft lip is a result that allows interaction with peers at a conversational distance without being detected as a cleft.

The complete bilateral cleft clip is a major deformity that remains difficult to reconstruct. Typically, the child has a projecting central lip that is repositioned preoperatively by some form of presurgical orthopedics. Most methods of repair use the skin from the central lip (prolabium) to reconstruct the philtrum, and skin from the lateral lip elements is advanced medially, closing the cleft with a straight-line closure.[17]

Repair of the cleft lip nasal deformity may be undertaken either at the time of lip repair (primary) or at some later stage in the child's development (secondary). The timing of nasal correction remains controversial. With several large series demonstrating no deleterious effects on nasal growth from primary repair, most surgeons adopt some form of primary nasal correction. This requires meticulous dissection of the small and fragile nasal cartilages to realign them in a more symmetrical position. Secondary nasal corrections are typically undertaken either at the age of 4 or 5 before the child enters school or in early adolescence. The goal, again, is interaction with peers at a conversational distance without the obvious stigmata of a cleft.

Cleft Palate

The secondary palate develops from the fusion of the two lateral palatine processes that close anterior to posterior be-

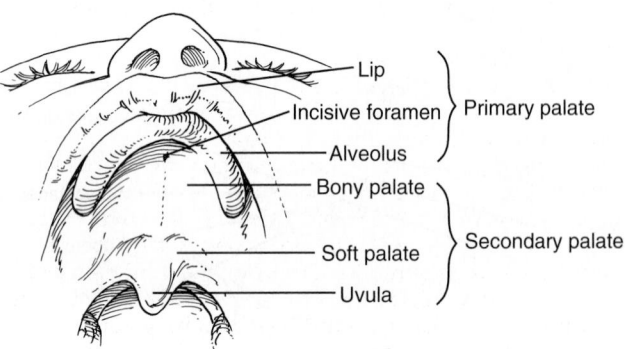

Figure 40–18. Anatomy of normal palate.

Lip
Incisive foramen } Primary palate
Alveolus
Bony palate
Soft palate } Secondary palate
Uvula

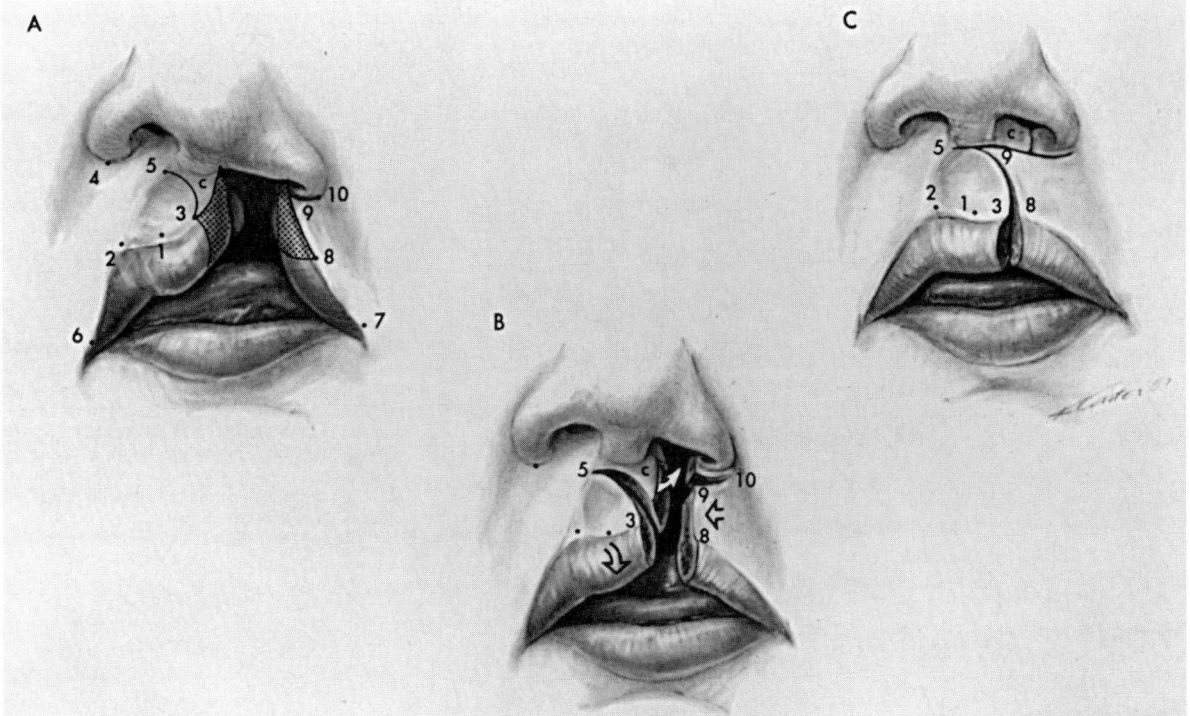

Figure 40–20. *A–C,* Millard rotation-advancement cheiloplasty. (Stippled areas are excised.) (From Jurkiewicz, M. J., et al.: Plastic Surgery: Principles and Practice. St. Louis, C. V. Mosby, 1990.)

ginning in the region of the incisor foramen, until the twelfth week of gestation when the uvula is formed. The left process rotates more slowly than the right; and, for this reason, it is thought that clefts are more common on the left than right.

The most common cleft of the secondary palate is a cleft uvula occurring in about 2% of the population.[18] It is often a marker for a submucous cleft of the palate. In this form of cleft palate, the mucosa is closed but there is a cleft or diastasis of the palatal musculature. This often causes palatal dysfunction. The second most common type of cleft palate is a unilateral left cleft of the primary and secondary palate (Fig. 40–21). The incidence of cleft palate alone is approximately 1 in 2000.

The etiology of cleft palate is also thought to be multifactorial and most are nonsyndromal. A variety of drugs, includ-

ing phenytoin (Dilantin), vitamin A, and corticosteroids have been associated with cleft palate.

Clinical and laboratory evidence suggest that surgical procedures to close the cleft palate negatively affect growth of the palate and maxilla. On the contrary, if the palate is not closed by 18 months of age, speech development is hindered. Early closure of the palate theoretically provides better speech development but poorer growth of the maxilla, whereas late closure of the palate would theoretically provide better maxillary growth but poorer speech and language development. Each surgeon must balance these considerations in timing closure of the cleft palate. In the United States, the cleft palate is typically closed at between 6 and 18 months of age.

Most techniques for palate closure involve elevation of the mucoperiosteum of the palatal shelves as flaps, based on the greater palatine arteries (Fig. 40–22). These flaps are then moved to the midline and sutured together with an everting stitch. Delicate flaps of nasal mucoperiosteum and vomer flaps are raised to provide closure of the nasal lining. Many surgeons believe it is important to reconstitute the muscular sling of the levator veli palatini. These muscles are important in posterior and superior movement of the soft palate to the posterior wall of the pharynx, partitioning the nose from the mouth. In the cleft palate, these muscles abnormally insert along the bony margins of the cleft.

Fistula formation and velopharyngeal insufficiency are two common complications after cleft palate closure.[19] A fistula, when present, is most often at the anterior aspect of closure or at the junction of the hard and soft palate. This may affect hygiene by allowing fluids and food to escape into the nose during feeding as well as negatively affect speech by allowing air to pass into the nose. Formation of fistulas has been reported as high as 6% to 16% in some series. These typically require closure, sometimes by raising adjacent mucoperiosteal flaps or by transposing local tissue from the tongue or cheek. Velopharyngeal insufficiency occurs when

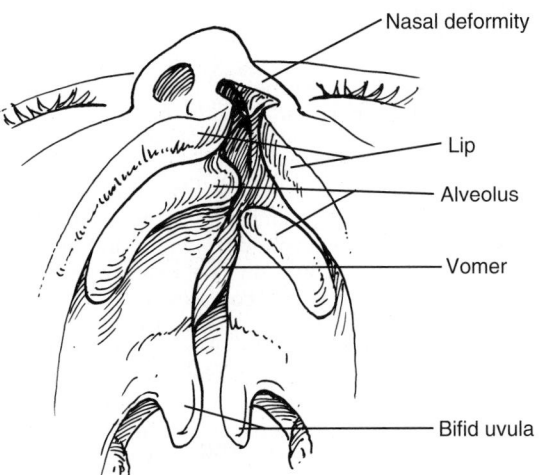

Nasal deformity

Lip

Alveolus

Vomer

Bifid uvula

Figure 40–21. Unilateral cleft of primary and secondary palate.

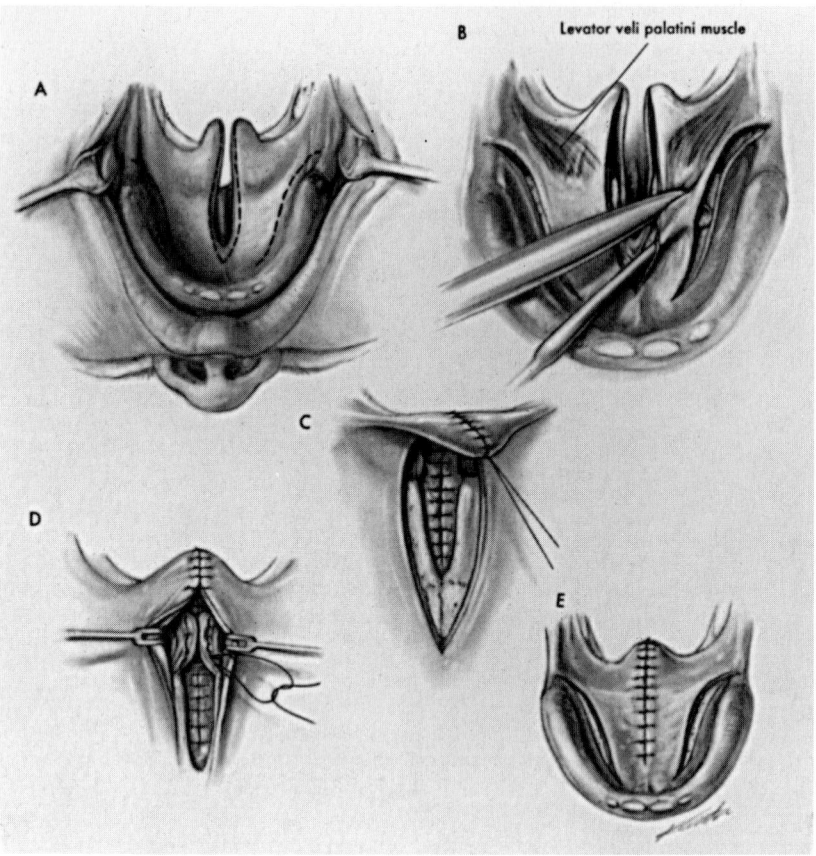

Figure 40–22. *A,* Von Langenbeck palatoplasty. *B,* Bipedicled mucoperiosteal flaps are elevated. Lateral relaxing incisions allow closure of midline cleft of secondary palate. *C,* Layered closure of nasal mucosa. *D,* Levator muscles (optional). *E,* Oral mucoperiosteum—complete repair. A drawback of the procedure is failure to provide lengthening in anteroposterior direction. (From Jurkiewicz, M. J., et al.: Plastic Surgery: Principles and Practice. St. Louis, C. V. Mosby, 1990.)

there is incomplete closure of the velopharyngeal sphincter. This allows for nasal air escape during speech, resulting in hypernasal speech. The palate forms a part of the velopharyngeal sphincter and even following appropriate surgical closure of the cleft palate there is a 15% to 20% incidence of velopharyngeal incompetence. Moderate to severe cases of velopharyngeal incompetence require a secondary palatal lengthening procedure or pharyngoplasty to correct the hypernasal speech.

Craniofacial Surgery

Craniofacial surgery involves the movement of segments of the craniofacial skeleton to reconstruct congenital or acquired defects. The field of craniofacial surgery did not exist before the pioneering work of Tessier. During the 1960s and 1970s, he not only clearly described most craniofacial anomalies but also provided what remains as the state-of-the-art techniques for reconstruction of these defects. Much of this work would have been impossible without the expansion of the fields of anesthesia and critical care.

Craniosynostosis

Craniosynostosis is the premature fusion of one or more of the sutures of the skull causing a limitation in cranial growth characteristic for each suture involved. When a suture is prematurely fused, compensatory growth occurs parallel to the long axis of the suture. The etiology of craniosynostosis is incompletely understood and has been considered multifactorial. There is some evidence that an abnormal cranial base, particularly in syndromal presentations, transmits abnormal forces through the dura to the sutures, causing premature fusion.

Craniosynostosis implies limitation of cranial vault growth.

If cranial vault growth does not keep pace with brain growth, this may result in increased intracranial pressure. This may be manifested by optic nerve atrophy, mental retardation, and death. Hydrocephalus may be secondary to a generalized stenosis of the cranial base and can be seen with craniosynostosis.

Craniosynostosis is often classified by cranial vault form. This clinical classification does not refer to particular sutures involved but rather describes skull morphology (Fig. 40–23). Plagiocephaly is an obliquity to one side of the skull. This creates a characteristic *swept back* appearance to the brow on the affected side. This is typically seen with coronal or lambdoid suture synostosis. Trigonocephaly is a keel-like form to the frontal bone and anterior calvarium. This is typically seen with synostosis of the metopic suture. Scaphocephaly refers to an abnormally long skull in the anteroposterior dimension with bitemporal narrowing. This is characteristically seen with sagittal suture synostosis. Brachycephaly refers to a shortened skull in the anteroposterior dimension and is commonly seen with synostosis of both coronal sutures. Turricephaly refers to excessive skull height and is commonly seen with multiple suture synostosis.

Treatment of craniosynostosis in the past relied on strip craniectomies to surgically create an open suture. This typically yielded uneven results and treatment failures. The surgically opened suture would quickly reossify, and this technique failed to address the complex other cranial vault deformities seen in craniosynostosis. Today, strip craniectomy is typically reserved for early treatment of sagittal synostosis. Most cases of craniosynostosis are treated by a formal cranial vault remodeling. For cases of metopic and coronal synostosis, the supraorbital rims and frontal bone are typically removed as two pieces, remodeled, and advanced into a slightly overcorrected position.[20] This not only corrects the craniofacial form but also increases intracranial volume,

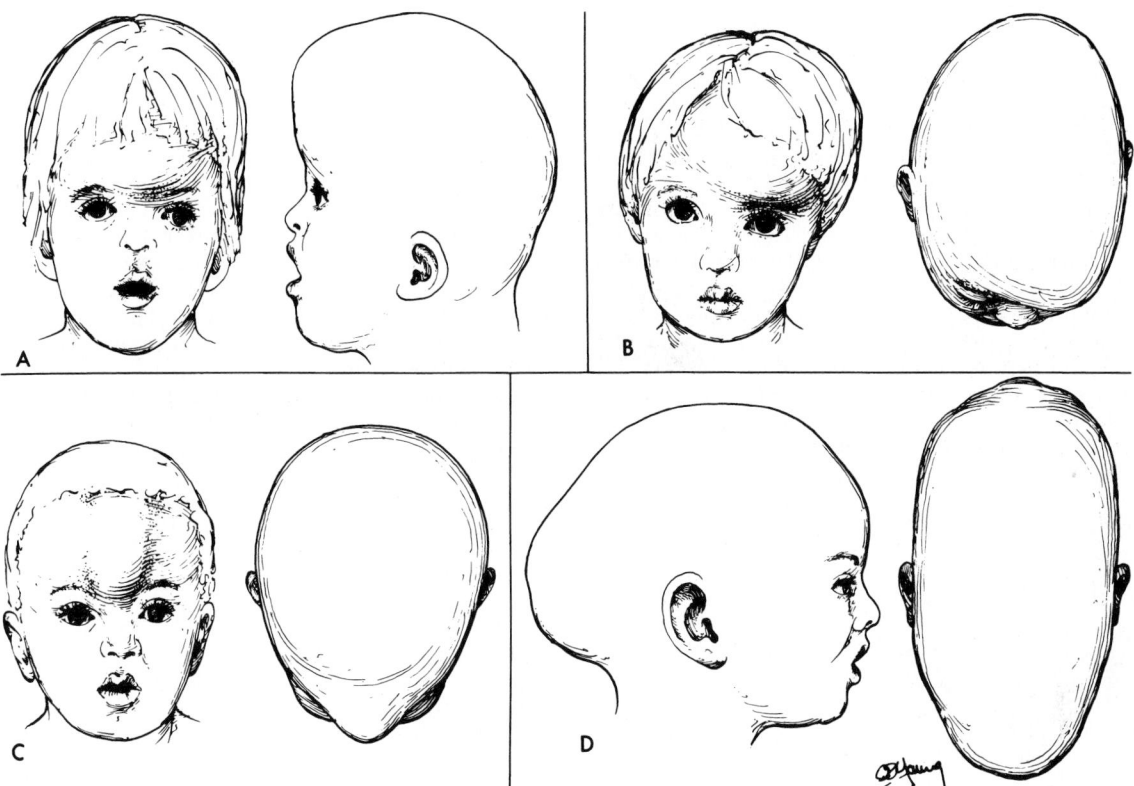

Figure 40–23. Typical patterns of craniofacial morphology associated with craniosynostosis. *A*, Turribrachycephaly. *B*, Plagiocephaly. *C*, Trigonocephaly. *D*, Scaphocephaly. (From Jurkiewicz, M. J., et al.: Plastic Surgery: Principles and Practice. St. Louis, C. V. Mosby, 1990.)

thereby decreasing intracranial pressure. Typically, the anterior cranial vault would also be remodeled at this time. In cases of craniosynostosis with a significant skull deformity but without signs of increased intracranial pressure, corrective operation is typically undertaken at 6 to 12 months of age. As more sutures become involved, the incidence of increased intracranial pressure increases and may necessitate earlier cranial vault remodeling.

Craniofacial Syndromes

A number of syndromes involve both craniosynostosis and deformities of the facial skeleton. There is typically retrusion of the maxilla and midface, which again may be secondary to an abnormal cranial base. This combination of cranial and facial skeletal deformities yields complex defects that are usually approached with staged procedures.

Crouzon's syndrome involves variable craniosynostosis, usually involving the coronal suture, and hypoplasia of the midface. The combined effect of these deformities is a very characteristic appearance, including brachycephaly from the coronal synostosis, exophthalmus, hypoplasia of the orbits, and generalized midface retrusion with hypoplasia of the maxilla and a Class III dental occlusion. The syndrome is transmitted in an autosomal dominant manner with variable penetrance.

Apert's syndrome is clinically similar to Crouzon's syndrome, with the addition of complex syndactyly. There is a high incidence of cleft palate in Apert's syndrome, and the midface hypoplasia is generally more severe than that seen in Crouzon's syndrome. Most cases are sporadic, but autosomal dominant transmission has been reported and some cases may be related to advanced parental age.

Treatment of Craniofacial Syndromes and Craniofacial Clefts

The initial concern for a child with a craniofacial syndrome is always maintenance of the airway and feeding. For those with more severe manifestations, particularly of the midface deformities, this may involve tracheostomy and possibly gastrostomy. The deformities are then partitioned and treated in a staged manner.

Craniosynostosis is treated as described previously. Once any craniosynostosis is addressed and adequate cranial vault volume is provided, the second stage of treatment typically involves the midface. In children with significant midface hypoplasia, osteotomies at the nasofrontal junction, floor of the orbit, lateral maxilla, and pterygomaxillary fissure mobilize the entire midface to be advanced anteriorly. This is known as a Le Fort III osteotomy, after the facial fracture of the same name. With the midface advanced, this not only provides a tremendous improvement in the syndromal appearance of these children but also typically provides salutary effects on the airway and correction of exophthalmus. The timing of midface operations is controversial. Early midface advancement can be performed at 3 to 4 years of age and provides early improvement in the airway and a decrease in the syndromal appearance of the preschool-age child. Some surgeons prefer to delay midface treatment until late childhood or adolescence, when the child is through the phase of mixed dentitia. A final phase of treatment typically involves a course of orthodontia followed by a jaw procedure to correct occlusion or any residual midface retrusion if necessary.

Orthognathic Surgery

Disproportion in the skeletal relationship of the maxilla and mandible can lead to malocclusion and difficulty with chewing and alimentation as well as a significant cosmetic deformity. Maxillomandibular disproportion is commonly associated with cleft lip and palate and craniofacial disorders. Maxillary retrusion with a cleft palate is likely to follow a combination of the mesodermal deficiency thought to exist in these children as well as growth restriction from previous procedures. Midface retrusion is a prominent feature of many craniofacial syndromes. Proper treatment of jaw deformities involves a multidisciplinary approach. These patients are typically evaluated by a craniofacial surgeon, orthodontist, speech therapist, and prosthodontist, as indicated. A routine evaluation involves posteroanterior and lateral cephalograms (standardized radiographs of the face and skull) and dental impressions, which allow plaster models of the alveolus and teeth to be made. The models permit the craniofacial surgeon and orthodontist to plan the bony movements necessary to provide proper dental occlusion. These models are cut and repositioned during a model operation.

Classification of the jaw deformities usually requires a description of both the dental and the skeletal relationships. When describing dental relationships, *mesial* means close to the dental midline; *distal* means distant from the dental midline; *lingual* means toward the tongue or the inner aspect of the inner arch; and *buccal* means toward the cheek or the outer aspect of the dental arch. Normally, the mesiobuccal cusp of the maxillary first molar lies within the mesiobuccal groove of the mandibular first molar. This is known as Class I occlusion, according to Angle's classification (Fig. 40–24). In Class II occlusion, the mesiobuccal cusp of the maxillary first molar is mesial to the mesiobuccal groove of the mandibular first molar. This occurs in a person with a small mandible or with overgrowth of the maxilla. Class III occlusion refers to the mesiobuccal cusp of the maxillary first molar, distal to the mesiobuccal groove of the mandibular first molar. This is typically seen with overgrowth of the mandible or retrusion of the maxilla.

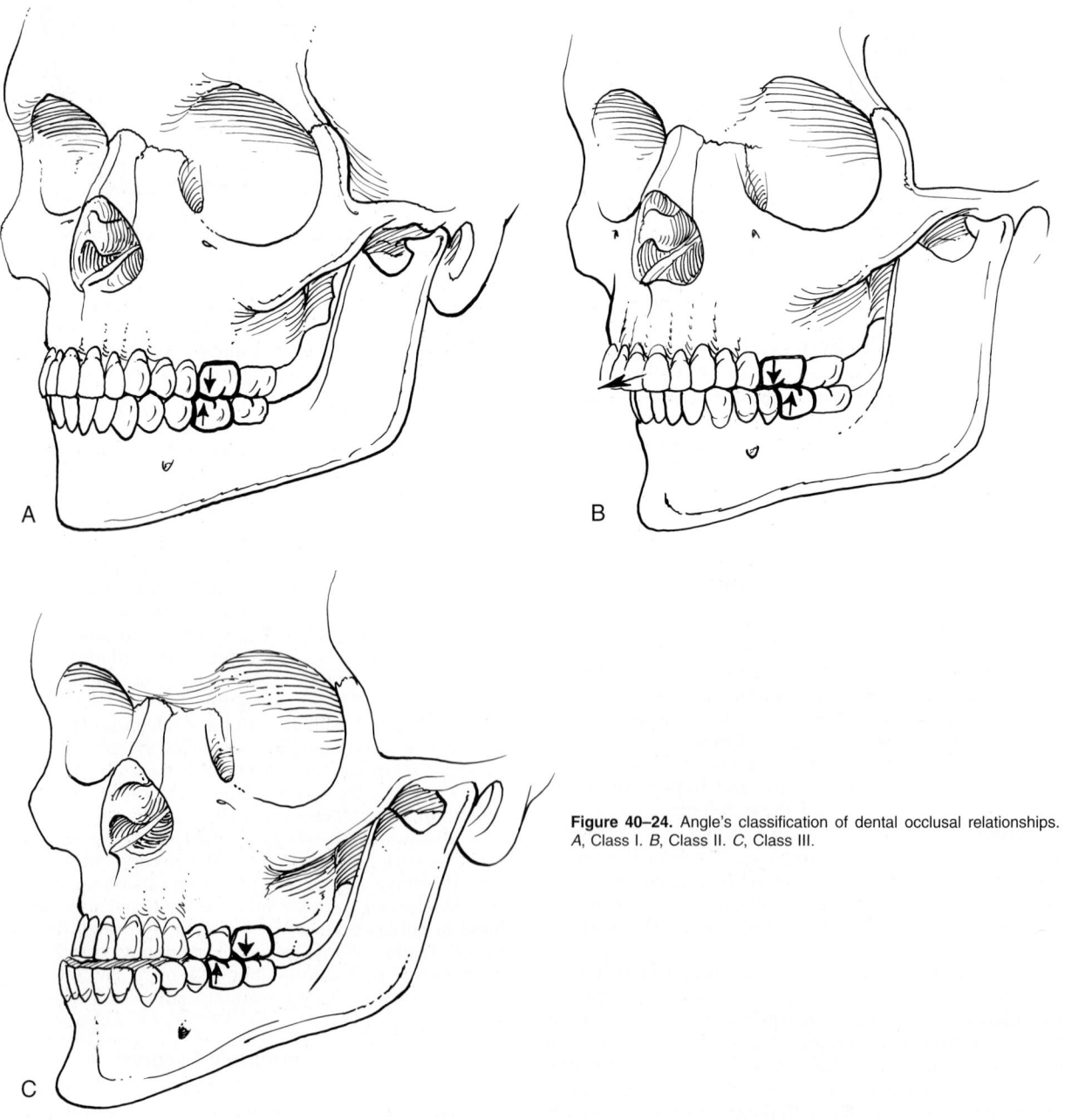

Figure 40–24. Angle's classification of dental occlusal relationships. *A,* Class I. *B,* Class II. *C,* Class III.

A number of clinical terms refer to the skeletal morphology of the jaws. *Maxillary retrusion* or *hypoplasia* refers to an abnormally small or posteriorly positioned maxilla, which is typically seen in patients with cleft palate and in those with craniofacial syndromes. *Maxillary hyperplasia* most often presents as excess vertical height of the maxilla and is also referred to as the long face syndrome. It presents with excessive exposure of the teeth at repose and gingival exposure when smiling. These patients may also have problems with lip competence. The primary treatment of maxillary deformities is the Le Fort I osteotomy, which transects the maxilla and allows for repositioning. The maxilla is then rigidly fixed in the new position with small plates and screws (Fig. 40–25).

Prognathia refers to an abnormally large lower jaw. These patients present with the appearance of a projecting chin point and Class III occlusion. This deformity is typically treated by osteotomies performed in the sagittal plane of both mandibular rami. The mandible is then set back into a more normal skeletal and occlusal relationship.

A horizontal osteotomy of the mandible or osseous genioplasty may be performed to further alter the soft tissue profile of the mandible and lower third of the face. This osteotomy is performed transversely across the bony chin, inferior to the foramen of the mental nerves. This bony segment then may be repositioned in all dimensions, either to add projection to the chin or alternatively to recess the chin point (Fig. 40–26). Chin augmentation can also be performed with a small silicone implant.

Micrognathia consists of an abnormally small mandible, and *retrognathia* is an abnormal posterior-positioned, more normally sized mandible. These deformities typically present as a weak chin and Class II malocclusion. The sagittal split osteotomy of the mandibular rami may be used with these deformities to advance the mandible into a more normal position.

Facial Fractures

Facial fractures commonly result from vehicular accidents, assaults, and other blunt trauma to the face. They are rarely surgical emergencies, and these patients first require an examination for other trauma. After the initial survey is complete and any life-threatening injuries are managed, a systematic examination of the craniofacial skeleton is undertaken. The scalp and calvarium should be examined for lacerations or bony irregularities, and the eyes and bony orbits should be evaluated for restrictions in gaze, enophthalmus, or bony irregularities of the orbital rims.

Nasal fractures often present as a frank external nasal deformity, and the nasal septum should be examined for the presence of a septal hematoma. Nasal septal hematomas warrant drainage to prevent possible septal necrosis and perforation.

Fractures of the midface may be assessed by grasping the upper incisors and alveolar ridge with one hand and palpating the nasofrontal junction with the other. The maxilla is then gently rocked back and forth, and any abnormal movements of the maxilla and the level at which these movements occur are noted. The bony margins of the mandible are also palpated, and the occlusion is examined by passively rotating the mandible into occlusion with the maxilla and also asking the patient if his or her teeth fit together normally.

Most patients with significant craniofacial trauma require anteroposterior, odontoid, and lateral views of the cervical spine through the first thoracic vertebra. Standard facial films include posteroanterior, lateral, and Waters views. Standard views of the mandible include oblique, Townes, and lateral views. The panorex, which is a panoramic radiograph of the entire mandible demonstrating both temporomandibular joints, is usually required in cases of suspected mandibular fracture (Fig. 40–27). Computed tomography is the most sensitive technique for imaging facial fractures and should include both standard axial cuts and coronal cuts through the orbits to demonstrate any fractures of the orbital floor.

The most common orbital fracture is the so-called blowout fracture of the orbital floor. The mechanism of injury is usually a direct blow to the orbit, which rapidly increases intraorbital pressure. This pressure is released through a frac-

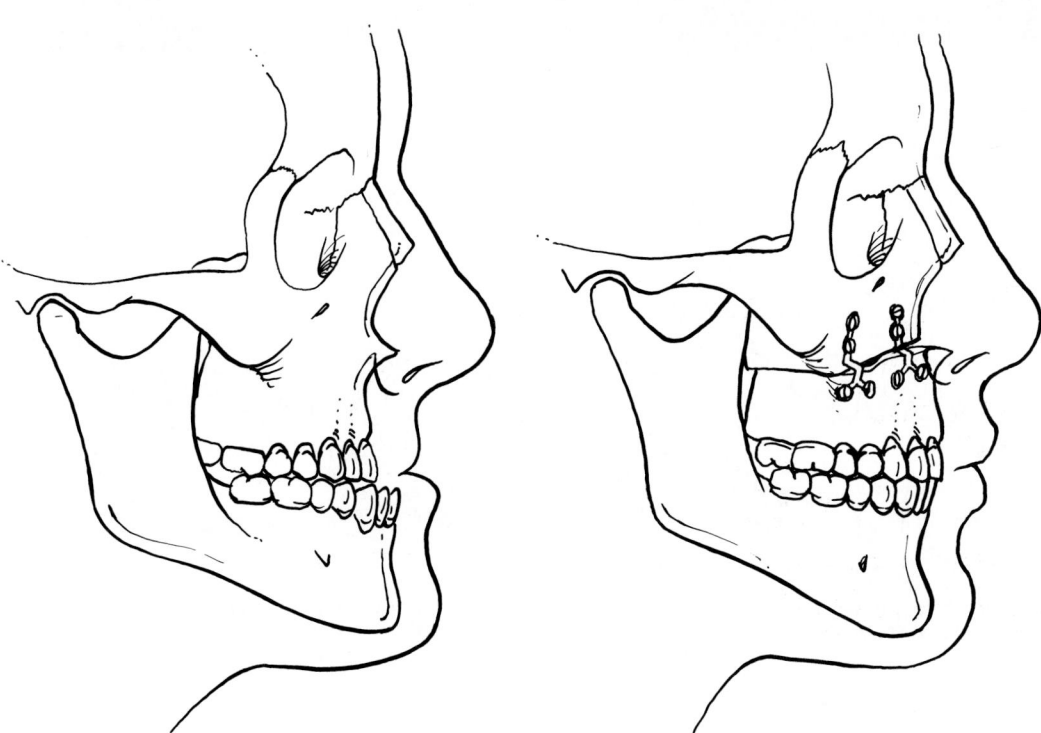

Figure 40–25. Le Fort I osteotomy with advancement of maxilla and fixation with miniplates.

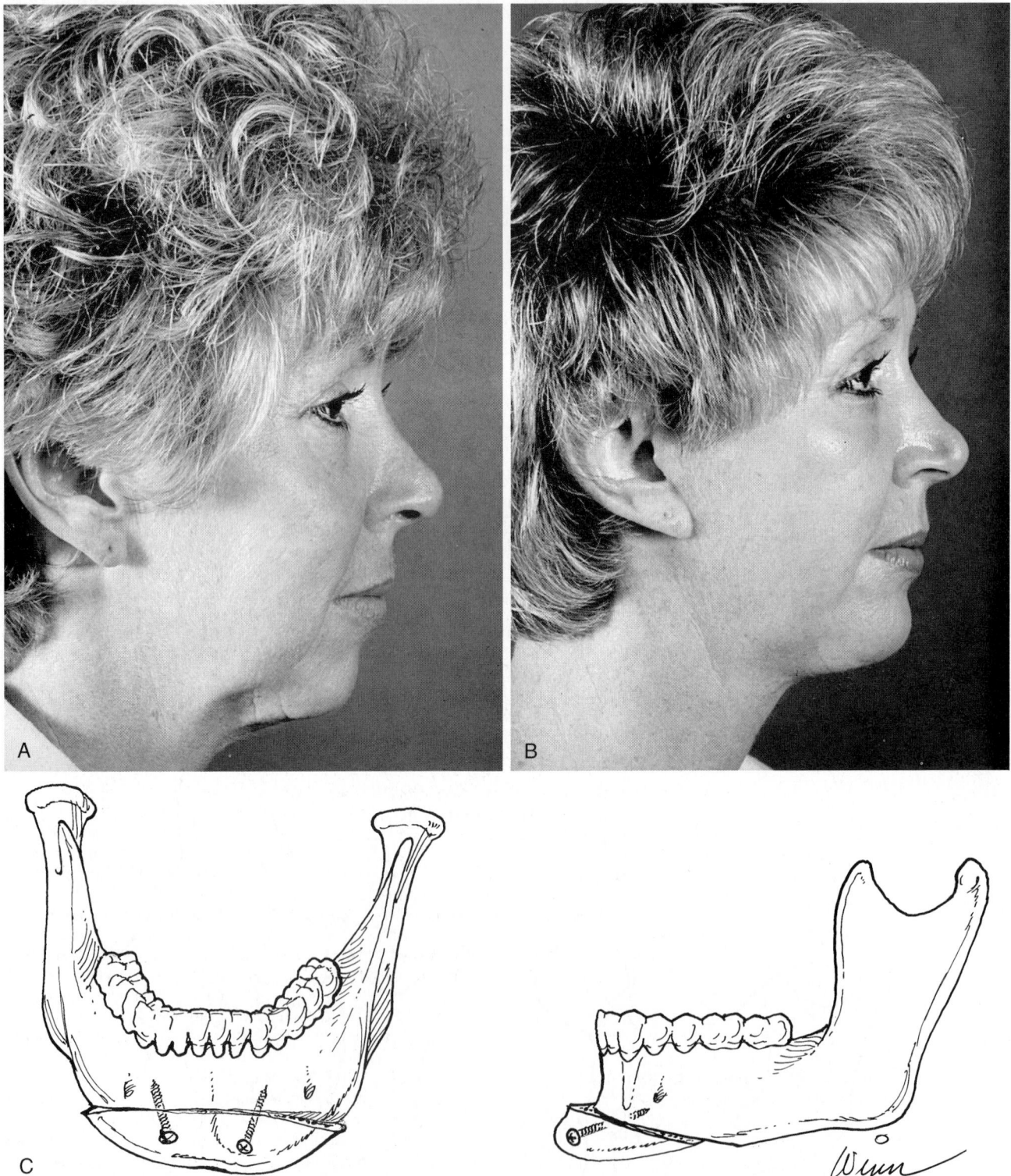

Figure 40–26. *A*, Preoperative photograph of patient with microgenia. *B*, Postoperative photograph following horizontal osteotomy of symphysis, advancement genioplasty, and facelift. *C*, Schematic representation of horizontal osteotomy of symphysis and advancement with lag screw fixation.

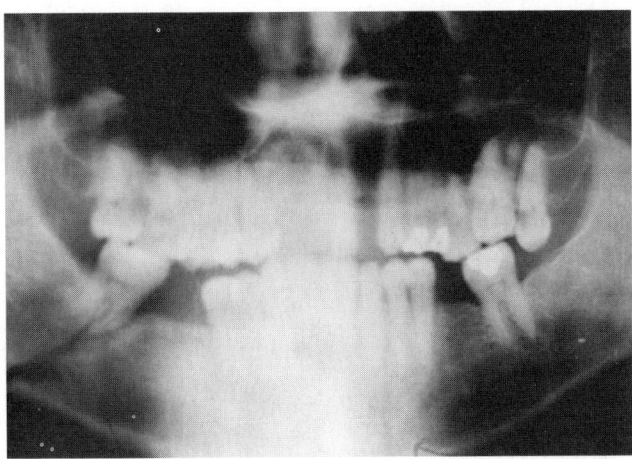

Figure 40–27. Panorex demonstrating a fracture through the body of the mandible and tooth root.

ture in the orbital floor. Orbital fat or the inferior rectus muscle may then become entrapped in this fracture, causing gaze restriction. Treatment of this fracture generally involves a transconjunctival incision and exposure of the orbital floor. The fracture is then reduced and bone grafts placed if necessary. Through the same exposure, any fracture in the orbital rim may also be reduced and plated.

Maxillary fractures often occur in a characteristic pattern first described by Le Fort (Fig. 40–28).[21] The Le Fort I fracture extends from the pyriform aperture to the pterygomaxillary fissure. This fracture presents as a mobile upper jaw and lower midface. The Le Fort II fracture extends from the pterygomaxillary fissure through the anterior maxilla to the nasofrontal junction. When examined as described previously, this fracture presents as a mobile midface and nose. The Le Fort III fracture separates the entire facial skeleton from the cranium. This fracture extends from the pterygomaxillary fissure through the zygomatic frontal sutures across the floor of the orbit to the nasofrontal junction. When these patients are examined, the entire face, including malar eminences, nose, and upper jaw, is mobile.

Maxillary fractures may be exposed by a combination of upper buccal sulcus incisions and lower eyelid incisions. The fracture fragments are typically reduced, and the patient is placed in intermaxillary fixation to re-establish occlusion. After rigid fixation of the fracture fragments, the intermaxillary fixation may then be released.

Mandibular fractures commonly occur through the body and neck of the condyle and the angle of the mandible (Fig. 40–29). Subcondylar fractures may be treated by intermaxillary fixation or a soft diet if they are not widely displaced. In those cases in which reduction cannot be accomplished or occlusion cannot be re-established, the condylar fracture may need to be opened and rigidly fixed. Fractures through the angle of the mandible are typically displaced by the powerful muscles of mastication. They usually require open reduction and internal fixation.[22] Fractures of the body and symphysis of the mandible are also frequently displaced by the muscles of mastication and require open reduction and internal fixation. If minimally displaced or nondisplaced, some of these may be treated by intermaxillary fixation or soft diet alone. Fractures of the alveolar process may occur as an isolated injury or in conjunction with other mandible fractures. These are typically displaced and fixed by ligating teeth in the fracture fragment to adjacent stable teeth. Alternatively, small plates and screws may be used for fixation.

HEAD AND NECK RECONSTRUCTION

Head and Neck Cancer

Epidemiology. The majority of head and neck cancers are squamous cell carcinomas of the upper aerodigestive tract. Generally affecting men in their fifth or sixth decade, squamous cell carcinoma accounts for about 8.5% of all malignancies in this age group. The male-to-female ratio is 4:1 but is decreasing because of an increase in tobacco use by women. In 1992, 42,800 new cases were diagnosed in the United States, with 11,600 deaths.[23] The vast majority of tumors are related to the use of tobacco and the risk of developing squamous cell carcinoma is proportional to the amount of tobacco smoked. Use of tobacco increases the risk at all sites except the salivary glands. Ethanol consumption potentiates tobacco-related carcinogenesis and is also an independent risk factor. Smokeless tobacco has become increasingly popular among young persons and has caused a rise in oral cavity cancers in this age group.

Occupational risk factors, including nickel refining, woodworking, and exposure to textile fibers, may predispose to cancers of the nasal cavity and paranasal sinuses. There also appears to be an inverse relationship between the consumption of fruits and vegetables and the incidence of head and neck cancer. Viruses may also play a role in head and neck carcinogenesis. DNA of the human papillomavirus has been detected in head and neck cancerous tissue. Additionally, infection with Epstein-Barr virus is associated with nasopharyngeal carcinoma. There is some genetic predisposition for head and neck cancer because of the sporadic occurrences in young adults and nonusers of tobacco and ethanol.

Biology. The carcinogens tobacco and ethanol affect the entire mucosal surface of the upper aerodigestive tract, lungs, and esophagus. This is termed *field carcinogenesis* and comprises the 5% to 7% incidence of synchronous cancers seen in the head and neck. Metachronous cancers develop in 30% to 40% of patients if they continue to smoke, but the risk decreases to 6% in those who stop smoking.[24]

Premalignant lesions can be observed during careful intraoral examination of high-risk patients. Leukoplakia, defined as a white, keratotic area that cannot be scraped off, is frequently seen in patients with head and neck cancer. Histologic examination of these areas reveals 11% to 15% of tissue to be dysplastic, and in 3% to 5% carcinoma eventually develops. Epithelial alterations are more common in leukoplakia found in the floor of the mouth or tongue compared with other sites. Reddened areas of oral mucosa, known as erythroplasia, are associated with *in situ* or invasive cancer in 54% to 64% of cases.

Diagnosis and Staging. The signs and symptoms of cancer of the upper aerodigestive tract vary with the location of the primary site and the stage of the cancer. Thirty-five per cent to 45% of patients present with early-stage disease and have vague symptoms and minimal physical findings.[25] A high index of suspicion is required in patients with a history of tobacco and ethanol use.

Cancer of the nasopharynx can present as nasal obstruction, epistaxis, or serous otitis media from obstruction of the eustachian tube. Advanced lesions present as cranial neuropathies and posterior cervical lymphadenopathy. Early cancers of the oral cavity can present as pain, ulcers that fail to heal, or a change in fit of dentures. Cancers of the oropharynx, hypopharynx, or supraglottic larynx rarely produce early symptoms and are usually diagnosed in the late stages. A persistent unilateral sore throat can be a manifestation of oropharyngeal cancer. Otalgia can result from referred pain pathways from the fifth, ninth, and tenth cranial nerves. Dysphagia and odynophagia may be a manifestation of hy-

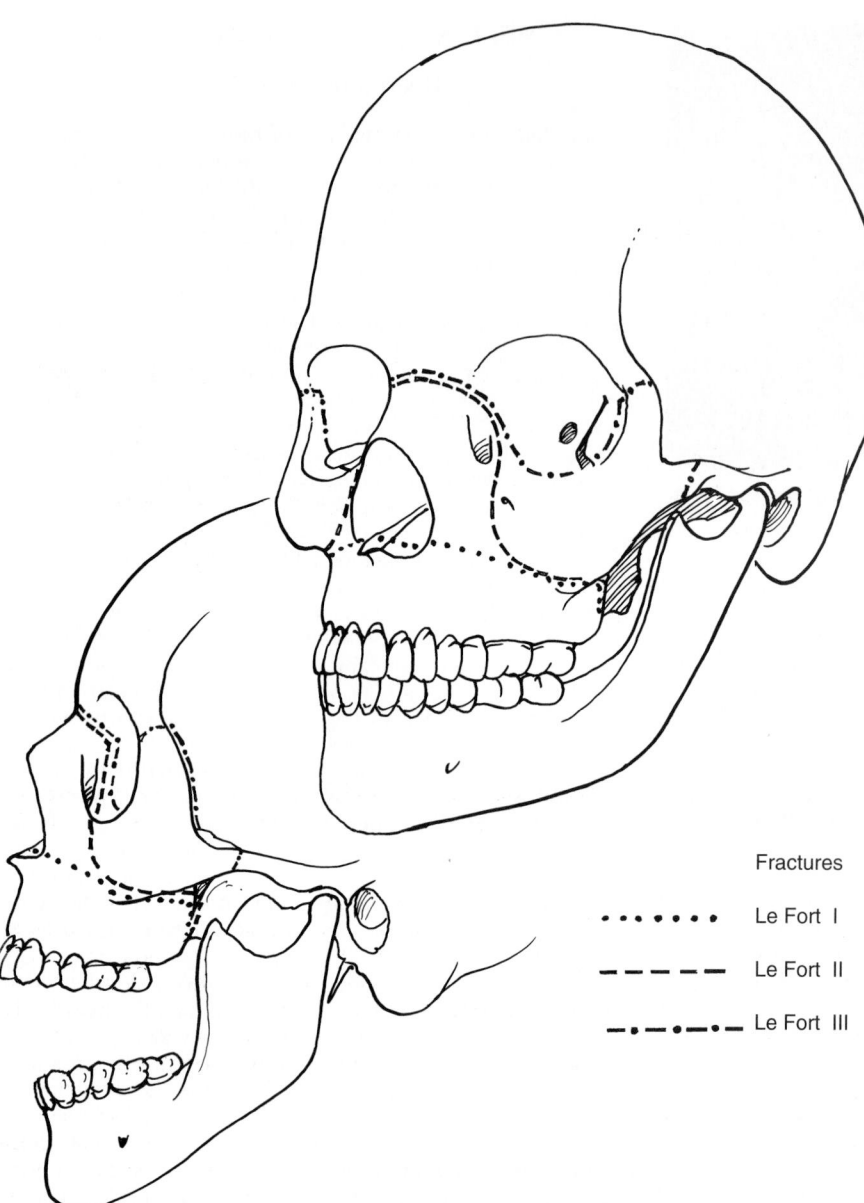

Figure 40–28. Le Fort fracture classification.

Fractures

••••••• Le Fort I

— — — — Le Fort II

—•—•—•— Le Fort III

popharyngeal or supraglottic laryngeal cancer. Hoarseness may be an early sign of glottic cancer.

Many patients with head and neck cancer present with a mass in the neck. Chronology, the patient's age, and the mass location are important diagnostic factors. Inflammatory lesions generally are of brief duration and are common in the pediatric and teenage population. A solitary mass in the neck of an adult that has been present for more than 6 weeks should be presumed to be cancer until proven otherwise. The vast majority of adult solitary nonthyroidal neck masses are metastatic cancers originating from a primary tumor above the clavicles. The location of the mass can be characteristic and frequently provides information as to potential locations of the primary cancer, as discussed later (Fig. 40–30 and Table 40–3).

Physical examination reveals more than 90% of cancers of the upper aerodigestive tract that have metastasized to the neck. Examination requires inspection of all visible mucosal surfaces. Palpation is useful for lesions of the floor of the mouth, tongue, and tonsils. Indirect laryngoscopy can be

TABLE 40–3. Levels of Cervical Lymph Nodes

Level	Location	Primary Site
Level 1	Submandibular, submental	Anterior tongue, floor of mouth anterior alveolar ridge
Level 2	Jugulodigastric, upper jugular	Oropharynx, nasopharynx
Level 3	Midjugular	Hypopharynx, larynx, lateral tongue
Level 4	Jugular	Usually subclavicular: breast, lung, kidney, gastrointestinal tract
Level 5	Posterior triangle, spinal accessory	Scalp, nasopharynx, parotid

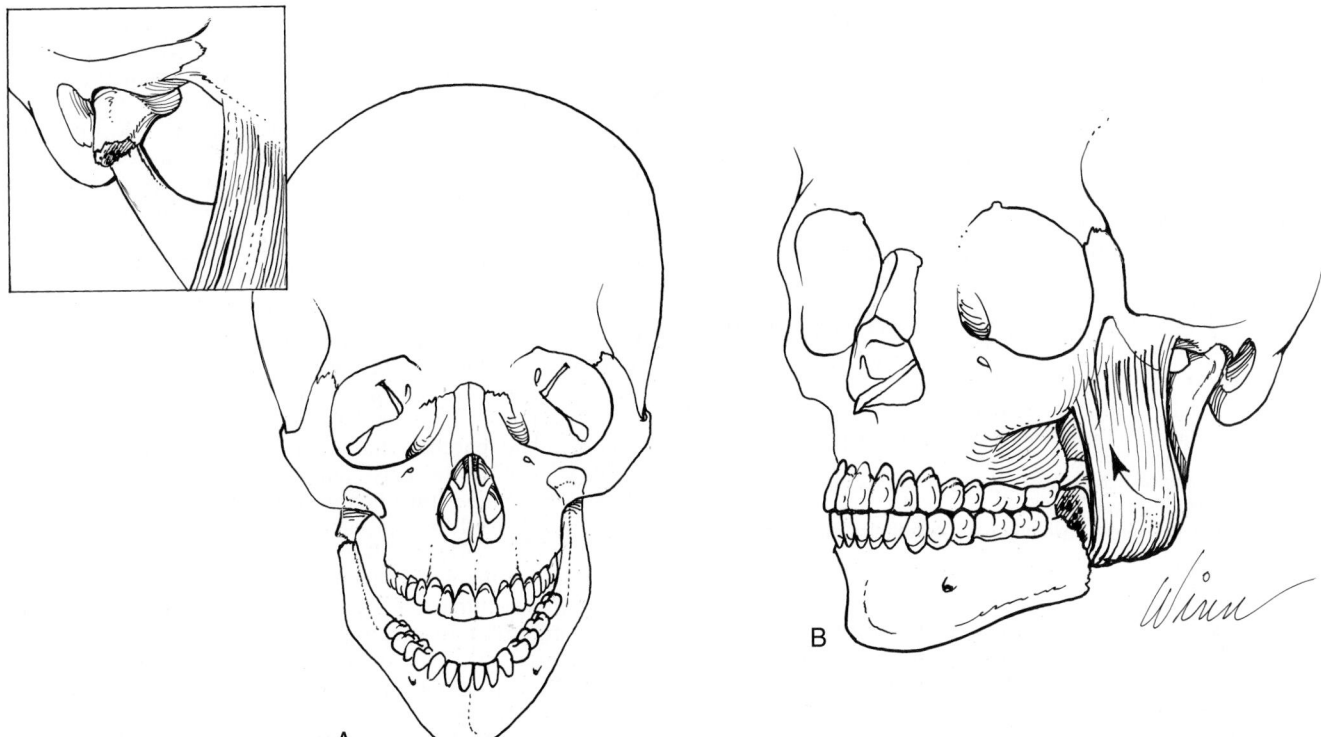

Figure 40–29. *A*, Subcondylar neck fracture of the mandible with displacement. Note the lateral deviation of the mandible toward the side of the fracture. *B*, Mandibular angle fracture with displacement of the posterior fragment by the powerful action of the masseter and pterygoid muscles.

accomplished with minimal topical anesthesia to evaluate the larynx. Occult malignancies frequently occur at the base of the tongue, at the tonsillar fossa, and in the pyriform sinuses and may be missed on cursory examination. Flexible nasopharyngoscopy can be performed without sedation and is useful in patients in whom indirect laryngoscopy is not possible or is equivocal.

Radiologic examination by computed tomography or magnetic resonance imaging can be useful to assess the extent of local or regional spread of tumor. It is especially helpful in

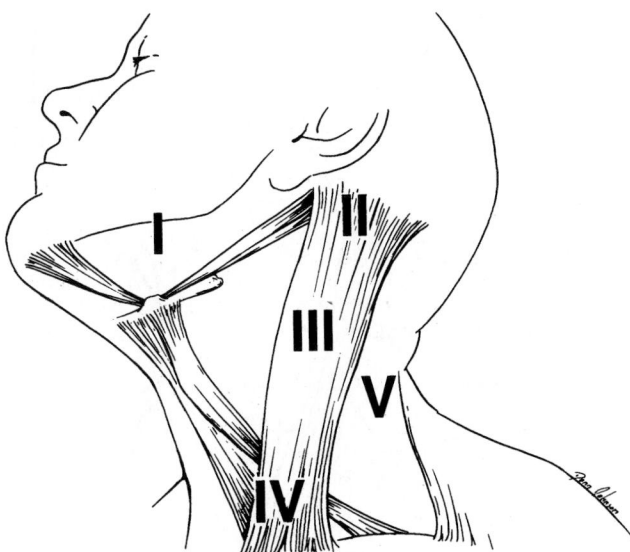

Figure 40–30. Levels of cervical lymph nodes as defined in Table 40–3. (Modified from Carlson G. W.: Surgical anatomy of the neck. Surg. Clin. North Am., *73*[4]:837, 1993.)

infiltrative cancers in which the depth of invasion is difficult to evaluate. Computed tomography provides a good assessment of possible lymphatic metastases. Lymph nodes suggestive of malignancy are usually greater than 1.5 cm. in diameter, are spherical, and have evidence of central necrosis. Plain radiographs, including panorex and soft tissue films, may be helpful for oral cavity lesions to evaluate possible mandibular involvement or calculus disease of the salivary glands.[26]

Examination with the patient under anesthesia is helpful to fully evaluate the primary cancer and to obtain biopsy specimens. Triple endoscopy—direct laryngoscopy, bronchoscopy, and esophagoscopy—to evaluate for synchronous malignancies is not cost effective and is not performed unless warranted by clinical suspicion.[27, 28] The diagnosis can be made by scraping accessible lesions for cytology. Excision biopsy is warranted only for small lesions. Fine-needle aspiration is simple and cost effective for masses in the head and neck, especially lymph nodes. It has a 96% to 100% accuracy, but a negative aspirate does not rule out cancer.[29]

Staging is critical for planning the appropriate treatment. The American Joint Committee of Cancer TNM staging has been adopted in the United States based on clinical and diagnostic tests (Table 40–4). *T* stands for tumor size and extent and has site-specific rules. *N* defines nodal involvement, and *M*, metastatic spread. The staging varies according to site: oral cavity by size, and larynx by involvement or fixation of the vocal cords. Unlike other cancers, labeling a head and neck cancer as Stage IV may not necessarily denote distant disease.

Natural History and Standard Therapy. The majority of patients with head and neck cancer present with locally and regionally advanced disease. Standard therapy usually combines surgical and radiation therapies, which has been shown to improve local and regional control over each modality used alone but has not produced an increase in survival. Chemotherapy is accepted as standard only for re-

TABLE 40–4. Classification of Head and Neck Cancers

Primary Tumor (T)

General–For All Sites

T_X	No available information of primary tumor
T_0	No evidence of primary tumor
T_{IS}	Carcinoma in situ

Oral Cavity, Oropharynx

T_1	Greatest diameter of primary tumor ≤2 cm.
T_2	> 2 cm. or = 4 cm.
T_3	> 4 cm.
T_4	Massive tumor, with deep invasion into maxilla, mandible, pterygoids, soft tissue of neck

Hypopharynx

T_1	Tumor confined to region of origin
T_2	Extension into adjacent region or site, without fixation of hemilarynx
T_3	Extension into adjacent region or site, with fixation of hemilarynx
T_4	Massive tumor, invading bone or soft tissue of neck

Larynx

Glottic

T_1	Confined to true vocal cords; normal mobility
T_2	Supra- or subglottic extension; normal or impaired mobility
T_3	Confined to larynx proper; cord fixation
T_4	Cartilage destruction and/or extension out of larynx

Supraglottic

T_1	Confined to site of origin; normal mobility
T_2	Extension to glottis or adjacent supraglottic site; normal/impaired mobility
T_3	Confined to larynx proper; cord fixation and/or extension hypopharynx or pre-epiglottic space
T_4	Massive tumor; cartilage destruction and/or extension out of larynx

Nodal Metastasis (N)

N_X	Nodes cannot be assessed
N_0	No clinically positive nodes
N_1	Single, clinically positive, ipsilateral node ≤3 cm.
N_{2A}	Single, clinically positive, ipsilateral node > 3 cm. or = 6 cm.
N_{2B}	Multiple, clinically positive, ipsilateral nodes; all ≤ 6 cm.
N_{3A}	Clinically positive, ipsilateral node(s); one > 6 cm.
N_{3B}	Bilateral, clinically positive nodes (each side subclassified)
N_{3C}	Contralateral, clinically positive node(s), only

Distant Metastasis (M)

M_X	Not assessed
M_0	No distant metastases identified
M_1	Distant metastases present

Stage Groupings

Stage I	$T_1N_0M_0$
Stage II	$T_2N_0M_0$
Stage III	$T_3N_0M_0, T_1, T_2,$ or $T_3N_1M_0$
Stage IV	T_4N_0 or N_1M_0
	Any T N_2 or N_3M_0
	Any T Any NM_1

current or metastatic disease.[30] Induction chemotherapy and radiation therapy have been used for organ preservation in cancer of the larynx.

Stage I and II disease can generally be treated equally by operation or irradiation, with a control rate of 60% to 80%. The choice of treatment modalities depends on potential morbidity as well as on the risk of developing a second malignancy, because irradiation can only be administered once.

Stage III and IV disease generally requires an extensive surgical procedure followed by irradiation. Disease control is usually less than 30%, and the majority of patients die of locally or regionally persistent or recurrent disease. Those unable to tolerate extensive operations or those with unresectable disease are treated with palliative radiation therapy.

Nasopharyngeal Carcinoma. This cancer is rare in the United States but is common in parts of China. Most patients present with nodal metastases in the posterior neck. A histologic variant, lymphoepithelioma has a better prognosis than squamous cell carcinoma. These tumors are highly radiosensitive (especially lymphoepithelioma), and irradiation is the treatment of choice. Neck dissections are performed for persistent nodal disease.

Oral Cavity. The oral cavity is the most common site of head and neck cancer. It is bordered by the lip vermilion anteriorly, the junction of the hard and soft palate, anterior tonsillar pillar, and the circumvallate papillae (Fig. 40–31). It includes the lip, floor of the mouth, anterior tongue to the circumvallate papillae, buccal mucosa, alveolar ridge, retromolar trigone, and hard palate. Treatment choice depends on the anticipated functional result, patient performance status, and the need for treatment of the neck.

Floor of the Mouth. Tumors in the floor of the mouth may involve Wharton's duct and cause submandibular gland enlargement, mimicking metastatic spread. Small cancers can be treated with transoral excision, radiation therapy through an intraoral cone, or brachytherapy. If the tumor abuts the mandible, a rim mandibulectomy can be performed. Advanced lesions may require a partial mandibulectomy. Large tumors are treated with surgery followed by irradiation.

Anterior Tongue. Carcinoma of the anterior tongue generally occurs as a chronic nonhealing ulcer along the lateral aspect. More than a third of patients have lymph node involvement at the time of diagnosis. Patients with ipsilateral lymph node spread have a 30% risk of metastases to the contralateral neck. Small lesions may be treated equally well with surgical therapy or irradiation. Larger lesions require

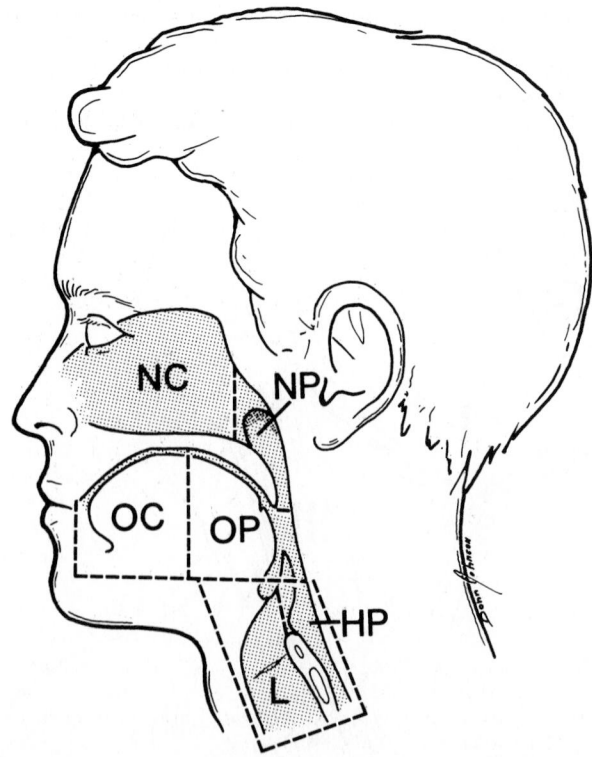

Figure 40–31. Sagittal section of the upper aerodigestive tract. OC, oral cavity; OP, oropharynx; NC, nasal cavity; NP, nasopharynx; HP, hypopharynx; L, larynx.

operative procedures, including neck dissection and flap reconstruction. Irradiation is administered if perineural lymphatic invasion is found.

Lip. The lip is the most common site of cancer in the oral cavity. The vast majority occur on the lower lip in males with a history of smoking and prolonged sun exposure. Primary lesions are usually treated by V-shaped surgical excision and primary closure after repair of the orbicularis muscle. Up to one third of the lower lip can be resected and closed primarily. Larger lesions can be closed with a staged lip switch, which transfers upper lip tissue pedicled on the labial artery by the Abbe technique. This procedure preserves the oral commissure and can close up to two thirds of the lower lip. Lesions of the oral commissure can be treated with radiation therapy to reduce morbidity. Lymph node metastases are uncommon, and elective node dissection is not indicated.

Buccal Mucosa. Cancer of the buccal mucosa is relatively uncommon in the United States, accounting for 5% of oral cavity cancers. It is common in areas, such as India, where chewing of tobacco and betel nuts occurs. The cancers tend to be well-differentiated, slow-growing tumors. Sixty per cent of patients present with Stage I or II disease. Tumor thickness of less than 6 mm. is associated with 85% survival, whereas patients with a tumor thickness greater than 6 mm. have a 35% to 45% 5-year survival. A variant, called verrucous carcinoma, exhibits an exophytic, frondlike growth pattern. It is a well-differentiated small cell carcinoma that rarely spreads to lymph nodes.

Oropharynx. The area known as the oropharynx is defined by the junction of the hard and soft palate anteriorly, extending to the level of the hyoid bone. It includes the soft palate, uvula, tonsil, pharyngeal wall, and the base of the tongue. In general, carcinomas of the oropharynx tend to be less differentiated, have a greater propensity for nodal metastases, and demonstrate lower survival than oral cavity cancer.

Soft Palate. The soft palate is the only site in the oropharynx where cancer is consistently diagnosed at an early stage. Approximately 30% of patients present with cervical node metastases. Radiation therapy gives excellent local control.

Base of the Tongue. This area is posterior to the circumvallate papillae, extending to the vallecula. Cancer of the base of the tongue is often occult, presenting as nodal spread in 75% of cases. The area is relatively inaccessible, making surgical therapy difficult and morbid. A mandibulotomy or lateral pharyngotomy is often required, frequently causing fistula formation, inability to swallow, and aspiration. The 5-year survival is around 50% for Stage I and 10% to 20% for Stage IV disease. Early exophytic lesions are usually treated with irradiation. Advanced, deeply invasive tumors are treated with operation followed by irradiation.

Tonsil. Cancer in this area can be exophytic or deeply invasive. Anterior tonsillar pillar lesions tend to have a better prognosis and are grouped with retromolar trigone cancers of the oral cavity. Tonsillar fossa tumors are the more common, and T_1/T_2 tumors can be successfully treated by irradiation in over 80% of cases.

Hypopharynx. The area from the level of the hyoid bone to the lower border of the cricoid cartilage is composed of three distinct areas. The pyriform sinus is the site of 60% of the cancers seen in the hypopharynx. Lesions remain occult until they achieve large size, invading the larynx and metastasizing to the cervical lymph nodes. The posterior surface of the larynx accounts for only 5% of hypopharyngeal cancers. The posterior pharyngeal wall is the site of the remaining 35% of these cancers.

Nodal spread occurs in over 66% of cases, and treatment of these lesions usually requires a laryngopharyngectomy

and bilateral neck dissections. The rare T_1/T_2 lesions may be treated with a partial laryngopharyngectomy.

Larynx. The larynx is the most frequent site of squamous cell carcinoma of the head and neck outside the oral cavity. It is composed of three anatomic areas with unique clinical features. The supraglottis is composed of the epiglottis, aryepiglottic fold, and false vocal cords. Cancers in this area may cause hoarseness when they reach a large size or involve the epiglottis. Unlike the intrinsic larynx, they tend to spread to lymph nodes at an early stage, frequently to the submental and submandibular nodes. Early-stage disease can be treated effectively with a supraglottic laryngectomy or radiation therapy.

The glottis comprises the true vocal cords. The area has a paucity of lymphatics, and patients tend to present early with hoarseness. Early glottic cancer can be treated effectively with irradiation. T_2 and T_3 lesions (cord fixation) can be treated by induction chemotherapy and irradiation, preserving the larynx in over 60% of cases.

The subglottis below the true vocal cords is an infrequent site of laryngeal cancer. These cancers are difficult to diagnose and usually present in a late stage. Treatment is usually operation followed by irradiation. The prognosis in primary subglottic cancer is generally poor.

Paranasal Sinuses. Cancer of the paranasal sinuses is unusual and difficult to treat. It most commonly occurs in the maxillary sinus, with the ethmoidal sinus being the second most frequent site. The vast majority are epidermoid carcinomas, 10% are of minor salivary gland origin, and 10% are lymphomas, sarcomas, or melanoma. T_1 and T_2 lesions of the maxillary sinus can be treated with operation or irradiation. More advanced lesions require a maxillectomy, frequently followed by irradiation. Lesions that invade or encroach on the skull base may require a craniofacial resection.

Management of the Neck. Detailed knowledge of the cervical lymphatics is necessary to diagnose and treat cancer of the head and neck.[31] One third of the lymph nodes in the body are concentrated in the head and neck region. At the junction of the head and neck are groups of nodes named for their location—the occipital, retroauricular, parotid, submandibular, submental, and retropharyngeal nodes. These nodes are frequently involved with metastatic skin cancer, such as melanoma. The second-echelon nodes course along the internal jugular vein and spinal accessory nerve. Levels of cervical nodes have been defined, which provides standardization of reporting and predicting sites of the metastatic primary tumor (see Fig. 40–30 and Table 40–3).

The risk of cervical node involvement is related to tumor stage and thickness, degree of vascular or neural invasion, and tumor angiogenesis.[32, 33] The management of the neck is not site specific. The goals are to stage the disease accurately and decrease the likelihood of regional recurrence. Metastatic involvement of the cervical lymphatics reduces survival by 50% for all sites and is the single best prognostic factor in head and neck cancer. The most common manifestation of recurrence is regional relapse, so adequate treatment of the neck is mandatory.

Radical neck dissection was described by Crile in 1906 for treatment of nodal metastasis in the neck. It involves excision of the sternocleidomastoid muscle, internal jugular vein, spinal accessory nerve, submandibular salivary gland, and the associated lymph node–bearing tissue in levels I to V. Regional control is related to control of the primary tumor and the amount of nodal disease. The regional recurrence after radical neck dissection for N_2 nodal disease is at least 30%. Postoperative irradiation can reduce neck recurrence to less than 10%. Radical neck dissection is associated with significant shoulder dysfunction and pain in at least 60% of patients. Nerve grafting the portion of the resected accessory nerve with the greater auricular nerve and aggressive physiotherapy can improve function in the majority of patients. Radical neck dissection is generally indicated in N_2 nodal disease, in spinal accessory node involvement, or after irradiation failure.

Various forms of modified neck dissections have been introduced that preserve some or all of the named structures excised during a radical neck dissection. The modified or functional neck dissection is designed to reduce the morbidity associated with neck dissection. The functional neck dissection was introduced by Bocca in 1980. This procedure spares the sternocleidomastoid muscle, internal jugular vein, and spinal accessory nerve. Shoulder dysfunction is reduced to 30% without compromise of local control in N_0 and N_1 disease. Adjuvant external beam radiation therapy is generally used if greater than one node is found to be involved or if there is evidence of extracapsular extension.

Elective node dissection is performed in cases with an increased risk of nodal metastases. It is controversial whether it improves survival over therapeutic neck dissection. Irradiation is effective in treating subclinical nodal disease and is used when the primary is treated nonsurgically.

Chemotherapy. Systemic chemotherapy continues to be controversial in the treatment of head and neck cancer. Despite high response rates, randomized trials have failed to demonstrate superiority of adjuvant chemotherapy when compared with local treatment alone. Response rates to single-agent chemotherapy—methotrexate, cisplatin, 5-fluorouracil, and bleomycin—range from 25% to 40% and are of short duration. Combination chemotherapy, usually cisplatin and 5-fluorouracil, has a response rate of greater than 60% and a clinical complete response rate of 10% to 15%. Paradoxically, randomized trials have not shown an improvement in survival over single-agent therapy, and drug toxicity is greater. Induction chemotherapy before local therapy is being evaluated in randomized trials but thus far has not shown improved survival.

The treatment of metastatic squamous cell carcinoma of the head and neck is largely palliative. Spread to the lung is common and, when solitary, can be difficult to differentiate from primary lung cancer.

Reconstruction. Reconstruction after extirpation of head and neck cancer continues to be a surgical challenge. The majority of patients are debilitated and present with locally advanced disease. Poor long-term survival and the need for adjuvant radiation therapy demand that the reconstruction be immediate, be single stage, allow a rapid restoration of function, and have a low morbidity.

The pectoralis major musculocutaneous flap has been a workhorse in head and neck reconstruction since its description by Aryian in 1978. It is a reliable, bulky flap near the operative field with a favorable rotation arc. It is based on the thoracoacromial artery, which supplies the muscle and overlying skin, and has been used successfully in many sites in the head and neck, including the oral cavity, oropharynx, and hypopharynx.

Microvascular free tissue transfer has supplanted the pectoralis major flap for the majority of head and neck reconstruction. Free tissue transfer provides restoration of form and function not possible using conventional flaps. Advantages include the ability to use unique, specialized tissue with an independent blood supply and the freedom from rotation arcs. Disadvantages include the demands for microsurgical expertise and equipment, long operative times, and a 5% to 10% risk of flap failure.

Oral Cavity Reconstruction. Reconstruction in this area must preserve tongue mobility for speech and swallowing. Small defects can be closed with skin grafts or local nasolabial flaps; tongue flaps are generally not used because of

potential interference with mobility. Defects larger than several centimeters require flap closure to prevent tongue tethering. The radial forearm free flap has become the flap of choice for intraoral reconstruction. It is a thin, pliable fasciocutaneous flap based on the radial artery and accompanying veins. The remote donor site is advantageous for a two-team operative approach, reducing procedure time. It can be used as a sensate flap by suturing the lingual nerve to the lateral antebrachial cutaneous nerve.

A pectoralis major musculocutaneous flap is used to restore tongue bulk when a total glossectomy or base of tongue resection is performed. The majority of patients maintain intelligible speech and swallow without aspiration.

Mandibular Reconstruction. The method of mandibular reconstruction depends on the defect size, location, and soft tissue involvement. Loss of the lateral mandible is generally well tolerated, but unopposed masticatory muscle pull can occasionally cause pain and dysphagia. Alloplastic reconstruction plates can restore the mandibular contour but will not permit dental restoration. They have a high extrusion rate when placed in the anterior dental arch. Autogenous bone grafts tolerate irradiation poorly and have a limited role in treatment of head and neck cancer.

Vascularized free bone flaps, such as from the fibula, iliac crest, radius, and scapula, have become the method of choice. They promote primary bone healing, resist radiation therapy, and allow dental restoration with osteointegrated implants. The fibular free flap can provide a long segment of sturdy bone and overlying skin. It is based on numerous segmental perforators from the peroneal artery. The remote donor site is advantageous, and loss of the fibula is well tolerated.

Hypopharyngeal Reconstruction. The pectoralis major musculocutaneous flap is useful to repair partial pharyngectomy defects and fistulas that develop after laryngectomy. Its bulk makes it a poor choice for total reconstruction of the hypopharynx and cervical esophagus. Free jejunal transfer has become the method of choice for circumferential reconstruction.[34] A segment of proximal jejunum is isolated on its mesentery, and bowel continuity is re-established. The segment is transferred to the neck and sutured to the base of the tongue and cervical esophagus in an isoperistaltic manner (Fig. 40–32). Microvascular anastomosis is then performed to vessels in the neck. A tubed radial forearm free flap can be used in instances in which a laparotomy is not possible. When an esophagectomy is required, a gastric transposition based on the right gastric and epiploic arteries can re-establish enteric continuity.

Salivary Gland Tumors

Neoplasms of the salivary glands are relatively uncommon, comprising 5% of hospital admissions for head and neck tumors. The major salivary glands include the parotid, submandibular, and sublingual glands. The minor salivary glands are scattered throughout the upper aerodigestive tract. In general, the larger the gland, the more likely a tumor will be benign. Seventy-five percent of salivary gland tumors involve the parotid.[35] Nonneoplastic processes account for 25% of parotid masses. These include cysts, inflammation, lymphoepithelial lesions of the acquired immunodeficiency syndrome, sarcoidosis, and granulomatous diseases.

Suppurative parotitis is seen in elderly, debilitated patients. Dehydration leads to stasis and infection, usually from *Staphylococcus*. Stimulation of salivary flow and therapy with antibiotics comprise the initial management. Surgical drainage is performed if medical management fails.

The causes of salivary gland tumors are unknown but may be related to radiation exposure, tobacco use, and occupational and genetic factors. Malignant degeneration of benign

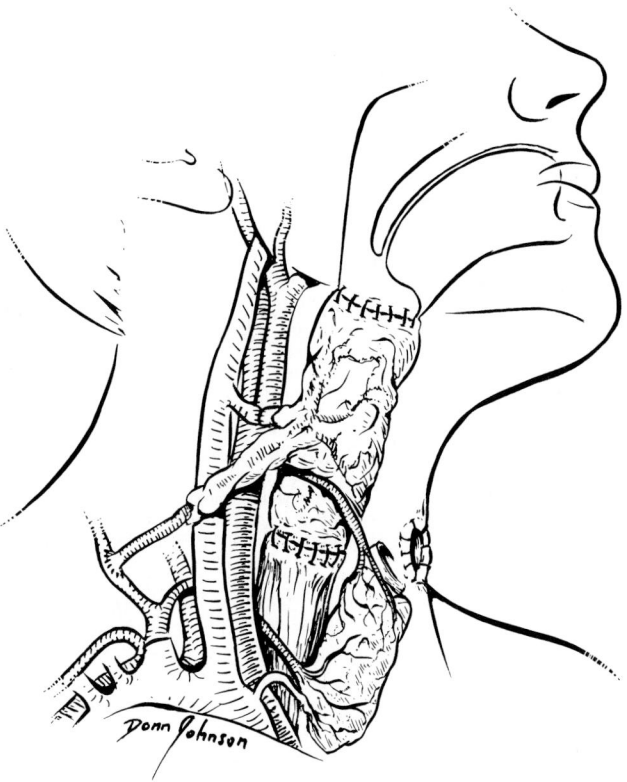

Figure 40–32. Free jejunal flap placed in an isoperistaltic manner to reconstruct the hypopharynx and cervical esophagus.

mixed tumors is occasionally reported, and parotid malignancy is associated with cancer of the skin, breast, thyroid, and colon.

The majority of parotid tumors are asymptomatic. Only 10% present with pain or facial nerve paralysis. Recurrent pain and swelling exacerbated by eating is indicative of calculous disease. Plain x-ray films may be helpful in stone identification. Sialography has been used but is seldom indicated because of the propensity to induce inflammation.

Tumors arise deep to the plane of the facial nerve in 10% of cases. Intraoral examination may show bulging of the tonsillar fossa or soft palate, which indicates parapharyngeal space invasion. Computed tomography or magnetic resonance imaging may delineate the position of the tumor with respect to the facial nerve. Preoperative scanning is indicated when cancer, deep-lobe involvement, or Warthin's tumor is suggested. Facial nerve paralysis and cervical lymphadenopathy are other indications for preoperative computed tomography or magnetic resonance imaging.

Fine-needle aspiration is helpful for cytologic study of a suggested inflammation or neoplastic process in the parotid lymph nodes. Fear of tumor seeding along the needle tract is unfounded. There is a 90% to 94% correlation between fine-needle aspiration and parotid histology.

Two thirds of parotid neoplasms are benign. Women are affected more often than men. Pleomorphic adenoma or benign mixed tumor is the most common parotid neoplasm, accounting for 50% of all parotid tumors. The clinical presentation is a discrete, slowly enlarging mass, rarely accompanied by pain or facial paralysis. Histologically, there is a mixture of mucoid, epithelial, and mesenchymal elements. They tend to have multiple projections, which account for the 30% to 50% recurrence rate after simple enucleation. Surgical treatment is complete excision with negative margins.[36] Tumors superficial to the facial nerve usually require

a superficial parotidectomy, whereas those deep to the nerve require a conservative total parotidectomy. The recurrence rate after complete resection should be 1% to 5%.

Warthin's tumor or papillary cystadenoma lymphomatosum is the second most common benign parotid tumor. It can be bilateral in up to 10% of cases. It usually presents as a discrete, painless, soft to semifirm mass. It is multifocal in up to 12% of cases, and malignant transformation occurs in less than 0.3% of cases. The surgical treatment is enucleation.

Benign lymphoepithelial lesions associated with human immunodeficiency virus (HIV) infection are becoming increasingly common. They are usually bilateral, multiple, and cystic. Lesions not associated with HIV are solitary and solid. Zidovudine is the treatment for HIV-positive patients, and irradiation has been shown to be effective in those with acquired immunodeficiency syndrome.

Mucoepidermoid carcinoma is the most common malignancy of the parotid. It has three histologic grades, which correspond to increasing proportion of epidermoid components and decreased cellular differentiation. The 10-year survival for all grades is 50%.

Malignant mixed tumor or carcinoma *ex pleomorphic* adenoma is the second most common parotid malignancy. A true malignant mixed tumor (carcinosarcoma) is relatively rare. In the majority of cases, only the epithelial element is malignant. These lesions may be low or high grade, and the treatment is usually aggressive—radical operation with postoperative radiation therapy. The 10-year survival is 30%, and death is usually from metastatic disease.

Acinic cell carcinoma comprises 15% of parotid malignancies. It has a low malignant potential, with a 10-year survival of 70%. Adenocarcinoma of the parotid can have various grades and histology. One third of patients present with nodal metastases, and survival is related to tumor grade.

Adenoid cystic carcinoma comprises less than 10% of parotid malignancy but is the most common cancer of the submandibular and minor salivary glands. It has a propensity to invade nerves and develop distant metastases. Long-term follow-up is needed because pulmonary metastasis 10 years after initial treatment is common.

Epidermoid carcinoma is a rare form of parotid cancer that can be confused with metastatic spread. It is a diagnosis of exclusion, and the survival tends to be poor.

The head and neck is the third most common site for lymphoma. It may involve the parotid and must be distinguished from Sjögren's syndrome and benign lymphoepithelial infiltration seen with HIV infection. A surgical procedure is appropriate for diagnostic purposes only.

The parotid gland is classically divided into superficial and deep lobes separated by the facial nerve. In fact, there is no anatomic separation between these two areas. The facial nerve branches must be identified before attempting to remove the parotid (Fig. 40–33). The main trunk can be seen exiting the stylomastoid foramen just medial to the insertion of the posterior belly of the digastric muscle. The nerve branches are traced distally until the superficial portion of the gland is removed.

Facial nerve injury occurs in up to 10% of parotidectomies, usually to the frontal or mandibular branches. Temporary paresis may occur from traction or ligation of a branch of the stylomastoid artery adjacent to the nerve trunk. Pain or numbness of the anterior ear can result from greater auricular nerve injury. Frey's syndrome or *gustatory sweating* is a not uncommon complication of parotidectomy. Sweating in the preauricular area during eating results from abnormal regeneration of auriculotemporal nerve fibers to the sweat glands of the skin.

The most common cause of a submandibular mass is ductal obstruction. History and physical examination, including

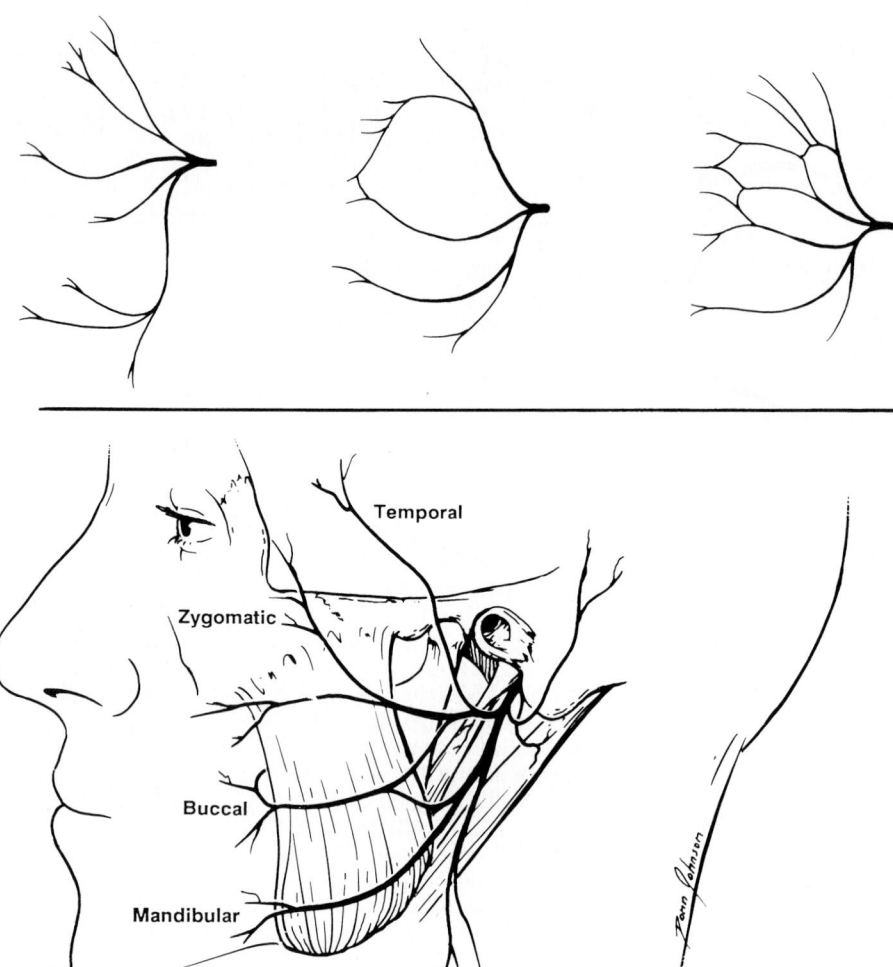

Temporal

Zygomatic

Buccal

Mandibular

Cervical

Figure 40–33. The facial nerve is depicted with the parotid gland removed. It exits the stylomastoid foramen just medial to the insertion of the posterior belly of the digastric muscle. Variations in the nerve branchings are depicted in the superior portion. (From Carlson, G. W.: Surgical anatomy of the neck. Surg. Clin. North Am., *73*[4]:837, 1993.)

plain x-ray films, can usually differentiate tumors from inflammation. Half of all submandibular neoplasms are malignant, and adenoid cystic carcinoma is the most frequent type.

Malignancy comprises 75% of minor salivary gland tumors. These tumors occur throughout the upper aerodigestive tract but most commonly in the hard palate and upper lip.

Other Head and Neck Neoplasms

Sarcomas are rare and comprise less than 1% of head and neck tumors but account for 15% of all soft tissue sarcomas. Treatment is surgical resection with negative margins. Irradiation is used for incompletely excised and high-grade lesions. The role of chemotherapy for adult soft tissue sarcomas is unknown.

Melanoma of the head and neck has a worse prognosis than in other anatomic sites. Metastatic melanoma must be considered in patients with parotid or cervical node enlargement. Mucosal melanoma is seen in the paranasal sinuses and has a very poor prognosis.

Chemodectomas or paragangliomas are rare tumors that arise from chromaffin tissue along the cranial parasympathetic nerves. They are slow-growing tumors of the chemoreceptor organs in the neck. They most commonly occur in the carotid body and along the vagus nerve. Carotid body tu-

mors present as asymptomatic pulsatile masses along the angle of the mandible. The diagnosis is suggested by computed tomography and confirmed by arteriography. Ten per cent of patients present with cranial nerve defects. The treatment is excision, and preoperative embolization may ease dissection and reduce blood loss. Patients with unresectable tumors and elderly patients may be treated by irradiation, which slows the growth of the tumors.

AESTHETIC SURGERY

The process of facial aging follows degenerative changes in the skin, often exacerbated by exposure to the sun and atrophy of the underlying muscles and subcutaneous tissue.[37] Wrinkles, deepened nasolabial folds, periorbital fat herniation, and a sagging jaw line all contribute to the tired and aged appearance. In the United States the public's emphasis on beauty and a youthful appearance has produced a significant increase in the number of surgical procedures to improve or enhance appearance. The facelift or rhytidectomy, blepharoplasty, liposuction, and chemical peel are surgical techniques commonly used by the plastic surgeon to re-create a more youthful appearance.

Rhytidectomy

The pathogenesis of wrinkles is related to the underlying histologic changes seen primarily in the dermis of aging and sun-damaged skin. The total amount of ground substance (glycosaminoglycans and proteoglycans) diminishes with age. The elastic fibers responsible for the physiologic recoil of skin become altered, and there is noted laxity. Normal adult collagen contains Type I and Type III collagen in a 6:1 ratio. Human aging studies have shown an increasing proportion of Type III collagen, which could be related to impaired synthesis of Type I collagen in aged skin. Sun-damaged skin, typified grossly by its worn, leathery appearance, shows under histologic examination thickened, degraded elastic fibers, described as elastosis.

In the aging face, the first appearance of significant morphologic changes begins at about age 30. The combination of the diminished thickness and elasticity of the skin, gradual resorption of subcutaneous tissue, gravitational descent of soft tissues, and formation of skin folds along the lines of skin adherence result in upper eyelid skin redundancy, lateral orbital crow's-feet lines, and prominence of the nasolabial folds. By age 50 the nasolabial folds are significantly deeper, and glabellar and forehead wrinkles are present. At age 70 there is significant atrophy of the fat in the temporal and buccal areas and marked thinning of the facial skin (Fig. 40–34).[38]

The facelift, which first originated in the early 1900s as a means of removing small areas of unwanted skin at the margins of the hairline, is today a more complex procedure designed not only to remove excess wrinkled skin but also to reposition the sagging atrophied muscles and re-create a more overall natural youthful appearance. The procedure can be performed under local anesthesia with intravenous sedation or with general anesthesia. It is often performed on an outpatient basis, depending on the patient's health and preference.

Preoperatively it is important to obtain appropriate photographs and discuss with the patient realistic expectations of what can be obtained with the procedure. Many computer-designed software programs are now available that image a patient's photograph. Alterations consistent with what might be obtained through plastic surgery can be graphically performed on the screen. Patients are generally asked to discontinue all aspirin-containing products as well as nonsteroidal anti-inflammatory drugs, which might cause a hematoma under the facial flaps after operation. Patients who smoke are warned that they are at a higher risk of skin necrosis after rhytidectomy, and they are generally advised to either stop smoking or at least discontinue smoking 2 to 3 weeks preoperatively.

Although multiple techniques have now been described for performing a rhytidectomy, including new endoscopic[39, 40] and subperiosteal approaches, the standard facelift involves an incision that extends from the hair-bearing area of the temporal scalp along the anterior margin of the ear around the lobe and along the posterior sulcus of the ear, terminating in the hair-bearing scalp (Fig. 40–35). Careful dissection of the skin of the face is then performed, creating skin flaps and removing any underlying excess subcutaneous fat. The skin flaps are generally extended to the nasolabial fold, onto the neck and submental area. A thin fascial layer overlying the facial musculature known as the superficial muscular aponeurotic system (SMAS) is then frequently dissected and

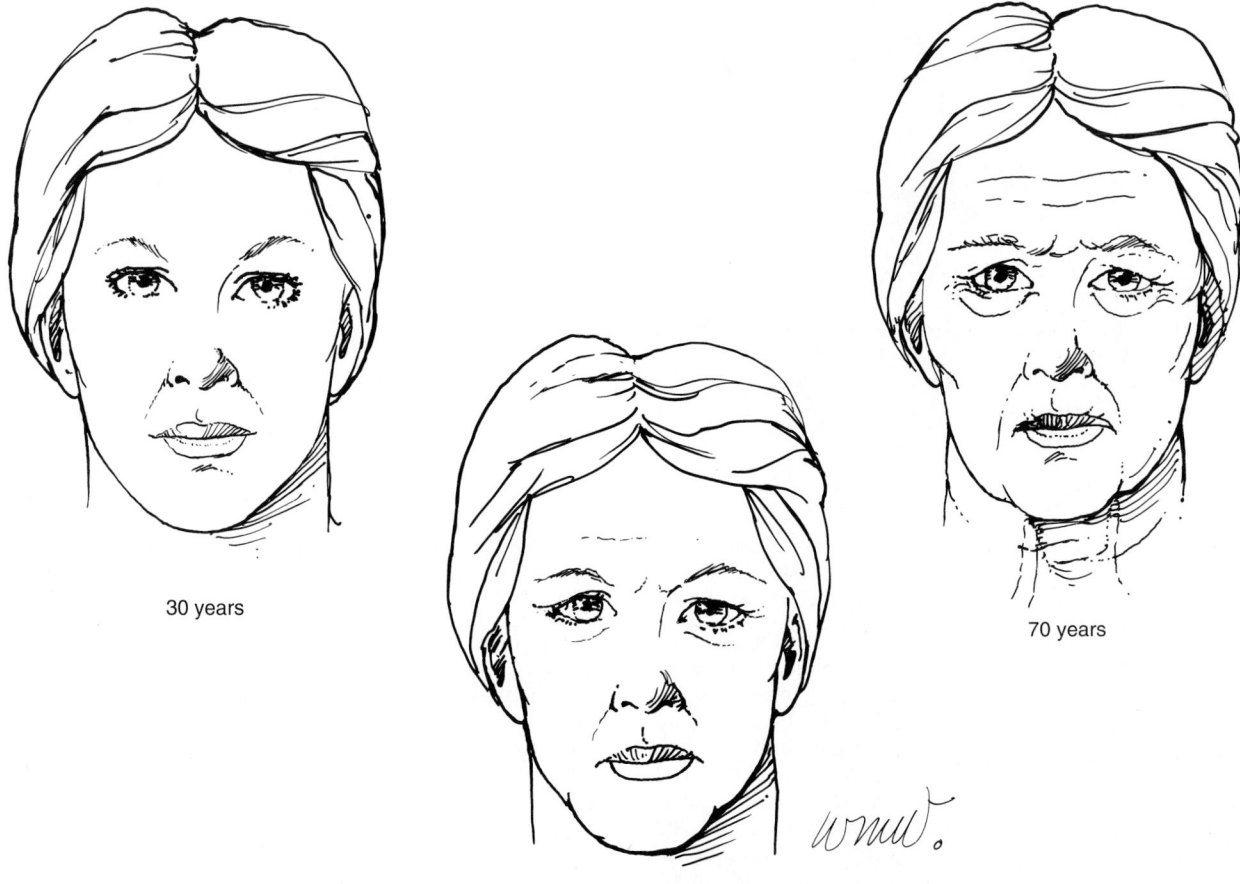

30 years

50 years

70 years

Figure 40–34. Schematic representation of the aging face.

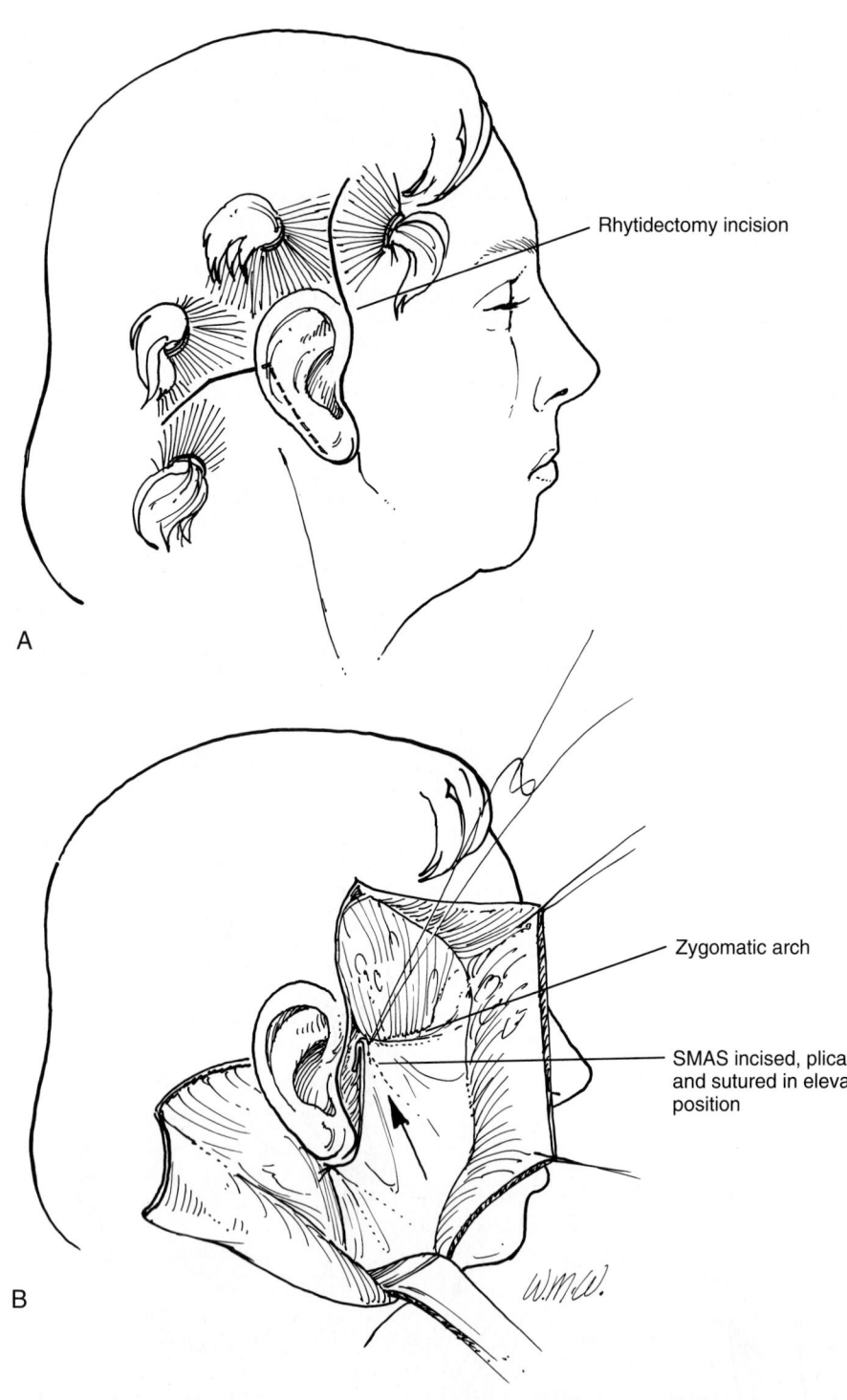

Figure 40–35. *A,* The conventional facelift incision. *B,* Superficial muscular aponeurotic system (SMAS) dissection and plication.

Rhytidectomy incision

Zygomatic arch

SMAS incised, plicated, and sutured in elevated position

A

B

sutured to the fascia anterior to the ear and over the mastoid. This SMAS plication is thought to help reposition the underlying musculature and reduce the amount of tension in the skin flaps. Many surgeons then proceed with suction-assisted lipectomy of selected areas in the face or chin and plication of the platysma muscle in the neck to create an improved jaw line. Lastly, the skin is redraped over the face, the excess skin is excised, subcutaneous drains are placed, and the incision sites are closed. A compression head dressing is usually left in place for 24 hours. Facial swelling and edema is generally present for 3 to 4 weeks postoperatively, but patients can be expected to return to normal activities in 2 weeks without noticeable bruising (see Fig. 40–26).

Complications of a rhytidectomy include development of a facial hematoma under the skin flaps, which, if large enough, may require postoperative drainage. Facial nerve injury is always a possibility, but reported incidences are generally less than 1% to 2%. Partial flap necrosis may occur and is more prevalent in tobacco smokers.

Blepharoplasty

The eyes are a pivotal point of human emotion and expression. As aging occurs in the face, the eyes are one of the first areas to demonstrate significant morphologic changes. Laxity in the soft tissue of the eyes causes excess lid skin in the upper and lower lids, often accompanied by periorbital fat herniation with the bulging, sagging appearance of tired eyes. The *bags* or festoons frequently referred to by patients desiring blepharoplasty are usually the result of the hypertrophy and subsequent laxity of the orbicularis oculi muscle. These age-related changes in the eyes can be altered by blepharoplasty, and this has become a very popular procedure, making it the third most commonly performed aesthetic procedure by plastic surgeons (Fig. 40–36). Careful preoperative evaluation of the patient who desires to undergo blepharoplasty is extremely important. Examination of the eye, orbit, and extraocular muscles and evaluation of lid laxity and visual acuity are performed. Any obvious lid ptosis, eye asymmetry, orbital bulging indicative of Graves' disease or thyroid dysfunction, excessive scleral show, or dry eye problems must be addressed. If significant lid laxity is noted, it may be necessary to perform a lid-tightening procedure concomitant with the blepharoplasty to prevent postoperative ectropion.

Blepharoplasty can be performed under local or general anesthesia. The technique involves excision of the redundant skin, underlying orbicularis oculi muscle, and excess bulging fat. The upper lid incision line is marked with the patient in the sitting position. The amount of excessive skin to be resected from the upper lid is determined and marked so that the incision line will be hidden in the supratarsal fold. A strip of orbicularis oculi muscle is generally removed after the skin is excised. Excessive fat beneath the orbital septum is carefully dissected free and then removed. The lower lid incision line is usually marked 2 to 3 mm. below the lash margin. If skin does not need to be excised from the lower lid and only fat removal is necessary, then the lower lid incision can be made in the transconjunctival position. Postoperative swelling and bruising usually begin to subside 2 to 3 weeks after the operation. The sutures are removed by 5 days postoperatively, because the rapidly growing epithelium of the eyelids will quickly move along the suture tract, leaving distinct suture marks.

Complications from blepharoplasty are rare if appropriate preoperative evaluation is adequate. Overexcision of skin from the lower lid can result in postoperative ectropion. Excessive fat removal from either the upper or lower lid can create a sunken or hollow appearance to the eyes. Although extremely rare, with a reported incidence of 0.04%, there has been an occasional report of associated blindness after blepharoplasty that is likely related to the development of a retrobulbar hematoma.

Chemical Peels

Fine wrinkles in the face noted about the perioral region and eyes and areas of uneven hyperpigmentation are generally not improved with a rhytidectomy. These are problems confined predominantly to the dermis and epidermis and are best addressed by dermabrasion or a chemical peel. Dermabrasion, a procedure using a high-speed, hand-held rotary wheel to remove the top layers of skin, is employed primarily for deep perioral wrinkles and acne scars. Chemical peeling is a procedure involving the application of chemicals, usually either phenol or trichloroacetic acid, to the skin to produce a superficial burn. After healing, the skin that re-epithelializes the area is smoother, is firmer, and demonstrates histologically increased amounts of collagen and abundant elastic fibers in the underlying dermis.

Proper patient selection is important to obtain optimal results. Fair-skinned, light-complected individuals are better candidates than darker, olive-skinned patients. Darker-skinned individuals tend to develop more obvious lines of demarcation between treated and untreated areas. Additionally, men with thicker, oily skin do not respond as well as thinner-skinned women.

The chemical peel is generally performed with the assistance of intravenous sedation. The peeling solution is applied to the skin with a cotton-tipped applicator. To deepen the penetration in a phenol peel, tape is applied over the area and left in place for 24 to 48 hours. The tape is then removed, and the underlying skin is left to crust over. Antibiotic ointments are generally applied to prevent superficial infection. As the chemical-induced burn heals, initially a pink-colored appearance to the skin is seen. After 2 to 3 months, the natural skin color will return. Patients must avoid sun exposure for several months after the procedure. Complications from chemical peels may include skin depigmentation with areas of bleaching and occasionally hypertrophic scarring.[41]

The ultrapulsed carbon dioxide laser has been introduced as a device for skin resurfacing. The laser vaporizes a precise, thin layer of skin. It has proved in early trials to be very valuable in removing fine- to medium-depth wrinkles and surface irregularities.

Liposuction

Suction-assisted lipectomy is a technique that removes unwanted fat from various areas of the body. In the past decade it has become the most frequently performed aesthetic procedure in the United States. Although not technically difficult,

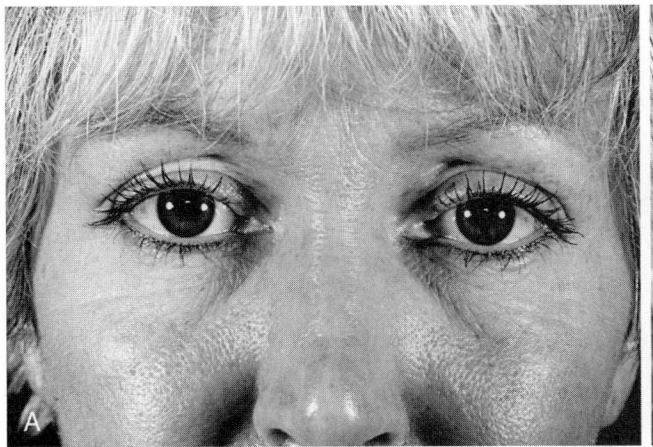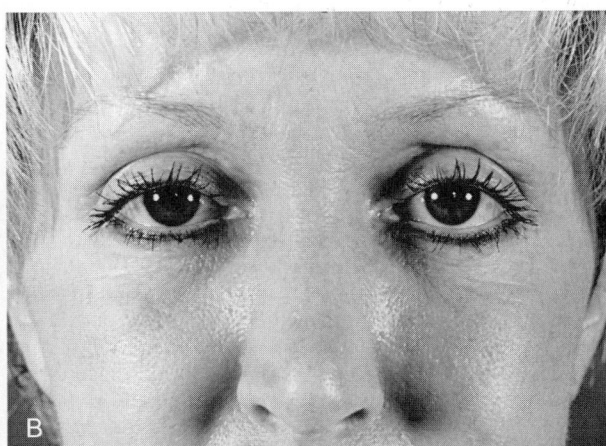

Figure 40–36. Preoperative *(A)* and postoperative *(B)* blepharoplasty.

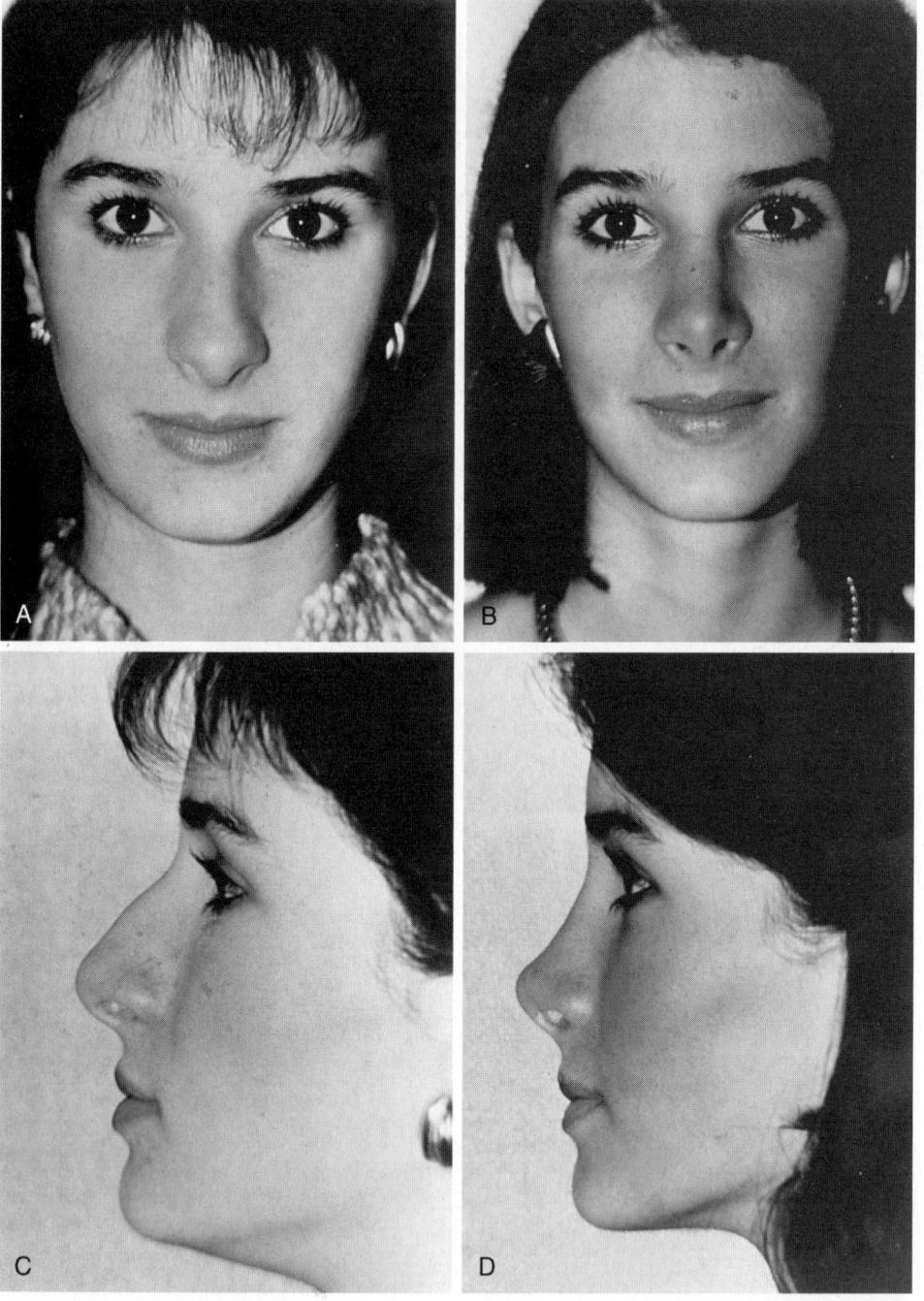

Figure 40–37. Preoperative *(A)* and postoperative *(B)* frontal views of a patient who underwent a corrective rhinoplasty. Also shown are preoperative *(C)* and postoperative *(D)* lateral views of same patient.

achieving consistent aesthetic results with minimal complications requires sound surgical judgment and appropriate intraoperative and postoperative care. The procedure is indicated primarily for patients who are close to ideal body weight but who have pockets of excess fat they wish removed and should not be considered a substitute for weight loss. In women, it is most often employed to remove fat from the buttocks, hips, thighs, and, occasionally, breasts. In men, common sites for liposuction include the waist, abdomen, and chin. Liposuction has also become popular for use in patients with gynecomastia, in removing lipomas, and for contouring and debulking flaps.[42]

The procedure can be performed with the use of local or general anesthesia. With a series of small incisions through which small blunt-tip cannulas can be inserted, the excess fat is removed under vacuum suction. Preoperative injection of large volumes of a saline-lidocaine solution into the excess fat pockets assists with the suction lipectomy and can greatly reduce blood loss. Postoperatively the patient is asked to wear compressive garments for 2 to 4 weeks. Initial bruising and edema subsides after the first 1 to 2 weeks, but sensory loss and associated paresthesia may persist for up to 3 to 6 months.

Complications after liposuction can range from mild aesthetic problems, including contour irregularities, hypertrophic or hyperpigmented scars, to frank skin slough. Fat emboli and pulmonary emboli, although extremely rare, have also been reported, and patients at increased risk include those who are grossly overweight and those who smoke or have a history of lung disease.[43] Results from liposuction can be very gratifying to both the patient and surgeon; however, the patient should maintain a proper diet after liposuction to prevent reaccumulation of the unwanted fat.

Rhinoplasty

Corrective nasal surgery is often performed as an aesthetic procedure to alter the contour of the external nose or as a reconstructive procedure to correct birth defects, breathing problems, or posttraumatic deformities. The procedure, which can be designed to modify the nasal tip, eliminate a large dorsal nasal hump, correct a septal deviation, or reshape the alar cartilages, is individualized to suit the patient's needs (Fig. 40–37). Rhinoplasty is usually performed on an outpatient basis with either local or general anesthesia. Depending on the surgeon's preference or complexity of the reconstruction, the procedure can be performed as a *closed* technique through incisions made inside the nostril rim, or as an *open* technique, which also includes a small incision made across the columella.

The procedure involves separating the skin envelope from the underlying cartilage and bony framework, so that these structures can then be reshaped to achieve the desired goals. For the patient with a large dorsal hump, a chisel or rasp is used to resect or file the excess bone and cartilage to improve the profile. If nasal bone repositioning is also indicated, an osteotome is used to infracture the nasal bones, separating them from the underlying maxilla and narrowing the root of the nose.

Cartilage or bone can be added as a nasal tip graft or as a columellar strut graft to improve tip projection. For the patient with very wide nostrils, a small wedge resection of the alar base can significantly decrease the overall width of the base of the nose and greatly enhance the patient's appearance.

A deviated nasal septum or hypertrophied inferior turbinates can occasionally result in obstructed nasal airways. Although septal procedures are not part of the routine aesthetic rhinoplasty, resection of the hypertrophied turbinates and resection or modification of the deviated septum can greatly improve nasal airway flow.

SELECTED REFERENCES

Rohrich, R. J., and Robinson, J. B., Jr.: Wound Healing and Closure, Abnormal Scars, Tattoos, Envenomation, and Extravasation Injuries, Vol. 3. Dallas, Selected Readings in Plastic Surgery, 1992.
This volume, from the Selected Readings in Plastic Surgery series, gives a superb overview of wound healing.

McCarthy, J. G. (Ed.): Plastic Surgery. Philadelphia, W. B. Saunders, 1990.
This is the classic textbook in plastic surgery. It provides excellent illustrations and is a complete and comprehensive eight-volume series.

Vokes, E. E., Weichselbaum, R. R., Lippman, S. M., and Hong, W. K.: Head and neck cancer. N. Engl. J. Med., 328:184, 1993.
This is an excellent review. It provides a succinct overview of the etiology, diagnosis, and treatment of squamous cell carcinoma of the head and neck.

REFERENCES

1. Gnudi, M. T., and Webster, J. P.: The Life and Times of Gaspare Tagliacozzi. New York, Herbert Reichner, 1950.
2. Majno, G.: The Healing Hand: Man and Wound in the Ancient World. Cambridge, MA, Harvard University Press, 1975.
3. Vasconez, L. O., Bostwick, J., III, and McCraw, J.: Coverage of exposed bone by muscle transposition and skin grafting. Plast. Reconstr. Surg., 53:526, 1974.
4. Mathes, S., and Nahai, F.: Clinical Atlas of Muscle and Musculocutaneous Flaps. St. Louis, C. V. Mosby, 1979.
5. Tessier, P. Osteotomies totales de la face, syndrome de Crouzon, syndrome d'Apert, oxycephalies, scaphocephalies, turricephalies. Ann. Chir. Plast., 12:273, 1967.
5a. Molina, F., and Ortiz-Monasterio, F.: Elongation and remodeling by distraction: A farewell to major osteotomies. Plast. Reconstr. Surg., 96:825, 1995.
6. McGrath, M. H.: Peptide growth factors and wound healing. Clin. Plast. Surg., 17(3), 1990.
7. Rohrich, R. J., and Robinson, J. B., Jr.: Wound Healing and Closure, Abnormal Scars, Tattoos, Envenomation, and Extravasation Injuries, Vol. 3. Dallas, Selected Readings in Plastic Surgery, 1992.
8. McGregor, I. A.: Fundamental Techniques of Plastic Surgery. New York, Churchill Livingstone, 1980.
9. Stahl, R. S., and Ariyan, S.: Microsurgery of the upper extremity. In Jurkiewicz, M. J., et al. (Eds.): Plastic Surgery: Principles and Practice. St. Louis, C. V. Mosby, 1990.
10. Jandauskas, S., Cohen, I. K., and Grabb, W. C.: Basic technique of plastic surgery. In Smith J. W., and Aston, S. J. (Eds): Grabb and Smith's Plastic Surgery, 4th ed. Boston, Little, Brown & Company, 1991.
11. Rudolph, R., and Ballantyne, D. L.: Skin grafts. In McCarthy, J. (Ed.): Plastic Surgery. Philadelphia, W. B. Saunders, 1990.
12. Jackson, I. T.: Local Flaps in Head and Neck Reconstruction. St. Louis, C. V. Mosby, 1985.
13. McCraw, J. B., and Arnold, P. G.: McCraw and Arnold's Atlas of Muscle and Musculocutaneous Flaps. Norfolk, VA, Hampton Press, 1986.
14. Shaw, W.: Microvascular free flaps: Survey. In Buncke, H., and Furnas, D. (Eds.): Symposium on Clinical Frontiers in Reconstructive Microsurgery. St. Louis, C. V. Mosby, 1984.
15. Fraser, F. C.: The genetics of cleft lip and palate. Am. J. Hum. Genet., 22:336, 1970.
16. Millard, D. R., and Latham, R. A.: Improved primary surgical and dental treatment of clefts. Plast. Reconstr. Surg., 86:856, 1990.
17. Mulliken, J. B.: Principles and techniques of bilateral complete cleft lip repair. Plast. Reconstr. Surg., 75:477, 1985.
18. Hartel, J., Kriens, O., and Kundt, G.: Incidence of cleft lip, alveolus and palate forms. J. Craniomaxillofac. Surg., 19:144, 1991.
19. Moore, M. D.: Complications of primary palatoplasty: A twenty-one-year review. Cleft Palate J., 25:156, 1988.
20. McCarthy, J. G., Epstein, F. J., and Wood-Smith, P.: Craniosynostosis. In McCarthy, J. G. (Ed.): Plastic Surgery, vol. 4, chap. 61. Philadelphia, W. B. Saunders, 1990.
21. Le Fort, R.: Etude experimental sur les fractures de la machoire superieure. Rev. Chir. Paris, 23:201, 1901.
22. Wood, R. J., and Jurkiewicz, M. J.: Plastic and reconstructive surgery. In Schwartz, S. I. (Ed.): Principles of Surgery, Chap. 44. New York, McGraw-Hill, 1994.
23. Bring, C. C., Squires, T. S., and Tong, T.: Cancer statistics, 1992. CA 42:19, 1992.
24. Gluckman, J. L.: Synchronous multiple primary lesions of the upper aerodigestive system. Arch. Otolaryngol. Head Neck Surg. 105:597, 1979.
25. Vokes, E. E., Weichselbaum, R. R., Lippman, S. M., and Hong, W. K.: Head and neck cancer. N. Engl. J. Med., 328:184, 1993.
26. Shaha, A. R.: Preoperative evaluation of the mandible in patients with carcinoma of the floor of the mouth. Head Neck, 13:398, 1991.
27. Leipzig, B., Sellmer, J., and Klug, D.: The panendoscopy study group: The role of endoscopy in evaluating patients with head and neck cancer. Arch. Otolaryngol. Head Neck Surg., 111:589, 1985.
28. McGuirt, W. F.: Panendoscopy as a screening examination for simultaneous primary tumors in head and neck cancer: A prospective sequential study and review of the literature. Laryngoscope, 92:569, 1982.
29. Schwartz, R., Chan, N. H., and MacFarlane, K.: Fine needle aspiration cytology in the evaluation of head and neck masses. Am. J. Surg., 159:482, 1990.
30. Sloan, D., and Goepfert, H.: Conventional therapy of head and neck cancer. Hematol. Oncol. Clin. North Am., 5:601, 1991.
31. Carlson, G. W.: Surgical anatomy of the neck. Surg. Clin. North Am., 73:837, 1993.
32. Jones, K. R., Lodge-Rigal, D., Reddick, R. L., Tudor, G. E., and Shockley, W. W.: Prognostic factors in the recurrence of Stage I and II squamous cell cancer of the oral cavity. Arch. Otolaryngol. Head Neck Surg., 118:483, 1992.
33. Williams, J. K., Carlson, G. W., Cohen, C., et al.: Tumor angiogenesis as a prognostic factor in oral cavity tumors. Am. J. Surg., 168:373, 1994.
34. Carlson, G. W., Coleman, J. J., and Jurkiewicz, M. J.: Reconstruction of the hypopharynx and cervical esophagus. Curr. Probl. Surg., 30:425, 1993.
35. Attie, J. N., Sciubba, J. J.: Tumors of major and minor salivary glands: Clinical and pathologic features. Curr. Probl. Surg., 18:68, 1981.
36. Spiro, R. H.: Diagnosis and pitfalls in the treatment of parotid tumors. Semin. Surg. Oncol., 7:20, 1991.
37. Barton, F. E.: Esthetic Surgery of the Face, Vol. 7. Dallas, Selected Readings in Plastic Surgery, 1994.
38. Gonzalez-Ulloa, M., and Flores, E. S.: Senility of the face: Basic study to understand its cause and effects. Plast. Reconstr. Surg., 36:239, 1965.
39. Mackay, G. J., and Nahai, F.: The endoscopic forehead lift: Operative techniques. Plast. Reconstr. Surg., 2:137, 1995.
40. Bostwick, J., III, Eaves, F. F., and Nahai, F.: Endoscopic Plastic Surgery. St. Louis, Quality Medical Publishers, 1994.
41. Baker, T. J., and Gordon, H. L.: Surgical Rejuvenation of the Aging Face. St. Louis, C. V. Mosby, 1986.
42. Baird, W., and Nahai, F.: The use of lipoplasty in contouring and debulking flaps. Clin. Plast. Surg., 16:195, 1989.
43. Gargan, T. J., and Courtiss, E. H.: The risks of suction lipectomy: Their prevention and treatment. Clin. Plast. Surg., 11:457, 1984.

I

PILONIDAL CYSTS AND SINUSES

Mark W. Sebastian, M.D.

Few conditions amenable to definitive cure have been debated as actively as pilonidal disease. Herbert Mayo in 1833 reported the case of a young woman with a hair-containing sinus in the sacrococcygeal region, and controversy has persisted since. In 1847, Anderson published "Hair Extracted from an Ulcer,"[2] which was followed in 1854 by Warren's report of incision and drainage of a sacrococcygeal abscess with extraction of a hair ball.[48] In 1880, Hodges introduced the term *pilonidal* (*pilus*, "hair," *nidus*, "nest") and proposed a theory of congenital origin of the disease.[27] Embryologic and autopsy studies by Mallory[34] found subcutaneous squamous epithelium–lined spaces in the tissues removed from the region of the sacrum and coccyx, which led some authors to conclude that a congenital origin was the primary and essential anatomic factor in the development of the clinical and pathologic entity.[12]

Since Patey and Scharff[41] reopened the debate concerning pathogenesis in 1946 the evidence has weighed heavily in favor of an acquired nature for all but the rare case of sacrococcygeal pilonidal disease. These investigators believed that the friction produced by the natal cleft was probably responsible for producing the sinus. Brearley[9] postulated that the hair becomes clustered in a drill-like form that enters the skin and that shedding causes the hairs to be drawn further into the sinus, thus increasing its depth. In 1959, Palmer[40] postulated that stretching of the integument at puberty, which was associated with rapid growth (particularly of the gluteal muscles), produced distention of hair follicles, sebaceous glands, and apocrine glands and sufficient spreading of their cutaneous orifices to allow the insinuation of foreign substances. There is growing evidence that these tiny midline holes or pits, sometimes termed *sinuses*, which are observed in the cleft of nearly all patients with pilonidal disease, are the source of the disease. It appears that these holes or pits represent distorted hair follicles that have enlarged. The pulling forces and the vacuum effect created in this area by gravity and by motion of the gluteal folds have been measured by Brearley and appear to be responsible for enlarging the follicles. The ingestion of hair by an existing pilonidal cavity was cleverly demonstrated by Page in 1969.[39] Thus, the emerging evidence is that enlarged hair follicles appear first, and the ingested hair is a secondary invader that prolongs disease and interferes with healing. These are the primary elements of Boscom's hypothesis (Fig. 40–38) of the evolution of pilonidal cysts from hair follicles, which offers a reasonable explanation for the fact that hair, which until now was considered the single source of pilonidal disease, is found in only one half of the patients.[6] In the other half, the follicles fill with keratin that becomes infected and ruptures into the deeper fat. Studies of large populations suggest an incidence of 26 cases per 100,000 inhabitants, with the disease occurring 2.2 times more often in men than women, and the average age of presentation centering around 21 years. Clinical characteristics associated with pilonidal disease include male sex, family predisposition, obesity, and sedentary lifestyle or occupation requiring prolonged sitting position leading to local trauma.[43]

Although pilonidal disease most commonly occurs in the region of the sacrococcygeal junction, it has been reported in the umbilicus, the axilla, the clitoris, the interdigital webs of barber's hands, the interdigital web of the foot of a worker in a hair mattress factory, the sole of the foot, and the anal canal. A recent report describes periareolar pilonidal abscesses in a hairdresser. Pilonidal sinuses containing wool, grass, animal hair, and hair of a color different from the patient's hair color all have been reported.[12, 17, 20, 22, 40, 46]

The condition was formerly believed to be common among army personnel (hence the name *jeep disease*)[11]; however, such a predilection has not been demonstrated with certainty in the recent literature. The ratio of male to female inpatients with pilonidal disease seeking treatment varies from 3:1 to 7:1. A survey of 31,497 male and 21,367 female students without symptoms observed at the University of Minnesota revealed 365 pilonidal sinuses among the males and only 24 among the females. The average age of both groups was 21 years. The affected students were more likely to be significantly overweight (45%:26%).[16] From his clinicopathologic study of 354 patients observed at the Mayo Clinic, Franckowiak derived a hypothetical pilonidal habitus as "the robust, fat, plethoric type of male with a narrow pelvis, a deep sulcus between prominent folds of the thick buttocks, an excessive glandular activity, and susceptibility to staph infection."[17]

Clinical Findings

Presentation. Patients with pilonidal disease may seek advice about asymptomatic pits or pores in the natal cleft. Tenderness after physical activity or a long drive that requires the patient to sit for a long time are common presentations. A tender or nontender nodule may be palpable. Twenty per cent of such patients seek care for the severe pain and tenderness of an acute abscess. Eighty per cent of patients with pilonidal disease present with moisture and drainage and occasional bleeding. They have usually not experienced previous difficulties, because the lesion is usually asymptomatic until the affected follicle becomes infected and ruptures

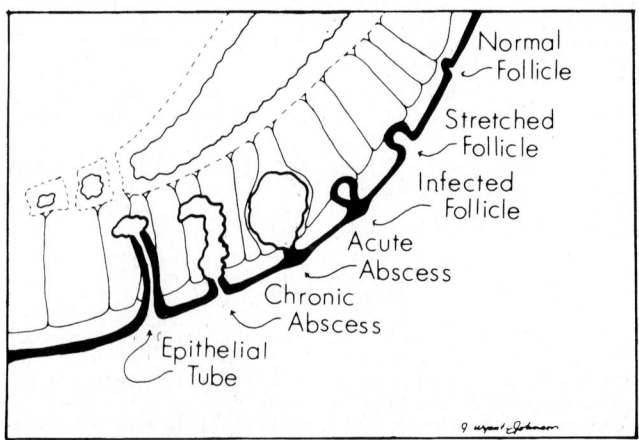

Figure 40–38. The stages of pilonidal disease (from top to bottom): (1) Normal follicle. (2) Follicle distended with keratin. Fibrous strands suspend follicle and skin from sacrum. (3) Infection of the distended follicle; edema closes the mouth of the follicle. (4) Rupture of infected follicle into fat, creating an acute pilonidal abscess. (5) Chronic pilonidal abscess. The ruptured follicle, which is now open at both ends, forms the mouth of the abscess. (6) Epithelial tube. Epithelium from the ragged end of a ruptured follicle has grown down the wall. (Adapted from Bascom, J.: Surgery, *87*:567, 1980.)

into the surrounding tissues[6] (Fig. 40–39). The findings of acute suppuration, tenderness, pain, swelling, and heat are similar to those of acute abscesses in other locations. In general, there is minimal cellulitis and induration surrounding the pilonidal abscess. Systemic reaction to the abscess is infrequent, but occasionally fever, leukocytosis, and malaise are found.

Because the abscess of an infected pilonidal cyst may be located deep to relatively thick skin, it enlarges rapidly and only rarely ruptures spontaneously. The abscess can extend in any direction but only infrequently extends to the perianal area. With enlargement of the abscess, tortuous, and usually multiple, sinuses develop external to the postsacral fascia. The inflammatory process may subside early or may progress until relief is obtained—usually by surgical means and rarely by spontaneous drainage. After drainage has occurred, the purulent discharge may cease completely, but more commonly it recurs intermittently with drainage from one or more sinuses as the disease enters its chronic phase.[12, 17, 25]

Pathology

The earliest stages of pilonidal *sinuses* demonstrate variously sized enlarged hair follicles in otherwise normal skin. Each follicle holds a single hair shaft surrounded by rings of keratin. The acute pilonidal *abscess* contains pus under pressure and a wall of edematous fat; polymorphonuclear cells predominate. The chronic abscess has a wall of fibrous tissue lined by granulation tissue of capillaries, lymphocytes, and giant cells. The cavity is laden with *Staphylococcus aureus* and

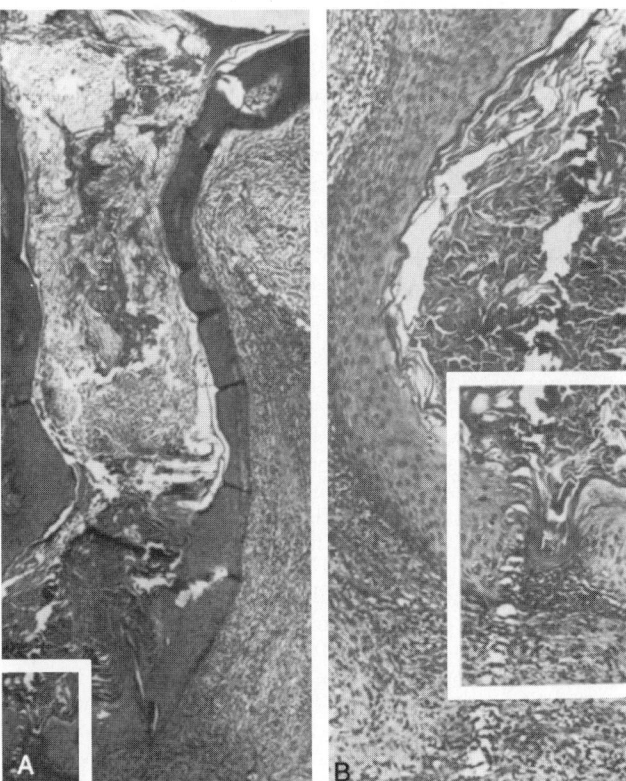

Figure 40–39. *A,* Early pilonidal disease. Section of a hole or pit from midline skin overlying a pilonidal abscess. This distended hair follicle is breaking out. Keratin is being evacuated. Inflammatory cells are gathering to meet the challenge and eventually form a pilonidal abscess. Original magnification, ×25. *B,* Magnification (×100) of area of hair follicle break-out and the resulting inflammatory response. See *A.* (From Bascom, J.: Pilonidal disease: Long-term results of follicle removal. Dis. Colon Rectum, *26*:800, 1983.)

other organisms, including anaerobes (particularly *Bacteroides* species).[35, 36]

Infiltration of hair occurs in one half of the specimens. No hair follicles have ever been found in the sinus tracts; this observation provided an early clue that hair found therein was of extraneous origin. Chronic abscesses of long duration begin to receive a thin and flat lining of epithelium that grows into the cavity from the skin surface, thus forming a cyst. Epithelial tubes or epidermal inclusion cysts may follow but are uncommon. Indolent wounds that fail to heal after surgical procedures resemble chronic abscesses.[7]

Differential Diagnosis

The diagnosis of pilonidal disease is usually apparent; however, the possibility of other conditions should be considered, including perianal abscesses arising from the posterior midline crypt, hidradenitis suppurativa, and a simple carbuncle or furuncle. Some other focus of infection, such as osteomyelitis, may produce a sinus in this area, but this is not common. If a probe inserted in the sinus follows a course away from the anus, this may be considered indicative of a pilonidal sinus. Care must be taken to exclude a complicated anal fistula, which may angulate posteriorly before passing into a retrorectal abscess. In this situation thorough examination of the anal cavity usually discloses the point of origin.

Rarely, pilonidal disease and anal fistula coexist. They arise independently and develop into the combined disorder because the anal fistula has extended posteriorly and has involved the pilonidal cyst or sinus. Most such patients have had previous operations, and it is likely that the surgeon connected the two pathologic processes by incision. However, well-documented instances of pilonidal cysts with the fistulous tract situated inside the anal canal have been reported.[1] In the pediatric and adolescent age group, coccygeal sinuses (congenital skin adherence to the coccyx) and sinuses overlying the sacrum in which there is pigmented and hairy skin have been mistaken for pilonidal disease. The sacral sinus is associated with a great risk of incurring meningitis in early life, but fortunately meningitis is easily distinguishable from pilonidal disease.

Treatment

There is a growing consensus that management of pilonidal disease should involve conservative approaches, because these approaches have yielded satisfactory results and lower recurrence rates.[28, 43] Treatment in an outpatient setting has gained acceptance and is widely practiced.[3]

Acute Pilonidal Abscess. In a prospective study of 73 patients, Jensen and Harling[29] considered the results of simple incision and drainage of a first-episode acute pilonidal abscess with special emphasis on cure rate and recurrence rate among patients with healing *per primam*. The abscesses were incised with a cruciform incision, and the four corners of the cruciform incision were excised to allow adequate drainage. The wound was not curetted. The patients shaved the area around the wound and were examined every 2 weeks for 12 weeks. Their treatment relieved symptoms, and all patients returned to work immediately after treatment. They demonstrated convincingly that healing *per primam* occurred in 58% of the patients within 10 weeks of treatment. Twenty-one per cent with healing *per primam* developed recurrence of their pilonidal abscess during the prospective follow-up period of 36 to 84 months; therefore, they had a constant cure rate of 76% after 18 months.[29] The best results were in patients with few pits and lateral tracts, whereas patients who developed recurrences had developed excessive granulation tissue and required later definitive surgical treatment. The decision to offer definitive treatment should be deferred for at least 10 weeks, and those patients with pits and lateral tracts should probably be selected for treatment using a more definitive procedure that includes evacuation of hair and curetting of granulation tissue with wide exposure of the posterior wall of the abscess cavity.[30] Some authors have advocated the use of sclerosing solutions such as phenol, silver nitrate, and Monsel's solution, but their use is probably not necessary and may be harmful.[6] With hair, hot tub baths, and use of Water Pik irrigation, healing by secondary intention is generally complete in 2 weeks, and recurrence is unusual.[28, 43] Antibiotics are not generally indicated, unless the patient has a medical condition such as rheumatic heart disease or is immunosuppressed.

Some clinicians have advocated aspiration of the abscess or a small lateral incision for evacuation of the acute abscess and appropriate antibiotic coverage, which is adjusted according to the results of bacteriologic culture, to control the acute process. An early date is then scheduled for outpatient excision of the cyst with curettage of the pits. This approach remains to be proved by wider experience.

CHRONIC PILONIDAL DISEASE

Eighty per cent of patients with pilonidal disease present with a chronic abscess and no history of a prior clinically apparent acute stage. Marks and others[10, 35, 36] have demonstrated the central role of infection, particularly by anaerobic bacteria, in the extreme difficulties of wound healing often associated with chronic pilonidal disease. Therefore, initial treatment involves providing an oral pain medication and an antibiotic regimen that is particularly directed against *Staphylococcus* and *Bacteroides* species. After administering local or regional anesthesia to the patient, the chronic abscess is opened widely by a long incision that is parallel to and 2 cm. to one side of the midline. Avoidance of the midline *ditch* containing the pits and sinuses is increasingly advocated.[30] The abscess cavity is scrubbed free of hair; this process removes portions of the cyst wall impregnated with hair (Fig. 40–40). In the rare patient with long-standing disease, the

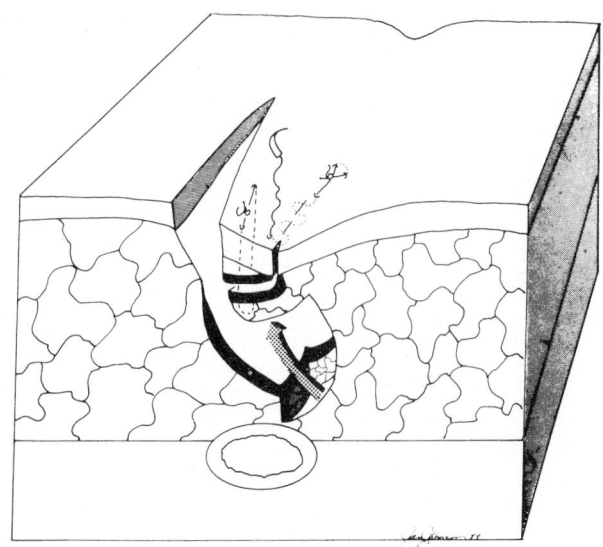

Figure 40–41. After procedures outlined in Figure 40–40, the lateral wound is left open to drain, but the midline wounds are sutured. Healing is enhanced by collapsing portion of the wall of the clean cavity against the underside and floor of the cavity.

abscess wall is covered with surface epithelium that has grown into the cavity. At this stage, it is no longer a chronic abscess; it becomes an epithelial inclusion cyst that is therefore excised. The lateral incision is left widely open to permit drainage, whereas all small holes from the midline skin are excised with minimal tissue loss (Fig. 40–41). The visible holes that represent enlarged follicles must be completely excised if recurrence is to be avoided.

Occasionally, multiple cavities may be seen under insignificant-appearing follicles. The amount of uninvolved tissue excised is kept to a minimum. The tiny midline openings are carefully closed with nonabsorbable suture material. Primary healing is aided by collapsing a portion of the *far wall* of the abscess against the underside of the closure (see Fig. 40–41). The loose stitch of nonabsorbable suture material that holds this flap in place is removed in approximately 1 week.

Antibiotics are continued for 24 hours. The patient is instructed to shower daily and is taught about local cleansing and care of the wound with frequent changes of absorbent cotton dressings. Half of the patients return to work the following day, and disability rarely exceeds 4 days for the other half. All wounds are usually found to be closed by the sixth postoperative week. In a few patients, a midline hole remains open or a new one appears. These patients require a weekly shave and/or daily packing with cotton gauze and an occasional silver nitrate cauterization of granulation tissue. A rare patient may return years after surgical therapy with an inclusion cyst.

Although a randomized trial comparing excision and excision with suture with and without antibiotics[32] and another comparing excision with marsupialization and phenolization[13] have been reported, the results confirm only the correctness of the present trend toward more conservative approaches. Asymptomatic patients who have sinuses that are dry and have never been painful should be observed. Patients who have large recurrent pilonidal disease may be treated by an *advancing flap operation*. This technique was applied in 7471 cases of pilonidal sinus during the period of 1966 to 1990 with a 95% rate of follow-up ranging from 2 to 20 years.[31] The principle of this treatment is an eccentric, elliptical excision; mobilization of a flap on the median side of the incision and fixation of the base of the flap to the

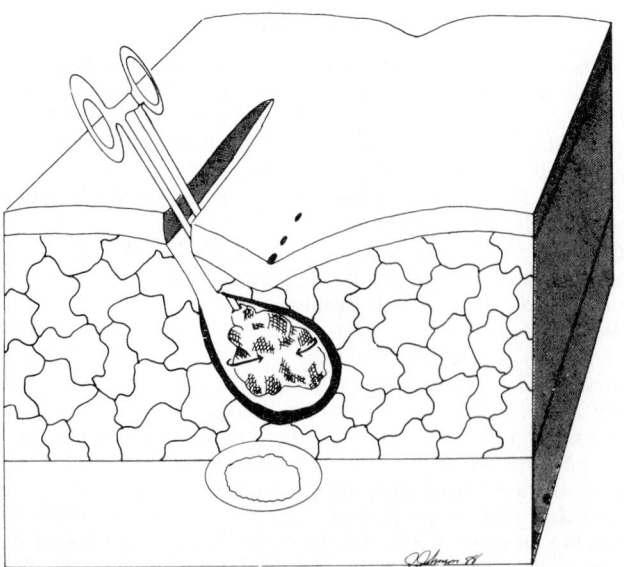

Figure 40–40. Principles of treatment of pilonidal abscess include (1) adequate incision *lateral* to the midline, (2) removal of hair and granulations, and (3) conservative removal of the midline holes and pits that sustain the abscess, minimizing tissue loss. (After Boscom, J.: Pilonidal sinus. *In* Sazio V. W. (Ed.): Current Therapy in Colon and Rectal Surgery. Toronto, B. C. Decker, 1990, p. 34.)

sacrococcygeal fascia; and the suturing of the flap to the lateral wound. The series included drainage, immediate ambulation with mean hospitalization of 3 days. The report cited a 1% rate of recurrence, with a recurrence of 3% in very young female patients.[31]

RECURRENT PILONIDAL DISEASE

It is evident from the proliferation of procedures advocated for pilonidal disease that no failure-proof operation has yet been discovered. All of the following procedures have been associated with significant failure rates: excision and packing with healing by open granulation[36]; marsupialization, which was championed by Buie[11, 13]; excision and closure[32]; injection[5, 26]; destruction of the tract[19]; irradiation[44]; and various plastic tissue flap rotational procedures[4, 45] and grafting.[23] Although the recurrence rate in some series is reasonably low, the procedures involved are long and complex, require prolonged hospitalization, or may cause potentially more morbidity than the disease itself. Beginning with the identification of infection as an important common denominator in the failure of these approaches,[10, 35, 36] future investigation of those factors that delay wound healing has been emphasized. Marks and others have identified basic principles, including wound reshaping to facilitate better drainage of pockets of uneradicated infection and the early use of specific antibiotic treatment, as being important to the achievement of cure in these patients.

After formal conservative primary treatment, most recurrences develop in the inferior portion of the scar. A blind cavity or sinus tract is frequently encountered through a midline opening. The posterior wall of the tract should be exposed and scraped free of granulation tissue, and the edges of the tract should be débrided. The epithelialized posterior wall of the tract should be left intact. Hot baths and Water Pik irrigation that is performed at least once daily keep the wound clean. Granulation tissue is removed, and the wound is cauterized with silver nitrate when the patient returns for weekly visits. The healing time averages 3 to 4 weeks, depending on the size of the wound.

Surgical débridement and retailoring of the wound[6] for better drainage and for elimination of loculations may be necessary in the rare patient, but they should probably not be performed until local measures have been exhausted. Rarely, malignant degeneration occurs in these lesions.[12, 22, 33, 42] Verrucous carcinoma (giant condyloma acuminatum[38]) developing within the pilonidal sinus has been described.

SELECTED REFERENCES

Boscom, J.: Pilonidal disease: Long-term results of follicle removal. Dis. Colon Rectum, 26:800, 1983.
> The author describes the results of therapy based on his hypothesis, which implicates hair follicles in the etiology of pilonidal disease. Convincing histopathologic support for the hypothesis is presented as the author describes the stages of development of a pilonidal cyst from a hair follicle. The theory implicates hair as a confounding "secondary invader" and provides ready explanation for the fact that hair, until recently considered the single source of the disease, is found in only one half of the patients.

Hurst, D. W.: The evolution of management of pilonidal sinus disease. Can. J. Surg., 26:603, 1984.
> An early advocate of conservative treatment, Hurst outlines a practical approach to pilonidal disease based on a comprehensive 10-year review of 72 consecutive patients who were successfully treated as outpatients with the use of local anesthesia.

Karydakis, G.: Easy and successful treatment of pilonidal sinus after explanation of its causative process. Aust. N. Z. J. Surg., 62:385, 1992.
> This article is an extensive review of the pathophysiology and surgical treatment of pilonidal sinus that reports a series of 7471 patients suffering from this disease who were followed for 2 to 20 years. This series was initiated in conjunction with the surgeons at St. Mark's Hospital, London.

REFERENCES

1. Accarpio, G., Davini, M. D., Fazio, A., Senussi, O. H., and Yakubovich, A.: Pilonidal sinus with an anal canal fistula. Dis. Colon Rectum, 31:965, 1988.
2. Anderson, A. W.: Hair extracted from an ulcer. Boston Med. Surg. J., 36:74, 1847.
3. Armstrong, J. H., and Barcia, P. J.: Pilonidal sinus disease: The conservative approach. Arch. Surg., 129:914, 1994.
4. Azab, A. S., Kamal, M. S., and El Bassyoni, F.: The rationale of using the Rhomboid fasciocutaneous transposition flap for the radical cure of pilonidal sinus. J. Dermatol. Surg. Oncol., 12:1295, 1986.
5. Biegeleisen, H. I.: Sclerotherapy for pilonidal cysts—sclerosing method of treatment. Arch. Surg., 37:112, 1938.
6. Boscom, J.: Pilonidal disease: Long-term results of follicle removal. Dis. Colon Rectum, 26:800, 1983.
7. Boscom, J.: Repeat pilonidal operations. Am. J. Surg., 154:118, 1987.
8. Boscom, J.: Pilonidal sinus. In Sazio, V. W. (Ed.): Current Therapy in Colon and Rectal Surgery. Toronto, B. C. Decker, 1990.
9. Brearley, R.: Pilonidal sinus: A new theory of origin. Br. J. Surg., 43:62, 1955.
10. Brook, I., Anderson, K. D., Controni, G., and Rodriquez, W. J.: Aerobic and anaerobic bacteriology of pilonidal cyst abscess in children. Am. J. Dis. Child., 134:679, 1980.
11. Buie, L. A.: Jeep disease (pilonidal disease of mechanized warfare). South. Med. J., 37:103, 1944.
12. Chamberlain, J. W., and Vawter, G. F.: The congenital origin of pilonidal sinus. J. Pediatr. Surg., 9:441, 1974.
13. Culp, C. E.: Pilonidal disease and its treatment. Surg. Clin. North Am., 47:1007, 1967.
14. Davis, K. A., Mock, C. N., Versaci, A., Lentrichia, P.: Malignant degeneration of pilonidal cysts. Am. Surgeon, 3:200, 1994.
15. Duchateau, J., DeMol, J., Bosten, H., and Allegaert, W.: Pilonidal sinus excision-marsupialization-phenolization? Acta Chir. Belg., 85:325, 1985.
16. Dwight, R. W., and Maloy, J. K.: Pilonidal sinus experience with 449 cases. N. Engl. J. Med., 249:926, 1953.
17. Franckowiak, J. J.: The etiology of pilonidal sinus. University of Minnesota, unpublished thesis, 1960.
18. Füzün, M., Bakir, H., Soylu, M., Tansug, T., Kaymak, E., and Harmancioglu, Ö.: Which technique for treatment of pilonidal sinus—open or closed? Dis. Colon Rectum, 37:1148, 1994.
19. Gage, A. H., and Dutta, P.: Cryosurgery for pilonidal disease. Am. J. Surg., 133:249, 1977.
20. Gannon, M. X., et al.: Periareolar pilonidal diseases in a hairdresser. Br. Med. J., 297:1641, 1988.
21. Goligher, J. C.: Surgery of the Anus, Rectum, and Colon, 3rd ed. Springfield, IL, Charles C Thomas, 1975.
22. Gupta, S., Kumar, A., Khanna, A. K., and Khanna, S.: Pilonidal sinus epidermoid carcinoma: A clinicopathologic study and a collective review. Curr. Surg., 38:374, 1981.
23. Guyuron, B., Dinner, M. K., and Dowden, R. R.: Excision and grafting in treatment of recurrent pilonidal sinus disease. Surg. Gynecol. Obstet., 156:201, 1983.
24. Hanley, P. H.: Symposium: The dilemma of pilonidal disease. Dis. Colon Rectum, 20:278, 1977.
25. Hanley, P. H.: Acute pilonidal disease. Surg. Gynecol. Obstet., 150:9, 1980.
26. Hegge, H. G. J., Vos, G. A., Patka, P., and Hoitsma, H. F. W.: Treatment of complicated infected pilonidal sinus disease by local application of phenol. Surgery, 102:52, 1987.
27. Hodges, R. M.: Pilonidal sinus. Boston Med. Surg. J., 103:456, 1880.
28. Hurst, D. W.: The evolution of management of pilonidal sinus disease. Can. J. Surg., 27:603, 1984.
29. Jensen, S. L., and Harling, H.: Prognosis after simple incision and drainage for a first-episode acute pilonidal abscess. Br. J. Surg., 75:60, 1988.
30. Karydakis, G. E.: New approach to the problem of pilonidal sinus. Lancet, 2:1414, 1973.
31. Karydakis, G. E.: Easy and successful treatment of pilonidal sinus after explanation of its causative process. Aust. N. Z. J. Surg., 62:385, 1992.
32. Kronborg, O., Christensen, J., and Zimmerman-Nielsen, C.: Chronic pilonidal disease: A randomized trial with a complete three-year follow-up. Br. J. Surg., 72:303, 1985.
33. Lineaweaver, W. C., Brunson, M. B., Smith, J. F., Franzini, D. A., and Rumley, T. O.: Squamous carcinoma arising in a pilonidal sinus. J. Surg. Oncol., 27:239, 1984.
34. Mallory, F. B.: Sacro-coccygeal dimples, sinuses, and cyst. Am. J. Med. Sci., 103:263, 1982.
35. Marie, T. J., Aylward, D., Keer, E., and Haldene, E. V.: Bacteriology of pilonidal cyst abscesses. J. Clin. Pathol., 31:909, 1978.
36. Marks, J., Hughes, L. E., Harding, K. G., Campbell, H., and Ribeiro, C. D.: Pilonidal sinus excision—healing by open granulation. Br. J. Surg., 72:637, 1985.
37. Mayo, H.: Observations on Injuries and Diseases of the Rectum. London, Burgess & Hill, 1833.
38. Norris, C. S.: Giant condyloma acuminatum (Buschke-Lowenstein tumor)

involving a pilonidal sinus: A case report and review of the literature. J. Surg. Oncol., 22:47, 1983.

39. Page, G. H.: The entry of hair into a pilonidal sinus. Br. J. Surg., 56:32, 1969.

40. Palmer, W. H.: Pilonidal disease: A new concept of pathogenesis. Dis. Colon Rectum, 2:303, 1959.

41. Patey, D. H., and Scharff, R. W.: Pathology of postanal pilonidal sinus: Its bearing on treatment. Lancet, 2:484, 1946.

42. Puckett, C. L., and Silver, D.: Carcinoma developing in pilonidal sinus: Report of two cases and review of the literature. Am. Surg., 39:151, 1973.

43. Salvati, E. P.: Symposium on outpatient anorectal procedures: Pilonidal disease. Can. J. Surg., 28:225, 1985.

44. Smith, R. M.: Roentgen irradiation as an adjunct to surgical treatment of pilonidal cyst. Am. J. Roentgenol., 38:308, 1937.

45. Søndenaa, K., Andersen, E., Nesvik, I., and Søreide, J. A.: Patient characteristics and symptoms in chronic pilonidal sinus disease. Int. J. Colorect. Dis. 10:39, 1995.

46. Toubanakis, G.: Treatment of pilonidal sinus disease with the Z-plasty procedure (modified). Am. Surg., 52:611, 1986.

47. Walsh, T. H., and Mann, C. V.: Pilonidal sinuses of the anal canal. Br. J. Surg., 70:23, 1983.

48. Warren, J. M.: Abscess containing hair on the nates. Am. J. Med. Sci., 55:113, 1854.

CHAPTER 41

NEUROSURGERY

I

HISTORICAL ASPECTS

Robert H. Wilkins, M.D.

American students who are interested in the history of neurosurgery have a unique advantage. This specialty is of relatively recent origin and has been developed mainly in the English-speaking countries. For this reason, classic works in neurosurgery are usually obtainable and understandable.[6, 7] In addition, there are several excellent reviews of neurosurgical history written in English.[2–5, 7] These reviews emphasize the fact that although the great majority of neurosurgical procedures have been developed recently, the history of trepanation dates back to the Neolithic period of the Stone Age. In widely separated geographic locations, archeologists have discovered human skulls containing craniectomy defects. Moreover, in many of these skulls, there is evidence of healing along the bony edges, indicating that the *patient* survived the operation. The rationale for these procedures is not known, because there are no written records from this era, but it is conceivable that skull deformities, injuries, or headaches might have led to this drastic form of treatment.

The oldest known writing concerning surgical topics, the *Edwin Smith Papyrus*, is of special interest to neurosurgeons. This treatise dates back to the seventeenth century B.C. and contains the first descriptions of the cranial sutures, meninges, external surface of the brain, cerebrospinal fluid, and intracranial pulsations. Brain injuries are related to changes in the function of other parts of the body, and hemiplegic contractures are well described. In addition, quadriplegia, urinary incontinence, and priapism are noted to occur in association with cervical vertebral dislocation. The Egyptian physicians of that period had a surprising knowledge of rudimentary neuroanatomy and neurophysiology, but their treatment of injuries of the central nervous system was only supportive. Significantly, trepanation is not mentioned in the *Edwin Smith Papyrus*.

The writings of Hippocrates contain the first recorded descriptions of trepanation, and his instruments and methods were very similar to their modern counterparts. In addition, Hippocrates considered other subjects of neurosurgical interest. He discussed epilepsy, the coexistence of spinal deformity and pulmonary tubercles, and the functional effects of compression of the spinal cord. He devised a method for reducing vertebral dislocations and described permanent and transient facial paralysis, sciatica, and the complex of headache, visual disturbances, and vomiting. Hippocrates' ability as an observer is well demonstrated by his descriptions of aphasia, unconsciousness, respiratory and cardiac irregularity, carphologia, pupillary inequality, and ophthalmoplegia associated with cerebral disease. He realized that a blow on one side of the head is occasionally followed by convulsions or paralysis of the contralateral side of the body, and he recognized the poor prognosis of a patient with a head injury complicated by a dural laceration. These and other observations made Hippocrates' contributions a beacon to surgeons for over 2000 years, until the development of anesthesia, asepsis, and the concept of cerebral localization in the nineteenth century established the foundation of modern neurosurgery.

The introduction of anesthesia and asepsis vastly increased the scope of surgery in general and made brain surgery feasible. Such operations were not performed often, however, because of the inability to locate lesions that did not involve the skull. The problem was resolved by the discovery of Bouillaud, Broca, Fritsch, Hitzig, Ferrier, and others that there is focal representation of bodily function in the brain. This third fundamental concept—cerebral localization—became an important part of the foundation upon which modern neurosurgery was established.[3]

Another vital advancement made during the late nineteenth century was the development of the technique of osteoplastic craniotomy by Wagner, which was later facilitated by the use of Gigli's wire saw. The introduction of this technique permitted the exploration of relatively large areas of cortex and, in so doing, significantly extended the limits of brain surgery.

British surgeons were among the first to take advantage of these new developments, and they guided neurosurgery through its infancy in the last two decades of the nineteenth century. William Macewen, professor of surgery at the University of Glasgow and a powerful figure in international surgical circles, was a pioneer in surgical therapy of the central nervous system. Macewen was a pupil of Joseph Lister, and he strongly believed in Lister's principles of antisepsis. His phenomenal success in treating intracranial abscesses was rarely equaled, despite the subsequent use of antibiotics, until the introduction of computed tomography scanning, which allows earlier and more accurate treatment.

Godlee also applied Lister's principles of antisepsis to neurosurgery in 1884, when he became the first surgeon to resect an intracranial tumor that had been localized solely by neurologic means. Bennett was another pioneering British surgeon. In 1888 he introduced the operation of posterior rhizotomy for the relief of pain.

The most outstanding surgeon in this field at the time, however, was Victor Horsley of London. He devoted the majority of his efforts to clinical and experimental neurosurgery, with exceptional results. Although he made myriad contributions, Horsley is best remembered today as the first surgeon to remove a neoplasm from the spinal canal (1887) and the first to attempt retrogasserian neurotomy for tic douloureux (1890). He and Clarke also described a stereotactic apparatus for intracranial procedures in 1908.

During the early development of neurosurgery, it was common for a neurologist to diagnose the disease, devise the operation, and direct the surgeon in its performance. For example, Hughes Bennett localized the brain tumor that was removed in 1884 by Rickman Godlee, and William Gowers diagnosed the spinal tumor that was removed by Victor Horsley in 1887. In the United States, similar situations were encountered frequently. William Spiller, at the University of Pennsylvania, directed Charles Frazier in the performance of a successful retrogasserian neurotomy in 1901, and 10 years later he directed Edward Martin in the performance of the first cordotomy. Similarly, Charles Dana at the Cornell University Medical College proposed posterior rhizotomy, which was performed a short time later by William Bennett in London and Robert Abbe in New York. Two outstanding neurologists of a later generation, Otfrid Foerster in Germany and Clovis Vincent in France, actually became neurosurgeons to facilitate the procedures they recommended. Foerster independently devised the operation of cordotomy; he also performed classic studies of human cortical function and peripheral sensory innervation during operations that he performed to treat epilepsy or pain.

A host of general surgeons attempted neurosurgical procedures during the formative years at the turn of the century. Most were soon discouraged by the innumerable difficulties accompanying this type of surgical therapy. For example, more than 500 surgeons reported performing brain operations between 1886 and 1896, but the number fell below 80 between 1896 and 1906.

Fortunately, during this time a young surgeon at Johns Hopkins Hospital became interested in neurosurgery and decided to devote his full attention to it. With little assistance, Harvey Cushing advanced neurosurgery from its infancy through its childhood.[1] He standardized operative technique and, by applying the rigid principles of William Halsted to neurosurgical procedures, was able to reduce operative morbidity and mortality significantly. Prior to this time, hemorrhage presented an almost insurmountable problem during brain surgery. In his typically thorough manner, Cushing mastered the techniques of compressing the scalp, waxing the diploë, and other approaches, and then introduced the vessel clips and electrocautery that have become indispensable in the control of intracranial and intraspinal bleeding.

Brain tumors also attracted Cushing's attention, and during the course of his career, more than 2000 patients with brain tumors were seen in his clinic. With the aid of several brilliant assistants, including Percival Bailey and Louise Eisenhardt, Cushing classified these tumors morphologically, described their biologic behavior, and formulated their surgical treatment. The standardization of technique and the classification of brain tumors were only two of Cushing's many contributions. There are few areas of modern neurosurgical interest that are not based to some extent on the important investigations of this one man.

Another such giant was Walter Dandy. He worked with Cushing for a short time at Johns Hopkins before the latter moved to the Peter Bent Brigham Hospital. Dandy remained at Johns Hopkins, and before he finished his residency in surgery, he made two important discoveries. In association with Kenneth Blackfan, he established the modern concept of hydrocephalus and developed the operations of choroid plexectomy and third ventriculostomy for the relief of communicating and obstructive hydrocephalus. A few years later, in 1918 and 1919, he introduced pneumoventriculography and pneumoencephalography, which proved to be of inestimable diagnostic value to neurosurgeons. As was true of Cushing, Dandy's contributions to neurosurgery were legion, and he profoundly influenced the subsequent course of modern neurosurgery.

A third such contributor was the Portuguese neurologist Antonio Egas Moniz. Moniz was unusually talented in a number of fields besides medicine, but he still found time to produce more than 300 medical publications. With neurosurgeon Pedro de Almeida Lima, he introduced the diagnostic technique of carotid arteriography in 1927 and initiated prefrontal lobotomy for psychiatric illness in 1936. For the latter work, Moniz received a Nobel Prize in 1949.

Despite the outstanding work of Cushing, Dandy, and Moniz, most advancements in neurosurgery have been made slowly by the patient efforts of many pioneers. The subsequent developments in the various areas of neurosurgery are outlined in the remainder of this chapter.

SELECTED REFERENCES

Walker, A. E.: History of Neurological Surgery. Baltimore, Williams & Wilkins, 1951.
This book is the standard history of neurosurgery, with 18 chapters on various aspects of the specialty by 12 contributors. It also contains 14 biographic sketches of pioneering neurosurgeons and a bibliography containing 2371 references.

Wilkins, R. H.: Neurosurgical Classics. New York, Johnson Reprint Corp., 1965. Reprinted in 1992 (see below).
This is a collection of 52 of the most outstanding written contributions in the field of neurologic surgery prior to 1940. These have been compiled into 38 groups, each of which is accompanied by a commentary and a list of related references. The 15 works originally printed in other languages have been translated into English.

REFERENCES

1. Fulton, J. F.: Harvey Cushing: A Biography. Springfield, Ill., Charles C Thomas, 1946.
2. Goodrich, J. T.: Landmarks in the history of neurosurgery. In Rengachary, S. S., and Wilkins, R. H. (Eds.): Principles of Neurosurgery. London, Wolfe, 1994, p. 1.1.
3. Green, J. R.: The concept of cerebral and spinal localization and the beginnings of neurological surgery. In Wilkins, R. H., and Rengachary, S. S. (Eds): Neurosurgery, 2nd ed. New York, McGraw-Hill, 1996, p. 3.
4. Scarff, J. E.: Fifty years of neurosurgery, 1905–1955. Int. Abstr. Surg., 101:417, 1955.
5. Walker, A. E.: History of Neurological Surgery. Baltimore, Williams & Wilkins, 1951.
6. Wilkins, R. H.: Neurosurgical Classics. Park Ridge, Ill., American Association of Neurological Surgeons, 1992.
7. Wilkins, R. H.: History of neurosurgery. In Wilkins, R. H., and Rengachary, S. S. (Eds): Neurosurgery, 2nd ed. New York, McGraw-Hill, 1996, p. 25.

II

NEURORADIOLOGY

Robert D. Tien, M.D., M.P.H.

In addition to plain films of the skull, sinuses, and spine, cerebral and spinal angiography, myelography, and pneumoencephalography, computed tomographic (CT) scanning has become the most important diagnostic modality in neuroradiology since its development in 1974. The advent of CT brought about a dramatic change in the evaluation of neurologic diseases and is able to visualize most disease processes of the brain and spine noninvasively. The addition of magnetic resonance imaging (MRI) further refined and expanded noninvasive neurologic imaging for the diagnostic evaluation of neurologic diseases. These noninvasive, advanced imaging modalities have made invasive and painful procedures such as pneumoencephalogram unnecessary. Today, diagnostic neuroradiologic examinations available for the evaluation of neurologic diseases include plain films of the skull, sinuses, and spine, water-soluble myelography, cerebral angiography, CT, and MRI.

PLAIN FILMS

At present, plain films are not very valuable in the evaluation of intracerebral diseases. Plain films may still be useful in detecting facial fractures or diseases of paranasal sinuses.

MYELOGRAPHY

Noninvasive procedures such as CT and MRI have taken the place of myelography in the evaluation of many neurologic diseases. Myelography is still performed, however, to evaluate diffuse disease of the subarachnoid space that may be difficult to identify on MRI or CT, such as diffuse subarachnoid seeding of tumor. Another situation in which a myelogram may be required is when the clinician cannot determine the exact level of disease involvement, often because it is too time-consuming or difficult to use MRI for the whole spine.

CEREBRAL ANGIOGRAPHY

Cerebral angiography is an invasive procedure with a 0.5 to 2% complication rate. CT scanning and MRI have taken over many of its former functions, but cerebral angiography remains an important or definitive examination in the evaluation of intracerebral aneurysm, arteriovenous malformation, vasculitis, vessel displacement or encasement by tumor when not readily apparent on CT or MRI, and atherosclerotic disease of the carotid bifurcation, as well as for intravascular neurointerventional procedures, such as embolization of feeding vessels responsible for uncontrollable bleeding, hypervascular tumor, or cerebral arteriovenous malformation.

In addition to conventional cerebral angiography, which employs routine radiographic film exposure and is used when fine radiographic detail in the work-up for cerebral aneurysm is required, digital subtraction angiography (DSA) has been developed over the past decade. DSA uses digital imaging with computer-assisted enhancement of images and is helpful when fine anatomic detail is not required, such as in the work-up for carotid artery disease.

COMPUTED TOMOGRAPHY

CT is a method of x-ray evaluation in which a thin slice or planar volume of tissues is examined. The patient is placed on a table inside the CT scanning machine, which records digitalized data from cross sections of variable thickness of the head and spine with the aid of a computer. Scans can be obtained at direct axial or coronal planes. Manipulation of controls on the computer console allows visualization of tissues on soft tissue or bone windows. With computer assistance, CT can differentiate various components of soft tissues in the brain such as gray matter, white matter, and cerebrospinal fluid (CSF). On plain films, these components have the same radiographic density and are therefore indistinguishable.

In interpreting the brain CT scan, it is important to visualize both the lesion itself and the surrounding soft tissue being affected by the abnormality. In addition, the position of the lesion should be localized in the brain or spine as best as possible, for example, intra-axial versus extra-axial (a lesion located within versus outside the brain parenchyma or spinal cord). On CT, two types of edema appear as more lucent areas than normal brain parenchyma. Cytotoxic edema is related to cell death from ischemia, such as in infarction, with increased intracellular water content. An infarct appearing as a lucency on the CT scan frequently corresponds to a vascular distribution and may involve both gray and white matter. Vasogenic edema (also termed interstitial or white matter edema) reflects increased water content in the interstitium and is nearly confined to the white matter. Vasogenic edema is usually associated with tumors, abscesses, hematomas, or other masses. Many tumors cause associated vasogenic edema and mass effect. Indeed, the associated findings, rather than the lesion itself, may be responsible for the symptoms.

Brain CT can be performed with or without iodinated contrast enhancement. A non-contrast-enhanced study is best in most acute situations; however, a contrast-enhanced study is usually necessary in chronic situations. In most acute situations, the clinical concern is either intracerebral hemorrhage or infarction. On a non-contrast-enhanced study, hemorrhage appears hyperdense (white) and is usually obvious. Calcification can also be detected easily on a non-contrast-enhanced study as a hyperdense area. Therefore, contrast administration is not necessary for the visualization of hemorrhage or calcification. Most acute infarcts appear as a lucency (darker gray or black) and do not show any contrast enhancement for 1 to 2 weeks. Therefore, any change that an infarct demonstrates acutely is apparent on a non-contrast-enhanced study. In chronic neurologic disease, such as tumor (primary tumor and metastasis) or abscess, the definition of the lesion can be obtained only on a contrast-enhanced study. The abnormal enhancement exhibited by intra-axial tumors and abscesses is caused by breakdown of the blood-brain barrier. Metastases and abscesses frequently appear as sharply marginated, noncalcified nodules or ring-enhancing lesions with massive white matter edema. They are often located peripherally in areas supplied by the large vessels, because most of them are spreading hematogenously. Primary brain tumors tend to be less well marginated, irregularly enhancing lesions, with or without calcification and white matter edema, which may be central or peripheral. Distinguishing a primary brain tumor from metastasis or abscess is not always possible.

CT scans of the spine without contrast are useful in examining lumbar disc disease, degenerative spinal disease, and spinal trauma. However, in the evaluation of cervical and thoracic disc disease or with involvement of the intraspinal contents by tumor, whether from metastatic disease or primary tumor of the spinal sac contents, opacification of the subarachnoid space on CT after intrathecal administration of water-soluble contrast via lumbar puncture is often necessary (the CT-myelogram). Contrast-enhanced CT scans of the spine may aid in differentiating herniated disc from scar material (a herniated disc is not enhanced; a scar is enhanced) and in defining an epidural abscess in the spine.

In addition, CT scans can be applied in paranasal sinus diseases, particularly for the evaluation of tumors in this region and as an aid to a functional endoscopic sinus procedure. CT is also useful for the location and staging of lesions of the base of the skull, particularly tumors, temporal bone and inner ear lesions, and facial trauma, and laryngeal and other neck and upper airway tumors.

Advances in CT Technology

Volume Scanning (Spiral CT, Helical CT). Progress in the field of CT has led to the development of volume scanning. In this method of obtaining imaging data from CT, the patient is moved continuously through the scanning gantry synchronously with continuous data acquisition.[1] The x-ray tube and detector within the gantry are moved continuously in a spiral or helical pattern as the patient is moved through the imaging zone. A key benefit of this technology is the markedly reduced scanning time needed for the acquisition of information. Scans can be performed in a single breath hold, with the elimination of motion-induced artifacts. The amount of contrast needed is also decreased, which increases patient safety and decreases cost. Because a volume of information is collected, reformatting images or three-dimensional reconstructions are smoother and more accurate. These changes have enabled the performance of accurate CT angiography.

Computed Tomography Angiography (CTA). The most accurate assessment of the carotid bifurcation remains carotid angiography. However, carotid angiography is an expensive and invasive procedure. Noninvasive techniques such as duplex and color Doppler sonography are operator dependent and may underdiagnose distal plaque or may yield a false diagnosis of carotid occlusion. Magnetic resonance angiography (MRA) has also been used to evaluate the carotid bifurcation, but it can overestimate the degree of carotid stenosis because of the turbulence dephasing at points of stenosis or irregularity. Recent advances in CT and in three-dimensional display have led to new vascular imaging methods that may overcome some of the limitations of sonography and MRI. The volume data obtained on spiral or helical CT can be reconstructed to produce a three-dimensional representation of the anatomic region scanned. Vascular structures can be selectively imaged by the use of a bolus intravenous infusion of contrast material. The potential utility of spiral CT with contrast is in imaging the carotid bifurcation and in evaluating aneurysms and other vascular malformations of the brain. The initial work comparing carotid CTA with conventional carotid angiography showed that the degree of carotid stenosis determined by CTA correlated with the carotid angiogram in 92% of cases.

MAGNETIC RESONANCE IMAGING

MRI is a relatively new development that is significantly different from other modalities of radiographic imaging. Certain abnormalities that cannot be detected on CT scans are evident on MRI because the information obtained by MRI reflects different properties of tissues (magnetic properties of the tissues versus their ability to attenuate irradiation). Therefore, CT and MRI have different sensitivities for detecting disease processes. Two types of images are traditionally included in an MRI examination. T1-weighted images are used to obtain anatomic detail. On these images, CSF is dark (hypointense) and fat is very bright (hyperintense). Abnormal contrast enhancement is also clearly demonstrated on T1 contrast-enhanced images. T2-weighted images demonstrate the water-related contents (CSF) as hyperintense and fat as relatively hypointense. Anatomy on T2 sequences is less well demonstrated than on T1 sequences, but T2 sequences are more sensitive in detecting focal abnormality. The contrast used with MRI is gadolinium chelating agent (Gd-DTPA), a paramagnetic substance administered intravenously that affects the magnetic properties of the tissues that accumulate the contrast. Gadolinium is different from iodinated contrast and has few of the systemic effects.

MRI has proved to be a better modality than CT scanning in the evaluation of disease of the central nervous system, such as diseases at the base of the skull, particularly the sellar and cerebellopontine angle cistern regions, and also for most tumors, white matter disease (e.g., multiple sclerosis), congenital abnormalities, vascular malformations, and spinal diseases (Fig. 41–1). This is mostly due to the absence of bone and dental artifacts on MRI, which are commonly seen in CT, as well as the presence of multiplanar images (sagittal, coronal, axial, and oblique) and MRI's high sensitivity for disease processes. However, CT is still better than MRI in the evaluation of patients with acute intracerebral hemorrhage, acute head trauma, subarachnoid hemorrhage, or disease processes requiring analysis with fine bone detail, such as facial or spinal fractures. Calcification is also poorly identified on all sequences of MRI. In addition, for patients who cannot cooperate for relatively long periods of time required for MRI or who have certain types of metal in their bodies (which may move because of susceptibility to the magnetic field and cause injury to the patient or significant artifact), CT scanning remains the better option. Consultation with a radiologist is often useful in determining which examination is the most appropriate for each patient.

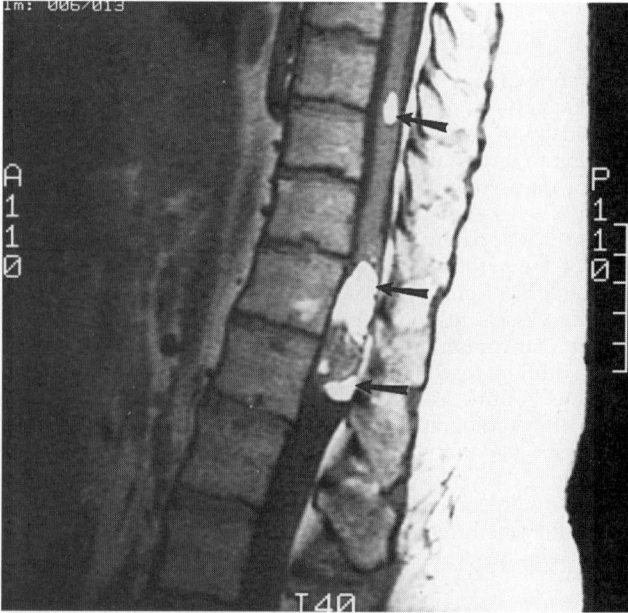

Figure 41–1. Teratomas of the spinal cord are well delineated on T1-weighted MRI without contrast. The high-intensity component of the tumors (arrows) is caused by the presence of fat contents.

Advances in MRI Pulse Sequence Design

There are many new MRI pulse sequences. The following two pulse sequences are mentioned as examples because of their clinical usefulness.

Fast Spin Echo (FSE) MRI. FSE is a pulse sequence technique that has recently been developed as an alternative to conventional spin echo (CSE) MRI sequences.[2, 3] The major advantage of this MRI pulse sequence is the marked reduction in acquisition time needed for long repetition time (TR) images; FSE images can be obtained in less than half the time required for CSE images. This significant time saving may be extremely useful when imaging uncooperative patients (infants, ill patients, etc.). FSE can be applied to both brain and spine studies.

Steady State Free Precession (SSFP). The MRI signal intensities of cystic masses of the brain on CSE images can be similar to the signal intensities of CSF. This is especially true on T2-weighted images. Using the SSFP technique,[4, 5] better lesion characterization is obtained compared with CSE images. With SSFP imaging, the signal intensities of all solid tissues are typically suppressed, leading to low signals from these tissues. However, the heavily T2-weighted SSFP images also show the high signal intensity fluid components of cystic masses, thereby differentiating solid from cystic (Fig. 41–2). Similarly, SSFP MRI can also distinguish between epidermoid and arachnoid cysts; epidermoid cysts appear to be of heterogeneous internal content, and arachnoid cysts have a homogeneous CSF-like internal signal. This may have implications for the surgeon planning the management of these lesions.

Advances in MRI Applications

MRI of the Hippocampus. The most frequent type of seizure is a complex partial seizure (CPS). In those patients with medically intractable CPS, mesial temporal sclerosis (MTS) is the most common pathologic abnormality, which is seen in approximately 60% to 80% of patients. Another 20% of patients have gross structural abnormalities such as tumor as the seizure focus. In cases of medically intractable CPS, surgical therapy (e.g., hippocampectomy) may be needed for seizure control. Before surgical therapy, accurate noninvasive evaluation of the seizure focus is essential. Recently developed FSE MRI has been shown to be useful in defining the anatomy and signal intensity of the hippocampus and in detecting both the atrophy and the signal abnormality associated with MTS (Fig. 41–3). The initial evaluation of FSE MRI has shown that this technique is both highly sensitive and specific (approaching 100%) in detecting MTS in this patient group.[6–8]

MRI in Hemifacial Spasm and Trigeminal Neuralgia. Hemifacial spasm and trigeminal neuralgia are frequently due to vascular loop compression by either the vertebral-basilar arteries or their branches.[9, 10] These disorders may be relieved by vascular decompression procedures. A new MRA technique has been developed that can better delineate the branches of the vertebral-basilar system. In this technique, a coronal three-dimensional time of flight MRA is obtained, centered on the vertebral-basilar system. The collapsed MRA is then superimposed on the routine spin echo T1-weighted images, which show the root entry zone of the seventh and eighth nerves and cisternal portions of the fifth nerve. With this technique, the compression is accurately identified, and a road map for the surgeon is obtained preoperatively.[11]

Diffusion-Weighted MRI. Diffusion-weighted MRI is an exciting new development and is sensitive to the microscopic motion of water protons (Brownian motion).[12–14] CSE MRI, conversely, is sensitive to the tissue water content and concentration. Initial applications of diffusion-weighted MRI have involved the imaging of early stroke and neoplasia, with increased sensitivity noted in the early detection of stroke. Early evidence also suggests that diffusion-weighted imaging can differentiate tumoral edema from tumor (Fig. 41–4); it can also distinguish necrotic tumor cells from living tumor cells and identify the nonenhancing part of the tumor. The implications for treatment evaluation and prognosis are obvious. Other possible areas of use include white matter diseases and multiple sclerosis.

MRA. Conventional angiography remains the definitive technique for evaluating cerebrovascular disease. New developments in MRI pulse sequences, however, have significantly improved the utility of MRA in the noninvasive evaluation of vascular structures. The identification of vasculature by MRA is achieved by showing the contrast between moving blood and stationary tissues. Both time of flight (TOF) effects and phase contrast (PC) effects can be exploited to generate an MRA. Currently there are four established MRA techniques available: two- and three-dimensional TOF, and two- and three-dimensional PC. All these techniques have different aspects that must be understood for both effective diagnosis and interpretation.

Two-dimensional TOF is useful in the carotid bifurcation, where a large volume of tissue must be scanned in a clinically acceptable time frame. A new application has been preoperative cortical venous mapping to localize major venous tributaries overlying areas of tumor. Three-dimensional TOF is the technique of choice when imaging small volumes that require high resolution. A frequent application is in the study of the circle of Willis for aneurysm evaluation. When compared with TOF, the major advantage of two- and three-dimensional PC techniques is the extreme degree of stationary tissue suppression, including methemoglobin or fat, which could confuse the interpretation of TOF images. These techniques are extremely useful in the setting of venous thrombosis. Determination of velocity is also possible with PC techniques.

Three-Dimensional Vessel Surface Rendering. This process creates three-dimensional images from the routine MRA (Fig. 41–5) by the use of perspective and shadowing to allow definite distinction of superimposed vascular structures, which are difficult to identify on routine MRA.

Magnetic Resonance Spectroscopy. With recent improvements in coil design and the resultant improved magnetic field homogeneity, it has become possible to perform high-resolution spectroscopy in addition to MRI. With MRI spectroscopy, metabolites within a selected region of interest can be investigated, and spectral peaks that reflect concentrations of the metabolite within the region of interest can be obtained. Metabolites such as lactate, amino acids (e.g., NAA [N-acetyl aspartate], a neuronal integrity marker), and phosphorus metabolites (e.g., adenosine triphosphate), can be measured noninvasively.[15–18] A multitude of projects are now under way to investigate spectroscopy in various neurologic applications. Reductions in the NAA level have been shown in multiple sclerosis plaques, MTS, ischemic brain lesions (Fig. 41–6), and brain tumors.

Dynamic MRI of the Lumbar Spine. MRI has the ability to define normal age-related changes in the vertebral marrow of the axial skeleton and has become the procedure of choice in evaluating many bone marrow disorders, including metastatic disease.[19, 20] However, CSE sequences have difficulty differentiating between malignancy and other causes of abnormal vertebral body signal, including inflammation, degenerative disease, and trauma (e.g., a new compression fracture versus a metastatic lesion in a patient with known primary carcinoma). A new technique called fast-SPGR (spoiled gradients-recalled acquisition in the steady state) pulse sequences with bolus gadolinium contrast infusion has

Text continued on page 1344

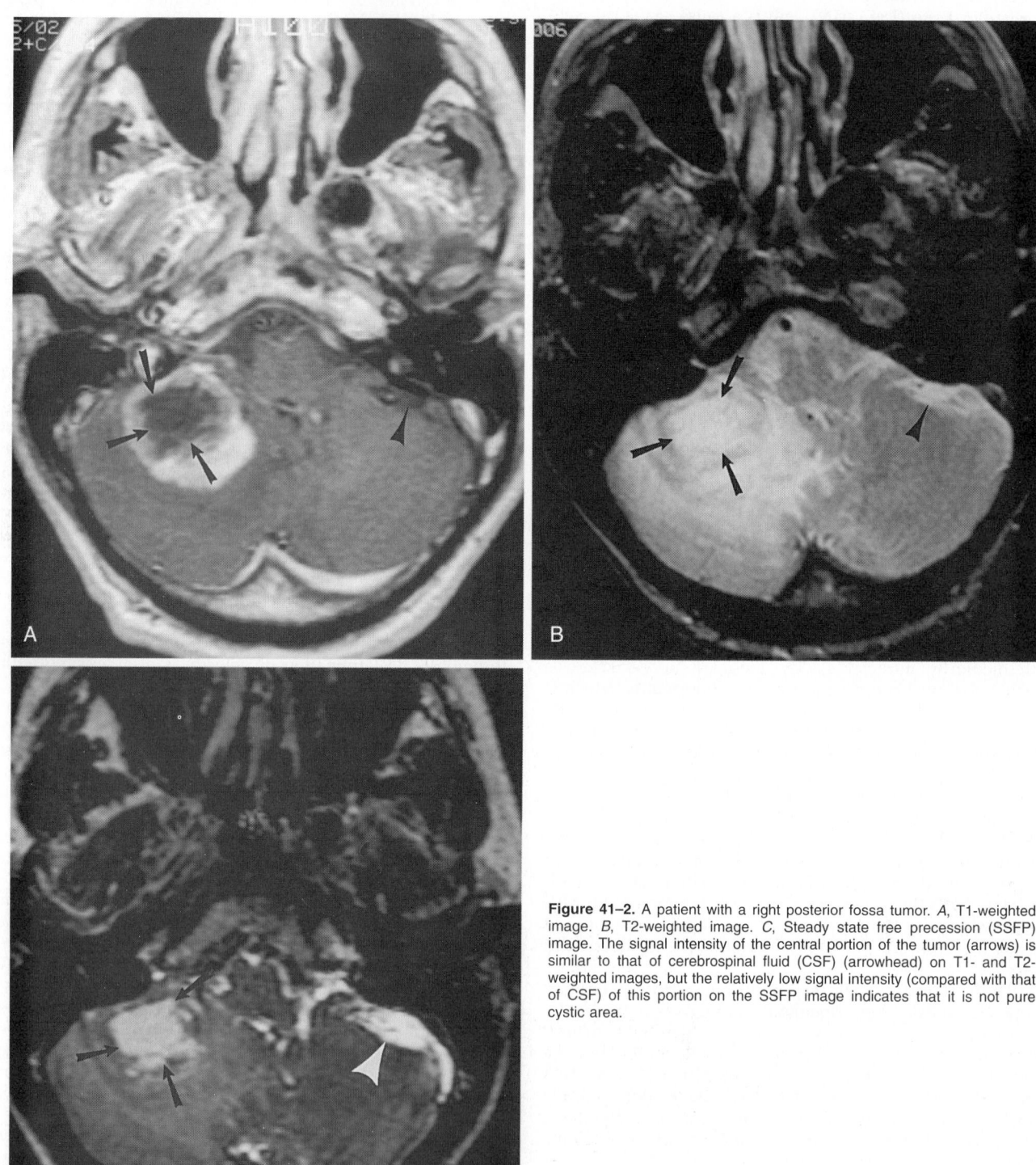

Figure 41–2. A patient with a right posterior fossa tumor. *A*, T1-weighted image. *B*, T2-weighted image. *C*, Steady state free precession (SSFP) image. The signal intensity of the central portion of the tumor (arrows) is similar to that of cerebrospinal fluid (CSF) (arrowhead) on T1- and T2-weighted images, but the relatively low signal intensity (compared with that of CSF) of this portion on the SSFP image indicates that it is not pure cystic area.

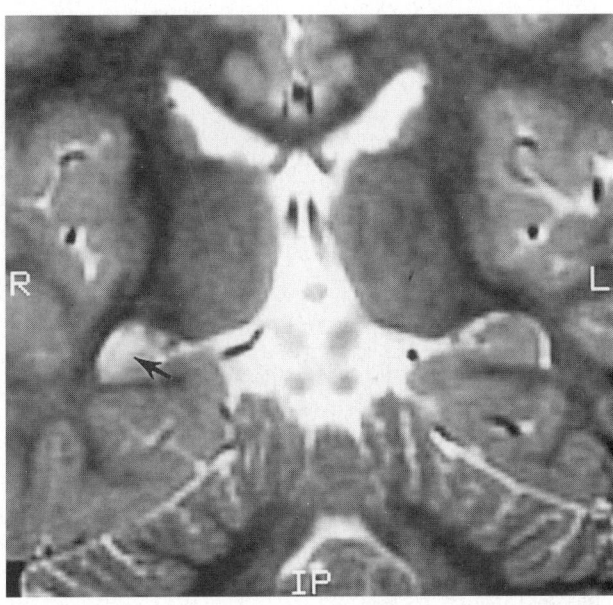

Figure 41–3. Oblique coronal fast spin echo MRI of the hippocampi of a patient with a left-side complex partial seizure shows decreased size of and increased signal in the right hippocampus (arrow). After hippocampectomy, the pathologic diagnosis is mesial temporal sclerosis.

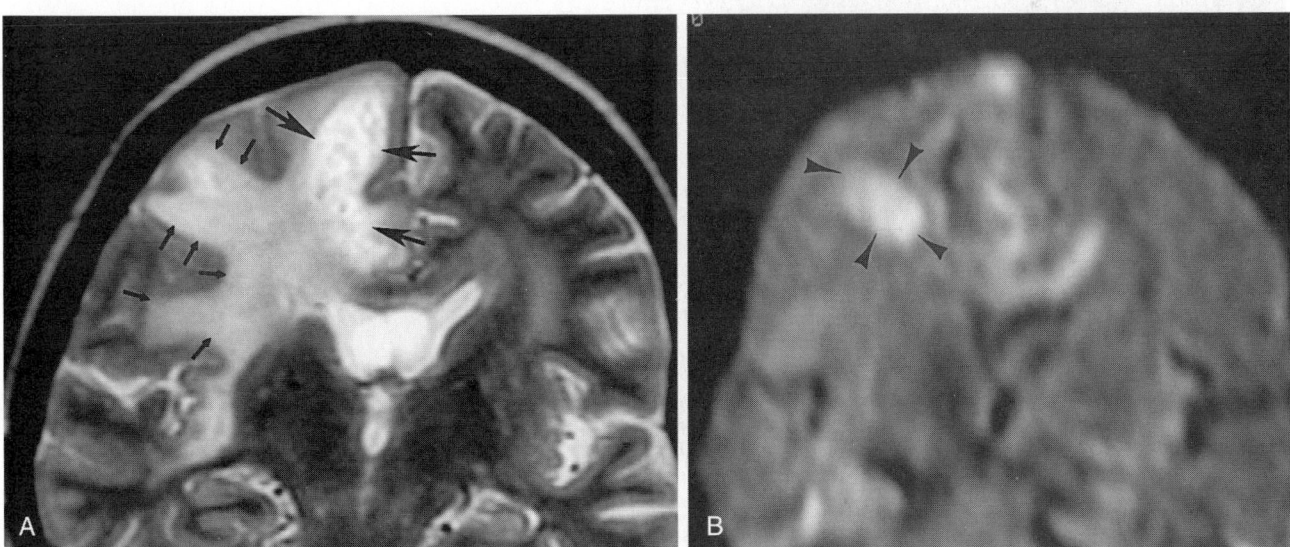

Figure 41–4. A patient with a glioblastoma multiforme. *A,* The T2-weighted image shows only the necrotic part of the tumor (large arrows) and peritumoral edema (small arrows). *B,* The solid parts of the tumor (arrowheads) are well demonstrated on the diffusion-weighted image.

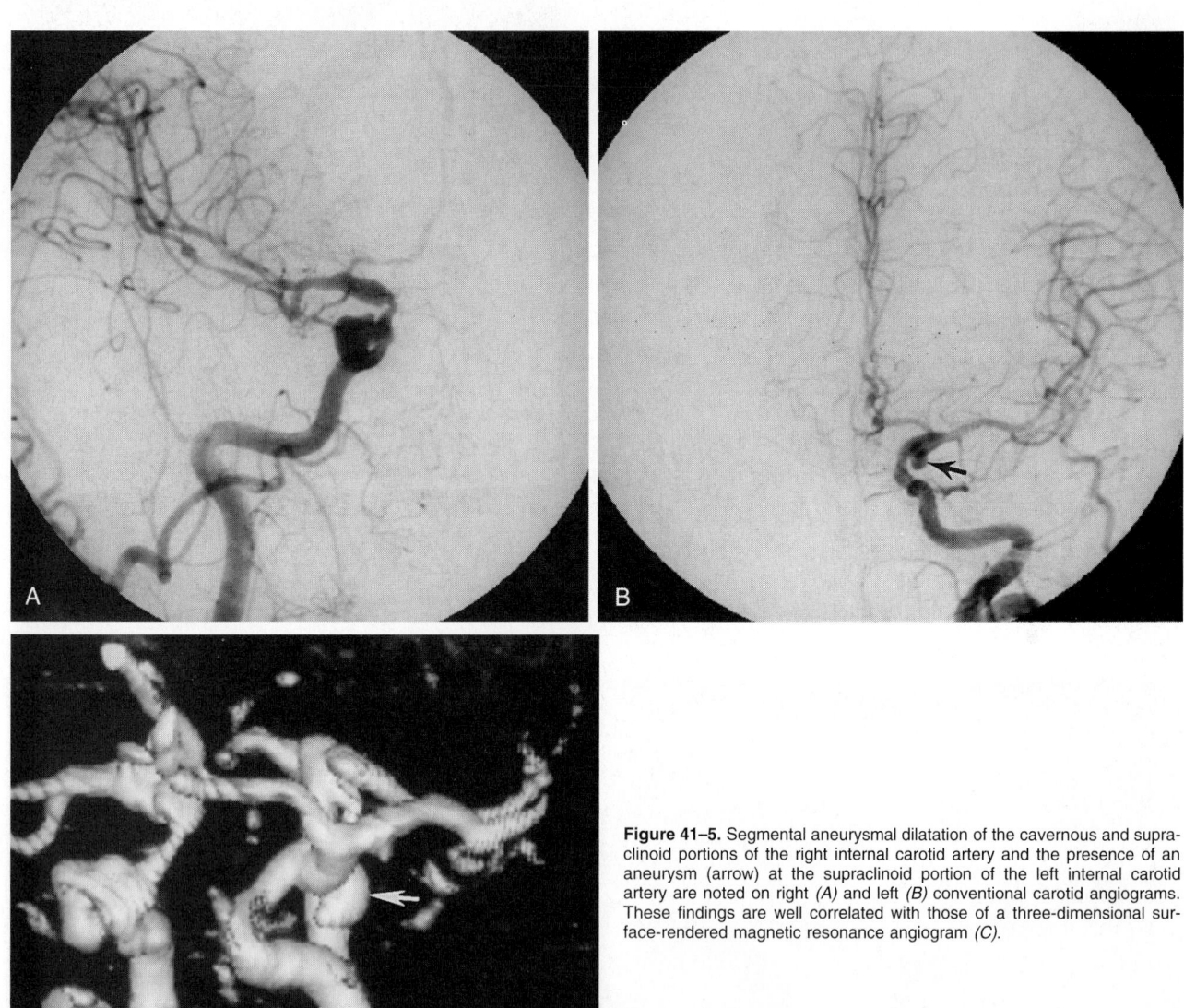

Figure 41–5. Segmental aneurysmal dilatation of the cavernous and supra-clinoid portions of the right internal carotid artery and the presence of an aneurysm (arrow) at the supraclinoid portion of the left internal carotid artery are noted on right *(A)* and left *(B)* conventional carotid angiograms. These findings are well correlated with those of a three-dimensional sur-face-rendered magnetic resonance angiogram *(C)*.

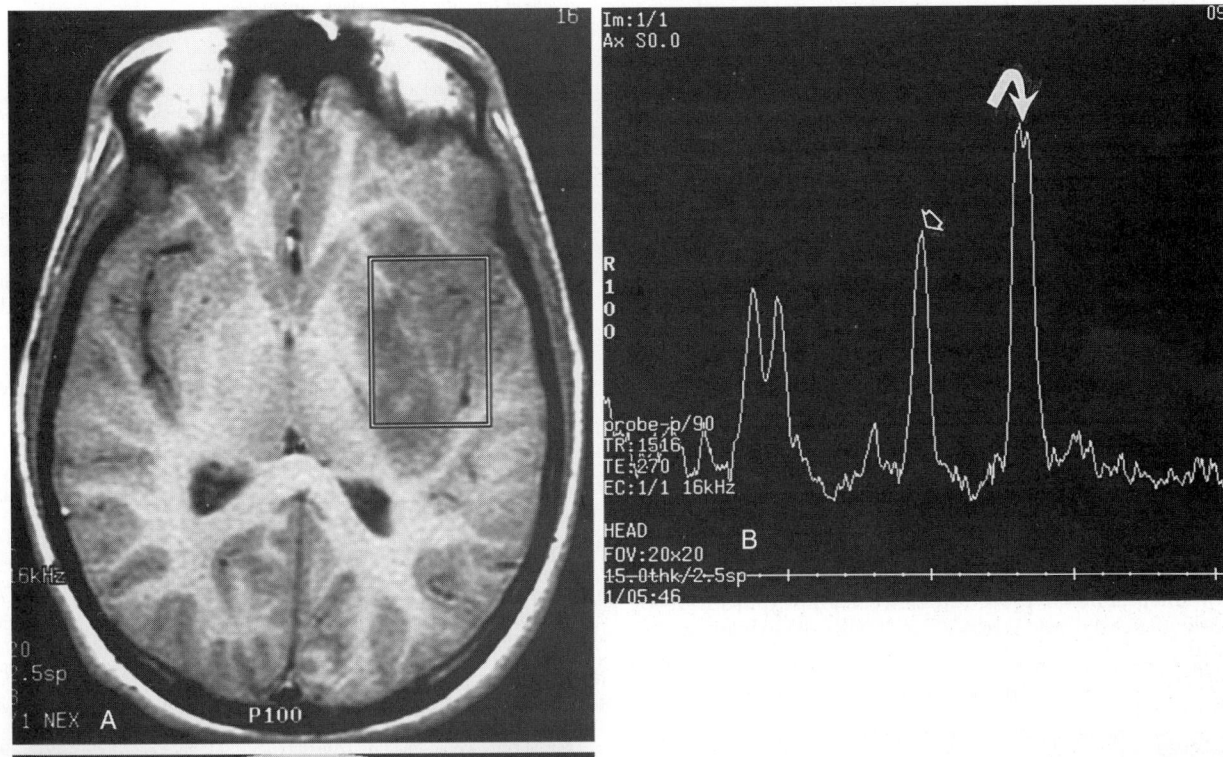

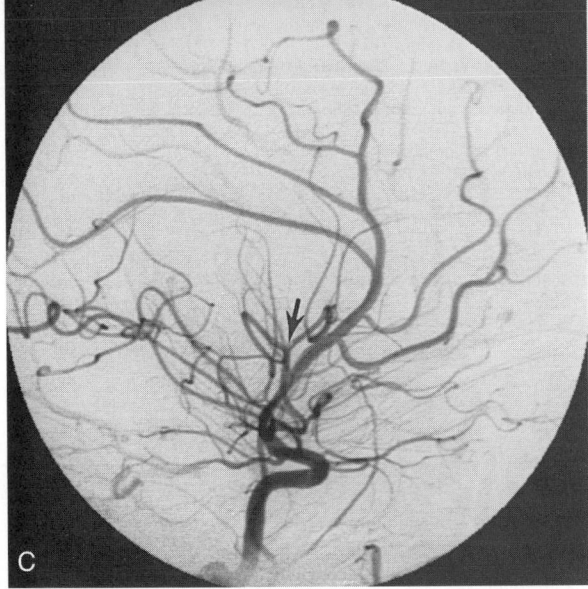

Figure 41–6. A 16-year-old patient with a young stroke. *A,* The spin echo MRI shows infarction of the left middle cerebral artery (MCA) territory. *B,* Magnetic resonance spectroscopy demonstrates a decreased amount of *N*-acetyl aspartate (arrow) and a markedly increased amount of lactate (curved arrow), indicating the change of infarction. *C,* The cerebral angiogram shows emboli in the branches of left MCA (arrow) and absence of a branch called the precentral sulcus artery.

been extremely useful in such cases. Initial outcomes indicate that most malignant processes causing vertebral body pathologic compression show abnormal enhancement early during the sequence of images, followed by a gradual decline in enhancement intensity over the time period studied. This differs from the findings in benign, osteoporotic compression fractures, which show no abnormal enhancement during the sequence of images. The identification of this marked difference between normal and abnormal marrow using this pulse sequence has clearly improved the detection of pathologic compression fractures.

Kinematic MRI of the Cervical Spine. MRI can also provide kinematic studies of the spine, although the motion must be able to be performed within the fairly narrow confines of the MRI gantry. The preliminary experience with cervical spine kinematic studies shows that this technique is useful, particularly for evaluating the amount of canal compromise in patients with disease involving the craniovertebral junction.

SUMMARY

Neuroradiologic imaging was greatly altered with the advent of CT and MRI, which provide quick, noninvasive, and accurate modalities for identifying pathologic conditions in the central nervous system. MRI provides better anatomic information and has greater sensitivity for diseases, but CT is frequently adequate for the evaluation of acute neurologic events and bone details. Cerebral angiography is reserved for specific diagnostic problems, such as the evaluation of cerebral aneurysms, carotid artery disease, and vasculitis, and for interventional procedures. Myelography has a significantly decreased role when CT and MRI are available.

SELECTED REFERENCES

Atlas, S. W.: Magnetic Resonance Imaging of the Brain and Spine. New York, Raven Press, 1991.
  This textbook is the best single volume devoted to MRI of the brain and spine and is the one most frequently read by neuroradiologists.

Lee, S. H., Rao, K. C. V. G., and Zimmerman, R. A.: Cranial MRI and CT. New York, McGraw-Hill, 1992.
  Of the several textbooks available on cranial CT, this is the most detailed and the one most worth reading.

Osborn, A. G.: Introduction to Cerebral Angiography. Philadelphia, Harper & Row, 1980.
  Although this book was written several years ago, it remains an excellent introductory text to cerebral angiography for every radiologist.

Osborn, A. G.: Diagnostic Neuroradiology. St. Louis, Mosby-Year Book, 1994.
  This textbook is the best and newest single volume devoted to diagnostic neuroradiology.

Som, P. M., and Bergeron, R. T.: Head and Neck Imaging. St. Louis, Mosby-Year Book, 1991.
  This textbook is the best single volume devoted to head and neck radiology.

REFERENCES

1. Vock, P., Jung, H., and Kalender, W.: Single-breath-hold spiral volumetric CT of the lung. Radiology, 176:864, 1990.
2. Hennig, J., Naureth, A., and Friedburg, H.: Rare imaging: A fast imaging method for clinical MR. Magn. Reson. Med., 3:823, 1986.
3. Tien, R. D., Felsberg, G. J., and MacFall, J.: Practical choices of fast spin echo sequence parameters: Clinically useful proton density and T2-weighted contrast. Neuroradiology, 35:38, 1992.
4. Tien, R. D., MacFall, J., and Heinz, E. R.: Evaluation of complex cystic masses of the brain: Value of steady state free-precession MR imaging. A.J.R. Am. J. Roentgenol., 159:1049, 1992.
5. Tien, R. D., Bernstein, M., and MacFall, J.: Pulsatile motion artifact reduction in 3-D steady-state-free precession-echo brain imaging. Magn. Reson. Imaging, 11:175, 1993.
6. Babb, T. L., and Brown, W. J.: Pathological findings in epilepsy. In Engel, J., Jr. (Ed.): Surgical Treatment of the Epilepsies, Vol. 5. New York, Raven Press, 1987, p. 511.
7. Tien, R. D., Felsberg, G. J., and Crain, B. J.: High resolution MR imaging of the normal human hippocampus. A.J.R. Am. J. Roentgenol., 159:1309, 1992.
8. Tien, R. D., Felsberg, G. J., de Castro, C. C., et al.: Complex partial seizures and mesial temporal sclerosis: Evaluation with fast spin-echo MR imaging. Radiology, 189:835, 1993.
9. Jannetta, P. J., Abbasy, M., Maroon, J. C., et al.: Etiology and definitive microsurgical treatment of hemifacial spasm: Operative techniques and results in 47 patients. J. Neurosurg., 47:321, 1991.
10. Wilkins, R. H.: Hemifacial spasm: A review. Surg. Neurol., 36:251, 1991.
11. Tien, R. D., and Wilkins, R. H.: MRA delineation of the vertebral-basilar system in patients with hemifacial spasm and trigeminal neuralgia. A.J.N.R., 14:34, 1993.
12. LeBihan, D., Breton, E., Lallemand, D., et al.: MR imaging of intravoxel incoherent motions: Applications to diffusion and perfusion in neurologic disorders. Radiology, 161:401, 1986.
13. Moseley, M. E., Kucharczyk, J., Mintorovitch, J., et al.: Diffusion-weighted MR imaging of acute stroke: Correlation with T2-weighted and magnetic susceptibility-enhanced MR imaging in cats. A.J.N.R., 11:423, 1990.
14. Henkelman, R. M.: Diffusion-weighted MR imaging: A useful adjunct to clinical diagnosis or a scientific curiosity? A.J.N.R. 11:932, 1990.
15. Husted, C. A., Duijn, J. H., Goodin, D. S., et al.: Normal appearing white matter changes in multiple sclerosis detected by proton and phosphorus MR spectroscopic imaging (Abstract). Soc. Magn. Res. Med., 1:1912, 1992.
16. Hugg, J. W., Laxer, K. D., Matson, G. B., et al.: H1 MR spectroscopic imaging detects neuron loss more sensitively than MRI in focal epilepsy (Abstract). Soc. Magn. Res. Med., 1:1913, 1992.
17. Knufman, N. M. J., Berkelbach van der Sprenkel, J. W., and Tulleken, C. A. F.: Differential diagnosis of ischemic cerebral disease by proton spectroscopic imaging (Abstract). Soc. Magn. Res. Med., 1:1910, 1992.
18. Lazeyras, F., Charles, H. C., Boyko, O., et al.: New perspectives in tumor grading by combined short echo/long echo 1H spectroscopic imaging (Abstract). Soc. Magn. Res. Med., 2:3604, 1992.
19. Ricci, C., Cove, M., Kang, Y. S., et al.: Normal age-related patterns of cellular and fatty bone marrow distribution in the axial skeleton: MR imaging study. Radiology, 177:83, 1990.
20. Daffner, R. H., Lupetin, A. R., Dash, M., et al.: MRI in the detection of malignant infiltration of bone marrow. A.J.R. Am. J. Roentgenol., 146:353, 1986.

III

INTRACRANIAL TUMORS

Robert H. Wilkins, M.D.

Primary intracranial tumors arise from tissues of the brain or pituitary gland or their coverings.[4, 5, 10, 13, 15–18] Often, these lesions are not clearly separable into benign and malignant forms. Some histologically benign pituitary adenomas, for example, may invade the adjacent dura mater and bone and grow into the cavernous sinus or the sphenoid sinus. As another example, the most histologically malignant of the astrocytomas, the glioblastoma multiforme, invades the brain locally but seldom spreads elsewhere.

Secondary intracranial tumors represent local extensions from regional tumors or metastases from primary malignancies elsewhere in the body.[4, 5, 10, 13, 15–18] Examples of regional tumors that can extend intracranially are chordomas and glomus jugulare paragangliomas. With regard to metastatic tumors, different malignancies vary in their propensity to metastasize to the brain and pituitary gland. Melanoma is especially prone to spread in this way. However, because carcinoma of the lung and carcinoma of the breast are more common lesions, these usually account for larger percentages of intracranial metastases in reported series.

The most common location of brain tumors in children is below the tentorium, within the posterior cranial fossa. In contrast, the most common location of brain tumors in adults is above the tentorium. Within the various intracranial locations, certain types of tumors occur more commonly than others, both in childhood (Fig. 41–7) and in adulthood (Fig. 41–8).

SYMPTOMS AND SIGNS

Intracranial tumors can present in several different ways. By their growth, they can cause an increase in intracranial pressure, either directly by the mass of the tumor or indirectly by obstructing the circulation of the cerebrospinal fluid (CSF) and producing hydrocephalus. In addition, bleeding may occur into the tumor, with a sudden increase in its mass effect. The symptoms that may be produced by a generalized increase in intracranial pressure are headaches (especially prominent in the morning, with a dependent head position, or during straining), nausea, vomiting, and a reduction in the level of consciousness. Patients may exhibit papilledema and unilateral or bilateral abducens paresis. A generalized increase in intracranial pressure may be tolerated for a period of time, but with further tumor growth, brain herniation may occur, with a rapid decline in the patient's neurologic function. Herniation of the medial aspect of the temporal lobe over the edge of the tentorium, with compression of the midbrain, downward brain stem displacement, or herniation of the cerebellar tonsils through the foramen magnum, may cause a progressive loss of consciousness, an elevation of the systemic blood pressure with widening of the pulse pressure, and the development of bradycardia.

A second way in which an intracranial tumor may present is by the loss of function of the portion of the nervous system involved by the tumor. In contrast to the symptoms and signs caused by an increase in intracranial pressure, those caused by the loss of nervous system function often permit an accurate presumptive diagnosis based on the neurologic history and physical examination. For example, if a patient presents with a progressive unilateral hearing loss that manifested initially as difficulty in understanding speech and demonstrates a unilateral reduction in pure tone hearing, with a disproportionate loss of speech discrimination and an ipsilateral reduction in corneal sensation, the suspected diagnosis would be an acoustic neuroma (vestibular schwannoma).

Finally, an intracranial tumor may present with hyperactive function. The tumor itself can be the cause of this hyperfunction, such as a pituitary adenoma that overproduces one or more hormones, or a choroid plexus papilloma that overproduces CSF. Alternatively, the tumor may stimulate seizures that arise from the adjacent or infiltrated brain.

DIAGNOSIS

The presence, location, and type of intracranial tumor can sometimes be suspected from the patient's symptoms and signs. In this case, the diagnostic studies are tailored to confirm the suspicion and to facilitate treatment. Often, however, the symptoms are vague and the signs are nonspecific, especially early in the course of the disease. In this circumstance, the initial diagnostic studies are of a general or screening type.

At present, the most common screening examination is computed tomography (CT). Most intracranial tumors are demonstrated by such scanning, especially if scans made

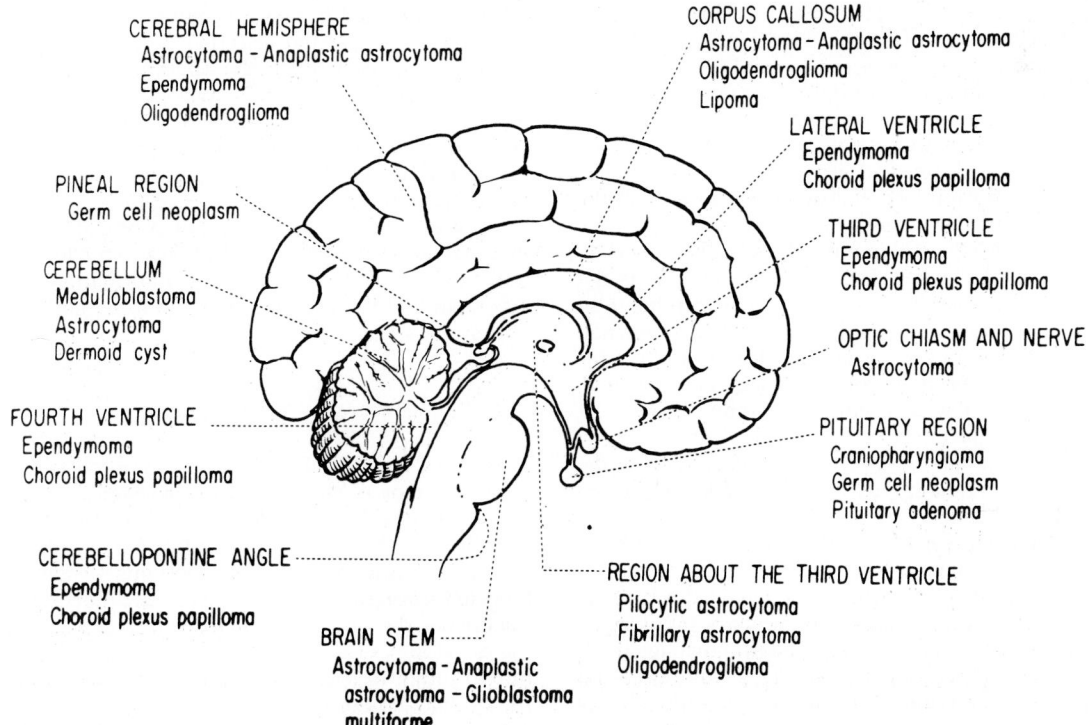

Figure 41–7. The most common types of intracranial tumors in childhood, by location. (From Burger, P. C., Scheithauer, B. W., and Vogel, F. S.: Surgical Pathology of the Nervous System and Its Coverings, 3rd ed. New York, Churchill Livingstone, 1991.)

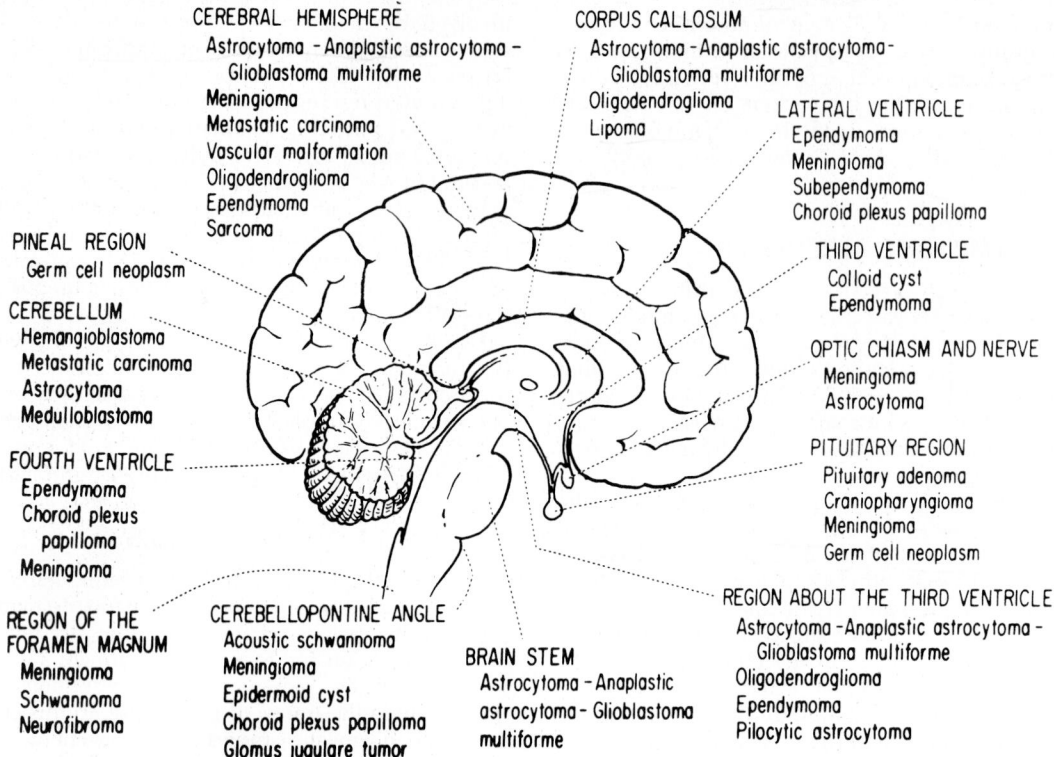

Figure 41–8. The most common types of intracranial tumors in adulthood, by location. (From Burger, P. C., Scheithauer, B. W., and Vogel, F. S.: Surgical Pathology of the Nervous System and Its Coverings, 3rd ed. New York, Churchill Livingstone, 1991.)

after the intravenous injection of an iodinated contrast agent (contrast-enhanced scans) are compared with analogous unenhanced scans. The bony structures forming the base of the skull are especially well demonstrated by CT. However, these same bony structures are often the source of artifacts that degrade the images of the adjacent portions of the brain. Magnetic resonance imaging (MRI) does not demonstrate bony detail, but it does provide excellent visualization of the brain at the cranial base and at the craniocervical junction. MRI also offers much clearer and more easily obtained coronal and sagittal views (Fig. 41–9). MRI does not expose the patient to x-rays, but the magnet may have adverse effects on certain metallic objects within a patient's body, such as an implanted cardiac pacemaker. This property, as well as the claustrophobia that some patients experience within the tight confines of the MRI device, limits its applicability somewhat. Among other types of radiologic studies are those done for specific purposes rather than for screening. For example, cerebral angiography may be useful to determine the vascularity of a tumor and its effect on the major adjacent vessels; with very vascular tumors, preoperative embolization of the tumor at the time of angiography can be used to reduce the intraoperative blood loss.

In certain circumstances, other types of studies may have diagnostic value. Electroencephalography may be helpful in analyzing patients with seizure disorders. Detailed hormonal assays can be useful in assessing the nature of a pituitary or hypothalamic tumor and in guiding its medical management. A thorough ophthalmologic examination, including visual field testing, is important in the pre- and postoperative evaluation of patients with tumors involving or adjacent to the visual or oculomotor pathways. Careful evaluation with audiometry, auditory evoked potential testing, and electronystagmography is ordinarily helpful in the assessment and

management of patients with tumors of the cerebellopontine angle or posterior skull base.

Preoperatively, the intracarotid injection of amobarbital sodium can be used to assess cerebral hemispheric dominance for speech. During the resection of a tumor, brain function can be tested directly (if the operation is done under local anesthesia and the patient is awake and cooperative) or indirectly by such techniques as electrical stimulation of the brain and cranial nerves (to determine areas that are important for motor function) or somatosensory and auditory evoked potential monitoring.

Lumbar puncture for examination of CSF has little role in the evaluation of intracranial tumors. This test usually does not provide significant diagnostic information, and it is dangerous in that it may precipitate brain herniation in a patient with a mass lesion.

TREATMENT

The mainstay of the treatment of intracranial tumors is surgical removal. Major advances in diagnostic and therapeutic technology have made this task easier and safer than ever before.[6, 15–17] With CT-guided or MRI-guided stereotactic techniques, tumors within the nervous system can now be biopsied through a burr hole, with low morbidity. The introduction of the operative microscope into neurosurgery and the development of neurosurgical microtechniques have permitted tumor exposure through a small cranial opening with the double aids of magnification and excellent illumination. The simultaneous evolution of bipolar electrical technology for tissue coagulation and cutting and the development of devices that employ laser energy, ultrasonic vibration, suction, or mechanical cutting to remove tissue permit the mod-

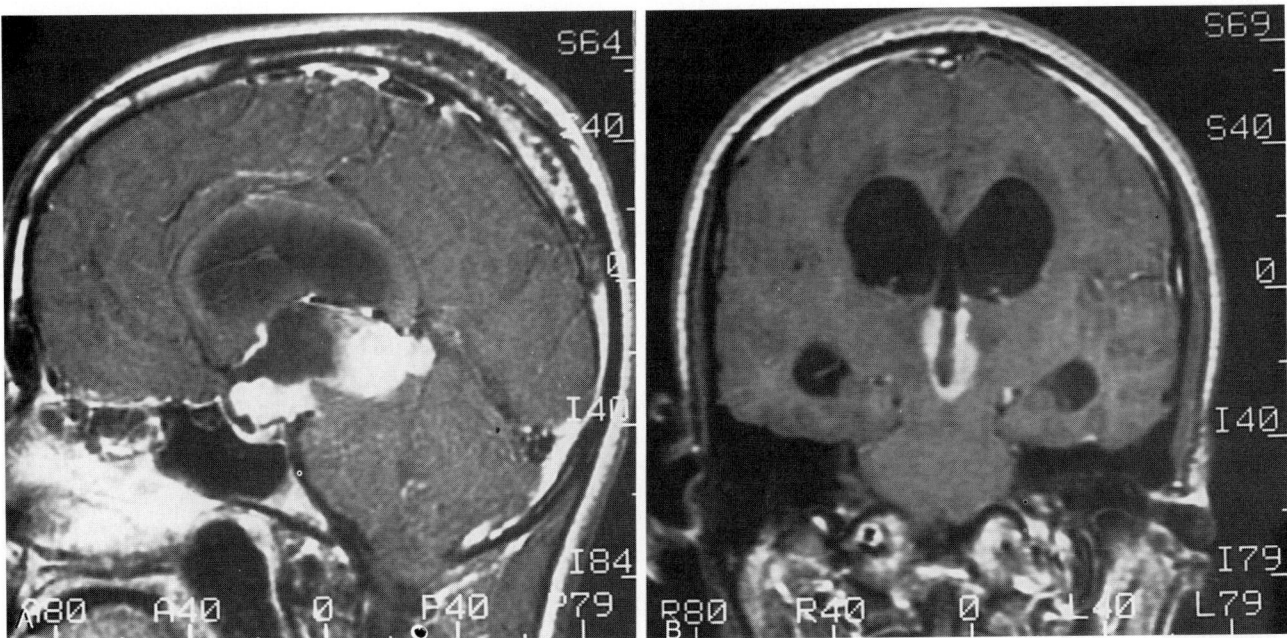

Figure 41–9. Sagittal *(A)* and coronal *(B)* magnetic resonance images, showing an enhancing germinoma in the pineal and suprasellar areas, with spread along the walls of the third ventricle. Obstructive hydrocephalus is also demonstrated.

ern neurosurgeon to resect intracranial tumors more easily and safely.

These technological advances have improved the prognosis for patients with certain types of intracranial tumors, such as meningiomas, pituitary adenomas, and schwannomas of the cranial nerves. However, they have not had a large impact on gliomas, which in most instances cannot be cured by surgical resection.

TUMOR TYPES

Various schemes have been used over the years to classify intracranial neoplasms, and in large part, these have been based on the presumed cell of origin. Among the tumors considered to arise from cells derived from the primitive neuroectoderm, the greatest number are attributed to the neuroglia and are called gliomas.

Intraparenchymal (Intra-axial) Brain Tumors

Among the primary tumors that arise within the brain, those of astrocytic, oligodendroglial, and ependymal origin are not divided sharply into benign and malignant forms; rather, they represent gradations on a spectrum from slowly growing to rapidly growing neoplasms. Moreover, with time, some tumors may shift from the benign end of the spectrum to the malignant end as the more aggressive cells replicate themselves to a greater extent than do the more indolent cells.

Brain tumors ordinarily exert their effects by progressive growth within one area of the brain, although some types, such as medulloblastomas, ependymomas, and certain pineal tumors, may spread via the CSF through the ventricular system or the subarachnoid spaces. Intraparenchymal tumors of the brain rarely spread outside the confines of the cranial cavity and spinal canal, unless an operative procedure has interfered with the normal meningeal barriers to such spread. Even though these tumors grow focally and recur focally after surgical resection, with few exceptions, they cannot be cured surgically.

Astrocytomas. Astrocytic neoplasms are the most common

of the primary brain tumors. Among Zülch's series of 9000 intracranial tumors, 6% were pilocytic astrocytomas, 6.6% were astrocytomas, and 12.2% were glioblastomas.[18] The peak age of occurrence for pilocytic astrocytoma is between 10 and 25 years; for astrocytoma, between 30 and 50 years; and for glioblastoma multiforme, between 50 and 70 years.

Astrocytic neoplasms of the cerebral hemisphere infiltrate the brain and have indistinct boundaries.[2–4] They tend to spread along white matter tracts and may cross the corpus callosum into the opposite hemisphere. The astrocytoma is more cellular than the normal brain and grows relatively slowly. The anaplastic astrocytoma is more cellular than the astrocytoma and has more of the cellular characteristics of malignancy; it also grows more rapidly. The most malignant form, the glioblastoma multiforme, exhibits additional histologic changes, including necrosis, neovascularity with endothelial proliferation, polymorphism, and hemorrhage.

Despite the many recent improvements in diagnostic, surgical, radiotherapeutic, and chemotherapeutic techniques, the prognosis for a patient with an astrocytic neoplasm of the cerebral hemisphere is poor. Even with the best current combination of these modalities, such tumors are seldom cured. Most patients with glioblastoma multiforme die within 1 year of diagnosis, and few survive beyond 2 years.[2, 4]

The pilocytic astrocytoma in the region of the third ventricle has a benign histologic appearance and grows slowly, but because of its location, it ordinarily cannot be cured, and the patient's life expectancy is usually less than 5 years from the time of diagnosis. Likewise, with few exceptions, astrocytic neoplasms arising within the brain stem cannot be cured, because of their location and their biologic behavior.

In contrast, astrocytomas of the cerebellum or optic nerve are usually amenable to surgical removal. There is a high probability of cure if the surgeon can remove the entire tumor mass. Why these tumors behave differently from the other astrocytomas is not well understood.

Oligodendrogliomas. Oligodendrogliomas typically grow within the cerebral hemisphere, especially within the frontal, parietal, or temporal lobe.[9] In Zülch's series, 9.6% were oligodendrogliomas.[18] The peak age of occurrence is between 40 and 50 years.

Ependymomas. Although intracranial ependymomas can occur throughout life, there is a peak incidence during childhood, at which time an infratentorial location is most common. In Zülch's series of intracranial tumors, ependymomas constituted 4.3%.[18] Surgical resection and postoperative radiotherapy are the mainstays of treatment but usually do not result in a cure. In one series, the median survival time from first symptoms was 36 months for 21 patients (mean age 7 years) with infratentorial ependymomas and 92 months for 22 patients (mean age 17 years) with supratentorial ependymomas.[12]

Medulloblastomas. The medulloblastoma is a malignant tumor of early life, with a peak incidence between 7 and 12 years of age. It seldom occurs in individuals over the age of 40. Among Zülch's 9000 intracranial tumors, 4.2% were medulloblastomas.[18] Medulloblastomas constitute approximately 20% of all brain tumors of childhood and adolescence. Most medulloblastomas involve the cerebellar vermis and extend into the fourth ventricle. Occasionally, and especially in patients over 15 years of age, they lie primarily in a cerebellar hemisphere.

When medulloblastomas were first studied in an organized manner between 1925 and 1930, the average survival was only 17 months.[18] With present-day treatment, the survival statistics have improved considerably. The current survival rates for patients of all ages are in the range of 50% to 60% at 5 years and 40% at 10 years.

Primary Lymphomas. Primary lymphomas constitute less than 2% of primary brain tumors, but their frequency of occurrence is increasing beyond that which can be attributed to improved diagnostic capabilities.[11] They appear to be related to immunosuppression and are encountered especially in recipients of transplanted organs and in patients with AIDS. Conventional management consists of a biopsy for pathologic confirmation of the diagnosis followed by radiotherapy, with or without chemotherapy. The median duration of survival is less than 2 years, and the 5-year survival is less than 5%.

Metastatic Neoplasms. The incidence of these tumors varies, depending on the source of the material being studied. The highest incidence would be expected if a pathologist with a special interest in the subject performed a prospective study of serially sectioned brains from patients dying at a cancer hospital. Neurosurgeons ordinarily become involved with metastatic brain tumors only if the diagnosis is not known, if the patient has a single brain lesion, or if it is thought that the removal of a metastatic tumor would provide significant palliation. Therefore, in surgical series of brain tumors, metastatic tumors constitute only a small segment, usually less than 5%.

The lung, breast, skin (malignant melanoma), kidney, and gastrointestinal tract are the most common primary sites of neoplasms that metastasize to the brain, contributing, respectively, approximately 35, 20, 10, 10, and 5% of all metastatic neoplasms.[14] Metastatic tumors ordinarily affect older adults and are distributed throughout the brain in accordance with the arterial supply. Management usually consists of biopsy or surgical resection (depending on the location and nature of the lesion) followed by radiotherapy and/or chemotherapy (depending on the exact tumor type). The prognosis depends on many factors, including the nature of the tumor, the completeness of the surgical resection, the sensitivity of the tumor to radiotherapy and chemotherapy, the status of the primary neoplasm, and the existence of other metastases.

Extraparenchymal (Extra-axial) Brain Tumors

Meningiomas. These benign tumors constitute a significant proportion of the intracranial neoplasms seen by neurosurgeons.[1, 14] In Zülch's series of intracranial tumors, 16.6% were meningiomas.[18] Although they can arise from the meninges at any place, meningiomas favor certain locations. They ordinarily indent or surround neural structures rather than invade them, but they often extend through the dura mater into the adjacent bone of the skull.

Meningiomas typically occur in the second half of life, and they are more common in women than in men. Because of their focal and benign nature, they offer the potential for a surgical cure. Yet the location of many of these lesions makes their exposure and removal a challenge. This problem, their tendency to involve adjacent bone, and the fact that multiple tiny meningiomas may exist near the main tumor all result in a high rate of recurrence. Even if the surgeon thinks that a complete removal has been achieved, there is a 10% to 15% recurrence rate by 5 years. However, even a recurrent meningioma ordinarily represents a focal benign neoplasm, and it can again be treated by surgical resection. Meningiomas are not very radiosensitive, so radiotherapy is usually reserved to treat certain inoperable lesions.

Schwannomas. Like meningiomas, schwannomas are benign tumors that constitute a significant portion of neurosurgical practice. Among the intracranial tumors reported by Zülch, 8.7% were schwannomas (neurinomas).[18] They typically form on sensory cranial nerves, in particular the acoustic nerve or, less frequently, the trigeminal nerve, and they usually appear in adult life.

If the surgeon can remove the tumor completely, which is usually the case, a cure can be achieved. The challenge is to excise the tumor without damaging adjacent structures such as the facial nerve. Radiotherapy ordinarily is not used, but in certain circumstances, small acoustic schwannomas are treated with a single treatment of focused high-energy radiation (stereotactic radiosurgery).

Pituitary Adenomas. These benign tumors are discussed in another chapter. In Zülch's series of 9000 intracranial tumors, pituitary adenomas constituted 6.6%.[18] They typically occur in adulthood.

Other Tumors. There are several other types of extra-axial intracranial tumors, including epidermoid and dermoid tumors, teratomas, craniopharyngiomas, and pineal region tumors. Each has its own characteristics and forms of therapy. As with meningiomas, schwannomas, and pituitary adenomas, many of these tumors are benign but are located in regions that are difficult to reach. They provide a challenge to the surgeon who wants to achieve total extirpation without an increase in neurologic dysfunction.

FUTURE DIRECTIONS

Further technical advances could improve the outcome of patients with benign extra-axial tumors but are unlikely to improve the prognosis of patients with primary intra-axial neoplasms. The hope in the latter area, as well as in the former, is that with an increased understanding of the molecular biology of intracranial tumors, some nonsurgical approach will be found to prevent or reverse their growth.[7, 8]

SELECTED REFERENCES

Tindall, G. T., Cooper, P. R., and Barrow, D. L. (Eds.): The Practice of Neurosurgery. Baltimore, Williams & Wilkins, 1996.

Wilkins, R. H., and Rengachary, S. S. (Eds.): Neurosurgery, 2nd ed. New York, McGraw-Hill, 1996.

Youmans, J. R. (Ed.): Neurological Surgery, 4th ed. Philadelphia, W. B. Saunders, 1996.

These three works contain numerous chapters about various intracranial tumors, with emphasis on their surgical management.

REFERENCES

1. Al-Mefty, O. (Ed.): Meningiomas. New York, Raven Press, 1991.
2. Apuzzo, M. L. J. (Ed.): Malignant Cerebral Glioma. Park Ridge, Ill., American Association of Neurological Surgeons, 1990.
3. Apuzzo, M. L. J. (Ed.): Benign Cerebral Glioma. Park Ridge, Ill., American Association of Neurological Surgeons, 1995.
4. Burger, P. C., Scheithauer, B. W., and Vogel, F. S.: Surgical Pathology of the Nervous System and Its Coverings, 3rd ed. New York, Churchill Livingstone, 1991.
5. Kaye, A. H., and Laws, E. R., Jr. (Eds.): Brain Tumors: An Encyclopedic Approach. New York, Churchill Livingstone, 1995.
6. Kelly, P. J.: Tumor Stereotaxis. Philadelphia, W. B. Saunders, 1991.
7. Lang, F. F., Miller, D. C., Koslow, M., and Newcomb, E. W.: Pathways leading to glioblastoma multiforme: A molecular analysis of genetic alterations in 65 astrocytic tumors. J. Neurosurg., 81:427, 1994.
8. Levine, A. J., and Schmidek, H. H. (Eds.): Molecular Genetics of Nervous System Tumors. New York, Wiley-Liss, 1993.
9. Ludwig, C. L., Smith, M. T., Godfrey, A. D., and Armbrustmacher, V. W.: A clinicopathological study of 323 patients with oligodendrogliomas. Ann. Neurol., 19:15, 1986.
10. Morantz, R. A., and Walsh, J. W. (Eds.): Brain Tumors: A Comprehensive Text. New York, Marcel Dekker, 1994.
11. O'Neill, B. P., and Illig, J. J.: Primary central nervous system lymphoma. Mayo Clin. Proc., 64:1005, 1989.
12. Rawlings, C. E., III, Giangaspero, F., Burger, P. C., and Bullard, D. E.: Ependymomas: A clinicopathologic study. Surg. Neurol., 29:271, 1988.
13. Salcman, M. (Ed.): Neurobiology of Brain Tumors. Baltimore, Williams & Wilkins, 1991.
14. Schmidek, H. H. (Ed.): Meningiomas and Their Surgical Management. Philadelphia, W. B. Saunders, 1991.
15. Tindall, G. T., Cooper, P. R., and Barrow, D. L. (Eds.): The Practice of Neurosurgery. Baltimore, Williams & Wilkins, 1996, p. 467.
16. Wilkins, R. H., and Rengachary, S. S. (Eds.): Neurosurgery, 2nd ed. New York, McGraw-Hill, 1996, p. 653.
17. Youmans, J. R. (Ed.): Neurological Surgery, 3rd ed. Philadelphia, W. B. Saunders, 1996, p. 2493.
18. Zülch, K. J.: Brain Tumors: Their Biology and Pathology, 3rd ed. Berlin, Springer-Verlag, 1986.

IV

SPONTANEOUS INTRACRANIAL AND INTRASPINAL HEMORRHAGE

Allan H. Friedman, M.D.

SPONTANEOUS SUBARACHNOID HEMORRHAGE AND INTRACRANIAL ANEURYSM

Subarachnoid Hemorrhage

Symptoms and Signs. Characteristically, this type of bleeding has an explosive onset, causing severe headache, nausea, vomiting, and perhaps loss of consciousness, with or without a concomitant seizure.[4] These symptoms are most likely due to the sudden increase in intracranial pressure caused by a jet of arterial blood at a mean pressure of 100 to 150 mm. Hg squirting into a space filled with cerebrospinal fluid having a pressure of about 10 to 15 mm. Hg. Fortunately, the bleeding ceases after a small amount of blood has escaped, perhaps as a result of a transient muscular spasm in the walls of the arteries adjacent to the site of bleeding or because the local intracranial pressure transiently is equal to the arterial pressure. Then, as the blood induces a sterile meningitis over the ensuing hours, stiff neck, minor fever, and photophobia develop. In approximately one third of cases, a particularly severe headache may precede the dramatic onset of subarachnoid hemorrhage, indicating a *small leak* of subarachnoid blood.[13] Unfortunately, these warning events may go unrecognized. The most prevalent remediable factor leading to mortality and morbidity following a ruptured intracranial aneurysm is misdiagnosis on presentation.

The ictus itself may be precipitated by physical stress, but more than one third of patients sustain the subarachnoid hemorrhage during sleep. An unusually high number of patients who have experienced a subarachnoid hemorrhage are noted to be hypertensive when they are brought to the hospital. However, in many instances, this systemic arterial hypertension simply reflects a physiologic response to increased intracranial pressure and pain.

Retinal hemorrhages may develop, because the blood in the subarachnoid spaces around each optic nerve compresses the central retinal vein at its exit from the nerve, causing retrograde venous distention back within the eye itself. Electrocardiographic changes, including prolonged QT intervals, elevated or depressed ST segments, and ventricular arrhythmias, reflect subendocardial ischemia and increased serum levels of catecholamines. Hyponatremia and hypovolemia result from elevation in serum atrial natriuretic factor.

Approximately 20% of patients die within 24 hours of their first major subarachnoid hemorrhage, largely as a result of the brain damage caused by intracerebral hemorrhage or by acutely increased intracranial pressure with cerebral herniation. The survivors frequently recover within a few days with little or no neurologic deficit, only to confront two more serious threats: cerebral arterial spasm and recurrent subarachnoid hemorrhage.

Cerebral Arterial Spasm. Vasospasm is the leading cause of death and morbidity in patients admitted to tertiary care centers with a ruptured intracranial aneurysm. Cerebral arterial spasm is demonstrated in cerebral arteriograms as a narrowing of previously normal arteries (Fig. 41–10).[22] This phenomenon is encountered in the arteriograms of at least 40% of patients with subarachnoid hemorrhage from a ruptured aneurysm. It almost never appears until the third day after the bleeding episode and rarely has its onset after the tenth day. Once it occurs, it lasts for days to weeks. Cerebral arterial spasm is frequently associated with decreased blood flow through the involved arteries;[23] depending on its severity, it may be manifested clinically as cerebral ischemia or infarction. A patient's propensity for developing vasospasm is proportional to the amount of subarachnoid hemorrhage visualized on the computed tomography (CT) scan.[5]

Intravascular volume expansion and systemic arterial hypertension are the most effective therapies for cerebral arterial spasm. Recently, some success has been reported in treating refractory vasospasm by mechanical balloon dilation of the contracted vessels. Some authors have reported a reduced incidence of vasospasm if intracisternal blood is dissolved within 48 hours of the hemorrhage using intracisternal injections of recombinant tissue plasminogen activator.[24] Nimodipine appears to protect patients from stroke following a subarachnoid hemorrhage.[18]

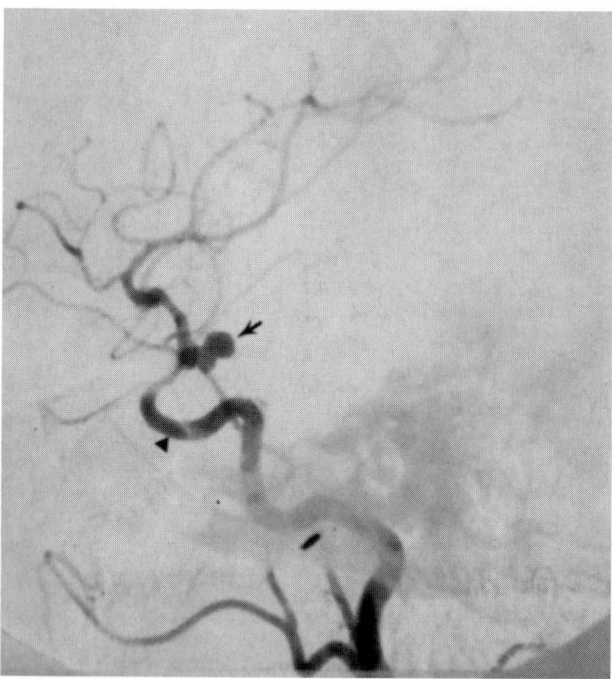

Figure 41–10. Angiographic demonstration of an aneurysm (dark arrow) of the internal carotid artery. Note the vasospasm of the internal carotid artery adjacent to the aneurysm.

Etiology. After the first bleeding episode, the patient's subsequent course depends a great deal on whether an aneurysm, arteriovenous malformation, or some other detectable lesion was responsible. In an extensive cooperative study involving 19 medical centers, the causes of spontaneous (i.e., nontraumatic) subarachnoid hemorrhage in 5834 cases were found to be intracranial aneurysm in 51%, cerebral angiomatous malformation in 6%, and both in 0.7%.[11] A small number of additional patients had hypertensive intracerebral hemorrhage, primary or metastatic brain tumor, cerebral embolus, blood dyscrasia, anticoagulation therapy, eclampsia, intracranial infection, spinal angiomatous malformation, or some other condition. Rarely, subarachnoid hemorrhage occurs secondary to a dissecting aneurysm.[6] In the remainder, the etiology of the hemorrhage was never satisfactorily explained.

Recurrent Bleeding. Patients in whom arteriography of both carotid and both vertebral circulations is normal seldom have any recurrence of bleeding, and their prognosis is good. However, intracranial aneurysms have a high propensity for recurrent hemorrhage. One in five patients experiences a second bleeding episode in the 2 weeks following the initial hemorrhage,[11] and the second rupture has a mortality of approximately 50%. The goal of surgical therapy is to prevent subsequent episodes of hemorrhage.

Antifibrinolytic agents have been shown to decrease the incidence of recurrent hemorrhage from cerebral aneurysms for the first 2 weeks following rupture.[11] Such agents are often employed by surgeons who delay intracranial operation. Unfortunately, patients treated with these agents have a higher incidence of posthemorrhage stroke, which negates their beneficial effect.

The incidence of rehemorrhage from an arteriovenous malformation is much lower than that from an intracranial aneurysm. A recent study reports a rebleeding rate of 6% in the year following a hemorrhage from an arteriovenous malformation and a 3% per year rate of hemorrhage in subsequent years.[8, 21]

Cerebral Aneurysm

Cerebral arterial aneurysms (sometimes referred to as berry aneurysms) account for slightly more than half of all cases of spontaneous subarachnoid hemorrhage. Unruptured congenital aneurysms appear to rupture at a rate of 1 to 2% per year.[10] An unruptured aneurysm's propensity to rupture is proportional to its size. Congenital cerebral aneurysms typically develop at vessel bifurcations and have been postulated to follow congenital deficiencies or degenerative changes in the vessel's wall. As the aneurysm enlarges, its internal elastic lamina frays, and its dome consists primarily of intima and the remaining adventitial connective tissue. The turbulent and irregular flow of blood entering the aneurysm through its relatively narrow neck contributes to its enlargement and also to the laminations of thrombus that are frequently deposited within its sac. These thrombi may be looked upon as the body's attempt to obliterate the aneurysm. However, they are usually inadequate to prevent rupture of the aneurysm, especially after it becomes larger than 1 cm. in diameter.

Aneurysms usually come to clinical attention as the source of a subarachnoid hemorrhage, but they may also give rise to an intracerebral or subdural hematoma. Giant aneurysms (greater than 2.5 cm. in diameter) can present as a tumor mass causing clinically detectable dysfunction in the adjacent brain. An aneurysm of the internal carotid artery may compress the adjacent oculomotor nerve or optic nerve. Similarly, an aneurysm of the internal carotid artery that occurs within the cavernous sinus may compress the adjacent ipsilateral third, fourth, fifth, and sixth cranial nerves as it enlarges. If such an aneurysm within the cavernous sinus ruptures, it causes a carotid cavernous fistula rather than a subarachnoid hemorrhage. Although this does not involve a serious threat to the patient's life, it may cause a series of disabling complications from an annoying bruit to bilateral blindness. Aneurysms are occasionally detected on an angiogram, CT scan, or magnetic resonance imaging (MRI) as an incidental finding.

Congenital berry aneurysms can occur almost anywhere along the components and larger branches of the arterial circle of Willis, but they are especially common at a few specific locations. Most of these aneurysms are located at the junction of the posterior communicating artery and the internal carotid artery (see Fig. 41–10), at the junction of the anterior communicating artery and one of the anterior cerebral arteries (Fig. 41–11), or at the first major branches of the middle cerebral artery (Fig. 41–12). Another, less common, site is the terminal bifurcation of the basilar artery. Multiple aneurysms can be found in approximately 20% of patients with aneurysms.

Management of Subarachnoid Hemorrhage

In a patient suspected of having a spontaneous subarachnoid hemorrhage, the diagnosis should be verified by a CT scan (or lumbar puncture if the scan is negative). The CT scan, if positive, may demonstrate the location or even the source of the hemorrhage (see Fig. 41–12). Subarachnoid blood is poorly seen on MRI, but this modality may demonstrate a clot of flowing blood within the aneurysm. If a lumbar puncture is done, a few milliliters of the bloody cerebrospinal fluid should be centrifuged and the appearance of the supernatant fluid noted. Oxyhemoglobin appears in the cerebrospinal fluid a few hours after the hemorrhage, and then bilirubin appears and persists for 2 to 3 weeks.[1] Therefore, the presence of xanthochromia in the supernatant fluid demonstrates that bleeding has occurred and that the bloody cerebrospinal fluid is not the result of a traumatic lumbar puncture. Similarly, when cerebrospinal fluid is ob-

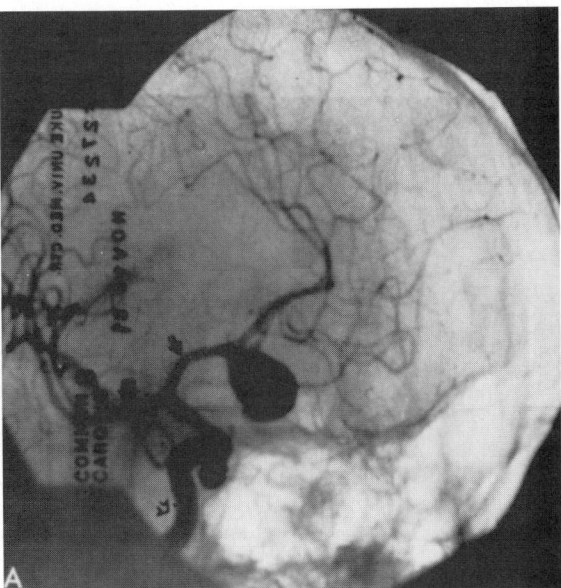
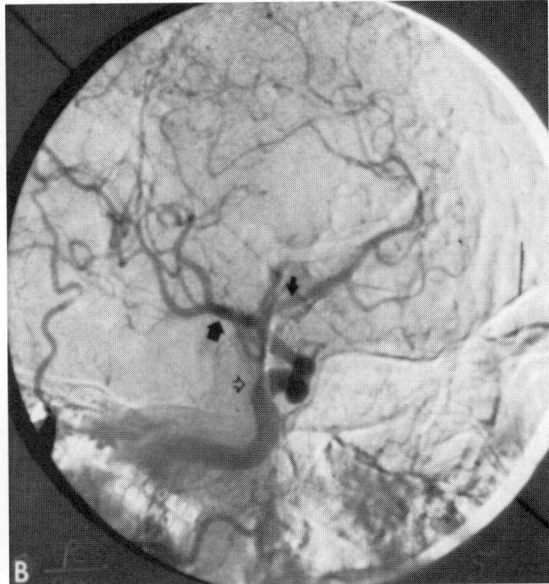

Figure 41–11. *A*, Oblique view of a right carotid angiogram demonstrating an aneurysm originating at the anterior communicating artery. *B*, The same angiographic view following surgical ligation of the aneurysm. Internal carotid artery, open arrow; middle cerebral artery, thick arrow; anterior cerebral artery, thin arrow.

tained more than 1 to 3 weeks after hemorrhage, the red blood cells are usually not present, and xanthochromia may be the only proof that bleeding occurred. The cerebrospinal fluid pressure is usually elevated, and the glucose content may be low. Although magnetic resonance angiograms and spinal CT scans hold promise, angiography remains the definitive test for demonstrating intracranial aneurysms.

After diagnosis, the patient should be transferred as soon as possible to a neurosurgical center equipped to treat intracranial aneurysms. The patient is maintained at strict bed rest in peaceful surroundings to minimize the danger of rebleeding, and cerebral angiography is performed to visual-

ize the cerebral arteries. If the angiogram is normal and focal hemorrhage has been identified on the CT scan, the angiogram should be repeated. When no source of hemorrhage can be identified, the patient is kept at bed rest for 2 weeks and then gradually returned to normal activities over the third week.[9] Patients in whom a source for the subarachnoid hemorrhage cannot be found have a low incidence of recurrent hemorrhage, but they are at risk for developing vasospasm, hydrocephalus, and cognitive deficits.

Surgical Treatment of Aneurysms

If an aneurysm is demonstrated arteriographically, the neurosurgeon must then decide when and how to treat it. The definitive treatment is surgical obliteration of the aneurysm. In the early days of aneurysm surgery, surgeons operated as soon as possible. At operation, they often confronted a swollen brain and premature rupture of the aneurysm; following the procedure, the patient often deteriorated from vasospasm. Soon it was noted that if the operation was delayed until the third week after the initial hemorrhage, the surgical morbidity and mortality were dramatically diminished. In many clinics, delayed surgical intervention became the standard method of therapy, with patients being given antifibrinolytic agents while awaiting surgical treatment. Unfortunately, patients were still exposed to the risk of a devastating recurrent hemorrhage or neurologic deficit secondary to vasospasm while waiting. Although operative complications have decreased dramatically, studies emphasize that patients who enter the hospital in relatively good condition following the rupture of an aneurysm have only a 50% likelihood of leaving the hospital in good condition if surgical therapy is delayed. For this reason, many authorities now advocate a reassessment of early surgical intervention for the treatment of intracranial aneurysms.[12] At present, most patients who survive their hemorrhage in good neurologic condition are operated on within 3 days after hemorrhage.

An aneurysm is best treated by removing it from the cerebral circulation while keeping the arteries from which it arises intact (see Fig. 41–11). If the aneurysm is accessible surgically and has a definable narrow neck that involves only a short segment of its parent artery, this goal can be accomplished by placing a metal clip or ligature about the

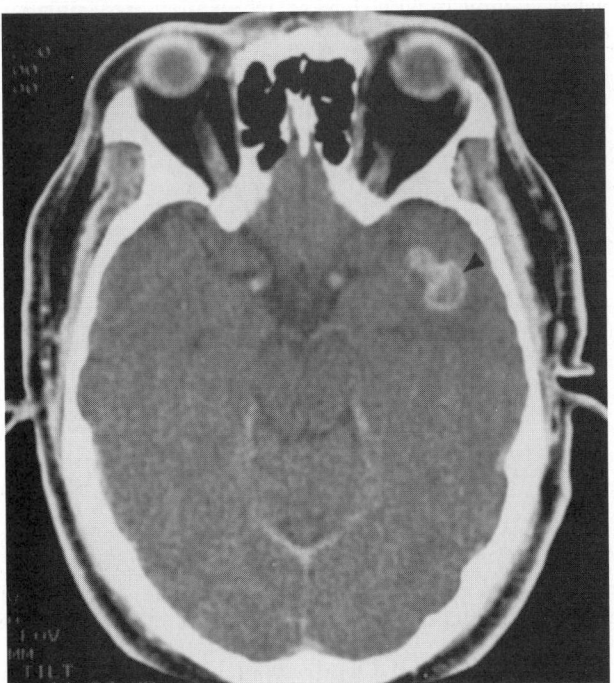

Figure 41–12. Iodine-enhanced computed axial tomogram (CT) of the brain demonstrating an aneurysm of the left middle cerebral artery (arrowhead). The large size of this aneurysm makes it visible on CT scan.

neck. Such procedures are attended by various hazards, such as the possible rupture of the aneurysm while it is being exposed. In experienced hands and with the use of the operating microscope, temporary occlusion of parent cerebral vessels, modern microsurgical instrumentation, and a wide array of removable aneurysm clips, the operative mortality should be less than 5%.

Some authors advocate reinforcement of the aneurysm by wrapping it with strips of muscle, fascia, cloth, or other material or by coating it with plastic. However, unlike cases in which just the neck of the aneurysm must be exposed to accept a clip or ligature, in these cases, the entire aneurysm, including its previous point of rupture, must be dissected free of the surrounding tissue before it can be adequately reinforced.

A third technique, proximal artery occlusion, reduces the pressure and promotes thrombosis within the aneurysm. This is accompanied by the danger of distal cerebral ischemia and infarction, especially if such treatment is complicated by cerebral arterial spasm. Gradual occlusion of the common or internal carotid artery has frequently been employed for the treatment of giant aneurysms of the internal carotid artery. Proximal artery occlusion has also been employed in the treatment of giant aneurysms throughout the cerebral vasculature.[3] However, as surgical technology improves, *second-best methods* such as proximal artery occlusion and aneurysm wrapping are employed less frequently.

Blood within the subarachnoid space from any cause obliterates the arachnoidal villi and other arachnoidal channels that are important in the normal absorption of cerebrospinal fluid. This frequently causes mild hydrocephalus for a few days or weeks until the blood has been absorbed. However, in some cases, the communicating hydrocephalus persists, and some type of shunt operation (e.g., ventriculo- or lumboperitoneal) may be required.

Operative complications represent only a small portion of the morbidity and mortality associated with ruptured intracranial aneurysms. Of the 28,000 patients who are expected to suffer from the rupture of an intracranial aneurysm each year in the United States and Canada, the major causes of morbidity and mortality will be misdiagnosis, rebleeding, and vasospasm.[10]

While unruptured, an aneurysm can be treated with a morbidity and mortality of under 5%. Once an aneurysm ruptures, its management mortality and major morbidity approach 60%. Since unruptured aneurysms of significant size have a propensity to rupture at a rate of 1% to 2% per year, a patient with an aneurysm of more than 5 mm. in diameter and an expected longevity of more than a few years should be considered for surgical therapy.

SPONTANEOUS INTRACEREBRAL HEMORRHAGE

Congenital berry aneurysms usually bleed primarily into the subarachnoid space and rarely bleed into the cerebral substance. Intracerebral hemorrhages are more commonly associated with hypertension, arteriovenous malformations, intrinsic clotting disorders, anticoagulants, brain tumors, and cerebral angiopathies.

Hypertensive Hemorrhage

Hypertensive intracerebral hemorrhages most frequently occur in the putamen, thalamus, cerebellum, or pons.[15] These hemorrhages follow bleeding from the small perforating arteries of the brain such as the thalamoperforating, lenticulostriate, or midline perforating basilar artery branches. Although these arteries can usually withstand high pressures,

when subjected to long-standing hypertension, their walls undergo fibrinoid necrosis, and miliary microaneurysms known as Charcot-Bouchard aneurysms appear. Rebleeding seldom occurs, although patients may deteriorate days after the first hemorrhage from perihematoma edema.

Hypertensive hemorrhages most frequently originate in the putamen. Patients harboring a hematoma in the putamen typically experience a rapidly progressive hemiparesis, hemisensory loss, and hemianopsia contralateral to the hemorrhage. If the hemorrhage involves the dominant hemisphere, aphasia is usually present. Patients suffering a thalamic hemorrhage usually manifest a hemisensory loss greater than their motor deficit. Small reactive pupils and downward eye deviation characteristically occur with this lesion.

Pontine hypertensive hemorrhages have a mortality of at least 75%.[14] In fatal cases, patients demonstrate small pupils, bilateral pyramidal signs, and a rapid loss of consciousness. In nonfatal cases, patients may complain of headache, vertigo, and transient visual hallucinations and demonstrate bilateral pyramidal dysfunction and various abnormalities of conjugate eye movements.

Cerebellar hemorrhage characteristically presents with headache, dizziness, nausea, and vomiting. Examination may demonstrate an early inability to walk, appendicular ataxia, facial weakness, and paresis of conjugate gaze. Hemiparesis, sensory deficit, homonymous field defect, and aphasia are conspicuous for their absence. Deterioration occurs secondary to progressive brain stem compression. In a patient with a rapidly progressive syndrome, prompt recognition of the cerebellar hematoma on clinical grounds is imperative to permit evacuation of the clot before the condition ends fatally.[17]

The diagnosis of a hypertensive intracerebral hematoma is corroborated by CT scan (Fig. 41–13). Angiography is performed in equivocal cases to identify surgically remediable lesions.

The neurologic deficit developing from the tissue destroyed directly by hemorrhage cannot be reversed. Therapy is directed at controlling edema and reducing mass effect to prevent brain herniation. Increased intracranial pressure is treated vigorously with steroids, mannitol, hyperventilation, and furosemide.

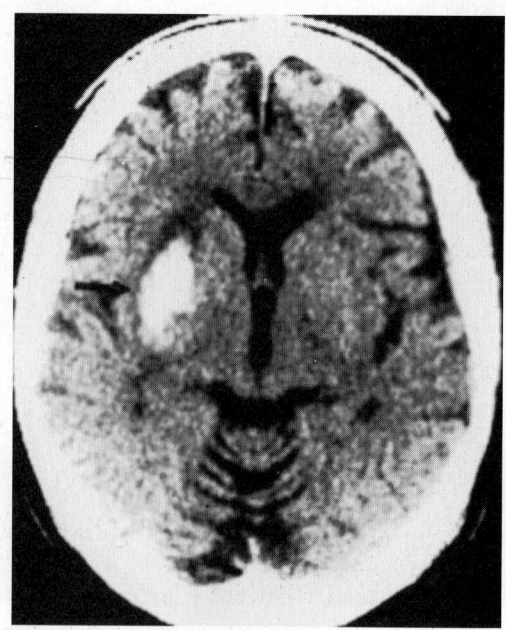

Figure 41–13. Computed axial tomogram from a hypertensive patient who suffered a spontaneous intracerebral hemorrhage in the basal ganglia (arrow).

Surgical therapy is routinely employed for the evacuation of cerebellar hematomas. Since the clot is quite tenacious, it cannot be simply evacuated through a burr hole with a needle and syringe. A suboccipital craniectomy and surgical evacuation of the hematoma with suction are required. When brain stem compression is allowed to progress to the point that the patient loses consciousness, the patient's prognosis drastically worsens.[17]

The indications for the evacuation of supratentorial hematomas are less clear. Surgical therapy is undertaken if the primary neurologic deficit is secondary to increased intracranial pressure and the neurologic examination does not demonstrate signs of irreversible brain stem damage. Patients with massive intracranial hemorrhages and signs of irreversible brain stem damage are generally not treated surgically.

Angiomatous Malformations

Pathologists differentiate vascular malformations into four categories: venous angiomas, telangiectasias, cavernous angiomas, and arteriovenous malformations.

Venous angiomas are characterized by an extensive network of veins separated by normal parenchyma. These lesions seldom bleed or give rise to clinical symptoms. Telangiectasias (capillary angiomas) are generally benign lesions of the brain stem. Cavernous angiomas are typically developmental malformations within the brain substance that are poorly visualized by angiography. They are best demonstrated by MRI (Fig. 41–14). Cavernous angiomas may manifest clinically as a growing mass, intracerebral hemorrhage, or intractable seizures. Symptomatic lesions are removed surgically.

Arteriovenous malformations are usually much larger than the other types, and most often they can be visualized angiographically (Figs. 41–15 and 41–16). Many occur in the distribution of the middle cerebral artery. The superficial portions of the malformation may cover part of the cerebral surface, but the lesion frequently extends like a cone down to the

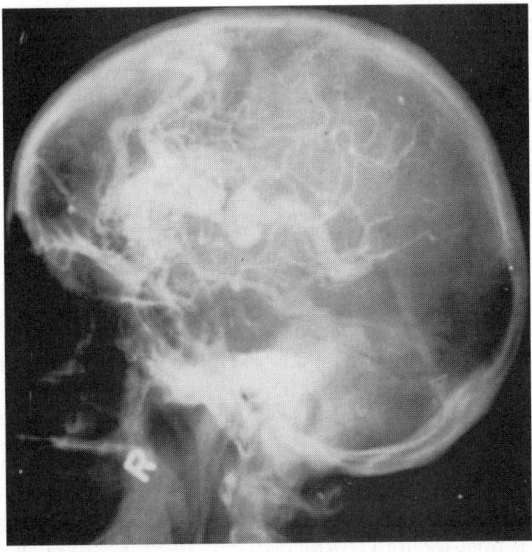

Figure 41–15. Arteriographic demonstration of an intracranial arteriovenous malformation.

ventricular surface. Therefore, the intracerebral hemorrhage occurring from these lesions may spill into the subarachnoid space or the ventricular system. Unruptured arteriovenous malformations bleed at a rate of 2% to 3% per year.[21]

In addition to bleeding, arteriovenous malformations may *steal* blood from the surrounding brain and may cause a

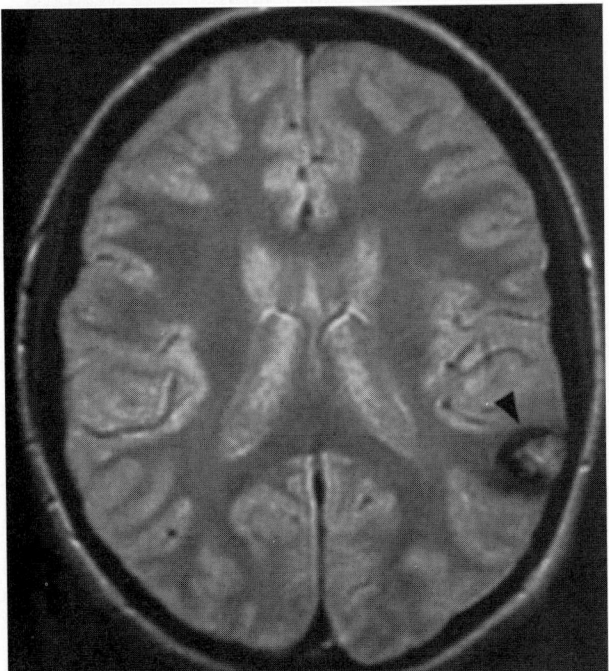

Figure 41–14. Magnetic resonance imaging scan demonstrating a left temporo-parietal cavernous angioma. The black halo around the lesion is the result of previous hemorrhage.

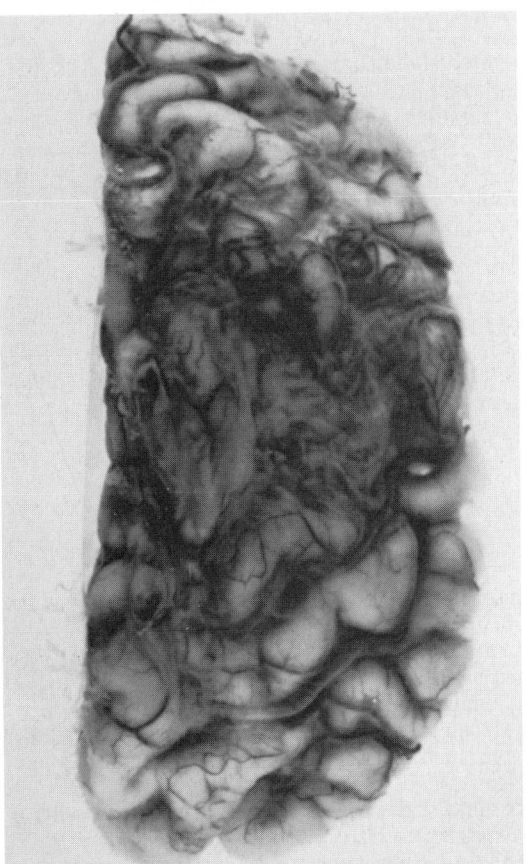

Figure 41–16. Superior aspect of the right cerebral hemisphere, showing a large arteriovenous malformation that had caused headaches and seizures during life.

significant increase in cardiac output. Likewise, patients with large arteriovenous malformations may have a variety of symptoms and signs aside from those directly related to bleeding, such as headache, cranial bruit, convulsive seizure, mental deterioration, or a hemispheric neurologic deficit. Therefore, in contrast to intracranial aneurysms, arteriovenous malformations can frequently be diagnosed by angiography before they bleed. However, arteriovenous malformations tend to bleed earlier in life than aneurysms, with a peak incidence in individuals between 30 and 39 years of age.

Surgical treatment by occlusion of the ipsilateral carotid arteries or of the arterial branches directly feeding the arteriovenous malformation does not have lasting value, since collateral feeding arteries quickly enlarge and the malformation persists. Repeated embolization of these malformations with glue or thrombogenic particles introduced through a percutaneously placed catheter or directly into the feeding arteries through a craniotomy has proved to be an effective method for reducing their size. Unfortunately, only a small number of malformations can be totally obliterated by this technique. Several investigators reported that focused radiation is effective in obliterating small arteriovenous malformations.[19, 20] It is sometimes necessary to perform a craniotomy to evacuate an intracerebral hematoma, even if the malformation cannot be resected.

The symptoms of untreated arteriovenous malformations tend to increase with time, and recurrent episodes of bleeding are common. The prognosis of lesions treated surgically depends on the size and location of the malformation and the extent of cerebral destruction from intracerebral hemorrhage, direct surgical trauma, and cerebral infarction due to arterial interruption.

Cerebral Arteritis

Intracerebral hematomas may occur in association with collagen vascular disease, methamphetamine abuse, or amyloid angiopathy. Amyloid angiopathy should be considered when a lobar hematoma occurs in a normotensive elderly individual. This entity may present with multiple discrete intracranial hemorrhages.

Clotting Disorders

Intracerebral hematomas may occur in association with primary hematologic disorders, such as idiopathic thrombocytopenia purpura or hemophilia, or as a complication of anticoagulant therapy. Surgical therapy for such a hematoma is hazardous when the patient's platelet count is below 50,000 cells per cu. mm. or the prothrombin time is prolonged.

SPONTANEOUS INTRASPINAL HEMORRHAGE

Angiomatous Malformations

Spinal arteriovenous malformations are best divided into those that are predominantly intramedullary, those that are extramedullary but intradural, and those that are extradural. Intramedullary malformations may be quite discrete, being fed by a small number of branches from the anterior spinal artery, or quite complex, with large feeding vessels. Intradural extramedullary lesions usually consist of congeries of vessels on the dorsum of the spinal cord (Fig. 41–17). In most instances, these vessels are the draining veins from a dural fistula.[16]

Spinal arteriovenous malformations occasionally present with a subarachnoid hemorrhage or sudden infarction of the spinal cord. More frequently, patients present with a progressive myelopathy.[7]

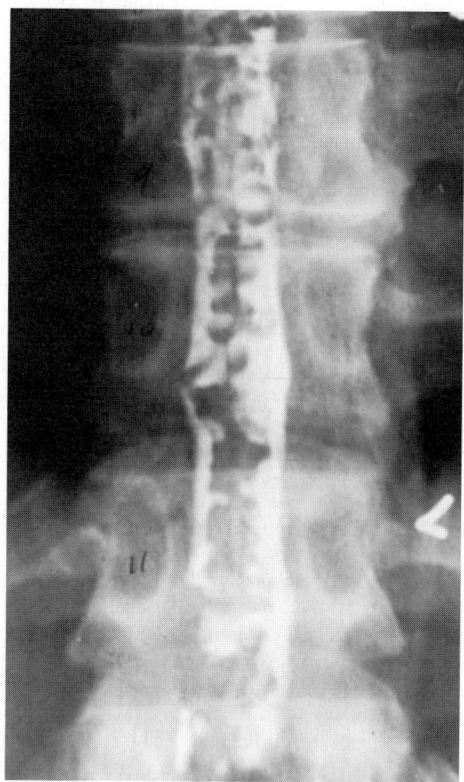

Figure 41–17. A low thoracic myelogram demonstrating the impression of a serpiginous vein of a spinal arteriovenous malformation.

Myelography often reveals an expansion of the cord with an intramedullary lesion. Dilated tortuous vessels are commonly visualized (see Fig. 41–17). The malformation is best delineated by spinal angiography.

Because of the predictable progressive deterioration suffered by most patients, surgical resection is indicated. Good results are routinely reported in patients with extradural and intradural extramedullary lesions. Although encouraging results have been reported in the treatment of small intramedullary lesions, larger lesions still remain a difficult challenge.

Neoplasm

Neoplasms of various types constitute a significant percentage of cases of spontaneous spinal subarachnoid hemorrhage, so they must be considered in the differential diagnosis, along with angiomatous malformations.

Spinal Epidural Hematoma

Epidural spinal hemorrhage can occur spontaneously or be associated with anticoagulation, a bleeding diathesis, or spinal trauma. Patients suffering from a spinal epidural hemorrhage typically experience the sudden onset of back pain followed by paralysis and loss of sphincter control.

The diagnosis is made by myelography, which demonstrates an extradural mass, or by CT scan, which reveals an epidural high-density lesion compressing the spinal cord.[2] Rapid operative evacuation of the hematoma is imperative. Good results are most likely to occur when the patient still has demonstrable neurologic function below the level of the hematoma prior to surgery.

SELECTED REFERENCES

Friedman, A. H.: Patients with ruptured aneurysm: Pre- and postoperative management. In Wilkins, R. H., and Rengachary, S. S. (Eds.): Neurosurgery. New York, McGraw-Hill, 1995.

Friedman, A. H.: Timing of aneurysm surgery. *In* Wilkins, R. H., and Rengachary, S. S. (Eds.): Neurosurgery. New York, McGraw-Hill, 1995.
These chapters review the pitfalls associated with the management of a patient who has suffered a subarachnoid hemorrhage from an intracranial aneurysm.

Kassell, N. F., Kongable, G. I., Torner, J. C., et al.: Delay in referral of patients with ruptured aneurysms to neurosurgical attention. Stroke, *16*:587, 1985.
The pitfalls of diagnosing a subarachnoid hemorrhage are reviewed in this article, as are the consequences of delayed diagnosis.

Wilkins, R. H.: Cerebral Vasospasm. New York, Williams & Wilkins, 1988.
This book contains the proceedings of the Third International Workshop on Cerebral Vasospasm.

REFERENCES

1. Barrows, L. J., Hunter, F. T., and Banker, B. Q.: The nature and significance of pigments in the cerebrospinal fluid. Brain, *78*:59, 1955.
2. Costabile, G., Husag, L., and Probst, C.: Spinal epidural hematoma. Surg. Neurol., *21*:489, 1984.
3. Drake, C. G.: Giant intracranial aneurysms: Experience with surgical treatment of 174 patients. Clin. Neurosurg., *26*:12, 1979.
4. Fisher, C. M.: Clinical syndromes in cerebral thrombosis, hypertensive hemorrhage, and ruptured saccular aneurysm. Clin. Neurosurg., *22*:117, 1975.
5. Fisher, C. M., Kistler, J. P., and Davis, J. M.: Relation of cerebral vasospasm to subarachnoid hemorrhage visualized by computerized tomographic scanning. Neurosurgery, *6*:1, 1980.
6. Friedman, A. H., and Drake, C. G.: Subarachnoid hemorrhage from intracranial dissecting aneurysm. J. Neurosurg., *60*:325, 1984.
7. Friedman, A. H., and Gray, L.: Clinical and radiological findings of spinal dural arteriovenous fistula. Perspect. Neurol. Surg., *3*:1, 1992.
8. Graf, C. J., Perret, G. E., and Torner, J. C.: Bleeding from cerebral arteriovenous malformations as part of their natural history. J. Neurosurg., *58*:331, 1983.
9. Juol, R., Fredriksen, T. P., and Ringkjob, R.: Prognosis in subarachnoid hemorrhage of unknown etiology. J. Neurosurg., *64*:359, 1986.
10. Juvela, S., Popias, M., and Heiskanen, O.: Natural history of unruptured intracranial aneurysms: A long-term follow-up study. J. Neurosurg., *79*:174, 1993.
11. Kassell, N. F., and Torner, J. C.: Aneurysmal rebleeding: A preliminary report from the Cooperative Aneurysm Study. Neurosurgery, *13*:479, 1983.
12. Kassell, N. F., Torner, J. C., and Jane, J. A.: The international cooperative study on the timing of aneurysm surgery. Part 2. Surgical results. J. Neurosurg., *73*:37, 1990.
13. Leblanc, R.: The minor leak proceeding subarachnoid hemorrhage. J. Neurosurg., *66*:35, 1987.
14. Nakajima, K.: Clinicopathological study of pontine hemorrhage. Stroke, *14*:485, 1983.
15. Ojemann, R. G., and Heros, R. C.: Spontaneous brain hemorrhage. Stroke, *14*:468, 1983.
16. Oldfield, E. H., DiChiro, G., Quindlen, E. A., Reith, K. G., and Doppman, J. L.: Successful treatment of a group of spinal cord arteriovenous malformations by interruption of dural fistula. J. Neurosurg., *59*:1019, 1983.
17. Ott, K. H., Kase, C. S., Ojemann, R. G., and Mohr, J. P.: Cerebellar hemorrhage: Diagnosis and treatment. A review of 56 cases. Arch. Neurol., *31*:160, 1974.
18. Pickard, J. D., Murray, G. D., Illingworth, R., et al.: Effect of oral nimodipine on cerebral infarction and outcome after subarachnoid haemorrhage: British aneurysm nimodipine trial. Br. Med. J., *298*:636, 1989.
19. Steinberg, G. K., Fabrikant, J. I., Marks, M. P., et al.: Stereotactic heavy-charged-particles Bragg-Peak radiation for intracranial arteriovenous malformations. N. Engl. J. Med., *323*:96, 1990.
20. Steiner, L., Lindquist, C., and Steiner, M.: Radiosurgery in arteriovenous malformations of the basal ganglia. J. Neurosurg., *70*:320A, 1989.
21. Wilkins, R. H.: Natural history of intracranial vascular malformations: A review. Neurosurgery, *16*:421, 1985.
22. Wilkins, R. H.: Cerebral Vasospasm. New York, Williams & Wilkins, 1988.
23. Yamakami, I., Isobe, K., Yamaura, A., Nakamura, T., and Makino, H.: Vasospasm and regional cerebral blood flow (rCBF) in patients with ruptured intracranial aneurysm: Serial rCBF studies with the xenon-133 inhalation method. Neurosurgery, *13*:394, 1983.
24. Zabramski, J. M., Spetzler, R. F., Lee, S. K., et al.: Phase I trial of tissue plasminogen activator for the prevention of vasospasm in patients with aneurysmal subarachnoid hemorrhage. J. Neurosurg., *75*:189, 1991.

V

CRANIOCEREBRAL INJURIES

Allan H. Friedman, M.D.

Accidental injury is the fourth leading cause of death in the United States and the leading cause of death in individuals between the ages of 1 and 44 years. Head injuries are present in more than 50% of trauma-related deaths. An estimated 400,000 patients with head injuries are admitted to the hospital each year, and an even larger number are evaluated and treated in emergency rooms.[12] Because head injuries are so ubiquitous, their primary management should be understood by all physicians.

The final neurologic status of a patient who has sustained brain trauma is the sum of the irreversible damage acquired at the time of the initial injury and the damage from secondary insults. At the time of the initial injury, a portion of the brain may sustain irreversible damage, and a second portion may sustain a lesser degree of damage from which it will recover over a period of months. Secondary insults that cause worsening of a patient's neurologic deficits include (1) systemic disorders, such as hypoxia or hypotension; (2) expanding intracranial mass, such as a subdural, epidural, or, rarely, intraparenchymal hematoma; and (3) sustained raised intracranial pressure with a concomitant decrease in cerebral perfusion pressure. Although several forms of intervention have been proposed to enhance the brain's normal repair processes, at this time, physicians can do nothing to either replace those cells that have suffered a fatal injury or accelerate the restoration of recovering tissue. The swift recognition or prevention of these secondary insults offers the best likelihood of improving the prognosis of a patient who has sustained a brain injury. In treating a patient with head injury, it is the physician's role to rapidly identify and correct these injurious influences.[23]

PRIMARY BRAIN INJURIES[10]

At the time of the initial head injury, the brain may suffer contusion, laceration, and shearing injuries. These injuries follow local direct brain trauma and brain acceleration and deceleration relative to the skull. Local direct brain trauma occurs when a stationary skull is struck by an object. If the force is sufficient, the skull indents, directly striking the underlying brain. More deleterious are injuries that follow acceleration or deceleration of the brain relative to the skull. At the time of impact, there is considerable movement of the brain. For example, when the skull is suddenly stopped by a windshield in an automobile accident, the brain continues to decelerate relative to the skull for approximately 20 msec. In a similar manner, at the time of impact, the brain may experience linear or rotational acceleration with respect to the sagittal, lateral, or vertical axis of the skull. This acceleration causes contusion of the brain, shearing of axons, and tearing of bridging veins. These mechanisms are responsible for the damage the brain incurs in a closed head injury.

Contusions occur in regions where the moving brain abruptly strikes the fixed skull, or under areas of impact where the skull is sufficiently bent inward to strike the underlying brain. Areas of contusion are marked by hemorrhage, which frequently spreads under the pia, and by swelling and necrosis of underlying tissue. If the impact is sufficiently severe, the pia is lacerated and the hemorrhage spills out into the subarachnoid or subdural space. After brain deceleration, areas of contusion tend to concentrate along the undersurface of the frontal lobes and the anterior poles of the temporal lobes, where the brain is relatively confined by bone. The neurologic deficit produced coincides with the region of direct brain injury; a contusion of the motor strip, for example, may produce a contralateral hemiparesis. The contusion is clinically silent when restricted to portions of the brain that have no clinically demonstable function, such as the anterior temporal lobes or the inferior aspect of the frontal lobes. These silent areas of contusion may become clinically significant days after the initial injury, as edema accumulates in areas where the blood-brain barrier has been destroyed and the swollen region begins to act as an intracranial mass. Occasionally, a hematoma of significant size accumulates in an area of contusion 24 to 72 hours after the initial injury.[27] These delayed traumatic hematomas are most likely to occur in older patients and may be responsible for deterioration in neurologic function days after the initial injury.

Rotation of the brain within the skull may lead to tearing of axons within the white matter of the brain, causing diffuse axonal injury.[1] According to the theory of Ommaya and Gennarelli, mild injuries damage only subcortical axons, but increases in the rotational force involve progressively deeper areas of brain.[20] There is little cerebral swelling and no increased intracranial pressure associated with this form of brain injury. A computed tomographic (CT) scan made immediately following such an injury may demonstrate hemorrhage in the corpus callosum and the superolateral aspect of the brain stem, but the remainder of the brain appears relatively normal, even though the patient may manifest severe neurologic damage. Months after the injury, the CT scan demonstrates that the bulk of the white matter is reduced. Magnetic resonance imaging (MRI) demonstrates diffuse, small, focal abnormalities limited to white matter tracts.[9]

Children may demonstrate rapid neurologic deterioration and a concomitant increase in intracranial pressure in the minutes to hours following a relatively mild head injury.[4] The clinical presentation can be mistaken as indicative of an enlarging intracranial mass. This increased pressure is thought to be secondary to vasodilation, with concomitant increased intracranial blood volume. These children often develop grave neurologic signs, but with control of their intracranial hypertension, their neurologic outcome is far better than that of adults who manifest the identical clinical findings.

The neurologic deficit that follows a penetrating brain injury is manifested only by a loss of function of the brain that is directly injured. Delayed deterioration in the patient's neurologic status following such an injury occurs secondary to a complicating hemorrhage or an infection induced by debris pushed into the brain at the time of injury. Penetrating injuries should be rapidly cleansed of bone fragments, necrotic brain, and debris. Recent data question the practice of pursuing bone chips spread deeply into the brain.[2] High-speed missile wounds produce a shock wave that cuts a wider area of damage than the bullet tract itself.

SECONDARY BRAIN INJURIES

Patients who have sustained head injuries must be monitored for factors that can produce further brain damage. Metabolic abnormalities are the most common secondary insults in patients who have suffered brain trauma. An evaluation of head trauma patients upon arrival at a university hospital emergency room demonstrated that approximately 35% have a PO_2 less than 60 mm. H_2O. Fifteen percent have a systolic blood pressure less than 95 mm. Hg, and 10% have a hematocrit of less than 30.[18] An unconscious patient has a diminution of the normal protective reflexes that may lead to mechanical obstruction of the oropharynx or to aspiration pneumonia. Pulmonary contusion, a flail chest, or, rarely, fat emboli or neurogenic pulmonary edema may further compromise a patient's oxygenation. Hypercapnia, although a rare concomitant of head injury alone, causes vasodilation and increased intracranial pressure. At the scene of the accident, the patient's mouth should be cleared of debris, and hypoventilation should be treated by the placement of an oral airway and the institution of positive-pressure ventilation. In the emergency room, all patients who are not verbalizing or following commands should be intubated. Care should be taken not to flex the spine, as a spinal injury may be present.

Hypotension is rarely a direct result of intracranial trauma and should alert the physician to the possibility of intra- or extracorporeal hemorrhage. A positive abdominal tap is reported to occur in 17% of patients who have sustained severe head trauma.[5] Serious scalp bleeding may also cause major blood loss and can be controlled by applying pressure to the lacerations. Life-threatening dural sinus bleeding can be slowed by placing the patient in the reverse Trendelenburg position. In rare cases, hypotension may develop in infants with large intracranial hemorrhage or in patients with high cervical fractures that produce medullary compression. Hypotension occurring later during the hospitalization of a patient with head injury may reflect hemorrhage from gastritis or a gastrointestinal ulcer, infection with secondary gram-negative sepsis, myocardial infarction, or pulmonary embolism. Hypotension is particularly deleterious in the setting of increased intracranial pressure, because it further diminishes cerebral profusion. Mean arterial blood pressure should be restored quickly to at least 80 mm. Hg.

Increased intracranial pressure produces neurologic dysfunction by decreasing cerebral blood flow and causing transtentorial herniation. Brain edema, an enlarging hematoma, a large cerebral contusion, or cerebrovascular engorgement can act as a supratentorial mass. An enlarging supratentorial mass is first partially compensated for by the displacement of intracranial venous blood and cerebrospinal fluid out of the skull. When these buffering systems are exhausted, any further increase in mass results in a marked increase in intracranial pressure.

Intracranial pressure is frequently monitored in patients who have sustained severe head injuries. Since the venous outflow pressure in the brain approximates the intracranial pressure, the cerebral perfusion pressure is equal to the mean arterial pressure minus the intracranial pressure. With elevation of the intracranial pressure, the cerebral perfusion pressure becomes compromised. By autoregulating its vascular resistance, normal brain can maintain a constant cerebral blood flow over a wide range of cerebral perfusion pressures. Pressure autoregulation is frequently disrupted in the setting of trauma, so a decrease in the cerebral perfusion pressure diminishes cerebral blood flow. Recent work suggests that jugular venous oxygen saturation and the pulsatility index of transcranial Doppler studies are helpful in determining the optimal cerebral profusion pressure in an individual patient.[6] In clinical practice, all patients who have an intracranial pressure greater than 40 mm. Hg have a significantly diminished cerebral blood flow. If the intracranial pressure becomes equal to the systemic arterial pressure, brain death quickly ensues.

Intracranial pressure can be monitored by measuring the

TABLE 41–1. Methods of Lowering Intracranial Pressure

Mechanical reduction of intracranial volume
  Reduction of intracranial venous blood by elevating head of bed
  Drainage of cerebrospinal fluid through ventricular drain
  Removal of intracranial mass
Induction of vasoconstriction
  Hyperventilation to $P_{CO_2} = 25$ to 36 mm. Hg
  Sedation and paralysis
  Intravenous barbiturates, lidocaine, etomidate, or propofol
Removal of intracerebral water using osmotic agents such as
  mannitol, urea, glycerol
Stabilization of membranes with steroids (steroids are rarely used in
  the treatment of head trauma)
Dehydration of brain with furosemide

pressure in the epidural space, subarachnoid space, intraventricular fluid, or in brain parenchyma. Normal intracranial pressure is less than 15 mm. Hg and becomes elevated with the appearance of an intracranial mass. The intracranial pressure is dynamic, and it is not unusual for a patient with a partially compensated intracranial mass to have a wave of pressure measuring 50 mm. Hg and lasting 5 to 20 minutes superimposed on a relatively normal pressure. Mortality is reduced without a concomitant increase in morbidity by aggressively lowering an increased intracranial pressure.[24] Methods used to lower intracranial pressure are outlined in Table 41–1.

An expanding intracranial mass not only causes a generalized increase in intracranial pressure but also distorts and shifts the brain. Focal mass lesions can cause brain herniations under the falx cerebri, through the tentorial notch, or through the foramen magnum. The most common form of herniation, transtentorial herniation, follows a supratentorial mass crowding the supratentorial contents into the tentorial notch, secondarily distorting the midbrain, third nerve, and posterior cerebral artery. Clinically, transtentorial herniation manifests as one of two clinical syndromes designated central and uncal herniation (Table 41–2).

Central herniation is most likely to occur following a nonfocal increase in the pressure above the tentorium, as seen in a multicentric supratentorial brain injury. The earliest warning of impending central herniation is a progressive depression in the patient's level of consciousness, followed by reflex flexor posturing of the patient's upper extremities to a painful stimulus (decorticate posturing) and Cheyne-Stokes respirations. This is followed by a progressive rostral to caudal brain stem ischemia, which manifests as a sequential dysfunction of successively lower brain stem levels. Midbrain dysfunction is marked by decerebrate posturing (abnormal extensor response to pain), fixed midposition pupils, and hyperventilation. As lower elements of the brain stem fail, the patient becomes flaccid, develops spasmodic respirations, and loses the oculocephalic reflexes.

Uncal herniation is most likely to develop from a focal, laterally placed mass, such as an epidural hematoma. Usually the examiner first notes a progressing contralateral hemiparesis. Early compression of the third cranial nerve causes miosis of the ipsilateral pupil, followed by ptosis and a limitation of motion of the ipsilateral eye. As the midbrain is compressed, the patient loses consciousness, begins to hyperventilate, and develops bilateral decerebrate posturing. If the intracranial pressure is not reduced, the patient will demonstrate signs characteristic of progressive rostral to caudal ischemia.

It is becoming apparent that damaged brain may be further injured by local processes brought about by the injury itself. Although interventions to halt these processes are still experimental, they are of interest to clinicians. Treating posttraumatic cerebrospinal fluid acidosis with tromethamine was beneficial in lowering patients' intracranial pressure.[26] Polyethylene glycol–conjugated superoxide dismutase, a scavenger of oxygen radical superoxide axions, has been shown to lower the need for mannitol and to improve the outcome in patients sustaining closed head injuries.[19] Moderate therapeutic hypothermia has been shown to reduce intracranial pressure and improve outcome.[15] These therapeutic modalities may prove beneficial in improving the outcome of patients suffering cerebral trauma.

PATIENT EVALUATION

After stabilization of the respiratory and cardiovascular systems, attention is turned to the central nervous system. Care is taken not to manipulate the neck prior to excluding cervical fractures. The initial examination must be recorded so that it can be compared with subsequent examinations in order to detect any deterioration in the patient's condition. The head is inspected for scalp lacerations, compound skull fractures, or signs of a basilar skull fracture. In an awake patient, a detailed neurologic examination should be performed, with special attention to abnormalities in mental status, asymmetry of pupillary size, unilateral weakness, changes in muscle tone, asymmetry of deep tendon reflexes, and the presence of pathologic reflex responses. In an uncooperative, stuporous, or comatose patient, the examiner must rely on the evaluation of reflexes to detect focal abnormalities

TABLE 41–2. Signs of Transtentorial Herniation

Type	Level of Consciousness	Respiratory Pattern	Pupillary Size; Response to Light	Oculovestibular Reflex	Motor Response to Pain
Uncal Herniation					
Early oculomotor nerve compression	Normal to obtunded	Normal	Unilaterally dilated; fixed	Full, conjugate	Appropriate
Late oculomotor nerve compression	Normal to obtunded	Normal	Unilaterally dilated; fixed	Unilateral third nerve palsy	Appropriate
Midbrain compression	Comatose	Hyperventilation	Bilaterally midposition; fixed	Dysconjugate gaze	Decerebrate posturing
Central Herniation					
Early diencephalon compression	Obtunded	Deep sighs, yawns	Small; reactive	Conjugate	Appropriate
Late diencephalon compression	Barely arousable to comatose	Cheyne-Stokes	Small; reactive	Conjugate without nystagmus	Cortical
Midbrain compression	Comatose	Hyperventilation	Midposition; fixed	Dysconjugate	Decerebrate

TABLE 41-3. Glasgow Coma Scale

Eye Opening	
Spontaneous	E4
To speech	3
To pain	3
Nil	1
Best Motor Response	
Obeys	M6
Localizes	5
Withdraws	4
Abnormal flexion	3
Extension response	2
Nil	1
Verbal Response	
Oriented	V5
Confused conversation	4
Inappropriate words	3
Incomprehensible sounds	2
Nil	1

Coma Score = E + M + V.

in the nervous system. Special attention is given to respiratory patterns, pupillary size and light response, oculocephalic reflexes, motor response to painful stimuli, and deep tendon reflexes.[8]

An assessment of mental status is particularly difficult to record in such a way that the patient's condition can be conveyed from examiner to examiner. The Glasgow Coma Scale is a standardized method of measuring the severity of a patient's neurologic deficits. It has a high concordance among different observers and should be employed to measure all patients who have sustained head injuries. The 15-point scale assesses the patient's neurologic responsiveness in three categories: eye opening, best motor response, and verbal response (Table 41-3).

Attention is then turned to the evaluation of the chest, abdomen, and extremities for other injuries. Many patients rendered comatose in an automobile accident have sustained other major injuries. The neurosurgeon must be aware of the presence of these injuries and their possible effect on the brain injury.

Mild, nonpenetrating head injuries are associated with a transient disturbance in vision, a transient period of confusion, and a loss of memory for the moment of impact. With progressively greater degrees of brain injury, the patient remains confused for proportionately longer periods of time and demonstrates a longer period of memory loss. Antegrade memory loss is loss of memory for events that follow the accident and may be the only type of memory loss present in milder head injuries. With more severe injuries, the patient may demonstrate retrograde memory loss, that is, loss of memory of events that preceded the accident. As the degree of brain injury increases, the patient experiences a longer loss of consciousness. Concomitant with the initial impact, there may be a period of apnea and systemic arterial hypertension and occasionally a generalized seizure.

Patients with mild head injuries and a brief loss of consciousness are often expected to make uneventful recoveries. In fact, these patients are found to have a surprising degree of postinjury disability in the form of persistent headaches, memory deficits, and difficulties with activities of daily living that persist for months following the accident. One study documented that one third of patients who had sustained minor head injuries had not returned to gainful employment in the 3 months following the injury.[21] Further studies corroborate the fact that early but not late neuropsychologic prob-

lems follow minor head injuries.[14] Patients who have sustained mild head injuries but have severe headache, lethargy, or restlessness should be observed for 24 hours. If the patient shows any deterioration in neurologic status or demonstrates any signs of a focal neurologic lesion on examination, a CT scan of the brain should be obtained.[7]

Patients who have sustained moderate head injuries are likely to be lethargic, stuporous, or combative when they first regain consciousness. Ten to 15% of patients entering the hospital with a moderate head injury are found to have a focal intracranial lesion. A CT scan of the brain is indicated in all patients with persistent lethargy. Nearly all patients who sustain an injury of this order of magnitude have persistent headaches, memory difficulties, and difficulties with activities of daily living for months following the injury.[22] Three months following a moderate head injury, two thirds of patients are still unemployed.[11]

A severe head injury is defined by a score of 8 or less on the Glasgow Coma Scale. Forty per cent of patients who have sustained severe brain injuries harbor a focal intracranial mass lesion. Signs of severe neurologic dysfunction such as an abnormal motor response, abnormal oculocephalic reflexes, or bilateral fixed pupils indicate a brain stem injury.

Each of these abnormal brain stem reflexes can be demonstrated in approximately one third of severely injured patients and is associated with an increased mortality. Mortality has also been shown to be proportional to the patient's age. Other factors associated with a poor outcome include the presence of a focal intracranial lesion, concomitant abdominal or chest injury, systemic arterial hypotension, and elevated intracranial pressure.[13]

A CT scan of the brain is indicated in all comatose patients. Frequent neurologic examinations are necessary to detect any change in the patient's neurologic status. These patients should be treated in an intensive care setting (Table 41-4).

SCALP AND SKULL INJURIES

Scalp lacerations frequently occur at the site of impact. Because of the scalp's rich vascular supply, most uncomplicated lacerations can be closed after cleansing and débridement. If a portion of the scalp is lost, the deficit may be repaired by rotating a portion of scalp. A large scalp deficit requires a skin graft or vascularized free flap for repair.

Although indicative of a relatively severe cranial blow, skull fractures are conspicuous for their absence in patients who have sustained severe brain trauma. The fracture fol-

TABLE 41-4. Basic Care of the Comatose Adult Patient

Position
    Elevate head 30 degrees
    Turn frequently
Respiratory care
    Endotracheal intubation
    Controlled respiration
    Pulmonary toilet
Management of intracranial pressure as indicated
Nutrition: 2500 kcal./day
Intravenous fluid: 0.45% normal saline and 5% dextrose—
    125 ml./hr.
Medications
    Antacid therapy
    Seizure prophylaxis
Monitor
    Arterial blood pressure
    Arterial Po_2 and Pco_2
    Serum sodium, glucose
    Serum osmolarity

lows inbending or outbending of the skull beyond its elastic tolerance. A linear, nondisplaced skull fracture in and of itself requires no special therapy but has stronger clinical implications when it extends into the air sinuses or base of the skull, crosses one of the meningeal arteries, is associated with an underlying dural tear, or underlies a scalp laceration.

Basilar skull fractures are difficult to detect on plain skull films. Because of the tenacity with which the dura adheres to the base of the skull, these lesions are frequently associated with a cerebrospinal fluid fistula. A basilar skull fracture of the anterior fossa should be suspected when the patient manifests the raccoon sign—periorbital ecchymosis limited at the edge of the orbit. A fracture involving the petrous portions of the temporal bone should be suspected when the patient is found to have blood or cerebrospinal fluid behind the tympanic membrane and when the patient demonstrates a Battle's sign, with ecchymosis of the mastoid prominence. A basilar skull fracture should also be suspected when an air-fluid level is seen on the lateral skull film in the frontal, sphenoid, or mastoid sinus. Most traumatic cerebrospinal fluid fistulas subside spontaneously if the patient's head is maintained elevated at 30 degrees, but a persistent fistula places the patient at risk for recurrent episodes of meningitis. It should be noted that the leak may be only temporarily closed with brain and then recur. If the leak persists longer than 10 days, craniotomy with reapproximation of the torn dura is indicated.

A linear fracture crossing the groove of the middle meningeal artery may be seen in patients with accumulating epidural hematoma. However, most patients with fractures in this location do not develop epidural hematomas, and some such hematomas are not accompanied by a skull fracture.

An infrequent complication of skull fracture seen exclusively in children is the progressive separation of the long edges of a seemingly benign linear skull fracture. The patient presents with a growing scalp mass or a dysfunction of the brain underlying the fracture. This type of fracture is always associated with an underlying dural tear. The most important aspect of the operative repair is the dural closure. A cranioplasty is usually performed.

If a hard blow is delivered to a small area of the skull, the fracture is comminuted, and the portion of bone lying under the area of impact is depressed. Depressed skull fractures may be associated with an underlying dural tear or lacerated cerebral cortex. These lesions are associated with a higher incidence of brain laceration and posttraumatic epilepsy. In the past, such fractures were routinely repaired surgically. Recent studies question whether surgical therapy decreases the neurologic deficit, incidence of epilepsy, or rate of infection associated with these lesions.

EPIDURAL HEMATOMAS

Acute epidural hematoma usually follows arterial hemorrhage between the skull and the dura.[11] At the time of impact, a dural artery is torn, and the inbending of the skull initiates the stripping of the dura from the bone. Occasionally, an epidural hematoma follows a torn venous sinus. Most frequently, acute epidural hematomas occur in the temporal or temporoparietal region as a consequence of hemorrhage from one of the branches of the middle meningeal artery, but the hematoma can collect under the cranium in any location.

The clinical presentation is variable. The trauma responsible for an acute epidural hematoma may create an immediate neurologic deficit following direct brain injury. The hematoma manifests as an enlarging intracranial mass that eventually precipitates transtentorial herniation. The classic clinical presentation is that of a brief loss of consciousness secondary to the initial cerebral concussion, followed by a lucid interval.

The patient eventually lapses from the lucid interval into a coma after the epidural hematoma enlarges to a size sufficient to precipitate tentorial herniation and midbrain compression. This classic triphasic clinical pattern is seen in only 20% of patients who have an epidural hematoma. More frequently, the initial concussion is insufficient to cause any loss of consciousness or it is so severe that the patient does not regain consciousness prior to the herniation. In either case, the *characteristic* lucid interval does not occur.

Although skull films frequently demonstrate a linear skull fracture, an epidural hematoma may accumulate without a concomitant fracture. The absence of a fracture is especially common in children. The CT scan demonstrates a biconvex high-density lesion that lies between the skull and the brain (Fig. 41–18).

The treatment for this lesion is early recognition and rapid surgical decompression. In a rapidly deteriorating patient who is suspected of harboring an epidural hematoma, a diagnostic burr hole is placed 1.5 inches above the zygoma on the side of the dilating pupil. Because of the jelly-like nature of the acute hematoma, a craniotomy must be performed to completely evacuate the mass. There is a strong correlation between the patient's preoperative level of consciousness and the outcome of therapy. With early diagnosis and rapid therapy, the mortality from this lesion approaches zero.[3]

Epidural hematomas occasionally accumulate in the posterior fossa secondary to bleeding from the transverse sinus or meningeal arteries. The patient may present with signs of acute brain stem compression, such as decerebrate rigidity and loss of consciousness, or a clinical pattern may slowly evolve that is characterized by altered mental status, headache, nausea, vomiting, and nystagmus prior to the patient's lapsing into unconsciousness. Posterior fossa epidural hematomas are frequently associated with occipital skull fractures and are easily demonstrated on CT scan. Rapid surgical decompression is indicated.

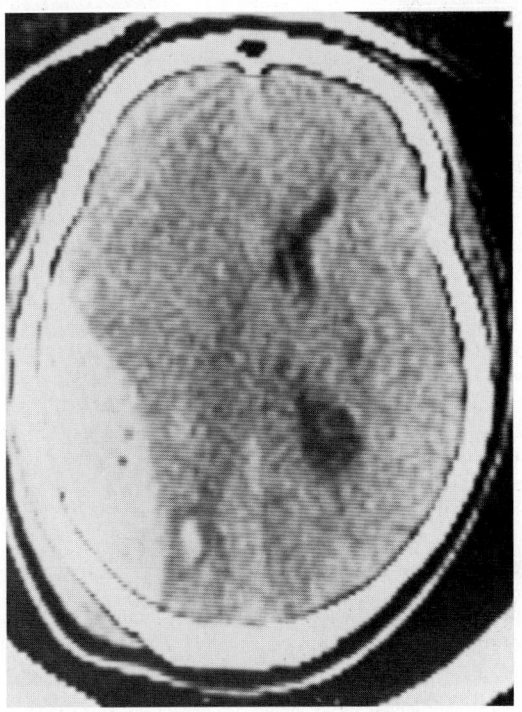

Figure 41–18. Computed axial tomogram of a patient who suffered a traumatic epidural hematoma. Note the shift of the ventricles off of the midline.

SUBDURAL HEMATOMAS

Subdural hematomas are blood collections that occur in the plane between the dura and the arachnoid. Unlike epidural hematomas, subdural hematomas most commonly develop from ruptured veins. Anterior or posterior acceleration of the skull with respect to the brain causes traction on the veins that traverse the subdural cleft as they pass between the cerebral cortex and the dural venous sinuses. Cerebral atrophy is seen in chronic alcohol abusers and in some elderly patients; this increases the size of the potential subdural space, thus enhancing this mechanism. Because of the lack of adhesions between the dura and the arachnoid, the venous blood spreads rapidly over the cerebral convexity. Rarely, a subdural hematoma may develop from a bleeding cortical artery, a ruptured aneurysm, or a superficial arteriovenous malformation.[17]

Acute subdural hematomas present with signs of rapid increase in intracranial pressure and herniation. A moderate-sized subdural collection may be compensated for initially but becomes clinically symptomatic after edema accumulates.

A subdural hematoma may develop from oozing following a brain laceration. In these cases, the problem is usually the intrinsic brain injury and not the subdural blood collection. In comparison with a massive primary brain injury, a rim of subdural blood is not clinically significant. Only when the hemorrhage is extensive enough to serve as an intracranial mass is it of clinical significance.

Less than 50% of patients harboring subdural hematomas have skull fractures demonstrable on skull roentgenograms. An acute subdural hematoma appears as a high-density spread over the convexity of the cerebral cortex on CT scan (Fig. 41–19). A chronic subdural hematoma, in which the blood clot has lysed, appears as a biconvex low-density area lying between the skull and the compressed brain. A subdural hematoma of intermediate age or a subdural hematoma in an anemic patient may appear isodense with the adjacent brain and is detected by noting a shift of the ventricular system or the adjacent cortex.

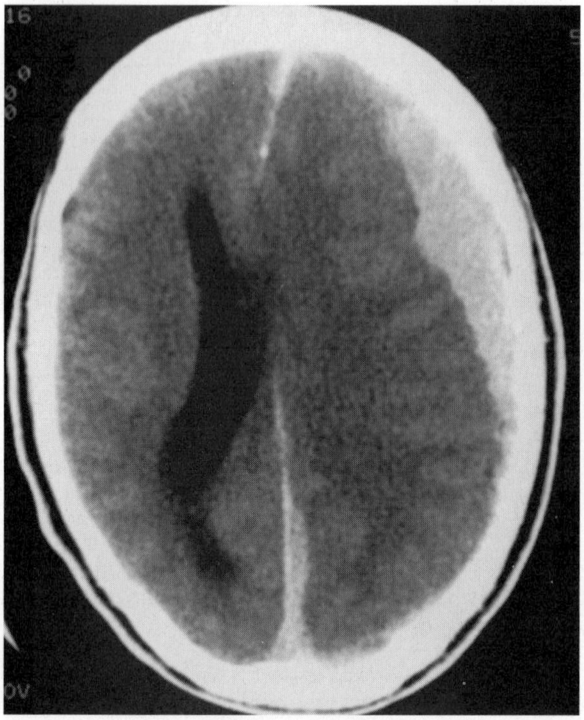

The mortality associated with acute subdural hematoma is 25% to 90%. This high mortality is due to the frequency of concomitant direct brain injury. If the patient has no primary brain injury, the mortality from the subdural hematoma is a direct function of the patient's age, neurologic status, and delay from time of trauma to surgical evacuation of the hematoma.[25] Although an acute subdural hematoma may first be detected through a diagnostic burr hole, its viscous nature necessitates a larger craniectomy or craniotomy for complete removal. Usually, the subdural hematoma is evacuated through a question mark–shaped flap that begins at the ear and continues to the midline.

An amount of subdural blood insufficient to cause a mass effect may accumulate following minor trauma. This is especially prone to occur in patients with cerebral atrophy. Although small amounts of subdural blood are usually spontaneously reabsorbed, the hematoma may occasionally become encapsulated by a membrane of fibrous tissue and friable capillaries emanating from the dura mater.[16] Small recurrent hemorrhages from the thin-walled vessels within the membrane cause the collection of liquefied blood to enlarge. This chronic subdural hematoma may come to clinical attention months to years after the initial insult, when it presents as an intracranial mass. The patient may complain of altered mental status, headaches, seizures, or a focal neurologic dysfunction (e.g., hemiparesis, aphasia), reflecting the position of the brain compressed by the hematoma.

The content of a chronic subdural hematoma is a thin liquid that can be washed out through multiple burr holes. In children, the liquid can be removed via a needle placed in the anterior fontanelle. If the chronic subdural hematoma recurs after simple drainage, a craniotomy with partial removal of the enveloping membranes or a shunting of the subdural cavity into the pleural or peritoneal cavity may be necessary.

DELAYED COMPLICATIONS

The likelihood of a patient's developing a seizure disorder following a head injury is proportional to the severity of the injury. It is estimated that 5% of patients admitted to the hospital with a head injury develop a seizure disorder. Early epilepsy, penetration of the dura, intracranial hematomas, and depressed skull fractures all predispose the patient to a delayed seizure disorder.

Several vascular complications associated with head injuries produce symptoms. A traumatic carotid cavernous sinus fistula may present as an audible bruit, conjunctival edema, chemosis, impaired extraocular motion, or loss of visual acuity. Dissecting aneurysms present as a sudden stroke or transient ischemic episode. Rarely, a traumatic intracranial aneurysm ruptures in the weeks following a head injury.

Figure 41–19. Computed axial tomogram of a patient who sustained a subdural hematoma from head trauma. The left subdural in this photograph appears isodense as compared with the adjacent skull.

SELECTED REFERENCES

Eisenberg, H. M., and Aldrich, E. F.: Management of head injury. Neurosurg. Clin. North Am. 2:251, 1991.
   This volume is an up-to-date review of the clinical aspects of head injury. The authors present the physiologic rationale behind the treatment of brain injuries.

Plum, F., and Posner, J. B.: The Diagnosis of Stupor and Coma. Philadelphia, F. A. Davis, 1980.
   This classic, now in its third edition, provides a detailed account of the assessment of the comatose patient.

REFERENCES

1. Adams, J. H., Graham, D. I., Murray, L. S., and Scott, G.: Diffuse axonal injury due to nonmissile head injury in humans: An analysis of 45 cases. Ann. Neurol., 12:557, 1982.

2. Brandvold, B., Levi, L., Feinsod, M., and George, E. D.: Penetrating cranio-cerebral injuries in the Israeli involvement in the Lebanese conflict, 1982–1985. J. Neurosurg., 72:15, 1990.
3. Bricolo, A. P., and Pasut, L. M.: Extradural hematoma: Toward zero mortality. A prospective study. Neurosurgery, 14:8, 1984.
4. Bruce, D. A., Alavi, A., Bilaniuk, L., et al.: Diffuse cerebral swelling following head injuries in children: The syndrome of "malignant brain edema." J. Neurosurg., 54:170, 1981.
5. Butterworth, J. F., 4th, Maull, K. I., Miller, J. D., and Becker, D. P.: Detection of occult abdominal trauma in patients with severe head injuries. Lancet, 2:759, 1980.
6. Chan, K. H., Miller, J. D., Dearden, N. M., et al.: The effect of changes in cerebral perfusion pressure upon middle cerebral artery blood flow velocity and jugular bulb venous oxygen saturation after severe brain injury. J. Neurosurg., 77:55, 1992.
7. Feuerman, T., Wackym, P. A., Gade, G. F., and Becker, D. P.: Value of skull radiography, head computed tomographic scanning, and admission for observation in cases of minor head injury. Neurosurgery, 22:449, 1988.
8. Friedman, A. H.: Head injuries: Initial evaluation and management. Postgrad. Med., 73:219, 1983.
9. Gentry, L. R., Godersky, J. C., and Thompson, B.: MR imaging of head trauma: Review of the distribution and radiopathologic features of traumatic lesions. A.J.R. Am. J. Roentgenol., 150:663, 1988.
10. Hardman, J. M.: The pathology of traumatic brain injuries. Adv. Neurol., 22:15, 1979.
11. Jamieson, K. G.: Epidural Haematoma: Handbook of Clinical Neurology, Vol. 24. Amsterdam, North-Holland Publishing Company, 1976.
12. Kalsbeek, W. D., McLaurin, R. L., Harris, B. S., 3rd, et al.: The national head and spinal cord injury survey: Major findings. J. Neurosurg. (Suppl.), 53:S19, 1980.
13. Klauber, M. R., Marshall, L. F., Luerssen, T. G., et al.: Determinants of head injury mortality: Importance of the low risk patient. Neurosurgery, 24:31, 1989.
14. Levin, H. S., Mattis, S., Ruff, R. M., et al.: Neurobehavioral outcome following minor head injury: A three-center study. J. Neurosurg., 66:234, 1987.
15. Marion, D. W., Obrist, W. D., Carlier, P. M., et al.: The use of moderate therapeutic hypothermia for patients with severe head injuries: A preliminary report. J. Neurosurg., 79:354, 1993.
16. Markwalder, T. M.: Chronic subdural hematomas: A review. J. Neurosurg., 54:637, 1981.
17. McDermott, M., Fleming, J. F., Vanderlinden, R. G., and Tucker, W. S.: Spontaneous arterial subdural hematoma. Neurosurgery, 14:13, 1984.
18. Miller, J. D., Sweet, R. C., Narayan, R., and Becker, D. P.: Early insults to the injured brain. JAMA, 240:439, 1978.
19. Muizelaar, J. P., Marmarou, A., Young, H. F., et al.: Improving the outcome of severe head injury with the oxygen radical scavenger polyethylene glycol–conjugated superoxide dismutase: A phase II trial. J. Neurosurg., 78:375, 1993.
20. Ommaya, A. K., and Gennarelli, T. A.: Cerebral concussion and traumatic unconsciousness: Correlation of experimental and clinical observations on blunt head injury. Brain, 97:633, 1974.
21. Rimel, R. W., Giordani, B., Barth, J. T., et al.: Disability caused by minor head injury. Neurosurgery, 9:221, 1981.
22. Rimel, R. W., Giordani, B., Barth, J. T., and Jane, J. A.: Moderate head injury: Completing the clinical spectrum of brain trauma. Neurosurgery, 11:344, 1982.
23. Rose, J., Valtonen, S., and Jennett, B.: Avoidable factors contributing to death after head injury. Br. Med. J., 2:615, 1977.
24. Saul, T. G.: Is ICP monitoring worthwhile? Clin. Neurosurg., 34:560, 1988.
25. Seelig, J. M., Becker, D. P., Miller, J. D., et al.: Traumatic acute subdural hematoma: Major mortality reduction in comatose patients treated within four hours. N. Engl. J. Med., 304:1511, 1981.
26. Wolf, A. L., Levi, L., Marmarou, A., et al.: Effect of THAM upon outcome in severe head injury: A randomized prospective clinical trial. J. Neurosurg., 78:54, 1993.
27. Young, H. A., Gleave, J. R., Schmidek, H. H., and Gregory, S.: Delayed traumatic intracerebral hematoma: Report of 15 cases operatively treated. Neurosurgery, 14:22, 1984.

VI

INTRACRANIAL INFECTIONS

Robert H. Wilkins, M.D.

The number of patients with infections amenable to neurosurgical treatment is relatively small, but because of the wide variety of infectious agents and the different pathologic lesions they can incite, this area remains a challenge for neurosurgeons.

CRANIAL OSTEOMYELITIS, EPIDURAL ABSCESS, SUBDURAL EMPYEMA[3, 4, 7, 10]

A cranial bone may be the site of hematogenous spread of a bacterial infection from another area of the body, but more often it becomes involved by adjacent spread from an infected paranasal sinus, by a penetrating wound, or by an operative infection involving a craniotomy flap. Pott's puffy tumor is such a frontal osteomyelitis, with marked overlying soft tissue swelling that is secondary to frontal sinusitis.

Treatment consists of the surgical removal of the infected bone, with simultaneous treatment of any coexisting sinusitis. Appropriate systemic antibiotics are administered, and an adequate margin of normal bone is removed with the specimen to minimize the risk of recurrent infection. A cranioplasty may be performed later for cosmetic and protective reasons, but at least a year should be allowed to pass, during which time there is no evidence of inflammation in the area, before the plate is inserted. Otherwise, this large foreign body can serve as a focus for a further inflammatory response.

An epidural infection is usually a well-confined bacterial abscess associated with one or more of the previously mentioned infections, and it is drained at the same time the coexisting osteomyelitis or sinusitis is treated. A subdural infection, however, is usually a more widespread empyema rather than a localized abscess, since the developing infection easily dissects open the subdural space to cover the surface of an entire cerebral hemisphere. Subdural empyema may begin by the extension of infection through the dura mater from without or through the arachnoid from within, or it may result from the operative infection of a subdural hematoma. In any event, subdural empyema is usually treated by immediate evacuation through multiple trephine openings or a craniotomy flap in order to avert death or serious neurologic morbidity. Drains are usually left in the subdural space for several days, until all drainage has ceased.

MENINGITIS[7, 9, 10]

Bacterial meningitis as such is not treated surgically, and all but the most resistant or unusual forms ordinarily respond to systemic antibiotics. However, if recurrent episodes of meningitis occur, the neurosurgeon may become involved in the search for and treatment of unrecognized cerebrospinal fluid rhinorrhea, a midline cranial or spinal dermal sinus tract, or some other portal of entry for organisms into the central nervous system.

Also, in some patients recovering from meningitis, effusions develop in the subdural spaces over the cerebral hemispheres, or hydrocephalus occurs as a result of the obstruction of subarachnoid pathways concerned with the normal absorption of cerebrospinal fluid. Subdural effusions ordinarily occur in infants and frequently may be cured by repeated aspiration with needle and syringe through the coronal suture. Rarely, unilateral or bilateral burr holes, craniectomies, or craniotomies are necessary for the evacuation of such effusions. Occasionally, the excessive fluid in the subdural space or ventricular system must be shunted into other areas of the body, such as the peritoneal cavity.

ENCEPHALITIS, CEREBRITIS, BRAIN ABSCESS[1, 2, 6–10]

The neurosurgeon may be deceived into exploring and resecting an area of severe viral encephalitis, mistaking it for a malignant glioma. Herpes simplex, for example, may cause a necrotic and cystic mass in the temporal lobe that closely resembles a brain tumor. However, even if the correct diagnosis is suspected preoperatively, biopsy of the lesion may be of value for verification. Moreover, resection of such a lesion, or some type of decompressive operation, may be necessary if steroids and other medical measures are inadequate to control the severe elevations of intracranial pressure that frequently accompany encephalitis.

The term *cerebritis* is usually reserved to describe the focal area of cerebral inflammation that immediately precedes the development of a brain abscess. Such areas of cerebritis may arise from:

1. Extension of an infection through the meninges. In this way, mastoiditis may lead to an abscess in the ipsilateral temporal lobe or cerebellar hemisphere, or frontal sinusitis may produce a frontal lobe abscess.

2. Hematogenous spread from some other site, especially from the lungs, pleura, or heart, or from other areas of the body via congenital heart defects that permit the paradoxical embolism of infected material. One form of hematogenous spread occurs in intravenous drug abusers who develop septicemia from the use of unsterile drugs, needles, and syringes. Brain abscesses that orginate by the hematogenous spread of bacteria are distributed among the various areas of the brain in proportion to the vascular supply, so a large number occur in the territory of the middle cerebral arteries.

3. Inoculation through the meninges, as by a compound depressed skull fracture.

Typically, a patient with a brain abscess uncomplicated by meningitis has no systemic signs of infection such as fever, tachycardia, or leukocytosis. The abscess presents clinically, and by computed tomography (CT) and magnetic resonance imaging (MRI), as an intracranial mass that must be differentiated from a neoplasm, hematoma, or some other type of space-consuming lesion (Fig. 41–20).

A brain abscess may contain one or more of a variety of organisms. Aerobic bacteria are often found. In addition, anaerobic or microaerophilic bacteria (frequently) or fungi (occasionally) can be discovered if appropriate cultures and staining techniques are employed. Even so, a significant percentage of brain abscesses are found to be sterile.

In the past, the preferred treatment of a brain abscess was total surgical excision. Now that such abscesses can be followed closely by CT or MRI, stereotactic aspiration and drainage are frequently employed, at least initially, to reduce the mass effect, provide information about the causative organism or organisms, and lower the risk of intraventricular rupture while the abscess is treated by systemic antibiotics. A patient with a brain abscess may also require treatment with a steroid medication to reduce reactive brain edema. No matter which operative technique is used, there is a high incidence of seizures among survivors of abscesses of the cerebral hemispheres, which justifies the prophylactic administration of anticonvulsants in most of these patients.

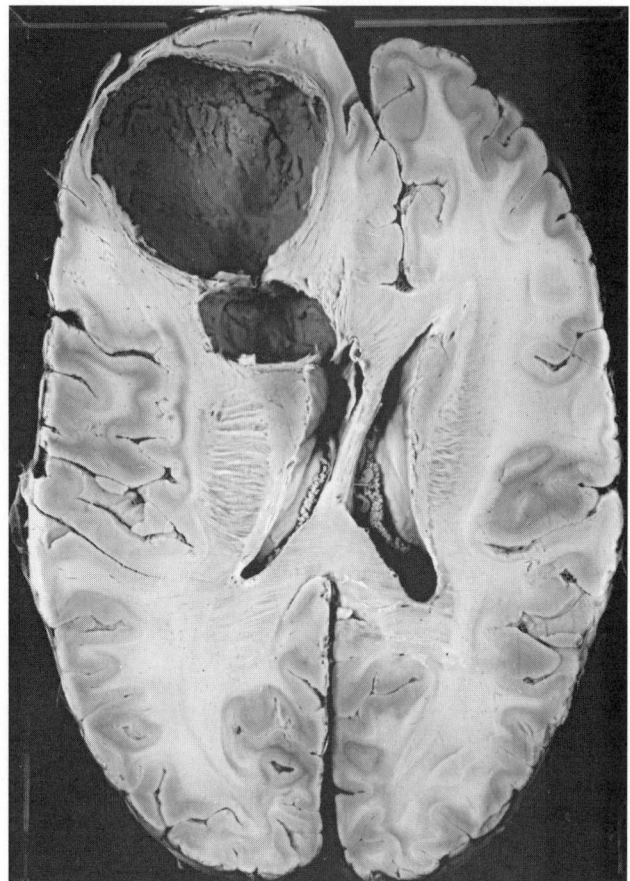

Figure 41–20. Brain abscess, left frontal lobe. A "daughter" abscess, posterior to the main lesion, had ruptured into the left lateral ventricle as the terminal event in this case.

OTHER TYPES OF INTRACRANIAL INFECTIONS[5, 7, 9–11]

Numerous organisms can cause lesions within the cranial cavity or spinal canal, varying from meningitis (sometimes accompanied by hydrocephalus) to one or more intraparenchymal granulomas or abscesses. In the setting of AIDS, lesions within the brain may be caused by opportunistic organisms such as *Toxoplasma gondii* and *Cryptococcus neoformans*.

The neurosurgeon's first task is often to establish the diagnosis by a stereotactic or open biopsy. Then the condition is ordinarily treated with the appropriate systemic medication; however, in certain circumstances, the neurosurgeon may be called upon to insert an intraventricular catheter attached to a subcutaneous reservoir to facilitate intraventricular drug administration. The neurosurgeon may also be required to drain or excise a fungal abscess or to shunt hydrocephalus resulting from the basal meningitis associated with tuberculosis, sarcoidosis, or a fungal infection.

Parasitic infections, especially echinococcosis and cysticercosis, present a problem to neurosurgeons in some countries, and although they are being encountered more often in the United States, they are still seen too infrequently to justify further discussion here.

SELECTED REFERENCE

Wilkins, R. H., and Rengachary, S. S. (Eds.): Neurosurgery, 2nd ed. New York, McGraw-Hill, 1996.

A section of this textbook (17 chapters) deals with infections of neurosurgical interest.

REFERENCES

1. Alderson, D., Strong, A. J., Ingham, H. R., and Selkon, J. B.: Fifteen-year review of the mortality of brain abscess. Neurosurgery, 8:1, 1981.
2. Artenstein, A. W., and Kim, J. H.: Antimicrobials for use in neurosurgical patients. *In* Wilkins, R. H., and Rengachary, S. S. (Eds.): Neurosurgery, 2nd ed. New York, McGraw-Hill, 1996, p. 3269.
3. Bok, A. P. L., and Peter, J. C.: Subdural empyema: Burr holes or craniotomy? A retrospective computerized tomography–era analysis of treatment in 90 cases. J. Neurosurg., 78:574, 1993.
4. Hlavin, M. L., Kaminski, H. J., Fenstermaker, R. A., and White, R. J.: Intracranial suppuration: A modern decade of postoperative subdural empyema and epidural abscess. Neurosurgery, 34:974, 1994.
5. Levy, R. M., and Rosenblum, M. L.: Neurosurgical aspects of human immunodeficiency virus (HIV-1) infection. *In* Wilkins, R. H., and Rengachary, S. S. (Eds.): Neurosurgery, 2nd ed. New York, McGraw-Hill, 1996, p. 3355.
6. Mampalam, T. J., and Rosenblum, M. L.: Trends in the management of bacterial brain abscesses: A review of 102 cases over 17 years. Neurosurgery, 23:451, 1988.
7. Scheld, W. M., Whitley, R. J., and Durack, D. T. (Eds.): Infections of the Central Nervous System. New York, Raven Press, 1991.
8. Stephanov, S.: Surgical treatment of brain abscess. Neurosurgery, 22:724, 1988.
9. Tyler, K. L., and Martin, J. B. (Eds.): Infectious Diseases of the Central Nervous System. Philadelphia, F. A. Davis, 1993.
10. Wilkins, R. H., and Rengachary, S. S. (Eds.): Neurosurgery, 2nd ed. New York, McGraw-Hill, 1996, p. 3267.
11. Young, R. F., Gade, G., and Grinnell, V.: Surgical treatment for fungal infections in the central nervous system. J. Neurosurg., 63:371, 1985.

VII

INTRASPINAL TUMORS

Robert H. Wilkins, M.D.

Intraspinal tumors can be divided into three groups according to location: extradural, intradural extramedullary, and intramedullary (Figs. 41–21 and 41–22). The neoplasms that occur in each of these three locations have different clinical and radiologic characteristics.

EXTRADURAL NEOPLASMS

Extradural (epidural) tumors are usually malignant.[1, 7, 8] The most common example is a metastasis to a vertebra from a primary carcinoma of the lung, breast, or prostate. Other examples of malignant extradural spinal tumors are lymphoma and myeloma.

Typically, such a tumor begins within the vertebral bone and extends into the epidural space or begins within the epidural space. In either case, the tumor gradually compresses the spinal cord or cauda equina and interferes with the blood supply to this neural tissue. On plain roentgenograms, destruction of the pedicles may be apparent on the anteroposterior views, and destruction and collapse of one or more vertebral bodies can be seen on the lateral views. Metastases of this sort are usually lytic but may be blastic (especially those from prostatic carcinoma). Computed tomography (CT) scanning permits the identification of bony involvement, epidural tumor extension, and neural compromise in the axial plane. Magnetic resonance imaging (MRI) permits similar identifications, but in sagittal and coronal planes as well as axial planes.

The most common location for an extradural neoplasm is in the thoracic area of the spine. The typical symptoms relate to the directions of tumor growth. The patient first develops back pain centered where the tumor involves the vertebral bone and then experiences radicular pain and dysfunction (radiculopathy) extending around the trunk at the same level

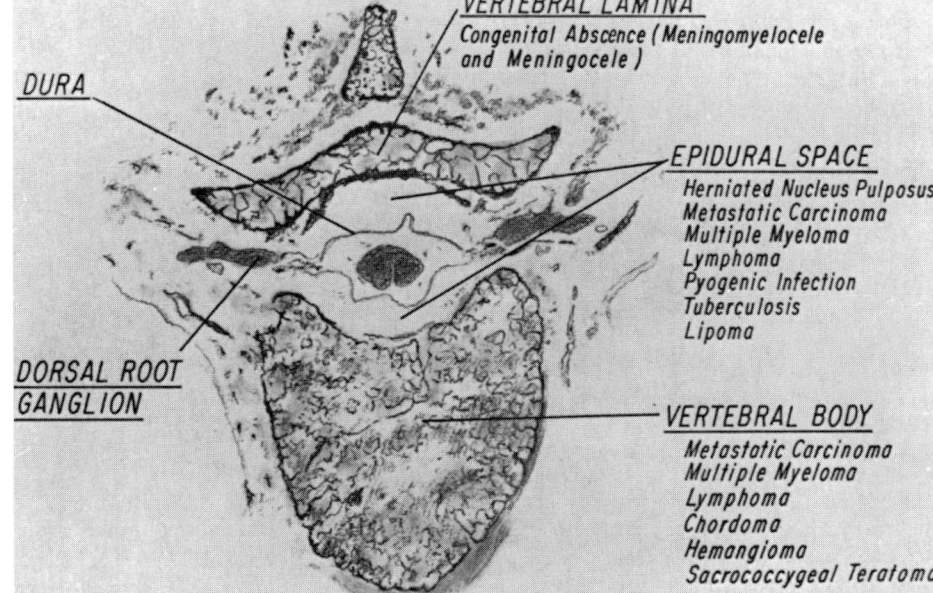

Figure 41–21. Topographic distribution of lesions of the spine and epidural space. (From Burger, P. C., Scheithauer, B. W., and Vogel, F. S.: Surgical Pathology of the Nervous System and Its Coverings, 3rd ed. New York, Churchill Livingstone, 1991.)

on one or both sides as the tumor involves the exiting spinal nerve roots. Finally, the patient develops a progressive interference with spinal cord function (myelopathy), with eventual paraplegia.

If a patient presents with progressive back pain (and especially pain that is not improved by recumbency), radicular pain, and neurologic loss, the preliminary assessment should include plain roentgenograms and CT scanning or MRI (Fig. 41–23), or all three. If such studies do not provide sufficient information, they can be supplemented by other studies such as radionuclide bone scanning and positive contrast myelography accompanied by postmyelographic CT scanning.

There are generally two treatment options: radiation therapy or surgical resection followed by radiation therapy. With either option, steroid administration is often advantageous; the steroid can be given immediately and reduces the bulk of the tumor (and the degree of neural compression) temporarily while the primary treatment modality is being accomplished. Surgical resection prior to radiotherapy is usually preferred if the patient is not known to have a malignancy or if the loss of neurologic function is proceeding rapidly. The goals of surgical treatment are to establish the diagnosis, to decompress the spinal cord or cauda equina, and to stabilize that area of the spine if the tumor has produced instability. Ordinarily, the tumor cannot be removed entirely, and radiotherapy is required postoperatively. Depending on the nature of the tumor, hormonal therapy or chemotherapy may also be beneficial.

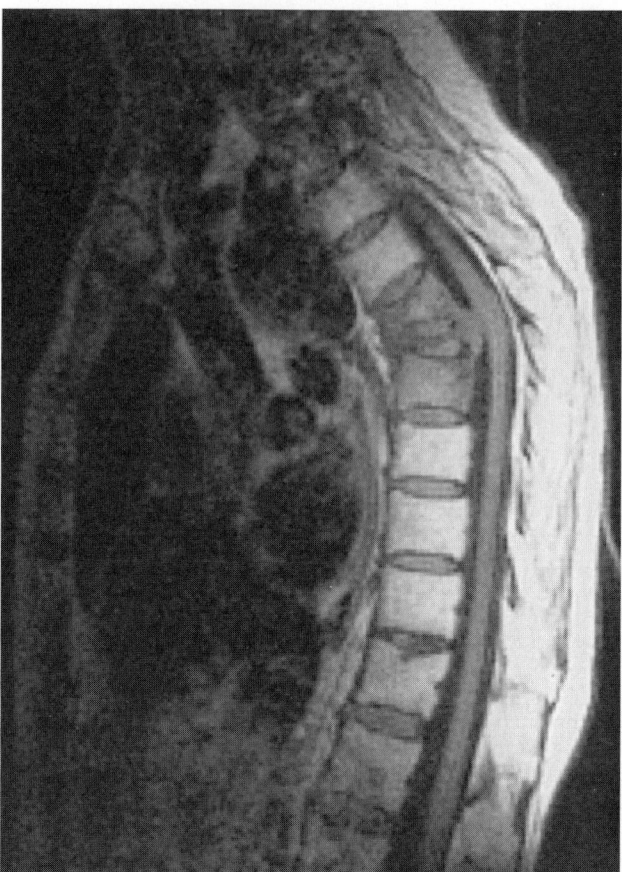

Figure 41–23. A sagittal magnetic resonance image of metastatic carcinoma of the breast in three contiguous thoracic vertebral segments, with vertebral marrow replacement, compression fracture, spinal angulation, and spinal cord compression. The epidural extension of the tumor anterior to the spinal cord is well demonstrated. (From Miller, K. D., Jr.: Magnetic resonance imaging of the vertebral column and spinal cord. *In* Wilkins, R. H., and Rengachary, S. S. [Eds.]: Neurosurgery Update I. New York, McGraw-Hill, 1990, p. 104. Copyright © 1990. Reproduced with permission of The McGraw-Hill Companies.)

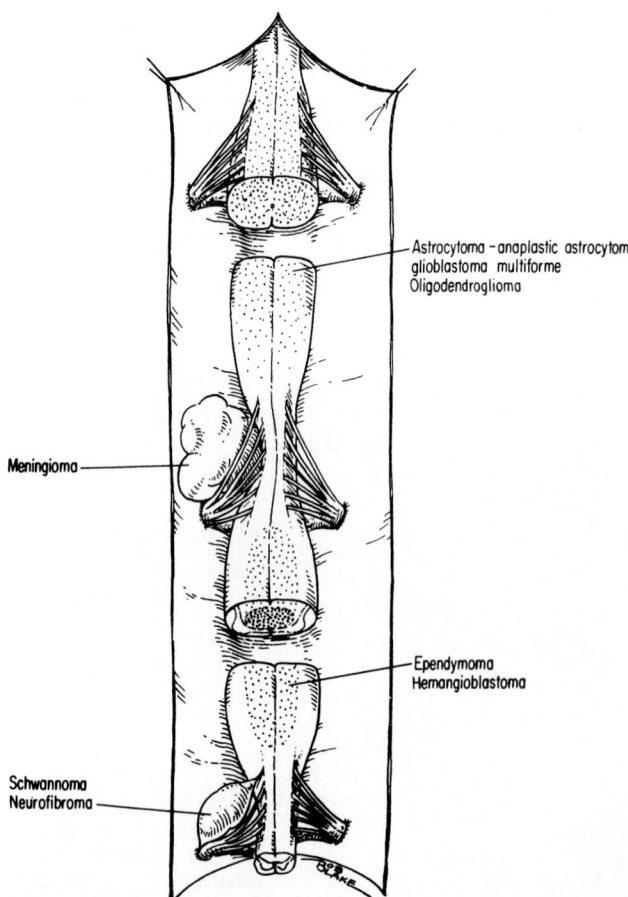

Figure 41–22. Topographic distribution of the common neoplasms of the spinal meninges, spinal nerve roots, and spinal cord. (From Burger, P. C., Scheithauer, B. W., and Vogel, F. S.: Surgical Pathology of the Nervous System and Its Coverings, 3rd ed. New York, Churchill Livingstone, 1991.)

INTRADURAL EXTRAMEDULLARY NEOPLASMS

Tumors that occur within the spinal subarachnoid space are of two types: benign neoplasms that arise from the meninges (meningiomas) or the nerve roots (neurofibromas, schwannomas),[1, 4–6, 8] or malignant tumors that have spread through the spinal subarachnoid space from a primary intracranial location (e.g., medulloblastoma, ependymoma, certain pineal region tumors) or from a malignancy elsewhere in the body (meningeal carcinomatosis). Fortunately, the first type is more common than the second.

Although nerve root tumors can arise at any spinal level, meningiomas rarely develop in the lumbar area. For reasons that are not clear, intraspinal meningiomas are 10 times more frequent in women than in men. A patient with a meningioma, neurofibroma, or schwannoma usually presents with myelopathy (if the tumor is located above the level of the cauda equina) but may also exhibit a radiculopathy in the distribution of the involved nerve root or roots. A nerve root tumor occasionally extends along the nerve, with one end within the dural sac, an isthmus extending through the intervertebral foramen (and enlarging it), and the other end outside the spine; a tumor with this configuration is called a *dumbbell tumor.*

Except for the occasional demonstration of an enlarged intervertebral foramen, plain roentgenograms and CT scans are not usually of value in the diagnosis of intradural extra-medullary tumors. Myelography and postmyelographic CT scanning and MRI with gadolinium enhancement are the most useful diagnostic studies. For meningeal carcinomatosis, the key diagnostic test is cytologic examination of cerebrospinal fluid removed by lumbar puncture.

The treatment of intraspinal meningiomas, neurofibromas, and schwannomas is surgical excision, which may include excision of the involved portion of the dura mater (meningioma) or the involved nerve rootlets or root (neurofibroma, schwannoma). At the level of involvement, neurofibromas and schwannomas typically grow on the sensory (dorsal) root in preference to the motor (ventral) root, and it may be possible to spare motor function during tumor removal. However, such tumors may be part of a more widespread process called neurofibromatosis, in which case there are similar tumors on other nerve roots and nerves. If the gross total removal of a solitary intraspinal meningioma, neurofibroma, or schwannoma can be achieved, which is usually the case, the patient is ordinarily cured. For example, Solero and associates followed 156 patients for an average of 15 years after the removal of spinal meningiomas.[5] The rate of recurrence was only 6% among the 150 patients who had gross total tumor removal.

Metastases within the subarachnoid space are not treated surgically. These are ordinarily managed with radiotherapy and hormonal therapy or chemotherapy.

INTRAMEDULLARY NEOPLASMS

Intramedullary tumors develop within the spinal cord, enlarging it in a fusiform manner.[1-3, 6, 8] The patient experiences a progressive myelopathy, and the radiographic studies demonstrate evidence of spinal cord expansion. Although plain x-ray films and CT scans may show enlargement of the spinal canal, MRI with gadolinium enhancement is the most useful test for demonstrating the tumor and any associated syrinx. Myelography and postmyelographic CT scanning may also be of value.

Intramedullary tumors are ordinarily treated surgically, through a laminectomy. If an ependymoma is encountered, it may be possible to excise it completely, with maintenance of the surrounding spinal cord. If only a partial resection can be achieved, radiotherapy can be given postoperatively. The outlook for a patient with an intraspinal ependymoma is significantly better than that of a patient with an intracranial ependymoma.[3]

As is true of most astrocytomas of the brain, an intramedullary astrocytoma ordinarily cannot be completely removed surgically. The decision about giving postoperative radiotherapy is based on the exact histology of the tumor, the degree of surgical resection, and the age of the patient. In contrast, intramedullary hemangioblastoma is a benign tumor that can

be cured by surgical excision, without the need for radiotherapy.

Intraspinal dermoid and epidermoid tumors are benign lesions that can be found within the subarachnoid space, the spinal cord, or both.[9] They are most common in the lumbosacral area, especially at the level of the conus medullaris. Either type of tumor can be associated with spinal dysraphism and, in particular, with a dermal sinus tract that opens onto the back, usually in the lumbosacral region. Lipomas are also benign spinal tumors that are often associated with spinal dysraphism. They can be found at any level from extradural to intramedullary and are most common in the lumbosacral region. These various benign tumors can be resected surgically, with the risks and difficulties of such treatment being related to the degree of tumor involvement with critical areas of the spinal cord and the extent of any associated dysraphic changes.

CONCLUSIONS

The spread of malignant neoplasms into the spinal canal has a poor prognosis. Successful treatment is usually defined as either an improvement in neurologic function or the maintenance of ambulation during the patient's short remaining life span. However, many intraspinal neoplasms such as meningiomas, neurofibromas, schwannomas, dermoid tumors, epidermoid tumors, lipomas, hemangioblastomas, and ependymomas have a high potential for surgical cure. Recent advances in neuroradiologic and neurosurgical technology have enabled neurosurgeons to achieve this potential to a greater degree than ever before and have also reduced the risks of such treatment.

REFERENCES

1. Burger, P. C., Scheithauer, B. W., and Vogel, F. S.: Surgical Pathology of the Nervous System and Its Coverings, 3rd ed. New York, Churchill Livingstone, 1991.
2. Cristante, L., and Herrmann, H. D.: Surgical management of intramedullary spinal cord tumors: Functional outcome and sources of morbidity. Neurosurgery, 35:69, 1994.
3. Epstein, F. J., Farmer, J.-P., and Freed, D.: Adult intramedullary spinal cord ependymomas: The results of surgery in 38 patients. J. Neurosurg., 79:204, 1993.
4. Levy, W. J., Latchaw, J., Hahn, J. F., Sawhny, B., Bay, J., and Dohn, D. F.: Spinal neurofibromas: A report of 66 cases and a comparison with meningiomas. Neurosurgery, 18:331, 1986.
5. Solero, C. L., Fornari, M., Giombini, S., Lasio G., Oliveri, G., Cimino, C., and Pluchino, F.: Spinal meningiomas: Review of 174 operated cases. Neurosurgery, 125:153, 1989.
6. Stein, B. M., and McCormick, P. C. (Eds.): Intradural spinal surgery. Neurosurg. Clin. North Am., 1(3):469, 1990.
7. Sundaresan, N., Schmidek, H. H., Schiller, A. L., and Rosenthal, D. I. (Eds.): Tumors of the Spine: Diagnosis and Clinical Management. Philadelphia, W. B. Saunders, 1990.
8. Wilkins, R. H., and Rengachary, S. S. (Eds.): Neurosurgery, 2nd ed. New York, McGraw-Hill, 1996, p. 1757.
9. Wilkins, R. H., and Rossitch, E., Jr.: Intraspinal cysts. In Pang, D. (Ed.): Disorders of the Paediatric Spine. New York: Raven Press, 1995, p. 445.

VIII

RUPTURED LUMBAR INTERVERTEBRAL DISC

Robert H. Wilkins, M.D.

Despite its common occurrence,[2–4, 6–9] intervertebral disc rupture escaped clinical recognition until just over 60 years ago. Low back pain and sciatica had been discussed in medical treatises for centuries, but it was not until Mixter and Barr's 1934 article in *The New England Journal of Medicine* that herniation of a lumbar intervertebral disc (formerly thought to be a rare result of severe spinal injury) was first linked clearly to the syndrome of low back pain and sciatica.[5] Today, this is one of the most common conditions treated by neurosurgeons in the United States.

NORMAL ANATOMY

The central portion of the intervertebral disc, the nucleus pulposus, is left as a remnant of the notochord as the spinal column is formed during embryonic life. It is ringed by the tough anulus fibrosus and is situated somewhat eccentrically toward the posterior aspect of the disc. It is bounded above and below by the cartilaginous plates covering the opposing surfaces of the two adjacent vertebral bodies. The nucleus pulposus is gelatinous in infancy but becomes more fibrous with age. The anulus fibrosus is supported anteriorly by the anterior longitudinal ligament and posteriorly by the posterior longitudinal ligament.

The bony arch that encircles the spinal canal posteriorly is formed by the two pedicles, the two transverse processes, the two laminae, and the spinous process. On each side of the midline, the laminal arches of adjacent vertebrae are connected by an elastic yellow ligament, the ligamentum flavum.

The tip of the spinal cord (conus medullaris) ends at the T12 or L1 level of the spinal canal. Caudal to the conus medullaris, the nerve roots of the cauda equina lie immersed in cerebrospinal fluid within the subarachnoid space, surrounded by concentric cylindrical sheaths, the arachnoid and the dura mater. The dural-arachnoidal sac usually ends at about the level of the first sacral vertebra. The space that surrounds the dura within the spinal canal, the epidural space, is filled with fat and is traversed by veins. The spinal nerves leave the dural sac in pairs, with one nerve on each side exiting at each vertebral level. Each nerve lies along the caudal border of the pedicle as it exits through the intervertebral foramen; in this position, it lies between the intervertebral disc anteromedially and the facet joint posterolaterally (Fig. 41–24). The nerve roots, however, do not exit directly transversely. Each nerve root exits from the main dural sac and then lies immediately lateral to it for 1 to 2 cm. before it turns further laterally to leave the bony spinal canal about one vertebral level below where it left the dural sac. For example, the left L5 nerve root ordinarily leaves the dural sac at the level of the L4–L5 intervertebral disc (where it is most likely to be involved by a left-sided L4–L5 disc herniation), but it leaves the bony spinal canal below the left L5 pedicle, opposite the L5–S1 disc (Fig. 41–25).

CLINICOPATHOLOGIC FEATURES

Degenerative changes in an intervertebral disc can take two main forms: (1) the nucleus pulposus can herniate out of its normally confined space (soft disc protrusion), or (2) the entire disc can lose substance, with loss of disc height and the formation of osteophytes that project outward from the adjacent rims of the vertebral bodies above and below the involved disc (hard disc protrusion).

Soft Disc Protrusion (Herniated Nucleus Pulposus, Herniated Disc, Ruptured Disc). The nucleus pulposus can herniate superiorly or inferiorly through the confining cartilaginous plate into the cancellous bone of the adjacent vertebral body. These are called Schmorl's nodules and are incidental radiographic or postmortem findings.

Disc herniation that is important clinically begins with the development of a posterolateral or posterior fissure through the concentric rings of the anulus fibrosus. The nucleus pulposus may then begin to extend into this fissure (Fig. 41–26, top). At this stage, the patient may experience low back pain and perhaps some referred pain into the buttock or hip on the affected side. Further protrusion of the nucleus pulposus may then occur, causing bulging of the outer layers of anulus and of the posterior longitudinal ligament sufficient to pinch the adjacent nerve root between the protruding disc and the lamina or the intervertebral facet (Fig. 41–26, lower left). Finally, a fragment of the disc may actually be extruded completely through the remaining layers of the anulus fibrosus and become wedged anterior to the nerve root; this is referred to as a free fragment (Fig. 41–26, lower right). When the nerve root is compressed by a protruding or extruded

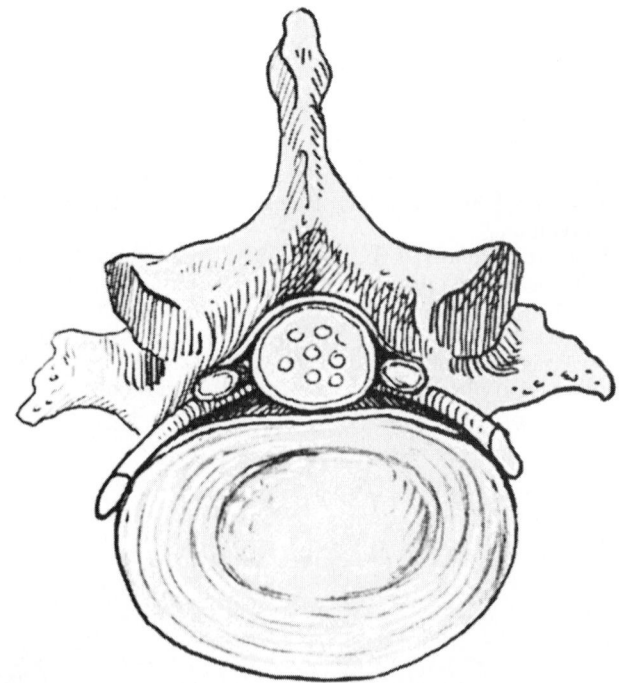

Figure 41–24. A lumbar vertebra, demonstrating the relationship of the exiting nerve root on each side to the intervertebral disc and the ipsilateral facet. (From Semmes, R. E.: Ruptures of the Lumbar Intervertebral Disc: Their Mechanism, Diagnosis, and Treatment. Springfield, Ill., Charles C Thomas, 1964.)

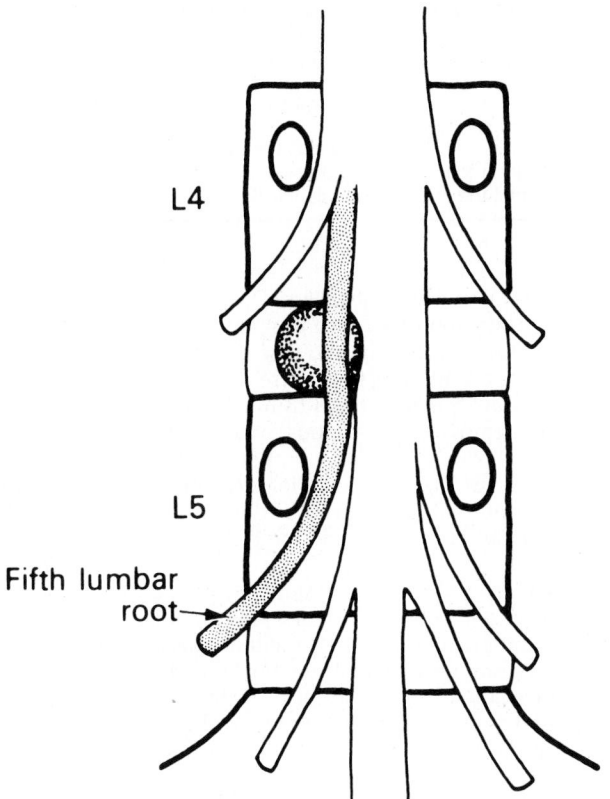

Figure 41–25. Herniation of the disc between the L4 and L5 vertebrae compresses the L5 nerve root. (From Macnab, I.: Backache. Baltimore, Williams & Wilkins, 1977.)

disc at the L4–L5 or L5–S1 levels, the patient develops radiating pain along the distribution of the sciatic nerve (sciatica) on the involved side, in addition to low back pain. The patient may also have neurologic deficits (hyperesthesia, weakness, or reduction of the deep tendon reflex) in the distribution of the involved nerve root. This clinical pattern of radiating pain, perhaps with neurologic deficits, is referred to as a radiculopathy.

If the disc herniation is quite large or in the midline (posterocentral rather than posterolateral herniation), it may compress many of the nerves of the cauda equina still within the dural sac at that level. Such compression may cause low back pain, bilateral sciatica, and interference with urinary and anal sphincter function and with sexual function. Fortunately, the latter neurologic deficits are rare; of these unusual dysfunctions, urinary retention is the most likely to occur.

Approximately 95% of lumbar disc herniations occur at the L5–S1 or L4–L5 level, with a slight numerical preponderance at one or the other level reported by various authors. About 4% occur at the L3–L4 level, and less than 1% at the L2–L3 or L1–L2 level.

Hard Disc Protrusion (Degenerative Disc Disease with Spinal Osteoarthritis, Lumbar Spondylosis). Degeneration in a lumbar intervertebral disc with narrowing of the disc space and generalized bulging of the anulus fibrosus is frequently associated with the formation of osteoarthritic bony ridges (osteophytes) along the rims of the vertebral bodies adjacent to the involved disc. The posterior elements (laminae, facet joints, ligamenta flava) may become thickened, and osteophytes may project anteriorly from the facets. All these changes tend to narrow the spinal canal (especially its lateral recesses) and the intervertebral foramina.[1] Such narrowing may cause compression of an individual nerve root or multiple nerve roots of the cauda equina. The resulting symptoms and signs are similar to those caused by disc herniation but tend to be more gradual in onset and more protracted in course. If significant narrowing of the spinal canal occurs (acquired spinal stenosis), the cauda equina may be compressed when the lumbar spine is placed into certain positions, such as extension; when the patient walks, he or she may develop disagreeable paresthesia, numbness, or weakness in the lower extremities (neurogenic intermittent claudication).

SYMPTOMS AND SIGNS

The typical patient with a posterolateral lumbar disc herniation has intermittent low back pain for several weeks to several years and then develops sciatica as well. The pain is usually aggravated by back movement, by sitting or standing for long periods, by lifting an object from the bent position, and by coughing or straining. It is ordinarily relieved tempo-

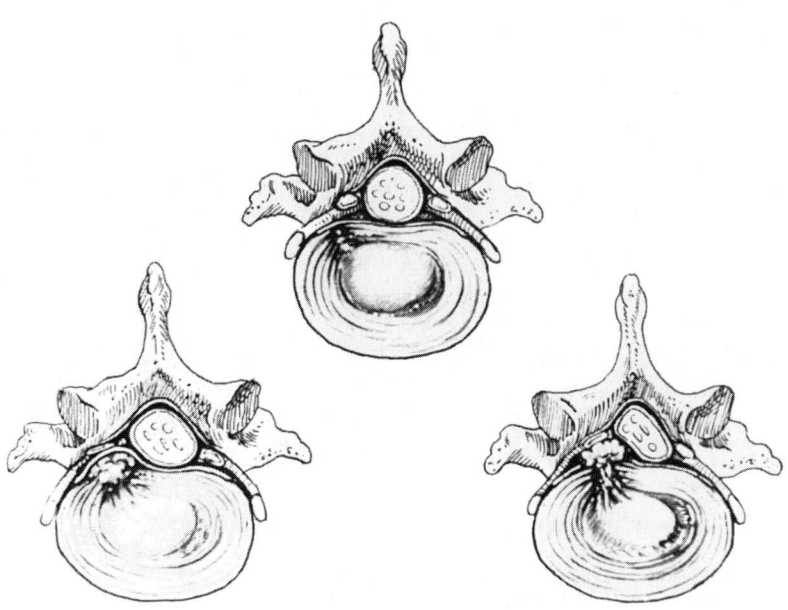

Figure 41–26. Soft disc herniation. Top, The initial tear in the rings of the anulus fibrosus. Lower left, Protrusion of the nucleus pulposus through the anulus. Lower right, Extrusion of a free fragment through the anulus and the posterior longitudinal ligament. (From Semmes, R. E.: Ruptures of the Lumbar Intervertebral Disc: Their Mechanism, Diagnosis, and Treatment. Springfield, Ill., Charles C Thomas, 1964.)

TABLE 41–5. Patterns of Neurologic Deficit Caused by Intervertebral Disc Herniation

Involved Disc	Involved Nerve Root	Reduced Neurologic Function		
		Sensory	Motor	Reflex
L3–L4	L4	Anterior thigh, anteromedial calf	Quadriceps femoris	Knee jerk
L4–L5	L5	Anterior calf, medial dorsum of foot, great toe	Foot dorsiflexors	Variable
L5–S1	S1	Lateral calf, lateral dorsum of foot, small toe	Foot plantar flexors	Ankle jerk

rarily by bed rest; the most comfortable position is horizontal, usually on the side, with the hips and knees flexed. The patient may also notice tingling paresthesia or numbness in certain aspects of the involved leg and foot, weakness in some muscle groups in that limb (less frequent), or, rarely, urinary retention.

On physical examination, the patient may demonstrate one or more of the following mechanical signs: lumbar scoliosis, paravertebral muscle spasm, tenderness over one or more of the lower lumbar spines, limitation of low back motion (especially forward flexion) by pain, limitation of straight leg raising on one or both sides by pain, or the initiation or intensification of sciatica and back pain by the popliteal compression test. Neurologic deficits, if present, have a typical pattern for each of the commonly involved lumbar discs (Table 41–5).

MANAGEMENT

The initial treatment of the acute symptoms of lumbar disc disease consists of bed rest on a firm mattress, with medication to combat pain and muscle spasm as needed. Locally applied heat, anti-inflammatory medication, pelvic traction, or the use of a lumbosacral corset may also be helpful. If these measures give relief of the acute episode, recurrences may be minimized by a daily maintenance program of low back exercises and avoidance of certain activities such as bending at the waist frequently or lifting heavy objects. Anti-inflammatory medication may be beneficial over a prolonged period to reduce the discomfort of lumbar osteoarthritis.

If conservative measures fail to relieve the patient's pain or if the patient develops significant weakness or urinary retention, a more aggressive approach to treatment should be taken. The patient should have diagnostic tests, such as magnetic resonance imaging or a lumbar myelogram followed by a computed tomography scan while the contrast agent is still within the spinal canal. If all available evidence indicates that a soft or hard lumbar disc protrusion is the cause of the patient's symptoms and signs, it should be treated surgically.

The aim of surgical treatment is to provide relief of existing nerve compression. The standard surgical treatment of a unilateral radiculopathy is via a partial hemilaminectomy. The surgeon makes a midline lower lumbar incision and retracts the paravertebral muscles away from the spines and laminae on the involved side. Then the surgeon removes portions of one or two laminae and the attached ligamentum flavum to gain entrance into the lateral aspect of the spinal canal. After retracting the affected nerve root and exposing the disc herniation immediately anterior to it, the surgeon incises any remaining fibers of the posterior longitudinal ligament and anulus fibrosus and extracts as much of the degenerated disc material (mainly nucleus pulposus) as is feasible. The wound is then closed in anatomic layers. The same technique is used for decompression of a nerve root entrapped by the changes of spondylosis, except that no disc material is removed.

If there is a central or transverse disc herniation or if there is generalized spinal stenosis from spondylosis, the surgeon generally removes the spinous process, both laminae, the ligamenta flava, and perhaps portions of the facets at one or more levels to provide posterior decompression. Any disc herniation present is removed in the manner previously described via an approach from one or both sides of the spinal canal.

The patient ordinarily leaves the hospital 2 to 5 days postoperatively and returns to work after another 3 to 6 weeks of recuperation at home. The patient is instructed in a maintenance program such as that mentioned earlier.

An alternative to open surgical treatment of a lumbar disc protrusion is the percutaneous removal of disc material by one of several techniques. However, such techniques cannot effectively treat a free-fragment disc extrusion.

Although disc herniation can usually be managed effectively, with resolution or improvement of the symptoms and signs, the underlying (and poorly understood) biochemical abnormality that led to the herniation continues. Therefore, some patients are destined to have future problems from disc disease at the same or a different spinal level.

SELECTED REFERENCE

Spurling, R. G.: Lesions of the Lumbar Intervertebral Disc. Springfield, Ill., Charles C Thomas, 1953.
This helpful little book (148 pages) is based on an earlier monograph on the intervertebral disc by F. K. Bradford and R. G. Spurling, also published by the Charles C Thomas Company. Although it was written more than 40 years ago, it is concise, practical, and readable; it provides the basic information that underlies the present management of a ruptured lumbar intervertebral disc.

REFERENCES

1. Anderson, G. B. J., and McNeill, T. W. (Eds.): Lumbar Spinal Stenosis. St. Louis, Mosby-Year Book, 1992.
2. Davis, R. A.: A long-term outcome analysis of 984 surgically treated herniated lumbar discs. J. Neurosurg., 80:415, 1994.
3. Dunsker, S. B.: Alternatives in the surgical treatment of herniated lumbar disks. Clin. Neurosurg., 35:459, 1989.
4. Hardy, R. W. (Ed.): Lumbar Disc Disease, 2nd ed. New York, Raven Press, 1993.
5. Mixter, W. J., and Barr, J. S.: Rupture of the intervertebral disc with involvement of the spinal canal. N. Engl. J. Med., 211:210, 1934.
6. Rothman, R. H., and Simeone, F. A. (Eds.): The Spine, 3rd ed. Philadelphia, W. B. Saunders, 1992.
7. Semmes, R. E.: Ruptures of the Lumbar Intervertebral Disc: Their Mechanism, Diagnosis, and Treatment. Springfield, Ill., Charles C Thomas, 1964.
8. Spurling, R. G.: Lesions of the Lumbar Intervertebral Disc. Springfield, Ill., Charles C Thomas, 1953.
9. Weinstein, J. N., Wiesel, S. W., and the Editorial Committee, International Society for the Study of the Lumbar Spine (Eds.): The Lumbar Spine. Philadelphia, W. B. Saunders, 1990.

IX

CERVICAL DISC LESIONS

Robert H. Wilkins, M.D.

Lesions of the cervical intervertebral discs are analogous to those that affect the lumbar discs. However, in the cervical region, the anatomy is somewhat different (Figs. 41–27 and 41–28), and those differences introduce variations in symptoms, signs, and treatment.

NORMAL ANATOMY

The cervical disc, like the lumbar disc, is composed of a tough outer anulus fibrosus and a softer inner nucleus pulposus and is separated from the vertebral bodies above and below it by cartilaginous plates. However, the entire cervical disc is much smaller than a lumbar disc.

The spinal canal in the cervical area contains the spinal cord rather than the cauda equina, so a reduction in the size of the spinal canal by spondylosis or a midline disc herniation causes compression of the spinal cord rather than of the cauda equina—a more serious form of neurologic involvement with a worse prognosis. The nerve roots of the cauda equina are more resistant to compression than is the spinal cord and are more likely to recover after surgical decompression.

In addition, the cervical spine contains the joints of Luschka, which are not present elsewhere in the spine. These joints, one on each side of the disc, can give rise to bony spurs or ridges (osteophytes), as can the main facet joints (apophyseal or interpedicular joints) and the edges of the vertebral bodies adjacent to the intervertebral disc (which is a symphysis type of articulation between vertebral bodies). The exiting nerve root on each side travels between these joints (see Fig. 41–27) and can be compressed by osteophytes extending into the intervertebral foramen from any or all of the three sources just mentioned (see Fig. 41–28).

In the cervical area, the nerves exit transversely. There are seven cervical vertebrae and eight pairs of cervical nerves. The nerve root exiting on each side at the level of the inter-

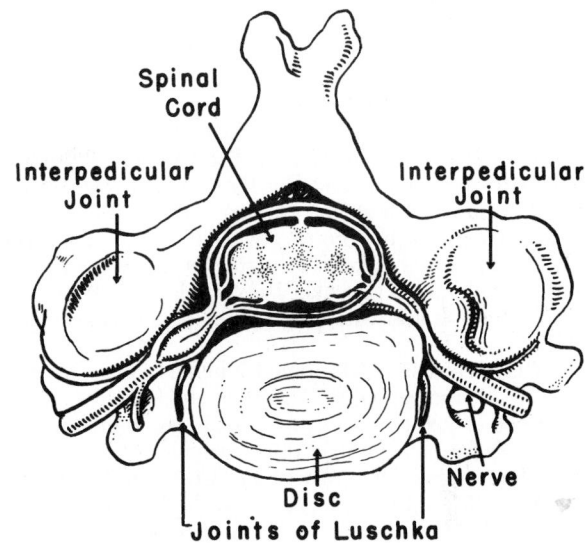

Figure 41–28. Mechanism of cervical nerve root compression by osteophytes extending into the intervertebral foramen. (From Spurling, R. G.: Lesions of the Cervical Intervertebral Disc. Springfield, Ill., Charles C Thomas, 1956.)

vertebral disc between the C7 vertebral body and the T1 vertebral body (the C7–T1 disc) is the C8 nerve root. The nerve root exiting on each side at the level of the C6–C7 disc is the C7 nerve root; the nerve root exiting on each side at the level of the C5–C6 disc is the C6 nerve root, and so on (Table 41–6).

CLINICOPATHOLOGIC FEATURES

As with a lumbar disc, degenerative changes in a cervical intervertebral disc can take two main forms: (1) the nucleus

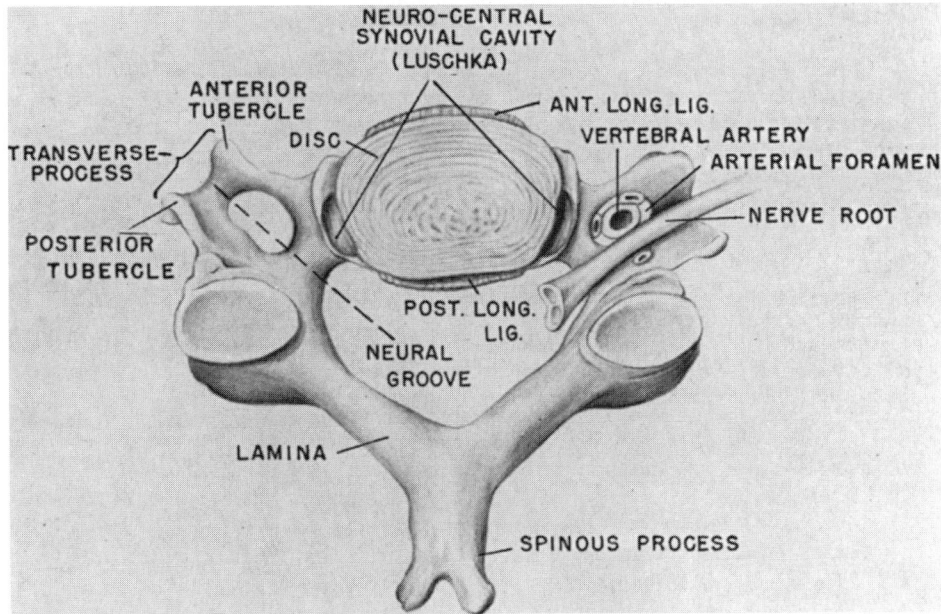

Figure 41–27. Semidiagrammatic representation of a vertebra from the midcervical region, viewed from above. (From Spurling, R. G.: Lesions of the Cervical Intervertebral Disc. Springfield, Ill., Charles C Thomas, 1956.)

TABLE 41–6. Patterns of Radiculopathy Caused by Cervical Disc Herniation or Osteophyte Formation

Involved Disc Level	Involved Nerve Root	Key Areas of Reduced Neurologic Function		
		Sensory	*Motor*	*Reflex*
C4–C5	C5	Deltoid area	Deltoid	—
C5–C6	C6	Thumb, index finger	Biceps	Biceps
C6–C7	C7	Index and long fingers	Triceps	Triceps
C7–T1	C8	Ring and small fingers	Grip	—

pulposus can herniate out of its normal confined space (soft disc protrusion), or (2) the entire disc can lose substance, with loss of disc height and the formation of osteophytes that project outward from the adjacent rims of the vertebral bodies above and below the involved disc. The second process is often combined with osteoarthritis of the apophyseal joints and the joints of Luschka. The combination of degenerative disc disease and osteophyte formation is called spondylosis.

Soft Disc Protrusion (Herniated Nucleus Pulposus, Herniated Disc, Ruptured Disc). The pathologic process and the steps in the development of a cervical disc herniation are similar to those of a lumbar disc herniation. Cervical disc herniations are most frequent at the C6–C7 level but also occur at C5–C6 and to a lesser extent at C4–C5 and other levels.

With the usual posterolateral disc rupture, the patient experiences pain in the neck. Then, as the nerve root is compressed, the patient develops pain radiating into the ipsilateral upper extremity and may also develop paresthesia, numbness, or weakness in an appropriate distribution (see Table 41–6). The pain and paresthesia may be intensified by neck movement, especially by extension or by lateral flexion to the side of the herniation, and by coughing or straining. They may be improved by bed rest.

On examination, the patient frequently exhibits restriction of neck movement, especially extension. Downward head compression by the examiner increases the patient's radicular pain and paresthesia, especially if the neck is simultaneously flexed to the side of the involvement. Hypesthesia, weakness, or the reduction of a deep tendon reflex may be present and should provide a clue to the level of the disc rupture and nerve root compression (see Table 41–6).

If the disc herniation occurs more toward the midline (i.e., is a more direct posterior herniation), it compresses the spinal cord in addition to, or instead of, a nerve root. This produces cervical myelopathy manifested by lower motor neuron dysfunction (muscle weakness and hypotonia, reduction or loss of appropriate deep tendon reflexes, dermatomal sensory impairment) at the level of the compression and upper motor neuron dysfunction (spasticity, clonus, increased deep tendon reflexes, Babinski's sign, reduction of sensation) below that level. Loss of voluntary control of bowel, bladder, and sexual function may also develop.

Hard Disc Protrusion (Degenerative Disc Disease with Spinal Osteoarthritis, Cervical Spondylosis). As in the lumbar area, these changes tend to narrow the spinal canal and the intervertebral foramina, which may result in the compression of one or more cervical nerve roots or of the spinal cord at one or more levels. The resulting symptoms and signs are similar to those caused by disc herniation but tend to be more gradual in onset and more protracted in course.

MANAGEMENT

Roentgenograms of the cervical spine are obtained to assess the presence and degree of spondylosis, but especially

to identify a cause of neck and arm pain other than disc disease, such as neoplasm or infection. The initial treatment of a patient with acute radiculopathy consists of bed rest, with medication for pain and muscle spasm. Locally applied heat may provide additional comfort. Intermittent cervical halter traction is often beneficial as well, but the direction of traction must be comfortable. Traction with the neck extended may actually increase the pain. Anti-inflammatory medication may be of value over a prolonged period to reduce the discomfort of cervical spondylosis.

If these measures do not provide adequate pain relief, or if the patient shows evidence of spinal cord compression, a more aggressive approach should be taken. The patient should have further diagnostic tests, such as magnetic resonance imaging (MRI) or a cervical myelogram followed by computed tomography (CT) scanning while the contrast material is still present in the cervical subarachnoid space.

Surgical treatment to provide nerve root decompression can be accomplished by a posterior approach through a hemilaminectomy (Fig. 41–29) or by an anterior approach through the intervertebral disc (Figs. 41–30 and 41–31).[1–4, 6, 8, 10–12] The posterior procedure is a smaller operation that takes less time, does not require a bone graft, and provides good results. For example, Henderson and associates reviewed the results of 736 consecutive patients who were treated by a posterior approach and followed for an average of 2.8 years;

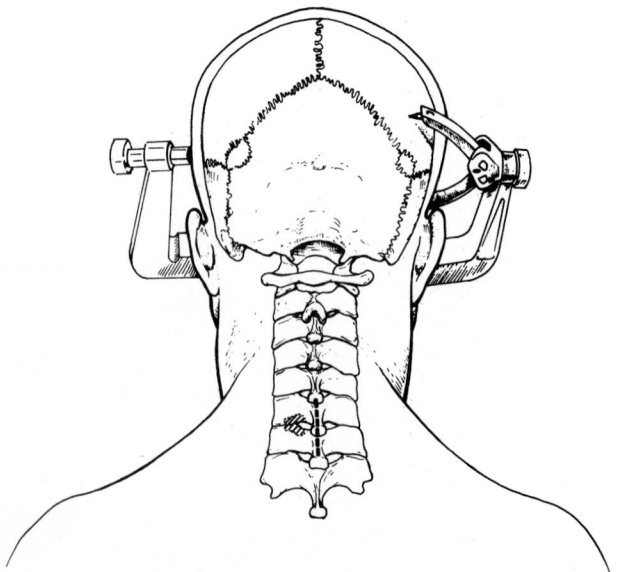

Figure 41–29. The posterior approach to a cervical nerve root decompression, in this case for the removal of a disc herniation at the C6–C7 level on the left. The interrupted line shows the position of the skin incision, and the oblique lines show the area of bone removal that exposes the left C7 nerve root and the disc herniation that is anterior to it. (From Wilkins, R. H., and Gaskill, S. J.: Cervical hemilaminectomy for excision of herniated disc. *In* Rengachary, S. S., and Wilkins, R. H. [Eds.]: Neurosurgical Operative Atlas. Baltimore, Williams & Wilkins, 1991, p. 37.)

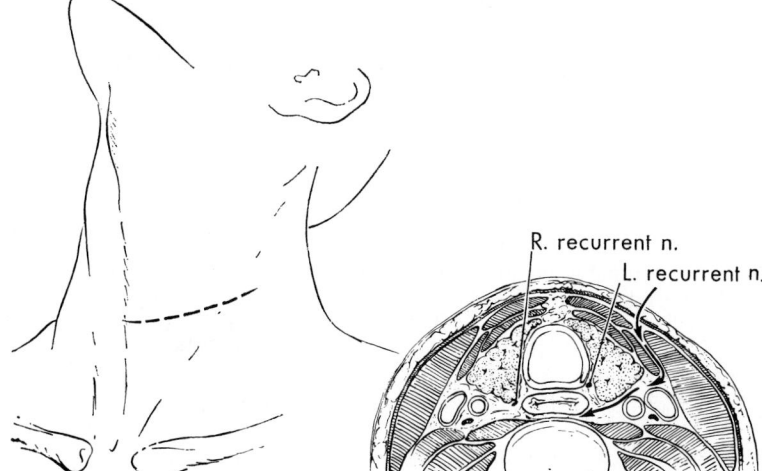

Figure 41–30. The anterior approach to the midcervical spine. A typical skin incision is shown on the left, and the route of approach is shown on the right. (From Aronson, N. I.: The management of soft cervical disc protrusions using the Smith-Robinson approach. Clin. Neurosurg., *20*:253, 1973.)

there was a 96% incidence of relief of significant arm pain and/or paresthesia and a 98% incidence of resolution of a preoperative motor deficit, with only a 1.5% minor complication rate and a 3% rate of recurrent radiculopathy.[6]

If a patient is being treated for the unusual circumstance of a single midline disc herniation with spinal cord compression, an anterior discectomy is the procedure of choice. Provided that the myelopathy is not too severe or too long-standing, improvement can be expected.

In contrast, the surgical treatment of spinal cord compression from spondylosis usually requires a larger operation, and the results are not as favorable.[1, 3–5, 7, 9] If the operation is done via a posterior approach, it necessitates a full laminectomy (removal of the spinous process and the lamina on each side) at multiple levels. If an anterior approach is chosen, it involves either a discectomy and osteophytectomy at one or more levels or the resection of the central aspects of one or more vertebral bodies, usually with the insertion of a bone

graft (and perhaps an overlying supportive metal plate held by screws) to ensure the postoperative maintenance of vertebral alignment and stability. These larger procedures carry additional risk, and, more importantly, the results are less satisfactory. For example, reports of the treatment of cervical spondylotic myelopathy by anterior discectomy and osteophytectomy typically indicate neurologic improvement in only 40% to 75%, with a significant percentage of patients showing further deterioration despite treatment.

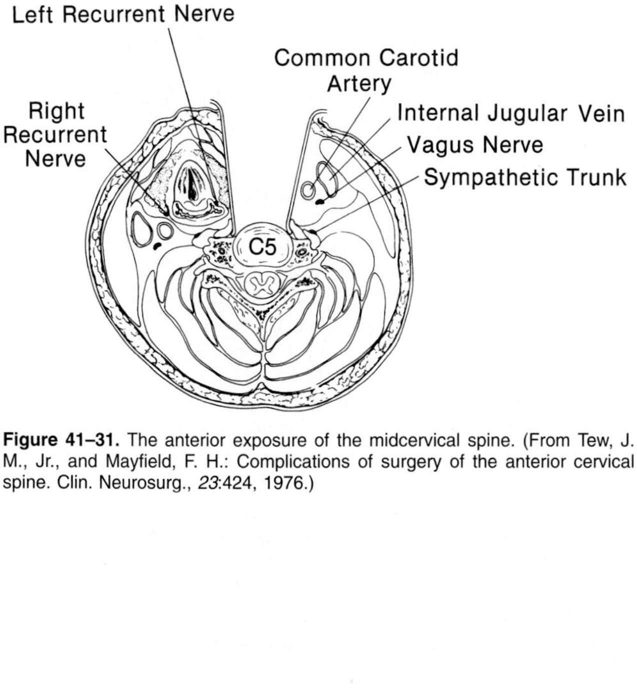

REFERENCES

1. An, H. S., and Simpson, J. M. (Eds.): Surgery of the Cervical Spine. Baltimore, Williams & Wilkins, 1994.
2. Bohlman, H. H., Emery, S. E., Goodfellow, D. B., and Jones, P. K.: Robinson anterior cervical discectomy and athrodesis for cervical radiculopathy: Long-term follow-up of one hundred and twenty-two patients. J. Bone Joint Surg. [Am.], *75*:1298, 1993.
3. Camins, M. B., and O'Leary, P. F. (Eds.): Disorders of the Cervical Spine. Baltimore, Williams & Wilkins, 1992.
4. Cooper, P. R. (Ed.): Degenerative Disease of the Cervical Spine. Park Ridge, Ill., American Association of Neurological Surgeons, 1992.
5. Fager, C. A.: Results of adequate posterior decompression in the relief of spondylotic cervical myelopathy. J. Neurosurg., *38*:684, 1973.
6. Henderson, C. M., Hennessy, R. G., Shuey, H. M., Jr., and Shackelford, E. G.: Posterior-lateral foraminotomy as an exclusive operative technique for cervical radiculopathy: A review of 846 consecutively operated cases. Neurosurgery, *13*:504, 1983.
7. Kojima, T., Waga, S., Kubo, Y., Kanamaru, K., Shimosaka, S., and Shimizu, T.: Anterior cervical vertebrectomy and interbody fusion for multi-level spondylosis and ossification of the posterior longitudinal ligament. Neurosurgery, *24*:864, 1989.
8. Lunsford, L. D., Bissonette, D. J., Jannetta, P. J., Sheptak, P. E., and Zorub, D. S.: Anterior surgery for cervical disc disease. Part 1: Treatment of lateral cervical disc herniation in 253 cases. J. Neurosurg., *53*:1, 1980.
9. Lunsford, L. D., Bissonette, D. J., and Zorub, D. S.: Anterior surgery for cervical disc disease. Part 2: Treatment of cervical spondylotic myelopathy in 32 cases. J. Neurosurg., *53*:12, 1980.
10. Raynor, R. B.: Anterior or posterior approach to the cervical spine: An anatomical and radiographic evaluation and comparison. Neurosurgery, *12*:7, 1983.
11. Spurling, R. G.: Lesions of the Cervical Intervertebral Disc. Springfield, Ill., Charles C Thomas, 1956.
12. Wilkins, R. H., and Gaskill, S. J.: Cervical hemilaminectomy for excision of herniated disc. In Rengachary, S. S., and Wilkins, R. H. (Eds.): Neurosurgical Operative Atlas. Baltimore, Williams & Wilkins, 1991, p. 37.

Left Recurrent Nerve

Common Carotid Artery

Right Recurrent Nerve

Internal Jugular Vein

Vagus Nerve

Sympathetic Trunk

C5

Figure 41–31. The anterior exposure of the midcervical spine. (From Tew, J. M., Jr., and Mayfield, F. H.: Complications of surgery of the anterior cervical spine. Clin. Neurosurg., *23*:424, 1976.)

X

PERIPHERAL NERVE INJURIES

Robert H. Wilkins, M.D.

ANATOMY AND PATHOPHYSIOLOGY

To correctly diagnose and treat peripheral nerve injuries, the surgeon must understand the anatomy and pathophysiology of peripheral nerves. The *wiring diagram* of the human body is complex,[3, 4, 8–10] in part because peripheral nerves contain varying proportions of motor, sensory, and sympathetic axons from diverse sources, and in part because of the mixing that occurs in the cervical, brachial, lumbar, and sacral nerve plexuses. In addition, the fascicles within a peripheral nerve divide and recombine along their course (funicular plexuses), and intercommunications between peripheral nerves (such as the ulnar and median nerves) are not uncommon. There also may be shared innervation by adjacent nerves and variations in nerve distribution in individuals. In assessing a patient with a peripheral nerve injury, the surgeon must bear in mind these facts about normal anatomy while evaluating the changes caused by the injury.

The axons within a peripheral nerve are myelinated to varying degrees; each is maintained by its neuronal cell body and by the Schwann cells along its lengthy course. The proportions are such that if a typical 50-μ neuronal cell body were 6 feet tall, its axon would be 3 to 4 cm. in diameter and about 2 miles long.[2]

In the Sunderland classification,[9, 10] there are five degrees of nerve injury:

1. Physiologic loss of axonal conduction.
2. Loss of continuity of the axons without interruption of their investing tissue, the endoneurium.
3. Disruption of the endoneurium.
4. Disruption of fascicles and their connective tissue sheaths, the perineurium.
5. Disruption of continuity of the entire nerve, including its connective tissue sheath, the epineurium.

Seddon[8] used only three terms to classify nerve injuries: neurapraxia, axonotmesis, and neurotmesis. Neurapraxia is equivalent to first-degree nerve injury. Anatomic continuity is preserved, but there is selective demyelination of large nerve fibers that typically causes complete motor paralysis with very little muscle atrophy and considerable sparing of sensory and autonomic function. Electrical conductivity of the nerve distal to the lesion is preserved. Surgical repair is not necessary, and recovery is rapid (within days or weeks). Recovery does not depend on regeneration, and there is no orderly sequence in the recovery of innervation. The quality of recovery is excellent.

Axonotmesis is equivalent to Sunderland's second-degree nerve injury. Anatomic continuity of the nerve and the Schwann sheaths is preserved, but the axons are interrupted and must recover by axonal regeneration. There is complete motor, sensory, and autonomic paralysis and progressive muscle atrophy. Surgical repair is not necessary. Recovery occurs at the rate of about 1 mm. per day (1 inch per month); it occurs according to the order of innervation, and the quality of recovery is excellent.

Neurotmesis is a more severe injury. There is significant disorganization within the nerve or actual disruption of its continuity, which precludes recovery without surgical repair. Wallerian degeneration occurs. In association with this, there is a gradual loss of electrical conductivity in the distal portion of the nerve over a period of up to 3 days. At 10 to 20 days,

fibrillations in the denervated muscles may first be detected by electromyography. From the time of the injury there is complete motor, sensory, and autonomic paralysis and progressive muscle atrophy.

At 10 to 20 days, axonal sprouting begins.[2] If scar tissue blocks their entrance into the distal portion of the nerve, these sprouts coil into a disorganized, painful neuroma. In contrast, if the nerve has been repaired, axonal regrowth proceeds at the rate of about 1 mm. per day. After the initial lag of 10 to 20 days, there is usually a further delay in the forward progress of nerve restitution if the regenerating axons have to bridge a narrow gap (e.g., where a divided nerve has been reapproximated) and another delay at the end organ before function resumes. The march of recovery occurs according to the order of innervation, and recovery is always imperfect.

The rate and success of nerve regeneration are influenced by several factors.[1–3, 5, 6, 8–11] Patient age is important. The younger the patient, the faster and more complete the recovery. The nerve involved is also important. *Pure* motor or sensory nerves recover better than mixed nerves. Recovery is better in the radial and musculocutaneous nerves than in the median nerve, and the tibial division of the sciatic nerve fares better than the peroneal division.

The level of the nerve injury and the duration of denervation also influence recovery significantly. If it takes more than 12 months for regenerating axons to reach a denervated muscle, a significant degree of muscular atrophy has occurred, and the muscle does not function. In contrast, sensory restitution may still be possible under these circumstances. Thus, from the standpoint of motor recovery, it is usually not worthwhile to suture the ulnar nerve near the axilla or the peroneal nerve above the midthigh; however, it may be worthwhile to suture the median nerve near the axilla or the tibial nerve above the midthigh to effect return of at least protective sensation.

Other factors that are significant in the rate and success of nerve recovery are the type of injury, the length of the defect in the nerve, the severity of associated injuries (to bones, blood vessels, muscles, tendons, and so forth), and the nature and timing of surgical treatment.

DIAGNOSIS

A standard neurologic examination reveals the extent of the neurologic deficits following a peripheral nerve injury.[4, 8–10] The examiner must not be deceived, however, by trick movements such as those that occur when an uninvolved muscle or gravity compensates for a paralyzed muscle, those permitted by an accessory tendon slip or an anomalous muscle insertion or nerve supply, or those caused by strong contraction and sudden relaxation of an antagonist. Because of the overlap of sensory nerve distributions and the tendency for fibers to grow from adjacent nerves into a denervated area after injury, the sensory deficits may involve smaller areas than the examiner expects. Unless the injury is old and trophic changes in the affected limb have developed, autonomic changes may be subtle and may escape detection on routine testing. In a warm room, the examiner can map the pattern of sweating with a magnifying lens or an ophthalmoscope.

The Hoffmann-Tinel sign refers to the radiating tingling paresthesia that is felt in the cutaneous distribution of an injured nerve when the nerve is percussed lightly. If the distal aspect of the nerve is percussed progressively proximally, the level at which the sign is first elicited marks the most distal point of small fiber regeneration. The progress of nerve regeneration may thus be followed over a period of days to months by periodic charting of the location of the most distal point.

Causalgia is a unique pain syndrome that may accompany a partial injury to a mixed peripheral nerve (especially the median or sciatic nerve).[7] The constant burning pain is quite severe and may be intensified by various stimuli, including cutaneous stimuli in the affected area and loud noises. It may be improved to some extent by soaking the affected part in water. Autonomic and trophic changes are common. The condition is diagnosed by history and physical examination. Although improvement may eventually occur over 6 to 12 months without treatment, an early trial of medical management, such as the administration of phenoxybenzamine, an alpha-adrenergic blocking agent, often provides some relief. If a medical approach is unsuccessful, causalgia may often be improved or relieved by an appropriate sympathectomy, especially if one or more preoperative sympathetic blocks have provided temporary relief.

A variety of electrical examinations may add significant diagnostic information to that gained from the history and physical examination. Electromyography shows changes of denervation (increased insertional activity, spontaneous fibrillation, positive waves, and absence of voluntary action potentials) and of early reinnervation (decreased insertional activity, decreased fibrillation, and nascent polyphasic potentials). Disappearance of fibrillations may antedate the reappearance of voluntary action potentials. Muscle contraction in response to electrical stimulation may precede voluntary recovery by weeks. Although electromyographic evidence of reinnervation may precede recovery, it does not guarantee recovery.

Other specialized tests for the evaluation of peripheral nerve injuries include various tests of sweating, diagnostic anesthetic nerve blocks, and elicitation of the axon reflex by scratching the skin or injecting histamine.

SURGICAL THERAPY

Since surgeons first began to repair injured nerves, there has been controversy about the timing of such repair. For many years, delayed repair was favored; the rare exceptions involved clean lacerations made by sharp objects. With the development of microsurgery and replantation surgery, there has been increased interest in primary nerve repair at the time of injury.

The arguments in favor of primary repair are that the structures are easier to identify and mobilize in the absence of scar, the nerve ends have not retracted as much as they will in the ensuing weeks, and the greatest time is allowed for regeneration before irreversible muscle atrophy occurs. The arguments against primary nerve repair are that the damage to the nerve may be more extensive than is apparent initially, the epineurium and perineurium are delicate at this stage and difficult to suture, infection may occur from the initial wound contamination, emergency conditions may be suboptimal for a careful and tedious operation, and 4 to 6 weeks are required for axons to cross the anastomosis because of the initial lag time.

With secondary repair at 3 to 8 weeks after injury, the extent of damage to the nerve can be better assessed and the correct amount trimmed off, the epineurium and perineurium are stronger and can be sutured more easily, optimal

operating room conditions can be arranged, and there is no lag time for wallerian degeneration (the involved neurons are capable of immediately regenerating new distal segments, and the regenerating axons can penetrate the repair site before a significant amount of scar forms). Even if secondary nerve repair is the treatment selected, the initial wound should be explored to document the extent of injury, to treat conditions that require acute attention (e.g., arterial injury), to débride and cleanse the wound, and to tag any divided nerve ends so that they can be found at later re-exploration or to loosely approximate the nerve ends with inert sutures to prevent their retraction.

If a clinically nonfunctioning nerve is in continuity when it is explored some weeks after the initial injury, the surgeon may find it helpful to electrically stimulate the nerve proximal to the injury and look distally for evidence of muscle contraction or transmission of nerve action potentials. If there is no evidence of transmission across the area of injury, the injured portion of the nerve should be excised and the cut ends of the nerve should be sutured together. If there is transmission across the area of injury, surgical treatment should be limited to an external neurolysis.

If the nerve was initially divided in the accident or is divided by the surgeon, it should be reapproximated carefully and without tension after each end has been trimmed back to healthy fascicles. To regain length so that the nerves can be sutured without tension, the nerve ends can be mobilized and rerouted, and the adjacent joints can be flexed. If the ends cannot be brought together even with these maneuvers, an interposed graft of an available cutaneous nerve, such as the sural nerve, can be used. Grafts of this type add another suture line that the regenerating axons must cross, and the results are not as good as with direct nerve reanastomosis.

SELECTED REFERENCES

Haymaker, W., and Woodhall, B.: Peripheral Nerve Injuries: Principles of Diagnosis, 2nd ed. Philadelphia, W. B. Saunders, 1953.
This book is a gem. It contains a wealth of material about the anatomy of peripheral nerves, the examination of the peripheral nervous system, and the causes and manifestations of peripheral nerve injuries. The last third of the book consists of a detailed analysis of injuries to each of the important nerve plexuses and peripheral nerves.

Sunderland, S.: Nerves and Nerve Injuries, 2nd ed. Edinburgh, Churchill Livingstone, 1978.
This is the bible of peripheral nerve injuries. The book is large and detailed. It is an excellent reference.

REFERENCES

1. Benzel, E. C. (Ed.): Practical Approaches to Peripheral Nerve Surgery. Park Ridge, Ill., American Association of Neurological Surgeons, 1992.
2. Ducker, T. B., Kempe, L. G., and Hayes, G. J.: The metabolic background for peripheral nerve surgery. J. Neurosurg., *30*:270, 1969.
3. Gelberman, R. H. (Ed.): Operative Nerve Repair and Reconstruction. Philadelphia, J. B. Lippincott, 1991.
4. Haymaker, W., and Woodhall, B.: Peripheral Nerve Injuries: Principles of Diagnosis, 2nd ed. Philadelphia, W. B. Saunders, 1953.
5. Kline, D. G., and Hudson, A. R.: Nerve Injuries. Operative Results for Major Nerve Injuries, Entrapments, and Tumors. Philadelphia, W. B. Saunders, 1995.
6. MacKinnon, S. E., and Dellon, A. L.: Surgery of the Peripheral Nerve. New York, Thieme, 1988.
7. Richards, R. L.: Causalgia, a centennial review. Arch. Neurol., *16*:339, 1967.
8. Seddon, H.: Surgical Disorders of the Peripheral Nerves, 2nd ed. Baltimore, Williams & Wilkins, 1975.
9. Sunderland, S.: Nerves and Nerve Injuries, 2nd ed. Edinburgh, Churchill Livingstone, 1978.
10. Sunderland, S.: Nerve Injuries and Their Repair: A Critical Appraisal. Edinburgh, Churchill Livingstone, 1991.
11. Woodhall, B., and Beebe, G. W.: Peripheral Nerve Regeneration: A Follow-up Study of 3,656 World War II Injuries (VA Medical Monograph). Washington, D.C., U.S. Government Printing Office, 1956.

XI

CONGENITAL ABNORMALITIES

Herbert E. Fuchs, M.D., Ph.D.

Congenital abnormalities of the central nervous system occur in 1% of live births[11] and account for more than 72% of fetal deaths prior to birth.[22] As knowledge of the normal embryology of the central nervous system improves, the mechanisms underlying these malformations are better understood. In addition, recent advances in diagnosis and therapy have greatly improved the prognosis for children with these congenital malformations.

EMBRYOLOGY OF THE BRAIN AND SPINAL CORD

The process of neural tube formation, termed neurulation, occurs during gestational days 18 to 27.[18] Defects occurring during this period result in the most severe forms of cranial and spinal dysraphism. In the later stages of embryonic development, the caudal neural tube is formed by canalization and regression. During these stages, the occult forms of dysraphism commonly develop. By the third week of gestation, the notochord induces the overlying ectoderm to form the neural plate.[23] During the next several days, the lateral portions of the neural plate begin to elevate and form neural folds, eventually fusing in the midline to form the neural tube (Fig. 41–32A and B). The closure of the neural tube begins in the cervical region and proceeds both cranially and caudally, with the anterior and posterior neuropores closing at 23 and 25 days, respectively. Following fusion of the neural folds, the superficial ectoderm fuses in the midline and separates from the neural tube (Fig. 41–32C). Mesenchymal cells then migrate between the skin and neural tube to ultimately give rise to the meninges, neural arches, and paraspinal muscles.

After neurulation is complete, the distal spinal cord begins to form as the caudal end of the neural tube blends into the caudal cell mass, a large mass of undifferentiated cells that eventually give rise to components of the nervous, urogenital, and digestive systems. This accounts for the common association of anomalies in these systems. Within the caudal cell mass, small vacuoles form, coalesce, and eventually connect with the central canal of the spinal cord, in the process known as canalization (Fig. 41–33). The distal spinal cord then begins the process of retrogressive differentiation, leaving a remnant of pia-arachnoid called the filum terminale. The spinal cord and developing vertebral column elongate, with the vertebral column growing faster than the spinal cord. The conus medullaris therefore ascends from its initial position in the coccyx to lie at the L2–L3 interspace by birth. By 3 months postpartum, the tip of the conus medullaris is nearly at the adult level of the L1–L2 interspace.[1]

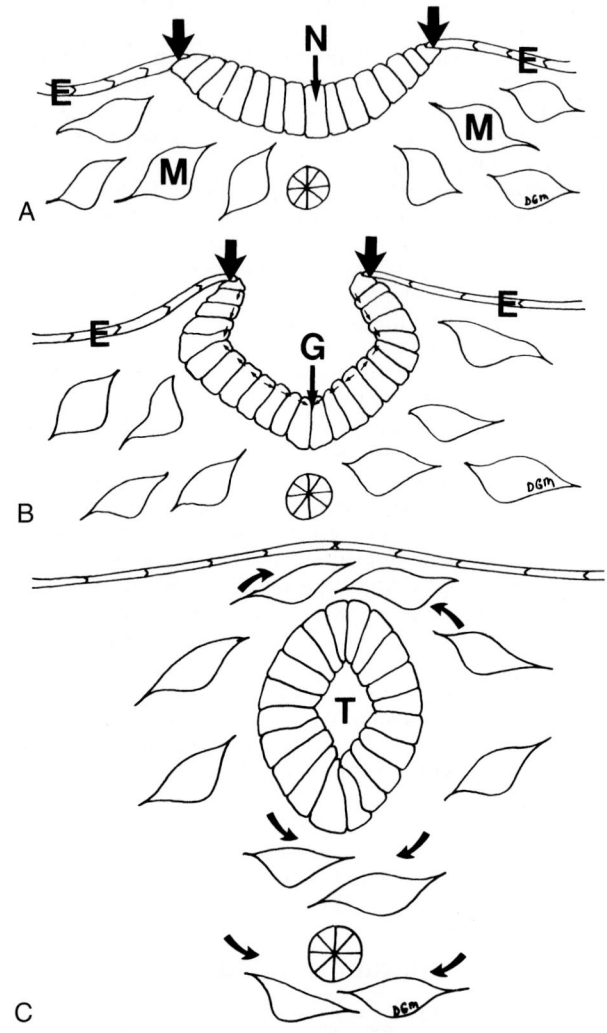

Figure 41–32. Schematic drawings of transverse sections through an embryo, showing the process of neurulation. *A,* Immediately beneath the neural plate (N) lies the notochord. Arrows demonstrate the junction of the ectoderm (E) with the neural plate. Mesenchymal cells (M) are also shown. *B,* As the neural tube begins to form, the neural groove (G) is seen. *C,* After neural tube (T) closure is complete, the ectoderm has fused in the midline, and mesenchymal cells (M) migrate between the neural tube and overlying ectoderm. (From McLone, D. G., and Naidich, T. P.: The tethered cord. *In* McLaurin, R. L., Venes, J. L., Schut, L., and Epstein, F. [Eds.]: Pediatric Neurosurgery: Surgery of the Developing Nervous System, 2nd ed. Philadelphia, W. B. Saunders, 1989.)

TABLE 41–7. Congenital Malformations of the Central Nervous System

Deranged Neurulation	Deranged Retrogressive Differentiation	Other Mechanisms
Myelomeningocele	Lipoma of filum terminale/ tight filum terminale	Diastematomyelia
		Neurenteric cyst
Lipomyelomeningocele	Terminal myelocystocele	Chiari malformations
Dermal sinus		Dandy-Walker malformation
		Meningocele
		Arachnoid cyst

The brain is formed in a complex series of folds giving rise to two cerebral hemispheres and the cerebellum. Each hemisphere contains a lateral ventricle, around which glial and neuronal precursors begin to form, and the cerebellum comes to overlie the fourth ventricle.[10] By day 47, cerebrospinal fluid (CSF) production begins, loosening the mesenchymal meshwork surrounding the brain to form the subarachnoid space.

Congenital malformations of the central nervous system are best understood as derangements in the events discussed above (Table 41–7).

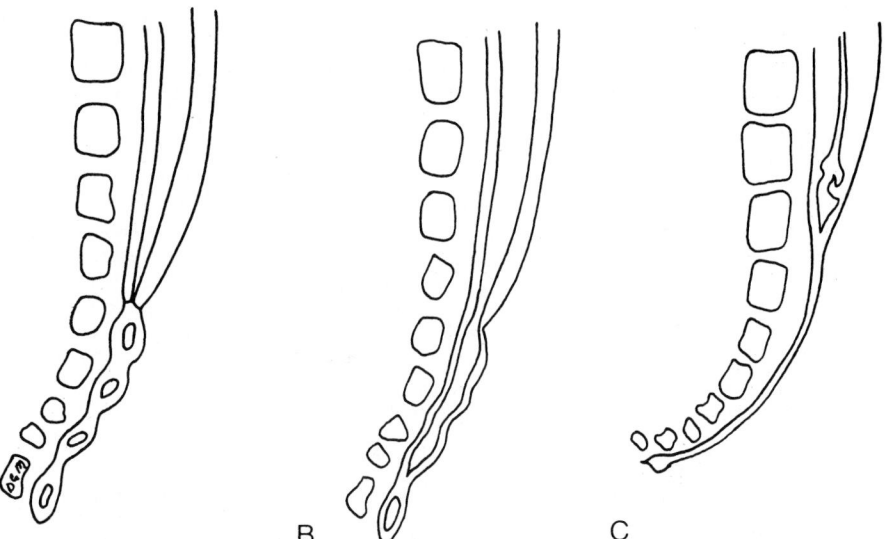

Figure 41–33. Schematic drawings of a sagittal section through an embryo showing the formation of the caudal spinal cord through vacuolization *(A)* and coalescence of the caudal cell mass *(B)*, and the formation of the filum terminale *(C)*. (From McLone, D. G., and Naidich, T. P.: The tethered cord. *In* McLaurin, R. L., Venes, J. L., Schut, L., and Epstein, F. [Eds.]: Pediatric Neurosurgery: Surgery of the Developing Nervous System, 2nd ed. Philadelphia, W. B. Saunders, 1989.)

A   B   C

DERANGEMENTS OF NEURULATION

Myelomeningocele is the most common derangement of neurulation, occurring in approximately 1 per 1000 live births. This incidence appears to be decreasing with the recent emphasis on prenatal maternal care, particularly folate supplementation. In this malformation, a focal segment of the spinal cord fails to roll up and form a tube. Since the neural tube does not fuse, the cutaneous ectoderm does not come to cover the neural tube but remains attached and lateral to the neural plate, leaving a cutaneous defect. The raw, exposed surface of the neural plate represents the interior of the spinal cord. Surrounding this neural placode is a thin layer of skin and arachnoid tissue, below which is the subarachnoid space (Fig. 41–34). The nerve roots lie inferior to the neural placode, with the ventral roots lying medial to the dorsal roots. A number of central nervous system anoma-

lies have been associated with myelomeningocele, including Chiari II malformation and hydrocephalus, which are discussed below.

Lipomyelomeningocele is believed to form by focal premature disjunction of neuroectoderm from cutaneous ectoderm, allowing access of mesenchymal cells to the dorsal surface of the unclosed neural tube.[14] The mesenchymal cells then give rise to fat. The anatomy is therefore very similar to that of myelomeningocele, with the exception that the cutaneous ectoderm is able to close over the neural tube. The lipoma may extend from the spinal cord and merge with the subcutaneous fat (Fig. 41–35).

In contrast to lipomyelomeningocele, a dermal sinus tract results from incomplete disjunction of the neural tube and cutaneous ectoderm. As the spinal cord becomes buried beneath the surface and elongates, the localized connection with the skin becomes an elongated tract (Fig. 41–36). The

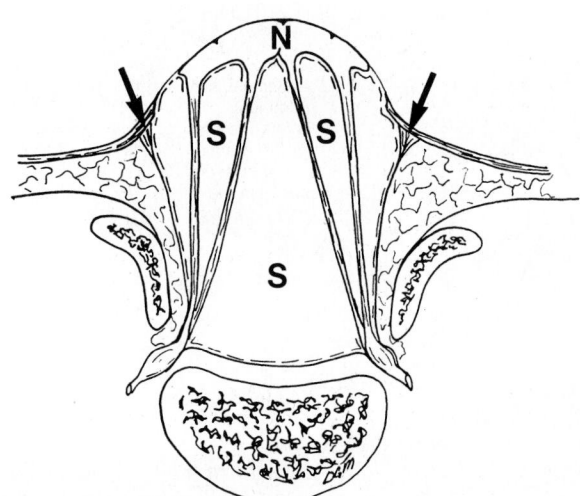

Figure 41–34. Schematic drawing of a transverse section through an embryo showing the anatomy of a myelomeningocele. Arrows demonstrate the junction of the neural placode (N) with the dura mater and skin. The subarachnoid space (S) is also shown. (From McLone, D. G., and Naidich, T. P.: The tethered cord. *In* McLaurin, R. L., Venes, J. L., Schut, L., and Epstein, F. [Eds.]: Pediatric Neurosurgery: Surgery of the Developing Nervous System, 2nd ed. Philadelphia, W. B. Saunders, 1989.)

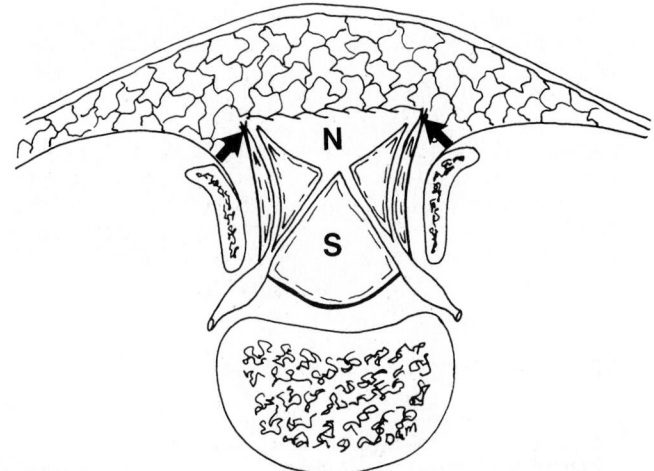

Figure 41–35. Schematic drawing of a transverse section through an embryo showing the anatomy of a lipomyelomeningocele. The neural placode (N) merges into the lipoma above the dorsal root entry zone (arrows). The subarachnoid space (S) is also shown. Note the similarity to the myelomeningocele shown in Figure 41–34. (From McLone, D. G., and Naidich, T. P.: The tethered cord. *In* McLaurin, R. L., Venes, J. L., Schut, L., and Epstein, F. [Eds.]: Pediatric Neurosurgery: Surgery of the Developing Nervous System, 2nd ed. Philadelphia, W. B. Saunders, 1989.)

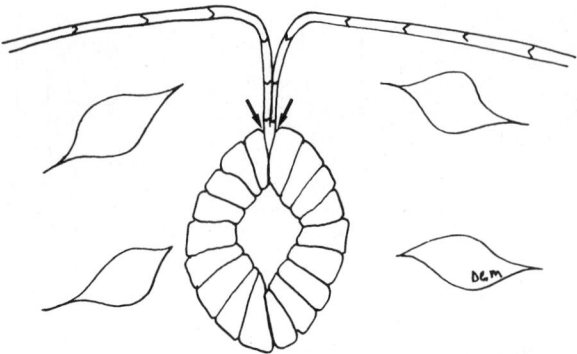

Figure 41–36. Schematic drawing of a transverse section through an embryo showing the formation of a dermal sinus through delayed disjunction of the neural tube from superficial ectoderm (arrows). (From McLone, D. G., and Naidich, T. P.: The tethered cord. In McLaurin, R. L., Venes, J. L., Schut, L., and Epstein, F. [Eds.]: Pediatric Neurosurgery: Surgery of the Developing Nervous System, 2nd ed. Philadelphia, W. B. Saunders, 1989.)

incidence of dermal sinuses is highest in the lumbosacral region, the site of posterior neuropore closure, but they may also occur in the cervico-occipital and nasal regions. They may extend to variable depths, ending in the subcutaneous tissues or the dura, or retaining their attachment to the spinal cord or the brain stem. Dermoid or epidermoid tumors may be found along the course of the dermal sinus tract.

DERANGEMENTS OF RETROGRESSIVE DIFFERENTIATION

The tight filum terminale/fatty filum terminale syndrome is a condition in which the spinal cord is tethered by an abnormally short, thickened filum terminale. Terminal myelocystocele is a complex malformation that is believed to form as a result of dilatation of the central canal in the caudal neural tube, forming a cyst.[15] This cyst distends the arachnoid lining of the distal spinal cord, forming a meningocele. This anomaly is commonly associated with extrophy of the bladder.

OTHER EMBRYOLOGIC DERANGEMENTS

Diastematomyelia is a condition in which the spinal cord is split in a sagittal plane into two hemicords that may or may not be symmetrical. Diastematomyelia is most common in females and is usually heralded by a hairy patch overlying the site of the cleft.[6] Recent studies by Dias and Walker[5] and Pang et al.[19] support the concept that these malformations are caused by disorders of gastrulation. Pang has classified these lesions as split cord malformation (SCM) Types I and II. Type I SCM is the classic diastematomyelia, with a bony septum lying between two hemicords, each in its own dural sac (Fig. 41–37A). Type II malformations consist of two hemicords in a single dural sac, with a thin sagittal fibrous septum (Fig. 41–37B). These malformations may be caused by splitting of the notochord, either by duplication or by persistence of the neurenteric canal, which effectively causes a localized split of the notochord. The development of mesenchymal elements between the two hemicords determines the type of SCM that forms. A thick mesenchymal tract could give rise to a bony septum and meninges, whereas a thin tract may form only a thin fibrous septum.

A neurenteric cyst may also be caused by persistence of the neurenteric canal and is often associated with an SCM. This rare lesion is most often seen as only a partial fistula and is most common in the cervicothoracic region of the spinal cord.

Meningoceles are thought to be caused by postneurulation disorders involving cutaneous ectoderm and mesenchyma, since the neural tube is normally formed beneath the cutaneous and mesenchymal defect, which contains CSF.

The embryology of encephaloceles has been reviewed by Chapman and colleagues.[4] Encephaloceles were originally thought to be caused by failure of closure of the anterior neuropore. However, these lesions contain well-developed neural and mesenchymal structures, which cannot be the cause of failure of neural tube closure. Therefore, these lesions are believed to be caused by herniation of fully neurulated neural tissue through a mesenchymal defect.

The Chiari II malformation is a complex disorder that is associated with myelomeningocele. This malformation consists of caudal displacement of the cerebellar vermis and

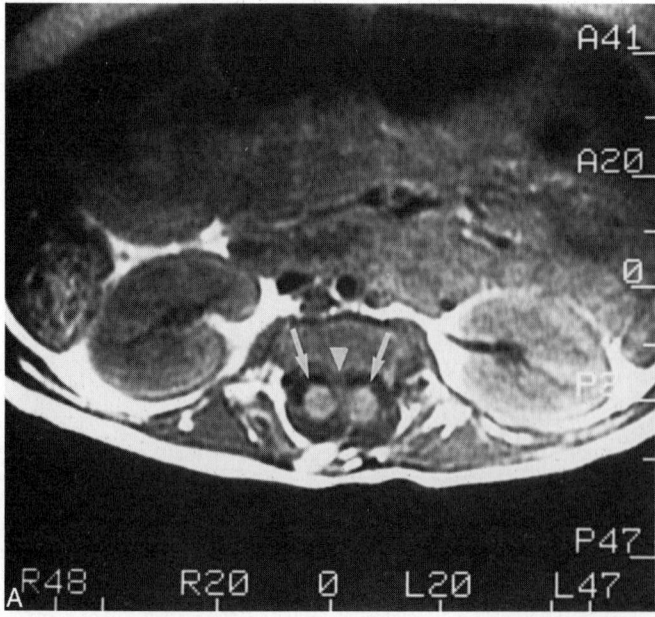
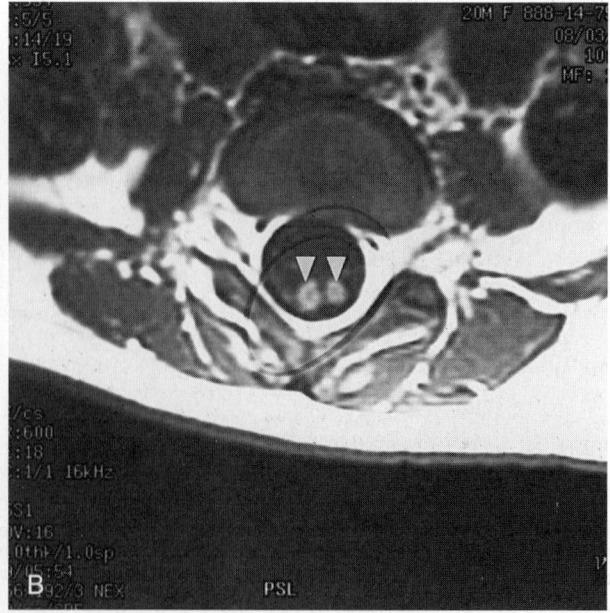

Figure 41–37. Axial magnetic resonance imaging scans of split cord malformations (SCMs). A, Type I SCM demonstrating two hemicords and two dural sacs (arrows), separated by a bony septum (arrowhead). B, Type II SCM demonstrating two unequal hemicords (arrowheads) contained in a single dural sac.

tonsils into the cervical canal; elongation, kinking, and caudal displacement of the lower brain stem into the cervical canal; and upward displacement of the superior cerebellum through a low-lying tentorial incisura, with a small posterior fossa. McLone and Knepper[13] proposed a unifying theory of the pathogenesis of these malformations: The open neural placode of the myelomeningocele allows the escape of CSF, which interferes with the normal distention of the ventricular system and development of the skull base. Incomplete distention of the fourth ventricle fails to stimulate growth of the skull base, causing a smaller posterior fossa, which is unable to respond during the later phase of rapid cerebellar growth and development. This produces herniation of neural tissue from the posterior fossa and impairs the flow of CSF, resulting in hydrocephalus. The Chiari I malformation, involving caudal displacement of the cerebellar tonsils with a normal posterior fossa, must have its embryologic origin at a later stage than the more severe Chiari II malformation, but the exact mechanisms responsible remain to be elucidated.

The Dandy-Walker malformation is a developmental abnormality in which the roof of the fourth ventricle fails to perforate to form the foramen of Magendie. The resultant cystic dilatation of the fourth ventricle expands the posterior fossa, elevating the tentorium and causing hydrocephalus because of obstruction of the aqueduct of Sylvius, with concomitant hypoplasia of the cerebellar vermis.

Arachnoid cysts are arachnoid-lined cavities filled with fluid similar in composition to CSF, which may create a disturbance in intracranial dynamics due to shift and displacement of surrounding structures and cause intracranial hypertension. Their pathogenesis is unknown. They appear to form early in development and may communicate to varying degrees with the surrounding subarachnoid space. The most common locations for arachnoid cysts are the sylvian fissure, suprasellar, and posterior fossa.[21]

DIAGNOSIS AND MANAGEMENT OF CONGENITAL MALFORMATIONS OF THE CENTRAL NERVOUS SYSTEM

The diagnosis of myelomeningocele is obvious at birth (Fig. 41–38). The lesion should be covered with sterile, saline-soaked dressings, and the patient is kept prone. After a general assessment, the location of the lesion is noted, and a neurologic examination is performed to assess sensorimotor function in the lower extremities. Anal sphincter tone should be assessed, as over 90% of children with myelomeningocele have bowel and bladder dysfunction. Head circumference should be measured and the anterior fontanelle palpated to assess for hydrocephalus. Following medical stabilization, and preferably within 24 hours of birth, the child should be taken to the operating room for closure of the myelomeningocele. This procedure involves meticulous anatomic reconstruction of the neural tube, dural sac, and overlying cutaneous tissues, with great care taken not to further injure the neural tissue. Postoperatively, the child is nursed prone while the closure heals and is monitored for the development of hydrocephalus, which is treated with a ventriculoperitoneal shunt. During this period, further orthopedic and urologic work-up can be completed, along with evaluation of brain stem function, to assess the associated Chiari II malformation. The long-term outcome of these children has been reported in depth by McLone et al.,[12] with an 85% survival rate for those children followed for 8 to 12 years, and 62% having IQs of 80 or greater. With the development of clean intermittent bladder catheterization, fully 85% of children with myelomeningocele can achieve social urinary continence. The development of improved leg braces has allowed children with motor levels of at least L3 function to be community

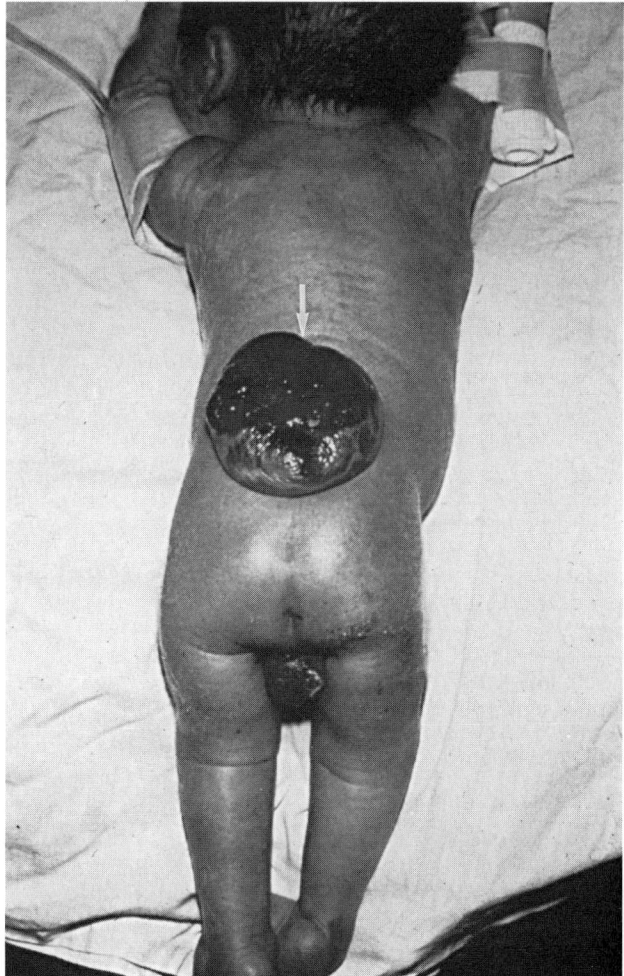

Figure 41–38. Photograph of a myelomeningocele in a newborn infant (arrow). Note the flaccid anal sphincter and the poorly developed lower extremity musculature.

ambulators. McLone's studies have shown that children with myelomeningoceles can be quite functional and that the natural history of such children is not one of relentless deterioration, as some prior studies had suggested. Any neurologic deterioration seen in a child with myelomeningocele should be promptly investigated and treated.

The congenital spinal cord lesions with intact skin are termed spina bifida occulta; they share a common presentation due to tethering of the spinal cord. These lesions also may be associated with an overlying skin lesion, such as a dermal sinus, subcutaneous lipoma, hemangioma, or hairy patch. The most common signs and symptoms of tethered cord include changes in gait, weakness, orthopedic deformity, and pain.[7, 9] The most common orthopedic deformities include varus and valgus and cavus changes of the foot. In addition, recurrent hip dislocation and scoliosis may be seen. Pain and sensory loss are common features of tethered spinal cord, and both may be asymmetrical and nondermatomal. Changes in bowel and bladder function may be missed in young children. Neurologic dysfunction results from traction on the conus medullaris, with stretching and deformation of vessels overlying the tethered cord, causing ischemia of the conus.[25] Spinal flexion or growth may result in chronic, repetitive ischemia to the spinal cord. With modern magnetic resonance imaging (MRI) techniques, the diagnosis of spina bifida occulta is straightforward. The treatment of all these lesions is centered around release of the tethered cord, with restoration of more normal anatomic relationships of the spinal cord and surrounding structures. With early recognition and treatment, pain, sensory loss, and motor weakness are likely to improve, but if treatment is deferred until bowel or bladder dysfunction occurs, improvement of these functions is unlikely.[24]

In the meningocele, the neural elements are intact, with a CSF-filled sac protruding through a cutaneous defect. Repair is accomplished by localizing the dural defect, amputating the herniating sac, and closing the dura. The remainder of the wound is then closed in layers.

The incidence of encephalocele varies according to geographic region, from as high as 1 in 5000 live births in Southeast Asia to as low as 1 in 10,000 live births in North America. The location of the encephalocele also exhibits geographic variability, with frontonasal encephaloceles more common in Southeast Asia and occipital encephaloceles more common in North America. The degree of herniation of neural tissue into the encephalocele sac may be highly variable. MRI scanning serves to classify the type of encephalocele, as well as to determine the presence of neural tissues within the sac. The treatment of encephaloceles is surgical resection of the lesion at its base, repair of the dura, and bone grafting to cover the calvarial defect. In some occipital encephaloceles, the sac may contain vital neural or vascular structures, and such repair is not possible. The outcome of surgical treatment depends on the location of the encephalocele and the amount of neural tissue remaining within the cranial vault. In general, occipital encephaloceles are more commonly associated with hydrocephalus and a worse cognitive outcome.

In children with myelomeningocele, the Chiari II malformation is invariably present. Despite impressive imaging studies, the patient may be asymptomatic. Typical Chiari II symptoms and signs include occipital pain, nystagmus, upper extremity weakness, lower cranial nerve dysfunction, hypotonia or spasticity, and scoliosis. Hydromyelia (dilation of the central canal of the spinal cord) may also be present. The surgical treatment of Chiari II malformation involves decompression of the brain stem and cervical spinal cord and restoration of normal CSF flow from the fourth ventricle. Chiari II malformations that become symptomatic in infancy are the leading cause of death in children with myelomeningocele. Respiratory wheezing and repetitive aspirations are particularly worrisome. Less severe symptoms frequently stabilize by 1 year of age. Older children with Chiari II malformations do better with cervical decompression. Results of Chiari II decompression have been good, with improvement reported in 60% to 80% of patients.[17]

The Chiari I malformation usually presents in a more delayed fashion than the Chiari II malformation, commonly late in the first decade or even into adulthood. Symptoms of Chiari I malformation include headache (often induced by coughing), upper extremity numbness and loss of pain and temperature sensation, lower extremity spasticity, and eventually lower cranial nerve dysfunction. MRI scan confirms the diagnosis and the extent of any associated hydromyelia. Surgical therapy consists of a suboccipital craniectomy, cervical laminectomy (usually involving C1), stent placement into the fourth ventricle, and duroplasty to restore normal CSF flow dynamics across the craniocervical junction; this usually results in resolution of the hydromyelia. Patients presenting with mild symptoms do quite well, with 70% to 80% reporting improvement in headache.[17]

The presentation of intracranial arachnoid cysts is dependent on the age of the patient. Infants commonly present with increased head circumference, full fontanelle, and signs of increased intracranial pressure. Older children may present with headache, seizures, or focal neurologic deficits. The signs and symptoms also vary with the site of the arachnoid cyst; posterior fossa cysts commonly present with obstructive hydrocephalus, sylvian fissure cysts present with seizures or hemiparesis, and suprasellar cysts present with visual disturbances. Sudden deterioration may be seen with the development of obstructive hydrocephalus, sudden cyst rupture, or bleeding into the cyst, either spontaneous or traumatic. Computed tomography (CT) or MRI scanning may provide the diagnosis, with MRI scan preferred due to its multiplanar imaging capability. Therapy of symptomatic arachnoid cysts is controversial, with some authors recommending simple shunting of the cyst, and other authors recommending cyst fenestration or excision.[21]

HYDROCEPHALUS

Hydrocephalus is a condition in which there is a discrepancy between the rate of formation and the rate of absorption of CSF, causing the cerebral ventricles to dilate.[2] CSF is normally formed from the choroid plexus in the lateral, third, and fourth ventricles. CSF flows through the ventricular system, exiting the fourth ventricle via the foramina of Magendie and Luschka, and circulates around the base of the brain, cerebral hemispheres, and spinal cord, to be reabsorbed into the bloodstream through arachnoid villi located primarily along the superior sagittal sinus. A block of CSF flow causes a noncommunicating hydrocephalus. A defect in the absorptive process leads to communicating hydrocephalus.

The clinical presentation of hydrocephalus is dependent on the age of the patient, as the open sutures of the infant skull allow cranial expansion, which helps dissipate increased intracranial pressure. An infant with hydrocephalus typically presents with increased head circumference and a full, bulging fontanelle; other symptoms include poor feeding, vomiting, and lethargy. Physical signs that may be detected include cranial sutural diastasis, prominence of scalp veins, and the *sunsetting sign*, with forced downgaze due to compression of the midbrain tectal plate. Macrocephaly in an infant may have a variety of causes, and the imaging studies discussed below can help distinguish them. Older children with fused sutures cannot dissipate increased intracranial pressure through cranial expansion and often have a more acute presentation of hydrocephalus. Severe headache, vomiting, and lethargy are common. Children with obstructive hydrocephalus secondary to a colloid cyst or tumor may require urgent intervention. Papilledema is commonly seen in patients with more chronic intracranial pressure elevation. The character of the headache is important; headache from increased intracranial pressure is characteristically worse at night or early in the morning, often waking the child from sleep, and is associated with vomiting. In such cases, cranial imaging studies should be done to rule out hydrocephalus prior to embarking on a gastrointestinal work-up. These symptoms may be seen prior to the development of other neurologic signs.

Radiologic imaging studies are essential in confirming the diagnosis of hydrocephalus. CT (Fig. 41–39) and ultrasonography are most commonly used. MRI has become more widely available over the past several years and provides imaging in axial, coronal, and sagittal planes. Recent advances have also allowed imaging of CSF flow, particularly through the aqueduct and the foramen magnum.

Examination of CSF by lumbar or ventricular puncture may reveal evidence of hemorrhage or infection prior to treatment with a shunt. In addition, in a shunted patient, a shunt tap may provide important information on shunt function or infection.

Neuropsychologic testing in older children and developmental assessment in younger children also provide useful information in the evaluation of hydrocephalus. Deteriora-

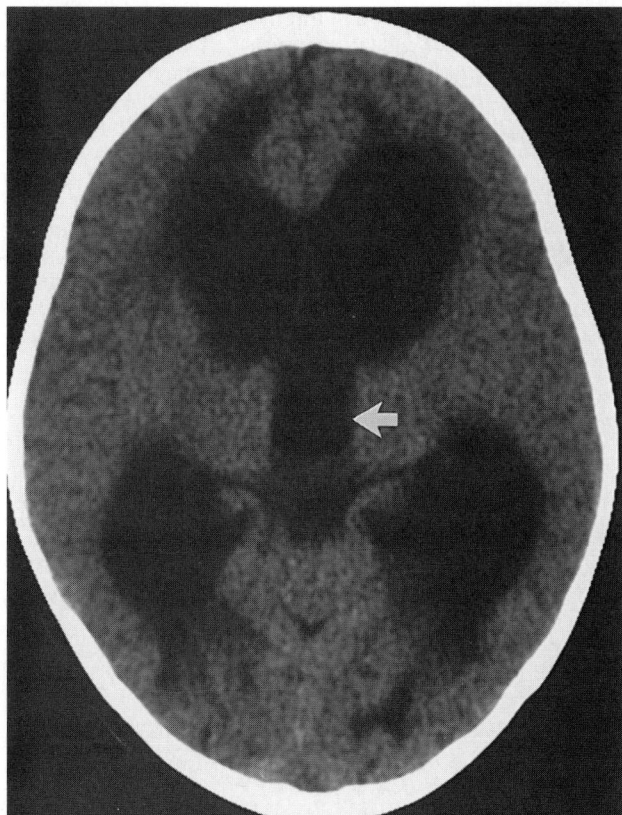

Figure 41–39. Axial computerized tomographic brain scan of patient with hydrocephalus. Arrow indicates the dilated third ventricle. Expanded occipital horns are posterior and lateral to the third ventricle, and dilated frontal horns are anterior and lateral to the third ventricle.

tion in performance on these tests could indicate progression of hydrocephalus or shunt malfunction.

Congenital hydrocephalus is associated with a variety of malformation syndromes discussed earlier. Children born with a myelomeningocele have an approximately 85% incidence of hydrocephalus. Ventricular enlargement may not be present at birth but may develop after closure of the myelomeningocele. Aqueductal stenosis may present in a newborn or young infant but can present at later ages as well. The Dandy-Walker syndrome may also present at later ages but is most frequently seen early in infancy.

Posthemorrhagic hydrocephalus is most commonly seen in premature infants. Meningitis is also a common cause of hydrocephalus. With postmeningitic hydrocephalus, ventricular loculations may be seen, complicating treatment of the resulting hydrocephalus. Tumors may cause obstructive hydrocephalus in a variety of locations, although fourth ventricular tumors are most common. Craniopharyngiomas may block flow at the level of the third ventricle. Choroid plexus tumors may oversecrete CSF, in addition to producing obstruction.

One condition that must be distinguished from hydrocephalus is external hydrocephalus. This condition is characterized by macrocrania, with the CT scan demonstrating a normal to mildly dilated ventricular system and pronounced extra-axial fluid spaces. This external hydrocephalus is believed to be caused by immaturity of the CSF absorption system at the level of the arachnoid villi, and it resolves in virtually every case.[3]

The development of valve-regulated shunt systems provided the major advance in the treatment of hydrocephalus. The key feature of all shunt systems is that drainage of CSF from the ventricle to a distant site (most commonly the peritoneal cavity or the right atrium of the heart) is controlled by a valve mechanism, to prevent overdrainage of CSF. The ventricular catheter is placed into the lateral ventricle from either a frontal or an occipital approach; the remainder of the system is tunneled subcutaneously either to the abdomen for a peritoneal shunt or to the neck for cannulation of the common facial vein to gain access to the right atrium for an atrial shunt. The goal of shunting is to normalize the intracranial pressure and to allow a re-expansion of the brain tissue to constitute a cortical mantle that is at least 3.5 cm. thick, to maximize the child's development. Patients with posthemorrhagic hydrocephalus are best managed initially with implantation of a subcutaneous reservoir system that may be tapped intermittently, until the CSF is cleared of blood products that could obstruct the shunt system.

In patients with compartmentalized hydrocephalus, such as the Dandy-Walker syndrome, or those with ventricular loculations, multiple ventricular catheters may be required. These catheters are usually connected to a single-valve system in order to equalize the pressures in the various compartments and avoid dangerous brain shifts.

Recently, with the development of fiberoptic ventriculoscopy, obstructive hydrocephalus has been treated with an endoscopic third ventriculostomy, creating an opening in the floor of the third ventricle into the subarachnoid space, thereby bypassing the obstruction to CSF flow. Reports have generally shown an approximately 70% success rate in treating aqueductal stenosis without the need for a shunt.

Shunt malfunction is the most common complication of shunting. This may be caused by obstruction of the shunt system, disconnection, or migration. The ventricular catheter may become obstructed due to choroid plexus, brain parenchyma, protein, or tumor cells. Protein plugs in either the proximal or the distal catheter are commonly seen in patients with posthemorrhagic hydrocephalus in the initial months after shunting. Disconnections are most common at sites of connection and mobility.

Shunt malfunctions associated with the distal catheter depend on the site chosen for distal drainage. The peritoneal catheter is the most common, due to the easy access to the peritoneal cavity and the ability to place redundant tubing into the abdomen to allow for future growth of the child. A CSF-filled pseudocyst may form around the distal catheter, causing shunt malfunction and abdominal pain. In addition, small bowel obstruction, abdominal viscus perforation by shunt tubing, and acute abdomen may be complications of abdominal shunting. Atrial shunts have their own associated complications. Although atrial shunts are very effective, they are more difficult to revise, and additional tubing cannot be inserted to allow for growth. In addition, pulmonary embolism, septicemia, shunt nephritis, cardiac arrhythmia, and pulmonary hypertension have been reported in patients with atrial shunts.

Shunt infection is the second most common complication of shunting, with the reported incidence ranging between 2.6% and 38%. The morbidity of shunt infection is severe, with a single episode lowering the IQ by 10 to 30 points.

CRANIOSYNOSTOSIS

Craniosynostosis, or premature closure of the cranial sutures, is commonly seen in the practice of pediatric neurosurgery. Most cases are sporadic, but up to 10% may be familial. Separation of the bones of the calvarium by the cranial sutures allows progressive enlargement of the skull to occur with growth of the brain. Brain weight doubles by 6 months of age, and triples by 10 months. Brain growth is virtually complete by 2 years of age, and the cranial sutures are fused by 6 to 8 years. When one or more sutures close prematurely, there must be compensatory growth at the remaining open sutures, producing recognizable patterns of deformity. When skull growth cannot keep pace with brain growth, increased intracranial pressure occurs, with the potential for cognitive impairment. Sagittal synostosis is the most common form of craniosynostosis and causes scaphocephaly. Coronal synostosis causes plagiocephaly if unilateral and brachycephaly if bilateral, metopic synostosis causes trigonocephaly, and multiple suture synostosis causes cloverleaf deformity (Kleeblattschädel). Multiple etiologies may be involved in craniosynostosis. Metabolic conditions affecting bone formation, intrauterine deformation, genetic abnormalities, and Crouzon's and Apert's syndromes have all been invoked in cases of craniosynostosis.[8]

The skull deformities resulting from closure of the various sutures are recognizable to the trained clinician. The abnormality is usually present at birth; with time, it may become more severe. Ridges along the fused sutures are obvious to palpation. Skull x-rays confirm the diagnosis of craniosynostosis (Fig. 41–40) and may show indentations of the inner table as evidence of increased intracranial pressure. CT scanning also demonstrates sutural fusion and allows examination of the underlying brain. Three-dimensional reconstruction of CT images may also facilitate surgical planning. The therapy of craniosynostosis varies with the involved suture, but in general, early surgical therapy provides the best cosmetic effects.[20]

VASCULAR MALFORMATIONS OF THE BRAIN

Vascular malformations of the brain are common causes of intracerebral hemorrhage in the pediatric age group. The classic arteriovenous malformation (AVM) is the most common, with cavernous angiomas and venous angiomas less commonly associated with hemorrhage. These lesions are discussed elsewhere in this text. The vein of Galen aneurysm deserves special mention, with its variable presentation dependent on the age of the patient. Infants presenting with vein of Galen aneurysms commonly present with high-output cardiac failure due to the tremendous arteriovenous shunting. This shunting may also cause cerebral ischemia. The dilated vein of Galen may cause obstructive hydrocephalus, and macrocephaly may be obvious. The treatment of these children is aimed at reduction of the arteriovenous shunt, thereby relieving the cardiac failure. This must be accomplished in a gradual fashion, or the risk of hemorrhage is high. Mickle and Quisling[16] reported on the transtorcular approach to embolization of these lesions and stressed the graded, multisession treatment approach. An older child with a vein of Galen malformation commonly presents with subarachnoid hemorrhage or hydrocephalus. In these children, direct surgical therapy is possible, but transtorcular embolization has also met with considerable success.

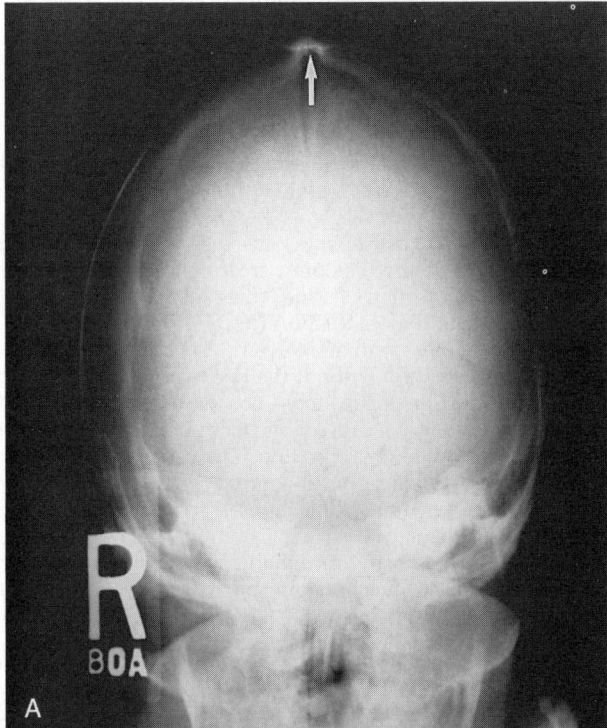

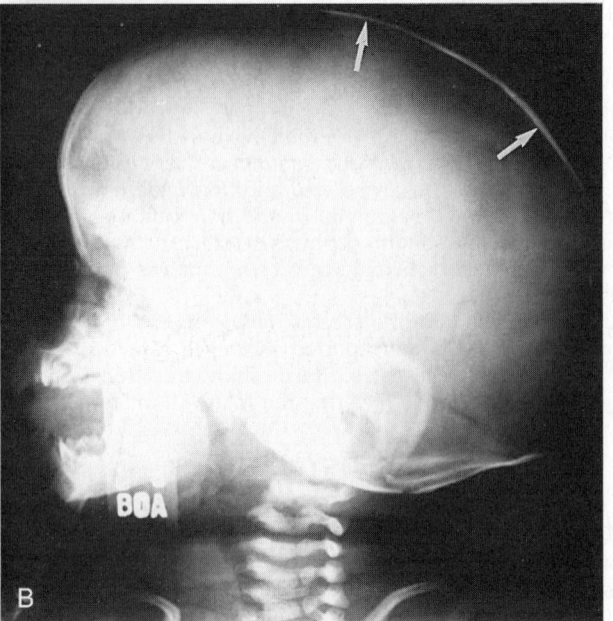

Figure 41–40. Preoperative skull x-rays of a patient with scaphocephaly demonstrating sclerotic sagittal suture (arrows) and elongated configuration of the skull. *A,* Anteroposterior view. *B,* Lateral view.

SELECTED REFERENCES

Butler, A. J., and McLone, D. G. (Eds.): Hydrocephalus. Neurosurg. Clin. North Am., 4, 1993.
  An excellent overview of the topic, addressing a number of current and controversial issues in the diagnosis and treatment of hydrocephalus.

Guthkelch, A. N.: Diastematomyelia with median septum. Brain, 97:729, 1974.
  A comprehensive natural history study of a group of patients with untreated diastematomyelia that gives strong support for the concept of early or prophylactic surgery to prevent neurologic deterioration.

McLaurin, R. L., Venes, J. L., Schut, L., and Epstein F. (Eds.): Pediatric Neurosurgery: Surgery of the Developing Nervous System, 3rd ed. Philadelphia, W. B. Saunders, 1994.
  The current standard text in pediatric neurosurgery.

McLone, D. G., Dias, L., Kaplan, W. E., et al.: Concepts in the management of spina bifida. In Humphreys, R. P. (Ed.): Concepts in Pediatric Neurosurgery, Vol. 5. Basel, S. Karger, 1985, p. 97.
  The authors review their experience with children with myelomeningocele, reporting an 85% survival rate for those children followed for 8 to 12 years, with 62% having IQs of 80 or greater. These data support an aggressive approach to the closure of myelomeningoceles.

Pang, D., Dias, M. S., and Ahab-Barmada, M.: Split cord malformation. Part I: A unified theory of embryogenesis for double cord malformations. Neurosurgery, 31:451, 1992.
  An excellent paper proposing a theory of embryogenesis for split cord malformations based on extensive clinical and laboratory data. Part II, which follows this article in the same journal, details the clinical care of these patients.

Warder, D. E., and Oakes, W. J.: Tethered cord syndrome: The low-lying and normally positioned conus. Neurosurgery, 34:597, 1994.
An excellent paper that reviews the tethered cord syndrome and describes patients with clinical signs and symptoms of the syndrome but with the conus in a normal position. This paper emphasizes that a thickened, fatty filum terminale may be the most important indicator of the tethered cord syndrome, regardless of the position of the conus medullaris.

REFERENCES

1. Barson, A. J.: The vertebral level of termination of the spinal cord during normal and abnormal development. J. Anat., 106:489, 1970.
2. Butler, A. J., and McLone, D. G. (Eds.): Hydrocephalus. Neurosurg. Clin. North Am., 4, 1993.
3. Chapman, P. H.: External hydrocephalus. In Humphreys, R. P. (Ed.): Concepts in Pediatric Neurosurgery, Vol. 4. Basel, S. Karger, 1983, p. 102.
4. Chapman, P. H., Swearingen, B., and Caviness, V. S.: Subtorcular occipital encephaloceles: Anatomical considerations relevant to operative management. J. Neurosurg., 71:375, 1989.
5. Dias, M. S., and Walker, M. L.: The embryogenesis of complex dysraphic malformations: A disorder of gastrulation? J. Pediatr. Neurosurg., 18:229, 1992.
6. Guthkelch, A. N.: Diastematomyelia with median septum. Brain, 97:729, 1974.
7. Hoffman, H. J., Hendrick, E. B., and Humphreys, R. P.: The tethered spinal cord: Its protean manifestations, diagnosis and surgical correction. Childs Brain, 2:145, 1976.
8. Hoffman, H. J., and Kestle, J. R. W.: Craniofacial surgery. In McLaurin, R. L., Venes, J. L., Schut, L., and Epstein, F. (Eds.): Pediatric Neurosurgery: Surgery of the Developing Nervous System, 3rd ed. Philadelphia, W. B. Saunders, 1994.
9. James, C. C., and Lassman, L. P.: Spina Bifida Occulta: Orthopaedic Radiological and Neurosurgical Aspects. London, Butterworth & Company, 1981.
10. Lemire, R. J., Siebert, J. R., and Warkany, J.: Normal development of the central nervous system. In McLaurin, R. L., Venes, J. L., Schut, L., and Epstein, F. (Eds.): Pediatric Neurosurgery: Surgery of the Developing Nervous System, 2nd ed. Philadelphia, W. B. Saunders, 1989.
11. Malpas, P.: The incidence of human malformations and the significance of changes in the maternal environment in their causation. J. Obstet. Gynaecol. Br. Commonw., 44:434, 1937.
12. McLone, D. G., Dias, L., Kaplan, W. E., et al.: Concepts in the management of spina bifida. In Humphreys, R. P. (Ed.): Concepts in Pediatric Neurosurgery, Vol. 5. Basel, S. Karger, 1985, p. 97.
13. McLone, D. G., and Knepper, P. A.: The cause of the Chiari II malformation: A unified theory. Pediatr. Neurosurg., 15:1, 1989.
14. McLone, D. G., Mutluer, S., and Naidich, T. P.: Lipomeningoceles of the conus medullaris. In Raimondi, A. J. (Ed.): Concepts in Pediatric Neurosurgery, Vol. 3. Basel, S. Karger, 1982.
15. McLone, D. G., and Naidich, T. P.: Terminal myelocystocele. Neurosurgery, 16:36, 1985.
16. Mickle, J. P., and Quisling, R. G.: The transtorcular embolization of vein of Galen aneurysms. J. Neurosurg., 64:731, 1986.
17. Oakes, W. J.: Chiari malformations, hydromyelia, syringomyelia. In Wilkins, R. H., and Rengachary, S. S. (Eds.): Neurosurgery. New York, McGraw-Hill, 1985.
18. O'Rahilly, R.: Developmental stages in human embryos, including a survey of the Carnegie collection. Part A: Embryos of the first three weeks (stages 1 to 9). Publ. 631. Washington, D.C., Carnegie Institution of Washington, 1973.
19. Pang, D., Dias, M. S., and Ahab-Barmada, M.: Split cord malformation. Part I: A unified theory of embryogenesis for double cord malformations. Neurosurgery, 31:451, 1992.
20. Persing, J. A., and Jane, J. A. (Eds.): Craniofacial disorders. Neurosurg. Clin. North Am., 2, 1991.
21. Raimondi, A. J., Choux, M., and DiRocco, C. (Eds.): Intracranial Cyst Lesions. New York, Springer Verlag, 1993.
22. Record, R. G., and McKeown, T.: Congenital malformations of the central nervous system. Br. J. Soc. Med., 4:183, 1949.
23. Schoenwolf, G. C., and Smith, J. L.: Mechanisms of neurulation: Traditional viewpoint and recent advances. Development, 109:243, 1990.
24. Warder, D. E., and Oakes, W. J.: Tethered cord syndrome: The low-lying and normally positioned conus. Neurosurgery, 34:597, 1994.
25. Yamada, S., Zinke, D. E., and Sanders, D.: Pathophysiology of tethered cord syndrome. J. Neurosurg., 54:494, 1981.

XII

NEUROSURGICAL RELIEF OF PAIN

John Gorecki, M.D.

Pain is the most common symptom that prompts patients to seek medical assistance. Neurosurgical intervention for the relief of pain is indicated when primary intervention for the disease in question does not lead to adequate comfort. Surgical procedures to reduce pain are grouped broadly into two categories: neuroablative and neuroaugmentative. Likewise, it is possible to describe two general patterns of pain. *Nociceptive* pain is caused by activation of peripheral receptors by a stimulus that is either stronger than normal or threatens the body. Patients with nociceptive pain who are referred to a neurosurgeon often suffer from cancer, although low back pain is probably the most common cause. *Neuropathic* pain is poorly understood and occurs in the absence of apparent ongoing stimulation. The best example is central pain following a stroke.

Anatomically distinct receptors located in the periphery code for various stimuli. The sensory experience is, however, a summation of the specific receptor activation and the modulation applied by the central nervous system to that resulting input. In general, nociceptors consist of free nerve endings, and painful sensations are transmitted in small, unmyelinated A delta and C nerve fibers. Cell bodies are located in the dorsal root ganglia, and axons enter the spinal cord through the dorsal roots. There is convergence of pain fibers more laterally in the root, and Lissauer's tract separates the dorsal horn from the cord surface. These axons synapse with second-order neurons in the dorsal gray of the cord. The majority of pain and temperature information is transmitted in the crossed spinothalamic tract to the thalamus, where third-order neurons are located. The paleospinothalamic tract, which includes multiple interneurons in the periaqueductal gray region of the brain stem, is involved in the perception of less well-localized, longer-lasting pain and, possibly, neuropathic pain. The central nervous system location for pain perception is not clearly defined (Fig. 41–41).

Ablative procedures can be done anywhere along this pathway. Neuroaugmentation refers to the use of chronic infusion of opioid agonists or stimulation, which is believed to activate intrinsic modulating systems that reduce or alter sensory input.

NEURAL DESTRUCTION

Neurectomy

Although conceptually appealing, there is little role for the transection of nerves to relieve pain. Neurectomy is used to treat painful neuromas, but these often recur. A number of procedures have therefore been described to prevent this recurrence, such as separating the two nerve ends, burying the nerve in muscle, burying the nerve in bone, or covering the nerve with Silastic. Most peripheral nerves are mixed, reducing the value of transection unless motor loss is accept-

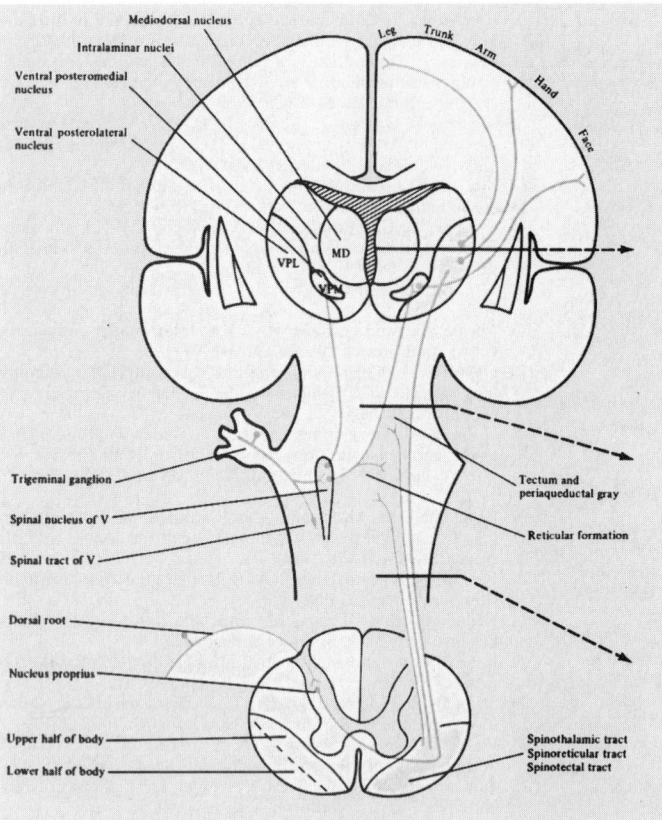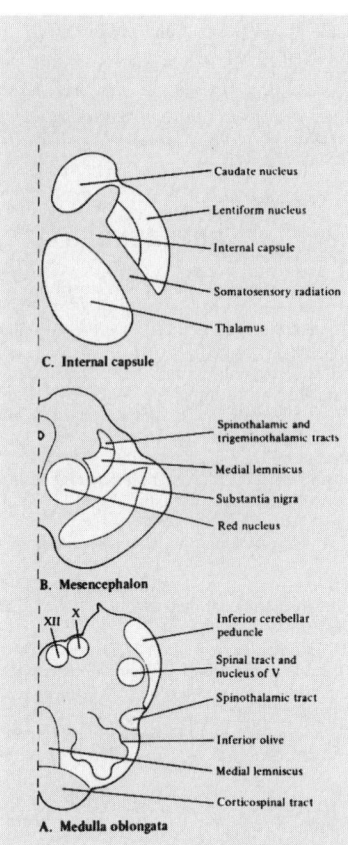

Figure 41–41. The course and termination of the main pathways for pain and temperature (i.e., the spinothalamic and trigeminothalamic tracts). Many of the ascending fibers in the anterolateral system of the spinal cord as well as from the trigeminal system terminate in the reticular formation, periaqueductal gray, and tectum. The spinothalamic tract is shaded on the cross section of the medulla oblongata *(A)*, mesencephalon *(B)*, and internal capsule *(C)*. (From Heimer, L.: The Human Brain and Spinal Cord. New York, Springer-Verlag, 1983.)

able. A notable exception is the superficial branch of the dorsal interosseous nerve in the forearm, which is best treated by transection rather than attempted repair following injury. It is a purely sensory nerve. Avulsion or alcohol ablation of the infraorbital, supraorbital, or mental nerve has a valuable role in the treatment of trigeminal neuralgia, although the benefit is often temporary. Denervation of the facet joints in the spine is sometimes attempted to relieve chronic low back pain, but this therapy is controversial.[23]

Rhizotomy

Rhizotomy refers to ablation of the sensory root. This can be done either as an open procedure, intradurally or extradurally,[22] or as a percutaneous procedure using radiofrequency coagulation[34] or injection with phenol. In spite of its long history, beginning with separate reports by Abbe and Bennett in 1889, the specific indications for this procedure remain elusive. Successful results have been reported in 30% to 80% of patients, with the majority of large series being disappointing. Patients selected for rhizotomy undergo a preoperative series of selective root blocks. Subsequent pain relief does not guarantee equally successful surgical outcome. There is considerable variability in the dermatomal distribution, with much overlap, and some sensory fibers travel in the ventral root. Therefore, several surgeons have turned to ganglionectomy to eliminate all sensory fibers at a specific level.[19] To produce any long-term sensory loss, at least three roots must be taken. Sacrifice of more than two sensory roots in an extremity can lead to loss of function, in spite of preserved motor capacity. In the sacral region, as long as S2

is preserved on at least one side, bladder control should be possible. In the upper extremity, preserving C6 or C7, or C5 and C8, is recommended to avoid proprioceptive difficulties. Similarly, in the lower extremity, L2, L3, or L4 should be preserved. Sacrifice of L5 and S1 increases the chance of dysfunction.

The most common indication is for rhizotomy pain following unsuccessful disc procedures. Leg symptoms are prominent and are presumably related to permanent root irritation. The results are not encouraging. Rhizotomy is useful for pain secondary to tumors involving a limited dermatomal region. It has been used with limited success in postherpetic neuralgia and postthoracotomy pain. Sometimes this causes discomfort at the denervation margin, producing a growing area of abnormal sensation and associated pain.

Technically the procedure is simple, but accurate localization is imperative. Stimulation in the lumbar region is usually used, since with the intra-arachnoid approach, the roots are identified near the conus at some distance from their exiting foramina. The roots or ganglia can be identified at the exiting foramen in an extra-arachnoid fashion, which is often easier. Care is taken to avoid vascular injury, as the blood supply to the cord enters along the roots.

Retrogasserian Rhizotomy for Trigeminal Neuralgia

Pain in the face that involves the distribution of the lower cranial nerves should be considered a distinct entity, and it responds to denervation more favorably. Trigeminal neuralgia consists of intermittent bouts of lancinating pain that is often triggered and is limited to the trigeminal distribution in a patient who is neurologically intact. Most patients are over 55 years of age. Retrogasserian ganglion compression,[6] glycerol ablation,[7] and radiofrequency lesioning[5] are variations of rhizotomy; however, results following these procedures are excellent. All three are performed percutaneously, with fluoroscopic control, while the patient is under sedation and they can incorporate specific localization by stimulation. In an elderly patient with idiopathic trigeminal neuralgia, these procedures represent the treatment of choice when medical management with carbamazepine, phenytoin, or baclofen has failed. In a younger patient, or one who considers sensory loss unacceptable, microvascular decompression of the trigeminal root entry zone is preferred,[8] but this has the added risk of open craniectomy. At times, vascular decompression is combined with open partial caudal root section.[38] The risks of denervation include recurrent pain, corneal anesthesia, and anesthesia dolorosa. At least six centers report series of over 1000 percutaneous procedures with no mortality.[31]

Dorsal Root Entry Zone Lesioning

Lesioning of the dorsal root entry zone (DREZ) with a radiofrequency current, using a 0.25-mm. diameter electrode with a 2.0-mm. exposed tip, was introduced by Nashold and Ostdahl in 1979.[18] Lissauer's tract and the dorsal horn gray matter are coagulated down to the Rexed V lamina, including the second-order neurons in the sensory and pain pathway. Lesions are made in line, close enough together so as to coalesce and produce a continuous zone of obliteration (Fig. 41–42). The greatest success is achieved for pain secondary to plexus avulsion and spinal cord injury. Intermittent spontaneous or induced pain, usually in a transition band located approximately at the level of the spinal cord injury, responds most consistently. Nashold refers to this as end-zone pain. DREZ lesions are notably less successful in relieving spontaneous steady burning pain covering the entire anesthetic area below the injury. The main complication of this procedure is injury to the adjacent long tracts, causing dorsal column dysfunction or weakness in the ipsilateral lower extremity; the incidence is about 30% transiently and 3% to 10% permanently. The experience at Duke includes over 800 cases.

The results following DREZ lesioning for failed back surgery syndrome have been poor, and this diagnosis is no longer an indication for surgery. DREZ lesioning is sometimes performed for postherpetic neuralgia but the risk of lesioning the thoracic cord is greater.

DREZ lesions have also been made with lasers. Sindou and co-workers introduced a technique in which a longitudinal incision is made into the cord at the lateral edge of the sensory root. This procedure was used mostly for spasms, but the authors report equal success in the treatment of pain.[26, 27]

Caudalis DREZ Coagulation

Nucleus caudalis DREZ coagulation was introduced as an extension of DREZ lesioning in 1982.[3] The trigeminal nucleus caudalis contains second-order neurons subserving pain, temperature, and crude touch from the fifth, seventh, ninth, and tenth cranial nerves. Sjoquist performed trigeminal tractotomy, and Hitchcock reported stereotactic nucleotomy. The latter causes destruction of only a portion of the nucleus caudalis.

The El-Naggar/Nashold electrode has been used since January 1990. It consists of two electrodes to accommodate the varying size of the nucleus caudalis and a right-angle bend to facilitate accurate lesion placement. Proximal insulation of the electrode tip protects the spinocerebellar tract, which overlies the nucleus. A small craniectomy is performed from just past the midline to the lateral edge of the foramen magnum, and the ipsilateral half of the atlas is removed. A single row of lesions is made at 75° C. for 20 seconds, in a gentle curve extending cephalad from C2, in line with the DREZ and remaining medial and dorsal to the rootlets of the eleventh cranial nerve. Approximately 10 lesions are made with the shorter electrode (1.8-mm. tip with 0.6-mm. proximal insulation), ending at the level of the motor rootlets of C1. The remaining 6 to 10 lesions are made with the longer electrode (2.6-mm. tip with 0.6-mm. proximal insulation) and extend up to the level of the obex, where the impedance decreases and the tissue is softer to penetration.

This procedure has been performed for anesthesia dolorosa secondary to multiple procedures for trigeminal neuralgia (14 cases), postherpetic neuralgia (8 cases), atypical facial pain (8 cases), pain following facial or dental trauma (4 cases), central pain following stroke (5 cases), cluster head-

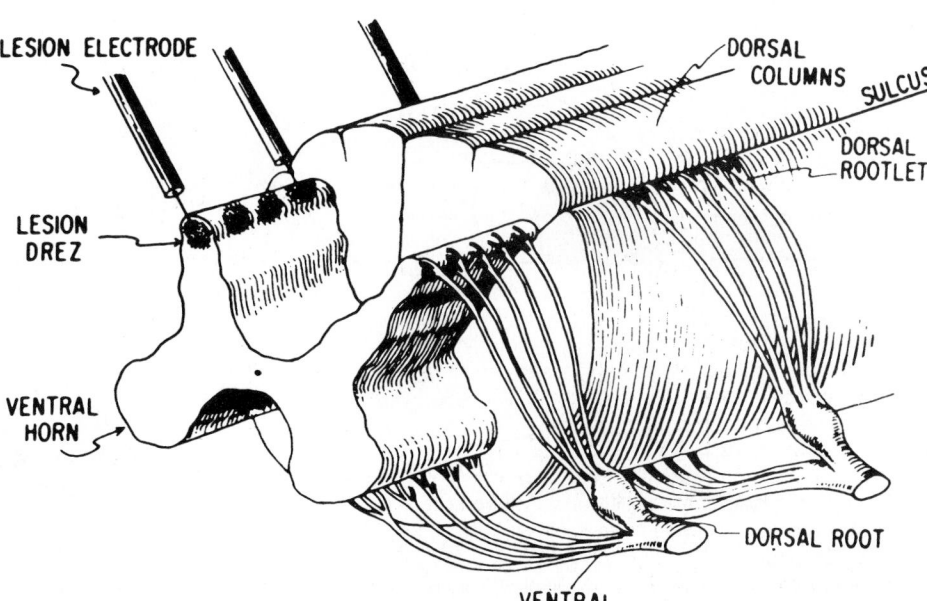

Figure 41–42. Dorsal root entry zone (DREZ) lesioning. (From Nashold, B. S., Jr., and Ostdahl, R. H.: Dorsal root entry zone lesions for pain relief. J. Neurosurg., *51*:59, 1979.)

ache (4 cases), multiple sclerosis (1 case), trigeminal tumor (1 case), and brain stem injury following stereotactic radiation (1 case).

Results for the first 18 procedures were described as good or excellent immediately afterward in 17 patients, but this fell to 11 (58%) on delayed follow-up.[3] Of seven patients with postherpetic neuralgia, 71% experienced a favorable response, and ataxia was identified in 90%. After a 1-year follow-up on 21 patients operated on with the current technique, pain relief was excellent in 48% and good in 5%; 33% developed ataxia.[17]

To date, 101 procedures have been performed at Duke, 46 with the El-Naggar/Nashold electrode.[10] Follow-up is available for 35 of the more recent cases, and pain relief was excellent in 12 and good in 14, for a total favorable response rate of 74%. Ataxia was identified in 39%. There was no significant difference in response rates between diagnostic categories. The substantially better response for postherpetic neuralgia (80% excellent)[17] was not confirmed in this larger group, where 71% experienced good or excellent pain relief. Very good results have been reported in four patients with headache, but follow-up is lacking.

Cordotomy

Edinger first described the spinothalamic tract in 1889, and in 1905, Spiller observed dissociated contralateral sensory loss in a patient with a tuberculoma, which compressed the anterior quadrant of the spinal cord. In 1912, Spiller was able to convince Martin to perform an open cordotomy in a patient with rectal carcinoma and intractable pain, with successful pain relief.[30] Mullan's[16] innovation led to the current technique of high percutaneous radiofrequency cordotomy.[13] This procedure is done with x-ray guidance in an awake patient and is therefore well tolerated, even by those who are very sick with advanced disease. The goal is to coagulate the spinothalamic tract in the anterior cord and ventral to the dentate ligament, which can be visualized myelographically. Impedance is used to identify penetration of the cord. Stimulation confirms localization within the cord when the patient describes hot, cold, or paresthesia on the contralateral side, in the absence of ipsilateral motor responses (Fig. 41–43).

Cordotomy is most useful in patients with cancer who have unilateral pain in the trunk or lower extremity; how-

ever, it is possible to treat upper extremity pain. Bilateral procedures should be separated by at least 2 weeks. Immediate pain relief is excellent in 95% of cases.[13] There is loss of pain relief with time, and the procedure has not proved to be effective in benign conditions such as failed back, shingles, or causalgia. Complications include ipsilateral leg weakness (10% temporary and 3% permanent), bladder dysfunction, respiratory alteration, and anesthesia dolorosa. Ondine's curse occurs almost exclusively following bilateral procedures and consists of a loss of involuntary respiratory drive, causing apnea and possible death. It is usually transient. Failure to respond to a CO_2 challenge with hyperventilation may predict this complication preoperatively. Some patients describe severe ipsilateral pain after their original contralateral pain is successfully eliminated. Open cordotomy is largely of historical interest.

Myelotomy

Myelotomy, first performed in 1927 by Armour,[1] also takes advantage of the crossed nature of the pain pathway. It consists of splitting the spinal cord in a midline sagittal plane, usually at and above the level of pain. Myelotomy is of particular value for bilateral and midline pain, especially pain involving the perineum. The resulting pain relief is widespread and often extends beyond the area of analgesia. A series of cervical myelotomies has been described for relief of pain in various locations, including the rectum.[21] Myelotomy has not gained popularity due to the extensive nature of the procedure and the risk of producing dorsal column dysfunction. Injury to the anterior spinal artery must also be avoided. This ablative procedure is effective for nociceptive pain, and its use is largely limited to pain secondary to malignancy.

Midbrain Tractotomy

Midbrain tractotomy consists of stereotactic ablation of the spinothalamic tract at the level of the midbrain, just below the superior colliculus. At this level, the tracts from the face and body are close to each other, with the face represented more medially. Tractotomy has been performed throughout the brain stem, including the pons and the medulla. The midbrain lesion is positioned so as to include part of the

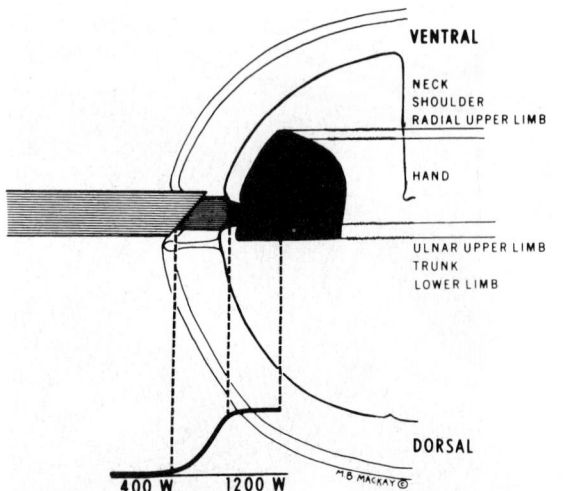
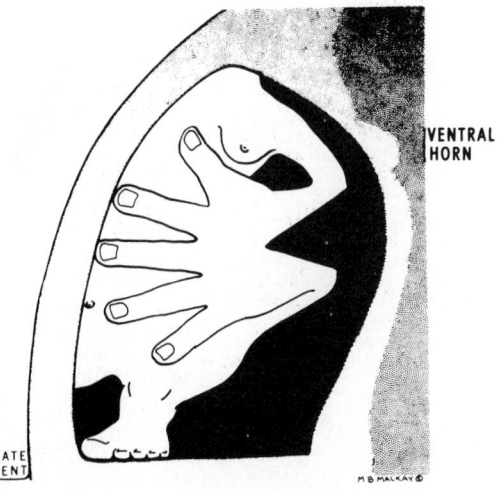

Figure 41–43. Left, Percutaneous cordotomy at C1–C2 by the lateral approach, illustrating the manner of penetration by the electrode needle assembly, the accompanying impedance changes, the location of spinothalamic tract (shaded) with reference to other structures, and the anteroposterior order of somatotopic representation within the tract. Right, The spinothalamic homunculus at C1–C2 in the spinal cord. (From Tasker, R. R.: Percutaneous cordotomy. *In* Schmidek, H. H., and Sweet, W. H. [Eds.]: Operative Neurosurgical Techniques. New York, Grune & Stratton, 1988.)

adjacent periaqueductal gray, which constitutes the paleospinothalamic pathway. This is believed to cause a greater reduction in the emotional suffering associated with chronic pain.[25] Midbrain tractotomy is most commonly indicated for head and neck cancer, with pain involving the face and shoulder region that cannot be successfully treated by cordotomy. The most common complication is diplopia and loss of upward gaze. Diplopia usually resolves within 3 to 8 weeks and is much less common following lesions that are made 5 mm. lower than originally described by Spiegel and Wycis.[29, 36] With magnetic resonance imaging (MRI) localization, the stereotactic procedure is much easier, since the target can be visualized directly rather than extrapolated from the posterior commissure, as seen on ventriculography (Fig. 41–44).

Thalamotomy

Along with the introduction of human stereotactic surgery, Spiegel and Wycis are credited with initiating thalamotomy for the management of pain.[29] In spite of the fact that the ventrocaudal nucleus of the thalamus constitutes the termination of the lateral spinothalamic tract, thalamotomy has not achieved widespread use. Lesions within the ventroposterior nucleus, where axons subserving other modalities are also present, cause numbness but do not reliably relieve pain. The most commonly selected target is in the medial thalamus, which consists of the intralaminar nucleus, parafascicular nucleus, and centromedian nucleus. These nuclei receive input from the brain stem reticular formation. Such lesions produce widespread pain relief without demonstrable analgesia and are indicated for pain secondary to cancer that is not amenable to procedures such as cordotomy. The early success rate approaches 80% but by 1 year falls to 30%; therefore, the procedure is rarely effective for benign pain syndromes. The risks are relatively small (1% to 3%) and include infection, hemorrhage, and confusion when done bilaterally.

An alternative target site involves the posteromedial thalamus and pulvinar, with lesions at this site producing no motor or sensory deficit. Little is known about pulvinar physiology. A fourth variation of thalamotomy consists of lesions made in the dorsomedial and anterior thalamic nuclei, which project to the frontal and limbic lobes. These lesions reduce suffering but do not produce detectable changes in the ability to appreciate noxious stimuli, a situation similar to cingulotomy. Lesions have also been made in the dorsal hypothalamus, as introduced by Sano, which is believed to receive C fiber input via a multisynaptic pathway. There are relatively few reports of this procedure, and Bonica suggests that it has limited indications.

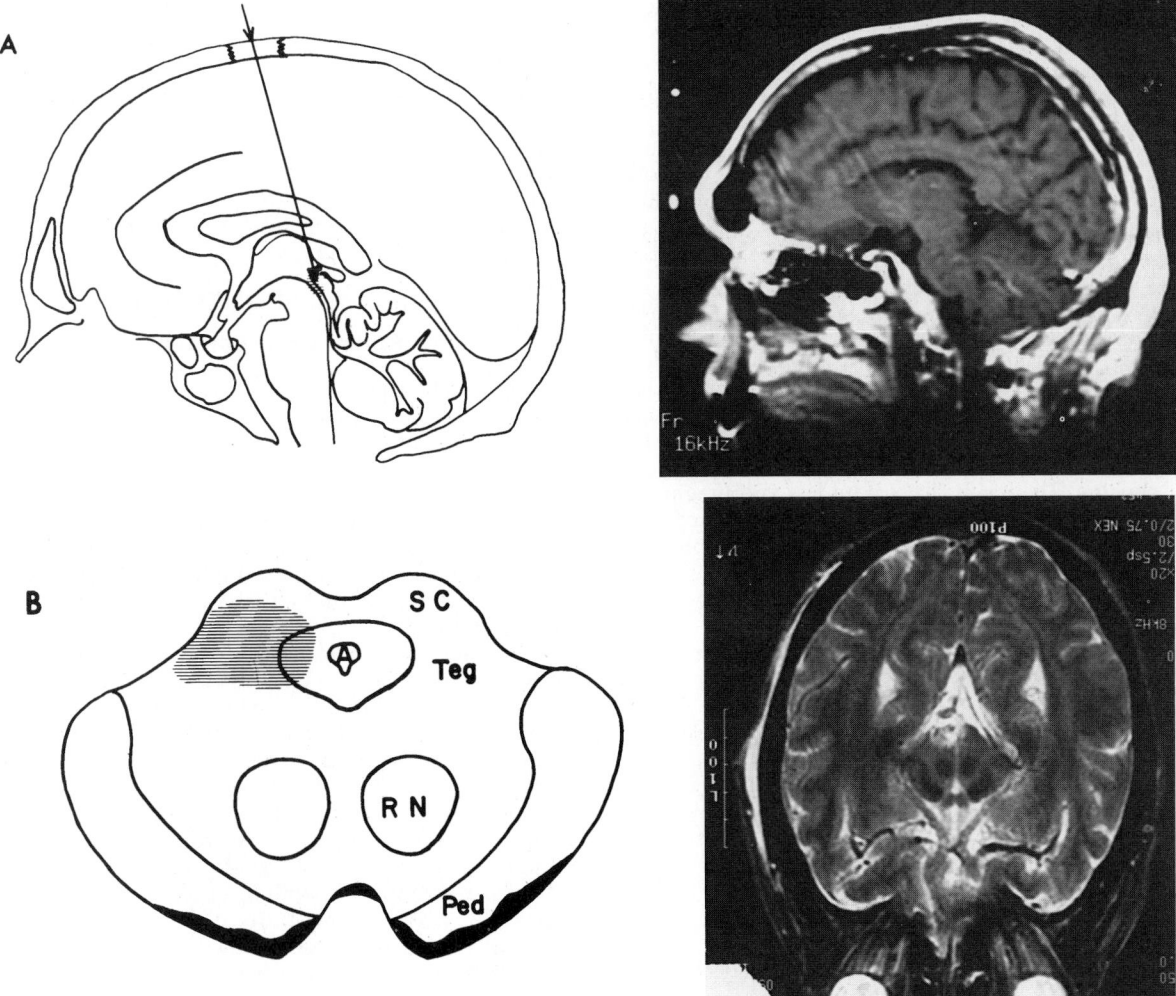

Figure 41–44. Stereotactic midbrain tractotomy. *A,* Sagittal section of the brain shows tract to the midbrain target. *B,* Cross section of mesencephalon at the superior colliculus, with the lesion shaded. The corresponding MRI is shown to the right.

Thalamotomy is performed stereotactically with the patient awake. Computed tomography (CT) is most commonly used for imaging,[33] but MRI is gradually becoming more useful, since the brain stem structures can be defined. Ventriculography has largely been replaced. Lesions are typically made with radiofrequency current, although in some series, gamma knife radiosurgery was employed. Electrophysiologic confirmation of the target site is believed to be essential. Comparing reported series is difficult because of varying pain etiologies and the frequent use of multiple lesions.[32]

Destructive lesions of the thalamus are probably useful in relieving diffuse pain secondary to cancer or the intermittent neuralgic pain or allodynia and hyperpathia present in some patients with neural injury pain. In general, however, stimulation is more beneficial for neural injury pain.

Hypophysectomy should be mentioned, although it is rarely performed. The mechanism for effectiveness of this procedure is unknown; it was introduced to treat hormone-dependent cancer and its pain. Levin[14] suggests a 70% to 95% succes rate for pain relief, with benefit even in non-hormone-sensitive malignancies.

Cingulotomy

Egas Moniz received the Nobel prize in 1949 for describing the results of prefrontal lobotomy in psychiatric illness. The result was that this psychosurgery was used indiscriminately in the United States prior to the introduction of major psychotropic agents. Consequently, this type of procedure came under considerable scientific and political scrutiny and is rarely performed today. It was, however, observed that some patients with complaints of pain as part of their mental illness lost their pain after prefrontal leukotomy.

Cingulotomy consists of lesioning the white matter deep to the cingulate gyrus, which represents the frontal lobe component of Papez's limbic lobe. An alternative procedure that is still actively performed, but less commonly for pain, consists of subcaudate capsulotomy, or lesioning the inferior medial frontal lobe.

Reports suggest that pain secondary to cancer is relieved in 30% to 90% of patients following cingulotomy or cingulotomy combined with midbrain tractotomy. Sweet is particularly enthusiastic about its use in selected cases. This procedure seems to be of most benefit when there is a major element of suffering and has been most commonly used for disseminated head and neck cancer with respiratory impairment or choking. The results have been less encouraging in nonmalignant chronic pain, but it has been suggested that cingulotomy may be useful in cases in which depressive symptoms dominate the clinical picture. There is substantial evidence to suggest that cingulotomy attenuates withdrawal symptoms in both animals and humans.

The procedure is performed stereotactically, with radiofrequency lesions targeted 2 to 4 cm. posterior to the tip of the frontal horn, 1 mm. above the ventricle, and 1.3 cm. lateral to midline; it is done bilaterally. Complications are relatively few; in fact, neuropsychologic testing suggests few changes and even an increase in IQ. Transient headache and fever, as well as transient incontinence, are common. Postoperative hemorrhage can be fatal but is rare, and seizures occur in a small proportion of patients.

Sympathectomy

Sympathectomy is a unique form of neuroablation that is indicated for the treatment of causalgia, reflex sympathetic dystrophy, or Raynaud's phenomenon; it is also used to relieve visceral pain, since afferent fibers from the viscera travel in the sympathetic nervous system. The explanations for pain relief following sympathectomy include the argument that afferent fibers to the extremities are present in the sympathetics, that abnormal efferent activity in sympathetic nerves maintains pain, or that ephaptic connections occur between sympathetic and somatic fibers. Two to 5% of peripheral nerve injuries cause causalgia. Reflex sympathetic dystrophy follows amazingly minor injuries. Left untreated for prolonged periods, both conditions progress through three phases that eventually lead to permanent conditions, with osteoporosis and trophic changes in skin and deeper tissues. If sympathetically mediated pain is treated early, usually by systemic sympathetic blockers such as phenoxybenzamine or a series of repeated sympathetic blocks, Bonica estimates an 80% cure rate.[4] Hannington-Kiff introduced regional sympathetic block using Bier's block and guanethidine to produce chemical sympathectomy,[11] but this technique lacks Food and Drug Administration (FDA) approval. In patients in whom repeated block achieves temporary pain alleviation but fails to produce progressive periods of remission, surgical sympathectomy is indicated. Early, aggressive treatment of these conditions is therefore justified.

For upper extremity pain, several approaches for sympathectomy of T2 and T3 are available, including supraclavicular, transaxillary, or posterior costotransversectomy. Limiting the resection to the lower stellate ganglion limits the incidence of Horner's syndrome (ptosis, miosis, anhidrosis, and apparent enophthalmos). Kux introduced endoscopic sympathectomy in Vienna in 1954,[12] and with modern endoscopic methodology, this should become the method of choice. For lower extremity pain, L1 and L2 sympathetic ganglia are typically removed. However, complete denervation may require section up to the T11 ganglion. Risks include regeneration, pain recurrence, pneumothorax, postsympathectomy neuralgia, and impotence following bilateral lumbar sympathectomy. Celiac plexus ablation, usually done percutaneously, is very effective for the pain of pancreatic cancer or pancreatitis.

NEURAL AUGMENTATION

Spinal Cord Stimulation

Based on the gate control theory,[15] spinal cord stimulation (SCS) was first attempted in 1966.[24] One year later, peripheral nerve stimulation (PNS) was documented. The basic concept involves the interplay between noxious and nonnoxious input in the spinal cord, which influences the ascending activity signaling pain. In experimental models, dorsal column stimulation inhibits the response to noxious stimuli. In humans, this effect generally does not produce analgesia, and it produces an effect that outlasts the paresthesia produced during stimulation.

SCS is generally indicated for neuropathic as opposed to nociceptive pain. Transcutaneous electrical nerve stimulation (TENS) was introduced as a method for screening patients; currently, patients are screened with a percutaneously placed temporary test electrode. The electrode, which may have multiple contacts that allow bipolar stimulation, is placed in the epidural space in close proximity to the dorsal column. When trial stimulation is successful, the electrode is connected to a subcutaneously implanted receiver that can be activated by the patient with an external unit or to a pacemaker-like pulse generator. Since the introduction of trial stimulation, short-term success has been reported in 80% of cases, but the long-term success is only about 50%. The majority of late failures occur within the first year; thereafter, the results are fairly stable.[20]

Stimulation is used for peripheral nerve injuries, reflex sympathetic dystrophy, postamputation pain, postherpetic neuralgia, arachnoiditis, deafferentation rhizopathy, spinal cord lesion, multiple sclerosis, and peripheral vascular disease. Stimulation is generally not effective for brachial plexus avulsion but is used for other plexus lesions. The most common indication is for the failed back syndrome or arachnoiditis, with leg symptoms responding better than back pain.[20] Paresthesia must be produced in the entire painful region. The electrode is placed in the mid to lower thoracic region for lower extremity pain and in the mid cervical region for upper extremity pain.

Complications are generally minor, and the most common is loss of effectiveness. Equipment malfunction can necessitate replacement. Some surgeons prefer to place larger electrodes through a small laminectomy in the hope of reducing migration. Infection occurs in about 5%, and injury to the spinal cord is rare, as is hematoma.

PNS uses the same concept but has the advantage of being more specifically applied directly to an individual nerve. Such specific injuries are relatively uncommon, however. There is usually sufficient differential threshold between motor and sensory effect.

Deep Brain Stimulation

Deep brain stimulation (DBS) has been performed since the mid-1970s. The specific mechanism that causes a reduction in pain is poorly understood. There are two general theories based on two different stimulation targets. Stimulation of the periaqueductal or periventricular gray (PVG) is believed to be effective by means of the endogenous opioid mechanism and is most effective for nociceptive pain. It is most commonly employed for failed back syndrome and is reversible with naloxone.[39] The other common target is the sensory thalamus, which is most effective for neuropathic pain. Its mechanism of action is believed to be based on the gate control theory of pain modulation. Indications include anesthesia dolorosa, central pain, postherpetic neuralgia, cord injury, and peripheral denervation. Due to small series and varied patient populations, reports are difficult to compare and summarize. Good long-term outcomes have been reported in up to 80% following PVG stimulation, whereas Tasker (personal communication) estimated 40% long-term benefit from sensory thalamus DBS. Just as in SCS, a trial period of stimulation is used prior to permanent implantation. Stereotactic technique is employed, with CT guidance and electrophysiologic confirmation by recording and stimulation. During the trial period, it is possible to compare the effectiveness of both targets.

As with SCS, equipment malfunction or displacement accounts for most of the complications, with some 20% of implanted patients requiring further procedures. Infection occurs in about 3%, and hemorrhage or stroke are rare. In many ways, this procedure can be considered reversible—a substantial advantage in these conditions, which are difficult to treat. At the time of this publication, the implanted device is not FDA approved.

Intraspinal Narcotic Analgesia

Intraspinal narcotic analgesia (INA) has affected pain management to the same extent that long-acting morphine altered the care of patients with terminal cancer. Consequently, neuroablative procedures are being done less frequently. Narcotics act directly on opioid receptors in the substantia gelatinosa of the DREZ of the spinal cord.[28] The potent analgesic effect of intrathecal morphine in rats was reported in 1976,[37] and results from human studies demonstrating the effectiveness of intrathecal[35] and epidural[2] morphine were reported shortly thereafter.

Following intrathecal injection, serum levels of morphine are negligible. The onset of action is 5 to 10 minutes, and the effect lasts 10 to 30 hours. Epidural drug administration leads to a slower onset of analgesia (1 hour) and exposes the drug to greater redistribution into the epidural vasculature; this causes higher serum levels but limits cerebrospinal fluid redistribution, producing a more regionalized effect.

Preservative-free morphine can be delivered into the intrathecal or epidural space by continuous infusion using an implanted programmable pump. This technique for the treatment of pain secondary to cancer has been available for 15 years. Quality of life is improved, and many patients are able to reduce or eliminate the intake of oral or parenteral narcotics.[9] Dosage requirements vary among individuals, but there is a trend to double or triple the dose over the life span of the patient. Early dose requirements for intrathecal morphine are about 5 mg. per day, and patients have been maintained for up to 3 years. This technique is indicated in those who have narcotic-responsive pain that is not adequately controlled, usually due to side effects, by systemic opioids. Continuous intraspinal infusion usually causes more potent analgesia with fewer unpleasant effects. A test dose is employed prior to implantation to demonstrate pain reduction of at least 50% sustained for 8 hours. The use of this technique in benign pain is controversial.

Complications are caused by the delivery system or specifically by the drug, and there is a 4% risk of infection. Catheter occlusion presents with loss of pain control. Drug-related complications consist of pruritis, nausea, urinary retention, dependent edema, and respiratory depression. Most side effects are not a problem during chronic drug delivery, and respiratory depression has been surprisingly rare. Reservoir refill constitutes a special risk, and most instances of respiratory depression have occurred with refill-related misadventure. Appropriate monitoring is recommended.

Tolerance can lead to diminished effectiveness, but a drug holiday is one method of dealing with this. Nonnarcotic agents that influence neural modulation, such as low-dose intraspinal bupivacaine, alpha agonists such as clonidine, drugs that increase serotonin such as fenfluramine, gamma-aminobutyric acid (GABA) agonists, somatostatin agonists, N-methyl-D-aspartate (NMDA) receptor antagonists, or calcium channel blockers, may become useful in the future.

SUMMARY

The decision to treat chronic pain by surgical means is a major and sometimes difficult one, quite apart from choosing the appropriate procedure. The pain of cancer can be effectively managed by progressive use of analgesics, adjuvant pharmacologic agents, and narcotics followed by intraspinal narcotic analgesia. Percutaneous cordotomy is preferred for selected patients, since it involves a single intervention, and midbrain tractotomy is the treatment of choice for pain above C5. Rare cases of low back pain respond to facet rhizotomy or selective dorsal rhizotomy; and SCS can be valuable for root deafferentation. PVG stimulation also appears to be appropriate. Neural injury pain has a 50% chance of amelioration by chronic stimulation. DREZ lesioning has a specific role in the treatment of brachial plexus avulsion and spinal cord injury.

SELECTED REFERENCES

Bonica, J. J.: The Management of Pain. Philadelphia, Lea & Febiger, 1990.
A comprehensive review of multidisciplinary pain management.

Gybels, J., and Sweet, W. H.: Neurosurgical Treatment of Persistent Pain. Basel, Karger, 1989.
An encyclopedic review of neurosurgical procedures for pain.

Wall, P. D., and Melzack, R.: Textbook of Pain. London, Churchill Living-stone, 1994.
  A comprehensive and up-to-date review of pain and its management.

White, J. C., and Sweet, W. H.: Pain and the Neurosurgeon: A Forty-Year Experience. Springfield, Ill., Charles C Thomas, 1969.
  A classic neurosurgical review dealing with pain.

REFERENCES

1. Armour, D.: Surgery of spinal cord and its membranes. Lancet, *1*:691, 1927.
2. Behar, M., Olshwang, D., and Magora, F.: Epidural morphine in treatment of pain. Lancet, *1*:527, 1979.
3. Bernard, E. J., Nashold, B. S., Jr., Caputi, F., and Moossy, J. J.: Nucleus caudalis DREZ lesions for facial pain. Br. J. Neurosurg., *1*:81, 1987.
4. Bonica, J. J.: Causalgia and other reflex sympathetic dystrophies. *In* Liebe-skind, J. C., and Albe-Fessard, D. G. (Eds.): Advances in Pain Research and Therapy, Vol. 3. New York, Raven Press, 1979, p. 141.
5. Broggi, G., Franzini, A., Lazio, G., Giorgi, C., and Servello, D.: Long-term results of percutaneous retrogasserian thermorhizotomy for "essential" trigeminal neuralgia: Consideration in 1000 consecutive patients. Neuro-surgery, *26*:783, 1990.
6. Brown, J. A., McDaniel, M. D., and Weaver, M. T.: Percutaneous trigeminal compression for treatment of trigeminal neuralgia: Results in 50 patients. Neurosurgery, *32*:570, 1993.
7. Burchiel, K.: Percutaneous retrogasserian glycerol rhizolysis in the manage-ment of trigeminal neuralgia. J. Neurosurg., *69*:361, 1988.
8. Burchiel, K. J., Clarke, H., Haglund, M., and Loeser, J. D.: Long-term efficacy of microvascular decompression in trigeminal neuralgia. J. Neuro-surg., *69*:35, 1988.
9. Gorecki, J. P.: Intrathecal narcotic analgesia. *In* Wilkins, R. H., and Ren-gachary, S. S. (Eds.): Neurosurgery. New York, McGraw-Hill, 1995.
10. Gorecki, J. P., and Nashold, B. S., Jr.: The Duke experience with the nucleus caudalis DREZ operation. Acta Neurochir., 1995.
11. Hannington-Kiff, J. G.: Intravenous regional sympathetic block with gua-nethidine. Lancet, *1*:1019, 1974.
12. Kux, M.: Thoracic endoscopic sympathectomy for treatment of upper-limb hyperhidrosis. Lancet, *1*:1320, 1977.
13. Lahuerta, J., Bowsher, D., Lipton, S., and Buxton, P. H.: Percutaneous cervical cordotomy: A review of 181 operations on 146 patients with a study on the location of "pain fibers" in the C-2 spinal cord segment of 29 cases. J. Neurosurg., *80*:975, 1994.
14. Levin, A. B.: Stereotactic chemical hypophysectomy. *In* Lunsford, L. D. (Ed.): Modern Stereotactic Neurosurgery. Boston, Martinus Nijhoff, 1988, p. 365.
15. Melzack, R., and Wall, P. D.: Pain mechanisms: A new theory. Science, *150*:971, 1965.
16. Mullan, S., Harper, P. V., Hekmatpanah, J., Torres, H., and Dobbin, G.: Percutaneous interruption of spinal-pain tracts by means of a strontium-90 needle. J. Neurosurg., *20*:931, 1963.
17. Nashold, B. S., Jr., El-Naggar, A. O., Ovelmen-Levitt, J., and Muwaffak, A.: A new design of radiofrequency lesion electrodes for use in the caudalis nucleus DREZ operation. J. Neurosurg., *80*:1116, 1994.
18. Nashold, B. S., Jr., and Ostdahl, R. H.: Dorsal root entry zone lesions for pain relief. J. Neurosurg., *51*:59, 1979.
19. North, R. B., Kidd, D. H., Campbell, J. N., and Long, D. M.: Dorsal root ganglionectomy for failed back surgery syndrome: A 5-year follow-up study. J. Neurosurg., *74*:236, 1991.
20. North, R. B., Kidd, D. H., Zahurak, M., James, C. S., and Long, D. M.: Spinal cord stimulation for chronic, intractable pain: Experience over two decades. Neurosurgery, *32*:384, 1993.
21. Schvarcz, J. R.: Stereotactic high cervical extralemniscal myelotomy for pelvic cancer pain. Acta Neurchir. (Suppl.), *33*:431, 1984.
22. Scoville, W. B.: Extradural spinal sensory rhizotomy. J. Neurosurg., *25*:94, 1966.
23. Shealy, C. N.: Percutaneous radiofrequency denervation of spinal facets. J. Neurosurg., *43*:448, 1975.
24. Shealy, C. N., Mortimer, J. T., and Reswick, J.: Electrical inhibition of pain by stimulation of the dorsal column: Preliminary clinical reports. Anesth. Analg., *46*:489, 1967.
25. Shieff, C., and Nashold, B. S., Jr.: Stereotactic mesencephalotomy. Neuro-surg. Clin. North Am., *1*:825, 1990.
26. Sindou, M., Fischer, G., and Mansuy, L.: Posterior spinal rhizotomy and selective posterior rhizidiotomy. Progr. Neurol. Surg., *7*:201, 1976.
27. Sindou, M., Jeanmonod, D., and Mertens, P.: Ablative neurosurgical proce-dures for the treatment of chronic pain. Neurophysiol. Clin., *20*:399, 1990.
28. Snyder, S. H.: Opiate receptors and internal opiates. Sci. Am., *236*:44, 1977.
29. Spiegel, E. A., and Wycis, H. T.: Mesencephalotomy in treatment of intrac-table facial pain. Arch. Neurol. Psychiatry, *69*:1, 1953.
30. Spiller, W. G., and Martin, E.: The treatment of persistent pain of organic origin in the lower part of the body by division of the anterolateral column of the spinal cord. JAMA, *58*:1489, 1912.
31. Sweet, W. H.: Complications of percutaneous rhizotomy and microvascular decompression operations for facial pain. *In* Schmidek, H. H., and Sweet, W. H. (Eds.): Operative Neurosurgical Techniques. New York, Grune & Stratton, 1988, p. 1139.
32. Tasker, R. R.: Stereotactic surgery. *In* Wall, P. D., and Melzak, R. (Eds.): Textbook of Pain. London, Churchill Livingstone, 1994, p. 1147.
33. Tasker, R. R., Dostrovsky, J. O., and Dolan, E. J.: Computerized tomography (CT) is just as accurate as ventriculography for functional stereotactic thalamotomy. Stereotact. Funct. Neurosurg., *57*:157, 1993.
34. van Kleef, M., Spaans, F., Dingemans, A., Barendse, G. A. M., Floor, E., and Sluijter, M. E.: Effects and side effects of a percutaneous thermal lesion of the dorsal root ganglion in patients with cervical pain syndrome. Pain, *52*:49, 1993.
35. Wang, J. K., Nauss, L. A., and Thomas, J. E.: Pain relief by intrathecally applied morphine in man. Anesthesiology, *50*:149, 1979.
36. Wycis, H. T., and Spiegel, E. A.: Long-range results in the treatment of intractable pain by stereotaxic midbrain surgery. J. Neurosurg., *19*:101, 1962.
37. Yaksh, L., and Rudy, T. A.: Analgesia mediated by a direct spinal action of narcotics. Science, *192*:1357, 1976.
38. Young, J. N., and Wilkins, R. H.: Partial sensory rhizotomy at the pons for trigeminal neuralgia. J. Neurosurg., *79*:680, 1993.
39. Young, R. F., and Chambi, V. I.: Pain relief by electrical stimulation of the periaqueductal and periventricular gray matter. J. Neurosurg., *66*:364, 1987.

XIII

NEUROSURGICAL RELIEF OF EPILEPSY

Allan H. Friedman, M.D.

HISTORY

Surgery for epilepsy in the modern era is an exceptional example of a harmonious joining of laboratory research, clini-cal observation, and medical practice. Prior to the late nine-teenth century, the entire cerebral cortex was thought to be homonymous, without regional differentiation. All regions of the cortex were thought to have the same functional capabili-ties, like the liver. Surgical procedures for the treatment of epilepsy were based on the unsubstantiated theory of "coun-terirritation" and included random trephination, brain cau-terization, appendectomy, and castration. Epileptics became double victims, suffering from both their epilepsy and the treatments rendered by physicians.

Although others theorized that specific functions were lo-calized to circumscribed regions of the cerebral cortex, it was Hughlings Jackson whose clinical pathologic correlations provided the foundation for localization of cerebral functions and focal cortical resections for the treatment of epilepsy. Employing Jackson's observations, Macewen in 1875 local-ized and resected a frontal meningioma based on the clinical manifestation of focal motor seizures.[6] In 1886, Victor Horsley reported the successful localization and removal of brain lesions responsible for epilepsy in three of Jackson's patients.[4] These cases initiated the modern era of epilepsy surgery.

Curative surgical therapy during this early period was limited to a small number of patients whose clinical seizures pointed toward a focal cortical origin and in whom a compatible cortical abnormality could be visualized at the time of surgical exploration. The number of epileptic patients who could benefit from seizure surgery expanded with the introduction of electroencephalography (EEG). EEG could localize the origin of some seizures whose clinical behavior was not indicative of a specific cortical origin or that did not result from a visible focal cortical abnormality. In 1951, Bailey and Gibbs reported a series of 25 patients undergoing anterior temporal lobe resection for seizures localized only by EEG data.

Although our diagnostic techniques have been improved by advances in technology, the cortical origin of seizures is established by observing the semiology of the patient's seizures, searching for a structural cortical lesion, and reviewing EEG findings.

PATIENT SELECTION

Although some palliative surgical procedures exist, most surgical therapy is aimed at resection of the epileptogenic area of cerebral cortex responsible for the patient's seizures. Surgical therapy for epilepsy is contemplated only when the patient's seizures are not adequately controlled by nontoxic amounts of anticonvulsant medications, and only when the patient's activities are limited by the seizures. Homebound patients who are not physically harmed by their seizures are not considered for surgical intervention. The epileptic focus responsible for the majority of the patient's seizures must be limited to a circumscribed area of cerebral cortex. The proposed cerebral cortical resection must not intentionally produce a significant neurologic deficit such as aphasia or hemiparesis.

CLASSIFICATION

Because the exact cellular pathology of epileptic disorders remains obscure, several classifications of epilepsy were developed to serve different purposes. The International League Against Epilepsy developed the most widely used classification system based on a review of videotaped seizures (Table 41–8).[1] For the epilepsy surgeon, the most important distinction is between partial seizures, which appear to begin with the activation of a limited portion of the cerebral cortex, and generalized seizures, in which there is an early activation of neurons throughout both hemispheres. A complex seizure

TABLE 41–8. Classification of Seizures[1]

I. Partial (focal, local) seizures
  A. Simple partial seizures (consciousness not impaired)
    1. With motor signs (focal motor, etc.)
    2. With somatosensory or special sensory symptoms (visual, auditory, etc.)
    3. With autonomic symptoms (pallor, sweating, etc.)
    4. With psychic symptoms (déjà vu, fear, anger, etc.)
  B. Complex partial seizures (impairment of consciousness)
    1. Simple partial onset followed by impairment of consciousness
    2. Impairment of consciousness at onset
  C. Partial seizures evolving to secondary generalized seizures (tonic-clonic, clonic, or tonic)
II. Generalized seizures (may be convulsive with motor movements, or nonconvulsive without motor movements)
  A. Absence (sudden interruption of activity with blank stare)
  B. Myoclonic (myoclonic jerks)
  C. Clonic
  D. Tonic
  E. Tonic-clonic
  F. Atonic (sudden loss of motor tone)

is one in which consciousness is lost; in a simple seizure, consciousness is retained. Simple partial seizures are those in which only one portion of the brain is affected and the patient remains conscious. A partial complex seizure is one in which the patient first manifests focal seizure activity and then, as the seizure activity spreads, loses consciousness, with or without tonic-clonic activity. Partial complex seizures or focal seizures with secondary generalization are the seizure type most amenable to surgical resection.

SURGICAL THERAPY

Surgical therapy is most commonly aimed at removing a circumscribed region of epileptic cerebral cortex. Occasionally, procedures such as hemispherectomy or corpus callosum section are employed to treat seizures of a less well-defined origin. Although these patients are usually young and in good health, surgical procedures for the treatment of epilepsy may be complicated by an adverse effect of anesthesia, infection, or intracranial hematoma.[8]

CLINICAL WORK-UP

The goal of the preoperative work-up is to identify those patients whose seizures emanate from a focal area of cerebral cortex, to identify the location of the cortex responsible for initiating the seizures, and to determine the extent of cortex that must be removed to stop the seizures. Although taking advantage of advances in technology, this selection of patients for surgical intervention is based on the principles set forth by Jackson, Horsley, and Penfield. The locus of the epileptic brain is determined by concordance of the clinical manifestations of the seizure, abnormalities demonstrated by cerebral imaging studies, and epileptic electrical activity demonstrated by EEG.

In the rare patient, the physical examination demonstrates a focal neurologic deficit or slight asymmetry in extremity size, indicative of an abnormality in the contralateral cerebral hemisphere. Neuropsychologic testing can detect subtle alterations in cognitive function, indicating a focal brain dysfunction. The most pertinent clinical information comes from analyzing the semiology of the patient's seizures. Initial symptoms or auras occurring prior to the loss of consciousness may reveal the locus of the cortex responsible for initiating the seizure. Episodes beginning with focal clonic or tonic movements indicate activation of the contralateral motor strip. Some auras, such as the perception of a foul odor or a tightness within the epigastric area that rises into the chest, raise the suspicion of epileptic activity within the mesial temporal lobe; other auras, such as vertigo and auditory hallucinations, indicate seizure activity within the lateral temporal lobe. Approximately 40% of seizures originating in the mesial temporal lobe begin with motionless stare followed by repetitive movements such as lip smacking, referred to as automatisms. Because seizure activity rapidly spreads within the brain, an aura does not necessarily denote where the seizure began but only that the focal area of cortex is stimulated early in the evolution of the seizure. Thus, a seizure that begins in the clinically silent anterior frontal lobe and spreads to the motor strip first manifests with contralateral clonic motor activity, although the motor strip was not the place where the electrical seizure began. Although clinical manifestations point toward the cortical region responsible for initiating the seizures, the accuracy of this prediction must be corroborated by other means.

Since the time of Horsley, when brain lesions could be detected only by overlying irregularities in the skull or by direct visualization of the cortex, a wealth of brain imaging techniques, including x-ray, computed tomography (CT),

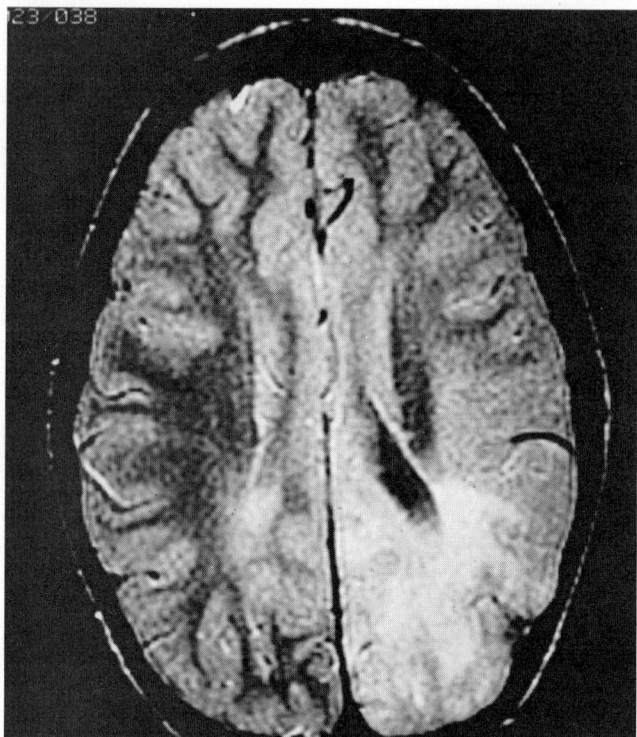

Figure 41–45. An MRI of an eight-year-old patient with intractable seizures. Note areas of dysplasia (white areas) most prominent in the left posterior hemisphere.

magnetic resonance imaging (MRI), positron-emission tomography (PET), and single-photon-emission computed tomography (SPECT), has become available to help ferret out intracerebral abnormalities. Neoplasia, atrophy, dysplasia, and trauma can all lead to epilepsy. X-ray CT, which was a major advance in brain imaging, has largely been replaced by MRI as the best test for detecting subtle epileptogenic brain abnormalities (Fig. 41–45). MRI often has the resolution to detect medial temporal sclerosis, the pathologic condition most frequently seen in temporal lobe epilepsy. Functional imaging had proved helpful in detecting seizures of temporal lobe origin. Other tests include interictal PET scanning of fluorodeoxyglucose, a marker of glucose metabolism, and ictal SPECT scanning of [99m]technetium-hexamethyl-propylene-amineoxime, a marker of blood flow. PET scanning correctly predicted a remission of seizures in 32 of 43 patients successfully treated with temporal lobectomy. A mesial temporal abnormality was identified on MRI scan in 37 of 39 patients whose seizures diminished following temporal lobectomy. The epileptogenic nature of an abnormality detected by neuroimaging must be corroborated by clinical and EEG data.

Empirically, EEG disturbances should be the hallmark of seizures. Unfortunately, EEG recordings collected from the electrodes placed on the scalp are distorted by the underlying scalp, skull, and dura. These electrodes do not record electrical activity emanating from the mesial and inferior surfaces of the brain, which are frequently the origin of the patient's seizures. Interictal EEG recordings may demonstrate abnormal electrical "spikes" indicative of a potentially epileptogenic area of brain. Simultaneous video monitoring and EEG recording of the patient's seizures allow for a correlation of the clinical manifestations of the seizure with the EEG. Electrographic activity that first appears after the onset of the clinical seizure cannot represent the origin of the seizure. In many cases, scalp EEG is insufficient to localize the origin of the patient's seizures.

INVASIVE EEG MONITORING

When clinical and noninvasive testing points to, but does not adequately prove, a focal origin of the patient's seizures, more precise electrical recordings are made from electrodes placed surgically within the cranium. Because of the risks and considerable costs of invasive intracranial monitoring, these techniques are employed only to answer specific questions raised during the noninvasive work-up.

Intracranial EEG recordings can be used to determine the side of origin of the patient's seizures. This question arises in seizures originating from the mesial or inferior frontal or temporal lobe surface far from the scalp electrodes. Intracranial EEG recordings can also be used to localize or delineate the extent of epileptic cortex once the general region of the seizure origin has been discovered. Electrical stimulation through electrodes placed on the surface of the brain can isolate eloquent areas of cortex that should not be encroached upon at the time of operation.

The electrode array utilized depends on the hypothesis posed regarding the onset of the epileptic seizures. Invasive techniques include depth electrodes that are placed in the brain, subdural electrodes placed on the brain, and, rarely, epidural electrodes placed inside the skull but outside the dura. Depth electrodes are most often used to lateralize temporal lobe epilepsy (Fig. 41–46). Although arrays of depth electrodes can be placed to tailor a resection, most centers use subdural electrodes placed along a linear strip or on a mat in a rectangular array for delineation of the epileptic cortex (Fig. 41–47).

Because these electrodes are recording from only a circumscribed area of brain, epileptic signals may indicate the starting point of the patient's seizures or propagation of epileptic activity that began elsewhere. Data accumulated from intracranial recording are used in concert with clinical and neuroimaging data to define the seizure's origin.

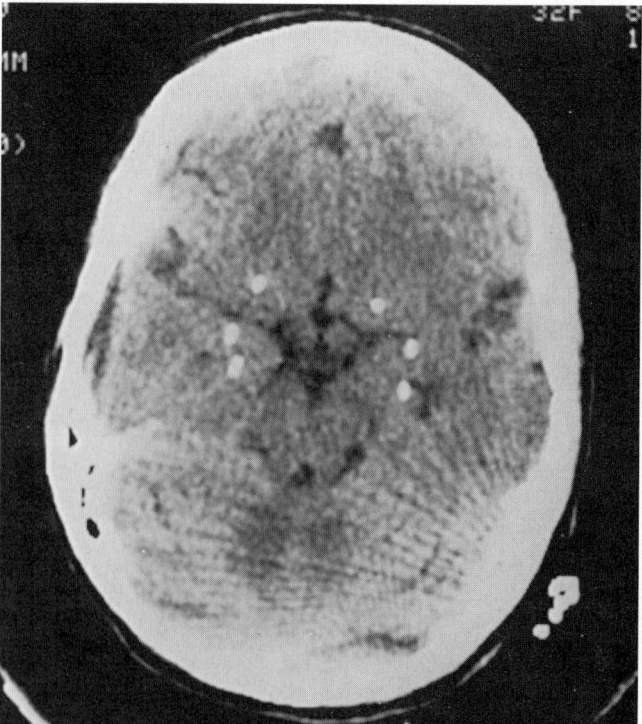

Figure 41–46. CT scan of patient with depth electrodes (intracerebral white dots). The electrodes are in the amygdala, anterior hippocampus, and inferior frontal lobes.

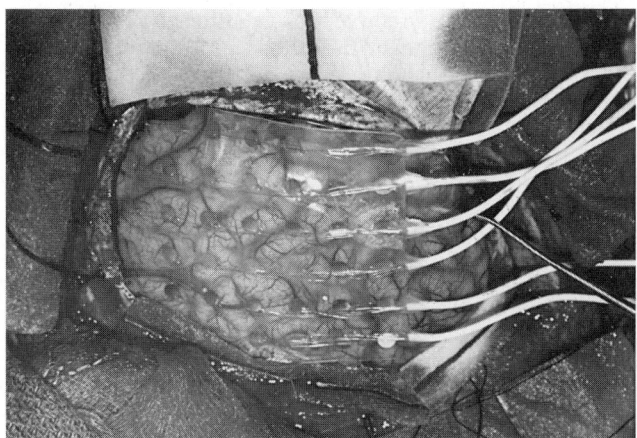

Figure 41–47. Electrode grid placed over the brain.

The most prevalent complications associated with invasive EEG monitoring are inadequate placement of electrodes, hemorrhage, and infection. Depth electrode placement is associated with a 1% to 3% risk of intracranial hemorrhage and a 1% to 5% risk of infection. Creutzfeldt-Jakob disease has been transmitted by the reuse of electrodes. Subdural grid and strip electrodes appear to be associated with a slightly lower incidence of complications.

TEMPORAL LOBECTOMY

The most commonly performed surgical procedure for the treatment of intractable epilepsy is temporal lobe resection. The origin of the patient's seizures is localized to the temporal lobe by concordant clinical, imaging, and EEG data.

The specific criteria for surgery vary among epilepsy centers, but the best results are obtained in patients in whom all methods of evaluation point toward a temporal lobe origin for the seizures. Prior to surgical therapy, the ability of the contralateral temporal lobe to sustain the patient's memory may be tested by the intracarotid injection of amobarbital (Amytal), a short-acting barbiturate. This procedure anesthetizes one side of the brain, allowing the evaluation of the other cerebral hemisphere in isolation. This same procedure can be used to determine the side of the brain dominant to speech.

The exact portion of temporal lobe removed varies with the technique of the surgeon. Most commonly, less than 6 cm. of lateral and inferior neocortex is removed, along with the inferior portion of the amygdala and anterior 2.5 to 5 cm. of hippocampus. Based on the theory that most temporal lobe seizures emanate from the mesial temporal structure, a few surgeons remove only the inferior amygdala and anterior hippocampus. Still other surgeons base the temporal lobe resection on intraoperative EEG recordings.[7] Despite the diversity of techniques, most centers find that almost 70% of patients are seizure free, and an additional 23% of patients achieve a significant reduction in the frequency of their seizures (Table 41–9).[2, 12] It is difficult to compare the efficacy of these surgical techniques, as the criteria for patient selection varies among surgeons. Histologic examination of the surgical specimens reveals mesial temporal sclerosis in approximately 60% of patients, low-grade primary brain tumors in 10% to 15%, and areas of cortical dysplasia in 10% to 15%.

Severe neurologic deficits such as hemiparesis or hemianopsia are reported to occur in approximately 2% of patients.[8] Although transient anomia frequently occurs following the resection of the language-dominant temporal lobe, 2% of patients suffer significant persistent dysphasia. Profound antegrade memory loss occurs if the contralateral temporal lobe cannot sustain the patient's memory. Transient loss of verbal memory performance commonly follows dominant temporal lobe resection, and temporary loss of visuospatial memory can follow nondominant lobe resection. Recovery of this function is directly proportional to seizure control.[5] Approximately 5% of patients suffer new postoperative seizures or depression.

EXTRATEMPORAL EEG RESECTION

Seizures arising outside of the temporal lobe are notoriously difficult to localize because of the rapid spread of electrical activity through the white matter pathways that interconnect areas of cerebral cortex. Clues reflecting the seizure origin can sometimes be found by observing the patient's auras and ictal or postictal activities. MRI scanning is a sensitive method for demonstrating potentially epileptogenic abnormalities in the patient's cerebral cortex. Cavernous angiomas, low-grade gliomas, cortical dysplasia, and cortical cicatrix are classic progenitors of epilepsy. Because extratemporal epilepsies are difficult to localize electrographically with electrodes placed on the patient's scalp, intracranial electrodes are frequently employed. The origin of a frontal lobe seizure, which rapidly disseminates to the contralateral frontal lobe, can be lateralized by placing intracranial electrodes in both frontal lobes. In a similar fashion, epilepsy tracked down to a single region of the brain can be localized by an intracranial grid electrode placed over that area.

Once the region responsible for the initiation of the patient's seizures has been identified, the surgeon must decide how much tissue must be removed. The area of cortex generating epileptiform spikes is generally larger than the radiographic abnormality. When a structural lesion can be identified in the epileptogenic region, some surgeons resect only the lesion. Other surgeons claim superior results resecting the lesion and the surrounding epileptogenic cortex as determined by EEG monitoring. Although the exact extent of resection is still debated, all surgeons agree that the procedure should not knowingly produce a neurologic deficit. If no lesion can be demonstrated by MRI or PET scanning, the extent of the cortex resected is generally guided by EEG recordings.

Forty-five percent of patients undergoing an extratemporal resection of neocortex for the treatment of epilepsy are rendered seizure free. If an extratemporal lesion is found and removed, 67% of patients become seizure free, a result comparable to that achieved by anterior temporal lobectomy. Specific neurologic deficits incurred as a complication of extratemporal lobe neocortical resection reflect the neurologic function of the locus of the procedure.

HEMISPHERECTOMY

Hemispherectomy is performed to treat hemiplegic patients suffering from intractable seizures emanating without

TABLE 41–9. Operative Results for Epileptic Seizures (1986–1990)[2]

Procedure	Number of Patients	Seizure Free (%)	Improved (%)	Not Improved (%)
Anterior temporal lobectomy	3579	67.9	24.0	8.1
Amygdala hippocampectomy	413	68.8	22.3	9.0
Extratemporal corticectomy	805	45.1	35.2	19.8
Lesion resection	293	66.6	21.5	21.1
Hemispherectomy	190	67.4	21.1	11.6
Corpus callosum section	563	7.6	60.9	31.4

focal origin from a single extensively damaged cerebral hemisphere. Diseases underlying hemiplegia and intractable seizures include extensive unilateral stroke, cortical dysplasia, infantile hemiplegia of unknown etiology, and chronic unilateral encephalitis. Because of late complications associated with removing a large volume of brain, anatomic hemispherectomy has given way to "functional" hemispherectomy, in which the diseased hemisphere is surgically disconnected from communication with the normal brain but is left in place.[9] Although the thought of removing or even disconnecting half of the patient's brain seems repulsive, the disconnection frees the normal brain from seizures and allows it to function optimally. Seventy percent of patients undergoing a hemispherectomy are rendered seizure free, and an additional 20% are significantly improved.

Although anatomic hemispherectomy is effective in controlling seizures, it is associated with a high complication rate. Early complications include infection and acute hydrocephalus. Late complications are caused by large and small hemorrhages into the cavernous surgical cavity and include hydrocephalus, subdural hematoma, and superficial cerebral hemosiderosis. Superficial cerebral hemosiderosis is a complication that is almost unique to patients undergoing anatomic hemispherectomy and occurs in one third of them.[11] This syndrome is clinically manifest by a gradual but devastating neurologic deterioration beginning years after the patient's surgical procedure. Autopsy studies demonstrate a hemorrhagic subdural membrane within the resected cavity, granular ependymitis along the ventricular walls, and superficial hemosiderosis of the remaining brain and cranial nerves. This complication is not seen in patients undergoing functional hemispherectomy.

CORPUS CALLOSUM SECTION

The corpus callosum is a major pathway by which focal epileptic discharges can spread to the opposite hemisphere. Sectioning of the corpus callosum has been proposed as a method to stop the spread of the seizure when the initiating focus or foci cannot be directly resected. Although corpus callosum section has been used to treat a number of different epileptic conditions, it has proved to be most effective in treating patients suffering from atonic seizures clinically manifested as sudden drop attacks.[10] This is a palliative procedure that rarely renders the patient seizure free. Only 8% of reported patients are rendered seizure free, but 60% are improved.[2]

Complications associated with corpus callosum sectioning are caused by trauma to the mesial cortex, disruption of bridging veins entering the sagittal sinus, retraction of the ipsilateral hemisphere, and sectioning of the corpus callosum itself. The transient syndrome of difficulty in initiating speech, leg paresis, and urinary incontinence following surgi-

cal section of the anterior corpus callosum is probably secondary to dysfunction of the parasagittal motor, premotor, and supplementary motor cortex. Complete section of the corpus callosum causes loss of the ability to read material presented in the left visual field and to name objects placed in the left hand. Interhemispheric antagonism or split brain syndrome occurs in 3% to 5% of operated patients.[3, 8]

CONCLUSION

Surgical treatment of intractable epilepsy is presently limited by our inability to localize the focus that initiates the patient's seizures. As functional imaging of the central nervous system improves, more patients may become candidates for this form of therapy.

SELECTED REFERENCES

Engel, J. (Ed.): Surgical Treatment of the Epilepsies, 2nd ed. New York, Raven Press, 1993.
This volume is an account of the Second International Conference on the Surgical Treatment of Epilepsy held in Palm Desert, California, February 1992. It defines the field of epilepsy surgery as it existed then.

Penfield, W., and Jasper, H.: Epilepsy and the Functional Anatomy of the Human Brain. Boston, Little, Brown, 1954.
This classic work outlines Wilder Penfield's experience treating epilepsy and stimulating the brain at the time of surgery. The observations provide the reader with a functional map of the human neocortex.

REFERENCES

1. Commission on Classification and Terminology of the International League Against Epilepsy: Proposal for revised clinical and electroencephalographic classification of epileptic seizures. Epilepsia, 22:489, 1981.
2. Engel, J., Jr., Van Ness, P. C., Rasmussen, T. B., and Ojemann, L. M.: Outcome with respect to epileptic seizures. *In* Engel, J. (Ed.): Surgical Treatment of the Epilepsies, 2nd ed. New York, Raven Press, 1993, p. 609.
3. Gates, J. R., Wada, J. A., Reeves, A. G., et al.: Reevaluation of corpus callositomy. *In* Engel, J. (Ed.): Surgical Treatment of the Epilepsies, 2nd ed. New York, Raven Press, 1993, p. 637.
4. Horsley, V.: Brain-surgery. Br. Med. J., 2:670, 1886.
5. Leonard, G.: Temporal lobe surgery for epilepsy: Neuropsychological variables related to surgical outcome. Can. J. Neurol. Sci., 18:593, 1991.
6. Macewen, W.: Tumour of the dura mater removed during life in a person affected with epilepsy. Glas. Med., 12:210, 1879.
7. Ojemann, G. A.: Different approaches to resective epilepsy surgery: Standard and tailored. Epilepsy Res. (Suppl.), 5:169, 1992.
8. Pilcher, W. H., Roberts, D. W., Flanigin, H. F., et al.: Complications of epilepsy surgery. *In* Engel, J. (Ed.): Surgical Treatment of the Epilepsies, 2nd ed. New York, Raven Press, 1993, p. 565.
9. Rasmussen, T.: Postoperative superficial hemosiderosis of the brain, its diagnosis, treatment and prevention. Trans. Am. Neurol. Assoc., 98:133, 1973.
10. Spenser, S. S.: Corpus callosum section and other disconnection procedures for medically intractable epilepsy. Epilepsia (Suppl. 2), 29:S85, 1988.
11. Villemure, J. G.: Hemispherectomy techniques. *In* Luder, H. O. (Ed.): Epilepsy Surgery. New York, Raven Press, 1992, p. 569.
12. Walczak, T. S., Radtke, R. A., McNamara, J. O., et al.: Anterior temporal lobectomy for complex partial seizures: Evaluation, results and long-term followup in 100 cases. Neurology, 40:413, 1990.

XIV

STEREOTACTIC NEUROSURGERY

Dennis A. Turner, M.D., M.A.

The goal of all stereotactic procedures is to provide accurate navigation to a point or region in space. Stereotactic methods provide guidance techniques to access deep structures within the brain without the necessity of direct visualization.[10, 23, 24] Two surgical indications provided the initial impetus for the development of a human stereotactic device (Fig. 41–48): improving frontal lobotomy procedures, and decreasing the risk of open (craniotomy) procedures to alleviate movement disorders.[33] The development of a stereotactic frame for human use required detailed maps of the human brain in standard and reproducible orientations (Fig. 41–49).[32] Initial stereotactic procedures were performed by defining radiographic landmarks close to the region of interest, such as the third ventricle for thalamic procedures. Further developments included frame-based, image-guided neurosurgical procedures for the biopsy and treatment of lesions[5, 15, 20] using primarily computed tomography (CT) or magnetic resonance imaging (MRI) (Fig. 41–50A and B), as well as the advent of frameless stereotaxis, which provides accurate localization based on various forms of three-dimensional digitization of the skull and brain.[3, 12, 17, 18, 21, 26, 31, 35, 36, 41, 42] Presently, there are two general indications for stereotactic procedures: approaches to structural lesions, such as tumors and vascular malformations; and treatment of functional abnormalities, such as movement disorders and pain conditions. Treatment using stereotactic methods has advanced considerably with the development of stereotactic radiosurgery for tumors and arteriovenous malformations (AVMs),[11, 13, 14, 28] brachytherapy for treatment of gliomas,[39, 40] stereotactic implantation of neural tissue and drug transplants,[1, 2, 16, 19, 22, 27, 29] and gene therapy techniques.[4, 6, 34]

STRUCTURAL FRAME-BASED STEREOTACTIC PROCEDURES

The concept of structural neurosurgery implies that a discrete abnormality such as a tumor, vascular lesion, or abscess

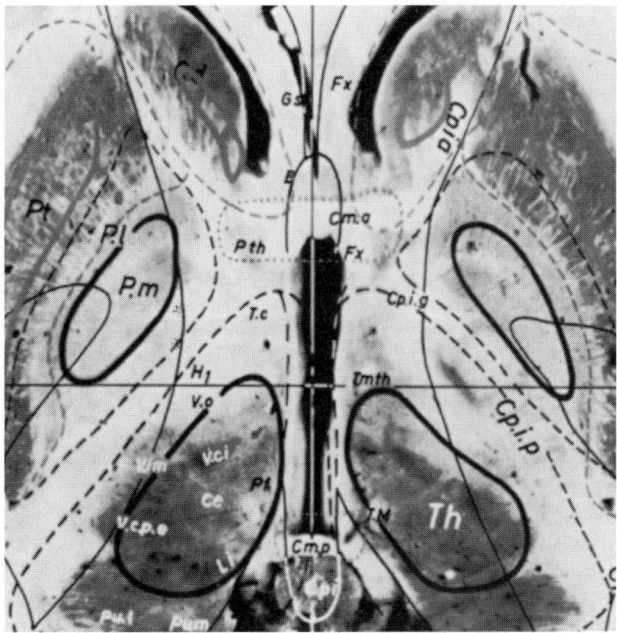

Figure 41–49. Stereotactic map of a horizontal section of the human brain through the diencephalon and basal ganglia showing the third ventricle (center) bordered by the anterior (Cm. a.) and posterior (Cm. p.) commissures. (From Schaltenbrand, G., and Wahren, W.: Atlas for Stereotaxy of the Human Brain. Stuttgart, Georg Theime Verlag, 1977, plate 17.)

can be detected on an imaging study (see Fig. 41–50).[8] This structural lesion can be approached for stereotactic biopsy using a stereotactic frame for guidance. The stereotactic frames developed for this purpose (notably the Brown-Roberts-Wells, Cosman-Roberts-Wells, and Leksell frames) require a further set of images to orient the lesion with respect to the coordinates of the frame after it has been fixed directly to the skull, usually with sharp points. Thus, the frame is applied; a repeat imaging study is performed to align the brain, lesion, and stereotactic frame; and then a biopsy is performed using an arc system attached to the frame (Fig. 41–51). The arc holds constant both the twist drill to penetrate the skull and the biopsy needle. Sequential biopsies of structural lesions are checked with frozen section to enhance the likelihood of a positive diagnosis on permanent sections.[5, 15, 20] Structural lesions that are amenable to biopsy include tumors and infections; vascular malformations and strokes are clearly to be avoided. The use of a larger skull entry and indirect endoscopic or direct microscopic visualization of the target may permit direct excision of the lesion, using specialized retractors in the form of an expanding cylinder.[25] The endoscopes available for the treatment of brain lesions are in the range of 1.5 to 2 mm. and can therefore be passed through small holes. However, the endoscope is quite limited in terms of treatment possibilities, both for dissection through brain tissue and coagulation of lesions; its use is thus usually restricted to the ventricular system.

Additional treatment options are possible using a stereotactic frame. Radiobrachytherapy involves multiple catheters that are placed in the brain for local radioactive treatment to inhibit local recurrences of a malignancy.[39, 40] An alternative

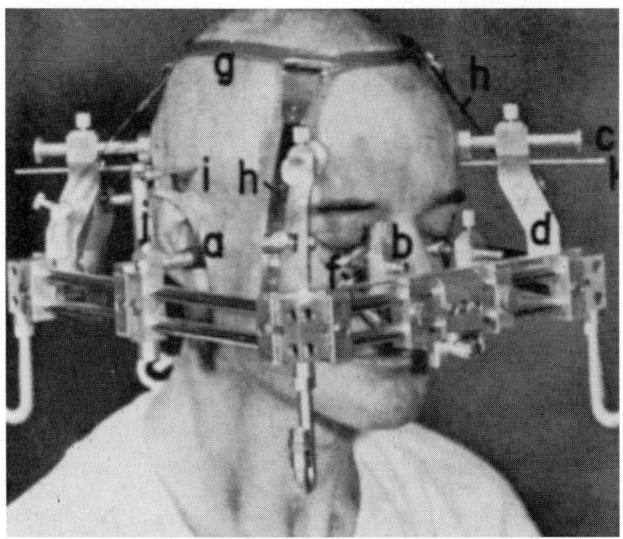

Figure 41–48. Human stereotactic instrument as devised by Spiegel and Wycis, showing base plate attached to patient's head. (Reprinted with permission from Spiegel, E. A., et al.: Stereotaxic apparatus for operations on the human brain. Science, *106*:349, 1947. Copyright © 1947, American Association for the Advancement of Science.)

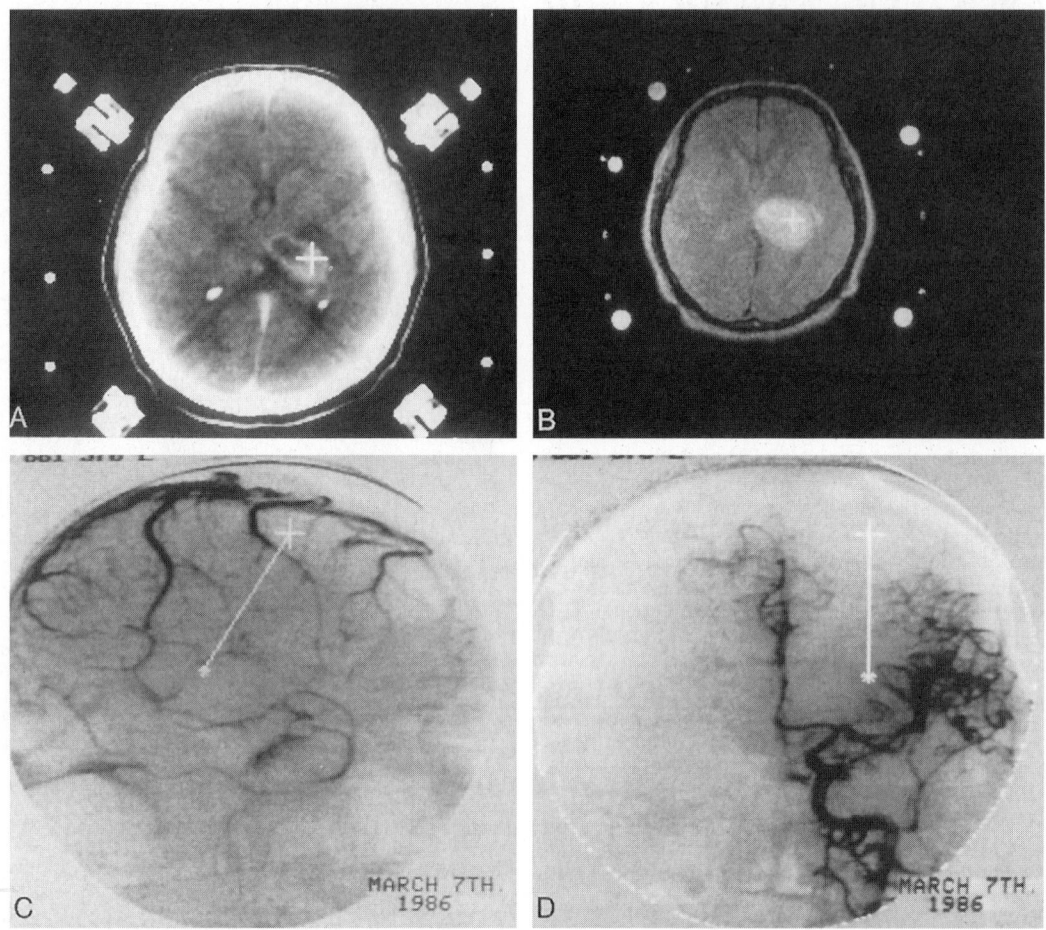

Figure 41–50. *A,* Example of a point digitized on a stereotactic computed tomography slice in the body of a lesion (note the points around the skull representing the stereotactic frame). *B,* A similar magnetic resonance image of the lesion. *C* and *D,* Companion cerebral angiography views with the lesion superimposed. (From Youmans, J. R.: Neurological Surgery, 3rd ed. Philadelphia, W. B. Saunders, 1990.)

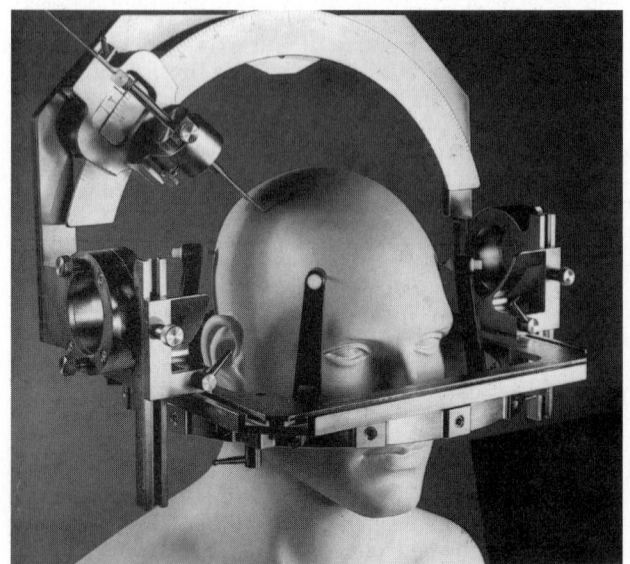

Figure 41–51. Cosman-Roberts-Wells frame fixed to a mannequin to demonstrate a stereotactic biopsy. This is a target-centered frame that allows considerable flexibility in trajectories and arc positions. (Courtesy of Radionics, Inc., Burlington, MA.)

developed over the last 30 years is the gamma knife, which involves the stereotactic delivery of multiple point sources of radiation using a stereotactic (Leksell) head frame. The radiation is delivered to a region in a single fraction (1200 to 2400 rads) for the treatment of lesions (primarily AVMs and tumors) smaller than 25 to 30 mm. in size. Approximately 75% of AVMs appear to be thrombosed within 2 years following this form of single-dose stereotactic radiation.[11, 28] This single, focused radiation dose may also be delivered using a Linac radiotherapy machine, but it gives arcs over multiple entry sites into the brain rather than multiple discrete delivery ports.

FRAMELESS STEREOTAXIS FOR LESION DIAGNOSIS AND GUIDANCE

The stereotactic frame translates coordinates obtained from an imaging study into operating room coordinates with respect to the frame. However, the application and use of a stereotactic frame can be inconvenient, and there are many regions of the body where a stereotactic frame cannot easily be applied. A relatively new concept is that of frameless stereotaxis, which relies on the rendering of scans (such as CT and MRI) into three-dimensional images, including scalp and skull contours. The rendering requires a powerful graphics workstation.[38] The rendered view of the patient can then be aligned with the actual patient using a three-dimensional digitizer, once the patient is fixed in a constant orientation in the operating room. The digitization can be performed using either fiduciary marks (such as skin staples or pins attached to the skull) or the surface of the scalp. The computer then aligns the actual patient (as digitized) with the computer representation obtained from the radiologic images.

The digitization can be performed by either a mechanical device (such as a robotic arm) or a line-of-sight device (such as a video camera or sound waves).[3, 12, 17, 18, 21, 31, 36] Line-of-sight devices require a clear, unobstructed path from the digitizing device to the patient. Mechanical arms can also reach into the patient, around corners, and through sterile drapes, but they are limited in terms of working distance (Fig. 41–52). The digitizing device can be used as a simultaneous pointer to actual brain structures and to the rendered image on the graphics workstation screen. For example, a tumor on the surface of the brain can be visualized prior to opening the skull, and an appropriately small craniotomy can be devised at the skin level to remove the tumor. Another example is the placement of a cerebrospinal fluid (CSF) shunt catheter; the angle and trajectory of the catheter can be imaged directly on the computer screen. Unfortunately, brain warping may occur following opening of the skull, CSF leakage, and partial tumor excision, affecting the accuracy of the device. A form of brain updating would be extremely helpful (such as three-dimensional ultrasound)[26] to circumvent the problems with landmarks moving during open procedures. Thus, frameless stereotaxis with accurate pointing and holding devices may eventually provide additional localization and guidance to neurosurgeons and may be extended to other regions of the body as well.[7, 37]

FUNCTIONAL STEREOTACTIC PROCEDURES

The concept of functional neurosurgery is to change the function of pathways in the brain by altering an intact aspect of the circuit, which may be upstream or downstream from the pathologically affected part of the circuit. The target is

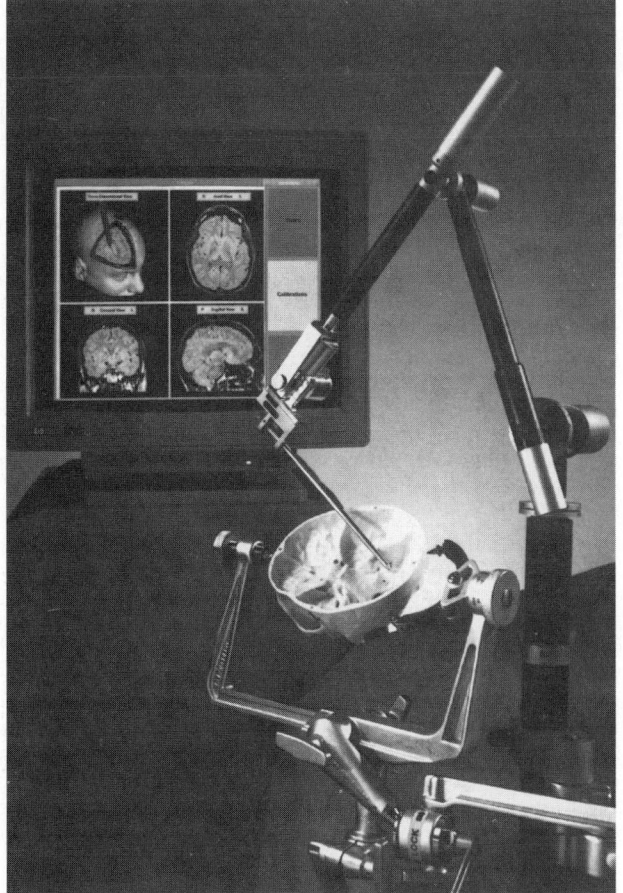

Figure 41–52. An example of a frameless digitizing and viewing system—the Operating Arm System from Radionics, Inc. The digitizing arm location can be viewed directly on the accompanying computer. (Courtesy of Radionics, Inc., Burlington, MA.)

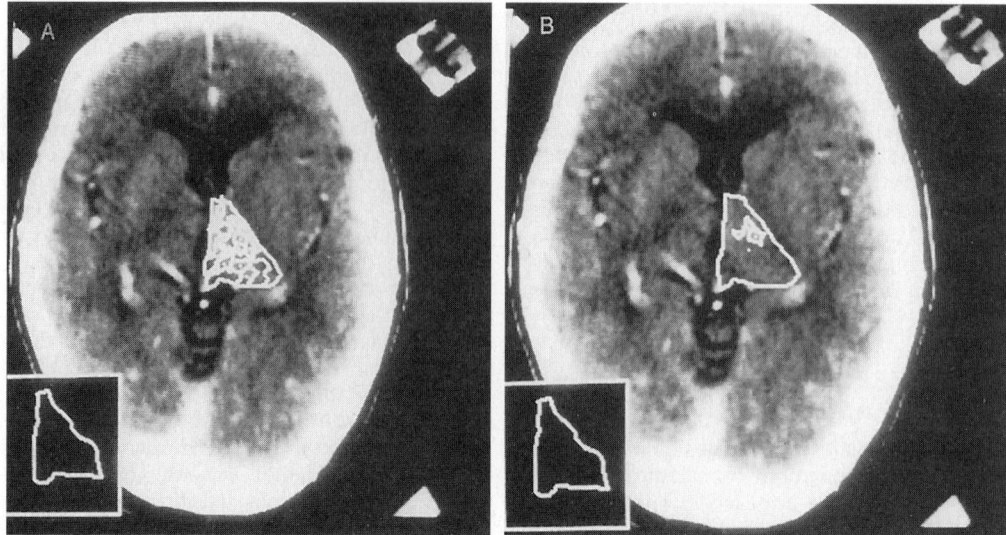

Figure 41–53. A computed tomography scan with a superimposed brain atlas, which has been stretched to fit the patient's own anatomy. Shown detailed are the thalamic substructures between the third ventricle and the internal capsule laterally; the defined area shows the ventralis intermedius externus nucleus. (From Youmans, J. R.: Neurological Surgery, 3rd ed. Philadelphia, W. B. Saunders, 1990.)

usually anatomically defined and requires precise localization by brain atlases, in coordination with the patient's own anatomy (see Fig. 41–49). For example, lesions in the globus pallidus may affect the overall function of the basal ganglia, thus improving the rigidity associated with Parkinson's syndrome.[19, 24] Other functional targets include the thalamus and midbrain to affect movement disorders and pain (Fig. 41–53). Other procedures include the placement of depth electrodes for localization of epileptic foci, stereotactic radiotherapy through the skull to lesion sites in the thalamus, and various anatomic methods of performing certain aspects of a frontal lobotomy.[9, 23, 24, 30, 32] Lesioning methods have included radiofrequency heat lesions, mechanical lesions (with a small wire loop), freeze lesions (cryolesions using liquid N_2), balloon lesions to percuss the surrounding brain on inflation, and chemical lesions. The radiofrequency lesion is the easiest to grade, using direct temperature control of the electrode tip. Temporary lesions can also be produced prior to causing permanent damage to the brain.

Other forms of stereotactic treatment include augmentative methods, such as cell or tissue transplants. These procedures can, in effect, replace lost cells, such as in Parkinson's disease or Huntington's disease.[1, 2, 16, 22, 27, 29] Gene transfer techniques involve the transfection of host cells (either glia or neurons) with novel genes, either to produce a missing enzyme or to modify cells to create sensitivity to treating agents.[6, 34] These methods require further investigation to delineate their specific role in treatment.

CONCLUSIONS AND FUTURE DIRECTIONS

Stereotactic procedures constitute a large part of clinical neurologic surgical therapy, particularly the diagnosis and treatment of structural lesions of the brain. Two basic types of stereotactic procedures are in common use—frame-based and frameless—and are used differentially, depending on the accuracy and type of stereotactic guidance required. Two common indications are the diagnosis and treatment of structural lesions and the treatment of abnormal functioning circuits. Stereotactic methods are expected to improve as computerized brain atlases, better imaging of individual patient's anatomy, and enhanced treatment options become available.

SELECTED REFERENCES

Heilbrun, M. P. (Ed.): Stereotactic Neurosurgery (Concepts in Neurosurgery, Vol. 2). Baltimore, Williams & Wilkins, 1988.
This monograph presents the background and practice of stereotactic surgery in a number of separate articles on various aspects of lesion diagnosis and treatment. This book is a classic resource for those interested in stereotactic neurosurgery from a number of different perspectives and is particularly useful as a starting volume.

Schaltenbrand, G., and Walker, A. E.: Stereotaxy of the Human Brain: Anatomical, Physiological and Clinical Applications, 2nd ed. New York, Georg Thieme Verlag/Thieme-Stratton, 1982.
This encyclopedic reference contains comprehensive chapters on both the basis of modern functional neurosurgery and the scientific rationale for stereotactic surgical procedures. The data presented arise from observations of functional neuroanatomy and neurophysiology during human procedures and thus augment data on the function and structure of the human brain. This is a critical background volume for those interested in the actual practice and development of stereotactic neurosurgery.

REFERENCES

1. Baetge, E. E.: Neural stem cells for CNS transplants. Ann. N. Y. Acad. Sci., 695:285, 1993.
2. Bakay, R. A., and Sladek, J. R., Jr.: Fetal tissue grafting into the central nervous system: Yesterday, today, and tomorrow. Neurosurgery, 33:645, 1993.
3. Barnett, G. H., Kormos, D. W., and Steiner, C. P.: Use of a frameless, armless stereotactic wand for brain tumor localization with two-dimensional and three-dimensional neuroimaging. Neurosurgery, 33:674, 1993.
4. Bellamkonda, R., and Aebischer, P.: Tissue engineering in the nervous system—review. Biotech. Bioeng., 43:543, 1994.
5. Bernstein, M., and Parent, A. G.: Complications of CT-guided stereotactic biopsy of intra-axial brain lesions. J. Neurosurg., 81:165, 1994.
6. Boviatsis, E. J., Chase, M., Wei, M. X., Tamiya, T., Hurford, R. K., Jr., Kowall, N. W., Tepper, R. I., Breakefield, O., and Chiocca, E. A.: Gene transfer into experimental brain tumors mediated by adenovirus, herpes simplex virus, and retrovirus vectors. Hum. Gene Ther., 5:183, 1994.
7. Brodwater, B. K., Roberts, D. W., and Nakajima, T.: Extracranial application of the frameless stereotactic operating microscope: Experience with lumbar spine. Neurosurgery, 32:209, 1993.
8. Bucholz, R. D., Ho, H. W., and Rubin, J. P.: Variables affecting the accuracy of stereotactic localization using computerized tomography. J. Neurosurg., 79:667, 1993.
9. Burchiel, K. J.: Image-based functional neurosurgery. Clin. Neurosurg., 39:314, 1992.
10. Clarke, R. H., and Horsley, V.: On a method of investigating the deep ganglia and tracts of the central nervous system. Br. Med. J., 2:1799, 1906.
11. Dion, J. E., and Mathis, J. M.: Cranial arteriovenous malformations: The role of embolization and stereotactic surgery. Neurosurg. Clin. North Am., 5:459, 1994.
12. Drake, J. M., Rutka, J. T., and Hoffman, H. J.: ISG viewing wand system. Neurosurgery, 34:1094, 1994.
13. Flickinger, J. C., Kondziolka, D., Lunsford, L. D., Coffey, R. J., Goodman,

M. L., Shaw, E. G., Hudgins, W. R., Weiner, R., Harsh, G. R., 4th, and Sneed, P. K.: A multi-institutional experience with stereotactic radiosurgery for solitary brain metastasis. Int. J. Radiat. Oncol. Biol. Phys., 28:797, 1994.

14. Flickinger, J. C., Loeffler, J. S., and Larson, D. A.: Stereotactic radiosurgery for intracranial malignancies. Oncology (Huntington), 8:81, 1994.

15. Franzini, A., Leocata, F., Giorgi, C., Allegranza, A., Servello, D., and Broggi, G.: Role of stereotactic biopsy in multifocal brain lesions: Considerations on 100 consecutive cases. J. Neurol. Neurosurg. Psychiatry, 57:957, 1994.

16. Freed, C. R., Breeze, R. E., and Rosenberg, N. L.: Survival of implanted fetal dopamine cells and neurologic improvement 12 to 46 months after transplantation for Parkinson's disease. N. Engl. J. Med. 327:1549, 1992.

17. Friets, E. M., Strohbehn, J. W., Hatch, J. F., and Roberts, D. W.: A frameless stereotaxic operating microscope for neurosurgery. IEEE Trans. Biomed. Eng., 36:608, 1989.

18. Giorgi, C., Luzzara, M., and Casolino, D. S.: A computer controlled stereotactic arm: Virtual reality in neurosurgical procedures. Acta Neurochir., S58:75, 1993.

19. Goetz, C. G., De Long, M. R., and Penn, R. D.: Neurosurgical horizons in Parkinson's disease. Neurology, 43:1, 1993.

20. Gomez, H., Barnett, G. H., and Estes, M. L.: Stereotactic and computer-assisted neurosurgery at the Cleveland Clinic: Review of 501 consecutive cases. Cleve. Clin. J. Med., 60:399, 1993.

21. Guthrie, B. L., and Adler, J. R., Jr: Computer-assisted preoperative planning, interactive surgery, and frameless stereotaxy. Clin. Neurosurg., 38:112, 1992.

22. Hansen, J. T., and Gash, D. M.: Functional aspects of mammalian neural transplantation. Crit. Rev. Neurobiol., 6:79, 1991.

23. Heilbrun, P. M. (Ed.): Stereotactic Neurosurgery (Concepts in Neurosurgery, Vol. 2). Baltimore, Williams & Wilkins, 1988.

24. Kandel, E. I.: Functional and Stereotactic Neurosurgery. New York, Plenum, 1989.

25. Kelly, P. J.: Stereotactic resection and its limitations in glial neoplasms. Stereotact. Funct. Neurosurg., 59:84, 1992.

26. Koivukangas, J., Louhisalmi, Y., and Alakuijala, J.: Ultrasound-controlled neuronavigator-guided brain surgery. J. Neurosurg., 79:36, 1993.

27. Lindvall, O., Widner, H., and Rehncrona, S.: Transplantation of fetal dopamine neurons in Parkinson's disease: One-year clinical and neurophysiological observations in two patients with putaminal implants. Ann. Neurol., 31:155, 1992.

28. Lunsford, L. D., Kondziolka, D., Bissonette, D. J., Maitz, A. H., and Flickinger, J. C.: Stereotactic radiosurgery of brain vascular malformations. Neurosurg. Clin. North Am., 3:79, 1992.

29. Menei, P., Benoit, J. P., Boisdron-Celle, M., Fournier, D., Mercier, P., and Guy, G.: Drug targeting into the central nervous system by stereotactic implantation of biodegradable microspheres. Neurosurgery, 34:1058, 1994.

30. Nashold, B. S., Jr., Wilson, W. P., and Slaughter, D. G.: Stereotactic midbrain lesions for central dysesthesia and phantom pain. J. Neurosurg., 30:116, 1969.

31. Roberts, D. W., Nakajima, T., and Brodwater, B.: Further development and clinical application of the stereotactic operating microscope. Stereotact. Funct. Neurosurg., 58:114, 1992.

32. Schaltenbrand, G., and Walker, A. E.: Stereotaxy of the Human Brain: Anatomical, Physiological and Clinical Applications. New York, Georg Thieme Verlag/Thieme-Stratton, 1982.

33. Spiegel, E. A., Wycis, H. T., Marks, M., and Lee, A. J.: Stereotaxic apparatus for operations on the human brain. Science, 106:349, 1947.

34. Suhr, S. T., and Gage, F. H.: Gene therapy for neurologic disease. Arch. Neurol., 50:1252, 1993.

35. Takizawa, T.: Isocentric stereotactic three-dimensional digitizer for neurosurgery. Stereotact. Funct. Neurosurg., 60:175, 1993.

36. Tan, K. K., Grzeszczuk, R., and Levin, D. N.: A frameless stereotactic approach to neurosurgical planning based on retrospective patient-image registration: Technical note. J. Neurosurg., 79:296, 1993.

37. Thomas, D. G., and Kitchen, N. D.: Minimally invasive surgery: Neurosurgery. Br. Med. J., 308:126, 1994.

38. Vannier, M. W.: Digital imaging, image processing, and three-dimensional computer graphics for radiology. Curr. Opin. Radiol., 4:1, 1992.

39. Wen, P. Y., Alexander, E., 3rd., Black, P. M., Fine, H. A., Riese, N., Levin, J. M., Coleman, C. N., and Loeffler, J. S.: Long term results of stereotactic brachytherapy used in the initial treatment of patients with glioblastomas. Cancer, 73:3029, 1994.

40. Woo, S., Butler, E. B., Grant, W., 3rd, Berner, B., and Gildenberg, P.: Fractionated high-dose rate brachytherapy for intracranial gliomas. Int. J. Radiat. Oncol. Biol. Phys., 28:247, 1994.

41. Zamorano, L. J., Nolte, L., and Kadi, A. M.: Interactive intraoperative localization using an infrared-based system. Neurol. Res., 15:290, 1993.

42. Zinreich, S. J., Tebo, S. A., and Long, D. M.: Frameless stereotaxic integration of CT imaging data: Accuracy and initial applications. Radiology, 188:735, 1993.

CHAPTER 42

FRACTURES AND DISLOCATIONS

I ——

GENERAL PRINCIPLES

Michael E. Berend, M.D., John M. Harrelson, M.D., and John A. Feagin, M.D.

There is no class of injuries which a practitioner approaches with more doubt and misgiving than fractures, or one which demands a greater amount of ready knowledge, self reliance, and consummate skill.

SAMUEL D. GROSS, 1882[1]

The treatment of fractures and dislocations requires a knowledge of anatomy, physiology, and biomechanics of the musculoskeletal system. Although a fracture represents a disruption in the continuity of a bone, it also represents a major soft tissue injury. The surgeon must be aware of the soft tissue structures adjacent to a fracture site and be particularly alert for neurologic and vascular components of the injury. Because many fractures occur in a setting of violent trauma, complete evaluation of each patient is necessary, and the surgeon must be prepared to consider major injuries in other organ systems.

MECHANISM AND CLASSIFICATION OF FRACTURES

Sufficient force applied to a bone causes fracture. A single fracture line is referred to as a *simple* fracture. When multiple fracture lines and bone fragments exist, the fracture is said to be *comminuted*. Penetrating injury producing a fracture, or fracture fragments protruding through the skin, constitute an *open* fracture. When no such wound is present, the fracture is classified as *closed* (Fig. 42–1). These distinctions are important because open fractures are likely to be contaminated with pyogenic bacteria. The treatment and prognosis of open fractures are significantly different from those of closed fractures.

The force necessary to produce a fracture may be transmitted to the skeleton in a variety of ways. The direction and rate of application of the force govern, to some extent, the pattern of the fracture and the associated soft tissue injury. A bending moment applied to bone usually produces a simple transverse or oblique fracture line. When a direct blow or crushing force is applied to bone, a comminuted, open fracture often results, accompanied by severe soft tissue injury. Torque force applied to bone produces a spiral or oblique fracture. Compression forces applied along the longitudinal axis of the bone cause an impacted fracture at the junction of the metaphysis and the diaphysis, where the cortex becomes thin; the diaphyseal portion of the bone usually impacts into the metaphyseal fragment. Traction force applied to a bone may also produce fracture. Vigorous or violent muscular contracture may produce avulsion of portions of bone where major tendons attach and may have associated ligamentous injury.

More subtle trauma such as the activities of daily living may also produce fractures in elderly patients with osteoporosis, in patients with metabolic bone-wasting disease, or in patients with tumor of the bone. Such injuries are referred to as *pathologic* fractures. The most common causes of pathologic fracture are osteoporosis and metastatic carcinoma. Healthy bone may fracture with the repetitive application of minor trauma, as in *fatigue* or *stress* fractures. These fractures are seen in the metatarsals after a long hike or in the tibia, fibula, femur, or other skeletal locations in individuals involved in regular athletic activities.

FRACTURES IN CHILDREN

Fractures in children deserve special consideration. The periosteum is extremely strong in children; children's bones are much more resilient and less brittle than those of adults. Bending moments applied to the bone of a child may cause a *greenstick* fracture, in which there is distraction of the cortex on the convex side and compression of bone on the concave side. There is angulation at the fracture site but no other displacement. Fractures may occur through the physeal plates and cause future growth disturbance. The parents should be cautioned accordingly. When fracture occurs entirely within the physeal plate and there is no displacement of the epiphysis relative to the metaphysis, anatomic reduction produces good results, with no disturbance in growth. When the fracture line extends partway through the physeal plate and then through either the adjacent metaphysis or the epiphysis, accurate anatomic reduction is mandatory to avoid future growth disturbance. When compression forces have produced a fracture across the physeal plate, growth disturbance is a likely result.

INITIAL EVALUATION

The initial evaluation of a fracture patient requires a careful history and physical examination. The history and mecha-

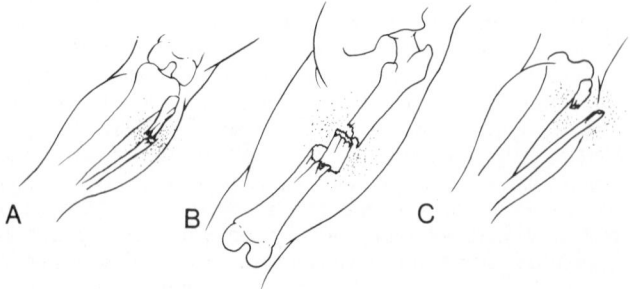

Figure 42–1. *A,* Closed simple fracture of the fibula. *B,* Closed, comminuted fracture of the femur. *C,* Open fracture of the fibula.

nism of injury should be obtained, as well as the patient's ambulatory status, occupation, and handedness. An examination of the overall body for associated injuries, including the axial skeleton, extremities, and skin, should be performed and documented. The examination should also determine the motor function, sensory deficit, vascular status, and firmness of the associated fascial compartments. The proximity of major nerves to bone makes them vulnerable to injury from adjacent fracture fragments. Direct arterial injury may also occur following penetration by a sharp bone fragment. More often, vascular insufficiency of a fractured limb is caused by swelling from the fracture hematoma, with compression of adjacent vessels.

Radiographs in at least two perpendicular planes should be performed of the fractured bone. The films should visualize the entire fractured bone with the associated proximal and distal articulations. Radiographs following reduction and splinting should also be obtained.

FRACTURE REDUCTION

The goal of reduction is restoration of length of the extremity, correction of angulation and rotation, and apposition of the bone ends. Fractures that are inherently stable and in acceptable alignment require no reduction. Once reduction of a displaced fracture has been accomplished, fracture healing requires that the bone ends be immobilized.

Fractures are displaced as a result of trauma, the pull of muscles crossing the fracture site, or both. The first step in reducing a displaced fracture is to relieve the patient of pain by either local anesthetic injection or systemic analgesics. It is then necessary to overcome the spasm of those muscles bridging the fracture site, allowing restoration of length of the fractured member and correction of angulation and rotation. The reduction of a fracture may be accomplished in several ways.

Manipulative reduction can be accomplished in fractures of the distal portion of the extremities, in which it is possible to manually overcome the pull of those muscles bridging the fracture site. When the fracture is more proximal (humerus, femur), muscle spasm is too great for manipulative reduction. In this situation, it may be necessary to apply continuous *skeletal traction* by inserting a transverse pin distal to the fracture site and placing the patient in bed with continuous pull on the pin. As muscle spasm is gradually overcome, length is restored and alignment is achieved. It is sometimes acceptable to use *skin traction* by applying strips of felt to the extremity with adhesive and attaching them to the appropriate amount of weight.

Some fractures are not appropriately treated by manipulative reduction or traction. Such fractures may require surgical therapy and *open reduction.* When open reduction is required, it is usually accompanied by some form of internal fixation of the fracture.

Some fractures require excision of a portion of bone rather than reduction and immobilization. Comminuted fractures of the patella are appropriately treated by excision of the patellar fragments and repair of the extensor mechanism rather than by attempts at reduction and fixation. Fractures of the radial head with severe comminution of the articular surface are best treated by excision and prosthetic replacement. More commonly, prosthetic replacement may be required in fractures of the femoral neck in the elderly, because healing is prolonged as a result of disrupted circulation to the femoral head. Rehabilitation of elderly patients may be significantly shortened by hip hemiarthroplasty in such situations.

IMMOBILIZATION

Impacted fractures with inherent stability may require only a sling or soft dressing for comfort. Most fractures of the extremities can be appropriately treated by plaster or fiberglass immobilization. Although the many advantages of plaster are well recognized, it should be borne in mind that improperly applied plaster can create more injury than it treats. The surgeon should be familiar with proper plaster technique. The cast should be appropriately padded and smooth on its inner surface and should not be constricting.

Because a bone participates in joint motion at both ends, it is necessary to immobilize the joint above and below the fracture site. Thus, forearm fractures require long-arm plaster immobilization of both the wrist and the elbow. Plaster maintains the reduction that has been achieved, provides rigid immobility, and relieves pain through stabilizing the fracture. A well-reduced, rigidly immobilized fracture should not require a significant amount of analgesic. Swelling occurs at a fracture site, and because a plaster cast is rigid, increasing pressure within the cast is heralded by increasing pain in the extremity and progressive numbness and diminished circulation to the digits. All patients should be cautioned to watch for these signs; they should be examined promptly for assessment of the cast and their neurovascular status upon developing clinical symptoms.

ACUTE COMPLICATIONS

Following fracture, bleeding from the bone ends and the adjacent soft tissues produces a rapidly enlarging hematoma that envelops the fracture site. Because most fractures occur following significant force, the bone ends are frequently displaced. This displacement is increased by the pull of those muscles that cross the fracture site and may further increase the extent of soft tissue injury. Bleeding within a closed compartment may cause significantly increased *compartment pressure*, which may cause muscular ischemia progressing to eventual muscle necrosis. This situation exists particularly when there is bleeding into the anterior compartment of the leg or into the volar compartment of the forearm. The surgeon must be aware of these syndromes and be prepared to do a decompressive fasciotomy.

Adjacent organ injury may occur with certain fractures. Fractures of the rib cage can rupture the lung, produce lacerations of the liver, or penetrate the spleen. Fractures of the pelvis, particularly those in which there is disruption of the symphysis pubis, can rupture the bladder. Spinal fractures often have associated spinal cord injury. With fractures of the femur or pelvis or with multiple fractures, the hemorrhage may produce hypovolemic shock.

Systemic manifestations such as *fat embolization* may occur following a fracture. Hypoxia, tachypnea, tachycardia, and confusion are some of the earliest signs of fat embolism. Large doses of corticosteroids, with supplemental oxygen administration, are usually of value.

OPEN FRACTURES

An open fracture should be treated as an emergency. Surgical débridement of the wound is required. Intravenous antibiotics should be administered, along with tetanus toxoid when appropriate. Because open fractures usually follow more violent trauma, other major injuries should be fully evaluated; when the patient is stable, débridement is performed in the operating room as a formal surgical procedure. All devitalized tissue is removed, with special attention given to devitalized muscle. Macerated skin edges are débrided, and the wound is thoroughly irrigated with saline-containing antibiotics, using pulse lavage if available. Fascia that is constricting should be released, and bone ends, which may contain embedded debris, are débrided by sharp dissection, with care taken to preserve nerves, vessels, and tendons.

Repair of nerves and tendons in an open fracture is rarely indicated. Vascular repair should be performed if circulation to the extremity is in jeopardy.

When débridement is completed, a decision must be made about stabilization of the fracture. Although some unstable fractures require internal fixation devices, the immediate use of such devices is generally not desirable in a contaminated wound. One alternative is skeletal traction with a transverse pin some distance from the wound. Cast immobilization with a window overlying the wound, delayed internal fixation, or external fixation may also be appropriate initial stabilization methods.

A decision must also be made regarding wound closure. When minimal penetration of the skin has occurred, no foreign body contamination is present, and no significant muscle injury is encountered, wound closure may be acceptable. If there is any question regarding viability of muscle tissue or degree of contamination, the wound should be dressed and left open. The morbidity from delayed closure at 3 to 5 days or free-tissue transfer coverage is minimal compared with the consequences of infection. When extensive skin loss has occurred, split-thickness skin grafts or pedicle or free-flap grafting may be required.

FRACTURE HEALING

Following fracture, a hematoma rapidly develops about the bone ends. As pressure from the hematoma increases, interstitial edema develops in the adjacent soft tissues, and there is some degree of venous congestion. Leukocytes invade the hematoma, producing a sterile inflammatory response. Primitive mesenchymal cells within the periosteum and the medullary canal differentiate into primitive osteoblasts and proliferate. These changes are appreciated microscopically at 48 to 72 hours. At this time there is also development of early granulation tissue about the periphery of the hematoma. This granulation tissue also contains pluripotent cells, which differentiate into osteoblasts. This proliferation of osteogenic cells and their subsequent primitive bone formation constitute the *fracture callus*. If the fracture fragments are in apposition and rigidly immobilized, bone growth progresses until the two fracture fragments are united by a network of primitive new bone. As the bone matures, constant remodeling occurs, and trabeculae become oriented in the long axis of the bone.

If there is motion at the fracture site, the mesenchymal cells may differentiate into chondroblasts. If the motion is not excessive or if the fracture site is subsequently rigidly immobilized, this cartilaginous tissue calcifies and is gradually replaced by new bone by the process of endochondral ossification. When distraction of the fracture fragments is present or when muscle is interposed between the fracture fragments, dense fibrous tissue develops between the fracture ends, causing *nonunion*. When motion is persistent at the fracture site, the differentiation of cartilage progresses. A cleft develops between the layers of cartilage covering the ends of the bones, and the cells at the periphery differentiate into synovial cells, producing a pseudarthrosis. If distraction at the fracture persists, a dense fibrous scar forms between the bone ends, causing a *fibrous nonunion*.

Compression of a fracture enhances fracture healing. This principle is used in treatment. Fractures of the tibial shaft may be treated in a walking cast, allowing the patient to bear weight across the fracture site. The compression principle also may be used through proper application of internal fixation devices.

Fracture healing is also affected by the available blood supply. In general, cancellous bone at the metaphyseal ends of long bones has a richer blood supply than the diaphysis;

fractures in these areas heal more rapidly than shaft fractures. Long bones with more overlying muscle have a greater blood supply. The shaft of the femur, enveloped by muscle, has a better blood supply than the distal tibia, which is subcutaneous in one third of its circumference. Therefore, fractures of the tibial shaft are traditionally slower to heal than fractures of the femoral shaft.

Perhaps the most notable advance in musculoskeletal research and fracture healing physiology in the last 20 years is the concept of *distraction osteosynthesis*, pioneered by Professor Ilizarov from Kurgan, Russia. The Ilizarov method consists of a thin wire external fixator with circumferential rings and is now used throughout the world in the treatment of acute fractures, nonunions, malunions, osteomyelitis, limb-length discrepancy, and angular deformities of both upper and lower extremities.

LATE COMPLICATIONS

The soft tissue injury that accompanies a fracture causes scarring of the adjacent muscles, ligaments, and tendons and produces limitation of motion of the joints adjacent to the fracture. Fractures occurring close to a joint produce more limitation of motion than fractures of the midshaft. Restoration of joint motion involves rehabilitation of the soft tissues. Physical therapy in the form of active and passive exercises may be necessary. Tendons may become adherent to the underlying bone, and subsequent surgical release may be necessary. Because of the muscle atrophy that follows inactivity, stasis edema is usually present after fracture and gradually diminishes as muscle tone and strength return.

Nonunion of a fracture, either as a pseudarthrosis or fibrous nonunion, may develop for the reasons previously mentioned. When an established nonunion is present, operative intervention is usually indicated. Surgical removal of the fibrocartilage or scar tissue that has formed at the fracture site and apposition of fresh bone ends are necessary. The addition of bone graft to the nonunion site at the time of surgical therapy is desirable. Bone is obtained from the patient (autogenous) or from a donor (homologous). The bone graft serves as a mineral lattice for new bone formation and becomes incorporated in the fracture callus. It is gradually replaced by osteoclastic resorption and subsequent new bone deposition, a process known as *creeping substitution*.

When a fracture heals with unacceptable angulation or rotation, a *malunion* has occurred. The disability from malunion may be immediately apparent (rotatory malalignment of a forearm fracture, which limits pronation and supination), or it may not develop for some time (valgus malalignment of a distal tibial fracture, producing subsequent degenerative arthritis of the ankle). Malunion may require surgical intervention. Osteotomy is performed at either the old fracture site or at a more appropriate level, and the angular or rotatory deformity is corrected. In almost all fractures, some degree of shortening occurs.

In the upper extremities, shortening is seldom noticeable and is rarely a functional disability. In the lower extremities, if shortening exceeds 0.5 inch, a shoe lift may be required. In some fractures, there is a loss of circulation to the involved bone, with subsequent *avascular necrosis*. This situation occurs in fractures of the femoral neck in elderly patients, in fracture-dislocations of the talus in any age group, and in fracture through the waist of the carpal navicular bone. Avascular necrosis usually causes collapse of the articular surface of the involved bone and the subsequent development of degenerative arthritis.

Fractures that involve articular surfaces may eventually cause *traumatic arthritis*. Even with accurate anatomic reduction, the process of healing may produce irregularities on the cartilaginous surface, with ingrowth of fibrous tissue, fracture callus, or both. Once the congruity of the joint has been lost, gradual deterioration usually occurs. The rate at which degenerative arthritis develops depends on the degree of incongruity, the age and activity level of the patient, and the amount of injury to the articular surface at the time of the fracture.

SUMMARY

The purpose of this section has been to emphasize the principles of fracture care and associated soft tissue management. Specific fracture treatments are discussed in the sections that follow. The primary principles emphasized in this section include:

1. An appreciation of fracture mechanics and a description of fractures—simple, comminuted, open, and closed.
2. The evaluation and treatment of adjacent soft tissue injury, including vessel, nerve, ligament, muscle, fascia, and skin.
3. The avoidance of local wound complications by appropriate débridement, fasciotomy, immobilization, and antibiotics.
4. That open fractures are an emergency and require formal surgical débridement.
5. That fracture healing proceeds most expeditiously with stabilization, compression, and function.
6. That late complications, such as nonunion, malunion, or traumatic arthritis, may require reconstructive surgery such as bone graft, osteotomy, or joint mobilization.
7. That new methods of fracture immobilization, such as

the Ilizarov method, require special skills but are based on the premise that anatomic alignment, constant compression, and early function enhance healing. These methods extend the armamentarium of the fracture surgeon, particularly in the restitution of multiply injured patients.

SELECTED REFERENCES

Browner, B. D., et al.: Skeletal Trauma, Vols. 1 and 2. Philadelphia, W. B. Saunders, 1992.
A current textbook of the care of fractures and dislocations—well illustrated.

Chapman, M. W.: Operative Orthopaedics, 2nd ed. Vols. 1–4. Philadelphia, J. B. Lippincott, 1993.
A current and complete textbook of operative orthopedics—well referenced.

Charnley, J.: The Closed Treatment of Common Fractures, 3rd ed. Baltimore, Williams & Wilkins, 1963.
An unparalleled, historic classic, which provides an anatomic basis for nonoperative treatment of a selected group of fractures.

Muller, M. E., et al.: Manual of Internal Fixation: Techniques Recommended by the AO Group, 3rd ed. New York, Springer-Verlag, 1991.
The techniques recommended by the AO Group (the Association for the Study of the Problems of Internal Fixation).

Rockwood, C. A., et al.: Fractures in Adults & Fractures in Children, 3rd ed. Vols. 1–3. Philadelphia, J. B. Lippincott, 1991.
Volumes 1 and 2 represent the definitive fracture text for orthopedic surgery, providing an in-depth discussion of the diagnosis, treatment, pitfalls, and outcome of adult fractures, with excellent references. Each section includes the author's preferred method of treatment for that fracture. Volume 3 is an excellent reference for children's fractures.

REFERENCE

1. Gross, S. D.: A System of Surgery: Pathologic, Diagnostic, and Operative, 6th ed. Vol. 2. Philadelphia, Henry C. Lea's Son and Company, 1882, p. 894.

II ——

FRACTURES OF THE SPINE

William T. Hardaker, Jr., M.D., and William J. Richardson, M.D.

The diagnosis of fracture of the spine ("broken neck" or "broken back") is terrifying to the patient and the family. When the fracture is associated with concomitant spinal cord injury, it represents one of the most physically disabling and economically devastating conditions seen in modern medicine. Few events are more tragic than a vigorous young adult being rendered para- or quadriplegic, with the likelihood of remaining forever dependent upon others for assistance in the activities of daily living.

Statistics regarding the precise incidence of spine injuries and their economic consequences are incomplete. Approximately 10,000 such injuries occur each year in the United States. Fifty per cent of these injuries occur in individuals 23 years of age or younger. The economic consequences of such injuries are enormous. The cost to society for the lifetime care of spinal cord–injured patients may approach 800 million dollars annually.[3, 22, 24, 26, 27] These figures are estimates, and they do not include the cost of care for people with spine injuries without attendant cord injury.

Fortunately, although fractures of the vertebral column are common, less than 10% of spine fractures are associated with neurologic deficit. Because the majority of spine fractures involve primarily the skeletal structures, proper treatment often leads to an excellent prognosis. Patients who present complaining of pain or tenderness in the neck or back following injury must be suspected of having a fracture of the spine until proved otherwise. The attending physician should determine the neurologic involvement in the initial assessment, because early neurologic status greatly influences both the course of treatment and the prognosis.

Trauma may subject the vertebral column to one or a combination of violent forces, including flexion, extension, axial compression, rotation, and shearing. If these forces produce motion greater than the physiologic range of the spine, a fracture or dislocation occurs. The spinal cord usually terminates between L1 and L2. In the cervical and thoracic spinal canal, it occupies approximately 50% of the available space. In the lumbar area, the cauda equina is the only neural element within the canal, so more free space surrounds the neural tube. The anatomic relationship of the vertebral supporting structures, the neural elements, and the types of forces producing the injury determines the amount of displacement, stability, and neurologic involvement in a given spine injury.

THE CERVICAL SPINE

When a patient complains of pain in the neck after an injury, a fracture or dislocation of the cervical spine should be suspected. A careful history concerning the mechanism of injury is important. If tenderness is present about the cervical region, a complete neurologic examination is followed by cervical spine roentgenograms. The roentgenographic examination should define the fractures and determine whether soft tissue swelling is present about the spinal column. Examination of plain films can often provide information on the stability of the spine. Plain films should include supine anteroposterior and lateral, open-mouth odontoid, and trauma oblique views. The patient's head should not be moved for conventional oblique examinations. If these studies are negative, supervised lateral flexion-extension views of the cervical spine may be obtained to exclude an unstable cervical spine secondary only to soft tissue injury.[17] However, because of severe muscle spasm, this evaluation may be initially unreliable. If the patient has pain, tenderness, and decreased motion of the neck, or neurologic symptoms or signs, the cervical spine must be immobilized pending a more complete roentgenographic evaluation.

Fracture of the Atlas (Jefferson's Fracture)

Jefferson described the mechanism of fracture of the first cervical vertebra.[13] The injury occurs from an axial load on the top of the head. The force is exerted laterally on the ring of C1, and the arches fracture at the thinnest and weakest points (Fig. 42–2). Usually the spinal cord is not damaged, because the canal of the atlas is normally large; with fracture, the fragments spread outward to further increase the dimensions of the neural canal. The fracture can usually be diagnosed on lateral cervical spine roentgenograms, but special plain films, such as the submental vertex view, may better delineate the injury. Computed tomography (CT) represents the best available roentgenographic study to evaluate such an injury. If the results of the neurologic examination are normal, this injury can be managed in an occipital-mandibu-

lar brace (Fig. 42–3A). In situations of considerable instability, the halo-vest system is preferred (Fig. 42–3B).

Fracture of the Odontoid

An understanding of the anatomic relationship of the first two cervical vertebrae is essential for a discussion of these injuries. Rotation of the atlas about the odontoid process of the axis represents about half of the rotatory movement of the head. The dens is held adjacent to the anterior arch of C1 by the transverse and alar ligaments. It is important to remember that the dens, spinal cord, and empty space each occupy approximately one third of the spinal canal at the arch of the atlas (the *rule of thirds*). On a lateral roentgenogram centered at C2, the predental space is 3 mm. or less in an adult. A predental space of greater than 5 mm. indicates rupture of the transverse ligaments, and a predental space of 12 mm. means that all ligaments about the dens have been ruptured.[10] Transverse or alar ligament ruptures are uncommon unless there are predisposing factors such as rheumatoid arthritis, posterior pharyngitis, or ankylosing spondylitis. If such a rupture occurs and the odontoid is intact, cervical myelopathy may be the presenting symptom. Fractures of the odontoid (dens), however, occur relatively frequently and represent about 10% of cervical spine fractures. Odontoid fractures as well as transverse ligament injuries occur following falls or blows to the head, in automobile accidents, and in sports such as gymnastics.

The diagnosis may be delayed because of difficulty in visualizing the dens on routine films. If the injured patient complains of neck or occipital pain or headaches, or has torticollis, the odontoid area should be examined thoroughly. Lateral views centered on the C2 vertebra and open-mouth views of the odontoid usually allow adequate visualization of the dens. However, tomograms in the anteroposterior and lateral views may be necessary to demonstrate the fracture.

Anderson and D'Alonzo[1] described three primary types of fractures based on the anatomic level of the injury.[1] Type I fractures are oblique and occur at the extreme upper level of the odontoid process (dens). These injuries do not lead to gross instability of the first cervical vertebra in relation to the second. A hard cervical orthosis provides satisfactory stability of this fracture. Type II fractures occur through the junction of the odontoid process and the C2 vertebral body. Type II injuries are the most common odontoid fracture and should be considered unstable injuries. Type II odontoid fractures may have nonunion rates as high as 50% if not treated effectively. Union occurs in most cases with prompt diagnosis, satisfactory reduction, and rigid external fixation. Operative arthrodesis using autogenous iliac bone grafts and wiring of C1 to C2 through a posterior approach is indicated if union is not achieved.[5, 18] Type III fractures extend through the cancellous bone of the C2 vertebral body. These injuries are rarely unstable and unite following 3 months of immobilization in a halo vest.[15]

Fracture of the Pedicles of the Axis (Hangman's Fracture)

A fracture through the pedicles of C2 usually occurs from a severe extension injury, such as an automobile accident or a fall.[25] This injury has been labeled the *hangman's fracture* because autopsy studies demonstrated that a long drop with a rope around the neck and a knot in the submental position produces a similar lesion. Frequently, the subjacent disc bond is broken, allowing varying degrees of anterior subluxation of C2 on C3 to occur. Cord compression is rare because the neural canal is enlarged with forward displacement of the body of C2. The posterior elements may rotate posteriorly,

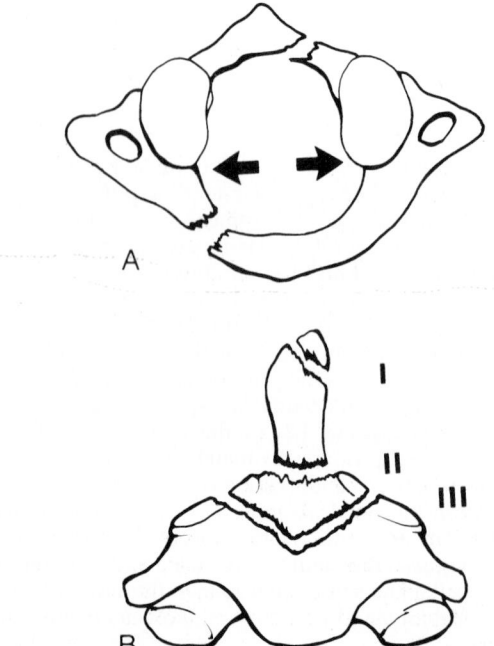

Figure 42–2. *A*, Jefferson fracture. Fractures of the arch of C1 are secondary to axial loads. The result of this force leads to expansion of the ring of C1 as indicated by the arrows, leading to a fracture of the narrow areas of the arch. *B*, Fractures of the odontoid may be Type I, oblique fracture of the tip of the odontoid process (dens); Type II, which occurs at the waist of the odontoid process; or Type III, which extends through the cancellous bone of the C2 vertebral body.

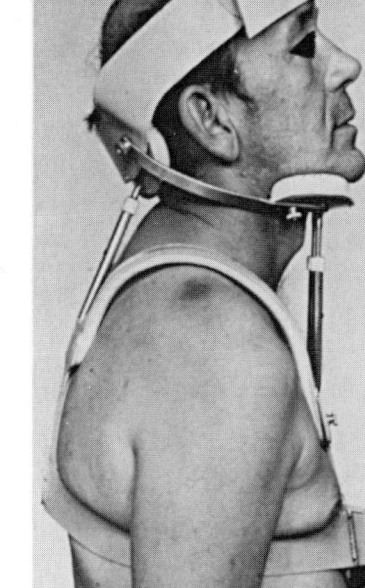
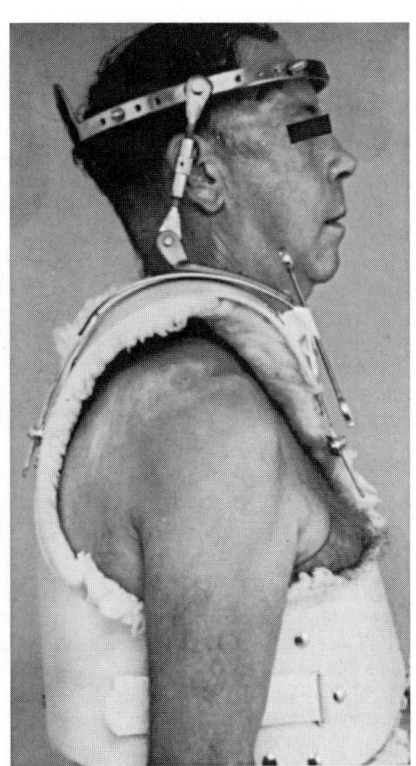

Figure 42–3. *A,* A four-poster brace. The uprights, the chin piece, and the occiput pad limit flexion and extension of the cervical spine, and the addition of the head band restricts rotation at C1–C2. The earlobe must be opposite the shoulder tip. *B,* Halo vest. The halo has four screws inserted into the outer table of the skull and provides very rigid external immobilization of the cervical spine. The halo may be used for cervical traction in the recumbent position or attached to a cast or body jacket lined with sheepskin. The patient may be ambulatory in the halo cast or vest.

A

B

but they generally remain in near anatomic alignment. Non-union is uncommon in this fracture. If the injury is stable with little or no displacement, an occipital-mandibular brace is usually satisfactory treatment. In unstable circumstances, more rigid stabilization using a halo vest may be required. Union usually occurs within 3 months, with spontaneous anterior interbody fusion. Operative intervention to achieve stability is rarely required.[16]

Fracture and Dislocation of C3–C7 Vertebrae

Fractures and dislocations of the lower cervical spine are common. The majority are caused by vehicular accidents, diving into shallow water, falls, and sports injuries. After the initial neurologic assessment, a patient with a suspected cervical spine injury should have complete roentgenograms. These should include studies from the occiput down to the C7–T1 junction. Adequate roentgenographic studies in some obese or muscular patients may require traction on the patient's upper extremities, the swimmer's view, or tomography.

Fractures of the lower cervical spine may be stable or unstable and may involve injury to the spinal cord and/or nerve roots. These fractures may follow the forces of flexion, extension, lateral bending, rotation, axial loads, or various combinations of these forces. The mechanism of injury is deduced from the analysis of the roentgenographic studies, enabling the physician to assess the stability of the cervical spine. Such information is paramount for selecting an appropriate method of treatment.

Compression Fracture of the Cervical Vertebral Bodies

Compression fractures of the cervical vertebral bodies can follow flexion, axial loading, or coupling of these two forces. The injuries can range from very mild to severe in terms of neurologic involvement. If there is minimal comminution of the vertebral body and no dislocation of the facets, the fracture is usually stable. Rarely are such injuries associated with neurologic deficits. These injuries can be adequately stabilized with minimal bracing such as a soft or hard cervical collar.

In contrast, comminuted *bursting* or *teardrop* fractures usually represent catastrophic injuries with a high association with significant spinal cord injury. These injuries are frequently caused by axial loading of the cervical spine, with varying degrees of concomitant flexion. The fragments of the vertebral body are displaced posteriorly into the spinal canal, with resulting injury to the spinal cord. This fracture is grossly unstable and requires skull traction with the halo or similar device for reduction and then application of the halo-vest system for satisfactory stabilization. Immobilization may be necessary for 3 to 4 months. In patients with incomplete neurologic injury and evidence of compression of the neural elements, operative anterior decompression with interbody bone grafting may be indicated. Such decompressions should not be attempted until adequate external stabilization is provided by the halo-vest system or until posterior stabilization has been performed.

Dislocation of the Cervical Spine

Dislocations of the cervical spine occur most commonly at the interspaces between C3 and C7. The C5–C6 level is most frequently involved. The injury is caused by a flexion-distraction force. These forces combine to dislocate the facet joints, with concomitant failure of the disc bond and varying degrees of failure of the longitudinal cervical ligaments. One or both facets may dislocate and interlock. Associated fractures of the facets or other posterior elements may occur at the time of dislocation. These injuries may be associated with a variable degree of neurologic loss, ranging from none to complete quadriplegia.

Because of supraimposition of the facet joints on lateral roentgenograms, dislocation of a single facet may be difficult

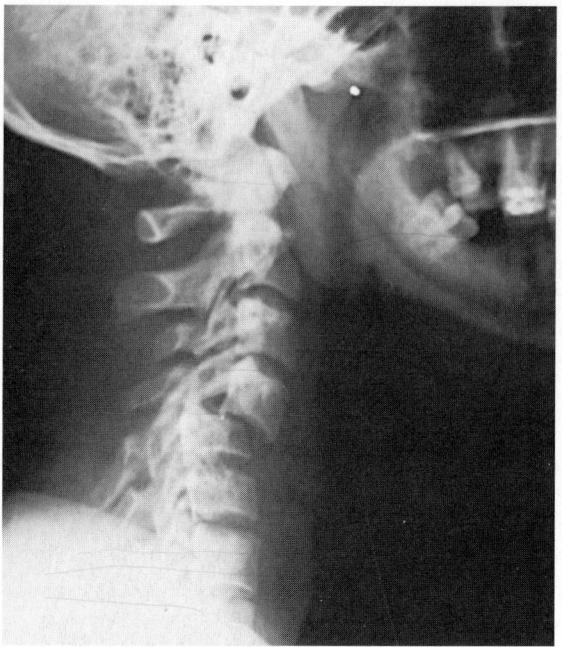

Figure 42–4. Bilateral facet dislocation of the cervical spine. This is a flexion-distraction injury and is often associated with complete quadriplegia at the level of the injury. Reduction is achieved by skull traction with tongs or halo. Surgical therapy may be necessary to achieve reduction and stabilization.

to directly visualize. A 25% anterior listhesis of a vertebral body on the body below in a neutral roentgenogram indicates probable fracture or dislocation of one of the posterior facet joints. An anteroposterior projection demonstrates displacement of the spinous processes from the midline as well as asymmetry of the uncovertebral joints, serving to corroborate the diagnosis of unilateral facet dislocation. Trauma oblique roentgenograms further delineate the subluxation or dislocation. Bilateral dislocation of the facets presents with forward subluxation of at least 50% on the lateral roentgenogram (Fig. 42–4). In the anteroposterior view, there is widening of the intervertebral disc space at the joint of Luschka.

Fractures and dislocations of the cervical spine are managed by prompt realignment. Many such dislocations can be reduced by serial traction under direct roentgenographic control and with concomitant serial neurologic examinations. Many dislocations reduce after brief periods of traction.[23] Prior to traction, magnetic resonance imaging (MRI) should be performed to ascertain whether concomitant disc rupture has occurred.[2] Initially, 15 pounds of traction is applied, and the weight is gradually increased while monitoring the cervical spine with serial lateral roentgenograms or with direct C-arm radiographic visualization. The weight is increased by 5-pound increments. If reduction is not achieved with 35 to 40 pounds of weight and with adequate muscle relaxation, bony or soft tissue interposition should be suspected. Increasing the weight usually does not cause a physiologic reduction and may produce cord or nerve root injury. Manipulation under general anesthesia is not recommended. If reduction cannot be achieved with the patient awake, operative reduction under direct vision followed by wire fixation and fusion using autogenous bone graft should be performed.

Following closed reduction, the patient should be maintained in the halo vest. In dislocations with marked instability, early posterior wiring and autogenous bone grafting are recommended. When disc herniation is demonstrated on MRI, anterior discectomy, fusion, and plating are indicated. In more stable situations, the patient may be maintained in the halo vest until spontaneous fusion occurs.

Fracture of the Posterior Elements

Lateral bending, tension, or compressive forces may cause mild fractures of a facet or pedicle. Avulsion fractures of the spinous processes are caused by sudden severe muscle contraction (clay shoveler's fracture) or by direct blows. These fractures are stable and are not associated with neurologic loss. They may be effectively managed by a soft collar until the patient is comfortable.

THE THORACOLUMBAR SPINE

It is important to recognize the relationship of the neural elements to the thoracolumbar skeletal structures when evaluating and treating injuries in this location. The spinal cord usually terminates at the lower margin of the L1 vertebra (Fig. 42–5). Caudal to L1, the spinal cord contains only spinal roots, the cauda equina. Whereas the spinal cord occupies nearly half of the spinal canal in the thoracic area, the neural canal has considerable free space below L1. Fractures or dislocations in the lumbar area require considerably more displacement to injure the neural elements than do fractures in the thoracic spine. Moreover, the cauda equina consists of nerve roots that have a greater capacity for recovery following an injury than does the spinal cord. A bursting fracture in the cervical or thoracic region may cause devastating neurologic loss, whereas a similar fracture in the lumbar area may produce no permanent neurologic deficit. Because of the anatomic structure of the terminal cord and roots, spinal injuries cephalad to T10 involve only the cord, those from T10 to L1 involve both the cord and roots, and those caudal to L1 involve only the roots. Individual spinal roots may be injured as they exit the intervertebral foramina by skeletal disruption. Because the sympathetic ganglia are located ante-

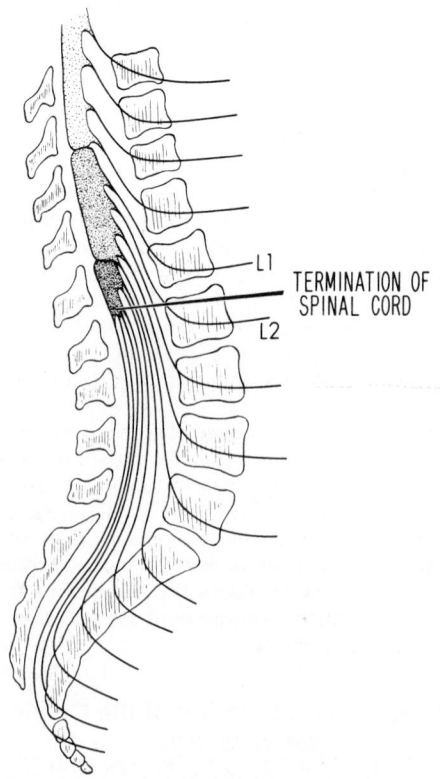

Figure 42–5. The spinal cord terminates at the L1 vertebra. The cauda equina, composed of spinal roots, is caudal to L1. These relationships are important in the diagnosis and treatment of fractures and fracture-dislocations of the thoracic spine, the lumbar spine, and the thoracolumbar junction.

rior and lateral to the vertebral bodies, fractures of the vertebral bodies or transverse processes frequently cause temporary paralytic ileus.

Diagnosis

The history of the mechanism of injury is helpful in the evaluation of a patient with a suspected thoracolumbar injury. Usually there is a clear history of sudden violence followed immediately by severe backache and muscle spasm. In an osteoporotic patient, a minimal incident such as bending, lifting an object, or a missed step may cause a compression fracture of the thoracic spine. However, most thoracolumbar fractures follow violent forces such as falls from heights, automobile collisions, or heavy objects falling onto the back.

Careful documentation of the onset of partial or complete loss of lower extremity motor or sensory function is essential for both management and determination of prognosis. If a spine injury is suspected, the patient should initially be examined in the position in which he is first seen. A brief neurologic examination to determine the motor and sensory status of the extremities should be performed first. The patient's clothing should be removed to allow a detailed inspection of the skin overlying the spine. If the patient is in the supine position, the examiner's hand may be gently positioned to palpate each spinous process for tenderness. The patient may then be gently rolled to the lateral position for inspection of possible swelling, abrasions, ecchymoses, or distortions, such as spasm, a *step-off*, or gibbus.

A complete neurologic evaluation is essential in all individuals with suspected spine injuries. This should be performed prior to any roentgenographic studies. The intercostal and abdominal muscles should be examined, and motor, sensory, and reflex testing of the extremities should be performed. The anal sphincter tone and bulbocavernosus reflexes must be included in the evaluation. During sensory testing, particular attention should be given to the perianal region, because many spinal cord levels are represented in this small cutaneous area.

Complete loss of motor and sensory function, including perianal sensation, during the first 24 hours after injury indicates complete cord injury. The bulbocavernosus reflex usually recovers within the first 24 hours. Recovery of this reflex together with complete anesthesia and paralysis is compelling evidence that the patient will not recover functional motor power of the lower extremity muscle groups innervated below the level of the fracture.

Anteroposterior and lateral roentgenographic views generally demonstrate fractures of the vertebral body (Fig. 42–6). CT and water-soluble contrast agents greatly improve the ability to thoroughly evaluate fractures and dislocations in the thoracolumbar area. A CT scan provides an extremely accurate assessment of the degree of spinal canal compromise, as well as valuable data for suspected fractures of the posterior elements. Myelography is not necessary in most cases of significant fracture-dislocation in which the results of the neurologic examination are consistent with the level of fracture. Metrizamide myelography or MRI is indicated, however, when there is no apparent fracture or dislocation and neurologic loss is present, or when the skeletal findings do not correlate with the neurologic findings.

Classification and Management

A spine fracture and dislocation is considered stable if the fragments are not likely to move and possibly cause neural damage when the spine is physiologically loaded. Conversely, if movement and neural damage are likely, the

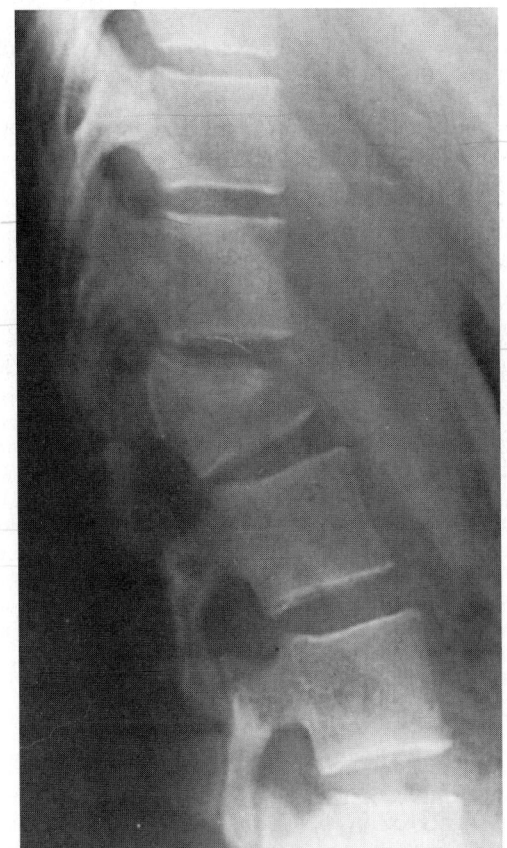

Figure 42–6. Burst fracture of T12, with anterior deformation, comminution, and retropulsion of bone fragments into the spinal canal.

injured spine is labeled unstable. The instability may be acute or chronic, depending on whether the displacement is immediately threatening or is a progressing deformity likely to occur during the extended healing process.

Denis developed a classification system for thoracolumbar spine injuries based on a *three-column* concept. In this system, the spine is divided into three longitudinal regions or columns: (1) the anterior column consisting of the anterior longitudinal ligament and the anterior half of the vertebral body, including the anulus fibrosus; (2) the middle column consisting of the posterior half of the vertebral body, disc elements, and the posterior longitudinal ligament; and (3) the posterior column consisting of the supraspinous and intraspinous ligaments, spinous processes, laminal arch, pedicles, facet joints, and capsule.

Although references to such columns are anatomically imprecise, the terms are clinically useful in assessing the stability of an injured spine. In general, instability results when significant disruption is present in two of the three columns. Although the classification of stable and unstable spine fractures and dislocations is not absolute, this scheme is practical from a management standpoint if the physician is cognizant that each injury must be individualized. A major goal of treatment is to maintain or achieve a painless functional back, which to a great degree means maintenance or restoration of spinal stability.

Flexion Injuries

Pure flexion injuries are the most common of all thoracolumbar skeletal fractures. Compression anteriorly, with or without distraction of the posterior ligaments, causes an anterior wedge compression fracture of the vertebral body (Fig. 42–7A). Most pure flexion injuries involve only the anterior column and, therefore, are acutely stable. Neurologic loss is uncommon. When there is greater than 50% anterior wedging or multiple contiguous anterior wedge compression fractures are present, progressive angulation may occur with time. This progressive flexion angulation during the healing phase would be considered an example of chronic instability.

These fractures can be painful, especially at the level of the injury. Paralytic ileus secondary to hemorrhage of the sympathetic ganglion is common. The patient should be admitted to the hospital and placed at bed rest on a firm mattress, with analgesics and muscle relaxants. Because there is an increased incidence of thromboembolic disease in patients with thoracolumbar fractures, anticoagulation therapy is indicated. The patient should be encouraged to move about the bed and may become ambulatory in an appropriate orthosis as soon as he is comfortable (3 to 5 days). If the compression is mild, a three-point brace is satisfactory. When wedging is greater than 50% of the anterior body height, a modified polypropylene jacket may be necessary to prevent progressive angulation. In severe cases with major anterior column comminution and significant posterior element disruption, posterior operative stabilization using Harrington or Cotrel-Dubousset instrumentation and autogenous iliac bone graft may be indicated.[7]

Lateral Compression Injuries

Lateral compression forces may produce a lateral wedge fracture of the vertebral body (Fig. 42–7B). These fractures are relatively uncommon and usually stable. Neurologic deficit is unusual. The initial symptoms are treated in a manner simi-

lar to anterior wedge compression fractures, and orthotic management for comfort is all that is usually required.

Axial Compression Injuries

Burst fractures result from axial compression of the spine, frequently associated with varying degrees of flexion. These injuries, which most commonly occur at the thoracolumbar junction (see Fig. 42–6), are characterized by circumferential expansion of the entire involved vertebra, with failure of the anterior, middle, and, in some cases, posterior spinal columns. Middle column failure in burst fractures causes retropulsion of the posterosuperior portion of the vertebral body into the spinal canal. With marked retropulsion, compression of the dural tube occurs, often with associated neurologic deficit (Fig. 42–7C).

Radiographically, burst fractures can be recognized on the anteroposterior roentgenogram with widening of the interpedicular distance. Severe burst fractures are three-column injuries with fracture of the posterior elements as well. Dural tears are commonly associated with posterior element fractures. Mild burst fractures with minimal anterior body deformation, minimal retropulsion of fragments into the spinal canal, no posterior element involvement, and minimal kyphotic angulation can be treated satisfactorily with a molded polypropylene body jacket. Healing of the fracture usually occurs within 3 to 5 months.[8]

If there is incomplete neurologic involvement, usually from fragments impinging on the cauda equina, surgical management may be indicated. The goal of surgical therapy is to provide an environment for spinal cord recovery. Fundamental to this goal are (1) decompression of the spinal canal to remove impinging bone and disc fragments, (2) restoration of the normal alignment of the spine at the thoracolumbar junction, (3) immediate stabilization of the spine with restoration of the normal vertebral body height, and (4) long-term stabilization of the fracture site through arthrodesis using autogenous iliac bone graft. At the time of operation, dural tears should be identified and repaired.[20] Not infrequently, portions of the cauda equina herniate through the dural defect; if this is not repaired, scarring and a chronic pain syndrome can ensue. When available, intraoperative somatosensory evoked potential monitoring is recommended.

Surgical procedures designed to decompress and stabilize thoracolumbar burst fractures can be performed through anterior or posterior approaches.[4, 9, 19] The major site of compression is anterior, and for this reason, laminectomy does little to relieve traction or compression of the spinal cord over an anterior lesion. Indeed, laminectomy may add to the instability of the spinal column. Anterior exposure of the vertebral body is gained by a transthoracic, transabdominal, or combined approach. Simple anterior fusion may be inadequate to prevent graft collapse and progressive angulation of the spine with weight bearing. Anterior or posterior instrumentation and fusion in a staged or combined procedure are usually required. Anterior decompression can also be achieved through a posterior lateral approach. Access is gained to the cephalad portion of the vertebral body through the pedicles. Transpedicular decompression is a technically demanding procedure, and meticulous attention to detail is necessary to achieve an adequate decompression without undue risk of further neurologic injury.

Posterior spinal instrumentation remains fundamental to the operative management of fractures and fracture-dislocations of the thoracolumbar spine.[11] Cotrel-Dubousset or similar implants can effectively restore height and realign the spinal column. In many cases, realignment of the spinal column and restoration of height may not effectively decompress the spinal canal. The procedure should therefore be

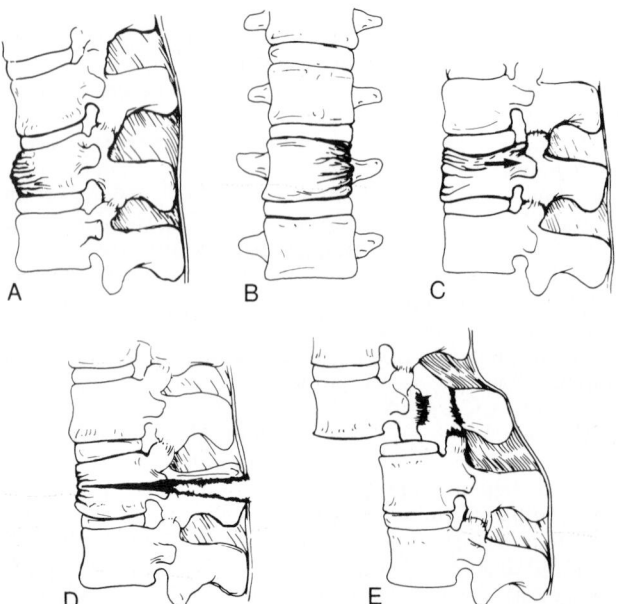

Figure 42–7. *A,* In an anterior wedge compression fracture, the posterior elements and ligaments generally remain intact. This fracture is usually stable, and neurologic loss is uncommon. *B,* A lateral wedge compression fracture of the vertebral body is a stable fracture and usually is not associated with neurologic loss. *C,* Burst fracture located at the thoracolumbar junction. These fractures are frequently unstable, and neurologic loss can follow posterior displacement or fractures into the spinal canal. *D,* A *chance* fracture is a horizontal splitting of the neural arch and vertebral body. This injury is secondary to a flexion-distraction force. Although three columns are involved, this injury is often classically stable. *E,* A fracture-dislocation of the thoracolumbar spine. Severe anterior translation is present. The injury is grossly unstable and requires open reduction and internal stabilization in most cases.

combined with definitive removal of bony and disc fragments under direct observation. Somatosensory evoked potentials are closely monitored during and following the realignment procedure.[21]

Fracture-Dislocations

Fracture-dislocations always involve translation of one spinal motion segment or a portion of one spinal segment in relationship to the remaining spine. Translation may be anterior, posterior, or lateral, but by definition, it always causes failure of all three columns. A variety of failure modes, including shear, compression, tension, and rotation, can occur within the individual columns, and various combinations of injury produce characteristic radiographic patterns. In most cases, the radiographic appearance of these injuries represents the recoiled position of some greater displacement at the time of the injury. The shear mode of failure of fracture-dislocations often causes severe injury to the neural elements and complete paraplegia.[14]

If the fracture occurs in the thoracic region, it may be relatively stabilized by the rib cage and heal without operative management. However, in the lumbar region (Fig. 42–7E), these injuries are usually grossly unstable, and great care must be exercised in managing these patients. Operative reduction and internal fixation are the most reliable means of creating a stable environment for potential maximal neurologic return.

Flexion-Distraction Injuries

Flexion-distraction forces classically occur in seatbelt injuries in which the individual is subjected to sudden deceleration and the torso is flexed forward over the restraining belt. Tension failure occurs in the posterior and middle columns.[12, 14] Failure of the anterior column also occurs. The mode of anterior column failure depends on the location of the fulcrum of rotation. If the fulcrum exists within the anterior column, compression failure of that column results. If the failure is anterior to the spine, tension failure of all three spinal columns occurs and the spine is literally pulled apart. These injuries may be associated with marked displacement and are usually very unstable. Open reduction with realignment and internal fixation is usually required in order to regain stability.

The *chance* fracture is a unique flexion-distraction injury in which there is a horizontal splitting of the neural arch, the pedicles, and the vertebral body (Fig. 42–7D).[6]

SELECTED REFERENCES

Bohlman, H. H.: Current concepts review: Treatment of fractures and dislocations of the thoracic and lumbar spine. J. Bone Joint Surg. [Am.], 76:165, 1985.
An excellent overview of management principles in treating thoracolumbar spine injuries.

Denis, F.: The three-column spine and its significance in the classification of acute thoracolumbar spinal injuries. Spine, 8:817, 1983.
A presentation of the three-column concept in the classification of thoracolumbar spine fractures.

Ferguson, R. L., and Allen, B. L.: A mechanistic classification of thoracolumbar spine fractures. Clin. Orthop. Rel. Res., 189:77, 1984.
A concise classification of thoracolumbar spine fractures based on modes of failure and their consequences for stability.

Hardaker, W. T., Jr., Cook, W. A., Jr., Friedman, A. H., and Fitch, R. D.: Bilateral transpedicular decompression and Harrington rod stabilization in the management of severe thoracolumbar burst fractures. Spine, 17:2, 1992.
The authors describe surgical techniques of decompression, stabilization, and fusion of thoracolumbar burst fractures through a posterior approach.

Holdsworth, F. W.: Fractures, dislocations, and fracture-dislocations of the spine. J. Bone Joint Surg. [Am.], 52:1534, 1970.
A classic description of spinal fractures and their management.

Kostuik, J. P.: Anterior spinal cord decompression for lesions of the thoracic and lumbar spine, techniques, and new methods of internal fusion, results. Spine, 8:512, 1983.
Surgical techniques of anterior decompression and instrumentation for spinal cord injuries.

Levine, A. M., and Edwards, C. C.: Treatment of injuries in the C1–C2 complex. Orthop. Clin. North Am., 17:31, 1986.
An excellent discussion of upper cervical spine injuries, emphasizing their unique presentation and treatment protocols.

McAfee, P. C., Yuan, H. A., and Lasda, N. A.: The unstable burst fracture. Spine, 7:365, 1982.
An excellent description of the posterolateral approach for decompression of fractures of the thoracolumbar junction.

REFERENCES

1. Anderson, L. D., and D'Alonzo, R. T.: Fractures of the odontoid process of the axis. J. Bone Joint Surg. [Am.], 56:663, 1974.
2. Arena, N. J., Eismont, F. J., and Green, B. A.: Intravertebral disc extrusion associated with cervical facet subluxation and dislocation. J. Bone Joint Surg. [Am.], 12:43, 1988.
3. Bracken, M. B., Shephard, M. J., Collins, W. F., et al.: A randomized controlled trial of methylprednisolone or naloxone in the treatment of spinal cord injury. N. Engl. J. Med., 322:1405, 1990.
4. Bradford, D. S., and McBride, G. G.: Surgical management of thoracolumbar spine fractures with incomplete neurologic deficits. Clin. Orthop., 218:201, 1987.
5. Brooks, A. L., and Jenkins, E. W.: Atlanto-axial arthrodesis by the wedge compression method. J. Bone Joint Surg. [Am.], 60:279, 1978.
6. Chance, C. Q.: Note on a type of flexion fracture of the spine. Br. J. Radiol., 21:452, 1948.
7. Cotrel, Y., Dubousset, J., and Guillaumat, M.: New universal instrumentation in spinal surgery. Clin. Orthop., 227:10, 1988.
8. Davies, W. E., Morris, J. H., and Hill, V.: Analysis of conservative management of thoracolumbar fractures and fracture-dislocations with neural damage. J. Bone Joint Surg. [Am.], 62:1324, 1980.
9. Dunn, H. K.: Anterior spine stabilization and decompression for thoracolumbar injuries. Orthop. Clin. North Am., 17:113, 1986.
10. Fielding, J. W., Cochran, G. V. B., Lawsing, J. F., and Hohl, N.: Tears of the transverse ligament of the axis. J. Bone Joint Surg. [Am.], 56:683, 1974.
11. Gaines, R. W., Breedlove, R. F., and Munson, G.: Stabilization of thoracic and thoracolumbar fracture-dislocations with Harrington rods and sublaminal wires. Clin. Orthop. Rel. Res., 189:195, 1984.
12. Gertzbein, S. D., et al.: Flexion-distraction injuries of the lumbar spine—mechanics of injury and classification. Clin. Orthop., 227:227, 1988.
13. Jefferson, G.: Fracture of the atlas vertebra: Report of four cases and review of those previously recorded. Br. J. Surg., 7:407, 1920.
14. Kaufer, H., and Hayes, J. T.: Lumbar fracture-dislocations. J. Bone Joint Surg. [Am.], 48:712, 1966.
15. Land, B., et al.: Odontoid fractures treated with halo-vest. Spine, 12:173, 1987.
16. Levine, A. M., et al.: The management of traumatic spondylolisthesis of the axis. J. Bone Joint Surg. [Am.], 67:217, 1985.
17. Levine, A., and Edwards, C.: Complications in the treatment of acute spinal injury. Orthop. Clin. North Am., 17:183, 1986.
18. McCraw, R. W., and Ruschi, R. N.: Atlanto-axial arthrodesis. J. Bone Joint Surg. [Br.], 55:482, 1973.
19. McEvoy, R. D., and Bradford, D. S.: The management of burst fractures of the thoracic and lumbar spine. Spine, 10:631, 1985.
20. Miller, C. A., Dewey, R. C., and Hunt, W. E.: Impaction fracture of the lumbar vertebra with dural tear. J. Neurosurg., 53:765, 1980.
21. Nash, C. L., et al.: Spinal cord monitoring. J. Bone Joint Surg. [Am.], 71:627, 1989.
22. Riggins, R. S., and Krause, J. F.: The risk of neurologic damage with fractures of the vertebra. J. Trauma, 17:126, 1977.
23. Sabiston, C., et al.: Closed reduction of dislocations of the lower cervical spine. J. Trauma, 28:832, 1988.
24. Schneider, R. C., and Kahn, E. A.: Chronic neurological sequelae of acute trauma to the spine and spinal cord. J. Bone Joint Surg. [Am.], 38:985, 1956.
25. Schneider, R. C., Livingstone, K. E., Cowe, A. J. E., and Hamilton, G.: Hangman's fracture. J. Neurosurg., 22:141, 1965.
26. Smart, C. N., and Sanders, C. R.: Cost of motor vehicle–related spinal cord injuries. Washington, D.C., Insurance Institute for Highway Safety, 1965.
27. Stover, S. L., and Fine, P. R.: The epidemiology and economics of spinal cord injury. Paraplegia, 25:225, 1987.

III _____

FRACTURES AND DISLOCATIONS OF THE SHOULDER, ARM, AND FOREARM

Robert D. Fitch, M.D., and Kevin P. Speer, M.D.

MECHANICS OF SHOULDER STABILITY

The glenohumeral joint is a unique articulation in that it has a high degree of mobility that is balanced with stability throughout the motion range. Both static and dynamic factors are involved in maintaining glenohumeral stability. The limited joint volume and negative intra-articular pressure are one such mechanism. It is apparent during cadaveric dissections that muscle activity is not required to hold the shoulder together, as long as the capsule is not vented. However, the magnitude of this negative intra-articular pressure is small. An estimate of this stability force is only 20 to 30 pounds, assuming that the maximal suction pressure can be only one atmosphere pressure (14.7 psi $\times$ glenoid surface area). In clinical studies, we have not seen the resumption of negative intra-articular pressure following an arthrotomy of the joint. The intra-articular joint pressure following an open capsular surgical procedure is about 0 mm. pressure (Speer and Urmey, 1992, unpublished data).

Another contributing mechanism to stability is concavity, or compression.[17] This is caused by dynamic compression of the humeral head into the glenolabral socket by the action of the muscle forces around the shoulder, predominantly the rotator cuff. This is likely the most important stability mechanism in the midrange of motion, since the capsule and ligaments are lax in this range. Matsen has estimated the efficiency of this mechanism to be approximately 40%: if the compression force into a glenoid is 100 units, then this mechanism can resist a translating force of 40 units.[28] If the labrum is excised, this mechanism's efficiency is reduced by half. In the typical clinical situation of glenohumeral instability, operative techniques do not address this stability mechanism. The enhancement or restoration of this stability mechanism is through neuromuscular conditioning and training. Dedicated rehabilitative exercise is essential for the optimal functional recovery of the shoulder following capsulorrhaphy operation.

ANTERIOR GLENOHUMERAL INSTABILITY

The primary stabilizer limiting anterior glenohumeral translation in the 90-degree abducted shoulder is the inferior glenohumeral ligament complex (IGHLC).[6] Using arthroscopy and histologic evaluation, O'Brien and associates have delineated the IGHLC into an anterior band, a posterior band, and an interposed axillary pouch. The role of the IGHLC as an anterior restraint becomes less important at lower degrees of abduction. At lower degrees of abduction, the middle glenohumeral ligament was found to act as a more significant stabilizer.

The detachment of the anterior band of the IGHLC from the anterior glenoid labrum is the Bankart lesion.[3] With an acute traumatic anterior shoulder dislocation, a Bankart lesion is present in over 90% of cases. However, the Bankart lesion is not only one specific anatomic defect; it reflects a cluster of similar lesions, all of which serve to defunctionalize the inferior glenohumeral ligament at the glenoid margin. Another common radiographic finding from an acute traumatic shoulder dislocation is a groove in the superolateral aspect of the posterior humeral head. This has been called a Hill-Sachs lesion. This compression lesion reflects a direct impact from the anterior inferior glenoid margin during the dislocation event.

The *in vivo* determination of the pathoanatomy of acute traumatic anterior shoulder dislocation can be readily accomplished with magnetic resonance imaging (MRI). The authors completed a study in which 20 patients who sustained first-time acute anterior traumatic dislocations of their shoulders underwent MRI. No patient had any shoulder symptoms prior to their accidents. All the injuries were traumatic and were reduced by physicians who documented the anterior dislocation. MRI was performed within 8 days of all injuries. Consistent findings included a moderate to large effusion in all the shoulders, as well as posterolateral bone bruises. In many cases, this area of posterolateral bone bruise actually had an indentation and qualified as a Hill-Sachs deformity on plain x-ray. An anterior inferior labral injury and detachment were seen in all the shoulders (Fig. 42–8). Seventy per cent of the patients had objective increased signal in the anterior capsule. This was interpreted as demonstrating edema in the capsule from sprain injury. Pertinent negatives included an intact rotator cuff musculature in all patients. These were young patients with an average age of 21 years. There was no evidence of muscle strain injury in any patient, even in the subscapularis.

The evaluation of an acute traumatic anterior shoulder dislocation should always include a neurologic and vascular examination, because injury to the brachial plexus, particularly the axillary nerve or axillary artery, can occur.[27, 30, 35] Radiographs show an anterior, posterior, and scapulolateral view of the shoulder. An axillary lateral view is helpful, but many times this is not practical in a patient who has experi-

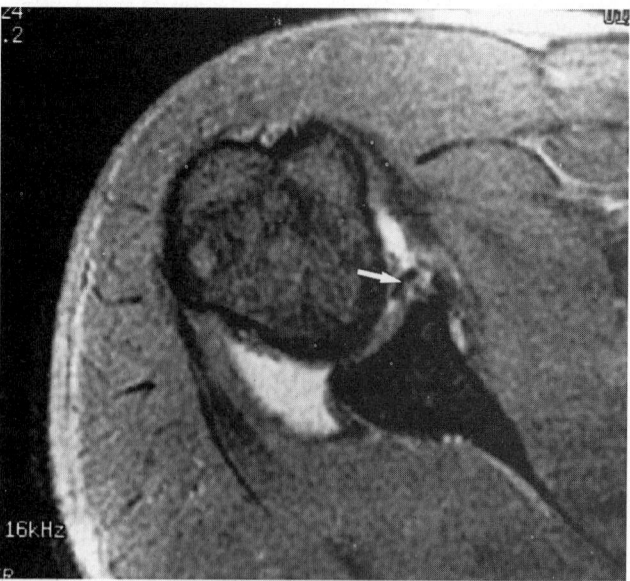

Figure 42–8. Axial magnetic resonance imaging (MRI) of the shoulder following a first-time traumatic anterior shoulder dislocation. Arrow points to the detached anterior inferior labrum, the Bankart lesion.

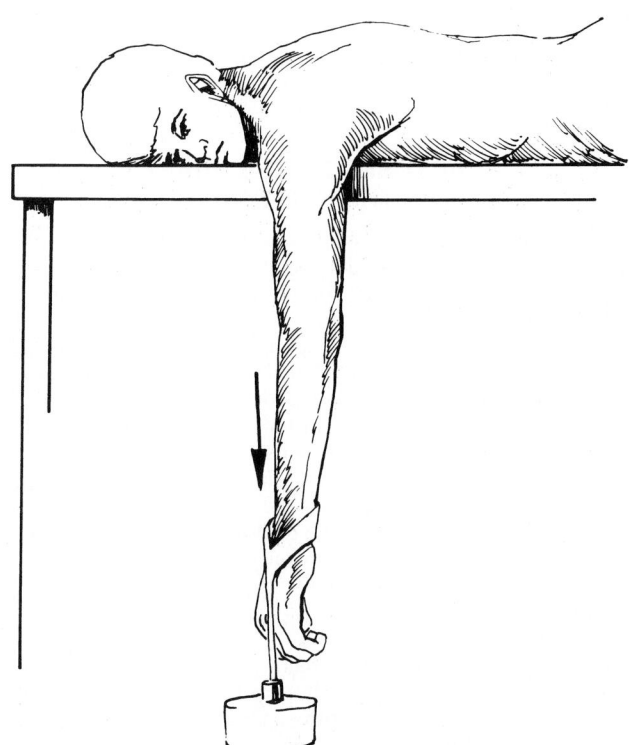

Figure 42–9. The modified Stimson technique of closed reduction. The amount of weight that is hung from the hand depends on the size of the patient. (From Rockwood, C. A., and Green, D. P.: Fractures, Vol. 1. Philadelphia, J. B. Lippincott, 1984, p. 750.)

enced an acute anterior shoulder dislocation. In younger patients, there may actually be a traumatic separation of the proximal growth plate, with placement of the metaphysis anteriorly.[16] This occurs because the weak link in the shoulder in this age group is the physeal plate.

The reduction of dislocation should be prompt. Numerous reduction techniques have been suggested, but all require gentle manipulation. Sedation is often required. Occasionally, a general anesthetic is needed. A safe method when trying to reduce the shoulder without assistance is the Stimson technique (Fig. 42–9).[36] Following reduction of the shoulder, the neurovascular status must be assessed again. The arm is then immobilized in a sling. Historically, sling wear for 3 to 6 weeks was recommended for these patients. No study has ever shown an advantage of immobilization of the shoulder based on subsequent recurrence rates for anterior shoulder instability; therefore, immediate mobilization of the shoulder is now recommended, along with attempts to regain full active motion of the shoulder as soon as possible following the dislocation. Recurrence is a common complication in young patients and probably occurs in over 90% of those under 20 years of age; it is less common as individuals get older. This is due to the varying activity levels of patients in different age groups.

With an acute anterior shoulder dislocation in a very young patient who is athletic and prone to dislocation, arthroscopic repair of the anterior labrum to the glenoid is considered. Although currently controversial, it takes advantage of the fact that the collateral injury in the anterior capsule can heal primarily, as long as the anterior labrum is reattached to the anterior glenoid. In recurrent anterior shoulder instability, an open surgical procedure is necessary. Historically, nonanatomic procedures have been employed. These have included the Putti-Platt procedure, which plicates the capsule and the subscapularis tendon; the Magnuson-

Stack procedure; and the Bristow procedure,[19] which transfers the coracoid process and the attached musculature to the anterior rim of the glenoid. The current state of the art is an anatomic reconstruction of the shoulder with stretching against the pathoanatomy of the current anterior shoulder instability. This pathoanatomy usually involves a detached anterior labrum and a classically deformed or patchless anterior inferior glenohumeral ligament and anterior capsule. A capsulorrhaphy is performed as well as a reattachment of the anterior labrum to the glenoid.

POSTERIOR GLENOHUMERAL INSTABILITY

The primary capsuloligamentous restraint to posterior translation in the 90-degree abducted shoulder is the posterior band of the inferior glenohumeral ligament.[33] However, studies have shown that even when the posterior capsule was completely incised, the glenohumeral joint did not dislocate posteriorly.[34] For dislocation to occur in the flexed, adducted, and internally rotated arm, in addition to the posterior capsule being incised, the anterior superior capsule had to be incised from the 12 o'clock to 3 o'clock position. Harryman and co-workers also demonstrated the importance of this anterior superior capsule, or rotator interval capsule, in posterior and inferior translation.[17] Incision of the rotator interval capsule increased posterior translation by nearly 50% and inferior translation by over 100%.

Posterior glenohumeral dislocations are much less common than anterior dislocations, representing approximately 2% of all glenohumeral joint dislocations.[31] The recurrence rate is also much lower than that for anterior shoulder dislocations. The greatest difficulty with posterior dislocation is actually diagnosing the injury. Up to 40% may be missed because of a fairly good axillary lateral radiograph at the time of the initial evaluation. An anterior posterior radiograph of the shoulder may not suggest any problem, even though the humerus is actually dislocated posteriorly behind the glenoid. Reducing a posterior dislocation involves traction and sedation with relaxation. The postreduction immobilization is quite different from that following an anterior dislocation, because with the arm in a sling, the shoulder is in a position of maximal instability. Instead, the shoulder needs to be placed in an abduction brace or external rotation brace that keeps the posterior capsule from being stretched. The shoulder needs to be kept in this position for 2 to 4 weeks.

INFERIOR TRANSLATION: STATIC STABILIZERS

The physical finding of a sulcus sign in the shoulder at 0-degree abduction reflects competence of the anterior superior capsular structures, predominantly the superior glenohumeral ligament.[38] The visible component of the sulcus sign in thin individuals likely also reflects negative intra-articular pressure in the joint.[6] In pressure-volume research on the shoulder, inferior translation of the adducted shoulder predictably generated the most negative intra-articular pressure, compared with every other position that the shoulder could attain (Speer and Urmey, 1992, unpublished data).

Warner and colleagues studied the static capsuloligamentous control of inferior translation of the shoulder in a selective cutting experiment.[38] They found that in the adducted shoulder, the superior glenohumeral ligament is the main capsular structure resisting inferior translation. The superior glenohumeral ligament in the shoulder has been found to be fairly constant. DePalma and associates noted its presence in 97% of anatomic specimens.[11] However, its size can be highly variable. The coracohumeral ligament has been found to have no significant suspensory role.[38] The coracohumeral ligament was a thin capsular fold in 10 of 11 cadaveric shoulders; in the one shoulder in which the coracohumeral ligament was more robust, it made a moderate contribution to inferior stability.

With abduction of the shoulder to 45 degrees and beyond, the anterior and posterior portions of the inferior glenohumeral ligament become the prime stabilizers to inferior translation. With rotation, the inferior glenohumeral ligament has an even greater role in resisting inferior translation. At 90-degree abduction, the posterior band of the inferior glenohumeral ligament was the prime restraint to inferior translation. The cutting sequence of Warner was reversed by Bowen and Warren, who sectioned the IGHLC alone to assess its contribution to inferior stability (Bowen and Warren, 1991, unpublished data). They found that at 0-degree abduction, the inferior glenohumeral ligament has only a minor role in inferior stability, but at greater degrees of abduction the sulcus sign basically reflects the status of the IGHLC.

Inferior glenohumeral instability as an isolated phenomenon is extraordinarily rare. An interior glenohumeral dislocation is called luxatio erecta. It usually occurs with significant glenohumeral capsular injury as well as tuberosity fracture. Generally, increased inferior translation or hyperlaxity is a component of either anterior or posterior instability of the shoulder, and the surgical procedure must restore the amount of the inferior translation to that of the opposite side. This is accomplished with a capsulorrhaphy, in which the excessive capsular volume or classic deformation of the capsule is imbricated, with reduction of the overall joint volume.

FRACTURES OF THE PROXIMAL HUMERUS

Many times, the identical trauma that causes an anterior shoulder dislocation in a young person causes a proximal humerus fracture in an older person. As with the proximal femur, loss of normal trabecular bone with aging makes this area more susceptible to injury. This fracture is observed in all age groups, however, and merges with epiphyseal separation injury of the proximal humerus, which occurs in individuals prior to skeletal maturity. In an elderly patient, fractures may occur following minor trauma, whereas fractures in younger individuals require considerable force, and fracture-dislocations may occur. In this group of fractures, the prognosis depends on the degree of displacement and the number of fracture fragments. In addition, the amount of soft tissue injury is an important variable. Proximal humerus fractures can be thought of as the visible tip of the iceberg. The whole iceberg as applied to the shoulder includes all the soft tissue injury that occurs in addition to the proximal humerus fracture. This makes stiffness a predictable and troublesome component for the postinjury management of this type of injury. A good way to classify such fractures is simply the anatomic description of the injury and the amount of displacement. In this way, every fracture line and injury is duly considered. It may take several weeks or months to restore passive motion to the shoulder. The soft tissue injury that exists with these proximal humerus fractures causes stiffness because of immobilization and scarring. Inability to restore full passive motion to the shoulder may affect shoulder mechanics and subsequent overhead function and may lead to clinical problems.

Two-part fractures usually involve either the greater or lesser tuberosity of the humerus or the surgical neck. If the greater tuberosity cannot be reduced and remains displaced more than 5 mm., open reduction and internal fixation are advisable, because malunion in a displaced position interferes with abduction and external rotation of the humerus and may be painful. Separation of the lesser tuberosity usu-

ally requires no treatment other than immobilization unless it is displaced 75 mm. or more. If significant angulation or displacement of the shaft is present, closed reduction should be performed. Open reduction is rarely necessary.

FRACTURES OF THE SHAFT OF THE HUMERUS

Anatomy. The humeral shaft is cylindrical proximally and broadens distally. The major neurovascular structures are located medially except for the radial nerve, which courses laterally. The muscles of the arm and gravity act on midshaft fractures to produce shortening and varus angulation. In fractures below the insertion of the deltoid muscle, the proximal fragment is abducted by the deltoid, while the biceps, triceps, and coracobrachialis adduct and shorten the distal fragment. In fractures above the insertion of the deltoid and below the insertion of the pectoralis major, the distal fragment is drawn into abduction by the deltoid, while the proximal fragment is adducted by the pectoralis major. In fractures above the insertion of the pectoralis major, the distal fragment is held in alignment, while the proximal fragment is abducted by the rotator cuff and internally rotated by the subscapularis.

Mechanism of Injury. The majority of these fractures are caused by direct trauma or a fall on the arm. Bending moments cause transverse fractures, whereas torsional forces cause spiral fractures.

Clinical and X-ray Findings. Pain, tenderness, and instability of the arm are obvious. Radial nerve involvement is relatively common and should be suspected in all cases.

Treatment. Open fractures are treated as emergencies with immediate débridement. Injuries to the vascular structures, either directly or indirectly, should likewise be treated as emergencies with appropriate arteriograms, internal injury exploration, and repair or grafting of the artery. Nerve trauma is usually treated by reduction of the fracture and not by immediate operation. After emergency treatment has been administered, the principles of treatment to be considered are the method of initial immobilization and alignment of the fragments. Treatment should allow the patient to perform shoulder and elbow motion exercise within 2 weeks.

Undisplaced Fractures. These fractures can be treated by padding the axilla and wrapping the arm to the chest. Early protective motion is started in 2 weeks, and healing occurs in about 10 weeks. Only the arm may be splinted, leaving the elbow free to move.

Displaced Fractures. Several methods have been used for the treatment of these fractures. The hanging arm cast is a lightweight cast applied to the arm from just above the level of the fracture to the hand. A sling is placed under the involved axilla and over the opposite trapezius through a loop or rope fixed to the forearm cast. A coaptation splint[10] consists of a single 10- to 15-thickness splint applied from the axilla, around the elbow, and over the deltoid, with light padding and nonelastic wrapping. This holds the fragments in alignment, and a sling is used for comfort. This has the advantage of allowing earlier elbow, wrist, and hand motion and often gives the patient more comfort initially than the hanging cast. Adjustment of fracture alignment is more difficult. Alternatively, orthotic management by the use of a functional brace utilizes the same principles as the coaptation splint. It can be adjusted frequently to maintain total contact and cylindrical compression, providing good control of the fracture. The orthotics are designed to allow early function of the extremity. In fractures associated with vascular injury, rapid internal fixation of the fragments is done prior to repair of the vessels if the time interval from injury to repair is no greater than 4 hours. Closed or open reduction and intramedullary nailing of humeral shaft fractures have gained popularity recently. This technique allows early restoration of function and is therefore most useful in multiply traumatized patients.[24]

In established nonunions or in fractures with soft tissue interposition, open reduction and fixation with metallic devices are indicated. Recently, external fixation devices have been used effectively in selected difficult humeral nonunions (Fig. 42–10).[9] The humerus is a common site of pathologic fractures caused by metastatic tumors, and these may be treated by local radiation and/or chemotherapy, and the fracture may heal. More commonly, however, there is a large defect in the bone with gross instability of the humerus. The patient is often uncomfortable, and open fixation is done followed by appropriate treatment of the tumor. Healing may be delayed in these patients. If there is extensive bone loss, methylmethacrylate supplements the metallic fixation.

Prognosis. Nondisplaced and minimally displaced fractures heal in 6 to 10 weeks and allow early functional use of the arm for light activities. In severely displaced or comminuted fractures associated with neurovascular injuries, the prognosis is guarded. Associated fractures of the elbow or shoulder worsen the prognosis.

Complications. The radial nerve may be injured in open fractures or fractures at the junction of the middle and distal thirds of the humerus. At this point, the nerve is in close proximity to the humerus. In most instances, the injury is caused by stretching or contusion, and function returns within several weeks to 6 months. It is safe to wait for at least 3 months to determine whether regeneration will occur. The electromyogram demonstrates early regeneration. In open fractures involving the radial nerve or in fractures with soft tissue interposition, exploration of the radial nerve is

indicated.[14] Delayed suture is acceptable, but the decision depends on the lesion.

FRACTURES OF THE DISTAL HUMERUS AND ELBOW

In this section, supracondylar fractures of the humerus, which account for 50% to 60% of all fractures about the elbow, plus intra-articular fractures of the distal humerus, fractures of the radial head, and fractures of the olecranon are discussed. Fractures about the elbow are common in children and frequently lead to malunion, growth disturbance, or joint incongruity. Adult fractures about the elbow, especially distal humerus fractures, tend to be comminuted and intra-articular and may cause permanent stiffness and posttraumatic arthrosis.

Anatomy of the Elbow. The distal humerus, in the transition from diaphysis to epiphysis, becomes progressively broad and fan shaped. The medial and lateral condyles of the humerus are kept apart by a thin membrane of bone that anatomically separates the coronoid fossa anteriorly and the olecranon fossa posteriorly. The lateral condyle consists of the lateral epicondyle (the origin of the extensor muscle mass) and capitellum. The medial condyle is formed by the medial epicondyle (the origin of the flexor muscle mass) and trochlea. The capitellum laterally and trochlea medially are covered by hyaline cartilage and form the humeral portion of the elbow articular surface. The trochlea has a central groove that is directed laterally in extension, and this determines the carrying angle (normally 7 to 15 degrees). The radial head articulates with the capitellum, and it is through this proximal radial-humeral joint that pronation and supination of the forearm occur. Flexion, extension, and rotation are

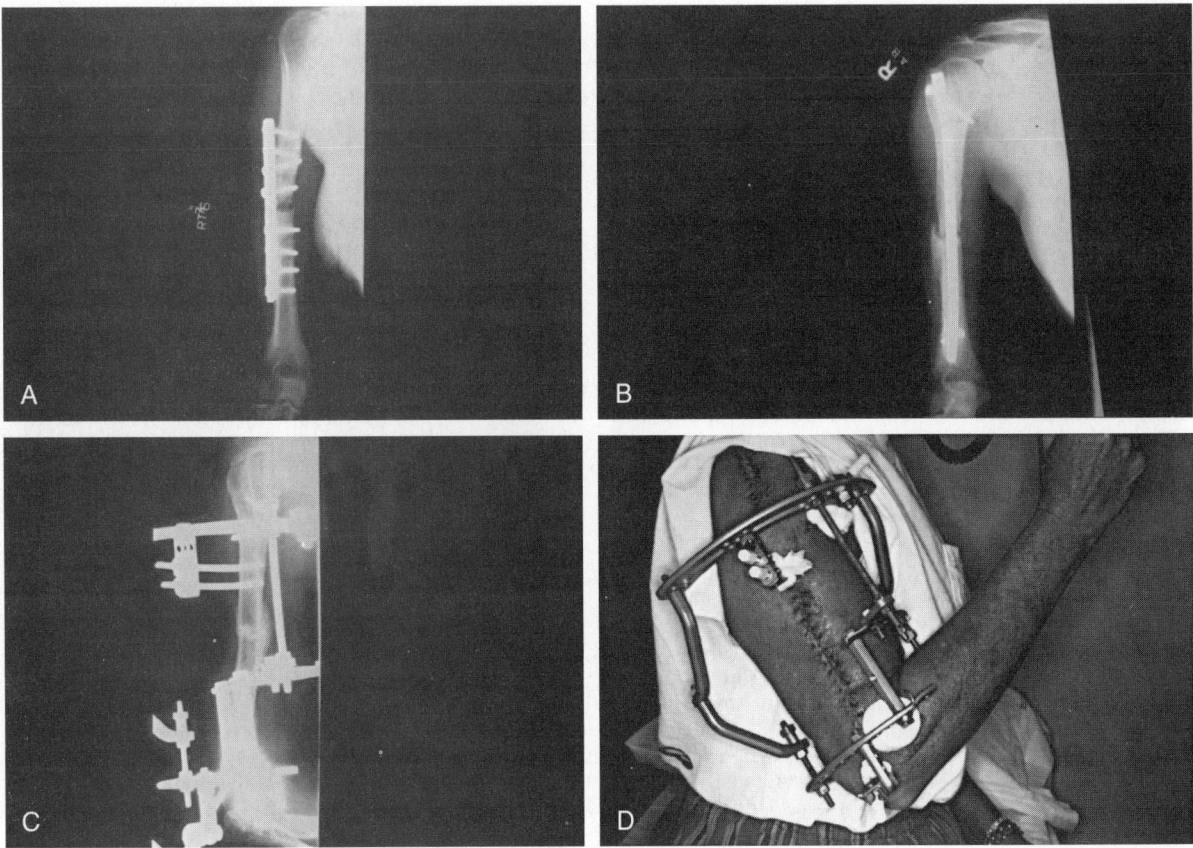

Figure 42–10. This patient has a nonunion of a humeral shaft fracture. Treatment was by plating and bone graft *(A)* and intramedullary nail *(B)*, which failed to achieve union. *C,* The application of an external fixation device allowed rapid bony consolidation. *D,* the device design allowed free shoulder and elbow motion.

dependent on the congruity among the three articulations: the humeral-ulnar joint, radial-humeral joint, and radial-ulnar joint. Any disturbance in the anatomy of these articulations leads to diminished elbow motion and function. When the elbow is flexed to 90 degrees, an isosceles triangle is formed posteriorly by the landmarks of the lateral epicondyle, medial epicondyle, and tip of the olecranon. Displaced fractures involving the elbow joint may lead to distortion of this relationship. The brachial artery and median nerve pass anterior to the elbow joint and can be damaged by displaced fractures, particularly supracondylar fractures of the humerus. The ulnar nerve, which is behind the medial epicondyle in close continuity with bone, is subject to early or late compression. The radial nerve courses laterally between the brachialis and brachioradialis, and distal to the elbow, it enters the supinator muscle mass.

Supracondylar and Intracondylar Fractures

Mechanism of Injury. Supracondylar fractures occur with a fall on the outstretched arm or flexed elbow. Two types of supracondylar fractures are distinguished: the flexion type and the extension type. The most common by far is the extension injury. This occurs with a fall on the outstretched arm, which leads to a compression and hyperextension force applied indirectly to the distal humerus. On the lateral radiograph, the normal anterior tilt of the distal humerus is lost, and there may be anterior angulation at the fracture site. Less commonly, compression and flexion forces cause a flexion type of injury. In this case, the fracture is angulated posteriorly, and there may be an increase in anterior displacement and angulation of the distal fragment. Transcondylar and intracondylar fractures are seen in adults, particularly in the elderly, related to significant trauma. Much comminution of the fragments is often noted.

Clinical Findings. Pain and swelling are present. Neurovascular status must be carefully assessed, because arterial or neurologic injury can occur by laceration and direct or indirect compression. Properly obtained radiographs are an important aspect of initial evaluation. In children, comparison films of the uninvolved distal humerus and elbow are helpful. During interpretation, one must look for obvious findings, such as degree of displacement and level and number of fracture fragments. In addition, particularly in children, one must look for subtle changes, such as rotary malalignment and varus impaction. Measurement of Baumann's angle on both the involved and the uninvolved extremity may be a helpful guide to preventing varus malunion.[7] In the anteroposterior radiograph, the presence of medial or lateral displacement should be recognized, because this must be corrected during treatment and should be a guide to positioning of the forearm.

Treatment. In children, undisplaced fractures are treated by immobilization of the arm with the elbow flexed to 90 degrees. The period of immobilization is approximately 3 weeks. However, care must be taken to be certain that an apparent nondisplaced fracture is not in fact a varus impacted fracture, which can lead to the late complication of cubitus varus. Varus impacted fractures should be manipulated, and this can usually be done with sedation. In a significantly displaced supracondylar humerus fracture without neurologic deficit, a reduction with anesthesia is warranted. Reduction is performed by traction of the forearm, with countertraction proximally. This maneuver is done with the elbow in slight flexion. Traction should never be applied with the elbow hyperextended, because this may cause further compression of the neurovascular structures anteriorly. The extension deformity of the distal fragment is then corrected by pressure applied posteriorly. Following this, any medial

or lateral angulation is corrected. The elbow is then flexed to 90 degrees and stability is tested. If this fracture is unstable with the elbow at 90 degrees, percutaneous pinning is recommended.[7] This is preferable to further flexion of the elbow to obtain stability, because the latter may cause vascular embarrassment and lead to Volkmann's ischemic contracture. If initial displacement in the anteroposterior plane is medial, this means that the medial periosteum is intact, whereas the lateral periosteum is disrupted. Soft tissue should be tightened laterally by pronation of the forearm. This allows reduction to be maintained against the medial periosteal hinge. Conversely, if initial displacement is lateral, the medial periosteum is disrupted and the medial soft tissue should be tightened, which requires supination of the forearm.

Occasionally, fractures cannot be reduced either by traction or by closed reduction because of soft tissue interposition. These fractures require open reduction and pinning. Likewise, in the case of neurologic deficit occurring after fracture reduction or vascular insufficiency, the fracture should be open reduced and the involved structures explored.

Supracondylar fractures in adults are often comminuted and have intra-articular extension; they are usually best managed by open reduction and internal fixation to allow early range of motion exercises of the elbow.[20]

Complications. The most serious complication is Volkmann's ischemia with subsequent contracture. Varus, valgus, or rotary malunion does not remodel and will persist. The most common malunion seen is that of cubitus varus, or gunstock deformity (Fig. 42–11). If significant, this may require a corrective supracondylar valgus osteotomy.[15]

Physeal Injuries

A variation of the supracondylar fracture in children is a transcondylar or transphyseal injury. The entire epiphysis of the distal humerus is displaced from the metaphysis, and the displacement can be anterior, posterior, or lateral, depending on the applied forces. In young children, this injury may be undiagnosed or may be confused with an elbow dislocation. Diagnosis is made by the abnormal relationship between the distal humeral metaphysis and the proximal ulna and radius and the preservation of a normal anatomic relationship be-

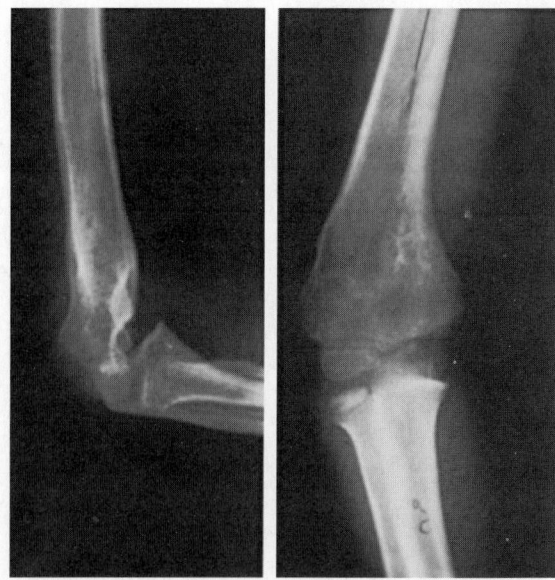

Figure 42–11. A malunion of a supracondylar humerus fracture has led to loss of the normal valgus carrying angle, because of a varus malunion leading to a gun-stock deformity.

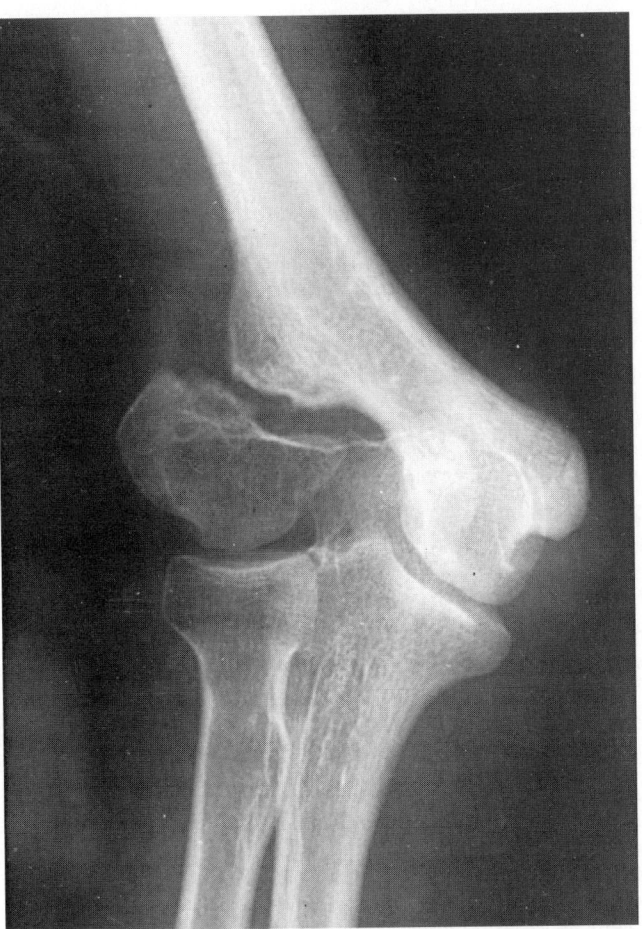

Figure 42–12. This elbow radiograph is of a 14-year-old girl with an old nonunion of a lateral condyle fracture. This has led to a cubitus valgus deformity, and the patient has developed tardy ulnar nerve symptoms.

tween the capitellum and proximal radius. One should also examine the radiographs closely for the presence of a small metaphyseal fragment arising from the distal humerus (Thurston Holland sign)[22] as a clue to the diagnosis. Normally, this injury can be managed by closed reduction, and reduction is usually stable. A posterior splint is then applied for 3 to 4 weeks.

Lateral Condyle Fractures

This fracture is a significant fracture of childhood and deserves special consideration. It may be misdiagnosed as a minor injury. The lateral condyle fracture is an intra-articular fracture, usually a Salter Type IV injury. Unlike most children's fractures, this fracture has a tendency to progress to nonunion (Fig. 42–12).[25] Even minimally displaced fractures may fail to unite if inappropriately managed.[13] This injury usually occurs with a fall on the outstretched arm with the elbow extended and the forearm abducted, leading to forces transmitted to the lateral condyle of the humerus through the radius. Displaced fractures must be treated by open reduction and internal fixation with smooth pins. Minimally displaced fractures, if determined radiographically not to be malrotated or significantly displaced, can be managed by plaster immobilization. However, if there is any question of malalignment, one should proceed to open reduction.

Medial Epicondyle Fractures

This fracture is usually caused by a traction injury from the flexor origin. This may be an isolated injury or may be

associated with dislocation of the elbow. Minimally displaced fractures require no treatment other than temporary immobilization; usually 3 weeks is sufficient. Fractures displaced more than 5 mm. warrant open reduction and internal fixation with pins. Pin placement should be under direct vision to avoid injury to the ulnar nerve.[12, 21]

Dislocations of the Elbow

Posterior dislocation is caused by a fall on the outstretched arm, with dislocation of the radius and ulna. Neurovascular structures are rarely affected, although arterial injury occurs occasionally. Anterior dislocations are caused by a blow on the flexed elbow. Dislocation of the radial head can occur as an isolated injury anteriorly or posteriorly. Dislocation of the ulna alone occurs rarely. Associated fractures of the coronoid process, medial epicondyle, or radial head may occur with dislocation.

Clinical Findings. Elbow motion is limited. There is deformity, and the neurovascular structures are usually intact. Median nerve injury occasionally occurs.

Treatment. Gentle pull on the olecranon followed by flexion usually relocates the dislocation. After reduction, the elbow should be extended through a reasonable range of motion to test stability. If the elbow is stable, immobilization is done for comfort, and motion exercises are begun as soon as they can be tolerated, preferably within the first week.

Complications. In simple dislocations, a functional range of motion usually occurs. Myositis ossificans, however, can produce mild or severe limitation of motion in a small percentage of patients. Neurovascular complications are occasionally seen.

Fractures of the Olecranon

The olecranon process constitutes the proximal ulnar articulation with the humerus and serves as a point of attachment for the triceps tendon. Because of the subcutaneous location on the extensor surface of the arm, it is susceptible to direct trauma. Fractures may also occur due to a traction-avulsion mechanism caused by the pull of the triceps tendon.

Clinical Findings. There is swelling and tenderness in the region of the proximal ulna. Because of the subcutaneous location, the fracture site may be palpable. Ulnar nerve function should be carefully tested, because contusion neurapraxia can be associated with this injury. Anteroposterior and lateral radiographs should be assessed for the size of the olecranon fragment, the degree of comminution, and the amount of displacement.

Treatment. Undisplaced fractures are treated by splinting with the elbow in 60 degrees of flexion. Fractures with any significant displacement should be treated by open reduction and anatomic realignment of the articular surface, when possible. Avulsion fractures usually involve only a small piece of the olecranon and can be excised or repaired. Comminuted fractures may be best managed by primary excision of the olecranon and repair of the triceps tendon. Internal fixation can be achieved by intramedullary screw fixation or a modified tension band wiring technique. Achieving an anatomic reduction with rigid internal fixation allows early active motion and should diminish the delayed complications of limited motion and degenerative arthritis.[29]

Fractures and Dislocations of the Radial Head

An isolated dislocation of the radial head in children or adults is uncommon. When a dislocation occurs, it is almost always associated with a fracture of the proximal ulna

(Monteggia's fracture-dislocation).[8] In young children, subluxation of the radial head through the anular ligament is common and is referred to as a *pulled elbow* or *nursemaid's elbow*. This is caused by forced distraction and pronation of the forearm.

Radial head fractures are common in both children and adults. Because of the normal valgus carrying angle, a fall on the outstretched arm causes transmission of forces along the radius, leading to impaction of the radial head against the capitellum. This occurs in three patterns of fractures in children. The most common injury is a compression fracture through the metaphysis, resulting in angular displacement. Less commonly, the injury is a physeal plate fracture (Type I or II); rarely, in adolescents, an intra-articular Type III fracture can occur. In adults, most fractures are intra-articular; therefore, it is important to determine the degree of displacement and depression and the amount of articular surface involved.

Clinical Findings. The diagnosis is made by noting direct tenderness over the radial head. There is pain and limited motion on pronation and supination of the forearm.

Treatment. The pulled elbow is often reduced by the time the child is examined by the physician, or it may be reduced when the arm is supinated to obtain a radiograph. Flexion and supination of the forearm allow the radial head to slip back under the anular ligament, facilitating a reduction.

Nonarticular radial head fractures in children require only temporary immobilization for pain if angular displacement is less than 30 degrees. If angular displacement is greater than this, an attempt should be made at closed reduction. Displaced epiphyseal fractures may require open reduction if a closed reduction fails to restore length and alignment. Radial head excision should never be performed in a child. In adults, minimally displaced fractures require temporary immobilization until pain subsides. If the fragment involves more than 50% of the articular surface and is comminuted, primary radial head excision is warranted. A silicone prosthesis may be a useful substitute if elbow instability is present. Articular fractures involving less than 50% of the articular surface should be treated by temporary immobilization and early range of motion exercises, including pronation, supination, and elbow flexion and extension. Occasionally, large articular fragments can be managed by open reduction and internal fixation.[26]

FRACTURES OF THE SHAFT OF THE RADIUS AND ULNA

The proximal and distal articulations of the radius and ulna allow the radius to rotate around the ulna, providing pronation and supination of the forearm. Proximally, this rotation is permitted through the complex articulation at the radial-ulnar and radial-humeral joints. Distally, the radial-ulnar relationship is maintained by the triangular fibrocartilage complex. The shaft of the radius and ulna is connected by the fibrous interosseous membrane, which serves as a hinge, allowing the radius to rotate around the ulna. Distortion of the anatomy by fractures or dislocations alters the biomechanics of the forearm. A change in the normal interosseous membrane space leads to limitation of pronation and supination. Distortion of the proximal or distal radial-ulnar joint similarly limits forearm rotation.

Mechanism of Injury. Isolated fractures of the radius or ulna and bone fractures of the shaft are usually due to a direct blow. A fall on the outstretched arm combined with a torsional stress may cause fracture of both the radius and the ulna. Monteggia's fracture,[8] a fracture of the proximal ulna associated with radial head dislocation, may also be caused by a fall on the outstretched arm and hyperpronation of the forearm. Similarly, the shaft of the radius may be fractured in the region of the distal third, with subluxation of the distal ulna—called the Galeazzi or Piedmont fracture.[23]

Clinical Findings. Pain and deformity of the forearm are present. Evaluation of the neurovascular condition of the extremity must be made, and the presence or absence of increased pressure within the muscle compartments of the forearm must be noted. Swelling within the tight muscle compartments of the forearm can lead to occlusion of venous and arterial circulation and may lead to Volkmann's ischemic contracture. Significant swelling of the forearm compartments associated with pain on passive extension of the fingers should alert one to this possibility.

Radiographs in forearm injuries should include views of the elbow and wrist. They define the location of the fracture, the degree of comminution, any rotational deformity, and the presence of associated radial head or distal ulna subluxation or dislocation.

Treatment. A compartment syndrome should be recognized and treated expeditiously to avoid irreversible muscle necrosis. Forearm compartment fasciotomy and median nerve decompression should be performed.

In adults, displaced fractures of the shaft of the radius and ulna, fractures of the proximal ulna associated with radial head dislocation (Monteggia's lesion), and fractures of the radius associated with disruption of the distal radial-ulnar joint (Piedmont fracture) are best managed by operative methods. With Monteggia's fracture, the radial head must be reduced, and the fracture of the ulna stabilized. Both bone forearm fractures are best managed by compression plating of the radius and ulna to restore a normal interosseous space.

Conversely, most forearm fractures in children can be managed by closed means.[39] The thick periosteum makes reduction of the fractures more stable than in adults, and the osteogenic potential in children allows for excellent remodeling of angular deformities. However, rotational malalignment does not remodel and must be avoided during closed treatment of these fractures. Occasionally with a Monteggia's fracture-dislocation, the radial head cannot be reduced, because of either a greenstick fracture of the proximal ulna or interposed tissue; in this instance, open reduction of the fracture and dislocation is indicated.

Complications. The most serious complication in forearm fractures, neurovascular compromise and subsequent ischemic contracture, must be avoided. Nonunion of forearm shaft fractures occurs in 5% to 10% of the cases in which closed treatment is used. Open treatment may be complicated by nonunion with or without infection. The most frequent complication is malunion and occurs more commonly with closed reduction of displaced fractures in adults. Malunion with compromise of the interosseous space leads to limited pronation and supination. Other complications include reflex sympathetic dystrophy and posttraumatic radial-ulnar synostosis.[4]

SELECTED REFERENCES

Boyd, D. W., and Aronson, D. D.: Supracondylar fractures of the humerus: A prospective study of percutaneous pinning. J. Pediatr. Orthop., 12:789, 1992.
This study demonstrates the safety and effectiveness of percutaneous pinning for the management of supracondylar humerus fractures in children.

O'Brien, S., Neves, M., Arnowsky, S., et al.: The anatomy and histology of the inferior glenohumeral ligament complex of the shoulder. Am. J. Sports Med., 18:449, 1990.
This classic study identifies the true anatomic and histologic features of this primary shoulder ligament stabilizer.

Ogden, J. A.: Skeletal Injury in the Child, 2nd ed. Philadelphia, W. B. Saunders, 1990.
This is an excellent reference text for fractures involving the immature skeleton.

Rockwood, C. A., and Green, D. P.: Fractures, 3rd ed. Philadelphia, J. B. Lippincott, 1991.
This textbook is a complete reference source. Two volumes cover adult fractures, and one volume is dedicated to pediatric fractures.

Speer, K., Deng, X., Altcheck, D., et al.: A biomechanical evaluation of the Bankart lesion. J. Bone Joint Surg. 76:1819, 1994.
This cadaveric study assesses a component of the pathoanatomy of an anterior dislocation. This study concerns the contribution of the detached labrum to the overall increased translation that the shoulder experiences.

REFERENCES

1. Altcheck, D., Warren, R., Wickiewicz, T., et al.: Arthroscopic labral debridement. Am. J. Sports Med., 20:702, 1992.
2. Arciero, R., Wheeler, J., Ryan, J., et al.: Arthroscopic Bankart repair versus nonoperative treatment for acute, initial anterior shoulder dislocations. J. Bone Joint Surg., 22:589, 1994.
3. Bankart, A.: The pathology and treatment of recurrent dislocation of the shoulder joint. Br. J. Surg., 26:23, 1938.
4. Bauer, G., Arand, M., and Mutschler, W.: Post-traumatic radioulnar synostosis after forearm fracture osteosynthesis. Arch. Orthop. Trauma Surg., 110:142, 1991.
5. Bigliani, L., Pollock, R., Soslowsky, L., et al.: Tensile properties of the inferior glenohumeral ligament. J. Orthop. Res., 10:187, 1992.
6. Bowen, M., and Warren, R.: Ligamentous control of shoulder stability based on selective cutting and static translation experiments. Clin. Sports Med., 10:757, 1991.
7. Boyd, D. W., and Aronson, D. D.: Supracondylar fractures of the humerus: A prospective study of percutaneous pinning. J. Pediatr. Orthop., 12:789, 1992.
8. Bryan, R. S.: Monteggia's fracture of the forearm. J. Trauma, 11:992, 1971.
9. Catagni, M. A., Guerreschi, F., and Probe, R. A.: Treatment of humeral nonunions with the Ilizarov technique. Bull. Hosp. Jt. Dis. Orthop. Inst., 51:74, 1991.
10. Connolly, J. F.: DePalma's Management of Fractures and Dislocations, 3rd ed. Philadelphia, W. B. Saunders, 1981.
11. DePalma, A., Callery, G., and Bennett, G.: Variable anatomy and degenerative lesions of the shoulder. Instr. Course Lect. (AAOS), 16:255, 1949.
12. Dunn, P. S., Ravn, P., Hansen, L. B., and Buron, B.: Osteosynthesis of medial humeral epicondyle fractures in children: 8-year follow-up of 33 cases. Acta Orthop. Scand., 65:439, 1994.
13. Flynn, J. C., and Richards, J. F., Jr.: Nonunion of minimally displaced fractures of the lateral condyle of the humerus in children. J. Bone Joint Surg. [Am.], 53:1096, 1971.
14. Foster, R. J., Swiontkowski, M. F., Bach, A. W., and Sack, J. T.: Radial nerve palsy caused by open humeral shaft fractures. J. Hand Surg. [Am.], 18:121, 1993.
15. Gaddy, B. C., Manske, P. R., Pruitt, D. L., Schoenecker, P. L., and Rouse, A. M.: Distal humeral osteotomy for correction of post traumatic cubitus varus. J. Pediatr. Orthop., 14:214, 1994.
16. Halliburton, R. A., Barbour, J. R., and Fraser, R. L.: Pseudodislocation: An unusual birth injury. Can. J. Surg., 10:455, 1967.
17. Harryman, D., Sidles, J., and Matsen, F.: The role of the rotator interval capsule in passive motion and stability of the shoulder. J. Bone Joint Surg. [Am.], 74:53, 1992.
18. Healy, W. L., White, G. N., Mick, C. A., Brooker, A. F., and Weiland, A. J.: Nonunion of the humeral shaft. Clin. Orthop. Rel. Res., 219:206, 1987.
19. Helfet, A. J.: Coracoid transplantation for recurring dislocation of the shoulder. J. Bone Joint Surg. [Br.], 40:198, 1958.
20. Helfet, D. L., and Schmeling, G. J.: Bicondylar intraarticular fractures of the distal humerus in adults (Review). Clin. Orthop. Rel. Res., 292:26, 1993.
21. Hines, R. F., Herndon, W. A., and Evans, J. P.: Operative treatment of medial epicondyle fractures in children. Clin. Orthop. Rel. Res., 223:170, 1987.
22. Holland, C. T.: Radiographic note on injuries to the distal epiphyses of radius and ulna. Proc. World Soc. Med., 22:695, 1929.
23. Hughston, J. C.: Fracture of the distal radial shaft, mistakes in management. J. Bone Joint Surg. [Am.], 39:249, 1957.
24. Ingman, A. M., and Waters, D. A.: Locked intramedullary nailing of humeral shaft fractures: Implant design, surgical technique, and clinical results. J. Bone Joint Surg. [Br.], 76:23, 1994.
25. Inoue, G., and Tamura, Y.: Osteosynthesis for long-standing nonunion of the lateral humeral condyle. Arch. Orthop. Trauma Surg., 112:236, 1993.
26. Kanlic, E., and Perry, C. R.: Indications and technique of open reduction and internal fixation of radial head fractures (Review). Orthopedics, 15:837, 1992.
27. Kirker, J. R.: Dislocation of the shoulder complicated by rupture of the axillary vessels: Report of a case. J. Bone Joint Surg. [Br.], 34:72, 1952.
28. Matsen, F., Harryman, D., and Sidles, J.: Mechanics of glenohumeral instability. Clin. Sports Med., 10:783, 1991.
29. Murphy, D. F., Green, W. B., and Dameron, T. B.: Displaced olecranon fractures in adults. Clin. Orthop. Rel. Res., 224:215, 1987.
30. Penn, I.: The vascular complications of fractures of the clavicle. J. Trauma, 4:819, 1964.
31. Rockwood, C. A., and Green, D. P.: Fractures. Philadelphia, J. B. Lippincott, 1984.
32. Rowe, C.: Dislocations of the shoulder. In Rowe, C. (Ed.): The Shoulder. New York, Churchill Livingstone, 1988, p. 165.
33. Schwartz, R., O'Brien, S., et al.: Capsular restraints to the abducted shoulder: A biomechanical study. Orthop. Trans., 12:727, 1988.
34. Schwartz, E., Warren, R., and O'Brien, S.: Posterior shoulder instability. Orthop. Clin. North Am., 18:409, 1987.
35. Stener, B.: Dislocation of the shoulder complicated by complete rupture of the axillary artery. J. Bone Joint Surg. [Br.], 39:714, 1957.
36. Stimson, L. A.: An easy method of reducing dislocations of the shoulder and hip. Med. Rec., 57:356, 1900.
37. Turkel, S., Panio, M., and Marshall, J.: Stabilizing mechanisms preventing anterior dislocation of the glenohumeral joint. J. Bone Joint Surg. [Br.], 67:1208, 1981.
38. Warner, J., Deng, X., Warren, R., et al.: Static capsuloligamentous restraints to superior-inferior translation of the glenohumeral joint. Am. J. Sports Med., 20:675, 1992.
39. Younger, A. S., Tredwell, S. J., Mackenzie, W. G., Orr, J. D., King, P. M., and Tennant, W.: Accurate prediction of outcome after pediatric forearm fracture. J. Pediatr. Orthop., 14:200, 1994.

IV

FRACTURE OF THE CARPAL SCAPHOID

Richard D. Goldner, M.D., and J. Leonard Goldner, M.D.

Because the scaphoid is the most frequently fractured carpal bone, the major emphasis of this section is on injuries involving the carpal scaphoid.

WRIST MOTION

Wrist dorsiflexion and palmar flexion occur at both the radial carpal and intercarpal joints. The relationships of the eight carpal bones are depicted in Figure 42–13. The axis of normal carpal movement is in the neck of the capitate. At the radial-carpal joint, the movement includes the scaphoid, lunate, and triquetrum. The scaphoid bridges the proximal and distal carpal rows. The motion of dorsiflexion and palmar flexion of the wrist joint occurs approximately half at the radial-carpal and half at the intercarpal joints. The scaphoid moves through an arc of approximately 40 degrees and articulates with the radius, lunate, capitate, and trapezium through the entire arc of flexion and extension.

Motion of the wrist is initiated by muscles that insert into metacarpals. As the wrist rotates from neutral to ulnar deviation, the proximal carpal row dorsiflexes and the profile of the scaphoid appears longer; from neutral to radial deviation, the proximal carpal row palmar flexes and the scaphoid appears foreshortened. For this reason, ulnar deviation radiographs are necessary for adequate visualization of the scaphoid. Because the scaphoid crosses both proximal and distal carpal rows, excessive dorsiflexion causes it to be pinned between the dorsal lip of the radius and the palmar sling of the strong radial capitate ligament. The scaphoid is the principal bony block to excessive dorsiflexion of the hand and wrist and is particularly susceptible to fracture during a fall on the outstretched hand.

HISTORY AND PHYSICAL EXAMINATION

A history and detailed physical examination are crucial in diagnosing wrist injuries. The amount of force sustained during the injury and the position of the wrist and upper

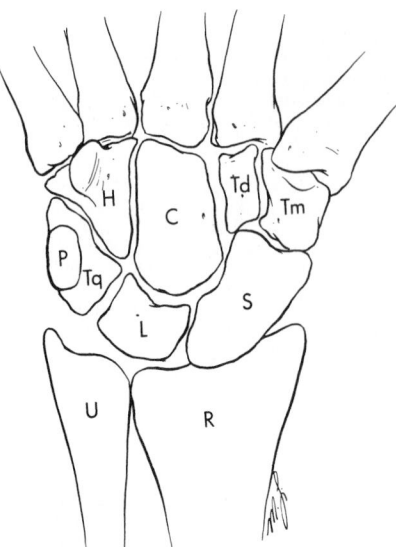

Figure 42–13. The carpal bones: scaphoid (S); lunate (L); triquetrum (Tq); pisiform (P), which is a sesamoid bone within the flexor carpi ulnaris; trapezium (Tm); trapezoid (Td); capitate (C); and hamate (H). (From Goldner, R. D., Ugino, M. R., and Goldner, J. L.: Injuries to carpal bones. *In* Edlich, R. F., and Spyker, D. A. [Eds.]: Current Emergency Medical Therapy. Norwalk, CT, Appleton-Century-Crofts, 1984.)

extremity while that force occurred should determine the physician's suspicion regarding significant carpal injury. An apparently minor injury is often associated with tremendous torque and twisting motion, and scaphoid fracture can occur even with an injury that the patient characterizes as minor.

The examination of patients with carpal injuries includes careful palpation to detect areas of tenderness, edema, or contusion; measurements of range of motion; motor and sensory assessment; and use of the Allen test to determine the integrity of the radial and ulnar arteries. The examiner should not overlook concomitant trauma, such as posterior dislocation of the elbow or radial head fracture.

CLINICAL ASSESSMENT

The most consistent sign of carpal injury is localized tenderness to digital pressure. Fracture of the carpal scaphoid produces tenderness to pressure in the anatomic *snuffbox* that is located between the extensor pollicis longus and extensor pollicis brevis–abductor pollicis longus compartments.

Radial and ulnar deviation produces pain on the radial side of the wrist. Forced dorsiflexion is the most painful maneuver. If the patient is asked to supinate and the examiner attempts to pronate the hand and wrist against resistance, and vice versa, pain may be stimulated. Pain can also be produced by having the patient put extreme pressure on the fingertips with the wrist in dorsiflexion.

RADIOGRAPHIC FINDINGS

Radiographic examination of a patient with carpal injury should include at least anteroposterior (AP), lateral, and supination and pronation oblique views. The lateral view must be a "true lateral," with the wrist in neutral position to demonstrate the linear relationship between the distal radius, lunate, and capitate.

When a scaphoid fracture is suspected and the clinical findings are strongly positive, a projection in ulnar deviation and pronation (posteroanterior [PA], palm down) may demonstrate the scaphoid clearly and reveal an undisplaced frac-

ture that is not evident on the other views (Fig. 42–14). During the ulnar deviation maneuver, excessive stress should not be applied; otherwise, displacement of a nondisplaced scaphoid fracture may occur.

A simultaneous radial styloid fracture is relatively common with a carpal dislocation, and a patient with a radial styloid fracture should have radiographs to exclude scapholunate dissociation (Fig. 42–15). These radiographs should include AP supination (palm up) and clenched-fist AP views in addition to the true lateral (Figs. 42–16 and 42–17).

Special Roentgenographic Considerations. Radiographic projections at the time of original injury may not demonstrate a fracture because of impaction and absence of resorption. Decreased bone density at the fracture site and physiologic resorption demonstrate a fracture line that is evident on a radiograph obtained 10 to 14 days after injury. If the clinical findings are strongly suggestive of fracture but routine radiographs are negative, special techniques and projections are considered. PA and lateral tomograms or direct sagittal and coronal computed tomography (CT) scans may demonstrate a fracture that is not visualized on a plain radiograph. Fluoroscopic visualization of the wrist in different positions may demonstrate a scaphoid fracture that is not visualized on a plain radiograph. If these special techniques do not detect a fracture, and if pain and tenderness persist, a [99m]technetium bone scan a few weeks after trauma may detect a fracture that plain radiographs would not necessarily demonstrate.

There are numerous instances of "sprained wrists" treated by simple soft dressings with subsequent nonunion of the carpal scaphoid. If these injuries were treated originally for 8 to 10 weeks in appropriate casts, the scaphoids probably

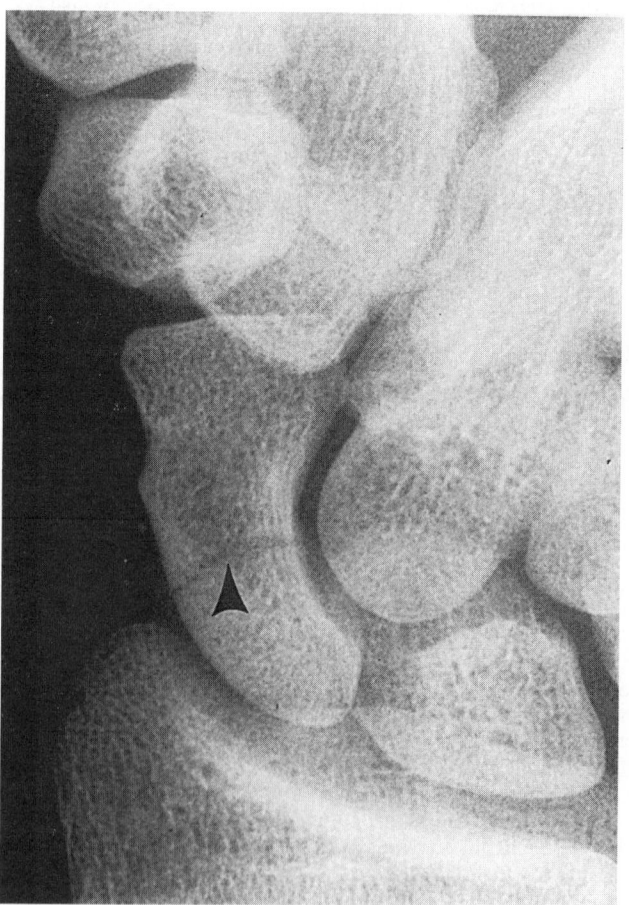

Figure 42–14. X-ray demonstrating a nondisplaced fracture of the carpal scaphoid (arrow). This fracture can be missed on other views of the scaphoid.

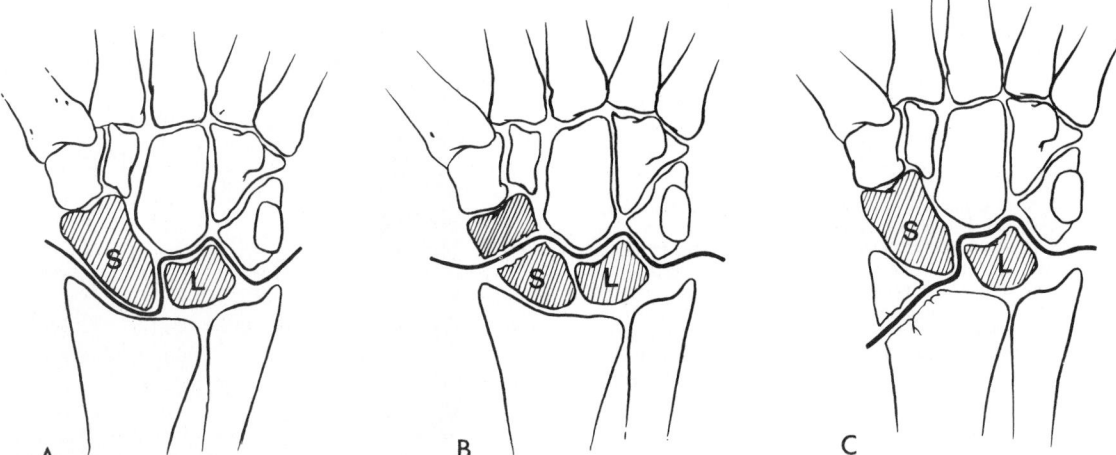

Figure 42–15. The scaphoid bridges the proximal and distal carpal rows. With a dislocation between these two rows, the scaphoid must either rotate or fracture. This produces *(A)* a perilunate dislocation, in which the remainder of the carpus dislocates around the lunate (L); *(B)* a transscaphoid perilunate dislocation, in which the distal half of the scaphoid (S) and the remaining carpus dislocate around the lunate; or *(C)* a transradial styloid perilunate dislocation, a fracture of the radial styloid with subsequent dislocation of it and the remaining carpus around the lunate. (From Goldner, R. D., Ugino, M. R., and Goldner, J. L.: Injuries to carpal bones. *In* Edlich, R. F., and Spyker, D. A. [Eds.]: Current Emergency Medical Therapy. Norwalk, CT, Appleton-Century-Crofts, 1984.)

would have united, eliminating the impairment that occurs with nonunion.

TREATMENT

When managing a scaphoid fracture, the major problems are lack of an early diagnosis and delayed initiation of appropriate treatment. If the initial radiographs are negative but tenderness to pressure exists in the anatomic snuffbox, a cast should be applied in slight radial deviation and 10 degrees of flexion, immobilizing flexion, immobilizing the thumb, and including the proximal phalanx, the wrist, and the forearm. This cast is removed after 2 weeks, and the radiographs are repeated. By that time, bone resorption usually allows the fracture line to be visible. If clinical findings persist but

the radiographs are negative, the special radiographs noted above or a technetium bone scan is obtained. A displaced, unstable scaphoid fracture usually does not heal with cast treatment and requires surgery for internal fixation.

The major blood supply to the scaphoid is from the radial artery. Branches have been demonstrated at the palmar surface (tubercle), but the majority enter through the dorsal surface. The distal location of the major blood supply has been considered to be the cause of the elevated incidence of nonunion and aseptic necrosis of the proximal fragment. The blood vessels passing distal to proximal are interrupted when the scaphoid fracture occurs, and the proximal segment becomes temporarily ischemic. The location and obliquity of the fracture line influence the average healing time of a scaphoid fracture.

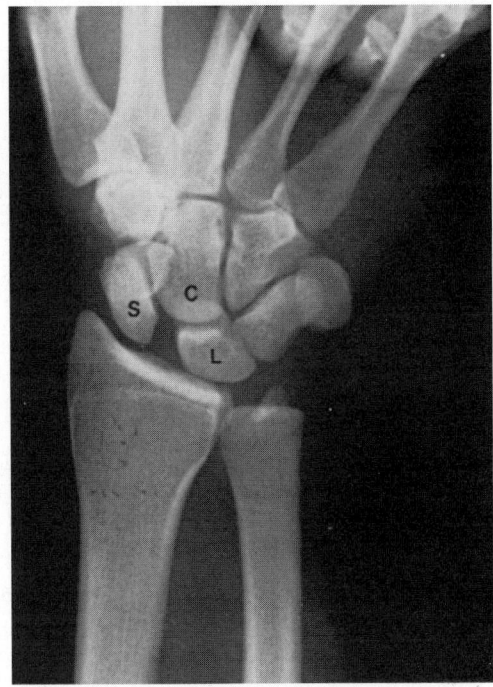

Figure 42–16. Clenched-fist view in a patient with scapholunate dissociation, demonstrating widening of the space between the scaphoid (S) and lunate (L) (Terry Thomas sign) and foreshortened appearance of the scaphoid. The anteroposterior (AP) view is taken with the forearm in supination (palm up), to demonstrate the scapholunate dissociation. This diagnosis is made by the following roentgenographic findings: (1) distance between the scaphoid and lunate (scapholunate gap) on the AP film greater than 2 mm. (Terry Thomas sign); (2) foreshortened appearance of the abnormally palmar-flexed scaphoid on the AP view; (3) cortical *signet ring* shadow, representing an axial projection of the abnormally oriented scaphoid; and (4) more vertical orientation at the scaphoid, as demonstrated by the increased angle between the scaphoid and lunate on the true lateral x-ray (normal, 30 to 60 degrees; see Fig. 42–18). Those patients suspected of having scapholunate dissociation should have a compression stress view, which is performed by having the patient clench his or her fist for the AP film. This view often demonstrates scapholunate widening not seen on the static view. (From Goldner, R. D., Ugino, M. R., and Goldner, J. L.: Injuries to carpal bones. *In* Edlich, R. F., and Spyker, D. A. [Eds.]: Current Emergency Medical Therapy. Norwalk, CT, Appleton-Century-Crofts, 1984.)

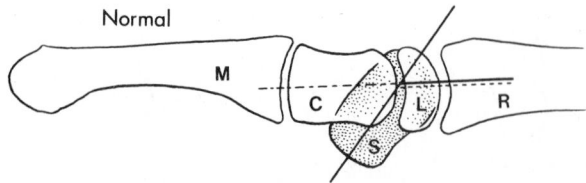

Figure 42–17. Diagram of a true lateral radiograph of the wrist. Lines are drawn through the longitudinal axis of the scaphoid (S), capitate (C), and radius (R) and through the midportion of the lunate (L). In a normal wrist in neutral position, the longitudinal axis of the center of the radius, lunate, capitate, and third metacarpal (M) is, in general, linear. The normal angle between the scaphoid and lunate is 30 to 60 degrees. The normal angles between the capitate and lunate and between the radius and lunate are 0 to 15 degrees. (From Goldner, R. D., Ugino, M. R., and Goldner, J. L.: Injuries to carpal bones. In Edlich, R. F., and Spyker, D. A. [Eds.]: Current Emergency Medical Therapy. Norwalk, CT, Appleton-Century-Crofts, 1984.)

Fractures of the distal third constitute 10% of the total number of scaphoid fractures and usually heal in approximately 8 weeks. Seventy per cent of scaphoid fractures involve the middle third of the bone, and the healing time at this location is generally 8 to 12 weeks, although many fractures require 16 to 18 weeks. In approximately 30% of middle-third fractures, aseptic necrosis of the proximal fragment develops because of the blood flow pattern. Fractures of the proximal third constitute approximately 20% of scaphoid fractures, and this group heals more slowly than the others. Healing time is 10 to 20 weeks, averaging approximately 16 weeks. In most of the fractures of the proximal fifth of the scaphoid, aseptic necrosis develops.

The orientation of the fracture and the alignment of the fragments affect healing. Horizontal oblique and transverse fractures are more stable and heal more rapidly than vertical oblique fractures, which have a high longitudinal shear component and less stability than horizontal fractures.

If the scaphoid fracture fragments are displaced or angulated, some degree of carpal instability exists. Displaced fractures and those with accompanying ligament injuries are treated under direct vision by open reduction and internal fixation. Fixation pins, a lag screw or the Herbert screw, are employed for fixation of scaphoid fractures.

Nondisplaced fractures of the scaphoid and those fractures without evidence of ligamentous instability are adequately

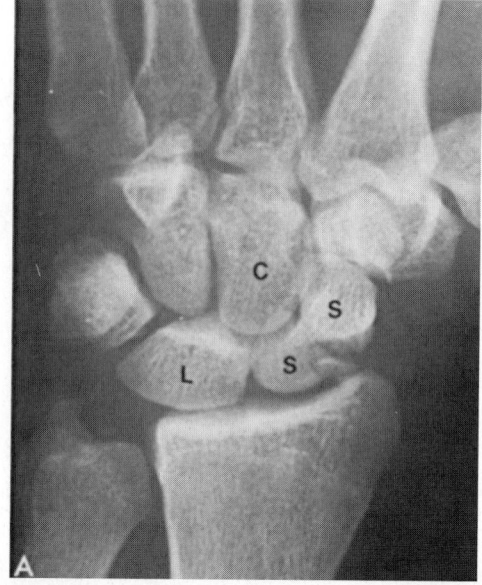

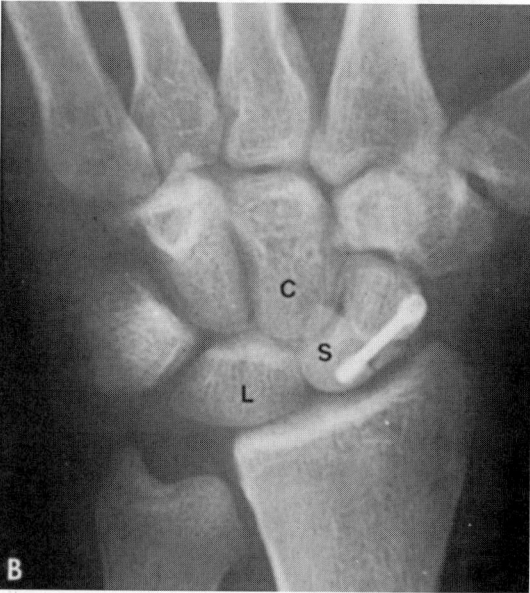

Figure 42–19. A, Fracture of the scaphoid with displacement and comminution. Closed reduction is not successful. B, Open realignment of the scaphoid through a palmar approach. The Herbert jig and screw were used for fixation. (See Fig. 42–13 for abbreviations.)

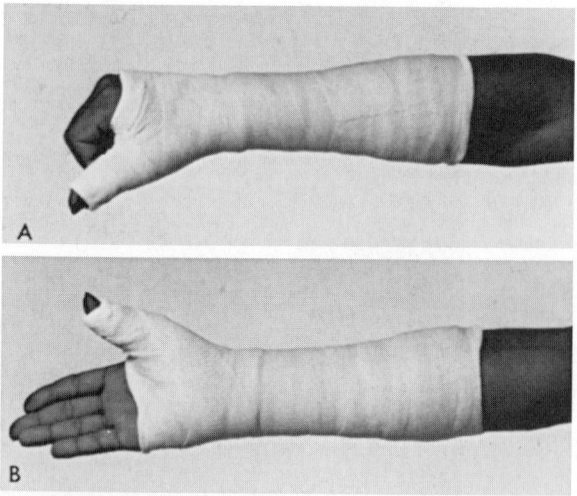

Figure 42–18. A, A well-fitting short-arm cast is sufficient to immobilize stable, nondisplaced carpal scaphoid fragments. The contour of the forearm is used to mold the plaster, thereby eliminating the need for a cast above the elbow. B, The thumb metacarpal and proximal phalanx are always included. In this example, the distal phalanx of the thumb was also included.

treated by external immobilization in a cast. However, there is no clear consensus concerning the necessity of a long-arm versus a short-arm cast in the treatment of stable scaphoid fractures. Also, there is limited consensus concerning the extent of the thumb and the digits to be included. Most surgeons agree that at least the forearm and the proximal phalanx of the thumb should be included in the initial cast. For a nondisplaced, stable fracture, the authors favor a gauntlet-type short-arm cast from the midpalmar crease and including the proximal phalanx of the thumb, with the wrist in 10-degree flexion and radial deviation to provide compression and apposition of the fragments (Fig. 42–18). This wrist position should maintain the anatomic alignment of the fracture fragments, which should be documented by radiographs after the cast is applied. If a short-arm cast is used and the patient is usually active, the cast should be changed every 10 to 14 days for the first 6 weeks so that it remains firm both around the forearm muscles and at the wrist.

PATHOLOGIC CHANGES ASSOCIATED WITH NONUNION OR MALUNION

Osteonecrosis of the fragment of the scaphoid proximal to the fracture occurs from inadequate blood supply and depends on the anatomic composition of the scaphoid and the relationship of the fracture to the distal arterial inflow.

Traumatic arthrosis follows cartilage damage at the time of the original injury, incongruity of cartilage surfaces secondary to malposition or malunion, or hypermobility from nonunion or ligament injury.

TREATMENT FOR NONUNION

The use of an iliac crest bone graft to bridge both proximal and distal segments of the scaphoid on the palmar surface, as described by Russe, has been 90% successful in treating scaphoid nonunion. Also, internal lag screw fixation has been employed. The development of the Herbert screw and jig has improved the fixation of fragments and diminished the time that a cast is necessary for postoperative immobilization (Fig. 42–19).

Another less predictable option for an established nonunion of the scaphoid without a synovial pseudarthrosis or malposition is pulsing electromagnetic field treatments applied over a cast for at least 3 months.

Radial styloidectomy is selected if the scaphoid is healed but has an exostosis on its surface that impinges on the radial styloid.

If scaphoid nonunion has led to radial-scaphoid arthritis in addition to arthritis between the carpal bones, one treatment option is excision of the scaphoid and arthrodesis of the lunate, capitate, hamate, and triquetrum. This procedure decreases pain and maintains some degree of radial-carpal motion.

Arthrodesis of the wrist eliminates pain, provides excellent strength and grip, and maintains pronation and supination, but the absent wrist motion causes limitation of certain activities of daily living.

SELECTED REFERENCES

Amadio, P. L., and Taleisnik, J.: Fractures of the carpal bones. *In* Green, D. P. (Ed.): Operative Hand Surgery. New York, Churchill Livingstone, 1993, p. 799.
This well-illustrated chapter covers the diagnosis, radiographic evaluation, and methods of treatment of carpal fractures.

Cooney, W. P., Linscheid, R. L., and Dobyns, J. H.: Fractures and dislocations of the wrist. *In* Rockwood, C. A., Jr., Green, D. P., and Bucholz, R. W. (Eds.): Fractures in Adults. Philadelphia, J. B. Lippincott, 1991, p. 563.
This comprehensive chapter includes a historical perspective, alternative methods of treatment, and the authors' preferred method of managing fractures and dislocations of the wrist.

Green, D. P.: Carpal dislocations and instabilities. *In* Green, D. P. (Ed.): Operative Hand Surgery. New York, Churchill Livingstone, 1993, p. 861.
Current concepts in the anatomy, kinematics, diagnosis, and treatment of carpal dislocations and instabilities.

Herndon, J. H. (Ed.): Scaphoid Fractures and Complications. Rosemont, IL., American Academy of Orthopedic Surgeons, 1993.
This monograph includes the anatomy, classification, diagnosis, and treatment of scaphoid fractures, in addition to chapters on nonunion and malunion.

Linscheid, R. L., Dobyns, J. H., Beabout, J. W., and Bryan, R. S.: Traumatic instability of the wrist: Diagnosis, classification and pathomechanics. J. Bone Joint Surg. [Am.], 54:1612, 1972.
These authors present a biomechanical background and classification of wrist instability after trauma. Difficulties associated with recognition of instability and treatment are emphasized.

REFERENCES

1. Bora, W. F., Osterman, A. L., and Brighton, C. T.: The electrical treatment of scaphoid nonunion. Clin. Orthop., *161*:33, 1981.
2. Cooney, W. P., Dobyns, J. H., and Linscheid, R. L.: Fractures of the scaphoid: A rational approach to management. Clin. Orthop., 149:90, 1980.
3. Cooney, W. P., Dobyns, J. H., and Linscheid, R. L.: Nonunion of the scaphoid: Analysis of the results from bone grafting. J. Hand Surg., 5:343, 1980.
4. Gilberman, R. H., and Menon, J.: The vascularity of the scaphoid bone. J. Hand Surg., 5:508, 1980.
5. Goldner, R. D., Ugino, M. R., and Goldner, J. L.: Injuries to carpal bones. *In* Edlich, R. F., and Spyker, D. A. (Eds.): Current Emergency Medical Therapy. Norwalk, CT., Appleton-Century-Crofts, 1984, p. 159.
6. Green, D. P.: The effect of avascular necrosis on Russe bone grafting for scaphoid nonunion. J. Hand Surg., 10:1, 1985.
7. Herbert, T. J., and Fisher, W.: Management of the fractured scaphoid using a bone screw. J. Bone Joint Surg. [Br.], 66:114, 1984.
8. Leslie, I. J., and Dickson, R. A.: The fractured carpal scaphoid: Natural history and factors influencing outcome. J. Bone Joint Surg. [Br.], 63:225, 1981.
9. Mack, G. R., Bosse, M. J., Gelberman, R. H., and Yu, E.: The natural history of scaphoid nonunion. J. Bone Joint Surg. [Am.], 66:504, 1984.
10. Mayfield, J. K., Johnson, R. P., and Kilcoyne, R. K.: Carpal dislocations: Pathomechanics and progressive perilunar instability. J. Hand Surg., 5:226, 1980.
11. Palmer, A. K., Dobyns, J. H., and Linscheid, R. L.: Management of post-traumatic instability of the wrist secondary to ligament rupture. J. Hand Surg., 3:507, 1978.
12. Swanson, A. B.: Silicone rubber implants for the replacement of the carpal scaphoid and lunate bones. Orthop. Clin. North Am., 1:299, 1970.
13. Taleisnik, J.: The ligaments of the wrist. J. Hand Surg., 1:110, 1976.
14. Taleisnik, J., and Kelly, P. J.: The extraosseous and intraosseous blood supply of the scaphoid bone. J. Bone Joint Surg. [Am.], 48:1125, 1966.
15. Vender, M. I., Watson, K. H., Wiener, B. D., and Black, D. M.: Degenerative change in symptomatic scaphoid nonunion. J. Hand Surg. [Am.], 12:514, 1987.
16. Watson, H. K., Goodman, M. L., and Johnson, T. R.: Limited arthrodesis. Part II. Intercarpal and radial carpal considerations. J. Hand Surg., 6:223, 1981.
17. Zemel, N. P., Stark, H. H., Ashworth, C. R., Rickard, T. A., and Anderson, D. R.: The treatment of selected patients with an ununited fracture of the proximal part of the scaphoid by excision of the fragment and insertion of a carved silicone-rubber spacer. J. Bone Joint Surg. [Am.], 66:510, 1984.

V

FRACTURES AND DISLOCATIONS OF THE HAND

Richard D. Goldner, M.D., and J. Leonard Goldner, M.D.

The hands are exposed to many forces that can cause bone or joint trauma. Fractures of the metacarpals and phalanges are estimated to constitute 10% of all fractures; of these, fractures of the distal phalanx are the most common, followed in order by fractures of the metacarpals, the proximal phalanges, and the middle phalanges.

Joints in each digit have a direct effect on the total function of the involved and the adjacent digits. An extension contracture of the metacarpophalangeal (MCP) joint limits the degree of flexion in the adjacent digits; if the MCP joint is held in flexion, the adjacent fingers cannot be extended completely. If the proximal interphalangeal (PIP) joint has been injured and fibrosis occurs, the fingertip cannot be flexed to the distal palmar crease. If the distal interphalangeal (DIP) joint has been affected by a ruptured extensor tendon, the distal phalanx remains in flexion and interferes with dexterity of the involved digit and usually the adjacent digits.

Hand and finger injuries can be avoided by preventive medicine. Admonitions to children about placing their hands near sharp, moving objects and the same advice to adults working with machinery and participating in athletics are part of this effort to prevent soft tissue trauma, joint injuries, and fractures. When an injury occurs, the physician must be able to diagnose the pathologic process and provide patient care or direct the patient to an appropriate source of treatment.

FUNCTIONAL ANATOMY OF THE HAND

To diagnose and treat bone and joint injuries of the hand, the physician must understand the functional anatomy of the hand. The distal transverse crease on the palmar aspect of the wrist corresponds to the carpal bones. The radial and ulnar arteries, median and ulnar nerves, and flexor tendons are frequently injured at that level.

The transverse crease in the distal palm corresponds to the MCP joints. The proximal crease of the fingers is located in the midportion of the proximal phalanx, the middle crease is opposite the PIP joint, and the distal crease is opposite the DIP joint. These joints are active in flexion and extension. The distal phalanx includes the pulp or pad of the finger, the fingernail (nail plate), the nail bed, the nail matrix (germinal layer), the attachment of the extensor tendon, and the insertion of the flexor profundus tendon.

The middle phalanx is located between the proximal and distal phalanges and is covered dorsally by the extensor mechanism; the flexor superficialis inserts on the palmar surface. The tendon of the flexor digitorum profundus passes palmar to the middle phalanx after passing through the superficialis chiasm.

The proximal phalanx articulates with the metacarpal head. The oblique fibers of the lateral bands and the intrinsic tendons cover it on the radial and ulnar surfaces. The flexor tendons are on the palmar surface. The extensor tendon covers the dorsum of the proximal phalanx but is not firmly adherent to bone at that level. The proximal phalanx is longer than the middle or distal phalanges.

The metacarpal head articulates with the proximal phalanx. The large articular surface provides a wide range of flexion, extension, abduction, and adduction. The joint is stabilized by the extensor hood, the collateral ligaments, the dorsal capsule, and the palmar capsule.

The fourth and fifth metacarpals are mobile, the second and third are relatively stable, and the first metacarpal is hypermobile in comparison with the others. The first metacarpal has an epiphysis at its proximal end, as do the proximal phalanges of the fingers. The second through fifth metacarpals have an epiphysis at the distal end. Each tubular bone is divided anatomically into the base, shaft, neck, and head (articular).

The first digit (thumb) has one metacarpal, two phalanges, and independent intrinsic muscles, as well as extensors and flexors (extensor and flexor pollicis longus). Stabilization of the thumb and the carpometacarpal joint is dependent on extrinsic and intrinsic muscles and tendons and the supportive ligaments.

With flexion of the fingers, their line of action converges,

with the center of each nail pointing toward the scaphoid. Since none of the fingers is flexed in a straight line, the fingers should not be immobilized parallel to the long axis of the hand. To avoid malrotation, the proper position of digit immobilization is determined by observing the position of flexion in the normal, uninjured digits.

Dressings, splints, and plaster should hold the digits in the "intrinsic plus" position. This may include 60 to 80 degrees of flexion at the MCP joints, 10 to 20 degrees of flexion at the PIP joints, and 5 to 10 degrees of flexion at the DIP joints. With MCP joint flexion and interphalangeal (IP) joint extension, the collateral ligaments at the respective joints are elongated, thereby decreasing the likelihood of ligament contracture and subsequent joint stiffness. At times, however, the IP joint is immobilized in greater flexion to correct palmar angulation or to maintain proper rotational alignment.

All fingers have a flexor profundus tendon that inserts into the proximal segment of the distal phalanx and a flexor superficialis tendon that inserts into the middle phalanx. The thumb has a single flexor pollicis longus. These extrinsic muscles originate in the forearm.

The interosseous muscles that abduct and adduct the finger and the lumbricals that assist in flexing the MCP joints and extending the IP joints originate within the hand and are termed intrinsic muscles. The thumb intrinsics include the opponens pollicis, abductor pollicis brevis, flexor pollicis brevis, and adductor pollicis.

The three ulnar fingers must be flexed and extended almost in unison. Full flexion of the index finger requires partial flexion of the long and ring fingers. Individual variations occur. The thumb may be flexed almost completely without simultaneous action of the adjacent fingers, although about 10% of the population has a connection between the flexor digitorum profundus of the index finger and the flexor pollicis longus.

The extensor aspect of the hand contains the subcutaneous extensor digitorum communis tendons and the anatomic snuffbox, which is visible at the base of the thumb. The radial border consists of tendons of the extensor pollicis brevis and abductor pollicis longus; the ulnar border is the extensor pollicis longus. Branches of the superficial radial nerve and the radial artery lie in the anatomic snuffbox. There are multiple skin creases over the finger joints so that skin stretches and is not excessively tense when all joints are flexed.

CLINICAL EXAMINATION OF THE HAND

The injured part may be examined before obtaining the history or after details concerning the injury have been elicited, but a pattern of assessment should be followed consistently. This includes ascertaining the patient's age, sex, occupation, and hand dominance and obtaining accurate data concerning the injury (when, where, how, why). What was the time interval between injury and examination? Who treated the injury initially, and what was this treatment? Was the injury in a dirty or clean environment? Was it a bite? Did it occur at work? What was the mechanism of injury (crush, direct blow, twist)? For example, was the ball that injured the hand large or small, and did it hit the tip or the middle of the finger? Was the thumb twisted in the loop of the ski pole, or was it caught on the rope attached to the boat that was pulling the water skier out of the water? Other factors to consider in determining the most appropriate treatment are associated diseases, patient motivation, and socioeconomic factors.

The resting position of the hand is initially observed. If a flexor tendon has been avulsed, the digit rests in more extension than usual. Also, the physician should refer to the wrist, thumb, and finger motion of the normal hand in both flexion and extension to perform a more meaningful assessment of the injured hand. Swelling may follow hemorrhage or extravasation of joint fluid or edema fluid and may be confused with prominence of a displaced segment of the articular surface of the involved bone.

The circulation is tested by compressing the distal pulp adjacent to the nail for capillary refill, observing the color of the digit, and comparing the surface temperature with that of the adjacent digits. Often, the digital artery compression test (Allen's) cannot be performed because of pain or swelling; therefore, capillary refill is particularly helpful. A pale finger is usually the result of diminished arterial blood flow. A blue finger indicates venous congestion. Elevating and lowering the extremity may provide information about venous and arterial flow. After a hand injury, all jewelry should be removed immediately from the hand before increased swelling occurs and subsequent compression causes compromise of the digital arteries and nerves.

Sensibility is tested by determining light touch, deep pressure, two-point discrimination, and sharp point. The sensory deficit may be profound if the digital nerve was lacerated completely, or it may be minimal if the digital nerve was contused by trauma. In an open fracture, the assumption is that the digital nerve has been lacerated or at least severely contused if a sensory deficit exists.

Limitation of motor function may be caused by soft tissue injury, bone deformity, or pain. However, an attempt is made to determine active flexion and extension of the IP and MCP joints and rotation of the base of the thumb. Wrist motion is also tested.

The motion of joints may be limited by intra-articular or extra-articular damage or by injury to the extensor or flexor tendons. The latter indirectly limits distal or proximal IP joint motion or both. Each joint is tested by isolating it from the adjacent joints. The patient voluntarily attempts to flex the DIP joint, the PIP joint, and the MCP joint. The examiner must differentiate rebound motion from voluntary motion. For example, if the distal phalanx is flexed actively, the tip rebounds to extension when the flexor is released. This implies that the extensors are functioning, but actually they may not be. Conversely, active digit extension may be possible, and rebound flexion occurs when the extensor muscle is relaxed. Intrinsic function producing extension of the IP joints should not be confused with extensor digitorum communis action causing extension of the IP joints when the MCP joints are held in 90 degrees of flexion.

The involved digit is examined carefully to determine the site of disruption of bone and soft tissue. Precise areas of tenderness are palpated, such as the central slip (dorsal), the collateral ligaments (radial and ulnar), the palmar plate (volar), and the flexor and extensor tendon insertions. Stability of the joint is determined. Alignment of the digits is noted, and any angular or rotational deformities are corrected, since slight metacarpal or phalangeal malrotation may cause significant digit overlap.

Open wounds should be assessed relative to the mechanism of injury. A foreign body should be expected in any open or penetrating injury. Many objects are not radiopaque, such as wood, clothing, some forms of glass, and certain plastics.

Open wounds are examined cautiously, and both sides of the hand are inspected. Swelling on the dorsum may follow penetration of the volar surface. The examiner should wear a mask, use sterile gloves and instruments, and do minimal probing until adequate peripheral anesthesia has been obtained and the patient is in a location where definitive treatment can be completed. Open wounds should generally be treated in an operating room where clean air and adequate assistance, instrumentation, lighting, and equipment are available; where the traffic is limited; and where the patient and medical personnel can be protected from airborne and other infections.

TERMINOLOGY

A description of the alignment is as follows. *Dislocation* means that the articular surfaces are not opposed or congruous and that the restraining ligaments and probably the capsule have been partially or completely torn. *Subluxation* means a partial displacement of one side of the joint on the other, but with less severe distortion than a dislocation. Soft tissue interposition may prevent complete reduction in either instance. The term *reduction* refers to the action required to obtain anatomic alignment.

Fractures are described as stable, unstable, displaced, nondisplaced, impacted, comminuted, intra-articular, extra-articular, transverse, oblique, or spiral. Angulation may occur in any direction: dorsal, volar, radial, ulnar, or combinations. Malrotation may also occur. If there is no wound, the fracture is referred to as closed; if the skin is broken, the fracture is referred to as open.

RADIOGRAPHIC EXAMINATION

The exact location of the fracture—articular surface, epiphysis, neck, metaphysis, shaft, or base of the digit—is determined by radiographs. They indicate the type of fracture—complete, incomplete, transverse, oblique, spiral, or comminuted—as well as the position of the fractured bones, the amount of displacement of one segment relative to the other, and the angulation of the segments compared with a straight line and with the apex of angulation, either dorsal or volar. Correct rotation of the digit may be assessed radiographically by the relationship of the proximal-to-distal fractured segment but is best determined clinically by comparison with adjacent digits.

Multiple radiographic views of the involved hand or digit are essential for an accurate diagnosis. The usual views are posteroanterior, pronation and supination oblique, and true lateral. True lateral exposures must be obtained of the individual digits rather than of the entire hand, since in the latter case, the digits are overlapping.

Magnification views and tomography are helpful in determining occult fractures of the metacarpals or the phalanges. Occasionally, an arthrogram is helpful in assessing capsular or ligamentous injury to the joint. The xeroradiogram may be useful in determining the presence of nonradiopaque foreign bodies such as glass or wood in soft tissues. Radiographs should be obtained prior to reduction of the fracture or the dislocation in the emergency room. If vascular supply is compromised by the dislocation, arrangements are made to obtain the radiograph immediately. Stress views taken with the joint forced open in a direction away from the injured ligaments provide more information about the extent of the dislocated joint than does a plain exposure.

Radiographs taken postreduction or posttreatment are usually obtained through a plaster or fiberglass cast, an aluminum splint, or a hand dressing. A portable radiograph taken before the dressing is applied but after reduction is helpful when an intra-articular fracture is being manipulated before determining whether open reduction is required.

ANESTHESIA

Relief of pain associated with trauma is essential if diagnosis and treatment are to be successful. Sensory and motor examination must be completed, however, before a local or regional anesthetic is administered. Manipulation and re-alignment of a fractured phalanx require relaxation of the extensor and flexor tendons of the forearm.

Fractures of the phalanx or an intra-articular injury in the digit can be managed by local infiltration or by digital nerve block using lidocaine without epinephrine in the metacarpal area. Digital block is accomplished by injecting the anesthetic agent into the web space, where there is adequate area for swelling, or dorsally on either side of the metacarpal neck, with the needle being inserted palmarward toward the digital nerve.

A circular injection at the base of the digit is not advisable, and epinephrine should not be used in the hand. In certain instances, median or ulnar nerve block at the wrist and superficial radial nerve injection at the level of the styloid process of the radius are most effective.

If open reduction is necessary, intravenous regional anesthesia or axillary block may be preferred, since this allows greater tolerance of the tourniquet. This can be supplemented with systemic analgesia.

Because of the occasional occurrence of pneumothorax, supraclavicular block should be avoided unless it is done by experienced personnel. With severe injuries that require extensive reconstruction or distant bone graft, nerve grafts, or soft tissue coverage, general anesthesia is preferred.

Complications associated with the use of local or regional anesthesia are rare, but they occur, and the physician must be prepared to manage a patient who develops syncope, hypotension, seizures, and anaphylactic reactions. This mandates that even with local infiltration, one must have oxygen, a positive-pressure bag, an airway, and intravenous medications immediately available. Intravenous regional anesthesia should not be used in children or adults unless the physician is prepared to leave the tourniquet elevated for approximately 45 minutes so that the anesthetic can be fixed in the tissues of the forearm.

OPEN WOUNDS

At the time of the initial wound excision, all tight fascial compartments must be opened, open joints irrigated, and circulation established. Meticulous excision of devitalized tissue and thorough irrigation are essential to prevent infection. If the wound has been caused by a high-velocity missile, severe crush, human or animal bite, or high-pressure injury, no primary effort is made to repair digital nerves or flexor tendons. If internal fixation is required, pins placed through the extensor retinaculum should be avoided, because this compromises joint motion.

An open fracture should be managed with consideration of the blood supply of the digit, nerve and tendon injury, intrinsic muscle injury, and skin injury. The circulation should be restored as quickly as possible by direct repair of digital arteries, by vein grafts to segmentally damaged arteries and veins, or by releasing edematous soft tissue to decrease external pressure or vascular spasm. Digital nerves and lacerated flexor tendons do not always require primary repair. Open joints must be irrigated and properly dressed but can be maintained open for 24 to 48 hours covered with saline dressings without damage to the articular surfaces. Severe injuries are inspected again at 24 to 48 hours.

A stable skeleton decreases persistent irritation to the adjacent vascular structures and diminishes the possibility of infection in open wounds. However, elongation of the digit to its original length may compromise the circulation. Bone angulation should be corrected early, but not at the risk of damage to adjacent soft tissues. The concept of leaving open wounds open until it is safe to close them with direct suture or additional skin, or by allowing secondary healing, eliminates many complications that occur in wounds treated by both expert and less experienced personnel.

Antibiotics should be administered for contaminated wounds. First-generation cephalosporins are given for most open hand fractures. Antibiotic coverage for human bite wounds includes penicillin. When there has been extreme contamination such as from farm injuries, aminoglycosides such as tobramycin or gentamicin should be given with a cephalosporin and penicillin. All open fractures are considered tetanus-prone wounds, and the patient's tetanus immunization should be updated.

Crush injuries demand a high index of suspicion for compartment syndrome. Signs of pain with passive stretch in addition to paresthesias in the digit may be secondary to nerve compression or to the pain from fractures, but compartment syndrome should be considered. In assessing a crushed, swollen hand, compartment pressure determination is appropriate. If the compartment pressure is above 40 mm. Hg in a normotensive individual, compartment release is advocated. Fasciotomy of the intrinsic muscles of the hand may be accomplished through two dorsal longitudinal incisions between the second and third and the fourth and fifth metacarpals.

ANATOMIC REGIONS OF FRACTURES

Distal Phalanx and Distal Interphalangeal Joint

Distal Phalanx Fracture. The distal phalanx is frequently fractured by a crush from a hammer, a heavy object, or a door. The fracture is splinted for 10 to 14 days to decrease discomfort and allow healing. The fingernail may be elevated by a painful hematoma that is trapped between the nail plate and nail bed. It is released after the digit has been cleansed with soap and water and antiseptic by making a hole in the center of the nail plate with the round end of an open paper clip that has been heated in a flame or by a disposable ophthalmic cautery. If the nail bed has been lacerated, the nail plate should be removed and the laceration repaired with fine absorbable sutures.

Open Fracture of the Distal Phalanx. The most important aspect of an open fracture of the distal phalanx is the skin and soft tissue damage. Initial treatment consists of wound débridement. If the wound is grossly contaminated, it is treated open; it is closed at 3 to 5 days with a skin graft or shifting of local flaps if direct closure is not possible. If the wound is clean or can be converted to a clean wound by débridement, immediate skin grafting or local flaps can be used to provide closure.

Dorsal Avulsion Fracture. A dorsal segment of bone is elevated when the extensor digitorum communis is avulsed by an acute flexion or hyperextension injury. The superior aspect of the articular surface may constitute part of the fragment after extensor tendon continuity is lost at the distal joint, and a *drop finger* or *mallet finger* occurs. If the fragment is small (less than 40% of the joint surface, displaced less than 2 mm.), slight hyperextension with a dorsal aluminum splint on the distal and middle phalanges provides sufficient apposition to allow healing. If blanching of the skin or increased pain is noted, the phalanx should be placed in neutral position. The splint is used for a total of 8 to 12 weeks. Similar treatment is used for a mallet finger of tendon origin in which no fracture or avulsion is noted.

A fracture fragment attached to the extensor tendon should be treated as early as possible after the injury. Alignment and function can be obtained as late as 2 to 3 weeks after injury, but each week decreases the likelihood of maximal recovery. If the fracture fragment is displaced and is greater than 40%

of the articular surface, with volar subluxation of the distal phalanx, open reduction with suture and pin or screw fixation may be necessary. This type of treatment is not often required.

Avulsion of a Fragment from the Flexor Surface. This occurs when the flexor digitorum profundus is forcibly pulled from its distal phalangeal insertion, such as when the digit is hyperextended as a result of a blow or fall or from catching the digit (usually a ring) in a football jersey. Physical findings are swelling, the patient's inability to flex the distal joint, and a palpable mass at the base of the finger or in the palm. Radiographs may show the bone fragment in the digit.

Operative treatment is required to reattach the flexor tendon to the point of avulsion. This is usually performed with a polypropylene suture through the distal end of the tendon and attached to the tendon just proximal to the bone fragment. The suture is directed through the distal phalanx on either side of the fingernail and is tied over a button on the dorsum of the nail. Two interrupted sutures are also placed through the tendon and the fragment into the adjacent soft tissues. A dorsal plaster splint is applied from the fingertip to the elbow. Although several postoperative rehabilitation protocols are available, the repair should be protected for 4 to 6 weeks. Early protected passive motion is recommended.

Middle Phalanx and Proximal Interphalangeal Joint

The extrinsic muscles such as the extensor digitorum communis, flexor digitorum profundus, and flexor digitorum superficialis all affect the position of the fragments after phalangeal fractures. The force of the initial injury directs the distal or proximal fragment either dorsal or palmar, and the natural pull of the attached tendons either aggravates this or neutralizes it, depending on the exact location of the fracture.

The intrinsic muscle attachments also affect the position of the fragments by extension of the lateral band mechanism across the proximal phalanx, onto the sides of the PIP joint, and over the dorsum of the middle phalanx to the insertion of the tendon into the distal phalanx. Active muscular contraction of the lumbricals and the interosseous muscles influences the position of the fragments and the deformity of the digit. Fractures through the distal portion (neck) of the middle phalanx are likely to have apex palmar angulation, because the proximal fragment is flexed by the superficialis tendon. A fracture through the proximal portion (base) of the middle phalanx is likely to have apical dorsal angulation caused by flexion of the distal fragment by the superficialis and extension of the proximal fragment by the central slip of the extensor. Fractures through the middle two thirds may be angulated in either direction or not at all. Rotary deformities and radial and ulnar deviation depend on the intrinsic tendon pull as well as the force of the original injury.

Stable fractures can be immobilized initially in a splint followed by adjacent digit taping (buddy taping). Fractures that are stable after closed reduction are immobilized for approximately 3 weeks. Although the fracture may be protected for 6 to 8 weeks, gentle motion should be initiated at 3 to 4 weeks. A displaced, unstable fracture of the middle phalanx that cannot be reduced or maintained by external immobilization requires fixation either by percutaneous pins or by open reduction and internal fixation. Spiral and long oblique fractures are well suited for internal lag screw fixation.

The PIP joint is stabilized by the main and accessory collateral ligaments. Tears of the collateral ligament or avulsions cause temporary instability. Fragments of bone avulsed with the collateral ligaments may be detected radiographically. The palmar capsule prevents excessive hyperextension and limits malrotation. A tear of the capsule can occur either with or without the bone fragment attached to it.

A chip fracture at the PIP joint indicates either collateral ligament tear or marginal capsular avulsion; this is a relatively common injury. This radiographic finding may be a subtle suggestion of more extensive instability, but as long as the phalanx can be placed in anatomic alignment, in the position that decreases tension and stress on the collateral ligaments, adequate healing usually occurs. Large, displaced avulsion fractures with the collateral ligament attached are repaired surgically.

A nondisplaced condylar fracture should be splinted for 2 to 3 weeks. These fractures are followed closely, because displacement can occur after motion has been initiated. Displaced condylar fractures often cannot be adequately reduced and held by closed methods. Open reduction corrects incongruity of the articular surfaces; if uncorrected, this would cause traumatic arthrosis.

Dorsal Dislocation of the PIP Joint. Dislocations of the PIP joint are classified by the location of the middle phalanx in relation to the proximal (palmar, dorsal, lateral).

Dorsal dislocation of the middle phalanx with avulsion of the volar plate from the middle phalanx is a common injury. The PIP joint is swollen and may be mistaken for a "sprained finger." The lateral radiograph demonstrates displacement and often a small volar fragment from the proximal end of the middle phalanx. Treatment consists of regional metacarpal block; the elbow is flexed at right angles, the wrist is dorsiflexed, and traction in slight extension is applied to the digit and held for about 1 minute. As traction is exerted, flexion is continued to about 70 degrees while gentle but firm compression is applied over the dorsum of the middle phalanx. After reduction, the stability is tested, with attention to collateral ligament instability. A splint is then applied with the PIP joint flexed 20 to 30 degrees and is left on for 2 to 3 weeks. If the joint is completely stable, taping the involved digit to the adjacent one provides assistive motion and protects the joint.

Irreducible PIP joint dislocation may follow interposition of the collateral ligament, lateral band, or volar plate. Late problems such as flexion contracture can be treated with dynamic splinting; hyperextension deformity with instability is treated by reattachment of the volar plate or by flexor digitorum superficialis tenodesis.

Dorsal Fracture-Dislocation of the PIP Joint. Dorsal dislocation of the middle phalanx with displaced fracture of the volar portion is a serious injury (Fig. 42–20). Fractures of greater than 40% of the articular surface are usually unstable. If the fracture is reduced and is stable, it can be treated by a splint that blocks extension but allows flexion. The PIP joint is blocked at 15 degrees short of the point of instability (approximately 40 degrees). The joint is then extended 25% (10 degrees) each week. If reduction is not maintained and alignment of the joint cannot be re-established, an operative procedure is indicated. If the base of the middle phalanx is comminuted, options are to remove bone fragments surgically and advance the volar capsule into the defect or to apply a distraction-mobilization device to allow early motion.

Palmar Dislocation of the PIP Joint. Palmar dislocation of the middle phalanx may disrupt the central slip and dorsal capsule in addition to the palmar plate and one collateral ligament. This may cause a flexion deformity of the PIP joint and hyperextension of the DIP joint (boutonnière deformity). The central extensor mechanism is disrupted, and the lateral bands, which are normally dorsal to the axis of rotation of the PIP joint, slip palmar to that axis. Thus, the lateral bands, which normally extend the PIP joint, now flex the PIP joint and hyperextend the DIP joint. If PIP active extension is absent after reduction, the central attachment of the extensor tendon from the base of the middle phalanx has been disrupted. The PIP is then immobilized in extension for approximately 6 weeks with the DIP free to flex. Dorsal bone avul-

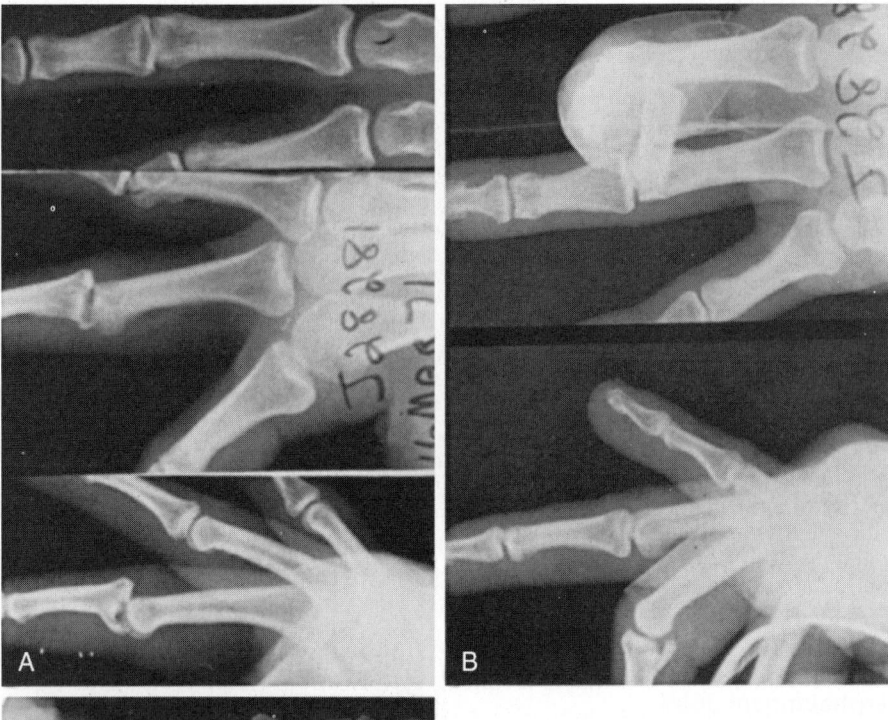

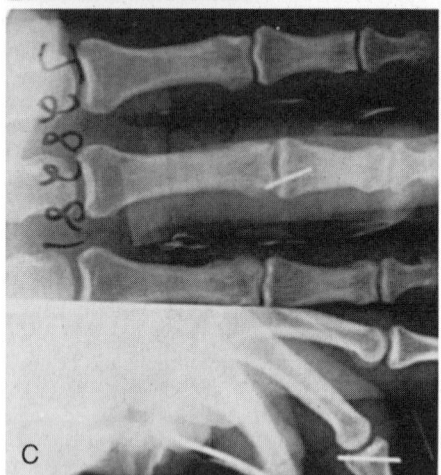

Figure 42–20. *A,* Proximal interphalangeal joint, dorsal fracture-dislocation with involvement of articular cartilage. Multiple views give a better representation of the fragments that are displaced. Both the dorsal capsule and the volar capsule are affected. *B,* The flexed lateral view shows where the volar capsule has been pulled off the proximal end of the proximal phalanx with a chip of bone, part of which is intra-articular. *C,* Fixation of the articular fragment with small fixation pins ensures articular congruity. However, cartilage damage and cartilage necrosis must be avoided in doing this kind of operation. The pins should not penetrate the joint, because this prevents early motion.

sion fractures from the middle phalanx with greater than 2 mm. displacement should be repaired.

Lateral Dislocation of the PIP Joint. Lateral PIP joint dislocation follows a lateral shear stress with collateral ligament disruption. The radial collateral is injured six times as frequently as the ulnar. Associated avulsion of the palmar plate and extensor mechanism at the base of the middle phalanx is noted. This is diagnosed clinically by stress testing and radiographically by assessing joint asymmetry. Whether operative treatment is necessary depends on the degree of lateral instability and the severity of the disruption of the extensor mechanism.

Proximal Phalanx

Fractures of the proximal phalanx can be oblique or transverse types. *Oblique* fractures through the shaft usually include a rotary component. The distal fragment may be displaced radially or ulnarly, and the condylar segment may be displaced either superiorly or inferiorly. An alternative type of injury is a *transverse* fracture, with resulting volar angulation. The interosseous muscles flex at the proximal fragment, and the extensor central slip extends the distal fragment.

Transverse Fracture of the Proximal Phalanx. A fracture through the midportion of the proximal phalanx with volar angulation presses the long flexor tendons and causes a flexion deformity at the PIP joint. Realignment of the fracture fragments restores active flexion at the PIP and DIP joints, whereas persistent palmar angulation causes adherence of the flexor tendons to the periosteum and bone fragments during healing and produces a fixed flexion contracture of the PIP joint and often of the DIP joint.

A shaft fracture with palmar angulation of the fragments is shown in Figure 42–21. Treatment requires adequate relaxation of the extrinsic and intrinsic muscles, usually achieved by regional nerve block. Manipulation is performed by flexing the distal segment of the phalanx while countertraction is applied to the proximal segment of the hand with the elbow flexed, the wrist dorsiflexed, and the MCP joint stabilized. Internal fixation, by percutaneous pins or by intraosseous wires, metal plate, and screws after open reduction, is required if the alignment cannot be maintained by plaster splint. A more proximal, malrotated, angulated fracture of the proximal phalanx is seen in Figure 42–22.

Oblique Fracture of the Proximal Phalanx. For treatment of an oblique fracture, the distal fragment is derotated and

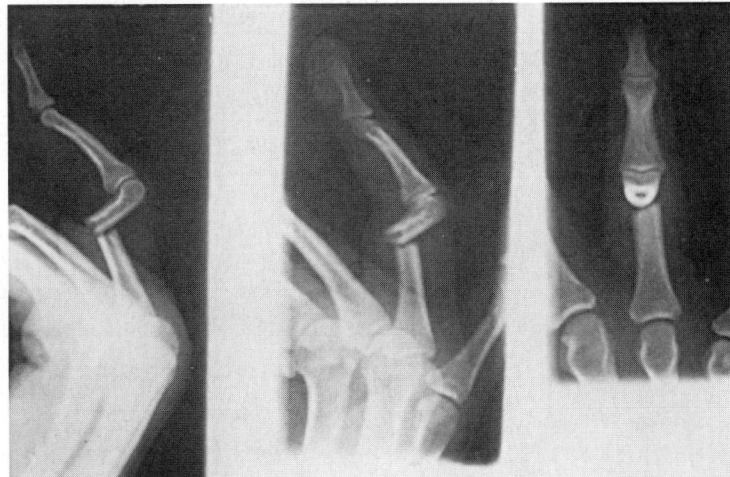

Figure 42–21. Fracture of proximal phalanx with apex volar angulation. Influence of the extensor tendon and intrinsic muscles affects the angulation.

the joints on either side of the phalanx are flexed. For dorsal angulation, the distal segment is extended and the MCP joint is flexed. When the angulation is palmar, the mobile distal fragment is placed in flexion, thereby bringing it into alignment with the proximal fragment. A metal dorsal splint incorporated in a short cast may be sufficient to maintain reduction. The wrist is held in dorsiflexion, and the MCP joints are flexed slightly. The rotation of the distal fragment is determined by the position of the fingernails when all joints are flexed. For fractures that can be reduced and held in a splint, immobilization for 3 weeks is necessary, after

which several weeks of protected motion are required. An interval change of splint ensures maintenance of position (Fig. 42–23). An oblique fracture of the proximal phalanx is likely to be unstable after closed reduction and often requires open reduction and internal fixation.

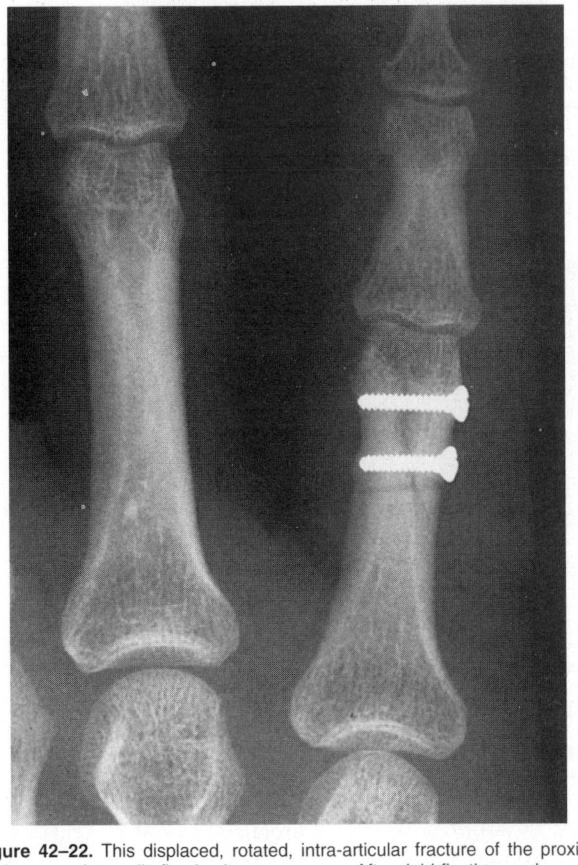

Dorsal Compression Fracture of the Proximal Phalanx. Proximal dorsal compression injuries of the proximal phalanx result when the distal fragment is forced dorsally and the proximal fragment is stabilized by the collateral ligaments. The dorsal cortex is compressed, and the angle between the articular surface and the shaft may be as much as 50 degrees. The muscle balance among the extensors, the flexors, and the intrinsic tendons is distorted. Edema on the dorsum of the digit causes additional deformity. A flexed position of the PIP joint occurs as a result of increased tension on the flexor digitorum superficialis. Radiographic diagnosis may be difficult because the anteroposterior film is misleading, since minimal radial or ulnar angulation occurs. The lateral view of the phalanges may be hidden by the adjacent digits, and the oblique view may not show the true extent of the deformity. A radiograph should be obtained with the digits in a position in which they are not overlapping completely, from both the radial and ulnar sides.

Treatment requires satisfactory regional block, counter- and straight traction, and a strong, forcible flexion manipulation with the collateral ligaments under tension when the MCP joints are flexed. The thumb of the physician should be directly under the proximal fragment as the fulcrum, and the index finger compresses volarly on the distal fragment. Immobilization is maintained with the MCP joints and the IP joints in flexion.

Intercondylar Fracture of the Proximal Phalanx. A condylar split fracture involving the distal end of the proximal phalanx is an intra-articular fracture. Collateral ligaments are attached to each of the condyles. Displacement of the condyles is demonstrated in Figure 42–24. Dorsal or palmar displacement of the condyles may complicate attempts to achieve alignment.

To reduce an intercondylar fracture of the proximal phalanges of the finger, direct longitudinal traction is applied to tighten the collateral and the retinacular ligaments and approximate the condyles. When the fragments are replaced and the middle phalanx is flexed, the position may be maintained by a palmar aluminum splint. A short plaster cast, to which is incorporated a palmar aluminum splint, is applied to the hand, the wrist, and the lower forearm (see Fig. 42–23). The involved digit is flexed at the MCP joint and the IP joint and held to the aluminum by tape, which is wrapped in

Figure 42–22. This displaced, rotated, intra-articular fracture of the proximal phalanx was internally fixed using two screws. After rigid fixation, early motion of the proximal interphalangeal (PIP) joint was begun to prevent stiffness of the joint.

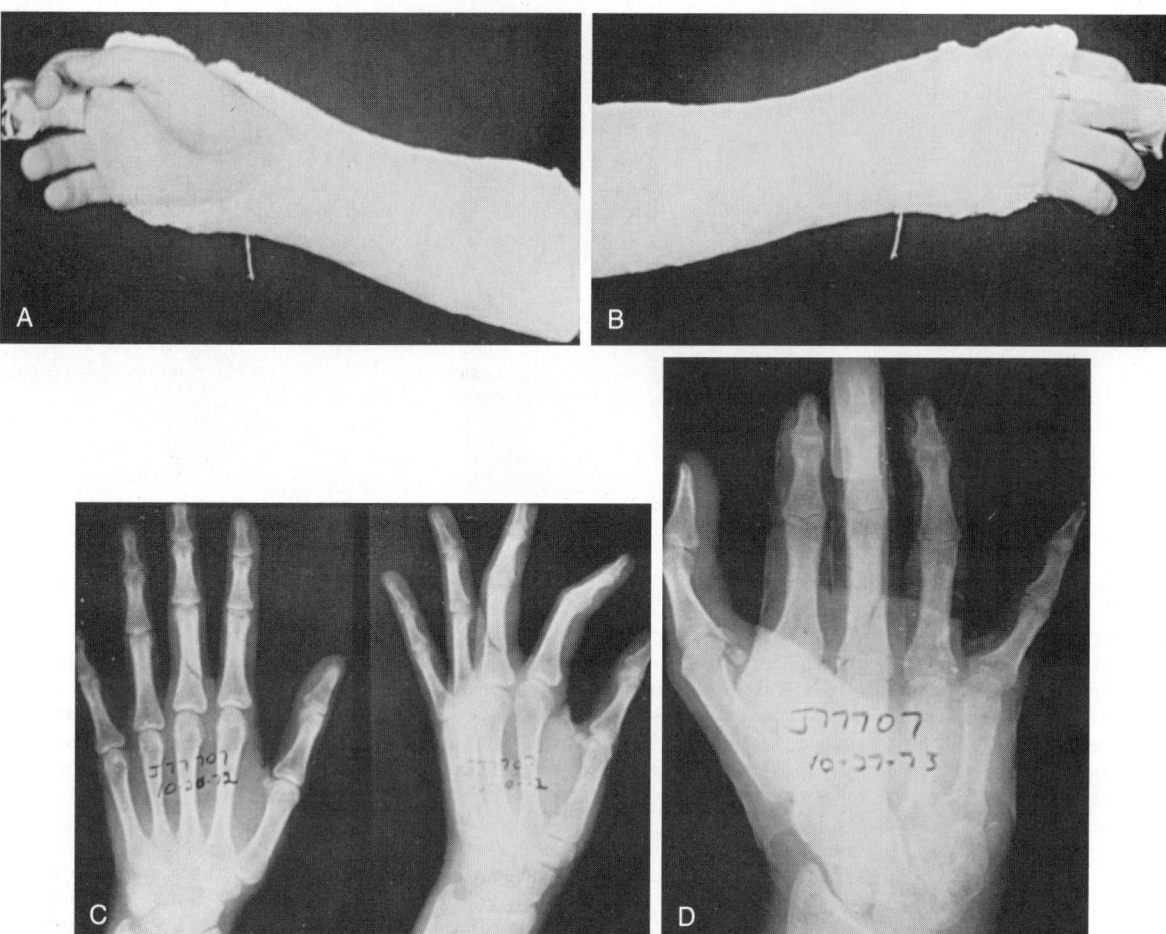

Figure 42–23. *A,* One method of managing phalangeal fracture. The plaster gauntlet serves as a base for the dorsal aluminum splint. The tape immobilizes the digit for a few days, and the dorsal splint blocks extension. The digital fragment of the phalanx is held in flexion, and early active motion is encouraged. *B,* Other digits are freely movable. The splint can be adjusted and the digit visualized throughout the entire treatment. *C* and *D,* Long oblique fracture with malrotation of the proximal phalanx. Pre- and postreduction and splinting. Open reduction and interfragmentary screw fixation allow anatomic alignment and early motion if the position cannot be maintained adequately in the splint.

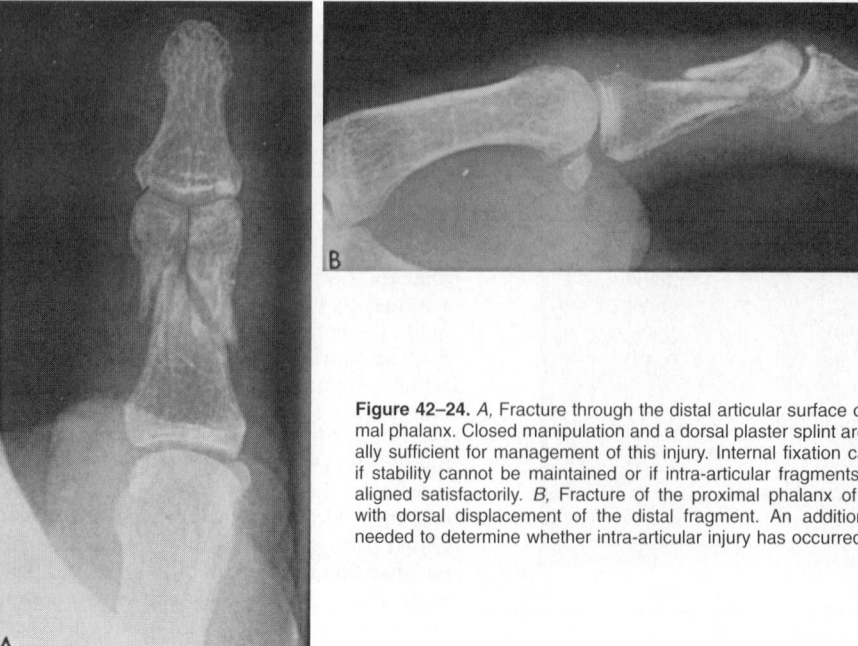

Figure 42–24. *A,* Fracture through the distal articular surface of the proximal phalanx. Closed manipulation and a dorsal plaster splint are occasionally sufficient for management of this injury. Internal fixation can be used if stability cannot be maintained or if intra-articular fragments cannot be aligned satisfactorily. *B,* Fracture of the proximal phalanx of the thumb with dorsal displacement of the distal fragment. An additional view is needed to determine whether intra-articular injury has occurred.

individual pieces, not under tension, and in such a way that each turn of tape overlaps the next most proximal turn to avoid edema. Rotation is corrected, and the nail plate is directed toward the radial aspect of the palm. The position is maintained for approximately 1 week, at which time the digit is retaped. Immobilization is continued for 3 weeks and the digit is protected for an additional 2 weeks, although an active range of flexion-extension is attempted several times a day.

If the condyles are malrotated and displaced greater than 2 mm., if adequate position cannot be obtained by manipulation, or if the reduction cannot be maintained, percutaneous pinning or open reduction with internal fixation of the condyles is performed. The latter procedure is usually necessary for fractures of one or both condyles of the proximal phalanx in order to prevent joint incongruity and angulation.

MCP Joint Dislocation. MCP joint dislocation follows a hyperextension force. The index finger is dislocated most frequently. If the palmar plate is avulsed from its origin and is trapped between the metacarpal head and the proximal phalanx, reduction is not possible by closed methods.

Open reduction is done through a palmar or dorsal approach. The palmar approach allows identification of the volar plate, the flexor tendons on the ulnar side, and the lumbrical on the radial side of the dislocated head. The radial digital nerve and artery to the index finger and the ulnar digital nerve and artery to the little finger are tethered over the metacarpal head and must be protected. Reduction is usually stable, and early motion with extension block splinting can be instituted.

Palmar MCP dislocation is uncommon and usually requires open reduction.

MCP Joint Collateral Ligament Injury. MCP joint collateral ligament rupture in the digits may occur with forced abduction. It most frequently affects the radial collateral ligament of the ulnar fingers but may also occur in the ulnar collateral ligament of the index finger. Discomfort to pressure is localized to the involved lateral aspect of the joint. The diagnosis is confirmed by stress radiographs. Treatment of acute injuries without ligament interposition consists of immobilization of the MCP joint in 30 degrees of flexion and slight overcorrection of the instability for 3 weeks, with 3 additional weeks of buddy taping.

Occasionally, an osteochondral fracture of the metacarpal head occurs and the segment is within the joint. If the avulsed chip of bone is displaced greater than 3 mm. or if the fragment involves greater than 20% of the articular surface and is displaced, operative treatment is indicated.

Epiphyseal Injury. Management of a fracture involving the physis requires knowledge about the different zones of the physis (region from which the bone grows). If the fracture damages the physis, growth can cease or can occur in an irregular manner. If the fracture is through the junction of the metaphysis and the diaphysis, growth is not disturbed and healing occurs rapidly. Displaced fragments of the epiphysis are assessed by appropriate radiographic studies. Anatomic reduction should be attempted so that the physeal plate is anatomically aligned and cartilage fragments are undisplaced for uniform healing and growth (Fig. 42–25).

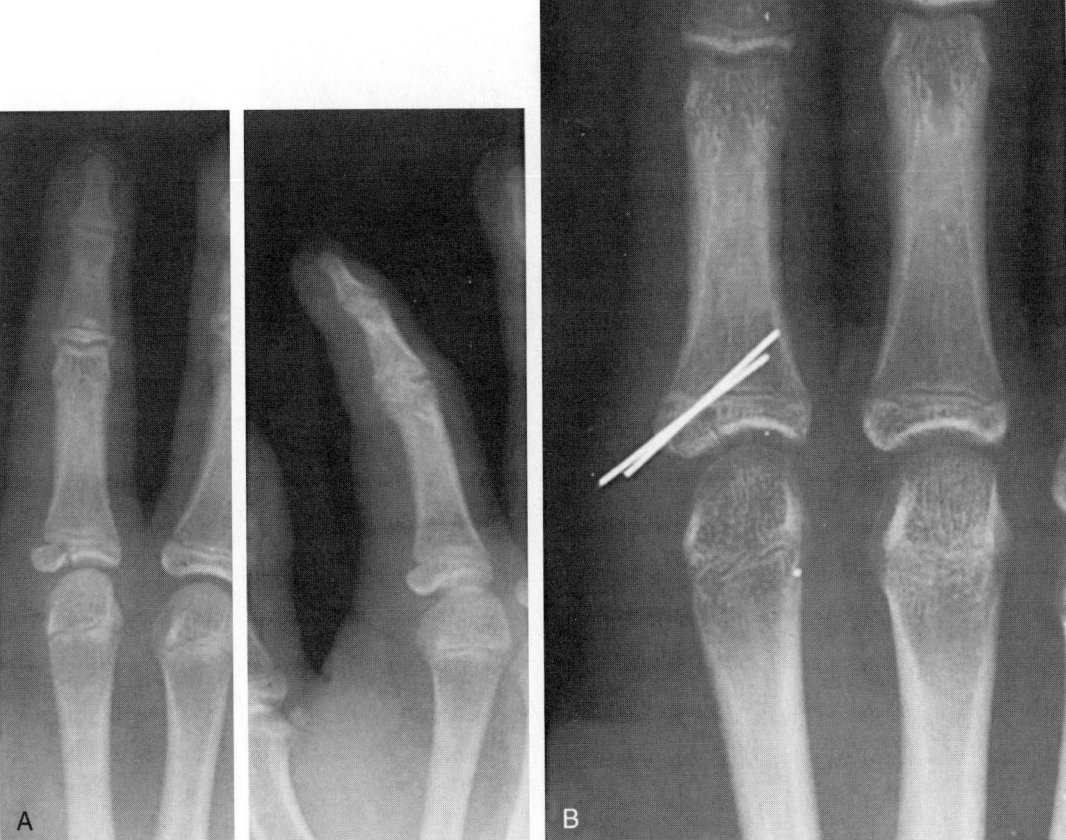

Figure 42–25. *A*, Intra-articular fracture of the proximal phalanx with osteochondral fracture attached to the collateral ligament. The lateral view shows probable rotation of the fragment. *B*, Open reduction and percutaneous pinning with 0.032 pins. The pins are subcutaneous and are left in place for approximately 3 weeks. Limited motion is initiated at 1 week, and active assistive motion is begun at 4 weeks.

The Metacarpals

Metacarpal fractures are divided as follows: (1) fractures of the metacarpal *head,* with intra-articular involvement and dorsal or palmar angulation of the fragments; (2) fractures of the metacarpal *neck,* with dorsal or palmar angulation and with a rotary element; (3) *transverse* fractures through the shaft of the metacarpal; (4) *oblique* fractures through the shaft of the metacarpal; and (5) *dislocation* at the base of the metacarpal. Nondisplaced metacarpal fractures are treated closed and immobilized for 3 weeks, followed by taping to the adjacent digit. Displaced fractures of the metacarpal head may require open reduction and internal fixation with small screws or wires. Severely comminuted fractures limited to the metacarpal head distal to the collateral ligament should be treated with early protected motion. Large articular fragments with collateral ligament avulsion may require open reduction and internal fixation. The Brewerton radiograph view is obtained with the MCP joint flexed 65 degrees, the dorsum of the hand next to the plate, and the x-ray apparatus angled 15 degrees ulnar to radial. This helps visualize fractures of the metacarpal head.

A fracture of the neck of the fifth metacarpal is a common injury caused by a direct blow. This is known as a boxer's fracture and occurs from a dorsal force applied directly to the metacarpal head. The head is displaced palmarward, the shaft bows dorsally, and the tip of the little finger rotates toward the radial side of the palm. Considerable soft tissue swelling usually occurs, and the alignment of the fragments cannot be determined from external examination. Radiographs show the angulation on the oblique and lateral views. Up to 40 to 45 degrees of dorsal angulation is acceptable in the fifth metacarpal, and approximately 30 degrees is acceptable in the fourth metacarpal; but in the index and long metacarpals, anatomic reduction is desirable because of the relative lack of mobility of the shaft. Angulation greater than 15 degrees is unacceptable secondary to the lack of compensatory carpometacarpal motion. Rotation alignment should be restored in all fingers.

Fractures with less than 15 degrees of angulation can be treated with an ulnar gutter splint for 10 to 14 days for the patient's comfort. Fractures with 15 to 40 degrees of angulation are reduced and splinted for 3 weeks with the MCP joint flexed 50 to 70 degrees and the PIP joint flexed no more than 20 to 30 degrees.

Closed reduction can be achieved with MCP and PIP joints flexed to tighten the collateral ligaments. Momentary pressure is exerted dorsally on the 90-degree flexed proximal phalanx, and counterpressure is directed palmarward on the metacarpal shaft. It is not desirable to immobilize the fracture in this position, however, because secondary stiffness, malrotation, clawing, angulation, and skin problems may be greater than the functional loss that occurs with no treatment.

For fractures with greater than 40 degrees of angulation and palmar comminution of the neck and extensor lag, percutaneous pinning or occasionally open reduction and internal fixation may be necessary (Fig. 42–26).

Transverse and Short Oblique Metacarpal Shaft Fractures. *Transverse shaft fractures* are often caused by a direct blow, with dorsal angulation secondary to exertion of palmar force by the interosseous muscles. The more proximal the fracture, the less the angulation. The intermetacarpal ligaments prevent shortening, and the interosseous muscles stabilize the digits. If the fracture is minimally displaced, it can be controlled with a well-molded short-arm cast with a dor-

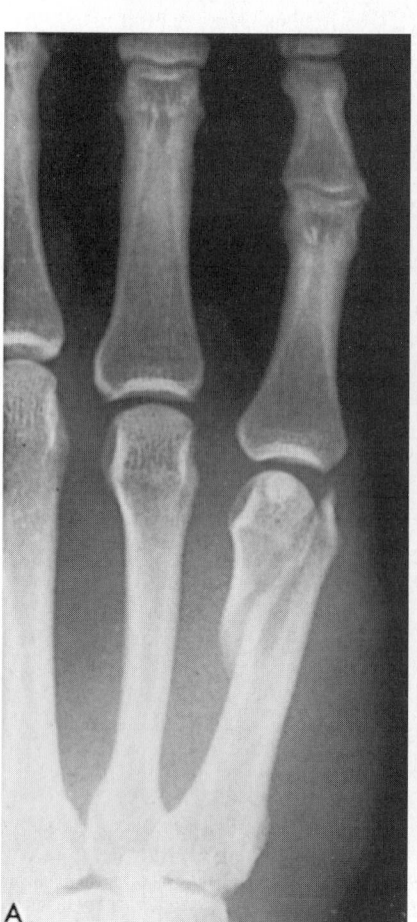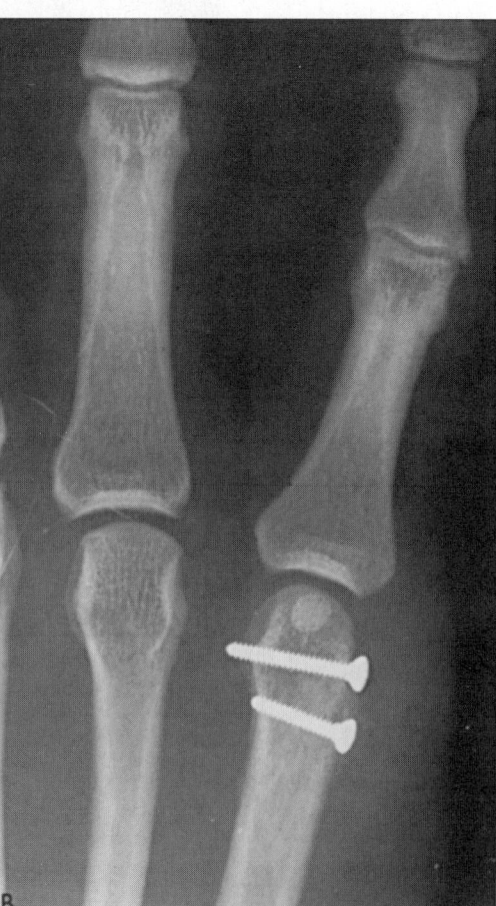

Figure 42–26. *A,* Spiral oblique intra-articular fracture with shortening and malrotation. The options for treatment are (1) manual traction and percutaneous pinning under image intensifier, (2) gauntlet plaster splint with aluminum extension on the volar aspect of the digit for slight traction and elongation of the fragments, and (3) open reduction and transfixation screw. *B,* In this instance, open reduction was selected, and anatomic alignment has been established.

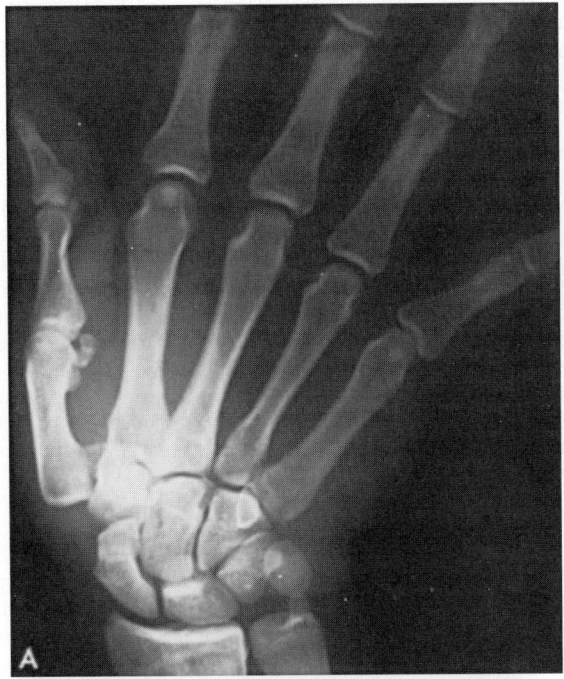

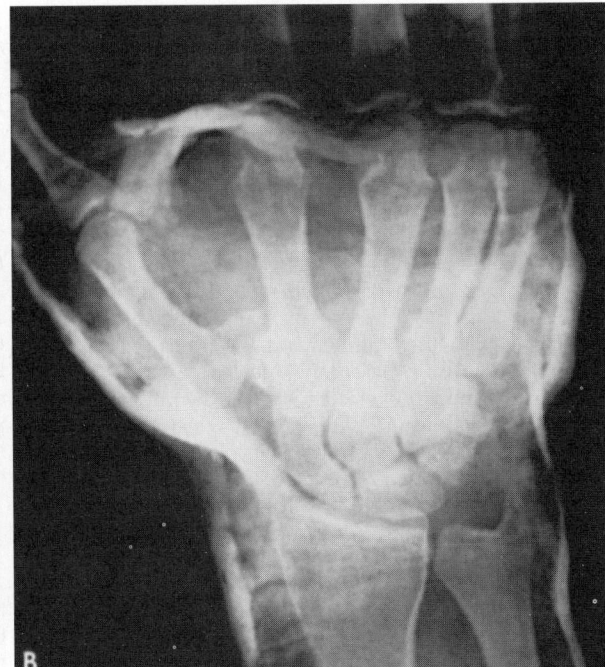

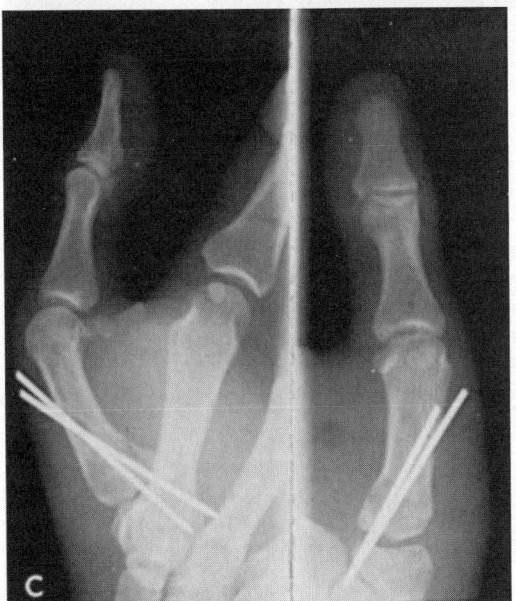

Figure 42–27. *A,* Bennett's fracture at the base of the first metacarpal. This involves the articular surface. The deformity is aggravated by pull of the abductor pollicis longus and the adductor pollicis. *B,* Realignment and reduction were attempted by extension traction. This is usually not successful if the metacarpal is displaced. The position for improving position is 45-degree abduction of the thumb from the palm rather than extension, external rotation. *C,* Anatomic position was regained by radial deviation and dorsiflexion of the hand and longitudinal traction abduction of the thumb. As traction was maintained, percutaneous 0.045 pins were inserted across the metacarpal and into the trapezium. At least two views are essential to document proper reduction. Pins are left in place for 4 weeks, and the thumb is protected for 6 weeks.

sal aluminum splint extending over the proximal phalanx with the MCP joints flexed 60 degrees. It is kept on for 4 to 6 weeks.

Indications for internal fixation include any persistent rotational deformity and uncorrected dorsal angulation greater than 10 degrees in the second or third metacarpal or greater than 20 degrees in the fourth or fifth metacarpal. Shortening more than 3 mm. or multiple displaced fractures usually require treatment of the adjacent soft tissues. Internal fixation of long oblique or spiral fractures with interfragmentary screw fixation controls excessive shortening and angulation and allows early motion of the digits.

Malunion of a metacarpal fracture with dorsal angulation that disturbs the intrinsic balance and produces metacarpal head prominence in the palm and pain on gripping requires an osteotomy. Other complications are nonunion, MCP extension contractures, intrinsic muscle contractures, and tendon adhesions.

Long, oblique, or spiral metacarpal fractures, minimally displaced, are treated by splinting. Displaced fractures that are not able to be reduced adequately or that are unstable after reduction are best treated by lag screw fixation.

Dislocation at the metacarpal-carpal joint usually requires pin stabilization.

Thumb Metacarpal Fractures. Fractures at the base of the thumb are usually caused by a fall on the hand, a twisting mechanism that involves the projected thumb, or a direct blow of the fist against a firm object. Lesions are classified as follows: (1) *intra-articular fracture* through the proximal end of the metacarpal, leaving a fragment held by the intermetacarpal ligament, and the base of the metacarpal displaced laterally out of the joint by pull of the abductor pollicis longus (Bennett's fracture, Fig. 42–27*A*); simultaneously, the adductor pollicis pulls the proximal phalanx and distal metacarpal toward the palm and the proximal metacarpal away from its base; (2) a *comminuted intra-articular fracture* of the proximal end of the metacarpal (Rolando's fracture); and (3) *fracture through the metaphysis,* extra-articular, with angulation dorsal or volar. Other variations may occur.

Treatment of a displaced thumb fracture depends on the type of injury. The *intra-articular fracture* with two segments (Bennett's) is managed as illustrated in Figure 42–27C. Force, directed inward, is applied at the base of the metacarpal. Traction is provided simultaneously, as is abduction and extension of the metacarpal head. A pin inserted percutaneously just distal to the articular surface of the first metacarpal and directed toward the base of the second metacarpal in line with the neck of the third metacarpal should allow the first metacarpal shaft, the fragment on the intermetacarpal ligament, and the base of the second metacarpal to be held adequately to maintain the reduction. This is followed by application of a light plaster splint or cast, which maintains the position described. The pin remains in place for 4 weeks, after which protected motion is initiated. Open reduction and internal fixation are indicated if soft tissue is interposed between the fragments or if a large fragment is malrotated and prevents joint congruity.

A comminuted fracture at the base of the metacarpal (Rolando's) may be treated either by percutaneous pin fixation or by traction obtained by placing a transfixion pin through the base of the proximal phalanx or neck of the metacarpal. If the palmar and dorsal fragments are large and cannot be reduced anatomically, open reduction and internal fixation can be considered.

A fracture at the proximal metaphysis of the thumb metacarpal, which does not include the joint, is managed by manipulation, realignment, and plaster fixation, with the thumb in wide abduction and the MCP joint in flexion. Extra-articular fractures of the thumb metacarpal are reduced and placed in a short-arm–thumb spica cast for about 4 weeks. Twenty to 30 degrees of angulation usually causes no functional loss. If plaster immobilization is unsuccessful in treating an oblique fracture, percutaneous pinning or interfragmentary screw fixation is considered.

Injuries to the MCP joint of the thumb include chip fractures of the ulnar collateral ligament; the fragment is avulsed from the proximal phalanx or from the distal metacarpal. The ligament can also rupture in its central portion or pull from bone without a fracture. In addition to the collateral ligament injury, the palmar plate and the dorsal capsule are usually torn, causing the phalanx to displace palmarward and radially. In most instances, these injuries are detected by clinical examination (carpometacarpal flexion, MCP flexion with stress). The stress radiograph is not essential, but if there is any question about the extent of soft tissue injury, a stress radiograph under local or regional block may be helpful.

If there is less than 30 degrees difference between the injured and uninjured thumb, incomplete tear is diagnosed. Treatment of an incomplete tear can be managed satisfactorily by application of a plaster or fiberglass cast that holds the phalanx in the neutral adducted position and realigns the metacarpal and the phalanx. A cast is applied for a minimum of 4 weeks, and protection with hand-based splints is necessary for 4 additional weeks, during which time range-of-motion exercises are performed several times a day.

If there is greater than 30 degrees difference, complete tear is diagnosed and operative repair is usually indicated. When examination indicates that the collateral ligament is torn completely and could be caught outside the adductor aponeurosis and not heal (Stener's), or when the individual is unwilling to undergo 6 weeks of immobilization with no guarantee of stability, open operation is recommended. Displaced intra-articular fractures involving more than 15% to 20% of the

articular surface and a small avulsion fracture displaced more than 5 mm. are relative indications for open reduction.

Dorsal subluxation of the proximal phalanx at the MCP level may cause a partial tear of the capsule and displacement of the dorsal capsule and extensor mechanism. Relocation is not difficult, and immobilization in the flexed position is usually sufficient. A serious articular and vascular injury may occur with complete dislocation of the metacarpal head and displacement of the proximal phalanx. The head protrudes through a tear in the capsule, and the palmar plate may be interposed in the joint (Fig. 42–28). If a dislocation is unrecognized, vascular insufficiency may occur. Amputation has followed this type of injury as a result of inadequate early reduction or failure to recognize the dislocation, which can occlude the digital arteries. One must be prepared to proceed with an open operation if replacement of the fragments is not done with relative ease and without excessive manipulative forces.

GENERAL PRINCIPLES OF TREATMENT

Stable fractures (undisplaced or impacted) without angulation or rotation may be treated by taping the injured digit to the adjacent one and beginning early, protected, active motion. Clinical and radiographic follow-up during the first several days is necessary. Joint dislocations require support after reduction to allow ligamentous healing for stability and to provide comfort. Less stable fractures are often treated by closed reduction and immobilization; when the fracture is unstable and cannot be maintained by external immobilization, open operation is recommended.

In many instances, athletes are treated by plastic tape and

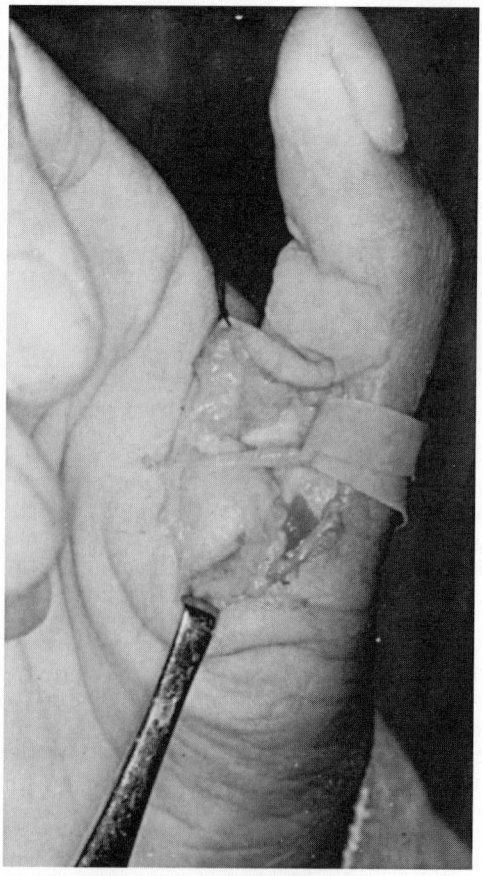

Figure 42–28. Dislocation of the metacarpophalangeal joint of the thumb with flexor tendon and capsule preventing relocation. Open operation is necessary.

splint fixation with strong immobilization. This allows them to continue their athletic endeavors without the interruption of an operative procedure.

Splints, plaster casts, and molded thermoplastic material provide support for certain fractures. A dorsal aluminum or plastic splint held by tape can be used for a mallet finger, a dislocated joint, a small chip fracture, or a stable oblique fracture. The splint need not be complicated or extensively padded. It is usually applied without padding and can be bent to contour, but it must be narrower than the width of the finger. It should be firm enough to require bending with a lightweight pair of wire benders or the arms of a pair of bandage scissors. If the splint can be bent easily by the fingers, it is not strong enough. When possible, a splint should be applied to the dorsal rather than the palmar surface of the digit so that the palmar tip of the finger can be used even with the splint applied. The end of the splint may be bent over the tip of the finger, depending on the type of injury. If a slight amount of elongation and traction of the fracture and the digit is needed, palmar or dorsal splints can be incorporated into a plaster gauntlet, and the digit can be held to the splint with tape after slight traction is applied and the splint is bent.

Plaster splints are useful and readily available for hand fractures. The position of the wrist, MCP joints, and IP joints determines the success of plaster splint treatment. The wrist is dorsiflexed to stabilize the metacarpals and relax the extensor tendons. The MCP joint should be flexed at least 60 degrees to ensure proper rotation and to avoid contracture of the collateral ligaments. The IP joints should be extended or flexed, depending on the type of injury. Plaster splints can be about six thicknesses, covered by sheet cotton, and applied directly to the skin with a small amount of protective padding over the involved area. The bony prominences are padded with felt. The splint is applied when wet, and the hand and the digit are held in the appropriate position. The splints are then wrapped by narrow sheet cotton and by bias-cut stockinette or more plaster. An uninvolved digit is usually included for additional protection. The hand should be elevated above the heart level for several days after the injury in order to decrease swelling. The initial plaster splint is often changed in 5 to 6 days when the swelling has decreased. Radiographs and clinical examination confirm adequate position of the fracture after changing of the splint or cast.

Prolonged periods of immobilization of fractures of the hand are not necessary. The radiograph is not a good guide to the length of time that the hand should be immobilized. Complete bone healing of hand fractures is not demonstrable by radiographs for approximately 5 months. With the exception of the mallet and boutonnière chip fractures, 3 to 4 weeks is usually sufficient time for immobilization of most fractures and ligamentous injuries. Protection is continued for an additional 3 to 4 weeks, but range-of-motion exercises are initiated promptly. Fractures of the midshaft region of the phalanges require protection for 5 to 7 weeks, and middle phalanx fractures even longer.

Dislocation of joints requires support after reduction to allow ligamentous healing for stability and to provide comfort to the patient. Fractures that are too unstable to be maintained by external immobilization usually require fixation of the fragments to allow healing with proper alignment and to permit early motion.

Open reduction is indicated in dislocations that are irreducible by closed means. Internal fixation, either percutaneous (K wires) or after open reduction (K wires, interosseous wiring, interfragmentary screws, miniplates and screws), is considered for irreducible or very unstable fractures, multiple-level fractures, displaced intra-articular fractures, and certain open hand injuries. External fixation with small threaded half-pins articulated with clamps and bars is used to stabilize fractures with extensive soft tissue injury. This provides access for wound care and maintains bone alignment even with extensive comminution or segmental bone loss. Certain severely comminuted intra-articular fractures cannot be reconstructed adequately and are best treated by arthrodesis of the joint. During internal fixation of a fracture, efforts are made to achieve stability of the fracture while deformities are corrected, including malrotation and angulation. Joints are not crossed by pins unless absolutely necessary.

The treatment of hand fractures is directed toward regaining flexible, properly aligned, strong digits with adequate vascular supply and sensibility. One common complication is decreased motion secondary to tendon adhesions or ligament and capsular contracture. This condition is often improved by active exercises and by dynamic splinting. Occasionally, however, these conditions require tendolysis or surgical release of joint capsules or ligaments. Malunion (malrotation, angulation) can be corrected by osteotomy, and nonunion can be corrected by bone grafting and rigid internal fixation if necessary. Infections may occur with open fractures or with those fractures treated by open reduction and internal fixation. The infection is usually treated by surgical débridement and antibiotics.

SELECTED REFERENCES

Dray, G. J., and Eaton, R. G.: Dislocations and ligament injuries in the digits. *In* Green, D. P. (Ed.): Operative Hand Surgery, 3rd ed. Vol. 1. New York, Churchill Livingstone, 1993, p. 767.
This chapter provides detailed information, illustrations, and a comprehensive bibliography on treating dislocations and ligament injuries in the digits.

Green, D. P., Rowland, S. A., and Buckely, R. W.: Fractures and dislocations in the hand. *In* Rockwood, C. A., and Green, D. P. (Eds.): Fractures in Adults, 2nd ed. Philadelphia, J. B. Lippincott, 1991, p. 441.
These authors detail the pathoanatomy of, the various methods of treating, and the preferred method of managing fractures and dislocations of the hand. Illustrations, photographs, and an extensive bibliography strengthen this comprehensive chapter.

Stern, P. J.: Fractures of the metacarpals and phalanges. *In* Green, D. P. (Ed.): Operative Hand Surgery, 3rd ed. Vol. 12. New York, Churchill Livingstone, 1993, p. 695.
This chapter provides detailed information, illustrations, and a comprehensive bibliography on treating hand fractures.

REFERENCES

1. Belsky, M. R., Eaton, R. G., and Lan, L. B.: Closed reduction and internal fixation of proximal phalangeal fractures. J. Hand Surg. [Am.], *9:*725, 1984.
2. Black, D. M., Mann, R. J., Constine, R. M., and Daniels, A. U.: The stability of internal fixation in the proximal phalanx. J. Hand Surg. [Am.], *11:*672, 1986.
3. Black, D. M., Mann, R. J., Constine, R. M., and Daniels, A. U.: Comparison of internal fixation techniques in metacarpal fractures. J. Hand Surg. [Am.], *10:*466, 1985.
4. Bowers, W. H.: The proximal interphalangeal joint volar plate II: A clinical study of hyperextension injury. J. Hand Surg. [Am.], *6:*78, 1981.
5. Conrad, R. W., and Goldner, J. L.: A study of the pathological findings and treatment in soft tissue injury of the thumb metacarpophalangeal joint. J. Bone Joint Surg. [Am.], *50:*439, 1968.
6. Dabezies, E. J., and Schutte, J. P.: Fixation of metacarpal and phalangeal fractures with miniature plates and screws. J. Hand Surg. [Am.], *11:*283, 1986.
7. Duncan, J., and Kettelkamp, D. B.: Low-velocity gunshot wounds of the hand. Arch. Surg., *109:*395, 1974.
8. Eaton, R. G., and Malerich, M. M.: Volar plate arthroplasty of the proximal interphalangeal joint: A review of ten years' experience. J. Hand Surg. [Am.], *5:*260, 1980.
9. Fyfe, I. S., and Mason, S.: The mechanical stability of internal fixation of fractured phalanges. Hand, *11:*50, 1979.
10. Goldner, J. L.: Trauma to the extensor mechanism at its attachment to the distal phalanx of the digits. *In* Current Practice in Orthopaedic Surgery. St. Louis, C. V. Mosby, 1964, p. 143.
11. Hunter, J. M., and Cowen, N. J.: Fifth metacarpal fractures in a compensation clinic population. J. Bone Joint Surg. [Am.], *52:*1159, 1979.
12. James, J. P.: Fractures of the proximal and middle phalanges of the fingers. Acta Orthop., *32:*401, 1962.

13. Kaplan, E. B.: Dorsal dislocation of the metacarpophalangeal joint of the index finger. J. Bone Joint Surg. [Am.], 39:1081, 1957.
14. Lister, G.: Intraosseous wiring of the digital skeleton. J. Hand Surg. [Am.], 3:427, 1978.
15. McCue, F. C., Honner, R., Johnson, M. C., Jr., and Gieck, J. H.: Athletic injuries of the proximal and interphalangeal joint requiring surgical treatment. J. Bone Joint Surg. [Am.], 52:937, 1970.
16. McElfresh, E. C., and Dobyns, J. H.: Intra-articular metacarpal head fractures. J. Hand Surg. [Am.], 8:383, 1983.
17. McElfresh, E. C., Dobyns, J. H., and O'Brien, E. T.: Management of fracture-dislocation of the proximal interphalangeal joints by extension-block splinting. J. Bone Joint Surg. [Am.], 54:1705, 1972.
18. Neviaser, R. J., Wilson, J. N., and Lievano, A.: Rupture of the ulnar collateral ligament of the thumb (gamekeeper's thumb): Correction by dynamic repair. J. Bone Joint Surg. [Am.], 52:1357, 1971.
19. Peimer, C. A., Sullivan, D. J., and Wild, D. R.: Palmar dislocation of the proximal interphalangeal joint. J. Hand Surg. [Am.], 9:39, 1984.
20. Meals, R. A. (Ed.): Problem fractures of the hand and wrist. Clin. Orthop. Rel. Res., 214, 1987.
21. Stark, H. H., Boyes, J. H., and Wilson, J. N.: Mallet finger. J. Bone Joint Surg. [Am.], 44:1061, 1962.
22. Stener, B.: Displacement of the ruptured collateral ligament of the metacarpophalangeal joint of the thumb. J. Bone Joint Surg. [Br.], 44:869, 1962.
23. Vanik, R. K., Weber, R. C., Matloub, H. S., Sanger, J. R., and Gingrass, R. P.: The comparative strengths of internal fixation techniques. J. Hand Surg. [Am.], 9:216, 1984.
24. Wehbe, M. A., and Schneider, L. H.: Mallet fractures. J. Bone Joint Surg. [Am.], 66:658, 1984.
25. Wilson, J. N., and Rowland, S. A.: Fracture-dislocation of the proximal interphalangeal joint of the finger. J. Bone Joint Surg. [Am.], 48:493, 1966.

VI

FRACTURES OF THE PELVIS, FEMUR, AND KNEE

Thomas Parker Vail, M.D., and Donald E. McCollum, M.D.

Major lower extremity trauma includes fractures of the pelvis and the femur as well as injuries to the knee joint. This chapter covers fractures of the pelvis, including injuries to the pelvic ring and sacrum, and the array of acetabular fractures. Fractures of the femur are divided into fractures of the femoral neck, the intertrochanteric region of the femur, the femoral shaft, and the distal femur. The divisions are not based simply on arbitrary anatomic differences but have a bearing on treatment and outcome. Finally, fractures of the intra-articular portion of the knee include not only fractures of the distal femur but also fractures of the patella and dislocations of the knee not associated with bone disruption.

High-energy trauma is usually responsible for fractures of the major weight-bearing bones. Massive trauma can follow motor vehicle accidents in which the passenger remains within the vehicle, is ejected from the vehicle, or is struck by a vehicle. In addition, a fall from a height or other types of blunt impact can produce these injuries. Elderly patients can sustain injuries to the pelvis and lower extremities from lesser trauma. These patients are predisposed to injury from senile or pathologic osteoporosis and from other less frequently observed conditions such as radiation-induced osteoporosis. The injuries associated with osteoporosis and lesser magnitudes of energy are frequently not life threatening, except for those patients who are debilitated from age or sickness. Major pelvic fractures associated with high-energy trauma are, however, frequently life threatening.[8, 12] Death may occur in as many as 20% of patients with high-energy pelvic trauma, especially with fractures associated with a large degree of displacement, hemorrhage, open wounds, and injury to the abdominal organs. Many organ systems can be involved in trauma associated with major lower extremity injuries, including retroperitoneal hemorrhage, neurologic damage from the lower end of the spinal cord to the peripheral nerves, genitourinary damage, and damage to major blood vessels. In addition, injury to the pelvis and lower extremities can be associated with head injury and injury to the upper extremities, making it mandatory that the initial examiner be diligent in looking for associated head and musculoskeletal trauma.

FRACTURES OF THE PELVIS

Pelvic Ring and Sacrum

Tile[17] has classified pelvic injuries by the mechanism of injury: anteroposterior compression, lateral compression, and vertical shear. An anteroposterior compression injury occurs when a patient is struck from the front by the bumper of a car, the dashboard, or the gas tank of a motorcycle in a straddle-type injury. There is disruption of the symphysis anteriorly and disruption of the anterior ligaments of the sacroiliac (SI) joint. The pelvis thus opens like a book, initially leaving the posterior ligaments of the sacroiliac joint intact and tearing those ligaments with higher-energy impact. Lateral compression injuries can result in fracture of one or both pubic rami, with concomitant fracture of the sacrum or iliac wing. Lateral compression injuries are also associated with a higher incidence of head injury compared with other types of pelvic ring trauma.[1] Vertical shear injuries follow axial loading, as in a fall from a height or a head-on collision, where energy is transmitted directly up the leg. A vertical shear injury may include fracture of one or both pubic rami or disruption of the symphysis pubis, along with associated disruption posteriorly through the SI joint, the ilium lateral to the SI joint, the sacrum, or a combination. A displaced vertical shear injury of more than 1 cm. is generally considered unstable (Fig. 42–29).

Other fractures of the pelvic ring that do not disrupt the continuity of the ring include fractures of the ilium, unilateral fractures of the pubic rami, and avulsion fractures at points of muscle attachments. Avulsion fractures can occur by forcible contraction of the associated muscle. These fractures include avulsions of the anterosuperior spine, the ischium, and the anteroinferior spine. These injuries are generally treated with restricted weight bearing, use of crutches, and pain control with medication. Swelling in the thigh from a retracted muscle can be massive and painful. A displaced avulsion fracture usually heals by fibrous union, with the patient generally resuming full activity with appropriate rehabilitation. Some patients are left with reduced athletic ability as a result of the injury.[15]

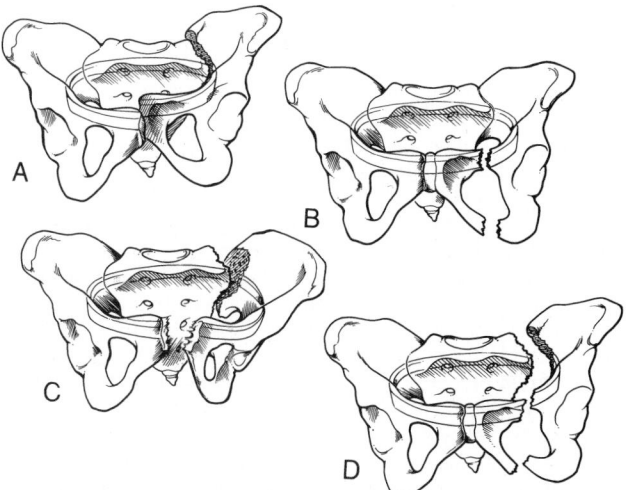

Figure 42–29. A and B, Stable fractures. C and D, Unstable fractures. The lateral compression fracture in A impacts the symphysis. The ligaments of the posterior sacroiliac joint are intact, and the fracture is stable. In B, the ring is disrupted on only one side at the superior and inferior ramus of the pubis. The sacroiliac joint is intact, and the fracture is stable. In C, the pelvis is opened as is a book. The symphysis is disrupted, and the anterior and posterior ligaments of the sacroiliac joint are disrupted. The fracture is unstable and is best treated by open reduction. In D, the fracture is caused by vertical shear; the ring is disrupted both anteriorly and posteriorly, and the fracture is unstable. This fracture should be treated by open reduction and internal fixation anteriorly and posteriorly.

Isolated fractures of the sacrum and coccyx are treated by bed rest and protected seating until the patient is comfortable and can be mobilized with crutches. Occasionally, fibrosis occurs around sacral nerve roots after a nondisplaced fracture of the sacrum, leading to persistent coccygeal pain. Treatment of chronic coccygeal pain following injury should consist of a foam rubber coccygodynia pad, which relieves pressure on the coccyx, and analgesics, including nonsteroidal anti-inflammatory medications if they are tolerated by the patient.

Fractures of the pelvic ring that cause mechanical disruption of the ring are of much greater clinical consequence. In a recently published study from Sweden,[13] the incidence of pelvic fractures treated in a hospital during the 10-year period from 1976 to 1985 was 20 per 100,000 people. The incidence of pelvic trauma increased among the elderly, especially women. Severe trauma dominated in age groups below 60 years. Eighty-one per cent of the fractures were stable fractures of the pubic rami; the remainder included 10% acetabular fractures and unstable pelvic ring injuries. There were associated injuries in 21% of the patients. These associated injuries included internal injuries to the urethra, bladder, and abdominal organs, as well as other distant neurologic trauma. The most common complication of these fractures is hemorrhage into the retroperitoneal space, occurring from the plexus of veins and arteries lining the inner pelvic wall. Several recent reviews emphasized the importance of associated injuries in the outcome of open pelvic fracture. A review of 27 patients with open pelvic fractures seen in a trauma center revealed a mean of 26 units of blood transfused, 9 operative procedures, and a length of stay of 43 days.[16]

Because of the life-threatening nature of disruption of the pelvic ring, the mainstay of therapy is stabilization in the acute setting. This can include such maneuvers as positioning the patient on his or her side to close an open book–type injury, application of pneumatic anti-shock trousers, or application of external fixation to close an open pelvis and decrease the intrapelvic volume. These procedures are performed in an effort to stabilize the clot within the pelvis

into a discrete and contained area and stop potentially life-threatening bleeding. A standard algorithm for resuscitation of a severely traumatized patient should be followed. Emergency evaluation of a patient with a pelvic fracture must include all the organ systems that are frequently involved. Careful neurologic examination should include evaluation of the spinal cord, sciatic nerve, obturator nerve, lumbosacral plexus, and peripheral nerves. Retroperitoneal bleeding may mimic gastrointestinal trauma, and diagnostic peritoneal lavage is extremely helpful in distinguishing between the two. Careful examination of the rectum and vagina may reveal blood—presumptive evidence of an open fracture of the pelvis via perforation of one of those structures.

Once the patient is stabilized, emergency radiographic evaluation includes an anteroposterior view of the pelvis as well as 40-degree inlet and outlet projections in the caudad-cephalad plane. In addition, for evaluation of the acetabulum, 45-degree oblique Judet views are helpful. Plain radiographs, however, are not adequate for evaluating fragments of bone within the joint or neural foramina and are often augmented by computed tomography (CT) with three-dimensional reconstruction, once the patient has been stabilized.[14] There have been some early reports of magnetic resonance imaging (MRI) being used to evaluate the pelvis in the acute setting. This may have some utility in evaluating articular surfaces and the condition of nervous structures, but at the present time, the use of MRI is still being evaluated.

Once resuscitation is achieved, patients are often initially placed in skeletal traction prior to surgical stabilization of the pelvic ring. Traction is seldom successful in reducing an unstable pelvic fracture and must be continued for 10 to 12 weeks if it is the only mode of treatment. Most authors experienced in the treatment of pelvic fractures now agree that open reduction of an unstable pelvic fracture is mandatory to achieve bony union and mobilization as quickly as possible. Persistent deformity can cause leg length inequality, pain, and difficulty in walking, sitting, and subsequent childbirth.

Complications of Pelvic Ring Disruption

Hemorrhage. The most common complication of displaced pelvic fractures is massive hemorrhage. Bleeding may occur from laceration of the hypogastric or gluteal vessels caused by fractures extending into the sciatic notch. Although a patient can initially appear stable, shock can rapidly ensue, as evidenced by changes in vital signs, urinary output, and central venous pressure. The patient must be massively transfused to correct shock and maintain urinary output. Application of an external fixator on an emergent basis can decrease the pelvic volume by a factor of four and contribute to the cessation of intrapelvic hemorrhage. If bleeding cannot be controlled, arteriography may be helpful to identify the source of the bleeding and allow embolization. In rare circumstances, packing of the pelvis through a laparotomy can be helpful. Attempts at open ligation of vessels are extremely hazardous.[6]

Lower Urinary Tract Injury. The bladder rests against the pubic bones and is seldom injured when empty. As the bladder fills and extends with urine or clot, it may fill most of the true pelvis and rise above the symphysis, where it becomes vulnerable to intra- or extraperitoneal rupture. Injuries to the lower urinary tract occur in 14% of all pelvic fractures. Injury can sometimes be diagnosed by blood at the meatus or blood on rectal examination. Occasionally, a high-riding prostate on rectal examination is a clue to injury to the lower urinary tract. In a recent review of 249 trauma patients with pelvic fractures, 50% had hematuria, and 7% had lower urinary tract disruptions.[2] Twenty-five per cent of the patients with unstable pelvic fractures had lower urinary tract disruption, compared with 6% of the patients with stable fractures. Retrograde urethrography followed by cystography is indicated in all cases of pelvic fractures with blood at the urethral meatus or with microscopic hematuria.

Intra-abdominal Visceral Injury. Internal injuries to the uterus, vagina, rectum, or abdominal viscera can create an open injury, which might require repair or intestinal bypass. In addition, intra-abdominal injury can be the source of bleeding. Diagnostic peritoneal lavage is therefore a helpful adjunct in evaluating intra-abdominal injury and remains a standard part of evaluation.[11]

Neurologic Injury. The sciatic nerve is most frequently damaged by fractures extending into the ilium or sciatic notch, by fractures of the ischium with displacement, or by posterior fracture-dislocations of the hip. The peroneal division of the sciatic nerve is damaged more often than the tibial division. The obturator and femoral nerves are less frequently injured.

Pulmonary Complications. Pulmonary complications can be associated with major pelvic trauma secondary to a pulmonary contusion, posttraumatic insufficiency related to embolism, or respiratory distress associated with fluid shift. Early mobilization through stabilization of the fracture is one of the mainstays of treatment for this potentially fatal complication. In addition, patients with multiple injuries that include pelvic fractures have an increased risk of deep venous thrombosis, which can lead to pulmonary embolism. The incidence of thromboembolism ranges from 1% to 9% in the current literature. Therefore, once the patient is hemodynamically and surgically stabilized, a regimen of mechanical and/or chemical prophylaxis should be instituted against deep venous thrombosis. In addition, patients treated with prolonged bed rest should be diligently observed for signs of deep venous thrombosis and receive chemical or mechanical treatment as prophylaxis.

Arthritis. Posttraumatic arthritis frequently develops after acetabular fractures. Although function after treatment with prolonged traction or surgery is often much better than the radiographic appearance, the joint space may narrow, and symptoms of pain may ensue. The radiographic signs of posttraumatic arthrosis include subchondral sclerosis, development of cysts in the acetabulum and the femoral head, and possible collapse of the femoral head with loss of sphericity. Range of motion gradually diminishes as pain increases. Treatment of this condition may require late osteotomy, fusion, or arthroplasty.

Heterotopic Ossification. Heterotopic ossification is another complication that frequently follows the operative treatment of acetabular fractures, particularly with the use of extended approaches.[4] Heterotopic ossification is graded by the Brooker classification, based on the amount of radiographically visible heterotopic bone. Recent information suggests that indomethacin may be helpful in diminishing the amount of new bone formation. Letournel[7] has published excellent results using 700-cGy single-dose postoperative radiation, with a very low incidence of new bone formation using the extended iliofemoral approach.

Treatment of Pelvic Ring Disruption

The objective of treating pelvic fractures after the patient's general condition has stabilized is to achieve bony union in a functional position as quickly as possible. Stable fractures of the pelvic ring, including nondisplaced ramus fractures and nondisplaced fractures of the sacrum, can be treated by closed means, including protected weight bearing and pain control. Serial radiographs are helpful to exclude subsequent displacement and to document healing. Some fractures are minimally displaced initially and appear to be stable but may ultimately displace. These include anterior ring disruptions with separation of the SI joint. The treatment of choice for this type of injury is reduction of the posterior component of the ring disruption through either an anterior plate or posterior fixation after plating of the symphysis disruption, if present (Fig. 42–30).

Stability of a pelvic fracture is influenced by the location of the injury and the presence of bony deformity or ligamentous injury. Pelvic instability is indicated by the amount of displacement of the posterior elements on either side of the SI joint. Displacement of the SI joint is a sign of instability when it is in excess of 1 cm. A fracture of the sacrum may be stable if it is minimally displaced. Any fracture or dislocation of the SI joint must be considered potentially unstable. A displaced fracture of the iliac wing may also be unstable. Anterior diastasis of the symphysis pubis, when it exceeds 3 cm., is considered an unstable injury requiring treatment. Diastasis of the pubic ramus does not usually occur when the rami on either side are fractured.

Unstable fractures of the pelvic ring—including displaced anteroposterior compression, vertical shear, and lateral compression injuries—require open reduction and internal fixation with plates and screws by an experienced surgeon in a medical center equipped to deal with multiple-trauma patients. When the SI joint is involved, the most common approach is a vertical incision 2 cm. lateral to the posterosuperior spine, extending from the iliac crest to the sciatic notch. This approach allows exposure of both the sciatic notch and the superior portion of the ala of the sacrum at the articulation with the ilium. Direct palpation of the SI joint reduction can therefore be achieved. Special care should be taken to avoid impingement of the L5 nerve root as it runs from its medial position in close proximity to the superior portion of the ala and just medial to the SI joint anteriorly. Once reduced, the SI joint can be stabilized by two screws passing from lateral to medial from the ilium into the sacrum under radiographic control with image intensification. There have been some recent reports of using CT guidance for the placement of screws. In addition, the SI joint can be plated from the front by working over the pelvic brim, using the most lateral portion of the ilioinguinal approach to the pelvis. One must keep in mind the close proximity of the lumbosacral plexus and not put retractors more than 1 cm. medial to the SI joint when approaching it from the front. Two three-hole plates placed from the front, with one 4.5-mm. screw placed medial to the joint and two lateral, are sufficient to provide

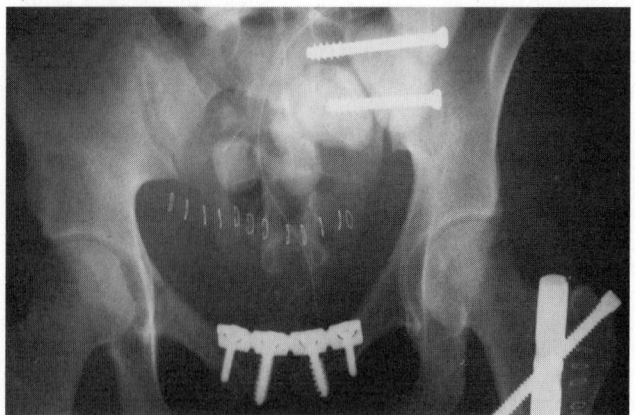

Figure 42–30. This pelvic x-ray demonstrates a symphysis disruption with displacement of the sacroiliac joint. The fracture is treated by open reduction and internal fixation using a four-hole plate anteriorly and cannulated lag screws, transfixing the iliac wing into the first sacral body posteriorly.

anterior fixation. Posterior fixation can be achieved with two 6.5-mm. screws. These screws can be augmented with a flexible plate extending from one iliac wing to the other above the sciatic notch. Alternatively, when both SI joints are disrupted, parallel sacral bars passing through the posterior iliac wing can be used once reduction has been obtained. Percutaneous passage of screws through the ilium into the first sacral body has been described using image intensification. This procedure requires a large amount of experience, because even with image intensification it is possible to place the screws in close proximity to vascular or neural structures. Because of the sacral promontory, image intensification can easily be misinterpreted.

For open reduction of anterior lesions, including the symphysis pubis or displaced fractures of the pubic rami, a transverse incision is made 2 cm. above the symphysis pubis. The linea alba is split between the two heads of the rectus abdominis, and the pubis is exposed by dissecting the rectus muscle from the symphysis. The spermatic cord is identified and protected. The symphysis is then reduced by using either ball-tipped pelvic reduction clamps or temporary placement of screws for clamp anchoring, followed by reduction. The pubis is then stabilized with a single four- or six-hole 3.5- or 4.5-mm. pelvic reconstruction plate. The plate is placed just dorsal to the rectus abdominis attachment (see Fig. 42–30). In general, the anterior disruption is fixed before the posterior disruption. However, if the diastasis is quite wide or if the fracture is being approached more than 12 weeks after injury, it may be necessary to reduce the posterior ring prior to putting on the anterior fixation and then revisit the posterior ring for permanent fixation. Patients can be mobilized within 4 to 7 days after fixation. Touchdown weight-bearing status is maintained on the affected side for a minimum of 6 weeks and often for as long as 3 months.

Acetabulum

Displaced fractures of the acetabulum require open reduction and internal fixation in most cases. Once a patient has undergone initial stabilization, any hip dislocation associated with an acetabular fracture should be reduced through gentle traction under anesthesia with radiographic visualization.[3] Because of the ongoing vascular compromise to the femoral head associated with a dislocated hip, it is in the best interest of the patient to reduce the hip as quickly as possible after dislocation. If early reduction is possible, it may decrease the incidence of late complications, including avascular necrosis of the femoral head.

The radiographic evaluation of acetabular fractures includes an initial anteroposterior view of the pelvis, demonstrating both hips. As with pelvic ring disruption, the ipsilateral femoral neck, the lumbar spine, and the ipsilateral lower extremity should be thoroughly evaluated for concomitant injuries. Forty-five-degree oblique views allow full view of the anterior and posterior columns of the pelvis. By utilizing the iliac and obturator 45-degree oblique views, one can apply the measurement of roof arc angles, as described by Matta and colleagues,[9] to aid in determining whether a particular fracture pattern requires open reduction and internal fixation. Displaced fractures through the roof of the acetabulum, which fall within a 45-degree arc from a line drawn vertically through the center of rotation of the femoral head, generally require open reduction and internal fixation. Once the patient's condition allows, CT evaluation with three-dimensional reconstruction is helpful in recognizing all components of the fracture. The fracture may involve the posterior wall, the anterior wall, the posterior column, the anterior column, or any combination of these four elements of the acetabulum (Fig. 42–31). The goal in treating fractures of the

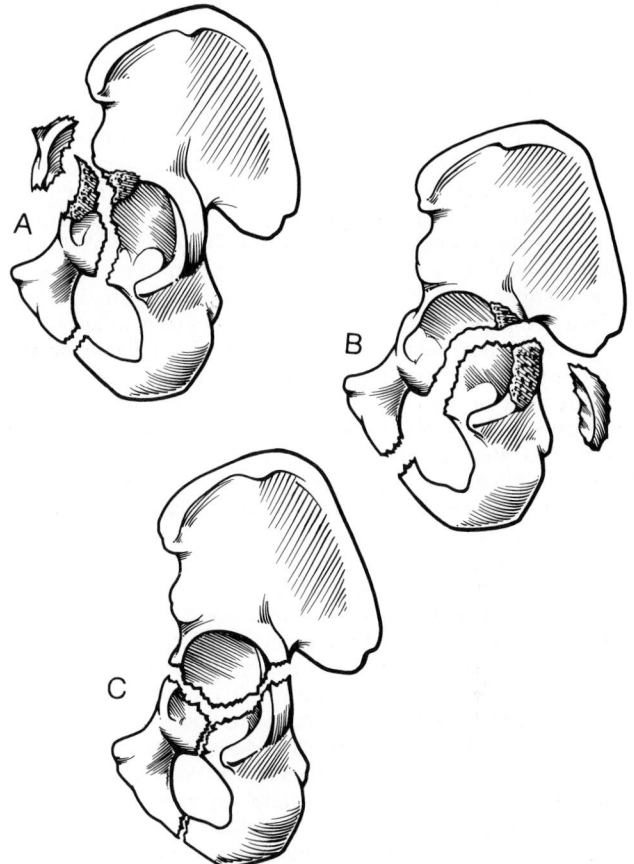

Figure 42–31. In *A*, the fracture involves the anterior column as well as the anterior wall. Open reduction and internal fixation are mandatory for restoration of anatomic alignment and painless function. This fracture could be approached through the ilioinguinal exposure. In *B*, the posterior column is fractured, as is the posterior wall. Open reduction and internal fixation can be accomplished through a Kocher-Langenbeck–type approach. In *C*, there is injury to both columns. This injury could be treated surgically by using an extended approach to visualize both columns; alternatively, either the anterior or the posterior approach could be used to achieve direct reduction of the visualized column and indirect reduction of the nonvisualized column.

acetabulum is to achieve as near an anatomic reduction as possible to prevent posttraumatic arthrosis. In general, open reduction is indicated if displacement of the articular surface is greater than 2 mm. If the displacement is minimal and does not involve the weight-bearing surface in the roof arc, fracture of the acetabulum can be treated nonoperatively. However, most displaced intra-articular fractures require open reduction and internal fixation. If manipulation under anesthesia in the presence of a posterior wall fracture indicates instability, the injury may require internal fixation. One recent article suggested that a fracture fragment of the posterior wall that constitutes greater than 40% of the posterior wall is an indication for open reduction and internal fixation.[5]

Understanding of the acetabular fracture patterns, operative approaches, and methods of internal fixation has progressed rapidly over the past 10 years. Classification of the lesions and results of treatment have been advanced through the work of Letournel, Matta, Mears, and others. Delay in treatment appears to have an adverse effect on the outcome of surgical procedures.[10] In patients who had surgical malreduction or secondary loss of fixation, only 57% had good or excellent results if reoperated within 3 weeks. This figure dropped to 29% when the delay exceeded 12 weeks. In contrast, patients with early anatomic reductions have a reported success rate of around 80%. Still, reported complications include infection, nerve palsy, heterotopic bone formation, and pulmonary embolus.

Exposure of the acetabulum is achieved through one of three general types of approach. The Kocher-Langenbeck approach is generally used for exposure of the posterior wall of the acetabulum and the posterior column from the ischial tuberosity up to and including a small area of the posterior column just above the sciatic notch (Fig. 42–32). However, this approach permits exposure of only the lower segment of the iliac wing. Attempts to stretch the exposure beyond the lower portion of the iliac wing can compromise the superior gluteal artery as it comes out of the sciatic notch. The approach involves a separation of the tensor fascia followed by the gluteus maximus muscle in the interval between the middle and posterior one third of the muscle. This allows visualization of the short external rotators, including the piriformis and the obturator internus, which require special attention. The sciatic nerve can be visualized passing beneath the piriformis and on top of the obturator internus, gemella, and quadratus femoris. The sciatic nerve can be protected during the approach to the posterior column by keeping the knee bent and by avoiding pressure from retractors. There have been several recent reports regarding the use of somatosensory evoked potentials for monitoring the tibial portion of the sciatic nerve during the procedure. Utilizing this type of precaution, it may be possible to eliminate some iatrogenic postoperative sciatic nerve palsy.

For fractures involving the anterior column and the anterior wall with hemitransverse-type lesions, an ilioinguinal approach may be preferred. An incision is made from the posterosuperior spine approximately 2 cm. below the iliac crest, proceeding anteriorly to a point just below the anterosuperior iliac spine and, from there, proceeding medially to a point approximately 2 cm. above the symphysis pubis. The ensuing dissection allows exposure from the SI joint all the way around to the symphysis pubis, if required. The inner portion of the pelvis is exposed first by elevating the iliacus muscle down to the sciatic notch region. The sartorius can be mobilized by elevating it with a bone block from the anterior superior spine. The lateral femoral cutaneous nerve should be identified and protected during this portion of the dissection. The anterior column exposure is then achieved through three separate windows. The first window is lateral to the iliopsoas; the second is between the iliopsoas and the vascular bundle; and the third is medial to the vascular bundle. This dissection and exposure are extremely complex and should be undertaken only by a surgeon experienced and trained in the operative approaches to the pelvis. Of particular note is the infrequent but potentially hazardous communication between the femoral and obturator vasculature. Failure to recognize this communication when mobilizing the femoral vasculature could lead to brisk bleeding that is difficult to stop because the origin cannot be easily visualized.

Extended approaches are also used for fractures of the acetabulum. These approaches include the extended iliofemoral as described by Letournel, the triradiate as described by Mears, and the modified iliofemoral as described by Mears. This type of approach allows visualization of the external iliac fossa as well as both columns of the acetabulum. It may be accompanied by osteotomy of the greater trochanter or division of the tendon of the gluteus medius muscle. The extended approach is dependent on an intact superior gluteal artery circulation to provide blood supply to the gluteal muscles and the entire flap when they are reflected off the pelvis. Failure to protect the vascular pedicle or ensure its patency prior to performing this approach can lead to disastrous wound complications. This approach is associated with the highest incidence of heterotopic ossification and should be accompanied by postoperative prophylaxis with either indomethacin or low-dose irradiation.

Reduction techniques and plate configurations are numerous and require a high degree of skill and knowledge of the local acetabular anatomy. In general, posterior wall injuries are best treated by configuration of a straight pelvic reconstruction plate (Fig. 42–33). Curved plates are reserved for use along the pelvic rim in the ilioinguinal approach. Techniques such as indirect reduction, lag screw fixation, buttress plating with undercontouring, and spring plating can allow reduction of fracture fragments while ensuring that screws do not pass into the articular portion of the hip joint. Antibiotics should be administered perioperatively. Suction drains should be continued for several days postoperatively, and thromboembolic prophylaxis should be included with prophylaxis for heterotopic ossification. Passive motion of the hip joint can be instituted within 24 hours for posterior wall injuries, but mobilization may be delayed for 4 to 5 days in large exposures with both-column injuries. Weight bearing is withheld until evidence of healing occurs, usually at least 6 weeks and frequently up to 3 months with complex and comminuted injuries.

FRACTURES OF THE HIP

Femoral Neck and Intertrochanteric Fractures

Hip fractures are an extremely common problem in the elderly. According to Armstrong and Wallace,[19] fractures of the hips affect one in four women by the age of 90 years, and one in eight men. A review of patients at a university hospital in the United Kingdom noted that hip fracture patients occupied a quarter of all orthopedic beds. Fifteen per cent of the patients died while in the hospital, and 33% died by 1 year after the injury. Of the survivors, only two thirds returned to their own homes. The rate of fractures of the hip in the United States appears to be highest in white women and lowest in black men, according to a retrospective study of 27,000 patients discharged from nonfederal Maryland hospitals from 1979 to 1988.[28] Review of mortality rates in Medi-

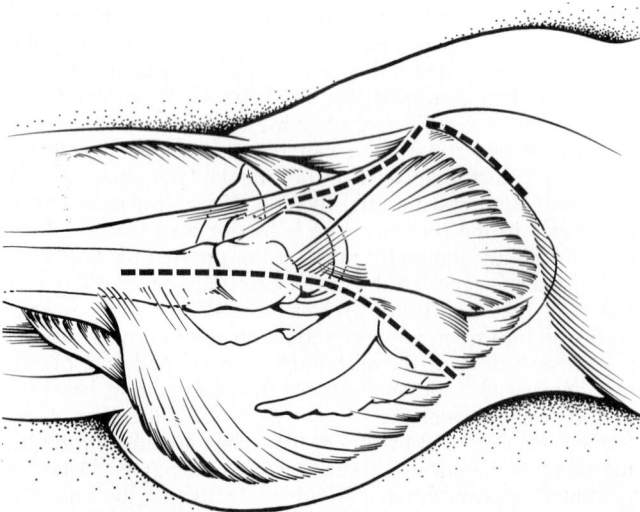

Figure 42–32. The extended approach passes along the crest of the ilium and then curves downward between the tensor and sartorius anteriorly. This approach can be extended both posteriorly and distally to allow exposure of both columns. The posterior approach passes along the trochanter, splits the gluteus maximus, and detaches the short external rotators for exposure of the posterior column and the posterior wall of the acetabulum.

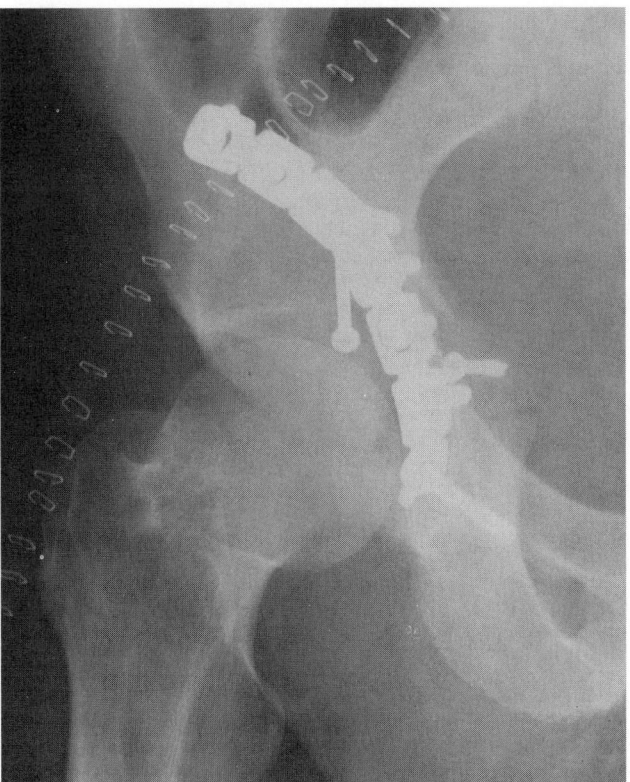

Figure 42–33. This posterior fracture-dislocation of the hip is treated by open reduction of the posterior wall with bone grafting and elevation of the compacted segment, followed by application of a buttressing pelvic reconstruction plate.

care patients sustaining hip fractures reveals that the lowest rates occur in white women, followed by black women, black men, and white men. The cause of these differences has not been well explained. Melton[32] made the interesting observation that half of the 1.66 million hip fractures reported in the year 1990 occurred in Europe and North America. Within these regions, there was substantial variation in incidence rates, suggesting that environmental factors may play an important role in the incidence of hip fractures. This observation has increased importance because of the cost of acute medical care and nursing home services associated with hip fractures, which Melton estimates at $8 billion annually in the United States.

Loss of bone density appears to be a risk factor for fracture of the proximal femur.[27] In addition to the normal, steady 1% to 2% loss of bone density after age 35 to 40 years in both sexes, there is accelerated loss after menopause in women as well as in patients who smoke, use alcohol, and are steroid dependent. In women, amenorrhea reduces bone density as well. In addition, a causal association has been demonstrated between osteoarthritis and osteoporosis of the hip.[22]

Hip fractures occur infrequently in children. A review from the University of Iowa revealed only 26 cases of hip fractures in children between 1926 and 1988.[23] Avascular necrosis of the femoral head complicated 47% of the fractures.

Before the twentieth century, fractures of the femur were almost universally fatal because of pulmonary, renal, and cardiac complications. Survival was only slightly better when elderly patients were treated by Whitman's methods of closed reduction and cast immobilization.[39] The healing rate of 30% was clearly unacceptable. Progress in the treatment of this very common injury was made by Smith-Peterson in the 1930s, when he developed the technique of open reduc-

tion and internal fixation with a triflanged nail. Advances have been rapid since then.

Classification of Hip Fractures

The most logical classification of hip fractures is one based on prognosis.[20] In any fracture, healing depends not only on fixation but also on blood supply. Blood supply is marginal and more subject to damage in the portion of the femur that is intracapsular, which makes the prognosis for intracapsular fractures worse than the prognosis for fractures occurring outside the capsule. Intracapsular fractures include fractures of the head of the femur, impacted subcapital fractures, and displaced subcapital and femoral neck fractures. Because there is no periosteum on the femoral neck, healing is by endosteal callus formation. Fixation must be rigid yet must allow impaction as the fracture line resorbs. The femoral head receives only a small amount of its blood supply from the pelvic side of the joint through the ligamentum teres. The major blood supply arises from the vascular ring at the base of the femoral neck. The retinacular arteries pierce the capsule and course up the posterior lateral portion of the femoral neck to enter the head in the subcapital area. These retinacular vessels may be damaged by torsion of fracture fragments or possibly by intra-articular pressure from a hematoma. Fractures of the femoral head occur most often in posterior fracture-dislocations of the hip.[26] Either the central portion of the head is avulsed by the ligamentum teres or a quadrant of the head is sheared off by the projecting lip of the acetabulum. This injury generally occurs when the knee strikes the dashboard of a car. The intra-articular fragment seldom heals, continues to cause pain, and can cause posttraumatic arthritis. The treatment of choice is open reduction of the hip with removal of loose fragments and repair of the capsule without disrupting the blood supply. If the dislocation is stable after repair, the patient can be mobilized rapidly on crutches.

Fractures of the subcapital portion of the femur and the femoral neck are generally classified by the Garden classification scheme. A Garden I fracture is an impacted valgus fracture, a Garden II fracture is a nondisplaced fracture, a Garden III is displaced less than 50% of the width of the neck, and a Garden IV is displaced greater than 50% of the width of the neck. Impacted subcapital fractures are relatively nondisplaced fractures in which the neck of the femur is telescoped into the femoral head (Fig. 42–34). Some authors believe that impacted fractures are actually collapsed stress fractures. There is some debate as to whether these fractures need internal fixation. Evidence supporting the stress fracture theory is the fact that a large number of united trabecular fractures have been found in the femoral necks of patients with senile-type subcapital fractures. Patients may present with minor groin pain and radiation of pain to the knee. Initial radiographs may not reveal the fracture line, which later becomes visible as the resorption phase of healing occurs. An elderly patient with hip pain must be treated for a fracture even though injury is not obvious on radiographs; otherwise, the nondisplaced fracture may become displaced, as demonstrated in Figure 42–34. Displacement increases the likelihood of disruption of the blood supply to the femoral head. The decision to treat an impacted valgus fracture with protected mobilization must be accompanied by close follow-up and frequent radiographs to rule out any interval displacement of the femoral head. An unstable or potentially unstable fracture of the subcapital region of the femur is best treated with application of internal fixation. One generally accepted surgical treatment is placement of three cannulated pins through the lateral cortex of the femur into the femoral head. Other options include placement of a compression-type screw with a side plate, in conjunction with a derotation

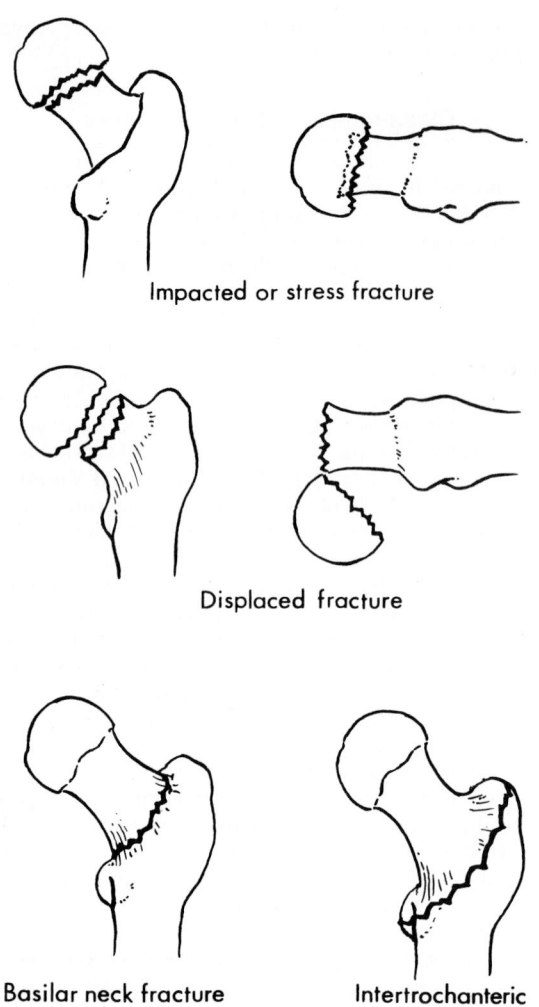

Impacted or stress fracture

Displaced fracture

Basilar neck fracture   Intertrochanteric fracture

Figure 42–34. An impacted subcapital fracture may heal without intervention, but there is a risk of the head slipping off the neck during the healing period. In younger patients, a displaced fracture should be reduced and fixed with multiple pins. In older patients, a displaced fracture is treated with prosthetic replacement. A basilar neck or intertrochanteric fracture must be fixed with a lag screw, which passes through the trochanter into the neck and the head and is attached to the femur by means of a side plate.

edly reducing the blood supply to the femoral head. These fractures should be treated as emergencies, with reduction being performed as quickly as possible with rigid internal fixation. One study suggested that reduction within 6 hours can lead to a lower incidence of avascular necrosis.[37] When moderate displacement is present, reduction can be accomplished by gentle abduction and internal rotation. The Leadbetter maneuver,[29] used for more severe displacement, is seldom necessary and may cause additional comminution of the neck. In younger patients, if anatomic reduction cannot be obtained by manipulation, the capsule should be opened anteriorly and the fragments reduced under direct vision. In general, achieving an anatomic reduction with expeditious internal fixation is chosen for younger patients. For elderly patients or patients with pre-existing arthritic conditions, osteoporosis, or medical infirmity, arthroplasty may be preferred.

Surgical Treatment of Hip Fractures

In young patients with good bone density, multiple-pin fixation provides good biomechanical fracture fixation (Fig. 42–36).[36] The risks and benefits of multiple small-screw fixation versus a screw and side plate have been debated in the literature. In older patients with osteoporotic bone, or in fractures lower in the femoral neck, fixation between the head and the shaft may be accomplished with a side plate. A guide pin is placed through the lateral cortex of the femur, through the inferior aspect of the neck, and into the head of the femur. The progress of the guide pin is followed by means of a fluoroscopic image intensifier. When the guide pin is in a satisfactory position on both anteroposterior and lateral projections, a lag screw is inserted over the guide pin through the lateral cortex of the femur, through the neck, and into the head of the femur. The side plate is then attached by means of a sleeve placed over the lateral shaft of the compression screw. The fracture is compressed using a screw, which shortens the lag screw into the sleeve of the side plate. Union of a displaced fracture may require a long time, with protected weight bearing lasting from 6 to 12 months.

In an elderly or debilitated patient, reduction and fixation of a subcapital fracture should be done when possible. If perfect reduction cannot be obtained, prosthetic replacement with a unipolar arthroplasty, a bipolar arthroplasty, or a

screw. Since only the metaphyseal and endosteal blood vessels are interrupted in a nondisplaced subcapital fracture, the retinacular vessels may remain intact. If this is the case, healing can occur without difficulty with adequate immobilization and protection from displacement. For this reason, aseptic necrosis of the femoral head occurs in only 5% to 10% of patients with impacted fractures, compared with a 30% rate of avascular necrosis in those with displaced Garden III– and Garden IV–type fractures of the femoral neck. Collapse of the femoral head with recurrence of pain secondary to avascular necrosis may develop as late as 5 or 6 years after injury.[38]

Displaced subcapital fractures and fractures of the neck of the femur are much more difficult to manage (Fig. 42–35). Nonunion and avascular necrosis occur much more frequently. In both of these fractures, bleeding occurs within the hip joint, and the resultant intracapsular pressure may rapidly exceed the pressure in intracapsular vessels if the capsule is not torn. This can cause thrombosis of the nutrient blood supply to the hip and possibly lead to the development of avascular necrosis. In addition, displacement of the fragments destroys the metaphyseal and endosteal vessels, mark-

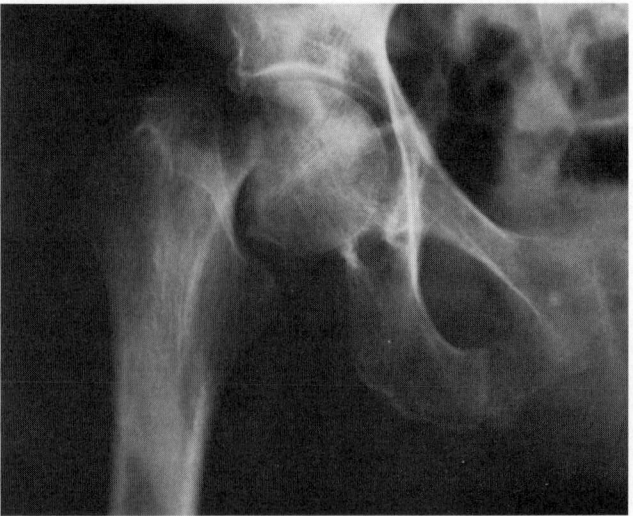

Figure 42–35. A displaced subcapital fracture in an elderly patient should be treated with prosthetic replacement, because nonunion and aseptic necrosis of the femoral head occur at a rate of 20% to 30%.

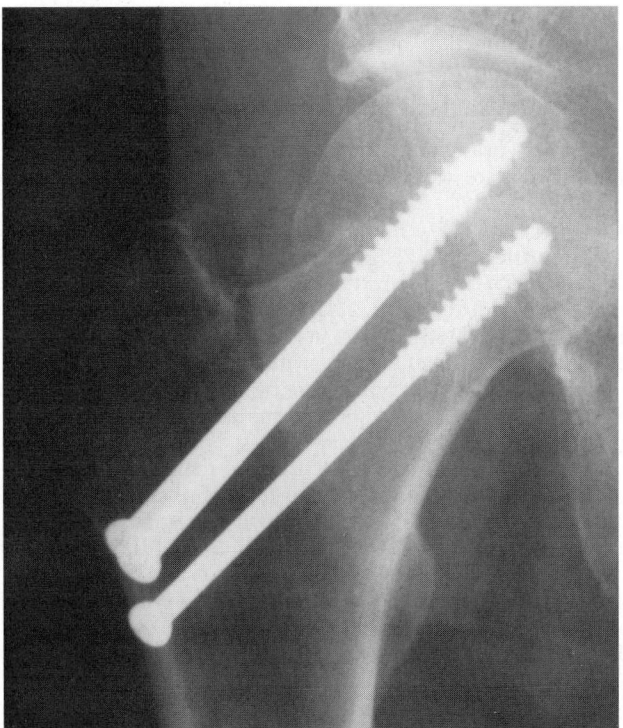

Figure 42–36. Fixation of a femoral neck fracture with three cannulated screws is the preferred method of treatment for nondisplaced or minimally displaced fractures. The screws can be placed with a small incision in a relatively atraumatic fashion.

total hip should be performed in an effort to achieve more expeditious mobilization of the patient. In a recent meta-analysis of outcomes after displaced fractures of the femoral neck, nonunion developed in 33% and avascular necrosis in 16% of the patients with internal fixation.[31] Conversion to an arthroplasty was the most common reoperation after internal fixation, and it accounted for two thirds of these procedures. The most common secondary operation after a hemiarthroplasty was conversion to a total hip arthroplasty. These potential complications requiring a secondary operation should be considered in the treatment algorithm at the time of the fracture. Endoprostheses should be used only as a last resort in younger patients, because of the limited life span of the bearing surface. Any patient with a hip fracture treated surgically should receive adequate prophylaxis for infection and thromboembolism. This includes perioperative antibiotics and either mechanical or pharmacologic anticoagulation in the perioperative period.

Intertrochanteric fractures occur below the inferior attachment of the hip capsule, outside of the vascular ring supplying the femoral neck and head. Blood supply in this area is excellent, so avascular necrosis rarely develops. If adequate stability can be obtained, union in a functional position generally occurs. Thus, the classification of intertrochanteric fractures is based on stability rather than blood supply.[24] The Boyd and Griffin classification of intertrochanteric fractures is based on the number of fragments and the anatomy of the fracture line (Fig. 42–37). Stability of an intertrochanteric fracture is dependent on support along the medial calcar and reduction of the posterior medial fragment. Proper reduction prevents the shaft from shifting medially, where it tends to be drawn by the pull of the adductor muscle groups. Muscle forces around the hip cause varus deformity at the fracture site in addition to medial displacement of the shaft. Reduction is accomplished by abduction and internal rotation. The

fracture is then stabilized rigidly with a compression screw and side plate.[33] A displaced posterior medial fragment may require additional lag screw fixation.

FRACTURES OF THE FEMUR

Fractures of the femur can be divided into four anatomically distinct areas: subtrochanteric, midshaft or diaphyseal, supracondylar, and condylar. Fractures at each level must be managed differently because of the deforming forces associated with the fracture fragments, which produce different patterns of displacement and require specific methods of internal fixation. Fractures in any of these areas can be either closed or open. Most open fractures not caused by gunshot wounds are compounded from within when the femoral shaft penetrates the subcutaneous tissue and skin. As the deformity is corrected either acutely or in the operating room, the exposed bone ends sink within the tissues, contaminating the deeper layers. Therefore, a small, benign-appearing wound still requires open irrigation and débride-

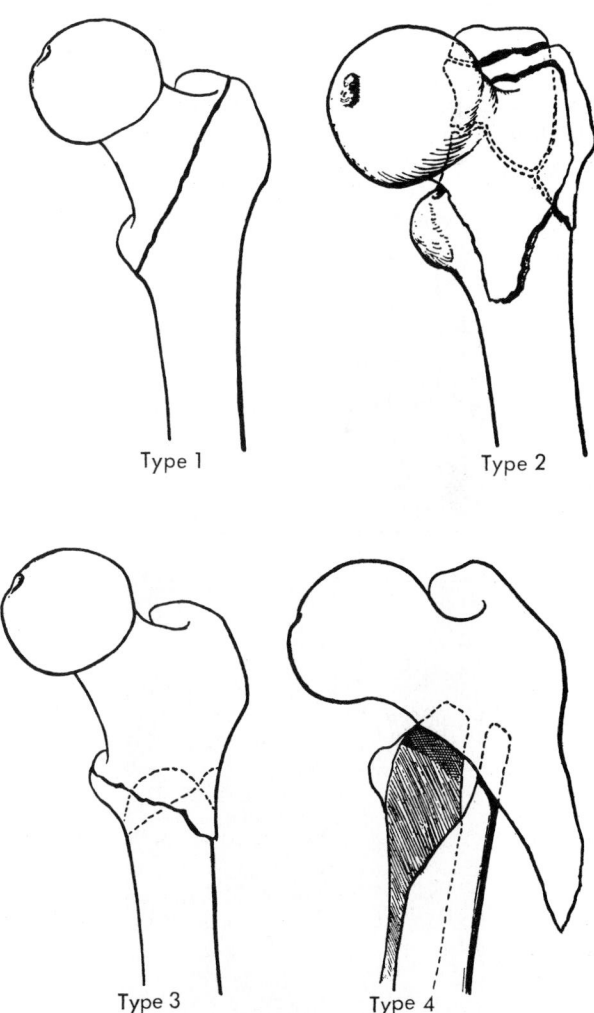

Figure 42–37. Intertrochanteric fractures. Type I is a stable fracture and can be fixed with a screw and side plate. Type II is an unstable fracture that can also be treated with a screw and side plate in addition to interfragmentary screw placement. In Type III intertrochanteric fractures, the shaft tends to displace medially, carrying the screw from the screw and side plate configuration into the head of the femur. This fracture, as well as Type IV fractures, can be treated with a screw and side plate apparatus but should be carefully protected. (From Boyd, H. B., and Griffin, L. L.: Classification and treatment of trochanteric fractures. Arch. Surg., 58:854, 1949. Copyright 1949, American Medical Association.)

ment, with removal of traumatized tissue and debris. Open fractures should be left open. Closing an open fracture may lead to serious infection, including clostridial myonecrosis.

A patient with a fractured femur has received a high-energy injury and must be evaluated carefully for associated injuries to the hip, knee, and spine, along with a standard trauma evaluation. Loss of 2 to 3 units of blood within the thigh may not be readily apparent, and hemodynamic instability can ensue without warning. In fractures of the lower third of the femur, nerves and vessels lie closely tethered to the bone and can be damaged either by the initial injury or during reduction.

Subtrochanteric Fractures

The subtrochanteric area of the femur is an extremely high-stress location, subject to displacement because of the high flexion and varus moment in the proximal femur.[25, 34] Displaced fractures in the subtrochanteric region (Fig. 42–38) in a skeletally immature patient can be treated with closed reduction and spica casting. Treatment of displaced fractures in a skeletally mature patient generally consists of closed reduction with intramedullary nailing using a standard proximal interlocking nail when the fracture line does not enter the piriformis fossa. Occasionally, traction is indicated for patients who are not operative candidates. However, the general trend has been toward early operative fixation and

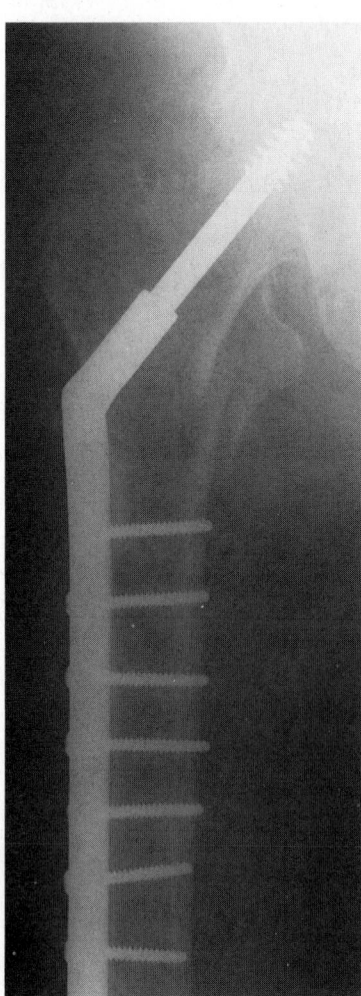

Figure 42–38. The screw and side plate construction can also be used for subtrochanteric fractures.

mobilization of the patient, which has beneficial effects on pulmonary function and general outcome.

Fractures of the Femoral Shaft

Fractures of the femoral shaft have been classified by Winquist and associates[43] into five basic patterns. A Winquist Type 0 femoral shaft fracture is transverse, with no butterfly fragment. A Type I fracture has a butterfly fragment that constitutes less than 25% of the width of the bone. A Type II fracture has a fragment greater than 25% but less than 50% of the width of the bone, and a Type III fragment is greater than 50% of the width of the bone. Finally, a Type IV fracture is extensively comminuted or segmental. The type of fracture has direct relevance to surgical treatment, with the larger butterfly fragments and the comminuted fracture types requiring locked intramedullary nailing.

Because fractures of the shaft of the femur can be associated with systemic complications such as respiratory distress syndrome, fat embolism, pulmonary embolism, and pneumonia, early stabilization and rapid mobilization of the patient are recommended. These are generally best accomplished by closed reduction of the shaft fracture and intramedullary fixation with one of a variety of nails available on the market (Fig. 42–39).[40, 42] The decision to perform either reamed or nonreamed nailing depends on the size of the patient, the pattern of the fracture, and whether the fracture is open or closed. Nonreamed nails are favored for open fractures of the femur, trading nail diameter and strength for a simpler procedure that does not require reaming of the medullary canal. However, as the more slender nonreamed nails are being redesigned with greater fatigue life and bending strength, they are coming into wider use in closed fractures of the femoral shaft.

Other types of operative treatment for fractures of the femoral shaft include external fixation and plate fixation. External fixation is occasionally chosen for open fractures with a large amount of contamination and soft tissue stripping. Plate fixation of displaced femur fractures has been used for children with multiple trauma because their open growth plates make them poor candidates for intramedullary nailing. Spica casting is less attractive in multiple trauma, where early mobilization is important. In patients with ipsilateral fractures of the neck of the femur and shaft of the femur, a reconstruction-type nail is an option that allows fixation of both fractures. Because the entry point of the intramedullary nail at the piriformis fossa is quite close to the retinacular vessels of the hip, use of image intensification, familiarity with the surgical protocol, and great care are required to achieve a favorable surgical outcome. The placement of an intramedullary nail requires a small incision made over the greater trochanter and extended to the piriformis fossa. When a reamed nail is chosen, a guide pin is inserted through the piriformis fossa into the medullary cavity of the femur and passed across the reduced fracture. This requires positioning of the patient on the fracture table in traction, with care to pad the perineum and to keep time in traction to a minimum to avoid the complication of pudendal nerve palsy. The femur can then be reamed to a diameter 1 to 2 mm. larger than the anticipated reamed nail. The length of the nail is determined using fluoroscopic guidance and radiographic measurement of the opposite noninjured femur. The decision to use interlocking screws is based on the fracture configuration. Unstable fractures that are Winquist Types II–IV generally require proximal and distal interlocking screws. Attention to the length and rotatory reduction ensures a favorable surgical outcome. Use of an interlocking nail has achieved excellent results in terms of fracture healing with appropriate length and rotation. Malunion and shorten-

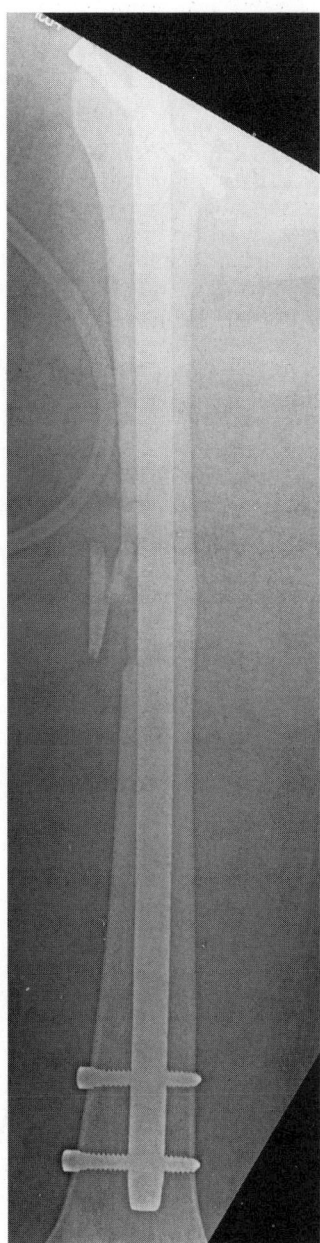

Figure 42–39. This radiograph of the femur demonstrates a comminuted fracture treated with an interlocking intramedullary nail. The interlocking screws enable the surgeon to maintain length and rotational control with an unstable diaphyseal segment.

ing are infrequent complications. The infection rates with closed intramedullary nailing have been 0.5% to 1.5%, in contrast with 2 to 4% for intramedullary nailing of open femoral shaft fractures.[41] As with fractures of the hip, perioperative antibiotics and an anticoagulation protocol are required. Patients are allowed mobilization and touchdown weight bearing initially, with institution of partial weight bearing at 6 to 8 weeks, depending on the fracture pattern and the rate of radiographically demonstrable healing.

Supracondylar Femoral Fractures

Supracondylar femoral fractures may follow automobile dashboard injuries, falls, or other types of trauma. Contraction of the gastrocnemius muscle pulls the distal fragments posteriorly into flexion (Fig. 42–40). Varus and internal rota-

tion can also occur, as the shaft of the femur rotates externally relative to the distal fragment. Displaced supracondylar fractures of the femur are best treated by open reduction, internal fixation, and early mobilization. Supracondylar fractures can extend into the knee joint. Displaced intra-articular fractures demand anatomic reduction. With an intra-articular fracture, reduction and early mobilization are imperative to avoid the complication of deformity and stiffness. In the case of condylar fragments, fixation is generally achieved through the use of lag screw fixation. The supracondylar portion of the fracture can be treated with a supracondylar compression screw and side plate, a blade plate configuration, or a buttress plate (Fig. 42–41). Treatment of these fractures is often accompanied by bone graft to avoid nonunion. The approach to the distal femur is generally achieved through an anterior midline skin incision, with a subvastus muscle exposure. A tubercle osteotomy or quadriceps turndown is occasionally required to obtain exposure.

FRACTURES OF THE PATELLA

The patella is vulnerable to injury, lying in its subcutaneous position in front of the femoral condyles. Fractures occur by direct injury to the knee from a blow or indirectly by contraction of the massive quadriceps muscle. Both mechanisms can occur simultaneously as the patient attempts to avoid falling by extending the knee; the patella separates, the knee collapses, and the patella strikes the ground. Fractures due to direct injury are most often stellate and comminuted and frequently compound. Displacement is usually minimal. Indirect fractures are frequently transverse, occurring in the upper, middle, or lower third; they may be

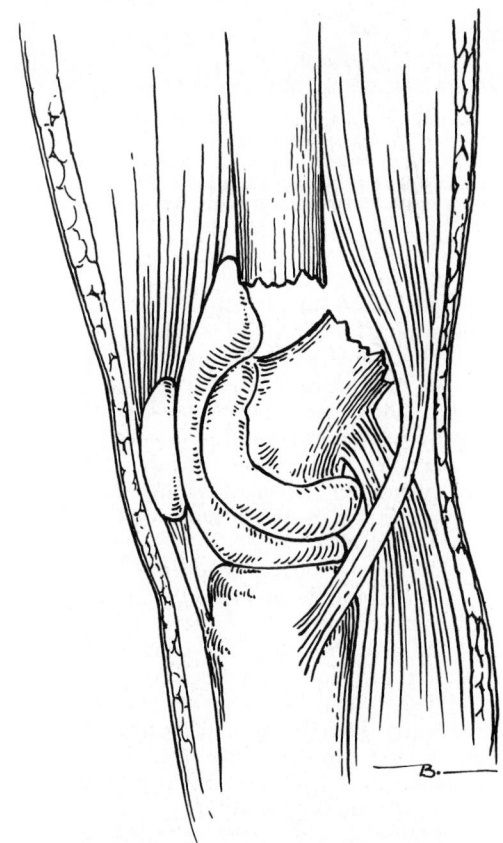

Figure 42–40. In a supracondylar fracture, the distal fragment of the femur is pulled posteriorly by the gastrocnemius. Complete displacement occurs when there is overriding of the fragments. Internal fixation is mandatory to restore early motion of the knee and healing of the fracture.

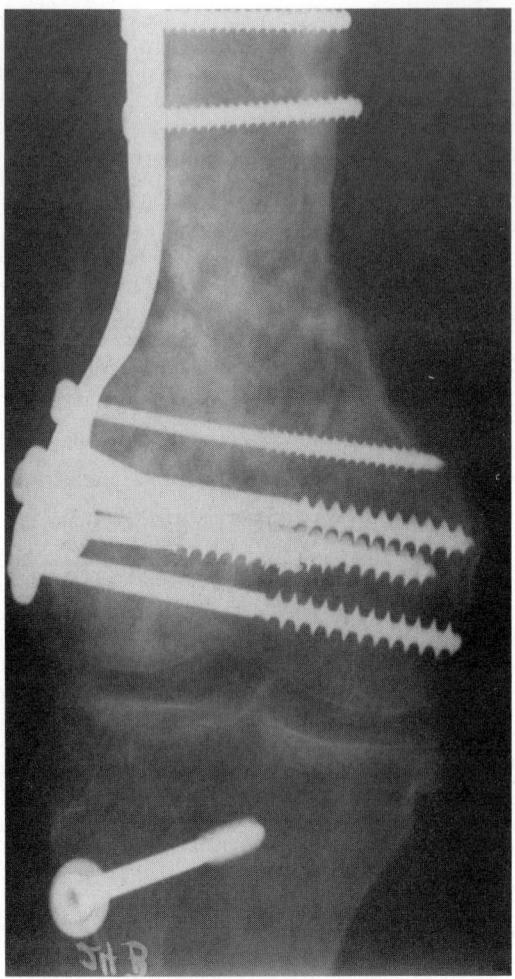

Figure 42–41. This comminuted supracondylar fracture in a young individual was treated with a condylar buttress plate, which is fixed to the shaft of the femur above and the condyles of the femur below with multiple screws. The screw in the tibia holds the tibial tubercle in place after it is removed to afford better exposure of the fracture. Early motion was begun, and the fracture healed rapidly.

widely separated, indicating extensive tearing of the retinaculum. If the extensor retinaculum is torn, active extension of the knee is not possible and open reduction is mandatory.

Fractures of the patella are relatively easy to diagnose because of the subcutaneous position of the fragments. Effusion is usually marked, and ecchymosis is extensive. Pain may be exacerbated by a tense effusion. If fragments are undisplaced, aspiration of hematoma and immobilization in a padded cylinder cast is sufficient treatment, with motion initiated at 3 to 4 weeks.

If large fracture fragments are separated and are approximately equal in size, open reduction of the fragments and repair of the retinaculum are indicated. The fragments can be reduced and held in place by two longitudinal Kirschner wires, and then a tension band wire loop is placed around the longitudinally oriented wires on the tension side to maintain the reduction (Fig. 42–42). It is frequently necessary to remove the tension band after the fracture is healed if the wire is a source of irritation to the subcutaneous tissues. Circumferential wiring is more difficult, and accurate reduction is less certain than with tension band wiring.

In comminuted or stellate fracture with displacement, partial patellectomy with repair of the retinaculum can produce an acceptable result. Immobilization must be maintained for 3 to 4 weeks, and forceful extension limited for another 4.

The most frequent complication of this difficult injury is late patellofemoral arthrosis. In fractures in which the superior or inferior fragment constitutes less than one third of the patella, the smaller fragment can be excised and the remaining quadriceps or patellar tendon repaired with interrupted nonabsorbable sutures.

Fractures of the patella must be differentiated from a bipartite patella. When the latter is suspected, radiographs of the opposite knee may reveal the same condition. In a bipartite patella, the fragments are surrounded by cortical bone with rounded margins, as compared with the jagged, sharp margins in a peripheral fracture.

DISLOCATION OF THE KNEE

Dislocation of the knee follows violent trauma, including motorcycle accidents, bumper injuries, athletic injuries, or falls. Knee dislocation can also follow relatively low-speed, high-torque twisting injuries, when the foot is fixed and the body is forced to pivot around the knee. The cruciate ligaments are torn as well as the joint capsule. Displacement of the tibia may be anterior, posterior, lateral, or medial. The anterior dislocation of the knee is the most common displacement pattern. Although partial disruption of the major ligaments of the knee must be present for dislocation to occur, many dislocations are stable after reduction. This should be documented with a postreduction lateral radiograph. Once reduction is achieved, the extent of the ligament injury can be evaluated through use of physical examination. MRI is helpful if the diagnosis is in doubt and there are no other

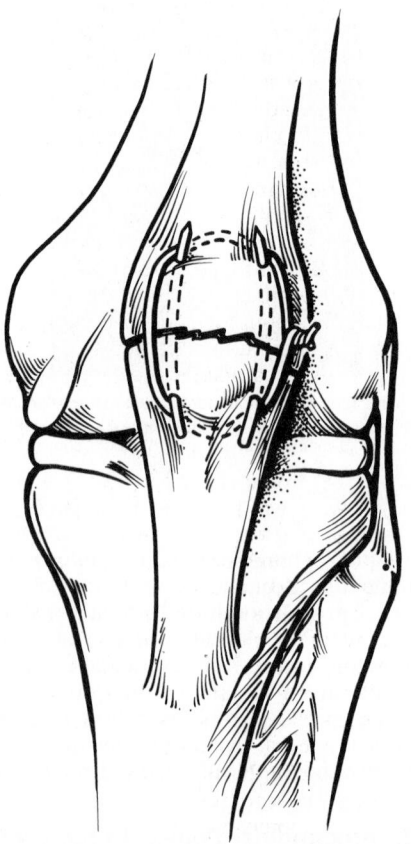

Figure 42–42. A preferred method of treating a transverse fracture of the patella is with the tension band technique. The fracture is reduced, two vertical Kirschner wires are placed across the fracture, and a circumferential wire is placed around the Kirschner wires and tightened to reduce the fracture completely. Early motion can begin 3 weeks after soft tissue healing has occurred.

considerations, such as vascular or neurologic injury, that require immediate treatment prior to any imaging study.

Most knee dislocations are easily reducible, sometimes spontaneously reducing prior to presentation in the emergency room. Alignment may be normal by the time the patient is first examined by a physician. Absence of a deformity may be misleading, so a high index of suspicion must be maintained in a patient with a knee that is unstable to anterior and posterior stress or varus-valgus stress in extension. This high index of suspicion is necessary because of the severe vascular and neurologic complications associated with a knee dislocation.[45, 46, 48] If the knee is still dislocated at the time of the first examination, the deformity should be corrected as soon as possible by gentle longitudinal traction. Occasionally, because of soft tissue interposition, a dislocated knee cannot be reduced closed. Soft tissue interposition within the joint can be recognized by the presence of a dimple over the medial joint line below the prominent medial femoral condyle. The condyle can project through a buttonhole deformity in the medial capsule. The dimple is produced by invagination of the medial ligament into the joint.

Dislocation of the knee is frequently associated with neurologic and vascular injury. Unrecognized vascular injury can lead to ischemia and loss of the leg. Ford and Goldner[44] found peroneal nerve palsy in half of the patients that presented with knee dislocation. Shields and co-workers[47] found vascular damage in 40% of 26 patients. The reason for frequent vascular injury is that the popliteal artery and vein are firmly fixed above and below the popliteal space. Hyperextension of the knee or anterior displacement of the tibia may either completely tear the popliteal artery or produce intimal damage, leading to thrombosis. Peripheral pulses must be assessed carefully on first examination and followed closely. If pulses are diminished or there is any question about the continuity of vessels, immediate exploration should be performed. Arteriography is time-consuming and unnecessary in a patient with a knee dislocation and an abnormal vascular examination after reduction. If a patient has a normal vascular examination after reduction, the surgeon in charge may elect to perform arteriography, or careful and frequently repeated vascular examinations, to rule out secondary thrombosis and ischemia from intimal damage. A patient with an abnormal vascular examination consisting of diminished pulses or abnormal capillary refill should be taken immediately to the operating room for exploration and bypass grafting if indicated. Delays in treatment while obtaining imaging studies in a patient with a documented knee dislocation and an abnormal vascular examination can negatively affect the salvage rate and success in obtaining adequate revascularization.

Compartment syndrome can follow knee dislocation and should be suspected when the patient continues to complain of severe pain in the leg after reduction. Tissue ischemia and elevated compartment pressures can be present, even though pulses are palpable. Documentation of the initial compartment pressures as well as the trend toward increasing or decreasing pressures provide information to a surgeon who is considering fasciotomy.[49] A judgment as to whether a fasciotomy is indicated depends not only on the measurement of the compartment pressure but also on the general condition of the patient. A mildly elevated compartment pressure on the order of 20 to 30 mm. Hg in a patient who has been hypotensive can result in tissue ischemia more readily than in a normotensive patient.

SELECTED REFERENCES

Balsano, N. A., and Reynolds, F. X.: Pelvic fractures. J. Trauma, 13:1011, 1973.
This comprehensive review of 273 fractures emphasizes the severity of pelvic frac-

tures. The complications are clearly outlined, and their management is well discussed. Open reduction of pelvic fractures with massive bleeding is discouraged. Preferably, bleeding points should be localized by arteriography, and hemorrhage controlled by the injection of autogenous blood clots unless major vessels are involved.

Burgess, A. R., Eastridge, B. J., Young, J. W., et al.: Pelvic ring disruptions: Effective classification system and protocols. J. Trauma, 30:848, 1990.
This article provides an excellent overview of the spectrum of pelvic ring injuries. A classification system is provided to allow application of specific protocols for each particular injury.

Lu-Yao, G. L., Keller, R. B., Littenberg, B., and Wennberg, J. E.: Outcomes after displaced fractures of the femoral neck. A meta-analysis of 106 published reports. J. Bone Joint Surg. [Am.], 76:15, 1994.
This meta-analysis covers the existing literature on displaced fractures of the femoral neck. It provides a retrospective look at results that now guide treatment and ongoing clinical protocols.

Matta, J. M., Anderson, L. M., Epstein, H. C., et al.: Fractures of the acetabulum: A retrospective analysis. Clin. Orthop., 205:230, 1986.
This review gives an in-depth explanation of the use of roof arc angles in evaluating acetabular fractures.

Winquist, R. A., Hansen, S. T., and Clawson, D. K.: Closed intramedullary nailing of femoral fractures: A report of 520 cases. J. Bone Joint Surg. [Am.], 66:529, 1984.
This classic article on closed intramedullary nailing of femoral fractures provides results and a classification scheme for treating the fractured femur. It is extremely valuable from the standpoint of understanding what constitutes a stable or an unstable fracture.

REFERENCES

Fractures of the Pelvis and Acetabulum

1. Burgess, A. R., Eastridge, B. J., Young, J. W., et al.: Pelvic ring disruptions: Effective classification system and protocols. J. Trauma, 30:848, 1990.
2. Chan, L., Nade, S., Brooks, A., and Deane, S.: Experience with lower urinary tract disruptions associated with pelvic fractures: Implications for emergency room management. Aust. N. Z. J. Surg., 64:395, 1994.
3. d'Aubigne, R. M.: Management of acetabular fractures in multiple trauma. J. Trauma, 8:333, 1968.
4. Ghalambor, N., Matta, J. M., and Bernstein, L.: Heterotopic ossification following operative treatment of acetabular fractures: An analysis of risk factors. Clin. Orthop., 305:96, 1994.
5. Keith, J. E., Jr., Brashear, H. R., Jr., and Guilford, W. B.: Stability of posterior fracture-dislocations of the hip: Quantitative assessment using computed tomography. J. Bone Joint Surg. [Am.], 70:711, 1988.
6. Klein, S. R., Saroyan, R. M., Baumgartner, F., and Bongard, F. S.: Management strategy of vascular injuries associated with pelvic fractures. J. Cardiovasc. Surg., 33:349, 1992.
7. Letournel, E.: Classification of acetabular fracture. In Judet, R. (Ed.): Fractures of the Acetabulum. Berlin, Springer-Verlag, 1981.
8. Malgaigne, J. F.: Treatise on Fractures. Philadelphia, J. B. Lippincott, 1859.
9. Matta, J. M., Anderson, L. M., Epstein, H. C., et al.: Fractures of the acetabulum: A retrospective analysis. Clin. Orthop., 205:230, 1986.
10. Mayo, K. A., Letournel, E., Matta, J. M., Mast, J. W., Johnson, E. E., and Martimbeau, C. L.: Surgical revision of malreduced acetabular fractures. Clin. Orthop., 305:47, 1994.
11. Mendez, C., Gubler, K. D., and Maier, R. V.: Diagnostic accuracy of peritoneal lavage in patients with pelvic fractures. Arch. Surg., 129:477, 1994.
12. Peltier, L. F.: Complications associated with fractures of the pelvis. J. Bone Joint Surg. [Am.], 47:1069, 1965.
13. Ragnarsson, B., and Jacobsson, B.: Epidemiology of pelvic fractures in a Swedish county. Acta Orthop. Scand., 63:297, 1992.
14. Resnick, C. S., Stackhouse, D. J., Shanmuganathan, K., and Young, J. W.: Diagnosis of pelvic fractures in patients with acute pelvic trauma: Efficacy of plain radiographs. A. J. R. Am. J. Roentgenol., 158:109, 1992.
15. Schlonsky, J., et al.: Functional disability following avulsion fracture of the ischial epiphysis. J. Bone Joint Surg. [Am.], 54:641, 1973.
16. Sinnott, R., Rhodes, M., and Brader, A.: Open pelvic fracture: An injury for trauma centers. Am. J. Surg., 163:283, 1992.
17. Tile, M.: Fractures of the Pelvis and Acetabulum. Baltimore, Williams & Wilkins, 1984.
18. Trunkey, D. D., et al.: Management of pelvic fractures in blunt trauma injury. J. Trauma, 14:912, 1974.

Fractures of the Hip

19. Armstrong, A. L., and Wallace, W. A.: The epidemiology of hip fractures and methods of prevention. Acta Orthop. Belg., 60:85, 1994.
20. Boyd, H. B., and Griffin, L. L.: Classification and treatment of trochanteric fractures. Arch. Surg., 58:858, 1949.
21. Coventry, M. B.: The treatment of fracture dislocation of the hip by total hip arthroplasty. J. Bone Joint Surg. [Am.], 56:1103, 1974.
22. Cumming, R. G., and Klineberg, R. J.: Epidemiological study of the relation

between arthritis of the hip and hip fractures. Ann. Rheum. Dis., *53:*707, 1993.

23. Davidson, B. L., and Weinstein, S. L.: Hip fractures in children: A long-term follow-up study. J. Pediatr. Orthop., *12:*355, 1992.
24. Dimon, J. H., and Hughston, J. C.: Unstable inter-trochanteric fractures of the hip. J. Bone Joint Surg. [Am.], *49:*440, 1967.
25. DiStefano, V. J., et al.: Stable fixation of the difficult subtrochanteric fracture. J. Trauma, *12:*1066, 1972.
26. Epstein, H. C.: Posterior fracture dislocation of the hip: Long-term follow up. J. Bone Joint Surg. [Am.], *56:*1103, 1974.
27. Freeman, M. A., et al.: The role of fatigue in the pathogenesis of senile femoral neck fractures. J. Bone Joint Surg. [Br.], *56:*698, 1974.
28. Hinton, R. Y., and Smith, G. S.: The association of age, race, and sex with the location of proximal femoral fractures in the elderly. J. Bone Joint Surg. [Am.], *75:*752, 1993.
29. Leadbetter, G. W.: A treatment for fracture of the neck of the femur. J. Bone Joint Surg. [Am.], *15:*931, 1933.
30. Lunceford, E. M.: Use of the Moore self-locking vitallium prosthesis in acute fractures of the femoral neck. J. Bone Joint Surg. [Am.], *47:*832, 1965.
31. Lu-Yao, G. L., Keller, R. B., Littenberg, B., and Wennberg, J. E.: Outcomes after displaced fractures of the femoral neck: A meta-analysis of 106 published reports. J. Bone Joint Surg. [Am.], *76:*15, 1994.
32. Melton, L. J., 3d: Hip fractures: A worldwide problem today and tomorrow. Bone, *14*(suppl.):S1–8, 1993.
33. Mulholland, R. C., and Gunn, D. R.: Sliding screw fixation of intertrochanteric femoral fractures. J. Trauma, *12:*581, 1972.
34. Shelton, M. L.: Subtrochanteric fractures of the femur. Arch. Surg., *110:*41, 1975.
35. Smith-Peterson, M. N., Cave, E. F., and Van Gorder, W.: Intracapsular fracture of the neck of the femur. Arch. Surg., *23:*715, 1931.
36. Swiontkowski, M., Harrington, R., Keller, T., et al.: Torsion and bending analysis of internal fixation techniques for femoral neck fractures: The role of implant design and bone density. J. Orthop. Res., *5:*433, 1987.
37. Swiontkowski, M., Winquist, R., and Hansen, S.: Fractures of the femoral neck in patients between the ages of 12 and 49 years. J. Bone Joint Surg. [Am.], *66:*837, 1984.

38. Vail, T. P., and Urbaniak, J. R.: Outcomes in surgical treatment of femoral neck fracture: Analysis of failures secondary to osteonecrosis. J. South. Orthop. Assoc., *4*(2):83, 1995.
39. Whitman, R.: A new method of treatment for fractures of the neck of the femur. Am. J. Surg., *36:*746, 1902.

Fractures of the Femur

40. Fitzpatrick, C. B.: The treatment of fractures of the shaft of the femur by closed intramedullary nailing. J. Bone Joint Surg. [Br.], *57:*255, 1975.
41. Johnson, K. D.: Femur: Trauma. *In* Frymoyer, J. D. (Ed.): Orthopaedic Knowledge Update 4: Home Study Syllabus. Rosemont, American Academy of Orthopaedic Surgeons, 1993.
42. Kunscher, G.: Intramedullary surgical technique and its place in orthopedic surgery. J. Bone Joint Surg.]Am.], *47:*809, 1965.
43. Winquist, R. A., Hansen, S. T., and Clawson, D. K.: Closed intramedullary nailing of femoral fractures: A report of 520 cases. J. Bone Joint Surg. [Am.], *66:*529, 1984.

Fractures of the Knee

44. Ford, G. L., and Goldner, J. L.: Dislocation of the knee joint. N. C. Med. J., *20:*463, 1959.
45. Kennedy, J. C.: Complete dislocation of the knee joint. J. Bone Joint Surg. [Am.], *45:*889, 1963.
46. Reckling, F. W., and Peltier, L. F.: Acute knee dislocations and their complications. J. Trauma, *9:*181, 1969.
47. Shields, L., Mital, M., and Cave, E. F.: Complete dislocation of the knee: Experience at the Massachusetts General Hospital. J. Trauma, *9:*192, 1969.
48. Taylor, A. R., Arden, G. P., and Rainey, M. H.: Traumatic dislocation of the knee: A report of 43 cases with special reference to conservative treatment. J. Bone Joint Surg. [Br.], *54:*96, 1972.
49. Whitesides, T. E., et al.: A simple method for tissue pressure determination. Arch. Surg., *110:*1311, 1975.

VII

FRACTURES OF THE TIBIA, FIBULA, ANKLE, AND FOOT

L. Scott Levin, M.D., and William E. Garrett, Jr., M.D., Ph.D.

FRACTURES OF THE TIBIA AND FIBULA
Historical Aspects

The tibia and fibula are two of the most frequently fractured long bones.[12, 22] High-speed motor vehicular trauma causes many injuries, producing open or *compound* fractures with soft tissue defects due to high-energy absorption. Treatment of fractures of the tibia and fibula has been the subject of much controversy for more than 2500 years. Hippocrates recognized in his treatise *Fractures:* "Of the bones of the leg, the inner one, called the tibia, is the more troublesome to manage, and requires the greater extension; and if the broken bones are not properly arranged, it is impossible to conceal the distortion, for the bone is exposed and wholly uncovered with flesh; and it is much longer before patients can walk on the leg when this bone is broken [as compared with the isolated fibula fracture]." In 300 B.C., Hippocrates wrote about the treatment of open fractures with methods of reduction and stabilization using a device quite similar to the mechanical design of the twentieth-century external fixator introduced by Hoffman and Vidal in the 1930s for management of the open tibia fracture. Ambroise Paré wrote on the treatment of open fractures, advocating débridement of exposed bone in compound fractures prior to reduction.

Despite sound principles of treatment for lower extremity fractures recognized years ago, above-knee amputation rates for tibia fractures were as high as 62% as reported by Mal-

gaigne in the nineteenth century, 82% during the Crimean War, and 54% during the Civil War. Mortality from such fractures was as high as 76% during the Franco-Prussian War (1870). Internal fixation for fractures was introduced at the turn of the century. The first recorded tibial plate fixation was attributed to Hansman (1886). The use of plates for tibial fractures was popularized by Lane in 1894.[30] Lambotte introduced the term *osteosynthesis* to describe primary fracture healing (1907). This began the modern era of fracture care.

Despite introduction of the external fixator by Hippocrates and early success in Europe in the 1930s, the external fixator was condemned by the Surgeon General of the Army, Colonel Cleveland, in 1943, because of the high incidence of pin tract infections, osteomyelitis, and nonunion. Alternative methods of treatment were devised, including the iron nail (Hey Groves) and the more popular Küntscher nail (1940), which established the intramedullary technique of fracture fixation. In 1949, Robert Danis introduced the *coapter* as a method to fix long bone fractures with compressive forces that would serve to enhance stability of fixation. This led to the development of the Arbeitsgemeinschaft Für Osteosynthesefragen/Association for the Study of Internal Fixation (AO/ASIF) group of Swiss surgeons, who consolidated sound mechanical and biologic principles that enable effective treatment of open and closed fractures with internal and/or external fixation.[27] Despite the evolution of modern fracture care of the tibia, surgeons today still debate the best methods of treatment.

Anatomy

The tibia is medial and stronger than the fibula. The upper end of the tibia is expanded particularly in the transverse axis to provide a bearing surface for the body weight transmitted through the femur. The upper tibia is divided into a medial and lateral condyle and has an anterior projection, the tibial tubercle, onto which the patellar tendon inserts. The lateral condyle articulates with the fibular head. The shaft of the tibia can be palpated along the medial subcutaneous border of the leg. The lower end of the tibia is slightly expanded and projects downward as the medial malleolus. The fibula can be divided into three regions: the head, the shaft, and the lateral malleolus. The two leg bones are connected by the interosseous ligament, a strong fascial band that supports the leg and serves as an origin for muscles of the anterior and posterior compartments.

Blood to the tibia and fibula is supplied by the popliteal artery, which branches into the anterior tibial, posterior tibial, and peroneal arteries. The posterior tibial nerve accompanies the posterior tibial artery and innervates the posterior compartment containing the gastrocnemius and soleus muscles superficially and the posterior tibial, flexor hallucis, and flexor digitorum longus muscles more deeply. The nutrient artery to the tibia is derived from the posterior tibial artery. The anterior tibial nerve innervates the anterior compartment, which includes the anterior tibial, extensor hallucis longus, extensor digitorum longus, and peroneus tertius muscles. The lateral compartment includes the peroneus longus and brevis muscles innervated by the peroneal nerve.

Mechanism of Injury

Tibial fractures can be caused by high- or low-energy injury. Prognosis is determined by the initial energy absorbed, and not necessarily by the location of the fracture.

Automobile-pedestrian accidents can impart up to 100,000 foot-pounds of energy to the victim in a bumper injury. These fractures are usually more comminuted than are low-energy injuries due to falls or skiing accidents, which tend to produce torsional deformity and oblique fracture patterns. Gunshot or shotgun injuries often produce soft tissue defects, depending on muzzle velocity and range. Pathologic fractures due to tumor may occur in any region. Stress fractures, as a result of chronic cyclic loading of long bones that do not receive sufficient muscle support, particularly in athletes, can evade diagnosis, with radiographic findings not revealed until late in the course of the fracture. Fibular fractures are usually observed with tibial fractures if sufficient energy is imparted. The fibula may be fractured by direct blow, or the head may fracture with an isolated medial malleolar fracture (Maisonneuve's fracture).

Classification of Fractures

Fractures of the tibia and fibula can be classified by anatomic region, whether they are open or closed, and by the fracture pattern or displacement. Tibial plateau fractures are commonly divided into six types according to Schatzker and McBroom (Fig. 42–43).[36] Type I is a wedge fracture of the lateral tibial plateau, usually occurring in young people. Type II is a wedge fracture combined with depression of the adjacent weight-bearing surface. Type III is a central lateral plateau depression fracture without a wedge fracture. Type IV is a medial tibial plateau fracture. Type V is a bicondylar fracture that consists of a wedge fracture of the medial and lateral plateau. Type VI fractures are the most complex fractures in that the metaphysis separates from the diaphysis of the tibia. An operative approach to Type V and VI fractures is generally required (Fig. 42–44). Tibial shaft fractures are usually classified into thirds, with delays in healing commonly observed in the middle third and the region between the proximal and middle thirds. Open tibial fractures commonly involve the shaft. Gustilo and Anderson classified open fractures into three categories that have significance

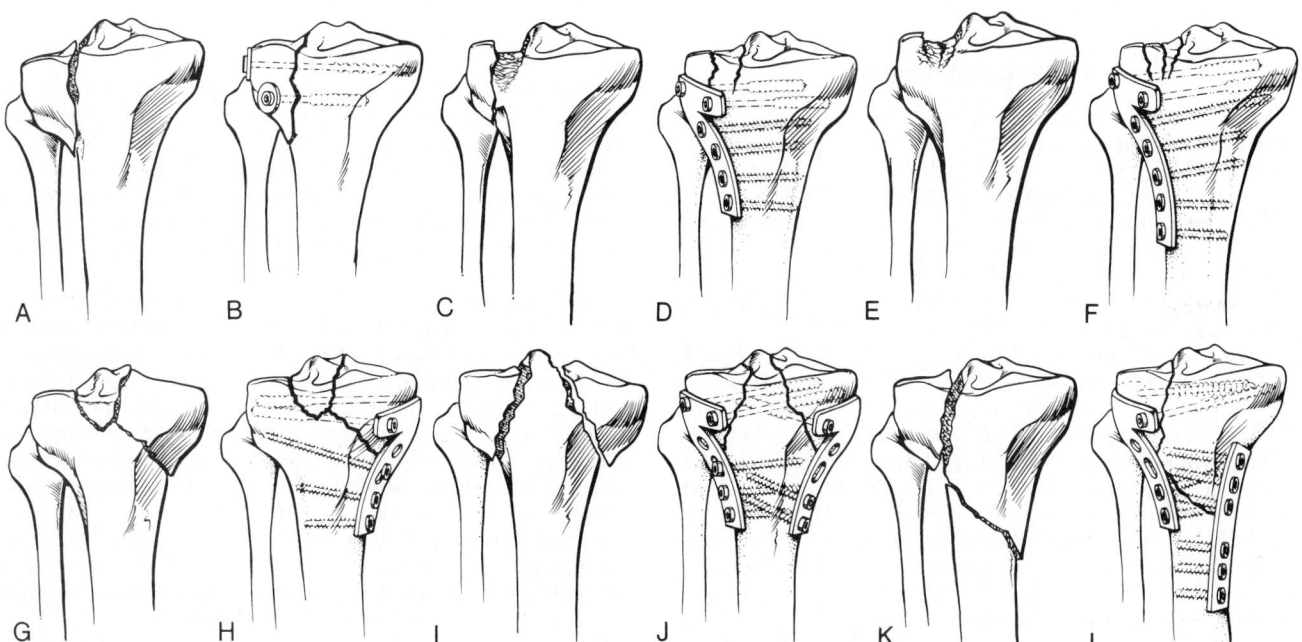

Figure 42–43. *A* and *B*, Type I tibial plateau fracture. *C* and *D*, Type II tibial plateau fracture. *E* and *F*, Type III tibial plateau fracture. *G* and *H*, Type IV tibial plateau fracture. *I* and *J*, Type V tibial plateau fracture. *K* and *L*, Type VI tibial plateau fracture. (From Schatzker, J., and Tile, M. [Eds.]: The Rationale of Operative Fracture Care. New York, Springer-Verlag, 1985.)

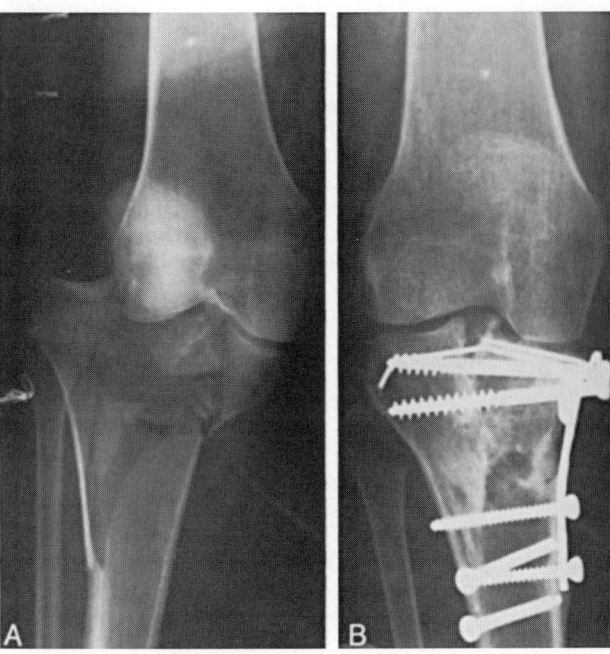

Figure 42–44. *A* and *B*, Type VI tibial plateau fracture. This patient was treated with open reduction and internal fixation using buttress plate and screws.

regarding the incidence of fracture union and risk for infection and/or amputation. Grade I fractures are those that have perforation of the skin from the inside; wounds are less than or equal to 1 cm. Grade II open fractures are produced by outside-to-inside forces, with soft tissue injury being greater than 1 cm. Grade III injuries involve significant soft tissue damage. These are further classified as Grade IIIa, soft tissue injury without periosteal stripping or vessel damage; Grade IIIb, soft tissue damage with periosteal stripping; and Grade IIIc, major vascular injury and soft tissue damage. Difficult fractures involving the lower tibia are tibial plafond fractures occurring in the lower tibia and frequently extending into the ankle joint.

Physical Examination

Examination of patients with tibial and fibular fractures requires knowledge of topographic, vascular, and neural anatomy of the lower extremity. In severely injured legs, simply positioning the leg in proper anatomic alignment may restore absent pulses. All open wounds should be noted and covered with a sterile dressing. *All punctures and lacerations of the integument should be considered open fractures until proved otherwise in the operating room, where irrigation and débridement of all open wounds are mandatory.*

Capillary refill, toe pulp turgor, and temperature should be assessed, in addition to posterior tibial and dorsalis pedis pulses. If pulses are not palpable because of shock or vasoconstriction, a Doppler examination should be performed. Vascular injuries commonly occur above the trifurcation of the popliteal artery, and vascular injury should be suspected if fractures occur in this area.[21] If capillary refill is slow or vessel damage is suspected, arteriography should be considered, particularly in cases of fracture-dislocation of the knee joint.

Palpation along the tibial crest may reveal a step-off or swelling that may represent a minimally displaced fracture. Examination of the ankle and knee joints should be performed to exclude any associated ligamentous injury, such as in lateral tibial plateau fractures, which often produce

injury to the medial collateral ligament. Notice should be taken of any excessive varus or valgus angulation of the knee, which may suggest tibial plateau fracture or distal femur fracture.[19]

A thorough sensory examination is required when one is evaluating tibial and fibular fractures. Proximal fibula fractures may cause peroneal nerve injury, with associated sensory and motor deficits. Anterior tibial nerve and deep peroneal nerve dysfunction may indicate compartment syndrome; similarly, diminished sensibility to light touch on the plantar aspect of the foot suggests posterior tibial nerve compression.

Compartment syndrome is defined as an increase in tissue pressure in the closed fascial compartments of the leg. It can occur in open or closed tibial fractures.[13, 15, 25] If intracompartment pressure exceeds capillary pressure, diminished tissue perfusion may cause anoxia and necrosis of tissue within the compartment. Signs include pain on passive stretching of muscles in the compartment, swollen compartments, diminished sensation, and motor weakness. A variety of methods are used in measuring compartment pressure. These include an arterial catheter inserted directly into the compartment, the wick catheter technique, the Whitesides technique, and a Stryker compartment pressure measurement device. Fasciotomy should be performed if clinical suspicion is high and pressures are elevated with respect to arterial pressure.

Radiographic Evaluation

Fractures involving the tibia and fibula should be visualized radiographically in the anteroposterior and lateral planes. It is imperative that the knee and ankle joint be visualized to avoid missing fractures that extend intra-articularly. Particularly in high-energy injuries, films of the ipsilateral femur and pelvis should be obtained to exclude the floating knee or pelvis injury. Forty-five-degree oblique radiographs may help in evaluating the tibial plateau. Tomography is helpful in fractures of the tibial plateau and plafond to define the extent of joint compression. Computed tomography (CT) with three-dimensional reconstruction has proved useful in planning open reduction and internal fixation of complex fractures.

Treatment

The principles of fracture care are classic: reduction of the fracture, stabilization of the limb to allow fracture healing, and proper care of the soft tissue envelope.[26] The actual application of these tenets has changed several times in the last 50 years. Understanding the mechanism of injury and the deformities of length, angulation, rotation, and displacement (LARD) enables the surgeon to obtain an acceptable reduction.

Nondisplaced fractures of the tibia are traditionally treated with casting.[28] Long leg casts are used initially to control forces above the knee joint. When fractures become consolidated with early callus, to ensure that they maintain their position, short leg casts are used until the mechanical strength of the callus can support the patient. Disadvantages of cast treatment include the possibility of creating fracture disease; the term *fracture disease* refers to disuse osteoporosis, muscle wasting, joint stiffness, and posttraumatic dystrophy. Below-knee casts have been advocated by Sarmiento.[34] The soft tissues act as hydrostatic supports for the bone in a total-contact patellar tendon–bearing cast.[35] Weight bearing gradually increases as the fracture stabilizes.

The external fixator was employed infrequently during World War II. However, with improvement in materials and pins and a better understanding of frame mechanics, it has been utilized for the majority of open tibial fractures where

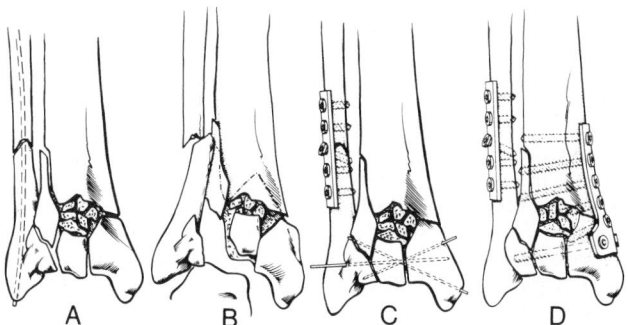

Figure 42–45. *A,* Schematic drawing of a fracture of the distal tibia at the ankle joint, also termed a pilon fracture. *B,* Temporary fibula fixation, regaining length of the tibia-fibula complex. *C,* Rigid fixation of the fibula with temporary Kirschner wire fixation of the tibial plafond. *D,* Rigid fixation of the tibia using a buttress plate supplemented with bone grafting, with restoration of the articular surface. (From Schatzker, J., and Tile, M. [Eds.]: The Rationale of Operative Fracture Care. New York, Springer-Verlag, 1985.)

gross contamination or severe soft tissue injury precludes the judicious use of internal fixation.[4]

Fracture treatment is dependent on the anatomic location of the fracture, whether it is intra- or extra-articular, whether it is open or closed, and whether it is amenable to nonoperative or operative management that requires internal fixation, external fixation, or a combination of both.

Plating is indicated for the treatment of tibial fractures in specific instances, such as preceding vascular repair or in fractures of the tibial plafond (Fig. 42–45).[9, 24, 32, 33] It is a technically demanding procedure owing to the risk of soft tissue compromise and impairment of vascularity to underlying bone.[2] Plates are also used as buttress devices when open reduction with internal fixation is performed for tibial plateau fractures, when the articular surface is elevated, and when medial or lateral support is required.

Segmental fractures have been fixed with interfragmentary compression of large butterfly fragments, followed by the application of a plate as a neutralization device (Fig. 42–46). Advocates of open reduction believe that fracture disease is avoided and that motion of joints and muscle units can be accomplished almost immediately, with earlier functional return than with traction or casting.

Intramedullary devices can be used for stabilization of tibial shaft fractures.[8, 23, 31, 40, 42] These are usually reserved for fractures that are difficult to control with closed methods

such as casting, or fractures that displace despite casting. They can be inserted with or without the locking screws that transfix the nail above and below the fracture to prevent shortening and to resist torque (Figs. 42–47 and 42–48). These devices traditionally required reaming of the medullary canal.[20] There are more flexible intramedullary devices that can be inserted without reaming and can be stacked in the canal to provide internal splinting of the fracture. They are less stable than plates or reamed nails, but their advantage is that the intramedullary blood supply is not disturbed, as in conventional reaming. Currently, locked nonreamed nails that provide good stability without reaming are available but with slightly less bending resistance when compared with conventional Küntscher-type devices. Most nailing is performed without opening the fracture, thereby reducing the risk of infection and vascular compromise to the fracture site.

The external fixator is commonly used to stabilize tibial shaft fractures. Although there is controversy surrounding its use, it affords excellent access to the soft tissue injuries that often accompany fractures of the tibial shaft. Its main purpose is to provide stability to the skeleton, which allows the soft tissue to heal.[4, 5] After the soft tissue envelope is restored, definitive treatment of the fracture can be undertaken. Often fractures involve bone loss that may require bone grafting, either vascularized (such as a free vascularized fibula) or nonvascularized (autogenous iliac crest).[39, 44] The external fixator can be used as definitive fracture treatment if there is evidence of callus formation and bone healing. When healing is not apparent, the external fixator should be removed and alternative methods of fracture fixation em-

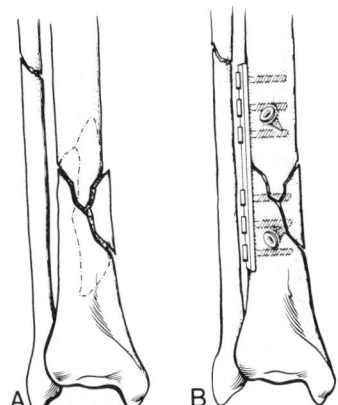

Figure 42–46. *A* and *B,* Schematic drawing of a tibial shaft fracture treated with open reduction and internal fixation using interfragmentary screw compression and a neutralization plate. (From Schatzker, J., and Tile, M. [Eds.]: The Rationale of Operative Fracture Care. New York, Springer-Verlag, 1985.)

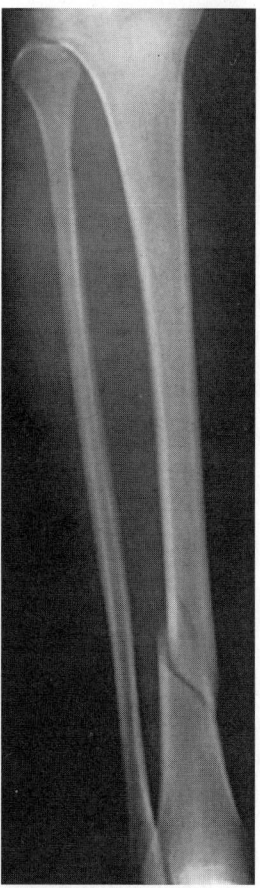

Figure 42–47. A closed oblique tibial fracture. Adequate closed reduction could not be maintained. The patient had to be treated with an intramedullary nail (see Fig. 42–48).

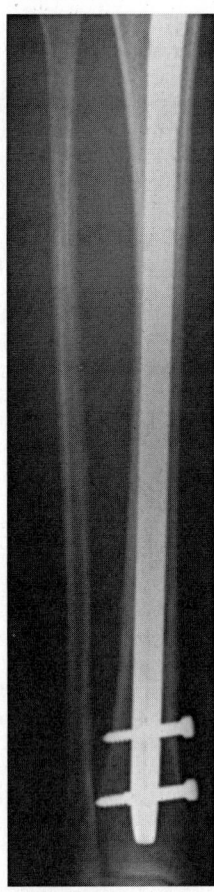

Figure 42–48. The fracture demonstrated in Figure 42–47 following closed reduction and intramedullary nailing. The screws shown in the distal tibia prevent shortening and rotational deformities.

ployed, such as casting, use of a cast brace, or internal fixation. Converting open fractures treated with external fixation to internal fixation (plates or intramedullary nails) has a high risk of infection and should be reserved for select cases.

The Ilizarov device, introduced from Kurgan, Russia, and originally used by Gavriil Ilizarov in the 1950s, has made its way to the United States after its introduction in Italy about a decade ago. The technical advantage of the Ilizarov device is that it utilizes thin wire fixators instead of larger Schanz screws to purchase bone and to attach to external circumferential rings connected with rods. The Ilizarov device has several applications in tibial fracture management. Because the tin wires can capture juxta-articular fractures without opening the fracture, the device is useful for pylon and tibial plateau fractures. It can be applied in instances of acute trauma and is similar to other external fixators, but it allows more uniform weight bearing than other fixators, such as anterior frames. Furthermore, the Ilizarov can be used in instances of bone loss to transfer bone by performing a corticotomy or a subperiosteal cut in the bone. This bone segment is pulled with wires over time, and a *regenerate* can be formed that is a distraction of callus. Finally, *docking* occurs, and the regenerate then matures to become similar to normal bone. This obviates the need for iliac crest bone grafting or vascularized bone grafting, and it can be useful in cases of large bone loss or segmental loss.

OPEN FRACTURES OF THE TIBIA AND FIBULA

These are usually high-energy injuries. The main treatment goal is to prevent acute and chronic infection. Management requires aggressive and thorough débridement of all nonvitalized tissue in the operating room, with provisional or definitive fracture stabilization, depending on the nature of the fracture. *All* wounds are left open. Staged soft tissue reconstruction is then performed, which may include delayed wound closure, bone and skin grafting, local muscle flaps, or distant free tissue transfer for large defects.[6, 14] Composite tissue transfer, using techniques of microsurgery, is highly effective in the treatment of these injuries. Entire muscles can be transferred for coverage and function. Bone with skin can be transplanted, which provides structural stability as well as coverage.

Principles for coverage of open tibial shaft fractures suggest that the gastrocnemius muscle be used as a rotational flap for proximal-third soft tissue defects, the soleus for middle-third defects, and microsurgical free tissue transfer for distal-third soft tissue defects.[43] Recently, based on anatomic dissections and anatomic studies performed in France, an increased awareness of vascular territories, called *angiosomes,* has led to the development of local flaps that are useful in the treatment of small soft tissue defects following trauma to the tibia. So-called fasciocutaneous flaps can be rotated based on perforating vessels to cover soft tissue defects either acutely or in chronic situations.

New external fixators, such as the pinless internal fixator developed by the AO group, obviate the need for pin placement into bone. Instead, they use a tenaculum-type clamp to hold the bone. This is particularly useful in converting external fixation to internal fixation, such as intramedullary nailing, early in the posttrauma course.

Complications

Complications include delayed union and nonunion.[1] Nonunion is usually defined as a fracture that does not demonstrate healing by 6 months. However, this is a somewhat arbitrary definition, in that the condition of the soft tissue, comminution, and blood supply to bone all have a bearing on healing. Nonunions can be treated by a variety of bone grafting procedures, by an increase in fracture stabilization, or by electrical stimulation, which remains controversial.[3] Bone augmentation includes corticocancellous grafts; free fibular microvascular transfers; fibular transpositions; deep circumflex iliac artery osteocutaneous composite transfers; bone substitutes such as calcium phosphate, allograft, or hydroxyapatite; and the Ilizarov method, which transports bone segments by callus distraction.[6, 16, 29]

Infection is perhaps the most severe complication of tibial fractures and usually follows open injuries.[10, 44] "Every man who develops separation has the right to ask his surgeon to justify it" (Alexis Carrel).[38] Current trends in aggressive management of soft tissue, with early coverage of exposed implants and bone, have reduced the incidence of infection-related morbidity and chronic osteomyelitis. One of the worst complications following open fracture of the tibia is infected nonunion.[37] Treatment goals in this situation require first achieving union, followed by eradication of the infection, if possible.

Malunion is defined as a fracture that heals in a significantly nonanatomic position. In fractures of the tibial shaft, up to 5 degrees of varus or valgus deformity in the anteroposterior and lateral plane is acceptable. Internal rotation of 5 degrees and external rotation of 20 degrees are accepted. Shortening of 8 mm. or less is functionally insignificant. Other complications include venous stasis disease, traumatic arthritis, claw toes due to unrecognized posterior compartment syndrome, refracture, and amputation. The role of the arteriogram is to define injury, to detect any abnormal anatomy or pathologic conditions, and to help determine the possibility of repairing vessels.

Indications for primary amputation of mangled limbs are now evolving because of the grave socioeconomic and personal consequences of limb salvage.[11] The process often requires several years and produces results that do not equal the gait and function of a conventional below-knee prosthesis.[7] Primary amputation is still a treatment option for some open tibial fractures. Indications for immediate amputation include disruption of the posterior tibial nerve, more than 6 hours of warm ischemia, and segmental bone defects greater than 20 cm.[17, 35]

FRACTURES OF THE FIBULA

Fractures of the fibula usually accompany fractures of the tibia and are usually not associated with the morbidity of tibial fractures. They heal rapidly. The fibula is important in providing a lateral buttress to the ankle joint and for optimal ankle function and requires accurate anatomic reduction. Proximal fibular fractures are indications that the medial malleolus may be injured and may involve injury to the peroneal nerve. A Maisonneuve fracture is a fracture of the proximal fibula, often with a fracture of the medial malleolus. If a medial malleolar fracture is identified, it is imperative that the entire tibia and fibula, including the knee joint, be identified to avoid missing this fracture. This may be accompanied by a peroneal nerve irritation or paresis. Isolated fibular fractures produced by external direct blows can be treated with casting for comfort or protected weight bearing until the fracture heals. Fractures of the fibula around the ankle are discussed in the next section.

FRACTURES AND FRACTURE-DISLOCATIONS OF THE ANKLE

The ankle joint derives its stability and function from the precise alignment of osseous and ligamentous structures acting together as a functional unit. The distal fibula and the medial aspect of the tibia extend beyond the larger articulation of the tibia with the talus. These extensions, or the malleoli, give medial and lateral stability to the ankle joint, allowing flexion and extension of the hindfoot within the mortise. Strong ligamentous structures ensure the stability of the bones. The syndesmotic and tibiofibular ligaments hold the tibia and fibula together, and medial and lateral ligaments extend from the respective malleoli to the hindfoot. The lateral malleolus extends farther than the medial malleolus for bone stability, and the medial ligament (or deltoid) provides stronger medial ligamentous stability. These structures have been considered together as a ring, with displacement of the hindfoot being possible only when at least two breaks occur in the ring.

Ankle injuries are among the most frequent conditions treated in orthopedic surgery.[41] Fractures occur from several mechanisms of injury. Most frequently, fractures involve *external rotation* of the foot in the ankle joint, which is most often due to an internal rotation or twisting of the leg on a foot fixed by weight bearing. The fibula fractures in an oblique or spiral plane and is often displaced posteriorly. The medial malleolus or, frequently, the deltoid ligament may be injured. When the foot is everted at the time of injury, the fibula fracture is high and the damage to the interosseous ligament is greater than when the foot is inverted. When the mechanism of fracture is an *abduction* force, the medial malleolus fractures transversely or the deltoid tears first. The fibula then fractures low in an oblique plane or proximally, following tear of the interosseous ligament. *Adduction* forces fracture the fibula or disrupt the lateral ligaments in combination with an oblique fracture of the medial malleolus, without injuring the interosseous ligaments. Finally, *vertical compression* forces may disrupt the articular surface of the tibia and leave the malleoli uninjured. All these fractures may be associated with an avulsion fracture of the posterior lip of the tibia.

Optimal treatment of ankle fractures should attain several goals. The talus must be located in its normal position in the ankle mortise. Even a slight amount of tilt or displacement can lead to early disabling arthritis. Joint congruity should be restored, as with intra-articular fractures in general. If these requisites are not present initially, then reduction should be obtained by closed or open means. Closed reduction requires awareness of the mechanism of injury, since an opposite stress is used to hold the fracture stable. Immobilization should then follow until the bony and ligamentous injuries are healed. This usually requires 6 weeks or longer in an adult. Initially, a cast is applied above the flexed knee to control rotational forces.

If the requisites for adequate treatment cannot be obtained by closed manipulation, open reduction and internal fixation techniques are employed. The procedure requires adequate reduction and stabilization of the fibular fracture. Screw fixation or plate and screw fixation is most commonly used. Fixation should be adequate to allow motion in order to prevent the need for casting and prolonged immobilization. The medial malleolus can usually be treated by screw or pin fixation. Oblique fractures of the tibia or fibula can be stabilized by interfragmentary screws. The screws are placed in a manner that allows compression between the fragments. Plates used for ankle fractures are neutralization plates; they hold the fracture stable after reduction, but they do not cause compression at the fracture site.

Ligamentous injuries should be considered and treated appropriately. The interosseous membrane may tear, leaving a diastasis between the distal tibia and fibula. Normal relationships must be re-established and maintained long enough to allow proper healing. Large associated fractures of the posterior lip of the tibia occasionally require fixation if the reduction of the malleoli and ligament stabilization do not achieve appropriate position of the fragment. Treatment following surgical therapy depends on the nature of the injury and the stability obtained. Total or partial immobilization for 4 to 8 weeks is frequent. An advantage of surgical fixation is the avoidance of prolonged immobilization. This can allow better ankle and subtalar joint motion recovery and a shorter rehabilitation time.

FRACTURES OF THE FOOT

Fractures of the hindfoot are serious injuries that frequently result in significant functional disability.[18] Chip fractures and small avulsion fractures of the talus are relatively common but do not cause substantial problems after the acute period. The most frequent major fracture of the talus is a transverse fracture through the neck of the bone, usually caused by forced hyperextension. Minimally displaced fractures of the talar neck can be treated by immobilization alone. Displaced fractures must be reduced for the best likelihood of a good result (Fig. 42–49). If closed means are unsuccessful, the fracture should be opened and reduced and held by internal fixation. Pins or longitudinal lag screws are used most often. Long-term results are related to the amount of displacement of the fracture. With displaced fractures or fracture-dislocations, there is a significant risk for avascular necrosis of the body of the talus. This may cause a poor result despite adequate stabilization and rehabilitation. The tenuous blood supply to the body may be interrupted by the fracture and cause eventual *collapse* of the body and disruption of the

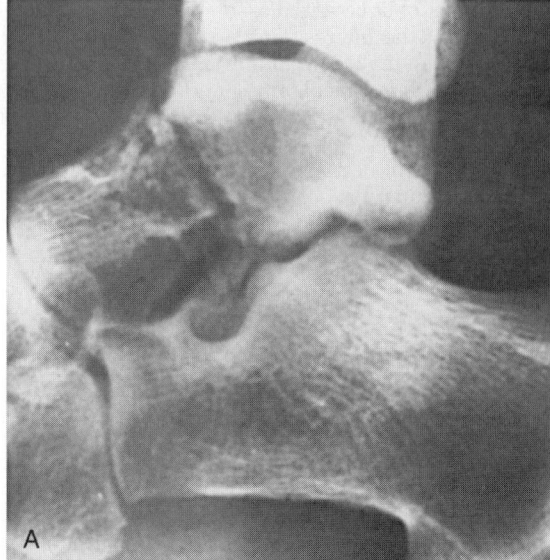

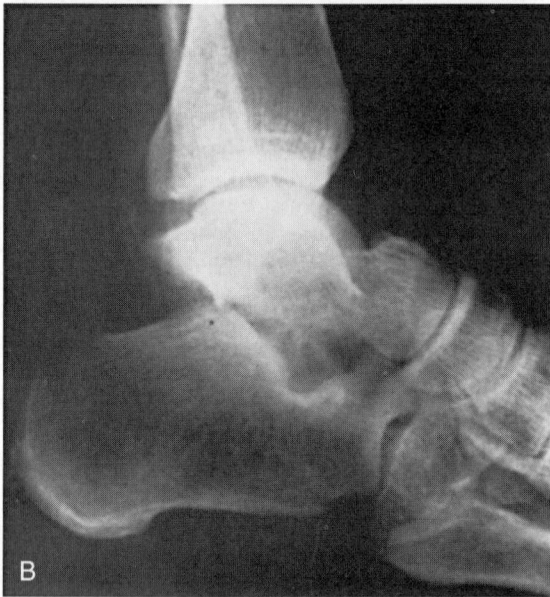

Figure 42–49. Fracture of the neck of the talus. *A*, Initial fracture line and the displacement. *B*, Satisfactory healing.

reduction and internal fixation. The aim of operative treatment is to restore the calcaneus to its original height and width and to restore the articular surface to its anatomic position. Operative treatment should be undertaken only by those with the requisite experience and skill.

Fractures of the calcaneus are better understood since the advent of CT scans, particularly the three-dimensional CT scan, which allows the surgeon to plan the placement of fixation and the realignment of the fracture fragments preoperatively. Lateral custom-designed buttress plates have been particularly helpful in restoring length and alignment of the calcaneus, leading to better functional results.

Fractures of the midfoot include fractures of the navicular, cuneiform, and cuboid bones. These bones are often fractured as a result of crush injuries; many are quite severe. These severe injuries are often open and can ultimately cause significant disability. Isolated fractures of bones of the midfoot may occur. The navicular bone can be fractured in several ways. Cortical avulsion fractures, tuberosity, and body fractures may occur. In addition, stress fractures of the navicular can occur, especially in endurance athletes.

Dislocations of the tarsometatarsal joints are usually the result of direct injury or twisting of the forefoot. This joint is known as Lisfranc's joint. The spectrum of dislocations of Lisfranc's joint ranges from complete dislocation of all five tarsometatarsal joints to the dislocation of one or two metatarsals. Occasionally, a divergent dislocation occurs, with dislocation of the first metatarsal medially and the other metatarsals laterally. Closed reduction of the dislocation is attempted by traction of the forefoot. If closed reduction is not possible, open reduction and K-wire fixation may be necessary. Recent trends lean toward the use of screw fixation. Soft tissue damage may be extensive and must be recognized and treated. These injuries frequently cause persistent pain and arthrosis in the foot, necessitating special shoes or inserts.

Fractures of the metatarsals can involve the necks, shafts, or bases, depending on the direction of the force and the mechanism of injury. Fractures of the neck of the metatarsals can be impacted as the result of a direct longitudinal force, or they can be oblique as the result of indirect twisting forces. Anatomic reduction is usually not necessary unless the metatarsal heads are displaced into the plantar surface of the foot, where future weight bearing would be painful. Fractures of the shaft of the metatarsals can be transverse, oblique, or

articular surfaces. Posttraumatic arthritis with or without avascular necrosis may ultimately require fusion of the ankle or subtalar joint. Additionally, there may be problems with skin necrosis and infection.

Fractures of the calcaneus can cause persistent problems. Unfortunately, most fractures of the calcaneus involve the joint surface, and these fractures often have a poorer prognosis. Better definition of the fracture can be obtained with oblique radiographs. The mechanism of injury is most often a fall with compressive loading of the heel. The talus acts as a wedge and is driven into the calcaneus. The articular surface of the calcaneus is driven into the underlying cancellous bone, usually with some disruption of the articular cartilage. In addition, the body of the calcaneus is compressed downward and expanded outward, which causes shortening and widening of the bone (Fig. 42–50). There are many treatment options but no consensus regarding the best methods for optimal results. Many accept nonanatomic alignment and begin early motion, avoiding weight bearing until healing. There are also many who treat these fractures with operative

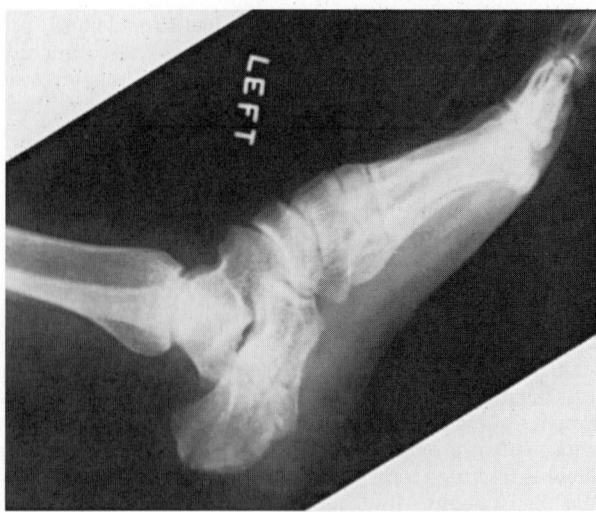

Figure 42–50. Calcaneus fracture. The fracture initially is depressed and involves the subtalar joint.

comminuted, depending on whether the trauma is direct or indirect. Fractures of the bases of the metatarsals, even when slightly displaced, usually produce no long-term ill effects and can be treated conservatively with a padded plaster cast. Avulsion of the styloid process at the base of the fifth metatarsal is the result of an inversion force, with avulsion following traction by the peroneus brevis tendon. Fractures of the diaphysis of the fifth metatarsal are considerably more difficult to treat because of their slower healing and potential for nonunion. These fractures may present as stress fractures or as pathologic fractures through a site of stress reaction in the bone. Immobilization and avoidance of weight bearing or open reduction and internal fixation are required. Stress and fatigue fractures of the metatarsals are common and should be suspected in any patient who presents with pain and puffiness in a foot following unaccustomed excess activity, such as walking or jogging. Such fractures are self-limited, and the goal of treatment is to create comfort. The second metatarsal is most frequently involved.

Fractures of the phalanges usually do not require reduction unless the toe is badly deformed. Longitudinal traction on the toe usually reduces the fracture. The toe can be strapped to an adjacent toe for some degree of comfort. At times a shoe with a firm sole, a cast, or an orthosis may help provide pain relief.

SELECTED REFERENCES

Bach, A. W., and Hansen, S. T.: Plate versus external fixation in severe open tibial shaft fractures: A randomized trial. Clin. Orthop. Rel. Res., 241:89, 1989.
Fifty-nine patients with Grade II or Grade III open tibial shaft fractures were randomized into external fixator or plate groups. Osteomyelitis occurred in 19% of the plate group and 3% of the external fixation group.

Bassett, C. A. L., Mitchell, S. N., and Gaston, S. R.: Treatment of ununited tibial diaphyseal fractures with pulsing electromagnetic fields. J. Bone Joint Surg. [Am.], 63:511, 1981.
The overall success rate in treating 127 ununited tibial diaphyseal fractures with pulsating electromagnetic fields was 87%. The exact mechanism by which the fractures heal is unknown.

Blick, S. S., Brumback, R. J., Lakatos, R., Poka, A., and Burgess, A. R.: Early prophylactic bone grafting of high energy tibial fractures. Clin. Orthop. Rel. Res., 240:21, 1989.
Fifty-three high-energy tibial fractures were treated with early prophylactic posterolateral bone grafting performed at 10 weeks following injury and 8 weeks following soft tissue coverage. Seventy-nine per cent of the fractures were Grade III open fractures, and 40% had bone loss greater than 50% of the cortical circumference. Chronic osteomyelitis was present in 1.9%.

Bone, L. B., and Johnson, K. D.: Treatment of tibial fractures by reaming and intramedullary nailing. J. Bone Joint Surg. [Am.], 68:877, 1986.
One hundred twelve fractures were treated by intramedullary nailing. The main complication was infection, treated in six of seven patients successfully.

Bourne, R. B.: Pilon fractures of the distal tibia. Clin. Orthop. Rel. Res., 240:42, 1989.
Pilon fractures are categorized into Ruedi and Allgower Type I, Type II, and Type III. Type I and Type II had 80% satisfactory function. In Type III, only 32% had satisfactory function. Seven per cent of tibial fractures are pilon-type fractures.

DeLee, J. C., and Stiehl, J. B.: Open tibia fracture with compartment syndrome. Clin. Orthop. Rel. Res., 160:175, 1981.
Among 104 open tibial fractures, compartment syndromes developed in six.

Golyakhovsky, V., and Frankel, V. H.: Operative Manual of Ilizarov Techniques. St. Louis, Mosby-Year Book, 1993.
A textbook reviewing principles and applications of the Ilizarov method for deformity correction of long bones.

Lange, R. H., Bach, A. W., Hansen, S. T., and Johansen, K. H.: Open tibial fractures with associated vascular injuries. Prognosis for limb salvage. J. Trauma, 3:203, 1985.
There was an ultimate amputation rate of 61% (22% primary, 39% delayed).

McAndrew, M. T., and Brick, A. L.: Initial care of massively traumatized lower extremities. Clin. Orthop. Rel. Res., 243:20, 1989.
In a review of Grade IIIb and Grade IIIc injuries, the amputation rate was 35%; 7 of 16, or 48%, were infected. There were 8 infections in 19 patients. Seven of the limbs were salvaged. Eighty-eight per cent returned to their previous or a more vigorous occupation, and 12 of 16 patients became ambulatory within 1 year.

Wist, D. A.: Medullary nailing of acute shaft fractures. Clin. Orthop. Rel. Res., 212:1122, 1986.
One hundred eleven tibial shaft fractures were treated with flexible intramedullary nailings. An advantage to this technique is less compromise to the medullary blood supply. There were four deep wound infections. Average healing time was 18.8 weeks, 5.4% had delayed union, and there was a 4.5% incidence of angulatory malunion between 6 and 10 degrees.

REFERENCES

1. Bach, A. W., and Hansen, S. T.: Delayed union, nonunion, and malunion of the tibia shaft. In Evarts, M. (Ed.): Surgery of the Musculoskeletal System. Vol. 3, Section 8. New York, Churchill Livingstone, 1983, p. 63.
2. Bach, A. W., and Hansen, S. T.: Plate versus external fixation in severe open tibial shaft fractures: A randomized trial. Clin. Orthop. Rel. Res., 241:89, 1989.
3. Bassett, C. A. L., Mitchell, S. N., and Gaston, S. R.: Treatment of ununited tibial diaphyseal fractures with pulsing electromagnetic fields. J. Bone Joint Surg. [Am.], 63:511, 1981.
4. Behrens, F.: Unilateral external fixation for severe lower extremity lesions: Experience with the ASIF (AO tubular frame). In Feligson, D., and Pope, M. U. (Eds.): Concepts in Internal Fixation. New York, Grune & Stratton, 1982.
5. Behrens, F., Comfort, P. H., Searls, K., Dennis, F., and Young, J. T.: Unilateral external fixation for severe open tibial fractures: Preliminary report of a prospective study. Clin. Orthop. Rel. Res., 178:111, 1983.
6. Blick, S. S., Brumback, R. J., Lakatos, R., Poka, A., and Burgess, A. R.: Early prophylactic bone grafting of high energy tibial fractures. Clin. Orthop. Rel. Res., 240:21, 1989.
7. Bondurant, F. J., Cotler, H. B., Buckle, R., Miller, P., and Browner, B. D.: The medical and economic impact of severely injured lower extremities. J. Trauma, 28:1270, 1988.
8. Bone, L. B., and Johnson, K. D.: Treatment of tibial fractures by reaming and intramedullary nailing. J. Bone Joint Surg. [Am.], 68:877, 1986.
9. Bourne, R. B.: Pilon fractures of the distal tibia. Clin. Orthop. Rel. Res., 240:42, 1989.
10. Burgess, A. R., Poka, A., Brumback, R. J., and Bosse, M. J.: Management of open Grade III tibial fractures. Orthop. Clin. North Am., 18:85, 1987.
11. Caudle, R. J., and Stern, P. J.: Severe open fractures of the tibia. J. Bone Joint Surg. [Am.], 69:801, 1987.
12. Chapman, M.: Fractures of the tibia and fibula shaft. In Evarts, M. (Ed.): Surgery of the Musculoskeletal System. Vol. 3, Section 8. New York, Churchill Livingstone, 1983, p. 5.
13. DeLee, J. C., and Stiehl, J. B.: Open tibia fracture with compartment syndrome. Clin. Orthop. Rel. Res., 160:175, 1981.
14. Ger, R.: Muscle transposition for treatment in prevention of chronic post-traumatic osteomyelitis of the tibia. J. Bone Joint Surg. [Am.], 59:784, 1977.
15. Gershuni, D. H., Mubarak, S. J., Yaru, N. C., and Lee, Y. F.: Fracture of the tibia complicated by acute compartment syndrome. Clin. Orthop. Rel. Res., 217:221, 1987.
16. Hansen, L. W.: Posterior bone grafting of tibia for nonunion. J. Bone Joint Surg. [Am.], 48:27, 1966.
17. Hansen, S. T., Jr.: The Type IIIc tibial fracture salvage or amputation (Editorial). J. Bone Joint Surg. [Am.], 69:799, 1987.
18. Hechman, J. D.: Fractures and dislocations of the foot. In Rockwood, C. A., Jr., and Green, D. P. (Eds.): Fractures in Adults. Philadelphia, J. B. Lippincott, 1984.
19. Hohl, M.: Fractures and dislocations of the knee. In Rockwood, C. A., Jr., and Green, D. P. (Eds.): Fractures in Adults. Philadelphia, J. B. Lippincott, 1984.
20. Johnson, K. D.: Indications, instrumentation, and experience with locked tibial nails. Orthopaedics, 8:1377, 1985.
21. Lange, R. H., Bach, A. W., Hansen, S. T., and Johansen, K. H.: Open tibial fractures with associated vascular injuries. Prognosis for limb salvage. J. Trauma, March:203, 1985.
22. Leach, R. E.: Fractures of the tibia and fibula. In Rockwood, C. A., Jr., and Green, D. P. (Eds.): Fractures in Adults. Philadelphia, J. B. Lippincott, 1984.
23. Lerud, S. O., and Karistrom, G.: The spectrum of intramedullary nailing of the tibia. Clin. Orthop. Rel. Res., 212:101, 1986.
24. Mast, J. W., Spiegel, P. G., and Pappas, J. M.: Fractures of the tibial pylon. Clin. Orthop. Rel. Res., 230:68, 1988.
25. Matsen, F. A., III, Winquist, R. A., and Kurgmire, R. B.: Diagnosis and management of compartmental syndromes. J. Bone Joint Surg. [Am.], 62:286, 1980.
26. McAndrew, M. T., and Brick, A. L.: Initial care of massively traumatized lower extremities. Clin. Orthop. Rel. Res., 243:20, 1989.
27. Muller, M. E., Allgower, M., and Willenegger, H.: Manual of Internal Fixation. New York, Springer-Verlag, 1979.
28. Oni, O. O., Hui, A., and Gregg, P. J.: The healing of closed tibial shaft fractures: The natural history of union with closed treatment. J. Bone Joint Surg. [Br.], 70:787, 1988.
29. Paley, D., Catagni, M. A., Argnanif, V. A., Benedetti, G. B., and Cattaneo,

R.: Ilizarov treatment of tibial non unions with bone loss. Clin. Orthop. Rel. Res., *241*:146, 1989.

30. Rang, M.: Anthology of Orthopaedics. New York, Churchill Livingstone, 1966.
31. Rolando, P. K., Teynor, J., Nagano, J., and Gustilo, R.: Critical analysis of results of treatment of 201 tibial shaft fractures. Clin. Orthop. Rel. Res., *212*:113, 1986.
32. Ruedi, T. P., and Allgower, M.: The operative treatment of intra-articular fractures of the lower end of the tibia. Clin. Orthop. Rel. Res., *138*:105, 1979.
33. Ruedi, T., Webb, J. K., and Allgower, M.: Experience with a dynamic compression plate (DCP) in 418 recent fractures of the tibia shaft. Injury, *7*:252, 1976.
34. Sarmiento, A.: Functional bracing of tibia fractures. Clin. Orthop. Rel. Res., *105*:202, 1974.
35. Sarmiento, A., Sobol, P. A., Sew Hoy, A. L., Ross, S. D. K., Sacette, W. L., and Tarr, R. R.: Prefabricated functional braces for the treatment of fractures of the tibial diaphysis. J. Bone Joint Surg. [Am.], *66*:1328, 1984.
36. Schatzker, J., and McBroom, R. B.: Tibial plateau fracture of the Toronto experience. Clin. Orthop. Rel. Res., *138*:94, 1979.
37. Seyfer, A.: Late results of free muscle flaps and delayed bone grafting in

the secondary treatment of open distal tibial fractures. Plast. Reconstr. Surg., *83*:77, 1989.
38. Shaw, W. (Ed.): Lower Extremity Reconstruction. (Clinics in Plastic Surgery.) Philadelphia, J. B. Lippincott, 1985.
39. Taylor, G. I., and Watson, M.: One stage repair of compound leg defects with free vascularized flaps of groin skin and iliac bone. Plast. Reconstr. Surg., *61*:494, 1978.
40. Trafton, P. G.: Closed unstable fractures of the tibia. Clin. Orthop. Rel. Res., *230*:58, 1988.
41. Wilson, F. C.: Fractures and dislocations of the ankle. *In* Rockwood, C. A., Jr., and Green, D. P. (Eds.): Fractures in Adults. Philadelphia, J. B. Lippincott, 1984.
42. Wist, D. A.: Medullary nailing of acute shaft fractures. Clin. Orthop. Rel. Res., *212*:1122, 1986.
43. Wood, M. B., Cooney, W. P., and Irons, G. P.: Lower extremity salvage and reconstruction by free tissue transfer: Analysis of results. Clin. Orthop. Rel. Res., *201*:1551, 1985.
44. Yaremchuk, J. M., Brumback, R. J., Manson, P. N., Burgess, A. R., Poka, A., and Weiland, A. J.: Acute and definitive management of traumatic osteocutaneous defects of lower extremity. Plast. Reconstr. Surg., *80*:1, 1987.

VIII

AMPUTATION AND LIMB SUBSTITUTION

Sean P. Scully, M.D., Ph.D., and John M. Harrelson, M.D.

The goals of patient care in cases of limb trauma, vascular disease, diabetic complications, infections, and neoplasms are to optimize patient function and minimize morbidity. Frequently, appropriate surgical care in these patients involves a tissue reconstructive procedure; in other cases, amputation is a better option for the patient, the surgeon, and the medical community. The destructive nature of an ablative procedure has produced a defeatist attitude among many surgeons, and some of these procedures are performed with haste and little forethought. This is reflected in the patient's attitude as well as in the postoperative course. In certain patients, an amputation shortens the period of convalescence, decreases financial burdens, and improves postoperative function. When a carefully planned amputation is performed with appropriate indications, goals, and patient education, it should be considered a reconstructive procedure. Moreover, rehabilitation should be supervised by those experienced in prosthetic fitting and rehabilitation.

An amputation is generally considered a resection through either the diaphysis or the metaphysis of a long bone of the extremities. This is distinct from a disarticulation, in which the resection passes through a synovial joint, preserving the articular surface. A disarticulation has some specific considerations, particularly in the pediatric population and with respect to prosthetic fitting. Since many of the same principles apply to both disarticulations and amputations, they are discussed jointly.

INCIDENCE AND INDICATIONS

The number of amputations performed in the United States is not easily determined, in part because of the wide variety of clinical conditions for which amputation may be indicated. Current estimates suggest that there are between 20,000 and 30,000 amputations performed in this country every year.[13] The highest incidence of lower extremity amputations is in the 50- to 75-year-old population, and these amputations are largely related to vascular disease and diabetes. This number is expected to increase as the population ages and the inci-

dence of vascular disease and diabetic complications increases. Amputations secondary to trauma tend to occur in a younger population. Although lower extremity amputations are the most common, the proportion of upper extremity amputations is highest in the younger population following trauma. Amputation secondary to neoplasm is relatively rare but occurs most commonly in an adolescent population with primary bone neoplasms and in an older population with soft tissue malignancies. Counting all causes, there are approximately 350,000 to 1,000,000 amputees to be cared for by the medical community.

The indications for amputation have evolved as surgical techniques have advanced with vascular reconstruction and microvascular surgery. The irreparable loss of blood supply is the only absolute indication for amputation. Sometimes an amputation is necessary to preserve life in the face of an uncontrollable infection, but with advances in antibiotic pharmacology and the use of adjuvants such as hyperbaric oxygen, such situations are rare. A relative indication for amputation is injury so severe that residual function would be inferior to prosthetic function. The physician's goal should be to optimize the patient's function and reduce morbidity.

Ischemia from peripheral vascular disease is the most common reason for amputation in the United States. Approximately 50% of patients who present with ischemic extremities from peripheral vascular disease also suffer from diabetes. Preoperative examination of these patients should include evaluation of perfusion as well as nutritional and immunologic status. Operations in these patients are complicated by poor tissue healing, infection, and sensory neuropathy. These factors similarly influence prosthetic fitting and rehabilitation.

The additional energy cost per meter traveled doubles for each amputation level and doubles again as a result of the age differential between 30 and 60 years. In ambulatory patients, the goal is to achieve healing at the most distal level feasible and to rehabilitate the patient. In the past, as many as 75% of successful amputations for this population were performed at the above-knee level. More recently, 75% to

80% of successful amputations are performed at the below-knee level, and this has produced a greater proportion of patients maintaining a functional ambulatory status. These considerations are heightened when it is realized that 15% of those who undergo amputation because of ischemia will lose the contralateral extremity within 2 years,[7] and 33% within 5 years.[9] It is clear that every effort should be made to keep the amputation as low as possible in a dysvascular patient, consistent with tissue viability and wound healing.

Trauma is the second most common indication for amputation overall and is the most common indication in patients less than 50 years old. An absolute indication for amputation in the posttraumatic setting is ischemia without a vascular reconstructive option. With the advent of microsurgical techniques and vascularized soft tissue transfer, many limbs have been salvaged that would otherwise have undergone early amputation. The price of limb preservation in a subset of these patients is multiple procedures, prolonged hospitalization, high financial costs, and impaired residual function. These considerations leave the patient and the surgeon with an emotional investment in limb preservation that can interfere with clinical judgment. Guidelines for early amputation differ for the upper and lower extremities. An insensate or dysfunctional foot is often less functional than a prosthetic leg. Trauma scoring systems have been developed for the lower extremity that estimate expected outcome and function. In the case of trauma to the upper extremity, a limb with reduced function but some residual sensation may be more functional than a prosthesis.

In treating patients with electrical and thermal injuries, the extent of tissue damage often cannot be appreciated from the outset. Frequently, serial surgical débridement and local wound care are necessary for a period of days to weeks to fully appreciate the extent of necrosis before a decision can be made about the need for and the level of amputation.

Acute infections may be unresponsive to surgical débridement, antibiotics, and adjuvant therapy such as hyperbaric oxygen. In such cases, amputation can be a lifesaving procedure. Alternatively, patients with traumatic or iatrogenic chronic osteomyelitis can coexist with infection for many years or even decades. For reasons that are unclear, the balance between host and pathogen can later shift such that the patient develops chronic pain, drainage, and an inability to bear weight. At a late stage, chronic infections may be unresponsive to medical and surgical management. In both acute and chronic infections, amputation and prosthetic fitting can provide improved function and cosmesis.

In tumor resection, levels of amputation are determined by the histologic grade of the neoplasm, the anatomic location, and the use of neoadjuvant therapy such as radiation or chemotherapy. With the increased effectiveness of adjuvant therapies and the advent of limb salvage procedures, patients with musculoskeletal neoplasms now have several reconstructive options. A study of functional outcome following distal femoral resection for tumor revealed no difference in velocity of gait or oxygen consumption among patients undergoing arthroplasty, arthrodesis, or amputation and prosthetic fitting.[6] Patients with amputations remained active and had less concern about damage to their limbs but had difficulty walking on uneven surfaces. Patients with arthrodesis were capable of strenuous work but had difficulty sitting in confined spaces such as airplanes and movie theaters. Patients with arthroplasty demonstrated a more sedentary lifestyle.

PEDIATRIC CONSIDERATIONS

Amputations in the pediatric population are commonly the result of congenital deformities, trauma, or neoplasm. Congenital deformities of the lower extremities, such as proximal femoral focal deficiency and hemimelia, treated with partial amputation of the limb can result in a more functional residual limb and improved prosthetic fitting. In contrast, amputation in the upper extremity is rarely indicated secondary to congenital deformities, since even rudimentary appendages with sensation usually have much better function than prosthetic options. Amputations due to trauma or neoplasm are governed by similar considerations as mentioned in the general discussion. There are two main issues specific to the pediatric amputee population irrespective of indications—terminal overgrowth and changing proportional limb lengths.

A diaphyseal or metaphyseal amputation, by definition, removes a physeal growth center so that the involved bone does not elongate as the contralateral extremity does. What appears to be a long above-knee amputation in a young child can produce a short residual limb at skeletal maturity. The changing proportional limb length can be avoided if a disarticulation can be performed rather than an amputation. But in few situations is the level of resection elective, permitting the choice of disarticulation over amputation.

Terminal overgrowth occurs when appositional growth of bone in pediatric diaphyseal fractures exceeds the growth of the surrounding soft tissues. This may be related to periosteal traction and scar formation. It takes place most frequently in the humerus, fibula, tibia, and femur, in descending order of occurrence, with an overall incidence of 8% to 12%. The stripping of periosteum has been suggested as one means of limiting terminal overgrowth. Several procedures have been devised to limit the appositional overgrowth by inserting a mechanical barrier, all of which have largely been unsuccessful. More recently, osteochondral capping has been described, which has had early promising results.[11]

Prosthetic fitting can be challenging because of ongoing growth and the need for frequent adjustments as well as family education. The emphasis is on attaining maximal function. Prosthetic fitting should be initiated to coincide with motor skill development. In upper extremities, prosthetic fitting should occur at 6 months of age to correlate with sitting balance—hence the adage "fit when they sit." Lower extremity fitting correlates with children's pulling themselves up to stand, which usually occurs at 8 to 12 months. Children are more adept than adults in developing efficient gait patterns as their motor development allows.

SURGICAL PRINCIPLES

Basic principles of surgery, especially with regard to soft tissue handling, are important in amputations because of the compromise of the local tissue by ischemia, infection, or trauma. The tissue compromise is balanced by the desire to preserve length, consistent with good surgical judgment. Attention to detail and gentle handling of tissue are important to creating a well-healed and functional residual limb. These surgical principles apply to each of the traditional amputational levels (Fig. 42–51).

The level of amputation is anatomically determined in oncologic, congenital, and traumatic cases. In dysvascular cases, clinical examination and evaluation of perfusion, nutrition, and immunocompetence need to be considered. Traditionally, Doppler examinations are used to provide information on the adequacy of blood flow to the extremity. This frequently employs the calculation of an ischemic index by dividing the systolic pressure at the level of a proposed amputation by the brachial artery pressure. Wagner reported greater than 90% successful wound healing in dysvascular patients with an index of 0.35 and in diabetic patients with an index of 0.45.[17] Arterial wall calcifications can artificially

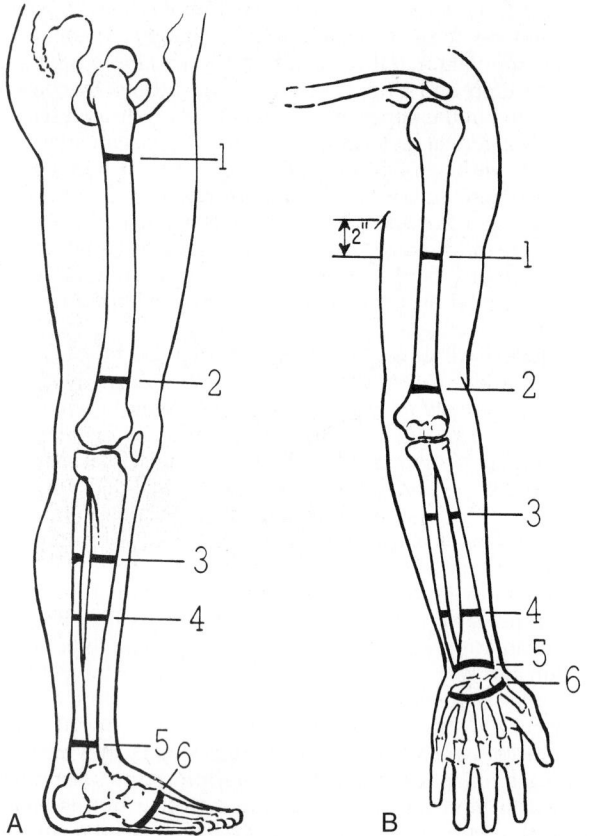

Figure 42–51. Traditional amputation levels. *A,* In the lower limb, amputation above 1 must be fitted with a hip disarticulation prosthesis because of the short stump. The area between 1 and 2 is fitted with the usual above-knee prosthesis with a quadrilateral socket and either pelvic band or suction suspension. Amputations between 2 and the knee joint do not have sufficient room in the prosthesis for a swing phase control knee mechanism and must be fitted with free-swinging outside joints. Areas 3 and 4 are the conventional "sites of election" for below-knee amputations. Amputations between 4 and 5 are more difficult for the prosthetist but offer some advantage to the amputee. Amputations below 6 require little in the way of a prosthesis; a toe filler and a steel shank in the shoe usually suffice. *B,* Amputations through the upper limb above 1 must be fitted with a modified socket over the shoulder, and active motion of the shoulder joint is not possible. Between 1 and 2, a conventional above-elbow prosthesis can be fitted. Between 2 and the elbow, an outside elbow joint must be used, but active humeral rotation is possible. Amputations through the forearm above 3 produce a very short forearm lever, and in some instances a geared elbow joint must be used to provide sufficient flexion of the forearm segment. Between 3 and 4, a conventional below-elbow prosthesis is used. Amputations below 4 allow some active pronation and supination. Transcarpal amputation (6) requires a prosthesis, but some hook function is provided by the stump alone.

increase the apparent perfusion pressure as determined by Doppler and auscultation, and in such cases, this measure is not predictive of wound healing. This is most problematic in older individuals with dysvascular extremities, which is the most common indication for consideration of ablative surgery.

[133]Xenon skin clearance has been used to improve the Doppler examination of perfusion but is technician dependent and expensive. Transcutaneous oxygen tension ($TcPO_2$) measurements have been used to supplement clinical data in determining the appropriate amputation level. The results demonstrate a correlation between increasing oxygen tension and the likelihood of successful primary wound healing; however, specific threshold value recommendations vary among treatment centers. Recommended measurements for predicting successful outcome range from 20 to 40 torr but are not absolutely predictive, even in the face of zero tension.[2, 3, 8, 18]

Nutrition and immunocompetence have been directly correlated with wound healing in residual limbs after amputation. Serum albumin greater than 3.5 g. per 100 ml. and total lymphocyte count greater than 1500 cells per cu. mm. are simple and inexpensive screening parameters indicative of adequate nutritional status. In elective situations, a period of nutritional supplementation may enhance wound healing.

It is apparent that there is no single clinical criterion on which to base the amputation level. Of the clinical signs, skin temperature and skin-edge bleeding are the most reliable predictors. Of the laboratory parameters, the Doppler-derived ischemic index is the most extensively utilized, but newer techniques such as $TcPO_2$ may avoid some of its shortcomings in the future.

The majority of amputations are closed primarily with suture. However, in patients with infectious indications or contaminated traumatic wounds, primary closure may compromise wound healing, and the amputation site should initially be managed open. This can be achieved either with appropriate tissue flaps in anticipation of early closure or with a circular or guillotine amputation. In the latter case, the muscles are cut and allowed to retract. The bone is subsequently cut at the level of muscle retraction. Skin traction is applied to prevent retraction. The wound can be revised later or allowed to heal by secondary intent.

Because wound infection leads to further morbidity and frequently to a higher amputation level, it is safer to leave a questionable wound packed open initially and return in 2 to 3 days for inspection and surgical débridement. If tissues appear healthy and viable at that time, the wound can undergo a delayed primary closure.

The decision-making process is facilitated by consideration of the five vital limb components: skin, muscle, nerve, bone, and blood vessels. The extent of compromise to these structures may collectively belie the potential for wound healing and function.

Skin Flaps. Regardless of the level of amputation, skin coverage is of paramount importance. The loss of skin, such as in a degloving injury, is usually not an indication for amputation. Skin grafts and vascularized soft tissue transfer make below-knee amputation possible rather than above-knee amputation. Soft tissue is frequently compromised, so to preserve existing tissue, skin flaps should be kept as thick as possible, avoiding unnecessary dissection between anatomic planes. Myocutaneous flaps should be fashioned when possible, thereby preserving the deep circulation to the skin. The skin at the end of the residual limb should be mobile and sensate. Scar location has become less important with the development of total-contact sockets, but a scar that is adherent to underlying bone may break down over time. Periosteum should be left intact on remaining bone, with the edges smoothed and rounded.

Muscles. A residual limb with functioning muscle seems less apt to develop pain syndromes. Muscle loses its contractile function when attachments are divided at the time of amputation. Stabilization of myotendinous structures can improve residual limb function. Muscles are sectioned longer than the expected limb length and then sutured to bone (myodesis) or opposing muscle groups (myoplasty). Proponents believe that such treatment improves residual function, decreases the incidence of painful bursa formation, and perhaps decreases subsequent phantom pain. Myodesis is contraindicated in patients with dysvascular extremities or if circulation has been compromised.

Nerves. The transection of a nerve always causes the formation of a neuroma; however, neuromas placed in soft tissues and away from areas of pressure irritation are usually not problematic. Surgical technique to diminish clinically symptomatic neuromas includes a clean transection under tension, allowing the nerve to retract into the soft tissues away from the scar and prosthetic pressure points. Larger nerves contain vasa nervorum and frequently require ligatures to ensure adequate hemostasis

Blood Vessels. Blood vessels should be isolated, clamped, transected, and ligated in a systematic fashion. Larger vessels may require double ligation proximally or perhaps suture ligation. Before the amputation wound is closed, the tourniquet should be deflated and hemostasis meticulously obtained with suture clips or electrocautery. The issue of postoperative drains remains controversial

Bone. Bony prominences such as in the distal anterior tibia should be beveled and smoothed with a rasp during a below-knee amputation. The bony prominences should be well padded with soft tissue when possible. Periosteum should be sectioned at the level of the bone. Proximal periosteal stripping may cause underlying bone devascularization and sequestrum formation.

POSTOPERATIVE MANAGEMENT

Immediately following amputation, the surgeon's efforts should be focused on establishing the optimal physical and metabolic circumstances for wound healing. The internal wound environment is dependent on the intraoperative result and on the physiologic state of the patient. Fluid balance, electrolytes, edema, nutrition, circulation, infection, and patient mobilization all affect postoperative wound healing. Postoperative patients, in particular elderly diabetic or dysvascular amputees, require great attention to detail to lower postoperative morbidity and mortality.

Postsurgical techniques that promote wound healing and the provision of immediate and preparatory functional prostheses have become standard. Wounds can be managed by soft dressings, semirigid dressings, rigid dressings, or controlled environment treatment (CET). There is no longer a perceived need to delay prosthetic fitting for residual limb maturation, and functional rehabilitation should proceed as soon as feasible.

With few exceptions, all long bone extremity amputations can be managed with a rigid dressing–early prosthesis technique. The rigid dressing consists of a plaster of Paris cast applied to the residual limb in the operating room at the conclusion of surgery. A rigid dressing provides support and protects the operative site. Early wound rest and infrequent dressing are thought to encourage wound healing. Joint contractures are prevented by correct positioning in the rigid dressing. Additionally, the patient's increased comfort allows early mobilization and movement. The rigid dressing should be removed and the wound inspected at 7 to 10 days. If the wound is healing well, consideration can be given to temporary prosthesis application.

Temporary prosthetic fitting and limited weight bearing are begun early, but timing is based on individual factors. Young patients can be fit immediately with a temporary prosthesis and begin weight bearing within the first few days following the operation. In older patients with dysvascular extremities, early weight bearing can further compromise ischemic tissues and lead to wound separation. In these patients, weight bearing is delayed to accommodate slower wound healing.

The immediate postoperative prosthesis (IPOP) is similar to a rigid dressing but employs residual limb socks, contoured felt padding, and suspension and is usually applied by a prosthetist. A metal pylon with prosthetic foot is attached to the postoperative cast at the conclusion of the operation (Fig. 42–52). The use of an IPOP not only allows early mobilization but also decreases the time to limb maturation and the time to definitive prosthetic fitting. The fitting

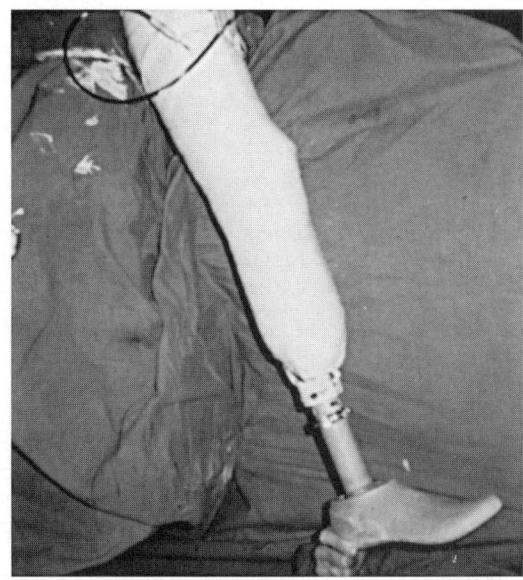

Figure 42–52. A long below-knee amputation with a rigid dressing and shin-foot unit applied in the operating room. Note the suction drainage tube. This is an excellent postoperative dressing, whether or not the shin-foot unit is used.

of an IPOP prosthesis may provide a psychologic advantage to an amputee who is faced with a difficult adjustment.

The CET was designed and has gained acceptance in Britain. The design of the unit provides pressure, humidity, temperature, sterility, immobilization, and visualization via a flow-through air bag attached to a mechanical console. The bag is placed immediately following the operation and suspended by a harness. Control of the temperature and oxygen tension in the wound healing environment may be of benefit, particularly in compromised tissues.

COMPLICATIONS

Patients treated with amputation are at increased risk for postoperative complications because of many factors, including bone marrow suppression and radiation soft tissue damage in patients with neoplasm. The ischemia of tissue in diabetic and dysvascular patients predisposes them to delayed wound healing and infection. Soft tissue compromise in traumatic amputations and wound contamination likewise can lead to infection and wound breakdown.

Hematoma. A postoperative hematoma can delay healing of the wound and serve as a culture medium for bacterial infection. Any hematoma should be aspirated, and firm compression should be applied to the residual limb over the affected area. If the hematoma is large and/or coagulated, surgical irrigation and débridement may be indicated.

Infection. Infection is a concern in dysvascular and diabetic patients because of ischemia and immunologic depression, and it is of concern in patients with neoplasm due to concomitant chemotherapeutic bone marrow suppression. In trauma patients, infection is of concern due to soft tissue compromise and wound contamination. The presence of a postoperative infection should be dealt with expeditiously with surgical irrigation, débridement of nonviable tissue, and delayed closure. Cultures should be obtained intraoperatively, and an appropriate antibiotic regimen administered. Because of further compromise of the soft tissue envelope, infection may require revision to a higher amputation level.

Contracture. Joint contracture tends to occur after amputation procedures but before prosthetic fitting. Long rigid dressings, early prosthetic fitting, and stretching can prevent most contractures. In above-knee amputations, the deforming forces are flexion and abduction. Patients should be started on early active range-of-motion exercises and prone stretching. In below-knee amputations, quad strengthening exercises can help avoid flexion contractures, which can interfere with prosthetic fitting.

Neuroma. All transected nerves develop a bulbous swelling, termed a neuroma. In certain anatomic locations and mechanical environments, a neuroma can become symptomatic. Surgical attempts to diminish postoperative symptoms include sharp transection under traction, thus allowing the cut end to retract into soft tissue away from scar and prosthetic pressure points. Ligature of larger nerves is often necessary to control bleeding from accompanying vessels.

Pain. Phantom sensation occurs in nearly all amputees and tends to decrease over time. In contrast, phantom pain is troublesome and is described as a burning pain in the amputated extremity. It occurs in less than 10% of acquired amputations, and its incidence is decreased by perioperative epidural and intraneural anesthesia. For patients experiencing phantom limb pain, surgical intervention has not been successful. Noninvasive techniques, such as massage and electrical stimulation, are sometimes beneficial. Reflex sympathetic dystrophy can occur in residual extremities and should be treated aggressively with a combined pharmaceutical and physical therapy regimen.

SPECIFIC CONSIDERATIONS
Lower Extremity

Foot Amputation. Frequently, partial foot amputations are necessary in the management of dysvascular and diabetic feet. A patient with a dry gangrene of the lesser toes can be adequately managed by observation with the expectation of autoamputation or can electively undergo a surgical resection. If a course of observation is elected, the foot should be kept clean and dry and should be examined frequently. In patients with cellulitis extending into the metatarsal phalangeal joint, a ray resection is a surgical option, but this has been associated with altered weight bearing and the development of plantar transfer ulcers. In diabetic patients who may have developed cellulitis because of neuropathic ulceration, this is a significant consideration.[12] Ray resection is generally contraindicated with involvement of the first or central ray. The alternative to ray resection is a transmetatarsal amputation performed through the metatarsal at any point from the head to the base. Wound closure is through either a long plantar flap or equal plantar and dorsal flaps. Patients with a web space infection can be managed with a transmetatarsal amputation and a delayed primary closure after 7 to 10 days. Healing has been as high as 75% in some series in the absence of pedal pulses detected by Doppler.[19]

Procedures described by Boyd, Chopart, Lisfranc, and Pirogoff involve disarticulations through the tarsal and intertarsal joints. The Chopart amputation preserves only the talus and calcaneus, removing the fore- and midfoot. Because of the resulting imbalance of dorsi- and plantar flexors, there is the potential for an equinus contracture, which can be prevented by either transection of the Achilles tendon or transfer of the extensors to the dorsum of the remaining tarsal bones. The Boyd and Pirogoff amputations involve a talectomy and tibiocalcaneal arthrodesis. Their primary indications are in children to preserve length and growth centers.

Ankle and Hindfoot Amputation. The Syme amputation removes the foot, talus, and calcaneus while preserving a portion of the plantar cortex of the calcaneus and the heel pad to act as a sensate and end-bearing surface.[16] The procedure has been used in congenital deformities, tumor resections, and dysvascular and insensate feet and following

trauma. Disadvantages include a bulbous residual limb and heel pad migration, both of which have been addressed by subsequent modifications of the original procedure.[14] Prosthetic fitting for patients with this amputation has made significant advances and utilizes an expandable wall prosthesis with a dynamic-response energy-storing foot.

Below-Knee Amputation. Preserving the knee joint enhances the rehabilitation potential in all age groups; younger patients can continue with athletic and active lifestyles, and older individuals can return to community ambulation. Moreover, the postoperative morbidity and mortality are significantly lower following a below-knee amputation than an above-knee amputation. The below-knee amputation is the most frequently performed and has reported healing rates of 85%, in spite of the fact that most patients who undergo this procedure have underlying vascular and immunologic compromise. Contraindications are an inadequate vascular supply to support healing and severely compromised function of the knee joint itself.

The surgical technique for this procedure is variable but generally differs only in the method of soft tissue closure—equal anteroposterior flaps, long anterior, long posterior, and medial-lateral flaps. Postoperative considerations are those mentioned previously, and this operation is well suited for IPOP. Prosthetic specifications should include a method of suspension, socket type, methods of construction (exoskeleton versus endoskeleton), and type of foot (Fig. 42–53).

Knee Disarticulation. When compared with an above-knee amputation, a knee disarticulation has the advantages of being end bearing, being amenable to supracondylar suspension, and having a longer lever, which may be especially important in the pediatric population. Disadvantages include a relatively thin soft tissue envelope and a resultant asymmetry in knee height. Derivations of the knee disarticulation include the Gritti-Stokes amputation, which involves a patellofemoral fusion.[10] Prosthetic considerations in addition to those described for a below-knee prosthesis include specifi-

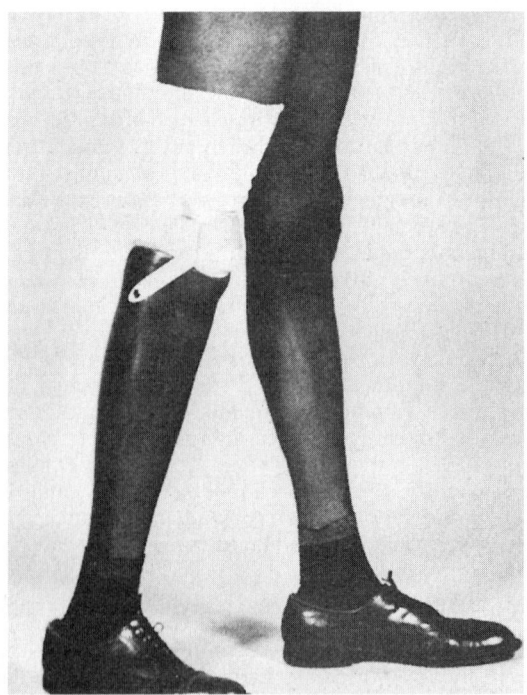

Figure 42–53. Patellar tendon-bearing prosthesis with a total-contact plastic socket. It is suspended by a supracondylar strap, as pictured, or by a removable wedge that clips over the medial femoral condyle. A solid ankle cushion heel (SACH) foot is usually used.

cation of a knee mechanism, the best of which is a polycentric or four-bar linkage knee.

Above-Knee Amputation. In the past, this was the most common level of amputation because of blood supply and healing in a high percentage of cases. In light of the recent appreciation for the ergonomic compromise associated with sacrifice of the knee joint, every effort is now made to spare the knee joint when possible. If an above-knee amputation is to be performed, length should be preserved as much as possible, because there is an increasing energy demand as limb length decreases. Additionally, as the residual femoral length is decreased, the strength of the hamstrings and adductors is decreased, leading to larger muscle imbalance. Surgical technique is based on the considerations mentioned previously, and postoperative function is improved by myodesis through drill holes in the distal femur. Postoperative care is notable for the difficulty of maintaining a rigid dressing and is best accomplished with a waistband suspension. Prosthetic considerations involve socket design, suspension, skeleton, knee mechanism, and foot specification. Recent advances in socket design have aided alignment and function (contoured adducted trochanteric–controlled alignment method, or CAT–CAM). The prosthesis is suspended by either a waist belt or a suction socket. The knee mechanism is individualized based on patient demands, but one recent enhancement is a hydraulic knee.

Hip Disarticulation and Hemipelvectomy. Resection of the entire lower extremity and sometimes the hemipelvis is most frequently indicated in the treatment of malignant neoplasms but is also infrequently used in cases of trauma and ascending infection. Surgical technique for hip disarticulation has been described by Boyd[1] and that for hemipelvectomy by Gordon Taylor and Monro.[5] Both are significantly disabling procedures with associated intra- and postoperative morbidity and mortality. Prosthetic considerations are similar for the two procedures—namely, a molded socket and hip, knee, and foot mechanism. They differ, however, in that a hip disarticulation prosthesis can bear weight through the ischial tuberosity, whereas a hemipelvectomy prosthesis relies on soft tissue support through the abdomen. Many patients forgo the use of a prosthesis and ambulate with crutches, which is faster and less cumbersome.

Upper Extremity

The hand is a primary tool of survival and acts through three basic functional elements: hook, grasp, and pinch. It also augments communication and is an integral component of self-esteem. Loss or amputation of all or part of the upper extremity is most common in young people and as a result of trauma. An amputation should be planned with as much forethought as possible, since replacement of the hand is difficult from a prosthetic standpoint. Patients are generally faced with a choice between cosmetic appearance and function. Function comes from either mechanical control, with voluntary opening or closing hooks, or a myoelectrical device. The mechanical terminal hook is functional for carrying, pinching, and holding objects but lacks the dexterity expected from a human hand. The myoelectrical prosthesis can provide cosmesis and a more physiologic function by way of electrodes that detect contraction of voluntary muscles and are used to activate electrical motors in the prosthesis. Myoelectrical prostheses are expensive, have an increased maintenance requirement, and have less sensory feedback than a mechanical prosthesis because of the absence of a harness.

Finger and Partial Hand Amputation. Traumatic finger and partial hand amputations have been objectively evaluated, and the functional results have been compared with those following replantation with microvascular techniques. Specific indications now exist for replantation, and it is recog-

nized that patients bypass an insensate digit for activities requiring manual dexterity. The surgeon should make every effort to preserve any digit with intact sensation and adequate skin coverage. Even the preservation of a single digit can be used to oppose a prosthetic post. Other reconstructive methods include pollicization, ray transposition, and toe-to-hand transfer.

Below-Elbow Amputation. An amputation through the forearm should be fashioned to use all available soft tissue coverage. Length provides improved leverage, and preservation of the distal radioulnar joint permits transmission of partial pronation and supination to the prosthesis and facilitates prosthetic suspension. Alternatively, when the distal radioulnar joint cannot be preserved, a passive pronation-supination device can be incorporated into the prosthesis. Tenodesis should be performed with the flexor-extensor tendons, which improves physiologic and possible myoelectrical function. In short below-elbow amputations, the prosthesis can be suspended on the humeral condyles with a Munster socket and can include a geared hinge, which increases the flexion that can be obtained. Prosthetic options include a myoelectrical terminal device that is activated by active contraction of the remaining dorsi- and palmar flexors. Such a prosthesis provides a cosmetic appearance and the ability to work overhead (which is difficult with a cable harness), but there is a loss of sensory feedback that the cable provides.

The Krukenberg kineplastic operation fashions the forearm into radial and ulnar pincers, which provide prehension and sensation and permit improved manipulative ability.[4] Although the physical appearance of the extremity has been cited as a disadvantage, a myoelectrical prosthesis can be worn satisfactorily. This procedure has been used predominantly for blind amputees, for whom sensory feedback is critical, but the indications may become broader in the future.

Above-Elbow Amputation. In amputation above the elbow, all possible length should be preserved. Amputation through the diaphysis of the humerus limits subsequent function because rotation of the shoulder cannot be transmitted to the prosthesis. Surgical technique is similar to that in the forearm, with anterior and posterior flaps. Preservation of triceps and biceps fascia with myodesis to the underlying humerus acts to improve subsequent prosthetic control, myo-

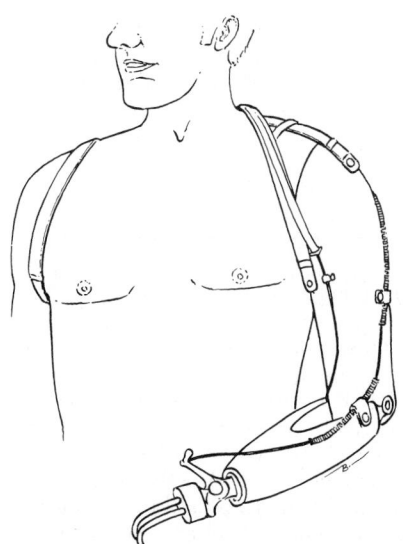

Figure 42–54. Prosthesis for the above-elbow amputee includes socket and arm segment, forearm, terminal device, harness, cable from harness that provides motion at the elbow and controls the terminal device, and control cable for the elbow lock.

electrical function, and strength and provides soft tissue coverage to the distal humerus. The prosthesis contains a socket attached to a mechanical elbow that provides flexion via a cable and extension by gravity (Fig. 42–54). The elbow contains a locking mechanism that is activated by a cable or a locking lever. A terminal device is fitted with or without a passive pronation-supination device.

Shoulder Disarticulation and Forequarter Amputation. Amputations are generally performed at this level for ascending severe infection or for neoplasm. The surgical technique is well described by Sugarbaker and is associated with significant postoperative morbidity and mortality.[15] Functional prosthetic fitting is difficult and prohibitively expensive. The use of a shoulder pad to aid in the fitting of clothing and a light flexible arm and hand for cosmesis are usually preferred.

CONCLUSION

In summary, amputation operations need to be viewed in a positive light, as a reconstructive procedure rather than as an objectionable chore that should be performed as rapidly as possible. Preoperative evaluation and planning should be as rigorous as for limb salvage procedures, giving forethought to rehabilitation. The surgical procedure should employ meticulous handling of usually compromised soft tissues. Postoperative rehabilitation should begin as soon as tissue healing permits and should involve a multidisciplinary group including a surgeon, a prosthetist, a physical therapist, a vocational rehabilitation counselor, and frequently a clinical psychologist. Patients' efforts play a large role in rehabilitation, and they should be given every opportunity to regain an optimal functional level following an amputation.

SELECTED REFERENCES

Harris, I. E., Leff, A. R., and Gitelis, S.: Function after amputation, arthrodesis, or arthroplasty for tumors about the knee. J. Bone Joint Surg. [Am.], 72:1477, 1990.
Functional outcome and psychologic impact were compared for 22 patients who underwent resection of a distal femoral sarcoma and were treated with above-knee amputation, arthroplasty, or arthrodesis. Each of the treatment options has specific advantages with respect to physical capabilities, activity levels, and psychologic impact, with the arthroplasty patients being the most sedentary and the amputation patients being least worried about damaging the limb. There were no differences detected in walking velocity or oxygen consumption.

Malone, J. M., Anderson, G. G., and Lalka, S. G.: Prospective comparison of noninvasive techniques for amputation level selection. Am. J. Surg., 154:179, 1987.
Doppler perfusion studies, transcutaneous oxygen measurements, and ¹³³xenon clearance were compared prospectively in 48 patients as predictors of healing

following lower extremity amputations. The authors concluded that transcutaneous oxygen tension was a better predictor than either ¹³³xenon clearance or Doppler pressure ratios.

Melzack, R.: Phantom limbs. Sci. Am., 266:120, 1992.
This article reviews phantom sensation and phantom pain in the context of the gate control theory of pain.

Robertson, P. A.: Prediction of amputation after severe lower limb trauma. J. Bone Joint Surg. [Br.], 73:816, 1991.
One hundred-fifty-two patients were retrospectively compared based on the Mangled Extremity Severity Score (MESS). The authors report a score of seven as being 100% predictive of an amputation, but the sensitivity is not reported.

REFERENCES

1. Boyd, H. B.: Anatomic disarticulation of the hip. Surg. Gynecol. Obstet., 84:346, 1947.
2. Dickhaut, S. C., DeLee, J. C., and Page, C. P.: Nutritional status: Importance in predicting wound healing after amputation. J. Bone Joint Surg. [Am.], 66:71, 1984.
3. Dowd, G. S. E.: Predicting stump healing following amputation for peripheral vascular disease using transcutaneous oxygen monitor. Ann. R. Coll. Surg. Engl., 68:31, 1986.
4. Garst, R. J.: The Krukenberg hand. J. Bone Joint Surg. [Br.], 73:385, 1991.
5. Gordon Taylor, G., and Monro, R. S.: Technique and management of hindquarter amputation. Br. J. Surg., 39:536, 1952.
6. Harris, I. E., Leff, A. R., Gitelis, S., and Simon, M. A.: Function after amputation, arthrodesis, or arthroplasty for tumors about the knee. J. Bone Joint Surg. [Am.], 72:1477, 1990.
7. Kihn, R. B., Warren, R., and Beebe, G. W.: The geriatric amputee. Ann. Surg., 176:305, 1972.
8. Kram, H. B., Appel, P. L., and Shoemaker, W. C.: Multisensor transcutaneous oximetric mapping to predict below-knee amputation wound healing: Use of critical Po₂. J. Vasc. Surg., 9:796, 1989.
9. Mazet, R., Schiller, F. J., and Dunn, O. J.: The Influence of Prosthesis Wearing on the Health of the Geriatric Amputee. Project 431. Washington, D.C., Office of Vocational Rehabilitation, 1963.
10. Newcombe, J. F., and Marcison, R. W.: Through knee amputation. Br. J. Surg., 59:260, 1972.
11. Pfeil, J., Marquardt, E., Holtz, T., Niethard, F. U., Schneider, E., and Carstens, C.: The stump capping procedure to prevent or treat terminal osseus overgrowth. Prosthet. Orthot. Int., 15:96, 1991.
12. Pinzur, M. S., Sage, R., Schwaegler, P.: Ray resection in the dysvascular foot. Clin. Orthop., 191:232, 1984.
13. Musculoskeletal injuries: Frequency of occurrence. In Praemer, A. (Ed.): Musculoskeletal Conditions in the United States. Rosemont, Il., American Academy of Orthopaedic Surgeons, 1992.
14. Sarmiento, A.: A modified surgical-prosthetic approach to Syme's amputation: A follow-up report. Clin. Orthop., 85:11, 1972.
15. Sugarbaker, P. H.: Forequarter Amputation in Musculoskeletal Surgery for Cancer. New York, Thieme, 1992.
16. Syme, J.: Amputation at the ankle joint. London Edinburgh Monthly J. Med. Sci., 2:93, 1843.
17. Wagner, F. W.: Partial foot amputations. In Bowker, J. H., and Michael, J. W. (Eds.): Atlas of Limb Prosthetics, 2nd ed. St. Louis, C. V. Mosby, 1981.
18. Wyss-Harrington, R. M., Burgess, E. M., and Matsen, F. A.: Transcutaneous oxygen tension as a predictor of success after an amputation. J. Bone Joint Surg. [Am.], 70:203, 1988.
19. Young, A. E.: Transmetatarsal amputation in the management of peripheral ischemia. Am. J. Surg., 134:604, 1977.

IX

INFECTIONS AND NEOPLASMS OF BONE

Sean P. Scully, M.D., Ph.D., and John M. Harrelson, M.D.

The rigid structure of bone and its periosteal covering determine how bone responds to both infection and neoplasia. In many instances, clinical and radiographic findings do not distinguish between these two conditions. The advice that every suspected tumor should be cultured and every suspected infection should be examined histologically is definitely applicable to bone.

INFECTIONS OF BONE

Osteomyelitis is the term used to denote infection of bone. Although any organism responsible for soft tissue infection can also produce osteomyelitis, the majority of bone infections are the result of *Staphylococcus aureus*. The clinical presentation and course of osteomyelitis vary with the location, offending organism, and age of the patient. *Staphylococcus* and other pus-forming bacteria usually produce an acute fulminating infection of bone, or *pyogenic osteomyelitis.* Tuberculosis and other nonpyogenic organisms produce a less aggressive granulomatous infection. These two types of infections are considered separately.

Pyogenic Osteomyelitis

Suppurative infection of bone occurs in one of two ways. Bacteremia from an active focus of soft tissue infection (furuncle, upper respiratory infection, urinary tract infection) may cause bacterial inoculation of bone and the development of an abscess. This mechanism is referred to as *hematogenous osteomyelitis.* More commonly, bacteria reach bone from the external environment via penetrating wounds, open fractures, or surgical incisions. This route of infection is known as *exogenous osteomyelitis.* Prior to the antibiotic era, the mortality from pyogenic osteomyelitis was 20% to 30%, and survivors could expect significant crippling effects of the disease. Antibiotics have greatly reduced the incidence of both types of osteomyelitis and have significantly improved the clinical outcome. Death from osteomyelitis is rare, and residual disability has been greatly reduced.

Hematogenous osteomyelitis is primarily a disease of childhood and occurs most frequently between the ages of 5 and 15 years. Males are affected three times more frequently than females.[3, 10, 19] In a growing child, the afferent arterial supply to bone enters through the nutrient artery and through small periosteal vessels that penetrate the cortex. As these vessels reach the arteriolar level at the metaphyseal end of the bone, they enter into numerous sinusoidal veins adjacent to the physeal plate. Flow in these veins is significantly slowed and provides an ideal location for the lodgement of bacteria. Accordingly, hematogenous osteomyelitis in childhood is most frequently seen in the metaphyseal ends of long bones. The adjacent epiphysis has a separate blood supply that enters through the joint capsule. After the first year of life, the physeal plate has no traversing blood vessels and acts as a barrier to the spread of infection from the metaphysis to the adjacent epiphysis and joint cavity. The metaphyseal portions of the distal femur, proximal tibia, and proximal humerus are most frequently affected. Other tubular bones and flat bones are less commonly involved.[5]

With bony maturity, ossification of the physeal plate occurs and the circulation of the epiphysis and metaphysis merges; the characteristics of sluggish blood flow are lost, and hematogenous osteomyelitis is less frequently encountered. Exogenous osteomyelitis is more common in adults and in those bones with the least soft tissue covering. The tibia, with only skin and subcutaneous tissues covering the anterior one third of its circumference, is often injured in high-speed trauma and is the most common bone involved in exogenous osteomyelitis.

Pathologic Considerations

When bloodborne bacteria lodge in the metaphyseal veins and multiply, the initial host response is an infiltration of polymorphonuclear leukocytes. The combination of bacteria and leukocytes constitutes an abscess. As a result of bacterial multiplication and interstitial edema, pressure increases within the rigid structure of bone, producing capillary occlusion and subsequent death of the trabecular bone within the abscess cavity. The increasing pressure is responsible for localized pain.

In the early stages of osteomyelitis, infarction of a portion of the metaphysis does not produce any observable radiographic change. As the process continues, granulation tissue develops about the periphery of the abscess, and there may be associated osteoclastic resorption of both living bone about the margin of the abscess and infarcted bone abutting the granulation tissue. The isolated necrotic bone within the abscess cavity is called a *sequestrum.* New bone formation occurring about the periphery of the abscess represents the body's attempt to wall off the infection. This new bone is called *involucrum.* Because of the pain and subsequent diminished activity, disuse osteoporosis develops in the affected extremity. Osteoporosis is further enhanced by increased circulation caused by the infection. Radiographs taken 14 days following the onset of infection show a central area of radiodensity (sequestrum) surrounded by a zone of relative radiolucency (granulation tissue) and varying amounts of increased radiodensity (involucrum).

If the host is successful in repelling the infection in its early stages, gradual obliteration of the abscess cavity with fibrous tissue may occur. This area is subsequently replaced by new bone, ultimately leaving no evidence of the infectious process. In some instances, a static abscess cavity remains without further enlargement. This equilibrium between host and organism is known as a Brodie's abscess. More frequently, the host is unable to contain the infectious process, and continued growth of bacteria occurs. New areas of bone become involved as the process spreads outward through the medullary canal. Upon reaching the cortex, purulent material permeates through the haversian and Volkmann's canals into the subperiosteal space. As intraosseous pressure increases, pus dissects along the subperiosteal plane and strips the periosteum from the underlying cortex. This periosteal stripping interrupts the blood supply and extends the area of infarction. The subperiosteal spread of infection is limited at each end of the long bone by the adherence of periosteum to the metaphyseal-physeal junction. The impermeability of the physeal plate impedes the spread of infection into the epiphysis. In severe cases, the entire shaft of the bone from one metaphyseal end to the other may be involved. From the inner surface of the elevated periosteum, osteoblasts begin to lay down new bone and form a periosteal involucrum (Fig. 42–55).

In untreated cases, the infection may rupture through the periosteum and the adjacent soft tissues, penetrate the der-

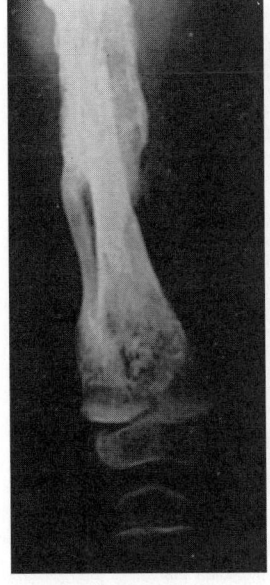
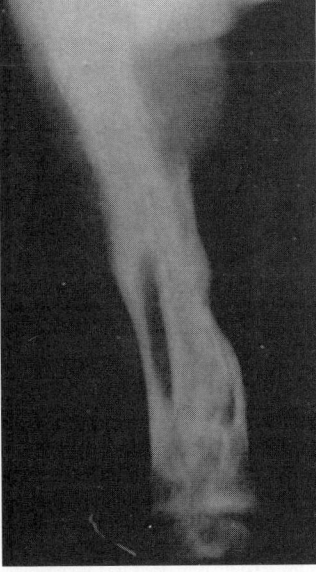

Figure 42–55. Notice the periosteal new bone (involucrum), which formed along the entire shaft of the femur. The central femoral cortex is necrotic and represents a sequestrum.

mis, and produce a draining sinus tract. Fragments of necrotic bone (sequestrum) may be extruded. If the sinus tract is large enough to extrude the entire sequestrum, subsequent healing may occur and the abscess cavity may be obliterated by fibrous tissue. However, this situation rarely occurs. The sequestrum is usually too large for complete extrusion, and the rigid nature of bone prevents collapse of the abscess cavity, greatly reducing the likelihood of obliteration of the infection.

Although the adherence of the periosteum to the metaphysis and the impermeability of the physeal plate usually protect the adjacent joint from infection, in the first year of life, there are vessels traversing the physeal plate, and osteomyelitis in this age group may produce an adjacent pyarthrosis. In the proximal femur, the physeal plate lies within the capsule of the hip joint. Osteomyelitis in the proximal metaphysis of the femur may thus permeate through the cortex directly into the hip joint, producing pyarthrosis (Fig. 42–56).

Clinical Considerations

The onset of hematogenous osteomyelitis is usually abrupt. Patients present with fever, generalized malaise, and local-

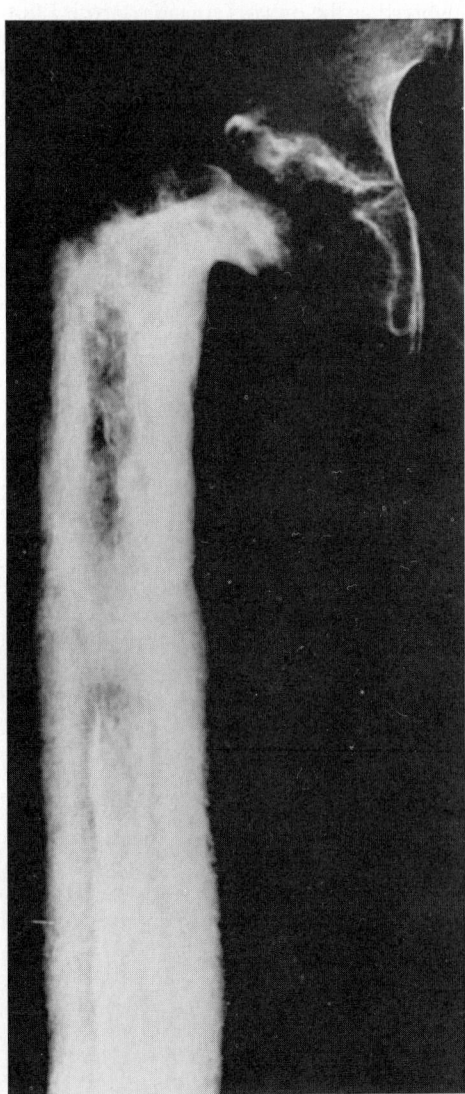

Figure 42–56. This child has osteomyelitis involving the entire femoral shaft. The central portion of the bone is the old femoral shaft, which is now necrotic and represents a sequestrum. Notice that the hip joint has been involved because the hip capsule extends beyond the capital femoral physeal plate.

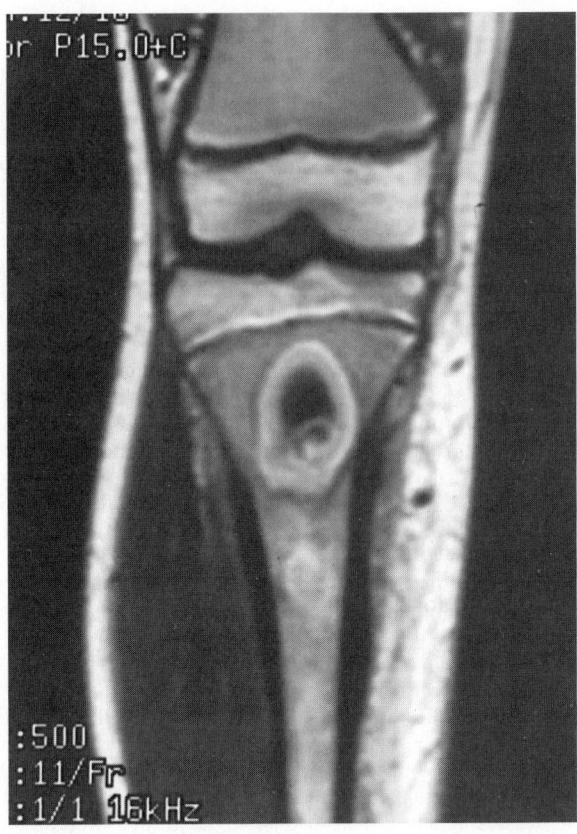

Figure 42–57. This T1 magnetic resonance image shows a metaphyseal abscess in a 13-year-old female. Notice the necrotic center. The peripheral granulation tissue enhances secondary to gadolinium contrast.

ized pain in the involved extremity. A history of a preceding infection may be obtained. Early in the course of the disease there is generalized swelling without erythema. A sterile sympathetic effusion of adjacent joints may be present. The patient appears toxic and irritable, and any manipulation of the extremity produces paroxysms of pain. Young children may demonstrate the phenomenon known as *pseudoparalysis*. These children refuse to move the involved limb, mimicking a neurologic deficit.

Laboratory examination reveals a leukocytosis exceeding 15,000 cells per ml., mild to moderate anemia, and a markedly elevated erythrocyte sedimentation rate. Blood cultures are positive in approximately 50% of cases. In the first 7 to 10 days of the disease there is no evident radiographic bony change. There may be loss of normal musculofascial soft tissue shadows produced by the accompanying edema. Radionuclide scan and magnetic resonance imaging (MRI) may be positive early in the course of infection when radiographs are still normal (Fig. 42–57). Within 10 to 14 days, bony changes are evident, consisting of mottled lucency followed by periosteal elevation and new bone formation.

Ewing's sarcoma, acute rheumatic fever, leukemia, scurvy, acute septic arthritis, and acute juvenile rheumatoid arthritis may all mimic the clinical pattern of acute osteomyelitis. Careful examination of the involved extremity is required to distinguish acute osteomyelitis from acute pyarthrosis. In osteomyelitis, tenderness is usually located over the metaphysis of long bone, and gentle manipulation of the adjacent joints is possible. In contrast, acute pyarthrosis produces swelling localized at the joint level, and the patient cannot tolerate any joint motion. In acute rheumatic fever and acute juvenile rheumatoid arthritis, the tenderness is similarly located at the joint level and more than one joint may be involved. In neonates and in some older children, aspiration of the joint may be required to rule out pyarthrosis.

Because of the widespread use of antibiotics, the pre-existing nidus of soft tissue infection may not be identified. When antibiotic therapy has been used for a preceding soft tissue infection, the subsequent clinical course of osteomyelitis may be considerably more benign than has been described, and the true diagnosis may not be recognized until the infection is well established. In adults, hematogenous osteomyelitis is characteristically more benign. Often the infection is limited to the metaphysis, with no spread to the adjacent subperiosteal space. Generalized toxicity is less, and symptoms are usually more localized to the site of infection.

Although *S. aureus* accounts for over 50% of the cases of osteomyelitis, in neonates and infants, *Streptococcus* infection occurs with greater frequency. These two bacteria produce the fulminating clinical presentation described. Less frequently, gram-negative organisms produce osteomyelitis. *Salmonella* osteomyelitis may be a complication of sickle cell anemia; curiously, it involves the diaphysis of the long bone rather than the metaphysis.[9] Gram-negative organisms characteristically produce a less virulent clinical course than gram-positive cocci.

Exogenous osteomyelitis is most frequently the result of open fracture. Any organism can be involved, and often the infections are polymicrobial. If the fracture wound has been closed, the subsequent development of infection may produce the same symptoms observed in hematogenous osteomyelitis, although to a lesser degree. Generally, the infection is limited to the site of injury and produces localized erythema and swelling. The continued multiplication of bacteria may cause spontaneous dehiscence of the wound, with a discharge of purulent material. When the periosteum has been disrupted, as in the case of fracture, infection does not produce periosteal elevation. Rather, there is local destruction of bone at the fracture site. Aggressive wound care and the use of prophylactic antibiotics, combined with early wound coverage using rotational or free vascularized muscle flaps, have greatly reduced the incidence of exogenous osteomyelitis.

Treatment

The treatment of acute hematogenous osteomyelitis begins immediately upon recognition. Once blood cultures have been obtained, antibiotics are administered intravenously without awaiting the culture results. Drugs effective against *S. aureus* are selected, since this is the most common offending organism. Blood cultures do not always reveal the etiologic agent. If there are enough localizing physical findings or confirmatory radiographic changes, the subperiosteal space may be aspirated with a large-bore needle and material obtained for Gram's stain and culture. Care must be taken not to contaminate an adjacent joint. If no material is obtained on penetration of the periosteum, the needle may be advanced through the cortex into the metaphysis and a marrow aspirate obtained for culture.

Supportive measures in the treatment of osteomyelitis include maintenance of fluid and electrolyte balance, correction of existing anemia, and use of antipyretics. Immobilization of the involved extremity is accomplished by the use of bivalved plaster or prefabricated splints. Immobilization allows the extremity to rest and reduces muscle spasm and pain. Removable splints are preferred to allow inspection of the extremity. In some instances, the administration of intravenous antibiotics produces dramatic improvement within 24 hours. However, surgical intervention is usually required.

The surgical principles in the treatment of osteomyelitis are the same as for the treatment of any soft tissue abscess and consist of incision and drainage. The surgical approach depends on the location and extent of the infection. When possible, the incision should be placed to allow subsequent dependent drainage. A cortical window is created in the metaphysis, and the pus under pressure, together with the necrotic sequestrum, is removed. Care must be taken not to damage the adjacent physeal plate and to avoid stripping the periosteum during débridement, since this interrupts the blood supply and may allow further extension of the infection. The wound is either packed open to allow drainage or, in some instances, closed over suction drains. When a repeat débridement appears advisable, beads of polymethylmethacrylate impregnated with antibiotics may be placed in the wound and left for up to 2 weeks. The beads are removed at subsequent débridement.

Antibiotics are continued for a minimum of 6 weeks. Some prefer intravenous antibiotics for a full 6 weeks. For sensitive organisms, 2 weeks of intravenous antibiotics and 4 weeks of oral antibiotics may be sufficient. Antibiotic treatment is discontinued when all clinical signs of infection are absent and the sedimentation rate has returned to normal. When the acute infectious process is under control, rehabilitation of the limb is accomplished by gentle motion of the adjacent joints to prevent arthrofibrosis. The resumption of activity with the involved limb depends on the extent of bone destruction and the healing response observed on serial radiographs. When large areas of bone have been involved, the return to full weight bearing and normal activities may require many months.

The best treatment of exogenous osteomyelitis is prevention. Open, contaminated fracture wounds should be débrided and packed open and then closed as a delayed procedure in 2 to 5 days if there are no signs of infection. When a fracture wound has been closed and infection develops, the wound must be opened and widely débrided to allow complete drainage. Any nonviable bone at the fracture site is removed. Immobilization of the limb is mandatory. Adequate cultures must be obtained and the appropriate antibiotics selected, based on bacterial sensitivity. When initial débridement results in a large wound, repeated débridement may be required. Wound sterilization may be facilitated by the use of polymethylmethacrylate beads containing antibiotics. The beads are placed in the wound and sealed with an adherent plastic drape. This *bead pouch* dispenses antibiotics directly into the wound. Once satisfactory control of the infection is obtained, wound closure usually requires split-thickness skin grafts or muscle flap coverage.[11, 13] In some instances, small wounds can be allowed to heal by secondary intention.

With the use of antibiotics, death from osteomyelitis is a rarity. The ultimate degree of disability depends on many factors. The location of the infection, the extent of bony destruction, the involvement of adjacent joints, the virulence of the organism, and the rapidity with which treatment is initiated all affect the outcome. In most cases, infection is successfully controlled by a combination of antibiotics and surgical therapy. In some instances, chronic osteomyelitis develops. The infection may be quiescent for many months or years only to recur periodically with drainage, fever, and swelling. Chronic sinus tracts may develop and become lined with squamous epithelium. In long-standing cases, squamous carcinoma may develop within the sinus tract. Patients with chronic osteomyelitis that cannot be adequately controlled by antibiotics and local surgical measures may require amputation of the extremity and fitting with a prosthesis to eradicate the infection and provide better function.

Tuberculous Osteomyelitis and Pyarthrosis

Like hematogenous osteomyelitis, the incidence of tuberculosis has decreased significantly in the last half of the twentieth century. The development of effective antimicrobial agents and an improved standard of living have contributed to the reduction of pulmonary tuberculosis. The identification of diseased cattle and the pasteurization of milk have reduced the incidence of bovine tuberculosis. In recent years, there has been an increase in the incidence of tuberculosis associated with HIV infections, and resistant strains of tuberculous organisms have been encountered.

Skeletal tuberculosis is the result of hematogenous seeding of tubercle bacilli from a pre-existing pulmonary or gastrointestinal focus. The organism most frequently inoculates joints and intervertebral discs rather than the metaphysis of long bones. The intervertebral discs of the lower thoracic and upper lumbar spine account for 30% of all cases of skeletal tuberculosis. The hip and knee joints are the second most frequently affected areas. Older statistics indicate that a majority of cases occurred in children between the ages of 5 and 15 years, but in recent years there appears to have been a decline in the number of childhood cases and an increase in the incidence of skeletal tuberculosis in adults.

Pathologic Considerations

Following hematogenous inoculation, tubercle bacilli lodge in the subchondral bone of the epiphysis, in the joint capsule, or in the synovial membrane. The initial host response is an infiltration of lymphocytes, plasma cells, and histiocytes. The histologic appearance of the tuberculous lesion in bone resembles that observed in visceral tuberculosis. Histiocytes, Langhans giant cells, and fibroblastic proliferation are all present. Caseous necrosis is less frequently seen in joint lesions than in pulmonary lesions. The destruction produced by granulomatous inflammation is characteristically slow. Within the joint, invasion of bone tends to occur at the margins where synovium is attached to bone, producing a characteristic marginal defect. The weight-bearing areas of the joint tend to be spared in the early phase of the disease, and there is preservation of joint width on early radiographs. As destruction proceeds, the joint becomes filled with necrotic products and fragments of articular cartilage, material called *rice bodies* because of its resemblance to grains of rice. In some instances, joint or disc space infection burrows into adjacent soft tissues, extends along fascial planes, and may eventually penetrate the skin, producing a draining sinus tract.

Clinical Considerations

The destruction of bone and articular cartilage by tuberculous infection is a slow process, and symptoms are correspondingly insidious in their development. The patient complains of a dull ache in the area of the affected joint. Pain is often worse at night than during the day. The patient often appears debilitated. A history of weight loss and easy fatigability may be obtained. There may be a history of close contact with a family member or friend with known tuberculosis.

Spinal involvement with tuberculosis produces diminished motion at the thoracolumbar level. Protective paraspinal muscle spasm holds the back hyperextended. If the tuberculous process has escaped the confines of the disc space and adjacent vertebrae, a large paraspinal abscess may result. As the spine becomes weakened, collapse of the vertebral column may occur, forcing caseous necrotic debris into the spinal canal and producing neurologic symptoms ranging from paresis to complete paraplegia. Prior to the development of effective antituberculous drugs, this clinical pattern of spinal tuberculosis was more common. The paraspinal abscess developing around a focus of tuberculous infection may extend some distance beneath the paraspinal muscle and present as a mass above the posterosuperior iliac crest, or it may extend down the psoas muscle and present as a mass in the medial thigh. On incision, these masses produce caseous necrotic material but characteristically do not have any associated erythema or increased heat. This clinical presentation is known as a *cold abscess*. The first radiographic change in tuberculous spondylitis is narrowing of the disc at the affected level. The outlines of the adjacent vertebral end plates become indistinct in appearance. As the disease progresses, the combination of interspace narrowing and vertebral collapse may produce a kyphotic deformity. If a paraspinal abscess is present, it usually produces a soft tissue shadow on plain radiographs. Calcification is occasionally observed within the abscess.

Tuberculous involvement of diarthrodial joints produces mild synovial thickening and effusion. Increased local heat may be felt over the joint, but erythema is usually lacking. Limitation of motion may be mild. Associated muscle atrophy and a limp are usually present. There may be enlargement of proximal regional lymph nodes.

Laboratory examination reveals a normal to slightly elevated white cell count, an elevated erythrocyte sedimentation rate, and mild anemia. The tuberculin skin test is usually positive. Synovial fluid from the involved joint is turbid, with a poor mucin clot and a low glucose level. The white cell count is elevated, with an increased number of mononuclear cells. The synovial fluid sediment should be examined for acid-fast bacilli and a portion retained for culture.

Radiographs of tuberculous joints demonstrate generalized osteoporosis, with preservation of the joint width and distention of the joint capsule. The earliest bony changes consist of erosion of the joint margins at the point of synovial attachment to bone. Similar defects may occur within the epiphysis, and infection may cross the physeal plate into the adjacent metaphysis. When the hip joint in children is involved, progressive capsular distention may interrupt the blood supply to the capital femoral epiphysis (Fig. 42–58).

Treatment

The development of effective antituberculous drugs has dramatically altered the treatment of this disease. Historically, a patient's primary defense against tuberculosis was his or her own immune system. If the lesion showed signs of healing, arthrodesis (fusion) of the joint was performed with the joint in the functional position. Today, arthrodesis is less frequently required.[1]

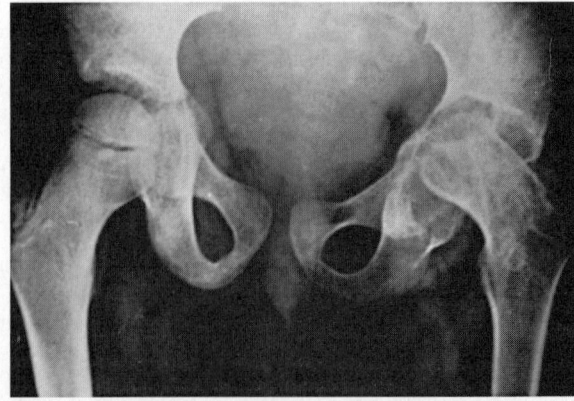

Figure 42–58. In this case of tuberculosis of the hip joint, the capital femoral epiphysis has been destroyed, probably because of loss of blood supply. Notice the narrowing of the joint space and osteoporosis of the pelvis and femur on the involved side. There is very little reactive bone formation.

The initial treatment of skeletal tuberculosis consists of appropriate antituberculous drugs (isoniazid, rifampin, p-aminosalicylic acid [PAS], streptomycin, ethambutol). Protection of the involved joint with splints or plaster is recommended. For spinal tuberculosis, bed rest or thoracolumbar bracing is effective. When tuberculosis spondylitis has resulted in paraparesis or paraplegia, surgical débridement of the infected disc space may be considered. Recovery of neurologic function may be somewhat quicker with surgical débridement than with antibiotic therapy alone. As healing occurs, resumption of activity is allowed. Joints in the lower extremity are rehabilitated by range-of-motion exercises. If there is no significant response after 6 to 8 weeks of antituberculous therapy, surgical débridement of diarthrodial joints may be necessary. Arthrodesis of the joint may be required if there is extensive joint destruction. In selected cases, total joint replacement may be effective.

Acute Pyogenic Arthritis

Joint infection with pyogenic organisms occurs as a result of hematogenous seeding of the joint, extension of adjacent osteomyelitis, or penetrating wounds of the joint. Hematogenous pyarthrosis is most commonly observed in children under the age of 5 years. *S. aureus* is the most common etiologic agent, followed by *Haemophilus influenzae*, *Streptococcus*, *Gonococcus*, and *Pneumococcus*. Acute pyarthrosis is almost always monarticular. Patients with immune deficiency may present with multiple joint involvement. The hip joint is the most frequently involved.[22]

Pathologic Considerations

The infiltration of polymorphonuclear neutrophils following inoculation of the joint is similar to that of pyogenic infection elsewhere. The initial irritation of the synovial membrane causes an increased production of synovial fluid and a joint effusion. As neutrophils and bacteria accumulate, the intra-articular pressure rises. The combination of toxic bacterial products, lysosomal enzymes, and increased pressure produces gradual destruction of the articular cartilage, beginning in the weight-bearing portion of the articular surface. If the full thickness of the articular cartilage is destroyed in any area, infection may gain access to underlying subchondral bone. Rupture of the joint capsule due to increased pressure may allow the infection to gain access to adjacent soft tissues. Penetration through to the overlying skin with the development of draining sinus tracts occurs rarely.

Clinical Considerations

The onset of pyogenic arthritis is acute, with fever, irritability, and pain. In the early stages of infection, a limp may develop, which rapidly progresses to severe pain, preventing ambulation. On examination, one observes swelling, overlying erythema, and exquisite tenderness to direct palpation. Any attempt at joint motion produces paroxysms of pain. It is necessary to distinguish between pyarthrosis and adjacent metaphyseal osteomyelitis, as discussed earlier.

Laboratory studies demonstrate an elevated white blood cell count and an elevated erythrocyte sedimentation rate. Aspiration of the involved joint under sterile conditions reveals a cloudy, turbid synovial fluid, with a cell count ranging from 50,000 to 200,000 polymorphonuclear neutrophils per cu. cm. A Gram's stain of the involved joint fluid shows organisms in 50% of cases. The joint fluid is sent for aerobic and anaerobic culture. Blood cultures are frequently positive. In performing joint aspiration, a large-bore needle should be used, since smaller needles may become plugged with edematous synovium or proteinaceous debris within the joint. Care should be taken to avoid damage to the underlying epiphyseal bone or articular cartilage.

Radiographs in the early stages of septic arthritis reveal no bony change. There is distention in the joint capsule secondary to increased pressure within the joint, and the joint may appear abnormally widened. In severe cases, there may be pathologic dislocation of the joint or pathologic separation of the epiphysis. In untreated or inadequately treated cases, destruction of articular cartilage eventually produces joint narrowing.

Treatment

Pyogenic arthritis is an emergency. When the diagnosis has been established, intravenous antibiotics are administered without awaiting the results of culture. A broad-spectrum antibiotic is begun initially and is changed based on the results of bacterial sensitivity testing. Supportive measures include fluid and electrolyte maintenance and the use of antipyretics. The affected joint must be put at rest to minimize further cartilage damage.

If the initial joint aspiration reveals a thin, serosanguineous fluid, the infection is in its early stages. In this situation, the joint may be irrigated with sterile saline through a large-bore needle and the patient observed during the initial 24 hours of antibiotic therapy. Alternatively, the joint may be inspected arthroscopically for thorough irrigation, and areas of abnormal synovium may be débrided. Usually this treatment produces marked improvement, with a fall in temperature and diminished local symptoms. Repeat aspiration or arthroscopic examination may be performed at intervals to confirm a reduction in the cell count. Repeat cultures are obtained on each aspiration to determine sterility. If improvement fails to occur, surgical incision and drainage should be undertaken.[19]

If the initial joint aspiration produces a thick, purulent material, antibiotic therapy and aspiration are unlikely to be adequate. At this stage, there is a thick, edematous synovial membrane and considerable intra-articular necrotic debris. Surgical incision and drainage with thorough joint lavage should be performed promptly. Many believe that all infections of the hip joint should be drained primarily in addition to instituting antibiotic therapy, since aspiration or arthroscopic examination of the hip joint is difficult and circulation of the capital femoral epiphysis is threatened by increased intra-articular pressure. Active and passive joint exercises are initiated as soon as the infection is under control.

NEOPLASMS OF BONE

Primitive mesenchymal tissue produces cartilage, bone, fibrous tissue, and marrow elements, the four basic tissue components of the mature skeleton. From each of these tissue types there may arise benign or malignant neoplasms. The skeleton also may be the site of neoplasms ordinarily associated with soft tissues. Hemangioma, angiosarcoma, lipoma, and liposarcoma are rare primary bone tumors. Although only primary neoplasms of bone are discussed in this section, metastatic disease from carcinomas of the breast, lung, thyroid, kidney, and prostate are the most common malignancy encountered in the skeleton. The most common benign and malignant primary skeletal neoplasms are listed in Table 42–1.

Staging

The treatment of skeletal neoplasms ranges from simple observation to radical surgical procedures and/or the use of chemotherapy and irradiation. To plan appropriate treat-

TABLE 42–1. Common Skeletal Neoplasms

Type	Cartilage	Bone	Fibrous	Marrow
Benign	Osteochondroma Enchondroma Chondroblastoma	Osteoid osteoma Osteoblastoma	Nonossifying fibroma Giant cell tumor Desmoplastic fibroma	Eosinophilic granuloma
Malignant	Primary chondrosarcoma Secondary chondrosarcoma	Osteosarcoma Periosteal osteosarcoma	Fibrosarcoma Fibrous histiocytoma	Ewing's sarcoma Lymphoma Myeloma

ment, accurate diagnosis and staging of skeletal lesions are necessary. Staging involves the determination of the local size and extent of the primary lesion, the histologic grade, and the presence or absence of visceral or nodal metastases. Evaluation begins with a careful clinical history, physical examination, and biplane radiographs. Since many benign bone lesions have a diagnostic appearance on routine radiographs, this initial evaluation may be sufficient for purposes of staging.[7]

Enneking has proposed a system for staging benign bone lesions in which the aggressiveness of the lesion is determined by its radiographic appearance. Stage 1 lesions tend to be contained completely within bone and are well marginated by reactive bone. Stage 1 lesions tend to remain static or regress. Stage 2 lesions may show some expansion of bone but remain contained within the original periosteum. The reactive bone surrounding these lesions may be less distinct. Stage 2 lesions are described as active and have the potential for further local growth. Stage 3 lesions demonstrate expansion or penetration through the overlying cortex and have little if any reactive bone at their interface with medullary cancellous bone. Stage 3 lesions have a potential for rapid growth and further bone destruction.

Stage 3 benign lesions of bone, primary malignant lesions of bone, and metastatic lesions of bone share many common radiographic characteristics. Penetration of the overlying cortex, destruction of medullary bone with no reactive bone formation, permeative destruction, and extension of tumor into the adjacent soft tissues are all signs of aggressive behavior. When plain radiographs suggest the possibility of a malignant lesion, more specific anatomic information is required. Radionuclide scanning, computed tomography (CT), and MRI may all be employed as staging studies. Imaging of suspected malignant lesions should always be accomplished prior to undertaking biopsy.

Enneking has also proposed a useful system for staging malignant skeletal neoplasms (Table 42–2). This system requires a determination of whether the lesion lies within an anatomic compartment or has extended outside the boundaries of the compartment of origin. The histologic grade must be assessed and a determination made about metastatic disease.

Biopsy

Biopsy is performed only after anatomic staging is completed. Asymptomatic lesions that are clearly benign by ra-

diographic evaluation may require no treatment. When biopsy of a lesion is required, several considerations should be borne in mind. Many skeletal neoplasms do not have a uniform histologic appearance. The biopsy specimen should be sufficient to obtain representative material for histologic examination. One must correlate the biopsy with the radiograph to make sure that neoplastic rather than reactive tissue is being obtained. Needle or trocar biopsy may be employed for lesions that are difficult to approach surgically.[6] The placement of the biopsy incision should take into consideration the possibility of future resection should the lesion prove to be malignant. Since the biopsy tract is contaminated, it must be removed *en bloc* with the surgical specimen at the time of resection.[24] Careful hemostasis following open biopsy is necessary to avoid contamination of adjacent normal tissues by hematoma. The pathologist should be consulted prior to biopsy and should be present in the operating room. The gross appearance of the lesion, the radiographic appearance of the lesion, and the histologic appearance of the tissue all contribute to the diagnosis. Tissue should be set aside for culture pending histologic examination. In many situations, infection mimics aggressive tumors.

Treatment

Four surgical procedures may be used in the treatment of skeletal neoplasms. *Intralesional* removal involves cureting the lesion from within. *Local resection* involves removal of the intact lesion through its capsule or the reactive tissues surrounding it. *Wide excision* removes the lesion with a cuff of normal surrounding tissue without ever entering the lesion. *Radical resection* removes the entire anatomic compartment in which the lesion arises. In general, Stage 1 benign bone tumors require no treatment if they are asymptomatic. If they are producing symptoms, intralesional curettage or local excision is appropriate. Stage 2 benign bone tumors are best treated by local excision without entering the lesion. Stage 3 benign bone tumors are most appropriately treated by local or wide excision without entering the lesion. For malignancies, Stage IA and IB lesions are adequately treated by wide excision, whereas Stage IIA and IIB lesions usually require radical margins.[8] Some high-grade malignancies may respond sufficiently to neoadjuvant chemotherapy or radiotherapy to allow surgical treatment by wide excision. It is worth noting that the surgical procedures described define the margins achieved at the time of resection and do not define whether amputation is necessary. If one were to amputate a limb through the reactive capsule surrounding a tumor, one would achieve only a local margin.

TUMORS OF CARTILAGINOUS ORIGIN
Osteochondroma

Osteochondroma is the most common benign neoplasm of bone and occurs with equal frequency in males and females. These tumors are usually discovered during adolescence as a result of local mechanical symptoms. Osteochondromas are composed of normal bone and cartilaginous tissue and are

TABLE 42–2. Staging for Malignant Tumors (Enneking)

Stage	Grade	Site	Metastasis
IA	Low	Intracompartmental	None
IB	Low	Extracompartmental	None
IIA	High	Intracompartmental	None
IIB	High	Extracompartmental	None
III	Any	Any	Present

thought to arise from ectopic rests of physeal plate cartilage. They arise at the metaphyseal ends of long bones, with 50% of lesions occurring in the distal femur. Osteochondromas have a characteristic radiographic appearance. A bony stalk is seen arising from the metaphysis, usually pointing away from the adjacent epiphysis (Fig. 42–59). The end of the stalk is irregular and covered with a cartilaginous cap of varying thickness. Osteochondromas tend to continue growing until skeletal maturity is achieved and fusion of the adjacent physeal plate occurs. The bony stalk is in continuity with the underlying cortex. The stalk may be thin, with a pedunculated cartilaginous cap, or it may be broad and sessile, with the cap closely adherent to the adjacent normal cortex. Grossly, the cartilaginous surface is lobulated, pearly white, and opalescent. Often a bursa overlies the cartilaginous cap. Although osteochondromas are usually solitary, there is a hereditary form of the disease known as multiple hereditary osteochondromatosis.

Osteochondromas are Stage 2 benign lesions during adolescence and become Stage 1 lesions after skeletal maturity. The treatment of an osteochondroma depends on symptoms. Lesions that are producing mechanical difficulty adjacent to a joint are best treated by local excision. Asymptomatic lesions may be treated by observation.

Malignant degeneration of the cartilaginous cap into a chondrosarcoma may occur rarely in solitary osteochondromas and with greater frequency in multiple hereditary osteochondromatosis. Lesions closer to the midline of the body (scapula, ribs, pelvis) are statistically more likely to undergo malignant degeneration. Evidence of growth of an osteochondroma after skeletal maturity should raise suspicions of malignant degeneration.

Enchondroma

An enchondroma is a benign growth of hyaline cartilage lying in the medullary cavity of a bone. Like an osteochon-

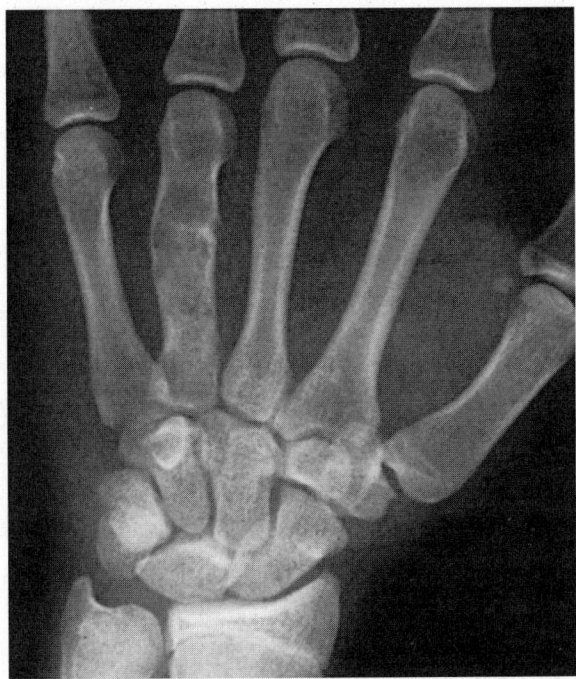

Figure 42–60. The lesion in the fourth metacarpal has expanded and thinned the overlying cortex. There is stippled calcification within the center of the lesion. This enchondroma was cured by curettage and bone grafting.

droma, the lesion is thought to arise from ectopic cartilaginous rests from the physeal plate. Enchondromas have an equal gender distribution and most frequently occur in the phalanges and metacarpals. Enchondromas also appear in other long bones, as well as the pelvis, scapula, and ribs. These lesions are rarely symptomatic and are most often discovered on radiographs obtained for other purposes.

Radiographically, enchondromas in the metacarpals produce a lucent defect with well-defined margins and surrounding sclerotic reactive bone (Fig. 42–60). The overlying cortex may be expanded and thinned. Varying degrees of stippled calcification may be seen within the lesion. When occurring in the metaphyses of larger long bones, the enchondroma may be less well defined. Subtle areas of stippled calcification may be the only indication of their presence. They may be better defined by CT scanning and MRI. Radionuclide scans usually show increased uptake that corresponds in extent to the size of the lesion identified on axial imaging. Endosteal erosion and expansion of the cortex are less common in enchondromas of the major long bones.

Grossly, enchondromas are blue-white and translucent. Microscopic examination reveals lobules of hyaline cartilage with a mild degree of increased cellularity compared with normal hyaline cartilage.[4]

Like osteochondromas, enchondromas have a potential for malignant degeneration. Because these are usually Stage 1 benign lesions, any clinical evidence of growth or the development of pain in the region of an enchondroma should raise suspicion of malignant degeneration. Radiographic evidence of cortical erosion or periosteal reaction is suspicious for malignant degeneration.

Enchondromas may occur as multiple lesions (Ollier's disease) and may produce growth disturbance in early childhood. Distortion in both length growth and angular growth may be observed. The likelihood of malignant degeneration in multiple enchondromas is higher than for solitary lesions. Periodic radiographic survey is indicated in patients with multiple lesions. On the rare occasion when enchondromas

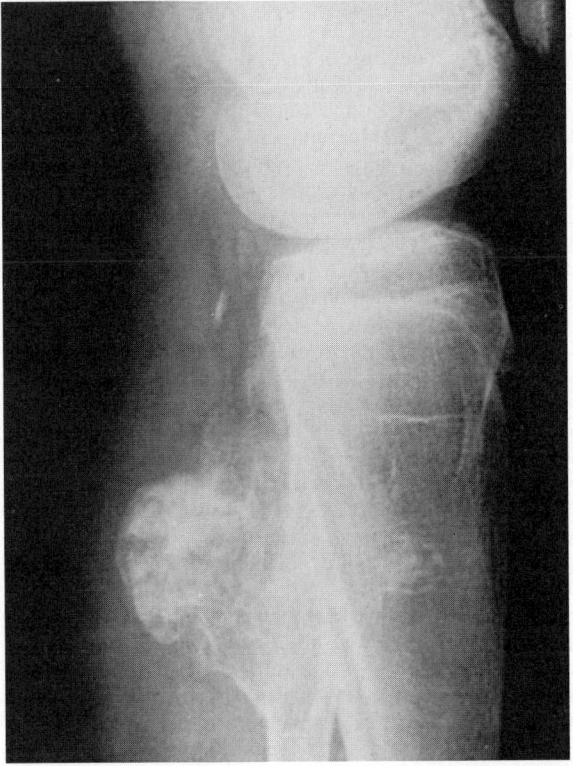

Figure 42–59. This child has multiple osteochondromatosis. Notice the lobulated bony stalk arising from the posterior portion of the fibula. This stalk is covered by a large cartilaginous cap not seen on radiographic examination.

require surgical treatment, intralesional curettage and bone grafting are appropriate.

Chondroblastoma

A chondroblastoma is a benign lesion of cartilaginous origin first identified by Codman in 1931. It has a peculiar affinity for the epiphyses of long bones or apophyseal equivalent areas. These tumors are most frequently encountered in the second decade of life and are most frequent in males (2:1). Symptoms are variable. Since these lesions occur adjacent to articular surfaces, aching pain in the joint, effusion, and some limitation of motion may be present.

The radiographic appearance of chondroblastoma is characteristic. These lesions occur within the epiphysis and have a smooth border and only a minimal sclerotic reactive margin. Central areas of calcific stippling may be seen and are often better appreciated on CT scan than on plain radiographs. Involvement of the adjacent physeal plate occurs occasionally, with extension of the lesion into the adjacent metaphysis (Fig. 42–61). Grossly, these lesions are gray-yellow in appearance and gritty to the touch because of calcification. Rarely, the articular surface of the adjacent joint may be penetrated by tumor.

Chondroblastomas are highly cellular. The primary cell can be described as polygonal in shape, with oval to round nuclei. Focal areas of chondroid matrix, multinucleated giant cells, and areas of focal calcification are observed throughout the tumor.

Chondroblastomas usually present as benign Stage 2 lesions, but aggressive behavior (Stage 3) is occasionally observed. Penetration into the adjacent joint or the adjacent periarticular soft tissues may be seen. There are scattered reports of pulmonary metastases from benign chondroblastomas.

Although other Stage 2 and Stage 3 lesions are usually

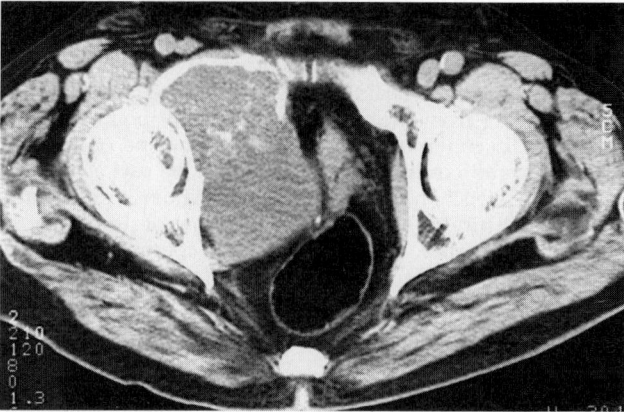

Figure 42–62. This pelvic CT scan demonstrates a large chondrosarcoma arising from the pubic ramus and extending medially and posteriorly. Notice the proximity to the rectum and the internal calcification of this cartilaginous lesion.

treated by local excision, the proximity of chondroblastomas to the articular surface would require sacrifice of joint function if local excision were employed. Accordingly, these lesions are most frequently treated by intralesional curettage and bone grafting. The recurrence rate with this treatment has been less than 10%. Recurrence may require more aggressive treatment.

Chondrosarcoma

Malignant cartilaginous tumors may arise from pre-existing benign neoplasms (secondary chondrosarcoma), may arise *de novo* in bone (primary chondrosarcoma), and are occasionally seen as primary soft tissue lesions. Chondrosarcoma is the third most common primary malignant neoplasm of bone.[4] The majority of chondrosarcomas are thought to be primary rather than secondary. This tumor occurs most frequently in the fourth to sixth decades of life and demonstrates a slight male predominance. Chondrosarcoma is most frequently encountered in the central flat bones (pelvis, scapula, sacrum), although any bone can be involved. Chondrosarcomas are rare in the small bones of the hand and foot. These tumors grow slowly, and patients with extremity lesions usually present with a history of local pain and swelling for months or years. Tumors arising in the pelvis often grow silently with no symptoms for a considerable time, and patients may present with tumors of massive size (Fig. 42–62). There are no specific laboratory data that aid in the diagnosis of chondrosarcoma.

The radiographic appearance of chondrosarcoma is variable. Focal calcification may be seen within the body of the tumor, outlining a lobulated pattern, or it may be sparse and located peripherally. Poorly differentiated, more aggressive lesions tend to demonstrate less calcification. CT and MRI are helpful in the evaluation of chondrosarcomas. The degree of bony destruction, the extension of tumor within the medullary canal of the bone, and the proximity of tumor to adjacent vital structures are all important in planning surgical treatment.

Grossly, chondrosarcomas have a lobulated, cauliflower-like surface. There may be invasion and entrapment of adjacent muscle fibers, and outgrowths of tumor may extend some distance along fascial planes. On cut section, the surface is white and opalescent. Focal areas of liquefaction necrosis and areas of calcification may be seen.

The histologic appearance of chondrosarcoma is variable. Some lesions demonstrate well-differentiated hyaline cartilage with mild cellular atypia. In such lesions, diagnosis of

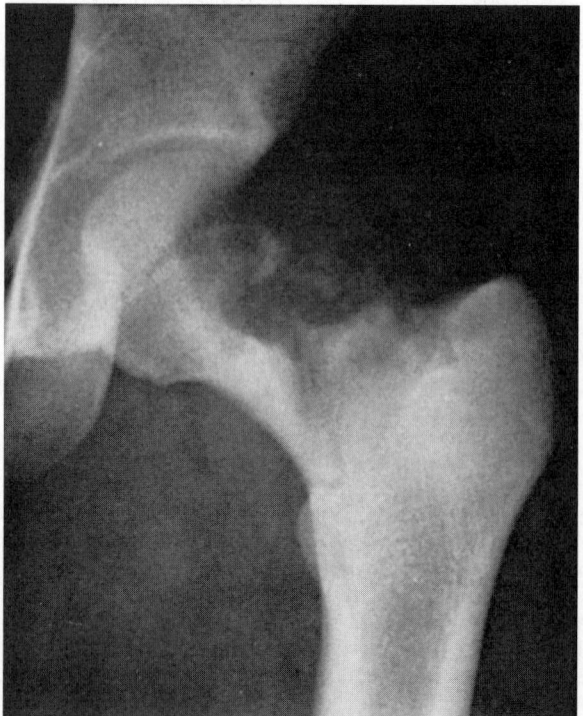

Figure 42–61. This rather aggressive chondroblastoma began in the epiphysis and subsequently involved the superior femoral neck. Notice the lack of sclerotic borders to the lesion. A pathologic fracture has occurred through the femoral calcar.

malignancy may be difficult. The radiographic appearance, the gross appearance, and the clinical behavior of the tumor must be considered in making the diagnosis. In less well-differentiated lesions, the usual characteristics of malignancy appear. Variations in nuclear size and shape, hypercellularity, multiple nuclei per cartilaginous lacunae, and mitotic figures are seen.

Most chondrosarcomas present as Stage IA lesions and are appropriately treated by wide excision, which includes removal of the biopsy tract. Because the lesions often arise in the pelvis and are close to neural and vascular structures, a wide margin may often be obtained only by hemipelvectomy.

TUMORS OF OSSEOUS ORIGIN

Osteoid Osteoma

Osteoid osteoma is a benign Stage 1 lesion of bone first described by Jaffe in 1935. Bones of the lower extremity are most frequently affected, although any bone can be involved. Osteoid osteomas are most frequently encountered in the first and second decades of life, demonstrate a slight male predominance, and are usually solitary. These lesions are exquisitely painful, and pain is the most common presenting symptom. Pain is described as a persistent discomfort unrelated to activity or rest and is often worse at night. Curiously, pain may be totally relieved for several hours by the use of aspirin or other nonsteroidal anti-inflammatory drugs. Some patients report exacerbation of pain upon consumption of alcoholic beverages.

Osteoid osteomas are small and may be difficult to demonstrate on routine radiographs. The use of radionuclide scanning has made their detection much easier. The radiographic appearance of an osteoid osteoma depends on location. When these lesions are located in cancellous bone, they present a central radiolucent defect surrounded by a dense cloud of sclerotic bone. In lesions of long standing, the sclerosis may obscure the radiolucent center on routine films. CT may be required to localize these tumors. Osteoid osteoma can also arise in cortical bone, where it produces a thickening of the cortex around a radiolucent nidus.

Osteoid osteoma is composed of a central nidus of closely packed trabeculae of woven bone. The surfaces of these trabeculae are lined with benign osteoblasts. Mineralization may be present in older lesions. The nidus is intensely vascular, with numerous capillary channels. Nerve endings have been demonstrated.

Osteoid osteoma usually presents as a Stage 2 lesion with the potential for continued pain, although its size rarely exceeds 1.5 cm. These lesions are most appropriately treated by *en bloc* excision. Because these lesions are small, radiographic control in the operating room is required to ensure proper localization. In some locations, localization may be enhanced by the use of intraoperative radionuclide scanning or by preoperative CT-guided placement of a needle into the center of the lesion.[16] In some locations, such as the femoral calcar or anterior tibial cortex, *en bloc* excision may produce unnecessary weakness and risk of pathologic fracture. In these locations, intralesional curettage may be performed. Incompletely cureted lesions may recur.

Osteosarcoma

With the exception of multiple myeloma, osteosarcoma is the most common primary neoplasm of bone, occurring in approximately 1 per 100,000 population in the United States. Osteosarcoma usually presents in the second decade of life (mean age, 15 years). It usually occurs in the metaphyseal ends of long bones, with the distal femur accounting for 30%

of cases. The proximal tibia and proximal humerus are the second and third most common sites of origin. There is a 2:1 male predominance.

Patients present with a 3- to 4-week history of pain in the region of the tumor. Local swelling and some increased heat are observed. There is often limitation of adjacent joint motion. A small percentage of patients present with pathologic fracture as the initial complaint.

The radiographic appearance of osteosarcoma is illustrated in Figure 42–63. Areas of lytic bone destruction mixed with areas of reactive and tumor bone formation are seen. This tumor rapidly permeates through the overlying cortex into the subperiosteal space and produces a characteristic *sunburst* appearance of trabecular bone oriented at right angles to the underlying cortical surface. Some tumors are almost purely lytic in nature, whereas others produce an abundant amount of both malignant and reactive bone. Histologically, osteosarcoma is composed of a disorderly deposition of osteoid produced by malignant osteoblasts. Nuclear pleomorphism and multiple mitoses are noted. In addition to malignant bone, there may be areas of malignant cartilage and fibrous tissue within the tumor. Osteosarcomas are, by definition, high-grade tumors, and almost all are extracompartmental at the time of presentation (Stage IIB).[12]

For the first half of the twentieth century, these Stage IIB lesions were treated by surgery alone. Amputation either

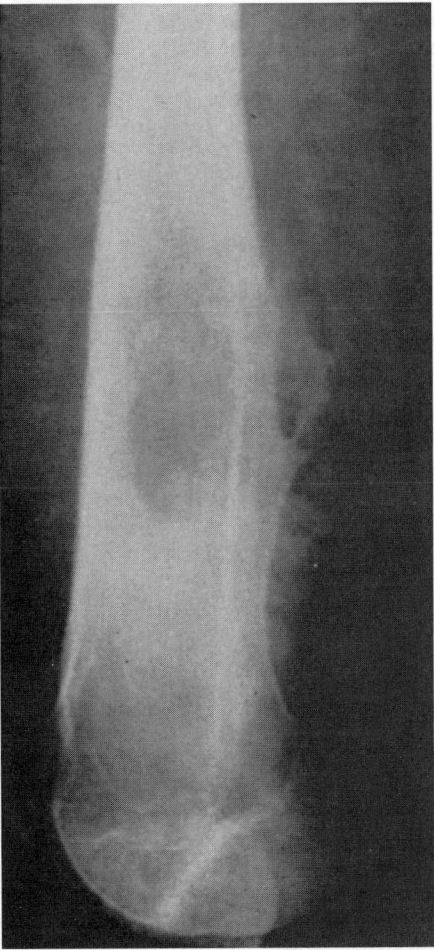

Figure 42–63. This lateral radiograph of the distal femur of a 14-year-old girl shows a central radiolucent defect in the femoral metaphysis, with periosteal elevation overlying the lesion. There has been erosion through the femoral cortex. Notice the *sunburst* appearance of the subperiosteal new bone along the posterior femoral cortex. This is the typical appearance of an osteosarcoma.

through the bone (wide margin) or through the joint above the involved bone (radical margin) was employed. In both instances, the 5-year survival rate was only 20%, with 80% of patients dying of metastatic disease, most within 2 years of diagnosis. In the late 1960s, chemotherapeutic agents were identified that had a beneficial effect in treating patients with pulmonary metastases of osteosarcoma. Although these agents did not increase ultimate survival in patients with metastases, their effect of prolonging life led to their eventual use as adjuvant chemotherapy following amputation in all patients with osteosarcoma. This adjuvant chemotherapy improved 5-year survival rates from 20% to 40%. As newer and more effective drugs were developed (Adriamycin, high-dose methotrexate, *cis*-platinum, ifosfamide), studies were undertaken to assess their effect on the primary tumor prior to surgical intervention. In many cases, the involution of the primary tumor in response to neoadjuvant chemotherapy was dramatic. For the first time, one could consider wide excision rather than amputation. Today, the standard approach to osteosarcoma is neoadjuvant chemotherapy followed by limb salvage surgery.[17, 20, 25] Approximately 80% of patients show a satisfactory response to neoadjuvant chemotherapy that allows limb salvage. In the remaining 20%, the primary tumor fails to respond, there is a pathologic fracture through the lesion, or the anatomic location is adjacent to viable structures, precluding limb salvage. Overall 5-year survival now approximates 65%.

With current chemotherapy regimens, pulmonary metastases tend to occur later and in fewer numbers than in the era prior to chemotherapy. In selected patients who present with small numbers of metastases more than 1 year from the time of diagnosis, pulmonary débridement may not only prolong life but in some instances result in apparent eradication of the disease.

TUMORS OF FIBROUS ORIGIN

Nonossifying Fibroma

Nonossifying fibroma is probably a focal developmental defect rather than a true neoplasm. Occurring primarily in children and located in the metaphysis of long bones, this lesion is also known as benign metaphyseal cortical defect or fibrous cortical defect. Nonossifying fibromas are usually an incidental finding on radiographs obtained for other reasons. Rarely, they are large enough to create a pathologic fracture. Nonossifying fibroma occurs with equal frequency in males and females. The lower extremities are most often involved, and there may be multiple lesions. Nonossifying fibroma is located eccentrically in the metaphysis of long bones lying immediately beneath the cortex. There may be cortical thinning, but a distinct sclerotic margin at both the cortical surface and the intramedullary interface is usually present. The central portion of the lesion is relatively radiolucent and appears to be divided by bony septa (Fig. 42–64).

Grossly, the contents of a nonossifying fibroma are soft and yellow to brown. On histologic examination, one sees swirls of fibrous tissue containing numerous multinucleated giant cells, lipid-filled histiocytes, and deposits of hemosiderin.

The natural history of nonossifying fibroma is gradual healing. These are Stage 1 lesions and require no treatment unless they reach a sufficient size to cause pathologic fracture. Intralesional curettage and bone grafting are curative.

Giant Cell Tumor

Giant cell tumor is an uncommon neoplasm arising in the third and fourth decades of life and occurring in the metaphyseal-epiphyseal area of long bone or in the apophy-

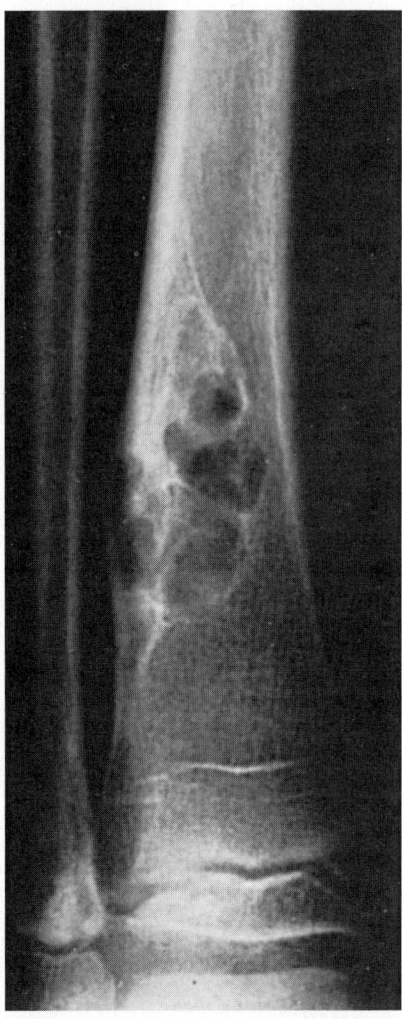

Figure 42–64. This eccentrically located metaphyseal lesion has smooth sclerotic borders on the medullary side and has expanded the overlying cortex. This appearance is typical of a nonossifying fibroma.

seal equivalent areas of flat and cuboid bones. In long bones, the tumor invariably extends to the subchondral bone of the adjacent joint. This radiographic characteristic distinguishes it from almost all other skeletal neoplasms. The radiographic aggressiveness of giant cell tumors ranges from Stage 1 to Stage 3. In Stage 1 lesions, one sees a radiolucent defect usually eccentrically located within the bone and thinning or expanding the adjacent overlying cortex. Thinned bony septa may be seen in the center of the lesion, producing a lobulated appearance. In more aggressive tumors, rapid growth of the lesion may produce a poorly demarcated medullary interface with little if any sclerotic bone peripherally. Resorption or penetration of the overlying cortex, with extension of tumor into the adjacent soft tissues, may be seen.

Grossly, giant cell tumor has a red-gray appearance, with areas of soft yellow material representing lipid deposits. There may be areas of cystic degeneration. The name of this tumor is derived from its microscopic appearance. Numerous multinucleated giant cells are found embedded within the fibrous stroma. Focal areas of hemorrhage and collections of lipid-filled histiocytes may be seen. Reactive bone formation may be present.

The treatment of giant cell tumor traditionally involves intralesional curettage. Although local excision or wide excision might offer lower recurrence rates, because of the proximity to the joint, significant disability results when this treatment is employed. Recurrence rates for intralesional curettage and bone grafting range from 40% to 60%. In recent years, there has been an emphasis on the use of some form of adjuvant treatment following curettage. The instillation of liquid nitrogen has lowered the recurrence rate to approximately 12%. This form of treatment may be difficult to use because of the proximity of adjacent neural and vascular structures, and it is associated with a higher rate of pathologic fracture. The use of phenol to coat the cureted surface has been shown to lower recurrence rates to the 8% to 20% range. Currently, the use of polymethylmethacrylate to fill the tumor cavity is advocated. The heat of polymerization is thought to reduce local recurrence, and this compound provides some instant stability for large lesions. Occasionally, extensive Stage 3 tumors require sacrifice of the joint surface and reconstruction with either cadaveric allograft or implanted prosthetic devices.[18, 23]

Fibrosarcoma and Malignant Fibrous Histiocytoma

Primary malignant fibrous tumors of bone are rare. Like osteosarcoma, these lesions occur more frequently in the lower extremity. There is a wide age distribution, with the highest incidence occurring in the third and fourth decades of life.

Fibrosarcoma produces a variety of patterns radiographically, depending on its aggressiveness. The lesion may present as a Stage IA or IB lesion with a moderately well-defined sclerotic border, or it may present with the more aggressive appearance of geographic or permeative destruction of Stage IIA and IIB lesions.

There is no established chemotherapy regimen for fibrosarcoma, and these lesions must be approached surgically based on their histologic and anatomic staging. Wide excision for Stage IA and IB lesions and radical excision for Stage IIA and IIB lesions are considered appropriate.

Malignant fibrous histiocytomas are characteristically high-grade lesions (Stage IIA and IIB). In some instances, they have been found to respond to chemotherapy in the same manner as osteosarcoma. It is probably advisable to treat malignant fibrous histiocytomas with neoadjuvant chemotherapy before formulating surgical plans.[27]

TUMORS OF MARROW CELL ORIGIN
Ewing's Sarcoma

Ewing's sarcoma occurs most frequently in the first and second decades of life. It is included here as a tumor of marrow cell origin, although some believe that it arises from endothelial cells. Although any bone can be involved, long bones of the extremities are the most frequent site of this neoplasm.

Patients present with complaints of local pain and swelling in the region of the tumor. There may be fever, leukocytosis, and an increased erythrocyte sedimentation rate. These findings, together with the early radiographic appearance, may lead to the mistaken diagnosis of osteomyelitis. In some cases, the onset is less abrupt, and patients may present with a large local tumor mass that has been present for many months.

The radiographic appearance of Ewing's sarcoma is highly variable. When these lesions occur in the diaphysis, a classic picture of *onion skin* periosteal elevation is seen because of permeation of the cortex by tumor. In this respect, the lesion may resemble osteomyelitis. In other locations, the radiographic changes may be less distinct. Varying degrees of bone destruction and varying degrees of reactive new bone formation create a wide range of radiographic appearances.

Grossly, Ewing's sarcoma is often necrotic, resembling purulent exudate, and areas of hemorrhage may be encountered. Microscopically, the tumor is composed of uniform round cells gathered in nests or cords and separated by thin fibrous septa. Histochemical staining and electron microscopy aid in the diagnosis of Ewing's sarcoma. Approximately 80% of Ewing's tumors are positive for glycogen on periodic acid–Schiff staining or electron microscopy.

Through 1960, the treatment of Ewing's sarcoma consisted of radical amputation. Five-year survival rates with this treatment were less than 10%. Subsequent identification of effective chemotherapy agents and the use of radiotherapy have resulted in improved survival. In selected locations, survival may also be improved by surgical excision of the primary lesion after chemotherapy. At present, 5-year survival rates for Ewing's sarcoma approach 50%. Patients less than age 10 and older than age 30 tend to have a poorer prognosis. Patients with lesions of the appendicular skeleton have a better 5-year survival rate (70%) than those with lesions of the axial skeleton (30%).[2, 14, 21, 26]

Myeloma

This malignant neoplasm of marrow cell origin is the most common primary malignant neoplasm of bone. Myeloma is often encountered in the late decades of life and is seen more frequently in males than in females. The disease varies from a solitary lesion (plasmacytoma) to widespread skeletal disease. The symptoms vary from local pain and discomfort to systemic symptoms of anemia, fever, hypercalcemia, and renal failure related to extensive skeletal involvement and the abnormal production of immunoglobulins.

Myeloma characteristically produces lytic destruction of bone with little if any reactive bone formation. These lesions are described as geographic or *punched out* in appearance. The absence of reactive bone formation is borne out by the observation that myeloma lesions are often silent on radionuclide scanning. Pathologic fracture is often the presenting symptom. The diagnosis of myeloma is made by marrow aspiration or the demonstration of abnormal plasma cells at the site of bony destruction. Fifty per cent of patients with disseminated disease have Bence Jones protein in their urine. Serum electrophoresis demonstrates an abnormal amount of immunoglobulins. Urine electrophoresis is also helpful when the diagnosis is in doubt and may demonstrate abnormal proteins in patients with a normal serum electrophoretic pattern. Microscopically, myeloma produces sheets of plasma cells. Usually these are well-differentiated cells in which the characteristic arrangements of nuclear chromatin can be recognized. With the exception of biopsy for diagnosis or the treatment of pathologic fracture or impending pathologic fracture, the treatment of myeloma is nonsurgical.

REFERENCES

1. Allen, A. R., and Stevenson, A. W.: A ten-year followup of combined drug therapy and early fusion in bone tuberculosis. J. Bone Joint Surg. [Am.], 49:1001, 1967.
2. Bacci, G., Toni, A., Avella, M., et al.: Long-term results in 144 localized Ewing's sarcoma patients treated with combined therapy. Cancer, 63:1477, 1989.
3. Boland, A. L.: Acute hematogenous osteomyelitis. Orthop. Clin. North Am., 3:275, 1972.
4. Dahlin, D. C., and Coventry, M. D.: Osteogenic sarcoma: A study of 600 cases. J. Bone Joint Surg. [Am.], 49:1010, 1967.
5. Dirschl, D. R.: Acute pyogenic osteomyelitis in children. Orthop. Rev., 23:305, 1994.
6. Dollahite, H. A., Tatum, L., Moinuddin, S. M., et al.: Aspiration biopsy of primary neoplasms of bone. J. Bone Joint Surg. [Am.], 71:1166, 1989.
7. Enneking, W. F.: Musculoskeletal Tumor Surgery. New York, Churchill Livingstone, 1983.
8. Enneking, W. F., Spanier, S. S., and Goodman, M. A.: A system for the surgical staging of musculoskeletal sarcoma. Clin. Orthop., 153:106, 1980.

9. Epps, C. H., Jr., Bryant, D. D., III, Coles, M. J., et al.: Osteomyelitis in patients who have sickle-cell disease: Diagnosis and management. J. Bone Joint Surg. [Am.], 73:1281, 1991.

10. Faden, H., and Grossi, M.: Acute osteomyelitis in children: Reassessment of etiologic agents and their clinical characteristics. Am. J. Dis. Child., 145:65, 1991.

11. Fischer, M. D., Gustilo, R. B., and Varecka, T. F.: The timing of flap coverage, bone grafting, and intramedullary nailing in patients who have a fracture of the tibial shaft with extensive soft tissue injury. J. Bone Joint Surg. [Am.], 73:1316, 1991.

12. Glasser, D. B., and Lane, J. M.: Stage IIB osteogenic sarcoma. Clin. Orthop., 270:29, 1991.

13. Gordon, L., and Chiu, E. J.: Treatment of infected non-unions and segmental defects of the tibia with staged microvascular muscle transplantation and bone-grafting. J. Bone Joint Surg. [Am.], 70:377, 1988.

14. Hustu, H. O., Pinkel, D., and Pratt, C. B.: Treatment of clinically localized Ewing's sarcoma with radiotherapy and combination chemotherapy. Cancer, 30:1522, 1972.

15. Lane, J. G., Falahee, M. H., Wojtys, E. M., et al.: Pyarthrosis of the knee: Treatment considerations. Clin. Orthop., 252:198, 1990.

16. Lenke, L. G., et al.: Osteoid osteoma of the proximal femur: CT-guided preoperative localization. Orthopaedics, 17:289, 1994.

17. Link, M. P., Goorin, A. M., Miser, A. W., et al.: The effect of adjuvant chemotherapy on relapse-free survival in patients with osteosarcoma of the extremity. N. Engl. J. Med., 314:1600, 1986.

18. Mankin, H. J., Gebhardt, M. C., and Tomford, W. W.: The use of frozen cadaveric allografts in the management of patients with bone tumors of the extremities. Orthop. Clin. North Am., 18:275, 1987.

19. Morrey, B. F., and Peterson, H. A.: Hematogenous pyogenic osteomyelitis in children. Orthop. Clin. North Am., 6:935, 1975.

20. Rougraff, B. T., et al.: Limb salvage compared with amputation for osteosarcoma of the distal end of the femur: A long-term oncological, functional, and quality-of-life study. J. Bone Joint Surg. [Am.], 76:649, 1994.

21. Sailer, S., Harmon, D. C., Mankin, H. J., et al.: Ewing's sarcoma: Surgical resection as a prognostic factor. Int. J. Radiat. Oncol. Biol. Phys., 15:43, 1988.

22. Shaw, B. A., and Kasser, J. R.: Acute septic arthritis in infancy and childhood. Clin. Orthop., 257:212, 1990.

23. Sim, F. H., Beauchamp, C. P., and Chao, E. Y.: Reconstruction of musculoskeletal defects about the knee for tumor. Clin. Orthop., 221:188, 1987.

24. Simon, M. A.: Biopsy of musculoskeletal tumors. J. Bone Joint Surg. [Am.], 64:1253, 1982.

25. Simon, M. A.: Current concepts review: Limb salvage for osteosarcoma. J. Bone Joint Surg. [Am.], 70:307, 1988.

26. Wilkins, R. M., Prichard, D. J., Burgert, E. D., Jr., et al.: Ewing's sarcoma of bone: Experience with 140 patients. Cancer, 58:2551, 1986.

27. Yasko, A. W., and Lane, J. M.: Current concepts review: Chemotherapy for bone and soft-tissue sarcomas of the extremities. J. Bone Joint Surg. [Am.], 73:1263, 1991.

X

THE HAND

TENDON INJURY AND REPAIR

James A. Nunley, M.D., and J. Leonard Goldner, M.D.

Tendon continuity is necessary for transmission of force from the muscle bellies to the hand or digits. Each muscle tendon unit has a vascular supply, a nerve supply, and a gliding mechanism, all of which ensure good nutrition and smooth activity. Disruption of a tendon causes loss of motion of the digit and diminished grip or pinch. The severity of tendon injury varies according to the location of the loss of continuity, the mechanism of injury, the conditions that exist at the time of the injury, the particular tendon involved, and the anatomic location of the laceration in relationship to the muscle-tendon unit. A tendon laceration directly over a joint is more serious than is an injury at the musculotendinous junction. Maximal tendon function requires full-thickness skin coverage, epitenon and peritenon to protect the tendon from surrounding adhesions, and muscle bellies of adequate strength. The annular ligaments should be reconstructed or spared. The method of suturing requires core and peripheral sutures large enough to tolerate controlled early motion. Postoperatively, a supervised, limited static and dynamic exercise program is undertaken with vigilance. In spite of all this, a perfect result is not guaranteed because of unforeseen occurrences.[1, 4-6]

BIOMECHANICS OF HEALING TENDONS

Within 3 to 7 days after the tendon is repaired, modified splints are applied so that modest active extension is possible, and limited active flexion is started. Continuous passive motion (CPM) initiated by a motorized apparatus has been successful in limiting the formation of adhesions. Controlled studies show that several methods have been successful. The major risk of these techniques is a wider-than-desired gap at the site of the repaired tendon or complete rupture of the repaired tendon. Strict monitoring and compliance diminish this complication. Wrist position is also critical in doing active flexion. Moreover, a dorsiflexed wrist gives the patient a greater risk of excess force of flexion than does a palmar flexed wrist.[8, 10, 13, 15]

The strength-duration curve shows that tendon healing is weak at 21 days but of sufficient strength to tolerate active contraction of the muscle. At 3 weeks, external elastic traction can be applied if the force is not excessive. At 3 months, moderate stress can be applied to the flexor tendon in both flexion and extension. At 8 months, full tensile strength has been recovered. The healing tendon forms a strong bond as fibroblasts realign, collagen matrices unite, blood vessels invade the area of healing, and fibroblasts migrate from the periphery to the centrum in order to establish a bond. The peripheral covering adheres to the tendon throughout its entire length early during the period of healing. A tenoma is formed, and this gradually matures. The degree of shortening or lengthening of the tendon should be within the limits of the tension-strength curve. If the tendon is shortened, too much stretch is applied to the muscle mass, and maximal strength is not obtained. A contracture results. A strong end-to-end suture with core and epitenon sutures or a woven technique for a free tendon graft proximally, along with firm, reliable fixation distally, allows early motion of the digit even when a free tendon graft is done.[7, 18]

CLASSIFICATION OF TENDON INJURIES

In order to clarify the results of tendon repair, it is necessary to define the different anatomic regions of the flexor tendon so that injuries in different locations can be readily compared.[3, 4] The flexor system of the digits consists of two tendons for each finger and one for the thumb. The muscle bellies of these tendons originate from the distal humerus and the proximal ulna. The musculotendinous junction is located in the distal portion of the forearm from which the tendons pass to the wrist, through the carpal canal, and into the hand and digits. The flexor digitorum superficialis divides into two tendon slips within the palm and inserts on the middle phalanx of each digit. The flexor superficialis is intimately associated with the flexor profundus tendon. The flexor digitorum profundus and the flexor pollicis longus tendons insert on the base of the distal phalanges of the fingers and the thumb, respectively.

Zone System for Defining Tendon Injuries

The modified Verdan zone system divides the entire length of the flexor tendons into five anatomic areas (Fig. 42–65).[2, 3] Zone I extends from the flexor superficialis insertion to the tip of the finger and involves only the flexor digitorum profundus. The skin laceration may lie anywhere distal to the midfinger crease. Zone II, which Bunnell termed "no man's land," begins proximal to the metacarpophalangeal joint and extends to the midportion of the middle phalanx. This corresponds to the distal palmar crease and the midfinger crease. In this location, there are two flexor tendons tightly enclosed within an unyielding fibro-osseous canal, which is critical to the mechanical function of these tendons. Zone III extends from the base of the palm or the distal end of the transverse retinacular ligament to the transverse crease in the palm. In this location, the lumbrical muscle belly is firmly attached to the flexor digitorum profundus, and both lie deep to the flexor digitorum superficialis. Zone IV extends from the distal end of the transverse retinacular ligament to the proximal margin. The lumbrical muscle belly thins out in this location, and the flexor tendons to the fingers and the one to the thumb make a compact mass of collagen over which the median nerve passes. Zone V extends from the proximal transverse carpal ligament at the wrist to the musculotendinous junction of the flexor tendons in the distal third of the forearm. When correlating injury to end result, the most critical zone is Zone II.[5]

The zone of injury and the severity of the original injury affect the end result. If the skin coverage is damaged, the digital nerves and vessels are injured, the annular ligaments

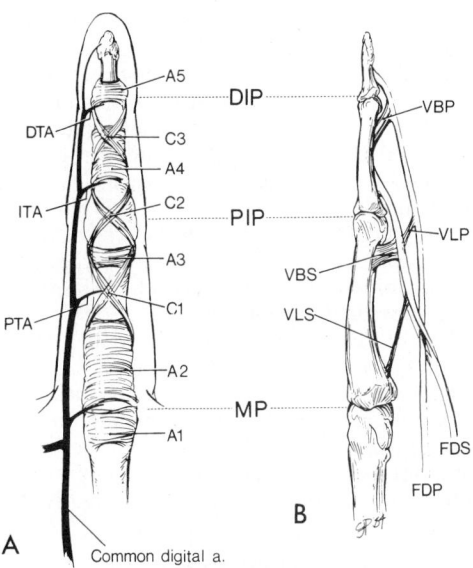

Figure 42–66. *A,* The annular ligaments covering the flexor tendons are represented by A1–A2 as the proximal pulley. The A3 pulley is opposite the distal end of the proximal phalanx, and the A4 pulley is opposite the middle of the middle phalanx. The A2 and A4 pulleys are essential. The cruciate ligaments are thin and fill the intervals between the heavier annular ligaments. The blood supply from the common digital arteries sends branches to the vincula, which at each level supply major segments of the tendon. *B,* The lateral diagram shows the long and short vincula, the flexor tendons, and the relationship between the vincula, the flexor tendons, and the adjacent joints. Function of the joints depends on the intact annular ligaments. DTA, distal tendon artery; PTA, proximal tendon artery; ITA, intermediate tendon artery; VBP, vinculum brevis profundus; VBS, vincula brevis superficialis; VLP, vincula longus profundus; FDS, flexor digitorum superficialis; FDP, flexor digitorum profundus; VLS, vincula longus superficialis; A5, pulley annular ligament.

are torn, the fibro-osseous gliding surface is injured, and a fracture occurs, the end result will be diminished in all the zones. Thus, outcome depends not only on the zone but also on the extent and severity of the original injury.[16, 24]

Flexor Retinaculum and Vincular Systems of Flexor Tendons

The complexity of early repair or late reconstruction of lacerated flexor tendons is best understood by having familiarity with the gliding and flexor retinaculum system and the intricacies of blood supply as well as a knowledge of the biologic method of healing.

The flexor retinaculum system consists of a firm fibrous sheath lined by synovium that holds the flexor tendons close to bone. This strong constraint provides a straight mechanical advantage so that a large arc of motion occurs for a relatively small applied force. The entire digital sheath includes annular and cruciate ligaments that act as pulleys. The heavy annular ligaments are thicker and stronger than the thinner cruciate pulleys. Anatomic dissections have shown that preservation of the A2 and A4 pulleys is necessary for complete tendon excursion (Fig. 42–66).[5]

Both recent and past investigators have shown that a physiologic pulley arrangement is essential for maximal function after tendon repair or grafting. The anatomic-physiologic pulley system does have segments that are compensatory, so part of the pulley system is nonessential, but the closer the repaired pulley is to the original condition, the better the traumatized tendon glides after repair.[14, 21, 28]

TENDON VASCULAR SUPPLY AND NUTRITION

Much information is available about the nutrition of flexor tendons. The vascular anatomy shows that each tendon re-

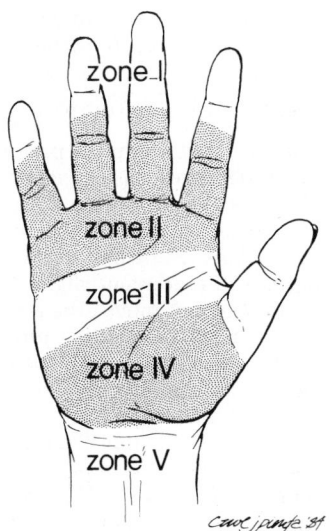

Figure 42–65. The hand zones are important in differentiating one tendon laceration from another and in determining how to treat single or double tendon lacerations that occur in the different zones. The annular ligaments vary according to the zones. They are most important in effecting postoperative function in Zone II. Zone I includes only the insertions of the flexor digitorum profundus, and Zone V contains median and ulnar nerves, median and ulnar arteries, the wrist flexor tendons, and all of the flexor digitorum profundus and flexor digitorum superficialis tendons.

ceives its blood supply from segmental vessels arising from the surrounding peritenon and extending from the forearm to the midportion of the proximal phalanx. In the digits, however, blood supply reaches the flexor tendons through the vincula.[19] These are folds of mesotenon through which course the small vessels that penetrate the tendons. One short and one long vinculum supply each flexor digitorum superficialis and flexor digitorum profundus tendon (see Fig. 42–66B). The vincula receive their blood vessels through the transverse communicating branches of the common digital artery located on the dorsal surface of the flexor tendons. The vincula provide the blood supply that participates in the early healing of flexor tendons and serve as a rein to limit proximal retraction of a lacerated tendon.

Additional blood supply to a tendon comes from small intrinsic longitudinal vessels that run parallel to the collagenous fibers of the tendon and extend from the muscle fibers to the bony insertions. The morphologic pattern of vascularization is the same for the index and ring fingers.[9, 26, 28]

Flexor Tendon Healing

Two forms of tendon healing occur within the *intrinsic* and *extrinsic* systems of the flexor tendons. Intrinsic healing occurs without direct blood flow to the tendon. Animal models have demonstrated that diffusion of synovial fluid around lacerated tendons allows intrinsic tendon healing without adhesion formation. The nutrition for tendon healing in that model comes indirectly from blood flow to the surrounding synovium. Moreover, the specimens that healed in a synovial pouch were not under stress.[19, 22] Extrinsic healing is known to occur by proliferation of fibroblasts from the peripheral epitenon. The fibrous proliferation forms a tenoma around the periphery of cut tendon ends and also invades the space between the tendon ends. Adhesions occur because of extrinsic healing of the tendon and limit tendon gliding within the fibrous and synovial sheaths. Both systems contribute to tendon healing and gliding. A healing tendon depends on nutrition from osmotic fluid that is high in protein and on granulation tissue that constitutes the tendon scar. The physiologic equilibrium between both systems allows healing without excessive scar.

The mechanisms of tendon healing are accompanied by early motion to elongate the adhesions and prevent fibrosis. To accomplish this, the healing tendon should have a strong core suture (at least four strands) as well as a peripheral epitenon suture placed at right angles to the longitudinal axis of the collagen fibers to maintain tensile strength and avoid an excessive gap. Nonsteroidal anti-inflammatory drugs (ibuprofen, indomethacin) may diminish adhesion formation.[16, 17, 19]

TENDON REPAIR

Concepts Concerning When and How to Repair an Injured Tendon

The timing and method of repairing a lacerated flexor tendon vary according to the existing conditions. There is agreement that either primary or delayed repair of all flexor tendons may be performed in Zones I, III, IV, and V. In Zone II, the options are primary repair of one or both lacerated flexor tendons, delayed repair, secondary repair, or tendon grafting 3 weeks or longer after injury.

Primary repair of a lacerated tendon is performed within 24 hours after injury. *Delayed repair* refers to a period up to 1 week after the initial injury, during which time the initial wound heals and repair of the tendon is performed, or delayed closure of the wound occurs and delayed repair of the tendon is performed at the same time as wound closure.[16] *Secondary repair* refers to any time longer than 1 week after the original injury when all wounds are healed and edema has subsided.

Primary repair of lacerated flexor tendons has several advantages compared with secondary repair: (1) accurate anatomic alignment, (2) no adhesions at the time repair is performed, and (3) no delay in initiation of recovery. Primary repair is appropriate if the surgeon is experienced in tendon repair, if the wound is exceptionally clean, and if there has been little or no crushing of the tendon or the surrounding tissues. The decision to perform delayed repair is made if the wound is contaminated, if trauma is severe, if the patient's general condition does not justify a prolonged operative procedure, and if the surgeon is not experienced in performing complicated tendon repair.

A delay of 2 weeks between injury and repair does not compromise the end result, and an even longer delay may be acceptable before the final repair is done. A delay of 6 weeks, however, may result in excess fibrosis, adherence of the tendon to the gliding canal, shortening of the muscle sarcomeres, and contracture of the muscle-tendon unit. These factors may diminish the final result. Although delay is not necessarily harmful, efforts should be made to complete the repair as early as possible. The severity of the initial injury is of greater importance than either the way the final repair is done or the period of delay. If an initial crush injury associated with a fracture and a lacerated tendon is repaired on the day of the injury, the result may not be as good as an 8-week delay for repair of a knife laceration of a tendon.[22, 27]

The delayed or secondary repair procedure involves initial wound exploration with excision of wound margins, removal of foreign material, and either primary or delayed wound closure at 3 to 5 days, depending on the mechanism of injury. The tendon may be repaired when delayed closure occurs 3 to 5 days after injury, or secondary repair may be performed 3 to 6 weeks after wound healing has occurred. Delayed repair has several advantages compared with immediate repair: (1) risk of infection is diminished, (2) an experienced physician is available to perform the repair, and (3) multiple injuries such as fracture, vascular trauma, or nerve damage can be treated prior to the definitive tendon repair. A severe injury managed by delayed repair requires early motion to prevent adhesions and diminish contractures.[20, 22]

Examination Prior to Tendon Repair

Before repair of a lacerated tendon is performed, an accurate diagnosis must be made. The examiner determines whether one, both, or neither of the flexor tendons is lacerated. The flexor digitorum superficialis is an isolated activator of the middle phalanx. Function of the superficialis is determined by holding the adjacent digits in extension so that the flexor profundi cannot move. The patient is asked to voluntarily flex the involved digit at the proximal interphalangeal joint (Fig. 42–67A). This is an accurate test for the index and long fingers and usually for the ring finger. The little finger, however, should be tested by simultaneously flexing the ring finger, since the little finger occasionally has a single muscle belly with tendons to each of the digits.

An isolated laceration of the flexor digitorum profundus is determined by the examiner's holding all finger joints in extension except the distal joint and then asking the patient to flex the fingertips (Fig. 42–67B). The flexor digitorum profundus to the index finger shows isolated function in 85% of the population but simultaneous function with the flexor pollicis longus in only 15%. The ulnar three digits act as a single unit and should be tested simultaneously.

Sensation, nail bed blanching, skin sweating, and tempera-

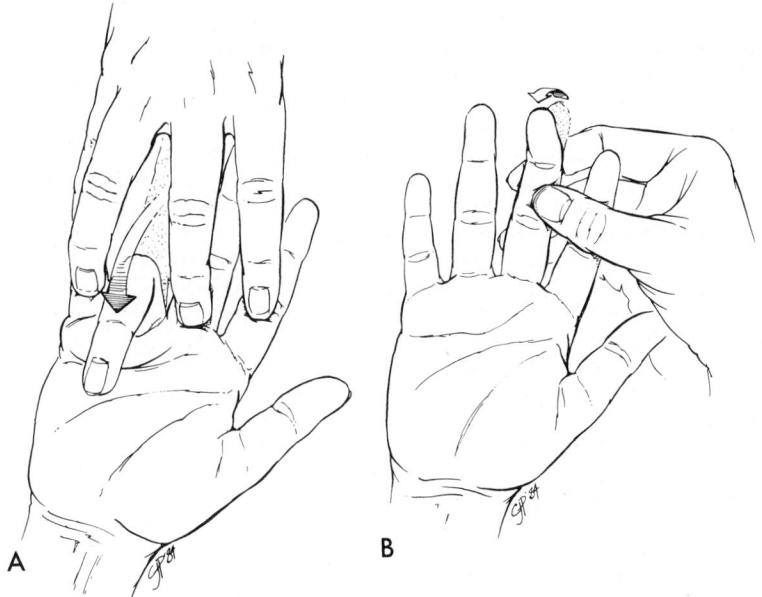

Figure 42–67. *A,* This technique is used to determine the strength of each individual flexor digitorum superficialis muscle. The adjacent digits are held in full extension to eliminate the action of the flexor digitorum profundus. The patient then voluntarily attempts to flex the proximal interphalangeal joint. Resistance is applied after flexion has occurred to determine the strength of the muscle. The distal phalanx of the same digit is tapped from the extensor side, and the flexibility of the joint is determined. If there is no tension on the flexor digitorum profundus and if all the action is through the flexor digitorum superficialis, the differentiation of the two tendons in the digits is evident. *B,* A method of testing the strength of the flexor digitorum profundus of the long finger. The proximal interphalangeal joint is maintained in extension, as is the metacarpophalangeal joint. The patient is then asked to voluntarily flex the distal phalanx at the distal joint. Accurate testing of the ulnar three digits requires that the distal joints of the long, ring, and little fingers be flexed simultaneously, after which each digit is tested individually. The thumb and index finger may be tested individually in 85% of the population and simultaneously in the remaining 15%.

ture are determined before a decision is made about degree of tendon injury, since they may represent injury to neurovascular structures that require repair as well.

Technique of Flexor Tendon Repair

Anesthesia for flexor tendon repair depends on the age of the patient, the condition of the extremity, the emotional status of the patient, and the patient's preference (awake or not awake) as well as the surgeon's preference. The choices are general anesthesia, axillary nerve block, supraclavicular brachioplexus block, or intravenous regional anesthesia with double tourniquet. The extremity is exsanguinated with an Esmarch rubber bandage, and a pneumatic tourniquet is elevated to a pressure of 230 to 250 torr. The skin laceration is extended proximally and distally, usually by zigzag extension. Medial or lateral digit incisions can be used if the repair is delayed. The lacerated flexor tendon ends are exposed, and the medial and lateral nerves and vessels are identified (Fig. 42–68). The lacerations of the flexor tendon and annular ligament are identified, and the edges are excised. All devitalized skin, fat, and fascia are removed. The wound is irrigated with antibiotic solution.

The severed distal stump of the tendon is then retrieved by flexing the middle or distal interphalangeal joints. At this time, the information previously obtained from the patient as to what position the fingers were in when the laceration occurred is valuable. If the fingers were flexed, the tendon was lacerated distal to the skin laceration. If the fingers were extended, the skin and tendon lacerations coincide. The distal tendon is then held in maximal flexion with a straight Keith needle, which is passed directly through the skin, annular ligament, and flexor tendons. The needle is usually dorsal to the neurovascular bundle. Proximally, the lacerated tendon stump is identified by compressing the muscle belly and tendons from proximal to distal while the wrist and metacarpophalangeal joints are in flexion. The location of the proximal flexor tendon is affected by the condition of the vinculum. If the vinculum has been lacerated, the tendon retracts proximally. If the proximal tendon cannot be retrieved by joint flexion and compression, an Esmarch rubber roll is wrapped from the elbow distally to force the tendons into the wound. An additional method of extracting the tendon is to pass a thin bent suction catheter into the fibro-osseous

canal. Suction is applied as the wrist and fingers are flexed, and the tendon, if cut within 24 hours, may be retrieved. If the tendon cannot be retrieved by these techniques, a separate incision is made in the palm, proximal to the A1 pulley. The flexor tendons are identified and brought out by the silicone rod technique. A 4-0 silk suture is then placed in the tip of the tendon, and a silicone rod tendon is passed from distal to proximal. The silk suture is tied to the silicone tendon, which is pulled distally. The proximal tendon is then held in position by a Keith needle, and the cruciate and annular ligaments are opened and trimmed so that the suture line is not affected by the fibro-osseous canal. The vincula, if intact, are not removed, since they bring blood to the tendon. Both ends of the tendon are held firmly, and the ends are sutured using nonabsorbable suture and circumferential reinforcing sutures. The tendons are brought together with minimal trauma.

Suture Techniques for Flexor Tendon Repair. Urbaniak

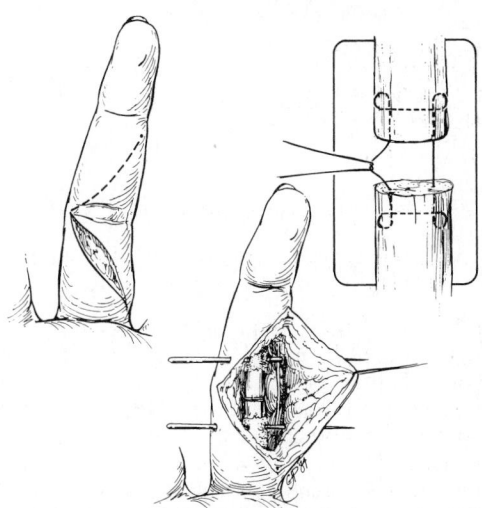

Figure 42–68. The zigzag incision on the volar surface allows exposure of the flexor tendons and annular ligaments. The nerves and vessels are on the radial and ulnar aspects of the tendons. This suture technique (Kessler) provides a strong grasp to the lacerated tendon ends. The major disadvantage is the knot between the tendon ends.

and Goldner noted that the modified grasping suture (Kessler) (see Fig. 42–68) and the figure-of-eight zigzag suture (Bunnell) were strongest at the time of initial repair.[22] A modification of these (Goldner) provided a crisscross without double knots and with good holding power (Fig. 42–69). A second vertical mattress suture is inserted so that there are at least four core strands holding the tendon ends. This initial suture is augmented by an additional vertical mattress suture from proximal to distal so that four strands of 4-0 suture pass across the gap. Suture material should be nonabsorbable and cause minimal reaction. The authors currently use 4-0 Ethibond (Ethicon, Johnson and Johnson), which satisfies all requirements. The modified Goldner or Kessler suture is used, and the knots are buried within the substance of the flexor tendon. A circumferential interrupted 6-0 nylon suture is used to smooth out the repair. The suture is placed at right angles to the fibers of the tendon, and the knot is buried (see Fig. 42–69). After tendon repair, the Keith needles are removed, and the digit is gently moved into flexion and extension to determine any binding of the suture lines on the annular ligaments. As much of the A2 and A4 pulleys (annular ligaments) is preserved as possible. Although closure of the annular ligament is desirable, stenosis must be avoided. A patch graft may be used to cover the tendon and fill the defect. If a strong, wide annular ligament is not present for both the A2 and A4 pulleys, a new annular ligament is constructed with a free tendon graft.

Zone II Laceration of Both Flexor Tendons. In Zone II injuries in which both flexor digitorum superficialis and flexor digitorum profundus tendons are lacerated, the authors believe that both flexor tendons should be repaired. A repaired flexor digitorum superficialis increases the strength of the digit, provides better and quicker flexion at the proximal interphalangeal joints, preserves the short vincula that provide blood supply to the flexor profundus, and acts as a pulley for the repaired profundus that provides improved excursion and strength. An intact functioning superficialis tendon has less tendency toward hyperextension or excessive flexion of the proximal interphalangeal joint.

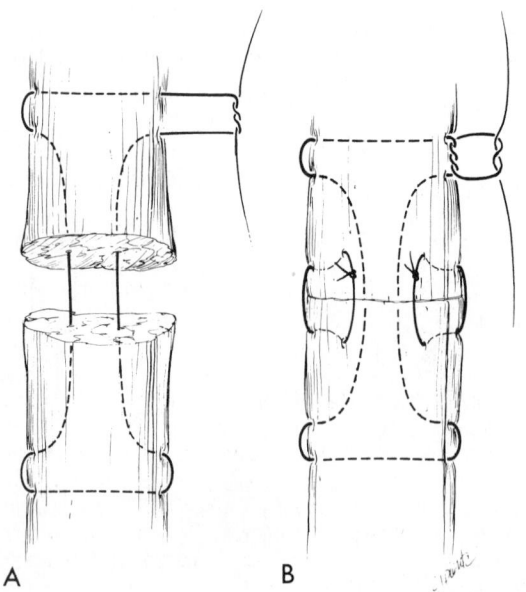

Figure 42–69. *A*, These structures are placed with either double-armed straight or curved needles. Minimal constriction occurs. Because the blood supply is primarily on the dorsum of the tendon, the suture should be placed so that it bisects the tendon or is slightly toward the volar surface. Only one knot is used for each suture. There is an option of single or double placement of the sutures both proximally and distally. *B*, After the single or double sutures are placed, the reinforcing sutures are placed to secure the cut edges of the tendon.

Post–Tendon Repair Program. In the operating room, when the tendons have been sutured, the tourniquet is released and bleeding points are controlled. The wound is closed with interrupted sutures, the capillary return is noted, and if the skin edges are dusky or pale, corner sutures are not used. A compression dressing is applied, covering all areas of the skin and extending above the elbow. The wrist is held in 25 degrees volar flexion, the metacarpophalangeal joints at 60 degrees flexion, and the proximal and distal interphalangeal joints at 25 degrees flexion. A dorsal plaster splint is used for rigid immobilization; no volar splint is used, because if this slips distally, there will be persistent traction on the repaired tendons and they will become separated. A drain may be inserted and is removed in 24 hours. The plaster is wrapped with a bias-cut stockinette bandage rather than an elastic bandage, which tends to wrap too tightly and increases in tension over time. The arm is suspended by an external support without pressure or wrapping around the wrist.

Tetanus prophylaxis is administered if necessary; preoperative and postoperative antibiotics are used for 48 hours, and the operation is performed in a clean air environment.

Extent of Early Motion After Tendon Repair: Current Investigations

There is a consensus that early but limited excursion of the repaired tendon diminishes peripheral adhesions during the postoperative healing period. However, the way to obtain this motion, the distance that the tendons are moved, and the frequency of motion are points about which there is no consensus. The frequency of rupture of repaired tendons following early forceful muscle contraction and passive motion has been as high as 35%. Conversely, absolute immobilization causes peripheral adhesions that may require several months for stretching. Pulvertaft's study showed no difference between early motion or absolute immobilization at 6 months after operation. Current studies, however, suggest that limited motion is a compromise. The authors' postoperative program includes a few millimeters of passive assistive motion three times a day while the extremity is in the dorsal splint. Duran and Houser[6] documented that 3 to 5 mm. of movement of the tendon at the suture line each day is sufficient to allow excursion of the fibroblastic scar during the healing period.

A study by Strickland indicated that active flexion and controlled extension, if carefully supervised, produced a greater range of motion and fewer ruptures. The actual difference at 1 year, however, was not determined. Kleinert and co-workers[16] recommended early postoperative rubber-band flexion and active extension. Flexion contractures and early ruptures are two of the complications that occur with this technique. However, if the procedure is well supervised, if the loop is placed on the proximal phalanx rather than on the fingernail, and if the proximal point of traction is in the midforearm, the technique has merit.

Recently, Gelberman and associates[10] demonstrated in a prospective randomized series that CPM improves the results of Zone II flexor tendon repairs when compared with rubber-band traction. Their series with CPM demonstrated very good results after tendon repair.

At 21 days, an active assistive exercise program is desirable, but the tendon should be protected for a minimum of 42 days. At that time, an outrigger extension splint is applied, and the patient is given specific exercises for elastic traction resistance against flexion, as well as Velcro splints at night to improve joint flexion and extension splints to stretch out the peripheral scar. The entire program of assistive flexion and extension must be performed meticulously, and the surgeon, patient, and therapist must be persistent. The greatest single complication associated with a vigorous postoperative therapy program is tendon rupture, which must be avoided. This is accomplished by a compromise between excessive exercise and no activity postoperatively.

Laceration of the flexor tendon at the wrist requires elbow flexion of 90 degrees for 21 days, wrist flexion of 45 degrees, metacarpophalangeal joint flexion of 30 degrees, and finger flexion of 20 degrees. Gradual extension is then allowed after 2 days, but the tendon is protected for 42 days.

Special Considerations According to the Anatomic Zone Involved

Laceration of Flexor Profundus Distal to Superficialis Insertion in Zone I. The pathologic lesion may be a laceration or an avulsion from the distal phalanx.

Management of Avulsion of the Flexor Profundus. The tendon retracts to the base of the digit or into the palm, depending on the force causing the avulsion; the vinculum prevents excessive retraction. Primary treatment is performed by isolating the tendon proximally and the phalanx distally and using a silicone flexible tendon as a guide to relocate the tendon to its usual position. A 3-0 Prolene suture is inserted into the distal end of the tendon as a double figure-of-eight, passed on either side of the phalanx through the periosteum, and tied over a rubber and plastic button insulator that is placed directly over the fingernail to avoid pressure on the tip of the digit (Fig. 42–70). Delayed repair after 21 days is managed similarly. However, if the tendon has retracted into the palm, it may become adherent to itself after 7 days and cannot be used for replacement. It must then be excised and a free tendon graft used.

Management of Laceration of the Flexor Profundus. The skin laceration may not coincide with the point of tendon laceration. Primary repair is performed if the wound is clean or can be converted to a clean wound. If not, delayed repair is completed at 7 to 21 days or even as long as 6 weeks after the original laceration. The tendon is mobilized proximally, the annular ligaments are maintained, and the tendon is advanced distally and sutured to the distal stump by end-to-end suture or by advancement if the distal stump is 1 cm. long or less. *Advancement greater than 1 cm. causes contracture.*

Laceration of Flexor Digitorum Profundus and Superficialis in Zone II. Primary repair of both tendons is performed only under ideal circumstances. The wound must be clean, there should be no element of crush to soft tissues or bone, and the tendon sheath should be at least partially intact. The surgeon must be experienced in all aspects of tendon repair. Otherwise, the safest approach is delayed or secondary repair. Even at 3 to 6 weeks after the initial injury, an end-to-end suture of both tendons is possible, the alternative being a free tendon graft. If a crush injury occurred, a silicone rod may be inserted. The surgeon should be prepared for these options with either a primary or a delayed procedure.

The technique used in primary repair is critical. Both ends are retrieved, the annular ligament is trimmed, and the ends are held in place with Keith needles. The flexor digitorum superficialis (which is deep) is repaired initially using a Goldner suture technique (see Fig. 42–69). The flexor digitorum profundus is then repaired end-to-end using 4-0 Ethibond suture with reinforcing peripheral sutures. An additional core vertical mattress suture is added with 4-0 Ethibond. An alternative technique is to use Prolene pull-out and circumferential sutures. A pull-out suture is placed over the middle phalanx, thereby obviating the need for extensive opening of the annular ligament or for extensive dissection in order to place the holding suture. Although closure of the

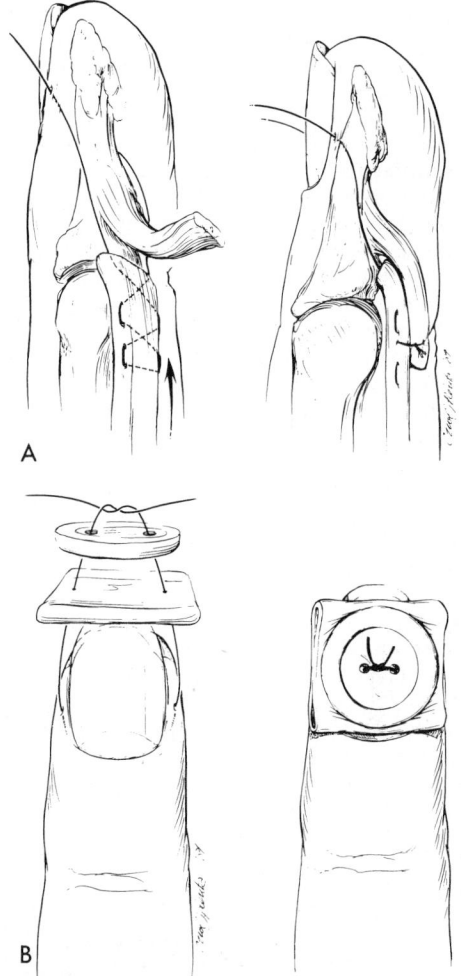

Figure 42–70. *A,* The technique for attaching the free tendon graft to bone and periosteum of the distal phalanx or to a remnant of lacerated flexor tendon. This technique is used for free graft or for an advancement of a previously lacerated tendon. The 3-0 Prolene suture is later extracted by cutting one segment of the suture distally and applying traction to the other. *B,* The pull-out sutures are placed adjacent to the nail plate as close as possible, or actually through the nail plate. A piece of firm rubber is applied against the nail plate, and a firm button prevents migration of the suture.

annular ligament is desirable, in most instances it is not possible. The proximal and middle pulleys are left intact to the extent possible, and if a pulley requires splitting, it is left in place, where it regenerates, or it is patched.

Lacerations of flexor tendons in Zone III (in the palm) involve injury to the lumbrical muscles as well as to the flexor tendons. A damaged lumbrical is either repaired or excised, depending on the severity of the injury and the location of the laceration. If the lumbrical muscle is intact, it is left adjacent to the flexor digitorum profundus repair. It is *not* wrapped around the repaired flexor. A lumbrical contracture is avoided if this muscle is not tightened or manipulated excessively during the repair. Both tendons, if lacerated, are repaired by end-to-end sutures with circumferential reinforcement, as already described. *Excision of the superficialis tendon is not advisable.*

Laceration of Flexor Tendons in Zone IV (Within the Carpal Canal). Lacerations of the flexor tendons within the carpal canal are usually associated with partial or complete laceration of the median nerve. Nerve repair is performed as a primary procedure if the wound is clean and after meticulous excision of nonviable tissue. The median nerve is aligned by the proximal and distal central arteries, by fascicular topography, or by proximal and distal electrical stimulation if the procedure is performed within 48 hours after the initial injury. Delayed electrical stimulation is possible with the patient awake. The distal nerve, however, may not demonstrate the motor and sensory fibers by electrical stimuli.

Nerve Injuries Associated with Flexor Tendon Laceration. Lacerations of the median or ulnar nerve in the carpal area or at the wrist, or of the digital nerves in the palm, may be repaired at the same time as the tendon repair. Tension is removed from the nerve suture line by flexing the wrist 30 degrees and the metacarpophalangeal joints 60 degrees. If nerves and tendons are lacerated, the tendon should be mobilized and the initial sutures placed in the proximal tendon. The distal tendon is isolated and held in place with a horizontal Keith needle. The nerves are then prepared for suture, but since more manipulation occurs during the tendon repair, that procedure should be completed first. After the tendons are sutured, the wrist is flexed, the digit is partially extended, and the digital nerves and vessels are repaired. The combined nerve-tendon procedure can be safely delayed for 21 days if the original wound is contaminated, if crushing trauma has occurred, or if the initial wound is not excised within 24 hours after injury.[22] The repair technique after that delay is more complex than an early repair.

If delayed repair is performed, there is clinical and experimental evidence that Surgicel wrapped around the nerve can temporarily delay the formation of adhesions between nerve and tendon. Occasionally, when an unusual amount of fibrosis exists, as in a delayed or secondary repair, a thin sheath of silicone is placed between the tendon and the nerve or between repaired tendons to prevent intertendinous adhesions. The silicone is removed several months later after healing has occurred and the range of motion has increased.

Laceration of Flexor Tendons in Zone V (Wrist and Lower Forearm Level). Laceration of the flexor tendons proximal to the carpal canal may be associated with median or ulnar nerve injury and laceration of the radial or ulnar arteries. Primary repair of the arteries is usually indicated. If the wound is contaminated, the arteries are repaired, and delayed repair of nerve and tendons is planned. The wound is left open for 3 to 5 days, at which time delayed closure is performed. The decision is made at that time whether to proceed with nerve and tendon repair in 5 days or to wait 21 days. Repair of the lacerated mixed nerve is readily accomplished as a primary procedure when anatomic alignment of the nerve, electrical stimulation, or both are used. However, delayed epineural repair of nerves or tendons is safe, is acceptable, and provides excellent results.

The nerves are repaired with 7-0 nylon as holding tension sutures and 9-0 nylon interval sutures. The tendons are repaired with nonabsorbable 3-0 polyester sutures in adults and 4-0 polyester sutures in children. Supplemental 5-0 circumferential sutures are used to reinforce the repair. However, anatomic constriction and gliding problems are less evident at the wrist than in the digits. Peritendinous adhesions occur, and controlled motion and elastic traction 21 days after repair are important. When nerves and tendons are repaired simultaneously, the problem of adhesions must be recognized. Forceful stretching after 21 days may cause nerves to stretch at the suture line if the nerves are adherent to the adjacent tendons. Thus, the postoperative management must be gentle, with use of elastic traction; forceful stretching must be avoided, and the program should be based primarily on the tensile strength of the nerve suture rather than of the tendon suture.

The wrist is maintained in volar flexion for 21 days and gradually brought to dorsiflexion during the subsequent 6 weeks. Tendon excursion is gradually increased with elastic traction and active exercise.

Improvement may occur for 6 to 12 months after the original repair. An elastic extension splint with outrigger rubber bands elongates the peritendinous adhesions and provides resistance when flexion is done. Finger flexion must be simultaneous in all digits. Flexion of the distal interphalangeal joint and the proximal interphalangeal joint is attempted with the wrist in 30-degree dorsiflexion 4 weeks after the repair.

Technique of Free Tendon Grafting— Fingers or Thumb

A midlateral or midmedial skin incision is made to expose the tendon involved. The neurovascular structures are reflected volarly with the flap. The dorsal branch of the digital nerve is spared. An alternative method of exposure is a zigzag incision with a 45-degree angle and the base of the flaps as wide as possible. For the index finger, for example, the proximal incision extends from the radial aspect of the proximal finger crease to the ulnar aspect of the middle crease and the radial aspect of the distal crease, and then to the ulnar aspect of the fingertip pad. The extension into the palm then follows the palmar creases. The tips of the flaps are rounded rather than pointed. The neurovascular structures are isolated with a rubber dam and retracted medially and laterally (Fig. 42–71). With the neurovascular structures and the flaps reflected, the annular ligaments are identified, and the proximal and distal ligaments are trimmed. The cruciate ligaments between the annular ligaments are opened so that the lacerated adherent tendons are retrieved and mobilized. As much of each annular ligament as possible is salvaged.

The distal stump of the profundus tendon is isolated and retracted so that a 6- to 10-mm. segment remains attached to the distal phalanx (see Fig. 42–70A). Proximally, the flexor digitorum profundus is identified at the base of the palm and cut back until healthy tendon is identified within the mass of the lumbrical. If it is fibrosed, the lumbrical is resected after it has been used to help identify the profundus. The flexor digitorum superficialis is removed at the wrist and may be used as a free tendon graft. This selection depends on the size of the profundus and the constriction of the annular ligaments in the digit.[2, 11, 12]

The distal end of the free tendon graft is placed within the fibro-osseous canal from the tip of the finger to the base of the digit. Distally, the graft is held in place with a 3-0 Prolene pull-out suture tied over a button placed on the fingernail as described for Zone I flexor tendon repairs (see Fig. 42–70). The remaining stump of the flexor digitorum profundus is sutured to the tendon graft with 4-0 nonabsorbable sutures. The distal incision is closed down to the base of the digit. Gentle traction is applied to the tendon, and the excursion and motion of the interphalangeal joints are tested.[2, 5]

An end-to-end or buttonhole suture is performed in the palm proximal to the annular ligament (A1 pulley). The tension of the final suture is determined by first observing the full excursion of the muscle belly of the flexor digitorum profundus by applying traction to the proximal tendon and measuring the distal and proximal excursion. The tendon graft is then sutured to the muscle belly, with the muscle belly at half resting length and under a sufficient amount of tension to cause the digit to be flexed at the metacarpophalangeal joint and at the proximal and distal joints approximately 10 degrees more than the normal resting position of the involved digit when the wrist is in neutral position. The resting attitude and position of the involved hand are used as a guide for determining the proper repair tension. The long finger, for example, is normally not flexed as much as

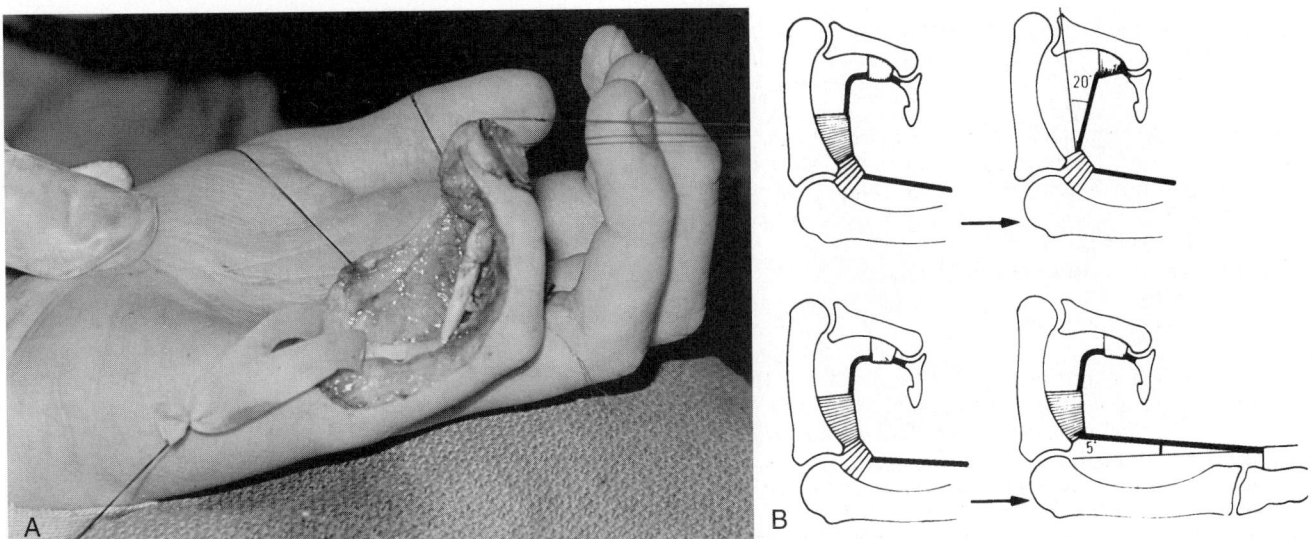

Figure 42–71. *A,* A free tendon graft to the little finger has been inserted. The original tendon was excised from the distal phalanx to the palm of the hand. A 14-cm. free tendon graft was taken from the extensor digitorum communis of the second toe. The A2 pulley is intact, and the A4 pulley has been partially reconstructed. An additional pulley was added at the level of the distal end of the middle phalanx in order to re-establish the restraints and friction. *B,* The pulleys must be constructed so that the flexor tendon is parallel with the proximal and middle phalanges and the metacarpal. (See Figure 42–66*A* for annular ligament and cruciate ligament arrangements.)

the ring finger but is flexed more than the index finger. After the graft is in place, the long finger is flexed approximately 5 degrees more than the adjacent ring finger and approximately 20 degrees more than the index finger.

Immobilization is completed by a compression dressing that extends from the fingertips to above the elbow. This is made by fluffing 2- by 2-inch gauze between the digits, with use of 4- by 4-inch gauze dressings for the palm and the back of the hand and the application of abdominal pads on the dorsal and volar aspects; the soft dressing is wrapped with 3-inch sheet cotton. A dorsal plaster splint extends 2 cm. beyond the fingertips to the olecranon process. A volar splint is *not* used, since this would cause undue tension on the flexor graft if the splint slipped. The plaster splint is then wrapped in place with a bias-cut stockinette in direct contact with the plaster so that it will not slip and will adhere to the plaster. The wrist is flexed 30 degrees, the metacarpophalangeal joints are flexed 60 degrees, and the interphalangeal joints are flexed 10 degrees. When this aspect of the dressing is applied, the elbow is included by posterior splints or U-shaped splints that hold the elbow at 90 degrees. This plaster is also wrapped with a bias-cut stockinette. A segment of tubular stockinette is then placed from the axilla to the fingertips, form fit distally, and cut to allow visualization of the fingers and the thumb. A second stockinette is then applied and is held to the arm by a bias-cut stockinette. The second stockinette is a suspension apparatus that is tied to an overhead pole with rope to provide constant elevation. Complete immobilization of the hand and forearm is maintained for 21 days, during which time the patient is shown how to flex the tips passively through a 5-mm. range of motion 10 times 3 times a day. Partial immobilization is then continued for an additional 21 days, after which assisted flexion and extension are initiated and an outrigger elastic splint is used.

If CPM is used, a dorsal extensor splint is shortened to the proximal interphalangeal joints so that the flexion loops can be applied to the digits. The motor is applied on the palmar surface, and the dressing is partially released so that finger flexion is possible at the interphalangeal joints. If an elastic outrigger program is used for all four digits, the splint is shortened on the dorsum so that extension is possible at the

proximal interphalangeal joints and passive flexion occurs as the extensor muscles are relaxed.

Silicone as an Adjunct in the Treatment of Tendon Repair and Tendon Fibrosis

Severe trauma, infection, or multiple tissue injuries may cause a fibrotic, adherent flexor tendon mechanism that adversely affects tendon gliding and digit function. The use of silicone sheeting, silicone rods, and, more recently, a permanent artificial silicone-Dacron tendon represents important advances in methods of reconstructing damaged flexor and extensor tendon complexes (Fig. 42–72). Attachment of the artificial tendon distally with a screw and proximally with Dacron ingrowth or bone-tendon junction is still under investigation.[14]

Silicone Rod Before Flexor Tendon Grafting. If the gliding surface of the involved digit is fibrotic and irregular, if annular ligaments require reconstruction because of damage to the major canals at the base of the finger, and if there is limited joint motion, a free tendon graft is usually not successful. A silicone rod (3, 4, or 5 mm.) provides an artificial tendon while pulleys are being reconstructed, joints are being mobilized, and a pseudosheath is forming. The rod orients collagen.[14] The flexor tendon sheath is exposed through a midlateral or palmar zigzag incision that extends to the base of the palm. A second incision is made at the wrist, and both the flexor digitorum superficialis and the flexor digitorum profundus of the involved digit are isolated. The profundus is cut, and the distal segment within the base of the palm is usually bypassed. The segment from the palm to the digit is removed. The silicone rod is inserted from the wrist to the fingertip, where the end of the rod is attached by a Dacron suture to the remaining stump of the profundus and into the distal phalanx (see Fig. 42–70).

The annular ligaments are reconstructed if they have been damaged. This is performed at the anatomic locations over the distal end of the proximal phalanx (A2) and over the middle of the middle phalanx (A4). Additional pulleys are made proximal to the metacarpophalangeal joint (A1), and cruciate ligaments are constructed to join the major A2 and

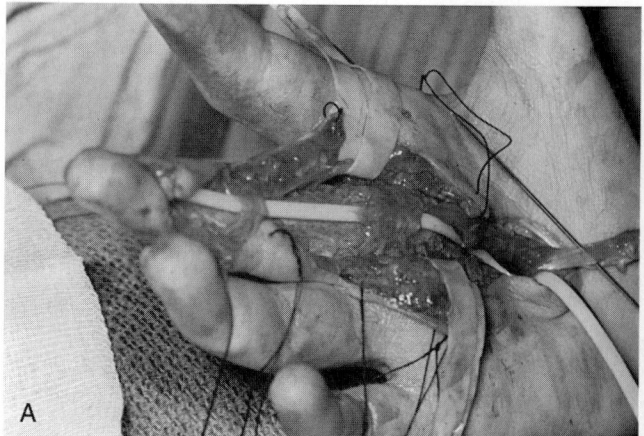
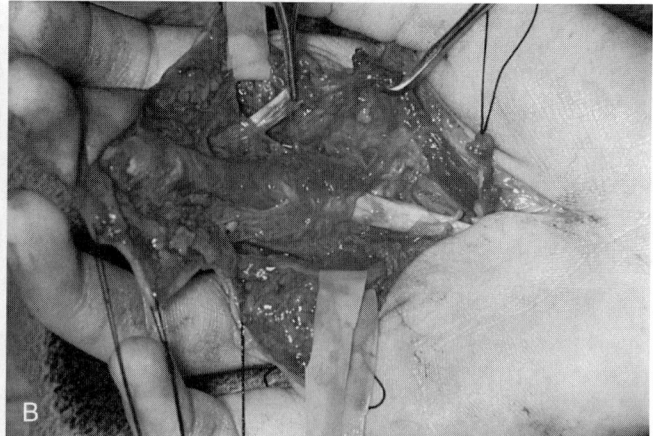

Figure 42–72. *A,* A complex flexor tendon injury resulted in severe fibrosis of the flexor tendon complex. The adherent, fibrosed, nongliding flexor tendon has been removed, the annular ligaments have been saved or reconstructed, and a silicone rod has been inserted from the tip of the digit to the palmar aspect of the wrist to stimulate a pseudosheath as the first step in providing a free tendon graft to the digit. The rod is left in place and full motion of the digit is obtained during a 6-week to 3-month period. A biologic autologous free tendon graft is inserted by attaching it to the distal end of the silicone rod and pulling it through the flexor complex to the wrist. *B,* The A2 and A4 pulleys and the cruciate ligaments between these pulleys have been reconstructed over the silicone rod.

A4 pulleys. The silicone rod is a structure over which the pulleys are formed; the distal end of the rod is attached to tendon and bone, but the proximal end moves freely so that passive motion forms an artificial fibrous synovium-lined sheath. The rod is ultimately in the same plane as the flexor digitorum profundus tendons.

The delay between the first-stage silicone rod insertion and the second-stage tendon insertion varies from 6 weeks to 6 months. The maximal range of passive motion must be recovered, and revascularization should be adequate in the sheath for tendon grafting. A segment of the extensor digitorum longus tendons from the second or third toe is selected as the graft, the involved hand digit is opened at the distal interphalangeal joint level where the pseudotendinous sheath and the silicone tendon are identified, and the tendons are exposed proximally at the wrist level. The silicone rod is identified proximal to the carpal canal, the free tendon graft is sutured to the proximal end of the silicone rod, the distal attachment of the rod is released, and traction is applied so that the free tendon graft enters the base of the palm, the midpalm, and the digit as the silicone rod is removed distally. The free tendon graft is then attached distally to the remaining stump of the flexor digitorum profundus tendon or, if the stump is absent, directly into the distal phalanx with a 3-0 nonabsorbable pull-out suture. Proximally, the tendon graft is woven through the musculotendinous junction of the flexor digitorum profundus under sufficient tension to maintain the digit in slightly greater flexion than the adjacent digits when the wrist is at neutral position. The position for immobilization is 30 degrees wrist flexion, 60 degrees metacarpophalangeal joint flexion, and 10 degrees proximal and distal interphalangeal joint flexion. An oblique 0.045 fixation pin is drilled across the distal interphalangeal joint in a position of 10 degrees flexion. This prevents hyperflexion of the distal joint as the graft is maturing.

Five days after insertion of the graft, passive motion is initiated. Stress on the suture line is avoided for 21 days, at which time active motion is initiated. The pull-out suture is left in place for approximately 4 weeks, and an elastic outrigger to provide limited extension is first used at 6 weeks after the insertion of the graft. A protective night splint in alternate flexion and extension is applied from the dorsum of the digit. Active motion is initiated at the interphalangeal joints by use of a wooden block and plastic putty.

Permanent Artificial Tendon

A silicone rod reinforced with Dacron is now available as a controlled clinical research implement. This is useful in providing motion for a digit affected by extensive multitissue damage in which a two-stage reconstructive procedure is unlikely to succeed. The digit tolerates the artificial tendon without developing excess fibrous proliferation. However, if biologic collagen is inserted, adhesions may cause flexion contracture and loss of joint motion. The distal attachment of the artificial tendon is into bone with a screw or metallic fixation that is invaded by bone. Proximally, the attachment is completed by bone-tendon junction with Dacron for ingrowth. A small number of patients have been treated in this manner, and the results are improving as the quality of the artificial tendon and its mechanism of attachment to biologic tissue improve.[14]

Silicone Tendons on the Extensor Aspect of the Hand

Severe damage to the dorsum of the hand may cause avulsion of the extensor tendons, damage to the extensor hood, and inability of the patient to actively elevate the digits, including the thumb. The skeleton is stabilized by pin fixation, the joints are mobilized, a split skin graft or pedicle skin graft is used to fill soft tissue defects, and autogenous tendons or fasciae latae or silicone tendons are then used, depending on the severity and extent of the previous injury. In many instances, silicone rods are inserted from the middle of the middle phalanx to the musculotendinous junction of the extensor digitorum communis. These tendons may be left in place for several weeks, and a pseudosheath forms around them. Occasionally, the pseudosheath acts as a tendon in itself, and the further addition of autogenous tendons can be delayed. In other situations, when greater strength and mobility are desired, the tendon graft is added through the pseudosheath in the same manner that the free tendon graft is used on the flexor surface. Combinations of silicone rods and silicone joints are now possible. A patient who has sustained a severe crushing injury to the metacarpophalangeal joint of the index finger and loss of the extensor tendon can be managed in this manner. Because of severe damage to the articular surfaces and because arthrodesis of that joint is not desirable, a silicone-Dacron joint is inserted to replace the damaged metacarpal head. The alternative to arthrodesis is resection, and the silicone-Dacron joint can be inserted for several years. If it fails to function mechanically, it can be resected, and the remaining pseudosheath provides a reasonably stable reaction. The combined tissue replacement also requires a silicone cord to replace the extensor tendon. The silicone rod serves as a replacement tendon for several months and eventually is replaced by an autogenous tendon graft.[2, 3]

SELECTED REFERENCE

Hunter, J. M., Schneider, L. H., and Mackin, E. J.: Tendon Surgery in the Hand. St. Louis, C. V. Mosby, 1987.

REFERENCES

1. Aoki, M., Manske, P. R., Pruitt, D. L., and Larson, B. J.: Tendon repair using flexor tendon splints: An experimental study. J. Hand Surg. [Am.], 19:984, 1994.
2. Bora, F. W., Jr.: Profundus tendon grafting with unimpaired sublimus function in children. Clin. Orthop. Rel. Res., 71:118, 1970.
3. Boyes, J. H., and Stark, H. H.: Flexor-tendon grafts in the fingers and thumb. J. Bone Joint Surg. [Am.], 53:1332, 1971.
4. Bunnell, S.: Repair of tendons in the fingers and description of two new instruments. Surg. Gynecol. Obstet., 26:103, 1918.
5. Doyle, J. R., and Blythe, W. F.: Anatomy of the flexor tendon sheath and pulleys of the thumb. J. Hand Surg., 2:149, 1977.
6. Duran, R. J., and Houser, R. G.: Controlled passive motion following flexor tendon repair in zones two and three. In AAOS Symposium on Tendon Surgery in the Hand. St. Louis, C. V. Mosby, 1975, p. 105.
7. Elliott, D., Moiemen, N. S., Fleming, A. F., Harris, S. B., and Foster, A. J.: The rupture rate of acute flexor tendon repairs mobilized by the controlled active motion regimen. J. Hand Surg. [Br.], 19:607, 1994.
8. Foucher, G., Lenoble, E., Ben Youssef, K., and Sammut, D.: A post-operative regimen after digital flexor tenolysis: A series of 72 patients. J. Hand Surg. [Br.], 18:35, 1993.
9. Gajisin, S., and Zbrodowski, A.: Local vascular contribution of the superficial palmar arch. Acta Anat. (Basel), 147:248, 1993.
10. Gelberman, R. H., Nunley, J. A., II, Osterman, A. L., Green, T. F., Dimick, M. P., Savio, L.-Y., and Woo, S. L.-Y.: Influences of the protected passive mobilization interval on flexor tendon healing: A prospective randomized clinical study. Clin. Orthop. Rel. Res., 264:189, 1991.
11. Goldner, J. L., and Coonrad, R. W.: Tendon grafting of the flexor profundus in the presence of a completely or partially intact flexor sublimus. J. Bone Joint Surg. [Am.], 51:527, 1969.
12. Honner, R.: The late management of the isolated lesion of the flexor digitorum profundus tendon. Hand, 7:171, 1975.
13. Horii, E., Lin, G. T., Cooney, W. P., Linscheid, R. L., and An, K. N.: Comparative flexor tendon excursion after passive mobilization: An in vitro study. J. Hand Surg. [Am.], 17:559, 1992.
14. Hunter, J. M., and Salisbury, R. E.: Flexor-tendon reconstruction in severely damaged hands. J. Bone Joint Surg. [Am.], 53:829, 1971.
15. Karlander, L. E., Berggren, M., Larsson, M., Soderberg, G., and Nylander, G.: Improved results in zone II flexor tendon injuries with a modified technique of immediate controlled mobilization. J. Hand Surg. [Br.], 18:26, 1993.
16. Kleinert, H. E., Kutz, J. E., Ashbell, T. S., and Martinez, E.: Primary repair of lacerated flexor tendons in "no man's land." J. Bone Joint Surg. [Am.], 49:577, 1967.
17. Lister, G. D., Kleinert, H. E., Kutz, J. E., and Atisoy, E.: Primary flexor tendon repair followed by immediate controlled mobilization. J. Hand Surg. [Am.], 2:441, 1977.
18. Noguchi, M., Seiler, J. G., III, Gelberman, R. H., Sofranko, R. A., and Woo, S.-L.: In-vitro biomechanical analysis of suture methods for flexor tendon repair. J. Orthop. Res., 11:603, 1993.
19. Potenza, A. D.: Tendon healing within the flexor digital sheath in the dog. J. Bone Joint Surg. [Am.], 44:49, 1962.
20. Silfverskiold, K. L., and May, E. J.: Gap formation after flexion tendon repair in zone II: Results with a new controlled motion program. Scand. J. Plast. Reconstr. Surg. Hand Surg., 27:263, 1993.
21. Uchiyama, S., Coert, J. H., Berglund, L., Amadio, P. C., and An, K. N.: Method for the measurement of friction between tendon and pulley. J. Orthop. Res., 13:83, 1995.
22. Urbaniak, J. R., and Goldner, J. L.: Laceration of flexor pollicis longus tendon: Delayed repair by advancement, free graft or suture. J. Bone Joint Surg. [Am.], 55:1123, 1973.
23. Vaughn-Jackson, O. T.: Rupture of the extensor tendons by attrition at the inferior radioulnar joint. J. Bone Joint Surg. [Br.], 30:528, 1948.
24. Verdan, C. E.: Primary repair of flexor tendons. J. Bone Joint Surg. [Am.], 42:647, 1960.
25. Wehbe, M. A.: Tendon graft donor sites. J. Hand Surg. [Am.], 17:1130, 1992.
26. Yalin, A., Cavdar, S., and Ercan, F.: Vascularization of the long flexor tendons. Okajimas Folia Anat. Jpn., 70:285, 1994.
27. Zbrodowski, A., Gajisin, S., and Bednarkiewicz, M.: Mesotendons of the flexor pollicis longus muscle. Acta Anat. (Basel), 151:131, 1994.
28. Zissimos, A. G., Szabo, R. M., Yinger, K. E., and Sharkey, N. A.: Biomechanics of the thumb flexor pulley system. J. Hand Surg. [Am.], 19:475, 1994.

COMPRESSION NEUROPATHIES OF THE HAND AND FOREARM

Richard D. Goldner, M.D., and
J. Leonard Goldner, M.D.

The diagnosis of abnormal compression of the median, ulnar, or radial nerves can easily be missed even though these syndromes occur relatively frequently. The diagnosis may be unnecessarily delayed if the physician waits until muscle atrophy is obvious or until sensory deficits are profound. An early diagnosis is preferable to allow the surgeon to provide pain relief and the patient to maintain complete motor power and full sensibility.

CLINICAL INVESTIGATION

An entrapped nerve is suspected if the patient complains of intermittent tingling, numbness, or functional impairment and if the symptoms are recurrent and affect a particular anatomic area of the hand or forearm. Historical details, such as occurrence of day or night paresthesias, frequency of complaints, and information about temporary recovery, are all helpful in making the proper diagnosis.

The physical examination consists of determining the patient's ability to recognize differences in light touch, sharp point, heat, cold, and two-point discrimination. Motor power of the hand and forearm muscles is tested manually, with the examiner cognizant of the fact that minimal substitution patterns affect the result. Adjunctive tests are helpful in establishing a diagnosis. These include the percussion test of the individual peripheral nerve from distal to proximal and from proximal to distal, the effect of wrist flexion or extension on paresthesias and pain production, and the effect of pressure applied over the median nerve in the carpal tunnel. Other methods of demonstrating changes in sensibility include the effects of a venous tourniquet on the arm, repetitive movement in the hand, and changes due to handheld vibrating objects.

Studies of nerve conduction, particularly sensory latency, are helpful in localizing nerve compression lesions. Sensory conduction studies are more sensitive than is motor conduction velocity. The amplitude of action potentials also indicates alteration of participating motor nerve axons.

Electromyography detects abnormal electrical action potentials following disruption of motor axons and wallerian degeneration. The denervated muscle fibers become spontaneously active, producing fibrillation potentials and positive sharp waves approximately 10 to 20 days after nerve injury. This test assists in differentiating neuropathic muscle atrophy from myopathic atrophy.

If electrical studies do not confirm the clinical diagnosis of focal nerve compression, a lesion may be present but is affecting the nerve minimally or intermittently. Nonoperative treatment is usually indicated in this instance.

DIFFERENTIAL DIAGNOSIS

A focal nerve compression must be differentiated from a neuropathy associated with systemic disease such as diabetes mellitus, hypothyroidism, rheumatoid arthritis, acromegaly, heavy metal toxicity, or paresthesias due to certain medications.

Paresthesias may be caused by lesions proximal to the hand or wrist such as cervical root irritation or brachial plexitis. Also, a spinal cord tumor or syringomyelia may cause distal symptoms and signs that resemble a nerve compression lesion.

DIGITAL NERVE COMPRESSION IN THE FINGERS OR THUMB

Compression of the digital nerves of the thumb by a bowling ball or harp string causes reactive perineural fibrosis. Thus, the patient's vocation or avocation must be determined in order to assess the cause of numbness, tingling, or paresthesias in the digits.

Bowler's Thumb. The edge of the hole in a bowling ball may irritate the ulnar or radial digital nerves of the thumb. The digital nerve nodule becomes painful to pressure, and the distal skin is hypesthetic. Bowling should be discontinued until the irritation subsides. A protective thumb guard, a change of grip, or a rounded edge to the hole may prevent recurrence. Surgical treatment is usually not indicated.

Harp Player's Thumb. Strings of a musical instrument may irritate the ulnar or radial nerves of the strumming digit. Painful hyper- or hyposensitivity may occur. The digit should be rested and the strumming pattern changed. A surgical procedure is not indicated.

Finger Compression. Digital nerve compression at the base of the finger by a palmar fibromatosis or a fascial band is usually recognized by history and examination. Surgical excision of the compressing tissue is indicated.

Arthritic Nodules. Digital nerves in the distal segments of the fingers may be irritated by arthritic nodules. Hypesthesia or paresthesias are due to compression or tethering of the nerve and secondary vasospasm. Anti-inflammatory medication, avoidance of excessive trauma to the fingertips, and the passage of time usually provide spontaneous improvement.

COMPRESSION OF THE MEDIAN NERVE WITHIN THE HAND

The median nerve may be compressed in the palm secondary to direct trauma. Occasionally, the motor branch of the median nerve is compressed by a fascial ring that surrounds the nerve as it enters the thumb muscles. Treatment is to avoid using the heel of the hand as a hammer and to wear gloves while repetitively squeezing tools or instruments. Surgical decompression is indicated when the lesion persists and when severity progresses after a reasonable period of observation.

COMPRESSION OF THE MEDIAN NERVE AT THE WRIST (CARPAL TUNNEL SYNDROME)

The median nerve is compressed within the carpal canal formed by the transverse carpal ligament on the palmar surface and the carpal bones on the dorsal side (Fig. 42–73). The flexor tendons lie in the carpal canal with the median nerve.

Compression of the median nerve within or adjacent to the carpal canal is the most common neuropathy of the upper extremity. Women are affected more frequently than men; the age range is wide but is usually between 40 and 60 years. The usual complaints are weakness or clumsiness of the hand and hypesthesia or paresthesias of the thumb or index or

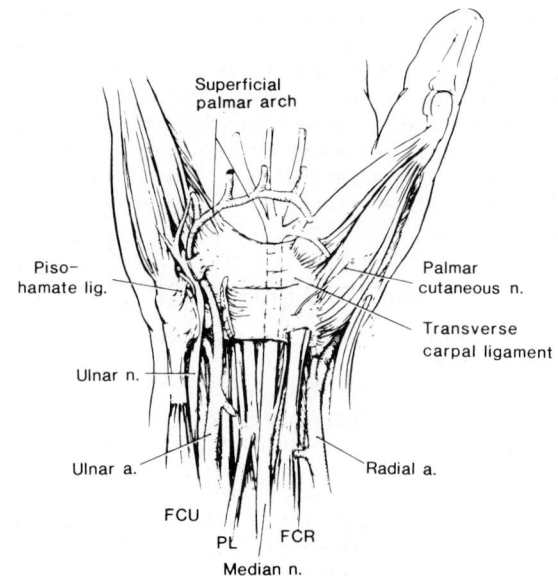

Figure 42–73. Volar aspect of wrist carpal tunnel showing flexor tendons to wrist and digits, course of median and ulnar nerves, and radial and ulnar arteries. (From Goldner, R. D.: Nerve compression in the upper extremity. Orthopaedic Surgery Update Series. Vol. 3, Lesson 28. Princeton, NJ, Bobbitt, 1984.)

long fingers, aggravated by grasping with the digits while the wrist is flexed or occasionally even extended. Nocturnal or early morning numbness is a frequent complaint that is quickly relieved by shaking the hand or moving the fingers. Tingling of the fingers may occur after holding an electric razor or after repetitive rotatory and flexion-extension movements of the fingers and hand. Cold intolerance may occur, and there may be vague discomfort in the hand or forearm or retrograde sensations. Other conditions such as rapid weight gain, fluid retention associated with pregnancy, or compression from tight watchbands or rubber gloves may initiate or aggravate the symptoms.

Examination may demonstrate sensibility changes in the thumb and in the index, long, and radial aspect of the ring fingers in certain patients, whereas others may have changes in only one digit. Percussion of the median nerve at the wrist proximal to the flexor retinaculum, over the carpal ligament, or in the palm may cause paresthesias. Tingling may be produced or aggravated by wrist flexion (Phalen's test) for 20 or 30 seconds and occasionally by wrist hyperextension. A venous tourniquet applied around the arm at 60 mm. Hg may cause tingling in the fingers of the involved hand. *Thenar muscle atrophy and profound sensory deficit occur only in the advanced stages of nerve compression.* Many patients with mild median nerve compression have intermittent complaints but normal motor and sensory examinations and electrical studies.

Factors that Contribute to Median Nerve Compression at the Wrist and in the Hand

1. Repetitive minor trauma such as grasping, squeezing, twisting, or hitting an object with the heel of the hand can produce symptoms of median nerve compression. If these actions are performed several hundred times a day, and if the frequency increases in an effort to increase production, median nerve compression may occur from tenosynovitis or trauma to the nerve from wrist flexion motions.

2. Synovial sheath hypertrophy of thumb and finger flexor

tendons within the carpal canal may cause secondary median nerve compression.

3. Trauma to the heel of the hand is often not recognized by the patient.

4. A palmar mass such as a ganglion, aberrant calcification, uric acid crystals, or hypertrophic fat may increase the contents of the carpal canal and cause compression of the median nerve.

5. If the muscle bellies of the palmaris longus or flexor digitorum superficialis pass over or extend into the carpal canal, the median nerve may be compressed after vigorous hand activity or repetitive use. *These muscle variations are the most common causes of median nerve compression in young, active individuals.*

6. A mass in the carpal canal such as a neurofibroma, a neurilemoma, a lipohemangioma, or another rare lesion of the median nerve may cause symptoms and signs resembling a median nerve compression syndrome.

7. Dislocation of the carpal bones, particularly the lunate, or severe displacement of a Colles' fracture may cause immediate damage to the median nerve or delayed nerve compression of the median and the ulnar nerves.

8. After a partial digit amputation, the digital nerve may adhere to bone or tendon either distally or in the palm. This adherence may cause proximal tethering of the median nerve, particularly during dorsiflexion of the fingers or the hand, and may cause secondary paresthesias. Also, the lacerated flexor tendons may retract proximally and increase the soft tissue volume at the wrist. The combined tethering, the tenosynovitis, and the increased mass in the canal compress the median nerve.

9. Systemic conditions such as amyloidosis, Raynaud's syndrome, and myeloma may affect the median nerve at the wrist by formation of abnormal soft tissue lesions or vasospasm of the vessels of the hand or the median nerve.

Treatment of Median Nerve Compression at the Wrist

Initial treatment consists of splinting the wrist in neutral position at night, weight reduction if indicated, and decreasing the repetitive activities of the hand and wrist. Anti-inflammatory agents are useful in treating tenosynovitis, and a diuretic may assist in partially dehydrating synovial sheaths. A soluble corticosteroid mixed with 1% lidocaine (1 ml. of steroid and 5 ml. of lidocaine) is injected into the tendon sheaths of the flexor digitorum profundus approximately 2 cm. proximal to the palmar flexor wrist crease and 1 cm. ulnarward to the palmaris longus. If the patient does not have a palmaris longus, the needle should be directed 1 cm. radial to the flexor carpi ulnaris at an angle of 30 degrees away from the ulnar nerve. The ulnar and median nerves should be avoided completely. Steroids should not be injected into or just adjacent to the median or ulnar nerve. The purpose of the injection is not to affect the median nerve directly but to inject the anti-inflammatory medication into the flexor tendon sheaths to decrease synovitis and swelling.

These procedures reduce the symptoms in at least 40% of patients who have mild compression lesions. Symptoms in those who have a moderate degree of compression are diminished but probably not eliminated. If symptoms worsen or demonstrate motor atrophy or more profound sensory change, surgical release is indicated.

Decompression. Median nerve decompression is performed by incision of the transverse carpal ligament at the wrist from just proximal to the ligament to the midpalmar extension at the superficial palmar arch. This eliminates the external compression, aids regeneration of compressed motor and sensory fibers, and improves muscle strength of the thumb and sensibility of the digits. Based on the authors' experience, the incision should begin in line with the long axis of the ring finger in the transverse crease at the wrist, course obliquely within the skin crease at the base of the palm, and extend within or adjacent to the midpalmar crease to the level of the superficial palmar arch. This incision avoids the palmar cutaneous branch of the median nerve, allows proximal isolation of the nerve, and provides adequate visualization of abnormal muscles or proliferative flexor sheath synovium. The nerve is carefully isolated proximally and protected as the transverse carpal ligament is incised along the ulnar border. This avoids damaging the motor branch of the median nerve that supplies the thenar muscles. At the distal palm, the superficial palmar arch crosses volar to the nerve and must be protected. Incising the ligament over an instrument placed in the carpal canal helps to avoid damaging the median nerve. Epineurial splitting is done occasionally, and intraneurolysis is not recommended.

Techniques are available for carpal tunnel release using an endoscope. Although this method has some potential advantages over the traditional open technique (smaller incision and possibly less postoperative discomfort and earlier rehabilitation), distinct disadvantages are also inherent. The role of this technique is currently under investigation.

At operation, the condition of the median nerve reflects the severity of the compression lesion. The nerve may have the appearance of an isthmus, with bulging masses both proximal and distal to the severe localized compression, or it may show only momentary obliteration of its vascular markings. The latter indicates minimal compression.

Tenosynovectomy Associated with Neurolysis. A tenosynovectomy may be desirable in patients with rheumatoid arthritis or other collagen diseases. The proliferating synovium may cause compression of the nerve even after the transverse carpal ligament has been incised. Also, hypertrophy of the synovium may be causing tendon damage, and invasion of the tendon may cause tendon rupture.

Bone Deformities Associated with Nerve Compression. If distal radial or carpal deformity persists, an osteotomy of the distal radius or reduction of the carpal bones may be performed in conjunction with median neurolysis.

Recurrent Median Nerve Symptoms. Recurrent median nerve symptoms may be due to persistent compression from perineural fibrosis or prior trauma to the palmar cutaneous branch of the median nerve; prior incomplete neurolysis because of inadequate exposure through a short transverse palmar incision; chronic tenosynovitis causing persistent median nerve compression; or persistent pain due to prior damage to the median nerve from injection of steroid or other substance directly into the nerve.

COMPRESSION OF THE MEDIAN NERVE BY THE PRONATOR TERES

The median nerve may be compressed as it passes through or under the pronator teres and/or collagen bands proximal or distal to that muscle (Fig. 42–74). The syndrome includes forearm pain and numbness in the median nerve distribution, and it may coexist with median nerve compression at the wrist. Initial treatment of the syndrome is to diminish the repetitive activity that may be causing the complaints, diminish stress on the wrist as well, and be certain that the median nerve is not irritated more proximally.

Other causes of median nerve compression around the elbow and the forearm are lacertus fibrosus, the proximal edge of the origin of the flexor digitorum superficialis muscle after exercise or secondary to prior compartment syndrome,

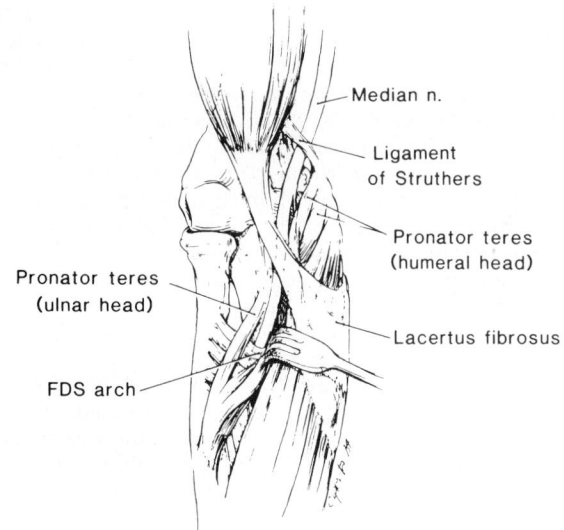

Figure 42–74. Diagram showing major points of possible median nerve compression. Above the elbow, the fibrous band from the humeral shaft to the epicondyle (ligament of Struthers) may be associated with a supracondyloid process. Distally, the humeral head of the pronator radii teres may compress the nerve if the muscle is hypertrophied and subject to repeated contractions many times each hour. Distally, the ulnar head of the pronator may compress the median nerve. The fibrous bands of the pronator radii teres or a large pronator muscle and a combination of nerve tethering by both proximal and distal compression may result in pain, paresthesia, and even motor weakness. The flexor digitorum superficialis (FDS) fascial arch may compress the median nerve if it is tethered or if the fascial band of the muscle is larger than average or is aggravated by repetitive activity. In the same way, the lacertus fibrosus may compress the median nerve in hyperextension, in direct extension, or in midflexion if the fibrous material shows minimal elasticity and if the contraction of the biceps is sufficient to shorten the lacertus. (From Goldner, R. D.: Nerve compression in the upper extremity. Orthopaedic Surgery Update Series. Vol. 3, Lesson 28. Princeton, NJ, Bobbitt, 1984.)

accessory muscle masses from the pronator teres, or a supracondyloid process from the distal end of the humerus to which the ligament of Struthers is attached.

Treatment of the elbow and forearm median nerve compression syndrome is initially nonoperative. If alteration of physical activity does not improve the syndrome, surgical release of the median nerve beginning proximal to the lacertus fibrosus and extending distally to the flexor digitorum superficialis is the treatment of choice.

COMPRESSION OF THE ANTERIOR INTEROSSEOUS BRANCH OF THE MEDIAN NERVE

The anterior interosseous nerve is a motor branch of the median nerve that is present in the proximal third of the forearm. It supplies the flexor pollicis longus, the flexor digitorum profundus of the index and long fingers, and the pronator quadratus. Specific causes of anterior interosseous nerve compression are an enlarged bicipital tendon bursa that affects the motor aspect of the median nerve; an aberrant or thrombosed radial artery in the midforearm; the tendinous origin of the deep head of the pronator teres; a fascial band at the origin of the flexor digitorum superficialis; and compression within the deep palmar compartment from aberrant accessory muscles such as the flexor pollicis longus (Gantzer's) muscle, a palmaris profundus mass, or an enlarged flexor carpi radialis brevis (Fig. 42–75).

Anterior interosseous nerve compression causes a vague pain in the proximal forearm that is aggravated by exercise and relieved by rest. The pinch between thumb and index finger is weak. Individual testing of the flexor pollicis longus

and the flexor digitorum profundus of the index finger demonstrates that these muscle bellies are weak. There is no sensory deficiency. This syndrome must be differentiated from a rupture of the flexor pollicis longus or the index profundus tendons.

Tendon ruptures are usually determined by placing the digits in different positions and applying tension to the flexor tendons; by electrical stimulation that indicates whether the muscle belly is partially denervated; or by a succinylcholine test, which may demonstrate *more* fasciculations of the flexor pollicis longus if there is partial or complete denervation.

If symptoms persist after a reasonable period of observation, and depending on the other diagnostic studies, an operative procedure is performed isolating the median nerve proximal to the lacertus fibrosus and dissecting it distally through the pronator teres to where the branches enter the flexor pollicis longus and flexor digitorum profundus of the index and long fingers. Electrical stimulation of the nerve during this decompression is helpful.

ULNAR NERVE COMPRESSION WITHIN THE HAND

Hook of the Hamate. Sensory branches of the ulnar nerve supply the palmar aspect of the little finger and half the palmar surface of the ring finger. The sensory and motor branches are separate at this site. Degenerative arthrosis or

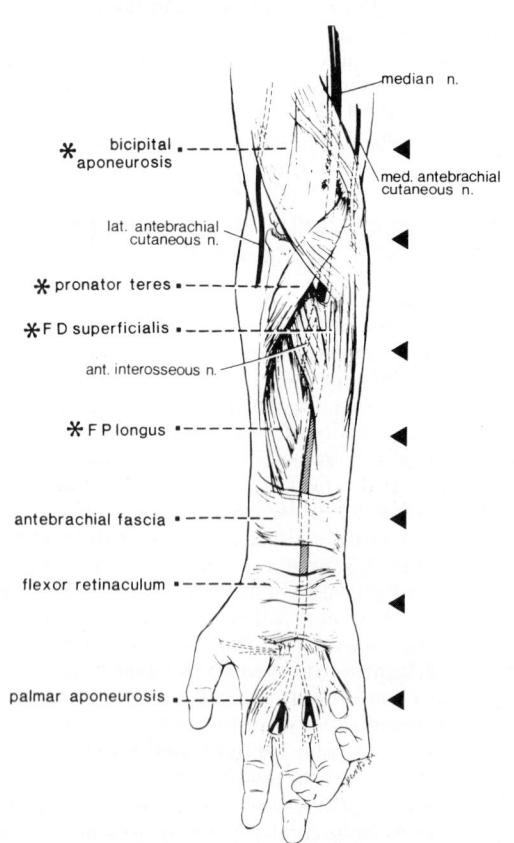

Figure 42–75. Composite diagram of multiple points of possible median nerve compression. The black points on the ulnar aspect of the elbow, forearm, and hand indicate sites of clinically recognized compression. The asterisks are adjacent to the names of structures that may cause compression of the median nerve, the lateral antebrachial cutaneous nerve, or the anterior interosseous nerve within the flexor pollicis (FP) longus. These points of compression are suspected by history and clinical examination and are usually documented by electrical studies. FD, flexor digitorum. (From Bull. Hosp. Jt. Dis. Orthop. Inst., 44:201, 1984.)

trauma around the pisiform or the hook of the hamate may cause irritation or tethering of the sensory nerves and pain or paresthesias.

The sensory branch of the ulnar nerve within the ulnar canal (Guyon's) may be compressed. Repetitive trauma from a stapler or a bicycle handle may cause ulnar compression. Also, space-occupying lesions such as tumor, ganglion, lipoma, or anomalous muscles traversing the canal may cause nerve compression. External compression of the ulnar nerve by a heavy watchband or by elastic garments may irritate the nerve.

Treatment. The diagnosis should be accurate. Daily activities should be investigated. Does the patient use the heel of the hand for a hammer, sleep on the palm, or use the hand repetitively on a chopping knife? When the diagnosis of nerve compression has been established, these movements should be discontinued and the patient observed. Electrical studies assist in establishing a baseline of muscle involvement, and nerve conduction velocities and especially sensory latencies are helpful in determining localization, gradual improvement, or regression.

If motor and sensory changes have occurred, the nerves should be decompressed and any subtle lesions removed.

ULNAR NERVE COMPRESSION AT THE ELBOW

Ulnar nerve compression occurs within the cubital tunnel or proximal or distal to it (Fig. 42–76). A dense fascia over the flexor carpi ulnaris distally or the fibrous ridge of the interosseous membrane proximally may cause nerve irritation with repetitive motion. Synovium or osteophytes within the cubital tunnel may irritate the nerve as a result of repetitive acute elbow flexion. A synovial cyst arising from the elbow joint and extending into the canal may compress the nerve. An ununited medial epicondyle of the humerus may irritate the nerve. Repeated subluxation of the nerve as it moves across the medial epicondyle causes nerve compression. Positional stress, such as prolonged elbow flexion during sleep, external pressure on the elbow during general anesthesia, or repetitive use of the flexed elbow against the mattress to change position while on bed rest can cause ulnar nerve compression. Other anatomic structures such as a fibrous arcade (arcade of Struthers) proximally or a combination of proximal tethering and distal muscle hypertrophy may irritate the nerve.

Symptoms and Signs. The symptoms of ulnar nerve compression at the elbow are aching or pain along the ulnar aspect of the proximal forearm and intermittent paresthesia, dysesthesia, or hyperesthesia of the little finger and the ulnar half of the ring finger. The patient usually complains that the "little finger is asleep." The heel of the hand may be *tingling*.

Anatomic localization of the compressed nerve is determined by percussion of the nerve beginning distally and advancing proximally, by demonstrating hypermobility of the nerve over the medial epicondyle, or by persistent or intermittent tingling and numbness in the ring and little fingers after voluntary forced elbow and finger flexion.

Early or mild nerve compression causes no intrinsic muscle atrophy, but nerve compression of a moderate or severe degree prolonged for several months causes atrophy of the hypothenar muscles and eventually the interosseous muscles of the hand.

Treatment. Nonoperative treatment depends on an accurate diagnosis. The patient is advised to avoid resting the elbow on chair arms, table surfaces, and airplane armrests. If the elbow is acutely flexed during sleep, a splint is applied to prevent this. An elbow pad worn during the day may diminish direct contusion of the nerve and limit repetitive

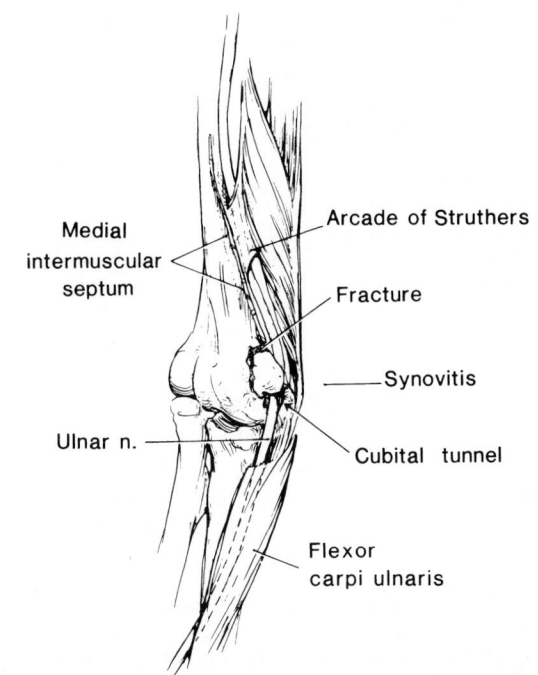

Figure 42–76. Ulnar nerve compression sites. The ulnar nerve is shown in the cubital tunnel. A fracture of the medial condyle, synovitis of the elbow joint, or compression by the arcade of Struthers may cause persistent compression of the ulnar nerve. The medial intermuscular septum may irritate the nerve proximal to the medial condyle. The nerve may slide anteriorly within the cubital tunnel, or it may be irritated by acute flexion of the elbow, which causes the nerve to displace forward. Synovitis of the elbow joint may cause indirect compression; fracture of the medial condyle affects the nerve because of condylar incongruity. The flexor carpi ulnaris covers the nerve as it enters the forearm. The fascial bands at the entrance of the nerve to the muscle may cause compression if the nerve is affected by progressive increase in muscle mass or decreased elasticity associated with aging. The nerve may migrate anteriorly from the cubital tunnel to directly over the medial epicondyle. The movement of the nerve during elbow flexion may result in chronic ulnar neuropathy. (From Goldner, R. D.: Nerve compression in the upper extremity. Orthopaedic Surgery Update Series. Vol. 3, Lesson 28. Princeton, NJ, Bobbitt, 1984.)

elbow flexion. Anti-inflammatory medications diminish connective tissue irritation and lessen the intensity of the complaints.

Surgical treatment is considered if hypesthesia and paresthesias persist for several months; rest, splinting, and other forms of treatment have not improved the persistent or progressive complaints after 3 months of observation; and electrophysiologic studies are positive in either motor or sensory conduction tests and/or abnormal action potentials are observed.

One method of surgical treatment is subcutaneous transfer of the ulnar nerve anteriorly. The important points to observe in order to prevent complications are a long posterior medial incision for adequate exposure; avoidance of the medial brachial and antebrachial cutaneous nerves; adequate proximal dissection to incise the arcade of Struthers and the interosseous fibrous ridge; distal mobilization of the nerve, including cutting the nerve branch to the joint and opening the flexor carpi ulnaris fascia; formation of a fat fascial flap that prevents the nerve from relocating; consideration of medial epicondylectomy if the bone is prominent and the nerve is very loose; avoidance of fascial compression of the nerve proximally and distally after the nerve is transferred; and release of tourniquet, coagulation of bleeding points, and use of suction drainage.

There are three alternative methods of managing the compressed ulnar nerve. First, the medial epicondyle of the humerus is excised without transferring the nerve anteriorly.

This is successful in some instances. Second, the nerve is placed anterior to the ulnar groove and within the forearm flexor muscles. This may be successful, but the muscle tissue may eventually constrict or compress the nerve. Third, the nerve is placed deep to the forearm muscles not only to warm the nerve, as in the case of leprosy, but also to protect the nerve during forceful exercise.

Recurrent ulnar neuropathy after prior transfer requires special experience and pre-, post-, and intraoperative electrical studies. In addition to neurolysis, local protection of the nerve is beneficial by means of fat, muscle, vascularized fascia, or circumferential vein wrap at the time of nerve decompression.

COMPRESSION NEUROPATHY OF THE RADIAL NERVE

With complete interruption of the radial nerve, there is no function of the muscles extending the wrist, thumb, or finger metacarpophalangeal joints (radial palsy). Anesthesia, hypesthesia, or paresthesia of the skin on the radiodorsal surface of the hand may occur. The radial nerve may be compressed by a displaced fracture of the distal third of the humerus or by prolonged external pressure associated with a *Saturday night palsy.* The anatomic area of compression may be opposite the humeral midshaft in the radial groove or in the distal third of the humerus, where the nerve courses from posterior to anterior. The radial nerve is directly adjacent to the humerus in the midshaft, and prolonged external pressure from the patient's head or a similar object compressing the nerve against bone may interrupt nerve conduction. If the patient has been asleep with the arm resting on the edge of a chair or bench, the nerve is also compressed.

An injury to the radial nerve associated with a proximal or midshaft fracture of the humerus usually follows trauma at the time of the injury. In 90% of patients, these lesions recover spontaneously within 3 to 5 months. A displaced distal oblique fracture of the humerus, however, may entrap the nerve between the fracture fragments and require operative decompression.

POSTERIOR INTEROSSEOUS NERVE COMPRESSION

The common radial nerve lies between the brachioradialis and brachialis muscles. This nerve divides into the posterior interosseous branch, which enters the radial tunnel between the superficial and deep heads of the supinator muscle, and the superficial radial nerve, which innervates skin over the dorsal thumb, index finger, and dorsoradial hand. The posterior interosseous nerve supplies all the radial nerve–innervated muscles except the brachioradialis, the extensor carpi radialis longus, and the extensor carpi radialis brevis. These muscles are innervated proximal to the origin of the posterior interosseous nerve. The posterior interosseous nerve may be compressed spontaneously in patients who perform repetitive pronation and supination several hundred times a day for months or years, or the lesion may occur between the radial head and the supinator after a fracture or dislocation of the proximal radius. Other causes are soft tissue tumor or synovial proliferation associated with rheumatoid disease.

Other sites of nerve compression within the radial tunnel are fibrous bands lying anterior to the radial head at the entrance of the radial tunnel; a leash of vessels (radial recurrent artery) lying across the radial nerve and branching to the brachioradialis and extensor carpi radialis longus; the proximal tendon margin of the extensor carpi radialis brevis compressing the posterior interosseous nerve and causing

pain associated with *tennis elbow*; and the arcade of Frohse, a ligamentous band spanning the posterior interosseous nerve as it enters the supinator muscle (Fig. 42–77).

Symptoms include aching of the extensor-supinator muscles and the entire dorsal forearm without muscle weakness (radial tunnel syndrome). If the lesion is confined to the posterior interosseous nerve but is not severe enough to cause motor weakness, pain without cutaneous sensory alteration may occur over the extensor muscle mass and is aggravated by forcible extension of the long finger against resistance when the wrist is held in neutral and the elbow is in a position of flexion from 45 to 90 degrees. Tenderness to digital compression is noted 4 cm. distal to the lateral epicondyle, and dorsal forearm pain is increased when the forearm is forcefully pronated and the wrist flexed. This condition can be confused with persistent lateral epicondylitis. This limited nerve compression does not cause motor weakness.

The clinical findings in an extremity with a complete lesion of the posterior interosseous nerve include active dorsiflexion of the hand in a position of radial deviation or a proximally innervated extensor carpi radialis longus and brevis. The hand cannot be ulnarly deviated in extension because the extensor carpi ulnaris does not function. The thumb or fingers cannot be voluntarily extended at the metacarpophalangeal joints. Sensibility is intact, since the compressive lesion is distal to the origin of the superficial radial nerve.

LESIONS SIMULATING RADIAL NERVE PALSY

Several conditions have an appearance similar to radial nerve injury. Rheumatoid arthritis may cause rupture of the extensor digitorum communis tendons of the ring and little fingers and the extensor digiti quinti (Vaughn-Jackson syndrome). The extensor pollicis longus tendon may separate by attrition or direct trauma after a distal radial fracture, or it may be ruptured by synovial invasion and erosion of collagen. An incomplete radial nerve injury proximal to the elbow

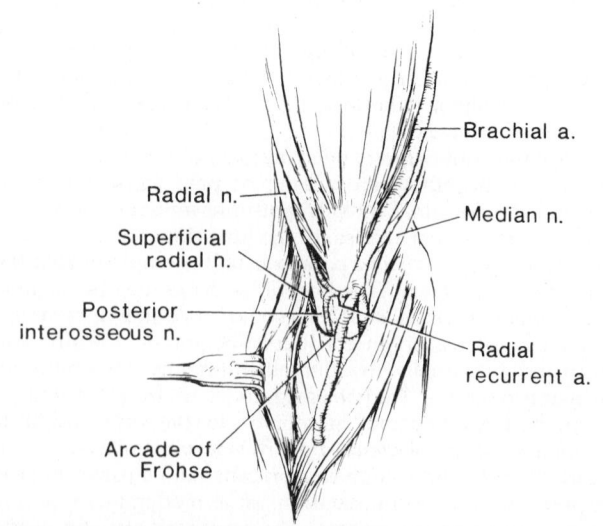

Figure 42–77. Diagram of the common radial nerve proximal to the elbow and lateral to the brachial muscle; the superficial radial nerve, which is primarily sensory; and the posterior interosseous nerve, which is almost entirely motor. This nerve enters the supinator muscle, within which the condensed fascia (the arcade of Frohse) and blood vessels may cause compression of the tethered nerve. Also, the sensory component of the radial nerve may be compressed proximally or distally as the nerve emerges from under the brachioradialis tendon. (From Goldner, R. D.: Nerve compression in the upper extremity. Orthopaedic Surgery Update Series. Vol. 3, Lesson 28. Princeton, NJ, Bobbitt, 1984.)

joint may be associated with neuralgic amyotrophy (Parsonage-Turner syndrome), usually causing pain and sensory diminution early in the syndrome. Asymmetrical weakness of the extensor muscles and diminished sensation along the course of the superficial radial nerve are noted. Lead poisoning affects the radial nerve or the posterior interosseous branch. Symptoms are observed in children eating lead-based paint or inhaling burning battery fumes. An adult may develop lead poisoning from retained lead-based metals within a joint. Diabetes mellitus or other neurotoxic systemic diseases may cause altered conduction of the radial nerve.

COMPRESSION OF THE SENSORY COMPONENT OF THE RADIAL NERVE

Hypesthesia or hyperesthesia on the dorsum of the thumb and/or the index finger may be related to compression of the cutaneous branch of the radial nerve at the point where the nerve exits beneath the brachioradialis and the shaft of the radius, or adjacent to an enlargement of the abductor pollicis longus annular ligament at the wrist. Also, direct trauma to the nerve at the wrist joint level or at the base of the thumb may affect sensory conduction of the radial nerve by primary compression. A careful history is important in establishing the diagnosis. For example, if the patient wears a tight bracelet or a heavy elastic watchband or has been cutting with large, dull scissors, the radial nerve may be compressed by external forces.

Clinical examination reveals an area of hyperesthesia or hypesthesia along the course of the nerve slightly proximal and always distal to the point of compression. The condition usually improves in time by eliminating the abnormal external compressive forces.

If the cutaneous symptoms persist, a neurolysis is performed from the proximal point of compression under the brachioradialis tendon, approximately 5 cm. proximal to the wrist joint, to the distal area of compression as determined by alteration of skin sensitivity and a positive percussion test.

PERIPHERAL NERVE REPAIR

An extension of the management of focal peripheral nerve lesions, entrapment syndromes, or old nerve injuries is consideration of resection and nerve repair to eliminate a damaged nerve segment. The concepts currently used in establishing continuity of lacerated nerves are primary direct epineurial or fascicular sutures, nerve grafts to bridge large gaps and provide continuity without suture line tension, and bone shortening to perform epineurial suture.

The conditions that cause severe intraneural damage are prolonged localized nerve compression lesions, nerve segment damage due to local injection of a toxic agent, traumatic crushing of a nerve, or nerve compression by a bone fragment. Localized resection of a 2- to 3-cm. neuroma may be repaired by direct end-to-end suture with moderate mobilization of the nerve, depending on the specific nerve and location of the defect. Defects that cannot be closed without tension after nerve mobilization usually require grafting. This decision depends on the length of the nerve gap, the ability of the adjacent nerve segments to be immobilized, and the diameter of the nerve segments.

Epineurial Repair, End-to-End. Epineurial or group fascicular repair is performed if the nerve gap allows end-to-end suture without tension. For example, a median nerve at the wrist with a total gap of 2 to 3 cm. after trimming and preparing for an end-to-end suture may require moderate mobilization of both proximal and distal segments, after which an epineurial end-to-end suture may be performed

without excessive tension. This would require the wrist to be in a position of flexion for several weeks.

Nerve Grafting. If the defect is greater than several centimeters, or when a full range of joint motion is desirable within 2 weeks after nerve repair, grafting of the defect should be considered. Nerve grafting requires a double suture line, and each junction site may interfere with axon flow. Moreover, the nerve graft is temporarily ischemic unless a vascularized graft is performed, and nerve regeneration and ultimate function after grafting are slower than after end-to-end epineurial suture. However, the goal of absence of tension on the suture line and the ability of nerve grafting to repair large defects are strong indications for grafting in certain patients.

Nerve Repair Technique. Adequate mobilization of both the proximal and the distal segments of the nerve should be accomplished without damage to the intrinsic blood supply of the nerve. Mobilization may require transfer of the median nerve anterior to the pronator teres muscle in the upper forearm or transfer of the ulnar nerve anterior to the medial epicondyle. Mobilization of each of these nerves may be accomplished to gain 2 to 3 cm. of length without actually damaging the blood supply. When the nerves are mobilized and the inherent elasticity is determined by gentle traction, a decision is made as to end-to-end epineurial or group fascicular repair or nerve grafting.

Nerve Suturing Procedure. The nerve segment being prepared is stabilized with a nerve holder and cut carefully at right angles with a sharp knife. Cuts are made so that the nerve ends are trimmed back to healthy *pouting* fascicles. Electrical stimulation, special nerve staining, and topographic alignment with magnification may be helpful in determining the proper orientation of the fascicles. Observation of peripheral vessels is helpful in aligning the fascicles. Adequate lighting and magnification in performing this maneuver are mandatory. Magnification may vary from 4 times for a large nerve to 10 times for a small nerve or graft. Topographic matching is attempted in order to bring proximal motor and sensory fibers to match with distal motor and sensory fibers. Microneedle holders and small forceps are used to handle the epineurium and adjacent tissue with relatively atraumatic technique. Sutures of 8-0 to 10-0 nylon are used to repair the nerve; the size of the suture depends on the size of the nerve and whether the repair is epineurial or group fascicular. Tension on the sutures should be sufficient to close the epineurium and prevent axons from escaping but not tight enough to wrinkle or cause malalignment of the fascicles.

The critical points to be remembered at the time of nerve repair are trimming of the nerve endings to nondamaged axons, adequate regional blood flow for nerve regeneration, anatomic topographic realignment of sensory and motor fascicles, apposition of nerve endings without tension, and adequate strength of apposition to avoid separation of the nerve segments.

SELECTED REFERENCES

Dahlin, L. B., and Rydevik, B.: Pathophysiology of nerve compression. *In* Gelberman, R. H. (Ed.): Operative Nerve Repair and Reconstruction. Philadelphia, J. B. Lippincott, 1991, p. 847.

Eversmann, W. W.: Entrapment and compression neuropathies. *In* Green, D. P. (Ed.): Operative Hand Surgery. New York, Churchill Livingstone, 1993, p. 1341.
Current, well-illustrated discussion of entrapment and compression neuropathies of the upper extremity.

Spinner, M.: Management of nerve compression lesions of the upper extremity. *In* Omer, G. E., Jr., and Spinner, M. (Eds.): Management of Peripheral Nerve Problems. Philadelphia, W. B. Saunders, 1980, p. 569.
This clearly written text provides detailed anatomic and clinical information concerning peripheral nerves of the upper extremity.

REFERENCES

1. Bell, G. E., Jr., and Goldner, J. L.: Compression neuropathy of the median nerve. South. Med. J., 49:966, 1956.
2. Blair, S. J.: Avoiding complications of surgery for nerve compression syndromes. Orthop. Clin. North Am., 19:125, 1988.
3. Bolesta, M. J., Garret, W. E., Ribbeck, D. M., Glisson, R. R., Seaber, A. V., and Goldner, J. L.: Immediate and delayed neurorrhaphy in a rabbit model; a functional, histologic, and biochemical comparison. J. Hand Surg. [Am.], 13:352, 1988.
4. Braun, R. M., Davidson, J., and Doehr, M. A.: Provocative testing in the diagnosis of dynamic carpal tunnel syndrome. J. Hand Surg. [Am.], 14:195, 1989.
5. Eason, S. Y., Belsole, R. J., and Greene, T. L.: Carpal tunnel release: Analysis of suboptimal results. J. Hand Surg. [Br.], 10:365, 1985.
6. Eversmann, W. W.: Entrapment and compression neuropathies. In Green, D. P. (Ed.): Operative Hand Surgery. New York, Churchill Livingstone, 1993, p. 1341.
7. Gelberman, R. H., Szabo, R. M., Williamson, R. V., and Dimick, M. P.: Sensibility testing in peripheral nerve compression syndromes. J. Bone Joint Surg. [Am.], 65:632, 1983.
8. Gelberman, R. H., Aronson, D., and Weisman, M. H.: Carpal tunnel syndrome: Results of a prospective trial of steroid injection and splinting. J. Bone Joint Surg. [Am.], 62:1181, 1980.
9. Gelberman, R. H., Rydevik, B. L., Pess, G. M., Szabo, R. M., and Lundborg, G.: Carpal tunnel syndrome: A scientific basis for clinical care. Orthop. Clin North Am., 19:115, 1988.
10. Goldner, J. L.: Biological principles of repair and regeneration of nerve and tendon. South. Med. J., 64:121, 1971.
11. Goldner, J. L.: Median nerve compression lesions, anatomical and clinical analysis. Bull. Hosp. Jt. Dis., 44:199, 1984.
12. Goldner, J. L.: Function of the hand following peripheral nerve injuries. Instructional Course Lecture. Vol. 10. Ann Arbor, MI, American Academy of Orthopaedic Surgeons, 1953.
13. Goldner, R. D.: Nerve compression in the upper extremity. Orthopaedic Surgery Update Series. Vol. 3, Lesson 28. Princeton, NJ, Bobbitt, 1984.
14. Goldner, R. D., and Koman, L. A.: Microsurgery of the hand. In Goldsmith, H. S. (Ed.): Practice of Surgery. Hagerstown, MD, Harper & Row, 1984, p. 1.
15. Groves, R. J., and Goldner, J. L.: Restoration of strong opposition after median nerve or brachial plexus paralysis. J. Bone Joint Surg. [Am.], 57:112, 1975.
16. Kelley, J. M., and Goldner, J. L.: Radial nerve injuries. South. Med. J., 51:873, 1958.
17. Lowry, W. E., Jr., and Follender, A. B.: Interfascicular neurolysis in severe carpal tunnel syndrome—a prospective, randomized, double-blind, controlled study. Clin. Orthop. Rel. Res., 227:251, 1988.
18. MacKinnon, S. E., and Dellon, A. L.: Experimental study of chronic nerve compression. Hand Clin., 2:639, 1986.
19. Ochoa, J., Fowler, T. J., and Gilliatt, R. W.: Anatomical changes in peripheral nerves compressed by a pneumatic tourniquet. J. Anat., 113:433, 1972.
20. Osterman, A. L.: The double crush syndrome. Orthop. Clin. North Am., 19:147, 1991.
21. Peimer, C.: Compression neuropathies in the upper extremities. Orthop. Rev., 16:41, 1987.
22. Roles, N. C., and Maudsley, R. H.: Radial tunnel syndrome: Resistant tennis elbow as a nerve entrapment. J. Bone Joint Surg. [Br.], 54:499, 1972.
23. Seddon, H. J.: Electrical Phenomena in Surgical Disorders of Peripheral Nerves. Baltimore, Williams & Wilkins, 1972, p. 577.
24. Seror, P.: Phalen's test in the diagnosis of carpal tunnel syndrome. J. Hand Surg. [Br.], 13:383, 1988.
25. Seror, P.: Tinel's sign in the diagnosis of carpal tunnel syndrome. J. Hand Surg. [Br.], 12:364, 1987.
26. Spindler, H. A., and Dellon, A. L.: Nerve conduction studies and sensibility testing in carpal tunnel syndrome. J. Hand Surg., 7:260, 1982.
27. Spinner, M.: Management of nerve compression lesions of the upper extremity. In Omer, G. E., Jr., and Spinner, M. (Eds.): Management of Peripheral Nerve Problems. Philadelphia, W. B. Saunders, 1980, p. 569.
28. Sunderland, S.: Nerves and Nerve Injuries. New York, Churchill Livingstone, 1978.
29. Szabo, R. M., and Gelberman, R. H.: The pathophysiology of nerve entrapment syndromes. J. Hand Surg. [Am.], 12:880, 1987.
30. Urbaniak, J. R.: Nerve repair in the upper extremity. Orthopaedic Surgery Update Series. Vol. 1, Lesson 31. Princeton, NJ, Bobbitt, 1981.

CHAPTER 43

REPLANTATION OF AMPUTATED LIMBS AND DIGITS

James R. Urbaniak, M.D.

HISTORICAL ASPECTS

The concepts of microsurgery and limb replantation developed in the early 1900s with the introduction of macrosurgical techniques for arterial and venous anastomoses in composite grafts and transplants. Hopfner, Carrel, and Guthrie began working on early animal limb replantation before 1905. However, it was not until the 1960s that Lapchinsky and Snyder succeeded in obtaining long-term results in dog replantations.

In 1922, Holmgren introduced the binocular operating microscope for middle ear surgery. The basic principles of anastomosing small vessels were described by Seidenberg and colleagues in 1958. The introduction of the operating microscope in 1960 by Jacobson and Suarez for the repair of small vessels had the greatest impact on the replantation of amputated hands and digits.

Microvascular surgery implies repair of small blood vessels (3 mm. or less in diameter) using an operating microscope, microsurgical instruments, and ultrafine suture material (usually approximately 20 μm. in diameter). The use of 10-0 (20 μm.) nylon or polypropylene suture, which is swedged on a needle of 50 to 130 μm. in diameter, is essential in anastomosing small vessels of 1 mm. or less found at the base of an adult digit (Fig. 43–1).

Replantation is defined as reattachment of a part that has been completely severed—that is, there is no connection between the amputated part and the patient. *Revascularization* is the reattachment of a part in which some portion of the soft tissue (such as skin, nerves, or tendon) is still connected. Vascular repair is necessary to prevent necrosis of a partially severed distal limb. This may require repair of the arteries, the veins, or both.

Malt in 1962 first successfully replanted a completely amputated arm in a 12-year-old male. The first successful replantation of an amputated digit by microvascular technique was performed by Komatsu and Tamai in Nara, Japan, in 1965. Digit and hand replantation using microvascular anastomosis of small arteries and veins has become an effective method of reconstructing hands that have sustained complete or incomplete amputations.

CARE OF THE AMPUTATED PART

Amputated or devascularized tissue survives for approximately 6 hours if the part is not cooled. Cooling lessens the metabolic needs of the tissues, and an amputated part may be successfully restored 12 hours after severance if it has been cooled. Because the digits have essentially no muscle tissue, they may be successfully replanted as long as 24 hours after amputation if they have been cooled.

Because most replantations are performed in centers with experienced microvascular teams, the referring physician must be given clear instructions regarding preservation of the amputated part and care of the injured patient. The amputated part should be placed in a plastic bag containing Ringer's lactate or saline solution; the plastic bag is placed on ice.[16] The amputated part must not be allowed to come in direct contact with the ice or to become frozen. The referring physician is instructed not to ligate or perfuse any of the vessels for fear of causing intimal damage. An alternative method of preserving the amputated part is to wrap it in a cloth or sponge moistened with Ringer's lactate or saline solution and place it in a plastic bag, which is put on ice.

PATIENT SELECTION

The decision whether to replant an amputated part is not always easy. An experienced replantation team can restore almost any amputated part and have it remain viable. However, success in viability must not be misconstrued as success in useful function of the replanted extremity. Guillotine-type amputations are obviously ideal for replanting; however, this type of amputation in uncommon. Most amputated parts are avulsed or crushed, making reconstruction more complex and viability more difficult to achieve.[1, 3]

Candidates for replantation are selected according to the following priorities: (1) thumb, (2) multiple digits, (3) partial hand (amputation through the palm), (4) almost any part of a child, (5) wrist or forearm, (6) above-elbow amputation (only sharp or moderately avulsed), and (7) isolated digit distal to the superficial insertion (distal to the proximal interphalangeal joint). This list is not necessarily in strict order of preference, but if other factors are favorable, replantation should be attempted. Replantation of thumbs, multiple digits, and the complete hand produces the best results; however, replantation of the other parts listed generally produces better function than can be obtained by prosthesis. In children, an attempt should be made to replant almost any part, since if the replanted extremity survives, excellent function can be expected.[13, 15]

Types of injuries that are not favorable for replantation are amputations involving (1) severely crushed or mangled parts, (2) multiple levels, (3) patients with other serious injuries or diseases, (4) arteriosclerotic vessels, (5) mentally unstable patients, (6) more than 6 hours of ischemic time, (7) severely contaminated parts, and (8) an individual finger in an adult when the amputation is proximal to the superficial insertion (proximal to the proximal interphalangeal joint). Replantations of isolated fingers at the base (proximal to the superficial insertion) generally produce a finger that *gets in the way* because of diminished tendon excursion.[19] If the isolated finger is amputated distal to the proximal interphalangeal joint, the flexor superficial tendon is still intact, and replantation produces a functional digit with good tendon excursion. Selection is also influenced by the patient's occupation, avocation, age, and sex. These contraindications to replantation

DIGITAL ARTERY

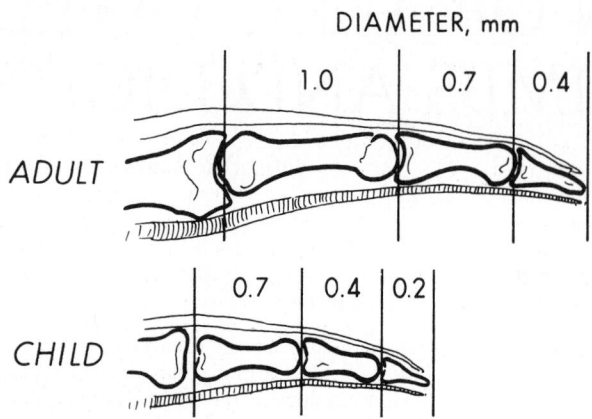

DIAMETER, mm

Figure 43–1. The comparative sizes of the human digital arteries in the adult and the child. Microsurgical anastomosis is possible in a vessel as small as 0.3 mm.

are not absolute. Often the final decision cannot be made until the status of the damaged blood vessels is determined under the operating microscope.

SURGICAL TECHNIQUE

When a patient with an amputated part arrives in the emergency room, the replantation team divides into two sub-teams. One team immediately takes the amputated part to the operating theater and prepares it for examination under the operating microscope. The vessels and nerves are located and labeled (with fine suture or hemoclips) under 10-power magnification. Microscopic evaluation determines the feasibility of restoration by revascularization. The other team assesses and prepares the patient for the operative procedure. Most replantations of upper extremity parts are performed under axillary block with a long-acting agent such as bupivacaine hydrochloride (Marcaine). General anesthesia is seldom indicated, and all the neural and vascular surgery is performed under the operating microscope.

The sequence of replantation of amputated digits or hands is as follows: (1) locate and tag the vessels and nerves, (2) thoroughly débride the amputated part and stump, (3) shorten and fix the bone with an intramedullary pin, (4) repair the extensor tendons, (5) repair the flexor tendons, (6) repair the arteries, (7) repair the nerves, (8) repair the veins, and (9) obtain loose skin coverage (split-thickness graft if necessary) (Fig. 43–2).

The bone is shortened to allow normal intima to be attached to normal intima.[18] Frequently, interposition vein grafts are necessary for arterial and/or venous repair when there is severe vascular damage.[8, 17] Usually two veins are repaired for each artery. An attempt is made to repair both digital arteries. Primary nerve grafts (from the medial antebrachial cutaneous nerve on the ipsilateral forearm) are used if the gap is large. None of the vascular or nerve repairs should be done under tension. *The most important factors in achieving permanent microvascular patency are easy coaptation of vessels with normal intima and the skill and expertise of the microsurgeon.*

MAJOR LIMB REPLANTATION

Since most amputations of the upper extremity occur at the digit or hand level, emphasis has been placed on describ-

ing the reattachment at these levels. Major limb replantation implies replantation of limbs proximal to the wrist or, in the lower extremity, proximal to the ankle. Replantation of limbs amputated at or proximal to the wrist level or amputations of the lower extremity below or above the knee involve similar principles with minor modifications. The major differences are related to the amount of muscle tissue involved. Because more muscle mass is involved, the duration of avascularity of the detached part is more critical.[5]

Whereas amputated digits may be successfully replanted 24 hours after amputation, an arm amputated at the elbow is in jeopardy if it has been avascular for 10 or 12 hours, even if it has been properly cooled. Extensive muscle débridement on both the detached part and the stump is essential to prevent myonecrosis and subsequent infection, which is the major problem in major limb replantation but is uncommon in digital reattachment. Major limbs are rarely sev-

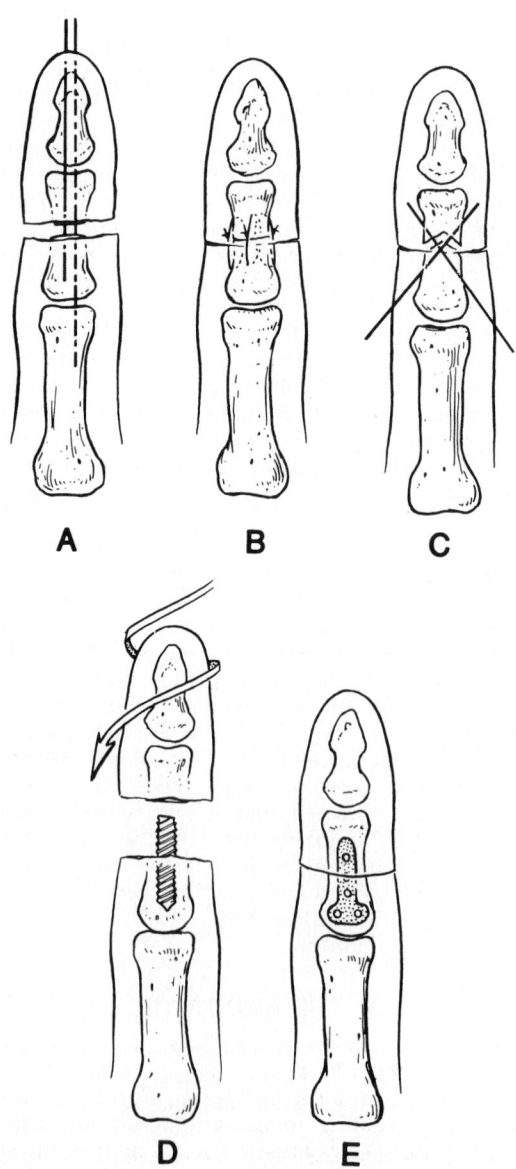

Figure 43–2. Methods of bone fixation. *A*, Intramedullary pins. *B*, Intraosseous wiring. *C*, Crossed pins. *D*, Intramedullary screw. *E*, Plate and screws. *A* is the preferred method. (From Goldner, R. D., and Urbaniak, J. R.: Replantation in the Upper Extremity. Orthopaedic Surgery Update Series, Vol. 2, Lesson 32, 1983.)

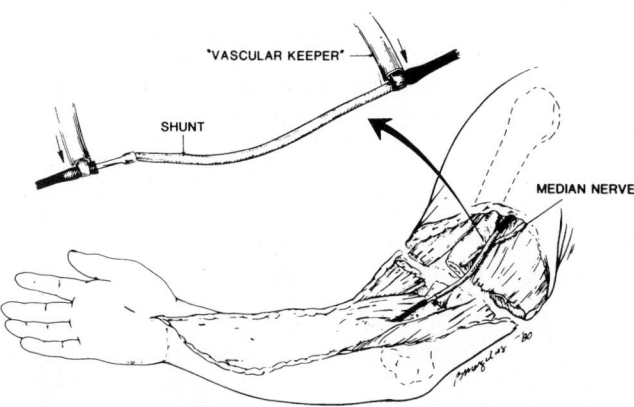

Figure 43–3. A Sundt shunt or a ventriculoperitoneal shunt is used to obtain rapid arterial inflow from the proximal vessel to the amputated part. (From Urbaniak, J. R.: Replantation. *In* Green, D. P.: Operative Hand Surgery, 2nd ed. New York, Churchill Livingstone, 1988, pp. 1105–1126.)

ered cleanly; therefore, the muscle damage is usually quite severe.

In replantations proximal to the metacarpal level, immediate arterial inflow is necessary to prevent or diminish myonecrosis. If the amputated part and the patient arrive in the operating room more than 4 hours after injury, it is desirable to initiate immediate blood flow to the detached part. This is best accomplished by using some form of shunt, such as a Sundt or ventriculoperitoneal shunt, to obtain rapid arterial inflow from the proximal vessel to the detached part (Fig. 43–3).[7] Shunting should be performed before bone fixation, unless the bone can be rapidly stabilized and early blood flow obtained. After the establishment of temporary blood flow, further débridement can be continued, the bone stabilized, the shunt removed, and a direct arterial repair or interposition vein grafting of the vessels performed.

Stable bone fixation is necessary for major limb replantation; however, the method should be rapid. Rigid plate and screw fixation of the long bones is preferable. As in digital replantation, bone shortening must be carefully planned relative to the type of injury and tissue damage. Usually, the plate may be secured to the amputated part after the initial débridement and then fixed to the stump after blood flow has been established through shunts, particularly if the ischemic time has been prolonged.

In major limb replantation, it is critical to perform the arterial anastomosis before the venous anastomosis. This sequence allows a physiologic washout of noxious agents such as lactic acid in the distal part. If this order is reversed, with the venous connection first, the return of toxic catabolites through the systemic circulation can cause serious consequences, even death. The administration of intravenous sodium bicarbonate before venous anastomosis is beneficial.

Extensive fasciotomies are always indicated in major limb replantations. *The two most common causes of failure in major limb replantation are myonecrosis with subsequent infection and failure to provide adequate decompression of the restored vessels.* Meshed split-thickness skin grafts may be used to provide coverage over the exposed vessels. Other areas may be closed primarily or grafted several days later.

In replantations of major limbs, the patient should be returned to the operating room within 48 to 72 hours for evaluation of the state of muscle tissue. The dressing should be changed with the patient under general anesthesia or regional block, and any necrotic tissue must be further débrided to prevent infection. In general, no anticoagulation is employed for major limb replantation. Whereas most patients with digital replantations are hospitalized for 6 to 7 days,

those with major limb replantations require longer periods, depending on the severity of the injury.

In major limb replantations, the likelihood of success occurs, in order, in replantations of the wrist, the arm, and the distal forearm. The poorest results occur in the proximal third of the forearm, an area where the motor branches of the radial, median, and ulnar nerves enter the extrinsic musculature of the hand.

There are few indications for replantation of the lower extremity.[6] The functional disability that follows a lower limb amputation is less than that sustained from an upper extremity amputation of a similar nature. Upper extremity prostheses poorly duplicate hand function because of a lack of sensory feedback; however, lower limb prostheses provide a stable stance and a functional gait.

In addition, lower extremity injuries are usually caused by an extensive crush or avulsion mechanism, and the skeletal shortening required to reapproximate undamaged tissue usually produces an unacceptable leg length discrepancy. It is usually prudent to revise the amputation of a lower extremity, sometimes using the amputated parts to serve as innervated free flaps to provide stump sensation and preserve more function—for example, preserving a below-knee amputation instead of an above-knee amputation. With the currently available lower extremity prostheses, considerable thought should be given before attempting replantation of the lower extremities, even in cases of cleanly severed limbs.

POSTOPERATIVE MANAGEMENT

A careful postoperative regimen is paramount in achieving a high viability rate in replantation.[9, 16] Most patients receive some type of anticoagulation. Intravenous heparin at 1000 units per hour for approximately 7 days is usually administered. This is monitored to maintain the activated partial

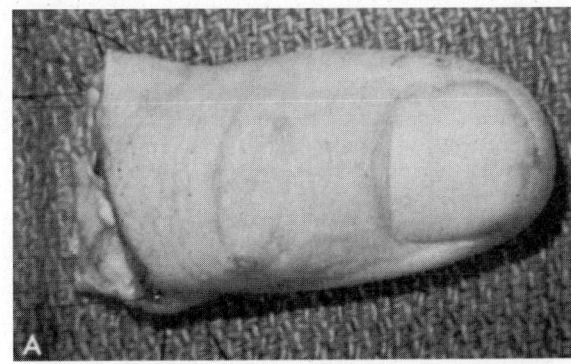

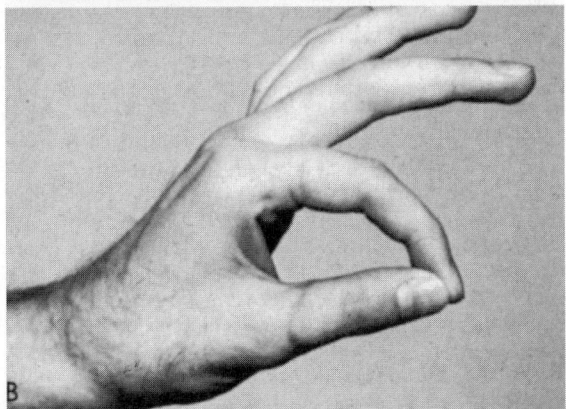

Figure 43–4. *A*, This clean thumb amputation was replanted in a 16-year-old male. *B*, Essentially normal sensibility, motor function, and pinch were achieved.

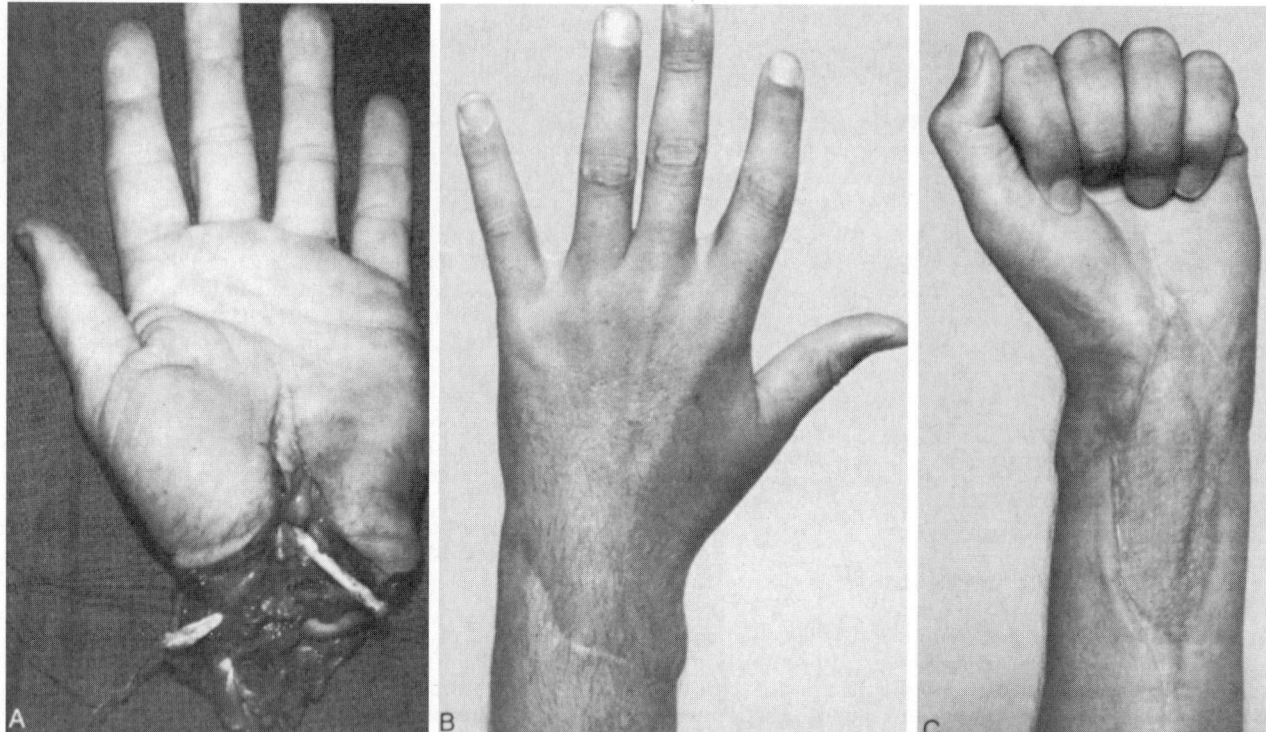

Figure 43–5. *A,* This 22-year-old male had replantation of a completely amputated hand. *B* and *C,* One year after replantation, he has nearly full flexion-extension of the hand. Intrinsic function has returned to the thenar and hyperthenar muscles. He has protective sensibility with a strong pinch and grip. (From Porubsky, G. L., and Urbaniak, J. R.: Limb and digital replantation. *In* Flye, M. W.: Principles of Organ Transplantation. Philadelphia, W. B. Saunders Company, 1989, pp. 453–477.)

thromboplastin time at one and a half to two times normal. Low-molecular-weight dextran, aspirin, chlorpromazine, and dipyridamole have all been used in difficult cases.[10, 14] Skin color, pulp turgor, capillary refill, and skin temperature are the most useful indicators. In general, if the skin temperature of the replanted part, which is continuously monitored by a small surface probe taped to the digit, drops below 30° C, poor vascular perfusion of the digit is certain, and a cause for the poor circulation must be found and corrected, if possible.[12] The dressing must be inspected for any constriction. Additional heparin may be indicated, and axillary or stellate blocks may be helpful. The hand may need to be elevated or depressed. Seldom is it necessary to return the patient to the operating room for a revision; however, if re-exploration is to be successful, it must usually be done within 24 to 48 hours after the primary procedure.

RESULTS OF REPLANTATION

The Duke Orthopaedic Replantation Team has attempted revascularization or replantation of more than 1500 partial or total amputations from 1972 to 1995. Ninety-two percent of the partial amputations have been successfully revascularized, and 81% of the complete amputations have remained viable. The viability rates have improved with experience of the team. Most major replantation centers are obtaining an approximate 80% viability rate in complete replantations.[11] The mechanisms of injury and patient selection significantly influence the survival and functional outcome of replantations.

Recovery of sensibility in replanted digits is similar to results of repair of an isolated peripheral nerve.[4] Cold intolerance is a problem in most patients, but this subsides in 1 to 2 years. Replanted thumbs produce the best functional results (Fig. 43–4).[2, 8] Strong pinch, adequate motion, excellent sensa-

tion, and almost normal appearance are to be expected. Replantation of digits distal to the superficial insertion produces good appearance with excellent results, good pulp turgor, and nonpainful digits.[19] Replantation of digits at the base of the finger (proximal to the superficial insertion) produces good sensibility but usually poor functional motion. Replantations of multiple digits, partial hands (through the palm), or complete hands provide good sensibility and useful function (Fig. 43–5).[20] Whereas amputations through the wrist or distal forearm provide good function of the hand, amputations at a more proximal level have varied results. Patients usually have weak pinch and grasp and poor sensibility. Amputations at the wrist or hand level seldom require additional secondary reconstructive procedures; however, amputations at a more proximal level, particularly above the elbow, usually require secondary nerve grafts and tendon or muscle transfers to achieve elbow and possibly digital flexion and extension.

SELECTED REFERENCES

Goldner, R. D., Fitch, R. D., Nunley, J. A., Aitken, M. S., and Urbaniak, J. R.: Demographics and replantation. J. Hand Surg. [Am.], *12*:961, 1987.
   This is an excellent demographic study of more than 1200 replanted upper extremities.

Goldner, R. D., Stevanovic, M. V., Nunley, J. A., and Urbaniak, J. R.: Digital replantation at the level of the distal interphalangeal joint and the distal phalanx. J. Hand Surg. [Am.], *14*:214, 1989.
   This study represents the largest collection of patients who have been followed after replantation of a single digit at or distal to the distal interphalangeal joint. It documents the value of distal replantation and describes the microsurgical techniques.

Lukas, F. N., Greenberg, B. M., Gallico, G. G., Panda, M., and May, J. W.: A socioeconomic analysis of digital replantations results from home use of power tools. J. Hand Surg. [Am.], *17*:1042, 1992.
   This article focuses on the home use of power tools as a cause of digital amputation and replantation. An analysis of the financial and emotional costs, additional surgical procedures, and rehabilitation periods for return to work is presented.

Saies, A. D., Urbaniak, J. R., Nunley, J. A., Taras, J. S., Goldner, R. D., and Fitch, R. D.: Results after replantation and revascularization in the upper extremity in children. J. Bone Joint Surg. [Am.], 76:1766, 1994.
This article reviews the results of revascularization and replantation in the upper extremities of 120 children. Techniques and expected results in children versus adults are discussed.

REFERENCES

1. Axelrod, T. S., and Buchler, U.: Severe complex injuries to the upper extremity: Revascularization and replantation. J. Hand Surg. [Am.], 16:574, 1991.
2. Beiber, E. J., Wood, M. D., Cooney, W. P., and Amadio, P. C.: Thumb avulsion: Results of replantation/revascularization. J. Hand Surg. [Am.], 12:786, 1987.
3. Bowen, C. V. A., Beveridge, J., Milliken, R. G., and Johnston, G. H. F.: Rotating shaft avulsion amputations of the thumb. J. Hand Surg. [Am.], 16:117, 1991.
4. Gelberman, R. H., Urbaniak, J. R., Bright, D. S., and Levin, L. S.: Digital sensibility following replantation. J. Hand Surg. [Am.], 3:313, 1978.
5. Kellis, G., Shaffer, J. W., and Field, G.: Development of collateral circulation in a replanted rat hindlimb model. J. Hand Surg. [Am.], 16:1070, 1991.
6. Kutz, J. E., Jupiter, J. B., and Tsai, T.-M.: Lower limb replantation—a report of nine cases. Foot Ankle, 3:197, 1983.
7. Nunley, J. A., Koman, L. A., and Urbaniak, J. R.: Arterial shunting as an adjunct to major limb revascularization. Ann. Surg., 193:271, 1981.
8. Nystrom, A., and Backman, C.: Replantation of the completely avulsed thumb using long arterial and venous grafts. J. Hand Surg. [Br.], 16:389, 1991.
9. Nystrom, A., Backman, C., and Backman, C.: Effects of cold exposure on the circulation of replanted fingers during the early postoperative period. J. Hand Surg. [Am.], 16:1041, 1991.
10. Parkhouse, N., and Smith, P. J.: The use of streptokinase in replant salvage. J. Hand Surg. [Br.], 16:53, 1991.
11. Russell, R. C., O'Brien, B. M., Morrison, W. A., et al.: The late functional results of upper limb revascularization and replantation. J. Hand Surg. [Am.], 9:623, 1984.
12. Stirrat, C. R., Seaber, A. V., Urbaniak, J. R., and Bright, D. S.: Temperature monitoring in digital replantation. J. Hand Surg. [Am.], 3:342, 1978.
13. Taras, J. S., Nunley, J. A., Urbaniak, J. R., Goldner, R. D., and Fitch, R. D.: Replantation in children. J. Microsurg., 12:216, 1991.
14. Tark, K. C., Kim, Y. W., Lee, Y. H., and Lew, J. D.: Replantation and revascularization of hands: Clinical analysis and functional results of 261 cases. J. Hand Surg. [Am.], 14:17, 1989.
15. Urbaniak, J. R.: Replantation in children. *In* Serafin, D., and Georgiade, N. G. (Eds.): Pediatric Plastic Surgery. St. Louis, C. V. Mosby, 1984, p. 1168.
16. Urbaniak, J. R.: Digital replantation: A 12-year experience. *In* Urbaniak, J. R. (Ed.): Microsurgery for Major Limb Reconstruction. St. Louis, C. V. Mosby, 1987, p. 12.
17. Urbaniak, J. R., Evans, J. P., and Bright, D. S.: Microvascular management of ring avulsion injuries. J. Hand Surg. [Am.], 6:25, 1981.
18. Urbaniak, J. R., Hayes, M. G., and Bright, D. S.: Management of bone in digital replantation: Free vascularized and composite bone grafts. Clin. Orthop., 133:194, 1978.
19. Urbaniak, J. R., Roth, J. H., Nunley, J. A., Goldner, R. D., and Koman, L. A.: The results of replantation after amputation of a single finger. J. Bone Joint Surg. [Am.], 67:611, 1985.
20. Zhang, Y. L., Yang, K. F., Li, C., and Wei, J. N.: Transmetacarpal replantation of the right hand onto the left. J. Hand Surg. [Br.], 16:392, 1991.

CHAPTER 44

GYNECOLOGY

The Female Reproductive Organs

Charles B. Hammond, M.D.

Gynecology is the branch of medicine that concerns function and diseases of the female reproductive system. Increasingly, this specialty includes not only the pelvic reproductive organs but also other areas, such as the primary health care of women, the adjacent pelvic structures (urinary system and bowel), and even diseases of remote, hormonally reactive organs, such as breast, bone, hypothalamus, and pituitary.

HISTORICAL ASPECTS

The art and practice of gynecology date from antiquity, when most thinking and practices were vested in superstition and based on empiricism. Early rules concerning sexuality and menstruation are recorded in the Bible in Leviticus 15:19–32. Soranus, Hippocrates, and Galen observed traits and attitudes in women and attempted to relate them to the "uterus and its humors." It was only with the emergence of scientific methodology in the Middle Ages that gynecology progressed by objective observation. Gynecology advanced as medical science as a whole prospered, but perhaps at a slower pace because of the persistence of the fantasies surrounding human reproduction, many of which remain as we near the twenty-first century.

Modern gynecologic surgery dates from 1809, when Ephraim McDowell performed the first ovariotomy for a large ovarian cyst. The operation was a success and established the foundation for abdominal and pelvic surgery. Many significant discoveries followed. In 1817, Langenbeck reported the first vaginal hysterectomy. Semmelweiss, in 1840, applied hypochlorite to all instruments, towels, and containers used during delivery and required thorough handwashing with soap, warm water, and hypochlorite rinse. His seminal work reduced the mortality of puerperal fever and introduced the concept of chemical antisepsis 20 years before Lister's first publication promulgating carbolic acid spray and 50 years before Lister capitulated completely to the concept of preventive antisepsis. Long, in 1842, and Morton, in 1846, introduced ether anesthesia. In 1849, Mattauer and, in 1852, Sims described successful closure of vesicovaginal fistula, a common complication at that time of obstructed labor. Hodge described the vaginal pessary for support of the prolapsed uterus in 1860. In 1861, Pasteur noted that living organisms led to fermentation and tissue destruction. In 1867, Freund performed the first successful abdominal hysterectomy for cancer of the uterus. Tait, in 1884, reported excellent success with abdominal operation for ruptured ectopic pregnancy. In 1895, Roentgen discovered x-rays, and 3 years later the Curies discovered radium. Also in 1898, Kelly described the operative cure of bladder and urethral prolapse and published a two-volume text of operative gynecology.

The twentieth century began with Wertheim describing a radical operation for cancer of the cervix and Landsteiner discovering the major human blood groups. In 1903, Cleaves first used radium to treat cancer of the cervix. In 1908, Hitsch-mann and Alder demonstrated the cyclic physiologic changes of endometrium. Sampson, in 1921, described pelvic endometriosis and published his theory of "retrograde menstruation." In 1923, Allen and Doisy isolated estrogen. In 1928, Aschheim and Zondek discovered human chorionic gonadotropin, and in the following year Allen and Corner isolated progesterone. Stein and Leventhal described the polycystic ovary syndrome in 1935, and in the following year Hamblen first induced human ovulation with gonadotropins of nonhuman primates and Colebrook and Kenny first used antibiotics (sulfanilamides) to treat human puerperal infections. Papanicolaou and Traut published their classic monograph on vaginal cytology for cancer screening in 1941. In 1949, Barr discovered the sex chromatin body and Li, Simpson, and Evans isolated human follicle-stimulating hormone. In 1951, Brunschwig reported exenterative pelvic operative procedures for advanced or recurrent cervical cancer. Li, Hertz, and Spencer first cured metastatic choriocarcinoma with chemotherapy in 1956, and in the same year Tijo and Levan identified the normal human karyotype as 46 chromosomes. In 1958, Gemzell reported successful ovulatory induction with human gonadotropins and Pincus introduced oral contraceptives. Ultrasonography and laparoscopy became necessary approaches in the 1970s in the assessment of obstetric and gynecologic patients. Rather amazingly, in 1978, the first child was born after *in vitro* fertilization.

In the 1980s and 1990s, many further advances have served to expand gynecologic practice. Gonadotropin-releasing hormone exists for medical therapies of selected patients by means of a *medical menopause*, for problems such as endometriosis and leiomyoma in selected individuals. Operative laparoscopy and hysteroscopy, with and without laser, have become increasingly important tools for surgical approaches to many gynecologic problems. Magnetic resonance imaging and computed tomography are increasingly important for noninvasive management of many problems. Most importantly, the expansion of sensitivity and usefulness of transvaginal ultrasound has dramatically improved our diagnostic abilities for pelvic disease. Tumor markers, such as CA 125, carcinoembryonic antigen (CEA), and human chorionic gonadotropin (hCG), are being further expanded to aid the diagnosis of malignancy, while a better understanding of hormonal receptor physiology allows novel therapeutic approaches to female disease. Menopause and other types of hormonal deprivation have been identified as major health factors in an aging population, and new methods of safely replacing deficient hormones have been developed. Sexually transmitted infectious diseases have rapidly become major problems for women in the 1990s. Although many such diseases are now perhaps better controlled by diagnostic and therapeutic improvements, others clearly are not and offer minor to major impacts (i.e., herpes simplex viruses, papillomaviruses, and the human immunodeficiency virus [HIV]). These pose threats not only to health and reproduction but even to life itself.

These accomplishments, plus many others, have enabled gynecology to become a broadly based discipline. Although this chapter is not intended to be a complete treatise on the diagnosis and management of gynecologic disorders, it is hoped that it provides a summation of the current and accepted knowledge of the specialty. Ideally, it will stimulate the reader to in-depth study regarding specific problems.[22]

EMBRYOLOGY AND ANATOMY

A knowledge of embryology is needed for proper understanding of gynecology, particularly because it relates to problems such as congenital malformation, hermaphroditism, endocrine interrelationships, and generative neoplasms. Minute details of this important series of embryologic changes are beyond the scope of this text but may be found in the work of Quigley and Gwatkin.[19] The external genitalia develop from the genital tubule, a group of cells found at the caudal end of the body. In week four after fertilization, it develops at the ventral tip of the cloacal membrane. The external genitalia of both sexes develop from this structure.

Androgens, produced by the testes, are responsible for masculinization of the undifferentiated external genitalia. In the absence of androgens, feminization of these structures occurs.

The internal reproductive structures and the lower urinary tract develop by the growth and resorption of primordial ductal systems (Fig. 44–1). The urogenital ridge forms on each side of the posterior body cavity. From these primordial cells develop the ovaries, the wolffian ducts and bodies, and the müllerian ducts. The müllerian ducts develop into the fallopian tubes, uterus, cervix, and upper vagina. To form these latter three structures, the müllerian ducts must fuse in the middle, and aplasia of one side or failure of fusion may result in congenital anomalies. Failure of resorption of the fused septum may result in vaginal or uterine septa or duplication.

The ovaries develop from coelomic epithelium covering the surface of the wolffian bodies. When ovarian development occurs, primordial follicles appear but remain inactive until gonadotropin stimulation begins. The wolffian ducts are the forerunner of the male reproductive system and undergo regressive changes in the female that cause them to become

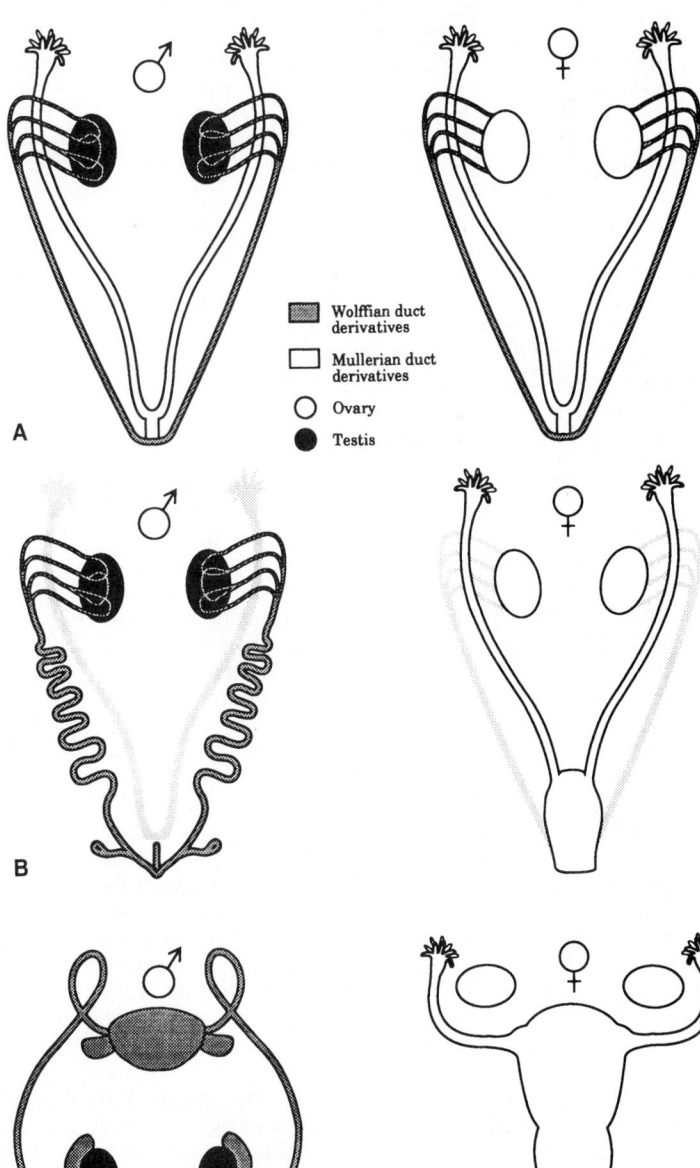

Figure 44–1. Development of the internal genital ducts. *A,* Indifferent stage. *B,* Intermediate stage. *C,* Definitive female and male. (From Quigley, M. M., and Gwatkin, R. B. L.: Embryology and developmental defects of the female reproductive system. *In* Scott, J. R., DiSaia, P. J., Hammond, C. B., and Spellacy, W. N. [Eds.]: Danforth's Obstetrics and Gynecology, 7th ed. Philadelphia, J. B. Lippincott, 1994.)

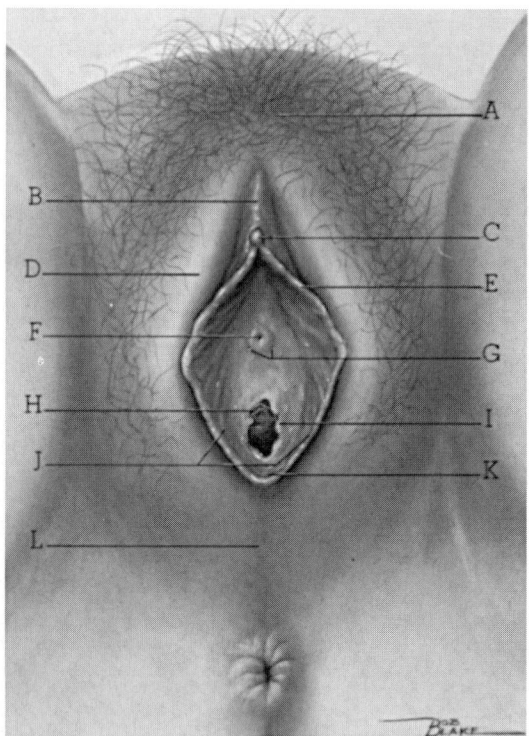

Figure 44–2. The external genitalia. A, mons pubis; B, prepuce; C, clitoris; D, labia majora; E, labia minora; F, urethral meatus; G, Skene's ducts; H, vagina; I, hymen; J, Bartholin's glands; K, posterior fourchette; L, perineal body.

vestigial. Remnants of the wolffian ducts persist in the normal female as ductal structures that may become clinically manifest as Gartner's duct cysts (lateral vaginal wall), parovarian cysts, and hydatid cysts of Morgagni.

The External Genitalia (Fig. 44–2)

The female external genitalia, or vulva, include the mons veneris, which is a fat pad over the pubic symphysis into which the labia majora blend. It is covered with skin that contains sweat glands and hair follicles. The labia majora are the most lateral structures of the external genitalia and do not acquire full growth until puberty. After menopause, atrophy may occur. These structures are covered with skin that contains sweat glands, hair follicles, and sebaceous and sudoriferous glands beneath the squamous epithelium. The underlying tissue is adipose, and the round ligaments of the uterus insert into the upper ends of the labia majora. The labia minora are medial to the majora and are covered with skin containing sweat glands but no hair follicles. The labia minora extend from the clitoris posteriorly and continue to the perineum. Anteriorly they pass over the top of the clitoris to form the prepuce and join below the clitoris to form the frenulum. Growth and configuration of the labia minora are influenced by estrogen. The clitoris is composed of two roots that traverse the pubic rami to unite beneath the symphysis in the clitoral body and terminate in the upper portion of the glans, which is exposed. The covering of the glans is modified cutaneous tissue. The clitoris contains two corpora cavernosa and is erectile.

The urethral meatus is situated below the clitoris and above the vaginal orifice. Lateral to this meatus open Skene's ducts, which lead from paraurethral glands. Bartholin's glands are located at 4 and 8 o'clock at the vulvovaginal orifice and are compound racemose glands that connect to the surface by a single tubule lined by transitional epithe-

lium. The gland acini are lined by a single layer of cuboidal epithelium. In its normal state the gland usually cannot be seen or palpated. The hymen divides the external and internal genitalia and may be a fibrous structure. The aperture varies greatly in size and shape and may on occasion be imperforate.

The Muscles and Fascia of the Perineum
(Fig. 44–3)

The superficial fascia of the perineum consists of outer and deep layers, both continuous with the layers of the anterior abdominal wall; the outer layer is called Cruveilhier's fascia and is continuous with Camper's fascia of the anterior abdominal wall; the deep layer of the superficial perineal fascia is called Colles' fascia and is continuous with Scarpa's fascia of the abdomen. The outer layer of superficial fascia forms the greater part of the labium majus and is continuous with the superficial fascia of the thigh. The deep layer of superficial fascia, Colles' fascia, is a strong membrane adding support to the urogenital structures. This fascia is firmly attached laterally to the medial surface of the thigh, being continuous with the fascia that covers the saphenous vein opening. It becomes attached to the deep fascia along the posterior border of the superficial transverse perineal muscle and blends on either side into the medial raphe of the perineum.

The deep perineal fascia consists of obturator fascia, infra-anal fascia, and fascia of the bulbocavernous, ischiocavernous, and transverse perineal muscles. The obturator fascia forms the lateral wall of the ischiorectal fossa and meets the infra-anal fascia deep in the fossa. The intra-anal fascia is the fascia of the levator ani and coccygeus muscles. The deep transverse perineal muscle is covered on both sides by fascia, and the three structures constitute the urogenital diaphragm. The urethra and vagina perforate this diaphragm, which stretches as a wall across the space between the ischiopubic

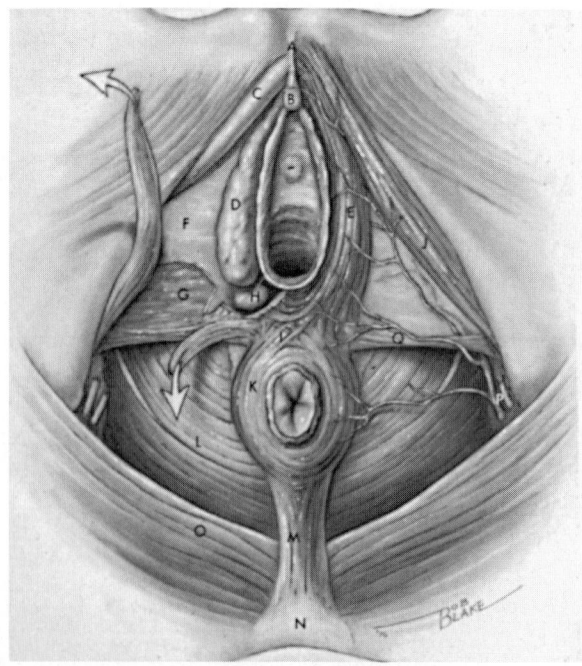

Figure 44–3. The muscles and fascia of the perineum. A, suspensory ligament of clitoris; B, clitoris; C, crus of clitoris; D, vestibular bulb; E, bulbocavernosus muscle; F, inferior fascia of urogenital diaphragm; G, deep transverse perineal muscle; H, Bartholin's gland; I, perineal body; J, ischiocavernosus muscle; K, external anal sphincter; L, levator ani muscle; M, anococcygeal body; N, coccyx; O, gluteus maximus muscle; P, pudendal artery and vein; Q, superficial transverse perineal muscle.

rami. The deep layer rests between the deep transverse perineal muscle and the pubococcygeal portions of the levator ani sling.

The perineal muscles divide into deep and superficial portions, sphincter urethrae, and bulbocavernosus and ischiocavernosus muscles. The superficial transverse perineal muscles arise from the ischial tuberosity on either side and insert into the central perineal tendon. They blend with the anal sphincter muscle and with fibers from the bulbocavernosus muscles. The bulbocavernosus muscles surround the vaginal orifice and have a sphincteric contractile effect arising anteriorly from the clitoris and inserting posteriorly into the perineal body. The ischiocavernosus muscles arise from the medial borders of the ischial rami and clitoris and course posteriorly and laterally to insert into the ischial tuberosity. The sphincter muscle of the urethra is attached to the periurethral structures and fans laterally on either side to attach to the pubic rami. The deep transverse perineal muscle lies below the superficial muscle and attaches in the midline of the perineal body.

The Internal Genitalia (Fig. 44–4)

The Vagina. The vagina is a muscular tube lined with stratified squamous epithelium that is histologically similar to the mucosa of the cervix and vulva. It does not contain glands or hair follicles, but individual cells produce mucus. The superficial layer is not keratinized. During menstrual life the vagina has transverse folds called rugae. After menopause, in the absence of estrogen, the vaginal walls become thin and atrophic, reflecting the lack of estrogen seen in the childhood years. The adult vagina measures 12 to 13 cm. in depth, and in nulliparous women there is coaptation of the anterior and posterior walls. The vaginal axis is toward the sacral promontory, and the cervix is suspended at the upper end, surrounded by the anterior, posterior, and lateral fornices. The upper two thirds of the vagina is supported by the paravaginal fascia and the paracervical tissues and the lower one third by the perineal body.

The Cervix. The inferior portion of the uterus, the cervix, is a fibromuscular organ covered with stratified squamous epithelium. The portio vaginalis of the cervix arises in the vaginal fornices and ends at the external cervical os at the entrance of the endocervical canal. This squamocolumnar junction is the most common site of origin of squamous cell carcinoma. The endocervical canal is lined by columnar epithelium, and racemose glands, lined with similar epithelium, are found in the fibromuscular stroma. Such glands, if obstructed, may form nabothian cysts on the cervical surface. The nulliparous cervical os is round, but parturition changes this to a horizontally flattened orifice. The cervix is the second most common site of genital malignancy in women.

The Uterus. The uterus is a hollow, fibromuscular-walled organ between the bladder and rectum and consists of the cervix and fundus. The organ is pear shaped and in nonpregnant women measures approximately 8 cm. in length and weighs 30 to 100 gm. The fallopian tubes and the cervical canal communicate with the uterine cavity, which is lined by the endometrium. The endometrium proliferates in response to estrogen, becomes secretory with progesterone, and bleeds as it sloughs when hormonal support is withdrawn or inadequate. The uterine fundus is covered by peritoneum except in the lower anterior portion, where the bladder is contiguous with the lower uterine segment and the peritoneum is reflected, and laterally where the folds of the broad ligament are attached. The uterus is supported by condensations of endopelvic fascia and fibromuscular tissue laterally at the base of the broad ligaments. The round ligaments provide

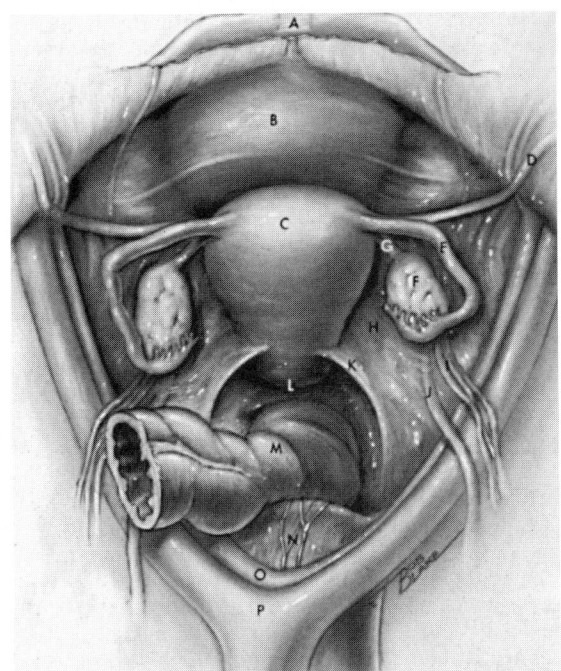

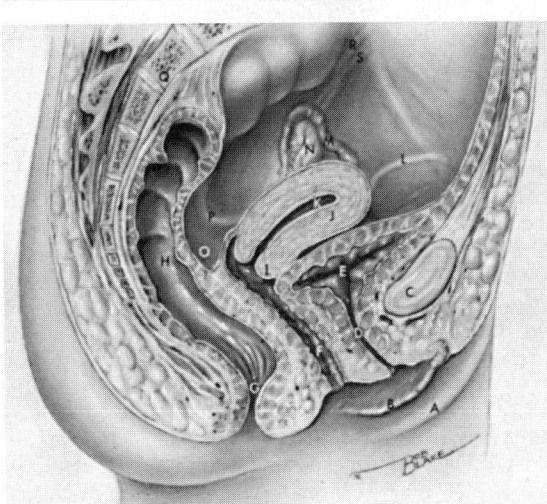

Figure 44–4. The internal genitalia. *Front view:* A, symphysis pubis; B, bladder; C, corpus uteri; D, round ligament; E, fallopian tube; F, ovary; G, utero-ovarian ligament; H, broad ligament; I, ovarian artery and vein; J, ureter; K, uterosacral ligament; L, cul-de-sac; M, rectum; N, middle sacral artery and vein; O, vena cava; P, aorta. *Side view:* A, labium majus; B, labium minus; C, symphysis pubis; D, urethra; E, bladder; F, vagina; G, anus; H, rectum; I, cervix uteri; J, corpus uteri; K, endometrial cavity; L, round ligament; M, fallopian tube; N, ovary; O, cul-de-sac; P, uterosacral ligament; Q, sacrum; R, ureter; S, ovarian artery and vein.

support laterally and the uterovesical fold, anteriorly. Neither of these two structures provides major uterine support.

The Oviducts. The fallopian tubes arise from the superior portion of the lateral borders of the uterus, superior to the attachment of the round ligaments, and are patent. The distal ends, the fimbriae, open into the abdominal cavity and the proximal ends open into the uterine cavity. The tubes are lined by a single layer of low columnar epithelium, some ciliated, arranged in a branching or frond pattern. This structure is divided into interstitial, isthmic, ampullar, and fimbriated portions. The wall is thin with two muscular layers and an outer layer of peritoneum within the upper borders of the broad ligament.

The Ovaries. The normal ovary is a white, almond-shaped structure measuring 2 × 3 × 3 cm. and is located on the posterior surface of the broad ligament and inferior to the fallopian tube. The nerves, lymphatics, and blood vessels enter the ovary at the point of attachment to the broad ligament, the hilus. Lateral support of the ovary is provided by the infundibulopelvic ligament, which extends to the pelvic side wall, and the medial support is to the uterus by the utero-ovarian ligament. The ovary has a cortex and a medulla. Germinal epithelium, a single layer of cuboidal cells, covers condensed fibrous tissue called the tunica albuginea. Follicles originate within the ovarian cortex and are composed of the basic embryonic complement; no new follicles are formed after birth. The medullary portion of the ovary is occupied by blood vessels, lymphatics, nerves, and connective tissue and contains remnants of wolffian body precursors. The ovary is an endocrine and a generative organ. Parafollicular granulosa cells produce estrogen and, after ovulation and corpus luteum formation, progestins. Androgens are produced by stromal cells, particularly in the hilus.

The Urinary System. The kidneys and ureters arise from the metanephros and a diverticulum from the wolffian duct in both sexes. The ureters vary from 28 to 34 cm. in length, with the right ureter 1 to 2 cm. shorter than the left. The ureter is not of uniform caliber. The abdominal part of the ureter lies behind the peritoneum on the medial part of the psoas muscle and is crossed obliquely by the ovarian vessels. It enters the pelvis by crossing either the termination of the common iliac vessels or the commencement of the external iliac vessels. The pelvic ureter courses at first downward on the lateral wall of the pelvic, then medially and forward toward the lateral aspect of the cervix, about 1.5 cm. from the exterior of the cervix. In this course, it is accompanied by the uterine artery. The uterine artery then crosses over the ureter and ascends between the leaves of the broad ligament to enter the uterus laterally. The blood supply of the ureter arises from branches of the renal, ovarian, hypogastric, and inferior vesical arteries.

In the female, the uterus, cervix, and upper vagina are behind the bladder, which is separated from the uterus by the vesicouterine fold. Below this peritoneal fold the bladder is connected to the cervix and upper vagina by areolar tissue. The bladder is stabilized by ligamentous attachments at its inferior portion or base, near the exit of the urethra, and at the vertex. The remainder is free to move. The basal attachment is to the internal investing layer of deep fascia on the pubic bone by strong fibrous bands. The arterial supply of the bladder is the superior, middle, and inferior vesical arteries, derived from the anterior hypogastric artery, the obturator and inferior gluteal arteries, and the uterine and vaginal arteries.

The female urethra is a narrow membranous canal about 4 cm. long, extending from the internal to the external urethral orifice. It is placed behind the symphysis, embedded in the anterior vaginal wall, and its direction is obliquely downward and forward. The resting diameter is about 6 mm. The urethra perforates the fascia of the urogenital diaphragm, where it acquires longitudinal folds. Many small paraurethral glands open into the urethra.

The Blood Vessels of the Pelvis (Fig. 44–5)

The ovarian arteries arise from the front of the aorta just below the renal arteries. The left ovarian vein empties into the left renal vein; the right ovarian vein empties into the vena cava just inferior to the renal vein. The ovarian vessels follow a downward course and pass between the layers of the infundibulopelvic ligament and the broad ligament to reach the ovary. Small branches divide to supply the ureter and fallopian tube. The main branches unite with the uterine

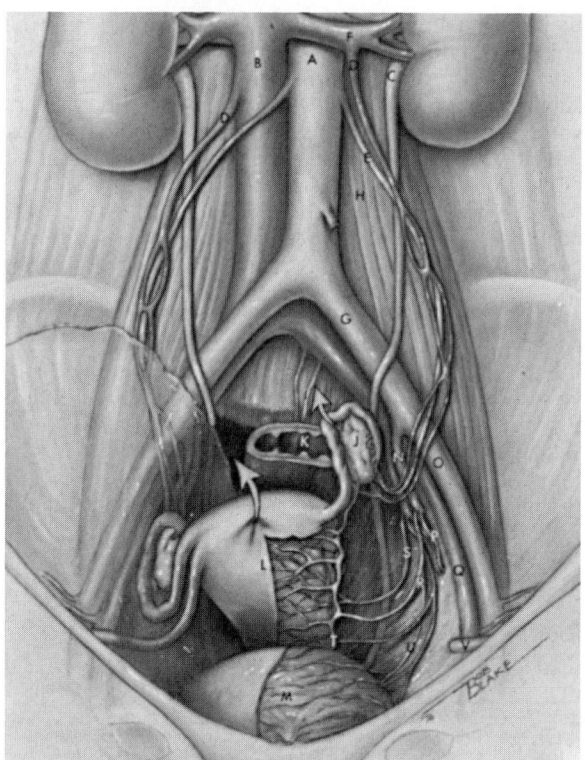

Figure 44–5. Blood supply of the pelvis. A, aorta; B, inferior vena cava; C, ureter; D, ovarian vein; E, ovarian artery; F, renal vein; G, common iliac artery; H, psoas muscle; I, middle sacral artery; J, ovary; K, rectum; L, corpus uteri; M, bladder; N, internal iliac (hypogastric) artery, anterior branch; O, external iliac artery; P, obturator artery; Q, external iliac vein; R, uterine artery; S, uterine vein; T, vaginal artery; U, superior vesicle artery; V, inferior epigastric artery.

vessels on the side of the uterus, and small branches supply the round ligaments.

The iliac vessels originate as the common iliac arteries from the aorta at the L4 vertebral level and slightly to the left of midline. Each is about 5 cm. long and, just below the S1 level, divide into the internal iliac (hypogastric) artery and the external iliac artery. The common iliac veins closely follow the arteries and join inferiorly and to the right of the aorta to form the vena cava. The external iliac vessels lie on the lateral walls of the pelvis above the psoas muscles, behind the peritoneum, to pass beneath the inguinal ligaments through the femoral canal to become the femoral artery and vein. The inferior epigastric vessels arise from the external iliac vessels immediately superior to the ligament. The hypogastric (internal iliac) vessels pass inferiorly and posteriorly along the border of the great sciatic notch. The hypogastric vessels are 3 to 4 cm. in length before they divide into anterior and posterior branches. The anterior branch provides the main blood supply to the bladder and forms the middle hemorrhoidal, obturator, internal pudendal, inferior gluteal, uterine, and vaginal arteries. An inferior branch of the uterine artery turns inferiorly on either side to form the cervical arteries. The vaginal artery arises from the hypogastric artery below the level of the uterine artery and sends branches to the vagina, bladder, and rectum. The internal pudendal artery is the most caudal extension of the hypogastric artery and supplies the internal genital organs. This vessel emerges from the pelvis between the piriformis and coccygeus muscles, crosses the ischial spine, and passes through the lesser sciatic foramen to enter the perineum. The artery traverses the lateral wall of the ischiorectal fossa and supplies the erectile tissue of the vulva.

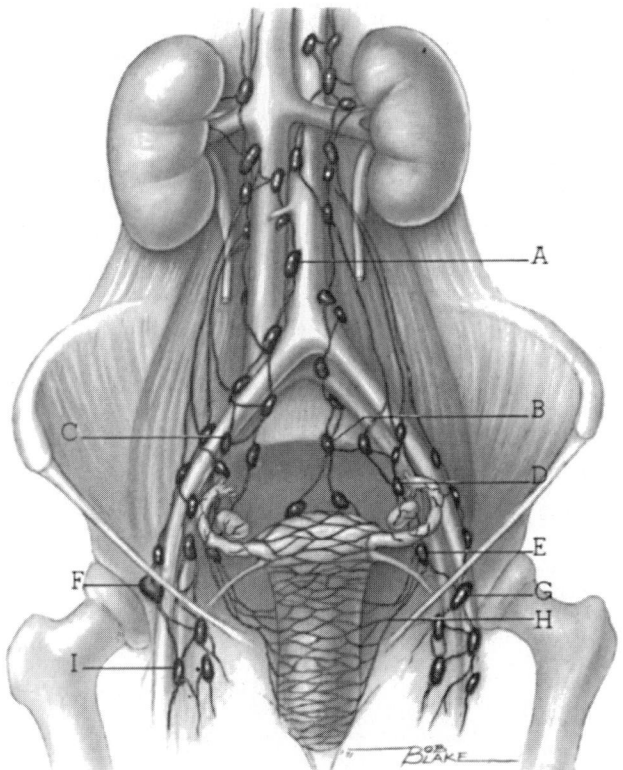

Figure 44–6. Lymphatics of the pelvic. A, aortic; B, sacral; C, common iliac; D, hypogastric; E, obturator; F, deep inguinal; G, Cloquet's node; H, parametrial; I, superficial inguinal.

The Lymphatics of the Pelvis (Fig. 44–6)

The lymphatics of the pelvis parallel the vascular channels. The external iliac nodes are interposed in the drainage pattern of the deep inguinal nodes, the fundus of the bladder, and the uterus, cervix, and upper vagina. The external iliac and hypogastric drainage occurs by means of the common iliac nodes. The hypogastric nodes surround the hypogastric vessels and receive drainage from the cervix, uterine fundus, upper vagina, bladder, urethra, and lower ureter. The obturator nodes reside in the obturator fossa, lateral to and surrounding the obturator nerve, and receive channels from the cervix, uterus, and part of the buttocks. The sacral nodes receive branches from the cervix and uterus and reside in the sacral concavity. The rectal lymphatics course posteriorly to the sacral nodes also. The vulvar drainage takes place through subcutaneous ascending lymphatics to the superficial and deep inguinal nodes and femoral nodes, which also receive the lymphatics from the lower portions of the vagina and urethra. The lower extremity lymphatics lead to the femoral and inguinal nodes. Cross drainage in this region may occur from Cloquet's node (femoral canal) to deep nodes of the pelvis.

The Nerve Supply of the Pelvis

The sacral plexus arises from the fourth and fifth lumbar and the first four sacral cord segments. The pudendal nerve originates from the second, third, and fourth sacral segments. The plexus rests in the hollow of the pelvis over the piriformis muscle. The branches of the plexus contain fibers of sympathetic and parasympathetic nerve trunks. The parasympathetic fibers are efferent and preganglionic to the pelvic viscera and afferent from the pelvic organs. The sympa-

thetic fibers arise from the hypogastric sympathetic plexus. The levator ani, coccygeus, and sphincter ani muscles receive branches from the pudendal plexus. The pudendal nerve leaves the pelvis through the greater sciatic foramen, crosses the ischial spine, and reenters the pelvis through the lesser sciatic foramen. It accompanies the pudendal vessels and sends branches to the sphincter ani muscle and sensory fibers to the labia majora, while another branch supplies the perineal muscles. The dorsal nerve of the clitoris also arises from the pudendal nerve.

PHYSIOLOGY AND ENDOCRINOLOGY

The interactions of physiologic and endocrinologic mechanisms cannot be separated in any adequate summary of the function of the female genital system. Numerous workers have identified the interrelationships among the central nervous system, hypothalamus, pituitary, ovary, and other endocrine systems. Dependence on estrogen and progesterone of the pelvic structures, breasts, skin, and other organs and on many metabolic processes has been demonstrated.

Hypothalamus, Pituitary, and Gonadotropins. The hypothalamus serves as the primary control center for the reproductive endocrine system. This system is essentially dormant until late childhood, when activation begins and certain hypothalamic cells become capable of releasing short-chain peptides to the anterior pituitary through the hypophyseal portal system. With the discovery of gonadotropin-releasing hormone (GnRH) by Schally and Guillemin, followed shortly thereafter by the synthesis of this compound, many new understandings of the hypothalamic control of gonadotropin secretion became possible.[5] In experimental animals and in humans, these humoral agents, or releasing factors, cause the anterior pituitary to produce and release follicle-stimulating hormone (FSH) and luteinizing hormone (LH). Physiologic, pathologic, and even psychologic problems can alter these interrelationships.

The pituitary gonadotropins, FSH and LH, are necessary for normal ovarian function and, through the hypothalamus, are in turn regulated through feedback mechanisms from ovarian estrogen and progesterone (Fig. 44–7). FSH is made in the anterior pituitary, is transmitted through the blood, and stimulates maturation of the ovarian follicle and parafollicular cells to produce estrogen. This gonadotropin, which can occasionally be found in small amounts in young girls, increases nocturnally just before puberty and is found in

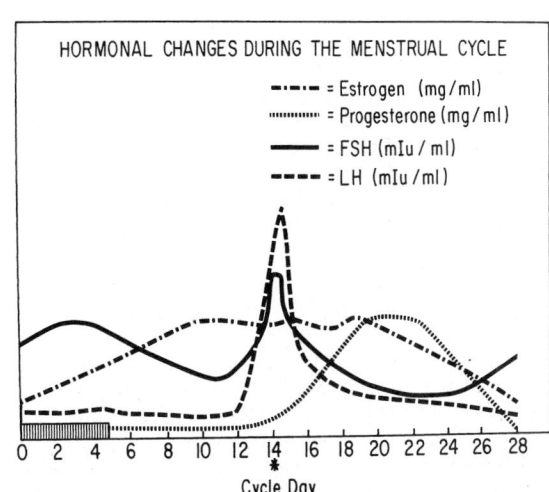

Figure 44–7. Hormonal changes during the menstrual cycle. Menses, days 0–5, ovulation, day 14.

large quantities in mature women. After the ovarian failure of menopause, there is a sharp rise in FSH as the hypothalamus attempts to correct resultant hypoestrogenism. In ovulating women, FSH is elevated during the follicular phase of the cycle, then rises sharply at mid cycle. FSH levels are relatively low during the luteal phase of the cycle. LH complements FSH secretion, and the two provide a synergistic effect on ovarian function. LH levels are relatively low during the follicular and luteal phases of the menstrual cycle but rise sharply for a 72-hour span surrounding ovulation. LH, acting on the FSH-stimulated follicle, can cause ovulation. LH also stimulates the interstitial cells of the ovary and may be an integral part of corpus luteum maintenance. Still another ovarian hormone, inhibin, is not yet fully characterized but appears to be a true ovarian secretory product. It appears that inhibin participates in regulation of FSH, in addition to estrogen, but its precise mechanisms are still being elucidated. Excessive amounts of sex steroid hormones, estrogen, progesterone, or androgens, inhibit hypothalamic control of pituitary secretion.

Neurotransmitters. Much work has been done during the past decade to study mechanisms of control of release of hypothalamic GnRH, as well as the pituitary gonadotropins, LH and FSH. The amplitude and frequency of the pulsatile release of GnRH not only are regulated by the feedback of two ovarian steroids, estradiol and progesterone, as well as by gonadotropins through the hormonal input pathway but are also modulated by several neurotransmitters and neuromodulators within the brain through a neural input pathway.[12]

The most important neurotransmitters involved in reproductive endocrinology are two catecholamines, dopamine and norepinephrine, as well as an indolamine, serotonin (Figs. 44–8 and 44–9). All three are monoamines. Dopamine is a neurotransmitter itself, as well as the precursor of another neurotransmitter, norepinephrine. Dopamine, in addition to stimulating prolactin-inhibiting factor and thus decreasing prolactin release, acts in the median eminence and appears to inhibit the release of GnRH. Several studies have demonstrated that dopamine inhibits LH secretion in humans. The role of norepinephrine is less clear; however, it may stimulate

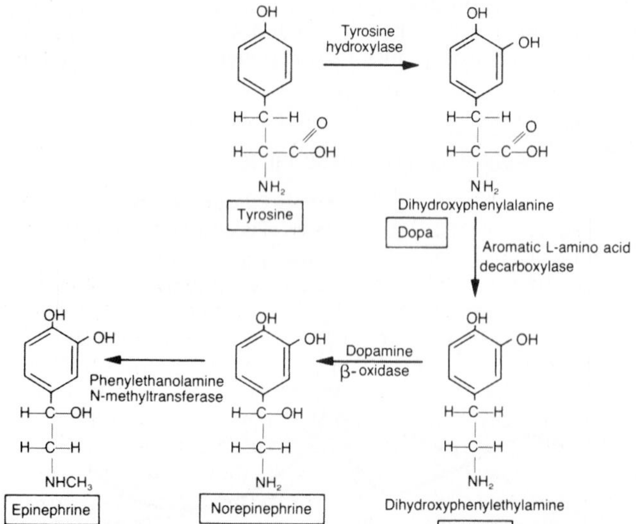

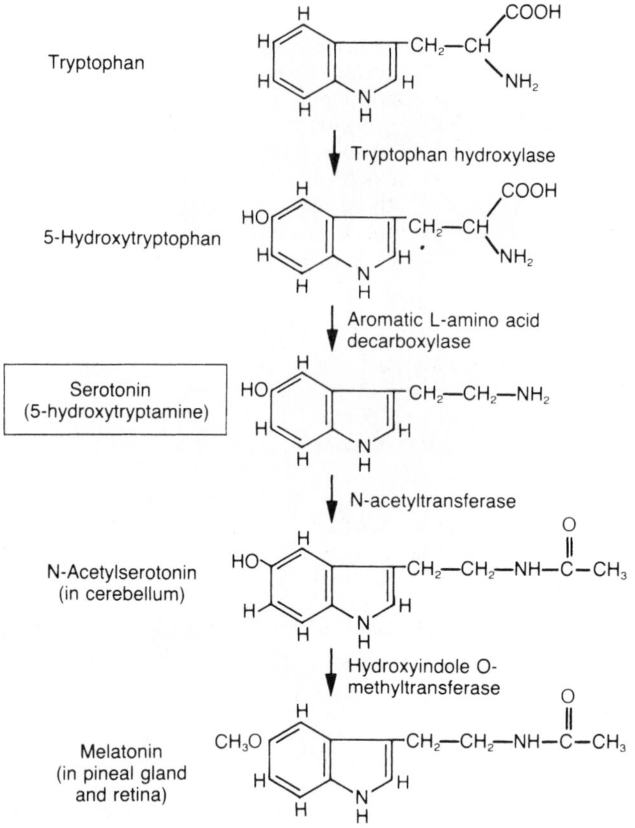

Figure 44–9. Metabolic pathways of serotonin synthesis. (From Kletzky, O. A., and Lobo, R. A.: Reproductive neuroendocrinology. *In* Mishell, D. R., Jr., and Davajan, V. [Eds.]: Infertility, Contraception and Reproductive Endocrinology, 2nd ed. Oradell, NJ, Medical Economics Books, 1986.)

the release of GnRH. Epinephrine has little effect on reproductive hormone release. Serotonin has not been shown to affect GnRH release, but it does stimulate the release of prolactin.

Neuromodulators

Opioids. Receptors for opioid peptides are present in the brain. There are three subgroups of opioids: enkephalins, endorphins (alpha, beta, gamma), and dynorphins. The concentrations of endorphins are approximately 1000 times higher in the pituitary than in the hypothalamus. Infusion of beta-endorphin results in an increase of prolactin and a decrease of LH.

Prostaglandins. Hypothalamic levels of prostaglandins may modulate the release of GnRH. Infusion of prostaglandin E$_2$ significantly increases GnRH levels in portal blood.

Catechol Estrogens. The compounds 2-hydroxyestradiol and 2-hydroxyestrone, as well as their 3-methyl derivatives, are present in the hypothalamus and are postulated to act as neuromodulators by altering the function of catecholamines.

Ovarian Function. During infancy and childhood, the ovary is dormant, owing to low gonadotropin production, but it is capable of being stimulated if these hormones are present. The beginning of puberty and the age of menarche vary considerably among individuals, but the usual age for the first menstrual period is from 12 to 15 years. The early menstrual periods are usually irregular and anovulatory. Later, regular ovulatory cycles usually ensue. At puberty there is a spurt in somatic growth. Later in adolescence, higher levels of estrogen result in epiphyseal plate closure.

Before puberty, the primordial follicles develop in the deeper portions of the ovary; and after puberty, the maturing follicle migrates to the surface of the ovary. After achieving

Figure 44–8. Metabolic pathways of dopamine, norepinephrine, and epinephrine synthesis. (From Kletzky, O. A., and Lobo, R. A.: Reproductive neuroendocrinology. *In* Mishell, D. R., Jr., and Davajan, V. [Eds.]: Infertility, Contraception and Reproductive Endocrinology, 2nd ed. Oradell, NJ, Medical Economics Books, 1986.)

full maturation, the graafian follicle ruptures and the ovum is extruded into the peritoneal cavity, usually around the fourteenth day of the cycle. With rupture of the follicle, the corpus luteum is formed. It persists for 14 days in a normal cycle. Should pregnancy occur, the corpus luteum will persist for approximately 12 weeks before beginning regression. After ovulation, the corpus luteum shows hypertrophy and vascularization of the theca lutein cells. The granulosa cells about the follicle become enlarged and polyhedral and are transformed into lutein cells. Progesterone, produced in small amounts just before ovulation, is now produced in large amounts. About 4 days before menses, the corpus luteum regresses and loses the ability to produce progesterone unless hCG from pregnancy sustains corpus luteum function.

Menopause occurs with waning of ovarian function, usually between 46 and 53 years of age. With intrinsic failure of the ovary, there is atresia of the follicles and failure of estrogen production, which is at first sharp but later becomes more gradual, with a minimal amount of estrogen production extending for several additional years. With the decline of estrogen, the breasts atrophy, the pelvic structures become smaller, and the vaginal mucosa becomes thin and smooth.

Estrogen. Many studies have demonstrated that oophorectomy performed on the immature female is followed by persistent infantile characteristics of genital tissues. If the gonads are removed from a mature female animal, the uterus and breasts atrophy. The human ovary produces estradiol-17β, the most potent naturally occurring estrogen, along with estrone and estriol. These estrogens are produced primarily in the theca interna cells. Preadolescent girls and women beyond the menopause secrete little estrogen. The adult cycling woman produces 10 to 55 μg. of the various estrogens each day, with a low level during menses, which increases steadily until ovulation. After ovulation there is a slight decline; then significant levels persist until 2 to 3 days before menses. The placenta and adrenal glands also produce estrogens.

The estrogens are lipids with the same phenanthrene nucleus as the other steroids, from which they are distinguished by a phenolic ring A. In addition to natural estrogens, chemicals with estrogenic activity have been synthesized. These include diethylstilbestrol, hexestrol, dienestrol, and, most recently, a group of ethinyl-17α steroids. The various estrogens are rapidly metabolized by the liver and are conjugated with glucuronic and sulfuric acid. These conjugated compounds are excreted 60% in urine and 40% in bile and feces by other routes.

The principal physiologic function of estrogen is stimulation of growth of the endometrium, the myometrium, other tissues of müllerian origin, the vulva, and breast. Estrogen is responsible for uterine and tubal contractility and is the feminizing hormone that at puberty brings about the secondary sex characteristics: mammary growth, primarily of ductal tissue, and the adult female fat pad distribution. A variety of metabolic processes are also influenced by estrogen, notably plasma protein production, bone matrix stabilization, and lipid metabolism.

Progesterone. Progesterone is the other steroid hormone produced by the ovary. The corpus luteum begins to secrete this hormone just before ovulation and throughout the luteal phase of the cycle. The placenta and adrenal glands also produce progesterone. It is synthesized in the body from cholesterol by means of pregnenolone and is converted by the ovary to estrogens and small amounts of testosterone. The production rate of progesterone from the ovary and adrenal glands of a normal adult woman is approximately 3 mg. per 24 hours during the follicular phase of the cycle and 22 mg. per 24 hours during the luteal phase. Progesterone is readily synthesized for both oral and parenteral use. Natural progesterone is deactivated by gastric secretions. Synthetic progestins are abundantly available and are useful for treating menstrual disorders, endometriosis, and inhibition of ovulation.

Progesterone is essentially for maintenance of pregnancy; initially it is produced by the corpus luteum and later by the placenta. It has not been of major use as a drug for quieting uterine activity or labor. There is some evidence that progesterone reduces tubal activity. Progesterone is responsible for the acinar and lobular development in the breast and characteristic changes seen in cervical mucus and in cervical and vaginal cytology. Progesterone is thermogenic, and basal body temperatures are 0.2° to 0.8° F. higher in the latter half of the ovulatory cycle.

Genital Structures. The female genitalia are responsive to estrogen. In the child, these structures are immature and thin and begin to mature only with pubescence and the onset of ovarian function. The vulva is thin and not prominent. The vaginal epithelium, which is quite thick at birth because of maternal gestational hormones, rapidly regresses to a thin membrane and is pH neutral. With puberty the vagina thickens, glycogen storage increases, and pH becomes more acid. The cycling woman's vagina normally contains diphtheroids and Döderlein's bacilli, which aid normal vaginal secretion and acidity. After menopause, the vagina again becomes thin and loses the normal rugal pattern, and pH slowly rises. Exfoliated vaginal cells may be stained and microscopically examined for histologic changes that occur with the varying hormonal patterns.

The cervix of the child is disproportionately larger than the fundus, but after puberty this ratio is reversed. As in the vagina, the cervical epithelium undergoes cyclic changes during the menstrual cycle, but these are less than those seen in the endometrium. The racemose glands of the endocervix are dormant in children but initiate secretion of mucus after puberty. Under the dominance of estrogen, the cervical mucus increases, is thin and watery, and forms a *fern* pattern when dried. When progesterone is present, cervical mucus is opaque, thick, and tenacious and does not fern. After menopause, cervical mucus production declines as estrogen production declines.

The myometrium of the adult woman normally undergoes spontaneous rhythmic contractions. The uteri of castrates lose this rhythmicity. Hypertrophy of myometrium occurs when higher levels of estrogen are present, and uterine atrophy occurs after menopause. The endometrium reflects generally the levels of estrogen and progesterone. Estrogen causes proliferation of the endometrium and its vascular channels. Progesterone transforms proliferative into secretory endometrium, with glandular and stromal features that promote possible implantation. Endometrial biopsy is a simple office procedure that may allow precise interpretation of ovarian hormonal production.

The fallopian tube epithelium also reflects ovarian hormonal changes through cyclic modification, maturation, and regression changes. The tubal musculature possesses an intrinsic peristaltic action believed to aid tubal transport. The action of cilia of certain tubal cells may also be involved in transport. Estrogen appears to influence these activities.

Of interest have been studies of the impact of chronic hypoestrogenism (menopause, castration, and other causes) on maintenance of bone density (osteoporosis) and arteriosclerotic cardiovascular diseases, particularly coronary artery disease. It appears that replacement of estrogen is the most potent prophylaxis to retard the development of age-related osteoporosis and fracture, as well as providing a significant benefit on these cardiovascular diseases, probably through direct effects and by beneficial modulation of plasma lipids.[11]

THE GYNECOLOGIC HISTORY AND EXAMINATION

An adequate history remains a prerequisite for intelligent diagnosis and treatment. All elements of a general medical history are essential to adequate evaluation of pelvic complaints.[14] This gynecologic history should include the following:

Present illness: A chronologic story of the patient's problem, relating symptoms, signs, dates, effects of other organ function, and prior investigation or therapy.

Menstrual pattern: Age at onset of menses; frequency, duration, and amount of flow; menstrual irregularities; date of the first day of the two most recent episodes of menstrual bleeding; history of pain with menses and its location, character, and duration; any vaginal bleeding between periods or any contact such as douching or coitus; and any other major physiologic or pathologic changes associated with menses.

Vaginal discharge: Amount, type, color, relation to menses, itching, and previous vaginal infections and therapy.

Obstetric history: Each pregnancy should be listed chronologically, with comments about duration, complications, delivery and the puerperium.

Marital history: The dates of marriages, contraceptive techniques and duration of use, frequency of coitus, and dyspareunia.

Other factors: Sensations of pressure, incontinence, urinary symptoms, bowel complaints, pelvic or abdominal surgery including findings and complications, and a thorough general and endocrine systems review.

The normal woman dislikes a pelvic examination and presents for examination with reservation. Gentleness, privacy, and dignity are necessary, and a female chaperon should always be present for assistance, patient reassurance, and protection from possible legal embarrassment. Each step in the pelvic examination should be explained briefly to the patient to gain her confidence and cooperation. The pelvic examination is done with the patient in the lithotomy position with the legs placed in stirrups. Before being placed on the table, the patient should empty her bladder. The chaperon aids in positioning of the patient and drapes her.

The first part of the pelvic examination consists of inspection of the external genitalia for evidence of infection, neoplasia, hypertrophy, atrophy, or trauma. Specific note is made about skin texture, hair patterns, clitoral size, Skene's ducts, and Bartholin's glands. The groin should be examined. The speculum examination is next, and a variety of instruments of different sizes and shapes are available. There is no substitute for adequate equipment and lighting. The instrument should be at approximately body temperature and lubricated slightly. The vaginal wall and cervix should be inspected for size, shape, and evidence of atrophy, infection, trauma, bleeding, or neoplasia. Specimens can be obtained for cancer cytologic study, hormonal interpretation, and bacteriologic examination. The vagina should be inspected again during withdrawal of the speculum, particularly the anterior and posterior surfaces, which may have been covered initially by the blades of the speculum. The patient then performs the Valsalva maneuver while the support of the bladder, rectum, and uterus is visualized, and note is made of any stress incontinence.

The examiner then proceeds to the bimanual part of the examination, introducing the first two fingers of one hand into the vagina and palpating above the symphysis with the outer hand (Fig. 44–10). The physician attempts to determine the consistency, size, shape, and mobility of the uterus. After the uterus is palpated, the adnexal regions are felt. Next, it is

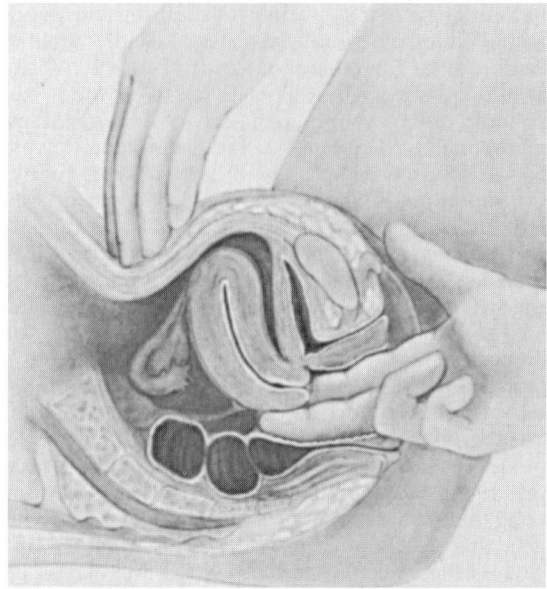

Figure 44–10. Bimanual pelvic examination. The examiner inserts two fingers into the vagina and places the other hand on the lower abdomen. The structures of the pelvis are then outlined between the two hands. (From Nelson, J. H., Jr.: Atlas of Radical Pelvic Surgery. New York, Appleton-Century-Crofts, 1969.)

important to palpate the parametrial and paracervical areas. Finally, a combined rectovaginal examination should be done. In children and virgins, a rectal examination may be all that is possible because of the intact hymen. A child's small speculum or Kelly cystoscope may aid visualization, and appropriate smears should be obtained.

LABORATORY AND CLINICAL TESTS

Cytologic Studies. Approximately 20% of cases of cancer in women arise in the genital tract. The most useful techniques for the early detection of genital malignant diseases are the pelvic examination and Papanicolaou studies. It should be routine to utilize these techniques for all women when they become sexually active or by 18 years of age and at least at yearly intervals thereafter. Not only can early malignancy be detected but also premalignant changes may frequently be discovered. Malignant and preinvasive lesions arising from the genital organs exfoliate tumor cells, which may traverse the intermediate structures and collect in the vaginal pool and on the surface of the cervix. Malignant cells from the cervix will often be present in patients with these lesions. If the tumor is of the vulva, it may be missed unless the external genitals are carefully examined and direct scrapings obtained from suspicious areas. For endometrial or uterine smears, best results are achieved by passing a fine probe, sound, or small brush into the uterine cavity and obtaining direct smears. Malignant tumors of the tubes or ovaries rarely exfoliate cells that can be collected on routine pelvic examinations.

Exfoliated cells are collected by aspiration or gentle scraping and are evenly spread onto glass slides, then immediately fixed in an equal solution of ether and 95% alcohol. Deeper scraping may yield basal cells of different cytologic patterns, which may confuse the unwary cytologist. Delay in fixation may allow drying and cytologic alteration. After fixation and Papanicolaou staining, slides should be studied microscopically by an experienced cytologist for cytologic changes compatible with malignancy.

Papanicolaou cervical cytology offers a high degree of accuracy but can be no better than the material collected. If gross infection or blood and mucus are present, care must be exercised to provide sufficient material for study. Such cytologic studies should be used in the detection of premalignant disease of hidden or occult malignant disease and for follow-up of patients after treatment of malignant disease. *Cytologic studies should rarely if ever be used as an indication for surgical or irradiative therapy;* rather, they should lead the examiner to diagnostic surgical studies to provide adequate tissue for histopathologic diagnosis.

Vaginal material obtained for study of the etiology of vaginal infection is mixed with saline, placed on a slide, and microscopically examined for the presence of *Trichomonas vaginalis* or *Candida albicans* (Fig. 44–11). Cultures may be required for positive identification of vulvovaginal fungus.

Cervical Studies. Although Papanicolaou cytology is the major approach in the screening for premalignant cervical or vaginal neoplasia, other techniques may be of use. Gross visualization of the cervix is mandatory, and any suspicious areas should be sampled; usually anesthesia is not required for this. The cervix may be painted with an iodine solution, such as Schiller's stain, with which normal cells rich in glycogen stain darkly, whereas neoplastic cells do not take the

stain. This technique, as well as colposcopy or colpomicroscopy (microscopic visualization of the cervix *in situ*), can serve to direct biopsies for histologic diagnosis. Endocervical curettage should also be used with this technique. If abnormal Papanicolaou smears have been reported, use must be made of either multiple biopsies or cold-knife conization of the cervix, which removes the exocervix, including the squamocolumnar junction, and the endocervical canal. The important fact is not to overlook the diagnosis of invasive carcinoma. Presumption of a benign or premalignant diagnosis on the basis of cytology alone may mean a patient with occult invasive carcinoma receives inadequate therapy.

The colposcope and colpomicroscope have increasingly become valuable tools for the evaluation of suspected neoplastic lesions. Magnification, coupled with various staining techniques, allows an accurate *in vivo* analysis and enables the examiner to properly direct biopsies from areas not noted in a nonmagnified evaluation. However, like most technology, proper education is mandatory to avoid missing detectable lesions and flawed evaluations may cause misdiagnosis and/or inadequate therapy.

Cervical smears and cultures are quite important for the diagnosis of gonorrhea and chlamydia, but all too often negative results are obtained because of faulty technique. To properly obtain cervical cultures, a vaginal speculum is inserted and the cervix is wiped clean with cotton swabs. Through compressive force of the blade of the speculum on the anterior and posterior cervix, the mucus of the endocervical glands is *milked* into the endocervical canal. A sterile culture swab is introduced into the endocervical canal, with care not to contaminate the swab with other vaginal secretions. One such swab is spread on a slide, dried, stained with Gram's stain, and examined under high microscopic power for the classic gram-negative intracellular diplococci. Another swab is immediately placed onto Thayer-Martin medium and then incubated in carbon dioxide for culture identification. One should never inform a patient that she unequivocally has gonorrhea on the basis of a smear, although therapy can be initiated. Diagnosis of this disease without culture identification might be fraught with legal hazard. In similar manner, cultures for chlamydia can be made. The presence of herpesvirus should be ascertained by opening vulvar or vaginal *blisters* and, after mild abrasion, placing swabs in appropriate transfer media.

Endometrial Studies. The endometrial biopsy is used to study hormonal effects, fertility, and ovulatory factors and, on occasion, to aid in the diagnosis of malignancy. The procedure is done without anesthesia, and discomfort is minimal. By the insertion of a fine curette, several samples of endometrium can be obtained for histopathologic examination. If the diagnosis for suspected neoplasia is negative, however, an indicated dilation and curettage with or without hysteroscopic guidance should seldom be replaced by endometrial biopsy, because the tissue sampled by curettage is considerably greater and diagnosis more accurate. Endocrine changes are reflected quite adequately through such endometrial biopsy techniques, and by timing the biopsy to the latter half of the menstrual cycle the presence of progesterone and ovulation can be detected.

Pregnancy Tests. Pregnancy may be determined by a variety of tests that detect the presence of hCG. Most immunologic tests give a positive result with a concentration of 20 to 40 mIU per ml. Such concentrations are usually achieved just before or near the time of the first missed menstrual period. Highly specific radioimmunoassays for the beta subunit of hCG can be even more sensitive and specific. Quantified levels of hCG are now readily available and are particularly useful in monitoring for ectopic gestation or other abnormal pregnancies.

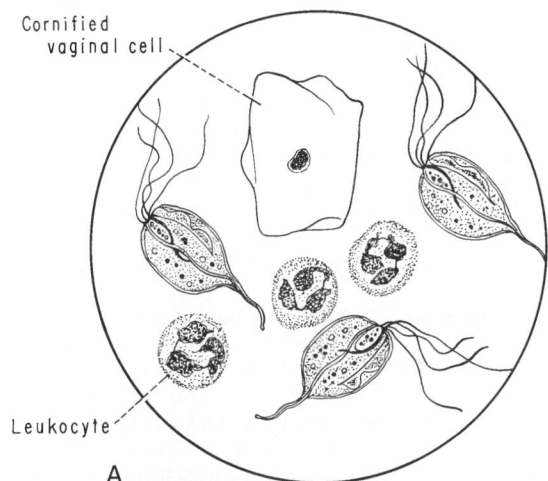

Cornified vaginal cell

Leukocyte

A

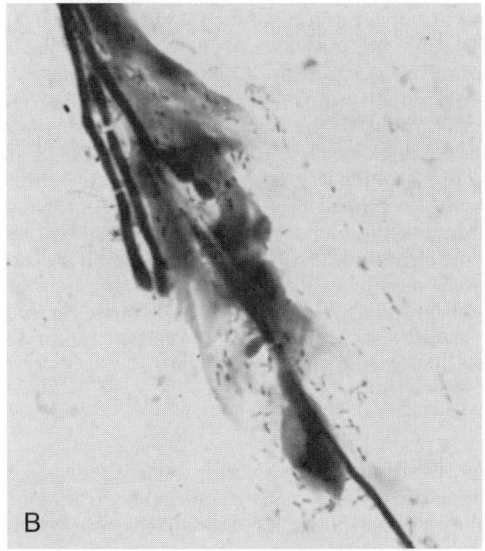

B

Figure 44–11. Preparations of vaginal secretions, showing in *A*, trichomonads, about one half the size of a cornified vaginal cell but larger than leukocytes, and *B*, the fiber-like mycelia of *Candida albicans*. (From Kistner, R. W.: Gynecology: Principles and Practice. Chicago, Year Book Medical Publishers, 1964. Used by permission.)

Other Studies. Several other diagnostic tests should be mentioned. Hysterosalpingography is a technique by which a cannula attached to the cervix allows the uterine cavity and fallopian tubes to be filled with radiopaque dye. By appropriate roentgenologic techniques the endometrial cavity and tubes can be outlined quite adequately. Laparoscopy is a technique by which the pelvic viscera can be directly visualized by a transperitoneal route and with a minimum of morbidity.

Hysteroscopy has become an increasingly useful technique in the assessment of intrauterine structures and pathology. This technique, which can be done under local anesthesia, offers an enhanced view of the endometrial cavity. Operative capabilities with the hysteroscope are now available. An additional technique that has received increasing usage in this specialty is ultrasonography, particularly transvaginal probe ultrasound examination. Through the use of real-time or sector-scanning techniques, pelvic pathology can be clearly demonstrated in a significant percentage of patients. This can be particularly useful in detecting the presence of a mass in a patient in whom examination was difficult, confirming the presence of an intrauterine pregnancy, or discerning the general characteristics of an adnexal mass as solid, cystic, or mixed. Computed tomography, magnetic resonance imaging, fine-needle aspiration (directed by ultrasound), and culdocentesis are other useful techniques.

CONGENITAL ANOMALIES

Imperforate Hymen

An imperforate hymen may lead to retention of mucus or blood, causing hematocolpos, hematometrium, hematosalpinx, and even hematoperitoneum. Such defects are rarely recognized until after puberty and the onset of menses and may present as primary amenorrhea, pelvic pain, or a palpable abdominopelvic mass. Diagnosis is based on careful examination of the external genitalia, which reveals a bulging hymen without communication with the vagina and a fluctuant pelvic mass that lies anterior to the rectum. Pelvic ultrasonography may be a particularly useful study. With adequate surgical drainage, the distended structures will promptly return to normal.

A transverse vaginal septum is rare but may present in a manner similar to that of imperforate hymen. A vertical vaginal septum occurs with failure of müllerian fusion. In both cases, the septum can be partial or complete. Therapy, if necessary at all, is surgical excision.

Defects of Müllerian Fusion

Other defects in müllerian fusion can present a spectrum of congenital anomalies. Because one tube and half of the uterine fundus, cervix, and upper vagina arise from each müllerian duct, improper fusion can result in duplication of part or all of the system. One abnormality is uterus didelphys, with two vaginas, cervices, and uteri, each with a separate tube and ovary. Such patients can present with pelvic pain due to obstruction of outflow of blood from one uterine horn, with an intra-abdominal crisis of pregnancy occurs in a rudimentary horn that cannot expand properly, or with an undiagnosed pelvic mass. Therapy, if indicated, is surgical excision or reconstruction.

Dysgenesis

A variety of defects of the female genital tract are due to hypoplasia or aplasia of its various components. Such defects may occur either primarily or as secondary underdevelopment because of lack of estrogen. Congenital absence of both ovaries is rare, but absence of one tube or ovary at birth is not unusual. There are cases of complete absence of the vagina, usually associated with absence of the uterus, and congenital absence of the uterus despite a normal vagina. In these patients, the androgen insensitivity syndrome should be suspected, in which case the gonads are testicular yet secondary sexual characteristics are feminine as the patient lacks the ability to respond to androgen. Most of these patients present with primary amenorrhea. Jacobs has shown that 40% of patients with primary amenorrhea have demonstrable chromosomal abnormalities or sex inversions of some type. Karyotypic studies are therefore important.

In patients with vaginal agenesis, a normally functional vagina can be surgically created by dissection of the potential space between the bladder and rectum or, in some, by progressive dilation. Skin grafting may be required. Such reconstruction should be delayed until the individual is mature and ready for coitus, because repetitive dilation is mandatory to retain patency. If the primary defect is due to ovarian abnormalities, replacement of estrogen provides a growth stimulus to the genital structures. In patients with androgen insensitivity, the intra-abdominal gonad should be removed in late adolescence because of the high rates of malignancy during the third and fourth decades of life. In such patients, the excision of the gonads and the vaginoplasty can often be done as combined procedures. A male pseudohermaphrodite has testes with the genitalia of a female.

During evaluation of patients with congenital anomalies of the female genital system, the physician should always evaluate the urinary system. Associated urinary tract anomalies are quite common, occurring in as many as 50% of patients with müllerian malformations.[10]

Wolffian Duct Persistence

Other congenital anomalies of the female genital system consist of those derived from remnants of the mesonephric duct or the wolffian duct and body, which normally regress during female genital development. The most common of these is the parovarian cyst, which arises from the upper wolffian duct and may grow to be as large as 20 cm. No symptoms are specific to a parovarian cyst to differentiate it from an ovarian cyst. The treatment is surgical excision, with preservation of the tube and ovary. A similar cyst, the hydatid of Morgagni, may also develop near the distal end of the fallopian tube. Significant enlargement of these cysts is rare, and only under unusual circumstances is their removal mandatory. Similarly, the wolffian system may give rise to Gartner's duct cysts. As the lower portion of the wolffian duct course along the lateral vaginal wall, remnants persist and may later form this tubular cystic tumor mass. Only if dyspareunia develops because of excessive size is surgical excision indicated. Finally, remnants of the mesonephric system may remain in the cervix, broad ligament, and ovarian hilus and rarely may develop into bizarre varieties of malignant neoplasms. These include clear cell tumors, adenocarcinomas, and mixed tumors.

THE VULVA

The physician faces an exceptional variety of problems in the area of female external genitalia. Trauma, allergy, inflammatory conditions, infections, degenerative changes, and neoplasia give rise to disorders ranging from minor annoyances to major hazards to life.

An important precept in the evaluation and management of any noted abnormality of the vulva is to be absolutely sure to exclude neoplasia. Punch biopsy with local anesthesia should be done at any time a suspicious or unusual vulvar lesion is noted.

The vulva is rich in pigment, which increases in pregnancy. Vitiligo of the vulvar skin is no different from the same lesion in other locations, nor does it require treatment. Vitiligo should not be confused with leukoplakia, in which the skin is whitish but thickened and leathery. Various skin eruptions involving the body as a whole may affect the vulva and appear as do other lesions elsewhere on the body. Varicose veins of the vulva are often found in association with varicosities of the lower extremities, and pregnancy may cause further hypertrophy. Therapy consists of lower extremity and vulvar support and ligation or injection in the nonpregnant patient. A severe direct blow to the vulva may be complicated by subcutaneous hematoma formation. Such a hematoma may dissect widely beneath the fascia of the vulva, and surgical evacuation is often necessary. It is frequently difficult to isolate bleeding points, and packing may be required. Vulvar lacerations should be cleaned and sutured as lacerations elsewhere on the body.

Glandular Lesions

The vulvar glands are subject to a variety of disorders. Skenitis usually occurs as a consequence of gonococcal infections. In the acute phase, the exudate may be expressed from urethral orifices and the patient often has dysuria and other symptoms of urethral irritation. In chronic infections, secondary organisms are usually present, and on occasion these glands may become abscessed and require surgical drainage. Antibiotic therapy is indicated for both acute and chronic infections. Infections and cysts of the Bartholin's glands are common. A Bartholin's abscess should be treated with heat until fluctuant and then sharply incised on the mucocutaneous junction between the vagina and vulva. Often, a small inflatable Word catheter may be inserted. If the abscess is drained by excision, the margins of the incision are marsupialized with interrupted sutures of fine chromic catgut. Bartholin's abscess may occur initially from gonococcal infection, but more commonly other organisms are also involved. Antibiotic therapy is indicated in cases of significant cellulitis or systemic symptoms, but drainage remains the treatment of choice. Bartholin's cysts may be marsupialized or excised, but the latter procedure is usually associated with significant blood loss. Small asymptomatic Bartholin's cysts usually require no treatment unless biopsy is necessary to exclude malignancy. The vulva is also a common site of sebaceous cysts. These may be removed if they become greatly enlarged or secondarily infected. Rarely, one may find vulvar apocrine tumors (hidradenomas) as raised, red, sessile masses less than 5 cm. in diameter. These are treated by wide local excision.

Vulvitis

Vulvar irritation occurs from a variety of causes: allergic, infectious, degenerative, or neoplastic. Pruritus accompanied by vaginal infection or vulvar skin change suggests allergy as the underlying cause. Usually the sensitivity is due to undergarments made of synthetic fibers or washed with harsh detergents. Other contact irritants can include soaps, vaginal lubricants or sprays, rubber condoms, and spermicidal foams or jellies. Other causes of vulvar irritation include pediculosis pubis or mechanical irritation from obesity, clothing, or menstrual pads. Intestinal parasites may remain on the vulva and cause irritation. Systemic diseases such as Hodgkin's disease, diabetes mellitus, leukemia, congestive heart failure, and anemia may cause vulvar irritation, along with inadequate nutrition, poor hygiene, and vitamin defi-

ciencies. The basic principles of management of a patient with vulvitis are to search thoroughly for a diagnosis, treat any specific infectious disease, investigate possible allergies, and then keep the area clean and dry and avoid trauma from scratching, harsh soaps, ointments, or rubbing with a towel.

The most common cause of vulvar irritation is an infectious vulvovaginitis caused by either *Candida albicans* or *Trichomonas vaginalis* or both. The vulva appears swollen and red and may be excoriated and secondarily infected. Mycotic vulvovaginitis is a common problem among diabetic patients, oral contraceptive users, and persons receiving systemic antibiotics. Diagnosis is based on fresh-preparation identification of yeast or *Trichomonas* (see Fig. 44–11). Therapy is discussed in the section dealing with vaginitis. For both types of infection, immediate relief is obtained by additional use of topical creams containing hydrocortisone or miconazole, as well as by following the general instructions for treatment of nonspecific vulvitis.

Follicular vulvitis may occur, and penicillin treatment and local therapy are recommended. Finally, condylomata acuminata, or venereal warts, occur as a presumed infectious vulvitis of viral origin (human papillomavirus [HPV]). Many different subtypes of HPV have been involved in pelvic infection. HPV types 16 and 18 may also be associated with premalignant and malignant lesions of the female genital tract. Such lesions are associated with an irritating vaginal discharge. These benign epithelial neoplasms may be few or many, in some cases even covering the entire perineum and extending onto the vagina or cervix (Fig. 44–12). Therapy is topical use of podophyllin or trichloroacetic acid. On occasion one may use 5-fluorouracil. Cautery is used for the more extensive forms of the disease but requires an anesthetic. Cryosurgery, laser therapy, and even interferon have all been used with increasing success in difficult cases and to treat venereal warts.

Recently, a near-epidemic of sexually transmitted vulvovaginitis has occurred, caused by herpes progenitalis (herpes simplex virus Type II). This infection is characterized by vesicular eruptions that are extremely painful and are often secondarily infected when the patient is seen. Current therapy includes warm baths in water containing potassium permanganate, drying, and systemic analgesics. The duration of

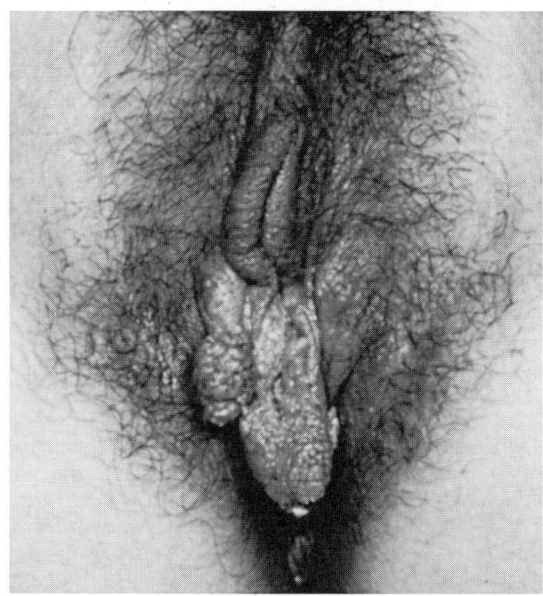

Figure 44–12. Condylomata acuminata. These growths may appear anywhere on the vulva. They may be either broad and confluent or papillary. (Courtesy of Mr. C. P. Jones.)

the infection is usually limited to 1 to 2 weeks, but it may recur. The antiviral agent acyclovir will reduce the severity of primary herpetic infections. Other data suggest that chronic use of acyclovir may reduce the frequency and severity of recurrences. However, there is no permanent cure, and approximately 20% of patients with a primary herpetic lesion will develop recurrent episodes.

Other venereal diseases may present as vulvar lesions. These include the primary chancre of syphilis or the moist, grayish patches (condylomata lata) of secondary syphilis. After darkfield examination for diagnosis, therapy consists of penicillin or its substitute. Granuloma inguinale is a rare infectious disease of the vulva caused by the Donovan bacillus. A scraping of the serpiginous lesion may reveal the intracellular Donovan body. Tetracycline and aminoglycosides are the most useful agents for this disease. Lymphogranuloma venereum is a disease of viral origin, associated frequently with inguinal adenitis, multiple draining sinuses, and rectal stricture. The diagnosis is made by the Frei skin test. Erythromycin and tetracycline are useful, as are the sulfonamides. Chancroid is caused by the gram-negative Ducrey's bacillus. It appears as a small papule 2 to 4 days after exposure and afterward becomes an indurated and punched-out lesion with soft edges and a purulent surface. Inguinal adenitis, often suppurative, is a frequent occurrence. Chancroid is treated with sulfonamides, although other broad-spectrum antibiotics may be useful.

Degenerative Diseases of the Vulva

There are three degenerative diseases of the vulva, all occurring most frequently after menopause. All cause itching, pain, dyspareunia, and frequent secondary infection. These diseases are more commonly seen after vulvar irradiation or premature menopause. The incidence of vulvar carcinoma is increased with these lesions, and biopsy should be employed when necessary to exclude neoplasia. Papanicolaou cytology of scrapings is of aid.

Kraurosis vulvae is a disease in which the vulva appears shrunken and dried. *Leukoplakia,* another degenerative vulvar disease, presents initially as a hypertrophic lesion and later as an atrophic problem. The skin is whitened and leathery. *Lichen sclerosis et atrophicus* may be difficult to differentiate from either kraurosis or leukoplakia. This is a slowly changing, chronic, localized lesion but, unlike the other two problems, tends to involve the skin of the thighs. In all three lesions an intense pruritus frequently occurs, and excoriation with secondary infection is often noted. Approximately 50% of vulvar carcinomas are found in areas of these degenerative lesions, and both cytologic smears and biopsy should be frequently used. Treatment of these three lesions is symptomatic, with relief of pruritus a primary goal. Systemic estrogens may offer limited aid. Local excision is frequently necessary, and with more extensive lesions simple vulvectomy may rarely be required. Topical 2% testosterone ointment may be of some benefit.[13]

Carcinoma in Situ of the Vulva

Bowen originally described a preinvasive cancer of the skin of the vulva, and others have noted a high incidence of this disease associated with previous sexually transmitted diseases. Carcinoma *in situ* of the vulva (vulvar intraepithelial neoplasia [VIN-III]) may appear in a woman who has leukoplakia, kraurosis vulvae, or lichen sclerosis et atrophicus, with or without pruritus. The diagnosis should be made only after adequate histologic study shows the criteria of intraepithelial changes characteristic of epidermoid carcinoma but without invasion. Treatment should be simple vul-

vectomy in most instances. In patients with carcinoma *in situ* of the vulva, up to 35% may have a second malignant genital lesion. In approximately 15% of patients with either intraepithelial or invasive carcinoma of the vulva, carcinoma of the vagina or cervix later develops. Thus, patients with carcinoma *in situ* of the vulva should be carefully followed.

Carcinoma of the Vulva (Fig. 44–13)

Vulvar cancers constitute about 3.5% of all genital cancers, and the peak incidence occurs in the seventh decade of life. DiSaia and Creasman reported that among patients with vulvar cancer, 20% were between 20 and 50 years old, 26% were in the sixth decade, and 40% were in the 61- to 70-year age range. In approximately half the patients, the cancer develops in areas of preexisting leukoplakia, kraurosis vulvae, or lichen sclerosis et atrophicus; others report a high incidence of syphilis and other vulvar venereal diseases among these patients. Most patients with vulvar carcinoma complain of a mass on the vulva or perineum, ulceration or vulvar irritation, or pruritus. Bleeding and pain may be additional findings. Any firm tumor or ulceration must be sampled, and the biopsy specimen should include the primary lesion and some adjacent normal tissue. There is an average delay by the patient of 20 months from discovery of some vulvar abnormality to examination and treatment.

Carcinoma of the vulva is usually squamous (95%) but adenocarcinoma, melanocarcinoma, basal cell carcinoma, and Paget's disease are reported. Squamous cancer may arise anywhere on the vulva, but lesions of the labia majora or labia minora are most frequent. Most squamous cancers of the vulva are rather well differentiated. Adenocarcinoma of the vulva usually arises from Bartholin's glands but may develop from paraurethral glands or embryonic cell nests. Melanocarcinoma is an infrequently found vulvar cancer, as is Paget's disease, which is a slowly spreading ulcerative eczematoid lesion of the vulvar skin that is thought to be an adenocarcinoma of the apocrine sweat glands of that region. Basal cell carcinoma of the vulva is most frequently seen on the labium majus but may appear on other structures. Microscopically, basal cell carcinoma shows extensive proliferation of the cells of the basal layer of the epidermis, which invade the dermis beneath and usually present as a crater-

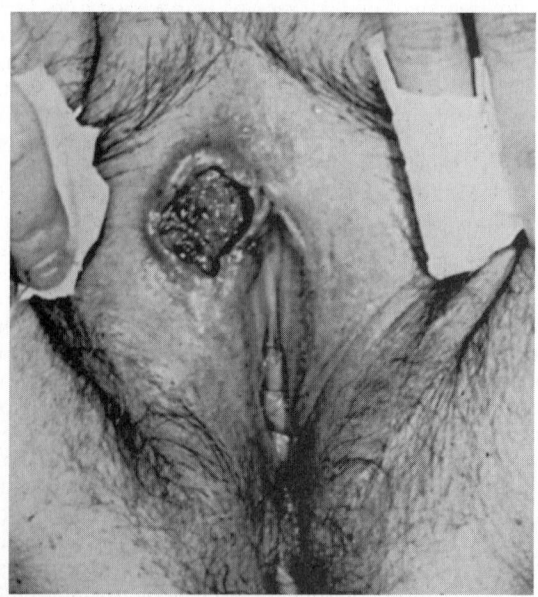

Figure 44–13. Carcinoma of the vulva. (Courtesy of Mr. C. P. Jones.)

like ulcer. Unlike other varieties of vulvar cancer, basal cell carcinoma usually does not metastasize but grows deeply into underlying or adjacent tissues. Some basal cell cancers have squamous cell carcinoma elements.

Vulvar cancer tends to spread by local extension and lymphatic metastasis. The frequency and sites of metastasis depend on the size, location, and differentiation of the vulvar lesion. Of patients in whom the primary lesion is less than 1.5 cm. in diameter, approximately 12% have positive lymph nodes. However, if the vulvar lesion measures 1.5 to 3.0 cm. in diameter, the incidence of lymph node metastasis is 45%. Way found lymph node metastasis in 62% of patients with anaplastic cancer, but if the primary tumor was well differentiated, the incidence of lymphatic metastasis was only 35%. The primary lymphatic drainage of the vulva is by means of superficial lymph nodes of that side. From there, the lymphatics drain through Cloquet's node to the external iliac nodes and up the aortic chain. Contralateral vulvar drainage may occur, however, even from well-lateralized lesions. The upper vulvar areas, principally around the clitoris, may drain directly to Cloquet's node, which then may be involved with tumor while the superficial inguinal nodes are negative. Vulvar lesions in the perineal, Bartholin's, or posterior fourchette areas may involve the rectovaginal septum, rectum, or vagina and may metastasize by means of the deep pelvic nodes. Way has demonstrated the difficulty of detecting inguinal node metastases by palpation, because many enlarged nodes will not contain metastases whereas nodes normal to palpation may have tumor cells when microscopically examined. In general, however, if the primary vulvar lesion is small and the superficial inguinal lymphatics and Cloquet's node are negative for malignancy, it is unlikely that the deeper nodes will be involved. Metastasis may also occur to the skin of the thigh, pubis, and groin and to the bladder, urethra, upper vagina, or rectovaginal septum. Blood-borne metastases are unusual.

The treatment of vulvar cancer is surgical.[25] Radiation therapy has been of little use for primary or recurrent disease and is contraindicated because of the risk of extensive vulvar necrosis. Basal cell carcinoma and Paget's disease of the vulva should be treated with wide and deep local excision of the tumor; and, if the tumor is large, hemivulvectomy should be done. Removal of regional lymph nodes is not indicated. The prognosis is generally excellent, but these patients should be followed closely for local recurrence. *Operations such as local excision, hemivulvectomy, and simple vulvectomy have proved, in general, to be inadequate therapy for vulvar cancer.* Most investigators have outlined appropriate therapy as including at least a block dissection of the vulva, in continuity, removing the skin, subcutaneous tissues, and lymphatic tissues of the groin, vulva, and perineum as one specimen. Controversy exists as to whether all patients should also have retroperitoneal node dissection to include removal of the femoral, iliac, and obturator nodes. These procedures are usually done as a one-stage operation but may be divided, with the deep node dissection performed later. When radical vulvectomy and node dissections are done, a 5-year cure rate of over 80% is noted in patients without positive nodes, with a 5-year survival rate of 47% even in patients with positive inguinal nodes. Overall, the 5-year cure rate after surgical therapy of cancer of the vulva is approximately 60%. If the vulvar lesion involves the vagina, rectum, or urethra, then pelvic exenteration may be the operation of choice. Recurrence of surgically treated vulvar cancer may occur at the skin margins of the primary operation or in the skin of the groin. Distant metastases may also develop. Treatment of recurrent vulvar cancer with local excision or chemotherapy may provide palliation. Irradiation to the vulva is usually very toxic and is rarely indicated.[9]

THE VAGINA

The stratified squamous epithelium of the vagina is histologically similar to epithelium of the cervix and the skin of the vulva and responds to estrogen by proliferation. The vagina of the child and that of the postmenopausal woman are similar in that the epithelial layer is thin, is easily traumatized, and is subject to a variety of infections. The normal adult vagina contains diphtheroids, Döderlein's bacilli, and anaerobic streptococci. This flora converts glycogen of vaginal cells to lactic acid, which maintains the vagina with an acid pH and enhances normal secretions.

Vaginitis

Vaginal inflammation can occur from protozoan, fungal, bacterial, or viral infection and also from deficiencies of estrogen. *Trichomonas vaginalis* is a common protozoan organism causing pruritus, tenderness, and dyspareunia. *Trichomonas* vaginitis is characterized by a foamy, greenish yellow vaginal exudate; the vaginal walls are erythematous and tender. The diagnosis of this infection is made by high-power microscopic examination of fresh preparations of the vaginal discharge and identification of the flagellated, motile organisms, which are the site of leukocytes (see Fig. 44–11). There is uncertainty about the epidemiology of *Trichomonas* vaginitis, but it is seen most commonly among sexually active women. The male sexual partner may harbor these organisms without symptoms and promptly reinfects the woman who has been treated successfully. This infection is also frequently seen in chronically ill and debilitated women and in women with other pelvic infections. Current therapy consists of oral metronidazole (Flagyl) for both sexual partners.

Candida albicans is probably the most frequent and bothersome cause of vaginitis. The wide use of antibiotics and oral contraceptives predisposes to this fungal infection, as does diabetes mellitus. Symptoms are vaginal discharge, vulvar and vaginal irritation, and itching. Inspection reveals a *curdy* white vaginal exudate, intense vaginal erythema, and a white, watery discharge. Diagnosis is made from fresh preparations of vaginal discharge, which microscopically reveal the mycelia as thread-like fibers or budding forms (see Fig. 44–11). Cultures on Sabouraud's medium may be necessary to identify the etiology of low-grade vaginitis. Therapy consists of the intravaginal application of the synthetic imidazoles—miconazole (Monistat), clotrimazole (Lotrimin), or butoconazole (Femstat). There is a tendency for vaginal candidiasis to recur, and in these patients the physician should consider evaluation for diabetes mellitus. If such a patient is taking oral contraceptives, their use may have to be halted temporarily until the infection is controlled.

Vaginal irritation can occur in the patient with insufficient estrogen to maintain normal vaginal thickness. Infection of this thin, atrophic, easily traumatized vagina is often nonspecific and caused by a variety of usually nonpathogenic bacteria. Treatment is systemic or topical administration of estrogen. In some women, there exists a nonspecific bacterial infection, now thought sexually transmitted, which most likely appears to be a symbiotic infection between anaerobic bacteria and *Gardnerella*. Both organisms contribute to produce clinical symptoms. This infection, now termed *bacterial vaginosis*, is confirmed by *clue cells* on wet preparations and is best treated with metronidazole or clindamycin.[15] Concurrent treatment of the male partner remains controversial.

Herpes simplex virus may produce an intense, painful vaginitis that is associated with a granular surface and vesicular eruption. The diagnosis is made clinically and by serial serum antibody determinations. Fresh preparations of ulcerations, stained as for a Papanicolaou slide, may show classic inclusion bodies that are highly suggestive but not diagnostic of herpes. Therapy is supportive but, fortunately, the episode usually terminates within 2 to 3 weeks. The antiviral agent acyclovir may reduce the severity of primary infections but is rarely indicated. More recent studies have suggested that chronic acyclovir therapy may reduce the frequency and severity of recurrent episodes after the primary infection.

Gonorrhea is an occasional cause of vaginitis in the child. The diagnosis is made by smear and culture, and therapy with penicillin is recommended. Children with vaginitis should be examined for intestinal parasites and intravaginal foreign bodies. Rarely do the causes of childhood vaginitis produce similar problems in the adult.

Dysplasia and Intraepithelial Carcinoma of the Vagina

Dysplasia of the vaginal epithelium may be the source of abnormal genital smears, even if the cervix is normal or absent. Treatment consists of excision or cryosurgery to remove abnormal epithelium. Intraepithelial carcinoma may also develop, most commonly in patients treated previously for other lower genital tract cancers. These lesions may occur at the apex of the vagina in patients after hysterectomy or may be multifocal in areas remote from the vaginal apex. As in dysplasia, intraepithelial carcinoma of the vagina causes no specific symptoms. Diagnosis is suspected from genital cytology and colposcopy and confirmed by biopsy. Therapy can be by irradiation or surgical treatment, either excision or partial or total colpectomy. The frequency of these lesions justifies the close follow-up suggested for patients, even after adequate treatment, who have had other lower genital tract cancers. Results of therapy are excellent.

Carcinoma of the Vagina

Primary carcinoma of the vagina is a rare lesion, and most are epidermoid. Postcontact bleeding is the usual presenting complaint. Many patients with invasive vaginal carcinoma have previously had other preinvasive or invasive epidermoid lesions of the lower genital system. Primary vaginal cancer may occur in any location, but the prognosis is considerably more grave if the lesion is situated anteriorly.

The current classification of primary vaginal cancer (International Federation of Gynecology and Obstetrics) includes Stage I, limited to the vaginal mucosa; Stage II, subvaginal tissue involved, but not to the pelvic wall; Stage III, tumor extending to the pelvic wall or to the symphysis, but not fixed to the symphysis; and Stage IV, tumor fixed to the symphysis, outside the pelvis, or proved by biopsy to involve the bladder or rectum. Treatment may be by irradiation or surgical therapy. Rutledge's review of radiation therapy of primary vaginal carcinoma describes the type of treatment, varied according to the location of the vaginal lesion. In general, it consists of 3000 to 5000 cGy of external irradiation followed by 3000 to 5000 cGy of intravaginal radium by sources specifically designed to deliver the radiation to the primary lesion. He reports survivors as follows: Stage I, 16 of 22 patients; Stage II, 19 of 25 patients; Stage III, 3 of 14 patients; Stage IV, 3 of 16 patients. Complications of therapy are relatively low but include radiation cystitis and proctitis. Individualization of therapy was recommended. Exenterative operation may be used as primary therapy or therapy for recurrence. Results of primary surgical therapy are not as good as those achieved with irradiation, and the operative and postoperative morbidity and mortality are significant.

The vagina may also be the site of other histologic types of cancer, including melanocarcinoma, sarcoma, and mesonephric adenocarcinoma. Melanomas of this organ have an extremely poor prognosis, regardless of the therapy utilized. Only 3 of 30 patients reported in the literature have survived 5 years of longer. Surgical therapy should be radical and usually exenterative and should include removal of the regional lymph nodes. Sarcoma of the vagina, the so-called sarcoma botryoides, is most frequently seen in children, and the prognosis is grave. Irradiation is ineffective, and radical operation is of only limited success. These tumors are thought to be of mixed mesodermal origin. Primary vaginal adenocarcinoma, while rarely seen in the past, is more common now in women who were exposed to diethylstilbestrol *in utero*. These tumors usually become symptomatic shortly after puberty. Older women may occasionally have similar lesions from mesonephric remnants or paraurethral glands. Treatment is usually exenteration or irradiation.

DEFECTS OF PELVIC SUPPORT

The major support of the uterus and vagina is provided by the cardinal ligaments, which are condensations of endopelvic fascia at the bases of the broad ligaments. The round, broad, and uterosacral ligaments are more important in maintaining uterine position than in providing support. Support from the vaginal side of the bladder and rectum is provided by the pubocervical fascia, which is not true fascia but condensed connective tissue in the vesicovaginal and rectovaginal septum. The distal vagina is also supported by the perineal body. Overdistention of these supporting structures, usually by childbirth, may give rise to a variety of defects in pelvic support. Frequently, these defects cause few symptoms until atrophy after menopause results in further weakness. Such defects include cystocele, urethrocele, rectocele, enterocele, and uterine descensus (Fig. 44–14).[1, 7, 16, 17]

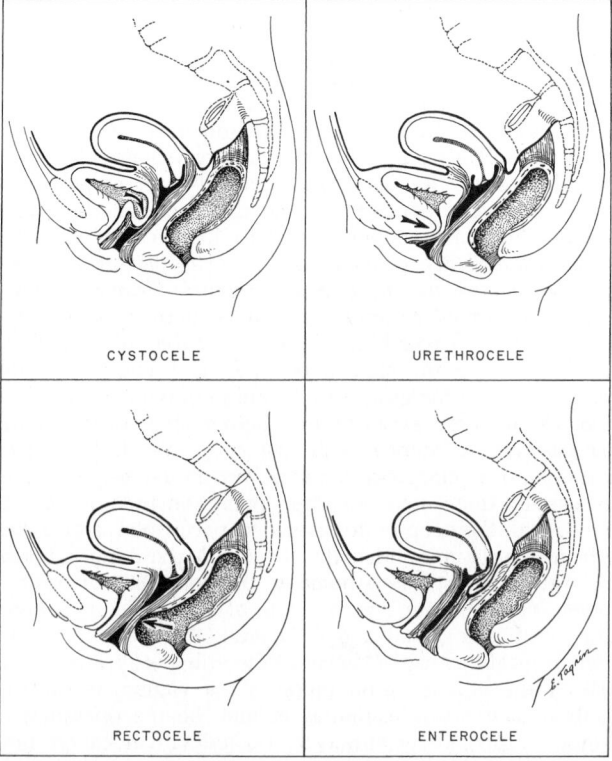

Figure 44–14. Diagrammatic representation of the four most common types of pelvic floor relaxation: cystocele, urethrocele, rectocele, and enterocele. Arrows depict sites of maximal protrusion. (From Kistner, R. W.: Gynecology: Principles and Practice. Chicago, Year Book Medical Publishers, 1964. Used by permission.)

Cystocele and Urethrocele and Stress Urinary Incontinence

A cystocele is a herniation of the anterior vaginal wall with secondary relaxation, descent, and protrusion of the bladder floor into the vaginal introitus. It is usually accompanied by some degree of uterine descensus or rectocele. The classic symptoms of cystocele are vaginal protrusion and recurrent cystitis, which occurs because of incomplete bladder emptying. A large cystocele may be relatively asymptomatic. Surgical repair is indicated not for the size of the cystocele but rather for its symptoms. A common problem associated with cystocele is urethrocele, and together they may produce flattening of the vesical neck, predisposing to stress urinary incontinence. There are a number of surgical approaches for the treatment of genuine stress urinary incontinence. These include anterior colporrhaphy, retropubic suspension, and urethral slings. Most important is the urodynamic evaluation of the patient, done by individuals with specific training in this area.

Urogynecology

The evaluation and treatment of the lower urinary tract have been the province of the gynecologist since Sims first successfully repaired a vesicovaginal fistula in 1846. However, it has only been since the late 1970s that a new understanding and approach has developed—using not only history and physical findings but also objective assessment with sophisticated endoscopic and urodynamic equipment, enabling the treating physician to develop a rational approach to patient management, particularly urinary incontinence. These therapeutic improvements, plus advances in reconstruction of pelvic floor disorders, have made major improvements in the life and function of women. This topic is beyond the scope of this chapter but is well addressed by the overview provided by Ostergard and Bast.[17]

Rectocele

Rectocele is protrusion of the rectal wall toward the vaginal canal. In this condition, the paravaginal tissue normally interposed between the vagina and rectum becomes attenuated and lacerated, usually during delivery. Symptoms of rectocele are vaginal protrusion and sacculation of the rectal wall when fecal material is propelled into the anal canal. Defecation may require digital pressure to the posterior vaginal wall to force the feces from the sacculation back into the ampulla. Such problems may be reduced by posterior colpoperineorrhaphy, by which the rectovaginal fascia is rebuilt and the pubococcygeus and lower levator ani muscles are joined. Most patients with rectocele also have some associated cystocele or uterine descensus. Thus, vaginal hysterectomy and anterior colporrhaphy often should be combined with the posterior repair for best results. In addition, combined repairs may be mutually supporting, because the posterior repair may provide extra support for cystourethrocele. Nonoperative treatment is usually unsuccessful.

Enterocele

Pelvic enterocele is a herniation of the peritoneum of the cul-de-sac with invagination of the sac into the rectovaginal septum. A sliding hernia may develop in this space, usually created by labor, delivery, or vaginal hysterectomy. An enterocele of considerable size may exist without symptoms, but most provoke pelvic pressure, pain, and posterior vaginal protrusion. Enterocele may be difficult to separate from rectocele, but combined rectovaginal examination, or examination with the patient in the standing position, usually clarifies the problem. Enterocele may be surgically repaired by vaginal or abdominal approaches, but the gynecologist usually utilizes the former to allow repair of other associated defects. From either approach, surgical repair of enterocele consists of plication of the uterosacral ligaments and obliteration of the cul-de-sac. If there is accompanying rectocele, it also should be repaired.

Prolapse of the Uterus

Uterine prolapse, or procidentia and uterine descensus, occurs when the uterus and its adjoining structures herniate through the vaginal canal. Prolapse is described as first, second, or third degree in severity, the last being protrusion of the entire uterus from the vagina, with the entire vagina everted as a consequence. Although congenital weakness of the supporting tissues may occasionally cause uterine prolapse, the most frequent cause is childbirth. The signs of uterine prolapse are protrusion of the cervix or uterus through the introitus. Prolapse is frequently associated with cystocele or rectocele, and these defects may cause presenting symptoms. Symptoms include backache, significant pelvic pressure, and ulceration or bleeding of the prolapsed structures. Uterine prolapse cannot be cured by nonoperative means, but some patients can be supported by a pessary if surgical therapy is not feasible. Uterine prolapse is best approached vaginally for surgical repair, because abdominal procedures are usually inadequate. Successful procedures include vaginal hysterectomy and repair of the pelvic diaphragm, procedures that preserve the uterus while resupporting these structures, and rarely total colpocleisis if coital function is never again anticipated.

BENIGN DISEASES OF THE CERVIX

The portio vaginalis of the normal cervix is covered with squamous epithelium that is similar to that of the vagina. In the nulliparous woman, the external cervical os is a centrally located, small, round opening connecting with the endocervical canal. After childbearing, the external os is longitudinally flattened. Mucus-secreting columnar epithelium lines the endocervical canal, and its junction with the squamous epithelium of the portio cervicis is the squamocolumnar zone.

Cervicitis

Cervical infection, in one form or another, is one of the most frequently encountered gynecologic lesions. Acute cervicitis is rarely seen except in gonorrhea, in patients with acute vaginitis from *Trichomonas vaginalis* or *Candida albicans*, in patients with puerperal endometritis, or in patients with retained vaginal foreign bodies. The cervix is erythematous and edematous, and leukocytic infiltration is prominent. Pain and tenderness are rarely prominent symptoms, but a purulent discharge is frequently seen. Diagnosis is made by appropriate smears and cultures, and therapy with topical or systemic antibiotics is usually curative.

In chronic cervicitis, the cervical mucus is mucopurulent and profuse. The histologic changes seen in chronic cervicitis are variable and are present to some extent in nearly all women. Cellular changes, such as metaplasia, epidermization, and hyperplasia of the basal cells, are frequently noted. Often seen are erosions or eversions of the cervix. An erosion is a true ulcer of the cervix, whereas the eversion is formed by columnar epithelium of the endocervical canal proliferating downward, forming a lowered squamocolumnar line. Orifices of the cervical mucus-secreting glands may become obstructed to form nabothian cysts. A mucopurulent discharge may be the only symptom of chronic cervicitis, although postcontact bleeding, infertility, and, rarely, pain may occur. Diagnosis is based on cytology and biopsy, but it should be remembered that while cervical cytologic studies are very effective in the discovery of early cervical cancer with an intact surface epithelium, they are much less reliable when an erosion is present. Colposcopy, colpomicroscopy, and iodine staining may be of aid in localizing areas for biopsy. Any suspicious or eroded area should be sampled before treatment. Therapy for chronic cervicitis is usually by electrodesiccation, ultrarefrigeration (cryosurgery), laser, or silver nitrate. Cautery should include the involved exocervix and endocervical canal and rarely requires an anesthetic. These methods destroy the infection of the columnar area and allow the squamous epithelium to grow over the area. Repeated cautery, surgical conization, and, on occasion, even hysterectomy (if childbearing is ended) may be necessary for severe chronic cervicitis.

Cervical Polyps

Polyps may arise from the endocervix and are rarely malignant. The usual symptom is postcontact bleeding. Polyps appear as single or multiple cherry-red growths protruding from the external cervical os. Such polyps may be removed by biopsy or dilation and curettage, with cauterization of the pedicle. One must not overlook uterine or other cervical causes of the abnormal bleeding, which may be the symptom of other, more severe, pelvic disease.

CANCER OF THE CERVIX

Invasive carcinoma of the cervix is now the second most common pelvic malignancy and comprises 15% of cancers of women. It is estimated that 10,000 women die in the United States each year from these neoplasms. It is encouraging that during the past 20 years, primarily through early detection, the death rate from cervical cancer has declined from 21.8 to 11.5 per 100,000 population. Invasive carcinoma of the cervix should be a preventable disease, because regular examinations and frequently use of today's diagnostic techniques should enable detection of nearly all patients with preinvasive cervical carcinoma, a totally curable disease.[9]

The average age at onset of carcinoma of the cervix is 49 years, with the majority of patients between 35 and 55 years of age. However, many workers have reported cervical cancer in women as young as the teens and as old as the eighth decade. Much has been written about the etiology of cervical carcinoma. Epidemiologic studies show peak occurrences among women of low socioeconomic status, those who begin coitus and childbearing at an early age, and those with multiple sexual partners. Heredity appears to have a small role. The theory of a viral relationship has been advanced, suggesting that a virus transmitted through intercourse may be at least partially responsible for cervical cancer.

Preinvasive Carcinoma or Carcinoma in Situ of the Cervix

Bowen, in 1912, described a preinvasive malignant lesion of the skin; and in the same year others described preinvasive carcinoma of the cervix. Thirty years later it was described as a precursor to invasive carcinoma. It remained for Papanicolaou and Traut, in 1941, to develop the cytologic evaluation of exfoliated cells that suggests the need for biopsy and adequate tissue study. Histopathologically, carcinoma in situ consists of cellular changes in the squamous epithelium of the cervix that are compatible with cancer but evidence of invasion in the underlying stroma is absent. Glandular epi-

thelial replacement by neoplastic cells may be mistaken for invasion, and it is important that the differentiation be made. Other benign conditions that may confuse diagnosis are atypical basilar hyperplasia or the metaplasia and hyperplasia of glandular elements frequently noted during pregnancy. The peak incidence of carcinoma in situ is at 35 to 40 years of age. *There are no gross lesions or symptoms of carcinoma* in situ *of the cervix.* The use of Papanicolaou cytology screening and adequate biopsy techniques is discussed in the Laboratory and Clinical Tests section of this chapter. The diagnosis of carcinoma in situ is made by histologic review of biopsy specimens (Fig. 44–15). It is of critical importance that patients who have an abnormal Papanicolaou smear be properly evaluated. DiSaia provides such an algorithm (Fig. 44–16).[9]

Many patients with dysplasia or carcinoma in situ of the cervix are now being treated with electrocautery, cryosurgery, or cone biopsy. Close follow-up after therapy is warranted, with repeat cytologic studies used frequently. If the lesion has been eradicated, as demonstrated on Papanicolaou stain smears and colposcopy, follow-up alone is indicated.

Treatment of extensive or recurrent carcinoma in situ of the cervix may be abdominal or vaginal hysterectomy, with excision of 2 to 3 cm. of upper vagina. The tubes and ovaries are usually left in place in younger women. Radical hysterectomy and pelvic lymph node dissection are not indicated. Results of therapy are uniformly good, and 5-year survival approaches 100%. Radiation therapy is rarely indicated for carcinoma in situ. Because carcinoma in situ is a disease of younger women, the question of allowing continued reproduction before hysterectomy has been raised. If the patient has normal smears after conization and desires to have more children, she is allowed to do so and have vaginal delivery. If the smears remain positive after conization, hysterectomy is usually suggested at that time. If abnormal smears are detected during pregnancy, cervical conization is used for diagnosis or quadrant biopsy is used later in pregnancy and when no obvious lesion is present. If carcinoma in situ only is detected, the pregnancy is allowed to continue with vaginal delivery. If invasive carcinoma is present, appropriate therapy is begun immediately.

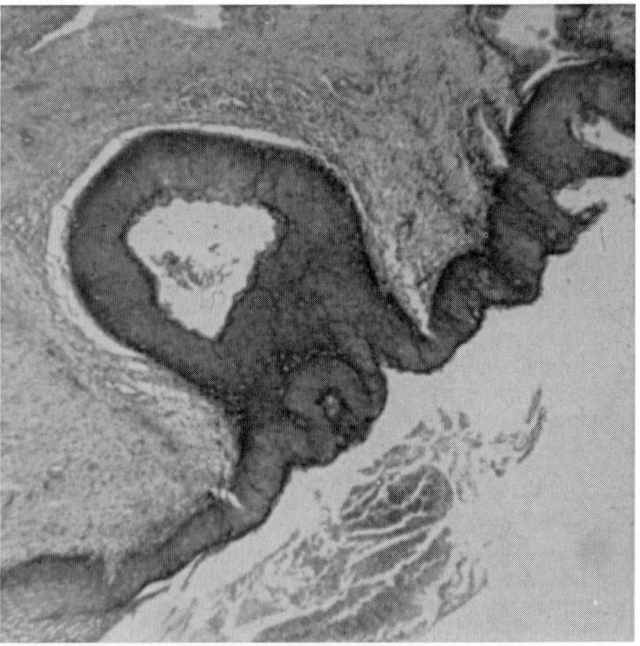

Figure 44–15. Carcinoma *in situ* of the cervix. Note sharp demarcation between normal and malignant epithelium (lower border) and the glandular epithelial involvement. (Courtesy of Dr. D. E. D. Jones.)

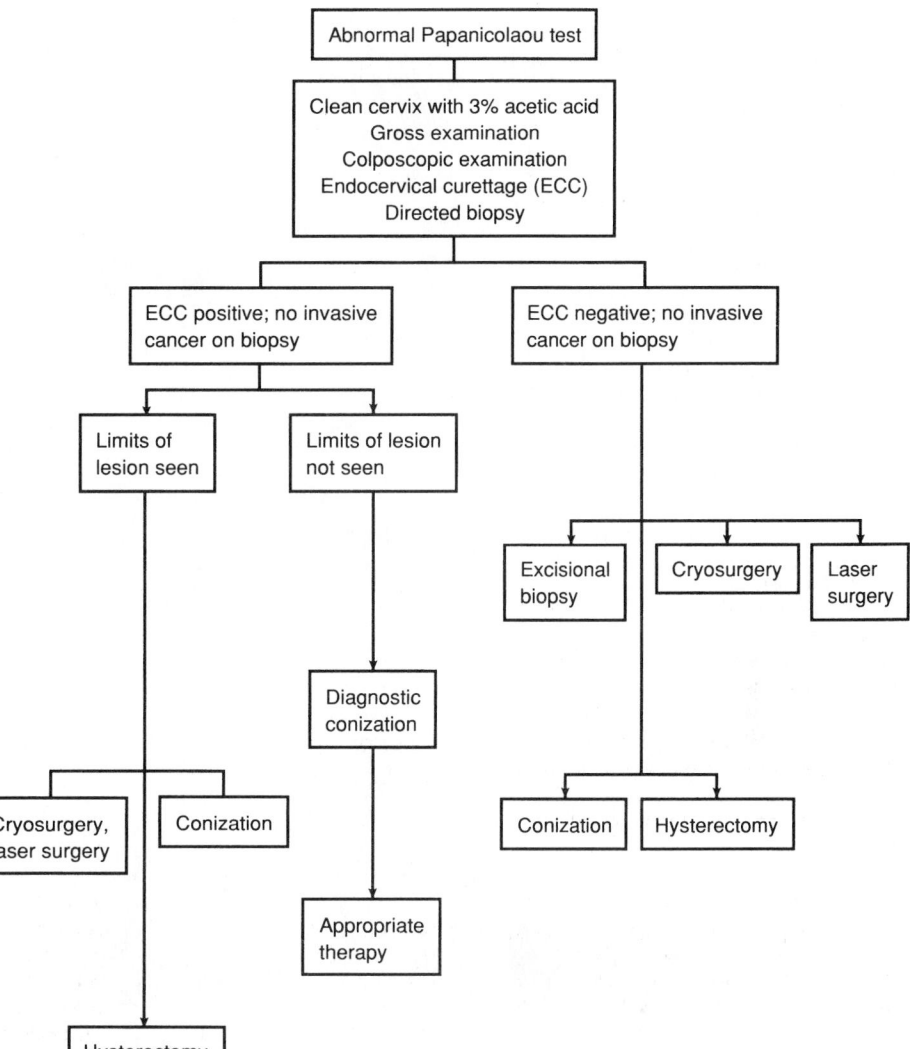

Figure 44–16. Evaluation and management of abnormal cytology. Patients with an abnormal Papanicolaou smear are given a colposcopic examination, and areas consistent with dysplasia or more advanced disease must be biopsied and an endocervical curettage (ECC) performed. Further therapy is determined on the basis of these results. (From DiSaia, P. J.: Disorders of the uterine cervix. *In* Scott, J. R., DiSaia, P. J., Hammond, C. B., and Spellacy, W. N. [Eds.]: Danforth's Obstetrics and Gynecology, 7th ed. Philadelphia, J. B. Lippincott, 1994.)

Microinvasive Cancer of the Cervix (Stage IA1)

There has been considerable debate as to both the diagnosis and the treatment of microinvasive carcinoma of the cervix, a condition in which carcinoma *in situ* exists and less than 3 mm. of invasion is present. Data showing lack of nodal metastasis have led to treatment of patients as if the lesions were only carcinoma *in situ*. Results of this treatment in microinvasive cancer of the cervix are equally as good as those of full radical therapy or irradiation, and morbidity has been much less.

Carcinoma of the Cervix

Approximately 95% of cervical cancers are squamous, the remaining 5% usually being adenocarcinoma. Most often the adenocarcinoma arises from the mucus-secreting epithelium of the cervix, but, rarely adenocarcinoma may arise in mesonephric duct remnants. Squamous cell, or epidermoid, carcinoma of the cervix usually arises at the squamocolumnar junction. Varying degrees of microscopic differentiation are found. A halo of carcinoma *in situ* is frequently found around the invasive cancer or on the vagina.

There are no symptoms of early carcinoma of the cervix; the first symptoms of bleeding, usually post contact, or a bloody discharge do not begin until ulceration is present.

More advanced cervical cancers cause symptoms referable to invasion of adjacent organs (bladder, rectum, ureter) or to distant metastasis. Pain is usually a sign of advanced cervical cancer.

Although cytologic findings and clinical appearance may strongly suggest carcinoma of the cervix, the diagnosis can be made only by histopathologic study. In the presence of an obvious exophytic lesion, as is found in more than 80% of patients with even early cervical cancer, tissue may be easily obtained by punch biopsy. If the lesion is endophytic, or if the punch biopsy shows carcinoma *in situ* (or less), conization may be mandatory to fully evaluate abnormal cytologic studies. Broken and ulcerated epithelium and proliferating tissue that bleeds easily on touch are most valuable clinical signs, particularly when such lesions involve the squamocolumnar junction. Colposcopy and staining techniques may aid direction of biopsies. Even if Papanicolaou smears are benign, the presence of an ulcerated lesion or exophytic cervical growth warrants biopsy.

If treatment of cervical cancer is adequate, the single most important factor in prognosis is the extent of disease when therapy is begun. For this reason, each patient should have a careful pelvic examination, cystoscopy, proctoscopy, intravenous pyelography, roentgenography of the chest, and possibly pelvic computed tomography or magnetic resonance imaging so that the extent of the disease may be established. Staging of cervical cancer is arrived at entirely by clinical

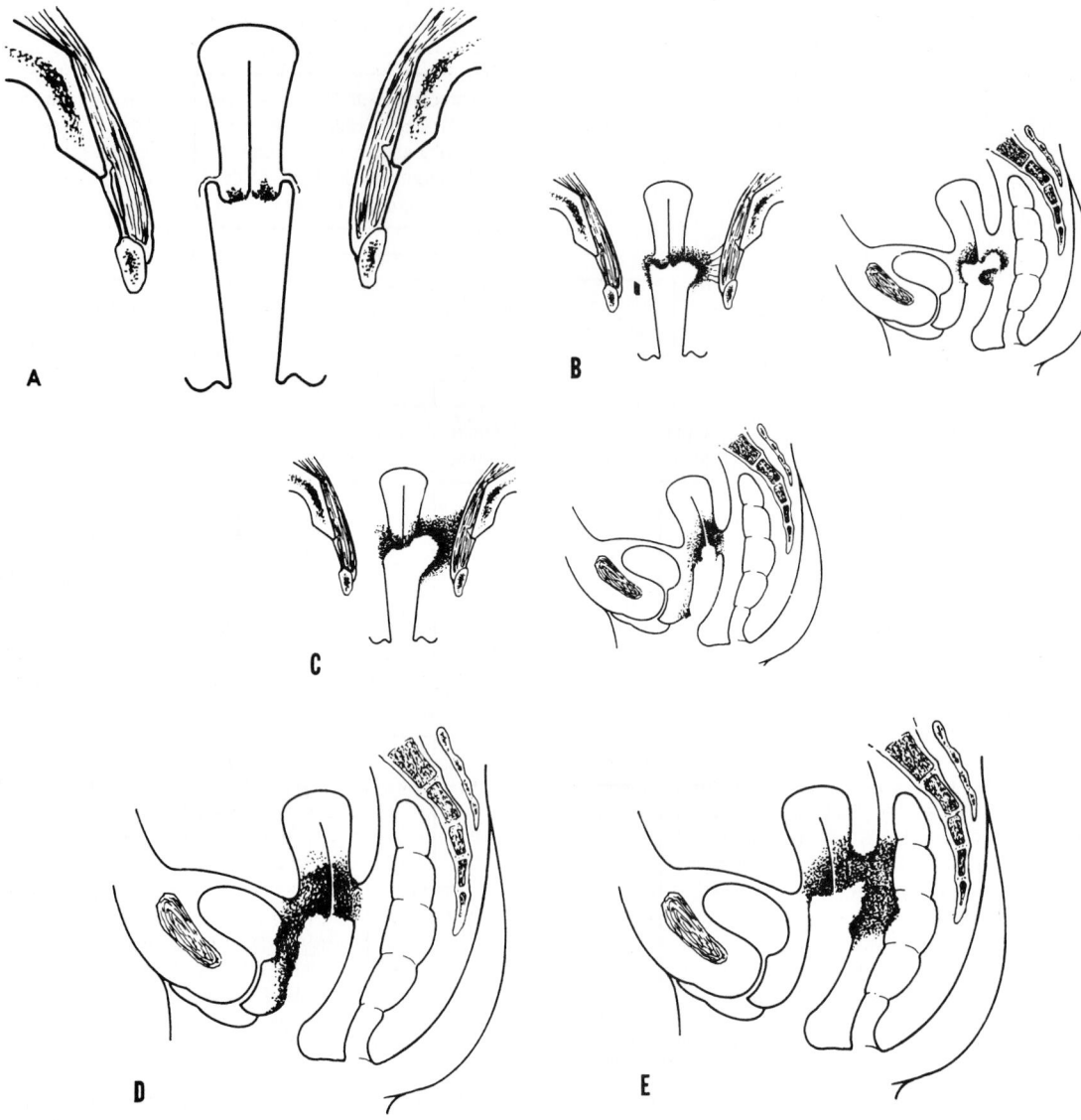

Figure 44–17. Stages of carcinoma of the cervix. *A*, Stage I: The cancer is confined to the cervix. *B*, Stage II: The cancer is confined to the parametrium on one or both sides and is not fixed to either pelvic wall, or the cancer involves the upper one third of the vagina. *C*, Stage III: The cancer has spread to one or both pelvic walls or has invaded the lower third of the vagina. *D* and *E*, Stage IV: the cancer involves the bladder or the rectum, or it has spread beyond the pelvis. (From Taylor, E. S.: Essentials of Gynecology, 4th ed. Philadelphia, Lea & Febiger, 1969.)

evaluation and is made before treatment is initiated (Fig. 44–17). Such staging should not be changed at a later time. The author uses the classification of staging of cervical carcinoma provided in 1987 by the Cancer Committee of the International Federation of Gynecology and Obstetrics:

Stage I
    Carcinoma is strictly confined to the cervix (extension to corpus should be disregarded)
    IA2 Preclinical carcinoma
    IA1 Minimal microscopically evident stromal invasion
    IA2 Microscopic lesions no more then 5 mm. in depth measured from base of epithelium, either surface or glandular, from which it originates, and horizontal spread not to exceed 7 mm.
    IB2 All other cases of Stage I; occult cancer should be marked "occ"
Stage II
    Carcinoma extends beyond cervix but has not extended to pelvic wall; it involves vagina, but not as far as lower third

    IIA No obvious parametrial involvement
    IIB Obvious parametrial involvement
Stage III
    Carcinoma has extended to pelvic wall; on rectal examination there is no cancer-free space between tumor and pelvic wall; tumor involves lower third of vagina; all cases with hydronephrosis or nonfunctioning kidney should be included, unless they are known to be due to another cause
    IIIA No extension to pelvic wall, but involvement of lower third of vagina
    IIIB Extension to pelvic wall, or hydronephrosis or nonfunctioning kidney due to tumor
Stage IV
    Carcinoma has extended beyond true pelvis or has clinically involved mucosa or bladder or rectum
    IVA Spread of growth to adjacent pelvic organs
    IVB Spread to distant organs

    Although clinical staging is done before therapy, it is useful to understand the significance of such staging on the spread of disease. The most common method of tumor spread, and the most frequent cause of patient death, is direct extension of cervical cancer to involve the vagina, uterus, bladder, and rectum. More than 50% of patients who die with cervical cancer die of ureteral obstruction and uremia. Fistula formation from the ureter, bladder, and rectum is frequent, and bleeding may be a serious complication. Carcinoma of the cervix also has a propensity for lymphatic metastasis. Lymphatic drainage of the cervix occurs by means of the hypogastric and obturator lymph chains to the iliac and then the aortic nodal systems. Vertebral lymphatic metastases may also occur. Morton and others have shown lymph node metastases in the following percentages of clinically staged cases of cervical carcinoma: Stage I, 15.5%; Stage II, 31.9%; Stage III, 46.7%; and Stage IV, 80.8%. In addition to the clinical staging, the size of the primary cervical lesion has also been shown to influence the frequency with which lymph node metastases are found: less than 1 cm., rare metastases; 1 to 3 cm., 17% with metastases; greater than 3 mm., 52% with lymph node metastases. These latter two factors of lymphatic node metastasis are variable and of little predictive value in the management of a given patient.

Other studies have shown that lymphatic spread beyond the pelvic nodal chains is present in more than 40% of patients who die of cervical cancer. Autopsy data demonstrate distant metastases in many patients dying of carcinoma of the cervix, and nearly every organ may be involved. The most common sites of distant metastases include liver, 16%; lung, 14%; vertebrae, 9%; and other bony metastases, 9%.

Treatment of Cervical Cancer. Carcinoma of the cervix can be effectively treated by surgical therapy or irradiation, *but treatment does not include simple hysterectomy or nonindividualized radiation therapy.* No other major lesion requires more critical selection of techniques and methods of therapy. The present operation for cancer of the cervix (Stages I and IIA) is an extended or radical hysterectomy (Wertheim) that removes the parametrial tissues, the upper third of the vagina, and perhaps the adnexa and a pelvic node dissection that removes the iliac, hypogastric, ureteral, obturator, and lower aortic lymph nodes. The radical operation for cancer of the cervix has two primary disadvantages. First, there is a 7% to 8% incidence of ureteral or bladder fistula; and, second, few surgeons are qualified to undertake the operation and perform it satisfactorily. Certain patients with Stage IV carcinoma, those with only rectal or bladder involvement, may be candidates for primary surgical therapy by pelvic exenteration. The results of primary surgical treatment for cervical cancer show 5-year survivals of 78% for Stage I, 53% for Stage II, 31% for Stage III, and 19% for Stage IV. The operative mortality should be under 1.0%, and a significant number of postoperative urinary fistulas occur. Most gynecologists now reserve the primary surgical treatment of carcinoma of the cervix for those operable patients with smaller Stage I or early Stage II lesions.[8]

Many favor primary radiation treatment of cancer of the cervix, especially those staged beyond IIA. The purpose of therapy is to deliver to the lesion and to areas of possible pelvic spread sufficient radiation to destroy the cancer and still not cause irreparable damage to surrounding tissues. Most therapists employ a combination of external supervoltage therapy, such as from cobalt-60, linear accelerators, and the betatron megavoltage units, as well as brachytherapy and intravaginal, contravaginal, and intracervical irradiation with radium or cesium. Usually, external radiation therapy is initially delivered in a dosage of 4000 to 6000 cGy. to the entire pelvis over a 4- to 6-week course. This is followed by one or two interval applications to deliver 4000 to 6000 cGy to the primary cervical lesion. Stage I and II disease tend to receive the higher dose by radium; in Stage III and IV disease, the higher dose is usually administered by external cobalt-60. Total dosage administered by the two routes approximates 10,000 cGy. As in surgical therapy, the prognosis with primary radiation therapy for carcinoma of the cervix varies with the clinical stage present at the time therapy is begun. The generally accepted figures for 5-year survival with this type of treatment are 86.4% for Stage I, 60.0% for Stage II, 26.3% for Stage III, and 8.8% for Stage IV.

Regardless of the type of therapy utilized, patients with carcinoma of the cervix must be followed frequently and regularly. One speaks optimistically of 5-year *cures*, but in significant numbers of patients, recurrent disease develops 10 to 20 years later or they later have other malignant lesions of the genital tract. Follow-up should include frequent cytologic study and appropriate biopsy. Secondary treatment for therapeutic failures, with surgical therapy or additional irradiation, has provided limited success. Chemotherapy has been of palliative aid only.

BENIGN UTERINE DISEASE

Various benign uterine diseases occur, including leiomyoma uteri, adenomyosis, endometrial hyperplasia, and polyps. Abnormal bleeding, uterine enlargement, and pain are the usual symptoms associated with these diseases, but the primary difficulty is to achieve an accurate diagnosis.

Leiomyoma Uteri

Uterine leiomyomas, also called myomas, fibromyomas, or fibroids, are the most common cause of benign uterine enlargement and are seen in 20% of women, with a higher incidence in blacks. Leiomyomas originate from the smooth muscle cells of the myometrium and vary from microscopic to large enough to fill the entire abdomen. Such tumors may be single but are more often multiple. On cut section these solid tumors have a white, glistening appearance with a characteristic whorl pattern. There is no true capsule; compressed peripheral fibers from a pseudocapsule are seen. Microscopically, smooth muscle cells are arranged in interlacing muscle bundles, interspersed with varying amounts of connective tissue and hyaline material. Such tumors may be submucous, intramural, subserous, pedunculated, parasitic, cervical, or interligamentous (Fig. 44–18).

The symptoms of leiomyoma vary according to location. Some may produce severe complaints and others may produce none at all. The three most common symptoms are abnormal bleeding, pain, and uterine enlargement. Abnormal bleeding, usually cyclic but profuse and prolonged, is most frequently due to submucous tumors that distort the overlying endometrium and interfere with normal hemostatic mechanisms. Occasionally a submucous or cervical myoma may be extruded and also cause abnormal bleeding. Abnormal bleeding is the most common indication for hysterectomy for leiomyoma, but caution must be taken to exclude other causes, because a malignant lesion may coexist with myoma. Often curettage may be mandatory to make this differentiation. Rapid enlargement is another symptom of concern in patients with leiomyoma; 1% to 2% of such tumors may undergo sarcomatous change or degeneration of other nonmalignant varieties. Estrogen, including the synthetic estrogens of oral contraceptives, may cause enlargement of myomas. Myomas tend to regress after menopause, and any enlargement of these tumors demands prompt removal of the uterus. Slow enlargement of leiomyomas during the menstrual years frequently occurs with a minimum of symptoms. Surgical removal is not mandatory for slow growth or moderate size unless other symptoms occur. Pelvic pressure, frequency of urination, and sciatic or hip pain from

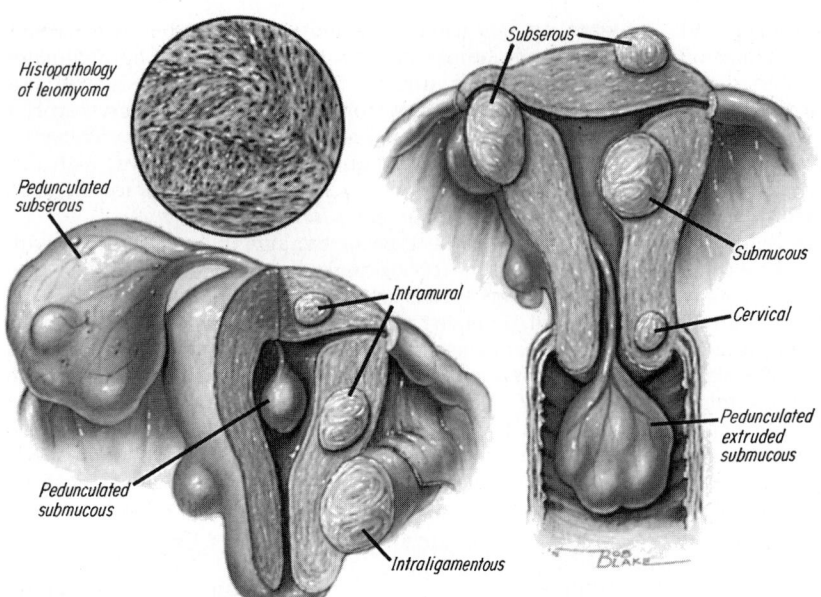

Figure 44–18. Leiomyoma uteri.

pressure on pelvic nerves can be symptoms of uterine leiomyoma. Tenderness in a myoma is usually caused by degeneration or by impairment of the blood supply. Cystic changes and calcification can follow degeneration. Significant pain or tenderness usually warrants hysterectomy. Infertility is not infrequently seen in patients with myomas, nor is abortion, but in the former it is not known whether the infertility or the myoma is primary. The increased rate of abortion is attributed to poor uterine distensibility and compression. Whereas uterine myomas are usually recognized without difficulty in the operating room, their preoperative diagnosis may be difficult, especially if the myoma primarily involves one of the adnexa.

The treatment of leiomyoma demands individualization for each patient. Some tumors require no treatment if small and asymptomatic, and only semiannual examination is warranted. If a young patient who desires further childbearing has symptomatic leiomyomas, then myomectomy may be a useful surgical procedure. For larger or more symptomatic myomas in a woman who has completed her reproduction, hysterectomy is the treatment of choice.

Recent work has focused on medical treatment of leiomyoma with gonadotropin-releasing hormone analog (GnRH-A). Significant size reduction has been made, presumably due to the acute hypoestrogenism that occurs with such therapy. However, regrowth rapidly occurs after treatment ceases, and this has not become a significant management method for long-term use. The attendant amenorrhea with GnRH-A treatment may allow rebuilding of hemoglobin before anticipated conservative surgical therapy or hysterectomy.[4]

Adenomyosis

Invasion of the myometrium by endometrium, known as adenomyosis, is a frequent cause of uterine enlargement and pain. Grossly, the uterus is enlarged, fibrotic, and thickened; and on cut section the areas of endometrial growth and loculated menstruation may be quite apparent.

The classic symptoms and signs of adenomyosis are acquired dysmenorrhea occurring in the 35- to 40-year age group, menstrual irregularities with cyclic, prolonged, and profuse flow, and an enlarged, tender uterus. Treatment is hysterectomy, although hormonal suppression (such as treatment with gonadotropin-releasing hormone) may provide relief without removal of the uterus.

Endometrial Hyperplasia and Polyps

Hyperplasia of the endometrium, causing abnormal uterine bleeding, is a common problem of women. Women near menopause or, less frequently, in early adolescence are most frequently affected. The basic problem is anovulation and failure of corpus luteum formation without production of progesterone. Continued stimulation of the endometrium by estrogen brings about proliferation, overgrowth, and hyperplasia of the endometrium. Areas of thickened endometrium may form polyps. Cycles become irregular, with intervals of amenorrhea associated with other intervals of intermenstrual spotting or bleeding. Pelvic examination is usually nonrevealing, and curettage produces copious amounts of endometrial scrapings. Microscopic examination shows hyperplasia of the epithelium and stroma. The cells lining the glands are nonsecretory, and the stroma often contains cells with frequent mitotic figures. Cystic changes of the glands may be present.

Curettage is useful in diagnosis and for treatment, because it removes the hypertrophied endometrium and leaves a fresh surface for endometrial regeneration. Because of the frequency of recurrence of hyperplasia, the administration of cyclic progesterone often aids in prevention of recurrence and promotes cyclic menses. If endometrial hyperplasia recurs, it may proceed to atypical or adenomatous hyperplasia and then to carcinoma *in situ*, which may lead to endometrial cancer. Recurrent abnormal bleeding requires repeated curettage for diagnosis and proper therapy.

Adenomatous hyperplasia is diagnosed when there is marked proliferation, with the glands being closely packed and the stroma quite dense and hyperplastic. This adenomatous pattern closely resembles adenocarcinoma and is thought to be a precancerous lesion. Diagnosis of this lesion is by curettage. Whereas cyclic progesterone is of aid for most patients, hysterectomy is probably the treatment of choice for the older patient who has completed her reproduction.

MALIGNANT DISEASES OF THE UTERUS
Adenocarcinoma of the Endometrium

Adenocarcinoma of the endometrium, now the most prevalent gynecologic cancer, is seen most commonly among postmenopausal women. The peak incidence occurs in the 50- to 70-year age group, but one must suspect the condition as early as the third decade if there is menstrual irregularity. Postmenopausal bleeding is the cardinal symptom of endometrial cancer and must be considered as due to malignancy until proved otherwise. Prolonged, profuse, or irregular bleeding may occur in the premenopausal woman. Papanicolaou cytologic study may yield negative results, because the exfoliated cells may not reach the vaginal pool. Cervical stenosis with secondary hematometrium or pyometrium is frequently present and can be identified by passage of an endocervical probe. Fractional curettage is the diagnostic method of choice, and only in this manner can the diagnosis be established as well as the degree of cervical involvement, an important factor influencing therapy. Histologically, adenocarcinoma of the endometrium has wide variations in differentiation and in stromal invasion by the glandular epithelial cells, and, finally, there is a highly undifferentiated type in which neither glandular nor stromal elements can be identified.

The etiology of endometrial cancer is unknown. There does appear to be a relationship to prolonged estrogenic stimulation, as in patients with estrogen-producing ovarian tumors. Newer studies also suggest a higher incidence of endometrial adenocarcinoma in women given high-dose estrogen replacement therapy for menopausal symptoms. Still other studies suggest that the sequential addition of progesterone to estrogen therapy significantly reduces the increased risk seen in patients who receive estrogen alone. Other frequently associated findings in patients with endometrial adenocarcinoma are obesity, diabetes, hypertension, and low parity.[3]

Endometrial cancer is usually a polypoid lesion growing into the endometrial cavity, and only late in the disease does myometrial or cervical involvement occur (Fig. 44–19). Uterine size is usually normal to slightly increased in women with early cancer of the endometrium. Uterine enlargement and menstrual irregularity occur in advanced disease or disease associated with hematometrium or leiomyoma. In addition to direct extension to adjacent structures, adenocarcinoma of the endometrium may spread through the extensive lymphatic anastomosis at the upper uterus between the tube and ovary. Thus, the tubes and ovaries are frequent sites of early metastases. In addition to this direct lymphatic extension of endometrial cancer, these tumors may spread by regional and distant lymph node metastasis to the pelvic and aortic nodal chains. The incidence of such lymph node metastasis is rare when only the uterine fundus is involved (2%), but it is frequent if the primary lesion is near the cervical junction (50%). Hematogenous dissemination may also occur; the most frequent sites are the peritoneal surfaces, lungs, liver, and skin. Local recurrence in the apex of the vagina, vaginal walls, and perineum occurs in 10% of patients who have been treated for endometrial cancer.

The usual clinical staging of endometrial cancer includes Stage 0, preinvasive carcinoma or carcinoma *in situ* of the endometrium; Stage I, in which the growth is confined to the uterine body; Stage II, in which the carcinoma involves the corpus and the cervix; Stage III, in which the tumor extends outside the uterus but not outside the true pelvis; and Stage IV, in which the carcinoma has extended outside the true pelvis or has involved the mucosa of the rectum or bladder. The location of the primary neoplasm in the uterus, the degree of anaplasia of the cells, and the gross size of the uterus influence the prognosis and the effectiveness of treatment.

The treatment of adenocarcinoma of the endometrium is primarily surgical. Survival for patients with cancer spread beyond the uterus is poor, regardless of whether surgical therapy, irradiation, or a combination of the two methods is used. Approximately 30% of patients with recurrent or metastatic adenocarcinoma of the endometrium benefit from large doses of parenteral progesterone (Megace or Depo-Provera)—usually those with tumors that are well differentiated histologically. Other forms of chemotherapy have been of little aid. External pelvic radiation therapy or transvaginal irradiation and intravaginal radium may provide palliation for locally recurrent adenocarcinoma of the endometrium.

The prognosis for adenocarcinoma of the endometrium is generally good, but results of larger series are frequently difficult to compare, owing to differences in tumor size, differentiation, stage, and type of treatment. Of those patients selected for surgical therapy because of an operable lesion, with or without preoperative irradiation, approximately 60% survive 5 years.

Sarcoma of the Uterus

Sarcomas may arise from the endometrium, myometrium, cervix, uterine blood vessels, or a leiomyoma. These diseases are most frequently seen in the fifth decade; a rare sarcoma of the cervix, sarcoma botryoides, is seen in infants. The incidence of corpus sarcoma is much higher than that of sarcoma of the cervix. Because all elements of the uterus are mesodermal in origin and ectodermal rests may be present, mixed tumors may occur. A wide spectrum of histopathologic types can be found. Rapid uterine enlargement is a prominent sign of uterine sarcoma, and abnormal bleeding may or may not be present. Pain, anemia, and weight loss are late symptoms. Pulmonary metastases frequently occur early. Surgical excision of the uterus, tubes, and ovaries is the recommended treatment for sarcoma of the uterus. The prognosis after treatment varies with the type and extent of the original tumor. The sarcomas arising in myomas generally appear to be of low grade and thus have a relatively good prognosis, with 45% to 50% of patients with operable lesions surviving. There are very few survivors among patients with the other types of uterine sarcoma, despite appropriate surgical therapy for patients with operable lesions. Radiation therapy may offer benefit. The author is currently exploring a combination approach, with extirpative surgical

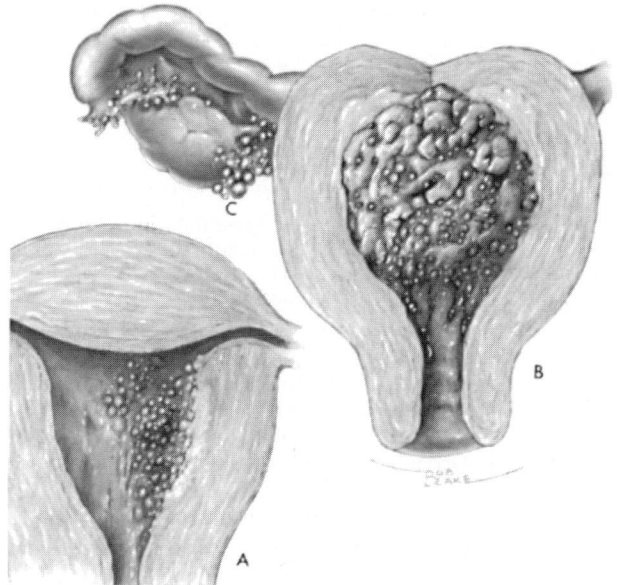

Figure 44–19. Carcinoma of the endometrium. *A*, Stage I. *B*, Stage III, myometrial invasion plus *(C)* ovarian extension of metastases.

therapy and combination chemotherapy, followed by external pelvic irradiation. The initial results are encouraging but warrant further investigation.

PELVIC INFECTION
Acute Pelvic Infection

Acute pelvic infection (pelvic inflammatory disease [PID]) may occur after pelvic surgery or result from other causes, but by far the most frequent causes are gonorrhea and chlamydial infection. The initial symptoms of acute PID usually occur within 3 to 6 days after inoculation and consist of urethritis, skenitis, bartholinitis, cervicitis, and vaginal discharge. Tubal involvement is often a later symptom and usually does not occur until after a menstrual period. At this time, the organisms spread rapidly from the endocervix and across the endometrium and involve the endosalpinx. The major infection and damage occur in the fallopian tube. The tube becomes acutely inflamed and edematous, and its lumen fills with a purulent exudate. The tubular, peritubular, ovarian, and pelvic peritoneal surfaces are rapidly involved. Secondary infection with anaerobic bacteria is common. Pelvic abscess may develop.[18]

The signs and symptoms of acute pelvic infection are those of pelvic peritonitis with bilateral lower abdominal pain and tenderness, temperature of 38 to 39° C., and signs of peritoneal irritation with direct and rebound tenderness and muscle spasm. On pelvic examination, one may be able to express pus from the paraurethral glands or cervix. Exquisite tenderness is present with cervical manipulation and in the adnexal areas, and there is a thickened, doughy feeling in the adnexa. Bilaterality of pain is an important point in differentiating acute pelvic infection from appendicitis, and the fever associated with PID is often higher. The diagnosis of acute pelvic infection may be made by cervical smear and culture (see Laboratory and Clinical Tests), but high clinical suspicion remains of primary importance, and laparoscopic examination may ultimately be necessary.

Therapy is based on the degree of peritonitis and fever. If significant peritonitis is present, compliance with outpatient therapy is uncertain, a pelvic mass is present, or the patient is HIV seropositive, hospitalization is indicated and intravenous antibiotic therapy recommended. For women with more serious episodes of pelvic infection, several therapeutic regimens are recommended. Included are doxycycline, 100 mg. orally or intravenously every 12 hours plus cefoxitin or ampicillin/sulbactam, 2.0 gm. intravenously every 6 hours. An alternative therapy includes clindamycin, 900 mg. intravenously every 8 hours, plus gentamicin or tobramycin, 2.0 mg. per kg. intravenously, then 1.5 mg. per kg. intravenously every 8 hours for patients with normal renal function. This intensive treatment, plus analgesia, elevation of the head to encourage pelvic localization of pus, and parenteral fluid replacement, is continued until the acute signs and symptoms have subsided; then oral therapy is begun and continued for at least a week using doxycycline, 100 mg. twice daily, or clindamycin, 450 mg. 4 times a day. If the presenting symptoms are not severe, one can treat the patient entirely as an outpatient, using either (1) ceftriaxone, 250 mg. intramuscularly, or cefoxitin, 2 gm. intramuscularly plus probenecid, 1 gm. orally, plus doxycycline, 100 mg. orally twice daily for 10 to 14 days, or (2) ofloxacin, 400 mg. orally twice daily plus either clindamycin, 450 mg. orally 4 times daily or metronidazole, 500 mg. orally twice daily for 10 to 14 days. Surgical therapy is not indicated for acute pelvic infection unless pelvic abscess drainage is required or adequate medical therapy fails. If the abdomen is opened for other preoperative diagnoses but acute pelvic infection is found, no further operative procedure is indicated, and the abdomen is closed and antibiotics are initiated. If significant pelvic contamination with pus is present, drains may be used.

The patient with relatively asymptomatic gonorrhea can be treated with either ceftriaxone, 125 mg. intramuscularly, cefixime, 400 mg. orally, ciprofloxacin, 500 mg. orally, or ofloxacin, 400 mg. orally (each as a single dose), plus presumptive treatment for genital chlamydial infection such as doxycycline, 100 mg. orally twice daily for 7 days, or azithromycin, 1 gm. orally as a single dose. An alternative regimen is a single intramuscular dose of spectinomycin, 2.0 gm. A syphilis serology is advised for these patients, as is determination of HIV and hepatitis B serostatus. *Test of cure* culture is unnecessary if one of the recommended regimens is used. A follow-up examination in 48 to 96 hours is important.

Pelvic Abscess

Abscess may follow acute pelvic infection, pelvic surgery, septicemia, puerperal endometritis, appendicitis, or peritonitis of any cause. It may be localized in the cul-de-sac or between the leaves of the broad ligament, or it may be tubo-ovarian. If gonorrhea is the primary cause, the purulent exudate usually does not contain the organism, because it is short-lived in such conditions. Secondary organisms such as colon bacilli and anaerobic organisms such as *Bacteroides*, streptococci, and staphylococci may be present in large quantities. The signs and symptoms of pelvic abscess are elevation of temperature and pulse, pelvic or lower abdominal pain, and leukocytosis. Ultrasound of the pelvis may be especially useful here. If the abscess is anteriorly placed, as in an interligamentous pelvic abscess, one may discover a tender, fluctuant mass on abdominal examination. Pelvic examination is usually quite helpful. A cul-de-sac abscess bulges into the posterior vaginal fornix and displaces the cervix anteriorly. Interligamentous abscesses may bulge into the lateral fornix and displace the cervix to one side.

Treatment of pelvic abscess consists of appropriate antibiotic therapy and, usually, some type of drainage procedure. If intraperitoneal rupture occurs, there is considerable morbidity and mortality from disseminated infection. Increasingly, patients with small, unruptured abscesses are treated for an interval with parenteral antibiotics and drainage, if needed, can be effected by ultrasound- or computed tomographic–guided aspiration or by laparoscopic aspiration. However, this takes considerable clinical judgment. In patients who have failed to improve with several antibiotic regimens, the uterus, tubes, and ovaries may have to be removed.

Chronic Pelvic Infection

Included among chronic pelvic infections are chronic salpingo-oophoritis, pyosalpinx, hydrosalpinx, and tubercular salpingitis. Chronic salpingo-oophoritis is one of the major complications of gonorrhea. The patient may have few complaints. Because the endosalpinx was intensely involved in the acute infection, the tube may be agglutinized. Pyosalpinx is one of the chronic destructive lesions of gonorrhea in which the tube is dilated, closed, and filled with pus. Hydrosalpinx results from pyosalpinx in which the purulent material is replaced by a serous fluid. Chronic oophoritis may develop after ovarian surface involvement, and often the tube and ovary are involved in a single inflammatory process. The classic pattern of chronic pelvic infection is one of quiescent intervals interspersed with episodes of more acute inflammation. After the initial, usually gonococcal, infection, anaerobic organisms invade and involve these tissues. Tuberculous salpingitis is now a rare problem in the

United States, and the process usually involves the endometrium and adjacent structures as well. The dense adhesions of pelvic viscera to bowel and omentum are outstanding features of this disease, and these structures may be covered with a caseous exudate.

Chronic pelvic infection may be treated medically or surgically. The important elements of medical therapy are rest, heat, and antibiotic therapy. Sedation and analgesia are usually required. Oral metronidazole, doxycycline, or tetracycline are the appropriate antibiotics utilized with modest increase of pain and symptoms from chronic pelvic infection. Those patients who have recurrent pain or abnormal uterine bleeding from reduced ovarian function caused by chronic pelvic infection are often difficult to relieve of symptoms.

This disease is a common gynecologic complaint, and surgical therapy is often required. The only cure for chronic, recurrent pelvic infection is surgical removal of the uterus, tubes, and ovaries. Surgical therapy should always be delayed, if possible, until maximal medical control has been obtained. Estrogen replacement is indicated for the younger woman if both ovaries are removed.

BENIGN DISEASES OF THE OVARY

Benign ovarian tumors may be solid or cystic and may represent a *functional* process or neoplasia. Although these growths are usually small, they may persist or become massively enlarged. The judgment about the necessity of surgical removal should be based on size, duration, or symptoms; the interval of persistence of the smaller lesions; and the age of the patient. Most classifications of such benign tumors include ovarian cysts (nonneoplastic and neoplastic) and solid ovarian tumors.

Many investigators report that more than 90% of ovarian growths discovered in women younger than 30 years old are benign. In the 30- to 50-year age group, 80% are benign. After 50 years of age, approximately half of such ovarian growths are malignant. Other investigators report the likelihood of the various benign ovarian growths, excluding the frequently seen follicular and corpus luteum cysts, as endometrial cysts, 33%; simple cysts, 26%; serous and mucinous cystadenomas, 19%; dermoids, 15.2%; and others, 2%. The most frequent sign of benign ovarian growths is slow abdominal enlargement. Other symptoms are pain and tenderness from torsion of the pedicle and interference with the blood supply. Less than 10% of such growths are associated with aberrations in the menstrual cycle. Amenorrhea or irregular bleeding may accompany follicular or corpus luteum cysts, polycystic ovaries, or endometrial cysts. Unless quite large, most benign ovarian tumors rarely cause pressure on adjacent pelvic structures. Most commonly, such ovarian growths are asymptomatic and discovered on routine pelvic examination.

The benign, nonneoplastic ovarian cysts are usually of *functional* origin. The follicular cyst represents failure of a developing follicle to rupture or regress and rarely exceeds 8 cm. in diameter. Corpus luteum cysts occur from hemorrhage into the corpus luteum; these blood-filled cysts have the yellow granular color of the normal corpus luteum, whereas the follicular cyst is filled with clear fluid. Both usually regress over a 4- to 8-week period. The theca lutein cyst and the luteoma of pregnancy are also functional cysts resulting from the high levels of circulating chorionic gonadotropin of normal pregnancy and trophoblastic disease. They regress after pregnancy is terminated. Germinal inclusion cysts occur in the cortex of the ovary and represent inward growth of the germinal epithelium that has undergone cystic change. These cysts are thought to be the origin of the neoplastic serous cystadenoma. Polycystic ovaries are enlarged with multiple small follicular cysts and luteinization of the stroma and have a thickened capsule. The etiology is unknown but may relate to tonic elevation of LH.

The benign neoplastic ovarian cysts are most frequently the endometrial cyst or *chocolate* cyst of pelvic endometriosis (Fig. 44–20) or the simple cyst. These may achieve large size, especially the latter. Serous and mucinous cystadenomas arise from neoplastic changes in germinal epithelium and often reach considerable size. These cystic tumors are multilocular, have smooth capsules, and usually replace the entire ovary. Histologic examination reveals an adenomatous pattern of tall columnar cells producing mucin. The benign teratoma, or dermoid cyst, is a common ovarian tumor, benign in more than 99% of patients. The gross appearance is that of a smooth-coated, gray tumor that usually replaces the ovary. Microscopically, ectodermal and mesodermal structures are found with hair, teeth, bone, and cartilage present. Approximately 20% of dermoids are bilateral; and thus if one ovary is involved, the other should be carefully inspected.

The solid benign ovarian tumors include the Brenner tumor, which is thought to arise from the Walthard inclusion rests in the cortex of the ovary. This tumor grossly resembles the ovarian fibroma, another benign solid tumor. Ovarian fibromas are occasionally the cause of Meigs' syndrome, with concomitant sympathetic pleural effusion and ascites. Other solid ovarian tumors include the rare androgen-producing Leydig cell tumor, or hilus cell tumor, and the neuroma, angioma, papilloma, and fibroadenoma. The most important decision facing the surgeon who finds a solid ovarian tumor is to differentiate benign from malignant.

The treatment of benign ovarian growths is primarily surgical removal with conservation of all possible normal ovarian tissue. The functional cysts of follicular and corpus luteum should regress in a relatively short interval and do not require removal unless rupture and hemorrhage have occurred. These are frequently found during surgical therapy for other reasons and do not require treatment. The majority of the other benign cystic and solid ovarian tumors usually replace or destroy any remaining ovarian tissue in the involved gonad; and oophorectomy, preserving the tube, is often indicated. Endometrial or chocolate cysts are an exception, and after all involved ovarian tissue is resected, one attempts to leave even a small amount of normal ovarian tissue for future fertility. In any event, bilateral oophorectomy is rarely indicated in the young woman unless one is *certain* that malignancy is present. If there is any doubt, the abdomen should be closed even if reoperation is needed at a later date. In general, it has been thought that if an undiagnosed ovarian mass is larger than 6 cm. or if it persists without

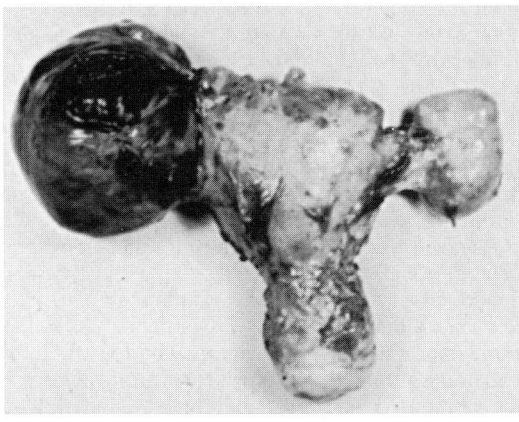

Figure 44–20. Endometrioma ("chocolate cyst") of ovary with attached hysterectomy specimen.

diminution in size for longer than 3 months, exploration should be done. Acute torsion or significant hemorrhage may require immediate operative intervention.

OVARIAN CANCER

The incidence of cancer of the ovary varies considerably in different reports because of the wide range of criteria accepted for making this diagnosis. Among the adenomatous tumors, there is a broad group of borderline cases. Most series report that ovarian cancer comprises 4% to 6% of all cases of malignant disease in women. Most investigators report incidences of histologic types as serous cystadenocarcinoma, 60%; pseudomucinous carcinoma, 15%; solid undifferentiated adenocarcinoma, 10%; granulosa cell carcinoma, 6%; dysgerminoma, 2%; and other rare types (arrhenoblastoma, teratoma, mesonephroma), 7%. The ratio of benign ovarian tumors to malignant ovarian tumors is 4 to 1, until the peak incidence of ovarian cancer at 40 to 60 years of age, when the ratio is 1 to 1.

The International Federation of Gynecology and Obstetrics has adopted the following clinical classification, based on clinical studies and surgical exploration, for staging primary carcinoma of the ovary. Further modification and expansion of this basic staging occurred in 1985.

Stage I
  Growth limited to the ovaries
Stage II
  Growth involves one or both ovaries with extension of the cancer to other areas within the pelvis
Stage III
  Growth involves one or both ovaries with widespread intraperitoneal metastasis to the abdomen
Stage IV
  Growth involves one or both ovaries with distant metastasis outside the peritoneal cavity

Several factors need to be emphasized in regard to ovarian cancer. First, the delay in diagnosis is reprehensible: 50% of ovarian cancers are neglected by the patient and 25% by the physician, who does not examine the patient in more than 60% of cases. Second, 30% to 50% of ovarian cancers are inoperable at the time of diagnosis, and in only 20% can the tumor be entirely removed surgically. Third, only 11% of patients have suspicious or positive Papanicolaou cytologic findings. Fourth, as expected, the survival is greater the earlier the stage of the disease at the time of diagnosis. Because the overall survival of patients with ovarian cancer has improved only slightly in the past 25 years, earlier diagnosis is mandatory.

Ovarian cancer occurs more frequently in white women, and the mean age at diagnosis is 51 years. Fifty-eight percent of patients are postmenopausal. Childbearing may have some effect in reducing the likelihood of ovarian cancer, as may use of oral contraceptives. It is suggested that a family history of cancer, exposure to pelvic irradiation, and previously existing benign ovarian tumors may increase the likelihood of development of cancer of the ovary.

Signs and Symptoms. The signs and symptoms of ovarian cancer may be only those of an enlarging tumor in the pelvis. Parker reported that 56% of patients complained of pain and 46% of abdominal swelling. He also reported that 31% had experienced at least a 10-pound weight change, usually loss, and 22% had either abnormal or postmenopausal bleeding. There may be ascites with unilateral or bilateral pleural effusion. Anemia is frequently seen in advanced disease. Pelvic examination may reveal firm, nodular implants of metastatic tumor in the cul-de-sac and pelvic viscera. As noted, often there are no early symptoms of ovarian cancer. Every woman should have an annual pelvic examination before age 40 and more frequently thereafter.

Diagnosis. The diagnosis is made histopathologically, and the differential diagnosis between benign and malignant ovarian tumors cannot be made until operation. The gross examination of the tumor at operation is usually helpful, because papillary growths on the surface of a cystic or semicystic tumor or papillations on the inside of the tumor are suggestive of malignancy (Fig. 44–21). Solid ovarian tumors that are lobulated or have hemorrhagic areas in the capsule are usually malignant. Peritoneal cell washings should be obtained with any suggestive ovarian tumor. Recent work has centered on evaluation of tumor markers for ovarian cancer (CA 125, CEA). Although not highly accurate for diagnosis, if present they may have a useful role.[21]

Treatment. The reader is referred to the many excellent reviews on the various types of therapy for ovarian cancer. Results of all therapy, however, remain poor, and various proponents report limited success with a variety of therapeutic regimens. There is general agreement that total abdominal hysterectomy, bilateral salpingo-oophorectomy, and omentectomy should be performed, even if some tumor is left behind. The abdomen, including the diaphragm, should be carefully inspected and appropriate lymph node sampling performed. The surgeon should routinely obtain peritoneal washings for cytology on entering the abdomen of patients suspected of having ovarian cancer. Because the 5-year survival for Stage I ovarian cancer is only 66%, and only 20% of patients explored have disease as limited as Stage I, most investigators believe supplemental therapy is mandatory for all patients with ovarian cancer. Radiation therapy and chemotherapy have both been used with moderate palliative success. Total pelvic and abdominal irradiation, intraperitoneal radioisotopes, alkylating agents, and combination chemotherapy are of significant palliative aid in nearly half of patients so treated.

MALIGNANT TROPHOBLASTIC DISEASE

Malignant gestational trophoblastic diseases are relatively rare cancers of women but are of major importance. Even if metastases are present, essentially all patients with these tumors can be cured. It is tragic for a woman to be given an erroneous diagnosis of *anaplastic metastatic cancer* and have the diagnosis of trophoblastic malignancy be overlooked. Because these tumors frequently present with the symptoms of metastases, it is useful for any physician who treats women of reproductive age to be aware of the patterns of these disease.

Malignant trophoblastic disease may follow any type of pregnancy, including abortion or term live birth, although more than half the tumors occur after hydatidiform mole.[6] Tissue diagnoses include invasive mole (chorioadenoma destruens), choriocarcinoma, and anaplastic trophoblastic tissue. Irregular uterine bleeding is a common presenting sign, but patients present with amenorrhea, uterine rupture or the sequelae of distant metastasis to the lung, vagina, brain, bowel, kidney or elsewhere. The anaplastic pattern of the placental trophoblast, with or without preservation of the pattern of the villus, may be seen histologically. Fortunately, all these tumors produce a hormone identical to human chorionic gonadotropin (hCG), which can be measured by sensitive radioimmunologic techniques. The finding of a suspicious metastatic lesion, with or without pelvic symptoms, should lead to hCG testing. If the hCG level is elevated and normal pregnancy can be excluded, one should strongly suspect malignant trophoblastic disease.[20]

Considerable assistance for physicians treating patients with suspected malignant trophoblastic disease can be ob-

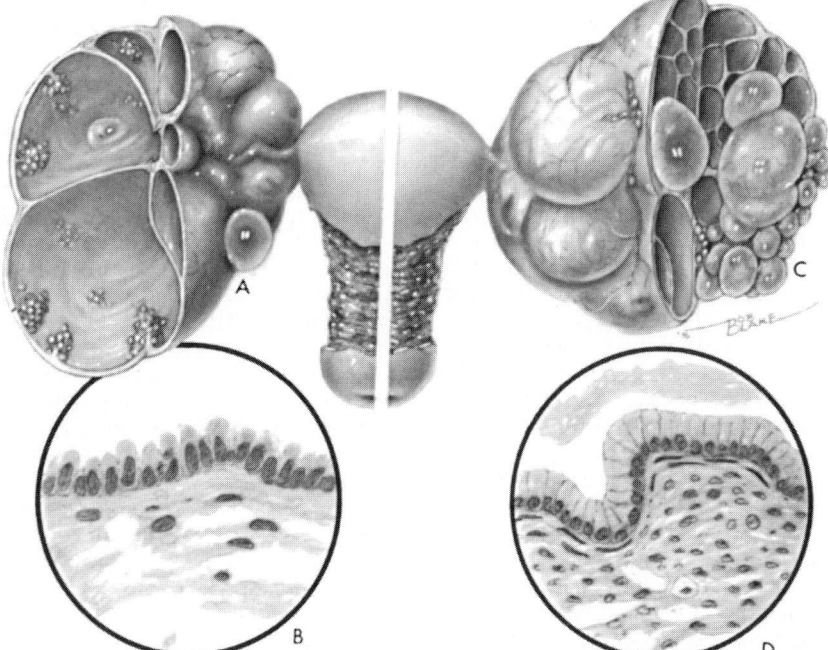

Figure 44–21. Ovarian carcinoma. *A*, Cystic, papillary. *B*, Microscopic view of *A*. *C*, Pseudomucinous. *D*, Microscopic view of *C*.

tained from any of the several trophoblastic disease centers in the United States. Treatment consists of intensive chemotherapy with methotrexate or dactinomycin, given alone or in combination with surgical therapy or irradiation. With appropriate and intensive therapy, essentially all patients with these diseases can be cured, even when metastases are present.[6]

AMENORRHEA

Amenorrhea is defined as the absence of menses at the time a woman should be menstruating and may be classified as primary or secondary. Most investigators believe a patient should be without menses for at least 6 months before the diagnosis of amenorrhea is made.[23] Amenorrhea occurs physiologically in pregnancy and lactation. Menstruation is based on the interaction of the central nervous system, hypothalamus, pituitary, ovary, uterus, and other glands and their hormones (see Physiology and Endocrinology).

Primary amenorrhea, in which the patient has never had menses, occasionally may be due to abnormalities of the central nervous system or the pituitary gland but much more commonly occurs from gonadal, adrenal, or uterine defects. Most girls begin menses by 18 years of age, and failure of menstruation by this age warrants careful examination, chromosomal testing, hormonal assays, and, on occasion, visualization of the gonad. Gonadotropin assays frequently provide the appropriate direction for further study, because these levels are increased in cases of ovarian failure or abnormal function and are usually reduced with central nervous system or pituitary gland diseases. Congenital absence of the uterus always, and endometrial disease frequently, results in amenorrhea, although gonadotropin levels are normal.

Secondary amenorrhea, or cessation of menses, may be due to a variety of problems. However, the most common cause of absence of menses is pregnancy. Space-occupying lesions of the central nervous system, hypothalamus, or pituitary result in absence or low levels of gonadotropins and amenorrhea. Pituitary tumors or infarction can also yield similar results. Skull films, visual field examinations, appropriate imaging, and hormonal studies may aid in making

these diagnoses. However, one must always remember that the symptom of amenorrhea may precede the diagnosis of such lesions by a span of years, and prolonged follow-up is mandatory.

Psychiatric illnesses may interfere with gonadotropin release and result in amenorrhea. Ovarian problems, such as polycystic ovaries and premature ovarian failure, may cause secondary amenorrhea, and in these patients gonadotropins are normal and elevated, respectively. Acquired failure of endometrial responsiveness may also cause secondary amenorrhea, as can significant dysfunction of the thyroid or adrenal glands. Treatment is based on the appropriate diagnosis.

ECTOPIC PREGNANCY

An ectopic pregnancy is one in which the ovum implants and develops outside the normal location, the uterine cavity. Ninety-five percent of ectopic pregnancies are tubal, with the greatest percentage of these occurring in the dilated ampulla, that portion of the distal tube immediately proximal to the fimbriated end. Less common sites of ectopic pregnancy are abdominal, ovarian, and cervical (Fig. 44–22). Abdominal ectopic pregnancy usually occurs after tubal abortion, with secondary reimplantation elsewhere in the abdominal cavity. The incidence of all types of ectopic pregnancy is increasing and is approximately 3 in 100 births.

Despite the fact that the ovum is implanted outside the uterine cavity, the uterine endometrium is converted into a decidua similar to that of normal pregnancy. The size and consistency of the uterus also change in ectopic pregnancy. The cervix and body of the uterus soften, and the corpus may enlarge to a size compatible with a 6- to 8-week intrauterine pregnancy. All these changes are due to the production of placental hormones from the ectopic embryo. As ectopic placental function declines, as usually occurs in tubal pregnancy, the hormonal support declines and irregular uterine bleeding begins. The decidua is usually discharged in fragments but may on occasion be expelled intact as a decidual cast.[2]

The duration and the eventual outcome of tubal ectopic pregnancy are determined primarily by the area of tube involved. If the ovum implants in the relatively large ampul-

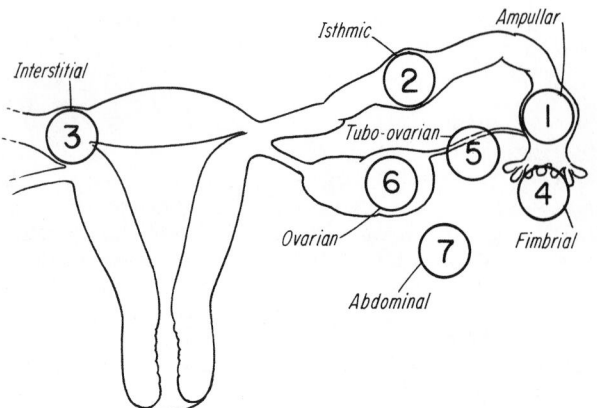

Figure 44–22. Ectopic pregnancy. Diagram shows the various implantation sites, numbered in order of decreasing frequency of occurrence.

lary region of the tube, the pregnancy usually continues longer than one in the narrow isthmus. Local bleeding from trophoblastic invasion continues and increases, and blood dissects the ovular sac from the tubal wall. With complete separation, the ovular sac is usually extruded from the end of the tube; and unless a major vessel is involved, bleeding is terminated. More often, however, the process is prolonged, and repeated bleeding episodes yield a pelvic hematoma. In other areas of the tube, the tubal wall is less distensible and the lumen narrower, and tubal rupture is inevitable as the trophoblasts invade and blood collects. Episodic pregnancies in the narrow isthmic segment usually rupture in 6 to 8 weeks, whereas those in the interstitial portion, where the tube traverses the uterine wall, continue for 14 to 16 weeks before rupture. Rupture is usually into the peritoneal cavity and is accompanied by sudden and significant bleeding. Tubal pregnancies may regress spontaneously, with the ovum either dying at an early age or being extruded from the tubal ostium without significant bleeding.

The classic symptoms of ectopic pregnancy are a history of infertility or pelvic disease, light vaginal bleeding within 2 to 4 weeks after the first missed period, and sharp and fleeting lower abdominal pain. Eventually the patient experiences sudden severe abdominal pain and shock as the tube ruptures. On examination, one usually notes the signs of early pregnancy such as cyanosis and softening of the cervix and uterine enlargement. The most important pelvic finding before tubal rupture is a unilateral tender mass. In patients with pelvic hematoma, the cul-de-sac may be *doughy* and distended. Signs of peritoneal inflammation may be present. Fever is a rare finding, but progressive anemia is frequently observed. Newer, more sensitive pregnancy tests are positive in most patients with unruptured tubal pregnancy.

The diagnosis of unruptured tubal pregnancy is not difficult to make when classic symptoms are present but, unfortunately, the symptoms are frequently atypical and the pelvic findings misleading. A high index of suspicion is the most valuable adjunct. Culdocentesis, or large-gauge needle perforation of the cul-de-sac, may reveal considerable dark old blood and strongly suggest pelvic bleeding. Laparoscopy may allow visualization of the ectopic pregnancy. Although it is usually possible to diagnose tubal pregnancy with reasonable accuracy, problems such as uterine abortion, salpingitis, appendicitis, or ruptured corpus luteum or follicular cysts may produce signs and symptoms causing confusion in diagnosis. In uterine abortion, the period of amenorrhea is usually longer, the amount of bleeding is greater, and pain is less severe, more midline, and cramping. No adnexal mass or tenderness is present. Salpingitis and appendicitis usually

present with signs of infection and without prior amenorrhea or irregular bleeding. Ruptured cysts, particularly those of the corpus luteum, are usually not associated with prolonged amenorrhea. Follicular cysts tend to rupture at mid cycle. In both varieties, an occasional patient may require surgical exploration for control of hemorrhage.

The diagnostic armamentarium for the assessment of ectopic pregnancy has changed dramatically. When the diagnosis is suspected, a sensitive pregnancy test should be done to determine whether hCG is present. If the test is positive, a quantified assay should be obtained. If the hCG titer is in excess of 2000 mIU per ml., an intrauterine pregnancy, if present, should be seen by transvaginal ultrasonography. The finding of an intrauterine pregnancy in such a setting likely excludes ectopic pregnancy in all but the very rare patient who might have simultaneous intrauterine and ectopic pregnancies. Failure to note an ectopically placed pregnancy with ultrasonography is not diagnostic of the absence of that problem. Likewise, if the hCG titer is less than 2000 mIU per ml., an intrauterine pregnancy may not be apparent with even well-done ultrasound examination. In patients in whom the initial value of hCG is less than 2000 mIU per ml., alternate-day assays should be performed. In normal gestations, hCG doubles every 48 hours during this portion of pregnancy. If this doubling is not observed, the diagnosis of an abnormal pregnancy—either a missed abortion, an incomplete abortion, or possibly an ectopic gestation—is supported. All these studies should be used in the subtle case.

The treatment of ectopic pregnancy remains surgical. In the event of tubal rupture and hemoperitoneum, the approach should be emergent pelvic laparotomy. In patients desiring to preserve reproductive options, hemostasis can be achieved by linear salpingostomy or *milking out* a fimbrial ectopic pregnancy. Hemostasis may be achieved by fine-point cautery or, if necessary, removal of a ruptured segment of the tube, leaving the residual proximal and distal segments for later, possible reanastomosis. Occasionally, a tube may be so destroyed that it cannot be salvaged and must be removed. Rarely is removal of the ovary a necessary part of the procedure.[2]

In unruptured tubal ectopic pregnancy, the therapy may be laparoscopic, also using linear salpingostomy or fimbrial expression. Rarely will salpingectomy be indicated. *In all cases—laparotomy or laparoscopy—serum hCG levels must be followed to zero if the involved fallopian tube is left in place.* Residual trophoblast may persist and later cause tubal rupture in up to 10% of such individuals. Lastly, there is an evolving role for methotrexate in the nonsurgical, medical treatment of unruptured, early ectopic pregnancy.[24]

Prompt correction of blood loss and surgical intervention are mandatory, but the patient's condition should be stabilized before operation if at all possible. General anesthesia should be used. Abdominal pregnancy is treated by removal of the fetus and ligation of the umbilical cord near its insertion into the placenta. Because of the vascularity of the placenta, it is usually best to leave this *in situ*. Prognosis with prompt management is good, and mortality from ectopic pregnancy has been reduced to 1% to 2%. Recurrence of ectopic pregnancy in the remaining tube occurs in about 10% of patients.

SURGICAL DISEASE IN PREGNANCY

The pregnant woman is subject to all the surgical diseases of the nonpregnant patient. Often, however, the diagnosis and management of such patients must be modified to allow for the physiologic changes that normally occur or to manage concerns generated about a second patient, the fetus. Added to these physiologic changes are the mechanical alterations associated with the enlarging uterus. Close collaboration between obstetrician, anesthesiologist, and surgeon is necessary if tragic consequences to the mother and child are to be avoided. This section can review only general concepts regarding common surgical diseases and pregnancy. It is to be hoped that the presentation of these concerns will stimulate the reader to consult the expanding literature on these topics. For further details, the reader is referred to the texts listed at the end of this chapter.

General Considerations, Including Anesthesia

Many remarkable physiologic changes occur in pregnant women, involving respiratory, circulatory, hepatic, renal, and gastrointestinal functions and acid-base balance. Most of the changes are induced by endocrinologic substances produced from the placenta and by the mechanical effects of the enlarging uterus.

Respiration. There is a progressive increase in minute ventilation, which, near term, is at a peak level of about 50% above normal. This effect is primarily through an increase in tidal volume and, to a much lesser extent, through a rise in respiratory rate. Consequently, alveolar ventilation is increased about 70% above normal at term. These changes are associated with a reduction in alveolar and arterial carbon dioxide tension to about 32 mm. Hg and an increase in oxygen tension to 95 to 105 mm. Hg. There is a progressive decrease in expiratory volume and residual volume, and consequently the functional residual capacity decreased to about 20% below that in the nonpregnant state. There is little or no change in vital capacity, maximal breathing capacity, or other pulmonary function parameters. Other physiologic changes occurring in pregnancy include edema and erythema of the nasopharynx, larynx, trachea, and bronchi. Chest films show increased lung markings, which may be of a degree to stimulate the features of mild congestive failure.

Circulation. Cardiac output increases progressively during pregnancy, reaching a maximum of 30% to 50% greater than normal by the seventh to eighth month, then falling to more normal levels during the thirty-sixth to fortieth week. Cardiac rate increases progressively until the last trimester, when it is approximately 10 beats per minute above the nonpregnant level. Arterial blood pressure decreases slightly during pregnancy, while venous blood pressure is normal in the lower extremities, where it becomes progressively increased as pregnancy advances. Hypotension may occur when the gravid patient assumes a supine position with concomitant venocaval obstruction. Operative positioning may thus be of major importance. The changes in arterial and venous pressure induced by pregnancy and the changes in the supine position may markedly influence anesthetic management. Vasomotor block, inherent in spinal and peridural anesthesia, often deprives the patient of the compensatory vasoconstriction and usually results in a much greater fall in arterial pressure than occurs in the nonpregnant state.

The increase in cardiac work is not a transient occurrence associated with activity but is maintained throughout the day. Although these increases are well tolerated by patients with normal hearts, they may present an excessive strain in patients with a low myocardial reserve and may precipitate pulmonary decompensation.

Hematologic Changes. There is a progressive increase in plasma volume, a lesser increase in red blood cell volume, and an intermediate increase in total blood volume. A resultant hemodilution occurs. There is an increase in total plasma protein, fibrinogen, and sedimentation rate. The oxygen and carbon dioxide dissociation curves of maternal blood are shifted to the right, while those of fetal blood are shifted to the left. During pregnancy, a significant decrease in cholinesterase activity may occur and may result in a prolonged paralysis and apnea after the administration of succinylcholine.

Acid-Base Balance. The total base decreases from the normal nonpregnant level of about 155 mEq. per liter to about 148 mEq. per liter. This is reflected in the decline of the plasma sodium level and a corresponding decrease in potassium, calcium, and magnesium levels. There is a commensurate total amnion diminution. The P_{CO_2} decreases to about 33 mm. Hg, and the plasma buffer base decreases from 47 to 42 mEq. per liter. In most patients, blood pH remains unchanged at 7.40.

Other Physiologic Changes. Pregnancy is associated with a diminution of gastric and intestinal motility, a relative hyperchlorhydria, and a slight delay in emptying time of the stomach. These changes are exaggerated by sedatives, general anesthetics, and labor. Regurgitation of acid stomach contents is a particular hazard of general anesthesia in the pregnant patient. Although some of the liver function tests are deranged during normal pregnancy, it appears that the liver is capable of functioning without difficulty in the normal individual. Hepatic blood flow is normal.

During pregnancy, there is a gradual dilation of the urinary collecting system and a progressive increase in glomerular filtration rate, affecting renal flow, filtration fraction, and tubular capacity for the rate of absorption.

A number of endocrinologic changes occur in pregnancy. Notable are hyperplasia of the thyroid and parathyroid glands, hypertrophy of the pituitary gland to nearly twice its normal size, enlargement of the adrenal gland to nearly twice its normal size, enlargement of the adrenal gland with increased plasma levels of glucocorticoids, and a threefold increase in aldosterone secretion. During pregnancy, there is a progressive increase in basal metabolic rate; in oxygen consumption; in retention and storage of water, protein, and minerals; in retention of salts; and in acquisition of fat.

Anesthetic Management. The objective of surgical anesthesia for the gravida is to prevent pain and emotional stress and to provide the surgeon with optimal operating conditions without undue risk to the mother and child. The ideal anesthetic for every surgical operation has not yet been developed, and the type of anesthesia must be selected for the needs of the individual patient. Preanesthetic medication in the form of a sedative, such as a barbiturate or an ataractic, is frequently used. If the patient is to receive a general anesthetic, it may be desirable to give atropine to reduce secretions within the respiratory tract.

Induction of general anesthesia should begin with the administration of 100% oxygen for at least 3 minutes before the induction. In maintaining anesthesia, the concentration of oxygen in the anesthetic mixture should never be less than 35%. Every precaution should be taken to avoid respiratory obstruction and hypoventilation, and often an endotracheal tube and assisted or controlled ventilation will be needed. If regional anesthesia is to be used, it is especially important that this procedure not be initiated unless all materials needed to treat cardiovascular and respiratory complications are ready for immediate use. The incidence and magnitude of arterial hypotension may be minimized by the prophylactic administration of 500 to 1000 ml. of lactated Ringer's solution. If hypotension develops, it should be treated promptly. Of the many vasopressors available, ephedrine is perhaps the best, because it has the least effect on uterine circulation. Obviously, in late pregnancy, the first maneuver is to displace the uterus to one side or to tilt the table to relieve venous compression.

General anesthesia is perhaps the most hazardous of the techniques of emergency surgical anesthesia, mainly because of the danger of aspiration of gastric contents. Pneumonia, cardiac arrest, and respiratory failure are also particular hazards. Again, the use of adequate preanesthetic oxygenation and the prompt placement of an endotracheal tube minimize these risks.

The Acute Abdomen in Pregnancy

As noted previously, a complex series of changes occur in pregnancy, and these may modify the manifestations of intra-abdominal disease processes. The continued growth of the uterus produces mechanical displacement of the gastrointestinal tract and a diminished motility. The stomach assumes a more horizontal position and comes to lie in the upper left quadrant beneath the diaphragm. Gastric emptying time is delayed and near term may be more than twice normal. Gastroesophageal regurgitation is common. Normally, the small intestine is displaced upward during pregnancy, with little alteration in its function. In the presence of incarcerated hernia or adhesion, however, the enlarging uterus may compound the obstructive process.

Because *acute appendicitis* is one of the most common and one of the most serious surgical complications of pregnancy, the anatomic changes in this area deserve particular attention. The colon is displaced by the enlarging uterus, so that the transverse colon deviates upward and the ascending and descending segments are displaced toward the flanks. The cecum and the base of the appendix rise from the iliac fossa and are displaced laterally, so that by the sixth month they are situated at the level of the iliac crest; at term the appendix is well up in the right upper quadrant, near the base of the liver.

The most frequent presenting symptoms in the pregnant patient with an acute abdomen are abdominal pain, nausea and vomiting, abdominal distention, and shock. Each of these may be attributable to or associated with the pregnancy or may herald the onset of an acute, nonobstetric emergency. In the assessment of a pregnant patient with a suspected acute abdomen, the usual signs of intra-abdominal disease remain valid—in particular, indications of generalized peritonitis, separate from uterine or adnexal tenderness *per se*. With recognition of the changing anatomic relationships of the abdominal contents occurring in pregnancy, one may usually rely on traditional symptoms and findings for acute appendicitis, cholecystitis, peptic ulcer disease, intestinal obstruction, and intra-abdominal hemorrhage. Radiologic and laboratory techniques generally retain their usefulness, although the relative leukocytosis and other hematologic changes seen in normal pregnancy may be confusing.

In general, laparotomy incisions heal well during pregnancy. The choice of an incision is dictated by the state of pregnancy and the nature of the problem, with the anatomic variations of pregnancy borne in mind. For acute appendicitis, a right lower quadrant, muscle-splitting incision is appropriate; in biliary tract disease, a high subcostal incision is usually desirable. Long vertical incisions may be indicated for intestinal obstruction. In all these procedures, adequate exposure is of paramount importance. The abdominal incision may be closed in the usual manner, preferably with interrupted sutures. If drainage or exteriorization is necessary, it is usually advisable to perform it through a separate stab incision.

In addition to the supportive postoperative measures usually employed, the following points should be emphasized in the care of the pregnant surgical patient: adequate efforts to ensure oxygenation and maintenance of an airway with supplemental oxygen as needed; accurate monitoring of blood volume and transfusion as necessary to maintain an adequate level; careful evaluation of fluid and electrolyte balance; adequate sedation to minimize the likelihood of premature labor (newer studies suggest prophylactic tocolysis may be of significant benefit); continuous gastrointestinal decompression; careful attention to an indwelling Foley catheter and the urinary retention to which the enlarged uterus predisposes; and careful attention to the extremities, particularly if varicosities are present. The incidence of phlebitis is considerably increased during pregnancy, because of venostasis. Unless specifically indicated, early ambulation is not advisable, nor is routine antibiotic prophylaxis indicated. Again, recent studies are exploring the use of tocolytic agents to reduce premature labor, and the practitioner would be well advised to consider these new approaches as they become further defined.

Cardiovascular Surgery in Pregnancy

The gestational changes of significance in cardiovascular disease have been mentioned earlier. In addition to the physiologic changes, there are anatomic changes with special relationships to the cardiovascular system. During pregnancy and the puerperium, there is a general loosening of the ground substance connective tissue, affecting the vascular system by reducing the tensile strength of blood vessels. The local anatomic change of importance in vascular disorders is the enlargement of the uterus, which results in compression of the vascular structures of the pelvis, obstructing venous return from the legs and setting the stage for venous thrombosis and its sequelae.

Acquired Heart Disease. Surgical treatment of acquired heart disease in pregnancy was first reported in 1952 by Cooley and Chapman. Within a short time, mitral valvulotomy during pregnancy was being performed in many centers, and by the mid-1950s sufficient data had accrued to indicate that mitral commissurotomy could be performed during pregnancy with a relatively low risk or harm to the mother or fetus. It should be emphasized that optimal medical management should precede the decision for operation. The operative risk to the pregnant patient in general is no greater than that to the nonpregnant patient. With increasing severity of disease, the risk of death increased in both the nonoperated and the operated patient. Candidates for operation during pregnancy are Class III and IV patients with mitral stenosis and those patients with mitral stenosis who during a previous pregnancy experienced an acute episode of cardiac decompensation. In addition, any patient who has sustained a systemic embolus associated with mitral valve disease should be considered for surgical intervention.

As to the timing of cardiac operation, commissurotomy is best done during the first trimester of pregnancy when the cardiac load has not yet increased appreciably. A contraindication to mitral commissurotomy is the presence of mitral insufficiency or coexisting aortic stenosis. These lesions are not now considered correctable by the technique of closed heart surgery. Closed mitral commissurotomy is unnecessary in asymptomatic patients but is an effective alternative to protracted bed rest and congestive heart failure in patients with functional limitations who become pregnant. Maternal and fetal mortality are lower in such patients operated on by the technique of closed commissurotomy than in the nonoperated patient. There are fewer data regarding open mitral operations than for closed mitral commissurotomies. Although a definitive statistical statement cannot be made at this time, published data indicate a favorable trend.

In an effort to provide optimal correction in patients whose valves were not amenable to closed or open heart reconstruction, newer techniques of valvular surgical repair have allowed restoration of cardiac function. There are relatively few reports of mitral valvular replacement procedures in pregnant women. It remains difficult to separate the hazards of anticoagulation from those of the surgical procedures in the long-term management of these gravidas.

Venous Thrombosis and Pulmonary Embolism. In pregnancy, as in the nonpregnant state, venostasis is a most controllable factor in preventing venous thrombosis and pulmonary embolism. Pregnant women are susceptible to venostasis in the lower extremities, because the gravid uterus interrupts flow through segments of the iliac veins and inferior vena cava. The primary means of alleviating venostasis is elastic compression of the legs, and it is thought that effective elastic compression should be used in all patients with varicose veins or a history of thrombophlebitis. Anticoagulation is important in limiting extension of thrombosis. The means of anticoagulation remains of great concern, however, because fetal hemorrhage and teratogenicity have been reported in patients treated with coumarins. Because heparin does not cross the placental barrier, its use is advisable in the interval before delivery. In general, heparin anticoagulation does not appreciably increase the blood loss associated with normal vaginal delivery (excluding bleeding from sites lacerated by trauma or episiotomy).

Venous thrombosis may be complicated by pulmonary embolism, and such embolism must be suspected as the cause of pleuritic chest pain or unexplained hemoptysis. Appropriate treatment is adequate heparinization with general supportive management for 10 to 14 days. At that time, the decision must be made to change to a coumarin anticoagulant or to continue the heparinization for the remainder of the pregnancy and puerperium. If pulmonary embolism recurs during heparin anticoagulation, ligation of the inferior vena cava and left ovarian veins by the transperitoneal route should be considered. Pulmonary embolectomy should be reserved for those patients in clinical shock with the appropriate clinical features and suggestive right-sided cardiac catheterization studies. In general, the usual diagnostic studies for pulmonary embolus are allowable in the pregnant patient.

Varicose Veins. Varicosities in pregnancy are a significant problem and usually have a fairly distinct pattern. They appear during the second or third month or pregnancy and become progressively larger until the last trimester. They may be unilateral or scattered over both lower extremities. Susceptible women have progressively larger varicosities with each successive pregnancy.

Many reports have described the surgical injection treatment of varicose veins during pregnancy. Many workers believe that pregnancy is no contraindication to injection or surgical therapy when such treatment is indicated. Others, however, believe that it is technically difficult to perform an adequate operation during pregnancy and that the danger of postoperative thrombosis and embolism is great. Before initiation of any therapy for varicose veins during pregnancy, several factors should be considered: (1) many of the dilated veins recede spontaneously after delivery; (2) although it is technically feasible to correct varices surgically, pregnancy often produces such distortion of the veins that the procedure can be difficult; (3) superior treatment is usually achieved when varices are treated in the postpartum state; and (4) in practically all cases, effective compression of the varicosities with elastic supports during pregnancy controls all symptoms and prevents complications.

Because elastic supports are effective, their use has become standard therapy for the enlarged varicosities in pregnancy. Elastic bandages are usually recommended to compress all varices from the time they appear until after delivery. The rubberized elastic bandages are considered preferable to rubber stockings to ensure adequate tension and compression. If there are large vulvar varices, a vulvar compressive support is available. In addition to elastic support, the patient is instructed to avoid prolonged standing. Frequent elevation of the legs and leg exercises have also been of help.

Trauma in Pregnancy

Trauma is responsible for a significant percentage of nonobstetric maternal deaths in the United States. Traumatic injury during pregnancy ranges from insignificant to catastrophic.

Effect of Trauma in Pregnancy. For many years there was thought to be a significant causal relationship between maternal injury and interruption of pregnancy. More current data, however, suggest that perinatal mortality does not appear appreciably increased in cases in which the mother has sustained noncatastrophic abdominal trauma during pregnancy. Yet even maternal injury that is less than catastrophic can alter the course of a pregnancy and jeopardize the fetus. The fetus in later pregnancy can be injured *in utero* as a result of blunt or penetrating trauma. The placenta, cord, or membranes can be damaged. Maternal injury can cause severe alterations in maternal homeostasis and severely compromise the fetus. Abruptio placentae and psychologic shock secondary to maternal trauma appear to have nonspecific roles.

Maternal Injury. Blunt injury is the most common form of abdominal trauma currently seen. It most frequently results in damage to a solid viscus, which is relatively thick and sustains injury either from direct blows to the abdomen or by contrecoup action. The spleen is the most commonly injured organ in pregnant women, followed by the liver and kidney. The pregnant uterus occupies a middle position between solid and hollow viscera. Rupture can occur, usually in the fundal portion.

Penetrating wounds of the abdomen and pregnant uterus have resulted from a variety of instruments. With penetrating wounds to the pregnant abdomen, multiple organ injury is the rule. The frequency with which an organ is injured is in direct proportion to the space it occupies in the abdomen. With increasing duration of gestation, the uterus tends to displace the small bowel into a smaller space in the upper abdomen and acts as a protective shield for other viscera. The mortality of penetrating wounds of the abdomen in pregnant patients is related to the number of organs injured. Only about one third of the patients who have sustained gunshot wounds in the pregnant uterus, however, have had other associated visceral injury. A review of gunshot wounds to the pregnant uterus revealed a perinatal mortality rate of 70%. Approximately half the infants sustained wounds that could have contributed to their demise; the remainder died as a result of premature delivery, often performed unnecessarily during the acute care of the mother.

Diagnosis and Treatment of Abdominal Trauma. As with any injured patient, those conditions that interfere with vital functions or threaten life require immediate attention. Hypotension and hypoxia must be corrected. Both experimental studies and clinical experience have shown that maternal shock has a deleterious effect on the fetus. The effect appears related to the period of gestation, because the fetus is better able to tolerate maternal hypotension in early pregnancy. The fetus becomes anoxic during periods of maternal hypotension as a result of decreased uterine blood flow. The mother responds to hemorrhage by attempting to maintain her blood pressure by decreasing perfusion to the uterine vascular bed.

As a result of the physiologic changes of pregnancy, the pregnant patient is better able to tolerate acute blood loss than is the nonpregnant one. Clinical signs and symptoms of blood loss may not appear in the obstetric patient until there has been a 30% to 35% reduction in blood volume. This would suggest that maternal blood pressure and pulse are not satisfactory parameters of fetal well-being. Adequate circulating blood volume, therefore, must be maintained, and therapy should be directed to restoring both maternal and fetal homeostasis. After emergency measures to control bleeding, restore blood volume, and maintain respiration have been instituted, diagnostic procedures must be accomplished systematically to spare the fetus unnecessary and hazardous exposure to radiologic and invasive procedures.

Roentgenograms have been proved useful in the care of accident victims with fractures and chest injuries, and contrast studies are essential in determining urinary tract status. The value of routine radiographic studies in abdominal trauma is limited. Arteriography is finding increased application in the detection of splenic, hepatic, and renal injuries. Roentgenograms must be used selectively during pregnancy, and their use should be supervised to reduce the hazard to the fetus. The fetus can be further protected by proper shielding and appropriate radiographic techniques.

Other hematologic studies, including leukocyte count, may be used in the assessment of the patient with abdominal trauma; the physician should exercise caution, however, because the normal leukocyte count in pregnancy is increased and may approach 20,000 per cu. mm. in the last trimester. Central venous pressure studies may be of use, but several investigators have shown a progressive fall in central venous pressure during pregnancy, with an average of 3.8 cm. H_2O in the third trimester in normal patients.

In general, conservatism may be recommended in patients with blunt abdominal trauma, and a conservative approach to penetrating abdominal trauma is receiving increased attention. The conservative approach is utilized when signs or symptoms do not definitely indicate visceral injury; these patients are observed closely for the presence of bowel sounds, direct or rebound tenderness, and abdominal rigidity. If blood is found in the peritoneum on paracentesis or in the urine, feces, or gastric aspirates, or if there is a worsening of vital signs, laparotomy is indicated.

Fractures. Fractures comprise 10% of accidental injuries during pregnancy. It has been suggested that fracture healing is less effective during pregnancy, but studies have not supported this contention. In general, these studies indicate that changes in the healing strength of fractures parallel those of connective tissue alterations, which become progressively greater in later pregnancy and are probably hormone related.

Fractures need have no deleterious effect on pregnancy, but their management is somewhat modified by the pregnancy and anticipated delivery. The number of roentgenograms taken should be limited, and the abdomen and pelvis shielded whenever practical to reduce the radiation hazard to the fetus.

Generally, simple fractures of the extremities present no problems in management. Internal fixation is preferable to prolonged traction in complicated fractures. Vertebral fractures that are stable require only bed rest and need no special attention in the pregnant patient. Fracture-dislocations requiring open reduction and spinal fusion do present significant problems. An abdominal window must be cut and the cast changed frequently to allow space for the growing uterus. Vaginal delivery is not contraindicated in stable fractures, but in patients with unstable fractures, abdominal delivery should be considered. Pelvic fractures, commonly seen since the advent of widespread automotive travel, now constitute a large percentage of fractures in women. Most pelvic fractures do not interfere with vaginal delivery, because distortions of the diameters of the birth canal are rare. Vaginal delivery usually can be anticipated in most cases of pelvic fracture after 8 weeks. In unhealed fractures with separation or displacement, the patient should be delivered by cesarean section.

Head Injuries. In general, the management of the pregnant patient with a head injury is no different from that of the nonpregnant patient. Immediate concerns include stabilization of the patient, evaluation of the patient's vital systems, assessment of the degree of damage incurred, and appropriate neurologic and other specific recommendations regarding the gestational status beyond support and maintenance of the patient.

SELECTED REFERENCES

Scott, J. R., DiSaia, P. J., Hammond, C. B., and Spellacy, W. N.: Danforth's Obstetrics and Gynecology, 7th ed. Philadelphia, J. B. Lippincott, 1994.
This is a standard text of both obstetrics and gynecology. It should serve the reader well for detailed information and further references for all topics relating to the specialty.

Speroff, L., Glass, R. H., and Kase, N. G.: Clinical Gynecologic Endocrinology and Infertility, 5th ed. Baltimore, Williams & Wilkins, 1994.
This textbook has become the "standard" for details regarding gynecologic endocrinology and infertility. It is superbly illustrated and useful in the care of such patients.

DiSaia P. J., and Creasman, W. T.: Clinical Gynecologic Oncology, 4th ed. St. Louis, C. V. Mosby, 1993.
This excellent book summarizes our knowledge of gynecologic malignancy, its diagnosis, care, and complications. It also deals with required surgical technique, staging, and adjunctive therapies.

Thompson, J. D., and Rock, J. A.: TeLinde's Operative Gynecology, 7th ed. Philadelphia, J. B. Lippincott, 1992.
This highly regarded surgical text is now in its seventh edition, attesting to its proven record as a useful source document for pelvic surgery. It presents very clear illustrations and many useful tips to enhance safely and effectively the practice of pelvic surgery.

Herbst, A. L., Mishell, D. R., Stenchever, M. A., and Droegemueller, W.: Comprehensive Gynecology, 2nd ed. St. Louis, Mosby–Year Book, 1992.
As entitled, this is a comprehensive gynecologic text that includes useful illustrations and algorithms to aid in the diagnosis of and therapy for gynecologic disorders.

REFERENCES

1. Bonney, V.: The principles that should underlie all operations for prolapse. J. Obstet. Gynecol. Br. Emp., 41:669, 1934.
2. Brenner, P. F., Roy, S., and Mishell, D. R.: Ectopic pregnancy: A study of 300 consecutive surgically treated cases. JAMA, 243:673, 1980.
3. Britton, L. C., Wilson, T. O., Gaffey, T. A., et al.: DNA ploidy in endometrial carcinoma: Major objective prognostic factors. Mayo Clin. Proc., 65:643, 1990.
4. Buttram, V. C., and Reiter, R. C.: Uterine leiomyoma: Etiology, symptomatology and management. Fertil. Steril., 36:443, 1981.
5. Casper, R. F.: Clinical uses of gonadotropin-releasing hormone analogues. Can. Med. Assoc. J., 144:153, 1991.
6. Curry S. L., Hammond, C. B., Tyrey, L., et al.: Hydatidiform mole: Diagnosis, management and long-term follow-up in 347 patients. Obstet. Gynecol., 41:1, 1975.
7. DeLancey, J. O. L.: Pelvic organ prolapse. In Scott, J. (Ed.): Danforth's Obstetrics and Gynecology, 7th ed. Philadelphia, J. B. Lippincott, 1994, p. 803.
8. DiSaia, P. J.: Surgical aspects of cervical carcinoma. Cancer, 48:548, 1991.
9. DiSaia, P. J., and Creasman, W. T.: Clinical Gynecologic Oncology, 4th ed. St. Louis, C. V. Mosby, 1993.
10. Fore, S. R., Hammond, C. B., Parker, R. T., and Anderson, E. E.: Urologic and genital anomalies in patients with congenital absence of the vagina. Obstet. Gynecol., 46:410, 1975.
11. Hammond, C. B.: The climacteric. In Scott, J. (Ed.): Danforth's Obstetrics and Gynecology, 7th ed. Philadelphia, J. B. Lippincott, 1994.
12. Jaffe, R. B., Plosher, S., Marshall, L., and Martin, M. C.: Neuromodulatory regulation of gonadotropin-releasing hormone pulsatile discharge in women. Am. J. Obstet. Gynecol., 163:1727, 1990.
13. Kaufman, R. H., Friedrich, E. G., and Gardner, H. L.: Benign Lesions of the Vulva and Vagina. Chicago, Year Book Medical Publishers, 1989.
14. Keye, W. R.: Gynecologic history, examination, and diagnostic procedures. In Scott, J. (Ed.): Danforth's Obstetrics and Gynecology, 7th ed. Philadelphia, J. B. Lippincott, 1994, p. 593.
15. Livengood, C. H., Thomason, J. L., and Hill, G. B.: Bacterial vaginosis: Treatment with topical intravaginal clindamycin phosphate. Obstet. Gynecol., 76:118, 1990.
16. Nichols, D. H., and Randall, C. L.: Vaginal Surgery, 3rd ed. Baltimore, Williams & Wilkins, 1989.
17. Ostergard, D. R., and Bast, A. E. (Eds.): Urogynecology and Urodynamics: Theory and Practice, 3rd ed. Baltimore, Williams & Wilkins, 1991.
18. Peterson, H. B., Galagid, E. I., and Zenilman, J. M.: Pelvic inflammatory disease: Review of treatment options. Rev. Infect. Dis., 12(S6):S656, 1990.

19. Quigley, M. M., and Gwatkin, R. B. L.: Embryology and developmental defects of the female reproductive system. *In* Scott, J. (Ed.): Danforth's Obstetrics and Gynecology, 7th ed. Philadelphia, J. B. Lippincott, 1994, p. 11.

20. Soper, J. T., Lewis, J. L., and Hammond, C. B.: Gestational trophoblastic disease. *In* Hoskins, W. J., Perez, C. A., and Young, R. C. (Eds.): Gynecologic Oncology: Principles and Practice. Philadelphia, J. B. Lippincott, 1992, p. 795.

21. Sparks, J. M., and Varren, R. J.: Ovarian cancer screening. Obstet. Gynecol., 72:787, 1991.

22. Speert, H.: Obstetric and Gynecologic Milestones. New York, Macmillan, 1958.

23. Speroff, L., Glass, R. H., and Kase, N. G.: Amenorrhea. *In* Clinical Gynecologic Endocrinology and Infertility, 5th ed. Baltimore, Williams & Wilkins, 1994, p. 401.

24. Stovall, T. G., Long, F. W., and Gray, L. A.: Methotrexate treatment of unruptured ectopic pregnancy: A report of 100 cases. Obstet. Gynecol., 77:748, 1991.

25. Thomas, G. M., Denbo, A. J., Bryson, S. C., et al: Changing concepts in the management of vulvar cancer. Gynecol. Oncol., 42:9, 1991.

CHAPTER 45

THE URINARY SYSTEM

David F. Paulson, M.D.

ANATOMY

The kidneys and ureters are paired structures. The kidneys are responsible for the formation of urine, and the ureters are responsible for conduit of the formed urine into the single midline bladder. Each kidney is 9 to 15 cm. long, 4 to 5 cm. wide, and approximately 3 cm. thick (Fig. 45–1). They are located on each side of the vertebral column between the parietal perineum and the fascia and musculature of the posterior abdominal wall and are embedded in a variable amount of fat and surrounded by a special layer of fascia (Gerota's fascia) (Fig. 45–2). They lie on the side of the psoas muscle, and for this reason they are not parallel, with the upper poles being approximately 2 cm. from the midline and the lower poles approximately 3.5 cm. from the midline. The anterior relationships of the two kidneys vary somewhat among individuals; however, an awareness of the structures overlying the kidneys when they are approached from the ventral surface is necessary for the surgeon to avoid damage to these structures (Fig. 45–3). The kidney may be approached from a transabdominal transperitoneal route; through a flank incision that enters directly into the retroperitoneal space, displacing the peritoneal envelope anteriorly; or through a posterior incision, which provides ready access into the renal pelvis.

EMBRYOLOGY OF THE URINARY SYSTEM[2, 8, 20, 23]

The adult human kidney develops progressively as three distinct entities: pronephros, mesonephros, and metanephros (Fig. 45–4). The pronephros is the most primitive form of renal development and disappears completely by the fourth week of embryonic life. The embryonic mesonephros corresponds to the mature excretory organ of higher fish and amphibians. It is the principal excretory organ during the fourth to eighth weeks of embryonic life, but it gradually disintegrates, although parts of its ductal system remain associated with the male reproductive organs. The final phase in the development of the nephric system originates from both the intermediate mesoderm and the mesonephric duct. The joining of the ureter, which arises from the wolffian duct, with the mesoderm of the nephrogenic cord is necessary for the final development of the collecting tubules and functioning nephrons. The development begins in the 5- to 6-mm. embryo with a budlike outgrowth from the mesonephric duct. This ureteral bud grows cephalad and collects mesoderm from the nephrogenic cord of the intermediate mesoderm. This mesoderm with the metanephric cap becomes larger and undergoes internal differentiation. As the kidney matures, it migrates upward from the region of the fourth to the first lumbar vertebra and progressively rotates so that the originally dorsal border becomes the convex lateral border. The ureter (metanephric duct) develops as a hollow outgrowth (ureteric bud) from the inferior end of the mesonephric duct. This metanephric duct grows cephalad, its blind end expanding to form the renal pelvis. As this primitive renal pelvis comes in contact with the undifferentiated metanephrogenic mass at the caudal end of the urogenital ridge, it branches into primary tubules, which in turn branch to form secondary tubules. The secondary tubules then form tertiary tubules, and the branching goes on until approximately 12 generations of tubules are formed. The primary tubules develop into the major calyces of the adult kidney,

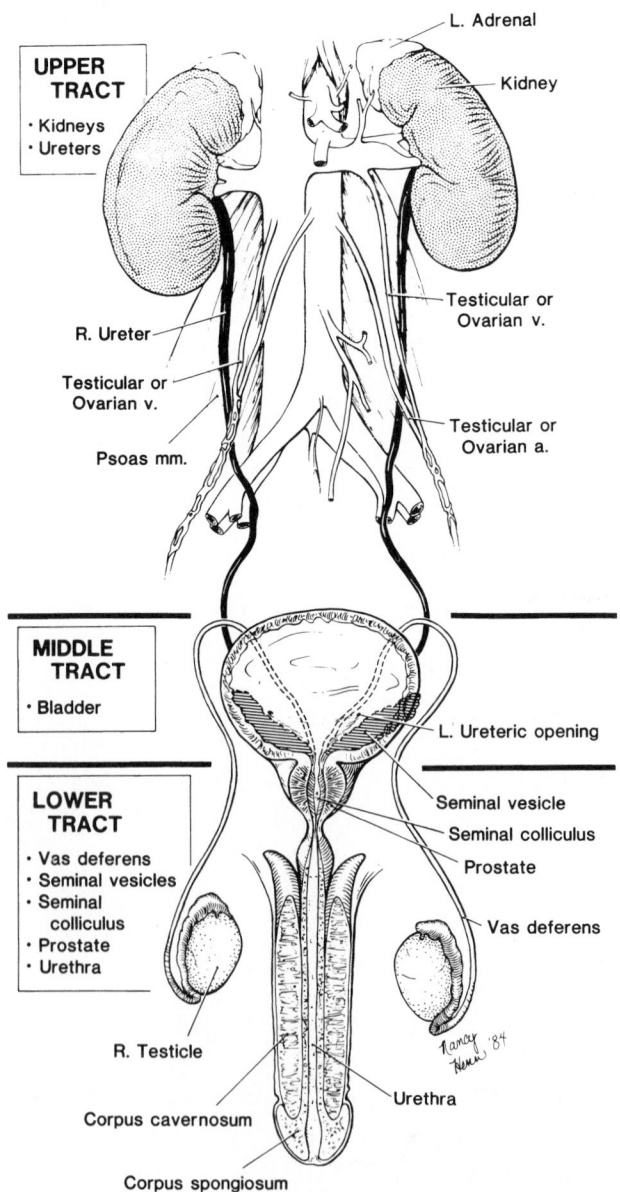

Figure 45–1. Anatomy of the male genitourinary tract. The upper and middle tracts have urologic function only. The lower tract has both genital and urinary functions.

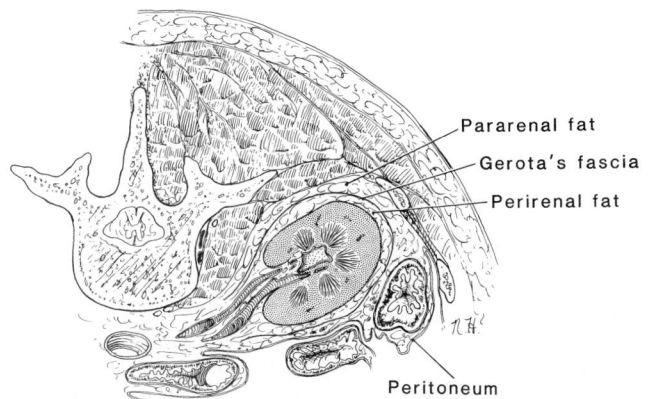

Figure 45–2. Diagram of the renal fascia in a cross section through the posterior abdominal wall.

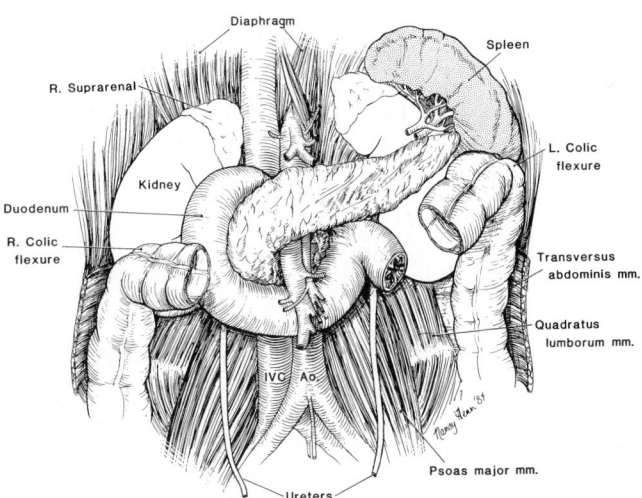

Figure 45–3. Some relations of the kidneys, anterior view. Compare with Figure 45–2.

the tubules of the second through the fourth generation fuse to form the minor calyces, while those of the fifth order form the papillary ducts and those of the higher orders form the several generations of collecting tubules. Each blind-ending collecting tubule develops into a secretory tubule with its associated Bowman's capsule and glomerulus.

During formation of the kidney by the union of the ureteric bud and the nephrogenic tissue, it progressively migrates out of the pelvis and into the upper portion of the retroperitoneum. Renal ectopia or the location of a kidney in a fixed position below its normal adult level must be viewed as a failure of normal ascent. The kidney may fail to leave the true pelvis, or it may remain at any higher level in its ascent to the retroperitoneum. As the kidney ascends, it is supplied by successively higher-located arteries. If the kidney fails to reach its normal adult position, it often retains an anomalous blood supply, which arises from the aorta or its branches below the level of the definitive renal arteries. Furthermore, as a kidney undergoes cephalad migration, it undergoes a *rotation* so that the renal pelvis, which in the embryo faces ventrally, comes to face medially with the major calyces projecting laterally. Ectopic kidneys, which have failed to ascend to the normal position, frequently fail to undergo rotation and their pelves still face forward.

Abnormal development of the kidneys leads to abnormalities that may provide difficulty in the clinical care of the patient. Failure of the metanephros to ascend properly leads to an ectopic kidney. The ectopic kidney may be on the proper side, or it may be on the opposite side (a cross-ectopy), with or without fusion to the contralateral renal mass. Failure of the kidney to rotate during ascent produces

a malrotated kidney. Fusion of the paired metanephric masses in the pelvis before ascent leads to various abnormalities, the most common being a horseshoe kidney.

During development the cloaca also undergoes subdivision, which changes the relationships of the mesonephric ducts and the ureter, and they come to have separate openings rather than a common one. As the cloaca is divided by the urorectal septum, the ureter migrates to empty into the larger ventral derivative of the cloaca, which becomes the urinary bladder. Growth of the bladder then leads to an absorption of the lower ends of the two mesonephric ducts, so that these ducts and ureters open separately into the bladder. Further growth produces additional separation between the openings of the ureters and the mesonephric ducts and occurs in such a fashion that the openings of the ureters remain some distance apart on the posterior wall of the bladder while the openings of the mesonephric ducts are shifted farther distally into the urogenital sinus. Once this has been accomplished, the urinary ductal system in the male is completely separate from the genital ductal system.

The ureteral bud, which arises from the mesonephric duct, may bifurcate, causing a bifid ureter at varying levels. An accessory ureteral bud may develop from the mesonephric duct, thereby forming a duplicated ureter. If the ureteral buds are close together on the mesonephric duct, they will open near each other in the bladder. When this occurs, the main ureteral bud, which is the first to appear and the most caudal

Figure 45–4. Schematic representation of the development of the nephric system. Only a few of the tubules of the pronephros are seen in the fourth week, while the mesonephric tissue differentiates into mesonephric tubules that progressively join the mesonephric duct. The first sign of the ureteral bud from the mesonephric duct is seen. At 6 weeks, the pronephros has completely degenerated and the mesonephric tubules start to do so. The ureteral bud grows dorsocranially and has met the metanephrogenic cap. At the eighth week, there is cranial migration of the differentiating metanephros. The cranial end of the ureteric bud expands and starts to show multiple successive outgrowths.

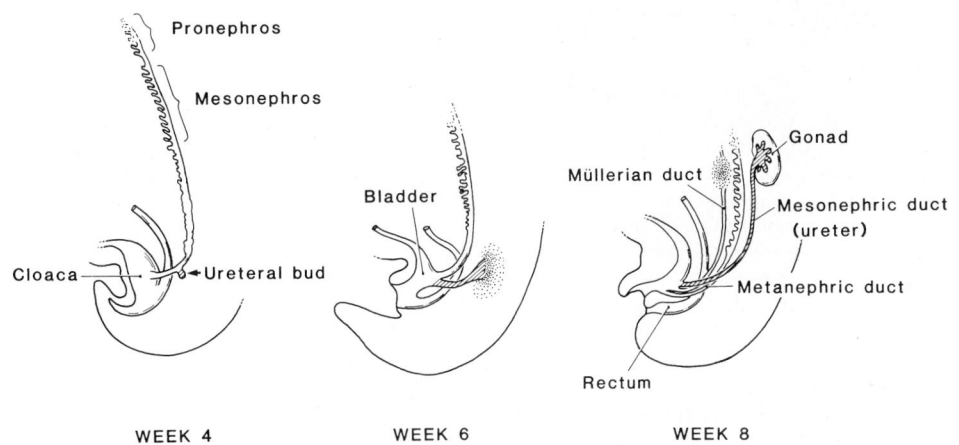

WEEK 4　　　　WEEK 6　　　　WEEK 8

of the mesonephric ducts, reaches the bladder first and then moves upward and laterally, followed later by a second accessory bud. When this occurs, the main ureteral bud drains the lower portion of the kidney, with the lower ureteral bud draining the upper portion of the kidney. The two ureteral buds will have reversed their relationship as they move from the mesonephric duct to the urogenital sinus. This is the reason why double ureters always cross (the Weigert-Meyer law). Failure of development of a ureteral bud leads to the production of a solitary kidney with a hemitrigone in the bladder.

PHYSIOLOGY OF THE URINARY TRACT[7, 18]

The kidney is divided into a cortex and a medulla. The cortex contains glomeruli and portions of the tubules and is located peripherally. The medulla, located centrally, is composed primarily of the remaining portions of the tubules and the collecting ducts (Fig. 45–5). Urine formation is initiated by filtration, which is accomplished within the glomerulus. The composition of the glomerular filtrate within the tubules is altered by reabsorption of specific solutes and water and by the secretion of specific substances.

SIGNS AND SYMPTOMS OF UROLOGIC DISEASE (Tables 45–1 and 45–2)

Frequently, pain is the initial indicator of disease involving the urinary tract. Renal pain, ureteral pain, and bladder pain

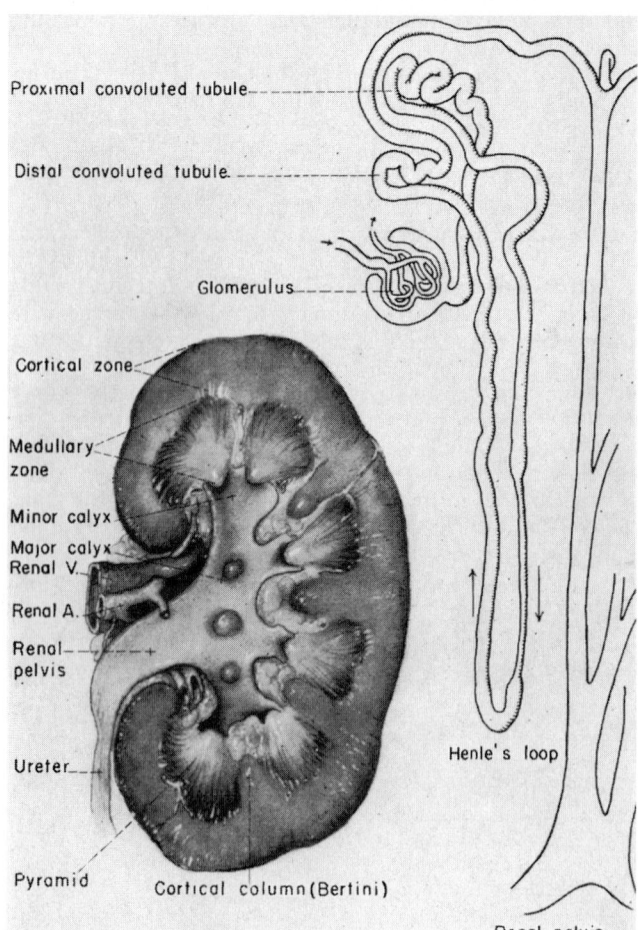

Figure 45–5. Cross section of kidney showing gross anatomic relationships. *Right*, Diagrammatic representation of the nephron shown joining a collecting duct. (From Dodson, A. I.: *In* Campbell, M. F. [Ed.]: Urology. Philadelphia, W. B. Saunders, 1954.)

have distinct characteristics, and a careful history will often hint of the diagnosis and direct the attention of the surgeon to a specific anatomic site. Renal pain may be dull and aching, localized to the flank. It may also be sharp, localized in the flank or radiating into the lower abdomen or the buttocks. It may be episodic, appearing in waves, or it may be persistent and result in loss of appetite with nausea and vomiting. Renal pain, when dull, often indicates a long-standing process, such as a chronic infection or slowly growing tumor. With severe renal discomfort, the patient tends to be restless and may hold his or her flank in an attempt to minimize the discomfort.

Ureteral pain may cause flank discomfort and may be associated with severe abdominal pain, nausea, and vomiting. As the clot or calculus moves distally in the ureter, the pain radiates from the flank to the lower abdomen and may radiate into the scrotum, the labia majora, or occasionally the thigh. A calculus in the lower ureter, or at the ureterovesical junction, may cause urinary frequency with urgency and pain on urination.

Bladder pain is usually dull and aching and localized to the suprapubic area. When caused by an acute infection, the pain is severe and precipitates a desire to void.

EVALUATION OF THE PATIENT WITH URINARY TRACT DISEASE

Patients who present with the signs and symptoms of urinary tract disease or with disordered urinary renal function deserve a complete evaluation, consisting of a physical examination, laboratory studies to determine the degree of renal functional impairment, and imaging studies that permit definition of the anatomy of the urinary tract.

Physical Examination

Inspection of the abdomen may disclose a lower midline mass when the bladder is full that flattens instead of accentuates the transverse lower abdominal crease. In adults, neither the distended bladder nor the hydronephrotic kidney is easy to define. However, in the child, the bladder is an intra-abdominal organ and is readily palpated and balloted. Similarly, the child's kidney is easily palpated and transilluminated. To palpate the kidney, the patient should be supine and the physician should place one hand posteriorly on the flank and press with another hand anteriorly on the abdomen. Careful observation of any alteration in position of the mass as the patient breathes or moves from a supine to a lateral or erect posture may identify the nature of the mass. When the kidney is tense or inflamed, sudden pressure in the costovertebral angle may produce pain.

Laboratory Studies

After completion of the physical examination, the physician should obtain laboratory studies that further define the nature of the abnormality (see Table 45–2).

Urinalysis.[13] Care should be taken to obtain the urine without contamination by the foreskin in the male or by the vulva and labia in the female. It is best to discard the first portion of the voided stream because this may contain urethral contaminant. The midportion of the stream usually reflects the pathologic process ongoing within the bladder. The third portion of the urinary stream may be discarded. In the male, the foreskin should be stripped from the glans penis and the glans cleansed with either saline or zephiran chloride. In the female, the labia should be separated and the female instructed to initiate voiding while the midportion of the urinary stream is collected in a wide-mouth container.

TABLE 45–1. Signs and Symptoms of Urologic Disease

Sign or Symptom	Definition	Disease Process
Hematuria	Blood in the urine (gross or microscopic)	Malignancy, calculous disease, iatrogenic, infection, trauma, foreign body
Pneumaturia	Air (gas) in the urine	Fistula between bowel and urinary tract, iatrogenic, infection
Pyuria	Pus in the urine	Infection
Nocturia	Awakening at night to void	Infection, obstruction (incomplete voiding), neurologic disease, metabolic disorder (diabetes mellitus, diabetes insipidus), congestive heart failure, renal failure, excessive fluid intake
Frequency	Voiding more than three to five times daily	Infection, obstruction, neurologic disease, metabolic disorder, excessive fluid intake, functional disease, psychogenic disorder
Polyuria	Greater than normal urine volume	Metabolic disease (e.g., diabetes mellitus, diabetes insipidus, adrenal insufficiency), renal disease, excessive fluid intake
Oliguria	Volume less than 400 ml. daily	Renal disease, cardiovascular disease, toxic drug effect
Anuria	No urine output	Obstruction, calculous disease, renal failure
Urgency	Precipitous desire to void	Infection, calculous disease, malignancy, idiopathic, neurogenic disease
Dysuria	Painful voiding	Infection, malignancy, calculous disease
Hesitancy	Delay and difficulty in beginning to void	Obstruction, neurogenic disease
Incontinence	Involuntary loss of urine	Anatomic loss of bladder support (stress incontinence), fistula, loss of sphincter control (urgent or iatrogenic)

The urine should be analyzed for specific gravity, pH, protein, sugar, acetone, red blood cells, white blood cells, bacteria, and casts; optional tests include measurement of bilirubin and osmolality and cytologic studies. Hematuria may be gross or microscopic and have either a glomerular or a nonglomerular origin (see Table 45–2). Nonglomerular hematuria more commonly reflects malignancy, stone, or infection. Diagnosis is mandatory to initiate proper therapy.

Evaluation of Renal Function. The clinician should determine the renal function of each patient with urinary tract disease. An evaluation of the total renal function is achieved by determining the amount of endogenous wastes in the blood, such as urea or creatinine, and the excretion of these substances in the urine. The serum creatinine level is a better indicator of renal function than is the blood urea nitrogen value. Both substances are excreted by glomerular filtration; however, the amount of urea available for excretion is variable. After hemorrhage, there may be excessive protein breakdown with a marked increase in the total urea production while creatinine production is essentially constant. The creatinine clearance test is a ready measure of glomerular filtration rate. The measured excretion of specifically administered substances such as insulin or p-aminohippurate assesses specific aspects of the renal function. Insulin clearance measures primarily glomerular filtration, while p-aminohippurate, secreted by the proximal tubule, is primarily a measure of renal plasma flow. All of the excretory tests (creatinine clearance, insulin clearance, and p-aminohippurate clearance) depend on a complete urine collection for accuracy.

Imaging of the Urinary Tract

Multiple methodologies are available to image the urinary tract.[16] In years past most of the imaging studies permitted only a structural or anatomic evaluation of the urinary tract; many of the imaging studies now also provide an assessment of function. Current methodology includes excretory urography with nephrotomography, retrograde ureteropyelography, retrograde cystography, arteriography, venography, digital venous arteriography, computed tomography (CT), ultrasonography, radioisotope renography, and magnetic resonance imaging (MRI). Each of these studies provides different information that can be used to compile a complete understanding of the urinary tract pathology.

Excretory urography is dependent on renal function and visualizes the urinary tract by concentration of an intravenous injection of organic iodine within the urinary tract. The contrast material is excreted primarily by renal function and is concentrated as the glomerular filtrate is reabsorbed. The kidney and its collecting system become radiopaque as the x-rays are absorbed by the iodinated agent (Fig. 45–6). Increasing the amount of the iodinated contrast material delivered to the patient or dehydrating the patient to increase absorption of water from the glomerular filtrate improves visualization. Excretory urography should be the first imaging study chosen for evaluation of the urinary tract. It is specifically indicated when the suspected diagnosis is a space-occupying lesion of the kidney such as a cyst or tumor, pyelonephritis, hydronephrosis, hypertension, or urinary tract calculi. Because the ability to visualize the kidney and urinary tract is dependent on renal function and the ability of the kidney to concentrate contrast medium, the quality of the urinary tract imaging may be markedly diminished in the patient with compromised renal function. Excretory urograms may be contraindicated if there is any evidence of hypersensitivity to iodinated contrast media or to foods or substances containing iodine. This contraindication is waived if this history is noted and the patient is appropriately pre-

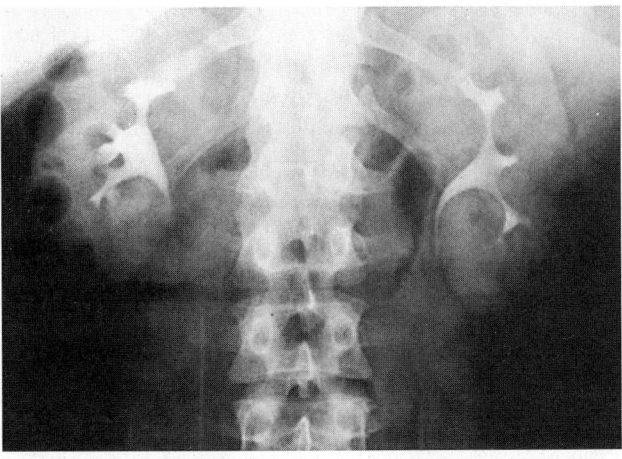

Figure 45–6. The iodinated contrast agent is excreted and appears in the collecting system. Note that the renal outline of the left kidney is sharp and distinct. The collecting system is delicate and shows no evidence of obstruction.

TABLE 45–2. Assessment of Glomerular and Nonglomerular Hematuria

Presentation	Studies	Diagnosis
Glomerular		
Dysmorphic erythrocytes and/or erythrocyte casts; ± proteinuria		
Infection?		
Recent upper respiratory or skin infection?	ASO titer Serum C3 level	Poststreptococcal GN
Multisystem diseases?		
Rash, arthritis?	C3, C4, ANA	Systemic lupus erythematosus nephritis
Hemoptysis?	Microcytic anemia	Goodpasture's syndrome
Bleeding tendencies?	Anti–double-stranded DNA	Schönlein-Henoch purpura
		Paraproteinemic disorders (e.g., multiple myeloma)
Hereditary?		
Glomerular	Urinalyses in family members	Familial hematuria
	Deafness? Audiogram	Familial (Alport's) nephritis
Other glomerulopathies?	Serum creatinine	Minimal change disease
	Creatinine clearance	Focal glomerulosclerosis IgA nephropathy (Berger's disease)
	Quantitative urine protein	Membranous glomerulopathy
		Proliferative glomerulonephritis
	ANA	
	C3, C4	
	Hb, Hct	
	Immunoglobulin level	Hemolytic-uremic syndrome
	Cryoglobulins	
	Skin, rectal, or renal biopsy	
	Tests negative	Early GN
		Benign "idiopathic" hematuria
Nonglomerular		
Tubulointerstitial, renovascular, or systemic disorder		
Circular erythrocytes; no erythrocyte casts; ± proteinuria		
Exercise?		
Prolonged running?		Runner's hematuria
Systemic coagulation disturbance?		
Hematuria-causing drug?		
Anticoagulant?	Stop drug	Drug-induced hematuria
Familial history of bleeding disorder?	Platelet values	Hemophilia
	PT, PTT	Thrombocytopenia
	Bleeding time	Disseminated intravascular coagulopathy
		Thrombotic thrombocytopenic purpura
Familial urolithiasis?	Urine calcium	Hypercalciuria
	Urine uric acid	Hyperuricosuria
Gross hematuria?		
Hereditary?		
Parenchymal	IVU	Medullary sponge kidney
	Renal ultrasound	Polycystic kidney
Papillary necrosis?		Papillary necrosis due to
Black?	Sickle cell screening	Sickle cell disease or trait
Analgesic abuse?	IVU	Analgesic nephropathy
Diabetes mellitus?		
Infection?	Culture; PPD skin test	Urinary tract infection, tuberculosis
Urinary tract abnormality?	IVU; cystoscopy	Tumor, obstructive or reflux nephropathy
Malignant hypertension?	Renal ultrasound	Malignant hypertensive nephropathy
Vascular?		
Atrial fibrillation?	IVU; renal ultrasound	
Recent myocardial infarct?	Renogram	Renal artery embolism and thrombosis
Umbilical catheter?	Renal angiography	
Trauma?		
Dehydration?	IVU; renal ultrasound	
	CT scan	Renal vein thrombosis
Bruit?	Renal angiography	Arteriovenous fistula
Renal biopsy?		

ANA, antinuclear antibody titer; ASO, antistreptolysin O; C3, C4, complement; CT, computed tomography; GN, glomerulonephritis; Hb, hemoglobin; Hct, hematocrit; IVU, intravenous urography; PPD, purified protein derivative; PT, prothrombin time; PTT, partial thromboplastin time.
From Walsh, P. C., et al. (Eds.): Campbell's Urology, 6th ed. Philadelphia, W. B. Saunders, 1992, p. 2067.

pared with corticosteroids and antihistamines before injection of the contrast agent. Excretory urography is best avoided during pregnancy.

Retrograde ureteropyelography requires specific training in urologic instrumentation and is done when excretory urography fails to provide adequate visualization of the collecting system and ureter. It is indicated when excretory renograms do not provide adequate ureteropelvic detail, when renal function is impaired to the point where it is anticipated that excretory urography will be inadequate, or when it is necessary to assess the level or degree of ureteral obstruction. It may also be used in patients who have a stated history of sensitivity to iodinated contrast agents.

Cystograms are performed by instilling the radiopaque contrast material into the bladder through the urethra. X-ray films are then taken to define the contour of the bladder. Cystography is indicated in patients who have a neurogenic bladder, who are suspected of having pelvic trauma sufficient to rupture the bladder, and who have recurrent infections or in whom a fistula between the bladder and bowel or other pelvic organ is suspected. Cystography should be avoided during acute urinary tract infection because the instillation of the contrast agent under pressure may precipitate systemic infection by forcing bacteria into the lymphatics and venules of the bladder or kidney.

Arteriography permits visualization of the main renal artery(s) and/or its branches. It is dependent on the delivery of a specific volume of iodinated contrast material into the renal arterial system and is independent of renal function. Renal arteriography is indicated whenever a vascular malformation, malignancy, or renovascular hypertension is suspected. Because most primary renal tumors are hypervascular, they are readily identified. Renal angiography may produce transient depression in renal function, particularly in patients who already have compromised renal function.

Digital venous arteriography uses computer-enhanced imaging of the renal vasculature after venous injection of contrast medium. This provides visualization of the arterial system of the kidney, but not in detail compatible with that of a direct arterial injection.

Venacavography is performed by the injection of iodinated contrast medium into the vena cava and is important for outlining enlarged retroperitoneal structures that may impinge on or displace the vena cava or to define extension of tumor from the renal vein into the vena cava itself.

CT uses technology in which the x-ray tube and the detection system are on opposite sides of the patient. During CT they rotate around the patient, recording information about the internal structure of the thin transverse cross sections through which the x-ray beam crosses. A computer then *reconstructs* each cross-sectional image as an array or grid of individual picture elements. The image bears a resemblance to a transverse anatomic section. The approximate density of any tissue within the image can be determined. CT provides information distinct from that obtained by arteriography or excretory urography. Its primary value is in determining the relationship of normal or abnormal anatomic structures to contiguous structures.

Ultrasonography uses vibrational energy generated at a frequency above the level of human hearing to produce information about the urinary tract. The primary advantage of ultrasonography is that it is independent of renal function. It permits identification of solid and cystic masses within the kidney and identification of calculi.

Radioisotopic techniques permit the clinician to evaluate both anatomic structure and function of the kidney without distorting normal physiologic processes. The radiopharmaceutical agents used to evaluate kidney function do not impose the hypertonic or chemical stress associated with intra-

venous iodinated contrast material, and the low iodine content of the iodinated radiopharmaceutical agents is not associated with any hypersensitivity risks. These drugs are detected by external instrumentation. The radiotracers provide information concerning renal position, anatomy, and function (Table 45–3). In the radioactive renogram, computer analysis of the critical areas is produced as a function of time after injection of the radiopharmaceutical agent. There are essentially three portions of the curve: a vascular phase, a functional phase, and a drainage phase. An analysis of the differential occurrence of these three portions of the radioisotopic renogram provides a differential assessment between the renal and ureteral function on both the right and left sides.

MRI permits the physician to image both bony and parenchymal structures in transverse and sagittal planes using information derived from hydrogen nuclei. Because hydrogen nuclei contain an odd number of nucleons, they demonstrate a property called spin, and each nucleon generates a magnetic field similar to that of a small bar magnet. Although normally oriented in a random manner to each other, in the presence of a strong, external magnetic field the protons become oriented in either a parallel or an antiparallel direction. From this new state of equilibrium, the protons can be deflected either 90 or 180 degrees from the magnetic field by an applied radiofrequency pulse, which causes the protons to resonate in a higher state of energy. Termination of the radiofrequency pulse allows the protons to return to the previous equilibrium, and the absorbed energy is reradiated as a radiofrequency that can be received by a detecting coil within the scanner. A computer processes the acquired information by a complex technique, known as Fourier transformation, and an image is constructed from a set of encoded signals. In this manner, transverse, sagittal, and coronal views may be obtained.

MRI also allows one to determine flow patterns within vascular structures, permitting accurate determination of the vasculature supplying tumors or occluded by tumors. This imaging modality has proved to be of great value in the staging of renal and prostatic malignancy (Figs. 45–7 and 45–8).

NONSURGICAL DISEASES OF THE URINARY TRACT

Nonsurgical diseases of the kidney can be divided into those medical renal diseases that may produce complications in the management of the patient undergoing surgery and those disease processes that may result from or be a concomitant of a surgical procedure. Most of the medical renal diseases produce specific alterations in the urinalysis and in the serum biochemical profile that are signal indicators that the etiologic disease process must be identified before surgery. Frequently, the abnormalities produced by these disease processes cannot be reversed, and the patient must be supported throughout the preoperative, intraoperative, and postoperative surgical periods by coordinated efforts of the surgeon and nephrologist.

Renal Failure

Renal failure may be prerenal in origin, may be primary due to parenchymal failure, or may be due to drug exposure (Tables 45–4 to 45–6).

Postrenal obstruction may occur in a patient with bilateral renal calculi or a single kidney and calculus obstruction. It is also noted in patients with retroperitoneal fibrosis, in patients with retroperitoneal malignancies, or in patients who have unanticipated surgical occlusion of the ureters.

TABLE 45–3. Radiopharmaceutical Agents for Urologic Diagnosis

Radiopharmaceutical	Usual Dose (μCi.)	Radiation-Absorbed Dose (Rads) from Usual Doses		Usual Scintiphoto Exposure Time and Imaging Time Post Dose	Use
		Renal	Whole Body		
99mTc-Fe ascorbate DTPA 99mTc glucoheptonate 99mTc methylsuccinate	20,000	1.0	0.008	Serial: 4-s. photos at 0–30 s.; static: 2–4 min. photos at 30 min.	Localized in renal cortex by deposition and retention in renal tubular cells. Uptake is proportionate to regional renal blood flow. Rapid serial photos show renal blood flow distribution.
99mTc (Sn)-DTPA	20,000	0.1	0.030	Serial: 1- or 2-min. photos at 0–20 min. or longer. Also useful to image blood flow.	Excreted solely by glomerular filtration. Useful for function imaging, but cortical definition vs. background less than with other 99mTc agents.
Sodium iothalamate 125I	50	Negligible	0.00015	Not useful for imaging.	Glomerular filtration rate measurement.
99mTc (Sn)-DTPA	1000	0.03 (bladder)	0.001	Static views during filling of bladder, 6-s. images during voiding.	Direct radionuclide cystography to detect and measure reflux.
Sodium iodohippurate 131I	200	0.080	0.0042 (assumes normal clearance)	2–10 min. photos (depending on renal function): 0–30 min. for normal function to 1–2 hours for poor function.	Excreted by tubular function (like p-aminohippurate); 70–80% extraction causes rapid clearance in normal tissue. Prolonged cortical transit time occurs in ischemic or other forms of tubular damage with increased water reabsorption.
Sodium iodohippurate 123I	2000	0.01	0.0005	Serial images for 30 min. or longer for poor function.	Excreted by tubular function. Same uses as for 131I hippurate.

From Smith, D. R.: General Urology, 10th ed. Los Altos, CA, Lange Medical Publications, 1981, p. 103.

Acute intrarenal obstruction occurs when the collecting tubules are blocked by crystals, debris, or Bence Jones protein. Certain drugs, such as the sulfonamides and methotrexate, have been known to produce acute crystalluria with obstruction if administered in excessive dosages. Acute obstructive oxaluria can be seen after anesthesia with methoxyflurane or in patients who ingest ethylene glycol, which is commonly used in antifreeze. Acute uric acid nephropathy may be precipitated by use of cytotoxic drugs, which cause nuclear lysis.

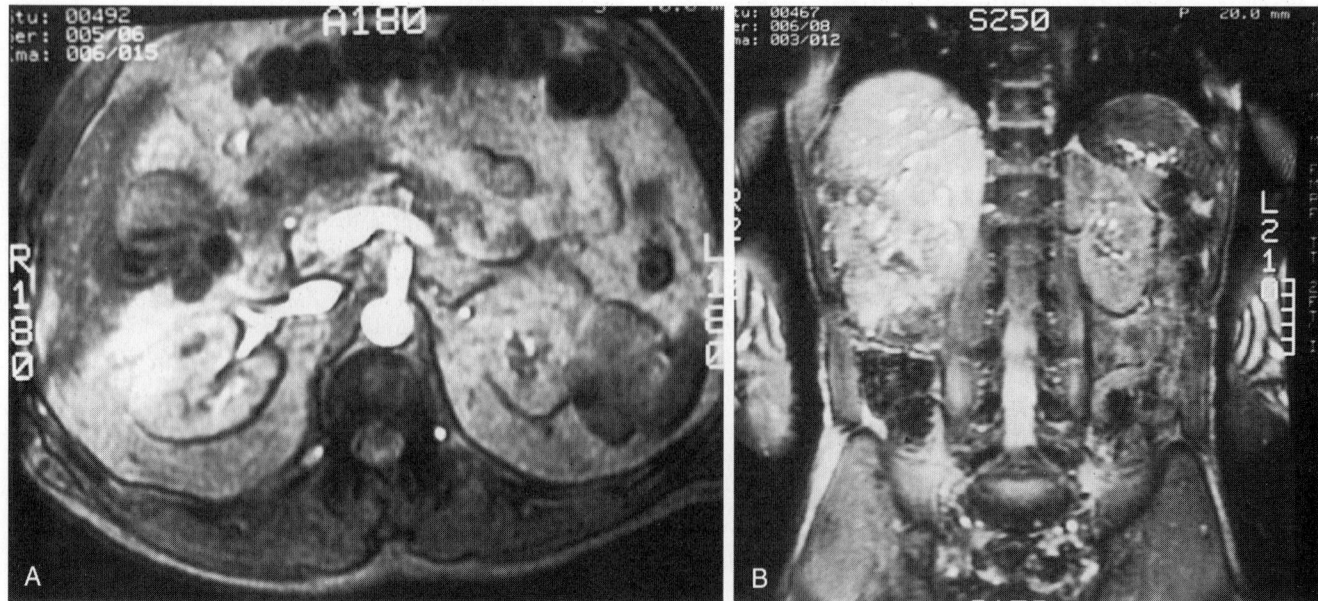

Figure 45–7. *A*, Transverse MRI at the level of the kidneys demonstrates a large left renal cancer and a normal right kidney. Note that the vascular structures are white on this T3-weighted image. *B*, The image has been oriented at a coronal section, again demonstrating a large left renal cancer with a normal right renal unit. The blood flow through the large left renal kidney causes this mass to be white on the T3-weighted image.

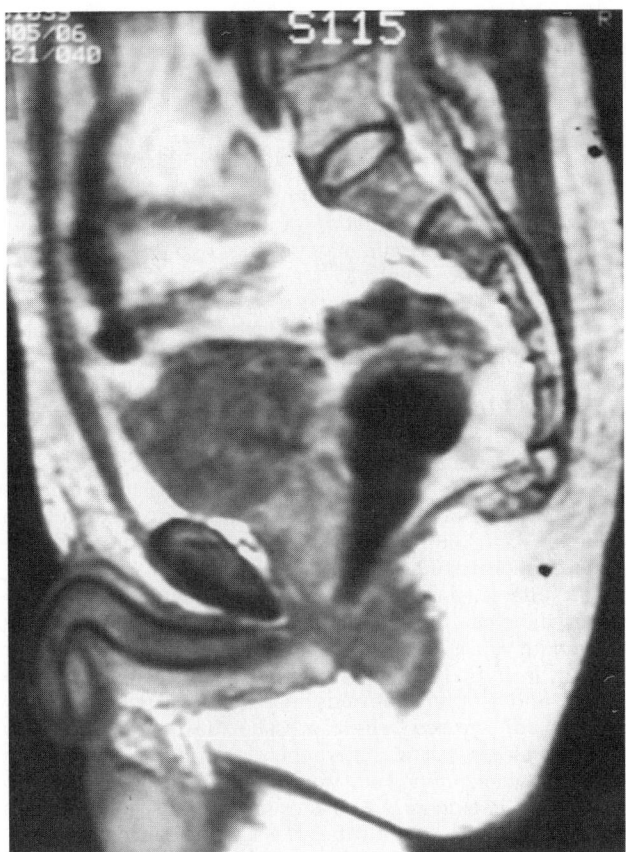

Figure 45–8. Sagittal MRI of the pelvis demonstrates the air-filled rectum posteriorly, the fluid-filled bladder anteriorly, and a large prostatic carcinoma.

Surgical patients may be susceptible to gram-negative sepsis, particularly while undergoing hepatobiliary or colonic surgery. Furthermore, there are certain specifically used drugs that are nephrotoxic and produce tubular necrosis.

TABLE 45–4. Major Parenchymal Causes of Acute Renal Failure

Primary Renal Disease

Glomerular

Primary acute glomerulonephritis

Tubulointerstitial

Acute interstitial nephritis
Acute tubular necrosis
Pyelonephritis
Transplant allograft rejection
Nephrolithiasis
Radiation nephritis

Systemic Disease

Glomerular

Vasculitis
Goodpasture's syndrome
Secondary acute glomerulonephritis (e.g., bacterial endocarditis)

Tubulointerstitial

Tumor lysis syndrome
Infiltration of kidney with tumor (rare)

From Shapiro, J. I., and Schrier, R. W.: Etiology, pathogenesis and management of renal failure. *In* Walsh, P. C., Retik, A. B., Stamey, T. A., and Vaughan, E. D. (Eds.): Campbell's Urology, 6th ed. Philadelphia, W. B. Saunders, 1992, p. 2047.

TABLE 45–5. Major Causes of Prerenal Azotemia

Decreased Cardiac Output

Decreased intravascular volume
　Dehydration
　Hemorrhage
　Anaphylactic shock
Decreased venous tone
　Autonomic neuropathy
　Spinal injury
Decreased contractile function
　Ischemic heart disease
　Cardiomyopathy
　Pericardial tamponade or constriction

Normal or Increased Cardiac Output

Systemic disorders
　Liver disease
　Sepsis
Local renal disease
　Renal artery stenosis

From Shapiro, J. I., and Schrier, R. W.: Etiology, pathogenesis and management of renal failure. *In* Walsh, P. C., Retik, A. B., Stamey, T. A., and Vaughan, E. D. (Eds.): Campbell's Urology, 6th ed. Philadelphia, W. B. Saunders, 1992, p. 2047.

Renal parenchymal failure occurs with rapidly progressive glomerulonephritis, acute interstitial nephritis, or the toxic nephropathies. These processes are not readily correctable on diagnosis; however, the etiology should be established so that patients are not subjected to other procedures that may exacerbate their renal failure.

TABLE 45–6. Drugs Commonly Associated with Acute Interstitial Nephritis

Antibiotics

Penicillins*
Cephalosporins
Trimethoprim
Sulfa derivatives
Rifampicin

Diuretics

Furosemide
Thiazides
Triamterene

Antihypertensives

Captopril
Alpha-methyldopa

Seizure Medications

Phenytoin
Carbamazepine
Phenobarbital

Nonsteroidal Anti-inflammatory Agents

Fenoprofen†

Miscellaneous

Cimetidine
Allopurinol
Azathioprine
Penicillamine

*Most often seen in methicillin.
†Virtually all nonsteroidal anti-inflammatory agents have been reported to cause acute interstitial nephritis, but the association is strongest with fenoprofen use.
From Shapiro, J. I., and Schrier, R. W.: Etiology, pathogenesis and management of renal failure. *In* Walsh, P. C., Retik, A. B., Stamey, T. A., and Vaughan, E. D. (Eds.): Campbell's Urology, 6th ed. Philadelphia, W. B. Saunders, 1992, p. 2048.

Urinary Tract Infection

The patient who presents with an acute urinary tract infection usually has symptoms related to the site and severity of the infection. The most frequent urinary tract infection is *cystitis*, an infection within the bladder. Patients with cystitis present with urinary frequency, painful urination, urgency, suprapubic pain, and hematuria. Pyelonephritis occurs when the infection involves the kidney. *Acute pyelonephritis* is accompanied by flank pain, fever, chills, and occasionally nausea and vomiting. It differs from acute cystitis in that most patients with bacterial cystitis do not have chills and fever. The diagnosis of the urinary tract infection is supported by urinalysis and confirmed by a positive urine culture. The urine in a patient with an acute urinary tract infection yields an increased number of white blood cells. In the uncentrifuged urine specimen, a finding of 10 white blood cells per high-power field indicates an infection. The presence of bacteria in the wet smear or Gram stain of the urine supports the diagnosis. The patient who is maintaining a high fluid volume and voiding frequently may have a urine sample that appears normal but that when cultured demonstrates bacteria. In the catheterized urine specimen, the presence of any pathogenic bacteria in the cultured specimen indicates infection. However, when the specimen is a midstream voided specimen, it is believed that the colony count must exceed more than 100,000 organisms per ml. to confirm a urinary tract infection. Testing of catheterized urine specimens is appropriate in the patient with a symptomatic and suspected urinary tract infection because the introduction of a new infection in a patient who is already infected is unlikely.

Most urinary tract infections in the nonhospitalized patients are ascending infections and occur by entrance of bacteria through the urethra into the bladder. This concept supports the observation that the incidence of urinary tract infections is greater in the female, whose urethra measures 4 to 5 cm., than in the male, whose urethra is much longer. Pyelonephritis is usually caused by the ascent of bacteria from the bladder up the ureter to the kidney. However, hematogenous spread of infection from other sites to the kidney can occur. The most commonly encountered organisms and the drugs of choice to treat infection are listed in Table 45–7. Dosages of commonly used drugs and their side effects are given in Table 45–8.

Gram-Negative Septicemia

The most serious accompaniment of an infection of the urinary tract is the production of gram-negative septicemia. Gram-negative septicemia may produce two distinctly different hemodynamic events. It is necessary that the physician recognize the differences between hypodynamic and hyperdynamic septic shock, because the management differs (Table 45–9). In both instances, identification of the organism involved and delivery of organism-specific antibiotics is the fundamental basis of treatment. For the patient with gram-negative shock whose intravenous pressure is low, fluids for intravascular expansion should be given rapidly to restore intravascular volume and pressure. When the hematocrit is decreased, intravascular volume should be expanded with whole blood. If central venous pressure rises, indicating progressive myocardial failure, a cardiac glycoside or isoproterenol is suitable. Isoproterenol, a beta-adrenergic agent, increases the force of contraction of the heart while relaxing the smooth muscles of the splanchnic bed to cause vascular dilation. In hypodynamic shock, peripheral resistance is increased and isoprenaline aids in shunting circulation back into the capillary bed, relieving tissue anoxia and helping to correct acidosis. An alpha-adrenergic blocking agent, such as phenoxybenzamine, will relax arterioles and venules to enhance the circulation. As this occurs, intravascular volume may be depleted, and further vascular expansion may be necessary. The use of corticosteroids to reduce peripheral resistance and increase cardiac output has been advocated, but their benefit is unproven. Associated abnormalities that accompany septic shock, such as acidosis and hypercalcemia, should be treated as they are recognized. The acidosis may be corrected with bicarbonate, and acute hyperkalemia may be managed by the simultaneous administration of glucose and insulin to increase potassium uptake by the cells.

TABLE 45–7. Choices of Drugs for Microorganisms Commonly Encountered in Infections of the Urinary and Genital Tracts

Microorganism	Drug(s) of Choice	Alternative Drug(s)
Gram-positive cocci		
Staphylococcus aureus (beta-lactamase producing)	Nafcillin or cephradine*	Vancomycin
Staphylococcus (non-beta-lactamase producing)	Penicillin G	Erythromycin
Streptococcus, group D		
Streptococcus faecalis (also *S. faecium*, enterococci)	Ampicillin plus gentamicin†	Penicillin G plus amikacin
Streptococcus bovis	Penicillin G	Vancomycin
Streptococcus, group B	Ampicillin	Cephalexin*
Gram-negative cocci		
Gonococcus	Penicillin G plus probenecid	Tetracycline
Gonococcus (beta-lactamase producing)	Spectinomycin	Cefoxitin plus probenecid
Gram-negative rods		
Escherichia coli	Sulfonamide or ampicillin	Gentamicin or probenecid
Klebsiella species	Gentamicin	Cefamandole
Enterobacter species	Gentamicin	Cefamandole
Proteus mirabilis	Ampicillin	Gentamicin
Proteus vulgaris and others	Gentamicin or amikacin	Cefoxitin or chloramphenicol
Pseudomonas aeruginosa	Gentamicin plus carbenicillin	Polymyxin or colistimethate
Serratia species	Co-trimoxazole and polymyxin	Gentamicin or amikacin
Haemophilus vaginalis	Metronidazole	Tetracycline
Chlamydiae (*Chlamydia trachomatis*)	Tetracycline	Erythromycin
Mycoplasmas (*Ureaplasma urealyticum*)	Erythromycin	Tetracycline

*Or other oral cephalosporin.
†Or amoxicillin.

TABLE 45–8. Antimicrobial Agents Often Used in Urology

Drug	Route	Daily Adult Dose	Daily Pediatric Dose	Untoward Effects
Soluble sulfonamide (sulfisoxazole, trisulfapyrimidines)	Oral	1 gm. four times	100–150 mg./kg.	Rashes, fever, nausea, vomiting, diarrhea, arthritis, stomatitis, thrombocytopenia, hemolytic or aplastic anemia, granulocytopenia, hepatitis, vasculitis, Stevens-Johnson syndrome, psychosis, etc. Crystalluria and hematuria rare.
Trimethoprim	Oral	100 mg. twice	15–30 mg./kg.	
Trimethoprim-sulfamethoxazole (co-trimoxazole)	Oral	4 tablets	Trimethoprim, 15 mg./kg., and sulfamethoxazole, 150 mg./kg.	
Ampicillin	Oral	2–4 gm.	50–100 mg./kg.	Hypersensitivity: rashes, fever, anaphylaxis, dermatitis, serum sickness, nephritis, eosinophilia, vasculitis, hemolytic anemia, granulocytopenia. Nausea, vomiting, diarrhea especially with oral penicillins. Central nervous system toxicity with very high doses and renal insufficiency.
	IV	2–10 gm.	100–300 mg./kg.	
Amoxicillin	Oral	0.75–1.5 gm.	20–40 mg./kg.	
Carbenicillin	Oral	1.5–3 gm.	50–70 mg./kg.	
	IV	30 gm.	100–600 mg./kg.	
Ticarcillin	IV	200–300 mg./kg.	200–300 mg./kg.	
Nafcillin	Oral	2–4 gm.	50–100 mg./kg.	
	IV	3–12 gm.	100–200 mg./kg.	
Dicloxacillin	Oral	1–2 gm.	25–50 mg./kg.	
Penicillin V or G	Oral	1.6–3.2 million units	0.05–0.1 million units/kg.	
Penicillin G	IV	1.2–20 million units	0.05–0.3 million units/kg.	
Cefazolin	IV	3–6 gm.	25–100 mg./kg.	Same as with penicillins
Cephalothin	IV	3–12 gm.	60–100 mg./kg.	
Cefoxitin	IV	3–12 gm.	?	
Cefamandole	IV	2–10 gm.	50–150 mg./kg.	
Cephalexin	Oral	1–4 gm.	25–50 mg./kg.	
Cephradine	Oral	1–4 gm.	25–50 mg./kg.	
Tetracycline	Oral	1–2 gm.	20–40 mg./kg.	Fever, rashes, anorexia, nausea, diarrhea, yellow mottling of teeth and bones, liver damage, vestibular reactions, renal tubular damage
Oxytetracycline	Oral	1–2 gm.	20–40 mg./kg.	
Doxycycline	Oral	200 mg.	2.5–4 mg./kg.	
Minocycline	Oral	200 mg.	2.5–4 mg./kg.	
Chloramphenicol	Oral	1–3 gm.	50 mg./kg.	Anorexia, nausea, diarrhea, aplastic anemia (rare), gray syndrome in neonates
	IV	2–4 gm.	50–100 mg./kg.	
Erythromycin	Oral	1–2 gm.	30–50 mg./kg.	Anorexia, nausea, diarrhea, cholestatic hepatitis as a hypersensitivity reaction
Gentamicin	IM or IV	3–5 mg./kg.	3–5 mg./kg.	Nephrotoxicity and ototoxicity
Tobramycin	IM or IV	3–5 mg./kg.	3–5 mg./kg.	
Amikacin	IM or IV	15 mg./kg.	15 mg./kg.	
Kanamycin	IM or IV	15 mg./kg.	15 mg./kg.	
Polymyxin B	IV	2.5 mg./kg.	1.5–2.5 mg./kg.	Paresthesias, dizziness, nephrotoxicity
Colistimethate	IM	2.5–5 mg./kg.	2.5 mg./kg.	
Nitrofurantoin	Oral	200–400 mg.	5–7 mg./kg.	Nausea, vomiting, rashes, pulmonary infiltrates, rare neurotoxicity
Methenamine hippurate	Oral	2 gm.	75 mg./kg.	Vesical irritation
Methenamine mandelate	Oral	4 gm.	75 mg./kg.	
Nalidixic acid	Oral	4 gm.	30–60 mg./kg.	Rashes, gastrointestinal disturbances, visual and central nervous system disturbances, photosensitization (rare).
Oxolinic acid	Oral	4 gm.	—	

THE KIDNEYS

Renal Calculi

The calcium oxalate calculus is the most common urinary stone in the United States, with 33% of recovered stones being pure calcium oxalate. Approximately 34% of all stones are mixtures of calcium oxalate and phosphate, approximately 15% are magnesium ammonium phosphate, 6% are pure calcium phosphate, 8% are uric acid, and 3% are cystine. Conditions that promote an alkaline pH of the urine (e.g., urinary tract infections, metabolic disease such as hyperparathyroidism, renal tubular acidosis, and medullary sponge kidney) predispose to an increased incidence of calcium phosphate stone. A discussion of the etiology and medical prevention of each specific type of stone is beyond the scope of this chapter. Nonetheless, the goal of each physician who treats the patient with renal calculi should be to identify the chemical composition of the stone, initiate therapy designed to remove the stone, establish medical therapy designed to prevent recurrence of the stone, and control any associated urinary tract infection.

Diagnostic Studies

An intravenous pyelogram should be obtained in all patients who present with the symptoms (flank pain, cramping, abdominal discomfort radiating to the groin, scrotum, or labia, microscopic hematuria) of urinary calculi. The plain scout film of the intravenous pyelogram identifies the location of the stone and directs the form of intervention. The

TABLE 45–9. Findings in Patients with Gram-Negative Septicemic Shock

	Circulatory States	
	Hypodynamic	*Hyperdynamic*
Arterial blood pressure	↓	↓
Pulse rate	↑	↑
Central venous pressure	↓	↑
Urine flow	↓	↓
Hematocrit	↑	May be normal
With arterial blood samples, the following are measured:		
Cardiac index	↓	↑
Blood gases:		
Po_2	↓	↓
Pco_2	↓	↓
Blood lactate	↑	↑
Blood pH	↓	Normal or ↑

intravenous pyelogram also reveals whether the stone is obstructing or partially obstructing and identifies any anatomic condition that produces stasis (e.g., ureteropelvic junction obstruction, pyelonephric scarring, or calyceal diverticulum), thereby promoting stone formation (Fig. 45–9).

Surgical Management

The presence of a calculus in the urinary tract is not an indication for open surgical therapy. Previously, many calculi in the urinary tract were observed only, either because they were asymptomatic or because they were small enough that spontaneous passage through the urinary tract was highly likely. However, in today's high-technology world, methodology exists for the nonsurgical removal of many of these calculi, using either ultrasonic energy delivered through a hollow probe or extracorporeal shock waves focused through a fluid medium on the offending calculi in such a way as to initiate dissolution of the calculus itself. It is axiomatic that all calculi producing obstruction, intractable pain, persistent urinary tract infection despite appropriate antibiotic therapy, or progressive renal deterioration should be removed. Only when there is an associated anatomic abnormality within the kidney, such as outflow obstruction at the ureteropelvic junction, such that this obstruction will promote future stone formation by promoting stasis, is it necessary to proceed with surgical exploration for removal of the stone with simultaneous correction of the defect. There are instances in which the amount of stone burden is such that open surgical removal is necessary; however, almost all stones can be managed by a combination of percutaneous ultrasonic lithotripsy and extracorporeal shock wave lithotripsy. Although previous texts dealing with the urinary system have devoted considerable space to the open surgical removal of calculi of the urinary tract, operative procedures are considered of historical interest and are deleted from this discussion.

Use of Extracorporeal Shock Wave Lithotripsy and Ultrasonic Lithotripsy

Ultrasonic Lithotripsy. Using a piezoceramic crystal to generate a high-frequency sound wave vibration (2300 to 2700 Hz.), this acoustical energy is transmitted through an acoustical horn, which focuses the sound wave longitudinally down a rigid hollow steel rod, concentrating the energy at the end of the rod. The renal stone is broken when the probe end contacts the stone as the end of the probe strikes the stone several thousand times per second, essentially battering

the stone until it fractures. Fluid circulates through the ultrasound probe and, with the circulation of this fluid, the small stone pieces are removed as they are created. Access to the stone in the kidney occurs by making a puncture wound in the skin and placing a long, sharp probe through the renal substance itself and into the collecting system. Through this hollow needle is passed a guide wire, and over the guide wire are passed either hollow dilating probes of increasing size or a dilating balloon. Once the access to the kidney has been created by progressive dilation, the rigid ureteroscope is passed through the flank and renal substance, and the stone is visualized. The ultrasound probe is then inserted and the stone is fragmented. Both stone and associated blood fragments are suctioned away (Fig. 45–10). Using this technique, stones of various sizes can be fragmented and removed from the kidney without the need for an open surgical procedure.

Extracorporeal Shock Wave Lithotripsy. Extracorporeal shock wave lithotripsy is based on the principle that shock waves, generated in a fluid media, can be focused through that fluid media and through the human body to impact and destroy calculi within the urinary tract. Currently, the shock waves are generated either by an underwater spark discharge unit, in which a capacitor stores electrical energy that is released within a microsecond, or by the simultaneous dis-

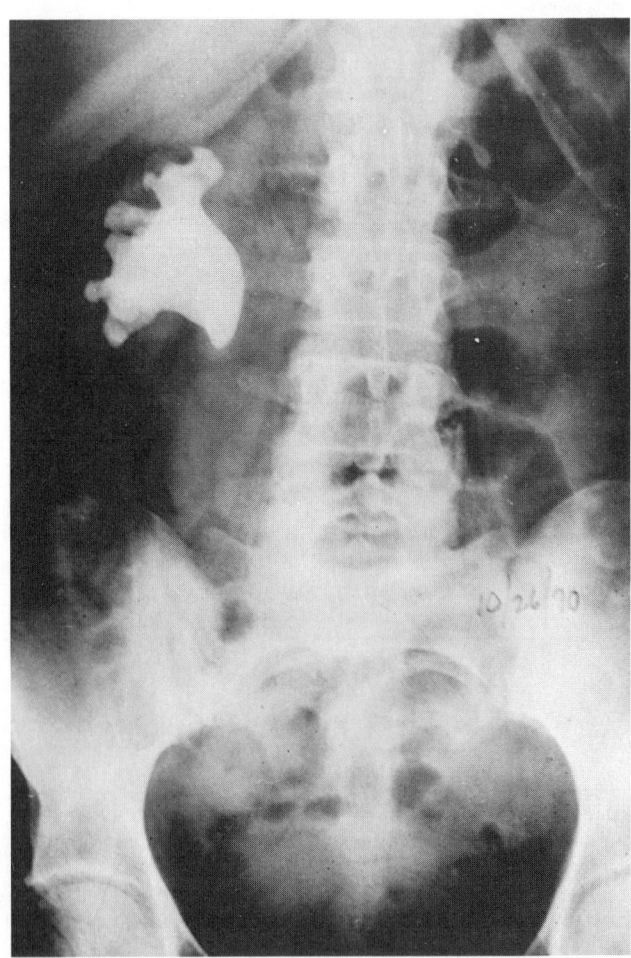

Figure 45–9. Kidney-ureter-bladder view demonstrating large right staghorn calculus. Although many surgeons may favor an anatrophic nephrolithotomy for removal of this calculus, it is feasible to remove calculi like these through an extended pyelolithotomy. The rather short unobstructed infundibulum seen in this case makes removal of the calculus through an extended pyelolithotomy possible. (From Paulson, D. F.: Genitourinary Surgery. New York, Churchill Livingstone, 1983, p. 62.)

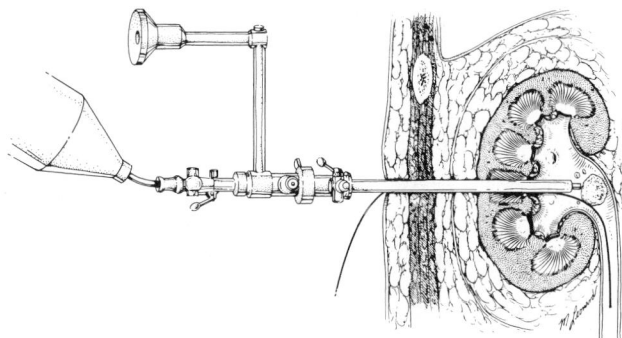

Figure 45–10. A percutaneous nephroscope has been placed through the body wall and the kidney. The stone that lies within the collecting system of the kidney can be visualized and destroyed by ultrasound waves.

charge of thousands of piezoelectrodes, similarly activated by an electrical discharge. This discharge gives rise to a shock wave in the surrounding fluid, which then propagates concentrically in a manner similar to sound waves in air, expanding from its organ of origin until it hits a solid structure. To transfer the pressure of these shock waves to the renal calculus, the shock wave created by the underwater spark discharge unit is focused using a rotationally specific semiellipsoid, whose walls are placed around the first geometric focus of this geometric configuration to direct the shock wave energy in a singular path. The electrode within the semiellipsoid and the patient are positioned so that the second geometric focus positioned by the shape of the ellipsoid is at the center of the calculus. Thus, reflection of waves from the ellipsoid walls transfers the maximum energy from the spark gap electrode to the center of the calculus itself (Figs. 45–11 and 45–12). Shock waves generated by the piezoelectrode are focused on the stone without use of the semiellipsoid but by specific focusing of the piezoelectrode crystals. The energy delivered by the spark gap generator and the area of entry of the energy through the patient's body are such that general anesthesia is required for pain relief during the treatment itself. However, with the piezoelectrode shock wave lithotriptors, the entry point of the shock wave is so diffuse that the treatments can be delivered without anesthesia; the patient essentially walks in, lies down on the instrument, and is able to arise after the treatment and walk from the treatment facility. It is believed that 75% to 80% of all patients with renal calculi can be managed by extracorporeal shock wave lithotripsy, and virtually all patients can be managed by a combination of extracorporeal shock wave lithotripsy and percutaneous ultrahydraulic lithotripsy.

Metabolic Evaluation of the Patient with Recurrent Calculi

The patient who presents with recurrent stone disease should be evaluated to determine if there is a correctable metabolic cause for the stone formation. Initially the physician should obtain a complete blood cell count and a Sequential Multiple Analyzer-12, including determination of levels of serum calcium, phosphorus, uric acid, creatinine, blood urea nitrogen, total protein with albumin-globulin ratio, and alkaline phophatase and serum electrolytes. A 24-hour urine collection should be obtained for calcium, uric acid, oxalate, mean pH, sodium concentration, and total volume. This 24-hour urine sample should be obtained on a random diet, and a second set of serum samples should be obtained at the conclusion of the 24-hour collection. The patient should then

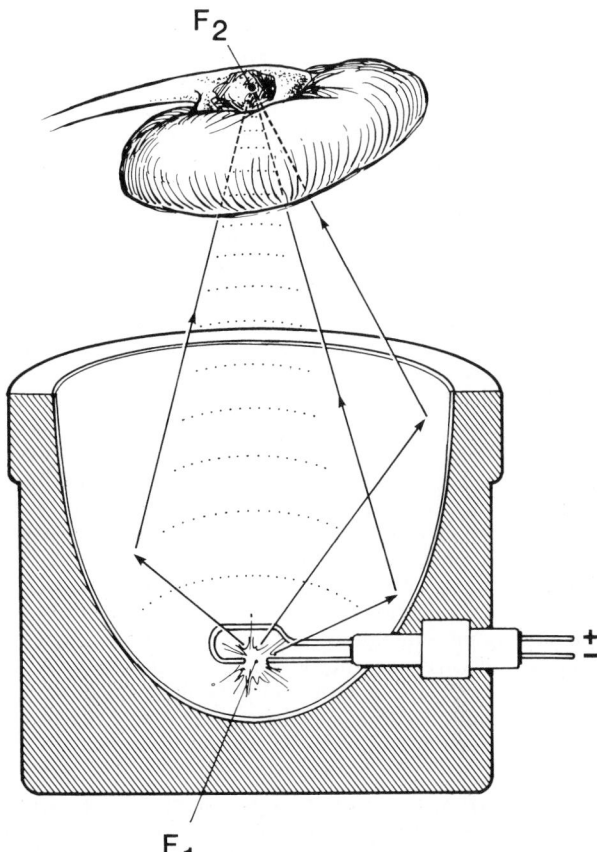

Figure 45–11. Spark gap electrode and semiellipsoid for focusing shock waves. Electrode is placed at first focus inside ellipsoid (F_1) with stone placed at second focus (F_2). (From Carson, C. C.: Endourology. New York, Churchill Livingstone, 1985, p. 310.)

be placed on a restrictive calcium and sodium diet of approximately 400 mg. of calcium and 100 mg. of sodium daily. A second 24-hour urine is then collected for uric acid, creatinine, oxalate, calcium, sodium, pH, volume, and cyclic adenosine monophosphate. A third set of serum samples is then collected for the previous studies plus a serum parathormone test. Patients with uric acid calculi, cystine stones, or struvite calculi with an associated urinary tract infection do not require this detailed metabolic evaluation. Although most calcium stone formers will respond to thiazide diuretics, it is important to determine the cause of recurrent stone forma-

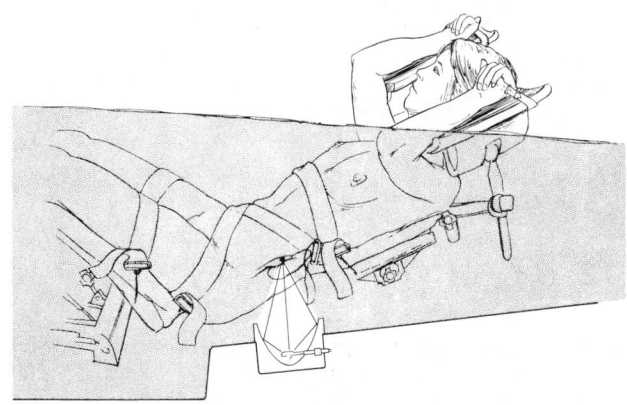

Figure 45–12. Patient positioned for extracorporeal shock wave lithotripsy. Area of flank is exposed for efficient shock wave conduction.

tion. It should be possible to establish the cause of more than 80% of calcium stone formers. *Hypercalciuria* is defined as the urinary calcium level that exceeds 200 mg. per 24 hours on a restricted calcium and sodium diet. An excretion of greater than 4 mg. per kg. for 24 hours on a random diet is also considered excessive. Patients with normal serum calcium values who are hypercalciuric are categorized in the idiopathic hypercalciuric group and may be further subdivided as having absorptive hypercalciuria and renal hypercalciuria.

A detailed outpatient evaluation of the hypercalciuric stone-forming patient should be done. A 24-hour urine sample is obtained after an overnight fast, with a 4-hour urine sample then obtained after the oral administration of 1 gm. of calcium. These two urine samples are then analyzed for creatinine, calcium, and cyclic adenosine monophosphate. To promote diuresis, 600 ml. of distilled water is ingested at the beginning of the test, followed by 300 ml. at the time of calcium ingestion with an additional 300 ml. 2 hours later. A high level of calcium excretion during the fasting state represents either impaired tubular absorption of calcium or excessive mobilization of calcium from bone. Intestinal calcium absorption can be assessed by measurement of renal calcium excretion after calcium load. Fasting urinary calcium and cyclic adenosine monophosphate are increased in renal hypercalciuria caused by renal leak and in secondary hyperparathyroidism. Patients with absorptive hypercalciuria have a normal calcium excretion in the fasting state with an elevated urine calcium level after an oral calcium load.

Surgical Management of Renal Obstruction

Occasionally the renal outflow tract may be obstructed by stone, tumor, or an iatrogenic complication of other surgery. When this occurs, drainage of the obstructed kidney must be accomplished. Current technology allows this to be accomplished either through an open surgical procedure or with a closed percutaneous technique. The preferred method is to drain the upper tract using percutaneous techniques, except when other events prompt open surgical exposure of the kidney (Figs. 45–13 and 45–14).

Renal Infections[6]

Severe infections of the kidney are not common today except in immunosuppressed patients, patients with diabetes mellitus, or those with other significant renal disease. These

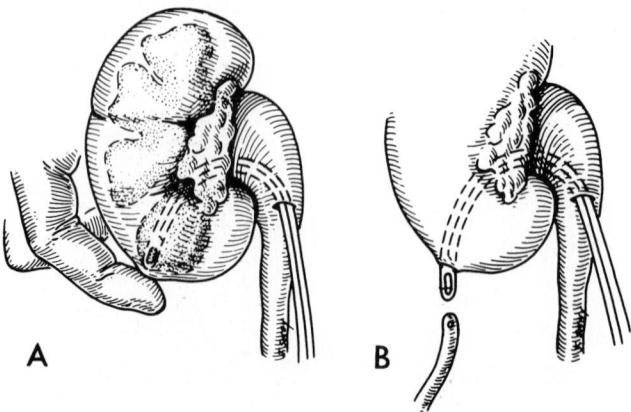

Figure 45–13. *A,* A sharply curved stone forceps was introduced into the interior calyx through an opening in the renal pelvis and guided to the thinnest point of the parenchyma. *B,* The end of the clamp is pushed through the renal parenchyma, and a small (12- or 14-French) red rubber catheter is tied to the end of the clamp. (From Paulson, D. F.: Genitourinary Surgery. New York, Churchill Livingstone, 1983, p. 37.)

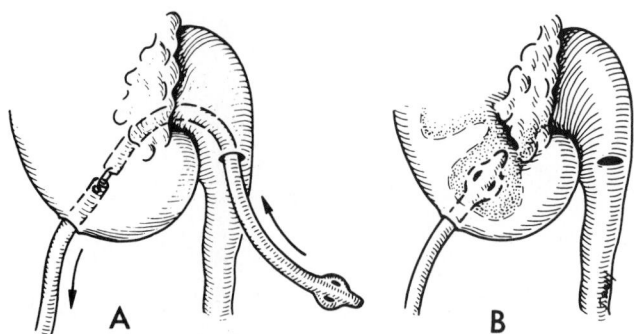

Figure 45–14. *A,* The external or distal end of a Malecot catheter is then sutured through the drainage end of the red Robinson catheter. A No. 16 or 18 Malecot catheter is usually suitable. *B,* The red Robinson catheter is then carefully withdrawn, pulling the Malecot catheter after it. The drainage end of the Malecot catheter is carefully positioned in the inferior calyx. The opening in the renal pelvis is then closed and drained and red rubber drains are also usually passed through a separate stab wound in the skin. (From Paulson, D. F.: Genitourinary Surgery. New York, Churchill Livingstone, 1983, p. 38.)

infections may be occult and go unrecognized until severe life-threatening symptoms appear. The perinephric abscess, a potentially fatal process, usually arises from rupture of a renal abscess, but it can be secondary to hematogenous dissemination from another site or from pyelonephritis. The patient may present with pyelonephritis or fever of undetermined origin. Diabetes mellitus or an antecedent history of recurrent urinary tract infection is frequently noted. Fever, abdominal or flank pain, and abdominal tenderness are present. When the diagnosis is suspected, blood and urine cultures should be obtained; blood cultures are positive in approximately 40% of patients and urine cultures are positive in 80% of patients. The organisms identified from these sites are frequently identical to the organisms isolated from the perinephric abscess, with the predominant organisms being *Escherichia coli, Proteus* species, and *Staphylococcus aureus.* Imaging studies may assist in diagnosis. The patient with a perinephric abscess usually has immobility of the kidney, and the renal shadow does not move with inspiration or expiration. There is a tendency to scoliosis as the patient splints the involved side. Loss of the psoas shadow may occur. Ultrasonography and gallium scanning may aid in making the diagnosis. Occasionally, percutaneous aspiration or lavage confirms the diagnosis. The treatment of a perinephric abscess is incision and drainage or nephrectomy (Fig. 45–15).

Renal Adenocarcinoma[15]

Adenocarcinoma is the most common malignancy involving the kidney. It most frequently occurs in the fifth decade of life, with the incidence three times higher in males than in females. These tumors are of tubular origin. Antibodies specific for microvilli of the convoluted proximal tubular cells cross-react with cells of both renal adenomas and renal adenocarcinomas. Renal adenomas can be segregated from renal adenocarcinomas on the basis of size; lesions smaller than 2 cm. are termed *adenomas,* with lesions larger than 2 cm. being termed *adenocarcinomas.* Whether renal adenomas are small renal carcinomas that have the potential for growth and subsequent metastases is debated. Three cell types can be identified: (1) the clear cell carcinoma composed of large polyhedral cells with distinct margins and clear to lightly vacuolated cytoplasm that is clear because it contains large amounts of triglycerides and phospholipids, which are removed during histologic processing, thus providing the *empty cell* appearance; (2) granular cell tumors, which are

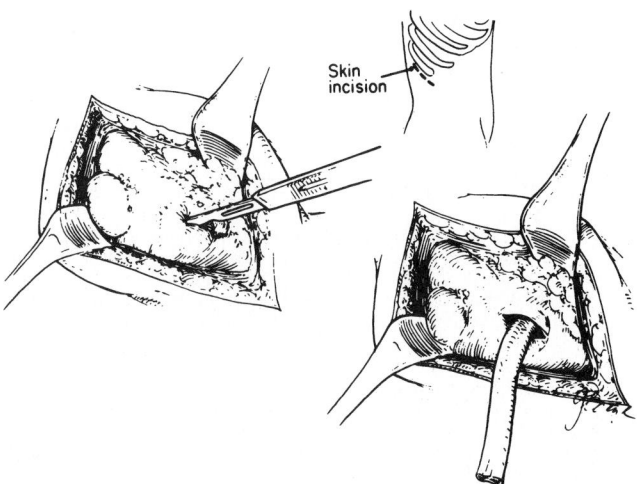

Figure 45–15. When exploring and draining an abscess or swelling in the kidney, it is important that the body cavities (intrathoracic and intraperitoneal) not be opened and violated. A small incision directly over the suspected areas usually suffices, preferably a subcostal or posterior one. The affected area is opened widely and drained with soft rubber drains. Cultures for anaerobic and aerobic bacteria should always be obtained. The skin incision may be closed, but in widespread infection they are best left open with packing, to be closed by secondary intention. (From Paulson, D. F.: Genitourinary Surgery. New York, Churchill Livingstone, 1983, p. 39.)

smaller and are round or cuboidal and with progressive anaplasia become more irregular; and (3) sarcomatoid tumors, composed of spindle-shaped cells resembling a fibrosarcoma often arranged in papillary or tubular structures. Mitotic cells are rare.

Signs and Symptoms of Renal Adenocarcinoma[15]

Renal carcinoma may present with a wide variety of symptomatic patterns (Table 45–10). The symptom-complex of reversible hepatosplenomegaly with hepatic dysfunction in the absence of liver metastases has been identified in some 10% of patients. The liver function parameters improve with disappearance of the hepatosplenomegaly after nephrectomy. Hypertension occurs in 14% to 40% of patients.

Evaluation of Renal Mass Lesions[12, 15]

Symptomatic or asymptomatic renal mass lesions of renal parenchyma should be evaluated by a series of sequential steps (Fig. 45–16). With a systematic approach to identification of renal mass lesions, 85% can be correctly identified by a combination of only two sequential examinations. Seventy per cent of all mass lesions identified by nephrotomography in the asymptomatic patient are benign renal cysts, with only 5.5% being malignant neoplasms. The most frequent asymptomatic renal neoplasm is metastatic tumor, with carcinoma of the breast being most common. Only 2.2% of asymptomatic space-occupying lesions of the kidney are renal cell malignancies.

The renal cyst presents a sharply defined interface against adjacent renal parenchyma. The lesions are thin walled in those areas that project outside the renal border. Ultrasonography may confirm the lesion as being cystic or solid. The benign cyst contains fluid that is clear, lightly straw colored, and low in fat, protein, lactic acid dehydrogenase, and amylase content. Cystic tumors have a darker, cloudy cystic fluid, which is high in fat, protein, and lactic acid dehydrogenase. When the urea nitrogen content of the cyst fluid is greater than 40 mg. per 100 ml., the cyst has a tendency to re-form. A cyst fluid pressure of less than 80 mm. H_2O indicates that the cyst will possibly regress if it is treated by aspiration alone. Should the opening pressure be greater than 160 mm. H_2O, the cyst is likely to re-form after aspiration. Should the intravenous pyelogram by bolus tomography demonstrate a hypervascular or mottled appearance, or if the ultrasound evaluation is indeterminate or represents a solid lesion, the patient should undergo angiography or CT. Approximately 85% of renal cell carcinomas are hypervascular by angiography and can be diagnosed with accuracy by selective renal artery angiography.

A more accurate method for evaluating renal cell masses is the use of CT. CT allows the determination of the extension of disease to associated structures, the presence or absence of associated adenopathy, and the definition of the density of the lesion. MRI is very useful in identifying the extent of associated vascular extension and is superior to venacavography in determining the degree of tumor thrombus extension into the vena cava and the level of such extension.

From a practical standpoint, once the renal mass lesion is identified by nephrotomography, most physicians move

TABLE 45–10. Presenting Symptoms, Laboratory Abnormality, or Abnormality on Physical Examination and Its Relation to Survival Rate in 309 Consecutive Patients Undergoing Nephrectomy for Renal Cell Carcinoma

Presenting Symptom, Abnormal Laboratory Finding, or Abnormality on Physical Examination	No. of Patients and Percent of Total	No. of Patients Surviving 5 Years
Classic triad (gross hematuria, abnormal mass, pain)	29 (9%)	9 (of 29) 31%
Hematuria	183 (59%)	74 (of 183) 40%
Pain	127 (41%)	56 (of 127) 44%
Abdominal mass	139 (45%)	49 (of 139) 35%
Fever	21 (7%)	8 (of 21) 38%
Weight loss	85 (28%)	29 (of 85) 39%
Anemia	64 (21%)	24 (of 64) 38%
Erythrocytosis	10 (3%)	4 (of 10) 40%
Hypercalcemia	11 (3%)	4 (of 11) 35%
Acute varicocele	7 (2%)	3 (of 7) 43%
Tumor calcification on x-ray film	39 (13%)	18 (of 39) 46%
Symptoms for metastases	31 (10%)	1 (of 31) 3%
Cancer, an incidental finding (silent)	20 (7%)	13 (of 20) 65%

Modified from Skinner, D. G., Colvin, R. B., Vermillion, C. D., et al.: Diagnosis and management of renal cell carcinoma: A clinical and pathologic study of 309 cases. Cancer, 28:1165, 1971. Copyright © 1971 American Cancer Society. Reprinted by permission of Wiley-Liss, Inc., a subsidiary of John Wiley & Sons, Inc.

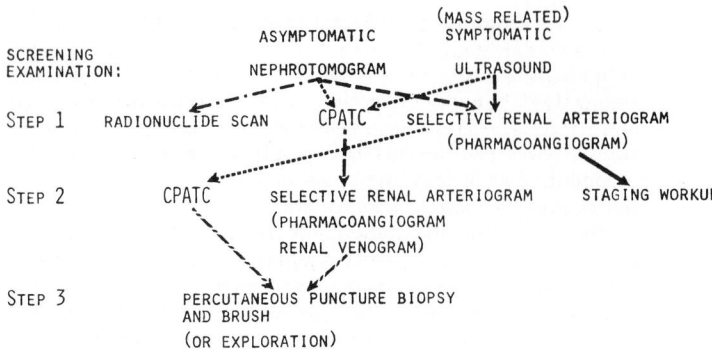

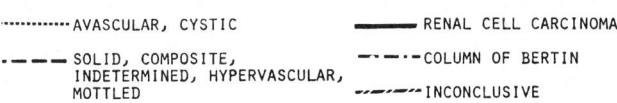

Figure 45–16. Steps in evaluating renal mass lesions. CPATC, computerized axial tomography. (From Paulson, D. F.: Genitourinary malignancies. *In* DeVita, V. T., Jr., Hellman, S., Rosenberg, S. [Eds.]: Cancer: Principles and Practice of Oncology. Philadelphia, J. B. Lippincott, 1982, p. 734.)

directly to CT to evaluate the nature of the mass lesion. CT is much more accurate in evaluating the lesion than a combination of ultrasonography and angiography.

Staging of Renal Adenocarcinoma[12]

Malignancies of the urinary tract are staged according to the anatomic distribution of disease. Two staging systems exist for identification of the anatomic distribution of renal cell malignancies (Table 45–11).

Surgical Therapy of Renal Adenocarcinoma[15, 28]

The management of renal cell carcinoma is based on the anatomic extent of disease, with treatment directed toward surgical removal of the kidney and associated tumor, the adrenal gland, the surrounding perinephric fat, and Gerota's fascia, along with the regional lymph nodes. Surgical removal of the kidney can be conducted through one of several incisions: transabdominal, modified flank, full flank, or thoracoabdominal. Irrespective of the incision used to gain access to the tumor, once the incision has been made, early control of the vascular supply of the tumor should be established to permit mobilization of the renal mass with minimal blood loss (Fig. 45–17). Surgical therapy is effective in controlling renal adenocarcinoma when the disease is confined to the kidney or when it has extended minimally outside the renal capsule. Surgical therapy is not effective once the disease has extended to adjacent structures or to regional lymph nodes or has invaded the renal vein or vena cava. When the tumor is confined to the renal substance beneath the capsule itself, survival rates greater than 90% in 10 years can be expected (Fig. 45–18).

The survival benefits of regional lymphadenectomy have not been established despite the occurrence of nodal spread in approximately 22% of patients. The node dissection may be performed in continuity with nephrectomy or after the renal mass has been removed. The dissection should include a minimum distance of 4 to 6 cm. above and below the renal vessels along with the lymphatic drainage posterior to the aorta and vena cava. The perfuse lymphatic drainage, the difficulty in removing all involved nodes, the frequency with which local nodes are bypassed with drainage directly to the cisterna chyli, and the frequency with which blood-borne metastases occur all mitigate against a therapeutically successful lymphadenectomy.

The benefit of surgical removal of the renal primary tumor in the presence of metastatic disease is controversial. Although it has been argued that removal of the primary renal malignancy may provide control of symptoms such as fever, pain, hematuria, anemia, and hypercalcemia, and that it may reduce the likelihood of further dissemination of disease, there is no evidence that removal of the primary tumor promotes spontaneous regression of metastases nor that removal of the primary renal malignancy improves the response of metastatic disease to either hormonal manipulation or chemotherapy.

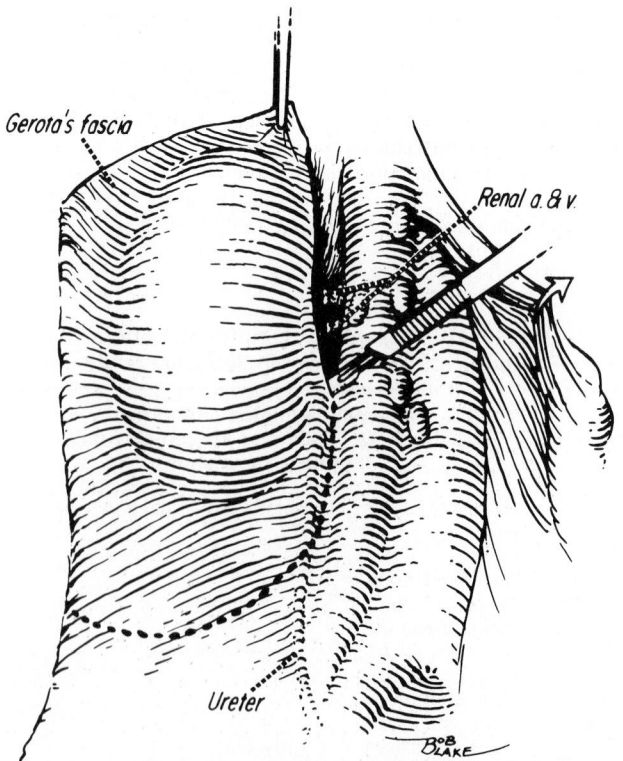

Figure 45–17. Radical nephrectomy. Kidney is removed within its investing fascia. (From Paulson, D. F.: Genitourinary malignancies. *In* DeVita, V. T., Hellman, S., Rosenberg, S. [Eds.]: Cancer: Principles and Practice of Oncology. Philadelphia, J. B. Lippincott, 1982, p. 737.)

TABLE 45–11. Comparison of Staging Systems*

TNM Clinical Classification

T	Primary tumor
T_X	Primary tumor cannot be assessed
T_O	No evidence of primary tumor
T_1	Tumor 2.5 cm. or less in greatest dimension, limited to the kidney
T_2	Tumor more than 2.5 cm. in greatest dimension, limited to the kidney
T_3	Tumor extends into major veins or invades adrenal gland or perinephric tissues but not beyond Gerota's fascia
T_{3a}	Tumor invades adrenal gland or perinephric tissues but not beyond Gerota's fascia
T_{3b}	Tumor grossly extends into renal vein(s) or vena cava
T_4	Tumor invades beyond Gerota's fascia
N	Regional lymph nodes
N_O	No identifiable nodes in a specified clinical assessment
N_1	Metastasis in single lymph node, 2 cm. or less in greatest dimension
N_2	Metastasis in single lymph node, 2 cm. but not more than 5 cm. in greatest dimension; in multiple lymph nodes, none more than 5 cm. in greatest dimension
N_3	Metastasis in a lymph node more than 5 cm. in greatest dimension
M	Distant metastasis
M_O	Tumors without distant metastasis
M_1	Tumors with distant metastasis
G	Histopathologic grading
G_1	Well differentiated
G_2	Moderately differentiated
G_3–G_4	Undifferentiated, anaplastic

Stage Grouping

Stage I	T_1	N_O	M_O
Stage II	T_2	N_O	M_O
Stage III	T_1	N_1	M_O
	T_2	N_1	M_O
	T_{3a}	N_O, N_1	M_O
	T_{3b}	N_O, N_1	M_O
Stage IV	T_4	Any N	M_O
	Any T	N_2, N_3	M_O
	Any T	Any N	M_1

*The regional lymph nodes are the hilar, abdominal para-aortic, and paracaval nodes. Laterality does not affect the N categories.

Adapted from International Union Against Cancer: Hermanek, P., Sobin, L. H. (Eds.): TNM Classification of Malignant Tumors, 4th ed. Berlin, Springer-Verlag, 1987.

Renal Trauma

Renal trauma may be classified as either blunt (nonpenetrating) or penetrating. Both blunt and penetrating trauma can be divided into two major classifications; those involving the parenchyma and those involving the renal pedicle. Patients with nonpenetrating injury who have microscopic hematuria are not candidates for intravenous pyelography because the incidence of identifying abnormalities requiring treatment is low. However, patients who have gross hematuria or who have penetrating injuries must be evaluated to determine the extent of the genitourinary injury. Much debate exists as to the optimum study. In patients who have blunt trauma, fracture of the lower ribs, fracture of the transverse vertebral processes, or scoliosis on the routine abdominal film, prompt urologic evaluation is indicated. An obliterated psoas margin or renal outline may indicate the presence of a large retroperitoneal perirenal hematoma. Unexplained ileus or abdominal pain also should raise the possibility of either retroperitoneal or renal injury. The patient who has sustained blunt renal trauma with gross hematuria or who has penetrating trauma and who presents with any of the signs or symptoms of vascular instability should undergo CT with contrast medium enhancement to determine the extent of the lesion and any associated perirenal hematuria. This study also allows the clinician to determine the bilaterality of renal function and the amount of gross urinary extravasation (Fig. 45–19). Any patient with nonvisualization of the kidney should undergo renal angiography to assess injury to the renal vasculature.

Blunt renal trauma can be classified according to the severity of injury (Fig. 45–20). The most common form of blunt renal injury is the renal contusion. Patients with renal contusion need no specific therapy other than observation for 48 to 72 hours. They may return to normal activity when the hematuria clears. Parenchymal lacerations that extend no deeper than the cortex may be treated nonsurgically with bed rest and broad-spectrum antibiotics. Patients who have a major parenchymal laceration may be treated conservatively; however, this patient population, when so treated, has a high incidence of infection, abscess formation, renal atrophy, hypertension, and secondary hemorrhage. Patients who have the more significant parenchymal lacerations should undergo surgical exploration and primary repair of these injuries.

When the decision is made to explore and repair—a decision often made only when the patient has persistent hemodynamic instability—the essential surgical principles are wide exposure and early vascular control. This is best done through a transabdominal transperitoneal approach. Gerota's fascia is left intact until the renal artery and vein are controlled. If Gerota's fascia is incised before vascular control, the tamponading effect of the fascia is lost and massive, life-threatening bleeding may occur. Once the renal vasculature is controlled, Gerota's fascia can be incised, the perirenal hematoma evacuated, and the renal injury assessed with intent to repair. Blunt trauma to the renal pedicle is usually produced by deceleration injury as the more mobile kidney moves away from the stationary aorta. As this occurs the media and adventitia stretch because of their elasticity; however, the intima, which is not as elastic as the other components of the vessel, tears. This intimal disruption leads to subsequent dissection and thrombosis. Salvage depends on early recognition, usually identified by failure of visualization on bolus nephrotomography, with perfusion failure confirmed by renal angiography.

Penetrating renal injuries are associated with other intra-

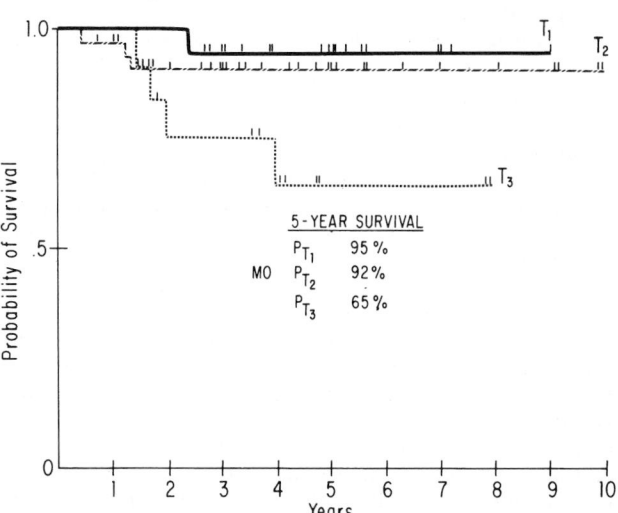

Figure 45–18. Survival of the nonmetastatic patients staged with the TNM classification. (From Selli, C., et al.: Cancer, 52:899, 1983. Copyright © 1983 American Cancer Society. Reprinted by permission of Wiley-Liss, Inc., a subsidiary of John Wiley & Sons, Inc.)

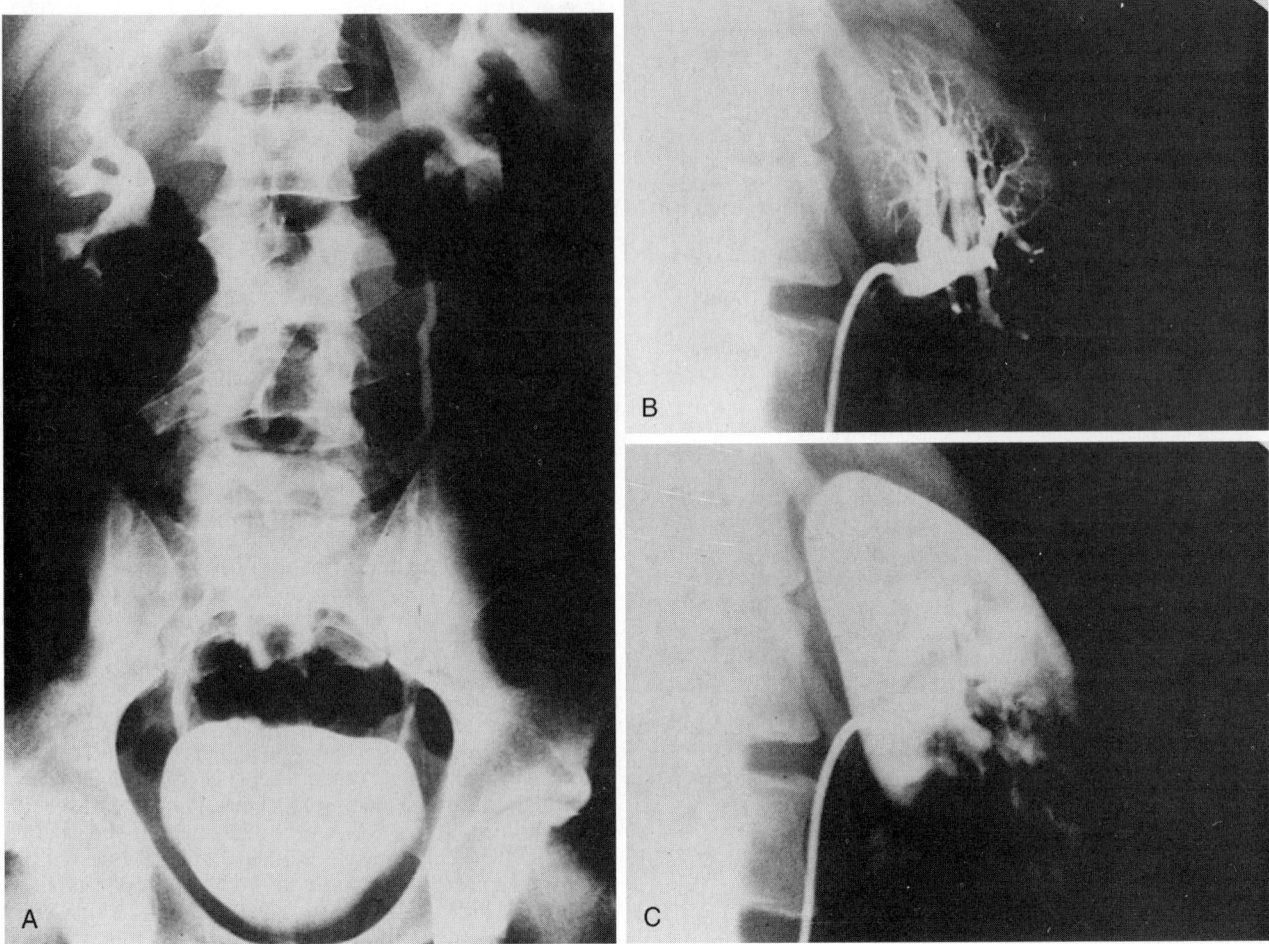

Figure 45–19. *A,* Intravenous pyelogram of a 26-year-old man with a fracture of the left kidney caused by a horseback riding accident. There is rather vague filling of the lower pole of the left kidney with evidence of extravasated contrast medium. (Note accentuation of left psoas margin secondary to extravasated urine.) *B,* Selective renal angiogram showing poor perfusion of the left lower pole. *C,* Delayed angiogram nephrogram phase showing disrupted parenchymal lower pole with deep laceration.

abdominal injuries in 80% of all patients. Thus, with the exception of superficial stab wounds, it is recommended that patients who have penetrating injuries near the kidney should have an intravenous pyelogram and be considered for surgical exploration. The principles for evaluation and management are similar to those discussed earlier for blunt renal trauma.

THE URETER

The ureter conveys urine from the renal pelvis to the bladder. It lies protected in the fibrofatty tissue of the retroperitoneum, and its integrity can be threatened by a variety of congenital, inflammatory, traumatic, iatrogenic, or neoplastic diseases. The ureters lie in the retroperitoneal space and are adherent to the posterior peritoneum. As they descend, they cross the common iliac vasculature to enter the true pelvis. The ureters then arc along the sacral promontory before converging toward the bladder trigone. The left ureter passes behind the pelvic mesencolon and the right ureter passes behind the root of the mesentery. In the male, the ureters cross the vas deferens ventrally to enter the wall of the bladder superior to the prostate and seminal vesicles, whereas in the female the ureters cross dorsally behind the uterine arteries and pass near the uterine cervix before entering the bladder.

The principles of management of ureteral injury include (1) gentle manipulation of ureteral tissue with noncrushing instruments or traction sutures to prevent damage to delicate ureteral vasculature; (2) adequate wound drainage in the site of urethral repair to remove any urine that may leak through the site of repair and inhibit the healing process; and (3) use of absorbable suture material, because use of nonabsorbable suture material provides a nidus that promotes the deposition of urinary salts and formation of calculi.

Ureteral injury or disease is diagnosed with intravenous pyelography, which permits visualization of the course of the ureter and identification of obstruction or deviation. When visualization of the ureter is not complete, cystoscopy and retrograde bulb occlusive ureteropyelography are required.

Calculus obstruction of the ureter is common, particularly in the more arid climates of the sunbelt. Open ureterolithotomy was at one time indicated by the following specific clinical situations: (1) a ureteral calculus greater than 1 cm. in diameter in a patient with a normal-sized ureter or in an individual who has not previously passed ureteral calculi; (2) sepsis associated with hydronephrosis secondary to obstruction by the calculus; (3) a jagged-hooded calculus that has impaled the ureteral mucosa and will not pass spontaneously; (4) a calculus in the upper ureter, which remains stationary for at least 2 weeks with hydronephrosis and hydroureter; and (5) increasing pain uncontrolled by oral pain medications, progressive nausea and vomiting, and associated fever in a patient with obstructive urinary calculus. These clinical situations may be managed by a combination

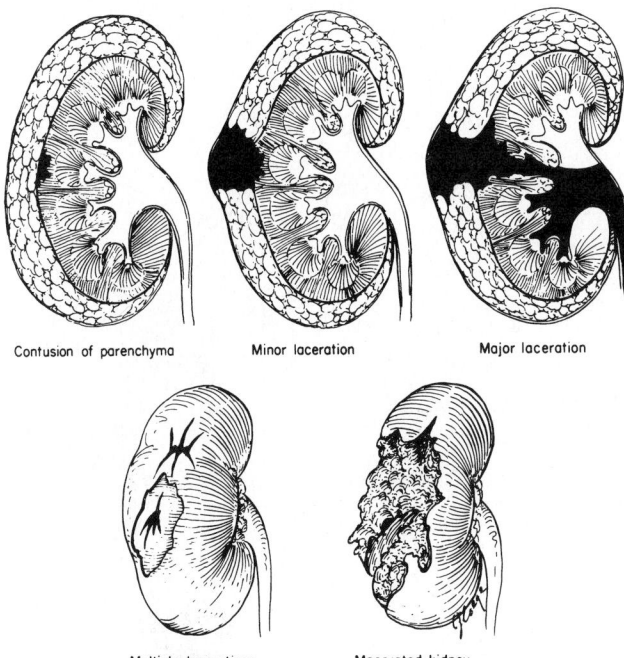

Figure 45–20. Categories of renal trauma. (From Paulson, D. F.: Genitourinary Surgery. New York, Churchill Livingstone, 1983, p. 112.)

Contusion of parenchyma   Minor laceration   Major laceration

Multiple lacerations   Macerated kidney

of ureteroscopy and basket extraction of the stone under direct vision ureteroscopy, with ultrasonic fracture of the stone followed by basket extraction of the fragments, or by percutaneous nephroscopy with basket extraction from above.

The ureteroscope may be passed through the urethra, through the ureteral orifice, and up the ureter all the way to the renal pelvis. In this manner the entire ureter and renal collecting system may be viewed (Fig. 45–21). Passage of the ureteroscope requires initial passage of floppy-tipped guide wire catheters through the ureteral orifice and up the ureter into the renal pelvis. The ureterovesical junction and distal ureter are then dilated to a caliber that can accept the ureteroscope. Then, under direct vision, the ureteroscope is passed over the working guide wire. Once the stone is visualized, it may be extracted under direct vision or fractured with the ultrasonic probe if it is too large for primary removal. With this technique, the majority of ureteral calculi may be removed without resorting to surgical incision.

When these methods of nonsurgical intervention do not allow removal of the stone, or when such technology results in damage to the ureter without removal of the stone, it may be necessary to proceed to open surgical procedure, both to remove the stone and to correct the ureteral injury. The ureter is divided into upper, middle, and lower segments. The surgical approach to the ureter depends on the anatomic site of the pathologic process. The upper ureter is best exposed through the anterior half of a full-flank incision; the midportion may be exposed through a Gibson, muscle-splitting, or hockey-stick incision; while the lower ureter is best approached through a midline infraumbilical incision, through a Pfannenstiel incision, or through an extension of the Gibson incision, with division of a portion of the rectus muscle.

Renal pelvic or ureteropelvic stones also may be removed through a posterior lumbotomy. The patient is placed prone or semi-prone, with the anterior rib cage elevated on blanket rolls. A vertical skin incision is made 2 cm. medial to the lateral edge of the sacrospinalis muscle, with the incision extended to the level of the twelfth rib superiorly and down-

ward toward the iliac crest. This posterior approach produces minimal postoperative pain. In addition, there is seldom postoperative adynamic ileus. No major muscle bundles are divided, and the patient is often up and about within 24 hours after surgery. Alternatively, a muscle-splitting incision may be used to remove upper ureteral calculi through a posterior flank approach.

Ureteral Obstruction Secondary to Malignant or Nonmalignant Disease[19]

The ureter may be obstructed secondary to either malignant or nonmalignant disease, and the obstruction may be either unilateral or bilateral. When it is bilateral, it is frequently associated with progressive loss of renal function. When it is unilateral, it is not frequently associated with any specific symptomatic presentation. In patients with known malignancies, a persistent urinary tract infection, proteinuria, or hematuria should suggest the possibility of retroperitoneal involvement. Any slow, progressive rise in the serum creatinine level or deterioration of renal function should be viewed with alarm. Early diagnosis is promoted by careful attention to these nonspecific signs and symptoms.

Obstruction of the ureter is best delineated initially by ultrasonography, intravenous pyelography with nephrotomography, or CT. Ultrasonography may suggest ureteral or renal pelvic enlargement and is a recommended initial study. Once ureteral or renal pelvic dilation is identified, the intravenous pyelogram with nephrotomography may further define the lesion. In those patients who have marked dilation of the upper urinary tract secondary to involvement of the middle to lower ureter and in whom a retrograde ureteropyelogram is not possible, percutaneous puncture of a dilated

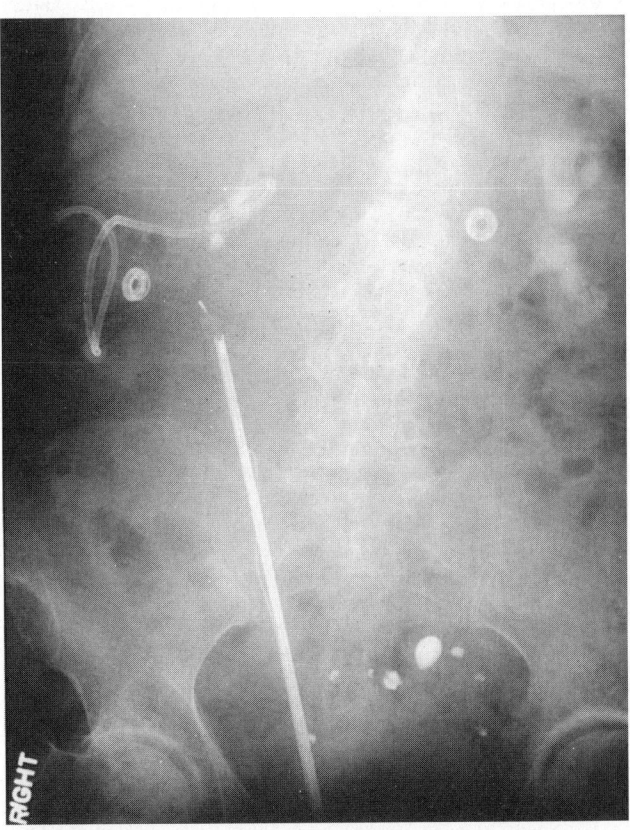

Figure 45–21. Ureteroscope in place, having been passed through the urethra and across the bladder up the ureter. The stone basket has engaged a fragment of stone in the upper ureter and the fragment will be extracted. (Courtesy of John L. Weinerth, M.D., Division of Urologic Surgery, Duke University Medical Center, Durham, North Carolina.)

collecting system with antegrade pyeloureterography may
identify the site of obstruction and the nature of the pathologic process. CT also shows the obstruction and may identify any surrounding anatomic disease. In patients with
known malignancy, the surgeon must be certain to be dealing
with obstruction secondary to recurrent malignancy, because
fibrosis from previous surgery or radiation therapy may
mimic malignancy. In previous years, ureteral obstruction
required either cutaneous ureterostomy or open nephrostomy. Today, current methodology can effect relief of the
obstruction without open surgical intervention. In the patient
with either unilateral or bilateral obstruction, internal drainage can be established using a double-J Silastic catheter (Fig.
45–22). These catheters may be inserted either transurethrally
from below or percutaneously from above. In either instance,
a guide wire is passed through the urethral lumen and a
soft Silastic catheter is threaded over the guide wire and
manipulated in place using a *pusher* catheter. When the
pusher catheter and guide wire are withdrawn, the preformed curves appear at either end of the indwelling ureteral
stent, holding it in place. The Silastic indwelling catheters
may be left in place for 6 to 12 months with minimal incrusta-
tion. They may be removed transurethrally and replaced
without difficulty.

Percutaneous Nephrostomy

When a transluminal ureteral catheter cannot be placed, a
percutaneous nephrostomy tube can be placed without the
necessity for open surgery. When the renal collecting system
is markedly dilated, the percutaneous tube may be placed
blindly, as described by Goodwin. However, by using ultrasonography or CT, the dilated collecting system can be visualized and a guide wire passed into the collecting system
under direct vision. Over the guide wire a series of dilating
catheters can be passed to progressively dilate the tract to a
9-French, after which an 8.5-French pigtail catheter can be
inserted over the guide wire and passed into the renal pelvis
to facilitate drainage. These techniques permit relief of obstruction and the placement of percutaneous catheters and
indwelling stents in patients with a variety of obstructing
lesions. They also permit the physician to stabilize renal
function and to approach definitive treatment under optimum physiologic conditions.

Ureteral Replacement[19]

In certain clinical situations, precipitated by either malignant or nonmalignant disease, it may be necessary to replace

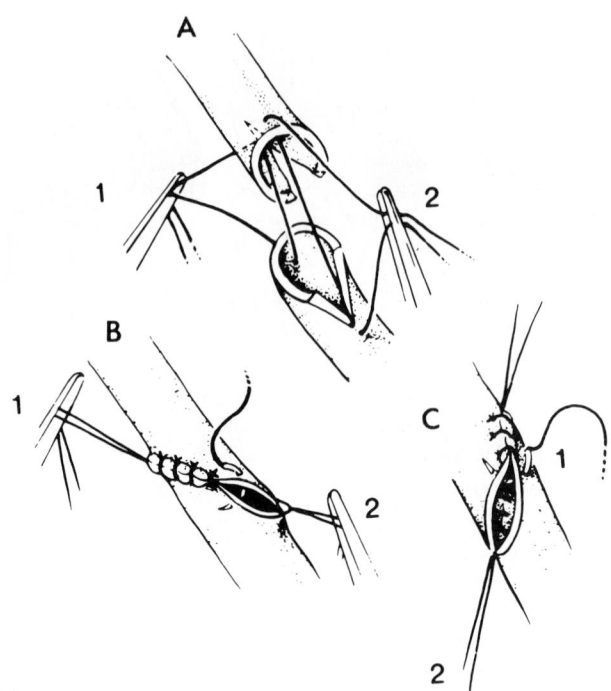

Figure 45–23. Technique for oblique spatulated end-to-end ureteroureterostomy. *A,* Initial suture placement. *B,* Ninety-degree rotation for closure of one
wall. *C,* One-hundred-eighty-degree rotation in the opposite direction to close
the other wall. (From Paulson, D. F.: Genitourinary Surgery. New York, Churchill
Livingstone, 1983, p. 179.)

the ureter either in part or *in toto.* Various surgical maneuvers
have been developed for ureteral replacement. When the
distal third of the ureter must be replaced, ureteroneocystostomy, with either a psoas hitch or bladder flap, may be the
treatment of choice. When there is a small segmental defect
of the ureter, ureteroureterostomy may be the simplest and
best procedure. When there is destruction of the major portion of any one ureter, transureteroureterostomy may be appropriate (Fig. 45–23). When there is involvement of all or
most of one ureter, replacement with a segment of ileum
may be considered. Autotransplantation with ureteroneocystostomy or vesicopyelostomy is an alternative procedure.

Carcinoma of the Ureter and Renal Pelvis[15]

Carcinoma of the renal pelvis constitutes 5% of all renal
carcinomas and is of transitional origin, arising from the
transitional epithelium that lines the calyceal system and
renal pelvis. Ninety per cent of all carcinomas of the renal
pelvis are transitional cell tumors, with the remaining being
either squamous cell carcinomas or adenocarcinomas. About
25% of all patients who have a single pelvic transitional cell
tumor develop malignancy at some other site in their urinary
tract at a future date. Patients who have multiple upper tract
tumors of transitional cell origin have a 50% probability of
the delayed appearance of invasive malignancy. Transitional
cell carcinomas spread both by direct extension and by blood
and lymphatic embolization. The malignant transitional cells
are shed into the urine, where they can be identified by
Papanicolaou's smear of the voided urine. Eighty to 90% of
all patients with renal pelvic tumors have either gross or
microscopic hematuria. Pain precipitated by ureteropelvic
junction obstruction secondary to the tumor mass produces
a symptom-complex similar to renal calculus disease. The
diagnosis is suggested by the appearance of a defect in the
collecting system or in the renal pelvis by excretory pyelogra-

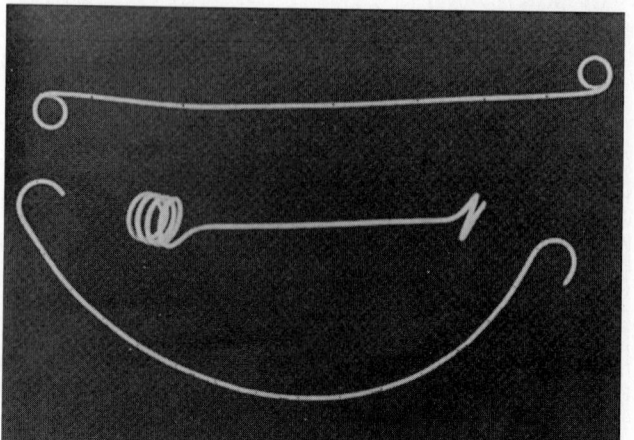

Figure 45–22. Various forms of double-J stents for internal ureteral drainage.

phy (Table 45–12). The classic surgical treatment of renal pelvic tumors is nephroureterectomy with excision of the ureteral orifice and a 1-cm. circle of surrounding bladder. Removal of the entire ureter is recommended, because approximately one fifth of all patients who have a residual portion of the ureter left in place develop tumors in the ureteral remnant. There are no data indicating that lymph node dissection at the level of the renal hilum provides enhanced disease control.

Carcinoma of the ureter is usually a transitional cell tumor. The characteristic ureteral dilation associated with ureteral tumors was described by Bergman and is said to distinguish ureteral tumors from ureteral calculi. The dilation that accompanies the ureteral tumor is the response of the ureter to accommodate a slowly expanding tumor mass and reflects the absence of renal spasm initiated by the presence of an irritating calculus. The differential diagnoses of the radiographic abnormalities associated with ureteral tumors include nonopaque calculi, blood clots, ureteritis cystica, ureteral varicosities, extraluminal malignancy with ureteral compression, periureteral fibrosis, and endometriosis. The diagnosis is suggested by the radiographic characteristics of the lesion in association with hematuria but is confirmed by the presence of urinary cytologic findings compatible with malignancy.

Treatment of ureteral tumors has traditionally been nephroureterectomy with removal of the entire renal unit and ureter. There is a trend to preserve the renal unit through local resection of the malignancy only. The relative advantages and disadvantages of these two philosophies remain undefined. However, the argument for less than nephroureterectomy springs from an interpretation that the salvage rate in patients with ureteral tumors is more dependent on the biologic aggressiveness of the tumor than on the aggressiveness of the chosen surgical procedure. It would appear that patients with high-grade lesions or lesions that have penetrated into or through the ureteral wall have little chance for cure, even with the most radical surgery, whereas patients with low-grade lesions have an excellent chance of cure with only a regional resection. Preservation of the renal unit allows use of nephrotoxic chemotherapeutic agents should the patient subsequently present with metastatic disease. The survival of patients with ureteral malignancy is influenced by the grade and stage of the tumor (Table 45–13).

THE URINARY BLADDER[4]

The urinary bladder can be carefully assessed by radiographic, physiologic, and endoscopic examination before the

TABLE 45–12. Differential Diagnosis of Cancer of the Renal Pelvis

Intrinsic Lesions

    Calculus
    Blood clot
    Cholesteatoma malakoplakia
    Inflammatory lesions of urothelium (e.g., pyelitis cystica)
    Benign ureteropelvic junction obstruction
    Benign (connective tissue) tumors of renal pelvis
    Renal cell carcinoma
    Suburothelial hemorrhage

Extrinsic Lesions

    Vascular impressions
    Parapelvic cyst

Modified from Fraly, E. E.: *In* Skinner, D. G., and deKernian, J. B. (Eds.): Genitourinary Cancer. Philadelphia, W. B. Saunders Company, 1978.

TABLE 45–13. Correlation of Survival Rate with Pathologic Characteristics of Ureteral Cancer

	5-Year Survival Rate (%)	
	Bloom et al[5] (54 Patients)	Batata et al[3] (41 Patients)
Histologic Grade		
I	83.0	78.0
II	52.0	50.0
III	18.0	0
IV	12.0	0
Pathologic Stage		
0, A	62.0	91.0
B	50.0	43.0
C	33.3	23.0
D	0	0

Modified from Skinner, D. G., and Lieskovsky, G. (Eds.): Diagnosis and Management of Genitourinary Cancer. Philadelphia, W. B. Saunders, 1987.

initiation of any therapeutic modality. This allows the surgeon to carefully select and plan appropriate treatment for a variety of disease processes. An awareness of the anatomy and physiology of the bladder is essential before undertaking any operative procedure, because the objectives of surgery should be resolution of the disease processes and restoration of normal storage and voiding function. The bladder in the adult lies in the true pelvis below the peritoneal cavity. It functions as a urinary reservoir and is under volitional control. The area surrounding the bladder contains loose areolar tissue, fat, and a plexus of veins that drain the pelvis, bladder, and anterior perineum. The bladder is covered superiorly by a reflection of the peritoneum. The arterial supply of the bladder is from the internal iliac artery, with three arterial branches called the superior, middle, and inferior vesical arteries. In the female, the uterine and vaginal vessels may have contralateral branches, which anastomose with the vesical blood supply. The arterial blood supply is not constant, and there are many variations. The veins of the bladder do not travel with the arteries. They tend to be short and unite to form the plexus of Santorini anteriorly and the pudendal plexus inferiorly. These two venous systems, which have numerous interconnections, communicate with the veins of the perineum and the dorsal vein of the penis or clitoris. The bladder receives innervation from both sympathetic and parasympathetic autonomic nerves. The sympathetic preganglionic nuclei are in the first and second lumbar segments and possibly the twelfth thoracic spinal cord segment. This sympathetic outflow proceeds through either the inferior mesenteric ganglia or the inferior hypogastric plexus. If the outflow is through the inferior mesenteric ganglia, fibers proceed down the aorta to the iliac vasculature and then follow the ureters before fanning out to enter the bladder. When the outflow is through the inferior hypogastric plexus, the fibers leave the ganglia in the lower pelvis and immediately fan out to enter the bladder. Although the course of the preganglionic sympathetic fibers is variable, the postganglionic fibers enter the bladder posterolaterally with the arteries and branch out to include the entire bladder. Parasympathetic preganglionic cell nuclei are in the second, third, and fourth sacral segments of the spinal cord and travel with the nervi erigentes or pelvic splanchnic nerves to enter the bladder in the same manner as the sympathetic fibers. Postganglionic cells arise in the wall of the urinary bladder proper. Afferent sensory fibers from the bladder can exit along either sympathetic or parasympathetic pathways.

The primary function of the bladder is to store urine until

TABLE 45–14. The International Continence Society Classification

Storage Phase	Voiding Phase
Bladder Function	**Bladder Function**
Detrusor activity	Detrusor activity
Normal	Normal
Overactive	Underactive
Unstable	Acontractile
Hyperreflexic	**Urethral Function**
Bladder sensation	Normal
Normal	Obstructive
Increased or hypersensitive	Overactive
Reduced or hyposensitive	Faulty mechanics
Absent	
Bladder capacity	
Normal	
High	
Low	
Compliance	
Normal	
High	
Low	
Urethral Function	
Normal	
Incompetent	

Adapted from Abrams, P., Blaivas, J., Stanton, S., and Andersen, J.: Standardization of terminology of lower urinary tract function. Neurourol. Urodynam., 7:403, 1988.

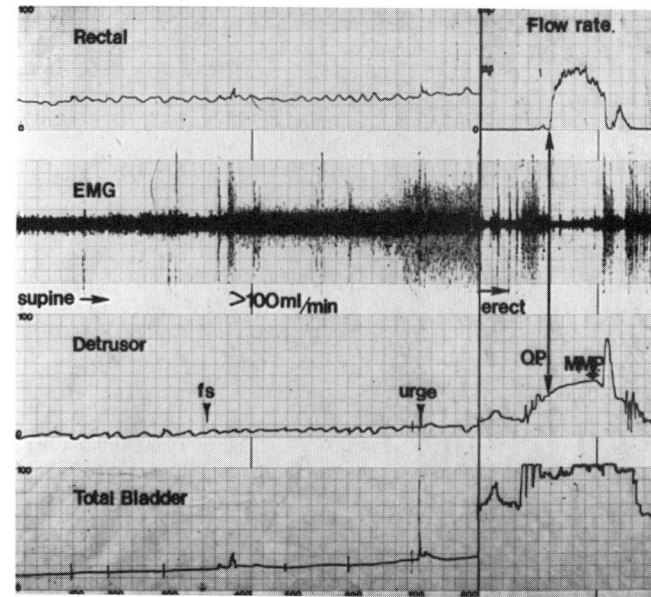

Figure 45–24. A composite urodynamic study showing rectal detrusor and total bladder pressures, plus the sphincter electromyogram. Note in the right hand panel that as urinary flow begins (marked by the upper arrow), the sphincter becomes electrically silent and detrusor pressure increases. (Courtesy of George D. Webster, M.D., Division of Urology, Duke University Medical Center, Durham, NC.)

volitional voiding is prompted. In its simplest terms, bladder dysfunction can be segregated into disorders of storage and disorders of emptying. The disease processes producing these disorders can be identified by a combination of contrast studies and urodynamic evaluation. Urodynamic evaluation is a physiologic study that determines the neuromuscular response of the bladder to filling and emptying (Tables 45–14 and 45–15). The urodynamic evaluation of the bladder consists of (1) a cystometrogram with a coordinated electromyographic evaluation of the urinary sphincter, (2) a urethral pressure profile, and (3) the urinary flow rate (Fig. 45–24).

TABLE 45–15. The Expanded Functional Classification

Failure to Store	Failure to Empty
Because of the Bladder	**Because of the Bladder**
Detrusor hyperactivity	Neurologic
Involuntary contractions	Myogenic
Suprasacral neurologic disease	Psychogenic
Bladder outlet obstruction	Idiopathic
Idiopathic	**Because of the Outlet**
Decreased compliance	Anatomic
Fibrosis	Prostatic obstruction
Idiopathic	Bladder neck contracture
Sensory urgency	Urethral stricture
Inflammatory	Functional
Infectious	Smooth sphincter
Neurologic	dyssynergia
Psychologic	Striated sphincter
Idiopathic	dyssynergia
Because of the Outlet	
Stress incontinence	
Nonfunctional bladder neck/proximal urethra	

From Walsh, P. C., Retik, A. B., Stamey, T. A., and Vaughan, E. D. (Eds.): Campbell's Urology, 6th ed. Philadelphia, W. B. Saunders, 1992, p. 600.

The cystometrogram is performed to determine bladder capacity, the presence of voluntary or involuntary contractions of the detrusor, and the compliance of the bladder (the ability of the detrusor muscle to stretch with filling) and to evaluate the integrity of the afferent (sensory) limbs of the detrusor reflex arc. The normal bladder will fill to a volume of 400 ml. with no increase in pressure, no uninhibited contractions, and normal bladder wall compliance. At this volume the patient states that the bladder feels full and, when asked to void, there will be a spiking increase in intravesical pressure and a coincidental relaxation of the sphincter mechanism. When rising intravesical pressure overcomes falling urethral resistance, voiding begins and the bladder empties. By measuring the electrical activity of the distal sphincter mechanisms during bladder filling and voiding, vesicosphincter dyssynergia (failure of sphincter reaction during detrusor contraction) may be identified. If uninhibited contractions of the detrusor muscle occur during periods of electrical sphincter silence, the patient will leak urine involuntarily. The urethral pressure profile is used to determine functional length, resting pressure, and maximal pressure (in response to stress) of the sphincteric mechanism. A normal urethral pressure profile shows an increase in pressure at the bladder neck, which normally corresponds to pressure exerted by the proximal urethral sphincter. Maximal pressure is recorded at the level of the distal urethral sphincter and is 70 to 90 cm. H_2O. The functional urethral length is the distance from the rise in pressure at the bladder neck to the point in the distal urethra where intraurethral pressure falls below intravesical pressure. In normal males without benign prostatic hypertrophy, this length is 2.5 to 4 cm. Urinary flow rates are physiologic, noninvasive, and informative. The volume of urine voided, voiding time, peak flow rate, and average flow rate usually are the determined parameters. A peak flow rate greater than 25 ml. per second is consistent with an unobstructed flow, provided the patient voids in less than 15 seconds. Peak flow rates below 10 ml. per second are consistent with obstruction, either functional or secondary to benign prostatic hypertrophy, or to stricture of the outflow passage. Although no blanket recommendation can be made as to the appropriate management of the various disorders of storage and emptying, when no specific anatomic defect that requires surgical correction can be identified, it may be possible to enhance emptying or facilitate storage by pharmaceutical manipulation (Table 45–16).

Bladder Fistulas[4]

Disorders of storage are occasioned by fistulas between the bladder and either the small or large bowel (enteric fistulas), the vagina, the uterus, or the skin. Vesical fistulas are usually of inflammatory, neoplastic, iatrogenic, or traumatic origin or secondary to radiation.

Vesicoenteric Fistulas

Fifty per cent of all vesicoenteric fistulas are secondary to sigmoid diverticulitis. Colorectal malignancy accounts for 16% to 20% of all enteric fistula, with 12% to 15% of fistula associated with Crohn's disease. Primary bladder malignancy is the cause of about 5% of all vesicoenteric fistula. Pneumaturia is not pathognomonic of an enteric fistula, because gas per urethra may result from fermentation of diabetic urine, from urinary tract infection by gas-producing organisms, or from urinary tract instrumentation. However, pneumaturia is the presenting symptom in two thirds of patients who present with a vesicoenteric fistula. Fecaluria is diagnostic of a vesicoenteric fistula; however, it occurs in only 20% to 50% of all patients. The differential diagnosis of vesicoenteric fistula should include recurrent urinary tract infections and interstitial cystitis. The diagnosis is usually established by cystoscopic examination of the bladder. However, contrast studies (intravenous pyelography, upper gastrointestinal study, or barium enema) may be necessary to identify the fistula. When a fistula is suspected but cannot be confirmed, the urine should be examined for barium after barium contrast studies of the bowel or for the appearance of charcoal granules in the urinary sediment after oral administration of charcoal.

Surgical repair may require resection of the offending bowel segment and bladder *en bloc* with primary restitution of the bowel and primary closure of the bladder. When possible, omentum should be interposed over the surface of the bladder closure to ensure against recurrence of the fistula and a breakdown of the closure.

Vesicovaginal Fistulas

Vesicovaginal fistulas are commonly seen as a complication of unattended childbirth. Today, in most of the civilized world, approximately 90% of vesicovaginal fistulas are secondary to gynecologic procedures. The remaining patients develop these fistulas as a consequence of urologic surgery, extensive pelvic trauma, or complications of internal or external radiation therapy for pelvic malignancies or by direct extension of a malignant process (most commonly squamous cell carcinoma of the cervix). The signs and symptoms of a vesicovaginal fistula depend on its size and location. Patients with small fistulas may have the intermittent appearance of a watery vaginal discharge and appear to void normally, while patients with large fistulas will have total urinary leakage through the vagina with no urethral voiding. Small fistulas located high in the vaginal vault may leak only when the bladder is full, whereas those located farther distal in the bladder base may leak constantly. Most patients complain of a malodorous watery vaginal discharge. When the fistula is secondary to recent vaginal or pelvic surgery, it usually becomes evident between 5 and 14 days postoperatively.

Identification of a vesicovaginal fistula may be difficult. Urinary leakage through the vagina may come from the ureter(s), bladder, or any of these three structures. Diagnostic evaluation should include an intravenous urogram with special attention to the lower ureters. The vagina should be viewed on lateral films for the appearance of intravaginal contrast medium. Cystography usually adds little to the diagnosis. A clean vaginal tampon should be placed in the vagina and methylene blue instilled in the bladder. The patient is then asked to retain the methylene blue within the bladder and be ambulatory for several hours. She then returns, a catheter is passed, and the bladder is drained. The tampon is removed. The presence of methylene blue on the upper end of the tampon confirms the working diagnosis of a vesicovaginal fistula. If the test is negative, the sequence of events is repeated after intravenous injection of indigo carmine. If staining of the tampon occurs after a negative intravesical methylene blue test, a ureterovaginal fistula is suggested.

TABLE 45–16. Therapy to Facilitate Bladder Filling and Urine Storage

Inhibiting Bladder Contractility/Decreasing Sensory Input/ Increasing Bladder Capacity

1. Timed bladder emptying
2. Pharmacologic therapy
   a. Anticholinergic agents
   b. Musculotropic relaxants
   c. Calcium antagonists
   d. Potassium channel openers
   e. Prostaglandin inhibitors
   f. Beta-adrenergic agonists
   g. Tricyclic antidepressants
   h. Dimethyl sulfoxide (DMSO)
3. Biofeedback, bladder retraining
4. Bladder overdistention
5. Electrical stimulation (reflex inhibition)
6. Acupuncture
7. Interruption of innervation
   a. Central (subarachnoid block)
   b. Peripheral (sacral rhizotomy, selective sacral rhizotomy)
   c. Dorsal
   d. Perivesical (peripheral bladder denervation)
8. Augmentation cystoplasty

Increasing Outlet Resistance

1. Physiotherapy, biofeedback
2. Electrical stimulation of pelvic floor
3. Pharmacologic therapy
   a. Alpha-adrenergic agonists
   b. Tricyclic antidepressants
   c. Beta-adrenergic antagonists
   d. Estrogens
4. Vesicourethral suspension
5. Bladder outlet reconstruction
6. Surgical mechanical compression
   a. Sling procedures
   b. Artificial urinary sphincter
7. Nonsurgical mechanical compression
   a. Periurethral polytef injection
   b. Periurethral collagen injection
   c. Occlusive devices

Circumventing the Problem

1. Antidiuretic hormone–like agents
2. Intermittent catheterization
3. Continuous catheterization
4. Urinary diversion
5. External collecting devices
6. Absorbent products

From Walsh, P. C., Retik, A. B., Stamey, T. A., and Vaughan, E. D. (Eds.): Campbell's Urology, 6th ed. Philadelphia, W. B. Saunders, 1992, p. 613.

Small vesicovaginal fistulas, which occur after either vaginal or pelvic surgery, may close spontaneously if the bladder urine is diverted by use of a Foley catheter. Larger fistulas may require surgical intervention for closure. Although it has been recommended that repair be delayed 4 to 6 months after the appearance of the fistula to allow tissues to soften and mature, become less inflamed, and thus enhance the possibility of repair, recent studies have demonstrated that immediate surgical closure of uncomplicated vesicovaginal fistula that occurs after hysterectomy or related procedures in otherwise healthy women may be accomplished with a high degree of success and thus spare the patient the prolonged morbidity and mental anguish of vaginal leakage. Vesicovaginal fistulas may be closed either perineally through a transvaginal route or suprapubically through a transvesical route (Figs. 45–25 and 45–26). The principles of surgical closure are similar: (1) total separation of the tissues of the wall of the vagina and the wall of the bladder; (2) sharp excision of the fistulous tract between the two structures; (3) closure of the defect in the vagina and the bladder with absorbable suture material with nonopposed, nonoverlapping suture line; and (4) where possible, interposition of alternative tissue (a myocutaneous gracilis flap or omentum) between the two suture lines.

Disorders of Storage[4, 11]

Disorders of storage may occur when an inadequate bladder volume exists and may require bladder augmentation to increase bladder volume. Currently, intestinal segments, of either ileum, cecum, or sigmoid colon, are used to increase bladder capacity (Fig. 45–27). Use of these bowel segments to augment bladder capacity and facilitate storage is contraindicated only in patients who have bladder outlet obstruction, an antecedent history of vesical malignancy, or border-

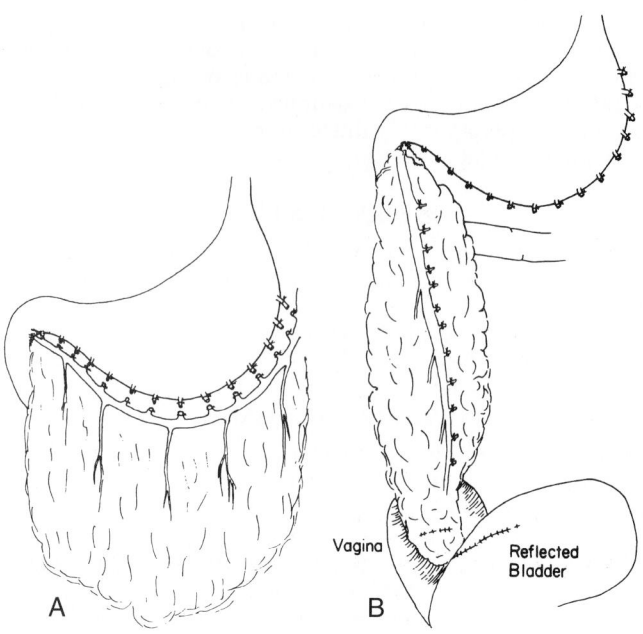

Figure 45–26. Omentopexy is useful in buttressing vesicovaginal fistula repairs. *A,* The omentum is detached from the transverse colon and subsequently from the greater curvature of the stomach by dividing the short gastric vessels. The omental pedicle can be mobilized from either the right or left. The greatest mobility is achieved when basing the omental blood supply on the right gastroepiploic artery as shown. *B,* The long omental pedicle brought down to interpose healthy, well-vascularized tissue between the vaginal and bladder closures (situated at right angles to one another). (From Paulson, D. F.: Genitourinary Surgery. New York, Churchill Livingstone, 1983, p. 235.)

line renal function with creatinine clearance of less than 40 to 50 ml. per minute.

A second disorder of storage is urinary incontinence secondary to damage of the sphincteric mechanisms, which provide the resistance to bladder emptying. Total incontinence is the continuous leakage of urine, with the bladder

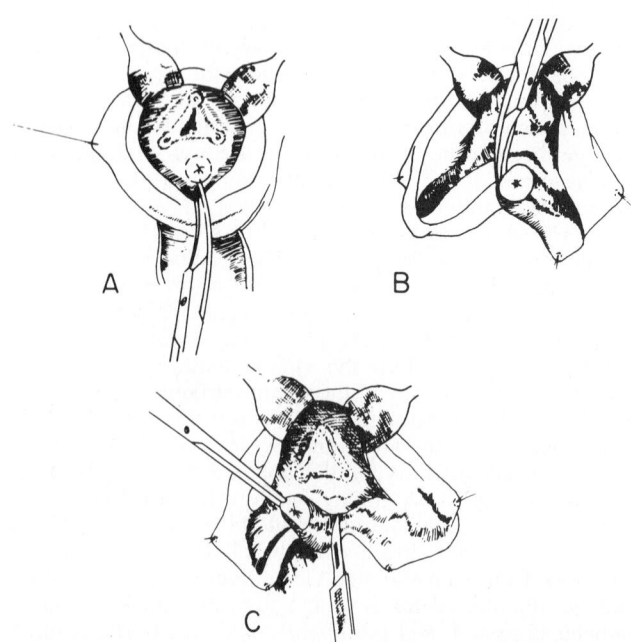

Figure 45–25. Extension of an anterior cystostomy in a racquet fashion to include excision of the posterior wall vesicovaginal fistula. *A,* Shows the continuation of the anterior cystotomy incision over the dome of the bladder. *B,* The incision is extended so as to circumcise the vesicovaginal fistula. *C,* The vaginal extent of the fistula is about to be excised. After completion of this racquet excision of fistula, the vagina and bladder are closed at right angles to one another. (From Paulson, D. F.: Genitourinary Surgery. New York, Churchill Livingstone, 1983, p. 233.)

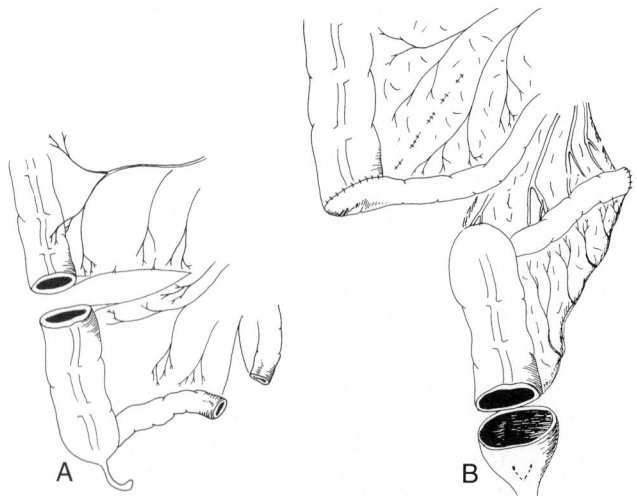

Figure 45–27. Ileocecal cystoplasty. *A,* The ascending colon is divided at a point just below the right colic artery. If it is intended to employ the distal ileum for ureteral anastomosis, an appropriate length of ileum is selected and its mesentery divided, taking care to ensure a good blood supply to the isolated ileocecal segment from the ileocolic artery. *B,* The isolated segment is rotated 180 degrees on its vascular pedicle, bringing the open end of ascending colon in apposition with the bladder remnant. Care should be taken that this rotation does not interfere with good vascular flow to and from the rotated segment. (From Paulson, D. F.: Genitourinary Surgery. New York, Churchill Livingstone, 1983, p. 252.)

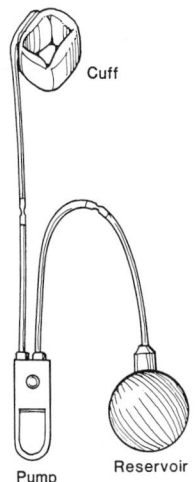
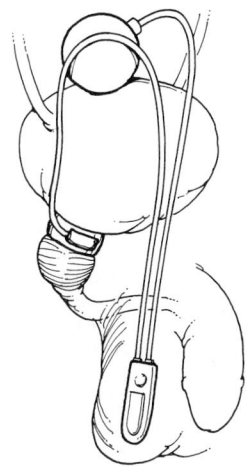
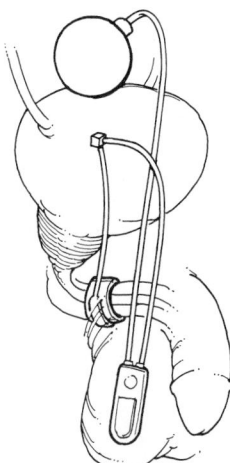

Figure 45–28. The implantable artificial urinary sphincter prosthesis is a three-component device (left to right): a pressure-regulating reservoir balloon, a control assembly deflation pump with a deactivation button, and an inflatable occlusive cuff. Each squeeze of the deflation pump transfers a bolus of fluid from the cuff to the reservoir balloon where the fluid is sequestered. (From Walsh, P. C., Retik, A. B., Stamey, T. A., and Vaughan, E. D., Jr. [Eds.]: Campbell's Urology, 6th ed. Philadelphia, W. B. Saunders, 1992.)

functioning only as a urinary conduit. In total incontinence, there must be incompetence of both the proximal and distal urethral sphincter mechanisms. This may be either neurologic or iatrogenic. Stress urinary incontinence refers to the intermittent leakage of urine associated with sudden increases in intra-abdominal pressure.

Incontinence occurs when there has been a disruption of the sphincter mechanism. In males this is most usually postsurgical, although it can be posttraumatic. In females, loss of closing urethral pressure occurs with loss of pelvic floor support and shortening of total urethral length. In males, the internal or proximal urethral sphincter routinely is destroyed by prostatectomy. The distal urethral mechanism, consisting of smooth muscle and fibroelastic tissue representing the intrinsic portion of the distal urethra as well as the surrounding skeletal muscle of the pelvic floor, is routinely undamaged during either transurethral or open prostatectomy. However, when the anatomy is such that the surgical procedure carries through both sphincter mechanisms or when a previous disease process, trauma, or surgical intervention has destroyed either the internal or the distal urethral sphincter, then either transurethral resection or open prostatectomy has a high likelihood of leaving the patient without urinary control in the postoperative period. When urodynamic studies demonstrate that anatomic incontinence is present in the male, then it may be necessary to intervene surgically to increase urethral closing pressure.

A single operative procedure is in vogue to increase intrinsic urethral closing pressures. This procedure uses a volitionally controlled occlusive device to provide increase in outflow obstruction to a point whereby this obstruction is greater than the voiding pressure created by the bladder. This device or the artificial inflatable sphincter functions in a more physiologic way, and the total closing pressure can be regulated so that regional tissue ischemia does not occur (Fig. 45–28).

The techniques that have been devised for control of urinary incontinence in the female in the presence of a supple, compliant, and nonhostile reservoir consist primarily of urethral lengthening procedures. These may be done transvaginally or suprapubically. The surgical principle to be followed in each of these procedures is to increase urethral length and thus enhance urethral closing pressure (Fig. 45–29).

Vesical Trauma[4]

Trauma to the bladder can be divided into trauma with and without pelvic fracture; penetrating injuries, either high or low velocity; and iatrogenic trauma. Each requires identification and repair. Blunt trauma without pelvic fracture damages the bladder only if the bladder is full. Rupture of the bladder with or without pelvic fracture may be extraperitoneal or intraperitoneal (Fig. 45–30). The patient who has lower abdominal trauma with or without bony fracture or who has penetrating trauma to the lower abdomen should have cystography to determine the nature and extent of the bladder rupture, followed by surgical exploration, identification of the traumatized site, sharp excision of the devitalized tissue, and primary repair using a two- or three-layer closure.

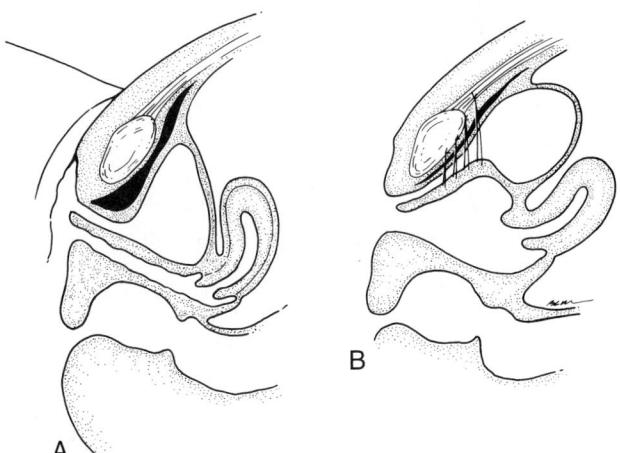

Figure 45–29. *A*, Preoperative cross section of the pelvis in stress incontinence. *B*, Correction of the anatomic defect by the Marshall-Marchetti procedure. (From Webster, G. D.: Female urinary incontinence. *In* Glenn, J. F. [Ed.]: Urologic Surgery, 3rd ed. Philadelphia, J. B. Lippincott, 1983, p. 673.)

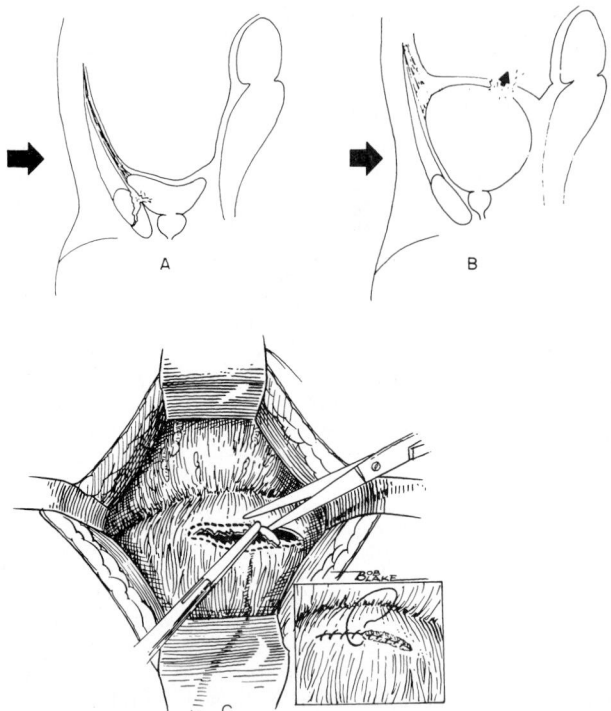

Figure 45–30. Types of bladder wall disruption associated with blunt lower abdominal trauma. *A,* When blunt injury results in pelvic fracture, associated bladder perforation is usually extraperitoneal and caused by mechanical perforation of the bladder by a bony spicule. *B,* If the bladder is full, the sudden increase in intravesical pressure may result in a disruption of bladder wall integrity at the dome, resulting in intraperitoneal extravasation. *C,* Limited débridement of edges of bladder rupture. (From Paulson, D. F.: Genitourinary Surgery. New York, Churchill Livingstone, 1983, p. 222.)

It is not necessary to drain the bladder with a suprapubic tube unless there has been severe bladder trauma and the likelihood of primary healing is diminished.

Carcinoma of the Bladder[15]

Ninety per cent of bladder malignancies are transitional cell tumors, reflecting their origin from the transitional cells that line the bladder. Squamous cell carcinoma accounts for 6% to 8% of bladder tumors, with only 2% being adenocarcinomas. Tumors are graded on a scale of 1 to 4, dependent on the degree of cellular atypia and nuclear abnormalities in association with the number of mitotic figures. The anatomic distribution of disease may be identified by one of several staging systems (Table 45–17).

Clinical Presentation and Diagnosis

Hematuria occurs in 75% of all patients with carcinoma of the bladder. Approximately 30% of patients may have an associated urinary tract infection, and the presenting symptom-complex is frequently dismissed as hemorrhagic cystitis. Bladder irritability alone is a presenting symptom in 30% of patients and is believed to be associated with muscle invasion. A presumptive diagnosis of transitional cell carcinoma of the bladder may be supported by urinary cytologic studies but is confirmed by cystoscopic examination and transurethral biopsy of the suspected area.

Treatment Considerations

Management of transitional cell carcinoma is directed to removal of the offending malignancy, with treatment based

TABLE 45–17. Staging Systems for Bladder Cancer

Finding	Jewett-Strong-Marshall Stage	1987 UICC Stage
No tumor in the specimen	0	T_0
Carcinoma *in situ*	0	T_{is}
Noninvasive papillary tumor	0	T_a
Submucosal invasion	A	T_1
Superficial muscle invasion	B_1	T_2
Deep muscle invasion	B_2	T_{3A}
Invasion of perivesical fat	C	T_{3B}
Invasion of contiguous organ	D_1	T_4
Regional lymph node metastases	D_1	(N_{1-3})
Juxtaregional lymph node metastases	D_2	—
Distant metastases	D_2	M_1

From Walsh, P. C., Retik, A. B., Stamey, T. A., and Vaughan, E. D. (Eds.): Campbell's Urology, 6th ed. Philadelphia, W. B. Saunders, 1992, p. 1119.

on the anatomic distribution of disease. Tumors that have not invaded the muscle (stage T_a, T_1 tumors) may be controlled by either transurethral resection or fulguration or by intravesical drugs that promote removal of the malignancy (Tables 45–18 to 45–20).[29] Whether the drugs placed within the bladder produce their effect by interdicting cell metabolism or whether these agents produce their effect through intravesical cauterization, which promotes sloughing of the offending malignant mucosa, is unknown. Nonetheless, these intravesical agents rid the patient of tumor with varying effectiveness. It should be recognized that, irrespective of treatment, patients with tumors that do not penetrate through the lamina propria have less than a 7% chance of ever dying of their malignancy. Once the tumor penetrates through the lamina propria (Stage A), the patient has a 30% chance of succumbing to the malignancy. The chance of death from the submucosally invasive tumor is a function of the pathologic grade of the malignancy, which seemingly reflects the biologic aggressiveness of the disease.

Controversy remains as to whether intravesical chemotherapy is appropriate for disease that penetrates through the lamina propria or whether these patients should be treated more aggressively, either with wide local transurethral resection, with aggressive partial cystectomy, or with total cystectomy and urinary diversion. Disease that penetrates into the muscle of the bladder is best managed by either partial or total removal of the bladder. The role of partial removal of the bladder (segmental cystectomy) in the management of this disease is controversial. Segmental cystectomy has fallen into disfavor because of high intravesical recurrence rates in the residual bladder. This probably reflects the biologic nature of the disease rather than the surgical procedure itself. In properly selected patients, patients who have no evidence of atypia or carcinoma *in situ* at other sites within the bladder

TABLE 45–18. Complete Response Rates of Intravesical Therapy

Agent	Number	T_a, T_1*	C_{is}*
Thiotepa	231/89	88 (38%)	34 (38%)
Doxorubicin	712/212	273 (38%)	101 (48%)
Mitomycin	627/147	270 (43%)	78 (53%)
Interferon alfa	16/62	4 (25%)	29 (47%)
Bacille Calmette-Guérin	188/718	115 (61%)	500 (70%)

*No. (%) of cases.
From Lamm, D. L.: Long-term results of intravesical therapy for superficial bladder cancer. Urol. Clin. North Am., *19*(3):573, 1992.

TABLE 45–19. Tumor Recurrence and Progression in Controlled Studies

Agent	Number (Patients/Series/Sig Results)	Recurrence			Progression		
		Control	*Treated*	*Benefit*	*C*	*Rx*	*Dif*
Thiotepa	1007/10/6	56%	44%	12%	6%	4%	NS
Doxorubicin	1241/5/3	47%	34%	13%	8%	9%	NS
Mitomycin	1157/6/2	50%	35%	15%	7%	4%	NS
Bacille Calmette-Guérin	496/5/4	72%	32%	40%	23%	13%	.03

Data from Lamm, D. L.: Long-term results of intravesical therapy for superficial bladder cancer. Urol. Clin. North Am., *19*:573, 1992.

either adjacent to or distant to the offending invasive malignancy may be appropriate candidates for partial cystectomy. However, the selection of patients for partial cystectomy is complicated by the tendency of the entire urothelial surface of the bladder to show premalignant change even in the presence of an isolated tumor.

Radical cystectomy is advised for patients whose tumors demonstrate muscle invasion and in the current thinking may very well be advised for patients who have high-grade disease that penetrates the lamina propria. Radical cystectomy in the male includes the bladder, prostate, seminal vesicles, and the immediate adjacent perivesical tissues; in women, radical cystectomy includes the bladder, uterus, tubes, ovaries, anterior vagina, and urethra. Pelvic lymphadenectomy is advocated by some; however, the poor survival identified when pelvic node mestastases exist makes the potential benefit of this additional procedure questionable. The value of preoperative radiation therapy before cystectomy is no longer under debate. However, this debate has been replaced by a debate over preoperative chemotherapy, currently called neoadjuvant chemotherapy. The purpose of preoperative chemotherapy is to reduce the volume of disease within the bladder and also to control any metastatic sites. However, no data exist to support the rationale for preoperative chemotherapy, and the current practice is to ablate the primary tumor by surgical removal of the bladder and associated structures and to treat metastatic disease secondarily with multiagent cisplatin-based chemotherapy when such disease appears.

Results of Treatment[15]

The survival rates appear dependent more on the grade, stage, and cell type of the tumor rather than maneuvers that occur at the time of removal (Fig. 45–31).

For radical cystectomy, the best approach is through a lower abdominal midline incision. After bladder removal, radical cystectomy of urinary diversion must be accomplished. The necessity for an effective and satisfactory bladder substitute has led to the development of multiple procedures to produce adequate drainage of urine. Initial attempts involved anastomosing the ureters to the sigmoid colon to rely on the intact anal sphincter to control both urinary and fecal streams. Ureterosigmoidostomy was popular until the early 1950s. However, the reflux of high-pressure colonic contents up the low-pressure ureter produced frequent upper urinary tract infections with coliform bacteria. Subsequent technologic improvements led to the development of an antirefluxing anastomosis between the ureter and the colon, which obviated the problem of reflux of colonic contents into the upper urinary tract. Nonetheless, even with the utilization of the antireflux anastomosis, the ureterosigmoidostomy has continued to be plagued with the electrolyte abnormalities of the hypercaloremic acidosis occasioned by the absorptive characteristics of the colon and the increased incidence of colonic malignancy in patients in whom there is a progressive series of technologic maneuvers for urinary diversion. In conduit diversion, a segment of either large or small bowel is selected and is used merely as a conduit to establish rapid transit of urine to the body surface where the urine is collected in a plastic collecting bag. This method adheres to the principle of separation of urine and fecal streams. The conduit diversion uses distal ileum, but a large bowel segment can also be utilized. The primary consideration in creation of a large or small bowel conduit is that the bowel tube be created sufficiently short to function merely as a conduit and not as a reservoir. The continent reservoir uses either large or small bowel and provides an internal storage device that is drained by intermittent catheterization of an external stoma

TABLE 45–20. Recurrence in Controlled Comparison Trials

Study	Bacille Calmette-Guérin	Thiotepa	Doxorubicin	Mitomycin C	p Level
Brosman	0	47%			<.01
Netto	7%	43%			<.01
Martinez	13%	36%	43%		<.01
Thiotepa avg.	7%	42%			
SWOG '91	63%		83%		<.02
Doxorubicin avg.	38%		63%		
Debruyne	30%			25%	NS
Finnblad	28%			62%	<.01
Rubben	35%			35%	NS
Witjes	29% (RIVM)			26%	NS
	34% (Tice)				NS
SWOG '93	20%			33%	<.01
Mitomycin avg.	29%			36%	
Bacille Calmette-Guérin avg.	25%				
Chemo. avg.	43%				

NS, not significant; SWOG, Southwest Oncology Group.
Data from Lamm, D. L.: Long-term results of intravesical therapy for superficial bladder cancer. Urol. Clin. North Am., *19*:573, 1992.

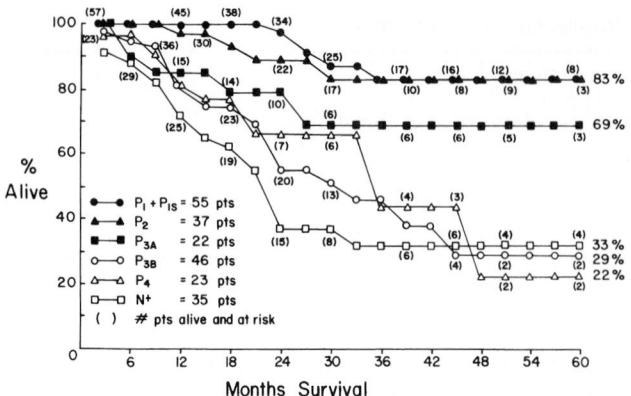

Figure 45–31. Actuarial survival (Kaplan-Meier) of 189 patients undergoing bilateral iliac pelvic lymph node dissection and *en bloc* radical cystectomy without preoperative radiation therapy. (From Skinner, D. G., and Lieskovsky, G.: Management of invasive and high-grade bladder cancer. *In* Diagnosis and Management of Genitourinary Cancer. Philadelphia, W. B. Saunders, 1988.)

created at the skin surface. The continent diversion attempts to create this internal reservoir using a nonrefluxing cutaneous stoma catheterized at intermittent intervals by the patient (Fig. 45–32).

An alternative to the continent diversion is orthotopic bladder replacement, in which an internal reservoir is created utilizing either large or small bowel and anastomosed to the native urethra at the level of the perineal diaphragm (Fig. 45–33). Such a maneuver allows the patient to void volitionally through the normal urinary tract. Modification of the cystectomy to preserve the nerves that innervate blood supply to the corpora cavernosum also permits these patients to be sexually active after removal of the bladder and prostate.

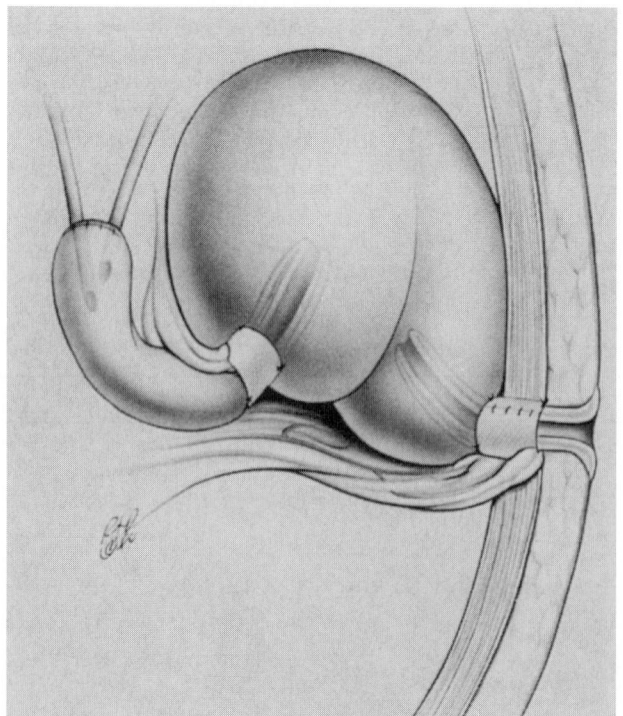

Figure 45–32. Diagram of completed Kock pouch with its proximal nipple valve draining the proximal terminus into which the ureters have been sutured. Distal terminus is brought flush to skin of abdominal wall. (From Olsson, C. A.: Kock continent ileal reservoir for urinary diversion. *In* King, L. R., Stone, A. R., and Webster, G. D. [Eds.]: Bladder Reconstruction and Continent Urinary Diversion. Chicago, Year Book Medical Publishers, 1987; with permission of C. V. Mosby.)

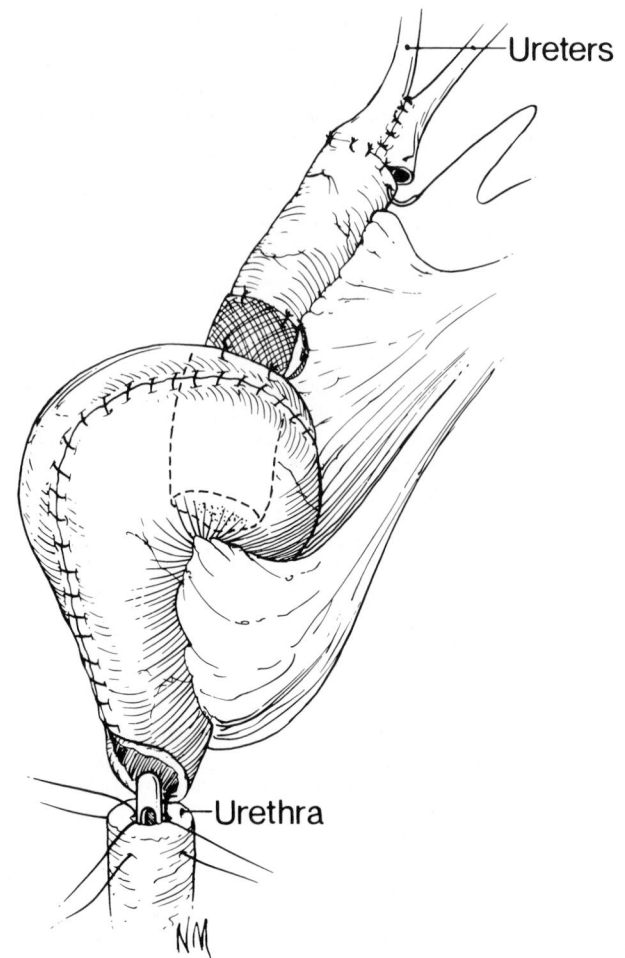

Figure 45–33. The open lower end of the pouch is approximated to the pelvic floor so that the length of the afferent ileal limb necessary for ureteroileal anastomosis without tension can be ascertained and any redundant ileal limb excised. A Wallace-type spatulated, stented, end-to-end ureteroileal anastomosis is performed. The urethral anastomosis is now performed between the membranous urethra and the residual opening at the inferior aspect of the pouch using interrupted sutures. A 20- to 24-French Foley catheter inserted per urethra across the anastomosis completes pouch construction. (From Webster, G. D., and Kreder, K. J.: Orthotopic bladder replacement in men. *In* Fowler, J. E. [Ed.]: Mastery of Surgery: Urology. Boston, Little, Brown & Co., 1992, p. 358.)

With this form of diversion, the long-term consequences of persistent infection of urine retained within this internal pouch and the probability of recurrent stone formation within this pouch are not yet established. However, the internal reservoirs that provide volitional control of the urinary stream are much desired by many patients.

The need to remove the urethra in males who undergo radical cystectomy continues to be debated. Approximately 7% of all males who undergo radical cystectomy eventually will develop a malignancy in the residual urethra. However, this figure may triple when diffuse carcinoma *in situ* exists within the bladder or prostatic urethra or when the primary tumor is at the level of the bladder neck. It is therefore recommended that patients with this form of malignancy undergo a simultaneous in continuity urethrectomy. Patients whose urethras are not removed should have follow-up urethral cytologic studies obtained either by urethral lavage or by direct swabbing of the retained urethra.

SELECTED REFERENCES

Gillenwater, J., Grayhack, J., Howards, S., and Duckett, J.: Adult and Pediatric Urology. St. Louis, Mosby–Year Book, 1995.

This comprehensive textbook provides in-depth discussion of the physiology and pathophysiology of the urinary tract along with detailed description of management of urologic disorders. It is well organized and is a comprehensive text that many find more readable than Campbell's Urology.

Glenn, J. F., and Graham, S. D.: Urologic Surgery, 4th ed. Philadelphia, J. B. Lippincott, 1990.
This text is a fine atlas of urologic surgery with 100 chapters by 100 different contributors. Advances in the surgical techniques necessary for the surgical management of urologic disease are detailed. Ample and detailed descriptions are provided of the surgical procedures. This text is strongly recommended for the individual who wishes to know in detail the methodology for the surgical management of urologic disease.

Paulson, D. F. (Ed.): Genitourinary Surgery. New York, Churchill Livingstone, 1983.
The goal of the editor was to identify contributors with recognized expertise in a single organ system and to have them present their philosophy of management of anatomic disease. The text is structured to present the normal anatomy and physiology of the kidney, ureter, and bladder and to identify abnormalities in development and other pathophysiologic processes that involve these organ sites. Special care has been taken by the contributors to provide a series of illustrations that describe step-by-step the technique of surgical control.

Skinner, D. G., and Lieskovsky, G. (Eds.): Diagnosis and Management of Genitourinary Cancer. Philadelphia, W. B. Saunders, 1987.
This is a comprehensive text that gives the clinician an in-depth reference to all aspects of genitourinary cancer. Sections on basic science, epidemiology, pathology, diagnosis, and management, as well as descriptive chapters on surgical techniques, present an overview of current concepts for urologists, oncologists, internists, pathologists, and radiologists. The contributors are acknowledged leaders in the field of genitourinary cancer, elaborating on topics in which they have considerable personal experience.

Walsh, P. C., Retik, A. B., Stamey, T. A., and Vaughan, E. D. (Eds.): Campbell's Urology, 7th ed. Philadelphia, W. B. Saunders, 1995.
This three-volume text has been the standard reference text in urologic surgery. Its contributors are recognized authors from various disciplines. Normal and abnormal anatomy and physiology are covered in detail, and each chapter is well referenced to assist the interested student in expanding his or her fund of knowledge.

REFERENCES

1. Andriole, V. T.: Renal and perirenal abscesses. *In* Schrier, R. W., and Gottschalk, G. (Eds.): Diseases of the Kidney, 4th ed. Boston, Little, Brown & Co., 1988, p 959.
2. Barrett, D. M., and Wein, A. J.: Voiding dysfunction: Diagnosis, classification, and management. *In* Gillenwater, J., Grayhack, J., Howards, S., and Duckett, J. (Eds.): Adult and Pediatric Urology. St. Louis, Mosby–Year Book, 1991, p 1001.
3. Batata, M. A., Whitmore, W. F., Jr., Hilaris, B. S., et al.: Primary carcinoma of the ureter: A prognostic study. Cancer, *35*:1626, 1975.
4. Benson, M., and Olsson, C. A.: The bladder. *In* Paulson, D. F. (Ed.): Genitourinary Surgery. New York, Churchill Livingstone, 1983, p 209.
5. Bloom, N. A., Vidone, R. A., and Lytton, B.: Primary carcinoma of the ureter: A report of 102 new cases. J. Urol., *103*:590, 1970.
6. Charlton, C. A. C.: Gram-negative septicaemia. *In* Chisholm, G. D., and Williams, D. I. (Eds.): Scientific Foundations, Urology, 2nd ed. London, William Heinemann Medical Books, 1982, p 212.
7. Drutz, D. J.: Fungal infections of the kidney and urinary tract. *In* Schrier, R. W., and Gottschalk, G. (Eds.): Diseases of the Kidney, 4th ed. Boston, Little, Brown & Co., 1988, p 929.
8. Garnick, M. B., and Richie, J. P.: Primary neoplasms of the kidney and renal pelvis. *In* Schrier, R. W., and Gottschalk, G. (Eds.): Diseases of the Kidney, 4th ed. Boston, Little, Brown & Co., 1988, p 785.
9. Gilbert, B. R., Leslie, B. R., and Vaughan, E. D., Jr.: Normal renal physiology. *In* Walsh, P. C., Retik, A. B., Stamey, T. A., and Vaughan, E. D. (Eds.): Campbell's Urology, 6th ed. Philadelphia, W. B. Saunders, 1992, p 70.
10. Hollingshead, W. H.: Anatomy for Surgeons, 2nd ed. New York, Harper & Row, 1971.
11. Maizels, M.: Normal development of the urinary tract. *In* Walsh, P. C., Retik, A. B., Stamey, T. A., and Vaughan, E. D. (Eds.): Campbell's Urology, 6th ed. Philadelphia, W. B. Saunders, 1992, p 1301.
12. Moffat, D. B.: Development of the urogenital system in the male. *In* Chisholm, G. D., and Williams, D. I. (Eds.): Scientific Foundations, Urology, 2nd ed. London, William Heinemann Medical Books, 1982, p 344.
13. Paganini-Hill, A., Ross, R. K., and Henderson, B. E.: Epidemiology of renal cancer. *In* Skinner, D. G., and Lieskovsky, G. (Eds.): Diagnosis and Management of Genitourinary Cancer. Philadelphia, W. B. Saunders, 1988, p 32.
14. Pasternack, M. S., and Rubin, R. H.: Urinary tract tuberculosis. *In* Schrier, R. W., and Gottschalk, G. (Eds.): Diseases of the Kidney, 4th ed. Boston, Little, Brown & Co., 1988, p 909.
15. Paulson, D. F.: Prognostic factors predicting treatment response. World J. Urol., *2*:99, 1984.
16. Paulson, D. F., Anderson, T., and Perez, C. A.: Genitourinary malignancy. *In* DeVita, V. T., Hellman, S., and Rosenberg, S. A. (Eds.): Cancer: Principles and Practice of Oncology. Philadelphia, J. B. Lippincott, 1982, p 731.
17. Powell, M. R., and Barnett, C. A.: Radioisotopic kidney stones. *In* Smith, D. R. (Ed.): General Urology, 10th ed. Los Altos, CA, Lange Medical Publications, 1981, p 101.
18. Redman, J. F.: Anatomy of the genitourinary system. *In* Gillenwater, J., Grayhack, J., Howards, S., and Duckett, J. (Eds.): Adult and Pediatric Urology. St. Louis, Mosby–Year Book, 1991, p 3.
19. Rees, A. J.: Pathophysiology of acute renal failure. *In* Chisholm, G. D., and Williams, D. I. (Eds.): Scientific Foundations, Urology, 2nd ed. London, William Heinemann Medical Books, 1982, p 81.
20. Richie, J. P.: The ureter. *In* Paulson, D. F. (Eds.): Genitourinary Surgery. New York, Churchill Livingstone, 1983, p 155.
21. Ronald, A. R., and Nicolle, L. E.: Infections of the upper urinary tract. *In* Schrier, R. W., and Gottschalk, G. (Eds.): Diseases of the Kidney, 4th ed. Boston, Little, Brown & Co., 1988, p 973.
22. Selli, C., Hinshaw, W. M., Woodard, B. H., and Paulson, D. F.: Stratification of risk factors in renal cell carcinoma. Cancer, *52*:899, 1983.
23. Shapiro, J. I., and Schrier, R. W.: Etiology, pathogenesis and management of renal failure. *In* Walsh, P. C., Retik, A. B., Stamey, T. A., and Vaughan, E. D. (Eds.): Campbell's Urology, 6th ed. Philadelphia, W. B. Saunders, 1992, p 2045.
24. Sobel, J. D., Kaye, D., and Reinhart, H.: Host defense mechanisms in urinary tract infections. *In* Schrier, R. W., and Gottschalk, G. (Eds.): Diseases of the Kidney, 4th ed. Boston, Little, Brown & Co., 1988, p 885.
25. Sosa, R. E., and Vaughan, E. D., Jr.: Renovascular hypertension. *In* Gillenwater, J., Grayhack, J., Howards, S., and Duckett, J. (Eds.): Adult and Pediatric Urology. St. Louis, Mosby–Year Book, 1991, p 853.
26. Stamm, W. E.: Cystitis and urethritis. *In* Schrier, R. W., and Gottschalk, G. (Eds.): Diseases of the Kidney, 4th ed. Boston, Little, Brown & Co., 1988, p 1007.
27. Waxman, S. W., and Webster, G. D.: Open surgery versus minimally invasive alternatives in the management of stress incontinence. Curr. Opin. Urol., *4*(4):201, 1994.
28. Williams, R. D.: Renal, perirenal and ureteral neoplasms. *In* Gillenwater, J., Grayhack, J., Howards, S., and Duckett, J. (Eds.): Adult and Pediatric Urology. St. Louis, Mosby–Year Book, 1991, p 571.

CHAPTER 46

THE MALE GENITAL SYSTEM

John L. Weinerth, M.D., and Cary N. Robertson, M.D.

The development of urologic surgery has its origins in Egyptian, Indian, Chinese, and Middle Eastern cultures thousands of years B.C.E. The establishment of the scientific basis for this subspecialty actually began in Greek and Roman medicine, only to wait until the eighteenth to twentieth centuries for refinement of endoscopic instruments and contrast media, which has allowed for investigation and treatment of disorders of the male genital system.[1-3]

The past 15 years have been an era of explosion in knowledge of urologic physiology, with advanced understanding of the physiology of the genital system, the endocrinology of sexual disorders, and the biochemistry of diseases of the prostate, seminal vesicles, and external genitalia. Recognition of the biochemical, neurologic, and hormonal capabilities of the male genital system has permitted accurate diagnosis and definitive therapy in a wide range of conditions, including carcinoma of the prostate, testicular tumors, infertility, sexual function, and urinary obstructive disease. The development of microsurgical techniques has allowed reconstructive processes on tiny structures within the male genitourinary system. The explosion in technology of endoscopic instruments, now with very small calibers and the capability for flexibility, has increased the diagnostic and therapeutic capabilities of the urologist.

ANATOMY[4-7]

Unlike the female, parts of the male genital system are conjoined with regard to sexual and excretory functions, specifically, the prostate and the urethra. The components of the male genital tract are the prostate gland, seminal vesicles, Cowper's glands, glands of Littre, the penis with its incorporated urethra, and the scrotum containing the testes, epididymides, vasa deferentia, and spermatic vessels. The male genitourinary system functions for the purposes of copulation, reproduction, hormone production, and urinary excretion (Fig. 46–1).

The prostate gland, seminal vesicles, Cowper's glands, and glands of Littre produce secretions that serve to lubricate the system and provide a vehicle for storage and passage of spermatozoa. Secretions of the seminal vesicles conjoin with enzymes from the prostate gland and Cowper's glands to produce coagulation and subsequent liquefaction of the ejaculate. The penis is composed of two vascular erectile bodies. The corpora cavernosa incorporates the corpus spongiosum, which contains the male urethra. The paired testes produce both male hormones, predominantly testosterone, and spermatozoa, the former in the interstitial cells and the latter in the seminiferous tubules. The epididymides, lying in intimate contact with the testes, serve as an area of maturation and storage of sperm, which are further transported along the efferent tract composed of the vasa deferentia and the ejaculatory ducts, emptying into the posterior urethra at the verumontanum of the prostate.

Testes.[8] The testes are the central organs of male reproduction. These two ovoid structures average 4 to 5 cm. in length and 2.5 to 3.5 cm. in width in the normal adult male. On the posterolateral surface of the testes, the epididymides are intimately attached to the surface and connected only by means of the tiny efferent ductules at the head of the epididymis to the interior portion of the testes. This is also the location of the terminal portions of the spermatic cord. The factors that control the descent of the testes from the abdominal cavity into the scrotum are probably mostly hormonal, but there may be some anatomic considerations associated with the poorly defined gubernaculum testis. The descent occurs predominantly during the later phase of gestation but may continue into early childhood. The peritoneum anterolateral to the testis invaginates into the scrotum, and after the descent of the testis this processus vaginalis is obliterated, leaving two layers of peritoneum around most of the testis to become the tunica albuginea, investing the testis itself and the tunica vaginalis and providing a potential cushioning space around the testis.

Because the testis arises from portions of the wolffian body on the genital ridge in close proximity to the kidney, it is not surprising that the major blood supply of the testis arises from the aorta just below the renal arteries. Further blood supply follows the course of the vas deferens and may be sufficient to maintain testicular viability in instances where the internal spermatic artery is divided. A third vascular supply, the external spermatic artery, a branch of the epigastric artery, probably forms during descent. Venous drainage of the testis is through multiple veins of the pampiniform plexus to the spermatic vein, which is usually single and emerges from the upper end of the cord and then follows the internal spermatic artery through the retroperitoneum. On the right the spermatic vein empties into the vena cava below the right renal vein, whereas on the left the spermatic vein empties into the main renal vein. Increased hydrostatic pressure, particularly on the left, may result in dilatation of the pampiniform venous plexus, producing a varicocele. The lymphatic drainage of the testis is through the spermatic cord and the inguinal canal and then to the common iliac and periaortic nodes, with the latter communicating across the midline at the level of the kidneys and also with the mediastinal and supraclavicular chains. Testicular nerves derive from the aortic and renal plexuses, which in turn communicate with the solar plexus. Traumatic injuries of the testis may produce acute abdominal pain because of these interdigitating pathways, and in a like fashion intra-abdominal disease may cause referred pain to the testes.

Histologically, there are two principal portions of the testis: the seminiferous tubules, which are responsible along with the Sertoli cells for spermatogenesis, and the interstitial or Leydig cells, which elaborate androgenic hormones, predominantly testosterone. Spermatogenesis appears to require relative hypothermia; seminiferous tubule function may be impaired in the cryptorchid or maldescended testes, whereas hormonal function may be unimpaired even in the intraabdominal undescended testis.

Epididymides.[9] The epididymides are coiled structures each containing a single epididymal tubule 12 to 19 feet long and attached to the posterolateral surface of each testis. The

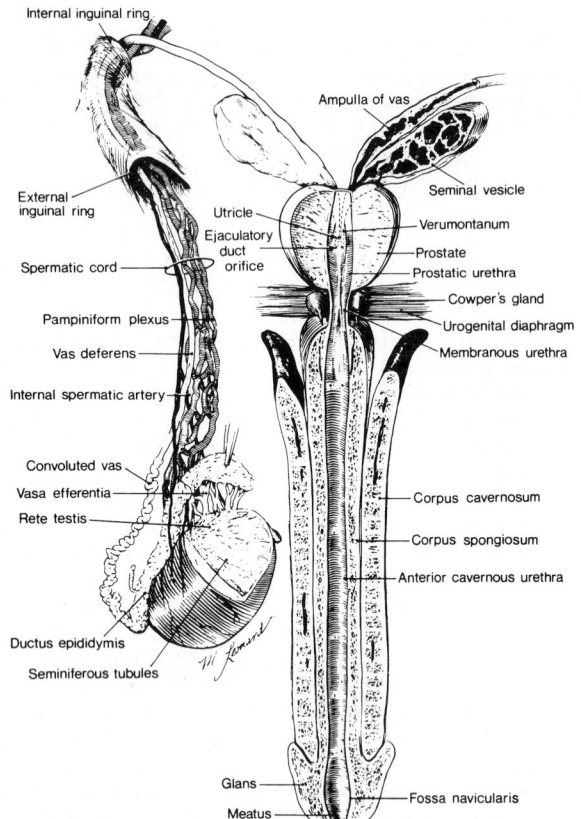

Figure 46–1. Schematic representation of the male genital system.

actual connection between the testis and the epididymis is the efferent ductules resting on the superior extremity of the testis, whereas the body of the epididymis is along the midportion of the testis, and the tail of the epididymis is attached to the inferior extremity of the testis. The medial surface of each epididymis attaches to the terminal portions of the spermatic cord, through which the blood, nerve, and lymphatic supply is received. After the spermatozoa pass from the rete testis through the dozen or more tiny tubular efferent ductules into the epididymis, they progressively pass through the entire length of the epididymis, undergoing maturation and finally storage in the more distal portions. From the tails of the epididymides sperm are transmitted into the vasa deferentia, which are direct continuations of the duct of the epididymides passing up the spermatic cord, across the inguinal canal, and then retroperitoneally to the ampulla of the seminal vesicles, with which they conjoin to form an ejaculatory duct on each side. The ejaculatory duct then empties directly into the prostatic urethra. The principal blood supply for the epididymis is from the internal spermatic artery, which also supplies the testis, but the deferential artery, arising from the superior inferior vesicle artery, follows the course of the vas deferens and provides some vascular supply to the epididymis. Venous drainage corresponds to the arterial supply, and the lymphatic drainage of the epididymis parallels that of the testis. The prime function of the epididymis is not only as a conduit for spermatozoa but also for biochemical and functional maturation and ultimate storage. Sperm recovered from the tail of the epididymis has exhibited a greater degree of maturation and fertilizing capacity than sperm recovered directly from the head or body of the epididymis.

Vas Deferens.[10] The vas deferens is an easily discernible structure within the scrotum and spermatic cord because

it is a heavily muscled tubular structure that aids in the transportation of the spermatozoa through contractions regulated by the autonomic nervous system. It has two main portions: (1) the straight portion that starts at about the level of the upper extremity of the testis and ends at the ejaculatory duct and (2) the convoluted vas, which joins the straight portion to the epididymal tubule at the lower extremity of the testis.

Spermatic Cord. The spermatic cord, suspending each testis and its attached epididymis, is composed of the vas deferens, the internal spermatic artery, the external spermatic artery, the pampiniform plexus of veins, the lymphatic drainage system of the contents of the scrotum, and the autonomic nerve supply to the testis. In addition, the cord is surrounded by fibers of the cremasteric muscle, which assist by contraction and relaxation in the maintenance of optimal testicular temperature and provide for testicular retraction with sexual excitation or in the primitive fright reaction.

The spermatic cord joins as a single unit at the internal ring of the inguinal canal. The spermatic vessels, the spermatic nerves, and the spermatic veins coming from higher retroperitoneal positions, and the vas deferens, with its artery coming from a more inferior retroperitoneal position, join at the internal ring and then are surrounded by the cremasteric muscle and extend into the scrotum, where all components terminate into the testis and epididymis.

Scrotum. The scrotal sac, consisting of two lateral compartments fused in the midline, denoted by the median raphe, encloses the testes, epididymides, and terminal portions of the spermatic cords. The dartos, consisting of elastic fibers, connective tissue, and smooth muscle fibers, is attached to the corrugated skin of the scrotum, rich in sebaceous glands, and provides for muscular contraction of the scrotal sac in response to temperature changes or sexual excitation. The principal function of the scrotum is to aid in temperature control of the testes for optimal spermatogenesis, which takes place at temperatures several degrees lower than those in the intra-abdominal cavity. The alternate contraction and relaxation of the scrotum in conjunction with a similar but separate contraction and relaxation of the cremasteric muscles of the spermatic cord allows for maintenance of testicular temperature within a narrow and precise range. The blood supply of the scrotum comes from the deep pudendal branches of the femoral artery and branches of the internal pudendal artery. The lymphatics of the scrotal halves anastomose freely, surround the penis, and drain to the inguinal and femoral nodes. There are no connections between the lymphatics of the scrotum and the testes; the scrotal lymphatics do not accompany the pudendal vessels.

Seminal Vesicles. The seminal vesicles are paired, monotubular, convoluted structures lying beneath the base of the bladder and trigone. Posteriorly they are invested by Denonvilliers' fascia, which separates them from the anterior wall of the rectum. One leaf of Denonvilliers' fascia separates the most cephalad portion of the seminal vesicles from the bladder. The two seminal vesicles fuse immediately with the ampullae of the vasa, forming the ejaculatory ducts, which open into the prostatic urethra at the level of the verumontanum. The seminal vesicles secrete a mucoid vehicle for the spermatozoa and also elaborate the body's only source of fructose, which is used as an essential nutrient for maintenance of spermatozoal viability. The muscular component of the seminal vesicle is contractile during ejaculation, expelling its contents through the ejaculatory ducts into the posterior urethra.

Prostate Gland.[11] The prostate gland is a fibromuscular, glandular organ that surrounds the vesicle neck and the proximal portion of the male urethra. The prostate of a normal young adult male is approximately 20 gm., consisting of two portions: an anterior (inner) group of glands intimately associated with the urethra and a posterior (outer) portion of more fibromuscular character. Embryologically, the gland derives from five to seven epithelial evaginations of the posterior urethra, producing alveolar glands emptying into the urethra. These lobes may be seen ultrasonographically as a periurethral zone (transitional zone), a central zone, and a peripheral zone of the prostate.

Normal prostatic function depends on androgens, principally testosterone, which is metabolized to dihydrotestosterone by the enzyme 5-alpha-reductase. The prostate is also affected by the adrenal androgens dehydroepiandrosterone and androstenedione. The prostate itself is capable of elaborating specific enzymes, principally acid phosphatase and prostatic specific antigen. The interrelated physiologic and endocrinologic functions of the prostate are necessary for normal reproductive function. Prostatic specific antigen is a serum protease believed to be important in ejaculate clot lysis.

The inferior vesical and internal pudendal arteries provide the blood supply to the prostate, entering the gland posterolaterally at the vesical neck. Venous drainage of the prostate is complex and diffuse, with plexuses over the anterior and lateral portions of the gland that drain into the internal iliac veins. The nerve supply is both secretory and motor, derived from the sympathetic fibers of the hypogastric plexus as well as the sacral plexus. Intercommunicating lymphatics of the prostate, bladder, seminal vesicles, vasa deferentia, and rectum provide drainage into both the internal and external iliac systems as well as the sacral promontory nodes.

The previously noted inner and outer portions of the prostate have now been clarified to contain distinct zones. These zones have physiologic and surgical significance because benign enlargement of the prostate occurs in the transition or periurethral zone and malignancy develops in the majority of cases in the peripheral zone. Anterior fibromuscular stroma constitutes one third of the total bulk of the prostate, and the central zone is situated between the transition zone and peripheral zone, comprising only 25% of the prostate mass. The peripheral zone comprises 75% of the total glandular tissue of the prostate, whereas the transition zone normally occupies less than 5% of the mass of the gland. In cases of significant benign enlargement of the prostate involving the transition zone, a cleavage plane is noted between the peripheral zone and the transition zone adenoma. This can be manipulated by open surgical technique to facilitate removal of the obstructing enlarged benign tissue. Such operations that deal with benign hyperplasia and hypertrophy leave the peripheral zone (posterior portion) of the gland intact. This tough tissue is frequently referred to as the surgical capsule.

The gland is supported anteriorly by the puboprostatic ligaments, inferiorly by the genitourinary diaphragm (external urinary sphincter), and posteriorly by the rectal wall, which is separated from the prostate by an obliterated pelvic reflection of the peritoneum called Denonvilliers' fascia. The urinary sphincters are located at either end of the prostate, with one at the vesical neck and the other at the external muscular sphincter of the urogenital diaphragm and the intrinsic urethral sphincter of the urethral muscle.

Urethra. The male urethra consists of two major portions, the posterior urethra and the anterior urethra, each with two subdivisions. Beginning most proximally at the bladder neck, the posterior urethra consists of the prostatic portion and the membranous urethra. The prostatic urethra is analogous to the entire urethra of the female and is liberally invested with periurethral glands. The verumontanum opens in the floor of the prostatic urethra proximal to the apex of the prostate gland. The membranous urethra lacks periurethral glands, although Cowper's glands are located in the urogenital dia-

phragm lateral to the membranous urethra, the site of external or voluntary sphincteric action. The prostatic and membranous portions of the urethra are relatively fixed by the puboprostatic ligaments and the inherent stability of the urogenital diaphragm, while the urethra distal to the urogenital diaphragm is relatively mobile.

The anterior urethra includes the bulbous or perineal portion of the urethra, beginning at the urogenital diaphragm and extending to the penoscrotal junction, and the distal penile or pendulous urethra. The bulbous urethra exhibits a larger caliber than the remainder of the male urethra and is richly invested with periurethral glands. The penile or pendulous portion of the anterior urethra begins at the penoscrotal junction and extends distally to the external urethral meatus, proximal to which is a bulbous enlargement, the fossa navicularis, which has a nozzle-like effect that produces a unified urinary stream.

Cowper's Glands. Cowper's glands (also called bulbourethral glands of Cowper) are small, paired glands lying between the layers of the urogenital diaphragm at the junction of the bulbous and membranous portions of the urethra. The ducts of the glands may be as long as 1.5 to 2 cm. and empty distally into the bulbous urethra traversing the corpus spongiosum. The secretions from this gland not only act as a lubricant but may also have factors that aid in seminal fluid coagulation after ejaculation.

Penis.[12] The penis serves the dual function of copulation and excretion of urine. It consists of two parallel erectile compartments known as the corpora cavernosa, which are situated dorsolaterally, and the corpus spongiosum, which invests the urethra ventrally, terminating distally in the erectile glans penis. Each corpus cavernosum and the corpus spongiosum are enveloped in fascial sheaths, and all three corpora are surrounded by dense fibrous Buck's fascia. The principal blood supply of the penis is through the dorsal arteries that course over the superior portion of the corpora cavernosa, lying deep to Buck's fascia and being derived initially from the internal pudendal arteries, which are branches of the internal iliac artery. An additional branch of the internal pudendal artery enters the crura on each side of the corpora cavernosa, traversing it lengthwise.

The venous drainage is through the dorsal veins, with the superficial dorsal vein emptying into the saphenous vein, and the deep dorsal vein emptying into the prostatic plexus known as the plexus of Santorini. Penile erection is induced by the engorgement of the erectile tissues of the corpora, principally the corpora cavernosa. The exact mechanisms of erection are not fully understood, but the competence of the pelvic blood supply as well as that of the autonomic nervous system is essential for complete erection. The corpora cavernosa take origin from the ischial pubic rami as the crura then fuse in the perineum. Further fixation of the penis is provided by the suspensory ligament, which connects the root of the penis to the underside of the pubis.

The erectile mechanisms respond to both psychic and tactile stimuli, which produce engorgement of the corpora cavernosa and, to some extent, the corpora spongiosum. Neurophysiologic studies indicate that there is a center localized to the medial frontal lobe that is a positive locus for penile erection. Certain anterior thalamic nuclei and mamillary bodies may also be involved.

Lymphatic drainage of the penis is abundant. The lymphatics from the shaft of the penis, the corpora cavernosa, and the skin pass through the superficial and deep inguinal nodes, communicating with the iliac nodes. Lymphatic drainage of the glans penis parallels that of the urethra to the subinguinal, external iliac, and deep pelvic nodes, while lymphatics from the urethral mucosa drain to the hypogastric nodes. The skin of the penis differs considerably from other skin of the body in its paucity of sebaceous glands, its elasticity, and its extensive blood supply.

TESTES

Function and Infertility[4, 13, 14]

The testes have two primary functions: the production of the major male sex hormone, testosterone, and the production of spermatozoa. Biochemical activity within the testes having to do with the production of testosterone and other androgens is extremely complex but is regulated in part through a feedback mechanism of the hypothalamus and pituitary gland by release of a luteinizing hormone. The production of testosterone and its release into the male environment enables the growth of secondary sex organs and maintenance of male body habitus and is essential for sexual and reproductive function. The production of spermatozoa by the testis is also influenced by pituitary hormones, namely, follicle-stimulating hormones in a similar feedback mechanism fashion. Adequate function of the cells of the seminiferous tubules, including the Sertoli cells, is essential for the production of adequate numbers and quality of the spermatozoa necessary for fertility.

Infertility, therefore, can be the consequence of disturbance in either one or both of the primary testicular functions. The inability of a couple to produce offspring is termed *infertility* or *sterility*. It is estimated that 15% of marriages in this country are initially barren, with approximately half of this number responding to various therapeutic measures.

Infertility may be attributed to the male in as many as 50% of barren marriages. Adequate evaluation of the marital unit for infertility demands assessment of the male partner. Infertility and sterility should not be confused with impotence. Impotence is the inability to achieve or sustain satisfactory erection for intercourse. The principal cause of male infertility is a spermatogenic defect, which is estimated to account for 95% of cases of male infertility or sterility. Most males with such spermatogenic defects produce sperm in some quantity, although there are usually diminished numbers of sperm, and those produced are of inadequate quality, exhibiting malformations and diminished motility. Oligospermia, by definition, indicates a sperm count of less than 20 million per ml., and under such circumstances fertility is difficult. The principal causes of defective spermatogenesis include congenital inadequacy of the seminiferous tubules; testicular damage as a consequence of infection, trauma, or infarction; chromosomal abnormalities such as Klinefelter's syndrome; hormonal defects as in hypopituitarism; varicocele; and cryptorchidism. Other causes of oligospermia may relate to the transport of spermatozoa. Chronic prostatitis and seminal vesiculitis may result in fibrosis and impede transport and delivery of sperm. Infection spreading into the vas deferens may induce fibrosis and stricture even to the point of total occlusion.

Azoospermia, complete absence of spermatozoa in the ejaculate, may be caused by total occlusion of the sperm transport system, vasa, seminal vesicles, or ejaculatory ducts. Congenital absence of the vas and seminal vesicles may occur as an isolated anatomic defect, and congenital absence of the vas is the rule in males with cystic fibrosis. An infection such as gonococcal epididymitis and vasitis may cause complete stenosis and azoospermia. Complete nonresponsiveness of the germinal epithelium as in primary gonadal failure may also produce a picture of azoospermia despite elevated follicle-stimulating hormone levels. Trauma to the vasa in the course of an inguinal hernia operation or orchidopexy may result in complete obstruction.

In some cases, infertility may be due to mechanical factors with no defects in spermatogenesis or delivery of spermatozoa. Procedures on the vesicle neck (particularly transurethral resection, open wedge resection, or plastic reconstruction) or treatment of a congenital contracture can result in an inability of the vesical neck to close with ejaculation, causing the ejaculate to pass in a retrograde fashion into the bladder rather than out through the urethra.

Physical examination of the infertile male should include careful examination of the genitalia, particularly to ensure the testes are of normal size and consistency, the epididymides and vasa are present, and there is no evidence of chronic inflammatory disease of the external genitalia. Prostatitis should be ruled out by digital examination, prostatic massage, and examination of the prostatic fluid. Appropriate cultures constitute the basis for antibiotic therapy, which is sometimes effective in alleviating chronic inflammatory processes as the cause of infertility. Other diagnostic modalities such as cystourethroscopic, ultrasonographic, and radiographic studies of the ejaculatory ducts, vasa, and seminal vesicles are occasionally helpful to identify obstructive problems in the transport system.

Laboratory studies that are helpful in the evaluation of infertility include complete semen analyses, usually obtained after a 3-day absence of sexual activity. The same sample can be tested for fructose, the absence of which would suggest either obstruction of the seminal vesicles or their absence. Serum levels of luteinizing hormone, follicle-stimulating hormone, and testosterone are helpful to identify pregonadal, gonadal, and postgonadal reasons for infertility.

Occasionally, scrotal exploration and testicular biopsy may be indicated, with the suggestion that identification of normal architecture of the seminiferous tubules and normal spermatogenesis strongly indicates an obstructive or inflammatory phenomenon, while inadequacy of the spermatogenic element indicates congenital or hormonal defects.

In mechanical obstruction, new microsurgical techniques have been of considerable help. Epididymal inflammatory lesions may be bypassed by vasoepididymostomy. Vas ligation or stricture may be treated by reanastomosis of the vas. Congenital or inflammatory obstructions at the level of the ejaculatory ducts are occasionally amenable to transurethral resection of the stenotic ducts at the level of the verumontanum in the prostatic urethra.

Orchidopexy cannot be expected to improve spermatogenesis if the patient is older than age 2 years. High ligation of the internal spermatic vein has been advocated in the treatment of oligospermia associated with a varicocele, although the final rationale is still unclear. It is suggested that the varicocele causes defective spermatogenesis on the basis of increased intrascrotal temperature and the possible backflow of inhibiting adrenal hormones from the adrenal and renal veins down the left spermatic vein. A high inguinal division of the left spermatic vein may occasionally cause an increased sperm count and often results in improved sperm motility and morphology. Pregnancy rates have been reported as high as 44% in partners of patients who undergo treatment for varicocele, although generally a figure of 30% is more widely accepted. Persistent semen abnormalities can frequently be overcome with advanced reproductive techniques with sperm processing.

Congenital Anomalies[15]

The most common congenital anomalies of the testes relate to anomalous location, although congenital absence of one or both testes may be observed. The testes develop within the abdominal cavity, differentiating from the primitive gonadal ridge in the early weeks of fetal life. Normally, the testis begins its migration and descent through the inguinal canal at the end of the first trimester of gestation, but various mechanical and hormonal events may impede or alter normal descent. The gubernaculum, previously thought to provide a fibroelastic cord for guidance of the testis into the scrotal compartment, probably adds little mechanical assistance in this process. It seems most likely that the inherent functions of the testis itself are primarily responsible for the necessary ductal differentiation and descent.

Anorchism. Classic experiments indicate that the primitive gonad must differentiate as a testis to produce androgens, which are the stimulus to normal male (wolffian) ductal development. In the complete absence of testes, female (müllerian) ductal development will differentiate in feminine configuration. However, one testis may fail to develop, occasionally in association with ipsilateral agenesis of kidney and ureter; monorchism is seen most often on the right and is termed the *right-sided syndrome.* Rare persons are seen who exhibit no evidence of viable testicular tissue, although the external genitalia are fully differentiated in masculine configuration. In these cases, internal male ductal structures, the vasa deferentia, can be identified, usually extending to the internal inguinal ring and terminating blindly in fibrous tissue. Such persons are apparently normal males, although with a completely empty scrotum; puberty is delayed and incomplete, with persistent elevation of gonadotropin levels and inadequate plasma testosterone levels. It is postulated that such persons with complete anorchism did indeed have normal testes at an early stage of gestation but that some time after the sixteenth week of fetal life the testes atrophied, possibly because of mechanical torsion or other interference with testicular blood supply in the course of the descent. Surgical exploration is required to establish a diagnosis, and a gratifying therapeutic response to continuing exogenous testosterone therapy will be observed: sexual maturation, cessation of growth, increased libido, and masculine redistribution of body fat and muscle mass are concomitants to treatment.

Cryptorchidism.[8] The term *cryptorchidism,* derived from the Greek *cryptos,* meaning *hidden,* should be reserved for those testes that are truly obscure, usually within the abdominal cavity and not palpable on examination. Testes lying in the course of normal descent in the inguinal canal or in ectopic locations can usually be palpated and are not truly hidden. Cryptorchid or intra-abdominal testes are observed unilaterally or bilaterally in 1% to 10% of male infants. Again, the cause of cryptorchidism is obscure, but a selective hormonal deficiency of the testis is suspected as a factor in such failure of descent. Occasionally, a truly cryptorchid testis descends spontaneously at puberty or in response to parenteral chorionic gonadotropin therapy, but this is not the rule, and surgical exploration with orchidopexy is generally required. The cryptorchid abdominal testis will fail in its spermatogenic function, although it may secrete adequate amounts of androgens. Spermatogenic failure is progressive, and transposition of an intra-abdominal testis to the scrotum should be accomplished before the age of 2 years to ensure production of normal quantity and quality of spermatozoa. Exploration may be accomplished through an extraperitoneal inguinal incision, but more adequate exposure is obtained through an abdominal approach, particularly if bilateral cryptorchidism exists. Planning of surgical incisions can be aided by laparoscopic examination to determine the actual location of the testes within the abdomen. Cryptorchid testes are usually found retroperitoneally deep within the pelvis and in proximity to the internal inguinal ring, but they may be located almost anywhere within the lower abdomen, even up in the renal fossa. It is necessary to isolate the testis with its vas and vessels, mobilizing these structures completely. When the spermatic artery is short, it may be possible to

bring the testis through the abdominal wall at Hesselbach's triangle, rather than through the inguinal canal, which necessitates a more devious course. Finally, because the testis may derive some blood supply from the small vessels coursing along the vas deferens, it may be feasible to divide the spermatic vessels and depend on this collateral blood supply, permitting scrotal placement of the testis. When it is impossible to bring the testis to a palpable location within the scrotum or low in the inguinal canal, it is generally thought best to remove the testis, because there is a very high incidence of carcinoma in abdominal testes, the incidence perhaps being as much as 20 times greater than that of carcinoma in a normally descended testis. When cryptorchidism is diagnosed after the age of 10 or 12 years, orchiectomy may be the preferred treatment, because such testes will rarely exhibit normal function despite adequate scrotal placement. In carefully chosen cases, translocation of the testis by complete division of the vessels and microsurgical reanastomosis of the artery and vein using the inferior epigastric artery may allow the salvage of a testis with placement in the scrotum where it might otherwise be surgically impossible to perform an orchidopexy.

Incomplete Descent. *Incomplete descent* or *maldescent of the testis* is the term reserved for those cases in which the testis is arrested at some point in its normal course of descent and is palpable on careful examination. The usual sites of arrest are at the internal inguinal ring, within the inguinal canal, or at the external ring. Often, there is an associated congenital indirect inguinal hernia, because the processus vaginalis has not been obliterated at its proximal extent; the accumulation of normal peritoneal fluid dependently within the processus vaginalis produces a communicating hydrocele. The presence of overt hernia prompts earlier surgical correction, and bilateral maldescent constitutes cause for earlier surgical intervention. Some authorities recommend the use of chorionic gonadotropin in dosages of up to 500 units three times weekly for 6 weeks as a stimulus to testicular descent, but in the truly arrested testis such treatment is generally ineffective. Further prolonged chorionic gonadotropin therapy may lead to premature pubescence and growth arrest. A brief course of chorionic gonadotropin therapy may, however, be employed in preparation before orchidopexy and herniorrhaphy because such stimulation may improve the vascular supply and augment the potential for surgical success. Exploration is accomplished through a high inguinal incision, exposing the entire cord to the internal inguinal ring. The testis and cord are completely freed from the surrounding structures; the patent processus vaginalis is identified, opened, stripped from the cord, and excised, so that the neck of the peritoneal sac is closed; and the spermatic vessels are carefully dissected extraperitoneally to afford maximal cord length. The testis is then positioned and fixed within the scrotum using a variety of techniques.

Ectopic Testis. Occasionally, one or both testes may undergo alternative excursion in the course of descent, coming to lodge in ectopic positions. The exact cause of such wandering ectopia is obscure but must relate to mechanical factors. Favorite sites of testicular ectopia are symphyseal, prepubic, femoral, crural, penile, or perineal positions. Surgical correction should be accomplished for cosmetic reasons as well as to ensure normal testicular function and patient comfort.

Trauma[6]

Surprisingly, the testes are relatively protected against trauma despite their external position. The primitive cremasteric reflex causes retraction of the testes to a protected inguinal position under extreme stress. Even in instances of avulsion of skin of the genitalia, the testes, appendages, and cords are usually undisturbed, remaining inviolate within their fascial coverings. Blunt external trauma may result in testicular hemorrhage and infarction, usually requiring surgical intervention. Penetrating wounds should be treated by surgical exploration. Torsion of the spermatic cord may occur as a result of external trauma, compromising blood supply and threatening viability of the testis, but such torsion is usually of spontaneous variety. Surgical intervention in instances of testicular trauma should be accomplished promptly because the risk of surgery is minimal and early surgical repair can prevent subsequent infarction, atrophy, and loss of testicular function.

Infections

Infections of the testis are almost always secondary to spread of infection through the male ductal system, the vas deferens, and the epididymis. Chronic urinary tract infection, particularly suppurative prostatitis and seminal vesiculitis, predisposes to the spread of bacteria through the vas into the epididymis and the testis. It is rare to observe pyogenic orchitis without associated epididymitis, while epididymitis may occur with virtually no involvement of the associated testis. In rare instances, systemic bacteremia may result in embolic metastatic foci of infection within the testis.

Orchitis may result from viral infection in association with mumps, usually not until after the patient has reached pubescence. Mumps orchitis produces severe local inflammatory reactions with excess accumulation of fluid within the compartment of the tunica vaginalis, the acute hydrocele of mumps. Supportive treatment is generally indicated, and aspiration of the hydrocele is avoided because there is a risk of introducing bacteria and initiating a secondary infection that can result in testicular atrophy. Mechanical support of the scrotum with an adhesive bridge, bed rest, analgesics, and antipyretics constitute the first line of treatment. Smallpox, varicella, measles, influenza, and other similar infections may occasionally induce a secondary orchitis.

Tuberculous orchitis is almost always secondary to tuberculous epididymitis, the primary focus within the urinary tract generally being within the kidneys, sometimes in the prostate. Genitourinary tuberculosis is responsive to intensive antituberculous medical management, and a surgical procedure is reserved for advanced cases of localized tuberculosis. Syphilitic gummas may occur within the testis, and surgical removal is almost always required, because chronic draining fistulas are the rule. Fungus infections such as blastomycosis and actinomycosis of the testis are rarely observed but usually necessitate orchiectomy and continued medical management.

The patient with an acute testicular infection is quick to appear for examination and treatment, because the condition is exquisitely painful. Orchitis must be differentiated from testicular tumor with hemorrhage and from torsion of the spermatic cord. Both conditions demand immediate surgical intervention.

Testicular Tumors[6, 7]

Neoplasms of the testis are almost always malignant, with the only exception being rare fibromas of the tunica vaginalis and pure Leydig's cell tumors, which are usually benign. In contrast, extratesticular tumors within the scrotum are almost always benign, such as the adenomatoid tumors of the epididymis and cord. Because of this sharp distinction in the potential of neoplasms within the scrotum, diligent physical examination is necessary in distinguishing the site of origin of a scrotal mass.

Malignant neoplasms of the testes may be of germinal or nongerminal origin, with the latter tumors arising from the interstitial cells and known as interstitial cell tumors, Leydig's cell tumors, or androblastomas. These are relatively rare tumors, producing excessive quantities of androgenizing hormones, which may cause virilism and precocious puberty in young males, impotence and gynecomastia in adults, and feminizing changes in the male that are analogous to those alterations observed with ovarian arrhenoblastomas in the female. Interstitial cell tumors of the testis must be differentiated from adrenal rest tumors, with cells of adrenal origin being of very similar histologic character. It has been suggested that many cases of testicular tumors identified as interstitial cell neoplasms may indeed have represented unrecognized rests of hyperplastic adrenal tissue.

The malignant germinal tumors of the testis arise from the totipotential cells of seminiferous tubules and constitute a serious threat to the male population, accounting for 2% of all malignant tumors, the dominant cause of death from genitourinary malignant disease in the younger adult male population. Testicular tumors are seen in all ages but predominate in persons between the ages of 20 and 35 years. Germinal testicular tumors are categorized according to the degree of cellular differentiation, which parallels malignant potential.

Seminoma. The most common of testicular malignant lesions, accounting for approximately 40% of germinal tumors, seminomas are uniform in gross and histologic appearance and are characterized by slow growth and late invasion. Metastatic spread is through the testicular lymphatics and dominates in the iliac, aortic, and renal hilar nodes. Because of the relatively slow growth of these tumors, they may be appreciated and removed surgically before the development of metastases. Metastatic seminoma of moderate tumor burden confined to the abdominal lymph nodes is responsive to radiation therapy, with 5-year survival rates in the range of 90%. Patients with more metastatic extension should receive multiagent chemotherapy in the same manner as for nonseminomatous tumors. In such patients, combination chemotherapy may still bring about complete remission in at least two thirds of the patients.

Embryonal Carcinoma. Of somewhat more malignant potential, embryonal carcinoma may also be seen in the younger age group and is usually thought to be the most common testicular tumor of childhood. The histologic pattern of embryonal carcinoma is of a less differentiated form than that of seminoma, and invasion and metastases occur earlier in the course of the disease. Because of the relatively rapid growth of the tumor, hemorrhage and necrosis are common. Metastases to the abdominal lymphatics and the lungs may occur as an early event.

Choriocarcinoma. Fortunately, pure choriocarcinomas account for only a small number of the germinal cell tumors. The tumor is extremely rapidly invasive, with trophoblasts invading the venous system early in the course of the disease. Metastasis may be both blood-borne and through lymphatics and has usually occurred by the time of diagnosis. Unlike choriocarcinoma in the female, which responds well to methotrexate, choriocarcinoma in the male is best treated with other agents such as cisplatin, bleomycin, and additional agents. The prognosis for these patients is usually far worse than for other patients because of the advanced stage at time of diagnosis.

Diagnosis and Management

The earliest symptom of testicular tumor is a mass in the testis, which unfortunately is unrecognized by most patients until there is associated dull, aching pain. Hemorrhage within the testis may follow minimal trauma, suggesting that traumatic injury is related to the tumor, which is probably not the case. Some of the more malignant tumors may produce hormones, measured as gonadotropins, which induce gynecomastia. In other instances, the more malignant tumors, relatively small in the primary location, may induce an abdominal mass as an early manifestation of disease.

The successful treatment of testicular tumors demands scrupulous physical examination, a high index of suspicion, and the willingness to accomplish prompt inguinal exploration when the diagnosis is suggested. The typical testicular neoplasm is stony hard with a suggestion of weightiness on palpation. When the suspicion of testicular tumor is raised, extensive laboratory evaluation should be deferred, with the exception of drawing serum for determination of beta-subunit human chorionic gonadotropin and alpha-fetoprotein levels, which are important tumor markers, and surgical exploration should be accomplished as a primary event. The approach is through a high inguinal incision, exposing the spermatic cord at its emergence from the internal inguinal ring where it is isolated. Rubber-shod clamps are applied, and the testis with its surrounding attachments can be mobilized for inspection and biopsy. If diagnosis of testicular neoplasm is confirmed, high inguinal orchiectomy is accomplished, removing the entire cord with the involved testis and leaving the stump of the cord within the retroperitoneum.

After orchiectomy, further diagnostic studies may be undertaken. Computed tomography of the chest, abdomen, and pelvis is generally the diagnostic imaging modality of choice and the basis for following the patient with regard to success of therapy. Beta-subunit human chorionic gonadotropin and alpha-fetoprotein should be re-collected after orchiectomy for comparison with the preoperative values. Elevations of gonadotropins are observed most commonly with choriocarcinoma, less frequently with embryonal carcinoma or teratocarcinoma, and only occasionally with pure seminoma. Bone survey and bone scan may rule out skeletal metastases, a relatively uncommon event in most testicular tumors, with the metastatic pattern being lymphatic and visceral.

Further treatment of testicular tumors after orchiectomy is dictated by the results of evaluation and by the philosophy of the urologic surgeon. It is thought in most instances that abdominal node dissection is of little value when pulmonary metastases have been demonstrated. If no pulmonary metastases are detected, radical retroperitoneal node dissection, usually through a transabdominal approach and less commonly through thoracoabdominal exposure, is advocated as an effective modality in the staging and control of the malignant process. Because metastatic seminoma is highly radiosensitive, many authorities question node dissection in treatment of seminoma. Any seminoma may contain a microscopic focus of more malignant germinal elements, and metastases may reflect embryonal carcinoma, teratocarcinoma, or even choriocarcinoma, which may not respond favorably to radiation therapy. Multiagent chemotherapy protocols rather than retroperitoneal node dissection appear to be the treatment of choice in this disease. It is the usual practice to accomplish transabdominal radical retroperitoneal lymph node dissections in all instances of nonseminomatous testicular tumor except when very large masses of nodes are discovered by computed tomography or there is tumor in the lung.

Patients with extensive abdominal tumor burdens or pulmonary metastases will more than likely undergo cyclical chemotherapy using multiple agents and then undergo retroperitoneal lymph node dissection and possible thoracotomy, if the computed tomographic scans are still positive or if there is suspected residual tumor once the tumor markers have normalized.

The efficacy of surgical node dissection has been elaborated irrespective of ancillary radiation therapy or chemotherapy. When node dissection is accomplished and there is no histologic evidence of metastatic disease, no further treatment is given. Survival rates in this group of patients irrespective of the histologic classification of the primary tumor are extremely good. On the other hand, when positive nodes are identified or removed at operation, adjunctive therapy is indicated, with chemotherapy depending on the cell type demonstrated in the nodes and the primary lesion.

A variety of chemotherapeutic agents have been developed over the past few years, resulting in dramatic responses. Historically, the antitumor agents have included dactinomycin, methotrexate, and chlorambucil. Some activity has also been noted with vinblastine. Cisplatin, bleomycin, and vinblastine with the addition of etoposide are now considered to be the primary therapeutic agents.

The ultimate prognosis in testicular malignant disease depends on the stage of the disease at diagnosis, the histologic character of the tumor, and the vigor with which therapeutic measures are pursued. With the advent of combination surgical, radiation, and chemotherapeutic regimens, the outlook for patients with testicular carcinoma is extremely optimistic. The follow-up should extend over a minimum of 5 years with regular and periodic examinations, monitoring of serum beta-subunit human chorionic gonadotropin and alpha-fetoprotein levels, chest radiographs, and other indicated modalities of evaluation in the hope of identifying recurrence of disease and initiating appropriate new therapeutic maneuvers.

SPERMATIC CORDS AND TUNICS

The entire spermatic cord is subject to inflammatory diseases, usually the result of trauma or pyogenic bacteria (termed *funiculitis*) and is occasionally seen with scrotal inflammation or epididymitis. Neoplasms of the spermatic cord are extremely rare, but sarcoma, usually rhabdomyosarcoma, and both invasive and metastatic malignant lesions from other structures may involve the cord. Benign tumors of the cord include adenomatoid tumors, lipoma, fibroma, and cysts, particularly hydrocele of the cord, a remnant of the processus vaginalis. However, the principal abnormality of the cord is torsion.

Torsion

Torsion of the spermatic cord is probably the result of an abnormally high attachment of the tunica vaginalis around the terminal cord, allowing the testis to twist freely within the compartment, the so-called bell-clapper deformity. When rotation of the testis on the end of the cord exceeds 90 degrees, there may be compromise of the blood supply, which causes exquisite pain and produces gangrene and subsequent atrophy of the testis unless the torsion is treated immediately. Incomplete torsion may cause partial strangulation, effects of which may be overcome if surgical intervention is accomplished within about 12 hours, whereas severe torsion with total compromise of the blood supply will result in loss of the testis unless an operation is effected within about 4 hours.

Torsion is usually seen in young males and most often occurs spontaneously, even during sleep. Physical and sexual activity may predispose to torsion and aggravate it by contraction of the cremasteric muscle. There is a rapid onset of severe pain and swelling accompanied by nausea, vomiting, abdominal pain, and occasionally fever.

On examination, the involved testis seems to ride high in the scrotal compartment and has a horizontal orientation. The differential diagnosis is between torsion and epididymitis, and epididymitis is almost always accompanied by evidence of prostatitis and pyuria. With torsion, the entire testis and appendages are involved in the swelling process, whereas with epididymitis the prominent induration is within the epididymides and not the testes; however, after a relatively short time this differentiation can often not be made.

Torsion must always be suspected with acute onset of scrotal pain, and prompt surgical intervention is required. Any delay in operation diminishes the prospects for salvage of the testis. Nuclear medicine blood flow scans and detection of testicular blood flow by a Doppler stethoscope have been used to differentiate epididymitis from torsion of the testis, but false-negative studies have been reported, and any question about the diagnosis should prompt surgical exploration.

When torsion is treated on one side, the contralateral scrotum should also be explored; the tunica vaginalis should be opened and inverted around the testis as with hydrocele repair, and steps should be taken to surgically correct any additional defect such as deficient attachment of the epididymis to the testis.

The appendix epididymis and the appendix testis (hydatid of Morgagni) are vestigial remnants of ducts attached to the head of the epididymis and to the superior pole of the testes, respectively. These small cystic structures may be twisted, producing acute and severe pain with generalized scrotal edema. Little permanent damage or disability is incurred by torsion of these appendages, but because of diagnostic confusion, it is often advisable to explore the scrotum when any doubt exists. It is possible to make the diagnosis without exploration if the process is very localized and the small area of tenderness can be seen as a *blue dot* through the scrotal skin.

VASA DEFERENTIA[10]

The vasa deferentia are the conduits for spermatozoa from the epididymis to the seminal vesicles and prostate. Thus, normal vasa are necessary to human reproduction. Because a single testis is capable of producing sufficient numbers of sperm for purposes of fertility, a single, normal, intact vas is all that is necessary to ensure the reproductive capacity of the male. The most common anomaly of the vas is congenital absence, seen almost universally in males with cystic fibrosis. There are other isolated instances of unilateral duct failure with the absence of the vas deferens. Discovery of bilateral absence of the vasa should alert the clinician to the possibility of other wolffian duct abnormalities, such as renal agenesis or renal ectopia.

Division of the vas for the purpose of sterilization (i.e., vasectomy) is the most popular means of elective sterilization. Millions of men have undergone vasectomy in the past few years, and most of these operations are being accomplished as outpatient procedures. Although vasectomy is very simple, it must be remembered that spermatozoa distal to the point of ligation and stored within the seminal tract and prostate may remain viable for many weeks.

Spermatozoa disappear from the ejaculate at a rate of 50% to 70% of the remaining sperm with each ejaculation, and most sexually active males will have emptied all viable spermatozoa from the seminal tract after 10 or more ejaculations. Microscopic examination of a freshly collected specimen of ejaculate should be accomplished 6 to 8 weeks after the procedure. The patient should not be pronounced surgically sterile until a negative specimen of ejaculate has been carefully examined. Vasectomy must be considered a permanent sterilization measure despite the fact that there are increasing successes in utilizing microsurgical reconstruction of the vasa. Even with excellent technical success rates of greater than 95% in terms of returning sperm to the ejaculate using microsurgical vasovasostomy techniques, the actual pregnancy rate may approximate only 50%.

SEMINAL VESICLES[10]

Abnormalities of the seminal vesicles are relatively uncommon. Rarely, one of the seminal vesicles may be congenitally absent or exhibit cystic anomalies, associated with the ipsilateral absence of kidney and ureter. Occasionally, with ureteral duplication one of the ureters will empty into the seminal vesicle, causing symptomatology. Because of the secluded and protected location of the seminal vesicles, they are infrequently involved in trauma.

The most common clinical problems related to the seminal vesicles are those of inflammation and involvement by malignancy, owing to the intimate connection of the seminal vesicles with the prostate and the base of the bladder.

Chronic lower urinary tract infection may cause seminal vesiculitis, usually seen in association with chronic prostatitis and obstruction of the ejaculatory ducts at the ampullae. This may predispose to an abscess of the seminal vesicle, although this is rare. A diagnosis of such inflammatory disease is made by digital examination; the dilatation and induration of the seminal vesicles can be readily appreciated, whereas the normal seminal vesicles are very difficult to palpate. A massage and stripping of the seminal vesicles produces purulent debris, confirming the diagnosis. Occasionally, pelvic computed tomography in association with vasography identifies an abnormal seminal vesicle.

Primary carcinoma of seminal vesicles is extremely rare. The surgical approach to seminal vesicles may be perineal, retropubic, transvesicular, or transperitoneal, with the method selected depending on the original diagnosis; benign cysts of the seminal vesicle are best approached abdominally, whereas removal of the entire seminal vesicles with the prostate may be most readily accomplished by perineal exposure. If the seminal vesicles alone are to be removed, leaving the prostate undisturbed and intact, a transvesicular, transtrigonal exposure may be most appropriate.

COWPER'S GLANDS

Under normal circumstances, Cowper's glands are not palpable, but occasionally infection may occur, usually secondary to urethritis, predisposing to enlargement that is palpable on rectal examination *distal* to the prostate in the genitourinary diaphragm in a paraurethral position. Dilated Cowper's ducts and glands may be demonstrated by retrograde urethrography, especially in association with stricture or urethral inflammatory disease. Treatment is usually conservative, although transurethral or perineal incision and drainage may be required. Carcinoma of Cowper's glands is extremely rare but produces perineal pain, difficult urination, and a stony hard mass that presents rectally and perineally. Rectal fistulas may occur, and a radical procedure is indicated for cure.

EPIDIDYMIDES[9]

The epididymides are more than simply transport tubules. The epididymis, which if dissected free is approximately 4.5 m. long, gradually increases in its lumen from the head of the epididymis to the tail of the epididymis, where it connects with the convoluted portion of the vas. An excellent review of the present knowledge and physiology of the epididymis has been presented by Howards. Not only is there a storage factor in the epididymis, but there is also a maturation phase changing physiologic conditions within the epididymal tubules. During ejaculation, sperm are actually brought from the very distal epididymis through the vas to the posterior urethra in the process called emission. Ejaculation then delivers the bolus of the semen from the posterior urethra to the outside.

The genital abnormalities of the epididymis include total absence with or without the absence of the associated vas. In addition, there may be defects in the fusion of the epididymis and the testis as well as defects in fusion of the epididymis and the vas, despite what appears by physical examination to be an entirely normal system. The incidence of epididymal defects appears to be higher in undescended testes. Defects may take the form of an extremely elongated epididymis, detached epididymis, or disruption of continuity.

Specific trauma to the epididymis is rare but certainly accompanies testicular injuries. The most common problem with the epididymis is infection, particularly after puberty; it is occasionally seen in a prepubescent male but usually in those with chronic urinary tract infection, obstructed urethras, or high voiding pressure.

Acute nonspecific epididymitis is nongonococcal and nontuberculous, secondary to suppurative infection, which usually has its origin in the prostate and seminal vesicles and then spreads in a retrograde fashion to the epididymis. Hematogenous and lymphatic spread of infection from a distant focus may occur but is rare. The inflammation is diffuse throughout the epididymis and may, or may not, involve the testis, depending on the severity.

The patient complains of severe pain and swelling with chills, fever, and other systemic symptoms, which may include headache, nausea, and vomiting. Symptoms of urinary tract infection such as frequency, urgency, burning, dysuria, pyuria, and hematuria may be present. The epididymis and surrounding structures, including the spermatic cord, may be thickened by edema, swollen, and exquisitely tender to palpation. It is important to differentiate testicular swelling from epididymitis (because a mass in the testis always suggests testicular tumor) and to differentiate acute epididymitis from torsion of the spermatic cord; torsion demands immediate surgical exploration, whereas epididymitis is treated by conservative measures.

In the very early phases of epididymitis, this distinction may be easy to make, but once the epididymitis has progressed to the point of causing inflammation of the surrounding tissue, distinction from torsion may be very difficult; and, because torsion of the testis can lead to total destruction, exploration may be needed to make the correct diagnosis. Other conditions that may confuse the diagnosis include inguinal hernia, with or without trapped bowel, and an acute hydrocele.

Treatment of epididymitis consists of bed rest, elevation and support of the scrotum, application of cold packs, antipyretics, anti-inflammatory agents, and appropriate antimicrobial agents, which are sometimes administered intravenously. Occasionally, suppurative epididymitis may localize into an abscess and drain spontaneously. Surgical intervention should be avoided unless a testicular abscess develops.

Chronic epididymitis is usually the sequel of acute epididymitis but may arise insidiously with few localizing symptoms except the sensation of epididymal enlargement and tenderness. The demonstration of an associated prostatic infection is an adjunct to differential diagnosis, but tumor must always be suspected when there is a relatively painless chronic enlargement of the epididymis. However, the most common neoplasms of the epididymis are benign and include adenomatoid tumors, leiomyomas, and cysts.

A spermatocele is a diverticulum of the epididymis that contains cloudy fluid with spermatozoa. It is unilocular or multilocular and often confused with hydrocele because both a spermatocele and a hydrocele can be transilluminated. Differential diagnosis of spermatocele and hydrocele is aided by the localization of the mass: hydrocele generally surrounds the testis, while the spermatocele is more eccentric, can often be palpated in direct conjunction with the epididymis, and is often tender.

Other epididymal abnormalities are less common. Gonococcal epididymitis, once seen with relative frequency, is less common now, and earlier treatment of gonococcal urethritis diminishes the tendency to development of subsequent gonococcal prostatitis, seminal vesiculitis, vasitis, and epididymitis. Similarly, tuberculous epididymitis is extremely rare today. Caseation necrosis may ensue, often involving the scrotal wall and skin with ulceration and fistula formation. In such cases, epididymo-orchiectomy with excision of the involved portion of the scrotal wall is usually necessary despite the use of newer antituberculous drugs. Other granulomatous reactions in the epididymis may be observed in association with syphilis or as a consequence of escape of spermatozoa with development of a sperm granuloma, which is sometimes painful and may require excision. This is occasionally seen after bilateral vasectomy for voluntary sterilization.

Varicocele

Varicocele is the term applied to dilatation and tortuosity of the veins of the pampiniform plexus, most commonly observed on the left. Later development of a varicocele may be an indicator of left renal tumor because the left spermatic vein system drains into the renal vein and obstruction at that point could produce dilatation of the veins of the left cord. Most varicoceles are idiopathic, although there may be a defect in the valve system of the spermatic vein, particularly on the left where the vein takes a longer course. Varicocele rarely causes symptoms, but there may be a heavy, dragging, aching sensation in the scrotal compartment. Discomfort or infertility may prompt surgical repair, accomplished by high ligation of the spermatic vein through an incision at the level of the internal inguinal ring, giving ready access to the single vein. After such ligation, venous collateral circulation is assumed by the deep pelvic venous system.

Hydrocele

The tunica vaginalis, derived from the peritoneum as the processus vaginalis at the time of testicular descent, is a secretory membrane. Fluid is generated by the serous surface of the tunica vaginalis, with fluid formation being enhanced by inflammation or trauma. Fluid within the tunica vaginalis is resorbed at a constant rate through the extensive venous and lymphatic systems of the spermatic cord. Hydrocele, the excessive accumulation of this serous fluid, results when there is increased production or decreased resorption, the latter condition usually being idiopathic (Fig. 46–2).

Congenital hydrocele may follow failure of obliteration of the processus vaginalis, and fluid formed within the peritoneal cavity may gravitate into the tunica vaginalis. Such congenital hydroceles may fluctuate in size, depending on position of the child, and there may sometimes be an associated palpable inguinal hernia; regardless of whether a hernia exists, the potential for herniation is present. Occasionally, spontaneous closure of the processus vaginalis occurs during infancy and surgical intervention may not be necessary. In instances of complete obliteration of the processus vaginalis along the spermatic cord, there may be excessive accumulation of fluid in the tunica vaginalis in the newborn, sometimes requiring aspiration or early surgical intervention for fear of mechanical compression and compromise of testicular

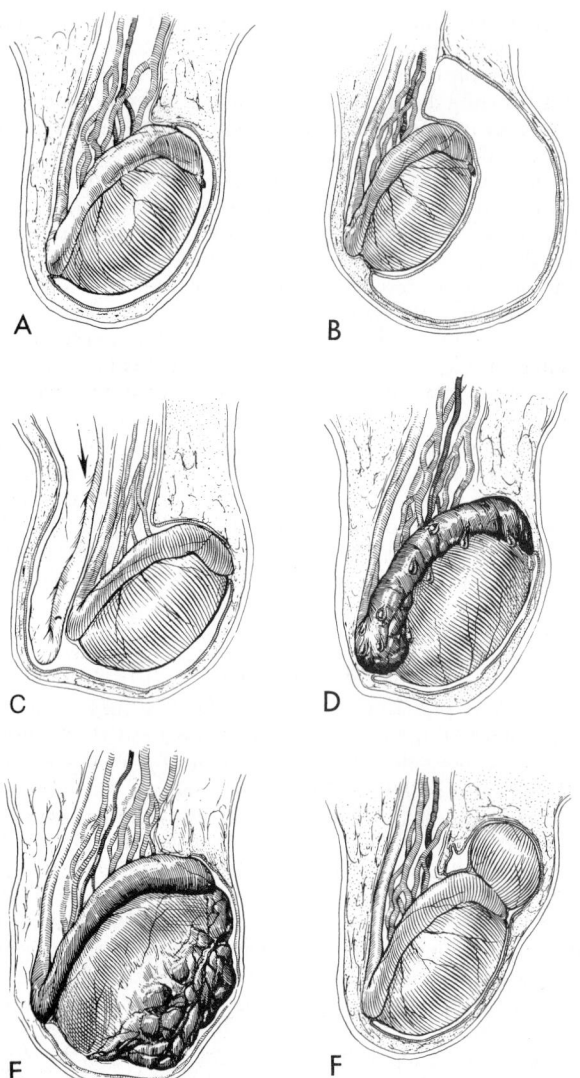

Figure 46–2. Common scrotal masses can be differentiated with knowledge of normal anatomy (A), as compared with hydrocele of the tunica vaginalis (B), inguinal hernia penetrating the scrotal compartment (C), epididymitis causing induration and enlargement of the epididymis but not the testis (D), testicular tumor causing an irregular mass intrinsic to the testis (E), and spermatocele or epididymal cyst arising extrinsic to the testis (F).

permanent cure is expected with this procedure. Aspiration and injection of sclerosing materials is condemned because of the risk of infection.

INGUINAL LYMPHATICS[6, 18]

The superficial and inguinal lymphatic intervals constitute the principal drainage system for the external genitalia. There is interdigitation of lymphatic drainage between the superficial inguinal nodes and the deep inguinal groups, which communicate with the hypogastric and iliac nodes. Lymphatics of the penis, penile skin, and scrotum drain to the superficial inguinal group, while drainage from the urethra is to the inguinal and hypogastric nodes and that from the glans penis is to the external iliac group. Inflammatory lymphadenitis occurs with many infections of the external genitalia and is usually treated conservatively with antimicrobial agents, bed rest, and other supportive measures. Suppuration may necessitate incision and drainage. Inguinal buboes may result from chancroid, the soft chancre that usually occurs primarily on the corona of the glans penis.

Lymphogranuloma Venereum

Probably of viral origin although possibly due to L-forms, lymphogranuloma is also known as lymphopathia venereum and lymphogranuloma inguinale. Transmission of infection is by sexual intercourse, either genital or anal. Severe adenitis is sometimes associated with elephantiasis of the genitalia. Diagnosis is established by an intradermal Frei test and complement fixation, although these are not positive early in the course of the disease. There may be spontaneous remission, but therapy is usually effective with sulfadiazine, tetracyclines, and chloramphenicol. Surgical excision of the involved node groups may be required, particularly if secondary infection supervenes.

Granuloma Inguinale

Granuloma inguinale is a superficial ulcerative skin lesion associated with inguinal adenitis due to the encapsulated gram-negative Donovan body, which is transmitted by sexual contact and is related to the Friedländer and *Klebsiella* groups of organisms. Granuloma inguinale is seen more commonly in the southern United States and among the black population. Multiple painless granulomatous lesions cause extensive scarring, which may necessitate surgical excision. Streptomycin and tetracyclines are effective in controlling the infectious process.

PROSTATE GLAND[6, 11]
Congenital Anomalies

Complete absence of the prostate gland in an otherwise normal male has not been observed. However, failure of normal development and maturation of the prostate may be associated with the intersex states and male gonadal failure. Congenital contracture of the vesical neck at the point of juncture of prostate and bladder may cause severe urinary obstruction. Congenital valves of the prostatic urethra—mucosal folds that may be diaphragmatic or alar—occur relatively frequently and cause profound obstructive uropathy in some cases. Congenital müllerian cysts predispose to obstruction and infection, present as midline masses beneath the gland and base of the bladder, and are treated by open surgical removal.

Trauma

Fracture of the bony pelvis may often result in laceration and transection of the membranous urethra just distal to the

viability. Congenital hydrocele, particularly with associated hernia, demands surgical repair. This is accomplished through a high inguinal incision, giving access to the internal inguinal ring, at which point the hernia sac or processus vaginalis is ligated.

In older persons, hydrocele is frequently the result of epididymo-orchitis or trauma. If there is active pyogenic infection, the hydrocele may become infected, demanding surgical incision and drainage. Compromise of venous and lymphatic return along the cord may occur with a large inguinal hernia or as a result of herniorrhaphy, with fibrosis of the inguinal canal obstructing venous and lymphatic drainage. Large intra-abdominal and pelvic masses may similarly compromise return and predispose to hydrocele. Although small hydroceles may require no treatment, the swelling may assume such proportions as to cause severe discomfort and interfere with physical and sexual activity. Hydrocelectomy is accomplished by scrotal exploration with excision of redundant tunica vaginalis and retroversion of the remaining sac around the testes, epididymis, and terminal portion of the cord. A

prostate, and urinary extravasation as well as bleeding may displace the prostate and bladder superiorly. Penetrating wounds of the prostate due to gunshot wounds or perineal straddle injuries have been reported. The most common cause of prostatic injury is inexpert urethral instrumentation, generally in the course of urethral dilation in treatment of stricture, although injury at the time of rectal operation is occasionally encountered. The usual concomitant of prostatic injury is damage to the external urinary sphincter, which lies in proximity to the distal portion of the gland, with fibrosis and stricture. Another major complication of prostatic trauma is impotence.

Infections

Prostatic infections constitute a significant fraction of urologic practice. Infectious agents that may involve the prostate gland include the spectrum of gram-negative organisms, gram-positive cocci, gonococci, various mycotic organisms, mycobacteria, trichomonads, *Chlamydia*, and *Candida* species. The ascending transurethral route of infection is usual, and exogenous infection is enhanced by urethral abnormalities. Hematogenous and lymphatic routes of access to the prostate as well as descending infection from the upper urinary tract have been described, especially with tuberculosis.

Acute Prostatitis. Suppurative acute prostatitis may be seen from pubescence throughout the life span. The organisms most commonly involved are the gram-negative group, principally *Escherichia coli*. Acute gonococcal prostatitis is relatively uncommon, but the involvement of the periurethral glands by gonorrhea predisposes to inflammation and stricture, which invite secondary gram-negative infection in the prostate.

Symptoms include urgency, frequency, dysuria, perineal aching, rectal discomfort, and even chills and fever with bacteremia. Edema may predispose to acute urinary retention. Examination discloses an exquisitely tender prostate that is diffusely indurated and enlarged. Urinalysis usually reveals pyuria, and often the offending organisms can be cultured. Prostatic massage should be accomplished most gently, if at all, seeking to avoid bacteremia. Prostatic secretions will be filled with purulent debris, and the stained smear may reveal bacteria.

Instrumentation should be avoided in the acute phase of prostatitis unless there is associated urinary retention that demands catheterization. Vigorous antibiotic therapy with a broad-spectrum agent should be initiated, pending culture and sensitivity studies. Bed rest, intermittent hot sitz baths, antipyretics, and restriction of sexual activity are necessary supportive measures. Antibiotic therapy should be continued for not less than 2 weeks.

Prostatic Abscess. Before the era of antibiotic therapy, prostatic abscesses were frequent sequelae of acute prostatitis, but they are encountered less frequently today. Surgical drainage of prostatic abscess is required and may be accomplished by transurethral incision and resection, perineal incision and drainage, aspiration, or massage. Transrectal drainage of prostatic abscess is effective and is attended by surprisingly few complications, with spontaneous healing of both the prostate and the rectal wall occurring in the majority of cases.

Chronic Prostatitis. Chronic inflammation of the prostate gland may ensue as a sequel of acute prostatitis or may occur as a complication of prostatic enlargement and obstruction. Presenting symptoms usually consist of dull, aching perineal discomfort with minimal but recurring symptoms of lower urinary tract irritation, frequency, and urgency with symptoms of fullness and irritability. Occasionally, urethral discharge occurs. Many patients may have chronic prostatitis without symptoms.

On examination, the prostate gland may be essentially normal in size and consistency, enlarged and boggy, or irregularly indurated and tender to palpation. Urinalysis may reveal red blood cells, white blood cells, and bacteria or may be entirely within normal limits. Prostatic secretions, elicited by gentle massage accomplished by a sweeping motion of the examining finger over the lobes of the prostate from lateral to medial, followed by antegrade stripping of the prostatic urethra in the midline, contain pus cells with or without demonstrable bacteria. Normal prostatic secretions contain a few white blood cells in the cellular elements of prostatic secretion, but greater numbers of pus cells, particularly leukocytes, trapped in mucoid clumps confirm the diagnosis of chronic prostatitis.

The treatment of chronic prostatitis is often less than satisfactory. Antimicrobial agents may or may not be effective, and unless the symptoms are extremely severe and a positive culture can be elicited, antibiotics are usually avoided. Regular and periodic prostatic massage is probably the most beneficial modality of treatment and must be accomplished over periods of several weeks or months. Warm sitz baths may offer symptomatic relief and encourage normal drainage of inspissated secretions. Anti-inflammatory agents may be of some help in selected patients. Surgical intervention is not often indicated. Calculi may occur in the glandular acini and ducts of the prostate gland, most often as the result of chronic inflammatory reaction with cellular necrosis, inspissation of debris, and deposition of calcific deposits. Although prostatic calculi may be scattered through the gland, they most often occur near the periphery of the prostate, lying in a cleavage plane between the adenomatous periurethral glands and the fibromuscular capsule; the stony hard induration produced may be mistaken for prostatic carcinoma. Bacteria may be trapped in the interstices of prostatic calculi, contributing to perpetuation of prostatitis. Treatment is dictated by the clinical course.

Tuberculous Prostatitis. Tuberculosis of the prostate gland does not occur as an isolated entity. Genitourinary tuberculosis is always secondary to a primary infection, either pulmonary or gastrointestinal. Tubercle bacilli are transmitted hematogenously, usually to the kidney and thence to the ureter, bladder, prostate, and other genitourinary organs. Digital examination of the prostate may disclose stony hard induration, reminiscent of carcinoma or prostatic calculi. The diagnosis is established by demonstration of tubercle bacilli in the urine or by prostatic biopsy. Medical management is indicated, employing various combinations of effective antituberculous drugs.

Miscellaneous Prostatic Infections. Other inflammatory processes in the prostate gland are encountered less frequently. Blastomycosis and actinomycosis have been reported as causes of chronic prostatitis, and treatment of these conditions may require surgical extirpation of the prostate gland. Candidiasis involving the urethra and prostate is usually alleviated by simple urinary acidification with concomitant treatment of the involved sexual partner. *Trichomonas vaginalis* may infest the prostate gland and produce symptoms and findings similar to those of chronic, nonspecific prostatitis, with the diagnosis being established by identification of trichomonads in the urine or prostatic secretions. A 10-day course of anti-*Trichomonas* chemotherapy for both sexual partners will usually eradicate the infestation. *Chlamydia* has been identified as the infecting organism by cell culture methods. Tetracycline derivatives are usually the treatment of choice.

Benign Prostatic Hypertrophy[6, 7]

Benign prostatic overgrowth is the most common cause of bladder outlet obstruction in men older than 50 years of age. Although exact mechanisms of prostatic hyperplasia are incompletely appreciated, it is recognized that adolescent development of the glandular acini and the fibromuscular matrix of the prostate is stimulated by gonadotropins and the androgens of the interstitial cells of the testes. After the age of 60, androgen production diminishes and glandular hypertrophy and hyperplasia of the prostate occur, progressing with advancing age. Typically, the glandular elements surrounding the prostatic urethra centrally—analogous to the periurethral glands of the female urethra—undergo spheroidal proliferation. The true acinar glands of the prostate and the fibromuscular capsule of the gland are displaced peripherally and compressed as the adenomatous hyperplasia progresses. A lobular pattern of growth is observed, with the hyperplastic process involving the two lateral lobes of the gland and the median lobe.

As the enlargement progresses, the prostatic urethra may become elongated and the caliber of the prostatic portion of the urethra may actually increase. However, the adenomatous process causes compression of the prostatic urethra, restricting the free flow of urine, sometimes associated with actual mechanical intrusion of a median lobe at the vesical outlet. Mechanical pressure phenomena then may include upward displacement of the base of the bladder, *fishhooking* of the lower ureters due to trigonal displacement, hypertrophy of the bladder wall with trabeculation, cellule formation, and even diverticula of the bladder. Complete bladder outlet obstruction may result in decompensation of the detrusor muscle and total urinary retention.

The symptoms of benign prostatic hyperplasia are those of mechanical obstruction and the consequences of urinary stasis. In the early stages of prostatic enlargement, the patient complains of diminished size and force of the urinary stream. As obstruction progresses, there is increasing frequency of urination, probably owing to pressure of the enlarging gland beneath the trigone of the bladder. Nocturia is a similar index of the mechanical pressure of the enlarging prostate. It should be noted that nocturia normally occurs in older patients, both men and women, partially as a result of the inability of the kidney to concentrate urine, with resultant excretion of larger nocturnal volumes. However, nocturia more than once or twice nightly in the elderly male suggests mechanical pressure of prostatic enlargement, as well as the possibility that the bladder is emptying incompletely with each voiding. Later, the patient with prostatic obstruction may note hesitancy and intermittency of the urinary stream, occasioned by intermittent fluttering occlusion of the prostatic urethra by the hypertrophic lateral lobes. Terminal dribbling suggests both residual urine and pooling of urine within the prostatic urethra.

Urinary bleeding may first bring the patient to seek a physician. Hematuria may be caused by prostatic enlargement with engorgement of the small mucosal vessels covering the adenomatous gland, ruptured as a consequence of straining to urinate. With progressive residual urine, infection may occur with purulent cystitis. Similarly, vesical stasis of urine can predispose to the formation of bladder calculi with severe symptoms of dysuria and stranguria. Occasionally, patients may have few symptoms of bladder outlet obstruction, the syndrome of silent prostatism. Residual urine volumes of 1000 ml. or more may produce a palpable lower abdominal mass before the patient experiences any particular symptoms, and it is not uncommon to observe bilateral hydroureteronephrosis and evidence of impending renal failure with azotemia and electrolyte imbalance.

The diagnosis of prostatic hypertrophy with bladder outlet obstruction is suggested by the history and is confirmed by careful physical and ancillary examinations. Rectal examination will reveal varying degrees of prostatic enlargement,

most often symmetric with the prostate and rubbery. As enlargement progresses, the gland protrudes posteriorly, compressing the anterior rectal wall and sometimes producing symptoms of constipation. The size of the gland may bear little relationship to the degree of symptomatic difficulty incurred by the patient, with a small gland often completely obstructing the bladder outlet whereas a large prostate, three or four times normal size, may produce few obstructive symptoms. Palpation of the distended bladder suggests incomplete emptying with significant residual urine. Cystourethroscopy confirms the presence of prostatic enlargement and permits assessment of the degree of occlusion of the bladder neck or prostatic urethra and the degree of bladder trabeculation and cellule or diverticulum formation. Azotemia may occur insidiously with bladder outlet obstruction, and the usual measurements of blood urea nitrogen, serum creatinine, and creatinine clearance provide indices of renal functional capacity. Thorough urodynamic study will confirm both the absence of primary bladder or neurologic problems and the presence of outlet obstruction. Occasional secondary bladder instability is also demonstrated by these studies.

Conservative and medical measures of managing benign prostatic enlargement with bladder outlet obstruction are generally unsuccessful. Prostatic massage and urethral dilation are of little value unless there is demonstrated substantial congestion and stricture formation, respectively. Anticholinergic drugs and antihistamines should be avoided because they may precipitate urinary retention. Occasionally, estrogens in small dosage may induce minimal improvement in the urinary stream, presumably through the mechanism of some prostatic shrinkage, but in general hormonal measures have been ineffective in benign prostatic hypertrophy.

The decision for surgical intervention in benign prostatic enlargement is reached after evaluation of a variety of factors. Indications for a surgical procedure include residual urine of more than 100 ml., particularly when there is associated azotemia of any degree; persistent or recurrent urinary infection refractory to usual therapeutic methods; gross hematuria on more than one occasion; acute urinary retention; and chronic urinary retention with overflow dribbling. Most urologic surgeons would add the factors of patient comfort and desire for an operation with nocturia more than two or three times nightly interfering with rest and diurnal urinary frequency.

There are four standard surgical procedures for removal of the obstructing enlarged portion of the prostate gland (Fig. 46–3). None of these procedures constitutes total prostatectomy; all of them are designed for removal of the adenomatous hyperplastic portion of the gland, lying centrally and periurethrally. Hence, these procedures should most properly be termed *prostatic adenectomy* rather than prostatectomy because the true prostate, compressed laterally into a fibromuscular and acinar surgical capsule, is retained after removal of the central adenomatous elements and may be the source of later carcinoma of the prostate.

Suprapubic Prostatectomy. Historically, the suprapubic or transvesical method of enucleating the prostatic adenoma was the first to be employed. Although used with less frequency today, this procedure still constitutes a fundamental method of surgical treatment in benign prostatic hypertrophy. A suprapubic incision, either vertical or transverse, gives access to the anterior surface of the bladder, which is then opened to give exposure of the vesical neck and the underlying prostate. From inside the bladder, the mucosa surrounding the bladder neck is incised and the adenomatous elements are removed by the establishment of a cleavage plane between the benign prostatic hypertrophy and the peripheral surgical capsule. Re-epithelialization occurs by growth of mucosa into the prostatic fossa from the trigone

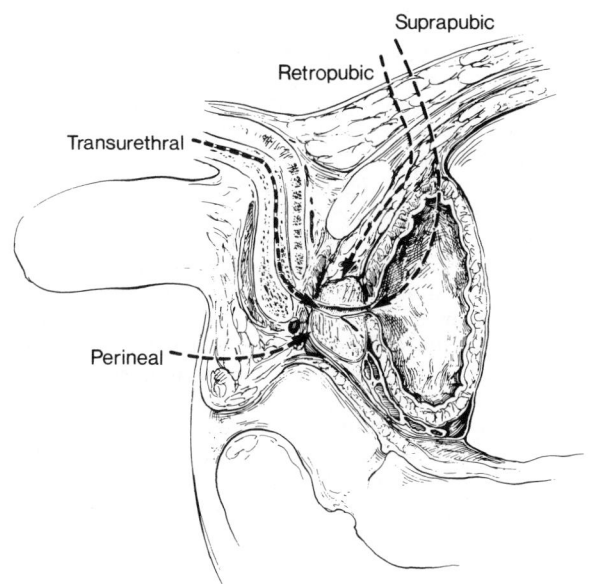

Suprapubic

Retropubic

Transurethral

Perineal

Figure 46–3. The four basic surgical enucleative procedures for benign prostatic hypertrophy: perineal prostatectomy, suprapubic prostatectomy, retropubic prostatectomy, and transurethral resection of the prostate.

and bladder neck, as well as from the membranous urethra below.

Perineal Prostatectomy. Perineal enucleation of the hyperplastic prostate was popularized at the turn of the century by Young. Perineal prostatectomy is particularly suitable to the large, low-lying prostate. The patient is placed in the extreme lithotomy position, giving access to the perineum, where a transverse incision in the shape of an inverted U is made anterior to the rectum. The rectum is separated from the posterior aspect of the prostate. The prostatic capsule is incised, and sharp and blunt dissection is employed to free the adenoma from the interior of the prostatic surgical capsule. The adenoma is amputated from the urethra distally and at the bladder neck. Hemostasis is effected with absorbable suture material at the vesical neck. A Foley catheter is inserted into the bladder through the urethra, and the capsulotomy opening is closed to re-establish continuity. The perineal procedure carries a lower mortality and morbidity rate than suprapubic prostatectomy. The procedure offers the advantage of good control of bleeding, and it is thought that the extreme lithotomy position promotes venous return and minimizes vascular complications.

Transurethral Prostatic Resection. The emergence of endoscopic transurethral surgery was dependent on the development of adequate lens systems, the incandescent bulb, and later fiberoptics, the refinement of electrical current for purposes of cutting and coagulation, and the ingenious combination of these advances into instruments satisfactory for surgical purposes. Transurethral prostatectomy has become the most commonly employed form of surgical treatment of benign prostatic hypertrophy with obstruction. Endoscopic resection of the enlarged prostate is most suitable for the smaller prostatic adenomas, those under 40 or 50 gm. in total resectable weight. It is better to resect the smaller fibrotic glands than to attempt difficult open surgical enucleative procedures.

The resectoscope sheath is introduced into the bladder, and the working element is positioned. Under direct vision, the wire loop is employed to cut away fragments of the obstructing adenoma. These fragments are subsequently evacuated from the urinary bladder. Constant irrigation is required, employing a nonelectrolytic, isotonic irrigant of satisfactory

optical properties. An isotonic solution must be employed, because fluid extravasated into the circulation may cause hemolysis with subsequent acute tubular necrosis. The electrical current passed through the wire loop may be modified as a high-frequency, high-amplitude cutting current or as a low-frequency, low-amplitude coagulating current for control of bleeding.

Retropubic Prostatectomy. The retropubic route to prostatic enucleation was popularized by Millin and is ideally suited to the high-lying larger gland with little if any intravesical component. The patient is placed in the supine position, and a transverse suprapubic incision is made. The anterior surface of the prostate is exposed, and the surgical capsule is incised transversely. Under direct vision, enucleation of the adenomatous portion of the gland is initiated by sharp and blunt dissection. After the adenoma is removed, the catheter is passed through the urethra and the prostatic capsule is closed. The procedure is modified by some surgeons who prefer to employ a vertical capsulotomy, extending the incision superiorly on the anterior surface of the bladder to gain added exposure of the bladder neck and the interior of the bladder itself. There are no contraindications to such an incision, which transects the region of the vesical neck, and exposure may be improved by this approach, particularly when there is a median lobe extending intravesically.

Long-term complications after a prostatic procedure for benign adenomatous hyperplasia are relatively minimal. Because the surgical capsule is retained, sexual potency is usually unaltered, sometimes even improved, by these enucleative procedures. Urinary incontinence may occur as a permanent result of any form of prostatectomy for benign enlargement, but the incidence of true and total urinary incontinence is minimal, probably no more than 1%. The retained surgical capsule may afford an opportunity for regrowth of further adenomatous tissue. A small percentage of patients undergoing transurethral resection may have recurrent prostatic obstruction at a later date, necessitating another operative intervention, whereas recurrent adenomatous obstruction is seen with less frequency after the open procedures.

Occasionally, a fibrotic process can involve the entire vesical neck without significant benign prostatic hypertrophy but can cause the same outlet obstruction. This may occur with or without surgical procedures involving the prostate or vesical neck. This bladder neck contracture can be treated both by open means such as a Bradford-Young YV-plasty and probably much more simply by a transurethral incision of the bladder neck down through the scar tissue to the muscle to allow complete opening of the vesical neck and relief of obstruction.

Carcinoma of the Prostate[6, 7, 19]

Adenocarcinoma of the prostate is the most common malignant disease of men. The incidence of this cancer has increased. Cancer of the prostate is now the most prevalent cancer in men by the most recent American Cancer Society statistics. It barely exceeds cancer of the lung, with 21% of all male cancers. Autopsy studies have established the fact that prostatic carcinoma, occult or overt, is present in about 15% of men older than 50 years of age. It is estimated that the prevalence rate of prostatic carcinoma may be up to 48 cases per 100,000 population, and as the geriatric population increases, an increase in the number of cases of this disease should be expected. Squamous cell carcinoma of the prostate remains a relatively rare occurrence, and sarcoma of the prostate, still rarer, is generally seen only in the first two decades of life.

The etiology of prostatic carcinoma remains unknown, and although carcinoma of the prostate frequently coexists with benign prostatic hypertrophy, they are not believed to be causally related. There are no definite carcinogens known to be responsible for prostatic carcinoma; a viral etiology has been suggested but not verified. There also appears to be no correlation between chronic prostatitis and prostatic calculi and the ultimate development of prostatic carcinoma. It is possible that alterations in the estrogen-androgen balance and metabolic alterations in the prostate may play a role, but the exact clinical significance of these changes remains to be established. Sexual activity is apparently not a factor, because prostatic carcinoma has been observed in both celibate groups and in men with histories of excessive sexual activity.

Prostatic carcinoma most often has its origin in glandular acini of the peripheral group of glands located in the posterior and posterolateral regions of the prostate. It appears that the adenocarcinoma of the prostate does originate in glands that are metabolically and biologically active, although the acinar elements of the fibromuscular surgical capsule of the peripheral prostate are often atrophic. There are variations in biologic activity of prostate cancers among those persons in whom the malignant lesion is peripheral as opposed to those who have a more centrally located paraurethral tumor, suggesting that different groups of glandular elements within the prostate may give rise to tumors of varying malignant potential.

One of the unique qualities of prostatic carcinoma is that many tumors produce an enzyme, acid phosphatase, which can be detected in the serum of patients with metastatic disease or at least a very large local lesion. Serum acid phosphatase has many sources, but the addition of tartrate to the serum inhibits over 90% of the prostatic contribution and thereby separates the prostatic acid phosphatase from the total acid phosphatase. Because acid phosphatase is richly concentrated in normal prostatic tissue, prostatic examination or massage may elevate the serum level for up to 36 hours after rectal examination. Normal levels of serum acid phosphatase do not rule out prostatic carcinoma, because patients with small local lesions may not exhibit acid phosphatase elevation, prostatic tumors of low order of metabolic activity or great dedifferentiation may not produce such elevations, and even patients with advanced osteoblastic metastatic disease may on occasion display normal serum acid phosphatase values.

The prostate gland is also known to be the source of fibrinolytic factors. Normal seminal fluid has significant fibrinolytic activity, possibly enhancing motility of the sperm and attributed to the release of fibrinolytic activators from prostatic epithelium. Plasminogen, the precursor of plasmin, is a fibrinolytic protease found in many tissues, including the prostate. In prostatic carcinoma, increased fibrinolytic activity predisposes to spontaneous bleeding and hemorrhage, particularly after prostatic surgery. Prostatic carcinoma may predispose to increased production of plasminogen, although the source of fibrinolytic activity in the blood of patients with prostatic carcinoma has not yet been identified.

Unfortunately, early symptoms of prostatic carcinoma are lacking. Because the majority of prostatic tumors occur in the periphery of the gland, encroachment on the urethra is a late manifestation of the disease. Irritative obstructive symptoms therefore do not signal the presence of the cancer, and it is only in advanced prostatic carcinoma that the lower tract symptoms occur. Occasionally, the patients may present with bone pain (usually lumbosacral) as a manifestation of metastatic disease long before local urologic symptoms occur. There is no satisfactory screening method for prostatic carcinoma other than routine and regular rectal examination.

In essence, the diagnosis of prostatic carcinoma must be based on suspicion. Every man older than the age of 50 should have a regular rectal examination, and the findings of areas of induration and irregularity should suggest the diagnosis. Characteristically, prostatic carcinoma is stony hard and must be differentiated from focal tuberculosis, granulomatous prostatitis, and prostatic calculi. The isolated prostatic nodule must be regarded with the highest suspicion and the appropriate diagnostic maneuvers be undertaken, including serum acid phosphatase and prostatic specific antigen determination, skeletal bone films, and radionuclide bone scan, but most importantly an appropriate form of biopsy. In advanced cases of local disease there is usually little doubt as to the diagnosis. The prostate becomes nodular and irregular with extension of the indurated process beyond the confines of the gland, culminating in fixation of the prostate to the surrounding pelvic structures. At this stage of the disease, the patient is often experiencing significant symptoms, not necessarily local urinary tract symptoms.

Definition of the stage of prostatic disease is aided by ancillary clinical and laboratory determinations. A long bone survey may disclose metastatic lesions. As an adjunct to a bone survey that may be negative, radionuclide bone scans are helpful in demonstrating tumor metastases. Serum acid phosphatase determination constitutes a necessary step in diagnostic evaluation because an elevated acid phosphatase value certainly suggests metastatic disease, precluding cure by local therapy, be it either radical prostatic surgery or radiation therapy. Prostatic ultrasonography has been developed as a technology useful for the staging of prostatic cancer patients if not the screening of selected populations of male patients.

Occasionally, intravenous urography and cystourethrography are useful in evaluating degrees of lower tract obstruction or obstruction of the ureters by advanced carcinoma.

The metastatic patterns of carcinoma of the prostate are unique and interesting. The most common manifestations of metastatic disease are bony lesions in the sacrum and lumbar spine, although it is thought that earlier metastases occur at the regional lymph nodes, supporting the rationale of staging pelvic lymphadenectomy to assess the obturator, hypogastric, and iliac nodes for the presence of disease as a method of establishing extent and anatomic stage of prostatic carcinoma. Paradoxical metastases to the brain and skull with no intervening metastatic lesions in the lung or other bones may occur through Batson's plexus, the spinal venous system that communicates directly with the periprostatic veins. Pulmonary lesions may be isolated nodular metastatic defects but are more often of an interstitial pattern or diffuse multiple seedlike lesions reminiscent of miliary tuberculosis. In advanced stages of the disease, metastatic adenocarcinoma of the prostate may be observed in virtually every organ, including such unlikely sites as the testes, the skin of the scrotum, and the adrenal glands.

Prostatic carcinoma can metastasize by either local extension, hematologic dissemination, or lymphatic invasion, and metastasis may occur early even with a very small lesion, although generally the size of the primary lesion correlates with degree of metastatic extent of the disease. The treatment of prostatic carcinoma at the present time is selected on the basis of accurate anatomic definition of the stage of the disease. It is the general feeling that local disease that has not escaped the confines of the prostate is best treated by surgical extirpation. The potential for surgical cure of early carcinoma of the prostate was clearly demonstrated shortly after the turn of the century. Radical prostatectomy involving removal of the entire prostate and the seminal vesicles can constitute cure only when the malignant process is confined to the prostate with no contiguous or distant spread. It is estimated that as many as 10% of the patients presenting with prostatic carcinoma are in such an early stage amenable to cure by radical operation. In general, the indications for radical prostatectomy include the isolated and localized prostatic malignant process, anticipated life expectancy of 10 years or more, good general health in the patient with no other life-threatening ancillary disease, and the absence of indication of metastatic disease evaluated by bone survey, radionucleotide bone scans, multiple serum acid phosphatase determinations, and negative pelvic lymphadenectomy.

Prostatectomy can be accomplished in the classic perineal fashion or by the retropubic approach during which both pelvic lymphadenectomy and radical prostatectomy can be carried out at the same time if the surgeon is willing to base his or her surgical decisions on frozen section. Complications of radical prostatectomy include impotence, a small percentage of urinary incontinence, occasional rectal injury, and a surgical mortality of approximately 1%. However, the efficacy of radical prostatectomy, given accurate tumor staging, is apparent in various reports recording a 60% 10-year survival after radical perineal prostatectomy as compared with a 22% 10-year survival with palliative therapy and a 30% 10-year survival with hormonal manipulation measures.

The use of radiation therapy for the curative treatment of local disease is attractive, and some evidence is available that suggests equivalent survivals for surgical versus radiation therapy for localized prostatic carcinoma. There are a number of studies that use external beam radiation therapy with various doses and fields, as well as interstitial radiation therapy with iodine-125 seed implantation. Careful follow-up is needed with regard to specific anatomic tumor staging, disease control failure, patient morbidity, and ultimate survival before these studies can be matched with a surgical series. Radiation therapy, however, does have an important role in the management of bone pain from metastatic disease and may offer palliation for patients with large local disease who are not candidates for radical surgery. The attractiveness of radiation therapy for the management of local disease creates hope that the precise place of this modality in the treatment of carcinoma of the prostate will be clearly defined in the near future.

Observations more than 50 years ago led to the recognition of the androgen dependency of a large percentage of prostatic tumors and the therapeutic response of these tumors to estrogen administration. These observations and subsequent investigations demonstrated the efficacy of hormonal management and provided the basis for the first genuinely effective chemotherapeutic approach to malignant disease. Although hormonal manipulation cannot affect cure of prostatic carcinoma, excellent prolonged tumor control can be achieved. The administration of exogenous estrogens, bilateral orchiectomy, pituitary ablation, or use of androgen synthesis inhibitors or antiandrogens may affect androgen-dependent tumors. The most efficacious methods are bilateral orchiectomy and the use of exogenous estrogens such as diethylstilbestrol. However, there is evidence that the use of combination drugs such as leuprolide and flutamide may be equivalent to orchiectomy and flutamide.

If exogenous estrogens such as diethylstilbestrol are considered, doses of diethylstilbestrol should be carefully managed because doses as small as 1 mg. per day do not produce anorchic levels of serum testosterone, but it is clear that doses as high as 5 mg. per day may have an adverse effect on the cardiovascular system. Therefore, the present recommended dose of diethylstilbestrol is approximately 3 mg. per day, but the long-term effects on the cardiovascular system have not been established. It is thought by a number of investigators that hormonal treatment, because of its potential side effects, should be withheld until the patient becomes symptomatic because it appears that on a statistical basis, longevity is not particularly affected by adjunctive therapies. Therefore, hormonal treatment should be reserved for symptomatic states. A new area of adjunctive therapy is the use of multiple chemotherapeutic agents. A number of drugs, including 5-fluorouracil, estramustine phosphate, and cisplatin, have been used in various protocols with some success in terms of partial objective and subjective responses. Major effects of these drugs are bone marrow suppression, gastrointestinal toxicity, and nephrotoxicity. Considering the rapid development of new chemotherapeutic agents, this is an area that may have the greatest impact over the next 10 years on the treatment of metastatic prostatic carcinoma and even as an adjunctive treatment for localized disease.

In summary, the treatment of carcinoma of the prostate is dependent primarily on establishment of correct anatomic definition of the disease. Disease that is confined to the single organ site of the prostate is best controlled by radical surgical removal. Disease outside of the prostate should be treated depending on the patient's symptomatology or physiologic abnormalities caused by the tumor. The timing of the treatment remains controversial. It seems reasonable to withhold adjunctive therapy, including androgen deprivation, until the rate of the disease progression is identified or the patient becomes symptomatic from his malignant disease.

MALE URETHRA[15, 17]

Congenital Abnormalities

Congenital abnormalities in the male urethra can occur anywhere—the bladder neck, prostatic urethra, membranous urethra, bulbous urethra, pendulous urethra, or meatus. The most common distal abnormality is urethral meatal stenosis, which can usually be recognized by inspection and suspected when the urinary stream is of poor caliber. Such stenoses may predispose to infection and be associated with enuresis. Simple meatotomy usually cures the stenosis. Other congenital strictures can be seen in the bulbous or pendulous urethra but are usually uncommon. Open surgical repair is preferred in longer strictures, whereas lesser areas of involvement can be satisfactorily handled by internal urethrotomy. In the area of the bulbous and membranous urethra there are also occurrences of diverticula, which may be a source of infection or by a flap valve effect obstruction. Open surgical incision in primary repair of the urethra is necessary. Duplication of the anterior urethra, either incomplete or complete, may occur with subsequent symptoms of potential obstruction, infection, or double stream.

In the area of the prostatic urethra, congenital valves occur, usually causing severe obstructive uropathy with decompensation of the urinary bladder, hydroureteronephrosis, infection, and renal insufficiency unless prompt and adequate treatment is instituted. Valves are mucosal or fibrous folds obstructing urethral urinary flow; they are usually in the distal portion of the prostatic urethra at the level of the verumontanum and occur in several configurations. Transurethral electroresection or destruction by fulguration is most often employed and is much preferable to the older retropubic transprostatic open exposure. The spectrum of secondary problems associated with urethral valves is wide but may be so severe that temporary or permanent urinary diversion is required.

Another anomaly of the urethra is called hypospadias, which involves varying degrees of failure of complete development of the distal urethra. The urethra may terminate just proximal to the glans (glandular hypospadias), at some point along the penile shaft (penile hypospadias), at the anterior margin of the scrotum (penoscrotal hypospadias), or in the perineum with a bifid scrotum (perineal hypospadias). Associated with this defect is a severe ventral curvature of the penis, or chordee, which results from a fibrous band occurring in the projected course of the urethra. The embryologic defect is a failure of closure of the urethral groove. In extreme cases, particularly if there is associated bilateral testicular maldescent, the configuration of the genitalia may be so ambiguous that an intersex state results.

Early and accurate diagnosis is imperative. Nearly all degrees of hypospadias demand surgical repair, for cosmetic as well as functional reasons. A variety of operative procedures are available depending on the severity of the defect and may involve single- or multiple-stage urethroplasties. The principal difficulty encountered in surgical repair of hypospadias with surgical chordee relates to achieving adequate penile straightening, which is imperative before urethral reconstruction is effected. The commonly employed techniques of urethroplasty involve construction of a skin tube from the original orifice to the coronal margin or the tip of the glans. Because hypospadias and chordee are universally associated with splaying of the glans and a hooded redundant dorsal foreskin, the glans can be reconstructed in conjunction with the urethroplasty, and the redundant dorsal foreskin can be mobilized and brought ventrally as a neourethra. The operative complications of urethroplasties of all sorts include fistula and stricture, both of which may be managed by relatively minor secondary surgical procedures.

Epispadias is the failure of development of the anterior wall of the urethra and concomitant failure of dorsal fusion of the penile corpora. Complete vesical exstrophy, a rare condition, is always associated with epispadias; epispadias alone with some degree of urinary continence is more commonly seen, although still infrequent. The urethral opening may lie anywhere from the vesical neck to the glans, but if it is distal to the prostatic urethra, urinary continence and control may be satisfactory. The severe cosmetic deformity and the associated difficulty in controlling the urinary stream demand surgical correction, usually accomplished in infancy. Plastic reconstruction and lengthening of the penis, closure and ventral inversion of the urethra, and reconstruction of the bladder neck are often satisfactory. Unless there is a complete failure of urinary control, urinary diversion is not necessary and with newer artificial urinary sphincters may never be necessary.

Trauma

Traumatic injury of the urethra commonly occurs in association with pelvic fractures but also can occur with injuries to the perineum, gunshot or stab wounds, or iatrogenic injury from instrumentation. Shearing injuries induced by external forces during blunt trauma cause rupture at the urogenital diaphragm in the region of the membranous urethra. Urinary extravasation is noted, often with extensive pelvic hemorrhage. The prostate and bladder may be displaced superiorly, well away from the distal urethra. Urethral catheterization is often impossible and is contraindicated in many centers under such circumstances because a partial tear could be converted to a complete tear if undue force is used. Depending on the circumstances, either open surgical repair or temporizing suprapubic urinary diversion should be accomplished promptly. The diagnosis of urethral rupture must be suspected in every instance of pelvic injury, and unless the patient is able to void clear urine in a normal fashion, a retrograde urethrogram should be undertaken in an aseptic fashion to determine the patency and competence of the urethra. If the urethra is normal, certainly a catheter can be passed to accomplish a cystogram, but if the urethra is abnormal, the bladder should be assessed either by the cystogram phase of an intravenous pyelogram or with an open surgical

procedure. Untreated urethral rupture, whether partial or complete, can result in urethral stricture and possible urinary incontinence.

Penetrating injuries of the urethra are also observed, most commonly due to gunshot or stab wounds. Immediate urethral reconstruction and urinary diversion by suprapubic cystostomy are appropriate. Similarly, straddle injuries to the perineum may cause urethral rupture on the ventral surface, which usually demands prompt surgical intervention and urethral stenting with a fenestrated catheter for at least 7 to 10 days. Iatrogenic perforation or rupture of the urethra may occur in the course of instrumentation, cystoscopy, or urethral dilation. Pre-existing urethral strictures due to trauma or gonococcal urethritis predispose to difficult instrumentation and potential perforation of the urethra, often followed by the establishment of a urethral diverticulum or false urinary passage. Periurethral abscesses and attendant complications may ensue unless urethral injury of this sort is recognized and promptly treated. In the incidence of iatrogenic injury, suprapubic cystostomy or urinary diversion should be initiated along with an antibiotic.

Infections[18]

The urethra is subject to both gonococcal and nonspecific infections. Abnormalities of the urethra such as urethral stenosis, acquired stricture, urethral diverticulum, or other structural abnormalities predispose to the development of urethritis and complicate management. It is often necessary to treat the anatomic abnormalities at the same time the infection is treated to achieve maximum control of the infectious process. Acute gonococcal urethritis occurs when gonococci are introduced into the urethra, finding an appropriate milieu in the relatively hypoxic recesses of the periurethral glands. Squamous cells are relatively resistant to infection so that the fossa navicularis is rarely involved. Infestation of the periurethral glands tends to lead to microabscesses, which may extend into the tissues of the corpus spongiosum. Characteristic symptoms of gonococcal urethritis include dysuria, frequency, and urethral discharge that is usually creamy white, exhibiting the typical gram-negative diplococci on the stained smear. Specific gonococcal cultures of the urethral discharge confirm the diagnosis. Treatment of acute gonococcal urethritis is with the use of penicillin, ampicillin, or relatively large doses of the tetracyclines. The rapid development of resistant organisms prompts perusal of the most up-to-date bulletin from the Centers for Disease Control and Prevention.

Secondary associated gram-negative infections may demand adjunctive antibiotic therapy. Untreated acute gonococcal urethritis may lead to urethral stricture through the mechanism of fibrosis and cicatrix formation, and such gonococcal strictures then predispose the development of posterior urethritis, prostatitis, and epididymitis, which may be refractory to general methods of management.

The term *nonspecific urethritis* refers to urethral infections in which no evidence of gonorrhea can be found. Nonspecific urethritis can be due to bacteria, a virus, *Chlamydia*, or a fungus. The typical complaint of the patient with nonspecific urethritis is the urethral discharge of clear mucus, particularly in the early morning, associated with some degree of urinary frequency and burning discomfort on urination. Prostatitis may or may not accompany the urethritis. Treatment is usually with one of the tetracycline derivatives.

Malignant Disease

Carcinoma of the male urethra is rare, with fewer than 1000 cases being documented in the English literature. Those malignant lesions occurring in the distal penile portion of the urethra are most often squamous cell carcinoma, while the more proximal tumors are transitional cell lesions. Symptoms of urethral malignant disease are hematuria, dysuria, frequency, and possible ultimate urinary retention. The diagnosis is established by endoscopic visualization of the lesion and appropriate biopsy either cystoscopically or by open biopsy of a palpable lesion. Spread of the malignancy is by lymphatics of the corpus spongiosum into the deep pelvic nodes and by venous channels. Because the diagnosis is usually established late in the course of the disease, the prognosis is poor despite radical surgical intervention. Depending on the location of the lesion, partial urethrectomy with or without penectomy may be effective as well as possible anterior exenteration and lymphadenectomy. Radiation therapy and chemotherapeutic measures are presently unproven as effective therapeutic modalities, but the development of new chemotherapeutic agents or combinations of agents may be helpful in the future. Because a high percentage of patients with carcinoma of the urethra give a history of previous venereal disease or urethral stricture, any stricture that fails to respond to appropriate therapy should be thoroughly investigated.

PENIS[6, 7, 15]

Congenital Anomalies

It is fortunate that congenital anomalies of the penis (other than hypospadias) are rare because abnormalities of the genitalia may be the cause of severe anxiety and psychologic stress not only to the patient but also to the parents of the male newborn. Rare anomalies of the penis include duplication (double penis), complete transposition of the penis and scrotum, and congenital absence of the penis in an otherwise normal male. The latter condition is probably best treated by a sex conversion operation, because there is no adequate surgical method for reconstruction of a satisfactory erectile phallus. A persistently small penis despite normal growth in an otherwise normal male is called microphallus and can be treated fairly successfully medically.

The most common congenital curvature of the penis is chordee, which is caused by a fibrous band along the ventral aspect of the penis and is usually associated with hypospadias, the congenital defect of the distal urethra. Epispadias, congenital absence of the upper portion of the urethra, causes dorsal deflection and curvature of the penis. In addition, abnormalities of the investing Buck's fascia may cause asymmetry with various lateral deviations. There is also an entity known as torsion in which the actual defect is in the investing skin and can be corrected by rotation of penile skin.

The normal foreskin of the penis provides a covering for the glans, the redundant portion of the foreskin being termed the *prepuce*. In many newborns, the prepuce cannot be retracted satisfactorily; infection and inflammatory reaction may occur as well as edema, fibrosis, and scarring, preventing retraction of the foreskin, or phimosis. Obstruction to urination may occur, causing urinary tract infection. Such chronic inflammation is believed to predispose to penile malignancy. In the past, prophylactic infant circumcision has been widely practiced, although in more recent years, universal necessity for such a routine circumcision has been questioned.

When phimosis leads to one of the previously mentioned complications, a dorsal slit of the foreskin may be required as an emergency measure, and circumcision should be accomplished at an appropriate time. Very often phimosis is accompanied by meatal stenosis, and a urethral meatotomy may be effected at the time of circumcision. If the contracted foreskin becomes retracted and trapped proximal to the glans, severe swelling and even necrosis of the glans may ensue, a condition known as paraphimosis. Emergency surgical intervention is necessary if the paraphimotic prepuce cannot be reduced manually; dorsal slit of the constricted foreskin is the procedure of choice.

Trauma

Trauma to the penis is relatively uncommon but can cause total sexual disability. In pelvic fracture, rupture of the urethra will cause extravasation of blood and urine in the penile tissues; treatment is indicated toward diversion of the urine. In the erect state, the penis is subject to dislocation or even fracture, the latter condition being rupture of one or both of the corpora cavernosa with severe bleeding and hematoma. Immediate surgical intervention is required to repair the laceration in the investing fascia.

Rupture of the veins of the penis may produce severe hemorrhage, and subcutaneous hematoma is usually best managed by urethral catheter drainage and compression dressings. Lacerations of the penile skin and the glans are not uncommon as a consequence of masturbation, manipulation, or sexual activity, and the frenulum of the penis occasionally tears with sexual intercourse. Avulsion of the penis and scrotal skin may occur when clothing is caught in various types of machinery, with the loose integument of the genitalia being avulsed rather readily. Split-thickness skin grafts to the penile shaft take well, and the cosmetic and functional results of such repairs are satisfactory, provided all distal loose skin is débrided at the time of the split-thickness grafting.

Complete traumatic amputation, whether intentional or unintentional, has occasionally been reported. It is treated by complete reanastomosis of all structures, including arteries, nerves, veins, and corporal bodies as well as the urethra, by microsurgical techniques.

Infections[18]

The penis is subject to infectious involvement by various venereal diseases as well as other pathogenic bacteria and viruses. The abundant blood supply of the penile skin predisposes to excellent healing of such lesions. However, furunculosis of the penis may lead to severe cellulitis and even infection of the erectile corpora of the penis; this is known as cavernositis and is most often due to urethritis of gonorrheal or nongonorrheal origin. Incision and drainage with appropriate antibiotic therapy constitutes the treatment of choice.

Inflammation of the glans penis and the prepuce constitutes balanoposthitis, which is most frequently the result of retained secretions and bacterial or fungal infection underneath the redundant prepuce, particularly when phimosis is present. Local irritative symptoms vary according to the severity of the infection, and it is thought that such chronic infections may predispose to squamous cell carcinoma of the penis. Dorsal slit of the foreskin, local measures, and antimicrobial agents are employed initially. After the inflammation has resolved, elective circumcision should be seriously considered.

Condyloma acuminatum is a cauliflower-like growth known as venereal wart, occurring singly or multiply on the prepuce and glans penis and within the urethra itself. The lesions are of viral origin and may be transmitted from one sexual partner to another. In cases of redundant foreskin, circumcision may be helpful in preventing recurrence, and in the past the topical application of 20% to 25% podophyllum in benzoin on superficial lesions on several successive occasions has been helpful. There appears to be an increased use of laser therapy for lesions on the glans or intraurethrally. Occasionally, the venereal warts may achieve such size that surgical excision is necessary. In advanced cases the differential diagnosis lies between condylomata acuminata and carcinoma of the penis.

Herpes progenitalis may appear as small reddened areas on the glans penis and dorsal surface of the penile shaft; these areas may become vesiculated, rupturing to leave superficial ulcerations as foci of secondary infection. These may be very small lesions, and in some cases, depending on the hematologic state of the patient, they may become extensive and debilitating. Small lesions, a common viral infection, are best managed by local cleansing and application of drying agents such as corn starch or baby powder, but the treatment of choice is acyclovir.

The principal venereal diseases (other than herpetic lesions) to involve the penis are syphilis and chancroid. The primary lesion of syphilis is a craterlike ulcer or chancre usually appearing around the corona of the glans penis. Darkfield smear of the lesion will reveal *Treponema pallidum*. Similar chancres may be caused by sporotrichosis and tularemia, but these lesions do not usually involve the penis. The penile lesion of chancroid is a soft ulcerated area, again usually on the distal portion of the penis and later associated with inguinal buboes. Gonorrhea does not produce external penile lesions, the primary involvement being of the urethra and periurethral glands. Granuloma inguinale and lymphogranuloma venereum involve the inguinal lymphatics.

Malignant Disease

Cancer of the penis is a rare tumor in the United States. It has a much higher proportion in populations where circumcision and personal hygiene are not well established. The most common form of cancer of the penis is squamous cell carcinoma, although basal cell carcinoma and melanoma have been described. Benign lesions such as nevi, hemangiomas, and papillomas are readily managed by local excision. Squamous cell carcinoma constitutes a more difficult challenge and is generally seen associated with chronic balanoposthitis from lack of circumcision, although occasional cases of penile carcinoma have been reported in circumcised persons. The lesion is frequently initially ignored by the patient or is hidden by the foreskin and possible phimosis. Treatment of the primary lesion is dependent on the extent identified at presentation and the status of the regional nodes. The Jackson classification defines Stage I, limited to the glans and prepuce; Stage II, invasion involving the shaft or corpora but without nodal or distant node metastases; Stage III, tumor confined to the shaft but with proven regional node metastases; and Stage IV, tumor invasive from the shaft with inoperable regional node metastases or with distant metastases.

Unfortunately, this classification does not allow cross comparison of results of different series, and a TNM classification is now under consideration for more accurately assessing the extent of the patient's disease at the time of diagnosis. Clearly, the lower the stage of tumor, the better the cure and survival rate, and this declines with increasing staging.

Diagnosis is established by biopsy. Treatment consists of partial or total penectomy; a proximal margin-free tumor of at least 1.5 cm. is desirable. Inguinal node dissection with excision of both superficial and deep inguinal nodes is advocated when clinically palpable nodes persist after amputation. Lymphadenopathy may occur from secondary infection seen in most cases of advanced penile carcinoma. Radiation therapy in squamous cell carcinoma of the penis is ineffective for large primary lesions but may be employed in the treatment of known lymph node metastatic disease; the primary

lesion should always be treated surgically. Chemotherapeutic efforts have been attempted with bleomycin either locally or systemically, in conjunction with other agents for very small lesions and carcinoma *in situ*, or as an adjunct to systemic disease. Cisplatin and methotrexate have been tested with some reasonable results; however, overall, with the exception of very small glandular lesions, the results have not been encouraging.

Special Conditions

Certain peculiar disorders of the penis or of penile function deserve special consideration, particularly because etiologic factors remain obscure in these disorders.

Peyronie's Disease. A localized induration of the fibrous investments of the penile shaft was first described by the French surgeon Peyronie more than 100 years ago. Despite adequate description and an abundance of clinical observation, the cause of the condition is unknown. A firm fibrotic thickening of the fascia of the corpora cavernosa is observed, usually involving the dorsolateral aspects of the penile shaft or the intracavernous septum between the corpora cavernosa, histologically similar to keloid or Dupuytren's contracture. The fibrous plaques themselves may be painless, but there is often compromise of erectile capacity of the penis with deviation of the penis on erection and pain as a consequence of this derangement.

Patients usually note the lesion by self-examination, and they may have experienced significant deviation of the penis that interferes with intromission and coitus. Progression is slow, and spontaneous remissions are observed. Treatment has been generally unsatisfactory, and recurrence, after local excision, has been noted. Therapy that has been used in the past includes vitamin E, potassium *para*-aminobenzoate (Potaba), systemic corticosteroid therapy, local injection of high corticosteroids, radiation therapy, and ultrasound therapy. Because the disease seems to remit on its own, there appears to be no clear evidence in any of these modalities of an advantage over time for natural resolution. However, if the patient is totally disabled and has long-term resistant disease, excision of the plaque with skin grafting, with or without the insertion of penile prostheses, has been advocated.

When the diagnosis of Peyronie's disease has been established, it is perhaps most important to reassure the patient that the process is not malignant and that in many cases the disease process is self-limiting with slow, if any, progression and perhaps resolution. Often anti-inflammatory agents alleviate some of the discomfort associated with the plaque for most patients, and although there is some penile deviation, sexual disability is not the rule.

Priapism. Prolonged pathologic and painful erection of the penis is termed *priapism*, in recognition of the Greek god of sexual excess, Priapus. Pelvic venous thrombosis predisposes to priapism, and such thrombosis is observed with certain metastatic malignant diseases, leukemia, pelvic trauma, sickle cell disease or trait, trauma to the corpora, or spinal cord injury. In the majority of patients, no definite etiologic factor can be identified and both local and neurovascular abnormalities have been incriminated as possible causes. Prompt recognition and therapy are essential because prolonged unrelieved priapism almost inevitably leads to subsequent permanent impotence from fibrosis of the corpora cavernosa.

Immediate sedation and analgesia sometimes relieves priapism, and continuous spinal anesthesia has been advocated as occasionally effective in the early hours of the condition. Current therapy consists of irrigating the corpora with vasoactive drugs. Failure of this treatment can be followed by the creation of a fistula between the corpora cavernosa and corpus spongiosum, opening the tunica between these bodies by incision through the glans penis because the corpus spongiosum is rarely obstructed in priapism.

Impotence. Although it is recognized that the aging process diminishes not only the libido but also the capacity of erection, many men remain potent throughout their lifetime. Potency in the elderly male may be related to psychologic factors as much as to general health. Disease processes may well affect the ability of any male to be potent, and male patients should be carefully questioned. Arteriosclerotic cardiovascular disease may compromise circulation to the corpora and, in addition, many of the drugs used to treat hypertension and cardiovascular disease may have a secondary effect on the ability to maintain an erection. Diabetes and other systemic disorders producing generalized neuropathies may diminish ability for erection. Impotence may be one of the earliest signs of Leriche's syndrome, which is thrombotic obstruction of the iliac arteries. The condition may be relieved by appropriate vascular operation. Spinal cord injuries may impair the capacity for erection as may prostatic operations, particularly perineal prostatic operation, which apparently compromises the pudendal nerves in some men undergoing such surgical treatment of benign prostatic enlargement. Most potent males undergoing prostatectomy remain potent postoperatively irrespective of the surgical method employed. Radical prostatectomy for malignant disease usually results in impotence, although there are modifications of radical prostatectomy that may leave the patients potent; the long-term results of radical prostatectomy as a cure for cancer have not been assessed.

Finally, certain drugs may impair erections and produce impotence, presumably by the adrenergic blocking effect of the medication. Despite knowledge of this spectrum of potential causes of the impotence, a large number of men who are otherwise healthy and who complain of an isolated problem of impotence must be suspected of having idiopathic or psychological difficulties. Psychological consultation is mandatory when the various physical causes of impotence have been eliminated. The use of nocturnal penile tumescence studies has been helpful in distinguishing some patients with purely psychological reasons for impotence from those with physiologic reasons for impotence. Injection of certain vasoactive drugs or penile prostheses may be possible choices of treatment.

Ejaculatory Disorders. One of the most distressing sexual disabilities of the young and middle-aged male may be premature ejaculation. Intromission may be scarcely achieved before ejaculation occurs, terminating the sexual act to the frustration of the patient and the partner. Certain organic and psychological factors can be incriminated; chronic prostatitis can increase irritability and predisposition to ejaculation, and long abstinence with attendant sexual excitation can initiate premature ejaculation. In most cases, however, the problem relates to inadequate sexual technique in the marital unit, and careful consultation and counseling may aid in overcoming premature ejaculation.

Another disorder of sexual function is retrograde ejaculation, occasionally seen as a consequence of neuromuscular disturbance of the vesical neck secondary to diabetes, spinal cord injury, and other causes of neuropathy but most often due to surgical alteration of the vesical neck. Prostatectomy by open and endoscopic means, transurethral resection of the bladder neck, vesical outlet reconstructive procedures, and even retroperitoneal surgery with autonomic nerve damage may diminish the capacity for closure of the bladder neck, an essential ingredient in normal ejaculation, with consequent retrograde flow of ejaculate into the bladder. Once such a surgical abnormality is incurred, little can be done to overcome retrograde ejaculation. In some patients, a trial of alpha-adrenergic drugs such as ephedrine or phenylpropanolamine may be tried to facilitate closure of the bladder neck. In some instances, gradual narrowing of the bladder neck over a period of 1 or 2 years after prostatectomy promotes more normal ejaculation. Retrograde ejaculation in no way diminishes sexual gratification, but it may, of course, be the cause of infertility because the sperm are deposited in the bladder rather than being expelled through the urethra.

Intersex States. The intersex state is a congenital condition in which there is ambiguity of the external genitalia or inadequate and incomplete differentiation in gonadal and ductal structures. The most common mode of presentation of the intersex patient is by request for sexual differentiation in the neonatal nursery. Ambiguity of the external genitalia necessitates prompt and definitive assignment of sex, reassurance of parents, and early mobilization of medical and surgical measures required to establish the appropriate sex of the child. On occasion, the intersex patient may be seen late, often because of microphallus, undescended testes, labial fusion, or clitoral hypertrophy noted as late as pubescence.

SELECTED REFERENCES

Bennett, A. H.: Impotence: Diagnosis and Management of Erectile Function. Philadelphia, W. B. Saunders, 1994.
The epidemiology, pathogenesis, psychological impact, and medical and surgical aspects of this common disorder are very well discussed with up-to-date concepts of management.

Gillenwater, J., Grayhack, J., Howards, S., and Duckett, J.: Adult and Pediatric Urology, 3rd ed. St. Louis, Mosby–Year Book, 1995.
This recently published two-volume compendium of adult and pediatric urology provides an excellent updating of current knowledge in both adult and pediatric urology. New sections have been added on specialized subjects such as gynecology, laser therapy, new imaging technologies, and new treatments for stone disease.

Glenn, J. F., and Graham, S. D.: Urologic Surgery, 4th ed. Philadelphia, J. B. Lippincott, 1991.
This text provides an excellent descriptive and artistic presentation of the vast variety of surgical techniques and procedures used in the treatment of urologic disease. The history, methods of diagnosis, indications, and complications of surgery are also well documented. This is an excellent reference text for all forms of urologic surgery.

Kelalis, P. P., King, L. R., and Belman, A. B.: Clinical Pediatric Urology, 3rd ed. Philadelphia, W. B. Saunders, 1992.
The complexities of sexual differentiation in the intersex states are fully presented in this compendium. The normal processes of sexual differentiation are emphasized, and the chromosomal and endocrinologic abnormalities associated with intersex are elaborated. A rational approach to the diagnosis and treatment of intersex patients is presented.

Walsh, P. C., et al.: Campbell's Urology, 6th ed. Philadelphia, W. B. Saunders, 1992.
This last edition far surpasses any effort made in the past for complete description of all areas of urology including physiology, embryology, diagnosis, and treatment. It constitutes one of the most exhaustive treatments of urologic surgery and its associated medical subspecialties. Excellent bibliographies within each subsection are up-to-date and pertinent.

REFERENCES

1. Murphy, L. J. T.: The History of Urology. Springfield, IL, Charles C Thomas, 1972.
2. Osborne, E. D., Sutherland, C. G., Scholl, A. J., and Rowntree, L. G.: Roentgenology of urinary tract during excretion of sodium iodide. JAMA, 80:368, 1923.
3. von Lichtenberg, A., and Swick, M.: Klinische Prufung des Uroselectans. Klin. Wochenschr., 8:2089, 1921.
4. Lipshultz, L. I., and Howards, S. S. (Eds.): Infertility in the Male, 2nd ed. St. Louis, Mosby–Year Book, 1991.
5. Spark, R. F.: Anatomic and development considerations. In The Infertile Male: The Clinician's Guide to Diagnosis and Treatment. New York, Plenum Medical Book Company, 1988, chap. 3, p. 15.
6. Walsh, P. C., et al.: Campbell's Urology, 6th ed. Philadelphia, W. B. Saunders, 1992.
7. Gillenwater, J. Y., Grayhack, J. T., Howards, S. S., and Duckett, J. W.: Adult and Pediatric Urology, 2nd ed. St. Louis, Mosby–Year Book, 1995.

8. Kelalis, K. P., King, L. R., and Belman, A. B.: Clinical Pediatric Urology, 3rd ed. Philadelphia, W. B. Saunders, 1992.

9. Yamamoto, M., and Turner, T. T.: Epididymis, sperm maturation, and capacitation. *In* Lipschultz, L. I., and Howards, S. S. (Eds.): Infertility in the Male, 2nd ed. St. Louis, Mosby–Year Book, 1991, p. 103.

10. Benson, G. S., and McConnell, J.: Erection, emission and ejaculation: Physiologic mechanisms. *In* Lipschultz, L. I., and Howards, S. S. (Eds.): Infertility in the Male, 2nd ed. St. Louis, Mosby–Year Book, 1991, p. 155.

11. Coffey, D. S.: The molecular biology, endocrinology and physiology of the prostate and seminal vesicles. *In* Walsh, P. C., Retik, A. B., Stamey, T. A., and Vaughan, D. E. Jr. (Eds.): Campbell's Urology, 6th ed. Philadelphia, W. B. Saunders, 1992, p. 221.

12. Bennett, A. H.: Impotence: Diagnosis and Management of Erectile Function. Philadelphia, W. B. Saunders, 1994.

13. Belker, A. M., et al.: Results of 1469 microsurgical vasectomy reversals by the vasovasostomy study group. J. Urol., *145*:505, 1991.

14. Goldwasser, B., Weinerth, J. L., and Carson, C. C.: Ejaculatory duct obstruction: A case for aggressive diagnosis and treatment. J. Urol., *134*:964, 1985.

15. Prentiss, R. J.: Anomalies of the male genitalia. *In* Amar, A. D., et al. (Eds.): Encyclopedia of Urology. Berlin, Springer-Verlag, 1968, p. 287.

16. Webster, G. D.: The urethra. *In* Paulson, D. F. (Ed.): Genitourinary Surgery. Edinburgh, Churchill Livingstone, 1983, p. 399.

17. Glenn, J. F. (Ed.): Urologic Surgery, 4th ed. Philadelphia, J. B. Lippincott, 1991.

18. Mellinger, D. C., and Smith, A. D.: STDs and other lesions of the external genitalia. Urol. Clin. North Am., *19*(1), 1992.

19. Oesterling, J. E. (Guest Ed.): Prostatic Tumor Markers. Urol. Clin. North Am., *20*(4), 1993.

DISORDERS OF THE LYMPHATIC SYSTEM

Richard L. McCann, M.D.

ANATOMY

The lymphatic system is composed of lymphatic capillaries that collect interstitial fluid, transporting vessels, and lymph nodes. Lymphatic capillaries are the site of interstitial fluid absorption throughout the body. These empty into the transporting vessels that traverse the extremities and body cavities to eventually empty into the venous system via the thoracic ducts. Lymph nodes periodically interrupt these transporting vessels. In the lymph nodes the lymph is filtered, and these structures serve a primary immunologic function.

Structurally, lymphatic capillaries are similar to blood capillaries except that the basement membrane is much less distinct. Large gaps exist between adjacent lymphatic endothelial cells that allow particles as large as bacteria, red blood cells, and even lymphocytes to pass through the vessel walls. A number of tissues have no lymphatic drainage, including the epidermis; the central nervous system; the layers of the eye; and skeletal muscle, cartilage, and tendon in the extremities. In contrast, the dermis is richly supplied with lymphatics, which are easily identified by intradermal injection of vital dyes. The capillaries are without valves, and they communicate directly with collecting vessels at the dermal subcutaneous junction. The superficial lymphatic channels of the extremities consist of several valved channels that pass primarily on the medial aspect of the limb toward the groin or axilla, where they end in one or more lymph nodes. These vessels are of uniform caliber as they ascend and form a plexiform network, with frequent intercommunications between the main channels. There is a separate deep lymphatic system with vessels that run deep to the muscular fascia coursing along with the neurovascular bundles. There is little if any communication between the superficial and deep lymphatic systems.

Lymph vessels have a well-defined adventitia, whereas the tunica media contains smooth muscle cells with a thin intima. These vessels are also innervated, and spasm as well as natural rhythmic contractions have been observed. Interposed throughout the course of the collecting lymphatic channels are lymph nodes. Typically, a lymph node has several afferent channels that enter the capsule, and lymph drains into sinuses that bathe the cortical and medullary areas of the lymph node. The lymph then exits by a single efferent channel. The cortical areas of the lymph node contain predominantly lymphocytes that are arranged in follicles separated by trabecular extensions of the capsule. Within the follicles are discrete germinal centers. The medulla may contain macrophages and plasma cells as well as lymphocytes, and these cells are believed to be in dynamic equilibrium within the lymph node. Each node also has a separate vascular and nervous supply, and lymphatic vascular interactions may occur within the node itself.

The lower-extremity lymphatic channels join with the visceral channels to form the *cisterna chyli* adjacent to the upper abdominal aorta. The cisterna passes through the diaphragm to become the thoracic duct. Within the mediastinum this duct ascends on the right anterior aspect of the vertebral column before crossing to the left side at the T5 level. The thoracic duct receives the intercostal and thoracic visceral lymph vessels and eventually enters the venous system by joining the left subclavian vein. A separate smaller right lymphatic duct drains the right upper extremity and neck and enters the right subclavian vein.

PHYSIOLOGY

The circulation of lymph is a complex and incompletely understood process. All the tissues of the body are bathed in interstitial fluid, and when an excess amount of this fluid accumulates, it is referred to as *edema.* Edema may result from excessive production of interstitial fluid or from inadequate removal. Interstitial fluid is formed by the flux of plasma across the semipermeable capillary membrane. Large molecules, such as plasma proteins, are retained within the capillary lumina and exert an osmotic effect. Excess production of interstitial fluid occurs when permeability of the capillary membrane increases, such as during local inflammation, or if the hydrostatic pressure is not counterbalanced by colloid osmotic pressure as might occur from hypoproteinemia. If the pressure on the venous side of the capillary is high, as in acute obstruction from venous thrombosis, less fluid is reabsorbed, and the volume of interstitial fluid increases and is observed as edema. Similarly, if the transport of interstitial fluid by the lymph system is inadequate, excess interstitial fluid accumulates. Excessive accumulation of interstitial fluid because of lack of lymphatic transport is termed *lymphedema.* Normally between 2 and 4 liters of interstitial fluid is filtered each day and must be returned to the vascular system by the lymphatic system.

Lymph propulsion is also a complex process. It is believed that, at rest, the intrinsic rhythmic contractions of the walls of the collecting ducts propel lymph toward the thoracic duct in a peristaltic fashion. Active skeletal muscle contraction increases tension within the subcutaneous compartment, producing compression of the lymphatic channels. Because of the presence of competent valves in these channels, lymph is propelled centrally. Increased intra-abdominal pressure, such as with coughing and straining, also compresses the lymphatic vessels, accelerating the flow of lymph upward. The phasic changes in intrathoracic pressure associated with respiration establishes another pumping mechanism to propel lymph through the mediastinum. Finally, the rapid flow of blood in the subclavian vein may exert a siphon effect on the thoracic duct. Another feature of the lymphatic system is to return macromolecules from the interstitial space to the vascular system. These large molecules cannot be readily absorbed in vascular capillaries because of the small pore size in the capillary walls. Actual gaps between endothelial cells of the terminal lymphatics readily admit these large molecules, however. It is estimated that 50% to 80% of the total intravascular protein circulates in this manner each day. The protein concentration of lymph depends greatly on the tissue being drained. In extremity lymph, protein concentration may be as low as 0.5 gm. per dl., whereas liver lymph may contain 6 gm. per dl.

Lymph draining the intestines following a fatty meal is opalescent in color owing to its content of fat in the form of chylomicrons. An additional function of the lymphatic system that has surgical implications is that of filtration and immunologic protection. Bacteria, foreign bodies, and malignant cells are known to be transported by the lymphatic system and carried to the regional nodes, where concentrations of macrophages, plasma cells, and lymphocytes can interact with them and initiate an immune response.

Formation of Lymphedema. Starling proposed that interstitial fluid was a filtrate of plasma across the capillary wall and that the rate of its formation depended on the pressure gradient across this membrane.[15] Pappenheimer and Soto-Rivera contributed the concept that the capillary pores were small and only partially permeable to large molecules such as plasma proteins.[13] These large molecules trapped within the capillaries exert an osmotic effect, tending to keep fluid volume within the capillary space. Thus, the exchange of fluid between the capillaries and interstitial space is dependent on four factors: the hydrostatic pressures within the capillary and within the interstitial space, and the osmotic pressures within these two compartments (Fig. 47–1). The oncotic pressure of normal plasma is about 25 mm. Hg, whereas the oncotic pressure of interstitial fluid approximates only 1 mm. Hg. The hydrostatic pressure at the arteriolar end of a capillary is estimated to be 37 mm. Hg and, at the venous end, 17 mm. Hg. The hydrostatic pressure of the interstitial fluid varies in different tissues, being –2 mm. Hg in the subcutaneous tissue and +6 mm. Hg in the kidney. There is a net flux of fluid out of the capillary into the interstitial space at the high-pressure arteriolar end of a capillary and a net flux inward at the venular end.

Net efflux normally exceeds net influx, and this extra fluid

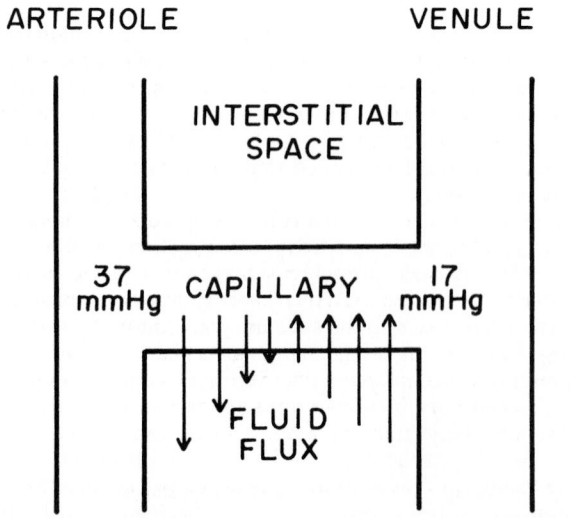

Plasma oncotic pressure = 25 mm Hg
Interstitial oncotic pressure = 1 mm Hg

Figure 47–1. Fluid flux across the capillary is dependent on the net hydrostatic and oncotic pressure gradient. This is positive near the arteriolar end leading to outflow of fluid and negative near the venular end, where most of the fluid returns to the capillary lumen.

returns to the circulation by way of the lymphatics. Normal lymph flow is 2 to 4 liters per day. The rate of flow is greatly influenced by a number of local and systemic factors, including protein concentration in plasma and interstitial fluid, local arterial and venous pressure relationships, and capillary pore size and integrity.

Edema formation occurs when there is an imbalance between the production of interstitial fluid and its transport by the lymphatic system. Excess production occurs when capillary pore size increases, such as during local inflammation, if the venous pressure becomes too high because of acute venous obstruction, or the colloid osmotic pressure becomes too low to reabsorb fluid across the capillary membrane, as in hypoproteinemia.

Lymphatic transport may become deficient when lymphatic vessels are absent, hypoplastic, or obstructed. This impairment of lymphatic flow may be congenital, as in lymphatic dysplasias, or acquired when lymphatics become obstructed as a result of disease or surgical extirpation.

CLINICAL EVALUATION OF THE SWOLLEN EXTREMITY

Clinical Evaluation. Extremity swelling may be due to a systemic disorder, to acute or chronic obstruction in the venous system, or to an abnormality of the lymphatic system. The systemic disorders that cause extremity edema include right-sided heart failure, constrictive pericarditis, many renal diseases, liver cirrhosis, and any other form of hypoproteinemia. These disorders are often detected during initial clinical evaluation. Acute deep venous thrombosis as a cause of extremity edema is often apparent because of the clinical setting and may be confirmed by duplex scanning, magnetic resonance imaging, or phlebography. Chronic deep venous insufficiency is often recognized by the characteristic eczema and stasis dermatitis with or without skin ulceration and also can be confirmed by noninvasive vascular laboratory studies or vascular imaging by phlebography, ultrasonography, or magnetic resonance imaging. Other causes of extremity swelling include acquired or congenital arteriovenous fistula and, occasionally, allergic disorders.

The clinical appearance of lymphedema is variable and depends on the severity and duration of the syndrome. Initially, protein-rich fluid accumulates in the affected tissues. Typically, this swelling is soft and pits easily with pressure. This early edema is often responsive to elevation and may decrease or disappear entirely with elevation of the limb. This type of swelling typically involves the distal aspect of the extremity and characteristically involves the dorsum of the foot and toes, which may help distinguish it from edema due to venous obstruction. Over a period of years, the edema becomes woody in texture because the presence of the protein-rich fluid incites an inflammatory fibrosis, and pitting becomes less prominent. Limb elevation and compression with elastic garments then are much less successful at reducing the extremity volume. The skin becomes thickened, hypertrophic, and hyperkeratotic. The eczema and ulceration seen in venous disease are not characteristic of swelling due to lymphedema. Approximately half of patients with lymphedema experience recurrent spontaneous attacks of bacterial cellulitis. These episodes are characterized by increased swelling due to local inflammation, pain, and high fever. This increased susceptibility to bacterial infection is believed to be related to loss of local immune defenses because of diminished lymphatic function.

Classification of Lymphedema. Extremity swelling due to abnormalities in the lymphatic system is classified as primary or secondary. The primary lymphedemas are relatively common, occurring at a rate of 1 in 10,000, and are classified by age at the onset of symptoms. *Lymphedema congenita* is a severe form of lymphedema that is usually apparent at birth or becomes so during early infancy. This condition most often involves the lower extremity, and the right side is affected more commonly than the left. However, in 25% of cases the condition is bilateral. In a few cases there is a familial history, termed *Milroy's disease*.[9, 10] This type of lymphedema most commonly involves the dorsum of the foot and lower extremity up to the level of the knee. Many of these patients, however, have associated lymphatic abnormalities, including involvement of the external genitalia, intestinal lymphangiectasia with protein-losing enteropathy, cystic hygroma in the neck, and pulmonary lymphangiectasia.

Lymphedema praecox is the most common form of primary lymphedema, accounting for more than 80% of the cases. In this form of the disease, swelling begins about the time of puberty. There is a 3:1 female predominance. Why swelling does not begin until adolescence is unclear. One hypothesis suggests that the lymphatic transport is marginally adequate at birth but decompensates with the increased demands associated with growth at the time of puberty. This disease usually involves the lower extremities only.

Lymphedema tarda refers to lymphedema that does not appear until the third or fourth decade. Approximately half of these are associated with an inciting event, such as infection and injury.

Radiographic Evaluation. The classic method of radiographic evaluation of the swollen extremity includes lymphangiography. This examination is performed by first identifying the lymphatics on the dorsum of the foot or hand by injection of a vital blue dye subcutaneously. This dye enters the lymphatic vessels, which can be identified by dissection in the subcutaneous tissue after cutdown. The vessels are extremely small, and optical magnification is required to successfully cannulate these tiny fragile structures. Once successfully cannulated, ethiodized oil contrast medium is slowly infused, and the transit of dye is observed by serial roentgenograms for 24 hours or longer. The absence of a cannulatable lymphatic vessel after subcutaneous injection of dye is considered evidence of lymphatic hypoplasia or aplasia.

Normal lymphangiographic anatomy includes several parallel channels coursing primarily on the medial aspect of the limb (Fig. 47–2). As these channels ascend, they branch and intercommunicate, but the diameter remains relatively constant throughout the extremity. Small ampullae are demonstrated every several millimeters representing the site of valves. The deep lymphatics below the muscular fascia are only rarely seen with a dorsal pedal injection. Normal lymph nodes have a uniform ground-glass appearance and may remain opacified for many weeks.

Several lymphangiographic patterns can be observed in patients with lymphedema. The most commonly observed pattern is hypoplasia, present in more than 90% of cases of primary lymphedema. In these patients, the lymph vessels are small and few in number. There usually are fewer than five trunks observed entering the inguinal region. In severe cases no major lymphatic trunks are identified (lymphatic aplasia). Hypoplasia may be limited to the distal portions of the limb so that limb swelling is mild and nonprogressive. Hypoplasia of the proximal lymphatic system in the upper thigh and pelvis produces a more severe clinical syndrome, with swelling of the entire limb that may be progressive. In this condition, *dermal back flow* is frequently seen, in which there is abnormal movement of dye out of the subcutaneous lymphatic channels into the dermal plexus (Fig. 47–3).

The second major lymphangiographic pattern seen in lymphedema is hyperplasia. It is believed that this pattern

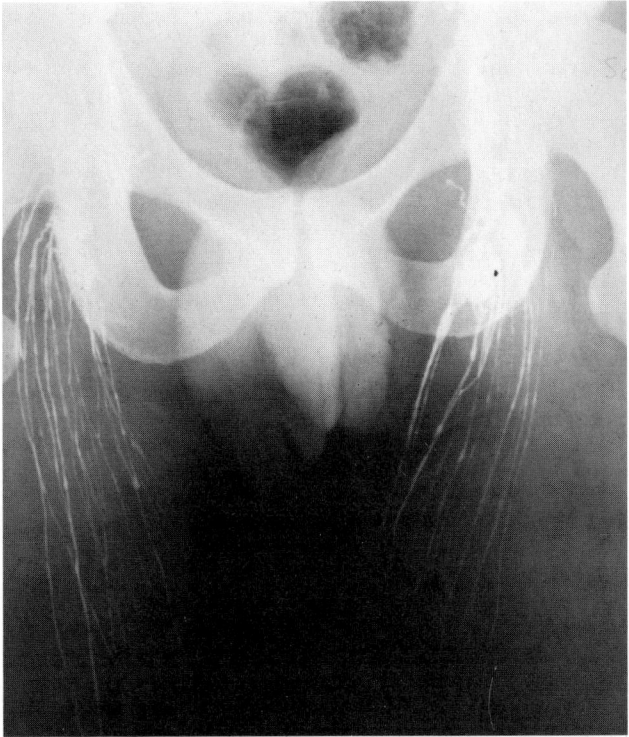

Figure 47–2. Normal lymphangiographic anatomy. Note the multiple branches, intercommunicating channels of uniform caliber. The bulges are ampullae at the site of valves.

follows lymphatic obstruction at the level of the abdominal cisterna chyli or thoracic duct; therefore, this disease is always bilateral. Numerous mildly dilated vessels are usually demonstrated in both lower extremities. This condition is distinct from a rarer unilateral form of hyperplasia, termed *megalymphatics*. In this condition, varicose valveless lymphatic channels are seen, usually in only one limb, and it is often associated with cutaneous angiomas. Chylous reflux may be prominent and may present as chylometrorrhea, chylous skin vesicles, or chyluria.

Because lymphangiography requires a surgical cutdown and microsurgical expertise, and because the risk of oil embolism and lymphangitis aggravates the syndrome, a better method of investigation has been sought. Lymphoscintigraphy requires only subcutaneous injection of technetium-labeled colloid and serial gamma camera imaging of the extremity. Although it does not provide as precise an image of the lymphatic system, it often is sufficient for diagnosis (Fig. 47–4).[2, 16] This technique is relatively noninvasive, and serial examinations can be obtained without significant risks or patient discomfort. Excellent sensitivity and specificity have been reported using this technique. Magnetic resonance imaging has also been employed to investigate the lymphatic system.[4] One advantage of magnetic resonance imaging is that it demonstrates lymph trunks, lymph nodes, and soft tissues proximal to sites of lymphatic obstruction (Fig. 47–5).

SECONDARY LYMPHEDEMA

Secondary lymphedema due to acquired lymphatic obstruction is commonly seen in surgical patients. The causes of acquired lymphatic obstruction are infiltration of regional nodes by tumor, surgical excision of regional nodes in treatment for malignancy, or fibrosis after infectious or inflammatory processes or radiation. The most common tumors infiltrating lymph nodes causing lymphatic obstruction are

promptly with effective antibiotics and bed rest with elevation of the involved extremity. Cellulitis is most frequently caused by gram-positive organisms, and antibiotics effective against these organisms should be given empirically and adjusted if necessary after the bacterial culture is known.

External compression with well-fitted elastic garments is the most useful method of controlling excessive fluid volume in the lymphedematous limb, and several brands of these stockings are available. The most effective garments are those that are custom manufactured and designed with a built-in pressure gradient from the toe to the groin. If begun before subcutaneous fibrosis has occurred, these garments, in combination with elevation of the foot of the bed, control edema and allow a functional limb in patients with mild to moderate swelling. In patients with severe swelling, the use of a mechanical pneumatic compression device may be considered.[12] This device consists of a sleeve containing several compartments. After the affected extremity is inserted into the sleeve, the compartments are serially inflated, driving the fluid out of the extremity. A period of intensive therapy is usually required followed by a maintenance program, using the device at night or several times a week. More recently, a similar effect has been achieved by special massage techniques, which are time consuming and expensive but effective in

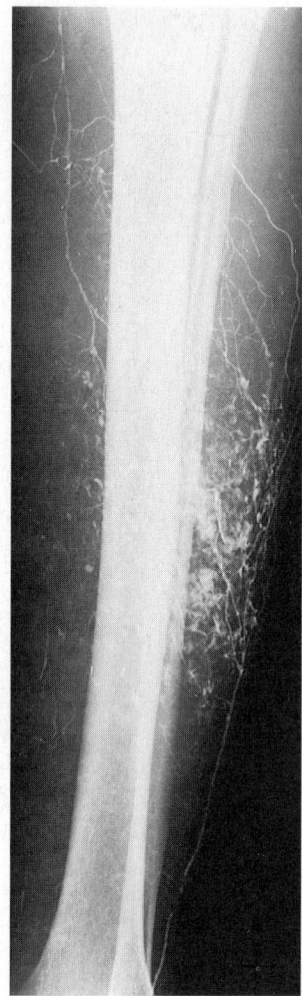

Figure 47–3. Lymphangiogram in a patient with primary lymphedema. There are few lymphatic channels that are not continuous. The blotchy areas represent the phenomenon of dermal backflow. The dye literally extravasates into the dermis because of the obstruction within the main channels.

carcinoma of the prostate in men and lymphoma in women. In Western countries, perhaps the most common cause of secondary lymphedema occurs in the arm after surgical excision of lymph nodes for carcinoma of the breast followed by axillary and chest wall radiation therapy. In tropical countries, infestation by filaria is the most frequent cause of secondary lymphedema. It estimated by the World Health Organization that 90 million people may be affected by filarial infections, most common being *Wuchereria bancrofti*. Tuberculous lymphangitis may also be a cause in areas where this disease remains prevalent.

TREATMENT OF LYMPHEDEMA

Nonoperative Therapy. Most patients with lymphedema can be managed with a program of meticulous skin hygiene, elastic support garments, extremity elevation, and avoidance of local injury. Most patients are able to maintain a functional extremity with these measures alone. Care should be taken to keep the interdigital spaces dry, and frequent use of an antifungal powder may be helpful. Local injury should be meticulously avoided as well as walking barefoot, especially outdoors, which is strictly forbidden. Interestingly, skin ulceration as observed in deep venous insufficiency is rarely seen in lymphedema. If cellulitis occurs, it should be treated

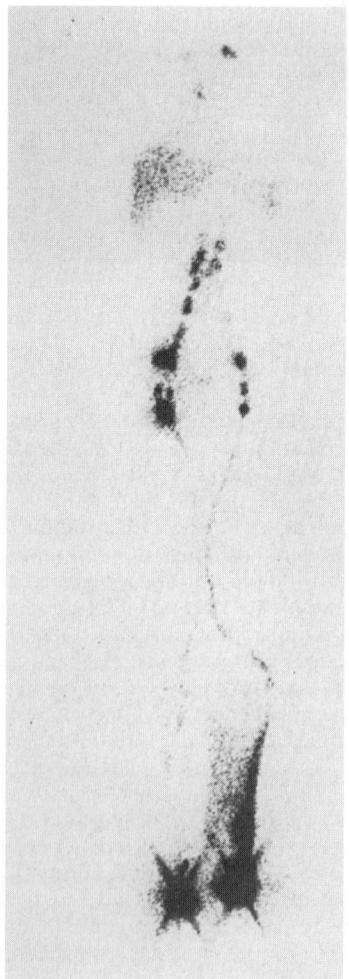

Figure 47–4. Lymphoscintigraphic pattern in primary lymphedema. Note area of dermal backflow on the left and the diminished number of lymph nodes in the groin. (From Cambria, R. A., Gloviczki, P., Naessens, J. M., and Wahner, H. W.: Noninvasive evaluation of the lymphatic systems with lymphoscintigraphy: A prospective, semi-quantitative analysis in 386 extremities. J. Vasc. Surg., 18:773, 1993.)

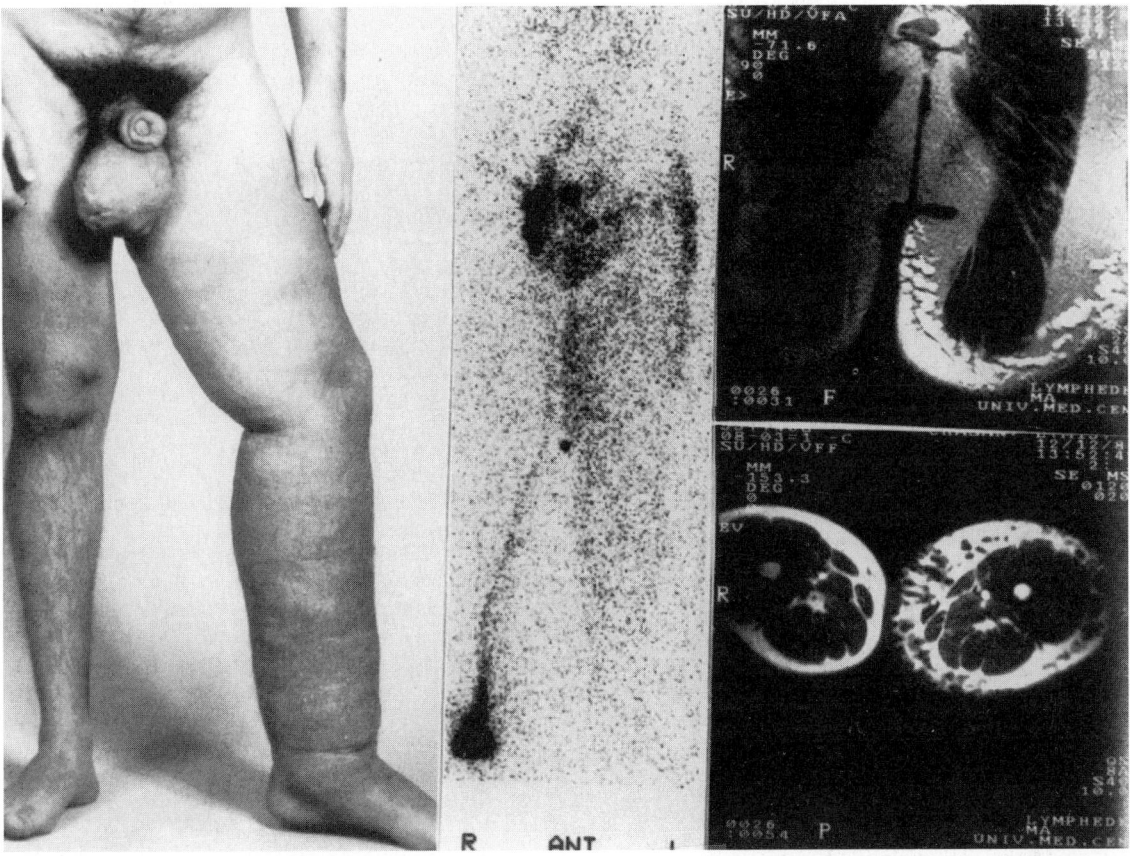

Figure 47–5. *Left panel,* Massive left leg swelling due to congenital lymphedema studied by lymphoscintigraphy and magnetic resonance imaging (MRI). Lymphoscintigraphy *(middle panel)* shows dermal backflow in the left thigh and a normal right side. The MRI *(right panel)* demonstrates massive subcutaneous swelling with lymph lakes and normal skeletal muscle. (Reprinted by permission of the publisher from Case, T. C., Witte, C. L., Witte, M. H., Unger, E. C., and Williams, W. H.: Magnetic resonance imaging in human lymphedema: Comparison with lymphangioscintigraphy. *Magn. Reson. Imaging, 10*:549, 1992. Copyright 1992 by Elsevier Science Inc.)

reducing the volume of lymphedematous limbs (Fig. 47–6).[5] The strategy is to massage the excess interstitial fluid from areas with deficient lymphatic drainage to areas with more normal lymphatic function. Medical therapy has been described, particularly the use of benzopyrones to reduce the formation of high-protein edema. These have shown promise in clinical trials but are not currently available in the United States.[6]

Surgical Therapy. Three surgical strategies have been used to treat severe disabling cases of lymphedema. Excision of the hypertrophic fibrotic subcutaneous tissues can be achieved by complete excision to muscle fascia with coverage of the surface by split-thickness skin grafts harvested from the excised tissue or from healthy skin more proximally on the same or on the contralateral extremity, known as the *Charles operation* (Fig. 47–7).[8] Conversely, relatively thick skin flaps can be mobilized in a staged fashion with excision of the underlying subcutaneous tissue, known as the *Kondoleon procedure.* To avoid slough of the flaps, this procedure is usually done in staged fashion. Usually the medial aspect is done first, followed in several months by a similar procedure on the lateral aspect of the limb. Although the cosmetic result of these procedures is marginal, the limb with true elephantiasis may be made more functional by this approach.

A second surgical strategy involves the pedicle transfer of lymphatic-bearing tissue into the affected limb with the intention of creating spontaneous connections to the dysfunctional lymphatic channels in the swollen limb. Pedicle transfers of defunctionalized bowel, omentum, and de-epithelialized skin have been attempted, but most of these attempts have met with disappointment.

The third surgical approach involves the microvascular bypass of obstructed lymphatic segments. Both creation of a lymphaticovenous fistula and the use of vein grafts to bridge lymphatic defects have been described, but few have been performed, and they should still be considered experimental.[1, 3, 11]

LYMPHATIC TUMORS AND MALFORMATIONS

Lymphangiomas. Lymphangiomas are congenital malformations of lymphatic vessels. More than half of these lesions are present at birth, and 90% are present by the end of the second year of life. The lesions usually grow slowly but may infiltrate the local tissues, although malignant degeneration is rare. Three types of lymphangiomas have been described: (1) lymphangioma simplex, consisting of small capillary-sized lymphatic channels; (2) cavernous lymphangioma, formed from dilated lymphatic channels, often with a fibrous capsule; and (3) cystic hygroma, a lymphatic malformation consisting of an endothelial-lined cyst, usually found in the neck or axilla. Because they form a disfiguring mass, many of these lesions are treated by surgical excision with preservation of surrounding vital structures. Radiation therapy is ineffective, as are attempts at injection of sclerosing solution.[7]

Chylous Syndromes. Chyle is formed in the lacteals of the small intestine by absorption of the products of fat digestion. Chyle is normally transported to the cisterna chyli and then to the thoracic duct. Chyle may be found outside of the normal channels if there is an acquired or congenital obstruction of the thoracic duct or incompetence of the lymphatic

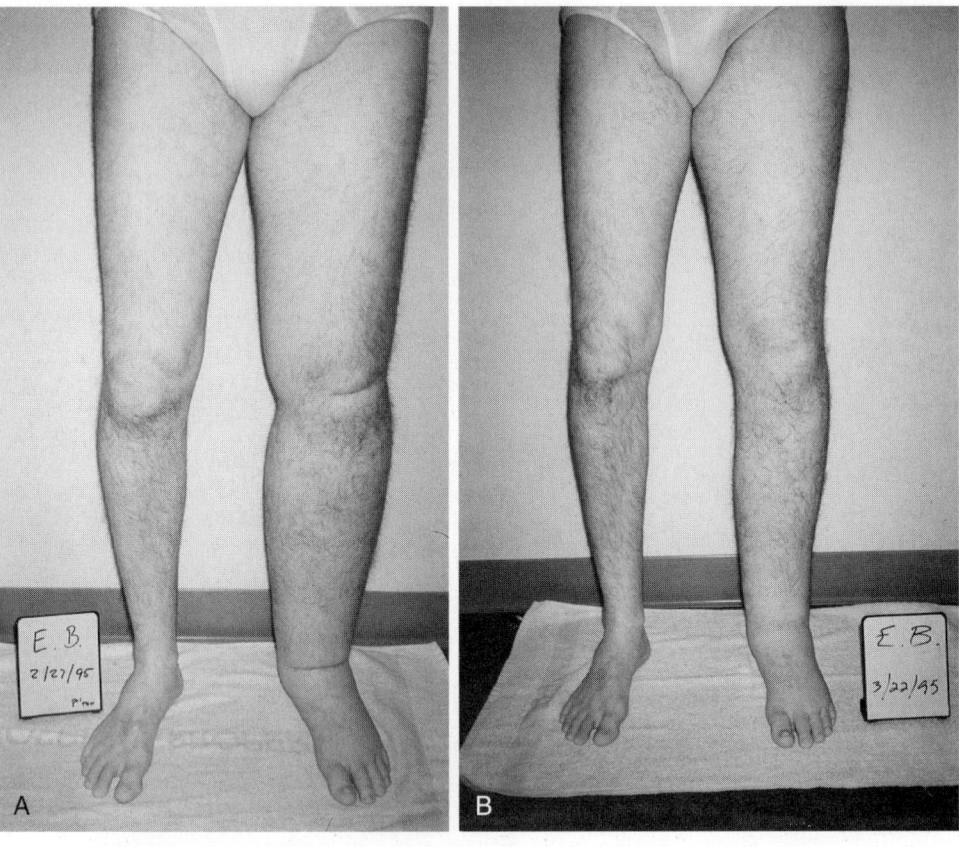

Figure 47–6. Results that can be obtained with massage therapy. Results are shown before *(A)* and 3 weeks after *(B)* initiating massage therapy.

valves. Fistulization may occur into the peritoneal, pleural, or pericardial cavities. Chylous ascites and chylothorax may respond to a medium-chain triglyceride diet, as these fats do not promote the formation of chylomicrons and thus reduce the volume of intestinal lymph secretion. Occasionally, direct suture closure of a chylous fistula is indicated if conservative measures fail. Chylous ascites developing spontaneously in an older patient is nearly always caused by an underlying malignancy, and this should be sought before therapy is initiated.

Lymphangiosarcoma. Lymphangiosarcoma is a rare lesion that may develop in a lymphedematous extremity regardless of the cause of the lymphedema. Malignant degeneration is more frequent in cases of secondary lymphedema. The lesion appears as purple-red nodules in the skin; it is an aggressive, rapidly fatal lesion.[14]

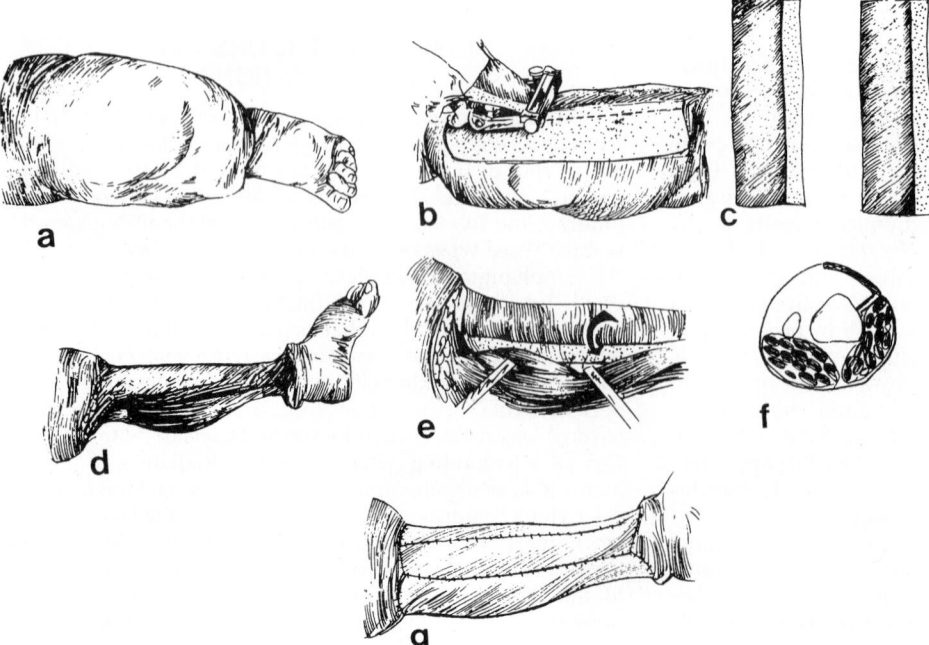

Figure 47–7. Schematic outline of the Charles operation in which the fibrotic thickened subcutaneous tissues are excised and the underlying muscle tissue is covered with split-thickness skin grafts harvested from the same leg. (From Mavilli, M. E., Naldoken, S., and Safak, T.: Modified Charles operation for primary fibrosclerotic lymphedema. Lymphology, *27*:14, 1994.)

SELECTED REFERENCES

Cambria, R. A., Gloviczki, P., Naessens, J. M., and Wahner, H. W.: Noninvasive evaluation of the lymphatic systems with lymphoscintigraphy: A prospective, semiquantitative analysis in 386 extremities. J. Vasc. Surg., 18:773, 1993.
This is the largest and most comprehensive evaluation of lymphoscintigraphy as a method of investigation of limb swelling. This study suggests that this noninvasive method can virtually replace lymphangiography in most cases.

Casley-Smith, J. R., and Casley-Smith, J. R.: Modern treatment of lymphoedema: I. Complex physical therapy: The first 200 Australian limbs. Australas. J. Dermatol., 33:61, 1992.
This is a large clinical evaluation of the use of special massage techniques for management of the swelling of mild to moderate lymphedema. This technique is likely to become increasingly popular for treatment of this condition.

Kantner, M. A.: The lymphatic system: An historical perspective. Plast. Reconstruct. Surg., 79:131, 1987.
This is the most comprehensive yet concise review of the history of knowledge of the lymphatic system. It also includes excellent reproductions of several important illustrations from key texts in the field, including Aselli and Pecquet from the seventeenth century.

Pappas Christos J., and O'Donnell, T. F. Jr.: Long-term results of compression treatment for lymphedema. J. Vasc. Surg., 16:555, 1992.
This paper succinctly outlines the conservative treatment for limb swelling due to lymphedema. It provides many practical hints and describes a commendable success rate.

REFERENCES

1. Baumeister, R. G., and Siuda, S.: Treatment of lymphedemas by microsurgical lymphatic grafting: What is proved? Plast. Reconstruct. Surg., 85:64, 1990.
2. Cambria, R. A., Gloviczki, P., Naessens, J. M., and Wahner, H. W.: Noninvasive evaluation of the lymphatic systems with lymphoscintigraphy: A prospective, semiquantitative analysis in 386 extremities. J. Vasc. Surg., 18:773, 1993.
3. Campisi, C.: Use of autologous interposition vein graft in management of lymphedema: Preliminary experimental and clinical observations. Lymphology, 24:71, 1991.
4. Case, T. C., Witte, C. L., Witte, M. H., Unger, E. C., and Williams, W. H.: Magnetic resonance imaging in human lymphedema: Comparison with lymphangioscintigraphy. Magn. Reson. Imaging, 10:549, 1992.
5. Casley-Smith, J. R., and Casley-Smith, J. R.: Modern treatment of lymphoedema: I. Complex physical therapy: The first 200 Australian limbs. Australas. J. Dermatol., 33:61, 1992.
6. Casley-Smith, J. R., Morgan, R. G., and Piller, N. B.: Treatment of lymphedema of the arms and legs with 5,6-benzo[α]-pyrone. N. Engl. J. Med., 329:1158, 1993.
7. Fonkalsrud, E.: Congenital malformations of the lymphatic system. Semin. Pediatr. Surg., 3:62, 1994.
8. Mavilli, M. E., Naldoken, S., and Safak, T.: Modified Charles operation for primary fibrosclerotic lymphedema. Lymphology, 27:14, 1994.
9. Milroy, W. F.: An undescribed variety of hereditary edema. NY Med. J., 56:505, 1892.
10. Milroy, W. F.: Chronic hereditary Milroy's disease. JAMA, 91:1172, 1928.
11. O'Brien, B. M., Mellow, C. G., Khazanchi, R. K., Dvir, E., Kumar, V., and Pederson, W. C.: Long-term results after microlymphaticovenous anastomoses for the treatment of obstructive lymphedema. Plast. Reconstruct. Surg., 85:562, 1990.
12. Pappas, C. J., and O'Donnell, T. F. Jr.: Long-term results of compression treatment for lymphedema. J. Vasc. Surg., 16:555, 1992.
13. Pappenheimer, J. R., and Soto-Rivera, A.: Effective osmotic pressure of the plasma proteins and other quantities associated with the capillary circulation in the hind limbs of cats and dogs. Am. J. Physiol., 157:471, 1948.
14. Scully, R. E., Mark, E. J., McNeely, W. F., and McNeely, B. U.: Case 18–1993: Case records of the Massachusetts General Hospital. N. Engl. J. Med., 328:1337, 1993.
15. Starling, E. H.: Classics in lymphology. Lymphology, 17:83, 1984.
16. Suat-Eng, T., Abass, A., Kim, C. K., and Merli, G.: Lymphoscintigraphy: A reliable test for the diagnosis of lymphedema. Clin. Nucl. Med., 18:646, 1993.

CHAPTER 48

VENOUS DISORDERS

M. Wayne Flye, M.D., Ph.D.

The pathophysiology of venous disease is, in many respects, more complex than that of arterial disease. With the exception of aneurysm formation, virtually all the physiologic aberrations characteristic of arterial disease are caused by obstruction. Venous pathophysiology, in contrast, involves both obstruction and valvular insufficiency. Moreover, the disability from venous disease includes not only regional problems but also those that result from the escape of thrombi into the pulmonary circulation. With the copious network of venous collaterals, the low intraluminal pressure, the collapsible nature of the venous wall, and the intermittency of venous flow, definition of the features of venous pathophysiology provides a real challenge.

Varicose veins and their associated symptoms and complications constitute the most common vascular disorder of the lower extremities. More than 20 million people in the United States alone are significantly affected. Most of these persons have either symptoms or complications from chronic venous insufficiency, and a substantial number suffer economic hardship from the resulting disability. Of all the earth's mobile creatures, only man, with his penchant for standing erect, is afflicted by this abnormal condition. No description of varicosities has been recorded in horses, dogs, cats, or other four-legged animals. In the upright position, blood from the leg must be returned to the heart against gravity. The delicate valves in the venous system break up the column of blood from the ankle to the atrium that, if unopposed, potentially exerts a gravitational force at the ankle of 110 to 120 mm. Hg. Even modest motion, however, such as shifting weight, contracts the calf muscles, forcing blood toward the heart in the valved venous system.

The term *varicose* is derived from the Latin word meaning dilated. It implies a dilated, tortuous, and elongated vein. Although varicosities may occur in any venous system, such as in the lower esophageal area, the anorectal area, or the spermatic cord, they occur most frequently in the lower extremity. They range in size from tiny cutaneous spider bursts to large protruding veins that may be confined to localized areas or may widely involve the venous system. Incompetence of venous valves by increasing segmental pressure predisposes to the development of varicosities. Although Fabricius' description of these venous valves in 1574 was instrumental in William Harvey's elucidation of the blood circulation, their importance in the integrity of the venous system was not recognized until almost 400 years later.

HISTORICAL ASPECTS

Although varicose veins were probably recognized in prehistory, the first written reference appears to be the Ebers papyrus, dated 1550 B.C.E. However, Hippocrates discussed their treatment at length about 2500 years ago and noted "that it was better not to stand in the case of an ulcer on the leg." A number of physicians during the Roman era, including Galen, Celsus, Aetuis of Amide, and Paulus Aegineta, advised avulsion and cauterization for the treatment of varicose veins and the use of bandages for the treatment of

leg ulcers. Over the centuries, numerous modes of therapy, including puncture, avulsion, excision, cautery, ligation, resection, injection, and stripping, were advocated, with different degrees of success. From the tenth to the eighteenth centuries, various physicians, including Haly, Abbas, Avicenna, Falopio, and Paré, attributed ulceration of the legs to the accumulation of black bile or bad humors and believed that ulceration in the legs served a useful purpose in getting rid of these vile substances.[37]

Recognition of Etiology

In the nineteenth century, writers including Brodie, Astley Cooper, Home, and Hodgson first stressed the importance of varicose veins in the etiology of leg ulceration, and the term *varicose ulcer* was coined. In 1868, two important books on venous ulcers, written by Gay and Spencer, stressed the role of deep venous thrombosis and other lesions of the arterial and venous systems (both deep and superficial) in the etiology of leg ulceration. Gay also described perforating ankle veins and suggested the use of the term *venous ulceration*. Subsequently, Homans found that deep vein thrombosis was frequently the cause of valvular damage. Linton drew attention to the incompetence of the communicating veins of the calf as a potential cause of venous ulceration.[21] Although both surgical and nonsurgical measures have proved generally therapeutic, the search for a more effective means of prevention and for the perfect cure for this common malady continues.

Methods of Treatment

Sclerotherapy of varicose veins began in Europe soon after Pravaz devised the hypodermic syringe in 1851. Injection therapy became widely accepted in most European countries as the best form of treatment after 1911, when Linser of the Tubingen Clinic discovered that intravenous injection of bichloride of mercury was less toxic than previously used sclerosing agents. However, it soon became evident that although the incidence of side effects was low, the recurrence rate was very high after sclerotherapy, particularly when the valves were also incompetent, and the varicosities would not remain occluded in the face of nature's efforts to recanalize the thrombosed veins.

Local excision of varicose veins was performed by early practitioners, but it was not until the advent of general anesthesia and aseptic surgery that a more extensive and definitive operation could be done successfully. In 1884, Madelung of Germany, in a radical surgical procedure, excised the greater saphenous vein through a long incision over the medial aspect of the leg and thigh. Although this formidable procedure was associated with a high morbidity and mortality, it remained the most favored of the early operations for varicose veins.

In 1905, Keller in the United States first reported the removal of varicose veins without extensive incisions. A wire was passed through the lumen of the saphenous vein, and the vein was pulled or stripped out by inverting the vein on itself. Homans, in 1916, emphasized that ligation of the saphenofemoral junction was a vital step in preventing the recurrence of varicosities, since tributaries to a patent proximal saphenous segment would often allow refilling of distal varicosities. Linton, in the late 1930s, emphasized the pathologic contribution of incompetent perforating veins to venous insufficiency and devised an operation to separate the deep and superficial venous system by dividing these perforating veins (Linton procedure).

Surgical treatment by venous stripping and excision now offers the best long-term prognosis in the treatment of superficial varicosities if the deep venous system is patent. However, for patients in poor general health or for those with trivial or cosmetic problems, other alternatives such as sclerotherapy, external elastic support, periodic leg elevation, and exercise are often used.

ANATOMIC AND PHYSIOLOGIC CONSIDERATIONS

The primary and most obvious function of the venous system is the return of blood to the heart from the capillary beds. In addition, veins play a predominant role in regulating vascular capacity (capacitance). They also assist the return of blood to the heart during exercise, by serving as part of the peripheral pump mechanism. Functioning together with the capillaries, veins also help control body temperature.

Anatomy of the Veins

Veins possess muscle and collagen but have considerably less elastic tissue than arteries. The smooth muscle is arranged in both a circular and a longitudinal manner. In general, the amount of circular muscle reflects the pressure exerted in that particular vein. As is expected, there is more muscle present in veins of the lower extremity than in those of the thorax. Unlike arteries, veins are divided into a superficial and a deep system. The superficial veins are large, relatively thick-walled muscular structures located just under the skin. Among the superficial veins are the greater and lesser saphenous veins of the leg (Fig. 48–1), the cephalic and basilic veins of the arm, and the external jugular veins of the

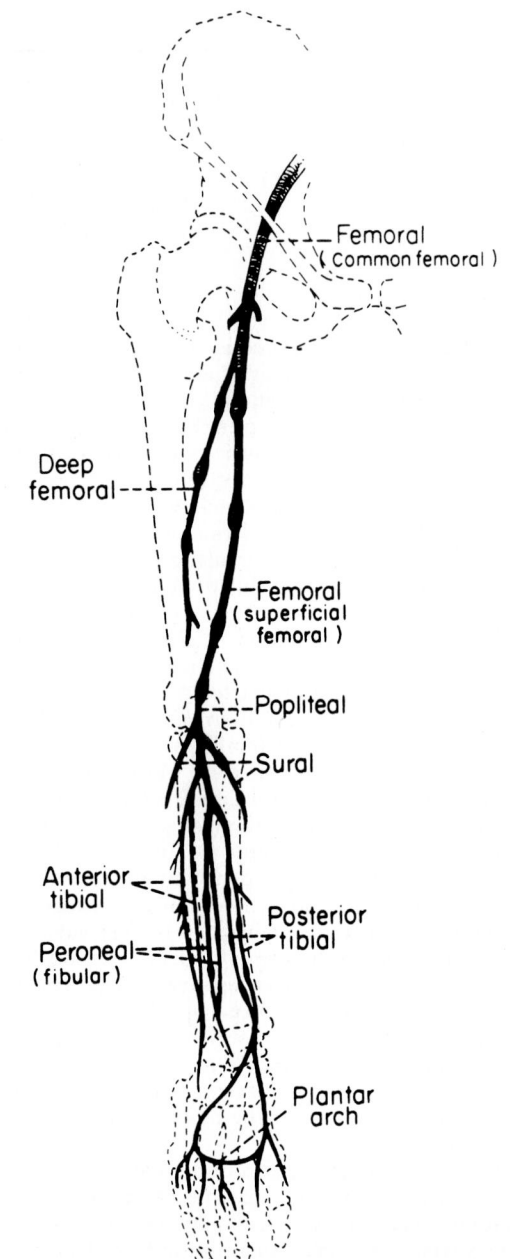

Figure 48–2. Deep venous system of the lower extremity that parallels the arterial supply. (From Juergens, J. L., Jr., Spittell, J. A., Jr., and Fairbairn, J. F., II: Peripheral Vascular Disease. Philadelphia, W. B. Saunders, 1980.)

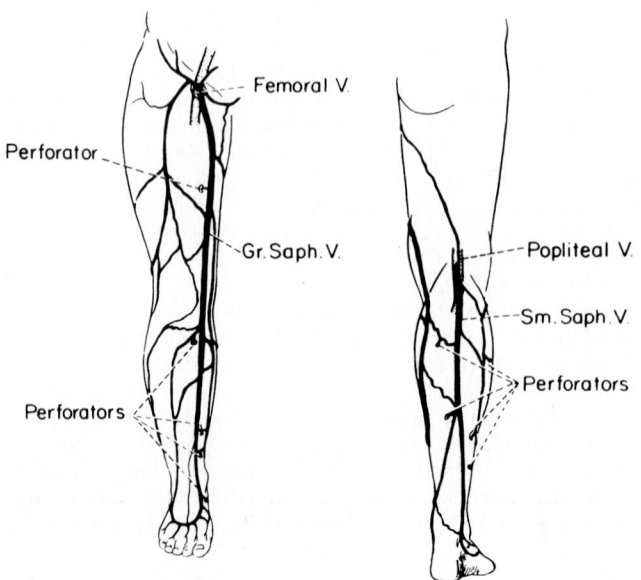

Figure 48–1. Greater and smaller saphenous superficial veins of the lower extremity and the perforating veins that communicate with the deep veins.

neck. The deep veins, in contrast, are thin walled and less muscular. These deep veins, unlike the superficial veins, are protected by the muscles and deep fascia; they accompany the arteries and bear the same names as the arteries they parallel (Fig. 48–2). The cross-sectional area of these veins is approximately three times that of the adjacent artery.

As part of the deep system, large, thin-walled veins are located within skeletal muscle and are referred to as *sinusoids*. They serve a particularly important function as part of the *bellows* of the muscle pump mechanism during exercise. For example, the soleal sinusoids of the lower leg empty into the posterior tibial vein, and the gastrocnemius sinusoids empty into the popliteal vein.

Perforating veins connect the deep and superficial systems by passing through the fascial layer that invests the deep venous system (Fig. 48–3). Of particular importance in the

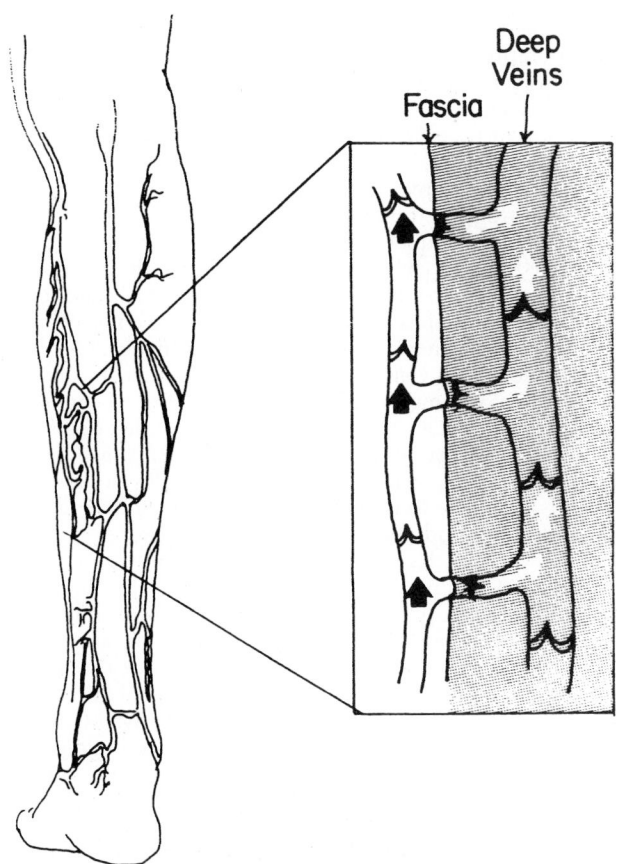

Figure 48–3. Direction of blood flow in the transfascial perforating veins between the superficial and deep venous systems. (From Burnham, S. J.: Operative treatment for varicose veins. *In* Rutherford, R. B. [Ed.]: Vascular Surgery, 2nd ed. Philadelphia, W. B. Saunders, 1984, p. 1348.)

pathophysiology of lower leg venous stasis is a series of about six medial calf perforators that join the posterior tibial vein to the greater saphenous vein. This area is most susceptible to venous hypertension and the development of ulceration. This characteristic *gaiter* area is located over the medial ankle between the instep and the lower leg. In the posterior calf, the superficial system is connected indirectly with the deep venous system via the large intramuscular sinusoids.

A most important anatomic and functional feature of veins is the presence of delicate but extremely strong bicuspid valves. An expanded sinus at the site of each valve allows the valves to open widely without making contact with the venous wall. Thus, when venous flow begins to reverse, rapid valvular closure is permitted. The deep veins contain more valves than the superficial veins. There may be nine to 19 valves in the distal posterior tibial or anterior tibial vein, but the number decreases more proximally, so that the common iliac vein and vena cava usually have no valves. Valves are present in venules as small as 0.15 mm. in diameter. In all areas of the legs and arms, valve cusps are oriented to direct flow centrally and to prevent reflux of venous blood. Although valves in perforating veins usually permit blood to flow only from the superficial to the deep venous system, valves in the foot, in contrast, allow flow from the deep to the superficial system. This anatomic pattern may exacerbate the venous hypertension and stasis changes that occur about the ankle with venous insufficiency.

The veins of the lower extremity are part of the postcapillary blood reservoir, which holds about 70% of the total blood volume. The venous system is not merely a passive conduit, however; the total potential venous volume is far

from filled, because some veins are always partially or completely collapsed. Because of a great venous capacitance, large fluctuations in venous volume are possible with little change in central venous pressure. When veins are filled sufficiently to assume a circular cross section, the venous smooth muscle contractile state plays an important role in regulating venous tone and volume and serves to regulate cardiac output. Regulation of hydrostatic pressure in the capillaries and regulation of temperature via the cutaneous veins are other functions of the venous system. It is estimated that since 80% of an increase in venous pressure is transmitted to the capillaries, whereas only about 10% of an increase in arterial pressure is reflected as an increase in capillary hydrostatic pressure, venous hypertension predisposes more to edema formation.

Venous Pump

The components of the venous pump are the skeletal muscle, the intramuscular venous sinusoids, and the superficial and deep veins. When skeletal muscles contract, blood forced from the intramuscular and surrounding veins is propelled toward the heart. As a consequence of this pumping action, venous pressures in the dependent portion of the leg are lowered, venous congestion is relieved, edema is reduced, and blood flow through exercising muscles is facilitated (Fig. 48–4). This venous pump is most highly developed in the calf, where the soleal and gastrocnemius sinusoids compose the major bellows of the muscle pump. Contraction of the calf muscles produces pressures in excess of 200 mm. Hg, which is sufficient to compress the intramuscular veins even in the standing position. With each muscle contraction, blood is, therefore, propelled centrally.

During the generation of higher pressures in the deep venous system during muscle contraction, valves in the connecting perforating veins prevent reflux flow from the deep to the superficial system.[26] The proper function of the venous pump depends on the presence of competent venous valves, particularly in the upright position. This valved venomotor pump mechanism is presumably an evolutionary adaptation

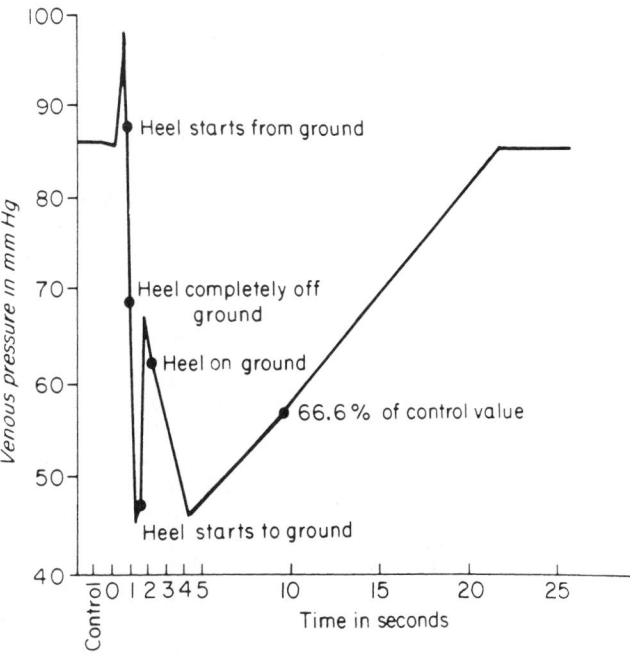

Figure 48–4. Pressure changes that occur in the deep venous pump of the lower extremity with each step.

to man's assumption of the upright position, because if a normal person were to stand motionless for a long enough time, venous pressures at the ankle would stabilize in the range of 80 to 100 mm. Hg, and swelling and petechiae would appear. Since competent venous valves prevent the reflux of blood, the venous pressure is reduced following venous emptying by muscle contraction. With even modest activity of the calf muscles, such as occurs in intermittently shifting one's weight, this venous pressure is transiently reduced to 20 to 30 mm. Hg before pressure again rises as the collapsed veins are refilled by inflow from capillaries or communicating veins.[26]

When venous valves are incompetent, the resulting hydrostatic column of venous blood is longer and there is immediate retrograde venous filling with muscle contraction. The venous pressure of the lower leg, therefore, remains high, which predisposes to the development of dependent edema. According to the Starling concept, return of fluid escaping from the arteriolar end of a capillary to the circulation at the venular end is facilitated by lower venous pressures. In the normal situation, any dependent swelling that accumulates during the day usually disappears overnight when the body is horizontal. However, with incompetent veins, the greater edema formation resolves more slowly, results in capillary underperfusion,[20] and predisposes to chronic stasis changes.

TREATMENT OF VARICOSE VEINS

Little more than visual inspection is required to diagnose varicose veins. However, before they can be treated intelligently, the surgeon should be aware of the functional status of the deep iliofemoral vein and perforating vein valves. Operation may be performed for cosmetic reasons or to relieve symptoms, but it should be intended to correct abnormal venous hemodynamics. The ideal patient for the elimination of superficial venous varicosities has patent deep veins and competent valves in both the deep and the perforator systems. The next most suitable patient is one who has a patent deep venous system with competent deep valves but incompetent perforator valves. In the latter patient, when the perforating veins are ablated along with the superficial venous stripping, good results can be expected. Patients with incompetence of all or most of the deep and perforator venous valves should not be considered for simple vein stripping, because recurrence of varicosities is likely. Restoration of deep venous valvular competency by venous valve reconstruction or transposition may be a logical choice for these patients. Finally, patients with deep vein obstruction, regardless of the condition of their venous valves, are the worst candidates for superficial venous ligation and stripping, because stripping of the superficial vein in such a patient may remove the major patent collateral vein and worsen the venous outflow problem.

Evaluation of the Venous System

Clinical Assessment. Prior to any operative treatment, the patency of the deep venous system and valvular competence should be determined. Historically, Perthes' test or some variant has been used to assess deep venous patency. With this test, superficial varicosities are compressed by wrapping the extremity with elastic bandages. Upon exercise, the development of increasingly severe crampy leg pain suggests a deep venous obstruction, if arterial occlusive disease has been ruled out.

The retrograde-filling test described by Brodie in 1846 and by Trendelenburg in 1890 (Brodie-Trendelenburg test) was the first scientific attempt to evaluate valve competence and function. With the patient in the supine position, the leg to be examined is elevated 30 to 45 degrees to ensure maximal venous emptying. An elastic tourniquet is adjusted around the thigh just below the saphenofemoral junction to occlude the superficial veins. The patient is allowed to stand while the pattern of superficial venous refill is noted. In the normal limb, refilling of the superficial veins will not be completed at 30 seconds, and removal of the tourniquet does not result in rapid retrograde filling. Rapid venous refilling upon release of the tourniquet suggests incompetent valves in the saphenous system, whereas rapid filling of the superficial veins prior to release of the tourniquet indicates that incompetent valves are present in some of the perforating veins.

Noninvasive Venous Assessment. Unfortunately, the diagnosis of the site of venous insufficiency by clinical examination is often incomplete and inaccurate. Since venous ulceration may result from incompetence of the deep, the superficial, or the perforating veins, appropriate management is dependent on a correct diagnosis. The development of venography allowed visualization of the deep and superficial venous systems and allowed assessment of patency and valvular competence (Fig. 48–5). Venography combined with the measurement of ambulatory venous pressure by direct venous cannulation provides a reliable diagnosis, but these invasive tests are uncomfortable, time-consuming, and potentially hazardous and are therefore used infrequently. Several noninvasive methods of assessment have been developed. These tests fall into two main categories: plethysmographic techniques[25] and those based on Doppler ultrasonography.

Plethysmography. Strain gauge plethysmography quantitates venous obstruction by measuring the rate at which the calf veins empty when the pressure in a proximally placed pneumatic cuff is released. Because the rate of maximum venous outflow is inversely proportional to venous resistance, venous obstruction can be detected and the functional disability can be estimated. During exercise, the efficiency of the muscle pump mechanism correlates with the decrease in calf volume. After cessation of exercise, the rapidity with which blood returns to increase the calf volume is also proportional to the degree of valvular incompetence.

Other plethysmographic techniques have also been developed. Impedance plethysmography works on the principle of electrical impedance. Since blood is a better conductor of electricity than is soft tissue, as blood volume increases, electrical impedance decreases. If a pressure cuff placed on the thigh is inflated between arterial and venous pressures, blood volume will increase and impedance will decrease proportionally. This technique is accurate only for proximal, occlusive venous thrombi. Photoplethysmography measures the decrease in skin blood content during exercise and the rapidity with which blood returns to the cutaneous circulation after exercise is terminated. Changes in venous volume, and therefore venous pressure, caused by leg elevation or exercise produce a change in the number of red cells in the dermis and in the photoplethysmographic recording. Proximal venous obstruction results in elevated venous pressures.[31] Direct measurement of pedal venous pressure via cannulation of a superficial vein on the dorsum of the foot is the standard with which various plethysmographic methods have been compared.

Phleborrheography, devised by Cranley and associates, is quite accurate for diagnosing deep venous obstruction proximal to the knee and may also detect many of the larger calf vein thrombi. Although phleborrheography is a plethysmographic test, it is based on an entirely different concept from that which governs venous occlusion methods. It, like Doppler ultrasonography, senses the effects of respiration and augmentation on venous flow. An abnormal study is characterized by the absence of respiratory waves and a rise in the baseline of the limb tracing with foot or calf compression.

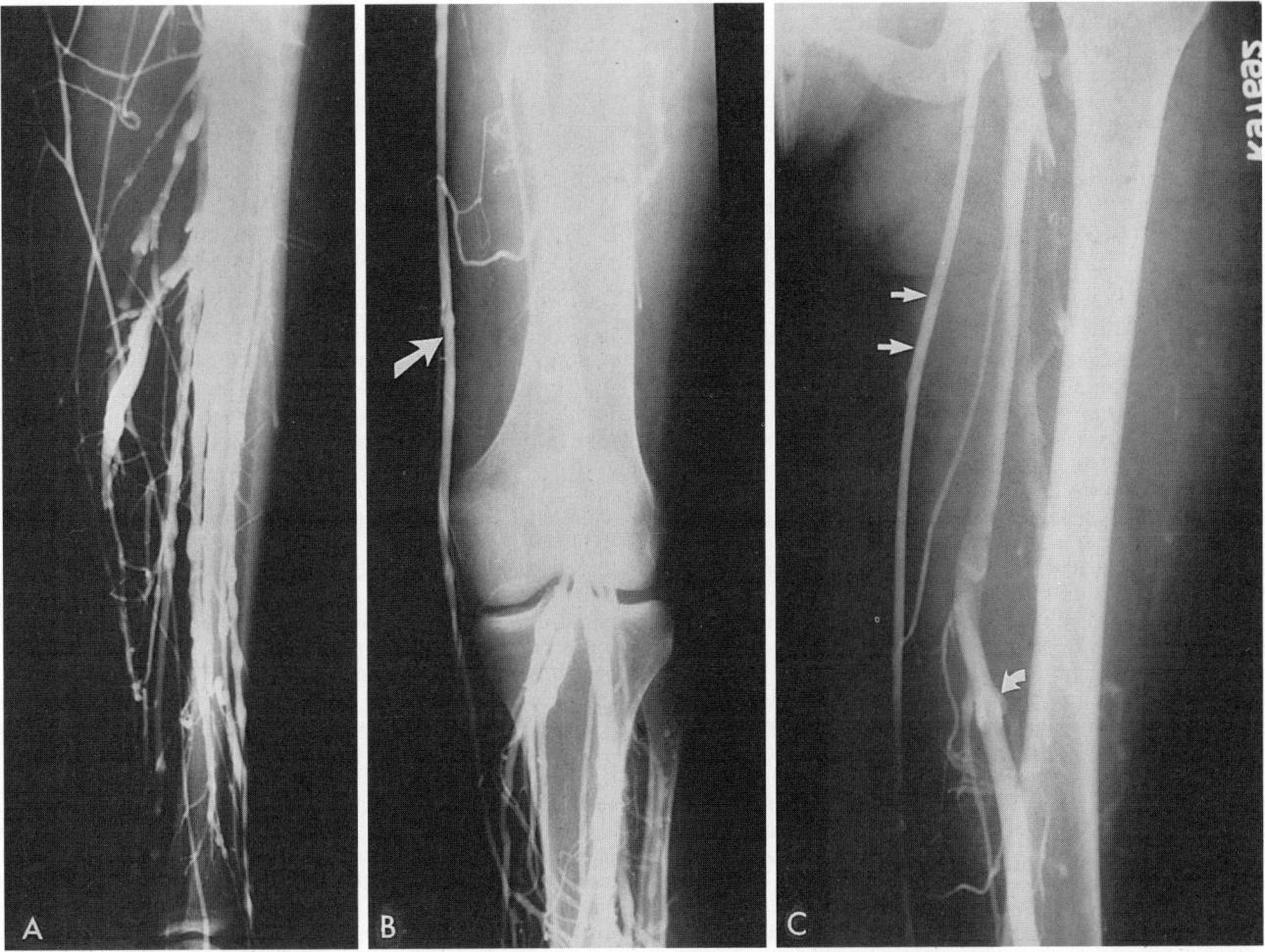

Figure 48–5. Normal leg venogram. *A,* Lower leg with multiple valves seen in the soleal and deep veins. *B,* Confluence of tributaries into popliteal and superficial femoral veins. The greater saphenous vein is well visualized (arrow). *C,* Superficial femoral vein with valves (arrow) joins the deep femoral vein in the upper thigh as components of the deep system. The greater saphenous vein (superficial system; double arrows) joins the common femoral vein at the saphenofemoral junction.

Duplex Doppler Ultrasonography. This technique combines B-mode real-time ultrasonography with pulsed Doppler ultrasonography. The B-mode image allows visualization of the underlying vessels so that a pulsed Doppler signal can then be specifically targeted to assess flow in a particular vessel.[25] Forward flow of venous blood toward the heart is augmented by a maneuver such as compression of the calf muscle; reverse flow of blood following this maneuver indicates that the vein is incompetent. Venous anatomy is notoriously variable, and duplex scanning eliminates the guesswork involved in venous assessment by all other methods except venography. Duplex Doppler ultrasonography has become the new gold standard for the assessment of venous incompetence.[38] Reflux studies have shown that if the sum of peak reflux in all veins is less than 10 ml. per second, skin changes or ulceration do not occur. However, these studies are not able to predict whether ulceration will occur for patients with a greater degree of reflux.[14] A limitation of this method is that the equipment is expensive and requires an experienced operator.

Treatment of Superficial Varicose Veins

Success in treating superficial venous insufficiency depends on the realization that effective treatment eliminates nonworking venous segments. This may be accomplished by both surgical and nonsurgical methods. In general, the surgi-

cal excision of incompetent veins is the more definitive treatment, because the results are more satisfactory and lasting. Nonsurgical methods are generally reserved for patients who have medical contraindications to surgical treatment, deep venous insufficiency, or minimal varicosities. Normal prominent superficial veins should not be disturbed or destroyed. These nonsurgical methods include sclerotherapy, elastic support, periodic elevation of the lower extremity, and exercise of the leg muscles. Advances in ablating symptomatic telangiectatic blemishes by sclerotherapy have now largely replaced minor surgical procedures. However, before any treatment is advised, the severity of the varicose problem must be carefully assessed.

Surgical Treatment

The philosophy in the treatment of varicose veins (superficial system) has changed from radical to selective in order to preserve the saphenous vein for reconstructive vascular procedures. Increased sophistication in localizing abnormal venous physiology justifies the use of more limited procedures. The surgical management of varicose veins involving the superficial venous system is based on the premise that the removed varicosity cannot recur, as may happen with sclerotherapy. Removal of symptomatic malfunctioning superficial veins restores the venous circulation to a more normal state and provides relief of symptoms of venous hypertension. Surgical procedures may also prevent progressive breakdown and incompetence of more distal but still normal tributaries of the saphenous system. However, operation on the superficial veins is not usually indicated unless definite venous incompetency and reflux are demonstrated by examination.

General indications for surgical treatment are (1) symptoms of aching, heaviness, and cramps; (2) complications of venous stasis, such as pigmentation, dermatitis, induration, superficial ulceration, and thrombosis of varicosities; (3) large varicosities subject to trauma; and (4) cosmetic concern. Procedures are not required for those patients who obtain relief by elastic stocking support, and surgical procedures should be recommended only for those patients who are in satisfactory general health.

The objectives of surgical treatment are to relieve symptoms, to alleviate stasis complications, to restore normal venous physiology, and to improve cosmetic appearance. All incompetent superficial veins and perforators should be thoroughly removed to prevent the tendency toward recurrence. Veins that have the potential to develop varicosities should also be removed, with particular attention directed to the smaller dilated tributaries in the thighs, calves, and feet. Special care should be taken not to damage or destroy normal competent greater or lesser saphenous veins, because they may be needed for future vascular bypass operations.

Operative Technique. One of the most important steps in the entire surgical procedure is the preoperative marking of the veins. This must be done carefully and accurately with an indelible skin pencil. It is best accomplished while the patient stands on a platform in front of a movable light source. By inspection and palpation, all varicosities, including the main saphenous channel, tributaries, and incompetent perforating veins, are marked. Particular attention should be focused on the identification of tortuous tributaries and perforating veins within fascial defects (Fig. 48–6).

On the day of operation, general, spinal, or epidural anesthesia is administered. Each leg is prepared with a suitable antiseptic solution, and the patient is draped from the ankle to the umbilicus. Venous bleeding may be minimized by elevating the legs 15 to 20 degrees during the operation. If the saphenous vein is not directly involved with varicosities, it may be preserved by removing only the varicose branches.[19] When a classic high ligation and stripping of the

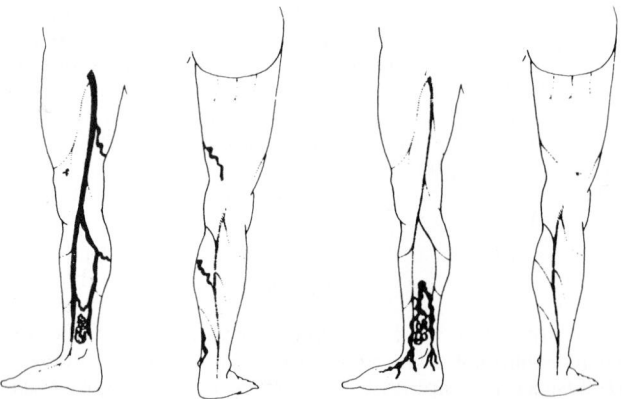

GROSS GREAT
SAPHENOUS
INCOMPETENCE

INCOMPETENT
ANTERO - MEDIAL
PERFORATORS

Figure 48–6. Patterns of superficial venous varicosities in the greater and lesser saphenous veins.

greater or lesser saphenous vein is performed, the operation should follow a systematic plan as follows: (1) high ligation at the saphenofemoral or saphenopopliteal junction, (2) insertion of a stripper into the greater or lesser saphenous vein, (3) ligation and removal of tributaries, (4) resection of incompetent perforating veins, (5) stripping of the saphenous vein, and (6) closure.

A groin incision is made just below the inguinal crease and medial to the femoral arterial pulse. The incision should be cosmetic but generous enough to allow dissection of the superficial tributaries that enter close to the greater saphenous bulb. These tributaries vary widely in number and distribution but classically include the medial and lateral femoral cutaneous tributaries and the superficial external pudendal, circumflex iliac, and inferior epigastric branches. Removal of these tributaries decreases the risk of recurrence and facilitates precise transfixion ligation of the saphenous vein at its junction with the deep femoral vein.

A small transverse incision is made over the distal greater saphenous vein just anterior and proximal to the medial malleolus. This segment of venous anatomy is consistent in its location and can be identified even in a morbidly obese patient. A distal ligature is placed, and the flexible intraluminal stripper is passed proximally. If the stripper encounters obstruction due to tortuosity of the varicosities or angulation at the sites of perforating veins, transcutaneous palpation of the tip allows cutdown at these sites and manipulation of the stripper. Caution is needed, however, because the stripper may enter the deep venous system through one of these venous connections. The tip of the stripper is brought out through the saphenous vein in the groin incision and anchored to the saphenous vein with a ligature. The stripper is left in place until just before closure. Care is taken to avoid damage to the saphenous nerve, which lies adjacent to the saphenous vein from the level of the ankle to the knee. Injury to the saphenous nerve causing sensory loss or a distressing traumatic neuritis involving the medial aspect of the ankle may occur in as many as one third of these patients.[33]

Although most tributaries have already been identified by the preoperative marking, additional ones will be found during the operation. The tributaries are exposed through multiple small transverse incisions and are removed by either stripping or excision. Perforating veins should, therefore, be ligated individually wherever they emerge through the deep fascial layer. The more important ones are found on the medial distal third of the lower leg. Associated incompetent perforating veins are found more commonly in the postphlebitic leg and in recurrent varicose conditions.

Stripping of the saphenous vein should be the last step before closure in order to minimize bleeding. All incisions are closed with absorbable subcutaneous and subcuticular sutures and are reinforced with sterile wound closure tapes. The assistant applies firm compression over the course of the stripper (with the leg elevated) while it is gently but forcefully removed, via the lower incision, proximally to distally. The compression is maintained while the ankle incision is closed. The leg is then wrapped with an elastic bandage with sterile gauze pads over the incisions. Adhesive tape placed in a spiral over the elastic wrap prevents bunching of the wrap to form tourniquets at the knee and ankle. The patient is encouraged to ambulate on the first postoperative day, and the bandages are removed on the second day for inspection of wounds prior to discharge. Ambulation is permitted only with elastic external support for the first 10 to 14 days. Continued use of support stockings is not necessary in patients who achieve a normal venous reflux time after removal of diseased superficial varicosities but is needed if the deep venous system is incompetent.

When performed as a separate procedure, operation on the

lesser saphenous system is most easily accomplished with the patient in the prone position. When combined with a procedure on the greater saphenous system, the patient is in a supine position, and the posterior incisions are made while the leg is extremely rotated and elevated. A small transverse incision is made just below the popliteal skin fold, and the lesser saphenous vein is doubly ligated at its junction with the popliteal vein. The distal lesser saphenous vein is exposed by an incision just posterior to the lateral malleolus. Interjoining tributaries between the greater and lesser saphenous veins and incompetent perforating veins are excised before the lesser saphenous vein is stripped. Care is taken to preserve the sensory sural nerve, which lies adjacent to the saphenous vein from the level of the ankle to the midcalf region.

Unsatisfactory Surgical Results. Outcomes of surgical treatment may be unsatisfactory because of inaccurate preoperative assessment or incomplete operative treatment. Inaccurate assessment can result from attributing venous incompetency to the wrong saphenous vein (greater instead of lesser, or vice versa), missing important tributaries, overlooking incompetent perforating veins, or failing to recognize concomitant deep venous insufficiency. An accurate diagnosis depends on a complete assessment of both the superficial and the deep venous systems, usually by Doppler duplex examination.

Incomplete operation is the leading cause of unsatisfactory results. Limiting the operation only to veins that can be easily stripped and neglecting to excise tortuous branches or incompetent perforating veins are considered major surgical mistakes. Recurrent varicose veins most often represent larger tributaries over the medial and lateral aspects of the thigh and leg that were not removed at the original operation. Parallel or duplicate saphenous channels must be recognized as a possible cause of recurrence. Small varicosities, for which initial removal was not necessary, sometimes develop as a true recurrence after an adequate and complete operation.

Because there is an intrinsic weakness of the superficial veins and a propensity for further varicosity development, periodic follow-up examinations are advisable after operation for uncomplicated primary varicose veins. For patients with stasis problems or postphlebitic conditions in which superficial vein operation does not restore normal venous physiology, follow-up examinations are even more important and should be performed at shorter intervals. In the early postoperative period, small varicosities can be extirpated under local anesthesia in the outpatient clinic or injected with a sclerosing solution. Surgical results are satisfactory (excellent or good) in 95% of patients after 5 years and in 85% after 10 or more years. The recurrence rate remains low, even many years after an adequate operation.

Nonsurgical Treatment

The aim of sclerotherapy is to inject a small volume of an effective sclerosant into the vein's lumen in order to destroy the venous intima. If external compression is not applied, a large thrombus forms, which soon recanalizes. The associated destruction of venous valves actually worsens the venous pathology. However, if the sclerosant is injected into an emptied vein and external compression is maintained until permanent fibrosis has obliterated the lumen, good results can be obtained.

Three per cent sodium tetradecyl sulfate has been found to be an effective and safe sclerosing agent. Disposable 2- or 3-ml. syringes fitted with 25-gauge needles are used to inject 0.5 ml. of the sclerosant into the empty vein at each of the *points of control.* These points of control are sites at which incompetent perforating veins join the superficial veins. The nearer the injection is made to the perforating vein, the more certain are the results. Repeated injections may be necessary for residual veins.

When larger veins are treated, the leg is elevated to 45 degrees and the segment of vein is isolated by pressure from the operator's index and ring fingers. As the injection is made, the top of the middle finger is placed over the tip of the needle to monitor the injection and to ensure that there is no perivenous leak of sclerosant. Cotton balls are then placed over each injection site, and the leg is firmly bandaged with 7.5-cm. cotton crepe followed by 10-cm. crepe with limited stretch (Elastocrepe, S.T.D. Export). This bandage must be smoothly applied so that there is less pressure over the proximal leg. Finally, these bandages are covered by a length of flesh-colored, size D, elasticized tubular stockinette (Tubigrip). The patient is instructed to walk immediately and to increase the distance daily. The compressive bandage is discontinued after 6 weeks (less for smaller veins), and two-way stretch elastic stockings are worn during the day for at least 4 more weeks.

The enthusiasm for sclerotherapy varies, but many authorities do not use it as the primary treatment for incompetent varicose veins, since the recurrence rate may be high, even after only a few years. Hobbs reported a recurrence rate of 29.5% with sclerotherapy, versus 7% with surgical therapy, at 3 years.[11] Recurrence is a particular problem when sclerotherapy is used for large-caliber veins. In addition, sclerosing solutions can cause allergic reactions. The inflammatory response can also cause local pain and periphlebitis, which is sometimes quite disabling. Repeated injections of large volumes can give rise to chronic swelling of the leg from inadvertent sclerosing of an otherwise normal deep venous system. Small prominent venules or minor varicosities causing cosmetic concern are generally unsuitable for surgical removal and are best treated by sclerotherapy. Small recurrent varicosities following surgery are often treated by this method as well.

SUPERFICIAL VENOUS THROMBOSIS

Unlike deep venous thrombosis, superficial thrombophlebitis is usually clinically obvious. The physical finding is commonly a linear, indurated, tender subcutaneous venous cord with local erythema. This type of thrombophlebitis most commonly occurs at the site of an intravenous infusion, as a result of the drugs being given or the intraluminal catheter itself. This condition also frequently occurs in the greater saphenous system below the knee in patients with varicose veins. If there is no predisposing cause in the superficial venous system, Doppler duplex examination may occasionally be necessary to rule out the presence of associated deep venous thrombosis.

The treatment of superficial venous thrombosis depends on its etiology, extent, and symptoms. Localized thrombophlebitis usually requires only a mild analgesic such as aspirin, and activity may be continued. More severe thrombophlebitis with pain and cellulitis should be treated with bed rest, elevation, and hot compresses. Upon resolution of symptoms, ambulation is begun with elastic stockings. Antibiotics are usually not necessary unless the process is suppurative, in which case adequate drainage must be achieved.

Surgical intervention is rarely indicated in nonsuppurative superficial venous thrombosis unless the process continues upward despite adequate nonoperative management, the inflammatory reaction is very severe, or a varicose vein is involved that will eventually require stripping. This disease rarely causes pulmonary embolism and, therefore, generally does not require anticoagulation. Although deep venous thrombosis rarely develops in association with superficial venous thrombosis, superficial involvement frequently occurs in patients with deep venous disease, especially in those with ankle ulceration.

Septic phlebitis usually occurs in association with infection of an intravenous cannula inserted for long-term administration of fluids or medications. Simple removal of the cannula and administration of systemic antibiotics are usually effective treatment. However, purulence within the vein or suppurative thrombophlebitis, often associated with generalized septicemia, is a more lethal condition. Treatment requires immediate and complete excision of all the involved veins. The wound is packed open for later closure, and appropriate systemic antibiotics should always be given.

Mondor's disease, or spontaneous thrombophlebitis of the superficial veins of the breast and anterior chest wall, is a rare condition. This self-limited condition usually involves a vein in the anterolateral aspect of the upper portion of the breast or in the region extending from the submammary fold toward the costal margin and epigastrium.

Migratory thrombophlebitis, or repeated thrombosis at varying sites in superficial veins, most commonly occurs in the lower extremity. No definite etiologic factor has been confirmed; however, in 1856, Trousseau reported an association with carcinoma. This condition has been noted to be especially prevalent with carcinoma of the tail of the pancreas.

DEEP VENOUS DISEASE

Whereas superficial venous thrombosis is usually a benign, self-limited disease, involvement of the deep venous system is a major cause of morbidity and mortality. Although any venous system may be involved (Fig. 48–7), the lower extremities are most frequently affected. The incidence of venous thrombosis is particularly high in older patients undergoing surgery. In the United States alone, Hume et al.[13] estimated that at least 140,000 fatal and 400,000 nonfatal cases of pulmonary embolism occur each year. The source of the emboli is almost always from the pelvis or lower extremities. In addition to the acute symptoms and risks, there may be long-term sequelae of the venous obstruction and valvular injury.

Chronic Venous Insufficiency

The edema that immediately follows deep venous thrombosis is purely obstructive in origin and quickly subsides

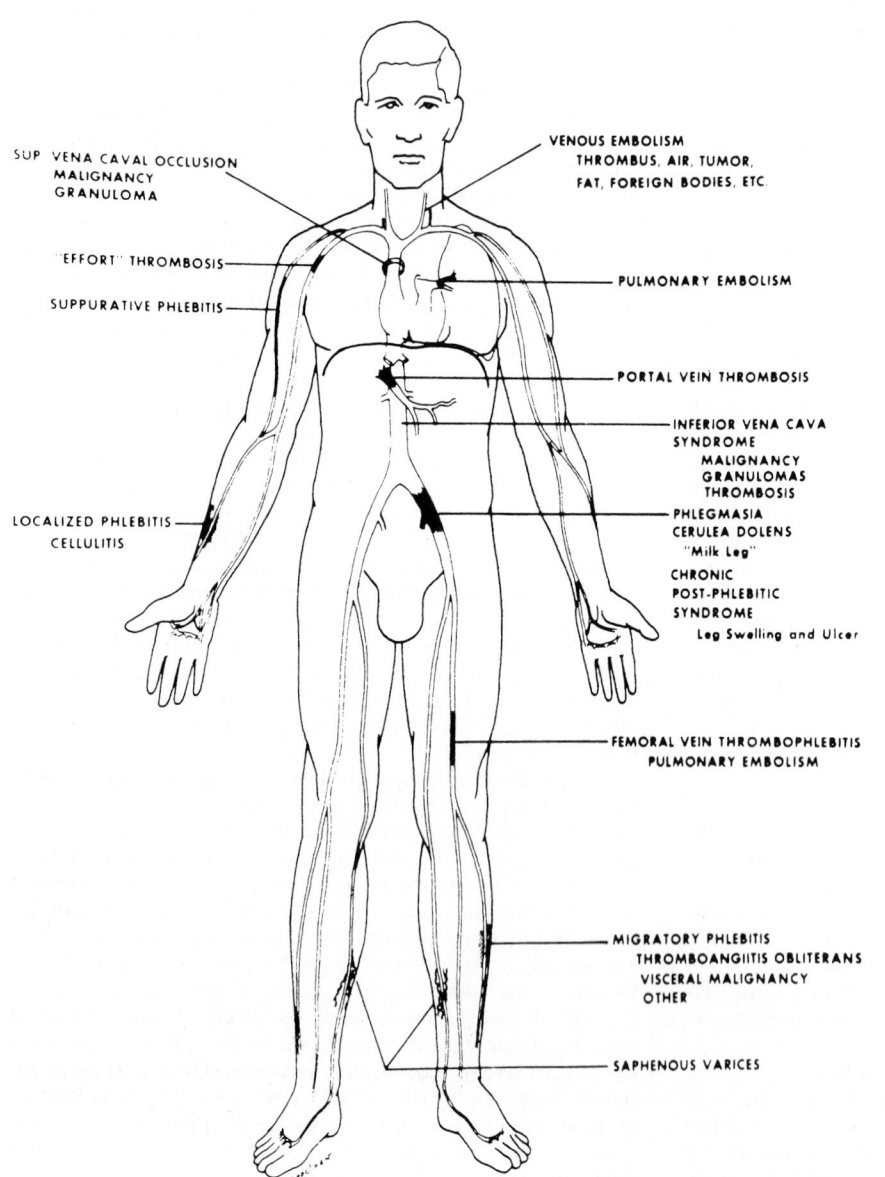

SUP VENA CAVAL OCCLUSION
MALIGNANCY
GRANULOMA

"EFFORT" THROMBOSIS

SUPPURATIVE PHLEBITIS

LOCALIZED PHLEBITIS
CELLULITIS

VENOUS EMBOLISM
THROMBUS, AIR, TUMOR,
FAT, FOREIGN BODIES, ETC.

PULMONARY EMBOLISM

PORTAL VEIN THROMBOSIS

INFERIOR VENA CAVA
SYNDROME
MALIGNANCY
GRANULOMAS
THROMBOSIS

PHLEGMASIA
CERULEA DOLENS
"Milk Leg"

CHRONIC
POST-PHLEBITIC
SYNDROME
Leg Swelling and Ulcer

FEMORAL VEIN THROMBOPHLEBITIS
PULMONARY EMBOLISM

MIGRATORY PHLEBITIS
THROMBOANGIITIS OBLITERANS
VISCERAL MALIGNANCY
OTHER

SAPHENOUS VARICES

Figure 48–7. Representative sites of venous disorders.

with bed rest and anticoagulants as venous collaterals develop. However, cessation of edema should not lull the physician into inadequately treating the underlying thrombophlebitis. Although the deep venous system is usually eventually recanalized, the delicate valves often remain imprisoned laterally in organized thrombosis. The resulting patent but valveless (completely or incompletely) deep venous system then transmits the gravitational pressure of the blood column unimpeded from the level of the heart to the ankles. This hypertensive venous state is the central predisposing feature in the pathophysiology of the postphlebitic state.[3]

Valvular incompetence alone is not enough to produce serious stasis sequelae, however. It must occur in combination with incompetent perforator veins through which the high deep venous pressure in the upright position is transmitted to the superficial tissues.[9] The location of these perforating veins from the malleoli up the lower half of the leg determines the predilection of this area to the development of stasis changes and ulcers. These venous perforators may have been involved in the initial thrombosis or may subsequently become incompetent by dilation resulting from the back pressure of the valveless deep venous system.[28] Within 10 years, 75% of patients with untreated thrombophlebitis develop advanced stasis changes, and 50% have stasis ulcers.[13]

This insidious process develops because the high ambulatory venous pressure within the calf muscle pump is transmitted through communicating veins to the superficial veins within the skin and subcutaneous tissues of the calf. The local capillary bed distends to widen the endothelial pores, thus allowing larger molecules to escape into the interstitial fluid. The most important molecule, fibrinogen, polymerizes to form insoluble fibrin in the extravascular space. The fibrin cannot be removed because of inadequate blood and tissue fibrinolysis,[4] and its accumulation acts as a barrier to the diffusion of oxygen and other nutrients. The subcutaneous tissue becomes thick, hard, and tender (liposclerosis) and develops the changes of stasis dermatitis (brawny edema, subcutaneous fibrosis, pigmentation, and cutaneous atrophy), which may lead to tissue death and ulceration.[5] Although varicosities are frequently associated with these changes, the opposite is not true; that is, uncomplicated varicose veins are rarely associated with ulcers.

Postphlebitic Syndrome

Both the calf muscle pump ejection fraction and the degree of deep venous reflux determine the propensity for venous stasis ulceration. A poor ejection fraction can be the primary cause of ulceration in limbs with minimal reflux. A good ejection fraction, however, significantly reduces the incidence of ulceration in limbs with marked reflux. Air plethysmographic measurements have been especially useful in identifying the predominant hemodynamic factor (ejection fraction, reflux, or both).[8]

Whereas the relatively simple hemodynamics of the arterial circulation are driven by the pumping function of the heart, the hemodynamics of venous return from the lower limbs against gravity is dominated by the pumping function of the calf muscle contraction and is more complicated and multifactorial.[35] In a limb with primary varicose veins, the calf muscle functions like a heart with a normal stroke volume but with increased preload because of venous reflux.[9] When deep venous disease is present, the limb is comparable to a reduced cardiac stroke volume, because the volume of the deep veins of the calf has been reduced, afterload has been increased by venous obstruction, and preload has been increased by venous reflux.[2] Associated superficial venous

insufficiency further complicates deep venous decompensation.

The venous pressure in normal patients not only quickly decreases with exercise but also takes several minutes to rise after exercise has been discontinued.[2] In contrast, a patient with postphlebitic syndrome has little decrease of elevated venous pressure during exercise.[34] The venous pressure changes in patients with primary varicose veins (superficial system) fall between these two extremes (Fig. 48–8).

The leg muscle pump, which consists of fascia against which the contained contracting muscles furnish a pumping force, normally prevents leg edema. In chronic venous insufficiency, the muscle pump has failed because (1) a leaking venous perforator system allows blood reflux and a rise in distal superficial venous pressure during muscle contraction, (2) narrowed or occluded subfascial veins retard the flow from the superficial to the deep venous system, or (3) the pumping muscles are inactive, paralyzed, or diseased.[22] When chronic venous insufficiency develops, the deep venous hypertension is transmitted into the superficial veins and tissues, and recurring edema develops when the patient is upright for any significant period of time.[24] Even in the early stage, this edema does not *pit* readily, and in the chronic stage, it is frankly *brawny* and associated with characteristic skin changes.[7] Unfortunately, these changes are subtle and gradual at first, and the patient comes to accept a degree of swelling, discoloration, and aching in the involved leg. It is often minor trauma leading to a skin break that precedes the development of an actual stasis ulcer.[36] Characteristically, the venous ulcer develops in the gaiter area of the lower leg, i.e., medially from the instep to above the ankle.

Venous insufficiency causes appreciable disability, resulting in an estimated 2 million lost workdays in the United States each year.[12] The time to begin treating chronic venous insufficiency is as soon as the diagnosis has been made. The patient must be made to understand that subsequent damage and ulceration of the leg are directly proportional to the swelling that is allowed to occur. Although the wearing of good, custom-fitted elastic stockings whenever the patient is out of bed provides external support, it should be combined with periods during the day when the ankles are elevated above the heart level. It is rarely necessary for a patient to wear the stockings above the knee, since ulceration does not occur above the knee, and higher stockings are so uncomfortable that most patients will not wear them for any extended period of time. The frequency of daily leg elevation must be individualized according to the degree of venous disease and the rapidity of edema formation. These measures control stasis sequelae in 100% of patients, if they are scrupulously followed. Unfortunately, patients who think that they are doing well are less attentive to this chronic problem.

When chronic venous stasis ulcers do develop, their natural history is to remain unhealed, often for years. The goals in treating chronic venous insufficiency complicated by ulceration must be the reduction of pain, protection against recurrence, low treatment cost, full maintenance of ambulatory outpatient status, and minimal interference with work schedules and regular activities. Good management is still aimed at improving the underlying calf pump dysfunction and the resultant increased venous pressure. Exercise, elevation, and compression are the most effective means of achieving healing and form the mainstay of treatment.[32] When external support is provided by elastic compression paste bandages (Unna's boot), about 80% of ulcers heal. The remainder can be healed by the application of split-thickness skin grafts with or without ligation of adjacent perforator veins. Unfortunately, these ulcers have a high rate of recurrence, which is dependent primarily on the patient's compliance in using effective elastic stocking support.[23]

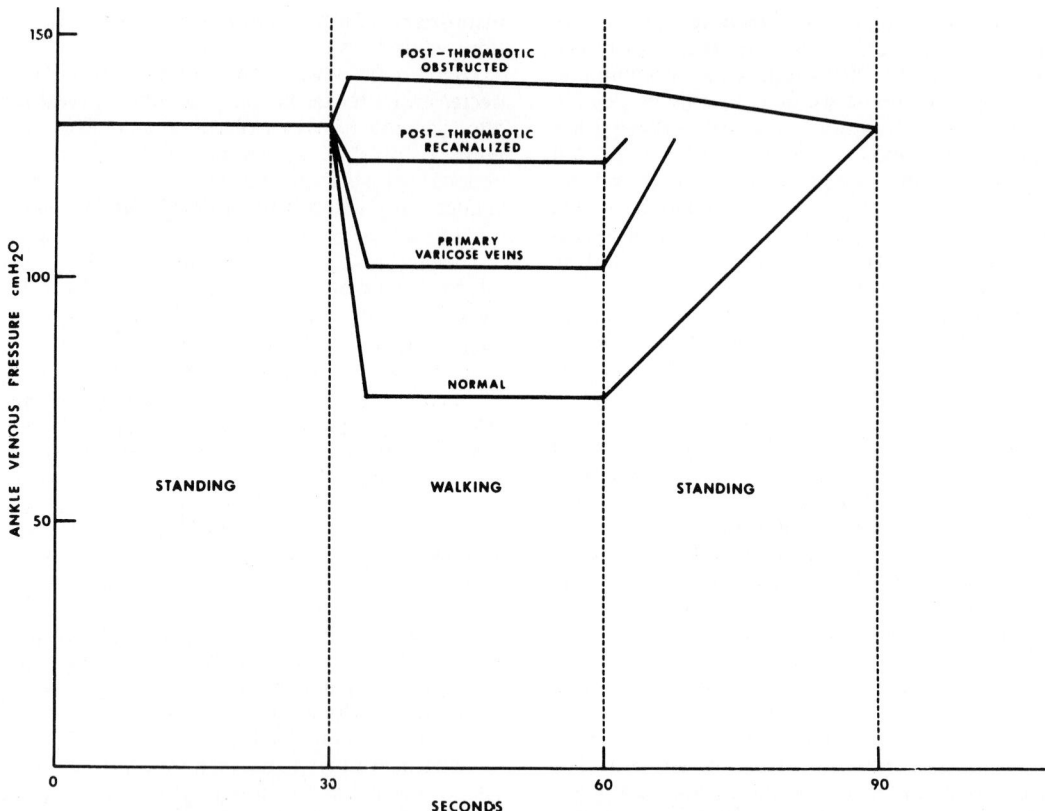

Figure 48–8. Ambulatory venous pressure in patients with postthrombotic obstructed veins, postthrombotic recanalized veins, primary varicose veins, or normal deep veins. (From Smith, D. E.: Surgical management of chronic obstructive venous disease of the lower extremity. *In* Rutherford, R. B. [Ed.]: Vascular Surgery, 2nd ed. Philadelphia, W. B. Saunders, 1984, p. 1414.)

The bandage described by Unna in 1885 (Unna's boot) is an around-the-clock substitute for a failing muscle pump. Its re-establishes a *pump* by fixing the volume compartment. The power of the moving ankle joint generates the pumping force, which compresses the lower leg against the nonelastic circumferential bandage. The therapeutic effect of Unna's boot appears to depend on control of edema by the resulting external pressure. By preventing leakage of fluid from the hypertensive capillary bed, edema is reduced and the damaged skin and subcutis are better perfused and nourished. The healing rate for first ulcers in compliant patients is 91% with Unna's boot application, but success decreases if further ulceration develops.[22] Unna's boot (Gelocast wrap, Beiersdorf, Inc., Norwalk, CT) are bandages impregnated with a paste of zinc oxide, calamine, glycerin, and gelatin. Although compressible during application, they harden to form rigid support bandages. Usually this dressing is changed weekly, although excessively exudative ulcers may require changes every 3 to 5 days. Elevation of the legs several times per day also decreases the associated limb edema.

Pruritus associated with stasis dermatitis can be controlled by topically applied corticosteroids and orally administered antihistamines. To control acute flares of stasis dermatitis, an intermediate-strength corticosteroid, such as 0.1% triamcinolone cream, may be used for 2 to 3 weeks. In addition, venous ulcers are usually heavily contaminated by aerobic and anaerobic bacteria. The predominant gram-positive *Staphylococcus aureus* and *Streptococcus pyogenes* usually respond to dicloxacillin and erythromycin; the major gram-negative bacteria, *Pseudomonas aeruginosa*, can be treated with orally administered ciprofloxacin (Cipro).[40]

Recurrent ulceration is prevented by wearing one-way stretch, woven-to-measure, heavy or medium-heavy, heel-covered, seamless, cotton-elastic, below-the-knee compressive stockings after the ulcer has healed. Surgical management should be needed only for large or persistent ulcerations.

Surgical Management

Although 90% of venous stasis ulcers can be managed nonoperatively, those patients who cannot follow this postphlebitic routine should be evaluated for an operative procedure.[6] It should be fully appreciated that in 15% to 20% of patients who develop venous ulcers, only isolated superficial venous disease is present, which can be treated simply by excision of the incompetent superficial venous system, with a high likelihood of cure.[28] The patent and competent deep venous system can then function normally.

Linton developed a radical technique for the subfascial ligation of incompetent perforators for the treatment of stasis dermatitis and ulceration.[21] He ligated and stripped all superficial varicosities, ligated the superficial femoral vein, subfascially ligated and divided all medial communicating (perforating) veins, and excised a strip of posterior calf fascia.[16] With increasing experience, it became apparent that removal of all superficial varicosities and complete subfascial ligation of all incompetent perforating veins were the essential parts of this operation. Following this procedure, the ulcer recurrence rate is 2% to 43%.[16]

The development of noninvasive techniques such as phlebography and duplex Doppler ultrasonography has made it easier to determine the contribution of incompetent superficial, perforating, or deep veins to the pathologic process.[39] Surgical therapy can now be directed toward correcting the specific abnormalities in these veins.[6] If there is incompetence of the superficial veins, they should be removed in combination with ligation of the incompetent perforators. The three major medial posterior arch vein perforators described by Cockett are especially important in the development of lower leg stasis changes.[9] If proximal deep venous occlusion is also present, it must be relieved before the incompetent perforators can be ligated; otherwise, reduction of the deep venous outflow is increased and symptoms will worsen.

Cross-Femoral Venous Bypass. The saphenous vein has been used to bypass proximal segmental venous occlusion in the iliofemoral or femoropopliteal veins. For iliofemoral occlusion, the contralateral saphenous vein is passed suprapubically and anastomosed to the affected side (Palma or Dale procedure.[10, 29] A temporary arteriovenous fistula distal to the anastomosis may ensure patency. If there is isolated iliac venous compression and entrapment by the right common iliac artery, this may be decompressed by completely mobilizing the arteries overlying the veins. Division of the right common iliac artery and reanastomosis behind the left common iliac vein may be necessary to prevent recompression of the vein.[11] When occlusive disease is limited to the femoropopliteal veins, the obstructed segment can be bypassed by anastomosis of the saphenous vein to the popliteal tibial trunk at the level of the knee (Husni or May procedure).

Venous Valvuloplasty. Occasionally, chronic venous insufficiency results from primary valvular incompetence of an otherwise normal valve. Descending venography shows the contrast agent regurgitating through a prolapsing valve cusp. Direct repair of these incompetent valves and ligation of any associated incompetent perforators have controlled induration and ulceration in 90% of the patients so treated.[18, 27] Only if there is marked deep venous reflux does venous valvular reconstruction improve the abnormal venous hemodynamics.

Venous Valve Transposition or Transplantation. In those patients in whom the valves of the superficial femoral and popliteal veins have been destroyed by thrombophlebitis, a competent valvular system can be produced by transposition of an adjacent vein containing a valve.[15] Anastomosis of a valve-containing segment to the incompetent superficial femoral or profunda femoris vein decreases the hydraulic venous hypertension. Free transplantation of venous valves is used infrequently because of the need to remove autogenous veins from elsewhere and their propensity for thrombosis.[39] However, the axillary vein has been used successfully, and creation of a distal arteriovenous fistula and postoperative anticoagulation are thought to improve patency.[39]

In some, but not all, cases of venous reconstruction, the initial physiologic response has been favorable. The ambulatory venous pressure has decreased, and the plethysmographic tracings have normalized. However, later follow-up studies in many of these patients have shown a disappointing return to the previously abnormal hemodynamic state, particularly when there is residual incompetence of the perforating veins or of the superficial venous system. Serial physiologic monitoring is essential to understand the results of venous operations and to design better operations and improve patient selection.[17]

External Popliteal Valve. In an effort to control deep venous reflux caused by incompetence of the popliteal veins without invasion of the vein, a technique has been developed to produce a valvelike external compression of the popliteal vein by an implanted silicone tendon attached to the gracilis muscle.[30] During walking, the popliteal vein becomes patent during contraction of the calf muscles when the knee is extended and the gracilis is relaxed. The popliteal vein is closed during relaxation of the calf muscles when the foot is off the ground because the knee is flexed and the gracilis muscle is contracted. Thus, the *valve* effect prevents or minimizes reflux in the deep veins during relaxation of the calf muscles. Preliminary success requires long-term confirmation.

Occlusion of Other Deep Veins

The axillary subclavian vein occupies a unique position in the thoracic outlet at the junction of three major anatomic regions of the body: the neck, the shoulder girdle, and the thorax. In this position, it is subject to pivotal motion and segmented stress between relatively stationary veins at either end. Motion subjects this vein to stretching and shearing trauma that may induce an inflammatory reaction in the vein wall. Additional factors may cause external compression and stasis of blood flow in the axillary subclavian vein, including an anomalous subclavius or anterior scalene muscle, congenital fibromuscular bands, callus from a fractured clavicle or first rib, or narrowing of the costoclavicular space from depression of the shoulder girdle while lifting or working overhead. These conditions may result in acute or chronic venous thrombosis.

The frequent association of thrombosis of the axillary subclavian vein with exertion has led to the phrase *effort vein thrombosis* (Pagen-Von Schroetter syndrome). This typically develops as an abrupt swelling of the upper extremity. Even with early medical treatment, complete resolution occurs in only 15 to 30% of patients, and most patients have residual symptoms or impaired use of the arm in the dependent position. Pulmonary embolism from an upper extremity source is not as rare as was originally thought. Adams and DeWeese found that it occurred in 12% of their patients.[1] Symptomatic occlusion of the subclavian vein, although not common, has also been noted with the use of permanent transvenous pacing electrodes, with the use of Swan-Ganz catheters in an intensive care setting, and as a result of the increased use of long-term central venous access catheters. Unlike in the lower extremity, it is highly unusual to develop ulceration of the arm with chronic venous obstruction. The development of collaterals and the presence of lower hydrostatic forces usually limit the degree of edema and stasis.

Superior Vena Caval Obstruction

Invasive malignant tumors, usually anaplastic lung cancers, are the most common cause of the distinctive superior vena caval syndrome. Occasionally, primary venous thrombosis, a chronic fibrosing mediastinitis, or a granulomatous lesion may be responsible. Depending on the rapidity of the development of vena caval obstruction, there are varying degrees of edema of the neck, head, and arms, with evidence of venous stasis. Acute obstruction of the superior vena cava, as during a thoracic operation, can result in fatal cerebral edema. However, when obstruction develops slowly, collateral circulation can develop, and the symptoms are mild.

Malignant involvement of the superior vena cava precludes curative surgical resection. However, significant palliation can be obtained with intensive radiation therapy. With benign obstructions, symptoms usually improve or subside completely as collateral circulation develops. Attempts to reconstruct the occluded superior vena cava have frequently been unsuccessful. The most favorable graft is a spiral or panel composite autogenous vein, which creates a graft of a sufficiently large diameter.

Inferior Vena Caval Obstruction

Anatomically, the inferior vena cava may be divided into thirds. The lower third extends from the confluence of the iliac veins that form the vena cava to the renal veins, the middle third extends from the renal veins to the hepatic veins, and the upper third extends from the hepatic veins to the right atrium. Obstruction of the inferior vena cava most commonly occurs by extension of pelvic and thigh vein thrombosis. Rapid blood flow from the renal veins usually stops the thrombus at this level. However, if the renal veins are involved, nephrotic syndrome may result. If renal vein obstruction is bilateral and acute, renal failure can ensue. If it is unilateral or slowly progressive, pain, hematuria, and proteinuria may result. If adequate collateral circulation develops, these findings may be reversible. When the upper third of the inferior vena cava is involved and the hepatic veins are occluded, portal hypertension and the Budd-Chiari syndrome cause ascites, hepatomegaly, and hepatic decompensation.

Renal carcinoma is the second most common cause of caval obstruction, usually by invasion rather than from external compression. Other causes include hepatomegaly secondary to a variety of hepatic diseases, ascites, primary leiomyosarcoma, retroperitoneal fibrosis, congenital membranes, hypercoagulable states, and expanding or leaking abdominal aortic aneurysms. In children, the causes of inferior vena caval obstruction are specific for this age group and include right-sided Wilms' tumor, adrenal carcinoma, neuroblastoma, hepatoma, and multicystic kidney. The site and extent of obstruction are determined by venography.

Treatment of an inferior vena caval obstruction varies according to the underlying cause, location, and extent of the process. The persistence of the edema of the lower body that usually develops depends on whether adequate collaterals develop. Thrombectomy and fibrinolytic therapy have occasionally been used for a benign process. Radiation therapy and/or chemotherapy are indicated when a malignant disease is involved. When Budd-Chiari syndrome of the membranous type occurs, dilatation of the hepatic vein membrane via the femoral vein or the transcardiac route may be effective. When more diffuse hepatic vein involvement occurs, a mesocaval shunt can decompress the portal system or, when associated with obstruction of the vena cava, a mesoatrial shunt can be constructed or the liver can be replaced with a transplanted organ.

SUMMARY

Prevention of initial venous thrombosis avoids the sequelae of deep venous thrombosis and prevents possibly fatal pulmonary embolism. However, venous diseases continue to cause death and incapacitate patients. The venous problems that arise are often managed nonoperatively. Nevertheless, there is now a definite role for surgical treatment in the management of many of these disorders. To optimize operative intervention, an effective venous assessment must determine whether the deep veins are competent. In the lower extremities, if there is deep vein reflux or obstruction, conventional surgery on the superficial venous system has a poorer outcome, and procedures aimed at the deep vein may be more appropriate. If the deep veins are competent and there is superficial vein reflux, saphenofemoral and saphenopopliteal incompetence should be corrected.

SELECTED REFERENCES

Christopoulos, D., Nicolaides, A. N., Cook, A., et al.: Pathogenesis of venous ulceration in relation to the calf muscle pump function. Surgery, 106:829, 1989.
An increase in the incidence of venous stasis ulceration occurs with increasing reflux and decreasing calf muscle pump ejection fraction, as measured by air plethysmography. These authors found that the residual volume fraction, which expresses the combined effect of venous reflux and ejection fraction with rhythmic

exercise, showed a good correlation with the incidence of ulceration and the measurements of ambulatory venous pressure.

Iafrati, M. D., Welch, H., O'Donnell, T. F., Belkin, M., Umphrey, S., and McLaughlin, R.: Correlation of venous non-invasive tests with the Society for Vascular Surgery/International Society for Cardiovascular Surgery clinical classification of chronic venous insufficiency. J. Vasc. Surg., 19:1001, 1994.
The lack of discrimination by noninvasive venous tests between the Society for Vascular Surgery/International Society for Cardiovascular Surgery staging criteria for Stage 2 (hyperpigmentation, brawny edema, and subcutaneous fibrosis without ulceration) and Stage 3 (ulcerated limbs) implies that the progression from lipodermatosclerosis to frank ulceration is not accounted for by large vessel hemodynamic changes but rather by microcirculatory alterations.

Lippmann, H. I., Fishman, L. M., Farrar, R. H., Bernstein, R. K., and Zybert, P. A.: Edema control in the management of disabling chronic venous insufficiency. Arch. Phys. Med. Rehabil., 75:436, 1994.
Over a 15-year period, edema control was achieved by the use of Unna's boot for leg ulcerations and by compressive hosiery for the prevention of ulcerations. Unna's boot is a functional substitute for the failing muscle pump in chronic venous insufficiency and resulted in 91% healing of first ulcers in compliant patients. Unna's boot is noninvasive and inexpensive and does not interfere with patients' activities.

Rutgers, P. H., and Kitslaar, P. J.: Randomized trial of stripping versus high ligation combined with sclerotherapy in the treatment of the incompetent greater saphenous vein. Am. J. Surg., 168:311, 1994.
Patients with isolated incompetence of the greater saphenous vein and local varicosities were randomized to standard saphenous stripping operation combined with surgical avulsion of varicosities or to high ligation of the saphenofemoral junction combined with sclerocompressive therapy of the varicosities. After 3 years, the cosmetic, clinical, and Doppler ultrasound results were significantly better after stripping than after high ligation combined with sclerotherapy.

Schanzer, H., and Pierce, E. C., II.: A rational approach to surgery of the chronic venous stasis syndrome. Ann. Surg., 195:25, 1982.
Since different mechanisms are responsible for the production of the chronic venous stasis syndrome, no one method of treatment is satisfactory for the entire population. Ambulatory venous pressure and ascending and retrograde phlebography were measured in 49 patients with chronic venous stasis to determine the specific venous abnormality. Significant improvement in the ambulatory venous pressure was obtained postoperatively when one of the following surgical procedures was correctly chosen: ligation of perforators, superficial femoral valvuloplasty, segmental venous transposition, ligation of the superficial femoral vein, cross femoral venous bypass, or high ligation and stripping of the long saphenous vein.

REFERENCES

1. Adams, J. T., and DeWeese, J. A.: "Effort" thrombosis of the axillary and subclavian veins. J. Trauma, 11:923, 1971.
2. Barnes, R. W., Collicott, P. E., Mozersky, D. J., Sumner, D. S., and Strandness, D. E., Jr.: Noninvasive quantitation of venous hemodynamics in postphlebitic syndrome. Arch. Surg., 107:807, 1973.
3. Bauer, G.: A roentgenological and clinical study of the sequelae of thrombosis. Acta Clin. Scand., 74:1, 1942.
4. Browse, N. L., and Burnand, K. G.: Hypothesis: The course of venous ulceration. Lancet, 2:243, 1982.
5. Burnand, K., Clemenson, G., Morland, M., Jarrett, P. E. M., and Browse, N. L.: Venous lipodermatosclerosis: Treatment by fibrinolytic enhancement and elastic compression. Br. Med. J., 280:7, 1980.
6. Burnand, K. G., O'Donnell, T. F., Thomas, M. L., and Browse, N. L.: Relation between postphlebitic changes in the deep veins and results of surgical treatment of venous ulcers. Lancet, 1:936, 1976.
7. Butler, C. M., and Smith, P. D. C.: Microcirculatory aspects of venous ulceration. J. Dermatol. Surg. Oncol., 20:474, 1994.
8. Christopoulos, D., Nicolaides, A. N., Cook, A., Irvine, A., et al.: Pathogenesis of venous ulceration in relation to the calf muscle pump function. Surgery, 106:829, 1989.
9. Cockett, F. B.: Ulcers of the leg. Adv. Surg., 12:327, 1978.
10. Dale, W. A., and Harris, J.: Cross-over vein grafts for iliac and femoral venous occlusion. Ann. Surg., 168:319, 1988.
11. Eriksson, I.: Reconstructive venous surgery. Acta Clin. Scand. (Suppl.), 544:69, 1988.
12. Fitzpatrick, J. E.: Stasis ulcers: Update on a common geriatric problem. Geriatrics, 44:19, 1989.
13. Hume, M., Sevitt, S., and Thomas, D. P.: Venous Thrombosis and Pulmonary Embolism. Cambridge, Harvard University Press, 1970.
14. Iafrati, M. D., Welch, H., O'Donnell, T. F., Belkin, M., Umphrey, S., and McLaughlin, R.: Correlation of venous noninvasive tests with the Society for Vascular Surgery/International Society for Cardiovascular Surgery clinical classification of chronic venous insufficiency. J. Vasc. Surg., 19:1001, 1994.
15. Johnson, N. D., Queral, L. A., Flinn, W. R., Yao, J. S., and Bergan, J. J.: Late objective assessment of venous valve surgery. Arch. Surg., 116:1461, 1981.
16. Johnson, W. C., O'Hara, E. T., and Corey, C.: Venous stasis ulceration: Effectiveness of subfascial ligation. Arch. Surg., 120:797, 1985.

17. Killewich, L. A., Martin, R., Cramer, M., Beach, W., and Strandness, D. E., Jr.: Pathophysiology of venous claudication. J. Vasc. Surg., 1:507, 1984.
18. Kistner, R. L.: Primary venous valve incompetence of the leg. Am. J. Surg., 140:218, 1980.
19. Large, J.: Surgical treatment of saphenous varices with preservation of the main great saphenous trunk. J. Vasc. Surg., 2:886, 1985.
20. Leutolf, O., Bull, R. H., Bates, D. O., and Mortimer, P. S.: Capillary under-perfusion in chronic venous insufficiency: A cause for leg ulceration? Br. J. Dermatol., 128:249, 1993.
21. Linton, R. R.: Postphlebitic ulceration of the lower extremity: Its etiology and surgical treatment. Ann. Surg., 138:415, 1953.
22. Lippmann, H. I., Fishman, L. M., Farrar, R. H., Bernstein, R. K., and Zybert, P. A.: Edema control in the management of disabling chronic venous insufficiency. Arch. Phys. Med. Rehabil., 75:436, 1994.
23. Mayberry, J. C., Moneta, G. L., Taylor, L. M., Jr., and Porter, J. M.: Fifteen year results of ambulatory compression therapy for chronic venous ulcers. Surgery, 109:575, 1991.
24. McEnroe, C. S., O'Donnell, T. F., and Mackey, W. C.: Correlation of clinical findings with venous hemodynamics in 386 patients with chronic venous insufficiency. Am. J. Surg., 156:148, 1988.
25. McMullin, G. M., and Smith, P. D.: An evaluation of Doppler ultrasound and photoplethysmography in the investigation of venous insufficiency. Aust. N. Z. J. Surg., 62:270, 1992.
26. Nicolaides, A. N., and Zukowski, A. J.: The value of dynamic venous pressure measurements. World J. Surg., 10:919, 1986.
27. O'Donnell, T. F., Mackey, W. C., Shepard, A. D., and Callow, A. D.: Clinical hemodynamic and anatomic follow-up of direct venous reconstruction. Arch. Surg., 122:474, 1987.
28. O'Donnell, T. F., and McEnroe, C. S.: Chronic venous insufficiency. Surg. Clin. North Am., 70:159, 1990.
29. Palma, E. C., and Esperon, R.: Vein transplants and grafts in the surgical treatment of the post-phlebitic syndrome. J. Cardiovasc. Surg., 1:94, 1960.
30. Psathakis, N. D., and Psathakis, D. N.: Surgical treatment of deep venous insufficiency of the lower limb. Surg. Gynecol. Obstet., 166:131, 1988.
31. Randhawa, G. K., Dhillon, J. S., Kistner, R. L., and Ferris, E. B.: Assessment of chronic venous insufficiency using dynamic venous pressure studies. Am. J. Surg., 148:203, 1984.
32. Riordan, C. A.: The management of venous ulcers of the legs. Australas. J. Dermatol., 32:111, 1991.
33. Rutgers, P. H., and Kitslaar, P. J. E.: Randomized trial of stripping versus high ligation combined with sclerotherapy in the treatment of the incompetent greater saphenous vein. Am. J. Surg., 168:311, 1994.
34. Schanzer, H., and Pierce, E. C., II: Pathophysiology evaluation of chronic venous stasis with ambulatory venous pressure studies. Angiology, 33:183, 1982.
35. Schmidt, C., Schmitt, J., and Scheffmann, J.: Haemodynamics of the post-phlebitic syndrome. Int. Angiol., 6:187, 1987.
36. Schull, K. C., Nicolaides, A. N., Fernandes e Fernandes, J., Miles, C., Horner, J., Needham, T., Cooke, E. D., and Eastcott, H. H. G.: Significance of popliteal reflux in relation to ambulatory venous pressure and ulceration. Arch. Surg., 114:1304, 1979.
37. Shami, S. K., Shields, D. A., Scurr, J. H., and Smith, P. D.: Leg ulceration in venous disease. Postgrad. Med. J., 68:779, 1992.
38. Struckmann, J.: Venous investigations: The current position. Angiology, 45:505, 1994.
39. Taheri, S. A., Pendergast, D. R., Lazar, E., Meenaghan, M. A., et al.: Vein valve transplantation. Am. J. Surg., 150:201, 1985.
40. Tam, M., and Moschella, S. L.: Vascular skin ulcers of limbs. Cardiol. Clin. 9:555, 1991.

CHAPTER 49

PULMONARY EMBOLISM

Mark W. Sebastian, M.D., and David C. Sabiston, Jr., M.D.

Pulmonary embolism is a significant source of hospital morbidity and mortality, and despite an improved understanding of the pathogenesis, diagnosis, and management of pulmonary embolism, there continues to be frequent and significant mortality. Although pulmonary embolism is a well-recognized postoperative surgical problem, many nonsurgical patients develop pulmonary embolism secondary to a serious medical disorder such as congestive heart failure, cerebrovascular accident, chronic pulmonary disease, systemic infections, and carcinomatosis. Nevertheless, pulmonary embolism remains a significant postoperative complication, and surgeons should constantly be aware of the associated problem of venous thromboembolism, especially in older patients. Current emphasis on the management of pulmonary embolism centers around identification of populations at risk, appropriate prophylaxis, and definitive diagnosis. Although high-risk populations continue to be defined, the overall incidence of pulmonary embolism in the United States is estimated at 600,000 cases annually, with up to 200,000 deaths reported (Fig. 49–1).[10] Routine autopsies in hospitalized patients over the age of 40 have shown that two thirds have either gross or microscopic evidence of pulmonary emboli, implying a high prevalence of subclinical emboli. Pulmonary embolism may be found only incidentally at death, but in many patients it either contributes to or is actually the principal cause of death.

HISTORICAL ASPECTS

Laennec described pulmonary embolism as "pulmonary apoplexy" in a treatise on the diagnosis of diseases of the lung and heart. He differentiated the lesion caused by pulmonary embolism from other pulmonary disorders causing hemoptysis. Cruveilhier said "all arterial branches which led to those lesions were filled with clots that branched according to the vascular tree." Despite these descriptions, neither investigator sought the origin of the thrombi and viewed them as arising as a primary process in the pulmonary arteries. Rokitansky confirmed Laennec's findings in 1842 and introduced the term *hemorrhagic infarct*.

The famed pathologist Rudolph Virchow first described the embolic concept of this disorder. He stated:

In the peripheral veins the danger proceeds chiefly from the small branches. By no means rarely do these become quite filled with masses of coagulum . . . new masses of coagulum deposit themselves from the blood upon the end of the thrombus layer after layer; the thrombus is prolonged beyond the mouth of the branch into the trunk in the direction of the current of blood, shoots out in the form of a thick cylinder farther and farther, and becomes continually larger and larger. From a lumbar vein, for example, a plug may extend into the vena cava as thick as the last phalanx of the thumb. These are the thrombi that constitute the source of real danger; it is in them that ensues the crumbling away which leads to secondary occlusion in remote vessels.[36]

Virchow also described two types of thrombus in the pulmonary arteries in such patients: (1) the embolus that arises as a thrombus in a systemic vein and is swept into the venous circulation through the heart and into the pulmonary arteries after being disloged from its site of origin, and (2) the thrombus that occurs in situ in the pulmonary artery distal to an occluding embolus following stagnant blood flow in that vessel. Responding to critics of his newly announced pathogenesis of pulmonary embolism and wishing to prove the embolic doctrine, Virchow inserted pieces of rubber and venous thrombi recovered from humans at autopsy into the jugular veins of dogs. When the animals were sacrificed, the emboli were found in the pulmonary arteries. An essential part of Virchow's studies centered around matching the assumed embolic particle with the apparent structure from which it had been detached. Embolism alone did not explain the development of a hemorrhagic infarct, and because he frequently found occluding emboli in pulmonary branches without an infarct, he considered the problem of infarction of pulmonary tissue difficult to explain. In 1872, Cohnheim provided additional basic data showing the importance of pulmonary congestion and left ventricular failure in the development of hemorrhagic infarction. Cohnheim also recognized that not all patients with pulmonary embolism have associated pulmonary infarction and that concomitant congestive heart failure is an important aspect of infarction.

In 1908 Trendelenburg first performed pulmonary embolectomy, describing emergency thoracotomy and removal of the emboli in three patients. The longest survivor lived for 37 hours and ultimately died of hemorrhage from an internal mammary artery. Kirschner did the first successful pulmonary embolectomy in 1924 with a long-term survivor, and the first successful pulmonary embolectomy using cardiopulmonary bypass was performed by Sharp in 1962.[31] As a medical student, McLean discovered heparin in 1916, and its value in the management of thromboembolism was confirmed by Murray and co-workers[27] in 1937 and later extended.[9]

PATHOGENESIS OF VENOUS THROMBOSIS

Venous stasis is the most important feature predisposing to venous thrombosis. Trauma or injury such as that following a surgical procedure is known to be associated with an increased incidence of venous thrombosis. Radiopaque contrast medium injected into the deep veins of the leg may take surprisingly long to clear when a postoperative patient remains flat in bed with little active movement due to pain. Allison showed that radiopaque dye may linger in the calf veins for as long as 25 minutes after injection in postoperative patients. Similarly, all ill patients are less likely to move the extremities, which predisposes them to intravenous thrombosis. Although knowledge of the pathogenesis of thrombosis evolved, scant attention was given to the basic features of venous thrombosis. Virchow concluded that primary thrombosis of the systemic veins was caused by three factors (Virchow's triad): stasis of blood flow, injury to the vein, and a state of hypercoagulability, factors still regarded as being important in the pathogenesis of venous thrombosis. The venous sinuses are especially vulnerable to stasis and

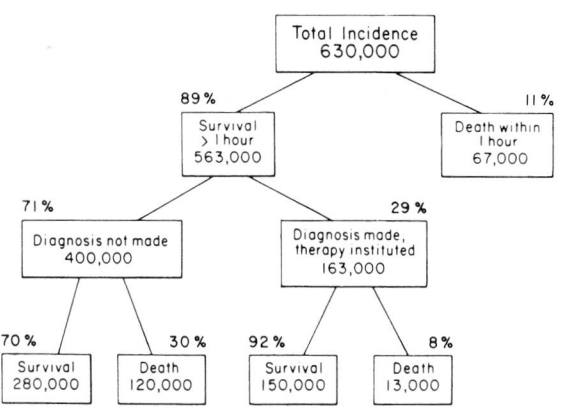

Figure 49–1. Annual incidence of pulmonary embolism in the United States showing the subsequent course of this complication with deaths and survivors. (From Dalen, J. E., and Alpert, J. S.: Natural history of pulmonary embolism. Prog. Cardiovasc Dis. *57*:259, 1975.)

thrombosis, and platelets become adherent at these sites. A thrombus develops and enlarges by successive deposition of aggregated platelets, leukocytes, and fibrin (Fig. 49–2). Propagation of the thrombus may then proceed upstream, or the process may spread retrograde (Fig. 49–3).

Hypercoagulability has been defined as the existence of an excessive amount of activity of one or more procoagulant substances, or a decrease in anticoagulant factors. Clearly, hypercoagulability has a multifactorial etiology. During pregnancy, the concentrations of fibrinogen, prothrombin, factor VII, Stuart factor, Christmas factor, and antihemophilic factor are elevated, and the risk of venous thrombosis is increased. Although the incidence of deficiencies in specific components of the coagulation cascade was thought to be rare, a recently identified deficiency in activated protein C (APC) among patients with familial hypercoagulability suggests a higher prevalence of 50%.[34] Protein C is a circulating factor that activates thrombin that is bound to thrombomodulin. Subsequently, APC acts as a natural anticoagulant in two ways: it controls conversion of factor X to Xa by inactivating factor VIIIa, and it controls conversion of prothrombin to thrombin by inactivating factor Va.. Early descriptions suggest a 10-

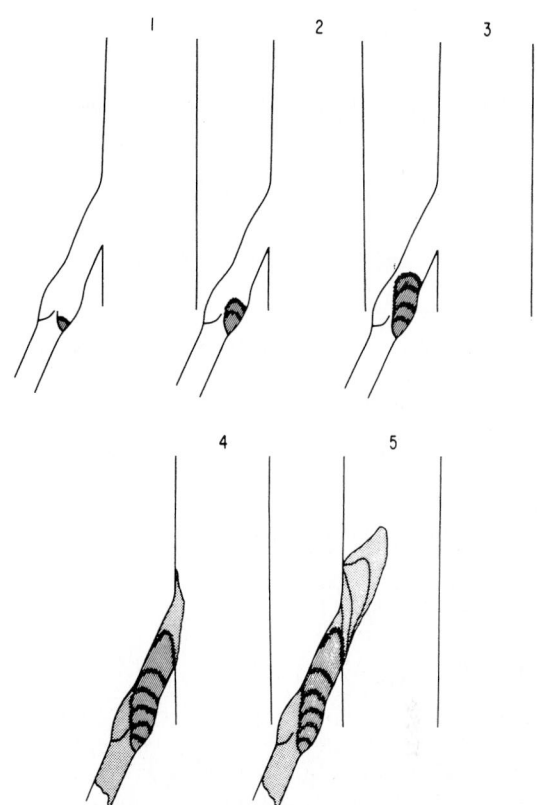

Figure 49–3. Illustration showing propagation of deep thrombus arising in a valvular pocket with deposition of successive layers and ultimate extension of the nonadherent red thrombus into the lumen of a larger parent vein. (From Cox, J. L., and Sabiston, D. C., Jr.: Phlebitis, thrombosis, and pulmonary embolism. *In* Condon, R. E., and DeCosse, J. J. [Eds.]: Surgical Care: A Physiologic Approach to Clinical Management. Philadelphia, Lea & Febiger, 1980.)

fold higher prevalence of deficiency in APC as compared with previously identified coagulation derangements, and deficiency in APC may prove to be a significant factor in the pathophysiology of deep venous thrombosis in the young and in patients with recurrent deep venous thrombosis. Other causes of hypercoagulable states predisposing to thrombosis include protein C deficiency, functional protein S deficiency, antithrombin III deficiency, lupus anticoagulant (antiphospholipid antibody), occult malignancy, documented malignancy, and carcinomatosis.

PATHOLOGIC ASPECTS

Pulmonary emboli are frequently present in the lungs at routine autopsy. This is emphasized by evidence that old or fresh pulmonary emboli are found at autopsy in 64% of patients over the age of 40. Unfortunately, the clinical diagnosis is frequently not established, and embolism is often first recognized at autopsy. Pulmonary embolism is a frequent cause of sudden death in the hospital setting as a result of near total occlusion of the pulmonary arterial circuit. This is demonstrated in the classic pathologic studies of Gorham[15, 16] on 100 consecutive patients with fatal pulmonary emboli. Among the 100 patients, 85 had emboli in both pulmonary arteries (Fig. 49–4). Only 15 had emboli restricted solely to one lung, and 12 of these patients were over 54 years of age, when underlying cardiac and respiratory disease is more frequent. Moreover, in patients with massive pulmonary embolism in whom embolectomy is done, it is common to find emboli in more than one pulmonary artery.[30] Other observations have shown that a marked reduction in pulmonary

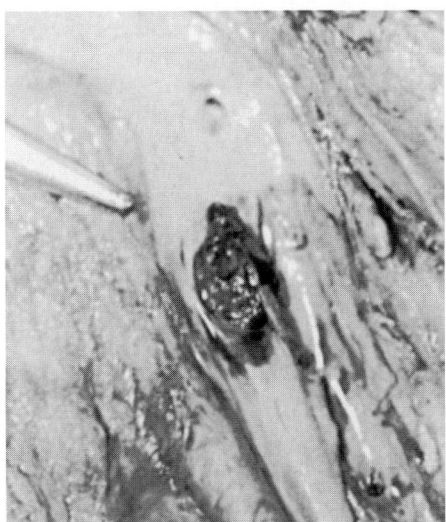

Figure 49–2. A primary thrombus forming in a valve sinus in the deep femoral vein. (Reprinted by permission of the publisher of VENOUS THROMBOSIS AND PULMONARY EMBOLISM by M. Hume, S. Sevitt, and D. P. Thomas, Cambridge, Mass.: Harvard University Press, Copyright © 1970 by the President and Fellows of Harvard College.)

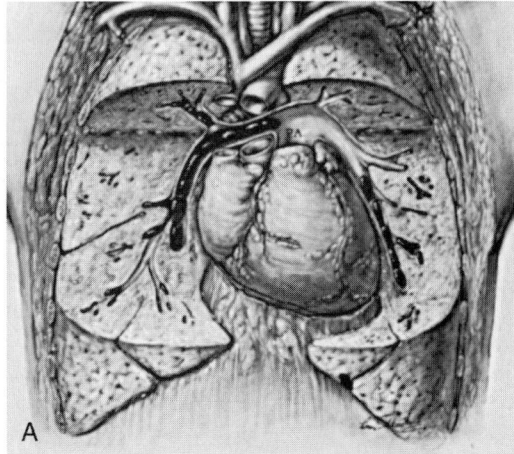

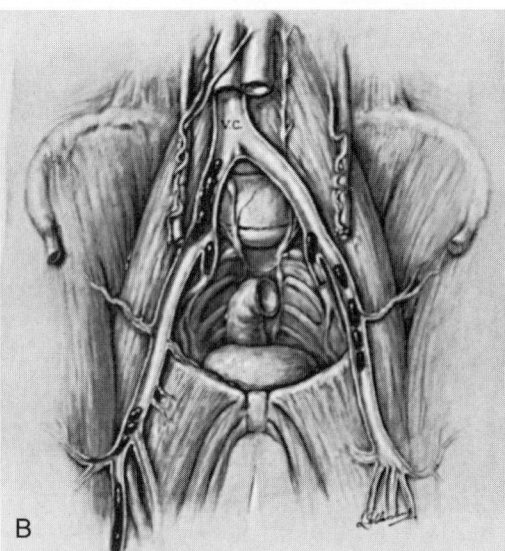

Figure 49–4. *A* and *B*, Illustration of the findings in a patient with massive pulmonary embolism at the time of postmortem examination. Multiple thrombi were present in the iliofemoral system. The right pulmonary artery and its branches are totally occluded by emboli. The left lower lobar pulmonary artery is also occluded. Under these circumstances, the entire output of the right ventricle must pass through the left lower lobe, which greatly increases pulmonary resistance and right ventricular work. The sudden development of this degree of pulmonary arterial occlusion produces a clinical state of severe shock, because the left ventricle receives a diminished amount of blood to supply the systemic arterial circulation. In otherwise normal patients, 50% or more of the pulmonary arterial circulation must be occluded before serious cardiovascular manifestations are produced. (*A* and *B* from Sabiston, D. C., Jr.: Pathophysiology, diagnosis and management of pulmonary embolism. Adv. Surg., *3*:351, 1968.)

blood flow by other causes, including arterial ligature, intravascular balloons, and pulmonary resection, is surprisingly well tolerated.[4] Following injection of experimental pulmonary emboli, reduced gas exchange function of the embolized lung follows immediately, but pulmonary gas exchange function returns to almost normal within several weeks.[30] Marked histologic changes occur in these thrombi with intravascular resolution, and most ultimately disappear. This resolution can be confirmed by serial pulmonary radioactive scans, arteriograms, and pulmonary function studies, as well as by gross and microscopic evaluation. Emboli found at postmortem examination as a cause of death are generally 1 to 1.5 cm. or more in diameter, providing evidence of having arisen in sizable veins. Their length can range to 50 cm., with a propensity to fragment into smaller pieces. The right pulmonary artery is more commonly involved than the left, and

the lower lobes are involved more often than the upper lobes. Emboli form primarily in the systemic venous circulation, and evidence suggests that most of the source thrombi arise in the iliac and femoral (proximal) veins.

Although pulmonary embolism usually occurs in adults, it has also been reported in children. In one study of children, the incidence was approximately 1% and was usually a secondary manifestation of a serious illness such as respiratory infection, phlebitis, systemic infection, or heart disease.[22] Although pulmonary embolism is rarely diagnosed before death in childhood, the clinical manifestations are similar to those in adults.

The iliofemoral and pelvic veins are commonly the sites of major thrombi, but other sources include the inferior vena cava and the subclavian, axillary, and internal jugular veins (Table 49–1). In addition to noninferior vena caval sources, emboli from neoplasms should also be considered in the differential diagnosis. Renal cell carcinoma is remarkable for early metastasis and involvement of the renal vein and inferior vena cava by direct extension. This causes pulmonary embolism in 10 to 54% of patients with this disorder. Primary pulmonary neoplasms can also mimic pulmonary embolism. Cardiac tumors arising in the right atrium and right ventricle may be the source of extensive pulmonary emboli, as can missiles such as bullets, which can embolize to the pulmonary arteries from systemic veins and via arteriovenous fistulas. The clinical manifestations of missiles lodging in the pulmonary arteries are usually related to associated complications, including erosion of the vessel, infarction of the distal lung, sepsis, and pulmonary vascular thrombosis. Among 18 patients, there were seven deaths (39%), all occurring in patients who did not undergo removal of the missiles. Therefore, removal of a missile embolus is recommended. When an embolus passes through an intracardiac defect from the venous to the arterial circulation with embolization of a systemic organ, it is termed a *paradoxical embolus*. The common cardiac defects responsible for such embolization include patent foramen ovale, atrial septal defect, and ventricular septal defect. This is more likely to occur with right atrial and right ventricular hypertension with right to left directional shunting.

It is currently believed that asymptomatic pulmonary embolism is a common event in the postoperative course of surgical patients. Resolution of large pulmonary emboli via the intrinsic lytic pathway, often in conjunction with systemic anticoagulation or systemic lytic therapy, is the usual course of events. Such observations have shown convincingly that the natural history of pulmonary embolism in most patients is resolution.[30] This concept is critical for a complete understanding of the principles of diagnosis and management. The areas of most active clinical and basic science research, and a source of ongoing controversy, involve risk stratification, the classification of patients at risk, optimization of prophylaxis, early diagnosis in suspected cases, and the treatment of symptomatic pulmonary embolism.

PHYSIOLOGIC RESPONSES

A primary feature of pulmonary blood flow is low vascular resistance. This enables flow in the vascular bed to increase several-fold with minimal elevation of pulmonary arterial pressure. The occasional finding of a small pulmonary embolus in a patient after sudden death has been cited as evidence that occlusion of a relatively small pulmonary artery can produce death, presumably as a result of reflex mechanisms. Currently, such an explanation is rarely tenable.

The concept of acute cor pulmonale contributed to an understanding of pulmonary embolism through physiologic features. Although the classic consideration of right ventricu-

TABLE 49–1. Site of Origin of Venous Thrombi

Investigator	No. of Cases with Thrombosis at Necropsy	Percentage of Cases with Thrombi in				
		Iliac Veins	Femoral Veins	Popliteal Veins	Soleal Veins	Any Deep Calf Vein
Rossle	94	—	49	—	—	92
Neumann	100	—	22	—	—	87
McLachlin and Paterson	34	9	82	—	—	41
Gibbs	149	—	42	—	—	65
Sevitt and Gallagher	81	70		33	67	74
Roberts	58	14	43	41	86	95

lar overload in pulmonary embolism involves electrocardiogram (ECG) changes, a minority of patients with massive pulmonary embolism exhibit an acute cor pulmonale pattern with the presence of Q waves in lead III, late inversion of T waves in lead III, and S waves in lead I (S1-Q3-T3), or right bundle branch block or right axis deviation. In 49 consecutive patients presenting with acute symptoms and subsequently proven pulmonary embolism, only 78% exhibited ECG criteria for right ventricular overload, but all patients exhibited tricuspid regurgitation and increased right ventricular end-diastolic diameter, suggesting right ventricular overload.[33] The acute physiologic response of a patient who suffers a pulmonary embolism is dependent on the patient's age, baseline physiology, comorbid diseases, and cardiopulmonary health. Since many postoperative patients lack significant concomitant cardiopulmonary dysfunction, obvious respiratory and cardiac compromise may not be apparent. This lack of overt physiologic compromise makes a firm clinical diagnosis more difficult in this population. A high index of clinical suspicion is essential to establish a diagnosis and institute appropriate treatment so that recurrent pulmonary embolism and potential hemodynamic compromise are avoided. It is currently thought that only 10% or less of emboli are associated with true infarction. An important clinical and pathologic feature is the observation that many patients with pulmonary embolism do not have evidence of infarction. Thus, the diagnosis of embolism can be missed by the clinician and, to a lesser degree, by the pathologist.

The physiologic changes following pulmonary embolism are related to the size of the emboli and can be divided into those that produce microembolism (obstruction of terminal small arteries and arterioles) and those that produce macroembolism (occlusion of the large pulmonary vessels). Considerable reduction in the diameter of the main pulmonary artery or the primary branches (at least 50%) is required to reduce pulmonary blood flow significantly or to produce pulmonary hypertension. Experimental thrombi of larger diameter produced in the inferior vena cava and embolized to either the right or the left pulmonary artery 10 to 14 days later produced minimal cardiovascular and respiratory responses. Specifically, occlusion of one pulmonary artery causes insignificant changes in the central venous pressure, right ventricular pressure, pulmonary arterial pressure, systemic arterial pressure, cardiac output, total oxygen consumption, and ECG, despite occlusion of half of the pulmonary arterial circulation. If one lung is normal or nearly normal, removal of the opposite lung is relatively well tolerated. Tidal volume and oxygen consumption at rest after resection of a lung change only a small degree.[4] Similarly, ligation of one pulmonary artery or occlusion by an intraluminal balloon is accompanied by few cardiodynamic changes.

Patients tolerate balloon obstruction of pulmonary flow to one lung for up to 2 hours,[3] and similar occlusion during exercise raises pulmonary arterial pressure only 12% to 50%. Cardiac output may increase as much as threefold. Such occlusion closely simulates the obstruction produced by large pulmonary emboli. It should be emphasized that these studies were conducted in normal subjects, and the presence of underlying cardiac or respiratory insufficiency alters this response appreciably. In patients with heart disease, exercise during unilateral occlusion of the right or left pulmonary artery by a balloon catheter produces a sharp elevation in pulmonary arterial pressure. Resection of less than one lung is followed by only minor changes in the pulmonary arterial pressure, whereas pneumonectomy produces elevated pulmonary arterial pressure.

Clearly, mechanical factors are most important in determining cardiodynamic effects of pulmonary embolism. Reflex effects may cause bronchoconstriction.[18] Moreover, tachypnea, pulmonary hypertension, and systemic hypotension can follow embolization with small particles (100 μ or less). However, this probably occurs infrequently, except after massive blood transfusion, when platelet, leukocyte, and fibrin emboli may occlude the pulmonary microcirculation. Embolization with larger particles requires considerably more blockage of the pulmonary arterial system to produce significant effects. Most believe that arterial emboli produce pulmonary hypertension by mechanical obstruction, whereas bronchoconstriction and vasoconstriction are produced by arteriolar embolism and are largely mediated by humoral factors.

INCIDENCE

Of the estimated 200,000 people who die from pulmonary embolism annually,[10] 10% may die within the first hour. The remaining patients survive for 1 hour or longer. If the diagnosis is made and appropriate treatment instituted, the mortality following pulmonary embolism is only 8% to 10%. However, autopsy studies estimate a missed diagnosis of clinically significant pulmonary embolism in 70% of patients. In this group of patients, the mortality of untreated pulmonary embolism may be as high as 30%. There has been a progressive increase in the incidence of death from pulmonary embolism and infarction in the United States, and similar data have been reported from England and Germany. Factors cited as being responsible for the increase in cases include the increasing age of the population, larger numbers and greater magnitude of operative procedures, increased recognition, and the use of oral contraceptives.

PREDISPOSING FACTORS

The patient's age is an important factor, since pulmonary embolism affects primarily the middle-aged and elderly (Fig.

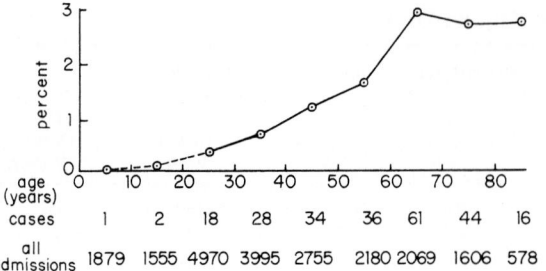

Figure 49–5. Graph showing the relationship of age and occurrence of thromboembolism. The ordinate represents the percentage of all hospital admissions in which a diagnosis was made clinically or at necropsy. (Reprinted by permission of the publisher of VENOUS THROMBOSIS AND PULMONARY EMBOLISM by M. Hume, S. Sevitt, and D. P. Thomas, Cambridge, Mass.: Harvard University Press, Copyright © 1970 by the President and Fellows of Harvard College.)

49–5). Inactivity, bed rest, and *reduced exercise* are well-established causes of pulmonary embolism. Cardiac disorders, especially congestive heart failure or atrial fibrillation, are particularly conducive to the development of pulmonary embolism. Acute myocardial infarction may be complicated by an increase in deep venous thrombosis, and the same occurs following cerebrovascular accidents, especially in patients with paralyzed lower extremities. Cancer, particularly carcinoma of the pancreas and prostate and carcinomatosis, is associated with a higher incidence of pulmonary embolism. Pregnancy increases the risk of pulmonary embolism, since pressure from the gravid uterus may retard venous flow from the legs and pelvis. Postpartum infection may also give rise to septic thrombophlebitis and embolism, and oral contraceptives have a positive association with the occurrence of venous thromboembolism.

Current literature emphasizes studies of deep venous thrombosis to identify patients at risk for pulmonary embolism (Table 49–2). A prospective study of venous thromboembolism after major trauma and the relative risk for pulmonary embolism was recently reported.[13] Prophylaxis against venous thromboembolism was not used. Approximately 50% of the 716 patients studied developed deep venous thrombosis, and proximal deep venous thrombosis developed in 63 of the 349 patients with documented deep venous thrombosis. Five independent risk factors were identified: age, history of transfusion, history of surgical intervention, femur fracture, and spinal cord injury. Emphasis should be placed on the fact that clinical diagnosis of deep venous thrombosis is reliable only half the time. Radioactive scanning of the lower extremities demonstrates deep venous thrombosis after operation in 54% of patients with hip fractures, 50% following prostatectomy, and 28% of general surgical patients over the age of 40.

DIAGNOSIS

Clinical Manifestations

The establishment of a diagnosis of pulmonary embolism is difficult due to signs and symptoms similar to a number of other cardiorespiratory disorders. Dyspnea, chest pain, hemoptysis, and hypotension are classic but are not sufficiently specific to make a definite diagnosis. Many patients have underlying cardiac disease, dyspnea and tachypnea are the most frequent clinical findings, and accentuation of the pulmonary second sound is common. Other suggestive signs such as hemoptysis, pleural friction rub, gallop rhythm, cyanosis, and chest splinting are present in a quarter or less of patients; clinical evidence of venous thrombosis is the exception and occurs in only one third of patients. The symptoms in 1000 consecutive patients at the Duke University Medical Center are shown in Table 49–3.[12]

TABLE 49–2. Risk for Pulmonary Embolism

	Low Risk	Moderate Risk	High Risk
Event or Condition			
General surgery	Age <40 yr, duration of operation <60 min	Age >40 yr; duration of operation >60 min	Age >40 yr; duration of operation >60 min and additional risk factors; previous deep-vein thrombosis or pulmonary emboli or extensive tumor
Orthopedic surgery	—	—	Elective hip or knee arthroplasty, prosthetic hip placement
Trauma*	—	—	Extensive soft-tissue injury; major fractures; multiple trauma, spinal cord injury
Incidence of thromboembolic events without prophylaxis (%)			
Distal deep-vein thrombosis calf veins	2%	10%–40%	40%–80%
Proximal deep-vein thrombosis pelvis, thigh, and popliteal veins	0.4	2–8	10–20
Symptomatic pulmonary emboli	0.2	1–8	5–10
Fatal pulmonary emboli	0.002	0.1–0.4	1–5
Recommended prophylaxis	Graduated-compression stockings and early ambulation	Heparin (5000 U subcutaneously twice daily), low-molecular-weight heparin, external pneumatic compression, or intravenous dextran	Heparin (5000 U subcutaneously three times daily), low-molecular-weight heparin, external pneumatic compression, intravenous dextran, warfarin (adjusted dose), vena caval interruption, or percutaneous insertion of intracaval filters

*Trauma has risk of fat emboli with long bone fractures.
Adapted from Weinmann, E. E., and Salzman, E. W.: Deep-vein thrombosis. N. Engl. J. Med., *331*:1630–1641, 1994. Copyright 1994. Massachusetts Medical Society. All rights reserved.

TABLE 49–3. Clinical Manifestations in 1000 Patients with Pulmonary Embolism at the Duke University Medical Center

Symptom or Sign	Percentage Afflicted
Dyspnea	77
Chest pain	63
Hemoptysis	26
Altered mental status	23
Dyspnea, chest pain, hemoptysis	14
Tachycardia	59
Recent fever	43
Rales	42
Tachypnea	38
Leg edema and tenderness	23
Elevated venous pressure	18
Shock	11
Accentuated P_2	11
Cyanosis	9
Pleural friction rub	8

Special Examinations

In patients with acute pulmonary embolism in the absence of other lung disease, the plain chest film is often normal. Diminished pulmonary vascular markings at the site of the embolus may be present (Westermark's sign).[37] The ECG is usually abnormal, but nonspecific changes such as sinus tachycardia are most common. Other ECG alterations include disturbances of rhythm (atrial fibrillation, ectopic beats, heart block), enlargement of P waves, ST segment depression, and T wave inversion. The most common abnormality is ST segment depression, which is a result of myocardial ischemia from reduced cardiac output and arterial pressure, as well as increased right ventricular pressure. An S1-Q3-T3 pattern, although highly suggestive of pulmonary embolism, is not universally present, even in patients with massive pulmonary embolisms whose ECGs were retrospectively analyzed, emphasizing the inadequacy of ECG for diagnosis.[33]

Impedance Plethysmography. Impedance plethysmography is a noninvasive method of assessing for the presence of proximal venous thrombosis, but it is not sensitive for calf vein thrombi. This test is infrequently employed due to operator dependence and a sensitivity of only 67%, even in the most experienced hands.

Doppler/Compression Ultrasonography. Ultrasonography of the lower extremities had over 95% sensitivity and specificity in one series of patients studied prospectively.[5] However, the series was small, and another series found it to be less sensitive and specific. Nevertheless, this is a reliable test for proximal deep vein thrombosis in the hands of an experienced operator. Furthermore, the test is portable and is commonly used in a high-risk patients in the intensive care unit, who are at increased risk when being transported to the radiology suite for diagnostic tests.[35]

Radioactive Pulmonary Scanning. Sabiston and Wagner[29] introduced radioisotope perfusion pulmonary scanning, and it remains the most frequently employed technique in the diagnosis of pulmonary embolism (Figs. 49–6 and 49–7). The principal method is measurement of intravenous injected particles such as [99m]technetium-labeled albumin, which become lodged in the pulmonary capilliary bed. Areas of nonperfusion on isotope scan suggest the absence of blood flow in that area. This scan was initially compared with a chest radiograph to identify areas of pulmonary parenchymal disease, which would imply a matched defect in ventilation and perfusion. The addition of xenon gas ventilation scan performed at the same time offers a more reliable way of comparing defects. Definitions commonly used for ventilation-perfusion (V-Q) scans concern the probability of embolism. For example, high probability indicates segmental or greater perfusion defects with a normal ventilation scan (V-Q mismatch). Moderate probability indicates multiple subsegmental perfusion defects with a normal ventilation scan or segmental perfusion defects without a ventilation scan performed. Indeterminate probability signifies chest film findings consistent with chronic obstructive pulmonary disease or other air-space disease in regions of perfusion defects. Intermediate probability refers to moderate- or indeterminate-probability scans. Low probability means subsegmental perfusion defects without a ventilation scan

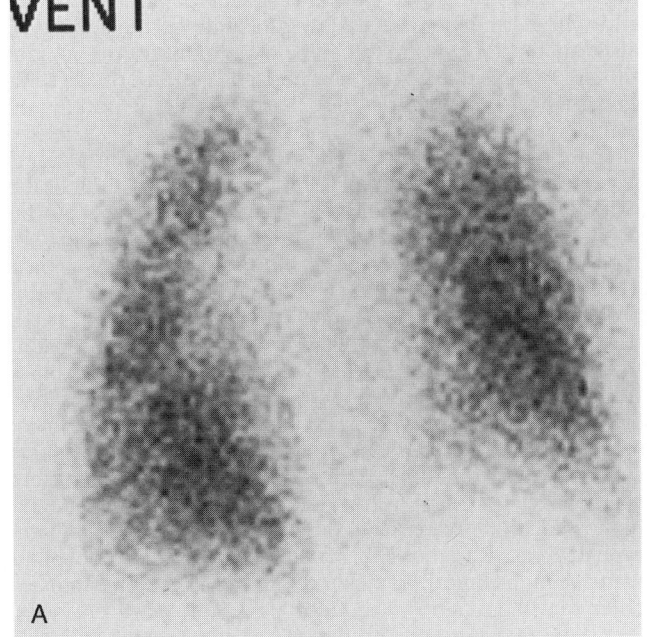
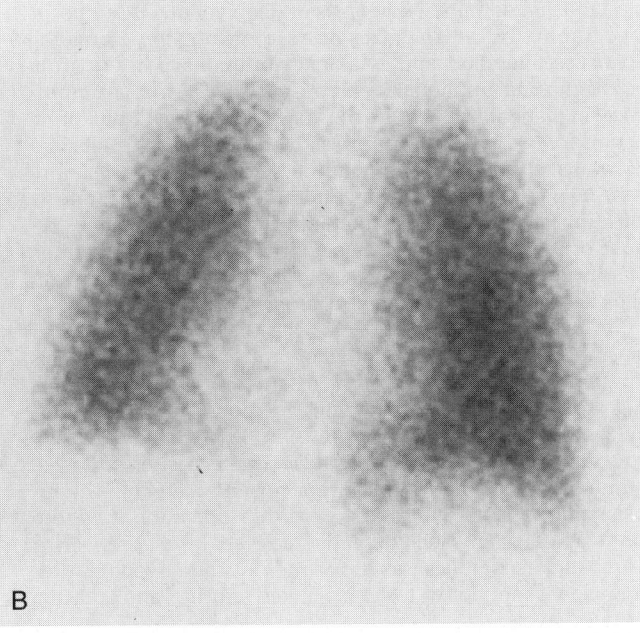

Figure 49–6. A normal ventilation *(A)* and perfusion *(B)* scan.

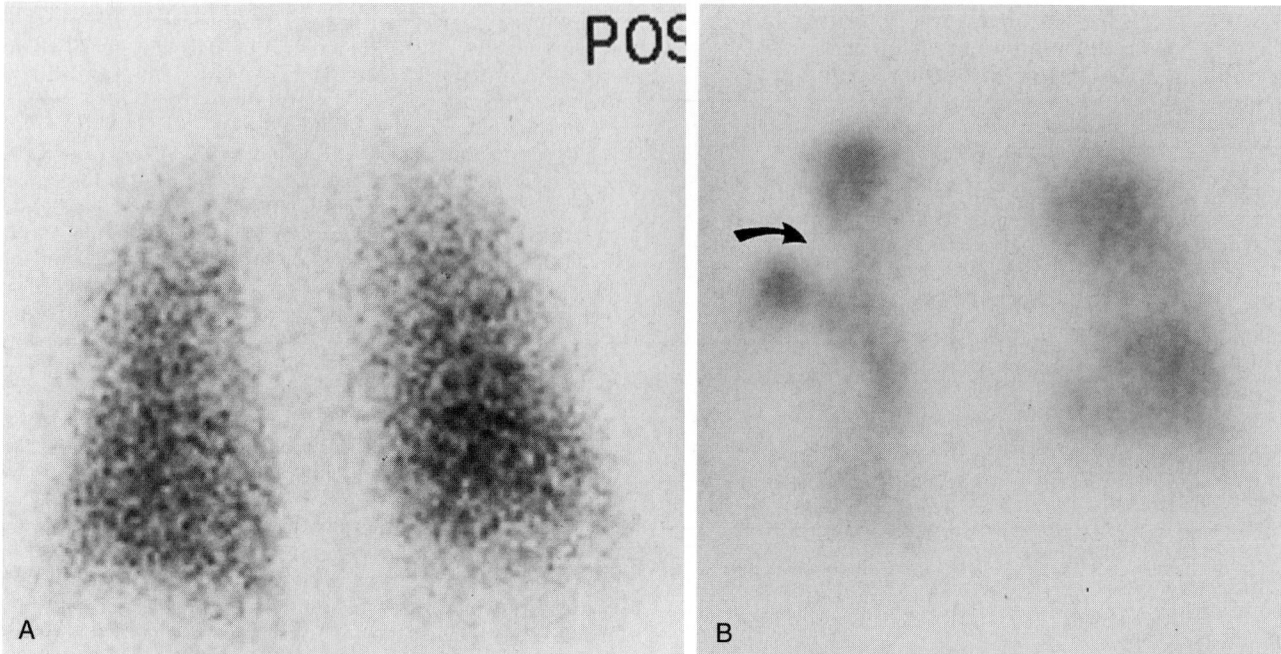

Figure 49–7. A high-probability ventilation *(A)* and perfusion *(B)* scan. Note the nonmatched areas of segmental perfusion. There are no corresponding defects of the ventilation component of the scan. The arrow in *B* points to an area of nonperfused lung.

performed or with small matched perfusion and ventilation defects.

Diagnosis of Deep Venous Thrombosis

An area of active analysis and study in the current literature centers around diagnosing deep venous thrombosis in a setting of clinical suspicion of pulmonary embolism and an indeterminate ventilation/perfusion scan. The performance of Doppler/compression ultrasonography to document proximal vein thrombosis is useful and has been recommended in the literature.[35] However, in a setting of high clinical suspicion of pulmonary embolism and an equivocal ultrasound examination of the deep venous system of the lower extremities and pelvic veins, contrast venography may be indicated to establish a definitive diagnosis of deep venous thrombosis. Venography for the diagnosis of deep venous thrombi is the most direct method and is akin to pulmonary arteriogram for diagnosing pulmonary embolism. It is of special importance in patients in whom the diagnosis is in doubt or in whom a vena caval procedure is being considered. Fibrinogen scans, although sensitive in the detection of the development of new thrombi in the extremities, are less accurate in detecting thrombi in the iliofemoral and pelvic regions, because of the background radioactivity in the urinary bladder. The fibrinogen scan has fallen into disuse because the tracer takes 24 hours to accumulate in propagating thrombi.

The definitive examination for the diagnosis of deep venous thrombosis remains phlebography. This technique is extremely effective is detecting distal thrombi in calf veins and proximal thrombi in popliteal, femoral and iliac veins. The major potential complication is a 0.067% rate of contrast-induced thrombophlebitis. This technique is cost-effective for symptomatic patients, those with recurrent deep vein thrombosis, and patients with a history of hip operation in whom noninvasive diagnostic methods may be insensitive. New diagnostic techniques include radionuclide venography, monoclonal antibody to cross-linked fibrin, and plasma D-dimer levels.

A major issue in the clinical management of pulmonary embolism centers around the identification of major risk factors for deep vein thrombosis and the stratification of patients into groups of relative risk for proximal (large vein) and therefore significant pulmonary embolism.[20, 21] Magnetic resonance imaging is now recognized as a reliable method of diagnosing venous thrombosis and visualizing the pelvic veins. A schematic outline of a plan to be followed in establishing the diagnosis of deep vein thrombosis and pulmonary embolism is shown in Figure 49–8.

Diagnosis of Pulmonary Embolism

The level of clinical suspicion, combined with the V-Q scan probability, is a powerful predictor of pulmonary embolism. In cases in which a high clinical suspicion persists in the face of an indeterminate or even low-probability scan, additional tests on the lower extremities or a pulmonary arteriogram should be considered. It is emphasised that a normal perfusion scan effectively rules out the diagnosis of pulmonary embolism.

The most consistently cited and studied cohort of patients was reported in 1990 in the PIOPED prospective study of the value of the V-Q scan in pulmonary embolism. The V-Q scan was followed by arteriogram in this study. The specificity of high-probability scans was 97%, but the sensitivity was only 41%. This emphasizes that nearly all patients with high-probability scans have pulmonary embolisms, but most patients with pulmonary embolisms do *not* have high-probability scans. Also, 33% of patients with intermediate-probability scans and 12% of patients with low-probability scans had arteriographically proven pulmonary embolisms. The most significant finding stemmed from the integration of clinical suspicion in the analysis. With a very high clinical suspicion, pulmonary embolism was found in 96% of patients with high-probability scans, 66% of patients with intermediate-probability scans, and 40% of patients with low-probability scans. A high clinical suspicion of pulmonary embolism mandates that the diagnosis be vigorously pursued, even in the face of equivocal results on the V-Q scan.

The most definitive method of diagnosing pulmonary em-

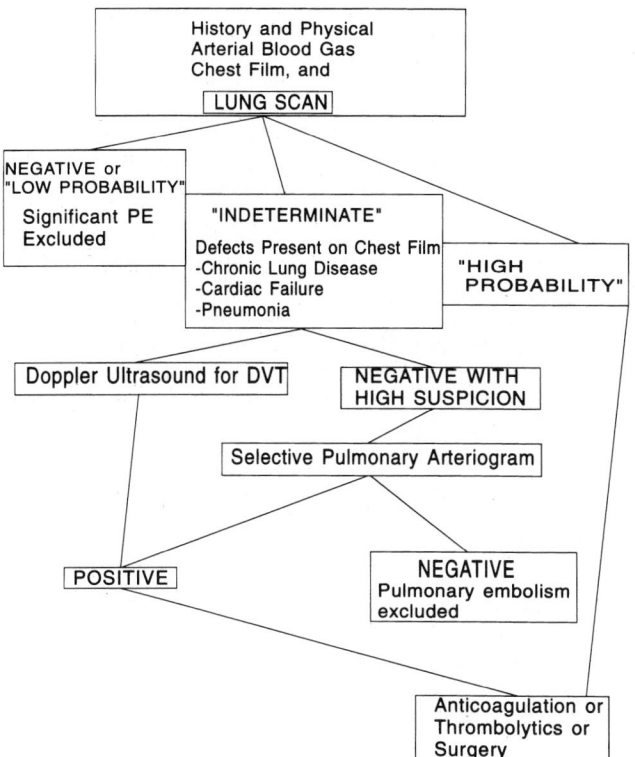

Figure 49–8. Schematic outline of plan to be followed in establishing the diagnosis of pulmonary embolism. PE, pulmonary embolism; DVT, deep vein thrombosis. (Redrawn from Duranceau, A., Jones, R. H., and Sabiston, D. C., Jr.: The diagnosis of pulmonary embolism. Compr. Ther., *2*:6, 1976.)

bolism is pulmonary arteriography. It is important to recognize the appearance of the normal pulmonary angiogram to permit appropriate interpretation of morphologic and physiologic changes. The arteries in the lower areas of the lung are normally larger due to a greater volume of pulmonary tissue. In most patients who survive the initial embolism, the obstruction in the pulmonary arteries involves lobar or segmental branches. The defect should remain constant on several successive films in the series, and the flow may be sluggish, resulting in a small pool of contrast medium that may persist in the artery above the obstruction after the venous phase of the angiogram. When pulmonary arteriography is done later in the course of embolism, contrast medium may pass around the obstruction, causing delayed opacification of the artery distally. The pattern in some areas may show avascular segments that represent unresolved thromboembolism. Oblique views of the pulmonary arteriogram should be obtained for maximal visualization and more accurate diagnosis.

MANAGEMENT

Prevention

Prophylaxis is an important aspect of postoperative care, since the incidence of pulmonary embolism is appreciable, and prevention of deep venous thrombosis is the best way to approach the problem of pulmonary embolism. Nevertheless, no proven method or combination of methods has been found that results in complete prevention of thromboembolism. Any prophylactic measure must address the pathophysiology of thrombus formation and must take into account possible morbidity from the therapy. Two factors of great importance are physical activity and position of the lower extremities, and these should be emphasized for their sim-

plicity, lack of morbidity, and proven association with a lower incidence of pulmonary embolism. Elevation of the lower extremities for gravity drainage of venous return has been shown experimentally to stop venous pooling in the lower extremities.[25] Elevation of the legs with flexion of the knee, as depicted in Figure 49–9, causes rapid runoff of the blood in the veins of the leg and thigh due to gravity. This is a simple, effective, and broadly applicable prophylactic measure. Likewise, exercise and early postoperative ambulation are simple, nonmorbid therapies. Early ambulation and resumption of physical activity after operation or bed rest for any reason have long been recommended. In a study evaluating the role of exercise, postmortem vein dissections showed that thrombi were found in only 18% of patients who had exercised before death, compared with 53% in controls (nonexercised and nonambulatory).

Sequential compression of the legs by pneumatic boots and prophylactic anticoagulation have been shown to be useful, but both remain controversial. In order for external pneumatic compression to be effective in the prophylaxis of deep vein thrombosis, proper timing and positioning of the devices are vital. The device should be placed preoperatively, and the proper position of the device must be verified. Sequential pneumatic compression of the lower extremities increases velocity of venous return and reduces stasis, stimulates regional and systemic fibrinolytic activity, and reduces endothelial cell damage by limiting intraoperative venodilation. In a recent study, failure of these devices was due primarily to improper placement and was seen in nearly 50% of patients examined on a regular surgical floor and in 22% of patients in the surgical intensive care unit.[8] The authors suggested that some of the controversy in the literature may stem from faulty use of the device and may not be related to the efficacy of the therapy.

Some patients benefit from prophylactic anticoagulation, especially those who experienced trauma or orthopedic disorders, including fracture of the hip. The concept of low-dose heparin as a prophylactic measure was introduced in 1966 but remains incompletely defined as a therapy for all patients. The usual recommendation is an initial dose of 5000 units subcutaneously every 8 to 12 hours until the patient is fully ambulatory. Routine coagulation tests are prolonged minimally, if at all, with a low risk of bleeding. The protective action may result from potentiation of a naturally occurring plasma inhibitor of activated factor X. A large number of trials with low-dose heparin given to surgical patients postoperatively have been reported using ^{123}I-labeled fibrinogen scanning, venography, or both for detecting venous thrombosis. With some exceptions, these studies have reported a decreased frequency of deep venous thrombosis compared with controls. Although it appears that the incidence of deep

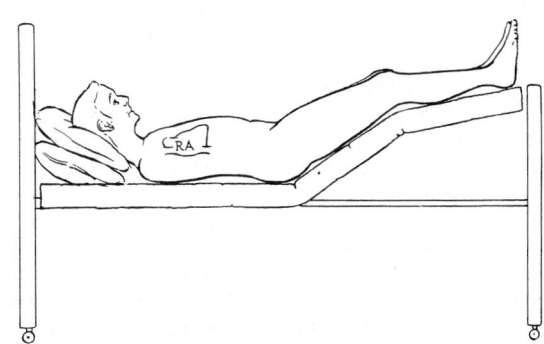

Figure 49–9. Correct position for lower extremities in prophylaxis of pulmonary embolism. Note the additional break at the knees. It is important that the level of the veins in the lower extremities be above the mean level of the right atrium (RA).

vein thrombosis is reduced, it has been difficult to firmly conclude that low-dose heparin is effective in the prevention of postoperative pulmonary embolism. A recent review comparing twice-daily low-dose heparin with no prophylaxis in over 4000 patients undergoing both elective and emergency procedures indicated a decrease in the incidence of fatal pulmonary embolism but a relatively high overall incidence (1%) of pulmonary embolism. The incidence of fatal pulmonary embolism among patients who received prophylaxis was 3.5%, compared with 11.2% in patients not receiving heparin prophylaxis. The authors concluded that pulmonary embolism can be documented in as many as 10% of patients who undergo abdominal operation in the presence of twice-daily prophylactic low-dose heparin administration. Other series indicate that subcutaneous heparin administered three times per day is more effective than twice-daily dosing.[21] Low-dose heparin prophylaxis is also inadequate for patients with an active thrombotic process. A serious complication of heparin administration is the development of a primary platelet dysfunction, leading to thrombocytopenia and occasionally to arterial or venous thrombi. This occurs in less than 1% of patients receiving heparin, however. Heparin-associated thrombotic thrombocytopenia may cause arterial thrombi, which may lead to gangrene of the extremities and other serious thrombotic problems.[23]

Low-molecular-weight heparins (LMWHs) are fragments of commercial-grade standard heparin produced by enzymatic or chemical depolarization, which leads to a more homogeneous population of molecules with mean molecular weights between 4000 and 6500 daltons. LMWH may have a more effective anticoagulant effect than standard heparin and may have a lower incidence of bleeding complications and heparin-associated thrombocytopenia.[19] Ongoing trials are evaluating LMWH as a prophylactic and therapeutic modality for deep vein thrombosis and pulmonary embolism.[1] LMWH appears to be more effective than placebo or standard low-dose heparin in the prevention of deep vein thrombosis following total hip replacement. A recent cost analysis comparing patients receiving once-daily LMWH in comparison with those receiving twice- and three-times-daily standard heparin administration suggested that LMWH is also a cost-effective prophylaxis.[11] In European contries, LMWH is routinely employed instead of standard low-dose heparin.

The 1988 National Institutes of Health consensus conference on the prevention of venous thrombosis and pulmonary embolism emphasized the prohibitive number of patients that would be required in a randomized clinical trial to accurately examine the effects of prophylaxis on pulmonary embolism. Due to the relatively low incidence of clinically significant pulmonary embolism, 5000 patients would be necessary to examine the effects of prophylaxis, and 100,000 patients would be needed to examine the effect on mortality. Therefore, the consensus conference chose to monitor the reduction of deep vein thrombosis as an appropriate marker for pulmonary embolism. The conference recommended tailoring prophylaxis to the individual patient. Recommended regimens include low-dose heparin, adjusted-dose heparin, external pneumatic compression, and gradient elastic stockings. The panel emphasized that effective regimens for the prevention of deep vein thrombosis differ according to the risk factors present in the individual patient. Prophylactic regimens for low-risk patients, such as a 40-year-old male with no known risk factors, no comorbid disease, and no hypercoagulability undergoing an uncomplicated operative procedure lasting under 1 hour, were not addressed. Prophylaxis was stressed for patients who could not be positioned to facilitate venous drainage and those with prolonged immobilization. A recent meta-analysis of general surgical patients favored low-dose heparin administered every 8 hours

for prophylaxis against deep vein thrombosis.[7] However, there was no apparent benefit among moderate-risk general surgical patients. Another meta-analysis of high-risk total hip replacement patients indicated that LMWH and compression stockings reduced the risk of pulmonary embolism.[21] Therefore, in low- and moderate-risk patients, the efficacy of prophylactic regimens to prevent pulmonary embolism remains controversial. Prophylactic methods to prevent deep vein thrombosis and pulmonary embolism in high-risk patients appears to be beneficial. Early mobilization and venous drainage must be coupled with adjunct prophylaxis in high-risk patients. Immobilized patients and high-risk patients with multiple comorbidities should be considered for external pneumatic compression beginning preoperatively, low-dose heparin, LMWH therapy, or combined treatment.

Medical Management

Anticoagulants

The management of documented venous thrombosis and pulmonary embolism is primarily by anticoagulant therapy. Heparin should be administered intravenously by constant infusion. Continuous intravenous infusion provides a more stable level of anticoagulation and a lower incidence of hemorrhage. Blood coagulation is affected by heparin in at least two ways: by preventing the activation of factor IX (Christmas factor) by factor XI (thromboplastin antecedent) in the early coagulation sequence, and by acting as a potent antithrombin in the presence of heparin cofactor. Therefore, heparin inhibits both the intrinsic and the extrinsic coagulation mechanisms by blocking the conversion of fibrinogen to fibrin by thrombin and, in high doses, by preventing the action of thrombin on platelets. Heparin is excreted mainly in the urine, and the enzyme heparinase is present in the liver, the site of some degradation.

Heparin should be administered in a concentration designed to prolong the activated partial thromboplastin time (aPTT) to 1½ to 2½ times the upper limit of normal. Heparin prevents both the extension of thrombus in the venous system and the formation of distal in situ thrombi in the pulmonary arteries. The duration of heparin therapy depends on the individual patient's response time to subsequent anticoagulation with coumarin. Oral coumarin anticoagulation is customarily begun several days before the cessation of heparin therapy to allow time for adequate prolongation of the prothrombin time. Delayed hemorrhage postoperatively may occur in patients receiving heparin therapy for pulmonary emboli, particularly those with recent prosthetic arterial grafts. There may be a continuous lysis and resorption of old thrombus and replacement with new thrombus in arterial prosthesis suture lines until it is sealed by regeneration of new intima. Thus, patients have suffered serious hemorrhage as long as 1 month after the placement of aortic arterial grafts when maintained on heparin therapy.

The coumarin drugs have an indirect and delayed action on the blood clotting mechanism. These agents act on the liver and inhibit the production of four of the factors involved in the transformation of prothrombin to thrombin—factors XII, IX, and X and prothrombin itself. The sum of these effects produces hypoprothrombinemia. These agents are rapidly absorbed from the gastrointestinal tract and are concentrated primarily in the liver. Although short-acting, warfarin sodium is one of the more commonly used coumarin drugs with only a slight cumulative effect. The average loading dose is 10 to 20 mg. on the first day and 10 mg. on the second day. The maximal effect is usually reached in 1½ to 2 days, and the average daily maintenance dose is usually between 5 and 10 mg. (range, 2 to 20 mg.). The dosage should be adjusted to maintain the INR at 2.0 to 3.0. The duration of coumarin therapy is controversial, but most believe that it should be continued for at least 6 weeks; others advocate treatment up to 6 months or longer. However, the presence of an ongoing predisposition to venous thromboembolism, a history of prior venous thromboembolic events, local responses, and subsequent course of the patient are the primary determinants of the duration of anticoagulation. Administration of vitamin K counteracts coumarin and can be used to reverse its effects. If active bleeding occurs, however, the administration of fresh frozen plasma is indicated, as vitamin K takes 24 hours or longer to show effect.

Thrombolytic Agents

Much effort has been directed toward defining the appropriate use of thrombolytic agents in the treatment of venous thrombosis and pulmonary embolism. Plasminogen is the inactive precursor of plasmin, the active fibrinolytic enzyme. Normally, plasminogen is present in the blood and tissues, and exercise, stress, and shock cause plasminogen to be activated to plasmin by a labile activator that is present in many tissues, including venous endothelium. Plasmin activity in the bloodstream is prevented by inhibitors, including an antiactivator and antiplasmins. Two thrombolytic agents, streptokinase (SK) and urokinase (UK), have been studied extensively. Both act by transforming plasminogen to plasmin. UK acts directly, and SK binds with plasminogen to form an SK-plasminogen complex, which then binds with unbound plasminogen and converts it to plasmin. SK is a soluble product of the metabolism of *Streptococcus pyogenes* (Lancefield Group A) and is available in a highly purified form. Since patients with recent streptococcal infections may have preformed antibodies to SK, it may produce toxic reactions (pyrexia, dyspnea, tachycardia, and anaphylaxis). UK is a strong thrombolytic agent found in human urine. The National Heart and Lung Institute conducted a multicenter study of the effects of these thrombolytic agents. Compared with heparin alone, UK followed by heparin therapy significantly accelerated the resolution of pulmonary thromboemboli at 24 hours as shown by pulmonary arteriogram, lung scans, and right-sided heart hemodynamics. However, no significant difference in clot burden was seen at 5 days, and there was no difference in the recurrence rate of pulmonary embolism or 2-week mortality. Bleeding was a prominent complication and occurred in 45% of patients receiving UK and heparin, compared with 27% of those given heparin alone.

To determine the long-term effects of thrombolytic treatment of acute massive embolism, seven patients with this problem underwent pulmonary angiography with pressure measurements before and after treatment with intrapulmonary infusion of UK (average dose 1724 units per kg. per hour) followed by heparin (average dose 17 units per kg. per hour). Treatment was monitored by daily measurement of pulmonary arterial pressure and was continued until the pressure had normalized (average of 6 days later). Patients later had pulmonary angiographic examinations, right heart catheterization at rest and during bicycle exercise, and phlebography of the deep veins of both legs. The pulmonary angiograms showed massive obstruction before therapy, with improvement occurring within 6 days after treatment. The mean pulmonary arterial pressure declined from an average of 37 ± 9 to 13 ± 5 mm. Hg after 6 days, and to 15 ± 3 mm. Hg after 15 months. No recurrence of pulmonary embolism was observed. All patients showed clinical signs of deep venous thrombosis. Fifteen months later, four patients had normal deep veins, and three had phlebographic signs of old thrombosis. Thus, after thrombolytic treatment of acute

massive pulmonary embolism, normal pulmonary arteriograms were obtained in six of seven patients studied. Moreover, the reserve capacity of the pulmonary vasculature during heavy exercise was normal. Although interesting, this is a small study lacking a control group, so widespread application of the data is not possible.

The role of SK therapy in the routine management of deep venous thrombosis in the lower extremities was evaluated in a retrospective study of phlebographic results and therapeutic complications. Among 108 patients with phlebographically verified deep venous thrombosis treated with SK, total or partial thrombolysis was demonstrated angiographically in 60 (55.6%). However, three died during treatment, each from pulmonary embolism, and six developed clinical signs suggestive of pulmonary embolism. Major bleeding complicated therapy in 16 patients (14.8%). Febrile reactions to SK occurred in 22 patients, and one had anaphylactic shock. The authors concluded that SK was effective in the management of deep venous thrombosis, but complications were significant.[28] SK may be indicated for the treatment of deep vein thrombosis in selected patients with large proximal clots and a low risk for bleeding complications. The putative benefit of lytic therapy in deep vein thrombosis is the preservation of venous valves and the prevention of postphlebitic syndrome, although results in the literature are mixed. The protocol involves admission to the intensive care unit with baseline coagulation studies, a small (22 or 23 gauge) heplock, acetaminophen and hydrocortisone premed, and administration of SK. SK is administered as a 250,000-unit loading dose over 30 minutes, with a constant infusion of 100,000 units per hour for 72 hours. Two to 4 hours after initiation of therapy, the (aPTT) is measured to ensure that it is at least two times normal. If it is not, the loading dose is doubled and repeated. If there is no change, SK is discontinued and UK or heparin is administered without a loading dose. After 72 hours, SK is discontinued and the aPTT is checked. If the aPTT is less than two times normal, heparin is begun without a loading dose, and oral warfarin therapy is begun. Patient selection for SK therapy of deep vein thrombosis includes documented proximal deep vein thrombosis symptom duration less than 7 days, no recent SK therapy or streptococcal infection, and no major contraindications such as recent major surgery, organ biopsy, puncture of noncompressible vessel, or cardiopulmonary resuscitation.[28] Relative contraindications include gastrointestinal bleeding, trauma, and hypertension.

A massive embolus in the right pulmonary artery from an indwelling catheter in the right atrium in a child receiving total intravenous hyperalimentation was shown in the chest film, with marked oligemia of the entire right lung (Westermark's sign). The pulmonary radioactive scan showed no perfusion of the right lung, and the pulmonary arteriogram demonstrated total occlusion of the right pulmonary artery. After 24 hours of intravenous SK, the pulmonary scan returned to normal. Such clinical cases further emphasize the importance of considering all the systemic veins and the right heart as potential sources of pulmonary emboli.

Other lytic agents with pending Food and Drug Administration (FDA) approval for use include recombinant tissue plasminogen activator (r-tPA), which has less systemic fibrinolysis due to a high affinity for fibrin within thrombi; scu-PA, which is a proenzyme single-chain UK with improved fibrin selectivity; and a monoclonal antibody to fibrin bound to conventional UK. Of these, the most extensively studied is r-tPA, and it is available for general use. In a study using r-tPA, Goldhaber and associates[14] reviewed a group of patients with angiographically documented pulmonary embolism. All had segmental or proximal pulmonary arterial obstruction within 5 days of the onset of symptoms or signs. The dosage consisted of 50 mg. of r-tPA every 2 hours, followed by repeat angiography and, if necessary, an additional 40 mg. every 4 hours. All 36 patients had angiographic evidence of clot lysis by 6 hours. Clot lysis was slight in four, moderate in six, and marked in 24. The fibrinogen levels decreased 30% from baseline at 2 hours and 38% from baseline at 6 hours. There were only two major complications. In a cooperative study to compare intrapulmonary and intravenous administration of r-tPA, pulmonary arterial infusion of r-tPA did not offer a significant benefit over the intravenous route. This study also suggests that a prolonged infusion of r-tPA over 7 hours (100 mg.) is superior to a single infusion of 50 mg. over 2 hours. Currently, the FDA-approved dose is 100 mg. over 2 hours.

The contraindications to thrombolytic therapy can be divided into those that are firm and those that are relative. Firm contraindications include internal bleeding (recent or active), recent neurosurgery, cranial trauma, and a history of hemorrhagic stroke. Relative contraindications include a recent surgical procedure (within 7 to 10 days), cardiopulmonary resuscitation (within 7 to 10 days), and the presence of a coagulopathy. Current recommendations for lytic therapy of pulmonary embolism emphasize its use in extreme settings of hemodynamic compromise that is refractory to inotropic support, with invasive hemodynamic monitoring and mechanical ventilation.

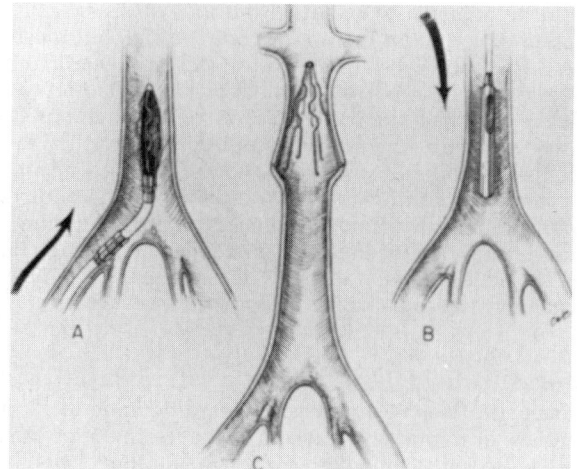

Figure 49–10. Insertion of the cone filter is accomplished by a carrier catheter inserted from the femoral vein *(A)* or retrograde from the jugular vein *(B)*. To avoid misplacement into the right renal vein, the jugular inserter should be passed down to the level of the pelvis and then withdrawn to the level of L3 for discharge *(C)*. Fixation is automatic, as the limbs spring open and the recurved hooks engage the wall of the inferior vena cava. (From Greenfield, L. J.: Pulmonary embolism: Diagnosis and management. Curr. Probl. Surg., *13*:1, 1976.)

Surgical Management

Although anticoagulant therapy for pulmonary embolism is most often successful, and lytic therapy is finding an accepted role in the management of patients with hemodynamic compromise, there are cases in which medical management fails. The role of surgical management of pulmonary embolism should then be considered individually for each patient.

Venous Thrombectomy

Although the direct removal of venous thrombi was previously recommended, it is now rarely done because of the high incidence of recurrent thrombosis postoperatively. One rare indication for thrombectomy, however, is in patients with phlegmasia cerulea dolens with secondary arterial spasm. Even though venous thrombosis may recur after thrombectomy, patency of the venous lumen may persist sufficiently long to relieve the arterial spasm and prevent a gangrenous limb. Systemic heparin is indicated to prolong venous patency following thrombectomy.

Interruption of the Inferior Vena Cava

Surgical interruption of the vena cava was previously recommended for selected patients with pulmonary embolism but is seldom done today.[32] Moreover, it does not necessarily prevent subsequent embolism, since evidence of recurrent pulmonary embolism is reported in as many as 20% of patients after ligation.

Several procedures designed to simplify caval interruption have been developed, with an emphasis on reducing perioperative morbidity and mortality. One device is a filter designed to trap large emboli arising from the branches of the inferior vena cava. A cone-shaped stainless-steel umbrella that causes minimal reduction in venous flow has been designed by Greenfield and Michna[17] and can be inserted under local anesthesia through the femoral or jugular vein (Fig. 49–10). Fixation of the filter is achieved by hooks that grasp the wall of the inferior vena cava. This design prevents proximal migration, and the filter becomes more securely fixed when emboli become trapped. Occasionally, complica-

tions of filter placement occur, including distal migration to the bifurcation of the inferior vena cava, perforation of the struts through the caval wall, and formation of thrombus on the filter. The most serious complication is filter migration into the iliac vein, renal vein, right atrium, right ventricle, or pulmonary artery, which can be fatal. Additional complications reported with these intraluminal devices include misplacement, retroperitoneal hemorrhage, perforation of the duodenum and the ureter, and development of a thrombus proximal to the filter, producing continued emboli. The filter may stimulate distal thrombosis in the vena cava, and late occlusion may occur. The precise rate of postplacement failure and asymptomatic migration is unknown. A recent case of asymptomatic filter strut migration into the left renal vein and filter disruption was discovered via an abdominal x-ray obtained for unrelated reasons (Fig. 49–11). The use of inferior vena caval filters was recently reported for a series of 84 patients at one institution. The patients ranged in age from 18 to 90 years of age. Sixty-four percent of patients had a contraindication to anticoagulation. The filter failed in 25% of patients. The authors concluded that filter placement in patients with multisystem organ failure and malignancy is not indicated, and they estimated that 25% of patients selected for filter placement exceeded an acceptable risk-benefit ratio.[24] Utilization of inferior vena caval filters is institutionally dependent, with indications including recurrent venous thromboembolism, recurrent pulmonary embolism, and venous thromboembolism or pulmonary embolism in a patient at high risk for heparinization and lytic therapy.

Pulmonary Embolectomy

In 1908, Trendelenburg performed the first pulmonary embolectomy and described three patients having the procedure.[2] The longest survivor lived for 37 hours and ultimately died of hemorrhage from an internal mammary artery. In 1924, Kirschner performed the first successful pulmonary embolectomy with long-term survival. Nevertheless, more patients have succumbed from this approach than have survived it, since significant brain damage due to cerebral hypoxia following interruption of the circulation was common. In a collective review, 22 patients managed by Trendelen-

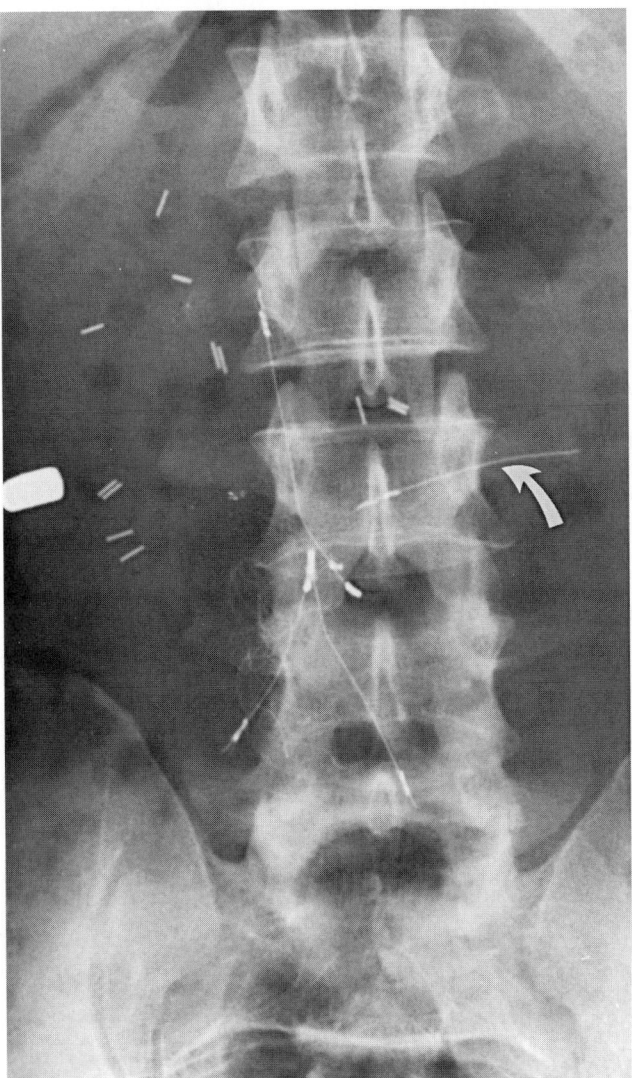

Figure 49–11. Migration and fragmentation of a bird's nest inferior vena caval filter. The superior struts are disloged from the inferior struts. The arrow points to a superior strut lodged in the left renal vein.

riogram. The immediate treatment of these patients includes systemic heparinization, administration of vasopressors and inotropic agents, and endotracheal oxygen, with consideration of lytic therapy. Every effort should be made to manage the patient by this approach. Many patients previously thought to require embolectomy now respond favorably, without the need for operation. Depending on the severity of the clinical condition, 1 or 2 hours may be taken in an effort to restore acceptable cardiopulmonary function. If this approach is effective in maintaining a blood pressure of 80 mm. Hg or more, as shown by a continuous intra-arterial recording, embolectomy may be deferred, particularly if acceptable renal and cerebral function is maintained. Massive pulmonary emboli may cause sudden death, but it has long been recognized that many patients, even those with massive embolism, survive for minutes or hours.[6] Among patients who were previously in good condition, 55% lived longer than 2 hours, and 48% survived for 8 hours or more. However, among those with terminal illnesses, only 32% lived for 2 hours. The pulmonary scan and the emboli removed from a patient with massive pulmonary embolism and intractable shock are shown in Figure 49–12. This patient was appropriately selected for the procedure, since all attempts to correct the severe state of hypotension failed, despite vigorous resus-

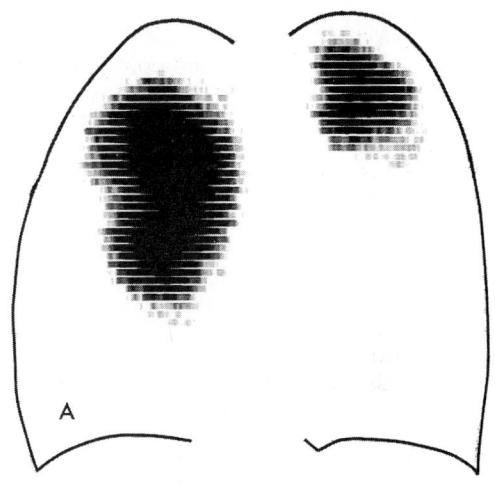

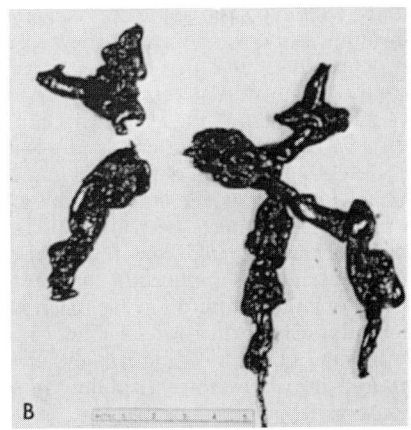

Figure 49–12. Illustrations from a patient with massive pulmonary embolism on the twelfth postoperative day after an orthopedic operation and accompanied by intractable shock. A, The pulmonary scan shows massive occlusion of the right lower and middle lobar pulmonary arteries as well as almost all of the pulmonary arterial circulation to the left lung. B, Emboli removed from both pulmonary arteries at the time of embolectomy. (From Sabiston, D. C., Jr.: Pathophysiology, diagnosis and management of pulmonary embolism. Adv. Surg., 3:351, 1968. Copyright 1968, Mosby-Year Book, Inc.)

burg's technique were reported.[2] Most had postoperative brain damage resulting from both pre-existing hypoxia and that occurring after embolectomy. Only 3 of the 22 patients were long-term survivors. In 1960, Allison performed a pulmonary embolectomy on a young athlete with massive pulmonary embolism secondary to traumatic thrombophlebitis. Total body hypothermia (20° C.) was used, the chest was opened, and both venae cavae were occluded. The pulmonary artery was opened, a massive embolus was removed, the pulmonary arteriotomy was closed, the caval occlusion was released, and the normal circulation was re-established. With the brain and heart protected by hypothermia while the circulation was temporarily occluded, the patient made a good recovery.

In 1961, Sharp was the first to perform pulmonary embolectomy using extracorporeal circulation.[31] This technique is now preferred, since it permits continuous perfusion of the entire body, with concomitant oxygenation while the emboli are removed from the pulmonary arteries.

The indications for emergency pulmonary embolectomy are persistent and refractory hypotension despite maximal resuscitation in a patient with massive embolism clearly documented by either a pulmonary scan or a pulmonary arte-

citative therapy. Often, high-dose catecholamine inotropic support is required, with the use of epinephrine. It is more common that appropriate inotropic support with optimization of intravascular volume affords 1 to 2 hours for localization and institution of anticoagulation, lytic therapy, or operation, as required.

That small amounts of pulmonary embolism in the presence of pre-existing cardiac and pulmonary insufficiency can produce serious cardiovascular manifestations is illustrated by the following case. Admitted for an ophthalmic procedure under local anesthesia, this 72-year-old male had a history of hypertensive cardiovascular disease and chronic respiratory insufficiency due to emphysema. Postoperatively, he was found in a state of cardiovascular collapse. A pulmonary scan showed evidence of obstruction to the pulmonary arterial flow in the left lower lobe. Under normal circumstances, this relatively small amount of embolism would not produce serious cardiopulmonary symptoms. In this patient, however, a persistent state of profound hypotension ensued that could not be corrected by vigorous resuscitative management. The presence of pre-existing cardiac and respiratory insufficiency obviously exacerbated the effects of this amount of obstruction. Ultimately, it was necessary to remove the emboli under cardiopulmonary bypass. All emboli were confined to the left lower lobe pulmonary artery. The patient made an uneventful recovery.

Technique. A median sternotomy provides excellent exposure of the pulmonary artery for pulmonary embolectomy. Once the pericardium is opened, cardiopulmonary bypass is established. The main pulmonary artery is exposed and incised and is usually free of emboli, although partial obstruction may be present. The emboli are removed from the right and left pulmonary arteries and their major branches with forceps. A Fogarty catheter is passed into the pulmonary arterial branches to remove smaller emboli. Finally, the entire pulmonary arterial tree is irrigated with saline. During this portion of the procedure, gentle compression of both lungs with the hand directs peripheral emboli toward the central arteries for more effective aspiration. The pulmonary artery is closed and cardiopulmonary bypass is gradually discontinued, allowing the heart and lungs to resume normal function.

When severe cardiovascular collapse is present, the patient can be supported by partial cardiopulmonary bypass using a femoral vein to femoral artery circuit for immediate resuscitation. If extracorporeal circulation is not available, a right or left thoracotomy, with exposure of the most severely involved pulmonary artery, can be done on the side of predominant occlusion, as determined by a scan or arteriogram. An anterior thoracotomy in the third interspace is appropriate for exposure of either the right or the left pulmonary artery. The artery can then be dissected, occluded, and opened distally for removal of emboli while the normal circulation and pulmonary function in the opposite lung continue. Successful results with this technique have been described. One of the complications that has been reported following pulmonary embolectomy is massive endobronchial hemorrhage. Successful management of this complication has been achieved by the use of an endotracheal tube for selective collapse of the lung and entrapment of the bleeding into either the right or the left main bronchus. Reperfusion pulmonary edema after pulmonary artery thromboendarterectomy has been described and may be a serious complication, often requiring prolonged mechanical ventilation. The syndrome is a cause of hypoxemia postoperatively with local pulmonary infiltrates.

Results. Among 24 patients having open pulmonary embolectomy with extracorporeal circulation, 17 patients (71%) had acute pulmonary embolism after a surgical procedure. In the remaining seven patients (29%), the embolism was secondary to a chronic medical disorder. The interval between clinical manifestations of acute pulmonary embolism and the embolectomy varied between 8 and 36 hours, and a definitive diagnosis of pulmonary embolism was made in each patient by pulmonary arteriography. All were in a state of shock, with an arterial oxygen tension less than 65 mm. Hg and the presence of acidosis. The definitive indication for embolectomy was occlusion of the right or left pulmonary artery. In the last 2 years of the study, the operative mortality in 17 patients was 23%. A recent series of pulmonary embolectomy in the literature involved a summary of 20 years of experience at one center utilizing cardiopulmonary bypass.[26] The indications included thrombolytic failure with ongoing hemodynamic compromise, contraindication to thrombolytics, and inadequate time for institution of thrombolytic therapy. Mortality among the 96 patients was reported as 37.5%. Mortality and morbidity were greatest among patients with a history of cardiac arrest or pre-existing cardiovascular disease.

SELECTED REFERENCES

Goldhaber, S. Z. (Ed.): Pulmonary Embolism and Deep Venous Thrombosis. Philadelphia, W. B. Saunders, 1985.
This updated monograph is quite complete and is highly recommended to students wishing to consult an authoritative and detailed series of presentations on all aspects of this subject.

Goldhaber, S. Z., Vaughan, D. E., Markis, J. E., et al.: Acute pulmonary embolism treated with tissue plasminogen activator. Lancet, 2:886, 1986.
An important series of patients managed with r-tPA.

Gorham, L. W.: A study of pulmonary embolism: Parts I and II. Arch. Intern. Med., 108:8, 189, 1961.
These companion papers emphasize the gross pathology of pulmonary embolism. Special emphasis is given to the fact that in most patients with fatal embolism, a substantial amount of the pulmonary arterial bed is occluded, generally more than half. This is one of the best pathologic studies in the literature.

Makhoul, R. G., Greenberg, C. S., and McCann, R. L.: Heparin-associated thrombocytopenia and thrombosis: A serious clinical problem and potential solution. J. Vasc. Surg. 5:522, 1986.
This reference provides an excellent presentation of heparin-associated thrombocytopenia and thrombosis (HATT). The pathogenesis, diagnosis, and management are discussed, including the high incidence of amputation of the extremities.

Marshall, R., Sabiston, D. C., Jr., Allison, P. R., Bosman, A. R., and Dunnill, M. S.: Immediate and late effects of pulmonary embolism by large thrombi in dogs. Thorax, 18:1, 1963.
In this experimental study, a variety of physiologic measurements were determined following pulmonary embolism. The study emphasizes the paucity of changes that occur when only one pulmonary artery is occluded and illustrates the wide margin of pulmonary reserve.

NIH consensus conference on prevention of venous thrombosis and pulmonary embolism. JAMA, 256:744, 1986.
This NIH consensus conference determined that deep vein thrombosis is an appropriate marker for pulmonary embolism and that prophylaxis should be tailored to the individual patient, based on risk factors for pulmonary embolism. Prophylaxis was stressed for patients who could not be positioned to facilitate venous drainage and those with prolonged immobilization.

PIOPED Investigators: Value of the ventilation/perfusion scan in acute pulmonary embolism. JAMA, 263:2573, 1990.
This multicenter prospective investigation determined the reliance on clinical suspicion for the proper use of the ventilation-perfusion scan in the diagnosis of pulmonary embolism. A high-probability scan is sufficient confirmation for institution of therapy, but most patients with pulmonary embolism do not have high-probability scans. Therefore, in a setting of high clinical suspicion and an indeterminate scan, arteriography is most likely indicated to confirm a diagnosis of pulmonary embolism.

Sabiston, D. C., Jr., and Wagner, H. N., Jr.: The diagnosis of pulmonary embolism by radioisotope scanning. Ann. Surg., 160:585, 1964.
This paper describes the original experimental and clinical studies introducing the technique of radioactive pulmonary scanning.

Sabiston, D. C., Jr., and Wolfe, W. G.: Experimental and clinical observations on the natural history of pulmonary embolism. Ann. Surg., 168:1, 1968.
In this paper, the natural history of pulmonary emboli in the experimental animal and man is discussed. The gross and microscopic features and their changes with the passage of time are illustrated. The gradual resolution of the emboli and their final disappearance are confirmed, in most instances, by serial scans and pulmonary arteriograms.

REFERENCES

1. Anderson, D. R., O'Brien, B. J., Levine, M. N., et al.: Efficacy and cost of low-molecular-weight heparin compared with standard heparin for the prevention of deep vein thrombosis after total hip arthroplasty. Ann. Intern. Med., *119*:1105, 1993.
2. Benichoux, R.: The surgical treatment of massive pulmonary embolism: Report of 22 cases of Trendelenburg's operation. J. Int. Chir., *11*:464, 1951.
3. Brofman, B. L., Charms, B. L., Kohn, P. M., et al.: Unilateral pulmonary artery occlusion in man: Control studies. J. Thorac. Surg., *34*:206, 1957.
4. Burnett, W. E., Long, J. H., Norris, C., et al.: The effect of pneumonectomy on pulmonary function. J. Thorac. Surg., *18*:569, 1949.
5. Burns, H. A., Cohn, S. M., Frumento, R. J., et al.: Prospective ultrasound evaluation of venous thrombosis in high-risk trauma patients. J. Trauma, *35*:405, 1993.
6. Carson, J. L., Kelley, M. A., Duff, A., Weg, J. C., Fulkerson, W. J., et al.: The clinical course of pulmonary embolism. N. Engl. J. Med., *326*:1240, 1992.
7. Clagett, G. P., and Reisch, J. S.: Prevention of venous thromboembolism in general surgical patients: Results of meta-analysis. Ann. Surg., *208*:227, 1988.
8. Comerota, A. J., Katz, M. L., and White, J. V.: Why does prophylaxis with external pneumatic compression for deep vein thrombosis fail? Am. J. Surg., *164*:265, 1992.
9. Crafoord, C., and Jorpes, E.: Heparin as a prophylactic against thrombosis. JAMA, *116*:2831, 1941.
10. Dalen, J. E., and Alpert, J. S.: Natural history of pulmonary embolism. Prog. Cardiovasc. Dis., *17*:259, 1975.
11. Drummond, M., Aristides, M., and Forbes, D.: Economic evaluation of standard heparin and enoxaparin for prophylaxis against deep vein thrombosis in elective hip surgery. Br. J. Surg., *81*:1742, 1994.
12. Duranceau, A., Jones, R. H., and Sabiston, D. C., Jr.: The diagnosis of pulmonary embolism. Compr. Ther., *2*:6, 1976.
13. Geerts, W. H., Code, K. I., Jay, R. M., Chen, E., et al.: A prospective study of venous thromboembolism after major trauma. N. Engl. J. Med., *331*:1601, 1994.
14. Goldhaber, S. Z., Vaughan, D. E., Markis, J. E., et al.: Acute pulmonary embolism treated with tissue plasminogen activator. Lancet, *2*:886, 1986.
15. Gorham, L. W.: A study of pulmonary embolism. Part I. Arch. Intern. Med., *108*:8, 1961.
16. Gorham, L. W.: A study of pulmonary embolism. Part II. Arch. Intern. Med., *108*:189, 1961.
17. Greenfield, L. J., and Michna, B. A.: Twelve-year clinical experience with the Greenfield vena caval filter. Surgery, *104*:706, 1988.
18. Gurewich, V., Sasahara, A. A., and Stein, M.: Pulmonary embolism, bronchoconstriction and response to heparin. *In* Sasahara, A. A., and Stein, M. (Eds.): Pulmonary Embolic Disease. New York, Grune & Stratton, 1965.
19. Hirsch, J., and Levine, M. N.: Low molecular weight heparin. Blood, *79*:1, 1992.
20. Hull, R. D., Hirsch, J. D., Carter, C. J., et al.: Pulmonary angiography, ventilation lung scanning, and venography for clinically suspected pulmonary embolism with abnormal perfusion lung scan. Ann. Intern. Med., *98*:891, 1983.
21. Imperiale, T., and Speerof, T.: A meta-analysis of methods to prevent venous thromboembolism following total hip replacement. JAMA, *271*:1780, 1994.
22. Jones, R. H., and Sabiston, D. C., Jr.: Pulmonary embolism in childhood. Monogr. Surg. Sci., *3*:35, 1966.
23. Makhoul, R. G., Greenberg, C. S., and McCann, R. L.: Heparin-associated thrombocytopenia and thrombosis: A serious clinical problem and potential solution. J. Vasc. Surg., *5*:522, 1986.
24. Magnant, J. G., Walsh, D. B., Juravsky, L. I., and Cronenwett, J. L.: Current use of inferior vena cava filters. J. Vasc. Surg., *16*:701, 1992.
25. McLachlin, A. D., McLachlin, J. A., Jory, T. A., and Rawling, E. G.: Venous stasis in the lower extremities. Ann. Surg., *152*:678, 1960.
26. Meyer, G., Tamister, D., Sors, H., Stern, M., et al.: Pulmonary embolectomy: A 20-year experience in one center. Ann. Thorac. Surg., *51*:232, 1991.
27. Murray, G. D. W., Jacques, L. B., Perrett, T. S., and Best, C. H.: Heparin and thrombosis of veins following injury. Surgery, *2*:163, 1937.
28. Rogers, L. Q., and Lutcher, C. L.: Streptokinase therapy for deep vein thrombosis: A comprehensive review of the literature. Am. J. Med., *88*:390, 1990.
29. Sabiston, D. C., Jr., and Wagner, H. N., Jr.: The diagnosis of pulmonary embolism by radioisotopic scanning. Ann. Surg., *160*:585, 1964.
30. Sabiston, D. C., Jr., and Wolfe, W. G.: Experimental and clinical observations on the natural history of pulmonary embolism. Ann. Surg., *168*:1, 1968.
31. Sharp, E. H.: Pulmonary embolectomy: Successful removal of a massive pulmonary embolus with the support of cardiopulmonary bypass—a case report. Ann. Surg., *156*:1, 1962.
32. Silver, D., and Sabiston, D. C., Jr.: The role of vena caval interruption in the management of pulmonary embolism. Surgery, *77*:1, 1975.
33. Sreeram, N., Cheriex, E. C., and Smeets, R. M.: Value of the 12-lead echocardiogram at hospital admission in the diagnosis of pulmonary embolism. Am. J. Cardiol., *73*:298, 1994.
34. Svensson, P. J., and Dahlback, B.: Resistance to activated protein C as a basis for venous thrombosis. N. Engl. J. Med., *330*:517, 1994.
35. Tapson, V. F., and Fulkerson, W. J.: Pulmonary embolism in the intensive care unit. J. Intensive Care Med., *9*:119, 1994.
36. Virchow, R.: Die Cellularpathologie in ihrer Begrudung auf physiologische und pathologische Gewebelhre. Berlin, A. Hirschwald, 1858.
37. Westermark, N.: On the roentgen diagnosis of lung embolism. Acta Radiol., *19*:357, 1938.

I

CHRONIC PULMONARY EMBOLISM

Mark W. Sebastian, M.D., and David C. Sabiston, Jr., M.D.

Although pulmonary embolism usually presents as an acute clinical problem, it can also be a chronic disorder. Most pulmonary emboli spontaneously resolve through intrinsic fibrinolysis.[11] In chronic pulmonary embolism, defective fibrinolysis begins a cycle of incomplete lysis of pulmonary emboli, partial recanalization of the obstructed pulmonary vasculature, organization and fibrosis of retained thromboembolic remnants, and proximal thrombotic extension. This leads to a gradual accumulation of thromboemboli within the pulmonary arterial vasculature. These thromboemboli gradually produce pulmonary hypertension and cause symptoms of progressive respiratory insufficiency, hypoxemia, and right ventricular failure.[11, 18] In most patients, medical management is unsatisfactory, with studies showing a poor prognosis.[18] The syndrome of chronic pulmonary embolism is distinct from primary pulmonary hypertension, which consists of distal pulmonary arterial and arteriolar occlusion with no evidence of a primary source of embolism. The treatment of patients with primary pulmonary hypertension is with appropriate pharmacologic agents. Although the number of patients with chronic pulmonary embolism remains comparatively small, the treatment of these patients has depended on and contributed to refinements in the understanding of pulmonary physiology, critical care, pulmonary and cardiac operations, coagulation, and arteriography.

In patients with chronic pulmonary embolic disease of the main lobar or segmental arteries, the presence of elevated pulmonary artery pressures is the most important clinical consideration, because it has been shown that the natural history of this syndrome is related to the magnitude of the pulmonary arterial hypertension. If the mean pulmonary artery pressure is more than 30 mm. Hg, survival at 5 years is only 30%. In those patients with a mean pressure greater than 50 mm. Hg, only 10% are alive at 5 years (Fig. 49–13). Fortunately, it is now established that pulmonary embolectomy in patients with proximal pulmonary arterial obstruction is likely to produce a reduction in pulmonary hypertension, with decreased respiratory insufficiency and

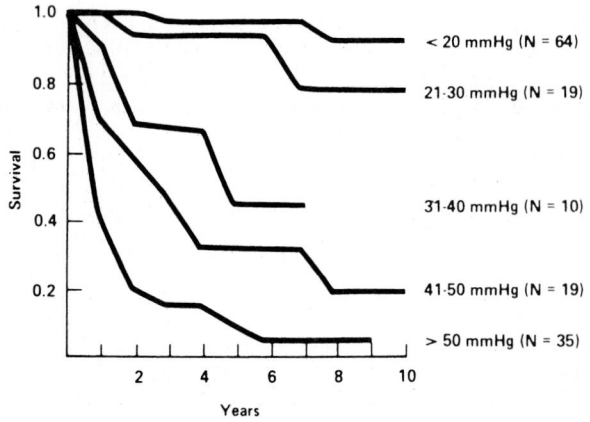

Figure 49–13. Survival in patients with pulmonary hypertension resulting from chronic recurrent emboli. Groups of patients are compared at different mean pulmonary artery pressures. (Modified from Riedel, M., Stanek, V., Widimsky, J., et al.: Long-term follow-up of patients with pulmonary thromboembolism. Chest, *81*:151, 1982.)

improvement in right-sided heart failure. The number of patients with documented chronic pulmonary emboli has risen in recent years, and the number of patients treated has also increased due to improved diagnostic techniques and documented clinical benefit in properly selected patients.

HISTORICAL ASPECTS

Virchow in 1847 suspected that the bronchial collateral circulation present in the pulmonary system prevented most pulmonary emboli from causing infarction. In 1948, Blalock confirmed this with the observation of bright red arterial perfusion of pulmonary vessels distal to chronic emboli. Collateral perfusion by bronchial vessels was confirmed angiographically by Viamonte in 1964.[27] The first antemortem diagnosis of chronic pulmonary embolism was made in 1950 by Carroll in a 30-year-old patient with progressive dyspnea, cardiac failure, and absence of vascular markings in the left lung field.[3] Although several early attempts at surgical therapy were made, the first successful embolectomy for recurrent pulmonary emboli was described by Allison and colleagues in 1960.[1] Chitwood and associates emphasized the importance of bronchial arteriography and the need to identify obstructing lesions in the proximal arterial system.[4] Daily and associates in 1987 reported bilateral thromboendarterectomy via median sternotomy and extrapericardial dissection of the pulmonary arteries, and in 1989 reported a series of 100 consecutive patients treated with cardiopulmonary bypass, deep hypothermia, and intermittent circulatory arrest to facilitate embolectomy.[8, 9]

CLINICAL PRESENTATION

Patients with the syndrome of chronic pulmonary embolism have a history of exertional dyspnea progressing to severe respiratory insufficiency over months to years. They may also complain of recurrent episodes of thrombophlebitis, chest pain, and hemoptysis owing to the presence of large bronchial collaterals (Table 49–4). Physical findings include signs of severe pulmonary hypertension, often combined with evidence of right ventricular failure. These signs may include an increased pulmonary second heart sound, a systolic murmur, hepatomegaly, and S3 or S4 gallop. Other physical findings are pulmonary rales, jugular venous distention, cyanosis, and clubbing of the fingers (Table 49–5).

TABLE 49–4. Symptoms of Patients with Chronic Pulmonary Emboli (*n* = 49)

Symptom (no.)	Percentage Afflicted
Dyspnea—exertion (45)	92
Thrombophlebitis (27)	55
Dyspnea—progressive (40)	82
Hemoptysis (13)	27
Chest pain (12)	24
Fatigue (12)	24

NATURAL HISTORY

The natural history of pulmonary embolism was studied by Moser and co-workers in a 1990 review of 250 consecutive patients.[20] In this group, 195 underwent surgical correction. Careful history usually revealed an acute event in most patients, often characterized by unilateral leg swelling, pneumonia, or dyspnea. Patients had often been diagnosed with primary pulmonary hypertension.

After the initial embolic event, improvement and increased functional ability ensue, largely independent of anticoagulation. It is during this period that the right ventricle hypertrophies in response to increased pulmonary vascular resistance. Experimental data indicate that noninvolved as well as occluded pulmonary vascular beds show pathologic change. Deterioration is exacerbated by proximal extension of thromboemboli. Right ventricular failure, hypoxemia, opening of the foramen ovale, and development of pulmonary arteriovenous fistulas ensue, with eventual death.[13]

PREOPERATIVE EVALUATION

The preoperative evaluation in appropriate candidates includes a chest film, which shows a dilated pulmonary artery with oligemic pulmonary fields in approximately half of the patients. A typical preoperative chest film is shown in Figure 49–14. Although some patients with chronic pulmonary emboli have been described as having normal chest films, this is unusual with proximal emboli. In one series, all plain films showed abnormalities, including cardiomegaly (84%), right-sided heart enlargement (55%), enlargement of the pulmonary artery (43%), azygous vein enlargement (27%), chronic volume loss (24%), atelectasis (22%), effusion (16%), and pleural thickening (12%) (Table 49–6).[32] Embolic involvement of the right lung was present in 96% of patients, and of the left lung in 80%; bilateral emboli were present in 82% of patients.[30]

Arterial blood gases at room air revealed evidence of severe respiratory insufficiency, with hypoxemia and arterial oxygen tension (PaO_2) values ranging from 55 to 60 mm. Hg and an arterial carbon dioxide tension ($PaCO_2$) of approxi-

TABLE 49–5. Physical Findings in Patients with Chronic Pulmonary Embolism (*n* = 49)

Finding (no.)	Percentage Afflicted
Increased P_2 (29)	59
Cardiac murmur (22)	45
Hepatomegaly (13)	27
S3 or S4 gallop (13)	27
Pulmonary rales (12)	24
Jugular venous distention (11)	22
Cyanosis (2)	4
Clubbing (1)	2

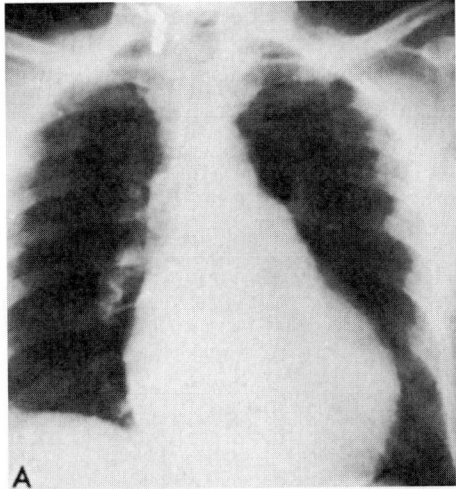

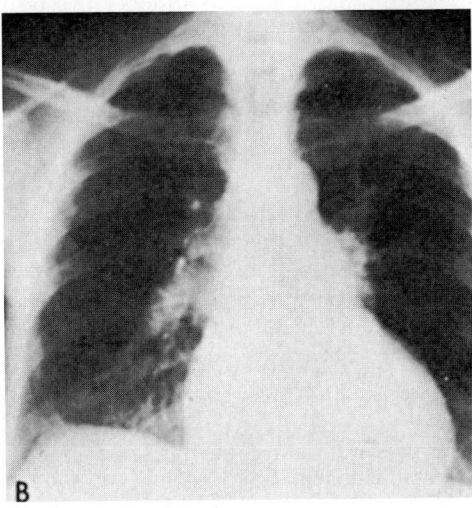

Figure 49–14. The anteroposterior chest film is shown before *(A)* and after *(B)* embolectomy of the right lower lobe pulmonary artery for chronic pulmonary emboli. Note an increase in parenchymal flow to the right lower lobe after operation. Also note the decrease in the size of both the right main pulmonary artery and the cardiac silhouette after embolectomy. (From Chitwood, W. R., Jr., Lyerly, H. K., and Sabiston, D. C., Jr.: Surgical management of chronic pulmonary embolism. Ann. Surg., *201*:11, 1985.)

mately 30 mm. Hg. Hypoxemia is a consequence of ventilation perfusion mismatch, pulmonary shunting, and a high oxygen extraction.

The electrocardiogram usually shows the presence of chronic cor pulmonale with a right axis deviation and right ventricular hypertrophy. ST segment and T wave changes are present in approximately a third of patients, and somewhat fewer have right bundle branch block.[15]

TABLE 49–6. Chest Film Findings in Patients with Chronic Pulmonary Embolism (*n* = 49)

Finding (no.)	Percentage Afflicted
Cardiomegaly (41)	84
Right-sided heart enlargement (27)	55
Enlargement of pulmonary artery (21)	43
Azygos vein enlargement (13)	27
Chronic volume loss (12)	24
Atelectasis (11)	22
Effusion (8)	16
Pleural thickening (6)	12

Peripheral venography usually indicates the source of emboli. Magnetic resonance imaging is now often used to demonstrate thrombi in the pelvic veins. Ventilation and perfusion scans show findings consistent with pulmonary emboli, and perfusion defects correspond to the oligemic regions on the plain film.

Pulmonary arteriography usually shows emboli in both lungs, with between 55% and 75% of the total pulmonary blood flow being obstructed. Pulmonary hypertension was present in all 48 patients with chronic pulmonary emboli evaluated at Duke University Medical Center. The systolic pulmonary arterial pressure was 75.0 ± 8 mm. Hg, and the diastolic pulmonary pressure was 26.0 ± 3.0 mm. Hg, with the mean pressure being 42.0 ± 5.0 mm. Hg.

A thorough preoperative evaluation is required before suitability for operation in individual patients can be determined. The most appropriate candidates for pulmonary embolectomy are those with severe respiratory insufficiency, a low PaO_2, and the demonstrated presence of enlarged bronchial vessels by arteriography (Fig. 49–15). Some patients are not candidates for embolectomy.[4] Contraindication commonly stems from distal pulmonary emboli with diffuse involvement of small pulmonary arteries. Other contraindications include severe cardiac failure and massive obesity. These patients are usually disabled, with a New York Heart Association (NYHA) classification of IV, or dyspnea at rest.

Pulmonary arteriography is crucial in the evaluation of any patient being considered for surgical intervention.[19] Auger and colleagues[2] in 1992 reviewed 250 patients being considered for embolectomy and identified five major arteriographic findings considered highly suggestive for chronic pulmonary embolism amenable to surgical correction (Figs. 49–16 and 49–17):

1. Pouching or concave configuration of pulmonary artery occlusion;
2. Pulmonary arterial webs or bands, defined as decreased opacity lines traversing a pulmonary vessel at the level of lobar or segmental vessels;
3. Intimal irregularity;
4. Abrupt narrowing of major pulmonary vessels secondary to recanalization, concentric narrowing, or reactive arterial contraction; and
5. Lobar vascular obstruction.

These characteristic findings are distinct from the sharply defined intraluminal defects of acute pulmonary embolism.

Finally, thoracic aortography or selective bronchial arteriography is used to demonstrate dilated, tortuous bronchial vessels. The bronchial circulation is often considerably augmented and communicates by collaterals with the distal pulmonary arteries. In patients in whom selective bronchial arteriogram is performed, patency of the distal pulmonary arteries is common.[28] When the *distal* pulmonary arteries are patent, the prognosis is favorable, because thrombectomy may be followed by pulmonary artery blood flow. Satisfactory distal back-bleeding can usually be predicted in advance in these patients from the information gained by the thoracic aortogram with selective injection of the bronchial arteries. These arteries are often dilated and tortuous and fill the distal pulmonary arterial circuit in a retrograde manner. Catheterization with endoluminal pulmonary arterial ultrasonography has been described as an adjunct diagnostic tool.[22] In a series of 11 patients, 10 pulmonary segments with suspected chronic pulmonary embolism were identified in seven patients, all of which were confirmed at operation. Nine pulmonary segments were discerned as being free of emboli, with one of these nine having embolism at operation. This technique was thought to aid in the assessment and precise location of the embolic distribution. Spiral computed

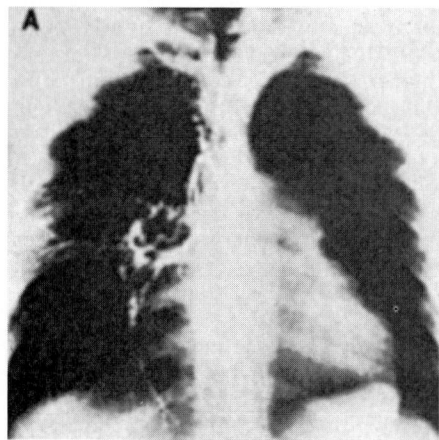
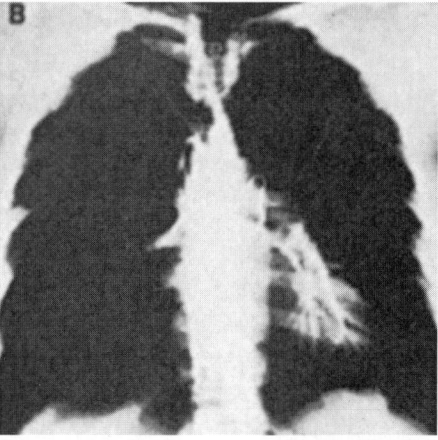

Figure 49–15. *A,* A selective bronchial arterial injection showing dilated bronchial collaterals on the right supplying the distal pulmonary parenchyma. *B,* A later phase of the same injection in which collaterals from the right side supply the distal pulmonary parenchyma in the left lower lobe. The left lower lobe pulmonary artery was noted to have a total proximal obstruction on the pulmonary arteriogram. (From Chitwood, W. R., Jr., Lyerly, H. K., and Sabiston, D. C., Jr.: Surgical management of chronic pulmonary embolism. Ann. Surg., *201:*11, 1985.)

tomography (CT) scans have also been advocated as sensitive for the detection of dilated bronchial arteries; they have a positive predictive value, with a lower risk of postoperative death in patients with dilated bronchial arteries.[16]

SURGICAL MANAGEMENT

Pulmonary embolectomy may be performed on one or both pulmonary arteries. In a number of patients, the pulmonary artery is occluded unilaterally and there are few, if any, proximal emboli in the contralateral lung. These patients usually improve dramatically after embolectomy. In those patients with primarily unilateral involvement, either a right or a left anterior thoracotomy can be used when there is proximal occlusion of the vessel. In patients with bilateral pulmonary emboli or in those with involvement of the main pulmonary artery, median sternotomy with extracorporeal circulation is indicated (Fig. 49–18).

Meticulous dissection is necessary, with removal of all distal emboli, to achieve optimal postoperative results. The procedure is a true endarterectomy, as the thromboemboli are well organized and densely adherent to the wall of the pulmonary artery. Great care must be taken in the dissection (Fig. 49–19). All distal emboli must be removed until adequate back-bleeding of bright red blood is seen. Even with circulatory arrest, back-bleeding obscures the latter stages of the operation. Daily and co-workers in 1991 described a thromboendarterectomy dissector designed to allow simultaneous dissection and suction of blood from the operative field (Fig. 49–20).[10] It may be preferable to close the arteriotomy with a pericardial patch to prevent luminal constriction. It is usually necessary to make a counterincision on the distal pulmonary artery to completely remove the adherent emboli in the secondary and tertiary branches of the pulmonary arteries. Typical specimens removed are shown in Figure 49–21.

Postoperative complications include severe right ventricular failure in patients with long-standing cor pulmonale and

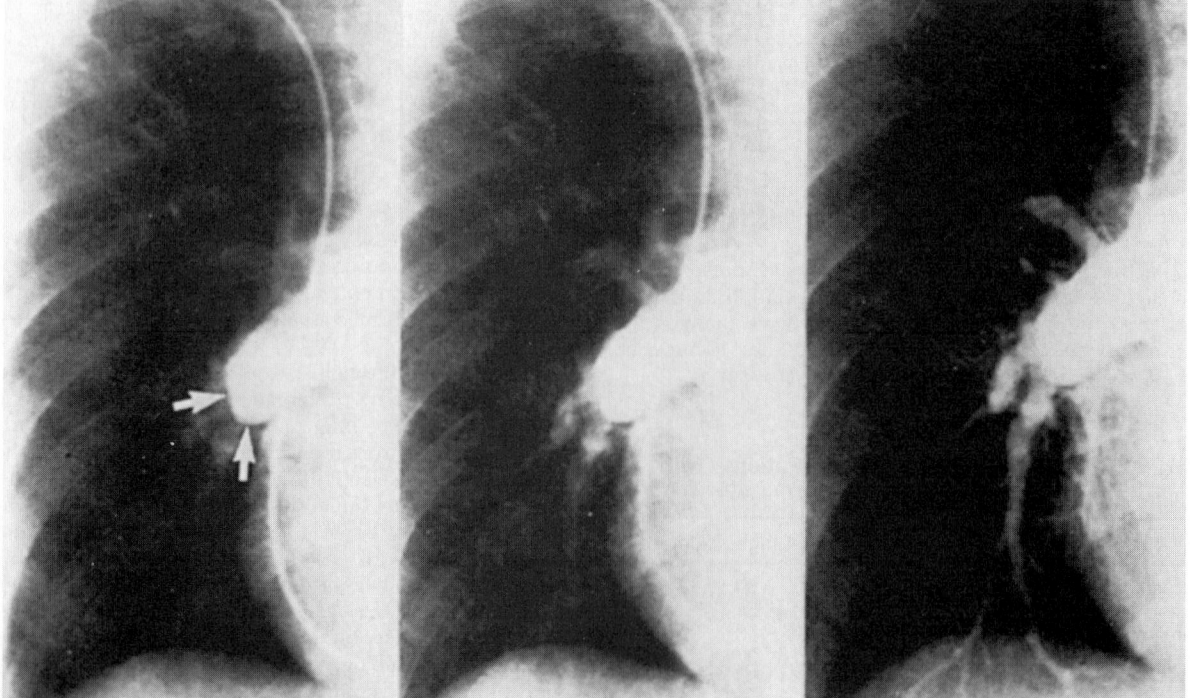

Figure 49–16. Right pulmonary arteriogram demonstrates a pouchlike defect in the sequence (arrows) that eventually gives rise to more distal vessels. This finding is consistent with partially occlusive chronic proximal thrombi. (From Auger, W. R., Fedullo, P. F., Moser, K. M., Buchbinder, M., et al.: Chronic major-vessel thromboembolic pulmonary artery obstruction: Appearance at angiography. Radiology, *182:*393, 1992.)

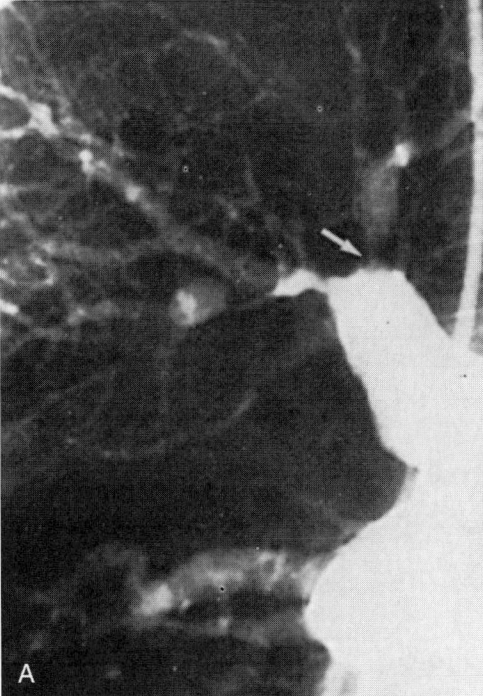
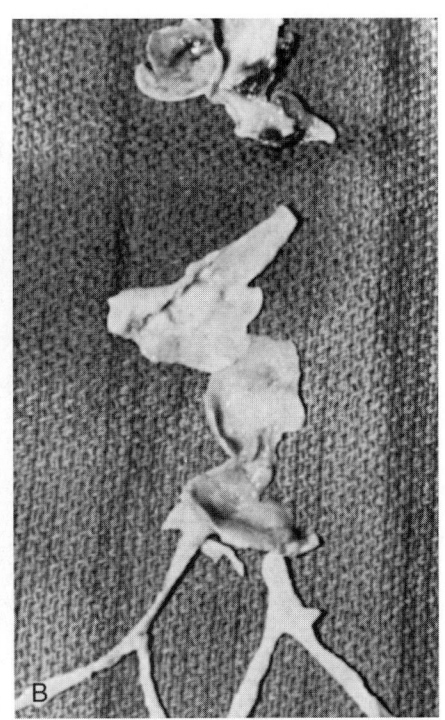

Figure 49–17. *A,* Pouch termination of the proximal right descending pulmonary artery. The arrow indicates bandlike narrowing and poststenotic dilatation of a right upper lobe segmental arterial branch. *B,* Chronic thrombus removed at surgery. (From Auger, W. R., Fedullo, P. F., Moser, K. M., Buchbinder, M., et al.: Chronic major-vessel thromboembolic pulmonary artery obstruction: Appearance at angiography. Radiology, *182:*393, 1992.)

pulmonary hypertension and hemorrhagic lung syndrome.[7] One patient in the author's series died of right ventricular failure 3 days after operation, despite removal of chronic pulmonary emboli.[23] After embolectomy and after re-establishment of pulmonary blood flow, massive parenchymal and intrabronchial hemorrhage may occur during or after cardiopulmonary bypass. Successful management of this complication can be achieved by the use of a Carlens (Broncho-Cath) catheter for tracheal intubations.[17] A Fogarty catheter is inserted transbronchially to occlude the right or left

main-stem bronchus and tamponade the blood within the lumen until appropriate blood coagulation can be achieved. The bleeding usually ceases when protamine is administered to counteract the heparin used during cardiopulmonary bypass.

POSTOPERATIVE RESULTS

After embolectomy for chronic pulmonary emboli, a decrease in pulmonary artery pressures occurs. An increase in PaO_2 and a return of PCO_2 to normal are expected reactions. Long-term follow-up data show that the NYHA function class of most patients changes dramatically, moving from Class III or IV to Class I in most cases, and to Class II in others (Fig. 49–22). These data, combined with other similar series in the literature, indicate favorable results. A long-term follow-up arteriogram is shown in Figure 49–23. In contrast, those patients who are unsuitable for embolectomy have a poor prognosis. In medically managed patients, many patients succumb to their disease, and most of the survivors are disabled.

DISCUSSION

Most patients with pulmonary embolism have an active fibrinolytic system responsible for rapid resolution of pulmonary emboli.[26] Therefore, most pulmonary emboli present as acute clinical problems that resolve with few long-term symptoms or residual effects. Experimental studies indicate that by 21 days after embolism, major perfusion defects have resolved.[30, 31] Clinical studies using pulmonary scans and arteriograms have shown that complete resolution of pulmonary emboli may occur as early as 8 to 14 days after the clinical event, although in some patients, this response may be delayed for several months, and the embolism may even persist, especially in patients with congestive heart failure.

A few patients may develop recurrent pulmonary emboli. As many as 16% of patients with pulmonary emboli have been shown to have continued pathologic evidence of emboli as a long-term phenomenon, although most of these chronic

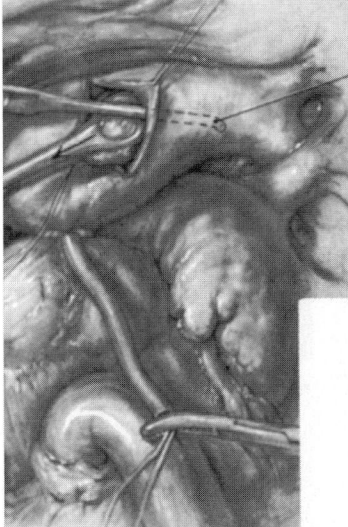

Endarterectomy instrument dissecting thrombus from intima left pulmonary artery

Figure 49–18. After occlusion of the proximal pulmonary artery by the tape when the patient is on cardiopulmonary bypass, an incision is made into the main pulmonary artery for removal of the chronic embolus. The thrombus is densely adherent to the wall of the pulmonary artery and requires exacting and tedious dissection. As much of the thrombus is removed through this incision as possible, preparatory to a counterincision in the distal left pulmonary artery. (From Wolfe, W. G., and Sabiston, D. C., Jr.: Pulmonary embolism. *In* Ebert, P. A. [Ed.]: Major Problems in Clinical Surgery, Vol. 25. Philadelphia, W. B. Saunders, 1980.)

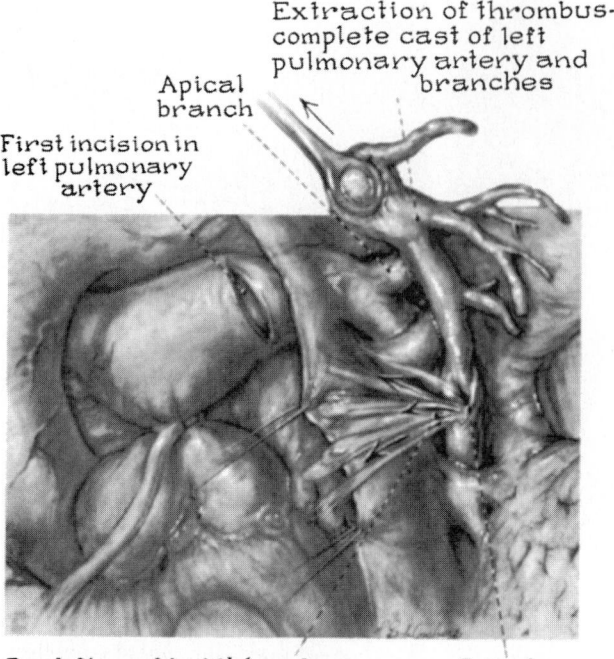

Figure 49–19. Through a counterincision in the distal left pulmonary artery, the branches of the chronic embolus are removed (as shown). Actually, the chronic embolus has formed a cast of the pulmonary arterial tree. After the cast has been removed, a large amount of back-bleeding occurs. The retrograde blood flow is bright red, which indicates that its source from the bronchial circulation is supplied by the aorta. The arteriotomies are closed. (From Wolfe, W. G., and Sabiston, D. C., Jr.: Pulmonary embolism. *In* Ebert, P. A. [Ed.]: Major Problems in Clinical Surgery, Vol. 25. Philadelphia, W. B. Saunders, 1980.)

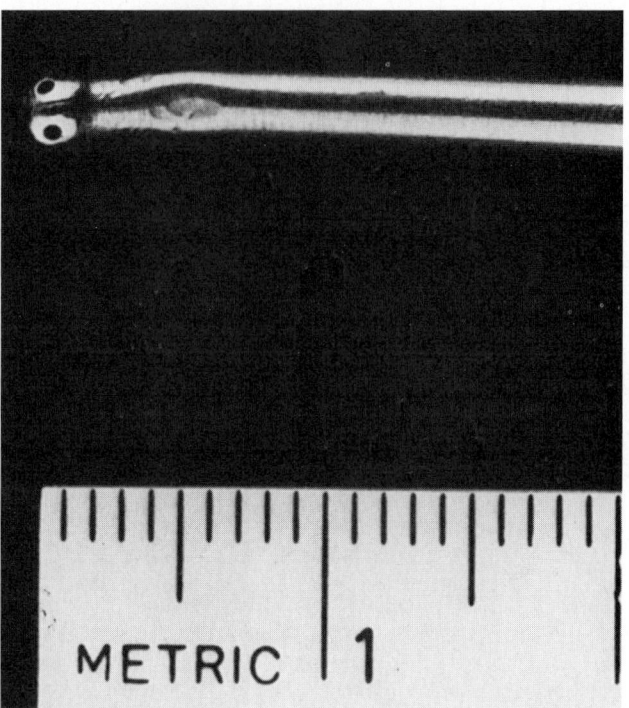

Figure 49–20. Dissector for use in surgical resection of chronic pulmonary embolism. (From Daily, P. O., and Daily, R. P.: Dissectors for pulmonary thromboendarterectomy. Ann. Thorac. Surg., *51*:842, 1991. Reprinted with permission from the Society of Thoracic Surgeons [The Annals of Thoracic Surgery, 1991, 51, 842].)

changes do not produce pulmonary hypertension. In one series, 22% of patients had findings of unresolved emboli, but in only 2% did chronic cor pulmonale actually develop.[21] Nevertheless, in this small number of patients, recurrent attacks of pulmonary emboli without resolution lead to a syndrome of chronic pulmonary hypertension and ensuing cardiac and pulmonary complications.

The failure of emboli to resolve is thought to be due to inadequate fibrinolysis. Deficiencies of coagulation inhibitors cause an inability to regulate intravascular clot formation. Congenital abnormalities of fibrinolysis include plasminogen deficiency, endothelial deficiencies of plasminogen activation, and abnormal fibrinogen. Diminished fibrinolysis has been described in coronary artery disease, cerebrovascular disease, and thrombotic thrombocytopenia purpura and with the use of oral contraceptives. Antithrombin III (AT-III) is essential for thrombin and other serine protease inactivation. Patients with a deficiency of AT-III have a hypercoagulable state that can manifest by recurrent thrombosis and pulmonary embolism. Deficiencies of activated protein C (APC), which inhibits factors V and IV, and of protein S, which serves as a cofactor for activated protein C, have also been reported to lead to an increased incidence of thromboembolism.[5]

Adequate anticoagulation in patients with chronic emboli decreases the number of recurrent episodes of pulmonary emboli. Despite anticoagulation, a few patients continue to have showers of emboli and an absence of significant resolution, which may proceed to major pulmonary arterial obstruction.[25] In patients with chronic pulmonary embolism, a major determinant of their appropriateness as surgical candidates is the response of the bronchial artery circulation. The adaptation of the bronchial circulation was demonstrated by

Sherrier and co-workers in 1989 with a model of hypertrophy of the bronchial vessels in response to chronic pulmonary embolism.[24] Other studies of the endothelium of the pulmonary vasculature have shown that the normal endothelium

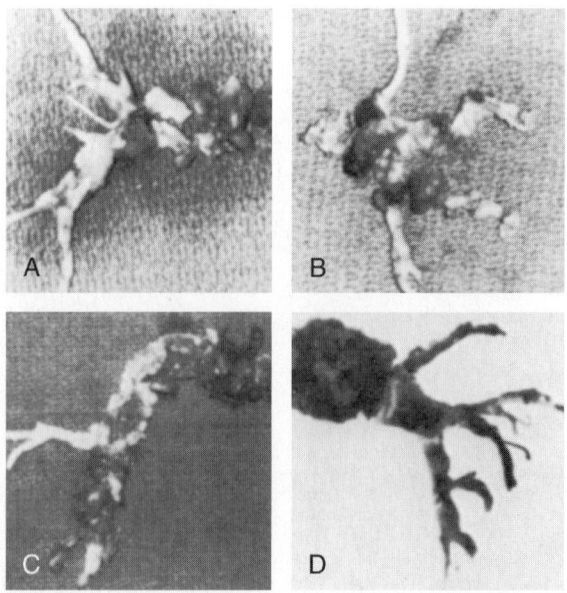

Figure 49–21. Chronic emboli removed from four patients undergoing pulmonary embolectomy. Three patients (specimens shown in *A* to *C*) had embolectomy via thoracotomy and localized lobar pulmonary artery occlusion. One patient (specimen shown in *D*) required cardiopulmonary bypass because of very proximal pulmonary artery involvement. Note the tenacious fibrotic material extended into the segmental vessels. In most patients, distal branches could be embolectomized. (From Chitwood, W. R., Jr., Lyerly, H. K., and Sabiston, D. C., Jr.: Surgical management of chronic pulmonary embolism. Ann. Surg., *201*:11, 1985.)

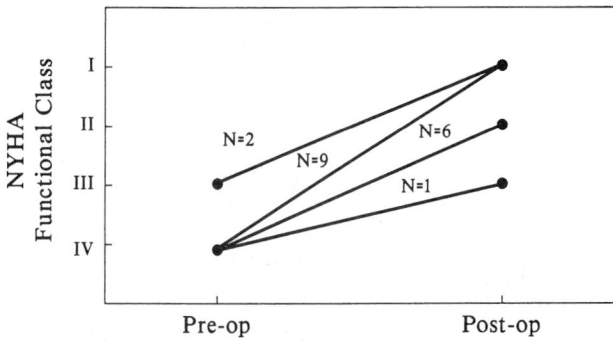

Figure 49–22. Preoperative and postoperative functional class of 13 patients having successful pulmonary embolectomy. NYHA, New York Heart Association. (From Lyerly, H. K., and Sabiston, D. C., Jr.: Chronic pulmonary embolism. *In* Sabiston, D. C., Jr., and Spencer, F. C. [Eds.]: Surgery of the Chest. Philadelphia, W. B. Saunders, 1990.)

can create a procoagulant environment that could lead to the development of thrombus in situ at the level of the large pulmonary vessels. Some patients may develop proximal pulmonary thromboemboli, which may cause retrograde propagation of thrombi after the initial pulmonary embolism. Other patients present with unexplained pulmonary hypertension secondary to thrombotic occlusion of the pulmonary microvasculature. A perfusion pulmonary scan should suggest the correct clinical diagnosis. Kapitan and colleagues examined the mechanism of hypoxemia in chronic pulmonary embolism. Through inert gas elimination analysis, the mechanism was shown to be a combination of ventilation-perfusion mismatching and a low mixed venous P_{O_2}. The level of inert gas dead space in these patients is less than expected, because areas of complete obstruction are removed from the dead space volume through anastomotic connection with bronchial arteries. The authors emphasized that the magnitude of hemodynamic compromise correlates only roughly with radionuclide scanning.[15] Although the ventilation-perfusion scan suggests the diagnosis, pulmonary arteriography is critical in the evaluation of chronic pulmonary embolism.

Medical management of chronic pulmonary embolism includes vasodilators in patients with obstruction at the arteriolar level. Patients with proximal obstruction and patients with arteriolar obstruction should be treated with chronic warfarin anticoagulation therapy to prevent progression of thromboembolism. Medical management also includes a number of fibrinolytic and vasodilating agents, although thus far they have been mainly ineffective.[12] Plasminogen activation has been shown to provide local thrombolysis of rela-

tively old thrombi in peripheral veins and could lead to resolution of chronic pulmonary emboli.[29] However, organized thrombi with fibroblastic ingrowth are resistant to any form of thrombolytic therapy. Surgical management is the most successful therapy in appropriate patients.[23]

Jamieson and associates reported the largest series in the literature. Since 1970, 323 thromboendarterectomies for chronic pulmonary embolism have been performed by this group.[14] Recently, they formulated a standard surgical approach to the management of chronic pulmonary embolism. They advocate simultaneous bilateral pulmonary thromboendarterectomy via median sternotomy, cardiopulmonary bypass, deep hypothermia with circulatory arrest, and intrapericardial dissection of the pulmonary arteries as the optimal surgical procedure. In 150 consecutive patients treated in this manner by a single surgeon, the mortality was 8.7%.[14] Significant risks for prolonged ventilator dependence have also been defined by this group; they are the presence of reperfusion edema and the transfusion of four or more units of packed red blood cells. The significant predictor of mortality was a failure to achieve a 50% reduction in pulmonary vascular resistance.[10]

In summary, selected patients with symptoms of severe respiratory insufficiency, hypoxemia, and pulmonary hypertension with proximal pulmonary arterial occlusion and adequate bronchial arterial collateral circulation with minimal impairment of right ventricular function are appropriate candidates for surgical embolectomy. However, patients who additionally have distal pulmonary emboli with patent proximal arteries, patients who are massively obese, and patients with severe right ventricular failure are generally unsuitable

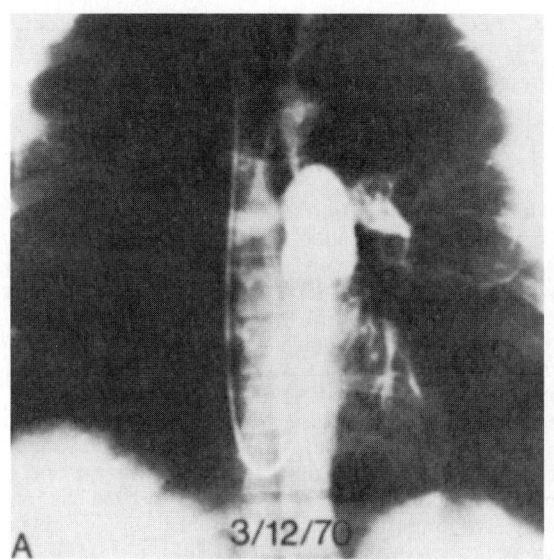
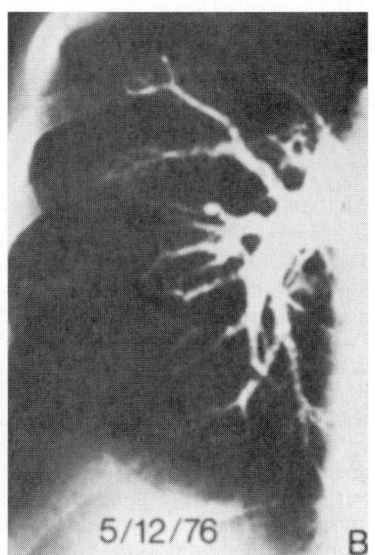

Figure 49–23. *A,* Pulmonary arteriogram in a patient before embolectomy. *B,* Six years after right lower lobe embolectomy. Note the continued perfusion of the right lower lobe after embolectomy. (From Chitwood, W. R., Jr., Lyerly, H. K., and Sabiston, D. C., Jr.: Surgical management of chronic pulmonary embolism. Ann. Surg., *201:*11, 1985.)

for surgical management. Long-term follow-up of patients with operable pulmonary emboli show favorable respiratory and cardiac dynamic changes. These patients have relief of incapacitating symptoms and maintain clinical improvement for prolonged periods.

SELECTED REFERENCES

Chitwood, W. R., Jr., Lyerly, H. K., and Sabiston, D. C., Jr.: Surgical management of chronic pulmonary embolism. Ann Surg., *201*:11, 1985.
  This report of a large series of patients in the United States managed surgically for chronic pulmonary embolism is extensively illustrated. The clinical manifestations, management, and results are evaluated in detail.

Jamieson, S. W., Auger, W. R., Fedullo, P. F., Channick, R. N., et al.: Experience and results with 150 pulmonary thromboendarterectomy operations over a 29 month period. J. Thorac Cardiovasc Surg., *106*:116, 1993.
  This article reports the most recent series of 323 thromboendarterectomies for chronic pulmonary embolism. The groups' standard surgical approach is discussed, as well as a more extensive discussion of 150 consecutive patients treated, with a mortality of 8.7%.

REFERENCES

1. Allison, P. R., Dunnill, M. S., and Marshall, R.: Pulmonary embolism. Thorax, *15*:273, 1960.
2. Auger, W. R., Fedullo, P. F., Moser, K. M., et al.: Chronic major-vessel thromboembolic pulmonary artery obstruction: Appearance at angiography. Radiology, *182*:393, 1992.
3. Carroll, D.: Chronic obstruction of major pulmonary arteries. Am. J. Med., *9*:175, 1950.
4. Chitwood, W. R., Jr., Lyerly, H. K., and Sabiston, D. C., Jr.: Surgical management of chronic pulmonary embolism. Ann. Surg., *201*:11, 1985.
5. Comp, P. C., and Esmon, C. T.: Recurrent venous thromboembolism in patients with a partial deficiency of protein S. N. Engl. J. Med., *311*:1525, 1984.
6. Cosgriff, T. M., Bishoop, D. T., Herrshgold, E. J., et al.: Familial antithrombin III deficiency: Its natural history, genetics, diagnosis and treatment, Medicine, *62*:209, 1983.
7. Couves, C. M., Makai, S. S., Sterns, L. P., et al.: Hemorrhagic lung syndrome. Ann. Thorac. Surg., *15*:187, 1973.
8. Daily, P. O., Dembitsky, W. P., Peterson, K. L., and Moser, K. M.: Modification of techniques and early results of pulmonary thromboendarterectomy for chronic pulmonary embolism. J. Thorac. Cardiovasc. Surg., *93*:221, 1987.
9. Daily, P. O., Dembitsky, W. P., and Iverson, S.: Technique of pulmonary thromboendarterectomy for chronic pulmonary embolism. J. Cardiac Surg., *4*:10, 1989.
10. Daily, P. O., Dembitsky, W. P., and Daily, R. P.: Dissectors for pulmonary thromboendarterectomy. Ann. Thorac Surg., *51*:842, 1991.
11. Dalen, J. E., and Alpert, J. S.: Natural history of pulmonary embolism. Prog. Cardiovasc. Dis., *17*:259, 1975.
12. Dash, H., Ballentine, N., and Zelis, R.: Vasodilators ineffective in secondary pulmonary hypertension. N. Engl. J. Med., *303*:1062, 1980.
13. Fleishner, F. G.: Recurrent pulmonary embolism and cor pulmonale. N. Engl. J. Med., *276*:1213, 1967.
14. Jamieson, S. W., Auger, W. R., Fedullo, P. F., Channick, R. N., et al.: Experience and results with 150 pulmonary thromboendarterectomy operations over a 29 month period. J. Thorac. Cardiovasc. Surg., *106*:116, 1993.
15. Kapitan, K. S., Buchbinder, M., Wagner, P. D., and Moser, K. M.: Mechanisms of hypoxemia in chronic thromboembolic pulmonary hypertension. Department of Medicine, UCSD Medical Center, San Diego, California, June 1988 and November 1988.
16. Kauczor, H. U., Schwickert, H. C., Mayer, E., et al.: Spiral CT of bronchial arteries in chronic thromboembolism. J. Comput. Assist. Tomogr., *18*:855, 1994.
17. Lyerly, H. K., Reeves, J. G., and Sabiston, D. C., Jr.: Primary sarcomas of the pulmonary artery and the management of intrabronchial hemorrhage. Surg. Gynecol. Obstet., *163*:291, 1986.
18. McIntyre, K. M., and Sarahara, A. A.: The hemodynamic response to pulmonary embolism in patients without prior cardiopulmonary disease. Am. J. Cardiol., *28*:288, 1971.
19. Mills, S. R., Jackson, D. C., Sullivan, D. C., et al.: Angiographic evaluation of chronic pulmonary embolism. Radiology, *136*:301, 1980.
20. Moser, K. M., Auger, W. R., and Fedullo, P. F.: Chronic major-vessel thromboembolic pulmonary hypertension. Circulation, *81*:1735, 1990.
21. Parakos, J. A., Adelstein, S. J., Smith, R. E., et al.: Late prognosis of acute pulmonary embolism. N. Engl. J. Med., *289*:55, 1973.
22. Ricou, F., Nicod, P. H., Moser, K. M., and Peterson, K. L.: Catheter-based intravascular ultrasound imaging of chronic thromboembolic pulmonary disease. Am. J. Cardiol., *67*:749, 1991.
23. Sabiston, D. C., Jr., Wolfe, W. G., Oldham, H. N., et al.: Surgical management of chronic pulmonary embolism. Ann. Surg., *185*:699, 1977.
24. Sherrier, R. H., Chiles, C., and Newman, G. E.: Chronic pulmonary emboli: Regional response of the bronchial circulation. Invest. Radiol., *24*:437, 1989.
25. Tilkian, A. G., Schroeeder, J. S., and Robin, E. D.: Chronic thromboembolic occlusion of main pulmonary artery or primary branches: Case report and review of the literature. Am. J. Med., *60*:563, 1976.
26. Tow, F. R., and Wagner, H. N., Jr.: Recovery of pulmonary arterial blood flow in patients with pulmonary embolism. N. Engl. J. Med., *276*:1053, 1976.
27. Viamonte, M.: Selective bronchial arteriography in man. Radiology, *83*:830, 1964.
28. Viamonte, M., Parks, R. E., and Smoak, W. M., III: Guided catheterization of the bronchial arteries. Radiology, *85*:205, 1965.
29. Weimar, W., Stibbe, J., VanSeyen, A. J., et al.: Specific lysis of an ileofemoral thrombus by administration of extrinsic (tissue type) plasminogen activator. Lancet, *207*:1018, 1981.
30. Wolfe, W. G., and Sabiston, D. C., Jr.: Radioactive ventilation scanning in the diagnosis of pulmonary embolism. J. Thorac. Cardiovasc. Surg., *555*:149, 1968.
31. Wolfe, W. G., and Sabiston, D. C., Jr.: Pulmonary Embolism: Major Problems in Clinical Surgery. Philadelphia, W. B. Saunders, 1980.
32. Woodruff, W. W., III, Hoeck, B. E., Chitwood, W. R., et al.: Radiographic findings in pulmonary hypertension from unresolved embolism. A.J.R., Am. J. Roentgenol., *144*:681, 1985.

II

FAT EMBOLI SYNDROME

Joseph A. Moylan, M.D.

The fat emboli syndrome is *one* of the causes of posttraumatic respiratory insufficiency. With sepsis, it remains the leading cause of morbidity and mortality following severe injury. During the first week following major trauma, the causes of posttraumatic respiratory insufficiency include pulmonary contusion, shock lung, and fat emboli. Complications of fat emboli syndrome were first described in 1862, when Bergmann reported a triad of confusion, dyspnea, and petechiae following long bone fractures.[5] Dennis, in his *Systems of Surgery,* emphasized fat emboli as a major cause of death, particularly in the first 3 days after injury.[10] A variety of therapies have been suggested, from ethyl alcohol[13] to the present-day administration of steroids.[1] The importance of morbidity and mortality from this complication was high-lighted during World War I and subsequent battles.[17, 27, 31] Some series describing civilian trauma have reported incidences of this syndrome as high as 80%,[28] although most reports have documented the incidence much lower, at approximately 35%.[9]

PATHOPHYSIOLOGY OF FAT EMBOLISM

The pathophysiology and classification of fat embolization have been studied, and there are two major theories concerning its pathogenesis. The mechanical theory offered by Gauss[12] in 1924 has many supporters, including Morton and Kendall[20] and Arnim and Grant.[2] This thesis supports mobilization of fat from the marrow at the site of a fracture, which

produces ischemia and hemorrhagic changes due to temporary occlusion of the pulmonary circulation. Pathologic and
animal studies have demonstrated gross fat particles in the
pulmonary capillaries.[33]

Lehmann and Moore[16] proposed the physiochemical theory, suggesting that neutral fat stores in the marrow cavity
release free fatty acids that have a toxic effect in a variety of
tissues, especially the lung. Refinement of the theory by
Peltier[24, 25] showed that free fatty acids, which derive from
either hydrolysis of neutral fats by lipase or mobilization of
fat stores by catecholamines, produce alterations in the capillary alveolar membrane as well as changes in lung surfactant
production. The end results of the phenomenon are hemorrhage, edema, and alveolar collapse. A correlation between
elevated free fatty acids and the severity of the fat emboli
syndrome has been documented in the literature (Table
49–7).[22]

The fat emboli syndrome has been classified and graded
both clinically and pathologically. One method is the respiratory distress index (RDI):

$$RDI = \frac{Po_2}{Fio_2} (VF + PF)$$

$$VF = 1 \text{ (without mechanical ventilation)}$$
$$= 1.5 \text{ (with mechanical ventilation)}$$

$$PF = 0 \text{ (PEEP} <5 \text{ cm. H}_2\text{O)}$$
$$= 0.5 \text{ (PEEP} >5 \text{ cm. H}_2\text{O)}$$

where Fio_2 = percent inspired oxygen, VF = ventilatory
factor, PF = positive end-expiratory pressure factor, and
PEEP = positive end-expiratory pressure.

A method for grading the severity of the fat emboli syndrome has been described. Correlation between increasing
levels of free fatty acids and the severity of pulmonary dysfunction has been statistically documented. The grading of
chest films and other parameters has not been satisfactory in
describing the severity of this disease process. Pathologically,
reliable grading of fat emboli has not been established. Attempts to classify embolic phenomena by size and distribution have been met with marked variance, making this
method ineffective. Use of a quantitative image analysis of
size and location of fat emboli is promising, but further work
in this area is needed.[7]

Unbound free fatty acids have been shown to produce
significant pulmonary decompensation in a variety of animal

TABLE 49–8. Free Fatty Acid (FFA) Levels in Patients with and without Albumin Administration

Group	Serum FFA (4 mmol./L.) on Postoperative Day (Mean ± SEM)				
	1	2	3	4	5
No albumin (n = 24)	356 ± 34	356 ± 31	280 ± 33	271 ± 38	239 ± 37
Albumin (n = 20)	354 ± 62	301 ± 48	260 ± 34	222 ± 30	153 ± 16

models. Studies by Kreis and associates[15] and by Cahill and
colleagues[8] have produced both radiologic and physiologic
abnormalities following oleic acid administration. In clinical
studies, the use of albumin as a method for binding free fatty
acids has been shown to be effective in decreasing their
levels, particularly during the second and third day after
injury (Table 49–8).[21]

DIAGNOSIS

Changes in the cerebral, pulmonary, and cutaneous organ
systems are involved in the fat emboli syndrome.[11] Patients
exhibit hypoxia, confusion, and petechiae. Classically, petechiae are found over the upper extremities and chest, particularly in the axillary areas, conjunctivae, and uvula. Cerebral
signs include confusion, agitation, stupor, and even coma.
Respiratory abnormalities begin with tachypnea and may
progress to profound hypoxia and cardiac arrest (Fig. 49–24).

The peak incidence of respiratory insufficiency from pulmonary embolization is on the second to fourth day after
injury. Other causes, such as contusion and shock lung, present either before or after this time. There is no predilection
for the development of this morbid complication based on
age or sex; however, the incidence is higher in male patients
due to the greater frequency of occupational and recreational
exposure to multisystem trauma.

The diagnosis is made using a combination of laboratory
and clinical parameters. Clinical indicators include a history
of skeletal trauma, the presence of posttraumatic shock, respiratory distress, change in cerebral function, and appearance
of petechiae in classic distribution. A number of laboratory
tests provide additional confirmation. Chest films demonstrate bilateral fluffy densities similar to those found following congestive heart failure with pulmonary edema (Fig.
49–25). Although the initial chest film may be abnormal
in only 30% of patients with respiratory distress, over the

TABLE 49–7. Free Fatty Acid (FFA) Inverse Relationship to the Respiratory Distress Index (RDI)*

FFA (mmol./L.)	RDI
88	3.0
110	1.8
134	2.8
165	3.2
166	3.2
173	4.1
175	1.6
185	2.1
198	1.8
235	1.0
321	1.7
352	1.7
360	1.4
384	1.5

*p <0.01.

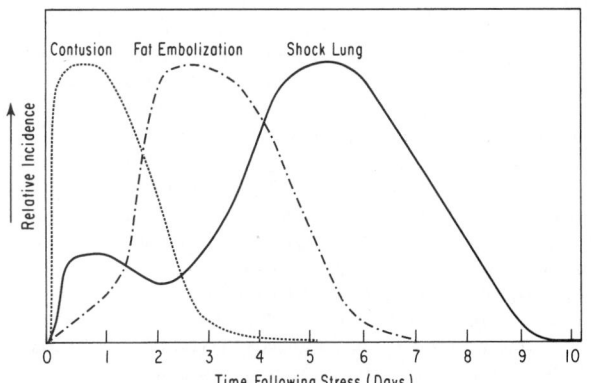

Figure 49–24. The peak incidence of respiratory insufficiency caused by fat
embolism is between 2 and 4 days after injury. Pulmonary contusion is functionally significant in the first day following chest trauma, and shock lung presents
later in the course.

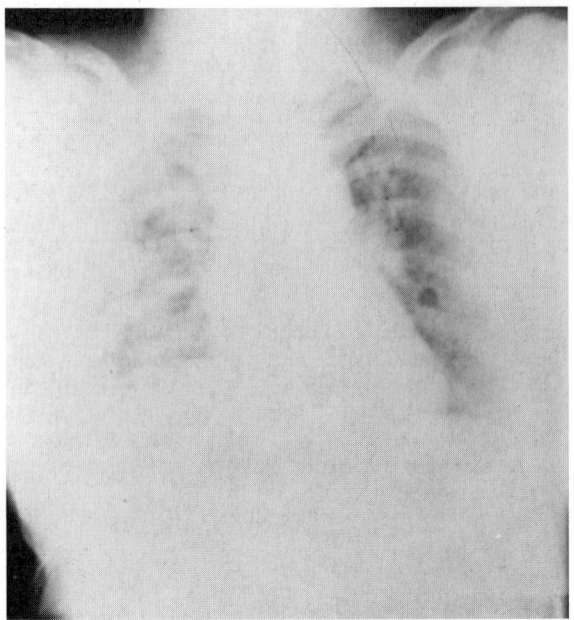

Figure 49–25. Diffuse, fluffy infiltrate at 72 hours after injury. Patient had progressive hypoxia during the preceding 12-hour period.

subsequent 24 hours, almost all patients develop radiologic abnormalities.

The arterial P_{O_2} is very important, and a measurement of less than 60 mm. Hg on room air is highly suggestive of respiratory distress. When coupled with a positive history and chest film, it is indicative of the fat emboli syndrome. This laboratory test is also valuable for following the course of the disease. Initially, the pH may be increased and the P_{CO_2} slightly decreased secondary to hyperventilation; however, further deterioration may produce serious hypoxia, hypercapnia, and respiratory acidosis.

The presence of fat globules in the urine was initially thought to be syndrome specific, but further investigations have shown that most patients with major trauma involving long bones have urinary fat globules, whether or not they develop the fat emboli syndrome.[19] However, the absence of fat in the urine makes the diagnosis of fat emboli unlikely.

Changes in the electrocardiogram are usually nonspecific and include prominent S waves in lead 1, prominent Q waves in lead 3, ST segment depression, and right axis strain, all indicative of increasing pulmonary resistance.

Thrombocytopenia, hypofibrinogenemia, and prolongation of the partial thromboplastin time have been reported in patients with the fat emboli syndrome. These changes, however, are not disease specific and may relate more to the primary problem of multisystem injury in major trauma.[18] Other serum tests, such as serum lipase and tributyrinase levels, do not appear to correlate well with either elevated free fatty acid levels or progressive respiratory failure.[14, 24] On an experimental basis, serum free fatty acid levels correlate very well with increasing severe pulmonary insufficiency. Unbound free fatty acids appear to reach their nadir at approximately 48 hours after injury, which correlates well with the onset of the fat emboli syndrome.

Fat emboli have been detected passing through the heart during intramedullary nailing of patients with femoral and tibial fractures. Early nailing was associated with smaller numbers of emboli.[23]

PREVENTION AND TREATMENT

The incidence of the fat emboli syndrome can be reduced and prevented by careful stabilization of fractures and the treatment of shock. The use of air splints at accident scenes and early operative intervention with intramedullary nailing and fracture plating have decreased the incidence of complications associated with the fat emboli syndrome.[18, 32] The aggressive treatment of hypovolemic shock has also contributed to the reduced incidence. The use of albumin to bind circulating free fatty acids has been particularly beneficial in the first 24 to 72 hours in reducing the incidence of posttraumatic respiratory distress secondary to this complication. Other agents, such as alcohol[20] and heparin, have never been effective and actually may produce significant complications, such as bleeding with heparin administration.

In the 1960s, steroids were thought to be effective in minimizing the morbidity and mortality of the fat emboli syndrome, but their use is controversial.[3, 30] Some have suggested the use of prophylactic steroids in high-risk patients.[29] Some side effects of steroids, including stress bleeding and increased infection due to suppression of immune competence, have made this prophylactic use questionable. Double-blind studies with high-dose methylprednisolone in patients with respiratory distress syndrome from a variety of causes, including fat emboli, did not show a beneficial influence on outcome.[6]

A volume respirator with an endotracheal tube and positive end-expiratory pressure (PEEP) remains a primary therapy in stabilizing or reversing posttraumatic pulmonary distress syndrome. PEEP produces an increase in the functional residual capacity and a decrease in pulmonary shunting.[4]

In one series of 20 cases of fat embolism, those with multiple fractures and high injury-severity scores had the highest mortality, with four deaths occurring among the 20 patients.[26]

By increasing awareness of the diagnosis and prevention of fat emboli, the high mortality and morbidity associated with this complication of major injury have been markedly reduced. But despite good therapy, vigilance for the development of this posttraumatic syndrome is mandatory.

SELECTED REFERENCES

Day, J. D., Walden, S. M., Stuart, S. R., Hutchins, G. M., and Hruban, R. H.: Fatal fat embolism syndrome after numerous vertebral body compression fractures in a lung transplant recipient. J. Heart Lung Transplant., 13(5):785, 1994.
It is interesting that transplanted lungs may be involved with fat emboli from traumatized donors and lead to death in the recipients. Obviously, every attempt should be made to avoid this error by careful preharvest evaluation of the status of the lungs.

Evarts, C. M.: The fat embolism syndrome: A review. Surg. Clin. North Am., 50:493, 1970.
This is a review of the entire topic of fat embolism.

Pell, A. C. H., Hughes, D., Keating, J., Christie, J., Busuttil, A., and Sutherland, G. R.: Fulminating fat embolism syndrome caused by paradoxical embolism through a patent foramen ovale. N. Engl. J. Med., 329:926, 1993.
Fulminating fat embolism can occur in association with paradoxical embolism through a patent foramen ovale following a fracture

Peltier, L. F.: The diagnosis and treatment of fat embolism. J. Trauma, 11:661, 1971.
This article discusses the historic background, the clinical presentation, and the course of fat embolism. Laboratory evaluation and treatment modalities are discussed.

Waller, D. A., Bennett, M. K., Corris, P. A., and Dark, J. H.: Donor-acquired fat embolism causing primary organ failure after lung transplantation. J. Heart Lung Transplant. 13:785, 1994.
This article details another case of fat embolism after lung transplantation.

REFERENCES

1. Alho, A., Saikkon, K., Eerola, P., and Koskinen, M.: Corticosteroids in patients with a high risk of fat embolism syndrome. Surg. Gynecol. Obstet., 127:358, 1978.
2. Arnim, J., and Grant, R. E.: Observations on gross pulmonary fat embolism in man and in the rabbit. Can. J. Surg., 9:286, 1966.
3. Ashbaugh, D. G., and Petty, T. L.: The use of corticosteroids in the treat-

ment of respiratory failure associated with massive fat embolism. Surg. Gynecol. Obstet., *123*:493, 1966.

4. Ashbaugh, D. G., and Petty, T. L.: Positive end-expiratory pressure: Physiology, indications and contraindications. J. Thorac. Cardiovasc. Surg., *65*:165, 1973.

5. Bergmann, E. B.: Ein Fall todlicher fetlenbolic. Berl. Klin. Wochenschr., 1873, p. 10385.

6. Bernar, G. R., Luce, J., Sprung, C. L., Rinaldo, J. E., Tate, R. M., Sibbaild, W. J., Kariman, K., Higgins, S., Bradley, R., Metz, C. A., Harris, T. R., and Brigham, K. L.: High-dose corticosteroids in patients with adult respiratory distress syndrome. N. Engl. J. Med., *317*:1565, 1987.

7. Bunai, Y., Yoshimi, N., Komorija, H., Iwasa, M., and Ohya, I.: An application of a quantitative analytical system for grading pulmonary fat emboli. Forensic Sci. Int., *39*:263, 1988.

8. Cahill, J. M., Daly, B. F. T., and Byrne, J. J.: Ventilatory and circulatory response to oleic acid embolus. J. Trauma, *14*:73, 1974.

9. Chan, K. M., Tham, K. T., Chiu, H. S., Chow, Y. N., and Leun, P. C.: Post-traumatic fat embolism—its clinical and subclinical presentations. J. Trauma, *24*:45, 1984.

10. Dennis, F. S.: Systems of Surgery, Vol. 1. Philadelphia, Lea Brothers & Company, 1895, p. 533.

11. Fenger, C., and Salisbury, J. H.: Diffuse multiple capillary fat embolism in the lungs and brain is a fatal complication in common fracture: Illustrated by a case. Chicago Med. J. Examiner, *39*:587, 1879.

12. Gauss, H.: The pathology of fat embolism. Arch. Surg., *9*:593, 1924.

13. Hermann, L. G.: Effect of dextrose alcohol mixture upon pulmonary fat embolism. Proc. Soc. Exp. Biol. Med., *30*:588, 1932–1933.

14. Herndon, J. H., Riseborough, E. J., and Fischer, J. E.: Fat embolism, a review of current concepts. J. Trauma, *11*:673, 1971.

15. Kreis, W. R., Lindenaur, S. M., and Dent, T. L.: Corticosteroids in experimental fat embolization. J. Surg. Res., *14*:238, 1973.

16. Lehmann, E. P., and Moore, R. M.: Fat embolism, including experimental production with trauma. Arch. Surg., *14*:621, 1927.

17. Malloy, T. B., Sullivan, E. R., Burnett, C. H., et al.: The general pathology of traumatic shock. Surgery, *27*:627, 1950.

18. Manning, J. B., Bach, A. W., Herman, C. M., and Carrico, C. J.: Fat release after femur nailing in the dog. J. Trauma, *23*:322, 1983.

19. Morton, K. S.: Fat embolism: Incidence of urinary fat in trauma. Can. Med. Assoc. J., *74*:441, 1956.

20. Morton, K. S., and Kendall, M. J.: The failure of intravenous alcohol in the treatment of experimental pulmonary fat embolism. Can. J. Surg., *9*:286, 1966.

21. Moylan, J. A.: Fat emboli syndrome. *In* Sabiston, D. C., Jr. (Ed.): Textbook of Surgery: The Biological Basis of Modern Surgical Practice, 13th ed. Philadelphia, W. B. Saunders, 1986, p. 1768.

22. Moylan, J. A., Evenson, M. E., and Birnbaum, M: Fat emboli syndrome. J. Trauma, *16*:339, 1976.

23. Pell, A. C., Christie, J., Keating, J. F., and Sutherland, G. R.: The detection of fat embolism by transesophageal echocardiography during reamed intramedullary nailing: A study of 24 patients with femoral and tibial fractures. J. Bone Joint Surg. [Br.], *75*:921, 1993.

24. Peltier, J. F.: The prophylactic value of a tourniquet. J. Bone Joint Surg. [Am.], *38*:385, 1956.

25. Peltier, L. F.: Fat embolism: The toxic properties of neutral and free fatty acids. Surgery, *40*:665, 1956.

26. Roberts, J. H., Hoffmeyer, P., Broquet, P. E., Cerutti, P., and Vasey, H.: Fat embolism syndrome. Orthop. Rev., *22*:567, 1993.

27. Scully, R. E.: Fat embolism in Korean battle casualties: Its incidence, clinical significance and pathologic aspects. Am. J. Pathol., *32*:379, 1956.

28. Sevitt, S.: Fat Embolism. London, Butterworths, 1962.

29. Shier, M. R., Wilson, R. F., James, R. E., et al.: Fat embolism prophylaxis: A study of four treatment modalities. J. Trauma, *17*:721, 1977.

30. Stitt, R. W., and Adler, F.: The effects of corticosteroids on lung surfactant activity in experimentally produced fat embolism in rats. Surg. Forum, *28*:492, 1977.

31. Sutton, G. E.: Pulmonary fat embolism and its relation to traumatic shock. Br. Med. J., *2*:368, 1918.

32. Talucci, R. D., Manning, J. B., Lampard, S., Bach, A., and Carrico, C. J.: Early intramedullary nailing of femoral shaft fractures. Am. J. Surg., *146*:107, 1983.

33. Zenker, F. A.: Bertrage zur normalen und pathologischen: Anatomie der Lunger. Dresden, Braunsdorf, 1862.

CHAPTER **50**

DISORDERS OF THE ARTERIAL SYSTEM

I

INTRODUCTION

David C. Sabiston, Jr., M.D.

The development of surgical control of the arterial system represents one of the most important achievements in the field of surgery. Within the past several decades, vascular surgery has reached an unusually high level of accomplishment. Direct operations on arteries and the use of autografts, arterial prostheses, and extracorporeal circulation form the basis for many significant surgical procedures.

Bandaging and the use of styptics were advocated for bleeding in the ancient Chinese literature. During the era of Hippocrates, ligation of vessels was rarely practiced, and amputations were done through a gangrenous extremity at a site where the vessels were thrombosed to ensure that significant bleeding did not occur. Celsus recommended amputation at the line of demarcation, but again, most of the vessels at this level were thrombosed. At that time he advocated limited use of ligatures of Celtic linen. In about A.D. 100, Archigenes was more daring and advanced the scope of amputation significantly by proposing that it be performed for "gangrene, necrosis, cancer, and certain callous tumors." Antyllus contributed by recommending surgical treatment of aneurysms by proximal ligation of the arteries. Despite these advances, the ligature was rarely used for amputations and then only as a last resort, preference being given to the hot, searing cautery to achieve hemostasis.

The ligature was rediscovered by Paré, who used it, rather than the hot iron, to control hemorrhage when amputating the leg of an officer wounded at the siege of Danvilliers in 1552. This procedure prompted Paré to state, "I dressed him and God healed him. He returned home gaily with a wooden leg saying that he had got off cheaply without being miserably burned to stop the bleeding." This operation initiated the standard use of the ligature to control arterial bleeding, and Paré deserves great credit for reintroducing a long forgotten principle. An excellent account of the historic facts concerning control of bleeding and the development of ligatures is found in *The History of Hemostasis* by Harvey.[11]

Recognition is due William Hunter for his dissections of aneurysms and recommendations for proximal arterial ligature to control them. He also was the first to recognize that an arteriovenous aneurysm represented a direct communication between an artery and a vein and was not a simple arterial aneurysm. In 1903, Matas first advocated endoaneurysmorrhaphy in the treatment of arterial aneurysms.[12] Another major advance was by Carrel, with the contribution of anastomosis of arteries.[4-6] It was for this and pioneering work in the transplantation of organs that he was awarded the Nobel Prize in 1912. Goyanes was the first to successfully use a venous autograft to replace a popliteal aneurysm in 1906.[10] The following year, Lexer inserted a segment of saphenous vein for reconstruction of a posttraumatic axillary-brachial aneurysm following trauma. The first successful venous autograft in the United States was by Bernheim, for the replacement of a popliteal aneurysm.[2] Halsted called it the "ideal operation" for this lesion. Despite these important early contributions, venous autografts were rarely employed until their use by Mobile Army Surgical Hospitals during the Korean War. At that time, venous autografts were used in the management of arterial wounds, especially those in the lower extremities that would have become gangrenous and required amputation unless venous autografts were inserted to restore arterial continuity.

The use of intra-arterial injection of contrast medium (sodium iodide) was introduced by Brooks, who published impressive arteriograms utilizing this technique in 1924.[3] In 1927, Moniz used intra-arterial injection of thorium dioxide to outline the cerebral vessels,[13] and dos Santos and associates injected contrast medium directly into the aorta.[14] An aortic abdominal aneurysm was successfully removed and replaced by an arterial homograft for the first time by Dubost in 1951.[8] Later, thoracic aneurysms were successfully attacked by DeBakey[7] and Bahnson,[1] and these procedures were greatly augmented by Gibbon's introduction of successful extracorporeal circulation in 1953.[9] The introduction of prosthetic arterial substitutes began in 1952, when Voorhees and Blakemore first used Vinyon-N; additional studies with other materials led to the present-day use of Dacron and Gore-Tex.

SELECTED REFERENCES

Edwards, W. S.: Alexis Carrel's contributions to thoracic surgery. Ann. Thorac. Surg., 35:111, 1983.

Edwards, W. S.: Alexis Carrel: A century later. Arch. Surg., 124:1014, 1989.
   The first of these articles is a concise review of Alexis Carrel's contributions to thoracic surgery. The same author updated this subject in the second paper cited above.

Harrison, L. H., Jr.: Historical aspects in the development of venous autografts. Ann. Surg., 183:101, 1976.
   This is a commendable and detailed description of the early use of venous autografts by Goyanes, Lexer, Bernheim, and others. These contributions are described and related to other associated achievements.

Harvey, S. C.: The History of Hemostasis. New York, Paul B. Hoeber, 1929.
   This excellent monograph concisely describes the history of surgical approaches to control bleeding and the development of ligatures. It is fascinating and makes excellent reading for all who desire a thorough understanding of this subject.

REFERENCES

1. Bahnson, H. T.: Definitive treatment of saccular aneurysms of the aorta with excision of sac and aortic sutures. Surg. Gynecol. Obstet., 96:382, 1953.
2. Bernheim, B. M.: The ideal operation for aneurysm of the extremity: Report of a case. Bull. Johns Hopkins Hosp., 27:93, 1916.

3. Brooks, B.: Intra-arterial injection of sodium iodide. JAMA, *82*:1016, 1924.
4. Carrel, A.: La technique operatoire des anastomoses vasculaires et la transplantation des viscere. Lyon Med., *98*:859, 1902.
5. Carrel, A.: Suture of blood-vessels and transplantation of organs. Nobel lecture, 1912. *In* Nobel Lectures in Physiology-Medicine, Vol. 1. New York, American Elsevier Publishing Company, 1967, p. 442.
6. Carrel, A., and Guthrie, C. C.: Uniterminal and biterminal venous transplantations. Surg. Gynecol. Obstet., *2*:266, 1906.
7. DeBakey, M. E., and Cooley, D. A.: Successful resection of aneurysm of thoracic aorta and replacement by graft. JAMA, *152*:673, 1953.
8. Dubost, C., Allary, M., and Oeconomos, N.: Resection of an aneurysm of the abdominal aorta: Reestablishment of the continuity by a preserved human arterial graft, with results after five months. Arch. Surg., *64*:405, 1952.
9. Gibbon, J. H., Jr.: Application of a mechanical heart and lung apparatus to cardiac surgery. Minn. Med., *37*:171, 1954.
10. Goyanes, D. J.: Substitution plastica de las arterias por las venae, ó arterioplastia venosa, aplicada, como neuvo metodo, al tratamiento de los aneurismas. El Siglo Medico, Sept. 1, 1906, p. 346; Sept. 8, 1906, p. 561.
11. Harvey, S. C.: The History of Hemostasis. New York, Paul B. Hoeber, 1929.
12. Matas, R.: An operation for the radical cure of aneurysm based upon arteriorrhaphy. Ann. Surg., *37*:161, 1903.
13. Moniz, E.: Injections intracarotidiennes et substances injectables opaques aux rayons. X. Press Med., *2*:969, 1927.
14. dos Santos, R., Lamas, A., and Caldas, J.: L'arteriographie des membres de l'aorte et des ses branches abdominales. Bull. Soc. Nat. Chir., *55*:587, 1929.

II

ANATOMY

David C. Sabiston, Jr., M.D.

Blood is delivered from the heart to the organs and tissues by the arterial system. Arteries may be categorized as large, medium-sized, or small. Arteries less than 100 μ. in diameter are termed *arterioles*. The histologic characteristics of the arterial wall are largely dependent on the size of the vessel. The large arteries must withstand the greatest stress and pressure and therefore contain considerable elastic tissue in their walls. The medium-sized arteries have less elastic tissue and more smooth muscle. At the level of the arteriole, elastic tissue is scant or absent. Collagen is present in all parts of the arterial system, the collagen ratio becoming dominant as the arteries become smaller.

Collateral circulation is of primary importance in all aspects of medicine, particularly in surgery. All organs have some collateral circulation, although it varies greatly in different tissues and organs. The subclavian artery can usually be ligated safely in the first portion, such as in the performance of a subclavian-pulmonary anastomosis for congenital cyanotic heart disease (Blalock operation), since the collateral circulation around the shoulder is excellent. It is rare for ischemic symptoms to follow ligation of the subclavian artery at this site; indeed, with the passage of time, a pulse frequently reappears in the radial artery as additional collateral circulation develops. Moreover, three of the four major arteries of the stomach (the left and right gastric and the left and right gastric epiploic) can be ligated without significant ischemia. With a number of other arteries, the extensiveness of collaterals varies considerably; ligation produces no ill

effects in some patients and ischemic symptoms in others. Finally, some arteries, such as the coronary, renal, and retinal arteries, have an inadequate natural collateral circulation. Acute occlusion of these vessels is usually followed by serious ischemia or infarction, and such arteries are referred to as *end arteries*.

Tissues and organs have a natural collateral circulation that is important in the sequence of events following acute occlusion. In addition, the time involved in occlusion of an artery is of considerable significance. For example, with slow, progressive occlusion of an artery, there is ample time for collateral vessels to develop and become larger. Generally, as a smaller vessel is subjected to a need for increased flow (primarily due to a pressure gradient), the vessel is apt to become thin-walled and tortuous. The latter characteristic is easily demonstrated by arteriography, as in chronic occlusion of the abdominal aorta (Leriche's syndrome). Under these circumstances, adequate arterial collaterals develop that join the branches above the occlusion with the iliac and femoral systems distally. It is surprising that total occlusion of the entire abdominal aorta over a period of time may produce minimal symptoms in some patients, whereas in others it produces the characteristic symptoms of intermittent claudication and impotence. Nevertheless, in Leriche's syndrome, it is rare for gangrene to occur until late in the disease. In contrast, acute occlusion of the abdominal aorta usually produces disastrous effects, including severe ischemia and gangrene of the lower extremities if untreated.

III

PHYSIOLOGY OF THE ARTERIAL SYSTEM, INCLUDING THE EFFECTS OF NITRIC OXIDE

Mark G. Davies, M.D., Ph.D., and Per-Otto Hagen, Ph.D.

The normal arterial wall consists of three layers: the intima, the media, and the adventitia. Endothelial cells are a confluent monolayer of thin, flattened, rhomboid-shaped cells lining the intimal surface of all blood vessels. Smooth muscle cells are found within the media in association with a matrix of connective tissue components (collagen, elastin, and occasional fibroblasts). The intima consists of a single layer of endothelial cells resting on a thin basal lamina. The intima and media are separated by a definite basal lamina in arteries; the demarcation between the intima and the media is less clearly defined in veins. There is a very slow turnover of both endothelial and medial smooth muscle cells in uninjured vessels.

In the adult human, the net mass of the endothelium is equivalent to approximately 1% of body mass and has a surface area of approximately 5000 sq. m. In many respects, the endothelium fulfills all the definitions of an *organ,* and perhaps it should be considered as such.[1] Normal endothelial cells maintain a delicate balance in the vasculature between growth promotion and inhibition,[2] vasoconstriction and vasodilation,[1, 3] blood cell adherence and nonadherence, and anticoagulation and procoagulation.[4, 5] In these ways, the endothelium controls vasomotor tone, regulates vascular structure, maintains blood fluidity, and mediates both inflammatory and immunologic responses.

The endothelium, as constituted by the endothelial cells and the subendothelium, forms a relatively impermeable surface that limits passive transfer of cellular and fluid elements between the circulating blood and the body's tissue. The net flow across the endothelium is less than 0.05% of daily cardiac output, and this flow occurs by ligand-specific and non-specific transcytosis and the passage of fluid between cells. Endothelial cells *in vivo* are attached to the surface of the blood vessels by their interactions with the underlying subendothelium, which consists of a highly organized matrix of molecules that includes collagen, elastin, fibronectin, laminin, glycosaminoglycans, thrombospondin, vibronectin, and von Willebrand's factor (vWF). The subendothelium provides structural integrity, mechanical strength, and elasticity to the vessel and contains primarily collagen fibers. Many of these collagens are secreted by the endothelial cells, and they are capable of either enhancing endothelial cell proliferation or inhibiting cell growth. In addition, the endothelial cells express VLA-2 and VLA-3, integrins that bind collagen and thereby act as attachment sites for the endothelial cells.

Both the endothelial cells and the subendothelium contain glycosaminoglycans such as dermatan sulfate, heparan sulfate, and chondroitin sulfate. Endothelial cells synthesize three subtypes of heparan sulfate that can bind to collagen and initiate endothelial cell attachment. In addition, heparan sulfates convey anticoagulant activity to the endothelial cells. Von Willebrand's factor is synthesized by endothelial cells and secreted in a functional form. Large multimers of this protein bind to collagens in the extracellular matrix of the subendothelium. A second factor produced during the intracellular synthesis of vWF, vWFII, mediates the assembly of the vWF multimers; vWF is found in the subendothelium and basement membrane and can be bound by several recep-

tors on the endothelial cells. Finally, vibronectin is another glycoprotein found in both the plasma and the subendothelium; it appears to support the attachment and spreading of endothelial cells and is necessary for the activity of plasminogen activator inhibitors.

Turnover is usually low within the subendothelium, even though endothelial cells secrete a variety of proteases such as metalloproteases, collagenases, elastases, and gelatinases. This is balanced by the secretion of a series of proteinase inhibitors to metalloproteases (TIMP), gelatinases, and collagenases. Furthermore, endothelium-derived plasminogen activators activate plasmin, which in turn activates endothelial cell collagenase. PAI-1, an endothelium-derived inhibitor of the plasminogen activators, inhibits the activation of plasmin. Modulation of the connective tissue matrix in the subendothelium by mediation of its synthesis and degradation allows the endothelium to control the activity of the underlying vascular smooth muscle cells and the structure of the vessel wall.

Smooth muscle cells are the principal cells found in the media of a vessel. They are embedded in a matrix of connective tissue elements and provide mechanical and structural support to the vessel. Physiologically active smooth muscle cells and the extracellular matrix provide intrinsic vascular dimensions and tone. In addition to their vasoreactive characteristics, smooth muscle cells are capable of synthesizing and secreting elements of the extracellular matrix, particularly proteoglycans. The biologic roles of the proteoglycans are diverse, including mechanical support functions, cell adhesion, motility, and proliferation. Most of these biologic actions are modulated by the binding of proteins to the glycosaminoglycan chains. There are three major groups of proteoglycans found in the extracellular matrix of the vessel wall: heparan sulfates, chondroitin sulfates, and dermatan sulfates; the latter two form the bulk of the proteoglycans found in the vessel wall. Heparan sulfates are localized on cell membranes, chondroitin sulfates are present principally in the interstitial matrix, and dermatan sulfates are confined to the periphery of collagen fibrils. Unlike endothelial cells, which synthesize primarily heparan sulfates, smooth muscle cells synthesize mainly chondroitin sulfates and dermatan sulfates. The exact mechanisms whereby smooth muscle cell proliferation is initiated, controlled, reduced, and eventually suppressed are not fully understood. Quiescent vascular smooth muscle cells are well-differentiated cells characterized by an abundance of contractile proteins—predominantly smooth muscle cell actin and myosin—but little rough endoplasmic reticulum. Once activated, smooth muscle cells lose their differentiated state; they acquire abundant endoplasmic reticulum and commence the synthesis of extracellular matrix.

Signal transduction is the process by which cell surface receptors convert external stimuli into the appropriate intracellular responses. There are two basic ligand-operated receptor mechanisms responsible for signal transduction: ligand-modulated release of a secondary intracellular mediator (G protein–coupled receptors), and ligand-regulated enzyme activity (tyrosine kinase–coupled receptors). Guanine nucleotide regulatory proteins (G proteins) are a superfamily of guanine triphosphate (GTP) binding proteins that range from the heterotrimeric forms to monomeric forms, GTPase activating protein (GAP), activated G proteins, and *ras*-associated nuclear proteins. Functionally related GTP proteins are involved in signal transduction, protein synthesis, microtubule assembly, and oncogene function. G proteins are also coupled to many pharmacologic receptors that mediate vascular smooth muscle cell contractile responses. The heterotrimeric G proteins are intrinsic membrane-bound proteins that act as transmembrane signal transducers in cells and activate intracellular secondary messengers, such as adenylate cyclases and phospholipases. These heterotrimeric G proteins consist of three distinct subunits: alpha, beta, and gamma; many are classified according to differences in their alpha subunits (α_i, α_s, α_q, and α_o). Receptor linked protein tyrosine kinases encompass a set of nine distinct families of receptor subtypes. Despite the number of subtypes, there is considerable commonality in the intracellular messengers stimulated by these receptors. These receptors are important in the responses of smooth muscle cells to many polypeptide growth factors. Upon binding to these receptors, the receptors phosphorylate themselves on the tyrosine residue. However, activation of the same receptor tyrosine kinase (fibroblast growth factor) in different cell types leads to different responses, and activation of the same receptor by distinct ligands results in different and diverse responses.

MAINTENANCE OF VASCULAR TONE

Seven families of compounds have been associated with endothelium-mediated vasomotor responses: prostanoids, nitric oxide (NO) and nitric oxide–containing compounds, oxy-

gen free radicals, endothelins, angiotensins, smooth muscle cell hyperpolarization factors, and other, as yet uncharacterized, endothelium-derived constriction factors (Fig. 50–1).[6–8]

Prostacyclin (PGI_2) production from endothelial cells was discovered in 1976 and has subsequently been shown to be a potent platelet antiaggregator, a vasodilator, and a profibrinolytic agent. It thus conveys both a thromboresistant and a vasodilatory property to the endothelium. The abluminal release from endothelial cells is small compared with its luminal release, suggesting that the primary function of prostacyclin is to inhibit platelet aggregation. Two serum factors influence prostacyclin synthesis: PGI_2 synthesis stimulating factor and PGI_2 stabilization factor. The former has not yet been characterized but is known to be absent in thrombotic microangiopathy, and the latter has been identified as Apo A-1, the major lipoprotein of high-density lipoprotein (HDL). PGI_2 acts on smooth muscle cells via receptor-mediated activation of adenylate cyclase. In the smooth muscle cell, increased cAMP concentrations activate intracellular kinases and bring about relaxation. However, in the platelet, PGI_2-mediated increases in cAMP concentrations inhibit adhesion and the release of vasoconstrictive, proaggregatory compounds such as thromboxane A_2 (TXA_2), adenosine diphosphate (ADP), and serotonin. PGI_2 synthesis can be increased by adenosine triphosphate (ATP), catecholamine, kinins, calcium antagonists, angiotensin converting enzyme (ACE) inhibitors, and nitrovasodilators through an increase in free intracellular calcium. The ratio of PGI_2 to PGE_2 generation is lower in the microcirculation than in major vessels. With PGI_2 production, endothelial cells also generate a small amount of TXA_2, a proaggregating vasoconstrictor. A variety of other eicosanoids, such as monohydroxy-, dihydroxy- and epoxy-derivatives of arachidonic acid, which are formed by

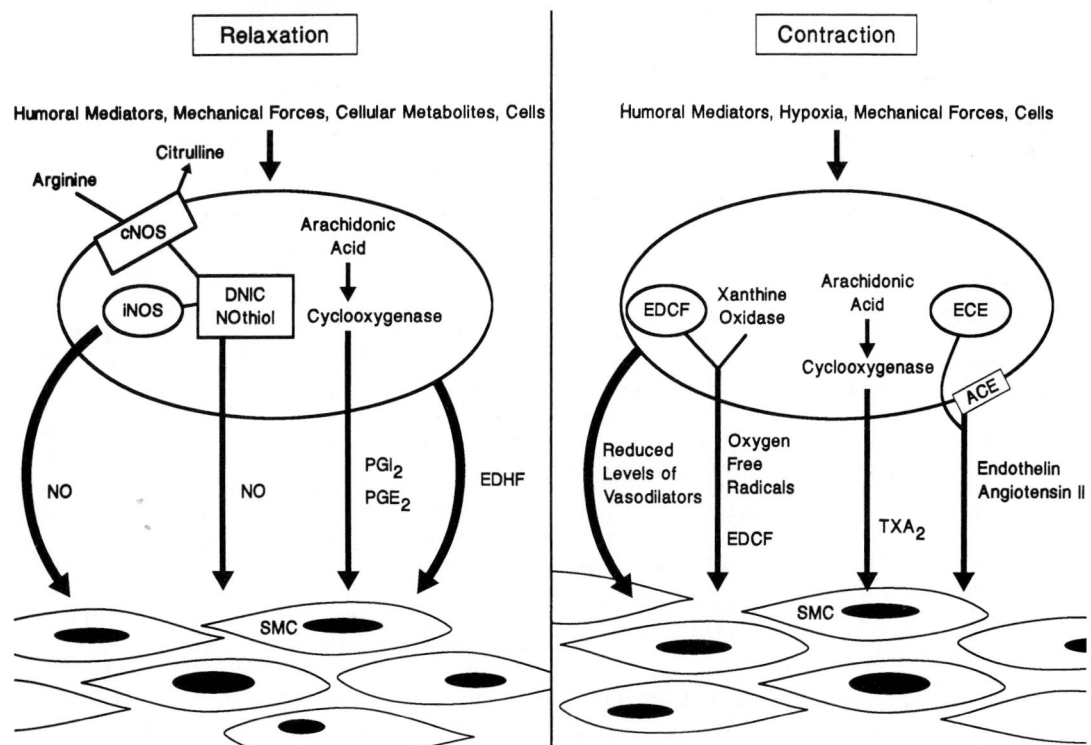

Figure 50–1. Maintenance of vascular tone. Relaxation is mediated by nitric oxide (NO) and other nitrosyl-containing compounds, prostacyclin (PGI_2) and prostaglandin E (PGE_2), and endothelium-derived hyperpolarization factor (EDHF). Vasocontraction can be induced by a reduction in the release of vasorelaxant factors and by thromboxane A_2 (TXA_2), oxygen free radicals, angiotensin II, endothelins, and endothelium-derived constriction factors (EDCFs). Both endothelium-derived relaxation and constriction can be influenced by alterations in local physical, chemical, humoral, and cellular factors. cNOS, constitutive NO synthase; iNOS, inducible NO synthase; DNIC, dinitrosyl iron cysteine; SMC, smooth muscle cell; ECE, endothelin converting enzyme; ACE, angiotensin converting enzyme. (From Davies, M. G., and Hagen, P.-O.: The vascular endothelium—a new horizon. Ann. Surg., *218*:593, 1993.)

the cyclo-oxygenase, lipo-oxygenase, and cytochrome P450–dependent mono-oxygenation pathways, also influence vascular tone.

Four years after the discovery of prostacyclin, Furchgott and Zawadzki in 1980 showed that acetylcholine-mediated relaxation of vascular rings was mediated by a nonprostanoid, endothelium-dependent factor later termed endothelium-derived relaxing factor (EDRF). Subsequent studies have shown that EDRF is NO. NO is synthesized from the conversion of L-arginine to citrulline by at least two categories of enzymes: constitutive NO synthases (cNOS; predominantly membrane bound) and inducible NO synthases (iNOS; predominantly cytosolic), both of which are calcium- and calmodulin-dependent and utilize at least five cofactors (NADPH, tetrahydrobiopterin, FAD, FMN, and heme). The various isoforms of NOS are shown in Table 50–1. It is now apparent that NOS activity is modulated by the Ca^{2+} flux into the cell, and recent studies suggest that NO can exert feedback inhibition on NOS to further control its synthesis. This feedback inhibition may be through the interaction of NO with the heme cofactor or by NO-mediated protein phosphorylation of the synthetase. Protein phosphorylation by the cGMP-dependent kinases that are activated by NO-mediated increases in target cell cGMP is the basis of many of the effects attributed to NO. NO shares many of the vasoactive properties of prostacyclin in that it can relax smooth muscle and inhibit platelet aggregation. In the appropriate circumstances, NO can be converted in the endothelial cell to peroxynitrite, a potentially toxic molecule that may play a pivotal role in the pathophysiology of several cardiovascular diseases. NO may be only one of several EDRFs present. Compounds such as nitrosothiols and dinitrosyl iron-cysteines, which are more stable than NO, may be responsible for a degree of the relaxation now attributed to NO. Additionally, such compounds would allow NO to be stored intracellularly. Before the discovery of endothelium-derived relaxation as mediated by EDRF or NO, several authors had demonstrated that acetylcholine and other transmitters could hyperpolarize vascular smooth muscle cell membranes. NO does not produce membrane hyperpolarization and thus is not responsible for this effect. These compounds have therefore been named endothelium-derived hyperpolarization factors (EDHFs). The EDHFs depolarize the membrane by opening ATP-sensitive potassium channels or by activating the sodium-potassium pump. The actual chemical nature of these compounds is as yet undetermined. The presence of other EDRFs is of biologic significance, as there is experimental evidence to suggest that not all the relaxation produced by stimulators of NO production can be attributed to NO or nitrosyl compound activity.

Endothelial cells contain xanthine dehydrogenase/oxidase, and the free radicals produced or transferred from the extracellular space are reduced by the endothelial cell superoxide dismutase, catalase, and glutathione redox cycle. Low intracellular levels of oxygen free radicals stimulate cyclo-oxygenation of arachidonic acid. Superoxide radicals can induce vasodilation in several tissue beds, and this is thought to be mediated by the release of prostacyclin from endothelial cells. However, increased intracellular concentrations of oxygen free radicals are able to inactivate EDRF or NO and can inhibit the production of prostacyclin in endothelial cells by inhibiting both PGG/PGH and PGI_2 synthetases. Higher levels result in the destruction of these enzymes. In contrast, TXA_2 synthetase is resistant to such free radical inhibition and destruction. The net effect of these interactions is vasoconstriction. Oxygen free radicals can lead to the formation of peroxides, and because of the difference in kinetics between the cyclo-oxygenase and peroxidase enzymes, lipid peroxides can accumulate; elevated concentrations of these compounds also destroy both PGG/H and PGI_2 synthetases. This damage can be prevented by antioxidants. In normal physiology, a balance exists between the production of PGI_2 and TXA_2 and between EDRF or NO and oxygen free radicals, which allows for the maintenance of vascular tone. Disruption of this delicate equilibrium leads to nonphysiologic blood cell adherence, vasoconstriction, and eventual pathophysiologic consequences.

The ability of the endothelium to produce vasoconstrictors was established by the discovery of the polypeptide endothelin-1 (ET-1) in 1988. This single polypeptide is now recognized as the proband of a family of endothelins that are considered to be the most potent vasoconstrictors yet identified. This family of peptides consists of ET-1, ET-2, and ET-3, and their rank contractile potencies are ET-1 = ET-2 > ET-3. Endothelins are formed by the conversion of big-endothelin to endothelin by one or two endothelin converting enzymes (ECEs). Although primarily thought of as vasoconstrictive agents, endothelins can also induce transient vasodilatation. Two classes of endothelin receptor have been identified in vascular tissue, ET_A and ET_B, both of which appear to be G protein linked. Recent evidence suggests that there may be two subtypes of the ET_B receptor. ET_A is found on vascular smooth muscle cells and is responsible for the vasoconstrictive response. ET_A-mediated vasoconstriction occurs through two distinct signal transduction systems. One is related to an enhanced influx of calcium ions through the activation of calcium channels, and the second is by phospholipase C and A_2 activation. ET_B receptors are located on vascular endothelial cells and exert their effects, in part, by stimulation of EDRF or NO and PGI_2 production. However, neither the inhibition of EDRF or NO synthesis nor the blockade of cyclo-oxygenase has been shown to reduce the vasodilatory action of endothelin. Endothelin-mediated relaxation is also mediated by a calcium-activated K^+ channel, which is activated by low doses of endothelin and inactivated by higher doses of endothelin. The long-lasting effect of endothelins on vascular preparations due to their prolonged receptor kinetics suggests that endothelins are more likely to be involved in longer-term responses regulating vascular tone and blood flow and may not be involved in the acute management of vascular homeostasis. In 1982, Vanhoutte and co-workers demonstrated that the endothelium could mediate not only rapid relaxation of the vasculature but

TABLE 50–1. Isoforms of Nitric Oxide Synthases

Isoform	Principal Tissue	Regulation	Cofactors
Soluble			
Ia	Brain	Ca^{2+}/calmodulin	NADPH, BH_4, FAD, FMN
Ib	Endothelial cells	Ca^{2+}/calmodulin	NADPH
Ic	Neutrophils	Ca^{2+}	NADPH, BH_4, FAD, FMN
II	Macrophages	Not defined	NADPH, BH_4, FAD, FMN
Particulate			
III	Endothelial cells	Ca^{2+}/calmodulin	NADPH, BH_4, FAD, FMN
IV	Macrophages	Not defined	NADPH

NADPH, nicotine adenine dinucleotide; BH_4, tetrahydrobiopterin; FAD, flavin adenine dinucleotide; FMN, flavin mononucleotide.
Adapted from Murad, F.: Regulation of cytosolic guanylyl cylase by nitric oxide: The NO-cyclic GMP signal transduction system. Adv. Pharmacol., 26:19, 1994.

also rapid contraction. Hypoxia and increased transmural pressure evoke the release of a nonprostanoid endothelium-derived constricting factor ($EDCF_1$) that is not an endothelin. This EDCF is likely to be involved in the more immediate responses required to modulate vascular tone.

It has recently become apparent that the local renin-angiotensin system in the vessel wall is important in the maintenance of blood pressure and the control of hypertension. Angiotensin I can be synthesized by endothelial cells and stimulates prostaglandin release in cultured endothelial cells. Angiotensin II, a potent vasoconstrictor, is formed from the conversion of angiotensin I by the endothelial cell ACE. Angiotensin II can bind to two receptor subtypes: AT_1, predominantly on smooth muscle cells, and AT_2, mainly on endothelial cells. ACE is a carboxypeptidase that not only converts angiotensin I to angiotensin II but also inactivates bradykinin, a peptide transmitter that stimulates the release of EDRF or NO and vasodilatory prostanoids. Inhibition of ACE thus leads to decreased angiotensin II–mediated vasoconstriction and increased bradykinin activity, with enhanced EDRF or NO release and the resultant reduction in vessel tone. In 1989, angiotensin I-7, which was once considered an inert by-product of angiotensin synthesis, was shown to be a potent stimulator of vasodilatory prostaglandin release (PGI_2 and PGE_2). It appears to act through its own specific receptor subtypes; these seem to be distinct from AT_1 and AT_2, although it has been reported that angiotensin I-7 can also activate AT_2. Angiotensin I-7 is produced from both angiotensin I and II by enzymes other than ACE. The enzymes in this alternative pathway are neutral and metalloendopeptidases and prolyl endopeptidases. ACE inhibition increases the production of angiotensin I-7.

MECHANOTRANSDUCTION

Positioned between the blood flow and the vessel wall, endothelial cells can function as mechanosensors and can transduce the physical forces produced by the flow of the blood into biochemical signals to which the vessel wall can respond. Rapid responses are mediated by changes in G protein activity, intracellular calcium concentrations, ion channel activity, adenylate cyclase activity, phosphatyl inosine turnover, and NO production. More delayed responses are characterized by protein kinase C–mediated mitogen-activated protein phosphorylation and subsequent alterations in gene expression for growth factors, proteolytic enzymes, and vasoactive peptides; there are additional changes in both cytoskeletal structure and cell topology in response to external stimuli. One of the principal proteins involved in transduction of mechanical signals to biochemical mediators is considered to be F-actin. The most recent data indicate that the NOS gene has a shear stress regulatory element (SSRE), which allows the cell to respond with an upregulation or a downregulation of NOS activity in response to altered external shear stresses. This finding may explain the phenomenon of flow-dependent vasodilation, which is seen in both the macro- and the microcirculation.

MICROCIRCULATION

In contrast to the macrocirculation, the microcirculation has distinctive vasomotor characteristics. Vessels of the microcirculation are the conduits responsible for the local delivery and transfer of cell substrates and metabolites. The endothelium regulates the microvasculature, reacting to the metabolic needs of tissue; it is essential in organ autoregulation and in the responses of these microvasculatures to changes in local blood flow. Increased tone in the microvascular circulation appears to be mediated by adrenergic stimu-

lation and by a decrease in cyclo-oxygenase production. Decreased cyclo-oxygenase production also results in an increased sensitivity of these vessels to norepinephrine. EDCF is likely to play a significant role in the positive modulation of microvascular tone. To maintain autoregulation, the microvasculature reacts to local concentrations of metabolic by-products and the local level of tissue oxygen. Metabolic by-products (e.g., ADP) can induce local vasodilatation to increase the supply of substrates and increase the removal of the by-products. Furthermore, microvascular vessels are sensitive to changes in oxygen levels within their local environment. Relaxation occurs in the presence of low oxygen tensions, and this response to hypoxia appears to be mediated by the release of prostaglandins. Hypoxia can mediate the release of EDHFs, which hyperpolarize the vascular smooth muscle cells, resulting in relaxation. Conversely, elevated oxygen concentrations can result in the production of leukotrienes, increased microvascular tone, and decreased blood flow. Finally, tissue oxygen tension and intracellular active oxygen species are related, but the role of these active oxygen species in hypoxic responses is presently poorly characterized. Many of the observations on the effect of oxygen free radicals on macrocirculatory vessels may be correlated (with some caution) to the microcirculation. Another feature of the microcirculation is reactive hyperemia. Reactive hyperemia appears to be dependent on the immediate production of endothelium-derived cyclo-oxygenase products—predominantly PGE_2 in the short term. PGI_2 does not appear to be involved in this rapid response. Oxygen free radicals such as superoxide anion, and secondary free radical products such as lipid peroxides, can induce vasodilatation in experimental microvasculature models and may also be involved in this response.

COAGULATION

The endothelium plays a primary role in the regulation of intravascular coagulation by four separate but related mechanisms: participation in and separation of procoagulant pathways, inhibition of procoagulant proteins, regulation of fibrinolysis, and production of thromboregulating compounds (Fig. 50–2). The focal point for the coagulation cascades is the generation of the enzyme thrombin, which cleaves fibrinogen to form insoluble fibrin clot. The endothelium participates in this cascade by producing a number of cofactors, including high-molecular-weight kininogen (HMWK), factor V, factor VIII, and tissue factor. Tissue factor is a procoagulant enzyme synthesized by the endothelium and is found mainly in subendothelium. Basal secretion of tissue factor is low compared with that of the underlying smooth muscle cells and fibroblasts. However, if stimulated or injured, the endothelial cells can increase tissue factor production by 10- to 40-fold. Moreover, there are binding sites for HMWK and factors VIII, IX, IX_a, X, and X_a on the endothelial cells. The presence of factors VIII and X on the endothelial cell surface lowers the affinity of endothelial cells for factor IX, which in turn allows the binding of factor IX_a and the formation of IX_a-VIII complexes on the endothelial surface. Once bound to the endothelium, factor IX_a decay is significantly inhibited in the presence of factors VIII and X, thereby providing an additional feedback mechanism for the perpetuation of cell-bound procoagulant activity.

The basic barrier function of the endothelium separates intravascular coagulation factors (factor VII_a) from tissue factor in the subendothelium and also prevents exposure of platelets to the proaggregating constituents of the subendothelium such as collagen and vWF. Furthermore, endothelial cells produce and express on their extracellular surfaces small amounts of the proteoglycan heparan sulfate, which serves

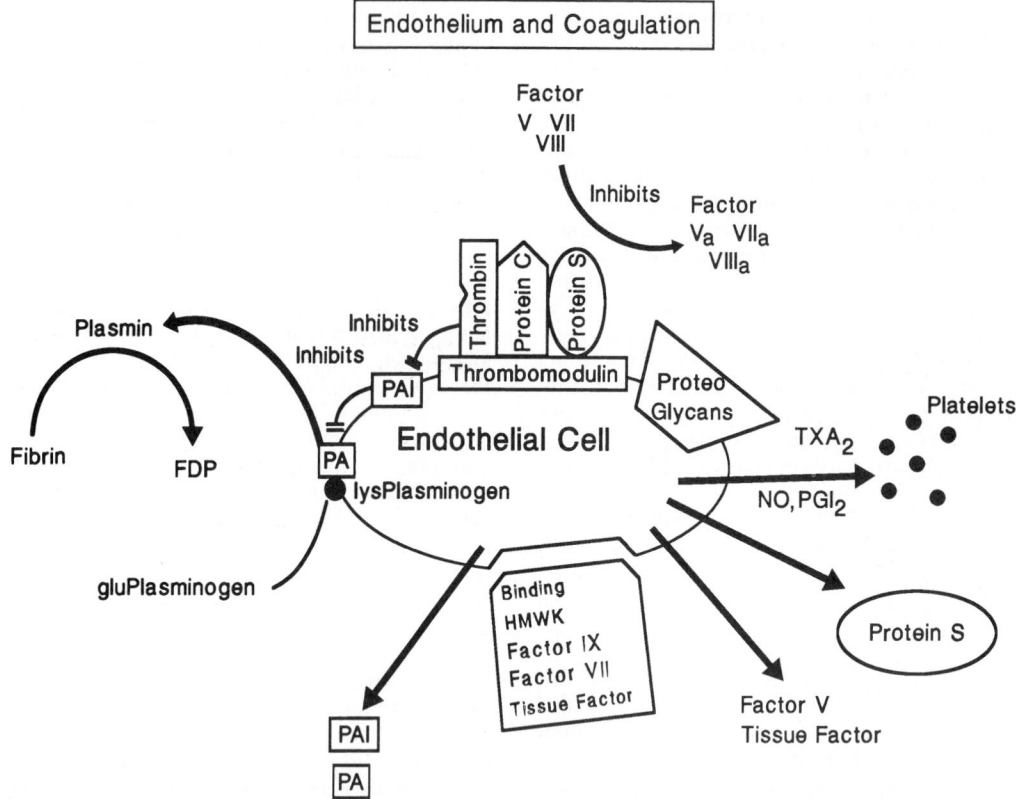

Figure 50–2. Coagulation. The endothelium plays a role in both the procoagulant and anticoagulant pathways. It synthesizes several factors: protein S, factor V, tissue factor, plasminogen activators (PAs), and plasminogen activator inhibitors (PAIs); in addition, the endothelium contributes to the proteoglycan pool, which influences coagulation and regulates platelet activation and adherence by producing prostacyclin (PGI$_2$), nitric oxide (NO), and thromboxane A$_2$ (TXA$_2$). Endothelial cells have binding sites for high-molecular-weight kininogen (HMWK), tissue factor, and factors VII and IV. Several pathways involved in fibrinolysis and anticoagulation reside on the membrane of the endothelial cells (plasminogen activators or inhibitors and the protein C pathway). FDP, fibrin degradation products. (From Davies, M. G., and Hagen, P.-O.: The vascular endothelium—a new horizon. Ann. Surg., *218*:593, 1993.)

to localize and increase the intrinsic activity of antithrombin III and lipoprotein-associated coagulation inhibitor (LACI). Although less than 1% of plasma antithrombin III is bound to the endothelium, this bound pool of antithrombin III is at least 1000-fold more reactive than the unbound pool. LACI is synthesized and released by the endothelium; it complexes with apolipoprotein A-II by a disulfide linkage. This complex is bound to heparan sulfate and other glycosaminoglycans on the endothelial cell surface and acts as a potent inhibitor of factor X_a. Through its interactions with factor X_a, it produces feedback inhibition of the factor VII$_a$–tissue factor complex.

Endothelial cells inhibit procoagulant proteins with the protein C pathway, an autoregulatory pathway that involves protein C, protein S, and thrombomodulin. Protein C is activated by thrombin, and protein C$_a$ inactivates factors V$_a$ and VIII$_a$. Protein C activation by thrombin is enhanced by thrombomodulin, an endothelial cell protein, and the activity of protein C$_a$ is potentiated by a second endothelium-derived peptide, protein S. Protein S promotes protein C$_a$ interaction with factors V$_a$ and VIII$_a$. Thrombomodulin is an integral membrane glycoprotein on the luminal surface of endothelial cells. In addition to its facilitating effects in the protein C pathway, thrombomodulin can effectively remove thrombin from the blood by complexing with thrombin, facilitating its internalization and subsequent degradation. Besides its direct effects on activated coagulant factors, protein C$_a$ also increases endothelial cell fibrinolytic activity by complexing with and decreasing the activity of the plasminogen activator inhibitory protein PAI-1, thereby increasing fibrinolysis. Finally, endothelial cells also secrete protease nexin I, a protease

inhibitor that inactivates thrombin and facilitates its degradation by the endothelium.

The endothelium also participates in the regulation of fibrinolysis. For fibrinolysis to occur, plasminogen must be converted to plasmin. Plasminogen (Glu-plasminogen) binds to endothelial cells and is converted to a form (Lys-plasminogen) that is more efficiently activated. Plasminogen activators, which are serine proteases, and inhibitors of these plasminogen activators are synthesized by the endothelium. Plasminogen-activating enzymes were first reported in 1959, and endothelium-derived inhibitors of these activating enzymes in 1978. Endothelial cells synthesize the plasminogen activators as single-chain proteins, secreting and then binding them to allow their assembly into functional complexes. There are two forms of plasminogen activators (PAs): the urokinase type (uPA), which activates plasminogen in the fluid phase, and tissue PA (tPA), which is most active when bound to fibrin. *In vivo*, normal endothelial cells express tPA only. However, if stimulated by a variety of cytokines and circumstances, endothelial cells preferentially synthesize uPA and downregulate tPA synthesis. In addition to these two fibrinolytic enzymes, endothelial cells secrete two PA inhibitors, PAI-1 and PAI-2. Both are serine protease inhibitors and form equimolar complexes with either active uPA or tPA molecules. PAI-1 requires the presence of vibronectin in the extracellular matrix to maintain its active conformation. It is inactive outside the matrix.

The endothelium is also a source of thromboregulators, which can be defined as physiologic substances that modulate the early phases of thrombus formation. Several groups of molecules have been identified as thromboregulators. First, there are the eicosanoids and, in particular, prostacyclin, which acts as a platelet antiaggregator, and TXA$_2$, which acts as a platelet proaggregator. A balance between these two prostanoids helps control platelet reactivity on the surface of the endothelial cells. The second group is EDRF or NO, which helps prevent platelet adhesion, activation, and recruitment. The third and final family of thromboregulators comprises the endothelial surface ectonucleotidases that metabolize ADP to prevent platelet recruitment and form adenosine, which can elevate platelet cAMP levels and further inhibit platelet reactivity.

INFLAMMATORY AND IMMUNOLOGIC RESPONSES

Due to its strategic position, the endothelium is important in the mediation and modulation of both inflammatory and immunologic responses. The process of cell adherence, cell activation, and cell migration involves an interplay between the expression of adhesion molecules by the endothelial cells, leukocyte activation, and local cytokine activity. The adhesion molecules involved in endothelial cell interactions with leukocytes are composed of three families: the selectins, which govern the interaction of lymphocytes and neutrophils; the immunoglobulins, which include antigen-specific receptors for T- and B-lymphocytes; and the integrins, which are important in platelet adhesion and cell migration. The presence of the cytokines IL-1, TNF-α, and TGF-β or the presence of bacterial endotoxin stimulates endogenous endothelial cell production of IL-1 and IL-6 and induces IL-8

secretion. IL-8 has been shown to regulate transendothelial migration of polymorphonuclear leukocytes through the endothelial barrier. Moreover, the action of IL-8 is enhanced by the fact that IL-8 is secreted preferentially into the vessel wall and is deposited in the subendothelial matrix by the endothelial cells, giving rise to a transmural chemotactic gradient.

In general, when endothelial cells are stimulated by either cytokines or thrombin, they also express endothelial cell leukocyte adhesion molecule-1 (ELAM-1) and intercellular adhesion molecule-1 (ICAM-1). Once activated, endothelial cells also produce an enhancement factor, platelet activating factor (PAF), which modulates the rapid expression of these adhesion molecules. The selectin, ELAM-1, is expressed on endothelial cells within hours and binds both PMNs and monocytes. The expression of ICAM-1, a member of the immunoglobulin family, is increased by interferon-γ, IL-1, and TNF-α. ICAM-1 facilitates the adhesion of both PMNs and lymphocytes. A second molecule in this series, ICAM-2, which is partly homologous to ICAM-1, mediates the binding of T and B cells to endothelial cells. Vascular cell adhesion molecule-1 (VCAM-1) is another inducible endothelial surface immunoglobulin that binds both lymphocytes and monocytes. Generally, endothelial cells express only major histocompatibility complex (MHC) Class I antigens. However, the expression of MHC Class II antigens modulates the interaction of endothelial cells with circulating lymphocytes. Although not constitutively present on the endothelium, MHC-II expression is induced by activated T cells, interferon-γ, and phytohemagglutinin. Once endothelial cells express

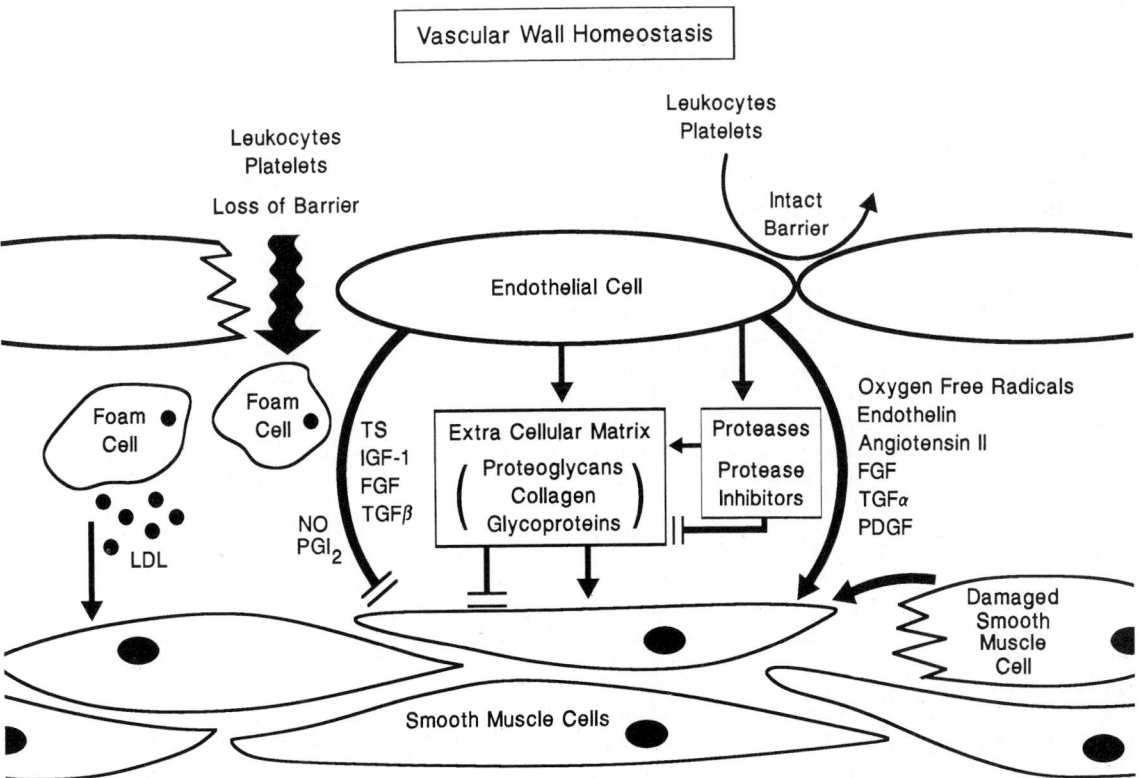

Figure 50–3. Vessel wall modeling. The endothelial cells regulate smooth muscle cell growth by producing both growth-promoting and growth-inhibiting factors. Growth-promoting factors include platelet-derived growth factor (PDGF), fibroblast growth factors (FGFs), transforming growth factor-α (TGF-α), oxygen free radicals, endothelin, and angiotensin II. Growth inhibitors include nitric oxide (NO), prostacyclin (PGI$_2$), FGFs, transforming growth factor-β (TGF-β), insulin growth factor-1, (IGF-1), and thrombospondin (TS). In addition, the composition of the extracellular matrix can either promote or inhibit smooth muscle cell growth. Extracellular matrix composition can be influenced by the mixture of proteases and protease inhibitors secreted by the endothelial cells. Intact endothelial cells form a barrier that helps prevent the accumulation of blood cells, foam cells, and low-density lipoproteins (LDL) in the subendothelium. Damaged activated smooth muscle cells can modulate the growth of their neighbors. (From Davies, M. G., and Hagen, P.-O.: The vascular endothelium—a new horizon. Ann. Surg., *218*:593, 1993.)

the MHC-II antigen, they can be considered to act as antigen-presenting cells and can induce a T-cell response. Finally, stimulated endothelial cells can express GMP-140, a surface receptor that preferentially binds platelets. The binding of platelets increases the local availability of PAF and further accelerates the endothelial cell expression of adhesion molecules.

VASCULAR WALL MODELING (Fig. 50–3)

In addition to the variety of extracellular matrix proteins that are produced by the endothelium, the endothelial cells also produce several regulatory substances that can be either growth promoting or growth inhibiting. Endothelial cells synthesize platelet-derived growth factor (PDGF), basic fibroblast growth factor (bFGF), and insulin-like growth factor 1 (IGF-1). The best characterized growth factor is PDGF, which is composed of the two polypeptide chains A and B. Both homodimers (AA and BB) and a heterodimer (AB) of PDGF can be synthesized by the endothelium. Analysis of the production and possible function of PDGF is complicated not only by the existence of these three isoforms but also by the presence of two forms of cell membrane receptors, alpha and beta. The alpha receptor subunit binds both the A and B PDGF chains, whereas the beta receptor binds only the B chains. It appears that PDGF activity is regulated by both the availability of the ligand and the receptor subunit on the target cell. Additionally, other factors such as thrombospondin and IGF-1 are required to stimulate smooth muscle cell proliferation. Interestingly, PDGF can induce both thrombospondin and IGF-1 expression in endothelial cells. IGF-1 acts as a progression factor for PDGF in smooth muscle cells, and both *in vivo* and *in vitro*, there is synergism between these two growth promoters. IGF-1 appears to act independently on connective tissue cells to increase cell growth, to increase production of hydroxyproline, and to enhance the organization and maturation of collagen fibers. Fibroblast growth factor (FGF) is part of a family of growth factors that bind heparin. The binding of FGF to heparan sulfate proteoglycans protects and stabilizes FGF *in vivo*. To date, there have been nine FGF peptides identified and six receptor subtypes for these growth factors. The precise action of each peptide and the localization of each receptor subtype are currently being defined, but it appears that many are required to regulate cell proliferation. In addition to these factors, other endothelium-derived factors, such as endothelin, angiotensin II, and oxygen free radicals, have been shown to be mitogenic for both endothelial and smooth muscle cells.

The endothelium inhibits cell growth in the wall by the production of the various extracellular matrix substances such as collagen (Type V), several glycoproteins, and the glycosaminoglycans. In addition, both EDRF or NO and prostacyclin inhibit cellular proliferation. Endothelial cells are capable of synthesizing and releasing transforming growth factor-beta (TGF-β) in one of several isoforms. These isoforms of TGF-β stimulate endothelial cell production of proteoglycans, collagen, and fibronectin and regulate the receptors for these proteins. Furthermore, TGF-β can also decrease the secretion of proteases and increase the formation of protease inhibitors by the endothelial cells, which results in the stabilization of the connective tissue matrix and the development of mature histologic features.

SELECTED REFERENCES

Davies, M. G., and Hagen, P.-O.: The vascular endothelium—a new horizon. Ann. Surg., *218*:593, 1993.
A broad overview of the physiologic function of the vascular endothelium.

Davies, M. G., and Hagen, P.-O.: Pathobiology of intimal hyperplasia. Br. J. Surg., *81*:1254, 1994.
This is a comprehensive review of intimal hyperplasia that covers all aspects of the biology of the vascular wall and its response to injury. The fields of physiology, pharmacology, pathology, cell biology, and molecular biology are integrated in this work.

Loscalzo, J., Creagher, M., and Dzau, V. J.: Vascular Medicine, 1st ed. Boston, Little, Brown, 1992.
This text, written by leaders in the field of applied vascular biology, provides a fundamental and comprehensive review of vascular biology, vascular pathology, vascular medicine, and vascular therapeutics.

Moncada, S., Palmer, R. M. J., and Higgs, E. A.: Nitric oxide: Physiology, pathophysiology and pharmacology. Pharmacol. Rev., *43*:109, 1991.
An extensive and well-referenced article that guides the reader through the myriad experimental and clinical data that are now available on nitric oxide.

Rubanyi, G.: Cardiovascular Significance of Endothelial-Derived Vasoactive Factors, 1st ed. Mount Kisco, N.Y., Futura, 1991.
This collection of monographs provides a well-referenced summary of the cardiovascular significance of endothelial cell function in normal vascular homeostasis and disease.

REFERENCES

1. Davies, M. G., and Hagen, P.-O.: The vascular endothelium—a new horizon. Ann. Surg., *218*:593, 1993.
2. Davies, M. G., and Hagen, P.-O.: Pathobiology of intimal hyperplasia. Br. J. Surg., *81*:1254, 1994.
3. Davies, P. F., and Tripathi, S. C.: Mechanical stress mechanisms and the cell: An endothelial paradigm. Circ. Res., *72*:239, 1993.
4. Eisenberg, P. R.: Endothelial cell mediators of thrombosis and fibrinolysis: Review in depth. Coronary Artery Dis., *2*:129, 1991.
5. Gertler, J. P., and Abbott, W. M.: Prothrombotic and fibrinolytic functions of normal and perturbed endothelium. J. Surg. Res., *52*:89, 1992.
6. Luscher, T. F., Rubanyi, G. M., Masaki, T., Vane, J. R., and Vanhoutte, P. M.: Endothelium as a regulator of tone and growth. Circulation, *87*(suppl. V):1, 1993.
7. Moncada, S., Palmer, R. M. J., and Higgs, E. A.: Nitric oxide: Physiology, pathophysiology and pharmacology. Pharmacol. Rev., *43*:109, 1991.
8. Rubanyi, G.: Cardiovascular Significance of Endothelial-Derived Vasoactive Factors, 1st ed. Mount Kisco, N.Y., Futura, 1991.

IV _____

ARTERIAL SUBSTITUTES

Gregory L. Moneta, M.D., and John M. Porter, M.D.

The explosive growth in arterial surgery over the last 45 years has in large part been dependent on the increased use of arterial substitutes. It has been estimated that in the United States alone, over 350,000 synthetic arterial grafts are implanted each year; the number of peripheral autogenous vein grafts exceeds 200,000 per year. This large use of arterial grafts indicates that development of the optimal arterial substitute is of great clinical importance. However, critical review of the present results of arterial grafting leads to the conclusion that the ideal arterial substitute has not yet been developed.

The optimal arterial substitute should (1) be strong, inexpensive, and capable of lasting the life of the patient; (2) be easily and permanently attachable to the host vessel; (3) be biocompatible with the host and have a nonthrombogenic luminal surface; (4) resist infection; (5) be readily available in appropriate sizes; (6) remain patent without subsequent intervention; and (7) have viscoelastic properties similar to those of a normal artery. An ideal vascular graft should not (1) leak blood or serous fluid with restoration of flow; (2) degenerate chemically or physically with time; (3) incite an abnormal proliferative response from the native vessel or the surrounding tissue; (4) promote thrombus formation or be a source of embolic material; (5) occlude when flexed; or (6) damage blood components. No currently available arterial substitute approaches these requirements; hence the large amount of clinical and basic research devoted to the development and evaluation of vascular grafts.

HISTORICAL ASPECTS

In 1906, Carrel and Guthrie first reported successful implantation of venous autografts into the arterial systems of dogs. They observed that these autografts underwent rapid structural change consisting primarily of a marked thickening of the connective tissue in the adventitia and media. They also noted improved patency when the calibers of the vein and the artery to which it was anastomosed were similar. This was soon followed by clinical use of the popliteal vein for arterial reconstruction after popliteal aneurysm excision by Goyanes in 1906. The first use of a saphenous vein graft in popliteal artery reconstruction after popliteal aneurysm excision in the United States was by Bernheim in 1915.

The first successful arterial allograft was reported by Hoepfner in 1903. Carrel performed a series of experimental arterial autografts and allografts several years later, accompanied by detailed microscopic studies. He found that fresh arterial autografts functioned well and remained microscopically normal during several months of observation. Viable, refrigerated allografts and nonviable, preserved allografts developed progressive wall thickening and hyalinization, depending generally on the type of preservative used and the duration of refrigeration. Nonviable grafts killed by heat, formalin, or glycerin showed rapid degeneration, accompanied by significant host fibrous reaction.

The monumental work of Carrel and Guthrie established the feasibility of arterial and venous autografts and allografts early in the twentieth century. Not until almost 50 years later, however, was widespread clinical application of arterial reconstruction feasible. The pioneering work of Murray on the intraoperative use of heparin, the work of Moniz and dos Santos and colleagues in establishing the technique of arteriography, subsequently combined with the concept of arterial substitutes to initiate the modern era of clinical vascular grafting.

EVALUATION OF ARTERIAL SUBSTITUTES

Patency is the most important end-point in the evaluation of the clinical performance of any arterial substitute. It is critical to distinguish between primary and secondary patency and assisted primary patency. Primary patency is that achieved without any additional graft-directed procedures. Secondary patency refers to grafts that have been maintained patent by one or more additional graft-directed procedures, regardless of whether the graft thrombosed prior to revision. If a later operation involves only the inflow or outflow of the graft and not the anastomoses of the graft or the graft itself, the graft may still be regarded as primarily patent. Assisted primary patency, a disputed term in limited use, refers to

secondarily patent grafts that undergo revision prior to actual graft thrombosis.

The concepts of primary, assisted primary, and secondary patency are all important. Primary patency reflects the natural history of individual arterial substitutes. Secondary patency is an indicator of the long-term functional effectiveness of a graft. Assisted primary patency has come to be an indicator of the effectiveness of a clinical follow-up program to detect failing grafts prior to thrombosis. Clearly, however, primary patency is the most important factor in assessing the true overall value of a graft.

Ideally, criteria for patency should be uniformly accepted and clearly stated. It is especially important that life-table analysis be used to display patency. Unfortunately, many reports of arterial substitutes have not employed uniform methods of obtaining and reporting data. Primary and secondary patencies are frequently confused, especially in older publications. However, standards for reports of lower extremity revascularization now exist.[26] Their uniform use will clearly result in more meaningful data in the future, permitting more accurate evaluation of arterial substitutes. In the following sections, the available arterial substitutes, including allografts, xenografts, autografts, and prosthetic grafts, are reviewed.

ALLOGRAFTS

Arterial Allografts

Arterial allografts were the first widely used arterial substitutes. Gross and associates reported the use of viable arterial allografts in patients in 1948. Early results were encouraging, and it was soon recognized that tissue viability was not essential for successful grafting, provided the vessels were properly preserved. This realization, in combination with increasing demand for allografts, led to the establishment of human arterial banks in the late 1940s, freeze-drying being the most popular method of allograft preservation.

Widespread clinical use of arterial allografts in the late 1940s and early 1950s produced a rapid increase in knowledge of the biology and natural history of this type of arterial substitute. Arterial allografts rapidly lose endothelium. A platelet-fibrin coagulum forms on the exposed basement membrane and slowly undergoes fibrous organization. This process begins in anastomotic sites and is frequently incomplete in the central area of the allograft, leaving this area permanently covered with only a fibrin coagulum and prone to ulceration. Allograft walls become less cellular with time. Progressive thinning of the wall, with loss of collagen and fragmentation of elastic fibers, typically occurs after several years. Similar degenerative changes affect both muscular and elastic arterial allografts, but they occur much more rapidly with the former. Thus, allografts of the aorta, composed predominantly of collagen and elastin, have been associated with fewer complications (thrombosis, calcification, aneurysm formation, rupture) and longer graft function than femoral artery allografts, which contain a large component of smooth muscle and elicit a more prominent rejection reaction. However, with the exception of short segment repairs for aortic coarctation, even aortic allografts have disappointing long-term results. They have a high closure rate after only a few years, occasionally accompanied by dilatation and/or rupture.

With the high incidence of complications, arterial allografts have been abandoned in favor of more satisfactory arterial substitutes. Allografts, however, occupy an important place in the history of vascular surgery. The modern era of vascular grafting began with the successful clinical use of arterial allografts by Gross. Oudot and Beaconsfield used an aortic allograft for the first aortic resection and replacement for occlusive disease; DuBost and colleagues used one for the first excision and grafting of an abdominal aortic aneurysm. Studies in animal models suggest that the immunologic rejection process that contributes to the degeneration of these grafts may be modified with low doses of cyclosporine.[27] Such studies raise the intriguing possibility of new applications for these grafts.

Saphenous Vein Allografts

Saphenous vein allografts from human cadavers generally have proved unsatisfactory in clinical practice. Initial encouraging reports were quickly overwhelmed by numerous studies demonstrating a high failure rate in the first postoperative year, as well as late aneurysmal degeneration.[20]

Like arterial allografts, venous allografts are normally antigenic and elicit an immunologic rejection response by the host (Fig. 50–4). Microscopic analysis of failed saphenous vein allografts reveals areas of wall necrosis and intimal disruption.[41] Cryopreservation alone does not alter allograft immunogenicity, and the suggestion by some that cryopreservation may enhance vein allograft function has not been confirmed. However, the ability to preserve veins, coupled with advances in immunosuppression, may eventually lead to the establishment of practical antigen-defined allograft vein banks. Currently, however, saphenous vein allografts have no significant clinical application. The only vascular allograft that has enjoyed widespread use is the umbilical vein allograft.

Umbilical Vein Allografts

Umbilical vein allografts have been used primarily for lower extremity revascularizations and were developed as an alternative to autogenous vein. The grafts are prepared from human umbilical cords and are subjected to glutaraldehyde tanning and multiple ethanol extractions and are externally reinforced with a polyester mesh tube (Fig. 50–5). This conduit has a bursting pressure approaching 1000 mm. Hg and is essentially nonantigenic. The largest clinical experience has

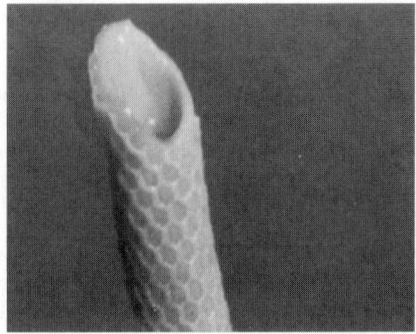

Figure 50–5. An umbilical vein graft. Note the external Dacron mesh.

been accumulated by Dardik and co-workers, who reported primary patency rates of 70% and 50% at 1 and 5 years for femoropopliteal grafts and 50% and 25% at 1 and 5 years for femorotibial grafts.[8] These results are distinctly inferior to patency rates for saphenous vein autografts in the same locations. Randomized prospective evaluation of umbilical vein grafts compared with polytetrafluoroethylene (PTFE) grafts (discussed later) indicates comparable patency rates for both grafts when used as below-knee femoropopliteal bypasses.[10]

Umbilical vein grafts have several disadvantages that have precluded widespread clinical use. The grafts exhibit degenerative changes over time and are prone to the development of aneurysms. They are technically difficult to implant, and the intima is easily damaged by clamps or attempts at thrombectomy. Infection of umbilical vein conduits requires their removal, and reoperative dissections are often difficult. At present, umbilical vein grafts have no well-defined role in the modern practice of vascular surgery, and they are used with decreasing frequency.

XENOGRAFTS

Unmodified arterial xenografts were used clinically in the early 1950s. These grafts elicited a prominent host immunologic reaction, leading to severe damage to the graft wall. Their use was associated with a high incidence of thrombosis and rupture, and it soon became obvious that unmodified arterial xenografts were not suitable for clinical use.

Rosenberg and associates produced modified xenografts by treating bovine carotid arteries with the proteolytic enzyme ficin, followed by tanning with dialdehyde starch. The result was an almost nonantigenic, collagenous tube that was devoid of smooth muscle and elastic tissue but possessing the same tensile strength as a normal artery. Modified xenografts were used frequently as arterial substitutes from the mid-1960s to mid-1970s but did not produce satisfactory clinical results, particularly in infrainguinal reconstructions. When used in the femoropopliteal position, these grafts were plagued by perioperative thrombosis and exhibited poor long-term patency rates of about 40% 3 to 6 years following implantation. In addition, aneurysms occurred in 3% to 6% of grafts, usually several years after placement. These figures represent aneurysm formation in all implanted grafts. The incidence of aneurysm formation in grafts that remained patent was undoubtedly considerably higher. Moreover, clinical use of these grafts was associated with an unacceptable infection rate of 3% to 7%, several times that associated with other arterial substitutes. Nevertheless, bovine xenografts have proved to function satisfactorily as hemodialysis access shunts and remain the preferred conduit for this purpose in some centers. They currently have no other well-defined role.

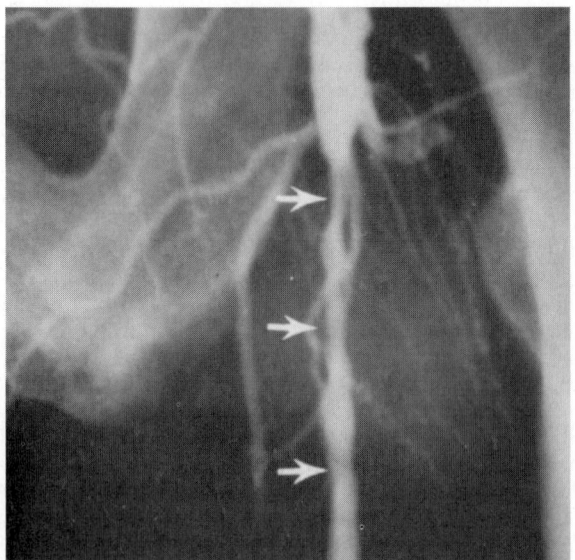

Figure 50–4. Angiogram of a femoropopliteal venous allograft in a patient 1 year after implantation. Diffuse stenosis of the proximal portion of the allograft is present (arrows). The graft subsequently thrombosed. Pathologic examination revealed diffuse fibrous thickening of all layers of the graft wall, accompanied by a striking mononuclear and giant cell infiltration.

AUTOGRAFTS

Arterial Autografts

The clinical use of arterial autografts was introduced by Wylie in 1965. Proponents of autografts cite their numerous advantages, including retention of viability associated with the maintenance of an intact intrinsic blood supply during grafting, absence of aneurysmal degeneration, resistance to infection, preservation of normal flexibility at points of joint motion, and possession of growth potential when used in pediatric patients. The obvious disadvantage is a lack of availability, including inadequate length of arteries for most potential applications.

The innermost 300 to 500 μ. of the arterial wall is nourished by luminal diffusion.[3] The outer layers of the arterial wall are nourished by a complex vasa vasorum system derived primarily from the most proximal portions of arterial side branches. If the proximal portions of side branches are excised or damaged during preparation of the autograft, spotty arterial wall necrosis may develop in that portion of the arterial wall more than 500 to 600 μ. from the lumen (Figs. 50–6 and 50–7).

The clinical use of arterial autografts is restricted primarily to coronary artery bypass grafting, renal artery bypass in children, and arterial substitutes in infected surgical fields. Radial arteries have been used as free grafts in coronary bypass surgery, but their use has been largely unsuccessful due to early graft closure associated with florid intimal proliferation. Currently, however, the internal mammary artery is frequently used as a conduit in coronary bypass surgery and provides patency rates that are clearly superior to those of saphenous vein grafts.

There is general agreement that children requiring renal artery reconstruction should have arterial autografts. The internal iliac artery has proved to be a suitable conduit, and its use obviates the high incidence of late aneurysmal graft dilatation in this age group when saphenous vein grafts are

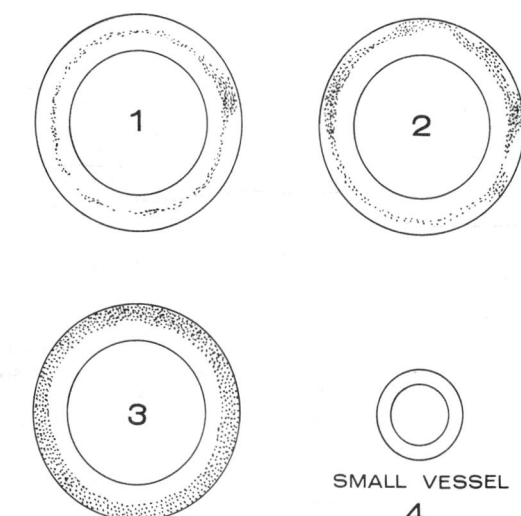

Figure 50–7. Diagrammatic summary of luminal diffusion and vasa vasorum zones of influence as observed in canine experiments. Necrosis is indicated by stippled areas. 1, Results from minor trauma exemplified by aortic-aortic anastomoses, namely, freeing of the vessel ends necessary for sewing them together. This is judged to be an example of overlap zone damage. 2, Irregular necrosis of outer wall following removal of thoracic aortic segment with only intercostals ligated. 3, Necrosis of the outer wall following removal of aortic segment, plus excision of intercostal ostia. In all three instances, the viable luminal diffusion zone remains at about the same order of thickness. 4, Full wall viability of a small transected and reanastomosed vessel, the wall thickness of which falls within the diffusion zone distance. (From Berger, K., Sauvage, L. R., Wood, S. J., and Sameh, A. A.: Endarterectomy and other surgical injuries to vascular walls. Pacific Med. Surg., 75:367, 1967.)

used. Iliac artery autografts have also proved to be remarkably effective in a limited number of adult patients undergoing renal vascular surgery. In a primarily adult population, Stoney and associates reported only two arterial autograft occlusions in 86 patients undergoing renal vascular surgery, with follow-up extending 16 years.[34] Use of the internal iliac artery is, however, limited in the adult population by its frequent involvement with advanced atherosclerosis. The external iliac artery may also be used as an arterial autograft, but it generally requires prosthetic replacement of the autograft donor site.

Arterial autografts are occasionally used to bridge short arterial defects in infected or contaminated surgical fields that preclude the use of synthetic grafts. Atherosclerotic arteries may be endarterectomized and used as either bypass conduits or, more frequently, patch grafts. These technical adjuncts are employed primarily in the management of traumatic wounds or infected prosthetic grafts. Unfortunately, the use of endarterectomized arteries as autografts has been associated with a disturbing incidence of fibrointimal hyperplasia leading to graft failure.

Venous Autografts

The routine clinical use of venous autografts began with the clinical report by Kunlin in 1949. Since that time, venous autografts have proved to be the most successful and clearly the most clinically important small-caliber arterial substitutes. They are the preferred graft for infrainguinal arterial reconstruction. The greater saphenous vein, lesser saphenous vein, cephalic and brachial veins, and superficial femoral and internal jugular veins have all been used as bypass conduits.

Greater Saphenous Vein. Greater saphenous vein autografts are by far the most widely used autogenous vascular graft in modern vascular surgery and are currently the standard with which all other small-caliber arterial substitutes

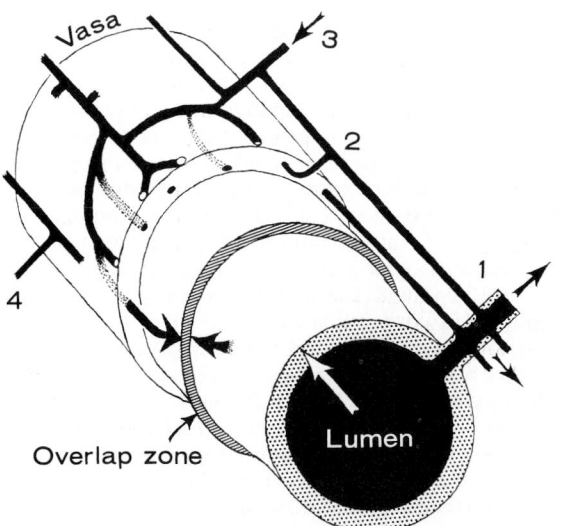

Figure 50–6. Diagrammatic conception of nutrition to the thoracic aortic wall. Luminal diffusion serves the inner portion of the wall. Vasa vasorum serve the outer portion. A narrower zone, the overlap zone, is served by both mechanisms. At 1, an intercostal artery emerges. This in turn gives off branches that travel in the outer medial layer of the wall, as well as along the adventitia. At 2, branches from the adventitial system traverse into the outer media. At 3, connections may occur at adventitial vessels other than those derived from intercostals. At 4, an adventitial vessel derived from the "nonintercostal" system. (From Berger, K., Sauvage, L. R., Wood, S. J., and Sameh, A. A.: Endarterectomy and other surgical injuries to vascular walls. Pacific Med. Surg., 75:367, 1967.)

are compared. Over 200,000 peripheral vascular operations are performed in the United States annually.

The normal greater saphenous vein averages 70 to 80 cm. in adult men. It begins at the medial malleolus at the junction of the medial marginal and internal malleolar veins. This vein is quite superficial in the leg but lies close to the deep fascia in the thigh. It is a single vessel in the thigh in 75% of patients; contains 8 to 12 bicuspid valves, mainly below the knee; and averages 5.5 mm. in diameter. The luminal surface consists of a monolayer of endothelial cells. The media is composed of an inner layer of longitudinally arranged smooth muscle cells and an outer layer of circumferentially oriented smooth muscle cells. The outer adventitial layer is composed of a loose mixture of collagen and elastic tissue.

The saphenous vein has been used as a replacement for small and medium-sized arteries in all parts of the body, with most being used for coronary artery bypass grafts and for lower extremity bypass of occluded superficial femoral, popliteal, and tibial arteries. Other less frequent uses include upper extremity bypass, as well as mesenteric and renal artery bypass. The coronary, mesenteric, and renal results are described in other sections and are generally excellent.

Lower extremity bypasses using autogenous saphenous vein may be performed using one of two basic techniques. An appropriate length of vein may be removed from either the ipsilateral or the contralateral lower extremity; it is then reversed in direction to permit arterial flow in the direction of the venous valves and sutured in place, usually in an end-to-side configuration. Alternatively, an intact ipsilateral vein of adequate quality may largely be left in its anatomic position and the valves destroyed using one of a variety of intraluminal devices, followed by similar proximal and distal arterial anastomoses. This technique has been termed *in situ* saphenous vein bypass. Both techniques are currently widely employed and generally produce similar results.

The primary patency of reversed femoropopliteal saphenous vein autografts ranges from 80% to 90% at 1 year, 55% to 86% at 5 years, and 38% to 46% at 10 years (Fig. 50–8).[38] Reversed saphenous vein grafting to tibial arteries produces

patency rates that are about 10% to 15% lower than those for femoropopliteal grafting at all time intervals.[38] Exhaustive analyses of variables affecting femoropopliteal patency indicate that patency is higher when bypass surgery is performed for claudication rather than limb salvage, and it is generally higher with a widely patent popliteal and tibial artery outflow tract. A patent outflow tract, however, is not an absolute requirement for long-term patency. Mannick and co-workers reported an intermediate-term patency rate of 65% when bypassing to an isolated popliteal segment without demonstrated angiographic patency of the popliteal artery trifurcation vessels.[19] A patient's continued cigarette smoking and the use of a small vein (less than 4 mm. after gentle distention) both decrease long-term patency. Curiously, vein graft patency appears to be slightly higher in diabetic patients.[38] The role of antiplatelet drugs in enhancing vein graft patency is unproven, although considerable anecdotal evidence supports their use.

Large series of *in situ* vein bypass initially suggested that the technique resulted in superior patency rates compared with the reversed vein technique.[18] Modern series of reversed vein bypasses, however, have demonstrated similar or superior patency rates to *in situ* bypasses in grafts to the popliteal and tibial arteries.[38] Clearly, reversed vein grafting is applicable to larger numbers of patients, because many patients do not have an intact ipsilateral saphenous vein, which is mandatory for an *in situ* bypass.

Alternative Venous Autografts. Venous conduits other than the greater saphenous vein are now recognized as being suitable for lower extremity bypass. As many as 20% to 30% of patients in need of leg bypass do not possess greater saphenous veins adequate for arterial grafting.[37] The vein is anatomically too small in 5% to 10% of patients and is unavailable or unusable in another 10% to 20% of patients because of prior removal, previous thrombosis, or varicosities. In such patients, alternative veins have been used for arterial grafting, including the lesser saphenous, basilic, cephalic, and superficial femoral. Various venous segments may be joined with venovenostomies to achieve an autogenous conduit of adequate length.[37]

Although the long-term effectiveness of these alternative conduits has been questioned, recent data suggest that they can serve as acceptable arterial substitutes. Harris and his associates reported 3-year patency rates of 82% and 65% using cephalic vein bypasses to the below-knee popliteal and tibial arteries, respectively.[14] The superficial femoral vein has been used as a femoropopliteal bypass conduit with a primary patency rate of 82% at 3 years.[28] Some report surprisingly little postoperative morbidity with the use of superficial femoral veins as bypass grafts, but most surgeons are reluctant to use them as a first-choice autogenous arterial substitute because of concerns about postoperative edema. Other investigators have also found alternative vein sources to be satisfactory arterial substitutes in the lower extremity.[37]

Pathology of Venous Autografts. Early postoperative vein graft failure can usually be attributed to technical flaws in the performance of the operation or the presence of an unrecognized hypercoagulable state. Late failures may follow progression of atherosclerotic disease above or below the vein graft. It is quite clear, however, that the vein graft itself is subject to a number of pathologic alterations that may contribute to occlusion of the bypass.

Carrel first noted that veins implanted into the arterial system that remain patent inevitably undergo significant thickening. This process, which has been erroneously termed "arterialization" of vein grafts, produces medial and subintimal fibrous hyperplasia, often in combination with fibrin deposition on the intimal surface.[31] The result is a variable thickening of the vein wall that may be minimal and remark-

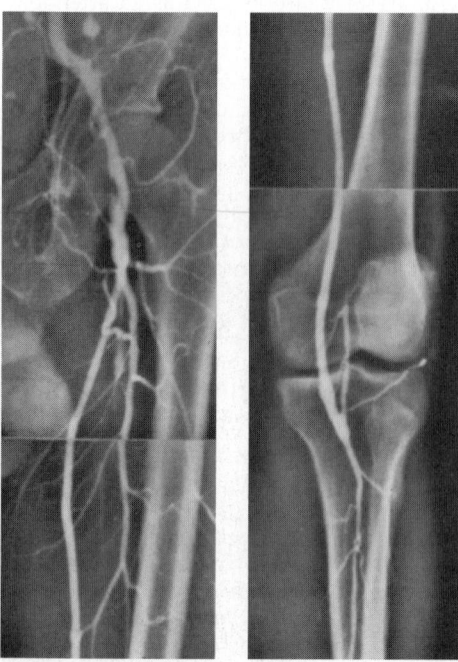

Figure 50–8. Angiogram of a well-functioning femoropopliteal venous autograft 2 years after implantation. Normal slight graft dilation at the site of the venous valves is still present.

ably localized or may involve the entire vein graft, with resultant diffuse obliteration of the lumen.

Szilagyi and colleagues, in a landmark review of the clinical outcome of peripheral arterial saphenous vein grafts, found that marked fibrointimal hyperplasia occurred in 8% of such grafts.[35] Interestingly, this process has been implicated as the cause of failure in 15% to 30% of aortocoronary grafts occluding during the first year[32] and is the probable cause of at least two thirds of all infrainguinal vein bypass graft failures. An intense search continues for the cause of fibrointimal hyperplasia and ways to prevent it.

Fibrointimal hyperplasia follows the conversion of normally quiescent myointimal and medial smooth muscle cells into actively proliferating secretory myofibroblasts. A number of factors appear to be important in stimulating this proliferative process. The predominant current theory regards fibrointimal hyperplasia as a response to vein injury occurring during and following grafting. Without doubt, veins are mechanically injured during removal and storage preparatory to arterial grafting. In addition, the vein wall is rendered ischemic during its dissection because of disruption of the vasa vasorum. Electron micrographs after vein harvest frequently show large areas of endothelial denudation and medial injury. Although there is agreement on the importance of gentle vein harvest techniques and the avoidance of excessive hydrostatic venous distention, there is little agreement on the optimal medium in which to store veins for reversed bypasses between harvest and arterial grafting. Some have found minimal endothelial disruption with storage in chilled autogenous blood. Others have recommended placing the vein in tissue culture medium at 37° C. with papaverine. Many surgeons simply leave the vein in a heparinized saline solution for the short time between vein excision and implantation.

In addition to the vein harvest itself, other mechanical factors may be important in inciting fibrointimal hyperplasia. These include increases in shear forces and venous wall stress induced by arterial pressure and compliance mismatch at anastomotic sites. The potential importance of the latter is suggested by the observation that failed saphenous vein grafts frequently have prominent fibrointimal hyperplasia at the proximal or distal anastomosis. Recent animal studies, however, suggest that although compliance mismatch may contribute to graft thrombosis, there does not appear to be any significant difference in anastomotic fibrointimal hyperplasia in compliant versus noncompliant grafts.[22]

Endothelial damage appears to be the final common pathway in the production of fibrointimal hyperplasia. Whereas in the past the endothelium was regarded as merely an inert nonthrombogenic surface lining, it is now clear that these cells are very active biochemical factories capable of responding to injury and producing a variety of substances involved in the regulation of vascular wall function.

Platelets, endothelium, smooth muscle cells, and macrophages can all produce similar growth factor proteins that can induce smooth muscle cell proliferation. Endothelial cells also produce growth-inhibiting factors (heparan sulfate), which suggests that endothelial cells may be able to modulate various mitogens capable of producing fibrointimal hyperplasia. The mechanisms by which alterations in cellular interactions and growth factor production combine to produce fibrointimal hyperplasia leading to a failing or failed vascular graft are currently the focus of intense investigation and have important clinical implications.

A number of other pathologic changes have been noted in vein grafts. Clamp trauma may produce localized stenosis associated with transmural fibrosis. This has been reported in 4% of lower extremity vein grafts.[35] About 9% of vein grafts develop localized stenosis following fibrosis of the

venous valves or suture narrowing caused by improper suture ligation of venous side branches. Significant vein graft atherosclerosis occurs after variable periods in approximately 7% of aortocoronary grafts and 15% of lower extremity grafts, causing localized stenosis in about 7% of the latter.[36] Atherosclerotic venous aneurysms develop in 3% to 8% of lower extremity vein grafts.[36] The incidence of nonatherosclerotic vein graft dilation or aneurysm formation varies significantly with the location of the graft and the age of the patient. Stanley and colleagues noted that although one third of aortorenal vein grafts become ectatic, actual aneurysmal degeneration occurs in only 1.5% of adults. In children, however, the incidence of aneurysmal degeneration with similar grafts is 20%, a finding that has led to the current preference for arterial autografts in children requiring renal artery reconstruction.[33]

About one third of vein grafts eventually develop recognizable structural defects.[36] The majority of these defects are stenotic lesions and develop within 1 year of graft implantation. If not corrected, many lead to failure of the graft. In the past, this has led some surgeons to recommend routine postoperative angiography at 1- to 2-year intervals.[36] Currently, however, it appears that noninvasive determination of blood flow velocity within the graft by means of duplex ultrasonography is quite accurate in predicting subsequent graft thrombosis. Patients with graft flow velocities in the midportion of the graft below 45 cm. per second or localized high peak systolic velocities (greater than 200 cm. per second) within the graft or at its proximal or distal anastomoses should undergo angiography to locate a potentially correctable lesion (Fig. 50–9).[1]

PROSTHETIC GRAFTS

Textile Grafts

The development of prosthetic arterial grafts was stimulated by the observation by Voorhees in the early 1950s that silk threads in the canine vascular system became covered by a glistening endothelium-like cellular coating. The hypothesis was then proposed that a fine mesh fabric would result in similar healing and thus function as a satisfactory arterial substitute. Voorhees and associates subsequently described successful replacement of arteries in animals with a porous

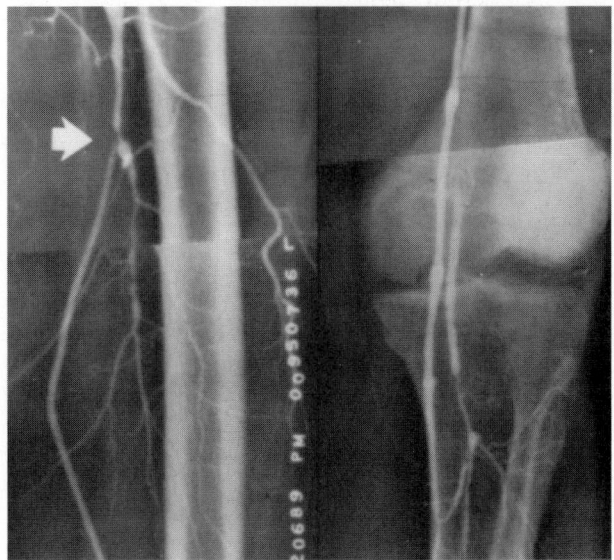

Figure 50–9. This high-grade stenosis (arrow) of a venous autograft was suggested by a duplex-determined low graft flow velocity.

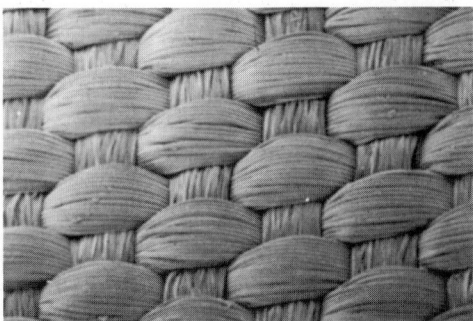

Figure 50–10. Close-up photograph (×50) of a woven Dacron prosthetic vascular graft. This graft is relatively impervious to blood because of the tightness of the weave.

textile graft made from the nylon derivative Vinyon-N. Two years later, the same graft was successfully implanted in humans. The field of prosthetic vascular grafts has since achieved enormous clinical and laboratory importance.

Composition and Fabrication. Both the material and its method of fabrication are important in the manufacturing of prosthetic arterial substitutes. Materials such as nylon, Orlon, Ivalon, and Marlex have all proved disappointing, primarily because of loss of tensile strength and kinking. The only textile materials thus far that have proved to function satisfactorily are Dacron and Teflon, neither of which loses significant tensile strength even after many years of implantation.

Dacron and Teflon grafts are manufactured by weaving or knitting multifilament texturized yarns (Figs. 50–10 and 50–11). Each process has advantages and disadvantages. Woven grafts must be tightly interlaced to prevent slippage and fraying of the yarn. This compact structure of the graft produces small interstices and low porosity. These grafts leak minimally at the time of implantation but are somewhat stiff and difficult to handle. In addition, the tight configuration of the graft theoretically reduces the potential for the development of a living neointima by connective tissue ingrowth through the graft interstices (see the following).

Knitted grafts are softer and more compliant than woven grafts, and the knit can be varied. The looser the knit, the more elastic and porous the graft. They have been widely used in vascular surgical operations below the diaphragm because of their excellent handling characteristics, including softness and lack of fraying at cut ends.

Knitted grafts are quite porous, between 1200 and 1900 ml. per cm. per minute, and must be preclotted prior to implantation. (Porosity for graft applications is defined as the amount of water that will pass through 1 sq. cm. of graft

wall per minute under a hydrostatic driving pressure of 120 mm. Hg.) A sample of the patient's own blood is forced repeatedly through the graft interstices. This causes platelet-fibrin deposition in the interstices, which renders the graft temporarily impervious to blood. After implantation, this platelet-fibrin material is slowly replaced by fibrous ingrowth from the host. Porous grafts must be used with great caution in patients with platelet or coagulation defects. Under these circumstances, the necessary initial coagulum may never properly form, and the patient may bleed excessively thought the graft interstices. A tightly woven graft is preferred in this setting. Woven grafts are also generally preferred in repairs of the thoracic aorta to limit hemorrhage through the graft interstices, especially in operations requiring full heparinization and cardiopulmonary bypass.

Innovative manufacturing modifications have been superimposed on the basic concepts of knitted and woven textile grafts. Velour surfaces can be added to the inside, outside, or both sides of knitted or woven grafts. Velour surfaces have loops of yarn extending almost perpendicular to the fabric surface (Fig. 50–12). Various porosities and thicknesses are possible. Velour surfaces improve the handling characteristics of woven grafts and provide a scaffold for fibroblast ingrowth, leading to firm graft adherence to surrounding tissue. The velour concept is widely accepted, and a large percentage of textile vascular grafts in current use have a velour surface.

Most textile grafts in clinical use are also crimped to impart greater flexibility without kinking. Although widely employed, this process has several potential disadvantages. Crimping diminishes luminal diameter, increases the thickness of the graft material, and may also cause deposition of thrombogenic fibrin in the crimped areas.[17] It is possible to manufacture externally supported grafts that avoid kinking with angulation and yield results equal or superior to those obtained with crimped grafts. These grafts have an incompressible large fiber wound around and adherent to the external surface.

Clinical Applications of Textile Grafts. The knitted Dacron graft has been the most frequently used prosthetic arterial graft during the past 30 years. Woven Dacron grafts have traditionally been used primarily in those settings in which interstitial bleeding would present major problems, but the addition of velour surfaces has prompted widespread application of woven grafts. Textile-fabricated Teflon grafts are presently used infrequently, but they generally appear to function satisfactorily, especially in large artery applications.

Textile grafts function most satisfactorily when used for arterial replacement proximal to the inguinal ligament (Figs. 50–13 and 50–14). Five- and 10-year patencies have been reported as high as 91% and 66%, respectively, for aortofem-

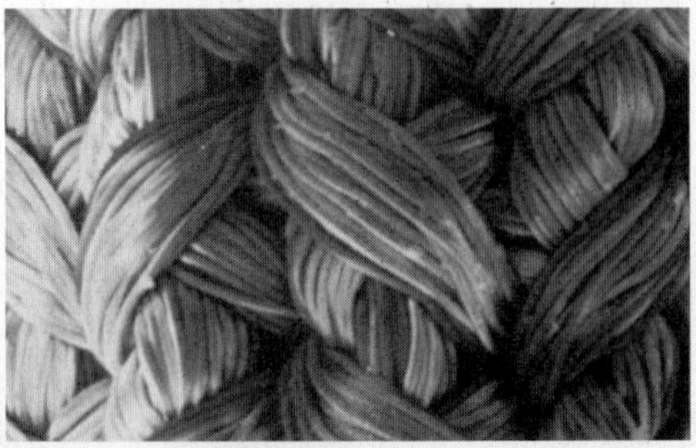

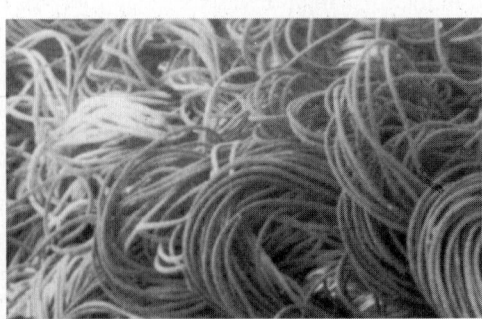

Figure 50–11. Close-up photograph (×50) of a knitted Dacron prosthetic vascular graft. The large openings between the knitted yarns make this graft relatively permeable to blood, and the graft must be preclotted before use in order to fill the interstices with fibrin.

Figure 50–12. Photograph (×50) of the external surface of a woven double velour Dacron graft. The striking difference in the surface texture compared with that of a standard knitted or woven Dacron prosthesis (Figs. 50–10 and 50–11) is obvious. The velour configuration promotes rapid fibrous anchoring of the graft to surrounding tissues.

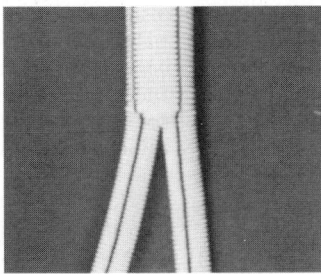

Figure 50–13. Photograph of a standard knitted Dacron bifurcation graft. The crimp pattern is clearly seen. The stripes aid the surgeon in proper graft positioning and diminish the likelihood of unrecognized axial rotation of the graft limb when placed in the aortofemoral position.

oral bypass.[5, 24] Axillofemoral bypass patency has been in the range of 75% to 77% at 5 years, and femorofemoral bypass patency at 5 years has similarly been 75% to 80%.[4, 13, 16] Textile grafts usually produce patency results distinctly inferior to those of saphenous vein bypass below the inguinal ligament. In the most favorable report, externally supported Dacron bypass to the above-knee popliteal artery produced a 5-year

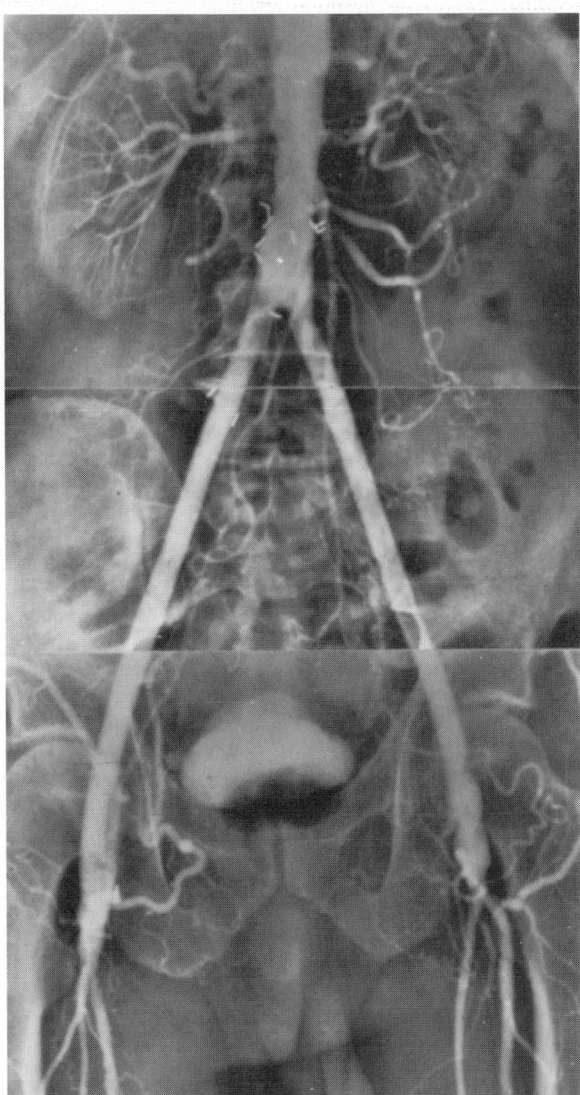

Figure 50–14. Angiogram of an aortofemoral knitted bifurcation Dacron graft. The graft extends from the infrarenal aorta to the common femoral arteries.

patency of 70%.[11] Textile grafts produce low patency results when used to bypass to arteries distal to the popliteal artery; therefore, their clinical use in this setting is not recommended.

Polytetrafluoroethylene (PTFE) Grafts

PTFE is a fluorocarbon polymer formed into sheets by a unique paste extrusion process. Extruded PTFE is not a textile but rather a semi-inert polymer consisting of solid nodes of PTFE with interconnecting small fibrils. The intranodal distance can be varied in the manufacturing process and is about 40 μ. for grafts in clinical use (Fig. 50–15). Although greater intranodal distances permit greater tissue ingrowth and, therefore, theoretically greater graft healing and increased patency, this has not proved to be the case in human trials.

PTFE grafts have a highly electronegative surface charge and are thus hydrophobic and resistant to thrombosis. The grafts are coated with an outer wrap of PTFE to avoid aneurysm formation, which occurred frequently with early clinical use of unwrapped grafts. PTFE grafts are available with external ring supports to avoid compression in subcutaneous locations and kinking with angulation. Wall thickness may be varied, with thin-walled grafts preferred for infrainguinal bypasses. Thick-walled grafts function well as hemodialysis shunts and, in most centers, have replaced bovine grafts as the preferred material for hemodialysis access when creation of a native fistula is not possible.

Clinical Applications of PTFE Grafts. PTFE grafts are available in a wide variety of sizes and configurations suitable for almost any arterial reconstructive procedure. They have been used most widely for construction of extra-anatomic bypasses and as a substitute for autogenous vein in infrainguinal bypasses.

Externally supported PTFE axillofemoral grafts provide 5-year patency rates of about 70%.[13] PTFE grafts in the axillofemoral position have been associated with occasional early postoperative disruption of the axillary artery anastomosis.[39] In some cases, the sutures have pulled through the graft. It is postulated that because PTFE grafts are formed from a continuous extruded polymer, penetration of PTFE grafts by

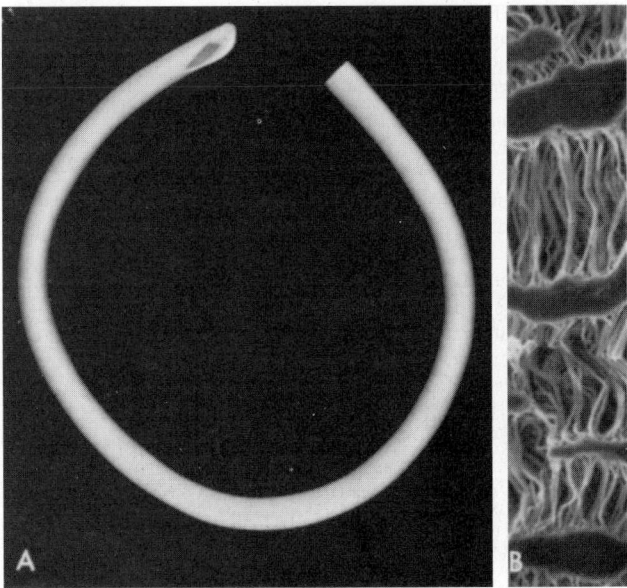

Figure 50–15. *A,* Photograph of a PTFE graft. *B,* Photomicrograph (×1000) of a PTFE graft. The dark areas are PTFE nodes interconnected by many PTFE fibrils. Average internodal distance in grafts in clinical use is now 40 μ.

needles may cause alteration of the polymeric structure and subsequent graft disruption when the anastomosis is stressed by shoulder elevation or arm abduction.[39] Positional operative modifications of the PTFE graft–axillary artery anastomosis have greatly reduced the incidence of this complication.

For infrainguinal bypass, initial reports of patency rates similar to those of saphenous vein grafts have been modified by larger series with more extended follow-up.[21] Cumulative patency of PTFE grafts used in the above-knee femoropopliteal position is about 75% at 1 year and 55% at 5 years. These results, at least in the short term, are sufficiently similar to those reported in certain series of saphenous vein grafts to prompt some to conclude that PTFE grafts should serve as the initial conduit for above-knee femoropopliteal bypass, especially in patients with limited life expectancy. PTFE grafts have performed poorly, however, in comparison with saphenous vein when used as bypass conduits to the below-knee popliteal and tibial arteries or in situations in which there is poor distal runoff. Although some have reported 50% to 60% intermediate patency of PTFE grafts performed for limb salvage, others have concluded that when such grafts must be anastomosed to tibial arteries, the results are so poor that primary amputation should be strongly considered.[9] Despite these considerations, PTFE grafts are widely employed as the prosthetic arterial substitute of choice for infrainguinal bypass when autogenous vein is not available. Patency of PTFE grafts may be extended through the use of routine warfarin anticoagulation. Although PTFE grafts are easily thrombectomized, it now appears that thrombosis of established infrainguinal PTFE grafts is best treated by placement of a new conduit.

Prosthetic Graft Healing

Shortly after prosthetic graft implantation, a thin layer of fibrin is deposited on the luminal surface. In grafts with high flow, the thickness stabilizes at about 1 mm. and is well tolerated. In a low-flow environment, however, the fibrin layer frequently continues to increase in thickness, proceeding to luminal occlusion.

In the experimental animal, the fibrin layer is progressively organized, resulting in the development of a lining consisting of fibroblasts, myofibroblasts, and fibrocollagenous connective tissue. The graft lining then becomes connected to the perigraft tissue by ingrowth through the interstices of the fabric. Prosthetic graft healing refers to the development of a living neointima inside the graft, connected to an external fibrous capsule around the graft by means of connective tissue ingrowth through graft interstices. *Well-healed* grafts offer the possibility of decreased thrombogenicity and increased resistance to infection.

The extent of graft healing is related to both the host species and the graft itself. With respect to the graft, the quality of healing reflects both the porosity of the graft and the thickness of the graft wall. Healing via tissue ingrowth is favored by increased porosity and decreased wall thickness. Healing may also occur at the graft margins via endothelial ingrowth from the host vessels. Healing by this mechanism is limited to the few centimeters adjacent to the anastomosis. Circulating blood cells, probably stem cells, also appear to aid in the healing of both Dacron and PTFE grafts.[29]

Complete graft healing routinely occurs in animal models when thin, porous grafts are used. However, such grafts, when implanted in patients, never develop a complete living neointima. An important clinical study by Berger and associates in 1972 first clearly demonstrated that prosthetic grafts in humans do not develop a living neointimal lining but rather maintain a permanent lining composed primarily of compacted fibrin.[2] These investigators later described detailed studies of prosthetic grafts removed from 64 patients months to years after implantation. The results showed that humans have a limited ability to organize fibrin deposits on the luminal surface of grafts, in sharp contrast to experimental animals. A small zone of luminal healing occurs adjacent to suture lines, but otherwise the graft is typically lined with compacted fibrin even years after implantation. Only two of the 64 grafts showed significant luminal healing, and even then endothelial cells could not be identified. Although this work involved primarily fabric grafts, others suggest a similar situation with PTFE grafts.[7]

The concept of limited graft healing in humans is supported by platelet survival and localization studies. Several investigators have correlated platelet survival and platelet-graft deposition with healing of the graft lumen. In the totally healed grafts of animals, both platelet survival and platelet-graft deposition return to normal. Harker and colleagues have shown that humans with aortic prostheses have shortened platelet survival for 9 months after graft implantation but have increased platelet deposition on the graft for at least 120 months.[12] Thus, all evidence clearly indicates that a large majority of prosthetic arterial grafts in man, unlike in experimental animals, never develop an organized internal lining and remain permanently lined with compacted fibrin. The relevance to man of animal-derived optimal graft design characteristics must be regarded as minimal.

Complications of Prosthetic Grafting

The most frequently observed prosthetic graft complications include anastomotic neointimal hyperplasia, graft infection, graft failure caused by fiber disruption or stretching, perigraft seromas, and development of anastomotic false aneurysms.

Neointimal Hyperplasia. This process is similar to that described for saphenous vein grafts and is present at both proximal and distal anastomoses. Clinically, the distal anastomotic process appears to be more significant and is frequently implicated as a cause of prosthetic graft failure. Both textile and PTFE grafts are affected. The aforementioned etiologic factors for neointimal hyperplasia associated with saphenous vein grafts also apply to prosthetic grafts. As with saphenous vein grafts, antiplatelet drugs are frequently prescribed for patients with prosthetic grafts in an effort to reduce the magnitude of anastomotic fibroplasia. Use of antiplatelet drugs, specifically aspirin, is clearly indicated in patients with peripheral vascular disease. These agents have been shown to decrease significantly the overall cardiovascular-associated morbidity and mortality.

Graft Infection. Infection is one of the most feared complications of prosthetic grafting. *Staphylococcus aureus*, *Staphylococcus epidermidis*, and *Escherichia coli* are the most frequently isolated organisms. The incidence is about 1.5% to 2.5%; it is slightly lower when the graft is completely intra-abdominal and higher when a groin anastomosis is present. Aortic graft infections may be associated with an operative mortality of 10% to 25% and an amputation rate of 15% to 20%.[43] Even infrainguinal graft infections are associated with high mortality and amputation rates. Graft infection may be decreased by careful patient selection, meticulous preparation of sites for surgical incision, and preoperative use of prophylactic antibiotics, usually a cephalosporin. Temporary bonding of antibiotics to prosthetic grafts is possible and is under evaluation in animal models.[30]

In a large majority of cases, an infected arterial graft must be removed to control infection. Anecdotal reports of successful treatment of graft infection by local drainage and antibiotic irrigation without graft removal are the exception. The basic principle of infected graft treatment remains graft excision and revascularization through a clean field, usually in an extra-anatomic configuration. It appears that both mortality and amputation rates can be improved if the revascularization is performed first, followed by removal of the infected prosthetic graft. Staging the operation in this manner lessens the complications of prolonged distal ischemia. On occasion, revascularization through the contaminated field may be successful if entirely autogenous tissue is used.

Graft Failure. Two distinct types of Dacron graft failure have been described. The first consists of gradual, diffuse graft dilatation, observed frequently with the ultralightweight knitted Dacron in widespread use in the early 1970s. The dilatation was caused by expansion of the knit rather than elongation or weakening of individual fibers. These diffusely dilated grafts frequently caused no trouble but were occasionally associated with delayed graft rupture or diffuse interstitial bleeding. The ultralightweight method of fabrication has been abandoned by all manufacturers.

The second type of graft failure follows specific defects, such as a dropped stitch in the manufacturing process, or fiber degeneration. This type of defect usually causes localized holes and leaks, with the potential for false aneurysm formation (Fig. 50–16).

Anastomotic False Aneurysms. An anastomotic aneurysm follows a partial or total separation of the prosthetic graft from the host artery. These are termed false aneurysms, because the blood is contained by the nonelastic surrounding fibrous capsule rather than the true vessel wall. The natural history of an anastomotic aneurysm is progressive expansion, with an eventual serious complication of rupture, thrombosis, or embolism. The incidence of false aneurysm with prosthetic grafting is estimated to be at least 3%. Both Dacron and PTFE grafts are affected.

Because a prosthetic arterial anastomosis is forever dependent upon the anastomotic suture line, many false aneurysms in the past followed degeneration and fragmentation of the silk sutures that were used for construction of the anastomosis. Since the recognition of this problem, silk sutures are no longer used for arterial anastomoses. The exact cause of currently encountered false aneurysms is unknown. Frequently, the suture line and sutures are found intact, with the aneurysm occurring through a tear in the host artery adjacent to the suture line. Obvious clinical infection can be implicated in only a small percentage of cases. With rigorous culture techniques, however, infectious organisms can be demonstrated in a large number of false aneurysms.[40] Whether these subclinical infections are the actual cause of the false aneurysms or merely incidental findings is unknown. Other suggested etiologies of false aneurysms include shallow suture placement or arterial degeneration associated with hypertension. Several interesting studies have suggested that anastomotic aneurysms may follow graft-artery compliance mismatches accentuated by graft dilation.[6] Placement of too short a graft with excessive anastomotic tension has also been implicated. With rare exception, anastomotic aneurysms should be repaired when discovered. The usual repair consists of a graft-artery reanastomosis, frequently with the insertion of a short additional piece of graft material.

Perigraft Seroma. A perigraft seroma is a sterile collection of clear fluid within a nonsecretory pseudomembrane surrounding a prosthetic vascular graft. It usually occurs in association with extra-anatomic bypasses, that is, an axillofemoral or femorofemoral graft. The incidence is probably around 2%, occurring with both Dacron and PTFE grafts. The etiology is unknown but may relate to relative fibroblast inhibition, with failure of graft incorporation into surrounding tissues. Treatment has included observation alone, multiple aspirations, graft removal, injection of perigraft sclerosing agents, excision of the fibrous pseudocapsule, or intraperitoneal drainage.

Graft Modifications and Experimental Arterial Substitutes

A number of modifications of knitted Dacron grafts have been proposed to eliminate the need for preclotting by rendering the grafts temporarily impervious to blood while maintaining desirable handling properties. Cooley and associates described soaking knitted Dacron grafts in the patient's own plasma, followed by steam autoclaving for 3 to 5 minutes. Other investigators have used albumin to temporarily coat knitted grafts. These grafts require special packaging and must be rehydrated prior to implantation, but they do handle somewhat better than standard low-porosity woven arterial substitutes. Dacron grafts may also be impregnated with bovine Type I collagen.[25] The grafts are leakproof and handle essentially the same as standard knitted grafts. Cross-linking of the collagen during the manufacturing process seems to eliminate the normal thrombogenicity of collagen, and the grafts appear to be no more prone to thrombosis than a standard preclotted, knitted prosthesis. In an effort to reduce intraoperative blood loss, collagen-impregnated knitted Dacron grafts have become the graft of choice for many surgeons performing aortic reconstructions.

Bovine carotid xenografts have been modified with a combination of amino acid carboxylation and glutaraldehyde tanning. The negative luminal electrical charge imparted by this process supposedly makes the grafts resistant to thrombosis but should be regarded as experimental and of unproven clinical efficacy. The same applies to autogenous fibrocollagenous tubes formed over a silicone mandril, pyrolytic

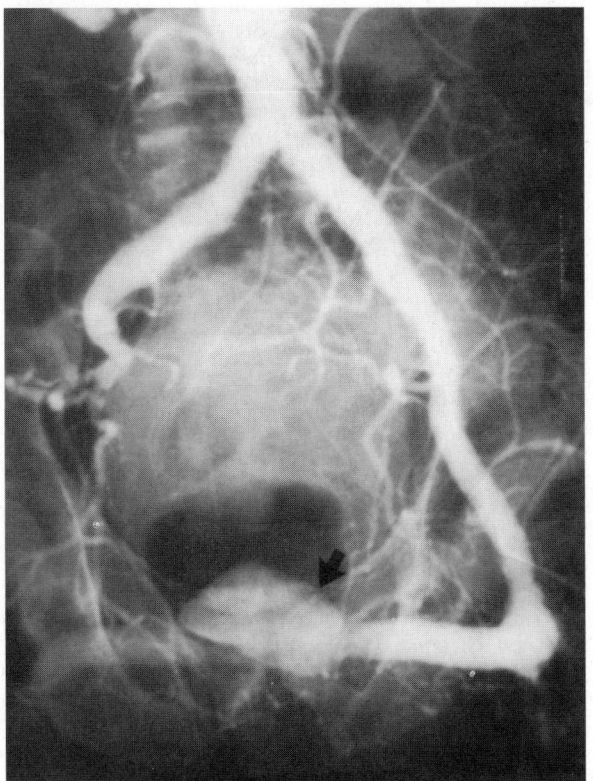

Figure 50–16. A defective knitted Dacron prosthesis resulted in this false aneurysm (arrow) of the midportion of a femorofemoral graft.

carbon-coated grafts, polyurethane grafts of various configurations, and Dacron-PTFE combinations.

Many studies have been published over the last 10 to 15 years concerning endothelial seeding of small-caliber synthetic vascular prostheses. It was hoped that the presence of a living neointima composed of viable endothelial cells would result in improved patency of prosthetic infrainguinal bypasses. The research is complex, including problems in harvesting viable endothelial cells, optimizing methods of seeding and cellular attachment to the graft, tracking of cells from harvesting to healing, and documenting normal function of seeded endothelial cells. Clinical trials of endothelialized PTFE grafts are beginning to be reported, with mixed but generally negative results. Zilla and colleagues randomized 49 patients with no saphenous veins who required femoropopliteal bypass to either endothelial seeded or standard PTFE grafts. After 32 months, life-table analysis revealed a patency of 85% for the endothelialized grafts and 55% for the control PTFE grafts.[44] Herring and colleagues compared 66 endothelial seeded femoropopliteal PTFE grafts with 53 autogenous vein femoropopliteal grafts. At 30 months, vein graft patency was 92%, and the patency of the seeded PTFE grafts was 38%.[15]

Another related and rapidly developing field involves the implantation of vascular grafts with genetically modified endothelial cells.[42] Researchers are exploring the possibility of using the vascular endothelial cell as a target for gene replacement therapy. The luminal location of the endothelial cell theoretically makes it ideal for the delivery of circulating gene products. In addition, this technology may prove important in prolonging graft patency by the delivery of gene products acting in a paracrine fashion to inhibit anastomotic intimal hyperplasia.

Currently, there is intense worldwide interest in the development of transluminally placed prosthetic arterial substitutes for the treatment of aneurysms. Dacron or PTFE grafts are mounted on expandable metallic stents (Fig. 50–17). An artery distal to the site to be grafted is surgically exposed. A coaxial delivery system under fluoroscopic guidance is then used to transluminally deliver the endoluminal stent graft to the desired location, where it either self-expands or is expanded with an angioplasty balloon, to exclude the flow stream from the aneurysm sac. The grafts are held in place by the outward pressure of the stent itself and/or by hooks attached to the proximal end of the stent portion of the prosthesis that engages the artery wall.

There are a number of potential problems with stent grafts, including the large size of the delivery systems currently required to place the grafts, the need for suitable anchoring sites, graft migration, arterial perforation, possible embolization of the luminal thrombus that is inevitably present within aneurysms, perigraft leakage such that the aneurysm is not completely excluded from the flow stream, and graft kinkage and axial twists in the limbs of bifurcated grafts. Despite these difficulties, a number of patients worldwide have had placement of endoluminal stent grafts for arterial disease.[23] The ultimate role of stent grafts as arterial substitutes awaits completion of careful clinical trials and further advances in the design of the grafts and their delivery systems.

OVERVIEW

Arterial grafting is of critical importance in modern vascular surgery. Available evidence clearly indicates that large artery bypass is best accomplished with textile-fabricated Dacron grafts or with PTFE grafts. For small artery bypass below the inguinal ligament, no arterial prosthesis has matched the performance and patency of autogenous saphenous vein grafts. To date, no arterial prosthesis 4 mm. or

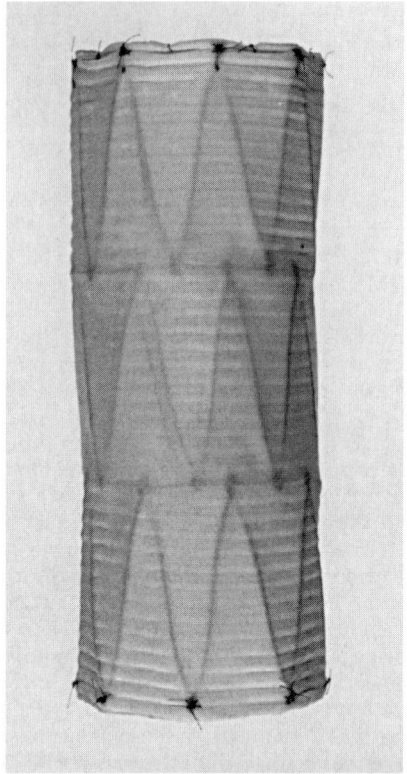

Figure 50–17. A *stent graft* for transluminal treatment of abdominal aortic aneurysms. A Dacron graft is mounted on an expandable metallic stent.

smaller in diameter has produced satisfactory clinical patency. Various prosthetic grafts to the above-knee popliteal artery have approached intermediate-term vein bypass patency, although none is as good as vein. No prosthetic graft has approached saphenous vein results for bypass to the below-knee popliteal artery or to tibial arteries.

Research in graft design and fabrication is currently directed toward the development of satisfactory prosthetic grafts for small artery bypass and endoluminally placed arterial substitutes. Most investigators believe that a satisfactory small artery prosthesis requires luminal healing and compliance characteristics that are considerably superior to those of grafts in present use, accompanied by improved understanding of the processes of atherosclerosis, thrombosis, and arterial healing.

SELECTED REFERENCES

Bandyk, D. F., Cato, R. F., and Towne, J. B.: A low flow velocity predicts failure of femoropopliteal and femorotibial bypass grafts. Surgery, 98:799, 1985.
This landmark paper paved the way for the use of duplex scanning in the postoperative evaluation of autogenous vein grafts. The use of noninvasive techniques has greatly facilitated understanding of the natural history of autogenous vein grafts.

Berger, K., Sauvage, L. R., Rao, A. M., and Wood, S. J.: Healing of arterial prostheses in man: Its incompleteness. Ann. Surg., 175:113, 1972.
This article reports detailed pathologic observations on arterial protheses removed from patients. It remains of pivotal importance in emphasizing the marked differences between man and animal in the healing of prosthetic arterial grafts.

Parodi, J. C., Palmaz, J. C., and Barone, H. D.: Transfemoral intraluminal graft implantation for abdominal aortic aneurysms. Ann. Vasc. Surg., 5:491, 1991.
With this publication, Dr. Parodi and colleagues launched an area of investigation that will dominate the field of arterial substitutes for a number of years.

Sawyer, P. N. (Ed.): Modern Vascular Grafts. New York, McGraw-Hill, 1987.
This multiauthored text contains literature reviews of various grafts by noted authorities.

Szilagyi, D. E., Elliott, J. P., Hageman, J. H., Smith, R. F., and Dal'Olmo, C. A.: Biologic fate of autogenous vein implants and arterial substitutes. Ann. Surg., 178:232, 1973.

This excellent reference clearly documents, with detailed clinical, angiographic, and pathologic follow-up, the long-term performance of autogenous vein grafts in man.

REFERENCES

1. Bandyk, D. F., Cato, R. F., and Towne, J. B.: A low flow velocity predicts failure of femoropopliteal and femorotibial bypass grafts. Surgery, 98:799, 1985.
2. Berger, K., Sauvage, L. R., Rao, A. M., and Wood, S. J.: Healing of arterial prostheses in man: Its incompleteness. Ann. Surg., 175:118, 1972.
3. Berger, K., Sauvage, L. R., Wood, S. J., and Sameh, A. A.: Endarterectomy and other surgical injuries to cardiovascular walls. Pacific Med. Surg., 75:367, 1967.
4. Brief, D. K., Brener, B., and Alpert, J.: Crossover femoro-femoral grafts followed up 5 years or more: An analysis. Arch. Surg., 110:1294, 1975.
5. Brewster, D. C., and Darling, R. C.: Optimal methods of aortoiliac reconstruction. Surgery, 84:739, 1978.
6. Clagett, G. P., Salander, J. M., and Eddleman, W. L.: Dilatation of knitted Dacron aortic prostheses and anastomotic false aneurysms: Etiologic considerations. Surgery, 93:9, 1983.
7. Clowes, A. W., Kirkman, T. R., and Reidy, M. A.: Mechanisms of arterial graft healing: Rapid transmural capillary ingrowth provides a source of intimal endothelium and smooth muscle in porous PTFE prostheses. Am. J. Pathol., 123:220, 1986.
8. Dardik, H., Miller, N., Dardik, A., Ibrahim, I. M., Saussman, B., Berry, S. M., Wolodiger, F., Kahn, M., and Dardik, I.: A decade of experience with the glutaraldehyde-tanned human umbilical cord vein graft for revascularization of the lower limb. J. Vasc. Surg., 7:336, 1988.
9. Dennis, J. W., Littooy, F. N., Greisler, H. P., and Baker, W. H.: Secondary vascular procedures with polytetrafluoroethylene grafts for lower extremity ischemia in a male veteran population. J. Vasc. Surg., 8:137, 1988.
10. Eickhoff, J. H., Broome, A., Ericsson, B. F., Hansen, H. J. B., Kordt, K. F., Mouritzen, C., Kvernebo, K., Norgren, L., Rostad, H., and Trippestad, A.: Four years' results of a prospective, randomized clinical trial comparing polytetrafluoroethylene and modified human umbilical vein for below-knee femoropopliteal bypass. J. Vasc. Surg., 6:506, 1987.
11. El-Massry, S., Saad, E., Sauvage, L., Zammit, M., Smith, J., Davis, C., Rittenhouse, E., and Fisher, L.: Femoropopliteal bypass with externally supported knitted Dacron grafts: A follow-up of 200 grafts for one to twelve years. J. Vasc. Surg., 19:487, 1994.
12. Harker, L. A., and Hanson, S. R.: Graft thrombus formation, detection, and resolution. In Stanley, J. (Ed.): Biologic and Synthetic Vascular Prostheses. New York, Grune & Stratton, 1983, p. 101.
13. Harris, E. J., Jr., Taylor, L. M., Jr., McConnell, D. B., Moneta, G. L., Yeager, R. A., and Porter, J. M.: Improved modern results of axillobifemoral bypass using externally supported PTFE. J. Vasc. Surg., 12:416, 1990.
14. Harris, R. W., Audros, G., Dulawa, L. B., Oblath, R. W., et al.: Successful long term limb salvage using cephalic vein bypass grafts. Ann. Surg., 200:785, 1984.
15. Herring, M., Smith, J., Dalsing, M., Glover, J., Compton, R., Etchberger, K., and Zollinger, T.: Endothelial seeding of polytetrafluoroethylene femoral popliteal bypasses: The failure of low density seeding to improve patency. J. Vasc. Surg., 20:650, 1994.
16. Kalman, P. G., Hosang, M., Johnston, K. W., and Walker, D. M.: The current role for femorofemoral bypass. J. Vasc. Surg., 6:71, 1987.
17. Kenney, D. A., Berger, K., Walker, M. W., and Sauvage, L.: Experimental comparison of the thrombogenicity of fibrin and PTFE flow surfaces. Ann. Surg., 191:355, 1980.
18. Leather, R. P., Shah, D. M., Chang, B. B., and Kaufman, J. L.: Resurrection of the in situ saphenous vein bypass: 1000 cases later. Ann. Surg., 208:435, 1988.
19. Mannick, J. A., Jackson, B. T., Coffman, J. D., and Hume, D. M.: Success of bypass vein grafts in patients with isolated popliteal artery segments. Surgery, 61:17, 1967.
20. Ochsner, J. L., DeCamp, P. T., and Leonard, G. L.: Experience with fresh venous allografts as an arterial substitute. Ann. Surg., 173:933, 1971.
21. O'Donnell, T. F., Farber, F. P., Richmond, D. M., Deterling, R. A., and Callow, A.: Above knee polytetrafluoroethylene bypass graft: Is it a reasonable alternative to the below-knee reversed autogenous vein grafts. Surgery, 94:26, 1983.
22. Okuhn, S. P., Connelly, D. P., Calakos, N., Ferrell, L., Man-Xiang, P., and Goldstone, J.: Does compliance mismatch alone cause neointimal hyperplasia? J. Vasc. Surg., 9:35, 1989.
23. Parodi, J. C., Palmaz, J. C., and Barone, H. D.: Transfemoral intraluminal graft implantation for abdominal aortic aneurysms. Ann. Vasc. Surg., 5:491, 1991.
24. Piotrowski, J. J., Pearce, W. H., Jones, D. N., Whitehill, T., Bell, R., Patt, A., and Rutherford, R. B.: Aorta bifemoral bypass: The operation of choice for unilateral iliac occlusion? J. Vasc. Surg., 8:211, 1988.
25. Reigel, M. M., Hollier, L. H., Pairolero, P. C., and Hallett, J. W., Jr.: Early experience with a new collagen-impregnated aortic graft. Am. Surg., 54:134, 1988.
26. Rutherford, R. R., Flanigan, D. P., Gupta, S. K., Johnston, K. W., Karmody, A., Whittemore, A. D., Baker, J. D., and Ernst, C. B.: Suggested standards for reports dealing with lower extremity ischemia. J. Vasc. Surg., 4:80, 1986.
27. Schmitz-Rixen, T., Megerman, J., Colvin, R. B., Williams, A. M., and Abbott, W. M.: Immunosuppressive treatment of aortic allografts. J. Vasc. Surg., 7:82, 1988.
28. Schulman, M. L., Badhey, M. R., and Yatco, R.: Superficial femoral popliteal veins and reversed saphenous veins as primary femoropopliteal bypass grafts: A randomized comparative study. J. Vasc. Surg., 6:1, 1987.
29. Scott, S. M., Barth, M. G., Gaddy, L. R., and Ahl, E. T., Jr.: The role of circulating cells in the healing of vascular prostheses. J. Vasc. Surg., 19:585, 1994.
30. Shue, W. B., Worosilo, M. S., Donetz, A. P., Trooskin, S. Z., Harvey, R. A., and Greco, R. S.: Prevention of vascular prosthetic infection with an antibiotic bonded Dacron graft. J. Vasc. Surg., 8:600, 1988.
31. Sottiurai, V. S., and Arson, R. C.: Ultrastructural studies of arterial grafts. In Bergan, J. J., and Yao, J. S. T. (Eds.): Evaluation and Treatment of Upper and Lower Extremity Circulatory Disorders. New York, Grune & Stratton, 1984, p. 371.
32. Spray, T. L., and Roberts, W. C.: Fundamentals of clinical cardiology: Changes in saphenous veins used as aortocoronary bypass grafts. Am. Heart. J., 94:500, 1977.
33. Stanley, J. C., Ernst, C. B., and Fry, W. J.: Fate of 100 aortorenal vein grafts; characteristics of late graft expansion, aneurysmal dilation, and stenosis. Surgery, 74:931, 1973.
34. Stoney, R. J., DeLuccia, N., Ehrenfeld, W. K., and Wylie, E. J.: Aortorenal arterial autografts. Arch. Surg., 116:1416, 1981.
35. Szilagyi, D. E., Elliott, J. P., Hageman, J. G., Smith, R. F., and Dall'Olmo, C. A.: Biologic fate of autogenous vein implants and arterial substitutes. Ann. Surg., 178:232, 1973.
36. Szilagyi, D. E., Hageman, J. G., Smith, R. F., et al.: Autogenous vein grafting in femoropopliteal atherosclerosis: The limit of its effectiveness. Surgery, 86:836, 1979.
37. Taylor, L. M., Jr., Edwards, J. M., Phinney, E. S., and Porter, J. M.: Reversed vein bypass to infrapopliteal arteries. Ann. Surg., 205:90, 1987.
38. Taylor, L. M., Jr., Edwards, J. M., and Porter, J. M.: Present status of reversed vein bypass: Long term results of a modern series. J. Vasc. Surg., 11:193, 1990.
39. Taylor, L. M., Jr., Park, T. C., Edwards, J. M., Yeager, R. A., McConnell, D. B., Moneta, G. L., and Porter, J. M.: Acute disruption of polytetrafluoroethylene grafts adjacent to axillary anastomoses: A complication of axillofemoral grafting. J. Vasc. Surg., 20:520, 1994.
40. Tollefson, D. F., Bandyk, D. F., Kaebnick, H. W., et al.: Surface biofilm disruption: Enhanced recovery of microorganisms from vascular prostheses. Arch. Surg., 122:38, 1986.
41. Williams, G. M., ter Haar, A., Krajewski, D., Parks, L. C., and Roth, J.: Rejection and repair of endothelium in major vessel transplants. Surgery, 78:694, 1975.
42. Wilson, J. M., Birinyi, L. K., Salmon, R. N., Libby, P., Callow, A. D., and Mulligan, R. C.: Implantation of vascular grafts lined with genetically modified endothelial cells. Science, 244:1344, 1989.
43. Yeager, R. A., Moneta, G. L., Taylor, L. M., Jr., Harris, E. J., Jr., McConnell, D. B., and Porter, J. M.: Improving survival and limb salvage in patients with aortic graft infection. Am. J. Surg., 159:466, 1990.
44. Zilla, P., Deutsch, M., Meinhart, J., Puschmann, R., Eberl, T., Minar, E., Dudczak, R., Lugmaier, H., Schmidt, P., Noszian, I., and Fischleiu, T.: Clinical in vitro endothelialization of femoropopliteal bypass grafts: An actuarial follow-up over three years. J. Vasc. Surg., 19:540, 1994.

V

ANEURYSMS

David C. Sabiston, Jr., M.D.

An aneurysm is the dilatation of an artery full of spiritous blood.
FERNEL, 1591

An aneurysm is a localized dilatation of an artery and occasionally of a vein. Most aneurysms are designated as *true aneurysms* and contain all three layers of the arterial wall (intima, media, and adventitia). *False aneurysm* (pulsating hematoma) is the term applied when only the adventitia is present, as is often the situation after traumatic rupture of an artery with subsequent aneurysmal formation. It is helpful to further classify aneurysms as *saccular* or *fusiform*. Saccular aneurysms usually arise from a distinct portion of the wall and have a mouth, whereas fusiform aneurysms involve the total circumference of the artery and represent a diffuse dilatation. Aneurysms tend to occur at certain anatomic sites, and the most common locations are shown in Figure 50–18.

Congenital and *acquired aneurysms* are both encountered, the latter being much more frequent than the former. Acquired aneurysms may be caused by atherosclerosis, trauma, infection (mycotic), medial cystic necrosis, and syphilis (rare today). Although aneurysms were once untreatable, nearly all can be managed now by surgical means and usually with highly satisfactory results.

ANEURYSMS OF THE SINUS OF VALSALVA

David N. Campbell, M.D.,
John H. Calhoon, M.D., and
Frederick L. Grover, M.D.

Sinus of Valvalsa aneurysms are dilatations of the aortic sinuses of Valsalva that may rupture into a cardiac chamber, the pulmonary artery, or the pericardium. These aneurysms occur secondary to acquired or congenital disease.

ACQUIRED ANEURYSMS OF THE SINUS OF VALSALVA

Causes of acquired sinus of Valsalva aneurysms include subacute bacterial endocarditis,[22] Marfan's syndrome, chronic dissection of the aorta and other degenerative lesions of the aortic root,[5, 26] atherosclerosis,[14] and syphilis.[13, 28] Those aneurysms associated with endocarditis are usually repaired at the time of aortic valve replacement and most commonly involve one sinus. The repair usually involves incorporating the mouth of the aneurysm with the valve sutures, thus obliterating the orifice, or patching the orifice of the aneurysm.[22] Atherosclerotic aneurysms are usually repaired with a Dacron patch.[14] Those aneurysms caused by cystic medial necrosis or degenerative lesions of the aortic root usually require total replacement of the aortic root and valve by a composite graft, with reimplantation of the coronary arteries (Bentall or Cabrol procedure) (Fig. 50–19).[5, 9, 26] This can now be accomplished with a 5% operative mortality rate and a 3-year actuarial survival of 81% to 88%.[26]

Acquired aneurysms are also discussed in other sections of this chapter.

CONGENITAL ANEURYSMS OF THE SINUS OF VALSALVA

Historical Aspects. The first described case of congenital sinus of Valsalva aneurysm was reported in 1835 by Hope in a patient whose condition was diagnosed at autopsy.[23] The first patient diagnosed during life by aortography was reported in 1953,[17] and the first surgical correction was performed by Lillehei and co-workers in 1956.[27] Since then, numerous reports of surgical corrections of ruptured sinus of Valsalva aneurysms have been made. They account for 0.23% to 0.69% of all cardiac procedures.[2, 28]

Etiology and Pathophysiology. Abbott believed that congenital aneurysms were caused by an abnormal fusion of the aortic-pulmonary septum with the ventricular septum.[1] Venning postulated that the aneurysms were caused by elastic tissue defects in the sinuses.[40] Edwards and Burchell demonstrated that the essential pathology was a separation between the aortic media and the heart at the anulus fibrosus of the aortic valve.[16] The reason for the unusually high incidence of ruptured aneurysms in the Asian population is unknown but may be related to the presence of a ventricular septal defect.[11, 34]

Congenital aneurysms frequently rupture into an intracardiac chamber, producing a sudden left-to-right shunt.[2, 6, 8, 11, 28, 29, 38, 41] The most common sinus involved is the right sinus, which usually ruptures into the right ventricle or, less frequently, into the right atrium. The noncoronary sinus is the next most frequent site, and it usually ruptures into the right

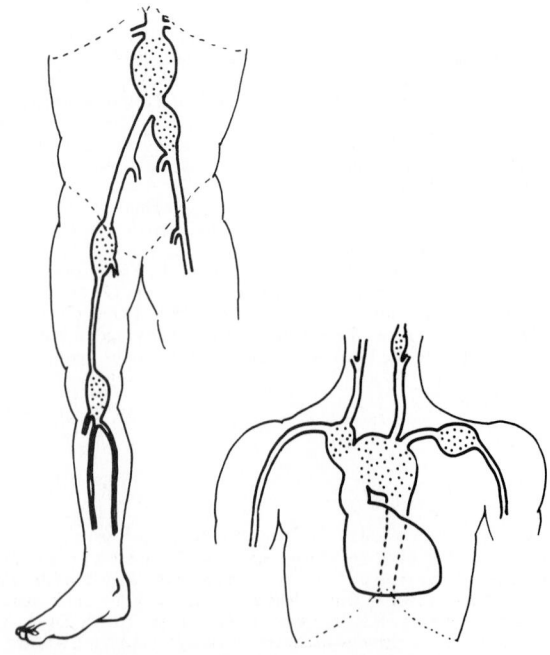

Figure 50–18. Common anatomic sites of arterial aneurysms. (From Ludbrook, J., and Elmsile, R. G.: An Introduction to Surgery: 100 Topics. New York, Academic Press, 1971.)

atrium. Unusual cases of rupture of the left sinus into all four chambers and the pulmonary artery have been reported. Nowicki and associates, in a collective review of 119 patients, noted that the right sinus was the origin of the fistula in 67% of patients, the noncoronary in 25%, and the left coronary sinus in 8%.[30] The anatomic location of the fistulas in these patients is demonstrated in Figure 50–20. Taguchi and colleagues developed 16 anatomic classifications based on the sinus involved and the location of the fistula.[37]

Associated intracardiac defects are frequently present, the most common being a ventricular septal defect. Aortic regurgitation may also be present to variable degrees and is most common in those patients who have a ventricular septal defect. Nowicki and associates found that 33% of patients had a ventricular septal defect, and 8% had an aortic valve abnormality.[30]

Clinical Presentation. The majority of patients are asymptomatic until the fistula ruptures. With rupture, the usual symptoms are dyspnea, palpitations, and chest pain. The

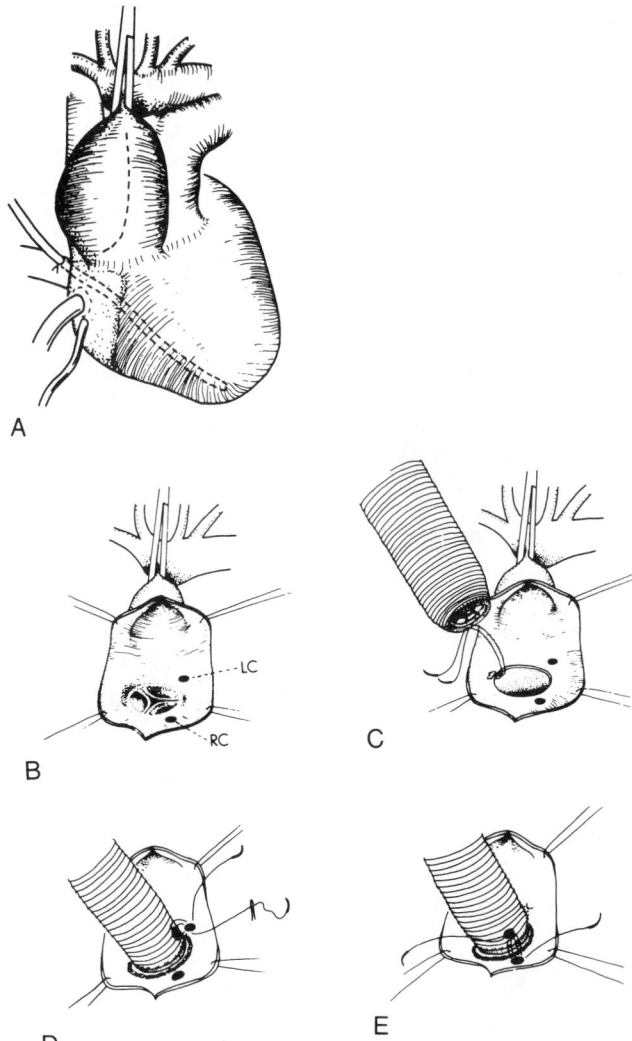

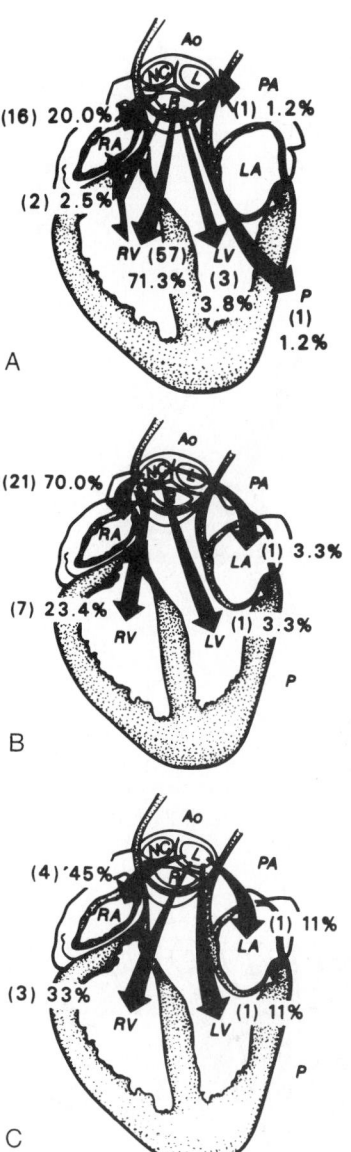

Figure 50–20. Origins and terminations of congenital sinus of Valsalva–cardiac fistulas in 119 patients. The chamber of termination for aortocameral fistulas is shown in *A* from the right sinus (80 patients); *B*, the noncoronary sinus (30 patients); and *C*, the left sinus (9 patients). (From Nowicki, E., Aberdeen, E., Friedman, S., and Rashkind, W.: Congenital left aortic sinus–left ventricle fistula and review of aortocardiac fistulas. Ann. Thorac. Surg., *23*:378, 1977.)

Figure 50–19. Insertion of a valved conduit into the aortic root (Bentall procedure). *A* and *B*, The aorta is opened longitudinally following institution of cardiopulmonary bypass and cross-clamping of the aorta. *C*, The valve conduit is sutured to the aortic valve anulus following removal of the aortic valve. *D* and *E*, The left and right coronary ostia are reimplanted into the sides of the graft. Following this, the distal anastomosis is performed to the aorta and the graft wrapped with residual aneurysm tissue. (From Kouchoukos, N. T., Karp, R. B., and Lell, W. A.: Replacement of the ascending aorta and aortic valve with a composite graft: Results in 25 patients. Ann. Thorac. Surg., *24*:142, 1977.)

symptoms are associated with signs of congestive heart failure, including peripheral edema, tachycardia, orthopnea, and elevated central venous pressure. A precordial thrill with a continuous murmur may be heard; it is loudest over the second to fourth intercostal spaces to the left of the sternal border for those that communicate with the right ventricle, and over the right third and fourth intercostal spaces for those that rupture into the right atrium. Pulse pressures are increased, and the murmur of aortic regurgitation may be present. Approximately one third of patients have a sudden onset of symptoms, sometimes associated with strenuous activity. Patients whose fistulas rupture into the pericardium present in cardiogenic shock with signs of cardiac tamponade.[8, 11, 25, 30, 41] Other diseases that may have a similar clinical presentation and should be considered in the differential diagnosis are patent ductus arteriosus, aortopulmonary window, coronary artery–cameral fistula, and ventricular septal defect with aortic insufficiency.

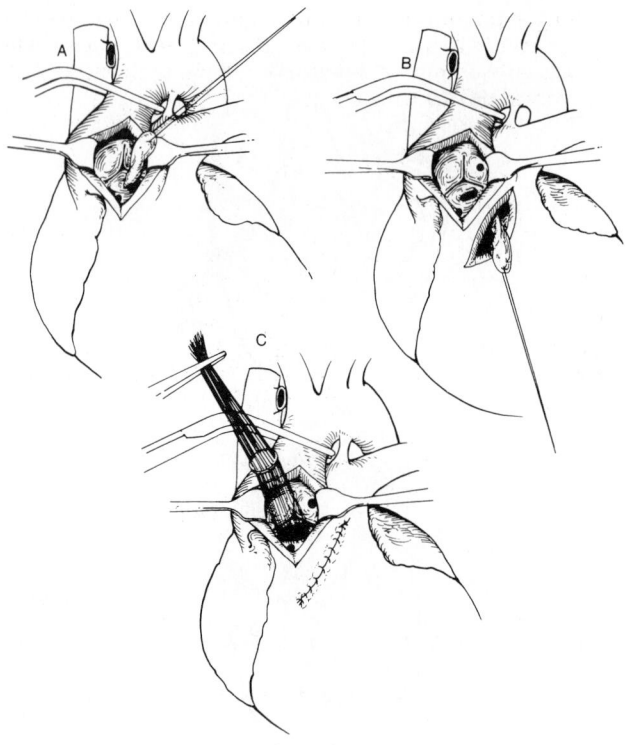

Figure 50–21. Repair of fistula from right sinus of Valsalva aneurysm into the right ventricle. The combined aortic and ventricular approach is shown, in which the fistula is identified from each end. The aortic opening is closed with a prosthetic patch and the cardiac end is closed separately. (From Arciniegas, E.: Pediatric Cardiac Surgery. Chicago, Year Book Medical Publishers, 1985, p. 383.)

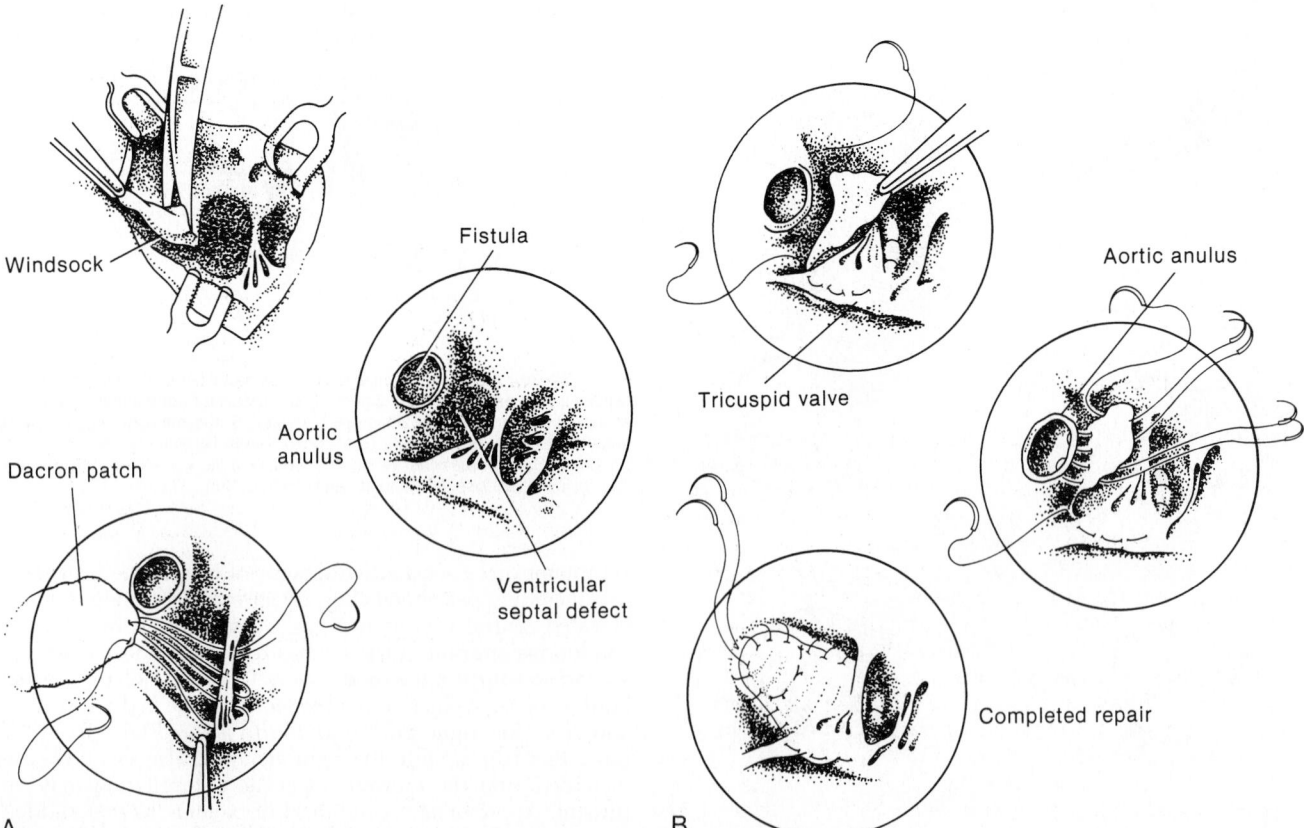

Figure 50–22. Closure of combined fistula and ventricular septal defect (VSD) through right ventriculotomy. *A,* The wind-sock deformity is excised, the fistula and VSD identified, and a common patch sutured to the inferior wall of the VSD. *B,* The patch is tacked to the septal-anulus tissue between the VSD and the orifice of the fistula and then also sewn over the fistula. This technique closes both orifices without allowing communication between the two. (From Doty, D. B.: Cardiac Surgery. Chicago, Year Book Medical Publishers, 1985.)

Nonruptured aneurysms can rarely cause signs and symptoms because of compression of adjacent structures. Obstruction of the right ventricular outflow tract produces an elevated jugular venous pulse and a systolic murmur increasing with inspiration and hepatomegaly secondary to tricuspid insufficiency.[18] Aneurysms can also cause acute myocardial infarction or unstable angina secondary to coronary artery compression.[21] In addition, left ventricular obstruction has occurred when the right coronary sinus of Valsalva protrudes into the left ventricle;[20] ventricular tachycardia[32] and heart block[3] have also been reported. Clot may form in the aneurysm and lead to emboli[36, 42] or thrombosis of the aneurysm.[33]

Chest films usually reveal increased pulmonary vascular markings, with enlargement of the right side of the heart and prominence of the main pulmonary arteries.[30] Common electrocardiographic changes are left ventricular hypertrophy, right ventricular strain, axis shift, and biventricular hypertrophy.[8, 11, 28, 30, 41] Cardiac catheterization is helpful in delineating the anatomy of the aneurysm and identifying and quantifying the shunt. Angiography is often not needed, because transesophageal color-flow Doppler echocardiography, magnetic resonance imaging, and radioisotopic angiography allow accurate visualization of the aneurysm and the fistula, if present, in greater than 95% of cases.[10, 15, 31, 34] The future role of intracardiac ultrasonographic imaging is unknown.[35] In the review by Nowicki and associates, the left-to-right shunt ranged from 1.2:1 to 5:1 liters per minute, with a mean of 2.2.[30]

Treatment. The presence of a fistula involving the sinus of Valsalva is considered an indication for operation, because progressive heart failure can lead to death.[2, 8, 30, 41] If severe heart failure is present, urgent operation should be undertaken. Patients with an asymptomatic nonruptured aneurysm of the sinus of Valsalva should be managed conservatively but followed closely with serial echocardiography because of the possibility of developing symptoms due to compression, embolization, or later rupture.[30, 36, 42]

The fistula can be approached via the chamber into which it ruptured[6, 8, 11] or through the aorta.[19] Most investigators now recommend a dual approach via the aorta and the chamber of entry of the fistula (Fig. 50–21).[4, 6–8, 28, 38, 41] Right ventricular fistulas can also be approached through the pulmonary artery.[2, 13] The advantage of the aortocameral approach is that the fistula can be probed from the aorta into the chamber involved and closed at both its origin and its termination, with an apparent decrease in recurrent fistula. The aortic valve can be inspected and protected from improperly placed sutures, which could distort the valve and create aortic insufficiency. The aortic valve can also be evaluated for insufficiency, which, if present, can be repaired using Trusler's technique[39] or replaced if necessary. The ventricular septum can be carefully inspected for the presence of a ventricular septal defect, which, if present, can be closed with a common patch covering the defect and the fistula; the patch is tacked to the septum between the ventricular septal defect and the fistula to eliminate communication between the two (Fig. 50–22). Small defects can be closed primarily.[6, 11, 38] A recent case report demonstrated nonoperative successful closure of a ruptured fistula using a transcatheter technique and a modified Rashkind umbrella device.[12]

Results. Nowicki and associates noted an operative mortality of 12.7%, a failure to close the fistula in 1.6%, and a good result in 85.7% of patients.[30] Seventy percent of the patients who died had an associated cardiac abnormality. Much of the mortality was in the early years, and more recent series report a mortality of 0 to 13%, with an almost negligible reoperation rate.[2, 18, 28, 38] Actuarial survival at 25 years has been reported at 86%.[2] Reoperation is rarely required for progression of aortic regurgitation, recurrent fistula, or residual ventricular septal defect. Death is more likely in the acquired group, particularly in those with endocarditis or myocarditis due to ongoing sepsis.[24]

SELECTED REFERENCES

Barragry, T., Ring, W., Moller, J., and Lillehei, C.: Fifteen- to thirty-year follow-up of patients undergoing repair of ruptured congenital aneurysms of the sinus of Valsalva. Ann. Thorac. Surg., 46:515, 1988.
This report reviews the long-term results of repair of ruptured congenital aneurysms of the sinus of Valsalva and includes the first patient to undergo operative correction.

Chih, P., Heng, T., Chun, C., and Chieh-Fu, L.: Surgical treatment of the ruptured aneurysm of the aortic sinuses. Ann. Thorac. Surg., 32:162, 1981.
This article reports the largest single institutional experience in the surgical treatment of ruptured aneurysm of the sinus of Valsalva. The report originates from the Shanghai Chest Hospital and reviews the higher incidence of this entity in the Asian population, patient characteristics, symptoms, associated defects, diagnostic studies, operative technique, and early and late results.

Edwards, J., and Burchell, H.: The pathological anatomy of deficiencies between the aortic root and the heart, including aortic sinus aneurysms. Thorax, 12:125, 1957.
This classic report concerns the anatomy of the aortic sinuses, the pathologic anatomy of those lesions that lie at the aortic root, and the deficiencies between the aortic media and the heart. It is a detailed pathophysiologic study of historic importance and remains the most important pathologic paper describing these abnormalities.

Kouchoukos, N., Karp, R., Blackstone, R., Kirklin, J., Pacifico, A., and Zorn, G.: Replacement of the ascending aorta and aortic valve with a composite graft. Ann. Surg., 192:403, 1980.
This is a detailed review of one institution's experience in replacing the ascending aorta and aortic valve with a composite graft using the Bentall technique.

Nowicki, E., Aberdeen, E., Friedman, S., and Rashkind, W.: Congenital left aortic sinus–left ventricle fistula and review of aortocardiac fistulas. Ann. Thorac. Surg., 23:378, 1977.
This paper offers a thorough review of 175 cases of aortocardiac fistulas from sinus of Valsalva aneurysms that were published in the English literature from 1839 to 1972.

REFERENCES

1. Abbott, M.: Clinical and developmental study of a case of ruptured aneurysm of the right anterior sinus of Valsalva. Contrib. Med. Biol. Res., 2:899, 1919.
2. Abe, T., and Komatsu, S.: Surgical repair and long-term results in ruptured sinus of Valsalva aneurysm. Ann. Thorac. Surg., 46:520, 1988.
3. Ahmad, R., Sturman, S., and Watson, R.: Unruptured aneurysm of the sinus of Valsalva presenting with isolated heart block: Echocardiographic diagnosis and successful surgical repair. Br. Heart J., 61:375, 1989.
4. Barragry, T., Ring, W., Moller, J., and Lillehei, C.: Fifteen- to thirty-year follow-up of patients undergoing repair of ruptured congenital aneurysms of the sinus of Valsalva. Ann. Thorac. Surg., 56:515, 1988.
5. Bentall, H., and DeBono, A.: A technique for complete replacement of the ascending aorta. Thorax, 23:338, 1968.
6. Bonfils-Roberts, E., DuShane, J., McGoon, D., and Danielson, G.: Aortic sinus fistula—surgical considerations and results of operation. Ann. Thorac. Surg., 15:492, 1971.
7. Bosher, L., Jr.: The combined surgical approach (transaortic and transatrial) for the correction of congenital aortic sinus fistula into the right atrium. J. Thorac. Cardiovasc. Surg., 50:243, 1965.
8. Burakovsky, V., Podsolkov, V., Sabirow, M., Nasedkina, A., Alekian, B., and Dvinyaninova, N.: Ruptured congenital aneurysm of the sinus of Valsalva: Clinical manifestations, diagnosis, and results of surgical correction. J. Thorac. Cardiovasc. Surg., 95:836, 1988.
9. Cabrol, C., Pavie, A., Gandjbakhch, I., Villemot, J., Guiraudon, G., Laughlin, L., Etievent, P., and Cham, B.: Complete replacement of the ascending aorta with reimplantation of the coronary arteries. J. Thorac. Cardiovasc. Surg., 81:309, 1981.
10. Chiang, C., Lin, F., Fang, B., Kuo, C., Lee, Y., and Chang, C.: Doppler and two-dimensional echocardiographic features of sinus of Valsalva aneurysm. Am. Heart J., 116:1283, 1988.
11. Chih, P., Heng, T., Chun, C., and Chieh-Fu, L.: Surgical treatment of the ruptured aneurysm of the aortic sinuses. Ann. Thorac. Surg., 32:162, 1981.
12. Cullen, S., Somerville, J., and Redington, A.: Transcatheter closure of a ruptured aneurysm of the sinus of Valsalva. Br. Heart J., 71:479, 1994.
13. DeBakey, M., Diethrich, E., Liddicoat, J., Kinard, S., and Garrett, H.: Abnormalities of the sinuses of Valsalva: Experience with 35 patients. J. Thorac. Cardiovasc. Surg., 54:312, 1967.

14. DeBakey, M., and Lawrie, G.: Aneurysm of sinus of Valsalva with coronary atherosclerosis: Successful surgical correction. Ann. Surg., *189*:303, 1979.

15. Dev, V., Goswami, K. C., Shrivastava, S., Bahl, V. K., and Saxena, A.: Echocardiographic diagnosis of aneurysm of the sinus of Valsalva. Am. Heart J., *126*:930, 1993.

16. Edwards, J., and Burchell, H.: The pathological anatomy of deficiencies between the aortic root and the heart, including aortic sinus aneurysms. Thorax, *12*:125, 1957.

17. Falholt, W., and Thomsen, G.: Congenital aneurysm of the right sinus of Valsalva, diagnosed by aortography. Circulation, *8*:549, 1953.

18. Gibbs, K., Reardon, M., Strickman, N., DeCastro, C., Gerard, J., Bycyna, J., Hall, R., and Cooley, D.: Hemodynamic compromise (tricuspid stenosis and insufficiency) caused by an unruptured aneurysm of the sinus of Valsalva. J. Am. Coll. Cardiol. *7*:1177, 1986.

19. Hamid, I. A., Jothi, M., Rajan, S., Monro, J. L., and Cherian, K. M.: Transaortic repair of ruptured aneurysm of sinus of Valsalva: Fifteen year experience. J. Thorac. Cardiovasc. Surg., *107*:1464, 1994.

20. Heydorn, W., Nelson, W., Fitterer, J., Floyd, G., and Strevey, T.: Congenital aneurysm of the sinus of Valsalva protruding into the left ventricle: Review of diagnosis and treatment of unruptured aneurysm. J. Thorac. Cardiovasc. Surg., *71*:839, 1976.

21. Hiyamuta, K., Ohtsuki, T., Shimamatsu, M., Ohkita, Y., Teresawa, M., Bekki, H., Toshima, H., Utsu, F., Ohishi, K., Koga, M., and Nagayama, K.: Aneurysm of the left aortic sinus causing acute myocardial infarction. Circulation, *67*:1151, 1983.

22. Holmes, E., Bredenberg, C., and Brawley, R.: Aneurysm of the sinus of Valsalva resulting from bacterial endocarditis. Ann. Thorac. Surg., *15*:628, 1973.

23. Hope, J.: A Treatise of Diseases of the Heart and Great Vessels, 3rd ed. London, John Churchill, 1839.

24. Hurley, J., and McGovern, E.: Rupture of a sinus of Valsalva aneurysm due to aspergillus endocarditis. J. Cardiovasc. Surg., *35*:75, 1994.

25. Killen, D., Wathanacharoen, S., and Pogson, G., Jr.: Repair of intrapericardial rupture of left sinus of Valsalva aneurysm. Ann. Thorac. Surg., *44*:310, 1987.

26. Kouchoukos, N., Karp, R., Blackstone, E., Kirklin, J., Pacifico, A., and Zorn, G.: Replacement of the ascending aorta and aortic valve with a composite graft. Ann. Surg., *192*:403, 1980.

27. Lillehei, C., Stanley, P., and Varco, R.: Surgical treatment of ruptured aneurysms of the sinus of Valsalva. Ann. Surg., *146*:459, 1957.

28. Mayer, E., Ruffmann, K., Saggau, W., Butzmann, B., Bernhardt-Mayer, K., Schatton, N., and Schmitz, W.: Ruptured aneurysms of the sinus of Valsalva. Ann. Thorac. Surg., *42*:81, 1986.

29. Meyer, J., Wukasch, D., Hallman, G., and Cooley, D.: Aneurysm and fistula of the sinus of Valsalva: Clinical considerations and surgical treatment in 45 patients. Ann. Thorac. Surg., *19*:170, 1975.

30. Nowicki, E., Aberdeen, E., Friedman, S., and Rashkind, W.: Congenital left aortic sinus–left ventricle fistula and review of aortocardiac fistulas. Ann. Thorac. Surg., *23*:378, 1977.

31. Ogawa, R., Iwama, Y., Hashimoto, H., Ito, T., and Satake, T.: Noninvasive methods in the diagnosis of ruptured aneurysm of Valsalva: Usefulness of MRI and Doppler echocardiography. Chest, *100*:579, 1991.

32. Raizes, G., Smith, H., Vlietstra, R., and Puga, F.: Ventricular tachycardia secondary to aneurysm of sinus of Valsalva. J. Thorac. Cardiovasc. Surg., *78*:110, 1979.

33. Reid, P. G., Goudevenos, J. A., and Hilton, C. J.: Thrombosed saccular aneurysm of a sinus of Valsalva: Unusual cause of a mediastinal mass. Br. Heart J., *63*:183, 1990.

34. Sahasakul, Y., Panchavinnin, P., Chaithiraphan, S., and Sakiyalak, P.: Echocardiographic diagnosis of a ruptured aneurysm of the sinus of Valsalva: Operation without catheterisation in seven patients. Br. Heart J., *64*:195, 1990.

35. Samaha, F. F., Lang, R., Abbo, K. M., Carroll, J. D., Weinert, L., and Follman, D. F.: Intracardiac ultrasonographic imaging to diagnose a ruptured sinus of Valsalva aneurysm. Am. Heart J., *128*:409, 1994.

36. Shahrabani, R. M., and Jairaj, P. S.: Unruptured aneurysm of the sinus of Valsalva: A potential source of cerebrovascular embolism. Br. Heart J., *69*:266, 1993.

37. Taguchi, K., Sasaki, N., Matsuura, Y., and Uemura, R.: Clinical studies: Surgical correction of aneurysm of sinus of Valsalva: A report of forty-five consecutive patients, including eight with total replacement of the aortic valve. Am. J. Cardiol., *23*:180, 1969.

38. Tanabe, T., Yokota, A., and Sugie, S.: Surgical treatment of aneurysms of the sinus of Valsalva. Ann. Thorac. Surg., *27*:133, 1979.

39. Trusler, G., Moes, C., and Kidd, B.: Repair of ventricular septal defect with aortic insufficiency. J. Thorac. Cardiovasc. Surg., *66*:394, 1973.

40. Venning, G.: Aneurysms of the sinuses of Valsalva. Am. Heart J., *57*:69, 1951.

41. Verghese, M., Jairaj, P., Babuthaman, C., Sukumar, I., and John, S.: Surgical treatment of ruptured aneurysms of the sinus of Valsalva. Ann. Thorac. Surg., *41*:284, 1986.

42. Wortham, D. C., Gorman, P. D., Hull, R. W., Vernalis, M. N., and Gaither, N. S.: Unruptured sinus of Valsalva aneurysm presenting with embolization. Am. Heart J., *125*:896, 1993.

TRAUMATIC ANEURYSMS OF THE AORTA

Walter G. Wolfe, M.D.

It is amazing that any patient survives traumatic rupture of the aorta. Among those who do, survival is dependent on the formation of a false aneurysm contained by the adventitia and the support of mediastinal structures. Such an aneurysm may rupture within minutes or persist for a prolonged period. In some patients who initially survive without evidence of aortic injury, an unsuspected aneurysm may be discovered or may rupture suddenly, months or even years later. In a review of 296 fatal cases of injury of the aorta, approximately 13% of the patients survived initially,[22] a finding confirmed in another study.[27] It was apparent that sudden death did not occur in all patients, with some 20% surviving longer than 30 minutes after injury.

INCIDENCE

The incidence of traumatic rupture of the aorta has increased markedly with the development of high-speed vehicles, and posttraumatic aneurysms now represent the most common thoracic aortic aneurysm in the younger age group (Fig. 50–23). The number of traffic accidents each year and the number of individuals sustaining thoracic injuries have risen sharply; acute aortic rupture occurs in 15% to 20% of individuals killed in vehicular accidents. Therefore, a history of sudden deceleration injury should immediately arouse the suspicion of acute aortic transection.

Improved methods of treating injuries and improved medical care of the injured have increased survival at the accident site.[6] The care of these patients is complicated by the fact that many suffer from multiple injuries,[4, 30] a factor that increases mortality. Because significant thoracic injury is often present without external evidence of an obvious superficial wound, attention is concentrated on problems that are apparent.

METHODS OF INJURY

Prior to high-speed travel, direct blows to the thoracic cage were common, but serious associated injuries were seldom seen. Such blows may produce rib or sternal fractures; pulmonary contusion and fractured ribs may secondarily cause pulmonary laceration with subsequent pneumothorax and hemothorax. Compression injuries of the chest, another common form of trauma, may cause rupture of the diaphragm, fractured ribs, and contusions of the lung. High-speed automobile accidents produce deceleration injuries, which are also seen in airplane or train accidents, as well as in falls from appreciable heights and compression by heavy objects.[4, 9, 22]

In general, such an injury is related to direct contact between the thoracic cage and a hard object, for example, the steering column or dashboard in a car. This type of injury follows rapid deceleration of the body and continued movement of the internal organs. The suspended heart and great vessels continue to travel, and tears occur at various attachments of fixed points within the chest.

The pathogenesis of thoracic aortic injury was first defined by Rindfleisch in 1893.[26] He surmised that the aortic arch and great vessels have relatively fixed attachments, whereas the heart and descending thoracic aorta are mobile. Sudden deceleration of the body at the time of impact, with differential rates of deceleration of the thoracic organs, the thoracic aorta, and the great vessels, can cause a tear involving the intima, the intima and media, or the entire wall. This tear is usually

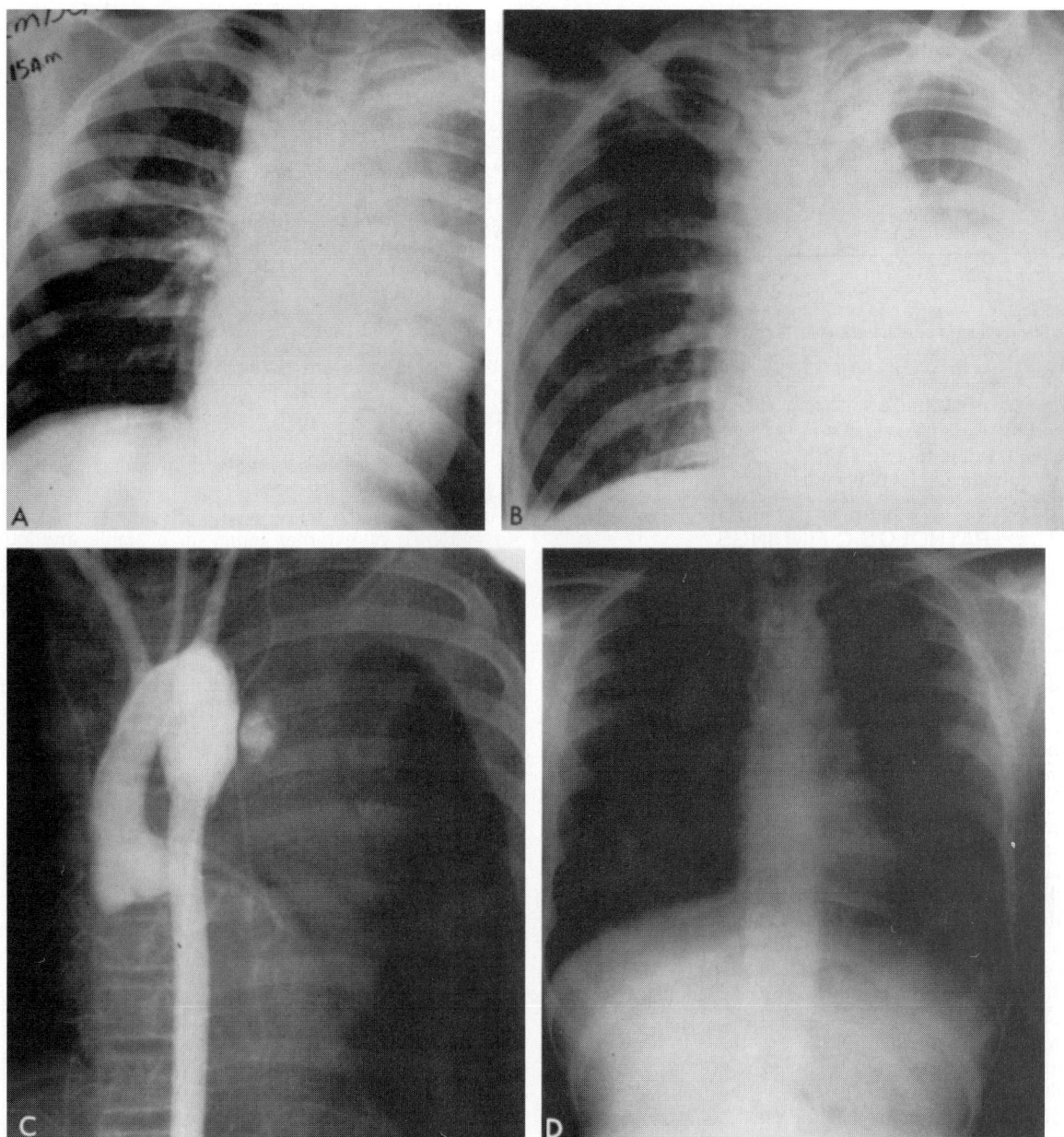

Figure 50–23. *A,* Chest film shows a large mediastinal hematoma in a 14-year-old boy after an accident involving a motorbike. Following chest x-ray examination at his local hospital, he was transferred. *B,* Chest film taken upon admission to the emergency room shows progression of the hematoma and pleural effusion in the left side of the chest, indicative of rupture. *C,* Aortogram demonstrating the pleural effusion and mediastinal hematoma as well as a complete transection of the aorta and mediastinal extravasation of contrast material. *D,* Radiograph 2 years following repair of the thoracic aorta with a Dacron graft.

transverse and may be partial or complete. The average age of these patients is in the third decade, and atherosclerosis is seldom a factor in the aortic injury. Since the adventitia provides 60% of the tensile strength of the thoracic aorta, survival of the patient depends on the continuity of this layer. The mechanism of aortic rupture with deceleration is related to different deceleration rates between fixed and mobile parts. Thus, in violent deceleration, the relatively free descending thoracic aorta snaps forward at a rate different from the fixed portion of the aorta. Such unequal forces subject the aorta to stretch, torsion, and shearing stress, with rupture at fixed points. An alternative interpretation is avulsion of the heart and aortic arch from the aorta at the ligamentum, which occurs as the heart is projected forward and upward in a violent deceleration. Therefore, the most frequent site of damage of the aorta is at its isthmus,[5, 22, 27, 29]

that is, the segment just distal to the left subclavian artery at the ligamentum arteriosum (Table 50–2). Injuries to the ascending aorta and aortic vessels are more likely to follow direct trauma than deceleration, and with such injuries, it is common to find fractures and fracture-dislocations in the

TABLE 50–2. Site of Injury

Isthmus
Arch
Ascending aorta
Descending thoracic aorta
Abdominal aorta
Multiple sites

TABLE 50–3. Associated Thoracic Injuries

Rib fractures
Sternal fractures
Thoracic vertebral fractures
Clavicular fracture
Scapula fracture
Pneumothorax
Hemothorax
Cardiac injury

region of the anterior chest wall overlying these vessels. This includes fracture of the first rib, fracture of the clavicle, and dislocation of the clavicle.

Landing feet first after a fall from a height may rupture the descending aorta by avulsion of the junction of the fixed aortic arch and the mobile heart. Such tears are usually associated with aortic valvular injury.

PATHOLOGIC FINDINGS

Traumatic rupture of the aorta has the appearance of an incised wound extending transversely or spirally. It may be partial or complete and involve the entire aortic wall. There is usually no evidence of existing disease such as medial necrosis, atheroma, or syphilitic aortitis, and the histologic appearance of the aorta in these patients, many of whom are young, is usually normal.

It has been shown that a pressure between 1000 and 3000 mm. Hg is required to rupture the aorta. If complete rupture of all layers occurs, immediate exsanguination is likely, but if the adventitia remains intact, 15% to 20% of patients survive the initial injury. In those who reach the hospital alive, the intima and media are usually ruptured, and continuity is retained by intact adventitia. Although this adventitia may contain the aortic pressure, rupture usually follows. If the diagnosis is not made in the acute situation and the patient survives, a chronic false aneurysm develops,[5] which may enlarge, rupture spontaneously, or later be demonstrated radiographically as a calcified aneurysm.

Although it is not unusual for these patients to have other major injuries, many patients sustaining rupture of the aorta have no other apparent injury. In those with severe associated injuries, it is not surprising that the aortic damage is often initially overlooked. Unfortunately, rupture of the traumatic aneurysm may be fatal.

ASSOCIATED INJURIES

There may be no external manifestations of a severe closed-chest injury; however, associated injuries may be obvious (Tables 50–3 and 50–4). These include serious head injuries, closed and compound fractures, hematuria from pelvic fractures or bladder and kidney injuries, and intra-abdominal bleeding from visceral trauma. Although associated thoracic injuries such as pneumothorax or hemothorax call attention to a chest injury coupled with fractured ribs, involvement of the thoracic spine confuses the situation, and the mediastinal changes seen on the chest film may be thought to be related to such injuries.

Management of associated injuries may be lifesaving in the resuscitative period. However, once stabilized, all severely injured patients should have adequate evaluation of the mediastinum and thoracic aorta if any abnormalities are present on the chest film.[3, 4, 6, 14, 21, 30]

CLINICAL PRESENTATION

Few conditions are of such sudden onset as the catastrophic outcome characteristic of traumatic rupture of the thoracic aorta. The single most important factor in considering the diagnosis of acute traumatic rupture is awareness of its occurrence in those involved in violent accidents that include sudden deceleration, regardless of external evidence of injury. The spectrum of the initial presentation ranges from no evidence of external injury in a stable and otherwise healthy-appearing patient with only minor complaints to multiple injuries in a patient with evidence of two or three life-threatening problems, including head injuries or intra-abdominal bleeding. It should be emphasized that there is a twofold increase in acute aortic transections in patients who are ejected from the vehicle, which explains the high incidence of aortic transection in patients thrown from motorcycles.[15, 16]

DIAGNOSIS

The diagnosis of acute aortic transection is made by the history of a violent, sudden, decelerating accident. The physical findings in this setting may be entirely negative but often include a history of severe chest pain, hypertension in the upper extremities, evidence of blood loss, and shock; in addition, a harsh systolic murmur may be present in the precordium or posterior scapular area.[21, 28] The patient may present with anuria and may be paraplegic (Fig. 50–24). More often, in those surviving acute transection, pulses may be equal. An important radiographic finding is widening of the mediastinum, often with blunting of the contour of the aortic knob.[3, 12, 21] Clearly, widening does not always indicate transection of the aorta, and there are instances of transection without this finding. Also, in acutely injured patients, the anteroposterior chest film frequently demonstrates a widened mediastinum. Therefore, posteroanterior chest films should be obtained if possible. The chest film may also demonstrate deviation of the trachea to the right, pleural effusion, and depression of the left main-stem bronchus. There may also be associated rib fractures and pneumothorax, along with contusion of the lungs. In the presence of any of these findings, or if there is suspicion of transection of the aorta, an aortogram must be obtained.[3, 12, 17, 21] Although this may lead to more frequent aortograms with a lower incidence of positive findings, the high mortality associated with a failure to diagnose makes the procedure justifiable. In the presence of first rib fracture, significant sternal injury, or posteriorly displaced clavicular fractures, aortography is generally indicated.

MANAGEMENT

Approximately 80% of patients with traumatic rupture of the aorta succumb before reaching the hospital.[22, 27] Without treatment, the majority of survivors die of secondary hemorrhage within the next 2 weeks. A small number survive and

TABLE 50–4. Extrathoracic Injuries

Facial lacerations
Facial fractures
Head injuries
Liver, spleen, pancreas injury
Bladder injury
Pelvic fracture
Kidney contusion and laceration
Dislocated hip
Long bone fracture

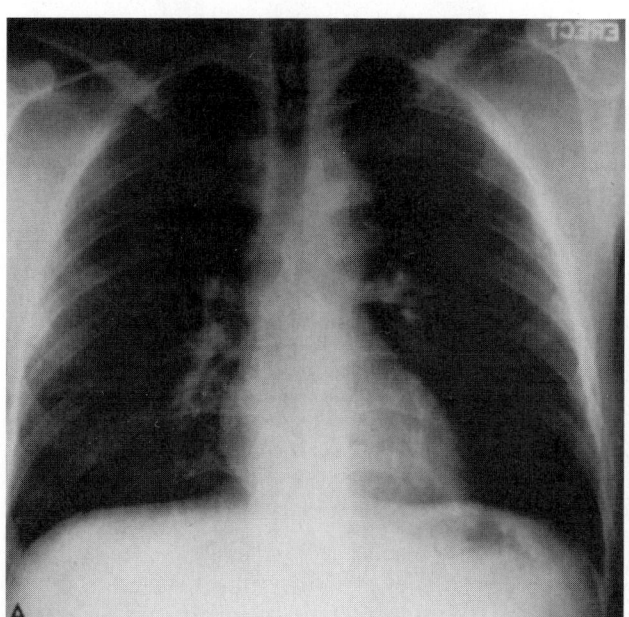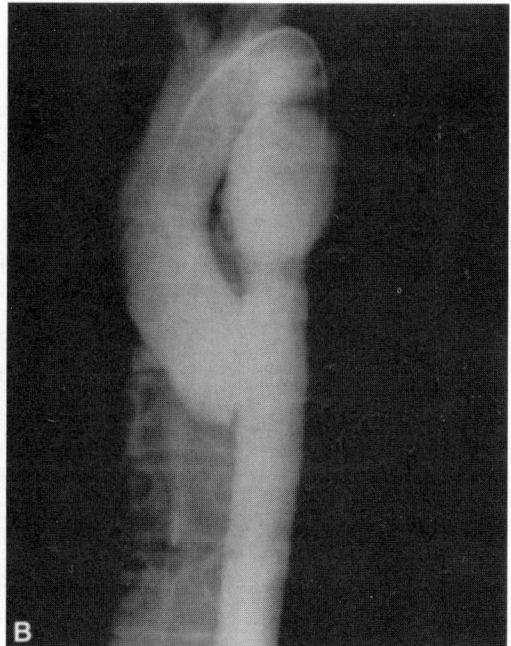

Figure 50–24. *A,* Chest film of a young man whose injuries in a severe auto accident resulted in paraplegia. This film shows a subtle widening of the mediastinum. He was admitted for evaluation and myelogram 4 years after the accident. *B,* Aortogram demonstrating chronic false aneurysm secondary to aortic transection.

develop chronic aneurysms and many future complications. For these reasons, early repair should be performed in most patients with acute traumatic rupture of the aorta.

When the diagnosis is established, preparation for operation should be made immediately.[12, 24] Resuscitation and supportive measures are initiated; other critical injuries may require prior or simultaneous treatment.[2] In some instances, surgery on the aorta may be delayed and treated medially with beta-blockers and hypotensive agents. The operation is complicated by the need to cross-clamp the aorta in the region of or above the subclavian artery and at the same time prevent left ventricular strain as well as protect the viscera and the spinal cord from ischemia.

In the first report of successful repair of traumatic rupture of the aorta, it was noted that following cross-clamping of the aorta of a 30-year-old man without bypass support for a period of 17 minutes, during which a 3-mm. tear was closed at the isthmus, the heart became grossly distended, the electrocardiographic pattern became bizarre, and the systolic blood pressure rose to 200 mm. Hg. Thus, this simple approach is inadequate.

There is current evidence that if the operation is performed expeditiously, bypass support is not necessary.[1, 11] Many, however, believe that it is preferable to give more attention to possible renal damage or the risk of paraplegia in these patients. Although paraplegia may be part of the process itself, reduction in arterial blood flow through the main branch of the anterior spinal artery supplying the spinal cord as it originates in the region of the lower thoracic and upper lumbar segmental vessels may produce spinal cord ischemia and can often be avoided. Since cardiac dilation and strain, ischemia to the visceral vessels, and paraplegia may occur, careful consideration must be given to these complications if operation is undertaken without bypass.[2, 4, 7, 19, 20, 31]

For correction of rupture of the descending thoracic aorta, a left lateral thoracotomy is performed, with entry into the chest through the fourth or fifth interspace. The mediastinal structures must be dissected, care being taken to preserve the vagus, phrenic, and recurrent laryngeal nerves. Proximal and distal control must be obtained without entering the hema-

toma. Although hypothermia alone was initially used, this was rapidly supported by cardiopulmonary bypass or left heart bypass. A troublesome complication of these types of bypass is postoperative bleeding secondary to the necessity of total-body heparinization. Femoral vein to femoral artery bypass with a pump oxygenator can also be used for partial cardiopulmonary support, but again, systemic heparinization is required.

Recently, left atrial to descending aorta or femoral artery bypass has been greatly improved and can support the distal circulation without the use of heparin; it is probably the preferred method of bypass today.[25]

Another method is the use of heparin-bonded shunts from the ascending aorta proximal to the aneurysm to the lower thoracic aorta or the femoral artery (or from the left ventricle to the femoral artery). The aorta should be clamped between the carotid and subclavian artery, the hematoma opened, and the aorta repaired either primarily or with the use of a Dacron graft. In most instances, primary repair is not feasible and the use of a graft is mandatory, since repair of the aorta may place undue tension on the suture line. A Carlen double-lumen endotracheal tube is usually used, with selective ventilation of the right lung and collapse of the left lung making exposure and dissection much easier.[17, 18, 31]

It is clear that these lesions can be safely operated on today with simple clamping of the aorta, pharmacologic support, and efforts to lower the left ventricular pressure with nitroprusside. Crawford and Rubio[11] and Appelbaum and colleagues[1] have presented data emphasizing the safety of this technique; they believe that the incidence of paraplegia is no greater in patients managed with bypass or a shunt and that operative time and blood loss are usually less with this direct approach.

As soon as the operative repair is completed, the chest is closed and ventilatory support is continued as necessary, depending on associated lung and other chest injuries as well as nonthoracic injuries. Long-term results have been excellent following repair of transection; in fact, the morbidity and mortality are usually related to other injuries rather than to the transection itself.

Management of Chronic Traumatic Aneurysms of the Aorta. Only 2% of patients with acute transection of the aorta survive to develop chronic aneurysms.[5, 13] Symptoms of such lesions include chest pain, hoarseness, cough, and dysphagia. In some patients, the lesion is found on routine roentgenogram as an enlarging aortic shadow. In general, a patient with a chronic aneurysm shows evidence of instability with the passage of time, usually due to the increasing size of the aneurysm. When a chronic traumatic aneurysm of the aorta is diagnosed, operative correction is recommended. This recommendation is based on the fact that over half of these patients ultimately show instability; in addition, there are no criteria to predict which aneurysms will remain stable. The majority of these lesions occur in young, healthy individuals; the operative mortality is low, and the results are quite successful.

The mortality related to management of acute transections is less then 10%, and the deaths are usually caused by associated injuries. In many series of chronic transections with aortic aneurysms, the mortality is less than 5%.[5, 11, 13, 31] The primary complications include recurrent laryngeal nerve injury and reoperation for bleeding. There is risk of a false aneurysm at the suture line, which is unusual, and phrenic nerve injury has been reported. In general, the morbidity in the management of these patients is related to the associated injuries and not to the operative procedure itself in either the acute or the chronic form of aortic aneurysm.

Management of Ascending Aortic Injury. The diagnosis of ascending aortic transection should be suspected in patients who have a fracture of the first rib.[9, 25] Mediastinal widening is usually evident on the chest film. A powerful and unique force is required for fracture of the first rib, and this force is transmitted throughout the thorax. Therefore, in addition to transection of a bronchus or of the ascending aorta, transection at the aortic isthmus may occur. The diagnosis is confirmed by arteriography (Fig. 50–25).

Management of ascending aortic injuries involving the aorta at its attachment to the heart or the great vessels is

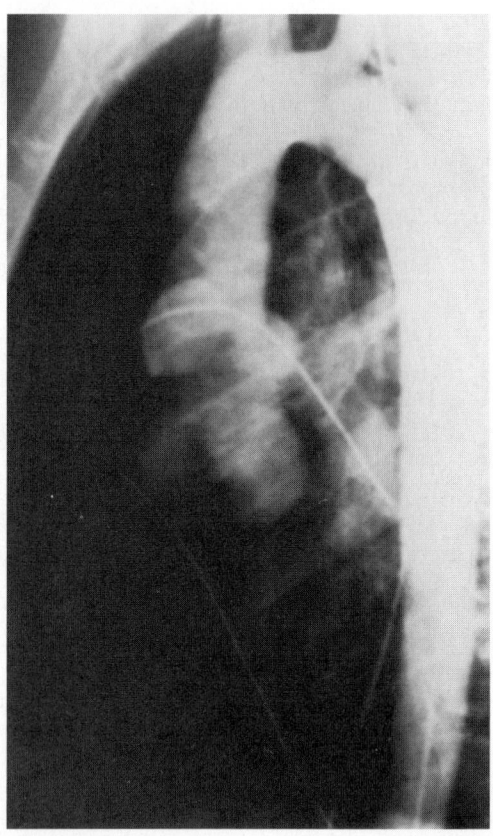

Figure 50–26. Film from a 20-year-old male involved in a motorcycle accident. He suffered a closed head injury, transection of the ascending aorta, and compound fractures of the left femur and tibia. The aortic injury was repaired successfully with primary suture through median sternotomy using cardiopulmonary bypass and cardioplegic arrest.

accomplished through a median sternotomy (Fig. 50–26). Full heparinization and cardiopulmonary bypass are usually required, although heparinized shunts may be utilized in some patients with great vessel injury.[9] Repair is accomplished with grafting of the ascending aorta or primary repair, depending on the extent of injury. Injury to the aortic valve may be such that valve replacement is necessary.

SELECTED REFERENCES

Bennett, D. E., and Cherry, J. K.: The natural history of traumatic aneurysms of the aorta. Surgery, *61*:516, 1967.
The incidence of chronic aneurysm following transection, the site, the time of death, and the prognosis of chronic aneurysms are discussed, with excellent references to the world literature.

Duhaylongsod, F. G., and Wolfe, W. G.: Traumatic thoracic aneurysms. *In* Moylan, J. A. (Ed.): Principles in Trauma Surgery, 2nd ed. New York, Gower Medical Publishing, 1991.
This edition incorporates color operation photographs along with the text.

Freed, T. A., Neal, M. P., Jr., and Vinik, M.: Roentgenographic findings in extracardiac injury secondary to blunt chest automobile trauma. A. J. R. Am. J. Roentgenol., *104*:424, 1968.
This thorough discussion of the diagnosis of traumatic injury of the aorta emphasizes the importance of routine chest films and arteriography.

Kirsh, M. M., Behrendt, D. M., Orringer, M. B., Gago, O., Gray, I. A., Jr., Mills, L. J., Walter, J. F., and Sloan, H.: The treatment of acute traumatic rupture of the aorta: A ten year experience. Ann. Surg., *184*:308, 1976.
This is one of the largest series published and thoroughly reviews the management of this problem and associated injuries.

Parmley, L. F., Mattingly, T. W., Manion, W. C., and Jahnke, E. J.: Nonpenetrating traumatic injury of the aorta. Cardiovasc. Surg., *17*:1086, 1958.
This classic reference to the pathology, clinical aspects, and management of nonpenetrating injuries of the aorta should be read by any surgeon involved with this problem.

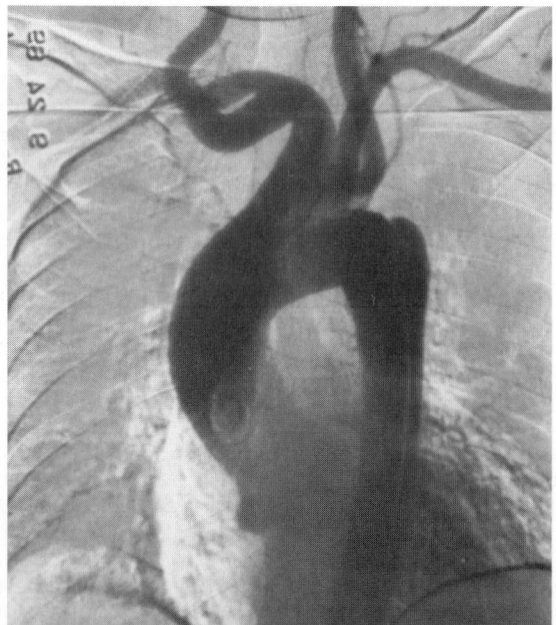

Figure 50–25. Aortogram demonstrates a transection of the ascending aorta with aortic insufficiency as well as transection at the isthmus. The patient's injuries were successfully managed, approaching the ascending aorta through a median sternotomy first; then the descending aortic tear was repaired via a left thoracotomy.

Pate, J. W.: Is traumatic rupture of the aorta misunderstood? Ann. Thorac. Surg., 57:530, 1994.
This editorial reviews problems in managing multiple injuries in patients with transection.

Spencer, F. C., Guerin, P. F., Blake, H. A., and Bahnson, H. T.: A report of fifteen patients with traumatic rupture of the thoracic aorta. J. Thorac. Cardiovasc. Surg., 41:1, 1961.
This article of an early series of 15 cases, 7 acute and 8 chronic, reviews the early problems with this lesion.

REFERENCES

1. Appelbaum, A., Karp, R. B., and Kirklin, J. W.: Surgical treatment for closed thoracic aortic injuries. J. Thorac. Cardiovasc. Surg., 71:458, 1976.
2. Aronstam, E. M., Gomez, A. C., O'Connell, T. J., Jr., and Geiger, J. P.: Recent surgical and pharmacologic experience with acute dissecting and traumatic aneurysms. J. Thorac. Cardiovasc. Surg., 59:231, 1970.
3. Attar, S., Ayella, R. J., and McLaughlin, J. S.: The widened mediastinum in trauma. Ann. Thorac. Surg., 13:435, 1972.
4. Ayella, R. J., Hankins, J. R., Turney, S. Z., and Cowley, R. A.: Ruptured thoracic aorta due to blunt trauma. J. Trauma, 17:199, 1977.
5. Bennett, D. E., and Cherry, J. K.: The natural history of traumatic aneurysms of the aorta. Surgery, 61:516, 1967.
6. Bodily, K., Perry, J. F., Jr., Strate, R. G., and Fischer, R. P.: The salvageability of patients with post-traumatic rupture of the descending thoracic aorta in a primary trauma center. J. Trauma, 17:754, 1977.
7. Burnsed, D. W., Weiss, J. B., Campbell, G. S., and Williams, G. D.: The relative merits of the heparin-bonded shunt vs. femorofemoral bypass for aortic arch injury. Surgery, 78:176, 1975.
8. Cammack, K., Rapport, R. L., Paul, J., and Baird, W. C.: Deceleration injuries of the thoracic aorta. Arch. Surg., 79:244, 1959.
9. Castagna, J., and Nelson, R. J.: Blunt injuries to branches of the aortic arch. J. Thorac. Cardiovasc. Surg., 69:521, 1975.
10. Connors, J. P., Ferguson, T. B., Roper, C. L., and Weldon, C. S.: The use of TDMAC-heparin shunt in replacement of the descending aorta. Ann. Surg., 181:735, 1975.
11. Crawford, E. S., and Rubio, P. A.: Reappraisal of adjuncts to avoid ischemia in the treatment of aneurysms of descending thoracic aorta. J. Thorac. Cardiovasc. Surg., 66:693, 1973.
12. DeMeules, J. E., Cramer, G., and Perry, J. F., Jr.: Rupture of aorta and great vessels due to blunt thoracic trauma. J. Thorac. Cardiovasc. Surg., 61:440, 1971.
13. Fleming, A. W., and Green, D. C.: Traumatic aneurysms of the thoracic aorta. Ann. Thorac. Surg., 18:91, 1974.
14. Freed, T. A., Neal, M. P., Jr., and Vinik, M.: Roentgenographic findings in extracardiac injury secondary to blunt chest automobile trauma. Am. J. Roentgenol., 104:424, 1968.
15. Gazzaniga, A. B., Khuri, E. I., Mir-Sepasi, H. M., and Bartlett, R. H.: Rupture of the thoracic aorta following blunt trauma. Arch. Surg., 110:1119, 1975.
16. Greendyke, R. M.: Traumatic rupture of aorta. JAMA, 195:119, 1966.
17. Kirsh, M. M., Behrendt, D. M., Orringer, M. B., Gago, O., Gray, L. J., Jr., Mills, L. J., Walter, J. F., and Sloan, H.: The treatment of acute traumatic rupture of the aorta: A 10-year experience. Ann. Surg., 184:308, 1976.
18. Kirsh, M. M., Kahn, D. R., Crane, J. D., Anastasia, L. F., Lui, A. H., Moores, W. Y., Vathayanon, S., Bookstein, J. J., and Sloan, H.: Repair of acute traumatic rupture of the aorta without extracorporeal circulation. Ann. Thorac. Surg., 10:227, 1970.
19. Krause, A. H., Ferguson, T. B., and Weldon, C. S.: Thoracic aneurysmectomy utilizing the TDMAC-heparin shunt. Ann. Thorac. Surg., 14:123, 1972.
20. Lawrence, G. H., Hessel, E. A., Sauvage, L. R., and Krause, A. H.: Results of the use of the TDMAC-heparin shunt in the surgery of aneurysms of the descending thoracic aorta. J. Thorac. Cardiovasc. Surg., 73:393, 1977.
21. Marsh, D. G., and Sturm, J. T.: Traumatic aortic rupture: Roentgenographic indications for angiography. Ann. Thorac. Surg., 21:337, 1976.
22. Parmley, L. F., Mattingly, T. W., Manion, W. C., and Jahnke, E. J., Jr.: Nonpenetrating traumatic injury of the aorta. Circulation, 17:1086, 1958.
23. Passaro, E., and Pace, W. G.: Traumatic rupture of the aorta. Surgery, 46:787, 1959.
24. Pickard, L. R., Mattox, K. L., Espada, R., Beall, A. C., Jr., and DeBakey, M. E.: Transection of the descending thoracic aorta secondary to blunt trauma. J. Trauma, 17:749, 1977.
25. Richardson, J. D., McElvein, R. B., and Trinkle, J. K.: First rib fracture: A hallmark of severe trauma. Ann. Surg., 181:251, 1975.
26. Rindfleisch, W.: Zur Entstehung und Heilung des Aneurysmsma dissecans aortae. Arch. Pathol. Anat., 13:374, 1893.
27. Spencer, F. C., Guerin, P. F., Blake, H. A., and Bahnson, H. T.: A report of fifteen patients with traumatic rupture of the thoracic aorta. J. Thorac. Cardiovasc. Surg., 41:1, 1961.
28. Symbas, P. N.: Great vessel injury. Am. Heart J., 93:518, 1977.
29. Symbas, P. N., Tyras, D. H., Ware, R. E., and Diorio, D. A.: Traumatic rupture of the aorta. Ann. Surg., 178:6, 1973.
30. Turney, S. Z., Attar, S., Ayella, R., Crowley, R. A., and McLaughlin, J.: Traumatic rupture of the aorta: A five-year experience. J. Thorac. Cardiovasc. Surg., 71:727, 1976.
31. Wolfe, W. G., Kleinman, L. H., Wechsler, A. S., and Sabiston, D. C., Jr.: Heparin-coated shunts for lesions of the descending thoracic aorta. Arch. Surg., 112:1481, 1977.

DISSECTING ANEURYSMS OF THE AORTA

Walter G. Wolfe, M.D.

CLASSIFICATION AND INCIDENCE

DeBakey classified aortic dissections into Type I, Type II, and Type III (Fig. 50–27) and urged emergency surgical intervention as the treatment of choice for nearly all patients. During the early 1970s, this original classification was reduced to two groups, those involving the ascending aorta and those originating in the descending aorta.[1, 3, 8] This was the result of evolving attitudes toward surgical therapy as well as the fact that only 10% of patients have involvement limited to the ascending aorta. Moreover, the clinical problems encountered in the patients with ascending versus descending dissections, the presence of hypertension, and the pathophysiologic aspects leading to the patient's death are somewhat different. Ascending and descending dissections should also be categorized as to whether they are acute or chronic. Ascending dissections can be termed Type A and descending lesions Type B. Type C indicates fatal, inoperable dissections.[1] The incidence of acute aortic dissection is two to three times more frequent than that of ruptured abdominal aortic aneurysms.

Acute aortic dissection is the most common catastrophic event involving the aorta.[24] There are approximately 60,000 patients who have dissecting aneurysms in the United States annually.[24] Aortic dissections are three times more frequent in males; however, 50% of the dissections seen in females younger than the age of 40 occur in pregnancy.[16] Acute dissection occurs most frequently between the ages of 45 and 70; the incidence appears to be greater in patients with Marfan's syndrome or congenital heart disease, such as coarctation of the aorta or bicuspid aortic valve disease.[18] A history of hypertension is present in 80% to 90% of patients. It is clear that the incidence of hypertension is over 95% in patients with descending dissections.[7]

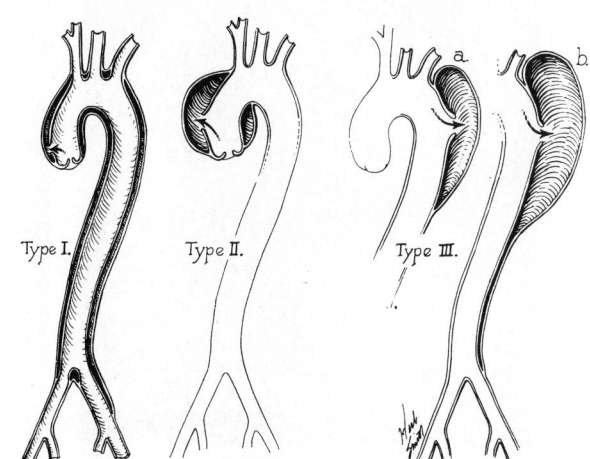

Figure 50–27. DeBakey's classification of dissecting aortic aneurysms: Type I, Type II, and Type III. (From DeBakey, M. E., Henly, W. S., Cooley, D. A., et al.: Surgical management of dissecting aneurysms of the aorta. J. Thorac. Cardiovasc. Surg., 49:130, 1965.)

ETIOLOGY AND PATHOPHYSIOLOGY

The aorta maintains a flexible blood flow pattern required for organ support under many different conditions and is subjected to 3 billion pulsations during an average life span. Unfortunately, there are several serious disease processes that have the potential to weaken the aortic wall. Although syphilitic aortitis has almost disappeared, atherosclerosis remains very common. In dissecting aneurysms, as in other diseases affecting the aortic wall, the underlying defect is the destruction of the medial layer that contains the elastic fibers. Although medial necrosis is associated with Marfan's syndrome, the relationship of this lesion to aortas with dissection or to aging without dissection is unknown. Hypertension, atherosclerosis, coarctation, epinephrine-induced dissection, and endocrine factors may cause medial necrosis. The epinephrine effect that produces a hyperkinetic heart may be important even through hypertension is not present. Pregnancy may incite the hypertension and hyperkinetic heart, and these responses may represent dissections in these patients. Trauma may also cause dissection. Medial necrosis is seen in congenital vessel anomalies in addition to Marfan's syndrome. Because, in most patients, acute aortic dissection occurs in the well-defined region of the aortic media, it may also be associated with necrosis, hemorrhage, or degenerative changes in this layer.

The aortic wall is elastic and constantly expanding during the pressure pulse wave and serves to dampen the suddenness of the compression wave. This is accomplished by the circumferential placement of intermingled collagen fibers and smooth muscle cells in the tunica media, which are arranged in laminar layers between layers of elastin fibers. The elastin allows expansion of the wall by its rubberlike nature, and muscle cells act as shock absorbers contracting in response to the acceleration of the systolic pulse. Collagen provides tensile strength to the wall and protection from rupture should high tension develop.

Another major stress acting on the inner aortic wall is longitudinal shear. Viscous blood flows through the aorta and places a considerable and continuous shearing force along the wall in the direction of flow. The high-risk shear points of the aorta are often most affected by proliferative changes in early atherosclerosis.

Most dissections occur in the inner one third to one half of the aorta wall. When medial degeneration of the wall of the thoracic aorta has occurred, the likelihood of dissection is increased by the diminished cohesiveness of the layers of the aortic wall. Medial necrosis leads to decreased intimal adherence, and specific mechanical factors may or may not cause dissection. Repeated motion of the aorta related to the beating heart causes flexion stresses, most marked in the ascending aorta and in the first portion of the descending aorta. This stress occurs some 35 to 40 million times per year. Along with this repeated motion of the aorta, patients with aortic stenosis, bicuspid aortic valves, and pure Marfan's syndrome have a greater risk of dissection. Hemodynamic forces in the bloodstream related to the pulse wave propagated by each cardiac systole act on the wall of the aorta and, most markedly, the proximal aorta. The combination of factors eventually leads to an intimal tear, following which there is a propagation of a dissecting hematoma of varying depth and length into the media of the aortic wall.

Most commonly, however, tears originating in the ascending aorta proceed along the entire length of the aorta, whereas those that originate distal to the left subclavian dissect distally into the descending thoracic aorta and abdominal aorta (Fig. 50–28). This hematoma dissects and commonly re-enters the lumen of the aorta. Multiple entry and re-entry points are seen throughout the aorta. Ascending dissection may proceed retrograde to involve coronary arteries and pericardium and to rupture into the mediastinum, leading to death. Dissection back toward the coronary arteries and aortic valve frequently produces aortic insufficiency, a situation that is poorly tolerated and is associated with cardiac failure and pulmonary edema.[1, 13] Those descending dissections that rupture into the pleural cavity are usually fatal.

The surgical approach to aortic dissection is based on the pathogenesis of this lesion.[30] An acute aortic dissection involving the ascending aorta usually affects the entire aorta. Only some 10% of the patients have involvement limited to the ascending aorta or the aortic arch. As the dissection advances distally, the visceral vessels are involved in varying degrees, as are the arteries to the brain. Usually, the noncoronary cusp becomes incompetent as the dissection proceeds toward the anulus, and this cusp prolapses into the left ventricle to produce acute aortic insufficiency (Fig. 50–29). Other cusps in spiraling dissections are usually spared as the

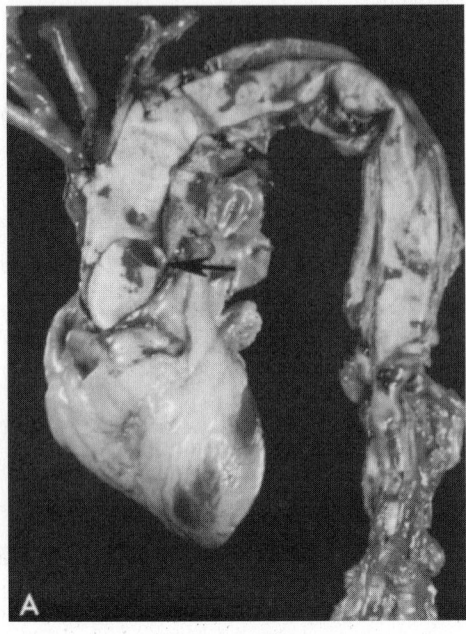

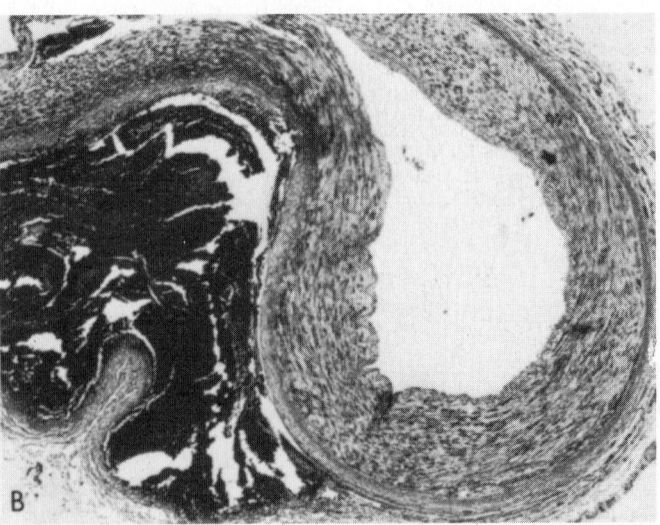

Figure 50–28. *A,* Pathologic specimen demonstrating an intimal tear in the ascending aorta distal to the aortic valve. The dissection involves the entire aorta. *B,* Example of the hematoma in the false lumen compressing the true lumen of a renal artery.

coronary arteries anchor the media, intima, and adventitia in this area and protect them from separation. If the dissection involves a coronary artery, sudden death is likely as a result of myocardial ischemia. Blood may enter the pericardium and cause tamponade or rupture into the mediastinum, either of which may lead to sudden death.

Dissections that involve the descending aorta with the point of origin distal to the subclavian artery may proceed to the subclavian artery and head vessels and often progress distally for the length of the aorta. Again, multiple re-entry points are not uncommon and the visceral vessels may be involved to varying degrees, these vessels originating from either the true or the false lumen of the aorta (Fig. 50–30).

Acute dissection of the ascending aorta usually produces aortic insufficiency and entry of blood into the pericardium, causing tamponade (Fig. 50–31). Varying degrees of coronary as well as cerebral insufficiency may also occur (Fig. 50–32). Many times, the blood flow to the visceral organs is spared through perfusion of the false lumen as the aortic dissection advances. It is not uncommon for one renal artery to be perfused by the true lumen and the other by the false lumen (Fig. 50–33). In both ascending and descending aortic dissections, the extremities may be involved, producing varying degrees of vascular insufficiency.

CLINICAL PRESENTATION

Pain is the most frequent symptom of patients presenting with acute aortic dissection. It is best described as cata-

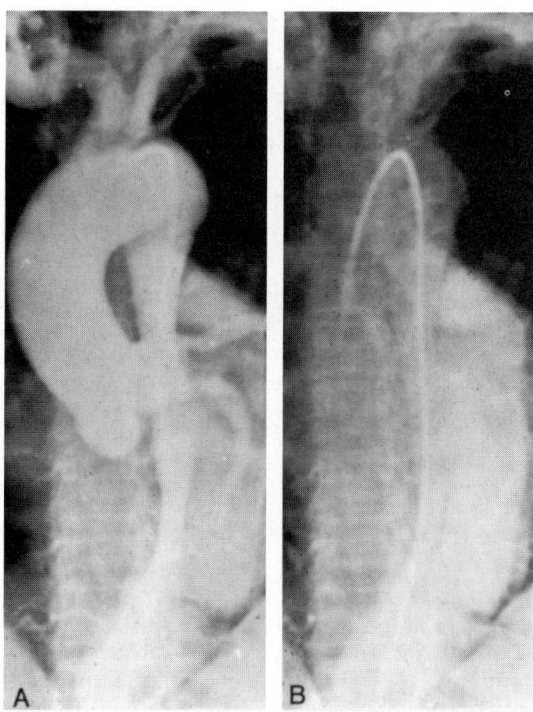

Figure 50–30. *A*, Example of a descending dissection showing marked compression of the thoracic aorta, normal aortic cusps, arch, and head vessels with marked compression of the descending thoracic aorta continuing on into the abdominal aorta. *B*, Late film shows opacification of the false channel.

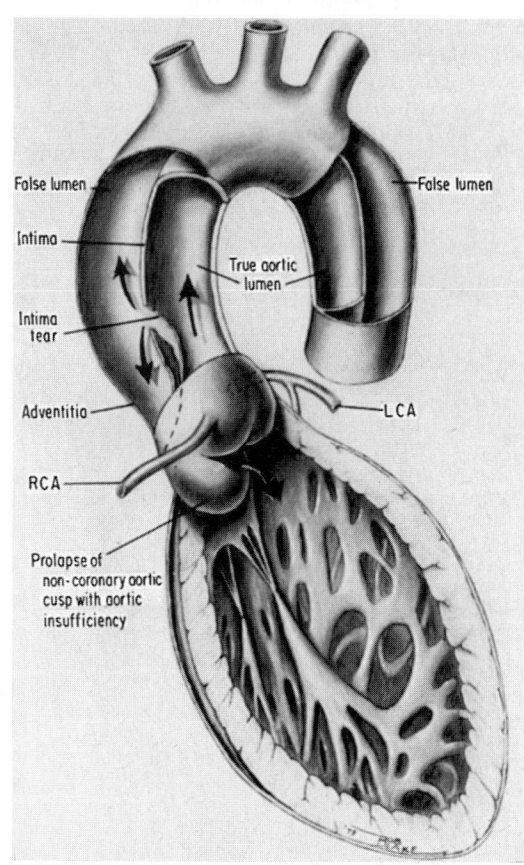

Figure 50–29. Illustration of the pathophysiologic mechanism of acute ascending dissection. The intimal tear originates above the aortic valve, and the dissection proceeds down the thoracic aorta and into the abdominal aorta. Mechanisms of aortic regurgitation in this situation were produced by circumferential widening of the aortic root and separation of the aortic cusp. There may be displacement of the aortic cusp substantially below the level of the anulus produced by the pressure of the dissecting hematoma. At times there may be actual disruption of the anular leaflet support leading to a flail cusp.

strophic chest pain, so severe that the individual almost immediately seeks medical attention. Although many terms are used to describe this pain, including *tearing, throbbing,* or *ripping,* the onset is almost always sudden. After the initial episode, the pain may be confined to the chest or may be substernal, in the back, along the route of the aorta, in the abdomen, or in a combination of these sites. Often the pain radiates into the upper or lower extremities. The point to be emphasized is the fact that the pain is catastrophic and may take one of several forms. Unless the history and physical examination are carefully considered, the correct diagnosis may not be made.

In 92% of patients with catastrophic pain who presented at one emergency clinic the pain was described as being located in the back, chest, or abdomen, and 30% of patients presented with pain in the extremity. A neurologic deficit was present in 30%, and 25% had nausea and vomiting. Dyspnea is not uncommon, and pulmonary edema may be present. Many patients may be normotensive or hypotensive in the aftermath of the acute episode, or this finding may be the result of pericardial tamponade.

Physical Examination. Frequently, the seriously ill patients present with shock despite previously known hypertension. Examination may demonstrate a differential blood pressure and pulse in the upper extremities or diminished or differential pulses in the legs. The patient who presents with both catastrophic chest pain and diminished pulses must be immediately considered to have had an aortic dissection. Neurologic findings are clearly related to the degree of dissection and to involvement of the arch vessels involved in the cerebral blood supply.

The differential diagnosis in this group of patients includes myocardial infarction, rupture of the sinus of Valsalva, cerebrovascular accident, acute surgical abdomen, pulmonary embolism, arterial thrombosis or embolism of the aortic bifurcation, or occlusion of the peripheral arteries. There may be

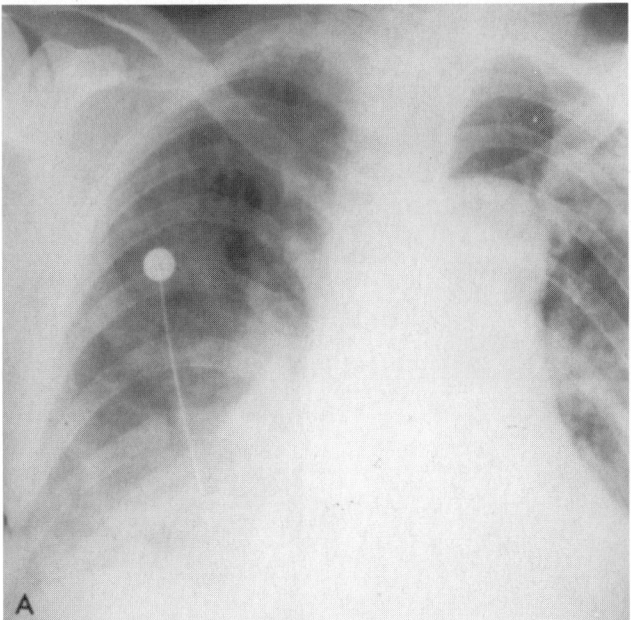

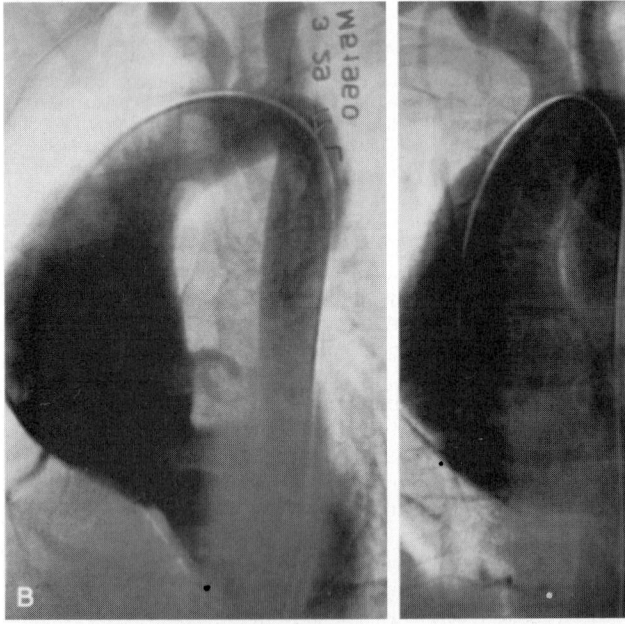

Figure 50–31. *A,* Chest film of a patient with acute ascending dissection illustrating massive pulmonary edema produced by aortic insufficiency. *B,* Arteriogram demonstrating aortic valve incompetence and filling of ventricle with contrast material.

a variety of murmurs and bruits varying from that of aortic insufficiency to those over major branches of the aorta, such as the carotid or renal arteries. Most significant is the difference in blood pressure that may be seen between two upper extremities. The patient may appear to be in shock while the pressure in the opposite extremity shows marked hypertension. When the condition is suggested, the patient is immediately prepared for arteriography to achieve an objective diagnosis.

DIAGNOSIS

Because severe chest pain is the common presenting symptom, the primary problem is that of differentiating acute dissection from acute myocardial infarction. The accessory

clinical findings are important. Electrocardiographic abnormalities include left-axis deviation, left ventricular hypertrophy, ischemic changes of varying degrees, conduction defects, and dysrhythmias. However, in none was the electrocardiogram diagnostic of acute myocardial infarction. In contrast, chest roentgenography yielded what was considered to be a normal chest film in only 10% of patients. The remainder of the patients had a dilated aorta, a widened mediastinum with cardiomegaly, pulmonary edema, or a mass effect with or without pleural effusion. Therefore, the plain chest film is of critical importance, and a normal film in this group of patients is extremely unusual.

Mediastinal widening is highly suggestive but not necessarily diagnostic of aortic dissection, because tumors can produce a similar change. Calcium in the wall of the aorta, with obvious widening beyond the calcium, is also suggestive but again is not diagnostic. Patients presenting with a combination of chest pain and abnormal chest film should have aortography. If this study reveals splitting of the contrast column, distortion of the contrast column, or aortic insufficiency, the test is positive. If a computed tomogram has been obtained, an aortogram may still be necessary to define the origin and extent of the dissection (Fig. 50–34).

In the majority of patients the aortogram localizes the origin of the dissection either distal to the left subclavian artery or in the ascending aorta. When the diagnosis has been confirmed, determination of whether the dissection is ascending or descending is important in deciding the type of management.

Survival of Untreated Dissection. The lethality of this condition makes early diagnosis and appropriate therapy mandatory. This is emphasized by Hirst's review, in which the 15-minute mortality was approximately 20%. At 24 hours, 40% of the patients had died and by 48 hours the death rate was 50%. At 2 weeks, only 20% of the untreated patients were alive; only 10% were alive at 1 year (Fig. 50–35). Therefore, a high index of suspicion is imperative in this group of patients.

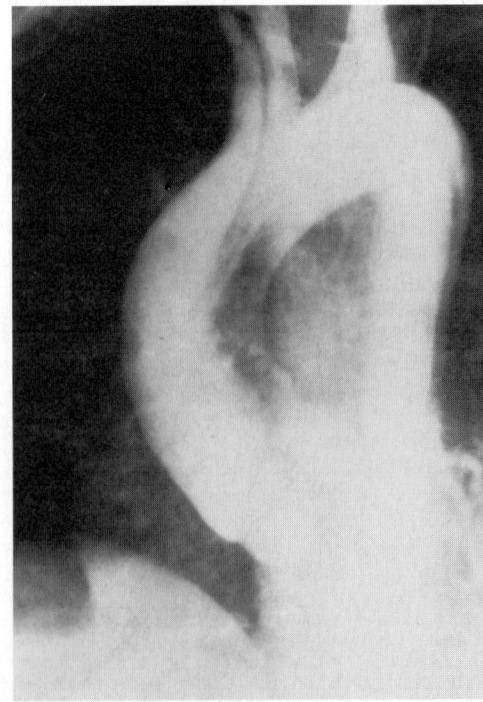

Figure 50–32. Arteriogram revealing ascending dissection with marked involvement of the innominate and arch vessels. The dissection continues distally into the abdominal aorta.

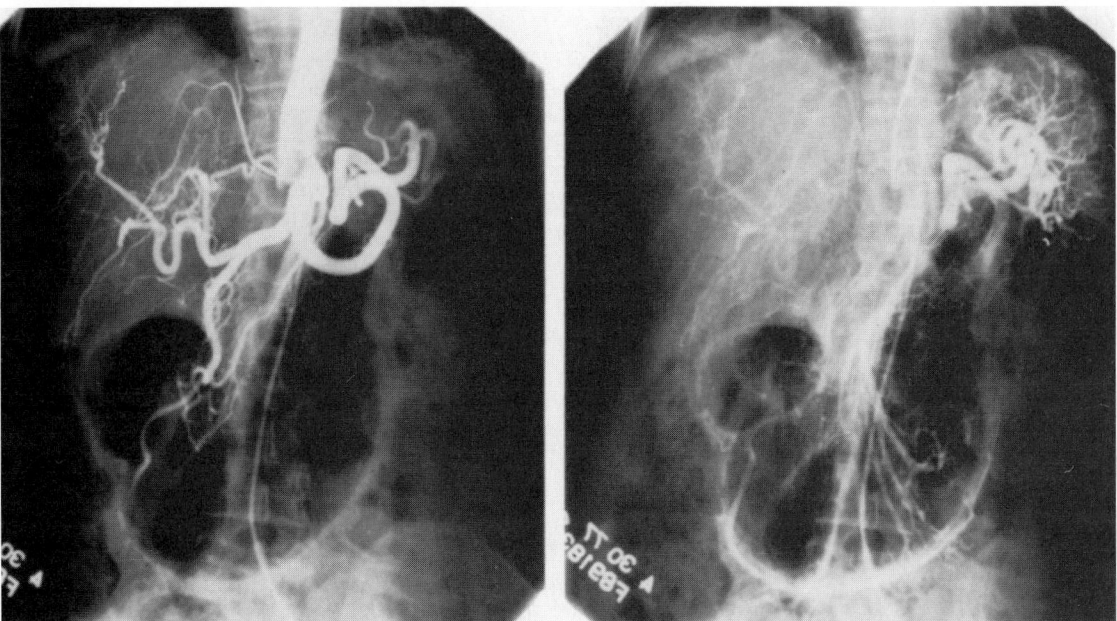

Figure 50-33. Abdominal aortogram revealing the celiac axis originating from the true lumen and no filling of either renal vessels or distal visceral vessels from the true lumen. Late film shows filling of the superior mesenteric vessels from the false lumen.

MANAGEMENT

Wheat and colleagues[28] pioneered modern pharmacologic hypotensive therapy for acute dissecting aneurysms of the aorta. They reduced both mean and systemic arterial pressure and maximum rate of tension development (dp/dt) through the administration of trimethaphan, reserpine, and guanethidine. The goal was conversion of all acute aortic dissections to subacute or chronic status. Then, after careful evaluation, treatment by elective operation was reserved for any complications that arose. They initiated this therapy for all patients with dissection, and early results showed an impressive 1-year survival of 84%. Nevertheless, there are clearly serious limitations to nonoperative therapy.[8, 27] Although many authorities originally employed pharmacologic therapy and reserved a surgical approach for patients with localized rupture, tamponade, or associated severe aortic insufficiency, it became evident that adoption of nonsurgical management did not ensure the high 1-year survival that was initially attained.[4, 17] One substantial advantage of induced hypotensive therapy is that it can be instituted in a community hospital after the initial diagnosis of dissecting aneurysm, with subsequent stabilization and transport to a cardiovascular surgical center.

Complications of an antihypertensive regimen, however, have included drug sensitivity and aggravation of concomitant renal failure. Sensitivity to drugs varies in each patient; trimethaphan may cause respiratory arrest, and the cerebral effects of reserpine are common. Nitroprusside has replaced these agents in the management of acute aortic dissection because of its effectiveness in lowering blood pressure, ease of administration, and rapid control.[21] However, some question has arisen as to its effectiveness in protecting against continued dissection despite lowering of the arterial pressure after the effect of increased aortic dp/dt. It is believed that intravenous nitroprusside is the agent of choice in controlling blood pressure in acute aortic dissection. Propranolol and methyldopa may be administered simultaneously, and when pressure is controlled the nitroprusside may be slowly discontinued. Although lowering of the blood pressure is mandatory in these patients, urinary output must also be carefully monitored and maintained. It is important that phy-

sicians who manage acute aortic dissection be familiar with the use of antihypersensitive drugs in this group of patients, because their roles in acute management and in the postoperative period are of great importance.

The consensus concerning the principles of management of acute aortic dissections has evolved from the collective experience of the past 20 years.[1, 3, 8, 14, 21, 26] After the initial presentation and diagnosis, time should be devoted to stabilization of the patient and utilization of antihypertensive therapy (usually nitroprusside) before and during aortography. During this time, all necessary preparations for operation can be made. Aortography should confirm the diagnosis of either an ascending or a descending dissection, at which point therapy, whether definitive or expectant, is chosen.

Ascending Dissections. Nearly all patients with ascending aortic dissection should be managed surgically immediately after the diagnosis is established. Acute aortic dissection of the ascending aorta almost invariably involves the entire aorta, except in 10% of patients (Fig. 50–36), in whom the involvement is limited to the ascending aorta or the aortic arch. Dissection begins proximal in the ascending aorta and continues around the arch to the iliac arteries. The visceral vessels are involved to varying degrees, as are the head vessels. The early causes of death in these patients are pericardial tamponade, rupture into the mediastinum, or acute aortic insufficiency with cardiac and renal failure. These are basically mechanical problems, and therefore surgical correction is mandatory.

Although the first successful treatment of dissecting aneurysm of the aorta using the fenestration operation was reported by DeBakey and colleagues in 1955,[7] this operation is now rarely used. DeBakey's group reported the most successful results with surgical therapy of the dissecting aneurysm in 179 patients, with a survival of 79%.[8] The most favored operative approach at present is a median sternotomy with cardiopulmonary bypass. Cannulation is made through the femoral artery; most patients have bloody fluid within the pericardium that may produce tamponade. The goal of the operation, then, is to correct the aortic insufficiency, either with aortic valve replacement or more often with resuspension of the aortic valve, and to graft the ascending aorta

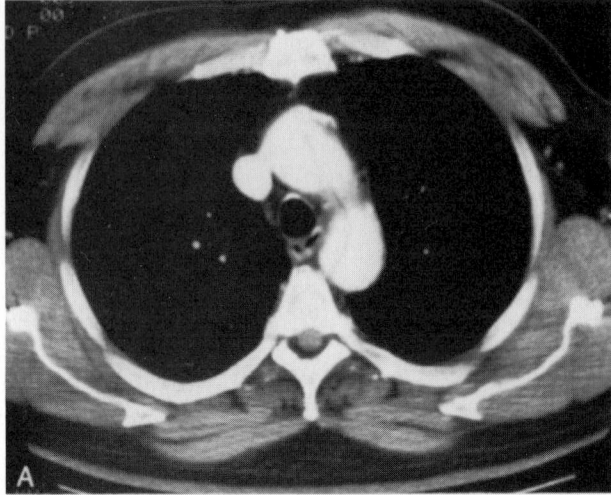
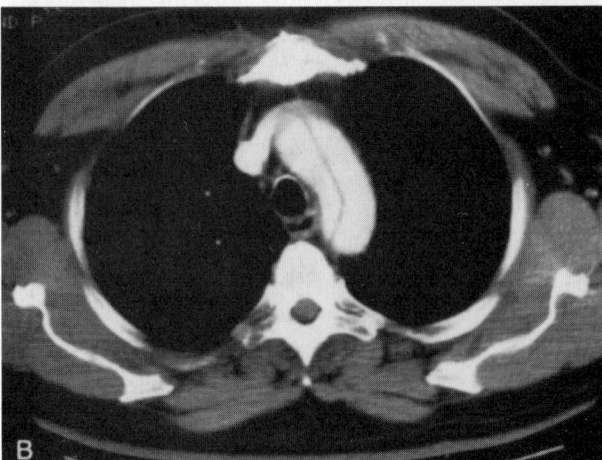
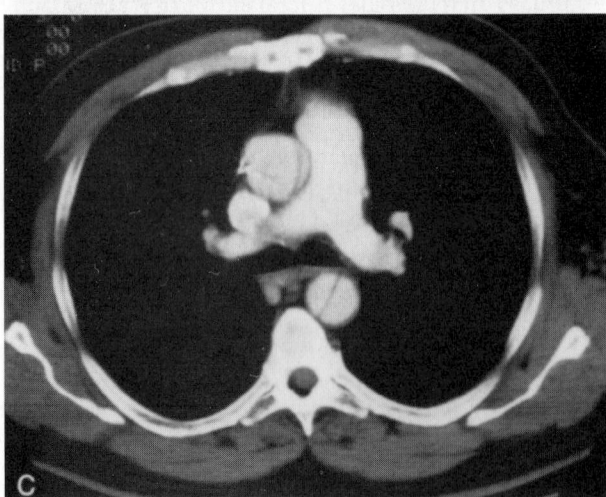

Figure 50–34. *A* to *C*, Computed tomography slices of a patient with a Type I dissecting aortic aneurysm demonstrating the dissection in the ascending aorta, arch, and descending aorta.

is then administered; most normotensive patients are given propranolol.

Descending Aortic Dissection. Dissections confined to the descending aorta can usually be carefully monitored. The life-threatening nature of descending aortic dissection is determined by, first, rupture into the pleural space, and, second, involvement of the visceral vessels. After the diagnosis has been confirmed and hypotensive therapy instituted, monitoring under close observation is imperative. Indications for immediate operative intervention include failure to control hypertension, continued pain, expansion of the aneurysm, or signs or symptoms of rupture such as pleural effusion, development of a neurologic deficit, or evidence of compromise of major visceral vessels or arteries to the lower extremities.

By use of a left lateral thoracotomy and either partial cardiopulmonary bypass or a heparin-bonded shunt, a graft is inserted into the thoracic aorta, obliterating the false lumen and redirecting blood flow into the true aortic lumen. In the absence of any of the previously mentioned indications, operation can be postponed. With the passage of time, edema around the aorta clears, and the development of fibrosis transforms initially friable adventitia of the aorta into less fragile tissue. The patient should be discharged from the hospital on antihypertensive therapy. These patients should be observed carefully by their personal physicians to be certain that the arterial blood pressure is maintained in an acceptable range. If with the passage of time there is enlargement of the thoracic aneurysm observed on the chest film, the patient must be considered a candidate for resection and grafting. It appears that approximately one third of these patients ultimately require operation, usually for an enlarging aneurysm. Late surgical procedures on descending aortic dissections are associated with a low mortality.[22, 23]

LONG-TERM FOLLOW-UP

DeBakey and colleagues reviewed their 20-year experience,[9] and patients have been followed at Duke University Medical Center more than 5 years.[32] Long-term survivors can be classified in two groups: those with DeBakey Type II dissections and those with DeBakey Type IIIA lesions. In

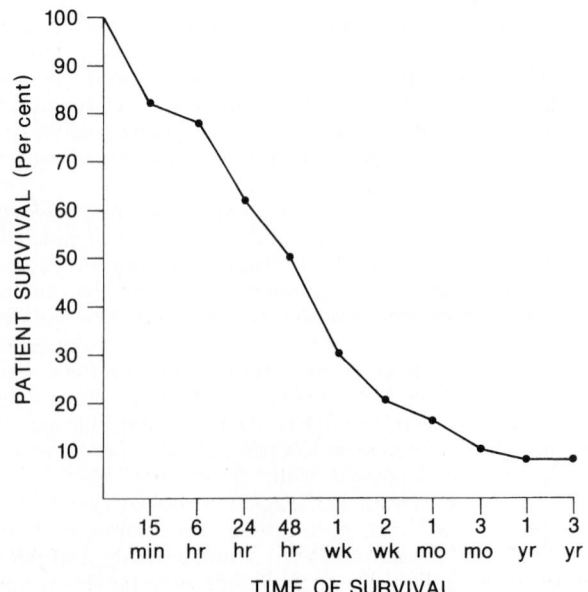

Figure 50–35. Graph indicating survival of patients with untreated acute dissecting aneurysms. (Adapted from Anagnostopoulos, C. E., et al.: Am. J. Cardiol., *30*:263, 1972.)

directing the blood into the true lumen with obliteration of the false lumen, thereby providing protection from rupture into the mediastinum or pericardium.[29, 32] When the operation is completed and cardiopulmonary bypass is discontinued, heparin is reversed with protamine and antihypertensive therapy is instituted (usually with nitroprusside). Propranolol, methyldopa, or hydralazine to control the blood pressure

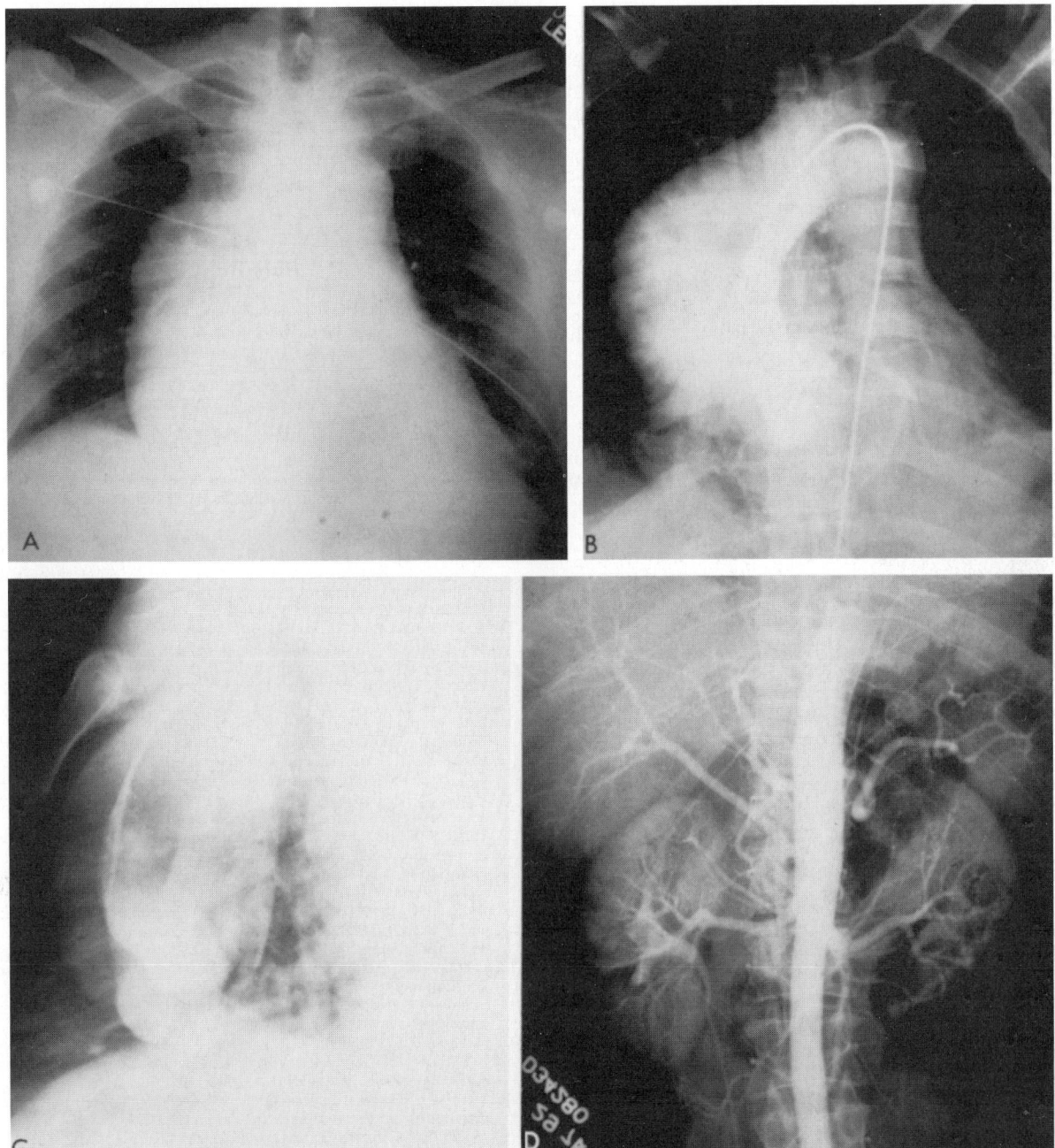

Figure 50–36. *A,* Chest film in a patient with an acute ascending dissection showing marked widening of the mediastinum without evidence of pulmonary edema. *B,* The aortogram shows an ascending dissection (Type II); the dissection does not involve the arch or descending thoracic abdominal aorta. *C,* Lateral view revealing the true and false lumens. *D,* Abdominal aortogram shows normal abdominal aorta and normal placement of the visceral vessels. Postoperative chest film reveals a Starr-Edwards prosthesis. A graft was inserted in the ascending aorta.

each group the disease process is localized and can be completely removed surgically. The DeBakey Type I lesion, which begins in the ascending aorta, and the Type IIIB lesion involve nearly total dissections of the aorta, including involvement of the visceral vessels; therefore, the prognosis is poorer for both surgical and medical management of these patients. The other classifications that have been suggested are helpful in distinguishing surgical versus medical management for dissecting aneurysms, that is, surgical management for almost all dissecting aneurysms that originate in the ascending aorta (DeBakey Type I and Type II) and initial medical therapy for descending aneurysms (DeBakey Type III). It is clear that more than 95% of patients with Type III descending dissection aneurysms are hypertensive contrasted to only

50% of those with ascending dissections (Type I and Type II). It also follows that the best results from therapy occur in patients with localized dissection (DeBakey Type II and Type IIIA). As stated earlier, surgical therapy in ascending dissections is performed to correct the aortic insufficiency that commonly accompanies it and to prevent rupture into the pericardium and mediastinum. Griepp and associates also believe that obliteration of the false lumen distally improves long-term progress in Type I (or A) dissection.[12] However, in descending dissections (DeBakey Type III), the indication for surgical intervention is impending rupture or continued pain. There are patients with chronic enlargement who require operation. The best long-term results occur in those patients with DeBakey Type IIIA lesions with the dissection localized

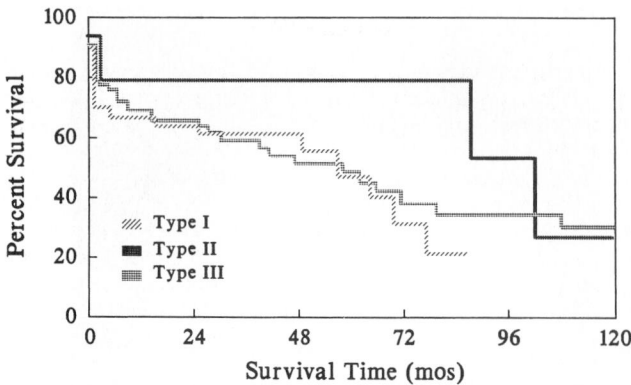

Figure 50–37. The 10-year survival at Duke University Medical Center for Type I, Type II, and Type III dissecting aneurysms.

to the thoracic aorta. As many as one fourth to one third may eventually require surgical management after successful medical therapy. The usual indication is an enlarging thoracic aortic aneurysm.

MORTALITY

The mortality of untreated aortic dissections is catastrophic, making immediate therapy of some type mandatory. Initially, antihypertensive pharmacologic therapy is generally employed. Although the early survival with antihypertensive therapy in Wheat's series was approximately 86%, it is now apparent that drug therapy alone (unless there are extenuating circumstances) should not be undertaken for long-term management of acute ascending dissections.[28] The control of descending dissections, however, is quite different.

The surgical mortality in acute ascending dissections should be between 10% and 20%, with long-term survival approaching 60%. The impact of coronary artery disease in patients with ascending dissection has been reviewed, and approximately 34% of patients may have significant coronary artery disease.[8] In patients with descending aortic dissections, the mortality for those in the surgical series and those managed with antihypertensive therapy is essentially the same. It is apparent that some patients with descending aortic dissections who are successfully managed with antihypertensive therapy will later be managed operatively for the reasons previously described, the most common indication being an expanding thoracic aneurysm. The operative mortality is less than 10%, and the long-term outlook is excellent.[23]

The ultimate prognosis of these patients is clearly related to the severity of the disease in the aorta and to the visceral involvement at the time of acute dissection. The survival over a 10-year period is shown in Figure 50–37.

SELECTED REFERENCES

Appelbaum, A., Karp, R. B., and Kirklin, J. W.: Ascending versus descending aortic dissections. Ann. Surg., *183*:296, 1976.
This article summarizes the surgical experience with dissecting aneurysms and indicates the importance of early surgical management.

Crawford, E. S., Svensson, L. G., Coselli, J. S., Safi, H. J., and Hess, K. R.: Aortic dissection and dissecting aortic aneurysms. Ann. Surg., *208*:254, 1988.
This is one of the most recent articles that summarizes one of the largest series of dissecting aneurysms in the literature.

Crawford, E. S., and Crawford, J. L.: Diseases of the Aorta. Tracy, T. M. (Ed.). Baltimore, Williams & Wilkins, 1984.
This classic is the state-of-the-art atlas for the surgical treatment of aneurysmal aortic disease.

DeBakey, M. E., McCollum, C. H., Crawford, E. S., Morris, G. C., Jr., Howell, J., Noon, G. P., and Lawrie, G.: Dissection and dissecting aneurysms of the

aorta: Twenty-year follow-up of five hundred twenty-seven patients treated surgically. Surgery, *92*:1118, 1982.
This classic article recounting DeBakey's experience at Baylor describes the largest series of dissecting aortic aneurysms. The superb follow-up makes this article a classic in surgical literature.

Glower, D. G., and Wolfe, W. G.: Management of dissecting aortic aneurysms. *In* Yao, J. S. T., and Pearce, W. H. (Eds.): Aneurysms: New Findings and Treatment. East Norwalk, Conn., Appleton & Lange, 1994.
This chapter highlights the long-term results after treatment of dissecting aneurysms.

REFERENCES

1. Anagnostopoulos, C. E.: Classification. *In* Anagnostopoulos, C. E. (Ed.): Acute Aortic Dissections. Baltimore, University Park Press, 1975.
2. Anagnostopoulos, C. E.: History. *In* Anagnostopoulos, C. E. (Ed.): Acute Aortic Dissections. Baltimore, University Park Press, 1975.
3. Appelbaum, A., Karp, R. B., and Kirklin, J. W.: Ascending versus descending aortic dissections. Ann. Surg., *183*:296, 1976.
4. Creswell, L. L., Kouchoukos, N. T., Cox, J. L., and Rosenbloom, M.: Coronary artery disease in patients with Type A aortic dissection. Ann. Thorac. Surg., *59*:585, 1995.
5. Daily, P. O., Trueblood, H. W., Stinson, E. B., Wuerflein, R. D., and Shumway, N. E.: Management of acute aortic dissections. Ann. Thorac. Surg., *10*:237, 1970.
6. Dalen, J. E., Alpert, J. S., Cohn, L. H., Black, H., and Collins, J. J.: Dissections of the thoracic aorta. Am. J. Cardiol., *34*:803, 1974.
7. DeBakey, M. E., Cooley, D. A., and Creech, O., Jr.: Surgical considerations of dissecting aneurysm of the aorta. Ann. Surg., *142*:587, 1955.
8. DeBakey, M. E., Henly, W. S., Cooley, D. A., Morris, G. C., Jr., Crawford, E. S., and Beall, A. C., Jr.: Surgical management of dissecting aneurysms of the aorta. J. Thorac. Cardiovasc. Surg., *49*:130, 1965.
9. DeBakey, M. E., McCollum, C. H., Crawford, E. S., Morris, G. C., Jr., Howell, J., Noon, G. P., and Lawrie, G.: Dissection and dissecting aneurysms of the aorta: Twenty-year follow-up of five hundred twenty-seven patients treated surgically. Surgery, *92*:1118, 1982.
10. Ergin, M. A., Phillips, R. A., Galla, J. D., Lansman, S. L., Mendelson, D. S., Quintana, C. S., and Griepp, R. B.: Significance of distal false lumen after Type A dissection repair. Ann. Thorac. Surg., *57*:820, 1994.
11. Harris, P. D., Bowman, F. O., Jr., and Malm, J. R.: The management of acute dissections of the thoracic aorta. Am. Heart J., *78*:419, 1969.
12. Hirst, A. E., Jr., Johns, V. L., Jr., and Kime, S. W., Jr.: Dissecting aneurysm of the aorta: A review of 505 cases. Medicine, *37*:217, 1958.
13. Hume, D. M., and Porter, R. R.: Acute dissecting aortic aneurysms. Surgery, *53*:122, 1963.
14. Kidd, J. N., Reul, G. J., Jr., Cooley, D. A., Sandiford, F. M., Kyger, E. R., and Wukasch, D. C.: Surgical treatment of aneurysms of the ascending aorta. Circulation, *54*:III-111, 1976.
15. Laennec, R. T. H.: Trait de l'Auscultation Mediate. Paris, J. A. Brosson and J. S. Chaude, 1819, p. 441.
16. Mandel, W., Evans, E. W., and Walsford, R. L.: Dissecting aortic aneurysm during pregnancy. N. Engl. J. Med., *251*:1059, 1954.
17. McFarland, J., Willerson, J. T., Dinsmore, R. E., Austen, W. G., Buckley, M. J., Sanders, C. A., and DeSanctis, R. W.: The medical treatment of dissecting aortic aneurysms. N. Engl. J. Med., *286*:115, 1972.
18. McKusick, V. A.: Cardiovascular aspects of Marfan's syndrome: A heritable disorder of connective tissue. Circulation, *11*:321, 1955.
19. Miller, D. C., Stinson, E. B., Oyer, P. E., Rossiter, S. J., Reitz, B. A., Griepp, R. B., and Shumway, N. E.: Operative treatment of aortic dissections: Experience with 125 patients over a sixteen-year period. J. Thorac. Cardiovasc. Surg., *78*:365, 1979.
20. Morgagni, G. B.: De Sedibus et Causis Morborum per Anatomen Indagitis (Venetiis, 1761): The Foundations and Causes of Disease Investigated by Anatomy, vol. 1. Alexander, A (Trans). London, A. Miller and T. Cadele, 1769, pp. 802–808.
21. Palmer, R. F., and Lasseter, K. C.: Sodium nitroprusside. N. Engl. J. Med., *292*:294, 1975.
22. Parker, F. B., Jr., Neville, J. F., Jr., Hanson, E. L., Mohiuddin, S., and Webb, W. R.: Management of acute aortic dissection. Ann. Thorac. Surg., *19*:436, 1975.
23. Reul, G. J., Jr., Cooley, D. A., Hallman, G. L., Reddy, S. B., Kyger, E. R., and Wukasch, D. C.: Dissecting aneurysm of the descending aorta. Arch. Surg., *110*:632, 1975.
24. Sorenson, H. R., and Olsen, H.: Ruptured and dissecting aneurysms of the aorta. Acta Chir. Scand., *128*:644, 1964.
25. Warren, W. D., Beckwith, J., and Muller, W. H., Jr.: Problems in the surgical management of acute dissecting aneurysm of the aorta. Ann. Surg., *144*:530, 1956.
26. Wheat, M. W., Jr.: Treatment of dissecting aneurysms of the aorta. Ann. Thorac. Surg., *12*:582, 1971.
27. Wheat, M. W., Jr., Harris, P. D., Malm, M. R., Kaiser, G., Bowman, F. O., Jr., and Palmer, R. F.: Acute dissecting aneurysms of the aorta. J. Thorac. Cardiovasc. Surg., *58*:344, 1969.
28. Wheat, M. W., Jr., Palmer, R. F., Bartley, T. D., and Seelman, R. C.: Treatment

of dissecting aneurysm of the aorta without surgery. J. Thorac. Cardiovasc. Surg., 50:364, 1965.

29. Wolfe, W. G.: Acute ascending aortic dissection. Ann. Surg., 192:658, 1980.
30. Wolfe, W. G., and Moran, J. F.: The evolution of medical and surgical management of acute aortic dissection. Circulation, 56:503, 1977.
31. Wolfe, W. G., Kleinman, L. H., Wechsler, A. S., and Sabiston, D. C., Jr.: Heparin-coated shunts for lesions of the descending thoracic aorta. Arch. Surg., 112:1481, 1977.
32. Wolfe, W. G., Oldham, H. N., Rankin, J. S., and Moran, J. F.: Surgical treatment of acute ascending aortic dissection. Ann. Surg., 197:738, 1983.

ANEURYSMS OF THE THORACIC AORTA

Walter G. Wolfe, M.D.

The thoracic aorta comprises the ascending thoracic aorta, the aortic arch, and the descending thoracic aorta that ends the diaphragmatic hiatus. Aneurysms of the ascending aorta may include the aortic valve, the sinuses, and the ascending aorta proper up to the innominate. The arch of the aorta includes the great vessels (the innominate, carotid, and subclavian) and ends in the area of the ligamentum. The descending thoracic aorta can be defined anatomically as that portion of the thoracic aorta from the subclavian to the diaphragm. Histologically, the aorta is composed of three layers: the intima, media, and adventitia. The intima is important because the etiologic factor of many thoracic aneurysms is atherosclerosis. The media is important because of the degenerative nature of cystic medial necrosis and its involvement in patients as well as in dissecting aneurysms. The adventitia is important because it is a strong supportive tissue that may protect patients from sudden death secondary to rupture into the mediastinum or free pleural space, which may be seen in dissecting aneurysms and/or traumatic transected aortas after high-speed automobile accidents.

ETIOLOGY

The etiology of thoracic aortic aneurysms includes atherosclerosis, cystic medial degeneration, myxomatous degeneration, dissection, infection, trauma, and post-stenotic dilatation. In the United States, syphilitic aortitis is unusual as a cause of thoracic aneurysms. Cystic medial necrosis was described by Erdheim in 1929,[18] and this finding is one of the prominent features in patients with Marfan's syndrome. The incidence of thoracic aneurysms increases with age. In the aging aorta, cystic medial necrosis is seen almost routinely and may accompany degenerative changes seen with atherosclerosis. Atherosclerosis that causes occlusion of the vasa vasorum produces medial necrosis and subsequent aneurysm formation. Aneurysm formation can be classified as either localized, as seen in saccular aneurysms, or fusiform, which produces a more generalized aneurysm.

PRESENTATION

Presenting symptoms of thoracic aneurysm depend on the area of the thoracic aorta involved. In general, compression, pressure, and chest pain are the main presenting symptoms. Often, a routine chest film reveals an asymptomatic thoracic aneurysm. Patients may experience hoarseness and superior vena caval syndrome. Cough and dyspnea from tracheobronchial obstruction may occur, and hemoptysis is a very serious sign, usually indicating erosion into the trachea, a mainstem bronchus, or lung tissue. Specifically, aneurysms in the ascending aorta may produce aortic insufficiency leading to cardiac failure and angina.

DIAGNOSIS

Although aortic aneurysms may be diagnosed on the plain chest film, the specific location of the aneurysm and the structures involved must be located using aortography. Computed tomography and now magnetic resonance imaging can be helpful in making specific anatomic diagnoses. Aortic aneurysms may also be detected by echocardiography and standard cardiac catheterization. In general, aortography including the entire thoracic aorta is the diagnostic procedure of choice in individuals with thoracic aortic aneurysms.

PROGNOSIS

The natural history of abdominal aortic aneurysms was well described by Estes.[19] One study indicated the seriousness of thoracic aortic aneurysms and the risk of rupture in this group of patients.[4] Consequently, a much more aggressive approach is taken toward thoracic aortic aneurysms, with resection and grafting of the aneurysms always being recommended unless there are extenuating circumstances that make the risk of operation prohibitive. Rupture is the common cause of death in these patients. Documented enlargement of an aneurysm is a clear indication for operation. MacDonald and colleagues believe that aneurysms of the ascending aorta over 5 cm. should be managed surgically even if they are asymptomatic.[26] Although the age of the patient and other clinical information must be evaluated before recommending an operation, the presence of an aneurysm and knowledge of the natural history (i.e., rupture and death) demand that strong consideration be given to resection in almost every case.

ASCENDING AORTIC ANEURYSMS

Aneurysms of the ascending aorta are almost always degenerative, with a high incidence of medial necrosis or myxomatous degeneration being present. The process may include the aortic root, the anulus, and the aortic leaflets. The diagnosis of ascending aortic aneurysms is suggested by prominence of the ascending aorta on the chest film and by the finding of a murmur of aortic insufficiency. Again, aortography is used to confirm the diagnosis. Treatment is basically resection and grafting of the ascending aorta with the other involved structures being managed separately or at the same time, as in the Bentall operation described later.

Aneurysms involving the sinus of Valsalva often rupture into one of the chambers of the heart (Fig. 50–38). Aneurysms originating from the right coronary sinus are common and may follow endocarditis, but in the Asian race there is evidence that this aneurysm may be congenital and that infectious processes are secondary.[27, 31] Right coronary sinus aneurysms may be asymptomatic until they rupture into the mediastinum or into a cardiac chamber, most frequently the right ventricle or the right atrium. Aneurysms of the left coronary sinus are relatively uncommon.

Anuloaortic ectasia is another common condition of the ascending aorta and can be seen with Marfan's disease (Fig. 50–39). Anuloaortic ectasia involves dilation of both the sinuses and the anulus of the aorta, usually often accompanied by aortic insufficiency. Therapy in this case is resection and grafting of the aneurysm, replacement of the aortic valve, and reimplantation of the coronary arteries.[20] This operation is named the Bentall procedure after the article by Bentall and DeBono in 1968 describing the technique for replacement of the ascending aorta and valve with a composite graft.[3]

Using homografts and cardiopulmonary bypass, Cooley, DeBakey, and Bahnson developed the early techniques for resection of ascending aortic aneurysms. By 1958, synthetic

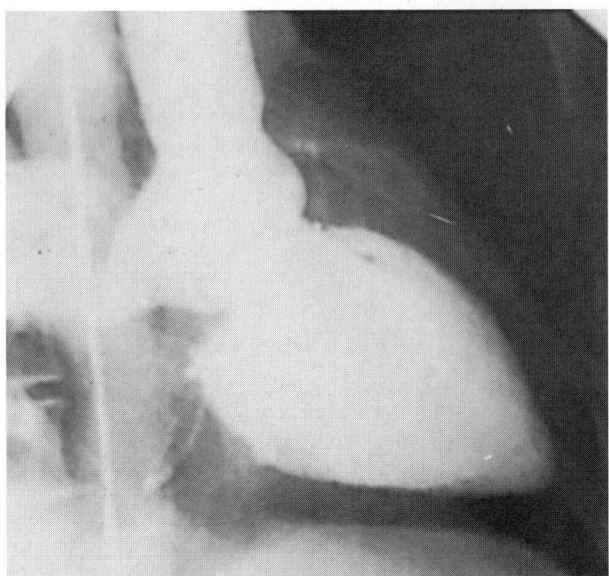

Figure 50–38. Aortogram demonstrates a sinus of Valsalva aneurysm and fistula that enters into the right atrium through the atrial septum. The lesion is repaired by approaching through both an aortotomy and an atriotomy.

grafts were used for most aortic operations.[31] Development of prosthetic heart valves in the early 1960s was a major advance in managing the valvular component of aneurysms in the ascending aorta. Currently, woven Dacron grafts are used in the ascending aorta, arch, or descending thoracic aorta. Recently, frozen homografts have been used as in the Bentall operation. The frozen homograft may may be the graft of choice in mycotic aneurysms in which the etiology is related to infectious complications.

Treatment. Aneurysms of the ascending aorta with or without aortic ectasia are managed using cardiopulmonary

bypass and resection and grafting of the aneurysms as standard techniques. Hypothermic circulatory arrest may be added when the aorta close to the innominate artery is involved. If the aortic sinuses and the aortic valve are involved, the Bentall operation is employed.[3, 23]

Results. The results of surgical treatment of these aneurysms are generally excellent. Mortality in general should be less then 10%, and serious complications are rare.[23, 27] Long-term results have been excellent.

TRANSVERSE AORTIC ARCH

The transverse aortic arch is that segment of the aorta from which the innominate, carotid, and subclavian vessels arise. As mentioned earlier, these aneurysms have a tendency to rupture into the pericardial mediastinum or into the pleural space and can compress airways, the pulmonary artery, and the great veins. The diagnosis is made with aortography (Fig. 50–40).

Treatment. Patients with aortic arch aneurysms are difficult to manage. In general, the operation is performed through a median sternotomy on cardiopulmonary bypass with deep hypothermic circulatory arrest[9, 12, 13, 15, 21] and a rectal temperature of 12° C. to 16° C. The aneurysm is resected and the segment reconstructed, usually with a Dacron graft, reinserting the brachiocephalic vessels usually as a button. When the arrest time is below 45 minutes, the incidence of central nervous system complications is less than 10%. In some cases, selected perfusion of the cerebral vessels can be performed under cardiopulmonary bypass. In 1957, DeBakey

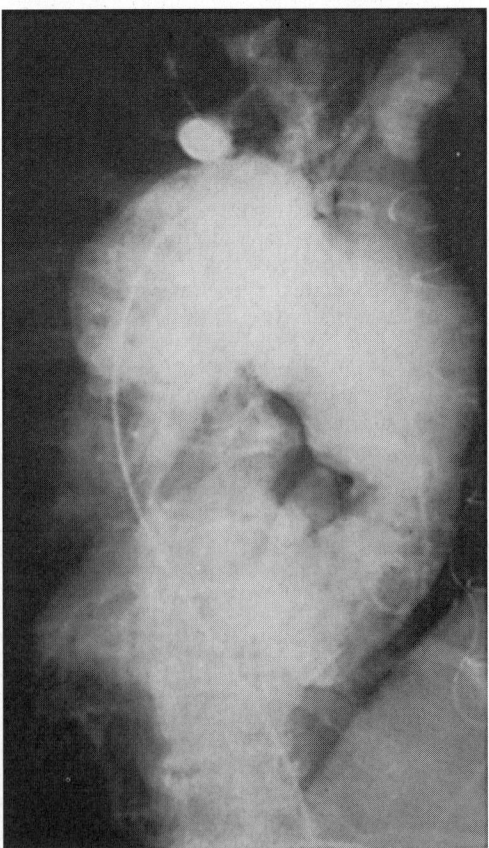

Figure 50–40. An aneurysm involving the aortic arch extends down into the proximal descending thoracic aorta. The operation in this case is done through a left thoracotomy with cardiopulmonary bypass and profound hypothermia so that the graft can be placed in the arch and then down through the descending thoracic aorta.

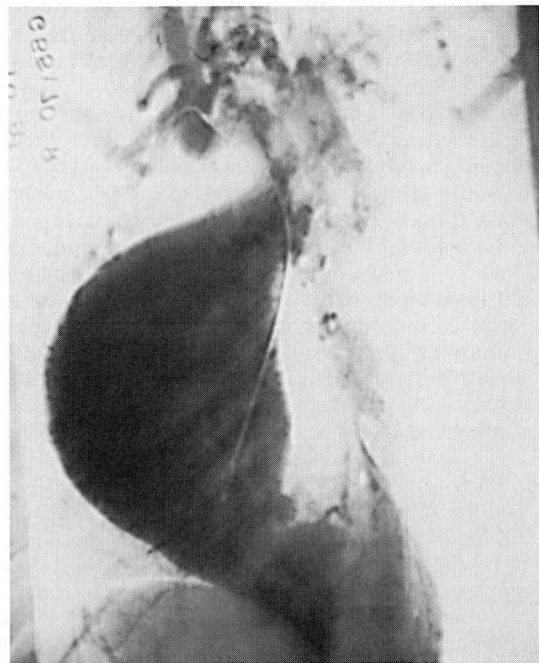

Figure 50–39. A large ascending aortic aneurysm with 4+ aortic insufficiency. Repair here is with the use of a composite graft with aortic valve replacement, reimplantation of the coronary arteries, and grafting of the ascending aorta, a Bentall operation.

and colleagues first successfully replaced an aneurysm involving the ascending and transverse arch with aortic homograft, using total cardiopulmonary bypass with innominate and left carotid artery perfusion.[17] Griepp and associates used cardiopulmonary bypass and total-body hypothermia with cerebral circulatory arrest to simplify the aortic reconstruction described.[21] Presently the use of retrograde cerebral perfusion may increase the protection of the central nervous system during the arrest period.[10]

Results. Results of therapy for arch aneurysms in most series have a mortality of 10% to 15%, with significant neurologic complications occurring in another 10%. Crawford and Crawford present one of the largest series and the best results in the management of this complex problem with an overall survival of approximately 90%.[11]

DESCENDING THORACIC AORTA

The descending thoracic aorta is that segment of the aorta from the left subclavian artery to the diaphragm (Fig. 50–41). The etiology is most commonly atherosclerosis, and the incidence of aneurysm in this area is second only to that seen in the infrarenal abdominal aorta. Patients with untreated aneurysms of the descending thoracic aorta usually die of rupture into the pleural space.[4] Perhaps 80% of these patients die within 5 years if the aneurysm is untreated. Aneurysms of the descending thoracic aorta compress and erode adjacent structures, including the spine, airway, lung, and esophagus. Patients may present with hoarseness, chest pain, cough, or hemoptysis as well as dysphagia. All of these symptoms represent late manifestations and serious complications of the aneurysm.

The diagnosis can be made by a plain chest film or computed tomographic scan. However, aortography is the best method of evaluating the entire aorta to demonstrate the extent of the disease and its relationship to the subclavian and arch vessels.

Treatment. The treatment is resection and grafting of the aneurysmal segment. The first successful segmental resection of the thoracic aorta was done by Alexander and Byron, who removed a segment involved with congenital coarctation and poststenotic aneurysm.[1] Shumacker[28] treated a similar case by end-to-end anastomosis in 1948, and Gross[22] and Swan[30] and their colleagues contributed to the management of these lesions using homografts to replace sections of the thoracic aorta. Lam and Arom[25] were the first to segmentally replace the descending thoracic aorta for acquired disease using a homograft to replace the syphilitic aneurysm of the descending thoracic aorta. Interestingly, an intraluminal shunt was used in this patient but partial paraplegia occurred and remains one of the most dreaded complications of operations on the thoracic aorta. In 1953, DeBakey and Cooley[16] successfully replaced a thoracic aortic aneurysm with an aortic homograft without using shunts or bypass.

Today these aneurysms are most commonly replaced with synthetic grafts made from woven Dacron. The patient may be operated on using partial femorofemoral bypass and a pump oxygenator with or without profound hypothermia.[15] Heparin-bonded shunts may be inserted to bypass the aneurysm from the ascending aorta, left ventricle, or subclavian artery to the distal circulation through the aorta or femoral artery. Finally, the Biomedicus pump can be used for left-sided heart bypass from the left atrium to the distal aorta.[5] These techniques have been developed in an attempt to reduce complications of clamping of the descending thoracic aorta, such as left ventricular strain and renal or spinal cord ischemia. Although shunting methods and cardiopulmonary bypass improve cardiac hemodynamics and protect the viscera (i.e., the gut and kidneys) from ischemia, no system completely prevents development of paraplegia with replacement of long segments of the thoracic aorta. Whereas aneurysms of the descending thoracic aorta in many instances are managed with clamping and supplemented vasodilation, the majority of surgeons continue to use some method of shunting with the belief that the incidence of paraplegia can be avoided.

Results. Aneurysms of the descending thoracic aorta can be treated with a mortality of less than 10% and the incidence of paraplegia approximately 5%.[15, 29] The leading cause of death in operated patients is coronary artery disease, with renal insufficiency also being a serious postoperative complication. Lower limb neurologic disturbance (i.e., paraplegia) is still the most catastrophic complication involving surgical procedures on the thoracic aorta. Other complications include recurrent laryngeal nerve injury, bleeding, and infection. Long-term survival is excellent, with the 5-year survival approaching 70%.[11]

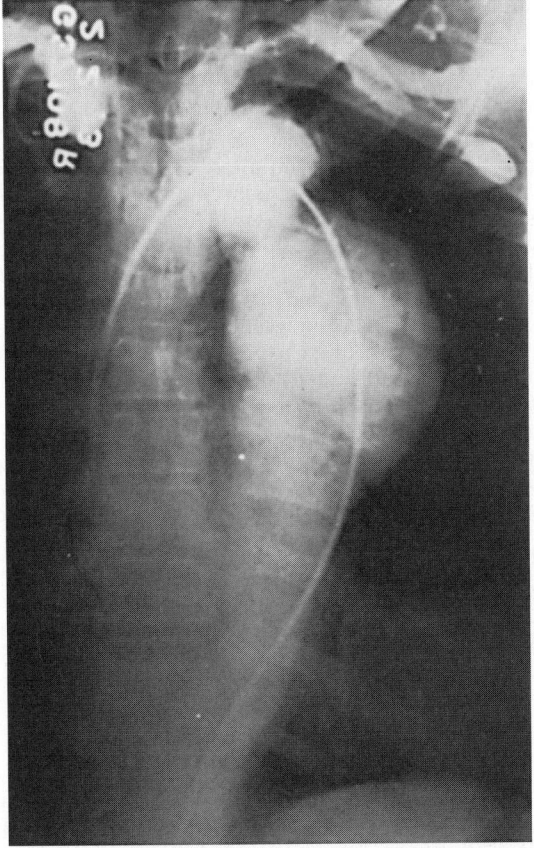

Figure 50–41. Aortogram demonstrates a standard descending thoracic aortic aneurysm originating below the subclavian artery. Approach is through a left thoracotomy with the use of a Dacron graft to replace the aneurysm segment.

SELECTED REFERENCES

Coselli, J. S.: Retrograde cerebral perfusion via a superior vena caval cannula for aortic arch aneurysm operations. Ann. Thorac. Surg. 57:1668, 1994.
This article presents the basic technical points for the use of retrograde cerebral perfusion in patients undergoing arch aneurysm repair.

Crawford, E. S., and Crawford, J. L.: Diseases of the Aorta. Tracy, T. M. (Ed.). Baltimore, Williams & Wilkins, 1984.
This classic is the state-of-the-art atlas for the surgical treatment of aneurysmal aortic disease.

Crawford, E. S., Coselli, J. S., and Safi, H. J.: Partial cardiopulmonary bypass, hypothermic circulatory arrest, and posterolateral exposure for thoracic aortic aneurysm operation. J. Thorac. Cardiovasc. Surg., 94:824, 1987.
This article describes a unique and important technique in the management of arch and descending thoracic aortic aneurysms.

Svensson, L. G., Crawford, E. S., Hess, K. R., Coselli, J. S., and Safi, H. J.: Experience with 1509 patients undergoing thoracoabdominal aortic operations. J. Vasc. Surg., 17:357, 1993.

REFERENCES

1. Alexander, J., and Byron, F. X.: Aortectomy for thoracic aneurysm. Univ. Mich. Hosp. Bull., 9:101, 1943.
2. Bahnson, H. T.: Definitive treatment of saccular aneurysms of the aorta with excision of sac and aortic suture. Surg. Gynecol. Obstet., 96:383, 1953.
3. Bentall, H., and De Bono, A.: A technique for complete replacement of the ascending aorta. Thorax, 23:338, 1968.
4. Bickerstaff, L. K., Pairolero, P. C., Hollier, L. H., Melton, L. J., Van Peenen, H. J., Cherry, K. J., Joyce, J. W., and Lie, J. T.: Thoracic aortic aneurysms: A population-based study. Surgery, 92:1103, 1982.
5. Carlson, D. E., Karp, R. B., and Kouchoukos, N. T.: Surgical treatment of aneurysms of the descending thoracic aorta: An analysis of 85 patients. Ann. Thorac. Surg., 35:58, 1983.
6. Cooley, D. A., and DeBakey, M. E.: Resection of entire ascending aorta in fusiform aneurysm using cardiac bypass. JAMA, 162:1158, 1956.
7. Cooley, D. A., and DeBakey, M. E.: Surgical considerations of intrathoracic aneurysms of the aorta and great vessels. Ann. Surg., 135:660, 1952.
8. Cooley, D. A., DeBakey, M. E., and Morris, G. C.: Controlled extracorporeal circulation in surgical treatment of aortic aneurysms. Ann. Surg., 146:473, 1957.
9. Cooley, D. A., Ott, D. A., Frazier, O. H., and Walker, W. E.: Surgical treatment of aneurysms of the transverse aortic arch: Experience with 25 patients using hypothermic techniques. Ann. Thorac. Surg., 32:260, 1981.
10. Coselli, J. S.: Retrograde cerebral perfusion via a superior vena caval cannula for aortic arch aneurysm operations. Ann. Thorac. Surg., 57:1668, 1994.
11. Crawford, E. S., and Crawford, J. L. (Eds.): Diseases of the Aorta. Baltimore, Williams & Wilkins, 1984.
12. Crawford, E. S., and Saleh, S. A.: Transverse aortic arch aneurysm: Improved results of treatment employing new modifications of aortic reconstruction and hypothermic cerebral circulatory arrest. Ann. Surg., 194:180, 1981.
13. Crawford, E. S., Saleh, S. A., and Schuessler, J. S.: Treatment of aneurysms of transverse aortic arch. J. Thorac. Cardiovasc. Surg., 78:383, 1979.
14. Crawford, E. S., Stowe, C. L., Crawford, J. L., Titus, J. L., and Weilbaecher, D. G.: Aortic arch aneurysm: A sentinel of extensive aortic disease requiring subtotal and total aortic replacement. Ann. Surg., 199:742, 1984.
15. Crawford, E. S., Walker, H. S. J., III, Saleh, S. A., and Normann, N. A.: Graft replacement of aneurysm in descending thoracic aorta: Results without bypass or shunting. Surgery, 89:73, 1981.
16. DeBakey, M. E., and Cooley, D. A.: Successful resection of aneurysm of thoracic aorta and replacement by graft. JAMA, 152:673, 1953.
17. DeBakey, M. E., Crawford, E. S., Cooley, D. A., and Morris, G. C., Jr.: Successful resection of fusiform aneurysm of aortic arch with replacement by homograft. Surg. Gynecol. Obstet., 105:657, 1957.
18. Erdheim, J., Jr.: Medionecrosis aorte idiopathica apitca. Virchows Arch. Pathol. Anat., 276:187, 1930.
19. Estes, J. E., Jr.: Abdominal aortic aneurysm: A study of one hundred and two cases. Circulation, 2:258, 1950.
20. Gott, V. L., Pyeritz, R. E., Magovern, G. J., Jr., Cameron, D. E., and McKusick, V. A.: Surgical treatment of aneurysms of the ascending aorta in the Marfan syndrome: Results of composite-graft repair in 50 patients. N. Engl. J. Med., 314:1070, 1986.
21. Griepp, R. B., Stinson, E. B., Hollingsworth, J. F., and Buehler, D.: Prosthetic replacement of the aortic arch. J. Thorac. Cardiovasc. Surg., 70:1051, 1975.
22. Gross, R. E., Hurwitt, E. S., Bill, A. H., and Pierce, E. C.: Preliminary observation in the use of human arterial grafts in the treatment of certain cardiovascular defects. N. Engl. J. Med., 239:578, 1948.
23. Kouchoukos, N. T., Karp, R. B., Blackstone, E. H., Kirklin, J. W., Pacifico, A. D., and Zorn, G. L.: Replacement of the ascending aorta and aortic valve with a composite graft. Ann. Surg., 192:403, 1980.
24. Krause, A. H., Ferguson, T. B., and Weldon, C. S.: Thoracic aneurysmectomy utilizing the TDMAC-heparin shunt. Ann. Thorac. Surg., 14:123, 1972.
25. Lam, C. R., and Arom, H. H.: Resection of descending thoracic aorta for aneurysm: Report of use of homograft in case and experimental study. Ann. Surg., 134:743, 1951.
26. McDonald, G. R., Schaff, H. V., Pyeritz, R. E., McKusick, V. A., and Gott, V. L.: Surgical management of patients with the Marfan syndrome and dilatation of the ascending aorta. J. Thorac. Cardiovasc. Surg., 81:180, 1981.
27. Sakakibara, S., and Konno, S.: Congenital aneurysm of the sinus of Valsalva: Anatomy and classification. Am. Heart J., 63:405, 1962.
28. Shumacker, H. B., Jr.: Coarctation and aneurysm of aorta: Report of case treatment by excision and end to end suture of aorta. Ann. Surg., 127:655, 1948.
29. Svensson, L. G., Crawford, E. S., Hess, K. R., Coselli, J. S., and Safi, H. J.: Experience with 1509 patients undergoing thoracoabdominal aortic operations. J. Vasc. Surg., 17:357, 1993.
30. Swan, H., Maaske, C., Johnson, M., and Grover, R.: Arterial homografts: Resection of thoracic aortic aneurysm using sternal human arterial transplant. Arch. Surg., 61:732, 1950.
31. Taguchi, K., Sasaki, N., Matsuura, Y., and Uemura, R.: Surgical correction of aneurysm of the sinus of Valsalva: A report of forty-five consecutive patients including eight with total replacement of the aortic valve. Am. J. Cardiol., 23:181, 1969.
32. Wolfe, W. G., Kleinman, L. H., Wechsler, A. S., and Sabiston, D. C., Jr.: Heparin-coated shunts for lesions of the descending thoracic aorta. Arch. Surg., 112:1481, 1977.

ANEURYSMS OF THE CAROTID ARTERY

Richard H. Dean, M.D.

Extracranial aneurysms of the carotid artery are extremely uncommon. Although the widespread use of cerebral arteriography probably has led to an increase in the discovery of carotid artery aneurysms over the past 25 years, McCollum and associates reported performing only 28 operations for carotid artery aneurysms among 8500 operations for aneurysms at all sites over a 21-year period.[8] Owing to the rarity of carotid aneurysms, details regarding their etiology, most common locations, natural history, presenting symptoms, and treatment cannot be discerned from any one surgeon's experience. Instead, collective reviews of reported cases are needed to provide those details.

The most frequent site of carotid artery aneurysms is the common carotid artery, particularly its bifurcation. The middle and distal portions of the internal carotid artery are the next most common sites. Aneurysms at the bifurcation are usually fusiform, whereas those located in the internal carotid artery are usually saccular. Atherosclerosis is responsible for 46% to 70% of all carotid artery aneurysms.[10] Trauma and previous carotid artery surgery are less common causes. Although syphilis was the most common cause 50 years ago, it is a rare cause today.

NATURAL HISTORY

Because most carotid artery aneurysms are identified because of the presence of symptoms, the true risk associated with the presence of an aneurysm is poorly defined. Nevertheless, it would appear that their natural history is generally unfavorable. In a 1937 collective review, Shipley and associates found a 71% mortality among 41 patients treated expectantly.[11] That review demonstrated that aneurysms may present as rupture, cerebral embolization, thrombosis, or expansion onto adjacent structures with pressure symptoms. Zwolak and associates underscored the frequency of embolization in their review, which reported a stroke rate of 50% for atherosclerotic aneurysms followed without operation.[14] In contrast, some small, posttraumatic, distal internal carotid artery aneurysms have been demonstrated to regress spontaneously. Therefore, therapy must be individualized, the major objective being prevention of the neurologic sequelae of the embolization of clot fragments from the aneurysm wall. Occasionally, progressive enlargement of the aneurysm may produce pressure on the vagus, the glossopharyngeus, the hypoglossus, or the sympathetic nerves in the region and thus cause dysfunction of any of these nerves.

CLINICAL MANIFESTATIONS

The clinical presentation of carotid artery aneurysms varies according to their location and size. Distal internal carotid artery aneurysms may be completely hidden. In contrast, almost every common carotid artery and bifurcation aneurysm is first discovered as a pulsatile mass just below the angle of the mandible. Occasionally, an aneurysm may present as a pulsatile mass in the tonsillar fossa or oropharynx without external manifestation. With either presentation, the aneurysms may have associated symptoms of pain and tenderness or they may be completely asymptomatic. Distal internal carotid artery aneurysms may produce recurrent facial pain, fifth or sixth cranial nerve palsy, deafness, or even a Horner's syndrome when they compress adjacent structures at the base of the skull. Even Raeder's paratrigeminal syndrome, the combination of intermittent facial pain and oculosympathethic paresis, has been caused by aneurysms situated at the base of the skull.[7]

The most common serious risks associated with carotid artery aneurysms are transient ischemic attacks and stroke.[9] Most such central nervous system defects are caused by embolization of laminated thrombus lining the wall of the aneurysm. Less commonly, cerebral symptoms are caused by diminished flow through the carotid artery secondary to its compression by the mass of an adjacent saccular aneurysm.

Although common in reports during the late nineteenth and early twentieth centuries, rupture of carotid artery aneurysms is rare today. When rupture does occur, it is manifested by hemorrhage from the pharynx, ear, or nose and may lead to death by suffocation.

DIFFERENTIAL DIAGNOSIS

Elongation with kinking of the carotid artery is the most frequently found lesion masking as a carotid artery aneurysm. Usually, this lesion presents as a pulsatile mass at the base of the right side of the neck, typically in hypertensive elderly women. This mass is easily distinguished from an aneurysm by the fact that the pulsation is along the long axis of the vessel. A prominent carotid artery bifurcation in a patient with a thin neck, carotid body tumors, enlarged lymph nodes, branchial cleft cysts, or other masses that overlie and transmit the carotid pulse can be mistaken for an aneurysm. Usually, careful palpation discriminates between these entities and a true aneurysm of the carotid bifurcation.

Duplex ultrasonography with B-mode imaging usually confirms or excludes the presence of an aneurysm of the extracranial carotid artery. Nevertheless, high internal carotid artery aneurysms cannot be diagnosed accurately by this method because of the limitations in visualizing that region. Computed tomography and magnetic resonance imaging are

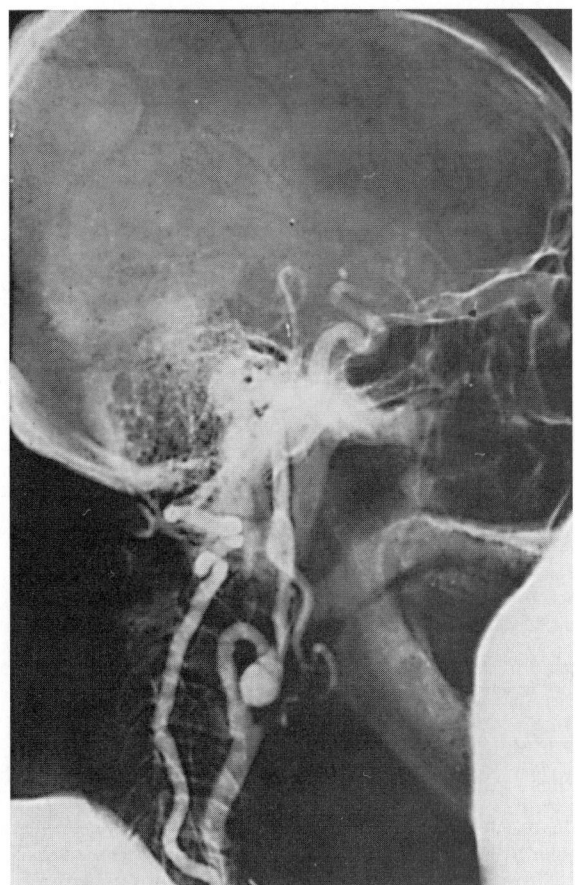

Figure 50–43. Carotid arteriogram showing distal internal carotid saccular aneurysm. (Courtesy of George Plum, M.D.)

useful substitutes for B-mode imaging for the diagnosis of such lesions located high in the neck.[4]

Angiography remains the definitive diagnostic test on which to base therapy, even when the diagnosis has been established by one of the noninvasive methods. Visualization of the entire length of both extracranial and intracranial components of the carotid artery and the vertebrobasilar system is required for any treatment strategies to be adequate. Examples of saccular and fusiform aneurysms of the carotid artery are depicted in Figures 50–42 and 50–43.

TREATMENT

Sir Astley Cooper introduced the operative treatment of carotid artery aneurysms by ligating one such aneurysm in 1805. Although that patient died in the immediate postoperative period, a second patient treated similarly in 1808 survived for 13 years.[1] Proximal ligation of the aneurysm remained the only treatment for the next 150 years, even though it was associated with a high rate of postoperative stroke and death. Even with that high morbidity and mortality, Winslow could report in 1926 that the 71% death rate from observational management alone was reduced to 30% after ligation of the aneurysm.[13]

Dimtza reported the first successful resection of an internal carotid artery aneurysm with reanastomosis.[3] Because most such aneurysms are associated with an elongated, tortuous vessel, this technique can be employed in about 50% of patients. Most other aneurysms are now treated by resection and interpositional placement of either a saphenous vein graft or a polytetrafluoroethylene graft. Occasionally, saccular

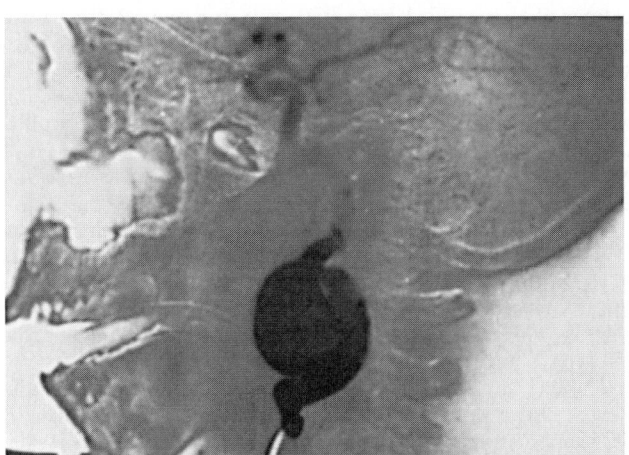

Figure 50–42. Carotid arteriogram showing typical appearance of an internal carotid artery aneurysm. (From Stoney, R. J., and Qvarfordt, P. G.: Accessible and inaccessible aneurysm of the extracranial carotid artery. *In* Moore, W. S. [Ed.] Surgery for Cerebrovascular Disease. New York, Churchill Livingstone, 1987, pp. 567–577.)

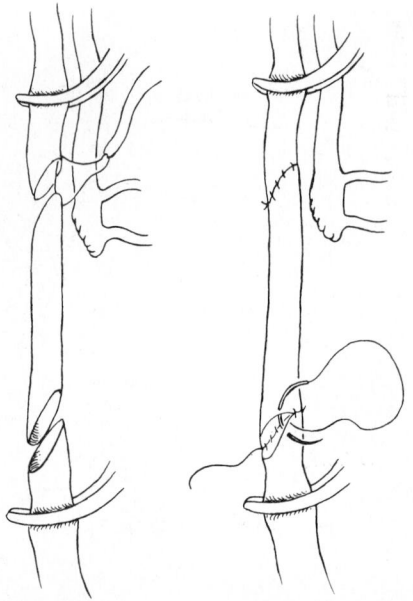

Figure 50–44. Drawings depicting technique of interposition grafting over a temporary shunt. (From Moore, W. S.: Reoperative carotid artery surgery. *In* Bergan, J. J., and Yao, J. S. T. [Eds.]: Techniques in Arterial Surgery. Philadelphia, W. B. Saunders, 1990, pp. 206–213.)

aneurysms can be treated by resection and lateral arteriorrhaphy or patch angioplasty.

The techniques for resection of the aneurysm and re-establishment of cerebral perfusion have been well described.[5, 8, 12, 14] Through the use of electroencephalography, stump pressure measurements, or test clamping of the carotid artery using regional anesthesia, the need for temporary shunting can be identified. When a neurologic deficit is produced by test cross-clamping or electroencephalographic monitoring or when the distal stump pressure is lower than 50 mm. Hg, resection, reanastomosis, or graft interposition is performed over a temporary shunt (Fig. 50–44). When these techniques of cerebral protection are used, along with intraoperative heparin anticoagulation and modern anesthetic techniques, the operative mortality should be no higher than 1% and permanent neurologic deficits should be less than 5%.

Occasionally, resection of the aneurysm is impossible owing to its distal location at the base of the skull. In this instance, ligation of the internal carotid artery remains the only therapeutic option. If test clamping of the vessel is tolerated, ligation can be performed at a single stage. If cross-clamping cannot be tolerated, extracranial-to-intracranial bypass using a microvascular technique can provide improved collateral perfusion to allow ligation.[6] Gradual occlusion (over several days) using a Crutchfield clamp also continues to be useful.[2] With either technique, anticoagulation for 10 days to 2 weeks is necessary to reduce the frequency of propagation of the distal clot into the collateral cerebral circulation.

SELECTED REFERENCES

Goldstone, J.: Aneurysms of the extracranial carotid artery. *In* Rutherford, R. B. (Ed.): Vascular Surgery, 3rd ed. Philadelphia, W. B. Saunders, 1989, p. 1418.
This review of the literature provides a complete résumé of the causes, clinical presentation, differential diagnosis, and treatment of carotid artery aneurysms.

Moreau, P., Albat, B., and Thévenet, A.: Surgical treatment of extracranial internal carotid artery aneurysm. Ann. Vasc. Surg., 8:409, 1994.
This is a detailed review of the literature with analysis of 38 cases of carotid aneurysm treated by excision and arterial restoration, including a breakdown showing the various methods of cerebral protection used during operation.

Zwolak, R. M., Whitehouse, W. M., Jr., Knake, J. E., Bernfeld, B. D., Zelenock, G. B., Cronenwett, J. L., Erlandson, E. E., Kazmers, A., Graham, L. M., Lindenauer, S. M., and Stanley, J. C.: Atherosclerotic extracranial carotid artery aneurysms. J. Vasc. Surg., 1:415, 1984.
This is an extensive review of the literature together with an analysis of the authors' experience treating 52 carotid aneurysms, 24 of which were atherosclerotic. Characteristics of this particular group are described in detail.

REFERENCES

1. Cooper, A.: Account of the first successful operation performed on the common carotid artery for aneurysm in the year 1808 with the postmortem examination in the year 1821. Guy's Hosp. Rep., 1:53, 1836.
2. Crutchfield, W. G.: Instructions for the use in the treatment of certain intracranial vascular lesions. J. Neurosurg., 16:471, 1959.
3. Dimtza, A.: Aneurysms of the carotid arteries: Report of two cases. Angiology, 7:218, 1956.
4. Duvall, E. R., Gupta, K. L., Vitek, J. J., Stanley, R. J., Luna, R. F., and Howieson, J.: CT demonstration of extracranial carotid artery aneurysms. J. Comput. Assist. Tomogr., 10:404, 1986.
5. Hardin, C. A.: Surgical treatment of extracranial carotid aneurysms with excision and arterial restoration. Vasc. Surg., 7:247, 1973.
6. Krupski, W. C., Effeney, D. J., and Ehrenfeld, W. K.: Fibromuscular dysplasia, aneurysms and spontaneous dissection of the carotid artery. *In* Bergan, J. J., and Yao, J. S. T. (Eds.): Cerebrovascular Insufficiency. New York, Grune & Stratton, 1983, p. 369.
7. Goldstone, J.: Aneurysms of the extracranial carotid artery. *In* Rutherford, R. B. (Ed.): Vascular Surgery, 3rd ed. Philadelphia, W. B. Saunders, 1989, p. 1418.
8. McCollum, C. H., Wheeler, W. G., Noon, G. P., and DeBakey, M. E.: Aneurysms of the extracranial carotid artery: Twenty-one years' experience. Am. J. Surg., 137:196, 1979.
9. Rhodes, E. L., Stanley, J. C., Hoffman, G. L., Cronenwett, J. L., and Fry, W. J.: Aneurysms of extracranial carotid arteries. Arch. Surg., 111:339, 1976.
10. Rittenhouse, E. A., Radke, H. M., and Sumner, D. S.: Carotid artery aneurysm: Review of the literature and report of a case with rupture into the oropharynx. Arch. Surg., 105:786, 1972.
11. Shipley, A. M., Winslow, N., and Walker, W. W.: Aneurysm in the cervical portion of the internal carotid artery: An analytical study of the cases recorded in the literature between August 1, 1925 and July 31, 1936: Report of two new cases. Ann. Surg., 105:673, 1937.
12. Welling, R. E., Taha, A., Goel, T., Cranley, J., Krause, R., Hafner, C., and Tew, J.: Extracranial carotid artery aneurysms. Surgery, 93:319, 1983.
13. Winslow, N.: Extracranial aneurysm of the internal carotid artery: History and analysis of cases registered up to August 1, 1925. Arch. Surg., 13:689, 1926.
14. Zwolak, R. M., Whitehouse, W. M., Jr., Knake, J. E., et al.: Atherosclerotic extracranial carotid artery aneurysms. J. Vasc. Surg., 1:415, 1984.

CAROTID BODY TUMORS

Richard H. Dean, M.D.

The carotid body is derived from both mesoderm and elements of the third branchial arch and neural crest ectoderm. It is a 3- to 4-mm. pinkish gray structure located within the adventitial layer of the posteromedial aspect of the common carotid bifurcation. Only very rarely is it involved in the medial layer. Tumors arising from this body were called chemodectomas originally, but they actually arise from paraganglionic cells and thereby should be classified as paragangliomas.

Normally, the cells of the carotid body sense changes in Po_2, Pco_2, and pH. In this regard, an unusually high incidence of carotid body tumors has been reported in individuals living at altitudes between 6900 and 14,000 feet, suggesting that chronic stimulation by chronic hypoxia may have a role in carotid body cell hyperplasia.[8]

The malignant potential of carotid body tumors is disputed, and reported figures range from 2.6% to 50%.[1, 6, 15, 16] Standard pathologic criteria for malignancy do not correlate well with the biologic behavior of the tumor. The metastatic rate of these tumors is approximately 5%.[9, 15] Regional lymph nodes are the most common site of metastatic spread.

Epidemiologic studies suggest that two types of carotid body tumors are seen. The first is a randomly occurring sporadic type, which has a 5% incidence of bilaterality.[11, 15] The second has an autosomal dominant pattern of familial occurrence, which is less common and has a 32% incidence of bilaterality.[7, 14]

CLINICAL PRESENTATION

Most commonly, a carotid body tumor presents as a painless, palpable mass over the carotid bifurcation region of the neck. Invasive and large benign tumors may produce associated hoarseness, dysphagia, stridor, or tongue weakness. Cranial nerve involvement has been estimated at 20%; most frequently, the vagal and hypoglossal nerves are involved.[3] Although dizziness is frequently described by the patient, it is rarely associated with identifiable cerebral ischemia. Hypertension is found in about 6% of patients[15] and has been associated with catecholamine secretion from the tumor in rare cases.[5] The differential diagnosis includes branchial cleft cyst, carotid artery aneurysm, enlarged lymph nodes, and metastatic tumor.

DIAGNOSIS

The definitive study for diagnosis of carotid body tumors is selective bilateral cerebral arteriography. Characteristically, these tumors appear as a hypervascular oval mass widening the angle of the carotid bifurcation (Fig. 50–45). Although the location of the mass can be identified with computed tomography, arteriography additionally identifies the sources and extent of *nonbifurcation* blood supply. In addition, arteriography is required to define the presence and need for treatment of concomitant atherosclerotic disease of the carotid artery bifurcation.

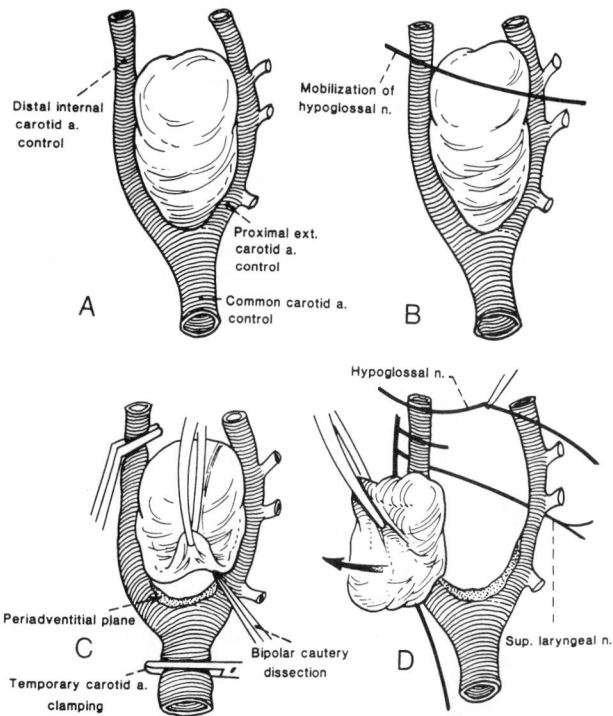

Figure 50–46. Artist's drawing of the technique of subadventitial resection of a carotid body tumor. (From Hallett, J. W., Jr., et al.: J. Vasc. Surg., 7:284, 1988, with permission from C. V. Mosby.)

TREATMENT

Current treatment of carotid body tumors is primarily operative, with excision of the tumor and maintenance of the integrity of carotid flow. The most important advancement in surgical therapy of these tumors has been recognition of and dissection along the subadventitial plane, which almost always allows complete removal of the tumor while maintaining carotid artery integrity (Fig. 50–46).

When there is deeper involvement of the carotid bifurcation wall or when combined endarterectomy of the carotid bifurcation is necessary, full-thickness excision of the base of the tumor with vein or synthetic patch closure of the defect facilitates the operation. Rarely, an interposition graft for replacement of the entire carotid bifurcation is necessary. When carotid artery cross-clamping is required, one should monitor cerebral function and be prepared to use an indwelling carotid shunt to maintain cerebral perfusion during the procedure.

When the tumor is very large, invasive, or malignant, the carotid artery may have to be sacrificed. If the artery is already occluded, this poses no hazard. If the artery is patent, carotid circulation may be restored by means of an arterial graft, using a shunt for cerebral protection. If no distal artery is available for anastomosis, attempts at resection should probably be abandoned unless the pressure in the carotid stump is higher than 65 mm. Hg, under which circumstance carotid ligation without reconstruction usually can be performed safely. For the rare tumor that is unresectable, radiation therapy may be of some value.[15, 17]

Seldom should simple excision of the tumor be associated with cerebral morbidity or mortality. In 1962, Rush[13] reported a mortality of 1.5% and a 2.9% incidence of hemiplegia. In several more recently reported series, which included cases of carotid replacement, there was no associated mortality or cerebral morbidity.[2, 4, 10, 12, 17]

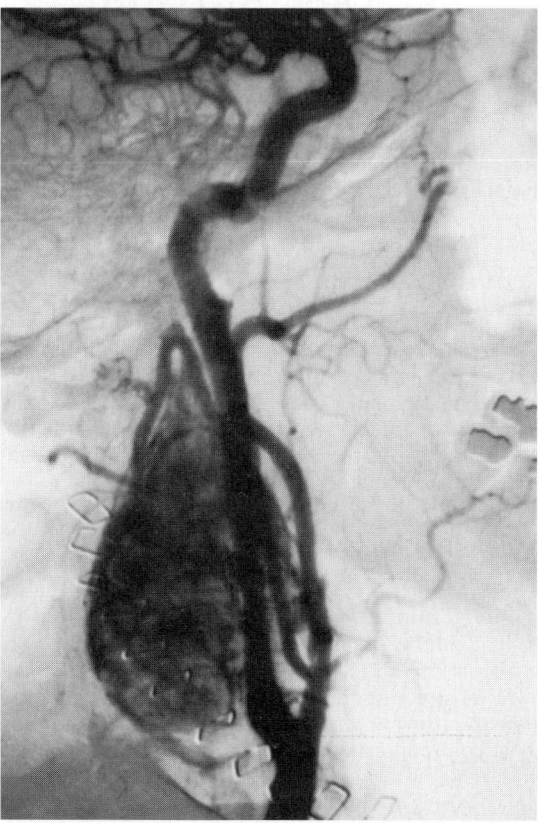

Figure 50–45. Characteristic arteriographic appearance of a carotid body tumor. Note the dramatic vascularity of the tumor. (From Hallett, J. W., Jr.: Carotid body tumor resection. *In* Bergan, J. J., and Yao, J. S. T. [Eds.]: Techniques in Arterial Surgery. Philadelphia, W. B. Saunders, 1990.)

SELECTED REFERENCES

Connell, J.: Carotid body tumours. Aust. N.Z. J. Surg., *47*:495, 1977.
   This article describes the details of the author's technique for simplified and safe removal of carotid body tumors, together with results of an extensive personal experience.

Hallett, J. W., Jr., Nora, J. D., Hollier, L. H., Cherry, K. J., Jr., and Pairolero, P. C.: Trends in neurovascular complications of surgical management for carotid body and cervical paragangliomas: A fifty-year experience with 153 tumors. J. Vasc. Surg., *7*:284, 1988.
   This article summarizes 50 years of experience in surgical management of carotid body tumors. It provides an up-to-date consideration of the technical problems with resection of all varieties of these tumors.

Rush, B. F., Jr.: Current concepts in the treatment of carotid body tumors. Surgery, *52*:679, 1962.
   This is a review of the subject up to 1962, with emphasis being placed on the natural history of untreated tumors and the mortality and morbidity associated with various types of surgical therapy.

Westbrook, K. C., Guillamondegui, O. M., Medellin, H., and Jesse, R. H.: Chemodectomas of the neck: Selective management. Am. J. Surg., *124*:760, 1972.
   This article clearly outlines signs and symptoms, the usefulness of angiography, indications for surgical therapy, and results of treatment in the authors' large series.

REFERENCES

1. Chambers, R. G., and Mahoney, W. D.: Carotid body tumors. Am. J. Surg., *116*:554, 1968.
2. Connell, J.: Carotid body tumours. Aust. N.Z. J. Surg., *47*:495, 1977.
3. Davidge-Pitts, K. J., and Pantanowitz, D.: Carotid body tumors. Surg. Annu., *16*:203, 1984.
4. Dent, T. L., Thompson, N. W., and Fry, W. J.: Carotid body tumors. Surgery, *80*:365, 1976.
5. Fries, J. G., and Chamberlin, J. A.: Extra-adrenal pheochromocytoma: Literature review and report of a cervical pheochromocytoma. Surgery, *63*:268, 1968.
6. Gaylis, H., and Mieny, C. J.: The incidence of malignancy in carotid body tumours. Br. J. Surg., *64*:885, 1977.
7. Grufferman, S., Gillman, M. W., Pasternak, L. R., Peterson, C. L., and Young, W. G., Jr.: Familial carotid body tumors: Case report and epidemiologic review. Cancer, *46*:2116, 1980.
8. High-altitude chemodectoma (Editorial). Lancet, *1*:1493, 1973.
9. Irons, G. B., Weiland, L. H., and Brown, W. L.: Paragangliomas of the neck: Clinical and pathologic analysis of 116 cases. Surg. Clin. North Am., *57*:575, 1977.
10. Lees, C. D., Levine, H. L., Beven, E. G., and Tucker, H. M.: Tumors of the carotid body: Experience with 41 operative cases. Am. J. Surg., *142*:362, 1981.
11. McIlrath, D. C., and ReMine, W. H.: Carotid-body tumors. Surg. Clin. North Am., *43*:1135, 1963.
12. Morris, G. C., Jr., Balas, P. E., Cooley, D. A., Crawford, E. S., and DeBakey, M. E.: Surgical treatment of benign and malignant carotid body tumors: Clinical experience with sixteen tumors in twelve patients. Am. J. Surg., *29*:429, 1963.
13. Rush, B. F., Jr.: Current concepts in the treatment of carotid body tumors. Surgery, *52*:679, 1962.
14. Rush, B. F., Jr.: Familial bilateral carotid body tumors. Ann. Surg., *157*:633, 1963.
15. Shamblin, W. R., ReMine, W. H., Sheps, S. G., and Harrison, E. G., Jr.: Carotid body tumor (chemodectoma): Clinicopathologic analysis of ninety cases. Am. J. Surg., *122*:732, 1971.
16. Staats, E. F., Brown, R. L., and Smith, R. R.: Carotid body tumors, benign and malignant. Laryngoscope, *76*:907, 1966.
17. Westbrook, K. C., Guillamondegui, O. M., Medellin, H., and Jesse, R. H.: Chemodectomas of the neck: Selective management. Am. J. Surg., *124*:760, 1972.

SUBCLAVIAN ARTERY ANEURYSMS

David C. Sabiston, Jr., M.D.

Subclavian arterial aneurysms are usually due to atherosclerosis, but trauma is also a cause. Poststenotic dilatation may cause an aneurysm as in the thoracic outlet syndrome. If thrombosis is present, there may be subsequent emboli in the arteries of the arm and hand. The lesions may be either intrathoracic (often asymptomatic) or supraclavicular (presenting as a pulsating mass). A review of the cases of true subclavian aneurysms of all cases reported in English has been published.[1] In a series of 31 patients with subclavian axillary aneurysms, the lesion was located on the right side in 20 patients and on the left in 10; and 1 patient had bilateral aneurysms. It is interesting that mural thrombi were present in 25 of the 31 patients and, of these, 23 presented with upper extremity pain. Thromboembolism occurred in five of the patients, and two had rupture of the aneurysm, followed by one death. A pulsatile mass was palpable in 20, including 8 patients who were asymptomatic. The cause was atherosclerosis in 12, trauma in 10, and poststenotic dilatation secondary to thoracic outlet obstruction in 6. At follow-up, there were no recurrences and no further complications appeared.[2] Treatment consists of excision with restoration of arterial continuity, but occasionally tangential aneurysmorrhaphy may be appropriate. Rarely, ligation of the artery proximally and distally with excision of the aneurysm can be performed if there is sufficient collateral circulation. However, excision with restoration of arterial continuity is the most desirable operation. This condition is also presented in the section on the thoracic outlet syndrome in which subclavian-axillary aneurysms are often seen.

REFERENCES

1. Dougherty, M. J., Calligaro, K. D., Savarese, R. P., and DeLaurentis, D. A.: Atherosclerotic aneurysm of the intrathoracic subclavian artery: A case report and review of the literature (Review). J. Vasc. Surg., *21*:521, 1995.
2. Pairolero, P. C., Walls, J. T., Payne, W. S., Hollier, L. H., and Fairbairn, J. F., II: Subclavian-axillary artery aneurysms. Surgery, *90*:757, 1981.

VISCERAL ARTERIAL ANEURYSMS

David C. Sabiston, Jr., M.D.

More common than usually appreciated, visceral arterial aneurysms may be asymptomatic or catastrophic. The fact that the condition is not rare is emphasized in a series of 45 patients with splanchnic arterial aneurysms seen in one center during a 12-year period. The most important visceral arterial aneurysms are those of the splenic, celiac, hepatic, superior mesenteric, and renal arteries. Similar aneurysms have also been reported of the gastroduodenal, pancreaticoduodenal, and gastroepiploic arteries. Selective arteriography of the visceral circulation has greatly aided the diagnosis of aneurysms of these arteries (Figs. 50–47 and 50–48), and a number have been discovered by this procedure when it is being performed for other reasons.

SPLENIC ARTERY ANEURYSMS

The most common visceral aneurysm is that of the splenic artery and constitutes about two thirds of all lesions in this group. In 1770, Beaussier[1] was the first to describe a splenic artery aneurysm, and since then many have been reported. They are most commonly found in women, and rupture of the aneurysm during pregnancy is a recognized complication. The most common cause is medial degeneration of the arterial wall, usually inducing a saccular aneurysm, which may contain calcium in the wall. Forty-five percent of women with these aneurysms have had six or more pregnancies. Splenic artery aneurysms may also be caused by fibromuscular dysplasia with involvement of the renal arteries. Atherosclerosis is also a cause of visceral aneurysms. Congenital

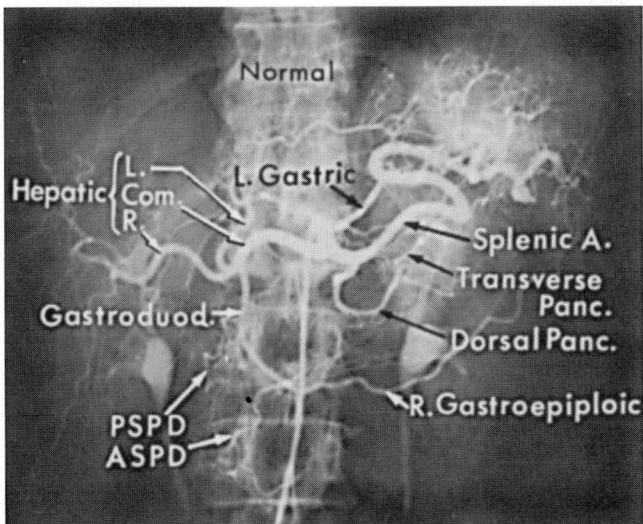

Figure 50–47. Selective injection of the celiac axis demonstrating normal anatomy. PSPD, posterior-superior pancreaticoduodenal artery; ASPD, anterior-superior pancreaticoduodenal artery. (Courtesy of Dr. Irwin Johnsrude.)

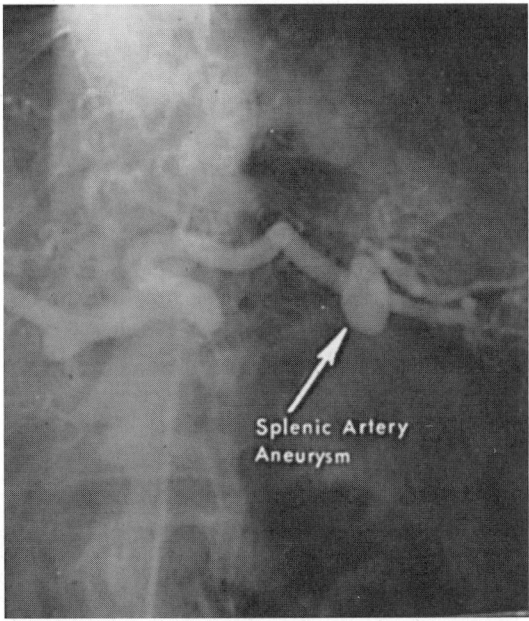

Figure 50–49. Splenic artery aneurysm demonstrated by selective arteriographic injection into the celiac axis. (Courtesy of Dr. Irwin Johnsrude.)

aneurysms are rare and when present are usually multiple. Mycotic lesions usually follow sepsis, often with splenic emboli, after subacute bacterial endocarditis.

Splenic artery aneurysms vary considerably in their clinical manifestations and many patients are asymptomatic. The most common complaint is vague pain in the left upper quadrant with radiation to the left subscapular region. In expanding aneurysms, the symptoms may be more prominent and become acute with rupture. The diagnosis is most often made by the discovery of a calcified lesion on abdominal films and proven by arteriography (Fig. 50–49). Physical findings are uncommon, although rarely a tender, pulsatile mass can be palpated in the left upper quadrant.

Splenic aneurysms are known to rupture, although the actual risk is difficult to assess, but some reports stress a high likelihood. In one study, among 40 ruptured splenic artery aneurysms, 10 were fatal (25%). Operation should be recommended for most splenic artery aneurysms, especially during pregnancy, in view of the risk of rupture, because mortality is high (68% in one group of 65 patients). Other complications caused by splenic artery aneurysms include portal hypertension and rupture into the stomach. The surgical procedure of choice is excision of the splenic artery with splenectomy or, if possible, preservation of the spleen. Spontaneous dissection of the splenic artery occasionally occurs and is characterized by severe substernal and epigastric pain. Urgent operation is lifesaving.[5]

CELIAC ARTERY ANEURYSMS

Although uncommon, celiac aneurysms may be arteriosclerotic, congenital, mycotic, or traumatic. The clinical manifestations are primarily those of vague abdominal discomfort, most previously reported cases having been recognized at rupture. Excision of the aneurysms with restoration of continuity either directly or with an interposed graft is the treatment of choice. In one report of 14 cases managed surgically, 13 had a good result.

Wilson first described a hepatic aneurysm in 1819. Causes include arteriosclerosis, infection (mycotic), trauma, medial degeneration, and, rarely, periarteritis nodosa. The most prominent clinical manifestation is right upper quadrant or epigastric pain, frequently similar to gallbladder disease. Hematemesis or melena may follow erosion of the aneurysm into the gastrointestinal tract, as may fever and jaundice. Free rupture into the peritoneal cavity is the most serious complication, and only five survivors have been reported after this complication.

Surgical extirpation is indicated when the diagnosis is made. Most of these aneurysms are discovered incidentally at operation. Eighty percent are extrahepatic and can be identified during abdominal operation, whereas 20% lie within the liver and are not easily discovered. The procedure of choice is excision of the aneurysm. If the aneurysm is located proximal to the gastroduodenal artery, the lesion may simply be excised with distal ligation, because the collateral circulation through the gastroduodenal artery to the liver is

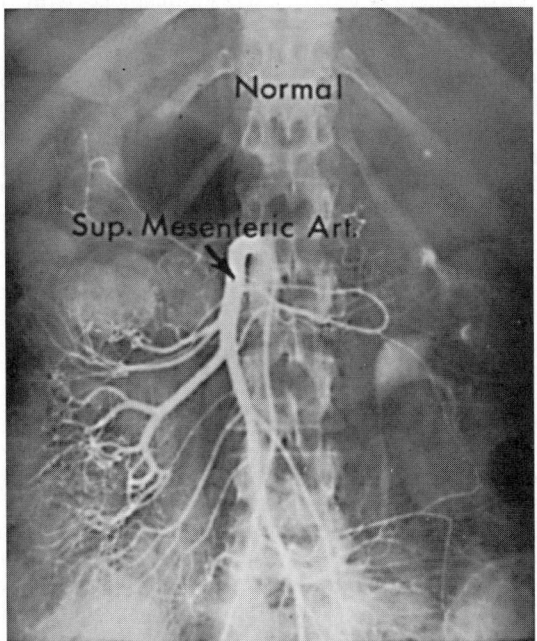

Figure 50–48. Selective injection of superior mesenteric artery demonstrating normal anatomy. (Courtesy of Dr. Irwin Johnsrude.)

excellent. If the aneurysm involves the hepatic artery distal to the gastroduodenal branch, preservation of arterial continuity to prevent liver necrosis is best managed by aneurysmorrhaphy or the use of a venous graft.

GASTRODUODENAL ARTERY ANEURYSMS

With the advent of wider use of arteriography, gastroduodenal arterial aneurysms are more frequently discovered. Acute pancreatitis may cause enzymatic destruction of the aneurysmal wall with rupture and ensuing hemorrhage. It is usually preferable to excise these aneurysms when they are discovered.

ANEURYSMS OF THE SUPERIOR MESENTERIC ARTERY

Superior mesenteric arterial aneurysms are often mycotic (57 in one series); atherosclerosis, trauma, and medial degeneration are other causes. In particular, this lesion should be suspected in patients with subacute bacterial endocarditis in whom abdominal pain develops in association with an expanding, tender mass. A high percentage of these lesions rupture. The first successful treatment was performed in 1949.[3] Since then, a number have been successfully managed by excision. Spontaneous dissection of the superior mesenteric artery also occurs, causing an aneurysm. Urgent operation is indicated and may be curative.[2]

ANEURYSMS OF THE GASTRODUODENAL AND PANCREATICODUODENAL ARTERIES

Aneurysms of the gastroduodenal and pancreaticoduodenal arteries are rare, with aneurysms of the gastric and gastroepiploic arteries being more common. The majority present as rupture either into the peritoneal cavity or into the upper gastrointestinal tract, with massive bleeding. Ligation of the aneurysm or partial gastric resection has been accomplished in some 30%.

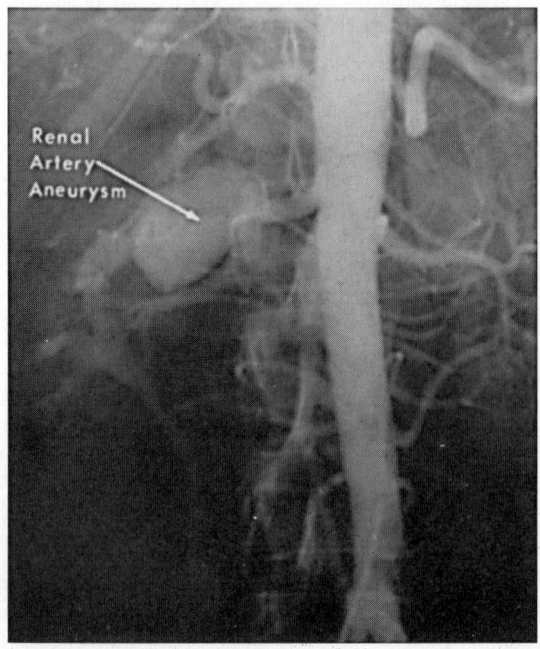

Figure 50–50. Aneurysm of the right renal artery. (Courtesy of Dr. Irwin Johnsrude.)

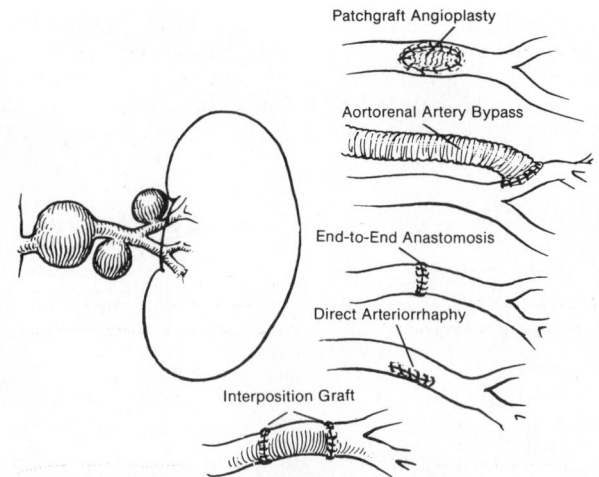

Figure 50–51. Surgical techniques employed in excision of renal artery aneurysms with preservation of the kidney. (From DeBakey, M. E., Lefrak, E. A., Garcia-Rinaldi, R., and Noon, G. P.: Aneurysm of the renal artery. Arch. Surg., *106*:438, 1973, with permission of authors and publisher. Copyright 1973, American Medical Association.)

ANEURYSMS OF THE RENAL ARTERIES

Although once considered rare, aneurysms of the renal arteries are being recognized with increasing frequency since the first description in 1770. These lesions constitute approximately 1% of all aneurysms and occur most frequently in patients with hypertension. They are located in the main renal artery or the bifurcation of the primary branches in approximately 60% (Fig. 50–50). Approximately 15% of the aneurysms are intrarenal, and in about 25%, calcification is present in the wall. Most of the lesions are due to atherosclerosis or medial necrosis, and occurrence distal to a renal arterial stenosis is not uncommon. Saccular aneurysms are the most frequent, and the primary risk is rupture. The clinical manifestations include the symptoms of hypertension, especially headache. Less common are symptoms of upper abdominal and flank pain. A bruit may be present over the flank, and hematuria may also occur. A palpable mass is rare (in less than 10% of cases). The diagnosis is made by arteriography.

The management of renal artery aneurysms includes careful demonstration of the size, type, and location of the aneurysm by arteriography. Rupture is an absolute indication for emergency operation. The majority, aneurysms with calcification, are more prone to rupture. For those aneurysms that are calcified, opinion is divided concerning management, since they are less likely to rupture, but there is no doubt that they may. At present, the majority of surgeons favor operation for these lesions, and it is usually possible to preserve the kidney. In a series of 72 patients, solitary aneurysms occurred in 53 and multiple lesions in 19. Arteriosclerotic changes were present in nearly 30%, and fibrodysplasia was an associated finding in 27 of the 72 patients; 57 of the group were hypertensive. Two patients experienced frank aneurysmal rupture, and rupture occurred into the renal veins twice. Aneurysmectomy was performed in 31 of the 72 patients; and nephrectomy, either partial or total, was the procedure in 17. In this series, the authors recommended operation for most lesions 1.5 cm. in diameter or greater. It was also emphasized that in many instances renal artery stenosis is present, requiring correction for associated hypertension. A renal artery aneurysm has also been removed successfully from a solitary kidney. In operative correction of all these defects, emphasis is placed on a vascular reconstructive approach, making every effort to avoid nephrectomy (Fig. 50–51).[4] Among a series of 8525 patients undergoing renal angiography, 83 had renal artery aneurysms, of which 6 were bilateral and 11 were multiple. Sixty-nine were not treated, and there were no deaths due to rupture of the aneurysm in a mean follow-up of 4 years. Fourteen patients underwent surgical correction.

SELECTED REFERENCES

Stanley, J. C., Rhodes, E. L., Gewertz, B. L., Chang, C. Y., Walter, J. F., and Fry, W. J.: Renal artery aneurysms: Significance of macroaneurysms exclusive of dissections and fibrodysplastic mural dilations. Arch. Surg., *110*:1327, l975.
In this review, the experience with 72 patients with renal artery aneurysms is presented. The majority of the patients were managed surgically, and the indications for operation and results are reviewed. This represents an unusually large series of patients from a single clinic.

Stanley, J. C., Thompson, N. W., and Fry, W. J.: Splanchnic artery aneurysms. Arch. Surg., *101*:698, 1970.
In this very good review of splanchnic aneurysms, the natural history, diagnosis, management, and results are described.

REFERENCES

1. Beaussier, M.: Sur un aneurisme de l'artere splenique dont les parois se sont ossifiees. J. Med. Toulouse, *32*:157, 1770.
2. Cormier, F., Ferry, J., Artru, B., Wechsler, B., Cormier, J. M.: Dissecting aneurysms of the main trunk of the superior mesenteric artery. J. Vasc. Surg., *15*:424, 1992.
3. DeBakey, M. E., and Cooley, D. A.: Successful resection of mycotic aneurysms of superior mesenteric artery: Case report and review of the literature. Am. Surg., *19*:202, 1953.
4. DeBakey, M. E., Lefrak, E. A., Garcia-Rinaldi, R., and Noon, G. P.: Aneurysm of the renal artery: A vascular approach. Arch. Surg., *106*:438, 1973.
5. Merrell, S. W., and Glovicski P.: Splenic artery dissection: A case report and review of the literature. J. Vasc. Surg., *15*:221, 1992.

AORTIC ABDOMINAL ANEURYSMS

David C. Sabiston, Jr., M.D.

It was not until 1951 that the first aortic abdominal aneurysm was successfully resected by Dubost and replaced with an aortic homograft.[10] Aortic abdominal aneurysms have since been resected very effectively with an appreciable extension of life.

PATHOLOGIC ASPECTS

Abdominal aortic aneurysms are caused by atherosclerosis in 95% of cases. Rarely, trauma, syphilis, mycotic infection, or Marfan's syndrome may be responsible. The majority of atherosclerotic aneurysms occur in the sixth and seventh decades. Inflammatory aneurysms have also been noted to have distinctive clinical and physical characteristics that separate them from typical atherosclerotic aneurysms. They appear to occur in 7% to 10% of patients undergoing aneurysmectomy. In one series of 19 patients with this problem, 63% were symptomatic, and all had dense periaortic inflammation. Adjacent structures most frequently involved were the duodenum, left renal vein, and ureter.[28]

NATURAL HISTORY

If untreated, abdominal aortic aneurysms have a natural history that is of much significance, especially in discussing with the patient the course of the disorder in relation to therapy to emphasize the role of surgical treatment. Before the advent of surgical therapy, Estes published a classic study of the natural history of abdominal aneurysms in 102 patients

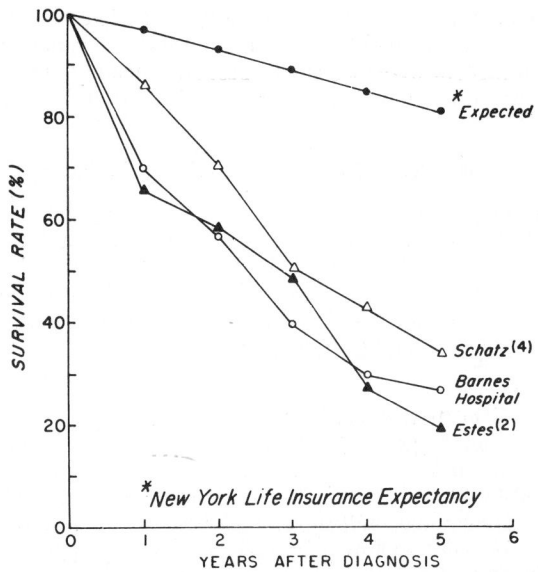

Figure 50–52. The natural history and survival rates among patients with untreated abdominal aortic aneurysms. (From Klippel, A. P., and Butcher, H. R., Jr.: The unoperated abdominal aortic aneurysm. Am. J. Surg., *111*:629, 1966.)

seen at the Mayo Clinic.[12] In this group, 64 patients died; and in 63% death was due to rupture. Only 67% of these patients survived 1 year, 49% survived 3 years, and 19% survived 4 years. Similar findings were reported by Schatz and associates[31] and Klippel and Butcher (Fig. 50–52).[20] In another study, emphasis was placed on patients with symptomatic aortic abdominal aneurysms. Thirty percent of these patients died within 1 month after onset of symptoms, 74% died by 6 months, and 80% died at 1 year.[14] Thus, the survival in this group was found to be much lower than that in a group of patients in whom aneurysms were asymptomatic. In the group in whom rupture of the aneurysm did not occur, other causes of death included coronary, cerebral, and renal complications of atherosclerosis (Fig. 50–53). Hypertension was present in 47% of the patients.

CLINICAL MANIFESTATIONS

Abdominal aortic aneurysms are most often discovered on routine examination and are asymptomatic. In the remainder, abdominal symptoms range from vague discomfort in the epigastrium to excruciating pain. Severe pain in the flank or back suggests leakage or rupture of the aneurysm and is usually accompanied by signs of blood loss.

A pulsating mass is usually found on abdominal examination. The smallest aneurysms are approximately 4 cm. in

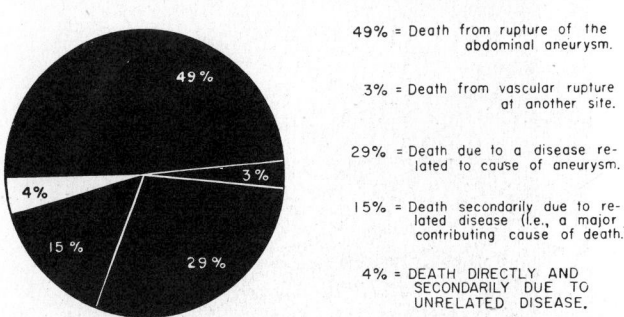

Figure 50–53. Cause of death in 68 patients with an untreated abdominal aneurysm. (From Gliedman, M. L., Ayers, W. G., and Vestal, B. L.: Aneurysms of the abdominal aorta and its branches. Ann. Surg., *146*:207, 1957.)

diameter, but the size may range upward to 20 cm. or more, and they may be tender on palpation. Fortunately, more than 95% of abdominal aortic aneurysms arise below the level of the renal arteries, the inferior mesenteric artery being the only important vessel arising from the aneurysm. The latter is usually completely occluded or severely stenotic, in which case the development of a prominent collateral circulation by means of the distal branches of the inferior mesenteric artery is stimulated. Bilateral examination of the femoral, popliteal, dorsal pedal, and posterior tibial pulses should be done, particularly in reference to possible postoperative changes.

DIAGNOSTIC STUDIES

Calcification is frequently evident on plain films of the abdomen in the wall of the aneurysm, often best observed on the lateral view (Fig. 50–54). The *eggshell* appearance is essentially diagnostic. The use of lateral films has also been helpful in those instances in which the calcification in the aortic aneurysmal wall is not clear on the anteroposterior abdominal films. Ultrasonography has become particularly useful and is a very simple, noninvasive technique that allows an accurate diagnosis and also provides information concerning the size and location of the aneurysm (Fig. 50–55). Moreover, this technique is quite helpful in following the progress of small aneurysms in patients who are not surgical candidates owing to specific medical contraindications.[22] Computed tomography is also valuable in the diagnosis and is a technique that allows delineation of the aortic lumen and intra-aneurysmal thrombus by the addition of contrast medium enhancement. It is helpful in following the size of small aneurysms in patients not considered ideal surgical candidates (see Fig. 50–55).[15] Arteriography can provide additional information, especially if there is concern about multiple aneurysms, peripheral vascular disease, or renal hypertension or when doubt exists concerning involvement of other branches of the abdominal aorta (see Fig. 50–55).[6] Important findings include suprarenal extension of the aneurysm; demonstration of stenotic lesions in the renal arteries, superior mesenteric artery, or celiac axis; the presence of thrombus in the aneurysm; and patency of the inferior mesenteric artery.[6] Arteriography is also of aid in the patient with a pulsating abdominal mass in whom a neoplasm or cyst must be seriously considered in the differential diagnosis. Arteriography is appropriate for evaluation of the distal circulation in patients who have evidence of obstruction in the iliac, femoral, or popliteal arteries, because additional procedures may be required for these lesions.

COMPLICATIONS

Untreated aortic abdominal aneurysms are associated with several significant complications that are largely dependent on the size of the aneurysm. In a collective survey, patients with aneurysms less than 7 cm. in diameter had a lower mortality from rupture (4% to 18%), whereas in those with aneurysms greater than 7 cm. in diameter mortality was 72% to 83%.[2] For these reasons, some believe that for asymptomatic aneurysms less than 5 to 6 cm. in diameter, observation without operation may be permissible. However, should symptoms appear, operation is indicated.

Rupture is the most frequent and serious complication of aortic abdominal aneurysms, but there are additional hazards, including (1) distal embolization of the peripheral arterial system by thrombi originating in the aneurysm[24]; (2) sudden complete thrombosis[19]; (3) infection, particularly with gram-negative organisms and staphylococci[18]; (4) chronic consumption coagulopathy[35]; (5) aortic intestinal fistula[23]; and (6) the development of an arteriovenous fistula from erosion of the aortic abdominal aneurysm into the inferior vena cava.[27] In this situation, hematuria frequently occurs and may be a sign of this complication.[5] Congestive heart failure may appear and require emergent operation.

Concomitant cholelithiasis can occur with an aortic abdominal aneurysm. In one series of 865 patients, 42 (5%) had this combination.[29] Although in that series simultaneous aneurysmectomy and cholecystectomy were advised provided no contraindications existed, this nevertheless remains a controversial subject and most surgeons prefer to perform aortic aneurysmectomy without an additional procedure that could

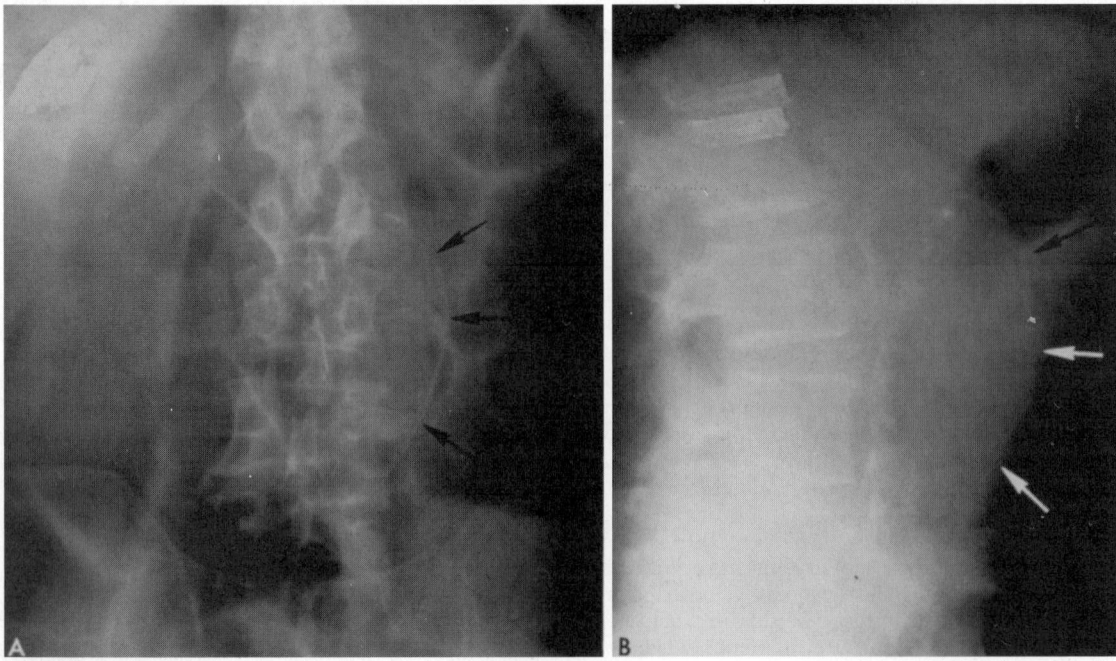

Figure 50–54. *A,* Plain film of abdomen of a patient with an abdominal aortic aneurysm. Note the calcium in the wall of the aneurysm outlining its border *(eggshell). B,* Lateral film showing calcified wall of the aneurysm.

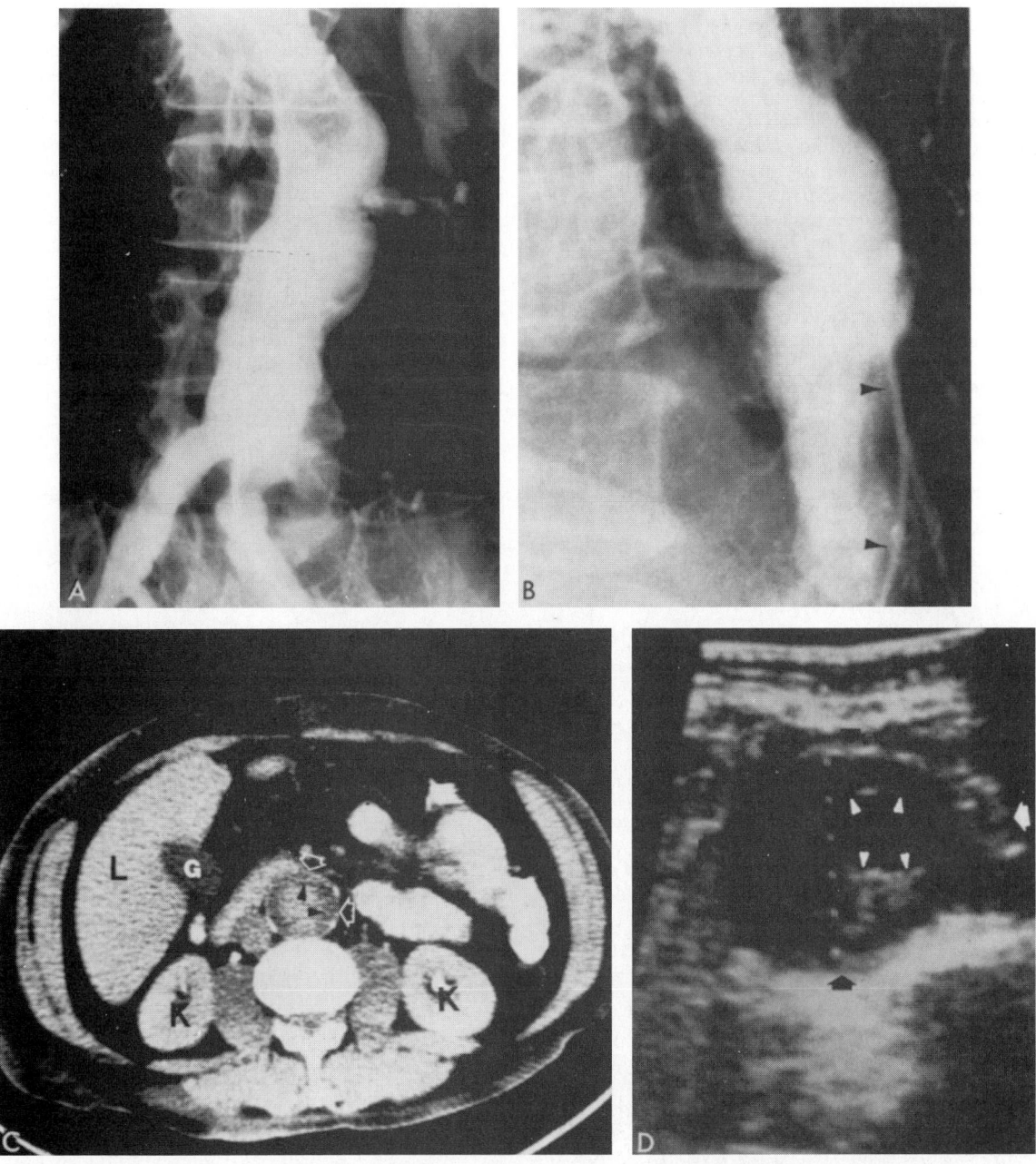

Figure 50–55. *A,* Angiogram in a patient with a pulsatile mass in the lower abdomen demonstrates atherosclerotic changes and mild aneurysmal dilatation of the abdominal aorta. There is some irregularity along the lumen of the common iliac arteries. The outer wall of the vessel is not demonstrated because only the patent portion of the lumen can be opacified with this study. *B,* Cross-table lateral view demonstrates stretching of a peripheral vessel (arrowheads) by a mass in the vicinity of the common iliac artery. *C,* Computed tomographic scan in a patient with an abdominal aortic aneurysm after intravenous contrast medium injection demonstrates the opacified lumen of the aorta (arrowheads define the outer limit of the aortic lumen). The outside wall of the aorta (open arrows) is calcified. The space between the lumen (arrowheads) and the aortic wall (open arrows) represents a clot in the aorta. The scan also demonstrates the liver (L), gallbladder (G), and kidneys (K). *D,* Cross-sectional ultrasonogram through the right common iliac artery demonstrates the vessel to be markedly dilated (arrows indicate outside diameter of vessel) and the lumen to be filled with a considerable amount of clot around the patent central lumen (arrowheads indicate margin of patent lumen). The distance between arrowheads and arrows represents clot-filled lumen. This case illustrates both the ability of ultrasonography to define the entire thickness of a vessel and its use in defining a clot within a vessel. Arteriography is limited to opacification of the patent vessel lumen.

potentially introduce infection into the graft. Of the 18 patients with gallstones in that series, 11 had aneurysmectomy without cholecystectomy and 13 had cholecystectomy only. For those in whom the gallbladder was removed at the time of aneurysmectomy, there was one instance of prosthetic infection that occurred in a patient in whom the graft was not retroperitonealized before cholecystectomy; this patient also had drainage of the liver bed and a gastrostomy. It was interesting that of the 11 patients who underwent aneurysmectomy only, 9 subsequently experienced an episode of acute cholecystitis in the mean follow-up period of 2.9 years.

Two patients had acute cholecystitis in the immediate postoperative period, 1 of whom died of biliary sepsis. It is difficult to be certain whether a combined procedure should be recommended and the issue remains controversial.

TREATMENT

Most abdominal aortic aneurysms should be managed by excision and restoration of arterial continuity with a prosthetic graft. Rarely, those with small aneurysms and those who are poor risks may be observed if asymptomatic. However, there is a growing view that most aneurysms should be excised, even small ones, because the operation has minimal current risk and most aneurysms enlarge with time.

Operative Technique. Operation for excision of abdominal aortic aneurysm is best accomplished through a midline incision extending from the xiphoid process to the symphysis pubis and providing excellent exposure. The abdominal aorta is mobilized proximally so that an arterial clamp can be placed across it for total occlusion (Fig. 50–56). Similarly, the iliac arteries are clamped below. The inferior mesenteric artery is ligated at its origin from the aneurysm and divided. The anterior portion of the aneurysmal sac, including any thrombus present, is then removed. Much of the aneurysmal sac is usually left in place to prevent unnecessary dissection and for use in wrapping around the prosthetic graft to separate it from the duodenum. The lumbar vessels entering the aneurysm usually bleed retrograde and are controlled with transfixion ligatures. A preclotted, straight prosthetic graft of woven Dacron is inserted, and a bifurcation graft is reserved for aneurysms with involvement of the iliac arteries.[9] Prophylactic antibiotics are administered several hours preoperatively and for several days after operation. The results of operation have been highly gratifying.

Certain special features of the operative approach deserve emphasis. During the procedure, it is possible to dislodge thrombi from the aortic aneurysm, which may embolize distally and cause arterial obstruction. Therefore, it is important to demonstrate good back-bleeding from both iliac arteries and to determine the presence of pulses in the femoral, popliteal, posterior tibial, and dorsal pedal arteries at the end of the procedure. Should discrepancy occur in postoperative pulses, compared with those present preoperatively, arterial embolectomy by the Fogarty technique should be considered. Anomalies are also important and include the presence of a retroaortic left renal vein in approximately 5% of patients. Therefore, the left renal vein should be identified routinely

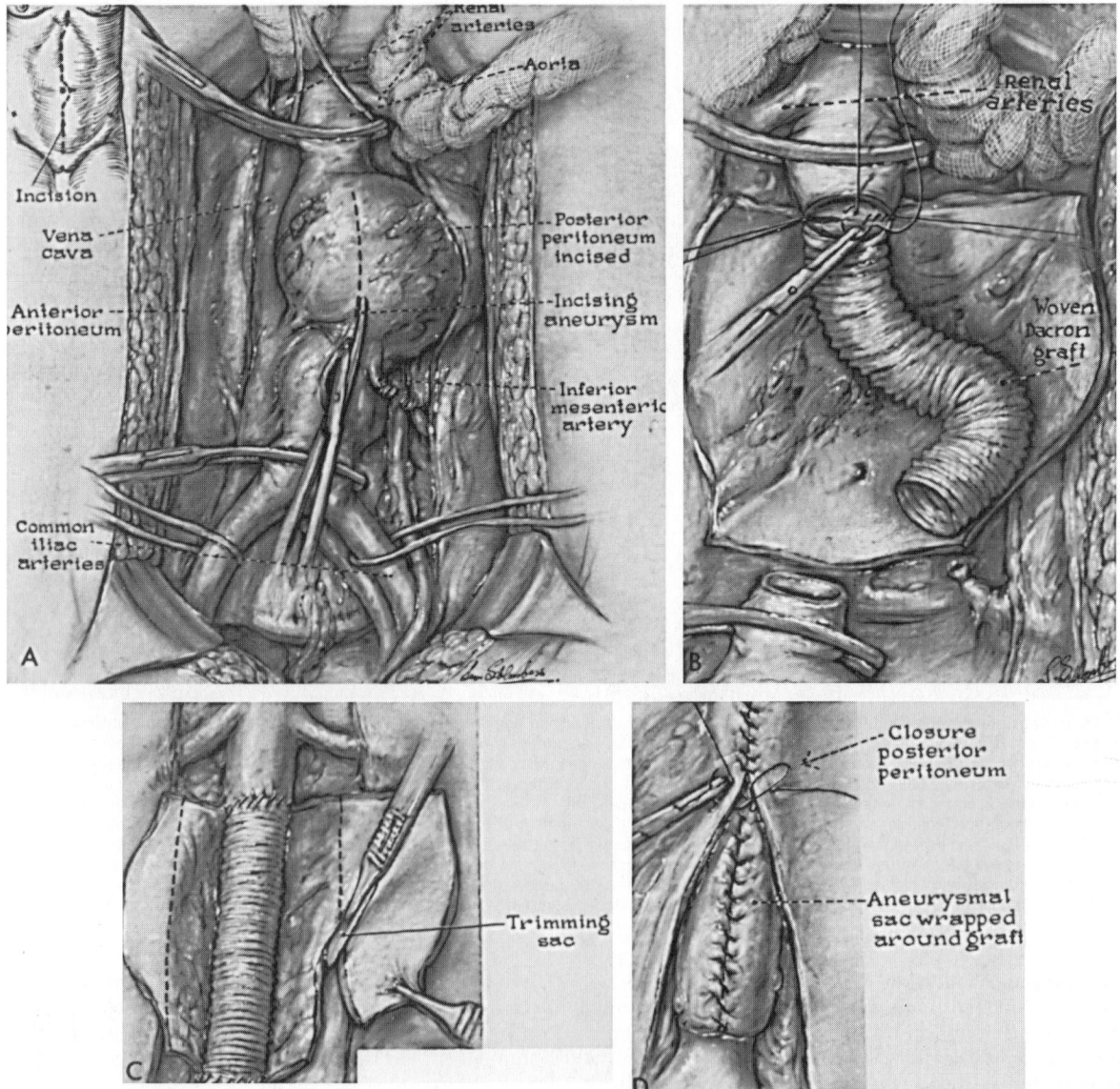

Figure 50–56. *A,* The retroperitoneal tissues are opened and the aneurysm is exposed. A tape is passed proximally around the aneurysm just below the origin of the renal arteries. The inferior mesenteric artery, which is usually obliterated at its origin, is ligated and divided. Tapes are passed around both common iliac arteries distally. Vascular occlusion clamps are placed across the abdominal aorta just above the aneurysm and also just below it. The aneurysm is then incised. *B,* The thrombus in the aneurysm, if present, is removed, and the excess aneurysmal sac is trimmed away. A woven, preclotted Dacron graft is then inserted and sutured end to end. *C,* The graft is shown in place with closure of the remaining aneurysmal wall around it. *D,* The posterior peritoneum is then closed.

in its normal anterior position; if it is not present, care must be taken to prevent injury to it in gaining proximal control of the abdominal aorta. The inferior vena cava may be transposed and found to the left of the aorta. In some instances, there is duplication of the inferior vena cava, which represents a persistent left inferior vena cava. The vena cava may cross the aorta in the region of the renal vessels and constitute a circumaortic renal collar.[4] If the latter is present, division of the left inferior vena cava provides adequate exposure. Although the inferior mesenteric artery can usually be ligated without concern, because its proximal portion is already severely stenosed or occluded, in a small number of patients (1% to 2%) serious ischemia of the sigmoid colon can result. Determination of inferior mesenteric arterial stump pressure has been advocated[11] but is usually unnecessary. If ischemia of the colon develops, the inferior mesenteric artery should be anastomosed to the graft whenever possible. If this is not possible, the colon may be exteriorized (Mikulicz procedure) with resection in several days after the wound has sealed to reduce the likelihood of infection of the graft; the colostomy can be closed later. In one series, in seven patients with ruptured aortic abdominal aneurysms who underwent aneurysmectomy, postoperative ischemic colitis developed. This emphasizes the high incidence of this complication in patients with rupture, and in this series 6 of the 7 patients died.[39] The cause is probably the prolonged hypotension that occurs with ruptured aneurysms before the time of correction. A fiberoptic colonoscopy is helpful in making the diagnosis. Patients with a horseshoe kidney associated with aortic abdominal aneurysm have been reported and present special operative problems.[3] Occasionally in patients with previous abdominal procedures who may have extensive adhesions, a retroperitoneal approach can be utilized through the left flank.[33] Some surgeons have emphasized that postoperative complications have been reported as being less with this approach with a reduction in hospital stay, but postoperative pain may be increased.[34]

More recently, transfemoral graft procedures have been introduced and are being evaluated. In this procedure, plastic grafts and stents are inserted through the femoral artery to treat aortic and peripheral arterial aneurysms and stenoses.

Data from the early series reported indicate the feasibility of the technique, but the complications are significant.[25] Illustrations of this approach are shown in Figures 50–57 and 50–58.

Aortic aneurysms may be extensive and involve the lower thoracic aorta; these thoracoabdominal aneurysms pose difficult problems in surgical treatment. The celiac axis, superior mesenteric artery, and renal arteries may arise from the aneurysm. Therefore, surgical correction requires extensive dissection and mobilization, with tedious restoration of blood flow to each of these critical vessels. By total resection of the aneurysm and stepwise insertion of appropriate grafts, these lesions can be successfully treated (Fig. 50–59).[8]

As a guide to the intraoperative replacement of fluid and blood, the preoperative insertion of a Swan-Ganz catheter for continuous measurement of pulmonary arterial pressures is helpful and is very frequently, if not routinely, used.[38, 40] It is clearly recommended in patients with a history of suspicion of cardiac disorders (Fig. 50–60).

A ruptured aortic abdominal aneurysm is an emergency, and operation should be undertaken immediately. The blood loss should be corrected rapidly; and as soon as the abdomen is entered, it is essential first to control the hemorrhage by proximal compression of the aorta. Large amounts of blood may be necessary in the resuscitation of these patients, and appropriate attention must be given to the temperature of the infused blood as well as to the administration of calcium. In those recovering from the immediate operative procedure, the effects of renal ischemia due to reduced perfusion associated with the low cardiac output state after rupture constitute the major cause of late death. Renal failure appearing postoperatively in these patients is usually associated with an unfavorable prognosis. However, aggressive management including the use of early hemodialysis, often necessary for a number of weeks, may reduce mortality and allow ultimate recovery of renal function.[7] The results after ruptured aortic aneurysms have steadily improved, and lower mortality figures have resulted.[32] Myocardial infarction may also occur, precipitated by hypotension. The mortality varies between 30% and 50% in operations for ruptured abdominal aortic aneurysms.[21]

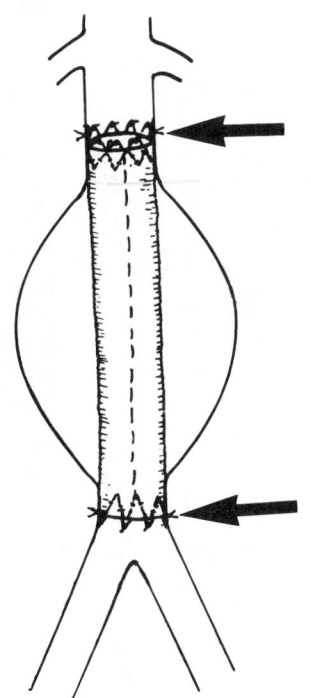
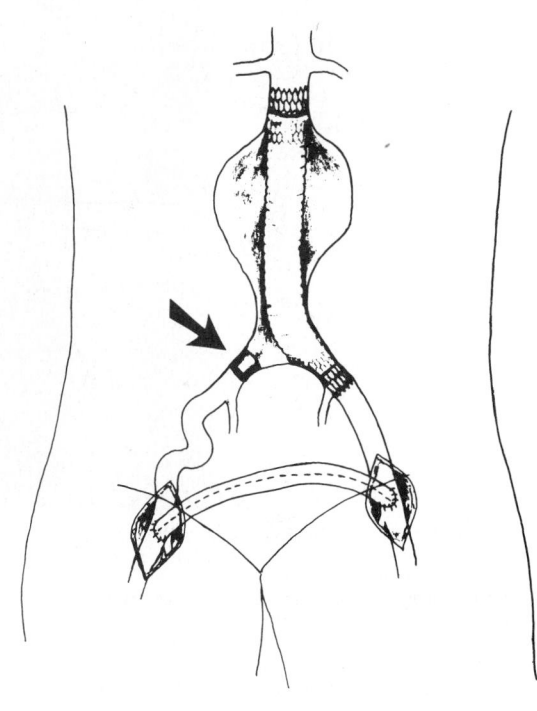

Figure 50–57. Drawing of an aortic reconstruction after transfemoral insertion of the Endovascular Technologies' self-expanding graft (Endograft), and sealing of the graft to the underlying arterial wall by self-expanding, hooked attachment to the arterial wall (arrows). For aneurysms extending to the bifurcation, an aortoiliac reconstruction is performed. Flow through the contralateral common femoral artery is occluded by an endoluminal occlusion device (arrow). A femorofemoral (FF) extra-anatomic bypass restores arterial flow to the contralateral limb. (From Marin, M. L., Veith, F. J., Cynamon, J., et al.: Initial experience with transluminally placed endovascular grafts for the treatment of complex vascular lesions. Ann. Surg., *222:* 449, 1995.)

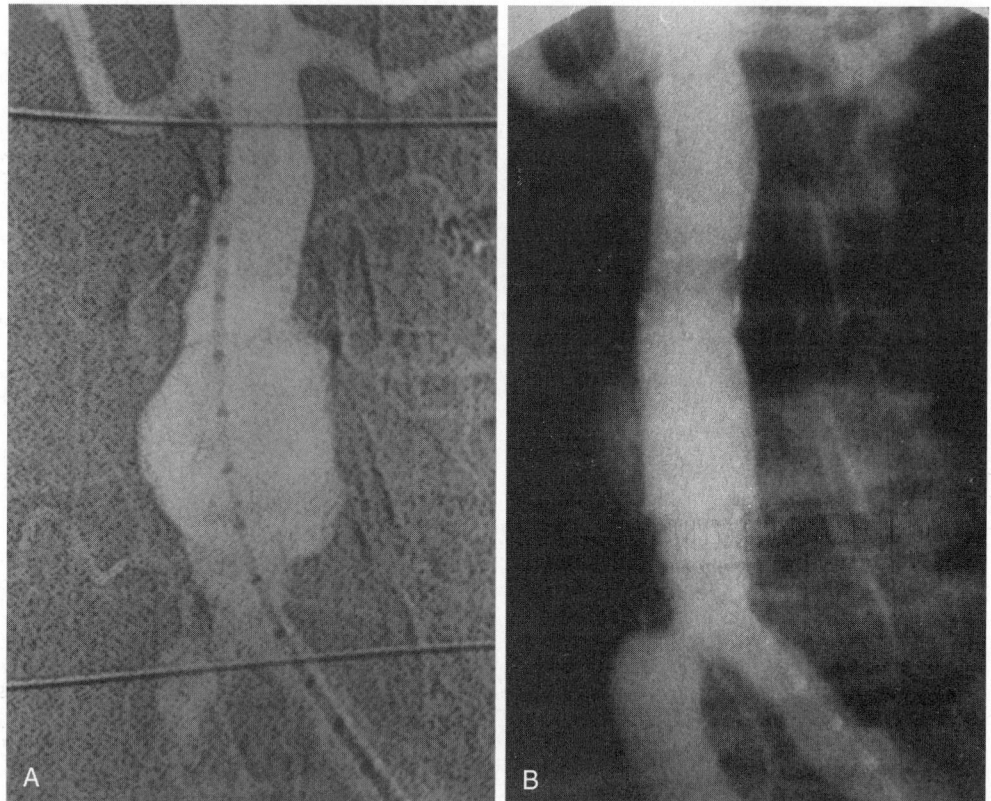

Figure 50–58. Transfemoral and endoluminal repair of aortic aneurysm with Endovascular Technologies' Endograft. *A,* Preoperative arteriogram. *B,* Insertion of the Endograft and exclusion of the aneurysm from the circulation. (From Marin, M. L., Veith, F. J., Cynamon, J., et al.: Initial experience with transluminally placed endovascular grafts for the treatment of complex vascular lesions. Ann. Surg., *222*:449, 1995.)

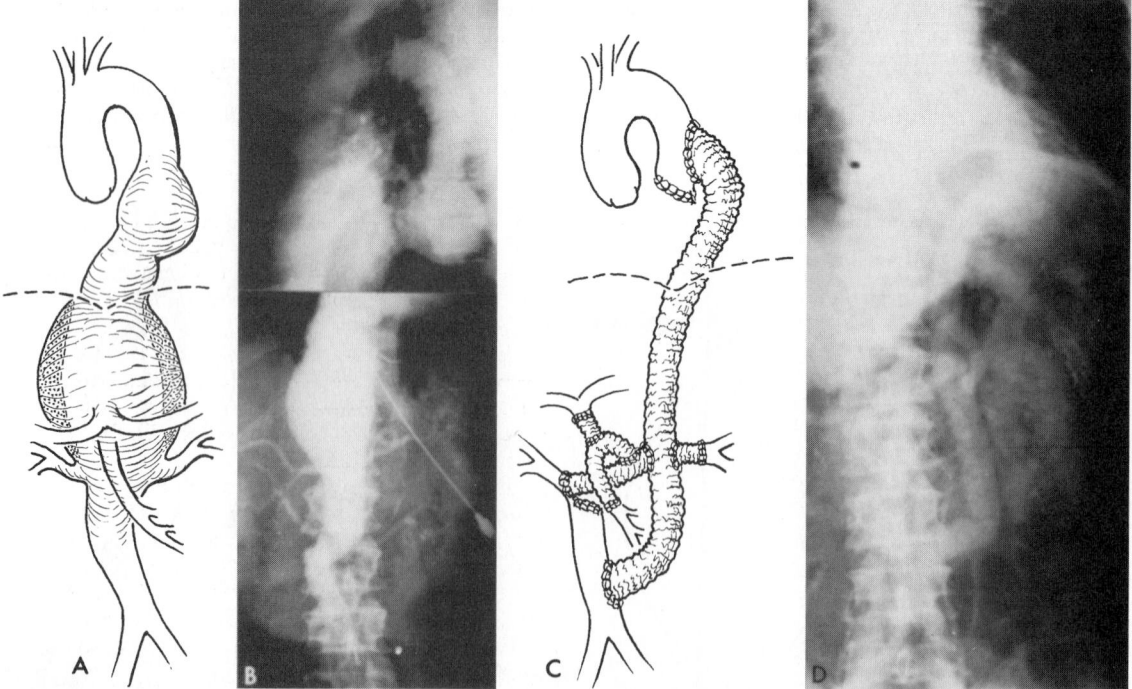

Figure 50–59. Drawing *(A)* and aortogram *(B)* before operation, demonstrating arteriosclerotic thoracoabdominal, aortic aneurysm in a 54-year-old man. *C,* Drawing illustrating method of resection and graft placement. *D,* Aortogram after operation, showing satisfactory function of graft replacements. Patient remains well 5 years after operation. (From DeBakey, M. E., Crawford, E. S., Garrett, H. E., Beall, A. C., Jr., and Howell, J. F.: Surgical considerations in the treatment of aneurysms of the thoraco-abdominal aorta. Ann. Surg., *162*:650, 1965.)

POSTOPERATIVE COMPLICATIONS

Aortic abdominal aneurysmectomy is recognized to be a major operative procedure, and a number of specific postoperative complications may occur. One of the most serious of these complications is acute myocardial infarction. Every effort is made to prevent this problem, either by preoperative correction of the myocardial insufficiency or careful monitoring during the operative procedure. In a series of 246 patients with aortic abdominal aneurysms, severe surgically correctable coronary artery disease was documented in 78 patients (32%), 70 of whom underwent myocardial revascularization before aortic aneurysmectomy. The mortality for this procedure was 5.7%. The authors believed that the data supported the view that selected patients who require elective resection of aortic abdominal aneurysms also warrant myocardial revascularization to reduce perioperative risk and improve late survival.[17] Fortunately, the majority of patients recover without significant problems and are usually discharged from the hospital within a week. Abdominal distention, usually due to postoperative paralytic ileus, may occur and is usually self-limited. Although some routinely use a nasogastric tube for several days postoperatively, this has proved unnecessary, because at least three fourths of patients never require it. However, if distention occurs or if a distended stomach or bowel is demonstrated on physical examination or the abdominal film, insertion of a nasogastric tube is indicated for immediate decompression and removal or maintenance until the distention is relieved and peristalsis returns.

Bleeding from the graft may occur at the suture line or through the interstices of the graft. Continuous measurement of the abdominal girth postoperatively is useful if this appears to be a problem, in addition to the usual measures for identification of reduced blood volume. Correction of blood loss may suffice if bleeding is minimal, but re-exploration should be performed if bleeding persists. Particular attention should be given to the arterial circulation of the lower extremities, because emboli and thrombi may occur after operation or during the postoperative period.

A very serious complication is infection of the graft, especially if it occurs at the suture lines.[16] Fortunately, this is rare and occurs in 1% or less in most series. Infection is particularly hazardous, because management is directed toward removal of the graft with occlusion of the terminal aorta by

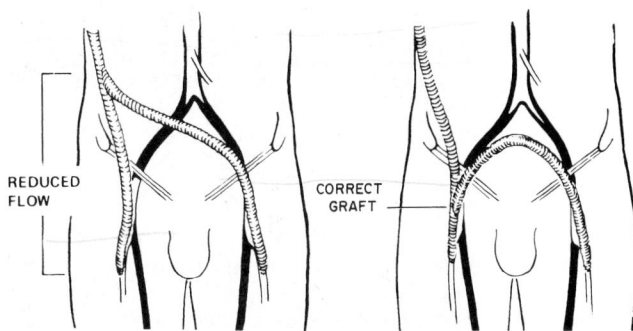

Figure 50–61. Optimal configuration of contralateral limb. *Left*, Diagram of incorrect "bifurcation" limb to contralateral artery, which subjects the distal portion of main limb to a sudden drop in flow. *Right*, Correct axillobilateral femoral bypass configuration, allowing the main limb to have the benefit of higher flow throughout the entire length. (From Ray, L. I., et al.: Axillofemoral bypass: A critical reappraisal of its role in the management of aortoiliac occlusive disease. Am. J. Surg., *138*:117, 1979.)

monofilament sutures or wire staples. Restoration of blood flow from an uninfected proximal area to the femoral vessels below, such as axillobifemoral grafting, is indicated (Fig. 50–61).[30] Unless a procedure of this magnitude is undertaken, ultimate massive hemorrhage from the infected anastomotic site usually follows. Thrombi in an abdominal aortic aneurysm are sometimes infected with various organisms, and in previous reports positive cultures have been found in 10% to 15%. In one study, 14% had positive cultures, but only rarely were specific antibiotics other than the routine prophylactic regimen given. There was no evidence of early or late prosthetic graft sepsis, and the conclusion was drawn that a positive culture may not imply clinical infection at the time of operation and that prolonged postoperative organism-specific antibiotic therapy does not appear necessary in patients who simply have a positive culture and no other clinical data to support the diagnosis of infection.[26]

The proximal suture line of the anastomosis may rupture into the duodenum or intestine and present an equally serious complication. Occasionally, chronic bleeding occurs in such a communication, allowing time for appropriate diagnosis and elective operation. In other instances, bleeding is sudden and massive, requiring emergency operation for control of the hemorrhage, closure of the duodenal or intestinal communication, and removal of the graft with appropriate reconstitution of blood flow through a noninfected area to the lower extremities.

False aneurysms also occur at the suture lines and may become manifest by pain or a pulsatile mass. In such instances, an appropriate diagnosis can be established by arteriography, whereas in other instances the first sign of such an aneurysm may be rupture.

Changes in sexual function are of considerable importance after resection of abdominal aortic aneurysms, and retrograde ejaculation has been reported in as many as two thirds of patients.[37] Loss of potency also occurs in as many as one third of patients, and these complications appear to be related to the extensiveness of dissection of the sympathetic plexus, which lies along the lower abdominal aorta on its left side and near the inferior mesenteric artery. If this is left undisturbed, interference with sexual function is minimized.

Although infrequent, spinal cord ischemia may follow abdominal aortic surgery.[13] This complication appears to be somewhat more common in association with *ruptured* aortic abdominal aneurysms, perhaps aggravated by the associated hypotension. However, rupture is not a prerequisite, and the phenomenon occurs after elective operations. The classic anterior spinal artery syndrome is characterized by paraple-

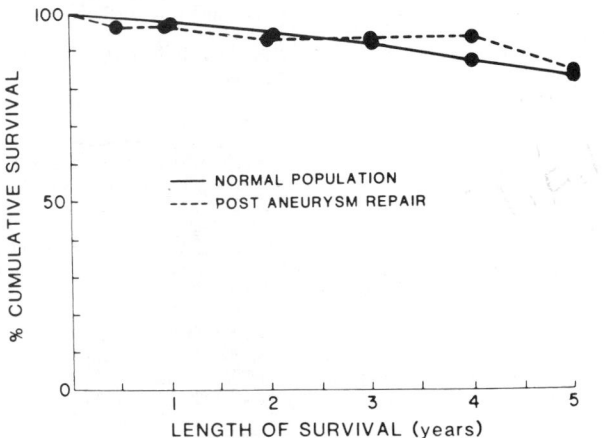

Figure 50–60. Five-year cumulative survival curve for 110 consecutive patients operated on for infrarenal abdominal aortic aneurysms compared with a similar curve for nonsurgical, age- and sex-adjusted populations derived from U.S. Department of Health, Education, and Welfare life-table statistics. The observed difference was not statistically significant (p = .157). (From Whittemore, A. D., Clowes, A. W., Hechtman, H. B., and Mannick, J. A.: Aortic aneurysm repair: Reduced operative mortality associated with optimal cardiac performance. Ann. Surg., *192*:414, 1980.)

gia, rectal and urinary incontinence, and loss of pain and temperature sensation below the lesion, but with sparing of vibration and proprioceptive sense. Patients sustaining neurologic deficits in the lower extremities after abdominal aortic procedures commonly have loss of posterior column modalities.

RESULTS

In earlier years the mortality was appreciable,[2] but it has diminished in recent years and is now 5% or less in most centers[36] and has been reported in a large series as low as 1%. The mortality is primarily due to associated lesions of atherosclerosis that complicate the postoperative recovery, including myocardial infarction, cerebrovascular lesions, and hypertensive cardiovascular renal disease. The long-term results of resection of abdominal aortic aneurysms showed that the 5-year survival was 72%; and for those younger than age 70 at the time of operation, the 5-year survival probability was 79%. These outstanding results are believed to be due to accomplishments following an aggressive policy of screening and selectively treating coronary disease and carotid stenosis preoperatively and utilization of such intraoperative adjuncts as routine Swan-Ganz monitoring, autologous blood transfusion with the cell saver, and the frequent use of tube grafts.[1]

SELECTED REFERENCES

Crawford, E. S.: Thoraco-abdominal aortic aneurysms involving renal, superior mesenteric, and celiac arteries. Ann. Surg., 179:763, 1974.

In this review, the management of 23 consecutive patients with thoracoabdominal aortic aneurysms, including those of renal, superior mesenteric, and celiac arteries, is presented. Emphasis is placed on surgical technique, which depended on the anatomic location of the aneurysm. A number of excellent illustrations are included and demonstrate the surgical procedures required. Of the 23 patients, 22 survived and did well for periods of up to 13 years, indicating the feasibility of the extensive operations required in the management of these lesions.

DeBakey, M. E., Crawford, E. S., Cooley, D. A., Morris, G. C., Jr., Royster, T. S., and Abbott, W. P.: Aneurysm of abdominal aorta: Analysis of results of graft replacement therapy one to eleven years after operation. Ann. Surg., 160:622, 1964.

Long-term follow-up of the fate of patients with removal of abdominal aortic aneurysms is presented in this paper. The favorable prognosis after operation is emphasized.

Estes, J. E., Jr.: Abdominal aortic aneurysm: A study of one hundred and two cases. Circulation, 2:258, 1950.

This is an often-quoted study of the follow-up of a large group of patients with aortic abdominal aneurysms before the advent of surgical treatment.

Pierce, G. E. (Guest Ed.): Abdominal aortic aneurysms. Surg. Clin. North Am., 69(4), 1989.

This is a review of the incidence, diagnosis, and management of abdominal aortic aneurysms. Considerable attention is given to special preoperative, intraoperative, and postoperative complications. It is a valuable reference source for the entire field.

Thompson, J. E., Hollier, L. H., Patman, R. D., and Persson, A. V.: Surgical management of abdominal aortic aneurysms: Factors influencing mortality and morbidity: A 20-year experience. Ann. Surg., 181:654, 1975.

The authors review a personal experience in a large group with aortic abdominal aneurysms undergoing elective resection over a 20-year period. The mortality diminished from 17% during the first 7 years of the study to 5.5% in the 1968–1974 period. Reasons for the diminishing mortality are presented.

REFERENCES

1. Bernstein, E. F., Dilley, R. B., and Randolph, H. F., III: The improving long-term outlook for patients over 70 years of age with abdominal aortic aneurysms. Ann. Surg., 207:318, 1988.
2. Bernstein, E. F., Fisher, J. C., and Varco, R. L.: Is excision the optimum treatment for all abdominal aortic aneurysms? Surgery, 61:83, 1967.
3. Bietz, D., and Merendino, K. A.: Abdominal aortic aneurysm and horseshoe kidney. Ann. Surg., 181:333, 1975.
4. Brener, B. J., Darling, R. C., Frederick, P. L., and Linton, R. R.: Major venous anomalies complicating abdominal aortic surgery. Arch. Surg., 108:159, 1974.
5. Brewster, D. C., Ottinger, L. W., and Darling, R. C.: Hematuria as a sign of aortocaval fistula. Ann. Surg., 186:766, 1977.
6. Brewster, D. C., Retana, A., Waltman, A. C., and Darling, R. C.: Angiogra-
7. Chawla, S. K., Najafi, H., Ing, T. S., Dye, W. S., Javid, H., Hunter, J. A., Goldin, M. D., and Serry, C.: Acute renal failure complicating ruptured abdominal aortic aneurysm. Arch. Surg., 110:521, 1975.
8. Crawford, E. S.: Thoraco-abdominal and abdominal aortic aneurysms involving renal superior mesenteric and celiac arteries. Ann. Surg., 179:763, 1974.
9. DeBakey, M. E., Crawford, E. S., Cooley, D. A., Morris, G. C., Jr., Royster, T. S., and Abbott, W. P.: Aneurysm of the abdominal aorta: Analysis of results of graft replacement therapy one to eleven years after operation. Ann. Surg., 160:622, 1964.
10. Dubost, C., Allary, M., and Oeconomos, N. M.: Resection of an aneurysm of the abdominal aorta: Reestablishment of the continuity by a preserved human arterial graft, with results after five months. Arch. Surg., 64:405, 1952.
11. Ernst, C. B., Hagihara, P. F., Daugherty, M. E., and Griffen, W. O., Jr.: Inferior mesenteric artery stump pressure: A reliable index for safe IMA ligation during abdominal aortic aneurysmectomy. Ann. Surg., 187:641, 1978.
12. Estes, J. E., Jr.: Abdominal aortic aneurysm: A study of one hundred and two cases. Circulation, 2:258, 1950.
13. Ferguson, L. R. J., Bergan, J. J., Conn, J., Jr., and Yao, J. S. T.: Spinal ischemia following abdominal aortic surgery. Ann. Surg., 181:267, 1975.
14. Gliedman, M. L., Ayers, W. G., and Vestal, B. L.: Aneurysms of the abdominal aorta and its branches: A study of untreated patients. Ann. Surg., 146:207, 1957.
15. Gomes, M. N., Schellinger, D., and Hufnagel, C. A.: Abdominal aortic aneurysms: Diagnostic review and new technique. Ann. Thorac. Surg., 27:479, 1979.
16. Hardy, J. D., and Conn, J. H. J.: Infected arterial grafts. In Hardy, J. D. (Ed.): Critical Surgical Illness. Philadelphia, W. B. Saunders, 1971.
17. Hertzer, N. R., Young, J. R., Beven, E. G., O'Hara, P. J., Graor, R. A., Ruschhaupt, W. F., and Maljovec, L. C.: Late results of coronary bypass in patients with infrarenal aortic aneurysms. Ann. Surg., 205:360, 1987.
18. Jarrett, F., Darling, R. C., Mundth, E. D., and Austen, W. G.: Experience with infected aneurysms of the abdominal aorta. Arch. Surg., 110:1281, 1975.
19. Johnson, J. M., Gaspar, M. R., Movius, H. J., and Rosental, J. J.: Sudden complete thrombosis of aortic and iliac aneurysms. Arch. Surg., 108:792, 1974.
20. Klippel, A. P., and Butcher, H. R., Jr.: The unoperated abdominal aortic aneurysm. Am. J. Surg., 111:629, 1966.
21. Lawrence, M. S., Crosby, V. G., and Ehrenhaft, J. L.: Ruptured abdominal aortic aneurysm. Ann. Thorac. Surg., 2:159, 1966.
22. Leopold, G. R., Goldberger, L. E., and Bernstein, E. F.: Ultrasonic detection and evaluation of abdominal aortic aneurysms. Surgery, 72:939, 1972.
23. Levy, M. J., Todd, D. B., Lillehei, C. W., and Varco, R. L.: Aorticointestinal fistulas following surgery of the aorta. Surgery, 120:992, 1965.
24. Lord, J. W., Jr., Rossi, G., Daliana, M., Drago, J. R., and Schwartz, A. M.: Unsuspected abdominal aortic aneurysms as the cause of peripheral arterial occlusive disease. Ann. Surg., 177:767, 1973.
25. Marin, M. L., Veith, F. J., Cynamon, J., Sanchez, L. A., Lyon, R. T., Levine, B. A., Bakal, C. W., Suggs, W. D., Rozenblit, A., and Parodi, J. C.: Initial experience with transluminally placed endovascular grafts for the treatment of complex vascular lesions. Ann. Surg., 222:449, 1995.
26. McAuley, C. E., Steed, D. L., and Webster, M. W.: Bacterial presence in aortic thrombus at elective aneurysm resection: Is it clinically significant? Am. J. Surg., 147:322, 1984.
27. Mohr, L. L., and Smith, L. L.: Arteriovenous fistula from rupture of abdominal aortic aneurysm. Arch. Surg., 110:806, 1975.
28. Moossa, H. H., Peitzman, A. B., Steed, D. L., Julian, T. B., Jarrett, F., and Webster, M. W.: Inflammatory aneurysms of the abdominal aorta. Arch. Surg., 124:673, 1989.
29. Ouriel, K., Ricotta, J. J., Adams, J. T., and DeWeese, J. A.: Management of cholelithiasis in patients with abdominal aortic aneurysm. Ann. Surg., 198:717, 1983.
30. Ray, L. I., O'Connor, J. B., Davis, C. C., Hall, D. G., Mansfield, P. B., Rittenhouse, E. A., Smith, J. C., Wood, S. G., and Sauvage, L. R.: Axillofemoral bypass: A critical reappraisal of its role in the management of aorto-iliac occlusive disease. Am. J. Surg., 138:117, 1979.
31. Schatz, I. J., Fairbairn, J. F., II, and Juergens, J. L.: Abdominal aortic aneurysms: A reappraisal. Circulation, 26:200, 1962.
32. Shumacker, H. B., Jr., Barnes, D. L., and King, H.: Ruptured abdominal aortic aneurysms. Ann. Surg., 177:772, 1973.
33. Shepard, A. D., Scott, G. R., Mackey, W. C., O'Donnell, T. F., Jr., Bush, H. L., and Callow, A. D.: Retroperitoneal approach to high-risk abdominal aortic aneurysms. Arch. Surg., 121:444, 1986.
34. Sicard, G. A., Reilly, J. M., Rubin, B. G., Thompson, R. W., Allen, B. T., Flye, M. W., Schechtman, K. B., Young-Beyer, P., Weiss, C., and Anderson, C. B.: Transabdominal versus retroperitoneal incision for abdominal aortic surgery: Report of a prospective randomized trial. J. Vasc. Surg., 21:174, 1995.
35. Siebert, W. T., and Natelson, E. A.: Chronic consumption coagulopathy accompanying abdominal aortic aneurysm. Arch. Surg., 111:539, 1976.
36. Thompson, J. E., Hollier, L. H., Patman, R. D., and Persson, A. V.: Surgical

management of abdominal aortic aneurysms: Factors influencing mortality and morbidity: A 20-year experience. Ann. Surg., *181*:654, 1975.

37. Weinstein, M. H., and Machleder, H. I.: Sexual function after aortoiliac surgery. Ann. Surg., *181*:787, 1975.

38. Weisel, R. D., Dennis, R. C., Manny, J., Mannick, J. A., Valeri, C. R., and Hechtman, H. B.: Adverse effects of transfusion therapy during abdominal aortic aneurysmectomy. Surgery, *83*:682, 1978.

39. Welling, R. E., Roedersheimer, L. R., Arbaugh, J. J., and Cranley, J. J.: Ischemic colitis following repair of ruptured abdominal aortic aneurysm. Arch. Surg., *120*:1368, 1985.

40. Whittemore, A. D., Clowes, A. W., Hechtman, H. B., and Mannick, J. A.: Aortic aneurysm repair: Reduced operative mortality associated with optimal cardiac performance. Ann. Surg., *191*:414, 1980.

FEMORAL ARTERY ANEURYSMS

Raymond G. Makhoul, M.D.

Aneurysms of the femoral artery may be grouped into two major categories: true aneurysms and false aneurysms. True aneurysms, which involve all three layers of the vessel wall, are largely due to atherosclerotic degeneration and are the second most common location for peripheral aneurysms. Atherosclerotic femoral aneurysms have a very high association with abdominal aortic and popliteal aneurysms (70%–95%), and approximately 50% occur bilaterally.[3, 5, 6, 8, 9, 25] Aneurysmal degeneration of the femoral artery almost always involves the common femoral artery. Those femoral artery aneurysms limited to the common femoral artery are known as Type I, whereas those involving the orifice of the deep femoral artery are termed Type II.[5] The type of femoral aneurysm has implications for the operative reconstructive approach. Isolated aneurysms of the superficial femoral artery and deep femoral artery have been reported, although they are rare.[19, 24]

False aneurysms of the femoral artery are most commonly iatrogenic, occurring after percutaneous cannulation of the femoral vessels or anastomotic and secondary to the gradual disruption of the anastomosis of a graft to the native artery. Iatrogenic false aneurysms occur when a puncture site does not seal and a perivascular hematoma forms, with a central area that remains fluid (Fig. 50–62*A*). With the introduction of complex percutaneous procedures such as angioplasty, valvuloplasty, atherectomy, and coronary stenting, there has

been a rise in the incidence of iatrogenic aneurysms to 0.6% to 1.0%.[2, 15, 17] Risk factors associated with the development of iatrogenic false aneurysms include the use of large-bore catheters, female gender, use of anticoagulant and thrombolytic agents, and unintentional cannulation of the deep femoral or superficial artery.[14, 17] Femoral anastomotic false aneurysms occur with an incidence of 1.5% to 3.0%.[16, 23] Possible etiologic factors include suture deterioration, infection, prosthetic dilation, and host vessel degeneration.[11, 16, 20, 23, 26] Interestingly, these aneurysms are more frequently associated with inflow procedures such as aortobifemoral bypass than with infrainguinal bypass (Fig. 50–63).

CLINICAL MANIFESTATIONS AND DIAGNOSIS

Patients with true femoral artery aneurysms may present with a painless, pulsatile groin mass (about 25%) or with symptoms of arterial ischemia, local compression of the femoral nerve or vein, or groin pain. The ischemic symptoms from a femoral aneurysm may vary from claudication to an acutely threatened limb and may be secondary to embolization of some of the laminated clot from within the aneurysm or from acute thrombosis of the aneurysm. Rupture of true, atherosclerotic femoral aneurysms is rare and occurs in less than 2% of patients. Because of their superficial location, diagnosis of femoral aneurysm is easily made by palpation. Ultrasonography is the most useful confirmatory test, enabling documentation of the size of the aneurysm and the presence or absence of mural thrombus. Computed tomography may occasionally be helpful, and arteriography is best reserved for those patients having operative repair.

Iatrogenic false aneurysms are usually symptomatic and may grow rapidly. They also present as a pulsatile groin mass that may be difficult to differentiate from a hematoma. Color-flow duplex ultrasonography is very useful in the diagnosis of these aneurysms, allowing for measurement of size, area of flow, and delineation of the track between the arterial injury and the pseudoaneurysm.[21] Femoral false aneurysms may thrombose spontaneously or may rapidly expand, rupture, or produce a femoral neuralgia or femoral venous thrombosis.[10, 12] Anastomotic false aneurysms produce symptoms related to local compression of the adjacent femoral nerve and vein. In addition, they may cause ischemia by embolism distally or by acute thrombosis. Ultrasonography is

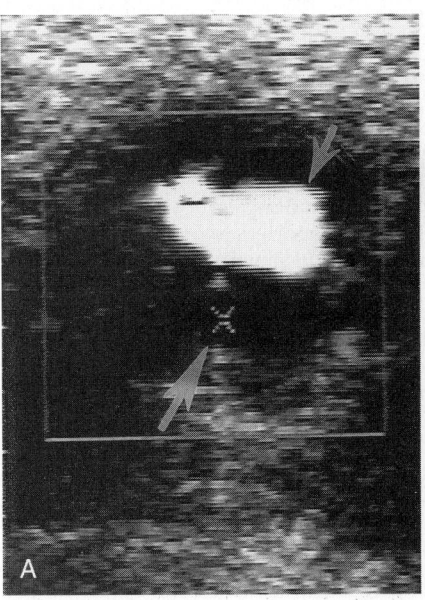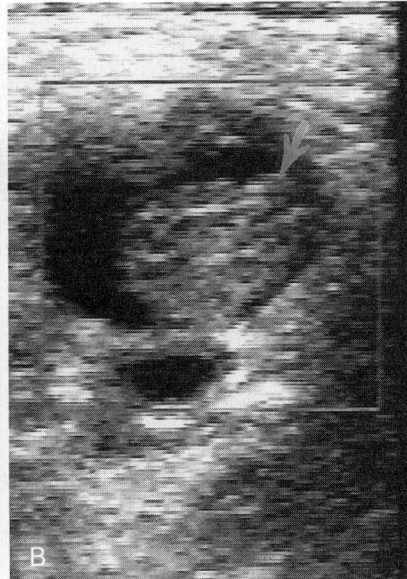

Figure 50–62. *A,* Color flow duplex scan (shown in black and white) of an iatrogenic femoral artery false aneurysm. The femoral artery (large arrow) is associated with a perivascular hematoma (small arrow). *B,* After 20 minutes of ultrasound-guided compression, the fluid center of the false aneurysm has been successfully thrombosed.

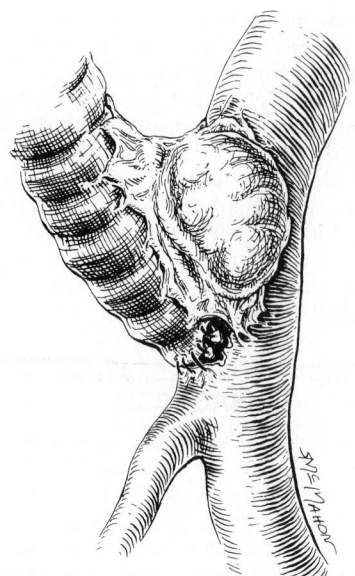

Figure 50–63. Femoral anastomotic aneurysm secondary to separation of the prosthetic graft from the native femoral artery. (From Rutherford, R. B.: Vascular Surgery, 3rd ed. Philadelphia, W. B. Saunders, 1989.)

useful to confirm the diagnosis, and arteriography is usually indicated before repair.

TREATMENT

All symptomatic atherosclerotic femoral artery aneurysms should be repaired surgically. The treatment of small, asymptomatic femoral aneurysms is somewhat more controversial owing to conflicting data regarding their natural history. In a report of 12 femoral aneurysms followed nonoperatively, there was a 42% rate of subsequent thrombosis.[25] In a much larger series of 105 aneurysms followed nonoperatively, only 3 were later associated with major limb-threatening complications.[9] Others have reported similar results.[1] Thus, it would seem that small, asymptomatic aneurysms can be observed safely, while surgical repair should be reserved for symptomatic aneurysms and asymptomatic aneurysms larger than 2.0 to 2.5 cm.

Iatrogenic false aneurysms were initially thought to be unstable lesions, and therefore surgical repair was recommended in all instances. More recently, however, there is evidence that a number of these pseudoaneurysms spontaneously thrombose with no residual complications. In addition, there are now numerous reports of nonoperative management of these lesions using ultrasound-guided compression.[7, 8, 13, 22] With this technique, the ultrasound probe is used to compress the aneurysm and aneurysm track, resulting in thrombosis (see Fig. 50–62B). The largest series reported to date is from the Cleveland Clinic, where successful closure was achieved in 94 of 100 patients with postcatheterization femoral pseudoaneurysms.[4] Thus, it appears that this is a safe, effective means of treating these iatrogenic injuries, with a high rate of success. For those pseudoaneurysms that are rapidly expanding, infected, very large, or ruptured, surgery remains the procedure of choice.

Surgical Technique

Surgical management of true atherosclerotic aneurysms of the femoral artery usually requires interposition grafting. These aneurysms are generally explored using a vertical inci-

sion and obtaining control of the common femoral artery below the inguinal ligament. If the aneurysm extends more proximally, the vertical incision can be extended laterally toward the anterior iliac spine. Alternatively, a separate retroperitoneal or *transplant* incision may be made for control of the external iliac artery. If the aneurysm is confined to the common femoral artery (Type I), an interposition graft of synthetic material is most commonly used, because autogenous vein is often too small for anastomosis to the artery. When the aneurysm involves the deep femoral (Type II) or a patent superficial femoral artery, the surgical technique must be modified to ensure perfusion of these vessels (Fig. 50–64). The long-term results for repair of femoral artery aneurysms are excellent, with a very low incidence of morbidity and mortality.[3, 18]

Repair of iatrogenic femoral false aneurysms usually involves a longitudinal groin incision over the femoral pulse with control of the common femoral artery. If the hematoma extends to or above the inguinal ligament, a retroperitoneal incision for proximal control of the external iliac artery may be needed. After the common femoral or external iliac artery is clamped, the hematoma is incised and evacuated. The puncture site in the artery is identified, gently controlled with finger pressure, and repaired with one or two sutures. Care must be taken during these repairs to avoid injury to

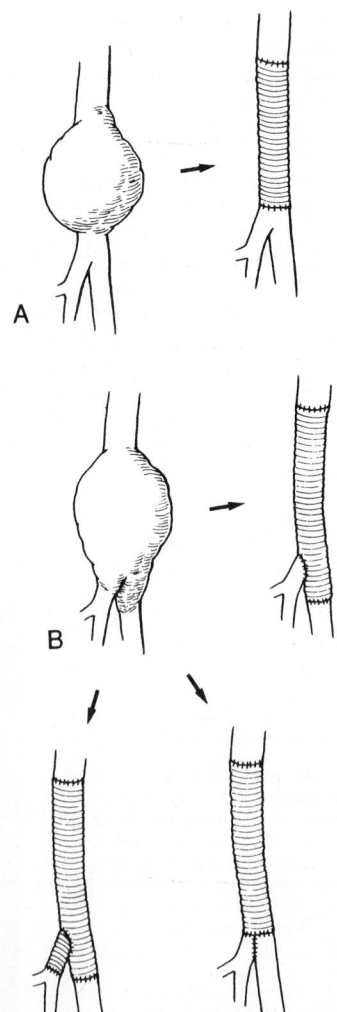

Figure 50–64. *A*, Repair of a femoral artery aneurysm (Type I) using prosthetic material. *B*, With involvement of the deep femoral artery orifice (Type II), reimplantation of this vessel may be necessary. (From Rutherford, R. B.: Vascular Surgery, 4th ed. Philadelphia, W. B. Saunders, 1995.)

the cutaneous branches of the femoral nerve, which may result in a painful femoral neuralgia.[10]

The repair of anastomotic false aneurysms requires proximal control of the graft limb, which may be obtained either through a vertical incision or through the retroperitoneum. Distal control of the deep femoral and superficial femoral arteries may be obtained directly or alternatively from within the aneurysm, using balloon tamponade. Usually a new graft segment is placed between the femoral artery and the old graft limb. Care should be taken to take deep bites of the artery and to avoid excessive tension on the anastomosis.

SELECTED REFERENCES

Cox, G. S., Young, J. R., Gray, B. R., Grubb, M. W., and Hertzer, N. R.: Ultrasound-guided compression repair of postcatheterization pseudoaneurysms: Results of treatment in 100 cases. J. Vasc. Surg., 19:683, 1994.
This is the largest series to date involving the use of ultrasound-guided compression in the treatment of iatrogenic femoral false aneurysms. The authors demonstrate the effectiveness of this modality in achieving successful thrombosis of these lesions.

Graham, L. M., Zelenock, G. B., Whitehouse, W. M., Erlandson, E. E., Dent, T. L., Lindenauer, S. M., and Stanley, J. C.: Clinical significance of arteriosclerotic femoral artery aneurysms. Arch. Surg., 115:502, 1980.
This is an often-cited review of the University of Michigan experience with femoral artery aneurysms over a 22-year period. This series includes 172 aneurysms in 100 patients and emphasizes the relatively benign natural history of small femoral aneurysms.

REFERENCES

1. Adiseshiah, M., and Bailey, D. A.: Aneurysms of the femoral artery. Br. J. Surg., 64:174, 1977.
2. Babu, S. C., Piccorelli, G. O., Shah, P. M., Stein, J. H., and Clauss, R. H.: Incidence and results of arterial complications among 16,350 patients undergoing cardiac catheterization. J. Vasc. Surg., 10:113, 1989.
3. Baird, R. J., Gurry, J. F., Kellam, J., and Plume, S. K.: Arteriosclerotic femoral artery aneurysms. Can. Med. Assoc., 117:1306, 1977.
4. Cox, G. S., Young, J. R., Gray, B. R., Grubb, M. W., and Hertzer, N. R.: Ultrasound-guided compression repair of postcatheterization pseudoaneurysms: Results of treatment in one hundred cases. J. Vasc. Surg., 19:683, 1994.
5. Cutler, B. S., and Darling, R. C.: Surgical management of arteriosclerotic femoral aneurysms. Surgery, 74:764, 1973.
6. Dent, T. L., Lindenauer, S. M., Ernst, C. B., and Fry, W. J.: Multiple arteriosclerotic arterial aneurysms. Arch. Surg., 105:338, 1972.
7. Feld, R., Patton, G. M., Carabasi, R. A., Alexander, A., Merton, D., and Needleman, L.: Treatment of iatrogenic femoral artery injuries with ultrasound-guided compression. J. Vasc. Surg., 16:832, 1992.
8. Fellmeth, B. D., Roberts, A. C., Bookstein, J. J., Freischlag, J. A., Forsythe, J. R., Buckner, N. K., and Hye, R. J.: Postangiographic femoral artery injuries: Nonsurgical repair with US-guided compression. Radiology, 178:671, 1991.
9. Graham, L. M., Zelenock, G. B., Whitehouse, W. M., Erlandson, E. E., Dent, T. L., Lindenauer, S. M., and Stanley, J. C.: Clinical significance of arteriosclerotic femoral artery aneurysms. Arch. Surg., 115:502, 1980.
10. Hallett, J. W., Wolk, S. W., Cherry, K. J., Gloviczki, P., and Pairolero, P. C.: The femoral neuralgia syndrome after arterial catheter trauma. J. Vasc. Surg., 11:702, 1990.
11. Hollier, L. H., Batson, R. C., and Cohn, I.: Femoral anastomotic aneurysms. Ann. Surg., 191:715, 1980.
12. Kent, K. C., McArdle, C. R., Kennedy, B., Baim, D. S., Anninos, E., and Skillman, J. J.: A prospective study of the clinical outcome of femoral pseudoaneurysms and arteriovenous fistulas induced by arterial puncture. J. Vasc. Surg., 17:125, 1993.
13. Khoury, M., Batra, S., Berg, R., and Rama, K.: Duplex-guided compression of iatrogenic femoral artery pseudoaneurysms. Am. Surg., 60:234, 1994.
14. Kim, D., Orron, D. E., Skillman, J. J., Kent, K. C., Porter, D. H., Schlam, B. W., Carrozza, J., Reis, G. J., and Baim, D. S.: Role of superficial femoral artery puncture in the development of pseudoaneurysm and arteriovenous fistula complicating percutaneous transfemoral cardiac catheterization. Cathet. Cardiovasc. Diagn., 25:91, 1992.
15. Kresowik, T. F., Khoury, M. D., Miller, B. V., Winniford, M. D., Shamma, A. R., Sharp, W. J., Blecha, M. B., and Corson, J. D.: A prospective study of the incidence and natural history of femoral vascular complications after percutaneous transluminal coronary angioplasty. J. Vasc. Surg., 13:328, 1991.
16. McCabe, C. J., Moncure, A. C., and Malt, R. A.: Host-artery weakness in the etiology of femoral anastomotic false aneurysms. Surgery, 95:150, 1984.
17. McCann, R. L., Schwartz, L. B., and Pieper, K. S.: Vascular complications of cardiac catheterization. J. Vasc. Surg., 14:375, 1991.
18. Pappas, G., Janes, J. M., Bernatz, P. E., and Schirger, A.: Femoral aneurysms: Review of surgical management. JAMA, 190:489, 1964.
19. Rigdon, E. E., and Monajjem, N.: Aneurysms of the superficial femoral artery: A report of two cases and review of the literature. J. Vasc. Surg., 16:790, 1992.
20. Schellack, J., Salam, A., Abouzeid, M. A., Smith, R. B., Stewart, M. T., and Perdue, G. D.: Femoral anastomotic aneurysms: A continuing challenge. J. Vasc. Surg., 6:308, 1987.
21. Sheikh, K. H., Adams, D. B., McCann, R., Lyerly, H. K., Sabiston, D. C., and Kisslo, J.: Utility of Doppler color flow imaging for identification of femoral arterial complication of cardiac catheterization. Am. Heart J., 117:623, 1989.
22. Sorrell, K. A., Feinberg, R. L., Wheeler, J. R., Gregory, R. T., Snyder, S. O., Gayle, R. G., and Parent, N. F.: Color-flow duplex-directed manual occlusion of femoral false aneurysms. J. Vasc. Surg., 17:571, 1993.
23. Szilagyi, D. E., Smith, R. F., Elliott, J. P., Hageman, J. H., and Dall'Olmo, C. A.: Anastomotic aneurysms after vascular reconstruction: Problems of incidence, etiology, and treatment. Surgery, 78:880, 1975.
24. Tait, W. F., Vohra, R. K., Carr, H. M. H., Thomson, G. J. L., and Walker, M. G.: True profunda femoris aneurysms: Are they more dangerous than other atherosclerotic aneurysms of the femoropopliteal segment? Ann. Vasc. Surg., 5:92, 1991.
25. Tolstedt, G. E., Radke, H. M., and Bell, J. W.: Late sequela of arteriosclerotic femoral aneurysms. Angiography, 12:601, 1961.
26. Youkey, J. R., Clagett, G. P., Rich, N. M., Brigham, R. A., Orecchia, P. M., and Salander, J. M.: Femoral anastomotic false aneurysms: An 11-year experience analyzed with a case control study. Ann. Surg., 199:703, 1984.

POPLITEAL ARTERY ANEURYSMS

Raymond G. Makhoul, M.D.

Popliteal aneurysms have been recognized for centuries and have played an important role in development of modern vascular surgery. Antyllus, in the fourth century, is credited with the first definitive operation for popliteal aneurysm. This consisted of doubly ligating both poles of the aneurysm and emptying the sac.[7, 25] Later, Philagrius modified this procedure to include excision of the entire sac. In 1785, John Hunter first performed his now-famous operation for popliteal aneurysm. The superficial femoral artery of a 45-year-old coachman was ligated in the thigh, with complete relief of symptoms. This operation was based on Hunter's experimental observations regarding the formation of collateral circulation after ligation of the external carotid artery of a stag.[7] In 1902, Rudolph Matas[20] introduced the technique of endoaneurysmorrhaphy to treat popliteal aneurysms, and by 1920 he had accumulated a series of 154 cases with remarkable results. Bertram Berheim,[4] in 1916, reported the use of a saphenous vein interposition graft for treatment of popliteal aneurysms, and in 1958 Crawford and associates[8] published their results using synthetic grafts for treating aortic and popliteal aneurysms.

Popliteal aneurysms frequently are the most common site of peripheral arterial aneurysms. Atherosclerosis is by far the most common cause, accounting for greater than 95% of aneurysms in most collected series[10, 12, 32, 33]; other causes include popliteal entrapment by the gastrocnemius muscle, bacterial infection, collagen disorders, and trauma. Popliteal aneurysms typically present in the seventh decade of life and occur 30 times more frequently in men.

Popliteal aneurysms occur bilaterally (38%–58% of cases); thus there is the need to examine carefully the contralateral side when an aneurysm is discovered.[9, 19, 26, 28] Additionally, there is a high incidence of other aneurysms in patients with popliteal aneurysm. In one series of 61 patients, abdominal aortic aneurysms were present in 62%, iliac artery aneurysms in 36%, and femoral artery aneurysms in 38% of patients.[32] When the popliteal aneurysms are bilateral, the incidence of concomitant extrapopliteal aneurysmal disease is even higher. Conversely, however, the incidence of popliteal aneurysm in a series of patients who initially presented with abdominal aortic aneurysm was only 6%.[3]

CLINICAL MANIFESTATIONS AND DIAGNOSIS

The majority (53%–79%) of popliteal aneurysms are symptomatic, the most common complaint being leg ischemia. The severity of the leg ischemia may range from mild claudication to severe limb-threatening gangrene. This ischemia develops because of thrombosis of the aneurysm itself, distal embolization to the tibial or pedal vessels, or a combination of the two. Less commonly, large popliteal aneurysms may cause local compressive symptoms such as venous obstruction or nerve impingement with pain and tenderness. Rupture is very rare, with a less than 5% incidence in most reported series.[1, 6, 14, 22, 23, 30, 31]

The diagnosis of popliteal aneurysm is principally clinical and evokes a high degree of suspicion. In one series, only 26% of symptomatic aneurysms were diagnosed by general practitioners, although 94% of these were easily palpable.[11] Particular attention should be paid to those patients with a contralateral popliteal aneurysm or a strong family history of aneurysmal disease. Most present as pulsatile popliteal masses or as firm, nonpulsatile masses if they are thrombosed. In the latter instance, they may be confused with a Baker's cyst. Popliteal aneurysms may be calcified and thus be identified on plain films. In one study of 233 aneurysms, the aneurysm or vascular calcifications suggestive of aneurysm were seen in 138 instances.[33] The diagnosis is confirmed by ultrasound, which will document the size of the aneurysm and the presence or absence of mural thrombus (Fig. 50–65). For those aneurysms not treated surgically, ultrasonography is also the best modality for serial follow-up. Arteriography should be performed before operative treatment of popliteal aneurysm. Although it may not accurately reflect the size of the aneurysm due to laminated thrombus, it is key in delineating the patency of the distal vascular tree and planning the operative approach (Fig. 50–66).

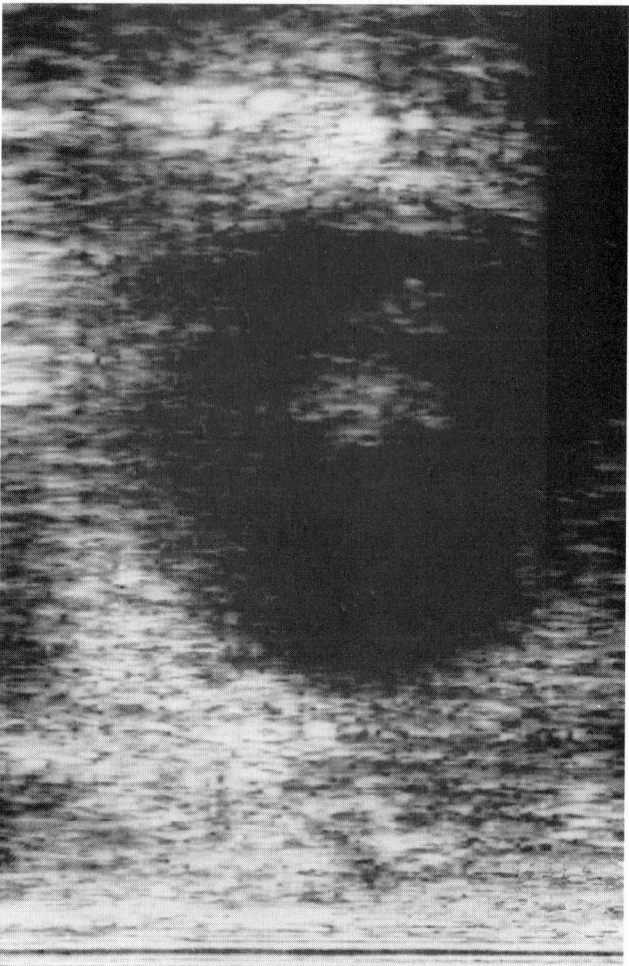

Figure 50–65. Ultrasound image of a popliteal artery aneurysm demonstrating the presence of an intraluminal thrombus.

TREATMENT

The preferred treatment of *symptomatic* popliteal aneurysms is surgical. For aneurysms that are *asymptomatic,* some controversy exists. Whereas some authors recommend surgical treatment for all asymptomatic aneurysms regardless of size, others advocate such treatment for those aneurysms greater than 2 cm. or containing mural thrombus.[5, 14, 21, 26] Factors in favor of the repair of all asymptomatic aneurysms include the high degree of morbidity associated with surgery for symptomatic aneurysms, the safety of elective repair, and the subsequent development of ischemic complications (approximately 30% in most published series). Furthermore, there is no evidence that small aneurysms are less benign and, in one report, they are even more prone to thrombosis.[17] In contrast, Schellack and associates[26] followed 26 patients with small, asymptomatic aneurysms and reported ischemic complications in only 2 (8%). Hands and Collin[15] found similar results in a smaller group of patients whom they observed. Overall, given the present available data, operative repair of asymptomatic aneurysms should be considered when they reach 2 cm. if the patient is a good operative risk and has adequate autogenous vein for use in bypass.

Surgical Technique. The aim of surgical treatment of popliteal aneurysm is to eliminate the aneurysm from the circulation and to restore blood flow to the leg. The procedure of choice is ligation of the aneurysm with bypass, preferably using a reversed saphenous vein (Fig. 50–67). This operation avoids the added morbidity associated with dissection in the popliteal space needed for resection of the aneurysm. Rarely, resection and grafting of the aneurysm may be necessary when it is large and is causing local compressive symptoms of the nerve or vein. In the elective, uncomplicated aneurysm, the patient is placed in the supine position and the upper end of the ipsilateral saphenous vein is harvested. The uninvolved popliteal artery is isolated below the adductor hiatus through a medial approach. Distally, the popliteal artery or, if necessary, a tibial vessel is isolated, and proximal and distal end-to-side anastomoses are constructed. Finally, the aneurysm is ligated, and a completion arteriogram is performed. In most cases the aneurysm thromboses, although there have been rare reports of continued expansion or rupture.[2, 13]

In patients with acute thrombosis of a popliteal aneurysm and limb-threatening ischemia, intra-arterial thrombolytic therapy in addition to operative repair is an option.[18] This thrombolytic therapy may be administered preoperatively or intraoperatively, depending on the degree of ischemia and the urgency for revascularization. In one report on the use of preoperative lytic therapy in seven patients presenting with a thrombosed aneurysm, complete clearing of the thrombus from the aneurysm and all runoff vessels was achieved in six cases, and from two of the runoff vessels in the remaining patient.[6] All of these patients electively underwent aneurysm ligation and bypass and had successful limb salvage. This was in contrast to an amputation rate of 24% for patients with thrombosed aneurysms treated with emergency surgery alone. Hoelting and colleagues[16] have achieved similar results using preoperative thrombolytic therapy in addition to surgery. Disadvantages of this technique include the prolonged time for lysis, the risk of distal atheroembolization, and the increased cost. Others have combined thrombectomy with intraoperative thrombolysis at the time of bypass in an attempt to clear the distal vessels and have achieved promising results in small numbers of patients.[29, 30]

RESULTS

The long-term results of popliteal aneurysm repair are influenced by a number of variables, including the nature of the aneurysm (symptomatic versus asymptomatic), the quality of the distal runoff vessels, and the type of graft employed. Large series with long-term follow-up exhibit overall graft patencies ranging from 50% to 76% at 5 years with a significantly better limb salvage rate (90%–95%).[17, 26, 28] In a

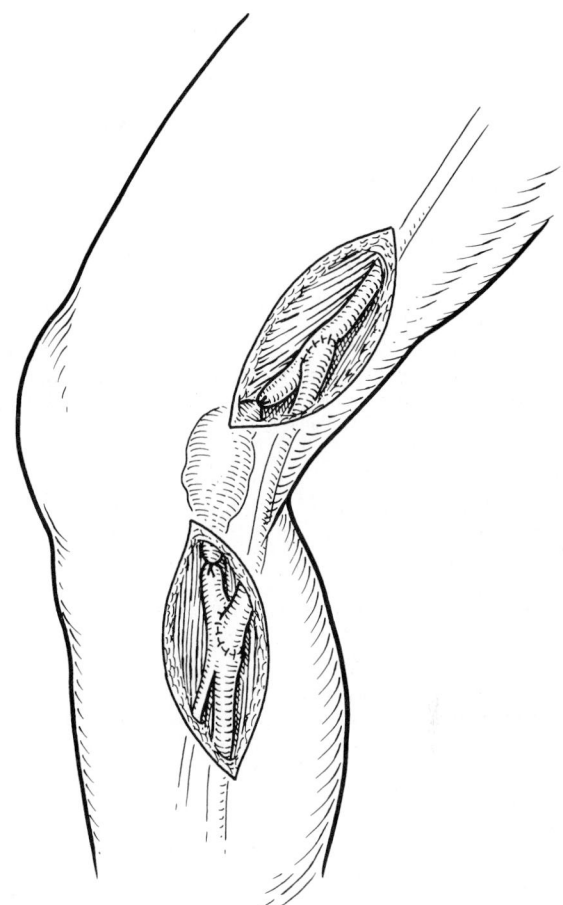

Figure 50–67. The preferred technique for treatment of popliteal aneurysm using a vein graft for bypass, followed by ligation of the aneurysm. (From Bell, P. R. F., Jamieson, C. W., and Ruckey, C. V. [Eds.]: Surgical Management of Vascular Disease. London, W. B. Saunders Company Ltd., 1992.)

large, retrospective series from the Cleveland Clinic, the 10-year graft patency for asymptomatic aneurysms was 82%, with a limb salvage rate of 93%.[1] In contrast, the 10-year patency for symptomatic aneurysms fell to 48%, with a limb salvage rate of 79%. This difference is likely on the basis of the patency of the distal runoff vessels, as has been demonstrated by Shortell and associates.[27] Finally, the superiority of autogenous saphenous vein over prosthetic grafts is well documented.[1, 10, 23, 24]

SELECTED REFERENCES

Anton, G. E., Hertzer, N. R., Beven, E. G., O'Hara, P. J., and Krajewski, L. P.: Surgical management of popliteal aneurysms: Trends in presentation, treatment, and results from 1952 to 1984. J. Vasc. Surg., 3:125, 1986.
This is a comprehensive review of the Cleveland Clinic's experience with popliteal aneurysm repair over a 32-year period. It emphasizes the difference in long-term results between symptomatic and asymptomatic aneurysms and the superiority of autogenous vein as a conduit.

Varga, Z. A., Locke-Edmunds, J. C., Baird, R. N., and the Joint Vascular Research Group, United Kingdom: A multicenter study of popliteal aneurysms. J. Vasc. Surg., 20:171, 1994.
A multicenter, prospective study of 200 popliteal aneurysms in 137 patients over a 4-year period is presented. The data demonstrate the value of intra-arterial thrombolysis in restoring distal runoff before bypass. The strength of this study is that it encompasses a large number of patients accumulated over a short period of time and treated with modern techniques.

REFERENCES

1. Anton, G. E., Hertzer, N. R., Beven, E. G., O'Hara, P. J., and Krajewski, L. P.: Surgical management of popliteal aneurysms: Trends in presentation, treatment, and results from 1952 to 1984. J. Vasc. Surg., 3:125, 1986.

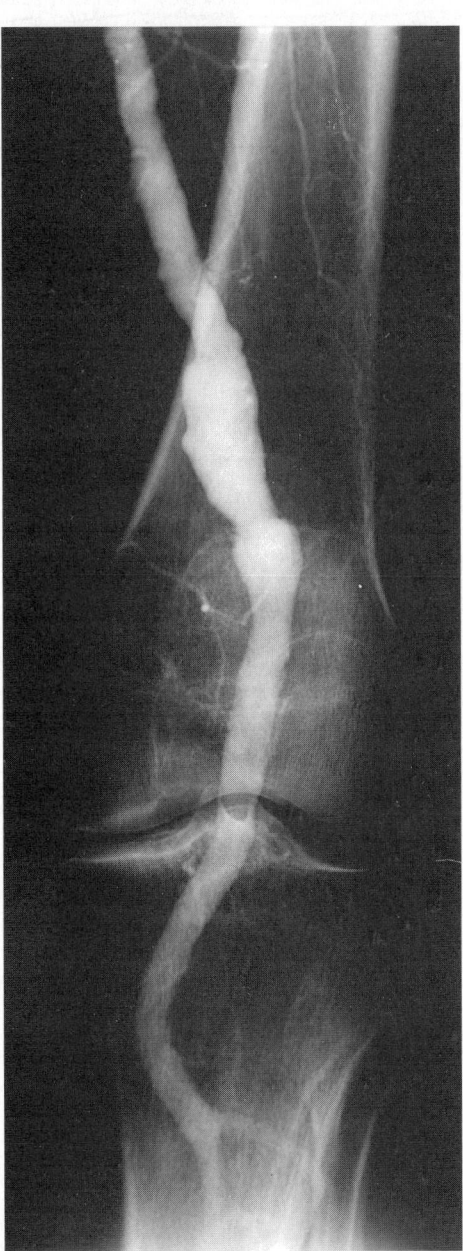

Figure 50–66. Preoperative arteriogram of a popliteal aneurysm in a patient who presented with an ischemic foot secondary to embolic occlusion of his posterior tibial and dorsalis pedis arteries.

2. Battey, P. M., Skardasis, G. M., and McKinnon, W. M.: Rupture of a previously bypassed popliteal aneurysm: A case report. J. Vasc. Surg., 5:874, 1987.

3. Bell, D. D., and Gaspar, M. R.: Routine arteriography before abdominal aortic aneurysmectomy: A prospective study. Am. J. Surg., 144:191, 1982.

4. Bernheim, B. M.: The ideal operation for aneurysms of the extremity. Bull. Johns Hopkins Hosp., 27:93, 1916.

5. Bowyer, R. C., Cawthorn, S. J., Walker, W. J., and Giddings, A. E. B.: Conservative management of asymptomatic popliteal aneurysm. Br. J. Surg., 77:1132, 1990.

6. Carpenter, J. P., Barker, C. F., Roberts, B., Berkowitz, H. D., Lusk, E. J., and Perloff, L. J.: Popliteal artery aneurysms: Current management and outcome. J. Vasc. Surg., 19:65, 1994.

7. Chitwood, W. R., Stocks, L. H., and Wolfe, W. G.: Popliteal artery aneurysms: Past and present. Arch. Surg., 113:1078, 1978.

8. Crawford, E. S., DeBakey, M. E., Cooley, D. A.: Clinical use of synthetic arterial substitutes in 317 patients. Arch. Surg., 76:261, 1958.

9. Crichlow, R. W., and Roberts, B.: Treatment of popliteal aneurysms by restoration of continuity: Review of 48 cases. Ann. Surg., 163:417, 1966.

10. Dawson, I., van Bockel, J. H., Brand, R., and Terpstra, J. L.: Popliteal artery aneurysms: Long-term follow-up of aneurysmal disease and results of surgical treatment. J. Vasc. Surg., 13:398, 1991.

11. Downing, R., Grimley, R. P., Ashton, F., and Slaney, G.: Problems in the diagnosis of popliteal aneurysms. J. R. Soc. Med., 78:440, 1985.

12. Farina, C., Cavallaro, A., Schultz, R. D., Feldhaus, R. J., and di Marzo, L.: Popliteal aneurysms. Surg. Gynecol. Obstet., 169:7, 1989.

13. Flynn, J. B., Nicholas, G. G.: An unusual complication of bypassed popliteal aneurysms. Arch. Surg., 111:118, 1983.

14. Halliday, A. W., Taylor, P. R., Wolfe, J. H., and Mansfield, A. O.: The management of popliteal aneurysm: The importance of early surgical repair. Ann. R. Coll. Surg. Engl., 73:253, 1991.

15. Hands, L. J., and Collin, J.: Infra-inguinal aneurysms: Outcome for patient and limb. Br. J. Surg., 78:996, 1991.

16. Hoelting, T., Paetz, B., Richter, G. M., and Allenberg, J. R.: The value of preoperative lytic therapy in limb-threatening acute ischemia from popliteal artery aneurysm. Am. J. Surg., 168:227, 1994.

17. Inahara, T., and Toledo, A. C.: Complications and treatment of popliteal aneurysms. Surgery, 84:775, 1978.

18. Lancashire, J. J. R., Torrie, E. P. H., and Galland, R. B.: Popliteal aneurysms identified by intra-arterial streptokinase: A changing pattern of presentation. Br. J. Surg., 77:1388, 1990.

19. Mangiante, E. C., Fabian, M. C., and Huffstutter, P. J.: Popliteal aneurysms: A clinical appraisal. Am. Surgeon, 50:469, 1984.

20. Matas, R.: Endoaneurysmorrhaphy. Trans. So. Surg. Assoc., 34:447, 1920.

21. Quraishy, M. D., and Giddings, A. E. B.: Treatment of asymptomatic popliteal aneurysm: Protection at a price. Br. J. Surg., 79:731, 1992.

22. Ramesh, S., Michaels, J. A., and Galland, R. B.: Popliteal aneurysm: Morphology and management. Br. J. Surg., 80:1531, 1993.

23. Reilly, M. K., Abbott, W. M., and Darling, R. C.: Aggressive surgical management of popliteal artery aneurysms. Am. J. Surg., 145:498, 1983.

24. Roggo, A., Brunner, U., Ottinger, L. W., and Largiader, F.: The continuing challenge of aneurysms of the popliteal artery. Surg. Gynecol. Obstet., 177:565, 1993.

25. Schechter, D. C., and Bergan, J. J.: Popliteal aneurysm: A celebration of the bicentennial of John Hunter's operation. Ann. Vasc. Surg., 1:118, 1986.

26. Schellack, J., Smith, R. B., and Perdue, G. D.: Nonoperative management of selected popliteal aneurysms. Arch. Surg., 122:372, 1987.

27. Shortell, C. K., DeWeese, J. A., Ouriel, K., and Green, R. M.: Popliteal artery aneurysms: A 25-year surgical experience. J. Vasc. Surg., 14:771, 1991.

28. Szilagyi, E. E., Schwartz, R. L., and Reddy, D. J.: Popliteal arterial aneurysms. Arch. Surg., 116:724, 1981.

29. Thompson, J. F., Beard, J., Scott, D. J. A., and Earnshaw, J. J.: Intraoperative thrombolysis in the management of thrombosed popliteal aneurysm. Br. J. Surg., 80:858, 1993.

30. Varga, Z. A., Locke-Edmunds, J. C., Baird, R. N., and the Joint Vascular Research Group, United Kingdom: A multicenter study of popliteal aneurysms. J. Vasc. Surg., 20:171, 1994.

31. Vermilion, B. D., Kimmins, S. A., Pace, W. G., and Evans, W. E.: A review of one hundred forty-seven popliteal aneurysms with long-term follow-up. Surgery, 90:1009, 1981.

32. Whitehouse, W. M., Wakefield, T. W., Graham, L. M., Kazmers, A., Zelenock, G. B., Cronenwett, J. L., Dent, T. L., Lindenauer, S. M., and Stanley, J. C.: Limb-threatening potential of arteriosclerotic popliteal artery aneurysms. Surgery, 93:694, 1983.

33. Wychulis, A. R., Spittell, J. A., and Wallace, R. B.: Popliteal aneurysms. Surgery, 68:942, 1970.

VI

THROMBO-OBLITERATIVE DISEASE OF THE AORTA AND ITS BRANCHES

David C. Sabiston, Jr., M.D.

Occlusive disease of the major branches of the aorta is most often the result of atherosclerosis. Certain arterial anatomic sites are especially susceptible to development of stenosis or total occlusion and the most common site is at the *origin* of the vessels where significant turbulence is present (Fig. 50–68).[7] When branches of the aortic arch (innominate, carotid, subclavian) become stenotic or occluded, the symptoms produced are caused by ischemic disturbances due to the reduction in blood flow.

CLINICAL MANIFESTATIONS

A large series of arterial occlusive lesions is shown in Table 50–5.[2] The symptoms depend on the nature and extent of the obstruction. Moreover, the natural development of collateral

TABLE 50–5. Location and Extent of 412 Lesions in 299 Patients

Location	Extent of Obstruction		
	Incomplete	*Complete*	Totals
Innominate artery	40	26	66
Right common carotid artery	5	19	24
Right subclavian artery	30	29	59
Left common carotid artery	24	37	61
Left subclavian artery	69	133	202
Total	168	244	412

From Crawford, E. S., DeBakey, M. E., Morris, G. C., Jr., and Howell, J. F.: Surgical treatment of occlusion of the innominate, common carotid, and subclavian arteries: A 10-year experience. Surgery, 65:17, 1969.

TABLE 50–6. Symptoms of Occlusion (299 Patients)

Type of Symptom	No. of Patients	%
Neurologic only	97	32
Neurologic and upper extremity ischemia	124	42
Upper extremity ischemia	63	21
Systolic ear noise	3	1
No symptoms	12	4
Total	299	100

From Crawford, E. S., DeBakey, M. E., Morris, G. C., Jr., and Howell, J. F.: Surgical treatment of occlusion of the innominate, common carotid, and subclavian arteries: A 10-year experience. Surgery, 65:17, 1969.

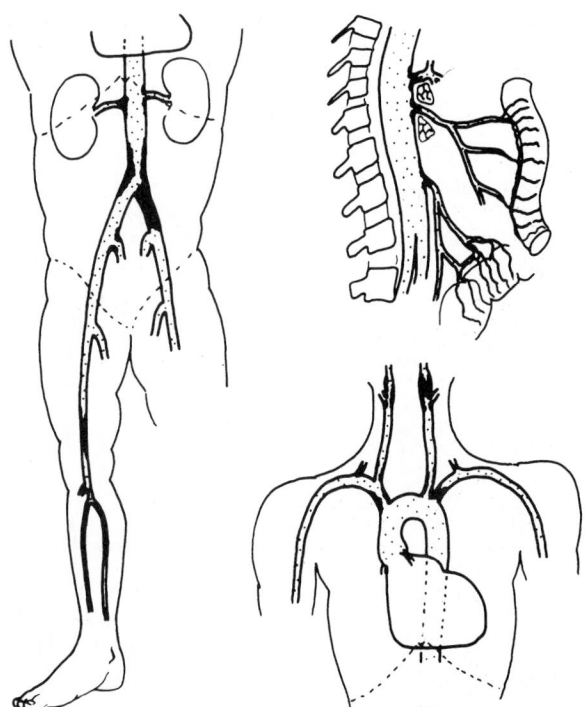

Figure 50–68. Anatomic sites particularly likely to become stenotic or occluded by atherosclerosis. (From Ludbrook, J., and Elmslie, R. G.: An Introduction to Surgery: 100 topics. New York, Academic Press, 1971.)

circulation that follows arterial stenosis and occlusion and the volume of blood flow through the collateral vessels are of prime importance. The symptoms and the distribution of symptoms are shown in Table 50–6.[2] The diagnosis is confirmed by arteriography, which demonstrates the lesion and the collateral channels around it.

SURGICAL MANAGEMENT

In patients with occlusive disease surgical management is primarily accomplished by bypass grafts (Fig. 50–69).[2] The results of surgical bypass are favorable as shown in Table 50–7.[2] In this series, obstruction was incomplete in 168 and complete in 244 of the arteries involved. Regardless of the extent of obstruction, the occlusive process was segmental in almost every instance. The surgical treatment is often a bypass graft, and endarterectomy is only occasionally applicable.

TAKAYASU'S ARTERITIS

David C. Sabiston, Jr., M.D.

A nonspecific arteritis affecting the thoracic and abdominal aorta and its major branches, Takayasu's disease was de-

scribed by a Japanese ophthalmologist in 1908.[10] Although uncommon in the United States, it is often seen in Asia and usually affects young females. It has also been described in older women and males, and the natural history of the disorder has been carefully documented.[5] The arteritis involves all layers of the arterial wall, with proliferation of connective tissue and degeneration of the elastic fibers, and may also involve the pulmonary arteries. Granulomatous lesions may be present with associated fusiform or saccular aneurysms. Three types of this disorder are now recognized (Fig. 50–70).[3]

Takayasu's disease is first characterized by fever, malaise, arthritis, and arthralgia. Pericardial pain, tachycardia, and vomiting may also occur. It has been suggested that the disorder may be an autoimmune disease,[8] and corticosteroids may be beneficial. The later manifestations are those of ischemia of both the cerebral and upper extremity circuits.

The long-term outcome in 120 patients with this disorder is reviewed with statistical analyses of related prognostic factors. Negative factors affecting outcome included retinopathy, hypertension, aortic regurgitation, the presence of an aneurysm, and a progressive clinical course. The overall survival at 15 years was 83%.[6] Surgical treatment of Takayasu's arteritis may prove disappointing, because the endarterectomy site and grafts are likely to reocclude later. Revascularization is recommended in appropriate patients, including those with aortic regurgitation, coronary stenosis, and aortic

TABLE 50–7. Functional Results in 299 Patients with Occlusion of Great Vessels of the Aortic Arch

Time of Follow-up	Asymptomatic, Improved		Unimproved		Worse		Dead	
	No. of Patients	%	No. of Patients	%	No. of Patients	%	No. of Patients	%
Immediate	268	89.6	10	3.3	5	1.7	16	5.4
Late	274	91.6	3	1.0	6	2.0	43	14.4

From Crawford, E. S., DeBakey, M. E., Morris, G. C., Jr., and Howell, J. F.: Surgical treatment of occlusion of the innominate, common carotid, and subclavian arteries: A 10-year experience. Surgery, *65*:17, 1969.

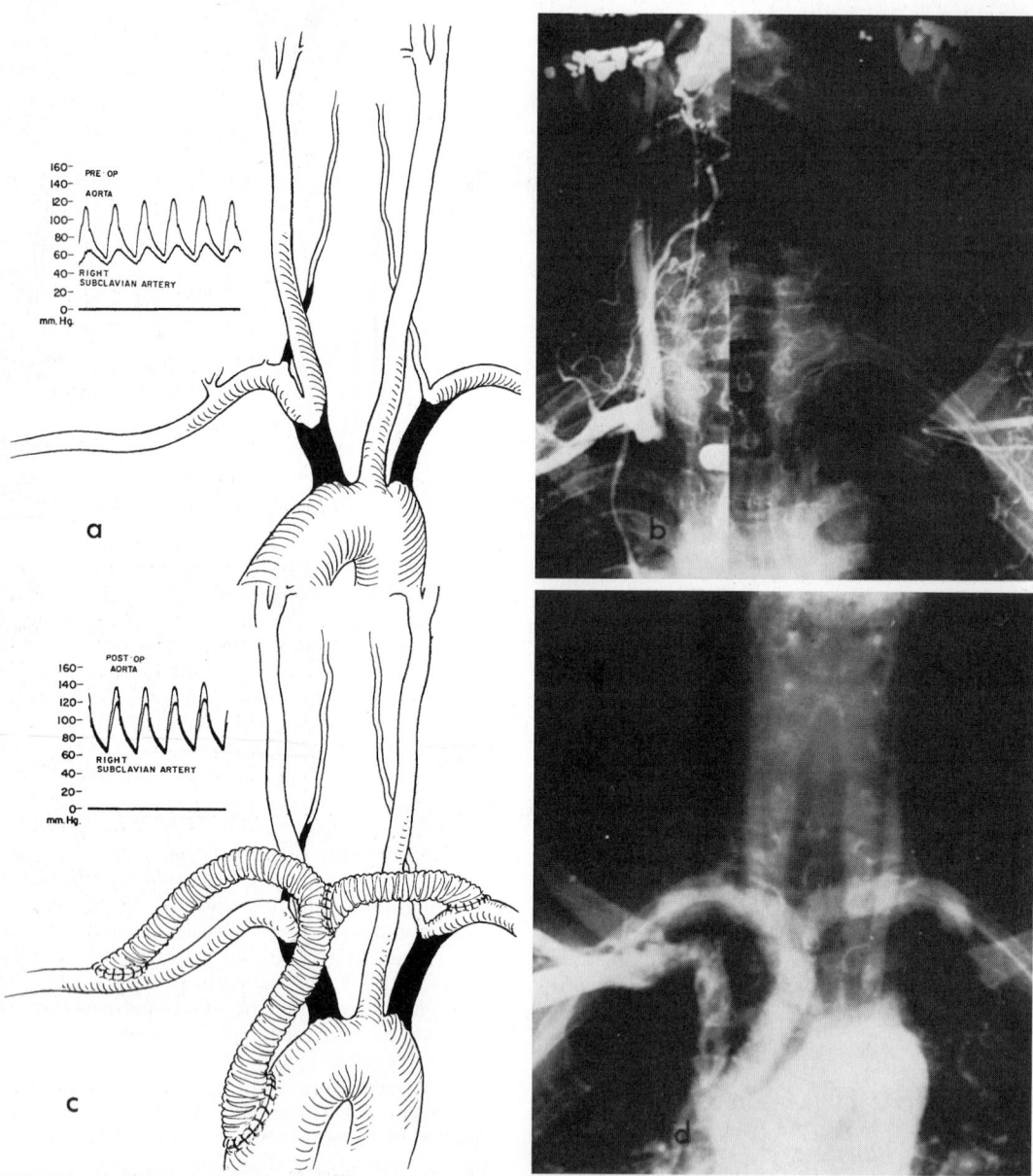

Figure 50–69. Patient with obstruction of innominate and left subclavian arteries, causing cerebral arterial insufficiency, and obstruction of the abdominal aorta and iliac arteries, causing both intermittent claudication and ischemic lesions of the feet. The patient was treated first at one operation by ascending aortobilateral subclavian bypass graft, and at a second operation by bilateral aortoexternal iliac artery bypass graft, relieving all symptoms. Diagram *(a)* and arteriogram *(b)* with pressure recording made before bypass show location and extent of innominate and subclavian lesions. Diagram *(c)* and aortogram *(d)* made 3 years after operation and pressure recordings made at operation after bypass show grafts in place and functioning.

Illustration continued on opposite page

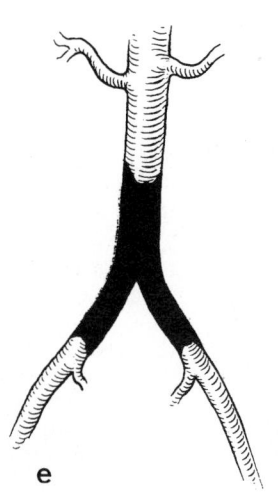

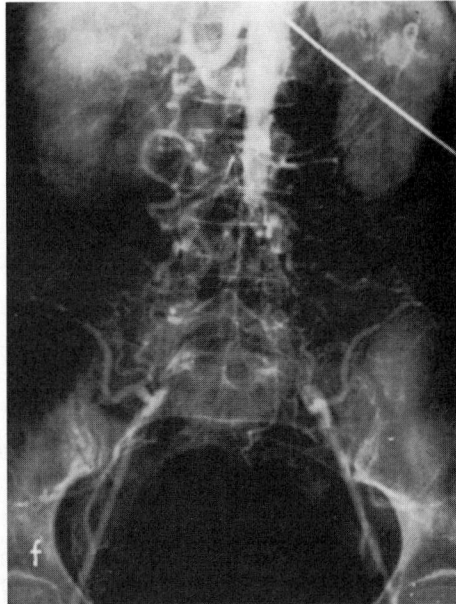

Figure 50–69 *Continued* Diagram *(e)* and aortogram *(f)* made before operation show location and extent of aortoiliac obstruction. Diagram *(g)* and aortogram *(h)* made 3 years after operation show graft in place and functioning. The patient is alive and well 5 years after operation. (From Crawford, E. S., DeBakey, M. E., Morris, G. C., Jr., and Howell, J. F.: Surgical treatment of occlusion of the innominate, common, carotid, and subclavian arteries: A 10-year experience. Surgery, *65*:17, 1969.)

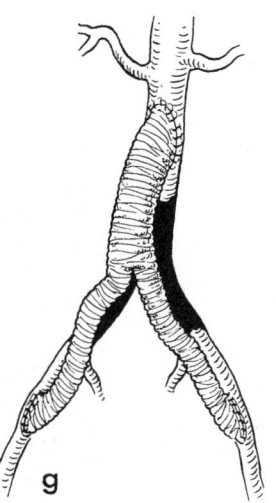

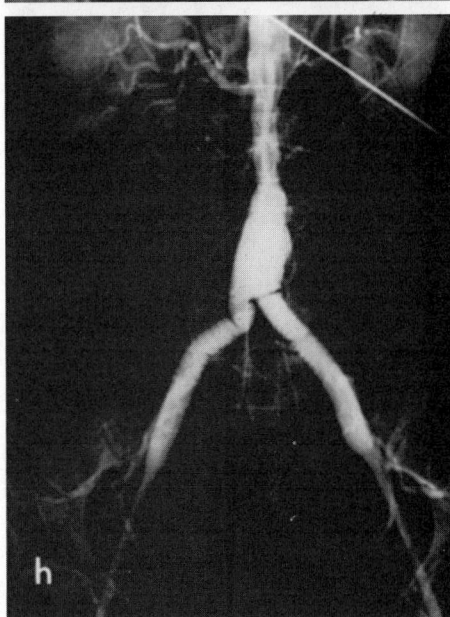

aneurysms.[4] Replacement of the aortic valve and coronary bypass can yield good results.[9]

In a collected series of 63 patients with 92 coronary lesions undergoing coronary artery bypass procedures, coronary ostial lesions were present in 73%. In this group, there were five early and three late deaths in the 63 patients.[1]

REFERENCES

1. Amano, J., and Suzuki, A.: Coronary artery involvement in Takayasu's arteritis: Collective review and guideline for surgical treatment. J. Thorac. Cardiovasc. Surg., *102*(4):554, 1991.
2. Crawford, E. S., DeBakey, M. E., Morris, G. C., Jr., and Howell, J. F.: Surgical treatment of occlusion of the innominate, common carotid, and subclavian arteries: A 10-year experience. Surgery, *65*:17, 1969.
3. Edmunds, L. H., Jr.: Trauma and occlusive disease. *In* Strandness, D. E., Jr. (Ed.): Collateral Circulation in Clinical Surgery. Philadelphia, W. B. Saunders, 1969.
4. Ekestrom, S., and Hansson, L. O.: Surgical treatment of "pulseless disease." Acta Chir. Scand., *128*:127, 1964.
5. Ishikawa, K.: Natural history and classification of occlusive thromboaortopathy (Takayasu's disease). Circulation, *57*:27, 1978.
6. Ishikawa, K., and Maetani, S.: Long-term outcome for 120 Japanese patients with Takayasu's disease: Clinical and statistical analyses of related prognostic factors. Circulation, *90*:1855, 1994.
7. Ludbrook, J., and Elmslie, R. G.: An Introduction to Surgery: 100 Topics. New York, Academic Press, 1971.
8. Nakao, K., Ikeda, M., Kimata, S., Niitani, H., Miyahara, M., Ishimi, Z., Hashiba, K., Takeda, Y., Ozawa, T., Matsushita, S., and Kuramochi, M.: Takayasu's arteritis: Clinical report of eighty-four cases and immunological studies of seven cases. Circulation, *35*:1141, 1967.
9. Ohteki, H., Itoh, T., Natsuaki, M., Minato, N., Ueno, T., Suda, H., Naito, K., Norita, H., and Sakai, H.: Aortic valve replacement for Takayasu's arteritis. J. Thorac. Cardiovasc. Surg., *104*:482:1992.
10. Takayasu, M.: Case of queer changes in central blood vessels of retina. Acta Soc. Ophthalmol. Jpn., *12*:2554, 1908.

CAROTID ARTERY OCCLUSIVE DISEASE

Richard H. Dean, M.D.

In 1856, Savory described the autopsy findings of an extracranial internal carotid artery occlusion and bilateral subcla-

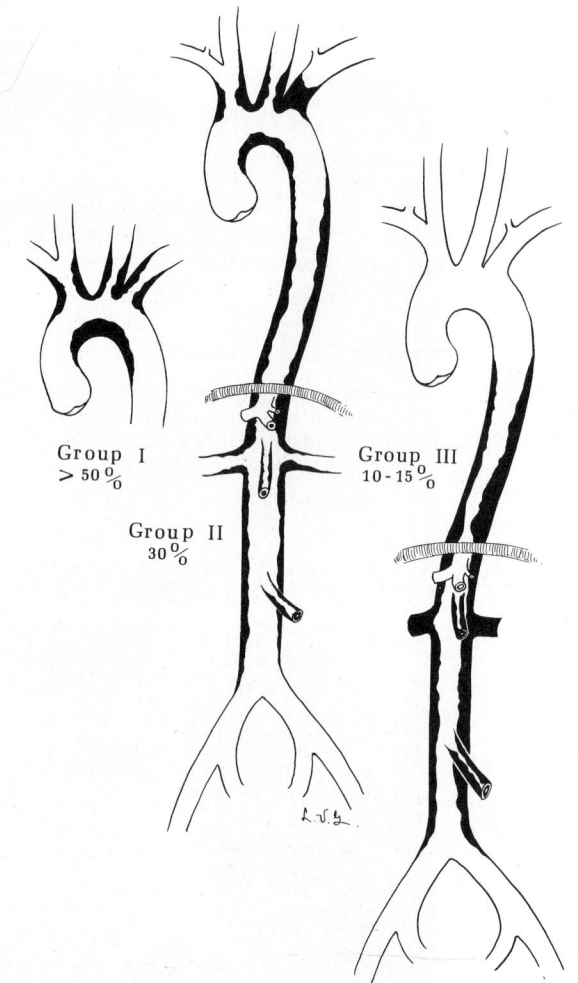

Figure 50–70. Clinical subdivisions of Takayasu's arteritis. The panarteritis may be localized to the aortic arch and great vessels (Group I), the distal thoracoabdominal aorta (Group III), or the entire aorta (Group II). (From Edmunds, L. H., Jr.: Trauma and occlusive disease. *In* Strandness, D. E., Jr. (Ed.): Collateral Circulation in Clinical Surgery. Philadelphia, W. B. Saunders, 1969.)

scanning regardless of the degree of the stenosis at the time of presentation.[13] Ten patients (6%) became symptomatic during follow-up; the development of symptoms was accompanied by disease progression in eight of those patients. By life-table analysis, the annual rate of symptom occurrence was 4%; however, the presence of progression to 80% stenosis was highly correlated with either total occlusion of the internal carotid artery or the development of new symptoms. Thus, 89% of the symptoms were preceded by disease progression to a greater than 80% stenosis. Progression to this extent was an important warning observation because the risk of ischemic symptoms or development of internal carotid occlusion was 35% within 6 months and 46% at 12 months. Conversely, only 1.5% of the lesions that remained in a less than 80% category developed such a complication. These data suggest that careful follow-up with repeated noninvasive evaluation is of great assistance in determining the appropriate management of the asymptomatic carotid lesion.

Other studies have suggested that the composition of the plaque influences the risk of stroke due to carotid artery lesions. In an analysis of 297 carotid arteries examined prospectively in asymptomatic patients, Johnson and colleagues concluded that patients with stenosis greater than 75% at the time of the initial study were at higher risk of developing symptoms ipsilateral to the lesion than were patients without significant narrowing.[7] However, even patients with less than 75% stenosis were at greater risk if their associated plaques were less organized, that is, soft. Plaque organization was determined by B-mode ultrasonography, and plaques were classified as soft, calcified, or dense. A definite trend toward higher risk was seen in plaques of lower density.

Moreover, it has been shown that the development of transient ischemic attacks (TIAs) also places patients at a higher risk of developing a stroke. In the Mayo Clinic population study,[15] 118 patients with TIAs were followed as a control group without therapy. The stroke rate at 1, 3, and 5 years was 23%, 37%, and 45%, respectively. Most permanent deficits occurred during the first year. This rate represents a 16-fold increased risk of stroke when compared with an age- and sex-adjusted population without TIAs. Some series[5, 9] have reported lower figures, but the average reported in the literature is 30% to 35% at 5 years, or 10% the first year, and 6% each year thereafter.

PATHOGENESIS OF TRANSIENT ISCHEMIC ATTACKS AND STROKE

Three causes of TIAs and stroke stem from occlusive disease of the extracranial carotid artery. These are thrombosis of the carotid artery, flow-related ischemic events, and embolization from the atherosclerotic lesion in the carotid artery.

Thrombosis of the internal carotid artery is the terminal event of progressive enlargement of the atherosclerotic lesion at the carotid artery bifurcation. If the distal propagation of the thrombus stops at the ophthalmic artery and remains stable, the event of total occlusion may be silent if collateral flow is sufficient. If the thrombus progresses beyond the ophthalmic artery into the middle cerebral artery, a hemispheric event varying from a TIA to a profound stroke occurs.

Flow-related ischemic events were once considered the most common cause of cerebral symptoms in conjunction with carotid artery disease. Although transient decreases in cerebral perfusion through a stenotic carotid artery can produce symptoms, the occurrence is rare. Owing to the rich collateral pathways for cerebral perfusion through the circle of Willis (Fig. 50–71) and the contralateral carotid artery and transcranial external-to-internal carotid artery connections,

vian occlusions in a woman with hemiplegia and dysesthesia—the first description of a link between stroke and extracranial carotid artery disease.[14] In 1914, Ramsay Hunt correlated the relationship between partial carotid artery occlusion and what he termed "cerebral intermittent claudication."[6] Further evolution in the understanding and management of extracranial cerebrovascular disease came with the use of carotid angiography in the diagnosis of carotid artery occlusion by Moniz, reported in 1927.[10] Although reports of the association between extracranial carotid disease and stroke continued to appear, acceptance of its relative importance and enthusiasm for pre-emptive management of the carotid disease awaited popularization of carotid endarterectomy during the late 1950s and early 1960s.

NATURAL HISTORY

There are approximately 500,000 new strokes in the United States each year; the direct and indirect cost of these is about 8 billion dollars a year.[16] Initial mortality from stroke is estimated to be between 20% and 30%.[12] The natural history of atherosclerotic occlusive disease of the extracranial carotid artery remains controversial.

In a report by Roederer and associates, 167 asymptomatic patients with cervical bruits were followed with serial duplex

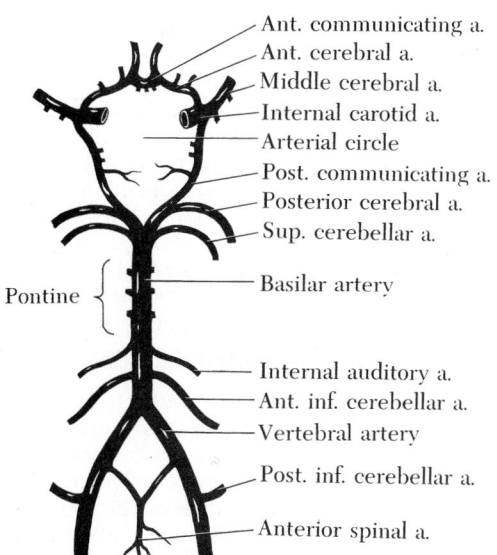

Figure 50–71. Diagram showing the most common configuration of the terminal branches of the vertebral and internal carotid arteries and their interconnections to form the circle of Willis. (From Wylie, E. J., and Ehrenfeld, W. K.: Extracranial Occlusive Cerebrovascular Disease. Philadelphia, W. B. Saunders, 1970.)

cerebral perfusion is rarely diminished to a critical level despite the presence of a severe carotid artery stenosis.

Cerebral embolization from the carotid artery lesion is the single most common cause of cerebral ischemic events. Embolization from the atherosclerotic plaque may occur by either of two mechanisms. First, the irregular surface of the plaque is thrombogenic and can accumulate platelet aggregates. If these platelet aggregates become large and embolize to an important cerebral branch, symptoms are produced. Second, as the atherosclerotic plaque becomes more advanced, it may undergo central degeneration. When this occurs, the plaque may rupture spontaneously, discharging its contents into the lumen, with subsequent embolization. In both of these instances, the type, severity, and permanency of the cerebral event is determined by the size and eventual location of the embolus.

CLINICAL MANIFESTATIONS

The clinical presentations of carotid artery occlusive disease can be categorized into three general groups: asymptomatic lesions, lesions producing TIAs, and those lesions that have produced cerebral infarction.

Asymptomatic patients are those who have a hemodynamically significant lesion or nonocclusive ulcerated lesion of the carotid artery but no history of cerebral symptoms. The presence of a bruit in an asymptomatic patient does not define this group; Kartchner and McRae[8] found that fewer than one third of patients with a cervical bruit had a hemodynamically significant lesion of the carotid artery by noninvasive criteria. Therapeutic intervention may be indicated in certain of these asymptomatic patients with high-grade lesions.

By definition, TIAs are temporary neurologic deficits lasting less than 24 hours and followed by complete recovery. In the area supplied by the carotid artery, they are usually discrete motor and/or sensory dysfunctions. Contralateral facial, arm, and/or leg motor weakness and sensory loss are the classic presentations. Because the left hemisphere is dominant in 95% of the population, left hemispheric TIAs may also cause either receptive or expressive aphasia.

Probably the most classic TIA of carotid artery origin is

transient loss of or blurred vision (amaurosis fugax) in the ipsilateral eye (Fig. 50–72). It is classically described as a curtain being drawn down over the eye or as a quadrant field defect and is caused by embolization to the retinal branches of the ophthalmic artery, the first major intracranial branch of the internal carotid artery.

The first clinical manifestation of carotid artery disease may be a permanent neurologic deficit or stroke. Depending on the area of cerebral cortex affected, the defect may range from minimal with ultimate recovery of the lost function to massive leading to death.

DIAGNOSTIC EVALUATION

A number of noninvasive diagnostic studies have been advocated in the preliminary evaluation of patients suspected of having cerebrovascular disease. The role of the respective diagnostic studies is dependent on the clinical presentation of the patient. Currently, evaluation of the

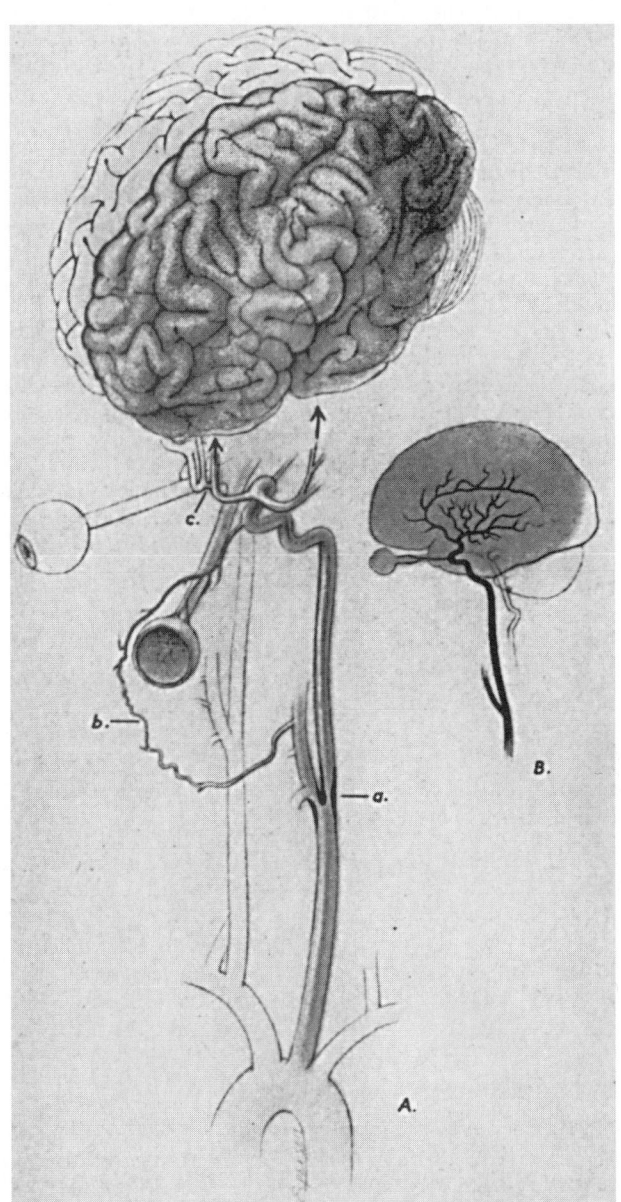

Figure 50–72. Atheromatous retinal embolus lodged at a bifurcation. (From Hoyt, W. F.: Some neuro-ophthalmological considerations in cerebral vascular insufficiency: Carotid and vertebral artery insufficiency. Arch. Ophthalmol., 62:262, 1959. Copyright 1959, American Medical Association.)

asymptomatic patient with a cervical bruit is best achieved by duplex scanning of the carotid artery. Through the combination of B-mode imaging of the vessel to identify the presence of lumen-narrowing plaques and pulse Doppler sampling of velocity spectra, a relatively accurate assessment for identification of hemodynamically significant disease can be obtained. If duplex scanning defines the bruit arising from an external carotid lesion or a mild or moderate internal carotid lesion, no further diagnostic evaluation is necessary and the patient should have a serial follow-up program of semiannual repeat scans. In contrast, if a severe lesion of the carotid bifurcation or the internal carotid artery is diagnosed, arteriography should be undertaken to determine more precisely the necessity of operative intervention.

Although duplex scanning may be performed in patients presenting with cerebral symptoms, it should not be used to determine the need for arteriography. Standard four-vessel carotid arteriography should be used in the evaluation of all patients presenting with TIAs or prior ischemic stroke in whom residual hemispheric function either remains or has been regained. The safest and most complete study is threefold: (1) assessment of the brachiocephalic trunks by intra-arterial digital subtraction arch aortography using the Seldinger technique from a femoral artery entrance site; followed by (2) selective cannulation and inspection of the carotid arteries for observation of both the extracranial and intracranial carotid arteries (Fig. 50–73); followed by (3) assessment of the vertebrobasilar system by subclavian inspection to visualize the origin and intracranial portions of the vertebral and basilar arteries.

Computed tomographic (CT) scanning of the head should be performed in all patients with cerebral symptoms. Intracranial space-occupying lesions such as neoplasms, vascular malformations, or subdural hematomas enter into the differential diagnosis of patients with even the most convincing symptoms of transient cerebral ischemia. CT scanning is a quick, noninvasive means of excluding alternative disease during patient diagnostic examinations.

The patient who presents with a TIA actually may have suffered a small cerebral infarction. CT scanning identifies an unsuspected cerebral infarction and establishes a baseline status before operative intervention.

Moreover, patients who present with a clinically overt cerebral infarction should have a CT scan to document infarct size and to differentiate between an ischemic and a hemorrhagic infarction. A hemorrhagic infarction is visible promptly on CT scan, whereas an ischemic infarction may take several days of evolution before its low-density mass is visualized. Data from CT scans are necessary in determining the proper timing of operative management after acute stroke in patients who have experienced a good neurologic recovery.

OPERATIVE MANAGEMENT

The first carotid artery operation for occlusive disease was performed in 1951 but was not reported until 1955. In that report, by Carrea and Murphy,[2] an atherosclerotic carotid bifurcation was resected with reanastomosis of the internal carotid to the external carotid artery. The first successful carotid reconstruction, performed by DeBakey and colleagues, was not reported until 1959.[3] The first report of carotid endarterectomy appeared in *Lancet* in November 1954. That article by Eastcott and associates[4] called the world's attention to the feasibility of managing this cause of TIAs.

Currently, carotid endarterectomy is indicated for treatment of patients with hemispheric TIAs and of patients with either retained or regained significant residual functional cortex after a completed stroke associated with carotid bifurcation occlusive disease. Although use of prophylactic carotid endarterectomy for asymptomatic patients remains debatable, it is probably indicated for patients with severe stenosis (greater than 80%) and complexly ulcerated plaques.

The technique of carotid endarterectomy is relatively simple but requires precision if the results are to be favorable. The important landmarks of the exposure are depicted in Figure 50–74. Technical details of the dissection are discussed elsewhere.[11]

Operative techniques to optimize cerebral perfusion during carotid cross-clamping vary according to the preference of the surgeon. Options include routine use of a shunt, selective use of a shunt based on a certain stump pressure or a change in electroencephalogram, and performing the operation under local anesthesia using a shunt if neurologic changes develop. Many cerebrovascular surgeons, including the author, have now begun using the last-named option in patients with the usual variety of carotid lesion.

Although some surgeons routinely use a patch to close the arteriotomy after completion of the endarterectomy, implementation of microvascular techniques and magnification allows most arteriotomies to be closed primarily.

Current results of carotid endarterectomy should include less than a 5% combined cerebrovascular morbidity and operative mortality. Most current series have combined morbidity and mortality in the asymptomatic patient group of less than 3%. Obviously, the preoperative neurologic status of the patient affects the incidence of immediate perioperative events as well as the late results. Bernstein and colleagues[1] reported a series of 456 carotid endarterectomies in patients followed for 1 and 11 years, with an average follow-up of 45.3 months. Operated asymptomatic patients had a 1.6% incidence of TIAs and a 3.2% incidence of stroke on late follow-up. Those operated on because of TIAs had a 19.5% and 5.2% incidence of recurrent TIAs or stroke, respectively. Patients with a permanent neurologic deficit preoperatively had an incidence of TIAs of 7.9%, and 11% developed a stroke during late follow-up.

Previously, the role of intervention for asymptomatic lesions has been controversial. Nevertheless, the recently com-

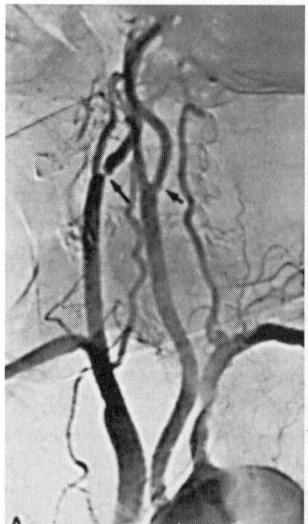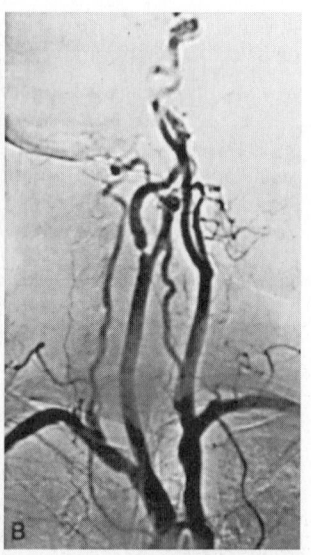

Figure 50–73. Arteriogram showing typical severe right internal carotid artery stenosis at its origin (long arrow). The left internal carotid artery has mild disease (short arrow). This particular study is a subtraction of an arch aortogram shown in the right posterior oblique *(A)* and left posterior oblique *(B)* projections. (From Gomes, A. S.: Aortic arch studies and selective arteriography. *In* Moore, W. S. [Ed.]: Surgery for Cerebrovascular Disease. New York, Churchill Livingstone, 1987.)

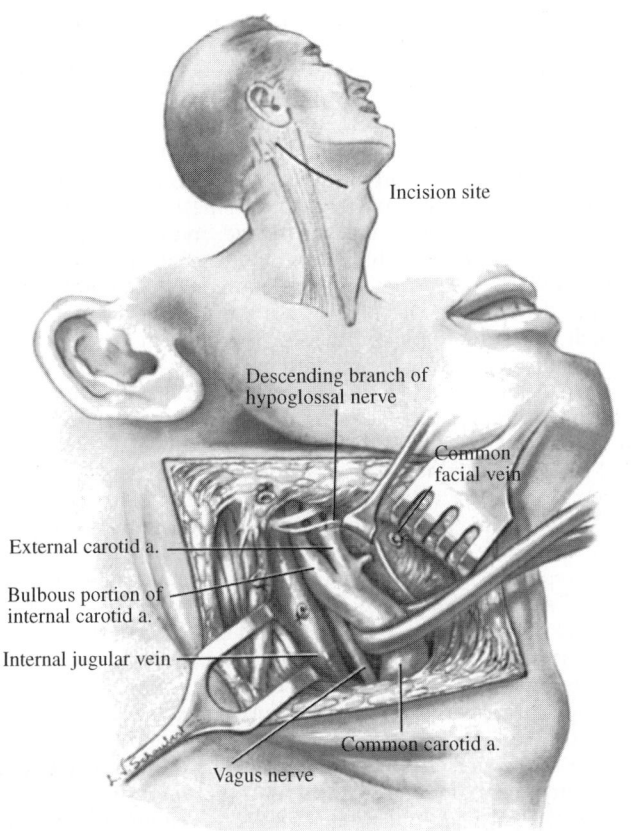

Figure 50–74. Incision site and exposure of the carotid bifurcation area. (From Wylie, E. J., and Ehrenfeld, W. K.: Extracranial Occlusive Cerebrovascular Disease. Philadelphia, W. B. Saunders, 1970.)

Labels in figure:
Incision site
Descending branch of hypoglossal nerve
Common facial vein
External carotid a.
Bulbous portion of internal carotid a.
Internal jugular vein
Common carotid a.
Vagus nerve

pleted prospective randomized multicenter trial has proven that carotid endarterectomy is the treatment of choice for symptomatic carotid artery disease and severe asymptomatic lesions.

SELECTED REFERENCES

Moore, W. S.: Surgery for Cerebrovascular Disease. New York, Churchill Livingstone, 1987.
This book provides a detailed description of cerebrovascular disease by multiple authors considered to be experts in the field. It includes excellent chapters that discuss the natural history of cerebrovascular disease and stroke. In addition, detailed descriptions of the indications for and techniques of operative intervention are included.

Moore, W. S., and Quiñones-Baldrich, W. J.: Extracranial cerebrovascular disease. *In* Moore, W. S. (Ed.): Vascular Surgery, 4th ed. Orlando, Fla., Grune & Stratton, 1993, pp. 532–576.
This review of extracranial cerebrovascular disease summarizes historical advances and provides an excellent summation regarding the current state of knowledge and controversy surrounding treatment of cerebrovascular disease. It also includes discussion of vertebrobasilar insufficiency and emergency management of stroke in progress.

Roederer, G. O., Langlois, Y. E., Jager, K. A., Primozich, J. F., Beach, K. W., Phillips, D. J., and Strandness, D. E., Jr.: The natural history of carotid arterial disease in asymptomatic patients with cervical bruits. Stroke, 15:605, 1984.
This report provides an excellent examination of factors influencing the subsequent incidence of symptoms in patients who present with asymptomatic carotid artery disease. It emphasizes the value of serial monitoring of patients with mild and moderate disease.

REFERENCES

1. Bernstein, E. F., et al.: Influence of preoperative factors on late neurologic events after carotid endarterectomy. *In*: International Vascular Symposium Programs and Abstracts. New York, Macmillan, 1981, p. 460.
2. Carrea, R., and Murphy, M. M.: Surgical treatment of spontaneous throm-
bosis of the internal carotid artery in the neck: Carotid-carotideal anastomosis: Report of a case. Acta Neurol. Latinoam., 1:71, 1955.
3. DeBakey, M. E., Crawford, E. S., Cooley, D. A., and Morris, G. C., Jr.: Surgical considerations of occlusive disease of innominate, carotid, subclavian, and vertebral arteries. Ann. Surg., 149:690, 1959.
4. Eastcott, H. H. G., Pickering, G. W., and Rob, C. G.: Reconstruction of internal carotid artery in a patient with intermittent attacks of hemiplegia. Lancet, 2:994, 1954.
5. Hass, W. K., and Jonas, S.: Caution falling rock zone: An analysis of the medical and surgical management of threatened stroke. Proc. Inst. Med. Chic., 33:80, 1980.
6. Hunt, J. R.: The role of the carotid arteries in the causation of vascular lesions of the brain, with remarks on certain special features of the symptomatology. Am. J. Med. Sci., 147:704, 1914.
7. Johnson, J. M., Kennelly, M. M., Decesare, D., Morgan, S., and Sparrow, A.: Natural history of asymptomatic carotid plaque. Arch. Surg., 120:1010, 1985.
8. Kartchner, M. M., and McRae, L. P.: Noninvasive evaluation and management of the "asymptomatic" carotid bruit. Surgery, 82:840, 1977.
9. Loeb, C., Priano, A., and Albano, C.: Clinical features and long-term follow-up of patients with reversible ischemic attacks (RIA). Acta Neurol. Scand., 57:471, 1978.
10. Moniz, E.: L'encéphalographie artérielle, son importance dans la localisation des tumeurs cérébrales. Rev. Neurol. (Paris), 48:72, 1927.
11. Moore, W. S.: Technique of carotid endarterectomy. *In* Moore, W. S. (Ed.): Surgery for Cerebrovascular Disease. New York, Churchill Livingstone, 1987, pp. 491–502.
12. Moore, W. S., and Quiñones-Baldrich, W. J.: Extracranial cerebrovascular disease. *In* Moore, W. S. (Ed.): Vascular Surgery, 4th ed. Orlando, Fla., Grune & Stratton, 1993, pp. 532–576.
13. Roederer, G. O., Langlois, Y. E., Jager, K. A., Primozich, J. F., Beach, K. W., Phillips, D. J., and Strandness, D. E., Jr.: The natural history of carotid arterial disease in asymptomatic patients with cervical bruits. Stroke, 15:605, 1984.
14. Savory, W. S.: Case of a young woman in whom the main arteries of both upper extremities and of the left side of the neck were throughout completely obliterated. Med.-Chir. Tr. Lond., 39:205, 1856.
15. Whisnant, J. P., Matsumoto, N., and Elveback, L. R.: The effects of anticoagulant therapy on the prognosis of patients with transient cerebral ischemic attacks in a community. Rochester, Minnesota, 1955–1969. Mayo Clin. Proc., 48:844, 1973.
16. Zarins, C. K., Giddens, D. P., and Glagov, S.: Atherosclerotic plaque distribution and flow velocity profiles in the carotid bifurcation. *In* Bergan, J. J., and Yao, J. S. T. (Eds.): Cerebrovascular Insufficiency. New York, Grune & Stratton, 1983, pp. 19–30.

SUBCLAVIAN STEAL SYNDROME

Anthony D. Whittemore, M.D.
John A. Mannick, M.D.

The subclavian steal syndrome occurs when there is reversal of flow in the ipsilateral vertebral artery distal to a stenosis or occlusion of the proximal subclavian, or, more rarely, the innominate artery. Because of the reduction of pressure in the subclavian artery distal to the obstruction, blood flows antegrade up the contralateral vertebral artery, into the basilar artery, and retrograde down the ipsilateral vertebral artery to supply collateral circulation to the upper extremity (Figs. 50–75 and 50–76). Thus, blood supply is presumably "stolen" from the basilar system and may compromise regional or total cerebral blood flow.

Contorni[3] is credited with reporting the first angiographic visualization of subclavian steal in 1960; however, the potential significance of this problem was not widely appreciated until Reivich and his co-workers reported in 1961 about two patients with clinical signs of cerebral vascular insufficiency associated with reversal of flow through the vertebral artery secondary to subclavian obstruction.[22] In their report, reversal of flow was demonstrated by angiography and with the electromagnetic flowmeter at the time of surgical correction. In a subsequent editorial discussing this case, Fisher introduced the term *subclavian steal syndrome*. Since that time, numerous reports have appeared in the literature describing

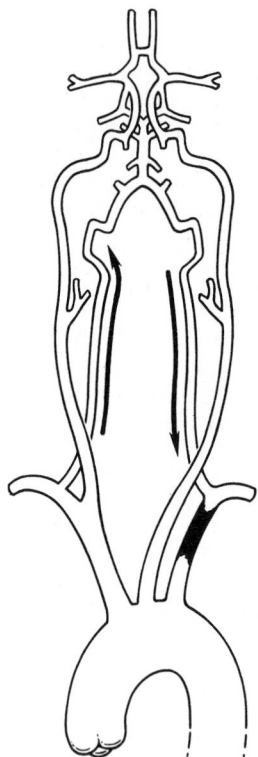

Figure 50–75. Diagram of the pattern of flow in the subclavian steal syndrome. Note the retrograde flow in the vertebral artery on the side of the lesion (after Weilbaecher).

patients found to have subclavian steal by angiography. There has been considerable variation, however, in assessment of the clinical significance of the observed phenomenon.

CLINICAL EVALUATION

Classically, the subclavian steal syndrome should be suspected in a patient who manifests symptoms of vertebral

basilar arterial insufficiency and is found to have a difference in the brachial systolic blood pressure of at least 30 mm. Hg between the two arms associated with a bruit in the supraclavicular area on the affected side. The cause of the proximal subclavian obstruction is atherosclerosis in most instances and more frequently affects the left side.[9] The neurologic symptoms reported in these patients most commonly include vertigo, limb paresis, and paresthesias. Bilateral cortical visual disturbances, ataxia, syncope, and dysarthria occur somewhat less frequently. The symptoms have been encountered initially as transient ischemic attacks of cerebral ischemia in the majority of patients, but a number of instances in which the symptoms progressed to complete stroke have been reported.[9, 22] In patients with innominate artery stenosis, any neurologic manifestations of subclavian steal may be obscured by those associated with concomitant carotid insufficiency.

North and associates reported in 1962 that symptoms of cerebral ischemia were produced by exercise of the affected arm in six of the seven patients encountered with subclavian steal syndrome.[18] Conflicting experimental evidence has since been reported concerning the effect of proximal subclavian occlusion on cerebral blood flow. Reivich and associates[22] and Sammartino and Toole[23] reported that the compensatory increase in forward flow through other major arteries supplying the brain was insufficient to compensate for the flow lost through the steal phenomenon and concluded that a net deficit in cerebral blood flow existed. Handa and associates, however, studied cerebral blood flow in monkeys with an electromagnetic flowmeter and found that reversal of flow in the ipsilateral vertebral artery was accompanied by a compensatory increase of flow in the remaining three arteries supplying the brain, causing a limited 6% decrease in total cerebral blood flow and no evidence of neurologic abnormality.[12] Whereas earlier reports suggested that subclavian steal syndrome was associated with disabling neurologic symptoms in most patients in whom it was encountered,[13, 14, 18, 22] increasing clinical experience suggested that this syndrome remained asymptomatic in most patients.[8] In an early report, Mannick and associates had suggested that the subclavian steal phenomenon was more likely to cause significant neurologic symptoms in patients with disease in other arteries supplying the brain.[14] The Joint Study of Extracranial Arterial

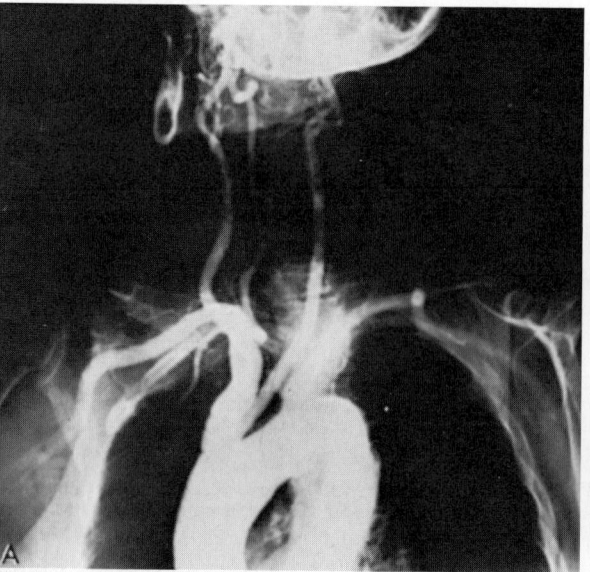 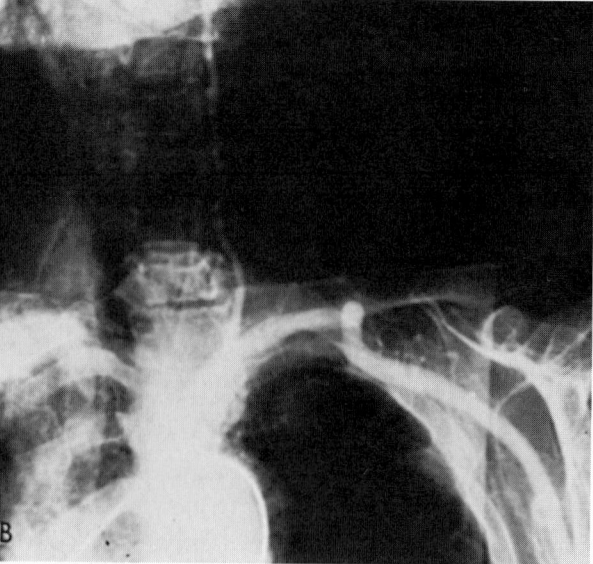

Figure 50–76. Early (A) and late (B) films of an angiogram of the aortic arch in a patient with the subclavian steal syndrome. In the early film, a stenosis of the origin of the left subclavian artery is seen. In the late film, there is retrograde flow of contrast material down the left vertebral artery, filling the left subclavian artery.

Occlusion subsequently reported that 80% of 168 patients with subclavian steal syndrome had demonstrable disease involving other extracranial vessels.[9] It is of interest that in patients in this study treated medically or receiving no treatment at all, the three (9%) who suffered strokes had associated carotid disease. Patients with subclavian artery disease alone did not have strokes during the follow-up period, whether they were treated medically, surgically, or not at all. It is now apparent that, paradoxically, only a few patients have manifested neurologic symptoms in response to exercise of the involved arm, which would be expected to increase the demand for collateral blood flow.

It appears reasonable to conclude, therefore, that the subclavian steal phenomenon may frequently be clinically asymptomatic but can produce or contribute to symptoms of cerebrovascular insufficiency when it exists in conjunction with other lesions of the extracranial vasculature, particularly carotid bifurcation lesions. Whether the subclavian steal phenomenon produces symptoms in a given individual probably depends on (1) the size of the vertebral artery on the uninvolved side and whether it is free from disease; (2) the variable anatomy of the circle of Willis; (3) the amount of collateral circulation from other sources (particularly the costocervical and thyrocervical trunks)[2, 17] that develops to supply the affected arm; and (4) the presence of other extracranial vascular lesions.

The diagnosis of subclavian steal is established with retrograde catheter angiography, during which the tip of the catheter is positioned in the aortic root and a delayed filming sequence demonstrates retrograde flow in the ipsilateral vertebral vessel. It has been noted that a forceful injection of contrast material with the catheter tip located close to the origin of the vertebral vessel may in fact produce a spurious demonstration of the subclavian steal syndrome.[21, 25]

SURGICAL CORRECTION

Indications. Because the subclavian steal syndrome is rarely symptomatic in the absence of associated extracranial lesions and, contrary to internal carotid artery lesions, rarely causes stroke, the more threatening extracranial lesions should be repaired either initially or concomitantly with reconstruction for subclavian steal.[9] In patients for whom the subclavian steal syndrome appears to be responsible for symptoms of vertebrobasilar insufficiency in the absence of other lesions in the extracranial cerebral arterial circulation, however, surgical correction of the lesion appears warranted and can result in amelioration of the symptoms. Surgical therapy cannot justifiably be urged for the prevention of stroke under these circumstances, because subclavian steal alone does not appear to cause stroke.[12] When the subclavian steal syndrome occurs in association with other extracranial arterial lesions, it is evident that the other significant lesions should be repaired as well. It appears likely that concomitant correction of the subclavian steal syndrome in certain of these patients should be undertaken; however, there are a number of reports of symptomatic relief in patients with subclavian steal in whom only the other arterial lesions were corrected.[9]

Operative Technique. A variety of surgical procedures have been recommended for correction of subclavian steal, including simple ligation of the ipsilateral vertebral artery, aorta–subclavian artery bypass graft, or subclavian endarterectomy using a mediastinal or transthoracic approach.[4, 5, 29] As the intrathoracic procedures were initially associated with impressive morbidity, several supraclavicular procedures emerged. By the late 1960s, most surgeons had adopted the carotid-to-subclavian artery bypass graft carried out through

a cervical incision as the procedure of choice.[4, 9] Subsequent experimental observations and widespread clinical application of this approach have demonstrated that significant reduction of internal carotid artery flow does not occur unless there is concomitant stenosis of the proximal common carotid artery.[1, 19] Under such circumstances, this operation is clearly not advisable, because a significant reduction in total cerebral flow may result from an associated carotid steal.

The optimal approach for carotid-subclavian bypass is through a transverse cervical incision superior and parallel to the clavicle (Fig. 50–77). The clavicular head of the sternocleidomastoid muscle is divided, and the exposed scalene fat pad swept inferiorly to expose the phrenic nerve coursing from lateral to medial over the anterior surface of the anterior scalene muscle. With gentle medial traction of the phrenic nerve, the scalene muscle is divided near its insertion on the first rib, exposing the mid-segment of the subclavian artery. The subclavian artery is then mobilized from the origin of the vertebral and mammary arteries to the lateral border of the first rib. The common carotid artery just deep to the sternal head of the sternocleidomastoid muscle and medial to the internal jugular vein is mobilized for a sufficient distance to accommodate a short arteriotomy and catheter tourniquets, in the rare event that an indwelling shunt is required. Although many surgeons prefer never to use a shunt, and others employ it routinely, some prefer to carry out this procedure with electroencephalographic monitoring, using the shunt on a selective basis. Whereas the choice of conduit is a subject of much debate, most surgeons prefer a short

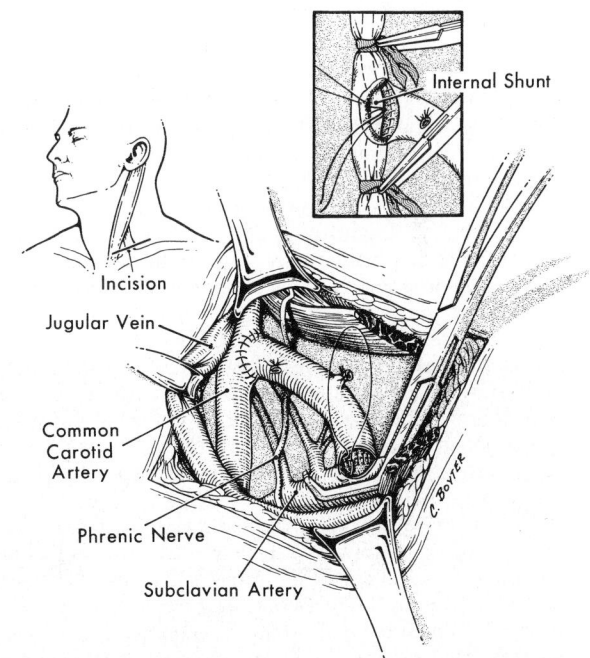

Figure 50–77. Diagrammatic illustration of the technique of carotid-to-subclavian bypass grafting. The incision is placed at the base of the neck. The clavicular portion of the sternocleidomastoid muscle is divided, exposing the anterior scalene muscle and phrenic nerve. The phrenic nerve is carefully spared and the anterior scalene is divided, exposing the fascia overlying the subclavian artery, which can be freed from the vertebral origin laterally beyond the margin of the first rib. The common carotid artery is exposed through the same incision as it lies beneath the sternocleidomastoid muscle posteromedial to the jugular vein. A graft of autogenous saphenous vein is sutured end-to-side to the common carotid artery. An internal shunt (inset) may be used to preserve flow in the carotid artery while the anastomosis is performed. The shunt is removed just before completion of the suture line. The vein graft is then trimmed to size and sutured end-to-side to the subclavian artery.

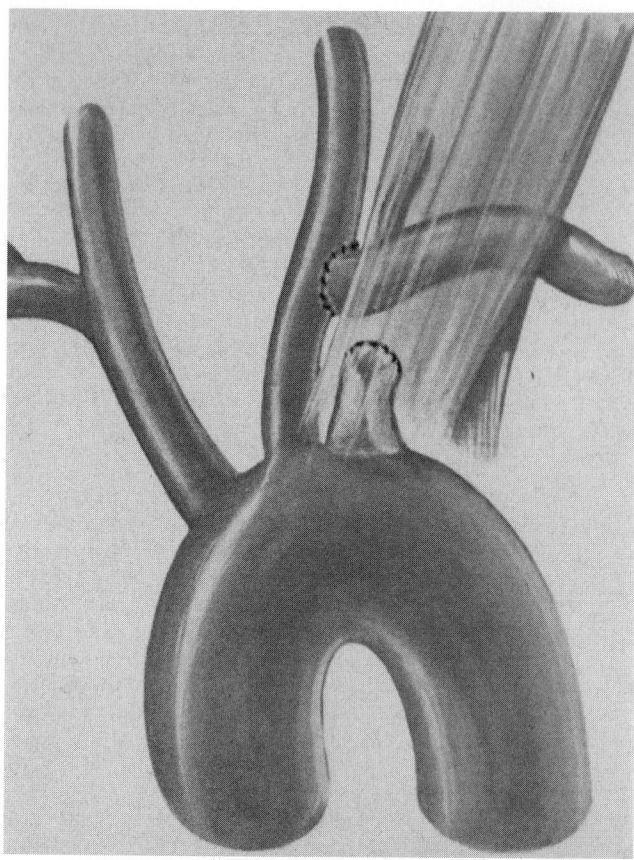

Figure 50–78. Diagrammatic illustration of the technique of subclavian–carotid artery transposition carried through the exposure described for Figure 50–77. The subclavian artery is transected distal to the stenotic or occlusive lesion and sutured directly end-to-side to the common carotid arteriotomy.

prosthetic graft.[30] A 6- to 8-mm. graft is sutured end-to-side to the common carotid artery, delivered deep to the internal jugular vein, and anastomosed end-to-side to the subclavian artery. Thirty-day operative mortality is generally in the range of 2%, and 5-year graft patency rates approach 95% with relief of symptoms in the vast majority.[7, 9, 20, 26–28]

The subclavian steal syndrome may also be corrected by a subclavian-subclavian artery bypass graft through bilateral supraclavicular incisions[10, 11] or by an axillary-axillary bypass graft carried out through two infraclavicular incisions.[16] Patency rates of these grafts have in general been favorable, and both avoid interfering with the anterior cerebral circulation. However, more extensive and therefore more time-consuming dissection is required: bilateral phrenic nerve palsy is a potential serious complication; and the axillary-axillary graft procedure places the graft in the undesirable superficial location as it crosses the sternum in the midline.

Since the mid-1980s an alternative procedure, the subclavian-carotid transposition, has become the procedure of choice for many surgeons. Initially recommended by Mehigan and associates in 1978 for patients exhibiting embolic complications from subclavian stenosis, the procedure is carried out through the supraclavicular approach.[15] The subclavian artery is divided just distal to its proximal stenosis or occlusion and the proximal end oversewn. The distal end is transposed and sutured end-to-side to the common carotid artery, converting the proximal common carotid vessel to a new innominate, perfusing both the subclavian and vertebral systems (Fig. 50–78). Although the procedure requires more extensive mobilization of the proximal subclavian vessel, it obviates the need for a graft and shortens the operating time considerably. Overall patency rates after 5 years approach 99%, with minimal operative morbidity and mortality.[6, 7, 20, 24, 26]

SELECTED REFERENCES

Crawford, E. S., Stowe, C. L., and Powers, R. W., Jr.: Occlusion of the innominate, common carotid and subclavian arteries: Long-term results of surgical treatment. Surgery, 94:781, 1983.
Report of the experience of the senior author with reconstructions for obstruction of the brachiocephalic arteries in 142 patients over a 23-year period points out that transthoracic and extrathoracic operations in recent years have carried an equally low mortality. In fact, 89% of all patients survived operation, including early deaths when new techniques were being applied. Nevertheless, for single-vessel occlusions on one side of the neck, the authors still prefer the simplicity of the carotid-subclavian bypass and report that extrathoracic operations were performed in this large series in 69% of their patients. Eighty-three per cent of the patients remained asymptomatic over a follow-up period that averaged 7.5 years.

Edwards, W. H., Tapper, S. S., Edwards, W. H., Sr., Mulherin, J. L., Martin, R. S., and Jenkins, J. M.: Subclavian revascularization: A quarter-century experience. Ann. Surg., 219:673, 1994.
The authors report their experience with subclavian-carotid transposition in 178 procedures. The mortality rate associated with the isolated subclavian-carotid transposition was 1.1%, and all but one remained patent after a mean follow-up of 46 months. A thorough discussion addresses the risks and benefits of both carotid-subclavian bypass and subclavian-carotid transposition and argues for the latter as the procedure of choice for routine subclavian carotid occlusive disease.

Mehigan, J. T., Buch, W. S., Tipkin, R. D., and Fogarty, T. J.: Subclavian-carotid transposition for the subclavian steal syndrome. Am. J. Surg., 136:15, 1978.
This paper was one of the first to describe the direct anastomosis of the divided distal subclavian artery to the side of the common carotid artery to correct cerebral symptoms of the subclavian steal syndrome and to relieve symptoms of arm claudication, which are often associated with proximal subclavian occlusive disease. The technique as described has the advantage of not requiring a graft to correct the subclavian steal and of eliminating the possibility of embolization of clot or atherosclerotic debris from the proximal subclavian stenosis, which theoretically can occur after repair of the subclavian steal by carotid-subclavian bypass.

Reivich, M., Holling, H. E., Roberts, B., and Toole, J. F.: Reversal of blood flow through the vertebral artery and its effect on cerebral circulation. N. Engl. J. Med., 265:878, 1961.
This is the classic report describing the subclavian steal syndrome clinically and experimentally. Two patients were studied who had neurologic symptoms and reversal of flow in the left vertebral artery secondary to proximal subclavian stenosis, as demonstrated by angiography. Reversal of flow in the ipsilateral vertebral artery was demonstrated for the first time in humans at the time of operation

in one of these patients by application of an electromagnetic flowmeter to the subclavian artery distal to the vertebral origin. The authors also report animal studies in which reversal of vertebral flow was demonstrated following subclavian artery occlusion. In the animal experiments, they conclude that total cerebral blood flow was markedly diminished by the subclavian steal.

REFERENCES

1. Barner, H. B., Kaiser, G. C., and Willman, V. L.: Hemodynamics of carotid-subclavian bypass. Arch. Surg., *103*:248, 1971.
2. Bosniak, M. A.: Cervical arterial pathways associated with brachiocephalic occlusive disease. AJR, *91*:1232, 1964.
3. Contorni, L.: Il circolo collaterale vertebraovertebrale nella obliterazione dell'arterio subclavia all sua origine. Min. Chir., *15*:258, 1960.
4. Crawford E. S., DeBakey, M. E., Morris, G. C., Jr., and Howell, J. F.: Surgical treatment of occlusion of the innominate, common carotid, and subclavian arteries: A 10-year experience. Surgery, *65*:17, 1969.
5. Crawford E. S., Stowe, C. L., and Power R. W., Jr.: Occlusion of the innominate, common carotid, and subclavian arteries: Long-term results of surgical treatment. Surgery, *94*:781, 1983.
6. Edwards, W. H., and Mulherin, J. L., Jr.: The surgical reconstruction of the proximal subclavian and vertebral artery. J. Vasc. Surg., *2*:634, 1985.
7. Edwards, W. H., Tapper, S. S., Edwards, W. H., Sr., Mulherin, J. L., Martin, R. S., and Jenkins, J. M.: Subclavian revascularization: A quarter century experience. Ann. Surg., *219*:673, 1994.
8. Ehrenfeld, W. K., Chapman, R. D., and Wylie, E. J.: Management of occlusive lesions of the branches of the aortic arch. Am. J. Surg., *118*:236, 1969.
9. Fields, W. S., and Lemak, N. A.: Joint study of extracranial arterial occlusion. JAMA, *222*:1139, 1972.
10. Finkelstein, N. M., Byer, A., and Rush, B. F., Jr.: Subclavian-subclavian bypass for subclavian steal syndrome. Surgery, *71*:142, 1972.
11. Forestner, J. E., Ghosh, S. K., Bergan, J. J., and Conn, J., Jr.: Subclavian-subclavian bypass for correction of the subclavian steal syndrome. Surgery, *71*:136, 1972.
12. Handa, J., Yoshida, K., and Meyer, J. S.: Hemodynamic effects of subclavian and innominate artery ligation. Surgery, *59*:1069, 1966.
13. Irvine, W. T., Luck, R. J., and Jacobey, J. A.: Reversed blood-flow in the vertebral arteries causing recurrent brain-stem ischaemia. Lancet, *1*:994, 1965.
14. Mannick, J. A., Suter, C. G., and Hume, D. M.: The "subclavian steal" syndrome: A further documentation. JAMA, *182*:254, 1962.
15. Mehigan, J. T., Buch, W. S., Pipkin, R. D., and Fogarty, T. J.: Subclavian-carotid transposition for the subclavian steal syndrome. Am. J. Surg., *136*:15, 1978.
16. Myers, W. O., Lawton, B. R., Ray, J. F., III, Kuehner, M. E., and Sautter, R. D.: Axillo-axillary bypass for subclavian steal syndrome. Arch. Surg., *114*:394, 1979.
17. Newton, T. H., and Wylie, E. J.: Collateral circulation associated with occlusion of the proximal subclavian and innominate arteries. AJR, *91*:394, 1964.
18. North, R. R., Fields, W. S., and DeBakey, M. E., et al.: Brachial-basilar insufficiency syndrome. Neurology, *12*:810, 1962.
19. Otis, S., Rush, M., Thomas M., and Dilley, R.: Carotid steal syndrome following carotid subclavian bypass. J. Vasc. Surg., *1*:649, 1984.
20. Perler, B. A., and Williams, G. M.: Carotid-subclavian bypass—A decade of experience. J. Vasc. Surg., *12*:716, 1990.
21. Pineda, A., and Smith, J. L.: True and false subclavian steal syndromes: Collateral circulation of the true subclavian steal syndrome demonstrated by angiography. Arch. Surg., *92*:258, 1966.
22. Reivich, M., Holling, H. E., Roberts, B., et al.: Reversal of blood flow through the vertebral artery and its effect on cerebral circulation. N. Engl. J. Med., *265*:878, 1961.
23. Sammartino, W. F., and Toole, J. F.: Reversed vertebral artery flow. Arch. Neurol., *10*:590, 1964.
24. Sandman, W., Kniemeyer, H. W., Jaeschcock, R., Hennerici, M., and Aulich, A.: The role of subclavian-carotid transposition in surgery for supra-aortic occlusive disease. J. Vasc. Surg., *5*:53, 1987.
25. Shockman, A. T.: Retrograde vertebral artery flow as an artifact of technique. AJR, *91*:1258, 1964.
26. Sterpetti, A. V., Schultz, R. D., Farina, C., and Feldhaus, R. J.: Subclavian artery revascularization: A comparison between carotid-subclavian artery bypass and subclavian-carotid transposition. Surgery, *106*:624, 1989.
27. Synn, A. Y., Chalmers, R. T. A., Sharp, W. J., Hoballah, J. J., Kresowik, T. F., and Corson, J. D.: Is there a conduit of preference for a bypass between the carotid and subclavian arteries? Am. J. Surg., *166*:157, 1993.
28. Vitti, M. J., Thompson, B. W., Read, R. C., Gagne, P. J., Barone, G. W., Barnes, R. W., and Eidt, J. F.: Carotid-subclavian bypass: A twenty-two-year experience. J. Vasc. Surg., *20*:411, 1994.
29. Vogt, D. P., Hertzer, N. R., O'Hara, P. J., and Beven, E. G.: Brachiocephalic arterial reconstruction. Ann. Surg., *196*:541, 1982.
30. Ziomek, S., Quinones-Baldrich, W. J., Busuttil, R. W., Baker, J. D., Machleder, H. I., and Moore, W. S.: The superiority of synthetic arterial grafts over autologous veins in carotid-subclavian bypass. J. Vasc. Surg., *3*:140, 1986.

THROMBOTIC OBLITERATION OF THE ABDOMINAL AORTA AND ILIAC ARTERIES (LERICHE'S SYNDROME)

David C. Sabiston, Jr., M.D.

Chronic occlusion of the aortic bifurcation by thrombosis was originally described by Leriche in French in 1923.[3] In 1948, Leriche and Morel wrote an excellent review in English.[4] Leriche emphasized that the disorder is a chronic one and is associated with a specific symptom complex. It typically affects men 35 to 60 years of age.

CLINICAL MANIFESTATIONS

Characteristic symptoms of thrombotic occlusion of the terminal aorta include (1) extreme liability to fatigue of both lower limbs, described as a weariness rather than the typical intermittent claudication; (2) symmetrical atrophy of both lower limbs without trophic changes in the skin or nails; (3) pallor of the legs and feet; and (4) inability to maintain a stable erection due to inadequate arterial flow to the penis from hypogastric arterial obstruction, thus reducing the blood flow through the internal pudendal artery and its blood flow to the corpora cavernosa. The physical findings include absence of pulses in the abdominal aorta and in the arteries distally. The changes in arterial pressure are shown

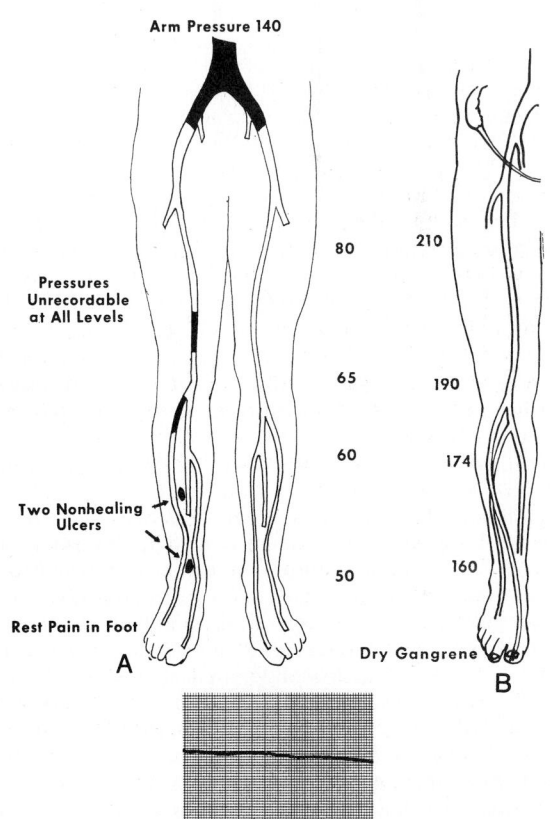

Figure 50–79. *A,* The extensive aortoiliac occlusion, combined with the superficial femoral artery and anterior tibial artery occlusion, reduced limb blood pressures below recordable levels. *B,* The normal ankle pressure of 160 mm. Hg and absent digit pulses placed the arterial occlusion between the ankle and digits. (From Strandness, D. E., Jr.: Collateral Circulation in Clinical Surgery. Philadelphia, W. B. Saunders, 1969.)

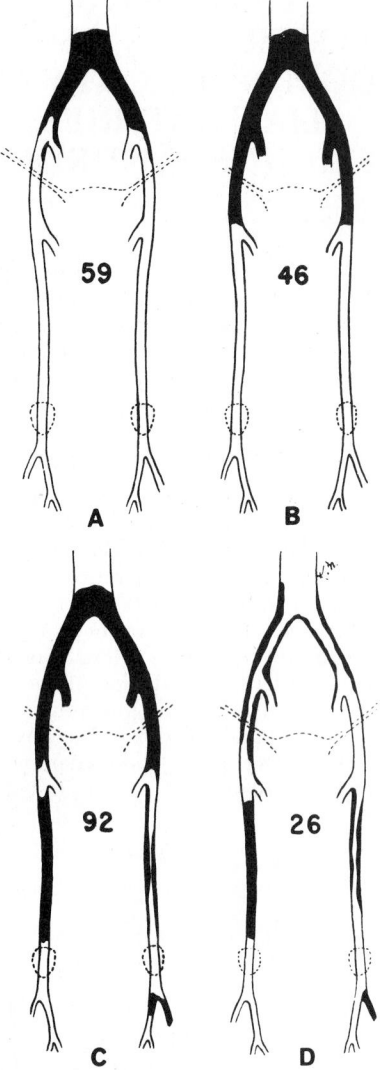

Figure 50–80. Classification of extent of involvement in a series of patients with aortoiliofemoral arterial occlusive disease. (From Perdue, G. D., Long, W. D., and Smith, R. B., III: Perspective concerning aortofemoral arterial reconstruction. Trans. South. Surg. Assoc., *82*:330, 1979.)

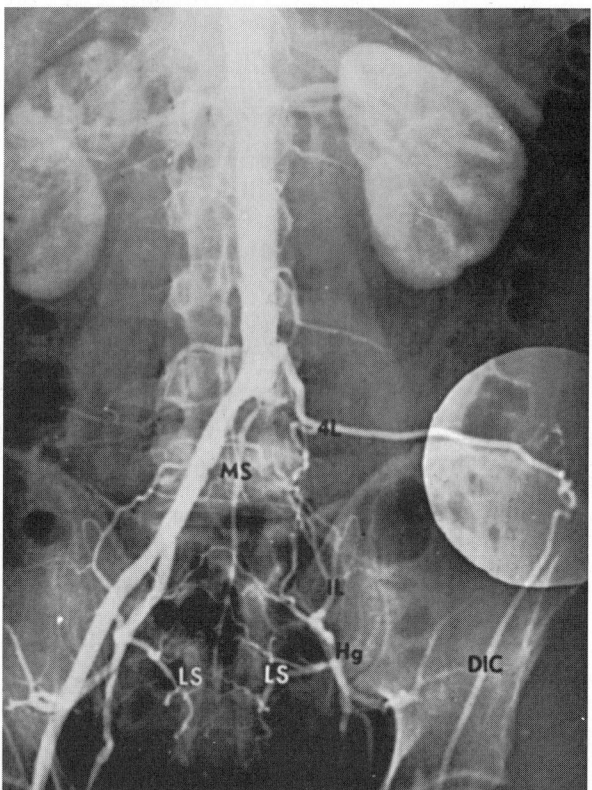

Figure 50–81. A 43-year-old man presented with left intermittent claudication. The fourth lumbar (4L) artery is the origin of a pathway to the femoral artery by means of the deep iliac circumflex (DIC) artery and to the hypogastric (Hg) artery through the iliolumbar (IL) artery. The middle sacral (MS) and lateral sacral (LS) arteries contribute to a transpelvic anastomosis to the hypogastric artery. (From Friedenberg, M. J., and Perez, C. A.: Collateral circulation in aortoiliofemoral disease: As demonstrated by a unilateral percutaneous common femoral artery needle injection. AJR, *94*:145, 1965.)

in Figure 50–79.[7] Distal sites of segmental occlusion produce a further fall in arterial pressure, and ischemic ulceration may appear.

This disorder is often well tolerated for 5 and even 10 years but usually terminates in gangrene of one or both legs. The pathologic findings include atherosclerosis of the arterial wall with superimposed thrombosis. The lumen usually narrows over a period of months and years such that acute symptoms are not likely to occur. Arteriography shows occlusion of the terminal abdominal aorta and often of one or both common iliac arteries (Fig. 50–80).[1, 5] The occlusion may involve any portion of the abdominal aorta from the renal arteries distally. The collateral circulation around the arterial blockage is shown in Fig. 50–81.[2] Patients should cease smoking after bypass grafts are performed because the evidence is clear that thrombosis of grafts is appreciably increased by continuance of smoking.[6] The relationship showing percentage of graft occlusion according to the smoking history is shown in Figure 50–82.

SURGICAL MANAGEMENT

Although thromboendarterectomy with direct reconstitution of flow is appropriate in a few patients, the majority of

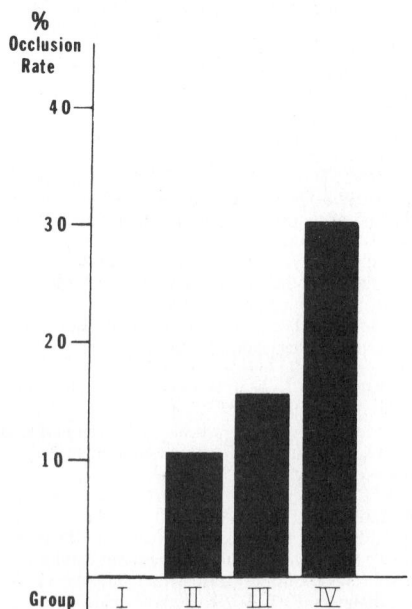

Figure 50–82. Occlusion rate of prosthetic grafts inserted for Leriche's syndrome according to smoking history. Group I: Patients who did not smoke either before or after operation. Group II: Patients who were cigarette smokers before operation but ceased smoking postoperatively. Group III: Patients who were cigarette smokers preoperatively and who continued to smoke up to one pack daily after operation. Group IV: Patients who remained heavy smokers after operation using more than a pack of cigarettes daily. (From Robicsek, F., Daugherty, H., Mullen, D. C., Masters, T. N., Narbay, D., and Sanger, P. W.: The effect of continued cigarette smoking on the patency of synthetic vascular grafts in Leriche syndrome. J. Thorac. Cardiovasc. Surg., *70*:107, 1975.)

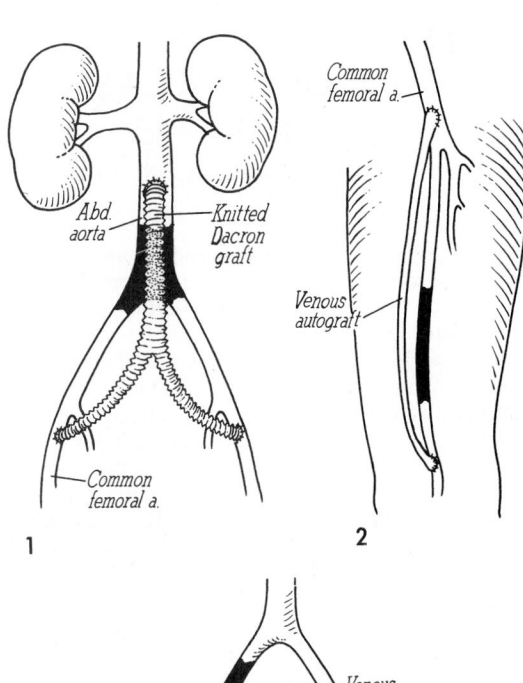

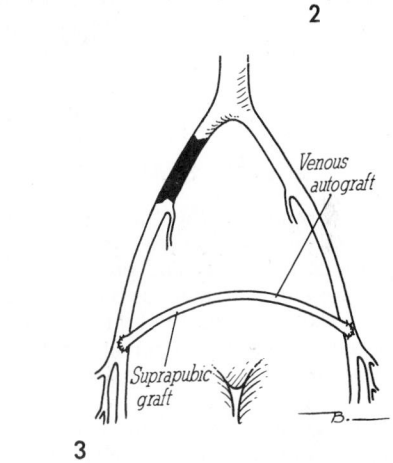

Figure 50–83. Diagram of various bypass grafts. *1,* For occlusion of the abdominal aorta, a bypass graft placed proximal to the occlusion can be inserted distally into each of the common femoral arteries in the groin. *2,* For occlusion of the superficial femoral artery, a venous autograft may be placed from the common femoral artery above to the femoral or popliteal artery distal to the obstruction. *3,* For unilateral iliac arterial occlusion, a suprapubic graft can be placed from one common femoral artery to the other in a subcutaneous suprapubic tunnel. Generally, under these circumstances a venous autograft is preferable to a plastic prosthesis, although the latter can be employed.

patients with occlusion of the abdominal aorta are managed by bypass grafts from the aorta to the iliac or more often the common femoral arteries (Fig. 50–83). It may be necessary to perform a thromboendarterectomy distal to the renal arteries to permit a patent lumen for the proximal anastomosis. However, it is important to minimize dissection in this region to prevent damage to the sympathetic and parasympathetic nerves. This helps to prevent postoperative retrograde ejaculation.

Balloon angioplasty can be effective therapy in selected patients.[8]

SELECTED REFERENCES

Foster, J. H.: Arteriography: Cornerstone of vascular surgery. Arch. Surg., *109*:605, 1974.
In this essay, the development of arteriography from its origin to the present is reviewed. Of particular significance is the fact that the author advocates more extensive use of arteriography.

Strandness, D. E., and Sumner, D. S.: Hemodynamics for Surgeons. New York, Grune & Stratton, 1975.
This is an excellent and quite thorough monograph concerning the hemodynamics of the vascular system. The determinants of cardiac output and arterial and venous flow as well as a variety of physical and physiologic aspects are discussed. In addition, a number of clinical problems are used as examples illustrating the basic physical and physiologic principles.

REFERENCES

1. Foster, J. H.: Arteriography: Cornerstone of vascular surgery. Arch. Surg., *109*:605, 1974.
2. Friedenberg, M. J., and Perez, C. A.: Collateral circulation in aorto-iliofemoral occlusive disease: As demonstrated by a unilateral percutaneous common femoral artery needle injection. AJR, *94*:145, 1965.
3. Leriche, R.: De la résection du carrefour aortico-iliaque avec double sympathectomie lombaire pour thrombose artéritique de l'aorta: Le syndrome de l'oblitération termino-aortique par artérite. Presse Médicale, *1940*:54, 1940.
4. Leriche, R., and Morel, A.: The syndrome of thrombotic obliteration of the aortic bifurcation. Ann. Surg., *127*:193, 1948.
5. Perdue, G. D., Long, W. D., and Smith, R. B., III: Perspective concerning aortofemoral arterial reconstruction. Trans. South. Surg. Assoc., *82*:330, 1979.
6. Robicsek, F., Daughterty, H., Mullen, D. C., Masters, T. N., Narbay, D., and Sanger, P. W.: The effect of continued cigarette smoking on the patency of synthetic vascular grafts in Leriche syndrome. J. Thorac. Cardiovasc. Surg., *70*:107, 1975.
7. Strandness, D. E., Jr.: Chronic arterial occlusion. *In* Strandness, D. E., Jr. (Ed.): Collateral Circulation in Clinical Surgery. Philadelphia, W. B. Saunders, l969.
8. Tadavarthy, A. K., Sullivan, W. A., Jr., Nicoloff, D., Castaneda-Zuniga, W. R., Hunter, D. W., Amplatz, K.: Aorta balloon angioplasty: 9-year follow-up. Radiology, *170*:1039, 1989.

ILIAC ARTERIAL OCCLUSION

David C. Sabiston, Jr., M.D.

The iliac arteries may be individually stenosed or occluded. The symptoms are usually those of claudication of the hip and thigh associated with diminished or absent pulses in that extremity. Arteriography is diagnostic. When symptoms are unilateral, involvement of the opposite leg can often be seen on the arteriogram. Indeed, symptoms may appear in the opposite leg after operation when the patient is able to exercise sufficiently. Bypass grafts from the aorta above to the common femoral artery below are usually indicated.

FEMOROPOPLITEAL AND FEMOROINFRAPOPLITEAL BYPASS

Richard L. McCann, M.D.

The treatment of vascular stenoses and obstructions by catheter dilatation techniques was reported by Dotter and Judkins in 1964.[1] Subsequently, Grüntzig popularized the transluminal balloon dilatation catheter technique for treatment of peripheral vascular stenosis.[2] There have been attempts to improve the results achieved with percutaneous treatment by employing miniature cutting devices mounted on catheters, using laser energy to assist in luminal disobliteration, and using expanding metallic stents to prop open the artery after balloon dilatation, but the role of these techniques has not been definitely established. Thus, the current practice of revascularization of the ischemic lower extremity has developed both from the experimental laboratory and from clinical contributions. A firm basis has been established, and continued improvements can be expected to occur.[3–12]

CLINICAL EVALUATION

An accurate diagnosis of the presence of vascular disease, as well as its location and severity, can often be made after completing a focused history and physical examination. Patients with peripheral vascular disease usually complain of pain. Careful analysis of the location, quality, and intensity of the pain and factors that aggravate and relieve it yields important information. Ischemic pain has a characteristic quality that is unlikely to be confused with other conditions. The term claudication (from the Latin verb *claudicare*, to limp) is applied to the cramping pain felt in specific muscle groups when nutritive blood flow is inadequate to meet the metabolic demands of exercise. The distance walked before onset of this leg pain is strikingly reproducible, and the pain is promptly relieved simply by cessation of ambulation. Claudication of the buttock and thigh muscles is indicative of an aortoiliac obstruction, whereas calf claudication usually indicates femoral artery disease. When blood flow is inadequate to meet metabolic requirements at rest, continuous pain (rest pain) may be described. This pain is usually felt in the toes and forefoot. It is often prominent at night. In the recumbent position, there is loss of the hydrostatic pressure component due to the gravitational force of the column of blood between the heart and the site of vascular obstruction. Loss of this component may cause the flow across a stenosis to decrease below a threshold value and awaken the patient with pain. Patients often discover that restoring a component of hydrostatic pressure by hanging the foot over the side of the bed or by standing relieves this pain. Rest pain is an ominous symptom and demands prompt evaluation, not only because of the considerable discomfort for the patient but also because it indicates such severe vascular compromise that the involved limb may soon progress to frank gangrene in the absence of intervention.

Ischemic ulceration refers to localized skin necrosis that is associated with arterial insufficiency and that fails to heal after a period of 6 weeks. It may be observed anywhere but is usually found on the plantar surface of the foot or between the toes; the toes themselves may become necrotic. This type of lesion occurs not so much from infarction of the skin as from local trauma, which in a well-vascularized extremity would be trivial. In a severely ischemic limb, healing may be so impaired that even minor lesions fail to respond to appropriate local therapy and often progress. The end stage of vascular insufficiency is frank tissue infarction or gangrene. If this is associated with infection, emergency treatment may be required to eliminate the source of the systemic sepsis.

Other historical aspects in the initial clinical evaluation may aid in the management of vascular patients. It is important to note the presence of vascular disease in other systems. Atherosclerosis is a systemic disorder, and overt manifestations of concomitant cerebrovascular or coronary artery disease may influence the management of lower extremity ischemia. Before embarking on a major operative procedure to alleviate calf claudication, it would be wise to ensure that the patient's cardiopulmonary reserves are sufficient to permit and support increased exercise tolerance. The importance of associated coronary and cerebrovascular disease in a patient with lower extremity ischemia cannot be overemphasized. The importance of this is indicated by studies that demonstrate that the 5-year survival rate following surgery for limb salvage is less than 50%, and maintenance of function and ability to ambulate have been reported in an even smaller percentage.[13]

The presence of other conditions associated with vascular disease, such as diabetes and hypertension, must be noted. The social history is also of great importance. Patients who continue to use tobacco have inferior results, and every effort should be made to convince these patients to stop.[14–16] In a patient with claudication, it is important to record the desired or necessary lifestyle. Claudication at a moderate distance is obviously of greater significance to a patient who is required to walk to earn a living than the same disability in an older, retired patient whose life may be limited very little by having to rest after walking a short distance.

Physical Examination

The physical examination often confirms the impressions formed by the history. Inspection of the limb may reveal muscular atrophy; skin changes associated with vascular insufficiency, such as a thin, brittle, shiny texture; and nails that are thick and opaque. Hair on the extremity may be absent or thinned, particularly over the toes and feet. Pallor may be present, particularly with elevation of the legs to 60 degrees for 1 to 2 minutes. This is often associated with rubor when the feet are then placed in a dependent position. Rubor is thought to be due to cutaneous reactive vasodilatation in response to chronic ischemia. Pallor of elevation and rubor of dependency are signs of advanced vascular insufficiency and are seldom seen if only claudication is present. Palpation of the extremities is important, along with searching for temperature changes and examining the pulses. An appreciation of the pulse amplitude and the presence and duration of turbulent flow may be obtained. Proximal obstruction affects the distal pulses not only by a decrease in the mean pressure but also by a decrease in the perceived pulse amplitude, because the pulse pressure is narrowed distal to a site of obstruction. Palpation of the pulses is best done by a warm hand in a warm room. In an obese patient, external rotation of the hip may aid in palpation of the femoral pulse. The popliteal pulse is often difficult to palpate in an obese patient, even by an experienced examiner. In fact, a prominent and easily palpable popliteal pulse should raise the question of a popliteal aneurysm. The dorsalis pedis and posterior tibial pulses are usually not palpable in patients with lower extremity ischemia owing to proximal obstruction. It should be remembered that in some normal extremities one of these ankle pulses may be absent due to anatomic variation in vascular supply to the foot. If ankle pulses are present, the effect of exercise should be noted, because if the pulses are not diminished directly following exercise, the diagnosis of vascular insufficiency is in doubt. Another important aspect of the vascular examination is an evaluation of the saphenous vein. The patient is asked to stand, and the vein is observed and palpated beginning at the medial malleolus and proceeding proximally. This is especially important when a long bypass to the tibial vessels is contemplated. This evaluation may be supplemented with duplex ultrasonography when the quality of a long saphenous vein is critical to the success of revascularization. Auscultation for bruits should be performed over the femoral area and also over the abdomen to detect the presence of potentially limiting iliac and distal aortic lesions. The vascular examination also includes palpation for the presence of an abdominal aortic aneurysm, auscultation for a carotid bruit, and a search for signs of cardiac disease. The general examination may also disclose other diseases that might influence the management of a vascular patient, such as orthopedic or pulmonary conditions.

Vascular Laboratory

An essential part of the initial evaluation of a vascular patient is noninvasive vascular laboratory testing. Although these examinations have many limitations, they are particularly useful for longitudinal comparisons over the course of operative or nonoperative therapy and as a semiquantitative examination for comparison between examiners. The most useful examinations are determination of segmental Doppler pressure, pulse volume recordings, duplex vascular imaging, and response to standardized exercise stress.

The Doppler instrument is a velocity detector rather than a flowmeter. It contains a piezoelectric crystal that emits a narrow ultrasound beam when electrically excited. The beam travels through a coupling gel and passes through the skin and tissues to an underlying blood vessel. The sound beam is then reflected by the moving red blood cells within the vessel lumen, and in this reflection the frequency of the sound wave is shifted (the Doppler shift) in proportion to the velocity of the blood. The reflected sound waves are sensed by a second crystal, and the shift in frequency is processed as an audible or analog signal. Commercial hand-held Doppler units are available with emitting frequencies of 3.5 to 10 MHz. Because the depth of penetration of the sound waves is inversely proportional to the emitted frequency, the higher-frequency units are most useful for examining the relatively superficial vessels of the lower extremity.

Doppler examination of the lower extremity vessels can be used to determine the presence or absence of detectable flow within a vessel. It requires a flow velocity of 5 cm. per second to obtain a reliable signal in most commercially available units. The quality of the signal may also provide additional information. The normal arterial signal is triphasic. This corresponds to the rapid flow during systole, the initial reversed flow in diastole, and the gradual return of forward flow during the late phase of diastole. When listening to a vessel distal to a site of obstruction, the signal first becomes biphasic, and as the degree of obstruction increases, the signal becomes increasingly damped and monophasic. This corresponds to the dampening of the velocity profile across the site of obstruction (Fig. 50–84). By inflating appropriately sized blood pressure cuffs placed on the thigh, below the knee, and above the ankle and listening with the Doppler unit over a distal artery, segmental systolic pressures can be obtained. A drop in pressure across a segment suggests the presence of a stenosis. Pressure values may be standardized by comparing the observed values with the brachial artery pressure, yielding an ankle-brachial index. Simultaneously, recordings of the pulse volume can be obtained by using the cuffs as volume plethysmographs. The response of these

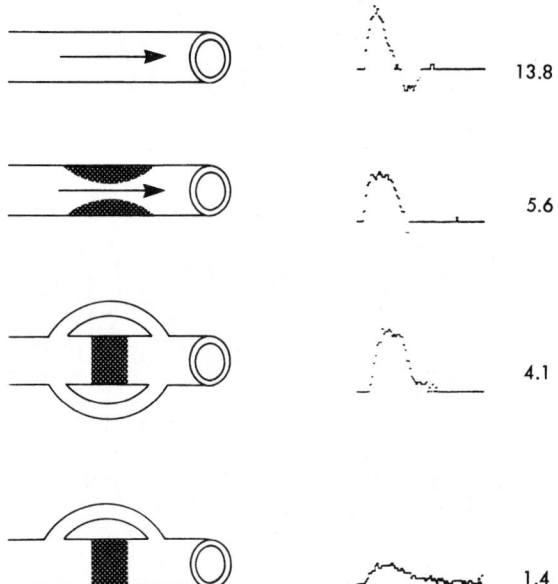

Figure 50–84. Progressive dampening of Doppler velocity waveform by proximal arterial stenosis. (From Johnson, K. W.: Doppler signal processing waveform analysis: Problems and solutions. *In* Bernstein, E. H. F. [Ed.]: Noninvasive Diagnostic Techniques in Vascular Disease. St. Louis, C. V. Mosby, 1982.)

parameters to exercise yields an evaluation of the functional significance of a stenosis. Exercise produces vasodilatation in the distal vascular bed. If inflow is restricted by a proximal stenosis, the pressure in the distal bed falls. Practically, the degree and duration of the fall in ankle-brachial pressure index following a standardized (10% grade, 2 miles per hour, 5 minutes) walking exercise are recorded. An added benefit of this test is a comparison of the exercise limitations imposed by lower limb vascular insufficiency with those of concomitant pulmonary, orthopedic, or cardiac disease. An example of a complete noninvasive laboratory examination report is shown in Figure 50–85.

A number of other techniques have been used for noninvasive evaluation of patients with peripheral vascular disease. Among these is the use of an oxygen electrode coupled directly to the skin to measure transcutaneous oxygen tension (TC_PO_2). However, oxygen tension in the skin does not decrease until ischemia is far advanced, so this examination has limited usefulness in a patient with claudication. The most promising new development in noninvasive vascular diagnosis is the continuing technical improvements in duplex ultrasound scanning. Modern duplex instruments are able to simultaneously display a real-time ultrasound image of the vessel structure and an analysis of the directionally segregated Doppler-detected flow within vascular channels. This permits visualization of areas of stenosis, identification of areas of turbulence due to vessel wall irregularity, and visualization of flow disturbances such as jet flow at sites of hemodynamically significant stenosis. As technology evolves and computer integration of the available images and data increases, advances and improvements are certain to continue.

The noninvasive vascular laboratory examination should not be used alone. Rather, it is used to complement the information obtained from the history and physical examination and helps establish a baseline for future comparison. This evaluation is useful whether the patient is treated medically or has an operation. These tests form an objective and semiquantitative method for following the success of revascularization and may also be helpful in detecting problems early in the postoperative period, when they may still be remediable (Fig. 50–86).[17]

Peripheral Arterial Exam

Resting Segmental Blood Pressures:

	RIGHT		LEFT	
	Pressure	Leg/Arm Ratio	Pressure	Leg/Arm Ratio
Arm	168		168	
Upper thigh	124	.74	127	.76
Above knee	99	.59	115	.68
Below knee	88	.52	100	.59
Ankle D.P.	82	.48	80	.48
P.T.	82	.48	74	.44
Toe .	60	.36	66	.39

Treadmill: 1.5 mph at 0% grade.

Stopped arbitrarily; no discomfort at 5:00 (202 meters)

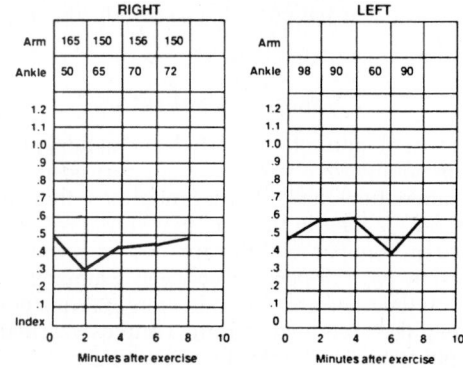

	RIGHT					LEFT			
Arm	165	150	156	150	Arm				
Ankle	50	65	70	72	Ankle	98	90	60	90

Figure 50–85. Information obtained from standard noninvasive peripheral arterial examination provides complete assessment of lower extremity circulation. (From Taylor, L. M., Jr., and Porter, J. M.: Natural history and nonoperative treatment of chronic lower extremity ischemia. *In* Rutherford, R. B. (Ed.): Vascular Surgery, 3rd ed. Philadelphia, W. B. Saunders, 1989.)

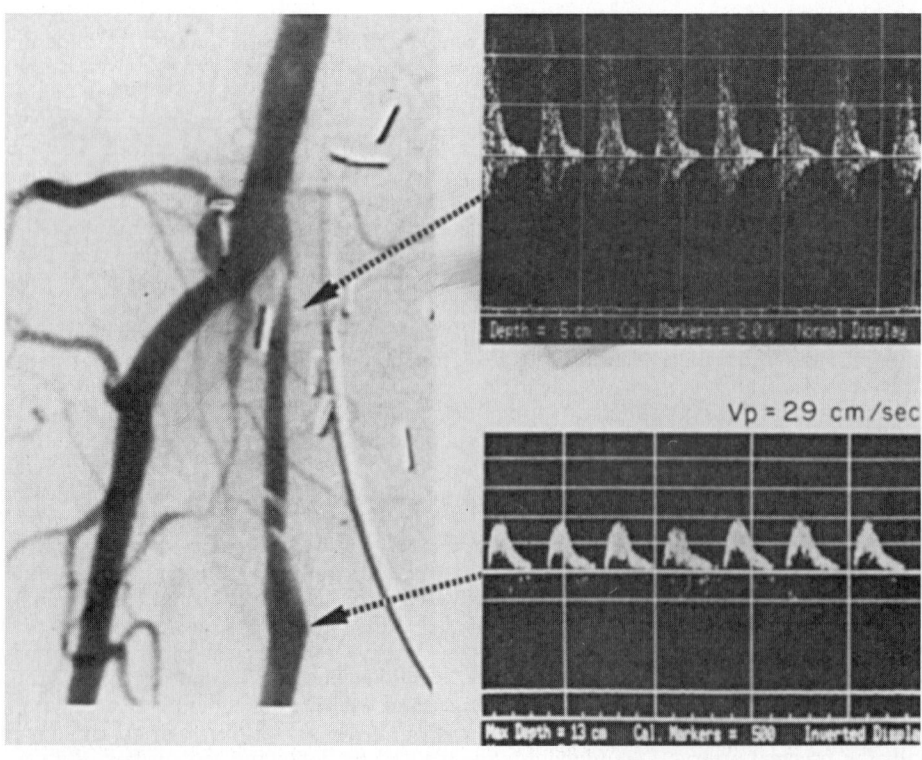

Figure 50–86. Use of duplex scan in postoperative surveillance detects graft stenosis before it progresses to graft thrombosis and while revision and graft salvage are possible. (From Bandyk, D. F.: Perioperative use of duplex scan. *In* Bergan, J. S., and Yao, J. S. T. [Eds.]: Arterial Surgery: New Diagnostic and Operative Techniques. Orlando, Grune & Stratton, 1988.)

Indications for Surgical Intervention

Treatment decisions in patients with vascular insufficiency of the lower extremity are based on an analysis of the potential risks and benefits. The goals of therapy are prevention of limb loss, relief of pain, maintenance of bipedal gait, and avoidance of disability. Studies of the natural history of intermittent claudication have shown that patients with this as the sole manifestation of lower limb ischemia have a low risk of limb loss. In fact, over 75% of these patients remain stable or even improve with conservative management alone. The amputation rate is less than 7% in patients treated medically and followed up to 8 years.[18, 19] Nonsurgical management consists of cessation of smoking, control of weight, and a graduated exercise program. The importance of total abstinence from tobacco cannot be overemphasized.[18] Men who smoke are nine times more likely to develop intermittent claudication than are nonsmokers. Importantly, patients who stop smoking have a much lower incidence of progression of disease from claudication to rest pain, require fewer bypass operations, and experience a significantly reduced risk of amputation and mortality. Although tobacco smoke produces demonstrable changes in vascular endothelial cell function and metabolism, and alteration of blood viscosity, platelet function, and the coagulation mechanism, the exact process by which it exerts its deleterious effect on the development of atherosclerosis remains undetermined.[19] It is important to note that the risk of limb loss in patients with chronic lower extremity ischemia who cease smoking has been found to be reduced in many studies. Also, it has been conclusively demonstrated that continued smoking following surgical lower extremity revascularization results in a dramatically lower success rate.[16]

A number of longitudinal studies have demonstrated that a program of regular walking exercise leads to a measurable improvement in walking distance in patients with intermittent claudication. The mechanism responsible for this improvement is not fully understood. The assumption that exercise leads to stimulation of the development of natural collaterals has not been supported by objective data examining exercise-induced changes in blood flow. Rather, it is now thought that improved performance following exercise is due to adaptive change in the muscle enzyme systems, leading to more efficient oxygen extraction and utilization.

Many agents have been prescribed for intermittent claudication, including platelet inhibitors, vasodilating agents, and hemorrheologic agents. There is some evidence that aspirin and other platelet-inhibiting drugs may slow the progression of lower extremity obstructive disease.[20, 21] In contrast, there is no objective evidence that any of the vasodilators, such as tolazoline, nicotinyl, or cyclandelate, improve blood flow or symptoms in an ischemic extremity.[22] The only class of drugs with objective evidence of improvement in walking distance is the hemorrheologic agents, such as pentoxifylline. Most objective studies of this agent show only a modest benefit in walking distance. Porter and colleagues' study of 82 patients showed only a 19% increase in walking distance, a clinically insignificant amount.[23] Furthermore, there is no evidence that any of these agents is of benefit in cases of severe ischemia with threatened or actual tissue loss.

For a patient presenting with intermittent claudication, initial recommendations include the complete discontinuation of tobacco use; participation in a regular exercise program of at least 1 hour's duration daily; walking to the point of claudication, resting, and then continuing again for another cycle; and weight control to minimize the amount of work required in ambulation. Adherence to this advice often leads to a doubling or greater of claudication distance and may be the only treatment required.

When nonsurgical treatment fails to alleviate the disability imposed by intermittent claudication, and when symptoms interfere with making a living or impose an intolerable limitation on lifestyle, surgical treatment can be offered, with the understanding that the goal is improvement in exercise capacity rather than salvage of the limb. In contrast, patients with rest pain, ischemic ulcerations, or limited gangrene are generally candidates for vascular reconstruction, because the threat of limb loss is much greater. In patients who present with gangrene, the necrotic tissue must be limited to the toes or distal metatarsal level. If the residual foot following débridement of the necrotic tissue is insufficient to function as a weight-bearing surface, the patient is more likely to maintain independent mobility and bipedal gait with amputation and a leg prosthesis.

Arteriography

Arteriography is necessary only if it has been decided that revascularization is indicated. It is used to determine whether balloon dilatation or other percutaneous catheter-based treatment is feasible and, in surgical patients, to confirm the adequacy of inflow at the femoral level and to select the sites for the proximal and distal anastomoses. The entire vascular tree from the distal aorta to the foot should be visualized. Biplane or oblique views are occasionally helpful and may reveal lesions not seen with a single projection. Inadequate visualization of the distal vascular bed may be due to the small amount of contrast material reaching the leg if the ischemic process is severe. Reactive hyperemia induced by inflation of blood pressure cuffs placed around the thighs and inflated for several minutes before injection may be helpful. It has been suggested that the new imaging modality of magnetic resonance angiography may be more sensitive than traditional contrast angiography in determining the status of the tibial vessels in cases of severe ischemia.[24, 25] If doubt remains concerning optimal placement of the distal anastomosis, prebypass intraoperative arteriography with direct injection into a patent runoff vessel may be of benefit in selected cases (Fig. 50–87). Adequate visualization of the entire arterial system of the lower extremity ensures that a bypass graft will not be placed proximal to a tandem stenosis, which might jeopardize long-term function of the graft.

PERCUTANEOUS METHODS OF TREATMENT

A number of catheter-based percutaneous treatment options are now available for patients with peripheral vascular obstructive disease in the lower extremities. These are largely based on the use of the dual-lumen catheter technique introduced by Grüntzig in 1974.[2] Balloon dilatation achieves an enlarged lumen by the mechanism of intimal fracture and stretching of the remaining vessel wall. This is a traumatic procedure and, as might be expected, causes a high rate of thrombosis if attempted over long vessel segments. It succeeds quite well for stenoses and even occlusions that are less than 10 cm. in length and that cause claudication, but the results with more severe disease that threatens limb viability have not been as favorable (Fig. 50–88). Metallic stents have recently been introduced in an attempt to reduce the considerable rate of restenosis. The role of these devices has not been firmly established. Techniques that have attempted to remove plaque by laser energy vaporization or by mechanical emulsification or shaving with miniature cutters based on catheter tips have not proved to be better than simple balloon dilatation and have been virtually abandoned.[26, 27] Of importance is the observation that no catheter-based system has been shown to be effective in treating the long and

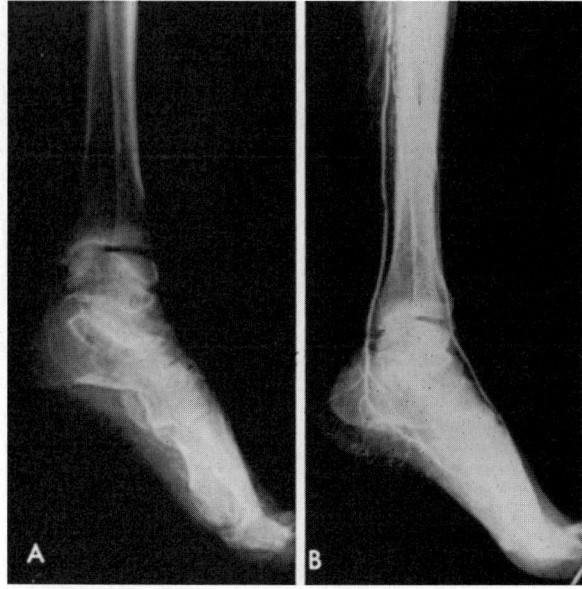

Figure 50–87. *A*, Preoperative arteriogram shows only faint visualization of the distal leg and foot vessels. *B*, Improved visualization of the distal vessels of the same patient by direct injection at operation. This visualization allowed subsequent femoral to posterior tibial bypass. (From Flanigan, D. F., Williams, L. R., Keith, J., Schuler, J. J., and Behrend, J. A.: Prebypass operative arteriography. Surgery, *92*:627, 1982.)

severe obstructive lesions that threaten limb viability and that remain best treated by surgical bypass.

SURGICAL LOWER EXTREMITY REVASCULARIZATION

Severe ischemia of the lower extremity due to femoral, popliteal, and tibial atherosclerosis is most frequently treated surgically by bypass grafting. Other options may be appropriate in highly selected cases. Endarterectomy may be used for localized disease in the superficial femoral artery, but it is unusual for the disease to be confined to a short segment of the vessel.[28, 29] When the origin of the major collateral vessel in the thigh, the profunda femoris, is stenotic, flow through this system may be improved by patch profundaplasty. Profundaplasty has been shown to be effective in treating claudication but is much less successful in treating limb-threatening ischemia in which improved blood flow to the foot must be achieved.[30]

Bypass procedures are usually performed under general or regional anesthesia. Continuous epidural blockade is favored by many surgeons and anesthesiologists because distal procedures may require considerable time; this method of anesthesia minimizes time limitations while providing effective analgesia with minimal cardiovascular stress. These catheters can be left in place for several days, providing both distal vasodilatation and effective analgesia. Some believe that early thrombosis rates of lower extremity bypass grafts are lower in procedures performed using this technique.[31, 32] It is also important to bear in mind that atherosclerosis is a systemic disorder, and nearly all these patients have some degree of associated coronary or cerebrovascular disease. When it is vigorously sought, as many as 40% of patients undergoing lower extremity revascularization are found to have episodes of myocardial ischemia in the perioperative period.[34] As many as 5% may experience myocardial infarction, and half of these may be fatal.[35]

Technique for Bypass Procedures

Successful bypasses for limb ischemia require mature surgical judgment and meticulous attention to technical details. Surgical candidates are selected on the basis of clinical presentation and undergo arteriography to determine the optimal site for placement of the proximal and distal anastomoses. These sites are selected to allow unobstructed flow distally to the foot if possible. If an adequate distal vessel is not visualized and the need for revascularization is clear, exploration and direct operative arteriography may reveal a patent distal vessel suitable for anastomosis. The common femoral artery has been considered the optimal site for the proximal anastomosis; however, more recently, more distal sites of origin in the superficial femoral and the profunda femoris have become acceptable if they provide unobstructed inflow and available graft length is limited.[36–38]

Choice of Graft Material

It has clearly been shown in several well-controlled, randomized trials that the autogenous saphenous vein provides the best long-term graft patency and limb salvage rates for patients with lower extremity vascular obstruction.[39–41] Although some authorities continue to argue that a first bypass in the thigh should be done with a prosthetic graft so that the saphenous vein can be preserved in the event that a secondary procedure becomes necessary,[42] most vascular surgeons believe that the greater saphenous vein, when present, should be used for infrainguinal reconstructions. In up to 30% of patients, the saphenous vein may have been used for previous bypass in the same leg or elsewhere in the body and may not be available. Alternative graft choices are the lesser saphenous vein from the posterior aspect of the leg, veins harvested from the arm, or synthetic grafts. Most authorities continue to believe that an autogenous venous graft, even if several segments must be spliced together to achieve adequate length, is the preferred graft and provides the best long-term patency rates.[41, 43, 44] Other graft materials have been tried, including Dacron, polytetrafluoroethylene (PTFE), and various biologic grafts, such as tanned, reinforced, human umbilical vein and even cryopreserved saphenous vein allografts harvested from cadavers. In a large, multicenter randomized trial, it was found that autogenous saphenous

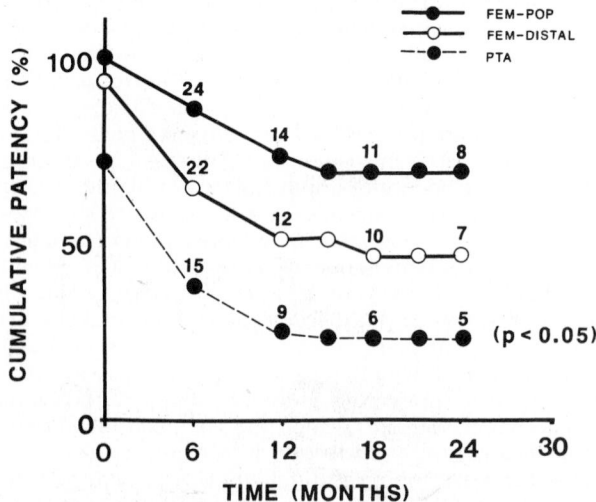

Figure 50–88. Cumulative patency by bypasses and percutaneous transluminal angioplasty by life-table method. Limbs at risk noted at each interval. (From Blair, J. M., Gewertz, B. L., Moosa, H., Lu, C. T., and Zarins, C. K.: Percutaneous transluminal angioplasty versus surgery for limb-threatening ischemia. J. Vasc. Surg., *9*:698, 1988.)

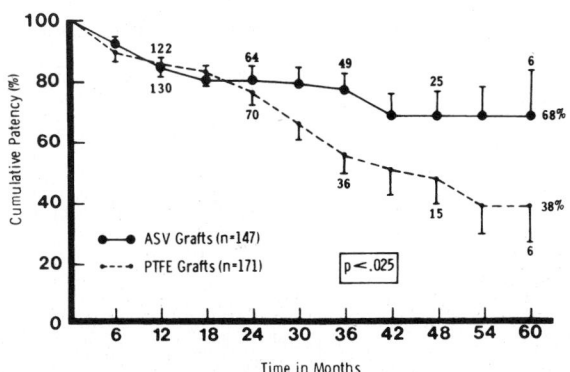

Figure 50–89. Cumulative life-table primary patency rates for all randomized bypasses performed to popliteal artery with autologous saphenous vein (ASV) and polytetrafluoroethylene (PTFE) grafts. Number with each point indicates number of patient grafts observed for that length of time. Standard error of each point is shown. (From Veith, F. J., Gupta, S. K., Ascer, E., et al.: Six-year prospective multicenter randomized comparison of autologous saphenous vein and expanded polytetrafluoroethylene grafts in infrainguinal arterial reconstructions. J. Vasc. Surg., 3:104, 1986.)

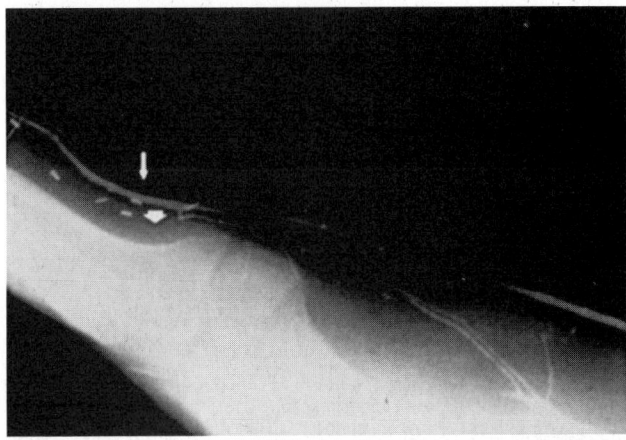

Figure 50–91. Operative arteriogram of *in situ* femoropopliteal saphenous vein graft (small arrow); large arrow points to residual arteriovenous fistula from a vein branch that requires ligation before wound closure.

vein and PTFE grafts to the popliteal artery yielded similar patency rates for the first 24 months postoperatively but diverged significantly thereafter (Fig. 50–89).[39] At 5 years, the patency rate for autogenous veins was 68%, compared with 38% for the synthetic grafts. Similar results have been found with human umbilical vein.[45] Other grafts appear to be inferior. Allograft veins have very poor long-term patency rates and are prohibitively expensive.[46, 47]

It therefore seems reasonable to recommend that prosthetic material be reserved for proximal lower extremity reconstruction, and only in those cases in which autogenous vein is not available or in which survival beyond 2 years is not expected. With respect to autogenous venous grafts, two alternative techniques have been established. Leather introduced the *in situ* saphenous vein graft in the late 1970s.[48] In this technique, only the proximal and distal saphenous vein segments are mobilized for the proximal and distal anastomoses. The intervening graft may or may not be exposed, but in either case, the vein is not dissected free from its bed. Valves may be rendered incompetent by a variety of valvulotomes introduced through the open end of the graft or through side branches (Fig. 50–90). The side branches of the saphenous vein must be ligated to prevent the occurrence of arteriovenous fistula postoperatively (Fig. 50–91). More accurate valve

cutting may be obtained under direct vision using an angioscope and modern video equipment.[49] The advantages of this technique are that it allows the use of smaller veins and allows anastomosis of the largest end of the vein graft to the largest artery and the smallest end of the vein graft to the smaller distal vessel. Excellent patency and limb salvage rates have been achieved with this technique (Fig. 50–92). However, comparable concurrent series using the more traditional reverse saphenous vein graft have also shown dramatic improvements in patency and limb salvage (Fig. 50–93).[50] Randomized studies have been unable to demonstrate a clear superiority of one technique over the other. Excellent results can be achieved using either technique as long as one adheres to the principles of graft spatulation, gentle vein handling, and avoidance of overdistention and prolonged storage in unphysiologic solutions. Moreover, the vein utilization is comparable or even higher using the reverse technique, because an inadequate length of vein can be augmented by splicing additional segments harvested from the opposite leg or from the arm or by using segments of lesser saphenous vein or major tributaries from the greater saphenous vein.

POSTOPERATIVE CARE

The elderly patient population and the systemic nature of the atherosclerotic process dictate careful intraoperative and

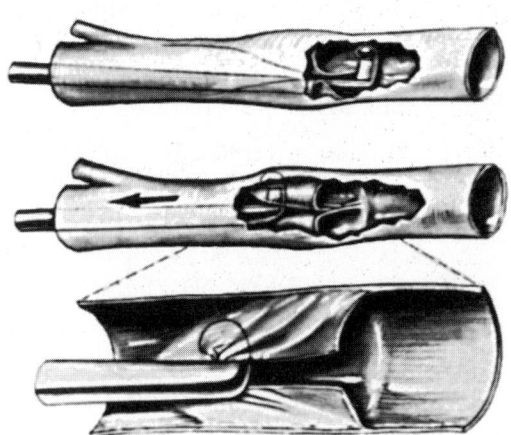

Figure 50–90. Valvulotome inserted through a side branch to cut the venous valve for an *in situ* vein graft. (From Leather, R. P., and Shah, D. M.: *In situ* saphenous vein arterial bypass. *In* Rutherford, R. B. [Ed.]: Vascular Surgery, 3rd ed. Philadelphia, W. B. Saunders, 1989.)

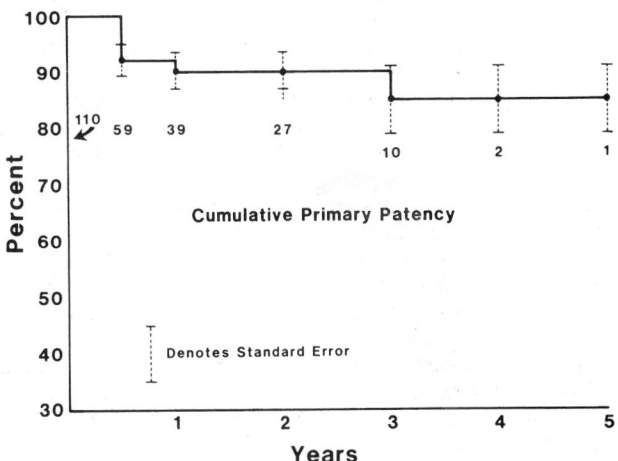

Figure 50–92. Primary and secondary patency rate for a large series of *in situ* grafts. (From Leather, R. P., Shah, D. M., Change, B. B., and Kaufman, J. L.: Resurrection of the *in situ* vein bypass: 1,000 cases later. Ann. Surg., 208:434, 1988.)

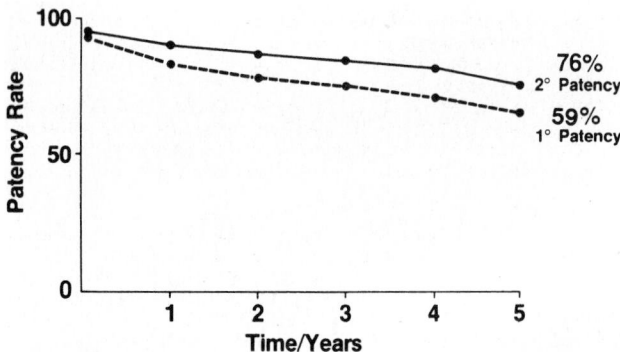

Figure 50–93. Life-table primary and secondary patency for a large series of reversed saphenous bypass grafts. Long-term results in this modern series are comparable to those achieved with the *in situ* technique. (From Taylor, L. M., Jr., Edwards, J. M., Phinney, E. S., and Porter, J. M.: Reversed vein bypass to infra-popliteal arteries: Modern results are superior to or equivalent to *in situ* bypass for patency and vein utilization. Ann. Surg., *205*:90, 1987.)

postoperative monitoring. This frequently includes an arterial pressure line and a urethral catheter. Heparin is not usually reversed and may be continued postoperatively, particularly if there is severe disease in the outflow tract. Intraoperative assessment of graft function is important and may include measurement of graft flow in the basal and papaverine vasodilated state, measurement of vascular input impedance, and visualization of the distal anastomosis and outflow tract by operative angiography or duplex ultrasound scanning.[41, 51]

Constant surveillance is maintained through periodic follow-up of all patients with lower extremity bypasses. This includes periodic noninvasive examinations and serial determinations of extremity blood pressure to detect any threat to the continued patency of the graft. Duplex scanning has been used in postoperative graft surveillance, with demonstrable improvement in secondary patency rate.[52] It has been conclusively demonstrated that repair of defects in vein bypass grafts before the onset of graft thrombosis has a much greater chance of graft salvage than interventions that occur following graft thrombosis.[53, 54]

RESULTS

Improvement in patency rates and limb salvage in patients treated for lower extremity peripheral vascular obstructive

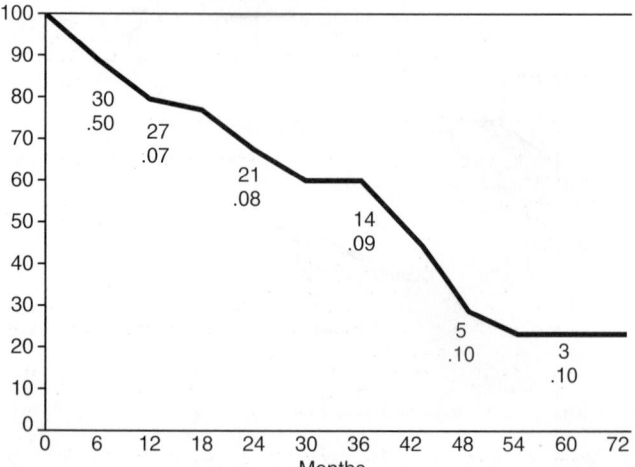

Figure 50–94. Life-table curve of survival for patients who required lower extremity bypass for limb salvage. Long-term survival in these patients is seriously compromised. (From Rosenbloom, M. S., Walsh, J. J., Schuler, J. J., et al.: Long-term results of infragenicular bypasses with autogenous vein originating from the distal superficial femoral and popliteal arteries. J. Vasc. Surg., *7*:691, 1988.)

disease has been dramatic in recent years. Contemporary series of saphenous vein grafts now report 90% 1-year and 70% multiyear patency rates, with 5% to 10% higher limb salvage rates.[41] Five-year primary patency rates for femoropopliteal bypass grafting using PTFE grafts now range from 25% to 55%, with even higher rates in patients operated on for claudication. These improvements have been achieved by an increased appreciation of the fragility of the saphenous vein, the importance of gentle technique in its preparation for use by either the *in situ* or the reverse technique, and the clear superiority of autogenous venous grafting over synthetic or modified biologic grafts. Technical advances, including improved coaxial fiberoptic lighting and optical magnification, have also had a role in this improvement. Furthermore, the increased appreciation for the importance of long-term graft surveillance and repair of graft defects prior to the occurrence of graft thrombosis has also contributed to the long-term graft success rate. Because of these improved results, it is more reasonable to offer treatment to patients with lifestyle-limiting claudication who were previously untreated. These patients can now be offered a reasonable likelihood of improved lifestyle with only minimal risk.

COMPLICATIONS FOLLOWING INFRAINGUINAL BYPASS

Because of the high incidence of concurrent coronary and cerebrovascular disease in patients with lower extremity ischemia, the postoperative mortality is 2% to 3%, with the majority of deaths caused by acute myocardial infarction. Frequent electrocardiographic monitoring and the liberal use of antianginal agents should be considered. Furthermore, the longevity of patients who require lower extremity bypass for limb salvage is seriously compromised. Fewer than 50% of these patients survive 5 or more years (Fig. 50–94).

One per cent to 2% of patients undergoing lower extremity bypass operation develop wound infection. When the vein graft itself becomes infected, it is subject to disruption and hemorrhage, and under these circumstances, the graft must be removed. The treatment for prosthetic graft infection includes graft removal and replacement, routing the new graft through uninfected planes. In the past, there was some consideration that a failed attempt at bypass would not only precipitate amputation but also jeopardize the length of the residual limb. There is, however, little objective evidence that an attempt at bypass jeopardizes the knee joint, and only patients who are obviously nonambulatory should be denied an attempt at limb salvage in lieu of primary amputation if suitable anatomy is present.

SELECTED REFERENCES

Ameli, F. M., Stein, M., Prosser, R. J., Provan, J. L., and Aro, L.: Effects of cigarette smoking on outcome of femoral popliteal bypass for limb salvage. J. Cardiovasc. Surg., *30*:591, 1989.
The importance of cigarette smoking cannot be overemphasized in discussing both the development of peripheral vascular disease and the success of its surgical treatment. This excellent study evaluated the long-term effects of smoking on cumulative patency rates and limb salvage rates and found that a measurable adverse effect is apparent with smoking as few as five cigarettes daily. Studies such as this re-emphasize the importance of convincing patients with peripheral vascular disease to completely discontinue the use of tobacco.

Christopherson, R., Beattie, C., Frank, S. M., Norris, E. J., Meinert, C. L., Gottlieb, S. O., Yates, H., Rock, P., Parker, S. D., Perler, B. A., Williams, G. M., and Perioperative Ischemia Randomized Anesthesia Trial Study Group: Perioperative morbidity in patients randomized to epidural or general anesthesia for lower extremity vascular surgery. Anesthesiology, *79*:422, 1993.
This study suggests that the immediate perioperative thrombosis rate may be lower in patients undergoing surgery using epidural anesthesia rather than general anesthesia. The rates of cardiac morbidity were similar between patients undergoing

general and epidural anesthesia, but there was a significant decrease in the rate of early graft failure in patients in whom epidural anesthesia was used.

Duggan, M. M., Woodson, J., Scott, T. E., Ortega, A. N., and Menzoian, J. O.: Functional outcomes in limb salvage vascular surgery. Am. J. Surg., *168*:188, 1994.
This interesting study describes a new method of evaluating the results of vascular bypass surgery. It describes the outcome of vascular surgery in terms of how patients are fundamentally benefited rather than in the more traditional terms of graft patency or limb retention. This type of analysis is particularly cogent and will become more frequent because of the evolving changes in the organization of medical care and the increasing importance of economic issues in medicine.

Friedman, S. G.: A History of Vascular Surgery. Mt. Kisco, N.Y., Futura, 1989.
This is a succinct monograph devoted entirely to the history of vascular surgery. It is particularly useful for review of the contributions made during the seventeenth and eighteenth centuries. It reproduces many classic illustrations as well as portraits of the pioneers in vascular surgery.

Veith, F. J., Gupta, S. K., Ascer, E., White-Flores, S., Samson, R. H., Scher, L. A., Towne, J. B., Bernhard, V. M., Bonier, P., Flinn, W. R., et al.: Six-year prospective multicenter randomized comparison of autologous saphenous vein and expanded polytetrafluoroethylene grafts in infrainguinal arterial reconstructions. J. Vasc. Surg., *3*:104, 1986.
This is the largest randomized trial comparing autologous saphenous vein with synthetic polytetrafluoroethylene (PTFE) grafts for infrainguinal arterial reconstruction. It is a well-controlled study of a difficult topic and conclusively demonstrates the superiority of the autologous saphenous vein graft for lower extremity reconstructions by careful analysis of patency rates over time.

REFERENCES

1. Dotter, C. T., and Judkins, M. P.: Transluminal treatment of arteriosclerotic obstruction. Circulation, *30*:654, 1964.
2. Grüntzig, A., and Kumpe, D. A.: Technique of percutaneous transluminal angioplasty with the Grüntzig balloon catheter. A. J. R. Am. J. Roentgenol., *132*:547, 1979.
3. Warren, W. D.: Presidential address: Reflections on the early development of portacaval shunts. Ann. Surg., *191*:519, 1980.
4. Callow, A. D.: Historical development of vascular grafts. *In* Sawyer, P. N., and Kaplitt, M. J. (Eds.): Vascular Grafts. New York, Appleton-Century-Crofts, 1978.
5. Carrel, A.: The surgery of blood vessels, etc. Johns Hopkins Hosp. Bull., *18*:18, 1907.
6. Harrison, L. H., Jr.: Historical aspects in the development of venous autografts. Ann. Surg., *183*:101, 1976.
7. Baird, R. J.: Presidential address: "Give us the tools . . ." The story of heparin—as told by sketches from the lives of William Howell, Jay McLean, Charles Best, and Gordon Murray. J. Vasc. Surg., *11*:4, 1990.
8. Friedman, S. G.: A History of Vascular Surgery. Mt. Kisco, N.Y., Futura, 1989.
9. Kunlin, J.: La traitement de l'artérite obliterance par la greffe veineuse. Arch. Mal. Coeur, *42*:317, 1949.
10. Martin, R. S., 3rd., Edwards, W. H., Mulherin, J. L., Jr., Edwards, W. H., Jr., Jenkins, J. M., and Hoff, S. J.: Cryopreserved saphenous vein allografts for below-knee lower extremity revascularization. Ann. Surg., *219*:664, 1994.
11. Blakemore, M. D., and Voorhees, A. B., Jr.: The use of tubes constructed from vinyon "N" cloth in bridging arterial defects—experimental and clinical. Ann. Surg., *140*:324, 1954.
12. Campbell, C. D., Brooks, D. H., Webster, M. W., and Bahnson, H. T.: The use of expanded microporous polytetrafluoroethylene for limb salvage: A primary report. Surgery, *79*:485, 1976.
13. Duggan, M. M., Woodson, J., Scott, T. E., Ortega, A. N., and Menzoian, J. O.: Functional outcomes in limb salvage vascular surgery. Am. J. Surg., *168*:188, 1994.
14. Cole, C. W., Hill, G. B., Farzad, E., Bouchard, A., Moher, D., Rody, K., and Shea, B.: Cigarette smoking and peripheral arterial occlusive disease. Surgery, *114*:753, 1993.
15. Krupski, W. C.: The peripheral vascular consequences of smoking. Ann. Vasc. Surg., *5*:291, 1991.
16. Ameli, F. M., Stein, M., Prosser, R. J., Provan, J. L., and Aro, L.: Effects of cigarette smoking on outcome of femoral popliteal bypass for limb salvage. J. Cardiovasc. Surg., *30*:591, 1989.
17. Dalsing, M. C., Cikrit, D. F., Lalka, S. G., Sawchuk, A. P., and Schulz, C.: Femorodistal vein grafts: The utility of graft surveillance criteria. J. Vasc. Surg., *21*:127, 1995.
18. Walsh, D. B., Gilbertson, J. J., Zwolak, R. M., Besso, S., Edelman, G. C., Schneider, J. R., and Cronenwett, J. L.: The natural history of superficial femoral artery stenoses. J. Vasc. Surg., *14*:299, 1991.
19. Imparato, A. M., Kim, G. E., Davidson, T., and Crowely, J. G.: Intermittent claudication: Its natural course. Surgery, *78*:795, 1975.
20. Hess, H., Mietaschk, A., and Deichsel, G.: Drug-induced inhibition of platelet function delays progression of peripheral occlusive arterial disease: A prospective double-blind arteriographically controlled trial. Lancet, *1*:415, 1985.
21. Anonymous: Collaborative overview of randomised trials of antiplatelet therapy. II: Maintenance of vascular graft or arterial patency by antiplatelet therapy. Anticiplatelet trialists' collaboration (Review). BMJ, *308*:159, 1994.
22. Duprez, D., and Clement, D. L.: Medical treatment of peripheral vascular disease: Good or bad? Eur. Heart J., *13*:149, 1992.
23. Porter, J. M., Cutler, B. S., Lee, B. Y., Reich, T., Reichle, F. A., Scogin, J. T., and Strandness, D. E.: Pentoxifylline efficacy in the treatment of intermittent claudication: Multicenter controlled double-blind trial with objective assessment of chronic occlusive arterial disease patients. Am. Heart J., *104*:66, 1982.
24. Owen, R. S., Carpenter, J. P., Baum, R. A., Perloff, L. J., and Cope, C.: Magnetic resonance imaging of angiographically occult runoff vessels in peripheral arterial occlusive disease. N. Engl. J. Med., *326*:1577, 1992.
25. Carpenter, J. P., Owen, R. S., Baum, R. A., Cope, C., Barker, C. F., Berkowitz, H. D., Golden, M. A., and Perloff, L. J.: Magnetic resonance angiography of peripheral runoff vessels. J. Vasc. Surg., *16*:807, 1992.
26. Cull, D. L., Feinberg, R. L., Wheeler, J. R., Snyder, S. O., Jr., Gregory, R. T., Gayle, R. G., and Parent, F. N., 3rd: Experience with laser-assisted balloon angioplasty and a rotary angioplasty instrument: Lessons learned. J. Vasc. Surg., *14*:332, 1991.
27. Vroegindeweij, D., Kemper, F. J., Tielbeek, A. V., Buth, J., and Landman, G.: Recurrence of stenoses following balloon angioplasty and Simpson atherectomy of the femoropopliteal segment: A randomised comparative 1-year follow-up study using colour flow duplex. Eur. J. Vasc. Surg., *6*:164, 1992.
28. van der Heijden, F. H., Eikelboom, B. C., van Reedt Dortland, R. W., van der Graaf, Y., Steijling, J. J., Legemate, D. A., and van Vroonhoven, T. J.: Endarterectomy of the superficial femoral artery: A procedure worth reconsidering. Eur. J. Vasc. Surg., *6*:651, 1992.
29. van der Heijden, F. H., Eikelboom, B. C., van Reedt Dortland, R. W., van der Graaf, Y., Steijling, J. J., Legemate, D. A., Theodorides, T., and van Vroonhoven, T. J.: Long-term results of semiclosed endarterectomy of the superficial femoral artery and the outcome of failed reconstructions. J. Vasc. Surg., *18*:271, 1993.
30. van der Plas, J. P., van Dijk, J., Tordoir, J. H., Jacobs, M. J., and Kitslaar, P. J.: Isolated profundaplasty in critical limb ischaemia—still of any use? Eur. J. Vasc. Surg., *7*:54, 1993.
31. Rosenfeld, B. A., Beattie, C., Christopherson, R., Norris, E. J., Frank, S. M., Breslow, M. J., Rock, P., Parker, S. D., Gottlieb, S. O., Perler, B. A., et al.: The effects of different anesthetic regimens on fibrinolysis and the development of postoperative arterial thrombosis: Perioperative ischemia randomized anesthesia trial study group. Anesthesiology, *79*:435, 1993.
32. Tuman, K. J., McCarthy, R. J., March, R. J., DeLaria, G. A., Patel, R. V., and Ivankovich, A. D.: Effects of epidural anesthesia and analgesia on coagulation and outcome after major vascular surgery. Anesth. Analg., *73*:696, 1991.
33. Christopherson, R., Beattie, C., Frank, S. M., Norris, E. J., Meinert, C. L., Gottlieb, S. O., Yates, H., Rock, P., Parker, S. D., Perler, B. A., Williams, G. M., and Perioperative Ischemia Randomized Anesthesia Trial Study Group: Perioperative morbidity in patients randomized to epidural or general anesthesia for lower extremity vascular surgery. Anesthesiology, *79*:422, 1993.
34. McCann, R. L., and Clements, F. M.: Silent myocardial ischemia in patients undergoing peripheral vascular surgery: Incidence and association with perioperative cardiac morbidity and mortality. J. Vasc. Surg., *9*:583, 1989.
35. Krupski, W. C., Layug, E. L., Reilly, L. M., Rapp, J. H., and Mangano, D. T.: Comparison of cardiac morbidity rates between aortic and infrainguinal operations: Two-year follow-up. Study of perioperative ischemia reset group. J. Vasc. Surg., *18*:609, 1993.
36. Mills, J. L., Taylor, S. M., and Fujitani, R. M.: The role of the deep femoral artery as an inflow site for infrainguinal revascularization. J. Vasc. Surg., *18*:416, 1993.
37. Brown, P. S., Jr., McCarthy, W. J., Yao, J. S. T., and Pearce, W. H.: The popliteal artery as inflow for distal bypass grafting. Arch. Surg., *129*:556, 1994.
38. Lyon, R. T., Veith, F. J., Marsan, B. U., Wengerter, K. R., Panetta, T. F., Marin, M. L., Goldsmith, J., Rivers, S. P., and Suggs, W.: Eleven-year experience with tibiotibial bypass: An unusual but effective solution to distal tibial artery occlusive disease and limited autologous vein. J. Vasc. Surg., *20*:61, 1994.
39. Veith, F. J., Gupta, S. K., Ascer, E., White-Flores, S., Samson, R. H., Scher, L. A., Towne, J. B., Bernhard, V. M., Bonier, P., Flinn, W. R., et al.: Six-year prospective multicenter randomized comparison of autologous saphenous vein and expanded polytetrafluoroethylene grafts in infrainguinal arterial reconstruction. J. Vasc. Surg., *3*:104, 1986.
40. Anonymous: Comparative evaluation of prosthetic, reversed, and in situ vein bypass grafts in distal popliteal and tibial-peroneal revascularization: Veterans Administration cooperative study group 141. Arch. Surg., *123*:434, 1988.
41. Yeager, R. A., Taylor, L. M., and Porter, J. M.: The present status of infrainguinal arterial reconstructive surgery for chronic lower-extremity ischemia. Curr. Probl. Surg., *28*:125, 1991.
42. Moore, W. S., and Quinones-Baldrich, W. J.: An argument against all-autogenous tissue for vascular bypasses below the inguinal ligament. Adv. Surg., *24*:91, 1991.
43. Neale, M. L., Graham, J. C., Lane, R. J., Cheung, D. S., and Appleberg, M.: The influence of graft type on patency of infrainguinal arterial bypass grafts. J. Am. Coll. Surg., *178*:155, 1994.

44. Londrey, G. L., Bosher, L. P., Brown, P. W., Stoneburner, F. D., Jr., Pancoast, J. W., and Davis, R. K.: Infrainguinal reconstruction with arm vein, lesser saphenous vein, and remnants of greater saphenous vein: A report of 257 cases. J. Vasc. Surg., 20:451, 1994.

45. Dardik, H., Miller, N., Dardik, A., Ibrahim, I., Sussman, B., Berry, S. M., Wolodiger, F., Kahn, M., and Dardik, I.: A decade of experience with the glutaraldehyde-tanned human umbilical cord vein graft for revascularization of the lower limb. J. Vasc. Surg., 7:336, 1988.

46. Faggioli, G., and Ricotta, J. J.: Cryopreserved vein homografts for arterial reconstruction (Review). Eur. J. Vasc. Surg., 8:661, 1994.

47. Martin, R. S., 3rd, Edwards, W. H., Mulherin, J. L., Jr., Edwards, W. H., Jr., Jenkins, J. M., and Hoff, S. J.: Cryopreserved saphenous vein allografts for below-knee lower extremity revascularization. Ann. Surg., 219:664, 1994.

48. Leather, R. P.: In situ bypass: Technical considerations. Overview: History and evolution of techniques. Semin. Vasc. Surg., 6:151, 1993.

49. Rosenthal, D., Dickson, C., Rodriguez, F. J., Blackshear, W. M., Jr., Clark, M. D., Lamis, P. A., and Pallos, L. L.: Infrainguinal endovascular in situ saphenous vein bypass: Ongoing results. J. Vasc. Surg., 20:389, 1994.

50. Taylor, L. M., Jr., and Porter, J. M.: Clinical and anatomic considerations for surgery in femoropopliteal disease and the results of surgery. Circulation, 83(2 suppl.):I63–9, 1991.

51. Schwartz, L. B., Purut, C. M., O'Donohoe, M. K., Smith, P. K., Hagen, P. O., and McCann, R. L.: Quantitation of vascular outflow by measurement of impedance. J. Vasc. Surg., 14:353, 1991.

52. Dalsing, M. C., Cikrit, D. F., Lalka, S. G., Sawchuk, A. P., and Schulz, C.: Femorodistal vein grafts: The utility of graft surveillance criteria. J. Vasc. Surg., 21:127, 1995.

53. Nehler, M. R., Moneta, G. L., Yeager, R. A., Edwards, J. M., Taylor, L. M., Jr., and Porter, J. M.: Surgical treatment of threatened reversed infrainguinal vein grafts. J. Vasc. Surg., 20:558, 1994.

54. Lundell, A., Lindblad, B., Bergqvist, D., and Hansen, F.: Femoropopliteal-crural graft patency is improved by an intensive surveillance program: A prospective randomized study. J. Vasc. Surg., 21:26, 1995.

PERCUTANEOUS TRANSLUMINAL ANGIOPLASTY

Jose A. Perez, M.D.
Alyson J. Breisch, R.N., M.S.
R. Duane Davis, Jr., M.D.

Since the performance of the first successful percutaneous transluminal angioplasty (PTA) by Dotter and Judkins in 1964,[6] this technique has rapidly evolved into an established treatment for obstructive disorders of the arterial and venous circulation. As a nonsurgical approach to peripheral arterial revascularization, PTA has gained widespread acceptance over the past 2 decades, due primarily to the following factors:

1. Advances in arteriographic and noninvasive vascular imaging
2. Improvements in balloon catheter and guidewire technology
3. The durability of PTA for treating short segmental lesions
4. Introduction of vascular stents
5. Patient acceptance of the decreased hospital stay, fewer risks, and shorter recovery time
6. The efficacy of combined PTA and surgical procedures to treat multisegmental disease
7. The potential for a cost-effective alternative to surgery in this era of cost containment and health care reform

This enthusiasm is somewhat tempered, however, by uncertainties about the long-term durability of these procedures when compared with surgical bypass. In general, PTA confers a lower long-term patency, but its use is justified by its reduced cost, lower risk, and excellent immediate success rate. This chapter discusses the current state of PTA for the treatment of peripheral vascular disease, including the role of newer endovascular technologies such as atherectomy, laser, and stents.

PATHOPHYSIOLOGY

When a balloon catheter is positioned across a stenotic lesion, a controlled injury is produced in the distended vessel wall, allowing a persistent increase in the luminal area. The increased luminal area following dilation is associated with disruption of the intima near the edges of the plaque, separation of the edges of the plaque from the media, stretching of the media and adventitia, and often rupture of the media (Fig. 50–95). Separation of the intima from the media occurs at the internal elastic membrane. The plaque separation extends from the lateral aspects of the plaque circumferentially toward the thickest portion of the plaque. This plaque separation also extends axially along the plaque within the vessel (Fig. 50–96). Plaques rarely become completely detached from the media, remaining adherent near the thickest portion of the plaque, where shear and tangential stresses are the least. The plaques also remain attached to the media proximally and distally to the region of dilation. These attachments between the plaque and the media explain the low incidence of clinically significant distal embolization with PTA. With concentric plaques, the disruption occurs in the region of the thinnest portion of the plaque, where shear and tangential stresses are greatest (Fig. 50–97). In addition, following the separation of the plaque from the media, the luminal circumference becomes more dependent on the media and adventitia. The increase in effective radius corresponds to an increase in the tangential tension in the medial and adventitial layers, which tends to maintain vessel patency. The plaque itself does not appear to undergo compression, deformation, herniation into the media, or remodeling. The resulting separation of the relatively rigid, cohesive plaque from the underlying arterial wall frequently appears as dissection and local flaps on arteriography. Intimal remodeling, however, occurs rapidly as the channels following separation become shorter and the vessel lumen regains its smooth contour. Arteriograms obtained in the weeks following PTA fail to demonstrate the ragged appearance typical of the immediate post-PTA arteriogram.

In contrast to dilation of a stenotic atherosclerotic lesion, other mechanisms are often utilized in recanalization of arterial occlusions. In circumstances in which there is a recent occlusion with fresh thrombus, the guidewire or other cathe-

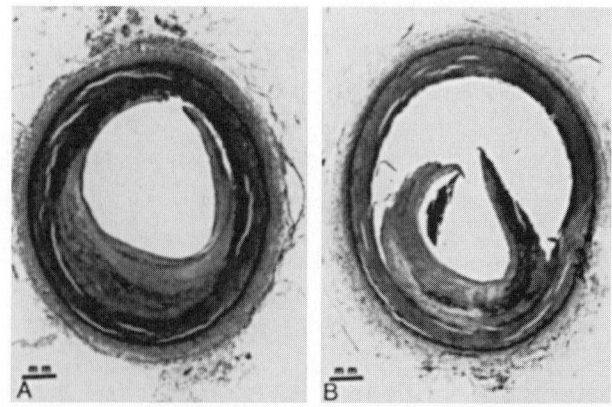

Figure 50–95. Histologic sections from adjacent vessel segments containing an obstructive atherosclerotic plaque. *A,* Nondilated segment. *B,* Dilated segment in which the plaque edges are separated from the media but the plaque is not disturbed. Although the lumen is increased in the dilated segment, lumen contour is distorted, assuming a mushroom-shaped contour. (From Lyon, R. T., Zarins, C. K., Lu, C. T., et al.: Vessel, plaque, and lumen morphology after transluminal balloon angioplasty. Arteriosclerosis, 7:306, 1987.)

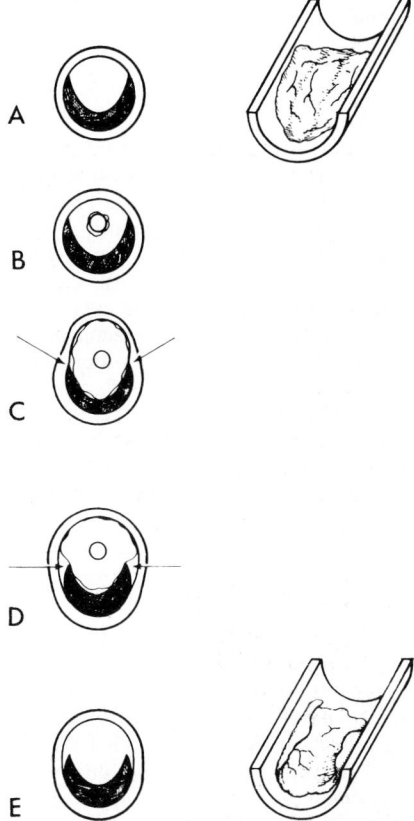

Figure 50–96. The physical mechanism of disruption that occurs during transluminal angioplasty. *A*, Cross-sectional view of an artery with an eccentric plaque. *B*, Deflated balloon catheter placed across the lesion. *C*, Partial inflation of the balloon causes deformation of the relatively normal artery wall, while the stiffer plaque retains its initial shape. Arrows point to the junction of the plaque and arterial wall and indicate regions where disruption starts. *D*, Full inflation of the balloon results in additional disruption of the plaque and artery. The tears have extended circumferentially along the plaque-artery border (arrows). *E*, Postdilation results show an enlarged lumen resulting from disruption of the plaque and artery. (From Kinney, T. B.: Transluminal angioplasty: A mechanical-pathophysiological correlation of its physical mechanisms. Radiology, *153*:88, 1984.)

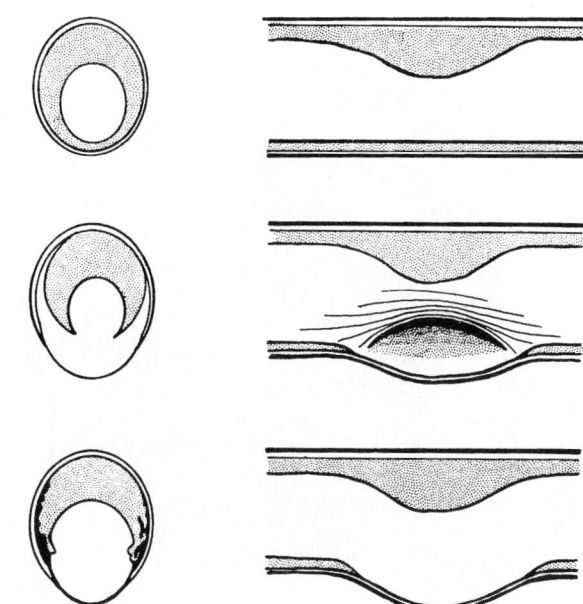

Figure 50–97. Disruption of intima and medial layers after balloon dilation. The increase in lumen size is reflected by bulging of the remaining medial and adventitial fibers opposite the plaque. Remodeling occurs with time, as the irregular lumen surface changes to a rounded, smooth contour. (From Zarin, C. K., Chien-Tai, L., Gewertz, B. L., et al.: Arterial disruption and remodeling following balloon dilatation. Surgery, *92*:1093, 1982.)

inherent in any surgical procedure. Because of the lack of postoperative fibrotic changes, PTA can be repeated easily. Added advantages of PTA are the preservation of the saphenous vein for future use as a conduit for coronary or other organ revascularization and the avoidance of impotence, which occasionally follows disruption of autonomic nerves during aortofemoral grafting.

ter devices usually pass through the thrombus, and the increase in luminal area occurs through the mechanisms previously described. However, as the thrombus becomes more organized, it becomes more resistant to instrument passage, which frequently leads to traversing the vessel wall. Often the passage is in the layer between the plaque and the arterial wall. Similarly, in the setting of obstruction secondary to a ruptured plaque, subintimal passage of the instrument is frequent (Fig. 50–98), and success depends on re-entrance into the true lumen. Remarkably, vessel perforation is uncommon in these settings, despite the fact that PTA often causes rupture of the media and stretching of the adventitia (Fig. 50–99).

COMPARISON OF PTA AND SURGICAL MANAGEMENT

PTA has many inherent advantages compared with surgical revascularization. With the technical simplicity of PTA and the need for only local anesthesia and mild sedation, the hospital stay, cost of the procedure, morbidity, and lost productivity are all greatly reduced. PTA can also be applied to patients whose general medical condition contraindicates surgical intervention. The transluminal approach avoids the disruption of local nerves, lymphatics, and blood vessels

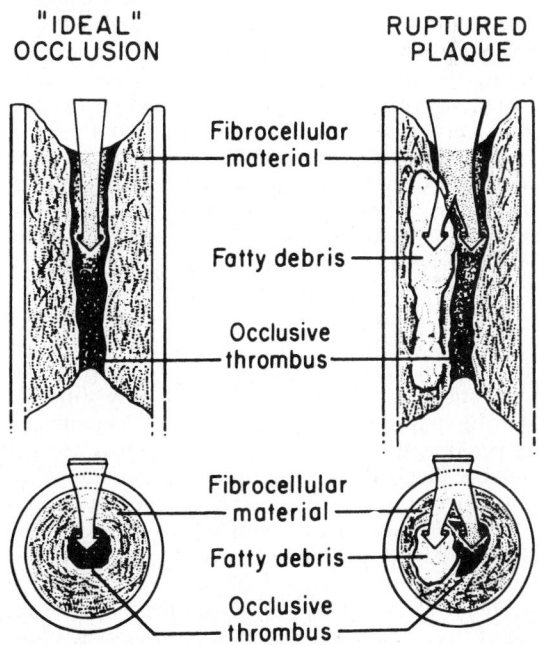

Figure 50–98. Pathways of recanalization in occluded vessels. In an ideal occlusion, a small, fresh central thrombus surrounded by a firmer fibrocellular narrowing provides the pathway of least resistance. When occlusion follows rupturing of an atherosclerotic plaque, the soft atheromatous debris may provide less resistance than the occlusive thrombus. (From Sanborn, T. A.: Recanalization of arterial occlusions: Pathological basis and contributing factors. J. Am. Coll. Cardiol., *13*:1559, 1989.)

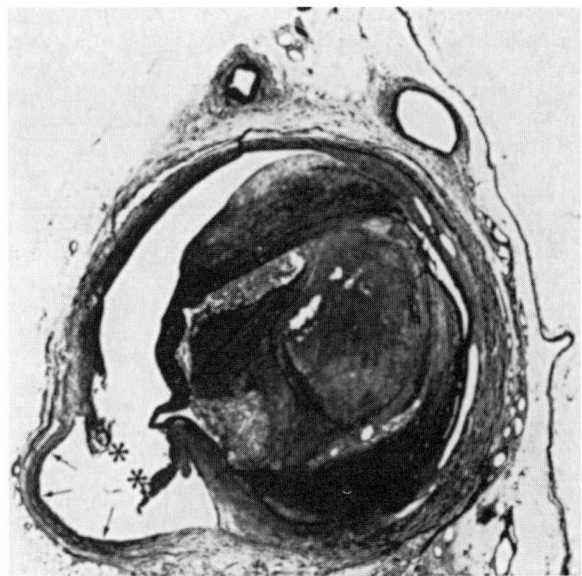

Figure 50–99. Histologic cross section of a long-standing superficial femoral artery occlusion after percutaneous transluminal angioplasty. The guidewire and balloon catheter pass in a plane between the plaque and the media, resulting in an extensive cleavage plane as the arterial wall is stretched away from the plaque. This causes rupture of the media (*) and stretching of the adventitia (arrows) to enlarge the lumen. (From Lyon, R. T., Zarins, C. K., Lu, C. T., et al.: Vessel, plaque, and lumen morphology after transluminal balloon angioplasty. Arteriosclerosis, 7:306, 1987.)

Using the available literature to directly compare the relative efficacy of PTA and that of bypass surgery is largely invalidated by intrinsic differences between the two patient populations. The lesions treated by PTA tend to be discrete, have better runoff, and appear in patients with milder symptoms and fewer comorbidities. Furthermore, the following problematic reporting practices make direct comparison of the two modalities impossible: not reporting initial failures, variable and nonobjective definitions of *success* and *long-term patency*, use of inappropriate statistical methods, and not reporting underlying risk factors or severity of clinical presentation.

To date, the only prospective randomized trial comparing PTA and bypass surgery has been reported by Wolf and associates.[35] The study included 263 men (73% claudicators) with stenoses or occlusions less than 10 cm. long in the iliac, superficial femoral, or popliteal arteries. Although the initial success rate for PTA was lower (85% versus 93% for operation), those patients with successful angioplasties had durable hemodynamic results at a median follow-up of 4 years (improvement in ankle-brachial index and functional status questionnaire). Interestingly, limb salvage favored PTA (89% versus 84% for surgery), although the difference did not reach statistical significance. There were only three deaths, all occurring in the bypass group, at 3 days, 3 months, and 11 months postoperatively. Those patients who required surgical intervention after a failed PTA attempt had a similarly good outcome when compared with PTA or a surgical procedure alone. This is in agreement with other investigators, who have found that an operative procedure can be safely and satisfactorily performed after a failed or complicated angioplasty. Therefore, in this subset of mostly claudicating men with short, focal peripheral arterial obstructions, both PTA and bypass surgery provided a similar sustained clinical benefit at up to 4 years of follow-up.

COMPLICATIONS

The true incidence of complications from PTA may not be accurately reflected in the current angioplasty literature due to marked variations in reporting practices as well as inherent limitations of retrospective surveys. Although most complications are minor, few studies have detailed the occurrence of adverse events that do not lead to surgical intervention or increased hospital stay.

The incidence of complications reported in a recent review of multiple angioplasty series representing a total of 3784 patients is summarized in Table 50–8.[23] PTA is associated with a total complication rate of about 5% to 10%. The number and extent of complications are dependent on the vascular bed being treated, the severity and diffuseness of the atherosclerotic disease process, the experience of the operator, and the completeness with which complications are reported. Fortunately, mortality is extremely rare (0.2%) and is usually caused by balloon-mediated rupture of a large vessel or a complicating myocardial infarction. Acute vessel closure or distal embolization results in limb loss in 0.2% of cases. PTA failures that cause acute limb ischemia or inadequate hemostasis require urgent surgical repair in approximately 2% of all cases.

INDICATIONS

Following Grüntzig's introduction of the balloon catheter, the indications for peripheral vascular angioplasty have gradually broadened as technological improvements and operator experience have resulted in increasing success rates and lower complication rates. Although PTA was originally envisioned as a simple and direct alternative to bypass surgery, after 15 years of widespread application, it is now more appropriately viewed as an independent therapeutic procedure with unique indications and contraindications. Currently this technique is performed in patients with lifestyle-limiting intermittent claudication that does not warrant operation, as well as in those patients with comorbidities that render them high surgical risks. The generally accepted indications for peripheral arterial angioplasty are as follows:

1. Lifestyle-limiting intermittent claudication
2. Ischemic rest pain
3. Ischemic tissue loss, including ulceration and gangrene
4. Impaired distal wound healing
5. Impending limb loss
6. Combined adjunct for simplification of surgical revascularization

TABLE 50–8. Complications of PTA

Complication	Incidence (%)
Bleeding	3.4
Pseudoaneurysm	0.5
Arteriovenous fistula	0.1
Thrombus	3.2
Vessel rupture	0.3
Dissection	0.4
Embolization	2.3
Renal failure	0.2
Myocardial infarction	0.2
Cerebrovascular accident	0.6
Consequences	
Urgent surgical repair	2.0
Limb loss	0.2
Death	0.2

Modified from Pentecost, M. J., et al.: Guidelines for peripheral percutaneous transluminal angioplasty of the abdominal aorta and lower extremity vessels. Circulation, 89:511, 1994.

7. Preservation of limb perfusion in patients with peripheral vascular disease requiring an intra-aortic balloon pump

As is true for surgical procedures, the use of percutaneous intervention to treat intermittent claudication should be offered only to patients who have significant functional limitations that are inadequately treated by conservative measures such as risk-factor modification, exercise rehabilitation, and pharmacologic therapy. Once the patient is appraised of the risk-benefit ratio, the decision to proceed with PTA becomes a value judgment jointly arrived at by the patient and the physician. Ischemic rest pain, ulceration, gangrene, impaired wound healing, and impending limb loss are clear indications for intervention when lesion morphology is deemed amenable to percutaneous techniques.

Adjunctive angioplasty to improve proximal inflow or distal runoff has proved to be a valuable technique for simplifying and enhancing the durability of surgical bypass grafts. This approach has been particularly useful in avoiding the risks of general anesthesia and intra-abdominal surgery in high-risk patients with iliac disease amenable to PTA, thus allowing for better tolerated and more distal femoropopliteal or femorofemoral bypass grafting that can be done under regional or local anesthesia.

Limb ischemia remains the most common complication after intra-aortic balloon pump placement. This is usually the result of thrombotic occlusion induced by the relatively large catheter shaft passing through a diseased iliac artery, frequently in the setting of hypotension or cardiogenic shock. Focal iliac stenoses found on angiography or noninvasive testing and suspected by weak femoral pulses, an aortofemoral gradient, or claudication symptoms have been safely dilated using a conservatively sized balloon diameter at least 1 mm. smaller than the reference vessel. Early experience in this setting suggests that PTA may indeed prove useful in alleviating limb ischemia, which occasionally complicates this already critical situation.

PREDICTORS OF SUCCESSFUL PTA OUTCOME

The following clinical factors have been identified as predictors of good outcome with PTA:

1. Adequate inflow to the dilated segment
2. Good distal runoff
3. Large, proximal vessels
4. Nonostial, concentric stenosis less than 7 cm. in length
5. Short segment occlusion less than 3 cm. in length
6. Occlusions converted to focal stenoses after thrombolysis
7. Nondiabetic patients
8. Symptoms of claudication rather than ischemic rest pain

Similar to results with peripheral bypass surgery, adequate inflow into the diseased arterial segment coupled with good distal runoff significantly enhances long-term patency after PTA.[8, 13] Large vessels, such as the aorta and common iliac artery, generally respond more favorably to PTA than the femoropopliteal or trifurcation vessels. Angiographic morphology of the treated lesion is also an important determinant of success, since long stenoses (greater than 7 cm.) and occlusions (greater than 3 cm.) indicate extensive and advanced atherosclerotic disease, and PTA has produced poor results in such situations.[8] Frequently, complete occlusion of a peripheral vessel in a patient with recent worsening of limb ischemia is the result of thrombus formation overlying a short, fixed stenosis, especially in patients with failing bypass grafts. The occluding thrombus can be successfully lysed by thrombolytic infusion. Thus the underlying stenosis

can be unmasked and dilated to yield results similar to those seen with other short focal lesions. The clinical indication for intervention also directly affects the likelihood of success, since patients with ischemic rest pain are more likely to be diabetic, with an increased risk for limb loss due to diffuse, multisegmental disease seriously impairing collateral distal flow. It is not surprising, therefore, that the pattern of disease encountered in this setting commonly includes tandem stenoses and occlusions, which limit both proximal inflow and distal runoff, leaving a vascular environment poorly suited for percutaneous revascularization.

RESULTS OF PTA IN PERIPHERAL VASCULAR DISEASE

Aortic

A small subgroup of relatively young patients with intermittent claudication presents with isolated stenosis of the infrarenal abdominal aorta (Fig. 50–100). These patients are usually middle-aged female smokers with small-caliber aortas, relatively free of additional peripheral vascular disease. Recent studies report a high initial success rate of 93% to 100% using PTA to treat these lesions.[4, 15, 20, 21, 32, 36] The long-term patency of 86% for up to 3 years compares favorably with the published results of aortoiliac reconstructive surgery (Table 50–9). The long-term results of aortofemoral bypass are well documented, with 5-year patency rates ranging from 76% to 91%. Although the operative mortality is acceptable at 2% to 5%, there remains significant associated morbidity, including impotence (11% to 33%), graft infection (1.8% to 4%), femoral neuropathy (3.4%), and spinal cord ischemia (0.25%). Given the excellent initial success rate and favorable long-term patency in the first 148 patients reported, aortic PTA should be considered the treatment of choice in selected patients with focal atherosclerotic stenoses of the nonaneurysmal infrarenal aorta.

Iliac

Angioplasty has become the procedure of choice for treating focal stenoses of the common and external iliac arteries

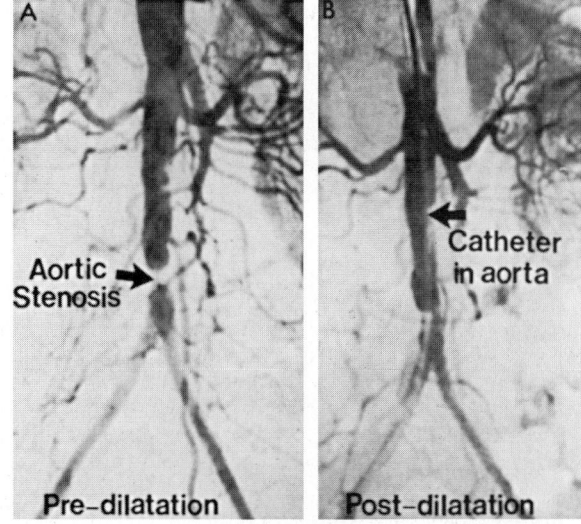

Figure 50–100. Percutaneous transluminal angioplasty (PTA) of an abdominal aortic stenosis. *A*, Concentric hourglass stenosis of the infrarenal aorta. Lumen diameter was 4 mm., with a gradient of 10 mm. Hg. *B*, Following PTA, the lumen diameter was 9 mm. and the pressure gradient was zero. Patient was asymptomatic at 6-month follow-up. (From Heeney, D., Bookstein, J., Danield, E., et al.: Transluminal angioplasty of the abdominal aorta. Radiology, *148*:81, 1983.)

TABLE 50–9. Results of Aortic Angioplasty

Study	Number	Initial Success Rate (%)	Follow-up Period (Yr.)	Clinical Patency (%)*
Tegtmeyer et al.[32]	32	94	1	90
Charlebois et al.[4]	14	93	1.5	100
Yakes et al.[36]	32	100	2	90
Johnston et al.[15]	17	94	3	75
Morag et al.[20]	14	100	3	92
Odurny et al.[21]	25	100	5	70
Hallisey et al.[9]	14	100	4	93
Total†	148	97	3	86

*Excluding initial failures.
†Total percentage expressed as weighted mean.

(Fig. 50–101). The initial success rate averages 90%, with good long-term durability after successful dilatation, as noted in several large studies reporting an average 4-year patency of 65% (Table 50–10).[8, 15, 16, 30, 34, 37, 38] Standard PTA of total iliac occlusions, however, has resulted in lower initial and long-term success rates, with most series reporting an average acute success rate of 65% (33% to 86%) and 2- to 4-year patency of 75% to 100%. Clinically significant emboli also complicate PTA of totally occluded iliac arteries in 3% to 20% of cases. Better results have been obtained through the use of lytics and stents. Although the 5-year patency of aortoiliac and aortofemoral bypass grafts is somewhat higher (74% to 95%), the surgical approach is also associated with a considerably higher morbidity and mortality, as noted in the above paragraph. Nonetheless, PTA is still best suited for patients with short, segmental iliac lesions, and surgical intervention is preferred for more complex aortoiliac disease, including long total occlusions, "shaggy" aortas, and aneurysms. In some earlier series, only 5% to 8% of patients presenting with lower extremity ischemia were considered candidates for iliac PTA. More recently, however, PTA of the iliac artery has been used more often as an adjunct to surgical therapy. In patients with inflow and outflow disease, PTA of focal iliac stenosis in conjunction with distal bypass has been successful. Similarly, in patients with bilateral iliac disease and one vessel containing a lesion ideally treated with angioplasty, PTA can be combined with femorofemoral artery by-

pass with good long-term patency. Aortobifemoral grafting, which requires an abdominal incision and carries greater morbidity and mortality, can thus be avoided.

In a retrospective comparison between PTA and aortofemoral bypass, PTA was found to be less durable, due to recurrence or progression of disease within the iliac vessels. Late failure occurred in 36% of PTA patients and 8% of surgery patients. Iliac stents are now considered to be the procedure of choice due to a significant improvement in long-term patency (discussed later).

Femoropopliteal

Pooled data from studies reporting at least 100 procedures followed up to 5 years are summarized in Table 50–11.[3, 8, 12–14, 17] Overall, femoropopliteal PTA can be expected to have an initial success rate of 89%, with a long-term patency of 65% at 2 years and 58% at 5 years. The largest decline in patency occurs within the first 6 to 12 months, with a much slower rate of attrition thereafter. Adar and co-workers[1] analyzed 12 studies from the PTA literature using the confidence profile method in an effort to quantitatively estimate the efficacy of PTA for femoropopliteal disease after adjusting for a variety of biases that might arise from patient selection, differences in expertise, or lack of standard reporting practices. They found combined estimates of long-term patency to be 73% at 6 months, 66% at 1 year, 61% at 2 years, 58% at

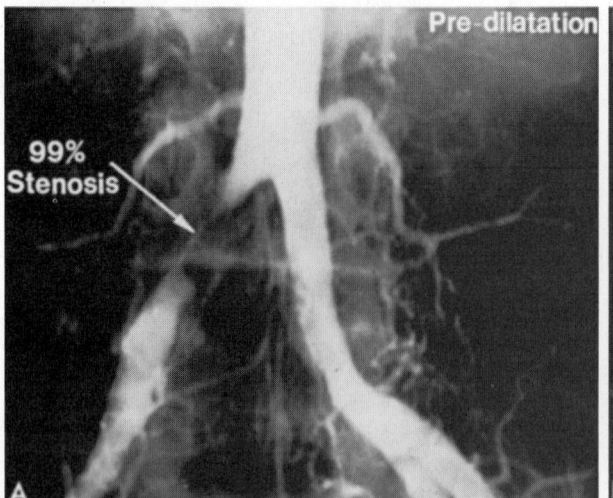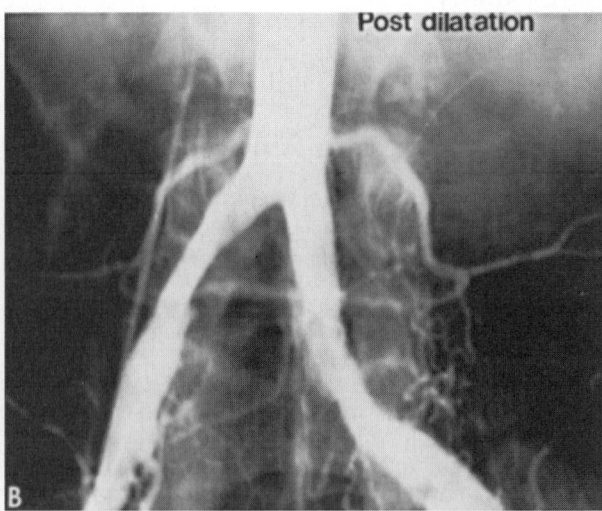

Figure 50–101. Arteriogram from a 68-year-old man with two-block claudication and a necrotic foot ulcer. *A,* Aortofemoral arteriogram demonstrates a 99% stenosis of the right common iliac artery. *B,* Percutaneous transluminal angioplasty (PTA) of the iliac artery resulted in marked improvement in the lumen diameter. The patient was relieved of his claudication, and the ulcer healed. Symptoms recurred 15 months later. Arteriogram revealed restenosis of the right common iliac artery. Repeat PTA was successful, and the patient has remained asymptomatic.

TABLE 50–10. Results of Iliac Angioplasty

Study	Number	Initial Success Rate (%)	Follow-up Period (Yr.)	Clinical Patency (%)*
Waltman[34]	100	97	3	92
Spence et al.[30]	160	93	3	80
Kadir et al.[16]	141	96	3	89
Zeitler[37]	88	NA	5	61
Zeitler et al.[38]	782	85	5	50
Gallino et al.[8]	153	95	5	83
Johnston et al.[15]	598	91	5	64
Total†	2022	90	4	65

*Excluding initial failures.
†Total percentage expressed as weighted mean.

3 years, and 60% at 5 years, similar to the weighted mean values depicted in Table 50–11.

The best results are obtained in femoropopliteal stenoses with two or three patent calf runoff vessels (78% patency at 3 years), and the worst results are obtained in femoropopliteal occlusions with one or no patent calf vessel (25% patency at 3 years).[13] Similarly, patients presenting with claudication and femoropopliteal stenoses have a 5-year patency of 55%, whereas patients presenting with critical rest ischemia and stenoses have a 5-year patency of only 29%.[12] Diabetics with peripheral vascular disease are known to have poor results and high complication rates with PTA. Attempts at limb salvage in diabetics with poor runoff were associated with a dismal 5-year femoral patency of 7% and popliteal patency of 0%. In contrast, several investigators have reported much more encouraging results in the general population, with 1- to 2-year limb salvage rates ranging from 34% to 76% in patients with limb ischemia treated with PTA.[7, 19] In current practice, many of these patients benefit from combined surgical procedure and angioplasty for optimal revascularization.

Comparisons between surgical bypass and PTA of the femoropopliteal system are difficult because of the different clinical variables in the patient populations treated. Femoropopliteal bypass using saphenous vein has an initial success rate of 85% to 90%, with 1-year patency rates of 61% to 100%, 2-year patency rates of 60% to 85%, and 5-year patency rates of 55% to 80%. In a randomized series of patients undergoing femoropopliteal bypass using either saphenous vein or polytetrafluoroethylene (PTFE), the patency rates using PTFE were 75% at 2 years and 38% at 5 years.[33] Similar to PTA, patency rates of bypass grafts are significantly affected by distal runoff and the indication for surgical therapy (claudication versus limb salvage).

Although comparisons of PTA and surgical revascularization are difficult, bypass procedures using saphenous vein appear to have better long-term patency and clinical benefits than PTA, particularly in patients with impaired outflow and increasing ischemia. However, PTA patency rates are comparable to those obtained using synthetic graft material for bypass. In addition, PTA is easier to repeat than surgical revision of a failed graft, and PTA preserves the saphenous vein for possible use as a conduit for coronary or other revascularization.

Tibioperoneal

Until recently, angioplasty of the distal tibioperoneal vessels was performed only in cases of threatened limb loss, in part because of the limitations of early angioplasty equipment, but also because salvage bypass surgery for failed tibioperoneal angioplasty is associated with an increased failure rate when compared with more proximal reconstructions. These factors led to an appropriately conservative approach to this vascular bed and limited published experience.[2, 11, 26, 28, 31] Using lower-profile, more flexible and steerable catheter equipment based on coronary angioplasty systems, recent investigators reported an initial success rate of about 90% in a total of 422 tibioperoneal procedures (Table 50–12). Although long-term follow-up data are scant, the average patency of 60% at 1.5 years is significantly lower than angioplasty results in the more proximal peripheral vessels.

Infrainguinal

A substantial number of infrainguinal venous and prosthetic bypass grafts fail within the first few years after operation. Although the durability of autogenous saphenous vein grafts is superior to PTFE reconstructions, a 20% to 40% vein graft attrition rate has nonetheless been documented during the first 5 years. Within the first 2 years after operation, the

TABLE 50–11. Results of Femoropopliteal Angioplasty

Study	Number	Initial Success Rate (%)	Clinical Patency (%)* 2 Yr.	5 Yr.
Krepel et al.[17]	164	88	80	74
Gallino et al.[8]	289	87	75	71
Hunink et al.[12]	131	95	55	50
Capek et al.[3]	217	90	62	52
Jeans et al.[13]	190	82	61	59
Johnston[14]	254	96	57	42
Total†	1245	89	65	58

*Excluding initial failures.
†Total percentage expressed as weighted mean.

TABLE 50–12. Results of Tibioperoneal Angioplasty

Study	Number	Initial Success Rate (%)	Follow-up Period (Yr.)	Clinical Patency (%)*
Bull et al.[2]	168	77	2	55
Horvath et al.[11]	103	96	1	80
Saab et al.[26]	14	100	1.5	64
Schwarten[28]	131	94	NA	NA
Sprayregen et al.[31]	6	83	1.5	40
Total†	422	90	1.5	60

*Excluding initial failures.
†Total percentage expressed as weighted mean.

obstructing lesion is frequently the result of intimal hyperplasia that develops focally within the graft, at anastomoses, or at the site of venous valves. Later graft failure is commonly the result of progressive atherosclerosis proximal and distal to graft anastomoses. Final graft occlusion is frequently an acute event caused by the rapid propagation of intraluminal thrombus (Fig. 50–102). In an effort to prolong the functional life of the graft, most vascular surgeons advocate close postoperative surveillance of these patients through the use of noninvasive vascular testing to monitor graft flow velocity. Early detection and repair of stenotic graft lesions prior to actual graft thrombosis yield far superior results when compared with the more complex approach warranted when attempting to salvage a totally occluded graft. Once thrombosis has occurred, complex thrombolytic and surgical procedures with relatively high procedural morbidity and mortality rates are commonly required.

The role of balloon angioplasty or other percutaneous techniques in the treatment of peripheral vein graft stenoses remains controversial, partly because of the relative paucity of data. Most of the available series reported on a small number of patients and produced conflicting results. Several studies noted recurrent stenosis in more than half of balloon-dilated graft lesions within the first 6 to 12 months, which

compares unfavorably with the durability of surgical revision, with a reported 5-year patency of approximately 60%. Other groups, however, have shown good results with PTA in vein graft lesions. Sanchez and associates, with the largest single-center experience, reported their experience with 285 peripheral graft lesions treated initially with either PTA (n = 156) or operation (n = 129).[27] The 5-year secondary patency rate for grafts initially treated with PTA (58%) was lower than but was not significantly different (p = 0.25) from that for grafts initially treated with operation (71%). These favorable PTA results are partly due to selection criteria limiting the use of angioplasty to stenoses less than 5 cm. in length. Stenoses greater than 5 cm. long and all occlusions were surgically revised. Further analysis of the PTA group revealed that the 2-year extended patency rate for lesions less than 1.5 cm. in length within vein grafts greater than or equal to 3 mm. in diameter (93%) was significantly better than the patency rate for lesions that were multiple, greater than 1.5 cm. in length, or within grafts less than 3 mm. in diameter (54%) (p = 0.001). These results perhaps partially reconcile the conflicting opinions regarding the efficacy of graft PTA by pointing out that good long-term results are likely to be achieved only with relatively short stenoses in larger grafts. Longer, more diffuse lesions and chronic occlusions in bypass grafts are best treated with surgical revision.

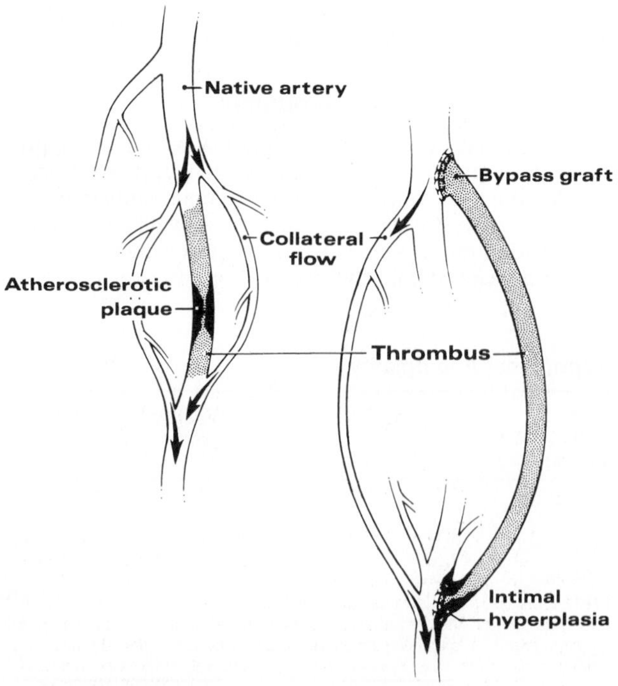

Renal

The large number of patients with renovascular hypertension and the reported increase in the survival of patients treated with revascularization compared with medical management have led to considerable interest in renal artery PTA (PTRA) (Fig. 50–103). Ten per cent to 15% of adults in the United States have hypertension. Of these 23 million people, approximately 4% have potentially correctable renovascular hypertension. In patients with accelerated or malignant hypertension, the incidence of a renovascular etiology is 30% and when present in conjunction with renal insufficiency, the incidence approaches 45%.

The indications for PTRA should be similar to those used for surgical intervention and include sustained hypertension, usually of a severe nature and poorly controlled medically, and evidence of renal artery stenosis by angiographic and hemodynamic data.

The likelihood of technical success is dependent on the nature and etiology of the lesion. Angioplasty of stenoses caused by fibromuscular dysplasia is technically successful in approximately 87% to 100% of patients. In comparison, angioplasty of atherosclerotic stenoses is technically successful in 37% to 90% of patients. The technical success rate in treating nonostial atherosclerotic lesions is 72% to 79%; for ostial lesions, technical success is achieved in 62% to 66%.[10] PTRA of ostial lesions has proved disappointing, due to the relatively low acute success rate and high restenosis rate.

Figure 50–102. Pathologic mechanism of total vascular occlusion in the peripheral native artery and infrainguinal bypass graft.

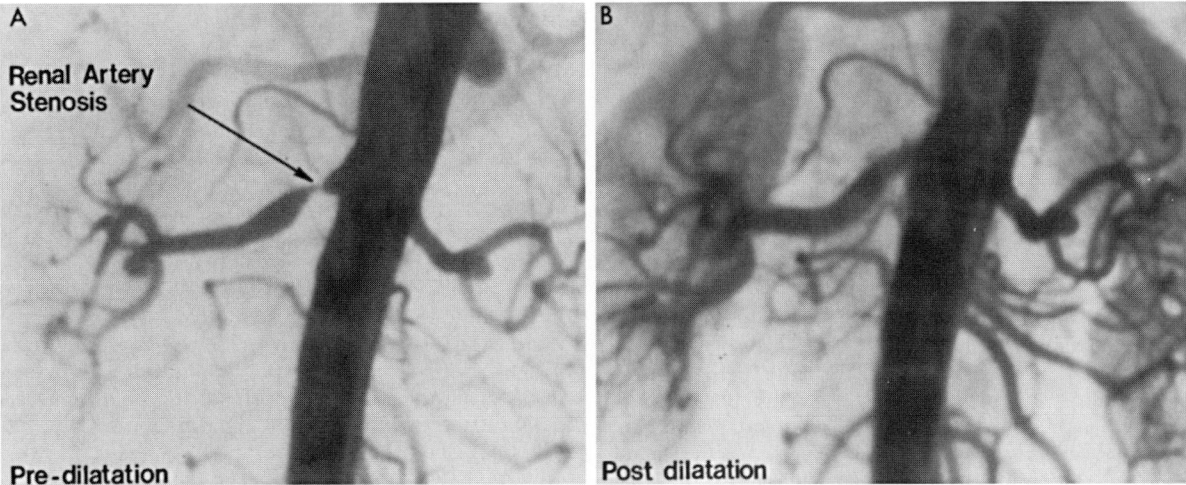

Figure 50–103. Arteriogram from a 44-year-old woman with multiple emergency room visits for uncontrolled hypertension. Her admission systolic and diastolic blood pressures ranged from 140 to 170 and 90 to 110 mm. Hg, respectively, on a three-drug regimen. *A,* Renal arteriogram demonstrates a 90% stenosis of the right renal artery. *B,* Postdilation arteriogram demonstrates marked improvement of the arterial stenosis. After percutaneous transluminal angioplasty, the patient was normotensive off all medications.

This has been attributed to the high elastic recoil of these lesions, which are composed primarily of aortic wall plaque (Figs. 50–104 and 50–105). Early experience with stenting of ostial lesions appears encouraging and is discussed later in this chapter.

Mortality associated with PTRA is approximately 1%, but mortality up to 7.3% has been reported.[10] Most deaths occur in patients with diffuse atherosclerotic disease, and myocardial infarction is the most common cause of death. Diffuse atherosclerotic emboli causing bowel infarction and peripheral ischemia, as well as retroperitoneal hemorrhage, are other common causes of mortality. Complications are more frequent than when performing PTA in other vascular beds—5% to 33%, with an average of 7% to 10% when treating fibromuscular dysplasia lesions and 15% to 25% when treating atherosclerotic lesions. The most common complications are renal insufficiency, renal artery dissection and perforation, renal artery emboli and other atheromatous emboli, myocardial infarction, and local complications at the femoral artery puncture site. Approximately 2% to 5% of patients require operative intervention, sometimes on an emergency basis. Following complications involving the renal artery or its branches that require surgical intervention, such as perforation and thrombosis, a reasonable likelihood of renal salvage is possible with immediate surgical revascularization, although a more complex vascular procedure is often necessary. In these cases, injury to the relatively short main renal artery complicates the technical aspects of surgical

revascularization. Because of these complications and the need for prompt intervention to optimize the clinical results, PTRA should be limited to centers with adequate surgical facilities to manage the complications.

Comparison of surgical revascularization and PTRA in the treatment of renovascular hypertension is complicated by the lack of controlled trials and the differences in patient characteristics. The National Cooperative Study on Renovascular Hypertension reported an overall surgical benefit of 78.7%, with a mortality of 5.9%. However, more recent reports utilizing better patient selection as well as improved technique and perioperative care have reported mortality of approximately 2% and clinical benefit in 90% to 97%. Forty per cent to 72% of the patients were cured of hypertension, and improved blood pressure control occurred in an additional 25% to 52%. Although cure of hypertension is less common with PTRA, the comparable success in patients with fibromuscular dysplasia (84% benefit rate) and in patients with nonstial atherosclerotic lesions (70% benefit rate), coupled with the procedure's lower morbidity, mortality, expense, and lost productivity time, allows PTRA to be an initial approach in these patients. Rarely does an unsuccessful angioplasty prevent or complicate a later surgical revascularization. However, the majority of patients with renovascu-

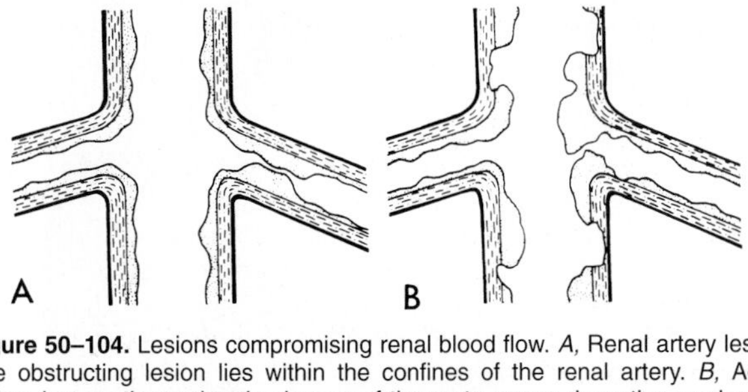

Figure 50–104. Lesions compromising renal blood flow. *A,* Renal artery lesion. The obstructing lesion lies within the confines of the renal artery. *B,* Aortic lesion. Large atherosclerotic plaques of the aorta encroach on the renal artery ostium, hindering blood flow. (From Cicuto, K. P., McLean, G. K., Oleaga, J. A., et al.: Renal artery stenosis: Anatomic classification for percutaneous transluminal angioplasty. A. J. R. Am. J. Roentgenol., *137*:601, 1981.)

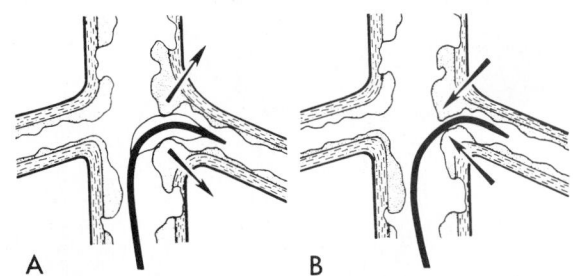

Figure 50–105. Displacement of aortic plaques rather than compression. *A,* Balloon catheter inflated in an area of narrowing. Large aortic plaques are displaced (arrows) rather than compressed because of the abundant elastic tissue underlying the diseased aortic intima and the orientation of the elastic and collagenous fibers of the aortic wall. *B,* After balloon deflation, aortic plaques return to original location (arrows). Although slight alteration of the plaque surface may occur, the stenosis remains relatively unchanged. (From Cicuto, K. P., McLean, G. K., Oleaga, J. A., et al.: Renal artery stenosis: Anatomic classification for percutaneous transluminal angioplasty. A. J. R. Am. J. Roentgenol., *137*:601, 1981.)

lar hypertension have atherosclerotic lesions that are not ideal for PTRA, and frequently these patients have diffuse atherosclerosis and other medical conditions that increase the risk of operative intervention. PTRA in these patients is associated with fewer technical successes, less clinical benefit, and more complications, which limit the overall utility of angioplasty.

NEW DEVICES FOR PERIPHERAL INTERVENTION

In an effort to improve the immediate and long-term results of percutaneous intervention in peripheral vascular disease, several new technologies are currently being tested clinically. Stenting, atherectomy, and laser angioplasty have generated widespread interest for their potential value in overcoming abrupt vessel closure and restenosis, the main limitations of balloon angioplasty. Except for stents, the role of these new devices remains largely speculative at this time. Given the low cost, simplicity, speed, and general efficacy of balloon angioplasty, it is unlikely that any of these newer devices will completely replace PTA. Rather, they are likely to be used in particular *niche* applications in the treatment of peripheral vascular disease.

Stents

Intravascular stents were first developed as an adjunct to balloon angioplasty for the purpose of scaffolding open the internal vessel lumen, thereby preventing acute closure due to elastic recoil and plaque dissection and leading to reduced restenosis rates. Several different types of stents have been developed for clinical application, including rigid, flexible, balloon-expanding and self-expanding varieties. The largest clinical experience to date in peripheral vessels has been gained with the use of the Palmaz balloon expandable stent (Johnson and Johnson), and the self-expanding Wallstent (Schneider). Only the Palmaz stent is currently approved by the Food and Drug Administration for iliac artery stenting in the United States. Most investigators have demonstrated that stents can be safely deployed in the iliac artery with a less than 1% risk of early thrombosis and long-term clinical success rates between 69% and 91%. In the only randomized study comparing primary iliac stenting with conventional PTA, Richter and colleagues found that use of the Palmaz

iliac stent not only resulted in a higher initial success rate but also produced a significantly higher 4-year angiographic patency (94% versus 69%) and clinical success rate (89% versus 67%).[25] Although iliac stenting is clearly indicated as an adjunct to salvage poor PTA outcomes, longer follow-up of Richter's data and additional independent randomized trials are needed before judging the efficacy of primarily stenting all approachable iliac lesions. Examples of Palmaz stenting in the common and external iliac arteries are depicted in Figures 50–106 and 50–107.

Rather limited experience has been reported with stenting of the femoropopliteal vessels. Nonetheless, early results demonstrate a significant rate of thrombosis within 30 days of stent implantation, occurring in 6% to 19% of patients despite full anticoagulation. This important complication is likely related to several factors, including the high percentage of total occlusions treated in the femoropopliteal region, longer mean lesion length (8 cm. versus 3 cm. for iliac stents), smaller vessel diameter, and larger stented surface area.[22] In addition to the danger of early thrombosis, the reported long-term patency of femoropopliteal stenting between 6 months and 3 years has been relatively poor (42% to 74%) and does not appear to be better than previously reported results with PTA alone. Late restenosis is caused primarily by intimal hyperplasia within the stented vessel segment. In a controlled comparison, Do and co-workers noted no significant difference between the secondary 1-year patency rates of femoral PTA alone (65%) and those of PTA plus stent (69%).[5] However, the 69% 1-year patency of stented vessels was achieved only at the expense of multiple repeat catheter interventions to treat the high rates of early thrombosis and late intimal hyperplasia. Therefore, these and other authors concluded that stents are not indicated for the primary treatment of femoropopliteal lesions. As is true in the iliac vessels, however, stents have been useful for salvaging PTA interventions complicated by severe occlusive dissections.

Early experience with stenting ostial renal artery stenoses appears encouraging. The limitations of routine PTA for treating bulky aortic plaque impinging on the renal ostium is well described and is primarily the result of aortic wall recoil. Theoretically, stents should have an important beneficial impact in the subgroup of renovascular hypertensive patients with ostial renal stenosis (Fig. 50–108). Rees and associates[24] reported preliminary results using Palmaz stents in ostial renal lesions of 28 hypertensive patients. The acute

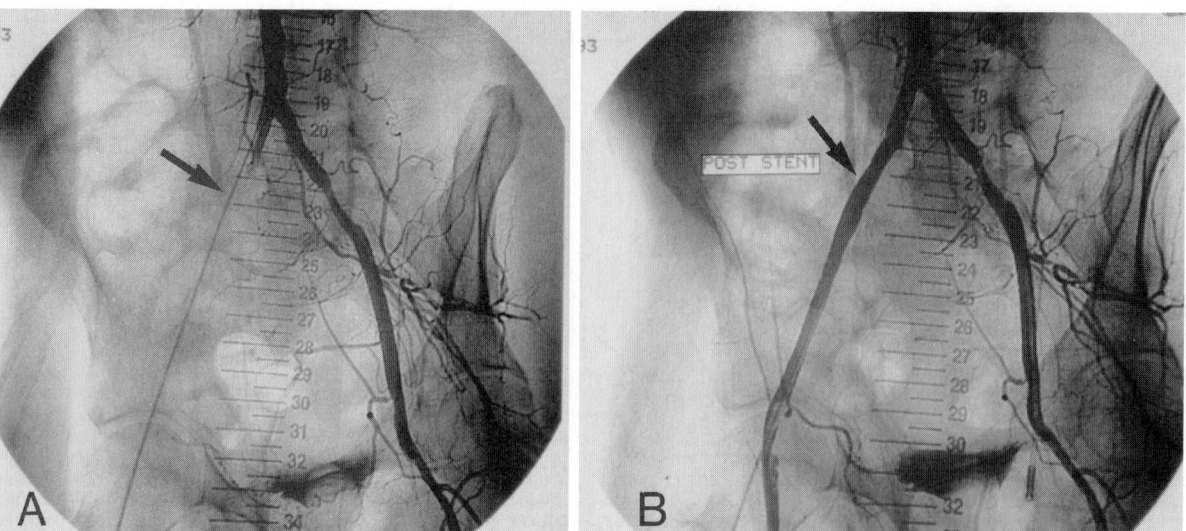

Figure 50–106. Aortoiliac arteriogram showing total occlusion of the right common iliac artery (arrow). *A,* Baseline. *B,* After deployment of Palmaz stent.

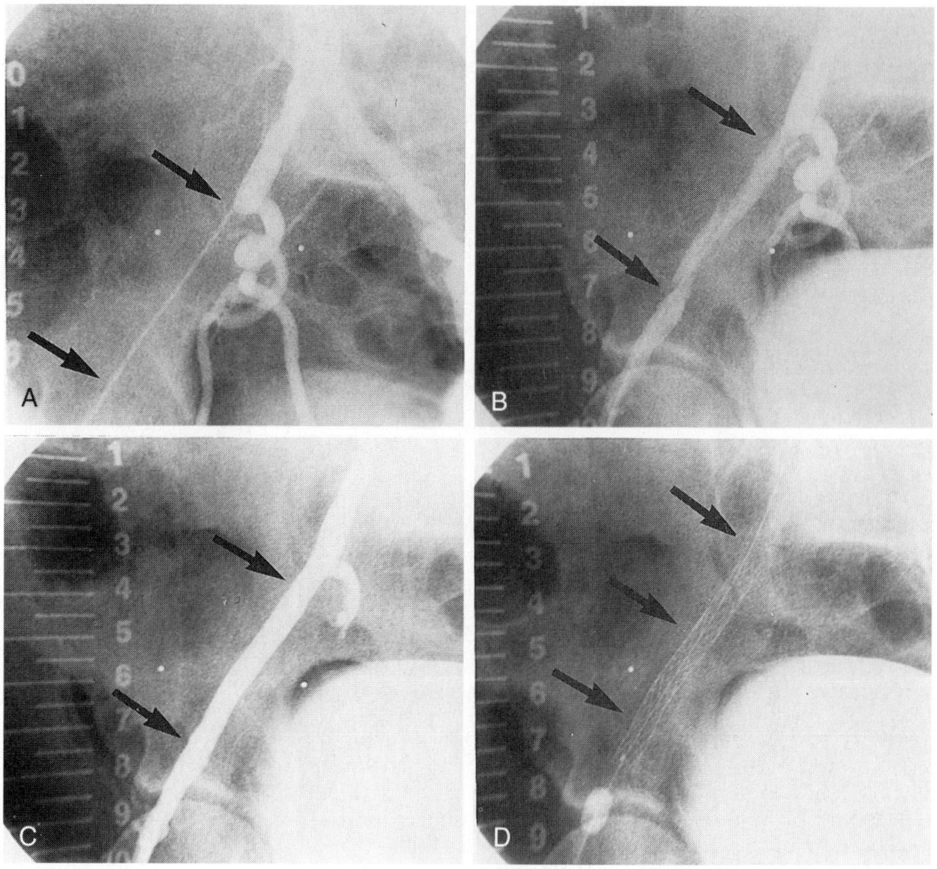

Figure 50–107. Arteriogram of the right iliac arterial system showing total occlusion of the external iliac artery (arrow). *A,* Baseline; a guidewire is seen coursing through the occlusion. *B,* After balloon angioplasty, a severe occlusive dissection is seen. *C,* After deployment of three Palmaz stents, a normal lumen is restored. *D,* The three Palmaz stents as seen under fluoroscopy.

technical success rate was 96%, and complications occurred in five patients. Cumulative clinical benefit at 6 months was 64%, with anatomic patency (less than 50% stenosis) in 61% (11 of 18 patients) when studied angiographically at 7 months. Other renal stent series have documented improved and sustained clinical benefit for up to 1 year, comparing favorably with the historically poor results of routine PTRA in the ostial location.[29]

Atherectomy

Atherectomy is defined as the removal of atheroma from diseased arteries. Although several devices have been designed to percutaneously perform atherectomy in peripheral vessels, only three have been approved for clinical use: the Simpson Atherocath (Devices for Vascular Intervention, Inc.), the Auth Rotablator (Biophysics International), and the Transluminal Extraction Catheter (TEC) (Interventional Technologies, Inc.). The present state of these technologies, however, greatly limits their general applicability and usefulness for the treatment of peripheral arterial disease. Except for unusual lesion morphologies, atherectomy has not proved superior to routine PTA.

The Auth Rotablator is an over-the-wire rotating catheter equipped with a football-shaped burr studded with diamond chips that act as microblades. At speeds of up to 200,000 r.p.m., hard and calcified atheroma is, in theory, preferentially pulverized and the microparticles sent harmlessly through the circulation.[2] The Rotablator is therefore best suited for hard, calcified atheroma, frequently encountered in the tibioperoneal arteries of diabetics.

Results have generally been poor when applied to peripheral vessels in patients with advanced disease and threatened limbs. Primary patency rates after rotablation were noted to be as low as 29% at 6 months and 10% at 2 years follow-up.[3]

The inability to burr through chronic thrombus or more elastic plaque and intimal hyperplasia limits the use of the Rotablator. Treatment of long lesions may generate a large particle burden capable of catastrophic distal embolization. If there is a potential niche for the Rotablator, perhaps it is for the treatment of undilatable, focal, heavily calcified stenoses in tibioperoneal vessels that are not amenable to bypass surgery.

Lasers

Despite tremendous efforts directed over the past decade toward the development of a clinically useful vascular laser system, results have generally remained discouraging. At great expense, various systems have been applied in the peripheral vasculature. Although acceptable acute success rates are attainable, many investigators noted an unacceptably high incidence of vessel perforation, in addition to poor long-term outcomes. Pulsed excimer laser energy theoretically offers advantages over previous laser systems and is currently being tested in the peripheral vasculature. To date, however, there are no conclusive data to support the use of lasers for the treatment of peripheral atherosclerosis.

SUMMARY

PTA, introduced in 1964 by Dotter and Judkins and popularized by Grüntzig, has become an established and effective technique in the treatment of vascular occlusive disease. Its role should not be considered competitive with but rather complementary to surgical therapy. Because angioplasty results are lesion-dependent and the procedure is most useful

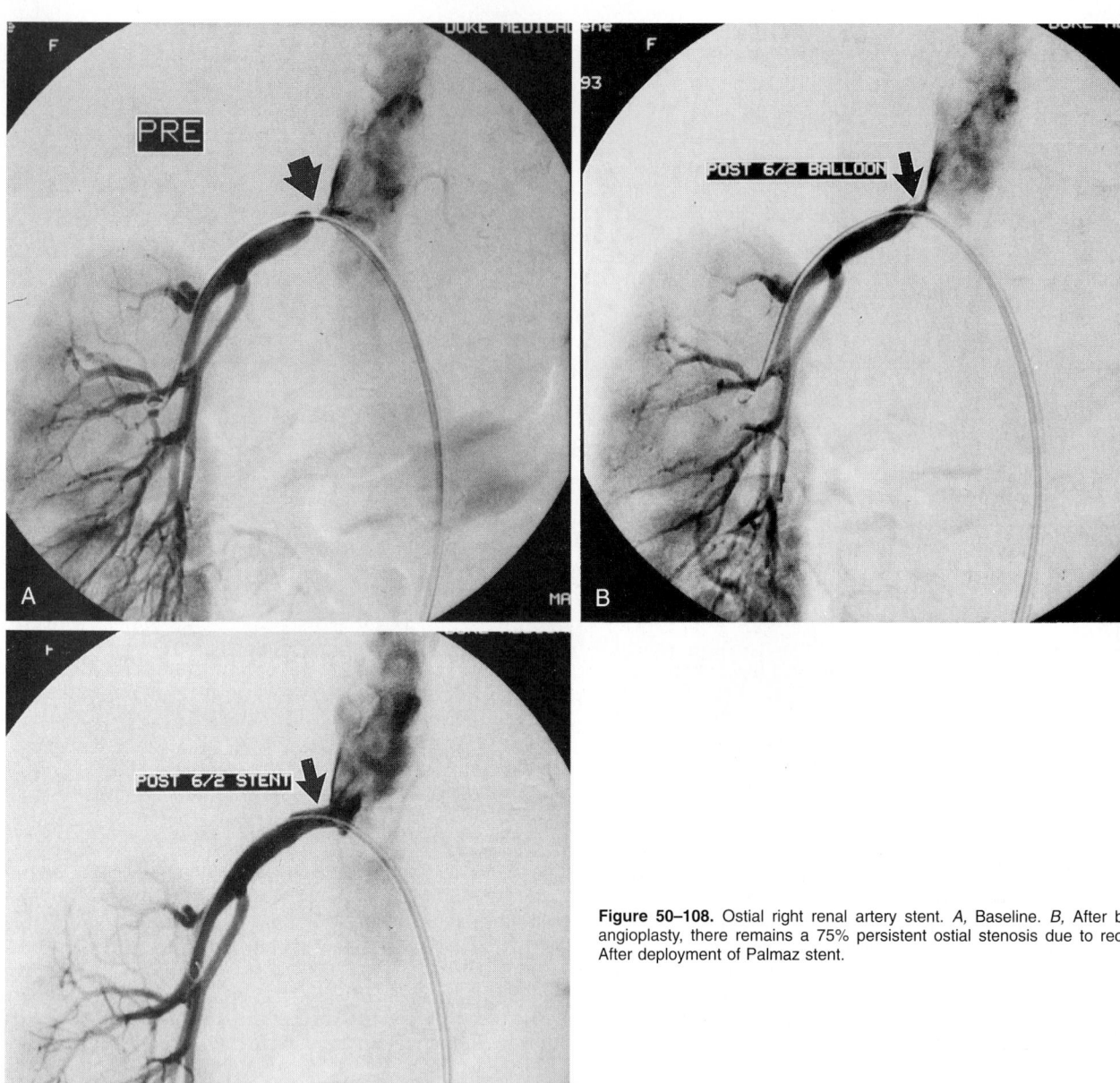

Figure 50–108. Ostial right renal artery stent. *A*, Baseline. *B*, After balloon angioplasty, there remains a 75% persistent ostial stenosis due to recoil. *C*, After deployment of Palmaz stent.

for the treatment of discrete stenoses and occlusions, PTA has much to offer when such favorable anatomy is present. The more frequent disease morphology of diffuse, long, or multiple lesions is often better treated with combined PTA and surgical revascularization. In addition, PTA can be applied to patients whose attendant surgical risk is great. The recent introduction of vascular stents has further expanded the role of percutaneous revascularization, particularly in the iliac vessels. However, enthusiasm for various atherectomy devices and laser ablation has been tempered by increased cost and disappointing long-term results. Future endovascular research efforts are now being focused on the development of ultrasound-guided devices, endovascular grafts, and pharmacologically impregnated biodegradable stents for local drug delivery.

SELECTED REFERENCES

Isner, J. M., and Rosenfield, K.: Redefining the treatment of peripheral artery disease: Role of percutaneous revascularization. Circulation, *88*:1534, 1993.
Excellent review and update on current technology available for peripheral vascular intervention and how this has affected our approach.

Johnston, K. W., Rae, M., Hogg-Johnston, S. A., Colapinto, R. F., Walker, P. M., Baird, R. J., Sniderman, K. W., and Kalman, P.: Five-year results of a prospective study of percutaneous transluminal angioplasty. Ann. Surg., *206*:403, 1987.
Presents the most accurate clinical results of PTA used for the treatment of occlusive vascular disease of the lower extremity. Life-table analysis of the 984 patients is presented, and predictors of success are discussed.

Palmaz, J. C., Laborde, J. C., Rivera, F. J., Encarnacion, C. E., Lutz, J. D., and Moss, J. G.: Stenting of the iliac arteries with the Palmaz stent: Experience from a multicenter trial. Cardiovasc. Intervent. Radiol., *15*:291, 1992.
Initial and largest reported experience with the only stent approved for peripheral arterial application.

Pentecost, M. J., Criqui, M. I., Dorros, G., Goldstone, J., Johnston, K. W., Martin, E. C., and Spies, J. B.: Guidelines for peripheral percutaneous transluminal angioplasty of the abdominal aorta and lower extremity vessels. Circulation, 89:511, 1994.
Current review of indications for PTA as recommended by a multidisciplinary consensus committee of the American Heart Association.

Wolf, G. L., Wilson, S. E., Cross, A. P., Deupree, R. H., Statson, W. B., and the principal investigators and their associates of Veterans Administration cooperative study no. 199: Surgery or balloon angioplasty for peripheral vascular disease: A randomized clinical trial. J. Vasc. Intervent. Radiol., 4:639, 1993.
The only prospective randomized trial comparing PTA with bypass surgery for the treatment of peripheral vascular disease.

REFERENCES

1. Adar, R., Critchfield, G. C., and Eddy, O. M.: A confidence profile analysis of the results of femoropopliteal percutaneous transluminal angioplasty in the treatment of lower extremity ischemia. J. Vasc. Surg., 10:57, 1989.
2. Bull, P. G., Mendel, H., Hold, M., Schlegl, A., and Denck, H.: Distal popliteal and tibioperoneal transluminal angioplasty: Long-term follow-up. J. Vasc. Intervent. Radiol., 3:45, 1992.
3. Capek, P., McLean, G. K., and Berkowitz, H. D.: Femoropopliteal angioplasty: Factors influencing long-term success. Circulation, 83(suppl. I):I-70, 1991.
4. Charlebois, N., Saint-Georges, G., and Hudon, G.: Percutaneous transluminal angioplasty of the lower abdominal aorta. Am. J. Radiol., 146:369, 1986.
5. Do, D. D., Triller, J., Walpoth, B. H., Stirnemann, P., and Mahler, F.: A comparison study of self-expandable stents vs. balloon angioplasty alone in femoropopliteal artery occlusions. Cardiovasc. Intervent. Radiol., 15:306, 1992.
6. Dotter, C.: Transluminally placed coil-spring endoarterial tube grafts: Long-term patency in canine popliteal artery. Invest. Radiol., 4:329, 1969.
7. Fletcher, J. P., Little, J. M., Fermanis, G. G., and Simmons, K.: Percutaneous transluminal angioplasty for severe lower extremity ischemia. Aust. N. Z. J. Surg., 56:121, 1986.
8. Gallino, A., Mahler, F., Probst, P., and Nachbur, B.: Percutaneous transluminal angioplasty of the arteries of the lower limbs: A 5 year follow-up. Circulation, 70:619, 1984.
9. Hallisey, M. J., Meranze, S. G., Parker, B. C., Rholl, K. S., Miller, W. J., Katzen, B. T., and Van Breda, A.: Percutaneous transluminal angioplasty of the abdominal aorta. J. Vasc. Intervent. Radiol., 5:679, 1994.
10. Hayes, J. M., Risius, B., Novick, A. C., Geisinger, M., Zelch, M., Gifford, R. W., Vidt, D. G., and Olin, J. W.: Experience with percutaneous transluminal angioplasty for renal artery stenosis at the Cleveland Clinic. J. Urol., 139:488, 1988.
11. Horvath, W., Oertl, M., and Haidinger, D.: Percutaneous transluminal angioplasty of crural arteries. Radiology, 177:565, 1990.
12. Hunink, M. G. M., Donaldson, M. C., Meyerovitz, M. F., Polak, J. F., Whittemore, A. D., Kandarpa, K., Grassi, C. J., Aruny, J., Harrington, D. P., and Mannick, J. A.: Risks and benefits of femoropopliteal percutaneous balloon angioplasty. J. Vasc. Surg., 17:183, 1993.
13. Jeans, W. D., Armstrong, S., Cole, S. E., Harrocks, M., and Baird, R. N.: Fate of patients undergoing transluminal angioplasty for lower limb ischemia. Radiology, 177:559, 1990.
14. Johnston, K. W.: Femoral and popliteal arteries: Reanalysis of results of balloon angioplasty. Radiology, 183:767, 1992.
15. Johnston, K. W., Rae, M., Hogg-Johnston, S. A., Colapinto, R. F., Walker, P. M., Baird, R. J., Sniderman, K. W., and Kalman, P.: Five-year results of a prospective study of percutaneous transluminal angioplasty. Ann. Surg., 206:403, 1987.
16. Kadir, S., White, R. I., Jr., Kaufman, S. L., Barth, K. H., Williams, G. M., Burdick, J. F., O'Mara, C. S., Smith, G. W., Stonesifer, G. L., Jr., Ernst, C. B., and Minken, S. L.: Long-term results of iliac angioplasty. Surgery, 94:10, 1983.
17. Krepel, V. M., van Andel, G. J., van Erp, W. F. M., and Breslau, P. J.: Percutaneous transluminal dilatation of the femoropopliteal artery: Initial and long-term results. Radiology, 156:325, 1985.
18. Kwasnik, E. M., Siouffi, S. Y., Jay, M. E., and Khuri, S. F.: Comparative results of angioplasty and aortofemoral bypass in patients with symptomatic iliac disease. Arch. Surg., 122:288, 1987.
19. Milford, M. A., Weaver, F. A., Lundell, C. J., and Yellin, A. E.: Femoropopliteal percutaneous transluminal angioplasty for limb salvage. J. Vasc. Surg., 8:292, 1988.
20. Morag, B., Rubeinstein, Z., Kessler, A., Schneiderman, J., Levinkopf, M., and Bass, A.: Percutaneous transluminal angioplasty of the distal abdominal aorta and its bifurcation. Cardiovasc. Intervent. Radiol., 10:129, 1987.
21. Odurny, A., Colapinto, R. F., Sniderman, K. W., and Johnston, K. W.: Percutaneous transluminal angioplasty of abdominal aortic stenoses. Cardiovasc. Intervent. Radiol., 12:1, 1989.
22. Palmaz, J. C., Laborde, J. C., Rivera, F. J., Encarnacion, C. E., Lutz, J. D., and Moss, J. G.: Stenting of the iliac arteries with the Palmaz stent: Experience from a multicenter trial. Cardiovasc. Intervent. Radiol., 15:291, 1992.
23. Pentecost, M. J., Criqui, M. H., Dorros, G., Goldstone, J., Johnston, K. W., Martin, E. C., and Spies, J. B.: Guidelines for peripheral percutaneous transluminal angioplasty of the abdominal aorta and lower extremity vessels. Circulation, 89:511, 1994.
24. Rees, C. S., Palmaz, J. C., Becker, G. J., Ehrman, K. O., Richter, G. M., Noeldge, G., Katzen, B. T., Dake, M. D., and Schwarten, D. E.: Palmaz stent in atherosclerotic stenoses involving the ostia of the renal arteries: Preliminary report of a multicenter study. Radiology, 181:507, 1991.
25. Richter, G. M., Roeren, T. H., Noeldge, G., Landwehr, P., Kauffmann, G. W., and Palmaz, J. C.: Superior clinical results of iliac stent placement versus percutaneous transluminal angioplasty: Four-year success rates of a randomized study, abstracted. Radiology, 181(suppl.):161, 1991.
26. Saab, M. H., Smith, D. C., Aka, P. K., Brownlee, R. W., and Killeen, J. D.: Percutaneous transluminal angioplasty of tibial arteries for limb salvage. Cardiovasc. Intervent. Radiol., 15:211, 1992.
27. Sanchez, L. A., Gupta, S. K., Veith, F. J., et al.: A ten year experience with one hundred fifty failing or threatened vein and polytetrafluoroethylene arterial bypass grafts. J. Vasc. Surg., 14:729, 1991.
28. Schwarten, D. E.: Clinical and anatomical considerations for nonoperative therapy in tibial disease and the results of angioplasty. Circulation, 83(suppl. I):I-86, 1991.
29. Shaw, D., White, C., Collins, T., Karsan, A., Facundus, R. M., and Ramee, S.: Acute and long-term effect of renal artery stenting on blood pressure control in patients with atherosclerotic renovascular hypertension (Abstract). J. Am. Coll. Cardiol., Special issue:381A, 1995.
30. Spence, R. K., Freiman, D. B., Gatenby, R., Hobbs, C. L., Barker, C. F., Berkowitz, H. D., Roberts, B., McClean, G., Oleaga, J., and Ring, E. J.: Long-term results of transluminal angioplasty of the iliac and femoral arteries. Arch. Surg., 116:1377, 1981.
31. Sprayregen, S., Sniderman, K. W., Sos, T. A., Vieux, U., Singer, A., and Veith, F. J.: Popliteal artery branches: Percutaneous transluminal angioplasty. Am. J. Radiol., 135:945, 1980.
32. Tegtmeyer, C. J., Kellum, C. D., Kron, I. L., and Mentzer, R. M., Jr.: Percutaneous transluminal angioplasty in the region of the aortic bifurcation—the two balloon technique with results and long-term follow-up study. Radiology, 157:661, 1985.
33. Veith, F. J., Gupta, S. K., Ascer, E., et al.: Six-year prospective multicenter randomized comparison of autologous saphenous vein and expanded polytetrafluoroethylene grafts in infrainguinal arterial reconstruction. J. Vasc. Surg., 3:104, 1986.
34. Waltman, A. C.: Percutaneous transluminal angioplasty: Iliac and deep femoral arteries. Am. J. Radiol., 135:921, 1980.
35. Wolf, G. L., Wilson, S. E., Cross, A. P., Deupree, R. H., Statson, W. B., and the principal investigators and their associates of Veterans Administration cooperative study no. 199: Surgery or balloon angioplasty for peripheral vascular disease: A randomized clinical trial. J. Vasc. Intervent. Radiol., 4:639, 1993.
36. Yakes, W. F., Kumpe, D. A., Brown, S. B., Parker, S. H., Lattes, R. G., Cook, P. S., Haas, D. K., Gibson, M. D., Hopper, K. D., and Reed, M. D.: Percutaneous transluminal aortic angioplasty: Techniques and results. Radiology, 172:965, 1989.
37. Zeitler, E.: Percutaneous dilatation and recanalization of iliac and femoral arteries. Cardiovasc. Intervent. Radiol., 3:207, 1980.
38. Zeitler, E., Richter, E. I., Roth, F. J., and Schoop, W.: Results of percutaneous transluminal angioplasty. Radiology, 146:57, 1983.

ARTERIAL INJURIES

William H. Baker, M.D.
Steven S. Kang, M.D.

The two leading causes of arterial injury in the United States are urban violence and automobile accidents. Penetrating injuries were once almost exclusively caused by knives but today are increasingly caused by gunshot wounds. High-speed automobile accidents propel both occupants and pedestrians in a manner that may tear an artery, stretch it beyond its limits of elasticity, or disturb its layers as a result of direct impact or associated bone fractures. These injuries are increasingly being treated in centers where there are the necessary skills and facilities for early diagnosis and definitive treatment. There remain, however, a distressing number of arterial injuries occurring in the home, on the athletic field, or at work that are unrecognized by physicians. Leg amputations in high school athletes with knee injuries and deformed and functionless hands in children with elbow fractures are clear evidence of the need for greater awareness of these injuries (see Table 50–13 for a list of arterial injuries).

TABLE 50–13. Specific Arterial Injuries

Artery	Common Mechanism of Injury	Possible Sequelae	Special Considerations
Common carotid	Penetrating wounds of neck, blunt trauma to neck	Airway obstruction due to hematoma, cerebral ischemia	Treatment controversial if neurologic deficit is present: if minor deficit, repair; if major or fixed deficit, ligation may be advisable
Internal carotid	Penetrating wounds, blunt trauma, hyperextension of neck	Cerebral ischemia	Similar to common carotid; anticoagulation for blunt dissection
Vertebral	Penetrating wounds	Hemorrhage	Exposure and repair difficult; surgical or radiologic occlusion usually well tolerated
Innominate	Penetrating wounds of neck and chest, tracheostomy erosions	Cerebral and arm ischemia	Ideally preserve innominate vein, right carotid, and vertebral artery flow
Subclavian	Fractures of clavicle and first rib, penetrating trauma, iatrogenic (needles, catheters, thoracic outlet surgery)	Intrathoracic bleeding, brachial plexus symptoms from associated injury or compression by hematoma	Proximal occlusions may steal vertebral flow for arm
Axillary	Fractures, dislocations of humerus, penetrating wounds	Gangrene (rare)	Repair desirable
Brachial	Catheter injuries, fractures and dislocations of elbow, especially in children	Gangrene (rare); ischemic symptoms (Volkmann's ischemic contracture)	Repair desirable
Radial and ulnar	Lacerations, iatrogenic, drug abuse	Gangrene may follow injections of thiopental and other drugs	May ligate; heparin used for injection injuries
Thoracic aorta	Blunt (rapid deceleration), fractures of sternum, clavicle, first and second ribs	Exsanguination, false aneurysm just distal to left subclavian	Angiography for mediastinal widening, tracheal shift, or diminished pulses
Abdominal aorta	Penetrating wounds, blunt	Exsanguination, visceral or lower extremity ischemia	Repair or prosthetic graft replacement
Common and external iliac	Penetrating wounds	Lower extremity ischemia	Repair
Internal iliac	Pelvic fractures	Pelvic hematoma, false aneurysms	Ligation or angiographic embolization
Renal	Blunt trauma—renal pedicle injury	Hematuria, renal ischemia	Early diagnosis important; unilateral nonvisualization on intravenous pyelogram requires angiography
Celiac and mesenteric	Penetrating wounds	Variable—may cause intestinal ischemia	Repair superior mesenteric; may ligate celiac, inferior mesenteric if necessary
Common femoral	Penetrating wounds, blunt, iatrogenic (catheters, aortic balloon pumps)	Leg ischemia	Repair
Superficial femoral	Penetrating wounds, femur fractures	Leg ischemia (may be minimal)	Repair
Profunda femoris	Penetrating wound, surgery (hip fractures)	Loss of valuable collateral for later life	No distal pulse point; preserve if feasible
Popliteal	Fractures of tibial plateau, dislocation of knee, surgery of knee joint	Amputation likely without prompt and expert repair	Repair; venous repair also advisable
Tibial and peroneal	Fracture of tibia and fibula	Loss of single artery usually well tolerated	Repair if feasible; try to preserve at least two arteries

MECHANISMS OF INJURY

There are three broad categories of arterial injury: penetrating, blunt, and deceleration. Knife wounds with low energy transect vessels much as a surgical scalpel does. Gunshot wounds, often related to urban violence, produce a much more devastating injury, with a direct correlation between the kinetic energy of the projectile and the resultant tissue destruction. Kinetic energy varies as the square of the velocity of the projectile; thus, more devastating injuries occur by increasing the velocity rather than the mass of the bullet. A high-velocity projectile causes cavitation in soft tissues and impact injury to bone. The involved arteries are frequently destroyed and/or thrombosed for several centimeters beyond the path of penetration, requiring extensive débridement of devitalized tissues.

Arterial injury from blunt trauma is caused by one of two mechanisms. Compressive forces can damage the arterial wall directly, or rapid deceleration, as occurs when an automobile hits a stationary object, can stretch an artery and cause an intimal tear, since the intima is the least elastic layer of the arterial wall. Blood dissects under this flap, frequently causing thrombosis of the vessel. Several points in the arterial system are relatively fixed and immobile. The ligamentum arteriosum is one such point just distal to the origin of the left subclavian artery joining the aorta to the pulmonary vessels. With rapid deceleration, the proximal aortic arch moves violently forward, and the distal descending aorta remains relatively stationary, producing a shearing force that disrupts the vessel at the fixed point. Other fixed points include the distal cervical internal carotid artery where it enters the skull, the proximal ascending aortic root, and branches of the thoracic or abdominal aorta.

PATHOPHYSIOLOGY

There are three basic patterns of arterial injury, as depicted in Figure 50–109. This simple classification provides a basis

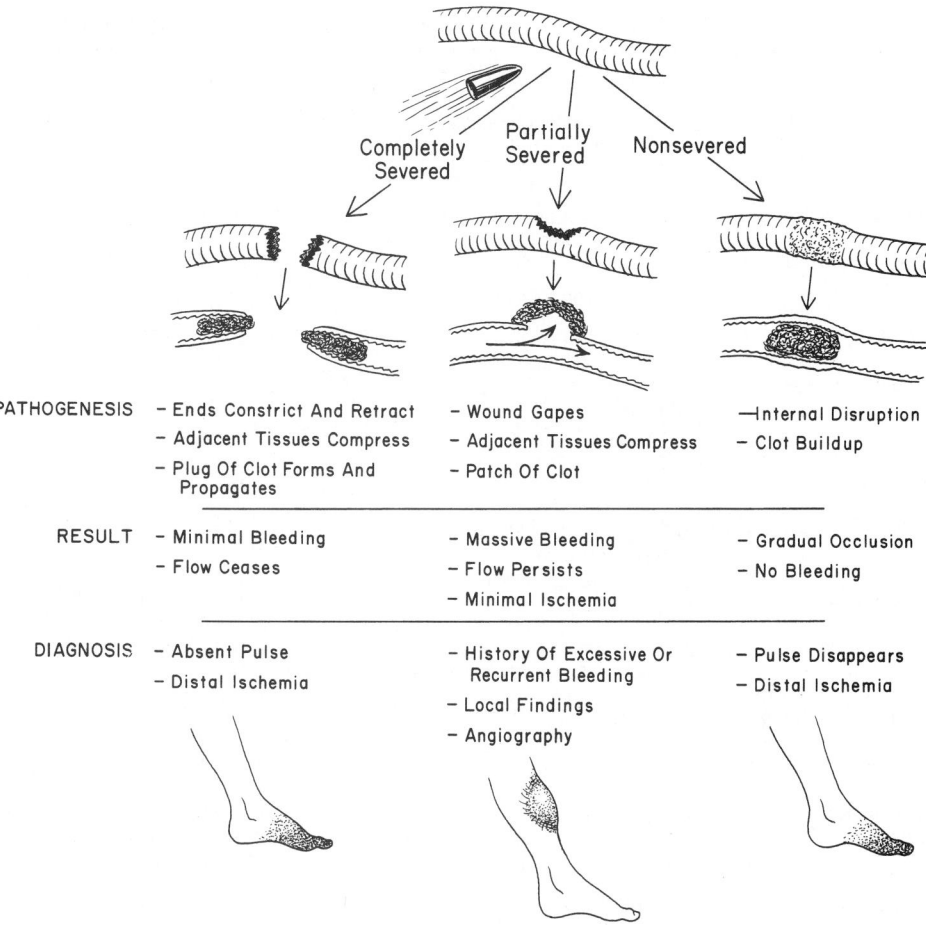

Figure 50–109. The three basic patterns of arterial injury. Careful and repeated examinations of the site of injury and the distal extremity usually establish the need for treatment.

PATHOGENESIS

- Ends Constrict And Retract
- Adjacent Tissues Compress
- Plug Of Clot Forms And Propagates

- Wound Gapes
- Adjacent Tissues Compress
- Patch Of Clot

- Internal Disruption
- Clot Buildup

RESULT

- Minimal Bleeding
- Flow Ceases

- Massive Bleeding
- Flow Persists
- Minimal Ischemia

- Gradual Occlusion
- No Bleeding

DIAGNOSIS

- Absent Pulse
- Distal Ischemia

- History Of Excessive Or Recurrent Bleeding
- Local Findings
- Angiography

- Pulse Disappears
- Distal Ischemia

for understanding the pathogenesis, clinical characteristics, and method of diagnosis of the various types of arterial injury.

Completely Severed Artery

Complete severance of an artery is commonly caused by penetrating wounds such as those inflicted by knives, missiles, or surgical instruments. The severed ends characteristically constrict and retract into the adjacent tissue, often leaving a considerable distance between them. Bleeding usually arrests spontaneously because of the tourniquet effect of vasoconstriction and the development of a firm thrombus in each of the two ends. These clots tend to propagate distally until flow is restored by collateral circulation. The thrombus that occludes the severed ends can be likened to a cork in a wine bottle owing to the narrowing following vasoconstriction. Disruption of the entire wall and loss of blood flow in a major artery cause immediate disappearance of distal pulsations, which is the usual basis for the diagnosis of this type of injury.

The severity of ischemia following complete severance of a major artery varies with the site of interruption; the number, size, and condition of the collateral vessels; and the demands of the supplied tissues. A severed carotid artery may cause irreversible damage of the involved cerebral hemisphere in a matter of minutes, whereas severance of a superficial femoral artery in the upper thigh may cause only muscle pain (claudication) during later exercise. For most major extremity arteries, the skin at some point distal to the injury is pale or mottled in color and cool to the touch when compared with the uninvolved side. In addition, there may

be loss of sensation, especially to light touch, or a feeling of numbness and tingling (paresthesias). Impairment of arterial supply to sensory nerves usually causes a stocking or glovelike loss of sensation in the involved skin, whereas loss of motor nerve function causes varying degrees of paralysis. In general, because of collateral circulation, the five Ps (pulselessness, paresthesias, paralysis, pallor, and pain) are noted at least one major joint below the site of arterial severance. The signs of ischemia are not always immediately apparent and may not develop until propagation of distal clot obliterates a large collateral; therefore, the loss of distal pulses is the earliest and at times the only sign of this type of arterial injury.

Although most completely severed arteries stop bleeding spontaneously, exceptions occur. Certain arteries (e.g., the intercostal and common iliac arteries) are surrounded by structures that either prevent their retraction into adjacent soft tissues or provide little compression of the severed ends. In patients with atherosclerosis, sufficient vasoconstriction does not always occur, and in patients with clotting disorders, the anticipated clot may not form or may dissolve spontaneously. In each of these circumstances, completely severed arteries may bleed excessively or recurrently.

Partially Severed Artery

Severance or disruption of only a portion of the arterial wall is perhaps the most important arterial injury to recognize and understand. This injury commonly produces serious or recurrent bleeding and is the forerunner of both false aneurysms and arteriovenous fistulas (Fig. 50–110). A wide variety of penetrating objects may be responsible, including

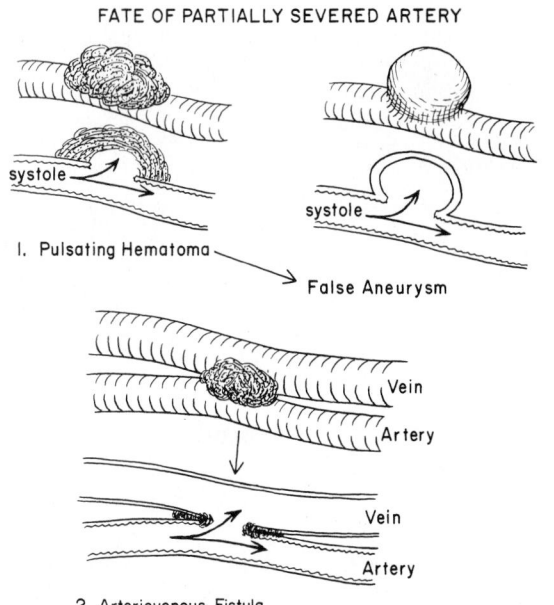

FATE OF PARTIALLY SEVERED ARTERY

1. Pulsating Hematoma

False Aneurysm

2. Arteriovenous Fistula

Figure 50–110. Partially severed arteries and those disrupted at their origin give rise to excessive or recurrent bleeding and the late development of false aneurysms or arteriovenous fistulas.

knives, missiles, drill points, needles, and catheters used in angiographic and cardiovascular monitoring techniques. Occasionally, partial severance occurs in association with closed injuries, usually as a result of bone fragments that lacerate a portion of the adjacent arterial wall.

A partially severed artery differs profoundly from a completely severed artery in many important respects. Since a portion of the arterial wall remains intact, constriction of the artery may cause retraction of the opened portion of the arterial wall, causing the arterial wound to gape. Blood loss may actually be increased in this type of injury, causing more rapid exsanguination. More often, the overlying muscles and skin tamponade the blood loss, particularly when the patient is hypotensive. This containment may be only a temporizing measure. The hematoma may gradually increase in size, particularly after the patient's blood volume has been restored and the blood pressure normalized. When the hematoma is carefully examined, it often has a pulsatile quality, since it communicates directly with the arterial lumen. Delayed or recurrent bleeding is a hallmark of a partially severed vessel. The blood clot that covers the arterial defect is more of a *patch* than a *plug*, although it occasionally protrudes into the lumen (see Fig. 50–110).

The arterial lumen is seldom narrowed initially by partial severance. Blood flow is maintained distally, and pulses may be palpated. End-organ ischemia is absent. These lesions are notoriously difficult to diagnose and are recognized only by physicians with an increased awareness of their possibility.

If the injury is unrecognized, the course of events is highly variable. Minimal wounds may heal much like the wounds that occur with diagnostic arterial punctures. However, the patient may present several days after the injury with discomfort in the region of the hematoma as it expands and stretches the overlying soft tissues. The mass may be warm and tender and the overlying skin erythematous. The mistaken impression that an abscess has developed at the site of penetration may have disastrous consequences if incision and drainage are attempted. The damaged intima may dissect some hours after injury, causing a delayed arterial occlusion. A late complication that occurs after internal resorption of

the hematoma is a false aneurysm. Arteriovenous fistulas can occur if both the artery and the vein are injured.

Nonsevered Artery

A third type of arterial injury is commonly seen when a blunt force or excessive stretch is applied to the arterial wall (see Fig. 50–109). A similar injury may follow the passage of a high-velocity missile adjacent to the vessel that causes intimal damage without actually severing the vessel's outer circumference. This form of injury is characterized by reduction or loss of flow through the artery but without external bleeding. Patients with blunt injury often have a normal examination initially, but signs of ischemia and loss of pulses develop over a variable period of time. This injury emphasizes the need for repeated evaluations of the arterial circulation in an injured patient.

This delayed obliteration of the arterial lumen may occur by one of several mechanisms (Fig. 50–111). The roughened or torn arterial intima attracts platelets, fibrin, and red cells, resulting in a traumatic thrombosis. On occasion, the flow of blood may elevate the torn distal end of the intima, creating a subintimal dissection and lifting an intimal flap that occludes the distal lumen. Moreover, even though the inner and outer coats of the artery remain intact, an intramural hematoma may form that obliterates the lumen of the artery.

Recognition that one or more of the preceding mechanisms is usually responsible for the loss of blood flow and disappearance of distal pulses has largely eliminated the concept of arterial *spasm* as a cause of arterial insufficiency. Although circular muscle fibers may contract segmentally or peripherally to narrow the arterial lumen and diminish blood flow, this phenomenon rarely obliterates pulses or causes ischemia. Spasm cannot be assumed unless angiographic evidence is irrefutable.

RECOGNITION OF ARTERIAL INJURY
History

The exact mechanism, time, and site of injury are helpful clues in recognizing arterial injury. The magnitude of a blunt force or the length of a knife blade and its direction and depth of penetration in a stab wound are important. Knowing the number and direction of bullets fired may be of benefit in assessing patients with missile injuries. The extent of bleeding, the methods used to control hemorrhage, and the amount of blood loss after injury should be ascertained from the patient or knowledgeable individuals in attendance. The patient may be aware of coolness, paresthesias (numbness or tingling), loss of sensation, or severe pain in an extremity with arterial insufficiency. All too often, however, the symptoms of ischemia are masked by the presence of other injuries.

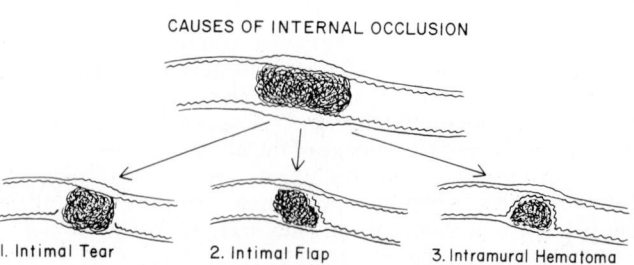

CAUSES OF INTERNAL OCCLUSION

1. Intimal Tear   2. Intimal Flap   3. Intramural Hematoma

Figure 50–111. Mechanisms of occlusion in injuries in which the outside wall of an artery is intact (nonsevered artery).

Examination

A full examination requires that the injured patient be fully disrobed to allow identification of all possible sites of injury and permit a comparison with uninjured body parts. A patient with a thready radial pulse in an uninjured arm can at best have a thready pulse in an injured extremity. The examination should include an assessment of the entire arterial system, including the presence and quality of all pulses of the neck, groin, and upper and lower extremities. In addition, auscultation is required to determine the presence or absence of bruits, especially in the area of suspected injury. The presence or suspicion of a fracture or dislocation requires a specific evaluation of adjacent vessels (Table 50–14). The extremity distal to the site of injury should be examined for pulse deficits or signs of ischemia. Fortunately, a proximal tourniquet is rarely applied by modern emergency medical technologists. If applied, its effect must be taken into consideration during the examination.

Many arteries do not have distal points for palpating pulsations, including the internal carotid, internal iliac, profunda femoris, and peroneal arteries. Other arteries such as the renal or mesenteric vessels can be assessed only by radiologic means or direct examination.

The temperature, color, degree of venous distention, and quality of pulses should be noted and compared with those in the uninjured extremity. In an ischemic extremity, distal motor function is first affected. For example, the intrinsic muscles of the hand cease to function before the extensors and flexors of the wrist. Loss of sensation to cotton touch or pinprick should be noted. In the case of a specific nerve injury, the loss of sensation follows the anatomic route of that nerve. Ischemic extremities have a stocking or glovetype pattern. If examination of the distal extremities shows definite evidence of arterial injury, angiography, operative repair, or both are done as soon as possible. It is both unwise and unnecessary to inspect the area of injury directly, since it risks contamination and rebleeding in a patient who most likely requires operative repair.

The diagnosis of arterial injury is obvious in a patient with loss or diminution of pulses distal to the site of injury, particularly when signs and symptoms of distal ischemia are present. Interestingly, several studies indicated that as many as 25% of injured peripheral arteries have palpable pulses on initial presentation,[32] thus a palpable pulse by no means excludes significant proximal arterial injury. In a patient with palpable pulses and no distal ischemia, the physician should suspect arterial injury when other *hard* signs are present: active bleeding from a penetrating wound, expanding or pulsatile hematoma, bruit, or thrill. These patients should be explored or undergo arteriography. In the past, most patients with *soft* signs of possible arterial injury from a penetrating extremity wound (history of hemorrhage or hypotension, small hematoma, adjacent nerve injury, or wound or missile track in proximity to a major artery) were also explored or had *exclusion* arteriography. Recently, several centers questioned the necessity of arteriography for occult arterial injuries of the extremities and stressed the reliability of physical examination[14, 16] and Doppler pressure measurements[21, 33] in excluding significant arterial injury. Doppler ultrasonography, when used with an ordinary blood pressure cuff, can be employed to obtain a blood pressure except under the most difficult circumstances. The pressure in the injured extremity should be the same as in the uninjured extremity. An ankle-brachial or wrist-brachial index that is less than 1.0 indicates arterial compromise. Doppler ultrasonography is also useful in detecting venous injuries and has been found to be of value in monitoring the patency of both arterial and venous reconstructions during the postoperative period. Those patients with possible occult injuries who are not studied with arteriography need close observation, and the most useful method may be duplex ultrasonography for both initial evaluation and follow-up.[5, 15]

Angiographic Study

By necessity, arteriography delays the surgical treatment of a traumatized patient. In patients with threatened uncontrolled exsanguination, immediate operative control of hemorrhage is indicated and angiography is not performed. If distal ischemia is present and the site of injury is obvious, arteriography is not required to plan the surgical procedure. If ischemia is not present, arteriography may provide a more precise diagnosis, but it is not required. If the site of injury is

---

TABLE 50–14. Vascular Injury Accompanying Skeletal Trauma

Bone Injury	Vascular Injury	Associated Findings
Fracture of first and second ribs	Transection of thoracic aorta	Widened mediastinum
Fracture of clavicle and first rib	Laceration and contusion of subclavian artery or vein; false aneurysm	Diminished pulse or blood pressure in involved arm
Dislocation of shoulder	Thrombosis of axillary artery	Diminished or absent distal pulse
Fracture of humeral shaft	Laceration of brachial artery	Diminished or absent distal pulse
Supracondylar fracture of humerus	Obstruction of brachial artery	Compartment hypertension of forearm (Volkmann's phenomenon)
Dislocation of elbow	Disruption of brachial artery	Absent radial pulse
Fracture of ribs	Laceration of intercostal artery	Hemothorax
Fracture of pelvis	Laceration of superior gluteal artery	Massive pelvic hematoma
Anterior dislocation of hip	Femoral artery contusion	Diminished or absent distal pulse
Fracture of hip	Deep femoral artery injury during operative repair	Excessive bleeding with no pulse deficit
Fracture of femoral shaft (mid or lower third)	Occlusion and laceration of femoral artery	Loss of distal pulsations; cold foot with loss of pulsation; cold foot with bleeding
Supracondylar fracture of femur	Laceration of popliteal artery or vein	Bleeding with diminished foot pulses
Dislocation of knee	Disruption and thrombosis of popliteal artery or vein	Diminished pulses with cold foot
Fracture of proximal tibia	Disruption or thrombosis of popliteal artery or vein	Diminished pulses with cold foot
Fracture of tibial shaft	Transection of anterior or posterior tibial artery	Diminished pulses with cold foot; compartmental hypertension
Dislocation of ankle	Transection and thrombosis of tibial arteries	Diminished pulses

not obvious (multiple fractures, multiple sites of penetrating injury, shotgun wounds), arteriography may be necessary to guide the surgeon to the proper injured area. Regardless of the circumstances, the patient must be accompanied by a member of the trauma team in case clinical deterioration suddenly occurs and prompt treatment is required. In an unstable patient, control of exsanguinating hemorrhage is of prime importance. An operative arteriogram can always be obtained.

In patients with arterial injury, the angiographic findings vary with the type of injury sustained. Completely severed arteries and complete occlusions arising from injuries in continuity show a sudden arrest of the column of contrast material (Fig. 50–112). In some patients, the collateral circulation may be sufficient to permit re-entry of dye into the more distal portions of the main artery, creating an angiographic gap at the site of injury. Although such collateral flow may be sufficient to prevent the development of signs of ischemia at rest, it rarely maintains a palpable distal pulse.

Angiographic studies of partially severed arteries may demonstrate the escape of contrast material from the arterial lumen. It is important to remember that the amount of contrast material outside the vessel may be relatively small in a patient with a large hematoma, because the palpable mass is composed largely of clot surrounding the arterial defect. In some patients, the resultant hematoma may actually protrude into the lumen and appear as a filling defect, not unlike an arteriosclerotic plaque (Fig. 50–113). Any distortion of the normally smooth column of dye in the vicinity of the injury should be viewed with suspicion. In patients who develop arteriovenous fistulas, visualization of the adjacent venous system as well as the sac of the false aneurysm or fistulous track confirms the diagnosis.

Patients with a pulse deficit on physical examination usu-

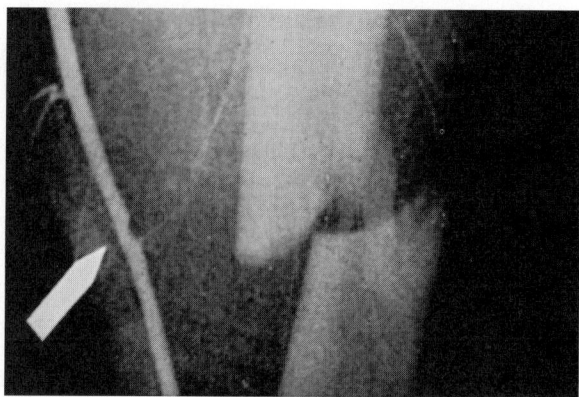

Figure 50–113. Femoral arteriogram in a patient with a closed fracture of the femur. Note the small filling defect at the site of injury, where sharp bone fragments had severed 60% of the circumference of the arterial wall.

ally have an angiographic pattern of acute occlusion. Prior to the complete loss of arterial flow, the site of injury in nonsevered arteries may be noted as an asymmetrical narrowing, a filling defect, or a point at which there is a sudden change in the diameter of the arteries. In the rare circumstance of arteriospasm causing a pulse deficit, the artery may be symmetrically narrowed, and the entire distal arterial tree may appear markedly constricted. A smooth lumen is maintained, however, and complete interruption of arterial flow does not occur.

TREATMENT

Emergency Treatment

Firm pressure applied over a site of arterial bleeding is the best method for its temporary control. Attempts to find the artery or control bleeding with clamps or ligatures usually dislodge clots and risk damage to adjacent neurovascular structures. Even well-applied but traumatic clamps may damage enough artery to convert a simple end-to-end reconstruction into a replacement graft. Proximal tourniquets other than inflatable blood pressure cuffs are rarely effective and usually only increase venous bleeding. Tourniquets that are inflated above arterial pressure occlude collateral flow, cause ischemic pain, and are not well tolerated by patients. Severe skeletal deformities with vascular compromise should be corrected and aligned as best as possible. The injured extremity should be splinted and kept level during transport. The use of military antishock trousers (MAST) or "G suits" in patients with hypotension should be recognized as potentially harmful to extremities with arterial injuries. Fortunately, these devices are usually removed after stabilization of the patient. Arterial injuries, particularly those associated with hemorrhage or, to a lesser degree, ischemia, should receive high-priority treatment. On occasion, other life-threatening injuries may require more immediate attention (restoration of airway, control of internal bleeding, intracranial hematoma). If the surgeon believes that limb loss is more likely because of these necessary delays in establishing arterial flow, the feasibility of simultaneous treatment should be considered.

Patients with partially severed arteries who are no longer bleeding and who have no evidence of distal ischemia have less emergent but nonetheless urgent problems. These pulsating hematomas are subject to recurrent bleeding. Delay of repair of large arteriovenous fistulas may cause acute, near-lethal congestive heart failure. Thus, these patients should be treated as soon as possible following diagnosis and localization of their injuries. Experience has shown that these early

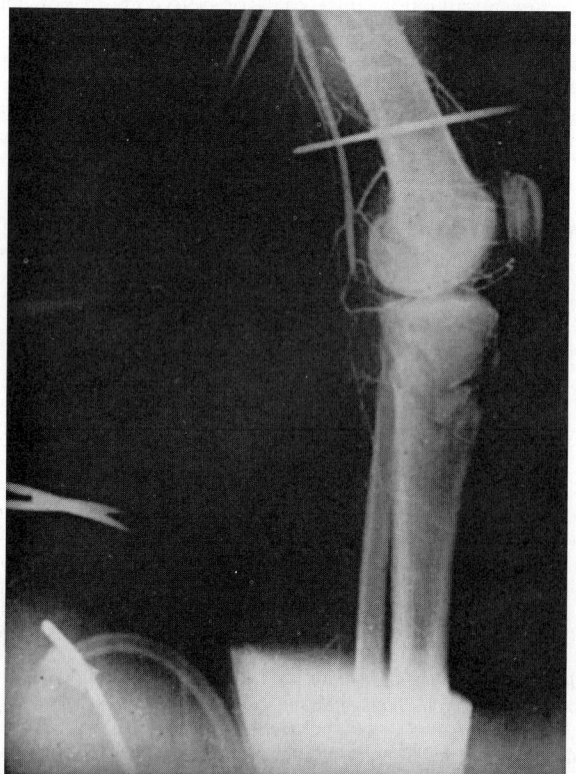

Figure 50–112. Arteriogram confirming complete occlusion of the popliteal artery associated with fracture of the tibial plateau. A fracture of the femur (not shown) and a pin previously placed for skeletal traction were other possible causes of the cold foot and loss of pulses in this patient.

repairs are more easily accomplished than are delayed repairs, and patient safety is enhanced.

Operative Repair

All major arterial injuries should be repaired when diagnosed, provided that the tissue they supply is viable, the general condition of the patient is satisfactory, and the risks of infection are not great. Notable exceptions include carotid injuries in a patient with a major fixed neurologic deficit and delayed renal pedicle injuries. In injuries to the extremities, the presence of distal cutaneous gangrene or stony hard musculature makes the benefits of revascularization questionable, but successful repair may preserve the viable tissue and permit amputation at a lower level.

Surgical repair should be undertaken promptly by a surgeon skilled in the techniques of emergency vascular surgery. Assuming hemorrhage is under control, the urgency of repair is directly related to the degree of ischemia. Re-establishment of arterial flow within 4 to 6 hours after arterial injury minimizes the possibility of permanent ischemic damage. Although every hour of delay may diminish success, there is no absolute period beyond which repair is contraindicated.

Although techniques of operative repair vary, special considerations are outlined in Table 50–13 and illustrated in Figure 50–114. In general, treatment proceeds as follows:

1. Hypovolemia and shock should be treated by controlling external blood loss and restoring blood volume. Ensure an adequate airway and ventilatory mechanism. Establish the presence and extent of all injuries and determine their priority of repair.

2. Initiate antibiotic and tetanus prophylaxis when indicated and arrange for assistants, equipment, arteriography, and the immediate availability of an adequate supply of type-specific and crossmatched blood.

3. Prepare a wide operative field and an uninvolved lower extremity for ready access to the saphenous vein, the best and safest arterial substitute for all but the largest arteries. In an extremity injury, the entire limb and proximal torso should be prepared to ensure access to all involved vessels and allow the operative evaluation of distal pulses by palpation or arteriography.

4. Localize the site of arterial injury by the location of the wound missile track, pulse deficits, or arteriography.

5. The usual incisions should be utilized for exposure of blood vessels. Sometimes the wound forces an eclectic skin incision. In these cases, the usual anatomic planes are developed so that unnecessary injury to associated structures is avoided. Proximal control is always obtained prior to entering the field of injury. In the case of groin, neck, or shoulder wounds, this may necessitate entering the abdomen or thorax.

6. Obtain control of the artery distal to the presumed site of injury to minimize the loss of blood by backbleeding. If the site of injury is inadvertently entered prior to control, balloon catheters of the Fogarty type may be inflated to control both proximally and distally. In the case of an aortic wound, a Foley catheter with a large balloon may be required.

7. Inspect or palpate the site of injury and determine the need for repair.

8. Proximal and distal control should be obtained at least 2 to 3 cm. from the site of injury so that the intima can be examined. In both penetrating and blunt trauma, the intima may be damaged beyond the obvious site of injury. This damaged intima requires resection.

9. Remove the proximal clot by flushing and the distal clot by milking the vessel, squeezing the distal limb, or passing a Fogarty balloon catheter.

10. Systemic heparinization is usually not employed in a multiply injured patient. In single wounds of an extremity requiring extensive reconstruction, the benefits probably justify the risk. In most instances, local heparinization with dilute heparinized saline (100 units per ml.) is enough to discourage local clot formation.

11. Prior to anastomosis, determine the need for graft replacement by estimating the amount of difficulty in approximating the severed ends. In general, 1 to 2 cm. of artery wall may be resected without graft replacement. This is especially true in some older patients with redundant arteries and in young patients who have healthy elastic arteries. Arterial anastomosis should not be performed under tension, but it is important not to interpret the retraction "gap" as a loss of arterial substance in making this decision.

12. Repair the injured artery using interrupted or continuous fine monofilament sutures. Smaller arteries and veins may be constricted using continuous suture techniques. In children, interrupted suture repair is preferred to ensure circumferential growth.

13. Reversed saphenous vein is the graft material of choice. Prosthetic graft material is avoided if possible because of risk of infection. In addition, late graft failure is thought to be increased when prosthetic material is used in an extremity. Prosthetic graft material, however, is preferred in the thorax and abdomen. Again, its use must be balanced against the threat of infection and the severe consequences of an infected prosthetic graft.

14. Prior to completion of the repair, the arteries are forebled and backbled. These final sutures are tied, and flow is restored. Pulses in the distal extremity should be palpable.

15. If distal pulses are not restored or the quality of arterial flow is unsatisfactory, a cause for these findings must be ascertained. If the repair is not adequate, it must be redone. If no cause is seen, an operative arteriogram that includes not only the operative site but also the distal circulation is obtained. The surgeon must assume that there is a mechanically correctable cause of this problem. The surgeon cannot assume that spasm exists unless mechanical causes have been excluded.

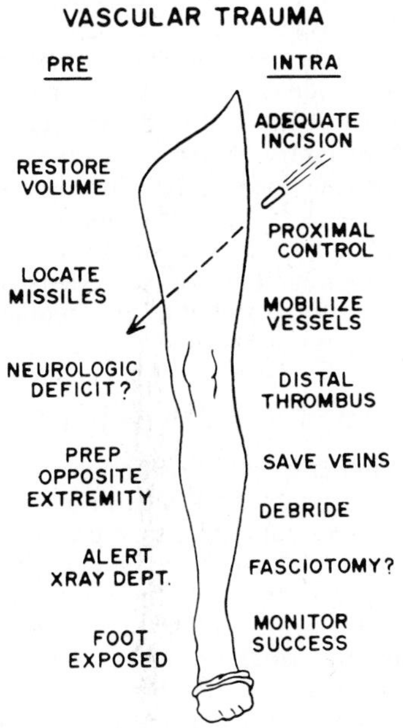

VASCULAR TRAUMA

PRE   INTRA

RESTORE VOLUME

LOCATE MISSILES

NEUROLOGIC DEFICIT?

PREP OPPOSITE EXTREMITY

ALERT XRAY DEPT.

FOOT EXPOSED

ADEQUATE INCISION

PROXIMAL CONTROL

MOBILIZE VESSELS

DISTAL THROMBUS

SAVE VEINS

DEBRIDE

FASCIOTOMY?

MONITOR SUCCESS

Figure 50–114. Important considerations prior to and during the operative treatment of a vascular injury to the lower extremity.

16. The wound should be thoroughly débrided and explored, and other injuries should be identified and repaired as necessary. Drains are occasionally employed for a period of 24 to 48 hours. Every effort is made to cover the repaired artery with viable muscle and fascia. Skin closure is dictated by the nature of the injury and risk of infection.

17. If systemic heparinization has been employed, its effects usually disappear over the several hours needed to complete the operation, and neutralization is not required. Dressings and splints should be well padded to protect anesthetic ischemic tissue. They should be applied in such a manner as to allow inspection of toes or fingers for capillary circulation, easy palpation of distal pulses, assessment of the musculature of the distal extremity, and ready access to the operative wound should bleeding occur. Any constriction of the limb should be avoided, and immobilization of fractures should be achieved by skeletal traction, posterior molds, or operative fixation (see later discussion).

POSTOPERATIVE CARE

Every effort should be made to maintain a normal intravascular volume following arterial repair. Maintenance of a satisfactory perfusion pressure is confirmed by systemic blood pressure and urinary output monitoring. Systemic anticoagulation is not required to ensure arterial patency and may be detrimental to other injuries.

Pulses distal to the site of arterial repair should be evaluated at frequent intervals by digital palpation or Doppler pressure measurements. Decreasing pulses and lowered ankle-brachial indices called for thrombosis of the arterial repair. Re-exploration is called for under these circumstances. Signs of compartmental compression syndromes and myoglobinuria should also be treated promptly.

SPECIAL PROBLEMS

Iatrogenic Arterial Injury

A frequent form of arterial injury occurs after the diagnostic or therapeutic insertion of a needle or catheter into an artery. Coronary arteriograms performed via the brachial artery at the elbow may cause a thrombosis rate as high as 25%.[27] Most thromboses involve the use of a large catheter in a small artery. Many of these injuries are benign and are unrecognized. Severe ischemia with gangrene of the finger is a rare complication. However, a significant number of patients experience pallor, coldness, numbness, or paresthesias. Depending on their occupations, many patients note diminished exercise tolerance in the forearm and hand. Cold intolerance is also increased after injury.

Iatrogenic arterial injury includes thrombosis of the radial artery following arterial blood sampling or pressure monitoring.[17] Such injuries have caused the loss of digits or the entire hand, even when the ulnar artery was present. This is most likely to occur in patients with an incomplete palmar arch. These patients can be identified before arterial cannulation by use of the Allen test. The subclavian and carotid arteries are occasionally injured during attempts to insert central venous catheters, during performance of brachial plexus or stellate ganglion anesthetic blocks, or in the course of surgical procedures to correct the thoracic outlet syndrome. Injuries to the common femoral artery and its immediate branches are also observed following catheterization of these vessels for a variety of angiograms, including coronary arteriography. The large diameter of these vessels makes thrombosis much less likely, but when it occurs, it is more likely to be associated with ischemic signs and symptoms. Withdrawal of the catheter may cause distal embolization of thrombus

that requires surgical thrombectomy or thrombolytic therapy. Bleeding after catheter withdrawal is usually controlled by direct pressure for 10 to 15 minutes. Delayed bleeding may be associated with pseudoaneurysm formation. Small pseudoaneurysms often close spontaneously. Recently, pseudoaneurysms have been successfully treated by duplex-guided manual compression, but surgical intervention is sometimes necessary, especially for anticoagulated patients.[9] Arteriovenous fistulas also occur after these studies.

The complications of transaxillary arteriography require a special note. The axillary artery is enclosed with the axillary vein and multiple nerves in a relatively inelastic neurovascular bundle. Relatively small amounts of bleeding within the sheath may cause a nerve compression syndrome. Unrecognized nerve compression may produce permanent neurologic sequelae. Therefore, special attention must be paid to patients following transaxillary arterial punctures, with hourly evaluation of strength and sensation. Even relatively minor complaints, particularly if they are new or increasing in severity, require prompt exploration.

Prompt exploration of the site of the catheterization should be done in any patient with continued bleeding, the loss of distal pulses, or the development of neurologic sequelae. Bleeding is ordinarily easily controlled with one or two sutures in the anterior puncture site. The arteries should always be explored on the posterior aspect to ensure that a second site of bleeding is not overlooked. Thrombosed arteries are opened through either a transverse or a longitudinally oriented arteriotomy. The intima must be inspected circumferentially to ensure that it has not been disrupted or dissected. The thrombus is extracted using a balloon catheter. If the posterior wall of the artery is extensively damaged, an arterial resection may be required. In small arteries opened via a longitudinal arteriotomy, a patch angioplasty may be required to ensure that the closure does not compromise the lumen of the explored artery.

Drug Abuse

Addicts who have progressively obliterated their venous channels or inexperienced *first-timers* may accidentally inject a variety of pharmacologic agents and particulate matter into arteries, with resultant ischemia and gangrene of the distal extremity. The mechanism of the ischemic changes is unclear. Although true vasospasm has been shown to be unlikely, sympathectomy has been employed as treatment. Anticoagulants and rheologic agents such as dextran are recommended but are unproven methods of treatment. Exclusion of other causes of vascular injury in drug abusers is also important. The most devastating complication in these patients is local infection at the site of injection, causing infected false aneurysms. Although some may be repaired *in situ* with autogenous tissue, other aneurysms are so extensive and infected with such virulent organisms that they require excision and extra-anatomic bypass, if possible.

Compartment Hypertension

Edema of or hemorrhage into the tight osseofascial compartment of the leg, thigh, and forearm may cause a marked increase in intracompartmental tissue pressure. The possibility of compartmental hypertension is especially great following a delayed arterial repair. During the period of ischemia, functional arterial integrity is damaged. After reconstruction and restoration of normal pressures, edema forms in the surrounding tissues. As tissue pressures increase, venous flow is first compromised. The resulting venous hypertension causes an increase in the formation of edema. These cascading events continue, with resultant nerve and muscle dysfunction. Arterial flow to the muscles of the compartment usually ceases when the tissue pressure rises to within 10 to 20 mm. of diastolic arterial pressure. Higher levels of intracompartmental pressure cause obliteration of flow in the major arteries, with reduction in distal pulses. Loss of audible Doppler flow distally is the last late finding.

A similar course has been described following venous occlusion, direct muscle trauma, vigorous exercise, deep burns, and application of MAST suits, or as a result of hemorrhage within a closed fascial space. The forearm and calf are most frequently involved. The involved compartment becomes firm to palpation, and loss of muscular function soon becomes apparent. Loss of cutaneous sensation may result when sensory nerves that pass through the compartment are subjected to increased pressure. In the lower extremity, loss of sensation may be noted in the web space at the base of the first and second digits or on the plantar surface of the foot. Distal pedal pulsations are maintained until the more advanced stages of the condition. The end result of severe untreated compartmental hypertension is the loss or replacement of ischemic muscle with fibrous tissue, causing deformity and loss of function.

Early recognition of the syndrome permits treatment before irreversible damage has occurred. Direct measurements of intracompartmental pressure by means of pressure transducers or a simple mercury manometer in line with an 18-gauge needle and plastic tubing should be made in susceptible patients. When the syndrome of significant compartmental hypertension is clinically or manometrically confirmed, it should be treated by an incision to release the trapped contents of the involved compartments (Fig. 50–115). The marked improvement in arterial flow that may follow fasciotomy in a patient with the anterior compartment syndrome is depicted in Figure 50–116. Delayed fasciotomy that exposes

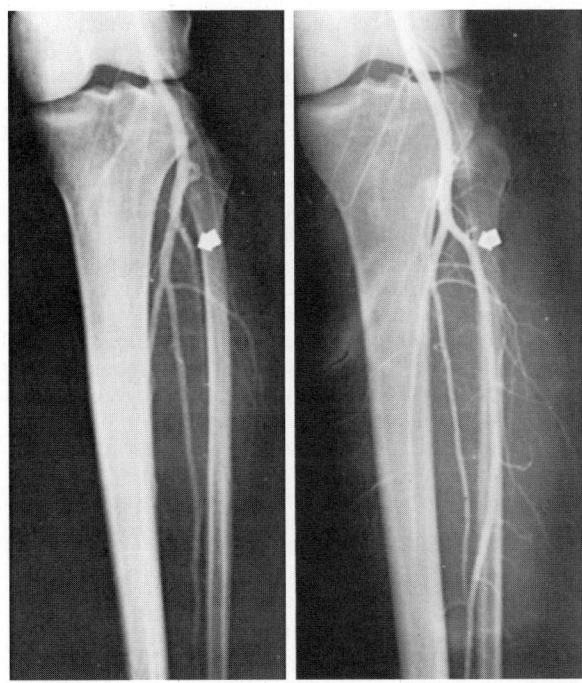

Figure 50–116. Pre- and postoperative femoral arteriograms in a patient with an anterior compartment syndrome secondary to femoral artery occlusion of over 6 hours' duration. The very small (occluded) anterior tibial artery (arrows) is much enlarged following anterior fasciotomy.

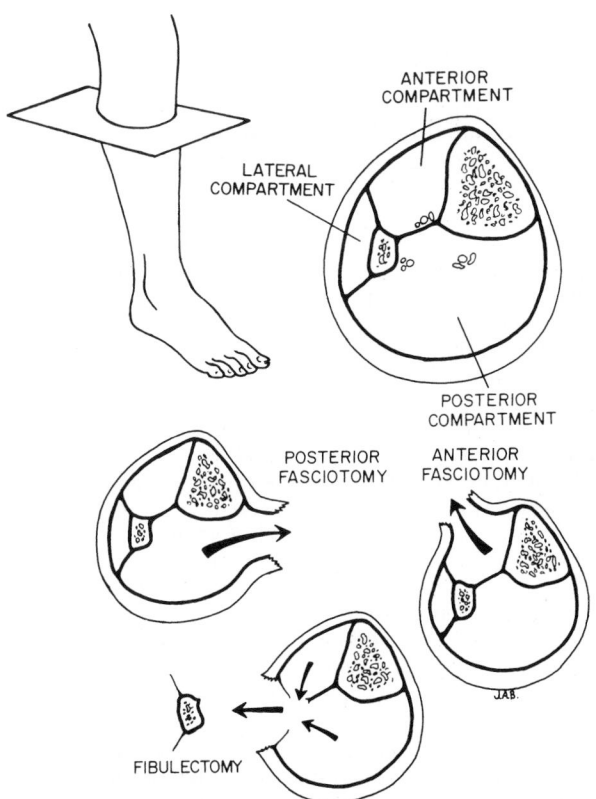

Figure 50–115. Diagram of the right calf, illustrating the muscular compartments and sites of incision to provide decompression when a rise in compartmental pressure occurs.

ischemic or necrotic muscle to hospital bacteria may induce uncontrollable infection and necessitate amputation. For this reason, some authors advocate prophylactic fasciotomy at the time of vascular repair in patients who are likely to develop compartmental hypertension, such as those with combined arterial and venous injuries or prolonged ischemia.[12]

Volkmann's ischemic contracture is a special syndrome of compartmental hypertension that develops in some children with supracondylar fractures of the humerus. Pain develops in the muscle of the forearm, with or without evidence of overt arterial injury. This pain is usually increased by efforts to extend the fingers. The radial pulse may or may not be diminished. This clinical condition must be promptly investigated. All constricting bandages or plaster should be removed and the fracture reduced by the use of skeletal traction or open reduction. Failure to obtain prompt relief of symptoms despite these maneuvers requires exploration of the brachial artery, evacuation of the hematoma, and fasciotomy of the forearm musculature.

VENOUS INJURIES

The wisdom of repairing venous injuries is being increasingly appreciated.[30] The ligation of major veins not only impairs venous return and contributes to the late development of chronic venous insufficiency but also acutely causes venous hypertension and may jeopardize the success of arterial reconstruction by contributing to the development of compartmental hypertension.

Chronic venous insufficiency is more common in patients with venous ligation as opposed to trauma victims who have had venous repair. The principles involved are the same as with arteries. Small stitches using fine monofilament suture material are required to produce the least venous constriction. Replacement of veins in the periphery is usually performed with saphenous vein taken from a contralateral or uninjured extremity. The use of a distal arteriovenous fistula to keep these sites open is usually not employed in a trauma victim. Although thrombosis at the site of repair commonly occurs, most authorities believe that even a temporary flow achieved by venous reconstruction is beneficial to the total circulation and outweighs the risks involved. Reports of pulmonary embolism from these thrombi are rare. Postoperatively, elevation of the extremity is usually employed. Fasciotomy is employed prophylactically if there is an excessive delay in repair. Postoperative anticoagulants and dextran may be used, depending on the extent of the original injury.

Reconstruction of the inferior and superior venae cavae is especially difficult. Most superior vena cava injuries are lethal. Control may require the use of cardiopulmonary bypass. The inferior vena cava is more easily controlled in its infrarenal position. The retrohepatic portion may require the use of an atriocaval shunt.[4] Replacement of the superior vena cava is usually performed with prosthetic material. Associated injuries involving the bowel and its contents may preclude the use of prosthetic material for repair of the inferior vena cava.

INJURIES TO THE AORTIC ARCH AND ITS BRANCHES

In the upper chest, arterial injuries are associated with particular difficulties in diagnosis and surgical repair. Approximately one third of these patients are hemodynamically unstable on admission and require immediate surgical intervention to control hemorrhage. This hemorrhage may reside in the thorax or in the mediastinum or may present as cervical bleeding, depending on the mode of injury. Compromise of the trachea is common.

A mortality in excess of 50% has been reported with injuries of the thoracic aorta. When blunt trauma is the mechanism of injury, only 15% of patients survive the initial insult to reach medical care.[22] Aortography is indicated in all hemodynamically stable patients suspected of having an aortic injury. Emergency thoracotomy without angiography is reserved for unstable patients with uncontrolled hemorrhage. With blunt trauma, a high clinical suspicion is necessary to diagnose the injury. Fifty per cent of the patients who reach the hospital with a blunt thoracic aortic injury have no external evidence of trauma to the chest. A widened mediastinum observed on the chest film in a patient with an appropriate mechanism of injury suggests aortic disruption. The authors recommend aortography to exclude this lesion. Computed tomography (CT) has been suggested in the past to screen high-risk patients for angiography, but a prospective study from Louisville found only a 55% sensitivity and 65% specificity for contrast-enhanced CT. The investigators thus concluded that there is no role for CT in the management of this injury.[25] Others, however, have shown that a normal CT scan effectively excludes aortic injury and suggest this study to screen stable patients with equivocal or suboptimal chest radiographs.[13, 29] Since transesophageal echocardiography can provide detailed images of the thoracic aorta and can be performed rapidly in a variety of settings, it may soon become the ideal method for screening for blunt thoracic aortic injury.[18]

A knowledge of thoracic anatomy is essential for the proper planning of surgical intervention. The ascending aorta, aortic arch, proximal innominate artery, and common carotid artery are best approached via a median sternotomy. The incision can be extended appropriately over the clavicle or into the neck. The left subclavian artery, however, is quite posterior in the upper mediastinum and is best exposed through a left third interspace anterior thoracotomy. Distal control of the subclavian arteries may require clavicular excision.

Cardiopulmonary bypass is required for ascending aortic and aortic arch reconstructions. In general, carotid shunts are not used unless both carotids or the aortic arch is being repaired. The operative repair of the descending thoracic aorta is via a generous left posterolateral thoracotomy. Placement of the proximal vascular clamp produces a marked elevation in cardiac afterload. This is usually managed pharmacologically, although left atrial-to-femoral bypass and a *Gott* shunt from the subclavian artery to the descending thoracic aorta have been employed for this purpose. The most dreaded complication is postoperative paraplegia. This complication has not been reduced by either technique. Recently, cerebrospinal fluid drainage has been used to improve spinal cord perfusion. In addition, naloxone and intrathecal papaverine have been used with some success.[1, 35] In general, suture repair of the descending aorta is impossible, and replacement grafting of a short segment is required.

CEREBROVASCULAR INJURY

The great majority (95%) of carotid arterial injuries are secondary to penetrating trauma, with over 80% of these caused by gunshot wounds. Penetrating injury is frequently associated with concomitant injury of the esophagus, pharynx, or respiratory tract. Patients with blunt carotid injuries often develop delayed neurologic symptoms, and the majority have either arterial dissection or complete thrombosis. Arterial dissections are usually effectively treated with systemic anticoagulation, but complete thromboses have high mortality rates and poor neurologic outcomes.[7]

The location of penetrating neck injuries in hemodynamically stable patients without expanding neck hematomas should alter the preoperative work-up. The authors find it helpful to divide the neck into three zones as originally described by Monson and colleagues.[26] Zone I extends from the sternal notch to the clavicles; Zone II extends from the clavicles to the angle of the mandible; Zone III extends from the angle of the mandible to the base of the skull. Proximal and distal control of the arterial system is somewhat more hazardous in Zones I and III. Thus, in a stable patient who is not bleeding, the authors routinely perform angiography to identify vascular injuries prior to surgical therapy. In Zone II, exploration may be performed without angiography, since arterial injuries in this location are readily controlled and repaired.

Although some surgeons advocate selective exploration of penetrating Zone II wounds based on clinical findings and diagnostic tests (arteriography, panendoscopy, barium swallow), the minimal morbidity of neck exploration and the high cost of missed injuries probably favor routine exploration.[24] However, both methods are acceptable.

The operation is begun with control of the airway. If extensive tracheal deviation or compression is present, fiberoptic orotracheal intubation or cricothyroidotomy may be required.[11] The chest and mediastinum are prepared in the operative field such that rapid sternotomy can be performed if needed. An incision is made that parallels the anterior border of the sternocleidomastoid muscle. Proximal carotid control is achieved first, followed by distal control. The need for heparinization is debated. Certainly in patients with multiple trauma or head injuries, its use is hazardous. Arterial repair is performed with either a primary anastomosis or an interposition graft. Autogenous vein is the graft of choice.

Hemorrhage is an obvious indication for operation, regardless of neurologic status. Patients with intimal flaps or nonoccluding thrombus who are neurologically intact undergo reconstruction; a good outcome is anticipated. A more controversial management problem involves a neurologically impaired patient with a carotid injury. Patients with neurologic deficits exclusive of coma seem to do better with reconstruction.[19] In a patient with coma, most surgeons repair a carotid artery if prograde flow is present. If the carotid artery is thrombosed, there is concern that restoration of flow may contribute to brain edema and worsening of the patient. Contrariwise, there are isolated cases of neurologic recovery in comatose patients after restoration of internal carotid flow.[3, 31] Thus, the treatment of unconscious patients remains controversial.

INTRA-ABDOMINAL VASCULAR INJURY

Abdominal vascular injuries are usually discovered at the time of emergency laparotomy. Exploration of midline hematomas is mandated to prevent the late sequelae of unrecognized aortic injury. Prior to exploration of these hematomas, proximal control is advisable. In a patient with precarious vital signs and a tense abdomen, control of the thoracic aorta at the level of the diaphragm through a low thoracic incision is advocated as a preliminary maneuver. When the abdomen is entered, proximal control of the aorta is obtained at the lowest possible level. Patients with prolonged hepatic and renal ischemia do poorly. Exploration of the upper abdominal aorta may be facilitated by the retroperitoneal approach from the left side with medial rotation of the viscera.[23]

Repair of intra-abdominal vascular injuries may require the use of the saphenous vein. Thus, one or both thighs should always be included in the preoperative preparation and draping. It is preferable to obtain saphenous vein in almost all cases of a contaminated abdomen rather than use prosthetic material, but for the aorta, prosthetic grafts may be unavoidable.

RENAL ARTERY INJURY

Trauma involving the renal artery is uncommon, with approximately 75% of these injuries being secondary to blunt trauma.[6] The mechanism of injury is usually a deceleration force, with the relatively mobile kidney pulling away from the fixed aorta. The diagnosis is usually established in multiple trauma patients by CT or intravenous pyelography, which demonstrates a nonfunctioning kidney. Arteriography is usually recommended in stable patients if time permits.

The kidney tolerates warm ischemia poorly. If the renal artery is occluded and collateral circulation is poor, probable irreversible renal damage occurs by 90 minutes. The management of these patients is controversial; the authors routinely explore patients who can obviously tolerate laparotomy and in whom early restoration of flow (within hours) can be anticipated. There are isolated reports of salvage of renal function many days to years after renal artery occlusion,[8, 36] but in general, these reports represent incomplete occlusion or occlusion of a stenotic lesion with well-developed collaterals. In patients with abrupt, complete renal artery occlusion without pre-existing stenosis, the salvage rate of kidneys is dismal.[6] Dean[10] suggested that a less aggressive approach toward attempted retrieval of renal function is appropriate, especially when there is no visualization of the distal artery (i.e., no collateral flow) on arteriography.

Exploration of the renal artery is usually performed via a midline laparotomy to allow examination of the intraperitoneal organs. The small bowel is packed to the right, and dissection is performed at the base of the mesentery, where the origin of the involved renal artery is controlled at the aorta. Alternatively, each kidney can be exposed, with anterior reflection of the colon. Dissection of the artery is extended distally past the injured segment. This segment is marked by a bluish discoloration of the wall secondary to the dissection. A longitudinal arteriotomy is made in the proximal artery and extended distally to normal lumen. The injured segment is resected. With mobilization of the kidney, a primary anastomosis is usually possible. If tension prohibits a primary anastomosis, a bypass graft is indicated. In the pediatric population, care must be taken not to use saphenous vein, since a high incidence of late aneurysmal degeneration occurs; most authors prefer hypogastric artery. Polytetrafluoroethylene or Dacron is suitable in adults if contamination is absent.

POPLITEAL ARTERY INJURY

Following dislocation of the knee, spontaneous reduction often occurs, and the radiograph reveals only soft tissue swelling. Early after injury, flow may be maintained in the injured popliteal artery. Thus, close observation or arteriography is recommended for all patients with either anterior or posterior dislocations of the knee. This injury is especially dangerous, because swelling associated with knee dislocation often obliterates the precarious collateral circulation around the knee. If distal pulses are absent, immediate operative repair is mandatory.[20] Confirmation by arteriography is usually unnecessary, but if deemed advisable, it can be performed on the operating table just prior to exploration of the popliteal vessels. Every effort should be made to restore flow in the distal arteries as soon as possible after injury.

The incision should be extended well up into the medial thigh for proximal control and distally into the calf to aid exposure and facilitate clot removal from the main branches of the popliteal artery. The incision also serves to decompress the muscles of the medial compartment of the leg. If the patient's condition, other injuries, or orthopedic considerations significantly delay immediate arterial reconstruction, a temporary shunt can be employed between the severed ends to maintain flow.[34]

Definitive arterial repair often requires a vein graft utilizing the saphenous vein from the opposite extremity. Both dorsalis pedis and posterior tibial pulses should return promptly; if not, a completion arteriogram should be obtained. The popliteal vein should be inspected, and if it is thrombosed or disrupted, it should also be repaired.

Postoperatively, careful monitoring of the distal pulses, preferably with the use of Doppler-derived pressures, should be done, as with any arterial reconstruction. Any loss of pulses or signs of ischemia should be evaluated immediately for the possibility of occlusion of the repair or the development of a compartmental syndrome, and appropriate treatment should be instituted.

VASCULAR AND ORTHOPEDIC INJURIES

Arterial injuries associated with open or closed fractures and dislocations are outlined in Table 50–14. Recognition of the vascular injury is often obscured by the difficulties of examining the painful, swollen extremity that accompanies bone injury. More often than not, however, it is the failure to assess the status of the distal extremity or to appreciate the significance of a large hematoma, recurrent bleeding, and distal ischemia that causes delay in recognition of arterial injury. A distressing preoccupation with bone abnormalities observed on the radiologic study is all too common in the care of extremity injuries and must be avoided to prevent the tragic consequences of overlooked arterial injury.

The diagnosis and principles of repair are similar to those for other arterial injuries, except for the problem of achieving stabilization of the fracture fragments adjacent to the arterial repair. Both orthopedic and vascular surgeons prefer to stabilize the bones prior to arterial repair.[2] This operative sequence provides a stable environment in which to perform arterial reconstructive surgery. To reverse the operative sequence invites disruption of the artery during orthopedic manipulation. However, this operative sequence promotes an increase in the ischemia time, which may not be tolerated in a truly compromised limb. Thus, the following plan has evolved. Patients with arterial injuries but with warm, pink feet are treated in the preferred manner. Patients who have severely ischemic feet have the orthopedic stabilization performed prior to arterial repair only when orthopedic stabilization can be achieved within a relatively short time (60 minutes). If stabilization will require a long time and there has been some delay in reaching the operating room, arterial repair is accomplished first.

Venous injuries should be repaired concomitantly. The combination of arterial injury, venous injury, and soft tissue injury associated with fracture makes these patients especially prone to develop compartment syndromes. Constricting bandages are avoided. Plaster casts are split longitudinally so that they do not contribute to the development of compression. Prophylactic fasciotomy is recommended if severe trauma exists, particularly if there has been a delay in restoration of flow.

SHOTGUN WOUNDS

Arterial injuries arising from shotgun wounds pose unique clinical problems. In close-range injuries (those in which the gun muzzle is adjacent to the area of injury), the amount of destruction to adjacent nerves, veins, and soft tissue often precludes successful restoration of function. Wide débridement of devitalized tissue, including skin and muscle, is required, and the remaining arterial ends usually have to be bridged by a long segment of reversed saphenous vein. The exposed arterial anastomoses and graft must be covered with viable tissue to prevent drying and disruption, and this often necessitates the transfer of adjacent uninvolved muscle or skin. The risk of infection is high, and the deleterious effects of bacteria on the suture lines and graft must be carefully monitored.

Shotgun wounds received at some distance from the muzzle cause minimal tissue damage, but the multiple pellets scattered beneath the skin may penetrate arteries over long distances and in multiple locations. Liberal use of arteriography is advisable to detect sites of injury and their late sequelae.

INTERVENTIONAL RADIOGRAPHY

Improved techniques of interventional radiography have widened the armamentarium for the treatment of vascular injuries. The ability to guide an arterial catheter into nearly every artery and its main branches permits a skilled radiologist to arrest bleeding or occlude false aneurysms by embolization techniques or the inflation of small detachable balloons. This method has proved particularly effective in controlling bleeding from severed branches of the internal iliac artery, which are often responsible for the massive blood loss accompanying pelvic fractures.[28] Difficulties with identifying and controlling vascular injuries at the time of laparotomy and the lack of serious sequelae from distal embolization of the internal iliac artery have made this the preferred method of control of this arterial injury. Similar applications have occasionally been utilized in injuries involving arteries to the abdominal viscera (e.g., traumatic hemobilia) and intra- and extracerebral vessels.

LATE SEQUELAE OF VASCULAR INJURY

Failure to recognize the existence of a vascular injury may cause acute or chronic ischemia. The most tragic examples are young men and women who sustain orthopedic injuries. Their fractures and dislocations are realigned, but amputation sometimes results. In some patients, amputation is avoided, but chronic ischemia causes intermittent claudication, ischemic rest pain, or Raynaud's phenomenon. Delayed arterial repair may cause ischemic neuropathy. This neuropathy is in a glove or stocking distribution and usually improves over months.

Partially severed arteries and those in which a major branch is completely detached at its junction with a main artery often develop false aneurysms. Initially, this may present as a pulsating hematoma, but eventually, the hematoma undergoes organization, with fibrous tissue replacement and the formation of a thick-walled sac. Since this wall is composed of fibrous tissue elements not derived from the artery and, as such, lacks elastic fibers, the continued expansion of this *false* aneurysm is inevitable. The distal extremity or organ supplied is seldom ischemic, and distal pulses are usually maintained unless thrombus within the aneurysm has embolized. The patient usually presents with a pulsating mass or because of signs or symptoms of compression on adjacent structures. Auscultation reveals a systolic bruit, and a systolic thrill may be palpable. Treatment is usually advisable and consists of surgical excision of the aneurysm, with restoration of arterial flow. Under special circumstances, angiographic embolization or thrombosis of aneurysms is occasionally undertaken. Compression of the fistula on physical examination slows the heart rate (Branham's sign). In large fistulas, high-output cardiac failure may occur.

It is important to auscultate areas of old injury or operation in any patient with unexplained heart failure to detect these lesions and correct the underlying cardiac problem. Treatment is surgical and requires permanent obliteration of the fistula, usually by excision of the involved segment of artery, with restoration of arterial flow and ligation or repair of the adjacent vein.

SELECTED REFERENCES

Bongard, F. S., Wilson, S. E., and Perry, M. O. (Eds.): Vascular Injuries in Surgical Practice. Norwalk, CT, Appleton & Lange, 1991.
    A concise text that offers a thorough review of the management of vascular injuries.

Flanigan, D. P. (Ed.): Civilian Vascular Trauma. Philadelphia, Lea & Febiger, 1992.
    This multiauthored text provides comprehensive coverage of all aspects of civilian vascular trauma in 47 chapters, beginning with the history of vascular trauma and wound ballistics and ending with litigation in and the epidemiology and economics of vascular trauma.

Moore, E. E., Mattox, K. L., and Feliciano, D. V. (Eds.): Trauma. Norwalk, CT, Appleton & Lange, 1991.
    This is the definitive, comprehensive textbook on trauma and has excellent, detailed chapters on vascular trauma written by top experts in the field.

Perry, M. O.: The Management of Acute Vascular Injuries. Baltimore, Williams & Wilkins, 1981.
    A personal perspective of the approach to vascular trauma based on an extensive civilian experience.

Rich, N. M., and Spencer, F. C.: Vascular Trauma. Philadelphia, W. B. Saunders, 1978.
    A comprehensive review of vascular trauma by military-oriented surgeons.

REFERENCES

1. Acher, C. W., Wynn, M. M., Hoch, J. R., et al.: Combined use of cerebral spinal fluid drainage and naloxone reduces the risk of paraplegia in thoracoabdominal aneurysm repair. J. Vasc. Surg., *19*:236, 1994.
2. Bishara, R. A., Pasch, A. R., Lim, L. T., et al.: Improved results in the

treatment of civilian vascular injuries associated with fractures and dislocations. J. Vasc. Surg., 3:707, 1986.

3. Brown, M. F., Graham, J. M., Feliciano, D. V., et al.: Carotid artery injuries. Am. J. Surg., 144:748, 1982.

4. Burch, J. M., Feliciano, D. V., and Mattox, K. L.: The atriocaval shunt—facts and fiction. Ann. Surg., 207:555, 1988.

5. Bynoe, R. P., Miles, W. S., Bell, R. M., et al.: Noninvasive diagnosis of vascular trauma by duplex ultrasonography. J. Vasc. Surg., 14:346, 1991.

6. Cass, A. S.: Renovascular injuries from external trauma: Diagnosis, treatment, and outcome. Urol. Clin. North Am., 16:213, 1989.

7. Cogbill, T. H., Moore, E. E., Meissner, M., et al.: The spectrum of blunt injury to the carotid artery: A multicenter perspective. J. Trauma, 37:473, 1994.

8. Cosby, R. L.: Traumatic renal artery thrombosis. Am. J. Med., 81:890, 1988.

9. Cox, G. S., Young, J. R., Gray, B. R., et al.: Ultrasound-guided compression repair of postcatheterization pseudoaneurysms: Results of treatment in one hundred cases. J. Vasc. Surg., 19:683, 1994.

10. Dean, R. H.: Management of renal artery trauma. J. Vasc. Surg., 8:89, 1988.

11. Feliciano, D. V.: A new look at penetrating carotid artery injuries. In Maull, K. I., Cleveland, H. C., Feliciano, D. V., et al. (Eds.): Advances in Trauma and Critical Care. Vol. 9. St. Louis, C. V. Mosby, 1994.

12. Field, C. K., Senkowsky, J., Hollier, L. H., et al.: Fasciotomy in vascular trauma: Is it too much, too often? Am. Surg., 60:409, 1994.

13. Fisher, R. G., Chasen, M. H., and Lamki, N.: Diagnosis of injuries of the aorta and brachiocephalic arteries caused by blunt chest trauma: CT vs. aortography. A. J. R. Am. J. Roentgenol., 162:1047, 1994.

14. Francis, H., Thal, E. R., Weigelt, J. A., and Redman, H. C.: Vascular proximity: Is it a valid indication for arteriography in asymptomatic patients? J. Trauma, 31:512, 1991.

15. Fry, W. R., Smith, R. S., Sayers, D. V., et al.: The success of duplex ultrasonographic scanning in the diagnosis of extremity vascular proximity trauma. Arch. Surg., 128:1368, 1993.

16. Frykberg, E. R., Dennis, J. W., Bishop, K., Laneve, L., and Alexander, R. H.: The reliability of physical examination in the evaluation of penetrating extremity trauma for vascular injury: Results at one year. J. Trauma, 31:502, 1991.

17. Johnson, F. E., Sumner, D. S., and Strandness, D. E., Jr.: Extremity necrosis caused by indwelling arterial catheters. Am. J. Surg., 131:375, 1976.

18. Kearney, P. A., Smith, D. W., Johnson, S. B., et al.: Use of transesophageal echocardiography in the evaluation of traumatic aortic injury. J. Trauma, 34:696, 1993.

19. Liekweg, W. G., Jr., and Greenfield, L. J.: Management of penetrating carotid arterial injury. Ann. Surg., 188:587, 1978.

20. Lim, L. T., Michuda, M. S., Flanigan, D. P., and Pankovitch, A.: Popliteal artery trauma. Arch. Surg., 115:1307, 1980.

21. Lynch, K., and Johansen, K.: Can Doppler pressure measurements replace "exclusion" arteriography in the diagnosis of occult extremity arterial trauma? Ann. Surg., 214:737, 1991.

22. Mattox, K. L.: Approaches to trauma involving the major vessels of the thorax. Surg. Clin. North Am., 69:77, 1989.

23. Mattox, K. L., McCollum, W. B., Beall, A. C., Jr., Gordan, G. L., and DeBakey, M. E.: Management of penetrating injuries of the suprarenal aorta. J. Trauma, 15:808, 1975.

24. Meyer, J. P., Barrett, J. A., Schuler, J. J., et al.: Mandatory vs. selective exploration for penetrating neck trauma. Arch. Surg., 122:592, 1987.

25. Miller, F. B., Richardson, J. D., Thomas, H. A., Cryer, H. M., and Willing, S. J.: Role of CT in diagnosis of major arterial injury after blunt thoracic trauma. Surgery, 106:596, 1989.

26. Monson, D. O., Saletta, J. D., and Freeark, R. J.: Carotid vertebral trauma. J. Trauma, 9:987, 1969.

27. Nicholas, G. G., and Demuth, W. E.: Long term results of brachial thrombectomy following cardiac catheterization. Ann. Surg., 183:436, 1976.

28. Panetta, T., Sclafani, S. J., Goldstein, A. S., Phillips, T. F., and Shaftan, G. W.: Percutaneous transcatheter embolization for massive bleeding from pelvic fractures. J. Trauma, 25:1021, 1985.

29. Raptopoulos, V., Sheiman, R. G., Phillips, D. A., Davidoff, A., and Silva, W. E.: Traumatic aortic tear: Screening with chest CT. Radiology, 182:667, 1992.

30. Rich, N. M.: Management of venous trauma. Surg. Clin. North Am., 68:809, 1988.

31. Robbs, J. V., Hum, R. R., Rajaruthman, P., et al.: Neurologic deficits and injuries involving the neck arteries. Br. J. Surg., 70:220, 1983.

32. Saletta, J. D., and Freeark, R. J.: The partially severed artery. Arch. Surg., 96:198, 1968.

33. Schwartz, M. R., Weaver, F. A., Bauer, M., Siegel, A., and Yellin, A. E.: Refining the indications for arteriography in penetrating extremity trauma: A prospective analysis. J. Vasc. Surg., 17:116, 1993.

34. Shah, D. M., Naraynsingh, V., Leather, K. P., Corson, J. D., and Karmody, A. M.: Advances in the management of acute popliteal vascular blunt injuries. J. Trauma, 25:793, 1985.

35. Svensson, L. G., Grum, D. F., Bednarski, M., Cosgrove, D. M., and Loop, F. D.: Appraisal of cerebrospinal fluid alterations during aortic surgery with intrathecal papaverine administration and cerebrospinal fluid drainage. J. Vasc. Surg., 11:423, 1990.

36. Weimann, S., Flora, G., Dittrich, P., Mikuz, G., and Bartsch, G.: Traumatic renal artery occlusion: Is late reconstruction advisable? J. Urol., 137:727, 1987.

ACUTE ARTERIAL OCCLUSION

Thomas J. Fogarty, M.D.
Amitava Biswas, M.D.

Reference to occlusion of the arterial circulation was first made by Harvey in 1628.[14] Labey has been credited with the first successful surgical removal of an arterial embolus in 1911.[16] Heparin—discovered in 1916 and made clinically available in 1936, when used by Best[4]—provided surgeons with a means of preventing thrombosis during the repair and manipulation of blood vessels. A review of the surgical literature prior to 1960 indicates that the operative approach to acute arterial occlusion was limited by the lack of a simple and effective method for removing the embolus and distally propagated thrombus. Some of the methods employed included retrograde flushing with saline, suction catheters, vein strippers, and local removal through multiple and lengthy arteriotomies. None of these surgical techniques was particularly effective in reducing the high morbidity (50%) and mortality (50%) associated with acute arterial occlusions. The introduction of the balloon catheter technique in 1963 dramatically simplified the technical aspects of surgical therapy for acute arterial occlusion.[11]

PATHOLOGY

Historically, the primary source of acute arterial occlusion has been embolization from the heart as a result of underlying rheumatic valvular disease. Today, the primary cardiac disorder is atherosclerotic heart disease. Manifestations of this disease include myocardial infarction, atrial fibrillation, congestive heart failure, and ventricular aneurysm. The decline in the prevalence of rheumatic heart disease has led to a decreased incidence of acute occlusion caused by embolization from mitral stenosis.[1, 22] At the same time, advances in cardiac procedures and an overall improvement in medical care have increased life spans, resulting in a significant increase in the incidence of systemic atherosclerosis and thrombotic occlusions of peripheral vessels. In the past 2 decades, occlusion from *in situ* thrombosis has surpassed occlusion from embolization as the major cause of acute arterial closure.[7]

Regardless of the source or histologic structure of an acute arterial occlusion, it is the location of and secondary events following the occlusion that determine the viability of the afflicted extremity. The majority of surgically treatable occlusions lodge in the lower extremities. Following occlusion, a softer coagulum of blood forms in the areas of decreased flow. In 1941, Linton[18] emphasized that this propagation of thrombus is of major importance in the outcome of the disease process. Distal and proximal propagation of the thrombus also occurs to varying degrees in situations of *in situ* thrombosis (Fig. 50–117).

Compromised oxygenation of tissue distal to the site of the occlusion leads to an anaerobic cellular metabolism in which tissue becomes acidotic. Elevated concentrations of potassium ions, lactic acid, P_{CO_2}, and the intracellular enzymes (creatine phosphokinase and lysozymes) are released into the bloodstream and interstitial tissue. The ischemic state affects the neural tissue, which induces the symptoms of localized pain and paresthesia. Without proper intervention, these symptoms are followed by muscle swelling and rigor. Tissue necrosis typically occurs after 6 to 12 hours of total ischemia. Further propagation of the distal clot can eventually lead to venous thrombosis (Fig. 50–118).

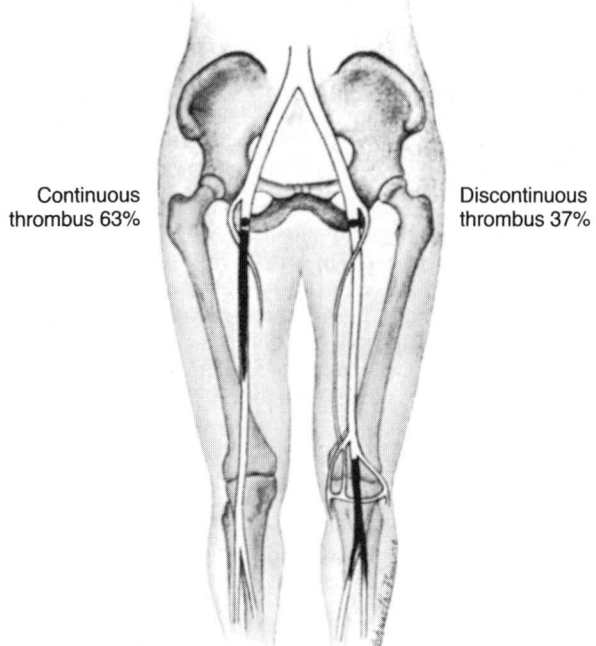

Continuous
thrombus 63%

Discontinuous
thrombus 37%

Figure 50–117. Incidence of discontinuous propagation of thrombus.

PREOPERATIVE EVALUATION AND CARE

Arterial emboli most commonly occur in elderly, seriously ill patients with multiple systemic diseases. Prolonged periods of surgical manipulation and general anesthesia have been considered valid deterrents to operative intervention in such patients—particularly when the clinical analysis indicates that conservative measures might preserve life at the cost of limb loss or functional impairment.

The possibility of a successful procedure is obviously dependent on the degree and extent of ischemia at the time of presentation. The condition of the extremity, rather than the duration of the occlusion, represents the primary determinant of operability. Reports in the literature are often confusing because the degree of ischemia has not been documented in assessing the outcome. In a series of 500 patients, every

TABLE 50–15. Time Interval in Relation to Advanced Ischemia (500 Patients, 570 Embolectomy Procedures)

Age of Embolus	Advanced Ischemia (%)	Amputation (%)
1–24 hr.	12	1.5
24–48 hr.	37	5.3
2–90 days	49	12.5

occlusion requiring emergent surgical intervention was characterized by loss of sensation and proprioception in the affected limb. Loss of motor function was present in 20% of the patients, and early rigor in 8%. In the absence of these three signs—loss of sensation and proprioception, loss of motor function, and early rigor—operation for acute occlusion may be considered urgent or even elective. In this same series, successful surgical intervention was possible even after prolonged periods of occlusion (Table 50–15). Even in the presence of established gangrene, a successful embolectomy often allows a lower-level amputation.

Patients presenting with an acute arterial occlusion should be assumed to have significant underlying heart disease. The large number of patients presenting with atherosclerotic heart disease reinforces the concept that evaluation of cardiac function should proceed simultaneously with evaluation of the peripheral vasculature. Digitalis, antiarrhythmic agents, morphine, diuretics, and heparin are essential to patient care. However, use of these agents should not delay surgical intervention.

Noninvasive Doppler ultrasound techniques and pressure and waveform measurements are useful in the preoperative setting. They can typically be performed in 5 to 10 minutes, and they provide a useful preoperative benchmark against which to compare postoperative results. In situations of overt advanced ischemia, a physical examination is sufficient. At the time of diagnosis of acute arterial occlusion, 5000 units of intravenous heparin is immediately administered. The presence of congestive heart failure, cardiogenic shock, and significant arrhythmias requires monitoring in the intensive care unit. Placement of a central venous catheter is required in the majority of patients. In addition to allowing rapid administration of drugs and fluids, the catheter permits mon-

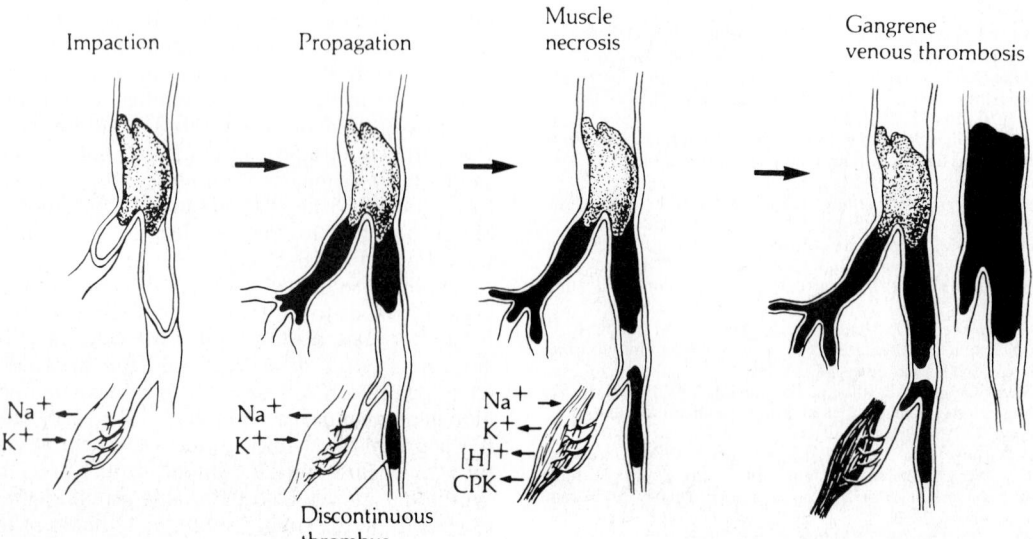

Impaction   Propagation   Muscle necrosis   Gangrene venous thrombosis

Na⁺
K⁺

Na⁺
K⁺

Discontinuous
thrombus

Na⁺
K⁺
[H]⁺
CPK

Figure 50–118. Process of discontinuous thrombus propagation.

itoring of central venous pressures. The pulmonary artery pressure should be monitored in those patients who present with hemodynamic instability or congestive heart failure.

In the presence of an embolus in a lower extremity, the possibility of simultaneous emboli in mesenteric or renal arteries should always be entertained. Hematuria or abdominal complaints indicative of a possible occlusion require preoperative visualization of these vessels. It should be kept in mind that involvement of more than one extremity occurs in approximately 10% of such patients.

INSTRUMENTATION

The balloon embolectomy catheter was constructed with specific adaptations for safe, effective extraction of arterial emboli (Fig. 50–119). It consists of a hollow, pliable catheter body in graduated sizes for use in major vessels of any caliber. At its proximal end, the syringe fitting provides the means for fluid exchange into a soft elastomeric balloon located at its distal tip. The instrument is inserted as far as possible into the acutely occluded vessel. The balloon is then inflated and withdrawn in the inflated position. By a mechanism of fluid displacement, the balloon maintains uniform, even contact with the vessel wall as it proceeds through areas of narrowing (Fig. 50–120). This mechanism allows removal of thrombotic material distal to stenotic areas. The surgeon manipulates both the syringe and the catheter during withdrawal. In this way, it is easy to judge both the amount of traction required for extraction of the occluding material and the quantity of fluid necessary to effect alternate inflation and deflation as the instrument proceeds through areas of atherosclerotic narrowing or vessels of increasing or decreasing diameter.

The concept of the balloon catheter for embolectomy has remained basically the same since its introduction in 1963. There have been only minor changes in the instrument to increase its effectiveness and reduce the incidence of complications. A variety of balloon configurations and catheter materials have been evaluated. Although balloon catheters with self-adjusting pressure mechanisms and spiked balloon catheters initially appeared to be improvements, their routine use has been associated with significant disadvantages. The utility and effectiveness of the original instrument are tied to its

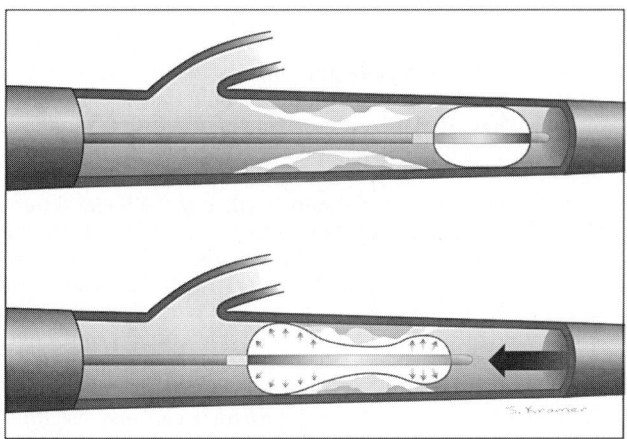

Figure 50–120. Depiction of Fogarty embolectomy catheter maintaining uniform fluid displacement as balloon is drawn through vessel lumen narrowed by atherosclerotic deposits.

simplicity, and attempts to incorporate nonessential refinements have not proved advantageous or practical. Double-lumen embolectomy catheters are now available, and they have significant utility when used in conjunction with fluoroscopy for selective placement into vessels below a bifurcation point. The thru-lumen catheters can be used for distal irrigation, particularly in situations in which fibrinolytic agents are required as an adjunct to surgical procedures (Fig. 50–121).

The significant increase of acute occlusions from *in situ* thrombus versus embolic events, combined with the association of such acute thrombotic occlusions with a high incidence of adherent thrombotic material, has produced a need for improved instrumentation for the removal of this more-adherent thrombus. Two new nonballoon catheter systems have been developed to address the problem of adhered thrombus, which is often found at the area of critical narrowing.

The first nonballoon catheter system, called the *adherent clot catheter* (ACC), was designed specifically for use in native vessels. The second system, called the *graft thrombectomy catheter* (GTC), was designed for use in synthetic grafts. The technique and use of these instruments are not dissimilar to those for the original balloon embolectomy catheter. These catheters were designed to allow the surgeon to respond to the requirements for removal of the more dense and adherent clot associated with *in situ* thrombosis.

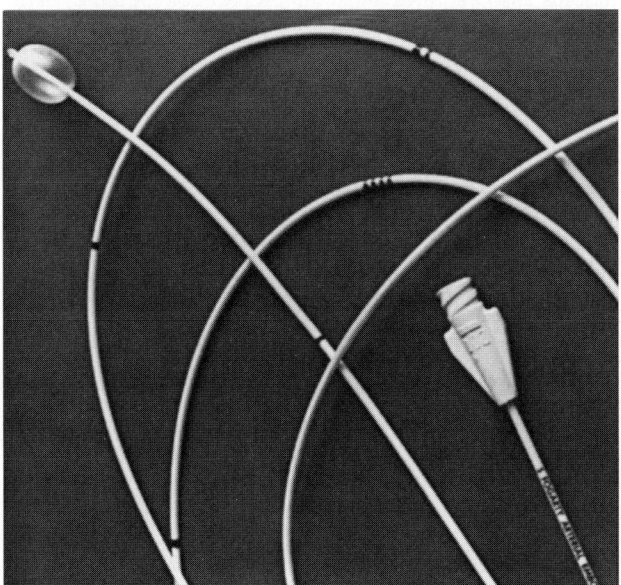

Figure 50–119. Fogarty catheter for extraction of arterial emboli and thrombus. Depth markings on catheter body indicate distance of balloon from arteriotomy.

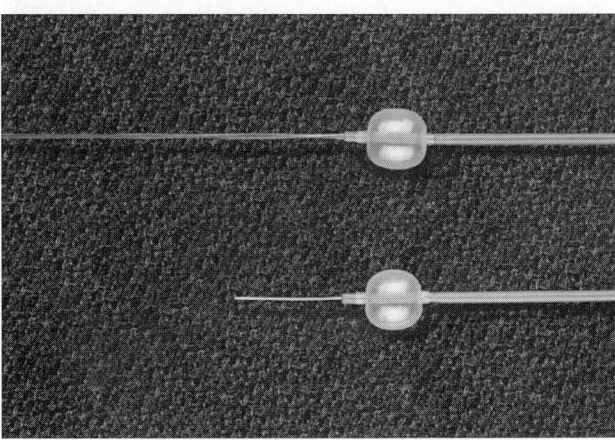

Figure 50–121. Thru-lumen catheter shown with balloon inflated. Fluid instillation or guidewire passage is facilitated with this catheter system.

The initial extraction of thrombus is performed with the standard balloon embolectomy catheter. A critical aspect that is often unappreciated is the information that can be obtained by examining the removed thrombotic material. The removed material should be laid on a towel for visual examination. By viewing this material as a cast of the artery from which it has been removed, one can gain significant insight into both the amount of material remaining and the linear length and location of that material vis-à-vis the arteriotomy. By the simple expedient of noting what is not present, one can safely assume that the residual material still lies within the vessel (Fig. 50–122).

After removal and examination of the softer propagated thrombus, the ACC is introduced in the low-profile configuration. Once past the area of residual material, the catheter is deployed by a button on the proximal end and assumes the shape of a corkscrew. This spiral configuration increases the surface area for traction on the clot without increasing the shear stress on the arterial wall. As with the balloon catheter, the surgeon can influence the diameter of the spiral by manipulating the proximal button. Moving the button back and forth increases or decreases the diameter in response to the force necessary to remove the adherent material (Fig. 50–123).

The GTC is similar in design to the ACC. Essentially, it can be viewed as a variable-diameter ring stripper, for use specifically in synthetic grafts. The body is pliable, and the surgeon can control the diameter of the helix during use. The technique employed is much like that for the ACC (Fig. 50–124). The balloon embolectomy catheter is initially used to remove the propagated thrombus. Again, one can determine the location of the residual densely adherent pannus by examining the removed thrombus. In the setting of aortic bifurcation grafts, the residual material usually lies at the bifurcation or in an area of sharp angulation. Another common area for residual material is the distal anastomotic site of the graft. Therefore, the incision is always made over the junction of the anastomotic site distally, which allows the surgeon to remove the adherent pannus directly or to do an endarterectomy.

After removal of the initial soft clot, an occlusion balloon is employed, followed by the GTC. The occluding balloon catheter is threaded through the helix of the bare wire of the GTC. Proximal occlusion using a balloon avoids the necessity for a proximal major abdominal incision and significantly reduces blood loss during the procedure (Fig. 50–125).

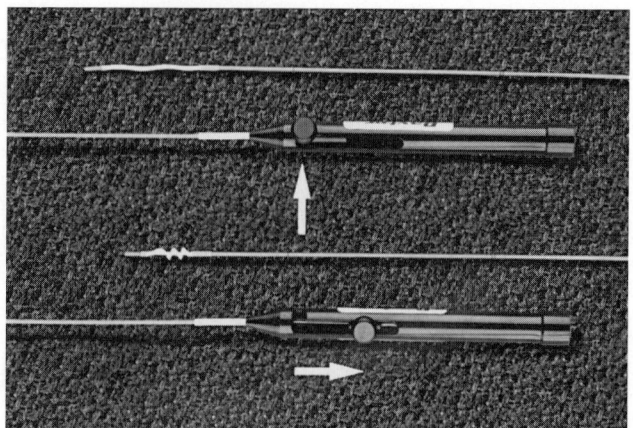

Figure 50–123. Upper arrow shows position of activator knob on the handle of the adherent clot catheter during insertion of the device in an extended, uncoiled position. Lower arrow denotes retracted knob position, which may be moved back and forth to increase or decrease the corkscrew diameter as necessary during removal of adherent material.

OPERATIVE PROCEDURE

The experience with acute peripheral arterial embolization has clearly indicated that successful management of these patients is related to well-defined factors. From a technical standpoint, it must be recognized that there are varying degrees of difficulty encountered in the attempt to re-establish the peripheral circulation. Patients with advanced ischemia and extensive distal propagation of the thrombus, and those with significant chronic occlusive disease, present the most difficult problems. A careful history and physical examination allow identification of these situations.

Preparation

The procedure is initiated with local anesthesia. An anesthetist should be in attendance to monitor vital signs and to administer a general anesthetic if required or appropriate. The extremity should be surgically prepared from the toes to the nipple line. A bilateral inguinal approach is utilized for aortic emboli, and both extremities are prepared. An iliac embolus also requires bilateral preparation because of the possibility of dislodging a high iliac embolus, with occlusion to the opposite extremity. Although this complication has not occurred in the author's experience, the possibility is always

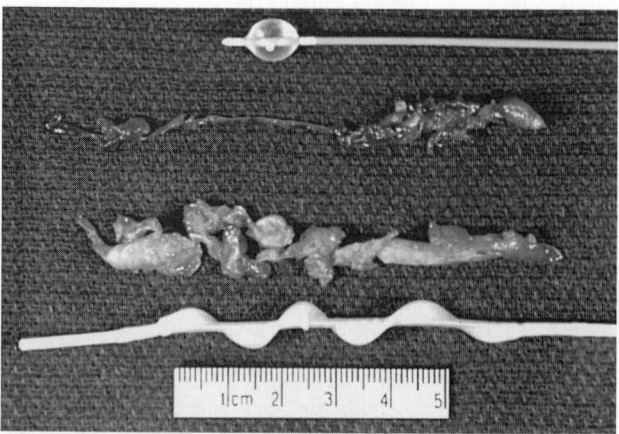

Figure 50–122. Examination of the cast of a clot removed by balloon embolectomy catheter may indicate a need for more aggressive instrumentation to complete the thromboembolectomy procedure. Soft clot retrieved with the balloon catheter is shown in upper picture; residual material removed with the adherent clot catheter is displayed below.

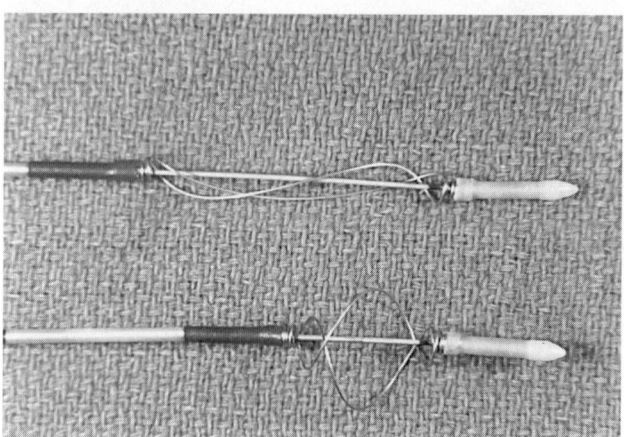

Figure 50–124. Graft thrombectomy catheter shown in extended position and (below) in the contracted wire position used to entrap adherent thrombotic clot during removal from synthetic grafts.

anticipated by preparing the opposite extremity to allow careful monitoring of the pulses. A continuous noninvasive pulse amplitude monitor is useful in the management of these patients.[12] Intraoperative angioscopy also has significant utility and has resulted in a decreased use of arteriography.

Technique

The initial approach to embolic occlusion, regardless of the anatomic location, has been through a common femoral incision (Fig. 50–126). The common femoral artery and deep femoral artery are isolated and occluded with atraumatic vascular clamps. The arterial incision is made in relation to the orifice of the superficial femoral artery and deep femoral artery. A distal exploration is performed initially, and catheters should be routinely placed in the superficial and deep femoral arteries. An open deep femoral circulation is capable of providing the margin necessary to maintain viability in many patients with advanced ischemia or in those who have had a prior chronic occlusion of the superficial femoral system. In the author's experience, instances of recovery of embolic material from the deep femoral artery, even in the presence of a patent common femoral artery, have been frequent. The 2-French and 3-French catheters are most commonly employed for exploration of the deep femoral system, whereas 3-French and 4-French catheters have been found suitable for exploration of the femoropopliteal systems.

The aim of surgical intervention is to restore the peripheral circulation to its preocclusive state. Evaluation of results is based on restoration of pulses, relief of symptoms, and return

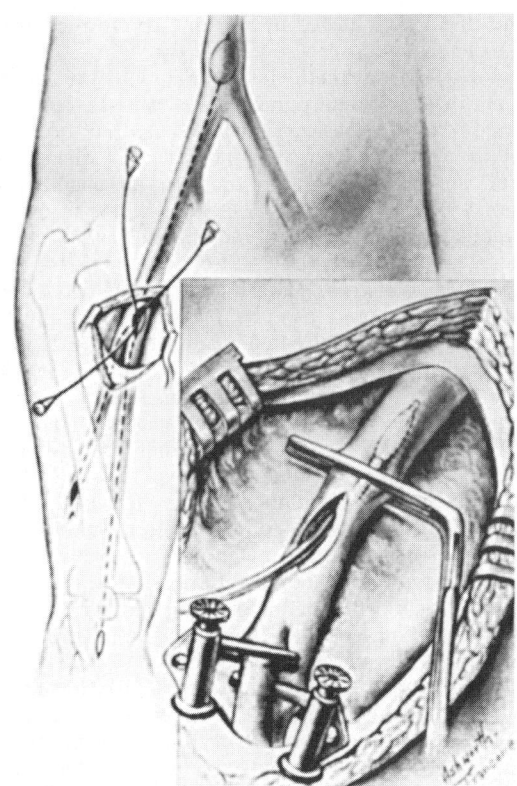

Figure 50–126. Balloon catheter extraction in the iliofemoral system via femoral incision. Use of padded clamps minimizes arterial trauma during instrumentation usage.

of normal color and temperature. It is sometimes difficult to assess results when the condition of the extremity of a given patient prior to the acute occlusion is unknown. Conditions such as mental confusion or concurrent illness obviously preclude a total and thorough evaluation. Outcome of therapy is best determined by mortality and amputation rates. The possibility of maintaining a viable, functional extremity following acute arterial occlusion should exceed 90%.

Regardless of the site of the occlusion, failure to recognize and automatically remove any distally propagated thrombus may cause less complete restoration of circulation and possibly amputation. Surgeons have often relied on the presence or absence of backbleeding from the peripheral arterial bed as a guide to distal patency. Repeated clinical observations have confirmed that backbleeding is an unreliable guide to distal patency. Discontinuous thrombotic material is present in approximately one third of cases. Under these circumstances, backbleeding may be quite forceful, despite the presence of total distal obstruction. The presence of adequate collateral vessels causes significant bleeding from the distal segment, despite the fact that the more peripheral arterial bed may be totally occluded. Failure to recognize this circumstance causes less than complete restoration of the circulation. For this reason, routine distal exploration with balloon catheters should be performed independently of the status of the backbleeding.

A physical finding that should be cause for considerable concern after an apparently successful embolectomy is the presence of a water-hammer–type pulse. An apparently stronger than normal pulse has been associated with a high incidence of reocclusion. Under these circumstances, obstruction is present at the small artery and arteriolar level. Re-exploration should include distal irrigation, in conjunction with the use of fibrinolytic agents that are directly introduced

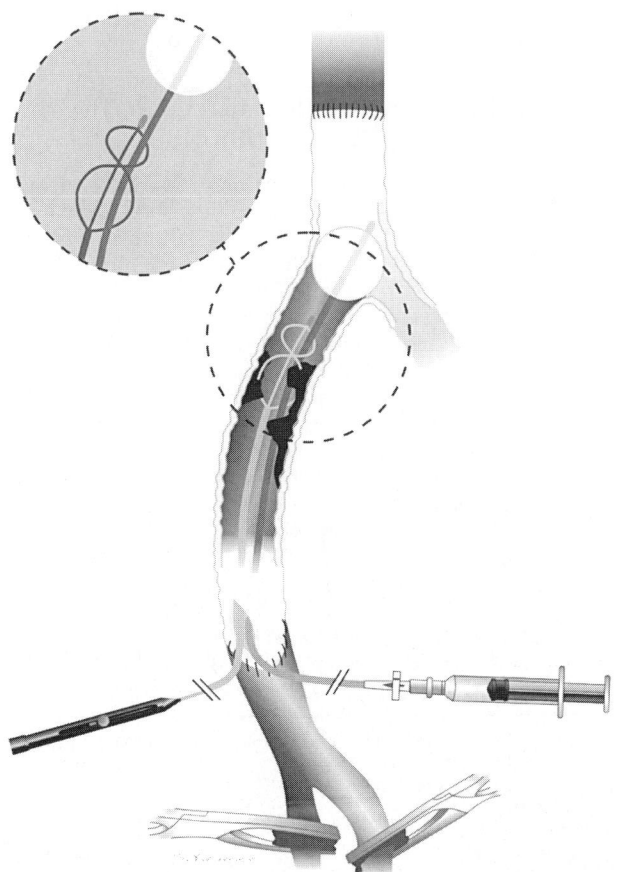

Figure 50–125. Proximal occlusion using balloon technique during thrombectomy procedure in aortobifemoral graft. Inset shows how the occlusion balloon catheter is threaded through the wire helix of the graft thrombectomy catheter.

into the distal arterial bed at the time of the second procedure.[5]

As previously indicated, clot examination is a critical and expedient means of determining distal patency. A sharp cut-off usually indicates residual material. A divot noted in the cast of the clot is likewise an indication of distal residual material. Smooth tapers with bifurcations are usually an indication of adequate clot removal. If there is uncertainty about the adequacy of distal clot removal, the vessel should be visualized. Angioscopy allows direct access to the femoro-popliteal and tibial vessels and minimizes the need for distal incisions and explorations. The proper use of angioscopy quickly documents distal patency and often avoids the need for intraoperative arteriograms.

In the presence of advanced ischemia—that is, in patients with early rigor—the simultaneous presence of major venous occlusion demands consideration. In these patients, the superficial femoral vein is isolated and explored prior to restoration of the arterial circulation. Large venous thrombi are removed by means of venous thrombectomy catheters. Prior to suture closure of the vein, the arterial circulation is re-established. After removal of the arterial occlusions, the distal arterial bed should be adequately irrigated with a heparinized saline solution. The distal venous clamp is then removed to allow smaller thrombi and the acidotic blood to be flushed out. Following completion of this copious heparin flush, the arteriotomy is closed. The vein is flushed once again and, finally, the venotomy is closed. Direct instillation of a fibrinolytic agent through an inflated thru-lumen balloon catheter is recommended in all patients presenting with advanced ischemia.

Immediately following restoration of arterial continuity in extremities with advanced ischemia, significant alterations in electrolytes and acid balance may occur. The venous efflux of ischemic extremities following restoration of arterial continuity was studied in 10 patients.[9] These data clearly indicated that following successful restoration of the circulation, there was a sudden return of acidotic blood with a high potassium content to the heart. This metabolic effect, in conjunction with pooling of blood in the revascularized extremity, can cause significant hypotension. In 8 of the 10 patients studied, adverse effects were associated with clamp release, in the form of significant electrocardiographic changes, hypotension, or both. The necessity of using buffering agents and antiarrhythmic agents should be anticipated at the time of clamp release. Electrolytes should be closely followed in the postoperative period. A high creatine phosphokinase level in the venous efflux indicates significant muscle damage. Both Fisher and co-workers[9] and Haimovici[13] have described the adverse systemic effects that may occur following revascularization of an extremity presenting with advanced ischemia.

ACUTE OCCLUSION IN THE PRESENCE OF SIGNIFICANT OCCLUSIVE DISEASE

A careful history and examination of the uninvolved extremity provide a reliable assessment of the peripheral circulation prior to the acute episode. The patient's general condition and prior level of activity and the extent of pathologic change encountered at the time of operation all have an important role in determining the extent of the surgical procedure. Initially, it is generally advisable to attempt only to return the circulation to its acute preocclusive state. Definitive reconstructive procedures are delayed until a more critical evaluation of the patient is possible. Major reconstructive procedures may be indicated, however, if the general condition is favorable when the patient is first observed. Definitive

procedures may be performed at the initial exploration, particularly if there is concern about the viability of the extremity and if the patient was active prior to the acute occlusion. Elderly patients in poor general condition are poor candidates for major reconstructive procedures. Local angioplasty or endarterectomy of the deep femoral system in these situations is simple and quick and can be done under local anesthesia. Frequently, it provides the margin necessary to maintain viability. Reconstructive procedures performed in conjunction with arterial embolectomy are listed in Table 50–16. Local endarterectomy and femorofemoral jump grafts are simple and can also be done under local anesthesia. Adjunctive dilation or atherectomy can easily be employed at the time of either thrombectomy or embolectomy.[10] Adjunctive endovascular procedures are being used with increasing frequency, and they are decreasing the magnitude of the operation in elderly and critically ill patients. In patients of advanced age, durability (although important) should be of secondary consideration.

UPPER EXTREMITY EMBOLI

The management of emboli in the upper extremities is identical to that described for the lower extremities. Proximal subclavian artery emboli can simply be removed under local anesthesia by retrograde extraction. However, the morbidity associated with upper extremity occlusions should not be underestimated. In their study, Baird and Lagos noted that more proximal emboli cause significantly more ischemia than the more distal brachial occlusions.[2] Recurrent emboli in the upper extremity are not uncommon. The cumulative effect of proximal occlusions can lead to significant ischemia and difficult reconstructions, particularly if the original embolus was not surgically removed.

RENAL, MESENTERIC, AND CAROTID ARTERY OCCLUSIONS

The principles of management of occlusion in organs outside the periphery are similar to those described for management of peripheral arterial emboli. It should be borne in mind, however, that the external support provided by adjacent tissue is significantly less with the vessels supplying the viscera and the brain than with the vessels of the peripheral vasculature. Considerable care should be taken in introducing a catheter into these vessels. The 2-French and 3-French catheters are of appropriate size for distal exploration of these vessels. These catheters have very flexible tips, which significantly diminishes the possibility of perforation. Only gentle inflation and traction should be used in removing occlusions in these areas.

Unless occlusions in the internal carotid system are ob-

TABLE 50–16. Peripheral Reconstructions Associated with Thromboembolectomy (500 Patients, 570 Reconstructions)

Procedure	No. of Patients
Common and deep femoral endarterectomy	24
Femorofemoral graft	14
Proximal endarterectomy	9
Aortofemoral graft	5
Adjunctive dilatation	22
Adjunctive atherectomy	17

TABLE 50–17. Morbidity and Mortality in 500 Patients, 570 Embolectomies

Outcome	No. of Patients	Percentage
Limb salvage	—	96
Patient survival	—	90
Death		
Myocardial infarction	25	5
Congestive heart failure	19	3.8
Pulmonary embolus	5	1
Cerebrovascular accident	4	.8
Renal failure	2	.04

served within the first few hours of onset, surgical intervention should not be considered. Hemorrhagic infarction represents a fatal complication when attempts are made to remove emboli to the cerebral circulation, especially when they are undertaken after a considerable lapse of time.

POSTOPERATIVE CARE AND MANAGEMENT

The value of heparin has been well documented. The indications should be individualized for each patient. The possible presence of simultaneous venous thrombosis and embolization following acute myocardial infarction represents an indication for heparinization in the postoperative period. In those situations in which it is recognized that heparin should be employed in the immediate postoperative period, the possible complications of hemorrhage and hematoma at incisional sites should be considered. A vacuum-type drainage system has proved effective in minimizing the postoperative hematoma.

The specific aspects of postoperative care are obviously dictated by the underlying pathologic condition responsible for the occlusion. The presence or absence of significant cardiac impairment and the presence or absence of associated diseases determine postoperative care. Concern about the status of the peripheral vasculature should not impair the management or care of these other critical disorders. Peripheral embolization following myocardial infarction should immediately direct one's attention to the underlying cardiac lesion. Catheterization of the left side of the heart and coronary artery visualization may be indicated. The presence of significant valvular heart disease obviously deserves diagnostic investigation and surgical correction. Timing of the intervention is determined by the overall condition of the patient.

MORBIDITY AND MORTALITY

Complications secondary to the use of embolectomy and thrombectomy catheters have been the same as those common to all catheter techniques, including plaque dissection, catheter tip separation, and vessel perforation. Vessel rupture can occur in the balloon if the instrument is overdistended in small vessels. Experience and an appreciation of instrument limitations are the most significant factors in reducing the incidence of complications. Recognition and appropriate surgical management of the more difficult technical problems associated with acute arterial occlusion decrease both morbidity and mortality.

Swelling of a revascularized, ischemic extremity can assume considerable proportions and requires treatment. Massive swelling that may embarrass arterial inflow is observed

ost frequently in those patients who present with advanced ischemia prior to surgical intervention. Capillary damage causes fluid exudation into ischemic tissues and is a factor in this swelling. Obstruction of the venous outflow tract aggravates the problem. Failure to immediately control this edema may cause reocclusion of the arterial inflow. Fasciotomy has been required in 10% of the patients who present with acute embolic occlusion. Initial decompression is accomplished through small skin incisions, as described by Rosato and colleagues.[21] If immediate improvement is not obtained by this limited fasciotomy, the skin incisions should be extended, and deeper fascial compartments should be widely opened. The use of a wound closure device, as described by Hirshowitz and associates[15] and Ersek and Vasquez-Salisbury[8] has significantly reduced the morbidity associated with fasciotomy. Radical decompression requiring fibular resection is rarely necessary in patients who have acute embolic occlusion. Patman and Thompson[20] provided an excellent review of the technique and indications for fasciotomy. Failure of the initial exploration after an apparent success is an indication for re-exploration. The most common cause of failure is related to technical factors that, if recognized, can sometimes be corrected. However, the possibility of reocclusion of the same extremity should not be overlooked. Its documented occurrence reinforces a second-look attitude.

The mortality associated with acute arterial occlusion is attributable primarily to the severe underlying disorder responsible for the occlusive event rather than to surgical intervention. Causes of death in patients with acute arterial occlusion almost always involve underlying cardiac disease and significant cardiac dysfunction (Table 50–17). Numerous studies have documented that recognition and correction of the cause of the underlying acute occlusion are important aspects of care for these patients.[6, 17, 23] It is only through aggressive treatment of the underlying pathology that mortality rates can be improved. With the increasing success of coronary artery procedures, patients who develop emboli after myocardial infarction should be considered for coronary visualization. The timing of such studies should take into consideration the general condition of the patient. Revascularization or aneurysmectomy, if indicated, should be done as soon as possible. The number and types of associated cardiac procedures in a group of 500 patients are listed in Table 50–18. Half of these procedures represented emergency situations and were performed at the time of arterial embolectomy. The remaining half were semiurgent, and all were accomplished within 1 month of the time of acute occlusion.

THROMBOLYTICS

Thrombolytic agents have been employed for the treatment of acute arterial occlusion for more than 25 years. The agents

TABLE 50–18. Thromboembolectomy-Associated Cardiac Procedures in 500 Patients

Procedure	No. of Patients
Replacement of prosthetic valve	
Aortic	2
Mitral	7
Replacement of mitral valve	
Ruptured papillary	8
Rheumatic	13
Triple valve	1
Resection of ventricular aneurysm and/or coronary artery bypass graft	27
Repair of infarcted ventricular septal defect	2

that have received the most widespread clinical use are streptokinase and urokinase. Streptokinase is a bacterial protein purified from beta-hemolytic streptococci. It combines with plasminogen through an intermediary complex to form plasmin. Because it is a foreign particle, it induces an antibody response that must be overcome by relatively large dose levels. Urokinase is a naturally occurring human enzyme produced by the kidney. It also combines with plasminogen to form plasmin, but without intermediary steps. Urokinase requires several smaller doses because it is not antigenic and it converts plasminogen to plasmin more efficiently than does streptokinase. After formation, plasmin degrades fibrin to effect fibrinolysis.

Although originally administered systemically, lytic agents are currently delivered directly to the occlusive site via an infusion catheter.[3] This approach reduces systemic exposure to the lytic agent. In recent years, urokinase has been favored over streptokinase because of its lower complication rate and improved efficacy.[19] The major disadvantage of urokinase is the cost of the drug itself.

The primary complication of lytic agents is hemorrhage, which can manifest in the form of bleeding at wound sites, hematomas of varying severity, stroke, and sometimes myocardial infarction. Another concern with the use of lytic agents is the uncertain duration of therapy. Additional embolization has been known to occur in fragmentation of embolic or thrombotic material from the lytic agent, and more distal embolization is a cause for concern. Lytic agents can be effective in some situations, particularly as a preamble to surgical intervention when dealing with autogenous grafts below the inguinal ligament. However, lytic therapy is rarely the only therapy required. The use of thrombolytics should be considered a preamble to a more definitive intervention, which could be an endovascular catheter-mediated approach, a direct arterial reconstruction, or a combination of the two. The use of thrombolytics as an adjunct has been advocated by Comerota and co-workers,[5] and it is an extremely effective approach—particularly when there is extensive distal propagation of thrombotic material associated with advanced ischemia.

Despite the considerable interest in thrombolytic agents during the last 2 decades, intra-arterial dissolution of thrombotic material still has limitations. The primary problems are time delay to reperfusion, cost, the need for multiple angiograms, and the potential for hemorrhage. These concerns have led to the development of lytic agents that convert plasminogen to plasmin specifically at the clot site rather than elsewhere in the circulation. Two such fibrin-specific lytic agents are tissue plasminogen activator (tPA), a naturally occurring protein produced in significant amounts via recombinant DNA technology; and pro-urokinase, a naturally occurring precursor to urokinase produced in quantity from modified human renal cells. Both of these substances are currently under clinical evaluation for a variety of acute thrombotic conditions.

CONCLUSION

Acute arterial occlusion continues to be a disease entity associated with patients of advanced age and multisystem disease. In general, treatment interventions should be noninvasive, predictable, and expedient. At present, however, heparinization with surgical balloon embolectomy remains the most effective form of treatment for acute arterial occlusion.

SELECTED REFERENCES

Fogarty, T. J., Daily, P. O., Shumway, N. E., and Krippaehne, W.: Experience with balloon catheter technic for arterial embolectomy. Am. J. Surg., 122:231, 1971.

The authors report a series of 330 embolic occlusions occurring in 300 patients. The paper emphasizes the necessity of identifying high-risk areas in terms of morbidity and mortality. An aggressive overall approach to the medical and surgical problems is presented.

Patman, R. D., and Thompson, J. E.: Fasciotomy in peripheral vascular surgery. Arch. Surg., 101:663, 1970.
The authors review their personal experience with 164 patients who required fasciotomy. The indications for fasciotomy and the technique employed are presented. Fasciotomy, performed correctly and with proper indications, is a valuable procedure that can increase limb salvage and decrease morbidity. The paper is well written, and a variety of clinical situations that may require fasciotomy are detailed.

Tawes, R. L., Jr., Harris, E. J., Brown, W. H., et al.: Arterial thromboembolism: A 20-year perspective. Arch. Surg., 120:595, 1985.
The authors review their experience in 739 patients with lower extremity thromboembolism. They detail the factors that have contributed to their overall 12% mortality and 95% limb salvage rate. They stress the importance of prompt diagnosis and treatment, postoperative heparinization, and the necessity of viewing thromboembolism within the context of the underlying cardiovascular disease process.

REFERENCES

1. Abbott, W. M., Maloney, R. D., McCabe, C. C., et al.: Arterial embolism: A 44 year perspective. Am. J. Surg., 143:460, 1982.
2. Baird, R. J., and Lagos, T. Z.: Emboli to the arm. Ann. Surg., 160:905, 1964.
3. Beard, J. D., Nyamekye, I., Earnshaw, J. J., Scott, D. J., and Thompson, J. F.: Intraoperative streptokinase: A useful adjunct to balloon-catheter embolectomy. Br. J. Surg., 80:21, 1993.
4. Best, C. H.: Heparin and vascular occlusion. Can. Med. Assoc. J., 35:621, 1936.
5. Comerota, A. J., White, J. V., and Grosh, J. D.: Intraoperative intra-arterial thrombolytic therapy for salvage of limbs in patients with distal arterial thrombosis. Surg. Gynecol. Obstet., 169:283, 1989.
6. Connett, M. C., Murray, D. H., Jr., and Wenneker, W. W.: Peripheral arterial emboli. Am. J. Surg., 148:14, 1984.
7. Englund, R., and Magee, H.: Peripheral arterial embolism: 1961–1985. Aust. N. Z. J. Surg., 57:27, 1987.
8. Ersek, R. A., and Vasquez-Salisbury, A.: A wound closure using a skin stretching device. Contemp. Orth., 28:495, 1994.
9. Fisher, R. D., Fogarty, T. J., and Morrow, A. G.: Clinical and biochemical observations of the effect of transient femoral artery occlusion in man. Surgery, 68:323, 1970.
10. Fogarty, T. J., Chin, A. K., Olcott, C., IV, et al.: Combined thrombectomy and dilation for the treatment of acute lower extremity arterial thrombosis. J. Vasc. Surg., 10:530, 1989.
11. Fogarty, T. J., Cranley, J. J., Krause, R. J., et al.: A method for extraction of arterial emboli and thrombi. Surg. Gynecol. Obstet., 116:241, 1963.
12. Fogarty, T. J., Biswas, A., Serra, K. L., and Hermann, G. D.: Monitoring distal extremity perfusion with the pulse amplitude monitor during vascular reconstruction. In Braverman, M., and Tawes, R. (Eds.): Surgical Technology International II: International Developments in Surgery and Surgical Research. San Francisco, Thomas F. Laszlo, 1993.
13. Haimovici, H.: Myopathic-nephrotic-metabolic syndrome associated with massive acute arterial occlusions. J. Cardiovasc. Surg., 14:589, 1973.
14. Harvey, S.: Exercitatio anatomica de motu cordis et sanguinis in animalibus (an English translation by Chauncey D. Leake). Springfield, Ill., Charles C Thomas, 1931, p. 37.
15. Hirshowitz, B., Lindenbaum, E., and Har-Shai, Y.: A skin-stretching device for the harnessing of the viscoelastic properties of skin. Plast. Reconstr. Surg., 92:260, 1993.
16. Labey: cited by Mosney, M., and Dumont, N. J.: Embolie femorale au cours d'un rétrécissement mitral pur. Artériotomie. Guérison Bull. Acad. Med., 66:358, 1911.
17. Levy, J. F., and Butcher, H. R.: Arterial emboli: An analysis of 125 patients. Surgery, 68:968, 1970.
18. Linton, R. R.: Peripheral arterial embolism. A discussion of the postembolic vascular changes and their relation to the restoration of circulation in peripheral embolism. N. Engl. J. Med., 224:189, 1941.
19. Motarjeme, A.: Thrombolytic therapy in arterial occlusion and graft thrombosis. Semin. Vasc. Surg., 2:155, 1989.
20. Patman, R. D., and Thompson, J. E.: Fasciotomy in peripheral vascular surgery. Arch. Surg., 101:663, 1970.
21. Rosato, F. E., Barker, C. F., Robert, B., and Danielson, G. K.: Subcutaneous fasciotomy. Description of a new technique and instrument. Surgery, 59:3, 1966.
22. Tawes, R. L., Jr., Harris, E. J., Brown, W. H., et al.: Arterial thromboembolism: A 20-year perspective. Arch. Surg., 120:595, 1985.
23. Thompson, J. E., Sigler, L., Raut, P. S., et al.: Arterial embolectomy: A 20-year experience with 163 cases. Surgery, 67:212, 1970.

ARTERIOVENOUS FISTULAS

H. Kim Lyerly, M.D.
David C. Sabiston, Jr., M.D.

One of the most fascinating lesions affecting the arterial system is the arteriovenous fistula. These may be either congenital or acquired and are also associated with numerous pathophysiologic changes, both at the local site and systemically.[12] Collectively, they represent some of the most challenging diagnostic and therapeutic problems in medicine.

The first description of an arteriovenous fistula was by William Hunter in 1758. He recognized that an arteriovenous aneurysm was characterized not only by the aneurysm but also by a direct communication between the involved artery and the accompanying vein.[16] Earlier, such lesions were interpreted as simple aneurysms, whereas Hunter designated these as aneurysms by anastomosis and placed emphasis on the communication between the two vascular systems.

An arteriovenous fistula is defined as a connection, other than the capillary bed, between the arterial and venous systems. This definition encompasses a vast array of conditions, including some occurring in the normal development of the circulation, congenital malformations, acquired lesions, and iatrogenic shunts. A classification based on the etiology of the fistula is helpful and is shown in Table 50–19.

CLASSIFICATION OF ARTERIOVENOUS COMMUNICATIONS

Arteriovenous fistulas are either *congenital* or *acquired*. For congenital communications, the terms *cirsoid aneurysms* and *cavernous angiomas* have also been used. Congenital lesions may have single or multiple communications and are denoted as arteriovenous fistulas and arteriovenous malformations, respectively.

Fistulas with a single communication usually represent normal fetal communications that fail to resolve or represent developmental abnormalities. Lesions with multiple communications usually represent persistent communications that normally exist during the early phase of the development of the arterial and venous systems. Both arteries and veins differentiate from a common capillary plexus during embryologic development. If failure occurs in differentiation of the common embryologic analog into arteries and veins, extensive communications may result between them. *Hemangiomas* are multiple abnormal venous malformations that do not have high-pressure arterial communications. Acquired lesions usually have a single communication and frequently consist of a distinct communication between an artery and a vein, bypassing the capillary bed. The causes of acquired arteriovenous communications include vascular tumors, such as angiosarcoma, glomus tumor, or hemangiopericytoma, and tumors associated with shunting, such as hepatoma or hypernephroma.

PATHOPHYSIOLOGY

Arteriovenous communications produce pathophysiologic changes locally, but frequently, especially in larger fistulas, the most significant and pronounced changes involve the body as a whole. The pathophysiologic changes are most impressive in fistulas in which enormous amounts of arterial blood pass directly into the venous circulation. A number of important systemic physiologic changes occur in an attempt to compensate for a major circulatory abnormality.

Direct communications between the arterial and venous systems are demonstrated by the presence of a *thrill* at the site of the lesion, especially if it is located near the surface. On auscultation, a *bruit* continuing through most if not all of the cardiac cycle is audible. An aneurysm or arterial and venous dilation is often seen or palpated. Large draining veins are also present—visible if they are subcutaneous, or apparent on angiography in more deeply located fistulas. Angiography demonstrates dilated arteries, rapid filling of veins, and tortuous arterial collaterals. Dilated arteries and veins may also be demonstrated by ultrasonic determination, and the addition of Doppler color-flow imaging allows the detection of small fistulas not only by direct detection of the anatomic defect but also by the turbulent flow in the vein from the jet of blood from the arterial side of the fistula (Fig. 50–127).[35]

Systemic symptoms are generally related to the size of the fistula and its proximity to the heart. These changes are maximal in fistulas involving a large artery that conducts massive amounts of blood. Under these circumstances, much blood is shunted through the fistula because the venous side offers very little peripheral resistance. With large volumes of blood being shunted directly into the venous circulation, a sequence of events follows that is directly related to the volume of blood flowing through the fistula (Figs. 50–128 and 50–129). The cardiac output increases, the heart rate rises, and the diastolic arterial pressure diminishes, usually with an increase in systolic pressure. The cardiac and pulmonary pressures also change, with increases in ventricular end-diastolic pressure, right and left atrial pressures, and pulmonary wedge pressure (Table 50–20). The blood and plasma volumes increase to compensate for the increased volume of blood in the venous circulation.

Moreover, with the high cardiac output, the heart increases in size, particularly the atrial and ventricular cavities; ultimately, cardiac hypertrophy results. A fistula may eventually cause congestive heart failure, especially if it is a large one. If the fistula is acute with a large volume of blood passing through it, the heart may not be able to compensate adequately, producing pulmonary edema and sometimes death. It is interesting that experimental and clinical studies have indicated that digitalis preparations are largely ineffective in the management of high-output cardiac failure.[34] These features can be dramatically illustrated experimentally after the creation of large fistulas and the determination of physiologic measurements.[32]

With a high cardiac output due to the fistula, the oxygen saturation in the mixed venous blood of the right heart is increased, because much of the blood bypasses the capillary bed. The central venous pressure is usually increased. Of considerable importance is the anatomic site of the fistula

TABLE 50–19. Classification of Abnormal Arteriovenous Communication

Congenital	Acquired
Single fistula	Single fistula
Multiple fistula—	Surgical
arteriovenous malformation	Pathologic
Hemangiomas	Aneurysm
	Iatrogenic
	Infection
	Neoplasia
	Spontaneous
	Traumatic
	Tumor-associated communications
	Vascular tumors
	Tumors associated with shunting

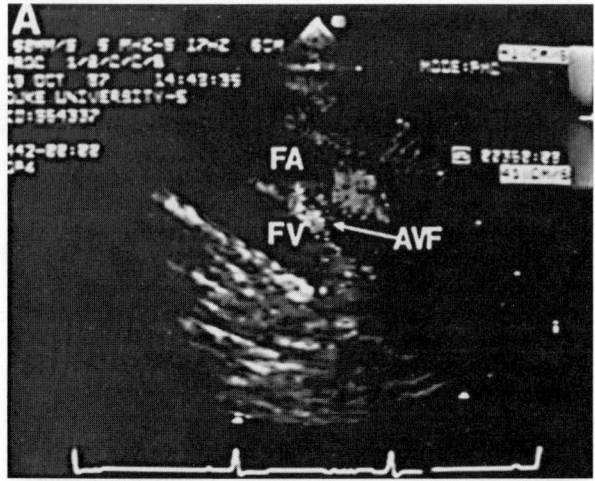

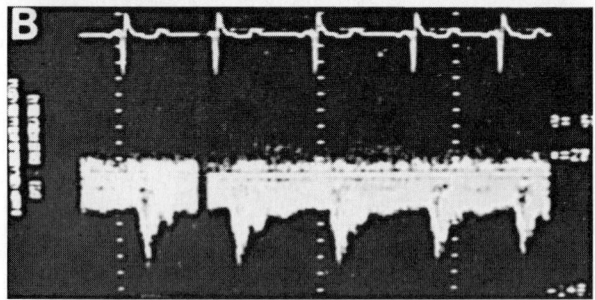

Figure 50–127. Color-flow imaging (*A*, reproduced in black and white) and pulsed-wave Doppler recording *(B)* of a patient with a right femoral arteriovenous fistula. Color-flow examination shows flow going from the femoral artery to the femoral vein. Doppler recording shows high-velocity systolic flow away from the transducer and lower-velocity diastolic flow also going away from the transducer. AVF, arteriovenous fistula; FA, femoral artery; FV, femoral vein. (From Sheikh, K. H., Adams, D. B., McCann, R., Lyerly, H. K., Sabiston, D. C., Jr., and Kisslo, J.: Utility of Doppler color flow imaging for identification of femoral arterial complications of cardiac catheterization. Am. Heart J., *117*:623, 1989.)

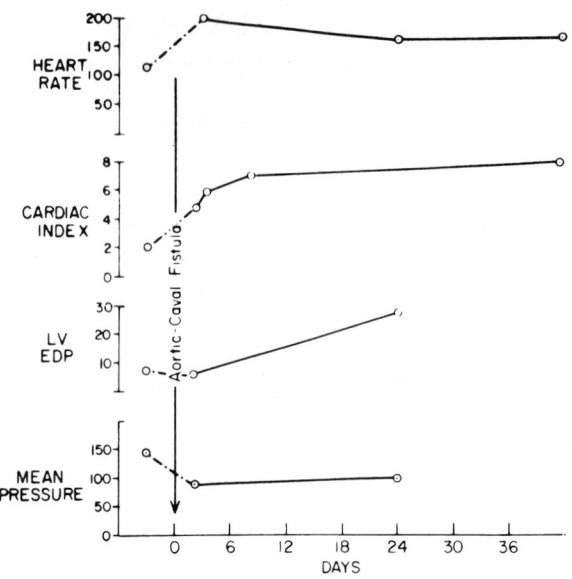

Figure 50–128. Changes in heart rate, cardiac index, left ventricular end-diastolic pressure (LV EDP), and mean arterial pressure in an experimental animal with a large aortocaval fistula.

and the systemic circulation, because the diameter of the involved vessel is of crucial importance. For example, much more blood flows through a fistula of a specific size from an artery with a large diameter than from one with a smaller diameter. It has been shown experimentally that small aortic fistulas can produce severe symptoms when they are centrally located near the heart, for example, between the ascending aorta and the pulmonary artery or the superior vena cava, contrasted with similar, more distal shunts, such as between the iliac or femoral vessels.[33] Structural changes in the vascular wall are also created by hemodynamic disturbances associated with arteriovenous fistulas.

In large fistulas, the venous wall becomes thin. The walls of small fistulas may become thickened and assume the appearance of an artery. Thrombi are apt to form in the dilated parts of these fistulas and may harbor bacterial organisms. Arteriovenous fistulas may be associated with the development of bacterial endocarditis. In fact, the first patient ever cured of a chronic bloodstream infection (*Streptococcus viridans*) before the introduction of antibiotics was managed by surgical closure of an iliac arteriovenous fistula. After the operation, the bloodstream infection disappeared, and the patient remained cured (Figs. 50–130 and 50–131).[30] Until that time, all such illnesses had been fatal. The turbulence at the site of the fistula usually causes *dilation* of the artery and vein, producing an aneurysm. In response to the low distal arterial pressure beyond the site of the fistula, an extensive collateral circulation develops, connecting the arteries above the fistula with those below. These collaterals become greatly

dilated and tortuous and deliver considerable blood distally as a result of a large pressure gradient (Fig. 50–132). This collateral circulation can become massive and often causes an increase in temperature in both skin and muscle. When the fistulas occur in an extremity, the limb may increase in length, a fact that has been confirmed by both experimental and clinical observations.[18] One explanation for this increased bone growth is the 1 or 2° C. elevation in the local temperature and resultant increase in metabolism. Typical changes in the arterial and venous pressures beyond the fistula are shown in Figure 50–133.[34]

Diagnostic measures employed in evaluating arteriovenous fistulas include measurement of venous oxygen tension in

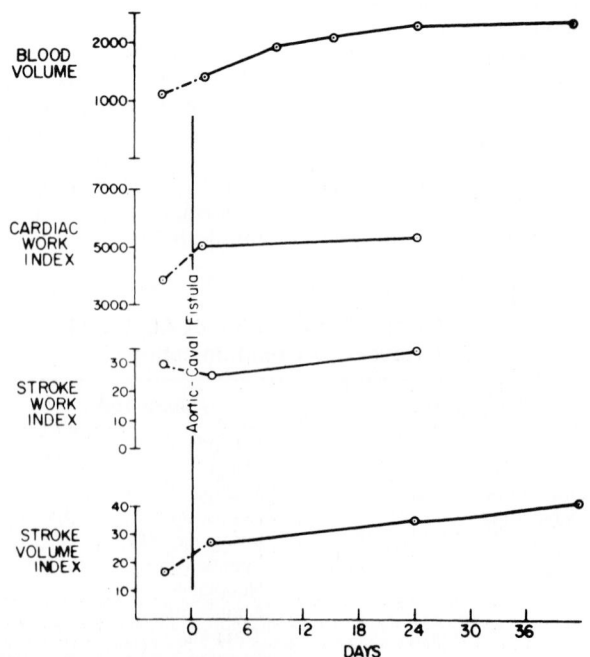

Figure 50–129. Changes in blood volume, cardiac work index, stroke work index, and stroke volume index in an experimental animal with a large aorto-caval fistula.

TABLE 50–20. Manifestations of Arteriovenous Fistula

Systemic

Pulse rate	↑	Diastolic arterial pressure	↓
Cardiac output	↑	Peripheral resistance	↓
Blood volume	↑		
Cardiac size	↑		

Local

Thrill
Continuous murmur
Increased arterial collaterals
Aneurysmal formation
Diminished pulse rate with occlusion

Physiologic changes occurring in the circulation with an arteriovenous fistula are most marked in the presence of a large fistula. These changes may be minimal to absent with a small fistula. Late manifestations of a large fistula include congestive heart failure, pulmonary edema, and death in untreated patients.

the limb with the suspected fistula. Oxygenated arterial blood passing through the fistula flows into the venous side with a high oxygen saturation, unlike normal venous blood.

In patients with arteriovenous fistulas, the cardiac output may be increased, and compression of the fistula, which diminishes the flow, is followed by a slower heart rate (Branham's or Nicoladoni's sign) and a lower cardiac output. Nicoladoni described a patient with an arteriovenous fistula in whom compression of the fistula (with cessation of flow through it) caused a decrease in the pulse rate from 96 to 64 beats per minute. This bradycardic reaction was later described by Branham and also bears his name (Fig. 50–134).[4, 15]

Angiography is the standard diagnostic study in the evaluation of an arteriovenous fistula. In acquired fistulas, a single communication often occurs at the site of the fistula and can be localized either by direct visualization of the communication or by the initial venous opacification at the site of the fistula (Fig. 50–135). Congenital lesions with multiple communications often have a radiologic appearance that is much more complicated. Indirect signs of an abnormal arteriovenous communication, including increased flow in the afferent arteries, decreased flow in the peripheral arteries, and rapid venous filling, are usually present. However, the multiple communications may not be visible, because they are often

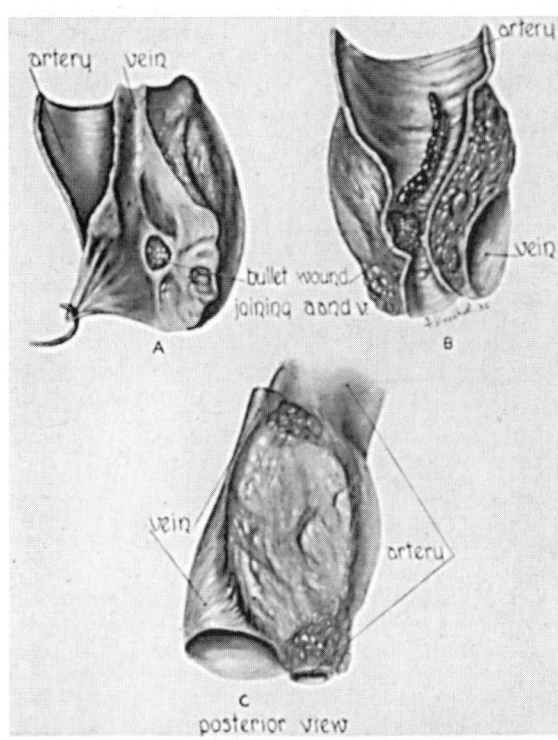

Figure 50–131. Drawings of specimens. *A,* Venous side of arterial venous aneurysm showing vegetation in the opening between the external iliac vein and aneurysmal sac. The upper or proximal portion of the vein has been cut across on the bias, giving the false impression that the lumen of the vein is narrowed in this drawing. *B,* Arterial side of specimen revealing the openings into aneurysmal cavity filled with vegetations and the protruding thrombus, which points cephalad. The dilated proximal portion of the artery is shown in the upper portion of the illustration. The external iliac artery of normal size is shown below. Along the right margin of the artery is the dark calcified wall of the aneurysm. The external iliac vein is on the opposite side lying directly behind the artery. *C,* Posterior view of the encysted varicose aneurysm. (From Rienhoff, W. F., Jr., and Hamman, L.: Subacute *Streptococcus viridans* septicemia cured by the excision of an arteriovenous aneurysm of the external iliac artery and vein. Ann. Surg., *102*:905, 1935.)

of microscopic size; overlying opacified arteries and veins add to the complexity of the radiographic pattern. Selective angiography of the afferent artery or arteries may be helpful in delineating the extent of the fistula. Localized dilated, contrast-filled spaces may indicate the site of the fistula with some precision. Small fistulas are usually revealed as faint, diffuse opacifications between major arterial and venous channels. Other indications include abnormal vessels arising from the parent artery and horizontal branches connecting parallel veins. Because radiopaque media tend to fill the most proximal fistulas and those with the greatest volume of flow, smaller and more distally located communications may escape detection. This is particularly unfortunate in congenital arteriovenous malformations, because of these lesions' tendency for multiple communications.

Arteriovenous fistulas can be readily identified by ultrasonic imaging.[9, 38] Although ultrasound may not be expected to reveal the actual fistula, the detection of aneurysms may show a previously unsuspected fistula as well as the diameter and morphologic features of the proximal vessels.[35] Color-flow imaging may also reveal patterns suggestive of increased turbulence at sites of increased flow.

Magnetic resonance imaging (MRI) and computed tomography (CT) can be used to demonstrate the location and extent of arteriovenous communications, including the involvement of specific muscle groups and bone.[6] Deep intramuscular lesions have a mottled appearance, and administra-

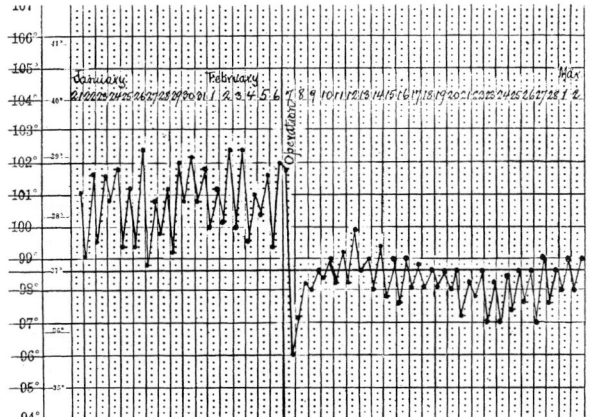

Figure 50–130. Condensed temperature chart, showing the maximal and minimal temperature each day before and after operation. The temperature, varying from 99° to 102.4° F., fell to subnormal on the day of operation and after a slight postoperative rise settled permanently at the normal level. (From Rienhoff, W. F., Jr., and Hamman, L.: Subacute *Streptococcus viridans* septicemia cured by the excision of an arteriovenous aneurysm of the external iliac artery and vein. Ann. Surg., *102*:905, 1935.)

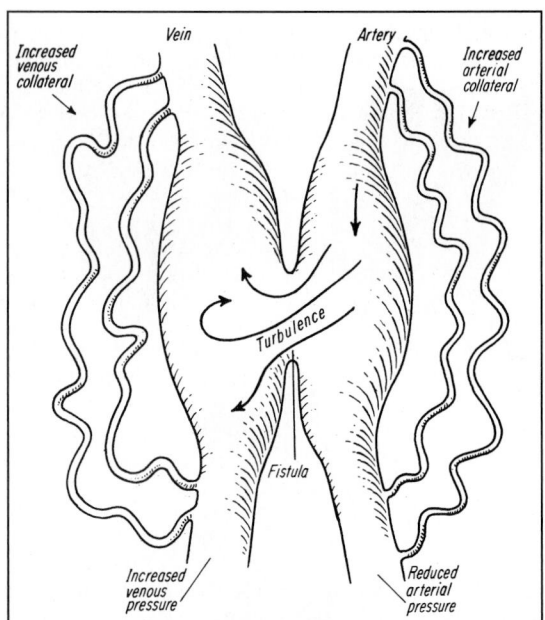

Figure 50–132. Diagrammatic illustration of the local changes that occur in the presence of an arteriovenous fistula. The changes shown are proportional to the size of the fistula. In a small fistula, these changes may be quite minimal.

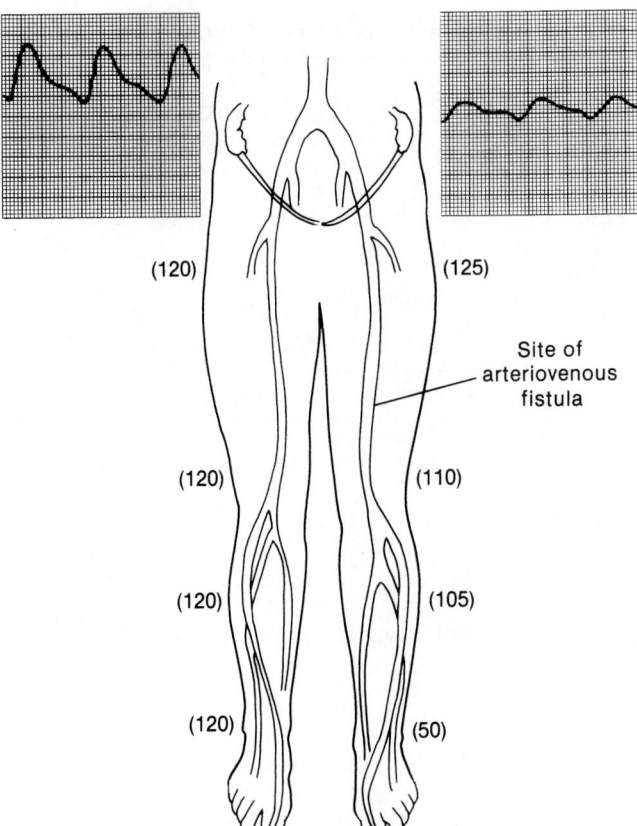

Figure 50–133. Plethysmographic record of a 35-year-old man with a traumatic superficial femoral arteriovenous fistula. Digit pulse contours are abnormal on the left, and there is a significant depression of the ankle pressure (50 mm. Hg) distal to the fistula. (Redrawn from Strandness, D. E., Jr. (Ed.): Collateral Circulation in Clinical Surgery. Philadelphia, W. B. Saunders, 1969.)

tion of contrast during CT scanning causes an enhancement that depends on the rate of arteriovenous shunting and the degree of cellularity of the lesion. Offsetting the desirable features of the CT scan are the need for intravenous contrast and the lack of an optimal protocol for its administration. MRI has distinctive advantages over CT in evaluating congenital vascular malformations, since contrast is not necessary and the anatomic extent is more clearly demonstrated.[27] Longitudinal as well as transverse sections may be obtained in the flow patterns, and the arteriovenous malformation may be characterized. MRI can identify high-flow vascular spaces and their feeding arteries and draining veins.[24] Other MRI techniques, such as even echo rephasing, can identify vessels with slow flow. In addition, MRI can identify hemorrhage into soft tissue because of the difference in signal intensity between blood and stromal tissue.

TYPES OF ARTERIOVENOUS COMMUNICATIONS

Arteriovenous communications of congenital origin in the extremities are quite common, especially in the legs, and varicose veins often result (Table 50–21).[12] Hemangiomas may involve a considerable part of the extremity and introduce serious cosmetic and physiologic problems. Congenital arteriovenous communications have been reported in all organs of the body and are frequently difficult to manage, because multiple communications exist between arteries and veins. Treatment by local interruption or arterial repair is rarely feasible. The dilated arteries and veins often encompass muscle and bone, with extensive involvement of subcutaneous tissues and skin, which makes *en bloc* resection impossible. Although surgical therapy has a role in specific types of arteriovenous communications, especially in localized lesions in which complete excision can be accomplished, some are too extensive for appropriate and complete surgical excision. For these, palliative surgical procedures are used to control disabling ulceration and infection or life-threatening hemorrhage. Ligation of major feeding arteries is not recommended because distal ischemia may result, and the intravascular

access required to allow embolization becomes limited. Alternative techniques of closure include selective intra-arterial embolization of autologous clot, wire coils, plastic balloons, or transcatheter coagulation.[20, 22, 29] Staged treatment with intervals between embolization allows portions of major malformations to be obliterated, with repeat treatment performed in persistent areas. Each of these techniques has been

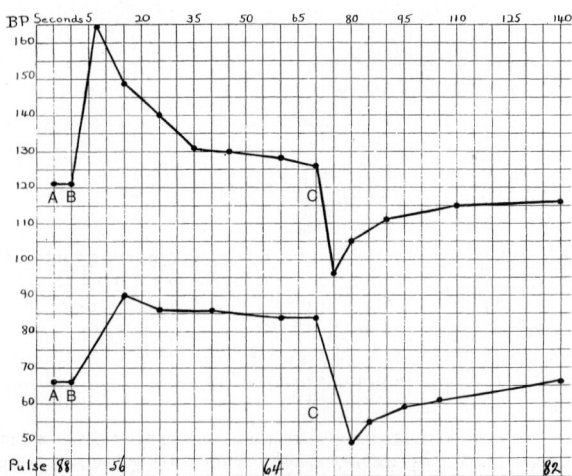

Figure 50–134. Demonstration of the Nicoladoni-Branham sign. Fluctuations in systemic blood pressure (left arm). *A*, Fistula open. *B*, Fistula closed by digital compression. *C*, Fistula reopened. (From Holman, E.: Abnormal Arteriovenous Communications. Springfield, Ill., Charles C Thomas, 1968.)

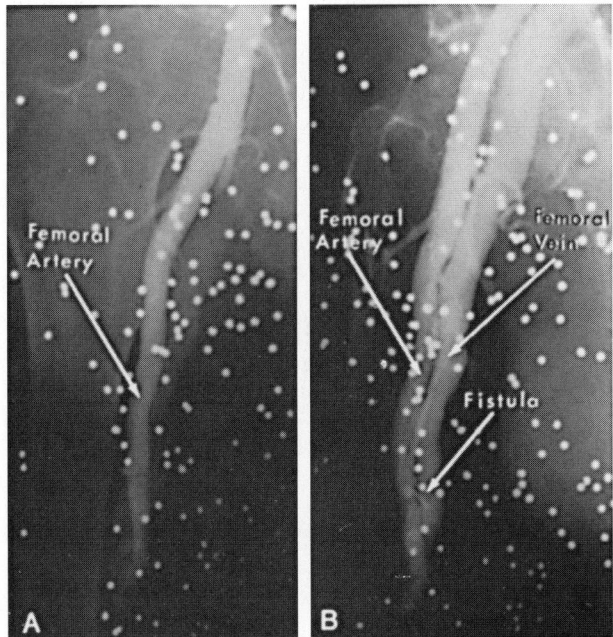

Figure 50–135. *A*, Femoral arteriogram in a patient with a gunshot wound of the thigh and a femoral arteriovenous fistula. *B*, The site of the fistula is seen, with rapid filling of the proximal femoral vein without filling distally.

successful in closing some of these fistulas that would be difficult, if not impossible, to manage surgically. Often this combination of embolization followed by surgical excision is effective in managing these difficult malformations. Other types of therapy include injection of sclerosing solutions or irradiation.

It is difficult to understand some congenital fistulas embryologically, such as those between the internal mammary artery and the pulmonary vessels.[31] Although such shunts may be small, closure of these lesions is recommended because of potential complications. Congenital pulmonary arteriovenous fistulas are common and are frequently multiple.[25] These are usually seen as well-circumscribed lesions on the chest film; if large, they may be accompanied by cyanosis due to the right-to-left shunting. Symptoms include exertional dyspnea, easy fatigability, cyanosis, and clubbing of the fingers. Approximately 10% to 15% of these lesions occur in children. Complications include cerebrovascular accidents, brain abscesses, hemoptysis, and intrapleural rupture.[40] A continuous bruit with systolic accentuation during deep inspiration is heard in approximately two thirds of patients. Pulmonary arteriography confirms the diagnosis. Hereditary telangiectasis (Rendu-Osler-Weber disease) is quite common and may be familial in origin. These patients also have a tendency to develop additional fistulas with the passage of time. Management of pulmonary arteriovenous fistulas is primarily surgical, and because only the lesion requires removal, most can be managed by either local or wedge resection. In the presence of bilateral fistulas, the site of major involvement is usually treated and the remaining one approached only if necessary. Some patients have also been managed by selective arterial embolization.[39] Penetrating pulmonary injuries can also produce this type of arteriovenous fistula, which should be corrected surgically.[37]

Acquired fistulas are most frequently found in the extremities and are often secondary to penetrating trauma, with accompanying varices, edema, and pigmentation. Unlike with congenital communications, a single or limited number of abnormal communications exist that can be demonstrated by angiography or color-flow Doppler. Vascular insufficiency

of digits and ulceration may also be present in the more severe forms. A palpable thrill and an audible machinery-like bruit are usually present at the site of the fistula. The affected extremity is generally warmer than is the control, and compression of the fistula usually causes a diminished heart rate and an increase in diastolic arterial pressure. A patient with a popliteal aneurysm and arteriovenous fistula is shown in Figure 50–136.

A number of surgical procedures, including operations on the kidney and intervertebral discs, can produce iatrogenic fistulas. Disc procedures may be associated with fistulas in the iliac vessels or with aortocaval fistulas.[19] Iatrogenic fistulas following thyroid procedures, coronary artery bypass grafting, distal splenorenal shunt, small bowel resection, Fontan's operation, and pelvic surgery have been described.[10, 11, 13, 28, 41] Cardiac catheterization and percutaneous transhepatic variceal embolization for bleeding varices have been complicated by arteriovenous fistulas.[2, 14] Renal arteriovenous fistulas after nephrectomy are usually large communications, and cardiac failure is not uncommon.[23] Increasing numbers of fistulas are observed after percutaneous biopsy or cardiac catheterization. Fistulas may also be present after *in situ* femoropopliteal bypass grafting if venous tributaries of the saphenous vein are not ligated. Fistulas also may occur with transplanted organs at the site of the vascular anastomoses.[21]

Erosion through the wall of an aneurysm at the site of atherosclerotic plaque into accompanying veins may also occur. An example is that of an aortocaval fistula from an abdominal aortic aneurysm (Fig. 50–137).[1] Such a lesion may produce congestive heart failure and require an emergent surgical procedure. In a series of six patients, symptoms of an abdominal bruit, widened pulse pressure, venous hypertension, edema, arterial insufficiency, and congestive heart failure were present in three. Proximal and distal control of the aorta allows the artery to be opened and the fistula controlled by a finger placed on the communication. Compression with sponge sticks proximal and distal to the fistula allows repair of the vein. After the vein is repaired, the preferred method for restoring arterial continuity is with a graft. A review of the literature cites 158 cases.[4] Aortocaval fistulas of neoplastic origin have also been reported.[7]

The most common acquired arteriovenous fistula is that associated with vascular access to permit renal dialysis in the management of renal insufficiency. Problems associated with this type of fistula are discussed in Chapter 19. Arteriovenous fistulas have also been surgically constructed to increase blood flow and patency to a vascular anastomosis, such as venous reconstruction and venous access procedures.[5, 8, 17]

Surgical closure of most arteriovenous fistulas is recom-

TABLE 50–21. Ten-Year Experience in Incidence of Congenital and Acquired Arteriovenous (A-V) Fistulas

	Congenital	Acquired
A-V fistulas of the extremities	80	17
Aorta–inferior vena cava fistulas	0	7
Pulmonary A-V fistulas	47	0
Renal A-V fistulas	0	6
A-V fistulas of the portal system	0	1
A-V fistulas of the neck and face	11	4
Pelvic A-V fistulas	1	5
A-V fistulas of the chest wall	0	2
Total	139	42

Adapted from Gomes, M. M. R., and Bernatz, P. E.: Arteriovenous fistulas: A review and ten-year experience at the Mayo Clinic. Mayo Clin. Proc., *45*:81, 1970.

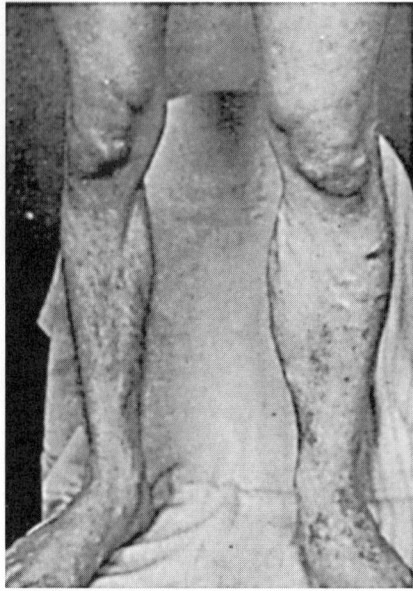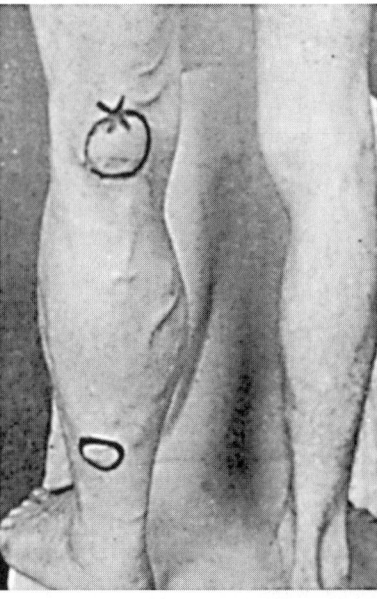

Figure 50–136. Appearance of patient with a left popliteal arteriovenous fistula of 25 years' duration located at X. Pulsating veins are circled. The palpated diameters of both femoral arteries are shown. (From Holman, E.: Abnormal Arteriovenous Communications. Springfield, Ill., Charles C Thomas, 1968.)

mended, since most are potentially symptomatic.[5] Early surgical attempts to correct these lesions consisted primarily of ligation of the involved artery proximal to the fistula. Whereas the threat of rupture of a classic arterial aneurysm might be diminished by ligating the artery proximally, this approach in the presence of an arteriovenous fistula is apt to end disastrously, because it is quite likely to be followed by gangrene of the extremity. Gangrene can result because blood reaching the distal extremity by arterial collaterals is apt to drain retrograde through the fistula directly into the venous system, thus depriving the limb of adequate distal arterial blood flow. The first successful treatment of an arteriovenous fistula was proximal and distal ligation of both the artery and the vein. This quadripolar ligation corrected the fistula and was not followed by peripheral vascular insufficiency of the limb, owing to the large number of arterial collaterals that had formed as a result of the fistula.

Surgical management includes accurate diagnosis and determination of the extent of the lesions. Acute fistulas with high flow causing cardiovascular collapse or distal ischemia require urgent repair, whereas long-standing lesions with extensive involvement of surrounding tissue require thoughtful preoperative planning. The site of the communication should always be carefully localized by arteriography; however, CT scanning, MRI, and color-flow Doppler imaging are increasingly utilized to diagnose arteriovenous communications. The ideal surgical management usually includes direct closure of the fistula, with restoration of arterial and venous continuity.[3] However, when this is not possible, quadripolar ligation is acceptable when there is sufficient arterial collateral circulation to adequately supply the tissues distally. Although gangrene usually does not occur, intermittent claudication frequently results, despite collateral circulation. However, in the majority of patients, it is possible to close the fistula without the need for amputation. Complete excision is reserved for fistulas involving small nonessential arteries, such as the radial or ulnar arteries, when adequate collaterals are present.

Small fistulas occasionally close spontaneously.[36] In congenital forms, excision of diffuse malformations may not be possible. The complex communications seen with congenital arteriovenous malformations often require a multidisciplinary approach, including selective intra-arterial embolization in conjunction with surgical therapy. Asymptomatic lesions may not require treatment, but any fistula represents a hazard. Absolute indications for treatment include hemorrhage, secondary ischemic complications, and congestive heart failure from arteriovenous shunting; relative indications include pain, nonhealing ulcers, functional impairment, and cosmetic deformity. If treatment is required, careful planning is mandatory. Patients with symptomatic lesions that are thought to be resectable should undergo surgical excision, since complete removal provides the best likelihood for cure. This is more suitable for superficial lesions on the trunk, scalp, face, and extremities, and the goal of surgical therapy should be complete excision of the lesion. Ligation of feeding vessels is only temporarily effective, and the rapid recruitment of collateral channels makes further treatment, especially embo-

Figure 50–137. Arteriovenous fistula between the abdominal aorta and the right common iliac vein due to erosion by atherosclerosis. IVC, inferior vena cava.

lization, difficult or impossible. Resection of large lesions may be associated with significant blood loss, and preoperative embolization may facilitate surgical resection and reduce operative blood loss.

Embolization by the transcatheter technique has a significant role in the treatment of many malformations. Numerous embolic materials have been developed, from simple Gelfoam pledgets to complex systems employing microcatheters and detachable balloons. Embolization procedures must be carefully planned, and a detailed, selective angiographic examination must be made initially to determine which vessels supply the lesion, likely sources of collateral resupply, and routes of venous drainage. Embolization is then performed as a separate procedure, usually under general anesthesia. Secondary feeder arteries are embolized first for conversion of the lesion into one supplied by a single vessel. The primary feeding vessel is then selectively catheterized and embolized, with the goal of penetration and obliteration of the lesion. Complex lesions may require multiple-stage embolization procedures because of limitations in anesthetic time and in the volume of contrast material that can be safely administered. Complications of embolization include tissue necrosis, inadvertent embolization of normal tissues, and passage of embolic materials through arteriovenous communications, causing pulmonary embolization. Recurrences after proximal ligation or embolization are extremely difficult to treat because of the recruitment of multiple new sources of blood supply to the lesion.

SELECTED REFERENCES

Calligaro, K. D., Savarese, R. P., and DeLaurentis, D. A.: Unusual aspects of aortovenous fistulas associated with ruptured abdominal aortic aneurysms (Review). J. Vasc. Surg., 12:586, 1990.
A review of 158 cases of aortocaval fistulas reported in the literature.

Gomes, M. M. R., and Bernatz, P. E.: Arteriovenous fistulas: A review and ten-year experience at the Mayo Clinic. Mayo Clin. Proc., 45:81, 1970.
A large series of patients with congenital and acquired arteriovenous fistulas is presented. It is a valuable reference and provides data on the many specific types of lesions.

Holman, E.: Abnormal Arteriovenous Communications. Springfield, Ill., Charles C Thomas, 1968.
This is a classic and authoritative reference on the subject of arteriovenous fistulas. All aspects of these lesions are considered from both physiologic and clinical viewpoints. Its author won the prestigious Samuel D. Gross Prize.

Tan, O. T., Sherwood, K., and Gilchrest, B. A.: Treatment of children with portwine stains using the flashlamp-pulsed tunable dye laser. N. Engl. J. Med., 320:416, 1989.
Thirty-five children, 3 months to 14 years of age, with disfiguring port-wine stains were treated with a flash-lamp-pulsed tunable dye laser. All had complete clearing of the stains after an average of 6.5 laser treatments to each lesional area.

REFERENCES

1. Baker, W. H., Sharzer, L. A., and Ehrenhaft, J. L.: Aortocaval fistula as complication of abdominal aortic aneurysms. Surgery, 72:933, 1972.
2. Bedell, J. E., Keller, F. S., and Rosch, J.: Iatrogenic intrahepatic arterial-portal fistula. Radiology, 151:79, 1984.
3. Branham, H. H.: Aneurismal varix of the femoral artery and vein following a gunshot wound. Int. J. Surg., 3:250, 1890.
4. Calligaro, K. D., Savarese, R. P., and DeLaurentis, D. A.: Unusual aspects of aortovenous fistulas associated with ruptured abdominal aortic aneurysms (Review). J. Vasc. Surg., 12:586, 1990.
5. Coburn, M. C., Carney, W. I., Jr.: Comparison of basilic vein and polytetrafluoroethylene for brachial arteriovenous fistula. J. Vasc. Surg., 20:896, 1994.
6. Cohen, J. M., Weinreb, J. C., and Redman, H. C.: Arteriovenous malformations of the extremities: MR imaging. Radiology, 158:475, 1986.
7. Crawford, E. S., Turell, D. J., and Alexander, J. K.: Aortoinferior vena caval fistula of neoplastic origin. Circulation, 27:414, 1963.
8. Dardik, H., Sussman, B., Ibrahim, I. M., Kahn, M., Svoboda, J. J., Mendes, D., and Dardik, I.: Distal arteriovenous fistula as an adjunct to maintaining arterial and graft patency for limb salvage. Surgery, 94:478, 1983.
9. Daxini, B. V., Desai, A. G., and Sharma, S.: Echo-Doppler diagnosis of aortocaval fistula following blunt trauma to abdomen. Am. Heart J., 118:843, 1989.
10. Decker, D. G., Fish, C. R., and Juergens, J. L.: Arteriovenous fistulas of the female pelvis: A diagnostic problem. Obstet. Gynecol., 31:799, 1968.
11. Diehl, J. T., and Beven, E. G.: Arteriovenous fistulas of the mesenteric vessels: Report of a case and review of the literature. J. Cardiovasc. Surg., 23:334, 1982.
12. Gomes, M. M. R., and Bernatz, P. E.: Arteriovenous fistulas: A review and ten-year experience at the Mayo Clinic. Mayo Clin. Proc., 45:81, 1970.
13. Gonzalez, E. M., Garcia, I. G., Blanch, G. G., Garcia, I. L., and Gonzalez, J. S.: Left gastric arteriovenous fistula after selective distal splenorenal shunt. Surgery, 93:510, 1983.
14. Hansbrough, J. F., Narrod, J. A., and Rutherford, R.: Arteriovenous fistulas following central venous catheterization. Intensive Care Med., 9:287, 1983.
15. Holman, E.: Abnormal Arteriovenous Communications. Springfield, Ill., Charles C Thomas, 1968.
16. Hunter, W.: The history of an aneurysm of the aorta, with some remarks on aneurysms in general. Med. Observ. Inquir., 1:323, 1757.
17. Jacobs, M. J., Gregoric, I. D., and Reul, G. J.: Prosthetic graft placement and creation of a distal arteriovenous fistula for secondary vascular reconstruction in patients with severe limb ischemia. J. Vasc. Surg., 15:612, 1992.
18. Janes, J. M., and Jennings, W. K., Jr.: Effect of induced arteriovenous fistula on leg length: 10 year observations. Mayo Clin. Proc., 36:1, 1961.
19. Jarstfer, B. E., and Rich, N. M.: The challenge of arteriovenous fistula formation following disk surgery: A collective review. J. Trauma, 16:726, 1976.
20. Kerber, C. W., Freeny, P. C., Cromwell, L., et al.: Cyanoacrylate occlusion of a renal arteriovenous fistula. A. J. R. Am. J. Roentgenol., 128:663, 1977.
21. Lowell, J. A., Bynon, J. S., Stratta, R. J., and Taylor, R. J.: Superior mesenteric arteriovenous fistula in vascularized whole organ pancreatic allografts. Surg. Gynecol. Obstet., 177:254, 1993.
22. McAlister, D. S., Johnsrude, I., Miller, M. M., Clapp, J., and Thompson, W. M.: Occlusion of acquired renal arteriovenous fistula with transcatheter electrocoagulation. A. J. R. Am. J. Roentgenol., 132:998, 1979.
23. McCutcheon, F. B., and Hara, M.: Arteriovenous fistula following nephrectomy. J. Cardiovasc. Surg., 8:253, 1967.
24. Mills, C. M., Brant-Zawadski, M., and Crooks, L. E.: Nuclear magnetic resonance: Principles of blood flow imaging. A. J. R. Am. J. Roentgenol., 142:165, 1984.
25. Moyer, J. H., Glantz, G., and Brest, A. N.: Pulmonary arteriovenous fistulas: Physiologic and clinical considerations. Am. J. Med., 32:417, 1962.
26. Nicoladoni, C.: Phlebarteriectasie der rechten oberen Extremität. Arch. Klin. Chir., 18:252, 1975.
27. Pearce, W. H., Rutherford, R. B., Whitehill, T. A., et al.: Nuclear magnetic resonance imaging: Its diagnostic value in patients with congenital vascular malformations of the limbs. J. Vasc. Surg., 8:64, 1988.
28. Przybojewski, J. Z.: Iatrogenic aortocoronary vein fistula. S. Afr. Med. J., 62:908, 1982.
29. Ricketts, R. R., Fink, E., and Yellin, A. E.: Management of major arteriovenous fistulas by arteriographic techniques. Arch. Surg., 113:1153, 1978.
30. Rienhoff, W. F., Jr., and Hamman, L.: Subacute *Streptococcus viridans* septicemia cured by the excision of an arteriovenous aneurysm of the external iliac artery and vein. Ann. Surg., 102:905, 1935.
31. Robinson, L. A., and Sabiston, D. C., Jr.: Syndrome of congenital internal mammary-to-pulmonary arteriovenous fistula associated with mitral valve prolapse. Arch. Surg., 116:1265, 1981.
32. Sabiston, D. C., Jr., Theilen, E. O., and Gregg, D. E.: Physiologic studies in experimental high output cardiac failure produced by aortic-caval fistula. Surg. Forum, 6:233, 1956.
33. Scott, H. W., Jr., and Sabiston, D. C., Jr.: Surgical treatment for congenital aorticopulmonary fistula. J. Thorac. Surg., 25:26, 1953.
34. Shadle, O. W., Ferguson, T. B., Sabiston, D. C., Jr., and Gregg, D. E.: The hemodynamic response to lanatoside C of dogs with experimental aortic-caval fistulas. J. Clin. Invest., 36:335, 1957.
35. Sheikh, K. H., Adams, D. B., McCann, R., Lyerly, H. K., Sabiston, D. C., Jr., and Kisslo, J.: Utility of Doppler color flow imaging for identification of femoral arterial complications of cardiac catheterization. Am. Heart J., 117:623, 1989.
36. Shumacker, H. B.: Arterial aneurysms and arteriovenous fistulas: Spontaneous cures. *In* Elkin, D. C., and DeBakey, M. E. (Eds.): Surgery in World War II: Vascular Surgery. Washington, D.C., Office of the Surgeon General, Department of the Army, 1955.
37. Symbas, P. N., Goldman, M., Erbesfeld, M. H., and Vlasis, S. E.: Pulmonary arteriovenous fistula, pulmonary artery aneurysm, and other vascular changes of the lung from penetrating trauma. Ann. Surg., 191:336, 1980.
38. Tafreshi, M., Steinbaum, S., Scarlett, K., and Alexander, L. L.: Ultrasonic demonstration of arteriovenous fistulas. J. Clin. Ultrasound, 12:299, 1984.
39. Taylor, B. G., Cockerill, E. M., Manfredi, F., and Klatte, E. C.: Therapeutic embolization of the pulmonary artery in pulmonary arteriovenous fistula. Am. J. Med., 64:360, 1978.
40. Waldhausen, J. A., and Shumacker, H. B., Jr.: Pulmonary arteriovenous fistulae. Heart Bull., 14:57, 1965.
41. Webster, M. W.: Arteriovenous fistula following thyroidectomy. J. Cardiovasc. Surg., 23:515, 1982.

THROMBOANGIITIS OBLITERANS (BUERGER'S DISEASE)

H. Brownell Wheeler, M.D.

In 1908, Leo Buerger published clinical and pathologic observations on young men with severe ischemia of the extremities.[2] These patients were addicted to cigarette smoking and often had migratory superficial phlebitis. Buerger called the syndrome thromboangiitis obliterans because the acute histologic picture was characterized by thrombosis in both arteries and veins and was associated with a marked inflammatory response. However, the condition became more commonly known as Buerger's disease.

CLINICAL MANIFESTATIONS

Thromboangiitis obliterans typically occurs in heavy smokers between 20 and 35 years of age. It was once thought to occur only in men, but several cases have been reported in women.[12] The diagnosis of thromboangiitis obliterans should be considered in any young smoker with peripheral ischemia. Unlike in atherosclerosis, the upper extremities are often involved and there is frequently a history of migratory superficial phlebitis. The ischemic areas are usually sharply demarcated, with relatively good circulation in adjacent tissues. The pain is often excruciating. Associated symptoms include cold sensitivity, Raynaud's phenomenon, and peripheral neuropathy. Foot claudication is particularly characteristic.[8] Exacerbations with smoking and remissions after abstinence from tobacco are typical of thromboangiitis obliterans. The disease has been described in patients who chew tobacco or use snuff[18, 25] as well as in those who smoke. It has also been reported infrequently in nonsmokers.[31] Careful clinical evaluation is necessary to rule out other causes of peripheral ischemia, especially atherosclerosis, hypercoagulable states, and autoimmune vasculitis. Unlike in atherosclerosis, the forearm, calf, or digital arteries are the main sites of occlusion.[19] Absence of a radial pulse, a positive Allen's test indicating ulnar artery occlusion, or superficial phlebitis may be clues to the diagnosis. The iliac, femoral, popliteal, and brachial arteries are usually not involved.

Arteriography early in the disease usually reveals segmental obliteration of small and medium-sized arteries, especially the arteries of the forearm and calf, with a strikingly normal appearance of other vessels. Digital arteries are frequently involved.[4, 6] Atherosclerotic plaques are absent, and collateral circulation in chronic cases is unusually well developed.

The clinical course of thromboangiitis obliterans is protracted and painful but relatively benign. If a patient ceases smoking, prolonged remission usually occurs. However, most patients continue to smoke despite the most emphatic advice. They have repeated attacks and may require multiple distal amputations. Life-endangering complications are uncommon, but infrequently the mesenteric or cerebrovascular circulation may be involved. Long-term life expectancy is only slightly less than that of the general population, unlike patients with comparable degrees of peripheral ischemia due to atherosclerosis (Fig. 50–138).[17, 26] In later life, patients with thromboangiitis obliterans often develop atherosclerosis and may exhibit features of both diseases.

PATHOLOGY

The most characteristic pathologic changes are seen early in the disease process. Thrombosis occurs in arteries and

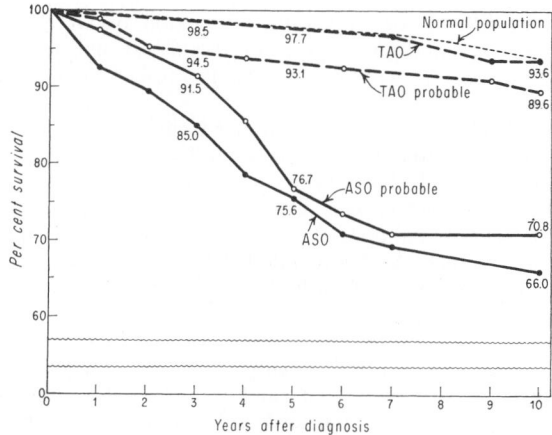

Figure 50–138. Widely differing 10-year survival rates in Buerger's disease (TAO) and arteriosclerosis (ASO). Confirmed cases of Buerger's disease show no significant difference from the normal population. (From McPherson, J. R., Juergens, J. L., and Gifford, R. W.: Thromboangiitis obliterans and arteriosclerosis obliterans: Clinical and prognostic differences. Ann. Intern. Med., *59*:288, 1963.)

veins of medium to small size, with dense aggregates of polymorphonuclear leukocytes within the thrombus. There is an associated panvasculitis, but the elastic lamina remains intact.[35] Unlike atherosclerosis or periarteritis nodosa, the disease does not cause necrosis of the arterial wall. Later, microabscesses occur, and giant cells appear within the granulation tissue. The thrombus is organized, and recanalization of the lumen may occur (Fig. 50–139). Older lesions show chronic inflammatory infiltrates and/or extensive fibrosis, which often involve peripheral nerves as well as arteries and veins. There is considerable variability in histologic findings, depending on the stage of the disease observed.[13]

ETIOLOGY

A specific cause for thromboangiitis obliterans has never been documented, although the striking association with cigarette smoking suggests a strong etiologic relationship.[14] Patients with thromboangiitis obliterans usually come from lower socioeconomic groups. They often have poor hygiene and a history of chronic fungal infection or cold injury.[7] Fibrinogen levels may be elevated, blood viscosity may be increased,[32] and a hypercoagulable state has been postulated. Hyperaggregability of platelets has also been reported during acute attacks. Familial predisposition has been reported, as well as a greater prevalence of specific leukocyte antigens.[23] An autoimmune etiology of the disease has been postulated, based on the finding of antibodies and lymphocyte-mediated sensitivity to collagen.[1, 30] Antibodies to rickettsial organisms have been reported in patients with thromboangiitis obliterans, as have circulating immune complexes.[5] A genetic factor is suggested by the fact that blacks are rarely affected, whereas the disease is common in Asia. Jewish men were originally reported to be particularly susceptible to the disease, although later studies failed to confirm this predisposition. Autonomic overactivity is suggested by the association with severe peripheral vasospasm and hyperhidrosis and has also been documented through cold pressor tests.[36] Any factor that causes vasospasm, thrombosis, or local inflammation may contribute to the development of thromboangiitis obliterans in a susceptible individual. It is likely that some immunologic process activated by smoking plays the primary etiologic role in thromboangiitis obliterans.[18, 21, 34]

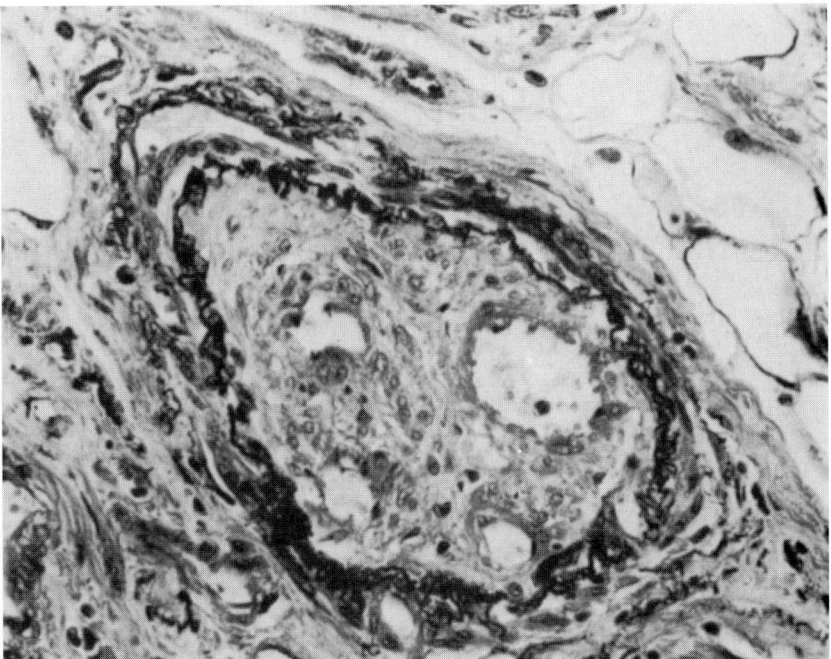

Figure 50–139. Chronic, well-organized arterial thrombosis in a 30-year-old man with Buerger's disease. Unlike arteriosclerosis, there is no degeneration or calcification in the vessel wall. The elastic lamina is intact, and the lumen has been partially recanalized. It would be unusual for arteriosclerosis to involve such a small artery (1 mm.). Van Giesen-elastic stain. ×570. (Courtesy of the Rev. Robert W. Bain, M.D., Department of Pathology, St. Vincent Hospital, Worcester, Mass.)

INCIDENCE

Based on data from World War II veterans, DeBakey and Cohen estimated the incidence of thromboangiitis obliterans at seven or eight cases per 100,000 white males 20 to 44 years of age.[3] However, the incidence of thromboangiitis obliterans has decreased markedly since World War II. At the Mayo Clinic, its prevalence declined 10-fold from 1947 to 1976, although there has been a slight upward trend in recent years.[11] The diagnosis of thromboangiitis obliterans was made in 24% of all young adults (age 35 or younger) presenting to the Mayo Clinic with lower limb ischemia from 1953 to 1981.[27]

In a retrospective review of 100 patients with ischemic finger ulcerations, thromboangiitis obliterans was the final diagnosis in 9%.[19] In patients with severe ischemia and digital gangrene, the incidence was 13%.[20] In another study of 700 patients with small-vessel arterial disease, thromboangiitis obliterans was the final diagnosis in 3.7%.[23] At present, thromboangiitis obliterans comprises less than 1% of all patients with severe peripheral ischemia in the United States. In Israel and Eastern Europe, the corresponding incidence is approximately 5%, whereas in Japan it is 16%. Patients with thromboangiitis obliterans are observed much more frequently in Asia, even in populations where atherosclerosis is rare.[16, 22]

MANAGEMENT

The major problem in treating patients with thromboangiitis obliterans is the management of pain, which is often excruciating. Narcotics are usually necessary but must be used cautiously because of the frequency of drug addiction. Peripheral or sympathetic nerve blocks may provide temporary pain relief, especially when the disease is accompanied by severe vasospasm. When nerve blocks prove beneficial, dorsal or lumbar sympathectomy may provide more lasting benefit, although experience is anecdotal. Meticulous conservative treatment of ischemic lesions may result in healing, especially in the upper extremity, but relief of pain sometimes requires amputation.[18, 21]

Every effort should be made to have the patient stop

smoking, since remission often follows abstinence from cigarettes. No specific medication has found wide acceptance. Anticoagulants, dextran, phenylbutazone, inositol niacinate, and corticosteroids have all been recommended. More recently, prostaglandin therapy[29] and defibrotide[33] have been advocated, as well as agents to prevent platelet aggregation. Pentoxifylline has also been advocated.[21] Severe hand ischemia due to acute thrombosis in thromboangiitis obliterans has been dramatically improved by intra-arterial infusion of urokinase, followed by small-vessel balloon catheter angioplasty and anticoagulation.[10]

Arterial reconstruction is usually impossible because of the distal nature of the disease, but it should be considered in segmental proximal occlusions. A successful mesenteric artery bypass has been reported in a 23-year-old man with visceral thromboangiitis obliterans.[28] Arterial reconstructions for thromboangiitis obliterans have a higher failure rate than comparable reconstructions for atherosclerosis. Microvascular transplantation of free omental grafts to areas not amenable to arterial reconstruction has been successfully employed,[24] as have pedicled omental grafts.[9, 15] When gangrene occurs, amputation at the lowest possible level is indicated. Digital amputations for thromboangiitis obliterans have a better healing rate than digital amputations for atherosclerotic gangrene.

SELECTED REFERENCES

Hagen, B., and Lohse, S.: Clinical and radiologic aspects of Buerger's disease. Cardiovasc. Intervent. Radiol., 7:283, 1984.
  This article combines a comprehensive description of the angiographic signs of thromboangiitis obliterans with excellent illustrations.

Lie, J. T.: Thromboangiitis obliterans (Buerger's disease) revisited. Pathol. Annu., 23:257, 1988.
  This article reviews the pathology of thromboangiitis obliterans and contains many excellent photomicrographs.

McKusick, V. A., Harris, W. S., Ottesen, O. E., Goodman, E. M., Shelley, W. M., and Bloodwell, R. D.: Buerger's disease: A distinct clinical and pathologic entity. JAMA, 181:5, 1962.
  This classic article documents that Buerger's disease is a distinct clinical and pathologic entity, based on arteriographic studies of both upper and lower extremities in 12 patients and histopathologic study of 10 biopsy and amputation specimens. No evidence of atherosclerosis was observed in any of these patients. Similar findings are also described in 28 Korean patients (in whom atherosclerosis is rare).

Mills, J. L.: Buerger's disease: Current status. Vasc. Med. Rev., 5:139, 1994.
This review article is the most comprehensive and authoritative recent summary of the medical literature on thromboangiitis obliterans.

REFERENCES

1. Adar, R., Papa, M. Z., Halpern, Z., Mozes, M., Shoshan S., Sofer, B., Zinger, H., Dayan, M., and Mozes, E.: Cellular sensitivity to collagen in thromboangiitis obliterans. N. Engl. J. Med., 308:1113, 1983.
2. Buerger, L.: Thromboangiitis obliterans: A study of the vascular lesions leading to presenile spontaneous gangrene. Am. J. Med. Sci., 136:567, 1908.
3. DeBakey, M. D., and Cohen, B. M.: Buerger's Disease: A Follow-up Study of World War II Army Cases. Springfield, Ill., Charles C Thomas, 1963.
4. Dible, J. H.: *In* Cameron, R., and Wright, G. P. (Eds.): The Pathology of Limb Ischemia. St. Louis, Warren H. Green, 1966, p. 79.
5. Gulati, S. M., Saham, K., Kant, L., Thusoo, T. K., and Prakash, A.: Significance of circulatory immune complexes in thromboangiitis obliterans (Buerger's disease). Angiology, 35:276, 1984.
6. Hagen, B., and Lohse, S.: Clinical and radiologic aspects of Buerger's disease. Cardiovasc. Intervent. Radiol., 7:283, 1984.
7. Hill, G. L., Moelino, J., et al.: The Buerger syndrome in Java. Br. J. Surg., 60:606, 1973.
8. Hirai, M., and Shionoya, S.: Intermittent claudication in the foot and Buerger's disease. Br. J. Surg., 65:210, 1978.
9. Hoshino, S., Nakayama, K., Igari, T., and Honda, K.: Long-term results of omental transplantation for chronic occlusive arterial disease. Int. Surg., 68:47, 1983.
10. Lang, E. V., and Bookstein, J. J.: Accelerated thrombolysis and angioplasty for hand ischemia in Buerger's disease. Cardiovasc. Intervent. Radiol., 12:95, 1989.
11. Lie, J. T.: The rise and fall and resurgence of thromboangiitis obliterans (Buerger's disease). Acta Pathol. Jpn., 39:153, 1989.
12. Lie, J. T.: Thromboangiitis obliterans (Buerger's disease) in women. Medicine, 66:65, 1987.
13. Lie, J. T.: Thromboangiitis obliterans (Buerger's disease) revisited. Pathol. Annu., 23:257, 1988.
14. Matsushita, M., Shionoya, S., and Matsumoto, T.: Urinary nicotine measurement in patients with Buerger's disease: Effects of active and passive smoking on the disease process. J. Vasc. Surg., 14:53, 1991.
15. Maurva, S. D., Singhal, S., Gupta, H. C., Elhence, I. P., and Sharma, B. D.: Pedicled omental grafts in the revascularization of ischemic lower limbs in Buerger's disease. Int. Surg., 70:253, 1985.
16. McKusick, V. A., et al.: Buerger's disease: A distinct clinical and pathologic entity. JAMA, 181:5, 1962.
17. McPherson, J. R., et al.: Thromboangiitis obliterans and arteriosclerosis obliterans: Clinical and prognostic differences. Ann. Intern. Med., 59:288, 1963.
18. Mills, J. L.: Buerger's disease: Current status. Vasc. Med. Rev., 5:139, 1994.
19. Mills, J. L., Friedman, E. I., Taylor, L. M., Jr., and Porter, J. M.: Upper extremity ischemia caused by small artery disease. Ann. Surg., 206:521, 1987.
20. Mills, J. L., and Fujitani, R. M.: Acute and chronic upper extremity ischemia: II. Small vessel arterial occlusive disease: Basic data underlying clinical decision making. Ann. Vasc. Surg., 7:195, 1993.
21. Mills, J. L., and Porter, J. M.: Buerger's disease: A review and update. Semin. Vasc. Surg., 6:14, 1993.
22. Mills, J. L., and Porter, J. M.: Buerger's disease (thromboangiitis obliterans): Basic data related to clinical decision-making in vascular surgery. Ann. Vasc. Surg., 5:570, 1991.
23. Mills, J. L., Taylor, L. M., Jr., and Porter, J. M.: Buerger's disease in the modern era. Am. J. Surg. 154:123, 1987.
24. Nishimura, A., Sano, F., Nakanishi, Y., Loshino, I., and Kassi, Y.: Omental transplantation for relief of limb ischaemia. Surg. Forum, 28:213, 1977.
25. O'Dell, J. R., Linder, J., Markin, R. S., and Moore, G.F.: Thromboangiitis obliterans (Buerger's disease) and smokeless tobacco. Arthritis Rheum., 30:1054, 1987.
26. Ohta, T., Shionoya, S.: Fate of the ischaemic limb in Buerger's disease. Br. J. Surg., 75:259, 1988.
27. Pairolero, P. C., Joyce, J. W., Skinner, C. R., Hollier, L. H., and Cherry, K. J., Jr.: Lower limb ischemia in young adults: Prognostic implications. J. Vasc. Surg., 1:459, 1984.
28. Schellong, S. M., Bernhards, J., Ensslen, F., Schaefers, H. J., and Alexander, K.: Intestinal type of thromboangiitis obliterans (Buerger's disease). J. Int. Med., 235:69, 1994.
29. Shionoya, S.: What is Buerger's disease? World J. Surg., 7:544, 1983.
30. Spittell, J. A.: Thromboangiitis obliterans—an autoimmune disorder (editorial)? N. Engl. J. Med., 308:1157, 1983.
31. Stojanovic, V. K., Marcovic, A., Arsov, V., Bujanic, J., and Lolina, S.: Clinical course and therapy of Buerger's disease. J. Cardiothorac. Surg., 14:5, 1973.
32. Szendro, G., Golcman, L., and Cristal, N.: Study of the factors affecting blood viscosity in patients with thromboangiitis obliterans: A preliminary report. J. Vasc. Surg., 7:759, 1988.
33. Ulutin, O. N.: Clinical effectiveness of defibrotide in vaso-occlusive disorders and its mode of actions. Semin. Thromb. Hemost., 14(Suppl.):58, 1988.
34. Vermylen, J., Blockmans, D., Spitz, B., and Deckmyn, H.: Thrombosis and immune disorders. Clin. Haematol., 15:393, 1986.
35. Williams, G.: Recent views on Buerger's disease. J. Clin. Pathol., 22:573, 1969.
36. Yamamoto, K., Iwase, S., Mano, T., and Shionoya, S.: Muscle sympathetic outflow in Buerger's disease. J. Autonom. Nerv. Syst., 44:67, 1993.

RAYNAUD'S SYNDROME

James M. Edwards, M.D.
Gregory J. Landry, M.D.
John M. Porter, M.D.

Raynaud's syndrome defines a condition characterized by episodic vasospasm resulting in closure of the small arteries and arterioles of the distal parts of the extremities in response to cold exposure or emotional stimuli. The fingers and hands are most frequently involved, although in many patients the toes and feet may be similarly affected. Classically, the episodes consist of intense pallor of the distal extremities followed by cyanosis and rubor on rewarming, with full recovery requiring 15 to 45 minutes. Many patients, however, develop only pallor or cyanosis during attacks, and it is now clear that the classic tricolor pattern occurs only in a small number of patients. A number of patients who complain of cold hands without digital color changes have abnormal arteriographic and blood flow findings identical to those of patients with classic digital color changes, thus leading to the suggestion that digital color change may not be essential for the diagnosis.

PATHOPHYSIOLOGY

The pallor in the early stage of Raynaud episodes is initiated by severe spasm of the arteries and arterioles, which causes cessation of capillary perfusion. Resultant hypoxia and the accumulation of the metabolic products of regional anaerobic metabolism cause the capillaries and probably the venules to dilate. This is followed by a slight relaxation of the arteriolar spasm with the entry of a small amount of blood into the dilated capillaries, which rapidly becomes desaturated, producing cyanosis. Rubor results from the entry of increasing amounts of blood into dilated capillaries. The episode terminates with the entry of a normal volume of blood through the relaxed arterioles and the return of the dilated capillaries to normal.

The mechanism of vasoconstriction that occurs during an episode of Raynaud's syndrome has interested investigators for more than a century. Raynaud's suggestion that the episodes represented sympathetic nervous system hyperactivity was largely disproved by Lewis in the 1920s and 1930s.[25] He concluded that the digital arteries in this condition close completely on exposure to cold and that this closure is responsible for the clinical symptoms. Based on failure to prevent cold-induced vasospasm by digital nerve conduction anesthesia, Lewis proposed the theory of local vascular wall hyperresponsiveness to cold exclusive of sympathetic innervation, a condition he termed *local vascular fault*. In the succeeding years, the nature of the local fault has never been defined.

Patients with Raynaud's syndrome may be divided into two distinct pathophysiologic groups: obstructive and spastic.[35, 43] Patients with obstructive Raynaud's syndrome have a significant obstruction of the palmar and digital arteries

Supported by Grant RR00334 from the General Clinical Research Centers branch of the Division of Research Resources, National Institutes of Health, and Grant 8839 from the Medical Research Foundation of Oregon.

caused by one of a variety of diseases, two of the more frequent being chronic arteritis associated with autoimmune disease and arteriosclerosis. To experience a Raynaud episode, the patient must have sufficiently severe arterial obstruction to cause significant reduction in resting digital artery pressure, a condition that requires obstruction of both arteries of a single digit. In such patients a normal vasoconstrictive response to cold is sufficient to overcome the diminished intraluminal distending pressure and cause arterial closure. This apparently correct theory predicts that all patients with arterial obstruction of the hand sufficient to cause resting digital hypotension experience episodes of cold-induced Raynaud's syndrome. Patients with spastic Raynaud's syndrome do not have significant palmar-digital artery obstruction and accordingly have normal digital artery pressure at room temperature. Arterial closure in these patients is caused by the markedly increased force of cold-induced arterial spasm.

A number of studies have suggested altered adrenoceptor activity as a mechanism of Raynaud's syndrome. Early studies with the sympathetic blocking drug reserpine demonstrated increased digital blood flow in patients with Raynaud's syndrome.[5] Laboratory studies showed a marked reduction in cold-induced digital artery vasospasm after the intra-arterial administration of reserpine.[39] This suggested that patients with Raynaud's syndrome may possess abnormal adrenergic receptors that become increasingly sensitive to stimulation after cold exposure.[19]

In recent years, knowledge of human adrenergic receptor function has increased markedly with the characterization of the alpha$_1$- and alpha$_2$-adrenoceptors. The alpha$_2$-adrenoceptors, which were initially thought to be presynaptic and inhibitory, are now known to occur both presynaptically and postsynaptically and may be facilitative as well as inhibitory. Alpha$_2$-adrenoceptors are present in a pure population on human platelets.[31] Although the precise relationship between platelet adrenoceptor activity and that of arteries has not been established, a clear precedent exists for a direct relationship between blood cell and tissue levels of adrenoceptors in biologic systems. Laboratory studies have demonstrated that platelets from patients with Raynaud's syndrome have elevated levels of alpha$_2$-adrenoceptors, a finding confirmed by others.[14, 21] Freedman demonstrated increased peripheral vasoconstriction in response to intra-arterial infusions of both alpha$_1$- and alpha$_2$-agonists.[12] An elevation in the number of alpha$_2$-receptor sites, receptor hypersensitivity, and alterations in the number of receptors exposed at any one time have been forwarded as possible mechanisms of alpha-adrenergic–induced Raynaud's syndrome.

Abnormalities in presynaptic beta-receptors and alterations in levels of the vasoactive peptide endothelin, a potent vasoconstrictor, and calcitonin gene-related peptide, a potent vasodilator, have been advanced as causes of Raynaud's syndrome.[2, 3, 47] These await further confirmation.

The role of the sympathetic nervous system remains unclear. In a series of papers by Lafferty and associates, abnormalities in the thermoregulatory response in patients with Raynaud's syndrome have been demonstrated by means of a test termed *thermal entrainment*.[24] In this test the blood flow patterns in one hand are measured while the contralateral hand is alternately dipped in baths of hot and cold water. There are clear differences in blood flow responses demonstrable between normals and controls. The obvious way to explain contralateral changes in blood flow is through the function of the sympathetic nervous system, although no research has been done to prove or disprove this hypothesis.

EPIDEMIOLOGY

The incidence of Raynaud's syndrome in the general population is not known with certainty. Several small studies indicate a remarkable incidence of 20% to 25% in cool, damp climates.[33] It is unknown whether these environmental conditions increase the true incidence of Raynaud's syndrome or merely make the underlying abnormality clinically apparent.

Of considerable interest is the prevalence of Raynaud's syndrome in certain occupational groups, especially those who use vibrating tools or experience chronic cold exposure. This has received considerable attention in recent years, because of both the impaired lifestyle of the patients and the potential impact of this finding on industrial compensation claims. The incidence of digital ischemia among chainsaw operators and miners using vibrating equipment ranges from 40% to 90%, the wide variation in incidence being generally related to the length of exposure.[15, 44] A 50% incidence of Raynaud's syndrome has been reported among food workers who work in cold areas.[28] The pathophysiologic mechanism underlying Raynaud's syndrome of occupational origin is unknown, because neither detailed sequential digital hypothermic tests nor angiography has been performed routinely. Available evidence suggests that the cases of short duration are probably vasospastic, whereas those of long standing may be primarily obstructive.

Women constitute 70% to 90% of most reported patients with Raynaud's syndrome.[9] Typically, younger women present with spastic Raynaud's syndrome, and idiopathic Raynaud's syndrome without associated disease is most common in this age and sex group. Some patients initially found to have no associated disease eventually are shown to have an autoimmune disorder, although the frequency of this occurrence remains unknown. Older men who develop Raynaud's syndrome usually have the obstructive variety associated with digital artery occlusion, usually due to atherosclerosis.

ASSOCIATED DISEASES

Raynaud's syndrome has been observed in association with a wide variety of disorders.[9, 27, 34, 36, 44] A general classification of these conditions appears in Table 50–22. Although in the past this array of apparently unrelated clinical entities obscured understanding of the nature of Raynaud's syndrome, it now appears clear that all these conditions produce either spastic or obstructive arterial phenomena or a combination. A detailed characterization of the associated diseases noted in the first 911 patients with Raynaud's syndrome examined at Oregon Health Sciences University appears in Table 50–23. Truly idiopathic Raynaud's occurred in 44% of patients, although the precise pathophysiologic relationships between the associated conditions and Raynaud's syndrome are not clear. In recent years, the number of patients with idiopathic Raynaud's syndrome has increased. In 1976, in a group of 100 patients, only 19% were given a diagnosis of idiopathic Raynaud's syndrome.[34] The percentage of patients with idiopathic Raynaud's syndrome has steadily increased since then. The increase in the proportion of patients presenting to this clinic with idiopathic Raynaud's syndrome has become much more rapid in the past 5 years. An explanation for the change is that interest in digital ischemia results in referral of increasing numbers of minimally symptomatic patients. Such patients are clearly less likely to have associated diseases than patients with severe vasospastic or obstructive symptoms.[10]

The data describing the percentage of patients presenting with Raynaud's syndrome who have an associated disease have been derived from tertiary referral centers. The obvious requirement for entry into such studies was that the patient have Raynaud's symptoms of sufficient severity to seek treatment. Although most of the published data clearly indicate that 70% of this group has some associated disease process, this association in all likelihood does not apply to the minimally symptomatic individuals in the population who have never sought medical care. In these individuals, the incidence of Raynaud's syndrome unassociated with other disease processes must be much higher.

CLINICAL DESCRIPTION

Most patients with spastic Raynaud's syndrome are women in whom the age at onset is typically younger than 30 years. Both hands are affected equally, and frequently the thumbs are spared. Although most patients have a mild associated vasospastic involvement of feet and toes, only about 10% of patients have a primary lower-extremity involvement. Obstructive Raynaud's syndrome appears to be about equally distributed between men and women, and the symptomatic onset occurs after age 40. The lower extremities are infrequently involved. A striking difference from the vasospastic variety is that the area of involvement is frequently limited to one or several fingers and often affects only one hand.

Most episodes of digital vasospasm are induced by environmental cold exposure, although emotional stimuli such as fear or anger may also produce episodes in about half the patients. The required stimulus may be as mild as a draft from an air conditioner or hand immersion in tap water. At the beginning of an episode, the patient usually experiences blanching or cyanosis of one or several fingers that may extend proximally to the metacarpophalangeal junction or even to the wrist. An episode is usually associated with an

TABLE 50–22. Disorders Associated with Raynaud's Syndrome

Immunologic and Connective Tissue Disorders

Scleroderma
Mixed connective tissue disease
Systemic lupus erythematosus
Rheumatoid arthritis
Dermatomyositis
Polymyositis
Hepatitis B antigen–induced vasculitis
Drug-induced vasculitis
Sjögren's syndrome

Obstructive Arterial Diseases

Arteriosclerosis
Thromboangiitis obliterans
Thoracic outlet syndrome

Environmental Conditions

Vibrational injuries
Direct arterial trauma
Cold injury

Drug-induced Raynaud's Syndrome Without Arteritis

Ergot
Beta-blocking drugs
Cytotoxic drugs
Birth control pills

Miscellaneous

Vinyl chloride disease
Chronic renal failure
Cold agglutinins
Cryoglobulinemia
Neoplasia
Neurologic disorders
  Central nervous system
  Peripheral nervous system
Endocrinologic disorders

TABLE 50–23. Associated Diseases in 911 Patients at Oregon Health Sciences University

Associated Disease	No. of Patients
Connective tissue disorders	290 (32%)
Progressive systemic sclerosis	108
Systemic lupus erythematosus	21
Rheumatoid arthritis	17
Sjögren's syndrome	21
Mixed connective tissue disease	17
Unknown connective tissue disease	16
Misc./unknown connective tissue disease	41
Other associated diseases	223 (24%)
Atherosclerosis	51
Cancer	10
Buerger's disease	16
Frostbite/cold exposure	31
Carpal tunnel syndrome	26
Hypothyroid disease	13
Vibration	15
Erythromelalgia	9
Hypersensitivity angiitis	21
Hematologic abnormality	15
Arterial/nerve trauma	16
No associated disease	398 (44%)

uncomfortable sensation of numbness. Severe pain is rare. The initial pallor or cyanosis persists for as long as the cold exposure continues and is followed by a gradual return to normal color 15 to 30 minutes after entering a warm area. Fingertip ulceration occurs only in the presence of widespread palmar or digital artery obstruction. Ischemic ulceration is never caused by vasospasm alone.

PATIENT EVALUATION

Historical information should be sought regarding symptoms of connective tissue disease, including arthralgia, dysphagia, skin tightening, xerophthalmia, or xerostomia. Symptoms of large-vessel occlusive disease, exposure to trauma or frostbite, drug history, and history of malignancy should also be sought. The skin of the hands and fingers should be inspected for ulceration or fingertip hyperkeratotic areas, suggesting healed ulcers. The hand and fingers should be examined for evidence of skin thinning, tightening, sclerodactyly, or telangiectasia, all of which may suggest associated autoimmune disease. The peripheral pulse status should be carefully noted, and special attention should be directed toward signs and symptoms of nerve compression syndrome. Carpal tunnel syndrome is seen with surprising frequency in Raynaud's syndrome patients, affecting about 15% of these individuals.[36] Patients who present with the sudden onset of digital ischemia should be questioned about coagulation abnormalities and a history of previous thrombotic episodes. It should be noted that the results of the physical examination are often completely normal in patients with Raynaud's syndrome. The diagnosis is made primarily from the history.

ANCILLARY EVALUATION

Hand arteriography was formerly used frequently in the evaluation of patients with Raynaud's syndrome. A detailed technique of cryodynamic arteriography provided important anatomic, pathophysiologic, and diagnostic information.[39] Representative arteriograms can be seen in Figures 50–140 and 50–141. Increasingly sophisticated vascular laboratory techniques have largely replaced arteriography in the routine evaluation of patients with Raynaud's syndrome. Currently,

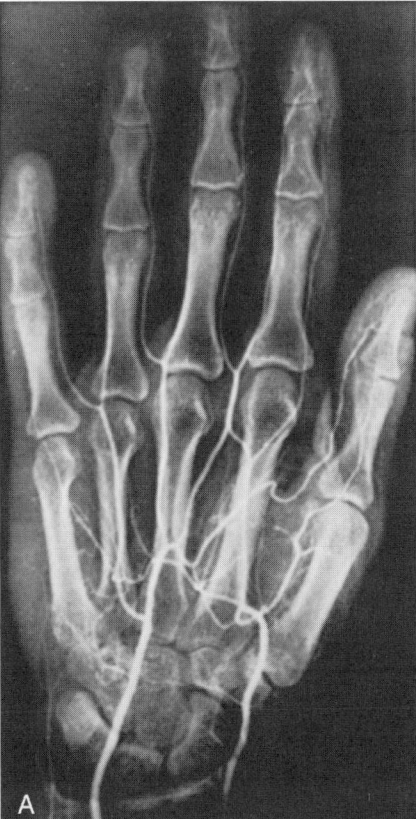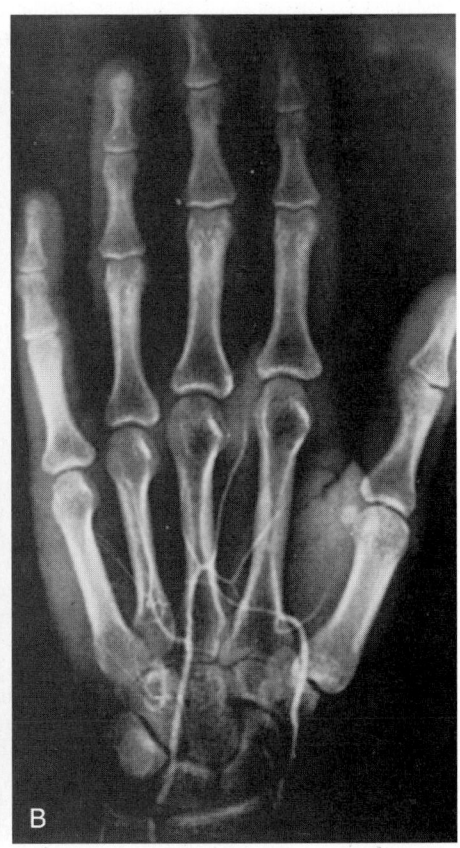

Figure 50–140. *A,* Hand arteriogram in patient with Raynaud's symptoms at room temperature. Significant vasospasm is present. *B,* Same patient after ice-water exposure for 30 seconds. A marked increase in vasospasm is present.

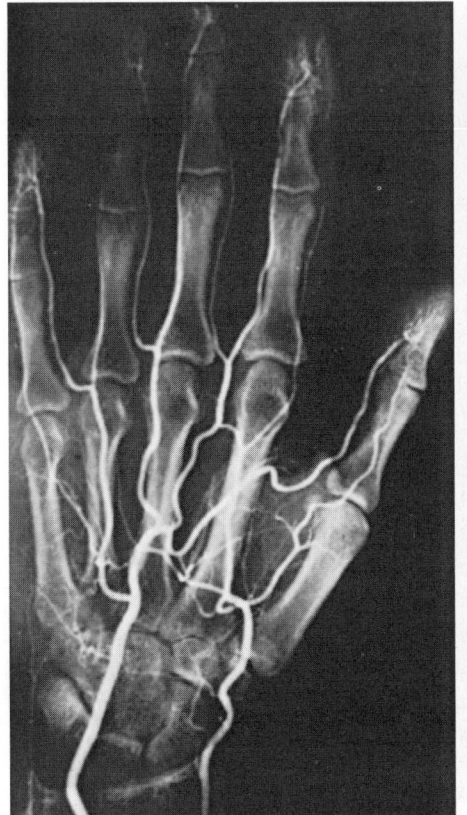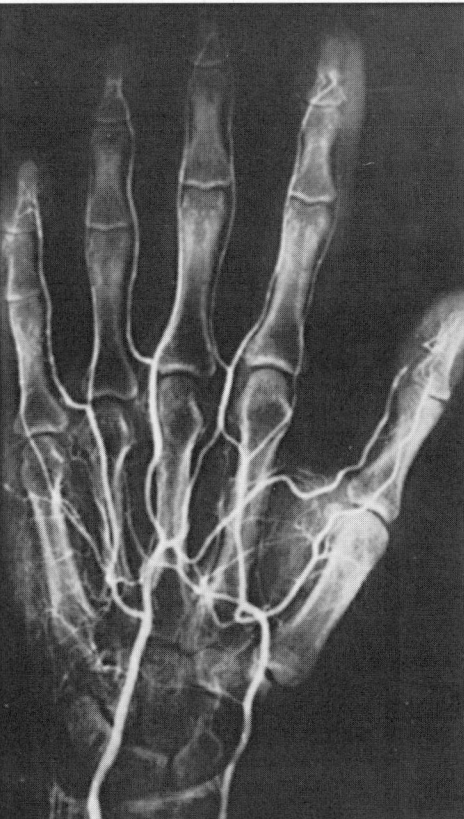

Figure 50–141. Left, Same patient as in Figure 50–140, 48 hours after sympathetic blockage, in this case accomplished by the intra-arterial injection of reserpine. A significant decrease in resting vasospasm is apparent. Right, After ice-water exposure. The vasoconstrictive response to cold is markedly diminished by sympathetic blockade.

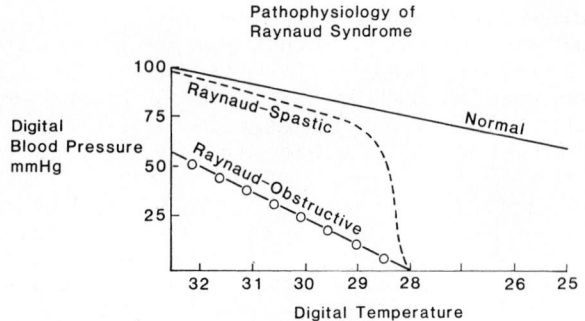

Figure 50–142. Alterations in digital blood pressure with decreasing digital temperature. See text.

arteriography is recommended only in patients presenting with unilateral ischemic digital ulceration to exclude embolization from a surgically correctable proximal arterial lesion.

The vascular laboratory has been of great help in objectively establishing the diagnosis of Raynaud's syndrome and allows a separation of spastic from obstructive Raynaud's syndrome. The change in digital blood pressure related to finger temperature is shown diagrammatically in Figure 50–142 for three groups: normal individuals, patients with vasospastic Raynaud's syndrome, and patients with significant digital artery obstruction. Normal individuals show only a modest digital pressure drop with decreasing temperature. Patients with vasospastic Raynaud's syndrome show a similar curve until a critical temperature is reached, at which time abrupt arterial closure occurs. Patients with severe arterial obstruction parallel normal but with a much lower pressure, with closure occurring at about 20 to 30 mm. Hg.

The first vascular laboratory test used widely for objective diagnosis of Raynaud's syndrome was the measurement of fingertip temperature recovery after digital exposure to ice water (Fig. 50–143).[36] Although normal individuals and patients with Raynaud's syndrome usually have similar resting digital temperatures and similar temperature drops after exposure to ice water, the time required for a return of digital temperature to normal averages 5 to 10 minutes in normal individuals and is prolonged to more than 20 minutes in most Raynaud's syndrome patients. Increasing experience has revealed that whereas this test is 100% specific, it is only about 50% sensitive and therefore is insufficiently accurate for clinical use.

The digital blood pressure response to 5 minutes of digital occlusive hypothermia as described by Lassen and associates has proved to be quite accurate in the vascular laboratory diagnosis of Raynaud's syndrome.[32] In an evaluation of 100 patients at this institution, the test was found to be 87% specific and 90% sensitive, yielding an overall accuracy of 92%.[13] This is the diagnostic test of choice in those occasional patients in whom a test is necessary. As noted previously, the diagnosis is usually established by the clinical history. However, the use of an objective test is most helpful in certain patient groups, including those in whom the diagnosis is in doubt, epidemiologic study groups, and those with pending litigation in whom historical accuracy is uncertain.

Digital photoplethysmography with digital blood pressure determination has become as accurate as arteriography in the detection of significant digital artery obstruction.[17] A finding of an obstructive digital plethysmographic waveform with a digital pressure of more than 20 mm. Hg below brachial pressure establishes the diagnosis of significant digital artery obstruction.[17] This, combined with the digital hypothermic blood pressure test described previously, allows ac-

curate characterization of obstructive or spastic Raynaud's syndrome.

The extent of laboratory evaluation varies somewhat, depending on the findings of the history and physical examination. Minimal evaluation includes a hand roentgenogram for calcinosis or tuft resorption, complete blood cell count, sedimentation rate, and rheumatoid factor and antinuclear antibody tests to aid in the diagnosis of any associated autoimmune disease. Additional information such as protein electrophoresis and antibodies to a variety of nuclear antigens may subsequently be obtained. Upper-extremity nerve conduction testing should be considered if there is any clinical suspicion of carpal tunnel syndrome. Cases with a history of the sudden onset of digital occlusion should be evaluated for hypercoagulable states. Current screen consists of antithrombin III, protein S, and protein C levels as well as screening for the presence of lupus inhibitor and anticardiolipin antibodies.

TREATMENT

Satisfactory results have been reported with many different agents empirically selected on the basis of the presumed pathophysiology of Raynaud's syndrome. Unfortunately, objective evaluation of every form of treatment, including surgical sympathectomy, has been made impossible by largely anecdotal reports and lack of controlled studies. Nearly every type of treatment has been used successfully in at least one study population. Few, if any, agents currently used have been subjected to rigorous randomized, double-blind trials with parallel-group placebo control.

Most patients with Raynaud's syndrome have only mild symptoms, which respond well to simple conservative treatment, including the wearing of warm clothes and gloves and cold and tobacco avoidance. Patients who work in cold areas may not respond to any treatment until their occupational exposure is reduced. Because of the adverse digital circulatory effects of ergotamine tartrate and beta-adrenergic blocking drugs, equally effective alternative treatment should be sought in patients with Raynaud's syndrome.[16]

Although a variety of vasodilator drugs have been used in the pharmacologic treatment of patients with Raynaud's syndrome, only about 10% of these patients require any treatment beyond avoidance of cold and of use of tobacco products. The primary difficulty with evaluation of the benefit of pharmacologic therapy in Raynaud's syndrome has been the lack of objective methods of assessing drug response. Currently no vascular laboratory test allows an objective assessment of drug benefit. It is unknown whether this reflects an actual absence of objective drug benefit or an insensitivity of the currently available vascular laboratory

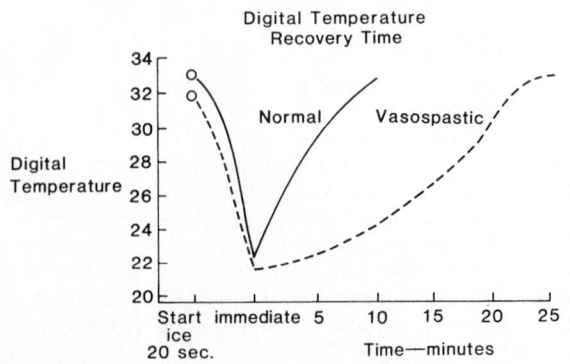

Figure 50–143. Digital temperature after cold exposure. The recovery time for patients with Raynaud's syndrome is markedly prolonged compared with normal individuals.

tests. Unfortunately, in the absence of adequate methodology, the assessment of efficacy of any drug devolves to the patient's subjective impression of benefit, an assessment that may be markedly affected by such variables as environmental temperature, the patient's emotional state, or concomitant medications.

Many patients require pharmacologic therapy only in winter months, with reserpine and guanethidine most commonly prescribed.[5, 36] A number of other adrenergic blocking drugs, including alpha-methyldopa, tolazoline, phenoxybenzamine, and prazosin, have been used occasionally with anecdotal good results.

Other vasodilators have proved unsuccessful in the treatment of Raynaud's syndrome. The beta-stimulating drugs have been ineffective, the two most widely used being nylidrin and isoxsuprine. The topical vasodilators papaverine and niacin as well as the topical application of nitroglycerine have been generally ineffective. The antifungal drug griseofulvin was initially thought to be helpful, but recent experience has not confirmed the early reports.

The calcium channel–blocking agents represent compounds that have found wide clinical application. Nifedipine is the most potent peripheral vasodilator in this group and has been moderately effective in the treatment of Raynaud's syndrome, producing clinical improvement in 50% to 60% of patients studied.[42] Headache is a frequently encountered side effect and is of sufficient severity to cause discontinuation of the drug in 10% to 20% of patients. At present, extended-release nifedipine is the first-line drug for Raynaud's syndrome. Patients with spastic Raynaud's syndrome are more likely to respond to medication than those with obstructive Raynaud's syndrome.

A variety of new drugs and unconventional treatments have been proposed for Raynaud's syndrome. Beta-blockers, which have been implicated in the causation of drug-induced Raynaud's syndrome, have been suggested for the treatment of Raynaud's syndrome in combination with a calcium channel blocker.[2] Several patients who have failed to respond to a calcium channel blocker alone have had a beta-blocker (atenolol, 50 mg./day) added with good results. Prostaglandin E$_1$ appeared to be beneficial in a number of anecdotal reports, but a randomized, double-blind, placebo-controlled study failed to show benefit. Ketanserin is a selective serotonin-2 receptor blocker that has been reported useful in the treatment of obstructive Raynaud's syndrome, particularly that seen in association with scleroderma.[23] Plasmapheresis has been attempted on occasion, as have agents that reduce blood viscosity, fibrinogen concentration, and platelet activity, with questionable benefit. Treatment of associated autoimmune diseases does not appear to benefit patients with Raynaud's syndrome. Temperature biofeedback is an area of active research and has been successfully used in alleviating symptoms in patients with Raynaud's syndrome.[12]

SURGICAL THERAPY

In a very small number of patients with Raynaud's syndrome, there is a proximal cause of upper extremity arterial insufficiency, sometimes associated with distal emboli to the palmar and digital arteries. The occasional patient with Raynaud's syndrome associated with subclavian, axillary, or brachial obstruction from arteriosclerosis; emboli; thoracic outlet syndrome; aneurysm; or trauma is an appropriate subject for vascular surgery and, in general, satisfactory results may be expected.[29, 40]

For the past half century, one of the frequent treatments for Raynaud's syndrome has been upper-extremity sympa-

thectomy. Typically the patient experiences a few months of good results followed by a gradual recurrence of symptoms.[26] It is unknown whether this represents an incomplete initial sympathectomy due to anatomic vagaries in the nerve distribution of the upper extremity or the development of receptor hypersensitivity to circulating catecholamines. Sympathectomy produces occasional anecdotal good long-term results, but in general these have been limited to patients with mild Raynaud's syndrome of the spastic variety. This is the same group of patients who respond best to pharmacologic treatment. Experiences with thoracoscopic sympathectomy have simplified the operative procedure, but equally disappointing long-term results in Raynaud's patients were obtained.[4] There is general agreement that sympathectomy of the upper extremity is of little or no benefit in patients with Raynaud's syndrome who have associated connective tissue disease.[26] At present, the modest surgical risk, expense, and mediocre long-term results of thoracic sympathectomy for Raynaud's syndrome constitute overwhelming arguments against its use; the procedure is not recommended. In contrast, lumbar sympathectomy for lower-extremity Raynaud's syndrome yields excellent long-term results.[20] The reason for the difference between the results of upper and lower sympathectomy is unknown.

In the treatment of Raynaud's syndrome, patients with painful digital ulceration are occasionally encountered. This almost always implies widespread palmar and digital arterial obstruction, since ischemic ulceration does not result from vasospasm. In one study a healing rate of 85% was achieved in a group of 100 such patients after scrubbing of the ulcer with soap and water, antibiotics as selected by culture, and conservative débridement.[30, 37] These results are equal to the healing rate achieved after thoracic sympathectomy and once again emphasize the critical lack of data supporting thoracic sympathectomy for either vasospasm or ischemia. A representative photograph of a painful digital ischemic ulcer that healed with conservative treatment is shown in Figure 50–144.

Periarterial digital sympathectomy has been suggested as an improved method of sympathectomy.[11, 46] Proof that this procedure produces results superior to randomized nonoperative therapy is conspicuously lacking. Direct microvascular bypass of occluded segments of palmar and digital arteries has been reported in recent years with occasional relief of symptoms.[41] These have been carefully selected cases, primarily traumatic in etiology, in patients with normal vessels elsewhere. There appears little likelihood that these techniques are of benefit in patients with generalized small-vessel disease. Arteriovenous reversal at the wrist has been advocated as a method of providing retrograde arterial perfusion to ischemic hands for limb salvage.[22] The usefulness of this procedure in patients with Raynaud's syndrome remains to be proved.

OVERVIEW

Raynaud's syndrome is the symptomatic expression of episodic digital vasospasm that has multiple causes and can be seen in association with many seemingly unrelated disorders. Most patients exhibit variable degrees of both vasospasm and palmar-digital arterial occlusions, although most cluster toward one end of the spectrum. Abnormal hemorrheologic parameters have been an inconsistent finding.

An objective evaluation of both medical and surgical treatments is hampered by a lack of controlled trials, poor definition of patient groups for the purpose of comparing results, variable follow-up, and a total unavailability of generally

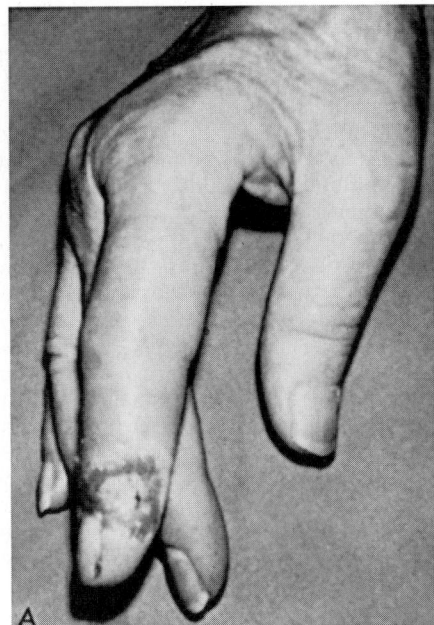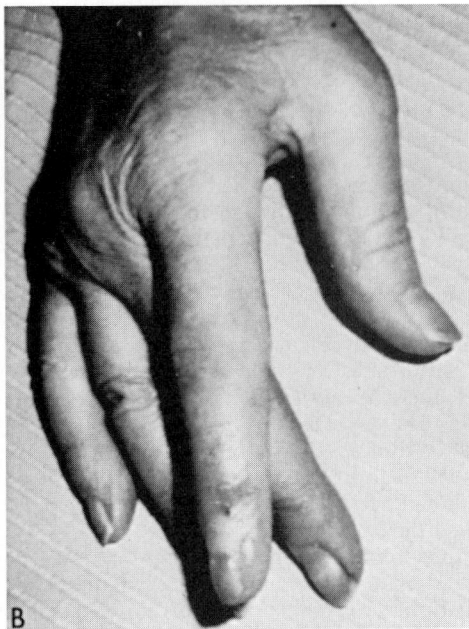

Figure 50–144. *A,* Painful digital ischemic ulcer in patient with scleroderma and massive digital artery obstruction. *B,* Total healing after 4 weeks of soap and water scrubs and antibiotics. Such healing with conservative treatment only may be expected in 85% of patients with digital ischemic ulcers.

applied and accepted objective tests of digital blood flow and digital artery closure characteristics. Conservative treatment consisting of cold and tobacco avoidance is adequate for the majority of patients with mild to moderate symptoms. About 10% of patients with Raynaud's syndrome have sufficiently severe and frequent or prolonged episodes to require drug therapy. Generally favorable anecdotal results have been achieved in about half of these patients after a variety of pharmacologic treatments. The one current preference is the use of extended-release nifedipine 30 mg. at bedtime. Conservative therapy is recommended, even in the difficult group of patients with severe pain or persistent digital ischemia with localized gangrene. Constant and meticulous attention to the fundamental principles of conservative therapy, including cessation of tobacco use and gentle cleansing and débridement of ulcers, leads to gratifying results in most patients.

Whereas upper-extremity sympathectomy undoubtedly causes dramatic improvement in occasional patients, the result in any single patient is unpredictable and usually disappointing. Sympathectomy appears to have its best long-term results in those mildly symptomatic patients who need it least. Similarly, digital artery sympathectomy or hand artery microvascular repair is not frequently used, and lumbar sympathectomy should be considered in the few patients who present with primary lower extremity Raynaud's syndrome and whose symptoms cannot be controlled by conservative measures and medical therapy.

SELECTED REFERENCES

Edwards, J. M., Phinney, E. S., Taylor, L. M., Jr., Keenan, E. J., and Porter, J. M.: Alpha₂-adrenergic receptor levels in obstructive and spastic Raynaud's syndrome. J. Vasc. Surg., 5:38, 1987.
The authors describe abnormalities in platelet alpha₂-adrenoceptor levels in patients with Raynaud's syndrome. The number of measurable receptors in patients with vasospastic Raynaud's syndrome is significantly elevated over those seen in normal controls and patients with obstructive Raynaud's syndrome. Additionally, a series of experiments in which normal platelets are incubated in the serum from patients with Raynaud's syndrome is described. A decrease in measurable platelet alpha₂-adrenoceptor levels is noted, from which the authors hypothesize the possibility of a serum receptor-blocking substance.

Edwards, J. M., and Porter, J. M.: Long-term outcome of Raynaud's syndrome. *In* Yao, J. S. T., and Pearce, W. H. (Eds.): Long-Term Results in Vascular Surgery. Norwalk, Conn., Appleton & Lange, 1993, pp. 345–352.
The authors summarize the long-term effects of Raynaud's syndrome, about which there is surprisingly little known. Patients presenting without evidence of digital artery obstruction, serologic abnormalities, or nailfold capillary abnormalities have a low rate of subsequent digital artery obstruction, digital ulcerations, or development of a connective tissue disease. Those who do present with one or more signs or symptoms of a connective tissue disease have a greater risk of subsequently developing a connective tissue disease and digital ulcerations. Current opinions on the management of digital ulcerations are discussed.

Mills, J. L., Friedman, E. L., Taylor, L. M., Jr., and Porter, J. M.: Upper extremity ischemia caused by small artery disease. Ann. Surg., 206:521, 1987.
One hundred patients with ischemic digital ulceration are described in this article. The healing rate with local wound care and conservative débridement was 85%. The authors conclude that the healing rate of digital ulcerations with conservative therapy is equal to or better than that reported after thoracic sympathectomy; thus, sympathectomy should not be a routine adjunctive treatment of digital ulceration.

REFERENCES

1. Allen, E. V., Brown, G. E.: Raynaud's disease: A critical review of minimal requisites for diagnosis. Am. J. Med. Sci., 183:187, 1932.
2. Brotzu, G., Falchi, S., Mannu, B., Montisci, R., Petruzzo, P., and Staico, R.: The importance of presynaptic beta receptors in Raynaud's disease. J. Vasc. Surg., 9:767, 1989.
3. Bunker, C. B., Foreman, J. C., and Dowd, P. M.: Calcitonin gene-related peptide and Raynaud's phenomenon. Lancet, 335:239, 1990.
4. Claes, G., Drott, C., and Göthberg, G.: Thoracoscopy for autonomic disorders. Ann. Thorac. Surg., 56:715, 1993.
5. Coffman, J. D., and Cohen, A. S.: Total and capillary fingertip blood flow in Raynaud's phenomenon. N. Engl. J. Med., 285:259, 1971.
6. deTakats, G., Fowler, E. F.: Raynaud's phenomenon. JAMA, 179:99, 1962.
7. Edwards, J. M., Phinney, E. S., Taylor, L. M., Jr., Keenan, E. J., and Porter, J. M.: Alpha₂-adrenergic receptor levels in obstructive and spastic Raynaud's syndrome. J. Vasc. Surg., 5:38, 1987.
8. Edwards, J. M., Harker, C. T., Taylor, L. M., Jr., and Porter, J. M.: Small artery disease of the upper extremity. *In* Machleder, H. I. (Ed.): Vascular Disorders of the Upper Extremity, 2nd ed. Mt. Kisco, N.Y., Futura Publishing, 1989, pp. 103–130.
9. Edwards, J. M., and Porter, J. M.: Long-term outcome of Raynaud's syndrome. *In* Yao, J. S. T., and Pearce, W. H. (Eds.): Long-Term Results in Vascular Surgery. Norwalk, Conn., Appleton & Lange, 1993, pp. 345–352.
10. Edwards, J. M., and Porter, J. M.: Associated diseases with Raynaud's syndrome. Vasc. Med. Rev., 1:51, 1990.
11. Flatt, A. E.: Digital artery sympathectomy. J. Hand Surg., 5:550, 1980.
12. Freedman, R. R.: Physiological mechanisms of temperature biofeedback. Biofeedback and Self-Regulation, 16:95, 1991.

13. Gates, K. H., Tyburczy, J., Zupan, J., Baur, G. M., and Porter, J. M.: The non-invasive quantification of digital vasospasm. Bruit, 8:34, 1984.
14. Graafsma, S. J., Wollersheim, H., Droste, H. T., ten Dam, M. A., van Tits, L. J., Reyenga, J., Rodrigues de Miranda, J. F., and Thien, T.: Adrenoceptor on blood cells from patients with primary Raynaud's phenomenon. Clin. Sci., 80:325, 1991.
15. Harris, E. J., Jr., Edwards, J. M., and Porter, J. M.: Vascular injuries caused by vibratory tools. In Flanigan, D. P. (Ed.): Civilian Vascular Trauma. Philadelphia, Lea & Febiger, 1990, pp. 306–315.
16. Henry, L. G., Blackwood, J. S., Conley, J. E., and Bernhard, V. M.: Ergotism. Arch. Surg., 110:929, 1975.
17. Holmgren, K., Baur, G. M., and Porter, J. M.: The role of digital photo-plethysmography in the evaluation of Raynaud's syndrome. Bruit, 5:19, 1981.
18. Hutchinson, J.: Raynaud's phenomenon. Med. Press. Circ., 123:402, 1901.
19. Jamieson, G. G., Ludbrook, J., and Wilson, A.: Cold hypersensitivity in Raynaud's phenomenon. Circulation, 44:254, 1971.
20. Janoff, A. J., Phinney, E. S., and Porter, J. M.: Lumbar sympathectomy for lower extremity vasospasm. Am. J. Surg., 150:147, 1985.
21. Keenan, E. J., and Porter, J. M.: Alpha-2 adrenergic receptors in platelets from patients with Raynaud's syndrome. Surgery, 94:204, 1983.
22. King, T. A., Marks, J., and Berrettone, B. A.: Arteriovenous reversal for limb salvage in unreconstructible upper extremity arterial occlusive disease. J. Vasc. Surg., 17:924, 1993.
23. Kirch, W., Linder, H. R., Hutt, J. H., Ohnhaus, E. E., and Mahler, F.: Ketanserin versus nifedipine in secondary Raynaud's phenomenon. Vasa, 16:77, 1987.
24. Lafferty, K., de Trafford, J. C., Roberts, V. C., and Cotton, L. T.: Raynaud's phenomenon and thermal entrainment: An objective test. Br. Med. J., 286:90, 1983.
25. Lewis, T., and Pickering, G. W.: Observations upon maladies in which the blood supply to digits ceases intermittent or permanently, and upon bilateral gangrene of the digits: Observation relevant to so-called "Raynaud's disease." Clin. Sci., 1:327, 1934.
26. Lowell, R. C., Gloviczki, P., Cherry, K. J., Bower, T. C., Hallett, J. W., Jr., Schirger, A., and Pairolero, P. C.: Cervicothoracic sympathectomy for Raynaud's syndrome. Int. Angiol., 12:168, 1993.
27. Maricq, H. R., McGregor, A. R., Diat, F., Smith, E. A., Maxwell, D. B., LeRoy, E. C., and Weinrich, M. C.: Major clinical diagnoses found among patients with Raynaud's phenomenon from the general population. J. Rheumatol., 17:1171, 1990.
28. MacKiewisz, A., and Piskorz, A.: Raynaud's phenomenon following long-term repeated action of great differences of temperature. J. Cardiovasc. Surg., 18:151, 1977.
29. McNamara, M. F., Takaki, H. S., Yao, J. S. T., and Bergan, J. J.: A systematic approach to severe hand ischemia. Surgery, 83:1, 1978.
30. Mills, J. L., Friedman, E. I., Taylor, L. M., Jr., and Porter, J. M.: Upper extremity ischemia caused by small artery disease. Ann. Surg., 206:521, 1987.
31. Motulsky, H. F., and Insel, P. A.: Adrenergic receptors in man. N. Engl. J. Med., 307:18, 1982.
32. Neilsen, S. L., and Lassen, N. A.: Measurement of digital blood pressure after local cooling. J. Appl. Physiol., 43:907, 1977.
33. Olsen, N., and Nielsen, S. L.: Prevalence of primary Raynaud's phenomenon in young females. Scand. J. Clin. Lab. Invest., 37:761, 1978.
34. Porter, J. M., Bardana, E. J., Jr., Baur, G. M., Wesche, D. H., Andrasch, R. H., and Rösch, J.: The clinical significance of Raynaud's syndrome. Surgery, 80:756, 1976.
35. Porter, J. M., Rivers, S. P., and Anderson, C. J.: Evaluation and management of patients with Raynaud's syndrome. Am. J. Surg., 142:183, 1981.
36. Porter, J. M., Snider, R. L., Bardana, E. J., Jr., Rösch, J., and Eidemiller, L.R.: The diagnosis and treatment of Raynaud's phenomenon. Surgery, 77:11, 1975.
37. Porter, J. M., and Taylor, L. M., Jr.: Limb ischemia caused by small artery disease. World J. Surg., 7:326, 1983.
38. Raynaud, M.: On Local Asphyxia and Symmetrical Gangrene of the Extremities. Selected Monographs. London, New Sydenham Society, 1888.
39. Rösch, J., and Porter, J. M.: Cryodynamic hand angiography in the diagnosis and management of Raynaud's syndrome. Circulation, 55:807, 1977.
40. Schmidt, F. E., and Hewitt, R. L.: Severe upper limb ischemia. Arch. Surg., 115:1188, 1980.
41. Silcott, G. R., and Polich, V. L.: Palmar arch arterial reconstruction for the salvage of ischemic fingers. Am. J. Surg., 142:219, 1981.
42. Smith, C. D., and McKendry, R. J.: Controlled trial of nifedipine in the treatment of Raynaud's phenomenon. Lancet, 2:1299, 1982.
43. Sumner, D. S., and Strandness, D. E.: An abnormal finger pulse associated with cold sensitivity. Ann. Surg., 175:294, 1972.
44. Taylor, W., and Pelmear, P. L.: Raynaud's phenomenon of occupational origin: An epidemiological survey. Acta Chir. Scand. (Suppl.), 465:27, 1976.
45. Taylor L. M., Jr., Rivers, S. P., Keller, F. S., Baur, G. M., and Porter, J. M.: Treatment of finger ischemia with Bier block reserpine. Surg. Gynecol. Obstet., 154:39, 1982.
46. Wilgis, E. F. S.: Evaluation and treatment of chronic digital ischemia. Ann. Surg., 193:693, 1981.
47. Zamora, M. R., O'Brien, R. F., Rutherford, R. B., and Weil, J. V.: Serum endothelin-1 concentrations and cold provocation in primary Raynaud's phenomenon. Lancet, 336:1144, 1990.

CIRCULATORY PROBLEMS OF THE UPPER EXTREMITY

Milton M. Slocum, M.D.
Donald Silver, M.D.

ARTERIAL INSUFFICIENCY

Approximately 1% of patients with peripheral vascular disorders have symptoms of upper extremity ischemia.[7] However, 17% of patients studied angiographically had a greater than 30% stenosis of the innominate and subclavian arteries.[4] The low frequency of symptoms in upper extremities with arterial stenoses is related to the rich collateral network, the small muscle mass, and the intermittent work requirements of the upper extremities.

Arterial flow to the upper extremity may be reduced by atherosclerotic stenoses or occlusions, thromboembolism, trauma, tumor, inflammatory processes (e.g., Takayasu's arteritis, Buerger's disease), and compression of the subclavian-axillary arteries in the region of the thoracic outlet. Atherosclerotic or embolic occlusions and aneurysms occur less often in the upper extremities than in the lower extremities, whereas vasospastic disorders and arteritis occur more frequently. Symptomatic atherosclerotic occlusions most commonly involve the subclavian or innominate arteries. Axillary and brachial arterial atherosclerotic occlusions are the next most frequent. The small arteries of the hands and fingers, in addition to being involved with atherosclerotic occlusions, are most often affected by vasospastic disorders, frostbite, drugs (e.g., ergot), hematologic disorders (e.g., thrombocytosis, polycythemia), and embolization.

Traumatic injuries to the upper extremity arteries occur about one fifth as often as do injuries to the arteries of the lower extremities.[3] Penetrating arterial injuries occur slightly more often in the upper extremities (53%),[12] whereas vascular injuries from blunt trauma, usually associated with fractures or dislocation, occur most often in the lower extremities (89%).[3] The injured arteries may be partially or totally disrupted or compressed. If the intima is torn by the sudden stretching of an artery, blood flow may lift the intima and produce a dissection, or *intimal flap* obstruction. Penetrating wounds to the arteries frequently penetrate adjacent veins and may produce arteriovenous fistulas. The true incidence of arteriovenous fistulas from penetrating trauma is difficult to ascertain; however, the incidence ranges from 2.3% in civilian vascular injuries to 10% in military injuries.

Emboli are an increasingly common cause of arterial insufficiency, with 3% to 5% of all arterial emboli lodging in the upper extremities. Emboli usually lodge at sites of arterial bifurcation or reduction of arterial diameter, with the majority of the emboli lodging in the axillary and brachial arteries.[2] A single embolus to the palmar or digital arteries is not likely to cause significant symptoms, but repeated embolization to these vessels may lead to ulceration and digital gangrene. Because most emboli arise in the heart, the incidence of thromboembolic occlusion of the upper extremity parallels the increasing number of geriatric patients with their cardiac problems. Brachial and axillary cardiac catheterizations also cause thrombotic occlusions of the respective arteries in approximately 0.5% of the cases.[13]

The subclavian or axillary arteries or both may be compressed as they course through the thoracic outlet and (1) may be asymptomatic; (2) may cause intermittent ischemia or symptoms similar to those seen in Raynaud's syndrome; (3) may develop poststenotic aneurysmal dilatation; and (4) when there is major compression or embolization of a mural thrombus, may cause significant ischemia of the distal portion of the extremity.

Arteritis is being recognized with increased frequency as a cause of upper extremity and hand ischemia. The larger proximal arteries may be obstructed by idiopathic medial arteriopathy, giant cell arteritis, or idiopathic arteritis, whereas the palmar and digital arteries are more frequently affected by collagen-related vasculitis (Fig. 50–145). The diagnosis may require arterial biopsy for confirmation. Management of the identified arteritis frequently includes the use of corticosteroids and, at times, other forms of immunosuppression. If significant ischemia of the fingers and/or hand persists, arterial bypass, usually with a vein graft, is indicated. The graft should not be placed in portions of the artery involved with the inflammatory process.

A careful history and physical examination, supplemented by appropriate roentgenograms, ultrasonograms, and angiograms, should document the site and extent of an arterial occlusion and provide some indication of the etiology of the insufficiency.

Asymptomatic or minimally symptomatic arterial occlusions usually require no therapy other than prolonged *antiplatelet therapy* (e.g., 325 mg. of aspirin daily) to reduce the incidence of thrombosis. The patient should be instructed to avoid injury to the ischemic parts and to use skin creams to keep the skin pliable. Symptomatic occlusions are treated according to the etiology (e.g., an embolus can usually be extracted using local anesthesia and an embolectomy catheter); compression in the thoracic outlet should be relieved, when necessary, with repair or replacement of the damaged artery; vein grafts may be used to bypass chronic occlusions; and vein patches may be used to enlarge short areas of stenoses. Infusions of fibrinolytic agents have restored patency to vessels obstructed by thromboembolism. The infusion is maintained until lysis occurs, but rarely longer than 3

to 4 days, and is followed with anticoagulant therapy. Causes of the thromboembolism should be corrected to prevent recurrences. If the source of the embolus cannot be eliminated, long-term anticoagulation with warfarin is required. Innominate and subclavian artery occlusions can be readily bypassed with extrathoracic grafts with a low mortality, lasting patency, and relief of symptoms.[5] Traumatic vascular injuries usually require prompt angiography and restoration of flow, because frequently there has not been a previous stimulus to the development of collateral blood flow.

Principles of repair of traumatic vascular injuries include reducing associated dislocations, stabilizing associated fractures, and débridement of the injured artery with an end-to-end repair or an interposition vein graft. The advent of percutaneous techniques for vascular intervention has made the treatment of intimal flaps with intravascular stents an acceptable option. All associated significant venous injuries should also be repaired, either primarily or with a vein graft.

VENOUS INSUFFICIENCY

The manifestations of venous insufficiency include edema, distention of superficial veins, tightness, aching, a reddish blue discoloration, and pain. Edema of the upper extremity from venous insufficiency is most often caused by occlusion of the axillary, subclavian, or innominate veins or the superior vena cava. More distal venous occlusions rarely produce significant edema or chronic symptoms.

Tumors, mediastinal fibrosis, and trauma are the usual causes of thrombosis in the large central veins. However, indwelling catheters for central cardiovascular monitoring, intravenous nutrition, hemodialysis, or chemotherapy are producing increasing numbers of thromboses of these veins. Thromboses of distal veins most often follow intravenous infusions.

Thrombosis of the axillary or subclavian vein that occurs after effort or strain has been called *effort thrombosis*.[9] This thrombosis occurs in the dominant arm of a young or middle-aged healthy individual. It usually occurs immediately after the effort, but onset may be delayed several hours. A history of effort or strain with the arm abducted can be obtained in most patients. Many of the cases of effort thrombosis are caused by compression of the axillary vein by the pectoralis minor tendon, by the costoclavicular ligament, by the subclavius tendon, or between the clavicle and first rib and are considered manifestations of the thoracic outlet syndrome.

Some patients in whom edema develops after effort do not have demonstrable thrombosis of veins. Their phlebograms usually demonstrate areas of compression of the axillary and subclavian veins in the area of the thoracic outlet. The edema, which primarily follows chronic compression and secondarily the patient's efforts, may be effectively treated by eliminating the site(s) of venous compression.

The presence and extent of venous thrombosis should be documented by phlebography. When proximal venous obstructions are present, the distal venous pressures, with the patient supine and the extremity at the right atrial level, are elevated above the normal pressure of 8 to 12 cm. of saline.

Management of the patient with venous obstruction without thrombosis includes eliminating the cause of the obstruction. For those patients with the thoracic outlet syndrome, this includes improvement of posture, avoiding positions of hyperabduction, and, if symptoms persist, offering a scalenectomy and/or first rib resection with, frequently, division of the compressing tendons. Those patients who present with acute thrombotic obstruction of their axillary-subclavian veins should receive fibrinolytic therapy (e.g., urokinase, streptokinase, or tissue plasminogen activator) to restore pat-

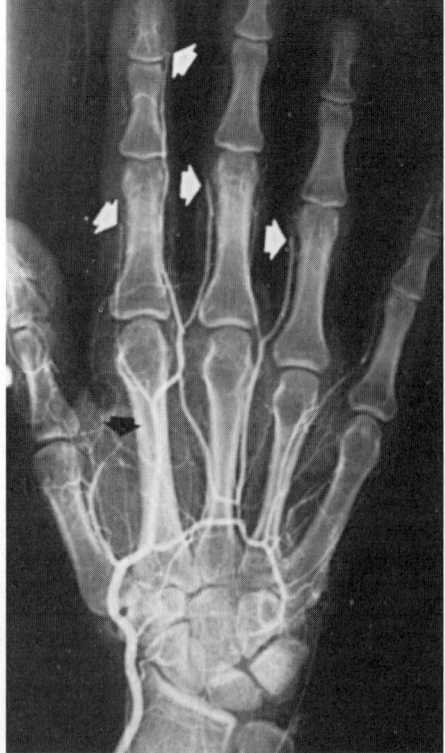

Figure 50–145. Arteriogram with magnification in a patient with scleroderma and Raynaud's phenomenon. Note absence of ulnar artery and superficial palmar arch. Several digital arteries are occluded (arrows).

ency of the veins. The fibrinolytic therapy is followed by heparin for a few days and then by long-term anticoagulation with warfarin until the causes of the compression can be eliminated. Many of these patients will require surgical decompression of the subclavian/axillary vein after the thrombolytic therapy.

Most patients with thromboses of the veins in the upper extremities are treated with elevation of the affected extremity and heparin (provided there are no contraindications) in sufficient amounts to prolong the activated partial thromboplastin time to twice the control value. Heparin is given as a constant infusion for 4 to 6 days; it is continued for a longer period if symptoms persist or the edema does not resolve. After the acute process is controlled, the patient is maintained on self-injected subcutaneous heparin, 5000 units every 8 hours, or warfarin for 3 to 4 months to allow recanalization to occur.

Although thrombectomy may be employed to reduce the sequelae of venous thromboses,[8] most vascular surgeons use thrombectomy only if fibrinolytic agents or elevation and anticoagulation fail to restore the circulation and tissue perfusion remains altered and if gangrene is imminent. Symptoms caused by proximal thrombotic obstructions can be relieved with saphenous vein bypasses of the obstruction (e.g., axillary-jugular bypass, brachial-subclavian bypass).

The superior vena cava may become stenotic or occluded by a variety of benign and malignant conditions. The superior vena cava syndrome consists of edema of the head, neck, and upper extremities; distended neck veins with dilated collateral veins of the upper extremities and thorax; headache; and confusion. The superior vena cava syndrome most commonly is caused by malignant disease (80%). Iatrogenic superior vena cava occlusions are increasing in frequency secondary to the increased use of indwelling central venous catheters. An occluded or stenotic superior vena cava may be treated with radiation or chemotherapy (malignant etiology). Thrombi may be treated with fibrinolytic therapy, operative reconstruction, or vascular stenting. Intravascular stenting is being used more frequently in superior vena cava obstruction secondary to malignancy because of the poor risk-benefit ratio of operative reconstruction in this setting. In patients with complete obstruction and thrombosis, fibrinolytic therapy is often utilized as an adjunct to stent placement.

LYMPHEDEMA

Primary lymphedema of an upper extremity is extremely rare. Secondary lymphedema has occurred in up to 10% of women who have had radical mastectomies, frequently followed by irradiation, for breast cancer and is a potential complication of any axillary dissection. The incidence of lymphedema of the upper extremity has decreased with the advent of less radical resections for breast cancer.

Most often lymphedema can be controlled with elevation, elastic sleeves, salt restriction, good skin care, and prompt management of infection. Lymphedema resistant to these simple measures most often can be controlled by frequent use, two to six times a day, of a lymphedema pump. Uncontrollable edema is usually treated with operative procedures for improving lymph flow and/or reducing the size of the extremity.

CAUSALGIA

In 1872, Mitchell coined the term *causalgia* to describe the burning, agonizing pain and vasomotor disturbances that occur in 2% to 5% of patients after peripheral nerve injuries.[10] The pain of causalgia varies in intensity and is exacerbated by touching or moving the involved body part, changes in

temperature, pressure changes, or local irritants. The pain may become so agonizing that complete cessation of motion of the involved extremity ensues.

Cervical sympathetic blockade is an excellent diagnostic and therapeutic procedure because it usually provides complete relief from pain and allows the use of the previously guarded limb. The vasomotor changes are also usually completely relieved by the blockade. In a few patients, lasting relief is provided by a single sympathetic blockade; other patients require repeated blocks to obtain complete relief. However, if sympathetic blocks provide only temporary relief, operative sympathetic denervation should be performed with the expectation that symptoms will be relieved. Active physical therapy is an important part of the postsympathectomy management.[11]

Posttraumatic Reflex Dystrophy

In some patients, causalgia-like pain develops after an injury to the soft tissues and/or a bone of the extremity in which there is no demonstrable nerve damage. In addition to the pain, there may be edema, vasomotor disturbances, soft tissue dystrophy, and atrophy of bone in the region or distal to the injury.

The process may follow minimal trauma, such as a sprain, or an infection and occasionally occurs after thrombophlebitis, burns, spinal anesthesia, or herniation of a nucleus pulposus. The syndrome has also been described after angina, myocardial infarction, stroke, and vascular disorders. The process is called posttraumatic reflex sympathetic dystrophy, or Sudeck's atrophy because of the description of bone atrophy by Sudeck in 1900.[16] Therapy consists of treating the local injury with supportive measures (e.g., local heat, analgesics). Cervical sympathetic blockade may be necessary to control the pain before physical therapy is initiated and may have to be repeated several times. Early sympathetic blockades and physical therapy are the mainstays of treatment. The majority of patients recover completely with these supportive measures. However, if the supportive measures do not completely relieve the symptoms, medical treatment with alpha-adrenergic blocking agents or surgical sympathetic denervation of the involved extremity is indicated. Physical therapy is a very important adjunct to sympathetic denervation.[11]

ACROCYANOSIS

Acrocyanosis is characterized by painless coldness and cyanosis of the distal portions of the extremities. It is caused by constant spasm of the small arteries in response to an overactive vasomotor system. The condition should be easily differentiated from Raynaud's disease by careful history and physical examination. Treatment consists only of protection from cold in mild cases or sympathectomy, which usually provides complete relief from symptoms, in severe cases.

ERYTHROMELALGIA

Erythromelalgia is characterized by a burning sensation in the extremities that is associated with local warmth and a reddish or cyanotic color of the skin of the affected part. It occurs most often in middle-aged men and women during times of exposure to increased heat and/or activity. It may be primary or secondary, occurring in patients with hypertension, myeloproliferative disorders, diabetes, or gout. Treatment of secondary erythromelalgia should be directed toward eliminating the underlying disorder. Treatment of primary erythromelalgia is symptomatic: local cooling and reduction of body temperature. Aspirin has been beneficial in relieving symptoms in patients with erythromelalgia and thrombocythemia.[6] Chemical sympathetic blockade may temporarily alleviate the symptoms. Surgical sympathectomy of the involved extremity provides favorable-to-excellent relief of symptoms.[14, 17]

SELECTED REFERENCES

Pearce, W. H., and Yao, J. S. T.: Upper extremity ischemia. Semin. Vasc. Surg., 3:207, 1990.
    This is an excellent review of the current techniques of evaluation and management of circulatory problems of the upper extremity.

Rich, N. M., and Spencer, F. C.: Vascular Trauma. Philadelphia, W. B. Saunders, 1978.
    This comprehensive text of vascular trauma has several nicely written and illustrated chapters devoted to trauma of the vessels of the upper extremity.

Rutherford, R. B.: Vascular Surgery, 4th ed. Philadelphia, W. B. Saunders, 1995.
    This comprehensive text of vascular surgery, which belongs in the library of all vascular surgeons, clearly defines many of the vascular disorders affecting the upper extremities.

REFERENCES

1. Adams, J. T., DeWeese, J. A., Mahoney, E. B., and Rob, C. G.: Intermittent subclavian vein obstruction without thrombosis. Surgery, 63:147, 1968.
2. Bernstein, E. J.: What's new in upper extremity ischemia. *In* Najarian, J. S., and Delaney, J. P. (Eds.): Advances in Vascular Surgery. Chicago, Year Book Medical Publishers, 1983, p. 435.
3. Bishara, R. A., Pasch, A. R., Lim, L. T., et al.: Improved results in the treatment of civilian vascular injuries associated with fractures and dislocations. J. Vasc. Surg., 3:707, 1986.
4. Fields, W. S., and Lemak, N. A.: Joint study of extracranial arterial occlusion. JAMA, 222:1139, 1972.
5. Finkelstein, N. M., Byer, A., and Rush, B. F., Jr.: Subclavian-subclavian bypass for the subclavian steal syndrome. Surgery, 71:142, 1972.
6. Harrison, R., Letz, G., Pasternak, G., et al.: Fulminant hepatic failure after occupational exposure to 2-nitropropane. Ann. Intern. Med., 107:466, 1987.
7. Jones, T. W., Thomas, G. I., and Edmark, K. W.: Thoracocervical occlusive disease. Am. Surg., 33:535, 1967.
8. Mahorner, H., Castleberry, J. W., and Coleman, W. O.: Attempts to restore function in major veins which are the site of massive thrombosis. Ann. Surg., 146:510, 1957.
9. Matas, R.: On so-called primary thrombosis of the axillary vein caused by strain. Am. J. Surg., 24:642, 1934.
10. Mitchell, S. E.: Injuries of Nerves and Their Consequences. Philadelphia, J. B. Lippincott, 1872.
11. Painter, P., and Blackburn, G.: Exercise for patients with chronic disease. Postgrad. Med., 83:185, 1988.
12. Pasch, A. R., Bishara, R. A., Lim, L. T., et al.: Optimal limb salvage in penetrating civilian vascular trauma. J. Vasc. Surg., 3:189, 1986.
13. Ross, R. S.: Cooperative study on cardiac catheterization: Arterial complications. Circulation, 37(Suppl. 3):67, 1968.
14. Shumacker, H. B., Jr.: Sympathetic denervation of the extremities. Curr. Probl. Surg., July 1965.
15. Snider, R., Porter, J. M., and Eidemiller, L. R.: Axillary-axillary artery bypass for the correction of subclavian artery occlusive disease. Ann. Surg., 180:888, 1974.
16. Sudeck, P.: Uber die acute entzudliche Knochenatrophie. Arch. Klin. Cir., 62:147, 1900 (cited in Allen, E. V., Barker, N. W., and Hines, E. A., Jr.: Peripheral Vascular Diseases, 3rd ed. Philadelphia, W. B. Saunders, 1962, p. 459).
17. Telford, E. D.: Discussion on peripheral vascular lesions. Proc. R. Soc. Med., 37:621, 1944.

VISCERAL ISCHEMIC SYNDROMES: OBSTRUCTION OF THE SUPERIOR MESENTERIC ARTERY, CELIAC AXIS, AND INFERIOR MESENTERIC ARTERY

William R. Flinn, M.D.
John J. Bergan, M.D.

Syndromes of mesenteric ischemia remain clinically challenging despite decades of surgical experience. The causes of mesenteric ischemia are well known, and its major complication, gangrenous necrosis of portions of the gastrointestinal tract, is well recognized by all surgeons. Nevertheless, diagnosis and effective treatment is often delayed in these patients; and when gut infarction occurs, the mortality rates range from 50% to 80%,[23, 39] making mesenteric ischemia one of our most lethal vascular problems. Even if patients survive such visceral catastrophes, they face permanent loss of gastrointestinal tract continuity or a loss of sufficient gut length to make normal alimentation impossible and may require life-long parenteral feeding. The prevalence of mesenteric ischemia is low compared with other vascular disorders, but it is clear that early diagnosis and effective treatment to prevent intestinal infarction is the only real hope for these patients.

The syndromes of mesenteric ischemia may be classified based on their symptomatic presentation (acute vs. chronic visceral ischemia) or on their vascular origins (arterial vs. venous). Acute mesenteric ischemia may be caused by mesenteric embolism, mesenteric arterial thrombosis, visceral arterial vasospasm (nonocclusive mesenteric ischemia), or mesenteric venous thrombosis. Syndromes of chronic mesenteric ischemia are produced in the majority of cases by atherosclerotic occlusive disease of the main mesenteric vessels: the celiac artery (CA), the superior mesenteric artery (SMA), and the inferior mesenteric artery (IMA). Chronic symptoms have also been attributed to isolated stenosis of the CA due to

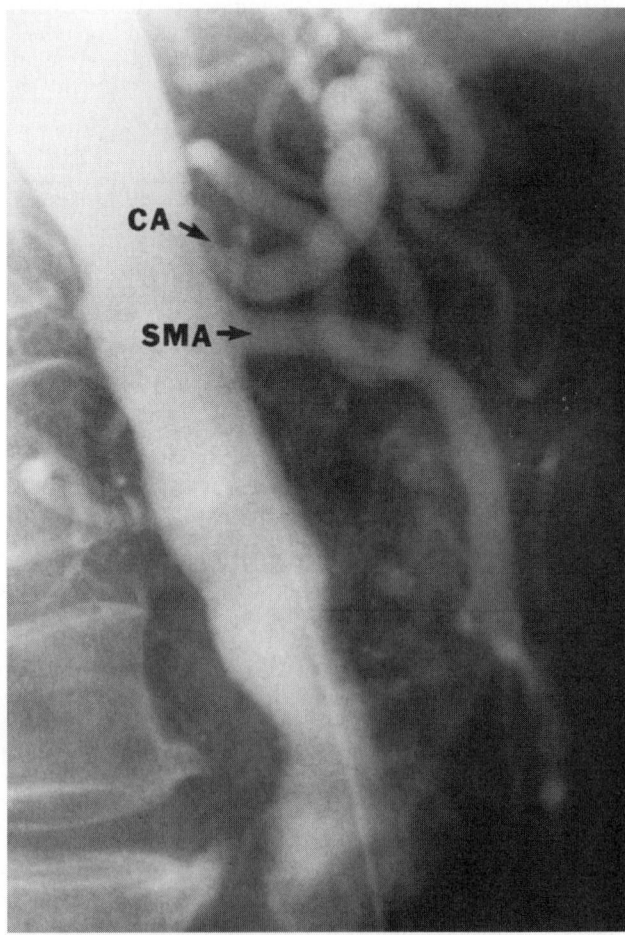

Figure 50–146. Lateral aortogram demonstrates the origins of normal celiac (CA) and superior mesenteric (SMA) arteries. Most occlusive lesions involve the first few centimeters of the main mesenteric vessels, and standard anteroposterior arteriographic views are inadequate to establish an accurate diagnosis.

extrinsic compression by the crura of the diaphragm, termed the *median arcuate ligament* or *celiac artery compression* syndrome. Finally, some cases of mesenteric venous thrombosis, like chronic gut ischemia of arterial origin, may produce indolent gastrointestinal symptoms over an extended period. Although components of these different syndromes (like the risks of eventual progression to gut infarction) may be universal, there are enough clinical differences to warrant individual discussion of these entities.

ANATOMY AND PATHOPHYSIOLOGY

Arterial perfusion is provided by the celiac trunk, the SMA, and the IMA. Anatomic variants abound, but the CA supplies the foregut, hepatobiliary system, and spleen; the SMA supplies the midgut (small bowel and proximal mid-colon); and the IMA supplies the hindgut (distal colon and rectum). The CA and SMA originate from the ventral surface of the suprarenal abdominal aorta, and the IMA has its origin from the left lateral aorta between the renal arteries and the aortic bifurcation. These anatomic relationships are important when arteriographic study of the main visceral arteries is performed. It is essential to obtain a lateral view of the aorta as well as the standard anteroposterior projection to assess adequately the CA and SMA (Fig. 50–146), because most arterial occlusive lesions occur in the first several centimeters.

The gastrointestinal tract has a sophisticated and luxuriant system of arterial collateral vessels between all three major visceral vessels that protect against gut ischemia. Collateral vessels between the CA and the SMA exist primarily through the superior and inferior pancreaticoduodenal arteries. The IMA may provide collateral arterial flow to the SMA through the marginal artery of Drummond, the arc of Riolan (Fig. 50-147), and other unnamed retroperitoneal collateral vessels termed *meandering mesenteric arteries* (Fig. 50-148). Additionally, systemic vessels may provide collateral visceral flow to the IMA and hindgut through the hypogastric arteries and the hemorrhoidal arterial system.

Regulation of intestinal blood flow is unique: hormonal and neural stimuli characteristically modulate blood flow throughout the body, and the mesenteric circulation responds to the intraluminal contents. Hormonal regulation is provided by splanchnic vasodilators, such as glucagon, vasoactive intestinal peptide, and nitric oxide, and by intrinsic vasoconstrictors, notably Pitressin. Neural regulation is provided by the extensive visceral autonomic innervation. However, autonomic regulation has been difficult to characterize because of the complex interrelationships between its effect on vasoreactivity compared with its more dominant effect on gastrointestinal motility.

Until recently, virtually all study of intestinal blood flow has been performed in experimental animals (because measurements were quite invasive), and extrapolations to humans have been uncertain. Mesenteric blood flow measurement in man has been performed using a dye-dilution technique requiring catheterization of the SMA and the portal or mesenteric venous system.[5, 36] Total splanchnic blood flow and SMA flow increase significantly after ingestion of a meal. In small numbers of patients with arteriographically proven major mesenteric arterial occlusive disease, this postprandial intestinal *hyperemia* was absent. After surgical revascularization procedures, these patients had postprandial intestinal blood flow responses that were similar to those of normal volunteers.[37]

Duplex ultrasound scanning has been used to study CA and SMA blood flow in man and to diagnose mesenteric arterial occlusive lesions. This technique has the advantage of being noninvasive and repeatable at intervals without risk or discomfort. Duplex scanning has allowed routine measurement of CA and SMA flow velocities in response to a variety of physiologic and pharmacologic stimuli. A number of early investigators[13, 20, 35, 42] observed increases in CA and SMA flow velocities after ingestion of a test meal, similar to the postprandial intestinal hyperemia evident in direct, invasive flow measurements. Mesenteric flow responses assessed by duplex scan could also be observed to vary with the nutrient and caloric content of a meal.[31] Lilly and associates[25] used mesenteric duplex scanning to compare postprandial CA and SMA flow responses to pharmacologically induced changes. Intravenous infusion of glucagon in normal subjects produced a significant increase in CA and SMA flow velocities, similar to observed postprandial flow increases. Infusion of

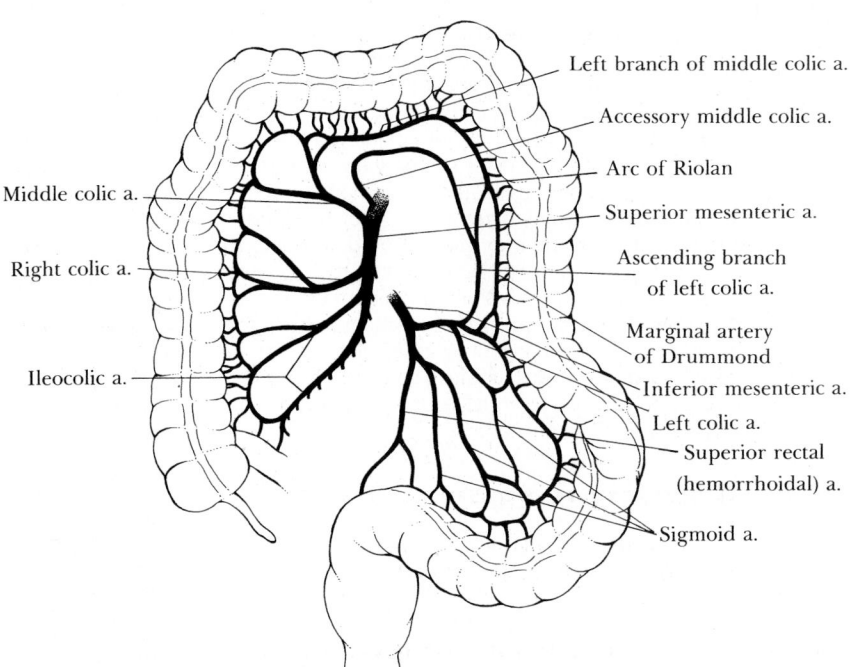

Figure 50–147. This diagram illustrates the normal anatomy of the superior mesenteric and inferior mesenteric arterial arborization. The arc of Riolan is indicated as separate from the marginal artery of Drummond. This latter vessel may be incomplete and allow colon necrosis to take place when inferior mesenteric artery occlusion occurs. From Ruzicka, F. F., Jr., and Rossi, P.: Normal vascular anatomy of the abdominal viscera. Radiol. Clin. North Am., *8:*1, 1970.)

Middle colic a.

Right colic a.

Ileocolic a.

Left branch of middle colic a.

Accessory middle colic a.

Arc of Riolan

Superior mesenteric a.

Ascending branch of left colic a.

Marginal artery of Drummond

Inferior mesenteric a.

Left colic a.

Superior rectal (hemorrhoidal) a.

Sigmoid a.

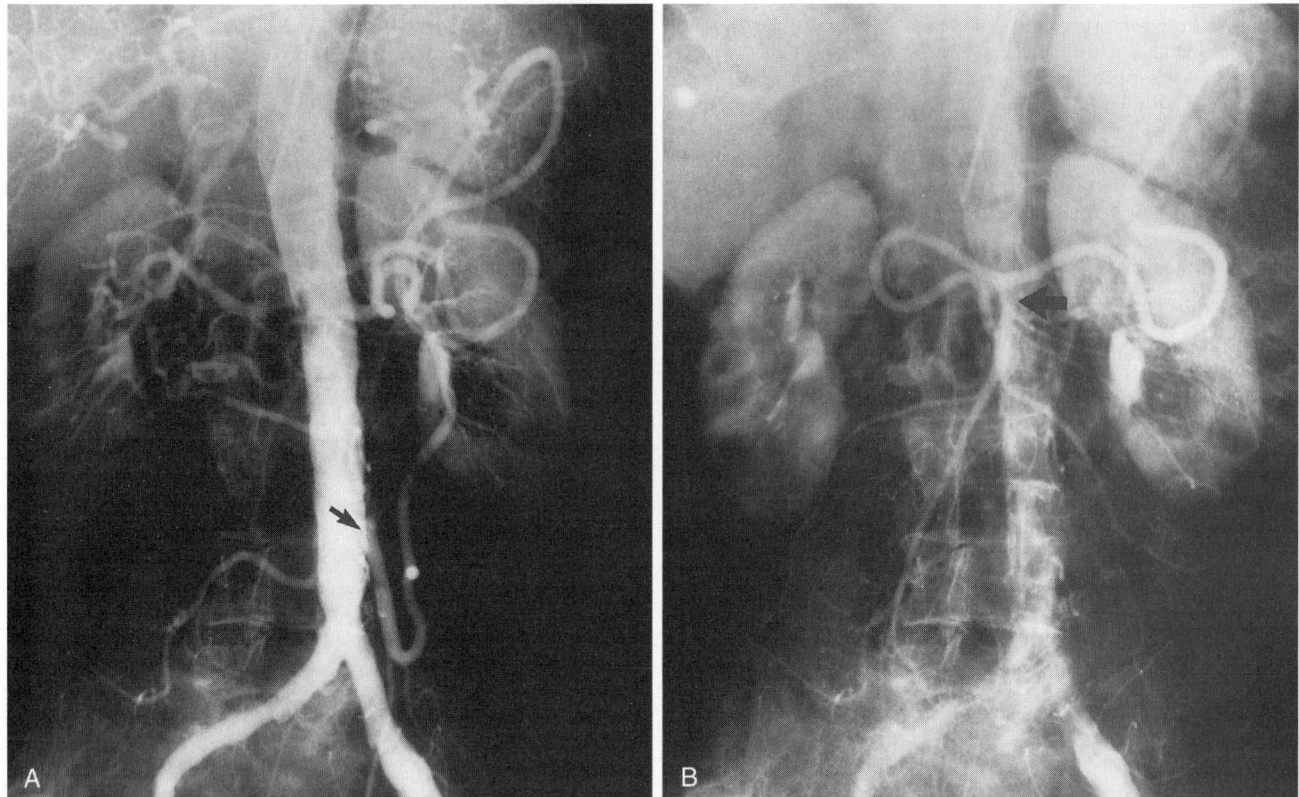

Figure 50–148. *A,* This flush aortogram demonstrates a markedly enlarged inferior mesenteric artery (arrow) with a "meandering mesenteric" collateral vessel. *B,* Delayed views demonstrate that this mesenteric collateral vessel fills the superior mesenteric artery (arrow), which was occluded at its origin.

the potent splanchnic vasoconstrictor Pitressin produced a significant reduction in CA and SMA flow velocities.

Duplex ultrasound scanning for the diagnosis of arterial occlusive disease has been most rigorously studied in the carotid system, where a very accurate estimation of the severity of arterial occlusive lesions is predicted by increasing systolic and diastolic flow velocities. Preliminary work has been done to develop similar diagnostic criteria for mesenteric arterial occlusive disease. Several investigators have performed retrospective comparisons of mesenteric duplex scanning with arteriography for the detection of CA and SMA occlusive lesions.[3, 32] Moneta and colleagues[33] used these duplex scan criteria to evaluate prospectively mesenteric occlusive lesions and achieved a sensitivity of 92% and a specificity of 96% for detection of 70% stenosis or occlusion. Although other investigators have called attention to factors that may compromise the diagnostic accuracy of mesenteric duplex scanning,[44] this technique may provide a helpful screening examination for patients suspected of having mesenteric ischemia. Arteriography is the most useful diagnostic examination for syndromes of mesenteric ischemia, but arteriography has been deferred in some cases because of its perceived risks. Under optimal clinical conditions, duplex scanning may provide a useful means of selecting patients for more invasive arteriographic study.

ACUTE MESENTERIC ISCHEMIA

The two basic stimuli that produce pain in the gastrointestinal tract are distention and ischemia. Acute gut ischemia produces diffuse abdominal (midgut) pain that is often quite severe. Experimentally, the initial reaction of the bowel to profound ischemia is intense spasm and, thus, patients with acute mesenteric ischemia are not markedly distended. This

initial spasm also contributes to the *gut emptying* that typically accompanies the acute ischemic insult, in the form of either vomiting or diarrhea. The mucosa of the bowel is the most sensitive to ischemia, and mucosal sloughing may occur with resultant bleeding into the gastrointestinal tract. This may produce an additional cathartic effect with bloody diarrhea, or blood may be detected in the stool on rectal examination. The lack of early involvement of the parietes produces few if any focal physical findings, and this *pain out of proportion to the physical findings* is the true hallmark of acute intestinal ischemia. Unfortunately, this often leads to an underestimation of the severity of the problem and a delay in diagnosis. When physical signs of focal or generalized peritonitis become evident, transmural necrosis of the bowel has already occurred, and this is inevitably associated with a marked worsening of the prognosis.

The results of routine, as well as very specialized, blood testing for the detection of intestinal ischemia have been clinically unrewarding; no single measurement nor any combination of electrolyte or enzyme studies has provided a reliable marker for gut ischemia. Patients may exhibit a profound leukocytosis (in the range of 25 to 40 $\times$ 10³/cu. mm.), or metabolic acidosis may develop. These findings are also nonspecific but are unusual in more prevalent intra-abdominal inflammatory processes (e.g., diverticulitis) that are being considered in a given patient. Considering the overall morbidity of acute mesenteric ischemia, definitive arteriographic study should not await serologic *screening* tests.

Duplex ultrasound scanning may be helpful for the evaluation of patients with suspected mesenteric ischemia. When a technologically satisfactory examination is possible, duplex scanning can identify major arterial or venous occlusions. However, when significant ileus has developed, bowel gas may obscure adequate ultrasound examination. Definitive diagnosis in most cases of acute mesenteric ischemia is established by arteriography. This includes a flush aortogram with lateral view to evaluate the origins of the CA and SMA (see Fig. 50–146). When the origins of the major mesenteric vessels are patent, selective CA and SMA injections are performed. When clinically indicated, the venous phase of selective mesenteric arterial injections is examined.

Mesenteric Embolism. Acute mesenteric embolism does not generally go unnoticed. The abrupt onset of *abdominal apoplexy* is associated with the most intense abdominal pain of all syndromes of mesenteric ischemia. Although the mesenteric arterial circulation possesses notable potential for collateral blood flow, sudden embolic occlusion of the SMA occurs in a previously normal vessel and produces a severity and acuity of ischemia that outstrips the short-term potential of these collateral vessels, a situation similar to that of acute embolic occlusion in the limbs or in embolic stroke. These emboli are almost all of a cardiac origin, and other clinical findings may help substantiate the diagnosis. These patients often have no significant history or physical evidence of severe peripheral arterial disease. Atrial arrhythmias or a history of previous myocardial infarction with a known ventricular aneurysm may confirm the obvious embolic source. In fact, 15% to 20% of these patients have a history of previous arterial emboli.

The diagnosis of mesenteric embolism is confirmed by arteriography. Selective catheterization of the SMA demonstrates the abrupt cutoff of contrast in an otherwise normal vessel with a *meniscus sign* or direct visualization of an intraluminal filling defect (Fig. 50–149). The thromboembolism occludes the main SMA trunk just beyond the origins of the middle colic artery and the first few jejunal branches, which accounts for the relative *sparing* of the proximal jejunum and distal colon that is seen at the time of surgical exploration in these cases (Fig. 50–150). In a patient without obvious signs of peritonitis, a consideration may be given to the infusion of thrombolytic agents such as streptokinase or urokinase.[12, 49] The arteriographic catheter facilitates direct infusion of the thrombolytic agent into the embolus, which facilitates rapid clot lysis; and this should result in some evident dissolution of the embolus, within minutes in some cases. In the

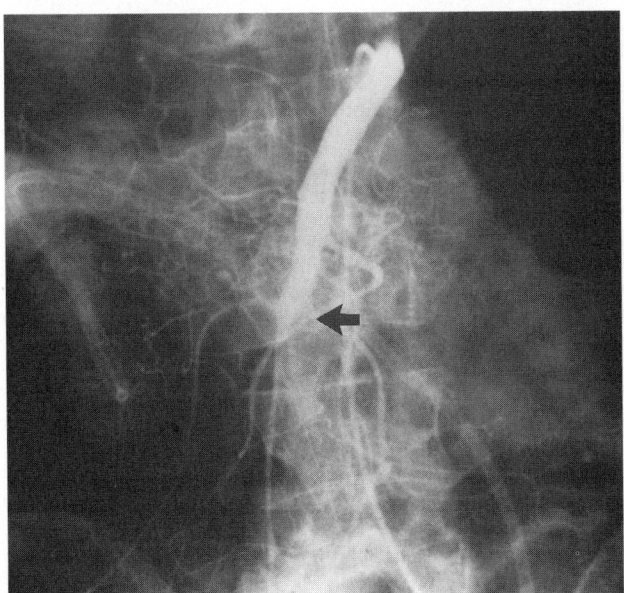

Figure 50–149. Selective superior mesenteric arteriogram demonstrates an abrupt occlusion of the SMA beyond the first jejunal branches diagnostic of mesenteric embolism (arrow). The patent jejunal branches explain the "sparing" of the proximal small bowel seen at the time of surgery.

absence of prompt lysis, or in the presence of any clinical deterioration, immediate surgical intervention is indicated. Significant gastrointestinal bleeding is obviously a relative contraindication to a consideration of thrombolytic therapy in such cases. In all cases, systemic heparin should be administered.

Surgical exploration is the treatment of choice in most cases of mesenteric embolism. Initial celiotomy reveals variable gut ischemia from the mid-jejunum to the ascending or transverse colon. In cases in which surgical exploration has been performed without arteriography, and thus without definitive diagnosis, this jejunal sparing is highly suggestive of an embolic event, and recognition may facilitate successful subsequent management. Initial exposure of the proximal SMA is similar to standard aortic surgery. The retroperitoneum is incised lateral to the fourth portion of the duodenum, which is mobilized to the patient's right. Dissection is then carried over the left renal vein. The proximal SMA is controlled where it emerges from beneath the pancreas in the root of the colonic mesentery, crossing superiorly and to the right over the left renal vein and then the duodenum. Extraction of the embolus is performed from this normal segment of SMA using standard balloon embolectomy catheters. In cases where the embolus has lodged more distally, exposure of the SMA may be elected more distally in the root of the small bowel mesentery. Here access to individual jejunal and ileal branches may allow a more comprehensive thromboembolectomy when required. After restoration of SMA flow, the viability of the affected segments of the gastrointestinal tract is reassessed. Nonviable bowel is resected and a decision is made concerning anastomosis or exteriorization.

Mesenteric Arterial Thrombosis. Acute mesenteric ischemia often occurs as a terminal thrombotic event of severe visceral atherosclerosis. The typical occlusive lesions of the CA and SMA occur at the origins of the vessels (Fig. 50–151), and patients often have diffuse atherosclerotic disease of even the distal visceral branches. Like those with mesenteric emboli, patients with acute thrombosis often have coronary artery disease; but most also have severe peripheral arterial disease and typically aortoiliac occlusive disease, which is a marker for visceral atherosclerosis of the renal and mesenteric arteries. In fact, patients who have unexplained abdominal complaints and a history of previous aortic grafting should be assumed to have mesenteric ischemia until proven otherwise, because this is by far the most morbid condition that can affect these patients.

The presenting symptoms of mesenteric thrombosis may initially be more insidious than those of mesenteric embolism. Mesenteric occlusive lesions have been present for a longer period in these patients, allowing maximal collateral development. A history of chronic mesenteric ischemia, with *abdominal angina*, is present in 20% to 50% of cases. The terminal thrombotic event may be precipitated by an unrelated intercurrent illness that results in dehydration from vomiting or diarrhea, which produces a confusing clinical picture. Complaints of abdominal pain are characteristically out of proportion to the physical findings and, in this elderly population, accurate diagnosis is delayed because these flulike symptoms are often misinterpreted as a benign condition. The downward clinical spiral includes progressive abdominal distention, oliguria, increasing fluid requirements, and metabolic acidosis. When peritoneal signs signal the development of a surgical abdomen, gut infarction and perforation have already occurred.

The diagnosis of mesenteric thrombosis is confirmed by arteriography, which demonstrates occlusion of the CA and SMA at or near their origins from the aorta. In most cases the IMA has been previously occluded secondary to diffuse infrarenal aortic atherosclerosis. Transcatheter therapy has

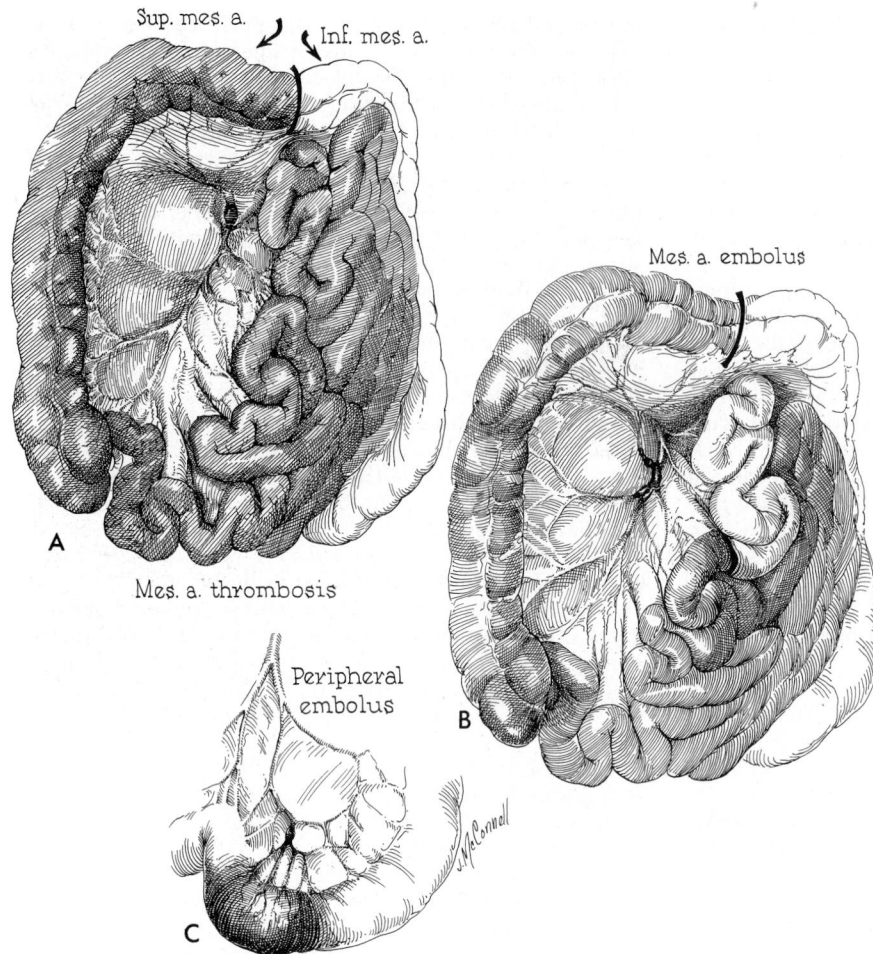

Sup. mes. a.   Inf. mes. a.

A

Mes. a. thrombosis

Mes. a. embolus

B

Peripheral embolus

C

Figure 50–150. This diagram illustrates differences seen at operation between patients with superior mesenteric artery thrombosis and those with mesenteric artery embolization. Notice the sparing of the upper jejunal arterial supply in mesenteric embolization and how this area is infarcted when the superior mesenteric artery is occluded by atherosclerotic thrombosis. Segmental infarction of bowel may also occur when emboli lodge in peripheral mesenteric branches. (From Bergan, J. J.: Recognition and treatment of intestinal ischemia. Surg. Clin. North Am., *47:*109, 1967.)

little role in the management of these patients. Successful thrombolysis requires selective cannulation of the vessels, and this is not possible in most cases. Additionally, even with successful initial thrombolysis, the critical occlusive lesions would require treatment, and endovascular strategies such as balloon angioplasty or stent placement for these lesions have been anecdotal. Additionally, these patients are often already in a relatively precarious clinical condition at the time of arteriography, and the time necessary for transcatheter therapy is unrealistic.

Surgical exploration is the treatment of choice for patients with mesenteric thrombosis. In fact, many patients come to surgical exploration before an accurate radiographic diagnosis has been established. Exploration in these patients often reveals a much more extensive intestinal necrosis than in patients with other forms of mesenteric ischemia. Because all three main mesenteric arteries are involved, gut ischemia extends from the duodenum to the distal colon. In many cases the remaining viable gut is insufficient to support life, and these patients cannot be salvaged. Successful surgical treatment will require mesenteric revascularization in all cases, and the appropriateness of these efforts must be critically assessed in each patient. When emergent, aortomesenteric vein bypass to revascularize the SMA provides the most expeditious management. Transaortic endarterectomy of the CA and SMA is also an alternative but involves more time for the required surgical exposure. When revascularization can be performed, a decision regarding bowel resection should be deferred until this has been completed. Even under optimal circumstances, the prognosis for these patients is grave.

Nonocclusive Mesenteric Ischemia. Acute mesenteric ischemia may be produced in some patients by diffuse, intense splanchnic arterial vasospasm. In such cases there are no major organic occlusive lesions in the mesenteric vessels and this entity has been termed *nonocclusive mesenteric ischemia* (NOMI). This disorder is typically seen in hospitalized patients with severe cardiopulmonary dysfunction due to other causes, such as cardiogenic or septic shock or a host of other life-threatening conditions. NOMI may also be seen postoperatively in cardiac surgery patients, especially those who have required extended vasopressor support.[1, 30] Because, like cerebral perfusion, visceral perfusion is generally preserved, this condition represents a failure of splanchnic autoregulation with paradoxical visceral hypoperfusion, often to the point of intestinal infarction. Past investigators believed that such visceral vasospasm might be related to digitalis therapy, but a precise causal relationship has been uncertain, especially considering the overall cardiodynamic status of these patients and the complexity of their other therapies. However, NOMI has been associated with other pharmacologic agents that produce splanchnic vasospasm, such as ergot or cocaine intoxication.[16, 34]

The diagnosis of NOMI can only be reliably established by mesenteric arteriography, which first serves to exclude other major organic occlusive lesions noted earlier. Selective SMA arteriography in cases of NOMI demonstrates a patent main vessel with severe vasospasm in the jejunal and ileal branches (Fig. 50–152). Direct catheterization of the SMA may also facilitate therapy in these cases by the direct intra-arterial infusion of papaverine, a splanchnic vasodilator. Ultimately, successful treatment of NOMI also requires stabilization and improvement of these patients' underlying hemodynamic dysfunction, regardless of its cause. As in all cases of acute mesenteric ischemia, the development of signs of peritonitis at any time during alternative therapy signals the need for surgical exploration. In these cases it may be useful to leave the arteriographic catheter in place in the SMA to allow continuous infusion of the vasodilator during and after the surgical procedure. Intestinal necrosis in these cases is often less extensive than in patients with mesenteric emboli or thrombosis, especially if successful pharmacologic therapy has been administered. Nevertheless, the mortality rates for NOMI remain high, because many patients succumb to their underlying medical problems.

Mesenteric Venous Thrombosis. Not all syndromes of mesenteric ischemia are produced by arterial occlusive diseases. Mesenteric venous thrombosis can produce intestinal ischemia that is clinically indistinguishable from any of the aforementioned arteriopathies; and when gut infarction occurs in these cases, the mortality rates are equally discouraging. Mesenteric ischemia in general is rare, and mesenteric venous thrombosis accounts for only about 8% of all cases. However, it can be one of the most clinically insidious of all syndromes of mesenteric ischemia, which explains why it is also classified as a chronic syndrome in this review. Mesenteric venous thrombosis lacks a *classic* prodrome or presentation and is more difficult to diagnose with conventional techniques. In addition, it can occur in young adults, which

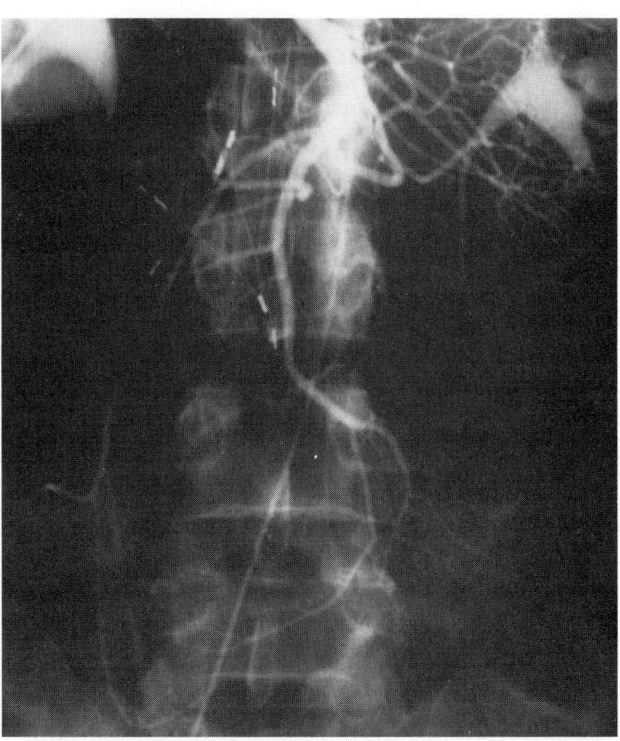

Figure 50–152. Selective superior mesenteric arteriography demonstrates patency of the main superior mesenteric artery and severe vasospasm of the jejunal and ileal branches diagnostic of "nonocclusive" mesenteric ischemia.

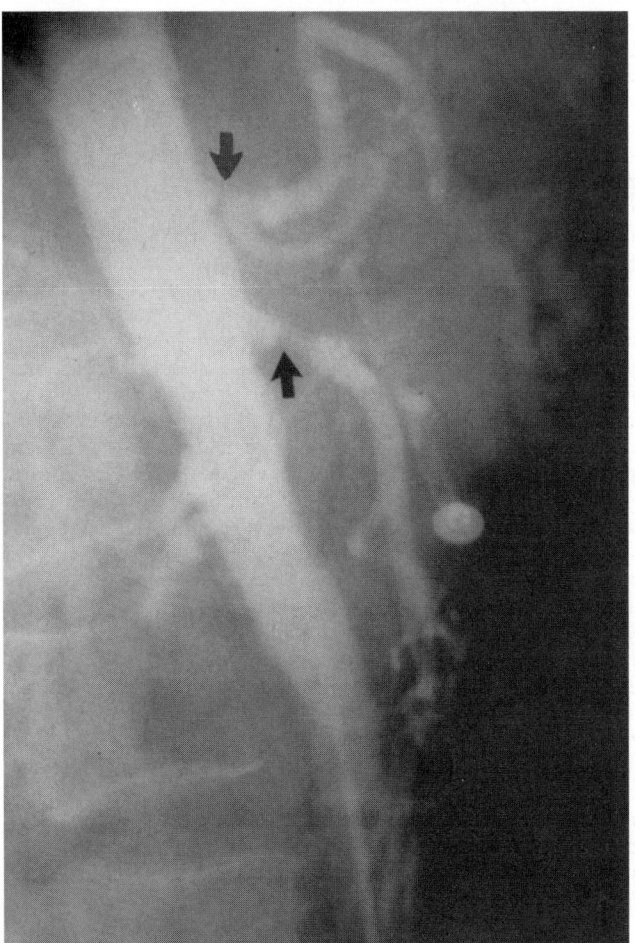

Figure 50–151. This lateral flush aortogram demonstrates severe atherosclerotic stenosis of both the celiac and superior mesenteric arteries (arrows). Such lesions may produce the symptoms of chronic mesenteric ischemia or progress to thrombosis, with resultant acute mesenteric ischemia.

is exceedingly rare for either mesenteric embolus or thrombosis.

Mesenteric venous thrombosis is considered primary when no other predisposing cause is found, but more than 80% of cases are secondary to some underlying disorder that produces abnormalities in mesenteric venous flow dynamics, which may predispose to thrombosis. Portal hypertension or congestive heart failure produces visceral venous stasis. Intra-abdominal sepsis may cause so-called pylephlebitis. Visceral malignancies may directly obstruct mesenteric venous flow and/or produce a relatively hypercoagulable state. In younger patients, mesenteric venous thrombosis may be a manifestation of an underlying congenital hypercoagulable state, such as deficiencies of antithrombin III, protein C, or protein S, or may be related to anticardiolipin antibodies.[4, 15, 17] In some series a significant number of these patients had a previous history of deep venous thrombosis.

The clinical presentation of mesenteric venous thrombosis can be identical to the arterial causes of acute mesenteric ischemia. Diffuse abdominal pain out of proportion to physical findings may progress rapidly to signs of peritonitis, requiring emergent surgical exploration. However, 27% of patients with mesenteric venous thrombosis had symptoms for more than 30 days.[26] Additionally, with the increased application of abdominal imaging by computed tomography or magnetic resonance imaging, it has been recognized that some patients with mesenteric venous thrombosis have minimal or no symptoms.

The presentation and complications of mesenteric venous thrombosis may be similar to those of acute splanchnic arterial disorders, but diagnostic strategies are somewhat different. Arteriography provides only indirect diagnosis in cases of mesenteric venous thrombosis, where the venous phase of selective SMA arteriography must be carefully examined. Rarely, thrombus may be visualized in the portal-mesenteric system, while in the majority of cases the diagnosis is established by a delayed or absent venous phase. Whereas arteriography is useful in these cases to exclude an arterial cause for mesenteric ischemia, computed tomography (Fig. 50–153), magnetic resonance imaging, and duplex ultrasound scanning provide a more direct examination of the mesenteric venous system.[18, 22, 53, 54]

Standard heparin anticoagulation is the initial treatment of choice for mesenteric venous thrombosis. Anticoagulation reduces the risk of progression, recurrence, and the overall mortality. Thrombolytic therapy has been used in anecdotal cases[45] and deserves consideration in stable, symptomatic patients where arteriographic access has already been established. When physical findings suggest an acute abdomen, exploration is indicated. Bowel necrosis, when present, is usually limited to the small bowel but may be patchy and segmental, making definitive resection challenging. Anticoagulation should be continued postoperatively, and surviving patients should receive long-term warfarin therapy.

The majority of patients with acute mesenteric ischemia, regardless of the cause, require surgical exploration at some point. In many, surgical exploration is necessary before a precise diagnosis has been established. Findings at exploration, like jejunal sparing, may clarify the diagnosis and the appropriate strategy for a revascularization attempt when indicated. As noted earlier, revascularization should be completed before a final decision is made regarding resectional treatment. In cases where it is believed that there will be (under ideal circumstances) sufficient bowel length to sustain life, gangrenous bowel is then resected. However, the surgeon ultimately faces the dilemma of distinguishing apparently viable or marginally viable bowel from nonviable bowel. A number of intraoperative techniques have been developed to assess bowel viability in these cases, including Doppler ultrasonography, intravenous administration of fluorescein, and photoplethysmography.[6, 38, 40] A sterile handheld Doppler probe is available in most operating rooms today, and the presence of pulsatile arterial Doppler signals on the antimesenteric surface of the bowel is a good indication of adequate arterial perfusion. Although all these techniques, including clinical judgment alone, have their proponents, none are universally reliable. This is not for a lack of technologic sophistication but because some additional intestinal necrosis may develop even after hemodynamically successful revascularization. This process represents an ischemia-reperfusion injury that may evolve many hours after the

original operation. The interaction of oxygen-derived free radicals, various cytokines, and leukocytes that mediate this reperfusion injury is being more accurately characterized by investigators in the laboratory and their work offers hope for pharmacologic modification of this reperfusion injury in the future.[2] In fact, a systemic effect of this reperfusion injury has been implicated in the development of multisystem organ failure in patients after intestinal revascularization,[19] which may also contribute to the unacceptably high mortality in patients even when intestinal viability has been successfully preserved.

The previous discussion would confirm the usefulness of a routine second-look operation 24 to 36 hours after initial treatment in patients with acute mesenteric ischemia who have had surgical exploration, especially when revascularization and/or bowel resection has been performed. Re-exploration of the abdomen is in itself unlikely to compromise patient survival, but untreated persistent or recurrent intestinal necrosis is uniformly fatal.

CHRONIC MESENTERIC ISCHEMIA

Mesenteric Atherosclerosis. Chronic mesenteric ischemia is produced most often by atherosclerotic occlusive disease of the main mesenteric vessels—the CA, SMA, and IMA. This syndrome is remarkably rare, considering the prevalence of other generalized atherosclerotic problems in our society. Conner, in 1933, speculated that misdiagnosed abdominal pain might have been a prodrome in some patients who suffered fatal intestinal infarction.[8] Later, Dunphy made a seminal contribution to the recognition of chronic mesenteric ischemia, observing that 58% of patients who died of intestinal infarction had well-documented histories of chronic, recurrent abdominal pain.[10] The typical ostial atherosclerotic occlusive lesions of the CA and SMA that led to mesenteric thrombosis were described in 1957 by Mikkelsen, who proposed that surgical treatment might relieve symptoms of *intestinal angina*.[29] In 1958, Shaw and Maynard reported the first cases of surgical revascularization by mesenteric endarterectomy for the treatment of chronic mesenteric ischemia.[46]

Chronic mesenteric ischemia occurs more commonly in women, with at least a 3:1 predominance, one of the only atherosclerotic ischemic syndromes to demonstrate such a pattern. The clinical hallmark of chronic mesenteric ischemia is postprandial, midabdominal, or epigastric pain. Postprandial pain occurs soon after eating and is generally disabling for the patient. Because initial medical evaluation rarely identifies the precise cause and prescribed remedies provide no relief, patients manage their own symptoms by meal avoidance. This *food fear* almost invariably results in significant weight loss in these patients, to the point of inanition in many cases. This combination of chronic abdominal pain and significant weight loss in patients with a mean age of 60 years is logically suspected to be due to an occult malignancy. Initial work-up then includes an extensive gastrointestinal diagnostic evaluation, including endoscopy, bowel contrast studies, and computed tomography scans. None of these reliably diagnoses mesenteric arterial occlusions, and in one series patients with chronic mesenteric ischemia were symptomatic for an average of 18 months before diagnosis.[48] These patients frequently have a history or physical evidence of peripheral vascular disease. Aortoiliac occlusive disease is particularly common and may account for occlusions of the IMA, which compromise visceral collateral flow.

The exact cause of visceral ischemic pain in these patients is not precisely known. Clearly, the normal postprandial hyperemic response is absent in these patients and the metabolic demands of nutrient absorption and increased intestinal motility may lead to the production of anaerobic metabolic

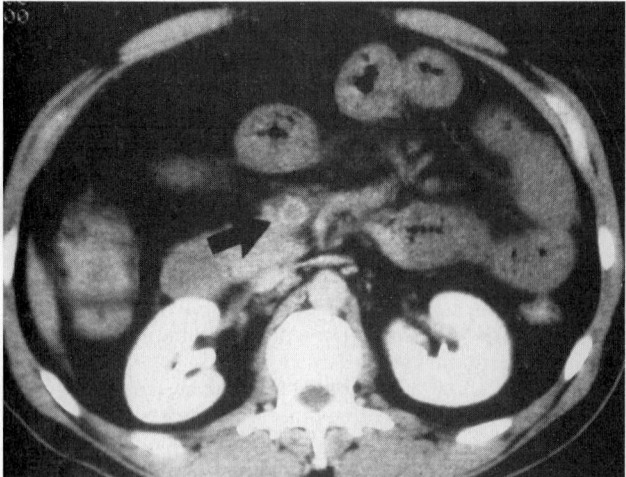

Figure 50–153. This computed tomographic (CT) scan demonstrates thrombus within a dilated superior mesenteric vein (arrow). Abdominal imaging techniques like CT or duplex ultrasonography provide a direct examination of the mesenteric and portal veins.

byproducts. Some clinicians have speculated that reduced gastric blood flow may induce increased acid production, peptic ulceration, and abdominal pain.[41] Although H_2-blockers and other antiulcer medications have not resulted in symptomatic improvement in patients with chronic mesenteric ischemia, successful revascularization has been associated with increased gastric mucosal pH.[11] Whatever the cause, clinical experience has indicated that a marked reduction in overall mesenteric perfusion must exist before symptoms develop. This has usually been associated with severe stenoses or occlusions of two or more of the main mesenteric vessels (CA, SMA, and IMA). Symptoms of chronic mesenteric ischemia have been associated with single-vessel obstruction of the SMA, but these cases probably represent patients with aberrant collateral anatomy.

The diagnosis of chronic mesenteric ischemia may be delayed by confusion with other more common ailments, but it is also often delayed because arteriography has previously been required. Occlusive disease of the main mesenteric vessels can now be identified by duplex ultrasound scanning, as described previously.[32, 33] The diagnostic usefulness of this technique is greatest in patients with suspected chronic mesenteric ischemia who can be examined electively under optimal conditions before the more acute complications of this disorder ensue. Duplex scanning in these cases has the potential to become more of an entry-level diagnostic test for patients with suspected mesenteric ischemia to select those who would truly benefit from arteriography. The diagnosis of chronic mesenteric ischemia is then confirmed by mesenteric arteriography (see Fig. 50–151). Arteriography also helps clarify the status of the supraceliac and infrarenal abdominal aorta, which is of use in planning subsequent surgical treatment. When significant aneurysmal or occlusive disease is present, concomitant aortic reconstruction may be indicated.

Successful resolution of symptoms and a return to normal alimentation in patients with chronic mesenteric ischemia requires mesenteric revascularization. Percutaneous transluminal balloon angioplasty has been used to treat severe stenosis of the SMA in small numbers of cases,[14, 24] but follow-up is limited. However, stenotic lesions of the SMA are frequently at the origin of the vessel, and percutaneous transluminal angioplasty is not technically feasible. Often, the mesenteric vessels are occluded, preventing catheter access. In general, surgical revascularization has been the most predictable and durable form of treatment.

Mesenteric arterial occlusive lesions have been treated successfully by either endarterectomy or bypass grafting. CA and SMA endarterectomy is most effectively performed using a transabdominal or thoracoabdominal exposure of the supraceliac aorta and a *trapdoor* transaortic exposure of the ostia of the visceral vessels.[50] This exposure is challenging for the uninitiated, but long-term success rates of 80% to 90% have been reported.[9] Bypass grafting may be performed either retrograde from the infrarenal aorta or antegrade from the supraceliac aorta. Both autogenous saphenous vein grafts and prosthetic grafts have been used successfully for mesenteric bypass. When infrarenal aortic replacement is required in these patients for aneurysm or occlusive disease, it would seem logical to use the aortic prosthesis as the origin for the bypasses and perform retrograde revascularization. Proponents of antegrade bypass note the relative absence of atherosclerosis in the supraceliac aorta, but, as mentioned earlier, the exposure is somewhat more demanding. Antegrade bypass is performed using a small-caliber aortic bifurcation graft, which is anastomosed to the supraceliac aorta in an end-to-side fashion. One limb of the graft is then carried directly to the CA, and the other limb is anastomosed to the SMA. The relative rarity of these cases has prevented prospective comparison of these different surgical procedures, but a number of reports have documented comparable excellent long-term success rates (80%–90%) with all these techniques.[9, 27, 52]

Generally, it has been the philosophy to perform a *comprehensive* revascularization for elective surgical treatment of chronic mesenteric ischemia (e.g., reconstruction of two or more of the main mesenteric vessels). This policy has been largely intuitive, recognizing that in the past, patients having single bypass grafts were more likely to develop recurrent symptoms when graft occlusion occurred. Because surgical treatment of all severely diseased mesenteric vessels does not increase the complexity of the procedure, comprehensive mesenteric revascularization remains a sound policy. However, in every case it is mandatory to perform revascularization of the SMA.

Mesenteric duplex scanning may also assist in the follow-up of patients requiring mesenteric revascularization for chronic or acute mesenteric ischemia. In the past, documentation of the patency of these reconstructions required arteriography or relied on the patient's continued freedom from recurrent symptoms. Early patency of visceral arterial reconstructions can now be performed noninvasively using duplex ultrasound scanning,[47] and the continued patency of these procedures can be objectively documented in a prospective fashion.[28]

Celiac Artery Compression Syndrome. Extrinsic compression of the CA may be produced by the median arcuate ligament of the diaphragm (Fig. 50–154). This anatomic variant has been observed in up to one third of cases in autopsy studies. However, CA compression syndrome has been implicated in some variants of chronic mesenteric ischemia. Symptomatic visceral ischemia due to isolated celiac compression has been difficult for many clinicians to reconcile. First, the compression is reversible. During deep inspiration the diaphragmatic crura relax and celiac anatomy and measured flow velocities return to normal, as has been documented by arteriography and duplex ultrasound scanning.[51] Second, foregut ischemia has rarely been described in patients with even the worst cases of mesenteric ischemia that require surgical exploration. Because symptomatic improvement has been reported after surgical division of the median arcuate ligament, there have been attempts to identify patients who would truly benefit from surgical treatment. Some have spec-

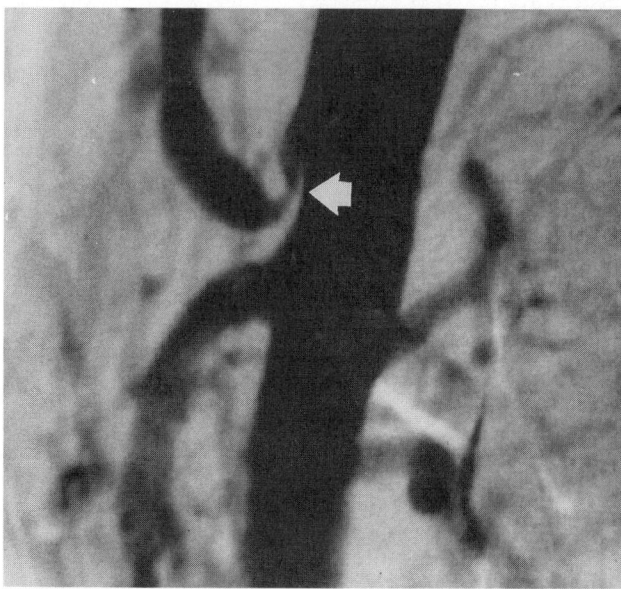

Figure 50–154. Extrinsic compression of the celiac artery (arrow) by the median arcuate ligament.

ulated that pain relief in these patients is due to lysis of the celiac ganglion splanchnic nerve fibers rather than to improvement in celiac blood flow.[7] Others have observed symptomatic improvement is more likely in women, patients with postprandial pain and weight loss, and those with an absence of drug abuse or psychiatric history.[43] Extrinsic compression of both the CA and SMA has been reported,[21] and certainly surgical treatment is clearly justified in such a case. However, the uncertain association of isolated celiac compression with gastrointestinal symptoms and the low risk of progression to gut infarction suggest that patients be very carefully selected for surgical treatment.

Rare Causes of Ischemia. Although atherosclerotic occlusion of the main mesenteric vessels is the most common form of chronic intestinal ischemia encountered by most surgeons, other more rare conditions are included in the differential diagnosis. These include polyarteritis nodosa, allergic or radiation-induced arteritis, scleroderma, and lupus erythematosus. Fibromuscular dysplasia may involve the CA or SMA, and intimal hyperplasia of the visceral arteries may occur in young women on oral contraceptives who smoke heavily. Mesenteric artery involvement may be a dominant part of the rare Cogan's syndrome or be seen in patients with Kawasaki's disease. Although rarely reported, these disorders may be challenging to treat with conventional techniques.

SUMMARY

In nearly half a century of modern vascular surgery, countless advances in surgical techniques, development of graft materials, and the perioperative management of patients with associated medical conditions have occurred. This has resulted in a progressive measurable reduction in surgical risk for almost every major vascular reconstructive procedure. There are two notable exceptions to this observation: ruptured abdominal aortic aneurysms and severe mesenteric ischemia. The mortality rates for these two vascular catastrophes remain almost universally 50% or greater. In the case of abdominal aortic aneurysms, the increased use of imaging techniques such as ultrasonography or computed tomography has resulted in more frequent elective repair of asymptomatic and smaller aneurysms. This has correspondingly resulted in a reduced percentage of ruptured aneurysms treated by any given institution or surgeon. Unfortunately the same has not yet been observed for syndromes of mesenteric ischemia. Few of these cases have been *routinely* diagnosed and treated, and there has remained uncertainty about the appropriate management of asymptomatic severe occlusive disease of the CA or SMA. It seems clear that early recognition of patients with intestinal ischemia combined with aggressive diagnostic testing to identify these lesions before they proceed to intestinal infarction is the only way to reduce these unacceptable mortality rates.

SELECTED REFERENCES

Bech, F. R., and Gewertz, B. L.: Pathophysiology of intestinal ischemia. *In* Strandness, D. E., Jr., and van Breda, A. (Eds.): Vascular Diseases: Surgical and Interventional Therapy. New York, Churchill Livingstone, 1994, p. 745.
This text presents a description of the hemodynamic, cellular, and biochemical events of mesenteric ischemia. This material is summarized by investigators actively involved in basic research in the field of ischemia-reperfusion injury to the gastrointestinal tract.

Cunningham, C. G., Reilly, L. M., Rapp, J. H., et al.: Chronic visceral ischemia: Three decades of progress. Ann. Surg., *214*:276, 1991.
This report is the summary of an extensive experience with surgical revascularization procedures for mesenteric arterial occlusion. The results of the two basic surgical procedures, endarterectomy and bypass, are compared. Important details of surgical techniques are provided.

Moneta, G. L., Lee, R. W., Yeager, R. A., Taylor, L. M., and Porter, J. M.:
Mesenteric duplex scanning: A blinded prospective study. J. Vasc. Surg., *17*:79, 1993.
This study presents a critical assessment of duplex ultrasound scanning for the noninvasive diagnosis of mesenteric arterial occlusive lesions. The authors have been in the forefront of the development of this technique, and the article and its references provide a complete summary of its evolution.

REFERENCES

1. Allen, K. B., Salam, A. A., and Lumsden, A. B.: Acute mesenteric ischemia following cardiopulmonary bypass. J. Vasc. Surg., *16*:391, 1992.
2. Bech, F. R., and Gewertz, B. L.: Pathophysiology of intestinal ischemia. *In* Strandness, D. E., Jr., and van Breda, A. (Eds.): Vascular Diseases: Surgical and Interventional Therapy. New York, Churchill Livingstone, 1994, p. 745.
3. Bowersox, J. C., Zwolak, R. M., Walsh, D. B., Schneider, J. R., Musson, A., Labombard, E., and Cronenwatt, J. L.: Duplex ultrasonography in the diagnosis of celiac and mesenteric artery occlusive disease. J. Vasc. Surg., *14*:780, 1991.
4. Broekmans, A. W., van Rooyan, W., Westerveld, B. D., et al.: Mesenteric vein thrombosis as presenting manifestation of hereditary protein S deficiency. Gastroenterology, *92*:240, 1987.
5. Buchardt-Hansen, H. J., Engell, H. C., Ring-Larsen, H., and Ranek, L.: Splanchnic blood flow in patients with abdominal angina before and after arterial reconstruction. Ann. Surg., *186*:216, 1977.
6. Bulkley, G. B., Zuidema, G. D., Hamilton, S. R., et al.: Intraoperative determination of small intestinal viability following ischemic injury. Ann. Surg., *193*:628, 1981.
7. Carey, J. P., Stemmer, E. A., and Connolly, J. E.: Median arcuate ligament syndrome. Arch. Surg., *99*:441, 1969.
8. Conner, L. A.: A discussion of the role of arterial thrombosis in visceral diseases of middle life, based upon analogies drawn from coronary thrombosis. Am. J. Med. Sci., *185*:13, 1933.
9. Cunningham, C. G., Reilly, L. M., Rapp, J. H., et al.: Chronic visceral ischemia: Three decades of progress. Ann. Surg., *214*:276, 1991.
10. Dunphy, J. E.: Abdominal pain of vascular origin. Am. J. Med. Sci., *192*:109, 1936.
11. Fiddian-Greene, R. G., Stanley, J. C., Nostrant, T., et al.: Chronic gastric ischemia: A cause of abdominal pain or bleeding identified from the presence of gastric mucosal acidosis. J. Cardiovasc. Surg., *30*:852, 1989.
12. Flickinger, E. G., Johnsrude, I. S., Ogburn, N. L., et al.: Local streptokinase infusion for superior mesenteric artery thromboembolism. AJR, *140*:771, 1983.
13. Flinn, W. R., Sandager, G. P., Lilly, M. P., Yao, J. S. T., and Bergan, J. J.: Duplex scan of mesenteric and celiac arteries. *In* Bergan, J. J., and Yao, J. S. T. (Eds.): Arterial Surgery: New Diagnostic and Operative Techniques. Orlando, Fla., Grune & Stratton, 1988, p. 367.
14. Furrer, J., Grüntzig, A., Kugelmeier, J., and Goebel, N.: Treatment of abdominal angina with percutaneous dilation of an arteria mesenterica superior stenosis. Cardiovasc. Intervent. Radiol., *3*:43, 1980.
15. Green, D., Granger, D. R., and Blei, A. T.: Protein C deficiency in splanchnic venous thrombosis. Am. J. Med., *82*:1171, 1987.
16. Green, F. L., Ariyan, S., and Stausel, H. C., Jr.: Mesenteric and peripheral vascular ischemia secondary to ergotism. Surgery, *81*:176, 1977.
17. Gruenberg, J. C., Smallridge, R. C., and Rosenberg, R. D.: Inherited antithrombin III deficiency causing mesenteric venous infarction: A new clinical entity. Ann. Surg., *181*:791, 1975.
18. Harward, T. R. S., Green, D., Bergan, J. J., et al.: Mesenteric venous thrombosis. J. Vasc. Surg., *9*:328, 1989.
19. Harward, T. R. S., Brooks, D. L., Flynn, T. C., and Seeger, J. M.: Multiple organ dysfunction after mesenteric artery revascularization. J. Vasc. Surg., *18*:459, 1993.
20. Jager, K., Bollinger, A., Valli, C., and Amman, N.: Measurement of mesenteric blood flow by duplex scan. J. Vasc. Surg., *3*:462, 1986.
21. Lawson, J. D., and Ochsner, J. L.: Median arcuate ligament syndrome with severe two-vessel involvement. Arch. Surg., *119*:226, 1984.
22. Levy, H. M., and Newhouse, J. H.: MR imaging of portal vein thrombosis. AJR, *151*:283, 1988.
23. Levy, P. J., Krauz, M. M., and Manny J.: Acute mesenteric ischemia: Improved results—A retrospective analysis of ninety-two patients. Surgery, *107*:372, 1990.
24. Levy, P. J., Haskell, L., and Gordon, R. L.: Percutaneous transluminal angioplasty of the splanchnic arteries: An alternative to elective revascularization in chronic visceral ischemia. Eur. J. Radiol., *7*:239, 1987.
25. Lilly, M. P., Harward, T. R. S., Flinn, W. R., Blackburn, D. R., Astlefor, P. M., and Yao, J. S. T.: Duplex ultrasound measurements of changes in mesenteric flow velocities with pharmacologic and physiologic alterations in intestinal blood flow in man. J. Vasc. Surg., *9*:18, 1989.
26. Matthews, J. E., and White, R. R.: Primary mesenteric venous occlusive disease. Am. J. Surg., *122*:579, 1971.
27. McAfee, M. K., Cherry, K. J., Jr., Naessens, J. M., et al.: Influence of complete revascularization on chronic mesenteric ischemia. Am. J. Surg., *164*:220, 1992.
28. McMillan, W. D., McCarthy, W. J., Bresticker, M., et al.: Mesenteric artery bypass: Objective measurement of primary patency. J. Vasc. Surg., *21*:729, 1995.

29. Mikkelsen, W. P.: Intestinal angina: Its surgical significance. Am. J. Surg., 94:262, 1957.
30. Moneta, G. L., Misbach, F. A., and Ivey, T. D.: Hypoperfusion as a possible factor in the development of gastrointestinal complications after cardiac surgery. Am. J. Surg., 149:648, 1985.
31. Moneta, G. L., Taylor, D. C., Helton, W. S., Mulholland, M. W., and Strandness, D. E.: Duplex ultrasound measurement of postprandial intestinal blood flow: Effect of meal composition. Gastroenterology, 95:1294, 1988.
32. Moneta, G. L., Yeager, R. A., Dalman, R., Antonovic, R., Hall, L. D., and Porter, J. M.: Duplex ultrasound criteria for diagnosis of splanchnic artery stenosis or occlusion. J. Vasc. Surg., 14:511, 1991.
33. Moneta, G. L., Lee, R. W., Yeager, R. A., Taylor, L. M., and Porter, J. M.: Mesenteric duplex scanning: A blinded prospective study. J. Vasc. Surg., 17:79, 1993.
34. Nalbaudiau, H., Sheth, N., Dietrich, R., et al.: Intestinal ischemia caused by cocaine ingestion: Report of two cases. Surgery, 97:374, 1985.
35. Nichols, S. C., Kohler, T. R., Martin, R. S., and Strandness, D. E.: Use of hemodynamic parameter in the diagnosis of mesenteric insufficiency. J. Vasc. Surg., 3:507, 1986.
36. Norryd, C., Dencker, H., Lunderquist, A., and Olin, T.: Superior mesenteric blood flow in man studied with a dye dilution technique. Acta Chir. Scand., 141:109, 1975.
37. Norryd, C., Dencker, H., Lunderquist, A., et al.: Superior mesenteric blood flow during digestion in man. Acta Chir. Scand., 141:197, 1975.
38. O'Donnell, J. A., and Hobson, R. W.: Operative confirmation of Doppler ultrasound evaluation of intestinal ischemia. Surgery, 87:109, 1980.
39. Ottinger, L., and Austen, W. G.: A study of 136 patients with mesenteric infarction. Surg. Gynecol. Obstet., 124:1251, 1967.
40. Pearce, W. H., Jones, D. N., Warren, G. H., et al.: The use of infrared photoplethysmography in identifying early intestinal ischemia. Arch. Surg., 122:108, 1987.
41. Poole, J. W., Sammartano, J. W., and Boley, S. J.: Hemodynamic basis of pain of chronic mesenteric ischemia. Am. J. Surg., 153:171, 1987.
42. Quamar, M. I., Read, A. E., Skidmore, R., et al.: Transcutaneous Doppler ultrasound measurement of superior mesenteric blood flow in man. Gut, 27:100, 1986.
43. Reilly, L. M., Ammar, A. D., Stoney, R. J., et al.: Late results following operative repair for celiac artery compression syndrome. J. Vasc. Surg., 2:79, 1985.
44. Rizzo, R. J., Sandager, G. P., Astlefor, P., et al.: Mesenteric flow velocity variations as a function of angle of insonation. J. Vasc. Surg., 11:688, 1990.
45. Robin, P., Gruel, Y., Lang, M., et al.: Complete thrombolysis of mesenteric vein occlusion with recombinant tissue-type plasminogen activator. Lancet 1:1391, 1988.
46. Shaw, R. S., and Maynard, E. P., III: Acute and chronic thrombosis of the mesenteric arteries associated with malabsorption: A report of two cases successfully treated by thromboendarterectomy. N. Engl. J. Med., 258:874, 1958.
47. Sandager, G. P., Flinn, W. R., McCarthy, W. J., et al.: Assessment of visceral arterial reconstruction using duplex scan. J. Vasc. Technol., 11:13, 1987.
48. Schneider, P. A., Eherenfeld, W. K., Cunningham, C. G., et al.: Recurrent chronic visceral ischemia. J. Vasc. Surg., in press.
49. Schoenbaum, S. W., Pena, C., Koenigsberg, P., and Katzen, B. T.: Superior mesenteric artery embolism: Treatment with intraarterial urokinase. J. Vasc. Intervent. Radiol., 3:485, 1992.
50. Stoney, R. J., and Cunningham, C. G.: Chronic visceral ischemia. In Yao, J., and Pearce, W. (Eds.): Long Term Results in Vascular Surgery. Norwalk, Conn., Appleton & Lange, 1993, p. 305.
51. Taylor, D. C., Moneta, G. L., Cramer, M. M., et al.: Extrinsic compression of the celiac artery by the median arcuate ligament of the diaphragm: Diagnosis by duplex ultrasound. J. Vasc. Technol., 11:236, 1987.
52. Taylor, L. M., Jr., and Porter, J. M.: Treatment of chronic visceral ischemia. In Rutherford, R. B. (Ed.): Vascular Surgery. Philadelphia, W. B. Saunders, 1995, p. 1301.
53. Tessler, F. N., Gehring, B. J., Gomes, A. S., et al.: Diagnosis of portal vein thrombosis: Value of color Doppler imaging. AJR, 157:293, 1991.
54. Vogelzang, R. L., Gore, R. M., Anscheutz, S. L., et al.: Thrombosis of the splanchnic veins: CT diagnosis. AJR, 150:93, 1988.

RENOVASCULAR DISEASE

J. Caulie Gunnells, Jr., M.D.
Richard L. McCann, M.D.

The observation that obstructive lesions of the renal arteries may produce hypertension is firmly established. Hypertension produced in this manner is referred to as renovascular hypertension, the most common form of potentially curable high blood pressure. Renovascular hypertension is usually difficult to control by medical means, and patients with this disorder are at a continuing potential risk for irreversible renal, as well as other critical organ, damage if inappropriate or ineffective pharmacologic modalities are used in an attempt to control blood pressure. More importantly, if the mechanical obstruction producing the hypertension is progressive, the inexorable loss of renal function is all too often an untoward and irreversible effect of inappropriate and untimely evaluation and treatment. So frequent and common has been such an occurrence that the term *ischemic nephropathy* has been used to describe the sequence of events.[1] It is now well accepted that mechanical intervention using revascularization techniques, either by surgical bypass or balloon angioplasty, provide a very appropriate and effective relief of this form of hypertension, and as well, often lead to preserved or improved renal function.[1, 2] Occasionally, a severely damaged kidney cannot be effectively revascularized, and nephrectomy may be equally successful in controlling hypertension and preserving function of the contralateral kidney.

Systemic arterial pressure is controlled by a number of factors, including cardiac output, peripheral vascular resistance, and blood volume, as well as the activity of the renin-angiotensin-aldosterone system together with the integrating function of the sympathetic nervous system. Among the features determining the mechanisms underlying certain forms of renal and renovascular hypertension is the critical interplay between the renin-angiotensin-aldosterone cascade, together with its important effect on systemic and renal vascular resistance as well as an influence over the intravascular volume and other fluctuations within the entire vascular tree. Many of these actions are manifested through the potent vasoconstrictor angiotensin II, producing increased vascular resistance, along with the action of aldosterone, produced and released from the angiotensin II–stimulated adrenal gland, with its resulting action on the kidney, leading to sodium retention and potassium excretion.

There are a number of specific causes of arterial hypertension. Among the forms of hypertension that are surgically correctable are those associated with coarctation of the aorta, pheochromocytoma, Cushing's syndrome (adrenal hyperplasia, cortical adenoma, or carcinoma), primary aldosteronism (adenoma), and unilateral renal parenchymal disease. In addition, and more importantly, renovascular hypertension is, as mentioned earlier, the most common form of hypertension amenable to surgical therapy. This form of hypertension may be caused by any lesion that produces a significant obstruction to renal arterial blood flow, either unilaterally or bilaterally. The majority of patients with this disorder have vascular lesions of the atherosclerotic variety or dysplasia involving the renal arteries.[2] The most common variety of dysplasia is the fibromuscular form.[3] Among other lesions that produce diminished arterial blood flow and may be associated with renovascular hypertension are renal artery aneurysms,[4] emboli, polyarteritis nodosa,[5] arteriovenous fistulas,[6] traumatic vascular injuries, radiation,[7] and a variety of extrinsic lesions that may compress the renal vascular supply, including neoplasms (metastatic or primary) and retroperitoneal fibrosis.

PHYSIOLOGIC ASPECTS

Occlusive lesions of the renal arteries are well recognized as a cause of sustained diastolic hypertension. The incidence of renal arterial lesions and coexistent hypertension has not been established with confidence. Estimates suggest their presence in from less than 5% to as much as 20% or more of the adult hypertensive population in the United States. It is difficult to determine the true incidence with accuracy because of wide variability in the criteria for selecting patients for clinical investigation leading to the anatomic and functional diagnosis of renovascular hypertension.

The now famous experiments of Goldblatt, in which hypertension was produced by unilateral narrowing of the renal artery, clearly documented the role of the ischemic kidney in the production of hypertension.[8] In the Goldblatt experiment, partial clamping of one renal artery resulted in transient hypertension, whereas sustained or persistent elevation in arterial pressure required constriction of both renal arteries or clamp restriction of one main renal artery with the removal of the contralateral kidney. This clamping of only one renal artery and removing the opposite kidney, the so-called one kidney, one-clip Goldblatt hypertension, produced a form of high blood pressure that was characterized by volume expansion, and the blood pressure in this setting was maintained by an entirely different mechanism than in the two-kidney, one-clip Goldblatt hypertension model. This latter animal model is the experimental counterpart of the renovascular hypertension in man that is classically recognized. With the understanding of the renin-angiotensin-aldosterone system in the functional maintenance of this vasoconstrictor form of hypertension produced by this model, the excess renin production by the ischemic kidney is believed to be largely responsible for the changes leading to the increased blood pressure observed clinically. The renal pressor mechanism initiated by renal ischemia, now known as the renin-angiotensin-aldosterone cascade, was first described by Tigerstedt and Bergman in 1898[9] and later amplified by Page and Corcoran.[10] Braun-Menendes and associates[11] and Helmer[12] followed the classic anatomic experiments of Goldblatt. The commonly accepted relationship of this important homeostatic control mechanism of the renin system is outlined in Figure 50–155, along with markers indicating the various sites at which this cascade may be interrupted to understand further its mechanism and participation in various clinical hypertensive states.

The introduction of the very important class of pharmacologic compounds known as angiotensin-converting enzyme inhibitors (ACEIs) and direct angiotensin II inhibitors has greatly expanded understanding of the renin cascade. ACEIs have also added to the diagnostic accuracy of patient evaluation for the presence of renovascular hypertension and the selection of candidates for further investigation leading to definitive invasive therapy.[13–16] In this cascade, renin is produced in excess from an ischemic kidney and released into

the circulation where it reacts with renin substrate, an alpha$_2$-globulin produced by the liver. This enzymatic reaction cleaves off the decapeptide angiotensin I, which has little physiologic activity. Angiotensin I, in the presence of converting enzyme, is rapidly converted primarily to the potent octapeptide angiotensin II. The effector limb of this cascade, angiotensin II, elicits a large and increasing number of actions, two of which directly relate to pressor control: (1) as a potent vasoconstrictor and (2) as a stimulator of the adrenal gland to produce and release aldosterone, thus indirectly increasing total vascular volume. It is the variable combination of these two actions that leads to the hypertension initiated by excess renin production by an ischemic kidney. The widespread availability of laboratory techniques to measure levels of plasma renin activity in both peripheral and renal venous blood, along with the appropriate utilization of ACEIs to enhance or augment renin secretion, has contributed greatly to the evaluation of patients suspected of having renovascular hypertension. In addition, research has defined a family of specific angiotensin II receptors that may play a significant role in many cardiovascular reactions.[17] Specific blockade of angiotensin II receptors is now in clinical trials and should add significantly to our understanding of the role of angiotensin II in cardiovascular disease.[18]

Convincing evidence has accumulated that in most patients with renovascular hypertension, a role exists for the renin-angiotensin cascade as a major pathogenic mechanism. It is generally agreed that measurement of one or more of the compounds involving the renin cascade provides useful information in the diagnostic evaluation and treatment of a patient suspected of having renovascular hypertension produced by the lesions previously described, either in unilateral or bilateral locations within the renal circulation.

PATHOLOGIC OBSERVATIONS

The most common cause of renovascular hypertension is atherosclerosis, which is the etiologic basis of the lesions in two thirds of the patients with this disorder. The lesions are most likely to occur near the origin of the renal vessels from the aorta (ostial) and are at times segmental and usually less than 1 cm. in length. Males, and often patients in the older age group, are more commonly affected, and bilateral lesions are present in approximately one third of these patients.

Fibrous and fibromuscular dysplasia is another cause of renovascular hypertension; these mural dysplasias may be classified according to the site and type of involvement (intimal, medial, or adventitial). The most commonly encountered variety is termed *medial fibromuscular dysplasia* or *hyperplasia* and occurs most often in young women.[3] The microscopic lesions consist of a thickening of the media with separation and distortion of the muscle fibers by a degenerative process involving myxomatous fibrous tissue. The lesions are likely to be multiple, and the term *microaneurysms* has been used to describe the appearance of serial constricted lesions interspersed with areas of greater diameter. On angiography this produces a corrugated effect, termed the *string of beads* phenomenon (Fig. 50–156).

Other vascular lesions, including aneurysms (congenital and acquired), arteriovenous malformations, renal artery dissections, renal artery thromboses, and emboli to the renal parenchyma, have been associated with, or productive of, renovascular hypertension and constitute an important reservoir of patients who can profit from angiographic study to define the particular site, etiology, and extent of vascular involvement that is necessary before any operative or angioplastic intervention.

In addition, a new group of vascular lesions has surfaced as an important consideration for surgical intervention as a

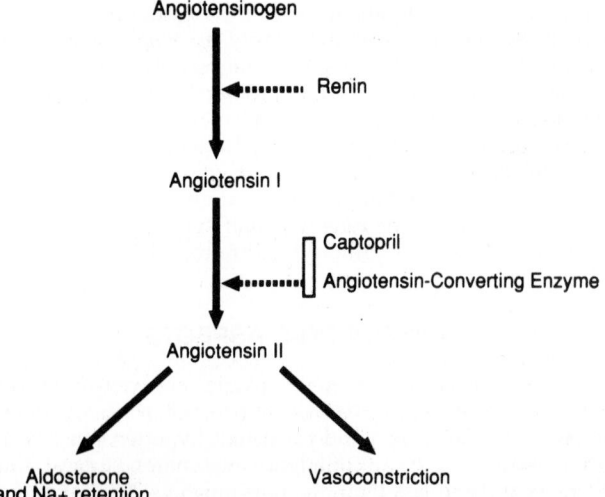

Figure 50–155. The renin-angiotensin system. (From Nally, J. V.: The captopril tests: A new concept in detecting renovascular hypertension? Cleve. Clin. J. Med., *56*:395, 1989.)

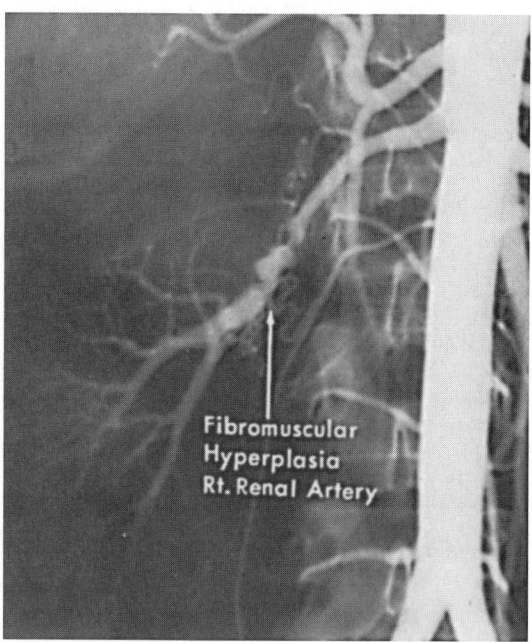

Figure 50–156. Arteriogram demonstrating fibromuscular dysplasia of the right renal artery producing hypertension. Note the characteristic "scalloping."

special form of renovascular hypertension, namely, atheroembolic renal disease in association with renal artery stenosis.[28] Renal cholesterol embolization may be an unsuspected cause of renal failure, particularly in the elderly and in patients with diffuse abdominal atherosclerosis in association with renal artery stenosis. Only recently has the close association of renal failure, renal arterial stenosis, and cholesterol emboli, leading to renal failure or an acute exacerbation of chronic renal insufficiency and hypertension, been considered a surgically approachable disease. However, the concomitant development of cholesterol emboli involving the renal circulation may contribute to hypertension as well as to compromised renal function, and this can be exacerbated or magnified in the presence of renal artery stenosis. The association of significant renal artery stenosis and its pivotal role or contribution to progressive renal failure, usually noted in association with cholesterol emboli, is being recognized with considerable frequency. There are increasing reports of this association along with the successful intervention after angiographic and biopsy demonstration, of the coexistent abnormalities. This constitutes a very important reservoir of patients who may benefit in two ways from correction of renovascular hypertension, namely, a reduction in their blood pressure as well as preservation or improvement of renal function.[1, 2, 14]

CLINICAL MANIFESTATIONS

Experience has demonstrated that there are a number of important clinical diagnostic features associated with renovascular hypertension; however, the dilemma concerning which patients should be evaluated for the presence of renovascular hypertension remains controversial.[13, 14, 20] Pauker and Kopelman[21] have correctly referred to this dilemma as a "which hunt"—which patients, which tests, which etiology, and which therapies. Important clinical diagnostic features include the sudden or abrupt onset of hypertension, often before the age of 35 or after the age of 55 and in the absence of a family history of hypertension.[22] In addition, there may be the onset or worsening of hypertension after an episode of flank pain. Another important feature may be the unex-

plained development or existence of accelerated or malignant hypertension at any age. Patients with renovascular hypertension often have what may be called *significant* levels of high blood pressure, namely, sustained, severe diastolic hypertension (greater than 115 mm. Hg) or, as noted previously, accelerated or malignant hypertensive disease.[23] Rarely do patients with functionally significant renovascular hypertension have mild levels of blood pressure. Other features that may be of importance are patients who exhibit antihypertensive drug failure and/or intolerable side effects of drug therapy; escape from previous control, particularly in patients in the older age group; and patients with deteriorating renal function despite good blood pressure control.

It is well known that there are serious limitations, insofar as the medical history and physical examination are concerned, in detection of renovascular hypertension. However, physical examination may reveal an important diagnostic feature associated with this entity, namely, an abdominal bruit located in the epigastrium or in either upper abdominal quadrant. This finding is present in 50% to 80% of patients with renovascular hypertension, whereas it occurs in less than 5% of those patients with essential hypertension. Patients with fibromuscular hyperplasia are more likely to have bruits than those with atherosclerotic lesions. Moreover, in fibromuscular disease, the bruits are soft, to and fro, and continuous, whereas higher-pitched systolic bruits are more characteristic of atherosclerotic disease.

Other clinical features emphasized and described in a large matched group of patients with proven renovascular hypertension, as compared with a similar group of patients with essential hypertension, have indicated that, in those patients with renovascular hypertension, there is a shorter duration of hypertension, a higher incidence of spontaneous, nondiuretic induced hypokalemia, and the presence of proteinuria. Patients exhibiting all of the previously mentioned historical findings are relatively rare; but when several of these findings are present, further investigation to establish a diagnosis of functionally significant renovascular hypertension must be strongly considered. However, all patients with significant hypertension must be initially considered as suspect for renovascular disease, and this high level of suspicion must be kept constantly in mind. Timely application of appropriate studies must be instituted to detect a higher incidence of renovascular hypertension in the large number of patients with primary hypertension who present for clinical evaluation.

At the outset, it is important to recognize that a general medical evaluation is necessary and that attention should be given to the presence or absence of coexistent systemic diseases. Emphasis must also be placed on a careful assessment of overall general health in addition to specific attention to the presence or absence of important involvement of other vascular beds, including the cerebral, coronary, and peripheral circulation.

LABORATORY EXAMINATIONS

The initial studies of importance include a urinalysis with culture, serum creatinine determination, chest roentgenography, electrocardiography, serum potassium determination, and possibly measurements of plasma renin activity, both in the peripheral and renal venous blood. The availability of ACEIs and their ability to increase the value of plasma renin measurement have greatly augmented the value of renin measurements.[13, 24] In addition, the extension of using converting enzyme inhibition in the performance of radioisotope studies has brought about new emphasis and interest in this particular technique as a screening test for renovascular disease.[2, 13] Wilcox[13] has pointed out that there are three aspects of responses to ACEIs that may be helpful in evaluating patients for renovascular hypertension: (1) the drugs may increase plasma creatinine levels during their administration, which when this occurs strongly suggests renovascular disease, particularly in patients with bilateral renal artery stenosis or arterial stenosis of a solitary kidney; (2) the exaggerated rise in plasma renin activity after an oral dose of an ACEI also suggests the presence of renovascular hypertension; and (3) the previously mentioned ACEI-induced changes in the radionuclide renogram may support the diagnosis after other preliminary studies have been performed and may also indicate the site of the functional stenosis.

In the hypertensive patient, in whom there is suspected renovascular hypertension, the presence of an increased peripheral plasma renin activity suggests that unilateral renal arterial disease may be present and that it is producing a hormonally dependent form of hypertension.[22, 24-28] However, peripheral venous plasma renin measurements may be quite variable, be elevated in a significant number of patients with the high-renin variety of primary hypertension, and be entirely normal in some 25% of patients with subsequently proven, functionally significant renal artery stenosis. The reliability of unstimulated peripheral measurements of renin activity as indicators of the presence of renal artery stenosis fell into some disfavor until the availability of captopril stimulation was used to differentiate these various subsets of patients undergoing investigation as to the etiology or mechanisms of their hypertension. The captopril stimulation of peripheral plasma renin activity uses the ACEI as a pharmacologic probe into the mechanism of the hypertension in the patient under investigation.[16, 26, 29] The patient should maintain a normal dietary sodium intake and also should not receive diuretic drugs for a minimum of 72 hours (preferably 2 weeks) before the test; and it is preferable, if possible, to discontinue other antihypertensive drugs other than betablockers because the former may depress the response of the renin cascade to captopril administration.[16, 29] At the time of the examination, 50 mg. of captopril is crushed and diluted in water and administered orally. Blood pressure is measured at 10- to 15-minute intervals over a 90-minute period. At the end of this time, blood pressure is again measured and a repeat venous blood sample is drawn for the measurement of the stimulated peripheral venous renin activity. In patients with renovascular hypertension, the induced fall in blood pressure after administration of captopril is greater than in patients with essential hypertension, but this is less reliable than the response of the plasma renin activity. A more reliable differentiating point between the presence of essential versus renovascular hypertension is related to the degree to which the administered captopril enhances the rise in plasma renin activity. The criteria for a positive response have varied from investigator to investigator; however, the results of Müller and colleagues[16] have been most useful, and they have proposed three criteria for a positive captopril test to distinguish between patients with renovascular hypertension and those with essential hypertension. Renovascular hypertension is considered to be present if one or more of the following conditions are met: (1) stimulated renin activity is 12 ng. per ml. per hour or more; (2) the absolute increase in plasma renin activity is 10 ng. per ml. per hour or more and the percentage increase in plasma renin activity is 150% or more; and (3) the percentage increase in plasma renin activity is 400% or more if the baseline plasma renin activity is less than 3 ng. per ml. per hour.[16, 29] A representative result of renin measurements after the oral administration of captopril in a number of patients with proven forms of hypertension is shown in Figure 50–157.[29] These data clearly indicate the efficacy and usefulness of this particular test as a screening maneuver in selecting patients for further study.

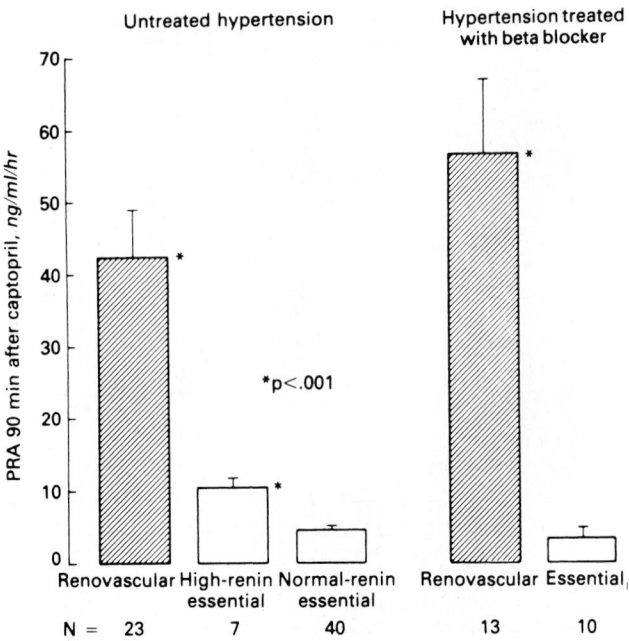

Figure 50–157. Levels of peripheral vein plasma renin activity (PRA) in hypertensive patients after a single dose of captopril. (From Case, D. B., et al.: Physiologic effects and diagnostic relevance of acute converting enzyme blockage. In Laragh, J. H., Buhler, F. R., and Seldin, D. W. [Eds.]: Frontiers in Hypertension Research. New York, Springer-Verlag, 1982, p. 546.)

The accuracy and diagnostic significance of renal vein renin measurement have considerable importance, and this is now one of the major diagnostic maneuvers in patients with renovascular hypertension to establish the functional significance of vascular obstructions.[24, 27] The accuracy and diagnostic significance of renal vein renin measurements have also been improved by the concomitant acute administration of captopril, utilizing the principles and action of this particular agent in a similar manner as noted in peripheral plasma renin measurements.[15, 24, 29] The use of this agent magnifies the difference in renal vein renin activity in patients with functionally significant renal artery stenosis. Measuring renal vein renin after the administration of captopril may minimize false-negative renin ratios that were previously seen in patients who subsequently may have responded well to surgical treatment. Patients with hypertension and abnormal renal arteries only rarely exhibit a renal vein renin ratio greater than 1.5 to 2.0:1, whereas in patients with functionally significant renal stenosis, renal vein renin concentrations are at least one and one-half to two times higher in renal venous blood of the involved or affected kidney than in the renal effluent of the contralateral venous drainage.[24, 27] The results of renal vein renin measurements in a group of patients assessed before and after the use of captopril are outlined in Figure 50–158, again demonstrating the usefulness of this particular technique in patients with renovascular disease.[29]

RADIOISOTOPE RENOGRAPHY

Before availability of ACEIs, the use of radioisotope renography was believed by many investigators to provide little additional information when performed before the consideration of more invasive-type studies, such as renal angiography. Radionuclide renal studies were at that time associated with a high incidence of false-negative and false-positive results, limiting their diagnostic usefulness except possibly in the preliminary investigation of those patients who exhibited an allergy to iodinated contrast media. However, the

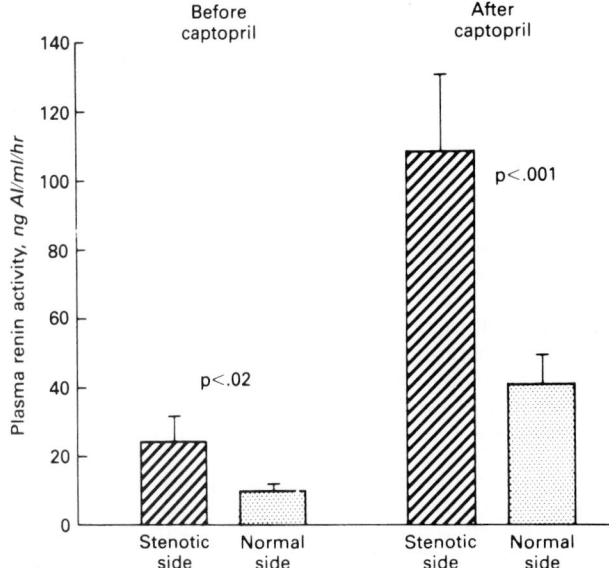

Figure 50–158. Levels of renal vein renin activity in patients with renovascular hypertension before and after captopril. (From Vaughan, E. D.: Clinical evaluation for renovascular hypertension and therapeutic decisions. Urol. Clin. North Am., *11*:383, 1984.)

By using technetium-labeled diethylenetriaminepentaacetic acid (DTPA), a measurement of glomerular filtration can be obtained at the time of the radionuclide angiogram, because DTPA is excreted by the kidney solely by way of glomerular filtration. Abnormalities in the conventional renogram suggesting the presence of renovascular disease include a reduction in kidney perfusion and size as well as a delay in the uptake and excretion of the radioactive label. The captopril-induced changes in the renogram that have been suggested as diagnostic criteria for the stenotic kidney include a reduction of delay in DTPA uptake of the stenotic kidney and a delay in the time of maximal activity of the labeled substance as well as the delay in the ^{131}I-Hippuran washout. It has been suggested that both DTPA and ^{131}I-labeled studies be performed to detect the maximal changes in renovascular disease after captopril administration. In addition, the use of another isotopic label, mercaptacetyltriglycine (MAG3), is being widely used as a diagnostic test material. The alterations in the renogram before and after the administration of DTPA with the associated time activity curves are shown in Figure 50–159.[32] Using similar studies, the nephrology group at the University of Florida has gathered data relative to the usefulness of these studies in the screening evaluation for renovascular hypertension.[33] There is a 20% incidence of false-positive tests, and the sensitivity of the test is in the range of 93% to 100%, with a specificity of approximately 80% in the population.

INTRAVENOUS UROGRAPHY

Minute-sequence intravenous urography is a simple and widely available test and continues to be a very good anatomic screening maneuver, mainly for the presence of suspected unilateral mainstem renovascular hypertension. The test is useful for several reasons: it is widely available; it can be performed using conventional radiographic equipment; it requires only a minimal exposure to contrast media; it is relatively inexpensive; and, when *properly interpreted* and in *highly selected* patients, it correlates well with conventional angiography and the response to surgical intervention.

Digital Subtraction Venous Angiography. A large bolus of iodinated contrast medium is rapidly injected in the central venous circulation and observed using digital subtraction

application and the appreciation of ACEI-induced changes in the renogram proved quite helpful in suspecting and confirming the diagnosis of renovascular hypertension.[2, 13, 20, 31–33] The rationale for the captopril stimulation in radionuclide studies is related to the functional activity of the angiotensin II–dependent action on efferent arteriolar resistance that produces a reduction in transcapillary forces driving glomerular filtration, thereby reducing function of the kidney distal to renal arterial stenosis. This decrement in individual kidney function may be noninvasively assessed using two-dimensional radionuclide studies.[2, 12, 14, 31, 32] Depending on the label and compound used, assessment of individual kidney function is possible using this noninvasive technology as well as making it possible to measure renal blood flow (^{131}I-Hippuran).

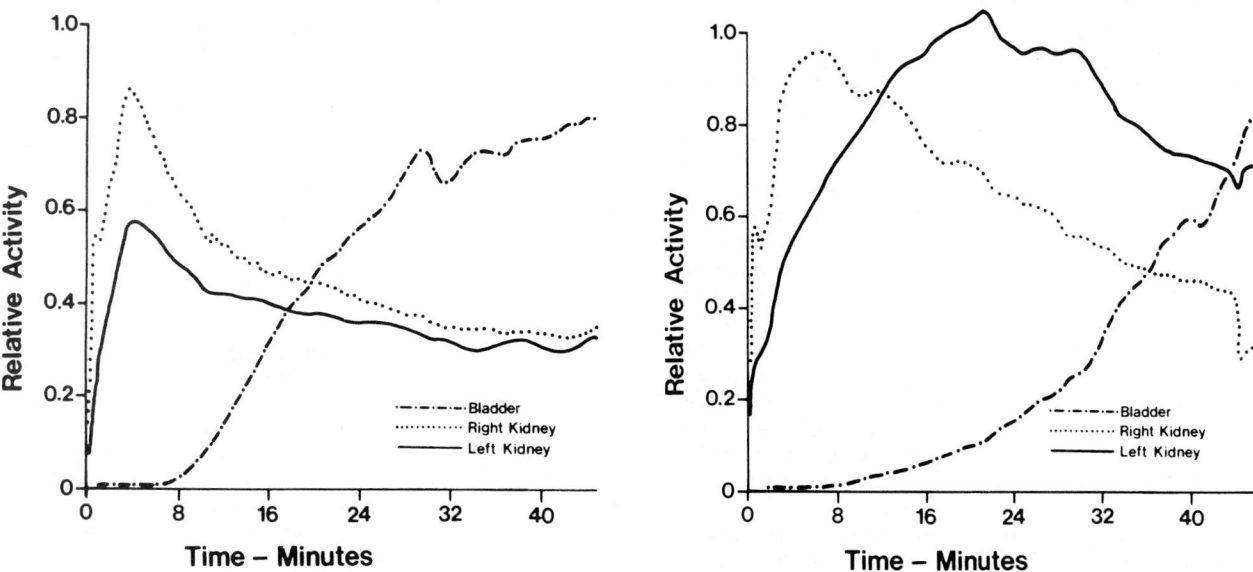

Figure 50–159. ^{99m}Tc-DTPA time-activity curves in a patient with unilateral left renal artery stenosis: Baseline on the left and after captopril stimulation on the right. (From Nally, J. V.: The captopril tests: A new concept in detecting renovascular hypertension? Cleve. Clin. J. Med., *56*:395, 1989.)

techniques as it passes through the arterial phase during its first pass through the circulation.[13, 34] This examination requires access to the central venous circulation, sophisticated radiographic equipment, and a good cardiac output, which maintains the bolus of contrast material as it passes through the arterial circulation. The main advantage of this technique is that it obviates an arterial puncture. However, the improvements and safety in outpatient angiography have largely displaced this technique in the study of the renal circulation.

Renal Arteriography. The definitive study for the anatomic localization of a renal artery lesion is arteriography.[2, 14, 35, 36] This study is indicated in patients judged to be eventual candidates for surgical or balloon angioplasty therapy in whom preliminary studies have suggested renovascular hypertension. The percutaneous retrograde transfemoral technique is widely used in the performance of *flush* aortography and, in conjunction with selective renal arterial injections of contrast media, adds diagnostic precision and greater vascular detail. In addition to demonstrating the main renal arteries, the study provides important additional information, including the extent of poststenotic dilatation, the presence of collateral circulation, and the visualization of other vessels that may be used for vascular repair and also makes possible the evaluation of the extrarenal and intrarenal arterial anatomy. After establishing the presence of a vascular lesion, it is then necessary to pursue further studies to determine whether the observed lesion is functionally responsible for the hypertension; this may then lead to the measurement of renal venous plasma renin activity as previously described. As noted earlier, these vascular studies can be performed with complete safety and accuracy in the outpatient setting, thereby avoiding the unnecessary expense and inconvenience of hospital admission. In addition, if a lesion is demonstrated and circumstances indicate, a procedure such as balloon angioplasty can be performed in a single setting, followed by a brief period of clinic or hospital observation.

TREATMENT

The treatment of patients with renovascular disease has two desired goals. The first is cure or amelioration of hypertension to prevent the long-term deleterious effects of elevated blood pressure on target organ systems, such as the eye; the cerebral, coronary, and peripheral circulations; and the renal parenchyma. The second goal is preservation and occasionally improvement in renal function.

The surgical management of the hypertensive patient with renal artery stenosis requires experienced clinical judgment. Although medical therapy may obviate the risk of operation, it requires a high degree of patient compliance, constant medical supervision, and life-long antihypertensive medication. Another consideration is that although medical therapy may be effective in controlling systemic blood pressure regardless of the cause, it is less effective than restoration of renal blood flow in terms of long-term preservation of renal function. In one study of patients treated with medical therapy, serial angiography has demonstrated progression of renal artery stenosis in 49% and progression to complete occlusion in 14% of patients.[37] In another study, 41% of patients with renovascular disease treated medically had significant loss of renal mass determined radiographically or significant decline in renal function despite adequate control of blood pressure.[38] Furthermore, it is estimated that renovascular disease may be responsible for as many as 15% of all patients developing end-stage renal disease.[37]

Correction of Renal Artery Stenosis. Renal artery stenosis may now be managed by percutaneous balloon angioplasty or by a variety of operative techniques for surgical revascularization. There has been no unbiased prospective comparison of these two approaches, and each has its strong advocates. In a review by Rimmer and Gennari,[37] it is suggested that whereas short-term effectiveness was similar, the surgical approach may be more durable. Interestingly, this review also found no difference in mortality rates between the percutaneous and surgical approaches.

Percutaneous Transluminal Angioplasty. Balloon catheter techniques for dilatation of renal artery stenosis were introduced by Grüntzig in 1978.[39] This technique requires passage of a guidewire under fluoroscopic control from a peripheral site across the stenosis in the renal artery (Fig. 50–160). A balloon dilating catheter is passed over the guidewire and positioned within the area of stenosis and inflated to produce a controlled disruption of the arterial wall. Completion angiography is usually performed to assess the immediate results.

The results of percutaneous balloon angioplasty of renal artery stenosis must be considered separately in the two principal disease processes causing renal artery stenosis. In patients with fibromuscular disease, particularly of the medial fibroplasia type, balloon angioplasty has a high rate of success and recurrence is uncommon.[40] Reported results with percutaneous transluminal renal angioplasty in patients with atherosclerotic lesions of the renal arteries range from 0% to 50% failure rate.[41] Even those who strongly advocate the percutaneous approach agree that this treatment is less effective in patients with ostial stenosis, with diffuse atherosclerotic disease, and with bilateral renal artery stenosis. For example, successful dilatation of ostial disease, which consists of aortic wall plaques that encroach on the lumen of the renal artery orifice, may be as low as 20%. In an effort to improve these results, new percutaneous techniques have been employed, including percutaneous atherectomy and the placement of transluminal intravascular stents.[42] Whether these approaches will improve the results of percutaneous treatment of ostial or nonstial atherosclerotic lesions of the

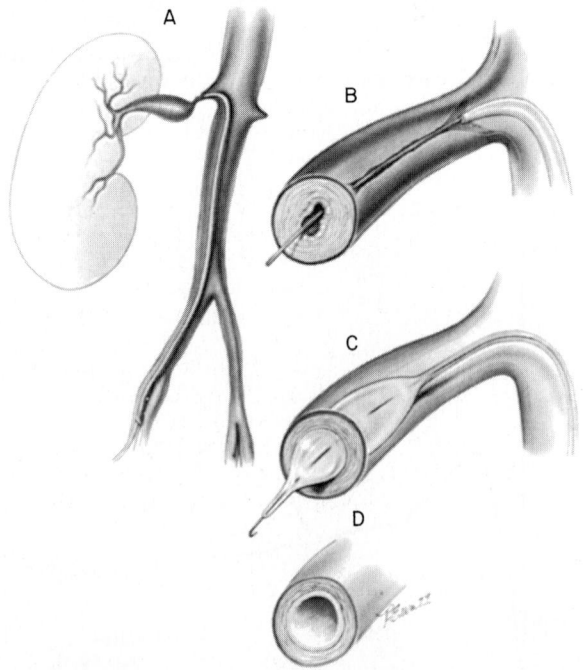

Figure 50–160. The technique of renal artery dilation with the dual-lumen balloon catheter system, using the femoral approach. *A*, The stenotic right renal artery is catheterized selectively. *B*, The guide wire is advanced through the stenosis. *C*, The selective catheter is exchanged for the dilation catheter and the balloon is inflated, dilating the stenosis. *D*, The obstruction is relieved. (From Tegtmeyer, C., Dyer, R., Teates, C., et al.: Percutaneous transluminal dilatation of the renal arteries: Techniques and results. Radiology, *135*:591, 1980.)

renal arteries requires considerable further objective evaluation. Furthermore, it should be kept in mind that the rate of major complications from percutaneous balloon dilatation of the renal arteries has been reported to be 10% to 21%. These include, in addition to puncture site complications common to angiography, uncontrolled renal artery dissection causing renal infarction, contrast medium–induced renal insufficiency, and renal artery rupture. Several deaths have also been reported.

Nephrectomy. Simple nephrectomy may be the appropriate procedure for patients with severe hypertension when the involved kidney has been so severely affected that it contributes little to total renal function. A renal length of less than 7 cm., complete renal artery occlusion with infarction, and severe arteriolar nephrosclerosis are indications for nephrectomy, especially if the opposite kidney is normal or reconstructible. In selected instances, a partial nephrectomy may be performed for localized infarctions, noncorrectable branch lesions, segmental renal hypoplasia, and intrarenal aneurysms and arteriovenous malformations when these are associated with hypertension.

In some patients, total renal artery occlusion may be of gradual onset, allowing maintenance of renal viability through development of collateral circulation from lumbar, ureteral, capsular, or mesenteric vessels. Factors suggesting potential salvage of the kidney with revascularization include urographic visualization of the kidney, renal length of 9 cm. or more, retrograde filling of the distal arterial tree, and lateralizing renal vein renin assay. Intraoperative renal biopsy may be helpful in these cases because severe sclerosis of all or most of the glomeruli indicates an unsalvageable kidney. Some centers have demonstrated significant retrieval of renal function with surgical revascularization of kidneys in patients with severe renal functional impairment or even in those patients who are dependent on dialysis.[43]

REVASCULARIZATION

A variety of operative techniques can be used to correct stenosis or occlusion of the renal arteries. The proper choice is based on the nature of the renal artery lesion, the presence or absence of associated aortic atherosclerotic disease, and the experience and preference of the surgeon treating the patient.

Aortorenal Bypass Grafts. Aortorenal bypass is the technique most frequently selected for surgical correction of renal

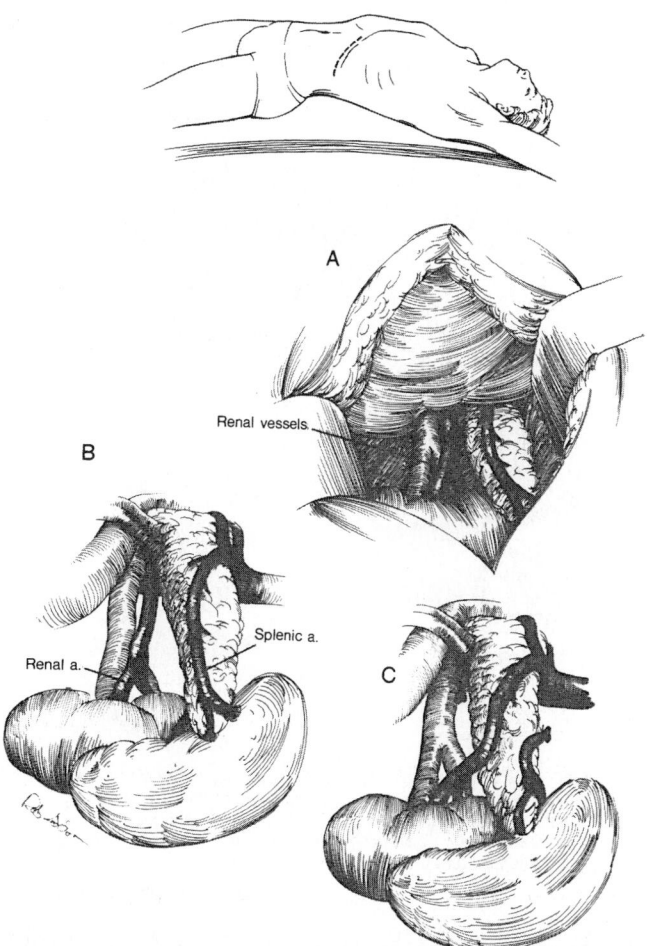

Figure 50–162. Technique of splenic-to-renal artery bypass. Inset at top shows the left subcostal incision. *A*, Retroperitoneal exposure of the renal artery and vein and the splenic artery on the inferior margin of the pancreas. *B*, The relationship between the renal artery and splenic artery is illustrated. *C*, The completed anastomosis is shown. The splenic artery should be kept as short as possible to prevent kinking. The spleen may be left in place because it is adequately nourished by the short gastric vessels.

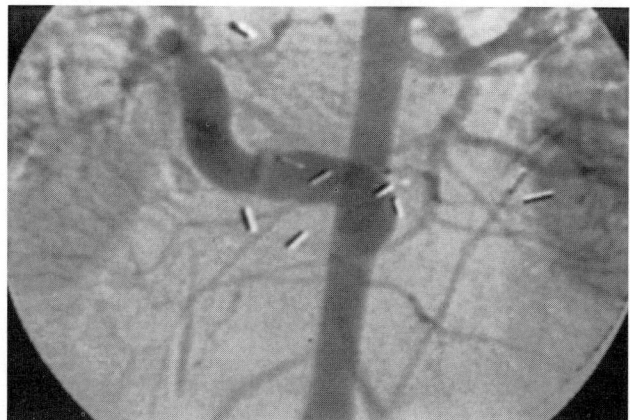

Figure 50–161. Aorta to right renal artery saphenous vein bypass graft done in an 11-year-old child. Routine follow-up angiography performed 1 year postoperatively demonstrates uniform expansion of the saphenous vein graft, which, despite its enlargement, continues to function well, and the patient remains normotensive with normal renal function.

artery stenosis. In most patients, the autogenous saphenous vein is the graft material of choice. Late follow-up of these grafts has sometimes demonstrated a tendency for uniform graft expansion (Fig. 50–161). In extreme cases, this may progress to aneurysmal proportions. This phenomenon is particularly prevalent in children, in whom many advocate the use of autogenous arterial grafts or renal artery reimplantation.[44] The internal iliac artery is often chosen as a graft because it is of appropriate size and, because the pelvis is well supplied with collateral vessels, it can be removed with little hazard. Synthetic grafts have been used successfully, particularly when the distal renal artery is large owing to poststenotic dilatation. However, long-term results have favored use of autogenous tissue grafts.[41] It is important to spatulate the graft when attaching it to the thick-walled aorta to ensure an adequate orifice for inflow into the graft. This technique is often facilitated by incorporating a large side branch of the vein in the spatulation to increase the size of the orifice.

Use of Branches of the Celiac Axis to Revascularize the Kidneys. A more difficult group of patients to treat are those with severe atherosclerotic disease of the wall of the aorta in combination with renal artery stenosis. These patients are recognized by the appearance of marked irregularity of the aortic wall on angiography. If there is occlusion or severe

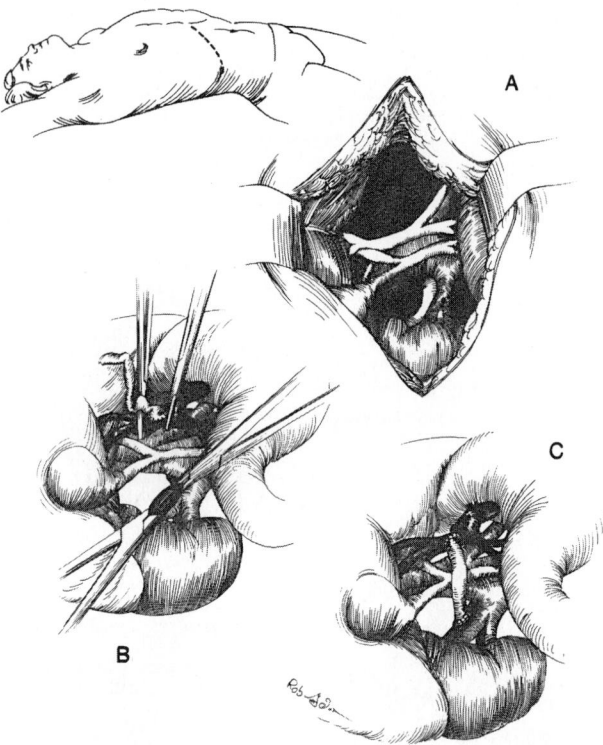

Figure 50–163. Technique of hepatic-to-right renal artery bypass. Inset at top shows the right subcostal incision. *A,* Exposure of the hepatic artery in the hepatoduodenal ligament. *B,* The proximal anastomosis is being placed on the common hepatic artery. *C,* The completed short vein graft in "H" configuration between the hepatic and the renal vessels.

luminal stenosis or aneurysm formation, consideration should be given to replacement of the aorta and simultaneous revascularization of the kidneys with vein autografts or synthetic grafts taking origin from the Dacron tube. If there is no intrinsic indication for aortic replacement, however, and if the lateral aortogram shows a widely patent celiac axis, then consideration can be given to using branches of the celiac axis for revascularization of the kidneys alone. On the left side, the splenic artery may be divided distally and rotated inferiorly to form an anastomosis with the left renal artery (Fig. 50–162). This procedure has the advantage of requiring only single vascular anastomosis but does require a nearly normal splenic artery. The spleen may be left in place and will be adequately nourished through the short gastric vessels. Splenic vessels that are extremely tortuous and calcified may not rotate inferiorly without kinking. In this instance, if the lumen is of satisfactory caliber, the vessel can still be used to supply blood to the left kidney using an interposition vein graft between the two vessels. On the right side, the hepatic or gastroduodenal artery serves as a convenient origin for a short vein graft to the right renal artery (Fig. 50–163). These techniques are particularly well suited for a staged approach to the surgical management of bilateral renal artery disease.

Bench Work Surgery. Disease of the small branch vessels may now be treated by *bench work surgery.* In these procedures, the vascular supply to the kidney is divided and the organ can be completely removed from the body or left attached only by the ureter. The kidney is flushed with cold preservative solution and is kept cold by packing in ice slush while delicate vascular repair of the branch vessels is performed with the aid of optical magnification using an operating microscope. When repaired, the kidney can be reimplanted into its original position or autografted to the pelvis using the iliac vessels for anastomoses. Using these techniques, the incidence of nephrectomy for *unreconstructible branch renal artery disease* is steadily diminishing.

RESULTS

Benefit from operative intervention in renovascular hypertension is directly related to accurate identification of surgical candidates and skilled performance of appropriate vascular reconstruction. Attention to these aspects in recent years has yielded improved long-term results. In experienced centers, cure or improvement of blood pressure has been reported in as many as 95% of patients, with very low mortality.[45] Mortality occurs almost exclusively in patients with widespread systemic atherosclerotic disease who require aortic or other arterial reconstruction in addition to renal revascularization.

SELECTED REFERENCES

Ram, C. V.: Southwestern Internal Medicine Conference: Current concepts in renovascular hypertension. Am. J. Med. Sci., *304*:53, 1992.
The epidemiology, pathology, and therapeutic options for management of patients with renovascular hypertension are reviewed. The importance of reperfusion of the kidney as a desirable long-term objective in the management of patients with renovascular disease is emphasized.

Semple, P. F., and Dominiczak, A. F.: Detection and treatment of renovascular disease. J. Hypertens., *12*:729, 1994.
The progress made in the past 40 years in the detection and treatment of patients with renovascular disease is reviewed. Careful history, physical examination, and repeated blood pressure measurements are simple but effective screening tools, and more detailed investigations can be reserved for groups identified with increased risks, such as those with known peripheral vascular disease or abnormal renal function.

Stanley, J. C., Zelenock, G. B., Messina, L. M., and Wakefield, T. W.: Pediatric renovascular hypertension: A thirty-year experience of operative treatment. J. Vasc. Surg., *21*:221, 1995.
This paper includes the largest single center experience with the management of renovascular disease in children. Excellent results can be achieved in this age group with appropriate contemporary surgical management, including direct reimplantation or bypass.

Textor, S. C.: Renovascular hypertension. Curr. Opin. Nephrol. Hypertens., *2*:775, 1993.
This article emphasizes the role of renovascular disease in the etiology of renal insufficiency. It reviews modern concepts of noninvasive and invasive diagnostic procedures, including captopril renography, duplex ultrasonography, magnetic resonance angiography, and contrast angiography. It emphasizes that contemporary advances in interventional radiologic procedures, including endovascular therapy as well as surgical revascularization, offer the ability not only to effect improved blood pressure management but also salvage of renal function.

REFERENCES

 1. Breyer, J. A., and Jacobson, H. R.: Ischemic nephropathy. Curr. Opin. Nephrol. Hypertens., 2:216, 1993.
 2. Textor, S. C.: Renovascular hypertension. Curr. Opin. Nephrol. Hypertens., 2:775, 1993.
 3. Hunt, J. C., Harrison, E. G., Jr., Kincaid, O. W., Bernatz, P. E., and Davis G. D.: Idiopathic fibrous and fibromuscular stenoses of the renal arteries associated with hypertension. Mayo Clin. Proc., 37:181, 1962.
 4. Cummings, K. B., Lecky, J. W., and Kaufman, J. J.: Renal artery aneurysms and hypertension retinopathy. J. Urol., 109:144, 1973.
 5. Dornfeld, L., Ledky, J. W., and Peter, J. B.: Polyarteritis and intrarenal renal artery aneurysms. JAMA, 215:1950, 1971.
 6. Oxman, H. A., Sheps, S. G., Bernatz, P. E., and Harrison, E. G., Jr.: An unusual case of renal arteriovenous fistula–fibromuscular dysplasia of the renal arteries: Report of a case. Mayo Clin. Proc., 48:207, 1983.
 7. Staab, G. E., Tegtmeyer, C. J., and Constable, W. C.: Radiation-induced renovascular hypertension. AJR, 126:634, 1976.
 8. Goldblatt, H., Lynch, J., Hanzal, R. F., and Summerville, W. D.: Studies in experimental hypertension: I. The production of persistent evaluation of systolic blood pressure by means of renal ischemia. J. Exp. Med., 59:347, 1934.
 9. Tigerstedt, R., and Bergman, J.: Neire und Kreislauf. Skand. Arch. Physiol., 8:223, 1898.
10. Page, I. H., and Corcoran A. C.: Hypertension: Review of humoral pathogenesis and clinical treatment. Adv. Intern. Med., 1:183, 1942.
11. Braun-Menendes, F., Fasciolo, J. C., Lelior, L. F., Munoz, J. M., and Taquini A. C.: Renal Hypertension. Dexter, L. (Trans.). Springfield, Ill., Charles C Thomas, 1946.

12. Helmer, O. M.: Presence of renin in plasma of patients with arterial hypertension. Circulation, 25:169, 1962.

13. Wilcox, C. S.: Use of angiotensin-converting enzyme inhibitors for diagnosing renovascular hypertension. Kidney Int., 44:1379, 1993.

14. Semple, P. F., and Dominiczak, A. F.: Detection and treatment of renovascular disease. J. Hypertens., 12:729, 1994.

15. Haber, E.: The renin-angiotensin system and hypertension. Kidney Int., 15:425, 1979.

16. Müller, F. B., Sealey, J. E., Case, D. B., Atlas, S. A., Pickering, T. G., Pecker, M. S., Preibisz, J. J., and Laragh, J. H.: The captopril test for identifying renovascular disease in hypertensive patients. Am. J. Med., 80:663, 1986.

17. Edwards, R. M., and Aiyar, N.: Angiotensin II receptor subtypes in the kidney. J. Am. Soc. Nephrol., 3:1643, 1993.

18. MacFadyen, R. J., and Reid, J. L.: Angiotensin receptor antagonists as a treatment for hypertension. J. Hypertens., 12:1333, 1994.

19. Meyrier, A., Buchet, P., Simon, P., Pernet, M., Rainfray, M., and Callard, P.: Atheromatous renal disease. Am. J. Med., 85:139, 1988.

20. Svetky, S. E., Himmelstein, S. I., et al.: Prospective analysis of strategies for diagnosing renovascular hypertension. Hypertension, 14:247, 1989.

21. Pauker, S. G., and Kopelman, R. I.: Screening for renovascular hypertension: "A which hunt." Hypertension, 14:258, 1989.

22. Maxwell, M. H., Bleifer, K. H., Franklin, S. S., and Parady, P. D.: Cooperative study of renovascular hypertension: Demographic analysis of the study. JAMA, 220:1195, 1972.

23. Davis, B. A., Cook, J. E., Vestal, R. E., and Oates, J. A.: Prevalence of renovascular hypertension in patients with a grade III or IV hypertensive retinopathy. N. Engl. J. Med., 301:1273, 1979.

24. Simon, G., and Coleman, C.: Captopril stimulated renal vein renin measurements in the diagnosis of atherosclerotic renovascular hypertension. Am. J. Hypertens., 7:1, 1994.

25. Dzau, V. J., Gibbons, G. H., and Levin, D. C.: Renovascular hypertension: An update on pathophysiology, diagnosis and treatment. Am. J. Nephrol., 3:172, 1983.

26. Gaul, M. K., Linn, W. D., and Mulrow, C. D.: Captopril-stimulated renin secretion in the diagnosis of renovascular hypertension. Am. J. Med., 80:633, 1986.

27. Gunnells, J. C., Jr., McGriffin, W. L., Jr., Johnsrude, I., and Robinson, R. R.: Peripheral and renal venous renin activity in hypertension. Ann. Intern. Med., 71:555, 1969.

28. Marks, L. S., Maxwell, M. H., Varady, P. D., Lupu, A. N., and Kaufman, J. J.: Renovascular hypertension: Does the renal vein renin ratio predict operative results? J. Urol., 115:365, 1976.

29. Vaughan, E. D.: Renovascular hypertension. Kidney Int., 27:811, 1985.

30. Pickering, T. G., Sos, T. A., Vaughan, E. D., Case, D. B., Sealey, J. E.,

Harshfield, G. A., and Laragh, J. H.: Predictive value and changes of renin secretion in hypertensive patients with unilateral renovascular disease undergoing successful renal angioplasty. Am. J. Med., 76:398, 1984.

31. Gates, G. F.: Glomerular filtration rate: Estimation from fractional renal accumulation of 99mTC-DTPA (stannous). Am. J. Radiol., 138:565, 1982.

32. Nally, J. V.: The captopril tests: A new concept in detecting renovascular hypertension? Cleve Clin. J. Med., 56:395, 1989.

33. Wilcox, C. S., Williams, C. M., Smith T. B., Frederickson, E. D., Wingo, C., and Bucci, C. N.: Diagnostic use of angiotensin-converting enzyme inhibitors in renovascular hypertension. Am. J. Hypertens., 34:S138, 1988.

34. Wise, K. L., McCann, R. L., Dunnick, N. R., and Paulson, D. F.: Renovascular hypertension. J. Urol., 140:911, 1988.

35. Eyler, W. R., Clark, M. D., Garman, J. E., Rian, R. L., and Meininger, D. C.: Angiography of the renal areas including a comparative study of renal artery stenosis in patients with and without hypertension. Radiology, 78:879, 1962.

36. Grim, C. E., Luft, F. C., Weinberger, M. H., and Grim, C. M.: Sensitivity and specificity of screening tests for renal vascular hypertension. Ann. Intern. Med., 91:617, 1979.

37. Rimmer, J. M., and Gennari, F. J.: Atherosclerotic renovascular disease and progressive renal failure. Ann. Intern. Med., 118:712, 1993.

38. Dean, R. N., Kieffer, R. W., Smith, B. M., Oates, J. A., Nadeau, J. H., Hollifield, J. W., and Dupont, W. D.: Renovascular hypertension: Anatomic and renal function changes during drug therapy. Arch. Surg., 116:1408, 1981.

39. Grüntzig, A., Kuhlmann, U., Vetter, W., Lutolf, U., Meier, B., and Siegenthaler, W.: Treatment of renovascular hypertension with percutaneous transluminal dilatation of a renal-artery stenosis. Lancet, 1:801, 1978.

40. Tegtmeyer, C. J., Selby, J. B., Hartwell, G. D., Ayers, C., and Tegtmeyer, V.: Results and complications of angioplasty in fibromuscular disease. Circulation, 83(Suppl. I):I-155, 1991.

41. Ram, C. V.: Southwestern Internal Medicine Conference: Current concepts in renovascular hypertension. Am. J. Med. Sci., 304:53, 1992.

42. Graor, R. A.: New techniques of percutaneous renal revascularization: Atherectomy and stenting. Urol. Clin. North Am., 21:245, 1994.

43. Hansen, K. J., Thomason, R. B., Craven, T. E., Fuller, S. B., Keith, D. R., Appel, R. G., and Dean, R. H.: Surgical management of dialysis-dependent ischemic nephropathy. J. Vasc. Surg., 21:197, 1995.

44. Stanley, J. C., Zelenock, G. B., Messina, L. M., and Wakefield, T. W.: Pediatric renovascular hypertension: A thirty-year experience of operative treatment. J. Vasc. Surg., 21:221, 1995.

45. Libertino, J. A., and Beckmann, C. F.: Surgery and percutaneous angioplasty in the management of renovascular hypertension. Urol. Clin. North Am., 21:235, 1994.

VII

VENOUS INJURIES

Norman M. Rich, M.D.

Simple ligation of injured veins is the classic method of management . . . . Lateral suture repairs is preferred to ligation . . . . Grafts to bridge venous defects are not advocated.

—M. R. GASPAR AND R. L. TREIMAN, 1960

Initially, when we started the Vietnam Vascular Registry we felt that the greatest interest would come from management of arterial injuries. We more or less pushed venous injuries to the background. But in the last year we have become more interested in repair of venous injuries and feel that this area needs to be pursued with great vigor.

—N. M. RICH, C. W. HUGHES, AND J. H. BAUGH, 1970

These quotations identify important changes in the management of injured veins during the past 35 years. In contrast to the management of injured arteries, in which repair rather than ligation has been widely and enthusiastically practiced in the years since the Korean conflict, the same approach has not been widely developed for the management of venous injuries. It is ironic that Murphy stated in 1897, when he described the first successful clinical end-to-end anastomosis

of an artery: "closure of wounds in the veins by suture is now an acceptable surgical practice."[26]

Two major concerns prevented the development of vein repair: belief that there would be an increased incidence of thrombophlebitis, and fear of pulmonary embolism. Morton, Southgate, and DeWeese summarized the general concern in 1966 when they stated: "Whether or not concomitant venous injuries should be repaired remains a point of contention."[26] It is recognized that many injured veins can be ligated with few or no immediate problems and no recognized long-term disability. Until recently, the effectiveness of venous repair remained uncertain. Thrombosis was recognized to be much more common in the lower-pressure venous system, compared with the good results achieved following repair of arterial injuries. Also, in contrast to arterial repair, in which simple palpation of a peripheral pulse is usually adequate to determine success or failure, effectiveness of venous repair is more difficult to evaluate because there is no simple method for determining the patency of a venous reconstruction. Acute venous hypertension in the extremities following ligation of major veins, particularly in the lower extremities, may contribute to an increased amputation rate.[21] In addition, the degree of disability from chronic venous insufficiency is not recognized by many.[20] This disability may not become evident for months or even 5 to 10 years or more following injury.[24]

It has been recognized throughout history that important surgical progress occurs during periods of armed conflict, when surgeons are required to treat large numbers of patients with similar injuries within a relatively short period of time. This corollary between military surgery and vascular surgery has been particularly noteworthy in the nineteenth and twentieth centuries. An analysis that included the importance and effectiveness of the repair of venous injuries during the American experience in Southeast Asia was started at Walter Reed General Hospital in 1966 as the Vietnam Vascular Registry. A preliminary report demonstrated a significant incidence of venous injuries: 27% (Table 50–24).[18] An early report emphasized the need for the repair of injured veins,[19] and a more aggressive approach for the repair of injured veins, particularly in the lower extremities, was advocated in 1974.[20]

Venous repair may be particularly important in large-caliber veins in the lower extremities, specifically the popliteal vein (Fig. 50–164). Venous repair may be necessary in the presence of massive soft tissue injury and is mandatory in replantation of extremities. Repair of injured large-caliber veins should be considered routinely to prevent acute or chronic venous insufficiency. Important central veins, such as the portal vein, the superior mesenteric vein, and the vena cava, should be included. Lateral suture repair of a lacerated vein is frequently the most rapid and safest method of halting hemorrhage. Although the general status of a patient with multiple injuries must be considered, it is often possible to repair veins by end-to-end anastomosis and by interposition grafts, including compilation and spiral venous grafts. The challenge of obtaining successful venous reconstruction remains. A major obstacle is identification of the ideal vein substitute that has a high degree of success with long-term patency in the venous system, where the pressure is lower than in the arterial system.

Recent studies have provided data that allay the fear of a higher incidence of venous thrombosis and pulmonary embolization following repair of injured veins.[27, 28, 30] Although this is a possible hazard, the dangerous sequence has been surprisingly absent. It is conceivable that small emboli may not be recognized clinically; however, the absence of clinically detectable pulmonary emboli has been uniformly documented both in the Vietnam Vascular Registry and in previous reports by others.[25] Civilian experience in the past decade has corroborated the previously cited military experience in some aspects; however, the difference in wounds in civilian practice has also been emphasized in a variety of experiences and results.[1–12, 14–17, 29–31, 33, 34]

INCIDENCE OF VENOUS INJURIES

Because many surgeons considered venous injuries to be unimportant and did not report them, the true incidence is undetermined. This is particularly true when venous injuries

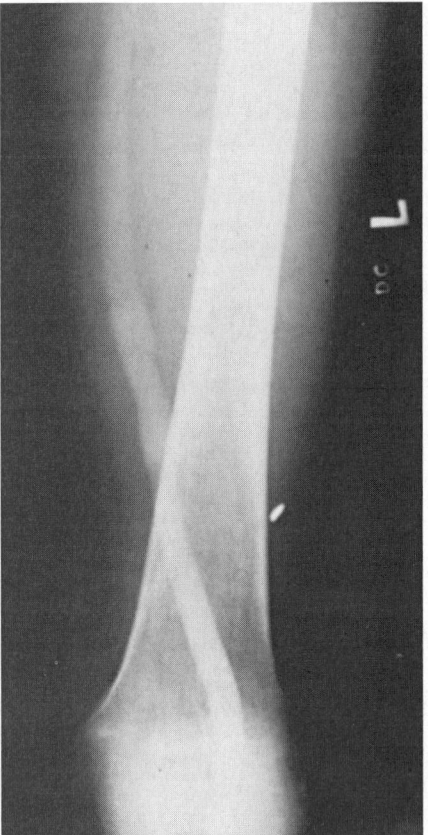

Figure 50–164. Venogram demonstrating patency of the popliteal vein at its junction with the superficial femoral vein. Note the metallic fragments that caused the injury. The vein had been repaired by lateral suture 3½ years earlier in Vietnam. Repair of concomitant venous injuries is advocated as one of the methods that help lower the relatively high amputation rate associated with popliteal artery trauma. (From Rich, N. M., Jarstfer, B. S., and Geer, T. M.: Popliteal artery repair failure: Causes and possible prevention. J. Cardiovasc. Surg., *15*:340, 1974.)

are associated with arterial injuries, with the emphasis given to arterial repair. In an analysis of the data in the Vietnam Vascular Registry, numerous cases were found in which venous trauma was not documented in the records; however, this documentation was possible through retrospective analysis. Considering reports from the civilian community regarding vascular injuries, the number of papers specifically addressing the management of venous injuries has increased over the past 15 years.

One notable exception to the lack of early reporting of venous injuries is the report by Gaspar and Treiman.[7] In a group of 228 patients with vascular injuries at Los Angeles County General Hospital over a period of 10 years, 51 patients (22%) had venous injuries. The superficial femoral vein was most frequently injured (nine cases). There were eight injuries to the inferior vena cava and eight to the internal jugular vein, and seven injuries of the brachial veins were noted. In 1966, an additional 40 patients were added to the original series in a supplementary report by Treiman and associates.

The frequency of venous injuries in the different anatomic locations is outlined in Table 50–25. There are also recent reviews.[1–5, 11, 12, 15, 29–31, 33, 34] Agarwal and colleagues reported in 1982 a retrospective analysis of 115 patients with venous injuries managed at Lincoln Hospital in New York City during a 7-year period.[1] Hardin and associates reported 83 patients with 86 venous injuries whose records were reviewed retrospectively at Tulane University Hospital.[11] During a 4-

TABLE 50–24. Incidence of Venous Trauma: Preliminary Vietnam Vascular Registry Report (500 Patients)

Total vascular injuries	718
Venous injuries	194 (27.0%)
Isolated	28 (14.4%)
Combined	166 (85.6%)

Modified from Rich, N. M., and Hughes, C. W.: Vietnam Vascular Registry: A preliminary report. Surgery, *65*:218, 1969.

TABLE 50–25. Incidence of Venous Injuries in Los Angeles

Vein	Number (1948–1958)	Number (1958–1963)	Total (1948–1963)	Percentage
Axillary-brachial	8	5	13	14.1
Innominate-subclavian	3	5	8	8.7
Superior vena cava	1	0	1	1.1
Inferior vena cava	8	4	12	13.0
Iliac	7	4	11	12.0
Femoral	11	6	17	18.5
Other	14	16	30	32.6
Total	52	40	92	100.0

Modified from Treiman, R. L., Doty, D., and Gaspar, M. R.: Acute vascular trauma. A fifteen year study. Am. J. Surg., *111*:469, 1966.

year period, 1979 to 1983, Hobson and colleagues reported a series of 81 venous injuries that were treated surgically. Thirty percent, or 24 cases, involved femoral veins—9 of the common femoral and 15 of the superficial femoral vein.[12] Meyer and colleagues identified 36 patients with major extremity venous injuries, with 34 also having major arterial injuries. Aitken and co-workers reviewed the cases of 26 patients with lower limb venous trauma.

The first major interest in identifying the frequency of venous injuries in military trauma was established during the Korean conflict. An analysis of 180 acute vascular injuries, showing that major veins were involved in approximately 40% of the total, is presented in Table 50–26. There were 71 major venous injuries and 79 major arterial injuries.[13] The preliminary Vietnam Vascular Registry report, which included approximately 25% of the patients with venous trauma, is shown in Table 50–27. There were only 28 isolated venous injuries, emphasizing that the majority of venous injuries are combined with adjacent arterial injuries.[18] The interim Vietnam Vascular Registry report documented a concomitant venous injury incidence of approximately 38% in patients with acute major arterial trauma.[19]

ETIOLOGY

Although numerous wounding agents have been identified as etiologic factors in venous trauma, specific documentation in published reports is limited. In the civilian report by Gaspar and Treiman, sharp instruments were responsible for the largest number of injuries—23, or approximately 44%.[7] The number of venous injuries caused by missiles was almost equal to the number caused by sharp instruments; only nine injuries were produced by blunt instruments. One iatrogenic laceration of the inferior vena cava occurred during abdominoperineal resection.

The number of iatrogenic injuries to the venous system has increased during the past 35 years as a result of the rapid development of vascular and cardiac angiography and

TABLE 50–26. Incidence of Acute Vascular Trauma in Korean Casualties

Vessel	Number	Percentage
Major arteries	79	43.9
Major veins	71	39.4
Minor arteries	30	16.7
Total	180	100.0

Modified from Hughes, C. W.: Acute vascular trauma in Korean War casualties: Analysis of 180 cases. Surg. Gynecol. Obstet., *99*:91, 1954.

TABLE 50–27. Location and Management of Concomitant Venous Injuries Associated with Arterial Injuries in the Vietnam Vascular Registry

Location	Arteries	Concomitant Veins	Ligation	Repair
Neck				
Carotid	50	14	10	4
Chest				
Innominate	3	1	0	1
Subclavian	8	4	1	3
Upper extremity				
Axillary	59	20	18	2
Brachial	283	54	42	12
Abdomen and pelvis				
Abdominal aorta	3	1	0	1
Common iliac	9	6	6	0
External iliac	17	5	3	2
Lower extremity				
Common femoral	46	17	8	9
Superficial femoral	305	139	83	56
Popliteal	217	116	82	34
Total	1000	377	253	124

Modified from Rich, N. M., Hughes, C. W., and Baugh, J. H.: Management of venous injuries. Ann. Surg., *171*:724, 1970.

catheterization. The reports of catheters that have been lost in the venous system are too numerous to review, emphasizing that this possibility must be fully appreciated. Thrombosis, sepsis, and phlebitis have also complicated the use of indwelling catheters. Iatrogenic venous injuries have been associated with most major operations at one time or another. Inadvertent injury to the common femoral vein during stripping of the greater saphenous system, usually caused by failure to recognize the common femoral vein, is one such surgical error. An unusual example of iatrogenic venous trauma is the report by Zabin in 1950 of an accidental tear of the inferior vena cava complicating cholecystectomy. Fractures have also been associated with venous injuries. The potentially lethal exsanguinating hemorrhage from venous trauma associated with pelvic fractures remains a challenge for surgeons.

In military casualties, as might be expected, fragments and high-velocity missiles are responsible for most venous injuries. In an analysis of 1000 acute major arterial injuries in soldiers in Vietnam, which included 377 concomitant venous injuries, 60% were produced by fragments from an assortment of exploding devices and 35% by bullets.[19]

PATHOPHYSIOLOGY

Most venous injuries that have been repaired have been lacerations. Despite the rather limited statistics, it is recognized that high-velocity missiles, as in military casualties, can be responsible for transection of veins. Considering the anatomic proximity of veins and arteries in most areas of the body, the possibility of concomitant arterial injuries should be suspected when a venous injury is found (Table 50–28).

Pertinent experimental research deserves mention.[22, 25, 26] An immediate decrease in femoral arterial blood flow was demonstrated as part of the evaluation of the hemodynamics of acute venous occlusion in the experimental model. It was demonstrated that femoral venous ligation in the canine hindlimb resulted in a 50 to 75% reduction in femoral arterial blood flow, with a marked increase in femoral venous pressure as well as in peripheral resistance.

As with arterial injuries, most venous injuries occur in the extremities (see Table 50–27). Many veins are vulnerable to

TABLE 50–28. Frequency of Concomitant Venous Injuries Associated with Acute Arterial Trauma

Artery	Number	Venous Injuries	Percentage
Axillary	59	20	33.8
Brachial	283	54	19.0
Iliac	26	11	42.3
Common femoral	46	17	36.9
Superficial femoral	305	139	45.5
Popliteal	217	116	53.5
Total	936	357	37.9

Modified from Rich, N. M., Hughes, C. W., and Baugh, J. H.: Management of venous injuries. Ann. Surg., *171*:724, 1970.

injury, because of their relatively superficial location. In contrast to the bright red, spurting blood of an arterial injury, there is usually dark, steady bleeding from a venous injury. In a closed wound, a massive hematoma may develop. It may not be possible to determine whether such a hematoma is due to trauma to multiple small vessels or arterial trauma. Consequently, many venous injuries are first recognized at the time of surgical exploration. It is particularly important to emphasize that acute venous insufficiency may develop within the first 12 to 24 hours following trauma. Massive edema and a cool, bluish extremity are principal clinical findings. The clinical pattern of chronic venous insufficiency—a familiar one because of the frequency of thrombophlebitis in surgical patients—includes edema, varices, brown pigmentation of the skin, and stasis ulcers.

DIAGNOSTIC CONSIDERATIONS

Doppler ultrasound may be useful as a diagnostic approach in the management of venous disease. Numerous clinical studies have documented variation in the accuracy of the Doppler technique, however. In the early experience of the Vietnam Vascular Registry follow-up, the Doppler technique was of value in determining the patency of venous repairs, particularly in the lower extremities. Color-flow duplex studies are of increasing value.

Impedance plethysmography, phlebography, and radionuclide studies have also had a degree of success in diagnosing venous occlusions. The phlebograph has been used in the long-term follow-up at Walter Reed Army Medical Center for patients with venous injuries. Whereas roentgenograms may be of value in identifying offending missile injuries or associated fractures, phlebography is the ultimate diagnostic means of determining the location and extent of venous injury, with or without associated thrombus formation. Gerlock and associates provided valuable information in performing phlebograms in patients with venous injuries.[8, 9, 16]

SURGICAL MANAGEMENT

General considerations in the management of injured patients should be of primary concern. Rapid assessment of multiple injuries, with establishment of priorities, is mandatory. Shock is common with major venous injuries, particularly when active hemorrhage is unabated. Concomitant arterial injuries may be part of the multiple-injury complex and can contribute to exsanguinating hemorrhage. Hemorrhage from injured veins can usually be controlled by judicious pressure or packing, except with penetrating injuries of the body cavities. This approach also helps prevent the entrance of air into the venous system. In some patients, particularly those with penetrating injuries of the body cavities, immedi-

ate operation may be necessary to control profound shock from exsanguinating hemorrhage. Shock should be treated by rapid infusion of whole blood and appropriate electrolyte solutions. Broad-spectrum antibiotics should be given routinely.

The principles of elective surgical procedures should be followed in the management of an injured patient who has sustained venous trauma. Elective incisions, usually longitudinal along the course of the vein, help provide adequate exposure for proximal and distal control of the vein to halt venous hemorrhage. A frequent question is whether an arterial or a venous injury should be repaired first. Normally, the injured artery should be repaired first to minimize anoxia in the distal extremity. In some instances, however, it may be more expeditious to repair the venous injury first, usually by lateral suture, to establish hemostasis and provide better exposure of the arterial injury. Copious irrigation with saline solution is useful for both visualization and removal of foreign material. Adequate wound débridement is essential, as is the removal of nonviable tissue following trauma.

Bleeding can usually be controlled temporarily with digital pressure until blood clot and foreign debris have been irrigated from the wound. The digital pressure can be augmented by stick sponges. A combination of encircling tapes around the vein, both distal and proximal to the area of injury, and a proximal temporary tourniquet affords simple, atraumatic control of hemorrhage. This is usually preferable to vascular clamps, particularly when the exposure is limited. With tangential injuries to large veins, however, a partial occluding vascular clamp may be used. This approach avoids the necessity of wider mobilization of the vein and also permits the flow of venous blood to continue unabated.

A venous injury can be managed by at least five different methods. In order of popularity, they are ligation, lateral suture repair, end-to-end anastomosis, venous patch graft, and venous replacement graft.[22, 23, 25]

Ligation has been used for many injured veins, but the use of lateral suture repair has been increasing. Most clinical data at present are concerned with techniques of lateral suture repair. Although the other methods of repair are theoretically satisfactory and there are anecdotal cases, few data are available for estimating the degree of success of venous reconstruction, particularly with venous replacement grafts inserted for injuries in different parts of the body.

Before repair is begun, the vein should be explored both proximally and distally for thrombi. A balloon catheter is most useful, although difficulty may be encountered during retrograde insertion because of competent venous valves. Gentle manipulation is necessary to avoid perforation. If thrombus is present, it can be expressed by gentle pressure peripherally toward the area of venous injury. If thrombus is present or if venous occlusion is necessary for more than a few minutes, heparin can be administered either locally or systemically to help prevent additional propagation of thrombus.

Meticulous technique is mandatory during venous reconstruction.[22, 30] Both experimental and clinical experience have demonstrated that meticulous technique is more critical in the management of injured veins than of injured arteries. Venous repairs have a greater tendency to thrombose. A fine synthetic vascular suture on a small needle minimizes bleeding. When a continuous suture is used, less tension is applied than in arterial anastomoses to avoid circular constriction. Leaving the loops of a continuous suture somewhat loose may create a few leaks, but bleeding usually stops with mild pressure.

The apparent simplicity of venous repair often deceives the inexperienced operator, who may think that the problem is simpler than the more complex arterial repair, with associated pulsatile hemorrhage and threatened viability of the extremity. With lateral suture repair, as with arterial repairs, the principal consideration is avoidance of undue constriction of the venous lumen. Occasionally, autogenous venous patches may be useful in preventing constriction. When the repair cannot be done by lateral suture, reconstruction by end-to-end anastomosis or by insertion of a vascular graft can be considered if the patient's general condition is stable. To date, autogenous venous grafts are the most satisfactory grafts. Synthetic grafts, particularly ringed, have been applied successfully in the repair of large-caliber veins. If there is great disparity between the size of the vein and the size of the venous replacement segment, turbulence and eddying result and contribute to thrombus formation.

Specific mention is made of injuries of the venae cavae because no acceptable autogenous vein grafts are available for the large-caliber cavae. Good results have been obtained by making composite grafts, such as those espoused by Doty and Baker in 1976. Quast and co-workers[17] in 1965 outlined a number of techniques that can be considered for lacerations in the vena cava (Fig. 50–165). Similar approaches can be utilized for other injuries of large-caliber veins. Schrock and colleagues in 1968 and Bricker and colleagues in 1971 described an internal vena caval shunt to maintain venous return during repair, with the shunt introduced through the right atrium; however, the clinical experience with this approach is limited.[25]

Operative phlebography is an adjunctive measure that may be of value after reconstruction, because palpation of distal pulses is not possible then, as it is after arterial reconstruction. A phlebogram performed in the operating room can help outline a stenotic area at the repair site or residual thrombus within the venous lumen.

POSTOPERATIVE CARE

Specific attempts should be made after the operation to minimize or eliminate edema of the involved extremity. This is particularly true when large veins, such as the vena cava, have been ligated. Early and vigorous postoperative care to prevent massive edema should be initiated as soon as possible, including elevation of the legs and careful wrapping of them or the use of elastic support hose when the patient is ambulatory. Disability from chronic venous insufficiency can be greatly minimized by early effective use of elastic support. This requires frequent inspection and periodic adjustment of both the type and the degree of support. These factors are probably mismanaged more often than any other form of supportive care in patients with chronic venous insufficiency.

RESULTS

In a summary of the experience in the Korean conflict, Hughes[13] reported that all 20 venous repairs were performed by lateral suture except for one end-to-end anastomosis. In Vietnam, approximately one third of the venous injuries were repaired. This was confirmed by both initial and interim registry reports. Interest was concentrated particularly on major veins in the lower extremities, and 85% of the repairs were performed by lateral suture technique. As experience increased, however, end-to-end anastomosis and autogenous venous grafts were used more frequently. Follow-up phlebo-

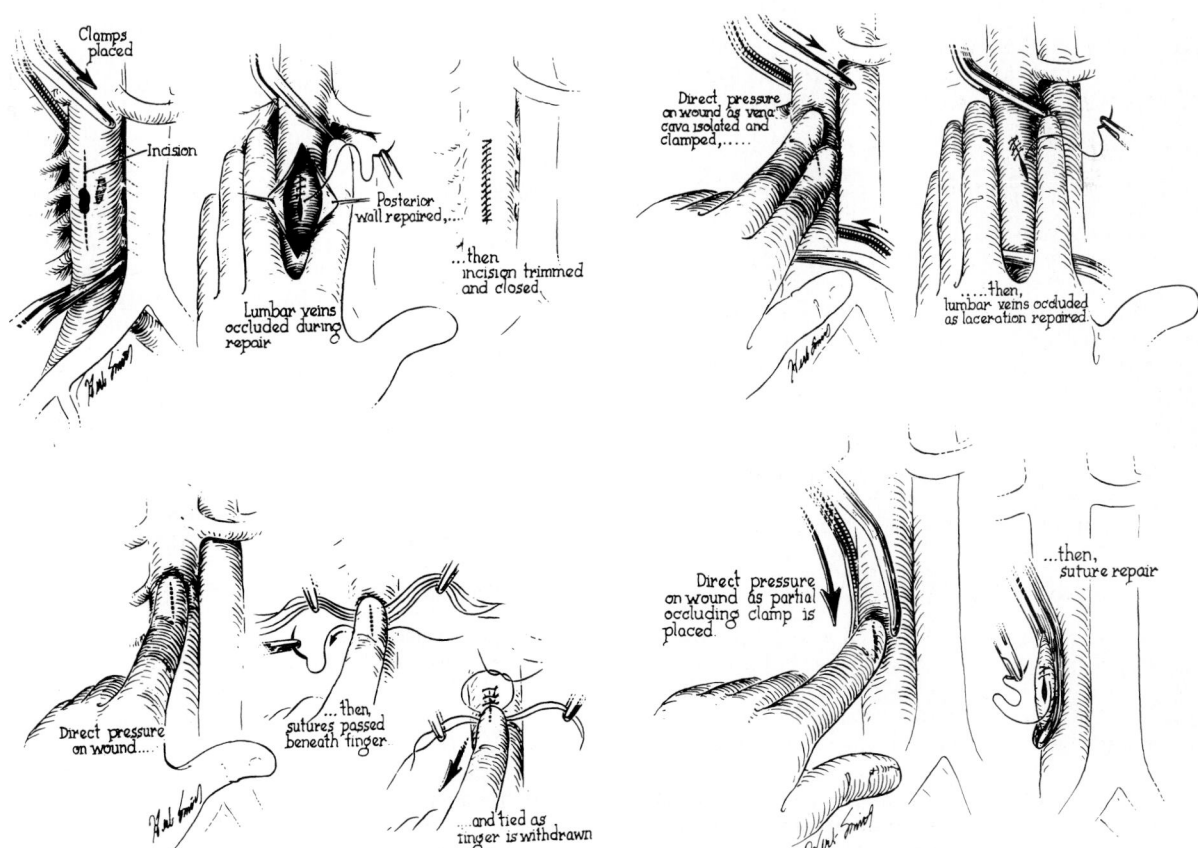

Figure 50–165. The management of vena caval injuries is outlined in these composite drawings. These methods can be utilized in injuries to large-caliber veins. (From Quast, D. C., Shirkey, A. L., Fitzgerald, J. B., Beall, A. C., Jr., and DeBakey, M. E.: Surgical correction of injuries of the vena cava: An analysis of sixty-one cases. J. Trauma, 5:1, 1965.)

grams (Fig. 50–166) demonstrate the success of the various techniques employed. Sullivan and co-workers performed a significant study on the management of injured popliteal veins at the Twelfth Evacuation Hospital in Vietnam.[32] There were 27 injuries to the popliteal vein among 35 popliteal vascular injuries, and 21 of the 27 venous injuries were repaired. Phlebograms performed on 11 patients within the first 72 hours after operation showed patent repair in eight. Success included patency of an autogenous venous graft in the popliteal vein. Probably of greatest importance was the finding that massive edema did not occur in any of 21 patients who had primary repair of a venous injury, which contrasted with severe venous insufficiency and morbidity in four patients in whom the popliteal vein was ligated. It is remarkable that no known cases of pulmonary emboli were recognized after venous repair in the initial Vietnam series, which included 124 reconstructions.[19] In later long-term follow-up, nonfatal pulmonary emboli have been seen infrequently. There is no statistically significant difference between these findings and those in patients who have had ligation of venous injuries.

One study from the Vietnam Vascular Registry evaluated the long-term follow-up of 110 patients with isolated popliteal venous trauma with the adjacent popliteal artery intact. Nearly an equal number were either ligated or repaired. Thrombophlebitis and pulmonary embolism were not significant complications in this series. Only one pulmonary embolus occurred after ligation of an injured popliteal vein.

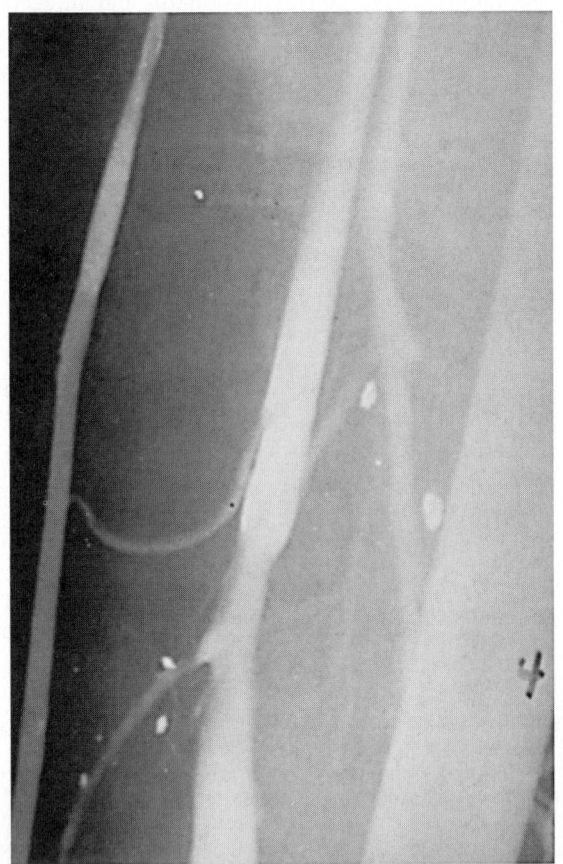

Figure 50–166. *A,* Patency of the superficial femoral vein is demonstrated by phlebography approximately 1 month after repair in a 20-year-old Vietnam casualty who developed a superficial femoral arteriovenous fistula from multiple fragment wounds. *B,* The distal superficial femoral vein in this patient was repaired with an autogenous greater saphenous vein patch graft. This venogram shows successful repair and patency of the vein at the junction with the popliteal vein. (From Rich, N. M., Hughes, C. W., and Baugh, J. H.: Management of venous injuries. Ann. Surg., *171:*724, 1970.)

TABLE 50–29. Incidence of Edema Following Ligation and Repair of Injured Popliteal Veins

Management	Number	With Edema	Percentage
Ligation	57	29	50.9
Repair	53	7	13.2

Modified from Rich, N. M., Hobson, R. W., II, Collins, G. J., Jr., and Andersen, C. A.: The effect of acute popliteal venous interruption. Ann. Surg., *183:*365, 1976.

There was a significant increase, however, in edema in the involved extremity following ligation of the popliteal vein, as contrasted with repair (Table 50–29). A second important study involved the 10-year follow-up of 51 Vietnam casualties whose lower extremity venous injuries were repaired by autogenous interposition venous grafts.[23] Only one patient (2%) developed thrombophlebitis in the postoperative period, and this was transitory (Table 50–30). Of particular significance is the relatively low edema rate of approximately 12%, as contrasted with the 51% edema rate following ligation of the popliteal veins.

In the civilian community, Gaspar and Treiman in 1960 documented lateral suture repair of 10 venous lacerations, representing only one fifth of the 52 venous injuries encountered.[7] Six of these 10 injuries were located in the inferior vena cava. All but one of the patients recovered, apparently with good results from the venous reconstruction. In the remaining patients, 27 ligations were performed, with good results in 21. Six could not be evaluated because of three deaths from associated injuries and three amputations due to concomitant arterial injuries. For various reasons, venous injury was not treated in 15 patients, eight of whom subsequently developed arteriovenous fistulas. In the supplemental report published by Treiman and associates in 1966, repair was utilized in approximately 50% of a total of 92 venous injuries.

Agarwal and associates, in their report of 115 civilian venous injuries, disclosed a total mortality of 15%.[1] In their experience, retrohepatic caval injury was uniformly fatal. They also documented that ligation of injured veins in upper extremities was not associated with any specific morbidity; however, ligation of larger-caliber lower extremity veins resulted in edema in 50% of patients, compared with edema in only 7% of patients who underwent repair of lower extremity veins.

Hobson and colleagues managed femoral venous injuries by lateral venorrhaphy in 10 patients (42%), venous patch angioplasty in 5 patients (21%), end-to-end anastomosis in 4

TABLE 50–30. Complications of Venous Repair Using Autogenous Venous Grafts (51 Patients)

Complications	Number	Percentage
Thrombophlebitis	1	2.0
Pulmonary embolism	0	0.0
Amputation	0	0.0
Death	0	0.0
Edema		
None	34	66.6
Early	11	21.6
Residual	6	11.8
Total	51	100.0

From Rich, N. M., Collins, G. J., Jr., Andersen, C. A., and McDonald, P. T.: Autogenous venous interposition grafts in repair of major venous injuries. J. Trauma, *17:*512, 1977.

TABLE 50–31. Assessment of Outcome in Lower Limb Vein Trauma

Procedure	Good	Fair	Poor
Ligation	1	1	4
Lateral pair	3	2	3
Vein patch	2		1
End-to-end anastomosis		1	2
Interposition saphenous vein graft	2	2	1
Panel graft		1	
Total	8	7	11

From Aitken, R. J., Matley, P. J., and Immelman, E. J.: Lower limb vein trauma: A long-term clinical and physiological assessment. Br. J. Surg., *76*:585, 1989. Reprinted with permission of Blackwell Science Ltd.

patients (17%), interposition autogenous saphenous vein grafts in 3 patients (12%), and ligation in 2 patients (8%).[12] They excluded one early death from associated injuries and one superficial femoral venous injury managed by ligation without postoperative complications, reporting that 17 of 23 femoral venous repairs (74%) were judged patent postoperatively, with 13 confirmed by venography and four by noninvasive testing. They believed that adjuvant use of intermittent pneumatic calf compression and low-molecular-weight dextran had some benefit in maintaining the patency of femoral venous repairs. Edema was treated in six of eight patients (75%) by ligation or was complicated by postoperative occlusion in patients with femoral venous trauma.

Additional evaluation of the management of injured veins in the civilian population will provide valuable information. An example is the valuable contribution by Phifer and colleagues, who evaluated the long-term patency of venous repairs with six femoral venous reconstructions.[16] Follow-up venography at 6 to 20 years demonstrated venous patency and functional valves in asymptomatic patients and no clinical evidence of venous insufficiency in all but one patient. Mullins and colleagues[15] from Detroit, as well as Timberlake and co-workers[33] from New Orleans, have had varying results but have not observed significant edema in civilian injuries following lower extremity venous ligation. Meyer and colleagues from Chicago reported a 61% success rate in maintaining the patency of lower extremity venous repair. Aitken and colleagues made a long-term clinical and physiologic assessment of lower limb vein trauma; their recommendation is that "vein ligation should be avoided unless another life-threatening injury demands priority" (Table 50–31).

TABLE 50–32. Management of Venous Injuries at Lincoln Medical Center, New York Medical College, 1981–1989

Type of Repair	Group I*	Group II†	Total
End to end	9	5	14
Lateral venorrhaphy	2	10	12
Vein patch	1	2	3
Vein compilation	2	2	4
Vein spiral	1	0	1
Vein bypass	2	0	2
Gore-Tex	0	1	1
Ligation	0	1	1
Total	17	21	38

*Meticulous repair group.
†Standard repair group.
From Sharma, P. V. P., Shah, P. M., Vinzons, A. T., Pallan, T. M., Clauss, R. H., and Stahl, W. M.: Meticulously restored lumina of injured veins remain patent. Surgery, *112*:928, 1992.

TABLE 50–33. Outcomes of Venous Injuries: Repair Versus Ligation

	Ligation (n = 44)		Repair (n = 30)	
	Hospital Day 4	Discharge	Hospital Day 4	Discharge
Edema				
0	31	38	24	24
Trace	0	0	1	1
+	8	6	3	3
+ +	5	0	1	1
+ + +	0	0	1	1
Vascular complications				
Arterial thrombosis	1		2	
Deep venous thrombosis	0		1	
Pulmonary embolus	0		1	

From Yelon, J. A., and Scalea, T. M.: Venous injuries of the lower extremities and pelvis: Repair versus ligation. J. Trauma, *33*:532, 1992.

Sharma and associates from New York City emphasized the importance of meticulous technique; they were able to maintain patency in all 17 repairs noted in Group I (Table 50–32) when the operating room microscope was utilized to ensure meticulous technique.

Although the final answer is not available at this time, it is obvious from both civilian and military experience that some patients, who may be difficult to identify at the time of injury, will have sequelae that might be anticipated from interruption of the lower extremity venous return if ligation is performed. Even in the more recent civilian reports with contrary views, repair of venous injuries has been accomplished. Table 50–33 outlines the results achieved by Yelon and Scalea.[34]

Eighty-six percent of the patients treated by ligation were totally free of edema at discharge. . . . Ligation is a safe alternative to repair in patients with injuries to the lower extremities or pelvis.

—J. A. Yelon and T. M. Scalea, 1992

Clinical or measured venous hypertension by stump pressure assisted in deciding for venous repair in 20 patients. A significant decrease in venous stump pressure (p < 0.000001) was noted after venous reconstruction. Thus the decision to ligate or repair venous injuries correlated primarily with (1) hemodynamic stability, and in stable patients, with (2) extent and location of injury and (3) clinical and measured venous hypertension.

—P. V. P. Sharma and associates, 1992

Additional studies, such as that by Aitken and co-workers, will provide additional data; however, those patients with lower extremity edema following ligation of injured veins attest to the challenge for some patients and their surgeons.

SELECTED REFERENCES

Aitken, R. J., Matley, P. J., and Immelman, E. J.: Lower limb vein trauma: A long-term clinical and physiological assessment. Br. J. Surg., 76:585, 1989.
This study reports long-term clinical and physiologic assessment of lower limb venous trauma and recommends that vein ligation be avoided unless another life-threatening injury demands priority.

Hobson, R. W., II, Rich, N. M., and Wright, C. B. (Eds.): Venous Trauma: Pathophysiology, Diagnosis and Surgical Management. Mount Kisco, N.Y.: Futura, 1983.
This monograph provides an informative review of the management of patients with injured veins in both civilian and military situations.

Meyer, J., Walsh, J., Schuler, J., et al.: The early fate of venous repair following civilian vascular trauma: A clinical, hemodynamic, and venographic assessment. Ann. Surg., 206:458, 1987.
Early fate of venous repair after civilian vascular trauma is reviewed from a major trauma center. A patency rate of 61% was documented.

Rich, N. M.: Management of venous trauma. Surg. Clin. North Am. *68*:809, 1988.

This review emphasizes differences between civilian and military experiences, noting the importance of repairing major injured veins in the lower extremity.

Rich, N. M., Hobson, R. W., II, Collins, G. J., Jr., and Andersen, C. A.: The effect of acute popliteal venous interruption. Ann. Surg., *183*:365, 1976.

This clinical study of Vietnam casualties provides long-term follow-up that emphasizes the contrasting results of ligation of injured veins (followed by a 51% incidence of disabling edema) and the improved results following repair of injured popliteal veins (with residual edema of less than 15%).

REFERENCES

1. Agarwal, N., Shah, P. M., Clauss, R. H., Reynolds, D. M., and Stahl, W. M.: Experience with 115 civilian venous injuries. J. Trauma, 22:827, 1982.
2. Barkun, J. S., Terazza, O., Daignault, P., Chiu, R. C.-J., and Mulder, D. S.: The fate of venous repair after shock and trauma. J. Trauma, 28:1322, 1988.
3. Bishara, R. A., Schuler, J. J., Lim, L. T., et al.: Results of venous reconstruction after civilian vascular trauma. Arch. Surg., 121:607, 1986.
4. Blumoff, R. L., Powell, T., and Johnson, G., Jr.: Femoral venous trauma in a university referral center. J. Trauma, 22:703, 1982.
5. Borman, K. R., Jones, G. H., and Snyder, W. H., 3d: A decade of lower extremity venous trauma: Patency and outcome. Am. J. Surg., 154:608, 1987.
6. Brigham, R. A., Eddleman, W. L., Clagett, G. P., and Rich, N. M.: Isolated venous injury produced by penetrating trauma to the lower extremity. J. Trauma, 23:255, 1983.
6a. Doty, D. B., and Baker, W. H.: Bypass of superior vena cava with spiral vein graft. Ann. Thorac. Surg., 22:490, 1976.
7. Gaspar, M. R., and Treiman, R. L.: The management of injuries to major veins. Am. J. Surg., 100:171, 1960.
8. Gerlock, A. J., and Muhletaler, C. A.: Venography of peripheral venous injuries. Radiology, 133:77, 1979.
9. Gerlock, A. J., Jr., Thal, E. R., and Snyder, W. H., 3d: Venography in penetrating injuries of the extremities. A. J. R. Am. J. Roentgenol., 126:1023, 1976.
10. Graham, J. M., Mattox, K. L., and Beall, A. C., Jr.: Portal venous system injuries. J. Trauma, 18:419, 1978.
11. Hardin, W. D., Jr., Adinolfi, M. F., O'Connell, R. C., and Kerstein, M. D.: Management of traumatic peripheral vein injuries: Primary repair or vein ligation. Am. J. Surg., 144:235, 1982.
12. Hobson, R. W., Yeager, R. A., Lynch, T. G., Lee, B. C., Jain, K., Jamil, Z., and Padberg, F. T., Jr.: Femoral venous trauma: Techniques for surgical management and early results. Am. J. Surg., 146:220, 1983.
13. Hughes, C. W.: Arterial repair during the Korean War. Ann. Surg., 147:555, 1958.
14. Jacobson, J. H., and Haimov, J.: Venous revascularization of the arm: Report of three cases. Surgery, 81:599, 1977.
15. Mullins, R. J., Lucas, C. E., and Ledgerwood, A. M.: The natural history following venous ligation for civilian injuries. J. Trauma, 20:737, 1980.
16. Phifer, T. J., Gerlock, A. J., Rich, N. M., and McDonald, J. C.: Long-term patency of venous repairs demonstrated by venography. J. Trauma, 25:342, 1985.
17. Quast, D. C., Shirkey, A. L., Fitzgerald, J. B., Beall, A. C., Jr., and DeBakey, M. E.: Surgical correction of injuries to the vena cava: An analysis of sixty-one cases. J. Trauma, 5:1, 1965.
18. Rich, N. M., and Hughes, C. W.: Vietnam vascular registry: A preliminary report. Surgery, 65:218, 1969.
19. Rich, N. M., Baugh, J. H., and Hughes, C. W.: Acute arterial injuries in Vietnam: 1,000 cases. J. Trauma, 10:359, 1970.
20. Rich, N. M., Hobson, R. W., 2d, Wright, C. B., and Fedde, C. W.: Repair of lower extremity venous trauma: A more aggressive approach required. J. Trauma, 14:639, 1974.
21. Rich, N. M., Jarstfer, B. S., and Geer, T. M.: Popliteal artery repair failure: Causes and possible prevention. J. Cardiovasc. Surg., 15:340, 1974.
22. Rich, N. M., Hobson, R. W., 2d, Wright, C. B., and Swan, K. G.: Techniques of venous repair. In Swan, K. G., Hobson, R. W., 2d, Reynolds, D. G., Rich, N. M., and Wright, C. B. (Eds.): Symposium on Venous Surgery in the Lower Extremities. St. Louis: Warren H. Green, 1975.
23. Rich, N. M., Collins, G. J., Andersen, C. A., and McDonald, P. T.: Autogenous venous interposition grafts in repair of major venous injuries. J. Trauma, 17:512, 1977.
24. Rich, N. M., Collins, G. J., Jr., Andersen, C. A., McDonald, P. T., and Ricotta, J. J.: Venous trauma: Successful venous reconstruction remains an interesting challenge. Am. J. Surg., 134:226, 1977.
25. Rich, N. M., and Spencer, F. C.: Vascular Trauma. Philadelphia, W. B. Saunders, 1978.
26. Rich, N. M., Hobson, R. W., 2d, and Wright, C. B.: Historical aspects of direct venous reconstruction. In Bergan, J. J., and Yao, J. T. S. (Eds.): Symposium on venous problems in honor of Geza de Takats. Chicago, Year Book Medical Publishers, 1978.
27. Rich, N. M.: Principles and indications for primary venous repair. Surgery, 91:492, 1982.
28. Rich, N. M., Gomez, E. R., Coffey, J. A., Hammond, S. L., Lauer, C. G., and Villavicencio, J. L.: Long-term follow-up of venous reconstruction following trauma. In Bergan, J. J., and Yao, J. S. T. (Eds.): Venous Disorders. Philadelphia, W. B. Saunders, 1991.
29. Richardson, J. B., Jr., Jurkovich, G. J., Walker, G. T., Nenstiel, R., and Bone, E. G.: A temporary arteriovenous shunt (Scribner) in the management of traumatic venous injuries of the lower extremity. J. Trauma, 26:503, 1986.
30. Sharma, P. V. P., Shah, P. M., Vinzons, A. T., Pallan, T. M., Clauss, R. H., and Stahl, W. M.: Meticulously restored lumina of injured veins remain patent. Surgery, 112:928, 1992.
31. Sharma, P. V. P., Ivatury, R. R., Simon, R. J., and Vinzons, A. T.: Central and regional hemodynamics determine optimal management of major venous injuries. J. Vasc. Surg., 16:887, 1992.
32. Sullivan, W. G., Thorton, F. G., Baker, L. H., LaPlante, E. S., and Cohen, A.: Early influence of popliteal vein repair in the treatment of popliteal vessel injuries. Am. J. Surg., 122:528, 1971.
33. Timberlake, G. A., O'Connell, R. C., and Kerstein, M. D.: Venous injuries: To repair or ligate, the dilemma. J. Vasc. Surg., 4:533, 1986.
34. Yelon, J. A., and Scalea, T. M.: Venous injuries of the lower extremities and pelvis: Repair versus ligation. J. Trauma, 33:532, 1992.

CHAPTER 51

DISORDERS OF THE LUNGS, PLEURA, AND CHEST WALL

I

ANATOMY

Walter G. Wolfe, M.D., and R. Eric Lilly, M.D.

EMBRYOLOGY

The primordia of the principal respiratory organs appear as a medial longitudinal groove in the ventral wall of the pharynx by the fourth week of gestation.[1, 19] The tube is lined with endoderm, from which the epithelium of the respiratory tract develops. The cephalic part of the tube becomes the larynx, followed by the trachea; from its caudal end, two lateral outgrowths arise that form the left and right lung buds. The right and left lung buds are initially symmetrical; however, by 6 to 7 weeks of gestation, the lung buds become lobulated, with three lobules appearing on the right and two on the left. Orderly bronchial development then proceeds such that by the end of the sixteenth week of gestation, the conducting portion of the airways, including the terminal bronchioles, has developed.[23] As development proceeds, the lungs migrate caudally, and by the time of birth the bifurcation of the trachea is opposite the fourth thoracic vertebra. As the lungs grow, they project into that part of the coelom that ultimately forms the pleural cavities.

In the seventh week of gestation, the left sixth aortic arch forms the main pulmonary artery, as well as the left and right pulmonary arteries.[3, 13] Each pulmonary artery is closely related to the main-stem bronchus and provides an arterial partner for each new bronchial ramification. These airway-artery pairs enter first the lobe, then the segments, and finally the lobules of developing lung tissue. As lung development progresses, these pairs assume a central location in each lobule and project branches toward that particular subdivision of the lung. The main pulmonary veins develop as outgrowths from the cardiac atria, and the intrapulmonary veins develop from mesenchyma. As the intrapulmonary veins develop, they receive tributaries from the pleura and the rich vascular networks that form about the growing tips of the respiratory tree. Intrapulmonary veins form interlobular veins as they arch across the base of the secondary lobules toward the periphery. These veins traverse the planes of connective tissue that separate adjacent pulmonary lobules. Interlobular veins unite to form intersegmental veins, which in most cases merge with the developing main pulmonary veins near the pulmonary hilus to form the superior and inferior pulmonary veins.[3]

ANATOMY

The respiratory system consists of the nose, nasal passages, nasopharynx, larynx, trachea, bronchi, and lungs. Associated structures—including the thorax, with its bony and muscu-lar components; the pleura; pleural cavity; and mediastinum—all contribute significantly to normal respiratory function. The relationship between the topographic anatomy of the thorax (Fig. 51–1) and the anatomy of the respiratory system is important.[19, 49]

Chest Wall and Pleura

Beneath the skin and subcutaneous tissue, the chest wall is covered by the pectoralis muscles anteriorly and the latissimus dorsi and serratus anterior muscles posterolaterally. In an anterior thoracotomy, the fibers of the pectoralis major are split, exposing the intercostal muscles. In the standard posterolateral thoracotomy, the latissimus dorsi is divided, and then the serratus anterior is divided or split. From the standpoint of preservation of normal chest wall mechanics, an anterior thoracotomy is usually better tolerated; however, exposure and control of intrathoracic structures are often better accomplished through the posterolateral approach, which is the standard thoracotomy incision.

There are 12 pairs of ribs, seven of which are *true ribs* and five of which are *false ribs*. True ribs have costal cartilage that directly articulates with the sternum. False ribs do not. The eleventh and twelfth ribs are called *floating ribs* because they are not attached anteriorly. The sternum is divided into the manubrium, the body, and the xiphoid. The clavicle articulates with the sternum and the first costal cartilage. This is an important anatomic relationship, because a posterior dislocation of the clavicle can cause respiratory distress secondary to compression of the trachea by the head of the clavicle.

Muscles associated with the intercostal space are the external, internal, and transversus thoracic muscles. There are 11 intercostal spaces. Each intercostal space contains a vein, an artery, and a nerve, which course along the lower edge of the rib. All the intercostal spaces are wider anteriorly than posteriorly, the widest being the third.

The parietal pleura is divided into four parts: costal, cervical, diaphragmatic, and mediastinal. The costal pleura lines the ribs, cartilages, and vertebral bodies and is the thickest portion of the parietal pleura. The visceral pleura covers the lungs so firmly that it is not possible to strip it from the lung tissue under normal circumstances. The pulmonary ligament is a fold of pleura that extends medially from the inferior hilum to the diaphragm.

The internal mammary artery and vein arise from the first portion of the subclavian artery opposite the thyrocervical trunk and descend along the sternum to anastomose with the superior epigastric artery. The lymphatics in the chest

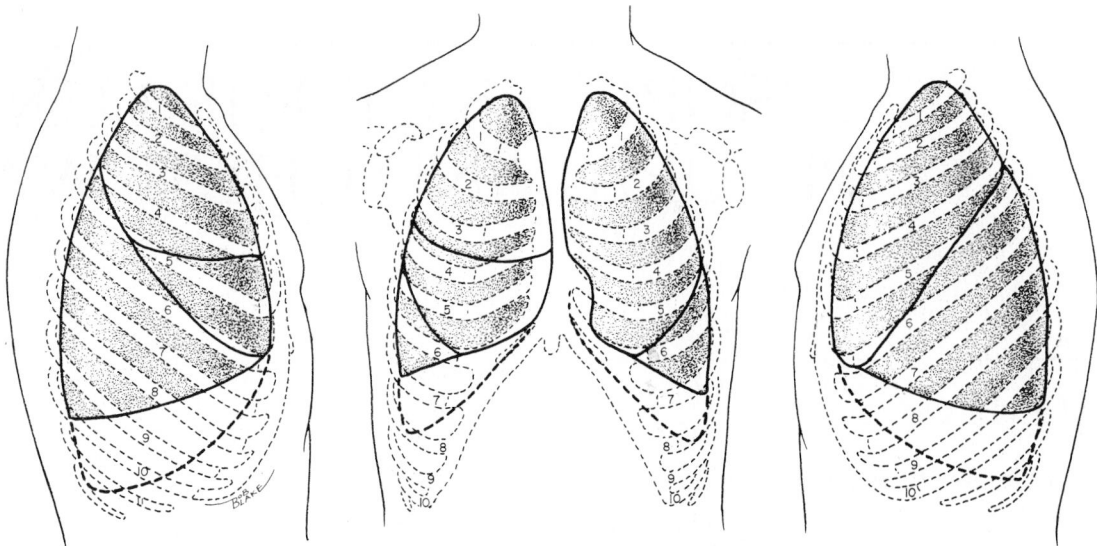

Figure 51–1. The relationships of the pleural reflections and the lobes of the lung to the ribs. The topographic anatomy and the relationship of the fissures of the lobes to ribs in inspiration and expiration are important in evaluation of the routine posteroanterior and lateral chest film.

wall and their drainage patterns are important and are discussed in the section on carcinoma of the breast.

Although considered associated structures of the respiratory system, the chest wall and pleura must function normally for maintenance of respiratory function. The recent resurgence of lung reduction operations in the treatment of emphysema, with the resultant improved chest wall mechanics and pulmonary function, is one example of this important interaction.[12]

Trachea

The entrance to the trachea is guarded by the larynx. It functions to prevent aspiration and facilitate phonation, and it has an important role in the production of the cough. The mucous membrane lining of the larynx is covered by ciliated epithelial cells and a few goblet cells. The epithelial surfaces in contact with food are covered by stratified squamous epithelium.[20] Except for the cricothyroid muscle, which is innervated by the external laryngeal branch of the superior laryngeal nerve, the larynx receives both motor and sensory innervation by way of the vagal accessory complex of nerve fibers. The intrinsic muscles of the larynx receive their motor innervation by way of the inferior laryngeal branch of the recurrent vagus nerve.[19]

The trachea is a fibromuscular tube 10 to 12 cm. in length and varying from 13 to 22 mm. in width. Approximately 20 U-shaped hyaline cartilages support the trachea laterally and ventrally. The trachea originates at the level of the cricoid cartilage and descends through the superior aperture of the thorax and the superior mediastinum to its bifurcation at the level of the sternal angle (lower border of the fourth thoracic vertebra). Here it divides into the right and left primary bronchi. The spur formed at the point of bifurcation is termed the *carina*. Half of the trachea lies in the neck and the other half within the thorax.[19, 29]

The dimensions of the trachea are constantly changing with the movement of the head and neck. It is attached to a moveable structure at both ends: the larynx cranially, and the pericardial sac and diaphragm caudally. During forced expiration, especially when the glottis is suddenly opened, as in coughing, the trachea is markedly narrowed. In young subjects, the lumen may be reduced to one tenth its original

size. Prior to cough, the bifurcation may ascend as much as 5 cm.[29]

The epithelial lining of the trachea is composed of pseudostratified columnar ciliated cells (30%), goblet cells (28%), and basal cells (29%). Basal cells are capable of differentiating into goblet or ciliated cells.[15] Other cells making up the epithelium include brush cells, serous cells, and Kulchitsky cells, all with uncertain function. The epithelium of the trachea rests on an unusually thick elastic basal lamina, beneath which is the submucosa. The submucosa varies in thickness, with the thinnest portion on the inner surface of the cartilage and the thicker, more loosely organized portion present on the muscular wall. This layer contains submucosal glands, blood vessels, nerves, and a plexus of lymphatics. The mucosa and submucosa are supported by a fibrous coat containing cartilage and smooth muscle. The dorsal membranous wall is fibromuscular, containing the only smooth muscle associated with the trachea; the trachea is unlike other areas of the respiratory tree, where smooth muscle is present in a helical arrangement about the airways.

Bronchi

At its termination, the trachea divides into the right and left principal bronchi. The right bronchus is shorter in length and deviates less from the axis of the trachea than does the left. This explains why foreign objects entering the trachea more often lodge in the right bronchus or one of its branches.[19, 29] The right bronchus is 12 to 16 mm. in diameter; the left, 10 to 14 mm. The combined cross-sectional area of the two main bronchi exceeds that of the trachea.

Within a primary lobe, the secondary bronchus soon divides into tertiary branches, which are remarkably constant in number and distribution. The segment of a lobe, aerated by a tertiary bronchus, is usually well delineated from adjoining segments by nearly complete planes of connective tissue. Knowledge of segmental anatomy is of great practical importance in radiology, bronchoscopy, and pulmonary surgery. Through the painstaking anatomic studies of Jackson and Huber[24, 25] and others, the description of the segments of the pulmonary lobes has been completed (Fig. 51–2). Each segment is identified by its position in the lobe of the lung, and the corresponding segmental bronchus is named for the

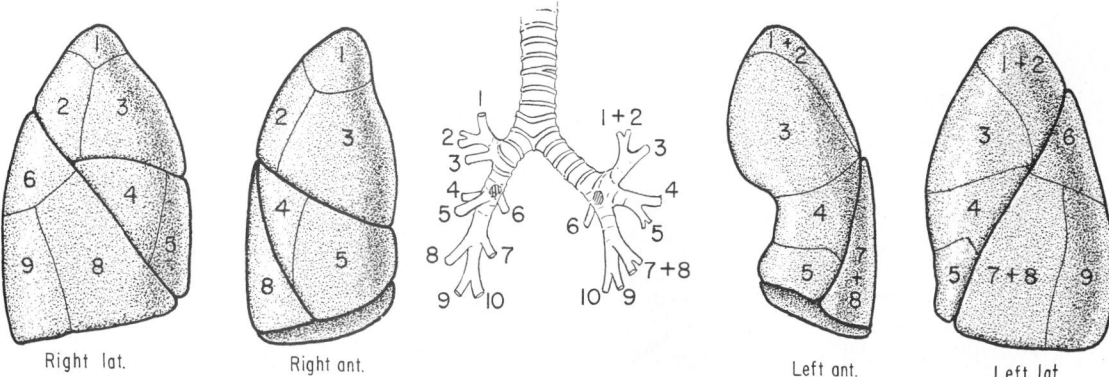

Figure 51-2. Segments of the pulmonary lobes. See Figure 51-3 for key to numbers. (Modified from Jackson, C. L., and Huber, J. F.: Correlated applied anatomy of the bronchial tree and lungs with a system of nomenclature. Dis. Chest, *9*:319, 1943.)

segment that it supplies (Fig. 51-3). A lobar abnormality, the azygos lobe, is illustrated in Figure 51-4. During fetal development, the precursor of the azygos vein, the posterior cardinal vein, penetrates the right upper lobe, drawing with it four layers of pleura. This action traps a part of the right upper lobe between the fissure and the mediastinum, creating the azygos lobe. It is ventilated by the apical or posterior segmental bronchus of the right upper lobe and is perfused by a corresponding pulmonary artery. According to one series, the azygos lobe occurs in 0.7% of normal individuals.[45]

In the human lung, bronchial branches usually arise from bifurcations, and although the resulting branches are smaller than the parent stem, their cross-sectional area is always greater by approximately six fifths. Structurally, large bronchi do not differ markedly from the trachea. Medium bronchi are distinguished by the large plates of cartilage, by the musculature, and by their relative abundance of glands. The most peripheral airways containing cartilage are the terminal bronchi. The smaller bronchi have fewer glands and are distinguished by rich venous plexuses between the muscular and cartilaginous fibrous layers. Bronchial muscle contraction probably has an important role in propelling venous and lymphatic drainage toward the hilus of the lung. These rich venous networks are also thought to be an important factor

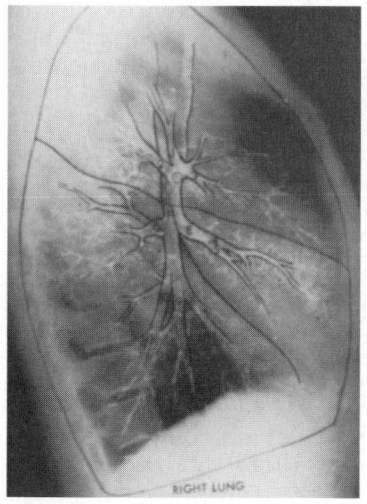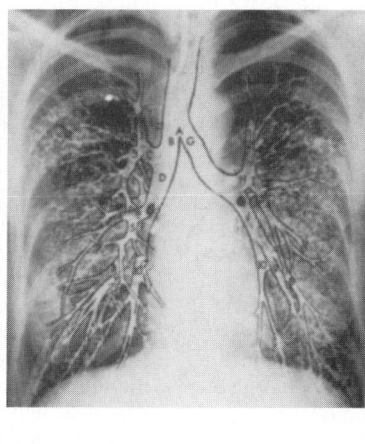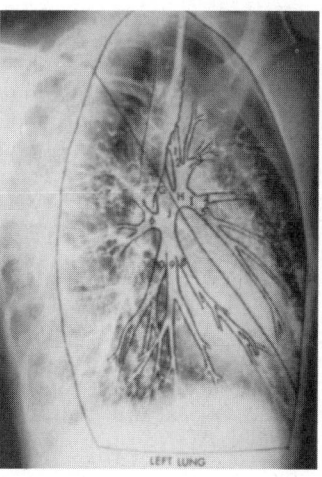

Figure 51-3. Normal bronchogram. The major bronchi are indicated by the letters; segmental bronchi are numbered. Key for Figures 51-2 and 51-3:

Right
1. Apical ⎫
2. Posterior ⎬ upper lobe
3. Anterior ⎭
4. Lateral ⎫ middle lobe
5. Medial ⎭
6. Superior ⎫
7. Medial (basal) RLL ⎪
8. Anterior basal ⎬ lower lobe
9. Lateral basal ⎪
10. Posterior basal ⎭

A. Carina
B. R. main stem bronchus
C. RUL bronchus
D. Bronchus intermedius
E. RLM bronchus

Left
1-2. Apical posterior ⎫
3. Anterior ⎬ upper lobe
4. Superior of lingula ⎪
5. Inferior of lingula ⎭
6. Superior ⎫
7. ⎪
8. Anterior-medial basal ⎬ lower lobe
9. Lateral basal ⎪
10. Posterior basal ⎭

F. RLL bronchus
G. L main stem bronchus
H. LUL bronchus
I. Lingula bronchus
J. LLL bronchus

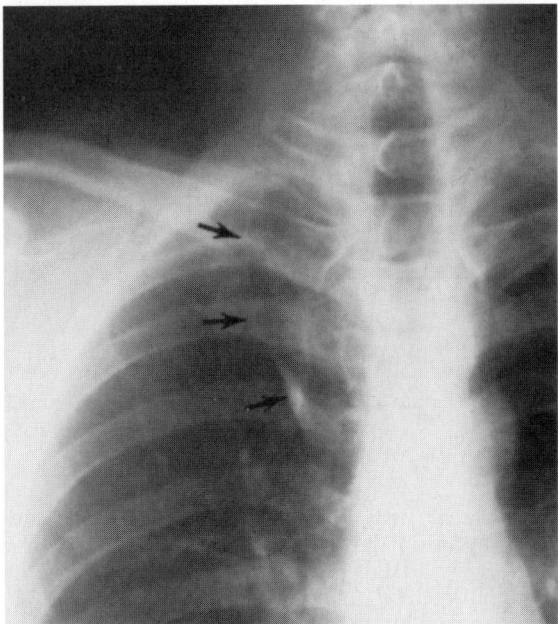

Figure 51–4. This posteroanterior chest film is normal except for the appearance of an azygos lobe, indicated by the arrow marking the course of the vein. The remaining lobar anatomy in this patient is normal. (From Weibel, E. R.: Is the lung built reasonably? Am. Rev. Respir. Dis., *128*:752, 1983.)

in the warming of air en route to the pulmonary parenchyma (Fig. 51–5).[29]

The epithelium of the bronchi, like that of the trachea, contains stratified ciliated columnar cells, basal cells, and goblet cells.[20] This epithelium rests on a basement membrane, which is surrounded by a richly vascular and fibrous lamina propria. Bronchial glands present within the submucosa secrete approximately 40 times as much mucus as do the goblet cells.[3] Peribronchial tissue consists of connective tissue that extends from the pulmonary hilus to the primary bronchioles. The peribronchium is continuous with the connective tissue investment of the arterial partners of the bronchi and the connective tissue sheath of the large veins. These connections form the basis for understanding the location and spread of certain types of edema and inflammation, as well as the paths followed by air in and about the lung in interstitial emphysema. Interestingly, the peribronchium occupies a space in which subatmospheric pressure prevails. Von Hayek[21] believes that this subatmospheric pressure has an

important role in the flow of venous blood, lymph, and alveolar fluid, as well as in the migration of inhaled particulate matter.

Ciliated, Goblet, and Brush Cells

It has been demonstrated that each cilium-bearing cell has approximately 270 cilia. Each cilium originates in a basal corpuscle just beneath the cell surface and measures approximately 0.5 μ. in length and 0.14 μ. in diameter. The cilium is round on cross section and contains a pair of separate central filaments and a peripheral ring of nine paired, closely branched filaments. Cilia are phylogenetically ancient structures. All cilia, whether in the plant or the animal kingdom, have the same basic structure.[27, 29, 48]

Although the many thousands of cilia present within the epithelium are borne by separate cells, they beat in an organized, coordinated manner. Studies have shown that they beat in a whiplike manner, the cycle of activity being divided into a rapid forward propulsive stroke and a slower recovery stroke.[27, 29, 48] This propulsion is effective in moving a superimposed carpet of mucus along with a variable number of trapped particles and cells upward toward the larynx. The rate at which particulate matter is propelled by cilia varies according to species and according to the portion of the respiratory tree involved and has been recorded at approximately 10 to 35 mm. per minute. The cilia do not beat within the viscous sheet of mucus but are bathed instead in fluid of considerably lower viscosity. The source of the fluid, factors controlling its viscosity, and the rate of production are not known.[27, 38, 46] The ciliated cells disappear gradually as respiratory bronchioles are approached.

The nonciliated cells are the goblet and brush cells. Goblet cells occur singly and in groups between the ciliated epithelial cells. When filled with secretion, they are conspicuous by their bulging walls. In cases of chronic irritation of the tracheobronchial mucosa, there is a marked increase in goblet cells at the expense of ciliated cells. It has been suggested that when mucus laden with particles of carcinogenic material has been carried to the branching point of an airway, there may be a temporary stasis at that site, owing to the local paucity of cilia.[29]

The brush cells are thin columnar cells with microvilli projecting into the lumen of the airway. Electron photomicrographs have demonstrated dovetailed cytoplasmic processes originating from their sides, which interlock with neighboring goblet cells. This arrangement may serve to add mechanical stability to the epithelial sheet. Other studies have demonstrated nerve endings associated with brush cells, leading to the theory that these cells may function as sensory receptors. Whether the brush cells are sensory cells or sustentacular in function is not known.[29, 47]

Bronchioles

Bronchioles are said to have a diameter of 1 mm. or less and to be devoid of cartilaginous support. Of all the airways, bronchioles have the highest proportion of smooth muscle in their walls relative to the diameter of the lumen. Small bronchi are also without connective tissue sheaths; therefore, the fibrous strands of the fibrocartilagines must extend peripherally into the mucous membrane of the bronchiole. These fibrous elements intermingle freely with the surrounding pulmonary parenchyma; therefore, the extent of inflation of surrounding pulmonary parenchyma determines the patency of the bronchiole.

The epithelium of the first-order bronchioles is composed of ciliated columnar cells and goblet cells. However, as the bronchi continue to divide, this epithelium is gradually re-

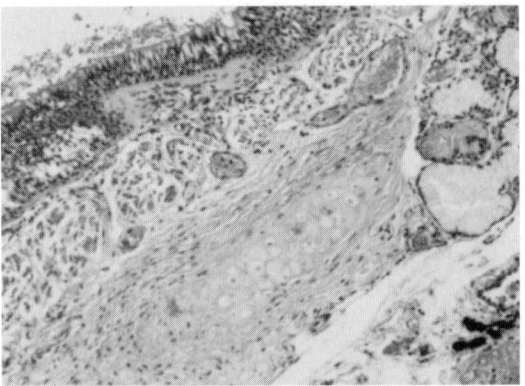

Figure 51–5. Section of a small bronchus. Note the prominence of the muscle layer, as compared with trachea and bronchi, and the rich vascular network between the muscular and cartilaginous fibrous layer. Magnification, ×100.

placed by Clara cells. These cells are columnar cells with a rounded, protruding apical cytoplasm, which on electron microscopic studies contains dense core granules and abundant smooth endoplasmic reticulum.[26, 56] The function of these cells is unknown, but they are believed to secrete a carbohydrate component of surfactant and an antiprotease.[57] In addition, they are capable of differentiating into mucous and ciliated cells.[26] As the bronchioles continue to divide, the Clara cells within the epithelium are replaced by a cuboidal epithelium. The last to be lined by this epithelium is the terminal bronchiole. Estimates of the number of terminal bronchioles from a single bronchus vary between 10 and 20 (Fig. 51–6).

A terminal bronchiole usually divides at an angle of 60 to 90 degrees into respiratory bronchioles, which may give rise to further divisions. The branching of the terminal bronchiole is not uniform: a single branch may be given laterally, and two or more may follow (Fig. 51–7). Respiratory bronchioles also vary in size (in humans ranging from 1 to 3.5 mm. in length and approximately 1.5 mm. in diameter). The cuboidal epithelium of the terminal bronchiole stops abruptly at the entrance of the alveoli, which are lined by extremely thin squamous epithelium that conventional light microscopes are unable to reveal. The last in a series of respiratory bronchioles usually bifurcates to produce the first in a series of alveolar ducts (Fig. 51–8).

Alveoli

The alveolar ducts terminate in one of several rotunda-like enclosures termed *alveolar sacs*. The sacs bear a small and variable number of terminal alveoli. Like the alveolar ducts, the sacs lack proper walls and open on all sides into alveoli. Each alveolus shares an entrance frame and a wall with its neighbor, similar to two rooms being separated by a single wall. Because the alveoli surrounding an alveolar duct are an integral part of the pulmonary parenchyma, they are subjected to all the stages of the respiratory cycle and to tractional forces that hold them open.

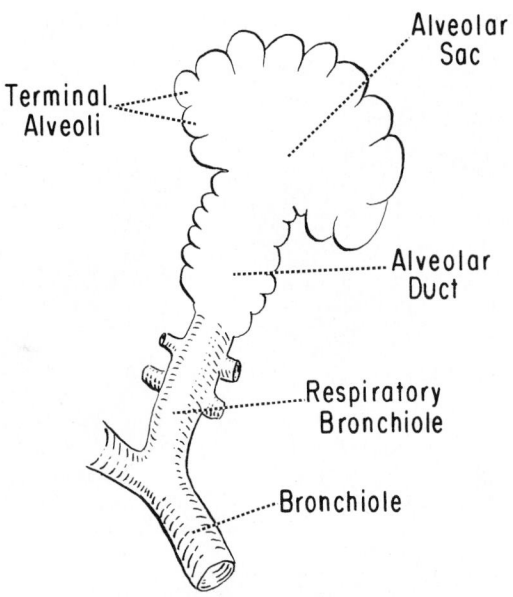

Figure 51–7. The relationship of the airway in the periphery of the respiratory tree. Bronchioles lead to the respiratory bronchioles, which then terminate in the alveolar duct and the alveolar sac.

Pulmonary alveoli vary considerably in shape and size among the various mammalian species, generally corresponding to body size. The determinants of the dimensions in specific species are not clearly understood but probably relate to a combination of factors, including the metabolic rate of the animal and the number and size of red blood cells. In humans, the alveoli are approximately 160 μ. in size (Fig. 51–9).[29] The number of alveoli present within two hu-

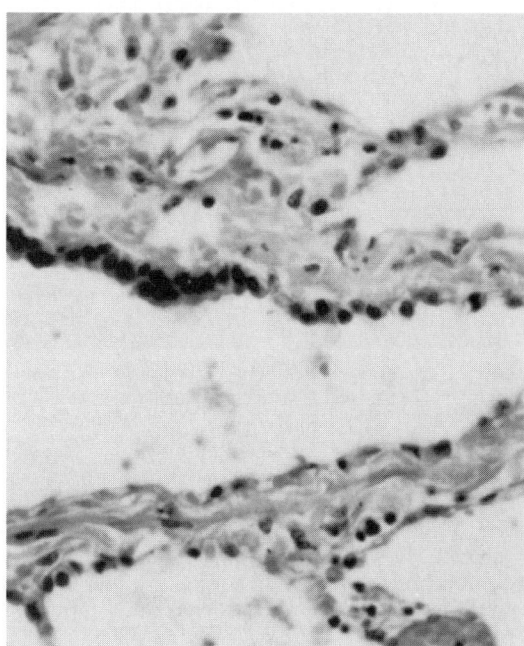

Figure 51–6. Section of a terminal bronchus, demonstrating the cuboidal epithelium, which grades off into a flat epithelium near the alveolar entrances. Also, a large amount of smooth muscle is evident. Magnification, ×400.

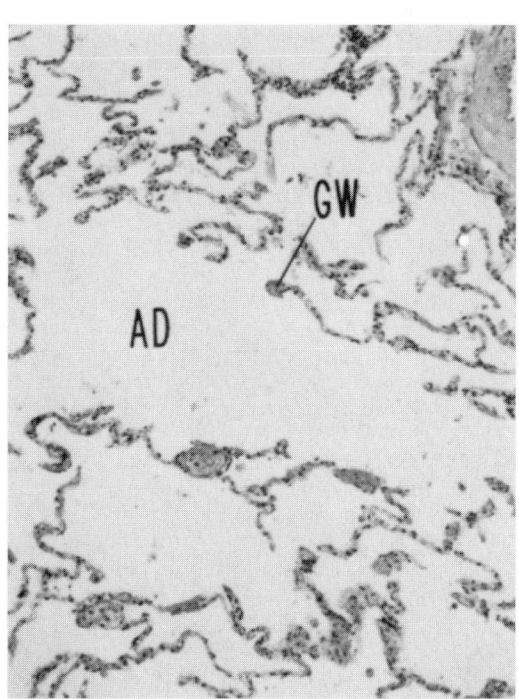

Figure 51–8. Section of lung demonstrating an alveolar duct (AD) with its contiguous alveoli. Note that the alveolar duct is not a structural entity in and of itself. Its walls are, in fact, alveolar septa. GW is a cross section of a collagen bundle. These bundles are important in maintaining patency of the alveolar ducts and the openings into the alveoli. They are analogous to guy wires.

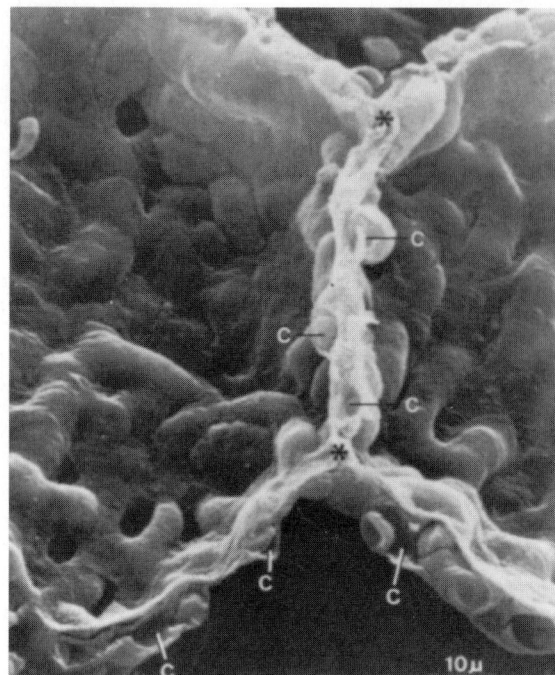

Figure 51–9. Scanning electron micrograph of *human lung* fixed near total lung capacity by instillation of fixative into the airways. Three alveolar septa and their triple junction line (*) are shown. Capillaries (C) alternate sides in the septal midplane marked by fibers. (From Weibel, E. R., and Bachoffen, H.: Structural design of the alveolar septum and fluid exchange. *In* Fishman, A. P., and Renkin, E. M. [Eds.]: Pulmonary Edema. American Physiological Society Clinical Physiology Series, 1979, pp. 1–20.)

man lungs has been estimated at 300 million, which provides a total area for gas exchange of approximately 140 m^2.[5]

Alveolar Epithelium

The alveolar epithelium is composed of two types of cells: the squamous alveolar cells (Type I) and the great alveolar cells (Type II). Type III alveolar cells are present in other mammals but have not yet been described in humans.[14] Type I alveolar cells constitute the overwhelming majority of the alveolar epithelial area (93% to 95% of the alveolar surface). These cells are extremely thin, with an average diameter of 0.2 μm., and serve as a protectant barrier between air and the alveolar septum.[15] Type II alveolar cells are cuboidal and occupy the remaining 5% to 7% of the alveolar surface. Type II alveolar cells are located at the junction of two alveolar septae, and they function to secrete pulmonary surfactant. The alveolar epithelium rests on a basement membrane, which is adjacent to the basement membrane of the alveolar capillary. A variable connective tissue layer separates these two basement membranes and composes the alveolar interstitium. The combination of this interstitium and the two basement membranes forms the alveolar septum. The air-blood barrier, therefore, is composed of the stratum of the alveolar epithelial cells, the alveolar basement membrane, the interstitium, the capillary basement membrane, and the alveolar capillary endothelium (Figs. 51–10 and 51–11).[5, 28, 36, 37, 44] The thickness of this barrier has been estimated as 0.57 to 1.25 μm.[55]

Both types of alveolar epithelial cells are known to be sensitive to the noxious fumes and foreign particles that may be carried by inspired air. Simple, rapid hypertrophy of the alveolar lining cell layer is possible and could be the source of the excessive cells found in alveolar cell carcinoma and in the lung disease of sheep, jaagsiekte.[21, 29, 40]

Although it was previously thought that alveolar epithelial cells were capable of undergoing metamorphosis into an alveolar phagocyte, recent DNA studies have clearly demonstrated that alveolar macrophages originate in the bone marrow and are carried to the alveolar interstitium as monocytes.[15] These monocytes, when activated, are transformed into alveolar macrophages, which then migrate into the alveolar lumen and serve as the primary phagocyte of the lung.

Alveolar Capillary Network

Pulmonary capillary networks are the richest in the body; they are so dense that openings in them are frequently

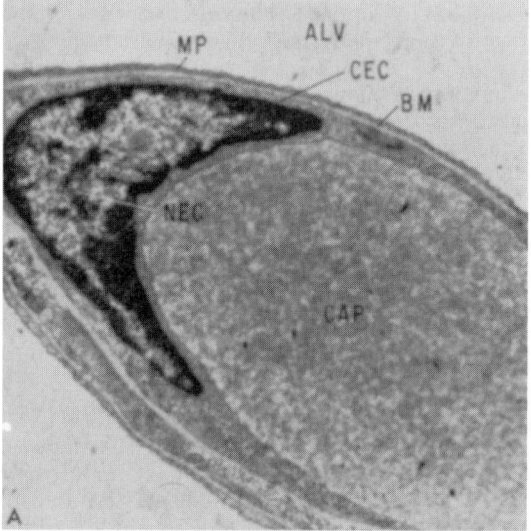

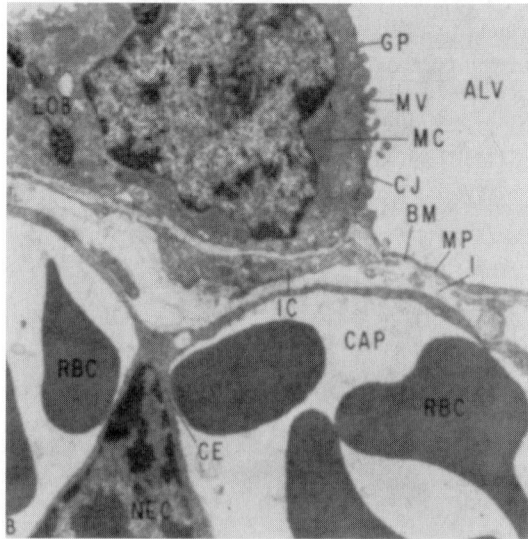

Figure 51–10. *A,* Electron photomicrograph of an alveolus. This demonstrates the structure of the thinnest part of the blood-air interface. Note that the blood is separated from the alveolar air only by the attenuated cytoplasm of an endothelial cell and a membranous pneumocyte joined by a basement membrane. Magnification, ×6700; print magnification, 13,725. *B,* Note the relationship of the granular pneumocyte to the alveolar wall. The granular pneumocyte is an integral part of the alveolar lining. This cell has been referred to as Type II cell, great alveolar cell, and alveolar phagocyte. It is thought to produce surfactant: the laminated osmiophilic bodies illustrated here may be surfactant or surfactant precursors. Magnification, ×6700; print magnification, 13,725. N, nucleus of granular pneumocyte; LO, laminated osmiophilic body (these cells are thought to be the site of surfactant production); GP, granular pneumocyte (sometimes called the alveolar Type II or the great alveolar cell); MV, microvilli; ALV, alveolus; MC, mitochondria; CJ, cell junction; BM, basement membrane; MP, membranous pneumocyte; I, interstitium; IC, interstitial cell; CAP, capillary; RBC, red blood cell; CE, capillary endothelium; NEC, nucleus of the endothelial cell; CEC, cytoplasm of the endothelial cell.

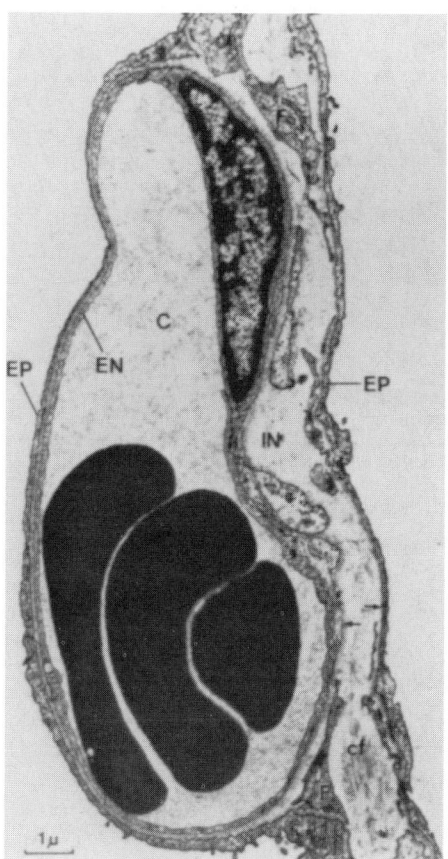

Figure 51–11. Transmission electron micrograph of the alveolar capillary (C) cross section from human lung. In the upper part of the air-blood barrier the basal laminae of epithelium (EP) and endothelium (EN) are fused, forming a restricted interstitial space; connective tissue fibers (cf) are found in the free interstitial space (IN) in the bottom part of the barrier, where the basal laminae (arrows) are separated. Note fibroblast processes (F) associated with fibers. (From Weibel, E. R., and Bachoffen, H.: Structural design of the alveolar septum and fluid exchange. *In* Fishman, A. P., and Renkin, E. M. [Eds.]: Pulmonary Edema. American Physiological Society Clinical Physiology Series, 1979, pp. 1–20.)

adapt longitudinally to surrounding parenchyma but cannot withdraw from it. The direct connection of the vein to adjacent lung tissue by connective tissue fibers is the anatomic device that makes its diameter largely dependent on lung volume. This arrangement provides the mechanism for promoting venous return in the special situation of the low-pressure pulmonary circuit.

Although blood from the rich pulmonary capillaries undoubtedly supplies the metabolic needs of the pulmonary parenchyma, the many servant tissues (conducting airways, pulmonary vessels, lymphoid tissue, and so forth) require their own circulation supplied by vessels derived from the systemic circulation, the bronchial arteries.

Leonardo da Vinci was perhaps the first to dissect the bronchial vessels. Deffebach recently reviewed the bronchial circulation, which has new importance with the resurgence of lung transplantation. The bronchials originate either directly from the aorta or indirectly via the intercostals. Bronchial arteries accompany the bronchial ramifications, eventually losing their identity along the respiratory bronchioles, where the capillaries that they supply drain into the alveolar capillary network and into the pulmonary veins (Fig. 51–16).

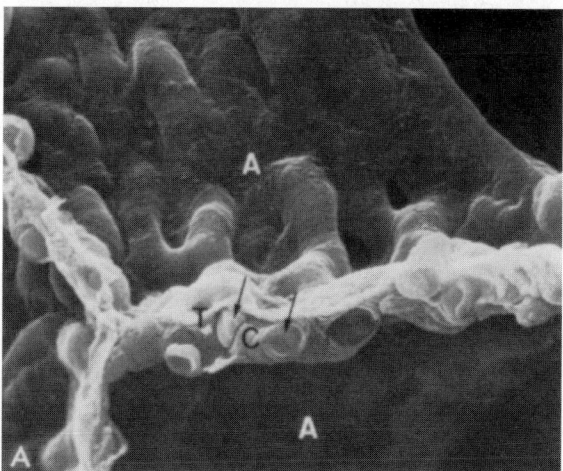

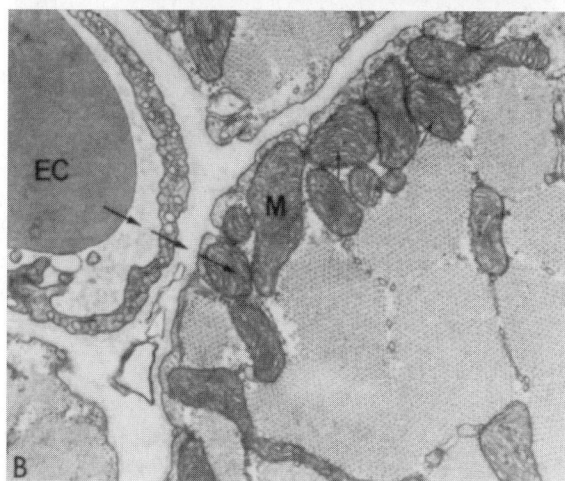

Figure 51–12. This figure demonstrates oxygen conductance in the lungs themselves. *A,* A scanning electron micrograph with gas exchanger of the human lungs consisting of capillary (C) between alveoli (A) with the blood separated from the air by a thin tissue barrier (T). *B,* The erythrocyte (EC) in the muscle capillary delivers oxygen to mitochondria (M) in the muscle cells. The oxygen transfer from the outside air is affected by convection in the pulmonary air spaces and in the bloodstream. Molecular diffusion is the process by which gas exchange occurs between air and blood and between blood and the cells. Finally, in the mitochondria, molecular oxygen disappears in water, the end product of oxidation.

smaller than the diameter of the capillaries. These capillary networks derive their principal support from the connective tissue that also supports the alveolus. Therefore, any disease state in which there is destruction of the alveolar wall and supporting framework, such as emphysema, would permit stretching, attenuation, and destruction of the entire capillary bed (Figs. 51–12 to 51–14).[33]

Pulmonary and Bronchial Vessels

The anatomy of pulmonary arteries and veins, particularly their relation to each other and to other structures of the pulmonary hilus, is of obvious importance in pulmonary surgery. Knowledge of the *anatomy* of the normal pulmonary angiogram is critical for recognition of pathologic conditions (Fig. 51–15).[7, 19, 49] The left main pulmonary artery is located above the left main bronchus, and the right is located slightly below the right main bronchus. Pulmonary arteries and their ramifications are invested in connective tissue sleeves, allowing continuous spatial adjustments to the changing position and volume of surrounding lung tissue. This permits marked dynamic changes in the arterial diameters without imposing direct mechanical change on lung tissue.

Pulmonary veins do not travel the same course as their arterial partners, as is the case in the systemic circulation. They course along interlobular connective tissue planes and

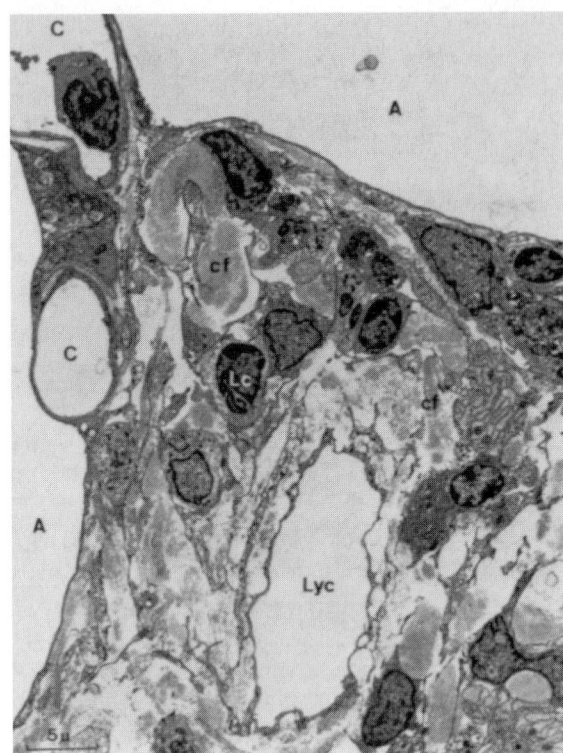

Figure 51–13. Juxta-alveolar fluid sump associated with connective tissue around small vessel from human lung. Note fluid-filled clefts among coarse fibers (cf) and free cells (Lc), as well a lymphatic capillary (Lyc) with irregular scalloped endothelial lining. (From Weibel, E. R., and Bachoffen, H.: Structural design of the alveolar septum and fluid exchange. *In* Fishman, A. P., and Renkin, E. M. [Eds.]: Pulmonary Edema. American Physiological Society Clinical Physiology Series, 1979, pp. 1–20.)

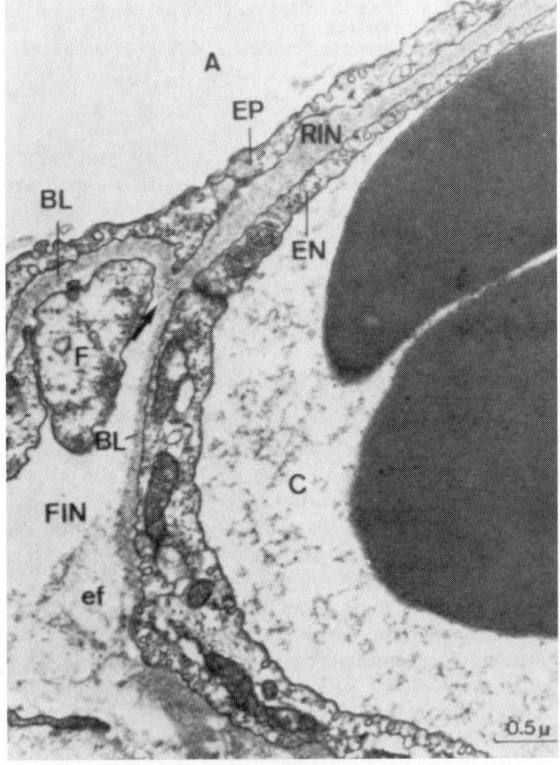

Figure 51–14. Higher-power view of air-blood barrier between an alveolus (A) and a capillary in human lung, showing transition (arrow) between free interstitial space (FIN) and restricted interstitium (RIN) due to fused basal laminae (BL) of epithelium (EP) and endothelium (EN). A small interstitial fluid pool is found between elastic fiber (ef) and fibroblast process (F). (From Weibel, E. R., and Bachoffen, H.: Structural design of the alveolar septum and fluid exchange. *In* Fishman, A. P., and Renkin, E. M. [Eds.]: Pulmonary Edema. American Physiological Society Clinical Physiology Series, 1979, pp. 1–20.)

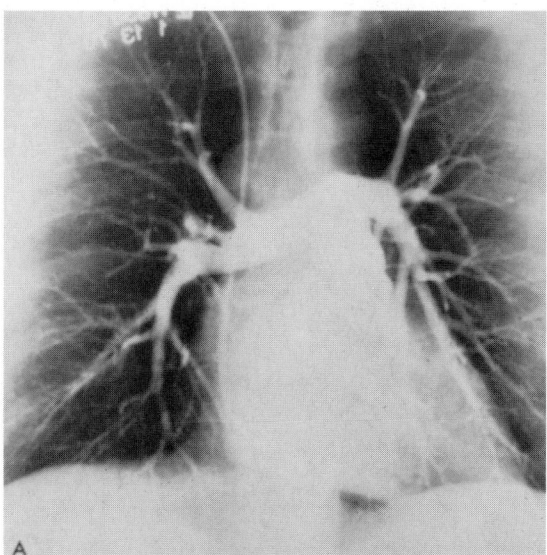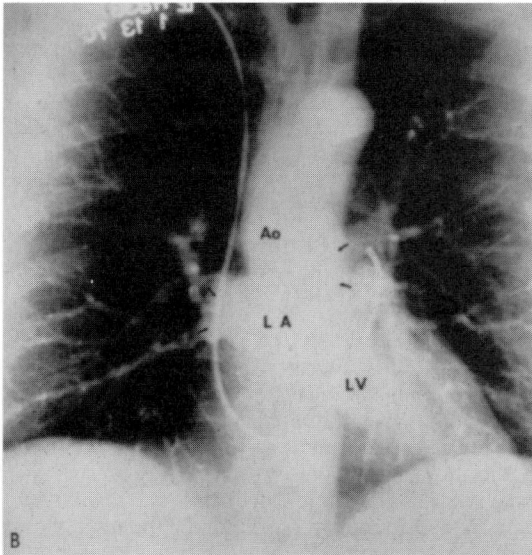

Figure 51–15. *A*, Normal pulmonary angiogram illustrating the branching of the pulmonary arteries in the right and left lungs to their respective lobes. *B*, Venous phase of the same arteriogram demonstrating the superior and inferior pulmonary veins entering the left atrium (arrows). Ao, aorta; LA, left atrium; LV, left ventricle.

There is no bronchial vein corresponding to the bronchial artery; however, there is a rich peribronchial venous network. The bronchial veins that drain the first several orders of bronchi empty into the azygos and hemiazygos system via mediastinal tributaries. The bronchial microvascular plexus serves as a link between the systemic and pulmonary veins in the periphery of the lung. Under normal conditions, most of the bronchial venous blood drains into the right side of the heart because of the orientation of the valves and the higher pressure in the left atrium as compared with the right. The pressure differences are slight, and if the valves become incompetent, flow can reverse. Although the bronchial veins are described, their presence in normal individuals has been questioned. In disease states such as pulmonary emphysema and mitral stenosis, however, these bronchial veins may appear as sizable vessels.[16, 33] In bronchiectasis, chronic obstructive pulmonary disease, or other conditions causing cor pulmonale, the bronchial venous plexus expands considerably, creating large shunts between systemic and pulmonary veins.[19]

Anatomic studies of pulmonary vascular anastomoses cover more than two centuries. In Weibel's studies,[54] it was concluded that pulmonary arteries and veins are end vessels and that there is no possibility for production of collateral circulation. He found no precapillary arteriovenous pulmonary anastomosis that might permit blood to bypass the alveolar capillary network. Extensive studies of pulmonary vasculature and its anastomotic connection have been made by von Hayek.[21] He described arterioarterial communications between pulmonary arteries and bronchial arteries, which are distinguishable by their remarkable thickness and unusual corkscrew course, in addition to the abundant longitudinal musculature. Nothing is known at present about their importance in the regulation of vascular perfusion in the lung.

Pulmonary Lymphatics

Pulmonary lymphatic vessels enter the hilar region in the second month of fetal life and continue to ramify and produce plexiform channels along the bronchi, pulmonary arteries, and veins, and within the subpleural connective tissue.[21, 29] According to Miller,[41] the lungs are more extensively supplied by lymphatics than the more metabolically active organs such as the liver and kidneys.

Studies by Tobin[50, 51] have demonstrated that pulmonary lymphatics extend as far as alveoli. In most instances, the distance between the alveolus and the nearest lymphatic is extremely small. In states of immunogenic stimulation, lymphoid aggregates may be found within the walls of the bronchi and bronchioles of humans, which are similar in appearance to intestinal Peyer's patches. These aggregates contain germinal centers and have been designated as bronchus-associated lymphoid tissue. Although normally in rabbits and other species, they are found in humans only after microbial stimulation.[4, 42] At the pulmonary hilus, the lymphatics, having gained both connective tissue and smooth muscle fibers, are relatively thick-walled and bear a histologic resemblance to the thoracic duct.

The lymph nodes collectively found along the lobar branches are termed *hilar nodes* and are included in the

Figure 51–16. Schematic of the systemic blood supply to the lung. Note that the flow from the extrapulmonary airways and supporting structures returns to the right heart, whereas intrapulmonary flow becomes anastomotic with the pulmonary circulation and returns to the left heart. (From Deffebach, M. E., Charan, N. B., Lakshminarayan, S., and Butler, J.: The bronchial circulation: Small but vital attribute of the lung. Am. Rev. Respir. Dis., *135*:463, 1987.)

greater group of nodes along the root of the lung. The tracheobronchial nodes are usually larger on the right. On the left, one or more nodes are commonly related to the ligamentum arteriosus, and thus to the recurrent laryngeal branch of the vagus nerve and to the vagal contributions to the anterior pulmonary plexus. Tracheal nodes form chains and are intimately related to the recurrent nerves.

Nerve Supply

Histologic studies and physiologic experiments have shown both afferent and efferent fibers in the nerves that follow the vessels and airways to the lung.[19, 29] Right and left vagus nerves send one or more bronchial branches to the smaller anterior pulmonary plexus and many others to the rich posterior pulmonary plexus dorsal to the pulmonary hilus. A great many ganglion cells are found scattered along the cervical and thoracic portions of the vagus nerves. Those in the cervical vagus are thought to be sensory, whereas the thoracic vagus is considered to be motor in function. Ganglion cells often lie adjacent to bronchial mucous glands and send short fibers with nonterminal twigs to cells of glandular epithelium.

Sympathetic nerves arise from the second to fourth thoracic sympathetic ganglia and join the vagi in formation of the pulmonary plexus. The clinical and experimental evidence points to the presence of sympathetic bronchodilator fibers having cells of origin in spinal cord levels T2 to T4.

In addition to the cholinergic and sympathetic nervous systems, a third system, termed the nonadrenergic and noncholinergic (NANC) system, has been described in the lung. This NANC system regulates airway smooth muscle tone through a variety of mediators, including nitric oxide, vasoactive intestinal polypeptide, and substance P.[2, 32, 34] It functions in both bronchoconstriction and dilation, and recent evidence suggests that an imbalance between these effects may play a role in asthma.[34]

The phrenic nerve, in addition to the usual fibers of origin in the third to fifth cervical nerves, has been found to receive various contributions from the cervical sympathetics. A number of afferent fibers from the diaphragm as well as the mediastinum also appear to ascend in the phrenic nerve (Fig. 51–17).

Collateral Ventilation

Airways less than 1 mm. in diameter (bronchioles) may be occluded secondary to a reduction of normal traction forces in the lungs by infection, inflammation, fluid accumulation, or secretions. The consequences of such occlusions may in some cases be offset by channels of collateral ventilation that form connections between well-aerated alveoli and those normally supplied by the occluded small airway. There are two principal mechanisms of collateral ventilation: interalveolar communications (pores of Kohn) and bronchial alveolar communications.

Alveolar pores are round to oval. Their shape and size are dictated by the delicate encirclements of elastic and other connective tissue fibers. As long as their fibrous framework is intact, the pores cannot enlarge beyond set limits. Alveolar pores may have the beneficial effect of preventing collapse of the lobules supplied by an occluded bronchiole. They may also serve as a temporary lodging place for alveolar phagocytes. Each communication may also provide pathways for the spread of fluid accumulations and for the transmission of bacteria between communicating pulmonary lobules.[22, 40, 52]

In the 1950s, Lambert[31] described short, epithelium-like communications between distant bronchioles and neigh-

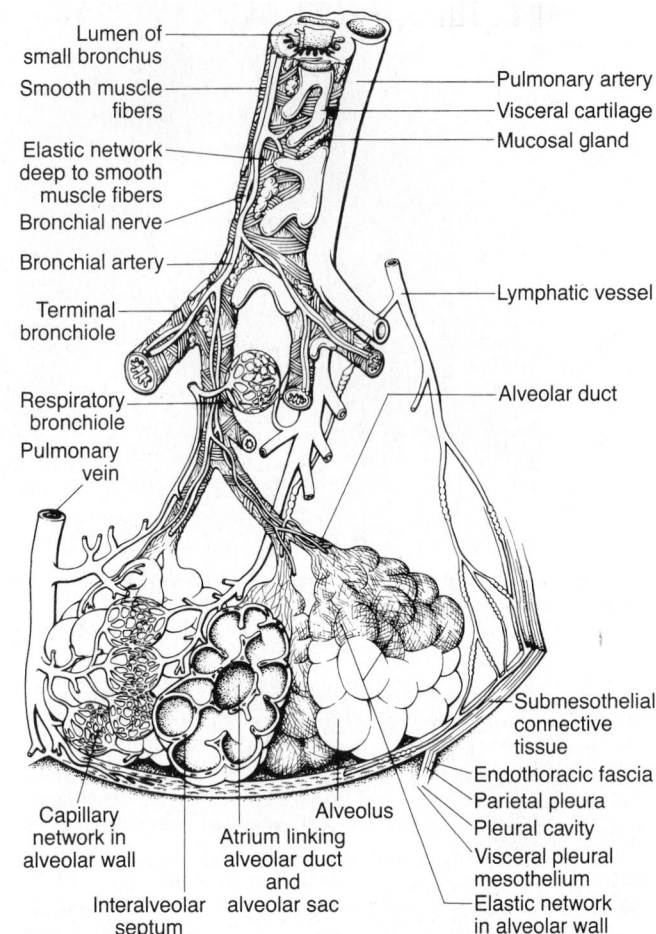

Figure 51–17. This illustration diagrammatically depicts and summarizes the interrelationships of all the anatomic structures involved in lung anatomy. (From Williams, P. L., Warwick, R., Dyson, M., and Bannister, L. H. [Eds.]: Gray's Anatomy, 37th ed. Edinburgh, Churchill Livingstone, 1989, p. 1279.)

boring alveoli. Such connections probably escaped earlier discovery because they are difficult or impossible to see in routine sections. They are approximately 30 µ. in diameter, thus three or more times the diameter of most interalveolar pores. These communications are evidently able to remain open regardless of the degree of contraction of the bronchiolar smooth muscle. The benefit of pores may be shared only by the immediately adjacent alveoli, whereas the bronchiole-alveolar communications provide means of aerating hundreds of alveoli.[31, 35, 52] Chen[10] has demonstrated the dynamic nature of the collateral ventilatory channels.

Radiographic Evaluation of Pulmonary Anatomy

The accurate preoperative evaluation of pulmonary anatomy is of critical importance for all surgical interventions involving the thorax. The chest roentgenogram remains the most widely used imaging modality for evaluation of the thorax; an anteroposterior view combined with a lateral view allows fairly accurate evaluation of most pathologic processes involving the pulmonary parenchyma. In clinical scenarios in which a more accurate evaluation of intrathoracic anatomy is required, computed tomography (CT) has become the procedure of choice. Routine CT employs contiguous collimated scans at 10-mm. intervals, whereas high-resolution CT employs 1.5- to 3-mm. scans. Used in combination or

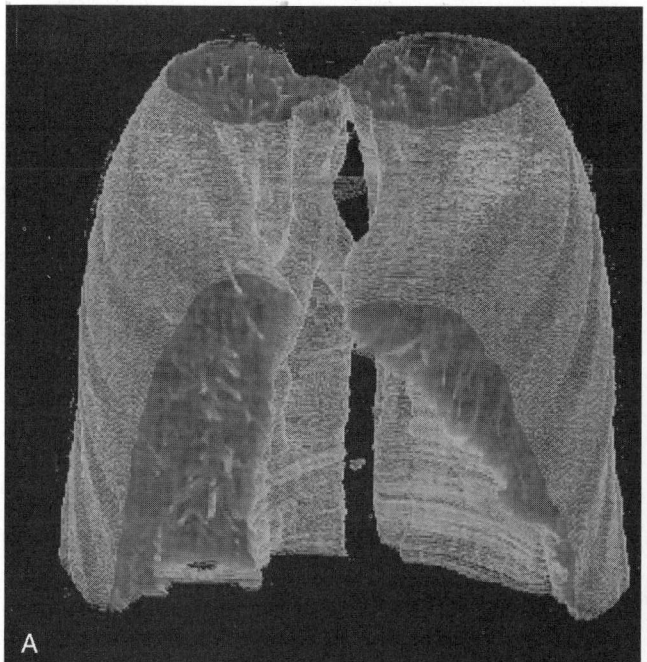

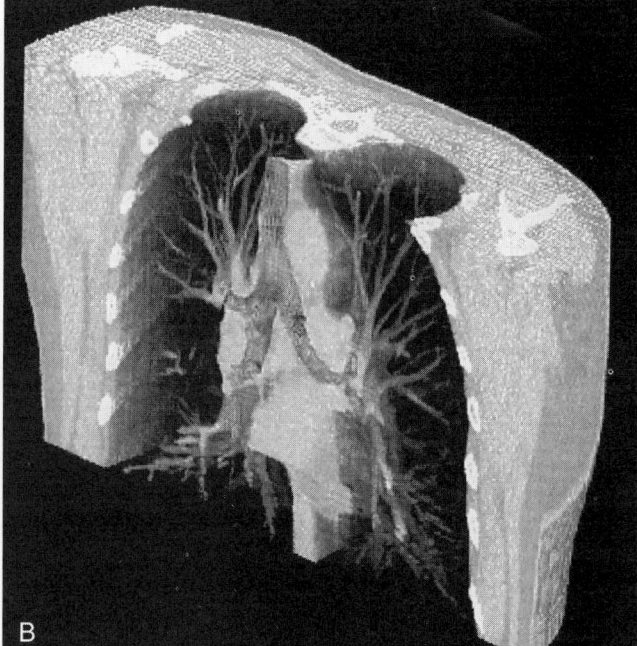

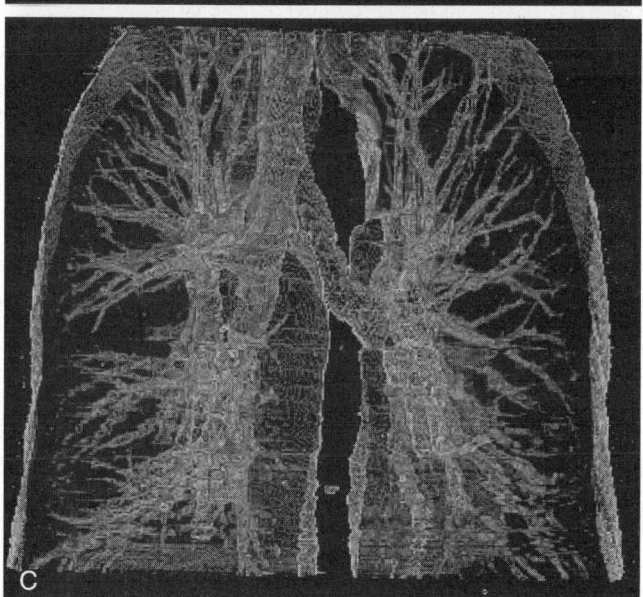

Figure 51–18. Helical computed tomographic data. *A, B,* Anterior views of the thorax demonstrating the spatial interrelationship between lung parenchyma and the chest wall. *C,* Anterior view of the thorax demonstrating normal bronchial anatomy. (*A* to *C* courtesy of G. A. Johnson, Ph.D., Department of Radiology, Duke University Medical Center, Durham, North Carolina.)

singly, these two tomographic modalities allow accurate localization of disease within the thorax; combined with an analysis of attenuation coefficients, they allow identification of various pathologic processes.[17, 53] Three-dimensional CT (Fig. 51–18) is a promising new modality for better localization of intrathoracic structures.

Evaluation of the pulmonary vascular anatomy is best accomplished using invasive pulmonary angiography. Radioisotope lung scanning, however, has proved to be a valuable adjunct, particularly in the evaluation of pulmonary embolism. Magnetic resonance imaging has recently gained popularity for the evaluation of the central pulmonary vessels and in many cases may obviate the need for invasive pulmonary angiography.[18]

SELECTED REFERENCES

Boyden, E. A.: Segmental Anatomy of the Lungs. New York, McGraw-Hill, 1955.
This excellent monograph not only reviews the historic development of the segmental anatomy of the lungs but also provides the groundwork for basic concepts of functional anatomy as it can be applied surgically and to the physiology of respiration.

Deffebach, M. E., Charan, N. B., Lakshminarayan, S., and Butler, J.: The bronchial circulation: Small, but a vital attribute of the lung. Am. Rev. Respir. Dis., *135*:463, 1987.
This article is clearly state-of-the-art, a comprehensive review of the structure and function of the bronchial circulation.

Galvin, J. R., Mori, M., and Stanford, W.: High-resolution computed tomography and diffuse lung disease. Curr. Probl. Diagn. Radiol., *21*:31, 1992.
This article combines a review of the basics of computed tomography with excellent illustrations in an examination of normal and pathologic lung anatomy.

Krahl, V. E.: Anatomy of the mammalian lung. *In* Fenn, W. O., and Rahn, H. (Eds.): American Physiological Society: Handbook of Physiology. Sec. 3, Respiration. Vol. 1. Baltimore, Williams & Wilkins, 1964, p. 213.
This chapter is one of the most complete treatises on the anatomy of the mammalian lung. It also contains more than 200 references, many of which are the original contributions that brought knowledge of the respiratory system to its present state.

Nagaishi, C.: Functional Anatomy and Histology of the Lung. Baltimore, University Park Press, 1972.
This magnificent volume combines studies of both the gross and the fine structures

of the lung. The author is a thoracic surgeon who clearly recognizes the importance of basic knowledge in understanding and approaching the many difficult clinical problems involving the pulmonary system.

Supplement: Comparative biology of the lung. Am. Rev. Respir. Dis., *128*, 1983.
This work reviews techniques in the study of gross, histologic, electron microscopic, and biochemical anatomy of the lung.

von Hayek, H.: The Human Lung. Trans. V. E. Krahl. New York, Hafner, 1960.
This monograph records the sophisticated anatomy of the respiratory system. It presents the concepts and findings in the functional anatomy of the lung and is one of the outstanding contributions to this field.

Webb, W. R.: High resolution lung computed tomography, normal anatomic and pathologic findings. Radiol. Clin. North Am., *29*:1051, 1991.
This is an excellent examination of computed tomography and anatomic correlates from a leader in the field.

Weibel, E. R.: Is the lung built reasonably? (The 1983 J. Burns Amberson Lecture). Am. Rev. Respir. Dis., *128*:752, 1983.
This article by a leader in the field makes the continuing research on the anatomy and function of the lung exciting.

Williams, P. L., Warwick, R., Dyson, M., and Bannister, L. H. (Eds.): Gray's Anatomy, 37th ed. Edinburgh, Churchill Livingstone, 1989.
This is the classic of anatomy books.

REFERENCES

1. Arey, L. B.: Developmental Anatomy, rev. 7th ed. Philadelphia, W. B. Saunders, 1974.
2. Barnes, P. J.: The third nervous system in the lung: Physiology and clinical perspectives. Thorax, *39*:561, 1984.
3. Baum, G. L., and Wolinsky, E. (Eds.): Textbook of Pulmonary Diseases, 5th ed. Boston, Little, Brown, 1994.
4. Bienenstock, M. R. C. P., Johnston, N., and Perey, D. Y. E.: Bronchial lymphoid tissue. I. Morphologic characteristics. Lab. Invest., *28*:686, 1973.
5. Blumenthal, B. J., and Boren, H. G.: Lung structure in three dimensions after inflation and fume fixation. Am. Rev. Tuberc., *79*:764, 1959.
6. Boyden, E. A.: Segmental Anatomy of the Lungs. New York, McGraw-Hill, 1955.
7. Boyden, E. A.: The nomenclature of the bronchopulmonary segments and their blood supply. Dis. Chest, *39*:1, 1961.
8. Brock, R. C.: The Anatomy of the Bronchial Tree with Special Reference to Surgery of Lung Abscess, 2nd ed. New York, Oxford University Press, 1954.
9. Brock, R. C.: The Anatomy of the Respiratory Tree. London, Oxford University Press, 1954.
10. Chen, C., Sealy, W. C., and Seaber, A. V.: The dynamic nature of collateral ventilation. J. Thorac. Cardiovasc. Surg., *59*:518, 1970.
11. Churchill, E. D., and Belsey, R.: Segmental pneumonectomy in bronchiectasis. Ann. Surg., *109*:481, 1939.
12. Cooper, J. D., Trulock, E. P., Patterson, G. A., Triantafillou, A., Sundaresan, R. S., Dresler, C. M., and Roper, C. L.: Bilateral pneumectomy (volume reduction) for chronic obstructive pulmonary disease. 74th annual meeting of the American Association for Thoracic Surgery, April 24–27, 1994.
13. Crelin, E. S.: Development of the respiratory system. Clin. Symp., *27*:3, 1975.
14. Dormans, J. A. M. A.: The alveolar type III cell. Lung, *163*:327, 1985.
15. Fawcett, D. W. (Ed.): Bloom and Fawcett: A Textbook of Histology, 12th ed. New York, Chapman & Hill, 1994.
16. Ferguson, F. C., Kobilak, R. E., and Detrick, J. E.: Varices of the bronchial veins as a source of hemoptysis in mitral stenosis. Am. Heart J., *28*:445, 1944.
17. Galvin, J. R., Mori, M., and Stanford, W.: High-resolution computed tomography and diffuse lung disease. Curr. Probl. Diagn. Radiol., *21*:31, 1992.
18. Gefter, W. B., and Hatabu, H.: Evaluation of pulmonary vascular anatomy and blood flow by magnetic resonance. J. Thorac. Imaging, *8*:122, 1993.
19. Goss, C. M. (Ed.): Gray's Anatomy of the Human Body, 28th ed. Philadelphia, Lea & Febiger, 1966.
20. Ham, A. W., and Wilson, T. S.: The Respiratory System in Histology, 4th ed. Philadelphia, J. B. Lippincott, 1961.
21. von Hayek, H.: The Human Lung. Trans. V. E. Krahl. New York, Hafner, 1960.
22. Hesse, F. E., and Loosli, C. L.: The lining of the alveoli in mice, rats, dogs, and frogs following acute pulmonary edema produced by ANTU poisoning. Anat. Rec., *105*:229, 1949.
23. Hislop, A., and Reid, L.: Development of the acinus in the human lung. Thorax, *29*:90, 1974.
24. Huber, J. F.: Practical correlative anatomy of the bronchial tree and lungs. J. Natl. Med. Assoc., *41*:49, 1949.
25. Jackson, C. L., and Huber, J. F.: Correlated applied anatomy of the bronchial tree and lungs with a system of nomenclature. Dis. Chest, *9*:319, 1943.
26. Jeffery, P. K., Gaillard, D., and Moret, S.: Human airway secretory cells during development and in mature airway epithelium. Eur. Respir. J., *5*:93, 1992.
27. Kilburn, K. H.: A hypothesis for pulmonary clearance and its implications. Am. Rev. Respir. Dis., *98*:449, 1968.
28. King, D. W. (Ed.): Ultrastructural Aspects of Disease. New York, Hoeber Medical Division, Harper & Row, 1966.
29. Krahl, V. E.: Anatomy of the mammalian lung. *In* Fenn, W. O., and Rahn, H. (Eds.): American Physiological Society: Handbook of Physiology. Sec. 3, Respiration. Vol. 1. Baltimore, Williams & Wilkins, 1964, p. 213.
30. Kramer, R., and Glass, A.: Bronchoscopic localization of lung abscess. Ann. Otol., *41*:1210, 1932.
31. Lambert, M. W.: Accessory bronchial alveolar channels. Anat. Rec., *127*:472, 1957.
32. Lammers, J. W. J., Barnes, P. J., and Chung, K. F.: Nonadrenergic, noncholinergic airway inhibitory nerves. Eur. Respir. J., *5*:239, 1992.
33. Liebow, A. A.: Pulmonary emphysema with special reference to vascular changes. Am. Rev. Respir. Dis., *80*:67, 1959.
34. Linden, A., and Skoogh, B. E.: NANC responses—role in control of airway tone. Respir. Med., *88*:249, 1994.
35. Loosli, C. G.: Intra-alveolar communications in normal and in pathologic mammalian lungs. Arch. Pathol., *24*:743, 1937.
36. Low, F. N.: Electron microscopy of the rat lung. Anat. Rec., *113*:437, 1952.
37. Low, F. N.: The pulmonary alveolar epithelium of laboratory mammals and man. Anat. Rec., *117*:241, 1953.
38. Luchsinger, P. C., LaGarde, B., and Kilfeather, J. E.: Particle clearance from the tracheobronchial tree. Am. Rev. Respir. Dis., *97*:1046, 1968.
39. Macklin, C. C.: Alveolar pores and their significance in the human lung. Arch. Pathol., *21*:202, 1936.
40. Macklin, C. C.: The alveoli of the mammalian lung: An anatomical study with clinical correlations. Proc. Inst. Med. Chicago, *18*:78, 1950.
41. Miller, W. S.: The Lung, 2nd ed. Springfield, Ill., Charles C. Thomas, 1947.
42. Pabst, R., and Gehrke, I.: Is the bronchus-associated lymphoid tissue (BALT) an integral structure of the lung in normal mammals, including humans? Am. J. Respir. Cell Mol. Biol., *3*:131, 1990.
43. Perkins, J. F.: Historical development of respiratory physiology. *In* Fenn, W. O., and Rahn, H. (Eds.): American Physiological Society: Handbook of Physiology. Sec. 3, Respiration. Vol. 1. Baltimore, Williams & Wilkins, 1964, p. 62.
44. Porter, K., and Bonneville, M. A.: Fine Structure of Cells and Tissues. Philadelphia, Lea & Febiger, 1968.
45. Postmus, E. P., Kerstjens, J. M., Breed, A., and Jagt, E. V. D.: A family with lobus venae azygos. Chest, *90*:298, 1986.
46. Quinlan, M. F., Salman, S. D., Swift, D. L., Wagner, H. N., Jr., and Proctor, D. F.: Measurement of mucociliary function in man. Am. Rev. Respir. Dis., *99*:13, 1969.
47. Rhodin, J. A. G.: An Atlas of Ultrastructure. Philadelphia, W. B. Saunders, 1963.
48. Spock, A., Heick, H. M. C., Cress, H., and Logan, W. S.: Abnormal serum factor in patients with cystic fibrosis of the pancreas. Pediatr. Res., *1*:173, 1967.
49. Thorek, P.: Anatomy in Surgery. Philadelphia, J. B. Lippincott, 1962.
50. Tobin, C. E.: Lymphatics of the pulmonary alveoli. Anat. Rec., *120*:625, 1954.
51. Tobin, C. E.: Pulmonary lymphatics with reference to emphysema. Am. Rev. Respir. Dis., *80*:50, 1959.
52. Van Allen, C. M., and Lindskog, G. E.: Collateral respiration in the lung: Role in bronchial obstruction to prevent atelectasis and to restore patency. Surg. Gynecol. Obstet., *53*:16, 1931.
53. Webb, W. R.: High resolution lung computed tomography, normal anatomic and pathologic findings. Radiol. Clin. North Am., *29*:1051, 1991.
54. Weibel, E. R., and Gomez, D. M.: Architecture of the human lung. Science, *137*:577, 1962.
55. Weibel, E. R., and Knight, B. W.: A morphometric study on the thickness of the pulmonary air-blood barrier. J. Cell Biol., *21*:367, 1964.
56. Widdicombe, J. G., and Pack, R. J.: The Clara cell. Eur. J. Respir. Dis., *63*:202, 1982.
57. Willems, L. N. A., Kramps, J. A., Jeffery, P. K., and Dijkman, J. H.: Antileucoprotease in the developing fetal lung. Thorax, *43*:784, 1988.

II

CLINICAL AND PHYSIOLOGIC EVALUATION OF RESPIRATORY FUNCTION

Richard A. Hopkins, M.D., Walter G. Wolfe, M.D., and Farid Gharagozloo, M.D.

The evaluation and treatment of pulmonary dysfunction, whether related to chronic obstructive pulmonary disease (i.e., emphysema and bronchitis), pulmonary edema due to cardiac failure, or pulmonary insufficiency secondary to either a surgical procedure or traumatic injury, demands a careful history, a physical examination, and a complete physiologic evaluation. In an elective situation, these can be obtained prior to the operative procedure. However, when there is an acute emergency or traumatic injury, even during resuscitation of the patient, the necessary pulmonary history should be acquired from a family member. Environmental pollution, exposure to asbestos and toxic chemicals, and a pulmonary history of allergies, emphysema, and bronchitis are extremely important, together with the patient's history of personal pollution, that is, cigarette smoking (measured in pack-years).

MEASUREMENT OF PULMONARY FUNCTION

Air flows into the lungs because of differences in pressure.[90] Knowledge of these pressures—oral, airway, alveolar, and pleural—is important in the management of respiratory insufficiency. The act of breathing is complex, and disease affecting any part of the airway has an effect on ventilation and therefore on the patient's physiologic performance after operation or injury.[92]

Understanding the factors that contribute to and alter pulmonary ventilation and gas exchange requires a detailed knowledge of lung function at the alveolar level.[69, 77] Ventilation serves to replenish the gas in the lungs to maintain the high oxygen–low carbon dioxide pressure, producing maximal gradients. Distribution of gas is the delivery of air to the alveolar units by way of the bifurcating tracheobronchial tree. Diffusion is the transfer of gas molecules across the alveolar membranes in the region of high concentration. The blood-air surface of over 90 sq. m. in adults is condensed in a lung volume of only 5 liters. This is made possible by the small radius and the large number of alveoli (300 million). Perfusion is the means by which desaturated blood is brought into intimate contact with the alveolar-capillary bed.

The need to measure lung function is usually obvious from the clinical evaluation. Initial tests are performed to determine whether there is functional impairment. Later, the preoperative studies are used as a guide for determining whether the patient's condition has improved, is unchanged, or has deteriorated after illness or operation. When the history and physical examination do not suggest any evidence of lung disease, measurement of the vital capacity and forced expiratory volume in 1 second, combined with a normal chest film and normal blood gas determination, is sufficient to support the clinical impression that there is no underlying pulmonary disease. However, in patients with obvious or suspected lung disease, more detailed studies are necessary.[9, 26, 76]

Pulmonary Function Tests. Pulmonary function tests are divided into static volumes, flow rates, compliance, and resistance, along with the measurement of arterial blood gases.[1, 9, 26, 76] At times, diffusion capacity (DLCO), right-heart catheterization, and measurement of pulmonary diastolic pressure (PAD) are necessary, as well as a ventilation-perfusion lung scan for the evaluation of overall lung function.

The vital capacity (VC) permits detection of small changes in lung function (Fig. 51–19). However, variations among individuals are so great that VC is not a very sensitive method for detecting disease, although improvement or deterioration can be demonstrated by sequential measurements. Measurement of lung volumes allows the physician to determine physiologically an approximate index of the severity of changes or dysfunction and to document the changes from time to time (Tables 51–1 and 51–2).

Respiratory excursion is the amount of air inspired and expired; this is termed tidal volume (V_T). The amount of gas contained in the lung at the end of quiet expiration is termed the functional residual capacity (FRC). When the patient makes a maximal inspiration and increases the lung volume, compared with that contained at the peak V_T, the inspiratory reserve capacity or volume (IRV) is reached. With forcible expiration—exhaling as much air as possible from the lung—the volume expired from maximal inspiration to maximal expiration is the VC. The amount of air remaining in the lungs after maximal expiration is the residual volume (RV). All these lung volumes can be measured in the spirometer, except for the RV and the FRC. The FRC can be measured by three different methods: inert gas dilution and washout, whole body plethysmography, and radioisotope techniques.

The RV is calculated by subtracting the expiratory reserve volume (ERV) from the FRC, since the respiratory midposition is believed to be more reproducible than the forced expiratory position. When the FRC is measured by inert

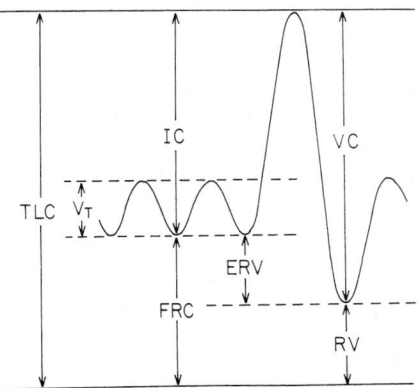

Figure 51–19. Spirometry. Subdivisions of lung volumes. TLC, total lung capacity; V_T, tidal volume; IC, inspiratory capacity; FRC, functional residual capacity, i.e., lung volume at end-expiration; ERV, expiratory reserve volume; RV, residual volume, i.e., lung volume after forced expiration from FRC; VC, vital capacity, i.e., the maximal volume of gas inspired from RV. For normal values in the adult, see Tables 51–1 and 51–2.

TABLE 51–1. Predicted Values for Pulmonary Function Tests: Men

Height (cm.)	Age (yr.)	VC	FRC	RV	TLC	FEV$_{0.75}$ X 40 (L./min.)	FEV$_{1.0}$ (L)	MMFR (L./sec.)	DLcoSS$_2$	Fico-Fexco / Fico	DLcoSB	ME%
155	20	3.97	2.72	1.13	5.10	136	3.6	4.3	23.8	0.56	26.7	70
	30	3.65	2.72	1.30	4.95	121	3.3	3.9	21.0	0.52	23.7	65
	40	3.35	2.72	1.45	4.80	106	3.0	3.5	18.2	0.49	20.7	60
	50	3.04	2.72	1.61	4.65	91	2.7	3.1	15.4	0.45	17.7	55
	60	2.73	2.72	1.77	4.50	76	2.4	2.7	12.6	0.42	14.7	50
	70	2.42	2.72	1.91	4.35	61	2.1	2.3	9.8	0.39	11.7	45
160	20	4.30	2.98	1.27	5.57	141	3.8	4.4	24.1	0.55	29.0	70
	30	4.00	2.98	1.42	5.42	126	3.5	4.0	21.3	0.52	26.0	65
	40	3.70	2.98	1.57	5.27	111	3.2	3.6	18.6	0.48	23.0	60
	50	3.40	2.98	1.72	5.12	96	2.8	3.2	15.8	0.45	20.0	55
	60	3.10	2.98	1.87	4.97	81	2.5	2.8	13.0	0.41	17.0	50
	70	2.80	2.98	2.02	4.82	65	2.2	2.4	10.1	0.39	14.0	45
165	20	4.62	3.23	1.42	6.04	145	3.9	4.5	24.5	0.55	31.3	70
	30	4.32	3.23	1.57	5.89	130	3.7	4.1	21.7	0.52	28.3	65
	40	4.02	3.23	1.72	5.74	115	3.3	3.7	18.9	0.48	25.3	60
	50	3.72	3.23	1.87	5.59	100	3.0	3.3	16.1	0.44	22.3	55
	60	3.42	3.23	2.02	5.44	85	2.7	2.9	13.3	0.42	19.3	50
	70	3.12	3.23	2.17	5.29	70	2.4	2.5	10.6	0.38	16.3	45
170	20	4.94	3.48	1.57	6.51	150	4.1	4.6	24.9	0.54	33.6	70
	30	4.64	3.48	1.72	6.36	135	3.8	4.2	22.1	0.50	30.6	65
	40	4.35	3.48	1.86	6.21	120	3.5	3.8	19.3	0.47	27.6	60
	50	4.05	3.48	2.01	6.06	105	3.2	3.4	16.5	0.43	24.6	55
	60	3.74	3.48	2.17	5.91	90	2.9	3.0	13.7	0.40	21.6	50
	70	3.44	3.48	2.32	5.76	75	2.6	2.6	10.9	0.37	18.6	45
175	20	5.26	3.74	1.72	6.98	155	4.3	4.7	25.2	0.53	35.8	70
	30	4.96	3.74	1.87	6.83	140	4.0	4.3	22.4	0.50	32.8	65
	40	4.66	3.74	2.02	6.68	124	3.7	3.9	19.6	0.47	29.9	60
	50	4.36	3.74	2.17	6.53	110	3.4	3.5	16.9	0.43	26.9	55
	60	4.06	3.74	2.32	6.38	94	3.1	3.1	14.1	0.39	23.9	50
	70	3.76	3.74	2.47	6.23	79	2.8	2.7	11.3	0.36	20.9	45
180	20	5.58	3.99	1.87	7.45	159	4.5	4.8	25.6	0.52	38.1	70
	30	5.28	3.99	2.02	7.30	145	4.2	4.4	22.8	0.49	35.1	65
	40	4.98	3.99	2.17	7.15	129	3.9	4.0	20.0	0.46	32.1	60
	50	4.68	3.99	2.32	7.00	114	3.6	3.6	17.2	0.42	29.2	55
	60	4.38	3.99	2.47	6.85	99	3.3	3.2	14.2	0.39	26.2	50
	70	4.08	3.99	2.62	6.70	83	2.9	2.8	11.6	0.35	23.2	45

Subdivisions of lung volume measured in seated subjects.
Ventilatory tests performed with subjects standing.
Diffusion capacity tests performed on seated subjects.

MMFR, maximal midexpiratory flow rate; DLcoSS$_2$, diffusion capacity, steady-state carbon monoxide uptake with alveolar carbon monoxide measured from an end-tidal sample of gas; VC, vital capacity; FRC, functional residual capacity; RV, residual volume; TLC, total lung capacity; FEV$_{0.75}$, forced expiratory volume at 0.75 sec. (the FEV$_{0.75}$ multiplied by 40 gives an approximate indication of the maximal breathing capacity in L/min.); FEV$_{1.0}$, forced expiratory volume at 1 sec.; Fico-Fexco/Fico, fractional uptake of carbon monoxide where Fico equals the inspired and Fexco equals the expired fraction of carbon monoxide; DLcoSB, diffusion capacity, single-breath method using helium and carbon monoxide, modified Krogh technique; ME%, closed-circuit helium index, measure of FRC.

From Bates, D. V., Macklem, P. T., Christie, R. V.: Respiratory Function in Disease, 2nd ed. Philadelphia, W. B. Saunders, 1971.

methods, helium or nitrogen is used. When helium is used, the patient rebreathes his own concentration of helium until it reaches a constant level (it equilibrates within the lung and spirometer). When nitrogen washout is performed to calculate the FRC, the patient breathes 100% oxygen. These two methods measure the residual volume of alveolar units in communication with an airway. The poorly ventilated units may be included in the overall calculation if helium equilibration and nitrogen washout are measured for sufficient periods of time. Although 7 minutes is usually sufficient when using nitrogen washout, more than 15 minutes may be necessary for patients with emphysema.

Body plethysmography measures all the gas in the lung and does not depend on communication with the airways. The volume is poorly termed thoracic gas volume (TGV), and the difference between TGV and the FRC measured by dilution techniques is an index of maldistribution of ventilation. The discrepancy between TGV and FRC is particularly striking in patients with bullous disease.

Boyle's law states that the product of the pressure and the volume of gas is constant for the same temperature. The patient is placed within a body plethysmograph, and the pressures within the plethysmograph and the mouth are measured. Any changes in the thoracic volume produce a reciprocal change in the plethysmograph volume, which changes the plethysmograph pressure. Thus, an increase in the thoracic volume decreases plethysmograph volume and increases plethysmograph pressure. At the end of quiet expiration, the airway is occluded by an electrically operated shutter, and the patient is asked to continue panting against the obstructed airway. Because gas does not flow during obstruction, the mouth pressure is assumed to be equal to alveolar pressure, and the increase is determined from the rise in the plethysmograph pressure.

Maximal Breathing Capacity. Maximal breathing capacity (MBC) is the largest volume of air that can be moved in and out of the chest per minute. The term *MBC* is reserved for the maximal breathing capacity of an individual, whereas

TABLE 51–2. Predicted Values for Pulmonary Function Tests: Women

Height (cm.)	Age (yr.)	VC	FRC	RV	TLC	$FEV_{0.75} \times 40$ (L./min.)	$FEV_{1.0}$ (L)	MMFR (L./sec.)	$DLCOSS_2$	FICO-FEXCO FICO	DLCOSB	ME%
145	20	2.81	1.96	1.00	3.81	88	2.6	3.6	20.7	0.58	19.5	70
	30	2.63	1.96	1.08	3.71	80	2.4	3.3	18.2	0.55	16.9	65
	40	2.45	1.96	1.16	3.61	72	2.1	2.9	15.7	0.51	14.2	60
	50	2.27	1.96	1.24	3.51	64	1.9	2.5	13.2	0.48	11.7	55
	60	2.09	1.96	1.32	3.41	56	1.5	2.2	10.7	0.44	9.0	50
	70	1.91	1.96	1.40	3.31	48	1.4	1.8	8.2	0.41	6.4	45
150	20	3.08	2.20	1.05	4.13	92	2.7	3.7	21.1	0.57	21.7	70
	30	2.89	2.20	1.14	4.03	84	2.5	3.3	18.6	0.54	19.1	65
	40	2.71	2.20	1.22	3.93	76	2.2	3.0	16.0	0.51	16.4	60
	50	2.53	2.20	1.30	3.83	67	2.0	2.6	13.5	0.47	13.7	55
	60	2.35	2.20	1.38	3.73	60	1.6	2.3	11.0	0.43	11.1	50
	70	2.17	2.20	1.46	3.63	52	1.5	1.9	8.5	0.40	8.5	45
155	20	3.34	2.43	1.19	4.53	95	2.8	3.8	21.5	0.56	23.9	70
	30	3.15	2.43	1.28	4.43	88	2.6	3.4	18.9	0.52	21.2	65
	40	2.97	2.43	1.36	4.33	79	2.4	3.1	16.4	0.49	18.5	60
	50	2.79	2.43	1.44	4.23	71	2.1	2.7	13.9	0.45	15.8	55
	60	2.61	2.43	1.52	4.13	63	1.7	2.3	11.4	0.42	13.1	50
	70	2.43	2.43	1.60	4.03	55	1.6	2.0	8.9	0.39	10.5	45
160	20	3.60	2.67	1.32	4.92	99	2.9	3.9	21.9	0.55	26.0	70
	30	3.41	2.67	1.41	4.82	91	2.7	3.5	19.4	0.52	23.3	65
	40	3.22	2.67	1.50	4.72	83	2.5	3.2	16.8	0.48	20.6	60
	50	3.05	2.67	1.57	4.62	75	2.2	2.8	14.3	0.45	17.9	55
	60	2.87	2.67	1.65	4.52	67	1.8	2.4	11.8	0.41	15.2	50
	70	2.69	2.67	1.73	4.42	59	1.7	2.1	9.2	0.39	12.5	45
165	20	3.88	2.90	1.44	5.32	103	3.1	4.0	22.2	0.55	28.1	70
	30	3.68	2.90	1.54	5.22	95	2.8	3.6	19.7	0.52	25.4	65
	40	3.50	2.90	1.62	5.12	87	2.6	3.3	17.2	0.48	22.7	60
	50	3.32	2.90	1.70	5.02	79	2.3	2.9	14.6	0.44	20.0	55
	60	3.14	2.90	1.78	4.92	71	1.9	2.5	12.1	0.42	17.3	50
	70	2.96	2.90	1.86	4.82	63	1.8	2.2	9.6	0.38	14.6	45
170	20	4.13	3.14	1.58	5.71	107	3.2	4.1	22.6	0.54	30.3	70
	30	3.94	3.14	1.67	5.61	99	2.9	3.7	20.1	0.50	27.6	65
	40	3.76	3.14	1.75	5.51	90	2.7	3.3	17.5	0.47	24.9	60
	50	3.58	3.14	1.83	5.41	82	2.4	3.0	15.0	0.43	22.2	55
	60	3.40	3.14	1.91	5.31	74	2.0	2.6	12.5	0.40	19.5	50
	70	3.22	3.14	1.99	5.21	66	1.9	2.3	9.9	0.37	16.8	45
175	20	4.38	3.37	1.80	6.18	111	3.3	4.1	22.7	0.53	32.3	70
	30	4.20	3.37	1.90	6.10	102	3.0	3.8	20.0	0.50	29.6	65
	40	4.02	3.37	2.00	6.02	94	2.8	3.4	17.7	0.47	26.9	60
	50	3.84	3.37	2.10	5.94	86	2.5	3.1	15.2	0.43	24.2	55
	60	3.66	3.37	2.20	5.86	78	2.1	2.7	12.7	0.38	21.5	50
	70	3.38	3.37	2.40	5.78	70	2.0	2.3	10.2	0.36	18.8	45

Subdivisions of lung volume measured in seated subjects.
Ventilatory tests performed with subjects standing.
Diffusion capacity tests performed on seated subjects.
For abbreviations, see Table 51–1.
From Bates, D. V., Macklem, P. T., Christie, R. V.: Respiratory Function in Disease, 2nd ed. Philadelphia, W. B. Saunders, 1971.

the term *maximal voluntary ventilation (MVV)* indicates the maximal volume of gas breathed per minute under testing conditions. The analysis of VC and MBC permits differentiation of ventilatory abnormality, such as obstructive versus restrictive disease, since MBC is markedly decreased in obstructive disease.

Specific Abnormalities of Lung Volume. In restrictive disease, the total lung capacity (TLC) and VC are small; in obstructive disease uncomplicated by fibrosis, the RV is large. In emphysema, the FRC and TLC are increased, but the VC may be equal to or less than normal. Certain restrictive diseases may decrease FRC; these include muscular weaknesses, pulmonary granulomatosis, heart failure, and mixed restriction and obstruction. A patient with kyphoscoliosis typically has a small FRC. Obstructive diseases such as mod-

erate asthma and acute bronchitis do not cause marked increases in FRC.[8, 68]

Patients with chronic emphysema and lung cysts have an increase in FRC. The ratio of RV to TLC is increased in emphysema but may also be increased in restrictive disease. Therefore, this ratio is of no value without simultaneous measurement of absolute figures for RV and TLC.

Flow Rates. Measurements of dynamic properties of the lungs, such as flow rates, are extremely important. The patient inhales maximally and then exhales forcibly into a spirometer while the device records the volume versus the time. A common test of maximal expiratory airflow is the volume of air expired in 1 second (FEV_1). This number is decreased in the presence of bronchial obstruction, but the value may also be decreased in restrictive disease. For this reason, the

FEV$_1$ is usually related to the total exhaled vital capacity. This ratio of FEV$_1$ to VC may be decreased in the presence of airway obstruction but normal in restrictive lung disease.

Diffusion of Gas. A single-breath carbon monoxide diffusion capacity (DLCO) measurement should be considered a screening test. In this test, the patient is required to inhale low, nontoxic concentrations of carbon monoxide, hold the breath for 10 seconds, and then exhale. This test is rapid, simple, safe, and painless. DLCO is an estimate of the pulmonary capillary surface area.[24]

There are several factors that affect diffusion in a single alveolus. The thickness of the alveolar lining membrane is important, as is the thickness of the layer of plasma between the capillary wall and the red blood cell. In addition, the permeability of the erythrocyte to carbon monoxide or oxygen must be considered, along with the reaction rate of hemoglobin with carbon monoxide or oxygen. In a single-breath diffusion capacity measurement using carbon monoxide, the presence of carbon monoxide hemoglobin in the pulmonary arterial blood diminishes the rate of carbon monoxide transfer.

A decrease in pulmonary diffusion capacity may be the earliest detectable abnormality in collagen disease, such as sarcoidosis, or in industrial diseases, such as asbestosis. Also, a decreased DLCO is found in patients with pulmonary emboli, and a perfusion lung scan and/or arteriogram may be indicated when this diagnosis is being considered. Diffusion capacity is increased in mitral stenosis, left heart failure, and polycythemia.

Airway Resistance and Lung Elasticity. In emphysema, the lung compliance is high, and therefore the FRC is large. These lungs exhibit little elastic recoil at the measured FRC. As a result, the resting intrapleural pressure is not as negative as it would be normally. This absence of negative intrapleural pressure allows the bronchi to collapse at a volume of only slightly less than FRC, because the bronchi do not have either a negative pleural pressure around them or the outwardly pulling forces of the lung tissues surrounding them to keep them open. With collapsed bronchi, the emphysematous patient has difficulty emptying the air from the lungs to reach a volume much lower than the large FRC. Adequate measurement of the lung's elastic properties is performed only by measurement of the static pressure-volume curve, in which absolute transpulmonary pressure is related to absolute lung volume over the whole vital capacity during both inflation and deflation. Airway resistance is increased in patients with emphysema and may also be increased in those with bronchitis. The degree of bronchitis is important, because with appropriate therapy, some of the increased resistance is reversible.

Arterial Blood Gases. Adequate pulmonary function is necessary to maintain delivery of oxygen to the periphery as well as to remove carbon dioxide, and the hemoglobin must function to absorb and release oxygen (Fig. 51–20). It is also important that the hemoglobin be fully saturated and sufficiently available so that the cardiac output can deliver the quantity of oxygen necessary for aerobic metabolism. The hemoglobin should be maintained at normothermia and normal pH so that it can transport adequate oxygen and unload it at the periphery.

The measurement of arterial blood gases is probably the most frequently used pulmonary function test. The interpretation of PaO$_2$ depends on the oxygen tension in the inspired air. After calculating the alveolar oxygen tension, the alveolar-arterial oxygen tension gradient can be determined; if the PaO$_2$ and the A-aDO$_2$ are normal, there is no disturbance in oxygen transport.

Arterial Oxygen Tension. The measurement of arterial PO$_2$ is useful in evaluating pulmonary function. An alveolar-

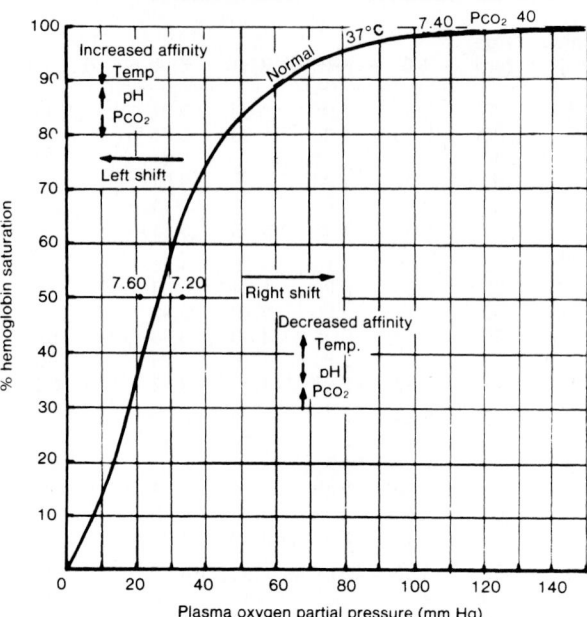

Figure 51–20. The oxygen-hemoglobin dissociation curve. This figure highlights the effects of temperature and acid-base as well as the effect of changes in the partial pressure of carbon dioxide on the curve. The points 7.6 and 7.2 represent the left and right shifts that occur secondary to pH. (From Margand, P. M. D., Brooks, C. G., Jr., and Hunter, J. W.: Preoperative Pulmonary Preparation: A Clinical Guide. Baltimore, Williams & Wilkins, 1981.)

arterial PO$_2$ difference of about 10 torr is customarily found in young healthy adults, and a 20-torr difference is found in healthy older adults. Greater differences—that is, an arterial PO$_2$ of less than 80 torr in the absence of hypoventilation—require explanation. Possibilities include a right-to-left shunt, a diffusion barrier, or an uneven distribution of ventilation to blood flow. To test for right-to-left shunt, the patient is given 100% oxygen, and the arterial PO$_2$ should increase to greater than 604. If the arterial PO$_2$ is less than predicted but greater than 150 torr, the percentage of right-to-left shunting can be calculated as follows:

$$\% \text{ shunt} = \frac{\dfrac{(673 - \text{PaO}_2)2.3}{760}}{\left(\dfrac{(673 - \text{PaO}_2)2.3}{760}\right) + 4.5} \times 100$$

This equation assumes 2.3 as the solubility of O$_2$ in plasma and 4.5 as the usual arteriovenous difference. The normal shunt is below 8%; in obese patients, this may approach 10%. Shunts greater than these are usually abnormal.

Arterial Carbon Dioxide Tension. Measurements of PaCO$_2$ provide an immediate indication of a patient's alveolar ventilation (Fig. 51–21). A PaCO$_2$ of less than 37 mm. Hg is hypocapnia, whereas hypercapnia is defined as greater than 43 mm. Hg (normal range is 38 to 42 mm. Hg). Any level of hypercapnia indicates severe disease, representing functional loss of more than 50% of the lung. Acidosis is defined as a pH of less than 7.37, and alkalosis is a pH of greater than 7.43. Evaluation of acid-base requires the interpretation of both respiratory and metabolic determinants of pH. Potential aberrations include respiratory acidosis, respiratory alkalosis, metabolic acidosis, and metabolic alkalosis.

Acid-Base. The principal buffering systems in the body are bicarbonate, phosphates, and cells. During acute changes, the

GAS EXCHANGE

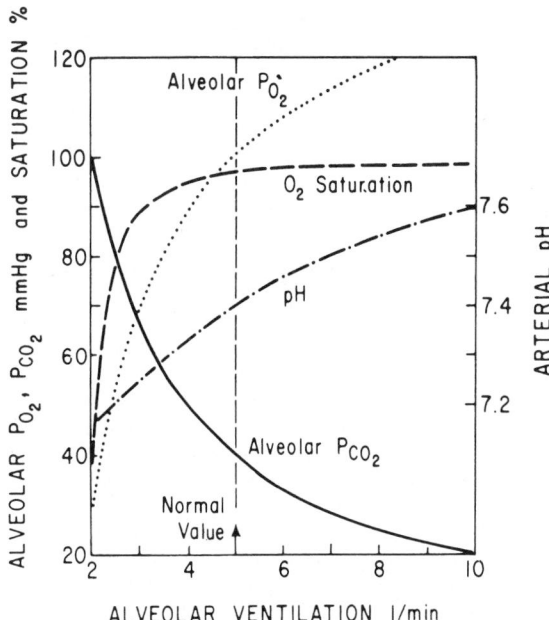

Figure 51–21. Changes in gas exchange during hypoventilation. Note the rapid rise in P_{CO_2} compared with the so-called slow fall in arterial oxygen saturation. (From West, J. B.: Pulmonary Pathophysiology: The Essentials. Baltimore, Williams & Wilkins, 1977.)

extracellular bicarbonate and the hemoglobin are the major buffers. In addition to chemical buffering, there are also physiologic responses to alterations in acid-base status that are critical in minimizing changes in pH for each of the four types of acid-base disturbances. Whenever compensation occurs for primary respiratory acid-base disturbances, there must be a physiologically induced metabolic alteration, usually renal. Conversely, metabolic disturbances must be corrected by using the respiratory mechanism. Renal acid-base adjustments occur slowly, because although urinary secretion of acid begins rapidly, it may take 2 hours to days to complete.

Respiratory Acidosis. Respiratory acidosis is compensated by renal retention of bicarbonate and excretion of acid. Renal compensation begins immediately upon the development of respiratory acidosis but takes days to weeks to become maximal. This mechanism can return blood pH to normal, given sufficient time, if the steady state of Pa_{CO_2} is 60 to 65 torr or less. Above this level of hypercapnia, the kidney cannot sufficiently increase its rate of reabsorption of bicarbonate. If the pH is low and the Pa_{CO_2} is below 60 torr, respiratory acidosis is likely to be acute or subacute.

The effect of respiratory acidosis on the sensorium is probably caused by a lowering of the pH of the cerebrospinal fluid (CSF), with which blood CO_2 equilibrates rapidly. Since the CSF is corrected toward normal by accumulation of bicarbonate in CSF, within a few days of the onset of hypercapnia, patients with chronic hypercapnia may have a clear sensorium at a level of Pa_{CO_2} that would cause coma if it should develop acutely. Thus, clinical observation of a patient with known hypercapnia often indicates whether hypercapnia is acute or chronic.

Respiratory Alkalosis. Controversy remains as to whether the kidney compensates for chronic respiratory alkalosis by excretion of bicarbonate and retention of acid. There is suggestive evidence that such compensation occurs, at least in chronic situations, but it is probably incomplete.

Metabolic Acidosis. Metabolic acidosis is corrected by in-

ducing respiratory alkalosis and stimulating chemoreceptors in both the aortic-carotid area and the floor of the fourth ventricle, which represents at least half (and possibly much more) of the respiratory stimulation occurring during metabolic acidosis. The aortic-carotid chemoreceptors are affected rapidly by changes in the pH of the CSF. The maximal respiratory response to an acid load is delayed for a matter of hours or days. For any given blood pH during chronic metabolic acidosis, there is an appropriate lowering of Pa_{CO_2}. A Pa_{CO_2} that is inappropriately above or below the response to uncomplicated metabolic acidosis suggests the presence of a superimposed primary respiratory acidosis or alkalosis.

Metabolic Alkalosis. Metabolic alkalosis is compensated by the development of respiratory acidosis, but under ordinary circumstances, Pa_{CO_2} does not increase above 50 torr no matter how severe the metabolic alkalosis; exceptional cases in which severe hypercapnia occurred have been reported, however. The usual minimal effect on Pa_{CO_2} appears to be related to the fact that ventilation is linked to the rate of oxygen consumption or CO_2 production in some unknown manner, and this link prevents the development of more severe hypercapnia by taking precedence over the compensatory mechanism.

PREOPERATIVE EVALUATION

Pulmonary complications are not infrequent after major operative procedures.[3, 4, 14, 16, 32, 76] Age, obesity, certain surgical procedures, cigarette smoking, and anesthesia impair pulmonary function and are preoperative risk factors.[45, 49, 50] With age, the lungs show gradual deterioration both in performance of the airways and in gas exchange (Fig. 51–22). Flow-volume curves and position, as well as blood gases, change with age (Table 51–3).[78] Although a nonsmoker's pulmonary function deteriorates only slightly with time, age remains a relative factor.[34, 35] An older patient with obstructive airway disease has a markedly increased risk. Obesity impairs lung and chest wall compliance. There may be a component of

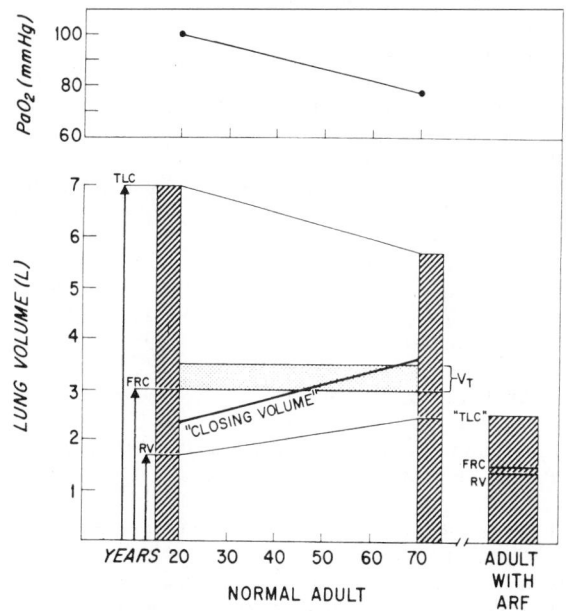

Figure 51–22. The changes in Pa_{O_2} and lung volumes with age in normal adults in the supine position and the typical values for FRC and vital capacity in an adult patient with adult respiratory failure (ARF). RV, residual volume; FRC, functional residual capacity; TLC, total lung capacity; V_T, tidal volume. (From Pontoppidan, H., Geffin, G., and Lowenstein, E.: Acute Respiratory Failure in the Adult. Boston, Little, Brown, 1973.)

TABLE 51–3. Effect of Age on Arterial Po₂ and Pco₂ While Breathing Ambient Air at Rest

Age Group (Years)	No. Observations	Mean Pao₂ (mm. Hg)	± SD	Mean Paco₂ (mm. Hg)	± SD
<30 (median = 23)	38	94.2	3.31	39.0	1.8
31–40 (median = 36)	30	87.2	3.47	38.5	2.0
41–50 (median = 46)	30	83.9	4.07	39.6	2.4
51–60 (median = 55)	30	81.2	3.74	39.0	1.9
>60 (median = 71)	24	74.3	4.43	39.8	2.1

From Sorbini, C. A., et al.: Arterial oxygen tension in relation to age in healthy subjects. Respiration, 25:3, 1968.

restrictive lung disease, and the work of breathing is increased. When abnormal closure of small airways occurs, this leads to significant ventilation-perfusion mismatches.[66] These changes become worse in the supine position, in which the weight of the abdomen and chest wall contributes to the impairment of pulmonary function (Fig. 51–23). These changes may be even more apparent if the patient is placed in a lateral position with one lung partially deflated. More effort is required for each breath, and the Paco₂ usually falls.

Smoking, even in the absence of detectable lung disease, is associated with increased postoperative atelectasis and infection.[17, 18, 31] The site of incision, whether abdominal or thoracic, also influences postoperative performance. With upper abdominal and thoracic incisions, the chest wall and diaphragmatic mechanics are altered. Incisional pain contributes to postoperative hypoventilation. These patients may cough ineffectively and experience difficulty in clearing secretions. With a lower abdominal incision, the changes in pulmonary function are less marked.[23]

Pulmonary function should be evaluated in relation to the operative procedure planned.[45–48, 57, 61] Patients can be divided into the following groups: (1) those undergoing thoracotomy for removal of lung tissue, (2) those undergoing thoracotomy without excision of pulmonary tissue, (3) those undergoing abdominal surgery, and (4) those undergoing procedures on extremities or elsewhere.[19, 23–25] It is apparent that each group responds differently to the effects of the operation, anesthesia, and pulmonary function, but postoperative expectations and problems can be predicted in view of the magnitude of the surgical procedure and the preoperative evaluation of the patient's pulmonary status (Table 51–4). Postoperatively, every effort should be made to obtain maximal pulmonary function as soon as possible, to ensure the rapid return of the FRC to the preoperative level. Supplemental oxygen should be used as necessary to prevent hypoxemia. If the vital capacity and the FRC are returned to the preoperative

level and hypoxemia is prevented, the ventilation-perfusion ratio is corrected. These are important guidelines, because all patients who are injured, undergo anesthesia, and have an operative procedure experience decreased lung volume with decreased ventilation, hypoxemia, and lowered FRC in the postoperative period. If these factors are not corrected and if hypoxemia progresses, respiratory insufficiency and failure may develop rapidly.[67, 69, 71]

Risk in Patients with Pre-existing Pulmonary Disease. Obstructive pulmonary disease is the most important risk factor in a patient undergoing surgical therapy. The more severe the disease, the greater the risk of postoperative complications (Table 51–5). Those with restrictive lung disease usually tolerate surgery better; however, these patients cannot afford to lose much functioning lung. Because of better expiratory flow rates, cough is better preserved in these patients than in those with obstructive disease. In general, an FEV₁ of 1 to 2 liters is not associated with an increased operative risk. With an FEV₁ of less than 800 ml., there is clearly an increased risk for severe pulmonary complications; those with less than 500 ml. have the greatest risk (Table 51–6). The presence of carbon dioxide retention is a marker for a patient at dramatically increased risk.[64, 65, 71, 80]

Thoracotomy and pulmonary resection are not well tolerated in patients with obstructive airway disease. There is a loss of functional tissue, and the thoracotomy alters the mechanical and gas exchange properties of the lung. This may be accentuated if lung tissue is removed during operation. Thoracotomy produces pain in the postoperative period, which reduces the patient's ability to cough to clear secretions. If the airway disease is severe, the patient may not be able to tolerate the loss of even a single pulmonary segment. Thus, in these patients, preoperative evaluation is extremely important, and preparation of the patient by cessation of smoking and the use of a variety of drugs to improve airway function and ventilation is extremely helpful in decreasing operative risk.[17, 18, 34, 61, 71]

In patients with pulmonary hypertension and carbon dioxide retention, resective procedures may be contraindicated. For example, when the FEV₁ is less than 2 liters and the MVV or MBC is less than 50%, patients do not usually tolerate pneumonectomy.[39, 50, 57, 64, 69, 80] Therefore, predicting postresection lung function can be helpful in preventing a surgically cured but pulmonary-challenged patient.

Evaluation of Tolerance for Thoracotomy and Lung Resection. Surgical resection is the preferred treatment for patients with localized non–small cell carcinoma of the lung. Most patients are elderly cigarette smokers, many of whom have cardiopulmonary disorders. The stress of thoracotomy and removal of lung tissue in a patient with an already compromised respiratory status may result in cardiopulmonary failure and death. In an attempt to predict the adequacy of postoperative pulmonary function, a number of tests have been proposed.[21]

The first preoperative test was spirometry. In 1955, Gaensler and co-workers demonstrated that those patients with an MVV of <50% of the predicted value and a forced vital

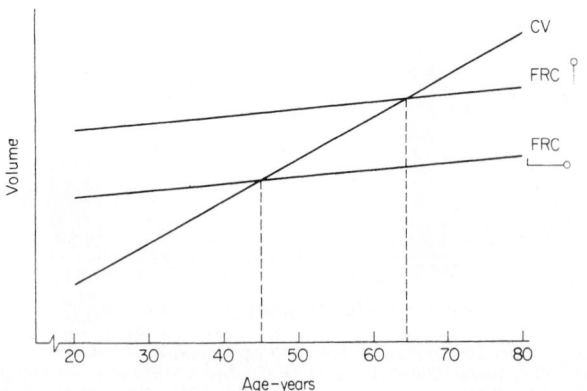

Figure 51–23. The effect of increasing age and closing volume (CV) in relation to functional residual capacity (FRC) in both the erect and supine positions. (From Sykes, M. K., McNicol, M. W., and Campbell, E. J. M.: Respiratory Failure, 2nd ed. Oxford, Blackwell Scientific Publications, 1976.)

TABLE 51–4. Effect of Moderate and Heavy Exercise on the Oxygen Required for Breathing

Condition	External Work (kg./m./min.)	Tidal Vol. (ml.)	Resp. Rate (breaths/min.)	Min. Vol. (L./min.)	O₂ Consumption (ml./min.)	Respiratory Work			
						Kg./m./min.	% Elastic	% Resistive	O₂ Cost (ml./min.)
Quiet breathing	0	500	15	7.5	300	0.3	66	33	3
Moderate exercise	620	1600	23	37.0	1500	5.2	57	43	52
Heavy exercise	1600	2400	48	115.0	3500	35.2	39	61	352
Maximal voluntary ventilation	0	1500	120	180	—	65.0	20	80+	—

Heavy exercise is accompanied by a 10-fold increase in oxygen consumption. The distribution of work is reversed as compared with quiet breathing (the elastic component falls from 66% to 39%, and the resistive component rises from 33% to 61%) and is associated with a fivefold rise in tidal volume but only a threefold increase in respiratory frequency. Maximal voluntary ventilation is achieved by a significantly greater increase in frequency than in tidal volume. An increase in minute ventilation during the postoperative period represents an increase in work to overcome resistance to gas flow. Thus an increase in respiratory rate is indicative of inefficient respiration and incipient respiratory failure.

capacity (FVC) <70% of the predicted value suffered a 50% mortality.[28] Since that time, pulmonary function testing has commonly been used to assess patients before thoracotomy.[94] The goals of preoperative pulmonary function testing include the identification of patients (1) with high surgical risk due to lung disease, (2) in whom preoperative pulmonary measures may decrease the risk of respiratory compromise, and (3) for whom further physiologic assessment is necessary to clarify the operative risk. Based on pulmonary function testing, thoracotomy is offered to patients with a preoperative FVC >50% of the predicted value, FEV₁ >2 liters, FEV₁-FVC ratio >50%, MVV >50% of predicted, and DLCO >50% of predicted. It has been shown that most cardiopulmonary complications develop in patients who fail these criteria.[63] Although a severe impairment of ventilatory function correlates with a high risk of postoperative morbidity and mortality, some patients with markedly abnormal routine pulmonary function tests do not have complications.[13, 28, 40, 49, 74] Furthermore, if these criteria are rigidly applied, many patients who could tolerate an operation will be denied the chance for a curative resection.

In an attempt to identify individuals with poor results on routine pulmonary function tests who would otherwise tolerate resection, a number of other tests have been proposed.[20, 42, 57, 75, 79] Bronchospirometry was developed to measure the function of each lung separately. Although the technique was helpful, it was not widely accepted due to its invasive nature and the considerable skill required to perform the procedure.[56] Quantitative ventilation and perfusion scintigraphic studies are more practical indices of postoperative lung function.[20, 38, 57, 58] Wernly and associates have shown that in patients undergoing a lobectomy, the predicted postoperative FEV₁ can be calculated by the following equation:

Expected loss of lung function = Preop FEV₁ × (no. of segments to be resected/total no. of segments in both lungs) × (estimated regional function of the lobe to be resected)

Calculation of the predicted FEV₁ by this equation, which considers the perfusion of the lobe to be resected, correlates closely with the observed postoperative FEV₁. Furthermore, in patients who underwent pneumonectomy, Wernly and associates estimated the predicted postoperative FEV₁ as the product of the FEV₁ and the percentage of perfusion, the percentage of ventilation at equilibrium, or the percentage of

TABLE 51–5. Evaluation of Risk of Pulmonary Resection in Patients with Pulmonary Disease

Function	Test	Patient at Risk—Needs Preoperative Optimization or Further Evaluation	Prohibitive Risk
Mechanical ventilatory	FEV₁ postoperative predicted	<1.01/sec.	<0.8 L./sec.
	FVC preoperative	<2.01	<1.5 L.
	MBC preoperative	<55%	<35%
Parenchymal pulmonary	Po₂ preoperative (rest)	50–60 mm. Hg	<50 mm. Hg
	Pco₂ preoperative (rest)	40–44 mm. Hg	>45 mm. Hg
	Qs/QT preoperative	10–20%	>20%
Cardiac	ECG at rest	Abnormal, especially ischemic changes	Acute MI, ventricular arrhythmias
	ETT	Stage IV + (consider cardiac cath.)	Early + ETT
	Ventricular function (rest-exercise ejection fraction by radionuclide studies)	EF < 50% or deterioration with exercise	EF < 30%
Cardiopulmonary capacity	Chronic Hgb level	>17 gm./100 ml.	>20% gm./100 ml.
	Cardiac: ETT	Unable to complete Stage IV secondary to dyspnea on exertion	Unable to complete Stage I (cardiac ischemia or arrhythmias)
	Stairwalking	Unable to complete three flights of stairs	Unable to walk one flight
	Postexercise arterial blood gases	Fall in Po₂	Fall in Po₂ to < 49 mm. Hg or CO₂ retention
	Cardiopulmonary exercise testing		

FEV₁, forced expiratory volume at 1 sec.; FVC, forced vital capacity; MBC, maximal breathing capacity; ECG, electrocardiogram; ETT, exercise tolerance test; Hgb, hemoglobin; EF, ejection fraction.

TABLE 51–6. Interpretation of Risk in Patients with Pulmonary Disease

Findings	Interpretation
Normal test	No increased risk demonstrated
Obstructive disorders	
FEV_1 >1.5 L.; MVV >50% Normal blood gases	Little increased risk if special precautions taken in patient management
FEV_1 = 1–1.5 L.; MVV = 35–50% Normal $Paco_2$; no more than slight hypoxemia; normal ECG	Definitely increased risk even with proper management; a relative contraindication to surgery
FEV_1 = 1–1.5 L.; MVV = 35–50% Normal $Paco_2$; slight hypoxemia; abnormal ECG	Greatly increased operative risk; a contraindication to major elective surgical procedures
FEV_1 = 1 L.; MVV <35% Normal $Paco_2$; mild hypoxemia; normal ECG	Greatly increased operative risk; a contraindication to major elective surgical procedures; probably precludes extensive lung resection
FEV_1 = 1 L.; MVV <35% Elevated $Paco_2$; severe hypoxemia or abnormal ECG	Extremely high operative risk; only mandatory surgery justifiable; probably precludes any pulmonary resection
Restrictive disorders	
VC >50%; DL >50% Normal blood gases	Little increased operative risk
VC = 35–50%; DL >50% Slight hypoxemia on exertion	Some increase in operative risk but not a serious contraindication to surgery, except extensive lung resection
VC <35%; DL <50% or frank hypoxemia	Greatly increased operative risk, especially contraindicating extensive lung resection
Cardiopulmonary exercise testing	
Vo_2max >20 ml./min./kg.	Low operative risk
Vo_2max 15–20 ml./min./kg.	Moderate operative risk
Vo_2max 10–15 ml./min./kg.	High operative risk
Vo_2max <10 ml./min./kg.	Unacceptably high operative risk

FEV_1, forced expiratory volume at 1 sec.; MVV, maximum voluntary ventilation; VC, vital capacity; DL, diffusing capacity; Vo_2max, maximum oxygen consumption; ECG, electrocardiogram.

Modified from Burrows, B., Knudson, R. J., and Kettel, L. J.: Respiratory Insufficiency. Chicago, Year Book Medical Publishers, 1975. Used by permission.

ventilation after a single breath in the remaining lung. They found all methods to be equally accurate.[89] Markos and colleagues have shown that estimates of the contribution of one lung or one lobe to the overall lung function by means of perfusion and ventilation scintigraphy correlate closely with the predicted postoperative FEV_1 and the diffusing capacity of the lung for carbon monoxide.[43] It has been suggested that a predicted postoperative FEV_1 of 0.8 to 1.0 liter by pulmonary scintigraphy correlates with an acceptable postoperative mortality of 15%.[15] Dunn and co-workers and others have suggested that due to the variability in pulmonary function seen on the basis of age, sex, and height, the acceptable postoperative FEV_1 should be corrected for these factors.[21, 29, 43] Such a *corrected* value is based on a percentage of the predicted normal value. Markos and co-workers have shown that a postoperative FEV_1 ≥40% of the predicted value was associated with no mortality, yet a value of ≤40% of the predicted amount was associated with a 50% mortality.[43] These results have been confirmed by other authors.[42, 57] In patients with a predicted postoperative FEV_1 of ≤40% who are being considered for curative resection, the measurement of pulmonary resistance by unilateral balloon occlusion of the pulmonary artery or by exercise testing can be used to further delineate the risk of thoracotomy and pulmonary resection.[53] The measurement of pulmonary artery pressure after occlusion of the vessel to the diseased lung requires right-heart catheterization, with its attendant morbidity. Therefore, this technique has not gained widespread acceptance.

In 1968, Van Nostrand and colleagues reported that routine pulmonary function tests could not predict which patients would develop complications following pulmonary resection. However, they observed that patients who could not climb one flight of stairs without dyspnea had a 50% mortality following pneumonectomy.[80] Reichel observed that patients who completed a preoperative treadmill exercise test did well postoperatively, and there was a 60% mortality and significant complications in patients who could not tolerate

level walking for 4 minutes.[65] With the development of rapidly responding oxygen and carbon dioxide analyzers that enable the measurement of oxygen uptake (Vo_2) and carbon dioxide production (Vco_2), the traditional stress test that measured only cardiac function was replaced with cardiopulmonary exercise (CPX). Clinically relevant issues that previously could not be adequately addressed from the measurement of hemodynamic parameters alone are examined in quantitative terms by CPX. With CPX, heart and lung function can be assessed simultaneously, allowing the evaluation of exercise response in patients with cardiovascular and respiratory disease. CPX can determine aerobic capacity, anaerobic threshold, the ventilatory response, and the onset of hypoxemia. In turn, this information can be used to determine the nature and severity of disease, the progression of disease over time, and the response to therapy.[84]

The observations made by Van Nostrand and Reichel underlined the inaccuracy of predicting complications or mortality of thoracotomy and pulmonary resection based on pulmonary function testing alone. The major determinant of the postoperative complications and mortality of thoracotomy stem from a functional defect in the cardiopulmonary unit. The heart and lungs, together with hemoglobin, constitute the integrated cardiopulmonary unit, which is responsible for sustaining O_2 availability for tissue metabolism. The successful functioning of the cardiopulmonary unit is determined by Vo_2 and Vco_2. In a patient with lung or heart disease, an impairment in the function of the cardiopulmonary unit may manifest in breathlessness, fatigue, or both. Such abnormalities in the cardiopulmonary unit may be detected by monitoring respiratory gas exchange during an incremental upright exercise test.[88]

Cardiopulmonary Exercise Testing. Incremental treadmill or upright cycle ergometry is used to maximally stress the cardiopulmonary unit. The latter is preferred in obese patients and those with severe ventilatory disease. During the test, the gas response data of the patient are monitored by a computerized on-line breath-by-breath stress test system. The visual display of the breath-by-breath monitoring allows reliable identification of the plateau in VO_2, which defines VO_2-max.

During incremental exercise, when O_2 delivery is inadequate to sustain oxidative metabolism, anaerobic pathways are used, leading to lactate production. Production of larger amounts of lactate or an earlier appearance of lactate production signals a deficiency in the cardiopulmonary unit. Wasserman and colleagues have recommended criteria for the detection of lactate (anaerobic) threshold during noninvasive monitoring of respiratory gas exchange.[81] One of the criteria, the disproportionate rise in VO_2 relative to VCO_2, can readily be applied when VO_2 and VCO_2 are monitored continuously during exercise testing. It has been observed that the anaerobic threshold generally occurs at 60% to 70% of the VO_2max. CPX has been used to evaluate the severity of circulatory failure; identify the cause of exertional dyspnea, monitor the response to medical treatment in patients with chronic congestive heart failure, and evaluate patients before they undergo thoracotomy or pulmonary resection.[36, 73, 85–88, 91]

Using CPX, the severity of circulatory failure can be categorized according to the patient's aerobic capacity:

Class A, patients with a mild impairment in aerobic capacity: maximal cardiac output (CO) >8 liters per minute per sq. m. and a VO_2max of >20 ml. per minute per kg. body weight

Class B, patients with mild to moderately severe impairment: CO 6–8 liters per minute per sq. m. and a VO_2max of 16–20 ml. per minute per kg.

Class C, patients with a moderately severe degree of failure: CO 4–6 liters per minute per sq. m. and a VO_2max of 10–16 ml. per minute per kg.

Class D, patients with severe failure: CO 2–4 liters per minute per sq. m. VO_2max <10 ml. per minute per kg.[85]

The severity of circulatory failure seems to correlate with the complication rate following thoracotomy and pulmonary resection.

In patients with exertional dyspnea, CPX testing can be used to differentiate between heart and lung disease as the primary cause of dyspnea. In these patients, VO_2 is determined when dyspnea occurs. In patients with a ventilatory cause of exertional dyspnea, VO_2max and the anaerobic threshold are not achieved, the maximal minute ventilation to incremental exercise (VEmax) is >50% of MVV, and hypoxemia often appears.

The role of CPX in the preoperative assessment of patients undergoing thoracotomy and pulmonary resection has evolved. In 1980, Eugene and colleagues reported that patients undergoing pulmonary resections with a VO_2max >1 liter per minute had no mortality, compared with a 75% mortality in patients with a VO_2max <1 liter per minute.[22] Smith and colleagues found that the VO_2max was more accurate in predicting complications than was the prediction of postoperative FEV_1 using quantitative lung scanning.[72] They reported no morbidity in patients with a VO_2max of 20 ml. per minute per kg., compared with a 100% complication rate in patients with a VO_2max <15 ml. per minute per kg. Bechard and Wetstein reported a 29% mortality and 43% morbidity in patients with a VO_2max <10 ml. per minute per kg. and a 10.7% morbidity and no deaths in those with a VO_2max >20 ml. per minute per kg.[10] Despite significant variation in techniques and methods of analysis, other investigators have reported a strong relationship between exercise performance and the frequency and severity of cardiopulmonary complications following lung resection.[11, 20]

In a recent study of CPX for the evaluation of patients at high risk for complications from lung resection, Morice and co-workers found no relationship between preoperative pulmonary function studies and exercise testing. Furthermore, these investigators found that 10% of patients with resectable lesions failed to qualify for resection on the basis of the results of routine tests, including split function lung scanning.[53] However, 38% of these patients were able to exercise to a VO_2max of >15 ml. per minute per kg., with no deaths and a 20% complication rate. Of the reported studies to date, some have used exercise to a maximal level, and others have used submaximal levels of stress. Submaximal testing is defined as exercise to a specific target heart rate. During submaximal testing, the ratio of VO_2 to basal surface area (VO_2/BSA) at a specific lactate level is used instead of VO_2-max. It has been suggested that submaximal steady-state exercise testing may be better tolerated by patients who are elderly and have poor cardiopulmonary function. Olsen and associates found that unlike VO_2max, which predicts complications, submaximal VO_2 is a predictor of survival following lung resection.[59] Similarly, Miyoshi and co-workers found that the blood lactate threshold, expressed as VO_2/BSA at a lactate level (LA) of 20 during submaximal levels of exercise, is a sensitive predictor of hospital mortality but not a predictor of patients who are likely to develop pulmonary complications.[51] Patients with a VO_2/BSA at LA 20 of 471 $\pm$ 53 survived; all patients with a VO_2/BSA at LA 20 of 296 $\pm$ 72 died.

Exercise testing is an attractive option in the preoperative evaluation of patients undergoing lung resection, because it simulates the postresection conditions of increased pulmonary blood flow, CO_2 excretion, and O_2 uptake required of the remaining lung. Based on the present knowledge about exercise testing, two separate parameters seem to be useful in predicting morbidity and mortality from thoracotomy and pulmonary resection. A higher lactate threshold, as defined by VO_2/BSA at LA 20 during submaximal exercise, is a strong predictor of survival following thoracotomy. In contrast, VO_2-max appears to be a useful determinant of morbidity in these patients. Patients with a VO_2max exceeding 20 ml. per minute per kg. have low morbidity following thoracotomy, patients with a VO_2max of 15 to 20 appear to be at moderate risk (25% complication rate), those with a VO_2max of 10 to 15 are at high risk (32% complication rate), and patients with a VO_2max less than 10 have an unacceptably high complication rate of 80%.

It is important to emphasize that exercise testing neither helps in determining the functional contribution of the lung tissue to be resected nor predicts the patient's postoperative pulmonary function. Exercise testing is useful primarily in the preoperative selection of patients who have severe pulmonary dysfunction and pulmonary lesions amenable to limited surgical resection. Exercise testing should be considered an important complement to conventional tests that are used in selecting patients for thoracotomy and pulmonary resection. Patients should be selected carefully to ensure the adequacy of long-term postoperative lung function.

PREOPERATIVE PREPARATION

When the risks have been defined, every effort should be made to eliminate or reduce postoperative complications. Patients should cease smoking; although the optimal time is unknown, there is a marked benefit from cessation of smoking, even after only 5 to 7 days. Preoperative respiratory muscle conditioning is important, as is patient education about breathing patterns and effective coughing. Patients should use bronchial dilators both preoperatively and postoperatively if their efficacy can be demonstrated (Table 51–7). Preoperative evaluation of the efficacy of or intolerance to medications is optimal. Many of these medications are associated with premature ventricular or atrial contractions; such

TABLE 51–7. Preoperative Pharmacologic Preparation

Category	Route	Typical Adult Dosage
Beta-agonist		
Isuprel	Nebulized	1/200 dilution 0.5 ml. in 4.5 ml. normal saline 2–4 times a day
Ephedrine	PO	12–24 mg. every 6 hr.
Racemic epinephrine	Nebulized	0.5 ml. in 4.5 ml. normal saline every 4–6 hr.
Beta-selective		
Metaproterenol	Nebulized	5.0% 0.33 ml. in 4.5 ml. normal saline 2–4 times a day
Metaproterenol	PO	10–20 mg. 4 times a day
Albuterol	Nebulized	2 (90-μg.) inhalations 2–4 times a day
Albuterol	PO	12–24 mg. every 6 hr.
Terbutaline	PO	2.5–5.0 mg. 3 times a day
Terbutaline	IM	0.25 mg. every 6–8 hr.
Theophylline		
Aminophylline	PO	200 mg. 3–4 times a day
Aminophylline	IV	load 5.6 mg./kg., then 0.9 mg./kg./hr.
Theophylline	PO	200 mg. 3–4 times a day
Oxytriphylline	PO	100–200 mg. 3–4 times a day
Diphylline	PO	200 mg. 3–4 times a day
Mucolytics and expectorants		
Acetylcysteine	Nebulized	20% 1–3 ml. every 4–8 hr.
Steroid		
Solu-Cortef	IM	100 mg. every 12 hr. for 6 doses, begin night before surgery
Solu-Medrol	IV	25–40 mg. every 6 hr. for 6 doses, begin with surgery
Prednisone	PO	10 mg. 4 times a day; begin 2–3 days prior to surgery
Beclomethasone	Inhalation	2 puffs (84 μg.) every 6 hr.

arrhythmias may become a serious postoperative problem and may be accentuated when hypoxemia is present. Therefore, it is important to administer intravenous antiarrhythmic agents to these patients. Every effort should be made to decrease the amount of secretions and assist the patient in coughing and deep breathing to clear secretions (e.g., postural drainage and chest percussion). In patients with asthma and severe chronic bronchitis, steroids may be used and can prevent the accentuation of postoperative bronchospasm.

OPERATIVE AND POSTOPERATIVE CHANGES

The effects of anesthesia may increase venous admixture, increase ventilation and perfusion mismatching, change the cardiac output, and alter the mechanical properties of the chest wall or the lung itself, whether or not paralysis is used during anesthesia. Mucociliary transport may be decreased, and the hemoglobin concentration and function may change.[19, 23, 47, 71, 92] Diaphragmatic function may be impaired, and the position of the patient during operation may compound some of these difficulties. The dependent basilar segments, for example, are usually underventilated and therefore have a greater tendency to develop atelectasis. In general, the patient is ventilated with positive pressure, and the dependent areas of the lung, which have the smallest airway diameters and are the least compliant, are poorly ventilated. The more compliant and less perfused areas receive the greatest ventilation. This leads to ventilation-perfusion mismatching and to hypoxemia and atelectasis. Also, as discussed earlier, the FRC decreases in almost all anesthetized surgical patients as well as in injured patients, regardless of whether the injury follows operation or trauma.[25] Therefore, the FEV_1 and VC are also reduced. These changes are maximal in the first and second postoperative days but remain abnormal for a week after operation. Decrease in the FRC leads to airway closure and ventilation-perfusion mismatching, with resulting hypoxemia, which may be accentuated in older patients.

To combat these changes, continuous airway pressure or positive end-expiratory pressure (PEEP) has been used.[6, 7, 19, 25, 37, 61, 68, 82] PEEP acts to increase the FRC, but it may also reduce cardiac output by limiting preload to the left ventricle.[70] Alveolar dead space generally increases with mechanical ventilation; therefore, increased minute ventilation is needed to maintain a normal $PaCO_2$. All these changes may lead to postoperative atelectasis, segmental lobar collapse, retained secretions, and pneumonia.[37]

The patient should be encouraged to sit upright as soon as possible. Lung function is clearly improved with early ambulation. This is especially important in the obese and the elderly. Early ambulation increases FRC and also reduces the risk of pulmonary embolism. Pulmonary embolism in the postoperative period is a dangerous complication in higher-risk patients with impaired pulmonary function. Moreover, care must be taken to prevent aspiration. Careful attention to these preoperative and postoperative details significantly reduces the risks of pulmonary complications.[8, 44, 46]

RESPIRATORY FAILURE

The adult respiratory distress syndrome (ARDS) has many definitions. Essentially, there is impairment of effective gas exchange, which is commonly defined in terms of findings on arterial blood gases. Usually there is arterial hypoxemia, a PaO_2 less than 60, or hypercarbia (i.e., a $PaCO_2$ greater than 50 that is not associated with metabolic alkalosis). The usual presentation includes hypoxemia, a PaO_2 less than 60, and respiratory alkalosis with a $PaCO_2$ less than 40. Other parameters associated with ARDS include increased dead space, decreased vital capacity, decreased FRC, and a decrease in inspiratory force that is less than 30 cm. of water (Table 51–8).[2, 27, 62]

Respiratory failure has two components: pulmonary parenchymal failure (failure of gas exchange), manifested by hypoxemia, and pulmonary ventilatory failure, manifested by hypercapnia. Both components have a role in the pathogenesis of respiratory insufficiency: (1) difficulty in ventilating and getting air (air hunger), (2) hypoxemia, (3) stiff lungs requiring increasingly high ventilatory pressures, and (4) evi-

TABLE 51–8. Indications for Respiratory Support

	Acceptable	PT/Monitor	Intubate
Mechanics			
Respiratory rate (breaths per min.)	12–25	25–35	>35
Vital capacity (ml./kg.)	70–30	30–15	<15
Inspiratory force (cm. H_2O)	100–50	50–25	<25
Parenchymal			
$AaDo_2$	50–200	200–350	>350
VD/VT	0.3–0.4	0.4–0.6	>0.6
$Paco_2$ torr	35–45	45–60	>60
Qs/QT	8–12%	12–20%	>20%
Pao_2 torr	100–75 air		<65 on mask O_2

Adapted from Wilson, R. S., and Pontoppidan, H.: Acute respiratory failure: Diagnostic and therapeutic criteria. Crit. Care Med., 2:293, 1974.

dence of infiltration and consolidation by radiographic evaluation.

Normally, there is an approximately 8% shunt within the lung. Factors that contribute to increased shunting are atelectasis, alveolar edema, abnormalities in hemoglobin, and the closing volumes of the airways.[5, 12, 55]

The FRC provides a mechanism for avoiding great fluctuations in arterial oxygen and carbon dioxide tensions. With a normal tidal volume, new air is added to the functional residual capacity, creating adequate alveolar ventilation. The normal lung has mismatched ventilation and perfusion. In the upright position, the upper segments are ventilated more effectively than they are perfused; the lower segments are ventilated less than the upper segments of the lung and have much greater perfusion. In the normal lung, although there are regional differences in ventilation and perfusion throughout, the net effect is a reasonable match of ventilation and perfusion. The pathologic changes of ARDS include increased capillary permeability, interstitial edema, and congestive atelectasis.[2, 26] With the development of interstitial edema, there is impaired gas flow to the fine terminal airways, and the FRC falls. With the reduction of the FRC, there is an increase in pulmonary shunting. As a result, when venous admixture increases, the arterial $Paco_2$ falls.

Awareness of the potential development of ARDS is a prerequisite for reducing morbidity and mortality.[54, 60] Often the chronic nature of pre-existing pulmonary disease is subtle. A history of increased sputum production, chronic cough, wheezing, orthopnea, multiple pulmonary infections, and smoking is extremely important. Smoking associated with chronic bronchitis or chronic obstructive lung disease is a major factor in determining the risk of postoperative and posttraumatic pulmonary problems. Cessation of smoking for 1 to 2 weeks prior to elective operation is one of the most important factors in managing any patient.[17, 18, 31, 32, 45, 67]

Pathophysiology. Whatever the etiology for respiratory distress syndrome—whether it is postsurgical, posttraumatic, or related to sepsis, hypovolemic shock, cardiogenic shock, or aspiration—the final common pathway is the same. Physiologically, there are two clinically significant components: an abnormal pattern of gas distribution related to alveolar closure, and interstitial edema caused by pulmonary vascular congestion or loss of endothelial integrity of the capillaries.[34, 35] There are decreases in both FRC and compliance as well as ventilation-perfusion abnormalities.

Pulmonary dysfunction becomes critical when the arterial oxygen content falls so low that elevations in cardiac output can no longer compensate to deliver sufficient oxygen to maintain aerobic metabolism. Many precipitating factors have been associated with progressive pulmonary insufficiency: fluid overload, pneumonia, shock, thromboembolism, massive blood transfusions, sepsis, peritonitis, prolonged

ventilatory therapy with high inspired oxygen concentrations, fat emboli, and prolonged cardiopulmonary bypass. Regardless of the precipitating factors, there are four general categories of abnormalities in pulmonary function: hypoventilation, ventilation-perfusion, diffusion defects, and arteriovenous shunts.[1, 54, 55, 60, 62]

Hypoventilation. The function of the pulmonary circulation is to expose the cardiac output to ventilation for the purpose of oxygenating hemoglobin and removing carbon dioxide. This gas exchange is less sensitive to variations in total pulmonary blood flow than to inequalities in the distribution of the blood flow as matched to regional alveolar ventilation. The relationship of the oxygen utilized by the body delivered to the periphery is known as the Fick principle:

$$O_2 \text{ utilized} = \frac{\text{cardiac output}}{a - vo_2 \text{ difference}}$$

This very simple but important relationship demonstrates the reciprocal behavior of the $a - vo_2$ difference and the cardiac output. As cardiac output declines, the amount of oxygen extracted from the hemoglobin must increase if aerobic metabolism is to be maintained. The total amount of oxygen delivered to the periphery depends on the cardiac output and the total oxygen content of arterial blood.

$$O_2 \text{ delivery at periphery} = (O_2 \text{ content})(\text{cardiac output})$$

$$O_2 \text{ content} = (Hgb)(O_2 \text{ sat})(1.34) + (.0031)(Pao_2)$$

It can readily be seen that most of the oxygen is transported by the hemoglobin molecule.

Hypoventilation exists when the volume of alveolar ventilation is reduced to the point at which normal gas exchange cannot occur. It is simply defined as an inability to maintain a normal Pco_2, and this definition is related to the rapid carbon dioxide dissociation that makes it more sensitive to alveolar Pco_2. As alveolar ventilation falls, alveolar Pco_2 rises rapidly, which is reflected in the arterial partial pressure CO_2 (see Fig. 51–21). In contrast, the oxygen saturation decreases only gradually until hypoventilation is quite severe.

Simply enriching the oxygen concentration of the inspired gas limits the hypoxemia of hypoventilation.[52, 77, 82, 93] The converse of this is true as well, in that pure hypoventilation does not cause a dramatic fall in the arterial oxygen partial pressure. Doubling the $Paco_2$, as a consequence of hypoventilation, decreases the arterial Po_2 by only 40 mm. Hg. Although the patient is moderately hypoxemic, he or she is markedly acidotic, and the CO_2 relationship dominates the clinical situation.

Although hypoventilation is by definition alveolar hypoventilation, it can follow a number of factors. In patients who are spontaneously ventilating, hypoventilation can be caused

TABLE 51–9. The Shunt Equation

A. Components of the shunt equation
1. Constant anatomic shunts (normal 2%)
   Bronchial veins
   Pleural veins
   Thebesian veins
   Abnormal AV connections
2. Variable intrapulmonary shunts ($2 \to 6\%$)
   $\dot{V}/\dot{Q}$ abnormalities (regional and changing)
   Alveolar wall interstitial edema
   RBC/capillary bed transit time
   Atelectasis
   Ventilation abnormalities

B. Shunt equation formula
1. $\begin{array}{c}\% \text{ intrapulmonary}\\ R \to L \text{ shunt}\end{array} = Qs/QT = \dfrac{Cc - Ca}{Cc - C\overline{V}} \times 100$

   Where $Cc = O_2$ content leaving alveolar capillary bed
   $Ca = O_2$ content of arterial bed
   $C\overline{V} = O_2$ content of mixed venous blood
2. Calculation of O_2 capacity

   $(Hgb.)\ \dfrac{(1.34\ cc.\ O_2)}{gm.\ Hgb.}\ (\% \text{ saturation}) + (Po_2)\ (.0031)$

3. e.g.,

   $Cc = \dfrac{(15\ gm.\ Hgb.)(1.34\ cc.\ O_2)}{100\ cc.\ blood\ gm.\ Hgb.}\ (1.00) + (673)\ (.0031)$
   $= 21.99\ vol.\ \%$

   $Ca = (15)(1.34)(.985) + (200)(.0031) = 20.30\ vol.\ \%$
   $C\overline{V} = (15)(1.34)(.670) + (35)(.0031) = 13.51\ vol.\ \%$

   $\dfrac{Qs}{QT} = \dfrac{21.99 - 20.30}{21.99 - 13.50} \times 100 = 19.8\%\ shunt$

C. Derivation of shunt equation
1. Amount of O_2 in arterial blood = amount of O_2 in blood that has traversed the pulmonary capillaries + the amount of O_2 in shunted blood.
2. Since the amount of $O_2 = Cc_2 \times Q$, then
3. $CaQT = (Cco_2) \cdot (Qc) + (C\overline{V} * Qs)$

   QT = total blood flow
   Qc = blood flow through pulmonary capillaries
   Qs = blood flow (of mixed venous blood) through shunt
4. Hence $Qc = QT - Qs$ or $QT = Qs + Qc$
5. Therefore,
   $CaQT = Cc(QT - Qs) + C\overline{V} * Qs$
6. Clearing

   $Qs = \dfrac{Ca - Cc}{C\overline{V} - Cc} \times QT$

   If QT has been measured, then Qs can be calculated in absolute quantities.

   If not, then
       Qs can be calculated as the fraction QT of the total cardiac output that flows through the shunt.

7. As before
   a. $\dfrac{Qs}{QT} = \dfrac{Cao_2 - Cco_2}{C\overline{V}o_2 - Cco_2}$

   This is the value of the "physiologic shunt," which includes not only the absolute anatomic shunts but also a quantity of blood coming from regions with low ventilation-perfusion ratios. The latter is included because the calculated "end-capillary" Po_2 is really a contrived end-capillary Pco_2.
   b. When ventilated with 100% O_2
      $PAo_2 = PB - Paco_2 - PH_2O$ (e.g., 673
             $= 760 - 40 - 47$)

      where $PAco_2 = (Hgb.)(1.34)(1.00) + (.0031)(PAo_2)$

D. Variations on the shunt equation
1. $\dfrac{Qs}{QT} = \dfrac{Cc - Ca}{Cc - C\overline{V}} = \dfrac{Ca - Cc}{C\overline{V}\ Cc}$

   if $Pao_2 > 150$, % Hgb. desaturation of Pao_2 may be disregarded and simplify the shunt equation to:
2. $\dfrac{Qs}{QT} = \dfrac{(.0031)(PAo_2 - Pao_2)}{(Cao_2 - Cvo_2) + (.0031)(PAo_2 - Pao_2)}$

   or
3. $\dfrac{Qs}{QT} = \dfrac{(.0031)(AaDo_2)}{(a - vo_2\ diff) + (.0031)\ (AaDo_2)}$

E. Alveolar-arterial O_2 gradient ($AaDo_2$)
1. $AaDo_2 = (PAo_2 - Pao_2)$
2. $PAo_2 = PB - Paco_2 - PH_2O$ as in the equation C-7b
3. Measure the gradient by ventilating the patient with $Fio_2 = 1.00 \times 20$ minutes and the above assumptions can be made
4. $AaDo_2$ correlates with Qs/QT
5. If the patient has a Swan-Ganz catheter in place and mixed venous samples are obtained simultaneously with Pao_2, and if the patient is preventilated with 100% O_2, then a specific $AaDo_2$:Qs/QT graphic relationship can be plotted and used after the Swan-Ganz catheter has been discontinued. This is better than making a-vo_2 diff assumptions unless cardiac outputs are obtained and an appropriate a-vo_2 diff is derived.
6. e.g.,

   $Fio_2 = 1.00$
   $Pao_2 = 200\ Pco_2 = 36$
   $AaDo - 2 = 760 - 36 - 47 - 200 = 477$
7. 40–50% shunt = 70% mortality
   >50% shunt = 90% mortality

---

by depression of the respiratory center by narcotics, neurologic damage to the neuromuscular respiratory axis, and mechanical abnormalities of the chest (e.g., pneumothorax, flail chest, paralyzed diaphragm). Muscular fatigue due to chronic disease or malnutrition, myasthenia gravis, or exhaustion can lead to hypoventilation and eventually airway obstruction to airway gas flow, which causes hypercarbia. Thus, the etiology of hypoventilation must be sought and corrected. Patients on ventilators can develop hypoventilation due to inappropriate adjustments or to mechanical problems with the gas exchange circuit, causing the expected delivery of gases not to occur.

Diffusion Impairment. Diffusion of oxygen between the alveolus and the pulmonary capillary blood is slower than that of CO_2. Even with increased cardiac output, sufficient transcapillary transit time exists for nearly total equilibration. However, if the blood-gas barrier is increased and diffusion is impaired, oxygen equilibration is slowed and pulmonary venous hypoxemia can occur, even at normal transit times. This usually occurs in chronic interstitial pulmonary diseases such as diffuse interstitial fibrosis, asbestosis, sarcoidosis, Goodpasture's syndrome, and collagen vascular diseases. Hypoxemia caused by diffusion impairment can be improved by administering higher Fio_2.

Arteriovenous Shunts. This category of causes for arterial oxygen desaturation includes congenital (anatomic) shunts that bypass the lungs, such as atrial or ventricular septal defects with right-to-left shunting or intrapulmonary shunts caused by arteriovenous fistulas. Perfusion of an unventilated portion of lung produces a physiologic shunt and is discussed in the next section on ventilation-perfusion abnormalities. With an anatomic shunt, no matter how high the FIO_2, the arterial PO_2 does not normalize. Physiologic shunting due to ventilation-perfusion abnormalities can be improved by altering the ventilation-perfusion ratio.

Ventilation-Perfusion Abnormalities. The major cause of hypoxemia in postoperative patients is physiologic shunting due to ventilation-perfusion mismatching. All lungs have some ventilation-perfusion mismatching due to the regional variation in pulmonary blood blow. Mismatches of ventilation and perfusion occur in the lung as a consequence of atelectasis, alveolar edema, interstitial edema, bronchial obstruction, acidosis, and alveolar collapse.

Variations in regional matching of perfusion and ventilation can occur in three different situations. An area can experience overventilation in comparison with perfusion, a situation that does not necessarily cause any abnormalities if the amount of perfusion to the rest of the lung is normal. An area can be overperfused in relation to the amount of ventilation, which can lead to hypoxemia. When severe or total alveolar hypoventilation occurs, PCO_2 begins to rise. Finally, the ventilation-perfusion matching can be essentially one to one, which leads to normal blood gas values. The first situation causes wasted work of breathing but may not necessarily lead to a change in arterial blood gases. A mismatch of overperfusion to underventilation is the most common clinical problem. Thus, ventilation-perfusion abnormalities cause variable degrees of intrapulmonary physiologic shunting that can be accurately measured by means of the shunt equation (Table 51–9):

$$Q_S/Q_T = \frac{Cc - Ca}{Cc - Cv} \times 100$$

This is an accurate measurement of the amount of blood traveling from the right heart to the left heart that does not equilibrate with the alveolar gases.

Closing Volumes. The closing volume is the remaining lung volume at the end of expiration, below which alveolar collapse begins to cause *physiologic* shunting. In a normal young individual, this closing volume is well below the FRC (see Fig. 51–23). Age alone is associated with a decrease in the elastic properties of the lung; although FRC gradually increases with age, so does the effective closing volume. At some point, these lines cross, and at end-expiration, portions of alveoli are underventilated, a physiologic right-to-left shunt occurs, and the total oxygen saturation decreases. This is why partial pressure of oxygen in the arterial blood gradually decreases with age. This process is accelerated by smoking and other causes of chronic pulmonary disease, leading to hypoxemia at a younger age. In addition, placing a patient (even a young one) supine, or other mechanical factors such as obesity, may lead to an elevation in closing volume and relative hypoxemia.[66, 78] Hypoxemia is common postoperatively because of this *closing volume effect*.[47, 60] The presence of interstitial pulmonary edema accentuates this effect. Applying end-expiratory pressure causes FRC to return to normal and corrects the closing volume abnormality.[12]

SELECTED REFERENCES

Bates, D. V., Macklem, P. T., and Christie, R. V.: Respiratory Function in Disease: An Introduction to the Integrated Study of the Lung, 3rd ed. Philadelphia, W. B. Saunders, 1989.
This outstanding text correlates respiratory physiology and pulmonary disease. Basic pulmonary function studies are reviewed, and individual disease processes that alter physiologic function are presented. It also contains one of the most complete and updated bibliographies on this subject.

Forster, R. E., II, Dubois, A. B., Briscoe, W. A., and Fisher, A. B.: The Lung: Physiologic Basis of Pulmonary Function Tests, 3rd ed. Chicago, Year Book Medical Publishers, 1986.
This is a classic text written for medical students and physicians. It explains, with excellent diagrams and illustrations, aspects of pulmonary physiology and presents the rationale for treatment of acute and chronic disease.

Tisi, G. M.: Pulmonary Physiology in Clinical Medicine, 2nd ed. Baltimore, Williams & Wilkins, 1983.
This outstanding monograph is well illustrated and provides an excellent clinical approach to the physiologic interpretation of pulmonary function in health and disease. This edition has been expanded and covers specific clinical situations commonly encountered in both medical and surgical patients.

REFERENCES

1. AHA Cardiopulmonary Council: Manual for evaluation of lung function by spirometry. Circulation, 65:644A, 1982.
2. Alexander, J. A., and Rodgers, B. M.: Diagnosis and management of pulmonary insufficiency: Symposium on noncardiac thoracic surgery. Surg. Clin. North Am., 60:983, 1980.
3. Ali, M. K., Mountain, C. F., and Miller, J. M.: Regional pulmonary function before and after pneumonectomy using ¹³³xenon. Chest, 68:288, 1975.
4. Ali, M. K., Mountain, C. F., Ewer, M. S., et al.: Predicting loss of pulmonary function after pulmonary resection for bronchogenic carcinoma. Chest, 77:337, 1980.
5. Ashbaugh, D. G., Bigelow, D. B., Petty, T. L., and Levine, B. E.: Acute respiratory distress in adults. Lancet, 2:319, 1969.
6. Ashbaugh, D. G., Petty, T. L., and Bigelow, D. B.: Continuous positive-pressure breathing (CPPB) in adult respiratory distress syndrome. J. Thorac. Cardiovasc. Surg., 57:31, 1969.
7. Ashbaugh, D. G., and Petty, T. C.: Positive end-expiratory pressure: Physiology, indications, and contraindications. J. Thorac. Cardiovasc. Surg., 65:165, 1973.
8. Barter, S. J., Cunningham, D. A., Lavender, J. P., Gibellino, F., Connellan, S. J., and Pride, N. B.: Abnormal ventilation scans in middle-aged smokers. Am. Rev. Respir. Dis., 132:148, 1985.
9. Bates, D. V., Macklem, P. T., and Christie, R. V.: Respiratory Function in Disease: An Introduction to the Integrated Study of the Lung, 3rd ed. Philadelphia, W. B. Saunders, 1989.
10. Bechard, D., and Wetstein, L.: Assessment of exercise oxygen consumption as a preoperative criterion for lung resection. Ann. Thorac. Surg., 44:344, 1987.
11. Berggren, H., Ekroth, R., Malmberg, R., Naucler, J., and William-Olsson, G.: Hospital morbidity and long-term survival in relation to preoperative function in elderly patients with bronchogenic carcinoma. Ann. Thorac. Surg., 38:633, 1984.
12. Bone, R. C.: Treatment of severe hypoxemia due to the adult respiratory distress syndrome. Arch. Intern. Med., 140:85, 1980.
13. Boushy, S. F., Billing, D. M., North, L. B., and Helgason, A. H.: Clinical course related to preoperative and postoperative pulmonary function in patients with bronchogenic carcinoma. Chest, 59:383, 1971.
14. Boysen, P. G., and Benfield, J. R.: Preoperative pulmonary evaluation and postoperative care. Clin. Challenge Cardiopul. Med., 3:1, 1980.
15. Boysen, P. G., Block, A. J., Olsen, G. N., Moulder, P. V., Harris, J. O., and Rawitscher, R. E.: Prospective evaluation for pneumonectomy using the 99m technetium quantitative perfusion lung scan. Chest, 72:422, 1977.
16. Bria, W. F., Kanarek, D. J., and Kazemi, H.: Prediction of postoperative pulmonary function following thoracic operations. J. Thorac. Cardiovasc. Surg., 86:186, 1983.
17. Buczko, G. B., Day, A., Vanderdoelen, J. L., Boucher, R., and Zamel, N.: Effects of cigarette smoking and short-term smoking cessation on airway responsiveness to inhaled methacholine. Am. Rev. Respir. Dis., 129:12, 1984.
18. Buist, A. S., Sexton, G. J., Nagy, J. M., and Ross, B. B.: The effect of smoking cessation and modification on lung function. Am. Rev. Respir. Dis., 114:115, 1976.
19. Craig, D. B.: Postoperative recovery of pulmonary function. Anesth. Analg., 60:46, 1981.
20. DeMeester, T. R., Van Heertum, R. L., Haras, J. R., Watson, R. L., and Hansen, J. E.: Preoperative evaluation with differential pulmonary function. Ann. Thorac. Surg., 18:61, 1974.
21. Dunn, W. F., and Scanlon, P. D.: Preoperative pulmonary function testing for patients with lung cancer. Mayo Clin. Proc., 68:371, 1993.
22. Eugene, J., Brown, S. E., Light, R. W., Milne, N. E., and Stemmer, E. A.: Maximum oxygen consumption: A physiologic guide to pulmonary resection. Surg. Forum, 33:260, 1980.
23. Fahey, P. J., and Hyde, R. W.: "Won't breathe" vs. "can't breathe": Detection of depressed ventilatory drive in patients with obstructive pulmonary disease. Chest, 84:21, 1983.
24. Ferguson, M. K., Little, L., Rizzo, L., Popovich, K. J., Glonek, G. F., Leff, A., Manjoney, D., and Little, A. G.: Diffusing capacity predicts morbidity and mortality after pulmonary resection. J. Thorac. Cardiovasc. Surg., 96:894, 1988.
25. Fiser, W. B., Friday, C. D., and Read, R. C.: Changes in arterial oxygenation and pulmonary shunt during thoracotomy with endobronchial anesthesia. J. Thorac. Cardiovasc. Surg., 83:523, 1982.

26. Forster, R. E., II, Dubois, A. B., Briscoe, W. A., and Fisher, A. B.: The Lung: Physiologic Basis of Pulmonary Function Tests, 3rd ed. Chicago, Year Book Medical Publishers, 1986.

27. Fulton, R. L., and Jones, C. E.: The cause of post-traumatic pulmonary insufficiency in man. Surg. Gynecol. Obstet., 140:179, 1975.

28. Gaensler, E. A., Cugell, D. W., Lindgren, I., Verstraeten, J. M., Smith, S. S., and Streader, J. W.: The role of pulmonary insufficiency in mortality and invalidism following surgery for pulmonary tuberculosis. J. Thorac. Cardiovasc. Surg., 29:163, 1955.

29. Gass, G. D., and Olsen, G. N.: Preoperative pulmonary function testing to predict postoperative morbidity and mortality. Chest, 89:127, 1986.

30. Hammon, J. W., Wolfe, W. G., Moran, J. F., Jones, R. H., and Sabiston, D. C., Jr.: The effect of positive end-expiratory pressure on regional ventilation and perfusion in the normal and injured primate lung. J. Thorac. Cardiovasc. Surg., 72:680, 1976.

31. Hammond, E. C., and Horn, D.: Smoking and death rates: Report on forty-four months of follow-up of 187,783 men. JAMA, 251:2840, 1984.

32. Harman, E., and Lillington, G. A.: Pulmonary risk factors in surgery. Med. Clin. North Am., 63:1289, 1979.

33. Heinemann, H. O., and Goldring, R. M.: Bicarbonate and the regulation of ventilation. Am. J. Med., 57:361, 1974.

34. Hoeppner, V. H., Cooper, D. M., Zamel, N., Bryan, A. C., and Levinson, H.: Relationship between elastic recoil and closing volume in smokers and non-smokers. Am. Rev. Respir. Dis., 109:81, 1974.

35. Hyatt, R. E., and Rodarte, J. R.: Modern medical physiology; "closing volume": One man's noise—other men's experiment. Mayo Clin. Proc., 50:17, 1975.

36. Kinasewitz, G. T.: Survival of the fittest: Exercise testing in the evaluation of thoracotomy candidates. Chest, 102:332, 1992.

37. Kirby, R. R., Downs, J. B., Civetta, J. M., et al.: High level positive end-expiratory pressure (PEEP) in acute respiratory insufficiency. Chest, 67:156, 1975.

38. Kristersson, S., Lindell, S. E., and Svanberg, L.: Prediction of pulmonary function loss due to pneumonectomy using ^{133}Xe-radiospirometry. Chest, 62:694, 1972.

39. Lipscombe, D. J., and Pride, N. B.: Ventilation and perfusion scans in the preoperative assessment of bronchial carcinoma. Thorax, 32:720, 1977.

40. Lockwood, P.: The principles of predicting the risk of post-thoracotomy function-related complications in bronchial carcinoma. Respiration, 30:329, 1973.

41. Lumb, P. D.: Perioperative pulmonary physiology. In Sabiston, D. C., Jr., and Spencer, F. C. (Eds.): Gibbon's Surgery of the Chest, 4th ed. Philadelphia, W. B. Saunders, 1983.

42. Marion, J. M., Alderson, P. O., Lefrak, S. S., Senior, R. M., and Jacobs, M. H.: Unilateral lung function: Comparison of the lateral position test with radionuclide ventilation-perfusion studies. Chest, 69:5, 1976.

43. Markos, J., Mullan, B. P., Hillman, D. R., Musk, A. W., Antico, V. F., Lovegrove, F. T., et al.: Preoperative assessment as a predictor of mortality and morbidity after lung resection. Am. Rev. Respir. Dis., 139:902, 1989.

44. Matthay, M. A., and Wiener-Kronish, J. P.: Respiratory management after cardiac surgery. Chest, 95:427, 1989.

45. McCarthy, D. S., Craig, D. B., and Cherniack, R. M.: Effect on modifications of the smoking habit on lung function. Am. Rev. Respir. Dis., 114:103, 1976.

46. Menkes, H. A., Beaty, T. H., Cohen, B. H., and Weinmann, G.: Nitrogen washout and mortality. Am. Rev. Respir. Dis., 132:115, 1985.

47. Meyers, J. R., Lembeck, L., O'Kane, H., and Baue, A. E.: Changes in functional residual capacity of the lung after operation. Arch. Surg., 110:576, 1975.

48. Miller, J. I., Grossman, G. D., and Hatcher, C. R.: Pulmonary function criteria for operability and pulmonary resection. Surg. Gynecol. Obstet., 153:893, 1981.

49. Mittman, C.: Assessment of operative risk in thoracic surgery. Am. Rev. Respir. Dis., 84:197, 1961.

50. Mittman, C., and Bruderman, I.: State of the art: Lung cancer—to operate or not. Am. Rev. Respir. Dis., 116:477, 1977.

51. Miyoshi, S., Nakahara, K., Ohno, K., Monden, Y., and Kawashima, Y.: Exercise tolerance test in lung cancer patients: The relationship between exercise capacity and post-thoracotomy hospital mortality. Ann. Thorac. Surg., 44:487, 1987.

52. Moran, J. F., Robinson, L. A., Lowe, J. E., and Wolfe, W. G.: Effects of oxygen toxicity on regional ventilation and perfusion in the primate lung. Surgery, 89:575, 1981.

53. Morice, R. C., Peters, E. J., Ryan, M. B., Putnam, J. B., Ali, M. K., and Roth, J. A.: Exercise testing in the evaluation of patients at high risk for complications from lung resection. Chest, 101:356, 1992.

54. Murray, J. F.: The adult respiratory distress syndrome: "May it rest in peace." Am. Rev. Respir. Dis., 111:716, 1975.

55. Murray, J. F.: Mechanisms of acute respiratory failure. Am. Rev. Respir. Dis., 107:115, 1977.

56. Neuhaus, H., and Cherniack, N. S.: A bronchospirometric method of estimating the effect of pneumonectomy on the maximum breathing capacity. J. Thorac. Cardiovasc. Surg., 55:144, 1968.

57. Olsen, G. N., Block, A. J., Swenson, E. W., Castle, J. R., and Wyne, J. W.: Pulmonary function evaluation of the lung resection candidate: A prospective study. Am. Rev. Respir. Dis., 111:379, 1975.

58. Olsen, G. N., Block, A. J., and Tobias, J. A.: Prediction of post pneumonec-

59. Olsen, G. N., Weiman, D. S., Bolton, J. W. R., Gass, D., McLain, W. C., Schoonover, G. A., and Hornung, C. A.: Submaximal invasive exercise testing and quantitative lung scanning in the evaluation for tolerance of lung resection. Chest, 95:26, 1989.

60. Peters, R. M.: Lifesaving measures in acute respiratory distress syndrome. Am. J. Surg., 138:368, 1979.

61. Peters, R. M.: Management of surgically treated patients with limited pulmonary reserve. Am. J. Surg., 138:379, 1979.

62. Pontoppidan, H., Geffin, B., and Lowenstein, E.: Acute Respiratory Failure in the Adult. Boston, Little, Brown, 1973.

63. Putnam, J. B., Jr., Lammermeier, D. E., Colon, R., McMurtrey, M. J., Ali, M. K., and Roth, J. A.: Predicted pulmonary function and survival after pneumonectomy for primary lung carcinoma. Ann. Thorac. Surg., 49:909, 1990.

64. Rams, J. J., Harrison, R. W., Fry, W. A., Moulder, P. V., and Adams, W. E.: Operative pulmonary artery pressure measurements as a guide to postoperative management and prognosis following pneumonectomy. Dis. Chest, 41:85, 1962.

65. Reichel, J.: Assessment of operative risk of pneumonectomy. Chest, 62:570, 1972.

66. Remolina, C., Khan, A. U., Santiago, T. V., and Edelman, N. H.: Positional hypoxemia in unilateral lung disease. N. Engl. J. Med., 304:523, 1981.

67. Shah, D. M., and Powers, S. R.: Prevention of pulmonary complications in high risk patients. Surg. Clin. North Am., 60:1359, 1980.

68. Shelhamer, J. H., Natanson, C., and Parrillo, J. D.: Positive end-expiratory pressure in adults. JAMA, 251:2692, 1984.

69. Smith, P. K., Fuchs, J. C. A., and Sabiston, D. C., Jr.: Surgical management of aortic abdominal aneurysms in patients with severe pulmonary insufficiency. Surg. Gynecol. Obstet., 151:407, 1980.

70. Smith, P. K., Tyson, G. S., Jr., Hammon, J. W., Jr., Olsen, C. O., Hopkins, R. A., Maier, G. W., Sabiston, D. C., Jr., and Rankin, J. S.: Cardiovascular effects of ventilation with positive expiratory airway pressure. Ann. Surg., 195:121, 1982.

71. Smith, T. C., Cook, F. D., DeKornfeld, T. J., and Siebecker, K. L.: Pulmonary function in the immediate postoperative period. J. Thorac. Surg., 39:788, 1960.

72. Smith, T. P., Kinasewitz, G. T., Tucker, W. Y., Spillers, W. P., and George, R. B.: Exercise capacity as a predictor of post-thoracotomy morbidity. Am. Rev. Respir. Dis., 125:604, 1982.

73. Spiro, S., Hahn, H., Edwards, R., and Pride, N.: An analysis of the physiologic strain of submaximal exercise in patients with chronic obstructive bronchitis. Thorax, 30:415, 1975.

74. Stein, M., Koota, G. M., Simon, M., and Frank, H. A.: Pulmonary evaluation of surgical patients. JAMA, 181:103, 1962.

75. Svanberg, L.: Bronchorespirometry in the evaluation of regional lung function. Scand. J. Respir. Dis. Suppl., 62:91, 1966.

76. Tisi, G. M.: Preoperative evaluation of pulmonary function. Am. Rev. Respir. Dis., 119:293, 1979.

77. Tisi, G. M.: Pulmonary Physiology in Clinical Medicine, 2nd ed. Baltimore, Williams & Wilkins, 1983.

78. Tucker, D. H., and Seiker, H. O.: The effects of change in body position on lung volumes and intrapulmonary gas mixing in patients with obesity, heart failure and emphysema. Am. Rev. Respir. Dis., 83:787, 1960.

79. Uggla, L. G.: Indications for and results of thoracic surgery with regard to respiratory and circulatory function tests. Acta Chir. Scand., 111:197, 1956.

80. Van Nostrand, D., Kjelsberg, M. O., and Humphrey, E. W.: Presectional evaluation of risk from pneumonectomy. Surg. Gynecol. Obstet., 127:306, 1968.

81. Wasserman, K., Hansen, J., Sue, D., and Whipp, B. J.: Principles of Exercise Testing and Interpretation. Philadelphia, Lea & Febiger, 1986.

82. Waxman, K., and Shoemaker, W. C.: Management of postoperative and posttraumatic respiratory failure in the intensive care unit. Surg. Clin. North Am., 60:1413, 1980.

83. Weber, K. T., Andrews, V., Kinasewitz, G. T., Janicki, J. S., and Fishman, A. P.: Vasodilator and inotropic agents in treatment of congestive heart failure: Clinical experience and responses in exercise performance. Am. Heart J., 102:569, 1981.

84. Weber, K. T., and Janicki, J. S.: Cardiopulmonary Exercise Testing: Physiologic Principles and Clinical Applications. Philadelphia, W. B. Saunders, 1986.

85. Weber, K. T., and Janicki, J. S.: Cardiopulmonary exercise testing for evaluation of chronic cardiac failure. Am. J. Cardiol., 55:22(A-31), 1985.

86. Weber, K. T., and Janicki, J. S.: Lactate production during maximal and submaximal exercise in patients with chronic heart failure. J. Am. Coll. Cardiol., 6:717, 1985.

87. Weber, K. T., Janicki, J. S., and Maskin, C. S.: Effects of new inotropic agents on exercise performance. Circulation, 73 (suppl. III):196, 1986.

88. Weber, K. T., Janicki, J. S., McElroy, P. A., and Reddy, H. K.: Concepts and applications of cardiopulmonary exercise testing. Chest, 93:843, 1988.

89. Wernly, J. A., DeMeester, T. R., Kirchner, P. T., Myerowitz, P. D., Oxford, D. E., and Golomb, H. M.: Clinical value of quantitative ventilation-perfusion lung scans in the surgical management of bronchogenic carcinoma. J. Thorac. Cardiovasc. Surg., 80:535, 1980.

90. West, J. B.: Ventilation/Blood Flow and Gas Exchange, 3rd ed. Philadel-
    phia, F. A. Davis, 1977.
91. Wilson, J. R., Martin, J. L., Ferraro, N., and Weber, K. T.: Effect of hydralaz-
    ine on perfusion and metabolism in the leg during upright bicycle exercise
    in patients with heart failure. Circulation, 68:425, 1983.
92. Wolfe, W. G.: Preoperative assessment of pulmonary function: Quantitative
    evaluation of ventilation and blood-gas exchange. In Sabiston, D. C., Jr.,

and Spencer, F. C. (Eds): Gibbon's Surgery of the Chest, 5th ed. Philadel-
    phia, W. B. Saunders, 1990.
93. Wolfe, W. G., Robinson, L. A., Moran, J. F., and Lowe, J. E.: Reversible
    pulmonary oxygen toxicity in the primate. Ann. Surg., 188:530, 1978.
94. Zibrank, J. D., O'Donnell, C. R., and Marton, K.: Indications for pulmonary
    function testing. Ann. Intern. Med., 112:763, 1990.

III

BRONCHOSCOPY

Mark Tedder, M.D., and Ross M. Ungerleider, M.D.

*In case of doubt as to whether bronchoscopy should be done or not,
bronchoscopy should always be done.*

CHEVALIER JACKSON, 1915

Fiberoptic technology has revolutionized the field of bronchoscopy by markedly expanding its diagnostic capabilities.
Initially performed only by pulmonologists, bronchoscopy
must now be part of the armamentarium of every anesthesiologist, otolaryngologist, and thoracic surgeon. A firm understanding of the indications for bronchoscopy, the various
anesthetic techniques, the technical aspects of the intervention (with both flexible and rigid instruments), and the management of potential complications is imperative.

HISTORICAL ASPECTS

Sensing the obvious desirability of extending the usual
limits of physical examination, Bozzini in 1806 created an
endoscopic instrument utilizing a wax candle as a light
source. Although he was able to examine the oropharynx, it
is doubtful that he saw distal to the cricopharyngeal sphincter. Following Edison's development of miniature electric
lamps came the first successful removal of an aspirated
foreign body. In 1897, Gustav Killian (the "father of
bronchoscopy") used an external light source and a head
mirror to remove an aspirated pork bone from a 63-year-old
farmer under cocaine anesthesia.[30] The worldwide sensation
that this operation created was caused not only by its success
but also by the demonstration that the tracheobronchial tree
could be safely intubated. Prior to this, these structures were
believed to be rigid and stiff, precluding safe instrumentation. The first American to successfully remove an aspirated
foreign body was Algernon Coolidge Jr. in 1898, using an
open urethroscope and sunlight reflected off a head mirror.[10]
Four years later, Einhorn produced an endoscope with illumination at the tip.[8] In 1904, Chevalier Jackson incorporated
suction at the end of a tip-illuminated bronchoscope. Thereafter, Jackson remained at the forefront of bronchoscopy, founding the Philadelphia School of Bronchoesophagology. At this
institution, Jackson trained all the leaders in the field and
subsequently published his *Bronchoesophagology*, which remains a fascinating landmark volume.[11]

Recent developments in fiberoptics[18, 26] and an interest in
the early diagnosis of lung cancer led Ikeda to develop a
prototype for the flexible bronchoscope in 1964.[8] After several
improvements over the next three years, he introduced the
first flexible bronchoscope. Given that its use requires only
topical anesthesia, flexible bronchoscopy was rapidly welcomed and gained widespread acceptance. Finally, the devel-

opment of the Hopkins rod-lens optical telescopes in 1976
revolutionized the optics of endoscopy by providing more
efficient light transmission, brighter images, improved resolution, greater depth of field, and a wider field of view.[7]

BRONCHOSCOPIC EXAMINATION

Adequately stocked portable carts have allowed bronchoscopy to be safely performed in the outpatient setting, the
intensive care unit, or the operating room, provided cardiopulmonary resuscitation equipment and medications are
present. Prior to the administration of any sedative or anesthetic agent, appropriate monitoring must be established.
This usually consists of pulse oximetry, telemetry, and blood
pressure assessment in the outpatient environment; more
invasive monitoring may be indicated in the intensive care
unit or operating room. Fluoroscopy is occasionally of benefit
in localization and should be available. Preoperative laboratory evaluation historically has included coagulation studies
and a platelet count, but the cost-effectiveness of performing these tests in otherwise healthy patients has been questioned.[5, 21]

Preprocedural preparation includes the patient consuming
nothing by mouth the night before bronchoscopy. Intravenous vagolytic agents (to decrease secretions and vasovagal
events) and anxiolytic or narcotic agents may be administered immediately prior to the procedure. The specific medications and doses vary among institutions and are highly
dependent on the patient's comorbidities.

In the ambulatory setting, topical anesthesia is preferred
and usually consists of either lidocaine (1% to 4%) or tetra-
caine (0.5% to 2%). The nasopharynx (or oropharynx) is first
anesthetized with an aerosolized topical agent. Topical anesthesia to the lower airway may be delivered transtracheally
but is more commonly administered through the bronchoscope under direct visualization.

The need for prebronchoscopic intubation must be individualized and should depend on the likelihood of a major
airway complication (e.g., presence of massive hemoptysis,
copious secretions), the patient's pulmonary status, and the
extent of the planned intervention. In addition, an ineffective
cough and altered mental status are relative indications for
bronchoscopic evaluation under general anesthesia. Although general anesthesia allows for simultaneous ventilation and bronchoscopic examination, care must be taken to
suction judiciously (based on the patient's pulmonary status)
and utilize laser therapy with great care (avoiding the concomitant use of flammable agents).

The indications for bronchoscopy are listed in Table 51–10,
with the most common being the assessment of preoperative
resectability or pulmonary lesions seen on chest films, re-

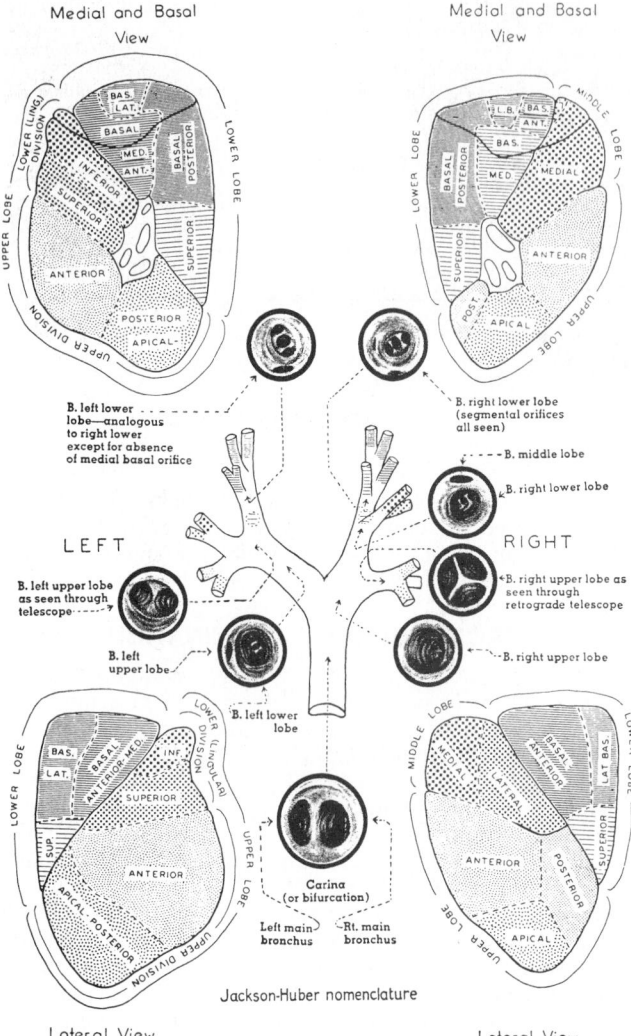

Figure 51–24. The pulmonary segments, with lobar bronchi and segmental branches. The insets depict various endoscopic landmarks. The bronchial tree is "upside down" to show the structures as the bronchoscopist sees them when the patient is examined in the usual position of dorsal recumbency. (From Jackson, C., and Jackson, C. L.: Bronchoesophagology. Philadelphia, W. B. Saunders, 1950.)

TABLE 51–10. Indications for Bronchoscopy

Diagnostic Bronchoscopy	Therapeutic Bronchoscopy
Hemoptysis	Foreign body removal
Pulmonary mass on chest x-ray	Difficult intubation
Recurrent or unresolved pneumonia	Lobar atelectasis
Air trapping or persistent atelectasis	Stricture dilation
Preoperative resectability	Lung abscess
assessment	Laser therapy
Diffuse lung disease	Phototherapy
Malignant pleural effusion	Cryotherapy
Suspicion of a foreign body	Brachytherapy
Suspicion of an opportunistic	Immunotherapy
infection	
Cough	
Localized wheeze	
Unexplained positive sputum	
cytology	
Inhalational injury	
Tracheobronchial trauma	
Diaphragmatic paralysis	
Upper esophageal carcinoma	
Recurrent laryngeal nerve paralysis	
Selective bronchography	
Bronchoalveolar lavage	

or transbronchial), which varies from institution to institution. This is particularly true for special studies such as electron microscopy and staining for tumor markers.

ACCESSORIES

Myriad instruments may be introduced through the bronchoscope's accessory port (Fig. 51–25). Standard biopsy forceps, brushes, curets, or needles are commonly used to evaluate endobronchial lesions. The accuracy of diagnosing carcinoma with bronchoscopy is dependent on the number and types of specimens obtained. Peribronchial tissues may be sampled by transbronchial biopsy (either forceps or needle aspiration). Transbronchial needle aspiration is performed with an ensheathed 21-gauge needle through the instrument channel and should be performed prior to brushings, washings, or lavage to decrease the false-positive rate. In addition, the false-negative rate is at least 15%.[20, 24] Brushings are generally performed after tissues have been directly sampled (Fig. 51–26). Use of the 7-mm. brush results in a higher yield of cellular material than does use of the 1.7-mm. brush. Removing the bronchoscope and brush as a unit increases the diagnostic yield; removing the brush through the instrument channel frequently loses tissue and may contaminate the channel for subsequent diagnostic interventions. Grasping forceps or a basket extractor is commonly used for the removal of airway foreign bodies. Suction traps facilitate recov-

moval of foreign bodies, persistent infiltrate, and difficult intubation. Prior to performing bronchoscopy, it is essential to understand the relationship and bronchoscopic appearance of the major lobar and segmental divisions (Fig. 51–24).

A careful examination is essential to maximize the amount of information gained from a bronchoscopy. Most bronchoscopists insert the flexible bronchoscope through the nasopharynx.[13, 16, 23] Prior to entering the trachea, the larynx and vocal cords should be carefully evaluated for all the information stated below and for cord mobility. The tracheobronchial tree must be inspected for airway position, branching pattern, and mucosal abnormalities (e.g., neoplasm, pronounced folds or corrugations, inflammation, laceration, vascular anomalies), extramucosal abnormalities (e.g., foreign body, secretions, blood, carbonaceous sputum), and airway patency (obstruction from neoplasm, foreign body, postoperative or inflammatory stricture or stenosis). Endobronchial washings (selective or nonselective) should be sent for appropriate studies (e.g., cytopathologic or microbiologic evaluation). One must know the preferred way to handle tissue samples obtained from bronchoscopic biopsies (forceps, brush, curet,

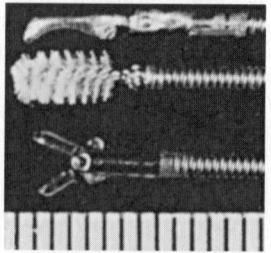

Figure 51–25. Curet, brush, and biopsy forceps for use through the flexible bronchoscope. (From Marsh, B. M.: Advances in bronchoscopy. Otolaryngol. Clin. North Am., 2:371, 1978.)

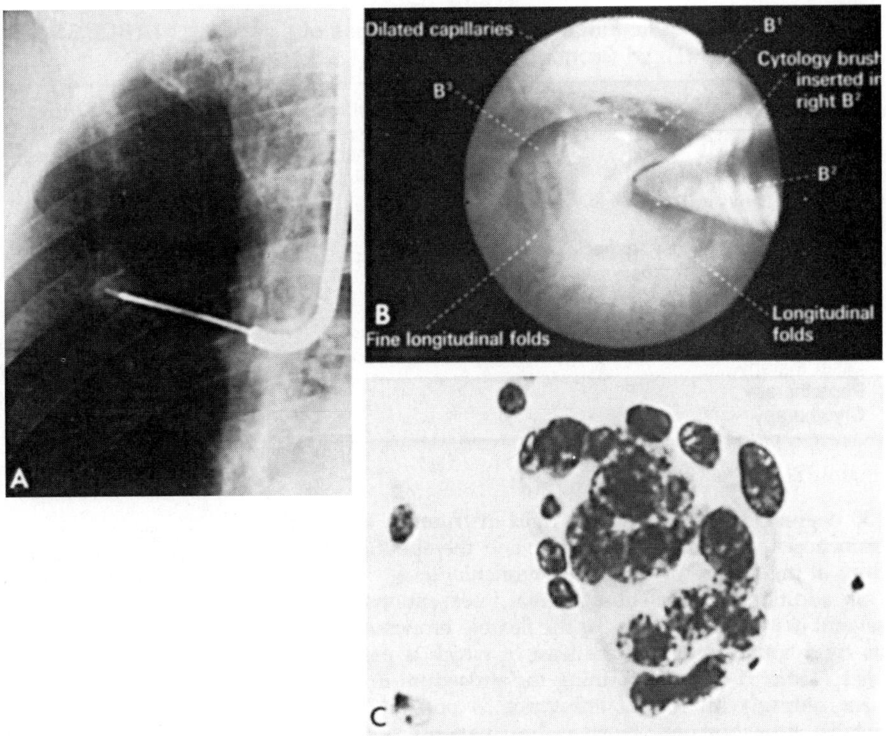

Figure 51–26. *A,* Film demonstrating the brush advanced under fluoroscopic guidance into the peripheral tumor in the right upper lobe. *B,* Fiberoptic view as the brush is advanced through the proper segmental bronchus. *C,* Confirmation of malignancy with a cytologic specimen obtained during maneuvers depicted in *A* and *B.* (From Oho, K., and Ryuta, A.: Practical Fiberoptic Bronchoscopy. New York, Igaku-Shoin, 1980.)

ery of samples for cytology, microbiologic stains, and culture and sensitivity. Several new bronchoscopic techniques have been applied, such as laser therapy, phototherapy, cryotherapy, immunotherapy, and brachytherapy.[17, 19, 22] Many of these techniques occasionally require fluoroscopy for localization prior to intervention. The ultimate roles of these modalities in treating various pulmonary diseases has yet to be determined.

RIGID BRONCHOSCOPY

Although only 2% of bronchoscopies are performed using the rigid bronchoscope, 90% of these are performed by surgeons,[16] necessitating adequate exposure to and training in this technique. The blunt and beveled tip of the rigid bronchoscope allows for safe insertion, and the proximal end allows for mechanical ventilation, a Hopkins telescope, and the introduction of various accessories (Fig. 51–27). The instruments are typically 20 to 30 cm. (pediatric) or 40 cm. (adult) in length, with internal diameters of 3 mm. and 7 to 8 mm., respectively. Rigid bronchoscopes have 0-, 30-, or 90-degree viewing ports and a 70-degree field of view. Diagnostic and therapeutic interventions in the distal tracheobronchial tree may be further enhanced by the insertion of a flexible bronchoscope through a rigid instrument.

Certain clinical scenarios are best approached with rigid bronchoscopy. This remains the procedure of choice for the majority of pediatric bronchoscopy (particularly foreign body removal) and for the evaluation of massive hemoptysis. Stricture dilation, stent placement, laser therapy, phototherapy, and cryotherapy may also be performed through the rigid bronchoscope (Table 51–11).[1, 2, 4, 12, 25]

FLEXIBLE BRONCHOSCOPY

Since its introduction less than 30 years ago, flexible bronchoscopy has become commonplace in the evaluation of numerous pulmonary disorders. The external diameters of the flexible bronchoscopes range from 2.2 to 6.2 mm., with associated instrument channel ports varying in size from 1.2 to 3.2 mm. (Fig. 51–28). The most commonly used flexible bronchoscope in the adult population is the 5.8-mm. external and 2.2-mm. internal diameter instrument. The field of view is 90 to 120 degrees, with an upward angle of deflection of 160 to 180 degrees and a downward angle of deflection of 100 to

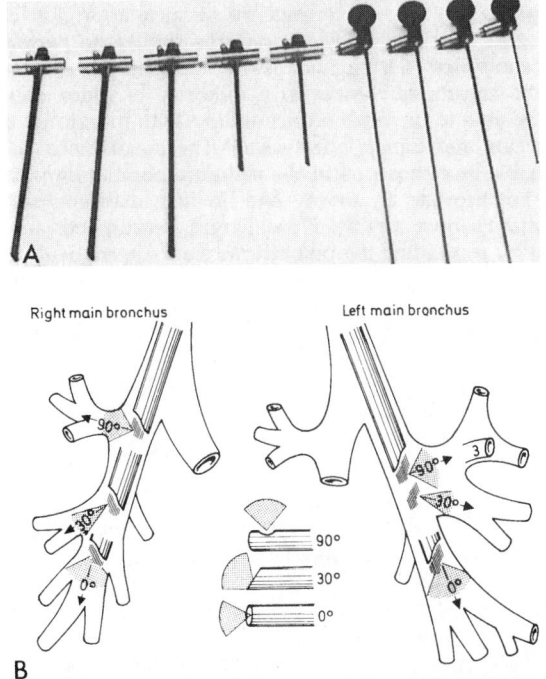

Figure 51–27. Array of bronchoscopes of varying sizes and standard telescopes with 0-degree, 30-degree, and 70-degree viewing angles. In addition, the small telescope is a 20-cm. forward-viewing model for use with the 3 mm. by 20 cm. bronchoscope (far right). (From de Kock, M. A.: Dynamic Bronchoscopy. New York, Springer-Verlag, 1977.)

TABLE 51–11. Advantages and Disadvantages of Rigid Bronchoscopy

Advantages	Disadvantages
Durability	General anesthesia
Large instrument channel	Limited distal visualization
Control of airway	Cost
Usefulness in:	
Pediatric bronchoscopy (especially foreign bodies)	
Massive hemoptysis	
Stricture dilation	
Stent placement	
Laser therapy	
Phototherapy	
Cryotherapy	

TABLE 51–12. Advantages and Disadvantages of Flexible Bronchoscopy

Advantages	Disadvantages
Patient tolerance	Instrument channel size
Topical anesthesia	Sterilization
Field of view	Maintenance
Angle of deflection	
Versatility	
Ambulatory setting	
Ventilator-dependent setting	
Usefulness in:	
Cervical spine disorders	
Subsegmental intervention	
Transbronchial needle aspiration	
Brachytherapy	
Immunotherapy	

130 degrees. In contrast to the rigid instrument, the flexible bronchoscope facilitates diagnostic and therapeutic interventions at the fourth- or fifth-order bronchial level.

In addition to these subsegmental interventions, there are several distinct advantages of the flexible bronchoscope over its rigid counterpart, not the least of which is patient tolerance (Table 51–12).[8] Performing the procedure in an outpatient setting with topical anesthesia is possible only with flexible bronchoscopy. Furthermore, patients with cervical spine disorders or aneurysms of the thoracic aorta can generally be evaluated with flexible bronchoscopy, whereas these diseases are contraindications to rigid instrumentation.

PEDIATRIC BRONCHOSCOPY

The Hopkins rod-lens telescopes have opened new vistas in the practice of pediatric endoscopy. Given the development of smaller equipment, indications for pediatric bronchoscopy parallel those outlined for adults.[15, 28] One unique indication is the localization of certain tracheoesophageal fistulas, as this helps determine the surgical approach (cervical versus thoracic). Most procedures should be performed in a controlled setting such as an operating room under general anesthesia; however, a minority of older children may be able to undergo bronchoscopy with monitored anesthetic care and topical anesthesia.[15] The major disadvantage of flexible bronchoscopy in the pediatric population is that it does not provide an airway and, in fact, may encroach on the infant's own airway. Hence, rigid instruments are preferred for evaluating the pediatric airway. Alternatively, some authors have used flexible instruments to remove secretions and localize foreign bodies.[15, 26, 27] The flexible bronchoscope may also be passed *through* a rigid scope for lesions in the more distal tracheobronchial tree.

Care must be taken intraoperatively to minimize trauma to the pediatric airway, as the resultant subglottic edema may obstruct the airway. Therefore, postoperative stridorous breathing should be aggressively treated with humidified supplemental oxygen, bronchodilators, and possibly steroids.

COMPLICATIONS

Bronchoscopy is generally considered a safe procedure.[3, 6, 9, 14] Most complications are preventable when appropriate attention is given to preoperative preparation, identification of high-risk patients, and performance of a careful bronchoscopic examination. Accordingly, the premedication and anesthetic care, duration of procedure, and degree of instrumentation must be individualized. A comprehensive survey of bronchoscopic complications (n = 24,521) revealed the morbidity and mortality to be 0.08% and 0.01%, respectively.[3] Complications are categorized in Table 51–13 as being related to anesthesia, technical difficulties, or biopsy. Endoscopy-related pneumonia has been reported, necessitating meticulous cleaning and sterilization procedures.[14] Appropriate

TABLE 51–13. Complications of Bronchoscopy

Premedication and Anesthesia

Respiratory depression/arrest
Transient hypotension
Seizures
Hyperexcited state
Laryngospasm
Syncope
Cardiac arrest

Technical Difficulties

Respiratory compromise
  Obstruction
  Perforation
Hemorrhage
Laryngospasm
Bronchospasm
Dysrhythmias
Syncope
Pneumonia
Hypoxemia
Pyrexia
Epistaxis

Biopsy

Hemorrhage
Perforation
  Mediastinal emphysema
  Pneumothorax
Air embolism

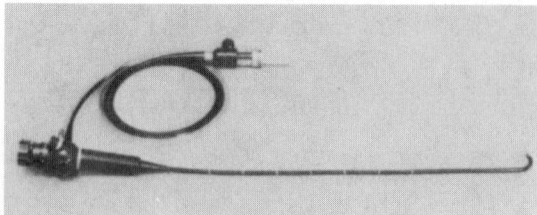

Figure 51–28. BF-B3–type fiberoptic bronchoscope (Olympus). (From Oho, K., and Ryuta, A.: Practical Fiberoptic Bronchoscopy. New York, Igaku-Shoin, 1980.)

therapy of bleeding and pneumothorax merits particular attention.

Most bleeding following bronchoscopy with biopsy is minor (less than 25 to 50 ml.) and self-limited. Patients are at particular risk for postprocedural hemorrhage if baseline coagulation parameters are abnormal. Although the volume of blood may not be large, the resultant airway compromise may be significant in a patient with minimal pulmonary reserve. Life-threatening hemorrhage may occur, most likely on the inferior aspect of the right upper lobe bronchus (which lies immediately superior to the right main pulmonary artery) or at the bifurcation of the bronchus intermedius.

Elderly patients[5] and those undergoing transbronchial biopsy are at an increased risk of bleeding (up to 10%).[29] Patients in the latter group are at a substantially higher risk of hemorrhage if they are immunocompromised or uremic. The more peripheral the biopsy, the less likely it is that significant bleeding will occur. With minimal to moderate hemorrhage requiring intervention, epinephrine injection or tamponade by lodging the tip of the bronchoscope into the appropriate segment may be indicated. Therapy may include exchange of a flexible instrument for a rigid bronchoscope, since the former yields poorer visualization in this scenario, and the suction is frequently incapable of handling the volume of blood. Following insertion of the rigid bronchoscope for massive hemoptysis, the opposite main-stem bronchus is preferentially intubated, and the patient is placed in the bleeding-side-down position. This allows for selective ventilation and a decreased risk of contaminating the uninvolved lung. Direct pressure, epinephrine washing, packing with prothrombotic agents, and selective balloon tamponade are other modalities that should be considered for moderate hemorrhage complicating bronchoscopy. Should these therapies fail, angiography with embolization and thoracotomy with pulmonary resection are more interventional therapeutic options.

Pneumothorax following bronchoscopy is an uncommon but potentially lethal complication. It occurs in less than 1% of patients who undergo transbronchial needle biopsy but in approximately 5% of those having a transbronchial forceps biopsy.[3] The routine use of fluoroscopic guidance in high-risk patients and procedures may decrease the incidence of pneumothorax. Frequent physical examination and radiographic evaluation are used to assess the need for decompression with either a dart or a chest tube, as nearly 50% of such pneumothoraces require such an intervention.[14]

SELECTED REFERENCES

Ikeda, S.: Atlas of Flexible Bronchofiberscopy. Baltimore, University Park Press, 1974.
Since his introduction of the bronchofiberscope in 1967, Ikeda has compiled excellent examples of pulmonary pathology amenable to bronchoscopic diagnosis. Recommended by experienced bronchoscopists, this atlas contains a detailed discussion of fiberoptic principles, including their application in visualizing fourth- or fifth-order bronchi.

Jackson, C., and Jackson, C. L.: Bronchoesophagology. Philadelphia, W. B. Saunders, 1950.
This classic monograph by the "dean of American bronchoscopy" and his son offers much insight into the diagnosis of and appropriate therapy for foreign body aspiration. It summarizes the work of the Philadelphia School of Bronchoesophagology and discusses a variety of endoscopic applications and their appropriate role.

Oho, K., and Ryuta, A.: Practical Fiberoptic Bronchoscopy. New York, Igaku-Shoin, 1984.
As proponents of the flexible instrument, the authors display brilliant pictures covering the entire spectrum of bronchoscopy. Its versatility and wide applicability are stressed.

Wood, R. E.: Medical progress: Endoscopy of the airway in infants and children. J. Pediatr., 112:1, 1988.
This article reviews over 1000 bronchoscopic procedures performed by one of the most experienced pediatric bronchoscopists. The roles of the flexible and rigid instruments are clearly stated. Specific differences between adult and pediatric bronchoscopy are also well summarized.

REFERENCES

1. Arroliga, A. C., and Matthay, R. A.: The role of bronchoscopy in lung cancer. Clin. Chest Med., 14:87, 1993.
2. Cavaliere, S., Foccoli, P., and Farina, P. L.: Nd: YAG laser bronchoscopy: A five year experience with 1,396 applications in 1,000 patients. Chest, 94:15, 1988.
3. Credle, W. F., Smiddy, J. F., and Elliott, R. C.: Complications of fiberoptic bronchoscopy. Am. Rev. Respir. Dis., 109:67, 1974.
4. Edell, E. S.: Bronchoscopic phototherapy with hematoporphyrin derivative for treatment of localized bronchogenic carcinoma: A 5-year experience. Mayo Clin. Proc., 62:8, 1987.
5. Haponik, E. F., Kvale, P., and Wang, K. P.: Bronchoscopy and related procedures. In Fishman, A. P. (Ed.): Pulmonary Diseases and Disorders. New York, McGraw-Hill, 1988.
6. Herf, S. M., Suratt, P. M., and Arora, N. S.: Deaths and complications associated with transbronchial lung biopsy. Am. Rev. Respir. Dis., 115:708, 1977.
7. Hopkins, H. H. Optical Principles of the Endoscope. New York, Appleton-Century-Crofts, 1976.
8. Ikeda, S.: Atlas of Flexible Bronchoscopy. Baltimore, University Park Press, 1974.
9. Inglis, A. F., and Wagner, D. V.: Lower complication rates associated with bronchial foreign bodies over the last 20 years. Ann. Otol. Rhinol. Laryngol., 101:61, 1992.
10. Jackson, C.: Bronchoscopy: Past, present and future. N. Engl. J. Med., 199:759, 1928.
11. Jackson, C., and Jackson, C. L.: Bronchoesophagology. Philadelphia, W. B. Saunders, 1950.
12. Jackson, C. V., Savage, P. J., and Quinn, D. L.: Role of fiberoptic bronchoscopy in patients with hemoptysis and a normal chest roentgenogram. Chest, 87:142, 1985.
13. Oho, K., and Amemiya, R.: Practical Fiberoptic Bronchoscopy, 2nd ed. Tokyo, Igaku-Shoin, 1984.
14. Pereira, W., Jr., Kovnat, D. M., and Snider, G. L.: A prospective cooperative study of complications following flexible fiberoptic bronchoscopy. Chest, 73:813, 1978.
15. Perez, C. R., and Wood, R. E.: Update on pediatric flexible bronchoscopy. Pediatr. Clin. North Am., 41:385, 1994.
16. Prakash, U. B. S., Offord, K. P., and Stubbs, S. E.: Bronchoscopy in North America: The ACCP survey. Chest, 100:1668, 1991.
17. Prakash, U. B. S., and Stubbs, S. E.: The bronchoscopy survey—some reflections. Chest, 100:1660, 1991.
18. Sackner, M. A. Bronchofiberscopy. Am. Rev. Respir. Dis., 111:62, 1975.
19. Sanderson, D. R.: Bronchoscopy. Br. Med. Bull., 42:244, 1986.
20. Shure, D., and Fedullo, P. F.: The role of transcarinal needle aspiration in the staging of bronchogenic carcinoma. Chest, 86:693, 1984.
21. Stradling, P.: Diagnostic Bronchoscopy—A Teaching Manual, 6th ed. Edinburgh, Churchill Livingstone, 1991.
22. Sutedja, G., and Postmus, P. E.: Bronchoscopic treatment of lung tumors. Lung Cancer, 11:1, 1994.
23. Wang, K. P.: Techniques in Pulmonary Disorders, 1st ed. New York, Raven Press, 1989.
24. Wang, K. P., Brower, R., Haponik, E. F., and Siegelman, S.: Flexible transbronchial needle aspiration for staging of bronchogenic carcinoma. Chest, 84:571, 1983.
25. Wolfe, W. G., Cole, P. H., and Sabiston, D. C., Jr.: Experimental and clinical use of the YAG laser in the management of pulmonary neoplasms. Ann. Surg., 199:526, 1984.
26. Wood, R. E.: Clinical application of ultrathin flexible bronchoscopes. Pediatr. Pulmonol., 1:244, 1985.
27. Wood, R. E.: The diagnostic effectiveness of the flexible bronchoscope in children. Pediatr. Pulmonol., 1:188, 1985.
28. Wood, R. E., and Postma, D.: Endoscopy of the airway in infants and children. J. Pediatr., 112:1, 1988.
29. Zavala, D. C.: Diagnostic fiberoptic bronchoscopy: Techniques and results of biopsy in 600 patients. Chest, 68:12, 1976.
30. Zollner, F.: Historical vignette. Gustav Killian: Father of bronchoscopy. Arch. Otolaryngol., 82:656, 1965.

IV

THORACOSCOPY

Joseph B. Shrager, M.D., and Larry R. Kaiser, M.D.

The availability of video-assisted thoracoscopic approaches in the management of diseases of the chest represents perhaps the greatest advance in thoracic surgery in the past decade. The rapid progress that occurred in the late 1980s in use of the laparoscope for abdominal surgery stimulated thoracic surgeons to rediscover the thoracoscope as a tool in the diagnosis and treatment of pulmonary and mediastinal pathology. Advances in video technology and surgical stapling facilitated the application of thoracoscopy to procedures previously not considered amenable to minimally invasive approaches. These new techniques, although not replacing conventional open techniques, in many circumstances allow the surgeon to accomplish the same goals with less morbidity. An entirely new field—video-assisted thoracoscopic surgery (VATS)—has arisen.

HISTORICAL ASPECTS

Thoracoscopy dates to 1910, when Hans Christian Jacobaeus (Fig. 51–29), a Swedish physician, noted that a simple

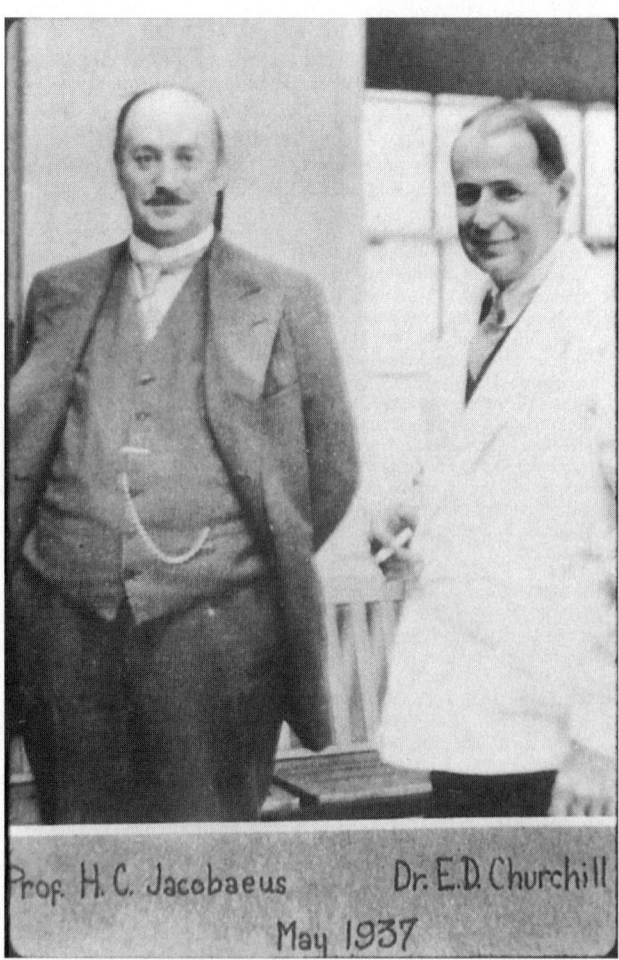

Figure 51–29. Professor H. C. Jacobaeus, the originator of thoracoscopy, pictured with Dr. Edward Churchill during a 1937 visit to the Massachusetts General Hospital. (From Kaiser, L. R.: Video-assisted thoracic surgery [VATS]: Current state of the art. Ann. Surg., *220*[6]:720, 1994.)

cystoscope could be passed into the thoracic cavity to aid in the diagnosis and treatment of pulmonary tuberculosis.[17] He later described the use of the thoracoscope to lyse pleural adhesions as an adjunct to the collapse therapy then in vogue for the treatment of tuberculosis,[18] and to localize and diagnose a variety of lesions of the pleura and lung parenchyma.[19] Although thoracoscopic procedures were sporadically performed in the United States during this era, they were never completely embraced. Lilienthal's 1925 textbook, *Thoracic Surgery*, warned against the routine use of the technique because of fear of bleeding and the risk of spreading infection.[27]

Outside of sporadic reports describing other uses, the major application of thoracoscopy until the past decade has been in the diagnosis of pleural pathology. *Pleuroscopy* has been most widely employed in the evaluation of pleural effusions of unknown etiology, when fluid cytology does not contain malignant cells and closed pleural biopsy is similarly nondiagnostic. It was found that with direct visualization of the pleural cavity in such cases, appropriate material could be obtained that facilitated the making of a diagnosis. A variety of endoscopes have been used for thoracoscopy, including rigid and flexible bronchoscopes and mediastinoscopes. A rigid thoracoscope employing a Hopkins rod-lens system was available but infrequently used. Because only the operator can visualize the field through these types of instruments, the surgeon is required to hold the instrument himself. As a result, complex procedures cannot be performed. In fact, the only therapeutic intervention carried out with any frequency by this technique has been pleurodesis, although the occasional lung biopsy has been reported.

The development of a light-sensitive silicon chip in the 1980s allowed sufficient video camera miniaturization to bring video imaging into the operating room. With a magnified image of the operative field on a video monitor that everyone in the operating suite can see, the surgeon is now able to work with an assistant, freeing his and the assistant's hands to work in concert in complex maneuvers. A further crucial innovation was the development of an endoscopic linear stapler, which cuts between parallel rows of staples that are both hemo- and aerostatic, allowing simple, safe stapling and removal of lung parenchyma. With these technological leaps forward, it is now possible to perform a wide variety of diagnostic and therapeutic procedures, which had previously required thoracotomy, through two to four small intercostal incisions. The lack of rib spreading has been shown in prospective, randomized studies to reduce postoperative pain, minimize pulmonary dysfunction, and shorten hospital stay,[39, 42] and it is likely to decrease overall morbidity related to thoracic surgical procedures.

PRINCIPLES AND GENERAL TECHNIQUE

Working within the abdominal cavity requires the insufflation of gas (carbon dioxide) to create a space in which to manipulate instruments, but the thorax, by virtue of its rigid bone structure, provides its own space once the lung is collapsed. Single-lung ventilation to the contralateral side through a double-lumen endobronchial tube allows collapse of the lung on the side of interest once the negative intrapleural pressure is lost by placement of the first intercostal incision. Use of an endobronchial tube obviously requires a general anesthetic, and most thoracoscopic procedures have been performed in this manner. The less complex techniques, however, have been performed using regional anesthesia, as the lung collapses even in a spontaneously breathing patient once the pleural space is opened to ambient pressure.[38] Exposure of the entire thoracic cavity is excellent after successful collapse of the lung. This includes exposure of posterior mediastinal structures such as the sympathetic chain and the thoracic duct, which may, in fact, be seen better with the magnification afforded by video thoracoscopy than by direct, open visualization.

For most thoracoscopic procedures, the patient is placed in the lateral decubitus position, and the chest is prepared and draped as for a thoracotomy. Arterial blood gas monitoring is recommended. The initial incision, through which the video telescope is placed, is generally positioned in approximately the posterior-axillary line in the seventh or eighth intercostal space. A 1-cm. transverse skin incision is made and deepened over the superior aspect of the rib to avoid the neurovascular bundle, as for placement of a chest tube. Once ventilation to the operative side is stopped, allowing the lung to fall away from the chest wall, the parietal pleura is penetrated carefully, and any adhesions are taken down bluntly with the index finger. A port to admit the video telescope is then placed in the chest, and the telescope follows. The placement of additional incisions is guided by direct visualization from within the thorax, as viewed on the video screen. Their positions depend to some extent on the procedure to be performed, but a triangular arrangement facilitates the performance of most operations (Fig. 51–30). An attempt is made to place these additional incisions in the line of a standard or muscle-sparing thoracotomy incision, so that if a thoracotomy is required, the incisions can simply be included. Two video monitors are generally employed, one on each side of the operating table. At the conclusion of the procedure, one or two chest tubes are placed through the operating ports; they are removed in the postoperative period according to standard thoracic surgical practice.

The surgeon and his or her assistants must become adept at working in three dimensions while visualizing the procedure on a video screen in only two dimensions. This takes some adjustment, but in this era of laparoscopic surgery, these skills are routinely acquired fairly early in a surgery residency. There are some three-dimensional video systems available, but they have not found widespread use. As long as the area where a surgeon is working is kept between the surgeon and the video screen, the orientation remains standard—that is, left remains left and right remains right.

The special requirements imposed by VATS have mandated the development of new instruments that can be placed through small incisions yet function like conventional handheld instruments. One specific problem of applying minimally invasive technology to thoracic surgery has been developing instruments that can grasp the lung tissue firmly without tearing it. Laparoscopic instruments have not proved useful in this regard. The ability to place instruments directly through incisions in the chest without the use of a trocar has allowed some conventional instruments to be modified for use in VATS, with significant success. Refinement of instruments for VATS continues.

CURRENT APPLICATIONS

VATS has been applied in virtually every disease process encountered by thoracic surgeons. Over time, the efficacy and cost-effectiveness of VATS in each of these areas will become clearer. Applications of the technology according to the degree of acceptance they have received are listed in

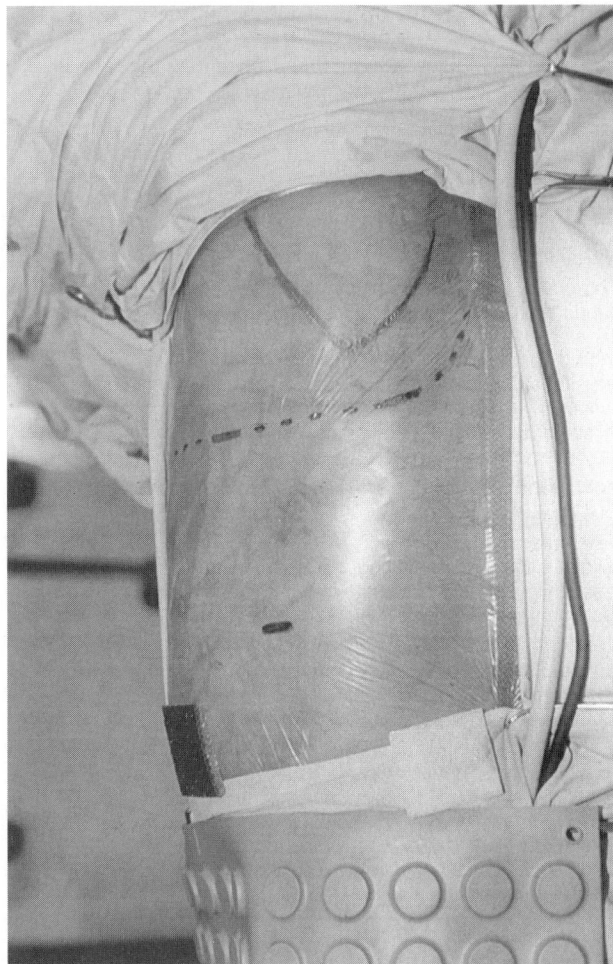

Figure 51–30. The triangular arrangement of intercostal incisions, which facilitates most thoracoscopic procedures. The camera is generally placed through the most inferior incision. The two superior incisions are placed along the course of a thoracotomy incision.

Table 51–14. Relative contraindications to VATS include inability to tolerate single-lung ventilation and severe pleural adhesions, preventing safe entry into the chest or precluding sufficient collapse of the lung to visualize the structures of interest.

Pleural Disease

As noted above, diseases of the pleura accounted for essentially the sole application of the thoracoscope in the era prior to the introduction of video technology, and they remain a major application of VATS.

Malignant Pleural Effusion. This is the most common indication for thoracoscopy in the management of pleural disease. Patients with recurrent effusion undiagnosed by fluid cytologic examination benefit from VATS. At operation, additional fluid is sent for cytologic, bacteriologic, and biochemical study. Direct examination of the pleural space to biopsy otherwise undetectable lesions frequently provides a diagnosis, and pleurodesis may be performed during the same procedure. Pleurodesis consists of the creation of inflammatory adhesions between the visceral and parietal pleural surfaces, such that the space into which pleural fluid accumulates is simply obliterated. At thoracoscopy, the necessary inflammatory process is created by insufflating powdered talc into the pleural space.

TABLE 51–14. Current Applications of VATS

Indications Generally Accepted and Commonly Performed

Diagnostic

Excision of indeterminate pulmonary nodule
Lung biopsy for interstitial disease in nonventilated patients
Biopsy of pleural lesion
Biopsy of mediastinal mass
Biopsy of lymph nodes in aortopulmonary window

Therapeutic

Pleurodesis for malignant pleural effusion
Débridement and drainage of loculated empyema or hemothorax
Excision of benign pleural lesions
Excision of benign pulmonary lesions
Excision of blebs with pleurodesis for spontaneous pneumothorax
Bullectomy for giant bullae with compressed lung
Sympathectomy for hyperhidrosis and upper extremity pain
    syndromes

Indications Not Generally Accepted but Commonly Performed

Excision of mediastinal tumors
Pericardial window
Wedge excision of early lung cancer as definitive treatment in
    patients with poor pulmonary reserve
"Volume reduction" for diffuse bullous lung disease
Treatment of disease of the thoracic spine

**Indications Not Generally Accepted and Not Commonly
Performed**

Lobectomy
Esophageal myotomy for achalasia
Excision of benign tumors of the esophagus
Total esophagectomy for esophageal cancer
Biopsy of mediastinal lymph nodes for esophageal cancer staging
Ligation of thoracic duct for chylothorax
Excision of mediastinal parathyroid adenoma
Closure of patent ductus arteriosus

Even after a diagnosis has been made, VATS may be indicated in a patient with malignant pleural effusion that is loculated and therefore cannot be adequately drained by a chest tube. The loculations can be easily broken up under direct vision, thereby providing complete drainage. Furthermore, any effusions that recur following an attempted chest tube drainage and chemical sclerosis are likely to respond to thoracoscopic pleurodesis with talc. Although a prospective, randomized trial has not yet been completed comparing thoracoscopic to chest tube pleurodesis, one nonrandomized trial demonstrated a significantly higher rate of successful pleurodesis with thoracoscopic insufflation of talc versus tetracycline or bleomycin introduced via a chest tube.[15] The only perceived disadvantage of thoracoscopic pleurodesis is the need for general anesthesia, which is not a requirement. The procedure can be performed with local anesthesia and intravenous sedation with the patient breathing spontaneously.

Empyema. If infected pleural fluid is not promptly drained, it stimulates the development of an inflammatory *peel* of fibrinous exudate around the lung, which ultimately prevents the lung's expansion, potentially creates an infected space, and compromises pulmonary function. In the past, this situation led to formal thoracotomy and decortication, or removal of the peel, to allow the *trapped* lung to re-expand. In the present era, VATS procedures should be performed in febrile patients with infected pleural fluid in whom complete drainage cannot be effected with tube thoracostomy. With early VATS débridement, at a time when a fibrinous exudate is present but no thick and rigid peel has formed, many of these patients are able to avoid thoracotomy.

Hemothorax. Posttraumatic hemothorax, if not drained

early and completely by tube thoracostomy, may organize and cause a *trapped lung*, similar to that seen with empyema. Early thoracoscopy has proved useful in these patients, as well as when chest tube drainage has been unsuccessful.

Pleural-Based Neoplasms. The occasional tumor arising from the pleural surface can be sampled by VATS and, if benign, may be amenable to VATS resection. Benign, solitary fibrous tumors, which usually arise from the visceral pleura, are ideal lesions for this approach.

Malignant pleural tumors such as mesothelioma are readily approached by VATS, and the ability to obtain relatively large tissue specimens often aids in establishing a precise histologic diagnosis. Unfortunately, often the only therapy for malignant mesothelioma is palliative pleurodesis, and this may be accomplished at the time of the diagnostic thoracoscopic procedure. Potential future gene therapy protocols for this neoplasm[40] will likely require VATS for documentation of histology and the extent of disease. The accessibility of the pleural space by a VATS approach makes these protocols feasible.

Parenchymal Disease

Thoracoscopic techniques have made, and will continue to make, significant inroads in the diagnosis and treatment of parenchymal disease.

Interstitial Lung Disease. Prior to the advent of VATS, many patients with diffuse or localized interstitial processes were treated empirically, often with steroids, because of the real or perceived morbidity of thoracotomy. The empiric approach is probably warranted in a non-neutropenic cancer patient with acute pneumonitis, for whom broad-spectrum antibiotic therapy is usually the treatment of choice.[34] In an immunocompetent patient with a chronic interstitial process, however, it is often beneficial to obtain a piece of lung tissue. Bronchoscopically obtained transbronchial biopsies have a low yield[2] and subject the patient to an additional potentially morbid procedure.

The recommended approach for surgical lung biopsies is controversial. A small inframammary incision through the fourth or fifth intercostal space may be done expeditiously, without single-lung ventilation, and with minimal morbidity. The authors prefer this approach in a critically ill, ventilator-dependent patient for whom even transport to the operating room may be a substantial risk. For those in more stable condition, however, VATS wedge lung biopsy offers a significant advantage. It provides excellent visualization of and access to the entire lung (impossible through a mini-thoracotomy), allowing biopsies of abnormal-appearing areas and likely increasing diagnostic yield. It also decreases postoperative pain and shortens hospital stay.

The VATS procedure is generally performed through the standard camera port in the seventh or eighth intercostal space at the posterior-axillary line and two additional ports—one in the fourth or fifth intercostal space at approximately the anterior axillary line, and one approximately two finger breadths below the inferior aspect of the scapula. The entire lung is visualized, and areas that appear abnormal are noted. A finger may be placed through the anterior port (where the ribs are more widely spaced), allowing a tactile assessment of the parenchyma. One or more abnormal areas are sampled by grasping the tissue with a ring forceps or similar instrument and excising that portion of lung with serial firings of the linear stapler. If there are no gross abnormalities apparent, areas that appear to be most involved on chest x-ray or computed tomography (CT) are chosen for biopsy. A chest tube is left in place as for any VATS procedure.

Ferson and colleagues compared thoracoscopic and open-wedge resection via limited thoracotomy in a retrospective study of nonventilated patients.[8] It was found that hospital stay was significantly shorter in the VATS group (4.9 versus 12.2 days) and that there were significantly more complications in the open group (50% versus 19%). In the authors' series of 50 similar patients, the mean hospital stay was only 1.9 days, there was no significant morbidity or mortality, and diagnostic tissue was obtained in all cases. Although one study showed that VATS cost more in patients undergoing lung biopsy for interstitial lung disease,[32] the benefits of the approach outweigh this financial consideration.

The availability of VATS lung biopsy has prompted the earlier referral of patients with interstitial lung disease who previously would have been treated empirically or referred in desperation at the time of severe decompensation. It is hoped that such early referral and tissue diagnosis will have an impact on long-term outcome in these patients.

Spontaneous Pneumothorax (Collapsed Lung). A young patient with congenital apical blebs may present with spontaneous rupture of such blebs, resulting in pneumothorax. The typical presenting features include sudden onset of chest pain and shortness of breath. Initial treatment consists of chest tube placement, unless the pneumothorax is very small and can be safely monitored. The risk of recurrent pneumothorax is approximately 30%.[3] Therefore, operation with resection of the blebs and pleurodesis is generally indicated only after a recurrence, in a patient with bilateral pneumothoraces, or in a patient who lives in a medically underserved area or has an occupation requiring frequent exposure to extremes of pressure. Although a transaxillary thoracotomy with excision of blebs and pleural abrasion or pleurectomy has been described,[6] this remains a substantial procedure.

VATS offers an alternative treatment for such patients with predictably less morbidity. The operative procedure entails excising the apical blebs and creating a pleural symphysis—the same goals of the open procedures. The blebs are easily visualized through the thoracoscope (Fig. 51–31) and excised by several applications of the linear stapler (Fig. 51–32). Although a number of techniques are likely to provide successful pleurodesis, we prefer to mechanically abrade the pleura with a gauze sponge. Talc is avoided in these usually young patients. Since the procedure is identical to that performed via open thoracotomy, one would expect

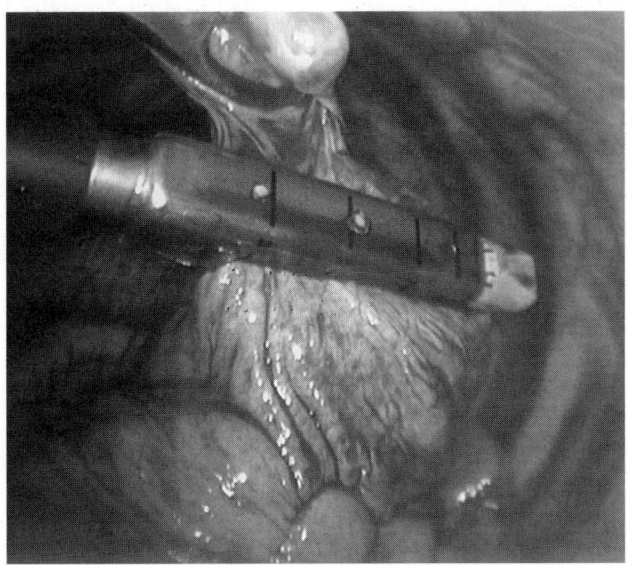

Figure 51–32. Initial application of a linear stapler in excision of an apical bleb.

similar (less than 5%) recurrence rates, although in practice, recurrence rates following the VATS procedure have been slightly higher.

In a randomized comparison of VATS and open bullectomy with pleurectomy, patients with primary spontaneous pneumothorax undergoing VATS benefited from decreased postoperative pain, shorter hospital stay, and less pulmonary dysfunction. No patient in either the VATS or the thoracotomy group suffered treatment failure.[42] In the authors' experience with 70 procedures in patients with spontaneous pneumothorax secondary to blebs, there has been one recurrence, and patients can leave the hospital on the first or second postoperative day.

Whereas the authors previously waited 7 days in these patients prior to proceeding to operation for prolonged air leak, the authors now recommend VATS apical blebectomy and pleurodesis at 48 to 72 hours, since this allows the patient to leave the hospital earlier and almost certainly prevents recurrence. In patients with bilateral spontaneous pneumothoraces, bilateral VATS procedures may be performed under a single anesthetic, as we have done in 12 patients.

Secondary Pneumothorax. Pneumothorax or air leak occurring secondary to a process other than congenital apical blebs—so-called secondary pneumothorax—may also be treated with a VATS approach. These patients, in fact, are particularly well suited to VATS; they often have significantly compromised baseline pulmonary function and therefore may benefit greatly by avoiding thoracotomy. The pathology in these situations is somewhat more complex, and the air leak should be identified prior to repairing it by stapling (the authors' preferred approach) or by the use of fibrin glue, the Nd-YAG laser, or the argon beam coagulator. In 13 such cases, the authors successfully managed the air leak in 12. One patient required conversion to open thoracotomy. These cases consisted of six patients with emphysema, two with *Pneumocystis carinii* causing bilateral pneumothorax, three with metastatic sarcoma, and two with persistent air leaks following lobectomy.

Giant Bullae. Surgery for bullous disease has undergone somewhat of a renaissance since the development of VATS. The primary indication for surgical treatment in these patients is the presence of a giant bulla causing compression of adjacent, relatively normal lung parenchyma (Fig. 51–33).

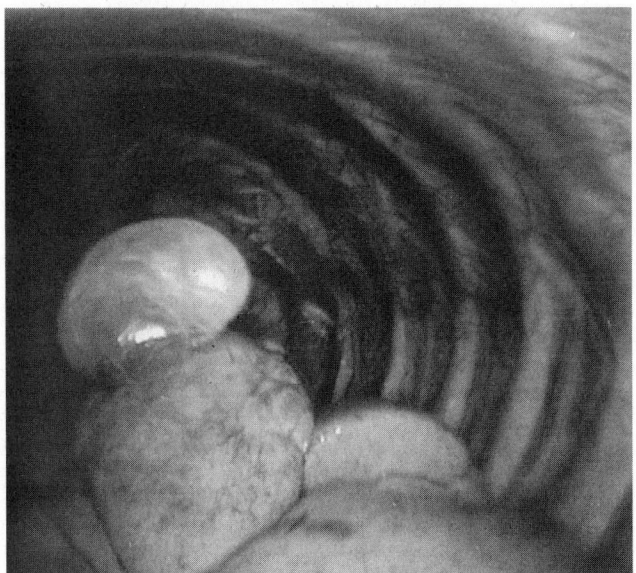

Figure 51–31. Thoracoscopic view of a typical apical bleb in a young patient who presented with spontaneous pneumothorax.

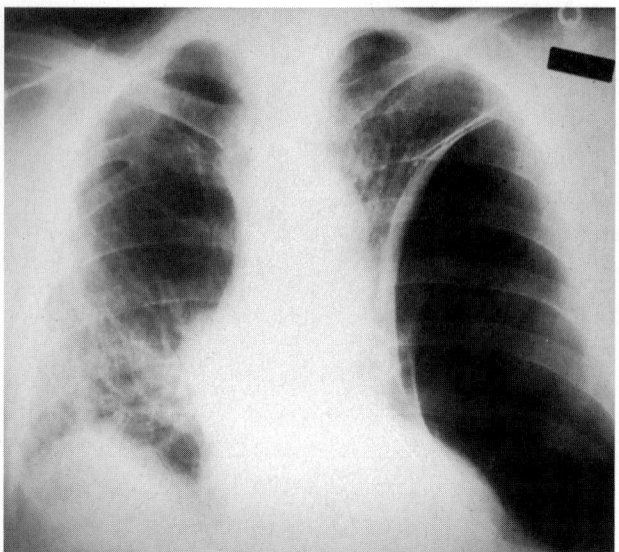

Figure 51–33. Chest x-ray showing giant bulla causing compression of adjacent lung parenchyma in a patient with bullous emphysema.

Simple bullectomy is likely to result in symptomatic improvement if there is enough lung parenchyma to expand and completely fill the space following the procedure. A residual space increases the chance of a prolonged air leak and further complications. Surgeons have been loath to perform thoracotomy in these compromised patients because of the fear that they might not survive the short-term effects of the incision on their already marginal pulmonary status. VATS techniques considerably attenuate this concern.

The recommended procedure involves application of the argon beam coagulator to the bulla under direct thoracoscopic visualization. As the surrounding, relatively normal lung collapses after the institution of single-lung ventilation, the bulla itself becomes prominent. At a low-power *spray* setting, the argon beam causes the wall of the bulla to contract but remain intact, thus avoiding air leaks. Once the bulla has shriveled, the base is more easily identified and stapled. To further decrease the risk of air leak, the staple line is buttressed with strips of bovine pericardium. Since postoperative pain management and chest physiotherapy are key to avoiding pneumonia in these patients, thoracic epidural analgesia with continuous infusion in the early postoperative period is used.

The authors have performed 23 consecutive VATS bullectomies, with no mortality and no conversion to thoracotomy. All patients showed symptomatic improvement. In the few patients in whom postoperative pulmonary function has been measured, forced expiratory volume at 1 second has at least doubled. Whether this procedure will improve the long-term outcome of these patients remains to be determined. However, bullectomy is considered as the initial procedure in some patients referred for lung transplantation in the hope that it may give them a few years before transplantation is necessary and allow the limited supply of donor organs to be used most efficiently.

Diffuse Bullous Disease. Surgery for *volume reduction* in patients with diffuse bullous or nonbullous emphysema but no dominant bullae or clearly compressed lung parenchyma has received considerable attention recently. This procedure sets out to improve pulmonary function in emphysematous patients by reducing the overall volume of the lung, thus shrinking the thorax and resulting in improved elastic recoil of the chest wall and improved motion of the diaphragm. Recent studies suggest dramatic improvement in objective

parameters of pulmonary function following bilateral volume reduction surgery performed via median sternotomy.[5] Although still controversial, these early data suggest a bright future for the procedure. If unilateral volume reduction proves to result in comparable improvement, there would clearly be a role for VATS in volume reduction surgery. Bilateral VATS for volume reduction, although more problematic because of the necessity of repositioning the patient and the endobronchial tube in the middle of the operation, may also find a role. It remains to be determined whether a VATS procedure for volume reduction has advantages over a median sternotomy, the currently preferred approach.

Pulmonary Nodules

A patient who presents with a solitary pulmonary nodule (a so-called coin lesion) presents a great challenge to the pulmonary physician and thoracic surgeon. VATS techniques have made a definite impact on the care of these patients. By allowing a reliable diagnosis to be made with a single, minimally morbid procedure, VATS has engendered a complete reassessment of the approach to this frequently encountered clinical problem.

The question that must be answered by the clinician when presented with a solitary pulmonary nodule is simple: is it malignant? Although no criteria are absolute, there are a number of factors that point to a benign diagnosis. If the lesion has not changed in size over several years, it is unlikely to be malignant. The importance of reviewing a prior chest radiograph cannot be overemphasized. This may be the only study that can spare the patient an operation. Lesions in young nonsmokers are unlikely to be malignant. Specific patterns of calcification on CT scan frequently point to the benign nature of a lesion. Despite all this, however, a benign diagnosis can never be guaranteed without tissue for histologic examination.

Furthermore, the preponderance of benign tissue fragments obtained from a nodule by one of the available nonoperative diagnostic studies—bronchoscopy or transthoracic needle biopsy—does not guarantee that a lesion is, in fact, benign. A specific benign diagnosis is made only 10% of the time at bronchoscopy,[21] and at a similar rate with transthoracic needle biopsy.[9] A negative result from one of these tests is of no benefit to the patient and mandates a further diagnostic procedure, whereas a diagnosis of malignancy merely tells us what is already known: that the lesion needs to be removed. For these reasons, transthoracic needle biopsy is not recommended except in a patient with multiple nodules in need of a tissue diagnosis that is highly likely to be malignant, or in a patient with an absolute contraindication to operation. The authors prefer to completely remove the lesion by thoracoscopic wedge resection.

Mack and colleagues looked closely at the role of VATS in the management of the indeterminate solitary pulmonary nodule.[28] They performed VATS excision on 242 patients as a primary diagnostic maneuver. A definitive diagnosis was obtained in all cases, and there was no mortality or major morbidity. Minor complications occurred in only 3.6%. In two patients the nodule could not be identified, and thoracotomy was required. When a primary lung cancer was identified, as it was in 48% of patients, formal open thoracotomy and anatomic resection were carried out. Thus, 127 patients were spared thoracotomy for a benign lesion. The average hospital stay for those undergoing thoracoscopy alone was 2.4 days. Santambrogio and colleagues performed a randomized, controlled clinical trial evaluating VATS excision of a solitary pulmonary nodule and excision via muscle-sparing thoracotomy. The diagnosis was made in 100% of both groups, but the VATS group had significantly less postoperative pain and a much shorter length of stay.[39] A prospective, nonrandomized study of 138 patients found that those undergoing VATS versus limited lateral thoracotomy for wedge resection benefited from a lower complication rate, reduced pain, less shoulder dysfunction, and less early impairment in pulmonary function.[25]

It is difficult to criticize a technique that has a sensitivity and specificity of 100% and may be done with no mortality and decreased morbidity. However, certain lesions are not considered for VATS excision. Since the likelihood of malignancy is greater than 90% in lesions over 3 cm. in size, in the absence of metastatic disease, thoracotomy and lobectomy should be the initial procedure in patients with these lesions. Lesions located centrally, in close proximity to hilar structures, are also unsuitable for VATS wedge excision and require open thoracotomy.

At operation, before manipulating the lung, the surgeon carefully inspects the visceral pleura. Visible irregularities of this normally smooth surface frequently allow the lesion to be identified. Additionally, a finger passed through one of the small incisions can often palpate the lesion. If the lesion is not visible on inspection, the preoperative CT scan can help locate the general area of the nodule, with final localization by palpation as the lung is grasped and moved toward the finger (Fig. 51–34). Once identified, the lung tissue containing the lesion is grasped and the lesion is wedged out with serial firings of the linear stapler. The specimen is placed in an endoscopic bag and then removed through one of the incisions. This practice of *bagging* the lesion should alleviate concerns that cancer could be spread to the incision through which the lesion is removed.[10, 43] Of note, all such catastrophic events occurred when the lesions were not bagged.

Carcinoma of the Lung

Controversy arises over the management of a solitary nodule that at VATS wedge excision proves to be a carcinoma. Based on current knowledge, wedge excision is not optimal therapy for primary lung cancer, even a T1 lesion, unless a patient is deemed too high a risk for thoracotomy and lobectomy. A body of work demonstrates the value of nonanatomic resections via thoracotomy for such patients with marginal pulmonary function,[7, 31, 35] and it is possible to extrapolate from this experience that VATS wedge excision

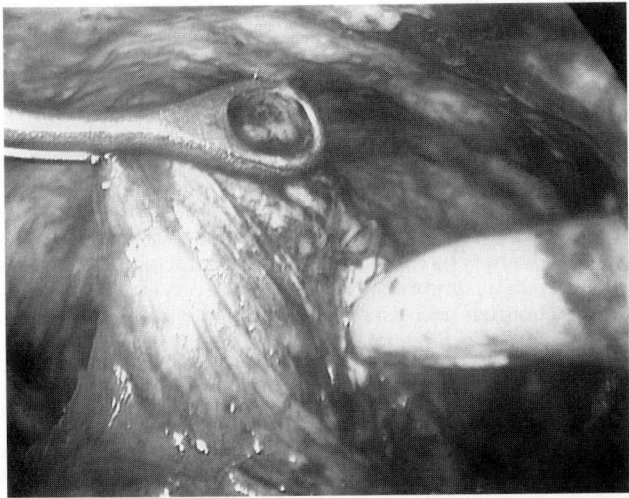

Figure 51–34. Localization of solitary pulmonary nodules is frequently achieved by palpating the lesion with a digit passed through one of the small intercostal incisions. The lung is moved toward the finger, with an instrument placed through a separate incision.

might be of still greater benefit to this population. However, the incidence of local recurrence following VATS wedge excision of carcinomas is not yet known.

In an ongoing study of great importance, the Lung Cancer Study Group is addressing the question of limited resection versus lobectomy for T_1N_0 lesions in a prospective randomized trial.[12] At 3 years, this study showed a significantly higher rate of local recurrence in those undergoing limited resection; most recently, it has been reported that this increased rate of local recurrence has translated into a definite 5-year survival advantage in the group that underwent resection with a lobectomy.[11] It is difficult, with this data available, to support a treatment plan consisting of VATS wedge excision alone in early bronchogenic carcinoma. Open anatomic resections for lung cancer are performed in all patients, except those in whom limited pulmonary reserve precludes thoracotomy. In such cases, the patient must understand that limited resection is a compromise.

It should be noted that some surgeons have performed VATS lobectomy, a technique requiring a 5- to 7-cm. *utility* incision in addition to standard 1- to 2-cm. thoracoscopy ports, although the ribs are not spread.[22, 26] McKenna reported performing a "complete cancer operation" by this VATS approach, including mediastinal lymph node dissection.[30] Although one might expect these techniques to reduce postoperative pain, in a limited number of these procedures, this has not been the case; the patients do not seem to be discharged any sooner than patients who have undergone lobectomy through a muscle-sparing incision. Two prospective trials comparing VATS lobectomy with standard muscle-sparing thoracotomy and lobectomy have confirmed this impression; they failed to show significant enough differences to justify the routine use of a VATS approach, which probably subjects the patient to a slightly greater risk of intraoperative catastrophe.[13, 23] Randomized trials are currently under way to assess the incidence of local recurrence and patient survival with VATS as compared with standard open lobectomy.

VATS has also been used as an adjunct to more established procedures to stage carcinoma of the lung. The gold standard for staging lung cancer is mediastinoscopy in all patients whose CT scans reveal mediastinal lymph nodes greater than 1 cm. in size. Patients who prove to have histologically positive lymph nodes in the ipsilateral mediastinum (N_2 disease) were previously thought not to benefit from operation; more recently, however, these patients have been entered into protocols in which they received preoperative chemotherapy followed by operation.[37] Patients with histologically positive lymph nodes in the contralateral mediastinum (N_3 disease) are still considered inoperable and generally do not undergo further operations.

Unfortunately, the posterior subcarinal lymph nodes (Level VII) and lymph nodes in the subaortic window (Level V) are not accessible by standard cervical mediastinoscopy. Therefore, involved lymphatic spread to these areas may be missed at mediastinoscopy, subjecting some patients to thoracotomy that may be of little benefit to them. VATS from the left side offers unmatched ability to visualize and sample nodes in the subaortic window, and the same is true for the subcarinal space from the right. Thus, if lymph nodes in these areas appear to be suspect on CT scan, a selected VATS staging procedure may be useful.

The utility of VATS for assessing resectability is limited. Dissection to document direct invasion of mediastinal structures can be hazardous, and there is no substitute for putting one's hand on a lesion of questionable resectability. It may be useful, however, to introduce the thoracoscope to document the absence of diffuse pleural metastatic disease if this possibility has been raised, usually by the presence of a pleural effusion without malignant cells on cytologic examination.

The Mediastinum

Primary Lesions of the Mediastinum. Although relatively rare, these lesions have proved to be ideal for VATS management, since they are often benign and easy to resect. The anterosuperior mediastinum most frequently houses thymomas, lymphomas, and teratomas; the middle mediastinal structures may give rise to pericardial or bronchogenic cysts; and the posterior mediastinum most frequently gives rise to neurogenic tumors or bronchogenic cysts. Lesions in all portions of the mediastinum are easily accessible, and whether biopsy or complete excision is the intent, VATS saves many patients from having to undergo thoracotomy or median sternotomy.

In the approach to an anterior mediastinal lesion, the patient is positioned with the operated side tilted up at approximately 30 degrees, instead of the full lateral position preferred for most other lesions. Often, a small inframammary or second intercostal space incision is necessary, but this is done without rib spreading. Although a VATS procedure is not appropriate for invasive thymomas, it may be used for encapsulated thymomas. In patients with myasthenia gravis and thymoma, total thymectomy is mandatory, and this is facilitated by combining a transcervical approach with VATS exposure. The gland is initially mobilized in the neck, and branches to the innominate vein are divided through the cervical incision. The dissection is then carried into the mediastinum until the thymoma is encountered. The gland is tucked down into the mediastinum, the neck is closed, and the patient is positioned as above for VATS. Dissection is completed in this manner, and the gland and tumor are bagged and removed through one of the chest incisions.

In a patient with a nondiscrete, diffuse mediastinal mass that is likely to be a lymphoma but may be a thymoma or germ cell tumor, a tissue diagnosis may be obtained by VATS. Although these lesions are frequently amenable to mediastinoscopy or a small parasternal incision and a completely extrapleural approach, lesions that are not in close proximity to the anterior chest wall can be reached more easily by the VATS approach. In all 14 patients in whom such an approach is used, adequate tissue was obtained and a definitive diagnosis was made. The surgeon must decide which procedure is most likely to provide the easiest approach to a given lesion and which approach is most sensible in each individual patient.

The posterior mediastinum may be the site of cystic or solid lesions, and these too are amenable to VATS resection. In one report, two cases of postoperative bleeding required repeat thoracoscopy in a group of 20 patients who underwent successful removal of a mediastinal tumor.[36]

Pericardial Effusion. Although easier from the right side, it is possible to perform a VATS pericardial drainage procedure for effusive disease from either the right or the left side. For diagnostic purposes, a simple needle aspiration of the pericardial space is indicated. With recurrent, symptomatic effusion, however, a pericardial window—the creation of a defect in the pericardium, with subsequent development of a fusion between the epicardial surface and the parietal pericardium—is indicated. This can be performed by either the traditional subxiphoid approach or a VATS approach. Care must be taken to identify and preserve the phrenic nerve in performing the VATS procedure. Although VATS is safe and effective, a subxiphoid approach is simpler, faster, and less invasive, and it accomplishes the same goals. If there is a need to create a large window, a thoracoscopic approach

may be more effective, as exposure of the pericardium is excellent through the video thoracoscope.

Patent Ductus Arteriosus. Ligation of patent ductus arteriosus has been reported in infants, with discharge in 72 hours and no postoperative complications.[1]

Mediastinal Parathyroid Adenoma. VATS excision of three parathyroid adenomas of the anterior mediastinum has been reported.[41] Since up to one third of cervical explorations for primary hyperparathyroidism fail because of ectopic mediastinal parathyroid tissue, this technique may prove to be of some value. The hospital stays of these patients averaged 3 days—considerably shorter than the typical stay following a median sternotomy, which is the alternative approach for removal of mediastinal parathyroid tissue.

Esophagus. Several European groups have taken an aggressive approach in using VATS procedures to perform total esophagectomy for carcinoma.[4, 14] The availability of a proven, minimally invasive approach for esophagectomy that avoids a chest incision—namely, transhiatal esophagectomy—renders the VATS approach an overuse of the technology. Although surgeons in the United States have not yet embraced VATS esophagectomy, some have used a VATS approach for staging esophageal cancer.[24] But since most patients with this tumor present with lymph node involvement and remain candidates for resection, this information is of dubious value, outside of stratifying patients prior to embarking on preoperative neoadjuvant therapy. Furthermore, as experience is gained with endoscopic ultrasonography—also a minimally invasive technique—it is likely to provide the same information. Perhaps of greater interest is the use of VATS as an adjunct to the performance of transhiatal esophagectomy, particularly for lesions at the level of the carina.

The role of VATS in benign disorders of the esophagus is much more clearly defined. Pellegrini and co-workers described the initial experience in 24 patients using VATS myotomy for achalasia,[33] and others have followed suit. After an early experience without it, they added the myotomy to simultaneous esophagoscopy. The median hospital stay was 3 days, and at late follow-up, swallowing was rated excellent in 17 patients and fair to good in 4. The ability to perform this procedure without a thoracotomy should pique the interest of gastroenterologists and prompt the earlier referral of these patients rather than subjecting them to repeated pneumatic dilation. The procedure is technically demanding and should be performed only by those with considerable thoracoscopic experience.

Esophageal leiomyoma is the most common benign tumor of the esophagus, lying in a submucosal location. The authors have performed two VATS leiomyoma excisions and have had no difficulty obtaining exposure or dissection of the lesion off the mucosa (Fig. 51–35).

Autonomic Nervous System. The sympathetic chain is readily visualized thoracoscopically where it courses along the vertebral bodies in the posterior mediastinum (Fig. 51–36). Dorsal sympathectomy may be indicated for palmar hyperhidrosis, reflex sympathetic dystrophy, or other upper extremity pain syndromes. The superior cervical ganglion is easily identified and preserved to avoid producing a Horner's syndrome. Bilateral lumbar sympathectomy has been used for the management of pancreatic pain.

Thoracic Duct. Chylous pleural effusion is a rare complication of thoracic surgical procedures and results from injury to the thoracic duct or its ramifications within the chest. It may also occur spontaneously or be associated with other diseases, particularly lymphoma. It is also occasionally seen following blunt chest trauma. The diagnosis is made by the presence of a high triglyceride level within the fluid and the presence of chylomicrons. Initial measures to stop the accumulation of fluid generally include placing the patient on a low-fat diet or a brief course of nothing by mouth and total parenteral nutrition, techniques that are rarely effective. When these fail, VATS offers a simple, effective cure. The thoracic duct is most readily identified as it courses through the aortic hiatus, where, in most patients, it is still a single trunk along the vertebral bodies running between the aorta and the esophagus. Ligation with clips at this point halts the flow of chyle from leaking points higher in the chest.

The Spinal Column

VATS provides excellent exposure of the thoracic spine. Procedures such as drainage of abscesses, biopsy of lesions of the vertebral bodies, discectomy, and anterior release for kyphoscoliosis have all been carried out successfully.[29] Because of the early successes in this realm and the significantly decreased morbidity, this approach to the spine is becoming quite common in a number of centers.

COMPLICATIONS

A review[20] of the complications that resulted from the 266 initial VATS procedures revealed the following: there were no deaths; 11 patients were electively converted to an open procedure when the intended VATS procedure was not able to be completed successfully; 10 patients had air leaks lasting longer than 7 days; bleeding requiring blood transfusion occurred in 5 patients; and 5 patients developed superficial wound infections. Data collected on 1358 patients from the VATS Study Group registry show a similar spectrum of complications and a 2% mortality.[16] No consistent pattern of major complications resulting from VATS has been reported. Given a probable learning curve, the fact that VATS proce-

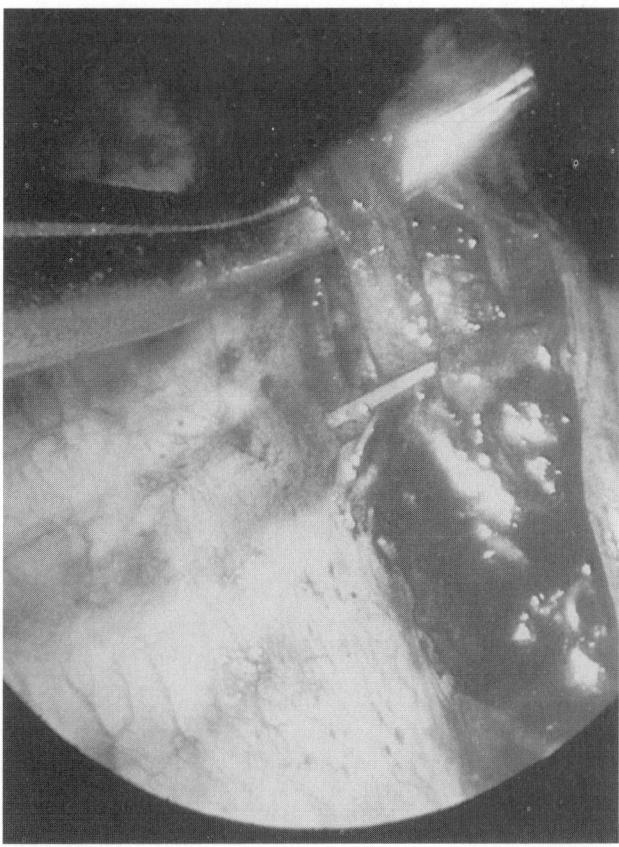

Figure 51–36. The sympathetic chain encircled with a hook probe after mobilization off the vertebral bodies. This structure is well seen along its entire course up to the level of the superior cervical ganglion.

dures have been performed with minimal major morbidity this early in most surgeons' experience is commendable. This record should only improve with time.

CONCLUSIONS

VATS procedures have proved to be extremely useful in the diagnosis and treatment of numerous thoracic diseases. There is now little doubt that many of these procedures can be performed as safely as, with efficacy equal to, and with less morbidity than the corresponding procedure performed via a thoracotomy. With the tremendous strides made in the development of equipment for VATS, there has been a rush on the part of thoracic surgeons to perform as many types of procedures as possible in this manner. Now that this initial rush is over, we are beginning to appreciate where these techniques have their greatest impact. Some procedures for which there was tremendous early enthusiasm are now being performed less frequently, whereas others have withstood the test of time. Critical comparisons between VATS procedures and corresponding open techniques are beginning to appear, and many are referenced herein, but more such studies are required before there are definitive answers to the many questions raised by these new procedures. In the current era of cost consciousness, cost issues may reign among these unresolved questions. VATS has clearly found a place in the modern practice of thoracic surgery and is likely to play an ever-increasing role in the management of diseases of the chest.

SELECTED REFERENCES

Kaiser, L. R., and Daniel, T. M. (Eds.): Thoracoscopic Surgery. Boston, Little, Brown, 1993.

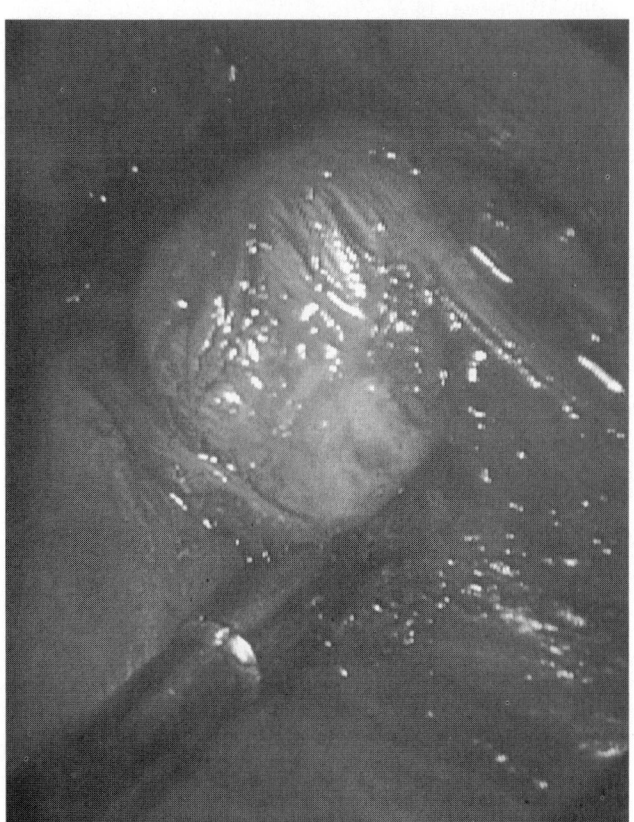

Figure 51–35. Dissection of an esophageal leiomyoma off the underlying mucosa.

This is the first comprehensive textbook describing in detail the application of VATS to all the currently acceptable indications.

Lewis, R. J., Kunderman, P. J., Sisler, G. E., and Mackenzie, J. W.: Direct diagnostic thoracoscopy. Ann. Thorac. Surg., 21:536, 1976.
This paper summarizes the state of the art of thoracoscopy prior to the current era of video thoracoscopy.

Waller, D. A., Forty, J., and Morritt, G. N.: Video-assisted thoracoscopic surgery versus thoracotomy for spontaneous pneumothorax. Ann. Thorac. Surg., 58:372, 1994.
This is the first prospective, randomized clinical trial demonstrating an advantage of VATS over thoracotomy for a particular disease with respect to pain, hospital stay, and postoperative pulmonary function. More studies like this one are needed to demonstrate the value of VATS techniques for specific disease processes.

REFERENCES

1. Alvarez-Tostado, R. A., Millan, M. A., Tovar, L. A., Shuchleib, S., Alvarez-Tostado, R., and Chousleb, A.: Thoracoscopic clipping and ligation of a patent ductus arteriosus. Ann. Thorac. Surg., 57:755, 1994.
2. Burt, M. E., Flye, M. W., Webber, B. L., and Wesley, R. A.: Prospective evaluation of aspiration needle, cutting needle, transbronchial, and open lung biopsy in patients with pulmonary infiltrates. Ann. Thorac. Surg., 32:1146, 1981.
3. Clark, T. A., Hutchinson, D. E., Deaner, R. M., and Fitchett, V. H.: Spontaneous pneumothorax. Am. J. Surg., 124:728, 1972.
4. Collar, J., Lengele, B., Otte, J., and Kestens, P.: En-bloc and standard esophagectomies by thoracoscopy. Ann. Thorac. Surg., 56:675, 1993.
5. Cooper, J. D.: Lung volume reduction surgery for chronic obstructive lung disease. Presented at the 31st annual meeting of the Society of Thoracic Surgeons, Palm Springs, Calif., Jan. 30–Feb. 1, 1995.
6. Deslaurier, J., Beaulieu, M., Depres, J. P., Lemieux, M., Leblanc, J., and Desmeules, M.: Transaxillary pleurectomy for treatment of spontaneous pneumothorax. Ann. Thorac. Surg., 30:569, 1980.
7. Errett, L. E., Wilson, J., Chiu, R. C., and Munro, D. D.: Wedge resection as an alternative procedure for peripheral bronchogenic carcinoma in poor-risk patients. J. Thorac. Cardiovasc. Surg., 90:656, 1985.
8. Ferson, P. F., Landreneau, R. J., Dowling, R. D., Hazelrigg, S. R., Ritter, P., Nunchuk, S., Perrino, M. K., Bowers, C. M., Mack, M. J., and Magee, M. J.: Comparison of open versus thoracoscopic lung biopsy for diffuse infiltrative pulmonary disease. J. Thorac. Cardiovasc. Surg., 106:194, 1993.
9. Fletcher, E. C., and Levin, D. C.: Flexible fiberoptic bronchoscopy and fluoroscopically guided transbronchial biopsy in the management of solitary pulmonary nodules. West. J. Med., 136:477, 1982.
10. Fry, W. A., Siddique, A., Pensler, J. M., and Mostafavi, H.: Thoracoscopic implantation of cancer with a fatal outcome. Ann. Thorac. Surg., 59:42, 1995.
11. Ginsberg, R. J.: The role of limited resection in the treatment of early stage lung cancer. Lung Cancer, 11 (suppl. 2):35, 1994.
12. Ginsberg, R. J., and Rubinstein, L.: A randomized comparative trial of lobectomy vs. limited resection for patients with T1 N0 non-small cell lung cancer. Lung Cancer, 7 (suppl.):83, 1991.
13. Giudicelli, R., Pascal, R., Lonjon, T., Ragni, J., Morati, N., Ottomani, R., Fuientes, P. A., Shennib, H., and Noirclerc, M.: Video-assisted minithoracotomy versus muscle-sparing thoracotomy for performing lobectomy. Ann. Thorac. Surg., 58:712, 1994.
14. Gossot, D., Fourquier, P., and Celerier, M.: Thoracoscopic esophagectomy: Technique and initial results. Ann. Thorac. Surg., 56:667, 1993.
15. Hartman, D. L., Gaither, J. M., Kesler, K. A., Mylet, D. M., Brown, J. W., and Mathur, P. N.: Comparison of insufflated talc under thoracoscopic guidance with standard tetracycline and bleomycin pleurodesis for control of malignant pleural effusions. J. Thorac. Cardiovasc. Surg., 105:743, 1993.
16. Hazelrigg, S. R., Nunchuck, S. K., LoCicero, J., and the Video Assisted Thoracic Surgery Study Group: Video assisted thoracic surgery study group data. Ann. Thorac. Surg., 56:1039, 1993.
17. Jacobaeus, H. C.: Possibility of the use of the cystoscope for investigation of serous cavities. Muench. Med. Wochenschr., 57:2090, 1910.
18. Jacobaeus, H. C.: The cauterization of adhesions in pneumothorax treatment of tuberculosis. Surg. Gynecol. Obstet., 32:493, 1921.
19. Jacobaeus, H. C.: The practical importance of thoracoscopy in surgery of the chest. Surg. Gynecol. Obstet., 34:289, 1922.
20. Kaiser, L. R., and Bavaria, J. E.: Complications of thoracoscopy. Ann. Thorac. Surg., 56:796, 1993.
21. Khouri, N. F., Mezisne, M. A., Zerhouni, E. A., and Siegelman, S. S.: The solitary pulmonary nodule: Assessment, diagnosis and management. Chest, 91:128, 1987.
22. Kirby, T. J., Mack, M. J., Landreneau, R. J., and Rice, T. W.: Initial experience with video-assisted thoracoscopic lobectomy. Ann. Thorac. Surg., 56:1248, 1993.
23. Kirby, T. J., Mack, M. J., Landreneau, R. J., and Rice, T. W.: Lobectomy: VATS vs. thoracotomy. A randomized study. Presented at the 74th annual meeting of the American Association for Thoracic Surgery, New York, Apr. 24–27, 1994.
24. Krasna, M. J., and McLaughlin, J. S.: Thoracoscopic lymph node staging for esophageal cancer. Ann. Thorac. Surg., 56:667, 1993.
25. Landreneau, R. J., Hazelrigg, S. R., Mack, M. J., Dowling, R. D., Burke, D., Gavlick, J., Perrino, M. K., Ritter, P. S., Bowers, C. M., Defino, J., Nunchuck, S. K., Freeman, J., Keenan, R. J., and Ferson, P. F.: Postoperative pain-related morbidity: Video-assisted thoracic surgery versus thoracotomy. Ann. Thorac. Surg., 56:1285, 1993.
26. Lewis, R., Caccavale, R. J., Sisler, G. E., and Mackenzie, J. W.: One hundred consecutive patients undergoing video-assisted thoracic operations. Ann. Thorac. Surg., 54:421, 1992.
27. Lilienthal, H.: Thoracic Surgery. Philadelphia, W. B. Saunders, 1925.
28. Mack, M. J., Hazelrigg, S. R., Landreneau, R. J., and Acuff, T. E.: Thoracoscopy for the diagnosis of the indeterminate solitary pulmonary nodule. Ann. Thorac. Surg., 56:825, 1993.
29. Mack, M. J., Regan, J. J., Bobechko, W. P., and Acuff, T. E.: Application of thoracoscopy for diseases of the spine. Ann. Thorac. Surg., 56:736, 1993.
30. McKenna, R. J., Jr.: Lobectomy by video-assisted thoracic surgery with mediastinal node sampling for lung cancer. J. Thorac. Cardiovasc. Surg., 107:879, 1994.
31. Miller, J. I., and Hatcher, C. R.: Limited pulmonary resection of bronchogenic carcinoma in the patient with marked impairment of pulmonary function. Ann. Thorac. Surg., 44:340, 1987.
32. Molin, L. J., Steinberg, J. B., and Lanza, L. A.: VATS increases costs in patients undergoing lung biopsy for interstitial lung disease. Ann. Thorac. Surg., 58:1595, 1994.
33. Pellegrini, C. A., Leichter, R., Patti, M., Somberg, K., Ostroff, J. W., and Way, L.: Thoracoscopic esophageal myotomy in the treatment of achalasia. Ann. Thorac. Surg., 56:680, 1993.
34. Potter, D., Pass, H. I., Brower, S., Macher, A., Browne, M., Thaler, M., Cotton, D., Hathorn, J., Wesley, R., Longo, D., Pizzo, P., and Roth, J. A.: Prospective randomized study of open lung biopsy versus empirical antibiotic therapy for acute pneumonitis in non-neutropenic cancer patients. Ann. Thorac. Surg., 40:422, 1985.
35. Read, R. C., Yoder, G., and Schaeffer, R. C.: Survival after conservative resection for T1 N0 M0 non-small cell lung cancer. Ann. Thorac. Surg., 49:391, 1990.
36. Roviaro, G. C., Rebuffat, C., Varoli, F., Vergani, C., Maciocco, M., and Scalambra, S. M.: Videothoracoscopic excision of mediastinal masses: Indications and technique. Ann. Thorac. Surg., 58:1679, 1994.
37. Rusch, V. W.: Neoadjuvant therapy for stage III lung cancer. Semin. Thorac. Cardiovasc. Surg., 5:258, 1993.
38. Rusch, V. W., and Mountain, C.: Thoracoscopy under regional anesthesia for the diagnosis and management of pleural disease. Am. J. Surg., 154:274, 1991.
39. Santambrogio, L., Nosotti, M., Bellaviti, N., and Mezzetti, M.: Videothoracoscopy versus thoracotomy for the diagnosis of the indeterminate solitary pulmonary nodule. Ann. Thorac. Surg., 59:868, 1995.
40. Smythe, R. S., Kaiser, L. R., Hwang, H. C., Amin, K. M., Pilewski, J. M., Eck, S. J., Wilson, J. M., and Albelda, S. M.: Successful adenovirus-mediated gene transfer in an *in vivo* model of human malignant mesothelioma. Ann. Thorac. Surg., 57:1395, 1994.
41. Smythe, W. R., Bavaria, J. E., Hall, A. R., Kline, G. M., and Kaiser, L. R.: Thoracoscopic removal of mediastinal parathyroid adenoma. Ann. Thorac. Surg., 59:236, 1995.
42. Waller, D. A., Forty, J., and Morritt, G. N.: Video-assisted thoracoscopic surgery versus thoracotomy for spontaneous pneumothorax. Ann. Thorac. Surg., 58:372, 1994.
43. Walsh, G. L., and Nesbitt, J. C.: Tumor implants after thoracoscopic resection of a metastatic sarcoma. Ann. Thorac. Surg., 59:215, 1995.

V

TRACHEOSTOMY AND ITS COMPLICATIONS

Hermes C. Grillo, M.D., and Douglas J. Mathisen, M.D.

Tracheostomy is one of the oldest operations and was long used for emergency management of upper airway obstruction. Tracheostomy was also employed to control secretions in severely ill patients. More recently, tracheostomy has provided a route for ventilatory support in respiratory insufficiency. This increased use of tracheostomy reawakened recognition of the large number of serious complications that may follow the procedure. A spectrum of lesions, principally associated with its use for ventilatory support, has been identified.

INDICATIONS

The occurrence of serious complications has caused critical reappraisal of the three classic indications for tracheostomy: (1) relief of upper airway obstruction, (2) control of secretions, and (3) ventilatory support in respiratory failure. Tracheostomy often cannot be avoided in organic upper airway obstruction, although in some situations a tube may be inserted beyond an obstruction until definitive treatment can be provided. Emergency management of airway obstruction is best effected by skillful dilatation of inflammatory stenosis[9] or *coring-out* of tumor.[17] These techniques are preferable, in terms of safety, efficiency, and cost, to the use of the laser.[3, 23]

The accumulation of secretions has increasingly been controlled by adequate humidification and by intensive pulmonary physiotherapy, consisting of expert instruction and assistance in cough, positional drainage, and thoracic percussion. Tracheal suctioning is used in conjunction with these measures, and, occasionally, transcricoid instillation of saline has been helpful. The flexible bronchoscope is frequently employed at the bedside. *Minitracheostomy*—the insertion of a relatively small-bore catheter percutaneously through the cricothyroid membrane for repetitive suctioning over a prolonged period of time—has increasingly been recognized as a simple alternative to conventional tracheostomy for this purpose.[19] Unlike conventional cricothyroidostomy, it is relatively free of complications when correctly used,[24] because damage to the larynx is minimal.

Patients with respiratory insufficiency or impending failure are usually supported by a respirator with an endotracheal tube for varying lengths of time. If it appears that more than a few days of support will be required, a nasotracheal tube is generally preferred for the patient's comfort. Patients may thus be supported for a brief period of needed ventilatory assistance postoperatively without tracheostomy. There is no firm indication regarding the length of time an endotracheal tube may be employed. If it becomes clear that long-term support is needed, a tracheostomy is usually done as an elective procedure within 5 to 7 days. Such a transfer becomes necessary because of the dangers of tube obstruction, the discomfort to the patient of a nasal or oral tube, and the considerable damage to the larynx that may follow prolonged intubation. This injury occurs especially in the posterior commissure, with damage to the arytenoid and interarytenoid area. In a prospective study of the sequelae of endotracheal intubation, Whited[25] found three reversible laryngeal stenoses and one chronic posterior stenosis in 50 patients intubated for 2 to 5 days, five chronic laryngotra-cheal stenoses in 100 patients intubated for 6 to 10 days, and six complex laryngeal stenoses in 50 patients intubated for 11 to 24 days. Early conversion to tracheostomy prevented these injuries. The data support a policy of conversion from endotracheal tube to tracheostomy after 7 days.

TECHNIQUE

Tracheostomy is only rarely an emergency procedure. The safest method of establishing an emergency airway is insertion of an endotracheal tube or, if that fails, introduction of a rigid ventilating bronchoscope. Even obstructing lesions can often be bypassed in this manner, or sufficient ventilatory force can be applied beyond an obstruction through a tube so that a patient can be maintained until a more carefully considered procedure can be accomplished. For this reason, the simplest emergency surgical airway, an opening in the superficially located cricothyroid membrane, is rarely required.

Tracheostomy may be done under local anesthesia, with the patient supine and the neck hyperextended. An anesthetist should be in attendance to maintain a clear airway, to adjust the positioning of the endotracheal tube during the procedure, and to supply oxygen or other support as needed. The procedure should be performed in the operating room, so that the most sterile conditions are maintained and the operator is impressed with the need for meticulous technique. Blind tracheostomy procedures are unneccessary and are condemned because of the high incidence of associated complications. Such procedures reappear irregularly but thus far have always been discarded due to serious complications. The rapidly made vertical cutaneous incision for emergency tracheostomy has been replaced by a carefully placed horizontal incision. This avoids the late tethering scars that may follow a vertical incision. Palpation of the extended neck always reveals the position of the cricothyroid membrane and the cricoid cartilage below. The incision is placed at the level of the second tracheal cartilage and extends through the platysma (Fig. 51–37). The strap muscles are separated vertically in the midline with minimal bleeding. The thyroid isthmus is usually divided between hemostats after careful dissection beneath it in the pretracheal plane. The thyroid tissue on either side is controlled with mattress sutures. Exact levels of the cartilaginous rings must be determined. The first cartilage must be left intact, and the opening in the trachea must be placed so that there is no tendency for the tube subsequently to erode the first ring or the adjacent cricoid cartilage by upward pressure. The second and third cartilages (and all or part of the fourth, if necessary) are incised vertically in the midline so that the potential danger of upward pressure by the outside of the elbow of the tube is minimized. If there is any question, incision of a lower cartilage avoids damage to a higher cartilage. Even after centuries of performance of tracheostomy, there is little controlled work to prove the superiority of the vertical incision over the cruciate or the horizontal incision, the excision of a disc or a segment of cartilage, or the turning of a flap. The tracheal opening probably enlarges to the size of the tube in most cases after some days. It is important not to make too

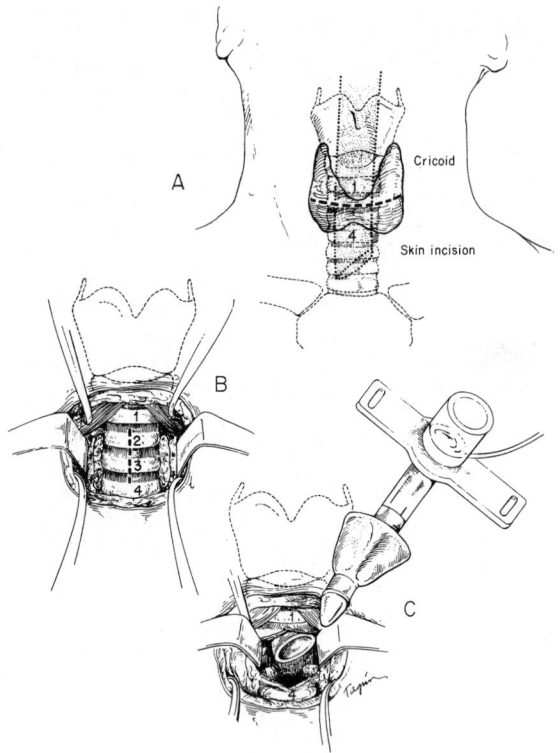

Figure 51–37. Technique of tracheostomy. *A*, An endotracheal airway is in place. With the patient's neck extended and centered in the midline, a short horizontal incision is made over the second or third tracheal ring after the level of the cricoid cartilage has been carefully palpated. The first and fourth tracheal cartilages are numbered. *B*, Following horizontal division of the platysma, the strap muscles are separated in the midline, the cricoid is identified, and the thyroid isthmus usually is divided and sutured to allow easy access to the second and third tracheal rings. The second and third rings are incised vertically. Occasionally an additional partial incision of the fourth ring is necessary. *C*, Smooth thyroid pole retractors are used to spread the opening in the trachea. The endotracheal tube is withdrawn to a point just above the incision. The tracheostomy tube is introduced with a small amount of water-soluble lubricant and with its large-volume cuff collapsed. The endotracheal airway is not removed until it is demonstrated that the tracheostomy tube is properly seated and permits suitable gas exchange. Closure is made with simple skin sutures. The flange of the tracheostomy tube is both sutured to the skin and tied with the usual tapes around the neck. On a rare occasion when an airway cannot be established from above, an emergency incision may be necessary over the cricothyroid membrane for rapid establishment of a temporary airway.

large an opening in the tracheal wall, whether with or without a flap, since the flap may well be destroyed or deformed. Any opening heals by cicatrization, and the larger the defect, the greater the likelihood of narrowing during stomal healing. If fine retractors are used in the open trachea, even a tube with a bulky low-pressure cuff may be inserted with ease with the assistance of water-soluble lubricant. Hemostasis should be precise throughout such an elective procedure.

Hypoxia and subsequent cardiac arrest, which formerly occurred during emergency tracheostomy, should not occur with this technique, because an airway has already been established. Formerly the site of tracheostomy was the suprasternal notch in the extended neck. In many patients, such an approach selects a midtracheal location and places the point of potential damage from cuff injury low in the trachea. The trachea is also farther away from the cervical skin surface at this level. In addition, it tends to further angulate the tube. In children and in some adults, a low incision also places the inner side of the elbow of the tube close to a high innominate artery, with greater potential for later erosive major hemorrhage.

Once the tube has been securely seated and the cuff is

functioning satisfactorily, the endotracheal tube is withdrawn and supportive oxygenation is given through a lightweight connector attached to the tube or to its inner cannula if it is a two-part tube. The skin is loosely closed with vertical mattress sutures on either side of the tracheostomy tube. Sutures on either side are passed through the flanges of the tracheostomy tube, securing it in place, in addition to the usual tracheostomy tapes. Such fixation is particularly important in the first few days, especially when a vertical incision in the trachea has been used, so that displacement of the tube does not occur at a time when replacement may be difficult. An overly long tube should be avoided to prevent placement in the right main bronchus. The precise location of the tip of the tube relative to any lesion and the carina is determined with a flexible bronchoscope. Cuffs must be firmly fixed or cemented, if they are not an integral part of the tube, to prevent dislodgement or prolapse over the end of the tube. Suctioning during tracheostomy and immediately after its completion helps avoid postoperative atelectasis. Prolonged suctioning, which may cause hypoxia, is avoided.

COMPLICATIONS

Conversion of tracheostomy to a carefully performed elective procedure has largely eliminated the immediate and early complications of the procedure.[21] The longer-term complications of tracheostomy present mainly in three ways: (1) sepsis, (2) hemorrhage, and (3) obstruction of the airway. Additional complications are tracheoesophageal fistula and persistence of the stoma. In general, the longer a tracheostomy is in place (especially with an inflated cuff), the greater the chance that complications will occur.

Sepsis. All tracheostomies are clinically contaminated, and *Staphylococcus aureus* (often a resistant strain), *Pseudomonas aeruginosa*, and a variety of other bacteria such as *Escherichia coli* and *Streptococcus* can be cultured. Despite this inevitability, sterile care and cleansing of the stoma and respiratory equipment must be maintained to minimize the possibility of invasive infection of the lower airway. Antibiotics are probably best reserved for use when there is evidence of tracheobronchitis, pneumonitis, or cellulitis, because premature use does not sterilize the stoma but may merely permit other flora to become established.

Hemorrhage. The curve of the tube may erode the innominate artery and produce late hemorrhage, especially in children, in whom the trachea is small and the artery high. Massive hemorrhage also occurs from erosion by tracheostomy cuffs or even by the tip of a tube through the trachea into the innominate artery as it passes obliquely over the trachea. Bleeding from granulations or more superficial tracheal erosions is more common and less massive. Only immediate tamponade of a major arterial leak, digitally when due to erosion at the stoma, or with an inflated cuff when caused by cuff or tip injury lower in the trachea, and prompt surgical treatment lead to salvage. Resection of the injured artery with suture closure of both ends is one of the few possibilities in such a contaminated field. In the small number of cases in which this has been done successfully, there have been no neurologic problems. The trachea requires only closure when arterial injury occurs at the stomal level. Injuries at the cuff level require resection and reconstruction.[7, 22]

Obstruction. Airway obstruction may occur while the tube is in place. If a tube with an inner cannula is used, crusts may be easily cleaned. With proper humidification, obstruction of single-lumen tubes is uncommon. Occasionally, a valve type of crust may form at the tip of a tube, so that a suction catheter may be easily passed without relieving the obstruction. If such a problem is found on flexible bronchoscopy, the tube must be changed. If change is necessary early after tracheostomy, it should be done over a guiding catheter, with adequate instruments and personnel available to reinsert an endotracheal tube or a rigid bronchoscope from above in the event that the tube is not easily replaced. Occasionally, obstructive granulations also form at the tip of a tube that is still in place.

A major syndrome of postintubation airway obstruction has been recognized (Fig. 51–38).[1, 5, 8, 11] Improvements in cuffs and awareness of the problems have reduced its incidence. *Every patient with signs of upper airway obstruction—wheezing or stridor, dyspnea on effort, episodes of obstruction from secretions—who has been previously intubated with either an endotracheal tube or a tracheostomy tube must be considered to have organic obstruction until it is proved otherwise.* Unfortunately, many such patients who have been discharged from the hospital are still treated for asthma to the point of death or subtotal obstruction before the lesion is recognized.

Obstructive *laryngeal lesions* from prolonged endotracheal intubation may occur at the vocal cord level and consist of granulation tissue or cicatrix, particularly in the posterior commissure.[5, 8, 16, 25] Large tubes relative to airway size may cause erosion at the subglottic and cricoid levels, with subsequent severe stenosis. Cricothyroidostomy, proposed to avoid the complications of tracheostomy,[2] fails to eliminate cuff lesions and transfers serious stomal lesions from the trachea to the subglottic larynx—where surgical treatment is more difficult, less satisfactory, and often impossible.[5, 13]

At the stomal level, obstruction may be due to a polypoid granuloma that forms on the healing surface of the stomal site. Narrowing and indentation at the point of cicatrization of the stoma are often seen after tracheostomy. When the stoma is large—because of overgenerous initial surgical therapy, erosion by local infection, or, most commonly, the prying action of heavyweight equipment that connects the tracheostomy to the ventilator—healing may produce clinically obvious obstruction. Such a stomal obstruction is usually three-sided, obstructing anteriorly and laterally, because the posterior wall is intact. Occasionally, some scarring occurs posteriorly as well. A combination of granuloma and stenosis may also produce obstruction. If the tracheostomy is placed too high, erosion of the cricoid cartilage may occur, with loss of substance and resultant subglottic stricture.

At the cuff site, pressure by the sealing cuff causes varying

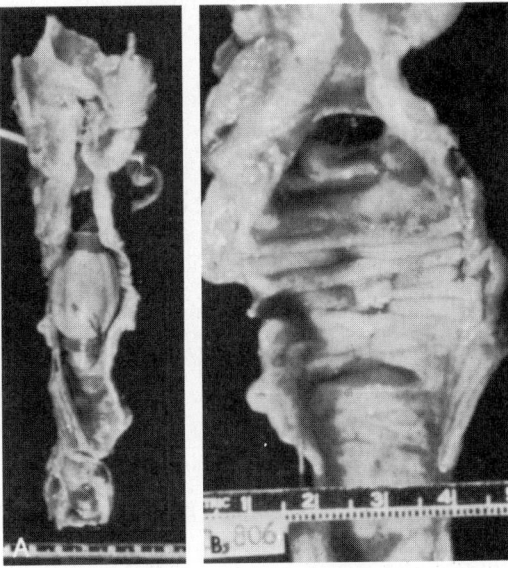

Figure 51–39. Tracheal injury due to a cuffed tracheostomy tube. Autopsy specimen of larynx and trachea. *A,* A metal tracheostomy tube with rubber cuff inflated had been in place for 16 days. *B,* Cartilaginous rings are exposed and fragmented at the cuff site. The tracheal wall is thinned and distended. (From Cooper, J. D., and Grillo, H. C.: The evolution of tracheal injury due to ventilatory assistance through cuffed tubes: A pathologic study. Ann. Surg., *169*:334, 1969.)

degrees of damage. Prior to the introduction of true large-volume, low-pressure cuffs, damage of varying degrees occurred in all patients in whom a cuff was inflated for more than 48 hours.[4] In the days and weeks following, erosion frequently bared numerous cartilages, leading to their fragmentation and, eventually, total destruction (Fig. 51–39). Occasionally, the erosion progresses anteriorly, through the wall of the innominate artery, or posteriorly, to produce a tracheoesophageal fistula. With lesser degrees of damage, healing occurs with variable deformity and narrowing. If the tracheal wall has been deeply eroded circumferentially, a circumferential stricture results during healing (Fig. 51–40). This may become arrested with partial closure and produce only dyspnea on effort, or it may go on to complete closure, with a fatal obstructive episode. The lengths of such strictures are extremely variable, extending from 0.5 to 4 cm. Such lesions may occur with either endotracheal tubes or tracheostomy tubes, because they are due to the cuff and not to the tube itself. A far greater number arise from cuffs on tracheostomy tubes, because there is greater long-term exposure to them. Other factors have been implicated in the etiology of cuff strictures, including periods of hypotension, which make it easier to compress the mucosal vascular supply; bacterial infection, which is always present; and toxic products from various materials and from ethylene oxide sterilization with inadequate aeration. However, clinical, pathologic, and experimental evidence clearly demonstrates that the common denominator is pressure.[1, 4]

The tracheal cartilages *between the stoma and the cuff level* are often thinned, presumably by inflammatory changes, and this segment may become malacic. With respiratory effort, the malacic segment tends to collapse, contributing to the obstructive process. Malacia may also occur at cuff level, instead of stenosis. Granuloma may form at the point of erosion by the *tip of the tracheostomy tube.* Children are more likely to show this lesion, because they are usually managed postoperatively without a cuff. Although most tracheostomies close spontaneously, a large *persistent stoma* may fail to close, requiring precise surgical repair.[15] This is apt to occur

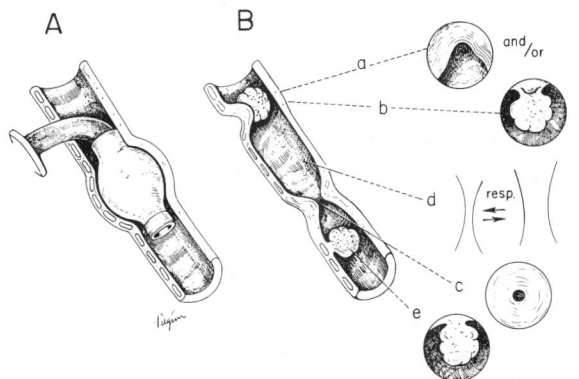

Figure 51–38. Obstructive lesions that may result from cuffed tracheostomy tubes. A conventional cuffed tube is in place at the left *(A).* Sagittal and cross-sectional (bronchoscopic) views of pathologic lesions are shown at the right *(B).* Anterolateral strictures are seen at the stoma (a), and granulomas also occur here (b). The lesions may occur concurrently. Circumferential stricture develops at the level of cuff injury (c). Between the stomal level and the cuff stricture, varying degrees of tracheal malacia may be seen; this leads to partial collapse during respiration (d). Granulomas may also occur at the level of the tip of the tube (e). (From Geffin, B., Grillo, H. C., Cooper, J. D., and Pontoppidan, H.: Stenosis following tracheostomy for respiratory care. JAMA, *216*:1984–1988, 1971. © by the American Medical Association.)

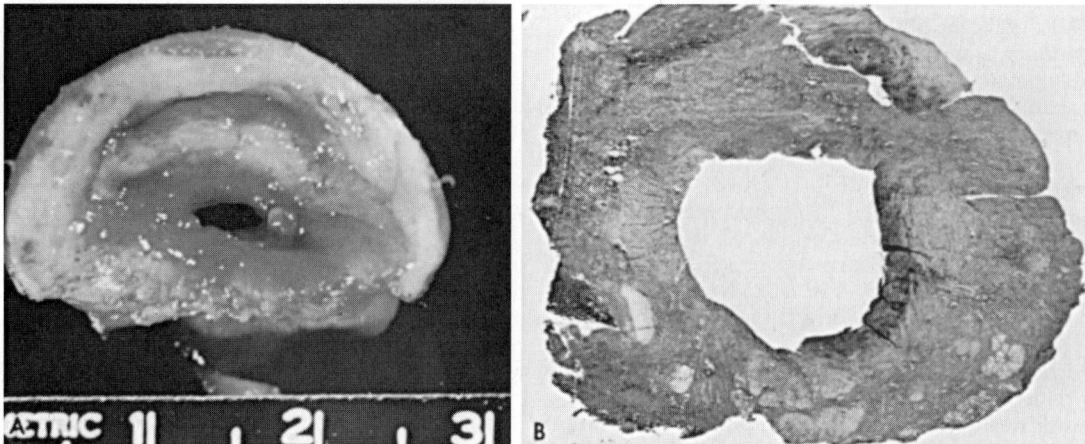

Figure 51–40. Tracheal stenosis from cuff damage. *A*, Gross specimen showing the typical circumferential fibrous and inflammatory lesion. *B*, Photomicrograph showing that the stricture in a severe case is composed almost entirely of scar tissue: little normal tracheal architecture is identifiable. Such strictures do not respond even to prolonged dilation or splinting. (From Grillo, H. C.: J. Thorac. Cardiovasc. Surg., *57*:52, 1969.)

after prolonged tracheostomy in aged or debilitated patients, in patients with metabolic disease, or in those who have been exposed to steroids.

Once a clinical diagnosis of obstruction is made, confirmation is easily obtained by simple radiologic studies (Fig. 51–41).[20] Routine chest films most frequently show clear lung fields. The unwary physician may treat the patient for adult-onset asthma or other vague diagnoses. Lesions are usually well defined by an anteroposterior radiograph of the airway from vocal cords to carina, using a copper filter for detail. Lateral neck roentgenograms reveal tracheal deformities at the stomal level. Oblique views of the chest, which rotate the mediastinum to the side, reveal the entire trachea and demonstrate areas of narrowing at cuff level or elsewhere. Fluoroscopy demonstrates the presence of malacia and describes vocal cord function. Tracheal laminagrams help define the character, level, and extent of a lesion, facts that are necessary for planning correction. Contrast medium produces a crisper picture but is not necessary. Computed tomographic scans of the airway contribute little useful information about postintubation stenosis.

TREATMENT

With the development of techniques of tracheal surgery that permit safe end-to-end anastomosis after resection of lengthy segments, the majority of these patients may be returned to normal function by surgical excision of the obstructing lesion and anatomic reconstruction of the upper airway.[5, 8, 11, 12]

If the patient is too ill for repair or has a disease that will soon require repeat tracheostomy, conservative management is recommended. This is possible in all but those patients in whom the lesion is immediately above the carina and is accomplished by reinstituting a tracheostomy, dilating the stricture, and passing a fenestrated tube or a Montgomery T-tube through it.[6] In a patient in whom the original damage was small in amount, repeated dilations or prolonged splinting with an inlying tube may produce a satisfactory airway over a long period of time. In most patients, however, conservative treatment does not succeed, despite prolonged attempts.

Five hundred three patients with postintubation tracheal injuries were submitted to surgical reconstruction at the Massachusetts General Hospital from 1965 through 1992.[11] A small number were treated conservatively because their basic diseases did not suggest that reconstruction would be toler-

ated or, more often, because they were likely to require tracheostomy again in the near future for diseases such as severe myasthenia gravis. Of the 503 surgical cases, there were 178 postintubation lesions at the *stomal* level and 251 at the *cuff* level; 38 patients had stenoses at *both* levels, and in 36 the lesion was of uncertain origin. One hundred twenty-three of the *cuff* stenoses were in patients who had had endotracheal intubation only, one for 18 hours.

The results of aggressive surgical treatment were good. Four hundred forty patients (87.5%) had good results; in 31 (6.2%), the results were clinically satisfactory, although not ideal if the patients were to be put under physical stress. Twenty (3.9%) represented failures. There were 12 (2.4%) deaths. A number of deaths and failures were in patients with supracarinal stenoses that were impossible to manage conservatively and necessitating high risks. Failure was treated by tracheostomy, T-tube, or dilation. Failure was much more likely to follow prior unsuccessful treatment, especially resectional.[11, 14] If the extent of tracheal damage is too great, usually as a result of prior failure of treatment, it is preferable to manage the patient with a T-tube rather than undertake hazardous reconstruction.[6]

Postintubation stenosis involving the subglottic larynx is much more difficult to correct than are tracheal injuries. Sixty-two of the 503 patients had involvement of the subglottic larynx. A multitude of mainly multistaged procedures have been applied, but one-stage laryngotracheoplastic procedures have been developed.[5, 13] Acquired tracheoesophageal fistulas are successfully managed in a single operation also, after the patient is weaned from the respirator.[18] Postintubation tracheoesophageal fistulas were successfully repaired in 18 of 20 patients.[11]

Although the laser is widely used to treat postintubation lesions, it rarely results in definitive correction, except for granulomas or in the case of rare and thin, weblike stenosis.[23] Scarring due to laser therapy, along with tracheal damage from a tracheostomy (often done in conjunction with laser therapy), frequently complicates surgical repair.

PREVENTION

Prevention of tracheal stenosis is of key importance. Diminution in the incidence of stomal strictures was noted at the Toronto General Hospital when heavy connecting tubing was abandoned for lightweight swivel connectors.[1] A relatively low incidence of stomal strictures in a corresponding period at the Massachusetts General Hospital, where lightweight connectors were in use, confirms this observation. Obviously, the surgical stoma should not be excessively large.

Strictures have been associated with tubes of every material and with cuffs of varying types of materials. At cuff level, the principal preventive factor is elimination of pressure necrosis.[1, 4, 10] The large-volume, low-pressure cuffs, which occlude the irregularly shaped tracheal lumen by conforming to the shape of the trachea rather than by expanding to distend and so seal the airway, may accomplish this. Such a cuff was devised initially in animal experiments and then tested clinically in patients (Fig. 51–42).[10] The introduction of such cuffs has markedly reduced the occurrence of cuff injury. However, the inextensibility of plastic materials permits conversion of most *low-pressure* cuffs to high-pressure ones if a small excess of air is introduced beyond the maximal resting volume of the unstretched cuff. Additional safeguards are direct pressure monitoring and side balloons with pop-off valves to bleed excessive air. The lesions continue to occur despite these advances.

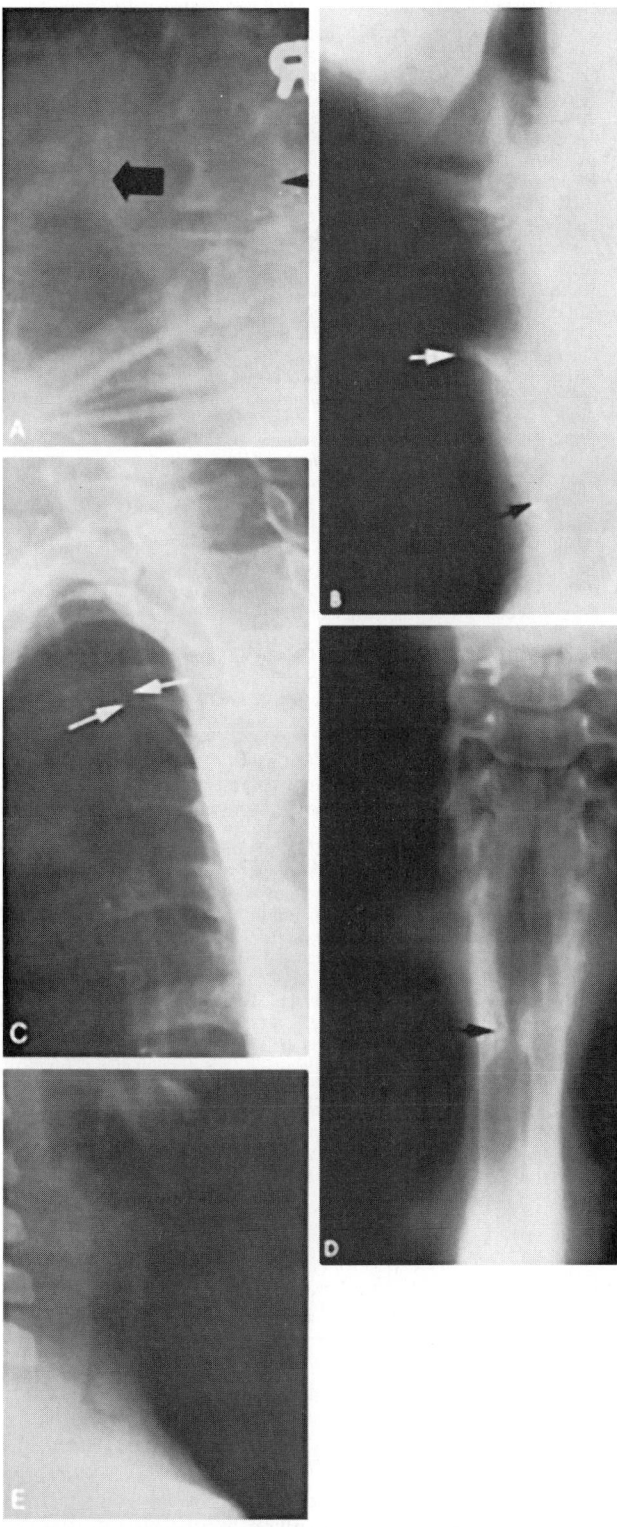

Figure 51–41. Roentgenograms demonstrating tracheal lesions. *A*, Granuloma at stomal site. Circular radiopaque marker is on skin at site of prior stoma. Large arrow points to partially narrowed air column with large anterior granuloma visible. *B*, Stricture at tracheostomy site, shown in detail of lateral neck view. Larynx is clearly seen above. Arrows mark longitudinal limits of anterior stricture. The posterior wall of trachea is not involved. *C*, Cuff-level stenosis is demonstrated on oblique view of chest, which rotates mediastinal structures away from the trachea and shows its full length. Arrows indicate the narrowness of the airway. The lesion is circumferential. *D*, Cuff stricture shown on laminagram. The exact length of the stenosis, degree of airway narrowing, and level of stricture in relation to larynx and carina are detailed. *E*, Granuloma at level of anterior erosion by tip of tracheostomy tube, shown in lateral neck roentgenogram. In this child, a cuff had not been used.

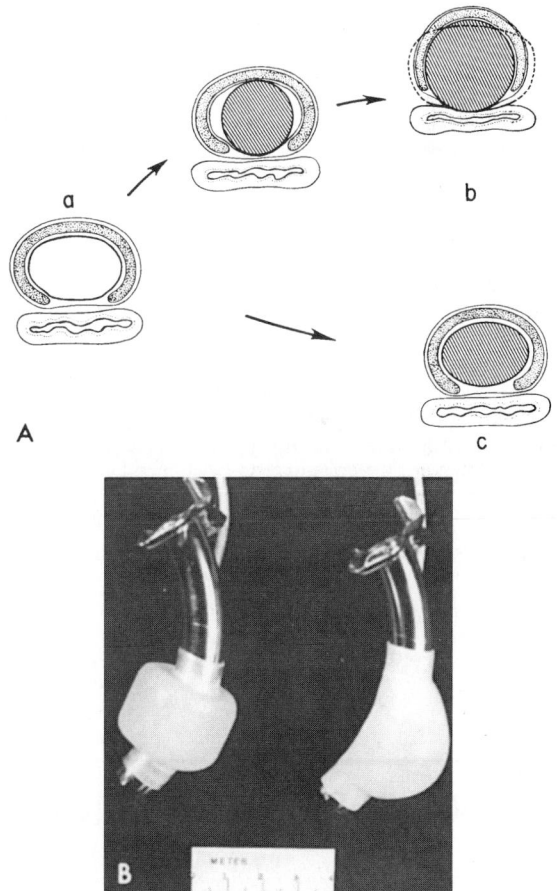

Figure 51–42. *A*, Diagram of the mechanism of cuff injury to the trachea and its avoidance. Above, a conventional cuff must be inflated under high pressure to effect a seal of the irregular tracheal airway. It distorts the trachea and exerts great pressure on the mucosa. Below, a cuff with large resting volume fills the irregular tracheal lumen by conforming to its shape at low intracuff pressures, below the point of elastic distention of the cuff. *B*, A low-pressure cuff and an old cuff mounted on standard Jackson tracheostomy tubes. The new cuff (left) is shown at its resting size. It must be collapsed with gentle syringe suction for insertion. The high-pressure cuff (right) has been inflated with 8 cc. of air. It has a high intracuff pressure, is asymmetrical, and is quite rigid. Unfortunately, overinflation of large-volume cuffs converts them to high-pressure cuffs if they are made of relatively inextensible plastic. (From Grillo, H. C., Cooper, J. D., Geffin, B., and Pontoppidan, H.: A low pressure cuff for tracheostomy tubes to minimize tracheal injury: A comparative clinical trial. J. Thorac. Cardiovasc. Surg., *62*:898, 1971.)

Substitution of cricothyroidotomy for tracheostomy[2] appears only to change the location of airway injury to a site more difficult to repair, despite the absence of complications in the experience of its original proponents. Endotracheal tubes obviously do not eliminate cuff lesions and may introduce glottic and subglottic laryngeal stenoses.

SELECTED REFERENCES

Andrews, M. J., and Pearson, F. G.: The incidence and pathogenesis of tracheal injury following cuffed tube tracheostomy with assisted ventilation: An analysis of a two-year prospective study. Ann. Surg., 173:249, 1971.
This excellent study correlates factors attendant upon respiratory therapy, gross pathologic observations at the time of extubation, and the subsequent appearance of stenosis.

Cooper, J. D., and Grillo, H. C.: The evolution of tracheal injury due to ventilatory assistance through cuffed tubes: A pathologic study. Ann. Surg., 169:334, 1969.
The pathogenesis of tracheal injuries is traced by the study of autopsy specimens of tracheas from patients who died while in respiratory therapy and surgically resected specimens of fully developed strictures. Pressure necrosis is identified as the major etiologic factor.

Grillo, H. C.: Congenital lesions, neoplasms, inflammation, infections, injuries, and other lesions of the trachea. *In* Sabiston, D. C., Jr., and Spencer, F. C. (Eds.): Gibbon's Surgery of the Chest, 6th ed. Philadelphia, W. B. Saunders, 1995.
The failure of conservative management is emphasized, and the successful application of techniques of surgical reconstruction in the management of postintubation lesions is described in this review of tracheal surgical problems.

Grillo, H. C., Donahue, D. M., Mathisen, D. J., Wain, J. C., and Wright, C. D.: Post-intubation tracheal stenosis: Treatment and results. J. Thorac. Cardiovasc. Surg., 109:486, 1995.
A 27-year experience in the management of 503 patients with postintubation injuries is described, detailing lesions, treatment, results, and complications.

Whited, R. E.: A prospective study of laryngotracheal sequelae in long-term intubation. Laryngoscope, 94:367, 1984.
Replacing largely retrospective prior data, this careful study documents the frequency and severity of laryngeal and subglottic injuries due to endotracheal intubation. It demonstrates the validity of limiting endotracheal intubation to 7 to 10 days.

REFERENCES

1. Andrews, M. J., and Pearson, F. G.: The incidence and pathogenesis of tracheal injury following cuffed tube tracheostomy with assisted ventilation: An analysis of a two-year prospective study. Ann. Surg., 173:249, 1971.
2. Brantigan, C. O., and Grow, J. B., Sr.: Cricothyroidotomy: Elective use in respiratory problems requiring tracheostomy. J. Thorac. Cardiovasc. Surg., 71:72, 1976.
3. Brutinel, W. M., Cortese, D. A., McDougall, J. C., et al.: A two-year experience with the Neodymium-YAG laser in endobronchial obstruction. Chest, 91:159, 1987.
4. Cooper, J. D., and Grillo, H. C.: The evolution of tracheal injury due to ventilatory assistance through cuffed tubes: A pathologic study. Ann. Surg., 169:334, 1969.
5. Couraud, L., Jougon, J., Velly, J. F., and Klein, C.: Sténoses iatrogènes de la voie respiratoire: Évolution des indications thérapeutiques. A partir de 217 cas chirurgicaux. Ann. Chir. Thorac. Cardiovasc., 48:277, 1994.
6. Gaissert, H. A., Grillo, H. C., Mathisen, D. J., and Wain, J. C.: Temporary and permanent restoration of airway continuity with the tracheal T-tube. J. Thorac. Cardiovasc. Surg., 107:600, 1994.
7. Grillo, H. C.: Complications of tracheal operations. *In* Cordell, A. R., and Ellison, R. G. (Eds.): Complications of Intrathoracic Surgery. Boston, Little, Brown, 1979.
8. Grillo, H. C.: Surgical treatment of post-intubation tracheal injuries. J. Thorac. Cardiovasc. Surg., 78:860, 1979.
9. Grillo, H. C.: The urgent management of tracheal obstruction. *In* Staudacher, V., and Bevilacqua, G. (Eds.): Eighth International Congress of Emergency Surgery. Milan, Monduzzi, 1987.
10. Grillo, H. C., Cooper, J. D., Geffin, B., and Pontoppidan, H.: A low pressure cuff for tracheostomy tubes to minimize tracheal injury: A comparative clinical trial. J. Thorac. Cardiovasc. Surg., 62:898, 1971.
11. Grillo, H. C., Donahue, D. M., Mathisen, D. J., Wain, J. C., and Wright, C. D.: Post-intubation tracheal stenosis: Treatment and results. J. Thorac. Cardiovasc. Surg., 109:486, 1995.
12. Grillo, H. C., and Mathisen, D. J.: Surgical management of tracheal strictures. Surg. Clin. North Am., 68:511, 1988.
13. Grillo, H. C., Mathisen, D. J., and Wain, J. C.: Laryngotracheal resection and reconstruction for subglottic stenosis. Ann. Thorac. Surg., 53:54, 1992.
14. Grillo, H. C., Zannini, P., and Michelassi, F.: Complications of tracheal reconstruction: Incidence, treatment and prevention. J. Thorac. Cardiovasc. Surg., 91:322, 1986.
15. Lawson, D. W., and Grillo, H. C.: Closure of a persistent tracheal stoma. Surg. Gynecol. Obstet., 130:995, 1970.
16. Lindholm, C. E.: Prolonged endotracheal intubation. Acta Anaesthesiol. Scand., Suppl. 33, 1969.
17. Mathisen, D. J., and Grillo, H. C.: Endoscopic relief of malignant airway obstruction. Ann. Thorac. Surg., 48:469, 1989.
18. Mathisen, D. J., Grillo, H. C., Wain, J. C., and Hilgenberg, A. D.: Management of acquired nonmalignant tracheoesophageal fistula. Ann. Thorac. Surg., 52:759, 1991.
19. Matthews, H. R., and Hopkinson, R. B.: Treatment of sputum retention by minitracheostomy. Br. J. Surg., 71:147, 1984.
20. Momose, K. J., and MacMillan, A. S., Jr.: Roentgenologic investigations of the larynx and trachea. Radiol. Clin. North Am., 16:321, 1978.
21. Mulder, D. S., and Rubush, J. L.: Complications of tracheostomy: Relationship to long term ventilatory assistance. J. Trauma, 9:389, 1969.
22. Nelems, B.: Tracheoarterial fistula. *In* Grillo, H. C., and Eschapasse, H. (Eds.): International Trends in General Thoracic Surgery. Philadelphia, W. B. Saunders, 1987.
23. Toty, L., Personne, G., Colchen, A., et al.: Laser treatment of postintubation lesions. *In* Grillo, H. C., and Eschapasse, H. (Eds.): International Trends in General Thoracic Surgery. Philadelphia, W. B. Saunders, 1987.
24. Wain, J. C., Wilson, D. J., and Mathisen, D. J.: Clinical experience with minitracheostomy. Ann. Thorac. Surg., 49:881, 1990.
25. Whited, R. E.: A prospective study of laryngotracheal sequelae in long-term intubation. Laryngoscope, 94:367, 1984.

VI _____

PULMONARY INFECTIONS

Stewart M. Scott, M.D., and Timothy Takaro, M.D.

LUNG ABSCESS

A lung abscess is a localized area of suppuration and cavitation in the lung. This definition includes such diverse etiologies as tuberculous, mycotic, or parasitic cavitation; bronchiectasis; infected cyst; and even pulmonary infarction with abscess formation. Cavitation of a tumor with an abscess may also occur. Most of these conditions are discussed in other chapters. This section concerns primarily pyogenic lung abscesses secondary to aspiration pneumonitis. These have been termed primary or simple lung abscesses to distinguish them from those abscesses occurring in association

with systemic diseases, malignant or nonmalignant, that follow the weakening of the body's natural defenses against infection.[9] The former are declining in incidence, whereas the latter have achieved increasing prominence in recent years.

Pyogenic lung abscess has been recognized and even treated surgically for centuries. However, accurate diagnosis of lung abscess awaited techniques of modern medicine, such as the chest roentgenogram. In 1927, David Smith at Duke University observed that organisms seen in the walls of lung abscesses were also present in patients' mouths, especially patients with bad oral hygiene. He demonstrated in experimental animals that aspiration of these bacteria could cause lung abscess. At that time, the mortality from this disease was approximately 30%, and treatment often required surgical drainage or pulmonary resection. Once penicillin became available, however, the need for surgical therapy rapidly declined.[1]

Pathogenesis

Pyogenic lung abscesses usually occur as a result of aspiration of septic debris from the oropharynx into the lung in a patient with gingivodental disease or oral sepsis, during a period when the cough reflex is suppressed. Dental or tonsillar operations also commonly precede the development of lung abscesses. Edentulous patients rarely have aspiration-type lung abscesses. Since episodes of aspiration occur during periods of unconsciousness from alcoholism, general anesthesia, epilepsy, cerebral vascular accident, or immersion, the victim is usually in a recumbent and often supine position. The most direct route for the airway embolus to travel is into the right main bronchus, and the first dependent bronchus in a supine patient is that to the superior division of the right lower lobe. The posterior segment of the right upper lobe is also dependent and accessible. These two segments are therefore the most common sites of lodgement of septic emboli and the usual sites of primary lung abscesses (Fig. 51–43). Esophageal disease that permits regurgitation and subsequent aspiration of esophageal contents into the lungs is another predisposing clinical setting. Rarely, septic pulmonary embolism causes infarction and lung abscess.

Following the development of severe pneumonitis in response to the embolus, liquefaction may occur. The microorganisms most commonly responsible are anaerobic bacteria, alpha- and beta-hemolytic streptococci, staphylococci, nonhemolytic streptococci, and *Escherichia coli*. Gram-negative rods and staphylococci are likely to occur in hospital-acquired lung abscess[27]; other organisms are isolated less often.[29] As the liquefied necrotic material empties through the bronchus, a necrotic cavity containing pus and air is formed. Clinically, lung abscesses present as indolent conditions in patients with a predilection for aspiration. Usually cough, foul-smelling sputum, fever, pleuritic chest pain, weight loss, and night sweats are noted.

In the suppurative pneumonias of infancy due to staphylococci, clinical symptoms and signs of abscess may be overshadowed by those of toxemia, dyspnea, cyanosis, and septic

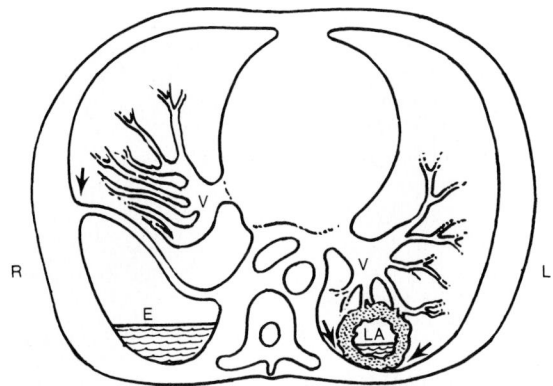

Figure 51–44. Diagram showing computed tomographic features of lung abscess and empyema. The lung abscess (LA) in the left lung is spherical, with thick, irregular walls and an irregular inner surface. The abscess forms acute angles with the chest wall (arrows). Pulmonary vessels (V) extend to the lung abscess. The empyema (E) in the right hemithorax is lenticular, with thin walls and smooth inner surfaces. It forms an obtuse angle with the chest wall (arrow). The pulmonary vessels (V) are compressed and distorted by the empyema. (From Williford, M. E., and Godwin, J. D.: Computed tomography of lung abscess and empyema. Radiol. Clin. North Am., *21*:575, 1983.)

shock. These may appear suddenly, or they may be greatly intensified if pyopneumothorax due to rupture of a subpleural abscess ensues.

The chest film in lung abscess is not pathognomonic in the early stages. An area or areas of dense pneumonic consolidation precede the appearance of the characteristic cavitary lesion. Multiple abscesses may form multiple cavities. A distinguishing roentgenographic feature of lung abscess, the air-fluid level, is seen only on thoracic roentgenograms exposed in the upright position (or the lateral decubitus, in a very sick patient). Accompanying pleural thickening, pneumothorax, or atelectasis may obscure or confuse this presentation. Computed tomography (CT) may be helpful in delineating the abscess (Fig. 51–44).[37] Staphylococcal pneumonia of infancy, which may lead to infected pneumoceles, differs in appearance from the classic lung abscess in that the lesions are characteristically thin-walled and cyst-like and are often accompanied by pleural effusion, empyema, or pyopneumothorax. Complete or partial opacification of the hemithorax may be the initial roentgenographic presentation under these circumstances. With adequate therapy, even the most dramatic roentgenographic features may disappear completely.

Because of the availability of effective broad-spectrum antibiotics such as penicillin, lung abscesses can often be aborted in the stage of pneumonitis; therefore, the incidence of this type of abscess has declined in recent years.[9] However, much more difficult clinical problems are presented by patients—often at the extremes of age—who have serious associated diseases, ranging from prematurity to malignant disease. In these patients the normal defense mechanisms for successfully combating infections are lacking,[9] and lung abscess may occur as a complication of a systemic disease. Prematurity, bronchopneumonia, congenital defects requiring surgical treatment, the postoperative state itself, and the presence of other infections, blood dyscrasias, or systemic diseases are common predisposing conditions in early infancy. In the older age group, postoperative states, systemic disease, malignant disease (especially of the lung and oropharynx), and prolonged use of corticosteroid, immunosuppressive, or radiation therapy are commonly associated with this type of lung abscess (Fig. 51–45). Such conditions often give rise to multiple abscesses, and the majority of these infections are acquired in the hospital. Bacteriologically, these abscesses differ somewhat from classic aspiration-type abscesses. *Staph-*

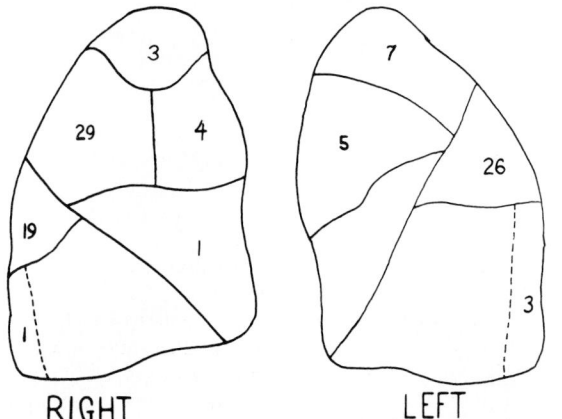

Figure 51–43. The segmental distribution of 98 lung abscesses caused by aspiration. Note the predilection for three principal sites: the superior segment of the right lower lobe, the posterior segment of the right upper lobe, and the superior segment of the left lower lobe. (From Bernhard, W. F., Malcolm, J. A., and Wylie, R. H.: Lung abscess: A study of 148 cases due to aspiration. Dis. Chest, *43*:620, 1963.)

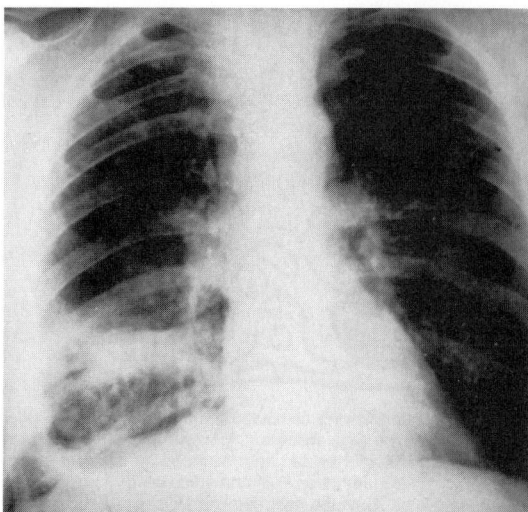

Figure 51–45. Thoracic roentgenogram of a patient with a huge lung abscess, right lower lobe, from which only the usually nonvirulent *Serratia marcescens* was cultured. This patient had had extensive corticosteroid therapy for severe asthma and multiple broad-spectrum antibiotics for superimposed infection, prior to operation. This type of abscess is currently being seen with greater frequency in similar clinical situations.

ylococcus aureus is a common causative organism, but alpha-streptococci, *Neisseria catarrhalis*, pneumococci, *Pseudomonas*, *Proteus*, *E. coli*, and *Klebsiella* are all recognized. Occasionally, after prolonged antibiotic treatment, rather unusual bacteria are all that remain to be cultured from the sputum.

The unpredictability of these organisms, coupled with the urgent need to identify them in a very sick patient, justifies the use of invasive means of obtaining secretions for bacteriologic examination, including transtracheal and occasionally even percutaneous needle aspiration.[11] These methods are not without hazard; alternative methods have been introduced using specially designed protected brush catheters in association with fiberoptic bronchoscopy. There is no predilection for particular sites for these abscesses. They can occur almost anywhere, but the right lung is more commonly involved than the left.

Treatment

The treatment of classic primary aspiration lung abscess is prolonged antimicrobial therapy.[29] Penicillin G has traditionally been the antibiotic of choice and can be initiated even before the results of sputum cultures are known. However, in one randomized controlled trial, clindamycin was found to be more effective for community-acquired putrid lung abscess. Other antibiotics are used as indicated by subsequent bacteriologic studies. Bronchoscopy for diagnostic purposes, to remove a foreign body if one is present, and to provide drainage of the abscess by aspiration of the appropriate bronchus through the bronchoscope is also usually indicated. The refinement of transbronchial drainage by catheterization of the appropriate bronchus with or without fluoroscopic guidance has also been helpful.

Surgical treatment is reserved for the complicated problems of massive hemoptysis, lack of response to antibiotics, and presence of a cavity that is thick walled or large (6 cm. or more) (Fig. 51–46).[9] When a malignant lesion is suspected or when empyema develops, surgical therapy may also be appropriate. In most instances, resective surgical treatment is performed. Occasionally, percutaneous catheter drainage of a large abscess in a poor-risk patient may be justified. The need for surgical resection for primary lung abscess has declined markedly in recent years, because the effectiveness of antibiotics has increased.[27]

The complications of lung abscesses include empyema, septicemia, metastatic brain abscess, and bronchogenic spread. The most common complication is the development of chronicity. A residual cavity may be an indication for resection if it is symptomatic or if infection recurs.

The mortality from aspiration-type lung abscess has declined appreciably in recent years and is currently reported at 5% to 6%.[28] Surgical treatment, if required, carries an 11% mortality.[9] In children, a 0% mortality is reported for lung abscesses treated medically. However, in patients whose abscesses complicate some other systemic disease, the mortality may be 35% to 90%. Prompt recognition and urgently applied appropriate antibiotic therapy may alter this dismal prognosis in the future.

FUNGAL INFECTIONS

Actinomycosis and nocardiosis have traditionally but mistakenly been classified as being caused by fungal organisms. The etiologic agents are actually bacteria belonging to the Actinomycetaceae. The distinction is important, because the treatment of infections caused by these two organisms differs from the therapy for mycotic infections.

Actinomycosis

Actinomycosis in man is usually caused by *Actinomyces israelii*. Actinomycotic organisms were described by von Graefe in 1854. The disease, known as "lumpy jaw," was more common in cattle (*Actinomyces bovis*) and in man before penicillin. It was associated with poor oral hygiene. The first description of thoracic actinomycosis was by Ponfic in 1882.[30]

The *Actinomyces* are anaerobic or microaerophilic organisms that require special techniques for culture and isolation. In pathologic material, organisms with branching filaments occur in clusters or microcolonies called granules. The much larger yellow-brown granules in draining material from abscesses or sinuses are called sulfur granules and are dense clusters of organisms. Since *A. israelii* is a normal inhabitant of the oral cavity, it must be recovered from closed tissue spaces, draining sinuses, or abscesses, or it must be shown to

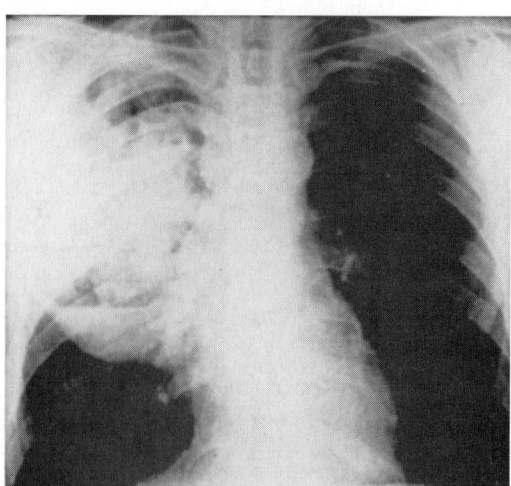

Figure 51–46. Posteroanterior thoracic roentgenogram of a patient with a pyogenic lung abscess, from which *Klebsiella pneumoniae* and alpha-streptococci were cultured. After a month of intensive antimicrobial therapy, a residual dense, thick-walled cavitary mass, 4 cm. in diameter, was resected by right upper lobectomy.

be invasive in histopathologic sections, to make a definitive diagnosis.

Cervicofacial, thoracic, and abdominal forms of actinomycosis are recognized. Thoracic actinomycosis is most commonly caused by bronchopulmonary invasion of infectious material from the oropharynx. The infection may be so indolent that there are few symptoms until pleural or chest wall involvement ensues.[17] Empyema and chronic draining chest wall sinuses, or roentgenographic evidence of involvement of the ribs or vertebrae, are characteristic. A nonspecific-appearing pulmonary infiltration, consolidation, or hilar mass strongly suggestive of bronchogenic carcinoma is also observed.[6] Primary actinomycetic empyema is rare.

The drug of choice is penicillin. Because of the dense fibrous tissue surrounding the colonies of organisms and the concentration of organisms in clusters, high doses of pharmacologic agents must be used for long periods, and radical surgical excision should accompany antibiotic therapy if possible. The difficulty of establishing a diagnosis in this disease frequently results in surgical excision of the pulmonary lesions of actinomycosis or of chest wall abscesses (Fig. 51–47). Empyema may require decortication or pleural drainage.

Nocardiosis

Like actinomycosis, nocardiosis was originally described in cattle (D. Nocar, 1888). Nocardiosis is usually caused by the aerobic actinomycete *Nocardia asteroides;* this organism has been isolated from the soil. It occurs in pathologic material in clumps or granules composed of short or long branching filaments that are gram-positive and acid-fast. This has led to confusion in the past with *Mycobacterium tuberculosis.*

Nocardiosis may mimic actinomycosis, tuberculosis, pneumonia, or lung abscess. In the last decade, most patients with nocardiosis have had some immunologic disorder associated with malignancy, organ transplantation, or immunosuppressive therapy. Thus, nocardiosis is often an opportunistic infection, with a grave prognosis. Nocardiosis occurs in patients with acquired immunodeficiency syndrome (AIDS), although the diagnosis may be concealed by the presence of *Pneumocystis carinii.*[5] The treatment is trimethoprim-sulfamethoxazole, continued on a long-term basis.[21] An alternative drug is minocycline. However, if the disease is resectable, a cure rate of 100% is reported. In many instances, the diagnosis is made for the first time from the resected specimen.

THORACIC MYCOTIC INFECTIONS

Formerly, blastomycosis, histoplasmosis, coccidioidomycosis, and cryptococcosis were considered to be rare, almost invariably fatal infections. Now it is recognized that benign, self-limited, and almost undetectable infections by all these organisms are much more common than had previously been thought. Millions of individuals exhibit evidence of subclinical histoplasmosis and coccidioidomycosis, with spontaneous healing.

The widespread use of antimetabolites, antibiotics, and steroids has given saprophytic fungi such as *Aspergillus, Candida,* and *Mucor* the opportunity to invade the host and cause disease. Thus, both true pathogens and saprophytes can cause opportunistic infection—that is, invade the host when body defenses have been weakened or altered by drugs or disease. The normally pathogenic fungi *Histoplasma, Blastomyces, Coccidioides, Paracoccidioides,* and *Sporothrix* are dimorphic. Because they exist in nature as molds that are not susceptible to phagocytosis by leukocytes, they cause infection. In hosts, in response to the 37° C. temperature, they change into yeasts or spherules *(Coccidioides)* that are susceptible to phagocytosis, allowing the host to heal the infection they cause. Fungi that exist only as opportunistic organisms probably do not cause disease in normal hosts because they are susceptible to phagocytosis, but they do cause disease in neutropenic patients. Both groups of fungi cause opportunistic infection in patients with suppressed cell-mediated immunity.[13]

The surgeon depends on the pathologist for a definitive diagnosis, but the pathologist must rely on the surgeon or physician to provide suspicion of fungal infection as well as appropriate samples of sputum or tissue to make positive identification possible. This is important, because for most of these diseases, serologic, immunologic, and skin tests cannot be relied on for a definitive diagnosis. Specific but rather

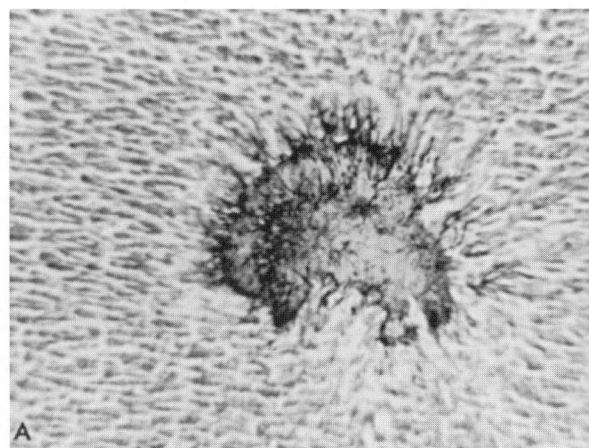
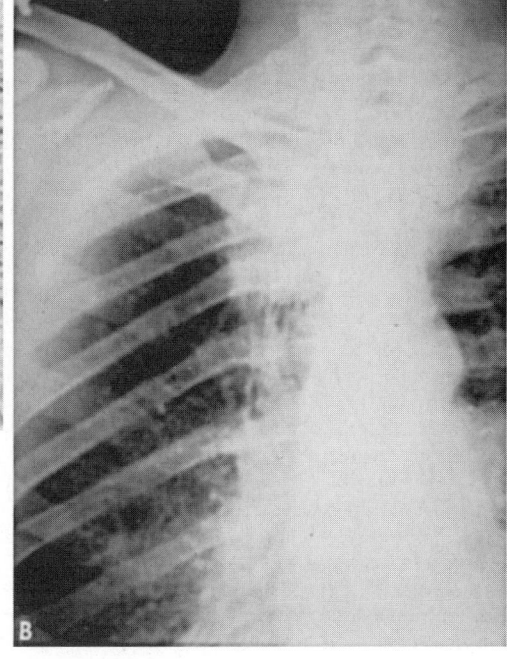

Figure 51–47. *A,* Actinomycotic granule showing branching filaments of a microscopic colony of *Actinomyces israelii.* Gomori's stain, ×250. *B,* Thoracic roentgenogram of a patient who subsequently underwent right upper lobectomy for a suspected malignant lesion. Actinomycosis was found in the resected specimen.

toxic antimycotic drugs are now available for treatment (Table 51–15).[21, 31]

Epidemiology

Many of the fungi that cause human infections are inhabitants of the soil. Most infections are believed to be caused by direct inhalation of the organisms in contaminated dust. Three of these organisms are known to occur in the soil of specific geographic areas in North America (Fig. 51–48). These are *Histoplasma capsulatum* (histoplasmosis), *Coccidioides immitis* (coccidioidomycosis), and *Blastomyces dermatitidis* (North American blastomycosis). A soil reservoir is also accepted for *Cryptococcus, Aspergillus,* and *Mucor.* Candidiasis is considered an endogenous infection, since the yeast *Candida* is part of the normal flora of human beings and animals.

Histoplasmosis

Histoplasmosis, the most common of the pathogenic fungal infections, occurs in the valley of the Mississippi River and its tributaries. *Histoplasma capsulatum* is found in soil contaminated by pigeon, chicken, or bat droppings. It was first observed in Panama in 1905 by Darling, who mistakenly thought that the organism was a plasmodium encapsulated in a histiocyte; hence its name. Some 30 million individuals have been infected, judging from skin reactions to histoplasmin.[15]

The pathologic findings resemble those of pulmonary tuberculosis, except for the finding of the yeast cells of *H. capsulatum* in macrophages or in the capsules of nonviable

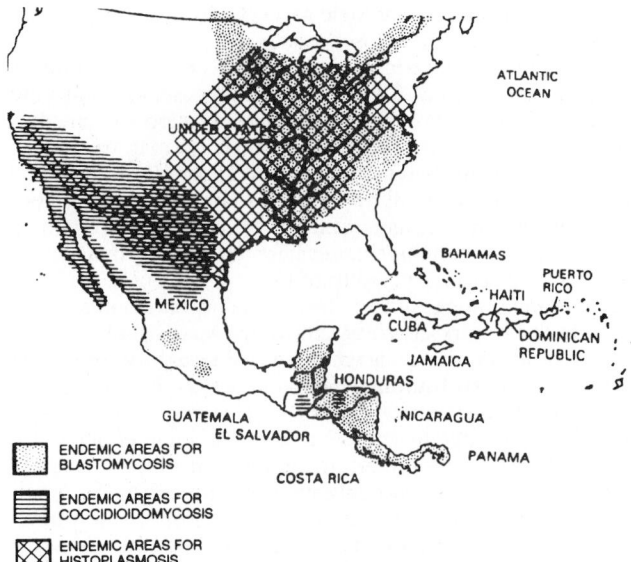

Figure 51–48. Areas of North America and Central America considered endemic for North American blastomycosis, histoplasmosis, and coccidioidomycosis.

organisms at the necrotic center of granulomas. Most cases of infection are asymptomatic. Acute pulmonic infection may be accompanied by diffuse pulmonary infiltration or scattered nodular densities and may be characterized by an acute febrile course. Whereas this disease is mild in normal hosts, in patients with AIDS it can be severe and even fatal unless aggressively treated.[18] By far the most common clinical presentation of histoplasmosis is an asymptomatic chronic granuloma, appearing on a thoracic roentgenogram as a solitary pulmonary nodule of undiagnosed etiology.

Chronic cavitary histoplasmosis resembles pulmonary tuberculosis both symptomatically and roentgenographically (Fig. 51–49), but it appears to progress more slowly. In a considerable percentage of cases, pulmonary tuberculosis has been found to coexist in such patients. A wide variety of

TABLE 51–15. Antibiotic Therapy for Actinomycetes and Fungi

Disease	Antibiotic
Actinomycosis	Penicillin (may require 1 yr. or more); erythromycin or tetracycline if patient is penicillin-sensitive
Nocardiosis	Trimethoprim-sulfamethoxazole or sulfadiazine for 3 to 6 mo.; minocycline if patient is sulfa-sensitive
North American blastomycosis	Itraconazole if not life threatening; amphotericin B is effective (2 or more gm.); 2-hydroxystilbamidine and ketoconazole are alternative drugs
Histoplasmosis	Itraconazole; amphotericin B is effective for most forms except endocarditis; ketoconazole for central nervous system disease
Coccidioidomycosis	Fluconazole for 6–12 mo.; amphotericin B, 0.5–2.5 gm.; ketoconazole
Cryptococcosis	Fluconazole; amphotericin B
Paracoccidioidomycosis	Itraconazole; amphotericin B; ketoconazole
Sporotrichosis	Itraconazole is primary drug; amphotericin B and 5-fluorocytosine are effective together
Aspergillosis	Amphotericin B; itraconazole for less ill patients
Candidiasis	Amphotericin B alone or with 5-fluorocytosine
Zygomycosis	Amphotericin B
Pseudallescheriasis	Ketoconazole; itraconazole

See references 21, 22, and 31.

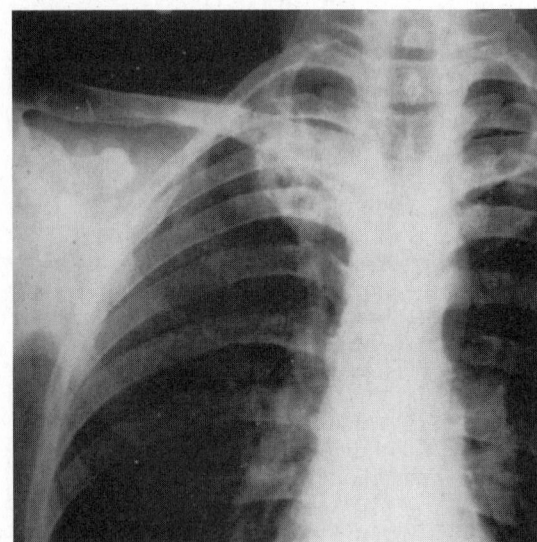

Figure 51–49. Thoracic roentgenogram of a patient with chronic cavitary histoplasmosis who underwent upper lobectomy prior to the availability of amphotericin B. (From Takaro, T.: Thoracic mycotic infections. *In* Lewis' Practice of Surgery. New York, Hoeber Medical Division, Harper & Row, 1968.)

clinical manifestations of chronic histoplasmosis involving the mediastinal structures is also seen.[15]

The treatment of histoplasmosis depends on the form of the disease encountered. For severe acute infections, therapy with amphotericin B, currently the only effective drug available, may be necessary. The solitary nodule may pose a problem in management. In a cooperative study of solitary pulmonary nodules resected in adult men, 53% were found to be granulomas and 36% malignant tumors. Fungi, either *H. capsulatum* or *C. immitis,* were isolated from the majority of these granulomas. Since malignancy was found in such a high percentage of cases, and since the presence of calcium in a nodule does not exclude carcinoma (unless calcification is concentric, dense, or unchanged for years), exploratory thoracotomy for an undiagnosed nodule is often indicated, especially in men over 40 years of age. If the diagnosis can be made by needle aspiration biopsy of the lesion, neither thoracotomy nor drug therapy may be necessary. Cavitary histoplasmosis, proved by culturing the organism in the sputum, should be treated primarily with either itraconazole (400 mg. per day for 6 months) or amphotericin B or ketoconazole.[31] Operative intervention is reserved for patients with large, thick-walled cavities who do not improve after treatment. If resectional surgery is undertaken, amphotericin B should be used until a total dosage of at least 2 gm. is reached over a period of a month before and a month after resection (if the diagnosis is established prior to operation). Surgical resection in Goodwin's series produced healed lesions in 95% to 100% of patients.[15] The treatment of mediastinal forms of histoplasmosis is variable, complicated, and beyond the scope of this text.[20] For disseminated forms of histoplasmosis, amphotericin B is urgently needed to prevent death.

Coccidioidomycosis

Coccidioidomycosis was first described by Posada in Buenos Aires in 1892, but in 1896, Rixford and Gilchrist in San Francisco incorrectly named the organism, believing it to be the protozoan *Coccidia.* Coccidioidomycosis is caused by the dimorphic fungus *C. immitis,* which may occur in tissues in the form of large spherules packed with endospores, as individual small endospores (following rupture of a spherule), or as mycelial elements or hyphae (in cavities) (Fig. 51–50).

Coccidioidomycosis is an exogenous infection occurring in certain well-defined regions of California, Nevada, Arizona, New Mexico, Texas, and Mexico.[26] These regions are characterized by a dry, windy, dusty, hot climate. Irrigation has made these areas important both agriculturally and epidemiologically, since population growth has been rapid in the past several decades. Extensive travel through these areas has helped spread coccidioidomycosis to every part of the United States, as well as to other countries. Some 10 million people in the United States are estimated to have been infected at some time in their lives with *C. immitis.*

The gross and microscopic lesions of coccidioidomycosis strongly resemble those of pulmonary tuberculosis, with two characteristic differences: the common occurrence of thin-walled cavities and chronic granulomas appearing as solitary nodules, as in histoplasmosis. Apical or subapical infiltrates or cavities (or both), indistinguishable roentgenographically from either chronic pulmonary tuberculosis or chronic pulmonary histoplasmosis, are also seen.

Classically, a history of *valley fever* during residence in an endemic area is obtainable, but often no clinical evidence is available as to the onset of the disease. With acute cavitation, hemoptysis is the most frequent symptom; with chronic infection, the presenting complaints are cough, weight loss, fever, and chest pain. Skin tests and complement fixation tests are almost always positive in active cases. The organisms can be recovered in the sputum and also by bronchial brushing.

The most effective specific therapy is amphotericin B, but many patients require no treatment at all. The drug should be reserved for acutely ill patients and those with cavitary disease and sputum cultures positive for *C. immitis.* Fluconazole is effective for certain forms of chronic coccidioidomycosis. Because coccidioidomycosis is particularly aggressive in patients with HIV infection, fluconazole may be required for life.[16]

Although the majority of undiagnosed solitary pulmonary nodules occurring in patients in the endemic area prove to be coccidioidomas, 26% to 35% are found to be malignant. Therefore, the indications for resection of solitary pulmonary nodules in this area may be difficult to define and must be individualized, as for histoplasmosis. For cavitary lesions, the indications are clearer. They include persisting cavities 2 cm. or greater in diameter; those that are enlarging, thick-walled, or ruptured; those associated with severe or recurrent hemoptysis; those occurring in diabetic or pregnant patients; and those coexisting with pulmonary tuberculosis. Drug coverage with amphotericin B is recommended by some, but it is not clear that the use of amphotericin B has resulted in significantly fewer complications of bronchopleural fistula, empyema, and recurrent cavitation.

North American Blastomycosis

North American blastomycosis is endemic not only in the central United States and Canada but also in parts of Central and South America, Africa, and Asia. It is caused by *Blastomyces dermatitidis,* a round, thick-walled, single-budding yeast first described by Gilchrist in 1894.[8] The disease often occurs in a cutaneous form, with chronic, indolent, usually enlarging papulopustules with thick adherent crusts and purple, raised edges. Biopsy in these areas may show microabscesses containing the organism. This form, with no evidence of systemic (including pulmonary) involvement, is the mildest. Pulmonary symptoms may be nonspecific. On the thoracic roentgenogram, cavitary, nodular, fibrotic, or disseminated lesions may be observed; the condition may mimic bronchogenic carcinoma. Occasionally, dissemination of blastomycosis occurs after operation on an undiagnosed blastomycotic lesion. Thus, a preoperative diagnosis is important to avoid an unnecessary operation. This may be aided by Papanicolaou smears of sputum and by serologic testing.[36] The standard therapy for blastomycosis is amphotericin B in a total dose of 0.5 to 0.6 mg. per kg. intravenously. Itraconazole is effective in curing patients with mild or moderately severe disease, and it is less toxic and can be taken orally.[21] Resectional operations are rarely needed except for diagnosis, especially when cancer is suspected.

Cryptococcosis

Cryptococcosis was once considered a rare and fatal disease, often accompanied by meningitis. Benign and subclinical bronchopulmonary infections are now recognized with increasing frequency, and even the dreaded meningeal form is controllable by drug therapy.

Cryptococcus neoformans is found in nature in soil, dust, and pigeon dung. The organisms are round, budding yeast cells with thick gelatinous capsules, which, until 1935, were confused with *Blastomyces.* Difficulty in classifying the organism has led to many confusing synonyms, such as *Torula histolytica.* Cryptococcosis is primarily an opportunistic infection. It is sometimes known as *malade signal,* because it often augurs significant underlying disease, such as cancer.[30] It is the most

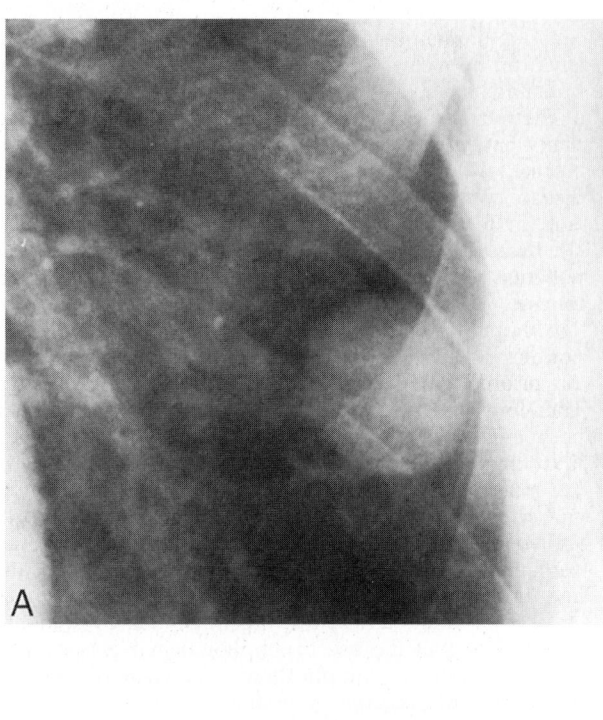
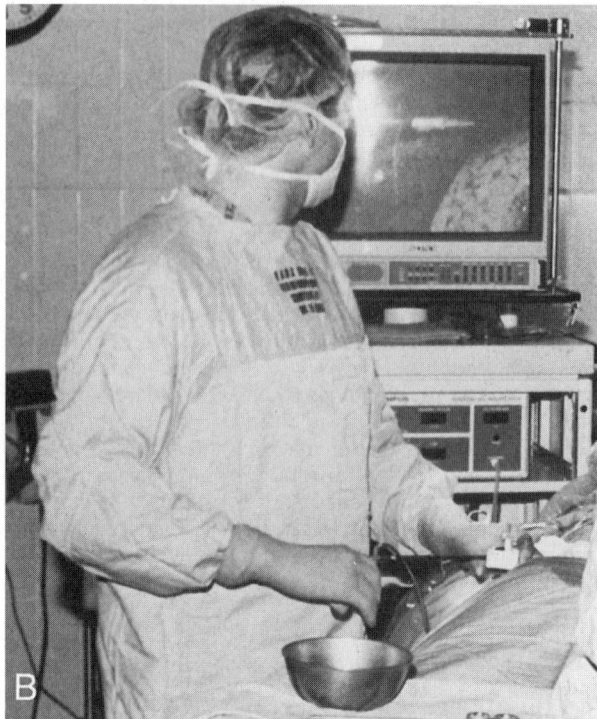
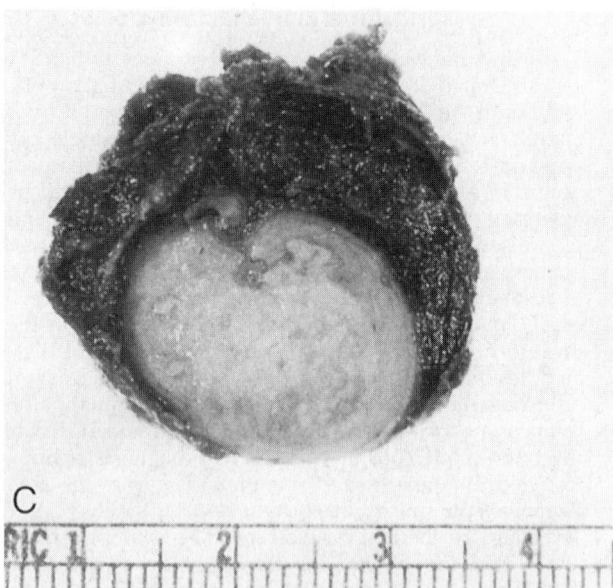
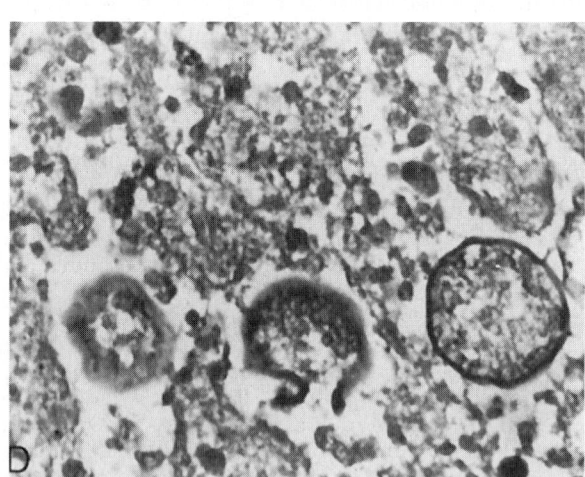

Figure 51–50. Coccidioidal granuloma. *A,* Thoracic radiograph showing a 2-cm. nodule in the left lower lobe of the lung of a 41-year-old man with a 75-pack-year smoking history. He had been stationed in the California desert while in the army. Bronchoscopy was negative. *B,* The nodule was resected thoracoscopically. Lung and instrument can be visualized on the television monitor. *C,* Resected specimen, which was a coccidioidal granuloma. *D,* Microscopic sections, ×400, showing spherules packed with endospores. (From Scott, S., and Takaro, T.: Thoracic mycotic and actinomycotic infections. *In* Shields, T. W. [Ed.]: General Thoracic Surgery, 4th ed. Baltimore, Williams & Wilkins, 1994.)

common fungus infection seen in renal transplant patients.[38] Colonization of otherwise healthy individuals, without tissue invasion, can also occur. The roentgenographic features are nonspecific and may even include pleural effusion.

If cryptococci are cultured from sputum and there is no demonstrable pulmonary lesion, or if they are isolated from lung tissue resected as an undiagnosed lesion but there are no symptoms or signs of active disease (the most common way the diagnosis is made), opinions differ regarding the need for antifungal therapy.[31] Active treatment may not be necessary if there is no evidence of central nervous system involvement and no organisms are found in spinal fluid.

However, now that effective agents are available (5-fluorocytosine, amphotericin B, and fluconazole), the proponents of treatment for proven disease have additional support.[31]

There is little controversy regarding the need for definitive treatment if the presence of active cryptococcosis can be shown by evidence of progression of a pulmonary lesion and continued sputum positivity, or by evidence of meningeal involvement.

Aspergillosis

Aspergillosis has become the third most common systemic fungal infection (after histoplasmosis and coccidioidomycosis) and, in recent years, the one with the most rapidly rising incidence.[12] It is usually caused by *Aspergillus fumigatus*, a filamentous organism with coarse, septate, fragmented hyphae. Of interest is the tendency for this organism to invade pre-existing pulmonary cavities and form a rounded necrotic mass of matted hyphae, fibrin, and inflammatory cells, called an *aspergilloma* or fungus ball. This mass usually lies free in the cavity and can change its location as the patient moves from an upright to a recumbent position. On the chest film, a crescentic radiolucency adjacent to a rounded mass within a cavitary lesion is almost pathognomonic of an aspergilloma (Fig. 51–51). Chronic cystic lesions of the upper lobes that remain as residua of pulmonary tuberculosis, sarcoidosis, lung cyst, or bronchiectasis commonly harbor such fungus balls; hemoptysis, occasionally severe, is the usual presenting symptom.

The medical management of aspergillosis is not always unsatisfactory. The primary drug is amphotericin B; itraconazole is recommended for long-term treatment. Surgical excision of an aspergilloma usually cures the symptom of hemoptysis and should be undertaken if the patient's condition permits and pre-existing disease has not produced generalized lung damage.[2, 7] However, there is no unanimity about the appropriateness of this treatment. If excisional surgery is contraindicated—as it often is because of pulmonary fibrosis and respiratory insufficiency—endocavitary or endobronchial treatment with sodium iodide or amphotericin B may be helpful. *Aspergillus* empyema is a serious complication requiring drainage and local instillations of amphotericin B or nystatin for effective management.[19] *Aspergillus* endocarditis occurs following cardiac surgery and on the valves of immunocompromised patients. Treatment includes surgical therapy; no patient has survived without valve replacement.[24, 39] *Aspergillus* pericarditis is a lethal infection.

Candidiasis and Fungal Endocarditis

The most common fungal infection is candidiasis.[33] It is usually caused by *Candida albicans*, an opportunistic organism first identified as a fungus by Bergin in 1841. *Candida* species normally inhabit the gastrointestinal tract and the female genital tract, but overgrowth occurs with prolonged use of antibiotics. Candidemia and systemic infection occur with glucocorticoid therapy and indwelling catheters and should be treated with amphotericin B, flucytosine, or fluconazole.[31] Candidiasis is of interest to cardiac surgeons because of the occurrence of *Candida* endocarditis in association with cardiac (usually valvular) lesions; over 100 such cases are already on record.[24] In a considerable number of patients, *Candida* endocarditis is diagnosed during or after prolonged and intensive antibiotic treatment for established subacute bacterial endocarditis. In another sizable group, fungal endocarditis (mainly caused by *Candida*, but in some cases caused by *Aspergillus*) has been reported following valve replacement. Heart operations offer a portal of entry through indwelling catheters, a damaged endocardial surface, and prolonged parenteral and antibiotic therapy, all of which favor the growth of this organism. The fungus is characterized by both budding yeast forms and mycelial elements (Fig. 51–52).

The clinical features of *Candida* endocarditis are almost indistinguishable from those of bacterial endocarditis, and suspicion and treatment of bacterial endocarditis may actually aggravate the fungal infection. The finding of sterile blood cultures when confronted with a clinical presentation of bacterial endocarditis should dictate a search for *Candida*; *Candida* species found on blood culture must be interpreted as an indication of a potentially lethal infection. Distinguishing features of *Candida* endocarditis are embolic episodes to major vessels, due to the unusually large size of the mycotic

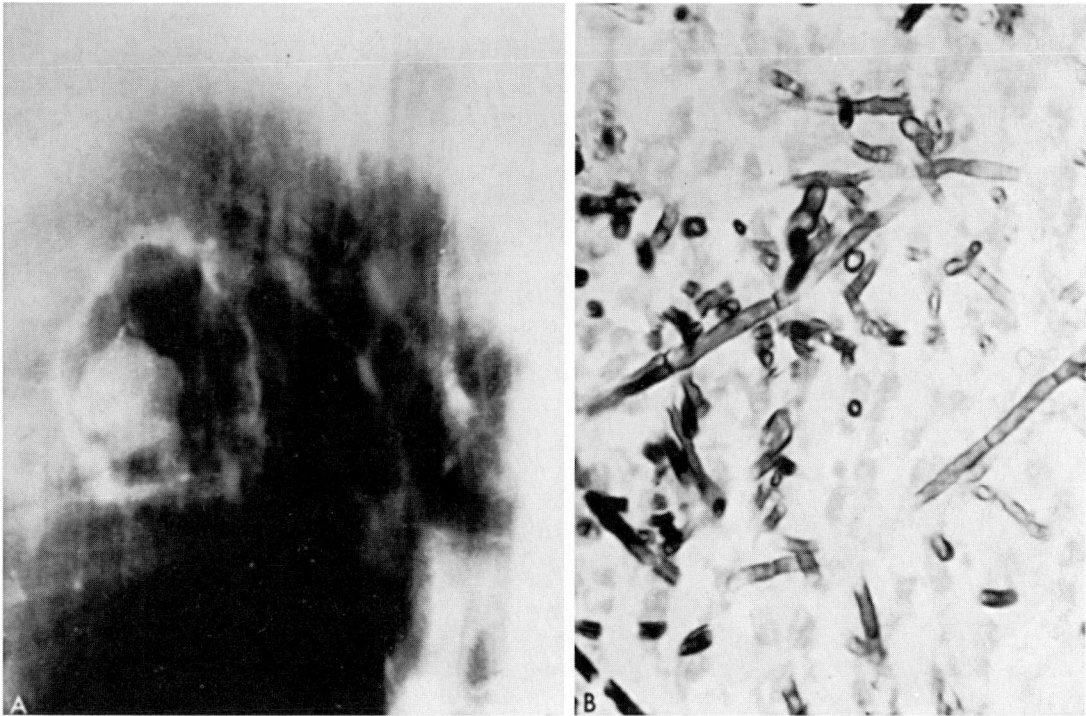

Figure 51–51. *A,* Laminagram showing typical aspergilloma ("fungus ball") lying free in a large cavitary lesion. This ball characteristically alters its location as the patient changes position. (From Aslam, P. A., Larkin, J., Eastridge, C. A., and Hughes, F. A., Jr.: Endocavitary infusion through percutaneous endobronchial catheter. Chest, *57*:94, 1970.) *B,* Coarse, fragmented, septate mycelia of *Aspergillus fumigatus.* (From Takaro, T.: Thoracic mycotic infections. *In* Lewis' Practice of Surgery. New York, Hoeber Medical Division, Harper & Row, 1968.)

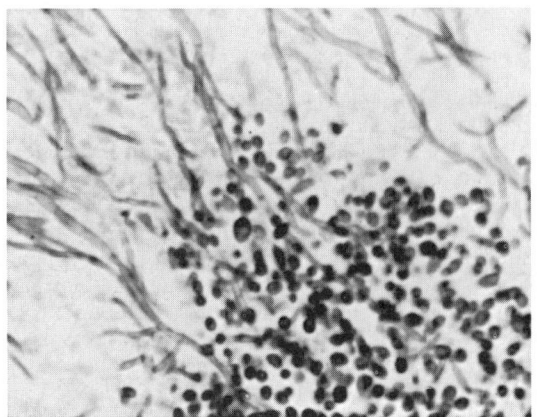

Figure 51–52. The organisms of *Candida albicans*, showing both mycelial and yeast forms. (From Takaro, T.: Thoracic mycotic infections. *In* Lewis' Practice of Surgery. New York, Hoeber Medical Division, Harper & Row, 1968.)

valvular vegetations. Despite potentially beneficial treatment with the combination of 5-fluorocytosine and amphotericin B, the medical cure rate is still very low, and the mortality is between 80% and 90%. Early surgical excision of vegetations or, when feasible, of an infected prosthetic valve, together with antifungal drug therapy, yields the best results (Fig. 51–53).[24] *Candida* lung abscess is uncommon and difficult to verify but has been diagnosed by needle aspiration biopsy and successfully treated with amphotericin B and flucytosine.[25]

Miscellaneous Fungal Infections

Sporotrichosis is caused by *Sporothrix schenckii*, and pulmonary involvement is rare; the condition is usually encountered in its cutaneous or lymphatic manifestations. Agricultural workers and florists are especially susceptible. Localized cavities and other forms of pulmonary disease have been reported in over 150 cases thus far.[30] Itraconazole is effective in lymphocutaneous sporotrichosis and some pulmonary forms.[21] However, surgical excision of localized disease appears to be the most reliable method of treating pulmonary sporotrichosis.[28]

Zygomycosis (mucormycosis) is another rare and serious infection by any of the members of the phylum of fungi known as Zygomycota.[30] The organisms are characterized by broad, nonseptate hyphae; characteristically, blood vessel invasion, thrombosis, and infarction of organs are seen. Extensive necrosis of face, lungs, or brain may occur. Debilitated persons and uncontrolled diabetics appear to be especially prone to this infection. Control of the underlying disease, amphotericin B administration, and surgical excision of necrotic or infected tissue may prove helpful.[34]

Pulmonary pseudallescheriasis, also known as monosporosis, is a rare mycotic infection caused by *Pseudallescheria boydii*.[30] This inhabitant of soil appears to act as a secondary invader of previously damaged lung tissue, such as a cavity, cyst, or saccule. Sometimes a fungus ball is formed. The organism is resistant to amphotericin B and 5-fluorocytosine. Ketoconazole and itraconazole have been effective in some instances, but pulmonary resection is indicated for cavitary lesions and sometimes to establish a diagnosis.

South American blastomycosis (paracoccidioidomycosis), a chronic granulomatous infection involving the skin, mucous membranes, lymph nodes, and visceral organs, is caused by *Paracoccidioides brasiliensis*, a soil saprophyte. Involvement of the lungs was once thought to be rare. It is now known that the infection occurs initially in the lungs and that, like histoplasmosis, subclinical and healed infections are common. It is endemic in South and Central America, and it has been recognized in the United States as well. The organisms resemble *Blastomyces dermatitidis* in tissues. Cavitary lesions occur in about 15% of patients with chronic pulmonary disease. Treatment with sulfonamides is suppressive but not curative. Amphotericin B, itraconazole, and ketoconazole are effective.[23] Surgical intervention is usually not required.

AIDS-ASSOCIATED PULMONARY INFECTIONS

AIDS is a complex disease caused by one or possibly several retroviruses that are collectively known as the human immunodeficiency virus (HIV). The major effect of HIV is to interfere with the function of T4 lymphocytes. The opportunistic infections that most often occur in AIDS patients are those caused by *Pneumocystis carinii*, cytomegalovirus, atypical mycobacteria, *Toxoplasma gondii*, *Candida*, herpes simplex virus, *Cryptococcus neoformans*, and *Cryptosporidium*. They involve the lung 80% of the time. *Pneumocystis*, the most common opportunistic infection, occurs in 80% of AIDS patients.[14]

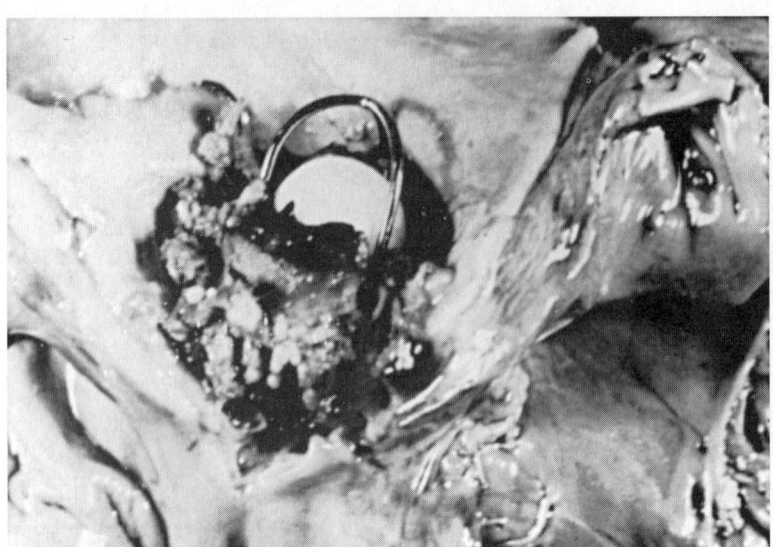

Figure 51–53. Fungal endocarditis caused by *Aspergillus* species, causing aortic prosthetic dehiscence due to perivalvular tissue necrosis. More commonly, *Candida albicans* is the etiologic agent in opportunistic fungal infections following cardiac surgery. (From Ostermiller, W. E., Jr., Dye, W. S., and Weinberg, M.: Fungal endocarditis following cardiovascular surgery. J. Thorac. Cardiovasc. Surg., *61*:670, 1971.)

Pneumocystis carinii Pneumonia

Pneumocystis carinii pneumonia is a diffuse interstitial pneumonitis that occurs as an opportunistic infection in marasmic or immunodeficient patients. It was first recognized in epidemic form in malnourished Central Europeans during World War II.

Until recently, most patients with *Pneumocystis* pneumonia were immunosuppressed by chemotherapy for malignancies or were congenitally immunodeficient infants and children. A resurgence of interest in the disease occurred in the early 1980s when a new syndrome of *Pneumocystis* pneumonia in immunosuppressed homosexuals, bisexuals, and more recently heterosexuals was recognized.[3, 10, 32, 38]

The disease is caused by *P. carinii,* a protozoan named for its discoverer, Carini, who described it in 1910. This organism occurs in thick- or thin-walled cystic forms, 5 to 12 μ. in diameter. It has a double-walled outer membrane, and within are three to eight intracystic bodies. The organism stains like a fungus with silver methenamine stains (Gomori's stain) but responds to antiprotozoan drugs. The pneumonitis almost invariably occurs in patients with impaired cellular immunity caused by intensive drug therapy, usually for malignancies, or after organ transplantation. However, patients with primary immunodeficiency states are also susceptible, and, as noted, it occurs in patients with AIDS.[3, 32]

In patients at risk, the combination of dyspnea, tachypnea, dry and nonproductive cough, fever, flaring of the nasal alae, intercostal retraction, and sometimes cyanosis, with minimal auscultatory signs, should raise suspicions. The roentgenographic findings of unilateral or bilateral diffuse infiltrates radiating from the hilus or even localized areas of pneumonitis or consolidation should lead one to suspect *Pneumocystis* pneumonia.

Since the diagnosis depends on the demonstration of the organisms in lung tissue by transbronchoscopic lung or brush biopsy, percutaneous needle biopsy, or transthoracoscopic or open lung biopsy, the thoracic surgeon is often called upon.[35] Neither needle biopsy nor open lung biopsy is entirely without risk in this disease. Therefore, bronchial brush biopsy, transbronchoscopic lung biopsy,[3] and bronchial lavage have been offered as less invasive and less risky techniques. Transthoracoscopic lung biopsy has also been advocated. However, open lung biopsy is still favored as the most certain method of making the diagnosis. In a series comparing transbronchial with open lung biopsy, 24 cases of a variety of pneumonias, including *Pneumocystis* pneumonia, were diagnosed by thoracotomy, compared with only 14 cases by transbronchoscopic lung biopsy. Moreover, bleeding, if it occurs, can be controlled under direct observation.

Clinical studies have shown two drug regimens to have therapeutic value: trimethoprim-sulfamethoxazole and pentamidine isethionate. Each is equally effective, but the former is preferred because of fewer side effects and less toxicity. Patients with AIDS require longer treatment and have higher relapse rates than do other adults with known causes of immunosuppression, but the outcome should be similar.[32]

Other opportunistic infections may coexist with *P. carinii* pneumonia or may be important differential diagnostic possibilities. They include cytomegalic inclusion virus infection, cryptococcosis, nocardiosis, and candidiasis. For some of these, the specific treatment is toxic; it is therefore important to make a definitive diagnosis so that appropriate drugs or combinations of drugs can be selected. One recommended strategy, however, is to treat all immunocompromised pediatric patients who develop pneumonitis with trimethoprim-sulfamethoxazole while routine diagnostic tests are being obtained and to reserve open lung biopsy for the diagnosis of those patients who do not respond to the drugs.[35] Un-

treated, *P. carinii* pneumonia is often fatal. In patients treated early and adequately, approximately 65% to 75% may survive.

Kaposi's Sarcoma of the Lung

Kaposi's sarcoma may be a viral-induced tumor.[4] It occurs in 47% of AIDS patients and is located in the lungs or airway in one third of afflicted patients. Kaposi's sarcoma appears as a painless purple or brown nodule. Biopsy of these lesions should be done with caution because of the risk of hemorrhage.

SELECTED REFERENCES

DeVita, V. T., Jr., Hellman, S., and Rosenberg, S. A. (Eds.): AIDS Etiology, Diagnosis, Treatment, and Prevention, 3rd ed. Philadelphia, J. B. Lippincott, 1992.
The third edition of this monograph on AIDS is thorough and up-to-date. The various chapters are written by authorities in the field. The text covers the basic virology, pathogenesis, epidemiology, clinical aspects, and prospects for future therapy.

Drutz, D. J., and Catanzaro, A.: Coccidioidomycosis. Parts I and II. Am. Rev. Respir. Dis., 117:559, 727, 1988.
A complete presentation of the ecology, immunology, and epidemiology of coccidioidomycosis, with an excellent section on clinical management and special emphasis on surgical aspects.

Goodwin, R. A., Loyd, J. E., and DesPrez, R. M.: Histoplasmosis in normal hosts. Medicine, 60:231, 1981.
A comprehensive treatise on the epidemiology, pathology, clinical characteristics, and management of acute and chronic forms of pulmonary histoplasmosis.

Rippon, J. W.: Medical Mycology, 3rd ed. Philadelphia, W. B. Saunders, 1988.
This outstanding reference provides in-depth descriptions of the pathogenic fungi and the actinomycetes.

Sarosi, G. A., and Davies, S. F.: Therapy for fungal infections. Mayo Clin. Proc., 69:1111, 1994.
This is the most current review of the principal antifungal agents available, their indications for use, and adverse effects.

Sarosi, G. A., and Davies, S. F. (Eds.): Fungal Diseases of the Lung, 2nd ed. Orlando, Grune & Stratton, 1990.
This volume is devoted to the diagnosis and management of pulmonary infections caused by fungi and actinomycetes. It provides a ready reference to the most recent experience with medical and surgical treatment of these diseases.

REFERENCES

1. Bartlett, J. G.: Anaerobic bacterial (aspiration pneumonitis and lung abscess). In Bone, R. C. (Ed.): Pulmonary and Critical Care Medicine. St. Louis, Mosby Year Book, 1993.
2. Battaglini, J. W., Murray, G. F., Keagy, B. A., Starek, P. J. K., and Wilcox, B. R.: Surgical management of symptomatic pulmonary aspergilloma. Ann. Thorac. Surg., 39:512, 1985.
3. Blumenfeld, W., Wagar, E., and Hadley, W. K.: Use of the transbronchial biopsy for diagnosis of opportunistic pulmonary infections in acquired immunodeficiency syndrome (AIDS). Am. J. Clin. Pathol., 81:1, 1984.
4. Chang, Y., Cesarman, E., Pessin, M. S., Lee, F., Culpepper, J., Knowles, D. M., and Moore, P. S.: Identification of herpesvirus-like DNA sequences in AIDS-associated Kaposi's sarcoma. Science, 266:1865, 1994.
5. Coker, R. J., Gignardi, H. P., et al.: Nocardia infection in AIDS: A clinical and microbiological challenge. J. Clin. Pathol., 45:821, 1992.
6. Conant, E. F., and Wechsler, R. J.: Actinomycosis and nocardiosis of the lung. J. Thorac. Imaging, 7:75, 1992.
7. Daly, R. C., Pairolero, P. C., Piehler, J. M., Trastek, V. F., Payne, W. S., and Bernatz, P. E.: Pulmonary aspergilloma. J. Thorac. Cardiovasc. Surg., 92:981, 1986.
8. Davies, S. F., and Sarosi, G.: Blastomycosis. In Sarosi, G., and Davies, S. F. (Eds.): Fungal Diseases of the Lung, 2nd ed. Orlando, Grune & Stratton, 1990.
9. Delarue, N. C., Pearson, F. G., Nelems, J. M., and Cooper, J. D.: Lung abscess: Surgical implications. Can. J. Surg., 23:297, 1980.
10. DeVita, V. T., Jr., Hellman, S., and Rosenberg, S. A. (Eds.): AIDS: Etiology, Diagnosis, Treatment, and Prevention, 2nd ed. Philadelphia, J. B. Lippincott, 1988.
11. Dobranowski, J., and Stringer, D. A.: Diagnosis of *Legionella* lung abscess by percutaneous needle aspiration. J. Can. Assoc. Radiol., 40:43, 1989.
12. Fraser, D. W., Ward, J. I., Ajello, L., et al.: Aspergillosis and other systemic mycoses: The growing problem. JAMA, 242:1631, 1979.
13. Fromtling, R. A., and Shadomy, H. J.: An overview of macrophage-fungal interactions. Mycopathologia, 93:77, 1986.

14. Gold, J. W. M.: Overview of infection with the human immunodeficiency virus: Infectious complications. Clin. Chest Med., 9:377, 1988.
15. Goodwin, R. A., Loyd, J. E., and DesPrez, R. M.: Histoplasmosis in normal hosts. Medicine, 60:231, 1981.
16. Graybill, J. R.: Treatment of coccidioidomycosis. Ann. N. Y. Acad. Sci., 544:481, 1988.
17. Jensen, B. M., Kruse-Anderson, S., and Andersen, K.: Thoracic actinomycosis. Scand. J. Thorac. Cardiovasc. Surg., 23:181, 1989.
18. Mandell, W., Goldberg, D. M., and Neu, H. C.: Histoplasmosis in patients with the acquired immune deficiency syndrome. Am. J. Med., 81:974, 1986.
19. Massard, G., Roeslin, N., Wihlm, J. M., Dumont, P., Witz, J. P., and Morand, G.: Pleuropulmonary aspergilloma: Clinical spectrum and results of surgical treatment. Ann. Thorac. Surg., 54:1159, 1992.
20. Mathisen, D. J., and Grillo, H. C.: Clinical manifestation of mediastinal fibrosis and histoplasmosis. Ann. Thorac. Surg., 54:1053, 1992.
21. Medical letter: Systemic antifungal drugs. Med. Lett., 36:16, 1994.
22. Medical letter: The choice of antibacterial drugs. Med. Lett., 36:53, 1994.
23. Negroni, R.: Azole derivatives in the treatment of paracoccidioidomycosis. Ann. N. Y. Acad. Sci., 544:497, 1988.
24. Norenberg, R. D., Sethi, G. K., Scott, S. M., and Takaro, T.: Opportunistic endocarditis following open-heart surgery. Ann. Thorac. Surg., 19:592, 1975.
25. O'Driscoll, B. R. C., Cooke, R. D. P., Mamtora, H., Irving, M. H., and Bernstein, A.: Candida lung abscesses complicating parenteral nutrition. Thorax, 43:418, 1988.
26. Pappagianis, D.: Epidemiology of coccidioidomycosis. Curr. Top. Med. Mycol., 2:199, 1988.
27. Pennza, P. T.: Aspiration pneumonia, necrotizing pneumonia, and lung abscess. Emerg. Med. Clin. North Am., 7:279, 1989.
28. Pluss, J. L., and Opal, S. M.: Pulmonary sporotrichosis: Review of treatment and outcome. Medicine, 65:143, 1986.
29. Rienhoff, H. Y., Jr. (Ed.): Clinical conferences at the Johns Hopkins Hospital. Johns Hopkins Med. J., 150:141, 1988.
30. Rippon, J. W.: Medical Mycology. Philadelphia, W. B. Saunders, 1988.
31. Sarosi, G. A., and Davies, S. F.: Therapy for fungal infections. Mayo Clin. Proc., 69:1111, 1994.
32. Smith, G. H.: Treatment of infections in the patient with acquired immunodeficiency syndrome. Arch. Intern. Med., 154:949, 1994.
33. Sobel, J. D.: Candida infections in the intensive care unit. Crit. Care Clin., 4:325, 1988.
34. Tedder, M., Spratt, J. A., Anstadt, M. P., Hegde, S. S., Tedder, S. D., and Lowe, J. E.: Pulmonary mucormycosis: Results of medical and surgical therapy. Ann. Thorac. Surg., 57:1044, 1994.
35. Trachiotix, G. D., Hafner, G. H., Hix, W. R., and Aaron, B. L.: Role of open lung biopsy in diagnosing pulmonary complications of AIDS. Ann. Thorac. Surg., 54:898, 1992.
36. Turner, S., and Kaufman, L.: Immunodiagnosis of blastomycosis. Semin. Respir. Infect., 1:22, 1986.
37. Williford, M. E., and Godwin, J. D.: Computed tomography of lung abscess and empyema. Radiol. Clin. North Am., 21:575, 1983.
38. Wilson, W. R., Cockerill, F. R., III, and Rosenow, E. C., III.: Pulmonary disease in the immunocompromised host. Mayo Clin. Proc., 60:610, 1985.
39. Woods, G. L., Wood, R. P., and Shaw, B. W.: Aspergillus endocarditis in patients without prior cardiovascular surgery: Report of a case in a liver transplant recipient and review. Rev. Infect. Dis., 2:263, 1989.

VIIA

THE PLEURA AND EMPYEMA

Stewart M. Scott, M.D., and Timothy Takaro, M.D.

THE PLEURA

The pleura is the serous membrane lining of two complete and independent pleural sacs or potential cavities. Each extends into the neck, the retrosternal area, and the costophrenic sinuses, and also into the interlobar fissures. Familiarity with these ramifications of the pleural cavity can be extremely important, since unwitting violation of the pleural space, with its special anatomic and physiologic attributes, can be followed by serious consequences. Thus, the earliest surgical experiences with wounds penetrating into the pleural cavities, or with deliberate attempts to open into them, often resulted in disaster or near-disaster from collapse of the lung, shift of the mediastinum, tension, pneumothorax, and, later, infection.

A major surgical achievement occurred when the potential space between the two layers of the pleural cavity, measuring 10 to 27μ., could at last be crossed safely. This was accomplished by Sauerbruch (1904), who placed his patient in a negative pressure chamber, leaving only the head and neck outside and exposed to atmospheric pressure, to achieve expansion of the lungs in the open chest. The entire surgical team had to operate within this chamber. This cumbersome method became obsolete when Melzer and Auer introduced positive-pressure insufflation of the lungs. The Empyema Commission's findings during World War I marked another milestone, when it became understood that opening the pleural cavity to atmospheric pressure to drain an empyema could be catastrophic if adhesions had not formed that limited the extent of the infection. In the years that followed World War I, intrathoracic surgical procedures gradually evolved. After World War II, this evolution progressed at a vastly accelerated pace. These surgical developments added greatly to the knowledge of pleuropulmonary physiology and pathology.[5, 9]

Anatomic Features. The pleural surface consists of a uniform layer of flattened mesothelial cells beneath which are layers of areolar connective tissue containing an abundance of blood vessels, nerves, and lymphatics. The visceral pleura is thinner, remarkably elastic, and intimately attached to the underlying lung by intrapulmonary fibrous prolongations of the deeper layer of connective tissue. The parietal pleura, however, is thicker and easily separable from the thoracic wall because of the loose layer of areolar tissue separating it from the endothoracic fascia. It is supplied by the intercostal arteries. The visceral pleura is supplied largely by the bronchial arteries. Sensory nerve endings are present in the costal and diaphragmatic parietal pleura. Sensory fibers are absent in the visceral pleura.[22]

Physiologic Characteristics. The two outstanding and interrelated features of the pleural cavities are the subatmospheric pressures in the normally nonexistent pleural space and the serous secreting and absorbing surface of the pleural membranes. The elastic recoil of the lungs produces intrapleural negative pressures of -6 to -12 cm. H_2O during inspiration, and -4 to -8 cm. H_2O during expiration. Extremes of $+40$ cm. H_2O during the Valsalva maneuver, or -40 cm. H_2O during inspiratory effort against a closed glottis, are also seen.

The secreting and absorbing properties of the pleura are substantial. Using special techniques, a rate of formation of 600 to 1000 ml. of fluid per day has been observed in patients, and an equal volume has been noted to be reabsorbed. Increased capillary hydrostatic pressure, or a greater negative intrapleural pressure, tends to increase transudation into the pleural cavities. Loss of intrapleural negative pressure diminishes transudation, whereas increased diaphragmatic and intercostal activity increases its absorption. Resorption is made possible by numerous microvilli present on the mesothelial cells lining the pleura, particularly the visceral pleura. Scanning electron microscopy has demonstrated microvilli and pores in the parietal pleura that communicate with the lymphatics, through which proteins, cells, and particulate matter pass (Fig. 51–54).[40] Particulate matter, such as red blood cells, can be absorbed directly by the normal pleura.[28] All these properties may be greatly altered by disease.

Pleural Effusions

Although pleural effusions are almost invariably secondary to some primary condition, they are often its first indication and therefore are always significant. Bloody effusions are ominous, for they may signify primary or secondary pleural tumor. Therefore, one should persist in attempts to make a precise diagnosis. The classic signs of fluid—flatness, absent tactile and vocal fremitus, diminished breath sounds, and mediastinal displacement—depend on the size of the fluid collection and on the care with which the signs are sought.

A pleural effusion of up to 500 ml. may not be apparent clinically or roentgenographically in an adult in the upright position, since it ordinarily gravitates into the costophrenic sinuses and is obscured by the diaphragm. Thus, when a *small* effusion is noted on a thoracic roentgenogram, usually considerable fluid is already present and can be removed by a carefully performed thoracentesis (Fig. 51–55). Fluid can collect almost anywhere from the apex to the base of the pleural cavity in one or more loculated pockets, either in contact with the parietal pleura or in an interlobar fissure. Often bizarre roentgenographic features result. Needle aspiration is sometimes necessary to establish the presence of an effusion and to differentiate it from other thoracic conditions.

Major causes of effusions and their differentiation are outlined in Table 51–16. Infection, tumor, and congestive failure account for 75% of effusions in most patient populations. Less common causes such as pharmacologic agents should be kept in mind. The differential diagnosis often depends on obtaining samples of the fluid, the parietal pleura, or the lung and subjecting these to appropriate examinations. This does not always resolve the problem, however.

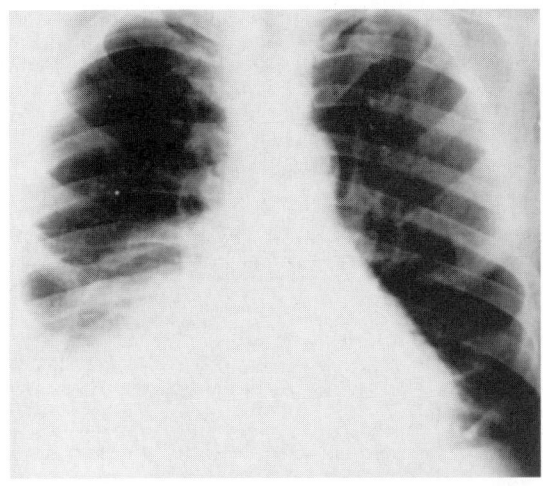

Figure 51–55. Pleural effusion, right base. After this thoracic roentgenogram was taken, 1300 ml. of straw-colored fluid was aspirated at thoracentesis. Surprisingly, large volumes of fluid may not be apparent clinically or roentgenographically when they gravitate into the costophrenic sinuses and are partially obscured by the diaphragm. A roentgenogram obtained in the lateral decubitus position may be more revealing.

Sometimes a diagnosis can be made either from the pleural fluid alone or from cultures and smears for pathogenic organisms or cell blocks for tumor cells. If the pleural fluid is a transudate—that is, one low in protein and lactic acid dehydrogenase—the effusion is probably caused by an underlying systemic disease such as congestive heart failure, cirrhosis, or renal insufficiency. An exudative effusion is more likely to be associated with diseased pleura, which results in increased permeability of the pleura to proteins and decreased lymphatic clearance, as seen in parapneumonic processes and malignancies. Pleural fluid analysis can be helpful even when not diagnostically specific. Normal pleural fluid glucose of less than 60 mg. per 100 ml. is seen only in tuberculosis, malignancy, rheumatoid disease, or parapneumonic effusion. A pleural fluid amylase greater than that which is normal for serum is present only in pancreatitis, malignancy, and esophageal rupture. Cytologic examination of pleural fluid is positive in 50% of patients with malignant disease. Chromosomal analysis of the malignant cells is particularly helpful in diagnosing pleural leukemia, lymphoma, and mesothelioma.[33]

Other studies of pleural fluid that may prove helpful include a white blood cell count and differential to help distinguish between a transudate and an exudate and to identify the presence of empyema. IgE should be determined for suspected paragonimiasis; carcinoembryonic antigen for suspected adenocarcinoma; lactic acid dehydrogenase as an indicator of the severity of pleural inflammation; complement, rheumatoid factor, and LE cells for suspected systemic lupus erythematosus and rheumatoid arthritis; lipid analysis for a diagnosis of chylothorax; and countercurrent immunoelectrophoresis for a diagnosis of *Streptococcus pneumoniae*, *Staphylococcus aureus*, or *Haemophilus influenzae* in children.[22]

Often a specific diagnosis cannot be made from pleural fluid alone, despite cultures and smears for pathogenic organisms and cell blocks for tumor cells. Biopsy by needle or trephine yields a specific diagnosis in fewer than half the cases in which it is attempted (Fig. 51–56). To obtain a definitive diagnosis, a small thoracotomy may be necessary to allow the surgeon to inspect both the visceral and the parietal pleura, as well as the lung, and to select the most promising areas for biopsy. Video-assisted thoracoscopy also provides excellent visualization of the thoracic cavity and its contents and is preferred by many surgeons for biopsy.[8] Decortication

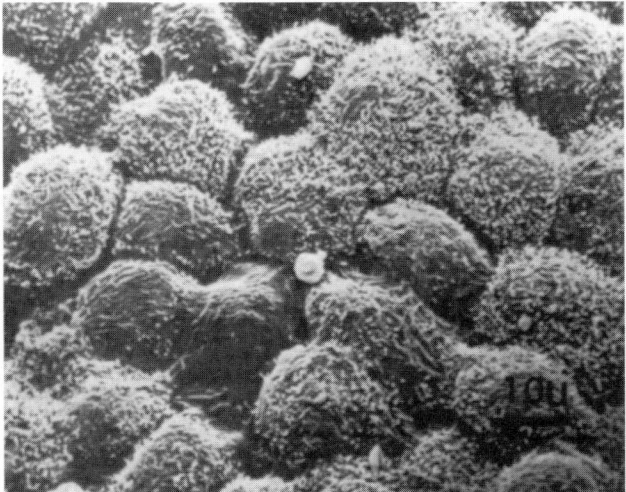

Figure 51–54. Many microvilli are present on the surface of cells forming the parietal pleura. Scanning electron microscopy. Original magnification ×1300. (From Wang, N. S.: The regional difference of pleural mesothelial cells in rabbits. Am. Rev. Respir. Dis., *110*:623, 1974.)

TABLE 51-16. Differential Characteristics of Pleural Effusions

	Congestive Failure	Malignancy	Pneumonia and Other Nontuberculous Infections	Tuberculosis	Fungal Infection, Actinomycosis, Nocardiosis	Rheumatoid Arthritis and Collagen Disease	Pulmonary Embolism	Trauma	Chylothorax	Esophageal Rupture
Clinical	Signs and symptoms of congestive failure	Older patient, poor health prior to effusion	Signs and symptoms of respiratory tract infection	Younger patient, exposure to tuberculosis, good health prior	Exposure in endemic area	History of joint involvement may or may not be present, subcutaneous nodules	Postoperative patient, immobilized patient, venous disease	History of trauma	History of trauma, known malignancy	History of instrumentation or of vomiting
Gross appearance	Serous	Often sanguineous	Serous	Usually serous, may be sanguineous	Serous or purulent	Turbid or yellow-green	Often sanguineous	Sanguineous	Chylous or milky	Serous, may contain food particles
Microscopic examination	0	Cytology positive in 50%	May or may not be positive for bacilli	Positive for acid-fast bacilli in 30 to 70% of cases, cholesterol crystals	May or may not be positive for fungi	0	0	0	Fat droplets	Squamous epithelial cells
Cell Count	10% 10,000 erythrocytes; 10% over 1000 leukocytes	65% bloody, over 40% over 1000 leukocytes, mainly leukolymphocytes	Polymorpho-nuclears predominate	Leukocytes mainly lymphocytes; eosinophils more than 10% excludes tuberculosis	Polymorpho-nuclear leukocytes or lymphocytes	Lymphocytes predominate	Erythrocytes predominate	Erythrocytes	0	Red blood cells and white blood cells
Culture	0	0	May or may not be positive	Less than 25% are positive	May or may not be positive	0	0	0	0	0
Specific gravity	90% under 1.016 (unless pulmonary embolism)	75% over 1.016	Over 1.016	75% over 1.016	Over 1.016	Over 1.016	Over 1.016	Over 1.016	Over 1.016	Over 1.016
Protein	75% less than 3 gm.	90% 3 gm. or more	3.0 gm. or more	Usually 5.0 gm. or more	3.0 gm. or more	3.0 gm. or more	3.0 gm. or more	3.0 gm. or more	Less than half plasma	3.0 gm. or more
Glucose	0	15% have 60 mg. per 100 ml. or less	Occasionally less than 60 mg. per 100 ml. or less	Less than 50% have 60 mg. per 100 ml. or less	0	78% below 30 mg. per 100 ml. (rheumatoid)	0	0	0	0
pH	Greater than 7.20	May be 7.20 or less	May be less than 7.20	May be less than 7.20	Greater than 7.20	May be 7.20 or less	Greater than 7.20	Greater than 7.20	Greater than 7.20	Usually less than 7.20; may be less than 6.00
Amylase	0	10% are elevated	0	0	0	0	0	0	0	Elevated
Lactic acid dehydro-genase	Not elevated	May be elevated	May be elevated	May be elevated	May be elevated	May be elevated	May be elevated	0	0	0
Other	Right-sided in 55 to 70%	If hemorrhagic fluid, 65% will be due to tumor, tends to continue to form after removed; hyaluronic acid >1 mg./ml. in mesothelioma	Associated with infiltrate on roentgenogram	Less than 5% mesothelial cells; will be the cause in 75% of men under 25 yr., 50% of men over 25 yr. Adenosine deaminase 70 I.U./L.	Skin and serologic tests may be helpful	Rapid clotting time; lupus erythematosus cell or rheumatoid factor titer >640	Source of emboli may or may not be helpful	0	Fat content higher than plasma	0

Modified from Bessone, L. N., Ferguson, T. B., and Burford, T. H.: Chylothorax. Ann. Thorac. Surg., 12:527, 1971; Light, R. W.: Pleural Diseases. Philadelphia, Lea & Febiger, 1983; and Kinosewitz, G. T.: Pleuritis and pleural effusions. In Bone, R. C. (Ed.): Pulmonary and Critical Care Medicine, St. Louis, Mosby-Year Book, 1993.

of the lung, if indicated, can be accomplished after enlarging the incision.

Pleural effusions may occur from subdiaphragmatic or intra-abdominal processes, such as subphrenic or hepatic abscesses, cirrhosis of the liver, nephritis, pancreatitis, or ovarian fibroma. The combination of pleural effusion and ovarian fibroma is called Meigs' syndrome. Whether passage of fluid from the peritoneal to the pleural cavities occurs through the lymphatics or through recognized or unrecognized openings in the diaphragm is a matter of debate.

Thoracentesis is best done after careful localization of the effusion by roentgenograms in frontal, lateral, or oblique planes, or by the use of the fluoroscopic image intensifier. A syringe no larger than 20 ml., with a three-way stopcock interposed between needle and syringe, affords the most satisfactory control. After thorough infiltration of skin, intercostal muscle, and parietal pleura with a local anesthetic agent, the needle of appropriate caliber and length is directed just above the superior border of the lower rib of the appropriate interspace. It is allowed to penetrate the parietal pleura until fluid is reached, with constant moderate negative pressure applied to the syringe. During aspiration low in the costophrenic sinus, the needle tip should be directed cephalad to avoid puncture of the diaphragm. One may place a clamp on the needle at the level of the skin to prevent further penetration and thus avoid injuring the lung after the appropriate depth has been reached. The removal of all available fluid usually presents no difficulty unless a massive acute effusion is being completely evacuated. Under these circumstances, pain, discomfort, and severe coughing may be initiated. Rarely, transient unilateral pulmonary edema occurs. Thus, it is wise to evacuate no more than 1500 ml. of a massive effusion at the initial attempt.

"Spontaneous" Pneumothorax

The accumulation of air in the pleural cavity without any apparent antecedent event, so-called spontaneous pneumo-

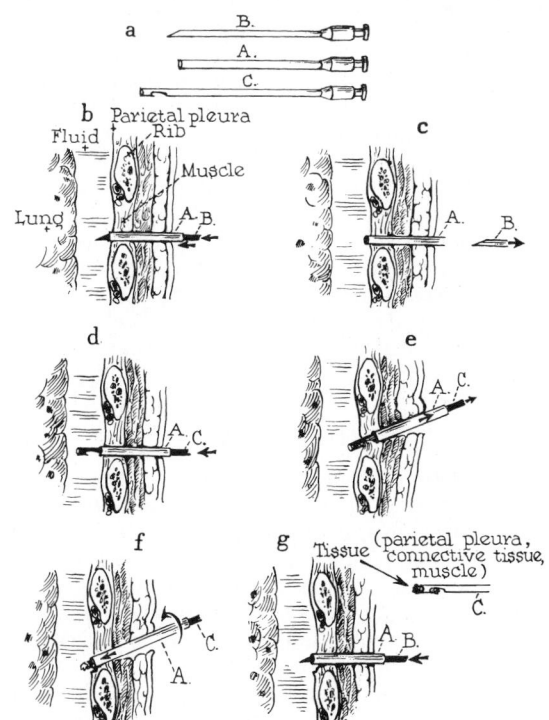

Figure 51–56. Diagrams illustrating methods of obtaining a pleural biopsy using the Cope needle. (From Levine, H., and Cugell, D. W.: Blunt-end needle biopsy of pleura and rib. Arch. Intern. Med., *109*:516, 1962. Copyright 1962, American Medical Association.)

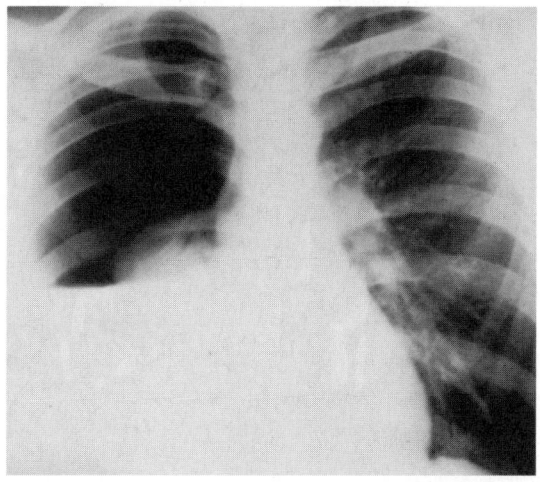

Figure 51–57. Thoracic roentgenogram illustrating spontaneous hemopneumothorax in a 22-year-old man. This was treated by closed-tube thoracostomy, and it responded with prompt and complete re-expansion of the lung. The etiology was undetermined.

thorax, is almost always caused by rupture of a subpleural cyst, bleb, or bulla, often in an otherwise apparently normal lung in a young adult (20 to 40 years of age), usually a male cigarette smoker (Fig. 51–57). Pneumothorax in the presence of normal lung tissue is often referred to as primary spontaneous pneumothorax (PSP), whereas pneumothorax occurring in patients with underlying lung disease such as bullous emphysema is called secondary spontaneous pneumothorax (SSP). Pneumothorax can occur in neonates, in whom it may result from vigorous resuscitation efforts, or in elderly and emphysematous patients, in whom it may pose a serious problem. Occasionally, primary or metastatic tumor is found in association with pneumothorax. Hemorrhage (hemopneumothorax) can accompany collapse of the lung due to a torn vascular adhesion and may be severe enough to warrant emergency thoracotomy for control.

Symptoms depend on the degree of collapse of the lung and on its previous condition. There may be no symptoms whatsoever, or there may be severe dyspnea, hypoxemia, and even shock. Chest pain may be prominent or absent. Hyperresonance and absent or diminished breath sounds are the characteristic physical findings.

The diagnosis is usually apparent from the chest roentgenogram. A film taken in expiration can help demonstrate a small pneumothorax more readily; appropriate laminagrams of the lung aid in the differentiation of localized pneumothorax from a large, thin-walled pulmonary cyst or pneumatocele.

Treatment depends on a variety of factors. An initial, small (5% to 20%) asymptomatic pneumothorax can be observed. Reabsorption of the pneumothorax is facilitated by the administration of supplemental oxygen, which, by lowering the P_{N_2} of capillary blood, increases the partial pressure difference between the pleural space and the pulmonary capillary. Intercostal tube thoracostomy with a closed drainage system is adequate for most patients with large pneumothoraces (Fig. 51–58). Prevention of recurrences is thought to be enhanced by keeping the tube in place for several days to foster a sterile pleuritis. Gentle suction on the catheter facilitates expansion of the lung. If air leakage persists or is larger than can be managed by a high-volume vacuum system, if the episode is a recurrent one, or if obvious bullae or cysts are seen in the collapsed lung, open thoracotomy is advocated, with suturing, ligation, or excision of the ruptured bleb or bulla and vigorous abrasion of especially the parietal, but

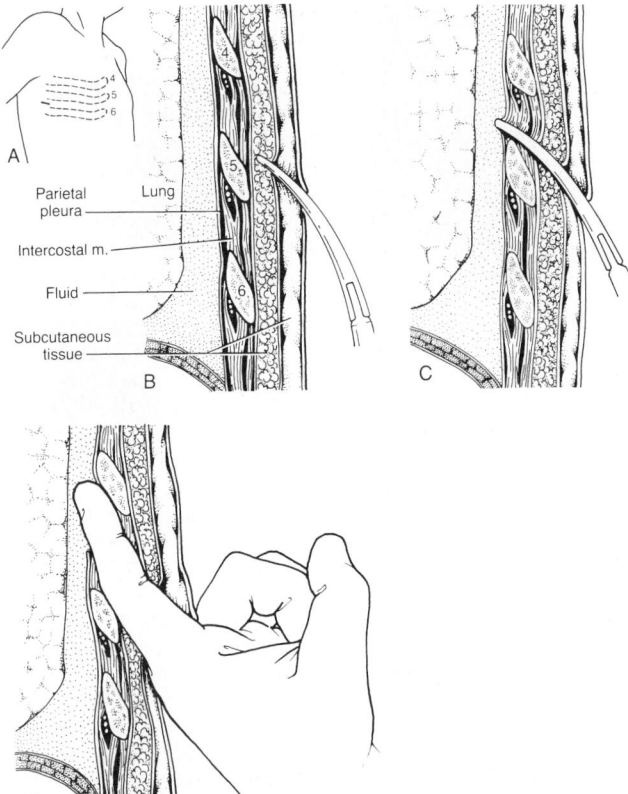

Figure 51–58. Insertion of a chest tube. *A*, Incision over intercostal space. *B*, Development of subcutaneous tract. *C*, Penetration of parietal pleura. *D*, Confirmation that lung is not adherent to the chest wall at the puncture site. (From Symbas, P. N.: Cardiothoracic Trauma. Philadelphia, W. B. Saunders, 1989.)

also the visceral, pleura. This produces filmy adhesions and helps prevent recurrences. Excision of the parietal pleura, which is advocated by some surgeons, is more traumatic and is associated with a higher complication rate.[10]

Video-assisted thoracic surgery (VATS) offers an alternative to open thoracotomy for the treatment of both primary and secondary spontaneous pneumothorax. VATS results in less perioperative pain and less postoperative respiratory dysfunction than thoracotomy. A slightly reduced hospital stay for VATS patients offsets the somewhat greater cost of the surgical procedure. The operative procedure includes ligation, suturing, stapling, and laser ablation of bullae. Pleurodesis is accomplished by pleurectomy or chemically with talc or quinacrine. Parietal pleurectomy is recommended, particularly for patients with secondary spontaneous pneumothorax. Failure occurs if air leak is not controlled and the lung does not expand against the chest wall.[4, 16, 18, 19]

Tension pneumothorax occurs when intrapleural pressure rises precipitously. This is due to a valvelike mechanism that allows air to enter the pleural spaces from the lung parenchyma or airway during brief episodes of markedly elevated airway pressure, as occurs during cough. Because of collapse of the lung and shift of the mediastinum, severe respiratory distress may develop, requiring emergency needle aspiration followed by tube thoracostomy drainage. Physical findings of hyper-resonance, absent breath sounds, and mediastinal shift away from the involved side are diagnostic.

Spontaneous pneumothorax—and especially tension pneumothorax—in an emphysematous patient with marginal respiratory function and cor pulmonale presents a grave man-

agement problem. Monitoring of blood gases and electrocardiogram, assisted ventilation, tracheostomy, appropriate cardiac drugs, multiple closed thoracotomies, and open thoracotomy may all be necessary. The prognosis in the average patient with pneumothorax, however, is very good, with few recurrences if a sterile pleuritis is produced by closed-tube thoracostomy.

Pneumothorax may occur in patients requiring mechanical ventilatory support (e.g., patients who have had cardiac surgery). This is more likely to occur in patients with emphysema or cystic or cavitary disease of the lung. High airway pressures and positive end-expiratory pressure (PEEP) should be used with caution in these patients.[14]

Rarely, as with pleural effusions, rapid re-expansion of a complete pneumothorax using high negative pressure may be followed by ipsilateral pulmonary edema. A slower decompression, using lower negative pressure, prevents this complication.

Closed pleural drainage systems range from the simple to the complex, depending on the particular clinical problem. Of primary importance is an understanding of the characteristics of the system by both the responsible physician and the attending nursing staff. When little or no continuing air escape is expected and only fluid drainage is required, a simple underwater seal apparatus, or only a rubber flutter valve with a plastic bag arrangement, is adequate.[12] In the past, a two-bottle system, with the first bottle being a dry trap, provided a separate reservoir for collection of fluid in addition to the underwater seal, but this added to the volume of dead space between the pleural space and the water-seal surface. In small patients this may be significant. When air leaks are expected, more complicated systems with active suction are recommended. The large glass bottles with rubber stoppers and glass tubes have been replaced by compact plastic drainage sets that require less space and are less likely to be damaged (Fig. 51–59). These sets may be used as simple underwater seals, or they may be attached to a vacuum source. They are made with three plastic compartments: a collecting chamber, a water seal, and a vacuum regulator with a long tube open to air and extending under water the specific distance that corresponds to the maximal negative suction in centimeters of water required (20 to 40 cm. H_2O).

Pumps with a low air-flow capacity should not be used when large air leaks, either continuous or intermittent (as during coughing), are expected. The drainage system should function to prevent ingress of air into the pleural cavity, even when the vacuum source fails. It is equally important that the system allow egress of large volumes of air suddenly, whether the vacuum source is functioning or not. Time spent in understanding the physiologic and physical principles of pleural drainage systems and in communicating this understanding to attending nurses is well spent.[38]

Hemothorax

An accumulation of blood in the pleural cavities (hemothorax) may result from trauma to the chest wall, the lung, the mediastinal structures, or the diaphragm. It is also seen in pulmonary infarction, pleural or pulmonary neoplasm, or following tearing of a pleural adhesion, as with spontaneous pneumothorax. It may occur as a complication of anticoagulant therapy. Hemothorax following thoracic surgery is also common. Partial defibrination of the blood occurs with deposition of fibrin on the pleural surface. A sterile hemothorax may be completely reabsorbed, but an infected hemothorax or hemothoracic empyema can lead to the development of a fibrothorax, with serious compromise of pulmonary function. This is more likely after war wounds and gunshot wounds with underlying lung damage; it is less likely after clean stab

Underwater Seal Drainage System

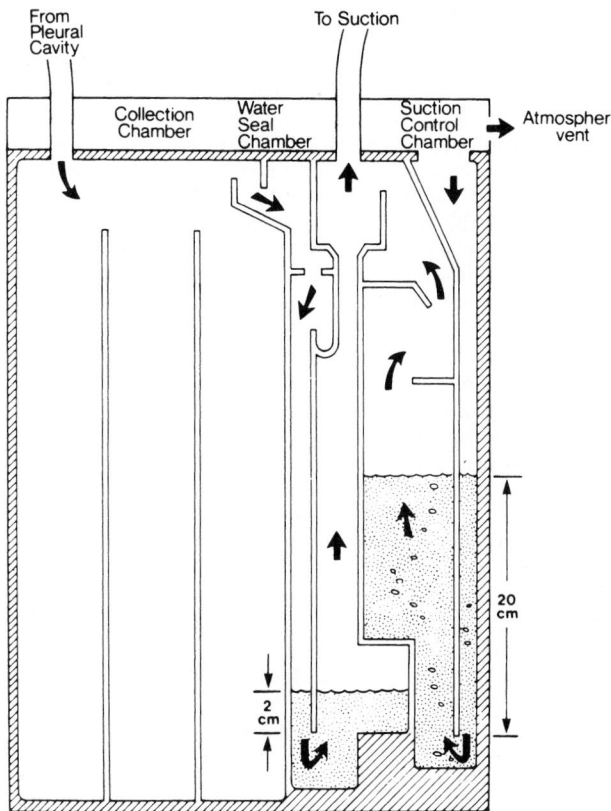

Figure 51–59. A commercial apparatus for chest drainage. (From Symbas, P. N.: Cardiothoracic Trauma. Philadelphia, W. B. Saunders, 1989.)

wounds. A hemopneumothorax is more likely to be followed by such a complication than is a hemothorax alone.

The management of hemothorax depends on the rate of bleeding and the total volume bled, as well as the underlying cause. If the hemothorax is small and bleeding has ceased, as determined by clinical signs and serial roentgenograms, only observation is required. For moderate amounts of estimated blood accumulation (500 ml. or more), a closed thoracostomy with intercostal tube drainage for complete evacuation of blood allows observation of its reaccumulation plus re-expansion of the lung and is preferable to needle aspiration. Continuing active bleeding (200 ml. per hour or more), as determined by serial thoracic roentgenograms, clinical signs, or output from chest tubes, demands open thoracotomy for control of hemorrhage. Massive bleeding, such as from an intrathoracic vascular injury, may require rigorous blood volume replacement. Because blood in the pleural space tends to be defibrinated and slow to clot, it can be collected in a sterile drainage system and reinfused into the patient.[17] Postoperative bleeding may cease upon re-exploration and removal of blood clots, even if no active bleeding point is found.

To prevent the development of an imprisoning fibrothorax and to gain re-expansion of a lung compressed by blood, early evacuation of clotted hemothorax and decortication are recommended.[26] Within 3 weeks of an injury, the fibrinous deposit peels off the visceral pleura readily, and pulmonary expansion can be restored. This can be accomplished by VATS or open thoracotomy.[3] One should not resort to thoracotomy precipitously, however, since most uncomplicated hemothoraces are completely absorbed.

Chylothorax

Chylothorax, or chyle in the pleural cavity, is most commonly caused by trauma or tumor. The thin, fibromuscular thoracic duct, which transports chyle along the length of the mediastinum from the cisterna chyli to the left subclavian vein, may be ruptured anywhere along its course. Rupture above the fifth or sixth thoracic vertebra generally results in left-sided collection. Because of excellent collateral pathways, the duct can be ligated with impunity.

Owing to the high fat and protein content of the milky white chyle (which aids in diagnosis), loss of this material into the pleural cavity can be serious from a nutritional standpoint. The large volume of the effusion can also cause severe respiratory embarrassment. Lymphangiography confirms the diagnosis and can locate the thoracic duct (although not the site of the rupture).

Chylothorax is readily distinguished from chyliform pleural effusion or pseudochylothorax by examining the milky pleural fluid for cholesterol crystals, which are absent in chylothorax. Pseudochylothorax occurs in long-standing pleural effusions and is usually caused by rheumatoid pleuritis or tuberculosis.[22]

Gunshot wounds, stab wounds, automobile accidents, and blunt injury are the usual causes of traumatic chylothorax. The rest of reported cases, about 20%, are iatrogenic; most are postsurgical, often following operations for congenital cardiovascular abnormalities.[31] Chylothorax rarely complicates pulmonary resection.[39]

Conservative therapy includes decompression of the thoracic lymphatics with parenteral hyperalimentation or oral medium-chain triglycerides and drainage of the pleural space by thoracentesis or intercostal tube drainage.[20] If chylothorax persists for 3 to 4 weeks, talc pleurodesis may be tried.[41] If conservative treatment fails, the thoracic duct should be ligated at the site of leakage. A fatty meal ingested just prior to the operation helps identify the leakage site, but this may not be effective for patients with malignancies. An external pleuroperitoneal shunt can be considered.[7] Pleuroperitoneal shunts have been used successfully for refractory chylothorax in infants following congenital heart surgery.[27] For adults with malignancies, surgical intervention may not be effective; in trauma cases and in infants, operation is usually unnecessary.

EMPYEMA

Pleural empyema is a collection of purulent fluid in the pleural space (Fig. 51–60). It may be localized (encapsulated), or it may involve the entire pleural cavity. Empyemas are classified as acute or chronic, depending on the duration and pathologic reaction, but there is no sharp division in either time or pathologic response between the two. A more informative differentiation among the stages of empyema is that proposed by the American Thoracic Society. Exudative empyemas are characterized by thin fluid with low cellular content and an underlying lung that re-expands readily. Fibrinopurulent empyemas are characterized by large numbers of polymorphonuclear leukocytes and by deposition of fibrin on both the visceral and the parietal surfaces of the involved pleura. In this transitional phase between acute and chronic empyema, there is a progressive tendency toward loculation and delimitation of the extent of the empyema space, accompanied by initial fixation of the lung. In organizing empyemas, fibroblasts appear in the now heavier fibrin coating of the pleural membranes, and the exudate is quite thick. Upon standing, over 75% to 80% of the fluid consists of sediment. These distinctions are important, because therapy differs with the stage of the disease.

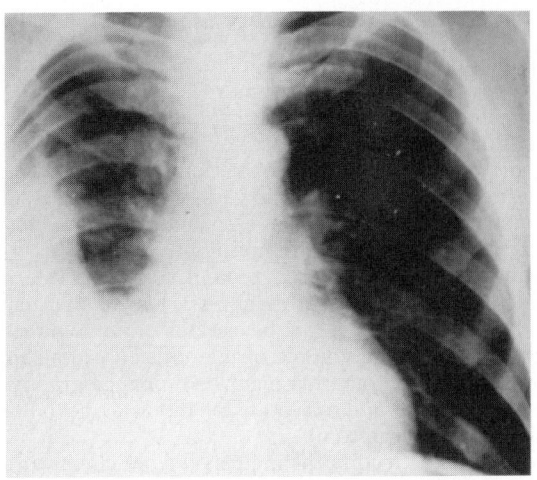

Figure 51–60. Roentgenogram of thoracic empyema of 2 months' duration, from which anaerobic streptococci and gram-negative *Bacteroides* bacilli were isolated. This patient was treated by open drainage following resection of a 2-inch segment of the seventh rib. The right lung re-expanded completely, and the empyema space was obliterated in approximately 2 weeks.

Despite antibiotics, there was an impressive increase in the incidence of both staphylococcal pneumonia and empyema in children in the late 1950s.[36] Such recrudescences of infections can be expected again. Today, because of the increasing age and debility of patients with empyema, and their underlying serious illnesses, this disease poses serious problems of diagnosis and management. The incidence of hospital-acquired empyemas appears to be increasing.

Etiology. Acute empyemas ordinarily result from primary disease elsewhere. Most commonly, the primary condition is a pneumonic process in the underlying lung, such as lobar pneumonia, pneumonitis, or lung abscess.[21] Extension to the pleura can occur directly, by way of the lymphatics, by hematogenous spread, or by rupture of necrotic pulmonary parenchyma. The pneumonic process itself may be secondary to other conditions, such as bronchial obstruction due to bronchogenic carcinoma or foreign body in an airway, or bronchial infection, as seen in bronchiectasis. A ruptured emphysematous bleb with spontaneous pneumothorax occasionally results in an empyema. Less commonly, the source of infection is a mediastinal structure, such as the trachea or bronchi (bronchopleural fistula); the esophagus (perforation, leaking esophagogastric anastomosis); an abscessed lymph node; or osteomyelitis of the dorsal spine. Subphrenic or intrahepatic abscesses can spread via the rich lymphatics of the diaphragm to cause empyema. Finally, infection can be introduced into the pleural spaces from without, for example, by trauma, needle aspiration, or operation. Chronic empyemas result from untreated or inadequately treated acute empyemas. This development should be prevented, if possible. Empyema necessitatis, an encapsulated empyema discharging into the subcutaneous tissues of the chest wall, is now rarely reported but still occurs.

The most common bacteriologic agents formerly responsible for empyemas—the pneumococci and streptococci—have been displaced in importance and frequency in recent years by *Staphylococcus aureus*, *Streptococcus*, and a variety of gram-negative organisms: *Pseudomonas*, *Klebsiella pneumoniae*, *Escherichia coli*, *Aerobacter aerogenes*, *Proteus*, *Bacteroides*, and *Salmonella*. Anaerobic flora are common, especially *Bacteroides*, and usually occur in mixed flora. Special techniques are needed for identification.[14, 21] Tuberculous empyema is uncommon except in hospitals with large indigent populations or those having a large number of immunocompromised patients.[14]

Diagnosis. The diagnosis depends on the detection of signs and symptoms of the underlying infectious process and the accumulation of purulent material in the pleural cavity. This is supported and localized by the clinical examination of the patient and the roentgenographic appearance of fluid, fluid and air, or a pleural or interlobar opacification compatible with fluid. It is confirmed by needle aspiration of the empyema with the demonstration of pus. Bacteria may not be identified if intensive antibiotic therapy has been employed previously or if the etiologic agent is not bacterial.

Treatment. The objectives of treatment for all stages of empyema are (1) control of the primary infection and its secondary manifestation, the empyema; (2) evacuation of the purulent contents of the empyema sac and eradication of the sac, to prevent chronicity; and (3) re-expansion of the underlying lung to restore function. The methods used to achieve these objectives depend on the stage of the empyema being treated and the nature of the primary infection or source of contamination. These objectives are realized by the use of appropriate antibiotic therapy, based on the bacteriologic diagnosis, and by prompt and adequate drainage.

Needle aspiration of an empyema when thoracentesis is done for diagnosis may be the only treatment necessary if the pus is the very thin variety that is seen with streptococcal infections. In this case, examination of the pus reveals a pH above 7.20, a glucose above 40 mg. per 100 ml., and a lactate dehydrogenase (LDH) concentration below 1000 I.U. per liter.

An *intercostal tube* for closed drainage should be employed promptly if the purulent fluid is thick and therefore cannot be completely evacuated by thoracentesis, if the fluid reaccumulates, or if infection and toxicity are difficult to control. Thoracentesis or intercostal tube drainage is adequate for most children with empyema associated with staphylococcal pneumonia.[36] When intercostal tube drainage is elected, negative pressure may have to be applied to hasten pulmonary expansion, especially in the presence of bronchopleural fistula. The tube should be of a generous caliber, commensurate with the material being evacuated, and should not be permitted to become occluded. It should be placed in the most dependent part of the empyema pocket, taking care to avoid perforation of the diaphragm. Accurate localization is greatly facilitated by the use of biplane roentgenograms of the chest or a fluoroscopic image intensifier. More than one tube may be necessary. Malecot or right-angle catheters, which can be inserted directly through a small incision and pulled flush with the parietal wall of the pleural cavity, are preferred by some surgeons.

Resection of a short segment of rib is necessary if the pus is thick and loculated or if the patient remains toxic after intercostal tube drainage. This technique provides adequate exposure, allowing one to evacuate the pus, break up loculations and adhesions, and assess the need for decortication. After washing the cavity, a tube may be placed in its most dependent portion and attached to underwater seal drainage. Open drainage may be necessary, in which case a wide-bore tube should be left in place, open to atmospheric pressure.[14, 21, 29] Another variation—the Eloesser skin flap, originally designed for tuberculous empyema—combines some of the virtues of open and closed drainage and eliminates the need for wide-bore tubes open to air. With open drainage, the appropriate site must be carefully localized roentgenographically or fluoroscopically, and by repeated exploratory thoracenteses, before the rib is resected. The drainage tube is removed only when the empyema sac has been eliminated, as determined by measurement of its capacity or radiographically, after the introduction of contrast material.

In some instances, *decortication* achieves the goals of therapy more efficiently than open drainage. This is more likely to be true in managing infected or noninfected hemothoraces in which the lung has become imprisoned by its nonelastic fibrinopurulent coat but presumably remains expandable, and the patient is not toxic. Decortication can follow closed-tube drainage. Although advocated by some as primary treatment for empyema, it is used by others only under unusual circumstances, as in immunosuppressed patients.[11] Even here, closed drainage is usually used as a preliminary step. The exact place of decortication in the treatment of empyema has not been clearly defined. Infrequently, conventional thoracoplasty to obliterate the pleural space or Schede thoracoplasty to unroof an empyema pocket may be necessary. Skin-flap open drainage or pedicled muscle flaps may be needed for complicated problems involving bronchopleural-cutaneous fistulas if simple open drainage fails to obliterate an empyema.

Approximately 25% of all empyemas follow thoracic surgical procedures, most commonly pneumonectomy.[1, 25] An empyema may or may not be associated with a bronchopleural fistula.[15] If a bronchopleural fistula occurs within the first week following operation, it is probably technical in origin, and an attempt should be made to close the fistula with a muscle flap. The pleural space should then be irrigated with antibiotics. A late-onset bronchopleural fistula is most likely associated with residual tumor or some condition predisposing to poor healing, and open drainage may be necessary. In the absence of an underlying bronchopleural or esophagopleural fistula, postpneumonectomy empyema can sometimes be sterilized with antibiotics. Successful endoscopic closure of bronchopleural fistulas with tissue adhesives has been reported.[34]

PLEURAL TUMORS

Pleural tumors are classified as primary or secondary. Primary pleural tumors are mostly mesotheliomas; localized benign and diffuse malignant types are recognized.[13] In both types, fibrous or fibrosarcomatous and epithelioid varieties are seen. Mixtures of the two histologic varieties also occur. Therefore, the pathologic classification of benign versus malignant, as well as the differentiation from carcinoma, is sometimes difficult.

Patients with localized fibrous mesotheliomas may be asymptomatic, or they may complain of arthralgia, clubbing of the fingers, or fever. Associated hypoglycemia has also been observed.[23] The solitary, often encapsulated, pedunculated, and usually easily removable tumor ordinarily arises from the visceral pleura. When it is excised, the symptoms and signs of arthralgia and pulmonary osteoarthropathy usually disappear, and longevity seems to be unaffected. These tumors may range in size from a few centimeters to 20 cm. or more in diameter.

Diffuse or malignant mesotheliomas cause chest pain and bloody pleural effusion containing malignant mesothelial cells. These tumors are characterized by findings ranging from multiple papillary projections on both visceral and parietal pleurae to encasement of the entire lung in a thick rind of tumor, with similar findings on the parietal side. Part or all of the pleural space may be obliterated. Metastases are uncommon, except late in the disease, and are often limited to the regional lymph nodes. Extrathoracic metastases do occur, however.

The evidence for a causal relationship between exposure to asbestos dust and the development of malignant mesothelioma is strong. It is based on occupational exposure, with a high incidence of both pleural mesothelioma and bronchogenic carcinoma in asbestos workers and those exposed to asbestos.[6]

Treatment of malignant mesothelioma has been unsatisfactory. There have been no cures. Palliation and a small number of long-term survivals have been achieved by *complete* pleurectomy or pleuropneumonectomy, but the great majority of patients succumb within 1 to 2 years of the diagnosis, regardless of the treatment.[37] Radiation and chemotherapy, or combined treatment, are recommended if excisional surgery is impossible or incomplete. Gene therapy is investigational but offers a new approach to treatment.[30] Gene transfer to human mesothelioma cells has been accomplished with recombinant adenovirus.[35] The prognosis of patients not only is related to the stage of the disease but also correlates with DNA ploidy pattern, S-phase fraction, and mean chromosome number. Patients with pleural fluid pH less than 7.30 have a decreased mean survival.[2, 24]

Pleural involvement by metastatic disease is far more common than primary pleural tumor and is usually associated with implants involving the lung or with blockage of or interference with the lymphatic drainage of the visceral, parietal, diaphragmatic, or mediastinal pleura. The most common sites of primary tumor are the lung, breast, pancreas, and stomach. With direct involvement of the pleura by tumor implants, bloody fluid containing neoplastic cells can often be obtained. Various types of palliative treatment are advocated, depending on the site of the primary tumor, the expansibility of the lung, the degree of disability from pleural effusion, and so forth.[32] Hormonal therapy, radiation or radioisotope therapy, multiple aspirations of the chest, closed-tube thoracostomy, the insufflation of talc, and the instillation of quinacrine have been reported, with varying degrees of palliation being achieved. Pleurectomy is the most effective treatment, but mortality (10%) and morbidity (20%) dictate careful patient selection.

SELECTED REFERENCES

Eloesser, L.: Milestones in chest surgery. J. Thorac. Cardiovasc. Surg., 60:157, 1970.
A brief but fascinating account of major landmarks in the development of thoracic and cardiovascular surgery, from Sauerbruch's chamber to Gibbon's pump-oxygenator.

Hood, R. M., Antman, K., Boyd, A., Naidich, D., and Shemin, R.: Surgical Diseases of the Pleura and Chest Wall. Philadelphia, W. B. Saunders, 1986.
Recommended for a detailed description of the surgical management of diseases of the pleura, with excellent illustrations of surgical techniques.

Kaiser, L. R., and Daniel, T. M.: Thoracoscopic Surgery. Boston, Little, Brown, 1993.
The authors provide an excellent overview of the rapidly developing field of video-assisted thoracic surgery. Techniques are clearly illustrated.

Light, R. W.: Pleural Diseases, 2nd ed. Philadelphia, Lea & Febiger, 1990.
The most complete exposition to date on pleural diseases. An excellent reference for both the student and the experienced clinician.

REFERENCES

1. Al-Kattan, K., Cattalani, L., and Goldstraw, P.: Bronchopleural fistula after pneumonectomy with a hand suture technique. Ann. Thorac. Surg., 58:1433, 1994.
2. Anand, A.: Prognostic factors of malignant mesothelioma of the pleura. Cancer, 72:755, 1993.
3. Battistella, F., and Benfield, J. R.: Blunt and penetrating injuries of the chest. *In* Shields, T. (Ed.): General Thoracic Surgery. Malvern, PA, Williams & Wilkins, 1994.
4. Brenner, M., Kayaleh, R. A., Milne, E. N., Bella, L. D., Osann, K., Tadir, Y., Berns, M. W., and Wilson, A. F.: Thoracoscopic laser ablation of pulmonary bullae. J. Thorac. Cardiovasc. Surg., 107:883, 1994.
5. Brock, L.: Evarts A. Graham: Recollections. Ann. Thorac. Surg., 9:272, 1970.
6. Craighead, J. E., Abraham, J. L., Churg, A., Green, F. H. Y., Kleinerman, J., Pratt, P. C., Seemayer, T. A., Vallyathan, V., and Weill, H.: The pathology of asbestos-associated diseases of the lungs and pleural cavities: Diagnostic criteria and proposed grading schema. Arch. Pathol. Lab. Med., 106:544, 1982.
7. Cummings, S. P., Wyatt, D. A., Baker, J. W., Flanagan, T. L., Spotnitz, W. D., Rodgers, B. M., Kron, I. L., and Tribble, C. G.: Successful treatment of postoperative chylothorax using an external pleuroperitoneal shunt. Ann. Thorac. Surg., 54:276, 1992.

8. Daniel, T. M.: Diagnostic thoracoscopy for pleural disease. Ann. Thorac. Surg., 56:639, 1993.
9. Dobell, A. R. C.: The origins of endotracheal ventilation. Ann. Thorac. Surg., 58:578, 1994.
10. Ferguson, L. J., Imrie, C. W., and Hutchison, J.: Excision of bullae without pleurectomy in patients with spontaneous pneumothorax. Br. J. Surg., 68:214, 1981.
11. Fishman, N. H., and Ellerston, D. G.: Early pleural decortication for thoracic empyema in immunosuppressed patients. J. Thorac. Cardiovasc. Surg., 74:537, 1977.
12. Heimlich, H. J.: Valve drainage of the pleural cavity. Dis. Chest, 53:282, 1968.
13. Hillerdal, G.: Malignant mesothelioma 1982: Review of 4710 published cases. Br. J. Dis. Chest, 77:321, 1983.
14. Hood, R. M., Antman, K., Boyd, A., Naidich, D., and Shemin, R.: Surgical Diseases of the Pleura and Chest Wall. Philadelphia, W. B. Saunders, 1986.
15. Icard, P., Fleury, J. P., Regnard, J. F., Libert, J. M., Magdeleinat, P., Gharbi, N., Brachet, A., Levi, J. F., and Levasseur, P.: Utility of C-reactive protein measurements for empyema diagnosis after pneumonectomy. Ann. Thorac. Surg., 57:933, 1994.
16. Inderbitzi, R. G. C., Leiser, A., Furrer, M., and Althaus, U.: Three years' experience in video-assisted thoracic surgery (VATS) for spontaneous pneumothorax. J. Thorac. Cardiovasc. Surg., 107:1410, 1994.
17. Jacobs, L. M., and Hsieh, J. W.: A clinical review of autotransfusion and its role in trauma. JAMA, 251:3283, 1984.
18. Janzing, H. M. J., Derom, A., Derom, E., Eeckhout, C., Derom, F., and Rosseel, M. T.: Intrapleural quinacrine instillation for recurrent pneumothorax or persistent air leak. Ann. Thorac. Surg., 55:368, 1993.
19. Kinosewitz, G. T.: Pleuritis and pleural effusions. In Bone, R. C. (Ed.): Pulmonary and Critical Care Medicine. St. Louis, Mosby Year Book, 1993.
20. Kosloske, A. M., Martin, L. W., and Schubert, W. K.: Management of chylothorax in children by thoracentesis and medium-chain triglyceride feedings. J. Pediatr. Surg., 9:365, 1974.
21. Lemmer, J. H., Botham, M. J., and Orringer, M. B.: Modern management of adult thoracic empyema. J. Thorac. Cardiovasc. Surg., 90:849, 1985.
22. Light, R. W.: Pleural Diseases, 2nd ed. Philadelphia, Lea & Febiger, 1990.
23. Mandal, A. K., Rozer, M. A., Salem, F. A., and Oparah, S. S.: Localized benign mesothelioma of the pleura associated with a hypoglycemic episode. Arch. Intern. Med., 143:1608, 1983.
24. Manzini, V. D., Brollo, A., Franceschi, S., DeMattaeis, M., Talamini, R., and

Bianchi, C.: Prognostic factors of malignant mesothelioma of the pleura. Cancer, 72:410, 1993.
25. Massard, G., Ducrocq, X., Hentz, J. G., Kessler, R., Dumont, P., Wihlm, J. M., and Morand, G.: Esophagopleural fistula: An early and long-term complication after pneumonectomy. Ann. Thorac. Surg., 58:1437, 1994.
26. Milfeld, D. J., Mattox, K. L., and Beall, A. C.: Early evacuation of clotted hemothorax. Am. J. Surg., 136:686, 1978.
27. Murphy, M. C., Newman, B. M., and Rodgers, B. M.: Pleuroperitoneal shunts in the management of persistent chylothorax. Ann. Thorac. Surg., 48:195, 1989.
28. Negrini, D., Venturoli, D., Townsley, M. I., and Reed, R. K.: Permeability of parietal pleura to liquid and proteins. J. Appl. Physiol., 76:627, 1994.
29. Orringer, M. B.: Thoracic empyema—back to basics. Chest, 93:901, 1988.
30. Pass, H. I.: Malignant pleural mesothelioma: The thoracic surgeon and gene therapy. Ann. Thorac. Surg., 57:1383, 1994.
31. Rheuban, K. S., Kron, I. L., Carpenter, M. A., Gutgesell, H. P., and Rodgers, B. M.: Pleuroperitoneal shunts for refractory chylothorax after operation for congenital heart disease. Ann. Thorac. Surg., 53:85, 1992.
32. Ruckdeschel, J. C.: Management of malignant pleural effusion: An overview. Semin. Oncol., 15:24, 1988.
33. Sahn, S. A.: The pleura. Am. Rev. Respir. Dis., 138:184, 1988.
34. Scappaticci, E., Ardissone, F., Ruffini, E., Baldi, S., and Mancuso, M.: Postoperative bronchopleural fistula: Endoscopic closure in 12 patients. Ann. Thorac. Surg., 57:119, 1994.
35. Smythe, W. R., Kaiser, L. R., Hwang, H. C., Amin, K. M., Pilewski, J. M., Eck, S. J., Wilson, J. M., and Albelda, S. M.: Successful adenovirus-mediated gene transfer in an in vivo model of human malignant mesothelioma. Ann. Thorac. Surg., 57:1395, 1994.
36. Stiles, Q. R., Lindesmith, G. G., Tucker, B. L., Meyer, B. W., and Jones, J. C.: Pleural empyema in children. Ann. Thorac. Surg., 10:37, 1970.
37. Sugarbaker, D. J., Mentzer, S. J., and Strauss, G.: Extrapleural pneumonectomy in the treatment of malignant pleural mesothelioma. Ann. Thorac. Surg., 54:941, 1992.
38. Symbas, P. N.: Chest drainage tubes. Surg. Clin. North Am., 69:41, 1989.
39. Vallieres, E., Shamji, F. M., and Todd, T. R.: Postpneumonectomy chylothorax. Ann. Thorac. Surg., 55:1006, 1993.
40. Wang, N. S.: The preformed stomas connecting the pleural cavity and the lymphatics in the parietal pleura. Am. Rev. Respir. Dis., 111:12, 1975.
41. Weissberg, D., and Ben-Zeev, I.: Talc pleurodesis. J. Thorac. Cardiovasc. Surg., 106:689, 1993.

VIIB

SURGICAL MANAGEMENT OF PULMONARY EMPHYSEMA

James R. Mault, M.D.

Pulmonary emphysema is a major health problem for more than 4.5 million Americans and is the most common cause of respiratory disability. In addition to causing severe restrictions in exercise tolerance, end-stage emphysema is associated with striking physical and radiographic abnormalities that impair chest wall mechanics and diaphragmatic motion. Supportive medical therapy is the mainstay of treatment for the majority of patients with dyspnea due to emphysema. However, in properly selected patients, surgical intervention may produce significant improvements in pulmonary function, chest wall mechanics, and corresponding exercise tolerance.

TERMINOLOGY AND CLASSIFICATION OF EMPHYSEMA

Air space enlargement is a term that encompasses all varieties of respiratory disorders with increased air space distal to the terminal bronchiole. This includes conditions of air space enlargement without evidence of destruction, such as in postpneumonectomy hyperinflation, as well as the pathologic conditions of pulmonary fibrosis and emphysema. Of a sam-

pling of 608 patients with air space enlargement, approximately 80% had emphysema.[6]

According to the standards established by the American Thoracic Society in 1962,[1] *emphysema* is defined as an anatomic alteration of the lung characterized by an abnormal and permanent enlargement of the air spaces distal to the terminal, nonrespiratory bronchiole, accompanied by destructive changes of the alveolar walls. Emphysema is subdivided into three categories based on its location in the acinus, which is the unit of bronchopulmonary tissue distal to the terminal bronchiole. These categories are termed *centriacinar*, *periacinar*, and *panacinar emphysema* and are illustrated in Figure 51–61.

Centriacinar emphysema develops in the proximal portion of the acinus and is associated with inflammatory destruction of respiratory bronchioles. It occurs most often in upper lung fields. The surrounding lung parenchyma may be preserved. Smoking is the most consistent cause of this type of emphysema.

Periacinar emphysema is due to disruption of subpleural alveoli. Initial small disruptions coalesce into larger air spaces called *blebs*. The outer wall of a bleb consists of visceral pleura whereas the underlying lung parenchyma is

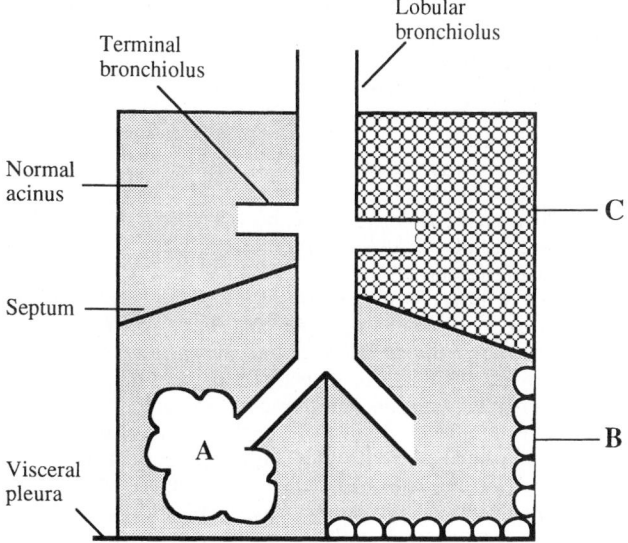

Figure 51–61. Terminology and classification of emphysema. According to the standards established by the American Thoracic Society,[1] emphysema is classified into three categories by its location in the pulmonary acinus: A, centriacinar (centrilobular) emphysema; B, periacinar (paraseptal) emphysema; and C, panacinar (panlobular) emphysema. Bullous emphysema (air spaces of greater than 1 cm. diameter in the inflated lung) can occur in any of these categories.

usually normal. The blebs are located in the upper lobes but occasionally occur along the superior segments of lower lobes. Blebs can either rupture or progress into giant subpleural bullae. This is the pathophysiology of primary spontaneous pneumothoraces that can occur in young adults with otherwise normal lung parenchyma.

In *panacinar* emphysema, all portions of acinus are uniformly destroyed. This diffuse emphysema occurs in all lung fields and is associated with low diffusing capacity, decreased arterial saturation with exercise, and pruning of peripheral pulmonary vasculature. Patients with alpha$_1$-antitrypsin deficiency can progress to panacinar emphysema, although smoking is again the overwhelming cause.

Pulmonary *bullae* are defined as emphysematous spaces of more than 1 cm. diameter in the inflated lung and can occur with any category of emphysema. The air space of a bulla is covered by visceral pleura, and the inner wall is composed of destroyed emphysematous lung crisscrossed by fibrous (cotton candy) strands—remnants of interlobular septa. A bulla that occupies one half of the hemithorax or greater is called a giant bulla.

Patients with emphysematous bullae are divided into two groups according to the status of their nonbullous lung parenchyma. In Group I, which comprises 20% of all bullous lung disease, bullae are associated with otherwise normal or preserved lung tissue. In these patients the bullae are well demarcated and are usually located at the apex of the upper lobes. The remaining 80% of patients with bullous emphysema have diffuse emphysema throughout the nonbullous lung tissue and are assigned to Group II. Bullae in these patients are considered local exaggerations of panacinar emphysema. They are often multiple, poorly demarcated, bilateral, and variable in size.

Indications for surgical management of patients with these various classifications of emphysema can be distinguished by the presence or absence of chronic dyspnea. In patients with emphysema who present *without* chronic dyspnea, surgical treatment is required for acute complications such as spontaneous pneumothorax, infection of bullae, and massive hemoptysis. In patients *with* chronic dyspnea due to bullous

(centriacinar) emphysema, a highly selected subset of patients may benefit from operation by resection of bullae that compress surrounding tissue and allow re-expansion of preserved lung parenchyma. In recent years, operative indications for emphysema have been expanded to include some patients with dyspnea due to panacinar emphysema. The rationale for operation in these patients is that reduction of total lung volume improves respiratory mechanics by restoring chest wall and diaphragmatic motion.

SURGICAL MANAGEMENT OF EMPHYSEMA WITHOUT DYSPNEA

Primary spontaneous pneumothorax (PSP) is due to rupture of a periacinar bleb in young patients with otherwise normal lung tissue and accounts for 85% of all spontaneous pneumothoraces. The incidence of PSP is 9 per 100,000 cases in the general population, and the typical patient is a 20- to 40-year-old, tall, thin man with a history of use of tobacco products. A positive family history of PSP is obtained in 10% of patients.

Secondary spontaneous pneumothorax (SSP) accounts for 15% of spontaneous pneumothoraces and occurs in patients with underlying lung disease.[13] Compared with PSP, this population of patients is much older, ranging from 45 to 75 years. The majority of cases are due to bullous emphysema (centriacinar and panacinar) but also include tuberculosis, cystic fibrosis, *Pneumocystis carinii* infection (commonly associated with the acquired immunodeficiency syndrome), primary or metastatic lung cancer, lung abscess, and catamenial pneumothorax (a spontaneous pneumothorax that occurs during menstruation in women aged 30 to 50 years).

Patients with PSP or SSP present with an acute history of chest pain and/or shortness of breath. Primary evaluation should include a careful history and physical examination. Any suggestion of tension pneumothorax should be treated immediately with needle decompression without further studies. Inspiratory and expiratory plain chest radiographs are diagnostic of pneumothorax.

Initial treatment for spontaneous pneumothorax is dictated by the patient's symptoms and extent of pneumothorax. The stable, nondyspneic patient with a unilateral pneumothorax estimated to be less than 15% of the hemithorax may be observed in the hospital and monitored by daily chest radiography. Supplemental oxygen administration may enhance resorption of pneumothorax, although the efficacy of this measure is limited if the pneumothorax occurred in room air.

Tube thoracostomy should be performed in patients with persistent symptoms; in those with a unilateral pneumothorax greater than 15% of a hemithorax; in all patients who present with simultaneous bilateral pneumothoraces or previous pneumonectomy; and in those who fail observation. The chest tube should be connected to a water-sealed drainage system with 20-cm. H$_2$O suction. With re-expansion of the lung and resolution of the air leak, the chest tube may be removed and the patient discharged after a follow-up chest radiograph confirms full lung inflation. The recurrence rate of spontaneous pneumothorax after nonoperative management of the first episode is 45% with PSP and 35% with SSP.[13] In patients with SSP who represent a significant operative risk, chemical pleurodesis (using sterile talc or other sclerosing agent) performed before chest tube removal has been shown to reduce recurrence of SSP by one half.[13]

Indications for operation after spontaneous pneumothorax are listed in Table 51–17. Patients with massive air leaks preventing lung re-expansion, patients with simultaneous bilateral pneumothoraces, as well as those with previous contralateral pneumothorax or pneumonectomy, should undergo operative intervention. Patients with a first recurrence

TABLE 51–17. Indications for Operation After Spontaneous Pneumothorax

Massive air leak preventing re-expansion of lung
Simultaneous bilateral pneumothoraces
Persistent air leak (>48 hours for primary spontaneous pneumothorax; >96 hours for secondary spontaneous pneumothorax)
Recurrent pneumothorax
Previous contralateral pneumothorax or pneumonectomy
First episode with occupational hazard for pneumothorax (pilot, scuba diver, parachutist)

of spontaneous pneumothorax have an excessively high risk of second recurrence and should be scheduled for operation. The optimal timing of operation for patients with unresolved, persistent air leaks has been demonstrated as 48 hours for both PSP and SSP.[12] However, because patients with SSP are generally at increased operative risk, Tanaka and colleagues advocate tube drainage with persistent air leak be continued for a longer period than in PSP.[13] Patients with occupational hazards for pneumothorax, such as pilots and scuba divers, should be treated operatively during hospitalization for the first episode.

Operative correction of spontaneous pneumothorax has traditionally consisted of open thoracotomy with resection of bleb(s) and mechanical pleurodesis with low morbidity and mortality and excellent long-term results. Over the past 5 years, videothoracoscopy has become an alternative approach for operative treatment of spontaneous pneumothorax with similar safety and efficacy.[10] In one prospective, randomized study,[15] videothoracoscopy resulted in less analgesic requirement, shorter length of stay, and similar postoperative recurrence rate as compared with open thoracotomy for the treatment of PSP. In patients with SSP, open thoracotomy remained the operation of choice. If a bleb or other anatomic source of pneumothorax cannot be identified thoracoscopically, conversion to open thoracotomy is recommended to reduce postoperative recurrence.[10] For PSP treated by either technique, operative morbidity and mortality are rare and freedom from recurrence of pneumothorax is greater than 95%. In SSP, the underlying pulmonary disease, age of the patient, and increased complexity of the operation result in greater morbidity and mortality as well as increased recurrence rate.[13]

Operative intervention in the patient without dyspnea is also indicated for an infected bulla that has failed to improve after a 6-week course of antibiotics as well as patients who present with massive hemoptysis secondary to bullous erosion into a pulmonary vessel. Preventive surgical treatment may also be considered for asymptomatic individuals with a bulla that occupies greater than one half of the hemithorax or has progressively enlarged over 2 to 3 years.

SURGICAL MANAGEMENT OF EMPHYSEMA WITH DYSPNEA

Although the majority of patients with dyspnea due to emphysema have a diffuse pulmonary disease that is best managed medically, a subset of patients may benefit from operation. In an analysis of 493 patients with bullous emphysema, 103 (21%) underwent operation.[6] Good outcome from surgical management of emphysema is achieved only from a detailed understanding of the pathophysiology of bullous disease and strict patient selection.

Pathophysiology of Bullous Lung Disease

The traditional rationale for surgical management of bullous emphysema is that removal of the bulla allows the normal, compressed lung to re-expand. This has been based on the hypothesis that bullae produce compression and collapse of surrounding pulmonary tissues by trapping gas under pressure from feeding airways that are obstructed by a one-way valve mechanism. Continued alveolar destruction and pressurized inflation of the air space are believed to be the cause of further expansion of the bulla and worsening function of the remaining lung.

However, these theories have been challenged by histologic examination of resected bullae as well as by direct *in vivo* measurements of bullous pressure and gas content.[9] Gross observation of the floor of bullae demonstrated a consistent broad base of airway openings that appeared widely patent. Histologically, the floor of bullae consisted of alveolar ducts and alveoli opening directly into the lumen without any evidence of valvular mechanism. During spontaneous tidal respiration, overall gas flow into and out of bullae was small and unimpeded with gas contents identical to that in alveoli and minimal contribution to dead space ventilation. Finally, the intrabulla pressure during inspiration was similar to pleural pressure during all phases of respiration. Together these findings suggest that an alternate physiologic basis must exist to establish the rationale for surgical management of emphysema.

A more accurate account of the pathophysiology of bullous disease is that bullae are analogous to a paper bag in that they are quite compliant until fully expanded.[9] The surrounding lung tissue is slightly less compliant and is inflated only after the bulla. Once a parenchymal weakness exceeds a certain size, it causes space that fills preferentially. Retraction of the neighboring lung away from the bullous space contributes to its enlargement. The resultant loss of elastic recoil on adjacent airways ultimately leads to occlusion and atelectasis (rather than compression) of the surrounding, preserved lung tissue. The degree to which bullae contribute to dyspnea depends more on the amount of lung they replace and the extent of underlying diffuse lung disease present than on the amount of lung they compress. Therefore, the physiologic benefit of bullectomy is not derived from elimination of the air space but rather from restoration of the architecture of the remaining lung parenchyma and re-establishment of mechanical linkage with the chest wall.

Patient Selection for Operation

Clinical Evaluation. Clinical parameters describing the ideal patient and relative contraindications for surgical management of dyspneic patients with bullous emphysema are listed in Table 51–18. The clinical evaluation begins with a careful history and physical examination to define the cause of dyspnea in the patient being considered for operation. Patients with alpha$_1$-antitrypsin deficiency, sarcoidosis, and even cardiovascular disease may present with dyspnea and bullae but would not benefit from bullectomy. A distinction must also be made between chronic obstructive pulmonary disease in patients who have primarily emphysema (pink puffers) and those with chronic bronchitis (blue bloaters). Patients with chronic bronchitis are characterized by a productive cough, frequent respiratory tract infections, carbon dioxide retention, and bronchospasm and are poor candidates for pulmonary surgical treatment.[6]

With smoking the common cause of this disease in more than 97% of patients in most series,[6] cessation of tobacco use at least 6 weeks before operation is essential. Further comorbidities associated with tobacco, such as coronary artery and cerebrovascular disease, must also be excluded. Cor pulmonale and mild, isolated right-sided heart failure are not strict contraindications because pulmonary hypertension may be caused by vascular crowding of the nonbullous lung.

TABLE 51–18. Clinical Indications and Contraindications for Bullectomy

Clinical Presentation	Ideal Case	Relative Contraindications
Age and medical status	Young age; no comorbidities	Advanced age; comorbidities
Cardiac status	Normal	Right-sided heart failure/cor pulmonale
Weight loss	None or <10%	>10%
Dyspnea	Rapidly progressive	Slowly progressive
Other respiratory symptoms	Pink puffer	Blue bloater

In these circumstances, right- and left-sided heart catheterization with pulmonary arteriography should be obtained to define the degree of right-sided heart failure and pulmonary vascular crowding and to exclude ischemic heart disease. Postoperative normalization of pulmonary arterial pressures is often observed after resection of bullous disease.

A somewhat subjective but essential aspect of the clinical evaluation is an assessment of the motivation and lifestyle of the patient being considered for surgical treatment. Individuals who appear fit and who are dedicated to returning to an active routine are more likely to benefit from surgery than obese individuals with a long-standing sedentary lifestyle. Patients should readily submit to a 4- to 6-week organized program of pulmonary rehabilitation before operation and commit to long-term exercise training and smoking cessation postoperatively.

Physiologic Evaluation. Physiologic parameters describing the ideal patient and relative contraindications for bullectomy are listed in Table 51–19. As part of the evaluation for consideration of operation, all patients should undergo standard pulmonary function testing with room air blood gas measurement. Small bullae occupying one third or less of radiographic volume with otherwise normal lungs have no measurable effect on lung volume or flow. A reduction of forced expiratory volume over 1 second (FEV_1) disproportionate to the size of the bulla suggests significant diffuse disease, whereas bullous compression of preserved, normal lung parenchyma is more consistent with a reduction of forced vital capacity almost equal to the reduction of FEV_1. Ohta and associates[11] examined a wide range of spirometric parameters and concluded that an FEV_1 greater than 50% of predicted with a nitrogen washout measurement less than 60% was predictive of long-term benefit from bullectomy. Lastly, a trapped gas volume greater than 2 liters, determined by the difference between spirometric and plethysmographic measured functional residual capacity, is considered a reliable indication for operation.

The diffusion capacity of carbon monoxide (DLCO) reflects the function of the nonbullous lung. Although a normal DLCO is encouraging relative to the status of reserve lung

tissue, a decreased DLCO is not a strict indication for operation. Decreases in DLCO may reflect generalized destruction of lung tissue or, conversely, may be due to compressed, atelectatic normal lung. However, DLCO is an excellent parameter for the purpose of preoperative and postoperative comparisons. Blood gas measurements are necessary to exclude patients with carbon dioxide retention and hypercapnia at rest. These patients are unlikely to benefit from pulmonary resection and represent a significant surgical risk.

Radiographic Evaluation. Radiographic parameters describing the ideal patient and relative contraindications for surgical management of dyspneic patients with bullous emphysema are listed in Table 51–20. In most cases, bullous disease identified on plain anteroposterior and lateral radiographs is usually the basis of initial referral for operation. Apical bullae occupying more than 50% of a hemithorax with lower crowding of lung marking and pulmonary vasculature predicts a good operative result. Review of previous radiographs provides additional information regarding the rate of progression of bullae. Expiratory films may be obtained to further distinguish bullae that are associated with diffuse emphysema versus preserved lung tissue.

Computed tomography (CT) is an essential component in the evaluation of these patients and can quantitatively define the size and number of bullous lesions. In addition, CT provides the best noninvasive assessment of the nature and extent of underlying lung disease.[8] Vascular crowding demonstrated by pulmonary angiography may provide additional confirmation of preserved lung tissue, although advances in dynamic CT capabilities have made angiography unnecessary except in cases where pulmonary artery pressure measurements are required. Ventilation-perfusion isotope scans are rarely necessary but may provide useful information in borderline cases.

Operative Technique

The operative strategy for bullous disease is directed at removal of the space-occupying disease while preserving all vascularized and potentially functional lung tissue. This is best accomplished by limited resections. Lobectomy and pneumonectomy are rarely indicated in the setting of emphysema. Small bullae can be obliterated by coagulation whereas narrow-necked bullae can be excised after ligation of their pedicle. Broad-based bullae should be oversewn or plicated. Giant bullae require excision of the thin wall down to the location of normal lung. The edges of visceral pleura are then sealed with a running mattress suture. With advances in stapling devices, resection and closure of bullae have been successfully accomplished with minimal air leaks when staple lines are reinforced by bovine pericardium or parietal pleura (Fig. 51–62).

In patients with bilateral bullous disease amenable to resection, simultaneous bilateral bullectomy can be performed safely through median sternotomy. This approach may enhance postoperative recovery because many patients experience less incisional pain and better pulmonary toilet with

TABLE 51–19. Physiologic Indications and Contraindications for Bullectomy

Pulmonary Function Tests	Ideal Case	Relative Contraindications
FVC	Normal–mildly decreased	Markedly decreased
FEV_1	>40%	<35%
DLCO	Normal	Decreased
PaO_2	Normal	Hypoxemia at rest/exercise
$PaCO_2$	Normal	Increased

FVC, forced vital capacity; FEV_1, forced expiratory volume in 1 second; DLCO, diffusion capacity; PaO_2 and $PaCO_2$, partial pressures of arterial oxygen and carbon dioxide.

TABLE 51–20. Radiologic Indications and Contraindications for Bullectomy

Imaging Study	Ideal Case	Relative Contraindications
Standard radiograph	Bulla occupying greater than one third hemithorax; large bulla with vascular crowding, localized disease	Multiple small bullae; diffuse disease, vanishing lung syndrome
Computed tomogram	Large and localized bulla with evidence of vascular crowding and normal pulmonary density and architecture around the bulla	Multiple bilateral bullae; evidence of emphysema in the underlying lung
Angiogram	Vascular crowding; preserved distal vascular branching	No crowding; winter-tree appearance
Isotope scan	Well-localized matching defect; normal uptake and washout from underlying lung	Diffuse multiple defects; poor washout in restricted lung

sternotomy than thoracotomy. With the introduction of video-assisted thoracic surgery over the past 5 years, resection of bullous emphysema has also been successfully accomplished using endoscopic stapling techniques as well as laser coagulation.[3] At the completion of bullectomy and elimination of all detectable air leaks, correct placement of at least two chest tubes per hemithorax is critical to achieve full expansion of the remaining lung and resolve postoperative air leaks.

Patients with giant bullae who are not suited for open or video-assisted thoracic resection may receive intracavitary drainage in a single-stage procedure.[14] A local anesthestic is administered, and then a small piece of rib is resected and an absorbable pursestring suture is placed through the parietal pleura and adjacent bulla wall. A large Foley catheter is inserted through the pursestring suture into the bullae and subjected to 10 mm. Hg suction for 36 to 48 hours, followed by water seal for 21 days. Bronchiolar leaks slowly resolve as the bulla contracts over this period.

Lastly, patients with end-stage emphysema may also undergo single or bilateral lung transplantation. Unfortunately, the availability of donor organs severely limits this option for the vast majority of eligible patients.

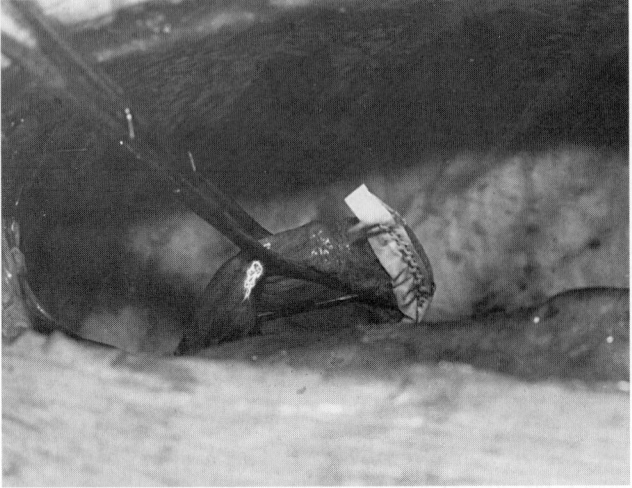

Figure 51–62. Bullectomy staple line reinforced by bovine pericardial strips. To optimize stapling success and minimize postoperative air leaks, a sheet of bovine pericardium is secured around each arm of the stapling device. When the device is fired, each side of the staple line is reinforced by a strip of pericardium. Parietal pleura or Teflon felt strips may also be used in place of bovine pericardium.

Outcome and Follow-up After Bullectomy

Mortality and Morbidity. In most series,[3, 5, 6, 8, 11] perioperative mortality averages 1% to 3% and is usually attributed to respiratory failure, pneumonia, or cardiovascular disorders. Morbidity is common (15%–40%) after operation for emphysema and primarily consists of prolonged air leaks, delayed lung expansion, and infection. With thoracostomy tube suction, antibiotics, and time, these complications uniformly resolve over an average of 2 weeks.[3]

Short- and Long-Term Follow-Up. In short-term follow-up, most patients demonstrate significant improvements in a host of spirometric parameters, whereas approximately two thirds of patients experience significant improvements in exercise tolerance and relief of symptomatic dyspnea.[3, 5, 8, 11] In a comprehensive long-term follow-up after bullectomy, FitzGerald and colleagues[5] obtained data on 80 of 82 patients operated on over a 25-year period. Fifty-three patients were examined, and there were 21 late deaths (12 unrelated to lung disease). The survivors were divided into three groups. The first had localized bullae occupying less than one third of a hemithorax, and, contrary to expectations, long-term decline in pulmonary function differed little from that expected with normal aging. In the second group, who had much larger, localized bullae, striking early improvement existed for the first 5 years but then rapidly declined to preoperative values within 7 to 10 years. The last group, characterized by diffuse emphysema, experienced a rapid decline in FEV_1 at a rate three times greater than that with normal aging. In this series, the best results occurred in patients with giant bullae who underwent simple excision or plication, while the poorest results were experienced in patients with diffuse emphysema.

Surgery for Diffuse Emphysema

Despite conventional teachings in the late 1950s, Brantigan[2] advocated surgical intervention for diffuse emphysema. He theorized that as the lung loses its elastic recoil, the respiratory system partially accommodates the expanding lung by enlarging the chest cavity. Clinically, this is demonstrated by development of a *barrel* chest wall and flattening of the diaphragms on chest radiograph (Fig. 51–63A). The consequence of this physical accommodation is worsening pulmonary mechanics. As the expanded chest wall and diaphragm become incapable of providing adequate respiratory excursions, the patient becomes increasingly dyspneic and functionally disabled. Brantigan proposed that reduction of overall lung volume would reduce airway collapse, restore

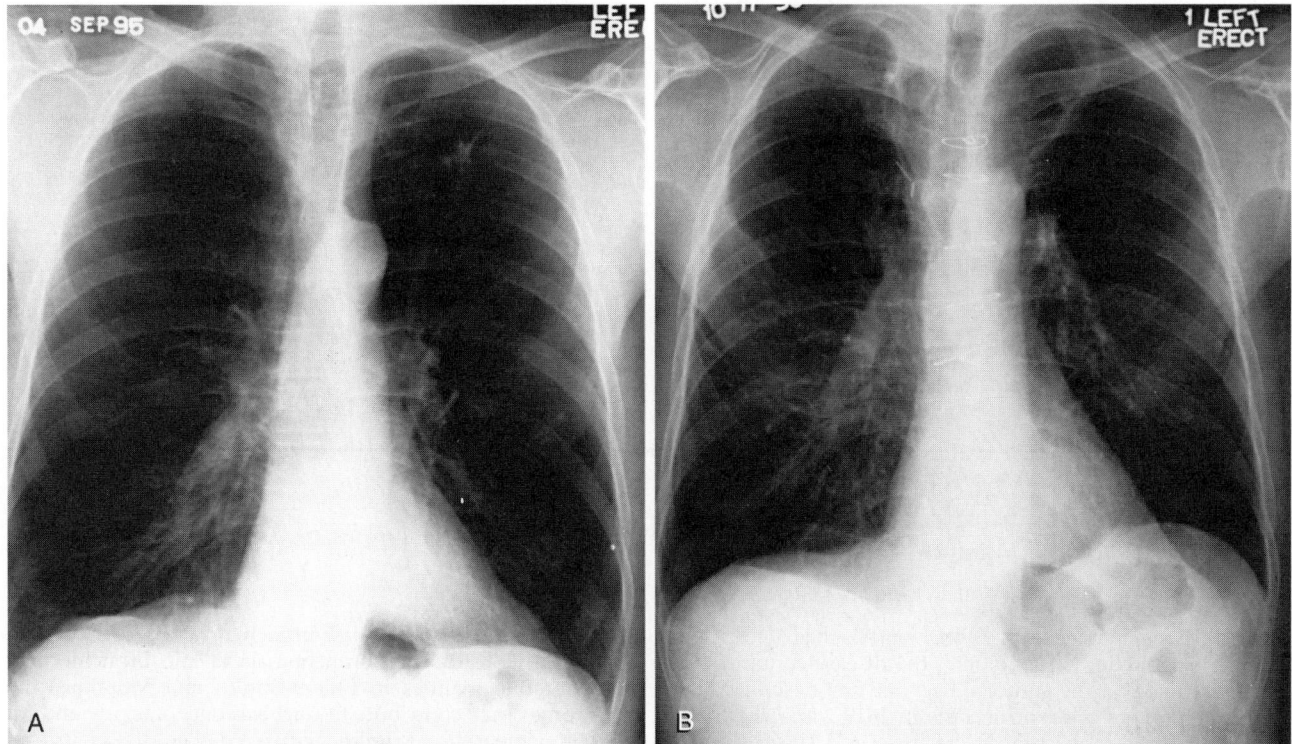

Figure 51–63. Anteroposterior chest radiographs before *(A)* and after *(B)* lung reduction. The preoperative radiograph shows the flattened diaphragms, reduced vascular markings, and hyperexpanded chest wall commonly observed with diffuse (panacinar) emphysema. After bilateral lung volume reduction surgery through a median sternotomy, the 1-month postoperative radiograph demonstrates recovery of normal diaphragmatic contour and decreased chest wall dimensions.

diaphragm and chest wall motion, relieve dyspnea, and improve lifestyle.

With an evolution in understanding of the pathophysiology of diffuse emphysema, this operative approach to the hyperexpanded respiratory system has received renewed attention in recent years. The goal of surgical therapy in this setting is to reduce total lung volume occupying the chest cavity and thereby re-establish diaphragmatic excursion and chest wall motion (see Fig. 51–63*B*). The lung reduction technique described by Cooper and coworkers[4] as *pneumectomy* is performed through a median sternotomy and involves excision of 20% to 30% of the volume of each lung. The most affected portions of lung were excised with the use of a stapling device fitted with strips of bovine pericardium. In this series of 20 patients with diffuse disease there was no early or late mortality and no requirement for immediate postoperative ventilatory assistance. Early (6-month) follow-up documented an 82% improvement in FEV_1 as well as significant reductions in total lung capacity, residual volume, and trapped gas. Clinically, all patients experienced marked relief of dyspnea and improvement in exercise tolerance.

Little and associates[7] have also published a separate series of 55 patients with diffuse emphysema treated unilaterally with a laser to achieve lung volume reduction. Postoperative mortality was 5.5%. Although the quantitative and qualitative results were not as marked as those reported after simultaneous bilateral lung reduction, these patients nonetheless experienced significant improvements in exercise capacity and relief of dyspnea. Improvements in pulmonary function directly correlated with reduction in lung volume by radiographic and spirometric measures. The long-term results of lung volume reduction remain to be determined.

SELECTED REFERENCES

Cooper, J. D., Trulock, E. P., Triantafillou, A. N., Patterson, G. A., Pohl, M. S., Deloney, P. A., Sundaresan, R. S., and Roper, C. L.: Bilateral pneumectomy

(volume reduction) for chronic obstructive pulmonary disease. J. Thorac. Cardiovasc. Surg., *109*:106, 1995.
This is the initial report of the leading experience with lung volume reduction surgery for diffuse emphysema. Patient selection criteria, preoperative rehabilitation programs, and specific operative technique are described in great detail.

FitzGerald, M. X., Keelan, P. J., Cugell, D. W., and Gaensler, E. A.: Long-term results of surgery for bullous emphysema. J. Thorac. Cardiovasc. Surg., *68*:566, 1974.
This paper provides a comprehensive analysis of the short- and long-term results of surgery for bullous emphysema. Eighty of 82 patients who received operations over a period of 25 years were accounted for at follow-up. The data obtained are critically analyzed and the conclusions remain the basis of surgical management more than 20 years since its publication.

Waller, D. A., Forty, J., and Morritt, G. N.: Video-assisted thoracoscopic surgery versus thoracotomy for spontaneous pneumothorax. Ann. Thorac. Surg., *58*:372, 1994.
These authors conducted a well-constructed prospective, randomized comparison of video-assisted thoracoscopy versus open thoracotomy for treatment of spontaneous pneumothorax. Subset analysis of the treatment results of primary versus secondary pneumothoraces provides additional insight regarding the surgical management of these patients.

REFERENCES

1. American Thoracic Society: Chronic bronchitis, asthma and pulmonary emphysema: A statement by the committee on diagnostic standards for nontuberculous respiratory disease. Am. Rev. Respir. Dis., *85*:762, 1962.
2. Brantigan, O. C.: Surgical treatment of pulmonary emphysema. Am. Surg., *23*:789, 1957.
3. Brenner, M., Kayaleh, R. A., Milne, E. N., Della, B. L., Osann, K., Tadir, Y., Berns, M. W., and Wilson, A. F.: Thoracoscopic laser ablation of pulmonary bullae: Radiographic selection and treatment response. J. Thorac. Cardiovasc. Surg., *107*:883, 1994.
4. Cooper, J. D., Trulock, E. P., Triantafillou, A. N., Patterson, G. A., Pohl, M. S., Deloney, P. A., Sundaresan, R. S., and Roper, C. L.: Bilateral pneumectomy (volume reduction) for chronic obstructive pulmonary disease. J. Thorac. Cardiovasc. Surg., *109*:106, 1995.
5. FitzGerald, M. X., Keelan, P. J., Cugell, D. W., and Gaensler, E. A.: Long-term results of surgery for bullous emphysema. J. Thorac. Cardiovasc. Surg., *68*:566, 1974.
6. Gaensler, E. A., Jederlinic, P. J., and FitzGerald, M. X.: Patient work-up for bullectomy. J. Thorac. Imaging, *1*:75, 1986.
7. Little, A. G., Swain, J. A., Nino, J. J., Prabhu, R. D., Schlachter, M. D., and

Barcia, T. C.: Reduction pneumonoplasty for emphysema: Early results. Ann. Surg., 222:365, 1995.

8. Morgan, M. D., Denison, D. M., and Strickland, B.: Value of computed tomography for selecting patients with bullous lung disease for surgery. Thorax, 41:855, 1986.

9. Morgan, M. D., Edwards, C. W., Morris, J., and Matthews, H. R.: Origin and behaviour of emphysematous bullae. Thorax, 44:533, 1989.

10. Naunheim, K. S., Mack, M. J., Hazelrigg, S. R., Ferguson, M. K., Ferson, P. F., Boley, T. M., and Landreneau, R. J.: Safety and efficacy of video-assisted thoracic surgical techniques for the treatment of spontaneous pneumothorax. J. Thorac. Cardiovasc. Surg., 109:1198, 1995.

11. Ohta, M., Nakahara, K., Yasumitsu, T., Ohsugi, T., Maeda, M., and Kawashima, Y.: Prediction of postoperative performance status in patients with giant bulla. Chest, 101:668, 1992.

12. Schoenenberger, R. A., Haefeli, W. E., Weiss, P., and Ritz, R. F.: Timing of invasive procedures in therapy for primary and secondary spontaneous pneumothorax. Arch. Surg., 126:764, 1991.

13. Tanaka, F., Itoh, M., Esaki, H., Isobe, J., Ueno, Y., and Inoue, R.: Secondary spontaneous pneumothorax. Ann. Thorac. Surg., 55:372, 1993.

14. Venn, G. E., Williams, P. R., and Goldstraw, P.: Intracavity drainage for bullous, emphysematous lung disease: Experience with the Brompton technique. Thorax, 43:998, 1988.

15. Waller, D. A., Forty, J., and Morritt, G. N.: Video-assisted thoracoscopic surgery versus thoracotomy for spontaneous pneumothorax. Ann. Thorac. Surg., 58:372, 1994.

VIII

BRONCHIECTASIS

Donald D. Glower, M.D.

Although the incidence of bronchiectasis has decreased since the introduction of antibiotics, the disease continues to have importance for the surgeon. Laënnec first described the pathologic findings of bronchiectasis in 1819,[10] and the term *bronchiectasis* was applied by Hasse in 1846.[17] The first successful operation for bronchiectasis was a partial lobe resection performed by Krause in 1898.[14] After Sicard introduced bronchography for diagnosis of bronchiectasis in 1922,[20] bronchiectasis became one of the most common diseases treated operatively in the early days of pulmonary surgery. The first successful total pneumonectomy was performed by Nissen in 1931 for bronchiectasis in a child.[16] By the 1940s, mortality fell to under 1%; and pulmonary resection for bronchiectasis remained a major portion of thoracic surgical practice in the 1950s. Whereas bronchiectasis has become relatively uncommon since the introduction of antibiotics, surgical treatment of this disease still has a role.

ETIOLOGY

Factors contributing to development of bronchiectasis may be categorized as either congenital or acquired. At least 74% of bronchiectasis cases can be attributed to acquired causes, specifically airway infection with impaired clearance of bronchial secretions leading to bronchial injury and subsequent bronchiectasis.[7] Responsible infections may be either bacterial or viral and include measles, whooping cough, pertussis, adenovirus infection, and tuberculosis. Bronchial obstruction from mucous plugging, foreign body, neoplasm, or enlarged peribronchial lymph nodes may produce bronchiectasis of the distal airway. Bronchiectasis is present in up to 39% of patients with chronic right middle lobe infection or *middle lobe syndrome*, which may involve impaired clearance of secretions secondary to anatomic configuration of the right middle lobe airway, extrinsic airway compression by lymph nodes, or inadequate collateral ventilation.[2] Aspiration, heroin ingestion, and inhalation injury with noxious gases or chemicals all can injure the airway, with resultant residual bronchiectasis. Recurrent pulmonary infection due to human immunodeficiency virus infection may also produce bronchiectasis.[9]

Although congenital bronchiectasis is unusual, several congenital disorders may produce bronchiectasis in up to 58% of children with bronchiectasis.[15] Congenital cystic bronchiectasis, with incomplete terminal airways, lack of alveolar tissue, and saccular bronchi, is now considered to be rare and the only truly congenital form of bronchiectasis. In Williams-Campbell syndrome, annular bronchial cartilage is congenitally absent, leading to bronchomalacia and bronchiectasis. Genetic abnormalities in Ehlers-Danlos and Mounier-Kuhn syndromes may contribute to tracheobronchomegaly and tracheobronchiectasis. Primary ciliary dysmotility with impaired mucociliary transport can produce bronchiectasis as an isolated abnormality or as part of Kartagener's syndrome (bronchiectasis, situs inversus, and sinusitis).[4, 15] In either partial or severe alpha₁-antitrypsin deficiency, enzyme deficiency may impair clearance of sputum elastase, producing airway damage and bronchiectasis in approximately 10% of patients. Patients with cystic fibrosis have abnormally viscid bronchial secretions and may be predisposed to bronchiectasis due to impaired clearance of bronchial airways. Intralobar bronchopulmonary sequestration may occasionally be complicated by bronchiectasis. Patients with panhypogammaglobulinemia have a clear predisposition to bronchiectasis, as may patients with human immunodeficiency virus infection or other forms of immunodeficiency.[8, 15]

PATHOPHYSIOLOGY

Bronchiectasis is defined as persistent, abnormal dilation of the bronchi, generally beyond the subsegmental level (Fig. 51–64). Reid classified the gross appearance of the bronchi into three types, cylindrical, varicose, and saccular, with the relative frequencies in surgically resected specimens of 27%, 62%, and 11%, respectively.[18] Early mucosal changes may include thickening, followed later by ulceration, inflammation, and fibrosis. The ultimate result may be bronchiolitis obliterans with little aeration of the distal alveoli and resultant atelectasis. Surrounding parenchyma is often involved with pneumonitis, and bronchial arteries may be enlarged with increased collateral blood flow into the pulmonary arteries.

In a review of 3000 bronchograms demonstrating bronchiectasis, LeRoux and associates[11] found the left lung to be involved more often than the right, with a ratio of 9 to 7. The left lower lobe was most frequently involved, followed by the right middle lobe, the lingula, the entire left lung, the right lower lobe, the entire right lung, the right upper lobe, and, finally, the left upper lobe, in descending order of frequency.

Sealy and coworkers[19] demonstrated that patients with bronchiectasis may be divided into two main groups—those with segmental disease and those with multisegmental dis-

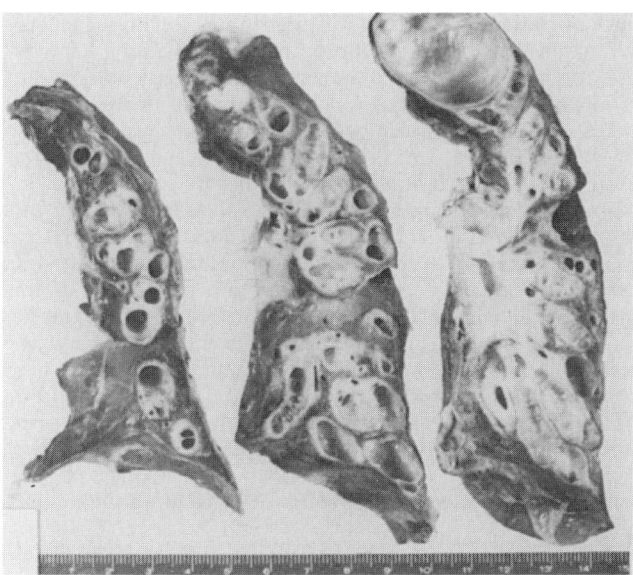

Figure 51–64. Lung specimen demonstrating grossly dilated subsegmental bronchi due to bronchiectasis. (From Bolman, R. M., and Wolfe, W. G.: Bronchiectasis and bronchopulmonary sequestration. Surg. Clin. North Am., *60*:867, 1980.)

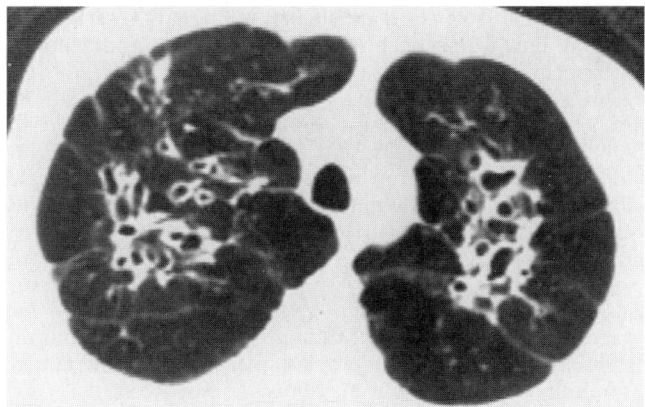

Figure 51–65. Computed tomogram of the chest of a 30-year-old man with multisegmental bronchiectasis involving both lungs. Note the abnormally dilated airways extending into the lung parenchyma bilaterally.

ease. Patients with bronchiectasis limited to a few isolated segments tended to have symptoms of shorter duration and more often related to a clear inciting event, such as pneumonia or bronchial obstruction. Patients with multisegmental disease tended to have a more chronic presentation, often with symptoms for more than 10 years. Multisegmental disease was associated with less symptomatic benefit from either medical or surgical therapy.

CLINICAL MANIFESTATIONS

In most cases, the onset of bronchiectasis is in childhood, whereas symptoms generally appear in the second or third decades of life.[5, 6] There is a female-to-male predominance of up to 2.5 to 1.[5, 19] Three fourths of the patients complain of a persistent cough productive of purulent sputum,[5, 6] with fetor oris often being present and producing social disability in up to 46% of patients.[5] As many as 50% of patients have hemoptysis, which may at times be massive secondary to the intense neovascularity that can be present in the inflamed airways.[6, 19] Repeated respiratory infection occurs in up to one third of the patients, with half of those relating episodes of pleurisy.[19]

The most common physical findings are audible rales over the involved lung fields, occurring in 55% to 91% of the patients.[19] Between 5% and 40% of the patients present with osteoarthropathy and some degree of clubbing, all of which may resolve entirely with adequate treatment.[11]

DIAGNOSIS

A clinical history of chronic, productive cough and repeated respiratory tract infection should cause one to suspect the diagnosis of bronchiectasis, but distinction from other disorders such as chronic bronchitis may be difficult. The plain chest radiograph is abnormal but generally nondiagnostic in up to 90% of patients with bronchiectasis, with common findings of increased lung markings, atelectasis, airfluid levels, or cystic spaces.[11]

After standard chest radiography, thin-section, high-resolution computed tomography has become the imaging method of choice to diagnose bronchiectasis by demonstrating abnor-

mally dilated bronchi extending into the lung parenchyma (Fig. 51–65).[13] Computed tomography has the advantage of being noninvasive, and the sensitivity and specificity of high-resolution computed tomography in diagnosing bronchiectasis can exceed 95%.

In patients who are surgical candidates, bronchography may have a role to define the bronchial anatomy for potential pulmonary resection (Fig. 51–66). Before bronchography, pulmonary toilet should be optimized with antibiotics and postural drainage, and any recent exacerbation should be allowed to clear for 4 to 6 weeks before bronchography. Reversible bronchodilation is known to occur after pulmonary infection and might be otherwise confused with bronchiectasis. Depending on institutional experience and preference, bronchography may be performed either with local anesthesia or general anesthesia. Likewise, bronchography may be performed bilaterally or at two different times, with each lung being studied individually.

Bronchoscopy may be performed in search of bronchial obstruction or endobronchial disease and to obtain sputum culture. Depending on institutional preference, bronchography may be done immediately after bronchoscopy or at a later date.[11] Bronchoscopy may also have some benefit in obtaining good tracheobronchial toilet and in assessing the

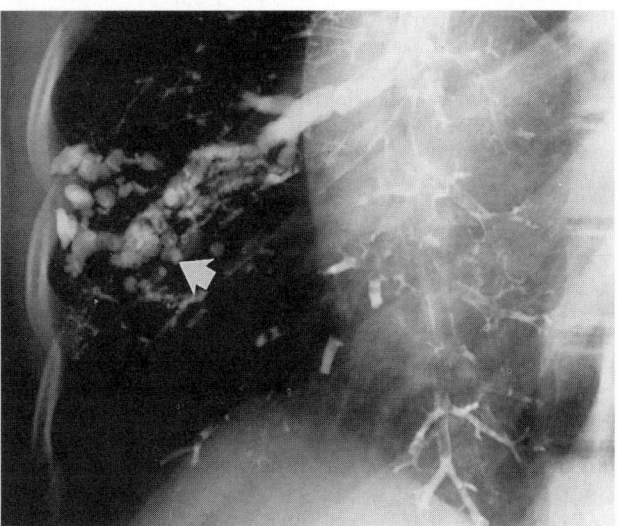

Figure 51–66. Bronchogram demonstrating saccular bronchiectasis of the right middle lobe (arrow) in an 18-year-old woman.

airway at the level of an anticipated pulmonary resection. In general, however, bronchoscopic findings are not diagnostic of bronchiectasis.[11]

An additional diagnostic procedure of potential use in bronchiectasis is sinus radiography, which can be used to look for evidence of sinusitis that may require treatment. Although pulmonary function tests in bronchiectasis generally do not demonstrate more than mild airway obstruction,[5] spirometry should be performed in surgical candidates to evaluate tolerance for lung resection. Lung ventilation and perfusion scans often show areas of relatively normal perfusion but impaired ventilation and may have some use for screening, particularly in children.[12] Quantitative immunoglobulins or sweat chloride determination may be obtained if immunodeficiency or cystic fibrosis is suspected.

TREATMENT

The mainstay of treatment for bronchiectasis is conservative medical therapy. A 2-week course of antibiotics such as amoxicillin is of proven benefit for acute exacerbations by decreasing the organism count in the sputum and by decreasing sputum protein and elastase content. Although long-term antibiotic therapy has been shown to decrease morbidity,[3] its use remains controversial and may follow the experience of cystic fibrosis with chronic nebulized antibiotic therapy being of some benefit.[21]

Chest physiotherapy and postural drainage are generally beneficial in bronchiectasis, but long-term compliance may be difficult. Patients should avoid tobacco, and consideration should be given to pneumococcal and influenza vaccine. Two neutrophil elastase inhibitors, Egin C and alpha$_1$-antitrypsin, are now available from recombinant DNA technology, and these may ultimately have some role in long-term medical management.[21]

Operative procedures should be reserved for those patients who continue to have significant symptoms despite a prolonged medical trial. Operation is seldom performed on children younger than the age of 2 years because of the likelihood of improvement on medical therapy as the child grows. In those patients who can tolerate pulmonary resection, priority is given to preservation of lung parenchyma, and a dual-lumen endotracheal tube may minimize spillage of secretions into the contralateral lung. Involved segments may be removed by either segmentectomy or lobectomy, as indicated by anatomic involvement. Pneumonectomy is rarely indicated for bronchiectasis today. For patients with bilateral disease, the side with greater involvement is resected first, with a common finding that symptoms are sufficiently improved to preclude resection of the opposite side.[19] In those patients ultimately requiring bilateral resection, an interval between procedures of 6 to 12 months is generally recommended to allow adequate recovery and evaluation of symptoms. Bilateral lung transplantation may improve the quality of life in selected patients with end-stage lung disease due to cystic fibrosis and resultant bronchiectasis.[1]

RESULTS

In studies before the use of antibiotics, life expectancy after the onset of bronchiectasis was 10 years. Death commonly ensued from septic complications such as meningitis and brain abscess.[17] After antibiotic therapy became prevalent, autopsy series[5] reported a mean age of patients dying of bronchiectasis of greater than 50. Those patients presenting with severe disease and debilitating symptoms often do progress despite therapy, with cor pulmonale or pulmonary infection as common causes of death.[5, 6]

Although data are difficult to obtain, between 18% and

36% of patients requiring hospitalization for bronchiectasis ultimately undergo operation, and the remaining majority are adequately managed with medical therapy. Of patients requiring operation for bronchiectasis, 95% of the 140 patients reported by Sealy were either asymptomatic or improved at follow-up.[19] Progression of disease to other previously uninvolved lung segments occurs in less than 5% of patients after either surgical or medical therapy.[5, 6] As demonstrated in the follow-up studies of Field,[6] children tend to experience definite improvement in the second decade of life after medical therapy alone, with persistence of this improvement into at least the third and fourth decades. Patients with bronchiectasis secondary to tuberculosis may be less likely to progress to severe symptoms than patients with bronchiectasis from other causes. Up to one third of children observed by Field after either medical or surgical therapy ultimately became free of symptoms.[6] Thus, selective application of modern surgical and medical therapy offers the patient with bronchiectasis opportunity for significant longevity and reduction in symptoms.[5]

SELECTED REFERENCES

Barker, A. F., and Bardana, E. J., Jr.: Bronchiectasis: Update of an orphan disease. Am. Rev. Respir. Dis., 137:969, 1988.
This is an excellent review of the etiology and pathophysiology of bronchiectasis with emphasis on a combination of host disorder and insult to the airways. A detailed protocol for diagnosis and evaluation of bronchiectasis is suggested.

LeRoux, B. T., Mohlala, M. L., Odell, J. A., and Whitton, I. D.: Suppurative diseases of the lung and pleural space: II. Bronchiectasis. Curr. Probl. Surg., 23:93, 1986.
The authors provide a thorough review of the history, anatomy, and surgical treatment for bronchiectasis. Supportive data come from a large South African experience of 2776 patients with bronchiectasis, of whom 1003 underwent pulmonary resection.

McGuiness, G., Naidich, D. P., Leitman, B. S., and McCauley, D. I.: Bronchiectasis: CT evaluation. AJR, 160:253, 1993.
Given the new role that computed tomography has assumed in the diagnostic evaluation of bronchiectasis, this paper thoroughly reviews the many findings and limitations of computed tomography.

Stockley, R. A.: Bronchiectasis: New therapeutic approaches based on pathogenesis. Clin. Chest Med., 8:481, 1987.
The author highlights recent developments in understanding both the pathophysiology of bronchiectasis and newer therapeutic approaches, such as nebulized antibiotics, elastase inhibitors, anti-inflammatory drugs, inhibitors of chemotaxis, superoxide scavengers, and modifiers of the immune response.

REFERENCES

1. Au, J., Scott, C., Hasan, A., Colquhoun, I., Gascoigne, A., Corris, P., Hilton, C., and Dark, J.: Bilateral sequential lung transplantation for septic lung disease: Surgical and physiologic advantages over heart-lung transplantation. Transplant Proc., 24:2652, 1992.
2. Bradham, R. R., Sealy, W. C., and Young, W. G.: Chronic middle lobe infection: Factors responsible for its development. Ann. Thorac. Surg., 2:612, 1966.
3. Currie, D. C., Garbett, N. D., Chan, K. L., Higgs, E., Todd, H., Chadwick, M. V., Gaya, H., Nunn, A. J., Darbyshire, J. H., and Cole, P. J.: Double-blind randomized study of higher-close oral amoxicillin in purulent bronchiectasis. Q. J. Med., 76:799, 1990.
4. Eliasson, R., Mossberg, B., Camner, P., and Afzelius, B. A.: The immotile-cilia syndrome: A congenital ciliary abnormality as an etiologic factor in chronic airway infections and male sterility. N. Engl. J. Med., 297:1, 1977.
5. Ellis, D. A., Thornley, P. E., Wightman, A. J., Walker, M., Chalmers, J., and Crofton, F. W.: Present outlook in bronchiectasis: Clinical and social study and review of factors influencing prognosis. Thorax, 36:659, 1981.
6. Field, C. E.: Bronchiectasis: Third report on a follow-up study of medical and surgical cases from childhood. Arch. Dis. Child., 44:551, 1969.
7. Glauser, E. M., Cook, D. C., and Hams, G. B. C.: Bronchiectasis: A review of 187 cases in children with follow-up pulmonary function studies in 58. Acta Paediatr. Scand., 165(Suppl.):1, 1966.
8. Hilton, A. M., and Doyle, L.: Immunological abnormalities in bronchiectasis with chronic bronchial suppuration. Br. J. Dis. Chest, 72:207, 1978.
9. Holmes, A. H., Trotman-Dickenson, B., Edwards, A., Peto, T., and Luzzi, G. A.: Bronchiectasis in HIV disease. Q. J. Med., 85:875, 1992.
10. Laënnec, R. T. H.: De l'Auscultation Mediate ou Traite du Diagnostic des Maladies des Poumons et du Coeur. Paris, Brosson et Chaude, 1819.

11. LeRoux, B. T., Mohlala, M. L., Odell, J. A., and Whitton, I. D.: Suppurative disease of the lung and pleural space: II. Bronchiectasis. Curr. Probl. Surg., 23:93, 1986.
12. Lewiston, N. J.: Bronchiectasis in childhood. Pediatr. Clin. North Am., 31:865, 1984.
13. McGuiness, G., Naidich, D. P., Leitman, B. S., and McCauley, D. I.: Bronchiectasis: CT evaluation. AJR, 160:253, 1993.
14. Meade, R. H.: A History of Thoracic Surgery. Springfield, Ill., Charles C Thomas, 1961, p. 47.
15. Nikolaizik, W. H., and Warner, J. O.: Aetiology of chronic suppurative lung disease. Arch. Dis. Child., 70:141, 1994.
16. Nissen, R.: Exstirpation eines ganzen Lungenflugels. Zentralbl. Chir., 58:3003, 1931.

17. Ochsner, A.: The development of pulmonary surgery, with special emphasis on carcinoma and bronchiectasis. Am. J. Surg., 135:732, 1978.
18. Reid, L. M.: Reduction in bronchial subdivision in bronchiectasis. Thorax, 5:233, 1950.
19. Sealy, W. C., Bradham, R. R., Young, W. G., Jr.: The surgical treatment of multisegmental and localized bronchiectasis. Surg. Gynecol. Obstet., 123:80, 1966.
20. Sicard, J. A., and Forestier, J.: Methode generale d'explanation radiologique par l'huile iodée. Bull. Soc. Med. Hop. Paris, 46:463, 1922.
21. Stockley, R. A.: Bronchiectasis: New therapeutic approaches based on pathogenesis. Clin. Chest Med., 8:481, 1987.
22. Varpela, E., Koistinen, J., Korhola, O., and Keskinen, H.: Deficiency of alpha-1 antitrypsin and bronchiectasis. Ann. Clin. Res., 10:79, 1978.

IX

SURGICAL TREATMENT OF PULMONARY TUBERCULOSIS

Jon F. Moran, M.D.

Pulmonary tuberculosis remains the leading infectious killer in the world, causing at least 3 million deaths annually. However, active tuberculosis has become an uncommon disease in North America and Europe. The introduction of effective chemotherapy shortly after World War II dramatically decreased the incidence of tuberculosis in the United States. This decline continued until the mid 1980s. Since 1985 the number of cases of tuberculosis has increased (Fig. 51–67). This reversal of the declining incidence of tuberculosis in the United States and Europe has been most noticeable in urban areas and seems to be coincident with the spread of human immunodeficiency virus (HIV) infection.[16] The 25,313 cases of tuberculosis reported in the United States in 1993 represented a 14% increase in total cases compared with 1985.[7] Tuberculosis involves only the lungs in 80% of cases.[20] The incidence of mycobacterial infections other than tuberculosis associated with acquired immunodeficiency syndrome (AIDS) has risen even more sharply since 1985. Despite modern antituberculous chemotherapy, approximately 2% of all cases of pulmonary mycobacterial infection require surgical treatment.

HISTORICAL ASPECTS

Throughout history pulmonary tuberculosis has been recognized as a devastating disease. Hippocrates (470–376 B.C.) wrote extensively about tuberculosis, or *phthisis* as the Greeks called it. *Phthisis* meant "a disease characterized by progressive weight loss and wasting." The Latin-based synonym was *consumption*. Tubercles, the characteristic gross pathologic changes seen in the lungs in advanced tuberculosis (Fig. 51–68), were described by the Greeks. Tuberculosis reached epidemic proportions in Europe and the United States during the eighteenth and nineteenth centuries. It is thought to have caused approximately 20% of all adult deaths in Europe during that time. In the United States in the 1920s tuberculosis was the second leading cause of death, and most victims were young adults.

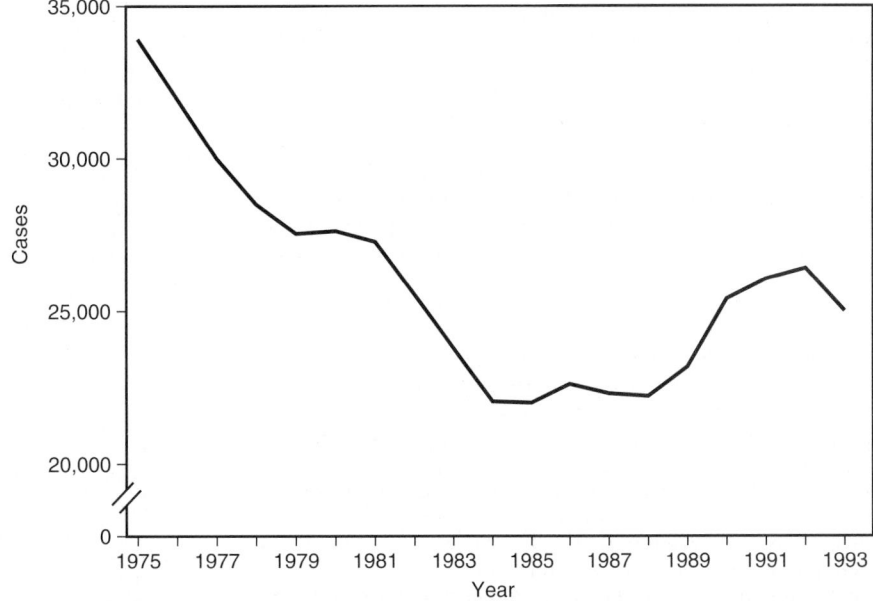

Figure 51–67. Number of reported new cases of tuberculosis in the United States, 1975–1993. During 1985 to 1993, there was an excess of approximately 64,000 reported cases, compared with the number predicted, based on the trend of decline from 1980 through 1984. (From Centers for Disease Control and Prevention: Expanded tuberculosis surveillance and tuberculosis morbidity—United States, 1993. MMWR, 43:362, 1994.)

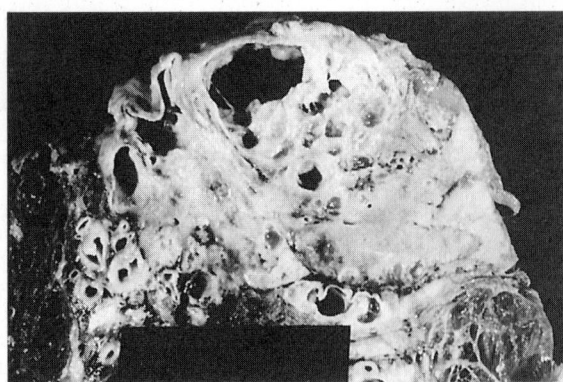

Figure 51–68. Section of the right lung with one large and numerous smaller tuberculous cavities (tubercles). The adjacent lung shows pneumonic consolidation with areas of caseous necrosis. (From Haque, A. K.: The pathology and pathophysiology of mycobacterial infections. J. Thorac. Imaging, 5:13, 1990.)

Understanding of the pathogenesis of tuberculosis evolved during the latter half of the nineteenth century. Rokitansky (1804–1878) observed that over 90% of individuals *not* dying of tuberculosis had evidence of prior tuberculosis in their lungs at autopsy. Koch's announcement in 1882 of his isolation of the tubercle bacillus was the key to understanding the etiology of tuberculosis.[21] This discovery marked the beginning of a medical crusade that led to the control of tuberculosis in developed areas of the world within 100 years. Simultaneously, Koch enunciated his *postulates* for proving bacterial causation of disease. "To prove that tuberculosis . . . is caused by invasion of bacilli and . . . the growth and multiplication of the bacilli, it was necessary to isolate the bacteria from the body; to grow them in pure culture . . .; and by administering the isolated bacilli to animals to produce the same morbid condition."

Tuberculin skin testing evolved from Koch's efforts to use "old tuberculin," a sterile filtrate of cultured tubercle bacilli, as therapy for tuberculosis.[3] His therapy failed, but Siebert altered the preparation of tuberculin, developing purified protein derivative (PPD) in 1934. By the 1940s, tuberculin skin testing and chest roentgenograms made mass screening for tuberculosis possible. It had already been shown that transmission of tuberculosis was almost exclusively by airborne bacilli; earlier case identification led to better case isolation and reduced the spread of tuberculosis. The Nobel Prize–winning discovery of streptomycin in 1944 by Waksman and the release of isoniazid in 1952 provided the first effective chemotherapy for tuberculosis.

The clinical treatment of tuberculosis changed dramatically during the century before the discovery of effective antimycobacterial drugs. The first sanatorium for tuberculosis opened in 1854 in Gorbersdorf, Germany. By 1952, there were over 100,000 sanatorium beds in the United States for the treatment of tuberculosis. The regimented routine of most sanatoria, stressing bed rest, diet, and fresh mountain air, was probably rarely effective in advanced cases. Forms of collapse therapy, including therapeutic pneumothorax, phrenic nerve division, and pneumoperitoneum, were developed and used widely during the early decades of the twentieth century. During this same period, Sauerbruch in Germany popularized thoracoplasty as treatment for pulmonary tuberculosis.[32] The yearly death rate from tuberculosis in the United States fell from 300 per 100,000 in 1880 to only 69 per 100,000 in 1935. Resectional pulmonary surgery for tuberculosis remained rare until the late 1930s. Before the development of antituberculous drugs, resectional operation for tuberculosis had a high mortality. Effective chemotherapy made resectional surgery far safer but simultaneously sharply reduced the need for surgical treatment of tuberculosis.

BACTERIOLOGY

The name *Mycobacterium* was given to this genus by Lehmann and Neumann in 1896 because of the moldlike appearance of the bacteria when grown on nutrient broth. Mycobacteria are no more related to fungi than are other bacteria. Mycobacterial cell walls have a high lipid content that prevents permeation by aniline dyes; but once a dye binds, decolorization is difficult. Koch discovered this "acid-fast" staining property of mycobacteria. The modern staining technique that bears the names of Ziehl and Neelsen is only slightly modified from Koch's original staining method. Acid-fast organisms stain red against a methylene blue counterstain.

Mycobacterium tuberculosis is responsible for the vast majority of pulmonary mycobacterial disease. *M. tuberculosis* is an obligate parasite, and humans provide its only reservoir. *M. tuberculosis* is an aerobic, nonmotile, slow-growing bacillus. Many other species of mycobacteria were isolated during the first half of the twentieth century. Several of these species can cause pulmonary infection, and they are referred to as *atypical mycobacteria*.[11] The atypical mycobacteria were divided by Runyon, a botanist, into four separate groups according to growth rate and pigment production (Table 51–21).[4, 35] Because atypical mycobacteria are frequently resistant to antituberculous drugs,[11, 38] patients with atypical mycobacterial infection represent a significant proportion of all patients referred for surgical therapy of mycobacterial disease.

Mycobacterium avium-intracellulare and *M. kansasii* are the atypical organisms that most frequently cause clinical pulmonary infection.[38] *M. avium-intracellulare* is usually resistant *in vitro* to most antituberculous drugs. It is a common cause of disease in patients with AIDS; however, it is rarely localized in these patients, and surgical treatment is rarely indicated in this patient group.[16, 38] Unlike *M. avium-intracellulare*, *M. kansasii* has not become a common pathogen in individuals with AIDS. In contrast to *M. avium-intracellulare*, *M. kansasii* more often shows *in vitro* susceptibility to antimycobacterial drugs; as a result, patients with *M. kansasii* pulmonary disease require surgical treatment less frequently.[11]

PATHOLOGY

The pathologic responses within the lung to the various common mycobacteria are identical.[15, 25] *M. tuberculosis* is a virulent organism requiring a *very small* inoculum for infection to occur *even* in normal lung tissue. Atypical mycobacteria are less virulent and more frequently cause infection either in previously damaged lung tissue or in immunocompromised individuals. Mycobacteria gain entry to the body by inhalation of droplet nuclei less than 5 μm. in diameter, containing only one to three bacteria. A first infection in an unsensitized host causes a localized necrotizing pneumonia.

TABLE 51–21. Classification of Atypical Mycobacterial Species (Runyon)

Group I	Photochromogens	*M. kansasii*
Group II	Scotochromogens	*M. scrofulaceum*
Group III	Nonchromogens	*M. avium-intracellulare*
		M. xenopi
Group IV	Rapid growers	*M. fortuitum*
		M. chelonei

Mycobacteria spread from this pneumonic focus through the lymphatics to the hilar lymph nodes. The peripheral pneumonic process is characterized by *caseous* necrosis, with formation of a granuloma containing mycobacteria with a rim of granulation tissue (Fig. 51–69). *Caseous* describes the gross appearance of the lesion with cheeselike material within a thin capsule. The peripheral lung lesion accompanied by hilar nodal enlargement is called the primary Ghon complex. Generally, the infection is contained at this stage by the body's immune responses.

Primary tuberculosis refers to the initial infection with *M. tuberculosis* in a previously unsensitized host. In the past this form of disease most frequently occurred in children and was referred to as *childhood tuberculosis.* As the prevalence of tuberculosis infection has declined, the incidence of primary tuberculosis in adults has risen. Primary tuberculosis may present as a large necrotizing pneumonia that progresses to cavitation with transbronchial spread. The areas of pneumonic infiltrate in primary tuberculosis tend to be in the lower lobes. Organisms may pass into the venous blood and be disseminated widely. When hematogenous spread is not stopped by cell-mediated immunity, the disease spreads most commonly to the lung apices, the kidneys, the epiphyses of long bones, or the brain. These locations are favored by the strict aerobic growth requirement of mycobacteria. Occasionally, hematogenous spread leads to miliary tuberculosis, which is massive hematogenous spread, giving rise to thousands of 1- to 2-mm. (millet seed–sized) tubercles throughout the body.

The most common pattern of mycobacterial infection is *reinfection* or *postprimary tuberculosis.* Postprimary tuberculosis begins as a segmental pneumonia in the apical or posterior segment of an upper lobe or the superior segment of a lower lobe. Bilateral lung involvement is common in postprimary tuberculosis. These pneumonic infiltrates progress to caseous necrosis, and cavity formation occurs when the area of liquefaction erodes into an adjacent bronchus. The size of the cavities formed varies from 2 to 12 cm., depending on the amount of lung destroyed before spontaneous drainage occurs. Erosion of a cavity into a bronchial vessel may cause severe hemoptysis. A Rasmussen aneurysm, an aneurysm of a pulmonary artery or arteriole within or adjacent to a cavity, is found in about 4% of advanced cavitary disease. These aneurysms may rupture, causing massive hemoptysis and asphyxiation. There is usually intense inflammatory reaction in the rim of lung surrounding tuberculous cavities. The

overlying visceral pleura tends to contract, decreasing the volume of the involved portion of the lung. The visceral and parietal pleurae are involved by this intense reaction, obliterating the pleural space and densely fusing the adjacent pleurae. This intense pleural reaction makes operative separation of the two pleural surfaces overlying the diseased portions of the lung essentially impossible.

Cavity formation permits spread of infection to the proximal bronchial mucosa. Endobronchial tuberculosis may cause bronchial stenosis with distal superimposed bacterial or fungal infection.[6, 23] Cavities can rupture into the pleural space and create a tuberculous or mixed tuberculous and bacterial empyema. Tuberculous empyema may also occur secondary to hematogenous or lymphatic seeding of the pleural space. Many pleural effusions associated with tuberculosis are the result of a hypersensitivity reaction in the pleural space and do not represent actual infection of the pleural space. Pure tuberculous effusions or effusions secondary to a hypersensitivity reaction tend to resolve very quickly after initiation of effective chemotherapy.

DIAGNOSIS

There is an important distinction between mycobacterial infection and mycobacterial disease.[13] Infection implies the entry of a mycobacterial organism into the body without symptoms or overt clinical evidence of disease. The diagnosis of mycobacterial pulmonary disease depends on the confirmation of active disease by radiographic and bacteriologic studies. Only 5% to 15% of individuals infected with *M. tuberculosis* develop clinically significant disease. The American Thoracic Society classifies tuberculosis infection into four categories: Category 0, no tuberculosis exposure (no exposure history, negative tuberculin skin test); Category I, tuberculosis exposure without infection (history of exposure, negative tuberculin skin test); Category II, tuberculosis infection without disease (positive tuberculin skin test without clinical disease); and Category III, tuberculosis disease proven by symptoms, roentgenographic studies, and bacteriologic studies.

The symptoms of pulmonary mycobacterial disease can be subtle. Symptoms include chronic productive cough, easy fatigability, weight loss, chest pain, hemoptysis, fever, and night sweats. Any history of exposure or membership in a high-risk group should increase the index of suspicion for mycobacterial disease. Pulmonary mycobacterial infection is more common in immunosuppressed patients (secondary to corticosteroids, cancer chemotherapy, transplant immunosuppression, or AIDS); in diabetics; after gastrectomy; and in individuals with silicosis, pneumoconiosis, or reticuloendothelial malignancies.[20, 31]

Mycobacterial disease in the lung can cause a variety of roentgenographic abnormalities.[5, 22, 33, 39] The most frequent radiographic findings in pulmonary tuberculosis are apical upper- or lower-lobe infiltrates with frequent cavitation (Fig. 51–70). The chest film findings in atypical mycobacterial disease are indistinguishable from those seen with tuberculosis.[40]

Skin Testing. Skin testing, using PPD from *M. tuberculosis* organisms, was widely adopted as a screening test for mycobacterial infection in the middle part of the twentieth century. Most patients are sensitized to the protein fraction of the tubercle bacillus within several weeks after the onset of infection. Current standard tuberculosis skin testing involves the intracutaneous injection of five tuberculin units (T.U.) of PPD on the volar aspect of the forearm. This is termed an *intermediate PPD,* and the extent of local reaction is evaluated after 48 to 72 hours. A positive test is defined as greater than 5, 10, or 15 mm. of induration depending on the likelihood of

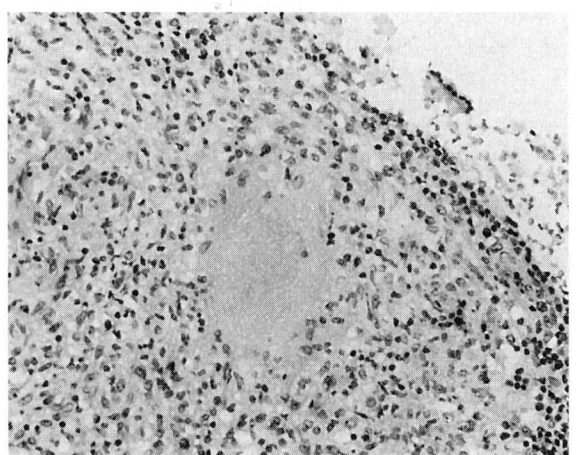

Figure 51–69. Caseating tuberculous granuloma showing a small area of central caseous necrosis (original magnification, ×200). (From Haque, A. K.: The pathology and pathophysiology of mycobacterial infections. J. Thorac. Imaging, *5*:9, 1990.)

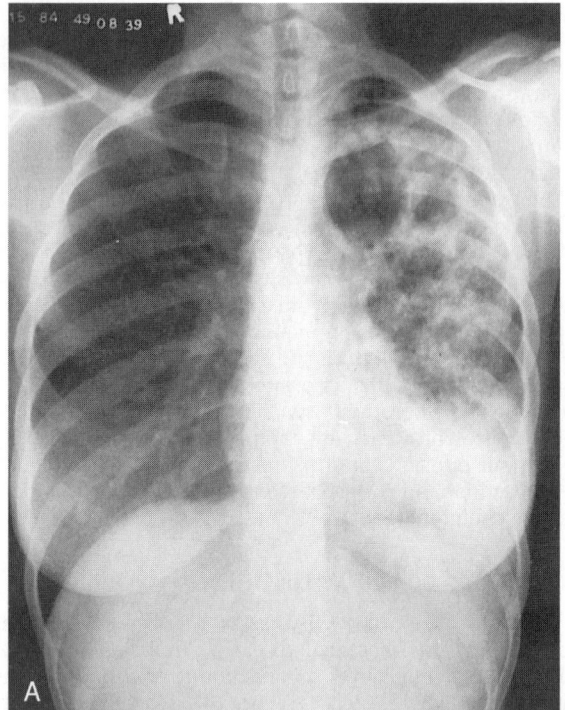

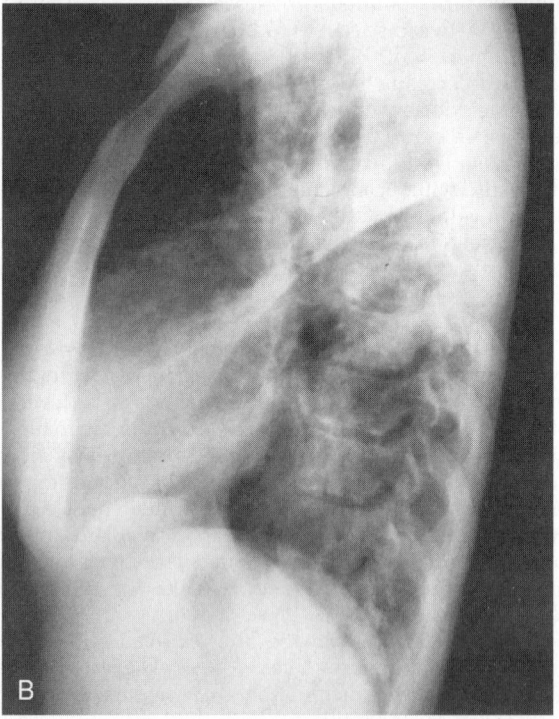

Figure 51–70. Posteroanterior (A) and lateral (B) chest radiographs showing typical appearance of postprimary tuberculosis. Extensive air space disease is evident in the left upper and lower lobes with multiple cavities. (From Buckner, C. B., and Walker, C. W.: Radiologic manifestations of adult tuberculosis. J. Thorac. Imaging, 5:35, 1990.)

infection.[3] For any population, the likelihood that a positive tuberculin test represents infection is influenced by the prevalence of infection. Tuberculin testing remains a useful test in populations with a prevalence of infection greater than 25%. Tuberculin reactions may be blunted in the elderly or in seriously ill individuals.

Smear and Culture. The isolation of mycobacterial organisms from the sputum or lung tissue is required to confirm the diagnosis of pulmonary mycobacterial disease. Early morning sputum specimens or washings obtained by fiberoptic bronchoscopy can be especially helpful in establishing a diagnosis. The presence of acid-fast organisms on smear allows a rapid presumptive diagnosis. Cultures are necessary to document the specific type of mycobacterial disease. Mycobacterial cultures require 3 to 6 weeks to grow, and it is often necessary to obtain multiple samples before a positive smear or culture is obtained. Smear positivity requires approximately 10,000 organisms per milliliter of sputum. When the clinical pattern supports the diagnosis of pulmonary mycobacterial disease, antimycobacterial chemotherapy is often begun as a 1- to 2-month therapeutic trial. Because patients referred for surgical treatment frequently are infected with organisms resistant to many antituberculous drugs, culture results with accurate sensitivity testing for most available antimycobacterial agents are particularly important in patients being considered for surgical intervention.

CHEMOTHERAPY

The vast majority of patients with pulmonary mycobacterial disease can be cured with appropriate chemotherapy. Many antimycobacterial drugs have been developed since Waksman's discovery of streptomycin in 1944.[2, 9, 10] Effective antimycobacterial drugs have made resectional therapy for mycobacterial disease relatively safe when it is required.

Initial treatment of pulmonary mycobacterial disease usually begins before the infecting organism is precisely identified and before the drug sensitivity pattern of the organism is known. Two or three antimycobacterial drugs should be administered initially to avoid the emergence of drug-resistant organisms.[2, 26] Compliance with the prescribed chemotherapy regimen is essential to a successful outcome. Mycobacterial organisms react differently to antimycobacterial drugs, depending on whether the organisms are extracellular or intracellular. Extracellular organisms tend to multiply rapidly in the hyperoxic neutral pH environment of the pulmonary cavity. Organisms within activated macrophages are in an acidic environment that slows growth. An effective treatment program halts mycobacterial growth intracellularly and extracellularly, converting the patient to a sputum-negative status within 6 weeks. The five most commonly employed antimycobacterial drugs are listed in Table 51–22. Atypical mycobacterial infections and drug-resistant M. tuberculosis infections may require the use of other antibiotics.[11, 14, 18]

During the 1960s and 1970s, the standard treatment regimen for pulmonary tuberculosis required 18 to 24 months of continuous therapy using two or three drugs throughout the treatment. Short-course therapy (6 to 9 months) has now been shown to be equally effective. The American Thoracic Society recommends two alternative regimens for treatment of pulmonary tuberculosis: 1) a 6-month regimen consisting of isoniazid, rifampin, and pyrazinamide given for 2 months, followed by isoniazid and rifampin for 4 months; 2) alternatively, a 9-month regimen of isoniazid and rifampin is acceptable for persons who cannot or should not take pyrazinamide.[2] With either regimen, ethambutol should be added initially until the results of drug susceptibility tests are available. Streptomycin should be used in place of ethambutol in children too young to be monitored for visual acuity. The major determinant of the outcome of treatment is patient adherence to the drug regimen, and consideration should be given to treating all patients with directly observed therapy. Multiple-drug–resistant tuberculosis (resistance to at least isoniazid and rifampin) presents a difficult treatment problem.[14, 18] The results of susceptibility studies should be used to individualize treatment in drug-resistant cases.[27]

The primary drug resistance rate for M. tuberculosis in the

TABLE 51–22. Commonly Used Antimycobacterial Drugs

| Drug | Daily Dosage | | Common Side Effects | Comments |
	Children	Adults		
Isoniazid	10–20 mg./kg., orally or intramuscularly	5 mg./kg., orally or intramuscularly	Hepatitis, peripheral neuritis	Bactericidal to both intracellular and extracellular organisms; pyridoxine, 10 mg./kg./day, as prophylaxis for neuritis
Rifampin	10–20 mg./kg., orally	10 mg./kg., orally	Hepatitis, febrile reaction	Bactericidal to both intracellular and extracellular organisms; colors urine orange; inhibits the effect of oral contraceptives, quinidine, digitalis, corticosteroids, and warfarin
Pyrazinamide	15–20 mg./kg., orally	15–30 mg./kg., orally	Hepatoxicity, hyperuricemia, arthralgia	Bactericidal to intracellular organisms; reduces total length of chemotherapy required
Streptomycin	20–40 mg./kg., intramuscularly	15 mg./kg., intramuscularly	Eighth cranial nerve damage, nephrotoxicity	Bactericidal to extracellular organisms within cavities; limit dose to 10 mg./kg. in elderly patients
Ethambutol	15–25 mg./kg., orally	15–25 mg./kg., orally	Optic neuritis (reversible), rash	Bacteriostatic to both intracellular and extracellular organisms

United States varies geographically and among ethnic groups but is generally about 14%.[18] Worldwide the prevalence of primary drug-resistant tuberculosis is generally higher than that found in the United States. The primary drug resistance rate for tuberculosis is estimated to be greater than 20% in China and India, and greater than 35% in Pakistan and the Philippines. The increasing frequency of primary drug-resistant tuberculosis and atypical mycobacterial pulmonary disease makes accurate sensitivity testing to a variety of chemotherapeutic agents important in order to optimize the selected drug regimen. Although atypical mycobacteria are frequently resistant *in vitro* to many or all of the usual drugs, four- and five-drug regimens may still be effective.[36, 38] Efficacy of any drug regimen is increased by selection of drugs to which the particular mycobacterial organism is susceptible.[14, 17] Because pulmonary mycobacterial disease caused by drug-resistant organisms is often referred for surgical intervention, accurate drug susceptibility testing and familiarity with the use of a variety of antimycobacterial drugs are important for the surgeon.

Coordination of chemotherapy and surgical intervention requires careful planning. Patients who have been converted to sputum-negative status preoperatively have fewer complications during and after resectional operation.[24, 29] Optimal pulmonary toilet, careful selection of chemotherapy, and the addition of one or two new drugs during the perioperative period are useful in reducing perioperative morbidity. Whenever possible, the patient should receive 1 to 2 months of appropriate chemotherapy before operation. In treating multiple-drug–resistant organisms (either *M. tuberculosis* or atypical mycobacteria), two or three drugs to which the infecting organism is susceptible should be given perioperatively and for 6 to 9 months postoperatively. In the case of organisms that exhibit resistance to all chemotherapeutic agents, the administration of isoniazid and rifampin for a period of 9 to 12 months postoperatively is still recommended.

SURGICAL TREATMENT

During the nineteenth century it was noted that when a pneumothorax occurred in a patient with pulmonary tuberculosis, the patient's symptoms seemed to improve, popularizing the concept that collapsing the affected portion of lung allowed the diseased area to rest and recover. The efficacy of collapse therapy probably derived from the lowering of oxygen tensions in the collapsed portion of the lung, thereby inhibiting growth of *M. tuberculosis*, a strict aerobe. A variety of techniques, including artificially induced pneumothorax, unilateral phrenic nerve division, extraperiosteal thoracoplasty with plombage, and standard paravertebral thoracoplasty, were developed to encourage collapse of the infected portions of the lung.[1] Before the discovery of effective chemotherapy for tuberculosis, extrapleural paravertebral thoracoplasty was the most frequently employed surgical procedure for the treatment of pulmonary tuberculosis. Thoracoplasty achieved closure of tuberculous cavities in more than 80% of patients without chemotherapy. Today thoracoplasty is rarely indicated as primary treatment for pulmonary tuberculosis.[28] Paravertebral thoracoplasty remains a reasonable operation for the treatment of selected bronchopleural fistulas and empyemas and for bronchopleural fistulas complicating surgical resections in other settings.

Surgical treatment of pulmonary mycobacterial disease is rarely necessary. When an operation is required, resection of the diseased or destroyed portion of the lung is the procedure of choice. Before the availability of effective chemotherapy, pulmonary resection for tuberculosis had an operative mortality of 20% to 40%. Once effective chemotherapy for pulmonary tuberculosis became available, pulmonary resection rapidly replaced thoracoplasty as the surgical treatment of choice. Compared with thoracoplasty, pulmonary resection has the advantage of achieving prompt conversion to sputum-negative status in a single stage without creating any chest wall deformity or severe limitation of ventilatory capacity. Elective pulmonary resection for mycobacterial disease now carries a low mortality and morbidity.[24, 29, 30]

The efficacy of modern antimycobacterial chemotherapy has reduced the commonly accepted indications for surgical intervention and pulmonary resection to the following:

1. *Persistently positive sputum cultures with cavitation after 5 to 6 months of continuous optimal chemotherapy with two or more drugs.* The chemotherapy should include isoniazid and rifampin, and the organism must be shown to be susceptible to both drugs. Otherwise, a change in the chemotherapy regimen is indicated. Relative indications for surgical intervention such as severe cavitation, bronchiectasis, or bronchial stenosis may contribute to the failure of chemotherapy in some individuals.

2. *Localized pulmonary disease caused by* M. avium-intracellulare *(or another atypical mycobacterium with a similar broad resistance to chemotherapy).* Localized pulmonary disease due

to drug-resistant *M. tuberculosis* is also an indication for pulmonary resection.[18] *Localized* disease is defined as any disease that can be encompassed by one or two pulmonary resections.

3. *A mass lesion of the lung in an area of tuberculous involvement.* This is an indication for resection for simultaneous diagnosis of the mass lesion and treatment of the mycobacterial disease. In the 1990s this is undoubtedly the most common indication for surgical resection of pulmonary mycobacterial disease.[37]

4. *Massive life-threatening hemoptysis or recurrent severe hemoptysis.* This is an indication for resection of the portion of the lung that is the source of the hemorrhage. Pulmonary hemorrhage is a rare, but frequently fatal complication of pulmonary mycobacterial disease. Tuberculosis continues to be the most common cause of massive hemoptysis. Massive hemoptysis is defined as greater than 600 ml. per 24 hours, whereas severe hemoptysis is defined as greater than 200 ml. per 24 hours. Asphyxiation, rather than hypovolemia, is the usual cause of death from hemoptysis. The site of bleeding is almost invariably a cavitary lesion. The bleeding arises from the abundant bronchial arterial circulation to the cavitated portion of the lung. Often the cavity that is the source of bleeding has been suprainfected with an opportunistic fungal organism such as *Aspergillus*.[6] Mild or moderate hemorrhage usually ceases with sedation, bed rest, and careful control of the patient's blood pressure. Bronchoscopy is performed to determine the lobe from which the bleeding arises, because these patients frequently have bilateral cavitary changes. Severe hemoptysis is unpredictable, and fatal hemorrhage can occur suddenly in seemingly stable patients. Various forms of nonoperative therapy frequently control bleeding for prolonged periods, but bleeding will recur in at least 30% of cases. In stabilized patients with a localized site of bleeding, lobectomy is the most definitive form of therapy for massive or recurrent severe hemoptysis.[8]

5. *A bronchopleural fistula secondary to mycobacterial infection that does not respond to tube thoracostomy.* This usually requires surgical treatment and may require pulmonary resection. The mixed tuberculous and pyogenic empyema that occurs when a bronchopleural fistula develops in a lung severely damaged by mycobacterial disease rarely responds to antimicrobial therapy alone. The efficacy of tube thoracostomy is limited in such cases by the dense pleural reaction that inhibits full re-expansion of the lung. Formal decortication can lead to full re-expansion of the underlying lung with excellent recovery of pulmonary function. Often, the pleural reaction is so intense that decortication is impossible. Open drainage of the pleural space by creation of an Eloesser flap is an excellent alternative procedure if the patient's overall condition is marginal.[12]

Several special situations may call for surgical treatment of pulmonary mycobacterial disease. Patients severely symptomatic from a destroyed lobe or bronchiectatic area of the lung may benefit from resection. Patients with thick-walled cavities who have reactivated mycobacterial disease or who cannot comply with prolonged chemotherapy may benefit from resection of the diseased area. A patient with a *trapped lung* with severely decreased ventilatory capacity after a tuberculous empyema may benefit from decortication to allow full expansion of the underlying lung.

There are a few specific contraindications to pulmonary resection for mycobacterial disease. Widespread pulmonary or endobronchial disease is generally a contraindication to resection. Children with mycobacterial disease rarely require lung resection. Mycobacterial disease in children often progresses to lobar tuberculous pneumonia with massive lymph node enlargement, but cavitation is rare. In children, chemo-

therapy is almost invariably curative, with complete resolution radiographically and excellent recovery of lung function.[19, 33, 34]

In planning an operation for mycobacterial infection, it is important that the patient's cardiopulmonary reserve be adequate to sustain the patient through the contemplated procedure. Every effort should be made to convert the patient to sputum-negative status before operation, including the administration of additional antimycobacterial drugs perioperatively. Adequate nutritional support and physical therapy to encourage overall physical conditioning and optimal pulmonary toilet are beneficial preoperatively. Preoperative bronchoscopy should be done on all patients considered for pulmonary resection to exclude active proximal endobronchial disease. Active endobronchial disease interferes with healing of the bronchial stump after resection. Generally, proximal endobronchial disease can be cleared by chemotherapy before pulmonary resection. The use of a double-lumen endotracheal tube can make operations for tuberculosis technically easier and safer. The dependent lung can be protected from contamination by secretions from the infected upper lung while the patient is in the lateral position. In cases of massive hemoptysis, a double-lumen tube partially protects the dependent lung during the resection of the bleeding site in the upper lung.

The extent of pulmonary resection depends on the extent of the mycobacterial disease and is guided by the principle that all gross evidence of disease should be resected. Conservation of pulmonary tissue and pulmonary function is desirable. For active mycobacterial disease, a lobectomy is usually required. The dense pleural reaction characteristic of mycobacterial disease makes separation of the segments in the upper lobes difficult. A generous wedge resection can be used for a mass lesion that is being excised to exclude the presence of carcinoma. Pneumonectomy is required only in the setting of a totally destroyed lung.

The operative techniques of lobectomy and pneumonectomy as presented elsewhere in this text do not need to be altered for the patient with tuberculosis. Because mycobacterial disease is a peripheral process with overlying dense pleural reaction, it is frequently necessary to mobilize portions of the lung in the *extrapleural* plane. Full re-expansion of the remaining lung tissue is important to avoid the complications of atelectasis, hemothorax, and apical space problems. Bronchoscopy may be required at the conclusion of the operation to clear infected secretions or blood from the airway.

Administration of effective antimycobacterial drugs, judicious timing of operation, careful operative technique, and attentive postoperative care are the important factors in avoiding serious complications from pulmonary resection for mycobacterial disease.[24, 29] Patients referred for operation generally have problems that predispose them to perioperative complications.[30] Good pulmonary toilet and careful attention to the pleural drainage system are necessary to ensure full re-expansion of the remaining lung. Two specific complications of resection for mycobacterial disease are particularly troublesome: *empyema*, with or without bronchopleural fistula, and *bronchogenic spread* of the mycobacterial disease. These complications occur more frequently when the patient is sputum-positive at the time of operation. The incidence of bronchopleural fistula after resection for mycobacterial disease is approximately 3%. An apical space problem occurs after approximately 20% of resections for mycobacterial disease, but only 10% to 15% of these patients develop a bronchopleural fistula or empyema. Judicious use of thoracoplasty or liberal use of muscle flaps in patients with positive sputa at the time of operation can minimize the incidence of bronchopleural fistula and apical space problems.[29] Appropriate treatment of empyema in this setting is tube thoracostomy with later conversion to open drainage if a lung remnant is present. Subsequent thoracoplasty may be required.

Careful patient selection, improved anesthetic techniques, the use of stapling devices, and better chemotherapy have contributed to the steadily decreasing morbidity and mortality associated with resectional operations for pulmonary mycobacterial disease. Resectional operations are now employed in a highly selected group of patients who have failed chemotherapy or who have suffered serious complications such as massive hemoptysis or bronchopleural fistula. Mortality for pulmonary resection is low, with a relatively low morbidity when surgical intervention is elective. The incidence of major complications is generally less than 15%. When resection is performed as an emergency procedure, mortality is significant and perioperative morbidity high. Long-term prognosis after successful resection is excellent, with 90% of patients who undergo operation for active mycobacterial disease surviving and remaining free of disease.

SELECTED REFERENCES

American Thoracic Society: Treatment of tuberculosis and tuberculosis infection in adults and children. Am. J. Respir. Crit. Care Med., 149:1359, 1994.
This official statement of the American Thoracic Society presents detailed recommendations for the treatment of tuberculosis in adults and children. This article reviews all of the available antituberculous drugs and the various dosage regimens that are effective. A wide variety of special situations in the treatment of tuberculosis are considered, and specific recommendations for each situation are given.

Friedman, L. N. (Ed.): Tuberculosis: Current Concepts and Treatment. Boca Raton, FL, CRC Press, 1994.
This multiauthored book covers recent advances in laboratory methods useful in the diagnosis and treatment of mycobacterial diseases. The epidemiology, pathophysiology, clinical presentation, and optimal treatment of tuberculosis are reviewed.

Pomerantz, M., Madsen, L. Goble, M., and Iseman, M.: Surgical management of resistant mycobacterial tuberculosis and other mycobacterial pulmonary infections. Ann. Thorac. Surg., 52:1108, 1991.
This article reports a large series of pulmonary resections for drug-resistant mycobacterial infections. Proper timing and guidelines for operative intervention are discussed.

Reichman, L. B., and Hershfield, E. S.: Tuberculosis: A Comprehensive International Approach. New York, Marcel Dekker, 1993.
This book exhaustively considers every aspect of tuberculosis and related mycobacterial infections. History, worldwide epidemiology, the role of HIV infection, appropriate diagnosis and treatment, as well as research and control strategies for the future are presented.

Rubin, S. A.: Tuberculosis—1990. J. Thorac. Imaging, 5:1, 1990.
This symposium reviews the microbiology, pathophysiology, and treatment of pulmonary mycobacterial infections with emphasis on the radiologic manifestations of these diseases.

REFERENCES

1. Alexander, J.: The Collapse Therapy of Pulmonary Tuberculosis. Springfield, Ill., Charles C Thomas, 1937.
2. American Thoracic Society: Treatment of tuberculosis and tuberculosis infections in adults and children. Am. J. Respir. Crit. Care Med., 149:1359, 1994.
3. Bass, J. B., Jr.: The tuberculin test. *In* Reichman, L. B., and Hershfield, E. S. (Eds.): Tuberculosis: A Comprehensive International Approach. New York, Marcel Dekker, 1993, pp. 139–148.
4. Boyars, M. C.: The microbiology, chemotherapy, and surgical treatment of tuberculosis. J. Thorac. Imaging, 5:1, 1990.
5. Buckner, C. B., and Walker, C. W.: Radiologic manifestations of adult tuberculosis. J. Thorac. Imaging, 5:28, 1990.
6. Butz, R. O., Zvetina, J. R., and Leininger, B. J.: Ten-year experience with mycetomas in patients with pulmonary tuberculosis. Chest, 87:356, 1985.
7. Centers for Disease Control and Prevention: Expanded tuberculosis surveillance and tuberculosis morbidity—United States, 1993. MMWR, 43:361, 1994.
8. Cahill, B. C., and Ingbar, D. H.: Massive hemoptysis, assessment and management. Clin. Chest Med. 15:147, 1994.
9. Cynamon, M. H., and Klemens, S. P.: Chemotherapeutic agents for myco-
10. Davidson, P. T., and Le, H. Q.: Drug treatment of tuberculosis—1992. Drugs, 43:651, 1992.
11. Davidson, P. T.: *M. avium* complex, *M. kansasii, M. fortuitum,* and other mycobacteria causing human disease. *In* Reichman, L. B., and Hershfield, E. S. (Eds.): Tuberculosis: A Comprehensive International Approach. New York, Marcel Dekker, 1993, pp. 505–530.
12. Eloesser, L.: An operation for tuberculous empyema. Surg. Gynecol. Obstet., 60:1096, 1935.
13. Glassroth, J.: Diagnosis of tuberculosis. *In* Reichman, L. B., and Hershfield, E. S. (Eds.): Tuberculosis: A Comprehensive International Approach. New York, Marcel Dekker, 1993, pp. 149–166.
14. Goble, M., Iseman, M. D., Madsen, L. A., Waite, D., Ackerson, L., and Horsburgh, C. R., Jr.: Treatment of 171 patients with pulmonary tuberculosis resistant to isoniazid and rifampin. N. Engl. J. Med., 328:527, 1993.
15. Haque, A. K.: The pathology and pathophysiology of mycobacterial infections. J. Thorac Imaging, 5:8, 1990.
16. Hopewell, P. C.: Tuberculosis and infection with the human immunodeficiency virus. *In* Reichman, L. B., and Hershfield, E. S.: Tuberculosis: A Comprehensive International Approach. New York, Marcel Dekker, 1993, pp. 369–394.
17. Horsburgh, C. R., Jr., Mason, U. G., III, Heifets, L. B., Southwick, K., Labrecque, J., and Iseman, M. D.: Response to therapy of pulmonary *Mycobacterium avium-intracellulare* infection correlates with results of *in vitro* susceptibility testing. Am. Rev. Respir. Dis., 135:418, 1987.
18. Iseman, M. D.: Treatment of multidrug-resistant tuberculosis. N. Engl. J. Med., 329:784, 1993.
19. Jacobs, R. F., and Eisenach, K. D.: Childhood tuberculosis. Adv. Pediatr. Infect. Dis., 8:23, 1993.
20. Jereb, J. A., Cauthens, G. M., Kelly, G. D., and Geiter, L. J.: The epidemiology of tuberculosis. *In* Friedman, L. N. (Ed.): Tuberculosis: Current Concepts and Treatment. Boca Raton, Fla., CRC Press, 1994, pp. 1–26.
21. Koch, R.: Die Aetiologie der Tuberculose, a translation by B. Pinner and M. Pinner. Am. Rev. Tuberc., 25:285, 1932.
22. Kuhlman, J. E., Deutsch, J. H., Fishman, E. K., and Siegelman, S. S.: CT features of thoracic mycobacterial disease. Radiographics, 10:413, 1990.
23. Lee, J. H., Park, S. S., Lee, D. H., Shin, D. H., Yang, S. C., and Yoo, B. M.: Endobronchial tuberculosis: Clinical and bronchoscopic features in 121 cases. Chest, 102:990, 1992.
24. Moran, J. F., Alexander, L. G., Staub, E. W., Young, W. G., Jr., and Sealy, W. C.: Long-term results of pulmonary resection for atypical mycobacterial disease. Ann. Thorac. Surg., 35:597, 1983.
25. Nardell, E. A.: Pathogenesis of tuberculosis. *In* Reichman, L. B., and Hershfield, E. S. (Eds.): Tuberculosis: A Comprehensive International Approach. New York, Marcel Dekker, 1993, pp. 103–122.
26. O'Brien, R. J.: The treatment of tuberculosis. *In* Reichman, L. B., and Hershfield, E. S. (Eds.): Tuberculosis: A Comprehensive International Approach. New York, Marcel Dekker, 1993, pp. 207–240.
27. Peloquin, C. A.: Pharmacology of the antimycobacterial drugs. Med. Clin. North Am., 77:1253, 1993.
28. Peppas, G., Molnar, T. F., Jeyasingham, K., and Kirk, A. B.: Thoracoplasty in the context of current surgical practice. Ann. Thorac. Surg., 56:903, 1993.
29. Pomerantz, M., Madsen, L., Goble, M., and Iseman, M.: Surgical management of resistant mycobacterial tuberculosis and other mycobacterial pulmonary infections. Ann. Thorac. Surg., 52:1108, 1991.
30. Reed, C. E., Parker, E. F., and Crawford, F. A.: Surgical resection for complications of pulmonary infections. Ann. Thorac. Surg., 48:165, 1989.
31. Rieder, H. L., Cauthen, G. M., Comstock, G. W., and Snider, D. E., Jr.: Epidemiology of tuberculosis in the United States. Epidemiol. Rev., 11:79, 1989.
32. Sauerbruch, F., and Schumacher, E. D.: Technik der Thoraxchirurgie. Berlin, Springer-Verlag, 1911.
33. Stansberry, S. D.: Tuberculosis in infants and children. J. Thorac. Imaging, 5:17, 1990.
34. Starke, J. R., Jacob, R. F., and Jereb, J.: Resurgence of tuberculosis in children. J. Pediatr., 120:839, 1992.
35. Timpe, A., and Runyon, E. H.: The relationship of "atypical acid-fast" bacteria to human disease: A preliminary report. J. Lab. Clin. Med., 44:202, 1954.
36. Tsukamura, M.: Evidence that antituberculosis drugs are really effective in the treatment of pulmonary infection caused by *Mycobacterium avium* complex. Am. Rev. Respir. Dis., 137:144, 1988.
37. Whyte, R. I., Deegan, S. P., Kaplan, D. K., Evans, C. C., and Donelly, R. J.: Recent surgical experience for pulmonary tuberculosis. Respir. Med., 83:357, 1989.
38. Wright, P. W., and Wallace, R. J., Jr.: Nontuberculous mycobacteria with and without HIV infection. *In* Friedman, L. N. (Ed.): Tuberculosis: Current Concepts and Treatment. Boca Raton, Fla., CRC Press, 1994, pp. 183–206.
39. Winer-Muram, H. T., and Rubin, S. A.: Thoracic complications of tuberculosis. J. Thorac. Imaging, 5:46, 1990.
40. Woodring, J. H., and Vandiviere, H. M.: Pulmonary disease caused by nontuberculous mycobacteria. J. Thorac. Imaging, 5:64, 1990.

X

BENIGN TUMORS OF THE TRACHEA AND BRONCHI

David H. Harpole, Jr., M.D.

Benign tumors of the trachea and bronchi consist of a variety of histologic masses that can be derived from any of the cells in the respiratory tract. Although these lesions were observed infrequently in large autopsy series of the past century,[10] Killian reported the initial premortem experience in 1897 soon after the introduction of indirect laryngoscopy.[10] Since 1900, several retrospective series have been published in the medical literature, including a 30-year experience at the Mayo Clinic with only 63 benign tumors or tumorlike conditions of the trachea and proximal bronchi.[3] In spite of the rarity of these tumors, a detailed description is warranted to aid in the early recognition of these potentially obstructive masses.

INCIDENCE

Most primary tumors of the tracheal and proximal bronchi are malignant, the majority being squamous cell or adenoid cystic carcinoma. In fact, Grillo observed only 23 benign tumors (12%) in a total series of 198 tumors of the trachea.[21] Benign tumors appear predominantly in males, with a peak incidence in the fifth and sixth decades of life. Squamous papillomas are observed in the second and third decades of life, and truly malignant lesions are unusual in youth.[3, 5, 6]

CLINICAL AND PATHOLOGIC FEATURES

Benign tumors of the trachea and bronchi develop over years, are usually less than 2 cm. in size, and tend to have a smooth contour. Occasional tumors may be ulcerated because of overlying inflammation or may have a large extrinsic component. Early symptoms of airway irritation include cough and hemoptysis, whereas later symptoms of dyspnea and wheezing occur once the mass has grown to a size that threatens the airway.[3, 5, 6, 19] The most proximal tracheal masses can cause stridor, and masses with a large extrinsic component may intermittently be obstructive as the individual's position is changed from prone to supine.[25] Although most patients with these tumors present early, occasionally one may present with recurrent pneumonia and atelectasis after chronic luminal obstruction.

Radiologic examinations aid in the diagnosis of a tracheal mass. The chest x-ray film can show tracheal or bronchial luminal narrowing, postobstructive atelectasis, or tumor calcification. Routine tomograms may localize the lesion, but calcification will not differentiate benign from malignant etiology.[13] Displacement or invasion of the esophagus can be demonstrated with a barium swallow; however, computed tomography is usually necessary to delineate the location

and extent of the lesion (Fig. 51–71).[30, 46, 48] Magnetic resonance imaging is useful to define a vascular etiology and allows anatomic correlation of the lesion in the coronal, sagittal, and axial planes. Differentiating benign lesions with cytology is difficult, so a definitive histologic diagnosis requires an endoscopic technique. This procedure should be performed in the operating room for the patients in whom airway obstruction is possible, because bronchoscopic manipulation can cause edema, hemorrhage, or bronchoconstriction and because visualization and biopsy using a rigid bronchoscope allow adequate control of the airway (Fig. 51–72).[11, 34, 41]

TREATMENT

Most lesions require a segmental resection of the airway for adequate treatment (Table 51–23). Pedunculated tumors resected with a bronchoscope often leave a foci of tumor, and recurrence is a significant problem. Therefore, after bronchoscopic resection, periodic surveillance of the airway is required. Treatment with fulguration, cryotherapy, or laser ablation seems to reduce recurrences compared with local bronchoscopic resection, and these procedures are recommended for large squamous papillomatosis (Fig. 51–73).[8, 9, 17, 18, 39, 42, 47, 50] Because squamous papillomas are caused by a virus, adjuvant treatment with interferon has had some success in reducing recurrence.[23] Systemic and local corticosteroid preparations have been used to control hemangiomas of the airway because of the risk of significant hemorrhage during endoscopic resection.[2, 14] However, the majority of these tumors regress over time and the remainder require segmental resection.

Segmental resection of the proximal airway requires special preparation and equipment to maintain ventilation during the operation. Once the trachea is divided, ventilation is accomplished through a sterile, armored endotracheal tube placed through the incision and into the distal airway. Either a standard volume ventilator or a high-frequency jet ventilator can be used.[7] Once the anastomosis has begun, the original endotracheal tube can be replaced past the lesion. The standardized technique used at the Brigham and Women's Hospital for resection of tumors in the proximal and distal major airway is an adaptation of techniques published in the literature.[22, 38, 39] Cervical and thoracic operations are illustrated in Figures 51–74 and 51–75. In summary, lesions of the trachea above the clavicle require a cervical incision; those of the midtrachea require a cervical and a proximal sternal division; and lower-tracheal lesions are approached through a serratus-sparing right posterolateral thoracotomy. Care must be taken to adequately localize the length of the lesion

TABLE 51–23. Treatment of Benign Tracheal and Bronchial Tumors

Series	Dates	No. Patients	Tracheal Resection	Endoscopic Resection	None
Mayo Clinic[3]	1930–1960	63	15	37	11
Mass. General[22]	1962–1989	23	21	2	
Suresnes, France[39]	1978–1985	47		47 (laser)	
Moscow, Russia[39]	1963–1983	27	23	4	

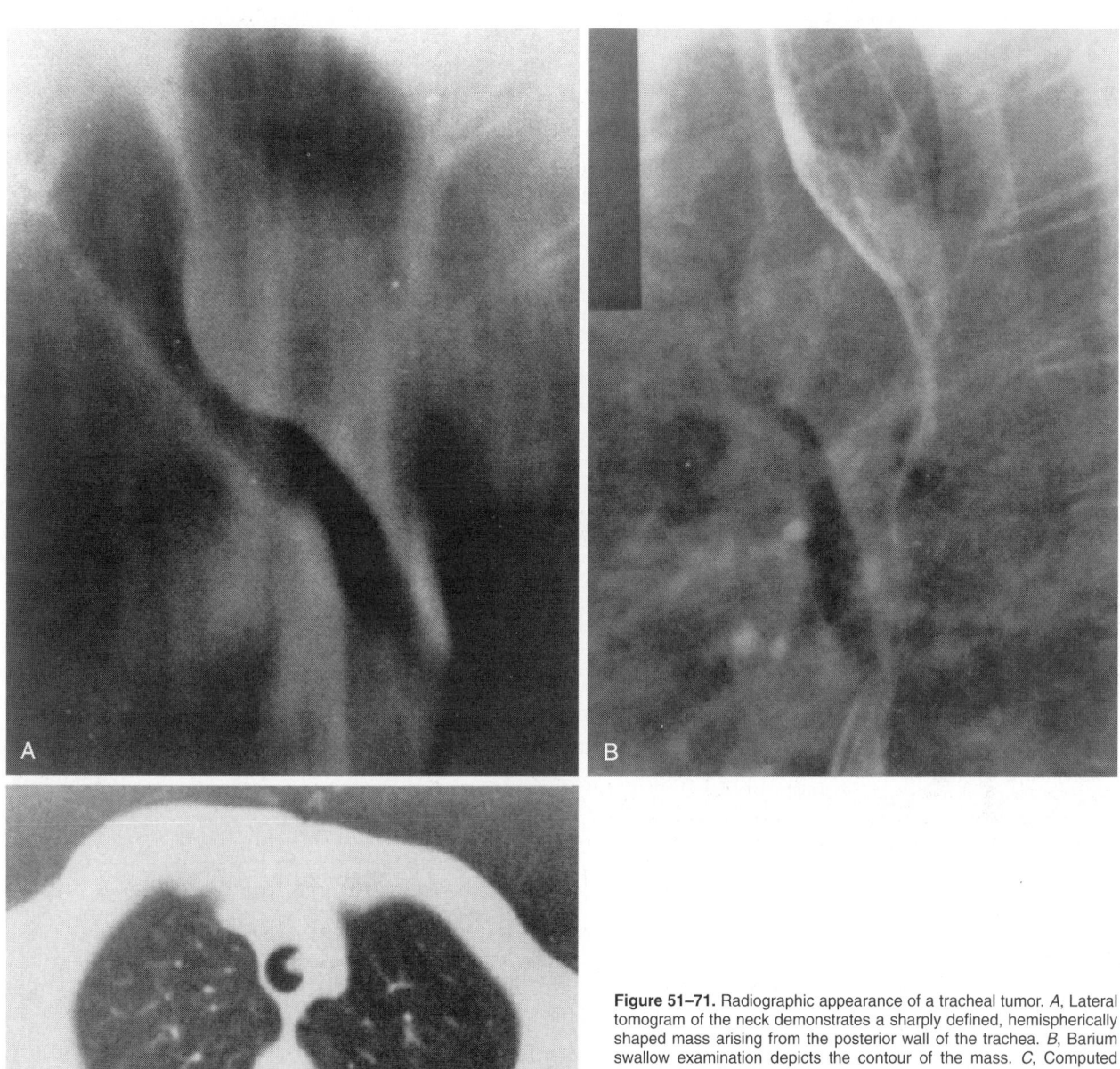

Figure 51–71. Radiographic appearance of a tracheal tumor. *A,* Lateral tomogram of the neck demonstrates a sharply defined, hemispherically shaped mass arising from the posterior wall of the trachea. *B,* Barium swallow examination depicts the contour of the mass. *C,* Computed tomogram from another patient demonstrates an intraluminal mass on the left wall of the trachea. (From Li, W., Ellerbroek, N. A., and Libshitz, H. I.: Primary malignant tumors of the trachea. Cancer, *66*:894, 1990.)

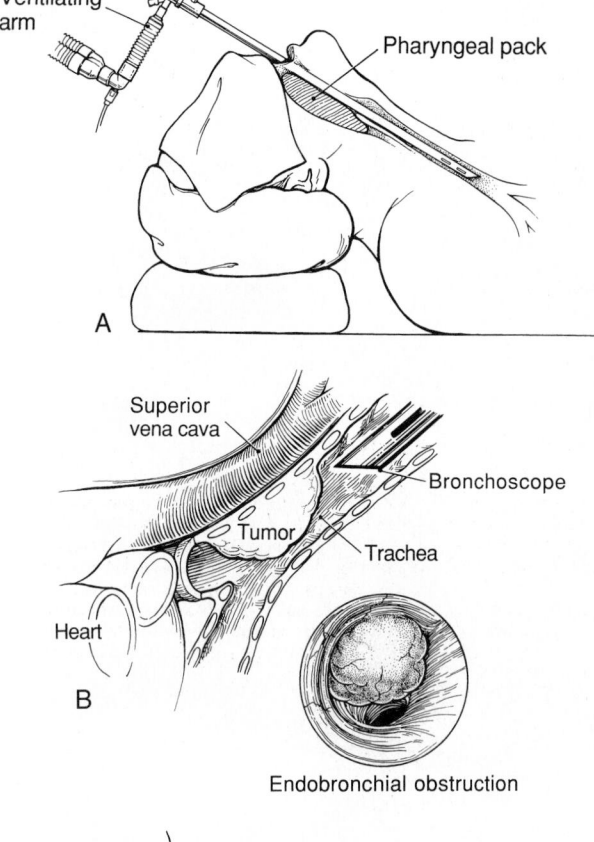

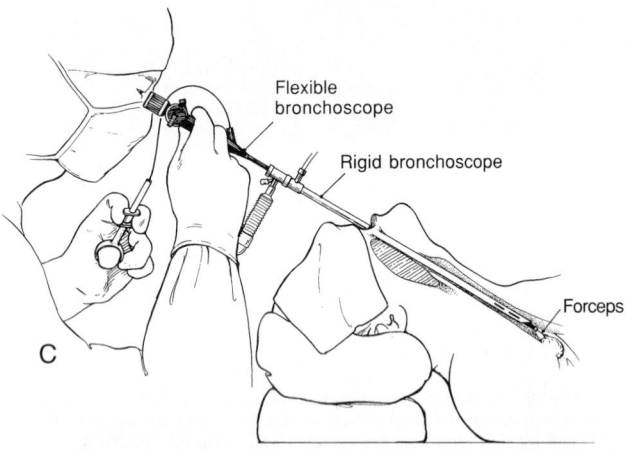

the serratus anterior.[1] The suturing technique has undergone an evolution since the widespread application of bronchial and tracheal anastomoses for lung transplantation. Many centers now use 3-0 polypropylene suture in place of polyglactin. The initial stitches are placed in the cartilaginous-membranous junctions and are simple mattress sutures. The membranous portions are then anastomosed using a continuous running technique, while interrupted, simple sutures between the cartilaginous portions complete the closure. The long-term results from this technique are good, with less granulation formation than observed with either silk or multistrand polyglactin. These techniques are appropriate for adults and children in most instances. Plastic stents and rotational skin flaps have been used in rare circumstances in the past.[20, 36, 45]

SELECTED BENIGN TRACHEAL AND BRONCHIAL TUMORS

Short descriptions of the six most common histologic types are included in this section (Table 51–24).

Squamous Papillomatosis. These are the most common benign lesions in adults and children, comprising 2% to 3% of all papillomatous disease. No obvious gender predomi-

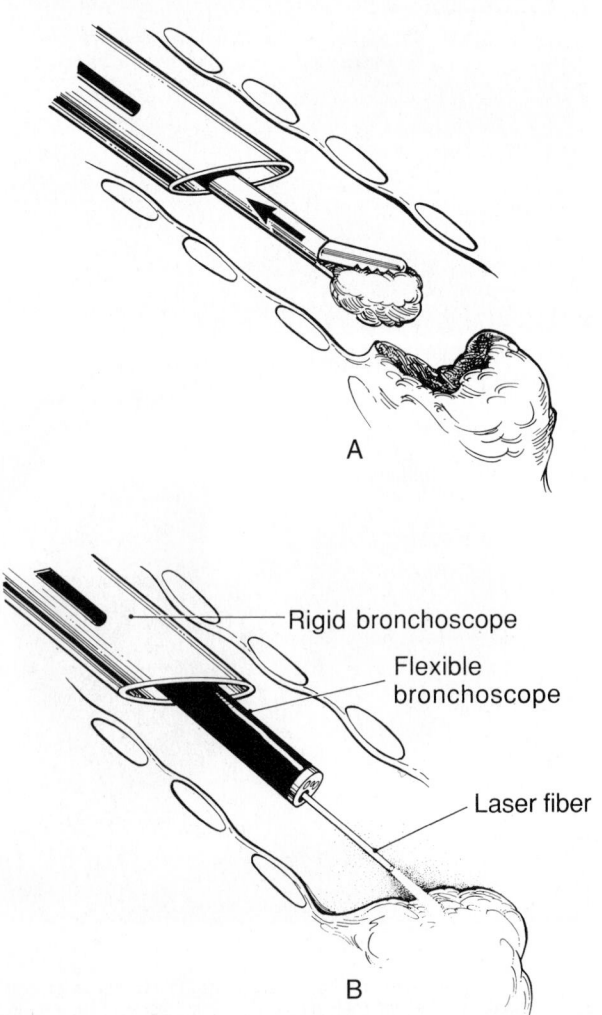

Figure 51–72. Proper technique for rigid bronchoscopy in a patient with a tracheal mass. *A,* Pharyngeal packing is used to protect the esophagus. *B,* A nearly obstructing tumor is shown. *C,* A flexible bronchoscope is placed into the rigid scope for the biopsy. This protects the airway. (From Sugarbaker, D. J., Mentzer, S. J., Strauss, G., and Fried, M. P.: Laser resection of endobronchial lesions: Use of the rigid and flexible bronchoscopes. Oper. Tech. Otolaryngol. Head Neck Surg., *3:*93, 1992.)

Figure 51–73. A technique for endoscopic resection of a tracheal mass with a rigid bronchoscope without *(A)* and with *(B)* use of the laser. (From Sugarbaker, D. J., Mentzer, S. J., Strauss, G., and Fried, M. P.: Laser resection of endobronchial lesions: Use of the rigid and flexible bronchoscopes. Oper. Tech. Otolaryngol. Head Neck Surg., *3:*93, 1992.)

and plan the operative approach; intraoperative bronchoscopy is often necessary. Primary anastomosis is possible after resection of 2 to 3 cm. of trachea; however, if a larger resection is necessary for an adequate margin, a tracheal mobilization procedure is needed. As much as 6 cm. can be resected with division of the inferior pulmonary ligament, complete mobilization of the right mainstem bronchus, or release of the larynx by separation of its thyrohyoid attachments. A tracheal anastomosis after an extensive resection should be covered with an appropriate myoplastic flap, such as from

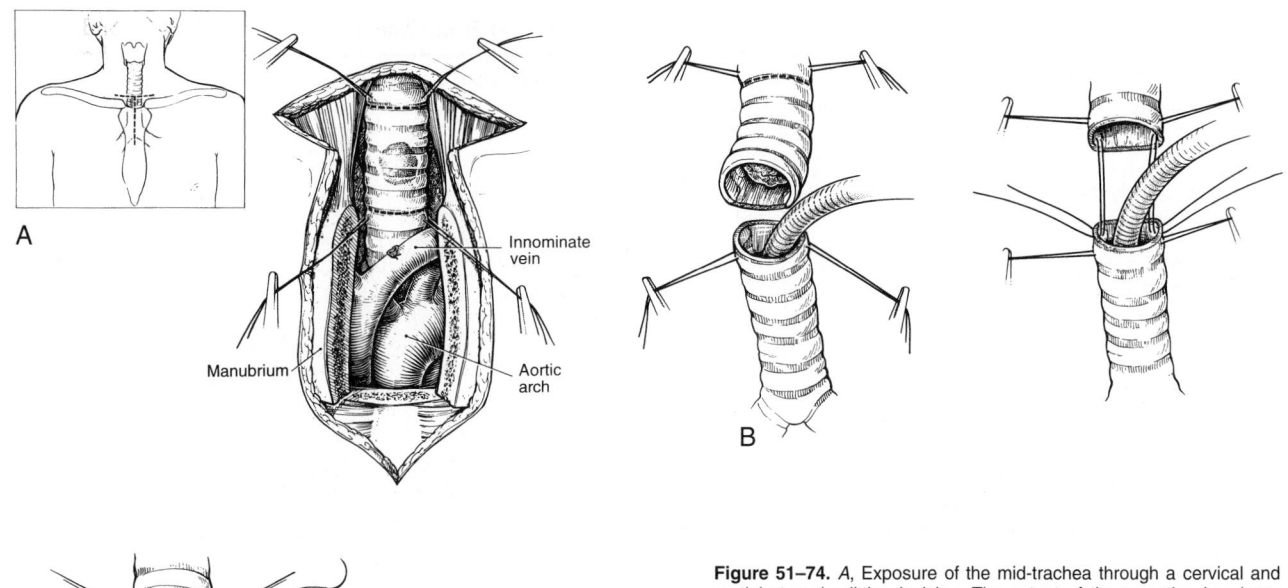

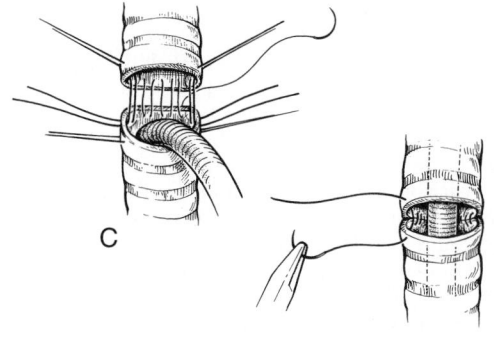

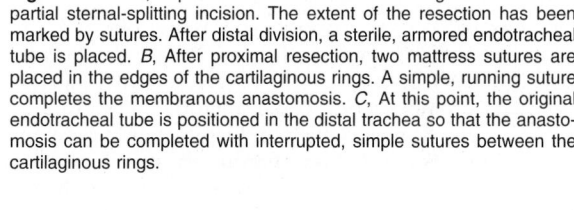

Figure 51–74. *A,* Exposure of the mid-trachea through a cervical and partial sternal-splitting incision. The extent of the resection has been marked by sutures. After distal division, a sterile, armored endotracheal tube is placed. *B,* After proximal resection, two mattress sutures are placed in the edges of the cartilaginous rings. A simple, running suture completes the membranous anastomosis. *C,* At this point, the original endotracheal tube is positioned in the distal trachea so that the anastomosis can be completed with interrupted, simple sutures between the cartilaginous rings.

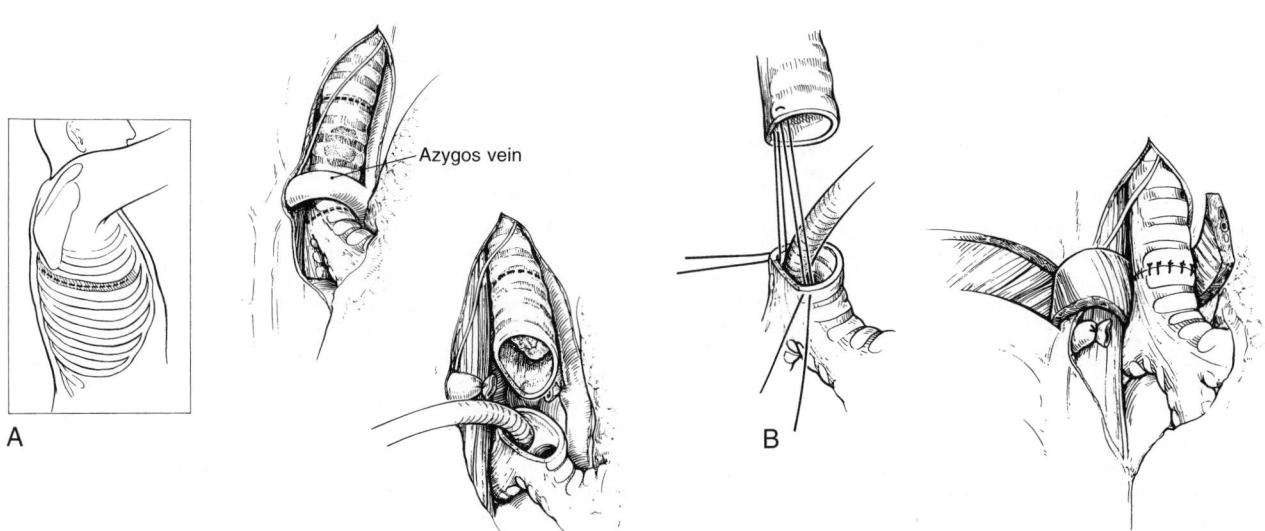

Figure 51–75. A right serratus-sparing posterolateral thoracotomy is extended behind the scapula. Proximal and distal exposure shows a tracheal tumor near the bifurcation. *A,* After division of the azygos vein and the distal trachea, a sterile, armored endotracheal tube is placed into the left mainstem bronchus. After proximal resection, the interrupted, mattress sutures are placed at the edges of the tracheal rings. *B,* After completion of the anatomosis (see Fig. 51–74), a vascularized intercostal muscle flap is placed around the anastomosis.

TABLE 51–24. Histology of Benign Tracheal and Bronchial Tumors

Histology	D'Aunov and Zoeller[6]	Culp[5]	Gilbert et al.[19]	Caldarola et al.[3]	Perelman and Korolwa[38]	Grillo and Mathisen[22]	Total
Squamous papillomas	59	63	65	26	9	5	227
Cartilaginous tumors	65	71	77	11		3	227
Fibroma/fibrous histiocytoma	33	36	39	7		2	117
Intratracheal thyroid	25	29	29				83
Benign mixed cell tumor	10	12	21		4	2	49
Vascular tumor/malformation	2	2	8		4	3	19
Lipoma	5	5	5	1	1		17
Hamartoma				7			7
Granular cell tumor						2	2
Leiomyoma			2		1	2	5
Nerve sheath tumor					6	2	8
Paraganglioma			5	2		2	9
Myoblastoma			1	2	1		4
Xanthoma				1	1		2
Undetermined benign	27	28	32				87
Series Total	226	246	284	57	27	23	863

nance is noted.[12] They are most commonly observed in the larynx, so a voice change is often apparent.[24] Lesions in the conducting airways can present with cough, hemoptysis, or airway compromise. Endoscopic anatomy reveals multiple cauliflower-like tumors, which on histologic examination are irregular papillary or villous fibrous masses covered with squamous epithelium. There is an association with human papillomatosis virus types 6 and 11.[26] Malignant transformation is unusual in children but is seen more commonly after radiation therapy.[12, 32] Adults with a single lesion must be observed carefully, because of a 50% rate of tumor degeneration to squamous carcinoma.[46] There is a tendency for regression for juvenile papillomatosis, and the lesions may regress and reappear during and after pregnancy.[29] The bronchoscopic appearance of multiple, smooth, thin-walled cavitary lesions is pathognomonic for papillomatosis.

Local bronchoscopic excision is complicated, with a 90% recurrence rate. Radical complete excision was the treatment of choice, but newer modalities have replaced this. Bronchoscopic fulguration, cryotherapy, and bronchoscopic laser ablation allow for multiple treatments with minimal morbidity and mortality.[17, 39, 42] Antiviral immunotherapy is being investigated; good short-term results have been seen with interferon therapy.[23]

Benign Cartilaginous Tumors. The second most common type of benign mass of the trachea and bronchi are cartilaginous tumors, which include chondromas, hamartomas, and tracheobronchopathia osteoplastica. Chrondromas of the conducting airways develop from the cartilaginous plates. The mucosa is usually intact over the lesion, and calcification may be evident on a chest radiograph. These tumors occur equally among men and women during mid-life (40 to 60 years). Histologic differentiation from a sarcoma is difficult on biopsy, and occasional tumors will degenerate into a chondrosarcoma.[49] This and the chance of recurrence after local excision emphasize the need for a complete surgical resection at diagnosis.[29]

Hamartomas contain cartilage along with lymph tissue, fat, and epithelial elements.[13] The most common presentation is an asymptomatic solitary pulmonary nodule that must be differentiated from bronchogenic carcinoma. Eighty percent of hamartomas are located in the periphery of the lung and occur less frequently as an endobronchial lesion in the more central airways. The peripherally located lesions are often immediately subpleural and are treated with thoracoscopic wedge excision. Because these lesions rarely recur, the margin of normal tissue resected may be small. Central endobron-

chial hamartomas are adequately treated with a minimal sleeve resection of the airway.

Tracheobronchopathia osteoplastica is a more generalized lesion that affects long segments of the distal two thirds of the trachea with multiple submucosal cartilaginous and bony tumors. Presentation with stridor and near-obstruction is common; however, many patients are initially seen who have a nonspecific cough and progressive dyspnea.[3, 5, 6] This process occurs equally among both sexes and has a peak incidence at an age of 50 years. Repeated rigid bronchoscopic excision is the treatment for symptomatic patients.

Fibroma/Fibrous Histiocytoma. Fibromas of the airways are typically discovered in the cervical trachea of children and are the third most common benign tracheal and bronchial mass. These solitary and well-defined masses are composed of either cellular or acellular fibrous tissue.[13] Most are located submucosally, so bronchoscopic excision is possible for primary and recurrent tumors. A fibrous histiocytoma is a benign proliferation of histiocytes and fibroblasts. Eighty percent occur on the extremities, but occasional submucosal tumors are seen in the trachea. Segmental, complete resection of the airway is necessary to limit recurrence.[33, 36]

Ectopic Thyroid. Although thyroid malignancies can invade the trachea, the fourth most common type of primary benign tumor of the trachea and bronchi is ectopically located, histologically normal thyroid tissue. There is a female predominance, and a goiter in the thyroid gland is usually present. Malignant degeneration occurs in 10% of cases, so surgical resection is recommended.[5, 6, 19, 40]

Benign Mixed Cell Tumors. Benign mixed cell tumors (pleomorphic adenoma) of the trachea are histologically similar to benign mixed tumors of the salivary glands and contain epithelial cells, cartilage, and mesenchymal cells. Although these lesions are less commonly found in the trachea or bronchi, they constitute the fifth most common type of benign mass. Recurrence is unusual, and treatment consists of complete excision with a segment of airway.[15, 27, 37]

Benign Vascular Tumors. Hemangiomas are the most common lesions of the trachea and bronchi observed in children. They may occur anywhere in the conducting airways but are most common in the subglottic region, where they may threaten the airway. Neonates who have a hemangioma of the airway usually become symptomatic with stridor and coughing within 3 months of birth. Like most vascular lesions, the size and symptoms may vary with engorgement, such that a misdiagnosis of croup may be made.[2] These lesions rarely occur without evidence of other congenital vascular lesions, such as hemangiomas of the skin, parotid gland, mediastinum, abdominal viscera, central nervous system, and retina.[32, 51] Hemangiomas often present in the supraglottic or laryngeal area in adults, causing hoarseness.[19] These lesions are more common in females and are typically of the cavernous type. The lesion is easily recognized, so bronchoscopic biopsy is unnecessary and may create severe hemorrhage. The treatment of choice for children and adults is observation, because many of these tumors spontaneously regress. Radiation therapy or corticosteroids are not recommended.[2, 4] Temporary tracheostomy may be necessary for airway preservation; and if the lesion persists, a tracheal resection may be necessary.[31] A limited tracheal resection may also be used if the lesion is a hemangioendothelioma. This slow-growing tumor appears as a solid polypoid mass and contains endothelial cells surrounded by microscopic vascular channels.[16]

TUMORLIKE CONDITIONS

Many systemic diseases can present as a tracheal or bronchial mass. Infectious disease such as tuberculosis, systemic histoplasmosis, or coccidiomycosis can form an intraluminal granuloma, such as a tuberculoma, which may simulate a primary tumor. Connective tissue disorders, including scleroderma, multiple xanthoma, amyloidosis, and Wegener's granulomatosis, can also cause tracheal lesions. Regression of these lesions involves systemic control of the disease process with chemotherapy.[43]

SELECTED REFERENCES

Caldarola, V. T., Harrison, E. G., and Clagett, O. T.: Benign tumors and tumor-like conditions of the trachea and bronchi. Ann. Otol., 73:1042, 1964.
This article details a large series of benign tumors of the trachea and bronchi from the Mayo Clinic. Clinical and pathologic information is included.

Gilbert, Y. G., Mazzarella, L. A., and Freit, L. J.: Primary tracheal tumors in the infant and adult. Arch. Otolaryngol., 58:1, 1953.
This manuscript is an extensive review of benign and malignant primary tumors of the trachea in adults and children summarized from the world's literature.

Grillo, H. C., and Mathisen, D. J.: Primary tracheal tumors: Treatment and results. Ann. Thorac. Surg., 49:69, 1990.
This paper summarizes a 25-year experience in tracheal resection for primary tumors of the trachea. Grillo's techniques for approaching a proximal and distal lesion are discussed.

Pearson, F. G., Todd, T. R. J., and Cooper, J. D.: Experience with primary neoplasms of the trachea and carina. J. Thorac. Cardiovasc. Surg., 88:511, 1984.
Pearson's large series of patients from the University of Toronto with benign and malignant tumors of the trachea is included. There is a description of the operative techniques, pathology, and long-term results.

Perelman, M. I., and Korolwa, N.: Surgery of the trachea. World J. Surg., 4:583, 1980.
An extensive experience of tracheal resections for benign and malignant tumors from the National Research Center of Surgery in Moscow is presented. Technical and prognostic information is included.

REFERENCES

1. Arnold, P. G., Pairolero, P. C., and Waldorf, J. C.: The serratus anterior muscle: Intrathoracic and extrathoracic utilization. Plast. Reconstr. Surg., 73:240, 1984.
2. Calcaterra, T. C.: An evaluation of the treatment of subglottic hemangioma. Laryngoscope, 78:1956, 1968.
3. Caldarola, V. T., Harrison, E. G., Clagett, O. T., et al.: Benign tumors and tumor-like conditions of the trachea and bronchi. Ann. Otol., 73:1042, 1964.
4. Cohen, S. R.: Unusual lesions of the larynx, trachea and bronchial tree. Ann. Otol. Rhinol. Laryngol., 78:476, 1969.
5. Culp, O. S.: Primary trachea tumors. J. Thorac. Surg., 7:471, 1938.
6. D'Aunoy, R., and Zoeller, A.: Tracheal and bronchial tumors. Arch. Pathol., 11:589, 1931.
7. Daum, R., Denecke, H. J., and Roth, H.: Tumour-induced intraluminal stenoses of the cervical trachea: Tumour excision and tracheoplasty. Prog. Pediatr. Surg., 21:50, 1987.
8. Dedo, H. H., and Jackler, R. K.: Laryngeal papilloma: Results of treatment
9. Diaz-Jimenez, J. P., Canela-Cardona, M., and Maestre-Alcacer, J.: Nd:YAG laser photoresection of low-grade malignant tumors of the tracheobronchial tree. Chest, 97:920, 1990.
10. Ellman, P., and Whittaker, H.: Primary tumors of the trachea. Thorax, 2:153, 1947.
11. Ellis, D. J., Millar, W. L., and Karagianes, T. G.: Anesthesia for laser resection of a tracheal tumor in a woman pregnant with twins. Anesthesiology, 68:629, 1988.
12. Fechner, R. E., and Fitz-Hugh, G. S.: Invasive tracheal papillomatosis. Am. J. Surg. Pathol., 4:79, 1980.
13. Felson, B.: Neoplasms of trachea and mainstem bronchi. Semin. Roentgenol., 18:23, 1983.
14. Ferguson, C. F., and Flake, C. G.: Subglottic hemangioma as a cause of respiratory obstruction in infants. Ann. Otol. Rhinol. Laryngol., 70:1095, 1961.
15. Ferguson, C. J., and Cleeland, J. A.: Mucous gland adenoma of the trachea. J. Thorac. Cardiovasc. Surg., 95:347, 1988.
16. Flege, J. B., Valencia, G., and Zimmerman, G.: Obstruction of a child's trachea by a polypoid hemangioendothelioma. J. Thorac. Cardiovasc. Surg., 56:144, 1968.
17. Frootko, N. J., and Rogers, J. H.: The treatment of juvenile multiple laryngeal papillomatosis by suction diathermy. J. Laryngol. Otol., 93:373, 1979.
18. George, P. J. M., Garrett, C. P. O., and Hetzel, M. R.: Role of the neodymium YAG laser in the management of tracheal tumours. Thorax, 42:440, 1987.
19. Gilbert, Y. G., Mazzarella, L. A., and Freit, L. J.: Primary tracheal tumors in the infant and adult. Arch. Otolaryngol., 58:1, 1953.
20. Grillo, H. C., Dignan, E. F., Miura, T., et al.: Extensive resection and reconstruction of mediastinal trachea without prosthesis or graft: An anatomical study in man. J. Thorac. Cardiovasc. Surg., 48:741, 1964.
21. Grillo, H. C.: Tracheal surgery. Scand. J. Thorac. Cardiovasc. Surg., 17:67, 1983.
22. Grillo, H. C., and Mathisen, D. J.: Primary tracheal tumors: Treatment and results. Ann. Thorac. Surg., 49:69, 1990.
23. Hendrickse, W. A., Irvin, B. C., Bailey, C. M., et al.: Regression of respiratory papillomatosis after treatment with interferon. BMJ, 289, 1984.
24. Irwin, B. C., Hendrickse, W. A., Pincott, J. R., et al.: Juvenile laryngeal papillomatosis. J. Laryngol. Otol., 100:435, 1986.
25. Karlan, M. S., Livingston, P. A., and Baker, D. C.: Diagnosis of tracheal tumors. Ann. Otol., 82:790, 1973.
26. Kashima, H., Wu, T. C., Mounts, P., et al.: Carcinoma ex-papilloma: Histologic and virologic studies in whole-organ sections of the larynx. Laryngoscope, 98:619, 1988.
27. Kay, S., and Brooks, J. W.: Benign mixed tumor of the trachea with seven-year follow-up. Cancer, 25:1178, 1970.
28. LeRoux, B. T., Williams, M. A., and Kallichurum, S.: Squamous papillomatosis of the trachea and bronchi. Thorax, 24:673, 1969.
29. Le-Tian, X., Zhen-Fu, S., Ze-Juan, L., et al.: Tracheobronchial tumors: An eighteen-year series from Capitol Hospital, Peking, China. Ann. Thorac. Surg., 35:590, 1983.
30. Li, W., Ellerbroek, N. A., Libshitz, H. I.: Primary malignant tumors of the trachea. Cancer, 66:894, 1990.
31. Maier, H. C.: Hemangiomas of the subglottic region, trachea, and mediastinum in infancy and childhood. Ann. Thorac. Surg., 3:514, 1967.
32. Matsuba, H. M., Thawley, S. E., Mauney, M., et al.: Laryngeal epidermoid carcinoma associated with juvenile laryngeal papillomatosis. Laryngoscope, 95:1264, 1985.
33. Miller, M. A. L., and Toma, G. A.: Fibroma of the trachea. Br. J. Dis. Chest, 53:177, 1959.
34. Monnier, P. H., Ravussin, P., Savary, M., et al.: Percutaneous transtracheal ventilation for laser endoscopic treatment of subglottic lesions. Clin. Otolaryngol., 13:209, 1988.
35. Nakayama, D. K., Harrison, M. R., deLorimier, A. A., et al.: Reconstructive surgery for obstructing lesions of the intrathoracic trachea in infants and small children. J. Pediatr. Surg., 17:854, 1982.
36. Pairolero, P. C.: Benign and malignant neoplasms of the trachea. In Roth, J. A., Ruckdeschel, J. C., and Weisenburger, T. H. (Eds.): Thoracic Oncology. Philadelphia, W. B. Saunders, 1989.
37. Pearson, F. G., Todd, T. R. J., and Cooper, J. D.: Experience with primary neoplasms of the trachea and carina. J. Thorac. Cardiovasc. Surg., 88:511, 1984.
38. Perelman, M. I., and Korolwa, N.: Surgery of the trachea. World J. Surg., 4:583, 1980.
39. Personne, C., Colchen, A., Leroy, M., Vourc'h, G., and Toty, L.: Indication and technique for endoscopic laser resection in bronchoscopy. J. Thorac. Cardiovasc. Surg., 91:710, 1986.
40. Randolph, J., Grunt, J. A., and Vawter, G. F.: The medical and surgical aspects of intratracheal goiter. N. Engl. J. Med., 268:457, 1963.
41. Richardson, M. A., and Cotten, R. T.: Anatomic abnormalities of the pediatric airway. Pediatr. Clin. North Am., 31:821, 1984.
42. Rogers, B. M., Moazam, F., and Talbert, J. L.: Successful cryotherapy of a benign tracheal neoplasm. J. Pediatr. Surg., 23:771, 1988.
43. Scully, R. E., Mark, E. J., McNeely, B. U.: Case records of the Massachusetts General Hospital, case 45–1986. N. Engl. J. Med., 315:1277, 1986.
44. Shaha, A., DiMaio, T., Money, S., et al.: Prosthetic reconstruction of the trachea. Am. J. Surg., 156:306, 1988.

with CO$_2$ laser and podophyllum. Ann. Otol. Rhinol. Laryngol., 91:425, 1982.

45. Spencer, H.: Rare pulmonary tumors. *In* Spencer, H. (Ed.): Pathology of the Lung, 3rd ed. New York, Pergamon Press, 1977.
46. Spizarny, D. L., Shepard, J. O., McLoud, T. C., et al.: CT of adenoid cystic carcinoma of the trachea. AJR, *146*:1129, 1986.
47. Sugarbaker, D. J., Mentzer, S. J., Strauss, G., and Fried, M. P.: Laser resection of endobronchial lesions: Use of the rigid and flexible bronchoscopes. Oper. Tech. Otolaryngol. Head Neck Surg., *3*:93, 1992.
48. Weber, A. L., and Grillo, H. C.: Tracheal tumors. Radiol. Clin. North Am., *16*:227, 1978.

49. Weber, A. L., Shortsleeve, M., Goodman, M., et al.: Cartilaginous tumors of the larynx and trachea. Radiol. Clin. North Am., *16*:261, 1978.
50. Wetmore, S. J., Key, J. M., and Suen, J. Y.: Complications of laser surgery for laryngeal papillomatosis. Laryngoscope, *95*:798, 1985.
51. Yousem, A. L., Wick, M. R., Singh, G., Katyal, S. L., Manivel, C. J., Mills, S. E., and Legier, J.: So-called sclerosing hemangioma of the lung. Am. J. Surg. Pathol., *12*:582, 1988.

XI

BRONCHIAL ADENOMAS

David H. Harpole, Jr., M.D.

In 1930, Kramer cited a group of lung cancers that appeared to be less aggressive and have a better prognosis for the patient than usual bronchogenic carcinoma.[21] These *bronchial adenomas* are classified into three distinct histologic types: bronchial carcinoid tumors, adenoid cystic carcinoma, and mucoepidermoid carcinoma, and they comprise 1% to 2% of lung cancers in most large retrospective series.[3, 8, 25, 34]

BRONCHIAL CARCINOID TUMORS

Although bronchial carcinoid tumors were described in the past century, Oberndorfer introduced the term *Karcinoide*, which means *resembles carcinoma*, in 1907.[29] These lesions were classified with cylindromas of the lung as bronchial adenomas by Kramer in 1930, because of their improved prognosis compared with bronchogenic carcinoma.[21] However, a subset of bronchial carcinoid tumors were observed to have a more rapid course and were termed *atypical* by Arrigoni and associates in 1972.[2] Carcinoid tumors comprise 1% to 2% of all malignant lung cancers and approximately 85% of all bronchial adenomas. They are seen in all ages (median age, 55 years) and are equally distributed in both sexes.[15, 26, 33]

Pathology

Bronchial carcinoids are members of the APUD (amine-precursor uptake and decarboxylation) family of Kulchitsky's neural crest cells, which are distributed throughout the oro-digestive tract. Characteristically, the cytoplasm contains neurosecretory granules, which may be identified by argyrophilic staining or electron microscopy.[6, 10, 23, 43] These cells have the capability to manufacture and store a number of active peptide hormones, including serotonin, bradykinin, leu-enkephalin, histamine, bombesin, vasoactive intestinal polypeptide, gastrin, growth hormone, corticotropin, glucagon, insulin, melanocyte-stimulating hormone, vasopressin, epinephrine, norepinephrine, somatostatin, substance P, calcitonin, and others.[6, 38, 44] As in small cell lung cancer, immunoreactivity to neuron-specific enolase is observed. Typical carcinoids consist of clusters of monotonous polyhedral cells in a fibrovascular stroma. Ten per cent to 15% of carcinoids have mitotic figures, nuclear pleomorphism, increased cellularity, increased nuclear-to-cytoplasmic ratios, prominent nucleoli with nuclear hyperchromatism, disorganized architecture, and necrosis. Arrigoni and associates observed a higher frequency of lymph node metastases and a more aggressive clinical course for these atypical carcinoid tumors.[2] As electron microscopy and immunohistochemistry have been utilized to type pulmonary malignancies, it has become appar-

ent that carcinoids share ultrastructure and immunoreactivity with small cell neuroendocrine cancer of the lung. Therefore, it is reasonable to group typical carcinoids, atypical carcinoids, and small cell lung cancer in a spectrum of neuroendocrine pulmonary malignancies as Kulchitsky Type I (typical carcinoid), Kulchitsky Type II (atypical carcinoid), and Kulchitsky Type III (small cell lung cancer).[31]

Clinical Presentation

Carcinoid tumors may be located anywhere in the tracheobronchial tree. However, a central location in the main airways has been observed in approximately 60% of cases.[15] The lesion can cause a variety of symptoms as the tumor enlarges in the bronchus, such as cough, hemoptysis, or wheezing and stridor (Table 51–25). Peripherally located carcinoids are often asymptomatic, unless they secrete an active peptide hormone. The carcinoid syndrome (flushing, facial skin pigmentation, and diarrhea) is observed in 10% of cases. Debate exists on which peptide causes the syndrome, but both serotonin and bradykinin have been implicated.[41] One series of carcinoid tumors of the lung revealed that levels of either serotonin or its breakdown product (5-hydroxyindoleacetic acid) were elevated in 35 of 106 patients (34%).[15]

Diagnosis

The routine chest radiograph is often abnormal (>90%), demonstrating a mass with or without distant atelectasis and a postobstructive pneumonia if the lesion is centrally located.[3, 13, 15] Computed tomography has replaced other radio-

TABLE 51–25. Presenting Symptoms of Bronchial Carcinoids

Symptom	% Population (n = 126)
No symptoms	39
Nonproductive cough	25
Productive cough	27
Hemoptysis	30
Dyspnea or wheezing	25
Chest pain	18
Sweating/flushing	12
Diarrhea	10

From Harpole, D. H., Feldman, J. M., Buchanan, S., Young, W. G., and Wolfe, W. G.: Bronchial carcinoid tumors: A retrospective analysis of 126 patients. Ann. Thorac. Surg. *54*:50, 1992. Reprinted with permission from the Society of Thoracic Surgeons.

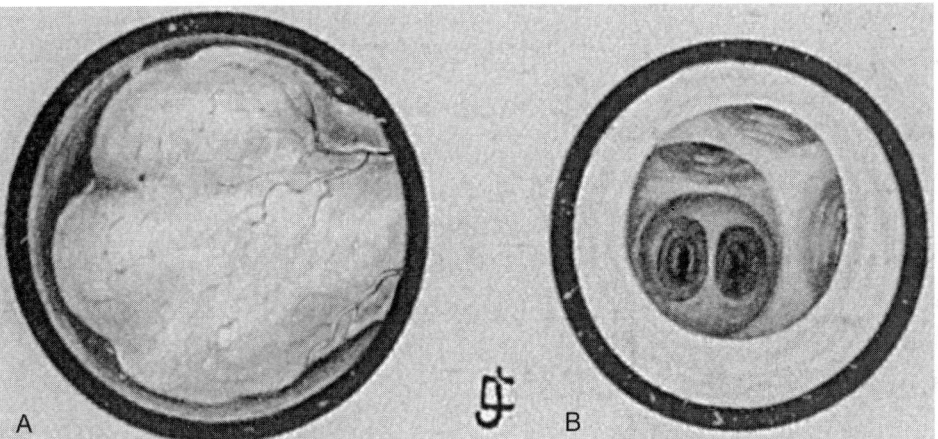

Figure 51–76. Original drawings by Jackson in 1917 demonstrating a carcinoid tumor in the right mainstem bronchus before *(A)* and after *(B)* bronchoscopic resection. (From Jackson, J.: Endothelioma of the right bronchus removed by peroral bronchoscopy. Am. J. Med. Sci., *153*:371, 1917.)

logic examinations as the primary method of evaluating the extent of the mass and possible extrapulmonary spread.

Histologic diagnosis is often possible utilizing bronchoscopy. The usual appearance of a carcinoid of the major airways was accurately described by Jackson in 1917 as *mulberry-like* (Fig. 51–76). He also noted that these lesions can sometimes bleed profusely.[18] Therefore, it is reasonable to biopsy these lesions in the operating room, where rigid bronchoscopy is available if bleeding ensues.

Treatment

Complete primary surgical resection is the treatment for all typical and most atypical carcinoids without mediastinal lymph node metastases. Peripheral lesions most often require a lobectomy to remove the regional lymph nodes. Central

lesions may require a larger resection if distal obstruction and parenchymal destruction exists or if there is involvement of the mainstem bronchus. In the past, a pneumonectomy was often required for carcinoid tumors of the mainstem bronchi. More recently there has been a trend toward a more conservative approach to preserve ventilatory function. If the mediastinal lymph nodes are not involved with cancer, central carcinoid lesions can be treated with a sleeve resection of the involved bronchus, but care must be taken to ensure histologically negative margins (Fig. 51–77).[15, 19, 24, 45]

Results

The overall prognosis after complete resection of a typical carcinoid is good, with at least a 90% 5-year survival (Table 51–26). Findings associated with a poor prognosis include the presence of symptoms, atypical histology (Fig. 51–78A), tumor size greater than 2 cm. in diameter (see Fig. 51–78B), expression of serotonin, central location, and lymph node metastases (see Fig. 51–78C).[15] Multivariate analysis has defined atypical histology, nodal metastases, and symptomatic presentation as the most important independent factors for a decreased survival.[15] There are no large series that define a significant role for either adjuvant radiation therapy or chemotherapy in advanced disease. However, most oncologists treat an aggressive carcinoid tumor as a small cell lung cancer, because these neuroendocrine tumors often respond well to combined radiation therapy and chemotherapy.[15, 26, 40]

ADENOID CYSTIC CARCINOMA (CYLINDROMA)

These tumors are common malignant tumors of the salivary glands. Although they grow slowly, there is a propen-

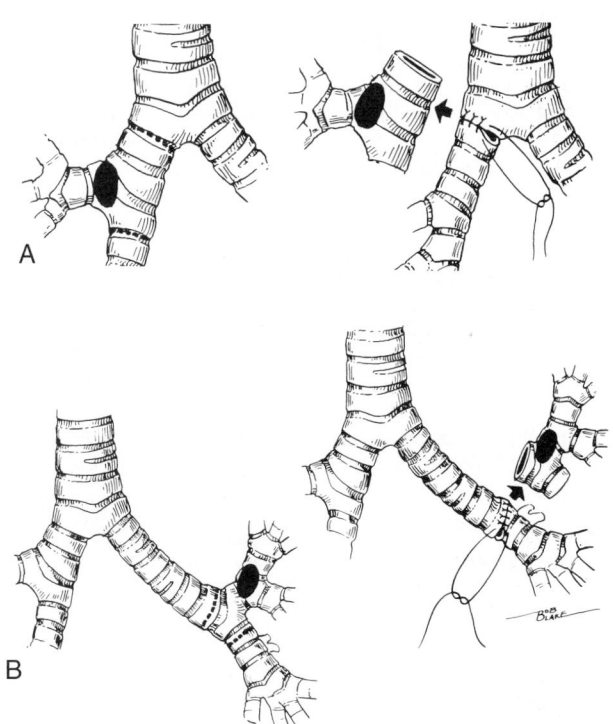

Figure 51–77. Technique for right *(A)* and left *(B)* upper sleeve lobectomy for a tumor of the upper lobe orifice. (From Lowe, J. E., Brigman, A. H., and Sabiston, D. C.: The role of bronchoplastic procedures in the surgical management of benign and malignant pulmonary lesions. J. Thorac. Cardiovasc. Surg., *83*:227, 1982.)

TABLE 51–26. Survival for Typical Carcinoid Tumors

Institution	Date	No. Patients	Survival % 5-Year	Survival % 10-Year
National survey (NCI)[11]	1974	151	96	
Mayo Clinic[30]	1976	190	94	87
Massachusetts General[45]	1984	111	90	82
Memorial Sloan-Kettering[26]	1985	95	92	87
Los Angeles County Registry[31]	1985	115	95	
Emory/State of Iowa[12]	1987	96	96	
Essen-Heidelberg, Germany[39]	1990	210	97	95
Duke University[15]	1992	106	93	90

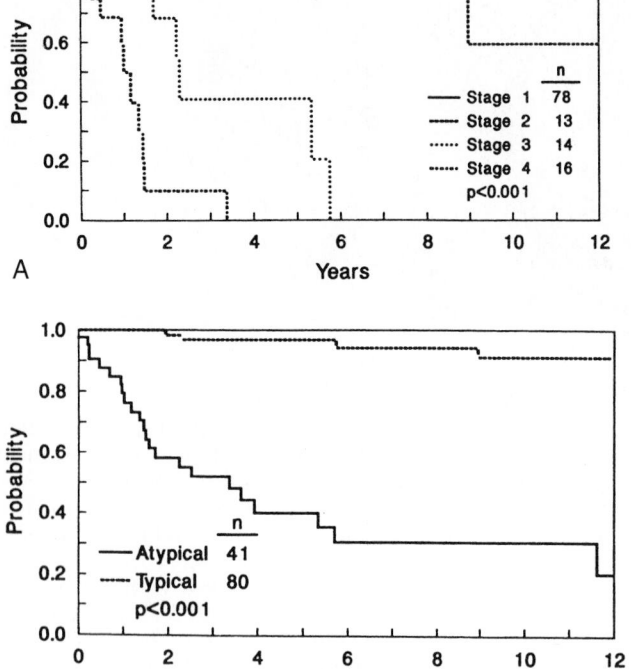

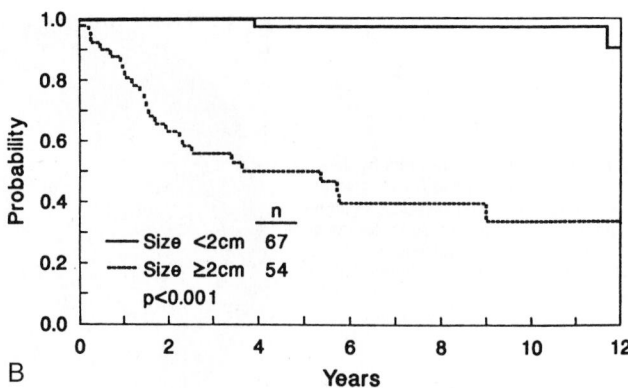

Figure 51–78. Kaplan-Meier survival is demonstrated for carcinoid tumors by stage *(A)*, size *(B)*, and histology *(C)*. (From Harpole, D. H., et al.: Bronchial carcinoid tumors: A retrospective analysis of 126 patients. Ann. Thorac. Surg., *54*:50, 1992. Reprinted with permission from the Society of Thoracic Surgeons.)

sity for submucosal and perineural invasion and distant metastases found at presentation.[17, 22, 41] They have been observed in all ages and comprise 10% of bronchial adenomas.

Pathology

Adenoid cystic carcinomas are usually located in the trachea or main bronchi. There are three distinct patterns of growth that occur with equal frequency and include the cribriform, tubular, and solid types (Fig. 51–79).[4, 5, 28] Perineural lymphatic and submucosal invasion is more often ob-

served in tubular and cribriform types, whereas the less differentiated solid type is associated with extraluminal growth into surrounding structures (esophagus or thyroid) and distant metastases.[28]

Presentation

The presence and the type of symptoms are related to the size and location of the tumor. Because most are found in the central airways, cough and hemoptysis, followed by stridor and respiratory distress, are observed as the tumor enlarges to fill the airway lumen. Occasional tumors can cause

TABLE 51–27. Adenoid Cystic Carcinoma of the Trachea and Bronchi

Author	Series	Dates	No. Patients	Age Range (y.)
Moran et al.[27]	Armed Forces Institute of Pathology	1970–1992	16	29 to 79

Results: No survival association by cell type, mitotic rate, atypia, or patterns of growth. Clinical stage was most important factor. Patients can live more than 5 years with recurrence. No nodal metastases observed, but distant metastases were seen in 7 patients before death.

| Pearson et al.[32] | Toronto, Canada | 1952–1972 | 16 | 15 to 70 |

Results: All cases were resected, and lymph nodes were positive in only 1 of 16 cases. Preoperative radiation therapy (3500–4000 cGy) in 10 allowed negative margins and no local recurrence. Eight patients lived more than 5 years free of disease; 4 died of distant metastases, and 4 with local recurrence lived several years.

| Nomori et al.[28] | Tokyo, Japan | 1964–1989 | 12 | 26 to 68 |

Results: All patients had their tumors resected, and all tumors had perineural invasion. Eight had positive resection margins and were treated with adjuvant radiation therapy (4000 cGy). Survival of more than 5 years was observed for three patients with known recurrence. Solid cell type recurred distantly, while the cribriform and tubular form recurred locally.

| Conlan et al.[7] | Mayo Clinic | 1927–1977 | 20 | 29 to 74 |

Results: Of 12 patients who had a complete resection, 7 were alive without disease and 5 had positive lymph nodes and died of cancer. Eight additional patients who presented with extensive disease were treated with palliative radiation therapy. All of these died of cancer an average of 3 years after diagnosis.

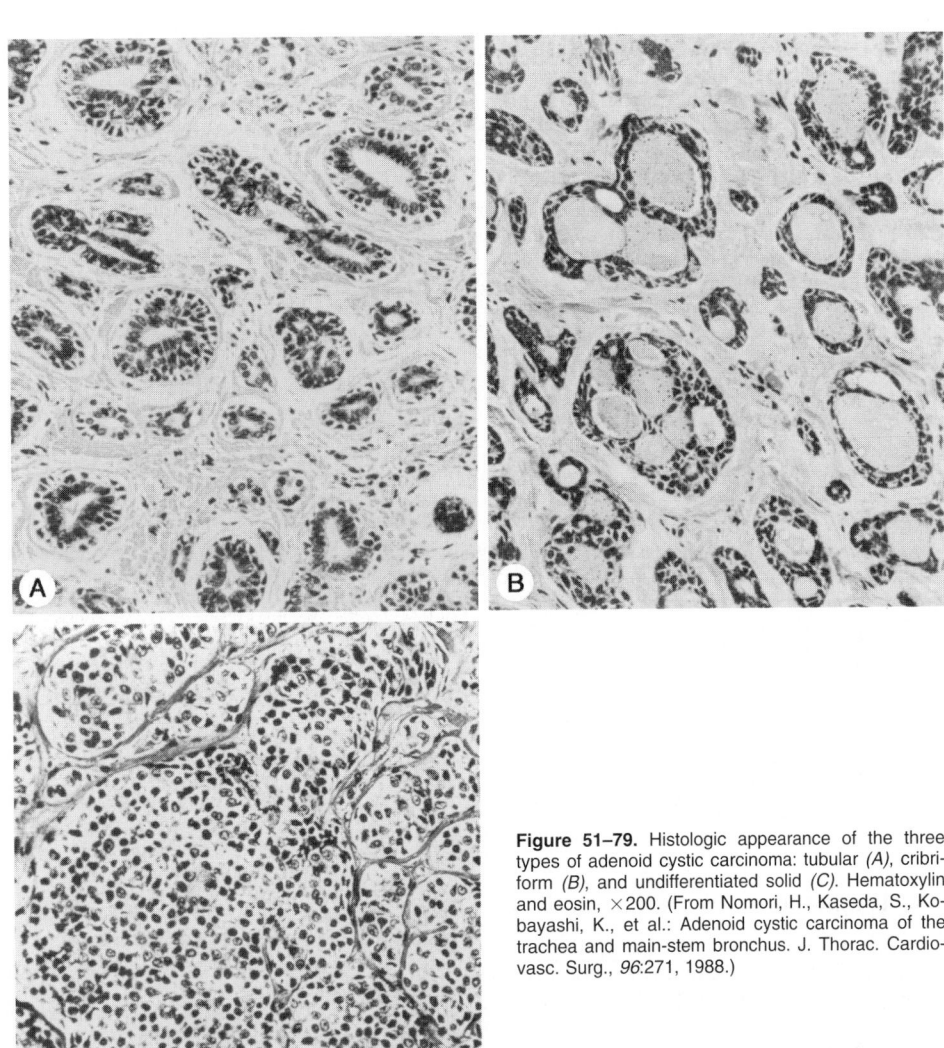

Figure 51–79. Histologic appearance of the three types of adenoid cystic carcinoma: tubular *(A)*, cribriform *(B)*, and undifferentiated solid *(C)*. Hematoxylin and eosin, ×200. (From Nomori, H., Kaseda, S., Kobayashi, K., et al.: Adenoid cystic carcinoma of the trachea and main-stem bronchus. J. Thorac. Cardiovasc. Surg., *96*:271, 1988.)

dysphagia as the tumor extrinsically blocks or directly invades the esophagus.

Diagnosis

Radiologic examinations reveal a centrally located mass, which is impossible to differentiate from bronchogenic carcinoma. Computed tomography and magnetic resonance imaging are used to define local extension of the tumor into contiguous structures.[35, 37] In addition, invasion into surrounding structures without obvious lymph node metastases may suggest adenoid cystic carcinoma. Definitive histologic diagnosis is obtained with elective flexible bronchoscopic biopsy in most cases.

Treatment

Surgical resection is the primary therapy for most adenoid cystic carcinomas. Tracheal resection requires special techniques for airway preservation during the operation (see Part X in this chapter). Preoperative radiation therapy has been used for large invasive tumors with a decrease in the rate of positive margins (Table 51–27).[32]

Results

These are uncommon tumors, accounting for a handful of cases even in the largest retrospective series of lung cancer. Therefore, it is difficult to form definitive conclusions on therapy and prognosis. Only 60% of cases can be completely resected, but the largest series in the literature suggests that patients can live many years with metastatic disease. Lymph node metastases are unusual for localized tumors (see Table 51–27). There is an increased rate of distant metastases with the solid type, resulting in a decreased survival.[28] The role for palliative radiation and chemotherapy has not been defined.[9, 17]

MUCOEPIDERMOID CARCINOMA

Mucoepidermoid carcinoma represents 0.1% to 0.2% of all lung tumors and 1% to 5% of bronchial adenomas.[1, 16] The first description was in 1952; however, cases from the early 1900s have been reclassified after a review of the pathology.[36]

Pathology

Mucoepidermoid carcinomas originate in the trachea and proximal bronchi. The tumor consists of squamous and inter-

TABLE 51–28. Mucoepidermoid Carcinoma

Author	Series	Dates	No. Patients	Mean Age (y.)
Yousem and Hochholzer[46]	Armed Forces Institute of Pathology	1960–1986	58	35

Results: All patients were completely resected. Of the 45 patients with a low-grade tumor, 44 were alive without cancer (97%). The remaining patient had positive lymph nodes and died of cancer. Thirteen additional patients had a high-grade tumor; 9 were alive without cancer (69%), and 4 with positive lymph nodes died of cancer.

Turnbull et al.[42]	Memorial Sloan-Kettering	1948–1968	12	56

Results: All of the tumors were high-grade. Two patients were completely resected and were alive without cancer. Five patients were resected with positive margins, and all died of cancer. An additional 5 patients presented with advanced disease, and all died of cancer after palliative radiotherapy and chemotherapy.

Heitmiller et al.[16]	Massachusetts General	1948–1988	18	37

Results: Twelve patients had a low-grade tumor and were completely resected. All were free of cancer. Six other patients with a high-grade tumor had an incomplete resection. Three died of cancer and 3 were alive with cancer.

Conlan et al.[7]	Mayo Clinic	1927–1977	8	44

Results: Eight patients were completely resected and were alive without cancer (7 of 8 tumors were low-grade). An additional 4 patients with a high-grade tumor presented with advanced disease. All died of cancer after palliative radiotherapy.

mediate elements with intracellular bridges or cytoplasmic membranes. Glandular elements are also present as individual mucous cells, glandular cells, or acini. Broadly, the tumors are classified as low grade or high grade by the mitotic activity, level of necrosis, and nuclear pleomorphism (Fig. 51–80).[16, 20]

Diagnosis

As with any tumor that exists in the conducting airway, symptoms of cough, hemoptysis, and airway obstruction predominate. A radiographic test demonstrates the location and extent of the tumor, but bronchoscopy is needed for a histologic diagnosis.

Treatment and Results

Complete surgical resection is curative for most low-grade lesions. Adjuvant radiation therapy after resection appears to improve survival in patients with high-grade cancers.[42, 46] Because most tumors are low grade, operative results are generally good (Table 51–28). Survival is decreased for high-grade tumors, which tend to be larger, have lymph node involvement, and have distant metastases.[16, 42] There is no proven role for either radiation therapy or chemotherapy for patients with advanced disease.

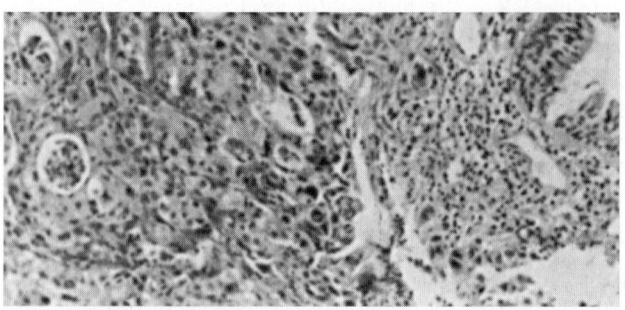

Figure 51–80. Histologic appearance of a low-grade mucoepidermoid carcinoma. Hematoxylin and eosin, × 125 before 3% reduction. (From Heitmiller, R. F., Mathisen, D. J., Ferry, J. A., et al.: Mucoepidermoid lung tumors. Ann. Thorac. Surg., *47*:394, 1989.)

SELECTED REFERENCES

Harpole, D. H., Feldman, J. M., Buchanan, S., Young, W. G., and Wolfe, W. G.: Bronchial carcinoid tumors: A retrospective analysis of 126 patients. Ann. Thorac. Surg., *54*:50, 1992.
A recently published series of patients with typical and atypical carcinoid of the lung reports multivariate analysis of factors, which negatively impacted survival, as well as a review of the literature.

Heitmiller, R. F., Mathisen, D. J., Ferry, J. A., et al.: Mucoepidermoid lung tumors. Ann. Thorac. Surg., *47*:394, 1989.
Data on 18 patients with mucoepidermoid carcinoma are presented, with a breakdown of results by tumor grade.

Moran, C. A., Suster, S., and Koss, M. N.: Primary adenoid cystic carcinoma of the lung. Cancer, *73*:1390, 1994.
Experience with 16 patients having adenoid cystic carcinoma is presented, with a detailed discussion of cell types and prognosis.

Warren, W. H., Memoli, V. A., and Gould, V. E.: Immunohistochemical and ultrastructural analysis of bronchopulmonary neuroendocrine neoplasms: I. Carcinoids. Ultrastruct. Pathol., *6*:15, 1984.
A description of light microscopic and ultrastructural anatomy of carcinoid tumors is presented.

Yousem, S. A., and Hochholzer, L.: Mucoepidermoid tumors of the lung. Cancer, *60*:1346, 1987.
An extensive series of patients with mucoepidermoid carcinoma from the Armed Forces Institute of Pathology is presented with a description of pathology, treatment, and long-term follow-up.

REFERENCES

1. Archer, R. L., Grogg, S. E., and Sanders, S. P.: Mucoepidermoid bronchial adenoma in a 6-year-old girl: A case report and review of the literature. Thorac. Cardiovasc. Surg., *94*:463, 1987.
2. Arrigoni, M. G., Woolner, L. B., and Bernatz, P. E.: Atypical carcinoid tumors of the lung. J. Thorac. Cardiovasc. Surg., *64*:413, 1972.
3. Attar, S., Miller, J. E., Hankins, J., et al.: Bronchial adenoma: A review of 51 patients. Ann. Thorac. Surg., *42*:126, 1985.
4. Azumi, N., and Battifora, H.: The cellular composition of adenoid cystic carcinoma. Cancer, *60*:1589, 1987.
5. Blalazs, M.: Adenoid cystic (cylindromatous) carcinoma of the trachea: An ultrastructural study. Histopathology, *10*:425, 1986.
6. Blodel, G. A., Gould, V. E., Moll, R., et al.: Coexpression of neuroendocrine markers and epithelial cytoskeletal proteins in bronchopulmonary neuroendocrine neoplasms. Lab. Invest., *52*:39, 1985.
7. Conlan, A. A., Payne, W. S., Woolner, L. B., and Sanderson, D. R.: Adenoid cystic carcinoma and mucoepidermoid carcinoma of the bronchus. J. Thorac. Cardiovasc. Surg., *76*:370, 1978.
8. Donahue, J. K., Weichert, R. F., and Ochsner, J. L.: Bronchial adenoma. Ann. Surg., *167*:873, 1968.
9. Dreyfuss, A. I., Clark, J. R., Fallon, B. G., Posner, M. R., Norris, C. M., and Miller, D.: Cyclophosphamide, doxorubicin and cisplatin combination chemotherapy for advanced carcinomas of salivary gland origin. Cancer, *60*:2869, 1987.
10. Feldman, J. M., Benning, T. L., and Saltzman, H. S.: Biochemical and

ultrastructural differences between mucoepidermoid and carcinoid tumors of the bronchus. J. Surg. Oncol., 37:227, 1988.

11. Godwin, D. J.: Carcinoid tumors: An analysis of 2837 cases. Cancer, 36:569, 1975.

12. Greenberg, R. S., Baumgarten, D. A., Clark, W. S.: Prognostic factors for gastrointestinal and bronchopulmonary carcinoid tumors. Cancer, 60:2476, 1987.

13. Halevy, A., Schachner, A., Nili, M., Moshe, N., et al.: Bronchial adenoma: Surgical experience with long-term follow-up (4–17 years). J. Surg. Oncol., 29:66, 1985.

14. Hamperl, H.: Über Gutartige Bronchialtumoren (Cylindrome und Carcinoide). Virchows Arch. Pathol. Anat., 300:46, 1937.

15. Harpole, D. H., Feldman, J. M., Buchanan, S., Young, W. G., and Wolfe, W. G.: Bronchial carcinoid tumors: A retrospective analysis of 126 patients. Ann. Thorac. Surg., 54:50, 1992.

16. Heitmiller, R. F., Mathisen, D. J., Ferry, J. A., et al.: Mucoepidermoid lung tumors. Ann. Thorac. Surg., 47:394, 1989.

17. Hosokawa, Y., Ohmori, K., Kaneko, M., Ahmed, M., Arimoto, T., and Irie, G.: Analysis of adenoid cystic carcinoma treated by radiotherapy. Oral Surg. Oral Med. Oral Pathol., 74:251, 1992.

18. Jackson, J.: Endothelioma of the right bronchus removed by peroral bronchoscopy. Am. J. Med. Sci., 153:371, 1917.

19. Jensik, R. J., Faber, L. P., Brown, C. M., et al.: Bronchoplastic and conservative resectional procedures for bronchial adenoma. J. Thorac. Cardiovasc. Surg., 68:556, 1974.

20. Klacsmann, P. G., Olsen, J. L., and Eggleston, J. C.: Mucoepidermoid carcinoma of the bronchus: An electron microscopic study of the low-grade and high-grade variants. Cancer, 43:1720, 1979.

21. Kramer, R.: Adenoma of bronchus. Ann. Otol. Rhinol. Laryngol., 39:689, 1930.

22. Le-Tian, X., Zhen-Fu, S., and Ze-Jian, L.: Tracheobronchial tumors: An eighteen-year series from Capital Hospital, Peking, China, Ann. Thorac. Surg., 35:590, 1983.

23. Linnoila, R. I., Mulshine, J. L., Steinberg, S. M., et al.: Neuroendocrine differentiation in endocrine and nonendocrine lung carcinomas. Am. J. Clin. Pathol., 90:641, 1988.

24. Lowe, J. E., Brigman, A. H., and Sabiston, D. C.: The role of bronchoplastic procedures in the surgical management of benign and malignant pulmonary lesions. J. Thorac. Cardiovasc. Surg., 83:227, 1982.

25. Markel, S. F., Abell, M. R., Haight, C., et al.: Neoplasms of bronchus commonly designated as adenomas. Cancer, 17:590, 1964.

26. McCaughan, B. C., Martini, N., and Bains, M. S.: Bronchial carcinoids. J. Thorac. Cardiovasc. Surg., 89:8, 1985.

27. Moran, C. A., Suster, S., and Koss, M. N.: Primary adenoid cystic carcinoma of the lung. Cancer, 73:1390, 1994.

28. Nomori, H., Kaseda, S., Kobayashi, K., et al.: Adenoid cystic carcinoma of the trachea and main-stem bronchus. J. Thorac. Cardiovasc. Surg., 96:271, 1988.

29. Oberndorfer, S.: Karzinoide. Ergeb. Allg. Pathol. Pathol. Anat., 13:527, 1909.

30. Okike, N., Bernatz, P. E., and Woolner, L. B.: Carcinoid tumors of the lung. Ann. Thorac. Surg., 22:270, 1976.

31. Paladugu, R. R., Benfield, J. R., Pak, H. Y., et al.: Bronchopulmonary Kulchitzky cell carcinoma: A new classification scheme for typical and atypical carcinoids. Cancer, 55:1303, 1985.

32. Pearson, F. G., Thompson, D. W., Weissberg, D., Simpson, W. J. K., and Kergin, F. G.: Adenoid cystic carcinoma of the trachea. Ann. Thorac. Surg., 18:16, 1974.

33. Rea, F., Binda, R., Spreafico, G., et al.: Bronchial carcinoids: A review of 60 patients. Ann. Thorac. Surg., 47:412, 1989.

34. Rozenman, J., Pausner, R., and Lieberman, Y.: Bronchial adenoma. Chest, 92:145, 1987.

35. Shaney, D. J., Daum-Kowalski, R., and Embry, R. L.: Adenoid cystic carcinoma of the airway. Am. J. Radiol., 156:1322, 1991.

36. Smetana, H. F., Iverson, L., and Swan, L. L.: Bronchogenic carcinoma: Analysis of 100 autopsy cases. Milit. Surg., 3:335, 1952.

37. Spizarny, D. L., Shepard, J. O., McCloud, T. C., Grillo, H. C., and Dedrick, C. G.: CT of adenoid cystic carcinoma of the trachea. Am. J. Radiol., 146:1129, 1986.

38. Stahlman, M. T., Kasselberg, A. G., and Orth, D. N.: Ontogeny of neuroendocrine cells in human fetal lung: II. An immunohistochemical study. Lab. Invest., 52:52, 1985.

39. Stamatis, G., Freitag, L., and Greschuchna, D.: Limited and radical resection for tracheal and bronchopulmonary carcinoid tumors. Eur. J. Cardiothorac. Surg., 4:527, 1990.

40. Todd, T. R., Cooper, J. D., Weissberg, D., et al.: Bronchial carcinoid tumors. J. Thorac. Cardiovasc. Surg., 79:532, 1980.

41. Toole, A. L., and Stern, H.: Carcinoid and adenoid cystic carcinoma of the bronchus. Ann. Thorac. Surg., 13:63, 1972.

42. Turnbull, A. D., Huvos, A. G., Goodner, J. T., and Foote, F. W.: Mucoepidermoid tumors of the bronchial glands. Cancer, 28:539, 1971.

43. Warren, W. H., Memoli, V. A., and Gould, V. E.: Immunohistochemical and ultrastructural analysis of bronchopulmonary neuroendocrine neoplasms: I. Carcinoids. Ultrastruct. Pathol., 6:15, 1984.

44. Warren, W. H., Memoli, V. A., and Gould, V. E.: Immunohistochemical and ultrastructural analysis of bronchopulmonary neuroendocrine neoplasms: II. Well-differentiated neuroendocrine carcinomas. Ultrastruct. Pathol., 7:185, 1984.

45. Wilkins, E. W., Grillo, H. C., and Moncure, A. C.: Changing times in surgical management of bronchopulmonary carcinoid tumor. Ann. Thorac. Surg., 38:339, 1984.

46. Yousem, S. A., and Hochholzer, L.: Mucoepidermoid tumors of the lung. Cancer, 60:1346, 1987.

XII _____

CARCINOMA OF THE LUNG

Thomas A. D'Amico, M.D., and David C. Sabiston, Jr., M.D.

Lung cancer is the most common cause of death from malignancy in both men and women (Table 51–29), and the age-adjusted death rate for lung cancer is increasing.[4] Staging of lung cancer by thoracic oncologists is essential for estimation of prognosis, selection of treatment, and evaluation of protocols. Advances in the understanding of the molecular biology of lung cancer are responsible for the development of novel immunotherapeutic strategies. Nevertheless, surgical resection represents the best chance for cure in most patients with lung cancer.

HISTORICAL ASPECTS

The first pneumonectomy was performed in 1895 by Sir William Macewen; he applied thermocoagulation in multiple stages to the chest wall, pleura, and lung in a patient with pleuropulmonary tuberculosis.[31] In 1933, Evarts Graham performed the first successful single-stage pneumonectomy in a patient with squamous cell carcinoma.[13] The patient recovered and survived two decades thereafter, to die eventually of an unrelated disease, free of cancer. This case demonstrated not only that pneumonectomy could be achieved but also that lung cancer was curable by adequate pulmonary resection.

PATHOLOGY

Lung cancer is divided into two categories for the purposes of staging, estimating prognosis, and selecting therapy: small cell and non–small cell carcinoma. Small cell lung cancer (SCLC) is characterized by more rapid growth, stronger likelihood of metastases being present at the time of diagnosis, and greater responsiveness to chemotherapy and radiation therapy. The remaining cell types, together considered non–small cell lung cancer (NSCLC), represent 75% to 80% of all lung carcinomas and are discussed collectively, because therapeutic approaches to patients with any of these cell types are identical.

The three major histologic types of NSCLC are adenocarcinoma, squamous cell carcinoma, and large cell carcinoma.

TABLE 51–29. Estimated Cancer Deaths by Sex and Type of Cancer

Type of Cancer	Percentage
Men	
Lung	33
Colon and rectum	10
Prostate	13
Leukemia/lymphoma	8
Urinary tract	5
Pancreas	4
Stomach	3
Melanoma	2
Oral	2
All other types	20
Women	
Lung	23
Breast	18
Colon and rectum	11
Leukemia/lymphoma	8
Pancreas	5
Ovary	5
Uterus	4
Urinary tract	3
Melanoma	1
Oral	1
All other types	21

From Boring, C. C., Squires, T. S., Tong, T., and Montgomery, S.: Cancer statistics, 1994. CA Cancer J. Clin., *44*:7, 1994.

Other less common histologic types include adenosquamous carcinoma, bronchoalveolar carcinoma (a subset of adenocarcinoma), bronchial carcinoids, and bronchial gland tumors. There has been a considerable shift in the incidence of histologic types of NSCLC over recent years: adenocarcinomas have been increasing in frequency and squamous cell carcinomas have become less common. Many pulmonary malignancies demonstrate more than one type of histologic differentiation pattern, suggesting the possibility of a pluripotential stem cell.

Adenocarcinoma is the most common histologic type, occuring in approximately 50% of patients with lung cancer. Adenocarcinomas are often peripheral lesions and tend to invade the pleura. Histologically, adenocarcinomas are subdivided into acinar, papillary, and bronchoalveolar forms. Bronchoalveolar carcinoma may present in two distinct manners, as a solitary pulmonary nodule or as a diffuse infiltrative process.[22]

Squamous cell carcinoma, once the most common cell type, now represents approximately 30% of all lung cancers. Squamous carcinomas originate centrally, grow toward the mainstem bronchus, and invade bronchial cartilage, pulmonary parenchyma, and lymph nodes. The epithelium in the normal tracheobronchial tree does not contain squamous epithelium; progressive histologic changes occur in the bronchial mucosa in the development of squamous cell carcinoma.[22]

Large cell carcinomas, peripheral lesions that are unrelated to bronchi, rapidly invade the parenchyma and tend to metastasize early. Histologically, large cell carcinomas exhibit no evidence for glandular or squamous differentiation; they are distinguished from small cell carcinoma by the presence of abundant cytoplasm, distinct borders, and enlarged nuclei containing prominent nucleoli. However, by electron microscopy, many large cell carcinomas demonstrate aspects of differentiation into adenocarcinoma, squamous carcinoma, or small cell carcinoma.[22]

The histologic features of SCLC are distinct. Within the nucleus, the distribution of chromatin is uniform, the nucleoli are unusually small and indistinct, and mitoses are frequent. The cells, which often contain scant cytoplasm, assume a spindle or fusiform shape, arranged in bundles.[12] An important distinguishing characteristic of small cell carcinoma is the presence of cytoplasmic neurosecretory granules on electron microscopy. Bronchopulmonary carcinoids are low-grade neoplasms characterized by neuroendocrine features: the presence of neurosecretory granules by electron microscopy and the production of peptide hormones. Carcinoids are characterized by cellular growth in solid sheets or in mixed patterns of sheets, cords, nests, and trabeculae. Atypical carcinoid tumors, which demonstrate cellular pleomorphism, frequent mitoses, hyperchromatic nuclei, and scant cytoplasm, confer poor prognosis.[22]

MOLECULAR BIOLOGY OF LUNG CANCER

Mutations in dominant and recessive oncogenes have been demonstrated in the pathogenesis of lung cancer. The presence of some oncogenic mutations is associated with shorter overall survival and disease-free survival compared with patients in whom no mutations have been identified. Advances in the understanding of the molecular biology of lung cancer may contribute to the development of strategies for prevention and treatment.

Oncogenes

Dominant Oncogenes. Dominant oncogenes are the mutated forms of cellular genes (proto-oncogenes) that control cellular proliferation. The genes involved are responsible for the production of growth factors, growth factor receptors, membrane proteins associated with signal transduction, and nuclear proteins involved in transcriptional control and gene expression. The three families of dominant oncogenes that are most commonly associated in the pathogenesis of lung cancer are the *ras*, *erb* B, and *myc* oncogenes.

The *ras* family of proto-oncogenes encode the membrane-associated proteins involved in signal transduction. The presence of the *ras* mutation is associated with shorter overall survival and disease-free survival compared with patients in whom no *ras* mutation has been identified.[44]

Another family of oncogenes mutated in human lung cancer is the *erb* B family, which encode membrane-associated tyrosine kinases that function as growth factor receptors. The *erb* B1 proto-oncogene is found to be amplified in all histologic variants of NSCLC; the *erb* B2 proto-oncogene was found to be overexpressed in 93% of patients with adenocarcinoma of the lung.[3] The presence of the *erb* B mutation has not been demonstrated to affect disease-free survival or overall survival in patients with lung cancer.

Transcriptional activation of the *myc* family of nuclear proto-oncogenes (c-*myc*, N-*myc*, L-*myc*) has also been demonstrated. The gene products of the *myc* family of oncogenes are nuclear phosphoproteins that are involved in cell-cycle regulation and are more frequently expressed abnormally in SCLC cells than in NSCLC cells.[5] Small cell lung tumors with c-*myc* amplified tumors confer a poorer prognosis, compared with other small cell tumors, among patients with advanced stage SCLC.

Recessive Oncogenes. The loss, inactivation, or transformation of the genes that function to suppress cellular proliferation may permit unregulated growth and contribute to the pathogenesis of lung cancer.[23] Such genes are termed *recessive oncogenes* (because both genes are deleted or mutated in transformed cells) or tumor suppressor genes (because the untransformed genes function to suppress cellular proliferation). The most common recessive oncogenes associated with the pathogenesis of lung cancer include *p53* and the retinoblastoma *(Rb)* gene.

Mutations of the *p53* gene, a tumor suppressor gene that normally codes for a nuclear phosphoprotein required to maintain a transformed (malignant) phenotype, are the most common genetic alteration identified in human cancer. Normal (wild-type) *p53* negatively regulates cell growth; mutated forms stimulate cell division and promote malignancy. Mutations in *p53* have been found in nearly all cell lines for patients with SCLC and in approximately 50% of cell lines from patients with NSCLC. There has been no association identified between the presence of *p53* mutation and survival.[18] The retinoblastoma *(Rb)* gene has been demonstrated to be mutated or deleted in up to 60% of SCLC primary tumors, and defective *Rb* gene product has been discovered in 95% of NSCLC tumors.

Immunotherapy

Various forms of immunologic modulation have been designed for the prevention and treatment of lung cancer. The strategies for therapeutic intervention at the cellular and molecular levels include administration of adoptive immunotherapy, delivery of monoclonal antibodies, development of antimetastatic vaccination, and modulation of oncogene expression.

Adoptive Immunotherapy. Adoptive immunotherapy with lymphokine activated killer (LAK) cells and high-dose systemic interleukin-2 (IL-2) has achieved tumor regression in some patients with advanced malignant disease but has not been shown to be effective in patients with NSCLC. Tumor necrosis factor-alpha (TNF) and IL-2 have poor antitumor activity as single agents, yet are synergistic for LAK activation. In a study from the National Cancer Institute, the synergistic activation of LAK with IL-2 and TNF demonstrated enhanced oncolytic activity against NSCLC tumor targets when compared with IL-2 alone.[47] The administration of the combination of IL-2 and TNF is biologically more active than either agent alone and may involve long-term stimulation of the immune system.

Monoclonal Antibodies. The generation of monoclonal antibodies using cell hybridization has been used for the production of specific molecular probes in the analysis of tumor cells. The characterization of tumor-associated antigens may provide a new approach to tumor-specific diagnosis and therapy. Tumor-associated antigens are expressed at significantly higher levels in neoplastic cells than in normal cells and may be used for site-directed delivery of therapy, including chemotherapy, radioisotopes, or elements of the antibody-dependent cellular cytotoxicity and complement-mediated toxicity cascades. Although no totally specific monoclonal antibody against human lung cancer has been developed, the tumor-associated antibodies that have been produced may contribute to better understanding of the molecular biology of lung cancer. A large panel of specific antibodies against lung cancer–associated antigens has been developed; these antibodies may be applied to tumor imaging, conjugation to radioisotopes, or conjugation to chemotherapeutic agents.

Tumor Immunization. Vaccination of tumor-bearing animals has been accomplished by introducing the interferon-gamma (IFN-γ) gene into tumor cells through retroviral vectors.[35] It has been demonstrated that IFN-γ augments the immune response by increasing the cellular antigen-presenting capacity and participates in the mediation of the inflammatory response by activating macrophages. The direct administration of IFN-γ to tumor-bearing animals has been shown to produce antitumor activity; however, adequate IFN-γ levels—necessary to provide sustained antitumor

activity—require constant infusions or repeated administrations.

In an experimental study from the Memorial Sloan-Kettering Cancer Center, the insertion (using retroviral vectors) of the IFN-γ gene into tumor cells of a metastatic, poorly immunogenic murine lung cancer model produced IFN-γ gene expression and high, sustained serum IFN-γ levels.[35] In this model, immunization of mice carrying an established lung tumor prevented metastatic dissemination. Furthermore, immunization of mice carrying established micrometastases produced significant regression of disease. The use of IFN-γ transferred tumor cells, by providing high, sustained levels of serum IFN-γ, may provide a therapeutic advantage for the treatment of advanced lung cancer.

Modulation of Oncogene Expression. Modulation of oncogene expression has heretofore been considered an ineffective method of treatment of carcinoma of the lung because most lung cancer cells prove to have multiple genetic abnormalities at the time of diagnosis. Recent studies, however, have demonstrated that it may not be necessary to reverse all of the genetic transformations in a lung cancer cell to be effective.[37]

Several strategies have been described to interfere with the expression of abnormal oncogenes. The antisense technique utilizes a nucleotide sequence that is complementary to the target mRNA to interfere with the translation of the abnormal protein (oncogene product) of the endogenous mRNA. The antisense approach is limited by the reliance of the technique on a continuous supply of the appropriate nucleotide sequence to interfere with the expression of the abnormal protein. However, if a recombinant construct expressing the antisense sequence becomes part of the cell genome, the antisense mRNA will be continuously produced.

Nucleotide sequences that specifically inhibit expression of oncogenes may be delivered by viral vectors. Retroviral vectors have been implemented, having the advantage of being incorporated in the genome of replicating cells exclusively, favoring integration into cancer cell DNA. Replication-defective retroviral vectors become integrated into the host genome and produce the protein encoded by the vector but do not replicate the virus. In one study, human lung cancer cells were delivered to immunosuppressed mice.[9] After the tumors were established, mice were inoculated with retroviral vectors, either with or without the antisense sequence. Tumor growth was suppressed in the group that received retrovirus expressing the antisense K-*ras* construct. A clinical protocol has been designed to test the efficacy of retroviral antisense K-*ras* constructs in inhibiting the growth of incompletely resected lung cancer.[37]

PATHOGENESIS

The relationship between environmental pathogens and the development of lung cancer was first observed in the 16th century in the workers in the mines of Schneeberg, Germany, and Joachimstal, Czechoslovakia. The combination of uranium and radon gas in these mines is thought to have been primarily responsible for the development of malignant pulmonary neoplasms. The most important agent in the pathogenesis of carcinoma of the lung is now recognized to be cigarette smoking, and evidence linking cigarette smoking and carcinoma of the lung is abundant. Several studies have established a clear relationship between the magnitude of tobacco use and the incidence of lung cancer. In a landmark postmortem study, Auerbach examined the entire tracheobronchial tree in 117 men.[1] In this study, 34 died of lung cancer, and all were smokers. Furthermore, progressive increases in the severity of cytologic transformation correlated with the amount of tobacco use. In a large prospective study of British male physicians, 114 cases of SCLC were observed in 155,708 man-years among smokers, compared with only 1 case in 103,383 man-years among nonsmokers.[8] This study also demonstrated a positive dose-response relationship between the number of cigarettes consumed each day and the incidence of SCLC.

Most carcinogens act synergistically with cigarette smoke as etiologic agents in the pathogenesis of lung cancer. Passive smoking, considered to account for 25% of carcinoma of the lung in nonsmokers, may increase the risk of cancer up to 50% among nonsmokers who live with smokers. Other carcinogens include arsenic, cadmium, chromium, radon, and workplace chemicals, such as chromoethyl ether. Chronic obstructive pulmonary disease (COPD) has also been demonstrated to be a predisposing factor in the development of carcinoma of the lung.

DIAGNOSIS AND STAGING OF LUNG CANCER

The primary objective in the diagnosis and staging of carcinoma of the lung is to identify patients who are candidates to undergo thoracotomy for curative pulmonary resection. A complete history is taken and a physical examination is performed, with particular attention to possible manifestations of the primary tumor. Symptoms relating to carcinoma of the lung depend on the anatomic location of the tumor, extension into surrounding structures, metastatic spread, and the systemic effects of paraneoplastic syndromes. Most patients found to have lung cancer present with symptomatic disease; only 6% of patients are asymptomatic at the time of diagnosis. By the time the diagnosis of carcinoma of the lung is made, most patients have regional lymph node involvement or distant metastases.

Thoracic Symptoms

Symptoms referable to the thorax may result from endobronchial growth, extrinsic growth, or regional spread of the primary tumor. Centrally located lesions may be associated with cough, stridor, wheezing, hemoptysis, dyspnea, and chest pain. The most common symptom is cough, which results from endobronchial erosion and irritation. Peripheral tumors may be associated with chest pain, cough, and dyspnea, secondary to pleural and chest wall involvement. Large peripheral tumors may undergo cavitation and present as lung abscesses.

Intrathoracic extension of lung tumors may involve surrounding structures. Invasion of the recurrent laryngeal nerve may be manifested as hoarseness, and involvement of the esophagus may present as dysphagia. Local extension of a tumor at the apex of the lung, involving the eighth cervical and first thoracic nerves, may produce the superior sulcus (Pancoast) tumor syndrome, characterized by ipsilateral shoulder and arm pain. Furthermore, paravertebral extension and sympathetic nerve involvement may result in Horner's syndrome: enophthalmos, ptosis, meiosis, and ipsilateral anhidrosis.

The development of malignant pleural effusion often results in exacerbation of symptoms of chest pain and shortness of breath. Recurrence after thoracentesis is a poor prognostic sign. Tumor involving the heart and pericardium may result in effusion, with subsequent pericardial tamponade, arrhythmia, or congestive heart failure.

Extensive tumor involvement of right mediastinal lymph nodes may result in superior vena caval syndrome, characterized by plethoric appearance, distention of the venous drainage of the arm and neck, and edema of the face, neck, and arms. Vena caval obstruction usually progresses gradually over a period of time, allowing the development of collateral venous drainage, detectable on physical examination.

Paraneoplastic Syndromes

Paraneoplastic syndromes, symptoms, or findings that are related to the primary tumor or its metastases by hormonal intermediates may accompany lung cancer. Systemic manifestations of NSCLC include cachexia, parathyroid-like hormone secretion with concomitant hypercalcemia, hypertrophic pulmonary osteoarthropathy, and various neurologic syndromes.[36] Weight loss and anorexia occur in up to one third of patients.

Paraneoplastic syndromes are frequently associated with SCLC and are more often present at the time of diagnosis than in patients with NSCLC. In addition to weight loss, anorexia, and neuromyopathies, paraneoplastic syndromes may result from tumor elaboration of antidiuretic hormone, adrenocorticotropic hormone, calcitonin, or parathyroid hormone.

Diagnostic Techniques

Chest Films. The diagnosis of lung cancer is often suggested by findings on chest radiography, and histologic confirmation may be accomplished by bronchoscopy, by percutaneous biopsy, or at thoracotomy for pulmonary resection. Most important, current chest radiographs are reviewed and compared with previous studies. A solitary pulmonary nodule, which may appear as either a smooth-bordered lesion or an irregular mass, is the classic radiographic presentation of carcinoma of the lung. The chest radiograph usually demonstrates a mass arising in the hilum or the lung field, although a pneumonic infiltrate, a pleural effusion, or an elevated diaphragm may additionally be present. Collapse of a pulmonary segment or lobe distal to an obstructing endobronchial lesion may be manifested as atelectasis. Gross nodal involvement is frequently evident as well.

Computed Tomography. Computed tomography (CT) of the chest is useful in the evaluation of the primary tumor, in the assessment of regional lymph node involvement, and in the detection of satellite nodules or mediastinal metastases. CT scans should include the apices of the thorax superiorly and extend inferiorly to include the liver and the adrenal glands. It is usually accepted that a maximum diameter of 10 mm. is acceptable for considering hilar and mediastinal nodes to be uninvolved, suggesting operability. However, even lymph nodes determined by CT scan to be enlarged will contain metastatic tumor in only 70% of cases. Thus, suspected inoperability on the basis of a positive CT scan should be confirmed histologically, unless evidence of inoperability is overwhelming. Patients without mediastinal lymphadenopathy on CT, and who are otherwise operative candidates, may proceed to thoracotomy; the false-negative rate in these patients is only 5%.[6]

Bronchoscopy. Flexible fiberoptic bronchoscopy is an important adjunct in the diagnosis of carcinoma of the lung. Bronchial biopsy, brushings, washings, and transbronchial aspiration may be used to establish the diagnosis of malignancy in a majority of cases. When the tumor is bronchoscopically visible, the yield for washings and brushings is approximately 75% and for biopsy the yield is approximately 85%, for a total yield of 94%. In contrast, for tumors that are not visualized, bronchoscopy with brushings and washings has a yield of 50% and bronchoscopy with biopsy has a yield of 60%.

Mediastinoscopy. The role of mediastinoscopy in the diagnosis and staging of carcinoma of the lung is controversial. In patients in whom noninvasive staging demonstrates evidence for mediastinal nodal involvement, mediastinoscopy will document involvement in approximately 70%. Mediastinoscopy with biopsy is recommended for selected patients whose CT scan demonstrates mediastinal lymph nodes greater than 10 mm. in diameter, who would not be candidates for pulmonary resection if the mediastinal nodes were positive for carcinoma. Several nodal groups (posterior subcarinal, pericardial, periesophageal, and para-aortic) are inaccessible by standard mediastinoscopy. Extended cervical mediastinoscopy, left parasternal mediastinoscopy (Chamberlain procedure), or thoracoscopy may be used for biopsy of enlarged nodes in these areas in some patients with carcinoma of the lung.

Thoracoscopy. Thoracoscopic staging of lung cancer has been demonstrated to be safe and effective in selected patients.[33] The most common application is the evaluation of indeterminate pulmonary nodules. However, thoracoscopy may also be used for complete evaluation of suspicious para-aortic, subaortic, tracheobronchial, carinal, paraesophageal, or hilar lymph nodes. Finally, thoracoscopy may also be used to confirm pleural invasion or dissemination.[45] The development of techniques to improve localization and characterization of pulmonary nodules (such as thoracoscopic ultrasound and preoperative needle-localization) may expand the indications for thoracoscopy in the staging of carcinoma of the lung.

Transthoracic Needle Aspiration. Transthoracic needle aspiration (TTNA), which may be performed using fluoroscopic, ultrasonographic, or CT guidance, may be useful in the diagnosis of lesions that are not visualized by bronchoscopy. TTNA need not be applied to every patient with a solitary pulmonary nodule to confirm the diagnosis of malignancy preoperatively. A benign or undetermined histologic diagnosis by TTNA (which has a significant false-negative rate) does not definitively exclude the possibility of malignancy. Regardless of the result of TTNA, a patient who is a candidate for thoracotomy should undergo pulmonary resection, for diagnosis and therapy. The indications for TTNA include pulmonary lesions in patients who are poor candidates for thoracotomy yet require definitive diagnosis; a new pulmonary lesion in a patient with a history of prior malignancy; and a lung mass that is suggestive of small cell carcinoma. The complications of TTNA include pneumothorax, hemothorax, and infection.

Magnetic Resonance Imaging. Magnetic resonance imaging (MRI) of the chest differentiates vascular from solid structures and demonstrates parenchymal, hilar, and mediastinal anatomy in both coronal and sagittal planes, without the use of contrast agents or ionizing radiation. MRI is nevertheless limited by long scanning times, motion artifacts, and inferior spatial resolution. The current role for MRI in the staging of carcinoma of the lung includes preoperative nodal staging in patients in whom the use of contrast agents is contraindicated and confirmation of spinal cord involvement in patients with metastatic disease.

Positron Emission Tomography. Positron emission tomography (PET) is a noninvasive imaging method that has demonstrated increased glucose metabolism in malignant cells. This technique has demonstrated a sensitivity of 94% and a specificity of 80% in distinguishing benign from malignant pulmonary nodules.[42] PET may prove to be especially useful in establishing the diagnosis of malignancy before thoracotomy in patients with high surgical risk. The application of PET in the evaluation of mediastinal lymph node involvement is being assessed in prospective trials.

Staging of NSCLC

The TNM staging system for carcinoma of the lung provides a consistent, reproducible description of the anatomic

TABLE 51–30. International TNM Staging System for Lung Cancer

Tumor (T)

T_x Occult carcinoma (malignant cells in sputum or bronchial washings but tumor not visualized by imaging studies or bronchoscopy)

T_1 Tumor 3 cm. or less in greatest diameter, surrounded by lung or visceral pleura, but not proximal to a lobar bronchus

T_2 Tumor >3 cm. in diameter, or with involvement of main bronchus at least 2 cm. distal to carina, or with visceral pleural invasion, or with associated atelectasis or obstructive pneumonitis extending to the hilar region but not involving the entire lung

T_3 Tumor invading chest wall, diaphragm, mediastinal pleura, or parietal pericardium; or tumor in main bronchus within 2 cm. of, but not invading carina; or atelectasis of obstructive pneumonitis of the entire lung

T_4 Tumor invading mediastinum, heart, great vessels, trachea, esophagus, vertebral body, or carina; or ipsilateral malignant pleural effusion

Nodes (N)

N_0 No regional lymph node metastases

N_1 Metastases to ipsilateral peribronchial or hilar nodes

N_2 Metastases to ipsilateral mediastinal or subcarinal nodes

N_3 Metastases to contralateral mediastinal or hilar or to any scalene or supraclavicular nodes

Distant Metastases (M)

M_0 No distant metastases

M_1 Distant metastases

From Mountain, C. F.: A new international staging system for lung cancer. Chest, *89*:225S, 1986.

extent of disease at the time of diagnosis.[32] In the TNM system, T represents the primary tumor and numerical suffixes describe increasing size or involvement; N represents regional lymph nodes with suffixes to describe levels of involvement; and M designates the presence or absence of distant metastases (Table 51–30). The TNM subsets are subsequently grouped in a series of stages of disease, to identify groups of patients with similar prognosis and therapy (Table 51–31 and Fig. 51–81). The value of the staging system in estimating prognosis is demonstrated by the 5-year survival statistics, as illustrated in Table 51–32.

Staging of SCLC

The TNM staging system has not proved to be as prognostically useful for SCLC, which usually presents as widespread metastases at the time of diagnosis. Even patients who present with small primary tumors and no evidence of nodal disease often have distant metastases. Currently, most

TABLE 51–31. Staging Groups for Lung Cancer

Stage	T	N	M
Occult	T_x	N_0	M_0
Stage I	T_{1-2}	N_0	M_0
Stage II	T_{1-2}	N_1	M_0
Stage IIIa	T_3	N_{0-1}	M_0
	T_{1-3}	N_2	M_0
Stage IIIb	T_4	N_{0-2}	M_0
	T_{1-4}	N_3	M_0
Stage IV	Any T	Any N	M_1

From Mountain, C. F.: A new international staging system for lung cancer. Chest, *89*:225S, 1986.

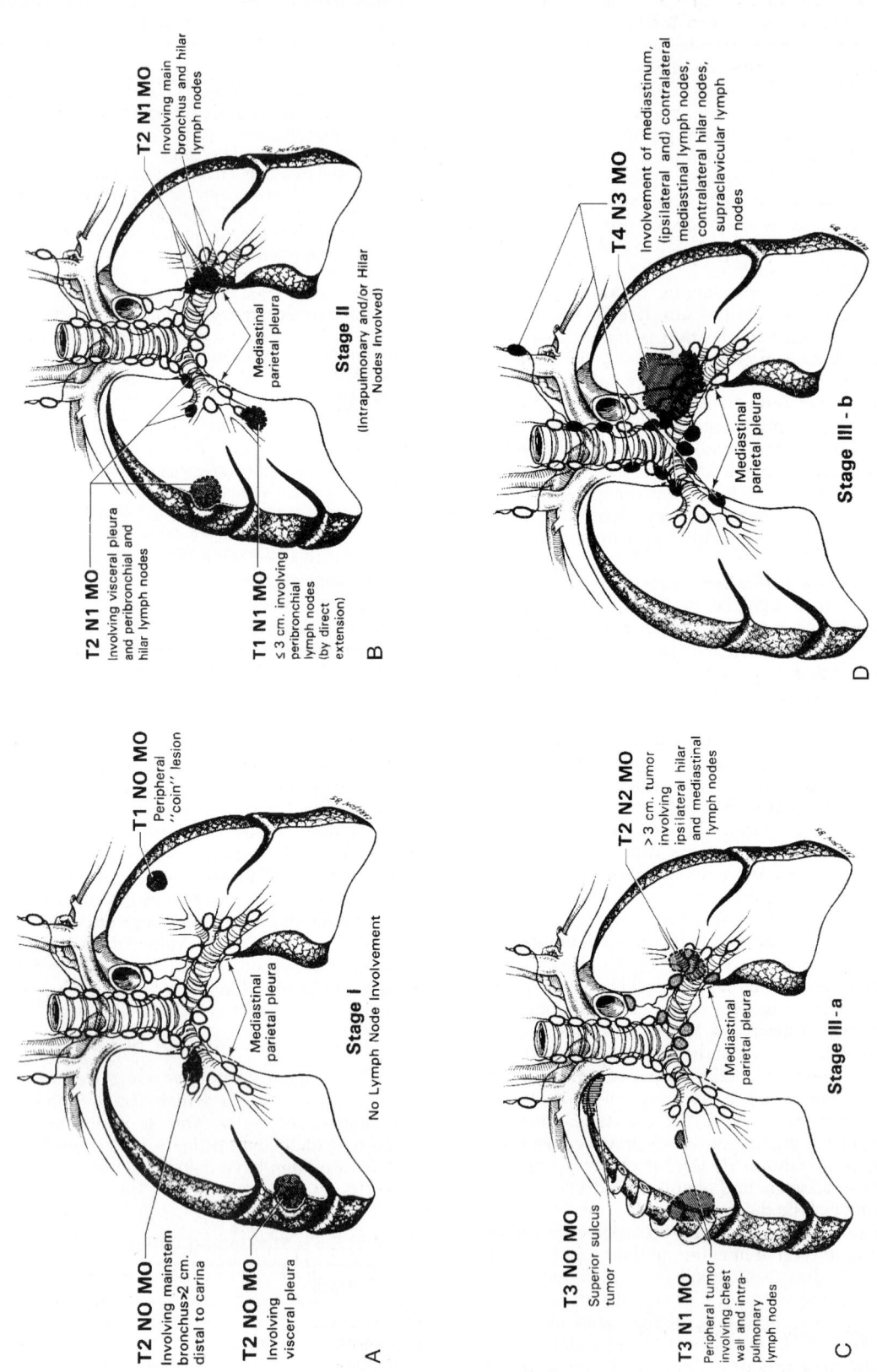

T2 N0 M0
Involving mainstem bronchus>2 cm. distal to carina

T2 N0 M0
Involving visceral pleura

Mediastinal parietal pleura

T1 N0 M0
Peripheral "coin" lesion

Stage I

No Lymph Node Involvement

A

T2 N1 M0
Involving visceral pleura and peribronchial and hilar lymph nodes

T2 N1 M0
Involving main bronchus and hilar lymph nodes

Mediastinal parietal pleura

T1 N1 M0
≤ 3 cm. involving peribronchial lymph nodes (by direct extension)

Stage II

(Intrapulmonary and/or Hilar Nodes Involved)

B

T3 N0 M0
Superior sulcus tumor

T2 N2 M0
> 3 cm. tumor involving ipsilateral hilar and mediastinal lymph nodes

Mediastinal parietal pleura

T3 N1 M0
Peripheral tumor involving chest wall and intra-pulmonary lymph nodes

Stage III - a

C

T4 N3 M0
Involvement of mediastinum, (ipsilateral and) contralateral mediastinal lymph nodes, contralateral hilar nodes, supraclavicular lymph nodes

Mediastinal parietal pleura

Stage III - b

D

Figure 51–81. *A* to *D,* Staging groups for carcinoma of the lung. (From Mountain, C. F.: A new international staging system for lung cancer. Chest, *89:*225S, 1986.)

TABLE 51–32. Five-Year Survival in Non–Small Cell Lung Cancer According to Stage

Stage	Five-Year Survival (%)
Stage I	66.7
Stage II	43.6
Stage IIIa	22.4
Stage IIIb	5.4
Stage IV	5.9

From Naruke, T., Goya, T., Tsuchiya, R., et al.: Prognosis and survival in resected lung carcinoma based on the new international staging system for lung cancer. J. Thorac. Cardiovasc. Surg., 96:440, 1988.

thoracic oncologists utilize a staging system that divides patients with SCLC into two major groups: those with *limited* disease and those with *extensive* disease. Limited disease is considered to be disease confined to the hemithorax (with or without ipsilateral hilar or mediastinal lymph nodes) and no detectable distant metastases. Extensive disease is characterized by involvement of the contralateral thorax or the presence of distant metastases.[5]

Solitary Pulmonary Nodule

A patient with a solitary pulmonary nodule—a single spherical lesion within the lung—represents an important and challenging diagnostic problem in thoracic oncology. A solitary pulmonary nodule is assumed to be primary lung cancer until proved otherwise; the differential diagnosis includes metastatic carcinoma, granuloma, and benign pulmonary tumors.

In most cases, solitary pulmonary nodules should be resected after thorough investigation to establish that systemic dissemination has not already occurred. Review of previous chest radiographs may assist in determining the growth pattern of the nodule. A malignant nodule will usually have a doubling time of 30 to 400 days. The demonstration of stability compared to previous films or the presence of visible calcification suggests a benign lesion, and a period of observation may be warranted.

CT scans of the chest, liver, and adrenals are obtained to confirm the location of the tumor, to evaluate the mediastinum, and to assess the abdomen for systemic disease. If there is no evidence of metastases on CT, the patient should undergo bronchoscopy. Bronchoscopic examination, with brushings and biopsy, may establish the histologic diagnosis and may determine resectability if an endobronchial lesion exists.

Pulmonary function studies are obtained preoperatively to assess the potential for pulmonary resection. A thorough review of systems is undertaken to exclude the presence of medical contraindications to thoracotomy. TTNA is not routinely performed and should be reserved for patients with marginal pulmonary function, for whom thoracotomy would only be performed after the verification of a malignant histologic diagnosis.

SURGICAL MANAGEMENT OF NSCLC

Every solitary pulmonary nodule should be resected unless the lesion is known to be benign or the patient's medical condition contraindicates surgical procedure. Thorough preoperative evaluation and preparation of a patient with carcinoma of the lung reduces the morbidity and mortality of thoracotomy and pulmonary resection. Surgical resection is the standard treatment of patients with Stage I or Stage II disease. In addition, a subset of patients with Stage III disease

have been demonstrated to have improved outcome with surgical resection.

Determination of Operability

Determination of operability must include assessment of the medical risk of thoracotomy as well as the risk of removal of the requisite pulmonary parenchyma. The degree of cardiopulmonary disease, usually a consequence of tobacco use, represents the most significant medical factor in determining operability and the major cause of postoperative morbidity and mortality. Patients with lung cancer have an increased risk of COPD: 90% have signs and symptoms of COPD, and 20% have severe pulmonary dysfunction.[24]

Preoperative Pulmonary Evaluation. Pulmonary function tests are used to determine the feasibility of pulmonary resection. Estimation of postoperative pulmonary function is based on the calculation of the preoperative function and the projected resection of pulmonary parenchyma. Patients are excluded from surgical therapy if estimated postoperative pulmonary function falls below the minimum acceptable values. In particular, when the forced expiratory volume at 1 second (FEV_1) and forced vital capacity are less than 30% of predicted values, thoracotomy is generally contraindicated. If the value of the predicted postoperative FEV_1 is at least 60% of the predicted value, the patient is considered able to tolerate resection. When the results of the preoperative pulmonary function studies are marginal, radionuclide ventilation (xenon-133 radiorespirometry) scans may be required to determine resectability. Postoperative FEV_1 may be calculated after assessing the contribution of either lung and specific pulmonary segments to overall pulmonary function.

Exercise oxygen consumption (VO_2max) studies may also be used to determine resectability in patients with borderline pulmonary function tests. In one study, high mortality was associated with VO_2max less than 10 ml. per kg. per minute; in patients with VO_2max greater than 20 ml. per kg. per minute, no deaths occurred.[2]

Resectability at Thoracotomy. Final determination of resectability is made at thoracotomy. Contraindications to pulmonary resection at the time of thoracotomy include pleural metastases, extensive mediastinal lymph node involvement (N_3 disease), or direct extension of the tumor (T_4 disease). In addition, pulmonary resection is aborted when complete resection would result in inadequate pulmonary reserve, as determined by preoperative pulmonary function studies.

Surgical Procedures

Complete resection of the tumor and all grossly involved regional bronchial and mediastinal lymph nodes, including *en bloc* resection of adjacent structures involved by direct extension of the primary tumor (such as chest wall and pericardium), is undertaken when feasible. Incomplete resection or resection that would leave a patient with an inadequate functional pulmonary reserve should not be performed. Intraoperative evaluation of tumor extent, in conjunction with the cardiopulmonary status of the patient, determines the particular surgical procedure employed. If histologic diagnosis has not been confirmed preoperatively, biopsy and frozen section examination are indicated, particularly if the planned resection is more extensive than lobectomy.

Standard surgical procedures employed in the management of carcinoma of the lung include pneumonectomy, bilobectomy, lobectomy, segmentectomy, and wedge resection. The procedure selected must provide removal of the entire tumor, with adequate margins, while preserving the maximum amount of functional lung tissue. Posterolateral thoracotomy, entering the thorax in the fifth or sixth intercostal space, provides adequate exposure in most cases. At the time of thoracotomy, a systematic lymph node evaluation is undertaken and recorded to ascertain complete pathologic staging.

The most commonly performed pulmonary resection for lung cancer is lobectomy. Functional loss after lobectomy is usually greater than predicted immediately after resection; however, over time, pulmonary function improves to the expected level. A sleeve lobectomy may be performed when the primary tumor encroaches on the lobar orifice, precluding complete resection with margins by standard lobectomy. In the right lung, a bilobectomy may be performed, conserving either the upper or lower lobe. The indications for bilobectomy include tumor extending across a lobar fissure, absent fissure, endobronchial tumor, or tumor invading bronchus intermedius.

Pneumonectomy is performed when lobectomy does not provide complete resection and when the loss of pulmonary parenchyma may be tolerated. Modifications of the standard pneumonectomy include intrapericardial ligation of the pulmonary vessels, supra-aortic pneumonectomy on the left, and tracheal sleeve pneumonectomy. After pneumonectomy, the ipsilateral pleural cavity is aspirated to prevent contralateral shift of the mediastinum and pulmonary compromise. Alternatively, a pressure-balancing pleural catheter may be placed.

Patients with small peripheral lesions may be candidates for segmentectomy. Segmentectomy has been advocated to provide complete resection while preserving more functional parenchyma. Wedge resection may be performed in high-risk patients or in patients with small lesions without lymph node involvement. Limited pulmonary resection is associated with a higher recurrence rate when compared with lobectomy.[11, 46]

Pulmonary resection of any magnitude may be combined with *en bloc* removal of structures contiguous with the visceral pleura, into which direct extension of the tumor has occurred (T_3 disease). Extended resection may include portions of the chest wall, diaphragm, or pericardium. The morbidity and mortality of the extended pulmonary resection is higher than that of standard resections. When appropriate patient selection is undertaken, the risk of the extended procedure is justified by the potential for complete resection.

Video-assisted thoracoscopic resection of carcinoma of the lung has been reported and is under evaluation.[19] Thoracoscopic management of a solitary pulmonary nodule may achieve specific histologic diagnosis, adequate nodal staging, and complete resection in selected patients. The Video Assisted Thoracic Surgery Study Group collected 1820 thoracoscopic procedures among 40 institutions for analysis.[14] The most common procedure performed was wedge resection (49%), and anatomic resection for carcinoma of the lung was achieved in only 38 patients (2%). Of 1820 cases, 439 (24%) were converted to open thoracotomy. In utilizing the thoracoscopic approach for evaluation and resection of primary pulmonary malignancy, complete excision and nodal staging must be ascertained and oncologic principles of thoracic procedure observed.

Results of Surgical Resection

Stage I. The treatment of choice, particularly for more centrally located tumors, is lobectomy, although wedge resection or segmentectomy may be performed for small peripheral tumors. A systematic lymph node dissection is performed at thoracotomy to ascertain that no hilar or mediastinal lymph node involvement is present. Patients with Stage I carcinoma of the lung can expect 3- and 5-year survival rates of approximately 85% and 70%, respectively. The most favorable group of patients with Stage I disease, those with T_1N_0 disease, experience 5-year survival rates of 80% to 85%.[27] Neither chemotherapy nor radiation therapy is recommended after complete resection of Stage I lung cancer.

Stage II. Surgical therapy for Stage II carcinoma includes resection of the primary tumor; *en bloc* resection of the hilar, interlobar, lobar, and segmental lymph nodes; and systematic mediastinal lymph node dissection to exclude the presence of mediastinal metastases. Patients with Stage II disease experience 5-year survival rates of 40% to 50%.[34] The rate of recurrence after resection of Stage II disease is greater than 50%, and most recurrences are distant metastases. Postoperative radiation therapy may reduce the incidence of local and regional recurrence but does not affect overall survival.[26]

Stage IIIa. Locally advanced carcinoma of the lung, in which the primary tumor is proximal to or has invaded adjacent structures (T_3) or in which ipsilateral mediastinal nodes are involved (N_2), is associated with a relatively poor prognosis. However, when surgical resection achieves total removal of the primary tumor and involved lymph nodes there is a reasonable chance for cure.

In patients with tumor invading the chest wall (T_3), complete resection of the tumor with involved adjacent tissue provides the most effective treatment. In a series of 111 patients with carcinoma invading the chest wall treated surgically, two thirds underwent complete resection and 5-year survival in this selected group was 40%.[27] In the subset of patients with T_3N_2 disease, 5-year survival after resection was approximately 30%. Postoperative irradiation does not appear to improve overall survival, although it has improved local control.[27]

The resectability of N_2 disease is controversial. Several series report 5-year survival rates of 10% to 20% in all patients undergoing thoracotomy and 20% to 30% in patients who have completely resectable disease.[28, 34] Other series investigating resection of N_2 NSCLC have demonstrated 5-year survival up to 40%.[7] Preoperative identification and histologic confirmation of N_2 disease usually contraindicates surgical resection; however, when unsuspected N_2 disease is encountered, pulmonary resection is performed if complete excision can be achieved. Multimodality protocols including neoadjuvant chemotherapy and surgical resection for patients with Stage IIIa (N_2) NSCLC are under evaluation.[20, 29]

Stage IIIb. Patients with Stage IIIb NSCLC (T_4 or N_3 disease) are generally considered unresectable. Occasionally, patients with unsuspected T_4 disease undergo thoracotomy and complete resection is attempted. Pneumonectomy with tracheal sleeve resection and direct reanastomosis of the trachea to the contralateral main bronchus has been advocated for proximal lesions, with 5-year survival approaching 20%.[30] Invasion of the vena cava has been treated by resection and graft replacement, with essentially no reported long-term survivors. In patients with invasion of the myocardium, aorta, esophagus, or vertebral body, complete resection is rarely possible; furthermore, palliative incomplete resection provides no survival benefit.

Multi-institutional prospective randomized trials have been undertaken to evaluate the safety and efficacy of induction chemotherapy in the treatment of Stage IIIb NSCLC. The Southwest Oncology Group has reported the results of preoperative cisplatin and etoposide, combined with concurrent radiation therapy, followed by surgical resection in patients with T_4 or N_3 disease.[39] After induction therapy, resection was achieved in 63% of patients, operative mortality was only 5%, and the 2-year survival for the entire group of patients was 39%.

Involvement of the contralateral hilar, contralateral mediastinal, scalene, or supraclavicular lymph node groups is considered N_3 disease. In most series, there are no 5-year survivors after surgical treatment for N_3 disease, which should be considered a definite sign of inoperability.

Patterns of Failure After Surgical Resection

The risk of recurrence after surgical resection according to the magnitude of the resection has been analyzed by the Lung Cancer Study Group (LCSG). In a prospective, randomized trial involving more than 400 patients with T_1N_0 lung cancer, lobectomy was compared with segmentectomy and wedge resection.[11] There was no significant difference in morbidity and mortality among the procedures. Furthermore, there was no difference observed in pulmonary function between patients who underwent lobectomy and those who underwent lesser procedures. The rate of locoregional recurrence was significantly lower in patients who underwent lobectomy (5%), compared with patients who underwent either segmentectomy or wedge resection (15%). In another study, segmentectomy was compared with lobectomy in patients with Stage I lung cancer.[46] In this study, the rate of locoregional recurrence was lower in patients who underwent lobectomy (5%), compared with those who underwent segmentectomy (23%). Furthermore, there was a survival advantage in the patients undergoing lobectomy for T_2 disease.

Distant metastases are the first site of recurrence in 80% of patients who undergo resection for NSCLC, with or without locoregional failure. Thus, improved locoregional therapy is unlikely to influence overall survival in patients with NSCLC who are not cured by surgical resection. In addition to lymph nodes, other sites of distant metastases include bone, adrenals, liver, kidneys, heart, lung, and brain.

Surgical Complications

Optimization of pulmonary status preoperatively in patients with borderline cardiopulmonary function and meticulous postoperative care contribute to minimizing morbidity and mortality in patients who undergo pulmonary resection for carcinoma of the lung. Atelectasis, the most common postoperative complication, is usually managed successfully with postural drainage, chest physiotherapy, and bronchodilators. Failure to clear secretions may progress to lobar collapse, requiring therapeutic bronchoscopy. Air leaks that are present after pulmonary resection usually resolve spontaneously. Persistence after 7 days may be due to bronchopleural fistula, requiring surgical exploration. Infection (pneumonia, empyema, sepsis) after thoracotomy is rare but should be aggressively sought and managed. Other complications after thoracotomy and pulmonary resection include myocardial infarction, atrial arrhythmias, pulmonary embolism, prolonged pulmonary insufficiency, chylothorax, and chronic thoracic pain. The LCSG, in a series of 2220 pulmonary resections, has reported an overall 30-day mortality of 3.7%. In this series, mortality varied with the extent of resection: 1.4% for wedge resection or segmentectomy; 2.9% for lobectomy; and 6.2% for pneumonectomy.[10]

ADJUVANT THERAPY FOR NSCLC

A minority of patients who present with lung cancer are considered potentially resectable. Systemic dissemination of cancer may be evident at presentation or after a resection for cure. The overall 5-year survival rate for lung cancer is 11% to 14%.[4] Although resection represents the best opportunity for cure, effective adjunctive therapy would be beneficial for many patients for whom complete resection is not possible. Current cooperative trials utilizing adjuvant and neoadjuvant

therapy for lung cancer have been summarized in the literature.[40]

Chemotherapy

Approximately 60% of patients with NSCLC have distant metastases at the time of initial diagnosis. Among the patients with apparently resectable disease, 5% are found at operation to have regional spread; the majority of the remainder later prove to have systemic disease. Thus, the establishment of effective chemotherapy would dramatically improve survival in patients with NSCLC. In contrast to chemotherapy for SCLC, in which many agents have been demonstrated to provide response rates up to 80%, chemotherapy in NSCLC induces tumor regression for a minority of patients.

Postoperative Chemotherapy. The LCSG has conducted several prospective randomized trials evaluating adjuvant chemotherapy for NSCLC. The first trial assessed the use of chemotherapy after resection for stage II or stage III adenocarcinoma or large cell undifferentiated carcinoma of the lung.[16] In this study, patients were randomized postoperatively to receive either a regimen of cyclophosphamide, doxorubicin, and cisplatin (CAP) or a regimen of immunotherapy with intrapleural Bacille Calmette-Guérin (BCG) and oral levamisole. Disease-free survival was significantly prolonged in the group receiving CAP chemotherapy. After 7 years of follow-up, the difference in time to recurrence and number of cancer deaths remained statistically significant in favor of the group receiving chemotherapy.[15]

The LCSG also evaluated postoperative chemotherapy and radiation therapy in patients with extensive lymph node involvement or with microscopic residual disease after resection.[21] Patients were randomized to receive CAP and radiation therapy or radiation therapy alone postoperatively. Patients who received chemotherapy and radiation therapy experienced significantly longer disease-free survival than those who received radiation therapy alone. Local recurrences occurred with equal frequency in each group; the difference in disease-free survival is attributed to the significant reduction in systemic recurrences in the group of patients who received both chemotherapy and radiation therapy.

In the third trial, the LCSG evaluated postoperative chemotherapy in patients with high-risk Stage I (T_2N_0 and T_1N_1) NSCLC.[15] After resection and lymph node evaluation, patients were randomized to receive CAP chemotherapy or no further treatment. In this study, there were no significant differences between the control and treatment groups with regard to survival or disease-free survival.

In summary, these trials demonstrate that postoperative chemotherapy may be responsible for significantly longer disease-free survival in patients with Stage III (and perhaps Stage II) NSCLC. The efficacy of postoperative chemotherapy and radiation therapy in patients with extensive lymph node involvement or positive surgical margins in reducing systemic recurrences and prolonging disease-free survival has also been demonstrated. Adjuvant therapy is not associated with improved overall survival and has not been shown to be beneficial in patients with Stage I NSCLC.

Preoperative Chemotherapy. The capability of induction therapy (consisting of chemotherapy alone or chemotherapy in combination with radiation therapy) to improve survival in marginally resectable patients and to allow resection to be performed in categorically unresectable patients is being evaluated in numerous studies.[40] In one series, patients with Stage IIIa (N_2) NSCLC received mitomycin, vinblastine, and cisplatin (MVP) preoperatively.[29] A major response was observed in 66% of patients and a complete response occurred in 10%. The overall complete resection rate was 65%, with a mplete resection rate of 78% in the subset of patients with a major response to chemotherapy. The overall 5-year survival rate was 17%; however, in patients who underwent complete resection, the 5-year survival rate was 26%.

In another study, researchers assessed the effect of neoadjuvant chemotherapy on resectability, stage of disease at resection, and patterns of recurrence and survival in patients with Stage IIIa (N_2) NSCLC.[20] After preoperative chemotherapy with one of various cisplatin-containing regimens, patients underwent thoracotomy, and 75% had complete resection. Pathologic analysis demonstrated that in 41% of patients the stage of disease was downstaged and only in 19% of patients did the disease progress. In patients with resectable disease, 2-year survival was 67%.

The Southwest Oncology Group reported a series of patients with Stage IIIa or Stage IIIb NSCLC who underwent preoperative chemotherapy (cisplatin and etoposide) and concurrent radiation therapy.[38] Complete resection was achieved in 73% of patients, and 2-year survival was 40% for both Stages IIIa and IIIb.

One review of the literature demonstrated 15 trials of induction chemotherapy (including 10 with radiation therapy as well) in patients with Stage III NSCLC.[42] Major response was observed in more than 50% of patients, but the complete response rate was less than 15%. Complete resection was achieved in 60% of patients. Overall 3-year survival was 25% to 30%. In summary, current survival is significantly better in patients with Stage III NSCLC who receive preoperative chemotherapy and undergo complete resection, as compared with historical controls. The evaluation of induction chemotherapy has demonstrated its feasibility; randomized trials are required to prove safety and efficacy.

Palliative Chemotherapy. The management of unresectable NSCLC, often complicated by large tumor burden and poor patient performance status, is largely unsuccessful, owing to poor response rates to chemotherapy. Nevertheless, selected patients should be offered the option of treatment with combination chemotherapy. Candidates for chemotherapy include patients with good performance status, minimal weight loss, and minimal bulk disease.

Radiation Therapy

Definitive Radiation Therapy. Patients with Stage I or II disease should undergo thoracotomy for pulmonary resection whenever possible. Thoracic irradiation for cure is reserved for patients with Stage IIIb disease, selected patients with Stage IIIa disease, and patients with medical contraindications to thoracotomy. Important considerations to the application of radiation therapy include tumor extent, volume of normal tissue, and cardiopulmonary reserve.[17]

Curative radiation therapy is limited to cases in which the entire tumor volume may be treated with an adequate dosage and with acceptable toxicity. Contraindications to definitive radiation therapy include malignant pleural effusion, distant metastases, inadequate pulmonary reserve, or active pulmonary infection. Tumor regression, defined as 50% or greater reduction in tumor mass as assessed by the chest radiograph, is accomplished in 50% to 60% of patients who receive radiation therapy for cure; complete regression is achieved in 20% to 25% of patients. Survival statistics for definitive radiation therapy vary with the clinical stage of the disease. Patients with Stage I or II disease who undergo definitive irradiation experience 5-year survival rates of 15% to 20%. For Stage III disease, 5-year survival rates of 3% to 10% have been reported, and median survival in most studies ranges from 9 to 12 months.[17]

Adjuvant Radiation Therapy. Radiation therapy is an effective adjuvant treatment in many patients with carcinoma of the lung. In patients with squamous cell carcinoma, the first site of recurrence is frequently local. Adjuvant radiation therapy, applied to patients with completely resected Stage II or Stage III NSCLC has been shown to decrease local recurrence but has no significant effect on survival. However, postoperative irradiation may provide a survival advantage in patients who have resection and are found to have metastases to hilar or mediastinal lymph nodes. Thus, the purpose of adjuvant radiation therapy is the prevention of local tumor recurrence, especially when lymph node sampling of the mediastinum at thoracotomy is incomplete.

Palliative Radiation Therapy. The use of radiation therapy in patients with unresectable disease has been reserved for those with symptoms. Few patients with advanced disease, however, are entirely asymptomatic. Symptoms of cough, chest pain, and dyspnea and the clinical signs and symptoms associated with the superior vena caval syndrome can be relieved in a majority of patients. At some centers, patients with unresectable disease are offered high-dose radiation therapy, which has resulted in cure rates of 5% to 10%.

Alternative Therapy

Several new modalities are in various stages of evaluation in the management of NSCLC. Interstitial and endobronchial brachytherapy have the ability to deliver high doses of radiation directly into the tumor, maximizing direct tumor irradiation and minimizing irradiation of surrounding normal tissue. Photoradiation with the neodymium:yttrium-aluminum-garnet (Nd:YAG) laser may provide palliative relief of airway obstruction by malignancy and may be used to deliver controlled hyperthermia. Photodynamic therapy, which involves the production of cytotoxic oxygen molecules, may also be useful in the amelioration of malignant tracheobronchial obstruction. Effective immunotherapy for carcinoma of the lung is being developed.[37]

MANAGEMENT OF SCLC

More than other solid tumors, SCLC behaves as a systemic disease. The natural history of SCLC is characterized by a relentlessly progressive course. Locoregional therapy directed toward the primary tumor is ineffective in prolonging survival because the majority of patients present with distant metastases or rapidly relapse with metastatic disease. Multimodal therapy including effective chemotherapy is therefore required for both locoregional control and systemic treatment of SCLC. The goals of therapy are to prolong survival and to alleviate symptoms, while minimizing treatment-associated toxicity. Despite encouraging response rates to aggressive combination chemotherapy, the 2-year survival rate is only 10%.

Major response rates can be achieved for 80% of patients with SCLC, regardless of stage. Complete response is produced in up to 50% of patients with limited disease and in 20% of patients with extensive disease. For patients with limited disease, median survival is greater than 12 months and survival beyond 5 years is attained in 10% to 20% of patients. For patients with extensive disease, median survival is 8 months, and survival beyond 5 years is attained in 3% to 5%.[12]

The adjuvant use of radiation therapy in SCLC is being examined in numerous clinical trials. In patients with limited disease, 5% to 15% improvement in disease-free survival at 2 years has been demonstrated when radiation therapy is added to combination chemotherapy. Despite improvement in disease-free survival and complete response rate, there is no clear advantage in overall survival for patients receiving chemotherapy and radiation therapy, as opposed to chemotherapy alone.[12]

Approximately 20% of patients survive 5 years after conventional management of SCLC, combination chemotherapy, and radiation therapy. With conventional therapy, the local recurrence rate is 30%. Complete resection in patients with limited disease may improve local control. In most surgical series, the rate of recurrence at the primary site is only 10%. Patients subjected to surgical management for SCLC should undergo complete resection, if possible, followed by postoperative chemotherapy and radiation therapy.

The primary goals in the management of a patient with SCLC are to prolong survival, improve disease-free survival, alleviate symptoms, minimize treatment-associated toxicity, and provide an estimate of prognosis. After ascertaining the histologic diagnosis of SCLC, staging is performed, including thorough neurologic examination and CT evaluation of the chest, abdomen, and brain.

For most patients with limited-stage disease, treatment is initiated with six cycles of combination chemotherapy. Radiation therapy to the chest is usually employed after three initial cycles of chemotherapy and is continued for 4 weeks. Among patients with limited-stage disease, thoracotomy for pulmonary resection is recommended in the subset of patients with Stage I SCLC. Postoperatively, patients receive six cycles of adjuvant chemotherapy and radiation therapy. Complete responders with limited-stage disease are offered prophylactic cranial irradiation. For patients with extensive-stage disease, six cycles of chemotherapy are administered. Therapy for local control is not employed; quality-of-life issues are paramount. Complete responders with extensive-stage disease receive prophylactic cranial irradiation.[43]

SUMMARY

Every solitary pulmonary nodule should be resected unless the lesion is known to be benign or unless operation is medically contraindicated. Accurate preoperative and intraoperative staging is essential in the management of carcinoma of the lung. Surgical resection represents the best chance for cure in patients with Stage I or Stage II NSCLC, provided that there are no medical contraindications to thoracotomy. Resection for cure may also be undertaken in selected patients with Stage III disease. Adjuvant therapy for patients with Stage III disease has been shown to improve disease-free survival without affecting overall survival. Neoadjuvant protocols are under evaluation in patients with N_2 NSCLC. Patients who have undergone resection for cure may nevertheless develop locoregional recurrence, metachronous primary lung cancer, or distant metastases; lifelong surveillance is required for all patients after pulmonary resection for carcinoma of the lung.

SELECTED REFERENCES

Bitran, J. D. (Ed.): Non–small cell lung cancer. Hematol. Oncol. Clin. North Am., 4:1023, 1990.
A multidisciplinary approach in the treatment of non–small cell lung cancer is emphasized, and the pathology, staging, and surgical approach to lung cancer is well described. In addition, adjuvant, neoadjuvant, palliative, and supportive modalities are presented.

Cook, R. M., Miller, Y. E., and Bunn, P. A., Jr.: Small cell lung cancer: Etiology, biology, clinical features, staging, and treatment. Curr. Probl. Cancer, 17:74, 1993.
This monograph summarizes the etiology, molecular biology, staging, and treatment of small cell lung cancer.

Ihde, D. C., and Minna, J. D.: Non–small cell lung cancer. Curr. Probl. Cancer, 15:65, 1991.
This superb monograph provides the current understanding of the molecular biology of non–small cell lung cancer.

Pass, H. I. (Ed.): Adjunctive and alternative treatment of bronchogenic lung cancer. Chest Surg. Clin. North Am., 1:1, 1991.
This review describes the use of adjunctive and alternative modalities in the treatment of bronchogenic lung cancer, including neoadjuvant chemotherapy, neoadjuvant radiation therapy, brachytherapy, photodynamic therapy, and endobronchial laser therapy.

REFERENCES

1. Auerbach, O., Gere, J. B., Forman, J. B., et al.: Changes in the bronchial epithelium in relation to smoking and cancer of the lung. N. Engl. J. Med., 256:97, 1957.
2. Bechard, D., and Wetstein, L.: Assessment of exercise oxygen consumption as preoperative criterion for lung resection. Ann. Thorac. Surg., 44:344, 1987.
3. Bongiorno, P. F., Whyte, R. I., Lesser, E. J., et al.: Alterations of K-ras, p53, and erb B-2/neu in human lung adenocarcinomas. J. Thorac. Cardiovasc. Surg., 107:590, 1994.
4. Boring, C. C., Squires, T. S., Tong, T., and Montgomery, S.: Cancer statistics, 1994. CA Cancer J. Clin., 44:7, 1994.
5. Cook, R. M., Miller, Y. E., and Bunn, P. A. Jr.: Small cell lung cancer: Etiology, biology, clinical features, staging, and treatment. Curr. Probl. Cancer, 17:74, 1993.
6. Daly, B. D. T., Faling, L. J., Bite, G. B., et al.: Mediastinal lymph node evaluation by computed tomography in lung cancer. J. Thorac. Cardiovasc. Surg., 94:664, 1987.
7. Daly, B. D. T., Mueller, J. D., Faling, L. J., et al.: N_2 lung cancer outcome in patients with false-negative computed tomographic scans of the chest. J. Thorac. Cardiovasc. Surg., 105:904, 1993.
8. Doll, R., and Peto, R.: Cigarette smoking and bronchial carcinoma: Dose and time relationships among regular smokers and lifelong non-smokers. J. Epidemiol. Community Health, 32:303, 1978.
9. Georges, R. N., Mukhopadhyay, T., Zhang, Y. J., et al.: Prevention of orthotopic human lung cancer growth by intratracheal instillation of a retroviral antisense K-ras construct. Cancer Res., 53:1743, 1993.
10. Ginsberg, R. J., Hill, L. D., Eagan, R. T., et al.: Modern thirty-day operative mortality for surgical resection in lung cancer. J. Thorac. Cardiovasc. Surg., 86:654, 1983.
11. Ginsberg, R. J., and Rubenstein, L. V.: Patients with T_1N_0 non–small cell lung cancer (Abstract 304). Lung Cancer, 7(Suppl.):83, 1991.
12. Goodman, G. E., and Livingston, R. B.: Small cell lung cancer. Curr. Probl. Cancer, 13:7, 1989.
13. Graham, E. A., and Singer, J. J.: Successful removal of an entire lung for carcinoma of the bronchus. JAMA, 101:1371, 1933.
14. Hazelrigg, S. R., Nunchuck, S. K., and LoCicero, J.: Video Assisted Thoracic Surgery Study Group Data. Ann. Thorac. Surg., 56:1039, 1993.
15. Holmes, E. C.: Postoperative chemotherapy for non-small cell lung cancer. Chest, 103:30S, 1993.
16. Holmes, E. C., and Gail, M.: Surgical adjuvant chemotherapy for stage II and stage III adenocarcinoma and large cell undifferentiated carcinoma. J. Clin. Oncol., 4:710, 1986.
17. Ihde, D. C., and Minna, J. D.: Non–small cell lung cancer. Curr. Probl. Cancer, 15:65, 1991.
18. Johnson, B. E., and Kelley, M. J.: Overview of genetic and molecular events in the pathogenesis of lung cancer. Chest, 103:1S, 1993.
19. Kirby, T. J., and Rice, T. W.: Thoracoscopic lobectomy. Ann. Thorac. Surg., 56:784, 1993.
20. Kirn, D. H., Lynch, T. J., Mentzer, S. J., et al.: Multimodality therapy of patients with stage IIIa, N_2 non-small cell lung cancer: Impact of preoperative chemotherapy on resectability and downstaging. J. Thorac. Cardiovasc. Surg., 106:696, 1993.
21. Lad, T., Rubenstein, L., Sedeghi, A., et al.: The benefit of adjuvant treatment for resected locally advanced non–small cell lung cancer. J. Clin. Oncol., 6:125, 1988.
22. Linnoila, I.: Pathology of non–small cell lung cancer: New diagnostic approaches. Hematol. Oncol. Clin. North. Am., 4:1027, 1990.
23. Marshall, C. J.: Tumor suppressor genes. Cell, 64:313, 1991.
24. Marshall, M. C., and Olsen, G. N.: The physiologic evaluation of the lung resection candidate. Clin. Chest Med., 14:305, 1993.
25. Martini, N.: Surgical treatment of non–small cell cancer by stage. Semin. Surg. Oncol., 6:248, 1990.
26. Martini, N., Burt, M. E., Bains, M. S., et al.: Survival after resection of stage II non–small cell lung cancer. Ann. Thorac. Surg., 54:460, 1992.
27. Martini, N., and Ginsberg, R. J.: Surgical approaches to non–small cell cancer stage IIIa. Hematol. Oncol. Clin. North Am., 4:1121, 1990.
28. Martini, N., and Flehinger, B. J.: The role of surgery in N_2 lung cancer. Surg. Clin. North Am., 67:1037, 1987.
29. Martini, N., Kris, M. G., Flehinger, B. J., et al.: Preoperative chemotherapy for stage IIIa (N_2) lung cancer: The Sloan-Kettering experience with 136 patients. Ann. Thorac. Surg., 55:1365, 1993.
30. Mathisen, D. J., and Grillo, H. C.: Carinal resection for bronchogenic cancer. J. Thorac. Cardiovasc. Surg., 102:16, 1991.
31. Meade, R. H.: A History of Thoracic Surgery. Springfield, Ill., Charles C Thomas, 1961.
32. Mountain, C. F.: A new international staging system for lung cancer. Chest, 89:225S, 1986.

Naruke, T., Asamura, H., Kondo, H., et al.: Thoracoscopy for the staging of lung cancer. Ann. Thorac. Surg., 56:661, 1993.

34. Naruke, T., Goya, T., Tsuchiya, R., et al.: Prognosis and survival in resected lung carcinoma based on the new international staging system for lung cancer. J. Thorac. Cardiovasc. Surg., 96:440, 1988.

35. Porgador, A., Bannerji, R., Watanabe, Y., et al.: Antimetastatic vaccination of tumor-bearing mice with two types of IFN-γ gene-inserted tumor cells. J. Immunol., 150:1458, 1993.

36. Richardson, G. E., and Johnson, B. E.: Paraneoplastic syndromes in lung cancer. Curr. Opin. Oncol., 4:323, 1992.

37. Roth, J. A.: Modulation of oncogene and tumor-suppressor gene expression: A novel strategy for cancer prevention and treatment. Ann. Surg. Oncol., 1:79, 1994.

38. Rusch, V. W., Albain, K. S., Crowley, J. J., et al.: Surgical resection of stage IIIa and stage IIIb non–small-cell lung cancer after concurrent induction chemoradiotherapy. J. Thorac. Cardiovasc. Surg., 105:97, 1993.

39. Rusch, V. W., Albain, K. S., Crowley, J. J., et al.: Neoadjuvant therapy: A novel and effective treatment for stage IIIb non–small cell lung cancer. Ann. Thorac. Surg., 58:290, 1994.

40. Rusch, V. W., and Feins, R. H.: Summary of ongoing cooperative group clinical trials in thoracic malignancies. Ann. Thorac. Surg., 57:102, 1994.

41. Scott, W. J., Schwabe, J. L., Gupta, N. C., et al.: Positron emission tomography of lung tumors and mediastinal lymph nodes using [18F]fluorodeoxyglucose. Ann. Thorac. Surg., 58:698, 1994.

42. Shepherd, F. A.: Induction chemotherapy for locally advanced non–small cell lung cancer. Ann. Thorac. Surg., 55:1585, 1993.

43. Shepherd, F. A., Ginsberg, R. J., Feld, R., et al.: Surgical treatment for limited small cell lung cancer. J. Thorac. Cardiovasc. Surg., 101:385, 1991.

44. Slebos, R. J. C., Kibbelaar, R. E., Dalesio, O., et al.: K-ras oncogene activation as a prognostic marker in adenocarcinoma of the lung. N. Engl. J. Med., 323:561, 1990.

45. Wain, J. C.: Video-assisted thoracoscopy and the staging of lung cancer. Ann. Thorac. Surg., 56:776, 1993.

46. Warren, W. H., and Faber, L. P.: Segmentectomy versus lobectomy in patients with stage I pulmonary carcinoma. J. Thorac. Cardiovasc. Surg., 107:1087, 1994.

47. Yang, S., Owen-Schaub, L., Grimm, E., and Roth, J.: Induction of lymphokine-activated killer (LAK) activity with interleukin-2 and tumor necrosis factor-alpha against fresh primary lung cancer targets. Cancer Immunol. Immunother., 29:193, 1989.

XIII

MESOTHELIOMA

David J. Sugarbaker, M.D., Michael F. Reed, M.D., and Scott J. Swanson, M.D.

Mesothelioma is an uncommon neoplasm that most frequently arises from the pleural mesothelium but also occurs in the peritoneum, pericardium, tunica vaginalis testis, and ovarian epithelium. In the National Cancer Institute's Surveillance Epidemiology and End Results (SEER) program, 81.8% of mesotheliomas were pleural (occurring in 87% among males and 64% among females), 14.4% were peritoneal, and 0.9% were pericardial.[9] Peritoneal mesothelioma is more common among patients with high occupational exposures to asbestos. The focus here is on the most frequently encountered form of the disease—pleural mesothelioma.

EPIDEMIOLOGY

Approximately 3000 patients with malignant pleural mesothelioma are diagnosed annually in the United States.[9] The well-established association between mesothelioma and asbestos exposure places certain individuals with occupational exposures at much higher risk for this disease. The incidence of mesothelioma is increasing.[21] Because of the mean latency period of 30 to 40 years between first exposure and diagnosis,[20] the incidence will likely continue to increase well into the next century.

The incombustibility of asbestos was recognized more than 2000 years ago, and asbestos fibers were used by ancient civilizations, including the Romans, Chinese, and Egyptians.[30] Commercial use of asbestos began early in the nineteenth century, and widespread industrial use emerged in the late 1800s. The health risks of asbestos exposure have only been elucidated during the past century. In 1898, respiratory failure was observed among asbestos workers, and in 1930 an association between asbestos exposure and asbestosis was noted.[3] A report in 1955 by Doll[14] identified lung cancer as a specific hazard of asbestos workers.

Asbestos is a generic term that refers to six minerals divided into two groups. Chrysotile belongs to the serpentine group, while crocidolite, amosite, anthophyllite, tremolite, and actinolite compose the amphibole group. The association between amphibole fibers and mesothelioma, as first described by Wagner and colleagues[41] in South Africa where crocidolite was mined, has been supported by numerous studies worldwide.[24] Even among patients with mesothelioma who are exposed primarily to chrysotile fibers, autopsy studies show an increased lung burden of amphibole fibers. Of note, recent studies demonstrate that carcinoma of the lung and severity of asbestosis also correlate with lung burden of crocidolite and amosite fibers, further supporting the *amphibole hypothesis*,[24] namely, that amphibole fibers are significantly more pathogenic than chrysotile fibers. Whereas cigarette smoking and asbestos act synergistically in causing carcinoma of the lung, cigarette smoking does not increase the risk of mesothelioma for either men or women.[27]

Commercial use of asbestos is due to its resistance to heat and acid, incombustibility, strength, and durability. Before the ban by the Environmental Protection Agency on its use asbestos was used as insulation and as a fire retardant. Over 3000 products still contain asbestos, including cement materials (pipes, flooring, and roofing products), brake linings, and thermal and electrical insulation.[25]

Asbestos fibers from ore are only released during mining and processing. Asbestos in buildings becomes respirable when its surface is damaged.[25] Fibers also become airborne when structures are demolished or during asbestos removal. Risk groups for asbestos-related diseases include insulators, pipe fitters, shipyard workers, brake mechanics, railroad workers, people in construction trades, and potentially those who work in buildings where disrepair has resulted in airborne asbestos fibers.[17]

The existence of a low incidence of mesothelioma unrelated to asbestos is supported by historical reports of malignant pleural tumors before the widespread industrial use of asbestos, as well as rare cases of mesothelioma among children. Most mesotheliomas afflict persons older than 60 years old. Among those diagnosed when 20 to 40 years old, the majority report exposure to asbestos during childhood. Familial clustering of mesothelioma appears to be a result of a common exposure to asbestos, such as dust on work clothes entering the home, rather than a genetic susceptibility.[13]

PATHOLOGY

Malignant pleural mesothelioma is typically a diffuse, spreading tumor. The cell type of origin is the pluripotent pleural mesothelial cell, which is of mesenchymal derivation. Initially, discrete grayish white nodules develop on the pleura. As they grow and merge into a rind that encompasses the visceral and parietal pleura, the lung becomes encased with tumor, frequently without significant parenchymal invasion until late in the disease course (Fig. 51–82). The diaphragm, pericardium, and fissures are commonly involved early in the disease process. This relentless local spread is typical and is usually the cause of death.

The three histologic types of malignant mesothelioma are epithelial, sarcomatous, and a combination of the two, also known as the mixed or biphasic type. The epithelial form is predominant, present in 50% of patients, while mixed tumors are observed in 34%, and the pure sarcomatous variant in 16%.[16] Epithelial mesothelioma (Fig. 51–83) is characterized by tubular, papillary, solid, or vacuolated patterns. Pseudo-acini are often observed. Light microscopy reveals acidophilic cytoplasm, and electron microscopy (Fig. 51–84) demon-

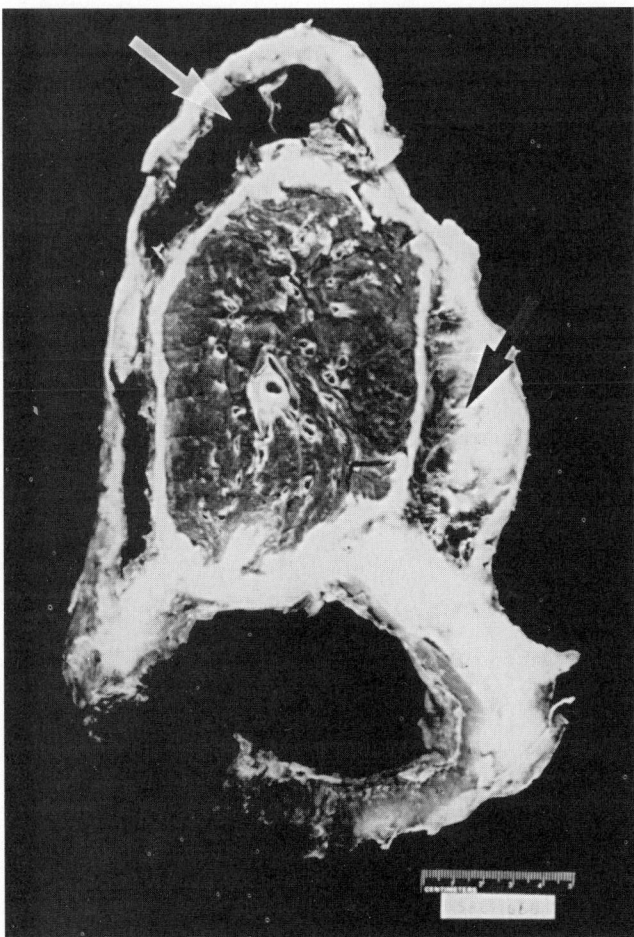

Figure 51–82. Gross pathologic specimen of a sagittal section of a left pleural mesothelioma demonstrating extensive involvement of the parietal and visceral pleura and diaphragm with superficial invasion into basal portions of the lung. The cavity between the parietal and visceral pleura represents the site of pleural effusion (white arrow). Organizing effusion invaded by tumor is also present (black arrow). The lung volume is diminished secondary to tumor encasement. (Courtesy of Joseph M. Corson, M.D., Boston, MA.)

strates specific cytostructural features, including branched microvilli with a large length-to-diameter ratio, intermediate filaments, and desmosomes. The sarcomatous variant (Fig. 51–85) exhibits spindle cells and hyperchromatism similar to sarcomas.

MOLECULAR BIOLOGY

The mechanisms by which asbestos leads to malignant transformation remain the subject of significant scientific scrutiny. Clues regarding the genetic changes that contribute to tumorigenesis can be elucidated by evaluating the cytogenetic alterations that occur in human tumors, in animal tumor models, and, to a certain extent, in cell lines. Chromosomal rearrangement or amplification can lead to oncogene activation, while deletions may result in the loss of tumor suppressors. Nonrandom cytogenetic alterations that have been reported to be associated with transformation of human mesothelial cells are located on a number of different chromosomes,[42] but the specific alterations that play a role in a significant percentage of mesotheliomas have yet to be identified. The retinoblastoma gene (Rb), a tumor suppressor that is deleted or mutated in a variety of human cancers, is the wild type in mesothelioma. The status in mesothelioma of the tumor suppressor p53, which is altered in over 50% of human cancers, is still unclear, with certain reports showing altered p53 expression[11, 18] and others demonstrating that loss of wild-type p53 expression does not play a role in the development of mesothelioma.[22] Oncogene amplification, using probes specific for N-myc, c-myc, H-ras, Ki-ras, v-myb, insulin-like growth factor-1, Her2/neu, v-fos, and the epidermal growth factor receptor, does not appear to contribute to malignant mesothelioma.[15]

Although chromosomal alterations specific to mesothelioma have yet to be demonstrated, the chromosomal number does correlate with survival. In one study,[38] patients with a normal mean chromosomal number of 46 survived 31 months, whereas individuals with a mean number less than 46 survived 26 months, and patients whose tumors had a mean number greater than 46 survived 13 months.

CLINICAL PRESENTATION

Malignant pleural mesothelioma most frequently affects men 50 to 70 years old. Common presenting symptoms are nonpleuritic chest pain, occurring in 60% of patients, dyspnea secondary to pleural effusion, seen in 50% to 70%, or both. Pleural effusion is present at some point in the course of the disease in over 90% of cases. Weight loss, fever, and cough also occur with high frequency. Physical examination is notable for dullness to percussion and diminished breath sounds. Advanced disease is often associated with wasting, ascites, and contracture of the involved hemithorax.

DIAGNOSIS

Accurate diagnosis of mesothelioma is difficult.[10] Mesothelioma should be suspected in any patient with a pleural effusion of unknown etiology. Thoracentesis usually resolves dyspnea unless the disease has progressed so that tumor encasement results in restrictive lung disease. The pleural fluid obtained during therapeutic thoracentesis is yellow, owing to the hyaluronic acid content. Alternatively, pleural fluid associated with adenocarcinoma is typically bloody. Pleural fluid cytology is inadequate for establishing a precise diagnosis, and obtaining tissue by open biopsy or thoracoscopy is essential. Appropriate placement of the biopsy incision along a future thoracotomy site is important if aggres-

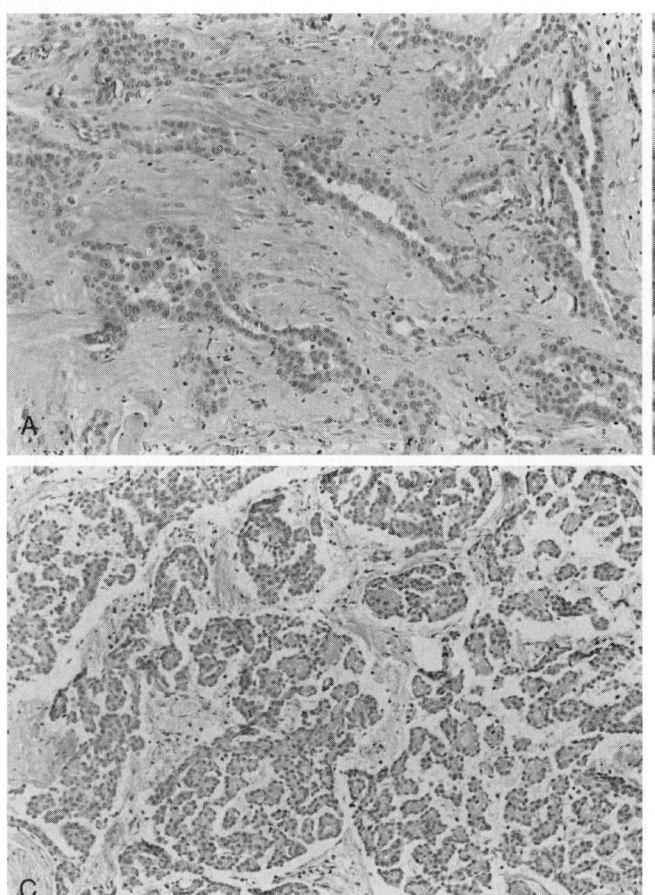

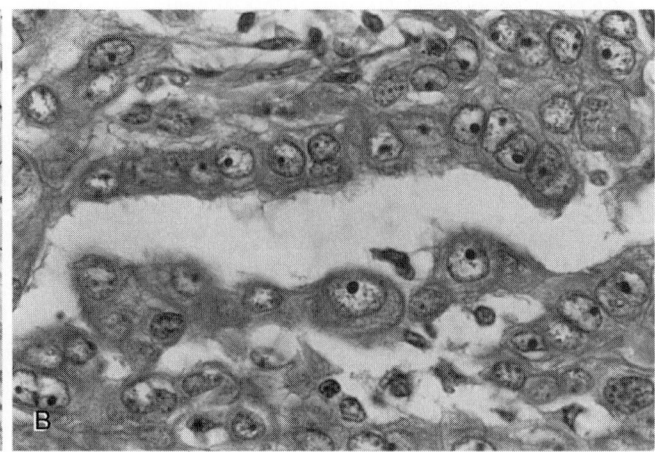

Figure 51–83. *A*, Low-power photomicrograph of a tubular epithelial mesothelioma invading fibromuscular tissue. *B*, High-power photomicrograph of a tubular epithelial mesothelioma showing rows of malignant cuboidal cells lining the tubule. Note the uniformly round nuclei with prominent central nucleoli. *C*, Low-power photomicrograph of a papillary epithelial mesothelioma. Uniform papillae composed of cuboidal mesothelial cells are set in a loose fibrous stroma. All specimens were stained with hematoxylin and eosin. (*A* to *C* courtesy of Joseph M. Corson, M.D., Boston, MA.)

sive surgical therapy is contemplated, because tumor seeding of the biopsy site is common.

The differential diagnosis of the sarcomatous type includes benign fibrous tumors of the pleura,[23] whereas the epithelial form must be differentiated from metastatic adenocarcinoma (Table 51–33).

Immunoperoxidase staining using a variety of antibodies should be performed whenever mesothelioma is suspected.[40]

Mesotheliomas always stain positive for keratin (Fig. 51–86; see also Fig. 51–85).[10] Whereas adenocarcinomas will almost always be positive for keratin, most sarcomas will be negative. Carcinoembryonic antigen is positive in 75% of adenocarcinomas but is negative in mesothelioma and some carcinomas (notably renal and prostate) (Fig. 51–87).[10] Likewise, Leu-M1 is characteristically positive for adenocarcinomas but negative for mesotheliomas. Mesotheliomas contain an acid

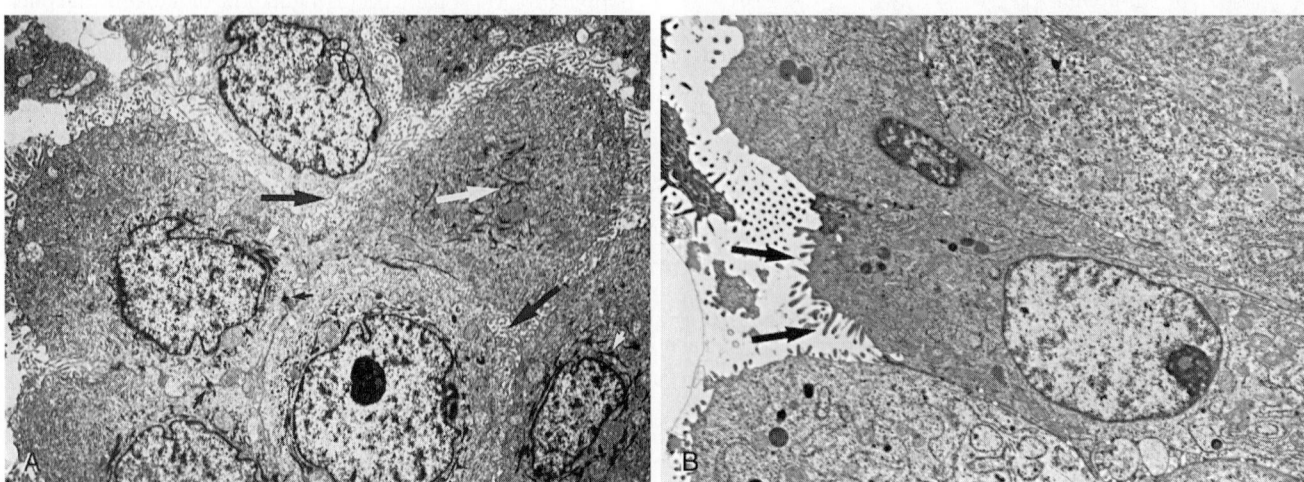

Figure 51–84. *A*, Electron micrograph of a mesothelioma demonstrating numerous long, thin, and branching microvilli projecting from the surface membrane into intercellular spaces and interdigitating with those of opposing cells (long black arrows). Densely aggregated keratin intermediate filaments (tonofilaments) encircle the nucleus (short white arrows) and are scattered within the cytoplasm (long white arrow). Desmosomal cell-cell junctions are present (short black arrows) and were confirmed under higher magnification (not shown). *B*, Electron micrograph of an adenocarcinoma exhibiting microvilli that are sparse, short, blunt, and straight (arrows). (*A* and *B* courtesy of Joseph M. Corson, M.D., Boston, MA.)

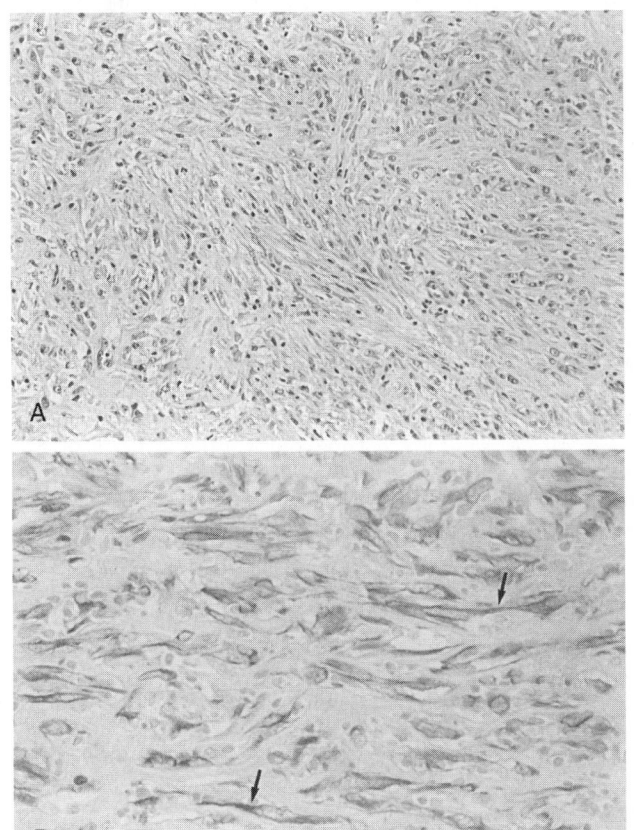

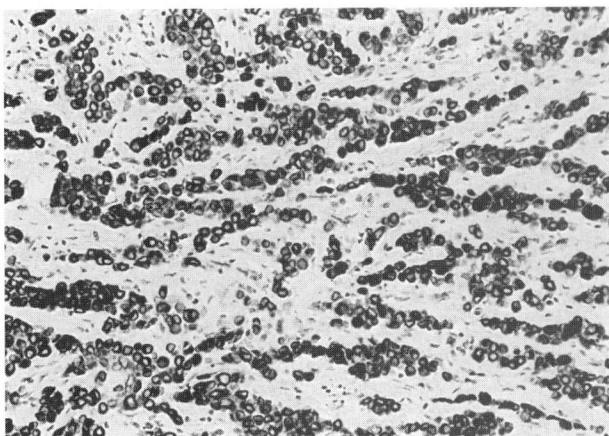

Figure 51–86. Immunohistochemistry is positive for keratin in an epithelial mesothelioma, with strong cytoplasmic staining. (From Corson, J. M.: Pathology of mesothelioma. *In* Antman, K., and Aisner, J. [Eds.]: Asbestos-Related Malignancy. Orlando, FL, Grune & Stratton, 1987:190.)

Figure 51–85. *A,* Photomicrograph of a sarcomatous mesothelioma with typical spindle-shaped cells. The tumor is quite cellular with nuclear atypia. *B,* Immunoperoxidase staining for keratin is positive in a sarcomatous mesothelioma. Dark areas reflect cytoplasmic and membrane immunolocalization of keratin (arrows). (*A* and *B* courtesy of Joseph M. Corson, M.D., Boston, MA.)

tinal shift (Fig. 51–88). Computed tomography can demonstrate extrapleural soft tissue invasion and rib displacement, tumor infiltration of mediastinal structures, and diaphragmatic involvement. Magnetic resonance imaging provides additional anatomic information, particularly in the sagittal and coronal planes, when resection is considered.[29]

mucin, hyaluronic acid, which is revealed by Alcian blue or colloidal iron staining of tissue sections. Pretreatment with hyaluronidase results in digestion of hyaluronic acid and absence of staining. In contrast, adenocarcinomas contain acid mucins other than hyaluronic acid, which stain positively despite hyaluronidase treatment. Laboratory findings are predominantly nonspecific, although thrombocytosis (>400,000/cu. mm.) is observed in over 60% of patients.

The plain chest film may show pleural plaques associated with asbestosis before the onset of mesothelioma. Later, as the tumor develops, pleural effusion may appear and pleural thickening can become evident. As lung encasement occurs, there is ipsilateral volume loss with a compensatory medias-

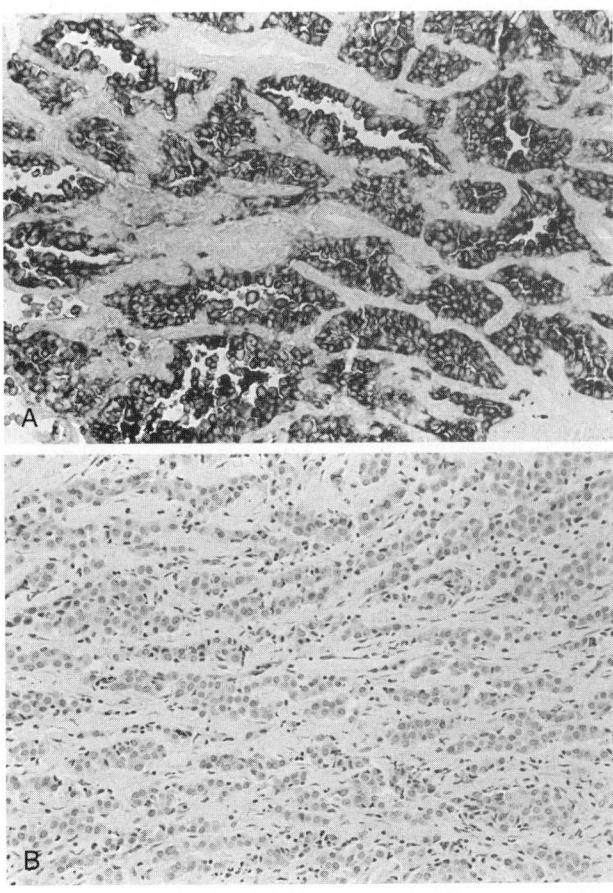

Figure 51–87. *A,* The cytoplasm of most of the adenocarcinoma cells stains strongly for carcinoembryonic antigen (CEA). *B,* The mesothelioma cells are completely negative for CEA. (*A* and *B* from Corson, J. M.: Pathology of mesothelioma. *In* Antman, K., and Aisner, J. [Eds.]: Asbestos-Related Malignancy. Orlando, FL, Grune & Stratton, 1987:189.)

TABLE 51–33. Pathologic Characteristics of Mesothelioma

Test	Mesothelioma	Adenocarcinoma
Electron microscopy (length-to-diameter ratio of microvilli)	>10:1	<10:1
Periodic acid–Schiff diastase	Negative	Positive
Alcian blue or colloidal iron		
Before hyaluronidase	Positive	Positive
After hyaluronidase	Negative	Positive
Mayer's mucicarmine	Negative	Positive
Keratin	Positive	Positive
Carcinoembryonic antigen	Negative	Positive
Leu-M1	Negative	Positive

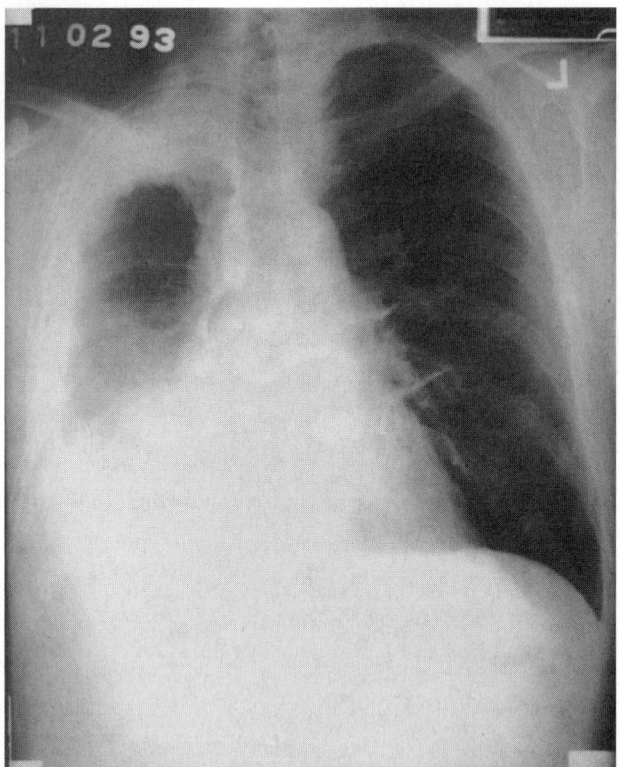

Figure 51–88. Chest radiograph of a patient with a right malignant pleural mesothelioma demonstrates a pleural mass, effusion, ipsilateral hemithorax volume loss, and a shift in the mediastinum. There is no evidence for a pleural mass or effusion on the left.

PROGNOSTIC FACTORS

Several centers have reviewed their series of mesothelioma patients to identify independent predictors of survival.[2, 35] As with other neoplastic diseases, younger age (<55 years old) and better performance status (ECOG performance status 0–1) correlate with longer survival. Female sex is a positive prognostic factor, and some series suggest that longer duration of symptoms is also favorable. Other diagnostic factors associated with an improved prognosis include Stage I disease, epithelial histology, the absence of malignant cells in the pleural fluid, tumor involving only the parietal pleura without visceral pleural spread, and the absence of evidence for lymph node metastases. Weight loss greater than 10% and chest pain at the time of diagnosis are negative prognostic factors.[2, 35]

STAGING

Pleural mesothelioma has been difficult to stage. Traditionally, staging systems are developed by following a cohort of patients treated in a like manner to produce a stratification of survival based on tumor characteristics. By grouping these characteristics, stages of a disease are developed.[26] This allows for rational treatment strategies and accurate prognoses. Ineffective therapy has, perhaps, led to the blurring of important features and resulted in a rather insensitive staging system for malignant pleural mesothelioma.

The first widely applied staging system, proposed by Butchart[8] in 1976, was based on experience with 29 patients. It suffers from the inability to accurately stratify survival. At presentation, 70% of patients with mesothelioma are clinical Butchart Stage I, yet survival in this group is only 5 to 14 months.

The Committee of the International Union Against Cancer (UICC) has proposed an empiric TNM staging system.[32] This staging system is new with respect to mesothelioma, and its stages as yet do not correlate with patient survival.

One staging system that has been developed based on patient survival is seen in Table 51–34.[1, 8, 37] This cohort of patients underwent trimodality therapy, including extrapleural pneumonectomy followed by chemotherapy and radiation therapy. Stratification of patients by stage is based on tumor involvement of the specific anatomic structures that determine resectability by extrapleural pneumonectomy and by nodal spread. Using this schema, a survival advantage was demonstrated in those patients who had their tumor resected and then went on to complete the protocol. A further advantage was suggested if there were no regional nodes involved, a heretofore unknown concept in mesothelioma. In summary, by carefully teasing out various aspects of this deadly disease, it is possible to create a useful staging system that provides for treatment strategies and gives reliable prognostic information.

THERAPY

If the disease is not treated patients usually survive less than 12 months. Single-modality therapy for malignant pleural mesothelioma has proved ineffective, and neither surgery, radiation therapy, nor chemotherapy alone significantly alters the rapidly lethal course of the disease.[4, 33, 39] The uniformly poor results of single-modality therapy have led many clinicians to adopt a pessimistic opinion regarding aggressive therapy for mesothelioma.

Surgical Management. Surgical procedures in the management of malignant pleural mesothelioma include biopsy for diagnostic purposes, pleurodesis, pleurectomy with decortication, and extrapleural pneumonectomy for cytoreduction. Once a definitive diagnosis has been made, radiographic evaluation of resectability includes computed tomography and, if necessary, magnetic resonance imaging to look for invasion of the diaphragm or mediastinal structures. Routine pulmonary function testing, including spirometry and functional oximetry, is also needed. If the forced expiratory volume in 1 second (FEV_1) is less than 2 liters or if the predicted postoperative FEV_1 is less than 1.2 liters, quantitative ventilation-perfusion scanning becomes necessary.

In patients who are unable to tolerate a major surgical procedure, pleurodesis through a small thoracotomy or utilizing thoracoscopy relieves the dyspnea associated with pleural effusion.[6] Talc pleurodesis has been used successfully.[43]

TABLE 51–34. Proposed Staging System for Mesothelioma Based on Survival Among 52 Patients

Stage	Description
I	Disease confined to within "capsule" of the parietal pleura: ipsilateral pleura, lung, pericardium, diaphragm, or chest wall disease limited to previous biopsy sites.
II	All of Stage I with positive intrathoracic (N_1 or N_2) lymph nodes.
III*	Local extension of disease into chest wall, mediastinum, or heart, or through diaphragm or peritoneum; with or without extrathoracic or contralateral (N_3) lymph node involvement.
IV	Distant metastatic disease.

*Stage III combines Butchart Stages II and II.
Adapted from Butchart, E. G., Ashcroft, T., Barnsley, W. C., and Holden, M. P.: Pleuropneumonectomy in the management of diffuse malignant mesothelioma of the pleura: Experience with 29 patients. Thorax, 31:15, 1976.

Pleurectomy with decortication should be considered if a radical resection is not feasible but the patient can tolerate an operative intervention. Two major debilitating symptoms associated with pleural mesothelioma are dyspnea secondary to lung encasement and chest wall pain from tumor invasion. Pleurectomy with decortication, in which grossly diseased pleura is resected while lung parenchyma is left intact, is a palliative procedure because while macroscopic disease remains, the restrictive disease is frequently relieved and chest wall pain often improves. In combination with chemotherapy and radiation therapy, pleurectomy with decortication may offer a potential for improved survival when radical resection is not possible.[31]

For individuals who have Butchart Stage I disease, are deemed resectable by noninvasive studies, and who possess an adequate cardiopulmonary reserve to tolerate radical pulmonary surgery, extrapleural pneumonectomy for local control can be offered. This procedure provides maximal cytoreduction, resolves the restrictive pulmonary symptoms, and, by resecting lung, allows higher dosage during radiation therapy. When transdiaphragmatic spread is suspected, laparoscopy or a small laparotomy should be performed before thoracotomy. If peritoneal invasion is excluded, extrapleural pneumonectomy is undertaken. As described by Sugarbaker and colleagues,[36] an extended thoracotomy is performed (Fig. 51–89)[36] and dissection proceeds in the extrapleural plane (Fig. 51–90).[36] Meticulous technique is essential to maintain hemostasis, to keep the pleural envelope intact, and to avoid damaging the subclavian and internal mammary vessels, the azygos vein, the esophagus, and the cavae on the right or the aorta and intercostal vessels on the left. The diaphragm is resected, and the pericardium is opened and subsequently resected, sacrificing the phrenic nerve. The main pulmonary artery and pulmonary veins and the mainstem bronchus are each divided (Fig. 51–91).[36] In a right-sided resection, the pericardium is reconstructed using a prosthetic patch to prevent cardiac herniation (Fig. 51–92).[36] The patch is fenestrated

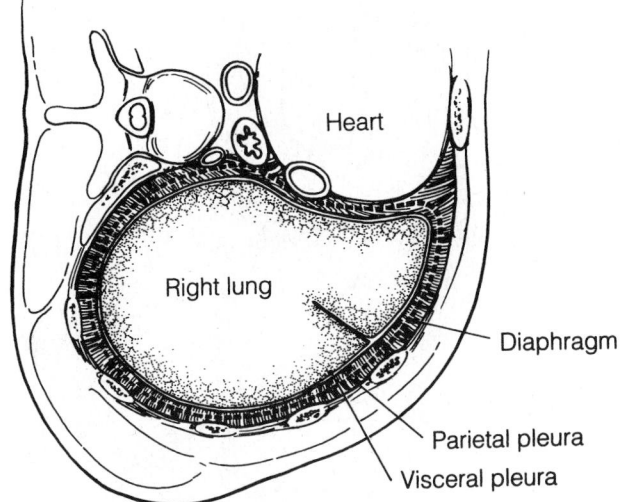

Figure 51–90. A dashed line in this cross-sectional view of the thorax shows the plane of dissection external to the pleura, with the diaphragm divided lateral to the esophagus and inferior vena cava. (From Sugarbaker, D. J., Mentzer, S. J., and Strauss, G.: Extrapleural pneumonectomy in the treatment of malignant pleural mesothelioma. Ann. Thorac. Surg., *54*:941, 1992. Reprinted with permission from the Society of Thoracic Surgeons.)

to avoid tamponade. Diaphragmatic reconstruction is carried out using a prosthetic patch (Fig. 51–93).[36] If gross tumor is unresectable, or if positive margins are noted by frozen section, surgical clips are placed to target postoperative radiation therapy.

Whereas early reports on extrapleural pneumonectomy documented a high operative mortality, in recent series[12, 34] the perioperative mortality rate is under 10%, comparable to standard pneumonectomy.

Radiation Therapy. As a single-modality treatment, radiation therapy is minimally effective, and radical radiation

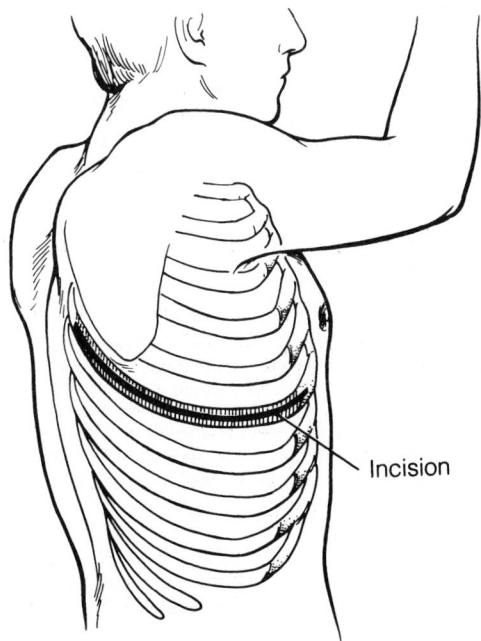

Figure 51–89. An extended thoracotomy (right-sided in this figure) incision is made in the sixth intercostal space. (From Sugarbaker, D. J., Mentzer, S. J., and Strauss, G.: Extrapleural pneumonectomy in the treatment of malignant pleural mesothelioma. Ann. Thorac. Surg., *54*:941, 1992. Reprinted with permission from the Society of Thoracic Surgeons.)

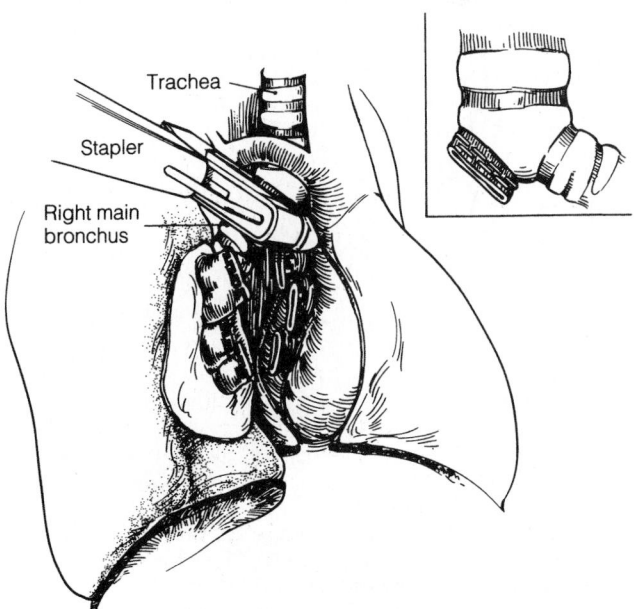

Figure 51–91. Hilar structures (the main pulmonary artery, the mainstem bronchus, and the superior pulmonary veins, on the right side in this figure) are divided. (From Sugarbaker, D. J., Mentzer, S. J., and Strauss, G.: Extrapleural pneumonectomy in the treatment of malignant pleural mesothelioma. Ann. Thorac. Surg., *54*:941, 1992. Reprinted with permission from the Society of Thoracic Surgeons.)

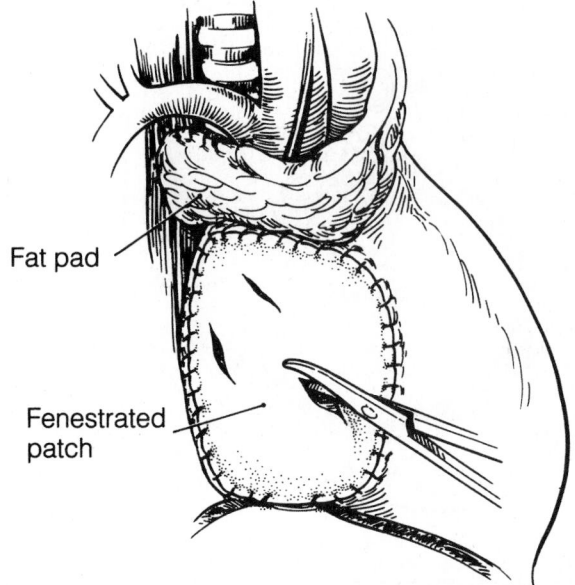

Figure 51–92. A pericardial prosthesis is fenestrated and placed when performing a right-sided resection. (From Sugarbaker, D. J., Mentzer, S. J., and Strauss, G.: Extrapleural pneumonectomy in the treatment of malignant pleural mesothelioma. Ann. Thorac. Surg., *54*:941, 1992. Reprinted with permission from the Society of Thoracic Surgeons.)

therapy carries a high risk of side effects, including pulmonary, cardiac, and hepatic toxicity.[4] Radiation therapy for local control may be effective after extrapleural pneumonectomy, using boosts to areas with positive margins. Palliative radiation therapy for pain control may provide temporary relief.[5]

Chemotherapy. Despite occasional reports of chemotherapeutic regimens with promising results, neither single-agent nor combination chemotherapy provides response rates greater than 20% when evaluated in a prospective, multicenter setting.[19] As with surgical and radiation therapy, chemo-

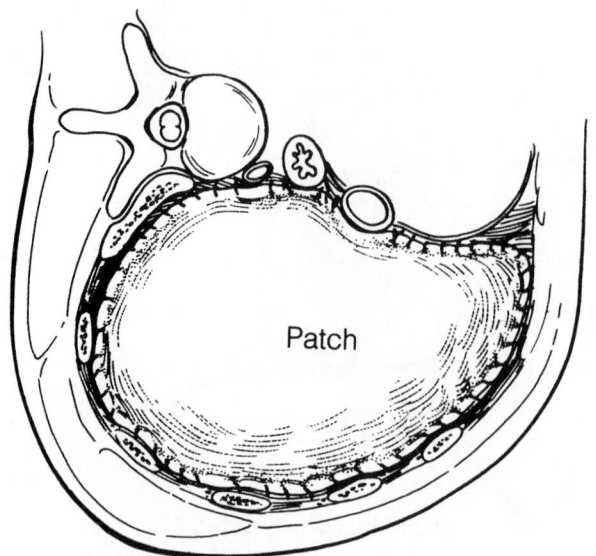

Figure 51–93. Right diaphragmatic reconstruction with a patch sutured in place. (From Sugarbaker, D. J., Mentzer, S. J., and Strauss, G.: Extrapleural pneumonectomy in the treatment of malignant pleural mesothelioma. Ann. Thorac. Surg., *54*:941, 1992. Reprinted with permission from the Society of Thoracic Surgeons.)

therapy offers potential benefit when used in a multimodality regimen.

Additional Therapies. Because of the poor results using conventional modalities, novel therapeutic strategies, such as immunotherapy and photodynamic therapy, have attracted attention. Systemic as well as intrapleural administration of interleukin-2 and gamma interferon demonstrated mixed results; however, in one study of 22 patients, intrapleural treatment with gamma interferon resulted in partial responses in 56%.[7] Intraoperative photodynamic therapy during resection or by means of thoracoscopy is another innovative technique under investigation.[28]

Multimodality Therapy. The inability of single-modality therapy to significantly alter the course of malignant mesothelioma has led a number of groups to advocate multimodality treatment. At the Brigham and Women's Hospital and the Dana-Farber Cancer Institute, a trimodality strategy employing extrapleural pneumonectomy followed by sequential chemotherapy with cyclophosphamide, doxorubicin, and cisplatin and up to 55 Gy. of radiation therapy was evaluated.[37] Perioperative mortality was 4.6%, and morbidity was 30%. Use of this multimodality regimen also demonstrated that patients with the epithelial variant and no nodal spread had a 5-year survival rate of 45%, suggesting that improved stratification of patients may allow selection of those individuals in whom aggressive multimodality therapy might significantly improve survival.

SELECTED REFERENCES

Butchart, E. G., Ashcroft, T., Barnsley, W. C., and Holden, M. P.: Pleuropneumonectomy in the management of diffuse malignant mesothelioma of the pleura: Experience with 29 patients. Thorax, *31*:15, 1976.
This classic paper is one of the earlier reports describing the use of extrapleural pneumonectomy in a large series of patients with mesothelioma. The first widely used staging system is also presented.

DaValle, M. J., Faber, L. P., Kittle, C. F., and Jensik, R. J.: Extrapleural pneumonectomy for diffuse, malignant mesothelioma. Ann. Thorac. Surg., *42*:612, 1986.
This report of 33 patients who underwent extrapleural pneumonectomy describes a number of critical points fundamental to the development of current treatment strategies for mesothelioma: Extrapleural pneumonectomy may be performed with a mortality comparable to that of standard pneumonectomy, palliation can be achieved in a significant percentage of patients, adjuvant therapy may improve survival, and careful selection of patients for aggressive therapy is critical.

Rusch, V., Saltz, L., Venkatraman, E., Ginsberg, R., McCormack, P., Burt, M., Markman, M., and Kelsen, D.: A phase II trial of pleurectomy/decortication followed by intrapleural and systemic chemotherapy for malignant pleural mesothelioma. J. Clin. Oncol., *12*:1156, 1994.
Some groups question whether radical resection by extrapleural pneumonectomy results in increased survival compared with limited resection. This controversial subject is studied by evaluating pleurectomy with decortication followed by intrapleural and systemic chemotherapy, which is shown to possibly improve survival. However, locoregional recurrence remains frequent (16 of 20 patients).

Sugarbaker, D. J., Mentzer, S. J., and Strauss, G.: Extrapleural pneumonectomy in the treatment of malignant pleural mesothelioma. Ann. Thorac. Surg., *54*:941, 1992.
This article presents a complete description of the technique of extrapleural pneumonectomy for diffuse malignant pleural mesothelioma. A right-sided resection is presented, and the important differences between right and left resections are highlighted. The experience with extrapleural pneumonectomies performed at the Brigham and Women's Hospital is reviewed, showing that the technique outlined in this paper has resulted in a significant decrease in operative mortality.

Sugarbaker, D. J., Strauss, G. M., Lynch, T. J., Richards, W., Mentzer, S. J., Lee, T. H., Corson, J. M., and Antman, K. H.: Node status has prognostic significance in the multimodality therapy of diffuse, malignant mesothelioma. J. Clin. Oncol., *11*:1172, 1993.
Three key issues regarding malignant pleural mesothelioma are addressed in this article. The prognostic value of lymph node spread is demonstrated, the role of trimodality therapy is outlined (extrapleural pneumonectomy with postoperative radiation therapy and chemotherapy), and a new staging system is proposed to improve on the deficiencies, described in this paper, of the Butchart system.

REFERENCES

1. Antman, K., Pass, H. I., and Recht, A.: Benign and malignant mesothelioma. *In* DeVita, V. T., Jr., Hellman, S., and Rosenberg, S. A. (Eds.): Cancer:

Principles and Practice of Oncology, 3rd ed. Philadelphia, J. B. Lippincott, 1989.

2. Antman, K., Shemin, R., Ryan, L., et al.: Malignant mesothelioma: Prognostic variables in a registry of 180 patients, the Dana-Farber Cancer Institute and Brigham and Women's Hospital experience over two decades, 1965–1985. J. Clin. Oncol., 6:147, 1988.

3. Antman, K. H., Pass, H. I., DeLaney, T., Li, F. P., and Corson, J.: Benign and malignant mesothelioma. In DeVita, V. T., Jr., Hellman, S., and Rosenberg, S. A. (Eds.): Cancer Principles and Practice of Oncology, 4th ed. Philadelphia, J. B. Lippincott, 1993.

4. Ball, D. L., and Cruickshank, D. G.: The treatment of malignant mesothelioma of the pleura: Review of a 5-year experience, with special reference to radiotherapy. Am. J. Clin. Oncol., 13:4, 1990.

5. Bissett, D., Macbeth, F. R., and Cram, I.: The role of palliative radiotherapy in malignant mesothelioma. Clin. Oncol. (R. Coll. Radiol.), 316:315, 1991.

6. Boutin, C.: Thoracoscopy in malignant mesothelioma. Pneumologie, 43:61, 1989.

7. Boutin, C., Viallat, J. R., Van Zandwijk, N., et al.: Activity of intrapleural recombinant gamma-interferon in malignant mesothelioma. Cancer, 67:2033, 1991.

8. Butchart, E. G., Ashcroft, T., Barnsley, W. C., and Holden, M. P.: Pleuropneumonectomy in the management of diffuse malignant mesothelioma of the pleura. Experience with 29 patients. Thorax, 31:15, 1976.

9. Connelly, R. R., Spirtas, R., Myers, M. H., Percy, C. L., and Fraumeni, J. F., Jr.: Demographic patterns for mesothelioma in the United States. J. Natl. Cancer Inst., 78:1053, 1987.

10. Corson, J. M.: Pathology of mesothelioma. In Antman, K., and Aisner, J. (Eds.): Asbestos-Related Malignancy. Orlando, FL, Grune & Stratton, 1987.

11. Cote, R. J., Jhanwar, S. C., Novick, S., and Pellicer, A.: Genetic alterations of the p53 gene are a feature of malignant mesothelioma. Cancer Res., 51:5410, 1991.

12. DaValle, M. J., Faber, L. P., Kittle, C. F., and Jensik, R. J.: Extrapleural pneumonectomy for diffuse, malignant mesothelioma. Ann. Thorac. Surg., 42:612, 1986.

13. Dawson, A., Gibbs, A., Browne, K., Pooley, F., and Griffiths, M.: Familial mesothelioma: Details of 17 cases with histopathologic findings and mineral analysis. Cancer, 70:1183, 1992.

14. Doll, R.: Mortality from lung cancer in asbestos workers. Br. J. Ind. Med., 12:81, 1955.

15. Foulke, R. S., Davidson, K., Zaloznik, A. J., and VonHoff, D.: Absence of oncogene amplification in malignant mesothelioma specimens (Abstract). Proc. Am. Soc. Clin. Oncol., 10:A1058, 1991.

16. Hillerdal, G.: Malignant mesothelioma 1982: Review of 4710 published cases. Br. J. Dis. Chest, 77:321, 1983.

17. Huncharek, M.: Changing risk groups for malignant mesothelioma. Cancer, 69:2704, 1992.

18. Kafiri, G., Thomas, D. M., Shepherd, N. A., Krausz, T., Lane, D. P., and Hall, P. A.: p53 expression is common in malignant mesothelioma. Histopathology, 21:331, 1992.

19. Krarup-Hansen, A., and Hansen, H. H.: Chemotherapy in malignant mesothelioma: A review. Cancer Chemother. Pharmacol., 28:319, 1991.

20. Lanphear, B. P., and Buncher, C. R.: Latent period for malignant mesothelioma of occupational origin. J. Occup. Med., 34:718, 1992.

21. McDonald, A. D., and McDonald, J. C.: Epidemiology of malignant mesothelioma. In Antman, K., and Aisner, J. (Eds.): Asbestos-Related Malignancy. Orlando, FL, Grune & Stratton, Inc., 1987.

22. Metcalf, R. A., Welsh, J. A., Bennett, W. P., et al: p53 and Kirsten-ras mutations in human mesothelioma cell lines. Cancer Res., 52:2610, 1992.

23. Moran, C. A., Suster, S., and Koss, M. N.: The spectrum of histologic growth patterns in benign and malignant fibrous tumors of the pleura. Semin. Diagn. Pathol., 9:169, 1992.

24. Mossman, B. T., Bignon, J., Corn, M., Seaton, A., and Gee, J. B. L.: Asbestos: Scientific developments and implications for public policy. Science, 247:294, 1990.

25. Mossman, B. T., and Gee, J. B. L.: Asbestos-related diseases. N. Engl. J. Med., 320:1721, 1989.

26. Mountain, C. F.: A new international staging system for lung cancer. Chest, 89(Suppl.):225S, 1986.

27. Muscat, J. E., and Wynder, E. L.: Cigarette smoking, asbestos exposure, and malignant mesothelioma. Cancer Res., 51:2263, 1991.

28. Pass, H. I., DeLaney, T. F., Tochner, Z., et al.: Intrapleural photodynamic therapy: Results of a Phase I trial. Ann. Surg. Oncol., 1:28, 1994.

29. Patz, E. F., Jr., Shaffer, K., Piwnica-Worms, D. R., et al.: Malignant pleural mesothelioma: Value of CT and MR imaging in predicting resectability. AJR, 159:961, 1992.

30. Pooley, F. D.: Asbestos mineralogy. In Antman, K., and Aisner, J. (Eds.): Asbestos-Related Malignancy. Orlando, FL, Grune & Stratton, 1987.

31. Rusch, V., Saltz, L., Venkatraman, E., et al.: A phase II trial of pleurectomy/decortication followed by intrapleural and systemic chemotherapy for malignant pleural mesothelioma. J. Clin. Oncol., 12:1156, 1994.

32. Rusch, V. W., and Ginsberg, R. J.: New concepts in the staging of mesothelioma: Invited comment to chapter 26. In Deslauriers, J., and Lacquet, L. K. (Eds.): Thoracic Surgery: Surgical Management of Pleural Diseases. Vol. 6, International Trends in General Thoracic Surgery, St. Louis, C. V. Mosby, 1990.

33. Rusch, V. W., Piantadosi, S., and Holmes, E. C.: The role of extrapleural pneumonectomy in malignant pleural mesothelioma: A Lung Cancer Study Group trial. J. Thorac. Cardiovasc. Surg., 102:1, 1991.

34. Sugarbaker, D. J., Heher, E. C., Lee, T. H., et al.: Extrapleural pneumonectomy, chemotherapy, and radiotherapy in the treatment of diffuse malignant pleural mesothelioma. J. Thorac. Cardiovasc. Surg., 102:10, 1991.

35. Sugarbaker, D. J., and Liptay, M. J.: Therapeutic approaches for malignant pleural mesothelioma. In Aisner, J., Arriagada, R., Green, M. R., Martini, N., and Perry, M. C. (Eds.): Comprehensive Textbook of Thoracic Oncology. Baltimore, Williams & Wilkins, 1996, pp. 786–798.

36. Sugarbaker, D. J., Mentzer, S. J., and Strauss, G.: Extrapleural pneumonectomy in the treatment of malignant pleural mesothelioma. Ann. Thorac. Surg., 54:941, 1992.

37. Sugarbaker, D. J., Strauss, G. M., Lynch, T. J., et al.: Node status has prognostic significance in the multimodality therapy of diffuse, malignant mesothelioma. J. Clin. Oncol., 11:1172, 1993.

38. Tiainen, M., Rautonen, J., Pyrhonen, S., Tammilehto, L., Mattson, K., and Knuutila, S.: Chromosome number correlates with survival in patients with malignant pleural mesothelioma. Cancer Genet. Cytogenet., 62:21, 1992.

39. Vogelzang, N. J.: Malignant mesothelioma: Diagnostic and management strategies for 1992. Semin. Oncol., 19(4):64, 1992.

40. Vortmeyer, A. O., Preuss, J., Padberg, B-C., Kastendieck, H., and Schroder, S.: Immunocytochemical differential diagnosis of diffuse malignant pleural mesotheliomas—a clinicomorphological study of 158 cases. Anticancer. Res., 11:889, 1991.

41. Wagner, J. C., Sleggs, E. A., and Marchand, P.: Diffuse pleural mesothelioma and asbestos exposure in the North Western Cape Province. Br. J. Ind. Med., 17:260, 1960.

42. Walker, C., Everitt, J., and Barrett, J. C.: Possible cellular and molecular mechanisms for asbestos carcinogenicity. Am. J. Ind. Med., 21:253, 1992.

43. Webb, W. R., Ozmen, V., Moulder, P. V., Shabahang, B., and Breaux, J.: Iodized talc pleurodesis for the treatment of pleural effusions. J. Thorac. Cardiovasc. Surg., 103:881, 1992.

XIV

THORACIC OUTLET SYNDROME

John G. Adams, Jr., M.D., and Donald Silver, M.D.

Thoracic outlet syndrome is the preferred term for those syndromes (e.g. the cervical rib syndrome, scalenus anticus syndrome, hyperabduction syndrome, costoclavicular syndrome, pectoralis minor syndrome, and the first thoracic rib syndrome) that result from compression of the neurovascular structures to the upper extremities. The syndrome is caused by compression of the brachial plexus or subclavian-axillary artery and/or vein in the region between the thoracic outlet and the insertion of the pectoralis minor muscle onto the coracoid process. Symptoms may arise from neural, vascular, or combined neural and vascular compression, with neural compression causing 90% to 95% of these symptoms.

HISTORICAL ASPECTS

One of the earliest descriptions of the thoracic outlet syndrome appeared in 1860 when Willshire reported a pulsating subclavian artery (possibly an aneurysm) that crossed a presumed cervical rib.[1] In 1861, Coote excised a cervical rib to relieve pressure on the axillary vessels and nerves.[6] Murphy, in 1905,[18] and Keen, in 1907, emphasized the role of cervical ribs in the compression of the neurovascular structures. In 1919, Stopford and Telford demonstrated that the brachial plexus and subclavian artery could be compressed by the first thoracic rib and indicated that resection of the rib would relieve symptoms.[30] In 1927, Adson and Coffey emphasized the role of the scalene muscles in neurovascular compression and popularized scalenotomy as a method of therapy.[2, 9] Various operative maneuvers were tried with varying degrees of success until 1962, when the role of the first rib and its ligamentous and muscular attachments in the pathogenesis of the thoracic outlet syndrome was re-emphasized.[5] Scalenectomy and/or resection of the first rib is offered to the approximately 40% of patients with the thoracic outlet syndrome who do not improve with a 4-month (or longer) trial of nonoperative management.

ANATOMY

An understanding of the sites of potential pressure in the thoracic outlet region is necessary for proper evaluation and management of this syndrome. The anterior rami of five spinal nerves, C5, C6, C7, C8, and T1 (C4 and T2 may also contribute to the brachial plexus), exit through the intervertebral foramina and form trunks that pass through the scalene triangle and then divide behind the clavicle. The divisions of the trunks reunite to form cords that surround the axillary artery as it passes behind the pectoralis minor tendon. The division of these cords into the major motor and sensory nerves of the upper extremity usually occurs distal to the pectoralis minor tendon.

Rami from C8 and T1 form the lowest trunk, which lies on the first rib behind the subclavian artery and is responsible for the groove in the rib (which is often attributed to the artery). The peripheral distribution of C8 and T1 fibers provides sensory perception from the fifth finger and medial half of the fourth finger and from the medial aspect of the forearm. The motor distribution of this trunk controls flexion of the wrist and fingers and innervates the intrinsic muscles of the hand.

Both subclavian arteries exit from the thorax behind the sternoclavicular joints and pass over the first ribs *between* the scalenus anticus and scalenus medius muscles. The arteries then course laterally behind the clavicles and become the axillary arteries. The axillary arteries pass posterior to the tendons of the pectoralis minor muscles and become the brachial arteries. The axillary veins pass behind the costocoracoid ligaments and pectoralis minor tendons. At the edge of the first rib, each axillary vein becomes a subclavian vein that passes over the first rib *anterior* to the scalenus anticus muscle to join its respective jugular vein at the base of the neck.

The arteries, veins, and nerves that form the brachial plexus may be compressed in any of several areas as they pass from the neck or the thoracic outlet into the upper extremity. The anatomic sites of compression from medial to lateral include (1) the interscalene triangle (arteries and nerves); (2) the space between the scalenus anticus muscle and the clavicle (vein); (3) the first rib, or between the first rib and clavicle (nerves, arteries, and veins); (4) the costocoracoid fascia (nerves, arteries, and veins); and (5) the pectoralis minor tendon (nerves, arteries, and veins).

Other causes of compression of the neurovascular structures include the following:

1. Cervical ribs occur in approximately 1% of the population and are bilateral in 80%. Cervical ribs or fibrous bands associated with them may compress or irritate portions of the adjacent brachial plexus and compress or elevate the subclavian artery. However, fewer than 10% of cervical ribs produce symptoms.

2. The long transverse process of C7 may function as cervical ribs.

3. Abnormal first thoracic ribs frequently fail to reach the sternum, may be attached to the sternum or to the second rib by ligaments, and may cause distortion or compression of the lower components of the brachial plexus.

4. Variations of the scalene muscles may occur. Roos has described at least 10 different fibromuscular anomalies in the thoracic outlet that may produce neuromuscular compression.[24] He has suggested that these various congenital bands and muscular abnormalities are "almost invariably" present in patients who do not respond to conservative management. In addition, spasm, fibrosis, or inflammation of the scalene muscles may produce symptoms.

5. Downward displacement of the upper extremity and shoulder girdle in occupations that require hyperabduction, carrying heavy loads, or working in narrow quarters, so that the upper extremities are drawn forward and down, is frequently associated with thoracic outlet syndrome symptoms.

6. Fractures of the first rib or clavicle with deformity or callus formation may be associated with thoracic outlet syndrome symptoms.

7. Compression by tumor in the outlet spaces may be causative.[36]

8. Osteoarthritis of the spine[33] or cervicothoracic scoliosis[32] may cause nerve root compression and mimic the symptoms of the thoracic outlet syndrome.

SYMPTOMS

The symptoms of the thoracic outlet syndrome vary, depending on the vessels or nerves compressed, and may be neurologic or vascular or both. The syndrome occurs most often in young to middle-aged women (70%–75%), although all age groups are affected.[7] The clinical manifestations rarely indicate the site of compression.

Neurologic symptoms consist of pain, weakness, paresthesias, and numbness, usually in the fingers and hands in an ulnar distribution, but they may occur anywhere in the upper extremity, neck, or shoulder girdle. Two different patterns of neurologic symptoms have been described and can be classified as *upper* and *lower* cord compression syndromes.[25] The upper cord compression syndrome results from compression or irritation of the upper nerves of the brachial plexus (C5, C6, and C7) and is usually associated primarily with pain. The pain usually occurs in the upper chest, anterior or lateral neck, mandible, face, temporal and occipital areas, and the scapular and deltoid regions; it may also occur in the lateral aspect of the arm and forearm and the dorsal surface of the hand between the thumb and index finger. The lower cord compression syndrome is the more common pattern of neurologic symptoms in patients with thoracic outlet syndrome. The lower nerves of the brachial plexus that form the ulnar nerve (C8 and T1) are affected. Pain typically occurs in the posterior neck, medial scapula area, medial aspect of the arm, ulnar aspect of the forearm and hand, and fourth and fifth digits. Weakness of the arm and hand may occur; paresthesias in the ulnar nerve distribution occur frequently. Rarely, a combination of upper and lower cord compression syndrome symptoms is encountered. Late neurologic sequelae of thoracic outlet syndrome include sensory loss, motor weakness, and atrophy.

Symptoms of arterial compression include ischemic pain, numbness, fatigue, paresthesias, coldness, and weakness in the arm or hand. These symptoms are accentuated by exercise and exposure to cold. Thromboses may occur in the compressed or poststenotic dilated, occasionally aneurysmal, areas of the subclavian or axillary arteries and, if occlusive, can produce distal ischemic changes. Recurrent, angina-like chest pain may occur in a few patients with the disorder. Distal embolization may be associated with vasomotor symptoms in the fingers, consisting of episodic pain with pallor and/or cyanosis. These symptoms are accentuated by cold exposure. If the embolization continues, advanced ischemia with ulceration or gangrene of the fingertips may occur.

Venous compression may produce upper extremity edema, pain, and cyanosis. The patients frequently complain of a sensation of heaviness and tightness in the arm.

DIAGNOSIS

A complete history and a thorough physical examination are essential in establishing the diagnosis of thoracic outlet syndrome. The symptom-complexes plus a history of trauma with fracture(s) of the clavicle or ribs or both, a history of unusual exercise or occupation, poor posture, and so forth should suggest the diagnosis. A careful history also indicates whether the symptoms are part of a generalized process such as occurs with spinal cord tumors, peripheral embolizations, osteoarthritis, and connective tissue or metabolic disorders. Cervical intervertebral disc disease and the carpal tunnel syndrome may be confused with thoracic outlet syndrome.

The physical examination should be thorough, with special emphasis given to detecting the neural, arterial, and venous signs. Neural signs include sensory deficits, weakness, and atrophy. Most often the sensory and motor deficits occur in the distribution of the ulnar nerve. Occasionally, the symptoms may be reproduced by percussion of the supraclavicular fossa. Signs of arterial compression and/or embolization include weakened or absent brachial and radial pulses, a bruit in the supraclavicular or axillary space, delayed capillary blush, petechiae of the hand or digits, or occasional areas of distal gangrene. Signs of venous compression include distended superficial veins on the chest, arm, or hand, distal edema, and cyanosis.

The physical findings are not constant. Therefore, several examinations may be required before the thoracic outlet syndrome is suspected. The findings may vary according to the patient's position during the examination. Except when reproduced by hyperabduction of the arm, neural and/or vascular compression is rarely detected when patients are examined in the supine position but is usually readily detected when the patient is sitting or standing. Diagnostic maneuvers for the thoracic outlet syndrome are listed below. The first three, which detect vascular compression *only*, may be abnormal in a large number (approximately 50%) of patients who are asymptomatic.

1. *Adson or scalene maneuver.*[2, 3] While the physician monitors the radial pulse, the patient takes a deep breath, extends the neck, and turns the chin toward the side being examined. Disappearance or reduction of the radial pulse constitutes a positive finding. During a positive test, a bruit frequently becomes audible in the supraclavicular fossa and the hand may become cool and pale. The deep breath causes elevation of the first rib and extending and turning the neck causes narrowing of the interscalene triangle. The symptoms are caused by compression of the subclavian artery and possibly of the brachial plexus by the first rib and scalene muscles. If the pulse is altered before the head is turned, one should suspect the presence of a cervical rib.

2. *Costoclavicular compressive maneuver.*[8] While the radial pulse is monitored, the patient places his or her shoulders back and downward into an exaggerated military position. Disappearance or reduction of the radial pulse or appearance of a subclavian bruit constitutes a positive finding. The pulse changes are produced by compression of the subclavian artery between the clavicle and the first rib.

3. *Hyperabduction maneuver.*[37] The radial pulse is monitored while the arm is passively moved into a hyperabducted position. Reduction or cessation of the radial pulse and the appearance of an axillary bruit indicate arterial compression by the pectoralis minor tendon.

4. *Three-minute elevated arm stress test.*[24] The patient is asked to slowly open and close the hands while keeping both arms abducted, externally rotated, and flexed to 90 degrees at the elbow. Normal patients may experience fatigue but rarely have pain or paresthesias. In patients with a thoracic outlet syndrome, this test may reproduce their symptoms.

Objective Examinations. Roentgenograms of the neck and chest may demonstrate cervical ribs, anomalous first ribs, prominent transverse processes, bony exostoses, calluses, abnormalities of the clavicle, and so forth. The roentgenograms also yield information about narrowing of the intervertebral foramina and tumors. Myelograms may be necessary to demonstrate a cervical disc or other causes of cervical cord compression.

Electromyography is useful in detecting sites of compression of peripheral nerves by recording the altered response of the distal muscles to proximal electrical stimuli. Nerve conduction times across the thoracic outlet to the elbow and wrist may be prolonged; they have returned to normal range after surgical relief of the compression.[34, 35] However, the variability and unreliability of the nerve conduction studies have limited their usefulness in establishing the diagnosis of thoracic outlet syndrome.[12, 24, 27] Nerve conduction velocities are most important in determining whether a more peripheral compressive lesion (e.g., carpal tunnel syndrome) is present.

Evidence suggests that somatosensory evoked potentials may be useful in identifying those patients likely to respond to surgical therapy for thoracic outlet syndrome.[16] In addition to their diagnostic value, somatosensory evoked potentials may provide objective evidence of persistent nerve dysfunction postoperatively. The technique consists of recording nerve action potentials at various sites along the central and peripheral nervous systems in response to electrical stimulation of the ulnar and median nerves at the wrist. By comparing the amplitudes of these various action potentials, the site of nerve dysfunction can be determined.

Arteriograms demonstrate sites of partial or complete arterial occlusion. Arteriography should be performed with the patient's arms by his or her side and while he or she is performing the Adson, costoclavicular, and hyperabduction maneuvers. Occasionally, poststenotic dilatation or aneurysms of the subclavian artery distal to the site of compression are demonstrated. A normal arteriogram does not eliminate neural compression as a cause of the syndrome and neither does narrowing or obstruction of the subclavian-axillary arteries during the maneuvers confirm the diagnosis, because some obstruction of these arteries can be demonstrated in approximately half of the patients without symptoms of thoracic outlet syndrome. Arteriography is usually reserved for those few patients with suspected arterial aneurysms, obstruction, or distal embolization. Plethysmography[28] has been used to document arterial compression. This technique records changes in digit volume that occur with each heartbeat and can demonstrate obstruction to arterial flow.[31] Phlebograms are useful to demonstrate sites of compression of the axillary or subclavian veins. If the veins become totally or partially occluded during the hyperabduction or costoclavicular compression maneuvers, support is obtained for the diagnosis of thoracic outlet syndrome.

Noninvasive direct visualization of the subclavian-axillary

vessels is being investigated as a means of evaluating vessel compression associated with the thoracic outlet syndrome. In a study composed of 16 patients suspected of having thoracic outlet syndrome, color duplex ultrasonography yielded a sensitivity and specificity for the diagnosis of thoracic outlet syndrome of 92% and 95%, respectively.[13] Magnetic resonance imaging is an additional noninvasive modality that is being used to evaluate neurovascular compression in thoracic outlet syndrome. In a study of 20 patients with symptoms consistent with thoracic outlet syndrome, magnetic resonance imaging was shown to have a sensitivity of 79% and a specificity of 87.5% for deviation of the brachial plexus. Magnetic resonance angiography has also been reported to be useful in the evaluation of vessel compression, but further studies are needed to evaluate its role in the diagnosis of thoracic outlet syndrome.[22]

MANAGEMENT

For all patients, except those with symptomatic arterial occlusion, distal embolization, a poststenotic aneurysm, or symptomatic venous occlusion, initial management should consist of a trial of weight reduction and an exercise program directed toward improving posture, strengthening the elevators of the shoulder girdle, and avoiding hyperabduction. These measures relieve symptoms in 50% to 70% of patients.[11, 19, 32] Nonoperative management appears to be the most successful in the obese, young to middle-aged woman with poor posture. When symptoms appear job-related, as in certain types of manual labor, a change in occupation may provide relief.

Patients with major neurologic or vascular complications and those who do not respond to a 4-month (or longer) trial of nonoperative management should be offered surgical intervention. Operative management has included excision of a cervical rib, division of the scalenus anticus muscle, resection of the clavicle, and division of the pectoralis minor tendon.[20, 29] Falconer and Li,[8] Clagett,[5] and Roos[24] emphasized that removal of the major portion of the first rib effectively decompresses the neurovascular structures. Subsequently, the removal of the first rib, and of a cervical rib if it is present, became the preferred surgical management for the thoracic outlet syndrome.

Clagett[5] suggested that the first rib be removed through a posterior incision along the medial border of the scapula. This approach provides good exposure for rib resection and for vascular reconstructive procedures. However, it produces a large scar and has increased morbidity. The posterior approach is uncommonly used today.

Nelson and Jenson[21] have employed an anterior extrapleural approach for excision of the first rib and have found this incision to be cosmetically acceptable with few complications. However, this approach is not suitable for removing cervical ribs or anomalous first ribs.

Roos[26] popularized the use of a transaxillary incision for removal of the first rib (Fig. 51–94). The vessels and nerves are lifted off the first rib when the arm is hyperabducted during operation. Of necessity, the scalene muscles are divided during removal of the rib. Although this procedure has proved effective for relieving neurovascular compression, it does not provide good exposure for vascular reconstructions. Brachial plexus injuries, injury to the long thoracic nerve of Bell, pneumothorax, pleural effusion, and infection appear to be more common with the transaxillary approach than with supraclavicular decompression.[4] Up to 20% of the operative injuries to the brachial plexus may be associated with significant residual disability.[6]

In recent years, increasing numbers of surgeons have chosen the supraclavicular approach for thoracic outlet decom-

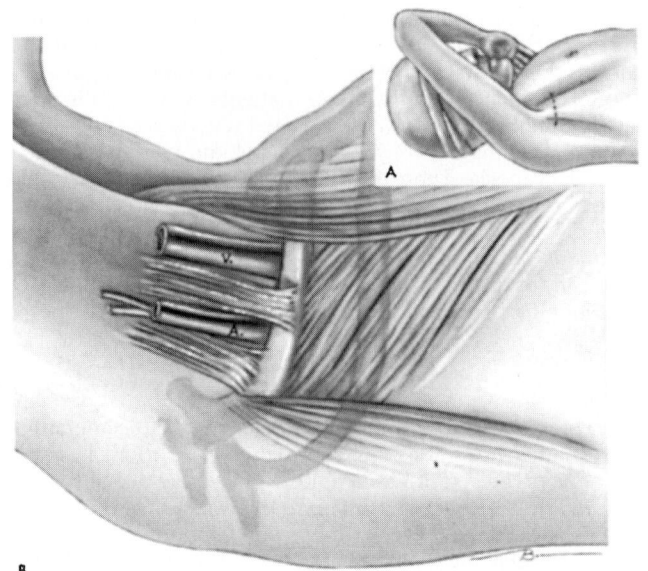

Figure 51–94. The transaxillary approach (A) to the first rib provides good exposure (B) of the first rib, scalene muscles, brachial plexus, and subclavian artery (A) and vein (V).

pression. This procedure consists of extensive anterior scalenectomy, middle scalenectomy, removal of the cervical rib if one is present, and, on occasion, first rib resection (Fig. 51–95).[28] Results of supraclavicular decompression are equivalent or superior to those achieved with transaxillary first rib resection. In a comparison of the two techniques by Cikrit and associates,[4] the supraclavicular procedure was accompanied by fewer complications, less blood loss, and shorter postoperative hospitalization. The average hospital stay is approximately 3 days, with most patients returning to work in 7 to 10 days. Supraclavicular decompression is becoming accepted as the preferred operation for the surgical management of the thoracic outlet syndrome. Symptomatic improvement may be achieved in over 90% of the cases.[4, 23, 25]

Recurrent symptoms severe enough to require reoperation may occur in 1% of patients after first rib resection.[34] Many of the patients with recurrent symptoms respond to physiotherapy and improvement in posture. A repeat supraclavicular decompression can be safely accomplished in the few patients who do not respond to physical therapy.[25]

Mild poststenotic dilatation of the subclavian artery usually does not progress once the compression is relieved and frequently remains of no clinical consequence. However, significant aneurysmal enlargement of the artery should be excised and replaced with a graft, preferably a vein graft. Thrombosis of the subclavian artery should be treated by thrombectomy and/or thrombolytic therapy or by replacement or bypass grafting of the involved segment.

Thrombosis of the subclavian-axillary vein has traditionally been treated with heparin and/or thrombolytic therapy, elevation, and an elastic sleeve until recanalization occurs. Currently, the subclavian-axillary vein thrombosis is treated with local infusion of urokinase by means of a percutaneous basilic vein approach.[10, 14, 15] An initial loading dose of urokinase consisting of 4000 I.U. per minute is infused for the first hour, followed by 1000 I.U. per minute until resolution of the thrombotic process has occurred. Systemic anticoagulation with heparin is maintained to keep the partial thromboplastin time at one and one-half to two and one-half times normal to prevent pericatheter thrombotic complications. After resolution of the thrombotic process with thrombolytic therapy, oral anticoagulation is instituted with warfarin and contin-

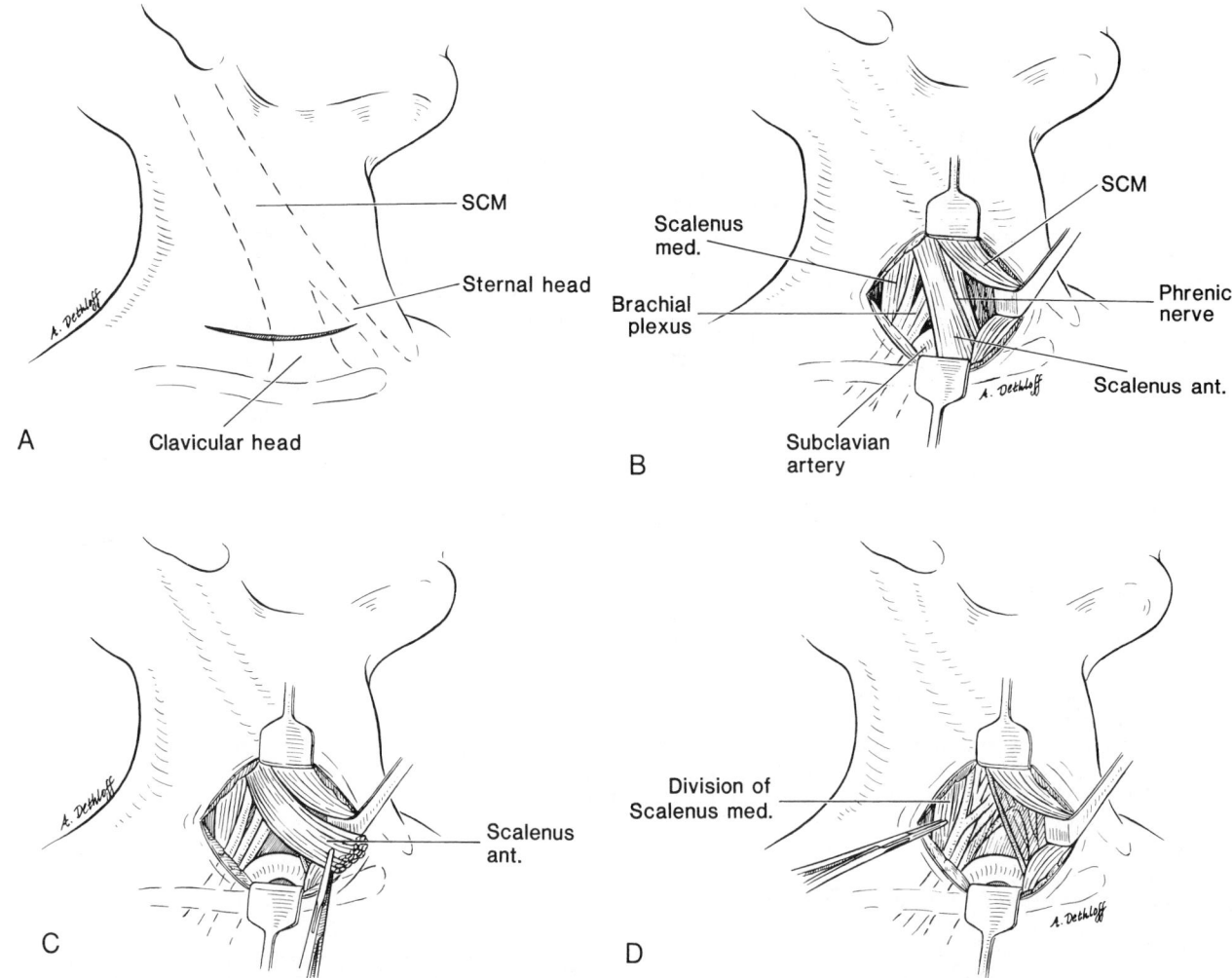

Figure 51–95. *A,* A 6- to 8-cm. incision is made 2 to 3 cm. above the clavicle. *B,* Exposure obtained after mobilization of the prescalene fat pad. *C,* Division of the scalenus anticus near its insertion on the first rib. The phrenic nerve must be protected. *D,* Exposure and division of the scalenus medius after excision of the scalenus anticus.

ued for a minimum of 3 months. In rare cases of acute, total thrombotic obstruction of the upper extremity, a thrombectomy may be useful to establish venous outflow.[17]

After recanalization of the subclavian-axillary venous system, an aggressive search is made for the causative factor. In patients in whom compression of the venous system is identified, a decompressive procedure is indicated. In a study of 38 patients with subclavian-axillary vein thrombosis treated with thrombolytic therapy followed by surgical decompression, there were no episodes of recurrent venous thrombosis at a mean follow-up of 3.1 years.[14] Residual vein stenosis after decompression has been treated by a variety of techniques, including patch angioplasty, placement of an interpositional graft, and percutaneous transluminal angioplasty.[10] In cases in which chronic symptomatic thrombosis persists, a saphenous vein bypass from the axillary vein to the jugular vein may provide symptomatic relief.

REFERENCES

1. A mirror of the practice of medicine and surgery in the hospitals of London: Clinical records; Supernumerary first rib. Lancet, 2:633, 1860.
2. Adson, A. W., and Coffey, J. R.: Cervical rib: A method of anterior approach for relief of symptoms by division of scalenus anticus. Ann. Surg., 85:839, 1927.
3. Adson, A. W.: Surgical treatment for symptoms produced by cervical ribs and the scalenus anticus muscle. Surg. Gynecol. Obstet., 85:687, 1947.
4. Cikrit, D. F., Haefner, R., Nichols, W. K., and Silver, D.: Transaxillary or supraclavicular decompression for the thoracic outlet syndrome: A comparison of the risks and benefit. Am. Surg., 55:347, 1989.
5. Clagett, O. T.: Research and prosearch: Presidential address. J. Thorac. Cardiovasc. Surg., 44:153, 1962.
6. Coote, H.: Pressure on the axillary vessel and nerve by the exostosis from a cervical rib: Interference with the circulation of the arm: Removal of the rib and exostosis. Recovery, Med. Times & Gaz., 2:108, 1986, cited in reference 5.
7. Dale, W. A.: Thoracic outlet compression syndrome: Critique in 1982. Arch. Surg., 117:1437, 1982.
8. Falconer, M. A., and Weddell, G.: Costoclavicular compression of the subclavian artery and vein: Relation to the scalenus anticus syndrome. Lancet, 2:539, 1943.
9. Falconer, M. A., and Li, F. W. P.: Resection of the first rib in costoclavicular compression of the brachial plexus. Lancet, 1:59, 1962.
10. Glanz, S., Gordon, D. H., Lipkowitz, G. S., Butt, K. M., Hong, J., and Sclafani, S. J.: Axillary and subclavian vein stenosis: Percutaneous angioplasty. Radiology, 168:371, 1988.
11. Haggart, G. E.: Value of conservative management in cervicobrachial pain. JAMA, 137:508, 1948.
12. Kremer, R. M., and Allquist, R. E., Jr.: Thoracic outlet compression syndrome. Am. J. Surg., 130:612, 1975.
13. Longley, D. G., Yedicka, J. W., Molina, E. J., Schwabacher, S., Hunter, D. W., and Letourneau, J. G.: Thoracic outlet syndrome: Evaluation of the subclavian vessels by color duplex sonography. AJR, 158:623, 1992.
14. Machleder, H. I.: Evaluation of a new treatment strategy for Paget-Schroetter syndrome: Spontaneous thrombosis of the axillary-subclavian vein. J. Vasc. Surg., 17:305, 1993.
15. Machleder, H. I.: The role of thrombolytic agents for acute subclavian vein thrombosis. Semin. Vasc. Surg., 2:82, 1992.
16. Machleder, H. I., Moll, F., Nuwer, M., and Jordan, S.: Somatosensory

evoked potentials in the assessment of thoracic outlet compression syndrome. J. Vasc. Surg., 6:177, 1987.

17. Mahorner, H., Castleberry, J. W., and Colemen, W. O.: Attempts to restore function in major veins which are the sites of massive thrombosis. Ann. Surg., 146:510, 1957.

18. Murphy, J. B.: A case of cervical rib with symptoms resembling subclavian aneurysm. Ann. Surg., 41:399, 1905.

19. Nelson, P. A.: Treatment of patients with cervicodorsal outlet syndrome. JAMA, 163:1570, 1957.

20. Nelson, R. M., and Davis, R. W.: Thoracic outlet compression syndrome. Ann. Thorac. Surg., 8:437, 1969.

21. Nelson, R. M., and Jensen, C. B.: Anterior approach for excision of the first rib. Ann. Thorac. Surg., 9:30, 1970.

22. Panegyres, P. K., Moore, N., Gibson, R., Rushworth, G., and Donaghy, M.: Thoracic outlet syndromes and magnetic resonance imaging. Brain, 116:823, 1993.

23. Reilly, L. M., and Stoney, R. J.: Supraclavicular approach of thoracic outlet decompression. J. Vasc. Surg., 8:329, 1988.

24. Roos, D. B.: Congenital anomalies associated with thoracic outlet syndrome. Anatomy, symptoms, diagnosis, and treatment. Am. J. Surg., 132:771, 1976.

25. Roos, D. B.: The place for scalenectomy and first rib resection in thoracic outlet syndrome. Surgery, 92:1077, 1982.

26. Roos, D. B.: Transaxillary approach for first rib resection to relieve thoracic outlet syndrome. Ann. Surg., 163:354, 1966.

27. Sadler, T. R., Jr., Rianer, W. G., and Twombley, G.: Thoracic outlet compression: Application of positional arteriographic and nerve conduction studies. Am. J. Surg., 130:704, 1975.

28. Sanders, R. J., Monsour, J. W., Gerber, W. F., Adams, W. R., and Thompson, N.: Scalenectomy versus first rib resection for treatment of the thoracic outlet syndrome. Surgery, 85:109, 1979.

29. Silver, D.: The thoracic outlet syndrome. In Goldsmith, H. S. (Ed.): Lewis' Practice of Surgery. New York, Harper & Row, 1975.

30. Stopford, J. S. B., and Telford, E. D.: Compression of the lower trunk of the brachial plexus by a first dorsal rib with a note on the surgical treatment. Br. J. Surg., 7:168, 1919.

31. Strandness, D. E., Jr., and Bell, J. W.: Peripheral vascular disease: Diagnosis and objective evaluation using a mercury strain gauge. Ann. Surg., 16(Suppl.):3, 1965.

32. Tomsick, T. A., Ahlstrand, R. A., and Kiesel, T. M.: Thoracic outlet syndrome associated with rib fusion and cervicothoracic scoliosis. J. Can. Assoc. Radiol., 25:211, 1974.

33. Urschel, H. C., Jr., and Razzuk, M. A.: Management of the thoracic outlet syndrome. N. Engl. J. Med., 286:1140, 1972.

34. Urschel, H. C., Jr., Razzuk, M. A., Albers, J. E., Wood, R. E., and Paulson, D. L.: Reoperation for recurrent thoracic outlet syndrome. Ann. Thorac. Surg., 21:19, 1976.

35. Urschel, H. C., Jr., Razzuk, M. A., Wood, R. E., Rarekh, M., and Paulson, D. L.: Objective diagnosis (ulnar nerve conduction velocity) and current therapy of the thoracic outlet syndrome. Ann. Thorac. Surg., 12:608, 1971.

36. Van Echo, D. A., Sickles, E. A., and Weirnik, P. H.: Thoracic outlet syndrome, supraclavicular adenopathy, Hodgkin's disease (Letter). Ann. Intern. Med., 78:608, 1973.

37. Wright, I. S.: The neurovascular syndrome produced by hyperabduction of the arms: The immediate changes produced in 150 normal controls, and the effects on some persons of prolonged hyperabduction of the arms, as in sleeping, and in certain occupations. Am. Heart J., 29:1, 1945.

XV

CONGENITAL DEFORMITIES OF THE CHEST WALL

Jeffrey S. Heinle, M.D., and David C. Sabiston, Jr., M.D.

Congenital deformities of the chest wall represent a spectrum of deformities ranging from minor cosmetic defects to gross deformities incompatible with life. The defects have both physiologic and psychologic consequences and are often associated with other abnormalities.[25] Although these deformities were recognized as early as the 1500s, surgical management was not considered until the early 1900s, and it was not until Ravitch's initial contributions beginning in the 1940s[29] that major advances in the repair of these defects were made. Surgical intervention offers excellent cosmetic results and symptomatic improvement with minimal morbidity and mortality, and therefore patients presenting with these defects should be considered for surgical repair.

EMBRYOLOGY OF THE CHEST WALL

During embryologic development of the chest wall, two events, development of the sternum and development of the rib cage, are occurring simultaneously and independently.[12] Abnormal development of one of these components does not imply abnormal development of the other. The sternum arises from two mesenchymal bands of lateral plate mesoderm at approximately 6 weeks of gestation.[12] These bilateral sternal bands become cartilaginous bars and fuse with each other in the ventral midline as the lateral embryonic walls fold inward.[25] This fusion takes place from cephalad to caudad, forming a median cartilaginous plate, and is normally complete by 8 weeks.[21] The sternum secondarily subdivides into segmental elements or sternebrae.[12] Multiple centers of ossification in the manubrium and body of the sternum ossify throughout childhood and young adulthood.

The pectoral muscles also arise from the lateral plate meso-

derm, and the sternum and pectoral girdle become part of the appendicular skeleton. During the same time period, the ribs are developing from mesenchyme of the somites, are contiguous with the intervertebral discs, and are components of the axial skeleton. The cartilaginous thoracic cage is present by 8 weeks,[21] and the ventral ends of the ribs remain to become the costal cartilages that fuse with the median cartilaginous plate of the sternum.[12, 25] At the same time that the appendicular and axial skeletons are forming, the heart and diaphragm are also developing, and intrauterine events may interrupt this simultaneous development and result in associated anomalies[25] such as Cantrell's pentalogy. The failure of midline fusion of the sternal bands leads to sternal clefts and the ectopia cordis syndromes described later. Abnormal growth of the costal cartilages can cause the sternum to be displaced posteriorly (pectus excavatum) or anteriorly (pectus carinatum).

PECTUS EXCAVATUM

Pectus excavatum, or funnel chest, is the most common of the congenital deformities of the chest wall, accounting for 90% of the defects and having an incidence of approximately 1 in 125 to 300 live births.[9, 27] It is characterized by a concave, posteriorly displaced sternum due to overgrowth of the costal cartilages (Fig. 51–96). Torsion and asymmetry of the sternum may also be present. Most commonly the defect begins at the junction of the manubrium and the body of the sternum and becomes progressively deeper toward the xiphoid. The most severe area of depression is usually just above the xiphoid. The manubrium and the first and second costal cartilages are typically normal. The defect is a progres-

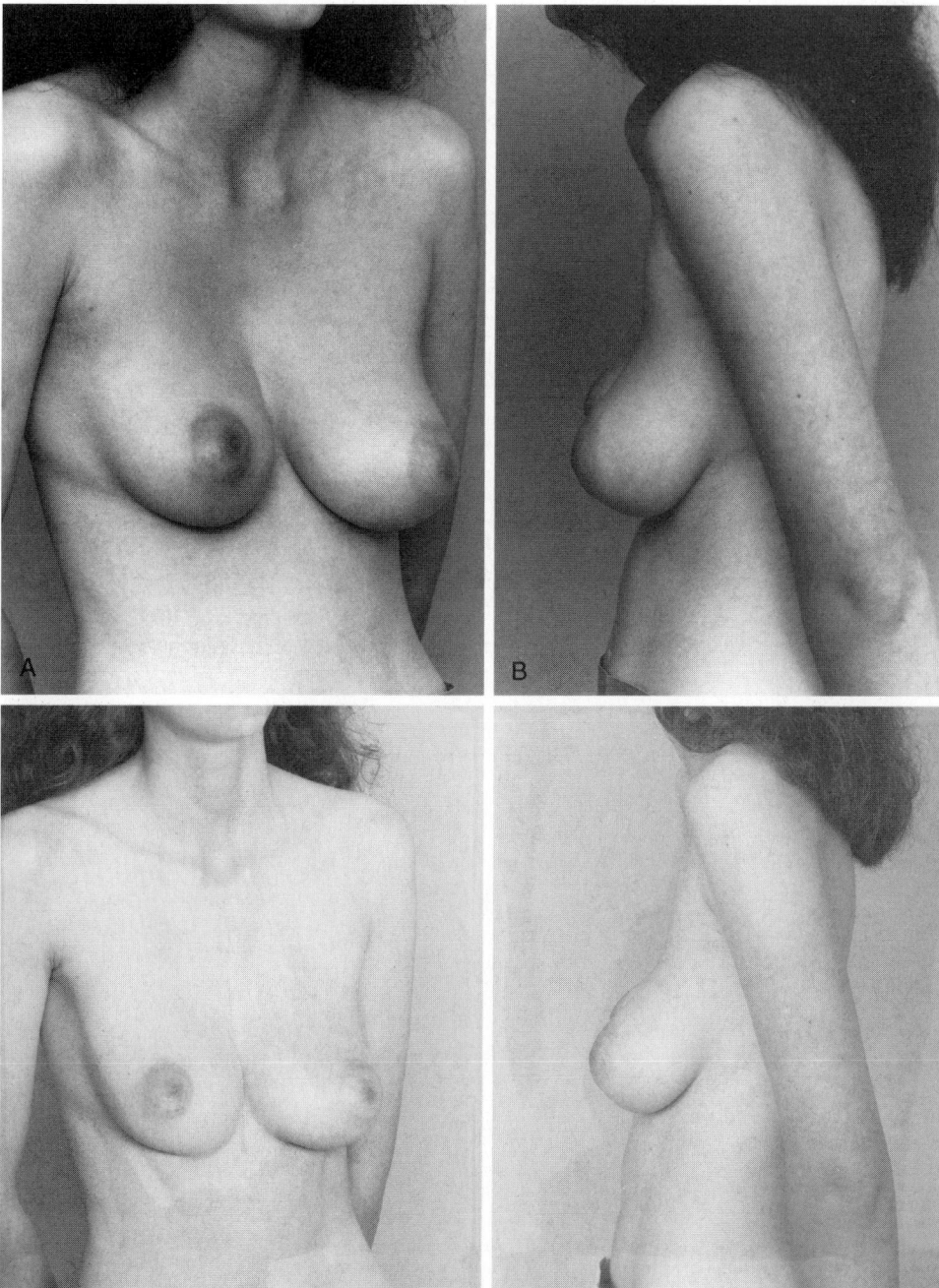

Figure 51–96. Pectus excavatum in a young adult female. *A* and *B*, Preoperative appearance. Note the characteristic central depressed sternum, rounded sloped shoulders, dorsal kyphosis, and protuberant abdomen. This patient also has an associated rotational deformity of the sternum with an asymmetric anterior chest wall. *C* and *D*, Postoperative appearance. Note the excellent cosmetic result with correction of the sternal depression and rotational deformity as well as associated improvement in posture.

sive deformity[27] usually presenting at birth or early in life[7, 20, 27] but can become manifest or exaggerated during growth surges.[27] Pectus excavatum runs the gamut from a mild and scarcely noticeable deformity to those that are severe and symptomatic. In the most severe cases, posterior concavity of the sternum leads to a decreased anteroposterior diameter of the chest, loss of retrosternal space with displacement of the heart to the left, and reduction in volume of the left pleural space (see Fig. 51–3). Severe defects often have additional rotation or torsion of the sternum, most commonly to the right side.[11, 20, 24, 27] Pectus excavatum is more common in males than in females, with a male-to-female ratio of approximately 2:1 to 3:1. It is most commonly sporadic, although familial occurrence has been reported.[7, 9, 20, 31] Although this deformity can be associated with congenital heart disease,

Marfan's syndrome, and other skeletal defects, it most commonly is an isolated finding.

Clinical Manifestations

The classic physical features were well described by Ravitch[29] and include the characteristic central depressed sternum, rounded sloped shoulders, dorsal kyphosis, protuberant abdomen, and paradoxic sternal retraction on inspiration (see Fig. 51–96). Patients most often present because of the cosmetic defect but are frequently found to have other symptoms (Table 51–35). Although a mild defect may have few manifestations and minimal symptoms, symptoms are not always related to the degree of the sternal deformity.[1] Older patients frequently note that they do not have the same

TABLE 51–35. Symptoms in Patients with Pectus Excavatum

Symptom	Percentage of Patients
Decreased exercise tolerance	51
Fatigability	43
Dyspnea on exertion	32
Upper respiratory tract infections	26
Lower respiratory tract infections	17
Asthma	7
Sternal pain	16
Palpitations	13

From Peterson, R. J., Young, W. G., Jr., and Godwin, J. D., et al.: Noninvasive assessment of exercise cardiac function before and after pectus excavatum repair. J. Thorac. Cardiovasc. Surg., *90*:251, 1985.

respiratory reserve or exercise tolerance as their peers when they are engaged in strenuous physical activities. After surgical correction, patients frequently note an improvement in respiratory reserve, although preoperatively they may not have been aware of exercise limitations.

The diagnosis of pectus excavatum is made by examination of the chest wall and identification of the posterior displacement of the sternum. Physical examination should also be directed toward the identification of possible associated anomalies. The deformity can clearly be seen on chest roentgenograms (Fig. 51–97), and radiologic severity can be determined by computed tomography (Fig. 51–98).

The most common reason for a patient with pectus excavatum to present to a physician is the significant cosmetic deformity.[27] Fonkalsrud found that 64% of patients in his study complained of an unattractive physical appearance,[7] whereas 50% of patients in Morshuis and associates' review paid conscious attention to the defect and took measures to hide it. Twenty-five percent of the patients believed that it altered their self-image.[20] Even when no other impairment or abnormality can be identified, the emotional and psychological component can be significant and is an indication for operation. These patients may also have subtle and not so subtle exercise intolerance that routinely improves postoperatively. In addition to the cosmetic and psychological factors, other significant findings include impaired cardiopulmonary function and associated skeletal defects such as scoliosis.

Heart murmurs are present in approximately one third of patients.[7] Systolic murmurs are most frequent and are probably caused by sternal compression on the pulmonary outflow tract. Congenital cardiac anomalies have been reported in 4%

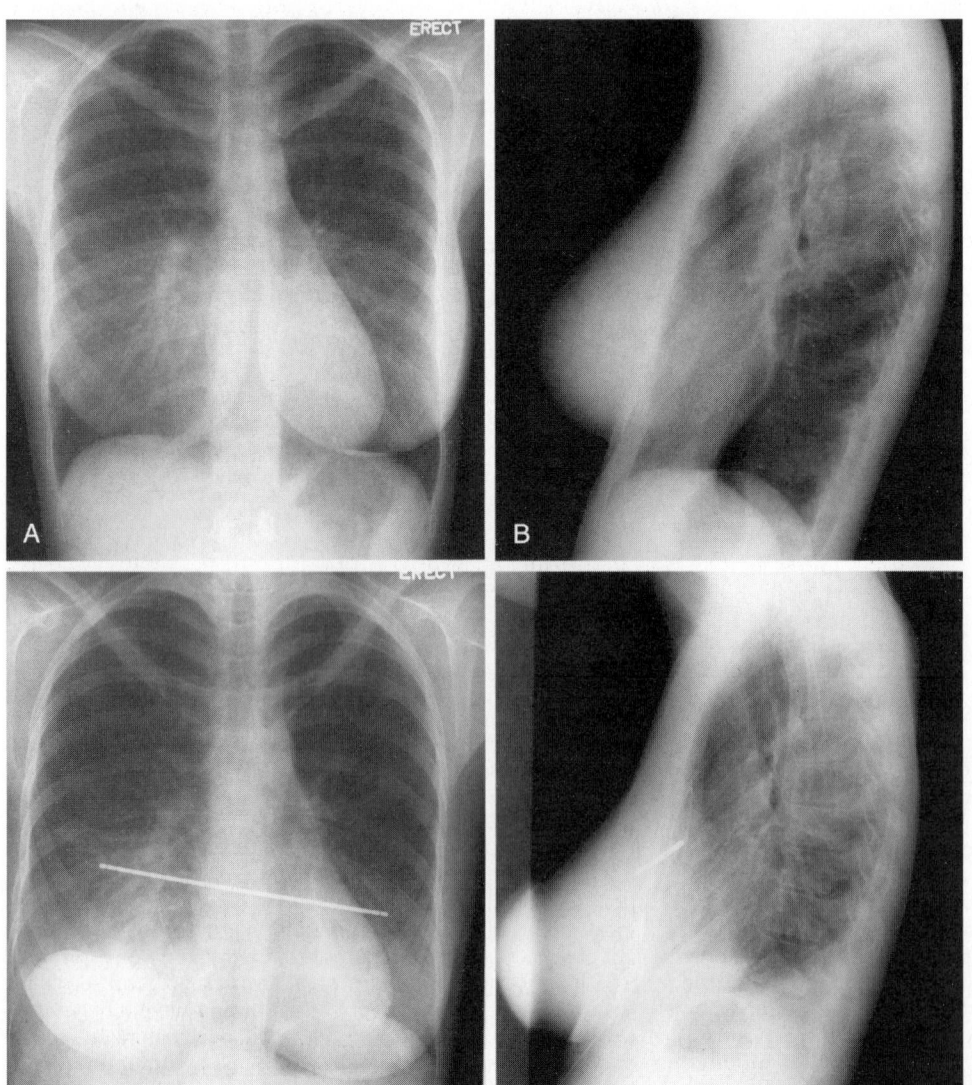

Figure 51–97. *A* and *B*, Preoperative posteroanterior and lateral radiographs of the patient in Figure 51–96. Note the significant posterior displacement of the sternum with subsequent decrease in anteroposterior diameter of the chest, displacement of the heart toward the left, and straightening of the heart border with the right heart border partially obscured by the sternum. *C* and *D*, Postoperative films of the same patient. Note the placement of a Steinmann pin to support the sternum and substernal drain to decrease seroma formation.

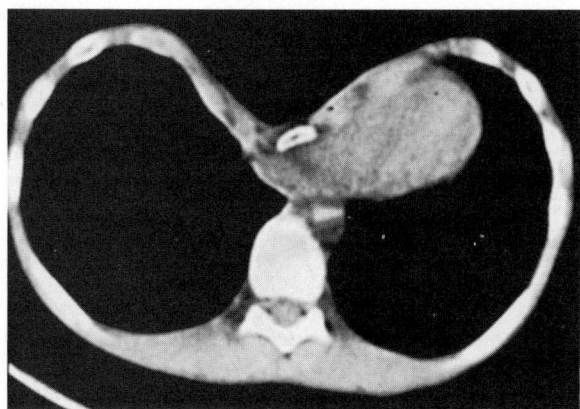

Figure 51–98. CT scan in a patient with pectus excavatum demonstrating the severe sternal depression with compression of the heart.

of patients,[7] whereas mitral valve prolapse has been found in 8%.[36]

The majority of patients with pectus excavatum report marked subjective improvement in exercise tolerance after repair. In addition, there are several studies that report objective evidence of cardiopulmonary dysfunction preoperatively and its subsequent improvement postoperatively. In a classic report in the 1950s, Ravitch[30] reported on patients with heart failure secondary to a pectus deformity. He provided early evidence of the effects of pectus excavatum on cardiac function in a patient with pectus excavatum and cardiac failure who preoperatively had elevated right-sided heart pressures and a cardiac output of one half of predicted normal. After surgical repair, the cardiac index doubled and cardiac failure resolved. Angiographic evidence of right ventricular compression was demonstrated by Howard[13] in 1959; the sternum was seen to be deeply indenting the wall of the right ventricle, and a right ventricular filling defect due to left ventricular compression was noted. This compression resolved postoperatively, and there was a marked symptomatic improvement in exercise tolerance.

Although some studies have failed to reveal hemodynamic changes in patients with pectus excavatum, this may be related to hemodynamic measurements being acquired while the patients were in the supine position. When patients with pectus deformities were studied while they were in the upright position, physical working capacity was significantly lower than when they were in the supine position.[3] In this same study, patients who were subjected to exercise in the sitting position had a higher pulse rate during exercise at the same workload than when they were in the supine position. Oxygen uptake at rest is higher than predicted in patients with pectus excavatum and is even higher when sitting, while mixed venous oxygen saturation at rest or exercise was lower in the sitting position. Although these patients have a normal stroke volume at rest and exercise in the supine position, there is less of an increase in stroke volume with exercise in the sitting position when compared with normal controls. These changes while in the upright position are thought to be due to impairment in ventricular filling secondary to compression and displacement of the heart by the sternum.

These changes were confirmed in Gattiker's study,[8] which revealed a slight decrease in cardiac index, heart rate, and mixed venous oxygen saturation in patients in the sitting position when compared with normals. Stroke volume during exercise and physical working capacity were reduced in the sitting position in those patients with pectus excavatum. Gattiker postulated that because of the altered position of the

heart behind the posteriorly displaced sternum, the right atrial capacity was reduced and complete and rapid filling of the right ventricle during exercise in the sitting position was not possible; however, in the supine position, the heart shifts away from the sternal depression and is no longer compressed. Stroke volume is then increased and is comparable to that of normal persons.

In a small study in older patients with pectus excavatum, Beiser and colleagues[2] found normal hemodynamic parameters at rest and exercise in the supine position, but cardiac output response to intense exercise in the upright position was below normal or at the lower end of normal. The pectus excavatum deformity impaired the cardiac output response in the upright position owing to a subnormal increase in stroke volume. Hemodynamic improvement occurred in patients after surgical correction of the deformity, with a significant enhancement of cardiac output during intense upright exercise postoperatively. Interestingly, there was no significant change in the supine hemodynamics postoperatively. All patients had significant subjective improvement in exercise tolerance after surgical correction of the pectus deformity.

Peterson and colleagues at Duke University examined non-invasive exercise cardiac function in 34 patients before and after surgical correction of pectus excavatum using radionuclide angiography.[22] Eight-five percent of patients in this study were symptomatic, with dyspnea on exertion being the most common complaint (54% of patients). As with other studies, the severity of the deformity did not correlate with symptoms. Postoperatively, all patients noted symptomatic improvement in their symptoms during a regulated exercise protocol. On physical examination postoperatively, four of five patients had resolution of their systolic murmur. By radionuclide imaging there were no changes in left ventricular ejection fraction, but left ventricular end-diastolic volume index consistently increased after pectus repair. Whereas rest and exercise right ventricular ejection fraction decreased after repair, right ventricular end-diastolic volume increased. This increase in end-diastolic volume suggests that sternal compression on the left and right ventricle is relieved postoperatively.

Pulmonary complaints are also common in patients with pectus deformities. In a recent review, 90% of patients younger than 6 years old who presented for surgical correction had functional pulmonary symptoms, including dyspnea or pulmonary infections.[24] In Fonkalsrud and colleagues' review,[7] over half of the patients reported mild to moderate exercise limitation and inability to keep up with peers in strenuous physical activity. In addition, recurrent pulmonary infections occurred in one third of patients, and asthmatic symptoms in 7%. Numerous studies have demonstrated restrictive alterations in chest wall mechanics and abnormalities in pulmonary function tests in patients with pectus excavatum including decreased vital capacity,[2, 4, 16, 18, 19, 44] decreased total lung capacity,[4, 18, 19, 44] decreased maximal ventilatory volume,[4, 18, 42] and decreased maximal breathing capacity.[2]

Improvement in pulmonary function postoperatively has been less clearly documented. In fact, several studies have documented worsening of the forced expiratory volume in 1 second,[6, 18, 19, 44] vital capacity,[6, 18, 19, 44] and total lung capacity[18, 19, 44] postoperatively, suggesting further chest wall restriction after correction of the deformity. However, Cahill and colleagues from the University of Washington,[4] in a prospective study of preoperative versus postoperative cardiorespiratory function, were able to show a significant improvement in maximal ventilatory volume, total progressive exercise time, and maximal oxygen consumption postoperatively. Most importantly, after surgical correction there was a consistent increase in maximal exercise capacity at every level of workload and a lower heart rate at every workload. Furthermore, in a Mayo Clinic study,[44] the exercise duration and percentage of predicted work performed increased significantly after operation. Despite the potential for an increase in chest wall restriction postoperatively, there appears to be a functional and subjective improvement in exercise tolerance, dyspnea, and respiratory tract infections. As Morshuis and coworkers[18] point out, factors other than changes in lung volumes may be responsible for the subjective physical improvement after surgery in most patients. Because of the satisfactory long-term results, surgical correction is justified in patients with pectus excavatum.

Also of interest is the association of scoliosis in patients with chest wall defects. After the age of 12, asymmetric deformities increase in number and are associated with scoliosis.[40] In patients with pectus deformities, this *thoracogenic scoliosis* is present in 15% to 30% of cases[7, 15, 20, 41] and appears to be due to the progressive asymmetric forces of the chest wall on the developing spine.[41] Most of these spinal deformities are single thoracic spinal curves between the fourth and ninth thoracic vertebrae. Furthermore, 18% of patients with pectus excavatum and 14% of patients with pectus carinatum with scoliosis will require intervention for their scoliosis.[41] Therefore, it is important to screen patients with chest wall deformities for the presence of scoliosis. Because these appear to be progressive changes with time, early operative intervention may prevent the development of scoliosis in these patients.

Indications for and Timing of Surgical Correction

Pectus excavatum itself has not been shown to be a contributing cause of death in those patients with the deformity,[1, 14] and therefore the long-term survival of these patients is not necessarily improved with surgical correction. However, because of the significant cosmetic and psychological improvement, subjective increase in exercise tolerance, documented changes in the cardiac and respiratory status, and prevention of the development of scoliosis after surgical intervention in these patients, surgical correction should be considered for all patients with a moderate to severe deformity. Because there may be spontaneous improvement in the pectus deformity in up to 40% of patients presenting in infancy,[14] these patients should be observed through infancy and early childhood; spontaneous improvement becomes much less frequent after 3 years of age and usually there is no improvement after 6 years of age.[14] Furthermore, long-term results are best in those patients operated on before age 6.[14] Therefore, the optimal age for repair appears to be in early childhood (age 3 to 5 years). Successful repair with good results can also be obtained in the older patient, and adolescents and young adults who present with the deformity should likewise be considered for repair.

In addition to the history and physical examination, preoperative evaluation should include a posteroanterior and lateral chest roentgenogram. Some authors have also advocated limited computed tomography of the chest; if the ratio of the transverse to the narrowest anteroposterior diameter is greater than 3.5, moderate to severe disease is present and the patient should undergo surgical therapy.[11] Preoperative pulmonary function tests should be obtained in symptomatic patients and pulmonary status optimized before operation. Prophylactic antibiotics are administered in the perioperative period.

Operative Technique

In 1949, Ravitch published a description of the operative technique used to repair pectus excavatum in eight children.[29]

The fundamentals of his repair included exposure of the sternum and costal cartilages, resection of all involved costal cartilages, correction of the posterior displacement of the sternum, and fixation of the sternum. Current surgical repairs are, for the most part, modifications of the original Ravitch procedure, avoiding the division of the intercostal bundles while using various maneuvers to support the repositioned sternum.

A midline or transverse inframammary incision is used for exposure. The pectoral muscle is elevated using needle-point electrocautery for hemostasis, and the costal cartilages are exposed. The perichondrium is elevated to expose the deformed cartilages, and a complete subperichondrial resection of all deformed cartilages is performed. The rectus attachments to the xiphoid and lower sternum are divided and the xiphoid is excised. Blunt dissection is used to free the substernal tissues and the pleura from the sternum, with care being taken to avoid entry into either pleural space. A transverse sternal osteotomy is performed, the posterior cortex of the sternum is fractured, and the sternum is mobilized anteriorly and fixed in place with nonabsorbable suture in a slightly overcorrected position. In older patients, internal fixation (Steinmann pin) should be used to support the sternum in the corrected position and is removed under local anesthesia in 3 to 6 months. The pectoral and rectus muscles are closed over the sternum and the skin edges are reapproximated. The technique of the repair is shown in Figure 51–99. Attention must also be directed at the rotational deformities of the sternum as well. Correction with partial osteotomies[26] or oblique wedge osteotomies[5] can be used to derotate the sternum. The use of a closed suction substernal drain will significantly reduce the incidence of seroma and fluid collections.[11]

An alternative technique for the repair of pectus excavatum is the sternal turnover technique (Fig. 51–100), as popularized by Wada in Japan.[40] The sternum and involved costal cartilages are removed *en bloc* with the intercostal muscles. This free graft is then turned over and sutured in place. If the internal mammary arteries are freed and preserved, this procedure provides excellent results with minimal morbidity and mortality.[39]

The use of silicone implants to correct the cosmetic aspects of the defect has been suggested[38]; however, this does not prevent the progression of the deformity nor the development of scoliosis. In addition, this approach may not be appropriate for use in children because of subsequent growth changes and may not be appropriate in general because of the concerns over the local effects and potential immunologic complications of silicone implants. Bracing of the sternum has been proposed as an effective nonoperative approach to the management of pectus excavatum.[10] Although short-term results are good, long-term follow-up is not yet available.

Postoperative Course

Operative mortality is rare (0%–0.5%),[7, 9, 11, 14, 20] and overall morbidity is quite low (5% to 6%).[11] Subcutaneous or substernal seromas and fluid collections occur in about 6% of patients,[7, 9] pneumothorax in 1% to 5%,[7, 9] wound infection in 1% to 2%,[9, 20] and pneumonitis in 4%.[7] The need for blood transfusion is uncommon. Pulmonary toilet needs to be encouraged postoperatively because of the common finding of atelectasis. Patients can often be admitted on the day of surgery, and the average hospital stay is usually 3 to 5 days.[7, 9, 11]

Postoperative cosmetic results are excellent or good in over 90% of patients.[9, 11, 20, 24] More than 90% of patients report a decrease in respiratory tract infections and 98% report improvement in exercise tolerance.[7] Recurrence of the defor-

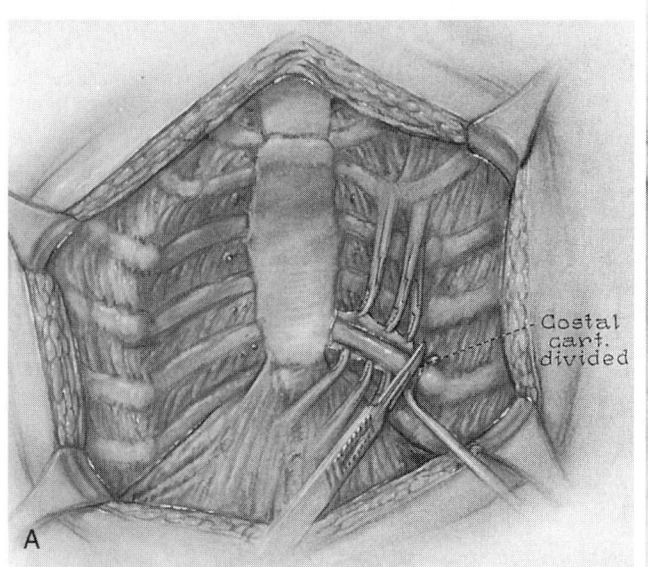

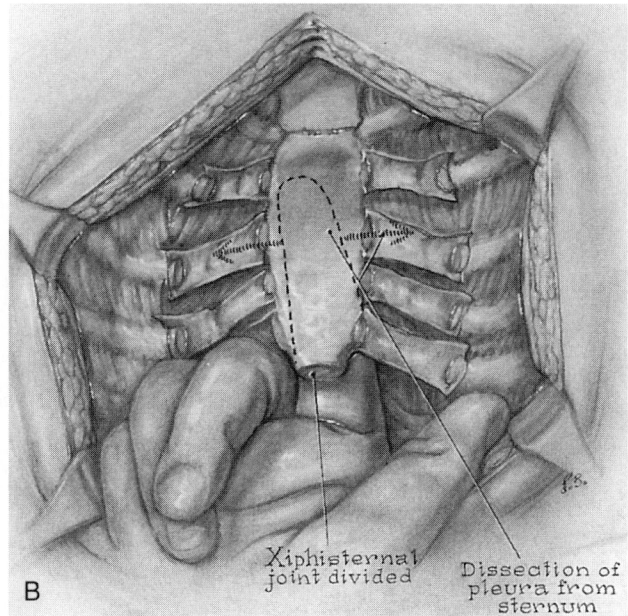

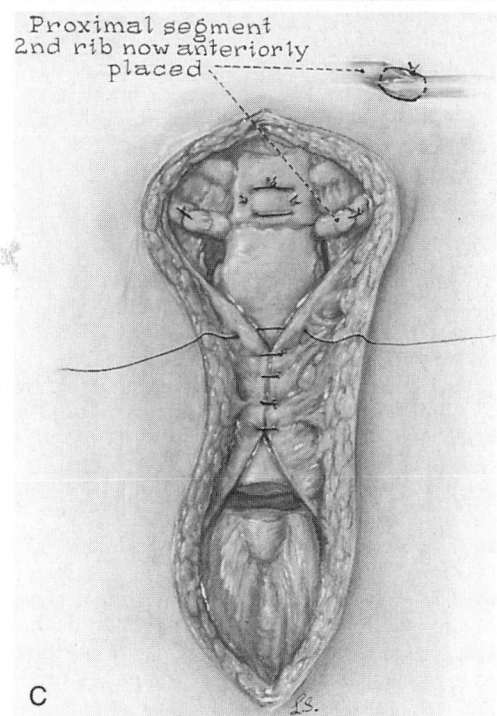

Figure 51–99. Repair of pectus excavatum (see text). *A,* After exposure of the sternum, subperichondrial resection of all affected costal cartilages is performed. *B,* The xiphoid is excised, the sternum is freed from the substernal tissue and pleura using blunt dissection, a wedge osteotomy is created, and the sternum is displaced anteriorly. *C,* After placement of a substernal drain (not shown), the pectoral muscles are closed in the midline and the subcutaneous tissue and skin are closed in layers. (From Ravitch, M. M., and Steichen, F. M.: Correction of pectus excavatum. *In* Atlas of General Thoracic Surgery. Philadelphia, W. B. Saunders, 1988.)

mity occurs less than 10% of the time and is related to the age at the time of repair. Late results are best in those patients who are younger than 6 years old at the time of operation.[14] Patients rarely require reoperation because of recurrence.[7, 24] Patients may return to physical activity within several weeks but should avoid direct trauma or contact sports for several months. Because of the excellent cosmetic results, psychologic and physiologic improvement, extremely low complication rate, and low likelihood of recurrence after the surgical procedure, all patients with significant pectus excavatum deformities should be considered for repair.

PECTUS CARINATUM

As opposed to pectus excavatum, pectus carinatum is a protrusion deformity of the breast. It represents a spectrum

of deformities and is less common than pectus excavatum.[27, 35] The deformity is due to an overgrowth of the costal cartilages, which forces the sternum anteriorly.[27] It usually manifests in mid childhood[27] and is a progressive deformity that worsens during the growth spurt of adolescence. Males are more commonly affected than females in a ratio of approximately 4:1.[35] It can be found as an isolated anomaly or associated with congenital heart disease or other skeletal anomalies. Scoliosis is present in approximately 20% of patients.[35, 41] A family history of chest wall deformities is present in one fourth of patients.[43]

Pectus carinatum represents a spectrum of deformities involving protrusion of the manubrium and body of the sternum. The anterior protrusion usually involves the lower portion of the sternum, and a lateral depression of costal cartilages accentuates the sternal prominence. This lateral

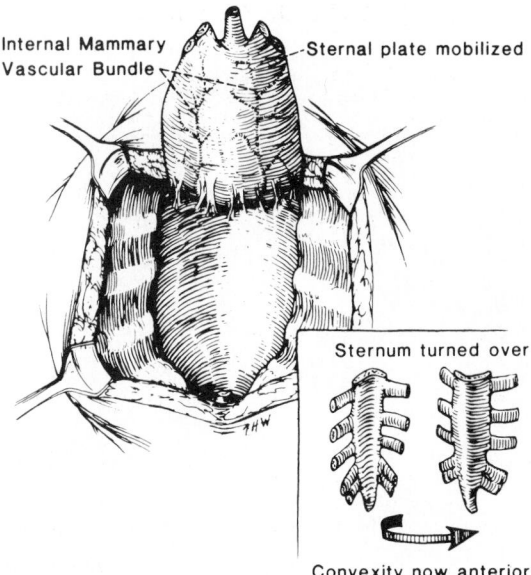

Figure 51–100. Sternal turnover technique for repair of pectus excavatum. After exposure of the sternum and subperichondrial resection of all affected costal cartilages, the sternum is divided and freed while preserving the internal mammary artery. The sternum is rotated 180 degrees, and this pedicle graft is then fixed in place. (From Hawkins, J. A., Ehrenhaft, J. L., and Doty, D. B.: Repair of pectus excavatum by sternal eversion. Reprinted with permission from The Society of Thoracic Surgeons [The Annals of Thoracic Surgery, 1984, Vol. 38, p. 368].)

depression can cause compression of the heart and reduce thoracic volume. Essentially two main types of deformity are described by Ravitch.[27] The first, *pouter pigeon breast,* or chondromanubrial prominence, is characterized by prominence of the manubrium and superior portion of the body of the sternum and a sharp depression of the body of the sternum with an upward deflection of the distal sternum. This form is less common than the typical pectus carinatum deformity, *chicken breast,* or chondrogladiolar prominence, in which the sternum is abnormally prominent especially in its mid or lower portion and is arched forward (Fig. 51–101). The manubrium in this deformity is not particularly prominent. The characteristic lateral depression of the costal cartilages to either side of the sternum accentuates the sternal prominence.[28] Asymmetry of the lesion is common, occurring in up to 35% of patients.[35] As with pectus excavatum, there is a significant psychological component to the deformity.[43]

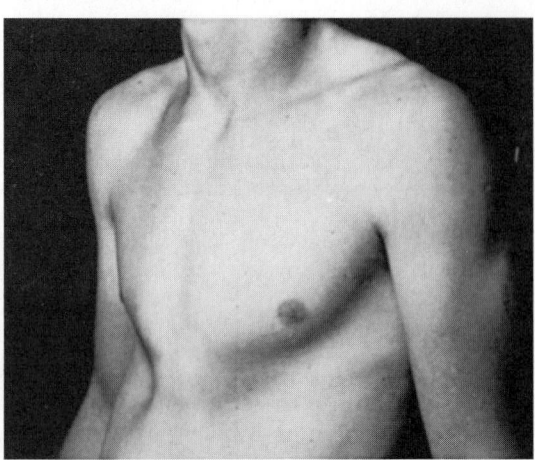

Figure 51–101. Pectus carinatum.

Characteristically, there is poor chest expansion with inspiration and although cardiorespiratory symptoms are not common early, they may manifest late owing to the rigid chest wall.

Because of the cosmetic appearance and psychological implications, surgical correction should be considered for all but the minimal deformities. Surgical repair is performed when the patient presents with the deformity[35] preferably before adolescence. The operative technique is similar to that of pectus excavatum, with exposure and subperichondrial resection of all involved costal cartilages. Reefing sutures are placed in the perichondrium to move the sternum posteriorly. Sternal osteotomies are not routinely performed in patients with carinatum deformities,[27] although transverse osteotomies may be needed to correct angulation deformities if they are present. A substernal drain is placed to prevent seroma formation.[35]

Excellent cosmetic results are obtained with essentially no mortality[43] and low morbidity. A complication rate of 3.9% was found in Shamberger's series[35] that included pneumothorax (2.6%), wound infection (0.7%), atelectasis (0.7%), and local tissue necrosis (0.7%). Recurrence of the defect, which requires operative revision, occurs in less than 2% of the cases.[35] Mean postoperative stay is approximately 6 days.[35] A recent series[10] of nonoperative management using an orthotic device noted improvement in the defect while avoiding disruption of the growth plates and subsequent interference in normal chest wall development. This form of treatment should be initiated early in life when the chest wall is still compliant and can be molded. The long-term success of this therapy is as yet unknown.

STERNAL CLEFTS

Sternal clefts are an uncommon but fascinating spectrum of defects of the sternum resulting from failure of midline fusion of the two sternal bands during embryologic development.[32] This failure of fusion can lead to defects ranging from simple sternal clefts to complete defects of the sternum and pericardium with herniation of the heart through the defect. This severe form of the defect, thoracic ectopia cordis, is believed to be the result of disruption of the amnion, chorion, or yolk sac during embryologic development.[17]

The spectrum of deformities has been classified by the group from Boston Children's Hospital.[34] Thoracic ectopia cordis, or so-called naked heart, involves a sternal cleft in which there are no overlying somatic structures and the heart is exposed. The apex of heart is characteristically positioned anteriorly and cephalad. Intrinsic cardiac anomalies are frequent, and this deformity is frequently fatal. Surgical management is aimed at construction of an anterior chest cavity with tissue coverage of the heart while avoiding posterior displacement of the heart back into the limited thoracic cavity and subsequent hemodynamic compromise.

Cervical ectopia cordis is a more severe form of this defect involving a more superior displacement of the apex of the heart, often with fusion of the apex of the heart to the mouth. The prognosis in these patients is dismal, but fortunately this defect is extremely rare. Thoracoabdominal ectopia cordis involves an inferiorly cleft sternum, in which the heart is covered by a thin layer of skin. The heart lacks the severe anterior and superior rotation of thoracic and cervical ectopia cordis, and successful surgical repair and long-term survival are possible. Associated abdominal wall defects, diaphragmatic defects, pericardial defects, and intrinsic congenital cardiac lesions are common (particularly tetralogy of Fallot, left ventricular diverticulum, and ventricular septal defect). Initial repair addresses the repair of the intracardiac defect as well as the skin defects overlying the heart and abdominal

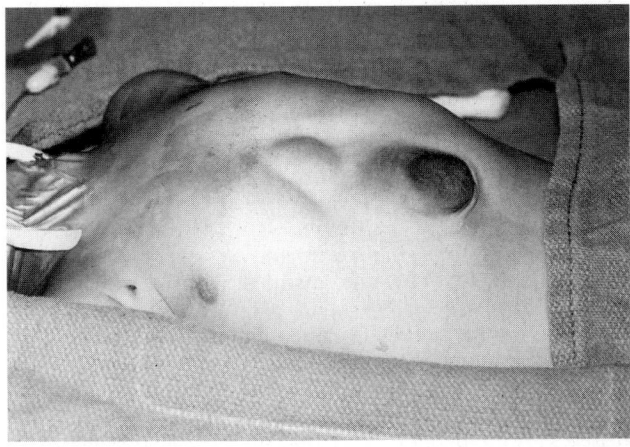

Figure 51–102. Cantrell's pentalogy with the characteristic lower sternal defect, abdominal wall defect, diaphragmatic defect, pericardial defect, and intracardiac defect (in this case, a ventricular septal defect). Note that only a thin layer of skin covers the heart.

cavity. In 1958, James Cantrell at the Johns Hopkins Hospital described five cases found to have the following common characteristics: (1) a lower sternal defect; (2) a midline, supraumbilical abdominal wall defect (omphalocele); (3) a diaphragmatic defect (hernia); (4) a pericardial defect; and (5) a congenital intracardiac defect. This association of defects has come to be known as Cantrell's pentalogy (Fig. 51–102). Finally, the simplest and least severe of these defects is the cleft sternum, which involves primarily the upper sternum and manubrium. Only the sternum is involved in this variant; there is an intact pericardium and normal skin coverage over the defect. Abdominal wall defects are not present, nor are intracardiac defects. This lesion is usually asymptomatic and uniformly correctable. Repair is performed to cover and protect the heart by separating the sternal bands from the posterior pleural attachments and reapproximating the sternal edges.[32]

POLAND'S SYNDROME

In 1841, Poland, a medical student at Guy's Hospital in London, published the first description in the English literature[23] of a cadaver with a peculiar spectrum of deformities, including unilateral hypoplasia of the thorax and upper extremity with absence of the ipsilateral pectoralis major muscle. This defect is an association of ipsilateral thoracic and hand anomalies and in its full expression Poland's syndrome includes (1) hypoplasia of the skin and subcutaneous tissue of the anterior chest; (2) absence or hypoplasia and upward displacement of the nipple and breast; (3) pectoral and axillary hypotrichosis; (4) absence of the sternocostal portion of the pectoralis major muscle; (5) absence of the pectoralis minor muscle; (6) absence of portions of costal cartilages two to four or three to five; (7) ipsilateral hand anomalies (*mitten hand*, or brachysyndactyly); (8) absence of latissimus dorsi and serratus anterior muscles; and (9) scoliosis.[25] It appears to occur more frequently on the right side of the body.[33, 37] These patients usually have little functional disability[33] but present because of the cosmetic deformity. The goal of reconstruction is to restore the natural contour of the chest wall while stabilizing the chest wall deficiency. This often involves rib transposition or grafting, mesh reconstruction, latissimus dorsi transposition, and breast reconstruction. This reconstruction can be performed with excellent cosmetic results and little or no morbidity or mortality.

SELECTED REFERENCES

Ravitch, M. M.: Congenital Deformities of the Chest Wall and Their Operative Correction. Philadelphia, W. B. Saunders, 1977.
This textbook reviews the embryology, symptoms, physical findings, physiologic implications, associated anomalies, and surgical correction of chest wall deformities. It is an excellent review based primarily on Ravitch's personal series and that of the Johns Hopkins Hospital. Although published in 1977, it remains one of the most definitive works in this area.

Ravitch, M. M., and Steichen, F. M.: Atlas of General Thoracic Surgery. Philadelphia, W. B. Saunders, 1988.
This excellent general thoracic surgical atlas devotes a large section to the correction of congenital deformities of the chest wall.

REFERENCES

1. Bay, V., Farthmann, E., and Naegele, U.: Unoperated funnel chest in middle and advanced age: Evaluation of indications for operation. J. Pediatr. Surg., 5:606, 1970.
2. Beiser, G. C., Epstein, S. E., Stampfer, M. D., et al.: Impairment of cardiac function with pectus excavatum with improvement after operative correction. N. Engl. J. Med., 287:267, 1972.
3. Bevegard, S.: Postural circulatory changes at rest and during exercise in patients with funnel chest, with special reference to factors affecting stroke volume. Acta. Med. Scand., 171:695, 1962.
4. Cahill, J. L., Lees, G. M., and Robertson, H. T.: A summary of preoperative and postoperative cardiorespiratory performance in patients undergoing pectus excavatum and carinatum repair. J. Pediatr. Surg., 19:430, 1984.
5. Choi, J. B., and Rim, T. G.: Oblique wedge osteotomy for correction of asymmetric pectus excavatum in young children. Ann. Thorac. Surg., 57:235, 1994.
6. Derveaux, L., Ivanoff, I., Rochette, F., and Demedts, M.: Mechanism of pulmonary function changes after surgical correction for funnel chest. Eur. Respir. J., 1:823, 1988.
7. Fonkalsrud, E. W., Salman, T., Guo, W., and Gregg, J. P.: Repair of pectus deformities with sternal support. J. Thorac. Cardiovasc. Surg., 107:37, 1994.
8. Gattiker, H., and Buehlmann, A.: Cardiopulmonary function and exercise tolerance in supine and sitting position in patients with pectus excavatum. Helv. Med. Acta., 33:122, 1966.
9. Golladay, E. S., and Wagner, C. W.: Pectus excavatum: A 15-year perspective. South. Med. J., 84:1099, 1991.
10. Haje, S. A., and Bowen, J. R.: Preliminary results of orthotic treatment of pectus deformities in children and adolescents. J. Pediatr. Orthop., 12:795, 1992.
11. Haller, J. A., Jr., Scherer, L. R., and Turner, C. S.: Evolving management of pectus excavatum based on a single institutional experience of 664 patients. Ann. Surg., 209:578, 1989.
12. Hanson, F. B.: The ontogeny and phylogeny of the sternum. Am. J. Anat., 26:41, 1919.
13. Howard, R.: Funnel chest: Its effect on cardiac function. Arch. Dis. Child., 32:5, 1959.
14. Humphreys, G. H., II, and Jaretzki, A., III: Pectus excavatum: Late results with and without operation. J. Thorac. Cardiovasc. Surg., 80:686, 1980.
15. Iseman, M. D., Buschman, D. L., and Ackerson, L. M.: Pectus excavatum and scoliosis: Thoracic anomalies associated with pulmonary disease caused by *Mycobacterium-avium* complex. Am. Rev. Respir. Dis., 144:914, 1991.
16. Kaguraoka, H., Ohnuki, T., Itaoka, T., et al.: Degree of severity of pectus excavatum and pulmonary function in preoperative and postoperative periods. J. Thorac. Cardiovasc. Surg., 104:1483, 1992.
17. Kaplan, L. C., Matsuoka, R., Gilbert, E. F., et al.: Ectopia cordis and cleft sternum: Evidence for mechanical teratogenesis following rupture of the chorion or yolk sac. Am. J. Med. Genet., 21:187, 1985.
18. Morshuis, W., Folgering, H., Barentsz, J., et al.: Pulmonary function before surgery for pectus excavatum and at long-term follow-up. Chest, 105:1646, 1994.
19. Morshuis, W. J., Folgering, H. T., Barentsz, J. O., et al.: Exercise cardiorespiratory function before and one year after operation for pectus excavatum. J. Thorac. Cardiovasc. Surg., 107:1403, 1994.
20. Morshuis, W. J., Mulder, H., Wapperom, G., et al.: Pectus excavatum: A clinical study with long-term postoperative follow-up. Eur. J. Cardiothorac. Surg., 6:318, 1992.
21. O'Rahilly, R., and Mueller, F.: Human Embryology and Teratology. New York, John Wiley & Sons, 1992.
22. Peterson, R. J., Young, W. G., Jr., Godwin, J. D., et al.: Noninvasive assessment of exercise cardiac function before and after pectus excavatum repair. J. Thorac. Cardiovasc. Surg., 90:251, 1985.
23. Poland, A.: Deficiency of the pectoral muscles. Guys Hosp. Rep., 6:191, 1841.
24. Prevot, J.: Treatment of sternocostal wall malformations of the child: A series of 210 surgical corrections since 1975. Eur. J. Pediatr. Surg., 4:131, 1994.
25. Ravitch, M. M.: Associated anomalies in infants and children with congenital defects of the thoracic wall. In el Shafie, M., and Klippel, C. H., Jr. (Eds.): Associated Congenital Anomalies. Baltimore, Williams & Wilkins, 1981.

26. Ravitch, M. M., and Steichen, F. M.: Atlas of General Thoracic Surgery. Philadelphia, W. B. Saunders, 1988.
27. Ravitch, M. M.: Congenital Deformities of the Chest Wall and Their Operative Correction. Philadelphia, W. B. Saunders, 1977.
28. Ravitch, M. M.: The operative correction of pectus carinatum. Ann. Surg., 151:705, 1960.
29. Ravitch, M. M.: The operative treatment of pectus excavatum. Ann. Surg., 129:429, 1949.
30. Ravitch, M. M.: Pectus excavatum and heart failure. Surgery, 30:178, 1951.
31. Sabiston, D. C., Jr.: Disorders of the sternum and thoracic wall. In Sabiston, D. C., Jr., and Spencer, F. C. (Eds.): Surgery of the Chest. Philadelphia, W. B. Saunders, 1990.
32. Sabiston, D. C., Jr.: The surgical management of congenital bifid sternum with partial ectopia cordis. J. Thorac. Surg., 35:118, 1958.
33. Seyfer, A. E., Icochea, R., and Graeber, G. M.: Poland's anomaly: Natural history and long term results of chest wall reconstruction in 33 patients. Ann. Surg., 208:776, 1988.
34. Shamberger, R. C., and Welch, K. J.: Sternal defects. Pediatr. Surg. Int., 5:156, 1990.
35. Shamberger, R. C., and Welch, K. J.: Surgical correction of pectus carinatum. J. Pediatr. Surg., 22:48, 1987.
36. Shamberger, R. C., Welch, K. J., and Sanders, S. P.: Mitral valve prolapse associated with pectus excavatum. J. Pediatr., 111:404, 1987.
37. Shamberger, R. C., Welch, K. W., and Upton, J., III: Surgical treatment of thoracic deformity in Poland's syndrome. J. Pediatr. Surg., 24:760, 1989.
38. Sorensen, J. L.: Subcutaneous silicone implants in pectus excavatum. Scand. J. Plast. Reconstr. Surg., 22:173, 1987.
39. Taguchi, K., Mochizuki, T., Nakagaki, M., and Kato, K.: A new plastic operation for pectus excavatum: Sternal turnover surgical procedure with preserved internal mammary vessels. Chest, 67:606, 1975.
40. Wada, J., Ikeda, K., Ishida, T., and Hasegawa, T.: Results of 271 funnel chest operations. Ann. Thorac. Surg., 10:526, 1970.
41. Waters, P., Welch, K., Micheli, L. J., et al.: Scoliosis in children with pectus excavatum and pectus carinatum. J. Pediatr. Orthop., 9:551, 1989.
42. Weg, J. G., Krumholz, R. A., and Harkleroad, L. E.: Pulmonary dysfunction in pectus excavatum. Am. Rev. Respir. Dis., 96:936, 1967.
43. Welch, K. J., and Vos, A.: Surgical correction of pectus carinatum (pigeon breast). J. Pediatr. Surg., 8:659, 1973.
44. Wynn, S. R., Driscoll, D. J., Ostrom, N. K., et al.: Exercise cardiorespiratory function in adolescents with pectus excavatum: Observations before and after operation. J. Thorac. Cardiovasc. Surg., 99:41, 1990.

LESIONS OF THE CHEST WALL

Cemil M. Purut, M.D.

Chest wall tumors are neoplasms primarily of bone and soft tissue. Malignant lesions slightly outnumber those that are benign, and most are primary rather than metastatic. Complete surgical excision of the tumor is usually required to effect a cure. The prognosis after surgical therapy is generally good if the margins are free of tumor but poor if resection is incomplete.

INCIDENCE

Tumors of the chest wall comprise approximately 2% of all tumors of the body[14] and may be primary or metastatic and benign or malignant. Approximately 60% are primary at the time of resection,[10, 18, 15] which is in contrast to earlier data showing metastatic lesions to be more common.[13] Tumors of genitourinary, thyroid, colonic, or mesenchymal cell origin are most likely to cause single metastatic lesions of the thoracic wall.[21]

Approximately 60% of primary tumors are malignant, and most are of bony origin. In a review of 11 collected series of patients in the literature, chondrosarcomas were the most prevalent malignant lesion, followed by fibrosarcoma, multiple myeloma, Ewing's sarcoma, and osteosarcoma.[16] Malignant fibrous histiocytoma, synovial sarcoma, liposarcoma, rhabdomyosarcoma, undifferentiated sarcoma, and malignant hemangioendothelioma were less common. The most common benign lesions of the chest wall are fibrous dysplasia of bone (30%), followed by chondromas/osteochondromas (20%), whereas desmoid tumors, neurofibromas, and rhabdomyomas compose the remainder.

SIGNS AND SYMPTOMS

Symptoms are variable, and most are related to the enlarging chest mass. Most tumors grow slowly and are initially asymptomatic; 75% of patients present with an asymptomatic, palpable chest wall mass.[10] Pain is often late and is usually present only after a palpable mass is detected. Some lesions of the ribs, however, manifest pain early without a palpable mass, especially when a pathologic fracture is present. These tumors are readily apparent on chest radiography. Metastatic tumors tend to produce symptoms earlier than primary lesions, presumably because of their more rapid doubling time.[10] A history of chest wall trauma may be elicited in some patients but is usually unrelated to the diagnosis.

In examining the patient, the size and location of the mass should be noted, as well as its firmness and mobility. Primary and metastatic tumors of the ribs and cartilage are usually hard and fixed, whereas tumors of soft tissue origin may be less firm and more mobile. The location of the tumor may provide a clue to its origin. For example, chondrosarcomas frequently arise along the costochondral junction anteriorly.[11]

Finally, constitutional signs and symptoms suggesting malignancy should be sought, including loss of appetite, malaise, fever, and weight loss.

DIAGNOSIS

Radiographic Tests. Standard posteroanterior and lateral chest radiographs should be the initial radiographic studies in all patients presenting with either a palpable chest wall mass or chest wall discomfort. The films should be examined carefully for bony destruction of the ribs, as well as any evidence of primary parenchymal disease of the lungs. If present, pleural effusions should be aspirated percutaneously and the fluid sent for cytologic examination. Lesions originating from the ribs of the lateral chest wall may be visualized most effectively by radiographic techniques directed specifically toward these bony structures. Plain tomograms are unnecessary if computed tomography is available.

Computed tomography is quite useful in the evaluation of chest wall tumors. It is superior to other radiographic modalities in distinguishing solid from cystic masses as well as in assessing the invasive extent of a tumor.[5] Knowledge of the extent of tumor invasion is useful when planning surgical resection as well as designing masks for radiation therapy. Note should be made of muscular invasion to help determine the feasibility of reconstruction of the chest wall with myocutaneous flaps.

Angiography should be employed to selectively evaluate major vascular invasion. It is also helpful if there is some question as to the adequacy of the vascular supply of an intended myocutaneous flap. For extremely large tumors, angiography may be helpful in defining the tumor blood supply with the intention of early arterial ligation during tumor excision. For the usual, modestly sized tumor, however, angiography is unlikely to yield important information. Bone scans should be performed in all patients presenting with bony lesions. Occasionally, synchronous, asymptomatic lesions elsewhere in the body may be found.

Other Tests. Bronchoscopy has little role in the evaluation of chest wall tumors except in those patients with direct extension of a primary pulmonary lesion into the thoracic wall. The indication for bronchoscopy in this setting is the same as for primary carcinoma of the lung.

Pulmonary function testing should be performed in all

patients with suspicion of pulmonary dysfunction or when pulmonary resection may be necessary. In addition, testing should be performed in those patients in whom an extensive resection of the chest wall is contemplated, even in the absence of pulmonary resection, because major chest wall reconstruction may have a detrimental effect on pulmonary function.

Biopsy. The choice of biopsy technique—needle, incisional, or excisional—is based largely on the size of the tumor. Small tumors (less than 4 cm.) should undergo excisional biopsy with wide margins (2 to 4 cm.).[20] This procedure may be considered both diagnostic and therapeutic. Although there is little danger in first performing a core needle or incisional biopsy, little is to be gained by it.

Controversy exists as to the appropriate role of biopsy in the diagnostic evaluation of large chest wall tumors. Complete resection of these tumors may involve considerable morbidity and mortality, and extensive preoperative preparation may be required. It seems reasonable that such preparations should be made only after a firm diagnosis is obtained. Therefore, large tumors should undergo incisional biopsy using a surgical approach, which does not compromise chest wall reconstruction later. The specimen obtained should be nonnecrotic and sufficient to permit special stains and electron microscopy.[6] Frozen sections are not necessary unless the adequacy of the specimen is questioned. Hemostasis should be obtained carefully, because a large and expanding hematoma may spread tumor cells.

TREATMENT

Benign Tumors

Osteochondroma. Osteochondromas are the most common neoplasm of bone and arise from the metaphases of the rib. These tumors typically begin before puberty and continue to grow until bone maturation is reached. Only painful or disfiguring osteochondromas in childhood require resection, while those osteochondromas arising in adulthood should always be resected.

Chondroma. Chondromas are slowly growing tumors that typically occur at the costochondral junction. Tumors less than 4 cm. in diameter may be considered benign, although exclusion of malignancy may sometimes be difficult. Therefore, all chondrosarcomas should be resected with wide margins.[11]

Fibrous Dysplasia. Most cases of fibrous dysplasia present as a solitary, slowly growing, painless mass localized on the posterolateral aspect of a rib. The tumor begins in infancy or childhood but is usually not detected until young adulthood. Malignant degeneration is rare. Some surgeons consider this tumor as the most common benign lesion of the chest wall, comprising as many as 30% of benign tumors.[9] Many lesions appear to stop growing at puberty. Excisional therapy may be offered to patients whose lesions are disfiguring or painful.

Malignant Tumors

Chondrosarcoma. Chondrosarcomas are slow-growing, painful tumors that typically arise from the costochondral junction or sternum. Tumors arising from the posterior cartilaginous junction of the ribs are rare. Men in the third or fourth decade are the most common victims. Histologically, the tumor may be difficult to distinguish from benign chondromas. Grossly, these tumors are typically lobulated, growing either inward toward the lung or outward toward the skin. Mottled calcification may be apparent on the chest x-ray film. Wide excision with 4 to 5 cm. margins is curative in 97% of patients at 10 years.[7]

Ewing's Sarcoma. Ewing's sarcoma is a highly vascular tumor occurring primarily in young males. This tumor comprises 10% to 12% of bone tumors in children and adolescents. The male-to-female preponderance is 2:1, and the tumors tend to produce symptoms early, primarily pain and generalized malaise. Physical signs such as fever, leukocytosis, and an elevated sedimentation rate may be present. Pleural effusions are common. Radiographically, the tumor may have an onion skin appearance caused by elevation of the periosteum and multiple layers of new bone formation. Pathologic fractures are uncommon. Because of the associated fever and leukocytosis, distinguishing Ewing's sarcoma from osteomyelitis may sometimes be possible only by biopsy.

Ewing's sarcoma spreads early, primarily by the homogeneous route, although lymph node metastases can occur. Approximately 50% of patients have metastatic disease at the time of presentation. Although Ewing's sarcoma is very radiosensitive, excision and chemotherapy are integral in treatment. In one retrospective study, the 10-year survival was 30% with resection and 8% without surgery.[17]

Osteogenic Sarcoma. Osteogenic sarcoma affects primarily male children and young adults. Presentation is usually characterized by a rapidly enlarging, painful, firm mass attached to the underlying bone. The radiographic appearance is one of a *sunburst* appearance caused by periosteal elevation by the nonossified tumor. The lungs are the usual first site of metastasis. The tumor is responsive to both chemotherapy and radiation therapy. The most common chemotherapeutic agents used to treat this tumor are vincristine, doxorubicin, and high-dose methotrexate.[12] Surgical resection with wide margins is appropriate for local control of disease. Surgical therapy should be preceded by chemotherapy if metastatic disease is evident at presentation; otherwise, chemotherapy should follow surgical removal. Survival with combined therapy is 15% to 20%.

PRINCIPLES OF CHEST WALL RESECTION

The patient is positioned on the operative table in the manner that provides the most direct access to the operative site. The supine position usually facilitates sternal resection, while the decubitus position is best for lateral chest wall tumors. Double-lumen endotracheal intubation should be considered routine when a lateral tumor is to be excised.

The skin incision should be planned carefully to include the old biopsy scar yet allow primary closure. Skin that has been invaded by tumor must be resected with at least a 3-cm. margin; uninvolved skin should be dissected free to the limits of resection. The tumor capsule must not be violated. The muscle is divided 4 cm. from the edge of the tumor. The rib margins should be 6 cm., and adhesions to the lung should not be divided but remain attached as the underlying lung is divided. At least one grossly normal rib should be excised above and below the primary tumor. Primary lung cancers that have invaded the chest wall are managed somewhat differently, as pulmonary resection is usually performed before the chest wall resection. In all patients, the achievement of negative margins is of utmost importance and resection should not be ceased prematurely because of concerns over the subsequent difficulty of chest wall reconstruction.

PRINCIPLES OF CHEST WALL RECONSTRUCTION

Chest wall reconstruction is undertaken to prevent paradoxical movement of the chest and to protect underlying organs. Defects of 5 cm. or less, or of three or fewer ribs, do not usually require special reconstructive closure techniques.[14] Rib resections covered by the scapula likewise require no reconstruction.

Large bony defects of the chest wall may be repaired with either autologous tissue such as fascia lata or harvested rib or with synthetic material such as Marlex mesh, Prolene mesh, or Gore-Tex soft tissue patch. Prolene mesh is considered superior to Marlex because the former is rigid in both vertical and horizontal directions while the latter is rigid in only one direction. Gore-Tex is preferred by some surgeons because of its imperviousness to both gas and fluid *in vivo* and because of its lack of adhesion formation with the underlying lung. Hard sandwich techniques, using layered Marlex mesh and methyl methacrylate, are not often used and are considered by some to be unnecessary.[14]

Soft tissue defects are most effectively approached with myocutaneous pedicle flaps, and the choice of flap depends on the extent and location of the defect. A latissimus dorsi flap based on the thoracodorsal neurovascular bundle is appropriate for large defects of the lateral and anterolateral thorax.[4] Defects of the upper sternum or lower neck may be covered with a pectoralis major flap. The transverse rectus abdominis flap, originally described for breast reconstruction,[19] may be used in any anterior or axillary location. Other flaps may be based on the serratus anterior or external oblique muscles. Free flaps of tensor fascia lata with fascia and skin have also been used successfully.[3] The omentum may be mobilized to reach the thorax, but its role in the repair of soft tissue defects is limited because of its inability to provide chest wall stability and the need to perform subsequent skin grafting.

POSTOPERATIVE CARE

Postoperative morbidity and mortality after resection of small tumors not requiring chest wall reconstruction should be quite low (<2%).[8] Operations that include chest wall reconstruction can be expected to be associated with a mortality of 3.8% to 4.5%.[1]

Procedures that violate the pleura can be expected to offer the same complications as a typical pulmonary resection, including persistent air leak, pneumonia, empyema, atelectasis, prolonged ventilator dependence, and hemothorax. When prosthetic material is used, there exists the added risk of infection of the prosthesis. Although an attempt may be made to treat mesh infections with local wound care and systemic antibiotics, it is usually necessary to remove the foreign material to effect a cure.[2]

SELECTED REFERENCES

Anderson, B. O., and Burt, M. E.: Chest wall neoplasms and their management. Ann. Thorac. Surg. 58:1774, 1994.
This excellent, up-to-date, and comprehensive review of benign and malignant neoplasms and their management also includes the management of locally invasive breast cancer and lung cancer.

REFERENCES

1. Anderson, B. O., and Burt, M. E.: Chest wall neoplasms and their management. Ann. Thorac. Surg., 58:1774, 1994.
2. Arnold, P. G., and Pairolero, P. C.: Chest wall reconstruction: Experience with 100 consecutive patients. Ann. Surg., 199:725, 1984.
3. Boyd, A. D., Shaw, W. W., McCarthy, J. G., et al.: Immediate reconstruction of full thickness chest wall defects. Ann. Thorac. Surg., 32:337, 1981.
4. Campbell, D. A.: Reconstruction of the anterior thoracic wall. J. Thorac. Surg., 19:456, 1950.
5. Leitmar, B. J.: The use of computed tomography in evaluating chest wall pathology. J. Comput. Tomogr., 7:399, 1983.
6. Linnoila, R. I., Tsokos, M., Triche, T. J., et al.: Evidence for neural origin and periodic acid–Schiff-positive variants of the malignant small cell tumor of thoracopulmonary region. Lab. Invest., 48:514, 1983.
7. McAfee, M. K., et al.: Chondrosarcoma of the chest wall: Factors affecting survival. Ann. Thorac. Surg., 40:535, 1985.
8. McCaughan, B. S., Martini, N., Bains, M. S., and McCormack, P. M.: Chest wall invasion in carcinoma of the lung: Therapeutic and prognostic implications. J. Thorac. Cardiovasc. Surg., 89:836, 1985.
9. McCormack, P.: Chest wall tumors. *In* Baue, A. E. (Ed.): Glenn's Thoracic and Cardiovascular Surgery. Norwalk, Conn., Appleton and Lange, 1991.
10. McCormack, P., Bass, M., Beathe, E. J., et al.: New trends in skeletal reconstruction after resection of chest wall tumors. Ann. Thorac. Surg., 31:45, 1981.
11. Marcone, R., and Hevos, A.: Cartilaginous tumors of the ribs. Cancer, 27:794, 1971.
12. Marcone, R., and Rosen, G.: *En bloc* resections for osteogenic sarcoma. Cancer, 45:30, 1980.
13. Ochsner, A., Lucas, G. L., and McFarland, G. B.: Tumors of the thoracic skeleton. J. Thorac. Cardiovasc. Surg., 52:311, 1966.
14. Pairolero, P. C.: Chest wall tumors. *In* Shields, T. (Ed.): General Thoracic Surgery. Philadelphia, Lea & Febiger, 1989.
15. Pairolero, P. C., and Arnold, P. G.: Chest wall tumors. J. Thorac. Cardiovasc. Surg., 90:367, 1985.
16. Pass, H. I.: Primary and metastatic chest wall tumors. *In* Roth, J. A., Ruckdeschel, J. C., and Weisenburger, T. H. (Eds.): Thoracic Oncology. Philadelphia, W. B. Saunders, 1989.
17. Pritchard, D. J., Dahlin, D., Dauphine, R., et al.: Ewing sarcoma. J. Bone Joint Surg., 57:10, 1975.
18. Rami-Porta, R., Bravo-Bravo, J. L., Aroco-Gonzales, M. J., et al.: Tumors and pseudotumors of the chest wall. Scand. J. Thorac. Cardiovasc. Surg., 19:97, 1985.
19. Robbins, T. H.: The rectus abdominus myocutaneous flap for breast reconstruction. Aust. N. Z. Surg., 49:527, 1979.
20. Sabanathan, S., Saloma, F. D., Morgan, W. E., et al.: Primary chest wall tumors. Ann. Thorac. Surg., 39:4, 1985.
21. Seltzer, P., and Gay, W. A.: Tumors of the chest wall. Surg. Clin. North Am., 60:779, 1980.

XVI

EXTRACORPOREAL MEMBRANE OXYGENATION

James R. Mault, M.D., and Robert H. Bartlett, M.D.

Since the first successful application of cardiopulmonary bypass by Gibbon in 1954, artificial replacement of the heart and lungs is performed on a routine basis for brief periods during cardiac surgery. With several modifications, extracorporeal circulation can be used for days or weeks to support the life of a patient with severe pulmonary or cardiac failure. Depending on the cannulation and clinical setting, this procedure has been called extracorporeal life support, extracorporeal CO_2 removal, extracorporeal heart assist, extracorporeal lung assist, and extracorporeal membrane oxygenation (ECMO). The differences between standard cardiopulmonary bypass and ECMO are contrasted in Table 51–36. ECMO involves extrathoracic cannulation of major vessels, carefully titrated partial anticoagulation with heparin, and continuous

TABLE 51–36. Comparison of ECMO with Standard Cardiopulmonary Bypass

	ECMO	Cardiopulmonary Bypass
Setting	Respiratory and/or cardiac failure	Intraoperative cardiac surgery
Location	Extrathoracic	Intrathoracic
Vascular Access	Venoarterial or venovenous	Venoarterial only
Anticoagulation	Partial	Total
Blood Reservoir	No	Yes
Bubble Traps	No	Yes
Blood Pump	Roller or centrifugal	Roller or centrifugal
Artificial Lung	Silicon-coated membrane	Bubble or microporous membrane
Temperature	Normothermic only	Hypothermic
Duration	Days to weeks	Hours

high-flow extracorporeal circulation through a membrane lung. ECMO is not a therapeutic modality but rather a mechanical support system that allows time for the damaged heart or lungs to heal in a milieu of normal perfusion and gas exchange, while *resting* the damaged organs from the effects of mechanical ventilation and inotropic drugs. Therefore, only patients with potentially reversible disease processes are considered candidates for this technology. ECMO has been widely successful in neonatal respiratory failure and is considered a standard of care in this setting. It has been applied to children and adults, although characterization and standardization of indications and techniques for these patient populations are ongoing.

PATIENT SELECTION

The most important criterion of patient selection for ECMO is reversibility of the underlying disease process. In this regard, neonates often experience severe but reversible forms of acute respiratory failure due to aspiration of meconium, neonatal sepsis, respiratory distress syndrome, or congenital diaphragmatic hernia. The common underlying pathophysiology (known as persistent pulmonary hypertension of the newborn [PPHN]) with each of these conditions is pulmonary arterial vasospasm causing pulmonary hypertension and right-to-left shunting through the ductus arteriosus or foramen ovale. Because of this pathophysiologic syndrome, vasospasm and right-to-left shunting results in postductal hypoxemia despite a high fraction of inspired oxygen (FIO_2). In most neonatal centers, PPHN is treated by hyperventilation to induce alkalosis and relax the vasospasm. Induced hyperventilation results in increased airway pressure, and therefore FIO_2 and airway pressure are indirect measures of the degree of pulmonary dysfunction. These factors have been combined into measurements to estimate the severity of pulmonary dysfunction in the alveolar-arterial oxygen gradient ($AaDO_2$) or the oxygenation index (OI). The normal $AaDO_2$ is approximately 10 mm. Hg. When the $AaDO_2$ is consistently higher than 600 to 620, the mortality risk is 80% to 90%. The OI is calculated as follows:

$$OI = \left\{ \frac{\text{Mean airway pressure} \times FIO_2}{PaO_2} \right\} \times 100$$

An oxygenation index consistently greater than 40 is generally associated with 80% or greater mortality risk. The usefulness of these measurements in any neonatal center is de-

pendent on the method and philosophy of ventilatory management, and each center must determine its own mortality risk using $AaDO_2$, OI, or some other objective measurement.

Contraindications to ECMO in newborns are prematurity of less than 35 weeks' gestational age, pre-existing intracranial bleeding or other major neurologic injury, mechanical ventilation longer than 10 days, and irreversible conditions such as pulmonary hypoplasia. Prematurity is associated with a high rate of intracranial bleeding.[8] Prior intracranial bleeding or neurologic injury may be made worse during ECMO. The incidence of severe bronchopulmonary dysplasia is high in children who have received mechanical ventilation with high airway pressures for a few days and is prohibitively high in infants who have been mechanically ventilated more than 10 days.

In adult patients, failure of standard therapy and high mortality risk with respiratory failure is identified by worsening right-to-left shunting and poor compliance. The criteria for randomization in the NIH ECMO study identified a group of patients with 90% mortality risk in 1977. These criteria can be summarized as transpulmonary shunt greater than 30% despite optimal treatment. This selects patients with mortality ranging from 60% to 90%, depending on how the qualifier *optimal therapy* is applied. In the pediatric population, epidemiologic studies have not yet defined high mortality risk criteria for respiratory failure. Patient selection for pediatric respiratory failure is usually based on the adult criteria just defined.

Contraindications to ECMO in older children and adults include age older than 65 years, major brain injury, conditions incompatible with a favorable long-term prognosis, and active bleeding. Relative contraindications are systemic sepsis and three or more organ systems failing (because of uniformly poor results), mechanical ventilation greater than 1 week (because of the high rate of irreversible pulmonary fibrosis), and irreversible immunosuppression (because of the risk of overwhelming bacterial infection).

THE EXTRACORPOREAL LIFE SUPPORT CIRCUIT

ECMO is performed by draining venous (deoxygenated) blood, pumping it through an artificial lung where carbon dioxide is removed and oxygen is added, and returning the blood to the circulation through an artery (venoarterial [VA] ECMO) or a vein (venovenous [VV] ECMO). The differences between VA and VV ECMO are contrasted in Table 51–37. In VA ECMO, the functions of both the heart and the lungs are partially or totally replaced. Deoxygenated blood is drained from the right atrium through cannulation of the right internal jugular or femoral vein, while oxygenated blood is pumped back into the circulation through the right common carotid artery. ECMO candidates who are hemodynamically unstable and require cardiovascular support in addition to gas exchange are placed on VA ECMO.

VV ECMO provides gas exchange but no cardiac support. Venous drainage and infusion cannulae are placed into the right atrium or vena cavae through the right internal jugular or femoral veins. Alternatively, a double-lumen catheter may be positioned in the right atrium through the right internal jugular vein for both drainage and infusion. In either case, blood is drained from and returned to the venous circulation at the same rate. With VV ECMO, systemic oxygenation saturations are slightly lower than with VA ECMO owing to a recirculation fraction. Most patients with acute respiratory failure who are hemodynamically stable are initially placed on VV ECMO. If hemodynamic instability develops, cannulation can be easily converted to VA ECMO.

TABLE 51–37. Comparison of Venoarterial and Venovenous ECMO

	Venoarterial ECMO	Venovenous ECMO
Organ Support	Gas exchange and cardiac output	Gas exchange only
Pulse Contour	Reduced or absent pulsatility	Normal pulsatility
CVP Monitoring	Unreliable	Reliable
PA Pressure Monitoring	Unreliable	Reliable
Circuit SvO$_2$ Monitoring	Reliable	Less reliable
Circuit Recirculation	None	15%–50%
Arterial O$_2$ Saturation	≥95%	75%–95%
CO$_2$ Removal	Sweep gas flow dependent	Sweep gas flow dependent
Ventilator Settings	Minimal	Moderate

CVP, central venous pressure; PA, pulmonary artery; SvO$_2$, mixed venous oxygen saturation.

Cannulation is performed at the bedside in the intensive care unit with an operating room team present. In neonates, the right common carotid artery and internal jugular vein are exposed through a small, right transverse cervical incision. Heparin (100 units/kg.) is administered intravenously after exposure of the vessels. The largest cannulae that may be easily advanced are placed with the tips in the aortic arch and the base of the right atrium. The internal diameter of the venous catheter is the limiting factor that determines maximal flow. The venous catheter must be large enough to allow total cardiopulmonary bypass. Rarely, a second venous access site is necessary to achieve adequate flow.

The components of a standard ECMO circuit are illustrated in Figure 51–103. Deoxygenated blood drains passively into a distensible silicone bladder that operates as the control point of a servo-regulated roller pump. If the pump flow exceeds the passive venous return, the bladder will collapse and the roller pump will automatically slow down or shut off until it re-expands. Blood is then pumped through a silicone-coated membrane lung designed to function for long durations. After passing through a counter-current heat exchanger, the warmed, oxygenated blood is then returned to the patient through the arterial or venous circulation. A tubing bridge is created between the drainage and perfusion catheters to allow recirculation of the blood during priming and weaning. Heparin and fluids are infused into the circuit immediately before the bladder.

The size of the artificial lung is selected to provide *total* cardiopulmonary support, even though partial support will be adequate for most patients. Each artificial lung has a *rated flow*, which specifies the blood flow rate at which 75% saturated venous blood leaves the oxygenator 95% saturated. The artificial lung chosen for a given case must have a rated flow equivalent to or greater than the cardiac output of the patient. Routine blood flow rates are 70 to 90 ml. per kg. per minute in adults, 80 to 100 ml. per kg. per minute in children, and 120 to 170 ml. per kg. per minute in neonates. As the blood is oxygenated, CO$_2$ and water vapor are removed into the gas phase of the artificial lung.

The circuit is primed sequentially with CO$_2$, electrolyte solution, albumin, and, finally, fresh blood. In neonates, the final prime is approximately 500 ml. in volume. This may be twice the newborn's blood volume, and the prime must therefore be carefully adjusted for electrolytes, pH, temperature, and hematocrit. After successful cannulation and circuit priming, extracorporeal life support is initiated and flow is gradually increased until adequate systemic oxygen delivery is achieved.

PATIENT MANAGEMENT DURING EXTRACORPOREAL LIFE SUPPORT

Because most of the clinical application of ECMO is currently in newborns, this description and discussion refers primarily to that group of patients. The basic principles of extracorporeal circulation, gas exchange, and systemic oxygen delivery apply to patients of all sizes and ages. However, the pathophysiology and clinical course of acute respiratory failure is quite different between newborns and older patients and is discussed separately.

Extracorporeal life support is usually conducted as partial venoarterial or venovenous bypass, taking 50% to 80% of the venous return into the drainage catheter. The amount of venous drainage is determined by the amount of support required; the extracorporeal flow rate is regulated to the minimum level that supports gas exchange and perfusion. Extracorporeal flow is balanced against normal flow through the right ventricle and pulmonary artery. If the lung is not functioning at all, 80% or more of the venous return must be diverted through the extracorporeal circuit. As lung function improves, the amount of extracorporeal support can be decreased.

The amount of oxygen that can be supplied through the extracorporeal circuit is a function of the flow, hemoglobin concentration, and saturation of the venous blood. Obviously the membrane lung can do no more than fully saturate the flowing blood; hence, the amount of oxygen that can be added per minute can be calculated as the difference in oxygen content from the inlet to the outlet of the membrane lung times the blood flow. For example, if the hemoglobin concentration is 15 gm. per 100 ml. and the venous blood is 75% saturated with oxygen, the venous (oxygenator inlet) oxygen content is 15.5 ml. O$_2$ per 100 ml. and the arterial (oxygenator outlet) oxygen content is 21.5 ml. O$_2$ per 100 ml. The amount of oxygen that can be introduced to the circulation is 6 ml. O$_2$ per 100 ml. of flow. The oxygen requirement for a 3-kg. newborn at rest is 15 ml. per minute, which would require 250 ml. per minute of blood flow. Oxygen delivery could be increased by increasing blood flow, by increasing hemoglobin concentration, or by decreasing venous saturation. If, for example, oxygen consumption increased to 20 ml. per minute because of muscular activity or catecholamine effect, venous oxygen saturation (SvO$_2$) would drop to approximately 50%, and the arterial-venous oxygen content difference (AVDO$_2$) would increase to 11 ml. O$_2$ per 100 ml. Oxygen delivery could be increased by increasing blood flow or increasing hemoglobin. Alternatively, oxygen consumption could be decreased by paralyzing or cooling the patient.

Although oxygen uptake is limited by the amount of unsaturated hemoglobin, CO$_2$ elimination is limited only by the gradient between the venous blood PCO$_2$ and the ventilating gas. With an artificial lung, CO$_2$ elimination during extracorporeal life support is always more efficient than oxygenation. Since this gradient is relatively constant at about 45 mm. Hg, the amount of CO$_2$ elimination is essentially a function of the membrane lung surface area. Therefore, if extracorporeal life support is conducted with the major intent of removing carbon dioxide, then extracorporeal circulation can be conducted at relatively low blood flow using a very large membrane lung surface area. This technique has been very successful in adult patients who retain most of the ability to oxygenate blood through the native lung.[9, 13] However, in newborns the lung usually goes through a stage of no gas

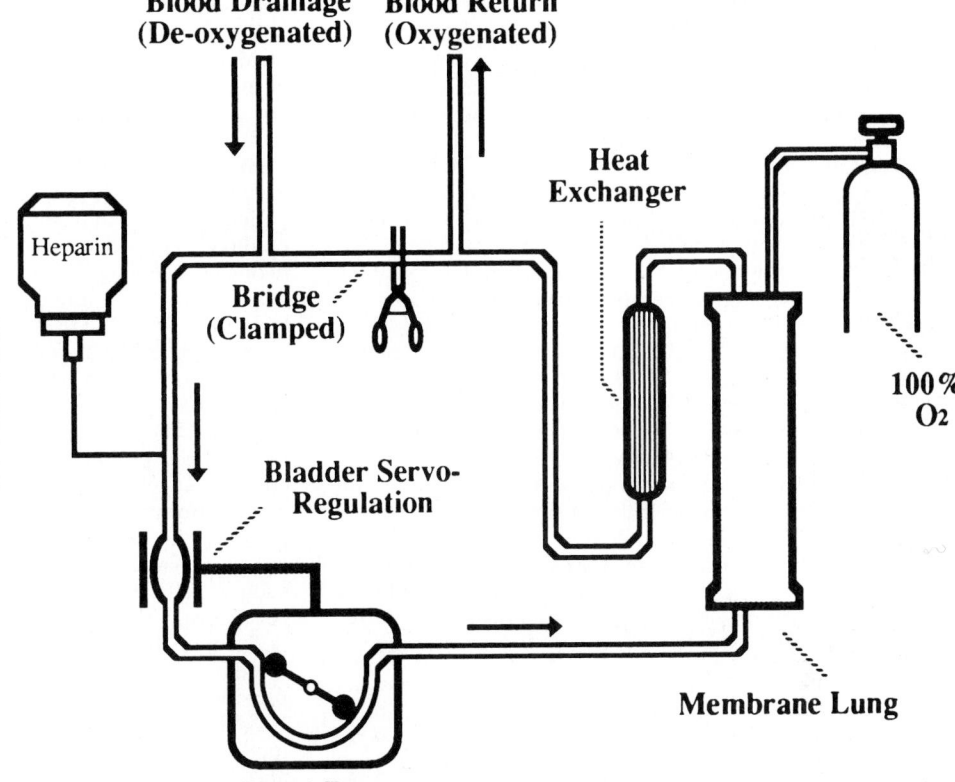

Figure 51–103. ECMO circuit schematic. Deoxygenated blood drains passively to a distensible bladder. If negative pressure occurs within the bladder, the roller pump is automatically shut off. After passing through the membrane lung, oxygenated blood is circulated through a countercurrent heat exchanger and back to the patient. Heparin is delivered into the circuit immediately before the bladder.

exchange; hence, both CO_2 and oxygen requirements must be supplied.

With VA extracorporeal life support, systemic perfusion is controlled in addition to gas exchange. The arterial pulse contour and pulse pressure are minimal, but as long as the flow is adequate this has no major physiologic side effects. During venoarterial bypass, blood flow is maintained at a level sufficient to keep the venous saturation at approximately 75%. Venous saturation is continuously monitored by a fiberoptic catheter in the venous line. A normal venous saturation ensures that the combined oxygen delivery from the patient's cardiopulmonary system and the circuit is adequate for oxygen consumption requirements. A continuous noninvasive arterial oxygen saturation monitor is placed on the patient in an area of postductal blood flow distribution. With this monitoring available, arterial blood gases need only be drawn occasionally once the patient is stable. The arterial saturation is maintained at 95% and is manipulated by adjusting the extracorporeal blood flow rate. The PCO_2 is maintained between 35 and 50 mm. Hg and is inversely proportional to the flow rate of gas ventilating the membrane lung.

When cardiac function is normal, it is possible to conduct extracorporeal life support in the VV mode. In this fashion, the oxygenated blood is returned to the venous circulation rather than the aorta, achieving prepulmonary gas exchange and leaving the patient totally dependent on his or her own cardiovascular system for systemic perfusion. It is relatively simple to achieve total CO_2 elimination during venovenous bypass for the reasons discussed previously. However, the ability to fully oxygenate the blood is limited by recirculation of circuit blood in the right atrium. During venovenous extracorporeal life support, the native lung provides a significant portion of the systemic gas exchange. However, even if there is no oxygen uptake across the native lung, the total oxygen

requirement can be supplied during VV ECMO by using higher extracorporeal flow and accepting a systemic arterial saturation between 80% and 90%. For example, if the venous drainage saturation is 90% and the hemoglobin is 15 gm. per 100 ml. and the $AVDO_2$ is 3.3 ml. O_2 per 100 ml., a VV ECMO flow of 450 ml. per minute supplies 15 ml. O_2 per minute. During VV ECMO, blood is drained and returned to the venous circulation at the same rate and thus has no influence on cardiac output or hemodynamics. Also, with recirculation, $S\bar{v}O_2$ monitoring is unreliable during VV ECMO. A recent multicenter comparison of VV ECMO (using a double-lumen catheter placed in the right internal jugular vein) demonstrated the safety and efficacy of this technique.[1]

Once on ECMO, support paralyzing agents, vasoactive drugs, and other infusions are generally discontinued. Ventilator settings are adjusted to minimal levels to allow *lung rest.* Typical neonatal settings are pressure limit, 20 cm. H_2O; positive end-expiratory pressure of 8 to 12 cm. H_2O; rate of 10 breaths per minute; and FIO_2 of 30%. The patient is usually awake and alert.

Heparin is infused continuously at 30 to 60 units per kg. per hour. The level of anticoagulation is monitored hourly by the whole-blood activated clotting time. The heparin dose is adjusted to maintain the activated clotting time between 160 and 180 seconds (normal is approximately 100 seconds). Platelet counts decrease at the onset of bypass, and platelet consumption continues during ECMO. In infants, platelet transfusions are required to maintain a level greater than 100,000. The hematocrit is maintained between 40% and 45%, and occasional red blood cell transfusion is required. In general, hemolysis is minimal and free serum hemoglobin levels are usually less than 30 mg. per 100 ml. during an ECMO course.

Patients are often edematous, and emphasis is placed on diuresis and return to approximate dry weight. If diuresis is

not adequate after administration of furosemide and mannitol, a hemofilter is placed in the circuit to supplement urine
output. Crystalloid administration is minimized and given
mostly in the form of parenteral nutrition. Red blood cells,
25% albumin, or plasma is infused when an increase in
intravascular volume is required. The patient is routinely
placed on antibiotics.

Weaning from ECMO. ECMO support is maintained until
the native lung recovers (4 to 7 days in neonates). Indications
of lung recovery include an increasing $S\bar{v}O_2$ and systemic PO_2
or decreasing PCO_2 while ECMO flow and ventilator settings
are constant. Other signs of improvement are noted by increased pulmonary compliance and a normalizing chest
x-ray. On documenting significant improvement in native
respiratory function during VA ECMO, blood flow is gradually reduced over a period of hours. When the native lung
and heart can provide adequate oxygen delivery and gas
exchange at 20% of the baseline VA ECMO flow, a brief trial
off bypass (cannulae clamped, bridge open) is attempted on
moderate ventilator settings. If this is successful, VA ECMO
is restarted and the patient is prepared for the sterile decannulation procedure. A trial wean from VV ECMO consists of
decreasing and capping the sweep gas flow to the membrane
lung without changing the pump blood flow. If the native
lungs provide adequate gas exchange, VV ECMO can be
discontinued.

RESULTS

ECMO is used for patients with very high mortality risk,
so the results are measured as survival. The outcome for
various age groups and diagnoses is shown in Table 51–38.
These data come from the ECMO Registry maintained by the
Extracorporeal Life Support Organization.[21]

Neonatal ECMO. The best results are in neonates with
respiratory failure, and the most experienced centers rou-

TABLE 51–38. Survival Rates in Various Categories of Patients Supported with ECMO*

	No. Patients	% Survival
Newborns	9911	81
Meconium aspiration syndrome	3607	94
Respiratory distress syndrome	1093	84
Primary pulmonary hypertension	1313	84
Congenital diaphragmatic hernia	1960	58
Sepsis	1528	76
Other causes	410	77
Children	883	52
Bacterial pneumonia	77	48
Viral pneumonia	273	56
Intrapulmonary hemorrhage	13	62
Aspiration	87	64
Pneumocystis carinii pneumonia	13	58
Adult respiratory distress syndrome	40	58
Other causes	380	47
Adults	171	42
Bacterial pneumonia	19	32
Viral pneumonia	18	72
Intrapulmonary hemorrhage	1	0
Aspiration	7	43
Adult respiratory distress syndrome	45	56
Other respiratory causes	29	48
Pre/post transplantation	17	29
Cardiac surgery	35	14

*ECMO is initiated when projected survival is less than 10%.
Data from the ELSO National ECMO Registry.[17]

tinely report survival rates over 80% in most diagnostic categories. Survival from congenital diaphragmatic hernia using
ECMO averages 58% but has been reported as high as 76%
in one series.[12] When death occurs during ECMO in a newborn, it is usually caused by anoxic brain injury from the
perinatal period or intracranial bleeding.[8]

Shanley and colleagues[26] identified several important
trends in a comprehensive review of 460 neonatal ECMO
patients (treated at a single institution over 20 years) and the
national experience with 9000 neonates. The proportion of
neonates receiving VV ECMO (single catheter, double-lumen)
has steadily risen and is now the preferred vascular access
technique. Over the past 5 years, the total number of patients
receiving ECMO has stabilized at 1200 to 1400 cases per year.
However, over the same period, the overall survival has
slowly decreased while complication rates have slightly increased. Others have confirmed these trends comparing the
results from periods 1985–1988 to 1990–1992 showing a decrease in survival from 84% to 80% and an increase in complications from 1.44 to 2.10 per case, respectively. In both papers, these changes are attributed to improved methods of
conventional rescue therapies for neonatal respiratory failure,
such as jet ventilation, nitric oxide, and surfactant therapy.
As a result, the population receiving ECMO are those patients who have failed these additional measures and are
therefore more severely ill than those receiving ECMO in
previous years.

Additional factors contributing to these directions is the
increasing application of ECMO to premature (≤35 weeks)
and low birth weight (<2.0 kg.) infants. Early experience
(pre-1985) with ECMO in this group of patients was dismal
owing to excessive rate of intracranial hemorrhage (100%)
and poor survival (23%).[8] These patients were therefore excluded from consideration for ECMO. As technical aspects
of ECMO have become more refined with a significant reduction in the level of anticoagulation during ECMO, these high-
risk populations have been reconsidered for ECMO with
reduced intracranial hemorrhage (37%) and improved survival (63%).[14]

Pediatric and Adult ECMO. With the favorable experience
of neonatal ECMO over the past 15 years, the application of
ECMO to children and adults has received renewed interest.
Moler and colleagues[18] reported a recent experience (1991–
1993) with ECMO for 25 pediatric patients with severe respiratory failure. The mean duration of ECMO was 373 ± 259
hours, and 88% survived their life-threatening respiratory
illness to be discharged home. This represented a statistically
improved survival rate, in comparison with the 58% survival
rate previously reported by the authors for an earlier group
of patients.

With the exception of Gattinoni and colleagues,[10] ECMO
for adult respiratory failure was essentially abandoned after
publication of the NIH-sponsored trial in 1977. Re-examination of the use of ECMO in adults began in 1988. Pranikoff
and associates[23] described their first 65 adult patients supported by ECMO for respiratory (n=51) and cardiac (n=14)
failure from 1988 to 1993. The etiology of respiratory failure
was evenly divided between pneumonia and ARDS, with an
overall survival of 59%. Mean duration of ECMO was 198 ±
177 hours for survivors and 343 ± 304 hours for nonsurvivors. Venovenous access was used in 40 of these patients.
The only prognostic indicator of survival from this experience was duration of mechanical ventilation before initiation
of ECMO (survivors 3.0 ± 2.4 days vs. 6.1 ± 4.0 days for
nonsurvivors). Recovery from cardiac failure was 29%.

The cumulative national experience with pediatric and
adult ECMO is listed in Table 51–38. Survival of these groups
supported by ECMO is 40% to 50% in all categories of respiratory failure (infection, aspiration, trauma, or capillary leak

syndromes). When death occurs, it is usually due to diffuse pulmonary fibrosis with obliteration of alveoli and vasculature or multiple organ failure and sepsis. ECMO has been used for cardiac support in approximately 1401 children, usually for cardiac failure after operation for congenital heart disease. Survival is 43%, and death is usually due to multiple organ failure from low cardiac output.

The reason that recovery occurs in 90% of newborns but only in 50% of children and adults relates to the pathophysiology of pulmonary dysfunction. In the newborn the problem is a functional problem related to pulmonary vasospasm and inadequate pulmonary blood flow. The lung parenchyma is intrinsically normal, and there is no factor that predisposes to fibrosis except for ventilator-induced lung injury. In children and adults, the primary disease usually affects the interstitium of the lung, leading to inflammation, fibrosis, and bacterial infection. All of these factors result in tissue destruction and scar formation, which obliterates lung parenchyma. The extent of fibrosis and necrosis determines the ability of the lung and the patient to recover.

Complications. The duration of the ECMO course is typically 4 days in neonates and 10 to 14 days in children and adults. Some patients have been supported by ECMO for more than 1 month with ultimate survival. The complication rate increases as the time on extracorporeal support increases. Approximately two thirds of patients experience some type of physiologic complication (Table 51–39). Bleeding is the most common complication because of the systemic heparinization and thrombocytopenia. Data from the Neonatal ECMO Registry[21] show that 13% experience intracranial bleeding (as detected by ultrasound examination), 6% have bleeding from the surgical site, and 11% have hemolysis. When bleeding occurs it is managed by decreasing the systemic heparin dose to activated clotting times below 160 seconds, transfusing platelets until the platelet count is greater than 150,000 per cu. mm., and surgical control of bleeding if these measures are unsuccessful. In newborns 13% experience seizures, which are common in critically ill newborns and not necessarily associated with poor neurologic outcome. Fourteen percent of newborns experience acute renal failure, and 6% have positive cultures. Organ failure (aside from respiratory failure) often occurs in chil-

dren and adults and is generally due to the primary disease. Most adult and pediatric patients have two or three organ systems failing before ECMO. As the comorbidities of ECMO patients have increased over the past 5 years, the complication rate has also increased.[31]

It is surprising that mechanical complications are unusual, considering the fact that all of the components of the ECMO circuit must work continuously for days or weeks. Twenty-three percent of neonates had mechanical complications,[21] but none were associated with a major decrease in survival. The most common significant mechanical complication is membrane lung failure requiring changing the device (5%) or cannulation problems (10%). Mechanical complications did not increase mortality because the system is continuously attended by an ECMO specialist who can recognize abnormalities and repair any circuit malfunction within minutes. The ECMO specialist is a unique medical professional who combines the role of nurse, respiratory therapist, perfusionist, bioengineer, and resident in managing the ECMO procedure.

Long-Term Follow-up. Most of the ECMO survivors are normal.[30] Abnormalities in follow-up are related to the neurologic and pulmonary system and are generally related to the primary disease rather than the ECMO procedure. In a recent long-term follow-up study,[25] 103 of 118 consecutive infants (older than 34 weeks' gestation) received ECMO and survived (87%) for follow-up. Ninety-two of these children were seen on at least one occasion at between 1 and 7 years of age. Each visit included a history and physical examination, an evaluation by a physical therapist, and developmental testing by a pediatric psychologist. Twenty percent of neonatal ECMO survivors have a detectable neurologic abnormality, including hearing loss, weakness, spasticity and other motor-tone abnormalities, and mental retardation. Interestingly, the incidence of neurologic handicap is generally less than that found in follow-up of other critically ill newborns who did not receive ECMO support. Neurologic injury occurs primarily in those children who have prolonged ischemic or hypoxic episodes in the perinatal period, but some cases of right-sided brain ischemic or hemorrhagic lesions have been identified that may be related to vascular ligation (either jugular vein or carotid artery). Pulmonary disability in the form of bronchopulmonary dysplasia, frequent pulmonary infection, or bronchospasm occurs in 10% of infants treated with ECMO. Pulmonary symptoms usually subside by 1 year of age. Other follow-up studies have confirmed these results.[32]

Follow-up examination in children and adults shows findings typical of recovery from severe pulmonary injury. Neurologic function is generally normal. Pulmonary function tests show a restrictive fibrotic pattern, which may be associated with bronchospasm. This pulmonary abnormality usually subsides within 1 year from the time of discharge.

Cost-Benefit Analysis of ECMO. A recent prospective randomized control trial compared early institution of ECMO ($20 \leq OI \leq 40$) with continued medical management in 41 patients.[24] ECMO duration averaged 4 days with corresponding hospital charge of approximately $2000 per day. The results demonstrated that ECMO patients averaged fewer ventilator days, fewer hospital days, and lower hospital charges than those who recovered with conventional ventilation. In the setting of neonatal respiratory failure, early institution of an "expensive" technology such as ECMO is not only efficacious but also cost effective.

TABLE 51–39. Physiologic and Mechanical Complications* in 9911 Newborns Treated with ECMO

	% of Series	% Survival†
Physiologic Complications		
Intracranial hemorrhage (ultrasound)	13	49
Intracranial hemorrhage (by CT/MRI)	4	83
Seizures	13	66
Surgical site hemorrhage	6	52
Cannula site hemorrhage	6	73
Renal failure (dialysis/hemofiltration)	14	58
Hemolysis	11	73
Arrhythmia	4	59
Positive culture	6	62
Hypertension	11	76
Mechanical Complications		
Oxygenator change	5	63
Tubing rupture	1	73
Pump failure	2	81
Cannula problem	10	75
Clots in circuit	24	76

*Physiologic complications are often associated with increased mortality, but mechanical complications are not.

†The overall survival rate in this series was 81%.

THE FUTURE OF EXTRACORPOREAL LIFE SUPPORT

Today, ECMO is the treatment of choice for infants with severe respiratory failure who fail to respond to conventional management. For children and adults, the indications for ECMO are being defined. In the next decade, conventional management will undoubtedly improve, resulting in less lung injury and less mortality, decreasing the need for radical approaches such as extracorporeal life support. At the same time, ECMO will become safer and simpler, so that management of the critically ill newborn will probably include both mechanical ventilation and extracorporeal support. ECMO will be simplified by the use of single-catheter venovenous access and perhaps arteriovenous access through the umbilical vessels in some infants. A major complication of ECMO is bleeding, which is in part related to heparinization. The use of heparin-coated circuits has been demonstrated to be effective in the laboratory.[20, 27, 28] Neonatal ECMO conducted with minimal systemic heparinization decreases the risk of bleeding and expands the indications for its use.

Aside from these applications in respiratory failure VA ECMO will be commonly used to support systemic perfusion. As outlined in this discussion, this application is used primarily for children with postoperative cardiac failure and is also being used to support the circulation in patients with sudden left ventricular failure induced in the cardiac catheterization laboratory during attempted angioplasty or arteriography. In the next decade this application will be extended to emergency department and intensive care unit resuscitation of patients in cardiac failure when the intra-aortic balloon pump is inadequate. In addition, the technique will be used for rewarming patients with systemic hypothermia and supporting patients with myocardial disease through difficult operations. The availability of ECMO without systemic heparinization will greatly expand the potential indications into areas such as trauma, intraoperative and postoperative support, and management of exsanguinating hemorrhage.

SUMMARY AND CONCLUSIONS

Extracorporeal life support has become standard treatment for term and near-term newborns with severe respiratory failure that is unresponsive to conventional ventilator and pharmacologic management. Pulmonary hypertension with right-to-left shunting is the underlying pathophysiology in these infants, regardless of the primary diagnosis. With the lung rest provided by extracorporeal support, pulmonary hypertension resolves in 3 or 4 days and lung recovery occurs in almost all of these infants. The survival rate for 9911 patients in the Neonatal ECMO Registry was 81%. The lesson learned from neonatal experience is that avoiding high-pressure, high-oxygen mechanical ventilation by means of extracorporeal life support results in recovery of the lung and patient survival.

In severe respiratory failure in children and adults the use of ECMO results in survival in approximately 50% of cases. The pathophysiology of lung injury produces tissue necrosis and fibrosis, causing irreversible progressive pulmonary injury in many cases. The use of ECMO earlier in the course of disease decreases whatever component of progressive lung injury is related to high-pressure, high-oxygen mechanical ventilation. The use of heparin-coated circuits to eliminate systemic anticoagulation, of automation of pump controls, and of simple percutaneous access catheters will expand the applications of all types of extracorporeal life support during the next decade.

SELECTED REFERENCES

Bartlett, R. H.: Extracorporeal life support for cardiopulmonary failure. Curr. Probl. Surg., 27:621, 1990.
   This monograph is a reference standard for ECMO. It is a useful source of information on the bioengineering of extracorporeal circuits, the physiology and pathophysiology of extracorporeal circulation, and the development of prolonged extracorporeal support.
Bartlett, R. H., Roloff, D. W., Cornell, R. G., Andrews, A. F., Dillon, P. W., and Zwischenberger, J. B.: Extracorporeal circulation in neonatal respiratory failure: A prospective randomized study. Pediatrics, 76:479, 1985.
O'Rourke, P. P., Krone, R., Vacanti, J., et al.: Extracorporeal membrane oxygenation and conventional medical therapy in neonates with persistent pulmonary hypertension of the newborn: A prospective randomized study. Pediatrics, 84:957, 1989.
   Both of these papers report the results of prospective randomized controlled studies of ECMO in newborn respiratory failure. Both showed that the results with ECMO were much better than the results of conventional treatment. Both studies used an adaptive design, and the statistical methodology is as interesting as the clinical studies themselves.
Pranikoff, T., Hirschl, R. B., Steimle, C. N., Anderson, H. L., et al.: Efficacy of extracorporeal life support in the setting of adult cardiorespiratory failure. ASAIO J., 40:M339, 1994.
   The success of ECMO in the neonatal population over the past decade has generated renewed enthusiasm for the application of this technology to adult respiratory failure. This paper is the most recent presentation of the modern application of adult ECMO to 65 patients between 1988 and 1993. The result for moribund patients with acute respiratory failure was an encouraging 59% survival.
Shanley, C. J., Hirschl, R. B., Schumacher, R. E., Overbeck, M. C., et al.: Extracorporeal life support for neonatal respiratory failure: A 20-year experience. Ann. Surg., 220:269, 1994.
   This paper is a comprehensive review of 460 neonates treated with ECMO over a 20-year period. In addition, the results from 9000 patients treated at other institutions are analyzed. Recent trends in patient population and implications of recently developed non-ECMO rescue therapies. It is the most complete description of the current state of the art of neonatal ECMO.

REFERENCES

1. Anderson, H., Snedecor, S. M., Otsu, T., and Bartlett, R. H.: Multicenter comparison of conventional venoarterial access versus venovenous double-lumen catheter access in newborn infants undergoing extracorporeal membrane oxygenation. J. Pediatr. Surg., 28:530, 1993.
2. Bartlett, R. H., Fong, S. W., Burns, N. E., and Gazzaniga, A. B.: Prolonged partial venoarterial bypass: Physiologic, biochemical and hematologic responses. Ann. Surg., 180:805, 1974.
3. Bartlett, R. H., Gazzaniga, A. B., Huxtable, R. F., Schippers, H. C., O'Connor, M. J., and Jefferies, M. R.: Extracorporeal circulation (ECMO) in neonatal respiratory failure. J. Thorac. Cardiovasc. Surg., 74:826, 1977.
4. Bartlett, R. H., Gazzaniga, A. B., Jefferies, R., et al.: Extracorporeal membrane oxygenation (ECMO): Cardiopulmonary support in infancy. Trans. ASAIO, 22:80, 1976.
5. Bartlett, R. H., Gazzaniga, A. B., Toomasian, J. M., et al.: Extracorporeal membrane oxygenation (ECMO) in neonatal respiratory failure: 100 cases. Ann. Surg., 204:236, 1986.
6. Bartlett, R. H., Isherwood, J., Moss, R. A., Olszewski, W. L., Polet, H., and Drinker, P. A.: A toroidal flow membrane oxygenator: Four day partial bypass in dogs. Surg. Forum, 20:152, 1969.
7. Bartlett, R. H., Roloff, D. W., Cornell, R. G., Andrews, A. F., Dillon, P. W., and Zwischenberger, J. B.: Extracorporeal circulation in neonatal respiratory failure: A prospective randomized study. Pediatrics, 4:479, 1985.
8. Cilley, R. E., Zwischenberger, J. B., and Andrews, A. F.: Intracranial hemorrhage during extracorporeal membrane oxygenation in neonates. Pediatrics, 78:699, 1986.
9. Dorson, W. Jr., Baker, E., Cohen, N. L., et al.: A perfusion system for infants. Trans. ASAIO, 15:155, 1969.
10. Gattinoni, L., Pesenti, A., Mascheroni, D., et al.: Low frequency positive pressure ventilation with extracorporeal CO_2 removal in severe acute respiratory failure. JAMA, 256:881, 1986.
11. Gille, J. P., and Bagniewski, A. M.: Ten years of use of extracorporeal membrane oxygenation (ECMO) in treatment of acute respiratory insufficiency. Trans. ASAIO, 22:102, 1976.
12. Heiss, K., Manning, P. B., Oldham, K. T., Coran, A. G., Polley, T. Z., Wesley, J. R., and Bartlett, R. H.: Reversal of mortality for congenital diaphragmatic hernia with ECMO. Ann. Surg., 209:225, 1989.
13. Hill, D., O'Brien, T. G., Murray, J. J., et al.: Extracorporeal oxygenation for acute post-traumatic respiratory failure (shock-lung syndrome): Use of the Bramson Membrane Lung. N. Engl. J. Med., 286:629, 1972.
14. Hirschl, R. B., Schumacher, R. E., Snedecor, S. N., Bui, K. C., et al.: The efficacy of extracorporeal life support in premature and low birth weight newborns. J. Pediatr. Surg., 28:1336, 1993.
15. Knoch, M.: Treatment of severe ARDS with extracorporeal CO_2 removal. *In* Gille, J. P. (Ed.): Neonatal and Adult Respiratory Failure. Paris, Elsevier, 1989, pp. 123–136.
16. Kolobow, T., and Boloman, R. H.: Construction and evaluation of an alveolar membrane artificial heart-lung. Trans. ASAIO, 9:238, 1963.
17. Kolobow, T., Zapol, W., Sigman, R. L., et al.: Partial cardiopulmonary bypass lasting up to seven days in adult lambs with membrane lung blood oxygenation. J. Thorac. Cardiovasc. Surg., 60:781, 1970.

18. Moler, F. W., Custer, J. R., Bartlett, R. H., Palmisano, J. M., et al.: Extracorporeal life support for severe pediatric respiratory failure: An updated experience 1991–1993. J. Pediatrics, 124:875, 1994.

19. Morris, A. H., Wallace, C. J., Menlove, R. L., Clemmer, T. P., et al.: Randomized clinical trial of pressure-controlled inverse ratio ventilation and extracorporeal CO_2 removal for adult respiratory distress syndrome. Am. J. Respir. Crit. Care Med., 149:295, 1994.

20. Mottaghy, K., Oedekoven, B., Schaich-Lester, D., and Poppel K.: Nonheparin and heparin bonded systems for $ECCO_2R$: An experimental study. In Gille, J. P. (Ed.): Neonatal and Adult Respiratory Failure. Paris, Elsevier, 1989, pp. 209–220.

21. ECMO Registry Report of the Extracorporeal Life Support Organization, Ann Arbor, Michigan, January 1995.

22. O'Rourke, P. P., Krone, R., Vacanti, J., et al.: Extracorporeal membrane oxygenation and conventional medical therapy in neonates with persistent pulmonary hypertension of the newborn: A prospective randomized study. Pediatrics, 84:957, 1989.

23. Pranikoff, T., Hirschl, R. B., Steimle, C. N., Anderson, H. L., et al.: Efficacy of extracorporeal life support in the setting of adult cardiorespiratory failure. ASAIO J., 40:M339, 1994.

24. Schumacher, R. E., Roloff, D. W., Chapman, R., Snedecor, S., et al.: Extracorporeal membrane oxygenation in term newborns: A prospective cost-benefit analysis. ASAIO J., 39:873, 1993.

25. Schumacher, R. E., Palmer, T. W., Roloff, D. W., LaClaire, P. A., et al.: Follow-up of infants treated with extracorporeal membrane oxygenation for newborn respiratory failure. Pediatrics, 87:451, 1991.

26. Shanley, C. J., Hirschl, R. B., Schumacher, R. E., Overbeck, M. C., et al.: Extracorporeal life support for neonatal respiratory failure: A 20-year experience. Ann. Surg., 220:269, 1994.

27. Shanley, C. J., Hultquist, K. A., Rosenberg, D. M., McKenzie, J. M., et al.: Prolonged extracorporeal circulation without heparin: Evaluation of the Medtronic Minimax oxygenator. ASAIO J., 38:M311, 1992.

28. Toomasian, J. M., Hsu, L.-C., Hirschl, R. B., Heiss, K. F., Hultquist, K. A., and Bartlett, R. H.: Evaluation of Duraflo II heparin coating in prolonged extracorporeal membrane oxygenation. Trans. ASAIO, 34:410, 1988.

29. Toomasian, J. M., Snedecor, S. M., Cornell, R. G., et al.: National experience with extracorporeal membrane oxygenation (ECMO) for newborn respiratory failure: Data from 715 cases. Trans. ASAIO, 34:140, 1988.

30. Towne, B. H., Lott, I. T., et al.: Long-term follow-up of infants and children treated with extracorporeal membrane oxygenation (ECMO): A preliminary report. J. Pediatr. Surg., 20:410, 1985.

31. Upp, J. J., Bush, P. E., and Zwischenberger, J. B.: Complications of neonatal extracorporeal membrane oxygenation. Perfusion, 9:241, 1994.

32. Wildin, S. R., Landry, S. H., and Zwischenberger, J. B.: Prospective, controlled study of developmental outcome in survivors of extracorporeal membrane oxygenation: The first 24 months. Pediatrics, 93:404, 1994.

33. Zapol, W. M., Snider, M. T., Hill, J. D., et al.: Extracorporeal membrane oxygenation in severe acute respiratory failure: A randomized prospective study. JAMA, 242:2193, 1979.

CHAPTER 52

THE MEDIASTINUM

R. Duane Davis, Jr., M.D., and David C. Sabiston, Jr., M.D.

The mediastinum is an anatomic division of the thorax extending from the diaphragm to the thoracic inlet. It is the site of many localized disorders and is involved in a number of systemic diseases. Localized disorders that occur in this region include primary tumors and cysts as well as infection, hemorrhage, emphysema, and aneurysms. Systemic diseases include metastatic neoplasms and granulomatous and other inflammatory disorders. Lesions that originate in the esophagus, great vessels, trachea, and heart may present as a mediastinal mass and are relevant in the differential diagnosis of the various primary mediastinal disease processes. Mediastinal disorders present as a number of clinical features. Many patients are asymptomatic, and the disorder is identified on routine chest films. However, most patients have clinical features related to local involvement of adjacent structures, tumor-secretory factors, or immunologic factors.

ANATOMY

The mediastinum is defined by the following borders: the thoracic inlet superiorly, the diaphragm inferiorly, the sternum anteriorly, the vertebral column posteriorly, and the parietal pleura laterally. Many mediastinal tumors and cysts occur in characteristic locations: therefore, the mediastinum has been subdivided artificially for the convenience of localizing specific types of lesions. Some subdivide the mediastinum into four compartments—superior, anterior, middle, and posterior; however, the frequency with which tumors occurring in the anterior or posterior extend into the superior mediastinum has prompted a division of the mediastinum into three subdivisions: the anterosuperior, middle, and posterior (Fig. 52–1). The anterosuperior mediastinum is anterior to the pericardium and the pericardial reflection over the great vessels. The posterior mediastinum is posterior to the pericardium and the pericardial reflection. The middle mediastinum is bordered anteriorly by the anterior pericardial reflection and posteriorly by the posterior pericardial reflection.

The contents of the anterosuperior mediastinum include the thymus gland, aortic arch and its branches, great veins, lymphatics, and fatty areolar tissue. The middle mediastinal contents include the heart, pericardium, phrenic nerves, tracheal bifurcation and main bronchi, hila of each lung, and lymph nodes. The posterior mediastinum contains the esophagus, vagus nerves, sympathetic nervous chain, thoracic duct, descending aorta, azygous and hemiazygous systems, paravertebral lymphatics, and fatty areolar tissue (Fig. 52–2).

MEDIASTINAL EMPHYSEMA

Air may enter the mediastinum from the esophagus, trachea, bronchi, lung, neck, or abdomen, producing mediastinal emphysema or pneumomediastinum. Injury to these structures can occur from blunt or penetrating trauma, intraluminal injury, such as during endoscopy, as well as barotrauma. Blunt trauma may produce fractured ribs or vertebrae, which may lacerate an air-containing structure. Barotrauma may be caused by either blunt trauma or positive-pressure ventilation. Blunt trauma due to compressive forces on the thorax, especially when the glottis is closed and ventilation is being achieved with high pressures (usually in the setting of decreased lung compliance), may cause sufficient pressures at the intra-alveolar region to rupture alveoli. Whereas dissection of air through the visceral pleura causes a pneumothorax, dissection of air along vascular structures into the hilum and mediastinum creates a pneumomediastinum. Mediastinal emphysema may also be caused by intra-abdominal air dissecting through the diaphragmatic hiatus.

Spontaneous pneumomediastinum is usually seen in patients with exacerbation of bronchospastic disease. In a similar manner to that caused by barotrauma, the pathophysiology of spontaneous pneumomediastinum is thought to involve the rupture of a bleb within the pulmonary parenchyma, creating interstitial emphysema. The air then dissects along vascular or bronchial planes into the mediastinum. The clinical manifestations of this include substernal chest pain, which may radiate into the back, and crepitation in the region of the suprasternal notch, chest wall, and neck. With increasing pressure, the air can dissect into the neck, face, chest, arms, abdomen, and retroperitoneum. Frequently, pneumomediastinum and pneumothorax occur simultaneously. Auscultation over the pericardium demonstrates a characteristic crunching sound that is accentuated during systole and is termed *Hamman's sign*. Rarely does sufficient pressure develop to cause compression of venous structures so as to impair venous return. Clinical manifestations similar to the superior vena caval syndrome occur, including cyanosis, prominence of neck and upper extremity veins, dyspnea, and, in severe cases, circulatory failure. The diagnosis of pneumomediastinum is confirmed by the presence of air in the mediastinum as visualized on the chest films or computed tomographic (CT) scans. Air is usually also present in the pectoral muscles, neck, and upper extremities. To evaluate the esophagus and large airways as potential sources, contrast studies of the esophagus, initially using a water-soluble contrast material, and bronchoscopy are best. Perforations of these structures usually require urgent surgical treatment. Spontaneous mediastinal emphysema and pneumomediastinum secondary to barotrauma usually respond to conservative measures that treat bronchospasm and minimize further barotrauma without sequelae. Surgical decompression is rarely necessary. In patients with pneumomediastinum and pneumothorax, tube thoracostomy is indicated in the affected pleural space. Patients with pneumomediastinum secondary to barotrauma continuing to require high levels of ventilator support may require bilateral tube thoracostomies to prevent the development of tension pneumothorax. In patients who are distressed by the inability to open their eyes, 5-mm. incisions in the skinfolds of the eyelids and neck can be made using local anesthesia. With gentle pressure on the surrounding soft tissue, sufficient air can be removed to provide symptomatic relief.

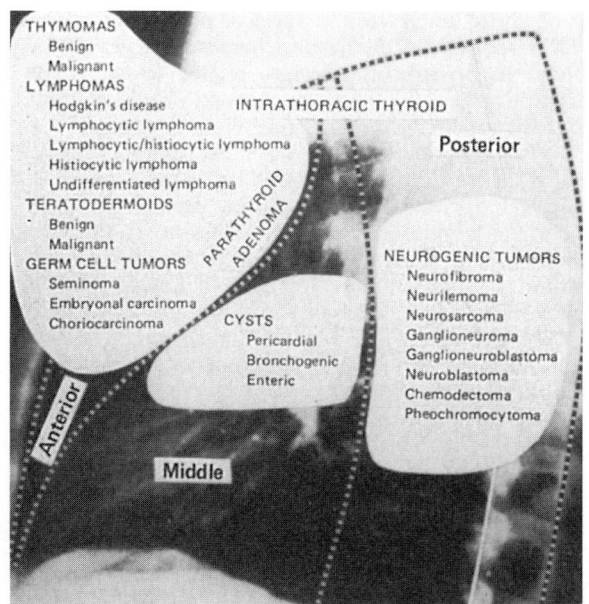

Figure 52–1. Lateral chest film divided into three anatomic subdivisions with the tumors and cysts that occur most frequently in each region. (From Davis, R. D., Jr., and Sabiston, D. C., Jr.: Primary mediastinal cysts and neoplasms. *In* Sabiston, D. C., Jr. [Ed.]: Essentials of Surgery. Philadelphia, W. B. Saunders, 1987.)

MEDIASTINITIS

Infection of the mediastinal space is a serious and potentially fatal process. Etiologic factors responsible for the development of acute mediastinitis include perforation of the esophagus due to instrumentation, foreign bodies, penetrat-

ing or, more rarely, blunt trauma, spontaneous esophageal disruption (Boerhaave's syndrome), leakage from an esophageal anastomosis, tracheobronchial perforation, and mediastinal extension from an infectious process originating in the pulmonary parenchyma, pleura, chest wall, vertebrae, great vessels, or neck. Mediastinitis occurs most often after median sternotomy for open-heart cardiac operations. Superficial wound infections occur in approximately 4% of patients after cardiac operations; in 1% to 2% of patients the infection involves the mediastinum. The risk factors for the development of mediastinitis identified in a number of series include prolonged operation, obesity, lengthy cardiopulmonary bypass, re-exploration for postoperative bleeding, dehiscence, external cardiac massage, postoperative cardiogenic shock, and the use of bilateral internal mammary arteries for coronary artery bypass grafting, especially in elderly patients or in patients with diabetes mellitus.

Mediastinitis is manifested clinically by fever, tachycardia, leukocytosis, and pain that may be localized to the chest, back, or neck, although in some patients the clinical course remains indolent for long periods. In postoperative patients, wound cellulitis and instability of the sternal closure is often present. The clinical presentation is usually 3 days to 3 weeks after the operation, although its development months later is not uncommon. When mediastinitis is secondary to esophageal perforation after instrumentation, the pain is most frequently localized to the neck because the most common site of perforation is at the level of the cricopharyngeal muscle. In these cases, subcutaneous emphysema is almost invariably present. The lateral chest film is useful in evaluating for air-fluid levels, abnormal soft tissue densities, and sternal dehiscence. CT may be useful when mediastinal gas is present, indicating the presence of gas-forming organisms or distinct abscess. It may also identify associated or contiguous infections such as an empyema, subphrenic abscess, or cervi-

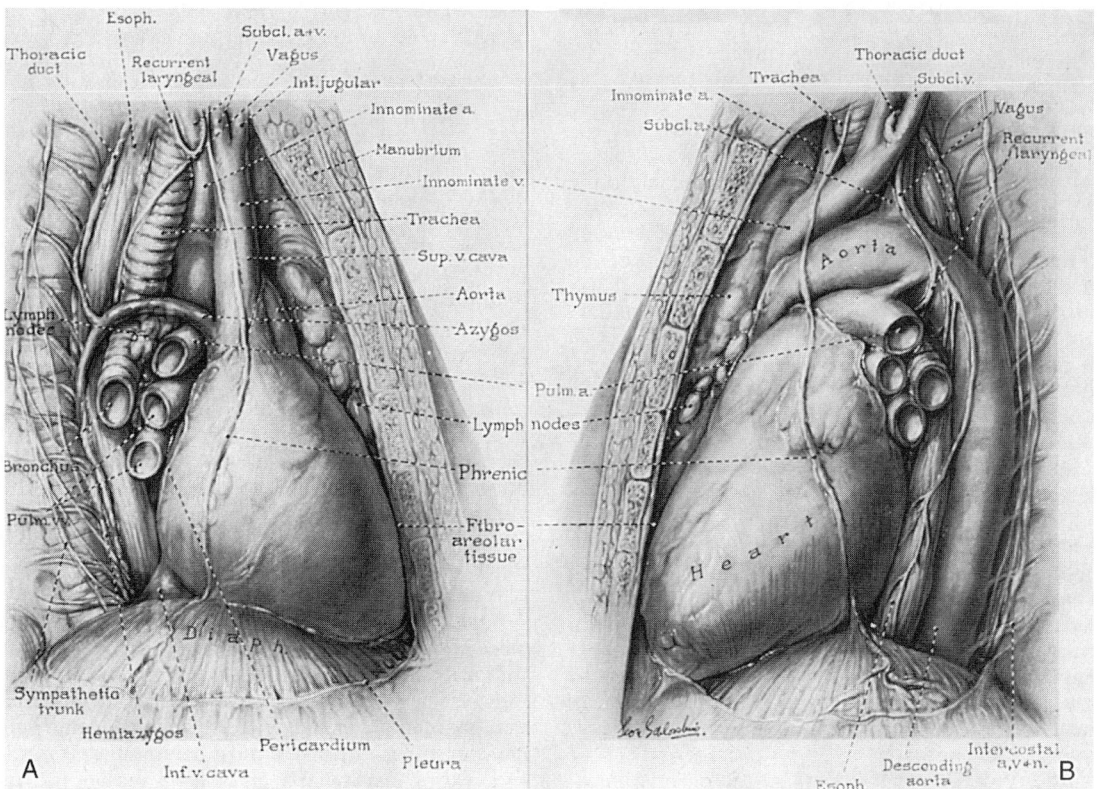

Figure 52–2. The anatomic structures of the mediastinum as seen from the right side *(A)* and from the left side *(B)*. (From Sabiston, D. C., Jr.: The esophagus and mediastinum. *In* Cooke, R. E., and Levin, S. [Eds.]: The Biologic Basis of Pediatric Practice. New York, McGraw-Hill, 1968. Copyright © 1968. Reproduced with permission of the McGraw-Hill Companies.)

cal soft tissue infection. Water-soluble contrast studies of the esophagus and esophagoscopy are important in evaluating a potential esophageal perforation or disruption. In patients with penetrating or blunt trauma, the use of both procedures has been necessary to minimize the number of overlooked esophageal injuries. Similarly, bronchoscopy is the optimal procedure to evaluate potential tracheobronchial disruption.

Treatment of mediastinitis requires correction of the inciting cause and aggressive supportive therapy. After obtaining cultures, appropriate antimicrobial coverage should be initiated with modification after results of culture and sensitivity testing are available. In patients with mediastinal infections in continuity or communication with empyema, subphrenic abscess, or neck abscess, drainage of the empyema with tube thoracostomy or percutaneous drainage of the abscess in conjunction with appropriate antimicrobial therapy is frequently successful. Similarly, mediastinitis associated with catheter sepsis can often be treated with removal of the catheter and antimicrobial therapy. However, in patients who do not respond to these initial measures or when mediastinitis occurs from most other causes, thorough débridement of necrotic and infected tissue is necessary in conjunction with surgical drainage. When costal cartilage is infected, it is necessary to excise the cartilage back to bleeding bone. In patients with descending mediastinitis originating from the oropharynx, cervical drainage and débridement may be adequate with infections limited to the superior mediastinum. However, when the involvement is more generalized, transthoracic débridement and drainage is necessary. Delays in making the diagnosis and subsequently initiating therapy, especially when the etiologic factor involves esophageal disruption, are associated with sharp increases in morbidity and mortality.

Postoperative mediastinitis after median sternotomy has been successfully treated with a number of different techniques. However, the best results have been obtained using a variety of tissue flaps to obliterate dead space and to provide immediate coverage of the heart, bypass grafts, and great vessels after effective surgical control of the wound. Débridement of infected and necrotic sternum, cartilage, and soft tissue in conjunction with wound care is necessary to provide a clean wound to optimize results. This therapy has further reduced morbidity and mortality, usually producing a good long-term functional result, and has significantly reduced the duration of hospitalization. The pectoralis major and rectus abdominis muscles have been the most commonly used tissue flaps. Because the rectus abdominis flap is based on the superior epigastric artery, this flap is only useful when the internal mammary artery remains viable. In situations in which both internal mammary arteries have been used for bypass conduits or have been sacrificed during débridement, the omentum has been used successfully.

Although chronic mediastinitis may be due to an indolent bacterial infection, more frequently chronic infections are granulomatous processes that follow tuberculosis or mycotic infections. Active infection requires treatment with antituberculosis or antifungal agents. With progressive cases of chronic infection, the granulomatous process within the mediastinal lymph nodes may compress adjacent structures, such as the vena cava, trachea, bronchi, or esophagus. Of the mycotic infections, histoplasmosis has the greatest predilection for severe involvement of the mediastinal lymph nodes. Active *Histoplasma* infections are treated with itraconazole in the immunocompetent patient and amphotericin B in the immunocompromised patient. Rarely, surgical decompression, excision, or bypass is necessary in addition to medical therapy to alleviate obstructive symptoms.

HEMORRHAGE

Mediastinal hemorrhage is most frequently caused by blunt or penetrating trauma, thoracic aortic dissection, rup-

ture of aortic aneurysm, or surgical procedures within the thorax. Spontaneous mediastinal hemorrhage is a recognized entity with predisposing factors related to the following: (1) complication of a mediastinal mass, of which thymoma, malignant germ cell tumor, parathyroid adenoma, retrosternal thyroid, and teratoma are the most common; (2) sudden sustained hypertension; (3) altered hemostasis due to anticoagulant therapy, thrombolytic therapy, uremia, hepatic insufficiency, or hemophilia; and (4) transient, sharp increases in intrathoracic pressure, which occur during coughing or vomiting, an entity initially described by Epstein and Klassen in 1959.[16] The pathophysiology of this disorder is thought to be associated with rupture of small mediastinal vessels. Usually, the clinical course is benign with resolution of symptoms without long-term sequelae.

The clinical presentation varies with the underlying etiology. Retrosternal pain radiating to the back or neck is common. With increased accumulation of blood in the mediastinum, signs and symptoms related to compression of mediastinal structures (primarily the great veins) develop, including dyspnea, venous distention, cyanosis, and cervical ecchymosis due to blood dissecting into soft tissue planes. Sufficient accumulation of blood causes mediastinal tamponade manifested by tachycardia, hypotension, reduced urinary output, equalization of right- and left-sided cardiac filling pressures, and diastolic collapse of the right ventricle. The development of mediastinal tamponade is more insidious than pericardial tamponade because of the larger volume of the mediastinum. Diagnostic measures include chest films, which may indicate superior mediastinal widening, loss of the normal aortic contour, and soft tissue density in the anterosuperior mediastinum; echocardiography; and CT scanning, which may better characterize a mass and its relationship to vascular structures, particularly if a false lumen is present. Arteriography may be useful in localizing the site of bleeding or intimal disruption. Therapy is directed toward evacuation of existing clot and repairing the underlying process. In patients who have suffered penetrating trauma with associated profound hypotension, emergency thoracotomy or sternotomy is indicated without initial arteriography.

SUPERIOR VENA CAVA OBSTRUCTION

A number of benign and malignant processes may cause obstruction of the superior vena cava, leading to superior vena caval syndrome. The pathophysiology of the syndrome involves the increased pressure in the venous system draining into the superior vena cava, producing the characteristic features of the syndrome, which include edema of the head, neck, and upper extremities; distended neck veins with dilated collateral veins over the upper extremities and torso; cyanosis; headache; and confusion. These findings are initially noted and remain more prominent when the patient is in a recumbent position. However, they are usually present to some extent even when the patient is upright. With processes that slowly cause obstruction, these features develop insidiously. However, with rapid or sudden occlusion, the clinical presentation is often striking, with rapid development of cerebral edema and intracranial thrombosis, which may lead to coma and death.

Superior vena caval obstruction may arise from compression, invasion, or thrombosis. The cause may be the primary tumor or mass or is often due to paratracheal lymph node metastases. Whereas in adults the most frequent cause is a malignant neoplasm, usually a bronchogenic carcinoma, in children the syndrome is most common after cardiac surgical procedures, particularly atrial level repairs for transposition of the great vessels. Malignant germ cell tumors and thymomas, lymphomas, and primary mediastinal carcinomas as well as metastatic lesions are the common malignant causes. In less than 25% of adults with superior vena caval obstruction is the cause benign. A large number of benign processes have been implicated, including mediastinal granulomatous diseases (particularly histoplasmosis and tuberculosis), idiopathic mediastinal fibrosis, mediastinal goiter, bronchogenic cyst, teratoma, pleural calcification, and thoracic aortic aneurysm. Superior vena caval obstruction secondary to indwelling catheters or trauma to the vessel when placing the catheter has become more common. However, rarely does the superior vena caval syndrome result.

Contrast medium–enhanced CT scanning or magnetic resonance imaging (MRI) is usually adequate to establish the diagnosis of superior vena caval obstruction and to assist in the differential diagnosis of probable cause. Although venous angiography is rarely required to establish the diagnosis, it does provide more accurate anatomic detail regarding the site of obstruction and collateral development, which is necessary if surgical bypass is required.

Rarely are the malignant processes responsible for the superior vena caval syndrome surgically resectable. Percutaneous needle biopsy is usually the initial diagnostic modality used to establish a histologic diagnosis, which is attempted before the initiation of empirical therapy because of the alteration of the morphologic appearance after therapy. In 42% of patients receiving prebiopsy radiation in one series, a histologic diagnosis could not be established.[28] Open biopsy in patients able to tolerate anesthesia may be necessary to establish a diagnosis. However, these patients are at an increased risk for cardiorespiratory compromise during general anesthesia. Preoperative screening and intraoperative management are discussed in a later section.

The most useful types of therapy include irradiation, corticosteroid therapy, and multiagent chemotherapy. The optimal therapeutic regimen is dependent on the histologic diagnosis. In patients in whom the syndrome develops rapidly or when neurologic symptoms are present, therapy may be necessary on an emergency basis. Improved success in the treatment of a number of the malignant causes of the superior vena caval syndrome has evolved, particularly with the lymphomas and germ cell tumors. Even when treating obstruction secondary to bronchogenic carcinoma, at least transient decompression can usually be obtained.

Historically, surgical bypass of obstructing lesions was associated with poor patency and high morbidity and mortality. In well-selected patients, bypass procedures using spiral vein grafts or polytetrafluoroethylene grafts have had acceptable patency rates.[12, 13] Of particular importance for success is the presence of adequate flow through either of the innominate veins, which is often not present when long-standing obstruction has induced collateral development. Although long-term survival is rarely possible in patients with bronchogenic carcinoma after resection with vascular reconstruction, in selected patients with primary mediastinal tumors 5-year survival of 60% is reported.[12] The usual approach to these mediastinal tumors is by means of a median sternotomy. Cross-clamping the superior vena cava is well tolerated if prior intravenous volume loading is performed. Heparin is administered before clamping. An 18- to 20-mm. polytetrafluoroethylene graft is suitable for superior vena cava replacement, while stented polytetrafluoroethylene graft between 10 and 14 mm. is preferable for replacement of the brachiocephalic vein. Postoperative anticoagulation for at least 6 months with warfarin (Coumadin) is recommended.

Superior vena caval syndromes that are caused by benign disease usually respond to medical therapy consisting of diuretics, upright positioning, and fluid restriction until collateral channels develop and allow clinical regression.

PRIMARY NEOPLASMS AND CYSTS

A large number of neoplasms and cysts may arise from multiple anatomic sites in the mediastinum and present as myriad clinical signs and symptoms. The natural history varies from those that are asymptomatic, to those with benign slow growth causing minimal symptoms, to aggressive, invasive neoplasms that are often widely metastatic, rapidly resulting in death. An increase in the number of patients diagnosed with a primary mediastinal mass has occurred. With improvements in treatment modalities, the observation of a mediastinal mass, except in rare circumstances, cannot be justified. A classification of primary mediastinal tumors and cysts is shown in Table 52–1. The relative incidence with which they occur in a series of 2431 patients is shown in Table 52–2. Although differences in the relative incidence of neoplasms and cysts exist in some series, the most common mediastinal masses are neurogenic tumors (20%), thymomas (19%), primary cysts (21%), lymphomas (13%), and germ cell tumors (10%).

Mediastinal masses are most frequently located in the anterosuperior mediastinum (54%), with the posterior (26%) and middle mediastinum (20%) being less frequently involved. Many of the mediastinal lesions occur in characteristic sites within the mediastinum. The masses that occur most commonly in each of the three anatomic subdivisions and the relative incidence with which they occurred in a series of 441 patients from the Duke University Medical Center are shown in Table 52–3. In the anterosuperior mediastinum, the most frequent neoplasms are thymoma (31%), lymphoma (23%), and germ cell tumor (17%). Posterior mediastinal lesions are usually neurogenic tumors (52%), bronchogenic cysts (22%), and enteric cysts (7%). Middle mediastinal masses are usually pericardial cysts (35%), lymphomas (21%), and bronchogenic cysts (15%). Because of the characteristic location of many

TABLE 52–1. Classification of Primary Mediastinal Tumors and Cysts

Neurogenic tumors	Mesenchymal tumors
Neurofibroma	Fibroma/fibrosarcoma
Neurilemoma	Lipoma/liposarcoma
Neurosarcoma	Leiomyoma/leiomyosarcoma
Ganglioneuroma	Rhabdosarcoma
Neuroblastoma	Xanthogranuloma
Chemodectoma	Myxoma
Paraganglioma	Mesothelioma
	Hemangioma
Thymoma	Hemangioendothelioma
Benign	Hemangiopericytoma
Malignant	Lymphangioma
	Lymphangiomyoma
Lymphoma	Lymphangiopericytoma
Hodgkin's disease	
Lymphoblastic	Endocrine tumors
Large cell diffuse growth	Intrathoracic thyroid
pattern	Parathyroid adenoma/carcinoma
T immunoblastic sarcoma	Carcinoid
B immunoblastic sarcoma	
Sclerosing follicular cell	Cysts
	Bronchogenic
Germ cell tumors	Pericardial
Teratodermoid	Enteric
Benign	Thymic
Malignant	Thoracic duct
Seminoma	Nonspecific
Nonseminomas	
Embryonal	Giant lymph node hyperplasia
Choriocarcinoma	Castleman's disease
Endodermal	
	Chondroma
Primary carcinomas	
	Extramedullary hematopoiesis

TABLE 52–2. Primary Mediastinal Tumors and Cysts in 2431 Patients

Type of Tumor	Sabiston and Scott 1952	Heimburger et al. 1963	Burkell et al. 1969	Fontanelle et al. 1971	Benjamin et al. 1971	Conkle and Adkins 1972	Rubush et al. 1973
Neurogenic tumor	20	21	13	17	49	8	36
Thymoma	17	10	12	17	34	11	42
Lymphoma	11	9	12	16	32	10	14
Germ cell neoplasm	9	10	3	7	27	2	14
Primary carcinoma	10	11	0	2	0	10	3
Mesenchymal tumor	1	4	4	0	24	2	10
Endocrine tumor	2	8	4	0	24	0	13
Other	14	0	0	0	0	0	0
Cysts	17	24	13	23	19	0	21
Pericardial	2	4	4	2	3	0	10
Bronchogenic	5	12	9	13	11	0	6
Enteric	2	5	0	4	1	0	2
Other	8	3	0	4	4	0	3
Total	101	97	61	82	209	43	153

mediastinal masses, the site of the mass establishes a useful differential diagnosis that aids in planning the diagnostic evaluation and possible operative procedure. In addition, the location of the mass explains some of the typical symptoms related to a mediastinal mass because of compression or invasion of adjacent mediastinal structures. Anterosuperior mediastinal masses are most likely to produce the superior vena caval syndrome; middle mediastinal masses are most likely to cause tamponade; and posterior mediastinal masses are most likely to cause spinal cord compression syndromes. The common symptoms related to mechanical involvement with mediastinal structures are listed in Table 52–4.

Malignant neoplasms represent 25% to 42% of mediastinal masses. Lymphomas, thymomas, germ cell tumors, primary carcinomas, and neurogenic tumors are the most common. The relative frequency of mediastinal mass malignancy varies with the anatomic site in the mediastinum. Anterosuperior masses are most likely malignant (59%), relative to middle mediastinal masses (29%) and posterior mediastinal masses (16%). The relative percentage of lesions that are malignant also varies with age (Fig. 52–3). Patients in the second through fourth decades of life have a greater proportion of malignant mediastinal masses. This period corresponds with the peak incidence of lymphomas and germ cell tumors. In contrast, in the first decade of life, a mediastinal mass is most likely benign (73%).

The incidence of mediastinal masses varies in infants, children, and adults. In a series of 838 children with mediastinal masses (Table 52–5), neurogenic tumors (34%), lymphomas (29%), germ cell tumors (10%), and primary cysts (15%) were diagnosed most frequently. The neurogenic tumors in children most commonly originate from sympathetic ganglion cells, gangliomas, ganglioneuroblastomas, and neuroblastomas. In contrast, neurilemomas and neurofibromas are the most common neurogenic tumors in adults. The childhood lymphomas are usually of a non-Hodgkin variety. The germ cell tumors are most frequently benign teratomas. Pericardial cysts and thymomas are uncommon in children.

Clinical Features

The clinical presentation varies from those patients who are asymptomatic (the diagnosis is made by routine chest film), to those with symptoms related to mechanical effects of invasion or compression, to those who have systemic symptoms. Of patients with a mediastinal mass, 56% to 65% are symptomatic at presentation. Patients with a benign le-

sion are more often asymptomatic (54%) than are patients with a malignant neoplasm (15%). The absence of symptoms is associated with a benign histologic diagnosis. In asymptomatic patients with a mediastinal mass at the Duke University Medical Center during the past 20 years, 76% had a benign lesion. In contrast, 62% of symptomatic patients had a malignant neoplasm during this period. The most common features in a series of 441 patients were chest pain, cough, and fever (Table 52–6). Infants and children are more likely to present with symptoms or findings (78%) because of the relatively small space within the mediastinum.[24] Paralleling the relative percentages of malignant neoplasms within the different anatomic regions, tumors of the anterosuperior mediastinum are most likely to cause symptoms (75%) relative to the posterior mediastinum (50%) and the middle mediastinum (45%).

Symptoms related to compression or invasion of mediastinal structures, such as the superior vena caval syndrome, Horner's syndrome, hoarseness, and severe pain, are more indicative of a malignant histologic diagnosis, although patients with a benign lesion, on occasion, present in this manner.

A number of primary mediastinal lesions produce hor-

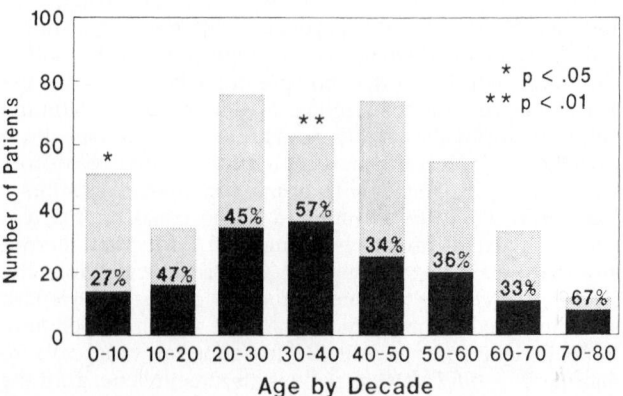

Figure 52–3. Age distribution and incidence of malignancy relative to age. The largest number of patients with a mediastinal mass were in the third through fifth decades. The fourth decade had a significantly greater proportion of malignant disease. The first decade had a significantly lower proportion of malignant disease. (From Davis, R. D., Jr., Oldham, H. N., Jr., and Sabiston, D. C., Jr.: Primary cysts and neoplasms of the mediastinum: Recent changes in clinical presentation, methods of diagnosis, management, and results. Ann. Thorac. Surg., 44:229, 1987.)

TABLE 52–2. Primary Mediastinal Tumors and Cysts in 2431 Patients *Continued*

Vidne and Levy 1973	Ovrum and Birkeland 1979	Nandi et al. 1980	Adkins et al. 1984	Parish et al. 1984	Duke Medical Center 1988	Total	Incidence
9	19	27	8	212	61	500	21%
9	10	18	4	206	68	458	19%
6	11	4	7	107	75	314	13%
3	5	7	11	99	44	241	10%
2	9	0	5	25	37	114	5%
4	4	2	0	60	29	144	6%
2	21	6	2	56	13	151	6%
1	2	1	1	36	10	65	3%
8	10	9	0	196	104	444	18%
2	7	2	0	72	37	145	6%
2	0	0	0	54	39	151	6%
1	0	0	0	29	11	55	2%
3	3	7	0	41	17	93	4%
44	91	74	38	997	441	2431	

mones or antibodies that cause systemic symptoms, which may characterize a specific syndrome (Table 52–7). Examples of these syndromes include Cushing's syndrome, caused by ectopic production of adrenocorticotropic hormone (ACTH), most frequently by carcinoid tumors; thyrotoxicosis, which is caused by a mediastinal goiter; hypertension and a hyperdynamic state caused by pheochromocytoma; and hypercalcemia secondary to increased parathyroid hormone release from a mediastinal parathyroid adenoma.

In other syndromes, the pathophysiology is not as well understood (Table 52–8), such as the association of large mesenchymal tumors with episodic hypoglycemia, presumably related to production of circulating factors capable of insulin-like action or of releasing insulin (Doege-Potter syndrome). Autoimmune mechanisms have been implicated in the association of myasthenia gravis and red cell aplasia with thymoma. In other cases the pathophysiology is less defined: osteoarthropathy and neurogenic tumors; pain after ingestion of alcohol and the cyclic Pel-Ebstein fevers associated with Hodgkin's disease; and the opsomyoclonus syndrome and neuroblastoma.

Diagnosis

The goal of the diagnostic evaluation in a patient with a mediastinal mass is a precise histologic diagnosis so that optimal therapy can be performed. The preoperative evaluation of a patient with a mediastinal mass should achieve the following: (1) differentiate a primary mediastinal mass from masses of other causes that have a similar radiographic appearance; (2) recognize associated systemic manifestations that may affect the patient's perioperative course; (3) evaluate for possible compression by the mass of the tracheobronchial tree, pulmonary artery, or superior vena cava; (4) ascertain whether the mass extends into the spinal column; (5) determine if the mass is a nonseminomatous germ cell tumor; (6) assess the likelihood of resectability; and (7) identify significant factors of medical comorbidity and optimize overall medical condition.

The initial diagnostic intervention should be a careful history and physical examination. The recognition of associated

TABLE 52–3. Anatomic Location of Primary Tumors and Cysts of the Mediastinum

Type of Tumor or Cyst	Percentage
Anterosuperior Mediastinum (n = 245)	
Thymic neoplasms	31%
Lymphomas	23%
Germ cell tumors	17%
Benign	9%
Malignant	8%
Carcinoma	13%
Cysts	6%
Mesenchymal	4%
Endocrine	5%
Other	1%
Middle Mediastinum (n = 83)	
Cysts	61%
Lymphomas	20%
Mesenchymal	8%
Carcinoma	6%
Other	5%
Posterior Mediastinum (n = 113)	
Neurogenic	52%
Benign	40%
Malignant	12%
Cysts	32%
Mesenchymal	10%
Endocrine	2%
Other	4%

TABLE 52–4. Clinical Manifestations of Anatomic Compression or Invasion by Neoplasms of the Mediastinum

Vena caval obstruction
Pericardial tamponade
Congestive heart failure
Dysrhythmias
Pulmonary stenosis
Tracheal compression
Esophageal compression
Vocal cord paralysis
Horner's syndrome
Phrenic nerve paralysis
Chylothorax
Chylopericardium
Spinal cord compressive syndrome
Pancoast's syndrome
Postobstructive pneumonitis

TABLE 52–5. Primary Mediastinal Tumors and Cysts in Children

Type of Tumor	Haller et al. 1969	Grosfeld et al. 1971	Whitaker and Lynn 1973	Pokorny and Sherman 1974	Heimburger and Batersby 1965	Bower and Kiesewetter 1977	King et al. 1982	Duke Medical Center 1988	Total	Incidence (%)
Neurogenic tumor	18	36	37	35	9	41	48	26	250	35
Lymphoma	9	20	9	27	3	12	87	13	180	25
Germ cell neoplasm	8	5	21	4	4	5	17	11	75	10
Primary carcinoma	10	0	0	6	0	0	0	1	17	2
Mesenchymal tumor	7	1	13	8	6	7	22	5	69	10
Other	0	0	0	0	0	6	4	6	16	2
Cysts	11	6	14	17	10	22	10	26	116	16
Pericardial	1	0	0	0	0	1	0	3	5	1
Bronchogenic	4	0	5	11	8	6	6	14	54	7
Enteric	6	6	7	3	2	11	2	5	42	6
Other	0	0	2	3	0	4	2	4	15	2
Total	63	68	94	97	32	93	188	88	723	100

systemic syndromes with many mediastinal neoplasms is necessary to avoid potentially serious intraoperative and postoperative complications. Although the majority of systemic syndromes listed in Table 52–8 may be of little consequence regarding the planned surgical management, the association of myasthenia gravis, malignant hypertension, hypogammaglobulinemia, hypercalcemia, and thyrotoxicosis with mediastinal neoplasms markedly impacts on appropriate management.

The posteroanterior and lateral chest films provide important information: location within the mediastinum, size of the lesion, displacement and alteration of anatomic structures in the mediastinum and adjacent regions, and the relative density of the mass with regard to whether the lesion is cystic or solid, whether calcifications are present, and the pattern of the calcifications. Information regarding the anatomic location of the mediastinal mass narrows the differential diagnosis. CT scanning with contrast medium enhancement should be obtained in the majority of patients with a mediastinal mass. In patients with a contraindication to the use of contrast dye, or in those patients with surgical clips in the anatomic region of interest, MRI is useful. Accurate anatomic information regarding the relationship of the mass to surrounding structures is provided. Considerable information can be obtained regarding the relative invasiveness and malignant nature of the mediastinal mass. Tumor disruption of fat planes, irregularity of pleural, vascular, or pericardial margins by tumor, and infiltration into muscle or periosteum are useful for differentiating tumor compression from invasion. Resectability is better assessed than nonresectability using CT or MRI. Additional information obtained using CT

includes the presence of chest wall invasion, differentiation of multiple masses from a single large mass (useful in differentiating lymphomas from other common solitary lesions), and possible extension from a posterior mediastinal mass into the spinal column. These posterior mediastinal masses should be further evaluated with CT-myelography or MRI.

CT or MRI reliably differentiates mediastinal tumors from mediastinal masses that are of a cardiovascular cause, such as aneurysm, dilation, and abnormal location of cardiac or vascular structures, and that may appear on a chest film as a mediastinal mass (Table 52–9). Similarly, abnormalities of the spinal column, such as meningoceles, are differentiated from neurogenic tumors and other posterior mediastinal masses. This differentiation is particularly important in patients with neurofibromatosis, who are at a greater risk for the development of both meningoceles and neurofibromas. CT or MRI will also differentiate other entities that may resemble a mediastinal mass, including esophageal lesions (e.g., esophageal diverticula, tumor, hiatal hernia, and achalasia), diaphragmatic herniations, pancreatic pseudocysts, herniations of peritoneal fat, mediastinitis, and a number of primary pulmonary parenchymal lesions and infections.

Several mediastinal masses can be diagnosed preoperatively using these imaging modalities based on their characteristic location, appearance, and attenuation values. For example, pericardial cysts usually occur at the cardiophrenic angle; they have smooth, circumscribed borders, and they have near-water attenuation values. Despite the accuracy of CT scanning, a precise histologic diagnosis is necessary to avoid mistreating a potentially curable neoplasm. Using CT, the correct preoperative diagnosis is made in only approximately 68% of patients.[36] Although CT scanning is sensitive in the evaluation of mediastinal masses and lymphadenopa-

TABLE 52–6. Presenting Symptoms in Patients with a Mediastinal Mass

Symptoms	Percentage of Patients (n = 441)
Chest pain	29%
Dyspnea	22%
Cough	18%
Fever	13%
Weight loss	9%
Superior vena caval syndrome	8%
Myasthenia gravis	7%
Fatigue	6%
Dysphagia	4%
Night sweats	3%

TABLE 52–7. Systemic Syndromes Caused by Mediastinal Neoplasm Hormone Production

Syndrome	Tumor
Hypertension	Pheochromocytoma, chemodectoma, ganglioneuroma, neuroblastoma
Hypoglycemia	Mesothelioma, teratoma, fibrosarcoma, neurosarcoma
Diarrhea	Ganglioneuroma, neuroblastoma, neurofibroma
Hypercalcemia	Parathyroid adenoma/carcinoma, Hodgkin's disease
Thyrotoxicosis	Thyroid adenoma/carcinoma
Gynecomastia	Nonseminomatous germ cell tumors

TABLE 52–8. Systemic Syndromes Associated with Mediastinal Neoplasms

Tumor	Syndrome
Thymoma	Myasthenia gravis
	Red blood cell aplasia
	White blood cell aplasia
	Aplastic anemia
	Hypogammaglobulinemia
	Progressive systemic sclerosis
	Hemolytic anemia
	Megaesophagus
	Dermatomyositis
	Systemic lupus erythematosus
	Myocarditis
	Collagen vascular disease
Lymphoma	Anemia, myasthenia gravis
Neurofibroma	von Recklinghausen's disease
Carcinoid	Cushing's syndrome
Carcinoid, thymoma	Multiple endocrine adenomatosis
Thymoma, neurofibroma, neurilemoma, mesothelioma	Osteoarthropathy
Enteric cysts	Vertebral anomalies
Hodgkin's disease	Alcohol-induced pain
	Pel-Ebstein fever
Neuroblastoma	Opsomyoclonus
	Erythrocyte abnormalities
Enteric cysts	Peptic ulcer

thy, it is not specific for tumor involvement. A histologic examination of abnormal mediastinal lymph nodes (>1.5 cm.) determined by CT scanning in patients with known malignancies demonstrates that in more than one third of patients the lymph node was benign.[11]

Echocardiography may be useful in the evaluation of mediastinal masses, especially tumors that occur in the middle mediastinum, or in patients with tamponade or pulmonary stenosis. Echocardiography delineates the cystic nature of lesions, and it has been used to guide needle biopsy, especially with lesions adjacent to the chest wall. Although echocardiography is not as sensitive as MRI or CT, it is useful in determining the physiologic effect of tumor involvement of the pericardium, heart, or great vessels.

Serologic evaluation is indicated in certain patients. Male patients with an anterosuperior mediastinal mass in the second through fifth decades should have alpha-fetoprotein and beta-human chorionic gonadotropin (beta-hCG) serologies obtained. A positive serology is indicative of a nonseminomatous germ cell tumor. Appropriate treatment with cisplatin-

TABLE 52–9. Diagnostic Evaluation of Mediastinal Masses

History	Ultrasonography
Physical examination	Radioisotope scanning
Radiology	Serology
Standard chest films	Endoscopy
Tomography	Bronchoscopy
Barium swallow	Needle aspiration and biopsy
Fluoroscopy	Operative procedures
Arteriography	Mediastinoscopy
Venography	Mediastinotomy
Computed tomography	Thoracotomy
Magnetic resonance imaging	
Myelography	

based chemotherapy may be initiated without surgical exploration.

Patients with a mediastinal mass and a history of significant hypertension or hypermetabolism should have measurement of urinary excretion of vanillylmandelic acid and catecholamines. This enables the initiation of appropriate perioperative adrenergic blockers in patients with hormonally active intrathoracic pheochromocytoma, paraganglioma, and neuroblastoma, limiting perioperative complications secondary to episodic catecholamine release. In these patients, nuclear scans using *meta*-iodobenzylguanidine (MIBG) are useful in tumor location and in identifying sites of metastatic disease, particularly when located in the middle mediastinum.

Asymptomatic patients with contrast-enhancing lesions in the superior mediastinum should be evaluated with an iodine-131 scan. In an asymptomatic patient with a positive scan indicative of a thyroid lesion and no identifiable active thyroid tissue elsewhere, careful observation without excision using serial CT scans to evaluate for growth is indicated.

Increased success has been reported in making a cytologic diagnosis preoperatively by using fine-needle biopsy techniques (22-gauge needle) with low morbidity and almost no mortality. Fluoroscopic visualization is usually used to guide the biopsy. CT and echocardiography, because of better localization of the mass and improved placement of the needle, have increased the sensitivity of the technique. Although a cytologic diagnosis of benign or malignant differentiation between masses can be made in approximately 90% of patients, a precise histologic diagnosis is not always possible in 20% to 40% of patients. Obtaining core biopsy specimens using cutting needles increases the accuracy of the precise histologic diagnosis and differentiation between benign and malignant lesions. Core biopsy techniques particularly are useful in the diagnosis of lymphomas, thymomas, and neural tumors.[30] Complications related to the procedure include pneumothorax in 20% to 25% of patients, with approximately 5% requiring tube thoracostomy; hemoptysis in 5% to 10%, with rare occurrences of significant hemorrhagic complications; and tumor seeding along the needle tract, which is a theoretical but extremely rare complication. Needle biopsy techniques are particularly useful for evaluating patients in which excisional therapy is not indicated. The use of electron microscopy to examine the cellular ultrastructure and immunohistochemical staining has increased the sensitivity of the various needle biopsy techniques. Needle biopsy techniques have limited yield in tumors with marked associated desmoplastic reaction, such as nodular-sclerosing Hodgkin's lymphoma. Additionally, needle biopsy rarely provides adequate tissue for precise immunotyping, which is necessary to determine optimal therapy, particularly with non-Hodgkin's lymphomas.

Poorly differentiated malignant tumors of the anterosuperior mediastinum, particularly thymomas, lymphomas, germ cell tumors, and primary carcinomas, can have remarkably similar cytologic and morphologic appearances. In addition to light microscopy using special staining techniques, immunostaining techniques and electron microscopy of multiple sections of the tumor may be necessary to establish an accurate diagnosis. The characteristic ultrastructural features as evaluated by electron microscopy are shown in Table 52–10. Monoclonal antibodies for surface antigens specific to a cell line of origin and for tumor-secretory products can be useful in establishing a precise diagnosis. Chromosomal analysis of tumor tissue is often useful at differentiating histology.[31] With poorly differentiated tumors, diagnoses based on examination of frozen sections may be incorrect, which can result in improper treatment. Immunotyping of non-Hodgkin's lymphomas has allowed accurate subtyping of these lesions,

TABLE 52–10. Ultrastructural Characteristics of Mediastinal Tumors

Tumors	Ultrastructure
Carcinoid	Dense core granules, fewer tonofilaments and desmosomes
Lymphoma	Absence of junctional attachments and epithelial features
Thymoma	Well-formed desmosomes, bundles of tonofilaments
Germ cell	Prominent nucleoli, even chromatin, scant desmosomes, rare tonofilaments
Neuroblastoma	Neurosecretory granules, synaptic endings

which has been important in predicting natural history and optimal therapy.

When needle biopsy techniques are contraindicated or do not produce sufficient tissue for the histologic diagnosis, more invasive procedures are often required, such as mediastinoscopy, mediastinotomy, thoracoscopy, thoracotomy, and median sternotomy. Mediastinoscopy is a useful technique to evaluate and biopsy lesions of the middle mediastinum, particularly those located in the anterior aspect of the subcarinal space, around the proximal mainstem bronchi, and around the lower trachea. Often this technique is used to evaluate associated lymphadenopathy in these particular regions. Lesions in the anterosuperior mediastinum that are unresectable are best biopsied using a limited anterior second or third interspace parasternal mediastinotomy or using thoracoscopy. Similarly, unresectable lesions in the superior mediastinum, hilar, or paratracheal regions can be sampled through a small lateral thoracotomy in the third or fourth interspace after retracting the apex of the lung inferiorly. Unresectable posterior mediastinal masses may be approached through a limited posterolateral thoracotomy. A representative section of the tissue obtained should be submitted for immediate frozen section to establish adequacy of the biopsy before closing. Importantly, the incision should not be made in the portals for potential radiation therapy. Lesions that appear resectable should be excised. Median sternotomy and anterolateral thoracotomy provide optimal exposure for lesions in the anterosuperior mediastinum. A transcervical approach using sternal elevators has been successfully used to resect tumors in the superior aspect of the anterosuperior mediastinum. Middle and posterior mediastinal masses are usually best excised through a posterolateral thoracotomy. Thoracoscopic and thoracoscopically assisted procedures have been used to sample and resect a variety of mediastinal lesions in carefully selected patients.

Although most patients undergo surgical procedures safely, patients with large anterosuperior or middle mediastinal masses, particularly children, have an increased risk of developing severe cardiorespiratory complications during general anesthesia. Exacerbation of superior vena caval obstruction or extrinsic airway compression occurs during general anesthesia because of (1) the loss of negative intrathoracic pressure during respiration, (2) bronchial smooth muscle relaxation that increases the compressibility of the bronchi, and (3) reduced tidal volumes used for ventilation. Patients with posture-related dyspnea and superior vena caval syndrome are at increased risk. Patients with a reduction in tracheal cross-sectional area of more than 35% as assessed by CT scanning or a reduction in peak expiratory flow assessed by pulmonary flow mechanics are at risk for airway compression.[2] In patients with airway compression or superior vena caval obstruction, the risk of general anesthesia is markedly increased and attempts to obtain a histologic

diagnosis should be limited to needle biopsies or open procedures done with local anesthesia. If a histologic diagnosis cannot be obtained, treatment with radiation, corticosteroids, and, when appropriate, chemotherapy based on a presumptive diagnosis is initiated. When such treatment is necessary before biopsy, a histologic diagnosis may not be obtainable in as many as 40% of patients. The majority of these lesions are malignant and unresectable. Occasionally, benign tumors, usually benign teratomas in young children and infants, may produce this clinical setting. In patients with large mediastinal masses who have an increased anesthetic risk but in whom a histologic diagnosis is needed before therapy, or for whom complete excision is the preferred treatment, recommendations for anesthetic management include (1) fiberoptic evaluation of the tracheobronchial system for evidence of severe extrinsic compression, (2) induction of anesthesia in a semi-Fowler position with the ability to change to the lateral or prone positions, (3) use of long endotracheal tubes to allow advancement of the tube beyond the site of obstruction, (4) standby rigid bronchoscopy to allow re-establishment of an adequate airway, (5) avoidance of muscle relaxants and use of spontaneous ventilation when possible, (6) lower extremity intravenous intubation to provide access to the systemic venous circulation if a sudden superior vena caval obstruction should occur, and (7) standby cardiopulmonary bypass with bilateral groin preparation.

Neurogenic Tumors

Neurogenic tumors are the most common neoplasm, comprising 21% of all primary tumors and cysts. These tumors are usually located in the posterior mediastinum and originate from the sympathetic ganglia (ganglioma, ganglioneuroblastoma, and neuroblastoma), the intercostal nerves (neurofibroma, neurilemoma, and neurosarcoma), and the paraganglia cells (paraganglioma). Only rarely are these tumors located in the anterosuperior mediastinum. Although the peak incidence occurs in adults, neurogenic tumors comprise a proportionally greater percentage of mediastinal masses in children (34%). Whereas the majority of neurogenic tumors in adults are benign, a greater percentage of neurogenic tumors are malignant in children.

Many of these tumors are found in asymptomatic patients on routine chest films. When present, symptoms are usually caused by mechanical factors such as chest and back pain due to compression or invasion of intercostal nerve, bone, and chest wall; cough and dyspnea due to compression of the tracheobronchial tree; Pancoast's syndrome; and Horner's syndrome due to involvement of the brachial and the cervical sympathetic chain. Approximately 10% of neurogenic tumors have extensions into the spinal column. These tumors are termed *dumbbell tumors* because of their characteristic shape due to the relatively large paraspinal and intraspinal portions connected by a narrow isthmus of tissue traversing the intervertebral foramen. Although 60% of patients with a dumbbell tumor have neurologic symptoms related to spinal cord compression, the significant proportion of patients without symptoms underscores the importance of evaluating all patients with a posterior mediastinal mass for possible intraspinal extension. CT, MRI, and vertebral tomography are useful for indicating enlargement of the foramen, erosion of bone, and intervertebral widening. If these findings are present, CT-myelography or MRI is indicated to evaluate the presence and extent of the intraspinal component. The recommended surgical approach to dumbbell tumors is a one-stage excision of the intraspinal component before resecting the thoracic component to minimize any spinal column hematoma. The incision used for the posterior laminectomy is extended into the appropriate interspace to allow resection of the mediastinal component.

Symptoms may be systemic and related to production of neurohormonal agents. Production of catecholamines by paragangliomas and neuroblastomas causes the constellation of symptoms that are characteristic of pheochromocytomas: hypertension, which is often severe and episodic; sweating; headaches; and palpitations. Production of vasoactive intestinal polypeptide by ganglioneuromas and neuroblastomas causes a syndrome of abdominal distention and profuse watery diarrhea. Secretion of an insulin-like factor or insulin-releasing factor by neurosarcomas causes the Doege-Potter syndrome characterized by episodic hypoglycemia. Some neurogenic tumors can be removed by the thoracoscopic approach (Fig. 52–4).

Neuroblastoma. Neuroblastomas originate from the sympathetic nervous system and therefore can occur wherever sympathetic nervous tissue is present. The most common location for a neuroblastoma is in the retroperitoneum; however, 10% to 20% occur primarily in the mediastinum (Fig. 52–5). These are highly invasive neoplasms that have frequently metastasized before diagnosis. Common sites of metastases are the regional lymph nodes, bone, brain, liver, and lung. A majority of these tumors occur in children and 75% occur in children younger than age 4 years. The tumor is composed of small, round, immature cells organized in a rosette pattern. On ultrastructural examination, the presence of neurosecretory granules is characteristic. Patients are usually symptomatic. Paraplegia and other neurologic symptoms related to spinal cord compression were present in a third of children with mediastinal neuroblastoma in one series.[39] A variety of paraneoplastic syndromes have been reported, including profuse watery diarrhea and abdominal pain related to vasoactive intestinal polypeptide production, the opsoclonus-polymyoclonus syndrome (an unexplained symptom-complex characterized by cerebellar and truncal ataxia with rapid, darting eye movements [dancing eyes] that is possibly related to an autoimmune mechanism), and *pheochromocytoma* syndrome due to catecholamine secretion. A 24-hour urine collection to measure catecholamines should be obtained in children with a posterior mediastinal mass.

Neuroblastoma and ganglioneuroblastoma are staged as follows: Stage I—well-circumscribed, noninvasive tumor; Stage II—tumor invasion locally without extension across the midline; Stage III—tumor spread across the midline; Stage IV—tumor with metastasis. Therapy is determined by the stage of the disease: Stage I—surgical excision; Stage II—excision and radiation therapy; Stage III and IV—multimodality therapy using surgical debulking, radiation therapy, and multiagent chemotherapy, as well as a second-look exploration to resect residual disease when necessary. The usual chemotherapeutic agents used include cisplatin, doxorubicin, cyclophosphamide, and etoposide. Children younger than 1 year of age have an excellent prognosis even when widespread disease is present. However, with increasing age and extent of involvement, the prognosis worsens. N-*myc* gene amplification and, particularly, N-*myc* protein expression are associated with an unfavorable prognosis.[38] Interestingly, mediastinal neuroblastomas appear to have a better prognosis than tumor occurring elsewhere. In patients with neuroblastomas resistant to therapy or in those who relapse, ablative chemotherapy with autologous bone marrow transplantation has been attempted with some success.

Ganglioneuroblastoma. Ganglioneuroblastomas exhibit an intermediate degree of differentiation between ganglioneuromas and neuroblastomas (Fig. 52–6). They are composed of mature and immature ganglion cells. Two different histologic patterns occur: composite ganglioneuroblastoma (predominantly mature neuroblasts with focal areas containing primitive neuroblasts) and diffuse ganglioneuroblastoma (diffuse mixture of well-differentiated and primitive neuroblasts). Patients diagnosed with a composite ganglioneuroblastoma have an incidence of metastatic disease between 65% and

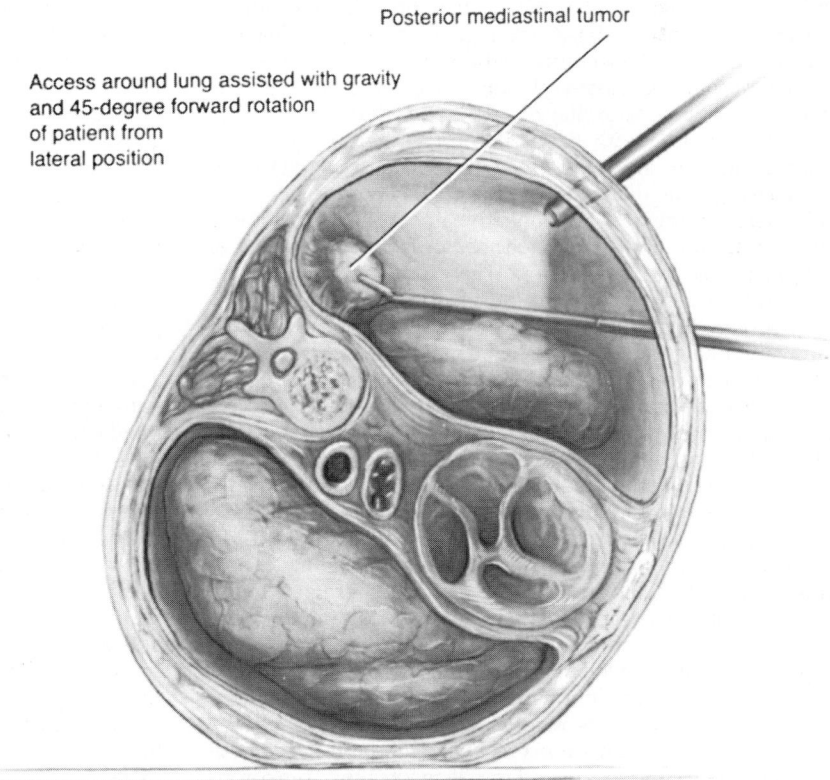

Posterior mediastinal tumor

Access around lung assisted with gravity and 45-degree forward rotation of patient from lateral position

Figure 52–4. The endoscopic dissector, scissors, and grasper can be introduced into the pleural cavity through the accessory intercostal space access sites to complete the tumor resection. The resected tumor can be put into a plastic bag and withdrawn through one of the access sites. The access site may have to be extended to allow tumor removal. Adequate hemostasis is essential. A chest tube (28 French) is inserted into the pleural cavity through the lowest access site for underwater sealed drainage. The other incisions are closed with sutures. (From Sabiston, D. C., Jr.: Atlas of Cardiothoracic Surgery. Philadelphia, W. B. Saunders, 1995, p. 560.)

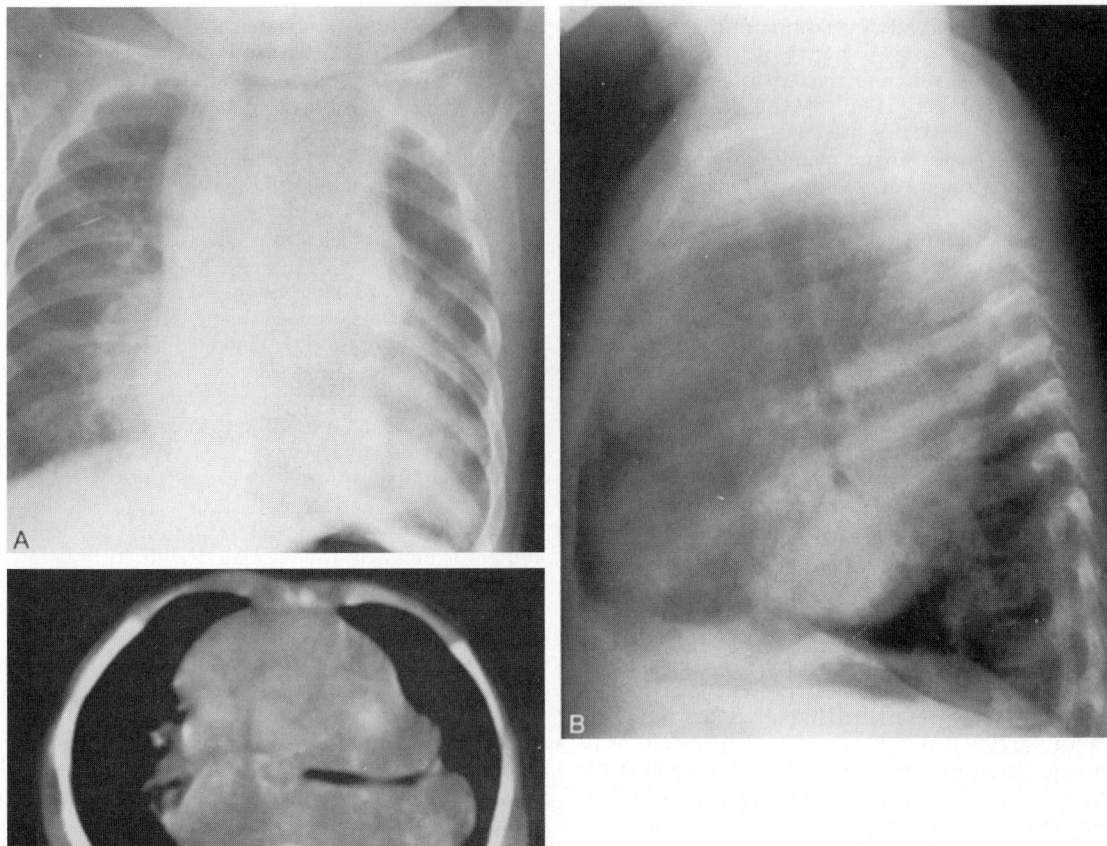

Figure 52–5. *A* and *B*, Chest films of a neuroblastoma in an 18-year-old female. *C*, CT scan demonstrates the extensive nature of the tumor.

75%. In contrast, less than 5% of patients with the diffuse variety develop metastases. Younger patients who have a diffuse histologic appearance and a lower-stage tumor have the best prognosis. Five-year survival of 88% has been reported in patients with Stage I or II disease treated solely by excision. Patients with Stage III or IV disease, composite morphology, or age older than 3 years are treated with multiagent chemotherapy.

Ganglioneuroma. Ganglioneuromas are benign tumors originating from the sympathetic chain that are composed of ganglion cells and nerve fibers. These tumors typically present at an early age and are the most common neurogenic tumors occurring during childhood. The usual location is the paravertebral region. These tumors are well encapsulated and, when cross-sectioned, they frequently exhibit areas of cystic degeneration. Surgical excision provides cure.

Neurilemoma, Neurofibroma, and Neurosarcoma. The most common neurogenic tumor is the neurilemoma, which originates from perineural Schwann's cells. These tumors are well circumscribed and have a defined capsule. There are two morphologic patterns: Antoni Type A, which has organized architecture with a cellular palisading pattern of growth, and Antoni Type B, which has a loose reticular pattern of growth. The peak incidence of these tumors is in the third through fifth decades of life.

In contrast to neurilemomas, neurofibromas are poorly encapsulated and consist of randomly arranged spindle-shaped cells. These tumors originate as a proliferation of all the elements of the peripheral nerve. Although both neurilemomas and neurofibromas occur as a manifestation of neurofi-

bromatosis (von Recklinghausen's disease), they must be differentiated from the two other common entities in the posterior mediastinum: meningioma and meningocele. With both neurilemoma and neurofibroma, surgical excision results in cure.

Neurosarcomas originate by malignant degeneration of either neurilemomas or neurofibromas, in addition to developing *de novo*. These tumors usually occur in adults. However, patients with neurofibromatosis may develop neurosarcomas as children. These are rapidly growing tumors that frequently invade vital structures, preventing attempts at resection. Unless tumor excision is possible, the prognosis is extremely poor owing to the unresponsiveness to adjuvant therapies.

Paraganglioma (Pheochromocytoma). Mediastinal paragangliomas are rare tumors, representing less than 1% of all mediastinal tumors and less than 2% of all pheochromocytomas. Although the majority are found in the paravertebral sulcus, an increasing number of middle mediastinal paragangliomas occur in the branchial arch structures, coronary and aortopulmonary paraganglia, the atria, and islands of tissue in the pericardium. The likelihood of functional activity of a paraganglioma is related to the site of origin: adrenal medulla—high likelihood; branchiomeric and intravagale—very low likelihood; and aorto-sympathetic and visceral autonomic—intermediate likelihood. Catecholamine production causes the classic constellation of symptoms associated with pheochromocytomas, including periodic or sustained hypertension, often accompanied by orthostatic hypotension, hypermetabolism manifested by weight loss, hyperhidrosis,

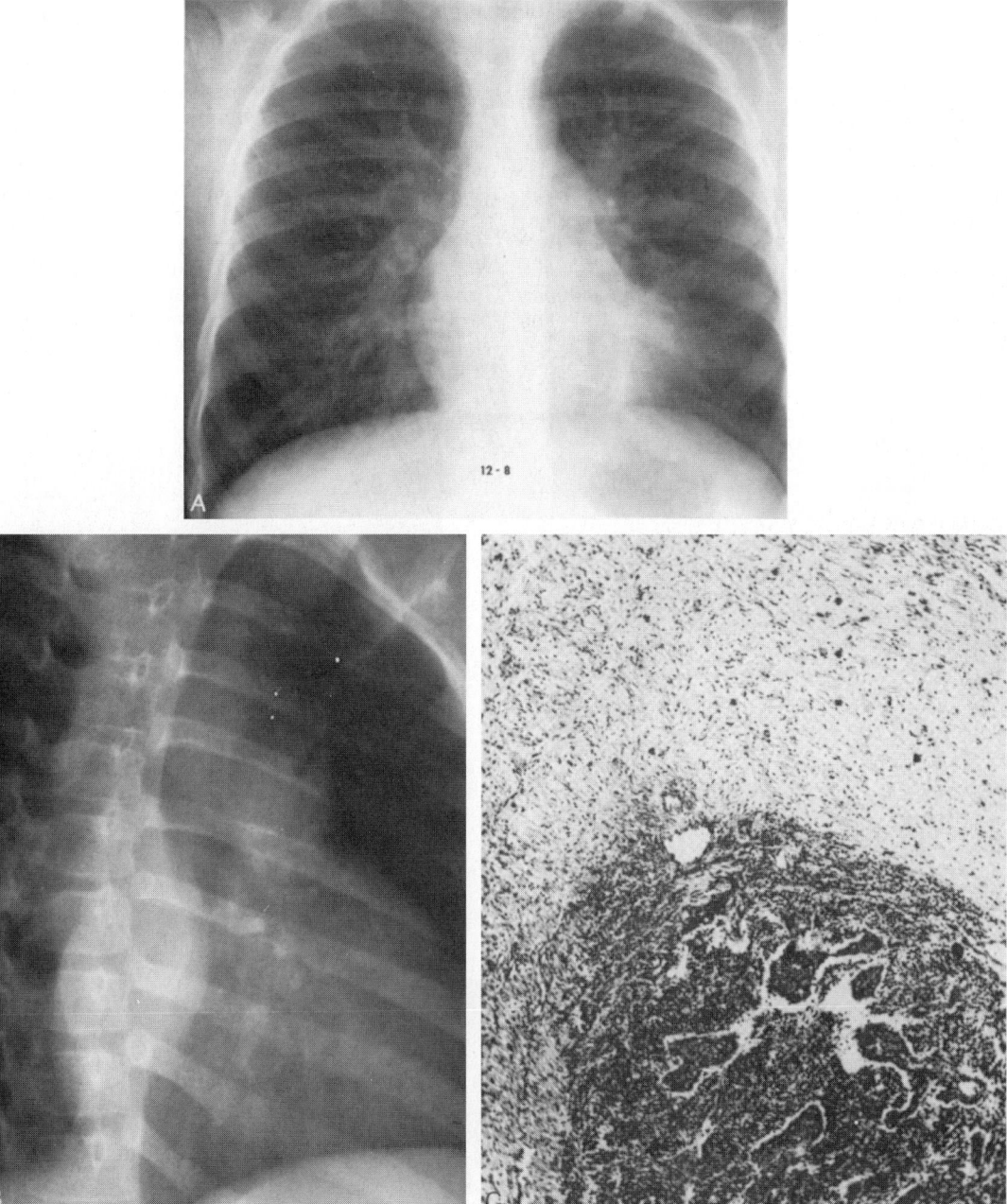

Figure 52–6. *A* and *B*, Chest films of a patient with ganglioneuroblastoma. *C*, Example of a histologic specimen demonstrating the focal area of primitive neuroblasts (arrow) characteristic of the composite ganglioneuroblastoma. (From Adam, A., and Hochholzer, L.: Ganglioneuroblastoma of the posterior mediastinum: A clinicopathologic review of 80 cases. Cancer, *47*:373, 1981. Copyright © 1981 American Cancer Society. Reprinted by permission of Wiley-Liss, Inc., a subsidiary of John Wiley & Sons, Inc.)

palpitations, and headaches. Measurement of elevated levels of urinary catecholamines or their metabolites, the metanephrines and vanillylmandelic acid, usually establishes the diagnosis. Although adrenal pheochromocytomas often produce both epinephrine and norepinephrine, extra-adrenal paragangliomas rarely secrete epinephrine.

Tumor localization has improved remarkably through the use of CT and ^{131}I-MIBG scintigraphy, particularly when the tumors are hormonally active. Hormonally active tumors may be located with an 85% sensitivity using the ^{131}I-MIBG scan. Because of the high vascularity of these lesions, enhancement with contrast medium administration occurs during CT scanning. Because of the accuracy of CT and MIBG scanning, rarely is selective venous angiography with serial sampling for catecholamine levels necessary for preoperative localization. Tumor localization using MRI has been reported.

When appropriate, surgical resection is the optimal therapy. In patients with tumors involving the middle mediastinum, cardiopulmonary bypass may be necessary to enable resection. Although 50% of tumors appear malignant morphologically, metastatic disease develops in only 3% of patients. In those with metastatic disease, alpha-methyltyramine, a tyrosine hydroxylase inhibitor that blocks the synthesis of catecholamines, is helpful in controlling symptoms.

Approximately 10% of patients have multiple paragangliomas. They are more common in patients with the multiple endocrine neoplasia syndrome, a family history of disease, and Carney's syndrome (pulmonary chondroma, gastric leiomyosarcoma, and extra-adrenal paraganglioma). In patients who have had excision of an adrenal pheochromocytoma and continue to have symptoms, a search for an extra-adrenal lesion should be undertaken, with careful attention directed to the evaluation of the mediastinum.

Thymoma

Thymoma is the most common neoplasm of the anterosuperior mediastinum and the second most common mediastinal mass (20%; see Table 52–2). The peak incidence is in the third through fifth decades but this tumor may occur throughout adulthood. Thymoma is rare in the first two decades. Roentgenographically it may appear as a small, well-circumscribed mass or a bulky lobulated mass confluent with adjacent mediastinal structures (Fig. 52–7). Patients are usually symptomatic at presentation, and symptoms may be

related to local mass effects causing chest pain, dyspnea, hemoptysis, cough, and the superior vena caval syndrome. However, thymomas frequently are associated with systemic syndromes caused by immunologic mechanisms. Although the most common syndrome is myasthenia gravis, many other syndromes have been associated with thymomas, including red cell aplasia, pure white cell aplasia, aplastic anemia, Cushing's syndrome, hypogammaglobulinemia and hypergammaglobulinemia, dermatomyositis, systemic lupus erythematosus, progressive systemic sclerosis, hypercoagulopathy with thrombosis, rheumatoid arthritis, megaesophagus, and granulomatous myocarditis.

The etiologic factors involved in these syndromes have not been fully elucidated. Myasthenia gravis is characterized

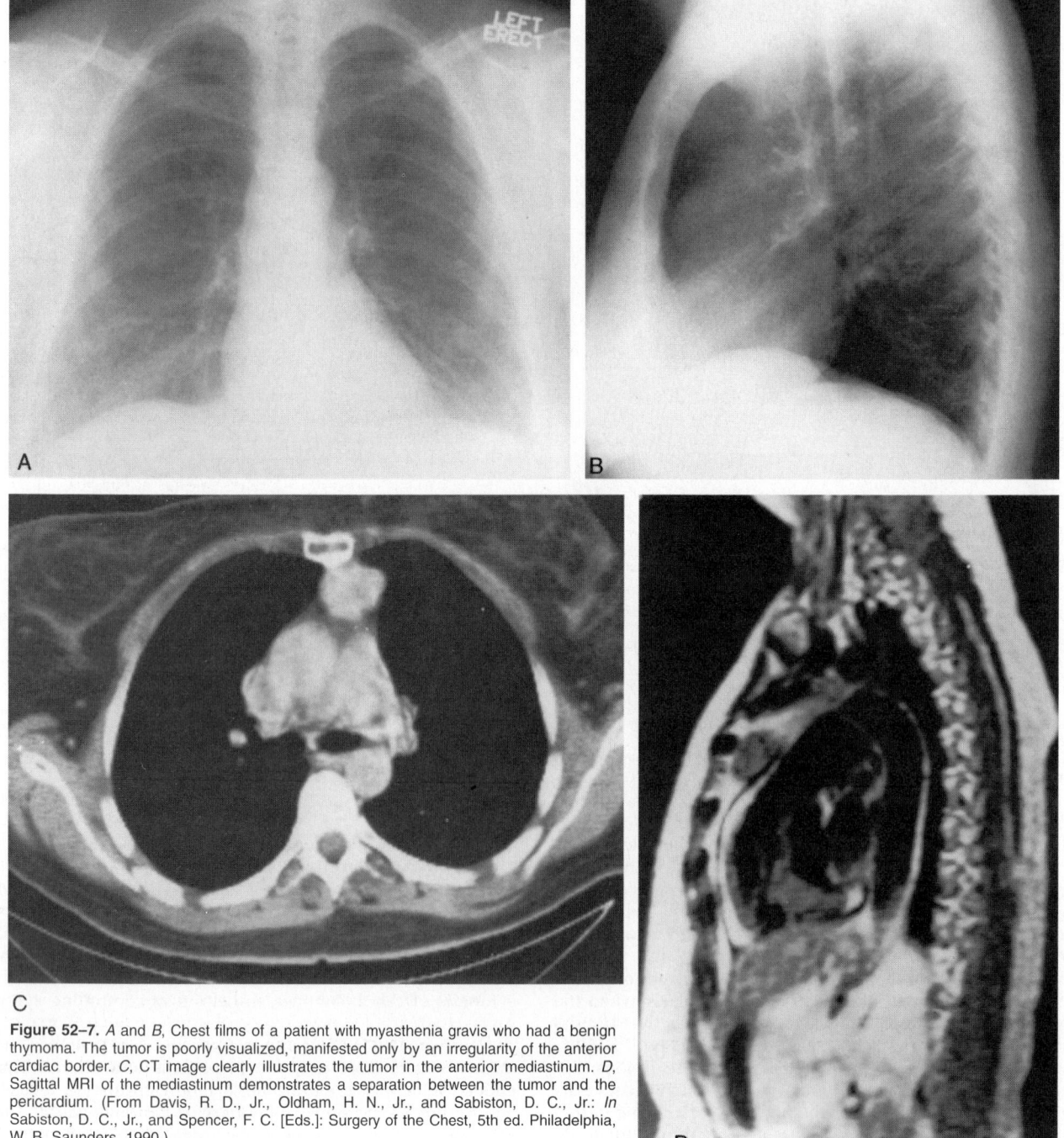

Figure 52–7. *A* and *B*, Chest films of a patient with myasthenia gravis who had a benign thymoma. The tumor is poorly visualized, manifested only by an irregularity of the anterior cardiac border. *C*, CT image clearly illustrates the tumor in the anterior mediastinum. *D*, Sagittal MRI of the mediastinum demonstrates a separation between the tumor and the pericardium. (From Davis, R. D., Jr., Oldham, H. N., Jr., and Sabiston, D. C., Jr.: *In* Sabiston, D. C., Jr., and Spencer, F. C. [Eds.]: Surgery of the Chest, 5th ed. Philadelphia, W. B. Saunders, 1990.)

pathologically by destruction of postsynaptic nicotinic receptors. In the majority of myasthenic patients, antiacetylcholine receptor antibodies are present in high titers. Thymic lymphocytes isolated from myasthenic patients produce significant amounts of antiacetylcholine receptor antibodies, and this production is enhanced by the addition of autologous or allogeneic thymic epithelial cells.[37] Similarly, the various hematologic abnormalities associated with thymomas appear to have an autoimmune basis. Serum from patients with red cell aplasia in the presence of complement, as well as T lymphocytes isolated from these patients are able to suppress erythropoiesis colonies in vitro.[40] The mechanisms related to the development and maintenance, as well as the clinical phenomenon related to these syndromes have not been completely elucidated. The systemic syndromes often do not improve after successful control of the thymoma. Multiple associated syndromes may be present in a patient with a thymoma, suggesting a possible common etiologic factor. In regard to myasthenia gravis, the number of complete remissions achieved increases with increasing length of follow-up after thymectomy. In addition, the change in the acetylcholine receptor antibody titer after thymectomy does not correlate well with the patient's clinical response.

Myasthenia gravis occurs in 10% to 50% of patients with thymoma and is characterized clinically by weakness and fatigue of the skeletal muscles, with sparing of cardiac or smooth musculature. Muscles innervated by cranial nerves are the most frequently involved, particularly the extraocular muscles. Generalized weakness may develop and myasthenia crisis may lead to respiratory failure. In only 14% of patients does the disease remain localized to the extraocular muscles. In patients in whom the disease becomes generalized, it does so within the first year after onset of symptoms in 87%. Peak severity is reached by 1 year in 55%, by 3 years in 70%, and by 5 years in 85%. Male patients have more rapid progression of disease, fewer remissions, and less improvement with treatment than females.[4]

The incidence with which myasthenia gravis occurs in patients with thymoma increases with the age of the patient. In men older than 50 and women older than 60, the incidence appears to be greater than 80%. The majority of patients with myasthenia gravis do not have thymoma. The incidence is 10% to 42%, depending on the reporting medical center. Men with myasthenia gravis are 1.8 to 2 times more likely to have a thymoma than women. Because of the significant association between thymoma and myasthenia gravis, an evaluation of the mediastinum with CT or MRI is recommended in all patients with myasthenia gravis.

The diagnosis of myasthenia gravis is usually confirmed by a transient increase in muscle strength after the administration of a short-acting anticholinesterase inhibitor such as edrophonium (Tensilon). Electromyographic testing is also used to make the diagnosis and to follow quantitatively the course of the disease. An abnormal loss of muscle contraction strength after multiple stimulations (usually three to five per second) of the appropriate motor nerve constitutes a positive test.

Since Blalock's pioneering work in 1939, thymectomy has been a significant component in the treatment of myasthenia gravis. The use of median sternotomy to perform extended thymectomy, which includes the removal of all anterior mediastinal fatty areolar tissue in addition to the thymus gland, has led to improved clinical benefit with fewer recurrences. In 85% to 96% of patients, clinical improvement, defined as decreased symptoms, decreased use of medications, or remission, occurs after thymectomy.[17, 21] Drug free remission is achieved in 46% to 63%. Remission rates increase with duration after thymectomy (up to 81% at 89 months). Improved results and earlier remissions are associated with

shorter duration of disease before thymectomy, decreased severity of disease, female sex (remission in 82% females, 46% males),[17] and absence of thymoma (remission rate of 13%; benefit rate of 60%).[21] Whereas red cell aplasia occurs in only 5% of patients with thymoma, 33% to 50% of adults with red cell aplasia have a thymoma.

Thymomas are histologically classified by either the predominance of epithelial or lymphocytic cells (lymphocytic, epithelial, mixed and spindle) or by the morphologic resemblance to cortical or medullary epithelium. Unfortunately, a wide variance in the cellular composition is often present within the tumor and a consistent relationship is not present between the microscopic appearance and biologic behavior, either with regard to tumor invasiveness or association with systemic syndromes. However, in one series an improved 10-year survival was reported in patients with spindle cell or lymphocyte-rich thymomas (75%) as compared with differentiated epithelial type (50%) and undifferentiated (0%).[41] Similarly, the differentiation into medullary and cortical types has been shown to offer no prognostic information in one series,[25] while in another series, the presence of cortical morphology was associated with a malignant clinical course.[15]

Differentiation between benign and malignant disease is determined by the presence of gross invasion of adjacent structures, metastasis, or microscopic evidence of capsular invasion. Fifteen to 65% of thymomas are benign. The relative percentage is partially related to early surgical treatment of myasthenia gravis; if thymectomy is performed early in the course of myasthenia gravis, a greater percentage of thymomas are benign.

Whenever possible, the therapy for thymoma is surgical excision without removing or injuring vital structures. Even with well-encapsulated thymomas, extended thymectomy with eradication of all accessible mediastinal fatty areolar tissue should be performed to ensure removal of all ectopic thymic tissue. This approach has been shown to lower the number of tumor recurrences. The best operative exposure is obtained using a median sternotomy. Because many thymomas are radiosensitive, the placement of surgical clips to outline the anatomic extent of disease aids in the determination of optimal radiation portals.

In patients with myasthenia gravis, perioperative patient management is extremely important to prevent complications. Anticholinesterase inhibitors are discontinued to decrease the amount of pulmonary secretions and prevent inadvertent cholinergic weakness. Plasmapheresis is used routinely within 72 hours of thymectomy. In the majority of patients, plasmapheresis is very effective in controlling generalized weakness. Also, careful attention to the maintenance of pulmonary function with chest physiotherapy, endotracheal suctioning, and bronchodilators is the mainstay of postoperative management. The decision to extubate is based on evidence of adequate respiratory mechanics (e.g., vital capacity greater than 15 ml. per kg. and expiratory pressures greater than 40 cm. H_2O) rather than evidence of adequate ventilation as determined by analysis of arterial blood gases. Although myasthenic patients with thymoma had a worse prognosis in past series, improvements in therapy for myasthenia gravis have allowed prognosis to be dependent on the stage of the disease rather than on the presence of myasthenia gravis.

Staging of thymoma is as follows: Stage I—tumor is well-encapsulated without evidence of gross or microscopic capsular invasion; Stage II—tumor exhibits pericapsular growth into adjacent mediastinal fat, pleura, or pericardium; Stage III—tumor invades adjacent organs or intrathoracic metastasis is present; Stage IV—extrathoracic metastatic spread occurs (uncommon). The adjunctive use of radiation therapy with a dose of 35 to 50 Gy. is the recommended treatment for Stage II and III disease. In one series with Stage II or III disease after complete resection, the 5-year actuarial mediastinal relapse rate was 53% in those patients not receiving radiation therapy, 0% in those receiving radiation therapy, and 21% in those with biopsy alone and radiation therapy.[10] In patients with resectable Stage III disease, excellent long-term results can be obtained with radiation therapy: 100% 5-year survival and 95% 10- and 15-year survival.[32] Preoperative radiation therapy is useful when superior vena caval obstruction is present or when extensive invasion is manifested by CT or MRI. Occasionally, tumors not resectable on initial exploration are resectable after therapy. In patients with Stage IV disease or recurrent disease that is unresponsive to prior therapy, multiagent chemotherapy has been used. Complete response rates of approximately 40% with 3-year survival of 34% have been achieved.[18] Aggressive multimodality therapy using irradiation, chemotherapy, and surgical resection has been advocated for aggressive thymomas by a number of groups. The prognosis for patients with thymoma is dependent on clinical stage; 5-year survival is as follows: Stage I—85% to 100%, Stage II—60% to 80%, Stage III—40% to 70%, and Stage IV—50%.[32, 41]

Germ Cell Tumors

Germ cell tumors are benign and malignant neoplasms thought to originate from primordial germ cells that fail to complete the migration from the urogenital ridge and come to rest in the mediastinum. These tumors are classified as teratomas and teratocarcinomas, seminomas, embryonal cell carcinomas, choriocarcinomas, and endodermal cell (yolk sac) tumors. Although these lesions are identical histologically to germ cell tumors originating in the gonads, they are not considered to be metastatic from primary gonadal tumors. The current recommendations for evaluating the testes of a patient with mediastinal germ cell tumor is careful physical examination and ultrasonography. Biopsy is reserved for positive findings. Blind biopsy or orchiectomy is contraindicated.

Teratomas are neoplasms composed of multiple tissue elements derived from the three primitive embryonic layers foreign to the area in which they occur. The peak incidence is in the second and third decades of life. There is no sex predisposition. These tumors are located most commonly in the anterosuperior mediastinum, although 3% to 8% occur in the posterior mediastinum. Symptoms when present are related to mechanical effects and include chest pain, cough, dyspnea, or symptoms related to recurrent pneumonitis. If a communication between the tumor and the tracheobronchial tree develops, the pathognomonic finding of a cough productive of hair or sebaceous material may result. Unusual presentations include recurrent pericarditis or pericardial tamponade after invasion or rupture into the pericardium. Rupture into the pleural space may cause respiratory distress owing to the markedly irritative nature of the cyst fluid. However, with the greater use of routine chest films, patients are diagnosed more frequently while asymptomatic and with much smaller tumors.

Although these tumors are rare, the diagnosis can be made on routine chest film by the identification of well-formed teeth. CT findings of a predominantly fatty mass with a denser dependent portion containing globular calcifications, bone, or teeth and a solid protuberance into a cystic cavity are considered specific. Despite occasional characteristic appearances using various imaging techniques, the diagnosis usually depends on microscopic examination.

The teratodermoid (dermoid) cyst is the simplest form. It is composed predominantly of derivatives of the epidermal layer, including dermal and epidermal glands, hair, and seba-

ceous material. However, careful examination of the cyst wall usually reveals endodermal and mesodermal elements (Fig. 52–8) that are usually unilobular but are occasionally multilobular. Teratomas are histologically more complex. The solid component of the tumor contains well-differentiated elements of bone, cartilage, teeth, muscle, connective tissue, fibrous and lymphoid tissue, nerve, thymus, mucous and salivary glands, lung, liver, or pancreas. Malignant tumors are differentiated from benign tumors by the presence of primitive or embryonic tissue. Diagnosis and therapy rely on surgical excision. For those benign tumors of such large size or involvement with adjacent mediastinal structures that complete resection is impossible, partial resection has led to resolution of symptoms, frequently without relapse. Late sequelae after excision of a childhood teratoma may include impaired spermatic function and decreased serum levels of testosterone and luteinizing hormone.[26]

Malignant Germ Cell Tumor

Malignant germ cell tumors also occur predominantly in the anterosuperior mediastinum and represent approximately 4% of the primary tumors and cysts in the collected series. Unlike benign teratomas, there is a marked male predominance. The peak incidence is in the third and fourth decades of life. The majority of patients are symptomatic with chest pain, cough, dyspnea, and hemoptysis; the superior vena caval syndrome occurs commonly. The chest film usually demonstrates a large anterior mediastinal mass that is often multilobular; frequently there is evidence of intrathoracic spread of disease. CT and MRI are most helpful in defining the extent of involvement for the purpose of providing a means of following response to therapy and diagnosing relapses. These imaging modalities are also useful in determining impingement on vital structures that may contraindicate the use of general anesthesia. Serologic measurements of fetal protein and hCG are useful for the following tasks: differentiating seminomas from nonseminomas, quantitatively assessing response to therapy in hormonally active tumors (plasma half-life of alpha-fetoprotein and beta-hCG is 5 days and 12 to 24 hours, respectively), and diagnosing relapse or failure of therapy before changes that can be observed in gross disease. Seminomas rarely produce beta-hCG (<7%) and never produce alpha-fetoprotein; in contrast, over 90% of nonseminomas secrete one or both of these hormones. This differentiation is important because of the marked radiosensitivity of seminomas and the relative radiosensitivity of nonseminomas. Chromosomal analysis of tumor tissue is useful at differentiating germ cell tumors from other tumors with a similar histologic appearance. A characteristic isochromosome of chromosome 12 has been identified as a karyotypic abnormality of all germ cells.[31]

Seminomas constitute 50% of malignant germ cell tumors and 2% to 4% of all mediastinal masses. These tumors predominantly occur in the anterosuperior mediastinum. Unlike other malignant germ cell tumors, seminomas usually remain intrathoracic with local extension to adjacent mediastinal and pulmonary structures. Although metastatic spread occurs first through lymphatics, hematogenous spread with extrathoracic involvement may develop late in the course of disease. Bone and lung are the most common sites of metastatic spread, although liver, brain, spleen, tonsil, and subcutaneous tissue can also be involved. Patients are usually symptomatic owing to the mechanical effects of the tumor on adjacent structures. The superior vena caval syndrome occurs in 10% to 20% of patients. The histologic appearance of this tumor is characterized by large cells with round nuclei, scant cytoplasm, and abundant glycogen.

Therapy is determined by the stage of the disease. Occasionally, excision is possible without injury to vital structures (22%) and is recommended when possible. When complete resection is possible, the use of adjuvant therapy is unnecessary. However, careful follow-up with serial CT examinations is required to diagnose recurrences. When excision is not possible, a biopsy sample of sufficient size to establish the diagnosis should be obtained. Owing to the radiosensitivity of this tumor and the excellent control of local disease with radiation therapy, cytoreductive resection before radiation therapy is unnecessary and is contraindicated when vital structures are involved or when the procedure is technically difficult. The basis of therapy is megavoltage radiation to a shaped mediastinal field including the supraclavicular and neck regions (sites of initial lymphatic spread of disease). When cervical lymph nodes are involved, the field is expanded to incorporate the axilla, the site of subsequent lymphatic spread. A dosage of 45 to 50 Gy. (midplane dosage) is usually given over a 6-week course. In patients with extrathoracic disease, relapse after appropriate therapy, or sufficient

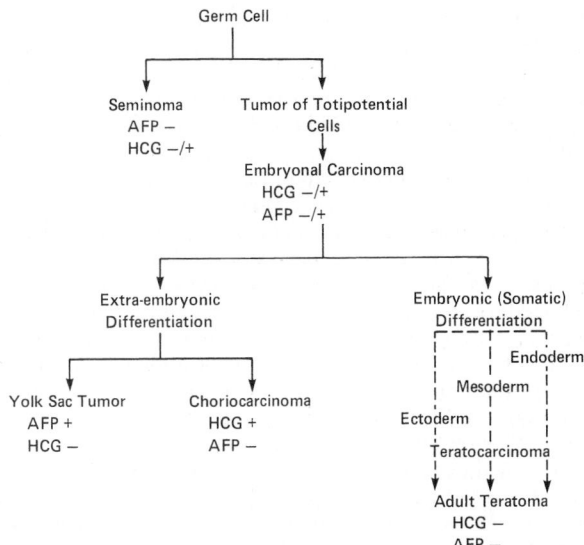

Figure 52–9. Interrelationships of germ cell tumors and tumor markers—alpha-fetoprotein (AFP) and beta-human chorionic gonadotropin (hCG). (Adapted from Sandhaus, I., Strom, R. L., and Mukai, K.: Primary embryonal choriocarcinoma of the mediastinum in a woman. Am. J. Clin. Pathol., *75*:573, 1981.)

intrathoracic disease to preclude the likelihood of a complete response using radiation therapy alone, cisplatin-based multiagent chemotherapy has successfully induced remission in a majority of patients.

Malignant nonseminoma tumors include choriocarcinoma, embryonal cell carcinoma, malignant teratoma, and endodermal cell (yolk sac) tumors, of which 40% are a mixture of tissue types. The nonseminomas differ from seminomas in several aspects: (1) they are more aggressive tumors that are frequently disseminated at the time of diagnosis; (2) they are rarely radiosensitive; and (3) over 90% produce either beta-hCG or alpha-fetoprotein. All patients with choriocarcinoma and some patients with embryonal cell tumors have elevated levels of beta-hCG; a hormone secreted by the syncytiotrophoblast alpha-fetoprotein is most commonly elevated in patients with embryonal cell carcinomas and yolk sac tumors. The presence of a significantly elevated titer of beta-hCG or an elevated titer of alpha-fetoprotein is indicative of a nonseminomatous germ cell component (Fig. 52–9). These tumors follow the natural history of a nonseminoma.

Like seminomas, the majority of patients with these neoplasms are symptomatic with chest pain, dyspnea, weight loss, cough, hemoptysis, fever, and chills and the superior vena caval syndrome (20%). Children with these tumors may present with precocious puberty. Patients are predominantly male and in the third or fourth decades. Chest films usually reveal a large anterior mediastinal mass with frequent extension into lung parenchyma and adjacent mediastinal structures. In addition to superior vena caval obstruction, they may cause pulmonary stenosis and coarctation of the aorta. Characteristically, these tumors have extensive intrathoracic involvement and frequently have metastasized outside the thorax. Frequent sites of metastatic disease include brain, lung, liver, bones, and the lymphatic system, particularly the supraclavicular nodes. Chest wall involvement is common.

A number of chromosomal abnormalities are associated with an increased incidence of germ cell tumors, including Klinefelter's syndrome, trisomy 8, and 5q deletion. In one series of patients with germ cell tumors, the incidence of Klinefelter's syndrome was 22%.[34] These patients were younger (median age of 15), and their tumors were nonseminomas. Additionally, mediastinal but not testicular germ cell

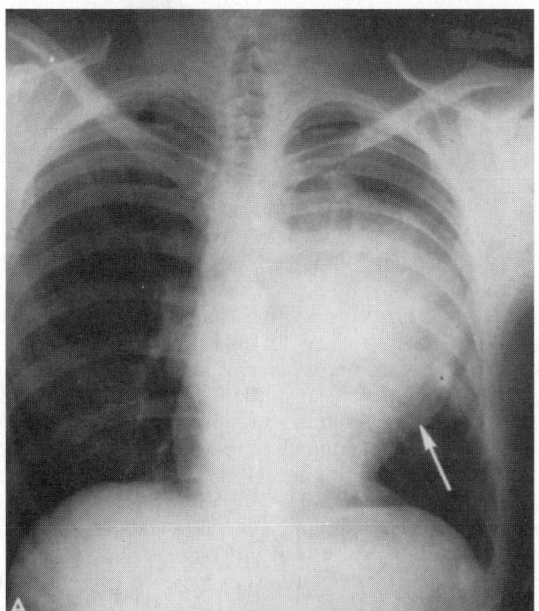

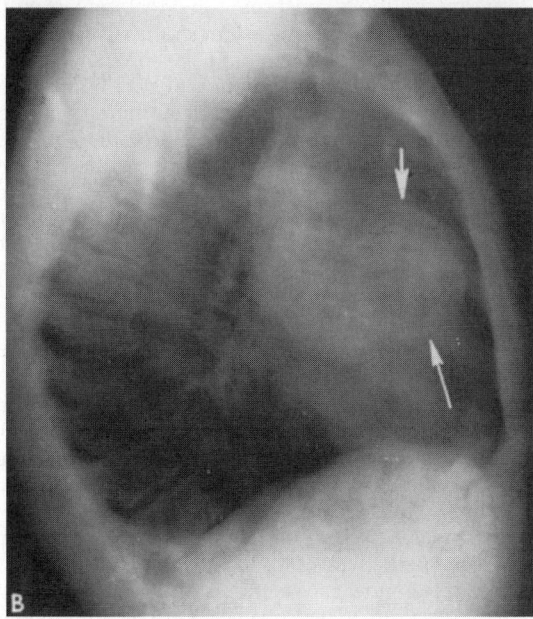

Figure 52–8. Chest films demonstrating teratoma of the anterior mediastinum.

tumors are associated with the development of rare hematologic malignancies such as acute megakaryocytic leukemia, systemic mast cell disease, and malignant histiocytosis, as well as other hematologic abnormalities including the myelodysplastic syndrome and idiopathic thrombocytopenia refractory to treatment.

The local invasiveness of these tumors and frequent metastases usually preclude surgical resection of all disease at the time of diagnosis. Initially, operative intervention is necessary only to establish the histologic diagnosis in patients without elevations in serum alpha-fetoprotein or beta-hCG. Multiagent chemotherapy, including cisplatin, is the basis of therapy. Other agents to which these tumors respond include vinblastine, bleomycin, methotrexate, etoposide, and doxorubicin. The serum markers, alpha-fetoprotein and beta-hCG are followed after administration of chemotherapy. When these markers return to normal values, operative exploration with removal of as much residual disease as possible without injuring vital structures is indicated. In patients in whom serum markers do not normalize after an initial course of chemotherapy, a second course using a different regimen of agents is indicated. In those patients who undergo surgical excision without normalization of the serologic markers, early relapse is characteristic. Patients with normalization of alpha-fetoprotein and beta-hCG after induction chemotherapy (achievable in up to 60%) have a good long-term prognosis.[23] The presence of residual disease after re-exploration portends an extremely poor prognosis. If viable tumor is present in the postchemotherapy resection specimen, additional chemotherapy is indicated due to the high relapse rate. A salvage chemotherapeutic regimen is usually employed. The postchemotherapeutic histology is often that of a mature teratoma. This is associated with a good long-term prognosis. Using surgical resection as an adjuvant to multiagent chemotherapy, complete responses of 20% to 80% have been reported. In patients with recurrent or refractory nonseminomatous germ cell tumors, salvage therapy with high-dose chemotherapy and autologous bone marrow transplant has not been successful.[6] Endodermal histology is associated with a worse prognosis compared with other germ cell tumors. Using an aggressive multimodality approach with cisplatin-based chemotherapy, followed by surgical resection of residual disease, 36% of patients were long-term survivors in one series.[23] However, of the patients who relapsed after therapy, no patients were salvaged despite aggressive chemotherapy. Mean survival in these patients was 6 months.

A subset of these tumors also contains malignant tissue characteristic for adenocarcinoma or sarcoma. Malignant teratomas or other germ cell tumors with mature differentiated teratoma within the primary are most commonly involved. Non–germ cell malignant transformation occurred in 29% of patients studied at autopsy.[1] Despite response of the germ cell component to chemotherapy, there is usually progression of the non–germ cell component. In these patients, the only effective treatment has been surgical resection, which is rarely possible. The overall prognosis is poor.

Lymphomas

Although the mediastinum is frequently involved in patients with lymphoma at some time during the course of the disease (40% to 70%), it is infrequently the sole site of disease at the time of presentation. Only 5% to 10% of patients with Hodgkin's and non-Hodgkin's lymphomas present solely with symptoms due to local mass effects, such as mediastinal involvement. Patients are usually symptomatic; chest pain, cough, dyspnea, hoarseness, and the superior vena caval syndrome are the most common clinical manifestations. Nonspecific systemic symptoms of fever and chills, weight loss, and anorexia are frequently noted and are important in the staging of patients with Hodgkin's lymphoma. Symptoms characteristic of Hodgkin's lymphoma include chest pain after consumption of alcohol and the cyclic fevers that were first described by Pel and Ebstein.

Characteristically, these tumors occur in the anterosuperior mediastinum or in the hilar region of the middle mediastinum. CT and MRI are useful in delineating the extent of disease, determining invasiveness into contiguous structures, differentiating the lesions from cardiovascular abnormalities, aiding the selection of radiation portals, and following the response to therapy and diagnosing relapse. Also, differentiation from thymomas and germ cell tumors, which usually are solitary masses, is possible because lymphomas are usually composed of multiple nodules that appear as separate masses by CT.

The Hodgkin's lymphomas are subdivided by histologic appearance into nodular sclerosing, lymphocyte predominant, mixed cellularity, and lymphocyte depleted. Mediastinal involvement is most common with nodular sclerosing (55% to 75%) (Fig. 52–10) and lymphocyte predominant (40%) lymphomas. Treatment of Hodgkin's lymphoma is determined by the stage of disease and is based on radiation therapy and chemotherapy. Surgical excision of all disease is rarely possible, and the surgeon's primary role is to provide sufficient tissue for diagnosis and to assist in pathologic staging, a process frequently requiring staging exploratory laparotomy. Although extrathoracic lymph nodes are frequently involved and available for biopsy, when the sole site of involvement is the mediastinum a needle biopsy is often unsuccessful because larger tissue samples are needed to make a histologic diagnosis, particularly with nodular sclerosing lesions. Thoracotomy, mediastinoscopy, or mediastinotomy may be necessary to obtain sufficient tissue. Although surgical excision, when possible, provides adequate therapy, more often Stage IA and IIA disease is treated with megavoltage external-beam radiation with a total dose of 45 Gy. Ten-year survival greater than 90% has been reported. Patients with Stage IIb, III, and IV disease are usually treated with chemotherapy. Patients with higher-grade tumor, advanced stage of disease, persistence of an abnormal erythrocyte sedimentation rate, extensive mediastinal disease, and advanced age (>50 years) are at an increased risk of disease relapse.

Controversy continues concerning the treatment of patients with extensive mediastinal disease as defined by tumor size greater than 35% of the cardiothoracic diameter. These patients have a higher relapse rate when treated with radiation therapy alone. Although combining chemotherapy with radiation therapy reduces the relapse rate, prolongation of survival has not necessarily resulted because of the efficacy of salvage chemotherapy and the significant risk of secondary malignancies after the use of alkylating chemotherapeutic agents.

Residual abnormalities within the mediastinum are commonly noted radiographically after treatment of Hodgkin's disease (64% to 88%).[22, 35] These abnormalities include minimal mediastinal widening in 44% of patients and widening greater than 6 cm. in 41%. In 27% to 41% of patients, radiographic abnormalities will persist for greater than a year. Residual radiographic abnormality is more common in patients with initial bulky mediastinal disease. Residual mediastinal abnormalities were not significantly associated with eventual disease relapse except when treatment was with chemotherapy alone. A negative gallium-67 scintigraphic scan has been predictive of absence of residual disease. Benign thymic cysts appear to be more common after radiation therapy for anterior mediastinal neoplasms. Optimal therapy is surgical excision without additional chemotherapy or radi-

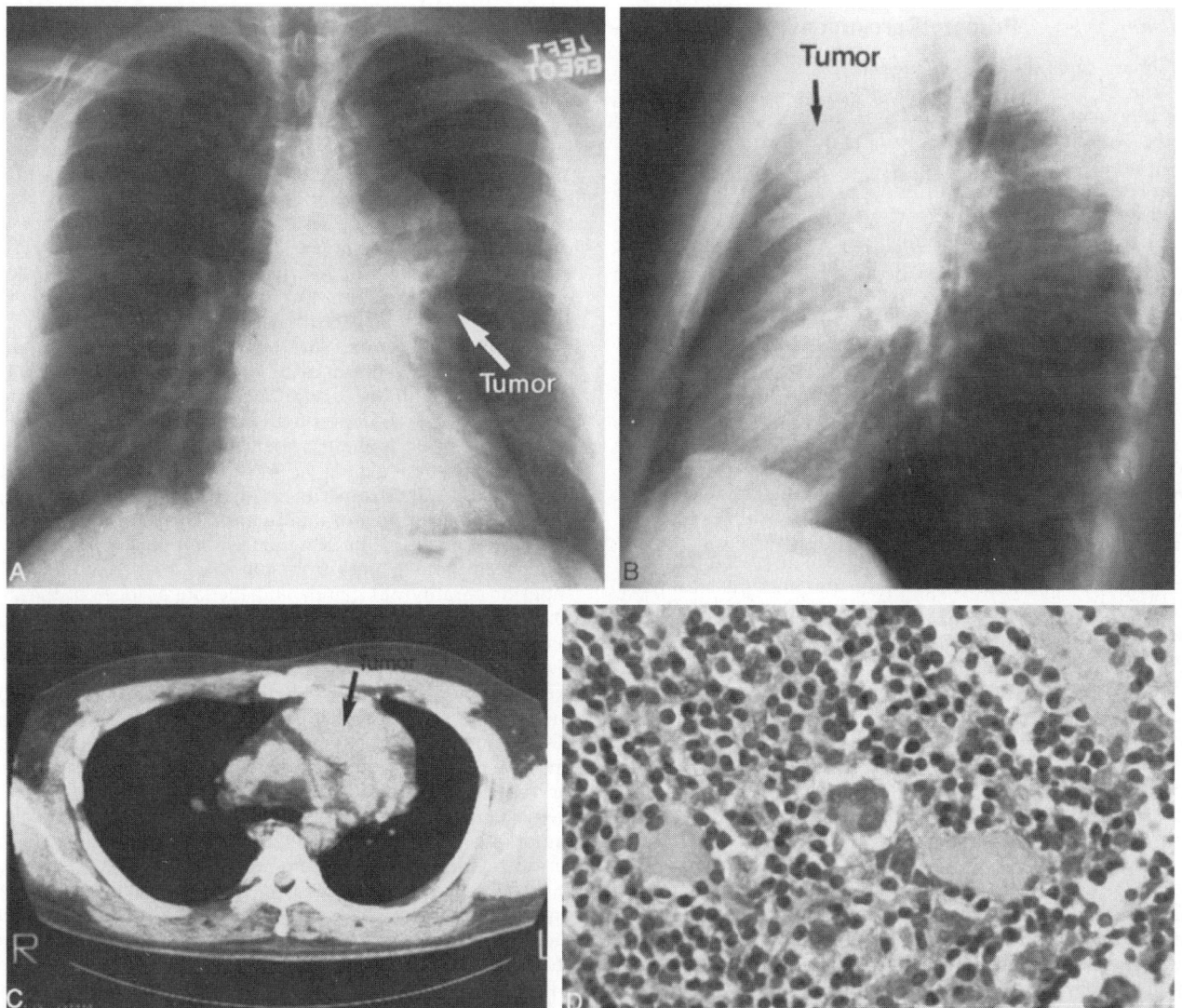

Figure 52–10. *A* and *B*, Chest films of an anterior mediastinal Hodgkin's tumor. *C*, CT image demonstrates the invasive nature of the tumor. *D*, The characteristic Reed-Sternberg cell is shown. (From Davis, R. D., Jr., Oldham, H. N., Jr., and Sabiston, D. C., Jr.: The mediastinum. *In* Sabiston, D. C., Jr., and Spencer, F. C. [Eds.]: Surgery of the Chest, 5th ed. Philadelphia, W. B. Saunders, 1990.)

ation therapy to determine whether residual disease is present.

Non-Hodgkin's lymphomas are usually either of lymphoblastic morphology (60%) or large cell morphology with a diffuse pattern of growth (40%). Patients with non-Hodgkin's lymphomas are usually symptomatic owing to involvement of adjacent mediastinal structures. The superior vena caval syndrome is relatively common. In 40% to 80% of patients with lymphoblastic lymphoma, the mediastinum is involved. Although all ages may be afflicted, the peak incidence is in the second and third decades of life. Operative intervention is limited to obtaining sufficient tissue to establish the diagnosis and, if necessary, to perform immunologic subtyping. The best results have been obtained using aggressive chemotherapy in conjunction with central nervous system prophylaxis.

The large cell lymphomas of diffuse growth pattern are a heterogeneous group differing in the cell type of origin, clinical presentation, natural history, and response to therapy. These tumors can be subclassified into at least three diseases: T-immunoblastic sarcoma, B-immunoblastic sarcoma, and sclerosing variants of follicular cell lymphoma. Operative intervention is useful in obtaining tissue for diagnosis, which

often requires immunotyping, but is rarely important with regard to therapy. These tumors may be confused with thymomas, germ cell tumors, anaplastic carcinoid tumors, and Hodgkin's lymphoma if the light microscopic appearance alone is used. This is especially true if prior radiation therapy or chemotherapy has been administered. Although needle biopsy frequently does not provide sufficient tumor specimen to establish the diagnosis, extrathoracic tissue is often available for biopsy. Therapy is based on doxorubicin-containing chemotherapeutic protocols, which can induce complete responses in over 90% of patients with relapse-free survival of 50% to 74% after 2 years.

A subset of patients with primary mediastinal lymphoma has been described with B-cell characteristics (MB2+).[27] The clinical course in these patients was remarkable for a prolonged phase in which the tumor remained confined to the mediastinum and thorax. Histology was notable for the amount of fibrosis and necrosis. In only 4 of 15 patients was a complete remission achieved. Initially, an aggressive chemotherapeutic regimen appears indicated. However, due to the prolonged period of strictly local involvement, surgical resection of residual disease appears indicated when technically feasible.

Primary Carcinoma

Primary carcinomas of the mediastinum comprise between 3% and 11% of primary mediastinal masses in most series and represent 4% of the mediastinal masses in the collected series. The origin of these tumors is unknown. However, it is important to differentiate them from malignant thymomas, germ cell tumors, carcinoid tumors, lymphomas, mediastinal extension of bronchogenic carcinomas, and metastatic tumors, which may have a similar light microscopic appearance. Metastatic disease in mediastinal lymph nodes is usually from bronchogenic or esophageal malignancies and rarely occurs with extrathoracic malignancies. The tumors most likely to metastasize to the mediastinum include those originating in the breast, head and neck, and genitourinary tract, as well as melanomas. Primary carcinomas are usually of the large cell, undifferentiated morphology, although small cell and squamous cell tumors have been described. The use of electron microscopic examination of the tumor ultrastructure and immunostaining for surface antigens and cellular proteins better defined the origin of some of these primary carcinomas and decreased the reported incidence.

These tumors occur with equal frequency in either sex. The majority of patients are symptomatic from the local mass effects of the tumor. Extensive involvement within the thorax and often metastatic disease outside the thorax characterize this disease. Surgical excision is rarely possible. Unfortunately, the routine use of radiation therapy and chemotherapy has been unsuccessful in prolonging survival. Only 2 of 32 patients treated at the Duke University Medical Center are alive at 6 and 11 years after surgical excision or biopsy and radiation therapy, respectively. Overall, the mean survival is less than 1 year.

Endocrine Tumors

Although substernal extension of a cervical goiter is common, totally intrathoracic thyroid tumors are rare and comprise only 1% of all mediastinal masses in the collected series. These tumors arise from heterotopic thyroid tissue, which occurs most commonly in the anterosuperior mediastinum but may also occur in the middle mediastinum between the trachea and esophagus as well as in the posterior mediastinum. Although there may be a demonstrable connection with the cervical gland (usually a fibrous connective tissue band), a true intrathoracic thyroid gland derives its blood supply from thoracic vessels.

The peak incidence is in the sixth and seventh decades. Women are more commonly affected. When these lesions occur in the anterosuperior or middle mediastinum, symptoms related to tracheal compression are often present, such as dyspnea, cough, wheezing, and stridor. When these tumors occur in the posterior mediastinum, esophageal compression manifested by dysphagia is common. Rarely, symptoms related to thyrotoxicosis may be the initiating factor for a patient to seek medical attention. On chest film, these lesions appear as sharply circumscribed, dense masses, occurring more frequently on the right. The administration of iodinated contrast material causes prolonged enhancement of thyroid tissue, and intrathoracic goiters are contrast enhancing lesions when visualized by CT. When functioning thyroid tissue is present, the ^{131}I scan is usually diagnostic. However, some of these neoplasms are functionally inactive and are not identified by ^{131}I scanning. In asymptomatic patients with anterosuperior or posterosuperior masses, ^{131}I scanning should be performed to document the presence of functioning cervical thyroid tissue to prevent the removal of the sole functioning thyroid tissue.

The majority of these tumors are adenomas, but carcinomas have been reported. If the lesion is identified as the sole functioning thyroid tissue and the patient is asymptomatic, surgical exploration and excision is not indicated. In these patients, frequent follow-up radiographic examinations are indicated to evaluate changes in the size or nature of the lesion. Otherwise, these lesions should be resected owing to their propensity to enlarge and compress adjacent structures. Because of the thoracic derivation of the blood supply, intrathoracic thyroid tumors should be approached through the thorax, using either an anterolateral thoracotomy or a median sternotomy for anterior lesions or a posterolateral thoracotomy for posterior lesions. Substernal extensions of a cervical goiter can usually be excised using a cervical approach.

Parathyroid Tumors. Although parathyroid glands may occur in the mediastinum in 10% of patients, they are usually accessible through the cervical incision. A sternotomy is necessary to excise a hyperfunctioning parathyroid gland in approximately 2.5% of all patients and in 15% to 30% of those with a mediastinal gland.[8, 9, 42] Most often these adenomas are found in the anterosuperior mediastinum embedded in or near the superior pole of the thymus. This anatomic relationship is the result of the common embryogenesis of the inferior parathyroid glands from the third branchial cleft. The superior parathyroid glands and the lateral lobes of the thyroid gland are derived from the fourth branchial pouch. Because they migrate with the lateral lobes of the thyroid gland to a paraesophageal position, they are found in the posterior mediastinum when they migrate further caudad. Factors contributing to the caudal movement of parathyroid glands into the mediastinum include negative intrathoracic pressure, gravity, and the movement of the pharynx and larynx with deglutition.

The clinical manifestations of a mediastinal parathyroid tumor are similar to those that occur with tumors of the cervical region; symptoms are related to the excess secretion of parathyroid hormone causing the hyperparathyroid syndrome. Because of their small size, these neoplasms rarely cause symptoms related to mechanical effects and are not often visualized using conventional roentgenography. Using CT, MRI, thallium and technetium scanning, and selective arteriography, preoperative localization of these tumors can be made in approximately 80% of patients. Venous angiography with selective sampling is useful at determining the side of the adenoma but is usually inadequate at defining the anatomic location. The utility of localization studies is variable between series. In a series reported from the National Institute of Health, the sensitivity of angiography, CT, and MRI at localizing a mediastinal parathyroid gland was 84%, 35%, and 19%, respectively. Ultrasound and technetium/thallium scans were very insensitive.[14]

Most frequently, the mediastinal adenoma may be excised after a negative exploration of the cervical region through the existing cervical incision. Usually, the vascular supply to the adenoma extends from cervical blood vessels. Mediastinal exploration using a median sternotomy is indicated in those patients with persistent hyperparathyroidism producing severe biochemical or metabolic disease after an unsuccessful cervical exploration in which four normal glands have been identified.[42] Preoperative attempts at anatomic localization is indicated. In patients whose preoperative studies have failed to locate the site of the responsible parathyroid gland, exploration of the mediastinum is often unsuccessful. Approximately 80% of mediastinal parathyroids are located in the anterior mediastinum, with the majority of the remaining 20% occurring in the posterior mediastinum.[8] Almost 75% of the mediastinal parathyroids are found within or adjacent to the thymus. If an adenoma is not found after a systematic exploration of the mediastinum, which may require incision of the pleura and pericardium, removal of the thymus and the parathymic fatty areolar tissue is recommended. Angio-ablation of mediastinal parathyroids can be performed with long-term success in 63% of patients.[14] In centers with appropriate expertise, angioablation may be indicated as the initial procedure of choice in patients with persistent or recurrent hyperparathyroidism if only one parathyroid gland was removed at the initial operation. In patients in whom two or more parathyroid glands were excised at the initial operation, persistent hypoparathyroidism often results after angioablation. In these patients, surgical exploration and excision with cryopreservation of excised parathyroid tissue is indicated.

Parathyroid carcinomas have been reported and are usually hormonally active. Patients differ in clinical presentation in that they often have higher serum calcium levels and manifest more severe symptoms of hyperparathyroidism. When possible, surgical resection is the optimal therapy.

Unlike parathyroid adenomas and carcinomas, parathyroid cysts are usually not hormonally active. These cysts are defined by the presence of parathyroid cells identifiable within the cyst wall. Because these lesions are frequently larger than adenomas, symptoms related to local mass effects are more common, as is visualization on chest film. Surgical excision yields a cure.

Carcinoid Tumors. Mediastinal carcinoid tumors arise from cells of Kulchitsky located in the thymus. Occurring more often in male patients, these tumors are usually located in the anterosuperior mediastinum. Owing to their origin from APUD cells, these tumors may be hormonally active, and they may occur as a variant of the multiple endocrine neoplasia syndromes. Mediastinal carcinoids have been most frequently associated with Cushing's syndrome due to production of ACTH and less frequently with multiple endocrine neoplasia Type 1 syndrome.

In patients with hormonally inactive tumors, symptoms are related to local mass effects, leading to chest pain, dyspnea, cough, and the superior vena caval syndrome. Hormonally inactive carcinoids tend to be larger and frequently are invasive locally. In addition, metastatic spread to mediastinal and cervical lymph nodes, liver, bone, skin, and lungs occurs in the majority of patients.

Often, these tumors are difficult to differentiate from other common anterior mediastinal masses, particularly thymomas and germ cell tumors. However, carcinoids are characterized by the ultrastructural findings of dense core neurosecretory granules. Positive immunohistochemical staining of these granules for ACTH is also characteristic.

Surgical removal of the tumor, when possible, is the preferred treatment. When local invasiveness or metastasis precludes the successful use of operative therapy, radiation therapy and multiagent chemotherapy have been used, although no consistent benefit has been documented.

Mesenchymal Tumors

Mediastinal mesenchymal tumors originate from the connective tissue, striatal and smooth muscle, fat, lymphatic tissue, and blood vessels present within the mediastinum, giving rise to a diverse group of neoplasms. Relative to other sites in the body, these tumors occur less commonly within the mediastinum. Mesenchymal tumors comprised 7% of the primary masses in the collected series. There is no apparent difference in incidence between sexes. The soft tissue neoplasms include lipomas, liposarcomas, fibrosarcomas, fibromas, xanthogranulomas, leiomyomas, leiomyosarcomas, benign and malignant mesenchymomas, rhabdomyosarcomas, and mesotheliomas. These tumors have a similar histologic appearance and generally follow the same clinical course as the soft tissue tumors found elsewhere in the body. Fifty-five per cent of these tumors are malignant. Surgical resection

remains the primary therapy, because poor results have been obtained using radiation and chemotherapy.

Similarly, the mesenchymal tumors derived from blood and lymph vessels are common elsewhere in the body but rare in the mediastinum. Although these tumors occur anywhere in the mediastinum, the most frequent location is in the anterosuperior mediastinum. They include capillary, cavernous, and venous hemangiomas; hemangioendotheliomas; hemangiopericytomas; lymphangiomas; and the derivatives of lymphangiomas. Symptoms are related to the size and invasiveness of the lesion. Occasionally, hemorrhage into the lesion may lead to a rapid increase in the size. Significant compression and obstruction of mediastinal structures may result, causing a variety of clinical manifestations, of which respiratory failure is the most dramatic. Rupture of hemangiomas into the pleural space may cause exsanguination; rupture into the mediastinum may cause tamponade.

Differentiation between the vascular tumors is based on the morphologic appearance: the size of the vascular space, the relative number and amount of pericytes, smooth muscle, and endothelial cells. Between 10% and 30% of vascular tumors are malignant, although the differentiation may be difficult because the histologic appearance, number of mitotic figures, and even the gross appearance are often similar. Vascular tumors are not well encapsulated, and even benign tumors may exhibit local invasion. However, the incidence of metastatic spread is low, approximately 3%. Hemangiopericytomas have the highest incidence of malignancy, and these tumors usually occur in older patients. Because these neoplasms are not supplied by large vessels, tumor opacification usually does not occur during angiographic studies. Excision remains the only effective means of therapy, although radiation therapy has been used with mixed results.

Tumors originating from lymph vessels are differentiated from tumors of blood vessel origin by using indirect evidence, such as the absence of red blood cells within the lumen of the tumor vasculature, extrusion of chylous fluid from the cut edges, and the tumor's relationship to documented lymphatic tissue. Also, these tumors usually occur in the anterior mediastinum, appearing as round or lobulated cystic densities on the chest films. The most common lymphatic tumor is the lymphangioma (also called cystic hygroma, lymphatic cyst, and lymphatogenous cyst), which in the majority of patients occurs in the superior mediastinum as an extension of a cervical lesion. Only 17% of mediastinal lymphangiomas are completely within the mediastinum, whereas 10% of cervical lymphangiomas have a mediastinal extension. Low-lying cervical lymphangiomas are more likely to have a mediastinal component. Lymphangiomas are usually diagnosed in children, and they frequently cause symptoms due to obstruction of the trachea, including stridor, dyspnea, recurrent pulmonary infection, and tachypnea. Prenatal diagnosis has been made using fetal ultrasonography. Lymphangiomas have characteristic appearances using ultrasonography or CT. Growth of these tumors is by proliferation of endothelium-lined buds that spread along tissue planes. The local ingrowth of vessels and fibrous reaction to the endothelial buds prevent easy surgical removal due to the lack of well-defined tissue planes. However, because radiation therapy and sclerotherapy have not been successful, operative resection is the optimal treatment. Total excision is not indicated when nerves and vital structures are involved. Multiple procedures may be necessary.

Extramedullary Hematopoiesis

Extramedullary hematopoiesis occurs in all age groups, usually as a result of altered hematopoiesis. In the adult, this is typically due to massive hemolysis, myelofibrosis, spherocytic anemia, or thalassemia. These lesions appear as bilateral, asymmetrical paravertebral masses and enhance with contrast medium. Because these tumors are composed of hematopoietic tissue, they are readily visualized using either radioactive iron (^{59}Fe) or radioisotope-labeled gold scanning. These scanning modalities are useful in differentiating these tumors from other mediastinal lesions in patients with known hematologic abnormalities. Surgical resection is unnecessary unless there is invasion or compression of mediastinal structures. Radiation therapy can produce rapid shrinkage of these masses.

Giant Lymph Node Hyperplasia (Castleman's Disease)

Giant lymph node hyperplasia was initially described by Castleman in 1954. Although the mediastinum was the site of disease in the initial report and in the majority of patients, these tumors may develop wherever lymph nodes are present; the retroperitoneum and cervical, axillary, and pelvic regions comprise the most frequent nonmediastinal sites. Although these tumors are usually located in the anterosuperior mediastinum, they are also found in the posterior mediastinum and at the pericardiophrenic angle where they may be confused with neurogenic tumors and pericardial cysts, respectively. Two distinct histologic entities exist: (1) hyaline vascular—characterized by small hyaline follicles and interfollicular capillary proliferation; and (2) plasma cell—characterized by large follicles with intervening sheets of plasma cells. The tumors most frequently appear as single, well-demarcated lesions. The hyaline vascular type represents 90% of Castleman's tumors, and these are most often discovered in the asymptomatic patient on a routine chest film. Patients with the plasma cell type often exhibit systemic features, including fever, night sweats, anemia, and hypergammaglobulinemia. Surgical excision effects cure, although resection of the hyaline vascular type may be associated with significant hemorrhage due to extreme vascularity.

Multicentric Castleman's disease is characterized by generalized lymphadenopathy with morphologic features of giant lymph node hyperplasia. Patients are most often symptomatic with fever, chills, weight loss, and hepatosplenomegaly and exhibit disordered immunity and autoimmune phenomena. Unlike the benign clinical course of classic Castleman's disease, multicentric disease is a much more malignant disease with death often occurring after infectious complications. It has also been reported in association with human immunodeficiency virus infection.

Chondroma

Chondromas are rare tumors that occur in the posterior mediastinum and originate from the primitive notochord. Males are affected twice as often as females, with the peak age of incidence in the fifth through seventh decades. Chest pain, cough, and dyspnea are the most common features. Spinal cord compression may follow extension into the spinal canal. Radical surgical excision is the only effective therapy; however, the majority of patients develop distant metastases. The mean survival is approximately 17.5 months.

Primary Cysts

Primary cysts of the mediastinum comprise 20% of the mediastinal masses in the collected series. These cysts can be bronchogenic, pericardial, enteric, or thymic or may be of an unspecified nature. More than 75% of patients are asymptomatic, and these tumors rarely cause morbidity. However, owing to the proximity of vital structures within the medias-

tinum, with increasing size even benign cysts may cause significant morbidity. In addition, these masses need to be differentiated from malignant tumors.

Bronchogenic cysts are the most common primary cysts of the mediastinum, comprising 6.3% of primary mediastinal masses and 34% of cysts. They originate as sequestrations from the ventral foregut, the antecedent of the tracheobronchial tree. The bronchogenic cyst may lie within the lung parenchyma or the mediastinum. The cyst wall is composed of cartilage, mucous glands, smooth muscle, and fibrous tissue with a pathognomonic inner layer of ciliated respiratory epithelium. When bronchogenic cysts occur in the mediastinum, they are usually located proximal to the trachea or bronchi and may be just posterior to the carina. Rarely, a true communication between the cyst and the tracheobronchial tree exists, and an air-fluid level may be observed on the chest film.

Two thirds of patients with bronchogenic cysts are asymptomatic. In infants, these cysts may cause severe respiratory compromise by compressing the trachea or the bronchus;

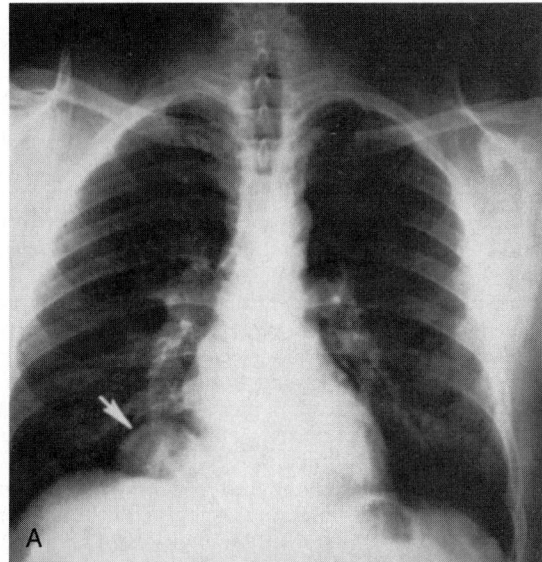
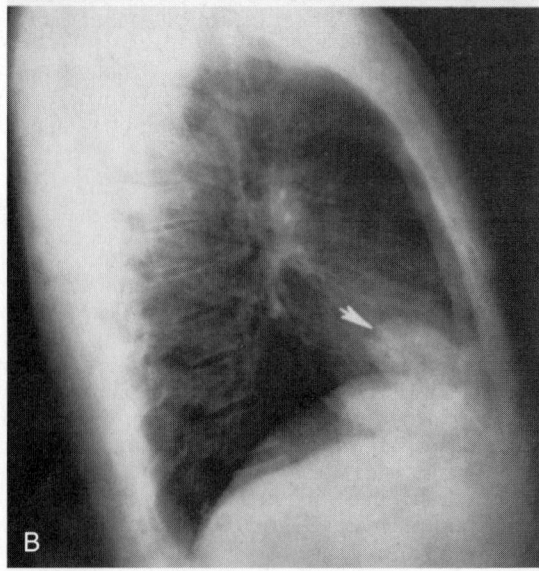

Figure 52–11. *A* and *B*, Chest films showing the typical location of a pericardial cyst in the right cardiophrenic angle. (From Sabiston, D. C., Jr., and Oldham, H. N., Jr.: The mediastinum. *In* Sabiston, D. C., Jr., and Spencer, F. C. [Eds.]: Gibbon's Surgery of the Chest, 4th ed. Philadelphia, W. B. Saunders, 1983.)

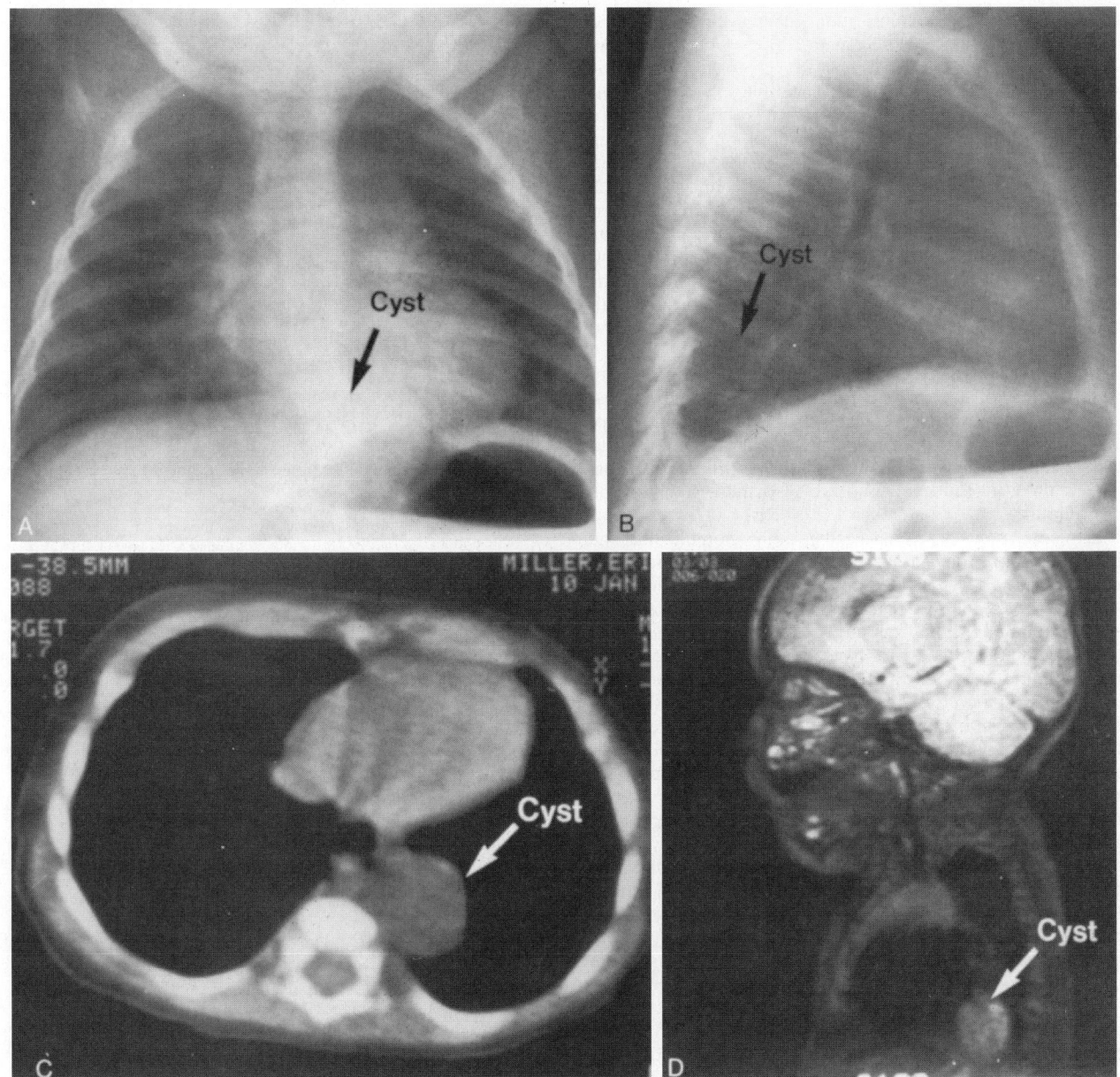

Figure 52-12. *A* and *B*, Chest films of a patient with an enteric cyst. *C*, CT delineates the anatomic location but does not further differentiate the mass from a neurogenic tumor. *D*, MRI demonstrates the cystic nature of the mass and its relationship to the esophagus. (From Davis, R. D., Jr., and Sabiston, D. C., Jr.: Primary mediastinal cysts and neoplasms. *In* Sabiston, D. C., Jr.: Essentials of Surgery. Philadelphia, W. B. Saunders, 1987.)

compression of the bronchus may cause bronchial stenosis and recurrent pneumonitis. In children with recurrent pulmonary infections, CT may be useful in assessing the subcarinal space for possible bronchogenic cyst, an area that is poorly visualized using standard roentgenography. More often, bronchogenic cysts occur in older children and adults, in whom these cysts may cause symptoms of chest pain, dyspnea, cough, and stridor. Bronchogenic cysts appear as a smooth density at the level of the carina that may compress the esophagus on barium swallow. Differentiation from hilar structures may be difficult.

Surgical excision is recommended in all patients to provide definitive histologic diagnosis, alleviate symptoms, and prevent the development of associated complications. Malignant degeneration has been reported, as well as the presence of a bronchial adenoma within the cysts.

Pericardial cysts are the second most frequently encountered cysts within the mediastinum and comprise 6% of all

lesions and 33% of primary cysts (see Table 52-2). These cysts classically occur in the pericardiophrenic angles (Fig. 52-11), with 70% in the right pericardiophrenic angle, 22% in the left, and the remainder in other sites in the pericardium. Pericardial cysts may or may not have a communication with the pericardium. Numerous reports have described the characteristic CT appearance of pericardial cysts: pericardiophrenic location, near-water attenuation value, and smooth borders. Patients with lesions demonstrating classic CT characteristics for pericardial cysts have been managed with needle aspiration and follow-up with serial CT rather than surgical excision. Surgical excision of pericardial cysts is indicated primarily for diagnosis and to differentiate these cysts from malignant lesions.

Enteric cysts (duplication cysts) arise from the posterior division of the primitive foregut, which develops into the upper division of the gastrointestinal tract. These cysts are found less frequently than bronchogenic or pericardial cysts and comprise 3% of the mediastinal masses in the collected series. They are also known as inclusion cysts, gastric cysts, or enterogenous cysts and are most frequently located in the posterior mediastinum, usually adjacent to the esophagus (Fig. 52–12).

These lesions are composed of smooth muscle with an inner epithelial lining of esophageal, gastric, or intestinal mucosa. When gastric mucosa is present, peptic ulceration with perforation into the esophageal or bronchial lumens may occur, producing hemoptysis or hematemesis. Erosion into the lung parenchyma may cause hemorrhage and lead to lung abscess formation. Gastric mucosa within enteric cysts may be visualized using technetium-99 scanning. Usually, enteric cysts have an attachment to the esophagus and may be embedded within the muscularis layer.

Symptoms are usually due to compression of the esophagus, leading to obstruction that commonly presents as dysphagia. Compromise of the tracheobronchial tree with symptoms of cough, dyspnea, recurrent pulmonary infections, and chest pain may also result. The majority of enteric cysts are diagnosed in children, who are also more likely to be symptomatic.

When enteric cysts are associated with anomalies of the vertebral column, they are referred to as neuroenteric cysts. Such cysts may be connected to the meninges, or, less frequently, a direct communication with the dural space may exist. In patients with neuroenteric cysts, preoperative evaluation for potential spinal cord involvement is mandatory. The vertebral anomalies associated with this syndrome include spina bifida, hemivertebrae, and a widened neural canal. CT and myelography are useful in delineating the vertebral deformities, extension into the spinal column, and the possibility of a connection with the dural space. Rarely, multiple mediastinal enteric cysts may occur, or there may be an association with a duplication of the abdominal portion of the alimentary tract. In the latter, there may be a transdiaphragmatic connection between abdominal and mediastinal components. Treatment is surgical excision, providing a definite histologic diagnosis as well as alleviating symptoms and preventing potential complication.

Nonspecific cysts include those lesions in which a specific epithelial or mesothelial lining cannot be identified. These lesions may originate in any of the aforementioned cysts by the destruction of the inner epithelial lining by an inflammatory or digestive process. Other causes include postinflammatory cysts and hemorrhagic cysts.

SELECTED REFERENCES

Lahdenne, P.: Late sequelae of gonadal, mediastinal, and oral teratomas in childhood. Acta Paediatr., 81:235, 1992.

This is a study of 32 patients with gonadal, mediastinal, and oral teratomas in childhood, with follow-up times ranging from 5 to 40 years. This long-term study is of considerable significance.

Lavabre-Bertrand, T., Donadio, D., Fegueux, N., Jessueld, D., Taib, J., Charlier, D., Rousset, T., Emberger, J.-M., Baldet, P., and Navarro, M.: A study of 15 cases of primary mediastinal lymphoma of B-cell type. Cancer, 69:2561, 1992.

This is a review of patients with primary mediastinal lymphoma of B-cell type, primarily involving the mediastinum. The poor prognosis is emphasized in long-term studies, with emphasis on chemoresistance and radioresistance.

Morrissey, B., Adams, H., Gibbs, A. R., and Crane, M. D.: Percutaneous needle biopsy of the mediastinum: Review of 94 cases. Thorax, 48:632, 1993.

This is a study of radiographically guided percutaneous biopsies of mediastinal masses with fine-needle aspiration and a comparison with cutting needles. The radiographically guided needle biopsy was found to be a safe procedure that provided useful diagnostic information. Fine-needle aspiration techniques generally provide adequate data, whereas a cutting needle biopsy should be performed whenever possible when lymphoma, thymoma, or neural masses are suspected to obtain larger specimens for more accurate diagnosis.

REFERENCES

1. Aliotta, P. J., Castillo, J., Englander, L. S., Nseymo, U. O., and Huben, R. P.: Primary mediastinal germ cell tumors: Histologic patterns of treatment failures at autopsy. Cancer, 62:982, 1988.

2. Azizkhan, R. G., Dudgeon, D. L., Buck, J. R., et al.: Life-threatening airway obstruction as a complication to the management of mediastinal masses in children. J. Pediatr. Surg., 20:816, 1985.

3. Bastianelli, R., quoted by Meade, R. H.: A History of Thoracic Surgery. Springfield, IL, Charles C Thomas, 1961.

4. Berrih-Aknin, S., Morel, E., Raimond, F., Safar, D., Gaud, C., Binet, J. P., Levasseur, P., and Bach, J. F.: The role of the thymus in myasthenia gravis: Immunohistological and immunological studies in 15 cases. Ann. N.Y. Acad. Sci., 505:472, 1987.

5. Blalock, A., Mason, M. F., Morgon, H. J., and Riven, S. S.: Myasthenia gravis and tumors of the thymic region: Report of a case in which tumor was removed. Ann. Surg., 110:544, 1939.

6. Brown, L. R., and Aughenbaugh, G. L.: Masses of the anterior mediastinum: CT and MR imaging. AJR, 157:1171, 1991.

7. Castleman, B., Iverson, L., and Menendez, V. P.: Localized mediastinal lymphoid hyperplasia resembling thymoma. Cancer, 9:822, 1956.

8. Clark, O. H.: Mediastinal parathyroid tumors. Arch. Surg., 123:1096, 1988.

9. Conn, J. M., Goncalves, M. A., Mansour, K. A., and McGarity, W. C.: The mediastinal parathyroid. Am. Surg., 57:62, 1991.

10. Curran, W. J., Kornstein, M. J., Brooks, J. J., and Turrisi, A. T.: Invasive thymoma: The role of mediastinal irradiation following complete or incomplete surgical resection. J. Clin. Oncol., 6:1722, 1988.

11. Daly, B. D. T., Faling, J., Bite, G., et al.: Mediastinal lymph evaluation by computed tomography in lung cancer: An analysis of 345 patients grouped by TNM staging, tumor size, and tumor location. J. Thorac. Cardiovasc. Surg., 94:664, 1987.

12. Dartevelle, P., Chapelier, A., Navajas, M., Levasseur, P., Rojas, A., Khalife, J., Lafontaine, E., and Merlier, M.: Replacement of the superior vena cava with polytetrafluoroethylene grafts combined with resection of mediastinal-pulmonary malignant tumors. J. Thorac. Cardiovasc. Surg., 94:361, 1987.

13. Doty, D. B.: Bypass of superior vena cava: Six years experience with spiral vein graft for obstruction of superior vena cava due to benign and malignant disease. J. Thorac. Cardiovasc. Surg., 83:326, 1982.

14. Doherty, G., Doppman, J., et al.: Results of a multidisciplinary strategy for management of mediastinal parathyroid adenoma as a cause of persistent primary hyperparathyroidism. Ann. Surg., 215:101, 1991.

15. Elert, O., Buchwald, J., and Wolf, K.: Epithelial thymus tumors—therapy and prognosis. Thorac. Cardiovasc. Surg., 36:109, 1988.

16. Epstein, A. M., and Klassen, K. P.: Spontaneous superior mediastinal hemorrhage. J. Thorac. Cardiovasc. Surg., 39:740, 1960.

17. Fischer, J. E., Grinvalski, H. T., Nussbaum, M. S., Sayers, H. J., Cole, R. E., and Samaha, F. J.: Aggressive surgical approach for drug-free remission from myasthenia gravis. Ann. Surg., 205:496, 1987.

18. Goldel, N., Boning, L., Fredrik, A., Holzel, D., Hartenstein, R., and Wilmanns, W.: Chemotherapy of invasive thymoma: A retrospective study of 22 cases. Cancer, 63:1493, 1989.

19. Harrington, S. W.: Surgical treatment of intrathoracic tumors. Arch. Surg., 19:1679, 1929.

20. Heuer, G. J., and Andrus, W. D.: The surgery of mediastinal tumors. Am. J. Surg., 50:146, 1940.

21. Jaretzki, A., Penn, A. S., Younger, D. S., Wolff, M., Olarte, M. R., Lovelace, R. E., and Rowland, L. P.: Maximal thymectomy for myasthenia gravis. J. Thorac. Cardiovasc. Surg., 95:747, 1988.

22. Jochelson, M., Mauch, P., Balikian, J., et al.: The significance of the residual mediastinal mass in treated Hodgkin's disease. J. Clin. Oncol., 3:637, 1985.

23. Kay, P. H., Wells, F. C., and Goldstraw, P.: A multidisciplinary approach to primary nonseminomatous germ cell tumors of the mediastinum. Ann. Thorac. Surg., 44:578, 1987.

24. King, R. M., Telander, R. L., Smithson, W. A., et al.: Primary mediastinal tumors in children. J. Pediatr. Surg., 17:512, 1982.

25. Kornstein, M. J., Curran, W. J., Turrisi, A. T., and Brooks, J. J.: Cortical versus medullary thymomas: A useful morphologic distinction? Hum. Pathol., 19:1335, 1988.

26. Lahdenne, P.: Late sequelae of gonadal, mediastinal and oral teratomas in childhood. Acta Paediatr., 81:235, 1992.

27. Lavabre-Bertrand, T., Donadio, D., Fegueux, N., et al.: A study of 15 cases of primary mediastinal lymphoma of B-cell type. Cancer, 69:2561, 1992.

28. Loeffler, J. S., Leopold, K. A., Recht, A., et al.: Emergency prebiopsy radiation for mediastinal masses: Impact on subsequent pathologic diagnosis and outcome. J. Clin. Oncol., 4:716, 1986.

29. Milton, H.: Mediastinal surgery. Lancet, 1:872, 1897.

30. Morrissey, B., Adams, H., et al.: Percutaneous needle biopsy of the mediastinum: Review of 94 procedures. Thorax, 48:632, 1993.

31. Motzer, R. J., Bosl, G. J., Geller, N. L., Peneberg, D., Yagoda, A., Golbey, R., Whitmore, W. F., Fair, W. R., Sogani, P., Herr, H., Morse, M., Carey, R. W., and Vogelzang, N.: Advanced seminoma: The role of chemotherapy and adjunctive surgery. Ann. Intern. Med., 108:513, 1988.

32. Nakahara, K., Ohno, K., Matsumura, A., Hirose, H., Mastuda, H., and Nakano, S.: Extended operation for lung cancer invading the aortic arch and superior vena cava. J. Thorac. Cardiovasc. Surg., 97:428, 1989.

33. Neuman, G. G., Weingarten, A. E., Abramowitz, R. M., et al.: The anesthetic management of the patient with an anterior mediastinal mass. Anesthesiology, 60:144, 1984.

34. Nichols, C. R., Heerema, N. A., Palmer, C., et al.: Klinefelter's syndrome associated with mediastinal germ cell neoplasms. J. Clin. Oncol., 5:1290, 1987.

35. Radford, J. A., Cowan, R. A., Flanagan, M., Dunn, G., Crowther, D., and Eddleston, B.: The significance of residual mediastinal abnormality on the chest radiograph following treatment for Hodgkin's disease. J. Clin. Oncol., 6:940, 1988.

36. Rendina, E. A., Venuta, F., Ceroni, L., Martelli, M., Gualdi, G., Caterino, M., and Ricci, C.: Computed tomographic staging of anterior mediastinal neoplasms. Thorax, 43:441, 1988.

37. Safar, D., Berrih, A. S., and Morel, E.: In vitro anti-acetylcholine receptor antibody synthesis by myasthenia gravis patient lymphocytes: Correlations with thymic histology and thymic epithelial-cell interactions. J. Clin. Immunol., 7:225, 1987.

38. Shamberger, R. C., Allarde-Segundo, A., Kozakewich, H. P., and Grier, H. E.: Surgical management of stage III and IV neuroblastoma: Resection before or after chemotherapy. J. Pediatr. Surg., 26:113; discussion 1117, 1991.

39. Simpson, I., and Campbell, P. E.: Mediastinal masses in childhood: A review from a pediatric pathologist's point of view. Prog. Pediatr. Surg., 27:93, 1991.

40. Taniguchi, S., Shibuya, T., Morioka, E., Okamura, T., Okamura, S., Inaba, S., and Niho, Y.: Demonstration of three distinct immunological disorders on erythropoiesis in a patient with red cell aplasia and autoimmune haemolytic anaemia associated with thymoma. Br. J. Haematol., 68:473, 1988.

41. Verley, J. M., and Hollman, K. H.: Thymoma: A comparative study of clinical stages, histologic features and survival in 200 cases. Cancer, 55:1074, 1985.

42. Wang, C., Gaz, R. D., and Moncure, A. C.: Mediastinal parathyroid exploration: A clinical and pathologic study of 47 cases. World J. Surg., 10:687, 1986.

I

ACUTE SUPPURATIVE MEDIASTINITIS

Thomas J. Krizek, M.D., and Lawrence J. Gottlieb, M.D.

The special construction of the chest wall serves a dual purpose: the rigid compartment *protects* the heart, lungs, and great vessels from injury and through *flexibility* allows expansion, which allows air to rush into the bronchi and alveoli with inspiration and to be forced out with expiration. The upper sternum and clavicles are important structurally and physiologically to elevate the upper rib cage and allow expansion of the chest volume. Removal of major portions of this part of the chest tends to promote collapse of the inferior ribs, resulting in functional loss. Loss of the lower two thirds of the sternum tends to restrict the ability of the abdominal muscles to aid in expiration and coughing. Movement of the area is less paradoxical. Depending on the covering over the absent sternum, varying degrees of protection of the heart are lost.

Although transecting the sternum to gain access to the heart and great vessels provides unparalleled access with minimal interference with respiration, at the same time it divides the superficially located sternum, a bone subject to the constant motion and stress of respiration. Techniques of closure have, in general, not involved rigid fixation as might be applied to other divided bones. The closed sternotomy wounds are large wounds, often incurred during long operations with considerable blood loss, often with hematoma, and with bone that is difficult to immobilize even with large amounts of foreign body (wire). That some wounds should become infected and that there should be dehiscence of bone is not surprising.

In the era before open heart surgery and antibiotic therapy, mediastinitis was found occasionally in conjunction with tumors of granulomatous infections, usually tuberculosis. Resolution of the infection occasionally produced mediastinal fibrosis and possible constriction of vessels. Suppurative mediastinitis has been reported after closed-chest cardiopulmonary resuscitation.[13] Sternal fracture from compression has been followed by hematogenous seeding (usually of *Staphylococcus aureus*) and has led to suppurative mediastinitis in the absence of any prior operation. Mediastinitis in the present time is almost entirely associated with surgical intervention.

Patients who have undergone cardiac surgery are often quite ill and prone to a variety of complications of infection. Patients may experience infections in leg wounds (as high as 11.3%), urinary tract (4.6%), and pneumonia (2.5%).[24] Superficial sternal wound infections occur in 4% to 6.3% of patients.[15] Although these are important, here the authors address the problem of deep sternal and mediastinal infections,

for which studies suggest an incidence of 2%, a percentage that has not changed for more than 20 years.[5, 6, 10, 11, 16, 18, 23]

A slight difference in the incidence of deep infection has been noted in patients undergoing various surgical procedures. The reported incidence of suppurative mediastinitis in children with congenital defects is less than 1%.[23] Valvular repairs carry a rate of infection of 1.8%, which is slightly higher than that of coronary artery bypass procedures. When these two procedures are combined the rate of mediastinitis is 2.5% to 3%.[16] Use of the internal mammary artery increases the incidence of infection; when both mammary arteries are used the infection rate nears 8%.[6]

PATHOGENESIS OF INFECTION

Surgical infections do not occur from the mere presence of bacteria but rather result from a complex interplay between the host (patient) and the available systemic and local host-defense mechanisms and pathogenic microorganisms. Experience in the management of burns and other contaminated wounds indicates that the presence of fewer than 10^5 microorganisms per gram of tissue is compatible with successful wound closure.[17] Levels higher than this result in wound breakdown, graft failure, and, as bacterial counts increase, invasive sepsis. Because 10^5 microorganisms per gram of tissue is the critical level, it is important to examine those factors in the patient and the operation itself, which might allow levels to reach 10^5 microorganisms per gram.

Predisposing Patient Factors. Many studies, both of infection in general and of mediastinitis in particular, have failed to identify specific patient factors such as age and sex as influencing the incidence of infection.[15] One prospective study, however, demonstrated that prolonged ventilation and female sex increased the risk of major sternal complications.[3] Obesity and diabetes both increase infection rates in general. Logic would dictate that those who are initially more ill, as manifested by poor nutrition and poor hemodynamics, and those who are undergoing reoperation have adverse factors that predispose toward infection.

Operating Factors. Patients with congenital heart defects appear to have a lower incidence of infection (less than 1%); those with coronary artery bypass have a higher infection rate, particularly when the internal mammary artery is used. A large series of operations on valves alone demonstrated an incidence of 1.4%. There is a correlation between how the sternotomy is made and infection. The change from Gigli (hand-driven) saws to high-speed mechanical devices have reduced infection rates.[14] As with other operations and infections, there is a linear increase in infection with prolonged duration of the operation (a reflection of complexity and duration of potential lodgment of bacteria). In a series of 17 patients with mediastinitis, the length of operative procedures ranged from 6 to 17 hours and 9 patients were operated on for more than 10 hours.[7]

Most studies show increased sepsis with prolonged bypass (more than 3 hours). As mentioned, the presence of bacteria does not correlate with infection. There is evidence that cardiopulmonary bypass affects phagocytic capacity and there is decreased ability to clear bacteria, a problem that increases with prolonged bypass time.[20]

The technique of immobilizing the sternum postoperatively has improved from nylon and silk sutures to more rigid approximation with wire. Union of bone elsewhere in the body depends on truly rigid fixation with plating or other techniques. Sargent and associates[19] demonstrated earlier sternal healing at 4 weeks after rigid fixation compared with cerclage wire closure in a primate model. Gottlieb and colleagues[9] reported successful healing with titanium miniplates in 29 patients; 24 of the 29 were in secondary closure after suppuration and 5 who were in high-risk groups were treated preventively.

Physiologic Factors

Low Flow. Low-flow states may cause decreased local host resistance to bacteria. Similarly, the use of both internal mammary arteries decreases the blood supply to the sternum and is accompanied by a fourfold to fivefold increase in mediastinitis.[2] As many as half of those with mediastinitis have had *low flow* phenomena.

Hemorrhage. All studies of infection support the fact that bleeding and hematoma predispose to bacterial growth. Data confirm that operative bleeding contributes to mediastinitis. More than 53% of patients with mediastinitis had postoperative blood loss of more than 1250 ml.[6] Reoperation (either early or elective) is also a predisposing factor, and 18% to 42% of patients with mediastinitis fit into this category.[6, 18] Similarly, postoperative cardiopulmonary resuscitation, which clearly may disrupt the repair and cause bleeding, increases complication rates two to four times.[2]

Other Factors

Technical Errors. Operating rooms rarely contain more than 60 to 70 microorganisms per cu. ft. in the air, a level far below the critical 10^5 microorganisms that must lodge in the tissue for infection to occur.[17] Studies of the operative environment showed positive cultures from the heart-lung machine in an astounding 71% of cases; 20% of patients had multiple positive sites of culture. Cultures of prosthetic valves were positive in 50%, and the cardiotomy site was positive in 64%. However, in only 2 of the 66 patients did clinical infection develop.[20] Other studies show *Staphylococcus epidermidis* grows from nasal cultures of 80% of operating room personnel, from 90% of the inside of gloves, and from 90% of wounds before closure,[17] yet the incidence of clinical infection from this organism is still low. Diphtheroids are also commonly found.

Distant Infection. It is well known that individuals with infection elsewhere in the body are predisposed to mediastinal infection.[17] Thus, it is not surprising that those with tracheotomies or those on prolonged mechanical ventilation are susceptible to infection.[24] Intravenous catheters, urinary catheters, and other drainage tubes are sources for entry of microorganisms and hematogenous seeding of operative sites.

MICROBIOLOGY

The most common microorganisms causing infection are those most indigenous to the patients and their environment;

Staphylococcus aureus and *S. epidermidis* are the most common and in a recent series accounted for 42% of infections.[9] Other gram-negative organisms and mixed infections accounted for another 25% of infections. In some infections no organisms can be recovered.

Quantitative cultures of biopsy specimens of contaminated or infected wounds are helpful diagnostically and therapeutically. In a recent series, 46% of the wounds contained more than 10^5 microorganisms per gram of tissue. About a third of the patients had persistent levels above 10^5 after débridement and required additional débridement before successful closure could be accomplished.[9]

ANTIBACTERIAL THERAPY

Many studies have indicated that antibacterial agents, to be more effective, must be administered in adequate doses, in a timely manner, and by the proper route.[17] In surgical wounds, a timely manner means before, during, and within the first several hours of the wounding. Although the antibacterial agents reach therapeutic tissue levels at the margins in well-vascularized tissue and prevent invasive wound sepsis, it is believed that most surgical wound infections and mediastinal infections are not preventable by antibacterial drugs administered after closure.

When infection has developed and when a wound is open, antibacterial agents are better delivered topically, because it is very difficult to achieve adequate tissue levels in the wound with systemic antibacterial agents. The opened sternotomy wound, the exposed mediastinum, and the granulating wound margins are biologically comparable to a burn wound, and lessons learned in burn therapy should be applied. Silver sulfadiazine and mafenide (Sulfamylon) are excellent antibacterial agents that penetrate well into granulating and infected tissue. Povidone-iodine (Betadine)-soaked materials deliver an agent that, albeit elegant for washing and skin decontamination, does not penetrate well into tissue. Many other agents can be delivered topically by constant or intermittent irrigation of the wound.

DIAGNOSIS

Suppurative mediastinitis does not present in the immediate postoperative period. Bacteria lodged in the wound must reach 10^5 microorganisms per gram to survive and then must reach levels of 10^8 per gram before they are clinically manifest. In actuality, prophylactic antibacterial agents, as part of the postoperative management, may delay the clinical appearance for 2 to 3 months; most mediastinitis will begin to be apparent between 4 days and 3 weeks.[20]

Although drainage of pus through the wound is an obvious sign, suspicion should be heightened in a patient whose pain begins to increase toward the end of the first week rather than decreasing and whose wound may become reddened and swollen. A spiking fever suggests the presence of an abscess. Fever and leukocytosis are almost always present.

Cardiac surgery is associated with other types of perioperative infection (e.g., leg, urinary tract), which may mask the systemic signs; careful attention to the chest wound itself is required to make an early diagnosis.

Patients who develop fever and leukocytosis must be suspected of harboring mediastinal sepsis, even if drainage has not appeared and the sternum is still stable. Aspiration of the mediastinum is a simple diagnostic maneuver that is of value when positive. Any drainage must be immediately cultured anaerobically as well as aerobically and antibacterial sensitivity determined.[20] Routine chest films are difficult to interpret; computed tomographic scans may be helpful, particularly if gas-forming organisms are seen.

THERAPY

All surgical complications compromise the quality of the result or in the case of suppurative mediastinitis represent a proximate and real threat to life. When subsequent to valve procedures, mortality as high as 70% has been reported.[10]

Nonoperative Therapy

Suppurative mediastinitis should be considered a surgical problem. Although nonsurgical supportive care to respiratory, vascular, and other systems is critical and although antibacterial agents given systemically are vital, they are strictly supportive and do not constitute definitive therapy, because few patients are treated nonsurgically. The nonoperative decision in the algorithm (Fig. 52–13) is usually a preliminary step. Some patients may develop a fever, leukocytosis, and other nonspecific signs and then have these features resolve with nonoperative measures. Purulent drainage is an indication for surgery.

Operative Technique

The fundamental surgical approaches to any surgical infection include adequate débridement, proper irrigation, appropriate use of antibacterial agents by the proper route, and timely closure.[17]

Débridement. Débridement has the dual purpose of removing dead tissue and foreign bodies and helping to restore bacterial balance. The wound should be opened completely and suture material, wire, blood clots, and any bits of bone removed. Costal cartilages are less vascular than bone and may require removal. Judgment is critical in determining the amount of tissue to be removed.

Irrigation. The intraoperative irrigation should be performed under pressure. Large amounts of irrigation fluid are not nearly so important as truly flushing out the microorganisms and debris from the interstices of the soft tissue where they are lodged. The pulsating jet lavage (70 psi.) is effective, as is a syringe with a fine needle directed to the wound. A bulb syringe is not adequate.

The term *irrigation* is also applied to a technique of postoperative management in which the contaminated but débrided wound is then closed over irrigation catheters into which antibacterial or other irrigating solutions may be instilled. These or other catheters are used to collect the effluent with or without suction. Introduced by Shumaker and Mandelbaum[22] in 1963, it is a technique of value in lesser infections, particularly where cavities (*dead space*) are not a feature of the wound.

Antibacterial Agents. Modern irrigating solutions include powerful antibiotics (e.g., polymyxin, bacitracin) not readily available for systemic use.[1, 4, 9, 21] The use of closed-system drainage has been a very effective management technique when performed early. Successfully used in the 1960s the technique has been expanded over the past two decades.[1, 3] Débridement and closed irrigation was used successfully in 16 patients with hospitalization ranging from 18 to 44 days.[4] A more recent study comparing closed irrigation with open techniques found no difference in outcome.[21]

Closure

Closure of the wound involves two steps: (1) rigid fixation of the sternum whenever possible and (2) adequate soft tissue coverage. The timing of closure is dependent on obtaining bacterial control of the wound.

Rigid Internal Fixation. Rigid sternal fixation has been demonstrated to be safe and effective when quantitative counts in the bone are less than 10^5 organisms per gram.[9] A rib approximator or circumferential wires are used to anatomically reduce and temporarily hold the remaining bone in place. Next 1.5-mm. holes are drilled in each sternal half. Titanium miniplates are secured with 2.4-mm. titanium *emergency* screws that act like wood screws. Miniplate fixation provides rigid fixation even to very osteoporotic bone. This technique was used successfully in 24 patients with suppurative mediastinitis; 20 (83%) were closed in one operation, and 4 required two stages of débridement before closure.[9]

The thorax is both semirigid and flexible; removal of large segments of the sternum, costochondral areas, and ribs may be accomplished without major functional loss. However, when instability leads to paradoxic motion, the defect may be bridged with autologous material such as fascia or rib. Alloplastic material such as Marlex may also be used. In general, both the cardiac and the reconstructive surgeon wish to preserve the sternum and to reconstitute continuity when the edges move. When bone is infected or marginally viable, it is far better to remove it. As final healing occurs, there is usually sufficient scarring to functionally stabilize the chest.

Soft Tissue Closure. Locally available tissue is the most desirable for closure. Additionally, muscle provides bulk and allows the soft tissue to obliterate *dead space*.

Muscle Flaps. The use of regional muscle to close the defect offers the exciting opportunity for filling the cavity with well-vascularized tissue and then either closing over the skin margins or applying a graft. Each of the muscle flaps provides vascularity to territories of skin of varying size and configuration overlying the muscle that may be transferred at the same time, thus serving a dual purpose.

Pectoralis Major Muscle. The pectoralis major muscle can

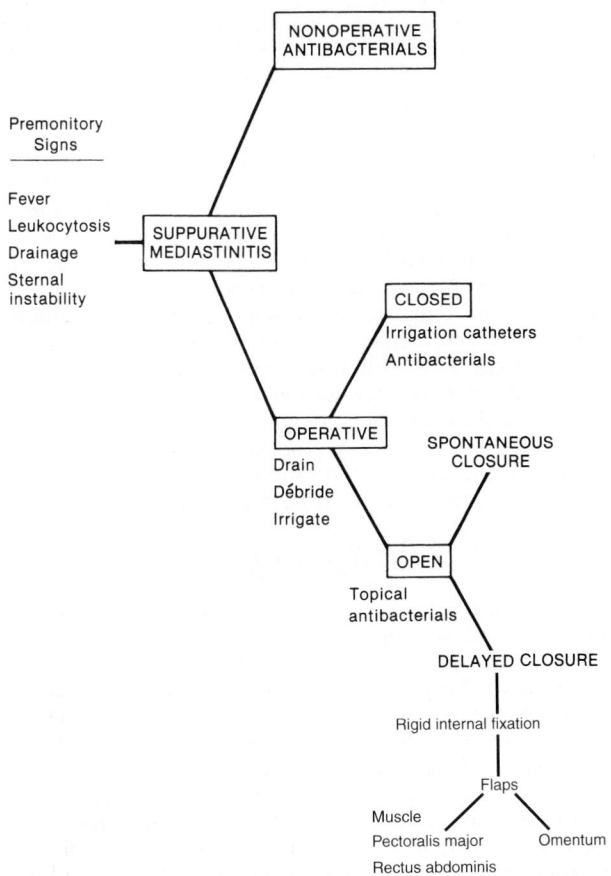

Figure 52–13. Algorithm of management of suppurative mediastinitis.

be elevated by separating it from its origin, thus taking tension off the sternal repair. The freed muscle edges can be joined in the midline (Fig. 52–14). When the humeral insertion is freed, the muscle is quite mobile and may be moved medially or turned over into cavitary defects.[2] The pectoralis major is particularly valuable in the upper three fourths of the anterior mediastinum but less so inferiorly because its arc of rotation is away from the xiphoid. The surface may be closed with chest skin if available or with skin grafts. In one study, 19 of 24 wounds were closed with pectoralis major muscle.[9]

Rectus Abdominis Muscle. A great deal of experience with this flap has been gained from its use for breast reconstruction after mastectomy. The unpredictability of its skin territories in patients who smoke or are obese is well known. This flap has become the flap of choice for some patients. Majure and co-workers[12] have used the rectus flap on 14 patients and prefer this flap because of ease of use, dependability, and aesthetic considerations. In Nahai and associates' large series,[14] the rectus was used on 145 occasions with only 3.3% complications.

Omentum. The *policeman of the abdomen* can be transposed to an extra-abdominal position. Many surgeons have demonstrated that the omentum could be freed from the colon and then rotated on either the left or the right gastroepiploic vessel (Fig. 52–15). The extent of the area of rotation is adjustable by subdividing the vascularity and thus lengthening it.

Open Technique. Open treatment is an alternative to débridement, and closure is done with or without irrigation catheters providing topical antibacterial therapy.[8] After débridement the wound is left open and treated with topical antibacterial agents.

The progress of the treatment can be monitored with real

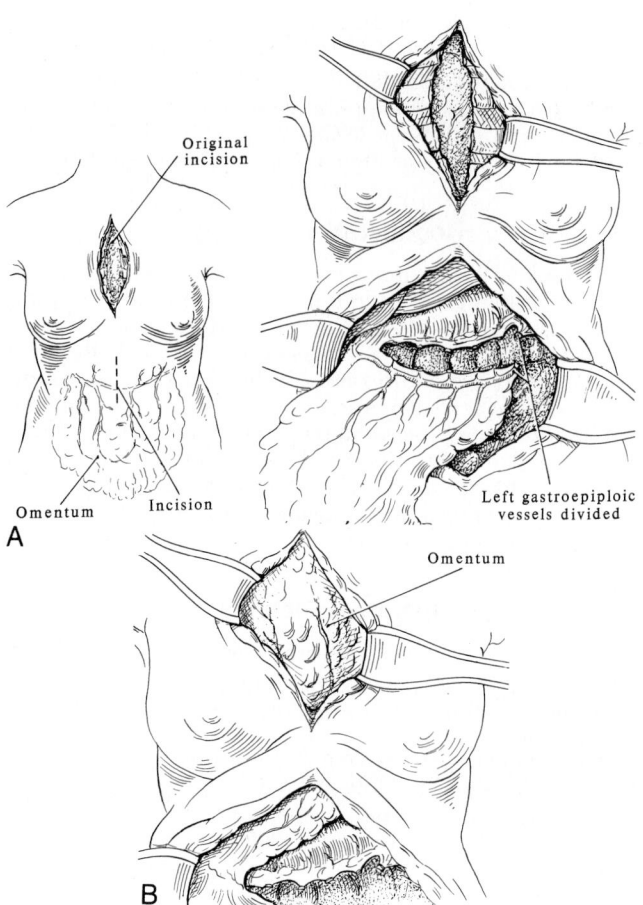

Figure 52–15. Omental flap technique. *A, left,* Relative position of omentum to defect. *A, right,* Omentum may be transferred on either right (illustrated) or left gastroepiploic vessel. *B,* Omentum in defect. The skin is then approximated, if possible, or a skin graft is applied.

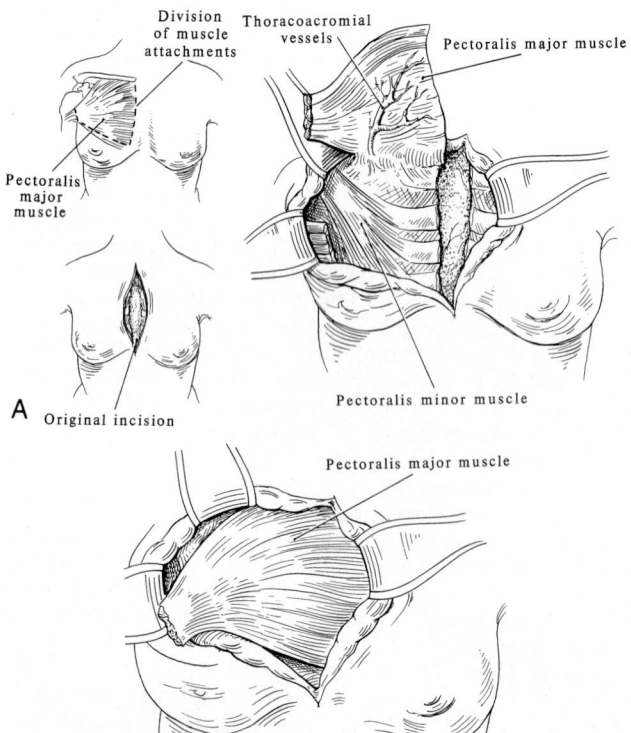

Figure 52–14. Pectoralis major transfer. *A, left,* Location of pectoralis sternal defect. *A, right,* Pectoralis major muscle with both origin and insertion released, carried on dominant vasculature, thoracoacromial vessels. *B,* Transferred into defects. Both pectoralis major muscles may be used.

diagnostic precision by quantitative microbiologic techniques. Small amounts of tissue are sampled to check the number and variety of microorganisms within the wound. The rapid slide technique provides information whether the wound has more or fewer than 10^5 microorganisms per gram of tissue.[17] This information can be available within 30 minutes and is of great value intraoperatively in determining the extent of débridement or deciding whether the wound can be closed. The traditional techniques will provide the number and variety of organisms as well as antibacterial sensitivity in 18 to 24 hours. Gottlieb and colleagues'[9] studies indicate that the quantitative techniques are useful for bone as well. When bacterial counts are controlled to less than 10^5 bacteria per gram, the wound should be closed.

RESULTS

The mortality from untreated suppurative mediastinitis is staggering, and no series includes these untreated controls. In one study, before early open débridement, 73% of the patients died. The accuracy of diagnosis and the precision by which superficial infections are differentiated from sternal dehiscence or true suppurative mediastinitis is often unclear. In one large series, 48 of 2579 cases were so diagnosed (1.86%) as having mediastinitis.[16] Of these patients, 19 (40% of infected cases, but only 0.7% of all cases) died. Because of selection of cases, it is difficult to compare *open* and *closed* techniques; certainly the more severe the infection the more likely it would be that open treatment would be used. In another large series of 2491 cases,[6] 36 patients developed suppurative mediastinitis (1.4%). Twelve of these were considered to be high risk because of other non–infection-related problems of whom 10 (83.3%) died. Of the remaining 24 patients, 8 were managed before techniques of débridement, open management, and flap closure were readily available and 2 of these patients (25%) died. The subsequent 16 patients were managed by débridement, topical therapy, and flap closure, and 3 underwent valve replacement. Of these only 1 (6%) died.

REFERENCES

1. Acinpura, A. J., Godfrey, N., Romita, M., et al.: Surgical management of infected median sternotomy: Closed irrigation vs. muscle flaps. J. Cardiovasc. Surg., 26:443, 1985.
2. Arnold, P. G., and Pairolero, P. C.: Use of pectoralis major muscle flaps to repair defects of anterior chest wall. Plast. Reconstr. Surg., 52:205, 1979.
3. Breyer, R. H., Mills, S. A., Hudspeth, A. S., Johnson, F. R., and Cordell, A. R.: A prospective study of sternal wound complications. Ann. Thorac. Surg., 37:412, 1984.
4. Bryant, L. R., Spencer, F. C., and Trinkle, J. K.: Treatment of median sternotomy infection by mediastinal irrigation with an antibiotic solution. Surgery, 169:914, 1969.
5. Cheung, E. H., Craver, J. M., Jones, E. L., et al.: Mediastinitis after cardiac valve operations. J. Thorac. Cardiovasc. Surg., 90:517, 1985.
6. Culliford, A. T., Cunningham, J. N., Zeff, R. H., et al.: Sternal and costochondral infections following open-heart surgery. J. Thorac. Cardiovasc. Surg., 72:714, 1976.
7. Engelman, R. M., Williams, C. D., Gouge, T. H., et al.: Mediastinitis following open-heart surgery. Arch Surg., 107:772, 1973.
8. Fanning, W. J., Vasko, J. S., and Kilman, J. W.: Delayed sternal closure after cardiac surgery. Ann. Thorac. Surg., 44:169, 1987.
9. Gottlieb, L. J., Pielet, R. W., Karp, R. P., Krieger, L. M., Smith, D. J., Jr., and Deeb, G. M.: Rigid internal fixation of the sternum in post-operative mediastinitis. Arch. Surg., 129:489, 1994.
10. Grmoljez, P. F., Barner, H. H., Willman, V. L., et al.: Major complications of median sternotomy. Am. J. Surg., 130:679, 1975.
11. Jurkiewicz, M. J., Bostwick, J., III, Hester, T. R., et al.: Infected median sternotomy wound. Ann. Surg., 191:738, 1980.
12. Majure, J. A., Albin, R. E., O'Donnell, R. S., et al.: Reconstruction of the infected median sternotomy wound. Ann. Thorac. Surg., 42:9, 1986.
13. Mensah, G. K., Gold, J. P., Schreiber, T., et al.: Acute purulent mediastinitis and sternal osteomyelitis after closed chest cardiopulmonary resuscitation: A case report and review of the literature. Ann. Thorac. Surg., 46:353, 1988.
14. Nahai, F., Rand, R. P., Hester, T. R., et al.: Primary treatment of the infected sternotomy wound with muscle flaps: A review of 211 consecutive cases. Plast. Reconstr. Surg., 84:434, 1989.
15. Nelson, J. C., and Nelson, R. M.: The incidence of hospital wound infection in thoracotomies. J. Thorac. Cardiovasc. Surg., 54:586, 1969.
16. Ottino, G., DePaulis, R., Pansini, S., et al.: Major sternal wound infection after open-heart surgery: A multivariate analysis of risk factors in 2,579 consecutive operative procedures. Ann. Thorac. Surg., 44:173, 1987.
17. Robson, M. C., Krizek, T. J., and Heggers, J. P.: Biology of surgical infection. In Ravitch, M. M., Austen, W. G., Scott, H. W., Thal, A. P., Wangensteen, O. H., and Steichen, F. M. (Eds.): Current Problems in Surgery. Chicago, Year Book Medical Publishers, 1973, pp. 1–62.
18. Rutledge, R., Applebaum, R. E., and Kim, B. J.: Mediastinal infection after open heart surgery. Surgery, 97:88, 1985.
19. Sargent, L. A., Seyfer, A. E., Hollinger, J., Hinson, R. J., and Graeber, G. M.: The healing sternum: A comparison of osseous healing with wire vs. rigid fixation. Ann. Thorac. Surg., 52:490, 1991.
20. Sarr, M. G., Gott, V. L., and Townsend, T. R.: Mediastinal infection after cardiac surgery. Ann. Thorac. Surg., 38:415, 1984.
21. Scully, H. E., Leclerc, Y., Martin, R. D., et al.: Comparison between antibiotic irrigation and mobilization of pectoral muscle flaps in treatment of deep sternal infections. J. Thorac. Cardiovasc. Surg., 90:523, 1985.
22. Shumaker, H. B., Jr., and Mandelbaum, I.: Continuous antibiotic irrigation in the treatment of infection. Arch. Surg., 86:384, 1963.
23. Stiegel, R. M., Beasley, M. E., Sink, J. D., et al.: Management of postoperative mediastinitis in infants and children by muscle flap rotation. Ann. Thorac. Surg., 46:45, 1988.
24. Verkkala, K.: Occurrence of and microbiological findings in postoperative infections following open-heart surgery. Ann. Clin. Res., 19:170, 1987.

II ───

SURGICAL MANAGEMENT OF MYASTHENIA GRAVIS

Jeffrey A. Hagen, M.D., and Joel D. Cooper, M.D.

Myasthenia gravis is a neurologic disorder defined clinically on the basis of weakness or fatigability occurring with repetitive exercise, which resolves with rest. It is believed to be an autoimmune disorder of neuromuscular transmission in which antibodies reduce the number of functional acetylcholine receptors at the neuromuscular junction. The clinical course in patients with myasthenia gravis is unpredictable, characterized by frequent spontaneous remissions and relapses. The response to treatment is also unpredictable; specifically, the response to thymectomy may be delayed.

Myasthenia gravis is relatively uncommon, occurring in 0.5 to 5 per 100,000 population. It can occur at any age, with a peak age at onset of 20 to 30 years in women and at older than age 50 in men. Overall, myasthenia gravis is more common in women, with a female-to-male predominance of 3:2. In young patients, the ratio of females to males approaches 5:1. The disease is nonfamilial in the majority of cases, but a genetic predisposition has been suggested. An association between HLA-B8 antigens and myasthenia gravis has been observed in young patients, as well as an association between HLA-A2 and HLA-A3 antigens in myasthenia associated with thymoma in older patients.[1] Myasthenia gravis has been shown to occur more commonly in those with other autoimmune disorders such as Graves' disease,

Hashimoto's thyroiditis, rheumatoid arthritis, systemic lupus erythematosus, and pernicious anemia.[2] There are no known racial or geographic predilections.

Although the prevalence of myasthenia gravis in the general population is low, it is one of the more common disorders of neuromuscular transmission, and it is one of the most clearly understood physiologically. However, controversy remains regarding the diagnosis and treatment of this disorder, much of which relating to the role of thymectomy.

HISTORY

The clinical disorder now known as myasthenia gravis was first recognized in 1877 when Wilks[3] reported a patient presenting with progressive weakness who ultimately died of respiratory paralysis. No central nervous system cause was found at autopsy. Over the next several years, similar case reports appeared in the literature. Goldflam[4] summarized these reported cases, along with his own collected series of patients, in 1893. He described the clinical findings that became known as the Erb-Goldflam symptom-complex. This symptom-complex was later termed *myasthenia gravis pseudoparalytica* by Jolly[5] in his classic description of the response to repetitive tetanic stimulation in these patients.

Although the clinical syndrome of myasthenia gravis and its often fatal nature were well described, little therapy was available until 1934, when Walker[6] first used physostigmine. The use of this anticholinesterase was prompted by the suggestion that the disease closely resembled curare poisoning. The dramatic improvement that followed physostigmine administration led Walker to try neostigmine therapy in a series of patients reported in 1935. This remained the standard treatment until Osserman and co-workers[7] reported the use of pyridostigmine (Mestinon) in 1954, which remains the standard medical therapy today.

The concept of surgical therapy for myasthenia gravis has its origin in observations by Weigert[8] and Bell[9] of the prevalence of thymic abnormalities in patients who died of myasthenia gravis. It was during this same time that the first thymectomy operations were being developed. In a series of 40 thymectomy procedures for Graves' disease reported in 1917, Von Haberer[10] noted that one patient who also suffered from myasthenia gravis had significant clinical improvement. This observation, along with their own experience reported in 1939, led Blalock and colleagues[11] to conclude that exploration of the thymus was indicated in all patients with severe myasthenia gravis. This was followed by a report of six intentional thymectomies in patients with myasthenia gravis without thymoma, demonstrating improvement in all five surviving patients.[12] By 1944, Blalock[13] had accumulated experience in 20 cases, firmly establishing the role of thymectomy in these patients. On the basis of this experience, he emphasized the importance of complete thymectomy as well as surgical intervention *early* in the course of the disease. These two observations remain important today.

The value of thymectomy in the *long-term* management of myasthena gravis was demonstrated by Buckingham and associates in 1967.[14] In this nonrandomized comparative study, they demonstrated that thymectomy resulted in higher remission rates and improved long-term survival when compared with medical therapy.

CLINICAL FEATURES

The clinical diagnosis of myasthenia gravis is based on the findings of weakness or early fatigue after repetitive exercise that improve with rest. The muscle groups involved, and the degree of their involvement, vary considerably over time. The ocular muscles are the most frequently involved, with approximately half of patients showing ocular muscle weakness at the time of diagnosis. Ocular muscles are ultimately involved in 90% of patients as the disease progresses. Ocular muscle involvement results in ptosis and diplopia, which can be exaggerated by sustained upward gaze (Cogan's sign). Involvement of other cranial nerves can result in dysphagia, nasal regurgitation, and aspiration.

Over time, 85% of patients develop generalized skeletal muscle involvement. This tends to involve the proximal more than the distal muscle groups. The shoulder girdle muscles are involved slightly more commonly than those of the hip girdle. The skeletal muscle weakness is often asymmetrical. Deep tendon reflexes are preserved, and results of the sensory examination are normal. A convenient system for classifying the pattern of clinical involvement was described by Osserman and Genkins[15] and is presented in Table 52–11.

NATURAL HISTORY

The natural history of untreated myasthenia gravis is not well documented, with early studies suggesting a mortality rate of between 30% and 60%.[16] These studies were performed before the existence of intensive care units and the use of mechanical ventilation, however. More recent data

TABLE 52–11. Summary of the Osserman and Genkins Classification System

I. Pediatric Myasthenia Gravis (MG)
  A. Neonatal MG (1%)
    1. Occurs in offspring of myasthenic mothers
    2. Self-limited (<6 weeks)
    3. Due to placental transfer of antibodies
    4. Progression to juvenile or adult form is rare
  B. Juvenile MG (9%)
    1. Onset from birth to puberty
    2. Tends to be permanent
    3. Differentiated from neonatal form by permanency and lack of maternal disease
    4. Subclassified by nature and degree of defect, as in adult forms
II. Adult MG
  A. Ocular MG (20%)
    1. Disease limited to ocular involvement
    2. Carries excellent prognosis
    3. Rarely progresses after 2 years of isolated ocular symptoms
  B. Mild generalized MG (30%)
    1. Initial ocular symptoms gradually progress to generalized symptoms
    2. Respiratory muscles are spared
    3. Good response to medical therapy
  C. Moderate generalized MG (20%)
    1. More severe generalized involvement
    2. Bulbar symptoms are common
    3. Relative sparing of respiratory muscles
    4. Less responsive to medical therapy
  D. Acute fulminating MG (11%)
    1. Rapid onset of severe generalized weakness
    2. Prominent respiratory symptoms
    3. High association with thymoma
    4. High mortality
    5. Poor response to treatment
  E. Late severe MG (9%)
    1. Patients with severe symptoms developing more than 2 years after onset of ocular or mild myasthenia gravis
    2. Thymoma common
    3. Poor response to therapy

From Osserman, K. E., and Genkins, G.: Studies in myasthenia gravis: Review of a twenty year experience in over 1200 patients. Mt. Sinai J. Med., *38*:497, 1971.

regarding the natural history of myasthenia gravis are lacking, because medical therapy with cholinesterase inhibitors became commonplace in 1934 and thymectomy has been used with increasing frequency since 1939.

The pattern and course of myasthenia gravis in the era of routine medical treatment were highlighted in a retrospective series by Grob and associates.[17] These researchers found that ocular complaints were the most common initial symptoms, occurring in 53% of patients. Bulbar dysfunction occurred as a presenting symptom in 11%, lower extremity weakness in 10%, and generalized muscle involvement in 9%. At the time of presentation, only 40% had purely ocular symptoms, and generalized muscular weakness was present in 40%. Over the long term, 14% continued to have ocular symptoms only. The time course of progression to generalized weakness varied, with 87% of patients experiencing progression within the first year. With medical therapy, these authors reported a spontaneous remission rate of 10%.

Similar findings regarding the natural history of medically treated patients were found by Bever and co-workers.[18] In their series, ocular symptoms were present in 84%, with roughly half of patients having only ocular symptoms at presentation. Forty-nine per cent of those who presented with isolated ocular symptoms progressed to generalized weakness, with 85% doing so in the first 2 years. Bever and co-workers also noted that 17 of 20 patients who developed myasthenic crisis did so within 2 years of the onset of disease. The rate of spontaneous remission was 17% in this series, with 30% of remissions occurring in the first year. However, spontaneous remission was reported as late as 13 years after the onset of illness.

DIAGNOSIS

Although suggested on the basis of symptoms, the diagnosis of myasthenia gravis is confirmed by electrophysiologic testing, pharmacologic testing, or immunologic testing of antibody levels. Although none of these tests is uniformly positive, in combination, they can establish the diagnosis in most patients.

Since the first description of the classic decremental response on electromyography (EMG),[19] the techniques of EMG have been refined, leading to improved accuracy in diagnosing myasthenia gravis. In a review of the diagnostic tests applicable to patients with myasthenia, Phillips and Melnick[20] found a sensitivity rate of 34% for standard EMG studies and a sensitivity rate of 76% in patients with generalized disease. The technique of single-fiber EMG, which detects the phenomenon of jitter or blocking, allows the identification of many subclinical cases of generalized myasthenia gravis. Single-fiber EMG studies may also improve the sensitivity and specificity of EMG testing, having been shown to be abnormal in 90% of patients with mild generalized symptoms and in virtually 100% of those with moderate to severe disease.[21] In patients with ocular myasthenia, single-fiber EMG studies are positive in 60% to 75%.[22]

Shortly after EMG was introduced as a diagnostic test, short-acting cholinesterase medications, such as edrophonium (Tensilon), were introduced by Osserman and Kaplan[23] as a diagnostic test for myasthenia gravis. When administered intravenously, edrophonium produces significant improvement in muscle strength, usually within 30 to 60 seconds. The sensitivity of the edrophonium test is approximately 85% for ocular myasthenia gravis and 95% for generalized myasthenia.

Finally, the diagnosis of myasthenia gravis can be confirmed on the basis of elevated acetylcholine receptor antibody titers. First detected by Almon in 1974, elevated titers of these antibodies are highly specific for myasthenia gravis. The sensitivity ranges from 64% in patients with ocular symptoms only to as high as 89% in patients with generalized myasthenia gravis.[20]

DIFFERENTIAL DIAGNOSIS

On the basis of symptoms of weakness and easy fatigability, myasthenia gravis must be differentiated from a variety of conditions that affect both muscle function and neuromuscular transmission. All types of muscular dystrophy, amyotrophic lateral sclerosis, a variety of ophthalmoplegias, and the weakness associated with psychoneurosis or hyperthyroidism can cause symptoms similar to those seen in myasthenia gravis. A thorough physical examination, including a detailed neurologic evaluation, usually differentiates these disorders from myasthenia gravis. The use of edrophonium as a diagnostic test also excludes these disorders, because no improvement in weakness occurs with its administration.

The differential diagnosis of myasthenia gravis also includes the myasthenia associated with organophosphate intoxication, certain snakebites, and drug-induced myasthenic syndromes. The drugs most commonly implicated include penicillamine, procainamide, and aminoglycosides in high doses. A detailed history is important to differentiate these causes of weakness from myasthenia gravis. Discontinuation of the offending medication is generally associated with reversal of the weakness within several weeks.

Two of the most common disorders of neuromuscular transmission in the differential diagnosis of myasthenia gravis include botulism and Lambert-Eaton syndrome. On the basis of history, physical examination, and edrophonium testing, these disorders may be indistinguishable from myasthenia gravis. EMG is essential to the differential diagnosis of these conditions.

Botulism is a disease of neuromuscular transmission caused by the toxin of the bacterium *Clostridium botulinum*. The bacteria involved can be either ingested in contaminated food or produced in anaerobically infected wounds. This toxin causes a descending-type paralysis, involving the eye muscles, then the other muscles of the head and neck, followed by generalized skeletal muscle weakness. The defect in neuromuscular transmission involves impaired acetylcholine release from the motor neuron,[24] in contrast to the impaired binding to receptors seen in myasthenia gravis. As a result, EMG reveals an incremental response to repetitive testing.

Lambert-Eaton syndrome is a myasthenic syndrome involving fluctuating weakness of the proximal muscle groups. The weakness may involve the facial muscles, but to a lesser extent than that seen in myasthenia gravis. This syndrome, also presumed to be autoimmune, is associated with an underlying malignancy in the majority of cases. Small cell cancer of the lung is the most common underlying malignancy, occurring in 70% of patients.[25] In contrast to patients with myasthenia gravis, those with Lambert-Eaton syndrome have diminished deep tendon reflexes, and autonomic symptoms are not uncommon. EMG shows an incremental response to repetitive stimulation, compared with the decremental response seen in myasthenia gravis.

Finally, patients presenting with isolated ocular symptoms of myasthenia gravis must be differentiated from those with intracranial mass lesions affecting the cranial nerves, as well as those patients suffering from progressive external ophthalmoplegia. Patients with ocular symptoms caused by mass lesions may be differentiated based on the presence of other neurologic symptoms or headache. Computed tomography (CT) or magnetic resonance imaging (MRI) also helps with this differentiation. Progressive external ophthalmoplegia can be differentiated on the basis of skeletal muscle biopsy. This rare condition is characterized by weakness of the extraocular muscles and occasionally proximal extremity weakness. It is, in most cases, also associated with abnormalities in mitochondrial function.

PATHOPHYSIOLOGY

Physiology of Neuromuscular Transmission

An understanding of the diagnosis and treatment of patients with myasthenia gravis requires familiarity with several fundamentals of the normal physiology of neuromuscular transmission. In contrast to the complex integration of impulses that occurs in other synapses, neuromuscular transmission involves a relatively simple relay process between a motor neuron terminal and a postsynaptic receptor on the muscle cell (Fig. 52–16). In response to stimulation of the nerve and calcium entry into the motor neuron axon, acetylcholine is released at the nerve terminal. The acetylcholine diffuses across the synaptic cleft, where it binds to receptors on the muscle cell. This binding creates an ion channel, which allows influx of positively charged ions, principally sodium, down the normal electrochemical gradient. This influx of positively charged ions causes a localized depolarization of

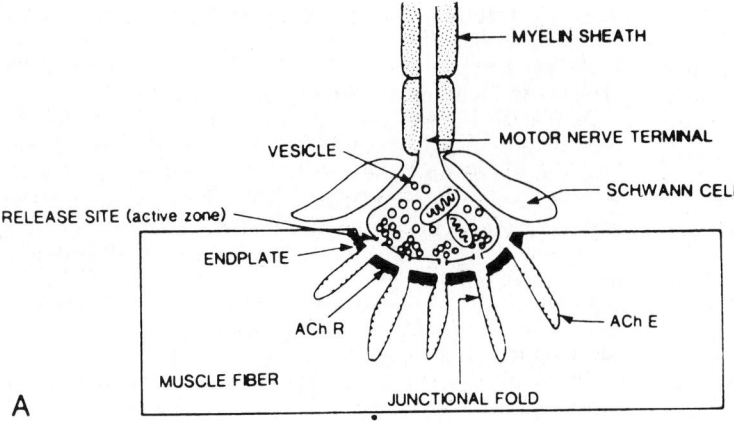

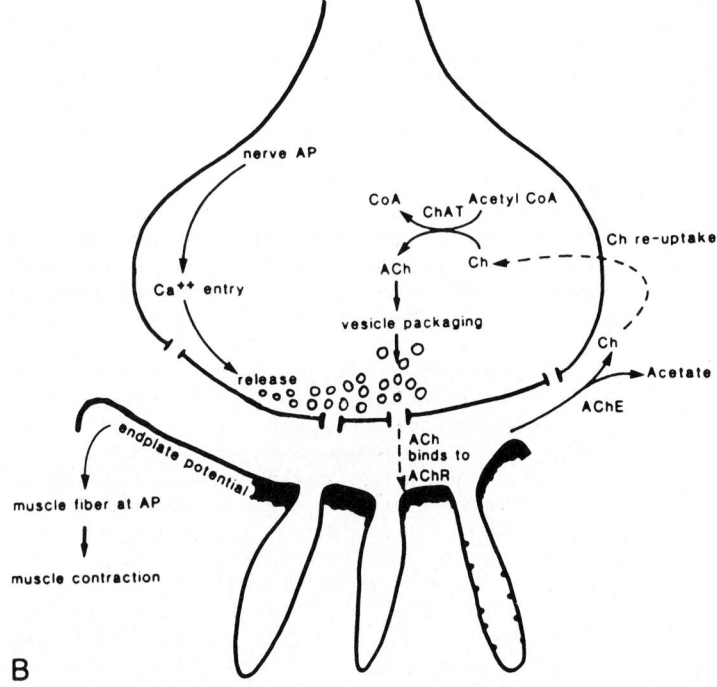

Figure 52–16. A, Schematic representation of the neuromuscular junction. B, Magnification of the neuromuscular junction showing details of acetylcholine release, degradation, and binding to receptors, leading to muscle contraction. (From Pascuzzi, R. M.: Introduction to the neuromuscular junction and neuromuscular transmission. (Reprinted with permission from Seminars in Neurology, *10*:1–5, 1990, Thieme Medical Publishers, Inc.)

the muscle cell membrane, which is referred to as a miniature end-plate potential. If the sum of several of these miniature end-plate potentials is of sufficient amplitude, which is dependent on the amount of acetylcholine bound to the receptors, the threshold for activation of the muscle cell is reached, resulting in generation of an action potential. Action potential generation causes calcium influx by the activation of membrane calcium channels, which results in muscle contraction.[26]

Under normal circumstances, far more acetylcholine is released from the motor neuron than is necessary to create an action potential in the muscle cell. In addition, many more acetylcholine receptors are present on the motor end plate than are needed for generation of action potentials. This provides a "safety factor,"[27] which ensures neuromuscular transmission under normal circumstances. Alterations in this safety factor give disorders of neuromuscular transmission such as myasthenia gravis their origin.

The basic pathophysiologic alteration producing defective neuromuscular transmission in patients with myasthenia gravis involves a reduction in the number of the functional acetylcholine receptors on the postsynaptic membrane. Thus,

although normal amounts of acetylcholine are released from the motor neuron, the number of resultant miniature end-plate potentials generated is reduced. As a result, the sum of miniature end-plate potentials may not reach the threshold for generation of action potentials. This causes failure of neuromuscular transmission.

The decrease in the number of functional acetylcholine receptors at the motor end plate is not uniform. As a result, the numerous muscle fibers innervated by a single motor neuron show variation in the number of miniature end-plate potentials occurring in response to acetylcholine release. This, in turn, produces a variability in the action potentials generated, resulting in the phenomenon referred to as *jitter*, seen on single-fiber EMG studies in patients with myasthenia gravis. When this variability in the timing of miniature end-plate potentials reaches 80 to 100 μs., the muscle fiber may fail to generate any action potential whatsoever. This phenomenon, called *blocking*, is the cellular cause for the decremental response to repetitive stimulation seen on standard EMG studies. This is the same phenomenon that is responsible for the fatigue following repetitive exercise that occurs in patients with myasthenia gravis.

Pathogenesis

The autoimmune nature of myasthenia gravis was first proposed by Simpson in 1960 and was subsequently confirmed by several clinical and experimental observations. The first of these observations was made by Chang and Lee,[28] who reported a specific, high-affinity binding of snake venom to acetylcholine receptors of skeletal muscle. This observation allowed precise identification and localization of these receptors and their subsequent purification. Once purified, the acetylcholine receptor function and structure were studied extensively.[29] Receptor turnover was also characterized as a process of endocytosis and of subsequent lysosomal destruction.

In the process of evaluating receptor structure and function, Patrick and Lindstrom[30] attempted to produce acetylcholine receptor antibodies in rabbits. In the course of these experiments, they noted that in addition to producing these antibodies after injection with purified acetylcholine receptors, the animals developed a pattern of weakness very similar to that seen clinically in patients with myasthenia gravis. This observation, along with a demonstrated response to anticholinesterase medication, led them to propose a relationship between this experimental model and clinical myasthenia gravis.

This model of experimental autoimmune myasthenia gravis (EAMG) was confirmed by Seybold to be similar to myasthenia gravis both clinically and electromyographically. By utilizing this model, it was demonstrated that acetylcholine receptors are reduced. In addition, autoantibodies to both receptors and complement fragments were isolated to the neuromuscular junction,[31] further implicating an autoimmune process.

Clinically, the autoimmune nature of myasthenia gravis was supported by the demonstration of acetylcholine receptor antibodies in the serum of 80% of patients with myasthenia gravis. These antibodies were subsequently localized to the neuromuscular junction.[31] In addition, the acetylcholine receptors were shown to be reduced in number.

The mechanism of the autoimmune process in myasthenia gravis is unknown. However, since the number of receptors is reduced in both EAMG and clinical myasthenia gravis, initial efforts were focused on the possibility of antibody-mediated destruction of the acetylcholine receptor. Studies performed in muscle cell cultures revealed that antibody-induced cross-linking of the acetylcholine receptors resulted in accelerated endocytosis and subsequent receptor degradation.[32] This mechanism was confirmed by studies of receptor half-lives in rats with EAMG, showing that the half-life was reduced approximately 50%.[33]

In addition to accelerated internalization and degradation of the receptors, evidence has accumulated to implicate complement activation in the development of myasthenia gravis. Along with IgG antibodies, complement fragments C3 and C9 have been isolated to the neuromuscular junction.[31] The potential role of complement has also been suggested by observations that passive transfer of EAMG from animal to animal is complement dependent.[34]

In addition to these proposed mechanisms, simple antibody binding to the receptor site and inhibition of acetylcholine binding may play a role. However, detailed studies of the autoantibodies present in both EAMG and clinical myasthenia gravis have shown that these particular antibodies are present in fewer than 30% of those affected.[35] The more common autoantibodies to the alpha subunit of the receptor, which result in accelerated degradation and not receptor blockade, suggest that the mechanism of simple competitive inhibition of the receptor may be of secondary importance.

ROLE OF THE THYMUS GLAND

Although the source of the autoantibodies in myasthenia gravis is unknown, the thymus gland is thought to have a major role for several reasons. First, it has been observed that the thymus gland is abnormal in up to 80% of patients with myasthenia gravis.[36] The most common abnormality is follicular lymphoid hyperplasia (Fig. 52–17), which is present in 60% of patients. These lymphoid follicles have been shown to contain B lymphocytes,[37] which produce antibodies to acetylcholine receptors. In addition to lymphoid hyperplasia, 10% to 20% have thymoma.[38] It has also been observed that 30% to 60% of patients with thymoma have or subsequently develop myasthenia gravis.

In addition to structural abnormalities of the thymus, the presence of acetylcholine receptor antibodies and antibodies to striated muscle has been demonstrated in the thymus of patients with myasthenia gravis.[35, 39] It is generally accepted that the thymic myoid cells, with their resemblance to embryonic muscle cells, serve as the antigen source for the development of these antibodies. Finally, the central role of the thymus in the pathogenesis of myasthenia gravis is supported by the observed beneficial effect of thymectomy.

TREATMENT

Therapeutic options for patients with myasthenia gravis include medical therapy with anticholinesterase medications and/or immunosuppression, plasmapheresis, and surgical treatment by thymectomy. There is considerable controversy

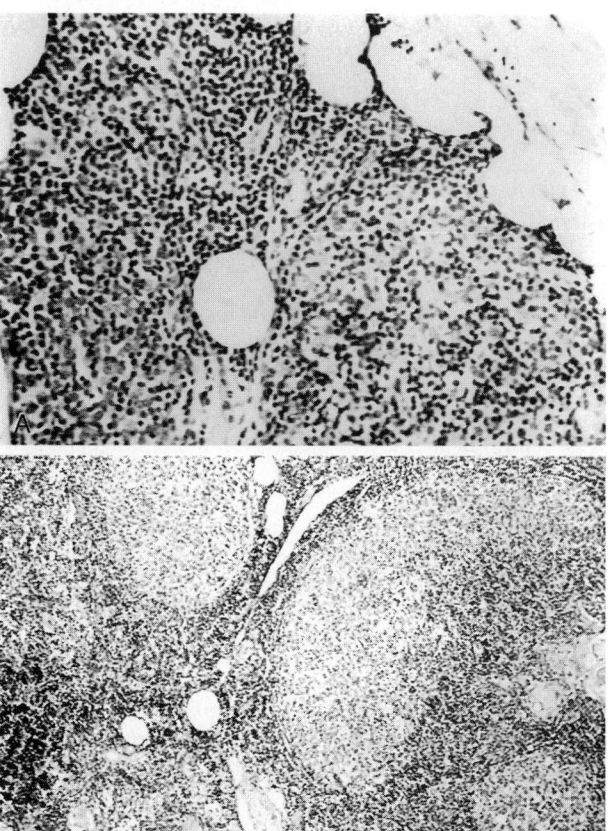

Figure 52–17. *A*, Photomicrograph of normal thymus. Note the absence of lymphoid follicles. Hematoxylin and eosin, ×80. *B*, Photomicrograph of thymus in a patient with myasthenia gravis. Pale germinal centers (arrows) represent follicular lymphoid hyperplasia. Hematoxylin and eosin, ×80.

with respect to the various combinations of these therapies and the sequence of their utilization. Much of this controversy centers around difficulties in classifying the extent of disease, to allow comparison of the various modes of therapy. In addition, the variable natural history of this disease, with its spontaneous remissions and subsequent relapses, makes discerning the benefits of any treatment modality difficult.

Anticholinesterase Therapy

Although it has no direct effect on the underlying disease, anticholinesterase therapy can lead to substantial improvement in symptoms. These drugs work by decreasing hydrolysis of acetylcholine in the synaptic cleft. Pyridostigmine (Mestinon) is the most commonly used agent and has a relatively long duration of action. Neostigmine (Prostigmin), with its more rapid onset and shorter duration of action, may be more useful in the perioperative period. Edrophonium (Tensilon) has a very rapid onset and short duration of action and is used mostly as a diagnostic test. The optimal dosage of these preparations varies widely from patient to patient. Therefore, careful adjustment is required to achieve the maximal response while minimizing the muscarinic side effects of abdominal cramping, diarrhea, excessive salivation, diaphoresis, and bradycardia.

A particularly feared complication of anticholinesterase inhibition therapy is the development of so-called cholinergic crisis. The mechanism of this profound weakness is unknown, but it may be related to excessive accumulation of acetylcholine at the neuromuscular junction. This would produce a depolarizing-type neuromuscular blockade. Differentiating drug-induced cholinergic crisis from myasthenic crisis on clinical grounds alone can be difficult. This differentiation can be made by administering the short-acting drug edrophonium, which results in improvement of strength in patients suffering from myasthenic crisis, with no improvement noted in those suffering from cholinergic crisis.

Corticosteroid Therapy

Corticosteroid therapy has been reported to produce improvement in symptoms in up to 80% of patients with myasthenia gravis,[40] although no controlled trials exist to document this benefit. Usually reserved for patients who fail to respond to anticholinesterase therapy or those who develop intolerable side effects, corticosteroids have also been used to prepare patients for thymectomy. The side effects of long-term corticosteroid therapy limit the usefulness of these agents, and relapses are particularly common after their discontinuation.

Immunosuppression

Immunosuppressive agents such as azathioprine (Imuran) have also been advocated as an alternative for patients who fail to respond to, or are intolerant of, anticholinesterase therapy. Again, there are relatively few controlled studies to document the usefulness of azathioprine, although response rates in retrospective studies range from 71% to 83%.[41, 42] Side effects are quite common, necessitating dosage reduction or discontinuation of therapy in many patients.

Plasma Exchange

Plasmapheresis to remove autoantibodies has been shown to produce improvement in symptoms in up to 90% of patients.[43] Because of the extravascular distribution of the majority of the primary pathogenic antibody (IgG), multiple exchanges are required. Typically performed every other day, five exchanges over 10 days reduce the IgG levels to 5% of baseline.[44] Levels return to within 10% of baseline by 28 days,[45] which effectively limits the use of plasmapheresis to the short term, such as to assist in the management of myasthenic crisis, to aid in weaning patients from the ventilator, and as a means of preparing patients with severe weakness for thymectomy.

Complications of plasmapheresis relate to the removal of plasma constituents other than the autoantibodies to acetylcholine receptors. Nonspecific reduction in immunoglobulins may predispose these patients to infection, leading many to administer human pooled gamma globulin after a course of plasma exchange. Theoretically, loss of coagulation factors during exchange may predispose to hemorrhage and antithrombin III removal may predispose to thrombosis. In addition, complement levels and platelet counts are reduced.[46, 47] Actual complications are rare, however, although the cost of plasmapheresis and the transient nature of the benefit limit the usefulness of the technique in the long-term treatment of myasthenic patients.

Surgical Therapy

Since Blalock's report in 1941, many series have been reported demonstrating a favorable response to thymectomy in patients with myasthenia gravis. Although it is generally agreed that thymectomy is of benefit to many patients, its precise role in treating patients with myasthenia gravis remains uncertain, owing to a lack of controlled studies identifying which patients are most likely to respond. The exact mechanism by which thymectomy exerts its beneficial effect is unknown, and the benefit following the procedure may not be apparent for years. Most physicians consider patients for thymectomy when medical treatment is unsuccessful or if side effects limit the usefulness of cholinesterase inhibitors. In addition, many consider patients for operation early in the presence of generalized symptoms. This concept is based on the observation, made initially by Blalock, that a patient with a short duration of illness is most likely to benefit from operation.

Before operation, the patient's symptoms should be controlled medically, usually by anticholinesterase therapy. In some cases, corticosteroids are used, although these should be avoided if possible; preoperative plasmapheresis can be used instead. Particular attention should be given to optimizing respiratory mechanics, especially if sternotomy is contemplated. A CT scan is performed in all cases to exclude the presence of thymoma.

The choice of operation varies from transcervical thymectomy, as advocated by Kirshner and associates[48] and Cooper and co-workers,[49] to a more radical thymectomy performed by means of a median sternotomy, as advocated by Jaretzki and colleagues.[50] Advocates of the transcervical approach emphasize the decreased morbidity associated with the less invasive procedure, which still achieves satisfactory remission and response rates. Furthermore, the minimal morbidity associated with the transcervical approach may facilitate acceptance of thymectomy early in the course of the disease, even if symptoms are well controlled with medication. Jaretzki and colleagues,[50] citing the common anomalies of thymic anatomy, emphasized the importance of removing all the adjacent cervical and mediastinal fat, which may contain aberrant thymic tissue. The remission and response rates from several series are shown in Table 52–12, indicating comparable results after transcervical and transsternal resection. Because there are no direct comparative studies, the optimal surgical approach remains to be identified. There is no doubt, however, that the single most important principle of surgical therapy, regardless of the approach taken, is complete re-

TABLE 52–12. Results of Thymectomy for Myasthenia Gravis

Series	Remission (%)	Benefit* (%)	Mortality (%)	Morbidity (%)
Jaretzki 1977–1985	40	94	0	7
Mulder 1954–1981	51	87	1	n/a
Mulder 1981–1987	36	80	0	n/a
Huang 1977–1984	46	95	0	12
Diehl 1972–1987	28	72	2	15
Cooper 1977–1986	52	95	0	2

*Improved symptoms or decreased medications.
n/a, Information not available.

moval of the thymus as early as possible in the course of the disease whenever generalized symptoms are present.

Surgical Technique

Transsternal thymectomy is performed using a standard median sternotomy. The mediastinal extension of the deep cervical fascia is identified on the undersurface of the sternothyroid muscle. This fascial layer is incised at the midline to expose the thymus gland. Each lower pole is then dissected bluntly from the undersurface of this fascia and from the pericardium posteriorly and the extrapleural fascia laterally. As the dissection proceeds superiorly, one or two arterial branches to the thymus arising from the internal mammary arteries are identified and divided. By continuing the dissection superiorly, with downward traction on the gland, the superior poles can be brought into the wound. At the apex of each superior pole, there is usually an arterial branch, arising from the inferior thyroid artery. Finally, blunt and sharp dissection posterior to the gland separates the thymus from the innominate vein. It is here that the venous drainage, by one or two branches draining directly into the innominate vein, can be ligated. The anterior mediastinum is drained, as are the pleural spaces if they are entered. The wound is closed with sternal wires and appropriate subcutaneous and skin sutures.

The *maximal thymectomy* approach described by Jaretzki and colleagues[50] combines a horizontal cervical incision with a median sternotomy to allow "removal of all thymic tissue predictably." This approach was based on observations regarding the variability of the anatomy of the thymus. In this operation, all mediastinal tissue anterior to the pericardium and great vessels is removed. The dissection extends laterally to a point located posterior to the phrenic nerves. The resection includes removal of the mediastinal pleura. In the neck, the upper poles are removed *en bloc* with the adjacent fatty tissue. Using this technique, the authors reported complete remission rates of 46% and an overall response rate of 96% in first-time operations.[50]

The transcervical approach, because of its less invasive nature, has continued to receive interest. Historically, this was the initial approach that was supplanted by the transsternal approach. Interest in the transcervical approach was rekindled by Carlens and colleagues,[51] Crile,[52] and Akakura.[53] In 1970, Kirshner reported 40 patients treated by transcervical thymectomy, and this was soon followed by a report by Papatestas and associates[54] involving more than 700 cases of myasthenia treated by transcervical thymectomy. The technique was further enhanced by Cooper's development of a specially designed retractor to improve exposure and ensure complete thymectomy.

The operative technique is as follows. The patient is placed supine with the shoulders elevated on an inflatable bag, with the head positioned at the top of the operating table resting in a "donut." The intravenous line is placed in the right arm, and the blood pressure is measured on the patient's left arm to avoid interference from intraoperative compression of either the innominate artery or the left innominate vein. The patient should be prepped as for a median sternotomy, should this become necessary. The anesthetic technique must avoid any use of paralyzing agents.

The skin incision is made along a skin crease approximately 2 cm. above the sternal notch, extending laterally to each sternocleidomastoid muscle. Flaps are raised in a plane beneath the platysma superiorly to the level of the thyroid cartilage and inferiorly to the level of the sternum. The strap muscles are split vertically at the midline, and the thymus gland is identified immediately beneath the sternothyroid muscle and anterior to the inferior thyroid vein. The uppermost aspect of the left upper pole is identified where it is ligated. The ligature is left attached to the upper pole for purposes of traction. The right upper pole is similarly dissected and ligated before division. The upper poles are then bluntly dissected free to the level of the sternal notch, where they typically fuse anterior to the innominate vein. A finger is inserted into the mediastinum anterior to the gland to dissect it from the undersurface of the sternum. Retraction of the superior pole anteriorly at this point allows the veins draining to the innominate vein to be easily identified, ligated, and divided.

At this point, a specially designed narrow right-angle retractor is placed beneath the sternum (Cooper Thymectomy Retractor, Pilling Company, Ft. Washington, PA) and attached to a Poly-Tract (Pilling Company, Ft. Washington, PA) overhead bar (Fig. 52–18). After the sternum is lifted with this apparatus, the inflatable pillow beneath the shoulders is deflated, which allows the shoulders to fall backward, improving exposure. With this technique, the entire mediastinal portion of the thymus can be dissected under direct vision. The dissection begins on the right lateral aspect of the gland, extending inferiorly to the limits of the right lower pole. The gland is then swept off the anterior surface of the aorta and pericardium, mobilizing the left lower pole, including the tail of tissue that often extends downward toward the aortopulmonary window. After the gland has been removed entirely

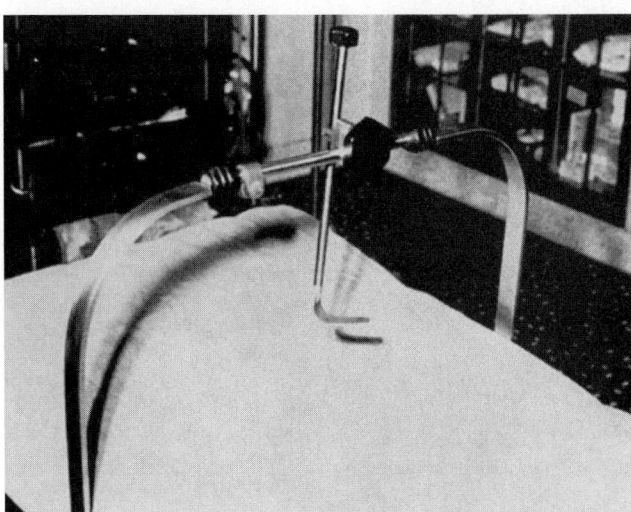

Figure 52–18. Specially designed right-angle retractor attached to an overhead bar. When placed behind the sternum, excellent exposure of the mediastinum is obtained. (From Cooper, J. D., Al-Jilaihawa, A. N., Pearson, F. G., et al.: An improved technique to facilitate transcervical thymectomy for myasthenia gravis. Ann. Thorac. Surg., *45*:242–247, 1988. Reprinted with permission from the Society of Thoracic Surgeons.)

(Fig. 52–19), the remaining mediastinal fat is removed on both sides, extending to the mediastinal pleura. The wound is then closed in layers over a red rubber catheter. This catheter is removed as the platysma is closed, with the lungs held in static inflation. A chest tube is rarely required, even if one or both pleural spaces have been entered.

The recent proliferation of video-assisted thoracic surgery (VATS) techniques has added yet another alternative to the surgeon's armamentarium. Because of the limited experience with this procedure, its role in the management of patients with myasthenia gravis remains uncertain. Thoracoscopic thymectomy, with the use of multiple access parts and the need for chest tube drainage, may not be less invasive than a transcervical procedure. There is little doubt, however, that this technique is easier to teach and to learn than the transcervical procedure.

The patient is positioned in the supine position with the left side of the chest elevated approximately 45 degrees on a small roll. The left arm is then secured overhead in a neutral (90-degree flexion) position. The thymus is then removed by a combined cervical approach and an anterior mediastinal dissection performed through three left-sided access ports.

The cervical dissection is performed in a manner similar to that described for transcervical thymectomy, mobilizing the left and right superior poles. After the upper portion of the gland is completely dissected, the three access ports are placed in the left chest. Two are placed in the fifth intercostal space at the anterior axillary line and at the midclavicular line. The third is placed in the sixth intercostal space parasternally. By utilizing the lateral port for traction and the medial port for dissection, the left lobe of the thymus is mobilized completely, including the extension into the aortopulmonary window. The venous drainage to the innominate vein is controlled with the application of endoscopic clips. The same process is used to mobilize the right lower pole, again identifying the venous drainage and controlling the veins by application of endoscopic clips. After the thoracoscopic mobilization is complete, the thymus gland is removed through the cervical incision. All incisions are then closed in an anatomic manner, and a single chest tube is left in place.

Postoperative Care

The essentials of postoperative care center around early extubation, aggressive attention to the patient's pulmonary status, and early ambulation, whether a transsternal or a transcervical approach has been used. Anticholinesterase medication is resumed when the patient is extubated, and the postoperative medical management is the same as that used preoperatively. Early postoperative results of this approach have been satisfying, with mortality in the range of 0% to 2% and morbidity occurring in 2% to 15% of patients in reported series (see Table 52–12).

RESULTS OF SURGICAL THERAPY

The long-term benefits of thymectomy for patients with myasthenia gravis are difficult to identify with precision because of the uncertainty regarding the natural history of the untreated disease, the unpredictable rate of disease progression, and the unpredictable occurrence of spontaneous remission. In addition, comparison between series is complicated by difficulties in classifying the extent of disease present in the various patient populations. In a large retrospective series, Buckingham and colleagues[14] reported a complete remission rate of 33% in patients who underwent thymectomy, compared with an 8% complete remission rate with medical treatment. They also noted a survival advantage associated with the performance of thymectomy. On the basis of this study and several subsequent studies, thymectomy is generally accepted for patients with generalized symptoms of myasthenia gravis.

The indications for thymectomy in patients with isolated ocular symptoms are less clear. Schumm and co-workers[55] reported a series of 18 patients with isolated ocular symptoms, noting clinical improvement after thymectomy in 80%, with a complete remission rate of 17%. Papatestas and associates,[54] in reporting the results in more than 2000 patients treated for myasthenia gravis, agreed with the concept of thymectomy for isolated ocular symptoms, noting that results after 10 years were not significantly different from the remission rates noted after thymectomy in patients with mild generalized disease. More importantly, thymectomy prevented the progression to generalized disease in these patients. They also showed that the results of thymectomy are best if the procedure is performed early in the course of the disease, before progression to severe generalized symptoms. Because the morbidity associated with the transcervical operation is minimal, an approach employing early transcervical thymectomy would avoid the risk of side effects from immunosuppressive drugs.

Finally, the series reported by Frist and co-workers[56] in 1994 included five patients with isolated ocular symptoms treated by thymectomy. In their experience, three of these patients were asymptomatic after surgery, one had no change in symptoms, and one deteriorated. They concluded that although the number of patients was small, the minimal morbidity associated with thymectomy, coupled with the propensity for patients with ocular symptoms to progress to generalized myasthenia gravis, suggests that the procedure should be considered for selected patients with ocular myasthenia.

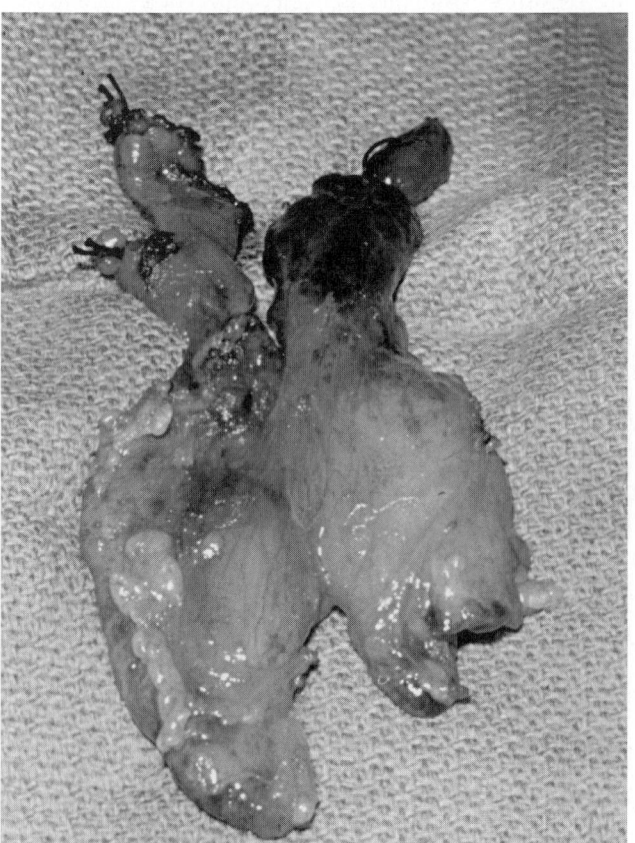

Figure 52–19. Representative specimen from a patient with myasthenia gravis, removed by transcervical thymectomy.

Specific predictors of improvement after thymectomy were addressed by the same authors in a series of 46 patients. An age younger than 45 years was found to be an independent predictor of favorable outcome after thymectomy. Age, however, was not found to be a predictor of outcome in series by Olanow and co-workers[57] and Papatestas and associates.[54] Female gender was identified in Frist and colleagues' series as an independent predictor of favorable response to operation. This was also observed in a series published by Hatton and co-workers[58] but not in the series by Jaretzki and colleagues[50] and Papatestas and associates.[54] In general, as was demonstrated in Frist and colleagues' series, the severity of symptoms at the time of operation is considered to be predictive of outcome, with the best results of thymectomy occurring in patients with mild generalized symptoms. Most series have demonstrated that the duration of symptoms alone does not appear to be an independent predictor of outcome.[50, 56, 59] The presence of a thymoma is associated with a higher likelihood of more severe symptoms and with less improvement after thymectomy.

SUMMARY

Although it has been nearly 100 years since myasthenia gravis was first recognized and 50 years since medical and surgical therapy have been available, a great deal of controversy remains regarding the ideal treatment strategy for these patients. Until proper controlled trials are performed, these controversies will remain. Recent advances in understanding the immunology of this disorder may help resolve this issue as specific immunotherapy becomes available. At present, the initial approach to a patient with myasthenic symptoms involves careful history and physical examination, along with a complete diagnostic evaluation to establish the diagnosis and to determine the pattern and severity of disease.

Patients presenting with isolated ocular symptoms can often be managed by low-dose pyridostigmine or corticosteroid therapy. They must be observed carefully, however, because the majority will go on to develop generalized symptoms. In those patients in whom conservative treatment fails, or in patients who progress to generalized disease, thymectomy should be performed. Alternatively, thymectomy may be used as primary therapy for ocular myasthenia to avoid the complications of conservative treatment. This produces remission in approximately 20% of patients, with minimal morbidity, especially if the transcervical approach is used. Patients who present with generalized symptoms should be offered thymectomy once the weakness is controlled by anticholinesterase therapy, corticosteroids, or plasma exchange. This approach maximizes the rate of remission while minimizing the side effects of long-term medical therapy.

The ideal operative technique remains to be defined. On the basis of available data, it appears that any technique that allows complete removal of the thymus gland is acceptable. As experience with newer strategies such as thoracoscopic thymectomy[60] increases, other surgical options may become available for these patients.

SELECTED REFERENCES

Finley, J. C., and Pascuzzi, R. M.: Rational therapy of myasthenia gravis. Semin. Neurol., 10:70, 1990.
  This comprehensive review of the natural history and treatment of myasthenia gravis includes more than 60 references covering all available treatment modalities.

Keesey, J. C.: Electrodiagnostic approach to defects of neuromuscular transmission. Muscle Nerve, 12:613, 1989.
  This is a comprehensive review of the mechanisms of neuromuscular transmission and the defects associated with various disease states, such as myasthenia gravis. Emphasis is placed on the role of electrodiagnostic testing.

Osserman, K. E., and Genkins, G.: Studies in myasthenia gravis: Review of a twenty year experience in over 1200 patients. Mt. Sinai J. Med., 38:497, 1971.
  This classic reference summarizes the important diagnostic and therapeutic aspects of myasthenia gravis. A patient classification system is included, as well as an outcome analysis of treatment in the largest series of myasthenic patients.

Pascuzzi, R. M.: Introduction to the neuromuscular junction and neuromuscular transmission. Semin. Neurol., 10:1, 1990.
  This concise, informative overview of the mechanisms of neuromuscular transmission includes details of the principles of electromyographic studies.

Phillips, L. H., and Melnich, P. A.: Diagnosis of myasthenia gravis in the 1990's. Semin. Neurol., 10:62, 1990.
  This overview of the diagnostic tests available for myasthenia gravis includes the rationale behind their use, as well as an interesting analysis of the clinical decision-making strategy.

REFERENCES

1. Seybold, M. E., and Lindstrom, J. M.: Immunopathology of acetylcholine receptors in myasthenia gravis. Springer Semin. Immunopathol., 5:389, 1982.
2. Seybold, M. E.: Myasthenia gravis: A clinical and basic science review. JAMA, 250:2516, 1983.
3. Wilks, S.: On cerebritis, hysteria and bulbar paralysis. Guy's Hosp. Rep., 22:7, 1877.
4. Goldflam, S.: Ueber einen scheinbar heilbaren bulbar paralytischen symptomen complex mit Beteiligung der Extremitaten. Dtsch. Z. Nervenheilkd., 4:312, 1893.
5. Jolly, F.: Ueber Myasthenia gravis pseudoparalytica. Berl. Klin. Wochenschr., 32:1, 1895.
6. Walker, M. B.: Treatment of myasthenia gravis with physostigmine. Lancet, 1:1200, 1934.
7. Osserman, K. E., Teng, P., Pahwa, S. G., and Good, R. A.: Thymic function in man. Thymus, 1:27, 1979.
8. Weigert, C.: Pathologisch-anatomischer Beitrag zur Erb-schen Krankheit (Myasthenia gravis). Neurol. Zentralbl., 20:597, 1901.
9. Bell, E. T.: Tumors of the thymus in myasthenia gravis. J. Nerv. Ment. Dis., 45:130, 1917.
10. Von Haberer, A.: Zur klinischen Bedentung der Thymus druse. Arch. Klin. Chir., 109:193, 1917.
11. Blalock, A., Mason, M. F., Morgan, H. J., and Riven, S. S.: Myasthenia gravis and tumors of the thymic region: Report of a case in which the tumor was removed. Ann. Surg., 110:544, 1939.
12. Blalock, A., Harvey, A. M., Ford, R. F., and Lilienthal, J. L., Jr.: The treatment of myasthenia gravis by removal of the thymus gland. JAMA, 117:1529, 1941.
13. Blalock, A.: Thymectomy in the treatment of myasthenia gravis: Report of twenty cases. J. Thorac. Surg., 13:316, 1944.
14. Buckingham, J. M., Howard, F. M., Jr., Bernatz, P. E., et al.: The value of thymectomy in myasthenia gravis: A computer assisted matched study. Ann. Surg., 184:453, 1967.
15. Osserman, K. E., and Genkins, G.: Studies in myasthenia gravis: Review of a twenty year experience in over 1200 patients. Mt. Sinai J. Med., 38:497, 1971.
16. Kennedy, F. S., and Moersch, F. P.: Myasthenia gravis: A clinical review of 87 cases observed between 1915 and the early part of 1932. Can. Med. Assoc. J., 37:217, 1937.
17. Grob, D., Arsura, E. L., Brunner, N. G., and Namba, T.: The course of myasthenia gravis and therapies affecting outcome. Ann. N. Y. Acad. Sci., 505:472, 1987.
18. Bever, C. T., Jr., Aquino, A. V., Penn, A. S., et al.: Prognosis of ocular myasthenia. Ann. Neurol., 14:516, 1983.
19. Harvey, A. M., and Masland, R. L.: The electromyogram in myasthenia gravis. Bull. Johns Hopkins Hosp., 69:1, 1941.
20. Phillips, L. H., and Melnick, P. A.: Diagnosis of myasthenia gravis in the 1990's. Semin. Neurol., 10:62, 1990.
21. Massey, J. M.: Electromyography in disorders of neuromuscular transmission. Semin. Neurol., 10:6, 1990.
22. Stalberg, E., and Sanders, D. B.: Electrophysiologic tests of neuromuscular transmission. In Stalberg, E., and Young, R. R. (Eds.): Clinical Neurophysiology. London, Butterworth, 1981.
23. Osserman, K. E., and Kaplan, L. I.: Rapid diagnostic test for myasthenia gravis: Increased muscle strength without fasciculations after intravenous administration of edrophonium (Tensilon) chloride. JAMA, 150:265, 1952.
24. Simpson, L. L.: Molecular pharmacology of botulinum toxin and tetanus toxin. Annu. Rev. Pharmacol. Toxicol., 26:427, 1986.
25. Lambert, E. H.: The Lambert-Eaton myasthenic syndrome: Clinical features and pathophysiology. Presented at the Seventh International Conference on Myasthenia Gravis, New York Academy of Sciences, 1986.
26. Keesey, J. C.: Electrodiagnostic approach to defects of neuromuscular transmission. Muscle Nerve, 12:613, 1989.
27. Waud, D. R., and Waud, B. E.: In vitro measurement of margin of safety of neuromuscular transmission. Am. J. Physiol., 229:1632, 1975.
28. Chang, C. C., and Lee, C. Y.: Isolation of neurotoxins from the venom of Bungarus multicinectus and their modes of neuromuscular blocking action. Arch. Int. Pharmacodyn. Ther., 144:241, 1963.
29. Seybold, M. E., Lambert, E. H., Lennon, V. A., et al.: Experimental autoim-

mune myasthenia: Clinical, neurophysiologic, and pharmacologic aspects. Ann. N. Y. Acad. Sci., 274:275, 1976.

30. Patrick, J., and Lindstrom, J.: Autoimmune response to acetylcholine receptor. Science, 180:871, 1973.

31. Engel, A. G., Lambert, E. H., and Howard, F. M., Jr.: Immune complexes (IgG and C3) at the motor end plate in myasthenia gravis: Ultrastructural and light microscopic localization and electrophysiologic correlations. Mayo Clin. Proc., 52:267, 1977.

32. Drachman, D. B., Adams, R. N., Stanley, E. F., and Pestronk, A.: Mechanisms of acetylcholine receptor loss in myasthenia gravis. J. Neurol. Neurosurg. Psychiatry, 43:601, 1980.

33. Fumagalli, G., Engel, A. G., and Lindstrom, J.: Estimation of degradation rate of acetylcholine receptor by external gamma counting *in vivo*. Mayo Clin. Proc., 57:758, 1982.

34. Lennon, V. A., Seybold, M. E., Lindstrom, J. M., et al.: Role of complement in the pathogenesis of experimental autoimmune myasthenia gravis. J. Exp. Med., 147:973, 1978.

35. Almon, R. R., Andrew, A. G., and Appel, S. H.: Serum globulin in myasthenia gravis: Inhibition of L. Bungarotoxin to acetylcholine receptors. Science, 186:55, 1974.

36. Buckberg, G. D., Herrmann, C., Dillon, J. R., and Mulder, D. G.: A further evaluation of thymectomy for myasthenia gravis. J. Thorac. Cardiovasc. Surg., 53:401, 1967.

37. Pahwa, R., Ikehara, S., Pahwa, S. G., and Good, R. A.: Thymic function in man. Thymus, 1:27, 1979.

38. Rivner, M. H., and Swift, T. R.: Thymoma: Diagnosis and management. Semin. Neurol., 10:83, 1990.

39. Williams, C. L., and Lennon, V. A.: Thymic B lymphocyte clones from patients with myasthenia gravis secrete monoclonal striational antibodies reacting with myosin alpha actin or actin. J. Exp. Med., 164:1043, 1986.

40. Pascuzzi, R. M., Coslett, H. B., and Johns, T. R.: Long-term corticosteroid treatment of myasthenia gravis: Report of 116 patients. Ann. Neurol., 15:291, 1984.

41. Matell, G.: Immunosuppressive drugs: Azathioprine in the treatment of myasthenia gravis. Ann. N. Y. Acad. Sci., 505:588, 1987.

42. Witte, A. S., Cornblath, D. R., Parry, G. J., et al.: Azathioprine in the treatment of myasthenia gravis. Ann. Neurol., 15:602, 1984.

43. Pinching, A. J., Peters, D. K., and Newsom-Davis, J.: Remission of myasthenia gravis following plasma exchange. Lancet, 2:1373, 1976.

44. Keller, A. J., and Urbaniak, S. J.: Intensive plasma exchange on the cell

separator: Effects on serum immunoglobulins and complement components. Br. J. Haematol., 38:531, 1978.

45. Hawley, C. J., Newsom-Davis, J., and Vincent, A.: Plasma exchange and immunosuppressive therapy in myasthenia gravis: No evidence for synergy. J. Neurol. Neurosurg. Psychiatry, 44:469, 1981.

46. Thorlacius, S., Mollnes, T. E., Garred, P., et al.: Plasma exchange in myasthenia gravis: Changes in serum complement and immunoglobulins. Acta Neurol. Scand., 78:221, 1988.

47. Keller, A. J., Chirnside, A., and Urbaniak, S. J.: Coagulation abnormalities produced by plasma exchange on the cell separator with special reference to fibrinogen and platelet levels. Br. J. Haematol., 42:593, 1979.

48. Kirschner, P. A., Osserman, K. E., and Kark, A. E.: Studies in myasthenia gravis: Transcervical total thymectomy. JAMA, 209:906, 1969.

49. Cooper, J. D., Al-Jilaihawa, A. N., Pearson, F. G., et al.: An improved technique to facilitate transcervical thymectomy for myasthenia gravis. Ann. Thorac. Surg., 45:242, 1988.

50. Jaretzki, A., Penn, A. S., Younger, D. S., et al.: "Maximal" thymectomy for myasthenia gravis. J. Thorac. Cardiovasc. Surg., 95:747, 1988.

51. Carlens, E., Johansson, L., and Olsson, P.: Thymectomy for myasthenia gravis with the aid of mediastinoscopy. Opuscula Med., 13:175, 1968.

52. Crile, G., Jr.: Thymectomy through the neck. Surgery, 59:213, 1966.

53. Akakura, I.: Mediastinoscopy. Presented before the Eleventh International Congress of Bronchoesophagology, Hakone, Japan, 1965.

54. Papatestas, A. E., Genkins, G., Kornfeld, P., et al.: Effects of thymectomy in myasthenia gravis. Ann. Surg., 206:79, 1987.

55. Schumm, J. F., Wietholter, H., Fateh-Moghadam, A., and Dichgans, J.: Thymectomy in myasthenia with pure ocular symptoms. J. Neurol. Neurosurg. Psychiatry, 48:332, 1985.

56. Frist, W. H., Thirumalai, S., Doehring, C. B., et al.: Thymectomy for the myasthenia gravis patient: Factors influencing outcome. Ann. Thorac. Surg., 57:334, 1994.

57. Olanow, C. W., Wechsler, A. S., Siratkin-Roses, M., et al.: Thymectomy as primary therapy in myasthenia gravis. Ann. N. Y. Acad. Sci., 505:595, 1987.

58. Hatton, P. D., Diehl, J. P., Daly, B. D. P., et al.: Transsternal radical thymectomy for myasthenia gravis: A 15 year review. Ann. Thorac. Surg., 47:838, 1989.

59. Huang, M., King, K., Ksu, W., et al.: The outcome of thymectomy in nonthymomatous myasthenia gravis. Surg. Gynecol. Obstet., 166:436, 1988.

60. Sugarbaker, D. J.: Thoracoscopy in the management of anterior mediastinal masses. Ann. Thorac. Surg., 56:653, 1993.

CHAPTER 53

SURGICAL DISORDERS OF THE PERICARDIUM

Michael E. Jessen, M.D.

Historical Aspects

Early descriptions of the pericardium date back to 460 B.C. when Hippocrates characterized the pericardium as "a smooth tunic which envelops the heart and contains a small amount of fluid resembling urine." Galen (A.D. 131–201) named the pericardium, suggested its protective role, and postulated the existence of pericardial diseases in man. It was not until the seventeenth century that Lower made the first accurate descriptions of cardiac tamponade in humans and Riolan suggested that relief of pericardial effusion might be achieved by pericardiotomy by trephination of the sternum. In the eighteenth century, Lancisi (in autopsy specimens) and Morgagni (in patients) reported the clinical and pathologic features of constrictive pericarditis.

Surgical attempts began in the early nineteenth century when Romero incised the pericardium of three patients through an incision in the left fifth interspace and reported recovery in two. Drainage of effusion was accomplished by blind insertion of a trocar by Schuh and by pericardiocentesis by Karanaeff, both in 1840. Excision of the thickened fibrous pericardium for relief of constrictive pericarditis was proposed by Weill in 1895 and by Delorme in 1898. It was not until 1913 that Rehn and Sauerbruch independently introduced pericardial resection. Churchill performed the first pericardiectomy for constrictive pericarditis in the United States in 1929. Later reports by Schumacker and Roshe, and by Fitzpatrick and associates, established the need for radical pericardiectomy to achieve the best results in this disease.

Many contributions to the pathophysiology of pericardial disease were made in the nineteenth and twentieth centuries. Chevers, in 1842, accurately described the physiologic basis of constrictive pericarditis, noting the prominent effects on diastolic function.[6] Kussmaul (1873) provided the first description of the paradoxical pulse found with cardiac tamponade[18] and noted the rise in venous pressure occurring with inspiration in constrictive pericarditis (Kussmaul's sign). Rose (1884) described the deleterious effects of effusion or hemorrhage on cardiac function and coined the term *herz tamponade*. Classic experimental studies by Isaacs[14] and by Parsons and Holman clarified the effects of localized compression of the heart on hemodynamics. Beck's experiments demonstrated that extensive pericardial fibrosis was needed to create the syndrome of constriction and proved that removal of the scarred pericardium could lead to hemodynamic improvement.

Embryology

The intraembryonic coelom appears during the third week of gestation as a coalescence of small isolated spaces within the lateral mesoderm and cardiogenic mesoderm in the developing embryo. This horseshoe-shaped cavity lined by mesothelial cells divides the lateral mesoderm into a somatic (parietal) layer and a splanchnic (visceral) layer.

During the second month of gestation, the intraembryonic coelom is divided into the body cavities. During transverse folding of the embryo, the lateral portions of the intraembryonic coelom are brought together on the ventral surface, and three distinct body cavities evolve: the pericardial cavity, two pleuropericardial (pleural) canals, and a peritoneal cavity. The formation of the head fold moves the developing heart and pericardial cavity ventrally. The pericardial cavity then opens dorsally into the pleuroperitoneal canals. Partitions known as *pleuropericardial membranes* separate the pericardial cavity from the pleural cavity and form the outer fibrous layer of the pericardium. Defective formation of these membranes can lead to congenital defects, whereby the pericardial cavity communicates with the pleural cavity, usually on the left side.[22]

Anatomy

The pericardium is often described in two layers: the visceral pericardium and the parietal pericardium. The *visceral pericardium* is the epicardial surface of the heart itself and consists of a thin layer of loose fibrous tissue covered by mesothelial cells. This layer encloses the entire heart and is continuous with the serous layer, which lines the inner aspect of the fibrous *parietal pericardium*. Thus, mesothelial cells line both opposing surfaces of the potential space known as the pericardial cavity.

External to the serous lining, the parietal pericardium is composed of a thick fibrous layer of collagen bundles and elastic fibers. Inferiorly, this layer blends with the central tendon of the diaphragm. Other ligamentous attachments serve to anchor the parietal pericardium to the sternum and xiphoid and to the vertebral column. The fibrous pericardium blends with the superior vena cava, the great vessels, the four pulmonary veins, and the ligamentum arteriosum. The aorta and pulmonary trunk are enclosed by a common sheath of the visceral pericardium, creating an opening behind the aorta and main pulmonary artery and in front of the left atrium and superior vena cava: the *transverse sinus*. Folds of serous pericardium surrounding the entrance of the right and left pulmonary veins are connected by an irregular pericardial reflection that creates a space termed the *oblique sinus*. Folds of fat often accumulate on the external surface of the pericardium at its junction with the diaphragm.

The pericardium is supplied by the pericardiacophrenic branches of the internal thoracic arteries and by branches of the bronchial, esophageal, and superior phrenic arteries. These vessels may collateralize with the coronary arteries. The epicardium is supplied directly by the coronary arteries. Branches of the phrenic nerve convey vasomotor and sensory fibers to the pericardium. Pericardial pain is felt diffusely behind the sternum and may radiate to the chest wall and abdomen. The epicardium is supplied with vasomotor and sensory fibers from the coronary plexuses, but stimulation of the epicardium does not cause pain.

The visceral pericardium secretes a clear serous fluid into the pericardial cavity, which may normally contain up to 50 ml. Reabsorption of this fluid occurs through lymphatics in the parietal and visceral layers, ultimately returning to the thoracic duct.

Pericardial Physiology

The pericardium serves three main functions: (1) it serves to fix the heart anatomically within the mediastinum despite changes in body position, (2) it reduces friction between the heart and surrounding organs, and (3) it acts as a barrier to spread of infection from local structures, particularly the lungs.[35] Under normal situations, the pericardium has minor effects on hemodynamics and congenital absence or surgical excision is not associated with clinical symptoms. Nevertheless, pericardiectomy results in decreased diastolic and developed pressures at any cardiac volume and more compliant diastolic pressure-volume curves.

Normal pericardial pressure varies between $+5$ and -5 cm. H_2O and equals the pleural pressure. The pericardium transmits respiratory effects: with inspiration, pleural and pericardial pressures fall, causing a decline in right atrial and ventricular pressures. As a result, right-sided heart filling is augmented and pulmonary flow increases. However, flow decreases in the aorta owing to a decrease in left-sided heart filling from temporary pooling of blood in the lungs.

The normal pericardium is noncompliant and restricts ventricular distention above certain limits. The presence of fluid within the pericardium may alter this process and further limit cardiac loading. Pericardial pressure-volume curves follow different courses during fluid addition and fluid removal,[23] a phenomenon known as *hysteresis* (Fig. 53–1). By limiting cardiac distention, the pericardium may help avoid cardiac rupture. Also, elevation of right ventricular filling pressure from any cause shifts the interventricular septum to the left, decreasing left ventricular volume and distensibility. This effect (*diastolic coupling*) is greatly enhanced by an intact pericardium.[27]

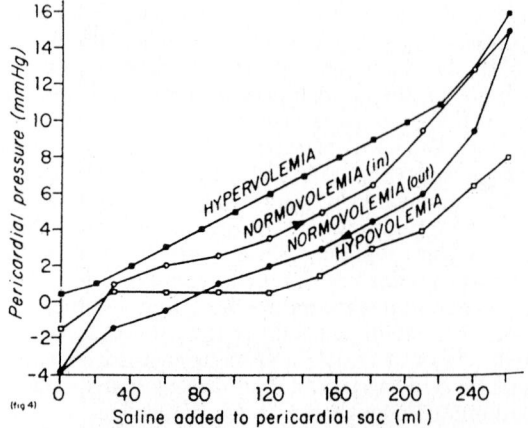

Figure 53–1. Pressure-volume relationships in the same animal in normovolemic state, after removal of 30 ml. blood per kg. body weight and after replacement of blood plus 30 ml. saline per kg. The two normovolemic curves represent infusion and withdrawal relationships, demonstrating mild hysteresis. (Reproduced with permission from Morgan, B. C., Guntheroth, W. G., and Dillard, D. H.: Relationship of pericardial to pleural pressure during quiet respiration and cardiac tamponade. Circ. Res., *16:*493, 1965. Copyright 1965, American Heart Association.)

PERICARDIAL DISEASES

Congenital Pericardial Defects

Congenital Absence. When one or both of the pleuropericardial membranes fail to form completely, deficiencies in the pericardium result.[22] Three main types are found: (1) a defect in the parietal pericardium that allows communication between the pericardial sac and pleural space, (2) the existence of a common cavity for the heart and left lung (most common form), or (3) total absence of the parietal pericardium. Defects occur more commonly on the left side, are more common in males, and are associated with congenital heart defects in 30% of patients. The heart is usually displaced to the left, more mobile, and frequently enlarged. With partial defects, herniation of the atrial appendices or entire heart has been described and may be life threatening. Total absence of the pericardium does not produce clinical symptoms.

Pericardial Cysts and Diverticula. The pericardial coelom forms from a coalescence of individual lacunae. Pericardial cysts may arise from lacunar cavities that failed to fuse. If they communicate with the pericardial cavity, they are usually referred to as diverticula. Most cysts are found incidentally on chest x-rays as masses in the cardiophrenic sulcus. They are generally unilocular and fluid filled. Most are asymptomatic, although in rare cases symptoms may arise from cyst torsion or compression of the adjacent structures. Cysts generally require no treatment, although surgical exploration may be needed to establish a diagnosis.

Acute Pericarditis

Acute inflammation of the pericardium is characterized by polymorphonuclear infiltration, increased vascularity, and formation of fibrinous pericardial adhesions. An exudative pericardial effusion may or may not be present. Most cases are idiopathic,[24] but a wide range of etiologic factors have been described.[33] Acute pericarditis may occur: (1) from a viral, bacterial, fungal, or tuberculous infection; (2) after mediastinal irradiation; (3) as a result of pericardial invasion by adjacent tumor (commonly breast, lung, or lymphoma); (4) in association with aortic dissection (when blood leaks into the pericardial space); (5) after transmural myocardial infarction; (6) after blunt or penetrating trauma; (7) after cardiac surgery; (8) in association with uremia; (9) with connective tissue diseases (usually rheumatoid arthritis, scleroderma, or systemic lupus erythematosus); or (10) from drug therapy (particularly hydralazine or procainamide).

Diagnosis
History. The patient with acute pericarditis complains of retrosternal chest pain that may radiate to the neck or left chest. The pain often worsens with deep inspiration, coughing, or lying supine and improves with sitting upright. Fever, chills, dyspnea, and weakness can be accompanying symptoms.

Physical Examination. A pericardial friction rub audible over the entire precordium is the pathognomonic finding. The rub is classically described as having three components, although it can appear and disappear from one minute to the next. If a large pericardial effusion is present, heart sounds may be muffled and the cardiac impulse difficult to palpate.

Electrocardiogram. In the early stage of acute pericarditis, diffuse ST segment elevation occurs and T wave flattening may be prominent (Fig. 53–2).[34] Unlike acute myocardial infarction, development of Q waves or loss of R waves does not occur, and the electrocardiogram may return to normal after the inflammation resolves. With significant pericardial effusion, QRS voltage may be diminished. Significant ar-

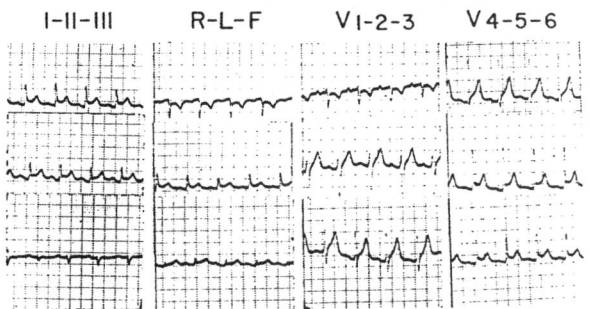

Figure 53–2. Electrocardiographic findings early in acute pericarditis. Diffuse ST segment elevation is seen. (From Spodick, D. H.: Differential characteristics of the electrocardiogram in early repolarization and acute pericarditis. N. Engl. J. Med., 295:523, 1976. Reprinted by permission of the New England Journal of Medicine.)

rhythmias are rare in this disorder and should prompt the search for other abnormalities.[36]

Imaging Studies. The chest x-ray is usually normal unless a significant pericardial effusion is present creating an enlarged mediastinal silhouette. The echocardiogram is the most sensitive test for confirming, localizing, and quantifying a pericardial effusion. Echocardiography, computed tomography, or magnetic resonance imaging may reveal thickening of the pericardium.

Natural History. Most cases of acute pericarditis are self-limited, with the inflammation and accumulated fluid resolving over 2 to 6 weeks. Recurrent episodes may occur weeks or months after the first episode, and relapses can continue for several months.[10] The course and prognosis are affected by the underlying disease process. Serious sequelae may result from pericarditis due to purulent infections or tuberculosis if aggressive therapy is not undertaken. Constrictive pericarditis is a rare complication of most forms of this disease.

Treatment. Symptomatic relief is usually achieved with nonsteroidal anti-inflammatory agents such as aspirin or indomethacin. The underlying cause should be determined and treated as well. When symptoms are severe or persistent, a short course of corticosteroids is often successful. Anticoagulants should be avoided. Recurrent pericarditis refractory to

anti-inflammatory agents or steroids may respond to colchicine.[12] Management of specific forms of acute pericarditis is described below.

Viral Pericarditis. Coxsackieviruses A and B are the most common viral causes of acute pericarditis, and acute and convalescent antibody titers may establish the diagnosis. The clinical course is generally benign. Even when a significant effusion is present, diagnostic pericardiocentesis is rarely helpful in establishing the diagnosis, although it may rule out purulent pericarditis.[24] Constrictive pericarditis rarely follows this process, and drainage of an asymptomatic pericardial effusion to prevent this complication is not indicated.

Purulent Pericarditis. Purulent pericarditis is caused by bacterial contamination of the pericardial space due to pneumonia, penetrating trauma, or hematogenous spread or after cardiac, pulmonary, or esophageal surgery. Rare cases have resulted from rupture of subphrenic or hepatic abscesses into the pericardial space. *Staphylococcus* and *Pneumococcus* species, *Haemophilis influenzae,* and gram-negative bacteria are common causative organisms.[16] Chest pain and fever may be more severe, and accumulation of pus can lead to signs of tamponade. Pericardiocentesis establishes the diagnosis and provides material for culture. Cases may be managed with repeated pericardiocentesis, but better drainage is usually achieved with open pericardiotomy and placement of drainage and irrigation catheters. If loculated pyogenic effusions persist, pericardiectomy may be required.

Tuberculous Pericarditis. Tuberculous pericarditis is found less frequently in modern series but has important features. It arises from tuberculosis at other sites that spreads to the pericardium by the bloodstream or by direct extension from the pleura, lungs, mediastinal lymph nodes, or lymphatics. Symptoms may be insidious in onset, and a large pericardial effusion may develop before the diagnosis is made. Both serous and bloody effusions have been described, and pericardiocentesis may reveal acid-fast bacilli within the fluid.

Once the diagnosis is made, treatment with antituberculous drugs (usually three-drug combinations) should be begun, and clinical improvement is expected within 2 to 3 weeks. With healing, fibrosis and calcification of the pericardium are common (Fig. 53–3) and constrictive pericarditis may result in up to one half of patients. This is more common when treatment has been delayed more than 4 weeks from

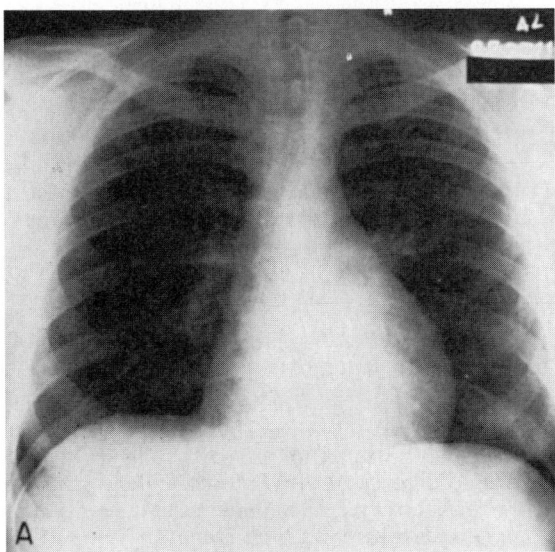
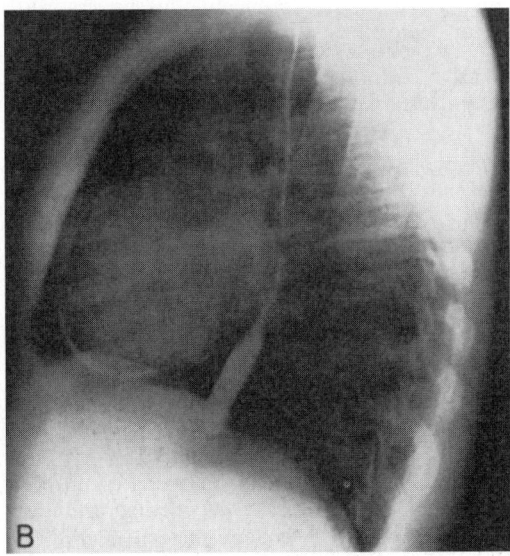

Figure 53–3. Chest films of a 45-year-old man with calcific constrictive pericarditis. The rim of calcium is clearly visible encircling the heart on the lateral film *(B)* but is not identifiable on the anterior view *(A)*. (From Ebert, P. A., and Najafi, H.: The pericardium. *In* Sabiston, D. C., and Spencer, F. C. [Eds.]: Surgery of the Chest, 5th ed. Philadelphia, W. B. Saunders, 1990, p. 1238.)

the onset of the disease. To prevent this complication, early operative resection is advised soon after the symptoms from the acute phase have resolved.[13]

Uremic Pericarditis. Pericardial inflammation and effusions develop in up to one half of patients with untreated chronic renal disease. Initiation of dialysis may lead to improvement, although dialysis patients with normal serum urea nitrogen and creatinine levels may develop this disorder. Some authors suggest that repeat anticoagulation during hemodialysis may exacerbate the inflammation because pericardial effusions are commonly bloody and the incidence is lower in patients undergoing peritoneal dialysis.[31] Treatment with anti-inflammatory agents or steroids is the first line of management, and pericardiocentesis is reserved for effusions associated with tamponade symptoms. Patients who develop recurrent cardiac tamponade or pericardial restriction should undergo pericardiectomy.

Postpericardiotomy Syndrome. The postpericardiotomy syndrome manifests as fever, malaise, pericarditis, and pleuritis appearing 2 to 4 weeks after cardiac operations. A pericardial friction rub is frequently present, and leukocytosis and elevated erythrocyte sedimentation rates are found. The electrocardiogram may demonstrate changes consistent with acute pericarditis. Antiheart antibodies have been demonstrated in the serum of patients after pericardiotomy, and the syndrome may represent an autoimmune reaction directed against the epicardium at a time of active or recurrent viral infection.[9]

The clinical course is similar to that in other forms of acute pericarditis, and rest, nutritional support, anti-inflammatory agents, or corticosteroids lead to resolution of most cases. Large effusions require pericardiocentesis or pericardiectomy in rare cases.

Constrictive Pericarditis

Constrictive pericarditis results from a thickened fibrotic pericardium that restricts diastolic filling of the heart. Tuberculosis was a leading cause in the past, but most cases now are idiopathic or follow prior radiation therapy or operation.[3, 7] Although uncommon after cardiac operations, constrictive pericarditis may develop even after a long lag period: in one large series the mean interval from surgery to presentation was 23 months.[15] Less frequently, restriction occurs after acute pericarditis secondary to viral, bacterial, or fungal infection; chronic renal failure; connective tissue disorders; drug therapy; or trauma.

Diagnosis

History. Patients with constrictive pericarditis may complain of fatigue or dyspnea from reduced cardiac output. Retrosternal chest pain may be present, and abdominal discomfort caused by ascites or passive hepatic congestion may occur. Symptoms of pulmonary venous congestion (orthopnea, nocturnal dyspnea) are rare.

Physical Examination. The principal finding is an elevated jugular venous pressure. The jugular veins are distended with prominent X and Y descents, and jugular venous pressure often increases with inspiration (Kussmaul's sign). Arterial blood pressure may be low or normal with a narrowed pulse pressure. The apical impulse may be soft and diffuse. On auscultation, S_1 and S_2 may be soft and a loud, early diastolic sound may be heard along the left sternal border (*pericardial knock*). This sound results from sudden cessation of left ventricular filling.[37] The liver is enlarged or pulsatile, and peripheral edema is common.

Electrocardiogram. The QRS voltage may be diminished, and nonspecific ST segment and T wave abnormalities are frequent. Atrial fibrillation may occur in up to one third of patients.

Imaging Studies. On chest x-ray, the cardiac silhouette may be normal or slightly enlarged. Dense pericardial calcification usually denotes a tuberculous etiology. Echocardiography may demonstrate characteristic left ventricular septal and posterior wall motion abnormalities and dilatation of the hepatic veins and inferior vena cava. Doppler echocardiography demonstrates abnormal flow velocities in the pulmonary and hepatic veins and an abnormal pattern of ventricular diastolic filling. The pericardium may appear thickened and immobile, but computed tomography and magnetic resonance imaging may provide more accurate assessment of pericardial thickness[32] (Fig. 53–4).

Catheterization. In constrictive pericarditis the diastolic pressures of all cardiac chambers are elevated and equal. Right atrial pressure demonstrates prominent X and Y descents. There is usually no respiratory variation because intrathoracic pressure changes cannot be transmitted to the obliterated pericardial space. Occasionally, venous pressure actually rises with inspiration. With high venous pressure, ventricular filling proceeds rapidly during early diastole. However, filling abruptly ceases when the intracardiac volume expands to the limit set by the noncompliant pericardium.[29] The result is an early diastolic dip followed by a high diastolic plateau (*square-root sign*) on the right and left ventricular pressure curves (Fig. 53–5). Left ventricular stroke volume is reduced, and cardiac output may be depressed, although left ventricular systolic function as assessed by ejection fraction is typically normal.

It may be extremely difficult to distinguish constrictive pericarditis from restrictive cardiomyopathy, but several features may be helpful: (1) respiratory variation is usually absent in constrictive pericarditis but may be present in restrictive cardiomyopathy; (2) pulmonary artery pressure is almost always below 50 mm. Hg with constriction, but frequently exceeds 50 mm. Hg in restrictive disease; (3) pulmonary capillary wedge pressure is usually below 18 mm. Hg in constrictive disease but may exceed this level in restrictive cardiomyopathy; (4) the right ventricular diastolic square-root sign is more prominent in constrictive pericarditis; and (5) right and left ventricular diastolic pressure are typically equal in constriction, but left ventricular diastolic pressure usually exceeds the right by more than 5 mm. Hg in restrictive processes. Despite these guidelines it is occasionally impossible to distinguish these two conditions. Endomyocardial biopsy may be helpful, or surgical exploration may be required.

Treatment. Patients with mild symptoms may benefit from diuretics. Corticosteroids have been used to treat constrictive pericarditis within the first 2 months of cardiac procedures and to prevent constriction from tuberculous pericarditis.[26] However, once irreversible pericardial fibrosis develops, total pericardiectomy is indicated. The operative mortality from this procedure averages 5% to 15%, with most deaths resulting from low-output states.[21] Long-standing constriction may produce myocardial atrophy, and constriction from radiation therapy may be associated with myocardial fibrosis: both factors may contribute to low-output states. Operative survivors generally get symptomatic relief (Fig. 53–6), and long-term survival is good.

Pericardial Effusion

Any of the causes of acute pericarditis may cause a pericardial effusion, as can biventricular congestive heart failure or hypothyroidism. In many patients, effusions accumulate slowly, allowing time for the pericardium to distend. Under these circumstances effusions of 1 to 2 liters may cause minimal or no symptoms. Symptoms referable to the underlying disease process (e.g., tuberculosis, rheumatoid arthritis, hy-

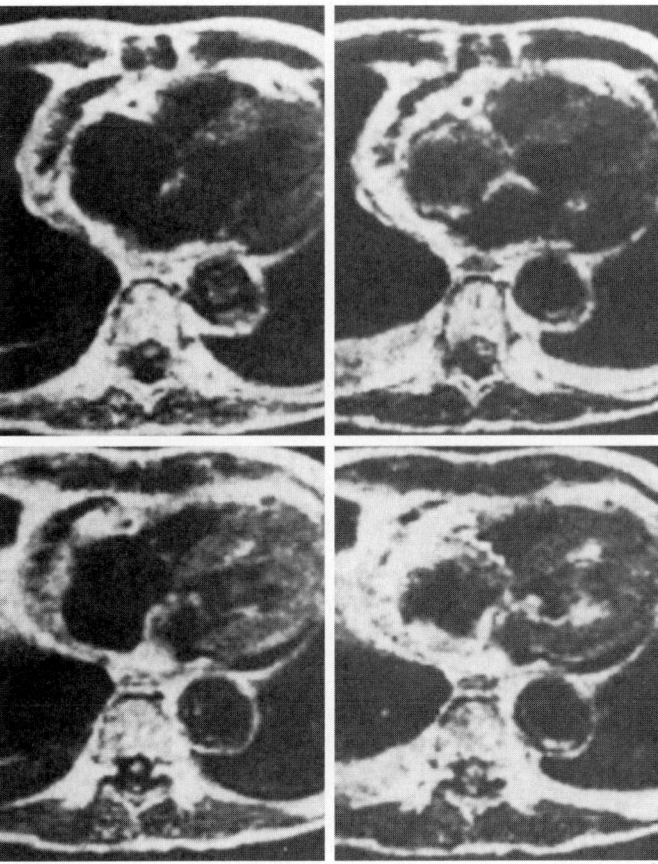

Figure 53–4. Constrictive uremic pericarditis. First (*left*) and second (*right*) spin-echo magnetic resonance images. Sequential axial images show irregularly thickened visceral and parietal pericardium of increased intensity, separated by low-intensity fluid, surrounding the enlarged right atrium. The second echo image shows a further increase in intensity, in keeping with a long T2. The right ventricle is normal in size, the left ventricle hypertrophied, the septum straight. Pericardial fluid is also seen behind the left ventricle where abnormalities of the pericardium itself are less marked. Bilateral pleural effusions are present. (From Soulen, R. L., Stark, D. D., and Higgins, C. B.: Magnetic resonance imaging of constrictive pericardial disease. Am. J. Cardiol., *55*:480, 1985.)

pothyroidism) may be present, or vague fullness in the anterior chest may occur. On physical examination, the apical impulse is difficult to palpate, heart sounds are muffled, and a friction rub may be audible. Signs of venous engorgement (distended neck veins, hepatomegaly, or peripheral edema) or decreased cardiac output are absent unless intrapericardial pressure is significantly increased. The electrocardiogram demonstrates diminished QRS voltage with T wave flattening. Electrical alternans (an alternation in height or direction of major deflection of the QRS complex) may also be found. Chest x-ray reveals an enlarged cardiac silhouette, and echocardiography is the most accurate diagnostic modality,

detecting as little as 20 ml. of fluid within the pericardial space (Fig. 53–7).

Treatment is directed at the underlying cause, and drainage of an asymptomatic effusion is not required. Pericardiocentesis or subxiphoid pericardial window (with pericardial biopsy) may be used to establish a diagnosis or relieve symptoms of tamponade. Patients with symptomatic malignant pericardial effusions may be treated with a variety of tech-

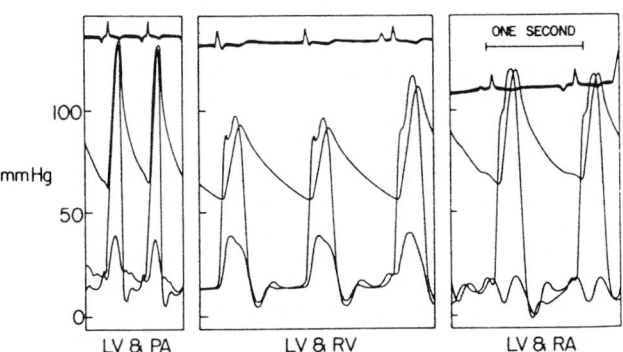

Figure 53–5. Simultaneously recorded left ventricular and right-sided heart pressures. The early diastolic dip and late diastolic plateau are recorded in both ventricles. Note the equilibration of the diastolic pressures in the left ventricle (LV), pulmonary artery (PA), right ventricle (RV), and right atrium (RA). The contribution of atrial systole to end-diastolic and to developed systolic pressure in this very noncompliant heart is illustrated by the transition from junctional to atrial rhythm *(middle panel)*. (Reprinted from American Journal of Cardiology: *34*:1; July, 1974; 107 to 110.)

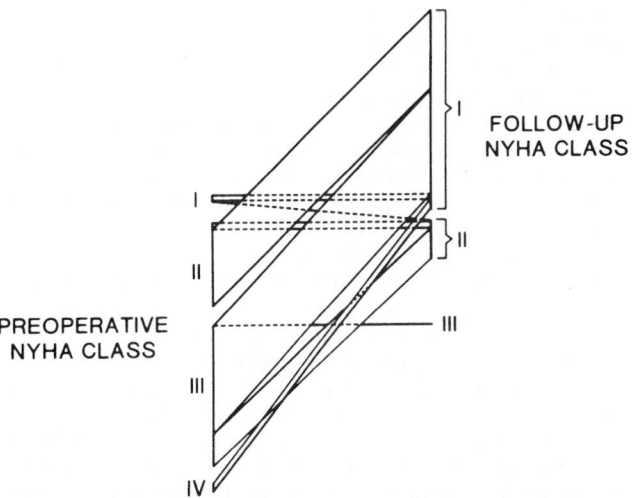

Figure 53–6. Long-term follow-up of 141 patients demonstrated marked symptomatic improvement after pericardiectomy for constrictive pericarditis. (From McCaughan, B. C., Schaff, H. V., Piehler, J. M., Danielson, G. K., Orszulak, T. A., Puga, F. J., Pluth, J. R., Connolly, D. C., and McGoon, D. C.: Early and late results of pericardiectomy for constrictive pericarditis. J. Thorac. Cardiovasc. Surg., *89*:340, 1985.)

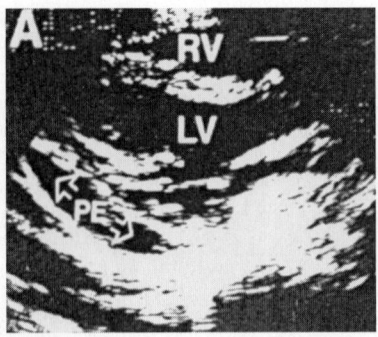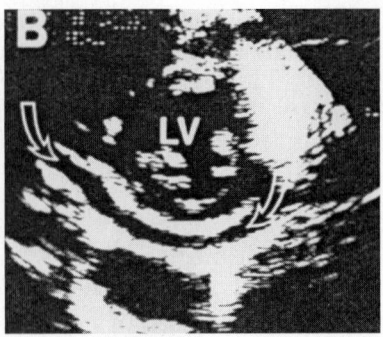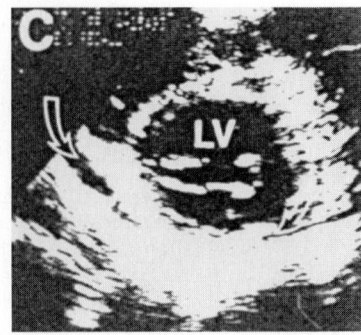

Figure 53–7. Representative frames from two-dimensional echocardiograms in a patient with a moderate pericardial effusion. Panels *A*, *B*, and *C* were recorded in end-diastole. Distribution of pericardial fluid appears relatively uniform in the long axis view (PE, in *A*) and the short axis view at the level of papillary muscles (arrows, in *B*). However, at a slightly more proximal level *(C)*, there is a marked decrease in the posterior echo-free space. (From Parameswaran, R., and Goldberg, H.: Echocardiographic quantitation of pericardial effusion. Chest, *83*:767, 1983.)

niques. Recurrences occur in over 50% of patients treated by pericardiocentesis alone.[5] Continuous drainage by an indwelling cardiac catheter for several days can reduce reaccumulation rates to around 25%.[38] Other strategies have been devised to prevent recurrence, including systemic chemotherapy or radiation therapy directed at the underlying tumor or intrapericardial instillation of sclerosing agents (tetracycline),[30] chemotherapeutic agents (bleomycin),[8] or radionuclides. These techniques are successful in about 70% of cases. Surgical approaches (pericardial window created by subxiphoid[4] or thoracotomy approaches and pericardiectomy) provide the highest success rates (80–90%) but are more invasive. Pericardiotomies have also been created by percutaneous balloon techniques.[40]

Pneumopericardium is a benign finding generally associated with air leaks from the lung and pneumothorax. Treatment is generally not required because air rarely causes hemodynamic compromise.

Cardiac Tamponade

Cardiac tamponade is caused by accumulation of fluid within the pericardial sac, leading to an increase in pericardial pressure. Intracardiac filling pressures rise until the intrapericardial and diastolic filling pressures of the heart equalize, resulting in diminished venous return to the right atrium. At this point, stroke volume declines and adrenergic activation attempts to compensate by increasing heart rate and contractility. As these compensatory mechanisms fail, systemic arterial pressure falls and perfusion of the coronary circulation and vital organs becomes impaired.[29]

As little as 100 to 200 ml. of fluid can cause tamponade if it accumulates rapidly and the pericardium has not had sufficient time to distend. In contrast, slowly accumulating effusions can reach large size without symptoms. Almost any cause of pericardial effusion can lead to tamponade, but chest trauma is a prominent cause.

The patient with cardiac tamponade may complain of dyspnea, fatigue, or syncope or may present in shock. On physical examination the patient is often anxious, restless, and pale, with a rapid thready pulse. Jugular venous pressure is elevated, heart sounds are distant or inaudible, and blood pressure is depressed: a constellation of findings known as *Beck's triad*.[1] Trauma victims with tamponade may lack one or more of these findings; for example, jugular venous distention may be absent in patients who are severely hypovolemic. The classic physical finding associated with tamponade is *pulsus paradoxus*, a fall in systemic arterial pressure of greater than 20 mm. Hg with inspiration. However, this finding may also occur in patients with severe congestive heart failure, chronic obstructive pulmonary dis-

ease, hypovolemia, acute pulmonary embolism, or shock. The fall in intrapericardial pressure caused by inspiration produces increased flow from the venae cavae to the right atrium, right ventricle, and pulmonary arteries. The resulting enlargement of the right side of the heart displaces the intraventricular septum to the left, decreasing volume on the left side of the heart and contributing to the fall in systemic output and arterial pressure.

The chest x-ray may show an enlarged cardiac silhouette, and the electrocardiogram may show a low QRS voltage, nonspecific ST segment and T wave abnormalities, and, rarely, electrical alternans. This last finding is highly specific for tamponade. Echocardiography can reliably demonstrate fluid within the pericardium and may suggest tamponade by signs such as diastolic collapse of the right atrium or ventricle.[25] If right-sided heart catheterization is performed, filling pressures of all cardiac chambers are found to be elevated and equal.

Cardiac tamponade is life threatening and must be treated immediately and effectively. Pericardial drainage by pericardiocentesis or subxiphoid window may stabilize the patient. If drainage cannot be achieved immediately, intravenous volume expansion may help transiently, but administration of inotropic agents or pressors is usually not helpful.[20] Once tamponade is relieved, the underlying cause must be identified and treated. For trauma victims or patients presenting after cardiac procedures, formal exploration by sternotomy or thoracotomy is needed.

Pericardial Neoplasms

Primary pericardial neoplasms are very rare tumors. About half are malignant, with mesothelioma the most common variant. Most mesotheliomas are diffuse and may encase the entire heart, infiltrate the superficial myocardium, or metastasize to mediastinal lymph nodes and lungs. These tumors may cause death by myocardial restriction. Benign tumors include teratomas (the most common), hemangiomas, leiomyofibromas, lipomas, and fibromas. When large they may produce symptoms from cardiac compression.

Secondary neoplastic spread to the pericardium is much more frequent, with up to 10% of patients with malignant neoplasms developing cardiac or pericardial involvement. Almost any tumor can metastasize to this site, usually by hematogenous spread. Among specific neoplasms the highest percentage of metastases to the heart is seen with melanoma (70%), leukemia (37%), and lymphoma (24%). However, in absolute numbers, the most common neoplasms with cardiac metastases are lung cancer and breast cancer. Pericardial metastases may be asymptomatic or may produce significant pericardial effusions. Treatment is directed at the underlying malignancy or drainage of symptomatic effusions.

SURGICAL TECHNIQUES
Pericardiocentesis

Pericardiocentesis, or aspiration of fluid from the pericardial cavity, may be performed (1) to establish a cause of pericarditis or pericardial effusion or (2) to relieve symptoms of cardiac tamponade. The procedure may be accomplished with local anesthesia, and positioning the patient upright may cause the fluid to pool anteriorly, where it is more accessible. A long needle is then inserted below and to the left of the xiphoid process and angled 30 to 45 degrees posteriorly and slightly to the left, while the operator gently aspirates with a syringe. The pericardium may also be approached through the left fourth or fifth interspace. Under emergency conditions, pericardiocentesis can be performed blindly, but complications can be reduced by monitoring the precordial electrogram with an electrode placed on the aspirating needle.[2] If the needle contacts the surface of the heart, a sharp deflection appears on the electrocardiogram and the needle may be withdrawn slightly (Fig. 53–8). Peri-

cardiocentesis can be performed under fluoroscopic or echocardiographic guidance. The latter is the preferred technique because loculated fluid collections can be identified and the cardiac structures visualized.[11] Generally, complete drainage of the pericardial space is attempted to relieve symptoms. A pigtail catheter may be inserted over a guidewire or through the introducer needle and left in place if continued drainage is needed.[17] For malignant effusions, sclerosants such as tetracycline[30] or bleomycin[8] may be instilled within the pericardium to prevent recurrence.

Complication rates of about 5% are reported with pericardiocentesis[39] and may be life threatening. Complications include ventricular arrhythmias (including ventricular fibrillation) and laceration of the heart, coronary arteries, lung, liver, or internal thoracic artery. If the aspirated blood forms clots, it likely was obtained from a cardiac chamber, because true pericardial blood is rapidly defibrinated by cardiac motion and does not clot.

Pericardiotomy and Pericardial Biopsy

Open pericardial drainage is indicated for treatment of purulent pericarditis and occasionally for chronic pericardial effusions. Examination of a biopsy specimen obtained during

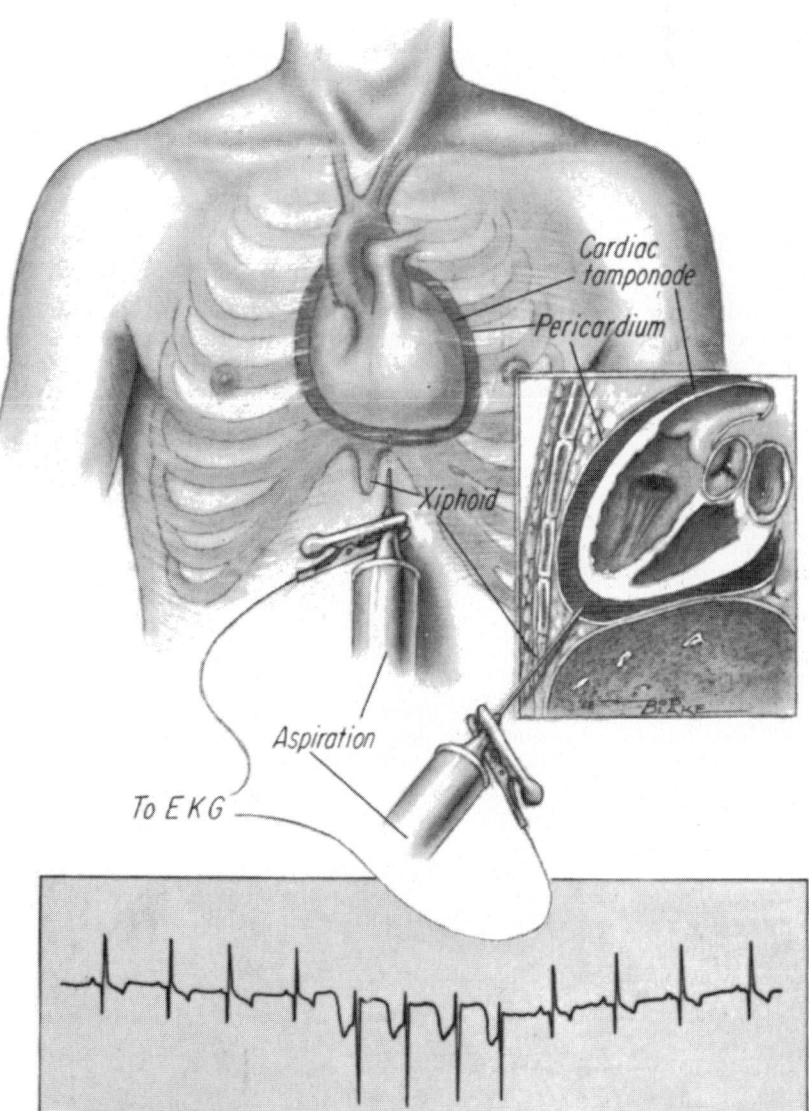

Figure 53–8. Technique of pericardiocentesis. Negative deflection of the QRS complex indicates contact with the epicardium. (From Ebert, P.: The pericardium. *In* Sabiston, D. C., and Spencer, F. C. [Eds.]: Gibbon's Surgery of the Chest, 4th ed. Philadelphia, W. B. Saunders, 1983, p. 996.)

the drainage procedure may be helpful for establishing a diagnosis.

When a subxiphoid approach is used, an incision is made to the left of the xiphoid process extending through a portion of the rectus muscle. By dissecting upward beneath the costal margin in a plane superficial to the transversus abdominis fibers, the inferior surface of the pericardium is encountered. Good drainage can be achieved through this dependent site, and two drainage catheters are usually placed within the pericardial sac (one anterior and one posterior to the heart), allowing chronic drainage or irrigation.

An alternate approach is through a left anterior thoracotomy through the fourth intercostal space. This achieves good exposure for removal of a portion of the pericardium to allow drainage of a chronic effusion into the left pleural space, where it may be absorbed. Temporary drainage catheters are left in both the pericardial and pleural spaces. This partial pericardial resection is frequently termed a *pericardial window*. The procedure can be performed as a video-assisted thoracoscopic technique.[19] Drainage of purulent pericarditis can cause costochondritis, and some authors have suggested complete excision of the fifth and sixth costal cartilages to avoid this complication.

Several centers have reported experience with *percutaneous balloon pericardiotomy* for malignant effusions.[40] In this technique, a subxiphoid pericardiocentesis is performed and a guidewire placed in the pericardial sac. A balloon dilating catheter is straddled across the pericardium and inflated to create a window. Fluid typically drains into the pleural space, relieving symptoms.

Pericardiectomy

Pericardiectomy is performed for treatment of constrictive pericarditis. A variety of surgical approaches have been described, including left anterior thoracotomy, bilateral thoracotomies, or median sternotomy. Best exposure is usually provided by the latter. The amount of pericardium to be removed is a matter of controversy, but most surgeons advocate a procedure that decorticates all of the right and left ventricles, including the anterolateral and diaphragmatic surfaces. Resection of pericardium overlying the atria or venae cavae probably adds little hemodynamic benefit but increases the risk of bleeding complications. The depth of the pericardiectomy is also important, and as much as possible of the constricting epicardial peel overlying the ventricles should be removed. Cardiopulmonary bypass is used in some instances to allow greater manipulation of the heart and to decompress the chambers during the dissection. It may help to control bleeding from friable areas of the heart. Regardless of the approach, care must be taken to avoid injury to the phrenic nerve.

Pericardiectomy has an operative mortality of 5% to 15%, with most deaths occurring from low cardiac output.[21] Chronic constriction may lead to myocardial atrophy, which contributes to this problem. Survivors, however, generally achieve significant hemodynamic and symptomatic improvement, and 5-year survival rates may exceed 80% for those discharged from the hospital alive. Results tend to be worse in patients who present with more advanced symptoms (New York Heart Association Class III and IV) and in those in whom constriction was secondary to mediastinal irradiation in which underlying myocardial fibrosis may be a factor.[28]

SELECTED REFERENCES

Cimino, J. J., and Kogan, A. D.: Constrictive pericarditis after cardiac surgery: Report of three cases and review of the literature. Am. Heart. J., *118*:1292, 1989.

These authors reviewed the world literature on constrictive pericarditis after cardiac surgery up to 1989, tabulating data on diagnostic testing, signs and symptoms, potential causes, and treatment options. They note an association with postpericardiotomy syndrome and suggest magnetic resonance imaging as the noninvasive procedure of choice, although they recommend cardiac catheterization to differentiate from restrictive cardiomyopathy. Pericardial stripping is advocated once irreversible pericardial fibrosis has developed.

McCaughan, B. C., Schaff, H. V., Piehler, J. M., et al.: Early and late results of pericardiectomy for constrictive pericarditis. J. Thorac. Cardiovasc. Surg., *89*:340, 1985.
This study reviewed outcomes after surgical treatment of 231 patients with hemodynamically significant constrictive pericarditis over a 47-year period at the Mayo Clinic. Operative mortality was 14%, with most deaths arising from low-output states. Long-term survival of surviving patients was good, with almost all experiencing symptomatic relief. These authors prefer the left anterior thoracotomy approach.

Shabetai, R., Fowler, N. O., and Guntheroth, W. G.: The hemodynamics of cardiac tamponade and constrictive pericarditis. Am. J. Cardiol., *26*:480, 1970.
This article describes the hemodynamic alterations that accompany cardiac tamponade and constrictive pericarditis. The effects on pressure and flow in the venous system, pulmonary arterial system, and systemic arteries are chronicled. The physiologic basis of pulsus paradoxus is discussed.

Spodick, D. H.: The normal and diseased pericardium: Current concepts of pericardial physiology, diagnosis and treatment. J. Am. Coll. Cardiol., *1*:240, 1983.
This concise review of pericardial disorders written by a leading authority reviews the anatomy and physiology of the pericardium and the differential diagnosis of pathologic entities. A discussion of electrocardiographic features and imaging modalities useful in pericardial disease is provided.

Vaitkais, P. T., Herrmann, H. C., and LeWinter, M. M.: Treatment of malignant pericardial effusion. JAMA, *272*:59, 1994.
This article reviews the world literature on the management of malignant pericardial effusion. The roles and effectiveness of pericardiocentesis, systemic chemotherapy and radiation therapy, intrapericardial sclerosis, subxiphoid pericardiotomy, pericardial window, pericardiectomy, and percutaneous balloon pericardiotomy are discussed. Although success rates are higher with the surgical procedures, operative risks are also greater. The authors suggest that treatment be individualized based on the patient's condition and tumor type.

REFERENCES

1. Beck, C. S.: Two cardiac compressor triads. JAMA, *104*:714, 1935.
2. Bishop, L. H., Estes, E. H., and McIntosh, H. E.: The electrocardiogram as a safeguard in pericardiocentesis. JAMA, *62*:264, 1956.
3. Cameron, J., Oesterle, S. N., Baldwin, J. C., et al.: The etiologic spectrum of constrictive pericarditis. Am. Heart. J., *113*:354, 1987.
4. Campbell, P. T., Van Trigt, P., Wall, T. C., et al.: Subxiphoid pericardiotomy in the diagnosis and management of large pericardial effusions associated with malignancy. Chest, *101*:938, 1992.
5. Celermajer, D. S., Boyer, M. J., Bailey, B. P., et al.: Pericardiocentesis for symptomatic malignant pericardial effusion. Med. J. Aust., *154*:19, 1991.
6. Chevers, N.: Observations on the disease of the orifice and valves of the aorta. Guy's Hosp Rep, *7*:387, 1842.
7. Cimino, J. J., and Kogan, A. D.: Constrictive pericarditis after cardiac surgery: Report of three cases and review of the literature. Am. Heart. J., *118*:1292, 1989.
8. Cormican, M. C., and Nyman, C. R.: Intrapericardial bleomycin for the management of cardiac tamponade secondary to malignant pericardial effusion. Br. Heart. J., *63*:61, 1990.
9. Engle, M. A., Ehlers, K. H., O'Loughlin, J. E. Jr., et al.: The postpericardiotomy syndrome: Iatrogenic illness with immunologic and virologic components. *In* Engle, M. A. (Ed.): Pediatric Cardiovascular Disease (Cardiovascular Clinics). Philadelphia, F. A. Davis, 1981, p. 381.
10. Fowler, N. O., and Harbin, A. D. III: Recurrent acute pericarditis: Follow-up study of 31 patients. J. Am. Coll. Cardiol., *7*:300, 1986.
11. Gatenby, R. A., Hartz, W. H., and Kessler, H. B.: Percutaneous catheter drainage for malignant pericardial effusion. J. Vasc. Interv. Radiol., *2*:151, 1991.
12. Guindo, J., Rodriguez de la Serna, A., Ramio, J., et al.: Recurrent pericarditis: Relief with colchicine. Circulation, *82*:1117, 1990.
13. Hageman, J. H., D'Esposo, N. D., Glenn, W. W. L.: Tuberculosis of the pericardium: A long-term analysis of forty-four cases. N. Engl. J. Med., *270*:327, 1978.
14. Isaacs, J. P., Carter, B. N. II, and Haller, J. A. Jr.: Experimental pericarditis: The pathologic physiology of constrictive pericarditis. Bull. Johns Hopkins Hosp., *90*:259, 1952.
15. Killian, D. M., Furiasse, J. G., Scanlon, P. J., et al.: Constrictive pericarditis after cardiac surgery. Am. Heart J., *118*:563, 1989.
16. Klacsmann, P. G., Bulkley, B. H., and Hutchins, G. M.: The changed spectrum of purulent pericarditis: An 86 year autopsy experience in 200 patients. Am. J. Med., *63*:666, 1977.
17. Kopecky, S. L., Callahan, J. A., Tajik, A. J., et al.: Percutaneous pericardial catheter drainage: Report of 42 consecutive cases. Am. J. Cardiol., *58*:633, 1986.

18. Kussmaul, A.: Uber schwielige Mediastion-Perikarditis und den paradoxen Puls. Berl Klin Wochenschr *10*:433, 1873.
19. Mack, M. J., Aronoff, R. J., Acuff, T. E., et al.: Present role of thoracoscopy in the diagnosis and treatment of diseases of the chest. Ann. Thorac. Surg., *54*:403, 1992.
20. Martins, J. B., Manuel, W. J., and Marcus, M. L.: Comparative effects of catecholamines in cardiac tamponade: Experimental and clinical studies. Am. J. Cardiol., *46*:59, 1980.
21. McCaughan, B. C., Schaff, H. V., Piehler, J. M., et al.: Early and late results of pericardiectomy for constrictive pericarditis. J. Thorac. Cardiovasc. Surg., *89*:340, 1985.
22. Moore, R. L.: Congenital deficiencies of the pericardium. Arch. Surg., *11*:765, 1925.
23. Morgan, B. C., Guntheroth, W. G., and Dillard, D. H.: Relationship of pericardial to pleural pressure during quiet respiration and cardiac tamponade. Circ. Res., *16*:493, 1965.
24. Permanyer-Miralda, G., Sagrista-Sauleda, J., and Soler-Soler, J.: Primary acute pericardial disease: A prospective series of 231 consecutive patients. Am. J. Cardiol., *56*:623, 1985.
25. Reydel, B., and Spodick, D. H.: Frequency and significance of chamber collapses during cardiac tamponade. Am. Heart J., *119*:1160, 1990.
26. Rooney, J. J., Crocco, J. A., and Lyons, H. A.: Tuberculous pericarditis. Ann. Intern. Med., *72*:73, 1970.
27. Santamore, W. P., Lynch, P. R., Meier, G., et al.: Myocardial interaction between the ventricles. J. Appl. Physiol., *41*:362, 1976.
28. Seifert, F. C., Miller, D. C., Oesterle, S. N., et al.: Surgical treatment of constrictive pericarditis: Analysis of outcome and diagnostic error. Circulation *72*(Suppl. II):264, 1985.
29. Shabetai, R., Fowler, N. O., and Guntheroth, W. G.: The hemodynamics of cardiac tamponade and constrictive pericarditis. Am. J. Cardiol., *26*:480, 1970.
30. Shepherd, F. A., Morgan, C., Evans, W. K., et al.: Medical management of malignant pericardial effusion by tetracycline sclerosis. Am. J. Cardiol., *60*:1161, 1987.
31. Silverberg, S., Oreopolos, D. G., and Wise, D. J.: Pericarditis in patients undergoing long-term hemodialysis and peritoneal dialysis: Incidence, complications, and management. Am. J. Med., *63*:874, 1977.
32. Soulen, R. L., Stark, D. D., and Higgins, C. B.: Magnetic resonance imaging of constrictive pericardial disease. Am. J. Cardiol., *55*:480, 1985.
33. Spodick, D. H.: Differential diagnosis of acute pericarditis. Prog. Cardiovasc. Dis., *14*:192, 1971.
34. Spodick, D. H.: Differential characteristics of the electrocardiogram in early repolarization and acute pericarditis. N. Engl. J. Med., *295*:523, 1976.
35. Spodick, D. H.: The normal and diseased pericardium: Current concepts of pericardial physiology, diagnosis and treatment. J. Am. Coll. Cardiol., *1*:240, 1983.
36. Spodick, D. H.: Frequency of arrhythmias in acute pericarditis determined by Holter monitoring. Am. J. Cardiol., *53*:842, 1984.
37. Tyberg, T. I., Goodyer, A. V. N., and Langou, R. A.: Genesis of pericardial knock in constrictive pericarditis. Am. J. Cardiol., *46*:570, 1980.
38. Vaitkais, P. T., Herrmann, H. C., and LeWinter, M. M.: Treatment of malignant pericardial effusion. JAMA, *272*:59, 1994.
39. Wong, B., Murphy, J., Chang, C. J., et al.: The risk of pericardiocentesis. Am. J. Cardiol., *44*:1110, 1979.
40. Ziskind, A. A., Pearce, A. C., Lemmon, C. C., et al.: Percutaneous balloon pericardiotomy for the treatment of cardiac tamponade and large pericardial effusions. J. Am. Coll. Cardiol., *21*:1, 1993.

CHAPTER 54

THE HEART

I

CARDIOPULMONARY RESUSCITATION

Donald D. Glower, M.D.

Cardiopulmonary resuscitation (CPR) includes a wide range of measures employed to salvage a person who has sustained cardiopulmonary arrest. In addition to the many persons who experience cardiopulmonary arrest due to progressive chronic disease, approximately 400,000 persons each year in the United States experience sudden cardiac death,[1] defined as unexpected circulatory arrest from cardiac causes with symptoms lasting for 1 hour or less. Approximately two thirds of sudden deaths occur outside the hospital. Survival from circulatory arrest has been shown to be influenced strongly by the availability and immediate institution of CPR. Rapid CPR may salvage more than 40% of out-of-hospital arrest victims and an even higher percentage of patients with in-hospital cardiac arrest.[2]

HISTORICAL DEVELOPMENT

Attempts have been made to restore life to the dead since biblical times.[4] Mouth-to-mouth resuscitation was well described during the eighteenth century, and Koenig reported successful resuscitation of six patients using external cardiac compression in 1885. Open-chest direct cardiac massage was successfully employed by Ingelsrud in 1901. Wiggers studied electrical defibrillation of the heart in animals in the 1930s and 1940s, Beck first successfully used internal electrical defibrillation in a patient in 1947, and Zoll developed external cardioversion in 1956. Kouwenhoven and colleagues[12] first instituted modern CPR by combining external cardiac massage with mechanical ventilation and electrical defibrillation.

ETIOLOGY

Ventricular fibrillation due to coronary artery disease is the most common cause of sudden death. Other causes of cardiac arrest include anoxia leading to ventricular fibrillation; electrolyte abnormalities such as hypokalemia or hyperkalemia; toxicity of such drugs as digitalis, procainamide, or quinidine; or other arrhythmias, such as severe bradycardia, asystole, heart block, or ventricular tachycardia.

PATHOPHYSIOLOGY

Cardiac arrest is characterized by cessation of the normal circulation, thereby halting delivery of oxygen and removal of tissue metabolic waste with progressive tissue hypoxia, anaerobic metabolism, acidosis, and, ultimately, cell death. The brain is probably the most susceptible organ to hypoxia, with permanent neurologic injury occurring after more than 5 minutes of cardiac arrest at normal body temperature.

Although CPR restores some degree of perfusion to the body, most techniques of CPR are characterized by inability to deliver normal amounts of blood and oxygen to tissues. Open-chest massage has been able to deliver nearly normal blood flow,[5, 10, 20] whereas closed-chest massage generally results in 25% or less of normal cardiac output, 5% of normal coronary blood flow, and 15% of normal cerebral blood flow.[2] Thus, CPR for more than 10 to 15 minutes generally fails to prevent some degree of organ injury, especially to the brain, heart, and kidneys.

Two main mechanisms have been proposed for the ability of CPR to restore the circulation. The simplest mechanism is direct cardiac compression, of which the best example is open-chest cardiac massage. External cardiac massage may also produce direct cardiac compression, as has been demonstrated in dogs undergoing closed-chest CPR.[14] In humans, direct cardiac compression is probably most prominent in persons with compliant chest walls and thin chests. Coronary blood flow in animals undergoing external cardiac massage is optimized by a compression rate of 120 beats per minute and by using a relatively rapid impulse type of compression.[24] As in the normal heart, coronary blood flow during CPR is maximal during diastole, and coronary blood flow in animals falls as the compression rate exceeds 120 beats per minute due to decreased diastolic time (Fig. 54–1). Early clinical studies have demonstrated some increased efficacy of high-frequency CPR.[9]

The second proposed mechanism for restoring circulation with external cardiac massage is the thoracic pump mechanism.[18] By this mechanism, external cardiac massage raises the pressure of all intrathoracic contents equally, thus expelling blood from the thorax with the heart serving as a mere conduit (Fig. 54–2). Collapse of veins at the thoracic outlet provides a one-way valve and maintains the direction of circulation. Animal studies have demonstrated that a thoracic pump mechanism is optimized by a compression rate of 60 beats per minute and a compression time that is 50% of the compression-release cycle.[2] The thoracic pump mechanism may be most prominent in patients with a large anteroposterior chest diameter, which makes direct cardiac compression unlikely. Adjunctive measures such as abdominal binding and synchronous ventilation augment the thoracic pump mechanism by decreasing chest wall compliance and augmenting intrathoracic pressure.[2]

DIAGNOSIS

The diagnosis of cardiac arrest requires documentation of total loss of consciousness, cessation of spontaneous breathing, and absence of a central arterial pulse. A 15-second period of observation is advisable to document the presence of cardiac arrest, to avoid the unnecessary application of

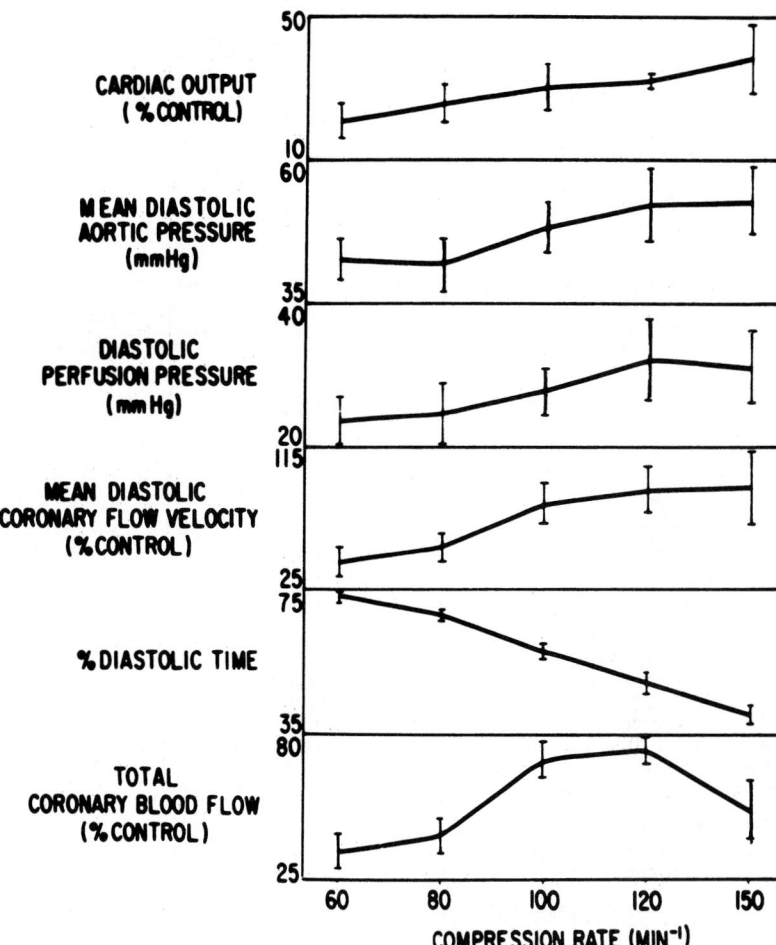

Figure 54–1. Cumulative hemodynamic data from compression rate study (mean +/− standard error). Changes in cardiac output, percentage diastolic time, and total coronary blood flow with increase in rate were significant by multivariate analysis (p<.05). Changes in other parameters were not significant. (From Wolfe, J. A., Maier, G. W., Newton, J. R., et al.: Physiological determinants of coronary blood flow during external cardiac massage. J. Thorac. Cardiovasc. Surg., 95:523, 1988.)

CPR, and to allow time to recruit additional individuals to administer CPR.

TREATMENT

The American Heart Association Subcommittee on Emergency Cardiac Care has divided CPR into two phases: (1) basic life support, which may be administered outside the hospital by nonmedical personnel; and (2) advanced cardiac life support, which generally requires trained medical personnel.[1]

Basic Life Support

Before basic life support is initiated, efforts should be made to quickly call for medical help because of the relatively short period of time that basic life support alone can sustain the body without organ damage.[23] After the diagnosis of cardiac arrest is established, the airway should be examined for obstruction by such material as food particles. If obstructed, the airway may be cleared digitally or by blows to the back or thrusts to the abdomen.[8] Airway obstruction by the tongue may be alleviated by placing the victim on his or her back, extending the victim's neck and tilting the head backward, and applying forward pressure to the jaw at the mandibular angle. A valved mask system is used to initiate ventilation, or mouth-to-mouth resuscitation is begun at a rate of 10 to 12 breaths per minute with the victim's nostrils held occluded. In single-rescuer CPR, 2 breaths should be given for every 15 chest compressions. In two-rescuer CPR, 1 breath is given after every 5 chest compressions.

Once an adequate airway has been established, the circulation is restored by external chest compressions. The heels of the hands are placed on top of each other and on the lower sternum with the arms straight and locked, and compressions are begun at a rate of 80 to 100 beats per minute (Fig. 54–3).

Advanced Cardiac Life Support

If mask ventilation is not satisfactory, endotracheal intubation may be performed either by placing a nasotracheal tube or by using a laryngoscope to pass an orotracheal tube. The tube should be advanced only 5 to 6 cm. beyond the vocal cords to avoid intubation of the right mainstem bronchus. The patient is placed on 100% oxygen and ventilated with a tidal volume of 10 to 15 ml. per kg. and a rate of 12 breaths per minute.

An electrocardiographic tracing from either the defibrillator or electrodes should be used to examine the cardiac rhythm. Ventricular fibrillation or tachycardia is treated by early electrical cardioversion with 200 J., 200 to 300 J., and 360 J. in rapid succession as necessary. Early defibrillation has been a determinant for survival after cardiac arrest. Good electrical contact of the external paddles may be improved by placement of one paddle on the back directly behind the heart and the other paddle directly anterior to the heart.

A large peripheral vein should be cannulated early during the resuscitation to allow administration of intravenous drugs. Each drug should be followed by a 20-ml. bolus to improve delivery of the drug to the central vascular compartment, which may take 1 to 2 minutes. If intravenous access is unavailable, epinephrine and lidocaine may be adminis-

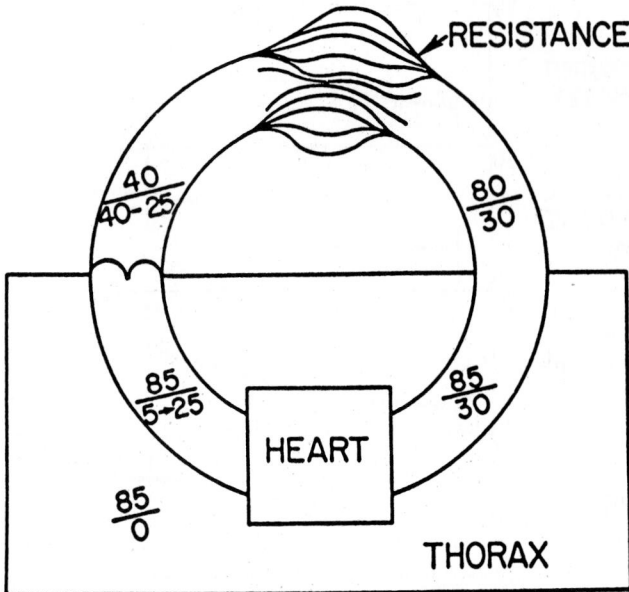

Figure 54–2. Representative pressures recorded during conventional CPR demonstrating the thoracic pump mechanism of forward arterial flow. Pressures are those recorded during compression, and intrathoracic pressures were indexed from esophageal pressures. There is no significant pressure gradient across the heart. The extrathoracic arterial pressure is similar to the intrathoracic aortic pressure. The extrathoracic venous pressure is markedly lower than the intrathoracic venous (right atrial) pressure. The extrathoracic arteriovenous pressure gradient results in forward flow. (From Chandra, N. C., and Weisfeldt, M. L.: Cardiopulmonary resuscitation and the subsequent management of the patient. In Schlant, R. C., and Alexander, R. W.: The Heart. New York, McGraw-Hill, 1994. Reproduced with permission of the McGraw-Hill Companies.)

tered by injection through a long catheter into the endotracheal tube beyond the endotracheal tube tip while briefly holding cardiac compressions. Endotracheal drug administration requires two to two and one-half times the standard intravenous dose and should be delivered in 10 ml. of saline or water. After initial resuscitation attempts, a central venous line (jugular or subclavian) allows more rapid drug delivery but may require temporary cessation of chest compression. Volume expansion with intravenous normal saline or lactated Ringer's solution is indicated only in those patients with volume depletion.

If initial defibrillation is unsuccessful, 10 mg. of 1:10,000 epinephrine should be given intravenously. Data suggest that epinephrine should be given frequently, every 3 to 5 minutes, until an effective cardiac rhythm is restored.[13] Hyperventilation and sparing intravenous sodium bicarbonate (1 mEq./kg.) may be used to correct acidosis. Recurrent ventricular fibrillation or ventricular tachycardia is treated with intravenous lidocaine (1–1.5 mg./kg. followed by 0.5–1.5 mg./kg. up to 3 mg./kg.), followed by defibrillation. Bretyllium (5 mg./kg.) is administered if ventricular fibrillation recurs after lidocaine administration, and bretyllium doses (5–10 mg./kg.) may be repeated up to a total of 30 mg. per kg. Procainamide (up to 17 mg./kg. as a slow infusion) or atenolol (5–10 mg.) may have use in treatment of refractory ventricular fibrillation. Asystole or profound bradycardia may be treated by atropine (0.5–1.0 mg.) given intravenously and may be repeated in 5 minutes up to a total dose of 0.04 mg. per kg. Asystole may also respond to 10 ml. of 1:10,000 solution of intravenously administered epinephrine. Temporary transvenous or external pacing may be instituted for profound bradycardia, asystole, or heart block. Hyperkalemia may require treatment with an infusion of 10 to 30 ml. of 10% calcium gluconate over 1 to 5 minutes, glucose and insulin

infusion, correction of acidosis, and administration of potassium binding resins. Electromechanical dissociation (electrocardiographic evidence of a ventricular rhythm without effective circulation) is a grave prognostic sign generally indicating severe, irreversible cardiac injury. Treatable causes that should be considered include cardiac tamponade, hypovolemia, tension pneumothorax, pulmonary embolism, and metabolic disturbances such as acidosis, hyperkalemia, hypoxia, and hypothermia.

If effective circulation cannot be restored after 10 to 15 minutes of CPR, consideration should be given to open-chest cardiac massage in selected hospitalized patients with cardiac arrest.[10, 23] In animal and human studies, open-chest massage has not benefited survival when total arrest time exceeded 20 to 25 minutes, and open-chest massage appeared to most benefit survival if it was instituted within 5 minutes of hospital arrival in patients with out-of-hospital arrest.[21] Patients in whom early open-chest massage should especially be considered include those with chest deformity or open body cavities that render closed-chest CPR ineffective; penetrating trauma to the chest or abdomen; abdominal hemorrhage;

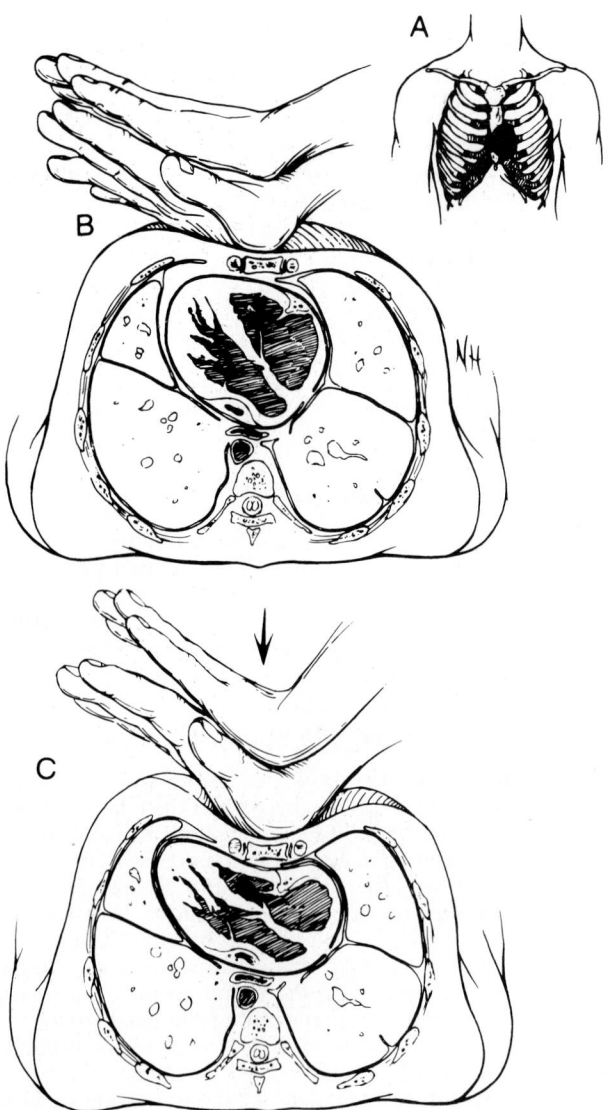

Figure 54–3. A, Manual compression is performed over the lower sternum. B, The position of the hands on the sternum is shown. C, External cardiac massage is performed with high-velocity compression of moderate force and brief duration.

pericardial tamponade; pulmonary embolism; or hypothermia. After application of antiseptic solution to the left side of the chest, a left anterior thoracotomy is performed through the fourth or fifth intercostal space, the pericardial sac is opened, and the heart is compressed at a rate of 60 to 80 beats per minute (Fig. 54–4). Defibrillation may be applied directly to the heart as necessary using a reduced energy of 10 to 15 J. After successful resuscitation, the thoracotomy incision is closed in the operating room. Even when the thoracotomy is performed under relatively nonsterile conditions, infections are rare.

Adjuncts to CPR that have benefited cerebral blood flow or coronary flow but have not been shown to influence survival after CPR include abdominal binding,[19] synchronous ventilation,[11] central administration of epinephrine,[15] use of a mechanical thumper device, and use of cardiopulmonary bypass.[7] A new external suction cup device may improve 24-hour survival over standard CPR.[22] No closed-chest technique has been able to match the ability of open-chest cardiac massage to restore the circulation to near-normal levels.[5]

MANAGEMENT AFTER RESUSCITATION

Successfully resuscitated patients generally require transfer to the intensive care unit, where monitoring with the use of an arterial pressure catheter, a continuous electrocardiogram, a urinary Foley catheter, and possibly hemodynamic monitoring with a Swan-Ganz catheter may be instituted. Serial electrocardiograms and determination of cardiac isoenzyme levels should be used to detect myocardial infarction. Appropriate patients demonstrating acute myocardial infarction may be treated with nitrates and thrombolytic therapy, followed by cardiac catheterization and consideration of coronary revascularization in several days if the patient remains stable. Coronary revascularization has been demonstrated to improve the survival of patients experiencing sudden death due to coronary disease. Patients with sudden death due to ventricular tachycardia or fibrillation in the absence of myocardial infarction should undergo 24-hour Holter monitoring and electrophysiologic stimulation study to detect arrhythmias that may be treatable with antiarrhythmic agents, revascularization, or automatic internal cardioverter-defibrillator implantation.

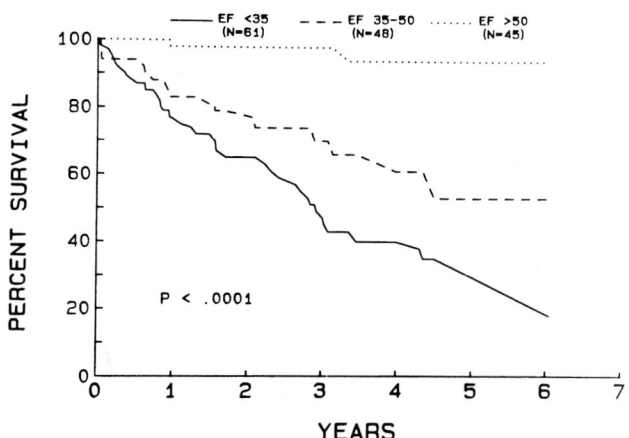

Figure 54–5. Survival of successfully resuscitated victims of sudden death as a function of resting left ventricular ejection fraction (EF). Survival decreased dramatically as ventricular function worsened. (From Ritchie, J. L., Hallstrom, A. P., Trobaugh, G. B., et al.: Out-of-hospital sudden cardiac death: Rest and exercise radionuclide left ventricular function in survivors. Am. J. Cardiol., 55:645, 1985.)

RESULTS

External cardiac massage may yield complications including costal or sternal fractures, liver or visceral laceration, or visceral contusion. The success of CPR out of hospital has been reported to be 30% to 60%, with 50% of the survivors subsequently dying in hospital, usually due to anoxic encephalopathy.[2] The primary determinants of outcome from CPR include patient age, underlying disease, and the time from arrest to defibrillation and resuscitation.[3, 16] Survival to discharge in patients older than 70 years old may be as low as 3%.[16] Successful resuscitation is unlikely after 30 minutes of unsuccessful CPR and is unlikely if ventricular electrocardiographic activity or peripheral perfusion cannot be restored after 10 to 15 minutes of adequate CPR.[23] Survival is extremely unlikely (<1%) in those patients for whom advanced cardiac life support is unsuccessful before arrival at the hospital. The in-hospital costs of resuscitating a patient with a 10% likelihood of successful resuscitation are estimated at $117,000.[6] Mean survival time after successful resuscitation is 3 to 6 years (Fig. 54–5).[17] Recurrent cardiac arrest may occur in 30% to 40% of survivors, emphasizing the need for thorough evaluation of survivors of CPR.

SELECTED REFERENCES

American Heart Association, Emergency Cardiac Care Committee: Guidelines for cardiopulmonary resuscitation and emergency cardiac care. JAMA, 268:2171, 1992.
This extensive and well-referenced document contains detailed guidelines for performing CPR. All practicing physicians should be familiar with this article.

Chandra, N. C.: Mechanisms of blood flow during CPR. Ann. Emerg. Med., 22:281, 1993.
This article provides an excellent review of the mechanisms involved in CPR and various modalities used to optimize CPR.

Kaye, W., and Bircher, N. G. (Eds.): Cardiopulmonary Resuscitation. New York, Churchill Livingstone, 1989.
The history, pharmacology, and techniques of CPR are presented in this excellent reference. Pediatric CPR and the educational aspects of CPR are also addressed.

REFERENCES

1. American Heart Association, Emergency Cardiac Care Committee: Guidelines for cardiopulmonary resuscitation and emergency cardiac care. JAMA, 268:2171, 1992.
2. Chandra, N. C.: Mechanisms of blood flow during CPR. Ann. Emerg. Med., 22:281, 1993.
3. Dautzenberg, P. L., Broekman, T. C., Hooyer, C., Schonwetter, R. S., and

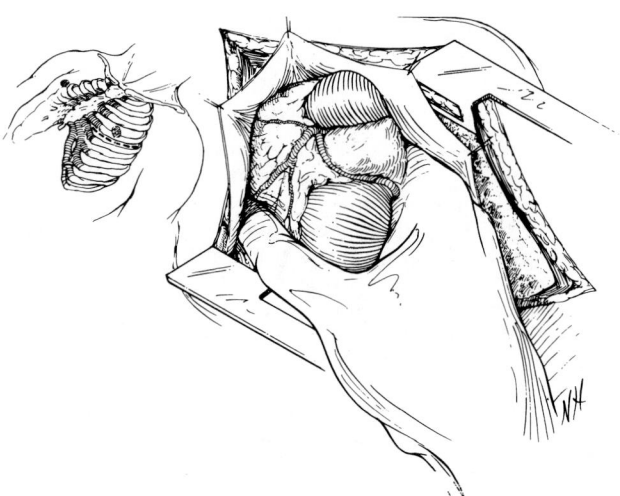

Figure 54–4. Open cardiac massage is performed through a short, left anterior thoracotomy. The ventricles are compressed directly with the hands 60 to 80 times per minute.

Duursma, S. A.: Review: Patient-related predictors of hospitalized patients. Age Ageing, 22:464, 1993.

4. DeBard, M. L.: The history of cardiopulmonary resuscitation. Ann. Emerg. Med., 9:273, 1980.

5. Del Guerci, L. R. M., Feins, N. R., Cohn, J. D., et al.: Comparison of blood flow during external and internal cardiac massage in man. Circulation, 31:1–171, 1965.

6. Ebell, M. H., and Kruse, J. A.: A proposed model for the cost of cardiopulmonary resuscitation. Med. Care, 32:640, 1994.

7. Hartz, R., LoCicero, J., III, Sanders, J. H., Jr., Fredericksen, J. W., Joob, A. W., and Michaelis, L. L.: Clinical experience with portable cardiopulmonary bypass in cardiac arrest patients. Ann. Thorac. Surg., 50:437, 1990.

8. Heimlich, H. J.: A life-saving maneuver to prevent food-choking. JAMA, 234:398, 1975.

9. Kern, K. B., Sanders, A. B., Raife, J., Milander, M. M., Otto, C. W., and Ewy, G. A.: A study of chest compression rates during cardiopulmonary resuscitation in humans: The importance of rate-directed chest compressions. Arch. Intern. Med., 152:145, 1992.

10. Kern, K. B., Sanders, A. B., Badylak, S. F., et al.: Long-term survival with open chest cardiac massage after ineffective closed-chest compression in a canine model. Circulation, 75:498, 1987.

11. Koehler, R. C., Chandra, N., Guerci, A. D., et al.: Augmentation of cerebral perfusion by simultaneous chest compression and lung inflation with abdominal binding following cardiac arrest in dogs. Circulation, 67:266, 1983.

12. Kouwenhoven, W. B., Jude, J. R., and Knickerbocker, G. G.: Closed chest cardiac massage. JAMA, 173:1064, 1960.

13. Lindner, K. H.: Adrenergic agonist drug administration during cardiopulmonary resuscitation. Crit. Care Med., 21:S324, 1993.

14. Maier, G. W., Tyson, G. S., Olson, C. O., et al.: The physiology of external cardiac massage: High impulse cardiopulmonary resuscitation. Circulation, 70:86, 1984.

15. Michael, J. R., Guerci, A. D., Koehler, R., et al.: Mechanisms by which epinephrine augments cerebral and myocardial perfusion during cardiopulmonary resuscitation in dogs. Circulation, 69:822, 1984.

16. O'Keefe, S., Redahan, C., Keane, P., and Daly, K.: Age and other determinants of survival after in-hospital cardiopulmonary resuscitation. Q. J. Med., 81:1005, 1991.

17. Ritchie, J. L., Hallstrom, A. P., Trobaugh, G. B., et al.: Out-of-hospital sudden cardiac death: Rest and exercise radionuclide left ventricular function in survivors. Am. J. Cardiol., 55:645, 1985.

18. Rudicoff, M. T., Maughn, W. L., Effron, M., Freund, P., and Weisfeldt, M. L.: Mechanisms of flow during cardiopulmonary resuscitation. Circulation, 61:345, 1980.

19. Sack, J., Kesselbrenner, M., and Bergman, D.: Survival from in-hospital arrest with interposed abdominal counterpulsation during cardiopulmonary resuscitation. JAMA, 267:379, 1992.

20. Sanders, A. B., Kern, K. B., Ewy, G. A., Atlas, M., and Bailey, L.: Improved resuscitation from cardiac arrest with open-chest massage. Ann. Emerg. Med., 13:672, 1984.

21. Takino, M., and Okada, Y.: The optimum timing of resuscitative thoracotomy for nontraumatic out-of-hospital cardiac arrest. Resuscitation, 26:69, 1993.

22. Tucker, K. J., Galli, F., Savitt, M. A., Kahsai, D., Bresnahan, L., and Redberg, R. F.: Active compression-decompression resuscitation: Effect on resuscitation success after in-hospital cardiac arrest. J. Am. Coll. Cardiol., 24:201, 1994.

23. Weaver, W. D., Cobb, L. A., Hallstrom, A. P., Fahrenbruch, C., Copass, M. K., and Ray, R.: Factors influencing survival after out-of-hospital cardiac arrest. J. Am. Coll. Cardiol., 7:754, 1986.

24. Wolfe, J. A., Maier, G. W., Newton, J. R., et al.: Physiological determinants of coronary blood flow during external cardiac massage. J. Thorac. Cardiovasc. Surg., 95:523, 1988.

II

PENETRATING CARDIAC INJURIES

Fred A. Crawford, Jr., M.D.

HISTORICAL ASPECTS

Penetrating chest injuries were described in the Edwin Smith Papyrus in 3000 B. C.,[20] and Homer clearly described wounds of the heart in *The Iliad* in the ninth century B. C.[14] The subsequent history of cardiac injuries and their treatment were beautifully reviewed by Claude Beck in 1926.[7] Hippocrates and Aristotle recognized the seriousness of cardiac wounds, and Galen noted that wounds of the heart in gladiators were often fatal. This concept persisted into the seventeenth century, when Boerhaave said, "All wounds of the heart deep enough to penetrate into either of the ventricles are mortal."[7] In contrast, as early as the sixteenth century, Hollerius postulated that all cardiac wounds might not necessarily be fatal. Morgagni, in 1691, pointed out the consequences of pericardial tamponade; and Larrey, in 1829, successfully treated a patient by drainage of pericardial tamponade.[7] By 1868, Fischer treated 452 patients with cardiac wounds, 10% of whom recovered. Block,[7] in 1882, was the first to experimentally suture wounds of the heart in rabbits. This concept was opposed by Billroth in 1883 with his famous statement, "The surgeon who should attempt to suture a wound of the heart would lose the respect of his colleagues."[5]

The first two attempts to suture a stab wound of the heart in humans by Cappalen in 1885 and Friria in 1896 were unsuccessful,[7] but these were followed subsequently by Rehn,[29] who in 1896 in Frankfurt successfully sutured a stab wound of the right ventricle with long-term survival. Ten years later, Rehn had compiled a series of 124 patients, 40% of whom recovered. The first American to perform this feat was Lister Hill of Montgomery, Alabama, who repaired a stab wound in a 13-year-old boy by the light of a kerosene lamp on a kitchen table.[13] Over the next several decades, a number of series with an increasingly larger number of patients were reported in which survival rates of 30% to 50% were obtained after thoracotomy and suture of a penetrating cardiac injury. In 1942, Blalock and Ravitch[8] advocated the somewhat more conservative approach of pericardiocentesis and close observation of selected patients. Several large series in the 1960s and early 1970s conclusively indicated that early thoracotomy and cardiorrhaphy is the most appropriate treatment in the management of patients with penetrating cardiac injury.[6, 31, 33]

INCIDENCE

The incidence of cardiovascular injuries has increased dramatically over the past several decades. In a series of 4459 patients with cardiovascular injuries treated over a 30-year period (1958–1987), the incidence increased from 27 patients per year in 1960 to 213 patients per year by the mid 1980s.[21] Paralleling this increase in numbers of injuries has been an increase in the relative frequency of injuries caused by gunshot wounds compared with stab wounds,[27, 32] due to the ready availability of inexpensive hand guns and, in some areas, to the increasing violence associated with illicit drug-related activities. According to Naughton and colleagues,[27] penetrating cardiac injuries occur most often in the home (70%), by a known assailant (83%), and are due to domestic or social disputes (73%). Victims are predominantly male (83%).

In the past, most reports of penetrating cardiac injuries originated from hospitals in large metropolitan areas. In the past decade, more series have been reported from smaller cities as well as from war zones.[27, 40] Trinkle[38] emphasized the difficulties inherent in comparing different clinical series. Significant differences in prehospital and in-hospital mortality may exist because of (1) differing modes of injury (gunshot wound vs. stab wound); (2) other associated injuries; and (3) variable availability of highly trained emergency medical personnel and well-organized rapid transport systems for trauma patients. For example, a series with a larger number of gunshot wounds as compared with stab wounds will usually have a higher mortality. Paradoxically, series from a city with an effective transport system may have a higher hospital or operative mortality because more seriously injured patients survive to get to the hospital. Ivatury and associates[15] have proposed an index for quantifying penetrating cardiac trauma (Penetrating Cardiac Trauma Index) and have shown that this index has a high correlation with survival. Factors influencing mortality from penetrating cardiac injury that are incorporated into this index include, in order of decreasing significance: (1) coronary artery injury; (2) multiple chamber injury or isolated left atrial or left ventricular injury; (3) comminuted tear of single chamber; (4) single right-sided chamber injury; and (5) tangential injuries that do not penetrate the endocardium. It is important to consider these factors when comparing results from different series. Most current series report survivals of 60% to 70% for those patients who reach the hospital with vital signs present.[16, 19, 39, 40]

ETIOLOGY

Penetrating injuries to the heart are most commonly associated with violence and are the result of stab wounds and gunshot wounds. However, such injuries have also been produced accidentally by nails, coat hangers, objects propelled by lawnmowers, and even iatrogenically by chest tubes and needles. Despite the increasing sophistication of emergency medical services and rapid transportation to the hospital, 60% to 80% of those injuries cause death at the scene or before arrival at a trauma facility.[32, 38]

DIAGNOSIS

Any patient with a penetrating injury to the chest, neck, upper abdomen, or back, and especially to the anterior chest and immediately adjacent to the sternum, should be suspected of having a cardiac injury. The right ventricle occupies approximately 55% of the anterior chest wall; the left ventricle, 20%; the right atrium, 10%; and the great vessels and venae cavae, 15%.[32] The relative frequency of cardiac chamber injury corresponds somewhat to the anatomy described previously. In a review of 20 series of penetrating cardiac injuries consisting of a total of 1802 patients,[20] the right ventricle was injured in 42.4%, the left ventricle in 32%,[9] the right atrium in 15.3%, and the left atrium in 5.8%. Great vessel injury occurred in 3.4%.

Presenting signs and symptoms may vary depending on the mode of injury, the location of injury, and other associated injuries. In general, these patients present in two quite difference states: cardiac tamponade or hemorrhagic shock.[38, 39] Patients with isolated stab wounds from smaller weapons (ice pick) to the left or right ventricle may present with normal hemodynamics and may have a relatively normal physical examination. Injuries to the ventricle may result in little or no bleeding or transient bleeding, followed by sealing of the injury by the muscle fibers of the ventricle or by cardiac tamponade. Injuries to the atrium may cause bleeding followed by sealing of the injury by clot because of the lower pressure in the atrium. However, atrial injuries can also result in exsanguination because of the inability of the thin-walled atrium to seal. Frequently in patients with stab wounds, the hole in the pericardium is small. If significant bleeding from the heart occurs, the blood is trapped in the pericardial cavity. These patients may present with classic cardiac tamponade with the typical findings of hypotension, elevated venous pressure (distended neck veins), and decreased heart sounds (Beck's triad).[5] These typical physical findings may be hard to detect, however, in patients who are uncooperative, combative, or intoxicated. In addition, the loss of a significant amount of blood from the cardiac wound or other injuries may cause flat neck veins despite the presence of significant pericardial tamponade. In these patients, evidence of increased venous pressure may only become obvious after volume resuscitation. When hypotension and distended neck veins are present in a cooperative patient with a penetrating chest wound, one must assume some degree of cardiac injury and proceed accordingly. However, the absence of the classic findings of tamponade does *not* allow exclusion of a cardiac injury.

Chest radiographs and fluoroscopy have been of little help in making the diagnosis and usually result in further delay of definitive diagnosis and treatment. The pericardium is relatively inelastic, and acute tamponade rarely causes significant cardiac enlargement on chest films. The electrocardiogram is rarely useful in making the diagnosis, but obvious ischemic changes may suggest an injury to a coronary artery.

The role of echocardiography in the diagnosis of penetrating cardiac injuries is controversial. Echocardiography requires a cooperative patient and a careful examination by a highly trained individual. Unfortunately, most patients with suspected penetrating cardiac injuries present at a time when it is difficult to quickly obtain a quality study. In addition, the patient's condition may not permit a delay in treatment until an echocardiogram can be obtained. Despite this, Aaland and associates used echocardiography in 53 hemodynamically stable patients with suspected cardiac injury and suggested that it was a sensitive method of evaluating suspected penetrating cardiac injury in this population.[1] Because further unnecessary operative procedures were prevented, these authors credited the techniques with substantial savings to the hospital. On the other hand, another report of 5 patients noted normal echocardiograms despite major intrapericardial injury in all 5.[9] It is likely that the echocardiogram is useful in a small number of these patients, but the logistics of obtaining a quality study in an uncooperative patient in the middle of the night limit its usefulness.

The role of pericardiocentesis in the diagnosis and treatment of penetrating cardiac injuries is also controversial. Pericardiocentesis is performed by inserting a large needle at the tip of the xiphoid and angling it posteriorly and superiorly toward the left shoulder. Some have advocated performing pericardiocentesis with the aid of electrocardiographic or echocardiographic monitoring, but this is not necessary. Pericardiocentesis is a difficult technical procedure under optimal circumstances in a cooperative patient; and in the setting frequently associated with this type of injury (shock, intoxication, shivering, hypoxia, combativeness), it may be impossible. Blood in the pericardial cavity is frequently clotted and cannot be aspirated through a small needle, thus causing a false-negative diagnosis. Perhaps of equal frequency, the return of nonclotting blood may be due to the needle penetrating a cardiac chamber or lacerating the heart or a coronary artery. In the acute setting, the pericardial cavity is nondistensible; and a relatively small amount of blood in this space can cause significant hemodynamic compromise. Accordingly, removal of a small amount of blood from the pericardial space can produce rapid improvement in blood pressure. This improvement is most often transient but may be helpful in stabilizing the patient until he or she is transported to the operating room.

Some authors have advocated creation of a subxiphoid pericardial window performed in the emergency department or the operating room with the patient under local or light general anesthesia as the diagnostic procedure of choice.[3, 10, 18, 25] If no blood is present in the pericardium, the cardiac injury can almost certainly be ruled out; and if there are no other injuries, the patient can be discharged with confidence in 24 hours. However, if injury is present, opening the pericardium can result in release of tamponade and, subsequently, exsanguinating hemorrhage. Therefore, when this technique is used, the surgeon should be ready to proceed immediately with a formal median sternotomy and/or thoracotomy for repair of the cardiac injury. A subxiphoid pericardial window is a particularly useful technique in patients undergoing laparotomy for penetrating injury when there is reason to believe that cardiac injury may have occurred in addition to the abdominal injuries.

Cardiac tamponade occurs in the majority (greater than 80%) of stab wounds of the heart but in only 10% to 20% of gunshot wounds. It is interesting that tamponade may have a protective effect and favorably influence survival. Moreno and associates found that survival occurred in 73% of patients presenting with tamponade as compared with 11% of those without it.[26] This was true regardless of the mode of injury or the chambers involved. Although all the diagnostic techniques just mentioned may be useful in selected patients who present in this manner, the emergency department physician and/or evaluating surgeon most often relies on his or her clinical skills and a high degree of suspicion in making the diagnosis.

The second mode of presentation is that of *hemorrhagic shock* (hypotension, decreased venous pressure), which is secondary to exsanguination from the penetrating injury of the heart. This occurs most commonly after gunshot wounds but also may be seen in 20% of patients with stab wounds. In these patients, the injury causes a large tear in the pericardium and in the underlying heart. As a result of the large defect in the pericardium, tamponade cannot occur. The more extensive injury to the heart is unable to seal spontaneously, and the patient may simply exsanguinate. Undoubtedly such patients account for a large percentage of those who die before reaching medical care. Moreno and co-workers documented higher hospital mortality in this group.[26] The diagnosis of a significant injury is usually not difficult in patients who present with evidence of penetrating injury to the chest, hemorrhage, profound hypotension, and flat neck veins. These conditions usually demand immediate definitive treatment, and the diagnostic techniques mentioned earlier (chest films, echocardiography, pericardiocentesis) are even less useful.

TREATMENT

Patients with penetrating chest trauma and suspected cardiac injury should undergo standard initial resuscitative measures on arrival in the trauma facility. These include appropriate airway control, insertion of large central intravenous lines, and fluid replacement.[20] If the patient is stable and the diagnosis of cardiac injury is strongly suspected, prompt transportation to the operating room is mandatory for thoracotomy and prompt repair of the injury. Blalock and Ravitch[8] advocated conservative management (pericardiocentesis and observation) in certain patients, and this continues to be advocated by others.[24] However, Sugg and associates[31] reported in 1968 in an analysis of 459 patients that in 23% no blood was obtained by pericardiocentesis despite the fact that at operation 100 to 660 ml. of blood was found in the

pericardium. In addition, 10 patients who had successful pericardiocentesis subsequently died of tamponade within 1 to 12 hours while being observed. All could have been saved by prompt thoracotomy. They recommended immediate operation for all cardiac injuries and noted a decrease in overall mortality from 36% to 14% after this policy was initiated. In 1972, in a series of 269 patients with penetrating cardiac injury, Beall and colleagues also advised immediate operation with cardiorrhaphy for penetrating injuries.[6] As a result of these two papers, most institutions have changed to a policy of early operation.[16, 20, 28, 32] As previously noted, however, successful pericardiocentesis may stabilize the patient temporarily until definitive thoracotomy can be performed.

Among patients with suspected cardiac injuries (1) some present initially *in extremis* with no blood pressure and agonal respirations; (2) some deteriorate rapidly immediately after arrival in the emergency department; and (3) some cannot be stabilized by the use of standard resuscitative measures. Emergency department thoracotomy has been advocated as offering the greatest chance of salvage in this group. In a group of 37 such patients, 67.5% survived emergency department thoracotomy, resuscitation, and repair of the cardiac wound. Survival was 82% with a stab wound and 68% with a gunshot wound.[22] In another series of 37 consecutive emergency department thoracotomies, 57% survived.[31] Baker and colleagues[5] noted 50% survival after emergency department thoracotomy in patients with cardiac injuries who had no vital signs on arrival. They also noted a significant cost-benefit ratio to emergency department thoracotomy, despite an extremely conservative method of calculating this benefit. Ivatury and associates[17] documented survival in approximately one third of patients who arrived *in extremis*. Survival in the entire series was directly related to the patient's status on arrival (73% survival with stable vital signs; 29% survival for those *in extremis*).

Most penetrating cardiac injuries occur in young, otherwise healthy individuals. Aggressive treatment including emergency department thoracotomy results in the survival of a significant number of these patients whose condition does not permit transportation to the operating room.[5, 17, 22, 32] Complications (wound infection, neurologic injury) occur with this approach, but they are relatively infrequent and must be accepted as the price that must be paid for the salvage of this population of patients.[17]

Operative Technique. The patient with a documented or suspected penetrating cardiac injury who responds appropriately to resuscitation and is relatively stable may be transported to the operating room for thoracotomy under controlled conditions. Caution must be exercised during induction of anesthesia because the initiation of positive-pressure ventilation in combination with an even moderate degree of tamponade may be sufficient to decrease venous return severely and cause rapid hemodynamic deterioration. Under such conditions, skin preparation and draping of the patient before induction may be useful. The operative approach may be through a left anterior thoracotomy in the fourth intercostal space or a median sternotomy. The anterior thoracotomy can be performed quickly and requires no special equipment. It provides perhaps better exposure to the posterior left ventricle as well as the aorta and esophagus, but exposure of the right ventricle and right atrium is not as good. The incision may be extended across the sternum into the right chest, thus giving adequate exposure to all cardiac chambers. Most elective cardiac procedures today are performed through a median sternotomy, and this is the preferred incision for most penetrating cardiac injuries. This approach requires division of the sternum; and although a sternal saw is preferred, the incision may also be made with a Lebsche knife. The cardiopulmonary perfusion team is routinely alerted as soon as a patient with suggested cardiac injury arrives in the trauma area so that cardiopulmonary bypass is available. However, its use is rarely necessary for most simple injuries. Autotransfusion may be helpful, and this may be facilitated by the pump team.

Once the patient's pericardium is opened and blood is evacuated, control of the point of injury is usually possible with digital pressure. The laceration or hole may be closed with several interrupted sutures of silk or synthetic material (Fig. 54–6B). Teflon felt bolsters may be used to prevent the sutures from tearing through the heart, but this is not always necessary. Shamoun and colleagues[30] have reported the usefulness of metallic skin staples as a way to rapidly control and close cardiac injuries in patients *in extremis*. For injuries to the atrium or great vessels, a tangential side-biting clamp may be applied and the injury sutured (see Fig. 54–6A). When the injury is adjacent to a major coronary artery, sutures should be placed beneath the coronary artery so that the injury is repaired without compromising blood flow in the coronary arteries (see Fig. 54–6C). More extensive or simple injuries that cannot be initially controlled by digital pressure may require prompt heparinization, institution of cardiopulmonary bypass, and more definitive techniques of repair. When small coronary artery branches or distal coronary arteries are injured, they may be ligated, producing only a localized area of myocardial ischemia (see Fig. 54–6D). More proximal coronary artery injuries require more definitive repair—either direct suture, which is rarely possible, or, more commonly, bypass, using a saphenous vein or internal mammary artery graft (see Fig. 54–6E). Such proximal injuries to coronary arteries may be fatal if not repaired, or if not fatal they may result in major myocardial infarction, subsequent loss of ventricular function, and/or development of a ventricular aneurysm.

In addition to simple external injuries to cardiac chambers and to coronary arteries, penetrating wounds may cause injury to intracardiac structures, such as valves as well as atrial and/or ventricular septum.[4, 21, 37] Arteriovenous fistulas or intracardiac shunts may occur in up to 5% of patients after penetrating cardiac injury.[4] Most commonly the shunt occurs between the left and right ventricles (ventricular septal defect), but it may also occur between the atria (atrial septal defect), between the aorta and vena cava, the aorta and pulmonary artery, or a coronary artery and a cardiac chamber. Occasionally the fistula is sufficiently large to produce a murmur heard on initial examination in the emergency department. Most commonly, however, the fistula is initially small and the associated murmur not appreciated at the time the patient is first evaluated. When a murmur is identified on initial assessment, preoperative evaluation by two-dimensional echocardiographic Doppler imaging may be extremely valuable in assessing any intracardiac pathology.[11]

If possible, intraoperative transesophageal echocardiography should be performed once the obvious external injury has been repaired and the patient is hemodynamically stable.[28] This permits identification of unsuspected injuries to the cardiac valves, atrial or ventricular septum with intracardiac shunts, or arteriovenous fistulas. Fortunately, many such intracardiac injuries are usually hemodynamically insignificant. The first goal is to have the patient survive the acute injury. Only when the intracardiac injury itself is life threatening or very significant hemodynamically should repair be attempted at the time of the emergency procedure.

Some intracardiac injuries first become obvious at some point after successful repair of the initial cardiac injury. Therefore, careful repeated physical examinations are required before and after discharge to pick up these defects. The physical examination should be supplemented by thorough two-dimensional echocardiographic Doppler study before discharge and subsequently if an intracardiac defect or

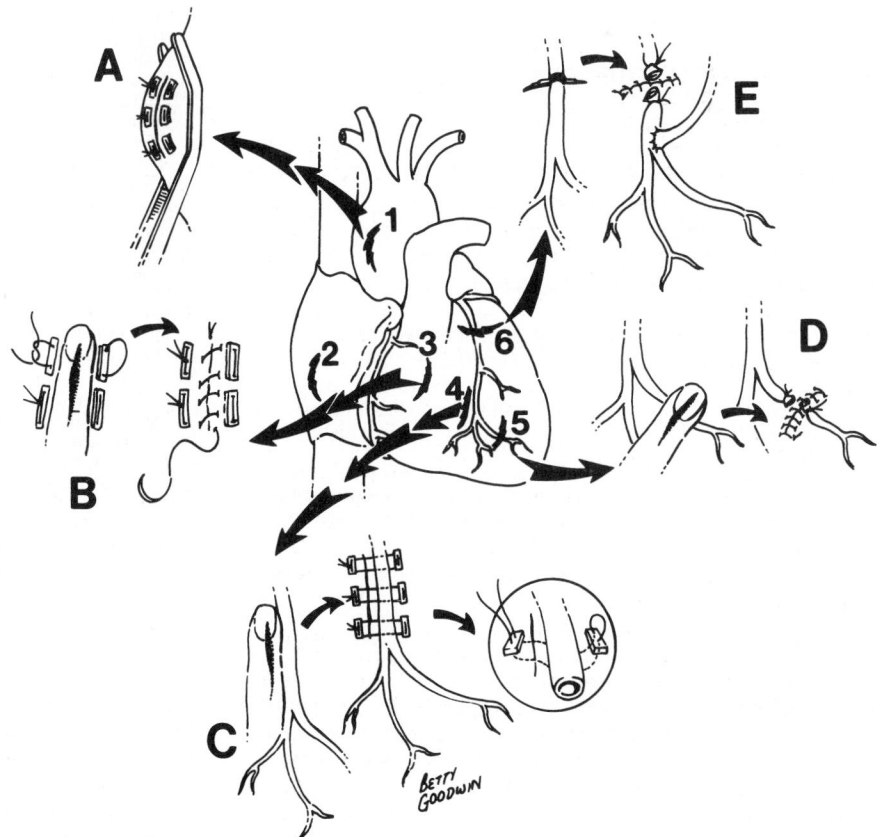

Figure 54–6. Penetrating injuries of the right atrium (2) or great vessels (1) may be initially controlled by digital pressure (B) and oversewn. An alternative way of handling this injury is to apply a tangential side-biting clamp and then to suture the laceration (A). Simple penetrating injuries to the left or right ventricle (3) may likewise be initially closed by digital pressure and oversewn (B). Injuries adjacent to a major coronary artery (4) may be closed with sutures placed in such a fashion as not to compromise coronary artery flow (C). Injuries to small coronary arteries (5) may be repaired in a similar fashion and the small coronary artery ligated (D). Injuries that involve a proximal major coronary artery (6) require both repair of the injury and a bypass to the distal vessel (E).

arteriovenous fistula is suspected. Small ventricular septal defects (less than 1.5:1 left-to-right shunt) may not require operative closure or may actually close spontaneously. Larger defects should be closed to prevent or to treat congestive heart failure. Standard techniques for the correction of such defects can be used at elective reoperation.

Gunshot wounds to the heart may result in the retention of bullets (whole or fragmented) in the pericardium, in the wall of the heart, or in a cardiac chamber. Such retained missiles may embolize, predispose to bacterial endocarditis, or erode into cardiac chambers or vessels. Harkin[12] described removal of retained foreign bodies from the heart in soldiers in World War II and generally believed that such foreign bodies should be removed. Symbas has reviewed the world literature on this topic and in addition has reported with co-workers the series from Grady Hospital.[32, 34] The fragment was removed in 7, could not be found in 1, and was left alone in another 12 patients. Symbas indicated that small fragments in asymptomatic patients could be left alone. Generally, indications for operative removal include (1) large missiles; (2) symptomatic patients; and (3) an intracardiac location, especially on the left side. It is clear that not all retained missiles in or around the heart warrant removal. Precise localization of the fragment may be helpful in the decision regarding removal of the missile. When a decision is made to remove the missile, careful preoperative localization, including fluoroscopy and echocardiography, is necessary. Intraoperative echocardiography may also be useful in the localization of retained missiles at the time of operation.

Finally, it has been shown that survivors of penetrating cardiac injuries may develop significant psychologic disturbances similar to those seen in other patients who have experienced severe trauma. In a study of 20 patients surviving penetrating cardiac injuries, Abbott and associates[2] found that all had cardiac complaints. Although stress testing showed work capacity to be normal in 90% of these patients, only 40% of them returned to work.[1]

SELECTED REFERENCES

Antunes, M. D., Fernandez, L. E., and Oliviera, J. M.: Ventricular septal defects and arteriovenous fistulas, with and without valvular lesions, resulting from penetrating injury of the heart and aorta. J. Thorac. Cardiovasc. Surg., 95:902, 1988.
This article describes intracardiac lesions that can occur at the time of a penetrating cardiac injury. Septal defects, arteriovenous fistulas, and valve lesions are described and discussed in detail along with the appropriate management.

Ivatury, R. R., Nallathame, M., Stahl, W., and Rohman, M.: Penetrating cardiac trauma. Ann. Surg., 206:61, 1987.
This is an analysis of 228 patients who sustained penetrating cardiac injury in a 20-year period from 1963 to 1983. All aspects of penetrating cardiac injury are reviewed.

Karrell, R., Shaffer, M. A., and Franaszek, J. B.: Emergency diagnosis, resuscitation, and treatment of acute penetrating cardiac trauma. Ann. Emerg. Med., 11:504, 1982.
This is an excellent review of all aspects of penetrating cardiac trauma. Included are a historical review, methods of diagnosis, techniques of treatment, and results that can be expected. Viewpoints of a variety of different authors are presented.

Naughton, M. J., Brissie, R. M., Bessey, P. Q., McEachern, M. M., Donald, J. M., Jr., and Laws, H. L.: Demography of penetrating cardiac trauma. Ann. Surg., 209:676, 1989.
This is a nice study covering a 2-year time span (1985–1986) in a medium-sized city. It includes all patients who sustained penetrating cardiac trauma, including those dying at the scene of their injury as well as those treated in a hospital. It documents nicely the increasing frequency of gunshot wounds as well as the fact that rapid transport, aggressive resuscitation, and definitive repair remain the best treatment for cardiac injuries.

Symbas, P. N.: Cardiothoracic Trauma. Philadelphia, W. B. Saunders, 1989.
The author reviews trauma to the contents of the thoracic cavity. The book is current and complete despite its brevity. All aspects of penetrating cardiac injury, including diagnostic techniques, different modes of treatment, and associated injuries (septal defects, retained missiles) are discussed in detail.

REFERENCES

1. Aaland, M. D., Bryan, F. C., and Sherman, R.: Two-dimensional echocardiogram in hemodynamically stable victims of penetrating precordial trauma. Am. Surg., 60:412, 1994.
2. Abbott, J. A., Cousineau, B. S., Cheitlin, M. D., Thomas, A. N., and Lim, R. C., Jr.: Late sequelae of penetrating cardiac wounds. J. Thorac. Cardiovasc. Surg., 75:510, 1978.
3. Andrade-Alegre, R., and Mon, L.: Subxiphoid pericardiac window in the diagnosis of penetrating cardiac trauma. Ann. Thorac. Surg., 58:1139, 1994.
4. Antunes, M. D., Fernandez, L. E., and Oliviera, J. M.: Ventricular septal defects and arteriovenous fistulas, with and without valvular lesions, resulting from penetrating injury of the heart and aorta. J. Thorac. Cardiovasc. Surg., 95:902, 1988.
5. Baker, C. C., Thomas, A. M., and Trunkey, D. D.: The role of emergency room thoracotomy in trauma. J. Trauma, 20:848, 1980.
6. Beall, A. C., Jr., Patrick, T. A., Okies, J. E., Bricker, D. L., and DeBakey, M. E.: Penetrating wounds of the heart: Changing patterns of surgical management. J. Trauma, 12:468, 1972.
7. Beck, C. S.: Wounds of the heart: The technic of suture. Arch. Surg., 13:105, 1926.
8. Blalock, A., and Ravitch, M.: A consideration of the nonoperative treatment of cardiac tamponade resulting from wounds of the heart. Surg., 14:157, 1943.
9. Bolton, J. W., Bynoe, R. P., Lazar, H., and Almond, C.: Two-dimensional echocardiography in the evaluation of penetrating cardiac injuries. Ann. Thorac. Surg., 56:509, 1993.
10. Brewster, S. C., Thirlby, R. D., Snyder, W. J., III: Subxiphoid pericardial window and penetrating cardiac trauma. Arch. Surg., 123:937, 1988.
11. Goldman, A., Kitler, M., Goldberg, S., Parameswaran, R., and Pairing, W.: The uses of two-dimensional Doppler echocardiographic techniques preoperatively and postoperatively in a ventricular septal defect caused by penetrating trauma. Ann. Thorac. Surg., 40:625, 1985.
12. Harkin, D. E.: Foreign bodies in, and in relation to, the thoracic blood vessels and heart: I. Techniques for approaching and removing foreign bodies from the chambers of the heart. Surg. Gynecol. Obstet., 83:117, 1946.
13. Hill, L. L.: Report of a case of successful suture of the heart. Med. Rec., November 29, 1902, p. 846.
14. Homer: The Iliad, book 16 (translated by Alexander Pope). New York, Heritage Press, 1934, p. 314.
15. Ivatury, R. R., Nallathame, M., Stahl, W., and Rohman, M.: Penetrating cardiac trauma. Ann. Surg., 206:61, 1987.
16. Ivatury, R. R., Rohman, M., Steichen, F. M., Gunduz, Y., Nallathambi, M., and Stahl, W. M.: Penetrating cardiac injuries: Twenty-year experience. Am. Surg., 53:310, 1987.
17. Ivatury, R. R., Shah, P. M., Ito, K., Ramirez-Shon, G., Suarez, R., and Rohman, M.: Emergency room thoracotomy for the resuscitation of patients with "fatal" penetrating injuries of the heart. Ann. Thorac. Surg., 32:377, 1981.
18. Johnson, S. B., Nielson, J. L., Sako, E. Y., Talhoon, J. H., Trinkle, J. K., and Miller, O. L.: Penetrating intra-pericardial wounds. Ann. Thorac. Surg., in press.
19. Kaplan, A. J., Norcross, E. D., and Crawford, F. A.: Predictors of mortality in penetrating cardiac injury. Am. Surg., 59:338, 1993.
20. Karrell, R., Shaffer, M. A., and Franaszek, J. B.: Emergency diagnosis, resuscitation, and treatment of acute penetrating cardiac trauma. Ann. Emerg. Med., 11:504, 1982.
21. Lindenbaum, G., Larrieu, A. J., Goldberg, S. E., Wolk, L. A., Ghosh, S. C., Ablaza, S. G. G., and Fernandez, J.: Diagnosis and management of traumatic ventricular septal defect. J. Trauma, 27:1289, 1987.
22. Mattox, K. L., Beall, A. C., Jr., Jordan, G. L., Jr., and DeBakey, M. E.: Cardiorrhaphy in the emergency center. J. Thorac. Cardiovasc. Surg., 68:887, 1974.
23. Mattox, K. L., Feliciano, D. V., Burch, J., Beall, A. C., Jr., Jordan, G. L., Jr., and DeBakey, M. E.: Five thousand seven hundred sixty cardiovascular injuries in 4459 patients: Epidemiologic evolution 1958 to 1987. Ann. Surg., 209:698, 1989.
24. Michelow, B. J., and Bremner, C. G.: Penetrating cardiac injuries: Selective conservatism—Favorable or foolish? J. Trauma, 27:398, 1987.
25. Miller, F. B., Bond, S. J., Shumate, C. R., Polk, H. D., Jr., and Richardson, J. D.: Diagnostic pericardial window: A safe alternative to exploratory thoracotomy for suspected heart injuries. Arch. Surg., 122:605, 1987.
26. Moreno, C., Moore, E. E., Majure, J. A., and Hopeman, A. R.: Pericardial tamponade: A critical determinant for survival following penetrating cardiac wounds. J. Trauma, 26:821, 1986.
27. Naughton, M. J., Brissie, R. M., Bessey, P. Q., McEachern, M. M., Donald, J. M., Jr., and Laws, H. L.: Demography of penetrating cardiac trauma. Ann. Surg., 209:676, 1989.
28. Porembka, D. T., Johnson, D. J., Hoit, B. D., Reising, J., David, K., and Koutlas, T.: Penetrating cardiac trauma: A perioperative role for transesophageal echocardiography. Anesth. Analg., 77:1275, 1993.
29. Rehn, L.: Veber penetrierer de Herzwunden und Herznaht. Arch. Klin. Chir., 55:315, 1897.
30. Shamoun, J. M., Barraza, K. R., Jurkovich, G. J., and Salley, R. K.: In extremist use of staples for cardiorrhaphy in penetrating cardiac trauma. J. Trauma, 29:1589, 1989.

31. Sugg, W. L., Rea, W. J., Ecker, R. R., Webb, W. R., Rose, E. F., and Shaw, R. R.: Penetrating wounds of the heart: An analysis of 459 cases. J. Thorac. Cardiovasc. Surg., 56:5312, 1968.
32. Symbas, P. N.: Cardiothoracic Trauma. Philadelphia, W. B. Saunders, 1989.
33. Symbas, P. N., Harlaftis, N., and Waldo, W. J.: Penetrating cardiac wounds: A comparison of different therapeutic methods. Ann. Surg., 183:377, 1976.
34. Symbas, P. N., Vlasis-Hale, S. E., Picone, A. L., and Hatcher, C. R., Jr.: Missiles in the heart. Ann. Thorac. Surg., 48:192, 1989.
35. Symbas, P. N.: Traumatic heart disease. Curr. Probl. Cardiol., 16:537, 1991.
36. Tavares, S., Hankins, J. R., Moulton, A. L., Attar, S., Ali, S., Lincoln, S.,

Green, D. C., Sequeira, A., and McLaughlin, J. S.: Management of penetrating cardiac injuries: The role of emergency room thoracotomy. Ann. Thorac. Surg., 38:183, 1984.
37. Thandroyen, F. T., and Matisonn, R. E.: Penetrating thoracic trauma producing cardiac shunts. J. Thorac. Cardiovasc. Surg., 81:569, 1981.
38. Trinkle, J. K.: Penetrating heart wounds: Difficulty in evaluating clinical series. Ann. Thorac. Surg., 38:181, 1984.
39. Trinkle, J. K., Toom, R., Franz, J., Jr., Arom, K., and Grover, F.: Affairs of the wounded heart: Penetrating cardiac wounds. J. Trauma, 19:467, 1979.
40. Zakharia, A. T.: Analysis of 285 cardiac penetrating injuries in the Lebanon war. J. Cardiovasc. Surg., 28:380, 1987.

III _____

PATENT DUCTUS ARTERIOSUS, COARCTATION OF THE AORTA, AORTOPULMONARY WINDOW, AND ANOMALIES OF THE AORTIC ARCH

J. William Gaynor, M.D., and David C. Sabiston, Jr., M.D.

PATENT DUCTUS ARTERIOSUS

Embryology and Pathologic Anatomy

The ductus arteriosus is derived from the sixth aortic arch and normally extends from the main or left pulmonary artery to the descending aorta just distal to the origin of the left subclavian artery. The ductus is usually 5 to 10 mm. long but varies in length, and the diameter varies from a few millimeters to 1 to 2 cm. The aortic orifice is usually larger than the pulmonary orifice. Rarely, the ductus may be right sided, bilateral, or completely absent. *In utero,* blood ejected by the right ventricle flows almost exclusively through the ductus to the lower extremities and placenta, bypassing the high-resistance pulmonary circulation.

Closure of the ductus occurs at birth during the transition from the fetal circulation. The lungs expand with the first breath, decreasing the pulmonary vascular resistance, causing increased pulmonary blood flow and arterial oxygen concentration. In normal full-term neonates, functional closure of the ductus occurs within the first 10 to 15 hours of life. Closure occurs after constriction of the smooth muscle layer, causing apposition of intimal cushions in the wall of the ductus, and is mediated by various substances that constrict or dilate ductal smooth muscle. Anatomic closure by fibrosis produces the ligamentum arteriosum connecting the pulmonary artery to the aorta.

Delayed closure of the ductus is termed *prolonged patency,* and failure of closure causes persistent patency. Final closure may occur at any age but is uncommon after 6 months. Intermittent closure and reopening of the ductus may also occur. Persistent patency of the ductus may occur as an isolated lesion or may be associated with a variety of other congenital defects. In infants with complex congenital heart disease, pulmonary or systemic blood flow may be dependent on the patency of the ductus, and these infants may suddenly decompensate as the ductus closes.

Prolonged or persistent patency of the ductus causes a left-to-right shunt of blood with pulmonary congestion and left ventricular volume overload. The magnitude of this shunt depends on the size of the ductus. With a large, nonrestrictive ductus, the level of pulmonary vascular resistance is important in determining the severity of shunting. Shunting occurs throughout systole and diastole and causes diastolic hypotension and possibly impaired perfusion of the heart, brain, lower extremities, and abdominal organs.

Incidence, Mortality, and Morbidity

Isolated patent ductus arteriosus (PDA) occurs approximately once in 2500 to 5000 live births. The incidence increases greatly with prematurity and with decreasing birth weight. The incidence may be more than 80% in infants weighing less than 1000 gm. and is related to several factors, including decreased smooth muscle in the ductal wall, diminished responsiveness of the ductal smooth muscle to oxygen, and possibly elevated circulating levels of vasodilatory prostaglandins. Persistent patency of the ductus occurs more commonly in females than in males, with a 2:1 ratio.

PDA is not a benign entity, although prolonged survival has been reported. The mortality of infants with untreated PDA may be as high as 30%. Forty per cent of patients with PDA died of bacterial endocarditis in the preantibiotic era, and most of the remainder died of congestive heart failure. Patients surviving to adulthood may develop congestive heart failure or pulmonary hypertension, with reverse shunting through the ductus. Young children with persistent patency of the ductus may demonstrate growth retardation. Infants with a large PDA may develop severe pulmonary hypertension at an early age. Calcification is often encountered in older patients and may complicate surgical repair.

Clinical Manifestations and Diagnosis

The signs and symptoms of PDA depend on the size of the ductus, the pulmonary vascular resistance, the age at presentation, and associated anomalies. Full-term infants usually do not become symptomatic until the pulmonary vascular resistance decreases at 6 to 8 weeks of life, allowing a significant left-to-right shunt. Because premature infants have less smooth muscle in the pulmonary arterioles, vascular resistance decreases earlier, and symptoms may develop during the first week of life.

A large, hemodynamically significant PDA usually presents in infancy as congestive heart failure. Afflicted infants are irritable, tachycardic, and tachypneic, and take feedings poorly. Physical examination usually reveals evidence of a hyperdynamic circulation, with a hyperactive precordium and bounding peripheral pulses. The systolic blood pressure is usually normal, but diastolic hypotension may be present secondary to the large left-to-right shunt. Auscultation reveals a systolic or continuous murmur, often termed a *machinery murmur,* which is heard best in the pulmonic area and radiates toward the middle third of the clavicle.

Absence of the characteristic murmur does not, however, exclude the presence of a PDA, especially in premature infants. A mid-diastolic apical rumble may indicate increased flow across the mitral valve. If cardiac failure is present, a gallop may also be heard. Hepatomegaly is frequently present. Cyanosis is not present in uncomplicated isolated PDA. Absence of these findings, however, does not exclude the presence of a significant PDA, especially in premature infants. In one study of infants with symptomatic PDA researchers found that the most sensitive clinical sign was a hyperdynamic precordium, which was present in 95% of patients. Bounding pulses and a murmur were absent in 15% and 20% of the patients, respectively.[26]

The diagnosis of PDA can often be made noninvasively, and the physical examination alone may be diagnostic. The chest film often shows cardiomegaly; and if cardiac failure is present, pulmonary congestion may be observed. However, 22% of infants with a symptomatic PDA show no increase in radiographic heart size.[21] In older infants, children, and adults, the electrocardiogram may reveal left ventricular hypertrophy. Two-dimensional echocardiography may demonstrate the ductus and associated anomalies. Continuous wave and pulsed Doppler echocardiography demonstrate abnormal aortic flow patterns and estimate the magnitude of ductal flow; and echocardiography may provide evidence of significant left-to-right shunting before it becomes clinically apparent.[18] Color-flow Doppler imaging also demonstrates flow in a PDA and reveals the direction of shunting. Formal cardiac catheterization is not required in children and young adults with classic findings and should be reserved for older patients and those with atypical findings, suspicion of associated anomalies, or pulmonary hypertension.

Patients with a moderate-sized PDA may remain asymptomatic until the second or third decade of life, when left ventricular failure occurs. The earliest symptom is usually dyspnea on exertion, followed by signs and symptoms of increasing congestive heart failure. Auscultation reveals the typical murmur. The electrocardiogram and chest film may show evidence of left ventricular enlargement and hypertrophy. A small PDA usually causes no symptoms or growth retardation. A systolic or continuous murmur is present, and the electrocardiogram and chest film usually appear to be normal. Some patients with PDA present with bacterial endocarditis as the first clinical manifestation of their disorder. Bacterial endocarditis usually develops at the pulmonary orifice of the ductus.

The development of pulmonary hypertension in a patient with PDA is a serious prognostic sign. Pulmonary hypertension may be encountered in children who are younger than 2 years of age and have a nonrestrictive ductus with greatly increased pulmonary blood flow; however, significant pulmonary hypertension is usually noted only in older patients with PDA. The elevated pulmonary artery pressures may be secondary to the increased blood flow and may become normal after surgical closure of the PDA. In some patients, irreversible pulmonary vascular changes occur and pulmonary hypertension persists after closure of the PDA. These patients usually have systemic pulmonary artery pressures and show evidence of Eisenmenger's physiology, with a bidirectional or right-to-left shunt resulting in cyanosis. Closure of the PDA in these patients is hazardous, and pulmonary hypertension frequently persists.

Management

The presence of a persistent PDA in a child or adult is sufficient indication for surgical closure because of the increased mortality and risk of endocarditis. In symptomatic patients, closure should be performed when the diagnosis is made. In asymptomatic children, intervention can be postponed, if desired, but should be done in the preschool years. Older patients should have the ductus closed when the diagnosis is made. However, if severe pulmonary hypertension has occurred with reversal of the ductal shunt, closure may not improve symptoms and is associated with a higher mortality. The management of PDA in premature infants remains controversial.

Surgical Procedures. Gross pioneered division of the PDA as a therapy of choice because of difficulties with recanalization after simple ligation.[17] In children, either division or multiple suture ligation of the ductus is appropriate. Ligation is usually done in neonates because of its simplicity and rare, if any, recurrences. In adults with a large ductus (10 mm. or more) or patients with pulmonary hypertension, division is indicated.

The operation may be done through either a left anterior or a posterior thoracotomy. The lung is retracted, and an incision is made in the pleura overlying the pulmonary artery between the phrenic and vagus nerves. The ductus is exposed, taking care to avoid damage to the recurrent laryngeal nerve. After the ductus has been mobilized, it may be obliterated with multiple suture ligatures (Fig. 54–7) or divided (Fig. 54–8). If division is planned, vascular clamps are placed across the ductus, which is then divided. Closure of each end is accomplished with two rows of nonabsorbable suture. If the ductus is particularly short and wide, it may be necessary to cross-clamp the aorta above and below the ductus as in a coarctation repair. The pulmonary end of the ductus is clamped, and the ductus is divided at the aorta, leaving a sufficient margin for closure. The opening in the aorta is closed, and the cross-clamps are removed. The pulmonary end of the ductus is closed, and the clamp is removed.

In neonates, single or double ligation is usually the procedure of choice. Closure of the ductus in neonates by applying one or two surgical clips has also been described.[1] There has been interest in video-assisted thoracoscopic interruption of PDA. Between 1991 and 1992, Laborde and colleagues[27] performed thoracoscopic PDA closure using surgical clips in 38 patients at a mean age of 23.3 months and a mean weight of 9.5 kg. The procedure was initially successful in 36 patients; however, 2 patients required a second procedure because of incomplete closure. No patient required open ligation, and there were no operative deaths.

Closure of a PDA in patients with pulmonary hypertension presents special difficulties. In patients with pulmonary vascular changes, closure may cause further elevation of the pulmonary pressures, causing right ventricular failure. John and co-workers,[22] in 1981, reported five deaths after PDA closure in 22 patients with pulmonary artery pressures greater than 70 mm. Hg. Patients with marked pulmonary hypertension and right-to-left shunt who survive closure may not improve, and progressive cor pulmonale may develop.

Surgical closure of a PDA may be complicated by hemorrhage, pneumothorax, chylothorax, left recurrent nerve damage, and infection. Phrenic nerve paralysis has also been reported after closure of a PDA. Great care must be exercised in dissecting or placing clamps on the ductus, because the ductal tissue may be friable and a tear may cause hemor-

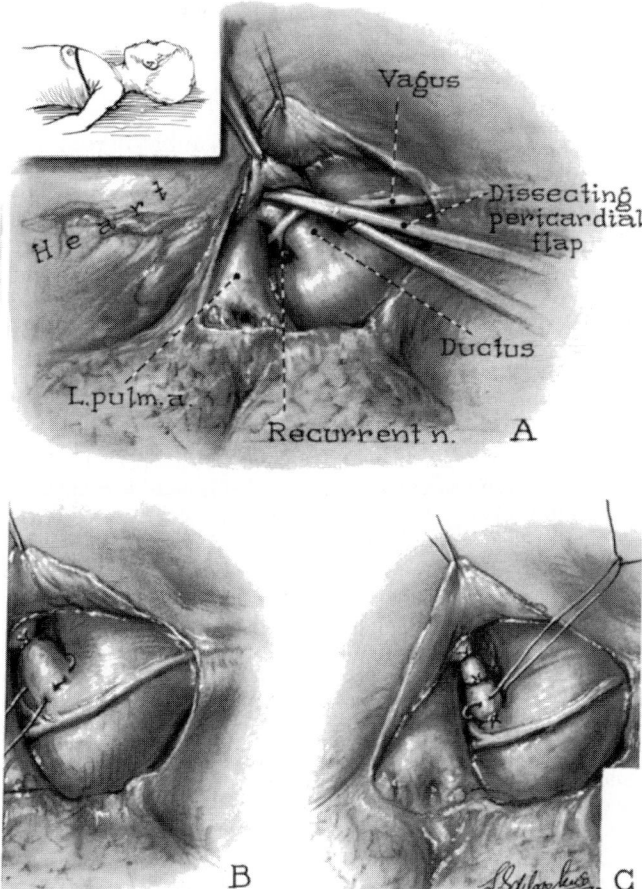

Figure 54–7. Operative treatment of patent ductus arteriosus by ligation. Incision is anterolateral in the third interspace. In females, the incision circles beneath the breast. Elevation of pericardial lappet exposes the ductus. A pursestring suture, which does not enter the lumen, is placed at each end, and perforating mattress sutures are placed in between. The ductus should be obliterated over an 8- to 10-mm. distance.

rhage that is difficult to control. In the current era the incidence of recurrent ductal patency should approach zero after division or multiple suture ligation.

Nonoperative Therapy. In 1986, Wierny and associates[45]

reported long-term follow-up of 208 patients who had closure of a PDA with an Ivalon plug. Ductal closure was successful in 94.7% of the patients. In 1987, Rashkind and colleagues[35] reported attempted ductal closure by using a double-umbrella device in 146 patients. The collective European experience was reported by the European Registry for Transcatheter Occlusion of Persistent Arterial Duct in 1992.[41] The study enrolled 686 patients, and the device was successfully implanted in 642 patients. The actuarial complete occlusion rate was 82.5% at 1 year. Forty-one patients have required a second device for persistent flow. Mechanical hemolysis occurred in 4 patients (0.5%), and there were two early deaths (0.3% mortality). Transcatheter occlusion of PDA has also been accomplished using Gianturco coils.[29] Complications of transcatheter closure include failure of occlusion, embolization, vascular complications, mechanical hemolysis, protrusion of the device into the aorta, and left pulmonary artery stenosis. Transcatheter techniques are potentially useful in patients who are poor candidates for surgical therapy. However, these techniques are still being investigated. In one multi-institutional trial in which catheter technique was compared with surgical treatment for closure of PDA, it was suggested that surgical closure was more effective and more cost effective; however, this finding is controversial.[16] The exact role of transcatheter techniques in the management of PDA has not been determined.[2, 16]

Management of PDA in Premature Infants. Premature infants face many problems, including immature lungs and hyaline membrane disease. These infants often require mechanical ventilation and oxygen therapy. An increased incidence of PDA is found with increasing prematurity and decreasing birth weight. The additional burden on the heart and lungs imposed by the left-to-right shunt may be poorly tolerated. The increased pulmonary blood flow causes increased pulmonary arterial pressures, decreased lung compliance, hypercarbia, and hypoxia, often necessitating prolonged mechanical ventilation, which may cause an increased incidence of bronchopulmonary dysplasia and retrolental fibroplasia. The abnormal hemodynamics may potentiate other problems of prematurity, such as necrotizing enterocolitis and intraventricular hemorrhage. It is sometimes difficult to differentiate the effects of a PDA from the underlying pulmonary disease. If the pulmonary disease is severe, ligation of the PDA may produce little or no improvement. A hemodynamically significant PDA is suggested by the presence of a hyperactive precordium, a continuous murmur, and

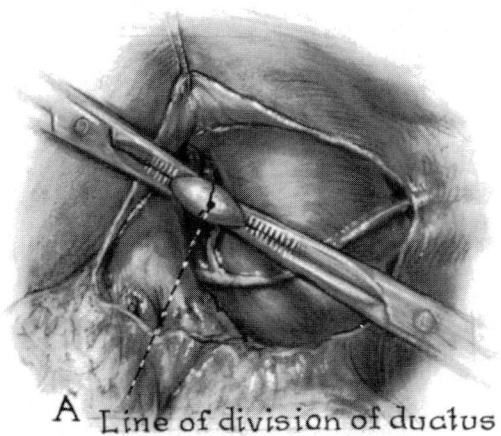

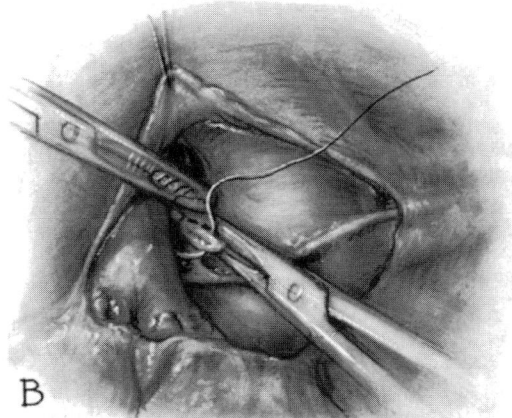

Figure 54–8. Treatment of PDA by division. Anterolateral third interspace incision is used for exposure, as for ligation. A thin occluding clamp is placed at each end, and the ductus is divided. Pressing the clamp against the pulmonary artery or aorta after division reduces the likelihood of slipping. Suture of the ductus is by a continuous mattress suture adjacent to the clamp, followed by whipstitch backup over the free edge. Suture of the pulmonary artery is easier when done from the patient's right side.

bounding pulses. The chest film usually reveals cardiomegaly, pulmonary congestion, and the changes of hyaline membrane disease.

Management of PDA in premature infants can be difficult.[14] If a child with evidence of left-to-right shunting demonstrates persistent congestive heart failure, need for continuing mechanical ventilation, or inability to receive adequate nutrition secondary to fluid restriction, further intervention is indicated. Two therapeutic options are available. Pharmacologic closure can be attempted with prostaglandin inhibitors such as indomethacin.[20] Final closure may be achieved in more than 70% of infants, although the ductus may reopen transiently in some children. Reopening occurs most frequently in the most premature infants and may be treated with a second course of indomethacin, but the success rate is lower. The success of therapy with indomethacin is related to the birth weight and postnatal age of the infant. Side effects of indomethacin include renal dysfunction, hyponatremia, impaired platelet function, and gastrointestinal hemorrhage. Impaired left ventricular diastolic function has been reported after administration of indomethacin and may worsen pulmonary edema. No adverse long-term sequelae of successful indomethacin therapy have been identified. Surgical closure can be used if there is a contraindication to indomethacin or failure of the PDA to close.

Early closure of a PDA in premature infants has been shown to decrease the need for mechanical ventilation and to decrease complications such as bronchopulmonary dysplasia, necrotizing enterocolitis, and intolerance of enteral feeding. Closure with indomethacin is as effective as surgical ligation in preventing these complications. There has been a trend toward earlier intervention in premature infants, and the prophylactic use of indomethacin before the development of a hemodynamically significant shunt has been suggested.

Results

Surgical closure of an isolated PDA has become a very safe procedure. Operative mortality approaches zero even in critically ill neonates. In premature infants, hospital mortality and long-term results depend primarily on associated pulmonary disease, coexistent anomalies, and the degree of prematurity. Mortality is increased and long-term results are poor in older patients with a calcified ductus and are poorest in those patients with severe pulmonary hypertension and reverse shunting. Most patients with PDA become functionally normal with a normal life expectancy after closure.

COARCTATION OF THE AORTA

Coarctation is defined as a narrowing that diminishes the aortic lumen and produces an obstruction to the flow of blood. The lesion may be a definite, localized obstruction or may be a diffusely narrowed segment, which is termed *tubular hypoplasia*. The most common location is at the site of the insertion of the ductus (or ligamentum) arteriosus. Coarctation of the abdominal aorta is present in approximately 2% of the patients. Externally the aorta appears to be sharply indented or constricted, and internally an obstructing diaphragm is present on the posterior wall (located preductally, postductally, or paraductally). The obstruction is usually more marked than is apparent by external appearance. The *shelf* consists of an infolding of the aortic media with a ridge of intimal hyperplasia. Tubular hypoplasia most often occurs in the aortic isthmus (the segment of aorta between the left subclavian artery and the insertion of the ductus arteriosus). Crafoord and Nylin performed the first surgical correction with resection of the coarctation and end-to-end anastomosis in 1944.[8] In recent years there has been increasing interest in the use of percutaneous transluminal angioplasty for native and recurrent coarctation.

Incidence and Associated Anomalies

Coarctation of the aorta represents 5% to 10% of congenital heart disease, and the autopsy incidence is 1 per 3000 to 4000 autopsies. With isolated coarctation, males predominate; but there is no sex difference in patients with more complex lesions. Several anomalies occur commonly in patients with coarctation of the aorta: bicuspid aortic valve, ventricular septal defect, PDA, and various mitral valve disorders. Patients with severe associated defects tend to have tubular hypoplasia, rather than isolated coarctation.

Clinical Manifestations

The age and the mode of presentation depend on the location of the coarctation and the associated anomalies. Infants with severe narrowing may appear normal at birth and have palpable femoral pulses if a PDA allows blood flow around the obstructing shelf. Symptoms usually develop as the PDA closes, resulting in significant aortic obstruction. The infant becomes irritable, tachypneic, and uninterested in feeding. A systolic murmur may be present over the left precordium and posteriorly between the scapulae. The blood pressure is difficult to record accurately in neonates; however, moderate upper-extremity hypertension and an arm-leg systolic pressure gradient may be present. These findings may be absent in critically ill infants with a low cardiac output. Hypotension, oliguria, and severe metabolic acidosis may be present in severely ill infants.

Older children and adults often present with unexplained hypertension or complications of hypertension. Some may be entirely asymptomatic for many years and lead active lives. Presenting complaints include headache, epistaxis, visual disturbances, and exertional dyspnea. Some patients present with a cerebrovascular accident (secondary to an aneurysm of the circle of Willis), aortic rupture, dissecting aneurysm, or bacterial endocarditis. Many cases are discovered during evaluation of hypertension or of a murmur heard on routine examination.

Diagnosis

The diagnosis of coarctation can usually be made clinically and depends on evidence of obstruction to blood flow in the thoracic aorta. The findings include hypertension, a systolic pressure gradient between the arms and legs, a systolic murmur heard over the left precordium and posteriorly between the scapulae, and diminished or absent femoral pulses with a delayed upstroke. Presence of an anterior diastolic murmur may indicate aortic regurgitation secondary to a bicuspid aortic valve. Anomalous origin of the right subclavian artery can occur with the orifice distal to the coarctation. Blood pressure measurements must be obtained in both arms because the orifice of either subclavian artery may be involved in the coarctation. There may be evidence of collateral circulation in older children and adults. The collateral circulation involves branches of the subclavian arteries that are proximal to the obstruction, including the internal mammary, vertebral, thyrocervical, and costocervical arteries. These vessels anastomose with intercostal vessels and other arteries distal to the obstruction. Enlarged collateral vessels may be observed or palpated in the infrascapular region; bruits may be audible as well.

In infants, the electrocardiogram may reveal right, left, or biventricular hypertrophy. In older children and adults, it may be normal or demonstrate evidence of left ventricular hypertrophy, often with a *strain* pattern. The chest film is usually helpful, demonstrating cardiomegaly with left ventricular hypertrophy. In infants with heart failure, extreme cardiomegaly and pulmonary congestion may be present. Rib notching secondary to the enlarged, tortuous intercostal vessels is almost pathognomonic of coarctation (Fig. 54–9). These are erosions that occur on the underside of the rib. Absence of rib notching in older patients may indicate a poor collateral circulation.

Angiocardiography can be used to demonstrate the coarctation, providing evidence of the location and extent of narrowing, the involvement of the great vessels, and the extent of collateral circulation. The pressure gradient can be measured, and associated cardiac defects can be evaluated by cardiac catheterization. Two-dimensional echocardiography with spectral and color-flow Doppler echocardiography is commonly used to demonstrate the site of obstruction, suggest or exclude associated anomalies, and provide an estimate of the pressure gradient.

Natural History

The natural history of untreated coarctation of the aorta depends on the age at presentation and associated anomalies. Symptomatic infants have a high mortality, depending on the severity of the coarctation and the presence of associated defects. Patients surviving until adulthood have a greatly decreased life expectancy. The most common causes of death in untreated coarctation are spontaneous rupture of the aorta, bacterial endocarditis, and cerebral hemorrhage. The advent of surgical therapy has significantly increased the life expectancy of patients with coarctation, although they do not become fully normal.

Physiology of Hypertension

The pathogenesis of hypertension in coarctation is multifactorial, and the most prominent causes appear to be mechanical and renal factors. In experimental coarctation, hypertension can be eliminated by transplanting one kidney to the neck (proximal to the obstruction) with contralateral nephrectomy. Renal blood flow is usually normal in patients with coarctation, and studies of the renin-angiotensin system have yielded conflicting results. Renin and angiotensin levels have been reported to be normal in both experimental animals and patients with coarctation. Abnormal rigidity of the prestenotic aortic wall, abnormal baroreceptor function, and abnormal vascular endothelial function have been demonstrated in patients with coarctation.

Management

Nonsurgical therapy has only a small role in the management of patients with coarctation, and the presence of coarctation is generally sufficient indication for surgical correction. The major questions are the timing and method of repair. Symptomatic infants usually require intervention, although a few improve with conservative medical treatment of congestive heart failure and can then undergo elective surgical correction. A major advance in the treatment of critically ill neonates with coarctation and interrupted aortic arch has been the introduction of prostaglandin E_1 therapy.[20] Infusion of prostaglandin E_1 can reopen and maintain patency of the ductus arteriosus in many neonates and allow perfusion of the lower body with correction of the severe metabolic acidosis and oliguria that are often present.

The timing of elective repair of coarctation of the aorta is perhaps the most important determinant of surgical outcome. Repair in late childhood or adulthood, although providing relief of some symptoms, has an increased incidence of persistent hypertension with its associated morbidity. The current trend is for elective repair at an early age to prevent development of complications.

Surgical Procedures. The classic method of repair of coarctation is resection of the area of obstruction with primary end-to-end anastomosis. A left thoracotomy is performed, and an incision is made in the pleura overlying the coarctation. The proximal aorta, the left subclavian artery, the area of coarctation, and the ligamentum arteriosum are dissected first, with an effort to avoid damage to the recurrent laryngeal nerve (Fig. 54–10). The ductus or ligamentum is divided, greatly increasing the mobility of the aorta. Care is taken not to injure any enlarged intercostal arteries during the dissection. It may be necessary to divide these arteries, especially if aneurysmal dilation has occurred, but it is preferable to preserve all collateral vessels. The aorta is cross-clamped proximally and distally and the area of constriction is excised. To obtain an optimal result, it is absolutely necessary to resect

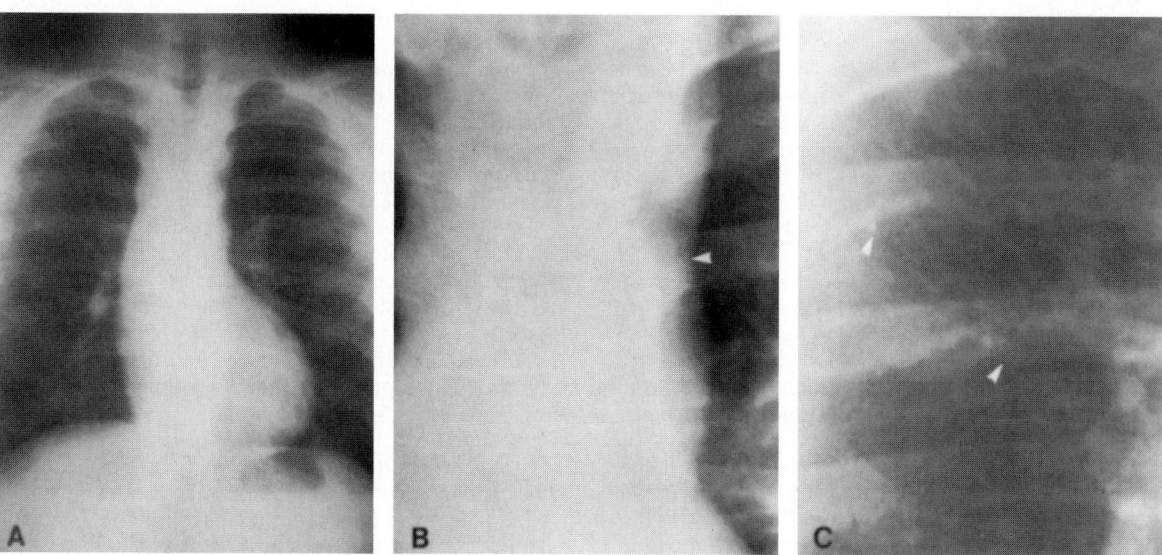

Figure 54–9. Patient with coarctation of the aorta. *A,* Chest roentgenogram. *B,* Detail demonstrating "3" sign formed by proximal dilated aorta, area of constriction (arrow), and distal dilated aorta. *C,* Detail demonstrating rib notching (arrows) secondary to dilated intercostal vessels. (Courtesy of Dr. James Chen.)

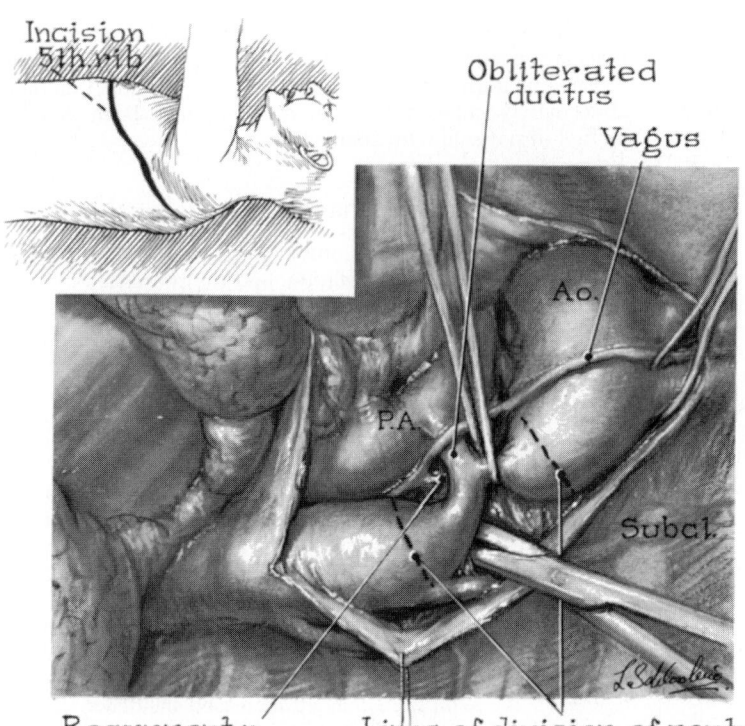

Figure 54–10. Operative exposure for resection of coarctation of the aorta is through the bed of the fifth rib. The entire rib is removed from neck to cartilage. The constricted segment is usually held medially by an obliterated ductus, division of which allows considerable mobility. The coarctation is held forward to facilitate dissection posteriorly. Large intercostal arteries must be carefully avoided. Division of the aorta should be through a point of normal diameter.

the entire constricted segment and construct the anastomosis without tension (Fig. 54–11). Even in infants with tubular hypoplasia, the aorta is elastic and can usually be mobilized sufficiently to allow primary repair. Advantages of the classic repair include complete resection of abnormal tissue, preservation of normal vascular anatomy, and no requirement for prosthetic material.

Because of early unsatisfactory results, especially in infants, other techniques were developed. In 1957, Vossschulte introduced the prosthetic patch onlay graft technique. The area of constriction is incised, and a Dacron patch is used to enlarge the lumen.[43] Advantages of the patch aortoplasty technique include decreased operative time, decreased dissection, maximal augmentation of the area of stenosis, preservation of the collateral vessels, and no need for sacrifice of normal vascular structures. Patch aortoplasty is highly effective in relieving the aortic obstruction, with a low incidence of restenosis and persistent hypertension (at rest and after exercise). The use of prosthetic material may predispose to infection. Aneurysmal dilation of the posterior aortic wall opposite the prosthetic patch has been reported with increasing frequency, but the true incidence is unknown.[4] Aneurysm formation may be related to weakening at the posterior wall after resection of the intimal shelf. All patients who have had patch aortoplasty must be observed closely to monitor for development of an aneurysm.

The subclavian flap aortoplasty was introduced by Waldhausen and Nahrwold in 1966 (Fig. 54–12).[44] A left thoracotomy is performed, and the pleura overlying the aorta is incised. The left subclavian artery is dissected free and ligated at its first branch. The vertebral artery should be ligated to prevent a subclavian steal phenomenon. A longitudinal incision is made through the region of coarctation and continued onto the subclavian artery, which creates a flap. The posterior obstructing shelf is resected, and the flap of subclavian artery is turned down to enlarge the constriction. It is important that the flap be of sufficient length to bridge the obstruction completely. Advantages of this technique include avoidance of prosthetic material, decreased dissection,

decreased aortic cross-clamp period, and increased anastomotic growth because there is no circumferential suture line. If the area of narrowing occurs proximal to the left subclavian artery, the flap may be directed proximally and a reversed subclavian flap aortoplasty done to enlarge the aortic arch.

Because of the risk of recoarctation after the classic repair, some authors have advocated use of an extended or *radically extended* resection and primary anastomosis.[28, 42] This technique is particularly applicable to infants with coarctation and associated hypoplasia of the transverse aortic arch. The coarctation is resected, and all visible ductal tissue must be excised. The underside of the aortic arch is incised proximally (in some infants the incision is carried proximal to the left common carotid artery). A spatulated anastomosis is performed augmenting the diameter of the aortic arch.

Management of Associated Anomalies. Outcome after surgical correction depends on the age at the time of operation, the method of repair chosen, and especially the presence of associated anomalies. The optimal management of infants with associated anomalies is still controversial. A PDA is frequently present and should be divided or ligated. A bicuspid aortic valve may be present but often requires no intervention at the time of correction of the coarctation. Appropriate management of an associated ventricular septal defect is less clear; several therapeutic options are available.[15, 31, 33] Formerly, the pulmonary artery was often banded at the time of repair of the coarctation in infants with a nonrestrictive ventricular septal defect. However, ventricular septal defects associated with coarctation are often of a type with a high incidence of spontaneous closure. In infants with coarctation, a ventricular septal defect, and no other associated anomalies, some experts advocate repair of the coarctation alone. If congestive heart failure does not resolve, the septal defect is closed at a second operation. Park and colleagues reported 23 infants younger than the age of 3 months with ventricular septal defect and coarctation managed with coarctation repair alone.[31] Nine needed no further surgical treatment, six required early closure of the ventricular septal defect, and eight required late repair of the ventricular septal defect. Eight

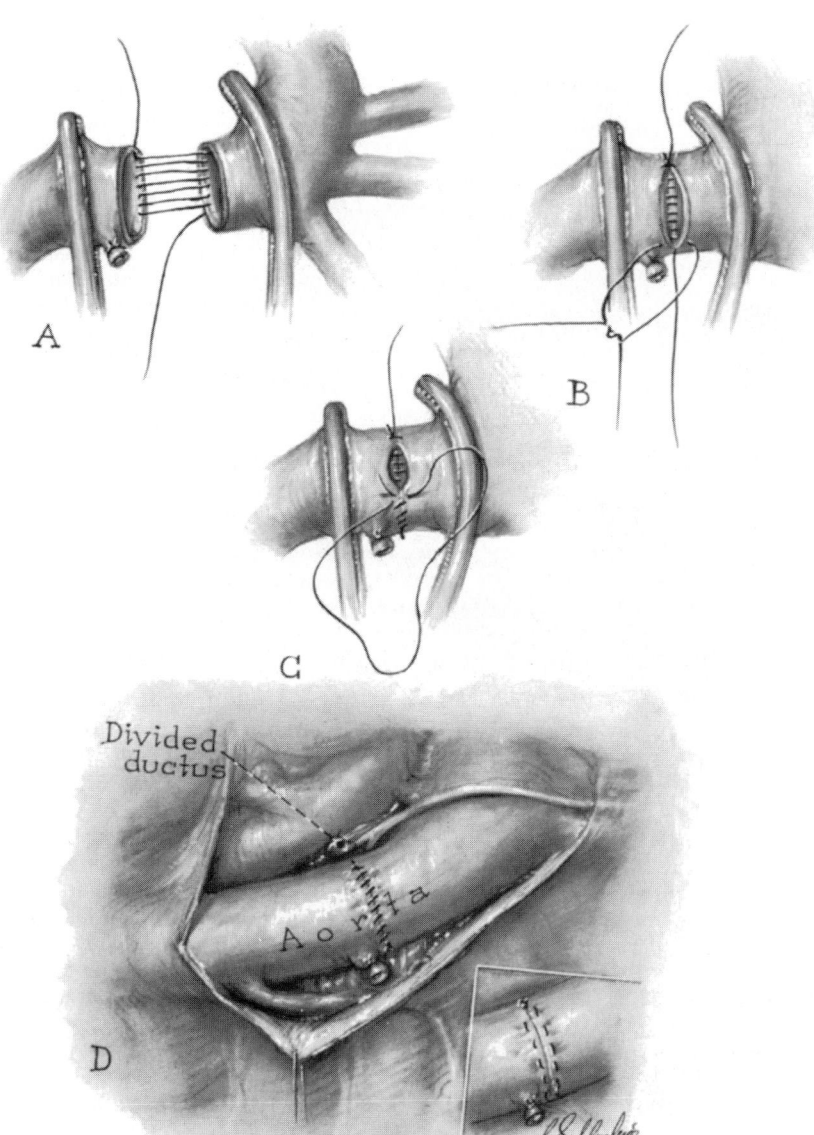

Figure 54–11. Anastomosis after excision of coarctation. *A,* An everting mattress suture is placed over about one third of the posterior row before the vessels are approximated and the suture is pulled up *(B). C,* The anastomosis is completed with continuous over-and-over suture. Inset in *D* shows the everting mattress suture sometimes used. In children, interrupted mattress sutures are used for the entire anterior row.

patients were treated after 3 months of age. Seven of these patients underwent coarctation repair alone, and none required a second operation for ventricular septal defect closure.

Nonoperative Therapy. In recent years, percutaneous transluminal balloon angioplasty has been introduced as an alternative therapy for coarctation.[34, 36] Initial results were encouraging; however, reports soon appeared of aneurysmal dilation of the aorta after balloon angioplasty. Balloon dilation of recurrent stenosis has been more successful, and there have been fewer reports of aneurysm formation, presumably secondary to surrounding scar tissue. Rao and Chopra reported balloon angioplasty of native coarctation in 20 neonates and infants younger than age 1 year.[34] The peak systolic gradient was reduced from 40 to 11 mm. Hg, and no patient required immediate surgical intervention. The residual gradient at a mean follow-up of 12 months was 18 ± 15 mm. Hg. No patient developed an aneurysm. Recoarctation developed in five infants and was successfully treated by surgical resection in two and by repeat angioplasty in three. The long-term results of balloon angioplasty for native coarctation in terms of recoarctation and especially aneurysm formation are unknown, and the technique must be considered investiga-

tional.[36] The results of angioplasty of postoperative recoarctation appear to be better, and angioplasty may be associated with less mortality and morbidity than reoperation; however, long-term follow-up is necessary.[13]

Complications

Correction of coarctation may be complicated by hemorrhage, chylothorax, recurrent nerve paralysis, infection, and suture line thrombosis. Postoperative paradoxical elevation of the blood pressure to greater than preoperative levels may occur. Up to 20% of patients having repair of coarctation experience the postcoarctectomy syndrome with abdominal pain and distention postoperatively. Laparotomy is occasionally indicated and may reveal evidence of mesenteric ischemia. On rare occasions, bowel resection may be necessary. Aggressive therapy of hypertension appears to prevent full manifestation of the postcoarctectomy syndrome. Many drugs have been successfully used to control the postoperative hypertension, including sodium nitroprusside, propranolol, and reserpine.

A dreaded complication of coarctation repair is paraplegia, which occurs in 0.5% to 1% of patients. Variations in the

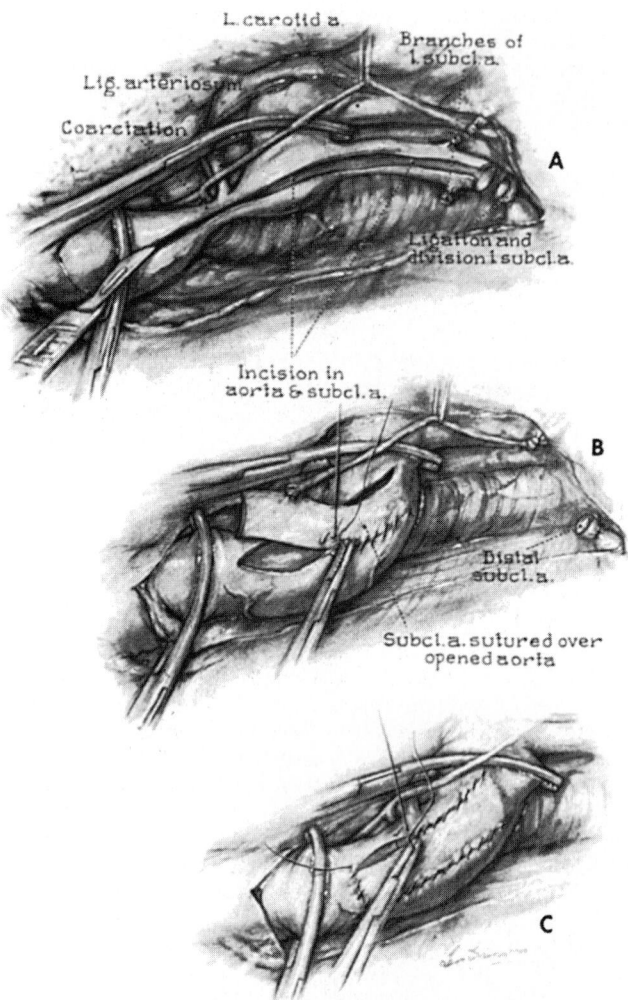

Figure 54–12. *A,* Through a left posterolateral thoracotomy, the proximal and distal aorta are mobilized and the aorta is cross-clamped between the left subclavian and left carotid arteries. The aorta is also clamped distally. The subclavian artery is divided, and a longitudinal incision is made through the entire length of the subclavian artery and the coarctation segment. *B,* The subclavian artery is rolled down over the coarctation to enlarge the segment. *C,* The suture line is completed. Care must be taken to ensure that the length of the subclavian artery is adequate to cover the entire coarctation segment. (From Elbert, P. A.: Atlas of Congenital Cardiac Surgery. New York, Churchill Livingstone, 1989.)

blood supply to the anterior spinal cord, poor collateral formation, anomalous origin of the right subclavian artery, distal hypotension during the period of aortic cross-clamping, and reoperation may predispose to paraplegia during the procedure. Neither sacrifice of intercostals nor duration of aortic cross-clamping can be related to the occurrence of paraplegia. There is marked variation in spinal cord blood supply, and measurement of distal pressure after cross-clamping of the aorta may be useful to assess adequacy of the collateral circulation.

Results

The results of surgical correction depend on the age at repair, the type of repair used, and the associated anomalies. Operative mortality in neonates has decreased to 5% to 10% and is lower in older children. Mortality is very low in patients with isolated coarctation. Classically, in patients who had resection and end-to-end anastomosis in infancy, the rate of recoarctation was as high as 60%. There is a decreased

incidence of recurrent coarctation with the subclavian patch aortoplasty and the prosthetic patch graft repair, compared with historical series. However, the most recent series using resection and end-to-end anastomosis show, even in neonates, results that compare very favorably with other methods in terms of mortality and recoarctation. Trinquet and associates in 1988 reported follow-up of 178 infants undergoing coarctation repair when younger than 3 months of age.[40] Sixty-three infants had isolated coarctation, 47 had associated ventricular septal defects, and 68 had other associated anomalies. Actuarial survival at 5 years was 90% for infants with isolated coarctation, 84% for those with associated ventricular septal defects, and 40% for those with complex anomalies. The rate of restenosis was the same for subclavian flap angioplasty, resection with primary anastomosis, and extended resection with anastomosis. Lacour-Gayet and colleagues reported results in 66 consecutive neonates treated with extended resection and anastomosis with reconstruction of the aortic arch.[28] The overall early mortality rate was 14%, and freedom from reoperation was 89.5% at 5 years. Van Heurn and associates, from the Hospital for Sick Children in London, reported 151 infants younger than the age of 3 months who underwent repair of coarctation between 1985 and 1990.[42] Over 50% of these children had hypoplasia of a portion of the aortic arch. The subclavian flap angioplasty was used in 15 patients, resection with a traditional end-to-end anastomosis in 43 and an extended end-to-end anastomosis in 77. The actuarial freedom from recoarctation at 4 years was 57% after subclavian flap angioplasty, 83% after extended end-to-end anastomosis, and 96% after radically extended end-to-end anastomosis (proximal to the origin of the left carotid artery). These authors believed that extended end-to-end anastomosis could be successfully applied to almost all types of arch anomalies and produced the lowest incidence of recoarctation. Sciolaro and associates reviewed 56 children with this disorder who were younger than 4 years of age.[37] Thirty-four had a subclavian flap angioplasty, and 22 had resection with end-to-end anastomosis. Among the 23 infants younger than 3 months of age, the 6-year actuarial freedom from recoarctation was 93% in the subclavian flap group compared with 53% in the end-to-end group. These investigators therefore recommended the subclavian flap angioplasty in patients younger than 3 months of age.[37]

Quaegebeur and associates have reported the results of a large multi-institutional study of 326 infants with coarctation.[33] The 1-month survival was 93%, and the 2-year survival was 84%. The most common procedure performed was resection with end-to-end anastomosis. There was an increased risk of death if the incision in the aorta was extended proximal to the left common carotid artery. Only the use of patch aortoplasty was associated with an increased incidence of need for reintervention. Knott-Craig and colleagues[25] reviewed 111 neonates undergoing repair of coarctation and found no difference in survival between resection with primary anastomosis, subclavian flap aortoplasty, and patch aortoplasty. There was no difference in the need for reintervention between resection with primary anastomosis and subclavian flap aortoplasty; however, the use of the patch aortoplasty was associated with an increased need for reintervention.

Any comparison of techniques for repair of coarctation must consider the historical time frame. Advances in the care of critically ill infants such as the introduction of neonatal intensive care units and prostaglandin therapy have provided dramatic improvements in the preoperative condition of patients that may affect mortality as much as the choice of repair. Advances in suture materials and vascular surgical technique also make it difficult to compare results of different time periods. Because a prospective, randomized trial of the various repair techniques has not been done, long-term results cannot be accurately compared. The optimal method for coarctation repair is unknown, and therapy should be individualized on the basis of each patient's anatomy, clinical condition, and associated anomalies as well as the experience of the surgeon.

Recoarctation usually manifests as persistent hypertension or arm-leg gradient. The arm-leg pressure gradient should be measured in the immediate postoperative period to differentiate residual stenosis secondary to an inadequate repair from true recoarctation. The causes of recoarctation include failure of growth of the anastomosis, inadequate resection of the narrowed segment, residual abnormal ductal tissue, and suture line thrombosis. Many patients who are normotensive at rest and who do not have a resting arm-leg gradient develop severe hypertension with a gradient after exercise.[9, 30] These patients may have significant restenosis. The long-term consequences of exercise-induced hypertension after the correction of coarctation are unknown but may adversely affect the prognosis.

Reoperation is indicated if significant hypertension or other symptoms occur and a pressure gradient is demonstrated.[12] Reoperation is more difficult secondary to scarring and is associated with an increased morbidity and mortality. Lack of collateral vessels may cause an increased incidence of paraplegia. In patients who have had previous resection and end-to-end anastomosis, subclavian flap aortoplasty and prosthetic patch onlay grafting are appropriate methods for repair of the recoarctation. Balloon angioplasty may also be used for treatment of recoarctation.[7]

Some patients who have had a technically excellent repair may not have complete resolution of hypertension. The cause of this persistent hypertension is unclear but is related to the age at repair and the duration of preoperative hypertension. Observation of surgical patients indicates that they are not rendered entirely normal. Increased coronary atherosclerosis is noted in patients with coarctation.[6] There is evidence of abnormal left ventricular function despite relief of the obstruction with a persistent increase in ventricular contractility after successful coarctation repair, possibly secondary to cardiac ultrastructural changes after congenital pressure overload.[24] Gardiner and colleagues[13] have documented abnormal endothelial response to nitroglycerine in normotensive patients after successful coarctation repair, suggesting damage occurs early in vessels proximal to the coarctation and may persist even after successful repair in the neonatal period. The relationship of abnormal endothelial function to persistent hypertension and coronary artery disease is unknown. Aortic stenosis or regurgitation secondary to a bicuspid aortic valve may develop and necessitate valve replacement. As has been emphasized, the long-term prognosis of many patients is determined primarily by the associated anomalies.

INTERRUPTION OF THE AORTIC ARCH

Incidence, Pathologic Anatomy, and Natural History

Interruption of the aortic arch (IAA) is a rare anomaly, constituting less than 1.5% of congenital heart disease.[23, 38] IAA may be an isolated defect but is usually associated with other anomalies, including a wide variety of cardiac anomalies, such as persistent truncus arteriosus and aortopulmonary window. The classification of IAA is based on the absent segment. In Type A, the interruption occurs distal to the left subclavian artery; in Type B, the interruption occurs between the left subclavian and left common carotid arteries; and with Type C, the interruption occurs between the left common carotid and innominate arteries.

The cause of IAA is unclear. As in coarctation, there is an association with defects that decrease ascending aortic flow and increase ductal flow, implying that abnormal fetal blood flow patterns are an etiologic factor. Type B IAA is frequently found in association with DiGeorge's syndrome (absence of the third and fourth pharyngeal pouches). In this syndrome the thymus and parathyroid glands are absent; thus, patients are hypocalcemic and suffer from defects in cellular immunity. Defects in the development of the neural crest may be responsible for DiGeorge's syndrome and Type B IAA.

The prognosis of uncorrected IAA is poor. The mean age at death has been reported to be 4 to 10 days. Ninety per cent of infants with IAA die in the first year of life unless they undergo surgical intervention. Only in the rare case of IAA with no associated anomalies is prolonged survival possible, presumably because of the development of a collateral circulation *in utero*.

Diagnosis and Management

Most infants with IAA present with congestive heart failure secondary to left-to-right shunting through a ventricular septal defect and increased left ventricular afterload. Lower-body perfusion is maintained by right-to-left shunting through a PDA. When the ductus closes, perfusion of the lower body essentially ceases; the infants become anuric and severely acidotic, with nonpalpable femoral pulses. The congestive heart failure and acidosis are resistant to medical therapy, and death occurs within a few days. Since the advent of prostaglandin E_1 therapy, however, it is possible to maintain ductal patency, improve lower body perfusion, reverse the acidosis, and increase urinary output. The physical examination is not specific for IAA, and there are no characteristic murmurs. The electrocardiogram is not useful, and the chest film reveals an enlarged heart with pulmonary congestion. Cardiac catheterization with angiography allows accurate diagnosis. Injection of contrast medium must be done in both the proximal and distal segments to define the anatomy adequately. Echocardiography is also useful to clarify the anatomy and exclude associated anomalies. When the diagnosis has been made and the infant has been stabilized with prostaglandin therapy, surgical correction is undertaken. In infants with Type B IAA, there is a high incidence of DiGeorge's syndrome and great care must be taken to avoid hypocalcemia. Because of their immunologic defect, these patients should receive irradiated blood products to prevent the development of graft-versus-host disease.

Various procedures have been used to either palliate or correct IAA. The ultimate goal is restoration of aortic continuity and correction of associated anomalies. Aortic continuity may be restored by direct anastomosis of the aortic segments, end-to-side anastomosis of an arch vessel to either the proximal or distal segment, or use of an interposition graft. If palliation is planned, a left thoracotomy may be used and aortic continuity restored by using one of the arch vessels as a conduit. In Type A IAA, a Blalock-Park anastomosis is used (the left subclavian artery is anastomosed to the distal aorta); in Type B, the left common carotid artery may be anastomosed to the distal segment or a *reversed* Blalock-Park anastomosis may be created; and in Type C, the left common carotid artery may be anastomosed to the ascending aorta. The use of ductal tissue in the anastomosis should be avoided, because obstruction may occur if the tissue contracts and fibroses. Alternatively, interposition of a Dacron or Gore-Tex graft may be used to restore continuity. Simultaneous correction of intracardiac anomalies is not possible through a left thoracotomy; however, pulmonary artery banding may be performed if indicated. Repair of a ventricular septal defect and other anomalies may be undertaken at a later date through a median sternotomy.

Improved results have been reported in patients with IAA when primary anastomosis is performed through an anterior approach. Cardiopulmonary bypass with biaortic cannulation is used for cooling, with profound hypothermia and circulatory arrest during the arch repair. The ductus is divided, the aorta is mobilized to the diaphragm, and aortic continuity is restored by direct anastomosis of the proximal and distal aortic segments. The ventricular septal defect is repaired through a right ventriculotomy. Development of subaortic stenosis has been reported after successful repair of interrupted aortic arch and may necessitate further surgical intervention.

Sell and associates reported 71 patients observed with IAA between 1974 and 1987.[38] In the early years of the series, tube graft repair was performed. More recently, direct anastomosis with repair of the ventricular septal defect was performed. Actuarial survival at 10 years was 47%, and mortality declined with increasing experience. Recurrent arch obstruction was managed with reoperation or balloon angioplasty. Two-dimensional echocardiography can be used to visualize the defect. Karl and colleagues have reported repair of IAA or coarctation plus hypoplastic arch in 55 infants through a median sternotomy.[23] The operative mortality for arch repair plus biventricular intracardiac repair was 9%. Mortality for arch repair plus palliative intracardiac repair was 40%, suggesting that primary repair of IAA and associated anomalies should be undertaken even when complex intracardiac anomalies are present.

IAA remains a difficult surgical problem. Advances in surgical techniques and neonatal intensive care as well as the introduction of prostaglandin E₁ therapy have greatly increased survival. After stabilization of these critically ill infants, total correction of the IAA and associated anomalies should be undertaken through a median sternotomy.

AORTOPULMONARY WINDOW

Aortopulmonary window is a rare congenital heart defect after abnormal septation of the truncus arteriosus into the aorta and pulmonary artery.[39] Various other terms have been applied to this anomaly, including aortopulmonary fistula, aortic septal defect, aorticopulmonary septal defect, and aortopulmonary fenestration.

An aortopulmonary window is usually a single large defect beginning a few millimeters above the aortic valve on the left lateral wall of the aorta. Multiple defects have been rarely reported. The defect may occasionally be found more distally overlying the origin of the right pulmonary artery; and, rarely, absence of the entire aortopulmonary septum may be encountered. Origin of the right coronary artery and rarely the left from the pulmonary artery may occur and can complicate surgical correction. Associated anomalies include Type A IAA, ventricular septal defect, tetralogy of Fallot, and PDA. An aortopulmonary window allows a large left-to-right shunt, causing pulmonary hypertension and congestive heart failure. Irreversible pulmonary vascular disease may occur at an early age.

Aortopulmonary window is a rare defect, and thus the natural history is not well defined. Patients with a large aortopulmonary window usually do not survive infancy. Children or young adults with an aortopulmonary window are encountered occasionally and usually have developed significant pulmonary vascular disease. The clinical course is thought to be similar to that of untreated patients with a large ventricular septal defect.

Diagnosis

Infants with aortopulmonary window usually present with congestive heart failure early in life. They often have growth retardation and recurrent pulmonary infections. Physical examination reveals a systolic murmur and occasionally a continuous murmur suggestive of PDA. The chest film reveals cardiomegaly, with pulmonary vascular engorgement or congestive heart failure. Aortopulmonary window must be differentiated from PDA, persistent truncus arteriosus, ventricular septal defect with aortic regurgitation, and ruptured aneurysm of the sinus of Valsalva.

Cardiac catheterization reveals an oxygen saturation step-up at the level of the pulmonary artery, and the course of the catheter may suggest the diagnosis. Retrograde aortography provides accurate visualization of the defect. It is necessary to document the presence of normal aortic and pulmonic valves to confirm the diagnosis, and the location of coronary ostia must be carefully demonstrated before surgical intervention. Echocardiography may also be used to diagnose aortopulmonary window.

Surgical Correction

The presence of an aortopulmonary window is sufficient indication for repair unless severe pulmonary vascular disease has occurred. The preferred technique for repair is transaortic closure, either by direct suture or patch closure. Simple ligation should not be done because of the risk of hemorrhage from the friable tissues. Division and primary closure may cause narrowing of the vessels. The transaortic approach is preferred to the transpulmonary method because it allows better visualization of the defect and the coronary ostia. The operation is undertaken through a median sternotomy, and either cardiopulmonary bypass or hypothermic circulatory arrest may be used. A transverse aortotomy at the level of the window is performed, and the anatomy is carefully defined. Particular attention should be given to the location of the coronary ostia and the origin of the right pulmonary artery. Small defects may be closed by direct suture; larger defects should be closed with a Dacron patch. Care must be taken to place the patch so that the coronary ostia are on the aortic side. If the defect involves the origin of the right pulmonary artery, a teardrop-shaped patch extending along the right pulmonary artery may be used to repair the defect. Repair of the aortopulmonary window may also be performed by opening the anterior wall of the defect, suturing a patch to the posterior wall, and continuing this suture to close the incision, incorporating the patch in the suture line. Division of the aortopulmonary window with patch closure of the aorta and pulmonary artery with either prosthetic material or a homograft may also be done.

Operative mortality is low for repair of isolated aortopulmonary window or aortic origin of a pulmonary artery in infancy. Long-term results are good if there are no associated anomalies. In older infants and children, the results depend on the severity and reversibility of the pulmonary vascular disease.

ANOMALIES OF THE AORTIC ARCH

Vascular rings are developmental anomalies of the aorta and great vessels that encircle and may constrict the esophagus and trachea (Figs. 54–13 and 54–14).[3, 5] In the embryo, six pairs of aortic arches arise sequentially from the truncus arteriosus and join paired dorsal aortas. Persistence or regression of various segments of these arches results in the normal pattern of the aorta, pulmonary artery, and great vessels. In normal development, the third pair of arches form parts of

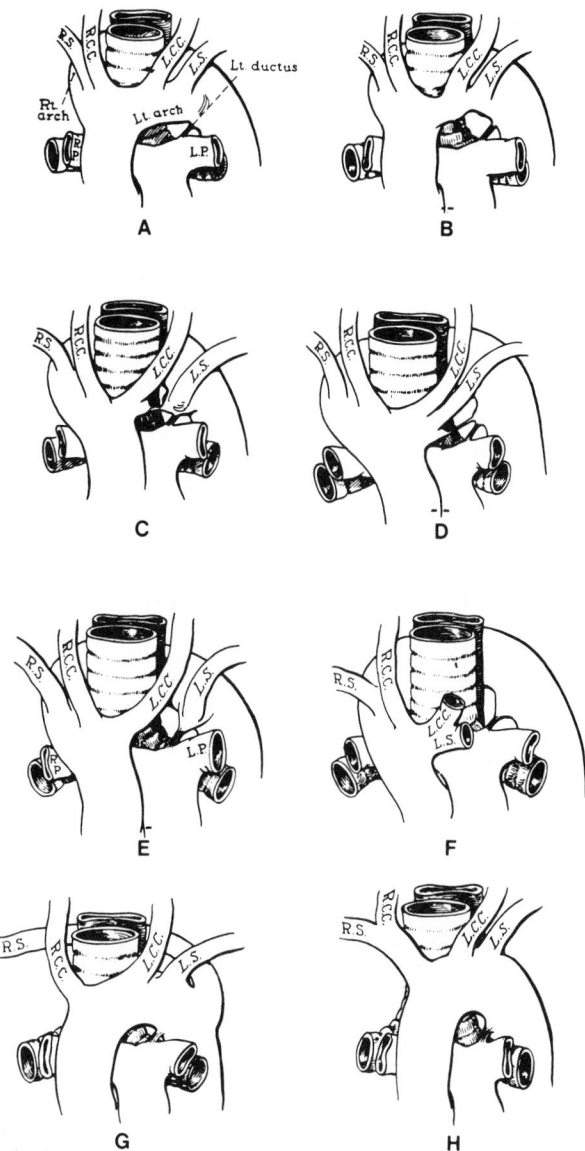

Vascular rings should be suspected in any infant with stridor, dysphagia, recurrent respiratory tract infections, difficult feeding, or failure to thrive. Vascular rings are not necessarily inconsistent with prolonged survival, and many patients are totally asymptomatic. Anomalies that become symptomatic usually present by 6 months of age, although some adults present when atherosclerosis causes dilation of the aorta and increasing constriction. Children with mild symptoms may show marked improvement as they grow. Afflicted infants most commonly present with respiratory difficulties; the breathing is stridorous and may be exacerbated by feeding. Hyperextension of the neck tends to reduce the constriction, and marked respiratory difficulties may occur if the neck is flexed. The physical examination is usually nondiagnostic,

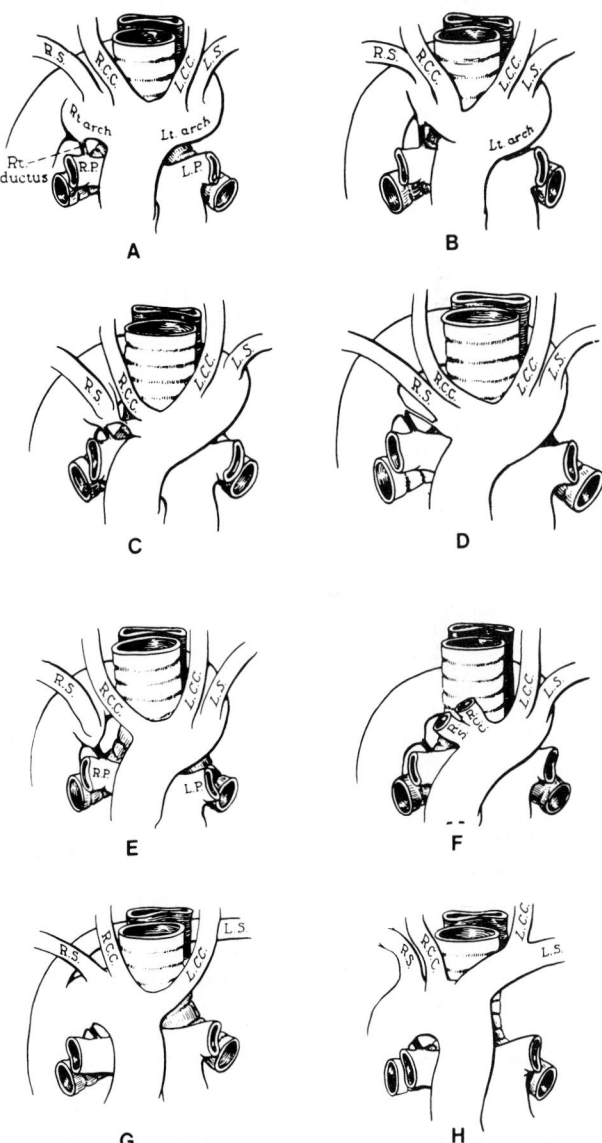

Figure 54–13. Aortic arch anomalies (left descending aorta and ligamentum arteriosum). *A,* Double aortic arch with equal anterior and posterior arches. *B,* Double aortic arch with smaller anterior (left) arch. *C,* Double aortic arch with atresia of anterior arch between the carotid and subclavian arteries. *D,* Double aortic arch with atresia of anterior arch distal to subclavian artery. *E,* Right aortic arch with retroesophageal segment and anomalous origin of the left subclavian artery from Kommerell's diverticulum. *F,* Right aortic arch with retroesophageal segment and mirror image branching. (Note the ligamentum arteriosum inserting onto the diverticulum of the descending aorta.) *G,* Left aortic arch with anomalous origin of the right subclavian artery. *H,* Normal pattern. (From Edwards, J. E.: Anomalies of the derivatives of the aortic arch system. Med. Clin. North Am., *32*:925, 1948.)

the common carotid arteries. The left fourth arch forms the adult aortic arch, and the proximal portion of the right fourth arch persists as the innominate artery. The pulmonary arteries develop from the proximal right and left sixth aortic arches. The distal left sixth arch develops into the ductus arteriosus, whereas the distal right sixth arch normally regresses. Failure of a segment to regress normally may cause a vascular ring. Associated cardiac defects may be encountered (often tetralogy of Fallot), especially in patients with a persistent right aortic arch.

Clinical Manifestations and Natural History

The natural history of vascular rings is obscured by the wide spectrum of anomalies and the range of symptoms.[3, 5]

Figure 54–14. Aortic arch anomalies (right descending aorta and ligamentum arteriosum). *A,* Double aortic arch with equal anterior and posterior arches. *B,* Double aortic arch with smaller anterior (right) arch. *C,* Double aortic arch with atresia of anterior arch between carotid and subclavian arteries. *D,* Double aortic arch with atresia of anterior arch distal to subclavian artery. *E,* Left aortic arch with retroesophageal segment and anomalous origin of right subclavian artery from Kommerell's diverticulum. *F,* Left aortic arch with retroesophageal segment. (Note the insertion of the ligamentum arteriosum onto the diverticulum of the descending aorta.) *G,* Right aortic arch with a normal origin of the left subclavian artery. *H,* Right aortic arch with mirror image branching. (From Edwards, J. E.: Anomalies of the derivatives of the aortic arch system. Med. Clin. North Am., *32*:925, 1948.)

although signs of associated cardiovascular defects may be found.

The plain chest film may be normal or may reveal pneumonia or occasionally compression of the air-filled trachea. A right aortic arch is observed in some anomalies. The barium esophagogram is a particularly valuable study. The combination of posterior compression of the esophagus on barium swallow and anterior tracheal compression is almost pathognomonic for a vascular ring. Angiocardiography accurately delineates the anatomy of vascular rings and allows evaluation of associated anomalies. Although most vascular rings can be divided without preoperative catheterization, many centers routinely perform catheterization because misdiagnosis can occur. Various other diagnostic modalities may occasionally be useful, including echocardiography, magnetic resonance imaging, and digital subtraction angiography. Bronchoscopy is indicated in some patients, especially those with suspected anomalous origin of the innominate artery.[11]

Management

Although a few patients with constricting vascular rings improve with growth, the long-term prognosis of medical therapy is poor in most symptomatic patients. Despite the wide spectrum of anomalies, the principles of surgical therapy are simple.[3, 5] Surgical intervention should be undertaken at the time of diagnosis and is designed to divide the vascular ring, relieve the constriction, and preserve circulation to the aortic branches. Adequate exposure is an absolute necessity.

The most common anomaly causing a true vascular ring is persistence of the right and left fourth aortic arches, forming a double aortic arch. In the usual situation, the right or posterior arch is larger and there is a left descending aorta with a left ductus arteriosus (see Fig. 54–13B). However, occasionally the arches are of equal size (see Fig. 54–13A) or the anterior (left) arch is larger. Rarely, a right descending aorta is encountered, in which case the right arch is anterior (see Fig. 54–13C and D). The right carotid and subclavian arteries arise from the right arch, whereas the left carotid and subclavian arteries arise from the left arch. Patients with double aortic arch usually present early in infancy and are severely symptomatic. The diagnosis of double aortic arch can be made easily from the barium esophagogram. In the most common situation, the anteroposterior projection shows right- and left-sided indentation of the barium-filled esophagus, with the right indentation being higher and larger. The lateral projection shows posterior esophageal compression from the retroesophageal posterior arch. Arteriography may also be used to make the diagnosis, although atretic segments are not visualized. Surgical correction is indicated at the time of diagnosis. In the usual situation, a left-sided thoracotomy is done and the smaller anterior arch is divided and oversewn at its junction with the descending aorta so that the left carotid and subclavian arteries arise from the ascending aorta or may be divided at an atretic segment, if present. The ligamentum arteriosum is also divided, and the constricting vessels are dissected away from the trachea and esophagus. If necessary, the divided left arch may be suspended from the posterior surface of the sternum to further relieve the constriction. In patients with atresia of the posterior (right) arch, a right-sided thoracotomy provides optimal exposure.

Aberrant origin of the right subclavian artery is a very common anomaly but rarely causes symptoms (see Fig. 54–13G). This defect follows regression of the right fourth aortic arch between the carotid and subclavian arteries, rather than distal to the subclavian. The artery may appear to arise from a diverticulum of the descending aorta (Kommerell's

diverticulum), which is actually a remnant of the distal right aortic arch. The artery most often courses posterior to the esophagus but may pass between the trachea and esophagus or anterior to the trachea. An anomalous right subclavian artery does not constitute a true vascular ring. However, the aberrant artery or occasionally the diverticulum may compress the esophagus, causing dysphagia. The diagnosis of aberrant origin of the right subclavian artery can be made by a barium esophagogram. The lateral esophagogram shows an oblique posterior impression coursing upward from left to right, and arterial pulsations may be observed. This anomaly may be an incidental finding at the time of barium study for other indications. In children, the artery may be simply ligated and divided without sequelae. In adults, a subclavian steal syndrome may follow simple division, and anastomosis to the aorta is usually necessary.

Compression of the anterior trachea may result from an innominate artery originating farther to the left on the aortic arch.[11] Children with anomalous origin of the innominate artery present with respiratory distress, stridor, and occasionally respiratory arrest. Dysphagia does not occur because the esophagus is not obstructed. Reflex apnea may follow irritation of the trachea by accumulated secretions or further compression of the trachea by a bolus of food in the esophagus. The physical examination is not helpful in the diagnosis of anomalous origin of the innominate artery. The chest film may reveal only pneumonia or atelectasis, and the barium esophagogram is normal. Bronchoscopy is the optimal method for confirming tracheal compression and reveals buckling of the tracheal cartilages in affected patients.[11] Many infants with innominate artery compression have mild symptoms and improve as they grow. Aortopexy may be donethrough a median sternotomy or a right-sided anterior thoracotomy. With the use of multiple adventitial sutures, the aorta and innominate artery are suspended from the posterior aspect of the sternum. The innominate artery is not dissected free from the trachea but is suspended and allowed to exert traction on the buckled tracheal cartilages.

Results

Results of surgical therapy in terms of both survival and relief of symptoms are good in infants with isolated vascular rings.[3, 5] Operative mortality is low. Postoperative morbidity is often related to tracheomalacia secondary to the vascular compression. Chun and associates[5] reported 39 patients treated at the Johns Hopkins Hospital between 1968 and 1990 for vascular rings. There were two hospital deaths, and one child had persistence of severe symptoms. At a median follow-up of 1 year, 97% of survivors were completely or nearly completely free from symptoms. Mortality is usually related to the severity of the tracheobronchial stenosis and associated defects. The infants may continue to have residual obstruction that causes recurrent respiratory distress and infection. These problems usually diminish as the child grows. In children with associated cardiac anomalies, the long-term outcome is related to the severity of the cardiac defect.

PULMONARY ARTERY SLING

Pulmonary artery sling is a rare cardiac anomaly occurring when the left pulmonary artery arises aberrantly from the right pulmonary artery and courses between the trachea and esophagus.[3, 32] A true vascular ring is not present; however, compression of the distal trachea and mainstem bronchi usually occurs. The aberrant left pulmonary artery arises from the posterior aspect of the right pulmonary artery (Fig. 54–15). It then courses posteriorly over the right mainstem bronchus and passes between the trachea and esophagus. The

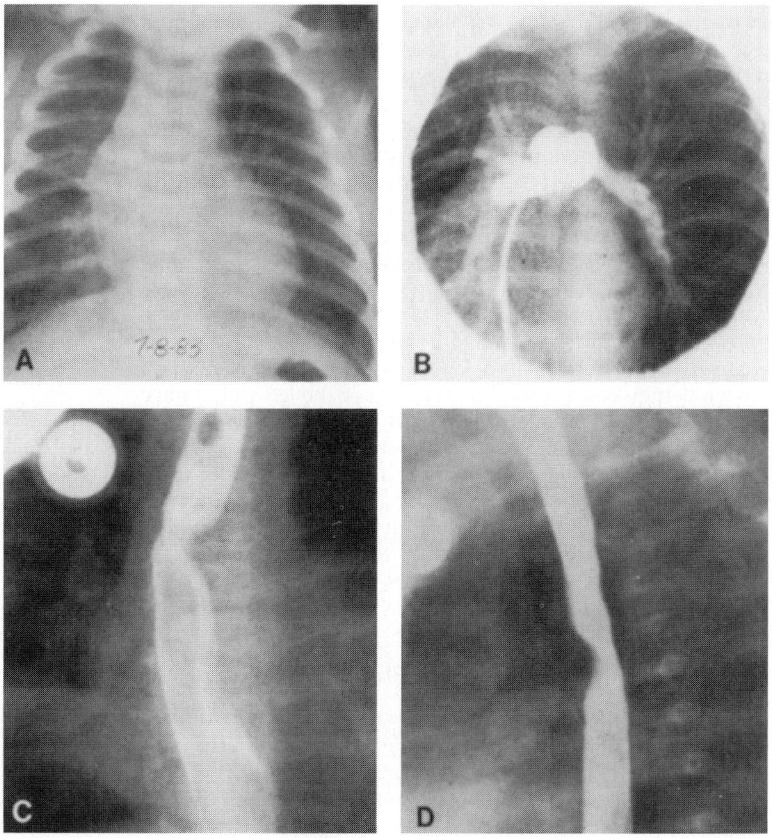

Figure 54–15. Infant with pulmonary artery sling. *A,* Plain chest film demonstrates hyperaeration of the left lung. *B,* Pulmonary arteriogram demonstrates anomalous origin of the left pulmonary artery from the right pulmonary artery. (Note the course of the left pulmonary artery around the tracheal air column.) *C,* Anteroposterior barium esophagogram showing compression of the esophagus. *D,* Lateral barium esophagogram showing characteristic anterior indentation of the esophagus behind the distal trachea. (*A* to *D,* Courtesy of Drs. Eric Effman and Bennett Pearce.)

hilum of the left lung is lower than normal. Tracheal stenosis with complete cartilaginous rings and absence of the membranous portion of the trachea occurs frequently. Tracheal stenosis may extend proximally, may include the right and left mainstem bronchi, and may be present in segments not actually compressed by the anomalous vessel.

Clinical Findings and Diagnosis

Infants with pulmonary artery sling often present with respiratory symptoms at birth, and many are symptomatic by 1 month. It is impossible to estimate the number of asymptomatic patients with pulmonary artery sling. The most common findings are respiratory distress, wheezing, and expiratory stridor. Acute respiratory failure secondary to obstruction may occur, requiring intubation. Signs and symptoms of esophageal obstruction are rare. Repeated respiratory tract infections may occur.

The physical examination is not helpful in the diagnosis of pulmonary artery sling. The chest film may be normal or may show a number of findings suggestive of pulmonary artery sling, including hyperinflation of one lung (most commonly the right, but occasionally the left), anterior bowing of the tracheal air column, and a low hilum of the left lung (see Fig. 54–15). Pulmonary artery sling may present in adults as a mediastinal or paratracheal mass. The barium esophagogram is particularly useful and shows anterior pulsatile compression of the esophagus (see Fig. 54–15). This finding strongly suggests a pulmonary artery sling but can be observed if an anomalous subclavian artery courses between the trachea and esophagus. Mediastinal tumors, cysts, or lymph nodes may occasionally cause anterior esophageal compression, but these lesions are nonpulsatile. Angiocardiography is useful to demonstrate the aberrant vessel and evaluate associated anomalies (see Fig. 54–15). Digital sub-

traction angiography, two-dimensional echocardiography, computed tomography, and magnetic resonance imaging may also prove useful in the diagnosis of pulmonary artery sling. Bronchoscopy is particularly useful in these patients for evaluation of associated tracheobronchial anomalies.

Natural History

The exact incidence of pulmonary artery sling is unknown. Patients may present with severe symptoms in infancy, but survival to an advanced age is also possible. The natural history of patients with pulmonary artery sling depends on the degree of respiratory obstruction and associated tracheobronchial and cardiac anomalies. Infants who present with respiratory obstruction may succumb to the acute event; if they survive, their prognosis is poor without surgical intervention.

Management and Results

Surgical intervention is indicated in any patient with a pulmonary artery sling and symptoms of significant respiratory obstruction. Nonsurgical management may be possible in patients with minor symptoms. Division of the anomalous artery with anastomosis to the main pulmonary artery may be performed using either a left thoracotomy or a median sternotomy with cardiopulmonary bypass. The management of associated tracheobronchial anomalies continues to be a difficult problem. If significant obstruction remains after correction of the pulmonary artery sling, resection of the stenotic segment of the trachea or tracheoplasty may be required.

Pawade and colleagues[32] from the Hospital for Sick Children in London reported 18 patients treated for pulmonary artery sling. Patients with isolated pulmonary artery sling underwent reimplantation of the left pulmonary artery through a left thoracotomy. Four patients with stovepipe tracheas and complete cartilaginous rings underwent tracheal resection and cardiopulmonary bypass and reanastomosis of the left pulmonary artery to the main pulmonary artery. There were no early deaths. There was one late death, and the pulmonary artery anastomosis was patent in 14 patients investigated postoperatively. Backer and colleagues[3] reported 12 infants who underwent surgical repair of pulmonary artery sling at a mean age of 5 months. Three patients had simultaneous pericardial patch tracheoplasty for complete tracheal rings. There were no operative deaths, and there were two late deaths. The pulmonary artery anastomosis was patent in 7 of 9 infants studied postoperatively.

Survivors of repair of pulmonary artery sling generally have a benign course despite occlusion of the left pulmonary artery, and residual symptoms tend to decrease as the patients grow. Although there has been concern that patients with an occluded left pulmonary artery might develop pulmonary hypertension in the right lung or hemoptysis secondary to bronchial collateral vessels, neither has been encountered. Attempts to restore patency to occluded pulmonary arteries have not met with success and are not generally recommended.

SELECTED REFERENCES

Chun, K., Colombani, P. M., Dudgeon, D. L., and Haller, J. A.: Diagnosis and management of congenital vascular rings: A 22-year experience. Ann. Thorac. Surg., 53:597, 1992.
A large series of congenital aortic arch anomalies treated at a single institution outlines the management principles for successful treatment of vascular rings.

Karl, T. R., Sano, S., Brawn, W., and Mee, R. B. B.: Repair of hypoplastic or interrupted aortic arch via sternotomy. J. Thorac. Cardiovasc. Surg., 104:688, 1992.
A large series from a single institution discusses infants with aortic arch obstruction and hypoplastic aortic arch who underwent a primary complete intracardiac repair with excellent results.

Pawade, A., de Leval, M. R., Elliott, M. J., and Stark, J.: Pulmonary artery sling. Ann. Thorac. Surg., 54:967, 1992.
A series of 18 patients with pulmonary artery sling were treated at the Hospital for Sick Children in London. Patients with isolated pulmonary artery sling were treated by division and reimplantation of the left pulmonary artery. Patients with tracheal stenosis were treated by tracheal resection as well as reimplantation of the left pulmonary artery. Methods for diagnosis and treatment of patients with pulmonary artery sling with and without complete cartilaginous tracheal rings are reviewed.

Quaegebeur, J. M., Jonas, R. A., Weinberg, A. D., Blackstone, E. H., and Kirklin, J. W.: Outcomes in seriously ill neonates with coarctation of the aorta: A multi-institutional study. J. Thorac. Cardiovasc. Surg., 108:841, 1994.

Sciolaro, C., Copeland, J., Cork, R., Barkenbush, M., Donnerstein, R., and Goldberg, S.: Long-term follow-up comparing subclavian flap angioplasty to resection with modified oblique end-to-end anastomosis. J. Thorac. Cardiovasc. Surg., 101:1, 1991.

Van Heurn, L. W. E., Wong, C. M., Spiegelhalter, D. J., Sorensen, K., de Leval, M. R., Stark, J., and Elliott, M. J.: Surgical treatment of aortic coarctation in infants age less than three months, 1985–1991. J. Thorac. Cardiovasc. Surg., 107:74, 1994.
These are reports of the recent experience with neonatal coarctation of the aorta including a large multi-institutional trial comparing the advantages and disadvantages of the different methods of repair. The conflicting results with these techniques obtained at different centers illustrate the difficulties in recommending one type of repair for coarctation of the aorta over another.

REFERENCES

1. Adzick, W. S., Harrison, M. R., and Delorimier, A. A.: Surgical clip ligation of patent ductus arteriosus in premature infants. J. Pediatr. Surg., 21:158, 1986.
2. Ali Khan, M. A., Al Yousef, S., Mullins, C. E., and Sawyer, W.: Experience with 205 procedures of transcatheter closure of ductus arteriosus in 182 patients, with special reference to residual shunts and long-term follow-up. J. Thorac. Cardiovasc. Surg., 104:1721, 1992.
3. Backer, C. I., Idriss, F. S., Holinger, L. D., and Mavroudis, C.: Pulmonary artery sling: Results of surgical repair in infancy. J. Thorac. Cardiovasc. Surg., 103:683, 1992.
4. Bromberg, B. L., Beekman, R. H., Rocchini, A. P., et al.: Aortic aneurysm

after patch aortoplasty repair of coarctation: A prospective analysis of prevalence: Screening tests and risks. J. Am. Coll. Cardiol., 14:734, 1989.
5. Chun, K., Colombani, P. M., Dudgeon, D. L., and Haller, J. A.: Diagnosis and management of congenital vascular rings: A 22-year experience. Ann. Thorac. Surg., 53:597, 1992.
6. Cokkinos, D. V., Leachman, R. D., and Cooley, D. A.: Increased mortality rate from coronary artery disease following operation for coarctation of the aorta at a late age. J. Thorac. Cardiovasc. Surg., 77:315, 1979.
7. Cooper, S. G., Sullivan, I. D., and Wren, C.: Treatment of recoarctation: Balloon dilation angioplasty. J. Am. Coll. Cardiol., 14:413, 1989.
8. Crafoord, C., and Nylin, G.: Congenital coarctation of the aorta and its surgical treatment. J. Thorac. Cardiovasc. Surg., 14:347, 1945.
9. Cyran, S. E., Grzeszczak, M., Kaufman, K., Weber, H. S., Myers, J. L., Gleason, M. M., and Baylen, B. G.: Aortic "recoarctation" at rest versus at exercise in children as evaluated by stress Doppler echocardiography after a "good" operative result. Am. J. Cardiol., 71:963, 1993.
10. Evans, N.: Diagnosis of patent ductus arteriosus in the preterm newborn. Arch. Dis. Child., 68:58, 1993.
11. Filston, H. C., Ferguson, T. B., Jr., and Oldham, H. N.: Airway obstruction by vascular anomalies: Importance of telescopic bronchoscopy. Ann. Surg., 205:541, 1987.
12. Foster, E. D.: Reoperation for aortic coarctation. Ann. Thorac. Surg., 38:81, 1984.
13. Gardiner, H. M., Celermajer, D. S., Sorenson, K. E., and Deanfield, J. E.: Abnormal endothelial response in the precoarctation vascular bed of young normotensive adults after successful coarctation repair. Br. Heart J., 69:18, 1993.
14. Gersony, W. M.: Patent ductus arteriosus in the neonate. Pediatr. Clin. North Am., 33:54, 1986.
15. Goldman, S., Hernandez, J., and Pappas, G.: Results of surgical treatment of coarctation of the aorta in the critically ill neonate, including the influence of pulmonary artery banding. J. Thorac. Cardiovasc. Surg., 91:732, 1986.
16. Gray, D. T., Fyler, D. C., Walker, A. M., Weinstein, M. C., and Chalmers, T. C.: Clinical outcomes and costs of transcatheter as compared with surgical closure of patent ductus arteriosus. N. Engl. J. Med., 329:1517, 1993.
17. Gross, R. E.: Complete surgical division of the patent ductus arteriosus: A report of fourteen successful cases. Surg. Obstet. Gynecol., 78:36, 1944.
18. Hammerman, C., Strates, E., and Valaitis, S.: The silent ductus: Its precursors and its aftermath. Pediatr. Cardiol., 7:121, 1986.
19. Heymann, M. A., Berman, W., Jr., Rudolph, A. M., and Whitman, V.: Dilatation of the ductus arteriosus by prostaglandin E_1 in aortic arch abnormalities. Circulation, 59:169, 1979.
20. Heymann, M. A., Rudolph, A. M., and Silberman, N. H.: Closure of the ductus arteriosus in premature infants by inhibition of prostaglandin synthesis. N. Engl. J. Med., 295:530, 1976.
21. Higgins, C. B., Rausch, J., Friedman, W. F., et al.: Patent ductus arteriosus in preterm infants with idiopathic respiratory distress syndrome. Radiology 124:189, 1977.
22. John, S., Muralidharan, S., Jairaj, P. S., et al.: The adult ductus: Review of surgical experience with 131 patients. J. Thorac. Cardiovasc. Surg., 82:314, 1981.
23. Karl, T. R, Sano, S., Brawn, W., and Mee, R. B. B.: Repair of hypoplastic or interrupted aortic arch via sternotomy. J. Thorac. Cardiovasc. Surg., 104:688, 1992.
24. Kimball, T. R., Reynolds, J. M., Mays, W. A., Khoury, P., Claytor, R. P., and Daniels, S. R.: Persistent hyperdynamic cardiovascular state at rest and during exercise in children after successful repair of coarctation of the aorta. J. Am. Coll. Cardiol., 24:194, 1994.
25. Knott-Craig, C. J., Elkins, R. C., Ward, K. E., Overholt, E. D., Razook, J. D., McCue, C. A., and Lane, M. M.: Neonatal coarctation repair: Influence of technique on late results. Circulation, 88:198, 1993.
26. Kupferschmid, Ch., Lang, D., and Pohlandt, F.: Sensitivity, specificity and predictive value of clinical findings, M-mode echocardiography and continuous wave Doppler sonography in the diagnosis of symptomatic patent ductus arteriosus in preterm infants. Eur. J. Pediatr., 147:279, 1988.
27. Laborde, F., Noirhomme, P., Karam, J., Batisse, A., Bourel, P., and Maurice, O.: A new video-assisted thoracoscopic surgical technique for interruption of patent ductus arteriosus in infants and children. J. Thorac. Cardiovasc. Surg., 105:278, 1993.
28. Lacour-Gayet, F., Bruniaux, J., Serraf, A., Chambran, P., Blaysat, G., Losay, J., Petit, J., Kachaner, J., and Planche, C.: Hypoplastic transverse arch and coarctation in neonates: Surgical reconstruction of the aortic arch: A study of sixty-six patients. J. Thorac. Cardiovasc. Surg., 100:808, 1990.
29. Lloyd, T. R., Fedderly, R., Mendelsohn, A. M., et al.: Transcatheter occlusion of patent ductus arteriosus with Gianturco coils. Circulation, 88(part 1):1412, 1993.
30. Markel, H., Rocchini, A. P., Beekman, R. H., et al.: Exercise induced hypertension after repair of coarctation of the aorta: Arm versus leg exercise. J. Am. Coll. Cardiol., 8:165, 1986.
31. Park, J. K., Dell, R. B., Ellis, K., and Gersony, W. M.: Surgical management of the infant with coarctation of the aorta and ventricular septal defect. J. Am. Coll. Cardiol., 20:176, 1992.
32. Pawade, A., de Leval, M. R., Elliott, M. J., and Stark, J.: Pulmonary artery sling. Ann. Thorac. Surg., 54:967, 1992.

33. Quaegebeur, J. M., Jonas, R. A., Weinberg, A. D., Blackstone, E. H., and Kirklin, J. W.: Outcomes in seriously ill neonates with coarctation of the aorta: A multi-institutional study. J. Thorac. Cardiovasc. Surg., *108*:841, 1994.

34. Rao, P. S., and Chopra, P. S.: Role of balloon angioplasty in the treatment of aortic coarctation. Ann. Thorac. Surg., *52*:621, 1991.

35. Rashkind, W. J., Mullins, C. E., Hellenbrand, W. E., and Tait, M. A.: Nonsurgical closure of patent ductus arteriosus: Clinical application of the Rashkind PDA occluder system. Circulation, *75*:583, 1987.

36. Ritter, S. B.: Coarctation and balloons: Inflated or realistic? J. Am. Coll. Cardiol., *13*:696, 1989.

37. Sciolaro, C., Copeland, J., Cork, R., Barkenbush, M., Donnerstein, R., and Goldberg, S.: Long-term follow-up comparing subclavian flap angioplasty to resection with modified oblique end-to-end anastomosis. J. Thorac. Cardiovasc. Surg., *101*:1, 1991.

38. Sell, J. E., Jonas, R. A., Mayer, J. E., et al.: The results of a surgical program for interrupted aortic arch. J. Thorac. Cardiovasc. Surg., *96*:864, 1988.

39. Tiraboschi, R., Salomone, G., Crupi, G., et al.: Aortopulmonary window in

the first year of life: Report of 11 surgical cases. Ann. Thorac. Surg., *46*:438, 1988.

40. Trinquet, F., Vouhe, P. O., Vernant, F., et al.: Coarctation of the aorta in infants: Which operation? Ann. Thorac. Surg., *45*:186, 1988.

41. Tynan, M.: Transcatheter occlusion of persistent arterial duct. Lancet, *340*:1062, 1992.

42. Van Heurn, L. W. E., Wong, C. M., Spiegelhalter, D. J., Sorensen, K., de Leval, M.R., Stark, J., and Elliott, M. J.: Surgical treatment of aortic coarctation in infants age less than three months, 1985–1991. J. Thorac. Cardiovasc. Surg., *107*:74, 1994.

43. Vossschulte, K.: Surgical correction of coarctation of the aorta by an "isthmusplastic" operation. Thorax, *16*:338, 1961.

44. Waldhausen, J. A., and Nahrwold, D. L.: Repair of coarctation of the aorta with a subclavian flap. J. Thorac. Cardiovasc. Surg., *51*:532, 1966.

45. Wierny, L., Plass, R., and Portsmann, W.: Transluminal closure of patent ductus arteriosus: Long-term results of 208 cases treated without thoracotomy. Cardiovasc. Intervent. Radiol., *9*:279, 1986.

IV

ATRIAL SEPTAL DEFECTS, OSTIUM PRIMUM DEFECTS, AND ATRIOVENTRICULAR CANALS

Ross M. Ungerleider, M.D.

An atrial septal defect (ASD) is an opening in the atrial septum that enables mixing of blood from the systemic and pulmonary venous circulations. This hole may develop in a variety of locations because the embryologic causes of ASDs are numerous. Although functionally the same with respect to the physiology of shunting, these defects present the surgeon with several considerations that differ depending on the precise nature and location of the defect.

Atrioventricular (AV) canal defects include defects in the atrial and ventricular septa immediately above and below the AV valves (tricuspid and mitral). These defects usually involve the valves to some degree, and the physiology of the lesion depends on the extent of shunting at both the atrial and ventricular levels as well as on regurgitation from the involved valves. Defects limited to the atrial septum are called ostium primum ASDs or partial AV canal defects. Complete AV canal defects (also referred to as complete AV septal defects or endocardial cushion defects) combine deficiency of both the atrial and ventricular septa with severe abnormality of the mitral and tricuspid valves—creating what is in essence a common AV valve that serves both ventricles.

ANATOMY

A wide variety of developmental factors influence normal development of the atrial septum, and some understanding of the embryologic development of this portion of the heart facilitates appreciation for the nature of these various anomalies. Partitioning of the AV canal and the atrium begins about the middle of the fourth week and is essentially complete by the end of the fifth week.[81] The atrial septum is initially partitioned by a thin membrane (septum primum), which seems to grow down toward the region of the AV valves from the superior aspect of the atrium. At the same time, endocardial cushion tissue grows in an upward direction to meet this septum and to close the intervening space (referred to as the ostium primum). Just before obliteration of the ostium primum, perforations appear near the middle of the

septum primum to allow free flow of blood between the right and left sides of the atrium. These perforations coalesce to form the ostium secundum. A second ridge of tissue (septum secundum) begins to grow in a downward direction from the top of the atrium and to the right side of the septum primum. This septum secundum covers the ostium secundum in such a manner that the septum primum attaches to the left atrial side of the superior aspect of the septum secundum and completes the atrial partitioning. Because of the nature of this septation, the septum primum can act as a flap valve to allow flow of blood from the right to left direction across the septum through a small potential defect referred to as the foramen ovale (Fig. 54–16). The septum primum, as seen from the right atrial side, is referred to as the fossa ovalis.

All defects in the atrial septum in the region of the fossa ovalis are referred to as secundum-type ASDs. In actuality, most of these are usually defects of the septum primum (Figs. 54–17*A*, *B*, and *D*), although they can also include deficient downward growth of the septum secundum and, in association with a normal septum primum, can be termed a foramen ovale defect (see Fig. 54–17*C*).

Concurrent with the septation of the atrium, thickenings of subendocardial tissue, called *endocardial cushions*, develop in the dorsal and ventral walls of the heart in the region of the AV canal. During the fifth week, the AV endocardial cushions grow toward each other and fuse, dividing the AV canal into right and left sides.[81] These cushions give rise to a portion of the atrial septum (the part that grows upward to fuse with the septum primum), the ventricular septum (immediately below the tricuspid valve in the inlet to the right ventricle), and the septal leaflets of both the mitral and tricuspid valves. Therefore, abnormal growth patterns in this region can produce a deficiency in the lowermost part of the atrial septum (often with associated abnormalities such as clefts of the mitral and tricuspid valves) (see Fig. 54–17*E*). The most extensive form of this developmental anomaly produces a ventricular septal deficiency as well (Fig. 54–18) and what essentially amounts to a hole in the middle of the

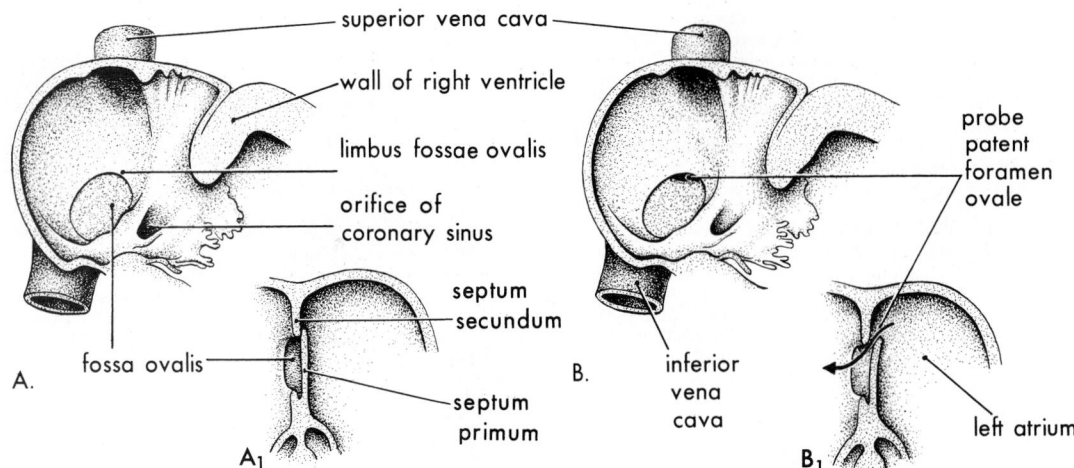

Figure 54–16. *A,* This depiction of the anatomy in the right atrium demonstrates that the fossa ovalis is closed by the septum primum, which attaches on the left atrial side of the septum secundum (A_1). The location of the fossa ovalis near the coronary sinus is a consistent anatomic feature. *B* and B_1, When the septum primum does not grow adequately to attach to the left atrial side of the septum secundum, a patent foramen ovale results that permits intra-atrial shunting. The distinction between the right and the left atrium is easily made by observing to which side the septum primum attaches, because that always identifies the left atrium. (From Moore, K. L., and Persaud, T. V. N.: The Developing Human: Clinically Oriented Embryology. Philadelphia, W. B. Saunders, 1993.)

heart (complete AV canal), with communication at this level between all four cardia chambers.

Defects can also occur high in the superior aspect of the interatrial septum and are referred to as sinus venosus defects. Initially, the sinus venosus is a separate chamber of the heart and opens into the caudal wall of the right atrium. The left side of the sinus venosus becomes incorporated into the coronary sinus, and the right side merges with the upper portion of the right atrium. The sinus venosus represents the confluence of venous drainage to the heart, and a defect in this region can produce communication between the posterior aspect of the superior vena cava and the top of the left atrium (see Fig. 54–17F). It is not uncommon for the right superior pulmonary veins to drain to the left atrium at the top of the sinus venosus and, if a sinus venosus defect is present, to appear to return anomalously to the right atrium at, or slightly above, its junction with the superior vena cava. In this sense, most sinus venosus ASDs are associated with partial anomalous pulmonary venous return. Other rare types of defects in the atrial septum do occur and are usually related to some definable abnormality during embryologic development. For example, a deficiency in the left horn of the sinus venosus, as it becomes incorporated into the coronary sinus, can result in an unroofed coronary sinus, which drains into the left atrium, or which enables communication between the left atrium and the right atrium in the usual region of the coronary sinus—a coronary sinus–type ASD. It is also possible to see a communication between the left and right atrium inferior to the substance of the septum primum and located between the inferior vena cava and the coronary sinus. This rare type of defect is probably in the inferior aspect of the sinus venosus and can be considered as a sinus venosus–type defect. It should be looked for in all cases of superior sinus venosus defects.

INCIDENCE AND ASSOCIATED DEFECTS

ASDs are among the most common congenital cardiac lesions and may be seen in association with almost any other type of cardiac anomaly.[25, 54, 74, 105] They are commonly found[121] in patients with ventricular septal defects, pulmonary stenosis, patent ductus arteriosus, coarctation of the aorta, mitral stenosis (which when associated with an ASD is described by the eponym of Lutembacher's syndrome),[107] and various

anomalies of systemic venous return such as a persistent left superior vena cava.[54] ASDs also seem to be more frequent with pericardial disease than would be accounted for by chance alone.[37] Approximately 30% of secundum ASDs occur with other cardiac defects.[121]

Physiologic flow communication at the level of the atrial septum is, in fact, essential for survival in some of the more complicated forms of congenital heart disease; and in this setting the occurrence of an ASD is not always considered to be part of the pathologic entity. Examples of this include pulmonary atresia (or critical pulmonary stenosis) with intact ventricular septum, tricuspid atresia, mitral atresia, and total anomalous pulmonary venous return. Furthermore, creation of an atrial level shunt (by balloon catheter or catheter-guided blade septostomy in the cardiac catheterization laboratory, or by surgical excision in the operating room) plays an important role in the treatment of certain lesions such as transposition of the great vessels and palliation for hypoplastic left heart syndrome. More recent investigators have even described methods by which the surgeon can leave an atrial level communication after surgery to optimize the postoperative convalescence in patients with right-sided heart dysfunction.[1]

When ASDs occur as isolated congenital lesions, they still comprise a common entity and may be the fifth most common congenital cardiac lesion, occurring in as many as 13,500 children younger than 14 years of age.[51] ASDs account for as many as 7% of all cases of congenital heart disease.[35] Furthermore, ASD is the most common heart defect detected in patients older than 20 years of age,[121] in large part owing to its benign and relatively obscure clinical course, which enables these patients to grow and develop normally with deceptively few clinical signs of heart disease.[33, 36, 44, 46, 85, 94, 104] It is of interest that secundum ASDs occur more frequently in females than males, with a ratio of 3:1.[121]

ASDs may also be correlated to some genetic factors and are clearly increased in incidence in certain syndromes such as Down's,[11] Turner's,[89] Ellis-van Creveld,[39] Marfan's,[37, 121] and Ehler-Danlos.[121, 123] It is not uncommon for the defects in these disorders to be extremely large, bordering on the appearance of a common atrium. Furthermore, familial inheritance on the basis of a dominant autosomal gene with incomplete penetrance has been reported and may help to explain the appearance of ASDs in a family lineage.[17] Varying degrees

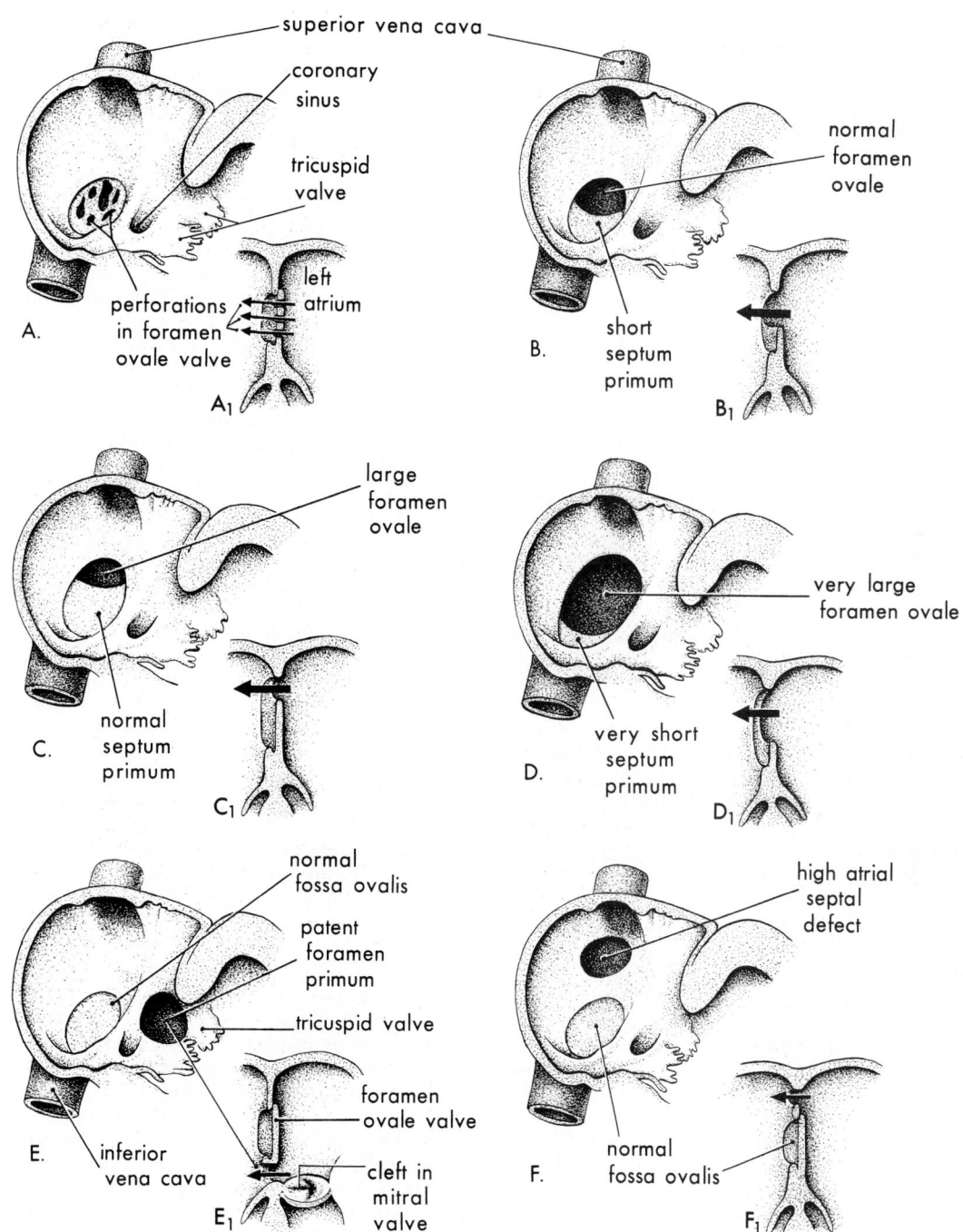

Figure 54–17. Drawings of the right aspect of the interatrial septum (*A* to *F*) and sketches of coronal sections of the septum (*A₁* to *F₁*), illustrating various types of atrial septal defect (ASD). *A,* Perforations in the substance of the septum primum create a deficiency in the foramen ovale that is commonly called a secundum type of ASD. *B,* A nonperforated but anatomically deficient septum primum allows communication between the atria below the limbus of the septum secundum, frequently referred to as foramen ovale type (secundum) ASD. *C,* A foramen ovale type ASD can also occur when a normal-sized septum primum is unable to attach to the left atrial surface of the septum secundum. *D,* Likewise, a very short septum primum leaves a large opening through the foramen ovale, resulting in a large ASD. *E,* Deficiency of the AV septum (endocardial cushion tissue) near the coronary sinus and immediately adjacent to the anulus of the tricuspid and mitral valve produces a partial AV canal defect or ostium primum ASD. In this situation, the fossa ovalis is intact and the atrial communication is just above the mitral and tricuspid valve orifices. These defects, as indicated, are often associated with a "cleft" in the mitral valve. *F,* A defect high in the limbus of the septum secundum can occur superior to the intact fossa ovalis and is referred to as a sinus venosus type ASD. This variety of ASD is commonly associated with partial anomalous pulmonary venous return of the right superior pulmonary veins. (From Moore, K. L., and Persaud, T. V. L.: The Developing Human: Clinically Oriented Embryology. Philadelphia, W. B. Saunders, 1993.)

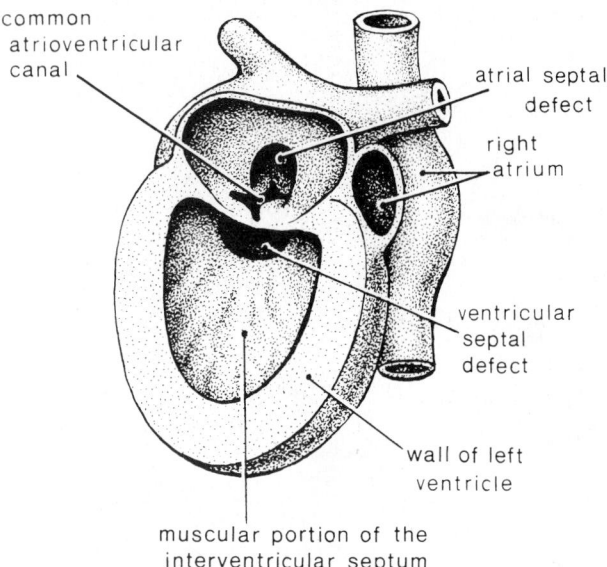

common
atrioventricular
canal

atrial septal
defect

right
atrium

ventricular
septal
defect

wall of left
ventricle

muscular portion of the
interventricular septum

Figure 54–18. When a defect of endocardial cushion tissue creates an atrial septal communication as well as a ventricular septal communication, the anomaly is referred to as a complete AV canal. This defect, depicted here as seen from the left side of the heart, creates communication between all four cardiac chambers at the level of a common AV valve orifice. (From Moore, K. L.: The Developing Human: Clinically Oriented Embryology. Philadelphia, W. B. Saunders, 1977.)

of AV block may be more common in the familial variety of ASD, and the risk to offspring of parents with ASD is 21 times higher than the risk to children of unaffected parents (although the overall risk is still less than 5%).[17, 121] Most ASDs are probably caused by unknown and random disturbances in development. This impression is based on the lack of association of most ASDs with known hereditary abnormalities, the high incidence of associated nongenetic abnormalities of other structures, and the lack of concordance of cardiac defects in identical twins.[113, 121] Exposure of the mother to rubella[103] or ingestion by the mother of thalidomide during the first few weeks of pregnancy seems to enhance the likelihood of an ASD developing in the fetus.[121]

Sinus venosus defects are much less common than secundum ASDs and account for about 10% of ASDs. Unlike a secundum-type ASD, a sinus venosus ASD is not commonly associated with other forms of congenital heart disease, aside from anomalies of pulmonary venous return, which really comprise part of the spectrum of this lesion. In some cases, the anomalies of pulmonary venous return constitute the most disturbing feature of the defect and may be associated with abnormalities of the ipsilateral lung.[54] Defects in the sinus venosus region are really a deficiency between the posterior portion of the superior vena cava and the anterior aspect of the left atrium where these two structures share a common wall (Fig. 54–19).

Endocardial cushion defects, which result in both partial and complete AV canal defects show no sex predilection with an equal incidence in both males and females. As is true with secundum-type ASDs, ostium primum ASDs (partial AV canal) and complete AV canals are frequently associated with other cardiac defects (ranging between 7% and 25%).[108, 121] AV canal defects (both partial and complete) are sometimes seen in association with more complex and severe forms of congenital heart disease, including the heterotaxy syndromes,[54] tetralogy of Fallot,[15, 55] double-outlet right ventricle,[15, 54] total anomalous pulmonary venous return,[108] and transposition of the great arteries.[15] It is very common for patients with complete AV canal to also have small secun-

dum-type ASDs.[118] A patent ductus arteriosus is seen in as many as 10% of these patients,[54, 108, 118] especially when the diagnosis is provided in infancy. There is clearly an association between Down syndrome and endocardial cushion defects, and some form of the defect may be present in as many as 30% of the children with this syndrome.[51]

NATURAL HISTORY

The natural history of untreated ASDs is related to the type of defect, the size of the shunt, and associated anomalies.[3, 22, 27] Young patients usually do not have symptoms, although a tendency for increased pulmonary infections due to the increased pulmonary blood flow, has been noted. As patients grow older, the impact of chronic intracardiac shunting can become apparent by development of congestive heart failure or atrial dysrhythmias. Pulmonary hypertension is a reported but unusual long-term complication that can occur in up to 14% of patients with ASDs.[27, 57] Because of the potential for bidirectional shunting at the atrial level, emboli from the systemic venous circulation (normally cleared by the lungs) can cross the atrial septum to the left-sided circulation and lead to systemic arterial embolization (paradoxical emboli)[111] and be the cause of a stroke, brain abscess, or renal failure. Long-term complications of an unrepaired ASD can also include mitral and tricuspid valve incompetence,[54] pulmonary valve incompetence,[65] and systemic hypertension.[104] Of particular note is the well-established fact that patients with ASDs have a shortened life expectancy compared with normal persons. Although over 99.9% of infants born with isolated ASDs reach the age of 1 year,[22, 54] there is a substantial decrement in survival by the time these patients reach the third and fourth decades of life, owing in large part to a combination of the various factors mentioned earlier (Fig. 54–20). Furthermore, the functional status of patients with ASDs deteriorates with age so that concomitant with the decline in life expectancy, patients begin to have increasing symptoms of easy fatigability, exercise intolerance, and palpitations. Children with ASDs are often noted by their parents to have increased sweating during eating and the tendency to appear chronically tired. ASDs are also a reason that children can begin to lag on their growth curve, and it is not infrequent for a child to have a marked increase in growth after repair of the defect.

The natural history for patients with AV canal defects depends on the extent of the lesion (partial vs. complete), the degree of mitral insufficiency, and the nature of any associated lesions (both cardiac and noncardiac). Expectations for patients with partial AV canal defects (ostium primum ASD) and only mild mitral insufficiency parallel those for ASDs.[102] There is an accelerated tendency for these patients to develop atrial arrhythmias, which may impact on the age at which they demonstrate symptoms. This may be due to the location of this defect near (and displacing) the AV node as well as to the fact that most of these patients have large left-to-right shunts with distention of the right atrium and ventricle. When an ostium primum defect is associated with moderate to severe mitral insufficiency, the impact on natural history is more pronounced. As many as one fifth of these patients are symptomatic (congestive heart failure, dyspnea, arrhythmias) in infancy,[54] and several of these die during the first decade of life. This reflects the degree of intracardiac shunting as well as the diminished forward cardiac output secondary to the mitral insufficiency.

The natural history for complete AV canal defect is not well understood because it is unusual for these patients to be treated without surgical intervention. Nevertheless, the addition of an intracardiac shunt at the ventricular level, combined with the atrial level shunt and AV valve insuffi-

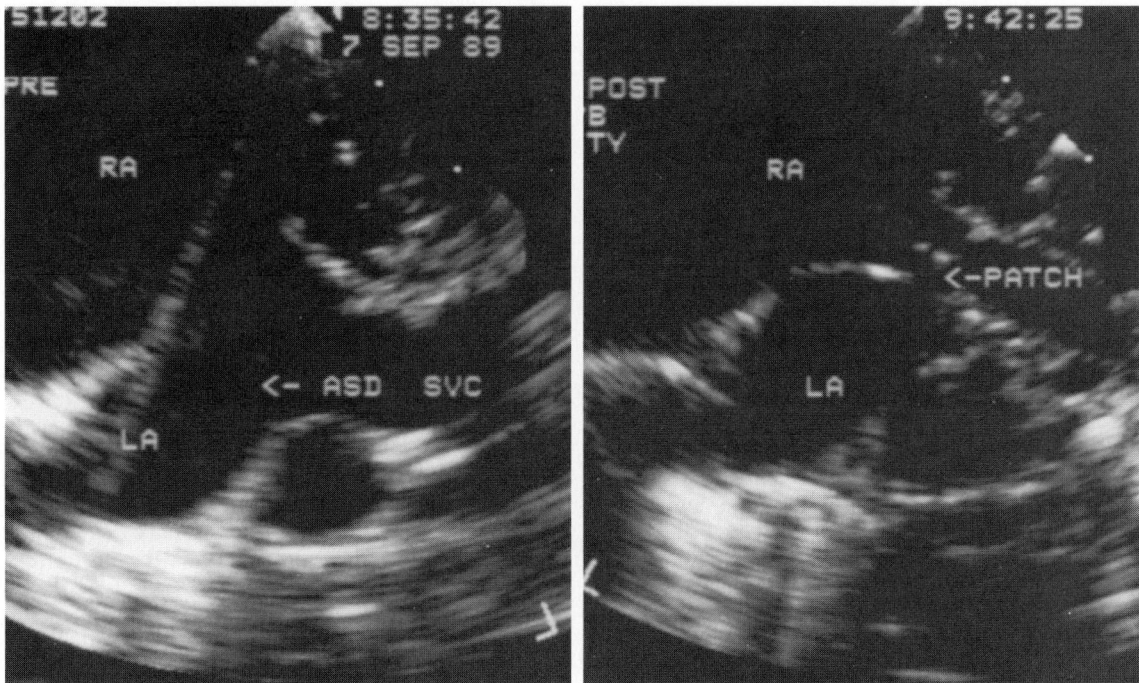

Figure 54–19. This two-dimensional echocardiogram obtained from the epicardial surface of the heart at the time of surgery nicely demonstrates a sinus venosus ASD. It is easily appreciated that the superior vena cava (SVC) and left atrium (LA) share a common wall (arrow) and absence of this wall creates the sinus venosus defect. The right panel demonstrates reconstruction of this wall (patch) so that the left atrium is separated from the overlying SVC and right atrium (RA).

ciency, makes this a particularly morbid lesion with low expectation for acceptable untreated survival. A few small series have confirmed this suspicion[13, 54, 79] and suggest that 80% of unoperated patients will die by 2 years of age. Even an infant who survives to be 1 year old has only a 15% chance of living to the age of 5 years. These patients die of the impact of overwhelming congestive heart failure with respiratory distress, arrhythmias, or pulmonary infections. Those infants who do survive do so by elevation of their pulmonary artery pressures to protect against the intracardiac shunt. They almost invariably go on to develop irreversible changes of pulmonary hypertension at a young age,[84, 128] and this can be expected in up to 90% of patients who survive until their first birthday. Patients with Down syndrome (a frequent association with complete AV canal de-

fects) may demonstrate more rapid development to irreversible changes of pulmonary hypertension, and this has been described to occur in these patients within the first 2 months of life.[2, 127, 128] Although patients who develop severe pulmonary hypertension have less intracardiac shunting and seem to be clinically improved, their outlook for the future is dismal since corrective surgery becomes extremely risky if not impossible. It is also of interest that 14% of women with repaired AV canal defects who survive to have children risk passing along a congenital heart defect (usually tetralogy of Fallot or an AV canal defect) to their offspring.[31] This is substantially higher than the 2% to 4% risk that mothers with other types of congenital heart defects have of giving birth to children with a heart lesion.[54]

PHYSIOLOGY

The natural history just described is created by abnormal blood flow patterns that result in excessive pulmonary blood flow, increased cardiac (especially right ventricular) work, and the potential risk of bidirectional intracardiac shunting with paradoxical emboli. The direction of an intracardiac shunt is predominantly determined by compliance of the downstream chamber. In the case of an ASD, the downstream chambers are the ventricles. Compliance is a reflection of distensibility or the amount of pressure necessary to add volume to a chamber. In infants, the right and left ventricles are essentially equivalent in muscle mass and equally distensible. However, because pulmonary vascular resistance falls shortly after birth, the right ventricle lags behind the left in hypertrophy of muscle mass and it becomes a more compliant, or distensible, chamber. Flow through an ASD that occurs during diastole, with the AV valves open, will move toward the direction of least resistance. The right ventricle offers less resistance to filling than does the left ventricle; and, therefore, most of the flow through an ASD moves from left to right across the atrial septum and causes volume loading of the right ventricle, which easily distends to accom-

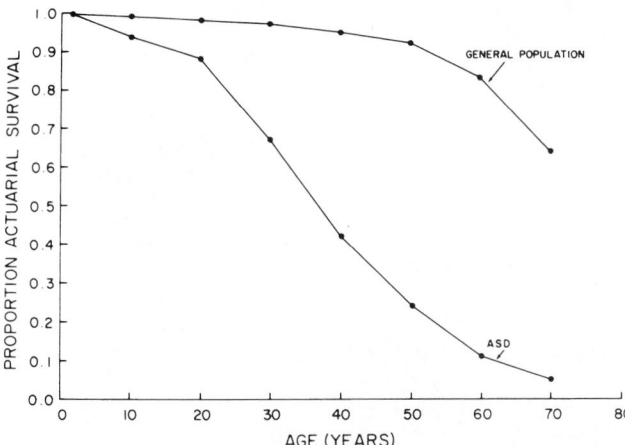

Figure 54–20. Actuarial survival for patients with unrepaired ASDs compared with an age-matched general population. These survival curves clearly demonstrate a marked increase in the mortality rate occurring beyond 20 years of age for these patients with unrepaired ASDs. (From Kirklin, J. W., and Barratt-Boyes, B. G.: Cardiac Surgery. New York, Churchill Livingstone, 1986.)

modate this load.[20] Even during systole, with the AV valves closed, pressure differences between the left and right atria favor flow from left to right.[63] Despite this predominant left-to-right shunt, there are moments during the cardiac cycle when the instantaneous pressure gradient favors right-to-left flow across an ASD. Furthermore, the dynamics by which the inferior vena cava empties into the right atrium will usually cause some *streaming* of inferior vena caval blood across the defect into the left atrium. This can be demonstrated easily with color flow Doppler mapping (Fig. 54–21) and is the reason that microcavitation studies are such a sensitive indicator of atrial septal shunts.[17, 34, 63] The total amount of shunt flow across the defect is determined by the compliance of the ventricles[20] and not by the size of the defect (unless the defect is small and restrictive to free flow). Thus, quantitation of the shunt does not predict the size of the defect.[63] Pulmonary blood flow may be three to four times systemic flow (Qp:Qs=3 or 4:1) in patients who are otherwise asymptomatic. In patients with large shunts, the right ventricular volume is usually increased and the interventricular septum may be displaced into the left ventricle. Although this may appear to create some diminished left ventricular function, left ventricular performance should be normal after closure of the defect,[19, 122] unless it is abnormally small and hypoplastic.[14] Right ventricular function, however, may be affected by the chronic volume loading and distention.[19, 129]

The long-term ability of the right ventricle to recover normal function is probably related to the age of the patient at the time of repair, with those undergoing ASD closure before 10 years of age having a better likelihood of achieving normal right ventricular function.[66, 86] In addition, the increase in right ventricular stroke volume causes relative stenosis across the pulmonary valve,[121] which can produce gradients as high as 40 mm. Hg (though usually only as high as 15–20 mm. Hg), and this can cause some degree of right ventricular hypertrophy over time. As the right ventricle hypertrophies,

it becomes less compliant and the size of the left-to-right intracardiac shunt decreases. Patients may then become less symptomatic, despite the fact that their heart is actually more impaired.

A small number of patients with ASDs develop pulmonary hypertension, and this also will lead to hypertrophy of the right ventricle and diminishment of the left-to-right shunt. Patients with ASDs living at lower altitudes can be expected to have comparatively lower pulmonary artery pressures than those living at higher altitudes. For example, the average mean pulmonary artery pressure in a group of patients younger than 20 years old living in regions below 2000 feet was 18.7 mm. Hg, whereas in a comparable group living at 4000 feet, the mean pressure was 30.4 mm. Hg.[28] As the right ventricular compliance begins to approach that of the left ventricle, the intracardiac shunt may dissipate and the patient may have a Qp:Qs equal to 1:1. This shunt ratio actually reflects net pulmonary versus net systemic blood flow and does not mean that there is no shunting across the defect. In reality, patients who develop pulmonary hypertension, which limits the left-to-right shunt flow, begin to develop right-to-left shunting during some phases of the cardiac cycle that balances out the left-to-right shunting that still continues during the remaining phases; even though they have no net increase in pulmonary flow versus systemic flow, they do have bidirectional shunting of blood inside the heart and the right-to-left component results in a significant quantity of desaturated (unoxygenated) blood crossing to the systemic circulation, which causes these patients to be mildly cyanotic. This is often a sign that the defect is no longer correctable.

Without the development of significant right ventricular hypertrophy from pulmonary stenosis or pulmonary hypertension, the intracardiac shunt continues to produce excessive pulmonary blood flow with increased blood return to the left atrium. Most of this blood shunts back across the ASD to produce volume loading of the right atrium and ventricle with signs of congestive heart failure. Atrial arrhythmias

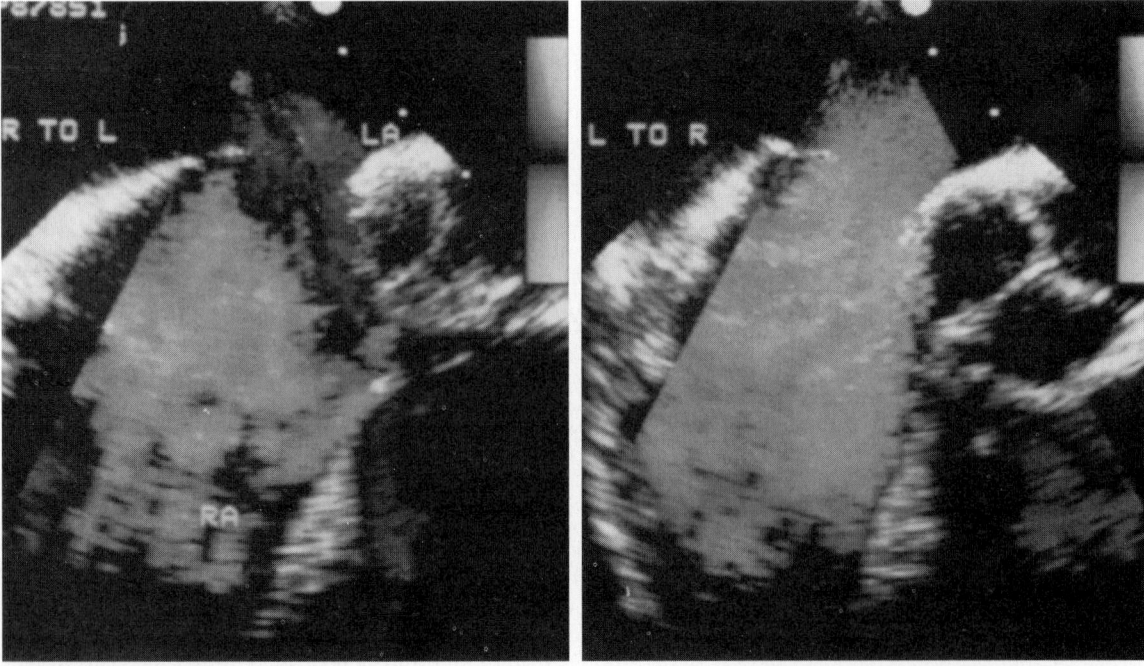

Figure 54–21. This transesophageal color flow Doppler image demonstrates the ability of ASDs to shunt right to left (left panel) as well as left to right (right panel) at various stages of the cardiac cycle. The phase of the cardiac cycle during which the image was obtained is demonstrated by placement of a bar over the electrocardiogram that is reproduced at the lower portion of each image. In this case, flow toward the transducer (which is represented by the white dot at the top of each panel) appears to be red whereas flow away from the transducer appears as blue. Therefore, right-to-left shunting appears as red flow (toward the transducer) and left-to-right shunting appears as blue flow (away from the transducer). RA, right atrium; LA, left atrium.

occur over time and seem to be related to the right atrial distention. Of interest is the fact that these arrhythmias do not seem to resolve after closure of the defect.[54, 71, 97, 104] As patients with ASDs grow older, they may begin to develop coronary artery disease; and the concomitant decrease of left ventricular function and compliance may actually result in an increase in left-to-right shunting across a previously insignificant ASD.[54] The increase in right ventricular work can also exacerbate symptoms from coronary artery lesions resulting in ischemia, infarction, or accelerated signs of congestive heart failure.[54, 121]

The physiology of sinus venosus ASDs is similar to that described for secundum ASDs. However, the fact that the pulmonary venous return is often directed into the right atrium in these patients contributes to the observation that sinus venosus ASDs are usually physiologically significant.

The physiology of shunting in partial AV canal defects (ostium primum ASDs) is also similar to that for secundum ASDs, though the degree of mitral valve insufficiency plays a large role in determining the severity of the lesion. The direction of the shunt is controlled by the differences between right and left ventricular compliance. However, when there is substantial mitral insufficiency, the regurgitant jet is often aimed directly into the right atrium across the absent AV septum (Fig. 54–22). This not only increases the shunt load to the right side but also requires an obligatory increase in left ventricular stroke volume to maintain forward cardiac output. The resultant demands on left and right ventricular function can hasten the onset of biventricular heart failure, and patients with ostium primum defects and moderate to severe mitral insufficiency usually present with symptoms early in life.

Patients with a complete AV canal defect also have a large interventricular communication, which dramatically alters the physiology of this lesion compared with isolated atrial level defects. Atrial shunting occurs for all of the reasons cited earlier, and this shunt is increased in patients with severe AV valve incompetence. However, it is the shunting at the ventricular level that produces the more serious problems. This shunting occurs at systemic pressures and leads to right ventricular and pulmonary artery pressures that equal left ventricular and systemic arterial pressures. To pro-

tect against torrential pulmonary blood flow, pulmonary vascular resistance quickly rises and may become fixed and permanent during the first months of life.[2, 127] Although elevated pulmonary vascular resistance decreases the net left-to-right shunt at the ventricular level (by decreasing compliance of the pulmonary vascular bed), permanent histologic changes prevent the pulmonary arteries from resuming normal resistance when the shunt is surgically repaired and these changes can impose an intolerable impedance to flow that prevents the right ventricle from performing acceptably as a pulmonary ventricle once the intracardiac defect is correctly partitioned. Once the pulmonary vascular resistance is allowed to attain this level (greater than 12 units per square meter),[54] the defects are usually considered to be inoperable, since the right ventricle will no longer be capable of supporting pulmonary blood flow once the ventricular septal defect is closed and the assistance of the left ventricle is blocked. Although the Qp:Qs of a complete AV canal defect may not be higher than in a patient with a secundum ASD, the increase in pulmonary artery pressure (and resistance) makes the impact of the shunt far more deleterious over the short term.

PHYSICAL FINDINGS

Patients with secundum, sinus venosus, or ostium primum ASDs may have few physical findings. They may be smaller than normal, as seen on serial growth charts. The patient may otherwise appear healthy and may have no disturbing complaints. Patients with sinus venosus defects may complain of palpitations, because it is not uncommon for this defect to be associated with supraventricular dysrhythmias. If the intracardiac shunt is greater than 1.8:1, there may be a visible left parasternal heave with a palpable right ventricular lift. In some patients, this can produce a localized chest wall deformity with protuberance of the costal cartilage in the left parasternal region. Auscultation reveals prominence of the first heart sound with fixed splitting of the second heart sound. (This fixed splitting of the second heart sound is not present in patients with partial anomalous pulmonary venous return if there is no associated ASD.) A soft (grade II or III) systolic ejection murmur is present in the second or

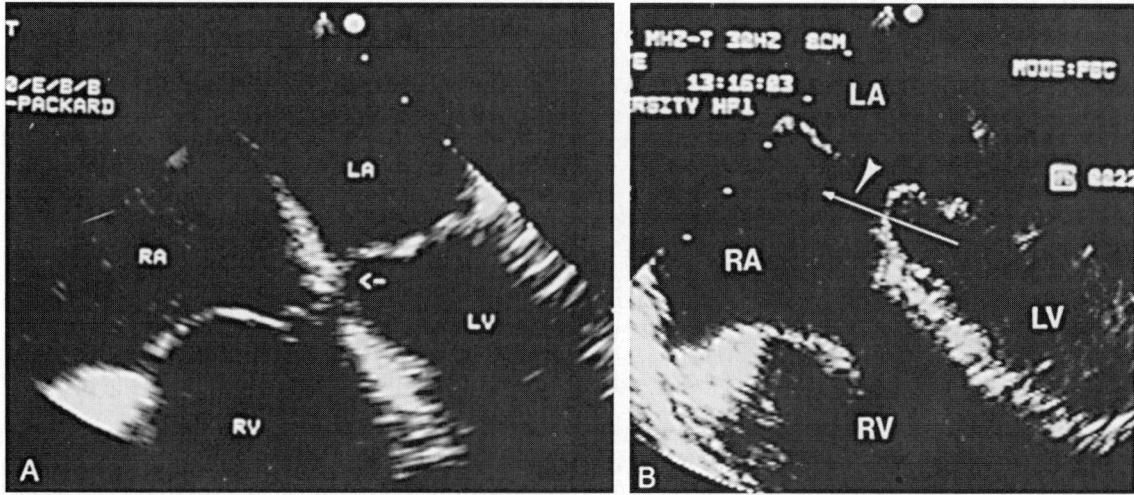

Figure 54–22. *A*, A four-chamber echocardiographic view of the heart obtained from a transesophageal probe demonstrates the left atrium (LA), right atrium (RA), right ventricle (RV), and left ventricle (LV). It is clearly appreciated that the tricuspid valve attaches closer toward the apex of the heart than the mitral valve in this normal situation. This creates a septum between the left ventricle and right atrium (arrow) that is the normal AV septum. *B*, When the AV septum is absent, as in an ostium primum ASD, the mitral valve attaches farther toward the apex at the crest of the ventricular septum. This displacement of the mitral valve is often associated with a cleft in the anterior leaflet that enables direct regurgitant shunting between the left ventricle to the right atrium (thin arrow). In addition, the absence of the AV septum enables intra-atrial shunting to occur as well (thick arrowhead). LA, left atrium; RA, right atrium; RV, right ventricle; LV, left ventricle; thick arrowhead, ostium primum ASD.

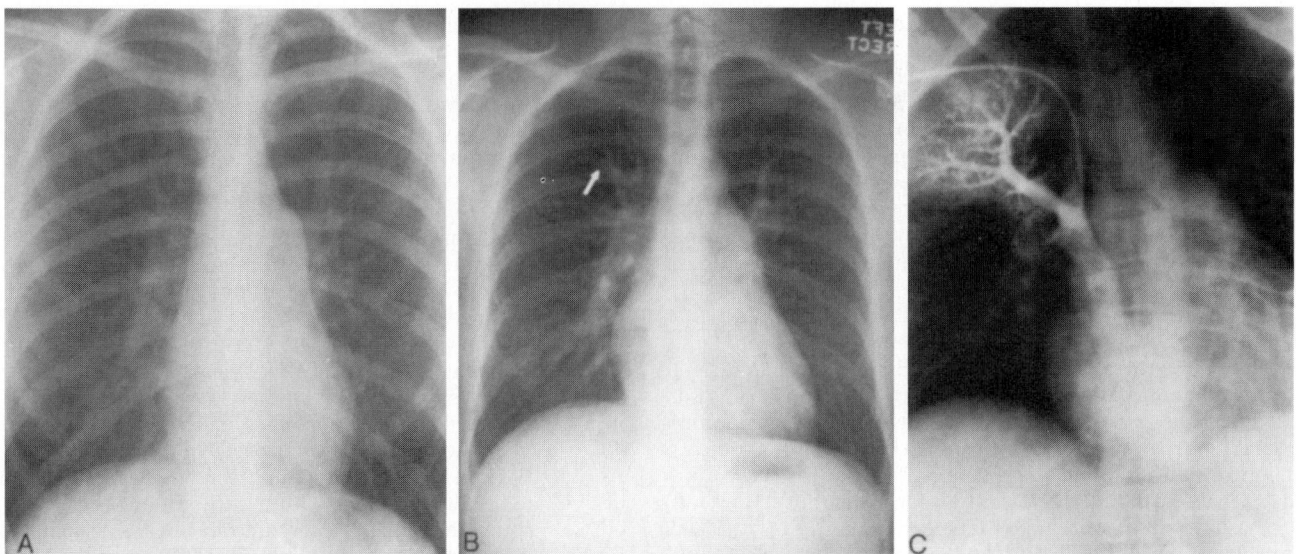

Figure 54–23. *A,* Posteroanterior chest x-ray film of a patient with a secundum ASD. Note the prominence of the pulmonary artery shadow and the increased pulmonary blood flow. *B,* This film is from a patient with a sinus venosus defect and suggests anomalous drainage of the right superior pulmonary vein to the superior vena cava (arrow). *C,* This latter suspicion is confirmed by direct injection of the anomalous right superior pulmonary vein.

third left intercostal space from the increased flow across the pulmonary valve. A mid-diastolic tricuspid flow rumble may also be audible in the fourth or fifth left intercostal space. If the patient is in congestive heart failure, there may be jugular venous distention, hepatomegaly, and cardiomegaly. Increased intensity of the right ventricular lift with accentuation of the second heart sound suggests the presence of elevated pulmonary artery pressures and alerts the clinician to the possibility of increased pulmonary vascular resistance. In patients with ostium primum defects and moderate to severe mitral insufficiency, there are usually more pronounced signs of heart failure and pulmonary edema may be present and detected by the appearance of bibasilar rales. These patients usually have pronounced cardiomegaly and auscultation discloses a distinct, apical pansystolic murmur of mitral regurgitation.

Patients with complete AV canal defects usually present in severe heart failure during the first year of life with tachypnea, poor feeding, failure to grow, and evidence of poor peripheral perfusion. This presentation usually parallels a normal postnatal fall in pulmonary vascular resistance. Occasionally, however, pulmonary vascular resistance does not fall to the point that the shunt becomes clinically apparent and as changes of fixed pulmonary vascular disease take over, the patient may seem clinically well. However, signs of right ventricular overload (parasternal lift with signs of a hyperactive precordium), interventricular shunting (loud systolic murmur), and pulmonary hypertension (loud second heart sound) should be obvious and should lead to correct diagnosis.

The risk of subacute bacterial endocarditis from a simple secundum or sinus venous ASD is slight; and when it occurs, it is usually on the pulmonary valve or right ventricular outflow tract.[121] Patients with partial or complete AV canal defects present a greater risk for subacute bacterial endocarditis because of the "jet" lesions created by the AV valve incompetence and the interventricular shunting. It is possible for these patients to first present with signs of intracardiac infection. Presentation with paradoxical emboli or cerebral infarction can also occur in any of the above defects but is unusual.[57, 88]

DIAGNOSIS

Patients in whom an ASD is suspected should have a chest film, which usually shows mild to moderate cardiomegaly, prominence of the pulmonary artery shadow, and increased pulmonary vascular markings (Fig. 54–23). The left ventricle and aorta should be normal or slightly smaller than normal. The roentgenographic appearance of a secundum ASD is indistinguishable from that of a sinus venosus ASD, unless the right superior pulmonary vein can be identified lying more superiorly than normal, in which case the diagnosis of sinus venosus ASD with partial anomalous pulmonary venous return can be entertained (see Fig. 54–23).[57] Patients with ostium primum ASDs have similar-appearing chest films, although moderate or severe mitral insufficiency may produce prominence of the left ventricle with distinctive biventricular cardiomegaly and signs of pulmonary edema (Fig. 54–24). Patients with complete AV canal defects usually have a chest x-ray consistent with severe heart failure during infancy with marked cardiomegaly and pulmonary overcirculation (Fig. 54–25). As pulmonary hypertension develops, the lung markings become clearer and the central pulmonary arteries appear larger.

The electrocardiogram shows distinctive differences between these lesions. Patients with secundum ASDs almost invariably have some degree of incomplete right bundle branch block in lead V_1. Prominent P waves may suggest atrial enlargement. The vectorcardiogram reveals a clockwise loop directed inferiorly and to the right in the frontal projection.[32] Patients with AV canal defects (partial or complete) usually demonstrate marked right ventricular hypertrophy with prolongation of the PR interval. There may be left ventricular hypertrophy as well. There is usually left axis deviation, and the vector loop in the frontal plane is counterclockwise. Although left axis deviation and a counterclockwise loop strongly suggest an AV canal defect, this pattern can occur in about 10% of patients with secundum ASDs.[57]

Diagnosis is clarified by two-dimensional echocardiography, and understanding of the physiologic alterations created by the defect is obtained with color flow mapping.[58, 100] Secun-

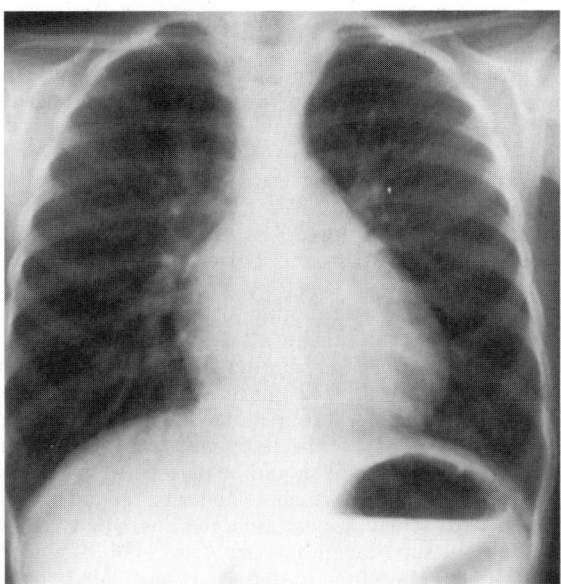

Figure 54–24. Posteroanterior chest x-ray film from a patient with an ostium primum ASD and moderate mitral regurgitation. Not only is the pulmonary artery shadow and pulmonary vascular pattern increased, but there is also left ventricular dilation as well, producing a pattern of biventricular hypertrophy and overall cardiomegaly.

dum defects are easily distinguished from ostium primum defects, and it is even possible to delineate both in the same patient. The direction of the intracardiac shunt can be visualized throughout the cardiac cycle (see Fig. 54–21). Although sinus venosus defects are difficult to visualize by transthoracic echocardiography, the addition of microcavitation to the examination assists in detection of these defects. Echocardiography can be performed from the chest wall or with the use of specially created esophageal transducers that are inserted transorally into the esophagus and advanced until

they lie directly posterior to the heart. Resolution from echocardiography is so good using currently available instruments (especially with the transesophageal approach) that precise details regarding the nature of the defect can be fully and uniquely appreciated. Echocardiography with color flow Doppler imaging is now the diagnostic modality of choice to demonstrate secundum and ostium primum defects and in most cases obviates the necessity for cardiac catheterization before surgery. In patients with ostium primum defects, the degree of mitral insufficiency is nicely demonstrated and the *cleft* in the mitral valve can usually be outlined.[10] Patients with complete AV canal defects can also be evaluated with echocardiography alone. It is easy to disclose the presence of a ventricular level shunt that distinguishes partial from complete forms of this lesion (Fig. 54–26).[117, 124] Although Doppler techniques can also predict gradients across areas of stenosis, patients suspected of having significant right or left ventricular outflow obstruction or aortic coarctation should probably receive cardiac catheterization. Infants with complete AV canal defects do not require cardiac catheterization before surgery, but patients older than 6 months of age (or older than 3 months in those with Down syndrome) should probably have cardiac catheterization to measure pulmonary artery pressures and resistances.[2, 127, 128]

Cardiac catheterization with angiography is being performed less frequently in patients with ASDs because of the superior information provided by two-dimensional echocardiography. Patients with secundum and sinus venosus defects usually can proceed to operative therapy based on results of echocardiography alone. However, patients with ASDs who are older than 40, especially if chest pain is one of the presenting complaints, should be catheterized to exclude pulmonary hypertension (usually not present if the color flow Doppler image shows predominantly left-to-right shunting) and undergo coronary angiography to evaluate the coronary arteries. Cardiac catheterization is also indicated for patients with secundum or primum defects who have a pronounced second heart sound. Catheterization provides data that enables calculation of pulmonary and systemic blood flow so that the magnitude of the intracardiac shunt can be quantified. A Qp:Qs of greater than 1.5:1 is usually considered an indication for surgical closure of an ASD.[40, 57] Moreover, the degree of pulmonary hypertension, when pres-

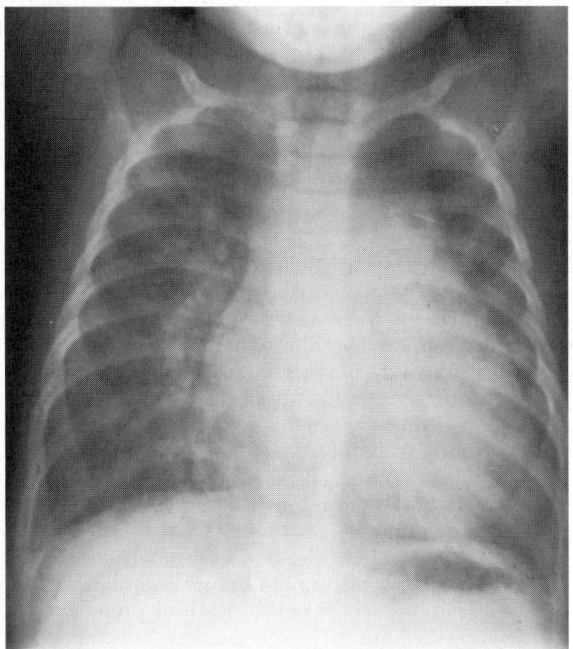

Figure 54–25. This infant with a complete AV canal defect shows cardiomegaly, pulmonary overcirculation, and congestive heart failure. This pattern seen early in infancy is highly suggestive of a complete AV canal defect.

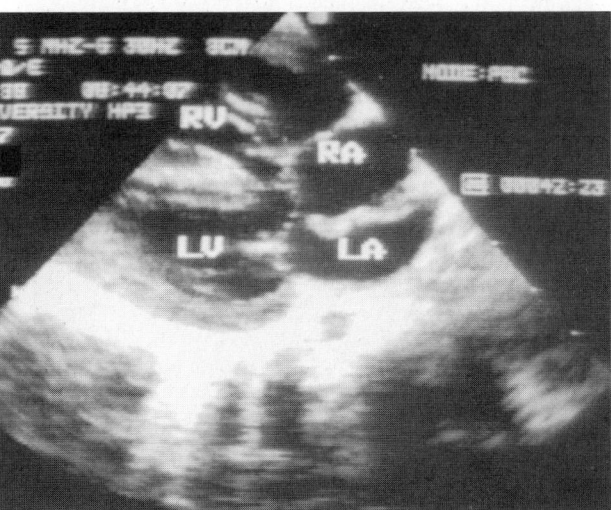

Figure 54–26. This four-chamber echocardiogram clearly reveals the distinguishing features of a complete AV canal defect with a large communication above the ventricular septum and below the atrial septum through which crosses the common AV valve. LA, left atrium; LV, left ventricle; RA, right atrium; RV, right ventricle.

ent, can be measured and an objective reflection of pulmonary vascular resistance can be calculated. Patients with pulmonary vascular resistance greater than 12 units per square meter are considered to be inoperable. If the pulmonary vascular resistance is less than 6 units per square meter correction can usually be done safely, although long-term survival may be less in patients with elevated resistance, compared with those with normal values. Patients with pulmonary resistances between 6 and 12 units may benefit from measurement of pulmonary and systemic arterial pressure changes during exercise with simultaneous calculation of shunt fractions. Patients whose systemic vascular resistance falls with an increase in right-to-left shunting during exercise may be best left uncorrected.[57] Finally, cardiac catheterization allows measurement of pressure gradients across the pulmonary and aortic outflow tracts so that in selected cases, repair of clinically relevant valvular heart lesions can be accomplished during ASD closure.[29, 60] In patients with AV canal defects, cineangiographic studies can demonstrate the elongation of the left ventricular outflow tract in relationship to the inflow tract, which produces a characteristic *goose-neck* deformity (Fig. 54–27). Although this finding is characteristic of AV canal defects, the anatomic detail provided by the less invasive echocardiographic technology has replaced the necessity of demonstrating this angiographic feature to establish the diagnosis of AV canal defect.

TREATMENT

Spontaneous closure of ASDs may occur at an early stage[21, 82] but is uncommon after the first year of life.[24, 78, 80] It is also unlikely to occur in patients with hemodynamically significant shunts that produce right ventricular enlargement and symptoms.[57] Specifically designed umbrella-like devices

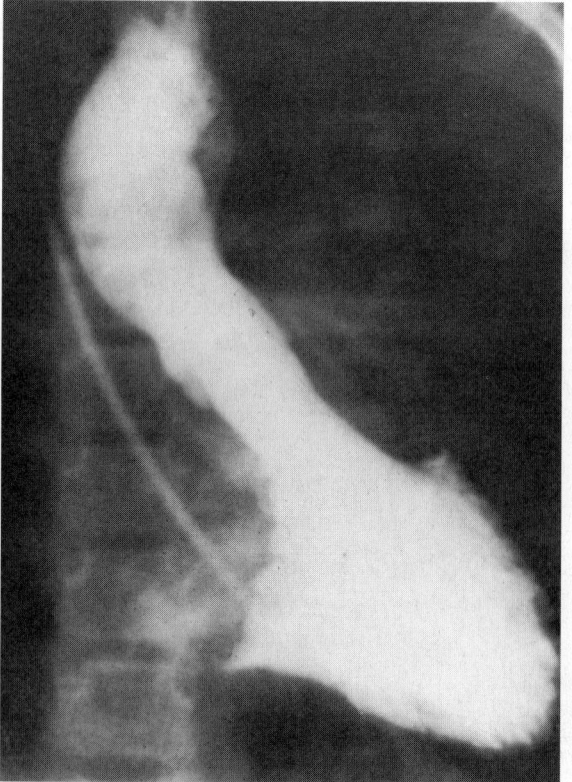

Figure 54–27. This cineangiogram of a patient with an AV canal defect shows scalloping of the AV valve and elongation of the left ventricular outflow tract (*goose-neck* deformity) that is characteristic of this lesion.

can be placed in secundum level ASDs in patients in the cardiac catheterization laboratory, but this procedure is largely experimental (in that no device is currently approved by the Food and Drug Administration) and is being used for special indications in patients who cannot otherwise safely undergo surgical intervention.[69] New devices, however, are awaiting approval, and it is very likely that catheter device closure of uncomplicated ASDs will become commonplace by the latter part of this decade. At this time, surgical closure continues to be the method of choice for hemodynamically significant ASDs.

The safety of modern cardiopulmonary bypass (CPB) techniques has antiquated previous approaches to ASDs. The most common approach is through a median sternotomy, though exposure through a right anterolateral thoracotomy does provide excellent exposure for correction of these defects. Once the chest has been opened and the anatomy exposed, careful inspection should be performed. Right atrial and right ventricular enlargement should be obvious and the pulmonary artery may appear enlarged compared with the aorta. The right superior pulmonary veins should be identified and their connection to the heart evaluated. If they appear to be more horizontal in position than normal, or if they seem to drain to the lateral aspect of the superior vena cava, then it is likely that the patient has a sinus venosus defect; and this information can help direct cannulation for CPB. Once the anatomy has been carefully examined and the pulmonary venous drainage evaluated, the patient is ready to be placed on CPB. Arterial perfusion is usually best obtained by direct cannulation of the aorta, although the femoral artery is an acceptable alternative, especially in older patients if a right thoracotomy approach is being used. In most cases, each vena cava should be cannulated so that the patient can be placed on total bypass to allow easy visualization of intracardiac anatomy. The venous return cannulae can be advanced into the vena cavae through insertion sites in the right atrium, or the vena cavae can each be cannulated directly. The decision of where to place the venous return cannulae depends, in part, on the nature of the defect being repaired. Before CPB, it is helpful to perform intraoperative echocardiography with Doppler color flow imaging to clearly evaluate the nature of the defect and its precise location. This can be done by either the transesophageal or the epicardial approach. This enables the surgeon to evaluate the anatomy of the particular defect, as well as ventricular function, mitral and tricuspid valve competence, and the pulmonary outflow tract anatomy before operative repair.[116, 117] It is not unusual for the pre-CPB echocardiogram to demonstrate previously unappreciated details of the patient's anatomy (including unsuspected associated defects) and to impact on the operative procedure.[117] Once the patient has been stabilized on CPB, the surgeon can open the right atrium to expose the defect. To avoid the risk of the heart ejecting air into the systemic circulation, the heart should be electrically fibrillated before atriotomy. An alternative technique is to cross-clamp the aorta and infuse cold cardioplegia solution to electrically and mechanically arrest the heart.

Repair of a secundum ASD is best performed through an oblique atriotomy, avoiding the sinoatrial node (Fig. 54–28). The intra-atrial anatomy is inspected for the presence of other defects. It is important for the surgeon to understand the anatomy of the conduction system so that injury to the AV node can be avoided (see Fig. 54–28). Secundum ASDs can be closed primarily with running suture technique (Fig. 54–29A) or by using a patch of pericardium or prosthetic material (see Fig. 54–29B and C). Large defects that require some tension to approximate the borders are best closed with patch material. Before completing the suture line, the left atrium is filled with saline to help reduce the risk of air embolus. The

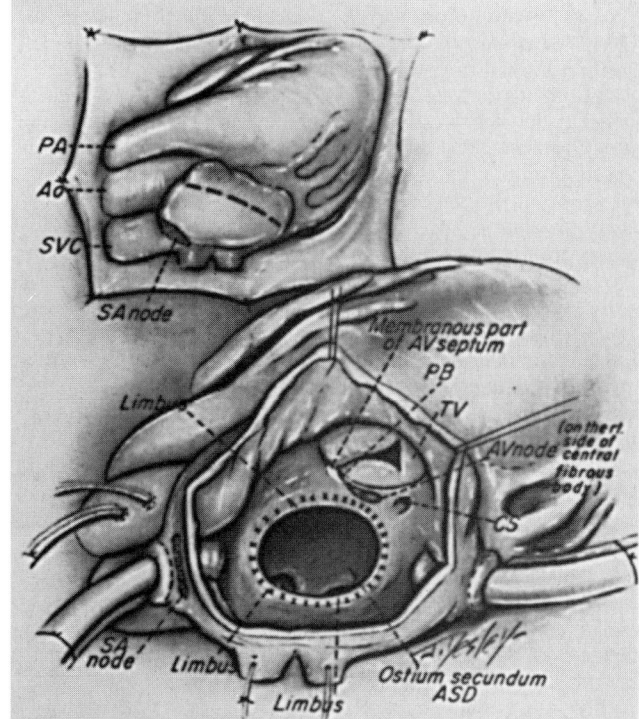

Figure 54–28. This diagram illustrates the location of the conduction tissue that must be appreciated by the surgeon during repair of an ASD. The sinoatrial node is located at the junction of the superior vena cava and right atrium and should be avoided by atrial incisions. The AV node lies in the AV septum between the coronary sinus and the tricuspid anulus. This illustration demonstrates a large secundum ASD and the Xs indicate the safe location for sutures placed to close this defect. (From Bharati, S., Lev, M., and Kirklin, J. W.: Cardiac Surgery and the Conduction System. New York, Churchill Livingstone, 1983.)

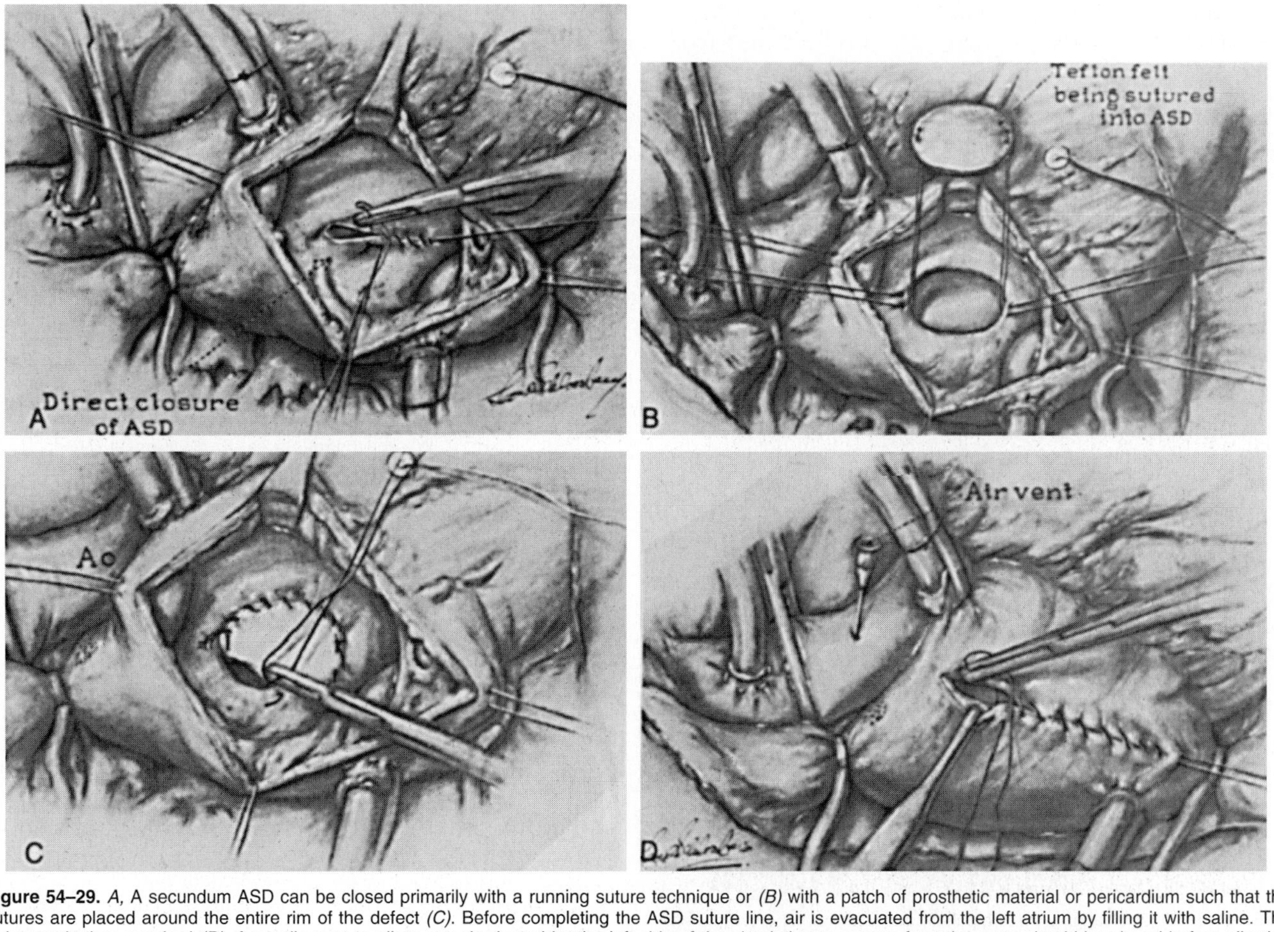

Figure 54–29. *A,* A secundum ASD can be closed primarily with a running suture technique or *(B)* with a patch of prosthetic material or pericardium such that the sutures are placed around the entire rim of the defect *(C).* Before completing the ASD suture line, air is evacuated from the left atrium by filling it with saline. The atriotomy is then repaired *(D).* A needle vent to allow any air ejected by the left side of the circulation to escape from the aorta should be placed before allowing the heart to resume normal sinus rhythm. (From Ebert, P. A.: Atlas of Congenital Cardiac Surgery. New York, Churchill Livingstone, 1989.)

right atrium is then closed, a needle vent hole is made in the aorta (to help vent any residual air that is ejected by the left ventricle), the aortic cross-clamp is removed and the heart is defibrillated (if necessary) (see Fig. 54–29D). The patient is then weaned from CPB, and the chest is closed in the usual manner over a chest tube. Since secundum defects are usually repaired with little difficulty, the CPB times are frequently short and these patients can often be extubated in the operating room.

Repair of sinus venosus ASDs is somewhat more complex. Because the defect is usually high in the atrium, over the top of the superior limbus of the septum secundum, it is sometimes helpful to directly cannulate the superior vena cava so that this venous return cannula does not interfere with exposure of the defect. With the use of this cannulation technique, most sinus venosus defects can be exposed by the same type of oblique atrial incision used to repair secundum defects (Fig. 54–30). Alternatively, the superior vena cava cannula can be placed through the tip of the right atrial appendage and the atrium can be opened with a low-lying horizontal incision that can be extended superiorly onto the superior

vena cava if necessary and still avoid the sinoatrial node (Fig. 54–31). In any case, it is essential to expose the orifices of the anomalous right superior pulmonary veins so that they can be redirected into the left atrium. These defects should always be closed with a patch (pericardium or prosthetic material) that is placed in such a manner that the superior pulmonary veins are kept below the patch and channeled through the venosus defect into the left atrium (see Figs. 54–30 and 54–31). If necessary, the superior vena cava is also patched to enable unobstructed venous flow to the right atrium over this patch.[30, 54] It is also possible to augment the superior vena cava with a flap of right atrial tissue.[54] If an oblique atriotomy is used, augmentation of the vena cava is rarely necessary. The other parts of this procedure are identical to those described earlier for secundum ASDs, although the potential that these patients have for supraventricular arrhythmias makes it advisable to leave temporary pacing wires on the heart before closing the chest. Because these procedures may take slightly longer than closure of an uncomplicated secundum defect, moderate hypothermia (28° C.) on CPB is usually recommended.

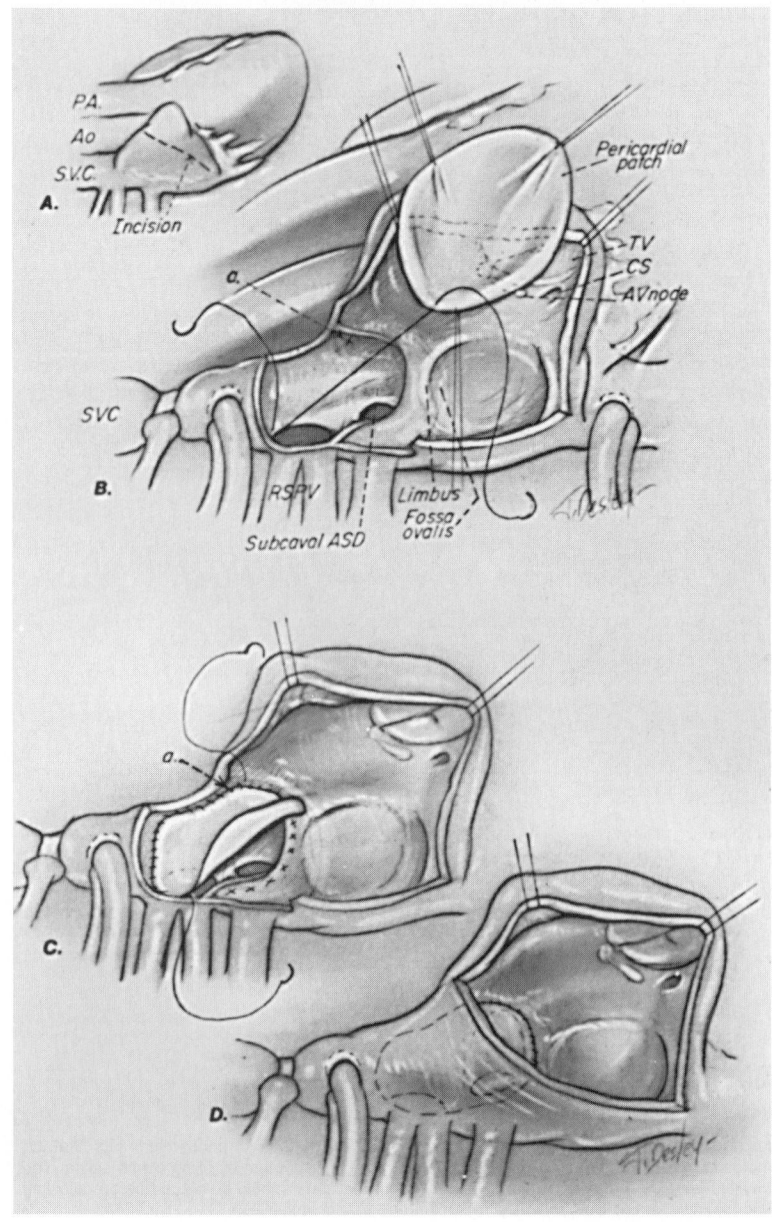

Figure 54–30. A sinus venosus ASD with anomalous return of the right superior pulmonary vein to the SVC *(A)* can be approached by an oblique atrial incision with direct caval cannulation. This defect is closed with a patch (usually of pericardium) that is placed in such a manner *(B to D)* as to redirect the pulmonary veins below the patch into the left atrium and to partition the posterior aspect of the superior vena cava so that there is no longer any atrial septal communication. (From Kirklin, J. W., and Barratt-Boyes, B. G.: Cardiac Surgery. New York, Churchill Livingstone, 1986.)

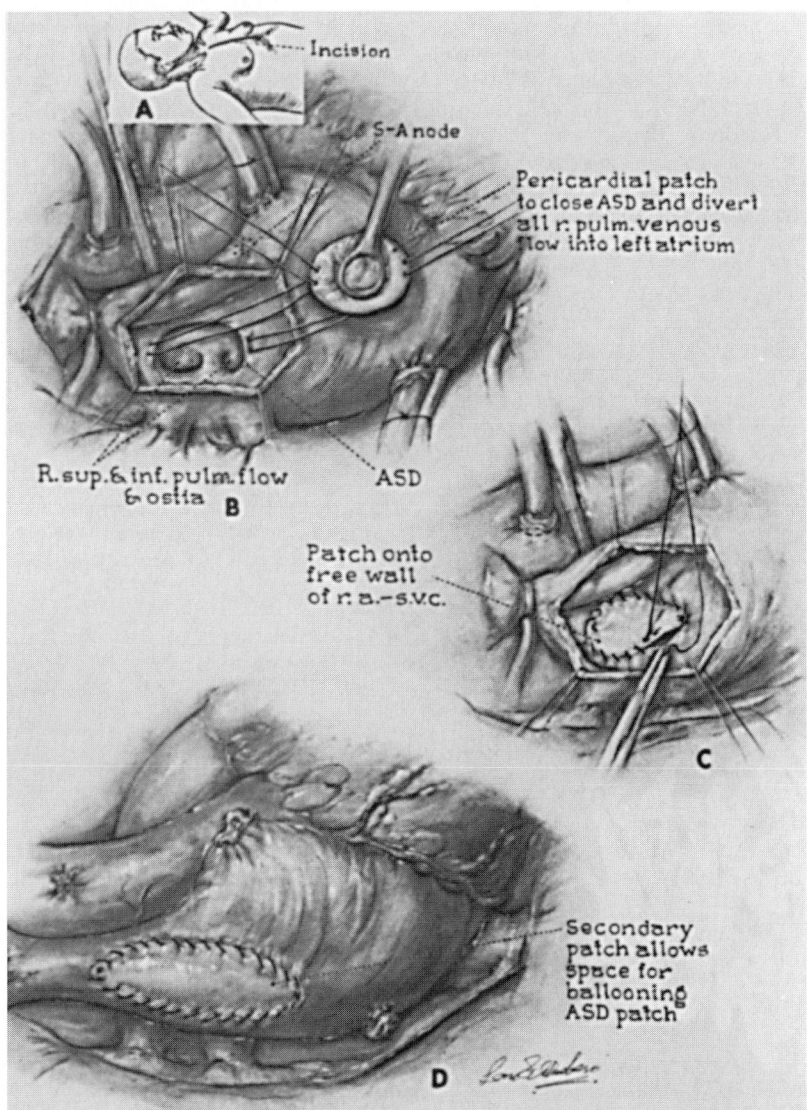

Figure 54–31. Another approach to a sinus venosus ASD is with a low, horizontally placed, atrial incision extending up onto the superior vena cava *(A* and *B).* This enables easy visualization of the defect and placement of a patch *(C)* to redirect the anomalous pulmonary venous return as well as to close the ASD. This type of incision should often be repaired with a patch of pericardium *(D)* to prevent constriction of the superior vena cava. (From Ebert, P. A.: Atlas of Congenital Cardiac Surgery. New York, Churchill Livingstone, 1989.)

Repair of AV canal defects can be even more complicated, depending on the extent of the defect. These defects are best approached through an oblique atriotomy (Fig. 54–32B). The intra-atrial anatomy is then carefully inspected because it is not unusual to have secundum level defects in association with defects of the AV septum. The mitral and tricuspid valves are inspected for clefts. The inlet portion of the ventricular septum is also carefully examined. If there is no ventricular septal defect, then the lesion is a partial AV canal (ostium primum ASD). The cleft in the mitral valve is repaired with interrupted sutures (Fig. 54–32B and C). Although there are some authorities who believe that the cleft does not require repair[4, 23, 57] and that the mitral valve will function well as a tri-leaflet structure, the long-term failure rate of this approach is not trivial, especially if there is significant preoperative valvular regurgitation, and careful approximation of the cleft anterior leaflet provides excellent long-term results.[30, 109] A recent large series reported no difference in outcome (with respect to mitral insufficiency) regardless of whether the cleft was repaired.[45] When repaired, the cleft should be closed with nonpledgeted sutures to diminish the risk of late valve dysfunction from calcification of the pledget material.[109] It is important that the surgeon be aware that hemodynamically significant left ventricular outflow obstruction can result after repair of this defect.[106, 109] The atrial septal communication is then carefully closed using a pericardial patch. Pericardium is the recommended material for this closure since residual mitral insufficiency directed against a patch made out of prosthetic material can cause significant hemolysis in the postoperative period.[51, 96, 119] Location of the AV node must be appreciated by the surgeon (Fig. 54–33), and there are several techniques available to limit damage to

this structure.[16, 62] It is advisable to leave temporary atrial and ventricular pacing wires in place to be used if necessary in the postoperative period. It is rarely necessary to leave permanent pacing wires on the heart, even if the patient is in complete heart block at the completion of the procedure (from injury to the AV node), because this damage is rarely permanent and normal conduction usually resumes within a few days following the operation.[54]

If the defect is a complete AV canal, the anatomy can look quite different than a partial AV canal. The single large AV valve bridges the canal defect and can be considered to have a superior and an inferior common leaflet (Fig. 54–34). Although the technique may vary depending on the precise anatomy of the common AV valve (Rastelli classification) (Fig. 54–35),[57, 90, 91] the principles are essentially to close the ventricular septal defect, to subdivide the common AV valves into a tricuspid and a mitral component, and to suspend these newly created valves from the top of the ventricular septal defect patch. The atrial defect is then closed in the same manner as an ostium primum defect (Fig. 54–36). As with partial AV canal defects, placement of temporary pacing wires is advisable before closing the chest.

Regardless of the type of defect repaired, it is recommended that the adequacy of the surgical repair be evaluated before the patient leaves the operating room. This can be done by obtaining a right atrial or pulmonary artery oxygen saturation or by performing a dye-dilution curve. The introduction of intraoperative echocardiography with Doppler color flow imaging to evaluate surgical results provides a more specific and sensitive method to assess the quality of the repair, to direct necessary revisions before allowing the patient to leave the operating room, and to provide prognos-

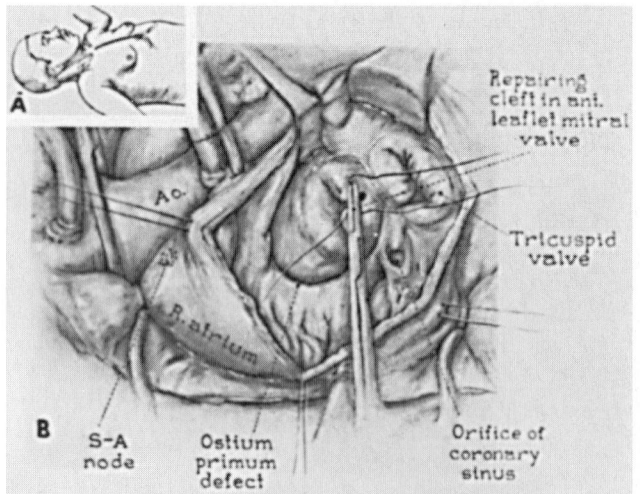

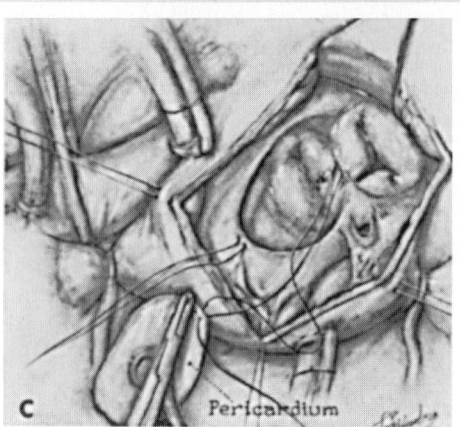

Figure 54–32. Exposure of an ostium primum ASD through an oblique atriotomy (A). The cleft in the anterior leaflet of the mitral valve is repaired with interrupted sutures (B). The defect is then closed with a patch of pericardium placed at the anulus between the mitral and tricuspid valves and sutured to the rim of the defect (C). (From Ebert, P. A.: Atlas of Congenital Cardiac Surgery. New York, Churchill Livingstone, 1989.)

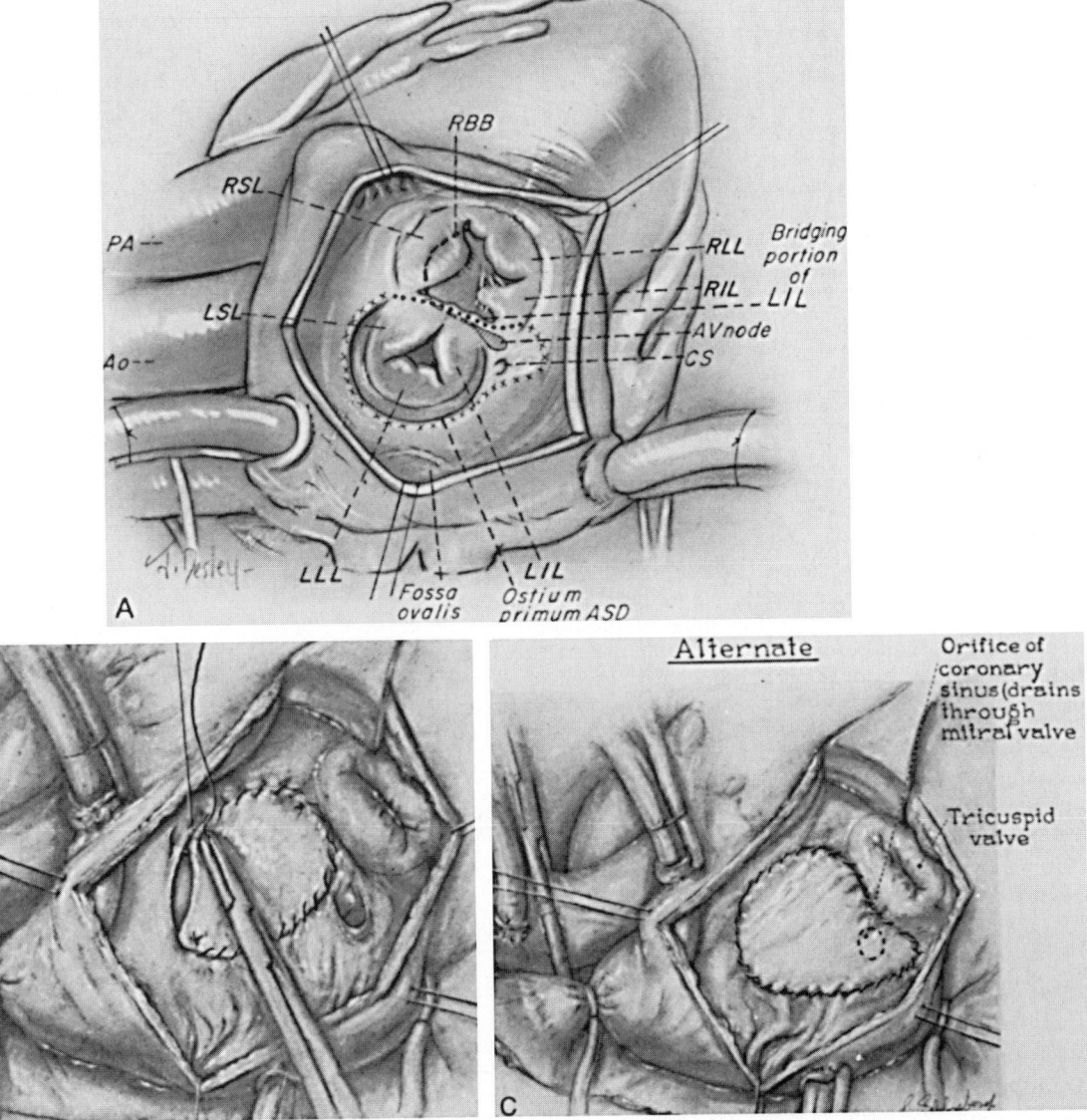

Figure 54–33. *A,* Location of the conduction system in an ostium primum ASD needs to be appreciated by the surgeon. The AV node is immediately adjacent to the coronary sinus and can be injured by sutures placed in this region. The Xs in this illustration demonstrate the location recommended by some for placement of sutures to secure the pericardial patch that closes the atrial level defect (see *C*). (From Bharati, S., Lev, M., and Kirklin, J. W.: Cardiac Surgery and the Conduction System. New York, John Wiley & Sons, 1983.) RBB, right bundle branch; RSL, right superior leaflet; LSL, left superior leaflet; LLL, left lateral leaflet; LIL, left inferior leaflet; RIL, right inferior leaflet; RLL, right lateral leaflet (all of these pertain to portions of the common AV valve); CS, coronary sinus; PA, pulmonary artery. *B,* Placement of a pericardial patch to close an ostium primum ASD can be secured in such a manner as to keep the coronary sinus on the right atrial side. Sutures can be carefully placed to avoid injuring the AV node. *C,* Alternatively (and as demonstrated by the Xs in *A*), a pericardial patch can be placed to avoid the AV node; and utilizing this technique, the coronary sinus remains on the left atrial side of the circulation. The small right-to-left shunt created by this procedure is hemodynamically and clinically insignificant unless a left superior vena cava drains to the coronary sinus. (*B* and *C* from Ebert, P. A.: Atlas of Congenital Cardiac Surgery. New York, John Wiley & Sons, 1983.)

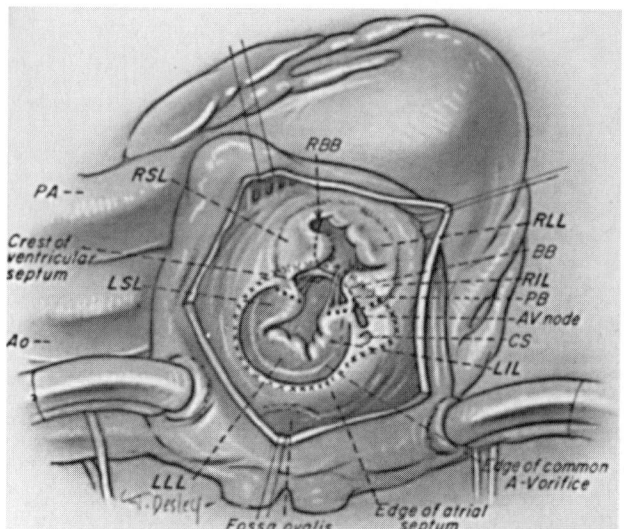

Figure 54-34. Location of the conduction system and anatomy of the AV valve in a patient with a complete AV canal defect. The abbreviations are the same as those in Figure 54-33A. The AV valve "bridges" the common atrial and ventricular chamber with free communication below and above the valve. (From Bharati, S., Lev, M., and Kirklin, J. W.: Cardiac Surgery and the Conduction System. New York, Churchill Livingstone, 1983.)

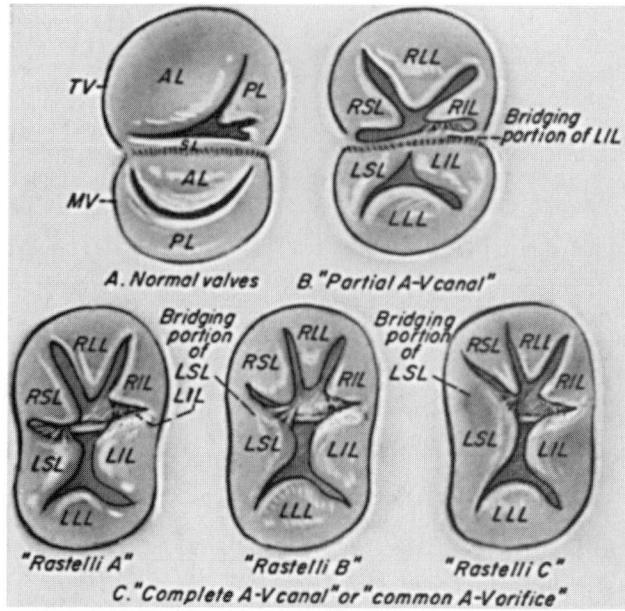

Figure 54-35. The anatomy of the AV valves as classified by Rastelli from the Mayo Clinic. A complete AV canal is classified as Rastelli Type A, B, or C depending on the attachment and nature of the superior bridging leaflet. Type A is distinguished by a superior bridging leaflet that is split in its middle and attached to the crest of the ventricular septum. A Rastelli Type B lesion has a superior bridging leaflet that is less evenly split but remains attached to the ventricular septal crest. A Rastelli Type C defect has an essentially unsplit superior bridging leaflet that is not attached to the crest of the ventricular septum. (From Kirklin, J. W., Pacifico, A. D., and Kirklin, J. K.: The surgical treatment of atrioventricular canal defects. In Arciniegas, E. [Ed.]: Pediatric Cardiac Surgery. Chicago, Year Book Medical Publishers, 1985.)

tic information regarding the likelihood for an optimal long-term outcome (Fig. 54-37).[114-117]

Special Situations. AV canal defects are frequently repaired in infants and small children because of the severe and life-threatening symptoms that can exist in the first year of life. In these small patients, the technique of profound hypothermia (18° C.) with periods of total circulatory arrest (TCA) has been used by many surgical groups with excellent results. This enables the surgeon to work in a bloodless field that is unencumbered by distortion produced from the cannulae necessary to sustain CPB. Although the effects of these techniques on long-term neuropsychiatric development remain obscure, there is an increasing body of information that prolonged periods of TCA, even at temperatures at or below 18° C., can be associated with impaired cerebral metab-

olism and altered neurologic outcome.[7, 42, 83] Nevertheless, using improved methodology, it appears that periods of TCA at 18° C. can be well tolerated by infants for periods as long as 60 minutes,[48, 49, 52, 53, 72, 73, 101] and perhaps even longer. These clinical and experimental investigations continue to elucidate our understanding of this fascinating alternative technique, and the role for deep hypothermic circulatory arrest in the future will in large part be determined by the effects of these alterations to the technique on eventual neurologic outcome.

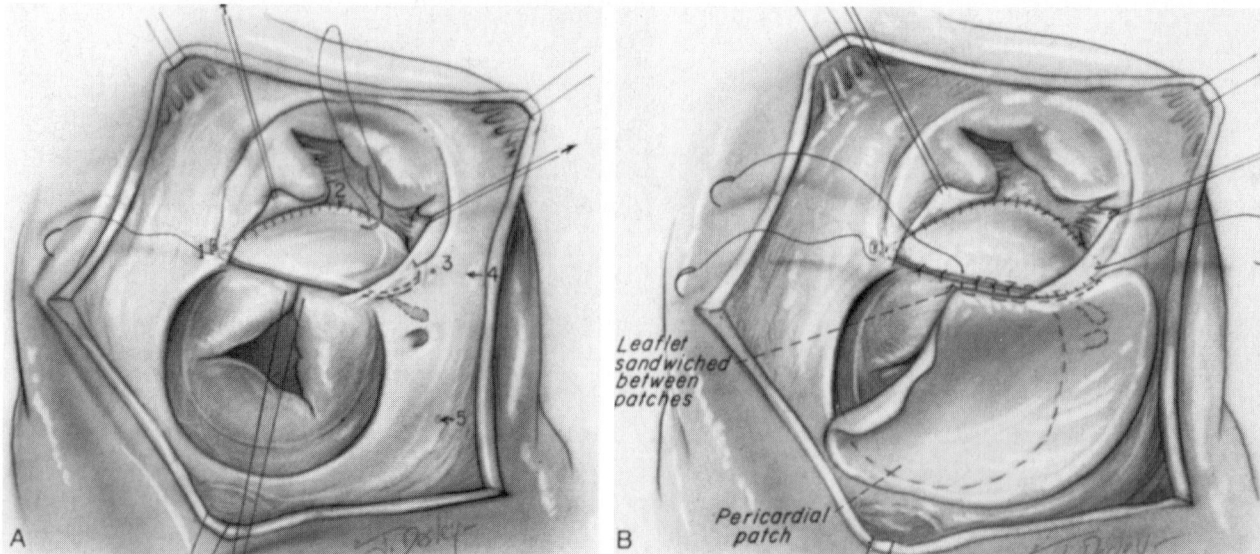

Figure 54-36. A complete AV canal can be closed by placing two separate patches to close the ventricular septal defect (A) separately from the ASD (B). The valve leaflets are suspended from the point where these two patches are attached. (From Kirklin, J. W., and Barratt-Boyes, B. G.: Cardiac Surgery. New York, Churchill Livingstone, 1986.)

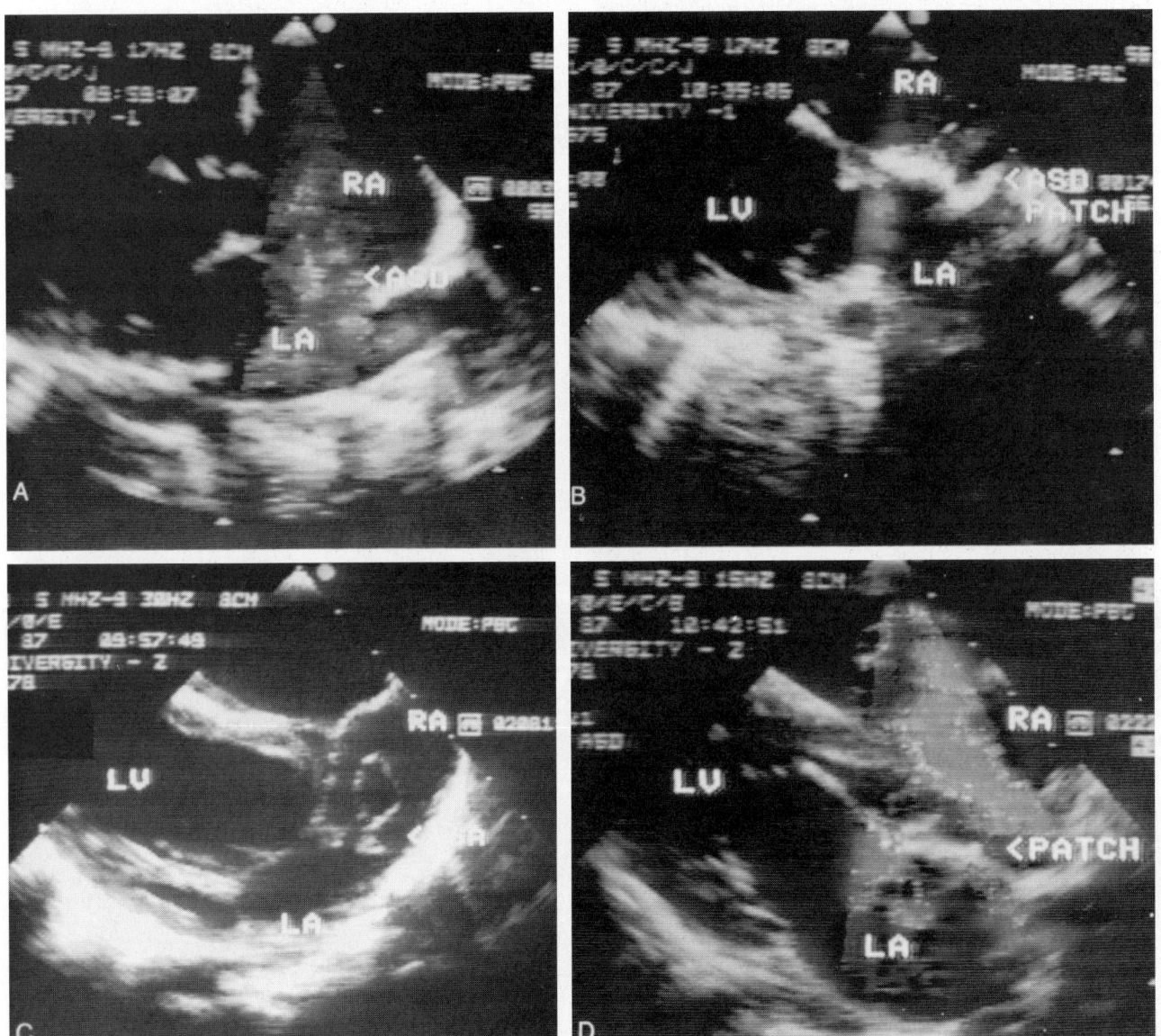

Figure 54–37. These intraoperative color flow Doppler examples illustrate the ability of this technology to provide anatomic detail of the defect before repair as well as to indicate the quality of the reconstruction before the patient leaves the operating room. *A,* A large secundum level ASD with a substantial left-to-right shunt shown as red flowing toward the transducer. *B,* The same patient after placement of a patch to close the defect. There is no longer any residual shunting. *C,* This intraoperative view nicely depicts a large aneurysm of the atrial septum that was also associated with an atrial level shunt. *D,* The same patient's heart before leaving the operating room. The aneurysm has been resected and the atrial septal defect has been successfully closed with a patch.

Illustration continued on following page

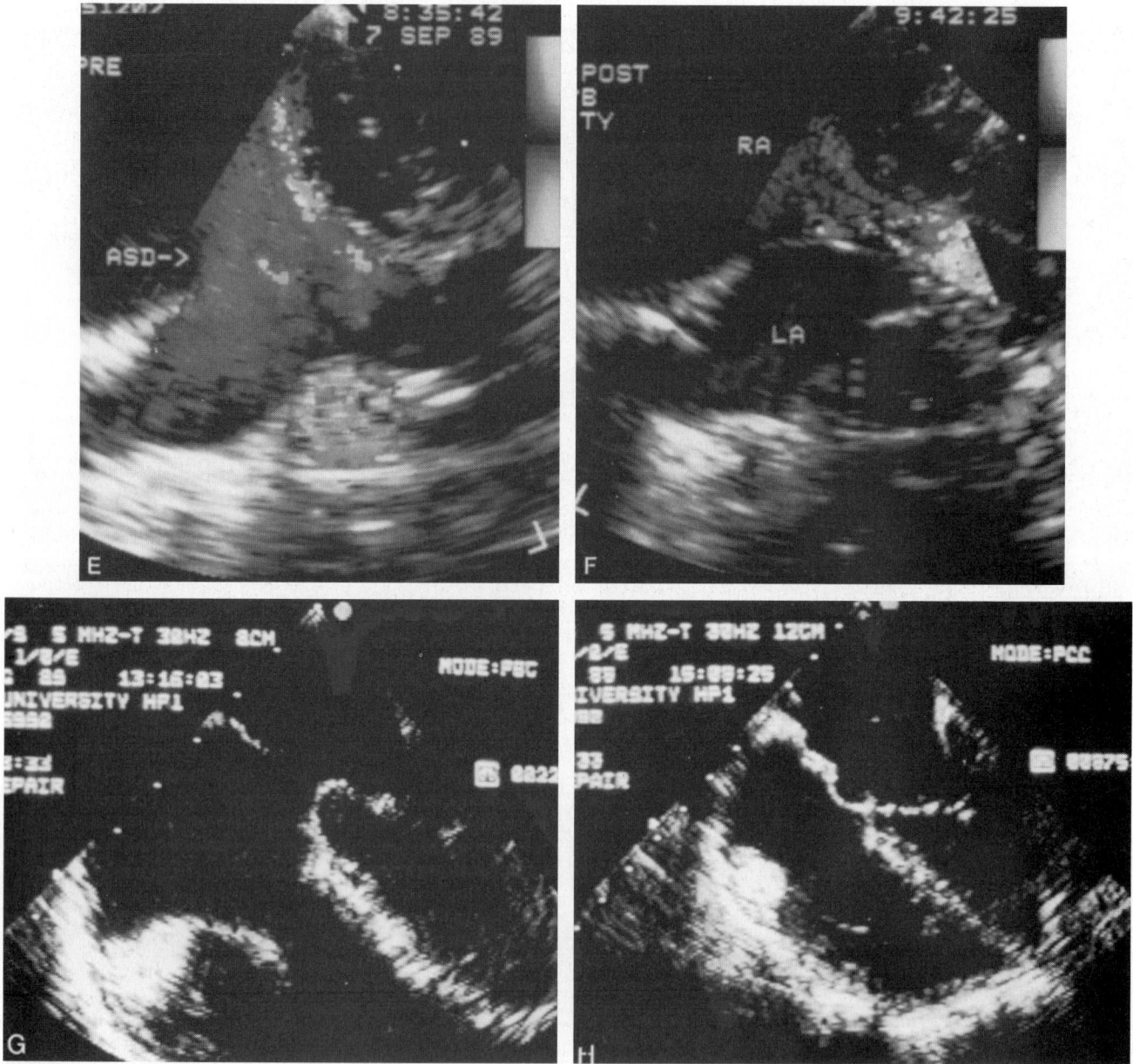

Figure 54–37 *Continued. E,* This patient has a large sinus venosus atrial septal defect with a significant left-to-right shunt. *F,* The same patient is seen after completion of repair. A pericardial patch now separates the left atrium from the overlying superior vena cava and right atrium. There is no residual shunting. *G,* A transesophageal image of an ostium primum ASD (see Fig. 54–22*B*) shown before repair and *(H)* after repair. There is now a pericardial patch closing the atrial level communication and the mitral valve has been reconstructed.

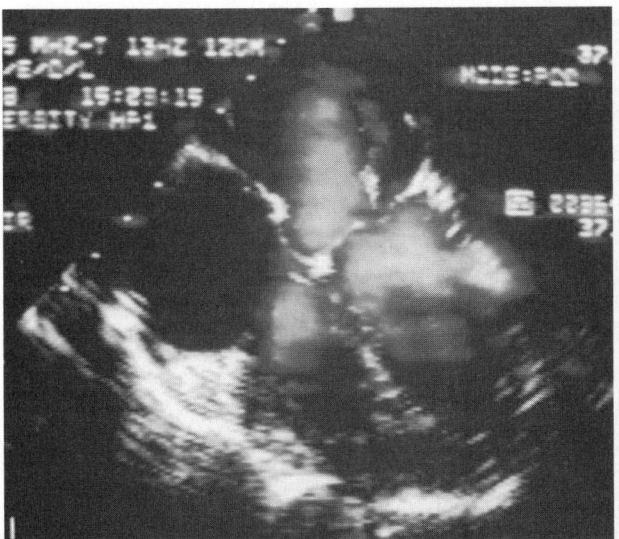

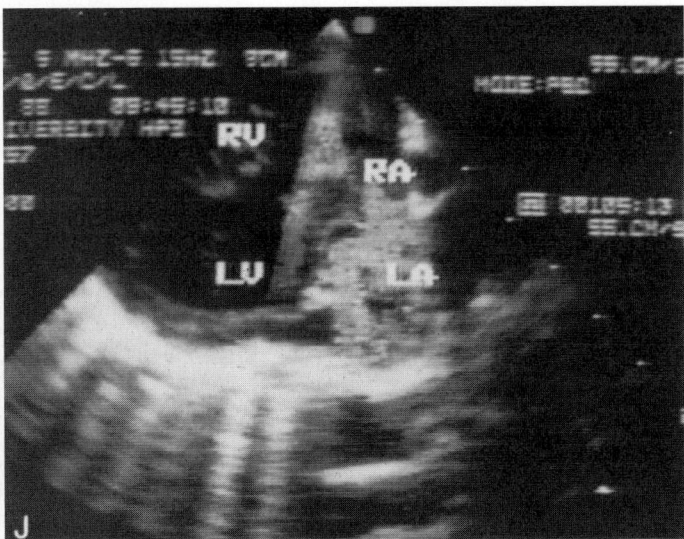

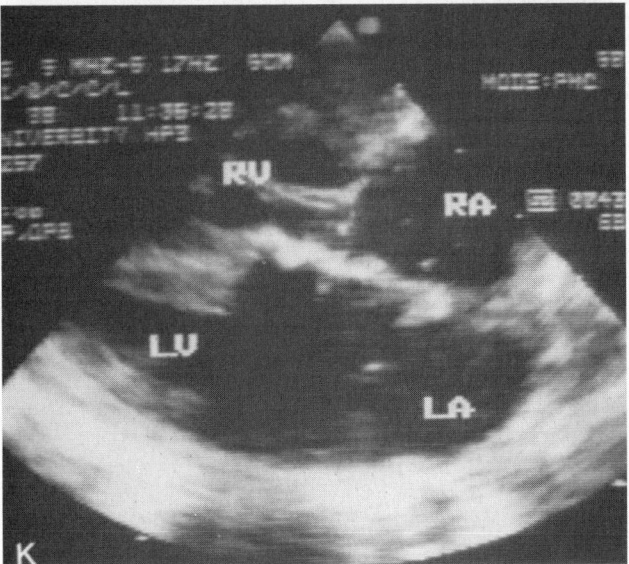

Figure 54–37 *Continued I,* This same patient shows no residual atrial level shunting and only mild residual mitral insufficiency (disclosed as the jet of red blood moving toward the transducer) after repair of the ostium primum defect. *J,* A color flow map of the large AV canal defect from the patient whose two-dimensional echocardiogram is show in Figure 54–26. This image nicely demonstrates the free communication of blood between all chambers of the heart. *K,* The same patient after removal from cardiopulmonary bypass shows that the patch now nicely divides the left and right sides of the heart and the valve is resuspended from this patch. This patient had no significant residual shunting or valvular insufficiency at the completion of the repair. (*J* and *K* from Ungerleider, R. M., et al.: Intraoperative prebypass and postbypass epicardial color flow imaging in the repair of atrioventricular septal defects. J. Thorac. Cardiovasc. Surg., *98*:90, 1989.)

Occasionally patients with ASDs have persistence of the left superior vena cava. This structure usually drains into the coronary sinus and can increase the intra-atrial venous return that confronts the surgeon once the right atrium is opened. Although this can usually be controlled with a cardiotomy sucker placed into the coronary sinus, it is an option to selectively cannulate the left superior vena cava—an alternative that might be considered if the technique of aortic cross-clamping is planned. With the patient on total CPB, the only blood that should be getting into the heart should be through the coronary sinus, and this can be eliminated by aortic cross-clamping to abolish coronary flow. If the surgeon encounters an excessive amount of blood return to the heart with the patient on total CPB, and there is no persistent left superior vena cava, then it is also important to look for a patent ductus arteriosus, a previously placed systemic pulmonary shunt, bronchial collateral vessels, a pulmonary (intralobar) sequestration, blood escaping around the snares on the vena caval cannulae, or (if the aorta is not clamped) a coronary fistula or aortic insufficiency.

Results. Operative mortality for closure of uncomplicated secundum and sinus venosus ASDs is extremely low, approaching 0% and should be no greater than 1% to 2% even in older patients.[6, 26, 31, 54, 59, 98, 120, 121] Morbidity is also extremely low. In addition to the typical problems that can occur after open-heart surgery such as bleeding or infection, potential problems more specific to repair of these particular defects include thromboembolism (usually seen in older patients with chronic atrial arrhythmias),[43] mitral insufficiency,[8, 61] neurologic deficits (most frequently from air embolism during CPB),[6, 54] and arrhythmias[18, 112] (especially in sinus venosus defects). The mortality risk is increased if the patient is older with advanced congestive heart failure[57] or when there is significant pulmonary hypertension with pulmonary vascular resistance approaching systemic resistance.[36, 121] Moreover, patients with preoperative arrhythmias are likely to have persistence of this problem even after successful closure of their defect.[6, 33, 47, 54] Long-term results are also very good, with survival statistics comparable to those of a normal, age-matched population. This is especially true if repair is undertaken before 5 years of age[57] and less predictable if repair is delayed past the age of 60.[104, 126] Symptoms, when present, almost invariably improve after repair and even patients who had no symptomatic complaints recognize a substantial improvement in their health.[28, 33, 54, 86, 87, 93, 94, 104] The likelihood of recurrence or the need for reoperation is less than 2%.[54]

Repair of AV canal defects carries a somewhat higher risk, depending on the nature and extent of the lesion, as well as the presence of any associated malformations. Uncomplicated partial AV canal defects, with minimal or no mitral incompetence, have a mortality risk that should approach 0% and that probably is no greater than 2%.[45, 57] The association of significant preoperative mitral insufficiency increases this risk to 4%.[64, 92] Long-term development of subaortic stenosis is reported and requires follow-up.[110] Overall long-term results are also affected by late mitral valve functional deterioration and arrhythmias.[41, 45, 70, 77] The operative mortality for repair of complete AV canal defects is highly inconsistent because of the wide variation in the anatomic patterns of this anomaly. Furthermore, many of these patients are operated on as infants at a time when they are critically ill. Although operative mortality in some small series is reported as 0% using current techniques to repair this defect in infants,[95] a more representative figure from larger series predicts the mortality risk to be between 3% and 13%.[24, 45, 54, 114] This risk is influenced by the nature of the common AV valve and the adequacy of the right and left ventricles.[45, 57] Pulmonary hypertension with elevation of pulmonary vascular resistance can be an early occurrence in the natural history of complete AV canal defects[2, 127, 128] and impacts on operative mortality for patients coming to surgical correction beyond 6 months of age (or even earlier in patients with Down syndrome).[35] Unless repair can be achieved by this age, it may be advisable to place a band around the pulmonary artery to limit pulmonary blood flow and protect the pulmonary vascular bed from progressing to irreversible damage. Although pulmonary artery banding is still applied with good success by some groups for small or seriously ill infants with complete AV canal defects (with repair then deferred for 1 to 2 years),[99, 125] current techniques allow safe and effective complete repair of this defect in most small infants as a one-state procedure.[9, 12, 24, 45, 54, 55, 75, 76, 114] Morbidity is similar to that cited earlier for repair of ASDs, although there are more problems with mitral valve failure and arrhythmias (including complete heart block). Failure of the AV valve occurs in as many as 7% to 10% of these patients,[45, 57] even if the preoperative valve function was good. Furthermore, this may be even more likely to result in patients after repair of partial as opposed to complete AV canal defects.[57] With enhanced appreciation of the location of the conduction tissue, permanent complete heart block is becoming an unusual complication after repair for these defects, but its likelihood is increased if AV valve failure results in the subsequent need for mitral valve replacement.[50] Long-term results are excellent, especially for patients with good mitral valve function, and survivors usually have excellent health with substantial improvement over their preoperative condition.

SELECTED REFERENCES

Bellinger, D. C., Jonas, R. A., Rappaport, L. A., et al.: Developmental and neurologic status of children after heart surgery with hypothermic circulatory arrest or low-flow cardiopulmonary bypass. N. Engl. J. Med., 332:549, 1995.
Although this article does not deal with AV canal, it addresses the outcome for patients whose operation includes a period of deep hypothermic circulatory arrest—a very common strategy employed during the repair of AV canal defects in infants. The association of some neurologic impairment with prolonged periods of circulatory arrest may lead to important alterations in the technique of repairing AV canal defects in small infants.

Bharati, S., Lev, M., and Kirklin, J. W.: Cardiac Surgery and the Conduction System. New York, John Wiley & Sons, 1983.
This carefully illustrated monograph depicts the location of important landmarks for conduction tissue in the normal heart as well as in a variety of common congenital heart defects. Careful review of these illustrations enables the surgeon to plan suture lines that will avoid damaging the important conduction tissue during intracardiac repair. This monograph is written by pioneers in this field.

Cardiology in the Young. Vol. 1. World Publishers, October 1991.
The entire issue of this journal is devoted to AV canal defects and includes numerous informative articles by several experts in the field. Topics range from anatomy to diagnosis to surgical techniques.

Ebert, P. A.: Atlas of Congenital Cardiac Surgery. New York, Churchill Livingstone, 1989.
This atlas contains exceptionally high-quality illustrations from Leon Schlossberg and combines these artistic treasures with the text written by a truly exceptional contributor to the field of congenital heart surgery. These illustrations, many of which are used in this chapter, make it easier for the student to visualize surgical methods for repair of these defects.

Hanley, F. L., Fenton, K. N., Jonas, R. A., Mayer, J. E., Cook, N. R., Wernovsky, G., and Castañeda, A. R.: Surgical repair of complete atrioventricular canal defects in infancy: Twenty year trends. J. Thorac. Cardiovasc. Surg., 106:387, 1993.
This overview of results for repair of 301 patients with complete AV canal defects between 1972 and 1992 nicely outlines the relevance of various parameters for increased risk. In this series, the risk of total correction has decreased from 25% before 1976 to 3% after 1987. Forty-six variables were examined and demonstrated that long-term results are good except for the continual risk for "mitral" valve failure requiring reoperation.

Kirklin, J. W., and Barratt-Boyes, B. G.: Cardiac Surgery, 2nd ed. New York, Churchill Livingstone, 1993.
This thorough and exhaustively complete textbook should be read by any student who is serious about the field of pediatric cardiac surgery. Drs. Kirklin and Barratt-Boyes present their extensive experience from several years of practicing surgical correction for these defects and provide important incremental risk tables describing the significance of various factors that might contribute to the overall outcome for patients with these defects.

Lillehei, C. W., Varco, R. L., Cohen, M., Warden, H. E., Patton, C., and Moller, J. H.: The first open-heart repairs of ventricular septal defect, atrioventricular communis, and tetralogy of Fallot using extracorporeal circulation by cross-circulation: A 30-year follow-up. Ann. Thorac. Surg., 41:4, 1986.
This paper provides 30-year follow-up for some of the first patients undergoing repair of atrial septal defects and AV canal defects as well as other intracardiac lesions using Lillehei's dramatic technique of cross-circulation. Of particular interest in this article is the discussion provided by many of Dr. Lillehei's students who went on to establish themselves as leaders in the field of congenital heart surgery. The poignancy of these remarks alone makes this article well worth reading.

Rastelli, G. C.: Atrioventricular Canal Defects. Philadelphia, W. B. Saunders, 1976.
This monograph was written by Dr. Rastelli shortly before his death. The Foreword by Dwight McGoon is a fitting memorial to this pioneer who contributed so much to the field of congenital heart surgery prior to his death at 39 years of age. In this monograph, Dr. Rastelli clearly describes the anatomy of this defect and delineates many of the anatomic features that have enabled surgeons to develop successful surgical corrections.

REFERENCES

1. Ad, N., Barak, J., Birk, E., Diamant, S., and Vidne, B. A.: A one-way, valved, atrial septal patch in the management of postoperative right heart failure. J. Thorac. Cardiovasc. Surg., 108:134, 1994.
2. Alt, B., and Shikes, R. H.: Pulmonary hypertension in congenital heart disease: Irreversible vascular changes in young infants. Pediatr. Pathol., 1:423, 1983.
3. Andersen, M., Lyngborg, K., Moller, I., and Wennevold, A.: The natural history of small atrial septal defects: Long-term follow-up with serial heart catheterizations. Am. Heart J., 92:302, 1976.
4. Ashraf, M. H., Amin, Z., Sharma, R., and Subramanian, S.: Atrioventricular canal defect: Two-patch repair and tricuspidization of the mitral valve. Ann. Thorac. Surg., 55:347, 1993.
5. Bailey, C. P., Nichols, H. T., Bolton, H. E., Jamison, W. L., and Gomez Almeida, M.: Surgical treatment of forty-six interatrial septal defects by atrio-septo-pexy. Ann. Surg., 140:805, 1954.
6. Behrendt, D. M.: Atrial septal defect. In Arciniegas, E. (Ed.): Pediatric Cardiac Surgery. Chicago, Year Book Medical Publishers, 1985, pp. 133–140.
7. Bellinger, D. C., Jonas, R. A., Rappaport, L. A., Wypij, D., Wernobsky, G., Kuban, K. C. K., Barnes, P. D., Holmes, G. L., Hickey, P. R., Strand, R. D., Walsh, A. Z., and Helmers, S. L.: Developmental and neurologic status of children after heart surgery with hypothermic circulatory arrest or low-flow cardiopulmonary bypass. N. Engl. J. Med., 332:549, 1995.
8. Ben-Zvi, J., Hildner, F. J., and Samet, P.: Development of mitral insufficiency following closure of ostium secundum atrial septal defect. Am. Heart J., 91:83, 1976.
9. Bender, H. W., Jr., Hammon, J. W., Jr., Hubbard, S. G., Muirhead, J., and Graham, T. P.: Repair of atrioventricular canal malformation in the first year of life. J. Thorac. Cardiovasc. Surg., 84:515, 1982.
10. Beppu, S., Nimura, Y., Sakakibara, H., et al.: Mitral cleft in ostium primum atrial septal defect assessed by cross-sectional echocardiography. Circulation, 62:1099, 1980.
11. Berg, J. M., Crome, L., and France, N. E.: Congenital cardiac malformations in mongolism. Br. Heart J., 22:331, 1960.
12. Berger, T. J., Blackstone, E. H., Kirklin, J. W., et al.: Survival and probability of cure without and with surgery in complete atrioventricular canal. Ann. Thorac. Surg., 27:104, 1979.

13. Berger, T. J., Kirklin, J. W., Blackstone, E. H., Pacifico, A. D., and Kouchoukos, N. T.: Primary repair of complete atrioventricular canal in patients less than 2 years old. Am. J. Cardiol., 41:906, 1978.

14. Beyer, J.: Acute left heart failure after surgical closure. Ann. Thorac. Surg., 25:36, 1978.

15. Bharati, S., Kirklin, J. W., McAllister, H. A., Jr., and Lev, M.: The surgical anatomy of common atrioventricular orifice associated with tetralogy of Fallot, double outlet right ventricle and complete regular transposition. Circulation, 61:1142, 1980.

16. Bharati, S., Lev, M., and Kirklin, J. W.: Cardiac Surgery and the Conduction System. New York, John Wiley & Sons, 1983.

17. Bizarro, R. O., Callahan, J. A., Feldt, R. H., et al.: Familial atrial septal defect with prolonged atrioventricular conduction: Syndrome showing autosomal dominant patterns of inheritance. Circulation, 41:677, 1970.

18. Bolens, M., and Friedli, B.: Sinus node function and conduction system before and after surgery for secundum atrial septal defect: An electrophysiologic study. Am. J. Cardiol., 53:1415, 1984.

19. Bonow, R. O., Borer, J. S., Rosing, D. R., et al.: Left ventricular functional reserve in adult patients with atrial septal defect: Pre- and post-operative studies. Circulation, 63:1315, 1981.

20. Brannon, E. S., Weens, H. S., and Warren, J. V.: Atrial septal defect: Study of hemodynamics by technique of right heart catheterization. Am. J. Med. Sci., 210:480, 1945.

21. Brody, H.: Drainage of the pulmonary veins into the right side of the heart. Arch. Pathol., 33:221, 1942.

22. Campbell, M.: Natural history of atrial septal defect. Br. Heart J., 32:820, 1970.

23. Carpentier, A.: Surgical anatomy and management of the mitral component of atrioventricular canal defects. In Anderson, R. H., and Shinebourne, E. A. (Eds.): Pediatric Cardiology. London, Churchill Livingstone, 1978, pp. 477–490.

24. Castañeda, A. R., Mayer, J. E. J., and Jonas, R. A.: Repair of complete atrioventricular canal in infancy. World J. Surg., 9:590, 1985.

25. Castañeda, A. R., Mayer, J. E. J., Jonas, R. A., and Hanley, F.: Cardiac Surgery in the Neonate and Infant. Philadelphia, W. B. Saunders, 1994.

26. Cayler, G. G.: Spontaneous functional closure of symptomatic atrial septal defects. N. Engl. J. Med., 276:65, 1967.

27. Cooley, D. A., Ellis, P. R., Jr., and Bellizzi, M. E.: Atrial septal defects of the sinus venosus type: Surgical considerations. Dis. Chest, 39:185, 1961.

28. Dales, J. E., Bruce, R. A., and Cobb, L. A.: Interaction of chronic hypoxia of moderate altitude on pulmonary hypertension complicating defect of the atrial septum. N. Engl. J. Med., 266:272, 1962.

29. Ebels, T., Meijboom, E. J., Anderson, R. H., Schasfoort-van Leeuwen, M. J. M., Lenstra, D., Eijgelaar, A., Bossinia, K. K., and Homan vander Heide, J. N.: Anatomic and functional "obstruction" of the outflow tract in atrioventricular septal defects with separate valve orifices ("ostium primum atrial septal defect"): An echocardiographic study. Am. J. Cardiol., 54:843, 1984.

30. Ebert, P. A.: Atlas of Congenital Cardiac Surgery. Skinner, D. B. (Ed.). New York, Churchill Livingstone, 1989.

31. Ellis, F. H., Jr., Brandenburg, R. O., and Swan, H. J. C.: Defect of the atrial septum in the elderly: Report of successful correction in five patients sixty years of age or older. N. Engl. J. Med., 262:219, 1960.

32. Evans, J. R., Rowe, R. D., and Keith, J. D.: The clinical diagnosis of atrial septal defect in children. Am. J. Med., 30:345, 1961.

33. Forfang, K., Simonsen, S., Anderson, A., and Efskind, L.: Atrial septal defect of the secundum type in the middle-aged: Clinical results of surgery and correlations between symptoms and hemodynamics. Am. Heart J., 94:44, 1977.

34. Fraker, T. D., Jr., Harris, P. J., Behar, V. S., and Kisslo, J. A.: Detection and exclusion of interatrial shunts by two-dimensional echocardiography. Circulation, 54:379, 1979.

35. Frescura, C., Thiene, G., Franceschini, E., Talenti, E., and Mazzucco, A.: Pulmonary vascular disease in infants with complete atrioventricular septal defect. Int. J. Cardiol., 15:91, 1987.

36. Gault, J. H., Morrow, A. G., Gay, W. A., Jr., and Ross, J., Jr.: Atrial septal defect in patients over the age of forty years. Circulation, 37:261, 1968.

37. Gerbode, F., and Carr, I.: Surgery of congenital lesions of the heart and great vessels. In Gay, W. A., Jr., and Goldsmith, H. A. (Eds.): Cardiovascular Surgery. Philadelphia, Harper & Row, 1981.

38. Gibbon, J. H.: Application of a mechanical heart-lung apparatus to cardiac surgery. Minn. Med., 37:171, 1954.

39. Giknis, F. L.: Single atrium and the Ellis-van Creveld syndrome. J. Pediatr., 62:558, 1963.

40. Glenn, W. W. L., Stansel, H. C., Jr., Talner, N. S., Deren, M. M., and Van Heeckeren, D.: Surgical treatment of atrial septal defect: Analysis of 150 corrective operations. Am. J. Surg., 121:485, 1971.

41. Goldfaden, D. M., Jones, M., Morrow, A. G.: Long-term results of repair of incomplete persistent atrioventricular canal. J. Thorac. Cardiovasc. Surg., 82:669, 1981.

42. Greeley, W. J., Kern, F. H., Mault, J. R., Skaryak, L. A., and Ungerleider, R. M.: Mechanisms of injury and methods of protection of the brain during cardiac surgery in neonates and infants. Cardiol. Young, 3:317, 1993.

43. Gross, R. E., Pomeranz, A. A., Watkins, E., Jr., and Goldsmith, E. I.: Surgical closure of defects of the interauricular septum by use of an atrial well. N. Engl. J. Med., 247:455, 1952.

44. Hairston, P., Parker, E. F., Arrants, J. E., Bradham, R. R., and Lee, W. H., Jr.: The adult atrial septal defect: Results of surgical repair. Ann. Surg., 179:799, 1974.

45. Hanley, F. L., Fenton, K. N., Jonas, R. A., Mayer, J. E., Cook, N. R., Wernovsky, G., and Castañeda, A. R.: Surgical repair of complete atrioventricular canal defects in infancy: Twenty year trends. J. Thorac. Cardiovasc. Surg., 106:387, 1993.

46. Hanlon, C. R., Barner, H. B., Willman, V. L., Mudd, J. G., and Kaiser, G. C.: Atrial septal defect: Results of repair in adult. Arch. Surg., 99:275, 1969.

47. Hawe, A., Rastelli, G. C., Brandenburg, R. O., and McGoon, D. C.: Embolic complications following repair of atrial septal defects. Circulation, 39(Suppl.):185, 1969.

48. Hindman, B. J., Dexter, F., Cutkomp, J., Smith, T., Todd, M. M., and Tinker, J. H.: Brain blood flow and metabolism do not decrease at stable brain temperature during cardiopulmonary bypass in rabbits. Anesthesiology, 77:342, 1992.

49. Jonas, R. A.: Review of current research at Boston Children's Hospital. Ann. Thorac. Surg., 56:1467, 1993.

50. Kadoba, K., and Jonas, R. A.: Replacement of the left atrioventricular valve after repair of atrioventricular septal defect. Cardiol. Young, 1:383, 1991.

51. Keith, J. D., Rowe, R. D., and Vlad, P.: Heart Disease in Infancy and Childhood. New York, Macmillan, 1978.

52. Kern, F. H., Ungerleider, R. M., Quill, T. J., Baldwin, B., White, W. D., Reves, J. G., and Greeley, W. J.: Cerebral blood flow response to changes in arterial carbon dioxide tension during hypothermic cardiopulmonary bypass in children. J. Thorac. Cardiovasc. Surg., 101:618, 1991.

53. Kern, F. H., Ungerleider, R. M., Reves, J. G., Quill, T., Smith, L. R., Baldwin, B., Croughwell, N. D., and Greeley, W. J.: Effect of altering pump flow rate on cerebral blood flow and metabolism in infants and children. Ann. Thorac. Surg., 56:1366, 1993.

54. Kirklin, J. W., and Barratt-Boyes, B. G.: Cardiac Surgery, 2nd ed. New York, Churchill Livingstone, 1993, p. 1779.

55. Kirklin, J. W., Blackstone, E. H., Pacifico, A. D., Brown, R. N., and Bargeron, L. M., Jr.: Routine primary repair vs. two-stage repair of tetralogy of Fallot. Circulation, 60:373, 1979.

56. Kirklin, J. W., Ellis, F. H., Jr., and Barratt-Boyes, B. G.: Technique for repair of atrial septal defect using the atrial well. Surg. Gynecol. Obstet., 103:646, 1956.

57. Kirklin, J. W., Pacifico, A. D., and Kirklin, J. K.: The surgical treatment of atrioventricular canal defects. In Arciniegas, E. (Ed.): Pediatric Cardiac Surgery. Chicago, Year Book Medical Publishers, 1985.

58. Kisslo, J. A., Adams, D. B., and Belkin, R. N.: Doppler Color Flow Imaging. New York, Churchill Livingstone, 1988.

59. Kyger, E. R., Frazier, O. H., Cooley, D. A., Gillette, P. C., Reul, G. J., Jr., Sandiford, F. M., and Wukasch, D. C.: Sinus venosus atrial septal defect: Early and late results following closure in 109 patients. Ann. Thorac. Surg., 25:44, 1978.

60. Lappen, R. S., Muster, A. J., Idriss, F. S., Riggs, T. W., Ilbawi, M., Paul, M. H., Bharati, S., and Lev, M.: Masked subaortic stenosis in ostium primum atrial septal defect: Recognition and treatment. Am. J. Cardiol., 52:336, 1983.

61. Leachman, R. D., Cokkinos, D. V., and Cooley, D. A.: Association of ostium secundum atrial septal defects with mitral valve prolapse. Am. J. Cardiol., 38:167, 1976.

62. Lev, M.: The architecture of the conduction system in congenital heart disease: I. Common atrioventricular orifice. Arch. Pathol., 65:174, 1958.

63. Levin, A. R., Spach, M. S., Boineau, J. P., Canent, R. V., Jr., Capp, M. P., and Jewett, P. H.: Atrial pressure-flow dynamics in atrial septal defects (secundum type). Circulation, 34:476, 1968.

64. Levy, S.: Long-term follow-up after surgical correction of the partial form of common atrioventricular canal (ostium primum). J. Thorac. Cardiovasc. Surg., 67:353, 1974.

65. Lewis, F. J., and Taufic, M.: Closure of atrial septal defects with the aid of hypothermia: Experimental accomplishments and the report of the one successful case. Surgery, 33:52, 1953.

66. Liberthson, R. R., Boucher, C. A., Strauss, H. W., Dinsmore, R. E., McKusick, K. A., and Pohost, G. M.: Right ventricular function in adult atrial septal defect. Am. J. Cardiol., 47:56, 1981.

67. Lillehei, C. W., Cohen, M., Warden, H. E., et al.: Direct vision intracardiac surgery by means of controlled cross circulation or continuous arterial reservoir perfusion for correction of ventricular septal defects, atrioventricularis communis, isolated infundibular pulmonic stenosis, and tetralogy of Fallot. In Lam, C. R. (Ed.): Proceedings of the Henry Ford Hospital Symposium. Philadelphia, W. B. Saunders, 1955, pp. 371–392.

68. Lillehei, C. W., Varco, R. L., Cohen, M., Warden, H. E., Patton, C., and Moller, J. H.: The first open-heart repairs of ventricular septal defect, atrioventricular communis, and tetralogy of Fallot using extracorporeal circulation by cross-circulation: A 30-year follow-up. Ann. Thorac. Surg., 41:4, 1986.

69. Lock, J. E., Rome, J. J., Davis, R., Van Praagh, S., Perry, S. B., Van Praagh, R., and Keane, J. F.: Transcatheter closure of atrial septal defects: Experimental studies. Circulation, 79:1091, 1989.

70. Losay, J., Rosenthal, A., Castaneda, A. R., Bernard, W. H., and Nadas, A. S.: Repair of atrial septal defect primum: Results, course, and prognosis. J. Thorac. Cardiovasc. Surg., 75:248, 1978.

71. Magilligan, D. J., Jr., Lam, C. R., Lewis, J. W., Jr., and Davila, J. C.: Late results of atrial septal defect repair in adults. Arch. Surg., 113:1245, 1978.

72. Mault, J. R., Ohtake, S., Klingensmith, M. E., Heinle, J. S., Greeley, W. J., and Ungerleider, R. M.: Cerebral metabolism and circulatory arrest: Effects of duration and strategies for protection. Ann. Thorac. Surg., 55:57, 1993.

73. Mault, J. R., Whitaker, E. G., Heinle, J. S., Lodge, A. J., and Ungerleider, R. M.: Intermittent perfusion during hypothermic circulatory arrest: A new and effective technique for cerebral protection. Surg. Forum, 43:314, 1992.

74. Mavroudis, C., and Backer, C.: Pediatr. Cardiac Surg., 1994.

75. Mavroudis, C., Weinstein, G., Turley, K., and Ebert, P. A.: Surgical management of complete atrioventricular canal. J. Thorac. Cardiovasc. Surg., 83:670, 1982.

76. McGrath, L. B., and Gonzalez-Lavin, L.: Actuarial survival, freedom from reoperation, and other events after repair of atrioventricular septal defects. J. Thorac. Cardiovasc. Surg., 94:582, 1987.

77. Meijboom, E. J., Ebels, T., Anderson, R. H., Schasfoort-van Leeuwen, M. J. M., Deanfield, J. E., Eijgelaar, A., and Homan van der Heide, J. N. H.: Left atrioventricular valve after surgical repair in atrioventricular septal defect with separate valve orifices ("ostium primum atrial septal defect"): An echo-Doppler study. Am. J. Cardiol., 57:433, 1986.

78. Menon, V. A., and Wagner, H. R.: Spontaneous closure of secundum atrial septal defect. N. Y. State J. Med., 1068, 1976.

79. Mitchell, S. C., Korones, S. B., and Berendas, H. W.: Congenital heart disease in 56,109 births: Incidence and natural history. Circulation, 43:323, 1971.

80. Mody, M. R.: Serial hemodynamic observations in secundum atrial septal defect with special reference to spontaneous closure. Am. J. Cardiol., 32:978, 1973.

81. Moore, K. L.: The Developing Human: Clinically Oriented Embryology. Philadelphia, W. B. Saunders, 1977.

82. Murray, G.: Closure of defects in cardiac septa. Ann. Surg., 128:843, 1948.

83. Newburger, J. W., Jonas, R. A., Wernovsky, G., and Ware, J. H.: A comparison of the perioperative neurologic effects of hypothermic circulatory arrest versus low-flow cardiopulmonary bypass in infant heart surgery. N. Engl. J. Med., 329:1057, 1993.

84. Newfeld, E. A., Sher, M., Paul, M. H., and Nikaidoh, H.: Pulmonary vascular disease in complete atrioventricular canal defect. Am. J. Cardiol., 39:721, 1977.

85. Pass, H. I., Crawford, F. A., Jr., Sade, R. M., Assey, M. E., and Usher, B. W.: Congenital heart disease in adults. Am. Surg., 50:36, 1984.

86. Pearlman, A. S., Borer, J. S., Clark, C. E., Henry, W. L., Redwood, D. R., Morrow, A. G., Epstein, S. E., Burn, C., Cohen, L., and McKay, F. J.: Abnormal right ventricular size and ventricular septal motion after atrial septal defect closure. Am. J. Cardiol., 41:295, 1978.

87. Phillips, S. J., Okies, J. E., Henken, D., Sunderland, C. O., and Starr, A.: Complex of secundum atrial septal defect and congestive heart failure in infants. J. Thorac. Cardiovasc. Surg., 70:696, 1975.

88. Rahimtoola, S. H., Kirklin, J. W., and Burchell, H. B.: Atrial septal defect. Circulation, 37,38(Suppl. V):V-2, 1968.

89. Rainier-Pope, C. R., Cunningham, R. D., Nadas, A. S., and Crigler, J. F.: Cardiovascular malformation in Turner's syndrome. Pediatrics, 33:919, 1964.

90. Rastelli, G. C.: Atrioventricular Canal Defects. Philadelphia, W. B. Saunders, 1976.

91. Rastelli, G. C., Kirklin, J. W., and Titus, J. L.: Anatomic observations on complete form of persistent common atrioventricular canal with special reference to atrioventricular valves. Mayo Clin. Proc., 41:296, 1966.

92. Rastelli, G. C., Weidman, W. H., Kirklin, J. W.: Surgical repair of the partial form of persistent common atrioventricular canal, with special reference to the problem of mitral valve incompetence. Circulation, 31,32:I-31, 1965.

93. Richmond, D. E., Lowe, J. B., and Barratt-Boyes, B. G.: Results of surgical repair of atrial septal defects in the middle-aged and elderly. Thorax, 24:536, 1969.

94. Saksena, F. B., and Aldridge, H. E.: Atrial septal defect in the older patient: A clinical and hemodynamic study in patients operated on after age 35. Circulation, 42:1009, 1970.

95. Santos, A., Boucek, M., Ruttenberg, H., Veasy, G., Orsmond, G., and McGough, E.: Repair of atrioventricular septal defects in infancy. J. Thorac. Cardiovasc. Surg., 91:505, 1986.

96. Sayd, H. M., Dacie, J. V., Handley, D. A., Lewis, S. M., and Cleland, W. P.: Hemolytic anemia of mechanical origin after open heart surgery. Thorax, 16:356, 1961.

97. Sealy, W. C., Farmer, J. C., Young, W. G., Jr., and Brown, I. W.: Atrial dysrhythmia and atrial secundum defects. J. Thorac. Cardiovasc. Surg., 57:245, 1969.

98. Sellers, R. D., Ferlic, R. M., Sterns, L. P., and Lillehei, C. W.: Secundum type atrial septal defects: Early and late results of surgical repair using extracorporeal circulation in 275 patients. Surgery, 59:155, 1966.

99. Silverman, N., Levitsky, S., Fisher, E., DuBrow, I., Hastreiter, A., and Scagliotti, D.: Efficacy of pulmonary artery banding in infants with complete atrioventricular canal. Circulation 68(Suppl. II):II-148, 1983.

100. Silverman, N. H.: Pediatric Echocardiography. Baltimore, Williams & Wilkins, 1993.

101. Skaryak, L. A., Chai, P. J., Kern, F. H., Greeley, W. J., and Ungerleider, R. M.: Combining alpha-stat and pH-stat blood gas strategies during cooling prior to circulatory arrest provides optimal recovery of cerebral metabolism. Presented at the American Heart Association 66th scientific sessions, November 1993.

102. Somerville, J.: Ostium primum defects: Factors causing deterioration in the natural history. Br. Heart J., 27:413, 1965.

103. Sondergard, T.: Closure of atrial septal defects: Report of three cases. Acta Chir. Scand., 107:492, 1954.

104. St. John Sutton, M. G., Tajik, A. J., and McGoon, D. C.: Atrial septal defect in patients ages 60 years or older: Operative results and long-term postoperative follow-up. Circulation, 64:402, 1981.

105. Stark, J., and de Leval, M.: Surgery for Congenital Heart Defects, 2nd edition. Philadelphia, W. B. Saunders, 1994.

106. Starr, A., and Hovaguimian, H.: Surgical repair of subaortic stenosis in atrioventricular canal defects. J. Thorac. Cardiovasc. Surg., 108:373, 1994.

107. Steinbrunn, W., Cohn, K. E., and Selzer, A.: Atrial septal defect associated with mitral stenosis: The Lutembacher syndrome revisited. Am. J. Med., 48:295, 1970.

108. Studer, M., Blackstone, E. H., Kirklin, J. W., Pacifico, A. D., Soto, B., Chung, G. K. T., Kirklin, J. K., and Bargeron, L. M., Jr.: Determinants of early and late results of repair of atrioventricular septal (canal) defects. J. Thorac. Cardiovasc. Surg., 84:523, 1982.

109. Sugimura, S., Okies, J. E., Litchford, B., and Starr, A.: Late results of mitral cleft closure for ostium primum atrial septal defect in adolescents and adults. Am. Surg., 45:670, 1979.

110. Taylor, N. C., and Somerville, J.: Fixed subaortic stenosis after repair of ostium primum defects. Br. Heart J., 45:689, 1981.

111. Thompson, T., and Evans, W.: Paradoxical embolism. Q. J. Med., 23:135, 1930.

112. Trusler, G. A., Kazenelson, G., Freedom, R. M., Williams, W. G., and Rowe, R. D.: Late results following repair of partial anomalous pulmonary venous connection with sinus venosus atrial septal defect. J. Thorac. Cardiovasc. Surg., 79:776, 1980.

113. Uchida, I. A., and Rowe, R. R. D.: Discordant heart anomalies in twins. Am. J. Hum. Genet., 9:133, 1957.

114. Ungerleider, R. M.: The use of intraoperative epicardial echocardiography with color flow imaging during the repair of atrioventricular septal defects. Cardiol. Young, 2:56, 1992.

115. Ungerleider, R. M., Greeley, W. J., Kanter, R. J., and Kisslo, J. A.: The learning curve for intraoperative echocardiography during congenital heart surgery. Ann. Thorac. Surg., 54:691, 1992.

116. Ungerleider, R. M., Greeley, W. J., Sheikh, K. H., Kern, F. H., Kisslo, J. A., and Sabiston, D. C., Jr.: The use of intraoperative echo with Doppler color flow imaging to predict outcome after repair of congenital cardiac defects. Ann. Surg., 210:526, 1989.

117. Ungerleider, R. M., Greeley, W. J., Sheikh, K. H., Philips, J., Pearce, F. B., Kern, F. H., and Kisslo, J. A.: Routine use of intraoperative epicardial echocardiography and Doppler color flow imaging to guide and evaluate repair of congenital heart defects: A prospective study. J. Thorac. Cardiovasc. Surg., 100:297, 1990.

118. Ungerleider, R. M., Kisslo, J. A., Greeley, W. J., Van Trigt, P., and Sabiston, D. C., Jr.: Intraoperative prebypass and postbypass epicardial color flow imaging in the repair of atrioventricular septal defects. J. Thorac. Cardiovasc. Surg., 98:90, 1989.

119. Verdon, T. A., Jr., Forrester, R. H., and Crosby, W. H.: Hemolytic anemia after open heart repair of ostium primum defects. N. Engl. J. Med., 269:444, 1963.

120. Verrier, E. D.: Secundum atrial septal defects. In Grillo, H. C., Austen, W. G., Wilkins, E. W., Jr., Mathisen, D. J., and Vlahakes, G. J. (Eds.): Current Therapy in Cardiothoracic Surgery. Philadelphia, B. C. Decker, 1989.

121. Waldhausen, J. A., and Tyers, G. F. O.: Atrial septal defects, ostium primum defects, and atrioventricular canals. In Sabiston, D. C., Jr. (Ed.): Textbook of Surgery. Philadelphia, W. B. Saunders, 1986.

122. Wanderman, K. L., Orsysheher, I., and Gueron, M.: Left ventricular performance in patients with atrial septal defect: Evaluation with noninvasive methods. Am. J. Cardiol., 41:487, 1978.

123. Wendet, V. E., Keech, M. K., Read, R. C., Bistue, A. R., and Bianchi, F. A.: Cardiovascular features of Marfan's syndrome: Family studies. Circulation, 32(Suppl. II):218, 1965.

124. Williams, R. G., and Rudd, M.: Echocardiographic features of endocardial cushion defects. Circulation, 49:418, 1974.

125. Williams, W. H., Guyton, R. A., Michalik, R. E., Jones, E. L., Rhee, K. H., Plauth, W. H., Jr., and Hatcher, C. R., Jr.: Individualized surgical management of complete atrioventricular canal. J. Thorac. Cardiovasc. Surg., 86:838, 1983.

126. Yalav, E., Brown, A. H., and Braimbridge, M. V.: Surgery for atrial septal defect in patients over 60 years of age. J. Thorac. Cardiovasc. Surg., 62:788, 1971.

127. Yamaki, S., Horiuchi, T., Sekino, Y.: Quantitative analysis of pulmonary vascular disease in simple cardiac anomalies with the Down syndrome. Am. J. Cardiol., 51:1502, 1983.

128. Yamaki, S., Yasui, H., Kado, H., Yonenaga, K., Nakamura, Y., Kikuchi, T., Ajiki, H., Tsunemoto, M., and Mohri, H.: Pulmonary vascular disease and operative indications in complete atrioventricular canal defect in early infancy. J. Thorac. Cardiovasc. Surg., 106:398, 1993.

129. Young, D.: Later results of closure of secundum atrial septal defect in children. Am. J. Cardiol., 31:14, 1973.

V _____

DISORDERS OF PULMONARY VENOUS RETURN

Erle H. Austin III, M.D.

Disorders of pulmonary venous return most commonly result from a developmental failure of the pulmonary veins to connect normally with the left atrium. If all four pulmonary veins fail to join the left atrium, the condition of total anomalous pulmonary venous connection (TAPVC) exists, whereas when some pulmonary veins connect normally and others anomalously, the condition is known as partial anomalous pulmonary venous connection (PAPVC). Obstruction to pulmonary venous return is a common component of TAPVC, significantly worsening its hemodynamic effects. Pulmonary venous obstruction may also occur rarely with normally connected pulmonary veins either at the level of the veins themselves (pulmonary vein stenosis) or within the left atrium (cor triatriatum).

TOTAL ANOMALOUS PULMONARY VENOUS CONNECTION

TAPVC occurs in 1% to 2% of all cardiac malformations. In this anomaly, the pulmonary veins do not join the left atrium but return saturated blood to the right side of the heart through connections into the right atrium or into its tributaries. The only inlet of blood into the left atrium is through a communication in the interatrial septum. Patients with this anomaly commonly present as critically ill infants requiring urgent evaluation and prompt surgical intervention.

Historical Review

Wilson was the first to describe TAPVC in 1798.[46] Clinical interest in this entity was renewed in 1942 when Brody reviewed 106 cases of anomalous pulmonary venous drainage, of which 37 were TAPVC.[3] The premortem diagnosis of this disorder became possible with the advent of cardiac catheterization. In 1951, Muller described successful palliation of a patient with TAPVC using a closed technique of anastomosing the left pulmonary vein to the left atrial appendage.[29] The first successful corrections of TAPVC were performed by Kirklin[5] in 1954 using the atrial well technique and by Lewis and associates[24] in 1955 using moderate hypothermia and venous inflow occlusion. Subsequent successful repairs were performed using cardiopulmonary bypass.[9] Despite these early successes, the surgical mortality for TAPVC remained high throughout the 1960s and early 1970s, especially in infants. Improvements in preoperative evaluation and management as well as the increased use of hypothermic circulatory arrest[1] have significantly reduced the risk of operation for this complex heart defect.

Embryology and Pathologic Anatomy

The lung develops as an outpouching of the foregut, and its venous plexus arises as part of the splanchnic venous system separate from the primitive heart. The pulmonary venous plexus initially connects with the cardinal and umbilicovitelline veins. These connections normally involute as the pulmonary venous plexus coalesces with the posterior region of the left atrium (Fig. 54–38). Failure of these primitive

connections to absorb produces anomalous communications between the pulmonary veins and the systemic venous system (Fig. 54–39). Failure of the pulmonary venous plexus to unite with the atrial portion of the heart results in TAPVC, and the route of pulmonary venous drainage is determined by the primordial pulmonary venous connections that persist. The classification of TAPVC is based on the anatomic level of the resultant anomalous venous connection[11]:

Type I (supracardiac type)—The common pulmonary vein drains by means of an anomalous left vertical vein into the left innominate vein (Fig. 54–40*A*). This left vertical vein represents a persistent remnant of the left cardinal vein. A less common form connects directly into the right superior vena cava. The supracardiac type is the most common form of TAPVC, representing 50% of the cases in most series.[17]

Type II (intracardiac type)—In the next most common type, comprising approximately 25% of the cases[17] the anoma-

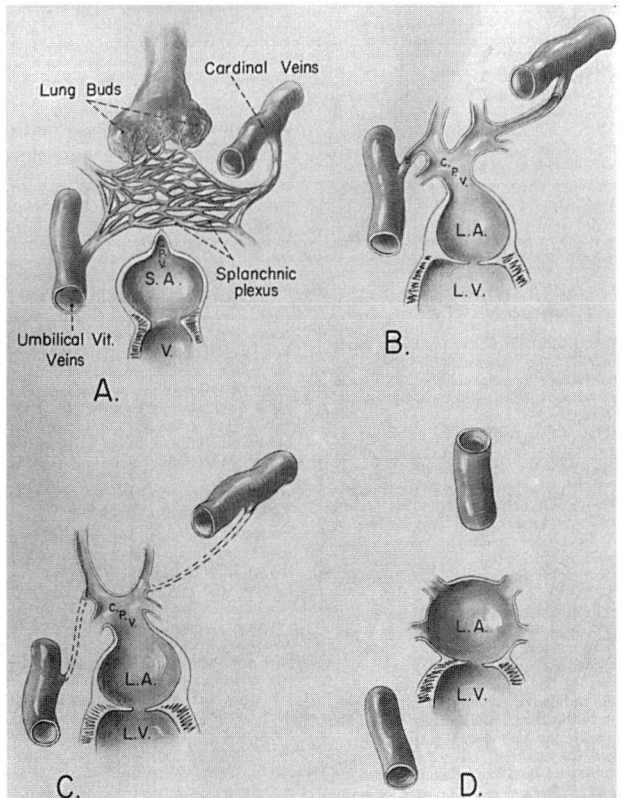

Figure 54–38. Normal pulmonary venous development. *A,* The lung buds are surrounded by the splanchnic plexus, which drains the foregut through the cardinal and umbilicovitelline veins. At this stage there is no direct connection between the pulmonary vascular bed and the heart. *B,* The common pulmonary vein (C.P.V.) from the back of the common atrium joins the splanchnic plexus, providing direct access of pulmonary venous blood to the left atrium. *C,* The primitive pulmonary venous connections disappear. *D,* With further development the common pulmonary vein is incorporated into the left atrium (L.A.). L.V., left ventricle. (From Lucas, R. V., Jr., Anderson, R. C., Amplatz, K., Adams, P., Jr., and Edwards, J. E.: Congenital causes of pulmonary venous obstruction. Pediatr. Clin. North Am., *10*:781, 1963.)

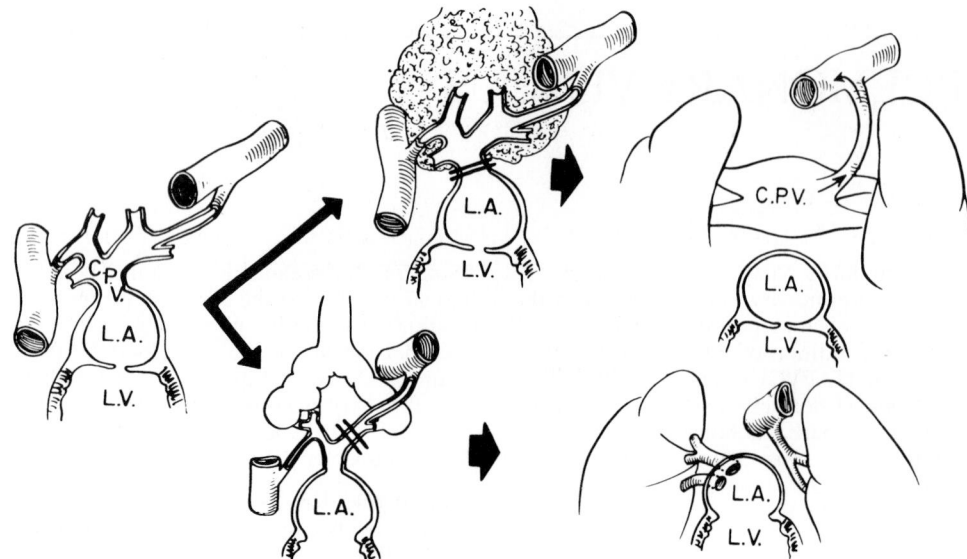

Figure 54–39. Embryogenesis of anomalous pulmonary venous connections. Upper right, Atresia or failed connection of the common pulmonary vein (C.P.V.) with the left atrium (L.A.) results in total anomalous pulmonary venous connection. In this case, persistence of the connection with the cardinal venous system results in the supracardiac form of the anomaly. Lower right, Atresia of a major branch of the common pulmonary vein results in partial anomalous pulmonary venous connection. In this case, the left lung drains anomalously to the innominate vein. L.V., left ventricle. (From Lucas, R. V., Jr.: Anomalous venous connections, pulmonary and systemic. In Adams, F. H., and Emmanouilides, G. C. [Eds.]: Moss' Heart Disease In Infants, Children, and Adolescents, 3rd ed. Baltimore, Williams & Wilkins, 1983.)

lous pulmonary drainage occurs at the level of the heart, either directly into the right atrium or, more commonly, through the coronary sinus (see Fig. 54–40B). Such a connection arises when the left common cardinal vein atrophies cephalad to its junction with the pulmonary veins and persists proximally, where it becomes the coronary sinus.

Type III (infracardiac type)—Drainage of the pulmonary veins is by means of a persistent connection with the umbilicovitelline venous system. This connection, encountered in 20% to 25% of TAPVC patients, occurs as a common trunk that passes through the diaphragm and joins the portal vein at the level of the sinus venosus (see Fig. 54–40C).

Type IV (mixed type)—The remaining patients, less than 5%, demonstrate independent connections at two or more levels.

The type of interatrial communication that exists and the potential presence of anatomic pulmonary venous obstruction are important factors affecting the pathophysiology and natural history of this anomaly. A patent foramen ovale occurs in approximately 75% of patients. The remaining 25% exhibit a secundum type of atrial septal defect. Pulmonary venous obstruction occurs most commonly at the site where the anomalous pulmonary venous connection joins the systemic venous system. All patients with infracardiac TAPVC, and as many as 50% of patients with the supracardiac type, have some degree of pulmonary venous obstruction.[12] Pulmonary venous obstruction has also been reported in 22% of patients with TAPVC to the coronary sinus.[19]

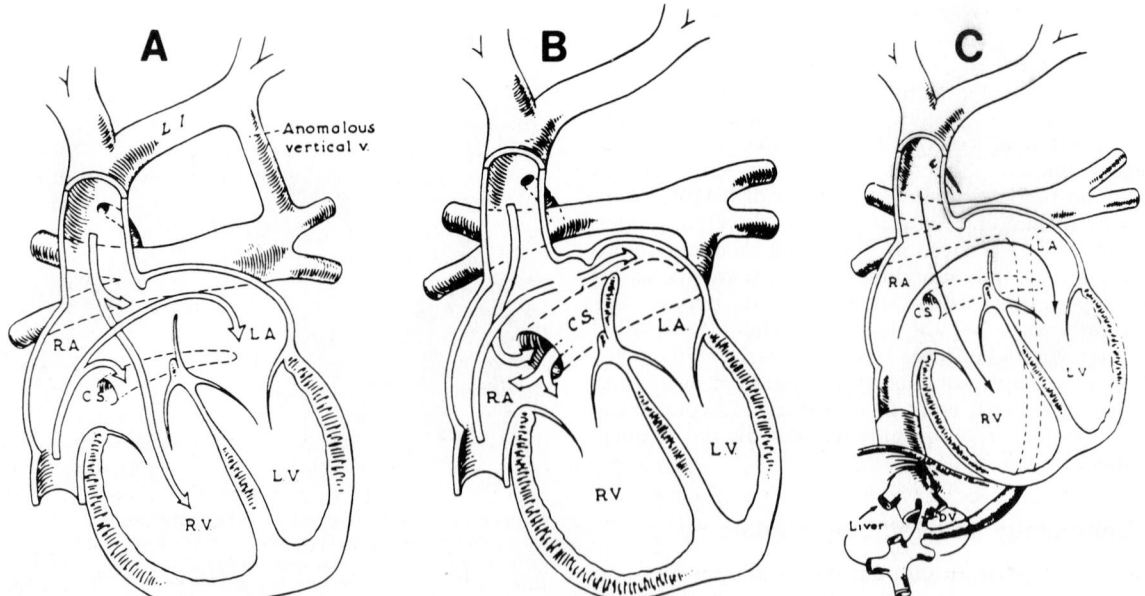

Figure 54–40. Types of total anomalous pulmonary venous connection (TAPVC). A, Supracardiac type with vertical vein joining the left innominate vein. B, Intracardiac type with connection to the coronary sinus. C, Infracardiac type with drainage through the diaphragm into the portal venous system. (From Hammon, J. W., Jr., and Bender, H. W., Jr.: Anomalous venous connections: Pulmonary and systemic. In Baue, A. E. [Ed.]: Glenn's Thoracic and Cardiovascular Surgery, 5th Ed. Norwalk, CT, Appleton & Lange, 1991.)

Associated cardiac defects are uncommon with TAPVC, but rare associations with tetralogy of Fallot and double-outlet right ventricle have been reported.[12] TAPVC is, however, a common component of right atrial isomerism with single functional ventricle.

Pathophysiology and Natural History

In TAPVC, all of the oxygenated pulmonary venous blood mixes with the desaturated systemic venous blood in the right atrium. Some of this mixed blood passes into the right ventricle and is circulated back to the lungs. The remaining portion crosses the interatrial septum to support the systemic circulation. The relative volumes that flow into the pulmonary and systemic circulations are determined by the presence and degree of pulmonary venous obstruction and the size of the interatrial communication. These factors affect the severity of the circulatory derangement and the resultant natural history.

In the absence of pulmonary venous obstruction, pulmonary blood flow is increased, and a large volume of oxygenated blood returns to the right atrium. The oxygen saturation of the right atrial and thus systemic arterial blood is relatively high in these patients (usually greater than 80%), and cyanosis is usually mild or unnoticed. The large left-to-right shunt produces enlargement of the right ventricle and pulmonary artery in addition to right ventricular hypertrophy. If flow into the left atrium is restricted by a small patent foramen ovale, adequate systemic circulation is achieved by an excessive load on the right side of the heart. A large atrial septal defect permits easy egress of blood into the systemic circuit and requires less work from the right ventricle.

When pulmonary venous obstruction is present, the increased hydrostatic pressure is transmitted to the pulmonary capillary bed, causing transudation of fluid into the lung parenchyma and increased pulmonary arterial pressure and resistance. Blood flow through the lungs is less, and the smaller proportion of oxygenated blood returning to the right atrium causes significant systemic arterial desaturation. The presence of a nonrestrictive atrial septal defect does not diminish the severity of the cyanosis but may lessen the right ventricular overload. The combination of pulmonary venous obstruction and a patent foramen ovale results in severe cyanosis, intractable congestive heart failure, and early death. These variations in pathophysiologic patterns explain the variations in clinical presentation from the rare noncyanotic adult with minimal disability to the more common cyanotic neonate who without surgical intervention dies in the first weeks of life.

Infants without pulmonary venous obstruction are usually tachypneic at birth but may not appear cyanotic. The presence of heart disease is often not considered until the child fails to thrive during the first 1 or 2 months of life, and reevaluation reveals a precordial bulge, a hyperactive heart, and hepatomegaly. Congestive heart failure becomes progressively worse, and without surgical therapy 75% will die before the age of 1 year.[4, 12, 22] Those patients who survive beyond 1 year usually have an atrial septal defect, in contrast to a patent foramen ovale. If the defect is large enough, the pathophysiology and natural history may resemble that seen in isolated atrial septal defects with survival into early adulthood.

Patients with pulmonary venous obstruction present with intense cyanosis soon after birth, and tachypnea and hepatomegaly may be marked. The course is usually stormy, with death from pulmonary edema or hypoxia. In the absence of surgical treatment, the median survival for this group is only 3 weeks, in contrast to a median survival of 3 months for the group without pulmonary venous obstruction.[12] The high prevalence of patent foramen ovales and pulmonary venous obstruction in the overall TAPVC group necessitates surgical intervention in early infancy in the majority of patients. Before the availability of successful surgical correction, 90% of infants with TAPVC were dead by 1 year of age.[22]

Clinical Features

TAPVC should be suspected in any infant with tachypnea and precordial bulging. Cyanosis may not be clinically apparent in the first weeks of life, but by the second or third month, cyanosis, a cardiac murmur (usually of pulmonary flow origin), and signs of congestive heart failure are noted. Failure to thrive is the most common presentation in infants diagnosed after 3 months of life.[36] The combination of mild cyanosis, cardiomegaly with increased pulmonary vascularity, and electrocardiographic evidence of right atrial and right ventricular hypertrophy indicates the presence of TAPVC without pulmonary venous obstruction. TAPVC with pulmonary venous obstruction is clinically diagnosed soon after birth by the presence of marked cyanosis, normal heart size, and congestive failure.

The definitive diagnosis of TAPVC is accomplished in many centers by two-dimensional echocardiography.[6, 16] Avoidance of the stress of cardiac catheterization and the osmotic load of angiography helps the critically ill infant with obstructed TAPVC arrive in the operating suite in optimal preoperative condition. However, when a satisfactory diagnosis cannot be made with two-dimensional echocardiography, cardiac catheterization must be employed. TAPVC is the only congenital cardiac malformation in which the oxygen saturation of the right atrium is equal to that of the systemic arteries. The presence of pulmonary venous obstruction can be expected when systolic pulmonary artery pressure exceeds 85% of systolic systemic arterial pressure.[20] Once the presence of TAPVC is confirmed by catheterization, contrast cineangiography is employed to demonstrate the location of the anomalous connection. Recent reports of electrocardiographic gated magnetic resonance imaging suggest that this modality may become a valuable noninvasive technique in the future and eliminate the need for cardiac catheterization.[7, 44]

Surgical Management

The presence of TAPVC is a clear indication for surgical repair. Timing of the operation is dependent on the presence of obstruction. If obstruction is absent, the surgical repair can be performed electively within the first months of life, although little is gained by waiting long after diagnosis because of the poor feeding and failure to thrive that can be expected before surgical correction. If obstruction is present, however, surgical repair becomes an emergency and should be performed within hours after the diagnosis is made and medical therapy initiated.

Success of surgical correction is directly related to the condition of the infant at the time of surgery. Initial medical therapy for the compromised infant is designed to optimize the patient's condition while preparations are being made for operation. Correction of metabolic acidosis is begun using sodium bicarbonate or tromethamine (THAM). The infant is intubated, sedated with fentanyl, paralyzed with pancuronium, and hyperventilated with 100% oxygen. These maneuvers eliminate the work of breathing, treat pulmonary edema, and help diminish pulmonary vascular resistance. The addition of prostaglandin E_1 (0.1 µg./kg./min.) may help open the ductus venosus in patients with infradiaphragmatic TAPVC, as well as open the ductus arteriosus to permit some decompression of the pulmonary circulation if pulmonary pressures have become suprasystemic. If arterial blood pres-

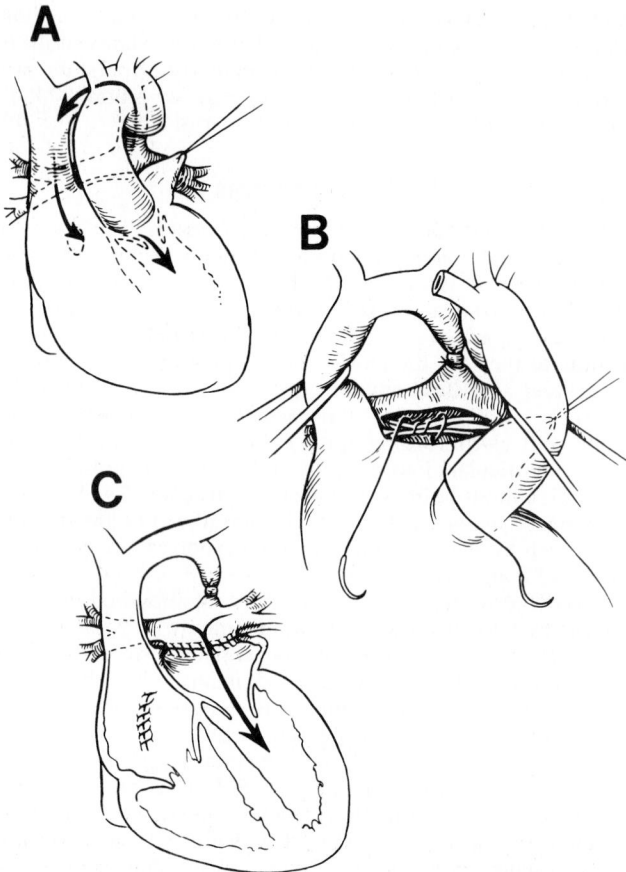

Figure 54–41. *A* to *C*, Repair of supracardiac TAPVC by exposing the common pulmonary vein between the aorta and superior vena cava. (From Lupinetti, F. M., Kulik, T. J., Beekman, R. H., III, Crowley, D. C., and Bove, E. L.: Correction of total anomalous pulmonary venous connection in infancy. J. Thorac. Cardiovasc. Surg., *106*:880, 1993.)

sure is diminished and ventricular function depressed, isoproterenol should be the first inotropic agent administered because of its tendency to decrease pulmonary vascular resistance. Ionized calcium and blood glucose should be monitored closely and corrected if necessary. Digoxin should be avoided at this stage because it increases the risk of ventricular fibrillation.

Operative correction of TAPVC requires anastomosis of the common pulmonary venous channel to the left atrium, obliteration of the anomalous venous connection, and closure of the interatrial communication. All types of TAPVC are approached through a median sternotomy. To achieve a widely patent and accurate anastomosis in neonates and infants, most surgeons currently employ the technique of deep hypothermia and circulatory arrest. With this method, the infant is placed on cardiopulmonary bypass with an aortic cannula and a single venous cannula placed in the right atrial appendage. At initiation of bypass it is important to dissect out and ligate the ductus arteriosus to prevent overperfusion of the lungs and possible air embolism in the systemic circulation during the period of arrest. The infant is then cooled on bypass until a rectal temperature of 18° C. and a tympanic membrane temperature of 16° C. is reached. At this point the aorta is cross-clamped and cardioplegia is infused into the aortic root. Cardiopulmonary bypass is then discontinued, blood is drained from the infant, and the venous cannula is removed. The technique of correction is then individualized for the type of TAPVC that exists.

In the case of supracardiac TAPVC, the vertical vein is ligated outside the pericardial reflection to avoid obstructing the left upper lobe vein. The common pulmonary vein and posterior aspect of the left atrium are easily exposed by retracting the superior vena cava and aorta (Fig. 54–41).[43] After making longitudinal incisions in both of these structures, a large side-to-side anastomosis is performed using 7-0 monofilament absorbable suture. Through a small right atriotomy the atrial septal defect is closed with 5-0 polypropylene suture. The heart is then refilled with blood, cardiopulmonary bypass is resumed, and the infant is rewarmed to 37° C. Another technique described for repair of supracardiac TAPVC employs leftward traction of the right atrium to expose the anterior aspect of the pulmonary confluence and the posterior aspect of the left atrium for anastomosis.[23] One other approach uses a long biatrial incision that extends across the interatrial septum into the back wall of the left atrium directly anterior to the pulmonary confluence.[19, 41, 47] With this approach the pulmonary confluence is easily incorporated into the left atrium but a pericardial patch is often required to close the interatrial septum. Whichever approach is chosen it is imperative that a large, tension-free anastomosis be created.

In patients with TAPVC to the coronary sinus the repair can usually be performed completely through the right atrium (Fig. 54–42). The atrial septum is widely opened and the coronary sinus unroofed into the left atrium. A large piece of pericardium or polytetrafluoroethylene is then placed to close the atrial septal defect and direct the coronary sinus return to the left atrium. In cases with obstruction at the junction of the coronary sinus with the pulmonary confluence, this technique will not relieve the obstruction, and an alternate method similar to that used for supracardiac TAPVC should be performed.

Repair of infracardiac TAPVC is similar to that for the supracardiac type, except that the vertical vein is divided at the diaphragm and the proximal portion is opened longitudinally for incorporation in a patulous anastomosis to the left atrium. By elevating the apex of the heart superiorly the pulmonary venous confluence and left atrium can be easily visualized and a large anastomosis performed between the two structures (Fig. 54–43). Again the atrial septal defect is closed through a limited right atriotomy. As with supracardiac TAPVC, some surgeons prefer a right-sided or biatrial approach for this lesion.

Proper perioperative management is crucial to the success of surgical repair, especially in infants with obstructed TAPVC. The placement of a pulmonary artery catheter permits monitoring pulmonary artery pressures on weaning

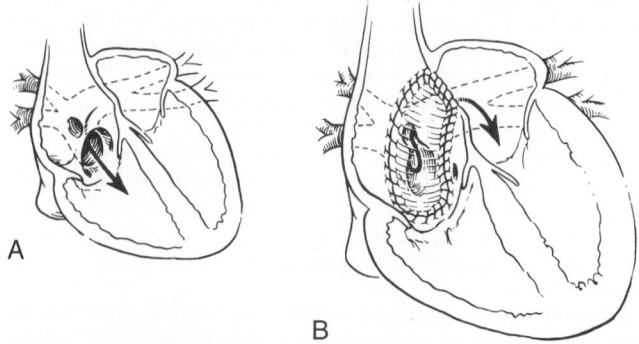

Figure 54–42. *A* and *B*, Repair of intracardiac TAPVC to the coronary sinus. The common wall between the coronary sinus and the left atrium is incised and a large patch closes the interatrial septum and directs all coronary sinus return into the left atrium. (From Lupinetti, F. M., Kulik, T. J., Beekman, R. H., III, Crowley, D. C., and Bove, E. L.: Correction of total anomalous pulmonary venous connection in infancy. J. Thorac. Cardiovasc. Surg., *106*:880, 1993.)

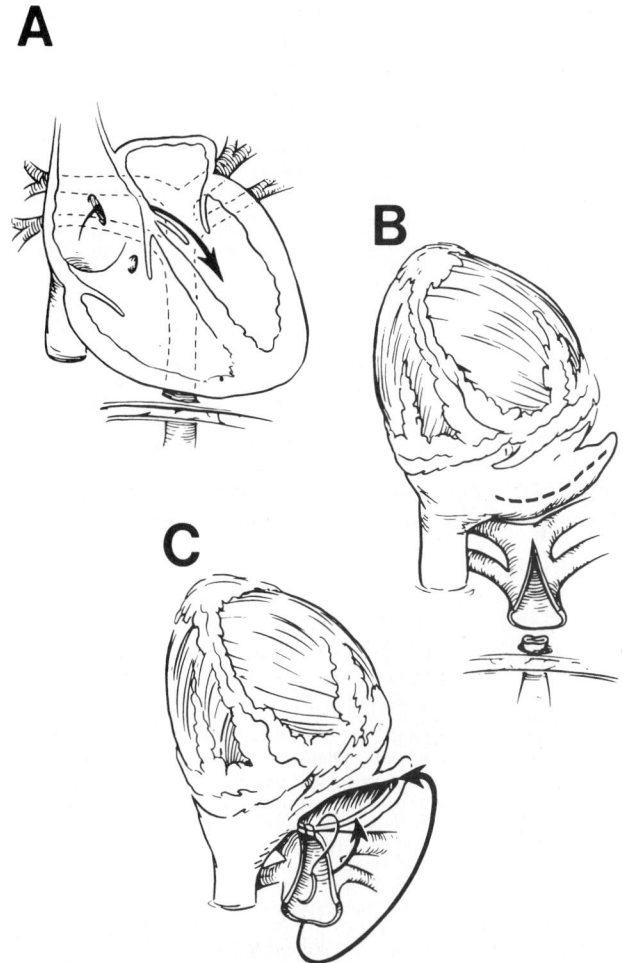

Figure 54–43. *A* to *C*, Repair of infracardiac TAPVC. Elevating the apex of the heart exposes the left atrium, and pulmonary confluence facilitates construction of a widely patent anastomosis. (From Lupinetti, F. M., Kulik, T. J., Beekman, R. H., III, Crowley, D. C., and Bove, E. L.: Correction of total anomalous pulmonary venous connection in infancy. J. Thorac. Cardiovasc. Surg., *106*:880, 1993.)

infants are at risk for developing episodes of pulmonary hypertension, which can be fatal. These episodes generally occur as a response to stress and develop as a result of severe constriction of heavily muscularized pulmonary arterioles. The combination of an acute pressure overload on the right ventricle and a lack of venous return to the left ventricle can result in sudden decompensation and death. To minimize stress in these infants, they are kept essentially anesthetized for the first 48 hours with a continuous infusion of fentanyl and hourly administration of pancuronium. A volume ventilator should maintain the PCO_2 between 25 and 35 mm. Hg, and the FIO_2 should be increased to a level that keeps pulmonary artery pressure less than two-thirds systemic. Should ventilatory maneuvers not suffice, pharmacologic agents such as isoproterenol, nitroglycerin, and nitroprusside should be considered. Experience with inspired nitric oxide suggests that it may be valuable in managing some cases of postoperative pulmonary hypertension.[21, 28] Endotracheal suctioning has often been associated with the initiation of pulmonary hypertensive crises and therefore should be minimized and performed with care only by expert nursing personnel. After 48 hours the muscle relaxant and sedation can be carefully tapered. If the infant is hemodynamically stable as he or she begins to react to his or her surroundings, ventilation can be weaned and the infant extubated within the ensuing 24 to 48 hours.

Surgical Results

The earliest surgical successes with TAPVC were in patients older than 1 year of age. By 1970 the operative mortality in this group was between 5% and 15%.[14, 48] The mortality in infants younger than 1 year of age, however, was in excess of 50%.[48] Since 1970 the surgical results for TAPVC correction in young infants have improved markedly. Reports published in the 1970s demonstrated a hospital mortality of approximately 25%.[31] More recent reports (Table 54–1) show hospital mortalities in the 5% to 10% range, with one report of only 2.3%.[38] It is especially notable in these reports that the median age at operation was as young as 13 days of life.

The most significant postoperative complication of TAPVC repair is pulmonary venous obstruction, which occurs in 5% to 10% of patients (see Table 54–1). This complication usually becomes manifest in the first weeks after operation with persistent pulmonary edema. Two-dimensional and pulsed Doppler echocardiography can identify the site of obstruction in most cases.[42] Early reoperation should be performed to relieve the obstruction. When the obstruction is at the level of the anastomosis, reoperation is likely to be successful.[40] Unfortunately some patients are found to have diffuse sclerosis and stenosis in the lobar veins both adjacent and distal to the anastomosis. Operative and transvenous attempts to relieve these obstructions have been disappointing.[18, 25, 38]

The prognosis is good for patients who survive operation without postoperative pulmonary venous obstruction. In a

from bypass and during the first 48 hours postoperatively. If there is no anastomotic narrowing, pulmonary artery pressures should be less than two-thirds systemic within 30 minutes of discontinuing bypass. Hyperventilation with 100% oxygen should minimize pulmonary vascular resistance and allow pulmonary pressures to fall to acceptable levels. Should pulmonary artery pressures remain systemic, an obstructed anastomosis or obstructed pulmonary veins are suggested. Intraoperative epicardial two-dimensional echocardiography may be helpful in examining these areas in question.

For the first 48 hours after repair of obstructed TAPVC,

TABLE 54–1. Repair of TAPVC in Infancy

Authors	Year Published	Years Reviewed	No. of Patients	Median Age	Hospital Mortality	Postoperative Obstruction
Sano, et al.[38]	1989	1979–1987	44	15 days	1 (2.3%)	4 (9.3%)
Corno, et al.[10]	1990	1983–1989	35	4.9 months (mean)	3 (8.6%)	Not reported
Wilson, et al.[47]	1992	Not reported	24	35 days	1 (4.2%)	2 (8.7%)
Raisher, et al.[34]	1992	1983–1990	20	32 days	1 (5%)	0 (0%)
Cobanaglu, et al.[8]	1993	1981–1991	30	28 days	4 (13.3%)	2 (7.7%)
Lupinetti, et al.[27]	1993	1985–1993	41	13 days	2 (4.9%)	2 (5.1%)
Total			194		12 (6.2%)	10 (6.7%)

follow-up study of 49 patients at the Mayo Clinic, 48 had survived from 1 to 14 years in good clinical condition.[15] Although the majority of patients are asymptomatic and on no medications, significant arrhythmias, including supraventricular tachycardia, intermittent heart block, and sick sinus syndrome, have been demonstrated in 30% to 40% of patients by 24-hour electrocardiographic monitoring, indicating a requirement for long-term follow-up.[39] Measurement of cardiopulmonary function during exercise has shown a mild reduction of aerobic capacity and an impaired heart rate response.[33] Despite these mild shortcomings, quality and quantity of life have been excellent in most patients after surgical repair.

PARTIAL ANOMALOUS PULMONARY VENOUS CONNECTION

PAPVC results when one or more, but not all, of the pulmonary veins fail to connect with the left atrium. PAPVC commonly occurs with an associated atrial septal defect and is often discovered during the evaluation or surgical repair of that defect. The physiologic effect of PAPVC is that of an atrial level left-to-right shunt with recirculation of oxygenated blood through the lungs. The degree of this effect is related to the number of anomalously connected veins, the site of the anomalous connection, and the presence, size, and location of any associated atrial septal defect. Although every possible combination of PAPVC has been reported, the three most common forms include connection of the right pulmonary veins to the superior vena cava, connection of the right pulmonary veins to the inferior vena cava, and connection of the left pulmonary veins to the left innominate vein (Fig. 54–44).

PAPVC with Right Pulmonary Veins to the Superior Vena Cava

The most common form of PAPVC occurs in association with a sinus venosus atrial septal defect. In this condition the right upper and middle lobe veins connect to the superior vena cava or high within the right atrium (see Fig. 54–44A). These veins are virtually never obstructed and thus only contribute to the left-to-right shunt that exists through the atrial septal defect. Most of these patients are asymptomatic; and, like other patients with atrial septal defects, the condition is detected when a systolic murmur and evidence of right-sided overflow is discovered.

Elective repair is best performed in the preschool years. Repair is effected with an intra-atrial baffle of pericardium that closes the high atrial defect and directs the flow from the anomalous veins into the left atrium. In cases in which placement of this baffle high within the superior vena cava threatens vena caval obstruction, the superior vena cava can be divided with the cardiac end oversewn and the cephalad end anastomosed to the right atrial appendage. A pericardial patch closes the atrial defect and allows the stump of the superior vena cava with its anomalous pulmonary veins to drain into the left atrium.[45]

PAPVC with Right Pulmonary Veins to the Inferior Vena Cava

In this condition the venous drainage of the right lung connects with the inferior vena cava near its junction with the right atrium (see Fig. 54–44B). Because of the crescentlike appearance that this abnormal pulmonary venous pathway displays on chest radiography, this particular form of PAPVC is often called the *scimitar syndrome*.[30] Hypoplasia of the right lung, a systemic arterial blood supply to the right lung,

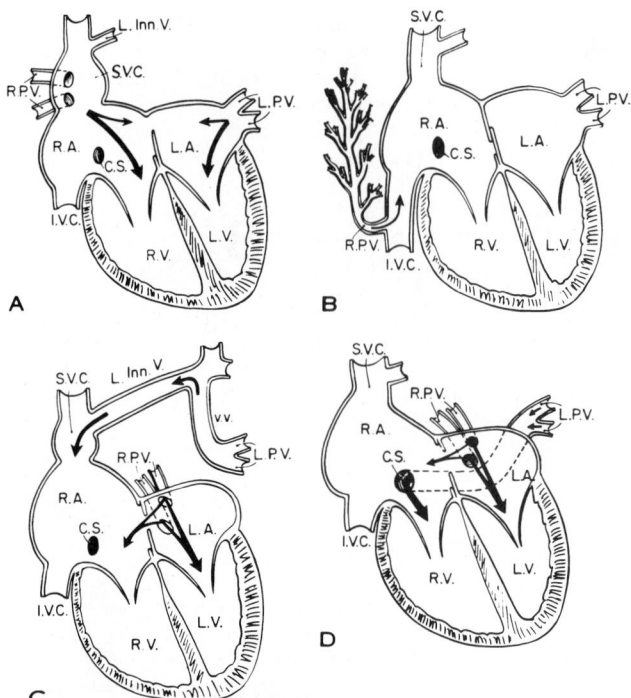

Figure 54–44. The most common forms of PAPVC. *A,* Anomalous connection of the right pulmonary veins (R.P.V.) to the superior vena cava (S.V.C.). This is commonly associated with a sinus venosus atrial septal defect. *B,* Anomalous connection of the right pulmonary veins to the inferior vena cava (I.V.C.). This is often referred to as the "scimitar" syndrome. *C,* Anomalous connection of the left pulmonary veins (L.P.V.) to the left innominate vein (L. Inn. V.) via a vertical vein (v.v.). A secundum atrial septal defect is also often present. *D,* Anomalous connection of the left pulmonary veins to the coronary sinus (C.S.). R.A., right atrium; L.A., left atrium; R.V., right ventricle; L.V., left ventricle. (From Lucas, R. V., Jr.: Anomalous venous connections, pulmonary and systemic. *In* Adams, F. H., and Emmanouilides, G. C. [Eds.]: Moss' Heart Disease In Infants, Children, and Adolescents, 3rd ed. Baltimore, Williams & Wilkins, 1983.)

and dextrocardia are variable components of this syndrome. Unlike most other forms of PAPVC, the interatrial septum is usually intact in these cases.[26] Surgical repair of this anomaly requires intra-atrial baffling of the right pulmonary vein orifice to an atrial septal defect created at the fossa ovalis.

PAPVC with Left Pulmonary Veins to the Left Innominate Vein

When the left pulmonary veins connect anomalously, they most commonly join the left innominate vein by means of a vertical vein derived from the left cardinal system (see Fig. 54–44C). If only the left upper lobe is so connected and no atrial septal defect exists, the physiologic and clinical consequences are minimal. However, if all of the left lung connects in this fashion, and especially if an atrial septal defect coexists, surgical correction is indicated. Operation includes ligation and division of the vertical vein and anastomosing the left pulmonary vein to the left atrial appendage in addition to closing any associated atrial septal defect.

CONGENITAL PULMONARY VENOUS OBSTRUCTION WITH NORMALLY CONNECTED PULMONARY VEINS

Pulmonary Vein Stenosis

This rare anomaly is characterized by localized narrowing of one or more pulmonary veins at or near their junctions with the left atrium. A fibrous intimal hyperplasia that can progress to complete occlusion is noted pathologically. Physiologically this condition resembles that of congenital mitral stenosis except that the pressure within the left atrium is normal and the pulmonary venous hypertension is unevenly distributed within the lungs. The severity of the clinical presentation relates to the number of veins involved and the degree of obstruction.

The condition usually presents in infancy as signs of pulmonary venous congestion (tachypnea, recurrent lower respiratory tract infections, hemoptysis) and failure to thrive. Chest radiography demonstrates asymmetrical pulmonary venous congestion, and electrocardiography reveals right ventricular hypertrophy without left atrial P wave abnormalities. Turbulent flow through the stenotic pulmonary veins is usually well delineated with two-dimensional echocardiography and Doppler flow imaging.

The prognosis of pulmonary vein stenosis is poor, with only a rare patient surviving beyond childhood. Methods of surgical repair have included the insertion of patches of pericardium or polytetrafluoroethylene to enlarge the stenotic area or excision of the stenotic segment and reimplantation of the pulmonary vein into the left atrium.[2] Unfortunately, in almost all of these attempts early restenosis has occurred, ultimately resulting in the death of the patient. A technique that employs autologous vascularized tissue to repair these stenoses involves using a flap of interatrial septum to enlarge narrowed right-sided pulmonary veins and applying an opened left atrial appendage to open stenoses of left pulmonary veins.[32] The initial report of this approach in a small number of cases is encouraging.

Cor Triatriatum

Cor triatriatum is a rare congenital heart malformation characterized by the presence of a diaphragm or membrane separating the left atrium into two chambers: an upper chamber into which all four pulmonary veins connect, and a lower chamber that communicates with the left atrial appendage and the mitral valve (Fig. 54–45). An atrial septal defect may also exist between the right atrium and the upper common pulmonary venous chamber or, less commonly, with the lower true left atrium. An incomplete incorporation of the common pulmonary vein into the left atrium is the most

commonly held theory for the embryogenesis of this anomaly.

The pathophysiologic effect of cor triatriatum is that of pulmonary venous obstruction similar to that seen in mitral stenosis. The clinical presentation is influenced by the size of the communication between the upper and lower chambers and the presence, location, and size of any associated atrial septal defect. The majority of patients present within the first year of life, but in some cases symptoms do not develop until the second or third decades. Presenting symptoms range from mild respiratory distress and fatigue to severe congestive heart failure. Physical signs are those of pulmonary hypertension and include a loud pulmonary S_2 sound and a right ventricular heave. Signs of right-sided heart failure, including hepatomegaly and distended veins, may be present. Cardiomegaly and increased pulmonary vascularity suggestive of pulmonary venous congestion are commonly noted on chest radiography. Electrocardiography often demonstrates right atrial and right ventricular hypertrophy. Definitive diagnosis can often be made with two-dimensional echocardiography. Apical four-chamber and subxiphoid atrial long-axis projections usually demonstrate the obstructing membrane between the confluence of pulmonary veins and the left atrial appendage and mitral valve. Doppler color flow imaging permits estimation of a gradient across the membrane. In some cases, however, cor triatriatum may be difficult to differentiate from total anomalous pulmonary venous connection to the coronary sinus or a persistent left superior vena cava connecting to the coronary sinus. Cardiac catheterization with selective pulmonary arteriography is performed when the echocardiographic evaluation is unclear.

As with presentation, prognosis is related to the degree of pulmonary venous obstruction. Patients with pulmonary edema or right-sided heart failure display a relentless downhill course and may die suddenly if the obstruction is not relieved surgically. Because even mild symptoms progress with time, the presence of cor triatriatum is an indication for surgical intervention.

Operative correction of cor triatriatum is relatively simple and straightforward. Cardiopulmonary bypass and cardioplegic cardiac arrest are employed. The obstructing membrane can be approached through the right atrium by incising the fossa ovalis or enlarging an existing atrial septal defect. The well-visualized left atrial membrane is then easily excised, and the atrial defect is then closed.[37] Good exposure of the membrane can also be achieved by opening the upper chamber just medial to the right pulmonary veins.[35] Recent experience with surgical correction indicates that operative mortality now approaches zero, especially if the lesion is identified early in its course and operation is performed in a timely fashion.[13, 35, 37] Survivors of surgical correction exhibit an excellent postoperative and long-term result.

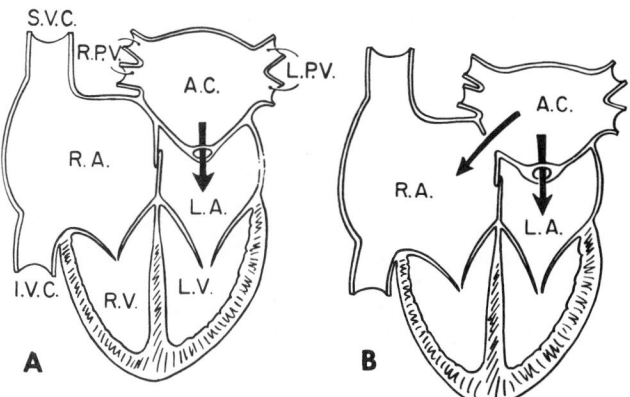

Figure 54–45. Cor triatriatum. *A,* In the classic form the only outlet of pulmonary venous blood from the upper accessory chamber (A.C.) is through the orifice in the intra-atrial membrane. *B,* When the upper accessory chamber communicates with the right atrium, the pulmonary venous system is decompressed and an atrial level left-to-right shunt results. S.V.C., superior vena cava; I.V.C., inferior vena cava; R.P.V., right pulmonary veins; L.P.V., left pulmonary veins; R. A., right atrium; L.A., left atrium; R.V., right ventricle; L.V., left ventricle. (From Lucas, R. V., Jr.: Anomalous venous connections, pulmonary and systemic. *In* Adams, F. H., and Emmanouilides, G. C. [Eds.]: Moss' Heart Disease In Infants, Children, and Adolescents, 3rd ed. Baltimore, Williams & Wilkins, 1983.)

SELECTED REFERENCES

Burroughs, J. T., and Edwards, J. E.: Total anomalous pulmonary venous connection. Am. Heart J., *59:*913, 1960.
This thorough analysis of TAPVC was written at the time when surgical repair first became possible.

Delisle, G., Ando, M., Calder, A. L., Zuberbuhler, J. R., Rochenmacher, S., Alday, L. E., Mangini, O., Van Praagh, S., and Van Praagh, R.: Total anomalous pulmonary venous connection: Report of 93 autopsied cases with emphasis on diagnostic and surgical considerations. Am. Heart J., *91:*99, 1976.
An exhaustive evaluation of a large collection of pathologic specimens is presented.

Kirklin, J. W., Barratt-Boyes, B. G.: Total anomalous pulmonary venous connection. *In* Kirklin, J. W., and Barratt-Boyes, B. G. (Eds.): Cardiac Surgery, 2nd ed. New York, Churchill Livingstone, 1993, pp. 645–673.
This thoroughly researched update on the subject has well-illustrated depictions of surgical techniques.

Lucas, R. V., Jr.: Anomalous venous connections, pulmonary and systemic. *In* Adams, F. H., and Emmanouilides, G. C. (Eds.): Moss' Heart Disease In

Infants, Children, and Adolescents, 3rd ed. Baltimore, Williams & Wilkins, 1983.
This chapter is a well-illustrated and comprehensive discussion of venous anomalies.

Lupinetti, F. M., Kulik, T. J., Beekman, R. H., III, Crowley, D. C., and Bove, E. L.: Correction of total anomalous pulmonary venous connection in infancy. J. Thorac. Cardiovasc. Surg., 106:880, 1993.
A recent surgical series demonstrates excellent results with modern techniques.

REFERENCES

1. Bailey, L. L., Takeuchi, Y., Williams, W. G., Trusler, G. A., and Mustard, W. T.: Surgical management of congenital cardiovascular anomalies with the use of profound hypothermia and circulatory arrest: Analysis of 180 consecutive cases. J. Thorac. Cardiovasc. Surg., 71:485, 1976.
2. Bini, R. M., Cleveland, D. C., Ceballos, R., Bargeron, L. M., Pacifico, A. D., and Kirklin, J. W.: Congenital pulmonary vein stenosis. Am. J. Cardiol., 54:369, 1984.
3. Brody, H.: Drainage of the pulmonary veins into the right side of the heart. Arch. Pathol., 33:221, 1942.
4. Burroughs, J. T., and Edwards, J. E.: Total anomalous pulmonary venous connection. Am. Heart J., 59:913, 1960.
5. Burroughs, J. T., and Kirklin, J. W.: Complete surgical correction of total anomalous pulmonary venous connection: Report of three cases. Staff Meet. Mayo Clin., 31:182, 1956.
6. Chin, A. J., Sanders, S. P., Sherman, F., Lang, P., Norwood, W. I., and Castañeda, A. R.: Accuracy of subcostal two-dimensional echocardiography in prospective diagnosis of total anomalous pulmonary venous connection. Am. Heart J., 113:1153, 1987.
7. Choe, Y. H., Lee, H. J., Kim, H. S., Ko, J. K., Kim, J. E., and Han, J. J.: MRI of total anomalous pulmonary venous connections. J. Comput. Assist. Tomogr., 18:243, 1994.
8. Cobanoglu, A., and Menashe, V. D.: Total anomalous pulmonary venous connection in neonates and young infants: Repair in the current era. Ann. Thorac. Surg., 55:43, 1993.
9. Cooley, D. A., and Ochsner, A., Jr.: Correction of total anomalous pulmonary venous drainage. Surgery, 42:1014, 1957.
10. Corno, A., Giamberti, A., Carotti, A., Giannico, S., Marnio, B., and Marcelletti, C.: Total anomalous pulmonary venous connection: Surgical repair with a double-patch technique. Ann. Thorac. Surg., 49:492, 1990.
11. Darling, R. C., Rothney, W. B., and Craig, J. M.: Total pulmonary venous drainage into the right side of the heart. Lab. Invest., 6:44, 1957.
12. Delisle, G., Ando, M., Calder, A. L., Zuberbuhler, J. R., Rochenmacher, S., Alday, L. E., Mangini, O., Van Praagh, S., and Van Praagh, R.: Total anomalous pulmonary venous connection: Report of 93 autopsied cases with emphasis on diagnostic and surgical considerations. Am. Heart J., 91:99, 1976.
13. Gheissari, A., Malm, J. R., Bowman, F. O., Jr., and Bierman, F. Z.: Cor triatriatum sinistrum: One institution's 28-year experience. Pediatr. Cardiol., 13:85, 1992.
14. Gomes, M. M. R., Feldt, R. H., McGoon, D. C., and Danielson, G. K.: Total anomalous pulmonary venous connection: Surgical considerations and results of operation. J. Thorac. Cardiovasc. Surg., 60:116, 1970.
15. Gomes, M. M. R., Feldt, R. H., McGoon, D. C., and Danielson, G. K.: Long-term results following correction of total anomalous pulmonary venous connection. J. Thorac. Cardiovasc. Surg., 61:253, 1971.
16. Goswami, K. C., Shrivastava, S., Saxena, A., and Dev, V.: Echocardiographic diagnosis of total anomalous pulmonary venous connection. Am. Heart J., 126:433, 1993.
17. Hammon, J. W., Jr., and Bender, H. W., Jr.: Anomalous venous connections: Pulmonary and systemic. In Baue, A. E. (Ed.): Glenn's Textbook of Thoracic and Cardiovascular Surgery, 5th ed. Norwalk, Conn., Appleton & Lange, 1991, pp. 971–993.
18. Jenkins, K. J., Sanders, S. P., Orav, E. J., Coleman, E. A., Mayer, J. E., Jr., and Colan, S. D.: Individual pulmonary vein size and survival in infants with totally anomalous pulmonary venous connection. J. Am. Coll. Cardiol., 22:201, 1993.
19. Jonas, R. A., and Castañeda, A. R.: Disorders of pulmonary venous return. In Sabiston, D. C., Jr. (Ed.): Textbook of Surgery: The Biological Basis of Modern Surgical Practice, 14th ed. Philadelphia, W. B. Saunders, 1990, pp. 1892–1898.
20. Jonas, R. A., Smolinsky, A., Mayer, J. E., and Castañeda, A. R.: Obstructed pulmonary venous drainage with total anomalous pulmonary venous connection to the coronary sinus. Am. J. Cardiol., 59:431, 1987.
21. Journois, D., Pouard, P., Mauriat, P., Malhere, T., Vouhe, P., and Safran, D.: Inhaled nitric oxide as a therapy for pulmonary hypertension after operations for congenital heart defects. J. Thorac. Cardiovasc. Surg., 107:1129, 1994.
22. Keith, J. D., Rowe, R. D., Vlad, P., and O'Hanicy, I. H.: Complete anomalous pulmonary venous drainage. Am. J. Med., 16:23, 1954.
23. Kirklin, J. W., and Barratt-Boyes, B. G.: Total anomalous pulmonary venous connection. In Kirklin, J. W., and Barratt-Boyes, B. G. (Eds.): Cardiac Surgery, 2nd ed. New York, Churchill Livingstone, 1993, pp. 645–673.
24. Lewis, F. I., Varco, R. L., Taufic, M., and Niazi, S. A.: Direct vision repair of triatrial heart and total anomalous pulmonary venous drainage. Surg. Gynecol. Obstet., 102:713, 1956.
25. Lock, J. E., Bass, J. L., Castañeda-Zuniga, W., Fuhrman, B. P., Rashkind, W. J., and Lucas, R. V., Jr.: Dilation angioplasty of congenital or operative narrowings of venous channels. Circulation, 70:457, 1984.
26. Lucas, R. V., Jr.: Anomalous venous connections, pulmonary and systemic. In Adams, F. H., and Emmanouilides, G. C. (Eds.): Moss' Heart Disease in Infants, Children, and Adolescents, 3rd ed. Baltimore, Williams & Wilkins, 1983.
27. Lupinetti, F. M., Kulik, T. J., Beekman, R. H., III, Crowley, D. C., and Bove, E. L.: Correction of total anomalous pulmonary venous connection in infancy. J. Thorac. Cardiovasc. Surg., 106:880, 1993.
28. Miller, O. I., Celermajer, D. S., Deanfield, J. E., and Macrae, D. J.: Very-low-dose inhaled nitric oxide: A selective pulmonary vasodilator after operations for congenital heart disease. J. Thorac. Cardiovasc. Surg., 108:487, 1994.
29. Muller, W. H., Jr.: The surgical treatment of transposition of the pulmonary veins. Ann. Surg., 134:683, 1951.
30. Neill, C. A., Ferencz, D., Sabiston, D. C., and Sheldon, H.: The familial occurrence of hypoplastic right lung with systemic arterial supply and venous drainage: "Scimitar syndrome." Johns Hopkins Med. J., 107:1, 1960.
31. Norwood, W. I., and Castañeda, A. R.: Disorders of pulmonary venous return. In Sabiston, D. C., Jr. (Ed.): Textbook of Surgery: The Biological Basis of Modern Surgical Practice, 13th ed. Philadelphia, W. B. Saunders, 1986.
32. Pacifico, A. D., Mandke, N. V., McGrath, L. B., Colvin, E. V., Bini, R. M., and Bargeron, L. M.: Repair of congenital pulmonary venous stenosis with living autologous atrial tissue. J. Thorac. Cardiovasc. Surg., 89:604, 1985.
33. Paridon, S. M., Sullivan, N. M., Schneider, J., and Pinsky, W. W.: Cardiopulmonary performance at rest and exercise after repair of total anomalous pulmonary venous connection. Am. J. Cardiol., 72:1444, 1993.
34. Raisher, B. D., Grant, J. W., Martin, T. C., Strauss, A. W., and Spray, T. L.: Complete repair of total anomalous pulmonary venous connection in infancy. J. Thorac. Cardiovasc. Surg., 104:443, 1992.
35. Rodefeld, M. D., Brow, J. W., Heimansohn, D. A., King, H., Girod, D.A., Hurwitz, R. A., and Caldwell, R. L.: Cor triatriatum: Clinical presentation and surgical results in 12 patients. Ann. Thorac. Surg., 50:562, 1990.
36. Rowe, R. D.: Anomalies of venous return. In Keith, J. D., Rowe, R. D., and Vlad, P. (Eds.): Heart Disease in Infancy and Childhood, 3rd ed. New York, Macmillan, 1978, p. 566.
37. Salomone, G., Tiraboschi, R., Bianchi, T., Ferri, F., Crippa, M., and Parenzan, L.: Cor triatriatum: Clinical presentation and operative results. J. Thorac. Cardiovasc. Surg., 101:1088, 1991.
38. Sano, S., Brawn, W. J., and Mee, R. B.: Total anomalous pulmonary venous drainage. J. Thorac. Cardiovasc. Surg., 97:886, 1989.
39. Saxena, A., Fong, L. V., Lamb, R. K., Monro, J. L., Shore, D. F., and Keeton, B. R.: Cardiac arrhythmias after surgical correction of total anomalous pulmonary venous connection: Late follow-up. Pediatr. Cardiol., 12:89, 1991.
40. Schafers, J. H., Luhmer, I., and Oelert, H.: Pulmonary venous obstruction following repair of total anomalous pulmonary venous drainage. Ann. Thorac. Surg., 43:432, 1987.
41. Shumacker, H. B., Jr., and King, H.: A modified procedure for complete repair of total anomalous pulmonary venous drainage. Surg. Gynecol. Obstet., 112:763, 1961.
42. Smallhorn, J. F., Burrows, P., Wilson, G., Coles, J., Gilday, D. L., and Freedom, R. M.: Two-dimensional and pulsed Doppler echocardiography in the postoperative evaluation of total anomalous pulmonary venous connection. Circulation, 76:298, 1987.
43. Tucker, B. L., Lindesmith, G. G., Stiles, Q. R., and Meyer, B. W.: The superior approach for correction of the supracardiac type of total anomalous pulmonary venous return. Ann. Thorac. Surg., 74:374, 1976.
44. Wang, J. K., Li, Y. W., Young, M. L., How, S. W., and Lue, H. C.: Delineation of obstruction in total anomalous pulmonary venous connection utilizing magnetic resonance imaging. Am. Heart J., 124:807, 1992.
45. Warden, H. E., Gustafson, R. A., Tarnay, T. J., and Neal, W. A.: An alternative method for repair of partial anomalous pulmonary venous connection to the superior vena cava. Ann. Thorac. Surg., 38:601, 1984.
46. Wilson, J.: A description of a very unusual formation of the human heart. Phil. Trans. R. Soc. Lond., 88:346, 1798.
47. Wilson, W. R., Ilbawi, M. N., DeLeon, S. Y., Quinones, J. A., Arcilla, R. A., Sulayman, R. F., and Idriss, F. S.: Technical modifications for improved results in total anomalous pulmonary venous drainage. J. Thorac. Cardiovasc. Surg., 103:861, 1992.
48. Wukasch, D. C., Deutsch, M., Reul, G. J., Hallman, G. L., and Cooley, D. A.: Total anomalous pulmonary venous return. Ann. Thorac. Surg., 19:622, 1975.

VI

VENTRICULAR SEPTAL DEFECTS

Henry L. Walters III, M.D., Albert D. Pacifico, M.D., and James K. Kirklin, M.D.

A ventricular septal defect (VSD) is a hole in the interventricular septum (IVS). It is most commonly single, but multiple defects may also occur. VSD, in its isolated form, is the most commonly recognized congenital heart defect.[35] It occurs at an approximate rate of 2 per 1000 live births and represents 30% to 40% of all congenital heart malformations at birth.[22] These defects vary widely in size and location and may be associated with a variety of related minor and major cardiac anomalies. When isolated VSDs are combined with VSDs associated with other congenital cardiac defects, the total group accounts for over 50% of patients with congenital heart disease. The focus here is on isolated VSDs in hearts with normal segmental connections without overriding of arterial or atrioventricular (AV) valves and also briefly on those VSDs associated with patent ductus arteriosus, aortic insufficiency, pulmonary stenosis, and coarctation of the aorta.

HISTORICAL ASPECTS

In 1879, Roger described the clinical manifestations of VSD and the underlying pathologic condition.[46] The development of cardiac catheterization techniques by 1950 allowed precise delineation of the hemodynamic alterations produced by such defects. Muller and Dammann[38] first surgically managed VSDs by banding the pulmonary artery to reduce the pressure and flow in the pulmonary vascular system and to reduce the likelihood of the development of irreversible pulmonary hypertension. Lillehei and colleagues,[33] in 1954, first successfully repaired a VSD using controlled cross circulation with an adult human as the oxygenator. Intracardiac repair using a pump oxygenator for cardiopulmonary support was first accomplished in 1955 by DuShane and colleagues.[12] Subsequent surgical refinements included the use of a transatrial approach to VSD closure in 1957 by Stirling and colleagues,[53] the use of profound hypothermia with total circulatory arrest followed by rewarming with a pump oxygenator by Okamoto in 1969,[40] the feasibility of primary repair of VSDs in infants by Kirklin and DuShane in 1961[29] and Sigmann and associates in 1967,[48] and the demonstration by Barratt-Boyes beginning in 1969 that routine primary repair of VSDs in symptomatic small infants was superior to pulmonary artery banding.[3]

ANATOMY

Orientation. A discussion of the morphology of VSDs is difficult to comprehend without an understanding of the positional terms that are used to describe the location, orientation, and relations of ventricular septal structures. The surgeon's view of the cardiac septum is usually from the right side of the operating table with the patient in the supine position. The patient's head is to the surgeon's left-hand side. Structures that tend toward the surgeon's left occupy the *superior* aspect of the cardiac septum. Conversely, structures that tend toward the surgeon's right (toward the patient's foot) occupy the *inferior* aspect of the septum. *Anterior* denotes location or extension in the cardiac septum toward the anterior interventricular groove away from the surgeon. *Posterior* denotes location or extension toward the insertion

of the septal leaflet of the tricuspid valve in the direction of the surgeon.

These same terms can be used to name the rims of any given VSD regardless of its location in the IVS. Hence, a muscular VSD located in the anterior portion of the apical-trabecular septum has anterior, posterior, superior, and inferior rims. These terms are also useful in describing the relationships of various lesions and normal cardiac structures to each other.

General. The ventricular septum can be subdivided into interventricular and AV components (Table 54–2). Because the tricuspid valve anulus inserts more apically on the cardiac septum than does the mitral valve anulus, a portion of the cardiac septum lies between the left ventricle and the right atrium. This is appropriately called the AV septum because a defect confined to this structure alone would result in a communication between the left ventricle and the right atrium and not between the two ventricles. Isolated VSDs, however, are classified according to their location within the IVS and according to the relationships of their borders to surrounding cardiac structures. A brief review of the normal anatomy of the IVS is essential to an understanding of the classification of VSDs (Fig. 54–46; see Table 54–2).

The IVS is divided into two components: membranous and muscular (see Table 54–2).

Interventricular Septum—Membranous Portion. The term *membranous septum* is an inclusive one that denotes the completely fibrous portion of the cardiac septum. The membranous septum is *not* entirely interventricular. It is divided into two components by the attachment of the tricuspid valve anulus to the cardiac septum. The interventricular component of the membranous septum is located on the right ventricular side of this tricuspid valve attachment. It separates the left ventricular outflow tract from the right ventricle and is, therefore, truly interventricular. The portion of the membranous septum on the right atrial side of the tricuspid valve insertion is the membranous portion of the AV septum (see General above). Thus, the membranous septum is partially interventricular (membranous portion of the IVS) and partially AV (membranous portion of the AV septum) (see Table 54–2). The membranous portion of the IVS is adjacent to the commissure between the anterior and septal leaflets of

TABLE 54–2. Anatomy of the Ventricular Septum

Interventricular Component

Membranous portion
Muscular portion
   Inlet
   Outlet (infundibular or conal)
   Apical-trabecular (trabecular or muscular)

Atrioventricular Component

Membranous portion
Muscular portion

The ventricular septum is divided into interventricular and atrioventricular components. Each of these components contains membranous and muscular portions. The muscular portion of the interventricular septum is further subdivided into inlet, outlet, and apical-trabecular regions (see text for details). Other terms commonly found in the literature are in parentheses.

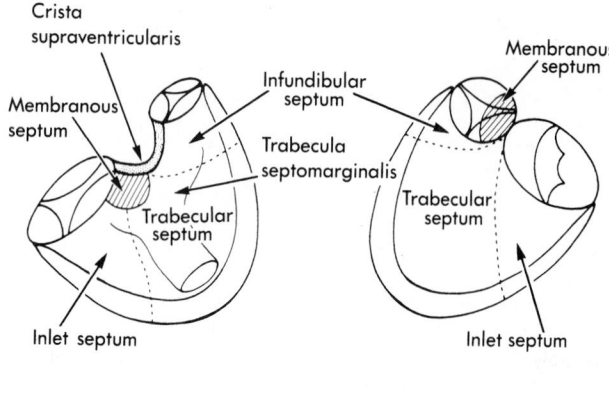

Figure 54–46. The components of the ventricular septum as observed from the right ventricle *(A)* and left ventricle *(B)*. (From Soto, B., Becker, A. E., Moulaert, A. J., et al.: Classification of ventricular septal defects. Br. Heart J., *43*:332, 1980.)

the tricuspid valve (anteroseptal commissure) (see Fig. 54–46). This serves as a useful landmark for the identification of the membranous portion of the IVS in a normal heart specimen.

Interventricular Septum—Muscular Portion. The right and

left ventricular septal surfaces are not identical, but the muscular portion of the IVS on both the right and the left ventricular sides can be subdivided into three portions termed the *inlet septum,* the *apical-trabecular* (also known as *trabecular*) *septum,* and the *outlet* (also known as *infundibular* or *conal*) *septum* (see Fig. 54–46 and Table 54–2). The inlet portion surrounds and supports the tricuspid valve on the right ventricular side and the mitral valve on the left ventricular side. It is typically smooth in its external appearance. The apical-trabecular portion is identified by its coarse trabeculations on the right ventricular side and by fine trabeculations on the left ventricular side. The outlet portion of the muscular IVS makes up the remainder of the IVS on both the right and left sides and lies beneath the arterial (pulmonary and aortic) valves.

Atrioventricular Septum. As described previously, the portion of the cardiac septum separating the left ventricle from the right atrium is termed the *AV septum* (see Table 54–2). The AV septum has a fibrous component anteriorly (membranous portion of the AV septum) and a muscular component posteriorly (muscular portion of the AV septum).

Normal Course of the Conduction Tissue. The AV node lies in the muscular portion of the AV septum within the triangle of Koch, the borders of the latter being formed by the coronary sinus, the tendon of Todaro, and the tricuspid anulus (Fig. 54–47). The bundle of His continues from the AV node and pierces the central fibrous body. It courses

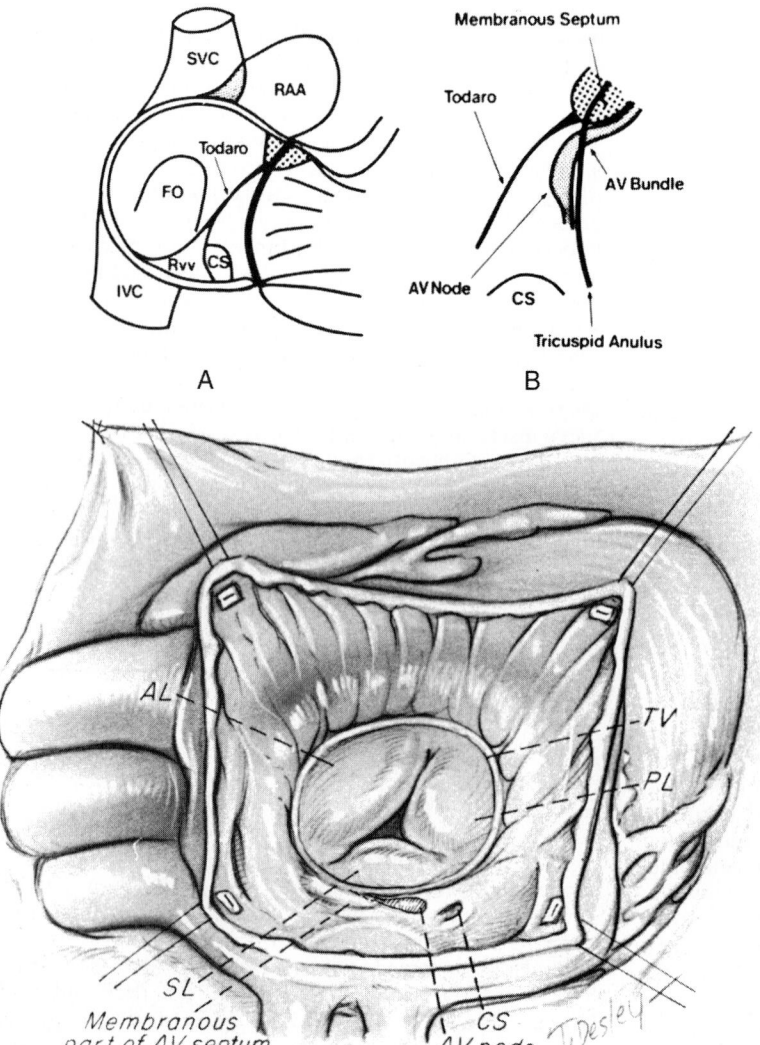

Figure 54–47. Anatomic and surgical aspects of the conduction system. *A,* Diagram of the triangle of Koch within the right atrium. The triangle is defined by the tendon of Todaro, the orifice of the coronary sinus, and the tricuspid anulus. *B,* Diagram showing the relationship of the AV node and AV bundle (His bundle) to the triangle of Koch. The AV node lies within the triangle, and the AV bundle is located at the apex of the triangle. *C,* Interior of the right atrium as seen at operation. AV, atrioventricular; CS, coronary sinus; SVC, superior vena cava; TV, tricuspid valve. (*A* and *B* adapted from Anderson, R. H., Becker, A. E., Wenink, A. C. G.: The development of the conducting tissues. *In* Roberts, N. K., and Gelband, H. [Eds.]: Cardiac Arrhythmias in the Neonate, Infant and Child. Norwalk, CT, Appleton & Lange, 1977, p. 19. *C* adapted from Kirklin, J. W., and Barrett-Boyes, B. G.: Anatomy, dimensions and terminology. *In* Cardiac Surgery, 2nd ed. New York, Churchill Livingstone, 1993, p. 14.)

along the posteroinferior border of the membranous IVS and along the crest of the muscular IVS in an area just inferior to the anteroseptal commissure of the tricuspid valve. During its course it gives off fibers forming the left bundle branch that fan out over the left ventricular septal surface. The remaining fibers of the bundle of His form the right bundle branch that fans out over the right ventricular septal surface.

MORPHOLOGY

Classifications. Many different classifications of VSDs have been proposed.[51, 52, 57, 60, 61] All of these classifications are helpful and share some common features. There is no consensus as to the superiority of one classification over another, and a familiarity with all of them is not only useful in understanding the literature but also in interpreting results.

One surgically relevant classification was proposed by Anderson and Wilcox[2] and builds on the principles developed in an earlier report by the same authors.[52] This classification was chosen because of the durability of its fundamental principles and because of the descriptive and simple nature of its terms. Because numerous terms have been used in the literature to categorize VSDs, many of them are included here to clarify their relationship to Anderson and Wilcox's classification and to minimize confusion. According to Anderson and Wilcox's classification, VSDs can be classified according to the (1) rims (or boundaries) of the defect and (2) region of the morphologic right ventricle, into which the defect opens. Variations in the rims of VSDs produce three general classes of defects: (1) perimembranous, (2) muscular, and (3) doubly committed/juxta-arterial (Fig. 54–48).

Perimembranous Defects. Perimembranous lesions (also known as paramembranous or Type II defects) occupy the area of the membranous portion of the IVS adjacent to the anteroseptal commissure of the tricuspid valve (see Fig. 54–48). Often a remnant of the membranous portion of the IVS (the membranous flap) is left hanging on the posteroinferior rim of the defect. These lesions border on the membranous portion of the AV septum (hence the name perimembranous) and are adjacent to the aortic valve, namely, to its right and noncoronary cusps. The anulus of the tricuspid and that of the aortic valves often form part of the rim of the defect, but in some patients they are separated from the VSD by a thin rim of muscular tissue. Perimembranous lesions can extend from the perimembranous region into the inlet portion of the right ventricle beneath the septal leaflet of the tricuspid valve (also known as AV canal type or Type III defects), into the outlet portion, into the apical-trabecular portion, or into a

combination of regions (confluent) (see Fig. 54–48, Table 54–3). These defects are accurately described as being perimembranous with inlet, outlet, or apical-trabecular extension, respectively. The conduction tissue in all of these perimembranous lesions passes along the posteroinferior rim of the defect (Fig. 54–49).

Muscular Defects. Lesions with an *exclusively muscular* rim are called muscular defects (also known as Type IV defects) (see Fig. 54–48). In the case of a muscular defect that does not extend into the perimembranous region of the IVS, the course of the conduction tissue remains as it is in the normal heart. The position of the conduction tissue relative to the defect therefore depends on where the defect actually opens into the right ventricle. For example, when the muscular defect opens into the right ventricle directly below the septal leaflet of the tricuspid valve (inlet muscular defect), the conduction tissue runs along its anterosuperior margin. When a purely muscular defect opens into the right ventricular outlet (outlet muscular defect or, alternatively, conal or infundibular muscular defect) the conduction tissue runs posteroinferiorly to the VSD but is protected by the muscular rim that forms the posterior edge of the defect. Muscular defects that open into the apical-trabecular region of the right ventricle (apical-trabecular muscular defects or, alternatively, trabecular muscular defects) can be either single or multiple. Most commonly, multiple defects are located in the anterior portion of the apical-trabecular septum. At times, defects that seem to be multiple when viewed from the right ventricular side have only a single opening when viewed from the left ventricular side. A multitude of these apical-trabecular muscular defects produces what is called a *Swiss cheese* septum. Apical-trabecular muscular defects are usually far removed from the central axis of the conduction tissue, with their proximity determined by the amount of muscle separating them from the perimembranous region of the IVS.

Doubly Committed and Juxta-arterial Defects. These defects (otherwise known as subarterial, subarterial infundibular, supracristal, or Type I defects) are described as being doubly committed because they open beneath both the aortic

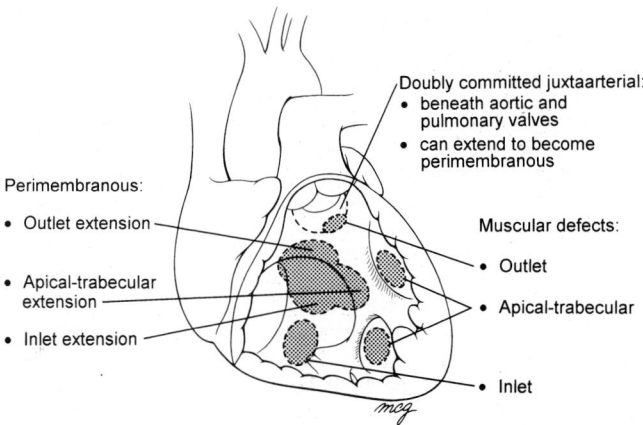

Figure 54–48. Classification of isolated ventricular septal defects. See text for details. (Courtesy of Professor Robert H. Anderson, Royal Brompton, National Heart & Lung Institute, London, England.)

Perimembranous:
- Outlet extension
- Apical-trabecular extension
- Inlet extension

Doubly committed juxtaarterial:
- beneath aortic and pulmonary valves
- can extend to become perimembranous

Muscular defects:
- Outlet
- Apical-trabecular
- Inlet

TABLE 54–3. Classification of Ventricular Septal Defects

Perimembranous Defects

Perimembranous* (paramembranous, Type II)
Perimembranous with
  Inlet extension (atrioventricular canal type defect or Type III)
  Outlet extension
  Apical-trabecular (trabecular or muscular) extension
  Confluent†

Muscular Defects (Type IV)

Inlet muscular
Outlet muscular (conal or infundibular muscular)
Apical-trabecular muscular (trabecular muscular)

Doubly Committed/Juxta-arterial (subarterial, subarterial infundibular, supracristal, Type I)

Without perimembranous extension
With perimembranous extension

---

*Isolated perimembranous VSDs without extension beyond the perimembranous region.

†"Confluent" denotes extension of the perimembranous VSD into any combination of inlet, outlet, or apical-trabecular regions.

Anderson's classification of isolated VSDs divides these lesions into perimembranous, muscular, and doubly committed/juxta-arterial lesions.[2, 52] This system attempts to categorize VSDs according to their rims (boundaries) and according to the region of the morphologic right ventricle into which these defects open.

The classification of VSDs can be confusing because of the lack of uniformity in the literature. Alternative terms, used in the literature and in the previous edition of this textbook, have been placed in parentheses.

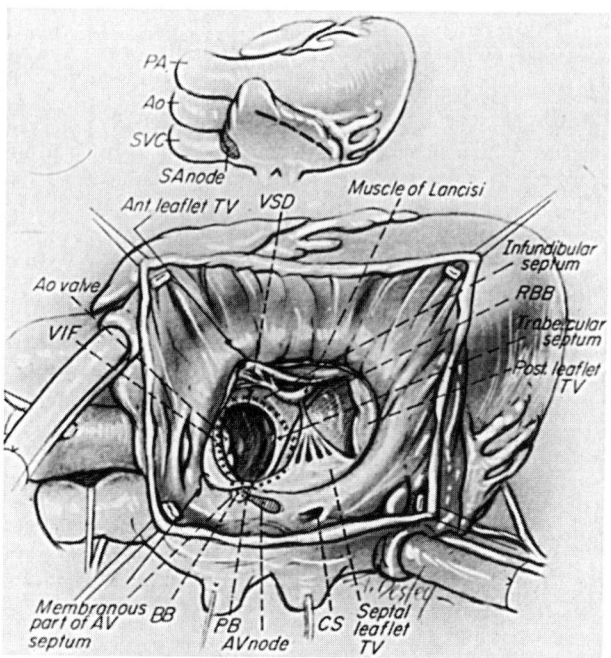

Figure 54–49. The sinus node and position of the right atriotomy are demonstrated above. Transatrial exposure of a perimembranous VSD is demonstrated below looking through the retracted tricuspid valve leaflets. The coronary sinus (CS) and the nearby atrioventricular (AV) node with the penetrating portion of the bundle of His (PB) and its branching portion (BB) as well as the right bundle branch (RBB) are demonstrated in relation to the VSD. The pathway of the suture line that secures the patch used to close the VSD is indicated by the Xs along the muscular portion of the ventricular septum as well as the ventriculoinfundibular fold (VIF) and the dots shown in the base of the septal leaflet of the tricuspid valve (TV). The suture line remains well away from the inferior free edge of the VSD and on the tricuspid leaflet near its base to avoid the surgical creation of heart block. Ao, aorta; PA, pulmonary artery; SVC, superior vena cava; SA, sinoatrial. (From Bharati, S., Lev, M., and Kirklin, J. W.: Cardiac Surgery and the Conduction System. New York, John Wiley & Sons, 1983.)

and pulmonary valves. They are juxta-arterial because their superior border is formed by fibrous tissue between the leaflets of the aortic and pulmonary valves (and not by muscle) (see Table 54–3 and Fig. 54–48). These defects, in particular, are associated with prolapse of the leaflets of the aortic valve, causing progressive aortic insufficiency. In most of these defects there is a muscular posteroinferior rim that protects the conduction tissue in its course. In a small number of hearts with doubly committed/juxta-arterial defects, this rim of muscle is not present so that the defect extends into the perimembranous region. These defects can be considered both doubly committed/juxta-arterial and perimembranous (doubly committed/juxta-arterial with perimembranous extension) (see Table 54–3).

ASSOCIATED LESIONS

Approximately 50% of patients undergoing surgical treatment for primary VSD have an associated lesion.[3, 5]

Patent Ductus Arteriosus. A moderate- or large-sized patent ductus arteriosus is associated with the VSD in approximately 6% of patients of all ages. In infants with VSD and concomitant heart failure, however, patent ductus arteriosus is present in approximately 25%.[3]

Coarctation of the Aorta. A VSD in combination with severe coarctation of the aorta occurs in approximately 17% of patients.[54] This combination is also more common among infants with a large VSD undergoing operation when younger than the age of 3 months.

Aortic Valve Incompetence. In some patients with a VSD, aortic valve incompetence develops over time, presumably as a result of progressive prolapse of the right aortic cusp through the defect.[39, 58] Abnormalities in the development of the aortic root may also contribute to the development of this aortic incompetence. In the United States, two thirds of patients with VSD and aortic valve incompetence have perimembranous lesions and one third have a doubly committed/juxta-arterial lesion. In Japan, however, the reverse is true: two thirds have doubly committed/juxta-arterial lesions, and one third have perimembranous lesions. Systolic pressure gradients between the inlet portion of the right ventricle and the pulmonary artery are present in approximately 50% of patients with VSD and aortic valve incompetence. This is related to displacement and hypertrophy of the infundibular portion of the septum and its parietal and septal insertions.[25] The prolapsed aortic valve leaflet may also contribute to the right ventricular outflow tract obstruction.[50]

Valvular/Subvalvular Aortic Stenosis. Congenital valvular or subvalvular aortic stenosis occurs in approximately 4% of patients undergoing an operation for VSD. Subvalvular stenosis is more common and may be present when there is associated infundibular pulmonary stenosis.[30] In addition, it may develop from the hypertrophy induced by pulmonary artery banding[14] and may be a discrete fibromuscular bar on the *inferior* edge of the VSD within the left ventricular outflow tract. When leftward (toward the left ventricular outflow tract) displacement of the infundibular (conal) septum occurs, the subaortic stenosis is *superior* to the location of the VSD. This type of subaortic stenosis is often associated with aortic arch anomalies, such as interrupted aortic arch.[10, 37, 59]

Other Associated Lesions. Associated lesions of minor anatomic or functional significance were present in 47% of patients undergoing closure of a primary VSD.[5] These included mild or moderate pulmonary stenosis in 20%; atrial septal defect in 17%; persistent left superior vena cava in 9%; and dextroposition of the aorta in 5%. Aneurysm of the membranous IVS, mild or moderate coarctation of the aorta, vascular ring, and tricuspid, mitral, or pulmonary valve incompetence occurred in less than 1% each.

PATHOPHYSIOLOGY

VSD Size. The size of VSDs varies considerably. A large VSD is approximately the size of the aortic orifice or larger and causes systemic (equal to left ventricular) right ventricular systolic pressure. In the absence of right ventricular outflow tract obstruction, the pulmonary artery systolic pressure is also systemic. Small VSDs have insufficient size to raise right ventricular systolic pressure, and the ratio of pulmonary to systemic flow (Qp:Qs) does not increase above 1.75. Moderate-sized VSDs are *restrictive* but have sufficient size to raise the right ventricular systolic pressure to approximately one half of the left ventricular pressure and may cause a Qp:Qs of 2 to 3.5. Several small defects may together appear as a large defect.

Shunting. The direction and size of the shunt in patients with VSD depend on the size of the defect and the differences in pressure between the ventricles during systole and diastole. When the VSD is small (restrictive), it offers considerable resistance to flow, and only a relatively large pressure difference between the two ventricles, such as occurs during mid- and late systole, causes significant flow across the defect. In this circumstance, because pressure is higher in the left ventricle than in the right ventricle, the direction of the shunt is left to right. In contrast, when the defect is large (unrestrictive) it offers little resistance to flow and similar peak pressures are present in both the left and right ventricles. The direction and magnitude of flow through the defect is dependent on the small pressure differences that are present during systole between the left and right ventricles.[24, 32] During mid- and late systole, when most of the shunting occurs, the pressure differences between the two ventricles are primarily due to the relative resistance to ejection offered by the systemic and pulmonary vasculature. In diastole and early systole, a number of additional factors, including the relative compliance of each ventricle, their diastolic pressures, and the presence of asynchronous contraction influence the magnitude and direction of the shunt.[32] The size of the VSD, which may vary during the various phases of the cardiac cycle, also may influence the degree of shunting.

When a left-to-right shunt is present at the ventricular level, pulmonary blood flow is increased above normal and above the systemic blood flow. Flow through the VSD into the right ventricle, pulmonary artery, pulmonary veins, left atrium, and mitral valve orifice into the left ventricle is similarly increased. Consequently, greater work is performed by both the left and the right ventricles. In the absence of a large atrial septal defect, the left atrium is enlarged in proportion to the magnitude of increase in pulmonary blood flow. A diastolic flow rumble may be heard over the apex of the heart, reflecting the increase in blood flow across the mitral valve. This left-to-right shunt also produces significant enlargement of the right ventricle, pulmonary artery, and left ventricle.

Pulmonary Vascular Resistance. Patients with a small (restrictive) VSD usually have normal right ventricular and pulmonary arterial pressures, slightly elevated pulmonary blood flow relative to systemic flow, normal pulmonary vascular resistance (PVR), and no histologic evidence of pulmonary vascular disease. Alterations in these variables occur according to the size of the VSD and are depicted in Table 54–4. When the VSD is large, the hemodynamic state is determined by the PVR. In these patients the PVR may be mildly, moderately, or severely elevated because of varying degrees of hypertensive pulmonary vascular disease. PVR (Rp) is numerically expressed in resistance units, normalized to body surface area:

$$Rp\ (units/sq.\ m.) = \frac{\text{Mean pulmonary artery pressure} - \text{mean left atrial pressure}}{\text{Cardiac output/body surface area}}$$

The absolute value for PVR may be a better predictor of operability than the ratio between the resistance in the pulmonary and systemic circuits because of variations in the systemic vascular resistance. Some patients with large VSDs have a low pulmonary resistance and hence a large pulmonary blood flow relative to systemic flow. In contrast, when the PVR is between 8 and 10 units per sq. m., indicating significant pulmonary vascular disease (see later discussion), pulmonary blood flow is only moderately elevated relative to systemic flow. When the PVR is greater than approximately 10 units per sq. m., the flow across the defect is usually bidirectional or right-to-left and the pulmonary blood flow is similar to or less than the systemic blood flow.

Physiology of Elevated PVR. Intense exercise in a normal individual may cause a fourfold increase in pulmonary and systemic blood flow without an increase in pulmonary artery pressure. In this circumstance, there is actually a decrease in PVR. In contrast, in patients with VSDs and moderate to severe pulmonary vascular disease, the pulmonary vasculature may lose the ability to accommodate to increases in pulmonary blood flow by a decline in PVR after physiologic stresses such as exercise. In this circumstance, the PVR may become *fixed.* When these patients exercise, the increase in systemic blood flow is derived from a reduction in left-to-right shunting or an increase in right-to-left shunting. Closure of the VSD when the PVR is *fixed* is hazardous, because the fixed PVR prevents an increase in systemic blood flow during exercise postoperatively.

Histology of Pulmonary Vascular Disease. The elevations of PVR in patients with VSDs are associated with anatomic changes in the small arteries of the lungs.[18, 19, 60] These changes follow a decrease in the ratio between the diameter of the lumen and the total diameter of the small muscular pulmonary arteries and arterioles. In patients with moderately elevated PVR, the increase in vessel wall thickness is primarily due to increased thickness of the muscle of the media and to intimal fibrosis, with actual occlusion of some of the vessels. In patients with severe elevation of PVR, intimal proliferation is more pronounced, with widespread occlusion of the muscular pulmonary arteries and arterioles and plexiform dilation of many of the remaining vessels.[19]

NATURAL HISTORY

Small VSDs. Many patients with VSDs have small defects and few or no symptoms, because the left-to-right shunt is small. Pulmonary hypertension with pulmonary vascular disease does not tend to develop in this group of patients. It is estimated that only 10% to 20% of patients have large defects leading to serious difficulties.[21]

Large VSDs. Infants born with large VSDs have moderate

TABLE 54–4. Alterations in Pulmonary Arterial Pressure, Pulmonary Blood Flow, and Pulmonary Vascular Resistance

Size of Defect	Pulmonary Arterial Hypertension		Pulmonary Blood Flow		Pulmonary Vascular Disease		Resistance Units
	Degree	$P_P{:}P_s$*	*Magnitude of Increase*	$Q_P{:}Q_s$†	*Severity*	$R_P{:}R_s$‡	
Small	None	<0.25	Mild	<1.4	None	<0.25	<5
	None	<0.25	Moderate	1.4–1.8	None	<0.25	<5
Large	Mild	0.25–0.45	Large	>1.8	Mild	<0.25	5–7
	Moderate	0.45–0.75	Large	>1.8	Mild	<0.25	5–7
	Severe	>0.75	Large	>1.8	Mild	0.25–0.45	5–7
			Moderate	1.4–1.8	Moderate	0.45–0.75	8–10
			Small	<1.4	Severe	>0.75	>10

*$P_P{:}P_s$ refers to the ratio between peak pressure in the pulmonary artery and that in a systemic artery (ratio between mean pressures is more commonly used and is similar).

†$Q_P{:}Q_s$ refers to the ratio between pulmonary and systemic blood flow.

‡$R_P{:}R_s$ refers to the ratio between pulmonary and systemic vascular resistance.

Modified from Pacifico, A. D., Kirklin, J. W., and Kirklin, J. K.: Surgical treatment of ventricular septal defect. *In* Sabiston, D. C., Jr., and Spencer, F. C. (Eds.): Gibbon's Surgery of the Chest, 3rd ed. Philadelphia, W. B. Saunders, 1976.

elevation of PVR owing to persistence of the medial thickening of the small pulmonary arteries present in the normal fetus. As the pulmonary vessels mature in the first few weeks of life, PVR declines. The magnitude of the left-to-right shunt across the defect increases, and symptoms develop. Such infants may die of severe congestive heart failure during this period.[36] If they survive and the hemodynamic state stabilizes, low cardiac output and breathlessness, which involve a large caloric expenditure and interfere with eating, can be the cause of severe failure to thrive. If surgical repair is not undertaken, death may occur from the sequelae of congestive heart failure, usually within the first year of life.[21]

In a small number of infants with large VSDs who survive the neonatal period, severe pulmonary vascular disease and a significant increase in PVR begin to develop by the age of 6 to 12 months. If an operation is not performed and this condition progresses over the ensuing months or years until it becomes severe, these patients can no longer be considered candidates for repair because of the severity of the pulmonary vascular changes. When the shunting becomes dominantly right to left across the defect as a result of the hypertensive pulmonary vascular disease, the patients become cyanotic and can be considered to have Eisenmenger's complex. Operation is then solidly contraindicated.

Another group of infants with large defects have only mild elevation in PVR in the first few years of life, although significant pulmonary hypertension and a large pulmonary blood flow are present. These children usually fail to thrive and have significantly impaired exercise tolerance. If the defect is still open or unrepaired by the time the patient is approximately 10 years old, the pulmonary vascular disease usually begins to progress. Eisenmenger's complex develops at the age of 15 to 20 years in these patients with severe elevation of the PVR and predominant right-to-left shunting across the defect. Occasionally severe pulmonary vascular disease does not develop, and heart failure may occur in the second or third decade of life. Patients with Eisenmenger's complex become polycythemic and eventually succumb to the complications of hypoxia and polycythemia, usually by the age of 25 to 30 years.

Spontaneous Reduction in Size of VSDs. In some infants, the VSD becomes smaller in size relative to the size of the heart as growth occurs. Pulmonary blood flow and pulmonary artery pressure decrease because of the resistance to flow imposed by the smaller defect. Although a left-to-right shunt is still present, severe pulmonary vascular disease does not develop. The growth and development of these children are quite normal. Rarely, bacterial endocarditis develops in these patients.[47]

Spontaneous Closure of VSDs. Spontaneous and complete closure of VSDs, even large ones, has been estimated to occur in 25% to 50% of patients during childhood.[21] The probability of eventual spontaneous closure is inversely related to the age at which the patient is observed (Fig. 54–50).[5] The mechanism of closure is usually related to ingrowth of fibrous tissue from the margins of the defect or adherence of the septal leaflet of the tricuspid valve to the margins of the defect.[21]

DIAGNOSIS

Presentation and Symptoms. Infants with large VSDs do not usually have symptoms until they reach the age of 6 weeks to 3 months. At this time the PVR has decreased from the elevated levels present at birth. Maximal left-to-right shunting of blood across the defect and a marked increase in pulmonary blood flow occur. Tachypnea, poor feeding, growth failure, recurrent respiratory tract infections, exercise intolerance, and severe cardiac failure may then develop.

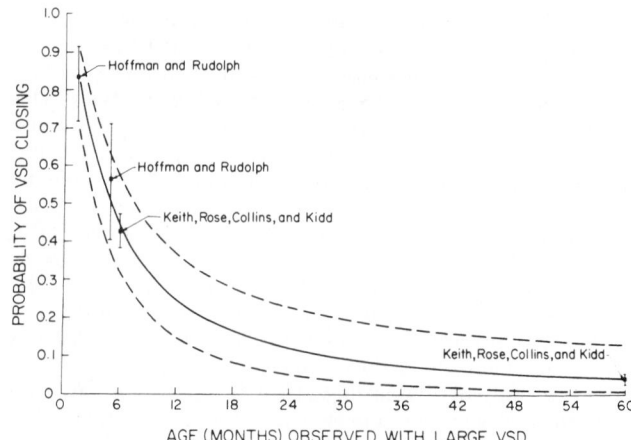

Figure 54–50. Probability of eventual spontaneous closure of a large VSD according to the age at which the patient is observed. The broken lines enclose the 70% confidence limits around the solid probability line. The specific ratios, with the 70% confidence limits reported by Hoffman and Rudolph[20] and Keith and associates[26] are demonstrated centered on the mean or assumed ages of patients in their reports (p < .0001). (From Blackstone, E. H., Kirklin, J. W., Bradley, E. L., et al.: Optimal age and results in repair of large ventricular defects. J. Thorac. Cardiovasc. Surg., 72:661, 1976.)

Patients with markedly elevated PVR and predominant right-to-left shunting across the septal defect (Eisenmenger's complex) are cyanotic, polycythemic, and severely limited in their activities.

Examination. The infant with a large VSD and increased pulmonary blood flow characteristically presents with tachypnea and marked subcostal retraction. Severe growth failure and a lack of subcutaneous tissue are often evident. The jugular venous pulses are prominent even when the infant is held erect. On palpation there is often a precordial bulge, and the heart is overactive with a rapid rate. A thrill is present in the third to fifth left intercostal space, and a loud systolic murmur is heard in this area. The second sound at the base is usually loud and may be split. The liver and spleen are usually enlarged, and the peripheral pulses are weak.

In older children with large VSDs, a protruding sternum or pigeon breast deformity is frequently present. Presumably this is caused by the enlarged right ventricle pushing the sternum anteriorly during the period of growth. The heart is hyperactive, there is a right ventricular lift, and the left ventricle is enlarged. A systolic thrill is often present over the left precordium. The characteristic murmur is harsh and pansystolic and is best heard in the left fourth interspace along the sternal border. If pulmonary blood flow is large, there may be a superimposed midsystolic ejection murmur in the area of the pulmonary valve.[31] A mid-diastolic murmur is present at the apex and indicates a large flow across the mitral valve. The first sound at the base is normal. The second sound is characterized by an abnormally wide split in expiration, and this splitting is accentuated during inspiration.[30]

Patients with small defects and small left-to-right shunts have only a systolic murmur. The heart is not hyperactive, and there is no enlargement of the left ventricle and no right ventricular lift. In patients with large defects and high PVR causing only small net left-to-right shunts or bidirectional shunts of equal magnitude, the systolic murmur is soft and short or may be absent. There is no apical diastolic rumble, and the second sound is markedly accentuated. There is no left ventricular enlargement, and a right ventricular lift is prominent.

Chest Radiograph. In patients with small VSDs and small

left-to-right shunts, chest radiographs are usually normal. Patients with large VSDs, mild elevation of PVR, and large left-to-right shunts have large pulmonary arteries, both centrally and peripherally (Fig. 54–51). The right and left ventricles are enlarged, as is the left atrium. When marked enlargement of the left atrium is present in a patient suspected of having a VSD, the presence of coexisting mitral valvular regurgitation should be considered.

In patients with large VSDs and severe elevation of the PVR, the chest radiograph is quite different (Fig. 54–52). The central pulmonary arteries appear normal or are enlarged, but the peripheral pulmonary arteries appear normal. This suggests a normal or decreased pulmonary blood flow. The right ventricle appears somewhat enlarged, but there is no evidence of significant left atrial or left ventricular enlargement. Aside from the enlarged central pulmonary arteries, the cardiac silhouette may appear normal.

Electrocardiogram. In patients with small VSDs, the electrocardiogram may be normal. When the defect and shunt are slightly large (Qp:Qs greater than approximately 1.8), the increase in left ventricular work from the large left ventricular stroke volume is evidenced by increased R wave voltage and tall peaked T waves from the left precordial leads. When the shunt is still larger, a pattern of mild right ventricular overload may be present, as suggested by an RSR pattern in the V_1 lead.

If the VSD is large and the left-to-right shunt is large (Qp:Qs greater than 2), but the PVR is significantly less than the systemic vascular resistance (Rp:Rs less than 0.75), then there is evidence of increased work for both ventricles. The R wave from the right precordial leads is tall, and when the right ventricular peak pressure is similar to the left ventricular peak pressure, it is notched on the upstroke. The left precordial leads in this situation have the pattern of left ventricular overload previously described, although there may be a deeper S wave.

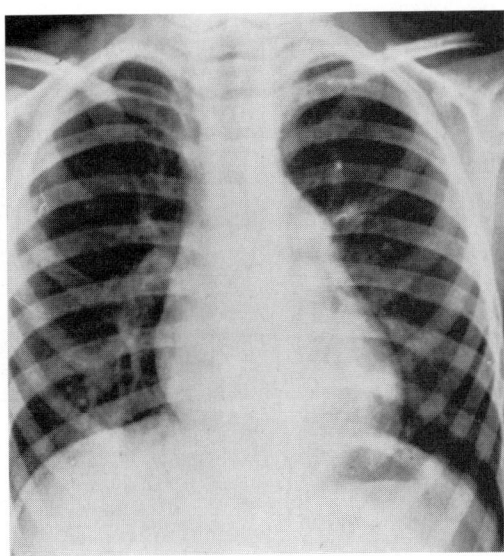

Figure 54–52. The chest roentgenogram is in contrast to that shown in Figure 54–51. The heart is not enlarged overall. The main pulmonary artery is enlarged; there is no evidence of increased pulmonary blood flow. This patient has a large VSD, pulmonary hypertension, severe elevation of PVR, and pulmonary blood flow that is less than systemic blood flow. The condition is inoperable. (From DuShane, J. W., and Kirklin, J. W.: Selection for surgery of patients with ventricular septal defect and pulmonary hypertension. Circulation, 21:13, 1960. By permission of the American Heart Association.)

When the VSD is large and the PVR is equal to or greater than the systemic resistance, right-axis deviation is usually present in the limb leads. The right precordial leads show the typical large, usually notched R waves of right ventricular hypertrophy, whereas the left precordial leads no longer show left ventricular overload.

The electrocardiogram supplements the physical findings and chest radiograph. Together they usually provide a useful categorization of patients as to the size of the VSD shunt and the magnitude of the PVR. Combined vectorgraphic and echocardiographic studies can provide additional noninvasive information and accurately identify infants with restrictive and nonrestrictive defects.[44]

Echocardiography. Doppler echocardiography with color-flow mapping allows the noninvasive display of intracardiac anatomy cross-sectionally and the simultaneous display of real-time blood flow. This technique has become invaluable in the noninvasive diagnosis of VSDs as well as other forms of congenital cardiac malformations. Unidirectional as well as bidirectional shunting can be demonstrated. This method provides important information regarding the size and location of a VSD (Fig. 54–53). Often, an estimate of the pressure difference between the two ventricles can be made from knowledge of the velocity of flow through the defect. Although the general location of the defect can be defined by this technique, the presence of additional VSDs may not be ascertained. Therefore, some groups continue to advise cardiac catheterization studies with axial angiography to provide definitive information regarding the location and number of defects as well as information about the hemodynamic state.

Cardiac Catheterization. Cardiac catheterization studies are useful to confirm the diagnosis and to detect secondary or multiple defects. In addition, the pulmonary and systemic arterial pressures and flows are measured and the PVR is calculated. These studies are also useful in excluding the presence of an associated cardiac defect.

Angiography. Injection of radiopaque contrast media into the left ventricle at the time of cardiac catheterization is

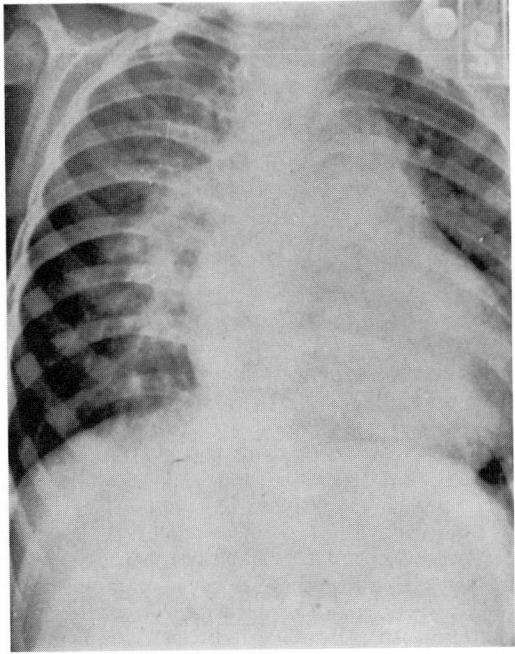

Figure 54–51. Chest roentgenogram of a child with a large VSD, large pulmonary blood flow, and pulmonary hypertension, but only mild elevation of PVR. This is reflected in the evidence of left and right ventricular enlargement, enlargement of the main pulmonary artery, and marked increase in pulmonary blood flow. (From Pacifico, A. D., Kirklin, J. W., and Kirklin, J. K.: Surgical treatment of ventricular septal defect. In Sabiston, D. C., Jr., and Spencer, F. C. [Eds.]: Surgery of the Chest, 5th ed. Philadelphia, W. B. Saunders, 1990.)

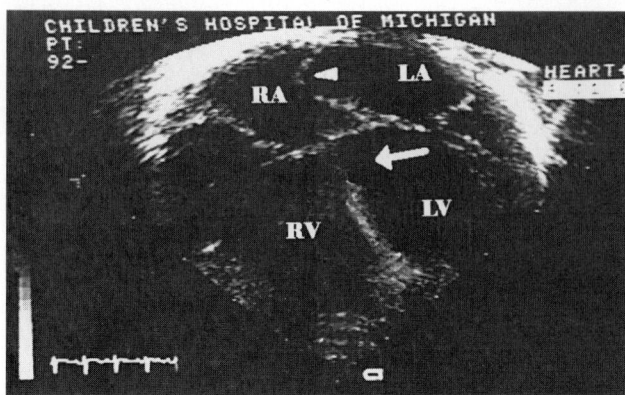

Figure 54–53. Apical four-chamber echocardiographic view of ventricular septal defect (large arrow). Small arrow points to interatrial septum. RA, right atrium; LA, left atrium; RV, right ventricle; LV, left ventricle. (Courtesy of Richard Humes, M.D., Associate Professor of Pediatrics, Director of Echocardiography Laboratory, Children's Hospital of Michigan, Detroit, Michigan.)

essential in any patient in whom operation is contemplated. This is particularly true for infants in whom information regarding the location and number of defects is of value in planning the technical details of the operation. Axial angiography to provide a profile of the ventricular septum beautifully defines the number and location of the defect(s) (Fig. 54–54). These studies are also of value in defining associated defects such as aortic valve incompetence or pulmonary valvular or infundibular stenosis.

INDICATIONS FOR OPERATION

The decision to recommend operation for an individual patient is based on knowledge of the natural history of similar untreated patients and of the results of surgical correction. Important considerations in the natural history include the presence of congestive heart failure or growth failure, the likelihood of development of severe pulmonary vascular disease, and the possibility of spontaneous closure. The results of surgical therapy depend on the risk of operation, its effect on pulmonary vascular disease, and the incidence of complications such as heart block or incomplete repair.

At any age, the presence of pulmonary vascular disease so severe that the PVR is greater than 10 to 12 units per sq. m. is considered a contraindication to operation. Closure of the

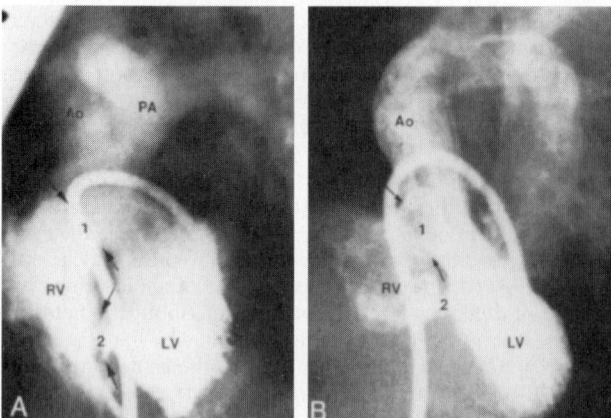

Figure 54–54. Axial angiography to profile the ventricular septum. A, Left ventriculogram in long axial view demonstrating a high perimembranous defect and a lower muscular defect in the trabecular septum. Ao, aorta; PA, pulmonary artery; RV, right ventricle; LV, left ventricle. B, Left ventriculogram in four-chamber view demonstrating a high perimembranous VSD and a lower muscular inlet VSD.

VSD, under these circumstances, would result in severe right ventricular hypertension due to the associated pulmonary vascular disease and would lead to death from low cardiac output. If the PVR is 8 to 10 units per sq. m., operation is generally advised but with full knowledge of a possible unsatisfactory long-term result owing to progressive pulmonary vascular disease.[7] The presence of severe pulmonary hypertension is not a contraindication to operation if the PVR is less than 10 units per sq. m.[4] Finally, operation may not be truly curative in older patients with established pulmonary vascular disease.

Prompt intracardiac repair is indicated in infants with large defects, large shunts, and pulmonary hypertension who present with severe and intractable left ventricular failure, recurrent pulmonary infections, severe growth failure, or evidence of rapidly increasing PVR. Pulmonary arterial banding does not have a place in the management of these patients unless a true Swiss-cheese septum is present.

VSDs have a tendency to close spontaneously, and this fact is relevant to decisions about the advisability of operation.[5, 8] Spontaneous closure can be complete by 1 year of age, or the defect may have only narrowed by then. The phenomenon of spontaneous closure or narrowing of VSDs explains the infrequency with which large VSDs are encountered in adults. An inverse relationship exists between the probability of eventual spontaneous closure and the age at which the patient is observed (see Fig. 54–50).[5, 20, 26] This is highly relevant to clinical decisions concerning individual patients. According to these data, approximately 80% of individuals observed at 1 month of age with large VSDs have eventual spontaneous closure, as do approximately 60% of those observed at 3 months of age, approximately 50% of those at 6 months of age, and 25% of those at 12 months of age.

A significant number of patients have moderate-sized VSDs associated only with modest elevations of pulmonary artery pressure, moderate cardiomegaly and pulmonary plethora, a Qp:Qs up to 3, and few symptoms. These patients can be observed until age 4, with the expectation of spontaneous reduction in size or closure of the defect. If the defect is closing gradually during this interval, operation can be deferred. If there is no change in the defect, operation is advised before the patient reaches school age.

Small VSDs not associated with symptoms, cardiomegaly, pulmonary plethora, elevated pulmonary artery pressure, or a Qp:Qs greater than 1.5 to 1.8 can be safely observed. When the patient reaches 10 to 12 years of age, the likelihood of spontaneous closure is remote, and the treatment is controversial. The risks of not operating in this subset of patients are small but include the risk of bacterial endocarditis, the psychologic impact of the VSD, and the ventricular dysfunction that may sometimes develop over time owing to the underestimation of the hemodynamic significance of the lesion. These small risks must be balanced against the low risk of surgical repair, and an individual decision must be made for each patient.

When aortic valvular incompetence develops in a child with a VSD, prompt closure of the defect should be undertaken to prevent further prolapse of the aortic cusps and to prevent progression of this aortic valve pathology. When coexisting pulmonary infundibular or valvular stenosis is present, the VSD is generally large; and if the stenosis is severe, right-to-left shunting may be present. In these situations operation is also advisable. Mild or moderate mitral incompetence in association with a VSD is not a contraindication to closure of the defect.

SURGICAL TREATMENT

External Anatomy. A median sternotomy is employed. Careful exploration within the pericardial cavity is done to determine the presence or absence of a patent ductus arteriosus, a left superior vena cava, possible anomalies of pulmonary or systemic venous connection, and the presence of other external anatomic variations. The size of each cardiac chamber is noted from the external examination. The presence of an enlarged left atrium and left ventricle generally indicates increased pulmonary blood flow.

Conduct of Cardiopulmonary Bypass (CPB). CPB is established by placing two appropriately sized, thin-walled angled metal cannulas directly into each vena cava for venous return. A cannula is placed in the ascending aorta for arterial return from the pump oxygenator. The perfusate temperature is adjusted to maintain moderate hypothermia at 24° to 28° C. The aorta is cross-clamped, and cold, hyperkalemic, dilute, sanguinous cardioplegia is injected into the aortic root to protect the myocardium during the period of global myocardial ischemia. Snares placed about the superior and inferior venae cavae are tightened around each respective venous cannula, and a right atriotomy is performed.

Exposure of the VSD. The right atrial approach is preferred for most perimembranous, inlet muscular and some apical-trabecular muscular, outlet muscular, and doubly committed/juxta-arterial defects. The right ventricular approach, through a transverse or longitudinal infundibular incision, provides consistently good exposure for outlet muscular and doubly committed/juxta-arterial defects, although these defects can sometimes also be closed through the pulmonary valve after making an initial pulmonary arteriotomy. A longitudinal, anterior right ventriculotomy, with or without extension around the apex, is useful for many apical-trabecular muscular defects that may not be well exposed through the right atrium. In general, the right atrial approach is preferred because it avoids an incision in the right ventricle. If an initial transatrial attempt to view the defect yields suboptimal exposure to perform an accurate repair, a right ventricular incision should be performed.

Technique of Repair. After performing the initial right atriotomy, the internal anatomy of the heart is carefully assessed to identify any undiagnosed associated lesions and to plan the approach (right atriotomy vs. right ventriculotomy) for surgical repair. After exposure of the VSD has been established, the lesion is repaired with a patch. Depending on the exposure of the defect, the repair is performed with either a continuous or interrupted (pledgeted, horizontal mattress) technique. The authors prefer a continuous suturing technique using polypropylene suture. The location of the specialized conduction tissue and its relation to the VSD must be clearly understood.

The right atriotomy used for transatrial repair and the exposure of a perimembranous VSD through the tricuspid valve are shown in Figure 54–49. The sinus node is shown in the intact heart above; the AV node and the course of the conduction tissue in relation to the tricuspid valve and VSD are shown below. The continuous suturing technique used to close the VSD with a patch is shown in Figure 54–55.

Perimembranous VSD Associated with Inlet Muscular VSD. In some cases, a perimembranous VSD is associated with a separate inlet muscular VSD, leaving an intact muscle bar between them (Fig. 54–56). Usually, these lesions are exposed transatrially by tricuspid leaflet retraction. When the tricuspid leaflet chordal pattern is particularly complex, thereby obscuring the margins of the defect, exposure is facilitated by incising the anterior and septal tricuspid valve leaflets near their base and retracting these leaflets anteriorly (see Fig. 54–56). In this particular defect, the conduction tissue courses in the muscle bar that separates the two defects. Injury to this conduction tissue is avoided by using a single patch to cover both defects, leaving the muscle bar

intact, and by placing the sutures in the path indicated in Figure 54–56.

Perimembranous VSD with Inlet Extension (AV Canal Type VSD). The perimembranous VSD with inlet extension and the course of the conduction tissue in relation to it are shown in Figure 54–57. No muscle tissue is present between the defect and the base of the tricuspid septal leaflet. This septal leaflet of the tricuspid valve is contiguous with the anterior mitral leaflet and usually with part of the aortic valve anulus superiorly. The conduction tissue is related to the inferior border of the defect, and the suture line used to attach the patch in this area is placed approximately 10 mm. inferior to the free edge of the VSD (see Fig. 54–57).

Apical-Trabecular Muscular Defect. The specialized conduction tissue is not related directly to the rim of a muscular VSD in the apical-trabecular septum (Fig. 54–58). In this case the patch suture line is placed circumferentially on the free edge of the defect.

Multiple anterior VSDs can be closed by mattress sutures placed over felt pledgets or strips operating transatrially through the tricuspid valve or through a vertical right ventriculotomy incision made near the septum.[6] A left ventriculotomy also provides excellent exposure[1, 49] but is not preferred in infants because it has been associated with left ventricular dysfunction both early and late postoperatively. Whereas avoidance of a left ventriculotomy appears to be less important in older children, the use of an incision in the systemic ventricle is advocated only when satisfactory exposure of the VSD is impossible through a right atriotomy or right ventriculotomy.

Swiss-Cheese Septum. The rare Swiss-cheese septum may at times not be totally correctable. Its repair occasionally needs a left ventricular approach and may require the placement of a patch over the entire muscular septum. An associated perimembranous defect should be repaired through the right atrium because its repair from the left ventricular side increases the risk of heart block.

Coexisting Pulmonary Stenosis. When pulmonary infundibular and/or valvular stenosis coexists with a VSD, performing the pulmonary valvotomy operating through a pulmonary arteriotomy incision is often preferred. The infundibular resection is started through the pulmonary arteriotomy and pulmonary valve, and it is completed through the right atriotomy and tricuspid valve. The VSD is then closed with a patch.[42]

Coexisting Aortic Insufficiency. When aortic valve incompetence coexists with a VSD, the severity of the incompetence should be fully assessed preoperatively. If the incompetence is mild, only closure of the VSD is indicated. If the aortic incompetence is moderate or severe, plication of the aortic leaflets should be performed through an aortotomy before closure of the VSD.[55]

Coexisting Coarctation of the Aorta. Neonates with a large VSD and coexisting severe coarctation of the aorta can be extremely ill. They are initially stabilized with an infusion of prostaglandin E_1 to maintain ductal patency and peripheral perfusion. Although there are several sequences in which these critically ill infants can be treated, some prefer to initially repair the coarctation through a left thoracotomy. Concomitant pulmonary artery banding is performed only if there are clinically significant multiple VSDs. If the patient, after coarctation repair, can be weaned from the ventilator with satisfactory work of breathing and can ingest adequate calories on a standard anticongestive medical regimen, no further surgical treatment is undertaken. The infant is then observed closely by the cardiologist for spontaneous narrowing and/or closure of the VSD. The usual indications for VSD repair, as discussed previously, would apply in this situation. If the patient, after coarctation repair, cannot be

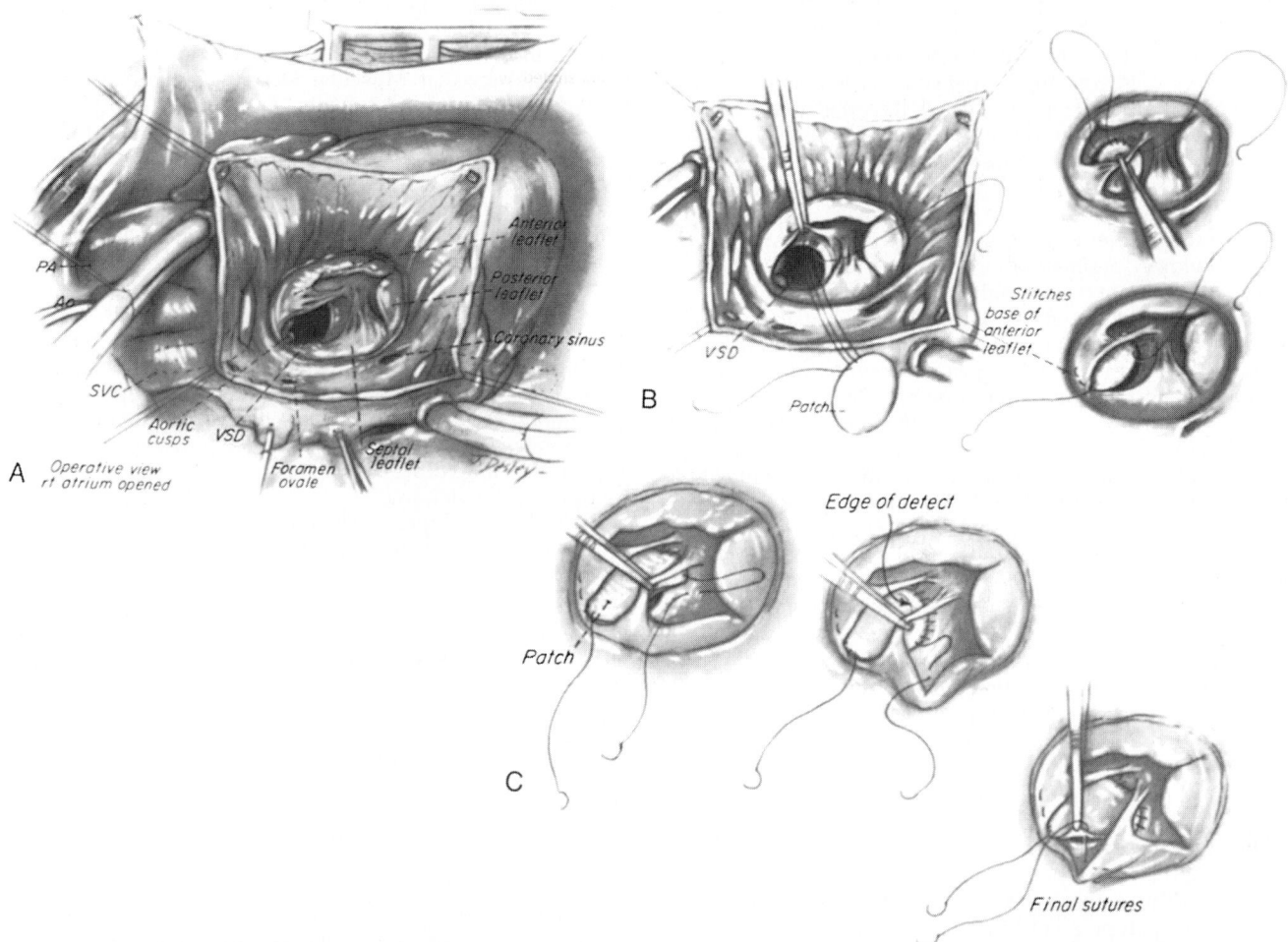

Figure 54–55. *A,* Right atrial incision and exposure of perimembranous VSD in the region of the tricuspid anteroseptal commissure. Stay sutures have been placed to slightly evert the atrial wall. Note that initially the superior edge of this typical perimembranous defect is not visible. The AV node is in the muscular portion of the AV septum, just on the atrial side of the commissure between the tricuspid septal and anterior leaflets. The bundle of His thus penetrates at the posterior angle of the VSD, where it is vulnerable to injury. *B,* The repair of the perimembranous VSD. This is initiated by placing a mattress suture of 4-0 Prolene with a small pledget at the 12 o'clock position in the defect as observed by the surgeon through the tricuspid valve. A piece of knitted Dacron velour is trimmed slightly larger than the approximate size of the defect, and one arm of the suture is passed through the Dacron patch, back through the septum, and again through the patch. Either now or after placing several more stitches, the sutures are snugged up as the patch is lowered into place. The suture line between the cephalad rim of the defect and the patch is continued. The traction on the suture exposes the next areas to be stitched and provides good visibility. When the junction of the superior muscular rim (ventriculoinfundibular fold) and tricuspid anulus has been reached, the suture is passed through the base of the contiguous portion of the tricuspid valve (usually the anterior leaflet) from the ventricular to the atrial side, then back from the atrial to the ventricular side of the valve and through the patch. After passing the stitch back through the leaflet, the suture is tagged. *C,* Operating now with the other limb of the suture, stitches are taken between the ventricular septum and the patch along the caudad side of the defect. These stitches are placed 3 to 5 mm. away from the edge of the defect to avoid the area most probably occupied by the bundle of His and more posteriorly 5 to 7 mm. back from the edge.

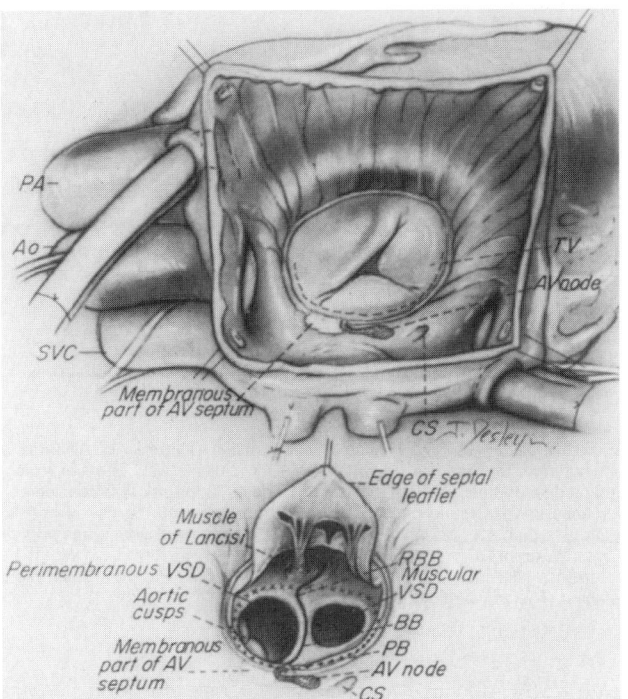

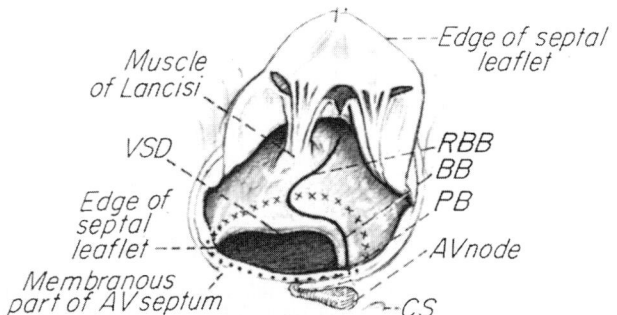

Figure 55–57. Transatrial exposure for repair of an AV canal type of VSD is demonstrated after incision of the base of the tricuspid valve and anterior traction as in Figure 54–56. The coronary sinus (CS), the AV node and its penetrating portion (PB) and branching portion (BB), and the right bundle branch (RBB) are shown in relation to the VSD. The Xs indicate the path of the suture line used to attach the patch to the muscular portion of the septum and the dots along the base of the tricuspid leaflet. Most defects of this type can be closed without incision of the tricuspid leaflets; however, when the chordal pattern is complex, this maneuver aids in exposure. (From Bharati, S., Lev, M., and Kirklin, J. W.: Cardiac Surgery and the Conduction System. New York, John Wiley & Sons, 1983.)

Figure 54–56. Transatrial exposure for closure of a perimembranous VSD associated with an inlet muscular VSD. The coronary sinus (CS) and atrioventricular (AV) node as well as an incision in the base of the anterior and septal tricuspid valve (TV) leaflets are demonstrated above. The leaflets are retracted anteriorly in the lower part of the illustration to expose the two VSDs. The penetrating portion of the bundle of His (PB), its branching portion (BB), and the right bundle branch (RBB) are demonstrated in relation to the VSDs. The pathway of the suture line used to attach the Dacron patch along the muscular portion of the septum is indicated by Xs and along the base of the tricuspid valve leaflet by dots. When repair is completed, the tricuspid leaflets are reattached to their basilar remnant by a continuous suture of fine polypropylene. PA, pulmonary artery; Ao, aorta, SVC, superior vena cava. (From Bharati, S., Lev, M., and Kirklin, J. W.: Cardiac Surgery and the Conduction System. New York, John Wiley & Sons, 1983.)

weaned from the ventilator, has increased work of breathing despite reasonable anticongestive therapy, or fails to feed satisfactorily, a VSD repair is undertaken through a median sternotomy during the same hospitalization.

Termination of Cardiopulmonary Bypass. When VSD closure is completed, rewarming is commenced, the vent is removed, and the atrial septal defect is closed after inflating the lungs to expel air from the left atrium. Air is aspirated from the ascending aorta, the aortic cross-clamp is released, and the right atriotomy is closed. De-airing is accomplished, and cardiopulmonary bypass is gradually discontinued. Decannulation is performed, and the incision is closed leaving temporary atrial and ventricular pacing electrodes.

Total Circulatory Arrest. Although some continue to prefer standard perfusion techniques even in small infants, others use a single venous cannula, deep hypothermia, and temporary total circulatory arrest during the repair.[3, 41]

Pulmonary Artery Banding

Indications. Although currently pulmonary arterial banding for uncomplicated VSDs is not often employed, it continues to have a place in the management of some infants with multiple cardiac anomalies and in some infants with severe heart failure from multiple (Swiss-cheese type) VSDs.[21, 56]

Technique. A left anterolateral thoracotomy incision in the third intercostal space or a median sternotomy is employed. The pericardium overlying the pulmonary artery is incised longitudinally, and a plane is developed between the pulmo-

nary artery and the aorta. A 4-mm. wide Teflon-coated band is passed initially about the aorta. A right-angle clamp is then passed through the transverse sinus, and the rightward limb of the band is grasped and delivered through the transverse sinus. By using this method, the band is placed around the entire circumference of the main pulmonary artery and the potential for exclusion of the right pulmonary artery is avoided. Although many methods are available to guide the degree of tightening of the band, the rule of Trusler and Mustard is often employed.[56] The circumference of the band in millimeters is determined from the weight of the infant in kilograms plus 20 mm. for an isolated VSD or plus 24 mm. for more complex cardiac anomalies. The calculated length is initially marked on the band before it is placed around the pulmonary artery. The marked points are joined with a mattress suture of 4-0 Prolene. The band is tightened to this circumference to produce a harsh thrill. The band circumference is adjusted to produce a 10- to 15-mm. rise in the

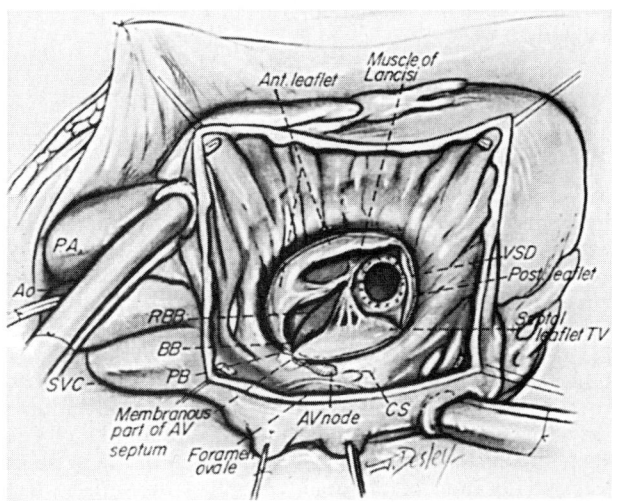

Figure 54–58. Transatrial exposure of a muscular defect in the trabecular portion of the septum is demonstrated. The pathway of the suture line used to attach the patch to close the defect is along its free edge and indicated by the Xs. CS, coronary sinus; AV, atrioventricular; PB, penetrating portion of the bundle of His; BB, branching portion of the bundle of His; RBB, right bundle branch; Ao, aorta; SVC, superior vena cava; PA, pulmonary artery; TV, tricuspid valve. (From Bharati, S., Lev, M., and Kirklin, J. W.: Cardiac Surgery and the Conduction System. New York, John Wiley & Sons, 1983.)

systemic pressure, a drop in the distal pulmonary artery pressure to less than 50% of the new systemic pressure, and a drop in the arterial saturations to approximately 85% on 50% inspired oxygen. The edges of the pericardial incision are then approximated, and the thoracotomy incision is closed in the usual manner, leaving a single chest tube for drainage.

POSTOPERATIVE CARE

The majority of infants and small children are extubated within 24 hours after the operation and do not require special supportive treatment. The outcome is primarily determined by events in the operating room and by the proper preoperative selection of patients.

Pulmonary Hypertensive Crises. Some sicker, small infants may be at risk for postoperative pulmonary hypertensive crises. These episodes are characterized by sudden marked increases in the PVR. When severe, these episodes may cause suprasystemic pulmonary artery pressure that may cause severe and acute cardiac failure. In these infants it is probably best to leave a monitoring catheter within the pulmonary artery for continuous measurement of postoperative pulmonary artery pressure. Management of pulmonary hypertensive crises can be difficult. The patient should be heavily sedated, paralyzed, and hyperventilated with 100% inspired oxygen to maintain an alkalotic serum pH. Pulmonary vasodilators including nitroglycerin, amrinone, prostaglandin E$_1$, tolazoline, and inhaled nitric oxide[13] may be helpful.[23]

Low Cardiac Output. In the unusual case of low cardiac output after operation, in addition to the usual supportive treatment,[27] consideration should be given to the possibility of an overlooked or incompletely closed VSD. This possibility must especially be considered if the left atrial pressure is considerably higher than the right atrial pressure. A Doppler examination with color-flow mapping should be performed. When secure information from this study is not obtained, urgent recatheterization is advisable.

Complete AV Dissociation. If complete AV dissociation was present for a time after CPB but sinus rhythm reappeared, a demand pacemaker attached to ventricular wires should be left in place for 1 week postoperatively. Rarely the AV dissociation recurs temporarily in the early postoperative period.

RESULTS OF SURGICAL REPAIR

Hospital Mortality. Even in very small infants, closure of VSDs can be safely accomplished in most centers properly prepared for this type of procedure.[3, 34, 43, 45] Hospital mortality and complications are directly related to the preoperative condition of the patient and to the conduct of the operative procedure. Hospital mortality now approaches 0%. In earlier years, younger age was an incremental risk factor in the authors' experience, as it was in many centers, but this effect was neutralized by 1978 (Fig. 54–59).[45] Multiple VSDs, in earlier years, were an important incremental risk factor for hospital death, but more recently the effect was only a minor one.[45] This improvement can be attributed primarily to better preoperative cineangiographic identification of the presence, size, and location of multiple VSDs that demand surgical closure. In earlier years, pulmonary artery pressure and PVR were determinants of hospital mortality.[7] Currently this is probably no longer true because the upper limit of acceptable *(operable)* PVR is better understood, and management has accordingly improved.

Effect of Major Associated Lesions. Major associated lesions, particularly when present in symptomatic infants with

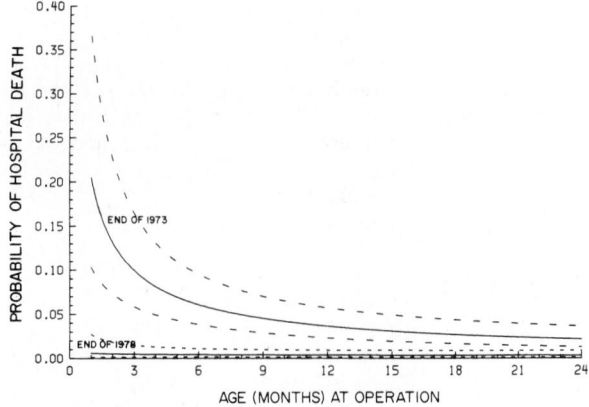

Figure 54–59. Probability of hospital death at the University of Alabama at Birmingham after repair of single large VSD in patients without major associated cardiac anomalies. Note that in 1971 and 1973 the risk was considerably increased in very young patients. By 1979, not only was the risk of hospital death less than 1%, but an incremental risk in patients of young age was no longer apparent. (From Rizzoli, G., Blackstone, E. H., Kirklin, J. W., et al.: Incremental risk factors in hospital mortality after repair of ventricular septal defect. J. Thorac. Cardiovasc. Surg., *80*:494, 1980.)

large VSDs, do have an incremental risk effect on hospital mortality. At the University of Alabama at Birmingham, in 312 patients operated on for VSD between 1967 and 1979, 16 (6.3%) hospital deaths occurred among 254 patients with single or multiple VSDs with no major associated lesion. This compared with 14 (24%) hospital deaths among 58 patients with major associated lesions (p <.0001).[45] Further scientific progress will probably reduce this incremental risk effect.

Effect of Route of Surgical Access. Although many VSDs can be closed through a right atrial approach, the precise route of surgical access, be it through the right atrium or right ventricle, has not been a determinant of hospital mortality after repair of a single VSD.[45] The same is true after repair of muscular or multiple VSDs through a left ventriculotomy, although many remain concerned about the long-term functional effects of a left ventriculotomy in infants.[28]

AV Dissociation. Although permanent heart block occurred after repair of VSDs in a large percentage of patients in the very early years of cardiac surgery, this complication is quite unusual at present. Its incidence in the current era continues to approach zero.[5]

Residual VSDs. High-quality left ventricular angiograms with angled views to profile the ventricular septum provide complete information regarding the size, location, and multiplicity of defects. Such studies minimize the chance of persistent (overlooked) defects after repair and have contributed significantly to the completeness of the surgical procedure.

Although small residual defects may sometimes be demonstrated by postoperative color Doppler studies, residual shunts of sufficient magnitude to indicate reoperation are uncommon. Only 1 (0.7%) of 138 patients undergoing operation for repair of a large VSD has required reoperation, and this was for an overlooked second muscular VSD.[5] The technique used for reoperation for a residual or recurrent VSD has been nicely described.[9]

Persistent Pulmonary Hypertension. Pulmonary artery pressure is more likely to be normal late postoperatively when operation is performed at a young age.[3, 5, 11] The relation is an inverse one. Postoperative progression of pulmonary vascular disease is uncommon when the VSD is repaired before the age of 2 years. Closure of a VSD in small infants should be advised when there is evidence of increasing PVR even in the absence of symptoms.

Severe pulmonary hypertension postoperatively can increase with time[15] and cause premature late death, usually within 3 to 10 years of operation.[11, 15, 17] However, some patients with pulmonary hypertension and elevated PVR late postoperatively have neither progression nor regression of their disease for as long as 20 years, although there is some limitation in exercise tolerance.[11, 16] It is presumed that life expectancy is reduced.

Late Results. Premature late death occurs uncommonly when PVR is low preoperatively. These rare deaths presumably follow arrhythmias, either ventricular fibrillation or the sudden late development of complete heart block. Patients with high PVR preoperatively have a tendency for this to progress and to cause premature death. Approximately 25% die within 5 years of operation when the preoperative PVR is more than 10 units per sq. m.

Nearly all patients with large VSDs and mild elevation of PVR have an excellent prognosis. Improved physical development is a prominent feature of the late postoperative course after repair of large VSDs in infants.[43] There is an impressive increase in weight and usually complete relief of symptoms.[7] Cardiac function late postoperatively is essentially normal when the repair is done in the first 2 years of life by modern techniques operating through the right atrium or right ventricle. Left ventricular end-diastolic volume, left ventricular systolic output, left ventricular mass, and left ventricular ejection fraction are normal approximately 1 year after operation in this subset. Persistent abnormalities of left ventricular size and function continue after repair of large VSDs at an older age, although patients remain asymptomatic. All of this information lends support to the advisability of surgical closure of a large VSD within the first 2 years of life.

SELECTED REFERENCES

Barratt-Boyes, B. G., Neutze, J. M., Clarkson, P. M., et al.: Repair of ventricular septal defect in the first two years of life using profound hypothermia—circulatory arrest techniques. Ann. Surg., *184*:376, 1976.
This classic paper describes the results of primary repair of VSD in 57 patients younger than 2 years of age, with many of the patients being younger than 6 months old. Hospital mortality was 4% in the patients without associated coarctation—a remarkable achievement. The late postoperative results are excellent. The method of profound hypothermia and total circulatory arrest and these superb results have had an important and worldwide impact on cardiac operations.

DuShane, J. W., and Kirklin, J. W.: Late results of the repair of ventricular septal defects on pulmonary vascular disease. In Kirklin, J. W. (Ed.): Advances in Cardiovascular Surgery. New York, Grune & Stratton, 1973, p. 9.
This paper analyzes the long-term course of 68 patients with large VSDs and severe pulmonary hypertension evaluated 5 or more years after operation with repeat cardiac catheterization, emphasizing the effects of operation on the pulmonary vasculature. Over 90% of patients younger than 2 years of age had normal or only mildly elevated PVR late postoperatively, even when it was severely elevated preoperatively. Over 50% of the older patients with moderate or severely elevated PVR preoperatively had moderate or severely elevated resistance late postoperatively and potentially unsatisfactory long-term results. On the basis of these findings, the authors advise closure of large VSDs before the age of 2 years.

Hoffman, J. I. E., and Rudolph, A. M.: The natural history of isolated ventricular septal defect with special reference to selection of patients for surgery. Adv. Pediatr., *17*:57, 1970.
This excellent article contains an enormous amount of information regarding the natural history of patients with isolated VSD. It extensively considers problems related to the severity of the disease, the frequency and the time course of spontaneous closure of VSDs, the incidence and importance of pulmonary vascular disease, and the changes in PVR that occur after surgical closure. In addition, a program is outlined for the management of patients with VSD, particularly infants, and the indications for operative intervention are given.

Rein, J. G., Freed, M. D., Norwood, W. I., and Castañeda, A. R.: Early and late results of closure of ventricular septal defect in infancy. Ann. Thorac. Surg., *24*:19, 1977.
The superb results obtained by Castañeda and colleagues in the operation of primary repair of VSD in the first year of life in 50 infants are reported. The Kyoto–Barratt-Boyes technique of profound hypothermia and total circulatory arrest was used. Hospital mortality was 6%, no late death occurred, and the late functional status was excellent. This paper provides strong supportive evidence for the excellence of the results that can be obtained from primary repair of VSD, even in very young infants.

Rizzoli, G., Blackstone, E. H., Kirklin, J. W., et al.: Incremental risk factors in hospital mortality after repair of ventricular septal defect. J. Thorac. Cardiovasc. Surg., *80*:494, 1980.
This paper describes the incremental risk of numerous factors in 312 patients having repair of VSD from 1967 to 1979. More importantly, it describes how these incremental risk factors have gradually been neutralized by scientific advances and minimization of human errors. Thus, in the era beginning in 1978, the hospital mortality of repair of single large VSDs is less than 1%, no matter how young the patient (neutralization of the previous incremental risk of young age). The mortality is approximately 5% for multiple VSDs, again without an incremental risk of young age. Major associated cardiac anomalies or procedures (large patent ductus arteriosus, simultaneous repair of coarctation or interrupted arch, and important mitral valve abnormalities) still increase risk.

Soto, B., Becker, A. E., Moulaert, A. J., et al.: Classification of ventricular septal defects. Br. Heart J., *43*:332, 1980.
Many anatomic studies of VSD have been reported through the years, but this study by Soto and colleagues has been particularly helpful to surgeons. They divide the ventricular septum into a membranous and muscular portion. The latter is divided into an inlet, trabecular, and infundibular (outlet) portion. This paper introduces the advisable phrase perimembranous VSD for those in the region of the membranous septum, proximal to the tricuspid anulus. It also clarifies the fact that the AV canal type of VSD is really a perimembranous one that extends beneath the septal tricuspid leaflet. Beautiful anatomic and cineangiographic plates clarify the description.

REFERENCES

1. Aaron, B. L., and Lower, R. R.: Muscular ventricular septal defect repair made easy. Ann. Thorac. Surg., *19*:568, 1975.
2. Anderson, R. H., and Wilcox, B. R.: The surgical anatomy of ventricular septal defect. J. Cardiac Surg., *7*:17, 1992.
3. Barratt-Boyes, B. G., Neutze, J. M., Clarkson, P. M., et al.: Repair of ventricular septal defect in the first two years of life using profound hypothermia–circulatory arrest techniques. Ann. Surg., *184*:376, 1976.
4. Barratt-Boyes, B. G.: Complete correction of cardiovascular malformations in the first two years of life using profound hypothermia. In Barratt-Boyes, B. G., Neutze, J. M., and Harris, E. A. (Eds.): Heart Disease in Infancy: Diagnosis and Surgical Treatment: Proceedings of the Second International Symposium on Surgical Heart Disease. London, Churchill Livingstone, 1973, p. 25.
5. Blackstone, E. H., Kirklin, J. W., Bradley, E. L., et al.: Optimal age and results in repair of large ventricular septal defects. J. Thorac. Cardiovasc. Surg., *72*:661, 1976.
6. Breckenridge, I. M., Stark, J., Waterston, D. J., and Bonham-Carter, R. E.: Multiple ventricular septal defects. Ann. Thorac. Surg., *13*:128, 1972.
7. Cartmill, T. B., DuShane, J. W., McGoon, D. C., and Kirklin, J. W.: Results of repair of ventricular septal defect. J. Thorac. Cardiovasc. Surg., *52*:486, 1966.
8. Collins, G., Calder, L., Rose, V., et al.: Ventricular septal defect: Clinical and hemodynamic changes in the first five years of life. Am. Heart J., *84*:695, 1972.
9. de Leval, M. R.: Reoperations after closure of ventricular septal defects. In Stark, J., and Pacifico, A. D. (Eds.): Reoperations in Cardiac Surgery. London, Springer-Verlag, 1989, p. 161.
10. Dirksen, T., Moulaert, A. J., Buis-Liem, T. N., and Brom, A. G.: Ventricular septal defect associated with left ventricular outflow tract obstruction below the defect. J. Thorac. Cardiovasc. Surg., *75*:688, 1978.
11. DuShane, J. W., and Kirklin, J. W.: Late results of the repair of ventricular septal defect on pulmonary vascular disease. In Kirklin, J. W. (Ed.): Advances in Cardiovascular Surgery. New York, Grune & Stratton, 1973, p. 9.
12. DuShane, J. W., Kirklin, J. W., Patrick, R. T., et al.: Ventricular septal defects with pulmonary hypertension: Surgical treatment by means of a mechanical pump-oxygenator. JAMA, *160*:950, 1956.
13. Fratacci, M-D., Frostell, C. G., Chen, T-Y., et al.: Inhaled nitric oxide: A selective pulmonary vasodilator of heparin-protamine vasoconstriction in sheep. Anesthesiology, *75*:990, 1991.
14. Freed, M. D., Rosenthal, A., Plauth, W. H., Jr., and Nadas, A. S.: Development of subaortic stenosis after pulmonary artery banding. Circulation, *47, 48*(Suppl. III):7, 1973.
15. Friedli, B., Kidd, B. S. L., Mustard, W. T., and Keith, J. D.: Ventricular septal defect with increased pulmonary vascular resistance: Late results of surgical closure. Am. J. Cardiol., *33*:403, 1974.
16. Hallidie-Smith, K. A., Edwards, R. E., Wilson, R., and Zeidifard, E.: Long-term cardiorespiratory assessment after surgical closure of ventricular septal defect in childhood (Abstract). Proc. Br. Cardiac Soc., *37*:553, 1975.
17. Hallidie-Smith, K. A., Hollmann, A., Cleland, W. P., et al.: Effects of surgical closure of ventricular septal defects upon pulmonary vascular disease. Br. Heart J., *31*:246, 1969.
18. Heath, D., Helmholz, H. F., Jr., Burchell, H. B., et al.: Graded pulmonary vascular changes and hemodynamic findings in cases of atrial and ventricular septal defect and patent ductus arteriosus. Circulation, *18*:1155, 1958.
19. Heath, D., and Edwards, J. E.: The pathology of hypertensive pulmonary vascular disease: A description of six grades of structural changes in pulmonary arteries with special references to congenital cardiac septal defects. Circulation, *18*:533, 1958.

20. Hoffman, J. I. E., and Rudolph, A. M.: The natural history of ventricular septal defects in infancy. Am. J. Cardiol., 16:634, 1965.
21. Hoffman, J. I. E., and Rudolph, A. M.: The natural history of isolated ventricular septal defect with special reference to selection of patients for surgery. Adv. Pediatr., 17:57, 1970.
22. Hoffman, J. I. E.: Natural history of congenital heart disease: Problems in its assessment with special reference to ventricular septal defect. Circulation, 37:97, 1968.
23. Hopkins, R. A., Bull, C., Sumner, E., et al.: Pulmonary hypertensive crises following surgery for congenital heart defects in children. Circulation, 72:259, 1986.
24. Jarmakani, M. M., Edwards, S. B., Spach, M. S., et al.: Left ventricular pressure-volume characteristics in congenital heart disease. Circulation, 37:879, 1968.
25. Keck, E. W. O., Ongley, P. A., Kincaid, O. W., and Swan, H. J. C.: Ventricular septal defect with aortic insufficiency: A clinical and hemodynamic study of 18 proved cases. Circulation, 27:203, 1963.
26. Keith, J. D., Rose, V., Collins, G., and Kidd, B. S. L.: Ventricular septal defect: Incidence, morbidity, and mortality in various age groups. Br. Heart J., 33(Suppl.):81, 1971.
27. Kirklin, J. K., Castañeda, A. R., Keane, J. F., et al.: Surgical management of multiple ventricular septal defects. J. Thorac. Cardiovasc. Surg., 80:485, 1980.
28. Kirklin, J. K., and Kirklin, J. W.: Management of the cardiovascular subsystem after cardiac surgery. Ann. Thorac. Surg., 32:311, 1981.
29. Kirklin, J. W., and DuShane, J. W.: Repair of ventricular septal defect in infancy. Pediatrics, 27:961, 1961.
30. Lauer, R. M., DuShane, J. W., and Edwards, J. E.: Obstruction of left ventricular outlet in association with ventricular septal defect. Circulation, 22:110, 1960.
31. Leatham, A., and Segal, B.: Auscultatory and phonocardiographic signs of ventricular septal defect with left to right shunt. Circulation, 25:318, 1962.
32. Levin, A. R., Spach, M. S., Canent, R. V., Jr., et al.: Intracardiac pressure-flow dynamics in isolated ventricular septal defects. Circulation, 35:430, 1967.
33. Lillehei, C. W., Cohen, M., Warden, H. E., et al.: The results of direct vision closure of ventricular septal defects in eight patients by means of controlled cross circulation. Surg. Gynecol. Obstet., 101:446, 1955.
34. Lincoln, C., Jamieson, S., Joseph, M., et al.: Transatrial repair of ventricular septal defects with reference to their anatomic classification. J. Thorac. Cardiovasc. Surg., 74:183, 1977.
35. Mitchell, S. C., Korones, S. B., and Berendes, H. W.: Congenital heart disease in 56,109 births: Incidence and natural history. Circulation, 43:323, 1971.
36. Morgan, B. C., Griffiths, S. P., and Blumenthal, S.: Ventricular septal defect: I. Congestive heart failure in infancy. Pediatrics, 25:54, 1960.
37. Moulaert, A. J., Bruins, C. G., and Oppenheimer-Dekker, A.: Anomalies of the aortic arch and ventricular septal defects. Circulation, 53:1011, 1976.
38. Muller, W. H., Jr., and Dammann, J. F., Jr.: Treatment of certain congenital malformations of the heart by the creation of pulmonic stenosis to reduce pulmonary hypertension and excessive pulmonary flow: A preliminary report. Surg. Gynecol. Obstet., 95:213, 1952.
39. Nadas, A. S., Thilenius, O. G., La Farge, C. G., and Hauck, A. J.: Ventricular septal defect with aortic regurgitation: Medical and pathological aspects. Circulation, 29:862, 1964.
40. Okamoto, Y.: Clinical studies for open heart surgery in infants with profound hypothermia. Arch. Jpn. Chir., 38:188, 1969.

41. Pacifico, A. D.: Cardiopulmonary bypass and hypothermic circulatory arrest in congenital heart surgery. In Grillo, H. C., et al. (Eds.): Current Therapy in Cardiothoracic Surgery. Toronto, B. C. Decker, 1988.
42. Pacifico, A. D., Sand, M. E., Bargeron, L. M., Jr., and Colvin, E. V.: Transatrial-transpulmonary repair of tetralogy of Fallot. J. Thorac. Cardiovasc. Surg., 93:919, 1987.
43. Rein, J. G., Freed, M. D., Norwood, W. I., and Castañeda, A. R.: Early and late results of closure of ventricular septal defect in infancy. Ann. Thorac. Surg., 24:19, 1977.
44. Riggs, T., Mehta, S., Hirschfield, S., et al.: Ventricular septal defect in infancy: A combined vectographic and echocardiographic study. Circulation, 59:385, 1979.
45. Rizzoli, G., Blackstone, E. H., Kirklin, J. W., et al.: Incremental risk factors in hospital mortality after repair of ventricular septal defect. J. Thorac. Cardiovasc. Surg., 80:494, 1980.
46. Roger, H.: Recherches cliniques sur la communication congenitale de deux coeurs: Pars inocclusion de septum interventriculaire. Bull. Acad. Med., 8:1074, 1879.
47. Shah, P., Singh, W. S. A., Rose, V., and Keith, J.: Incidence of bacterial endocarditis in ventricular septal defects. Circulation, 34:127, 1966.
48. Sigmann, J. M., Stern, A. M., and Sloan, H. E.: Early surgical correction of large ventricular septal defects. Pediatrics, 39:4, 1967.
49. Singh, A. K., de Leval, M. R., and Stark, J.: Left ventriculotomy for closure of muscular ventricular septal defects. Ann. Surg., 186:577, 1977.
50. Somerville, J., Brandao, A., and Ross, D. N.: Aortic regurgitation with ventricular septal defect: Surgical management and clinical features. Circulation, 41:317, 1970.
51. Soto, B., Ceballos, R., and Kirklin, J.W.: Ventricular septal defects: A surgical viewpoint. J. Am. Coll. Cardiol., 14:1291, 1989.
52. Soto, B., Becker, A. E., Moulaert, A. J., et al.: Classification of ventricular septal defects. Br. Heart J., 43:332, 1980.
53. Stirling, G. R., Stanley, P. H., and Lillehei, C. W.: Effect of cardiac bypass and ventriculotomy upon right ventricular function. Surg. Forum, 8:433, 1957.
54. Tawes, R. L., Jr., Aberdeen, E., Waterston, D. J., et al.: Coarctation of the aorta in infants and children: A review of 333 operative cases, including 179 infants. Circulation, 39(Suppl. I):173, 1969.
55. Trusler, G. A., Moes, C. A. F., and Kidd, B. S. L.: Repair of ventricular septal defect with aortic insufficiency. J. Thorac. Cardiovasc. Surg., 66:394, 1973.
56. Trusler, G. A., and Mustard, W. T.: A method of banding the pulmonary artery for large isolated ventricular septal defect with and without transposition of the great arteries. Ann. Thorac. Surg., 13:351, 1972.
57. Van Praagh, R., Geva, T., and Kreutzer, J.: Ventricular septal defects: How shall we describe, name and classify them? J. Am. Coll. Cardiol., 14:1298, 1989.
58. Van Praagh, R., McNamara, J. J., and Gross, R. E.: Anatomic types of ventricular septal defect with aortic insufficiency. Circulation, 36(Suppl. 2):256, 1967.
59. Van Praagh, R., Bernhard, W. F., Rosenthal, A., et al.: Interrupted aortic arch: Surgical treatment. Am. J. Cardiol., 27:200, 1971.
60. Wagenvoort, C. A., Neufeld, H. N., DuShane, J. W., and Edwards, J. E.: The pulmonary arterial tree in ventricular septal defect: A quantitative study of anatomic features in fetuses, infants and children. Circulation, 23:740, 1961.
61. Wells, W. J., and Lindesmith, G. G.: Ventricular septal defect. In Arciniegas, E. (Ed.): Pediatric Cardiac Surgery. Chicago, Year Book Medical Publishers, 1985.

VII

TETRALOGY OF FALLOT

Ross M. Ungerleider, M.D.

Tetralogy of Fallot (TOF) is one of the most common congenital heart malformations. Depending on the criteria used to define this entity, it can be present in three to six infants for every 10,000 births. It is probably proper to consider TOF within the spectrum of pulmonary stenosis (or atresia) with an accompanying ventricular septal defect. The condition usually presents as cyanosis shortly after birth, attracting early medical attention. Diagnosis can be made with two-dimensional echocardiography or cardiac catheterization. Most patients are candidates for surgical repair, and several options exist that can provide excellent immediate and long-term outcomes for many of these children.

ANATOMY AND PHYSIOLOGY

A wide morphologic variability exists in the spectrum of TOF. This can encompass the size of the right ventricle (RV), the size and distribution of the pulmonary arteries, the location of the pulmonary stenosis (i.e., subvalvular, valvular, or peripheral), and additional sources of pulmonary blood flow (i.e., systemic-pulmonary collateral vessels).

The lesion described by Fallot was believed by him to consist of four major defects: (1) infundibular pulmonary stenosis, (2) a ventricular septal defect, (3) dextroposition of the aorta, and (4) hypertrophy of the RV. It is now recognized

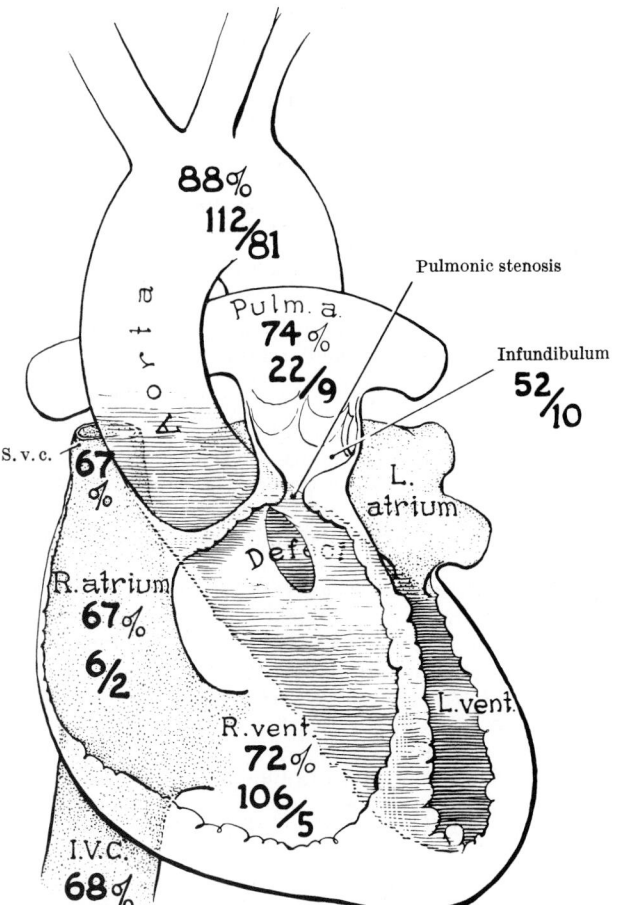

Figure 54–60. This schematic of typical cardiac catheterization findings in a patient with TOF demonstrates both the anatomy and the physiology of the defect. The pulmonary stenosis below the pulmonary valve causes shunting of desaturated blood from the right ventricle into the left ventricle, thus lowering the systemic arterial oxygen saturation. The pulmonary artery pressures are usually normal, but the pressures in the right ventricle are high and often are as high as the systemic pressures because the ventricular septal defect is usually large and nonrestrictive. (S.v.c., superior vena cava; I.V.C., inferior vena cava.)

by most authorities that the two most important features of TOF are the RV outflow tract obstruction, which is nearly always infundibular and/or valvular; and the ventricular septal defect, which is usually large, subaortic, adjacent to the membranous septum (perimembranous), and associated with malalignment of the conal septum. A working definition of the tetralogy includes the basic principle that it is a congenital cardiac malformation with a large ventricular septal defect and with significant pulmonary stenosis (that may be valvular, subvalvular, or supravalvular), which can severely restrict pulmonary blood flow (Fig. 54–60).

These anatomic features nicely explain the basic physiology of the lesion. Shunting across the ventricular septal defect is determined by the degree of RV outflow obstruction. Those patients with severe pulmonary stenosis (regardless of the level of the RV outflow obstruction) will shunt right to left across the ventricular septal defect and will have a degree of cyanosis that reflects the volume of their shunt. When the pulmonary stenosis is less severe, bidirectional shunting may occur. In some patients, the infundibular stenosis is minimal and the predominant shunt is from left to right, producing what is termed the *pink tetralogy.* Although such patients may not appear cyanotic, they often have oxygen desaturation in the systemic arterial blood. A sudden decrease in systemic

vascular resistance or an increase in the pulmonary outflow resistance (which can vary in some patients due to the tone of the infundibular—or subvalvular—muscle) can produce sudden alterations in the amount of right-to-left shunting and result in a hypercyanotic (or "tet") spell.

The pulmonary arteries can also be variable in size and distribution. Occasionally, the left pulmonary artery may be absent (3%), although this is rare for the right pulmonary artery. Many patients have some degree of stenosis of the peripheral pulmonary arteries, which further restricts pulmonary blood flow. There may be no communication between the RV and main pulmonary artery (pulmonary atresia), and in this case pulmonary blood flow is maintained by a ductus arteriosus or some other form of bronchopulmonary collateral vessel.

Aortic overriding is caused by true dextroposition and abnormal rotation of the aortic root, resulting in an aorta that arises from the RV to a varying degree. The aorta itself may have a right arch in as many as 25% to 30% of patients with TOF; and in these situations the branching pattern of the arch vessels may be abnormal (Fig. 54–61). Occasionally, the ductus arteriosus persists on the side opposite the arch or it may be completely absent. An aberrant subclavian artery running in a retroesophageal location may be present (5%–10%), although it is quite rare for the retroesophageal subclavian vessels to cause dysphagia. A persistent left superior vena cava occurs with about the same incidence.

Coronary artery anatomy may have important variability. Most notable is the origin of the left anterior descending coronary artery from the proximal right coronary artery, resulting in the RV outflow tract being crossed by this important coronary artery at variable distances from the pulmonary valve annulus. Occasionally, all coronary arteries may arise from a single main coronary ostium (usually the left) or the left coronary artery may arise from the pulmonary artery.

Associated defects are not uncommon with TOF. The existence of an atrial septal defect is frequent enough to prompt its inclusion as *pentalogy* of Fallot. Other defects of impor-

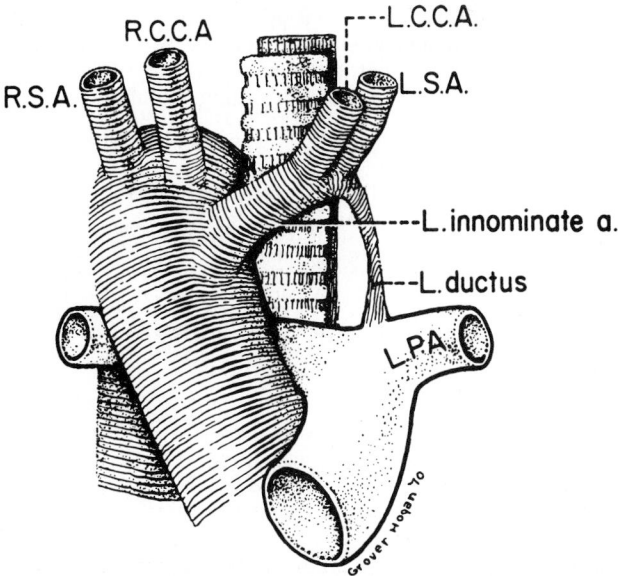

Figure 54–61. In patients with a right aortic arch there is usually mirror image branching of the head vessels. If the aorta descends on the right, it will be located posterior to the right pulmonary artery. If the aorta descends on the patient's left (not shown), it will pass behind the trachea and the esophagus. It is unusual for a right aortic arch to cause symptoms of a vascular ring, but it is possible and needs to be evaluated in symptomatic patients. (From Shuford, W. H., and Sybers, R. G.: The Aortic Arch and Its Malformations. Springfield, Ill., Charles C Thomas, 1974.)

tance include atrioventricular septal defects, muscular ventricular septal defects, anomalous pulmonary venous return, and aortic insufficiency.

DIAGNOSIS
Clinical Manifestations

The clinical presentation is dependent on the severity of the anatomic malformation. Infants with pulmonary atresia may become intensely cyanotic as the ductus arteriosus closes unless they have numerous bronchopulmonary collateral vessels. Heart failure is usually not a feature unless collateral vessels are extensive. Patients with RV to pulmonary continuity are cyanotic in relation to the degree of pulmonary stenosis and consequent pulmonary blood flow. Occasionally, children will have enough pulmonary blood flow that they will not appear cyanotic, and the lesion may go undetected until they begin to outgrow their pulmonary blood flow. A common way for these older children to increase pulmonary flow is to squat, thus increasing peripheral vascular resistance and decreasing the size of their right-to-left shunt across the ventricular septal defect. This position had diagnostic significance and was highly characteristic of TOF in a previous era. It is now distinctly unusual for these children's defects to remain unrepaired beyond infancy, and this *important* descriptive sign of TOF will be less frequently, if ever, observed in the future. Nevertheless, this same physiology is the basis for hypercyanotic or *tet* spells that can be observed in any patient with unrepaired TOF and constitutes the rationale for flexing affected infants into a tight *ball* in an effort to increase systemic vascular resistance and break the spell.

The natural history of unrepaired TOF is heavily influenced by the severity of the anatomic defect. Statistics demonstrate a 30% mortality by age 6 months that increases to 50% by 2 years. Only 20% of patients can be expected to reach 10 years of age, and not more than 5% to 10% live to reach 21 (Fig. 54–62).[27] Patients with pulmonary atresia and ventricular septal defect (TOF with pulmonary atresia) have an even worse prognosis for survival without surgical intervention,[27] with a mortality that approaches 50% in the first year of life and that can be as high as 84% by 5 years of age.

The greatest risks that these patients face (if left unrepaired) are paradoxical emboli (leading to stroke or end-organ failure), cerebral or pulmonary thrombosis (from increasing polycythemia), and subacute bacterial endocarditis. Heart failure is uncommon in surgically untreated patients but does pose a greater risk after creation of a systemic-to-pulmonary artery shunt, especially if pre-existing collateral vessels are not dealt with.

Physical Examination

Infants with TOF may appear to be of normal size and otherwise healthy except for a mild-to-moderate duskiness related to their degree of cyanosis. Older patients may appear to be smaller than expected for their age, and cyanosis of the lips and nail beds is usually apparent. The fingers and toes usually show clubbing (hypertrophic pulmonary osteoarthropathy). On palpation of the chest, a thrill is usually present anteriorly. A harsh systolic murmur is audible over the pulmonary area and along the left sternal border. Absence of a murmur in a patient suspected of having tetralogy is suggestive of pulmonary atresia. In fact, the harsher the murmur, the more likely that the patient has substantial pulmonary blood flow (since the murmur reflects the flow across the stenotic outflow tract). A murmur that has dissipated in intensity may reflect deficient antegrade flow across the pulmonary outflow tract and may be accompanied by intense cyanosis unless pulmonary blood flow is provided by a patent ductus arteriosus (or by a previously placed aortopulmonary shunt). The second heart sound is usually single and rarely increases in intensity. A continuous murmur suggests a collateral source of pulmonary blood flow (either a patent ductus arteriosus, a significant bronchopulmonary collateral vessel, or a surgically created shunt).

Laboratory Studies

In infants, the laboratory studies are ordinarily unremarkable for age, except for systemic arterial oxygen desaturation. In older patients, who have remained cyanotic for some time, the hemoglobin, hematocrit, and erythrocyte count are usually elevated. The magnitude of the increase is generally proportional to the cyanosis, with hematocrit values varying from normal to as high as 90% (in extreme cases). Similarly, the oxygen saturation in the systemic arterial blood is variable, usually between 70% and 90%. However, in severe forms of the malformation, the arterial oxygen saturation during exercise or stress may fall to as low as 25%.

Diagnostic Evaluation

In the early stages, the chest film may be normal, but as the ductus arteriosus closes shortly after birth, the chest film in TOF usually shows diminished vascularity in the lungs and absence of prominence of the pulmonary artery. The shadow of the great vessels in the superior mediastinum is narrow, owing to the diminished caliber of the pulmonary artery. If cyanosis and dyspnea are quite prominent, the pulmonary vascular markings are usually markedly diminished. Later, the classic boot-shaped heart (*coeur en sabot*) may develop, and it is recognized as a hallmark of TOF (Fig. 54–63). RV enlargement is present and is best demonstrated in the left anterior oblique position. Approximately one fourth of the patients with TOF have a *right* aortic arch (see Fig. 54–63); and although this can be demonstrated with a barium swallow, it is now common practice to diagnose most anatomic features of the lesion with echocardiography.[45] In fact, the presence of a right aortic arch with cyanosis is strong evidence that the malformation is indeed TOF, or some variant of ventricular septal defect with pulmonary stenosis or atresia.

The electrocardiogram shows right ventricular hypertro-

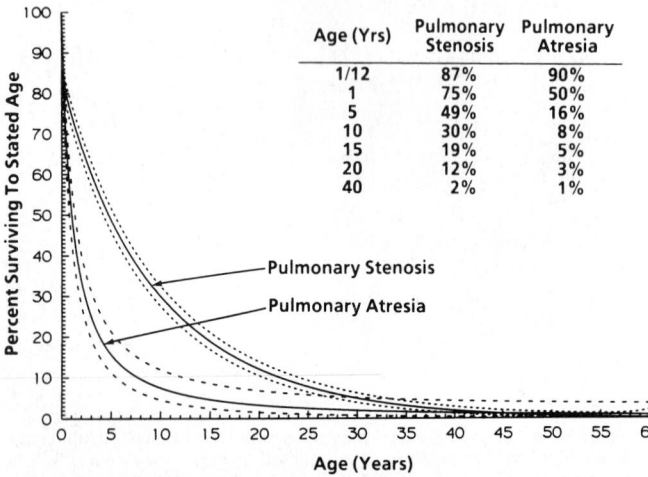

Age (Yrs)	Pulmonary Stenosis	Pulmonary Atresia
1/12	87%	90%
1	75%	50%
5	49%	16%
10	30%	8%
15	19%	5%
20	12%	3%
40	2%	1%

Figure 54–62. Nomogram depicting the survival of surgically untreated patients with TOF. The smooth lines represent the survival of each group, and the dashed lines enclose the 70% confidence limits around each of these. (From Kirklin, J. W., and Barratt-Boyes, B. G.: Cardiac Surgery, 2nd ed. New York, Churchill Livingstone, 1993.)

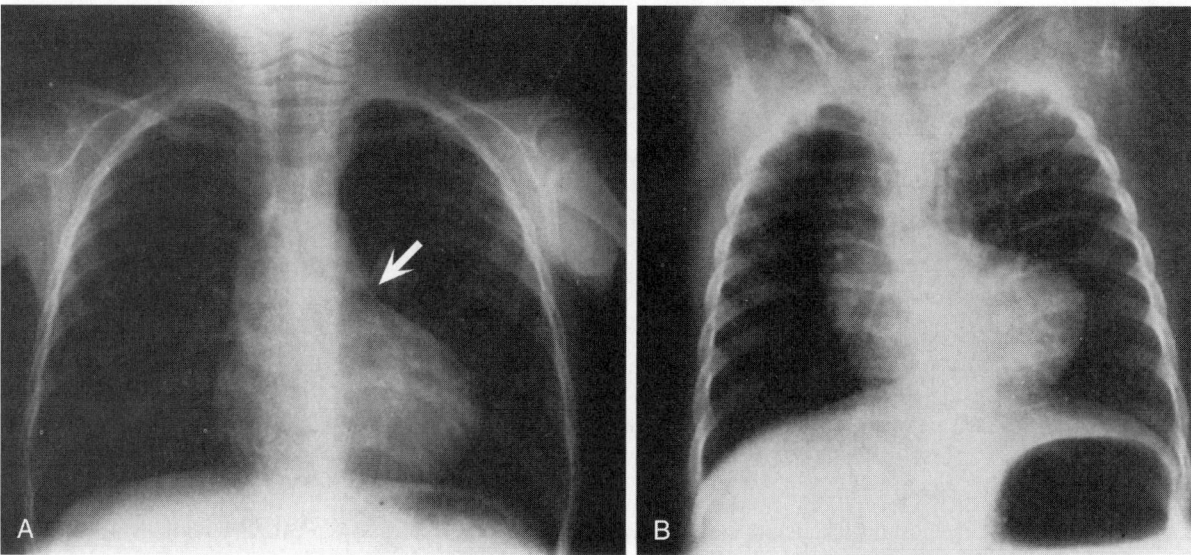

Figure 54–63. *A,* Chest film of a patient with TOF and a left aortic arch. The absence of the pulmonary artery shadow (arrow) gives the heart a characteristic boot-shaped appearance. *B,* In this patient, the boot-shaped appearance of the heart is made even more prominent because of the right aortic arch accentuating the absence of the pulmonary arterial shadow.

phy, usually apparent in the standard leads and most consistently found in the unipolar leads. The more commonly encountered findings include tall and peaked T waves, reversal of the RS ratio, and a normal PR interval and QRS complex duration. If RV hypertrophy is absent, a diagnosis of TOF should be seriously questioned and pulmonary atresia with hypoplastic RV should be considered.

Advances in two-dimensional echocardiography with color-flow Doppler imaging have elevated the diagnostic capabilities of this technology.[45] It is not uncommon for infants and children to be accurately diagnosed by echocardiography before the performance of any laboratory tests, radiographs, electrocardiograms, or angiograms. The addition of color-flow mapping can sensitively detect the presence of a patent ductus arteriosus, an additional muscular ventricular septal defect, or a small atrial septal defect. Echocardiographic documentation of the physiology of a cyanotic spell with right-to-left shunting across a ventricular septal defect that is reversed by elevation of peripheral vascular resistance has been nicely demonstrated.[20] The coronary anatomy can be revealed with remarkable accuracy, and abnormalities of valvular apparatus (i.e., straddling chords) may be best delineated with this technology. It is not uncommon to take patients to the operating room for palliation or correction based on preoperative echocardiographic data alone.[11, 32, 33] In most centers, cardiac catheterization is performed only for those patients in whom there is still some uncertainty remaining following the echocardiogram regarding the coronary anatomy, the pulmonary artery anatomy, or other sources of pulmonary blood flow.

Cardiac catheterization provides angiographic demonstration of ventricular size, pulmonary artery size, and, with aortic root injection, sources of pulmonary blood flow, as well as anomalies of coronary artery anatomy. Some authors base prediction of the postrepair RV/left ventricle (LV) pressure ratio on data obtained from catheterization, thus assisting operative planning of the type of repair that should be performed.[5, 21] Other pressure measurements should demonstrate equal pressures in both ventricles (distinguishing this condition from isolated pulmonary stenosis with intact ventricular septum in which the RV pressure may be considerably greater than that in the LV). Angiograms are especially helpful before complete repair in those patients who have

received palliative shunt procedures. These pictures define the anatomy of the pulmonary arteries as well as any iatrogenic distortion caused by the shunt that might need attention (Fig. 54–64). If pressure data (i.e., cardiac catheterization) are not needed, magnetic resonance imaging can provide excellent views with minimal invasion—a worthwhile consideration because it is not unusual for cyanotic spells and seizures to occur in these children during intracardiac catheter manipulation.

INDICATIONS FOR OPERATION

As suggested by the natural history of this lesion, most patients will require surgical intervention. Current trends are to provide surgical correction as soon as possible (often electively before the first year of life) and generally by the

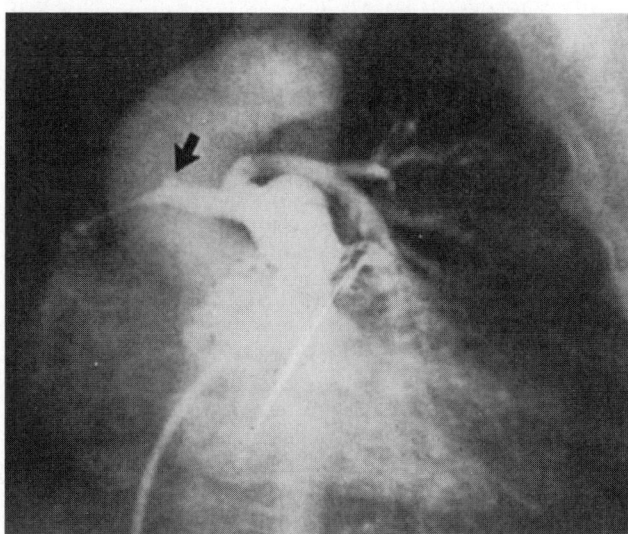

Figure 54–64. The arrow depicts the insertion site of a previously placed (but now occluded) Blalock-Taussig shunt. Distortion from surgery has obstructed blood flow to the distal right pulmonary artery, which is now no longer salvageable. The majority of the pulmonary blood flow in this patient is directed toward the left lung.

time the patient has reached the age of 18 months. The urgency with which a procedure is performed is affected by numerous variables, which include the symptoms at presentation, age at presentation, and associated lesions. The use of prostaglandin E_1 to stabilize patients with diminished pulmonary blood flow has greatly influenced the emergent care of these patients.[13, 17] Rather than performing emergency systemic-to-pulmonary artery shunts on critically ill, hypoxemic, and acidotic neonates, surgeons have the luxury of more fully evaluating the patient's anatomy, while prostaglandins maintain ductal patency (and thus pulmonary blood flow). This grants the surgical team time to arrive at the most appropriate decision for each individual patient and to plan a procedure aimed at correction of the underlying lesion as opposed to palliation alone. Although controversy continues concerning the preferential operation during infancy, there has been a general trend toward open correction in early infancy.[9-11, 21, 27, 48, 54] The groups that urge early total correction at any time emphasize that it prevents the necessity for a second operation and that the current results are sufficiently good to support this judgment. Furthermore, palliation has its own inherent risks, which include death after the procedure or before the time the patient can return for complete repair.[9, 28, 55] Palliation, in the form of aortopulmonary shunts, can also result in significant distortion of the pulmonary arteries, which can complicate and increase the risk of subsequent complete repair.[55] Therefore, some groups currently believe that a corrective procedure should be performed in all patients with TOF, irrespective of age or weight, including those with TOF with pulmonary atresia.[9, 55] Opposed to this group are those who believe that palliation is preferable in infancy because they believe that the overall mortality is lower.[25, 28, 55] In addition, these observers are concerned about whether the small heart in infancy will remain corrected as growth continues, thinking perhaps that outflow tract obstruction of the right ventricle may recur. Finally, there is some suggestion that the pulmonary valve annulus may continue to grow after shunt palliation and, thus, allow the eventual repair to be accomplished with less likelihood of a transannular patch.[54] These data, however, are inconclusive and have not been characteristic of the experience of others.[11, 49] This issue would probably require a randomized prospective trial for more accurate evaluation.

Two articles have addressed this issue of palliation versus repair[28, 55] by examining the outcome for patients with TOF from the time they are diagnosed as opposed to from the time they have surgical intervention. The information reported by these studies is important in understanding the natural history of the disease in the first years of life using various treatment protocols. Risk factors for death (for all patients diagnosed with TOF) include the presence of multiple ventricular septal defects, Down syndrome, large aortopulmonary collateral vessels, complete atrioventricular canal defects (especially if the patient also has trisomy 21), and early age at presentation.[28] There can be significant mortality that occurs before surgical repair, especially in infants chosen for palliation. For 237 patients diagnosed with TOF at Toronto Sick Children's Hospital,[55] there were eight deaths in 216 patients undergoing complete repair (3.7%). This very acceptable surgical mortality seems to support a protocol of early shunting followed by subsequent complete repair (in this study, patients received aortopulmonary shunts if they were diagnosed and were symptomatic before 18 months of age). However, there were an additional 15 patients who died before complete repair, either as a direct effect of attempted palliation or as an effect of waiting for surgical intervention after palliation. This brings the total mortality to 23 of 231 patients (10%) and is considerably higher than mortality of early repair in infancy without previous palliation

(0%–6%).[11, 21, 28, 48, 49, 54] In one series,[28] it appeared that surgical repair after previous palliation had a slightly higher mortality (12%) than primary repair (6%), and this might be due to identified risk factors for operative mortality, which include pulmonary artery distortion from previous shunts (see Fig. 54–64) and more than one previous palliative procedure. Other risk factors for operative mortality include need for a transannular patch, high (>0.65) postrepair (measured in the intensive care unit) RV/LV pressure ratios,[28] and persistent, uncontrollable tet spells at the time of repair. Although "comparative study has shown primary one-stage repair to be preferable to the two-stage approach,"[27] good outcomes with this protocol, especially in small infants (<6 months old) requires a team and institution experienced with and dedicated to all aspects of neonatal and infant congenital heart operations, including pediatric cardiac anesthesia and pediatric critical care medicine. Although the institutions that are properly equipped for specialized neonatal cardiac procedures can obtain good outcomes with early, one-stage repair of TOF, the application of primary palliative procedures may be beneficial. Furthermore, palliation may be considered in unusual circumstances, such as in patients with an anomalous coronary artery crossing the RV outflow tract, in patients with extremely small pulmonary arteries, in patients who have been having severe, unrelenting tet spells for several hours, or in patients with significant and severe associated lesions that may preclude total repair. Therefore, it is important for surgical teams to be familiar with current options for palliation as well as with the techniques for complete repair.

SURGICAL TECHNIQUES

Palliative Procedures

Various factors that increase the risk for early repair have been described and include pulmonary artery problems, major associated anomalies, more than one previous operation, and absent pulmonary valve syndrome. Small size and young age, which at one time was believed to also be a risk factor for early repair, may not be a true risk factor when patients are examined with multivariate analysis that corrects for other anatomic risks.[9, 27, 28]

The presence of pulmonary atresia or an anomalous left anterior descending coronary artery across the RV outflow tract may preclude the possibility of establishing transannular RV to pulmonary artery continuity if necessary and require placement of a conduit. Although conduits can be used in infants, some surgeons prefer to defer conduit placement until the infant is older and of a size that can permit placement of a larger conduit. Nevertheless, the availability of cryopreserved homografts has made conduit placement in infants safer. Each case must be individualized but these considerations can provide adequate justification for performing a palliative rather than a corrective procedure when the patient is first diagnosed.

There are a number of systemic-to-pulmonary artery shunts being performed by various surgeons, but the most common shunts (Fig. 54–65) include a classic Blalock-Taussig shunt, the modified Blalock-Taussig shunt,[47] and a central aortopulmonary shunt[11] using prosthetic graft material. In addition, there seem to be advantages to performing an RV outflow patch instead of a shunt in properly selected patients, such as those with extremely small pulmonary arteries. Recently, there has been enthusiasm for establishing continuity between the RV and pulmonary artery in patients with TOF and small pulmonary arteries by placement of either a conduit from the RV to pulmonary artery (with the ventricular septal defect left open), or direct anastomosis of the pulmonary artery (if the branch pulmonary arteries are

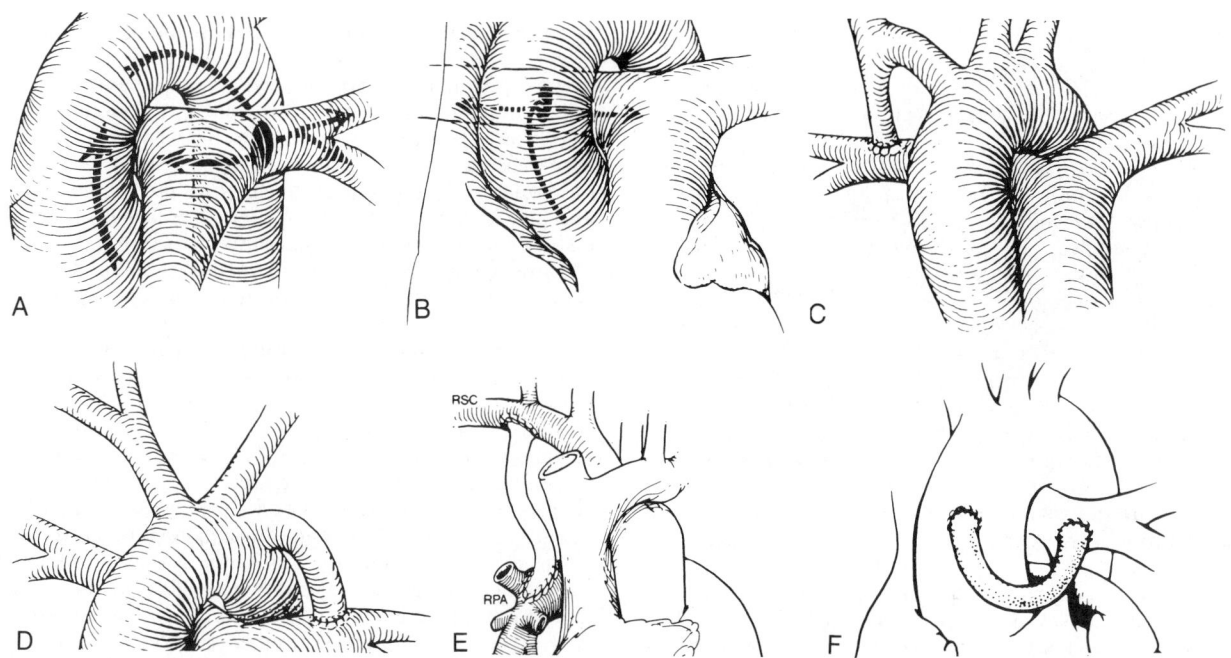

Figure 54–65. The most commonly encountered palliative shunts for increasing pulmonary blood flow in TOF. *A*, Potts' shunt. *B*, Waterston shunt. *C*, A classic Blalock-Taussig shunt. *D*, A Blalock-Taussig shunt performed on the side of the aortic arch. *E*, A modified Blalock-Taussig shunt (After Cooley, D. A.: Techniques in Cardiac Surgery, 2nd ed. Philadelphia, W. B. Saunders, 1984.) *F*, A central aortopulmonary shunt with prosthetic graft material. (From Turley, K., Tucker, W. Y., and Ebert, P. A.: The changing role of palliative procedures in the treatment of infants with congenital heart disease. J. Thorac. Cardiovasc. Surg., *79*:194, 1980.)

less than or equal to 1.5 mm. in diameter) to the side of the aorta. In both of these instances, the small size of the pulmonary arteries limits the amount flow into the pulmonary vascular bed and the pulmonary arteries can achieve symmetrical and uniform growth. Furthermore, the establishment of continuity of RV and pulmonary artery (with a conduit) enables the interventional cardiologist access to the pulmonary arteries for balloon dilation or intravascular stent placement to relieve areas of distal stenosis before complete repair.

The shunts popularized by Potts (see Fig. 54–65), Waterston (see Fig. 54–65), and Glenn are no longer being widely used. This is because the Waterston anastomosis (ascending aorta to right pulmonary artery) can cause kinking and stenosis at the anastomotic site and that may make subsequent open correction difficult. The Potts anastomosis (descending aorta to left pulmonary artery) can enlarge with time, producing an excessive shunt with pulmonary hypertension and often aneurysm formation at the site of the anastomosis. Moreover, a Potts anastomosis is more difficult to close at the time of subsequent correction. The Glenn anastomosis (which is between the superior vena cava and the right pulmonary artery) can produce good effects initially, with respect to symptoms in some patients, but more difficulty is experienced in the subsequent total correction. Irrespective of the type of palliation chosen, the goal is simply to increase pulmonary blood flow, independent of ductal patency, to allow for pulmonary artery growth and eventual total correction.

Blalock-Taussig Operation. In performance of a subclavian-pulmonary anastomosis, the incision is generally made on the side opposite that on which the aorta descends. Ideally, the subclavian branch of the innominate artery is used for the anastomosis because the angle produced at its origin from its parent vessel is better than that formed when the subclavian artery is used. The latter arises directly from the aorta and is likely to kink at its origin when deflected inferiorly for an anastomosis to the pulmonary artery. Experimental studies have shown that approximately three fourths of the blood passing through a subclavian pulmonary shunt is

directed to the lung on the side of the anastomosis.[16] There is evidence to suggest that growth of the pulmonary arteries after shunting is influenced by their structural composition and proportion of elastin as well as by differential blood flow.[43] Detailed attention must be given in performing the Blalock shunt, especially in the construction of the anastomosis. Every effort must be made to prevent constriction of the anastomosis, and meticulous technique is essential. The advantages of the Blalock shunt are that it produces a reliable shunt with excellent flow characteristics and shunt flow that is ordinarily well-matched to the size of the patient. Significant complications from transection of the subclavian artery are unusual and occur in less than 1% of patients,[2, 27] but numerous reports[2, 22, 31, 56] have suggested that subtle changes in arm strength and growth do occur in these patients with regularity. The shunt employs no prosthetic material and is fairly easy to take down at the time of total correction. Disadvantages are that the shunt requires meticulous and time-consuming dissection that may be difficult to justify in a severely ill infant. In addition, a Blalock shunt can cause distortion of the peripheral pulmonary artery even if no technical difficulty is encountered during performance of the procedure. This tendency for the normal healing and scarring process to produce pulmonary artery distortion significant enough to require pulmonary angioplasty at the time of subsequent TOF repair has been reported to be approximately 15%[55] and reaches 50% in patients who receive two palliative shunts before repair. As patients grow, one pulmonary artery may develop better than the other owing to flow characteristics, especially if there is anastomotic distortion. This pulmonary artery distortion may make subsequent total correction more hazardous.

Modified Blalock-Taussig Shunt. With the advent of reliable prosthetic graft material, technically easier forms of systemic-to-pulmonary artery shunting as a means of palliation have become popular. In addition, because most patients return within 2 years for total correction, the temporary nature of *palliation* justifies the use of an artificial conduit that may not have optimal longevity but that does allow for

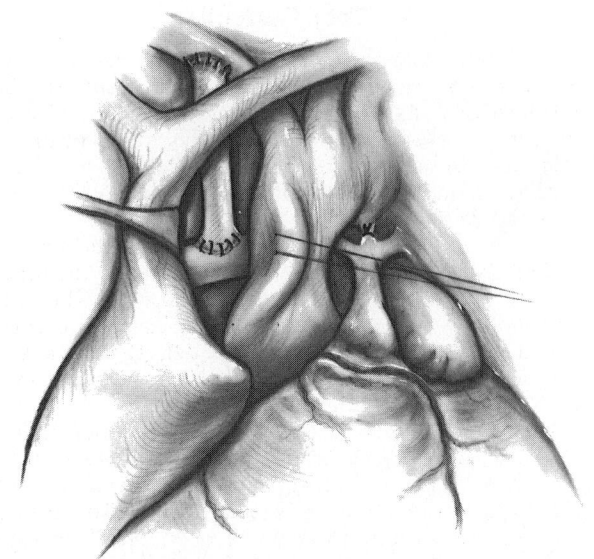

Figure 54–66. A modified Blalock-Taussig shunt using Gore-Tex can be placed through a median sternotomy without difficulty. This shunt has the advantage of being more centrally located on the pulmonary artery in a region that will eventually be incorporated into the future surgical plan. Furthermore, this shunt is easy to take down at a future operation.

preservation of the subclavian arterial supply to the arm. This "Great Ormond Street"[47] or modified Blalock-Taussig shunt requires interposition of a segment of polytetrafluoroethylene graft material (usually 4 or 5 mm. in diameter) between the subclavian artery and the pulmonary artery (see Fig. 54–65). Each anastomosis can be performed with a partial occlusion clamp and continuous monofilament suture. The shunts can be easily constructed on either side, since kinking of the subclavian artery is no longer a problem. Placement on the side of the aortic arch descent through a thoracotomy may be technically easier to construct but is more difficult to take down at the time of eventual repair. Although flow through this shunt is still controlled by the size of the subclavian artery, a long segment of prosthetic graft nevertheless provides its own unique amount of resistance so that flow through these shunts can be more variable. Furthermore,

because the graft is fixed in size, distortion of the pulmonary artery by the shunt can be anticipated as the patient grows, though this has not been a universal experience. Placement of a modified Blalock-Taussig shunt through a median sternotomy (Fig. 54–66) is gaining increasing favor because it enables the shunt to be placed more centrally on the right pulmonary artery so that it may be less likely to cause distortion and so that it is in a location that makes eventual shunt takedown quite simple. Regardless of the surgical approach employed, GoreTex interposition shunts have become the shunt of choice for some groups in infants who require palliation.

Central Aortopulmonary Shunt. Several groups have been proponents of interposing a short segment of prosthetic graft material between the ascending aorta and main (or right) pulmonary artery (see Fig. 54–65). This is an easy shunt to construct and, in older children, can usually be performed without cardiopulmonary bypass (using partial occlusion clamps while pulmonary blood flow is maintained by the ductus arteriosus). Although subsequent total correction requires a repeat sternotomy, this is not usually a problem and the shunts are easy to take down because of their anterior location. In patients who are surviving from antegrade blood flow across the RV outflow tract, occlusion of the main pulmonary artery may not be tolerated and placement of a central shunt in those patients requires cardiopulmonary bypass. Nevertheless, even if cardiopulmonary bypass support is necessary, these shunts usually work well and provide symmetrical pulmonary artery growth while avoiding the problems of distorting the branch pulmonary arteries.

RV Outflow Tract Patch. An alternative method for increasing pulmonary blood flow and palliating patients with TOF is to relieve the pulmonary stenosis but leave the ventricular septal defect open. This is usually done by a combination of infundibular muscle division and then placement of a patch (pericardium or prosthetic material) across the pulmonary valve annulus (Fig. 54–67). This converts the physiology to that of a ventricular septal defect alone. Most infants with TOF can tolerate this physiology without going into uncontrollable heart failure, since their *small* pulmonary arteries offer some resistance to limit the left-to-right shunt across the ventricular septal defect. However, it is this left-to-right shunt across the ventricular septal defect that provides increased pulmonary blood flow and that palliates the cyano-

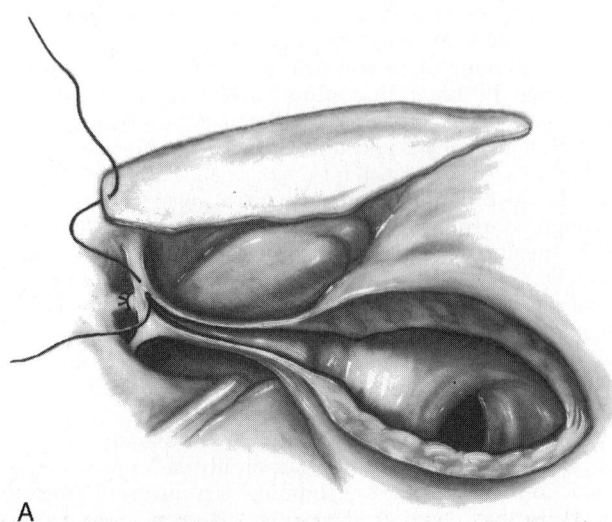

A

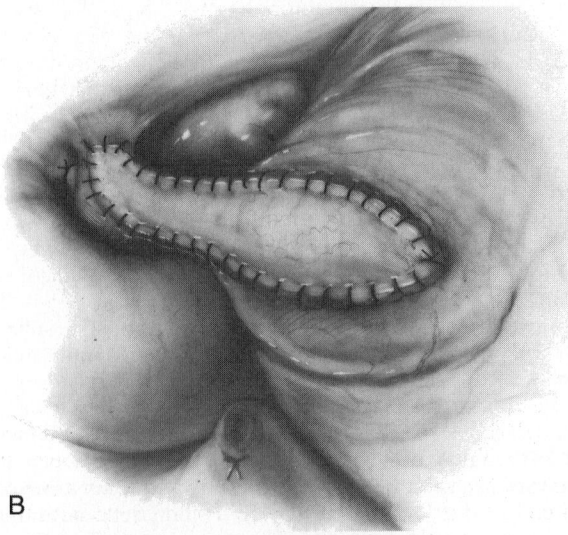

B

Figure 54–67. *A,* In patients with TOF and extremely hypoplastic pulmonary arteries, an RV outflow patch can be constructed by extending an incision from the RV to the small pulmonary arteries. A patch is then placed without closing the ventricular septal defect so that there is unobstructed continuity between the RV and pulmonary artery. *B,* Blood will then shunt from the LV toward the pulmonary artery to augment pulmonary blood flow. The resistance imposed by the small pulmonary arteries will control the flow and prevent the patient from having excessive pulmonary blood flow.

sis of severe TOF. This *intracardiac* shunt (as opposed to the *extracardiac* shunts described earlier) offers the theoretical advantage of symmetrical pulmonary artery blood flow with excellent potential for pulmonary artery growth and no risk of shunt thrombosis. Furthermore, in light of the poor experiences with conventional shunts in infants with very small pulmonary arteries,[55] RV outflow tract patches may be the palliation of choice for this group of patients. This procedure must be performed through a median sternotomy and on cardiopulmonary bypass. However, it does not require long cardiopulmonary bypass times and can be performed during aortic cross-clamping or electrical fibrillation with the use of moderate hypothermia (32° C.). The surgeon should carefully inspect the anatomy and note the presence of any important anatomic anomalies, such as persistent left superior vena cava. If an anomalous coronary artery is identified (e.g., left anterior descending arising from the right coronary artery and crossing the RV outflow tract) then the procedure must be abandoned and, if palliation is still desired (vs. total correction), a more conventional aortopulmonary shunt should be performed. To achieve adequate palliation with an RV outflow patch, the ventricular incision should extend far enough onto the proximal portion of the infundibulum so that after transection of the parietal bands, the RV chamber is easily viewed. The distal extent of the patch should extend to the pulmonary artery bifurcation, and the shape of the patch distally should be *squared* or *blunt* as opposed to *tapered* to limit the likelihood of late stenosis.[27] In patients who receive a good outcome from this procedure, the produced physiology causes a dramatic increase in pulmonary blood flow. Over time, and with growth of the pulmonary arteries, these patients gradually experience increased congestive heart failure from excessive left-to-right shunting across the ventricular septal defect. They are then returned to the operating room where the ventricular septal defect is closed (either through the atrium or by making an incision in the lower portion of the outflow patch).

Balloon Angioplasty of RV Outflow Tract. Recent experience and enthusiasm for balloon angioplasty techniques has encouraged some groups to experiment with balloon angioplasty of the RV outflow tract in symptomatic infants with TOF.[8, 30, 46] Although these procedures risk stimulating a severe hypercyanotic spell when the catheter is manipulated across the narrowed outflow tract, and although the anatomy of TOF (with hypoplasia of the muscular infundibulum) does not seem that it would be amenable to balloon angioplasty, initial effects with this technique in properly selected patients have been encouraging and may have a role in the treatment of patients who present a high surgical risk or in those in whom it might be preferable to delay surgical correction. The advantage of these techniques is that they can increase pulmonary blood flow (and thereby relieve cyanotic symptoms) without distorting the anatomy in a way that might interfere with an eventual complete repair.

The decision of which procedure to use can be based on many factors, including the experience and comfort that a particular surgeon has with each procedure. It must also be recognized today that these procedures in most cases are temporizing and that eventually total correction will be performed. Therefore, the shunt should be chosen that gives the best preparation for repair. Individual problems with anatomy (such as proximal stenosis of the right or left pulmonary artery) should be considered, for in such an instance it may be more advantageous to perform a central aortopulmonary shunt or an RV outflow patch (even if cardiopulmonary bypass is necessary) to enable concomitant enlargement of the area of pulmonary artery stenosis. Creation of a peripheral subclavian-to-pulmonary shunt in such a setting might otherwise limit flow to the contralateral pulmonary artery.

Total Correction

Total correction is the ideal operation for treatment of TOF and is accomplished with extracorporeal circulation. Before establishing cardiopulmonary bypass, previously placed systemic-to-pulmonary artery shunts should be identified so that they can be easily controlled. The patients are placed on cardiopulmonary bypass and usually cooled to 25° C. (unless a period of deep hypothermic circulatory arrest is anticipated, such as might be the case in infants. In these instances, patients are usually cooled to 18° C.). During this time previously placed shunts are divided or ligated. The goals of operation once cardiopulmonary bypass has been established are to close the ventricular septal defect, to relieve right ventricular outflow obstruction, and to repair any stenoses in the pulmonary arteries (Fig. 54–68).

Ventricular Septal Defect Closure. Several methods have been employed for closing the ventricular septal defect in patients with TOF and reflect the variety of choices available for closure of any perimembranous defect.[27] The most time-honored approach has been to close the defect through the incision that is commonly made in the RV outflow tract to relieve the infundibular stenosis. Closure of the defect through this incision is similar to closure of any ventricular septal defect through a transventricular approach except that the presence of hypertrophied muscle in the infundibulum and the desire to limit the extent of the incision add some difficulty to exposure. The incision should be vertical so that it can be extended across the valve annulus if necessary to relieve pulmonary stenosis (Fig. 54–69). In neonates and young infants, the parietal extension of the infundibular sep-

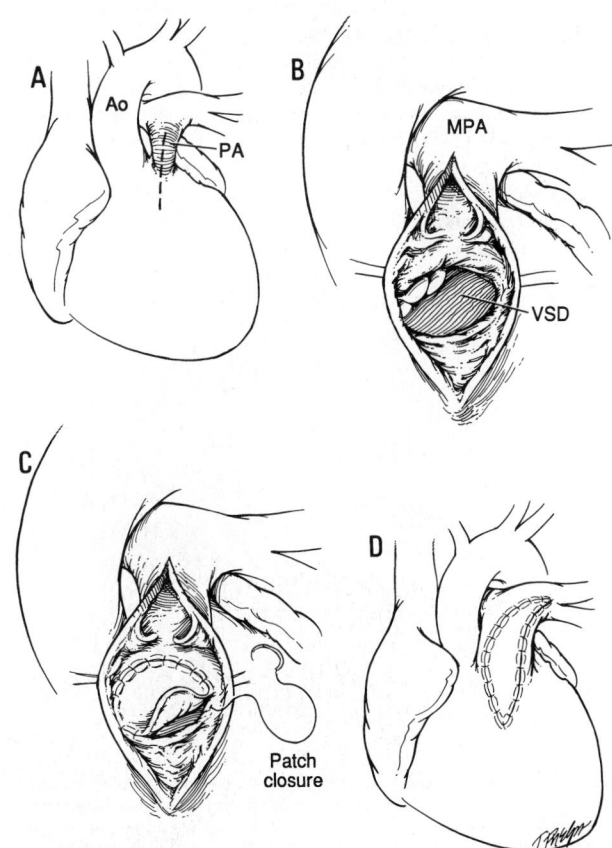

Figure 54–68. The goals of surgery in TOF are to enlarge the connection between the RV and main pulmonary artery using a transannular incision (as shown) if necessary *(A)*; to identify the ventricular septal defect by resecting extra muscle from the infundibular portion of the RV *(B)*; to close the ventricular septal defect with a patch *(C)*; and to augment the RV to pulmonary artery connection with a patch (transannular) if necessary *(D)*.

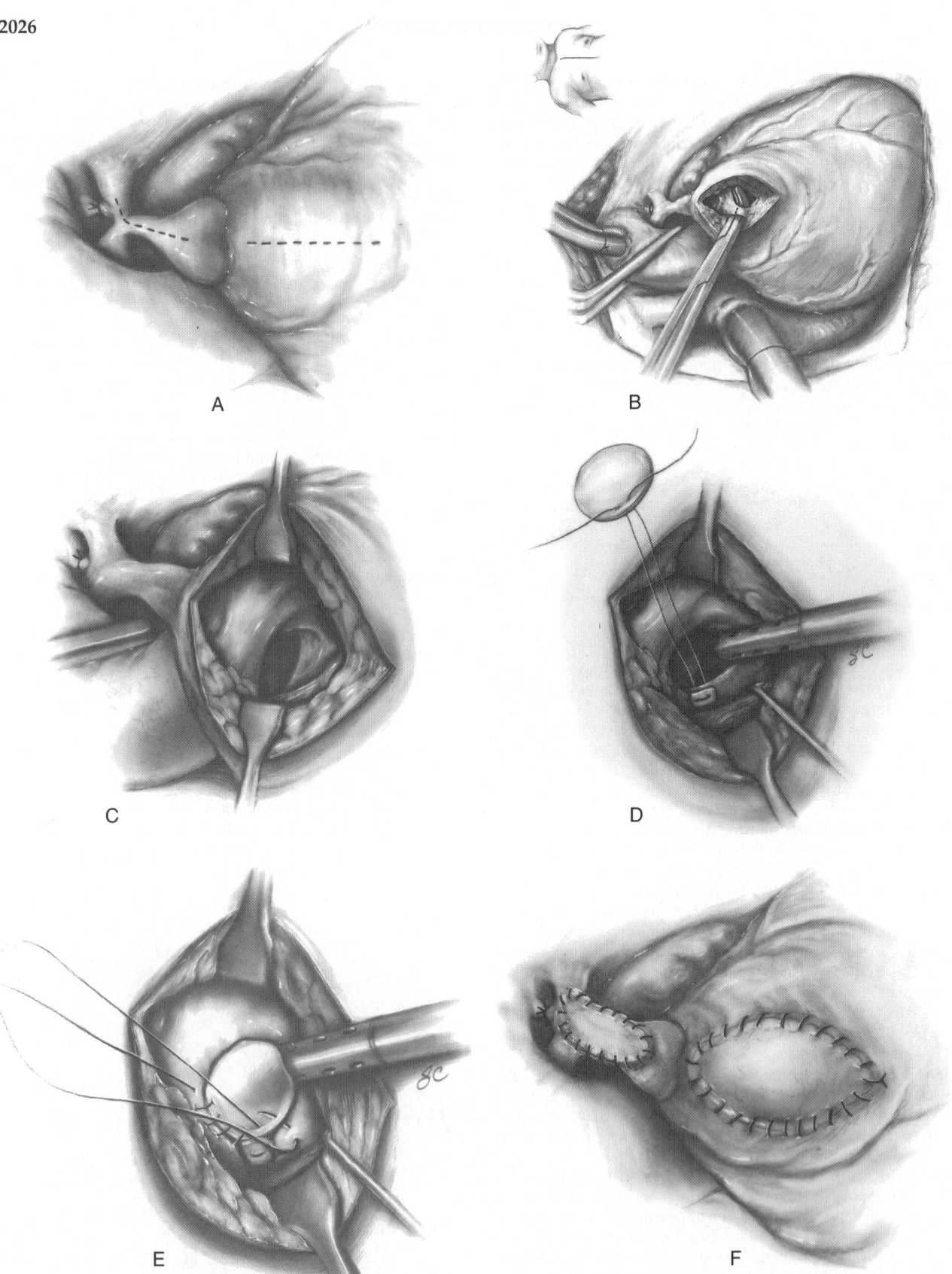

Figure 54–69. A variety of incisions can be used for repair of TOF. *A,* When a ventricular incision is planned, it is usually made just below the pulmonary valve in the infundibular portion of the heart. It should be longitudinal (or vertical) so that it can be extended to the main pulmonary artery if necessary. In patients with small main pulmonary arteries, a second incision can be made in the main pulmonary artery. This will provide exposure of the pulmonary valve for valvotomy. *B,* Once the ventricle is opened, a right-angle clamp can be passed around the parietal bands and these can be divided. This will open the RV outflow area. Division of the parietal bands will help provide exposure of the ventricular septal defect *(C),* which is then closed with a patch of prosthetic material *(D).* The suture line for this patch can be placed in a continuous fashion *(E)* or with an interrupted technique if desired (not shown). Care should be taken along the inferior border to keep the sutures away from the edge of the ventricular septal defect (as shown by the needle) and on the right ventricular surface of the defect to avoid injury to the conduction system. *F,* After closure of the ventricular septal defect and resection of the ventricular muscle, the incisions are patched with pericardium or prosthetic material. When the pulmonary valve annulus is small, the incision can be extended to the main pulmonary artery and the entire incision closed with one patch as shown in Figure 54–67*B.*

tum can be divided to expose the underlying defect. It is usually not necessary to resect very much, if any, muscle when performing repair through the RV outflow tract in infants.[21] It is also possible to perform this part of the procedure through a much more limited ventricular incision than has been described in earlier reports. The ventricular septal defect should be closed with a patch because it is usually large and unrestrictive. It can also be closed through a transatrial approach (Fig. 54–70) by exposing it through a right atriotomy and either by retracting the tricuspid valve leaflets[27] or by incising the tricuspid valve annulus to lift the tricuspid valve out of the way.[42] Personal preference of the surgeon determines whether the patch is placed with continuous or with interrupted sutures. The suture line can be inspected and buttressed where necessary with additional sutures. The best way to evaluate the ventricular septal defect

closure is with the use of intraoperative echocardiography at the end of the procedure after the patient has been removed from cardiopulmonary bypass.[41, 51, 53]

Proponents of the transatrial approach indicate that the entire repair (including relief of RV outflow obstruction) can often be performed through the right atrial incision, and this limits the extent of any incision—if one is needed at all—in the RV, thus preserving long-term RV function and limiting the chance for future ventricular dysrhythmias. Furthermore, the transatrial approach to the ventricular septal defect also gives the surgeon access to the atrial septum and the ability to close the frequently associated atrial septal defect at the same time as ventricular septal defect closure. In infants, most surgeons have found it advantageous to leave a small atrial septal defect (see section on postoperative management), thereby reducing the advantage of using a transatrial

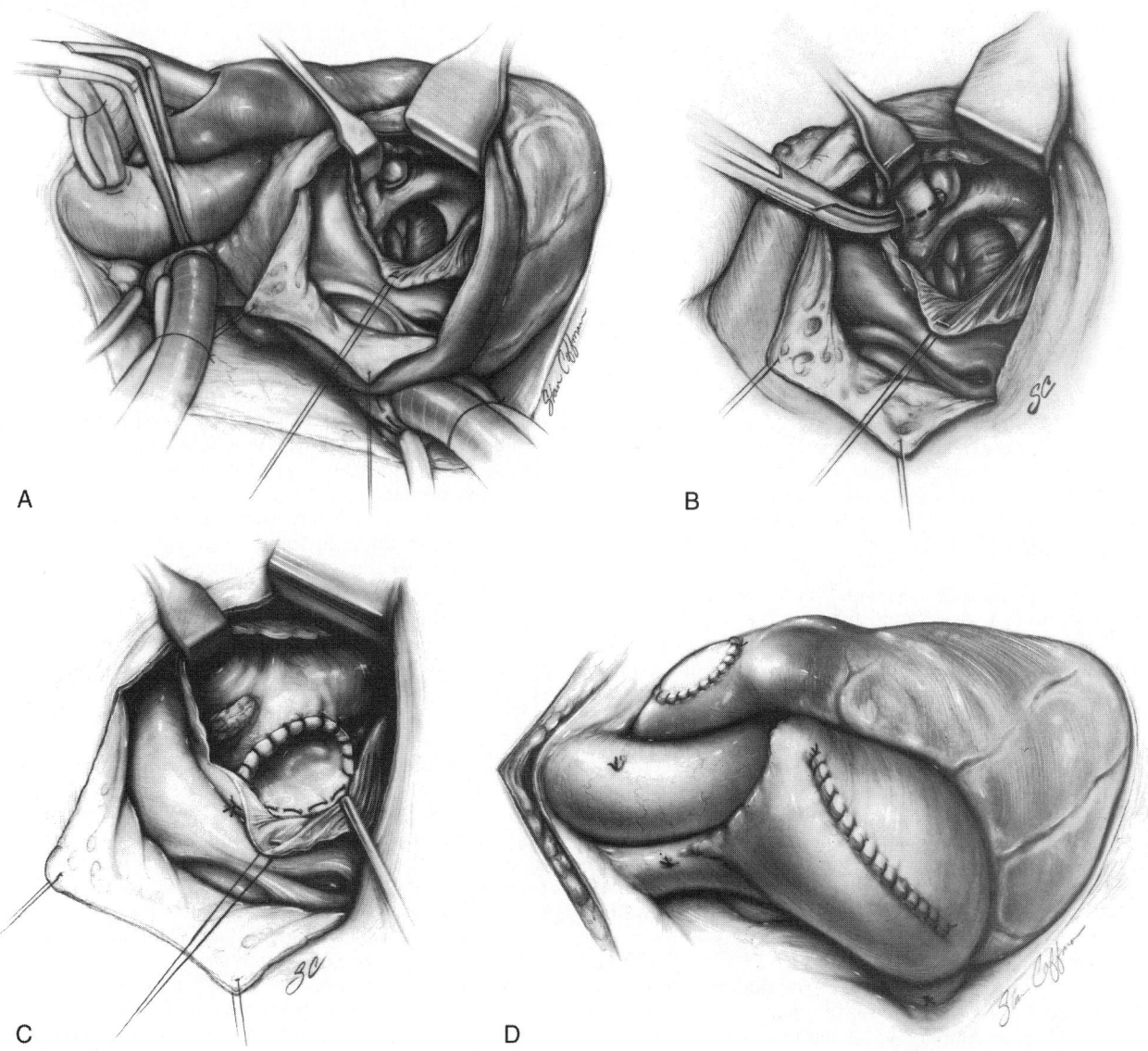

A

B

C

D

Figure 54–70. *A,* The anatomy in TOF can also be exposed through an incision in the right atrium. A dilator can be passed through the main pulmonary artery and pulmonary valve into the right ventricular outflow tract to help delineate the outflow tract in selected cases. The tricuspid valve leaflets should be gently retracted to expose the ventricular septal defect. *B,* The parietal extension of the infundibular septum can be divided by retracting the anterior leaflet of the tricuspid valve. It is important to resect the parietal extension as far superior as possible to avoid injury to the infundibular septum. *C,* Once the infundibular muscle is divided it should be possible to view the pulmonary valve through the RV outflow tract by inspecting through the tricuspid valve. Division of the parietal muscle will cause the infundibular septum to drop posteriorly and will allow the ventricular septal defect to be easily closed with a patch through the tricuspid valve. *D,* In selected cases, with a normal size pulmonary valve annulus it is possible to completely repair TOF without any incision on the RV surface. If a pulmonary arteriotomy was performed (either for exposure of the pulmonary valve or enlargement of the main pulmonary artery), it should be closed with a patch. It is possible to perform this operation successfully even in small infants.

incision in these patients. Those who prefer the ventricular incision claim that ventricular septal defect closure is possible through a very limited ventriculotomy and that the nature of the anatomy of TOF with hypoplasia of the infundibular septum usually also requires patch enlargement in the infundibulum immediately subjacent to the pulmonary valve. Closure of the defect can be safely and easily performed by either approach, and selection probably depends on preference of the surgeon and the unique anatomic features of each individual defect. Knowledge of the location of the conduction tissue is important, and sutures placed along the posteroinferior border of the defect should take this anatomy into account.

Relief of RV Outflow Obstruction. As mentioned earlier, RV outflow obstruction can occur at several levels. Hypoplasia of the infundibular septum almost invariably produces some element of subpulmonary stenosis that must be relieved. This is done by division of the parietal and septal bands (see Fig. 54–69) that bind the infundibular septum to the lateral and septal boundaries of the RV outflow tract. Because of the extremely restricted dimensions of the subpulmonic outflow area, it is often desirable to place a patch (pericardium or Gore-Tex) to "raise the roof" over the subvalvular area and to enlarge the outflow from the RV chamber. Initial attempts to perform complete repair were often described in older patients and included considerable resection of muscle from the RV outflow tract. Furthermore, these procedures were performed through fairly extensive incisions in the RV, and the combination of extensive muscle resection and long ventriculotomies has raised concern about the long-term outcome of patients undergoing transventricular repair.[36, 50] For this reason, a number of surgeons have begun favoring a transatrial approach to muscle resection in relief of the outflow obstruction in TOF repair.[25, 27, 40] This approach can be very successful as long as the intracardiac outflow chamber is enlarged. In some patients, a small ventricular incision is still necessary to allow patch enlargement of the hypoplastic infundibular outflow area. The appropriateness of a transatrial repair is probably determined most importantly by the anatomy of the particular lesion. In some patients, the RV outflow tract can be easily enlarged by transatrial division of the parietal band, whereas in others the subpulmonary infundibular area is so narrow that extension of a transannular incision onto the proximal right ventricle is a necessity to provide relief of the RV outflow stenosis. In actuality, the ventricular incision can be kept quite small even if used for ventricular septal defect closure and the advantages of transatrial versus transventricular repair may not appear to be as great if patients from the current era are compared with one another, as opposed to comparing current transatrial repairs to older transventricular repairs.[50]

Despite the methods and approach used to enlarge the subvalvular outflow area, the pulmonary valve and annulus should also be inspected and enlarged if necessary. Severe narrowing of the RV–pulmonary trunk junction seems to correlate with risk of mortality as well as with likelihood for elevated postrepair RV/LV ratios, despite generous patch enlargement.[26–28] Many patients with TOF have bicuspid valves, and an incision in the main pulmonary artery provides excellent exposure of the pulmonary valve to enable valvotomy. The pulmonary valve annulus should be sized; and if it is too small, the surgeon should not hesitate to perform a transannular incision with enlargement of the RV outflow tract onto the pulmonary artery (Fig. 54–71). Although transannular patches have not been previously considered to be an incremental risk factor for late surgical failure, more recent evidence suggests that the need to place a transannular patch identifies a higher risk anatomy that does tend to correlate with higher long-term mortality.[26–28]

This may be due to geometric limitations to pulmonary blood flow found in patients with small RV–pulmonary trunk junctions that cannot be corrected simply by performing an adequate transannular patch.[26, 28, 44] Thus, the risk imposed by placement of a transannular patch may be related to the risk of elevated postrepair RV/LV pressures (that can persist despite transannular patches in many of these patients) and not necessarily to the transannular patch itself. Nevertheless, there is also concern that transannular patches can increase long-term risk by leading to progressive RV dysfunction, and it is clear that the likelihood of requiring reoperation in the future (e.g., for important pulmonary insufficiency) is significantly greater in patients with transannular patches.[23, 26, 55] Current practice is that transannular patching should not be employed unless necessary to provide adequate RV outflow and, when performed, should be constructed in such a manner as to limit the degree of pulmonary insufficiency to preserve long-term RV dynamics. Furthermore, there is evidence to suggest that although initial postoperative recovery may be slowed by leaving a gradient between the RV and the pulmonary arteries,[12] long-term exercise performance of the patient may be improved by restrictive RV–pulmonary artery physiology.[19] When performing a transannular patch, many surgeons fashion a monocusp valve (out of pericardium) to limit pulmonary insufficiency in the short term. Pulmonary homografts have provided excellent long-term pulmonary valve function for many patients who are limited by significant pulmonary insufficiency.[1]

Relief of Pulmonary Artery Stenoses. The presence of important obstructions in the main pulmonary artery branches should also be recognized and dealt with at the time of complete repair. These stenoses may be from previous shunts,[55] they may be related to tissue from the ductus arteriosus,[14] or they may be part of the spectrum of the anatomy of the defect. Most often, extending the transannular patch past the pulmonary artery bifurcation and onto the left pulmonary artery is sufficient to relieve most significant obstruction (see Fig. 54–70). It is important that the distal aspect of the transannular patch be blunt and not tapered[27] to limit the likelihood of recurrent stenosis at the distal patch site. Obstruction in the main pulmonary arteries can sometimes be treated by local angioplasty at the time of surgical correction, but if the stenosis is more distal in the pulmonary artery (especially the left pulmonary artery that is difficult to expose at operation), excellent outcomes have been obtained with the placement of intravascular stents at the time of surgical correction.[35, 39]

Several groups prefer to perform the procedure under conditions of moderate hypothermia (25° C.) with cold potassium cardioplegic arrest, although the procedure can also be accomplished on the cold, non–cross-clamped, electrically fibrillating heart, or during a period of total circulatory arrest under profound hypothermic conditions (18° C.). The optimal method of myocardial protection remains controversial and probably depends on numerous factors related to the anatomy and physiology of each patient's lesion as well as to their age at repair and the conduct of the operation itself.[21, 27, 49] Once the ventricular septal defect has been closed and all levels of obstruction have been relieved the patient is rewarmed and removed from cardiopulmonary bypass. Even if conduction problems are not present, it is recommended that temporary atrial and ventricular pacing wires be left in place for the perioperative period. After the patient has been successfully weaned from cardiopulmonary bypass and cannulae have been removed, several methods are available to test for adequacy of the repair. These include selective atrial, ventricular, and pulmonary artery oxygen saturations or pressure measurements. Recent experience with intraoperative echocardiography with color-flow Doppler imaging,

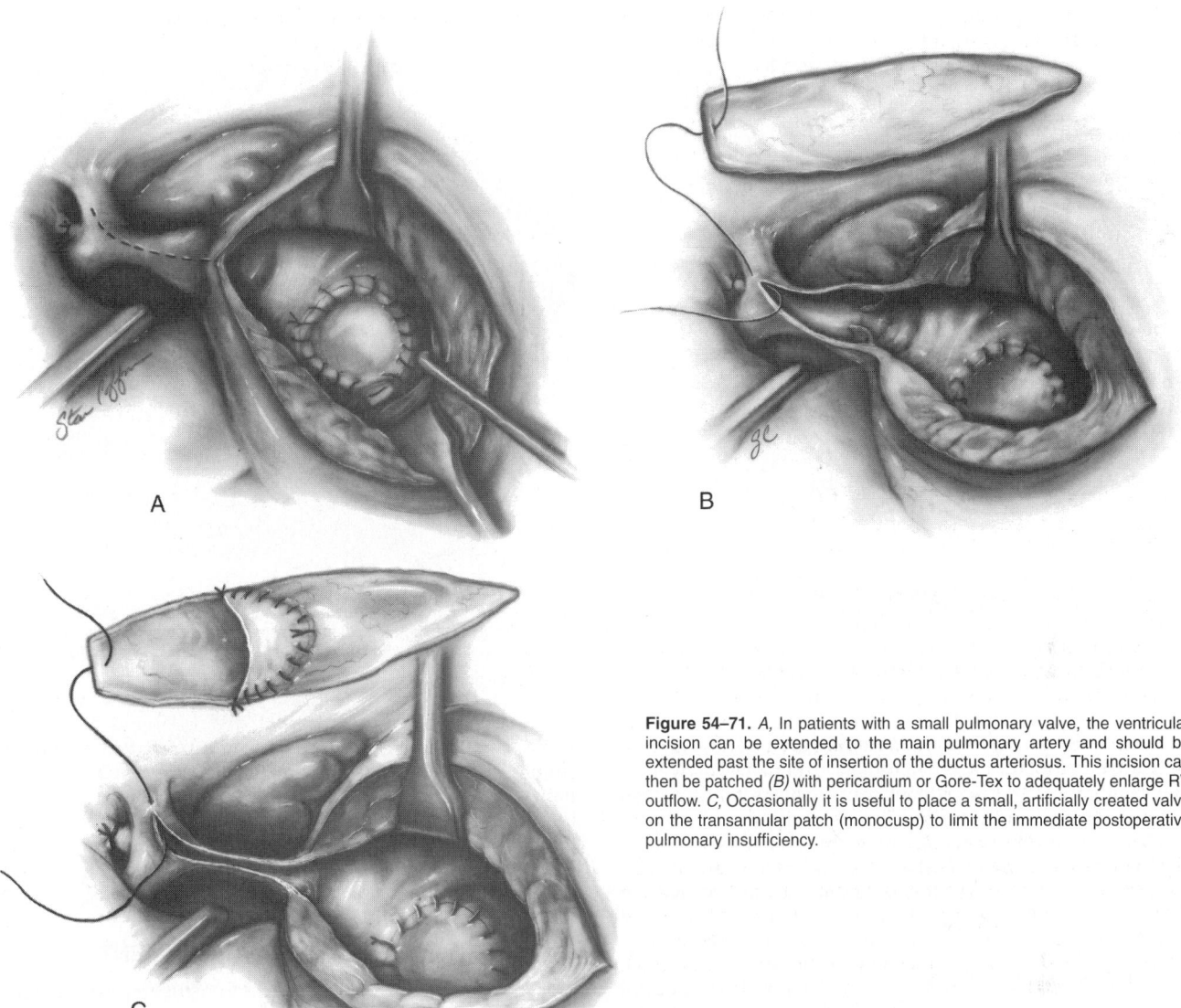

Figure 54–71. *A,* In patients with a small pulmonary valve, the ventricular incision can be extended to the main pulmonary artery and should be extended past the site of insertion of the ductus arteriosus. This incision can then be patched *(B)* with pericardium or Gore-Tex to adequately enlarge RV outflow. *C,* Occasionally it is useful to place a small, artificially created valve on the transannular patch (monocusp) to limit the immediate postoperative pulmonary insufficiency.

however, suggest that this technique may provide for a more sensitive and accurate ability to assess the quality of the intracardiac repair, especially in relation to long-term outcome.[37, 41, 52, 53] When the surgeon is satisfied with the effects of the repair, the chest is closed and the patient is returned to an intensive care setting.

Special Situations

Because of the variability of anatomy in patients with TOF, numerous special situations deserve comment. When the left anterior descending coronary artery crosses the RV outflow tract a standard transannular enlargement is not feasible because this would cause transection of that coronary artery. In these instances (depending on the location of the stenosis) it may be possible to perform a transverse incision in the infundibulum below the coronary artery for closure of the ventricular septal defect and resection of the infundibular stenosis (Fig. 54–72). If the pulmonary valve requires commissurotomy or the pulmonary artery requires additional enlarging, this can be performed through a separate incision

above the pulmonary annulus with patching of the pulmonary artery after valvotomy has been performed (see Fig. 54–69*F*). These two separate incisions are preferable to dissecting the coronary artery off the outflow tract with placement of the patch beneath the coronary artery. This is because RV distention can cause coronary ischemia by stretching of the overlying coronary artery. In some patients with a major coronary artery crossing the infundibular outflow tract, and who have otherwise favorable anatomy, the lesion can be repaired by the transatrial approach without the need for any incision in the RV. Another alternative in patients with coronary anomalies that prohibit transannular patching, but whose outflow tract is too hypoplastic to allow a transatrial resection, is to place a systemic-to-pulmonary artery shunt and allow the patient to grow until such a time that the patient can accept a large enough conduit between the RV and pulmonary artery that total correction by this method can be achieved. However, the availability of cryopreserved homografts, which provide excellent conduits for infants, has encouraged most groups to perform complete repair in infancy, even if a conduit is required (see Fig. 54–72).

Patients with pulmonary atresia and ventricular septal de-

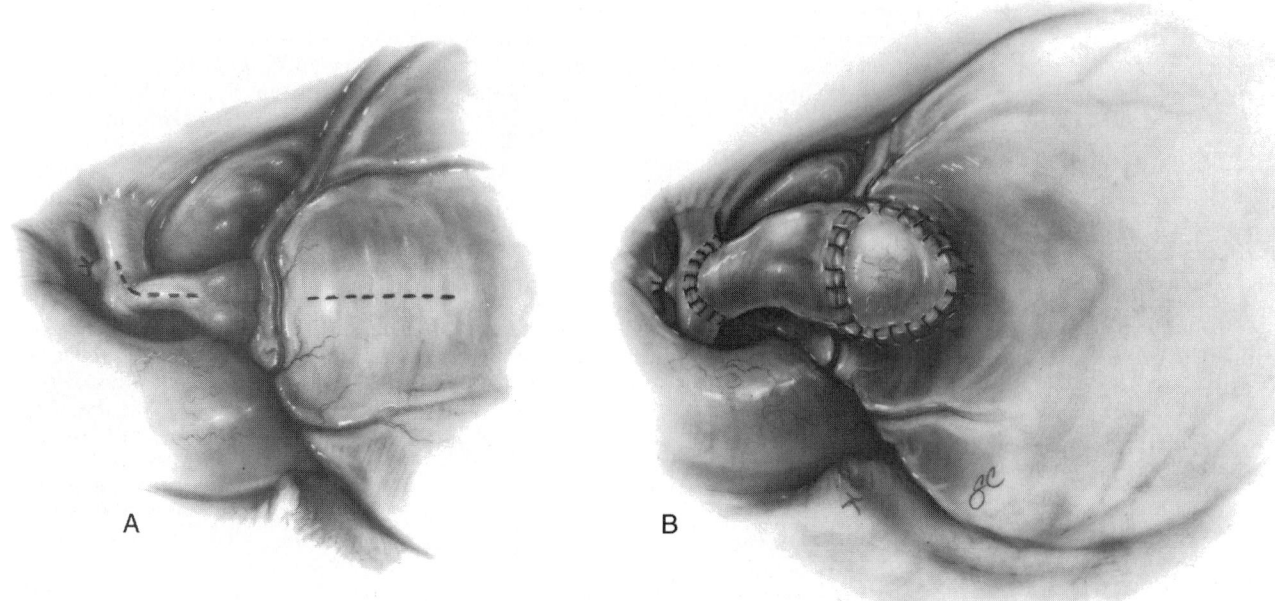

Figure 54–72. *A,* In patients with an anomalous coronary artery crossing the RV outflow tract, it is not possible to make a transannular incision. If the pulmonary valve annulus is adequate, these patients can be repaired with an incision in the ventricle and main pulmonary artery as shown. Alternatively, it is possible in many of these patients to use a transatrial approach instead of a ventricular incision for the subannular pathology. *B,* When the pulmonary valve annulus is hypoplastic in the presence of an anomalous left coronary artery, the area of obstruction can be bypassed by connecting the ventricular incision to the pulmonary artery incision with a homograft conduit after the ventricular septal defect has been closed.

fect who have otherwise normal pulmonary arteries can also be repaired in infancy. In the author's experience, as well as that of others,[9, 27, 28] these patients can receive total correction in infancy following initial stabilization with prostaglandins to enable accurate diagnosis. In many instances (personal experience), correction of *tet atresia* in infancy can be performed without the need for a conduit merely by creating RV-to-pulmonary artery continuity with an RV outflow patch. This is possible when there is a main pulmonary artery segment in proximity to the atretic RV outflow tract. If this procedure is not performed in infancy, it is doubtful that repair without a conduit would be possible at a later time. The author prefers to use a monocusp valve in the RV outflow patch in these patients. Although it is acceptable to perform initial palliation (in the form of an aortopulmonary shunt) for patients born with tet atresia, total repair in infancy can be safely performed with very low mortality and constitutes an excellent option that avoids the long-term problems associated with staged correction.

Infants who present with intractable tet spells that cannot be controlled despite aggressive intensive care unit attention (with sedation, intubation, and Neo-Synephrine) may represent a high-risk group of patients that warrant consideration for palliation. Some have suggested placing these patients on extracorporeal membrane oxygenation for 24 to 48 hours before operative correction.

Overall, it appears that the following technical considerations should be emphasized regarding repair of TOF. Patients should receive early correction, and there is no advantage and a possible disadvantage to strategies that employ initial palliation (or delay of repair past 12 months of age), except in specific circumstances (e.g., patients with intractable tet spells or patients with severely hypoplastic pulmonary arteries and multiple associated defects). Repair should be performed through limited ventricular incisions or through the right atrium. Minimal, if any, RV muscle should be resected, especially if the procedure is being performed through a limited ventriculotomy. Indiscriminate use of a transannular patch should be avoided and the pulmonary valve preserved

whenever possible. When a transannular patch is used, it should not be overly abundant (to limit the amount of pulmonary insufficiency) and a monocusp valve can be useful in some cases. The distal portion of the patch should extend onto the left pulmonary artery and should not be tapered. Repair quality should be assessed before leaving the operating room with intraoperative echocardiography.

POSTOPERATIVE MANAGEMENT

Many variables must be followed postoperatively. Pulmonary function is maintained by the use of an endotracheal tube and respirator until the patient's cardiac and respiratory status is stable, maintaining relatively normal values for the arterial PO_2, PCO_2, and pH. Maintenance of an adequate cardiac output is also of crucial importance. In small children, cardiac output may be difficult to measure, and it is essential that peripheral perfusion be followed as well as urine output and acid-base status. It is not uncommon for these patients to have elevated RV pressures postoperatively, and some inotropic support may be necessary. Patients with this disease have small RV volumes and can increase their cardiac output more effectively by increasing heart rate rather than stroke volume. Therefore, atrial pacing to improve heart rate or the use of dopamine or dobutamine may be useful. The patients should be maintained on a ventilator until they are hemodynamically stable and show good evidence of no longer requiring ventilatory support. Poor peripheral perfusion, indicative of low cardiac output, should be aggressively treated. Mechanical causes, such as cardiac tamponade, should be ruled out and, if necessary, echocardiography performed in the intensive care unit can immediately assess ventricular function and/or the presence of pericardial fluid. Central venous pressure should be adequate, and in these patients with poor RV compliance, central venous pressure may be maintained at slightly higher than normal values. Following acid-base status is an excellent way to monitor the clinical convalescence of patients after repair of TOF.[34] Patients who continue to produce lactic acid can be considered to have a cardiac output that is too low to meet tissue oxygen demands, and these patients require aggressive intervention to improve their clinical state. Occasionally, these patients may benefit from a short period of support with extracorporeal life support (e.g., extracorporeal membrane oxygenation).[29]

If echocardiography demonstrates a significant residual defect, this may need to be dealt with by the surgical team. If intraoperative echocardiography is performed before leaving the operating room, the presence of a residual defect that necessitates return to the operating room should occur in less than 2% of patients.[51] However, occasionally, a suture may tear, causing a residual ventricular septal defect, or RV outflow obstruction may become more apparent in the hours after repair, and the critical care team should not hesitate to recommend urgent cardiac catheterization and/or return to the operating room if appropriate for the patient whose convalescence is abnormal. In some patients, stenosis of distal pulmonary artery branches can be treated with placement of intravascular stents in the catheterization laboratory, obviating the necessity of returning to the operating room.[39] If a patient whose recovery is not normal has a documented high RV/LV ratio 24 hours after repair, and if a transannular patch was not part of the repair, it may be prudent to return the patient to the operating room for this procedure.[26, 27] In infants, it is advisable to leave the foramen ovale open and these infants may exhibit some degree of systemic arterial oxygen desaturation in the days immediately after repair. This provides them with physiology similar to that for a fenestrated Fontan procedure and enables them to maintain their cardiac output (by right-to-left shunting across the foramen) until the RV becomes more normal and the foramen closes. Although this may take several days after repair, it prevents a scenario in which the patient has high central venous pressure and low cardiac output because of poor RV compliance.

It is not uncommon for these patients to increase their need for inotropic support throughout the course of their first postoperative night. Daily weights of the patient should be obtained to help follow volume status. It is typical for these patients to show a tendency toward fluid retention, and diuretics may be useful. Because prosthetic materials are routinely used for palliation or correction of this lesion, perioperative broad-spectrum antibiotics should be commonplace. Arrhythmias, when they occur, can often be diagnosed by use of the temporary pacing wires to allow treatment directed specifically at each individual arrhythmia. Patients in heart block should be sequentially paced until conduction returns to normal through the atrioventricular node. If conduction has not returned in 7 to 10 days, it is likely that the patient will require placement of a permanent pacemaker. However, with properly performed surgical closure of the ventricular septal defect, the incidence of conduction disturbances requiring permanent pacing should approach 1%.[27, 28] The hemodynamic results after intracardiac repair of the TOF have been assessed in several series. Surgical repair of infants under deep hypothermia has been compared hemodynamically with correction by conventional cardiopulmonary bypass, with the finding that the results are equal or better with deep hypothermia.[38] In a companion study, LV dysfunction as determined after an afterload stress was found to be present postoperatively for those patients who had open correction at an older age but not in patients who underwent repair during infancy. This raises the possibility that early definitive repair may help to preserve postoperative left ventricular function.[7] Ventricular function in the immediate postoperative period is probably related to several factors, including the myocardial preservation, the surgical technique used, and the ability of the heart to adapt to sudden changes in loading conditions. Neurologic injury is uncommon after

correction of TOF, but seizures and major motor impairment can be seen in any patient who has had an operation with the left side of the circulation open (as in TOF). Although these findings may occur irrespective of whether deep hypothermic circulatory arrest was used during the repair, there is increasing evidence that prolonged periods of circulatory arrest may lead to some long-term neurodevelopmental dysfunction.[4]

OUTCOME

Tetralogy of Fallot is now being corrected with an ever-diminishing mortality. The outcomes with open correction during the recent past have been impressive. Nevertheless, it is important to realize that the spectrum of this disease with respect to the age at presentation as well as the severity of the anatomic derangements can greatly affect the outcome. Overall, the mortality rate in most series is less than 6% when the repair is done primarily or after a single systemic-to-pulmonary artery shunt.[9, 11, 21, 25, 27, 28, 41, 48, 49, 54] Improved techniques of myocardial protection with hypothermia, cold cardioplegia, and even total circulatory arrest are enabling more precise anatomic repairs in younger infants with excellent results.

Late outcome is reasonably good with 85% to 94% of patients living 16 to 28 years after repair.[23, 27, 57] Eighty per cent of the patients live a normal life without impairment of intellect, exercise tolerance, or fertility.[18] Data suggest that with good repair, long-term pulmonary and cardiac function can be excellent.[19, 24]

Data regarding long-term outcome after one-stage correction of TOF in early infancy are not yet available, but indications are that these patients are growing and developing extremely well.[11, 27] TOF is a lesion that has reflected the growth and development of the field of pediatric cardiac procedure. It is the lesion that stimulated creation of the first shunt for cyanotic heart disease, and it now provides a barometer for progress that has been made in neonatal cardiac surgery. The success that has been achieved in treating this lesion has been a testimony to the entire multidisciplinary field of subspecialists dedicated to the field of congenital heart disease.

SELECTED REFERENCES

Bellinger, D. C., Jonas, R. A., Rappaport, L. A., Wypij, D., Wernovsky, G., Kuban, K. C. K., Barnes, P. D., Holmes, G. L., Hickey, P. R., Strand, R. D., Walsh, A. Z., Helmers, S. L., Constantinou, J. E., Carrazana, E. J., Mayer, J. E., Hanley, F. L., Castañeda, A. R., Ware, J. H., and Newburger, J. W.: Developmental and neurologic status of children after heart surgery with hypothermic circulatory arrest or low-flow cardiopulmonary bypass. N. Engl. J. Med., 332:549, 1995.

Although this article examines patients with transposition of the great arteries (and not TOF), it addresses the outcome for patients who present with cyanosis and whose operation includes a period of deep hypothermic circulatory arrest—a very common strategy employed during the repair of TOF in infants. The association of some neurologic impairment with prolonged periods of circulatory arrest may lead to important alterations in the technique of repairing TOF and related defects in small infants.

Blalock, A., and Taussig, H. B.: The surgical treatment of malformations of the heart in which there is pulmonary stenosis or pulmonary atresia. JAMA, 128:189, 1945.

In this paper, Dr. Blalock's first three operations for creation of a systemic-pulmonary anastomosis are reported. The first patient, a 15-month-old infant with severe cyanosis, had a history of multiple episodes of loss of consciousness. An anastomosis of the left subclavian artery to the left pulmonary artery was made, and the clinical improvement was striking. Two additional patients with successful results are also described. It is of interest that Dr. Blalock refers to earlier experimental work in which subclavian pulmonary anastomoses were performed in the dog in an effort to produce pulmonary hypertension. Although these experiments did not succeed in producing an elevated pulmonary arterial pressure, the operation was subsequently used for an entirely different purpose. This procedure was the first of many additional cardiac surgical advances.

Groh, M. A., Meliones, J. N., Bove, E. L., Kirklin, J. W., Blackstone, E. H.,

Lupinetti, F. M., Snider, A. R., and Rosenthal, A.: Repair of tetralogy of Fallot in infancy: Effect of pulmonary artery size on outcome. Circulation, 84(Suppl. III):206, 1991.

In this review of 58 infants younger than 1 year old with tetralogy of Fallot and pulmonary stenosis or atresia and without important pulmonary artery collateral vessels, hospital mortality was 0% despite several patients with pulmonary artery McGoon ratios less than 1.0. The authors also remark that transanular patching was used in only 36% of patients; and in 50% of patients, muscle resection was avoided (whereas it was minimal in the remaining 29 patients). The authors conclude that repair of TOF should not be denied to infants solely on the basis of small pulmonary arteries.

Karl, T. R., Sano, S., Pornviliwan, S., and Mee, R. B. B.: Tetralogy of Fallot: Favorable outcome of nonneonatal transatrial, transpulmonary repair. Ann. Thorac. Surg., 54:903, 1992.

This excellent series of patients from Royal Children's Hospital in Melbourne, Australia, suggests that early aortopulmonary shunts can be performed with extremely low risk and allow patients to grow until they are large enough to undergo repair of TOF without ventriculotomy. The authors suggest that the long-term outcome from this protocol will be favorable.

Kirklin, J. K., Kirklin, J. W., Blackstone, E. H., Milano, A., and Pacifico, A. D.: Effect of transannular patching on outcome after repair of tetralogy of Fallot. Ann. Thorac. Surg., 48:783, 1989.

In this series of 814 patients undergoing repair of TOF with pulmonary stenosis between 1967 and 1986, transanular patching was a weak risk factor for death in the early postoperative period but not late postoperatively. Transanular patching was a risk factor for reoperation for pulmonary regurgitation late postoperatively. This very large and well-analyzed series provides an important perspective on the effects of transanular patching in repair of TOF.

Kirklin, J. W., and Barratt-Boyes, B. G.: Ventricular septal defect and pulmonary stenosis or atresia. In Cardiac Surgery, 2nd ed. New York, Churchill Livingstone, 1993.

This remarkable book catalogs the extraordinary experience of these two well-known experts in the field of congenital heart surgery. The material included in this chapter is among the most up-to-date, comprehensive, and well-organized presentations available and should be read by anyone who desires in-depth reading in this field.

Kirklin, J. W., Blackstone, E. H., Jonas, R. A., Shimazaki, Y., Kirklin, J. K., Mayer, J. E., Pacifico, A. D., and Castañeda, A. R.: Morphologic and surgical determinants of outcome events after repair of tetralogy of Fallot and pulmonary stenosis: A two institution study. J. Thorac. Cardiovasc. Surg., 103:706, 1992.

Outstanding comparison of two different protocols for the management of TOF (with pulmonary stenosis) in infants, comparing the strategy of early infant repair (100 patients from Boston Children's Hospital) to a strategy of initial palliation and delay of complete correction until the patient is older than 6 months (or more) (100 patients from the University of Alabama). The findings from this study demonstrated no advantage and a possible disadvantage to initial palliation as opposed to early repair.

Lillehei, C. W., Varco, R. L., Cohen, M., Warden, H. E., Patton, C., and Moller J. H.: The first open heart repairs of ventricular septal defect, atrioventricular communis and tetralogy of Fallot using extracorporeal circulation by cross-circulation: A thirty-year follow-up. Ann. Thorac. Surg., 41:4, 1986.

More than just a 30-year follow-up of the first patients to successfully receive open cardiac correction of complex cardiac lesions, this article provides a poignant recapitulation of the early days of open-heart surgery. Dr. Lillehei's historical account of the frustrations and ingenious attempts by the intrepid individuals who began the era of open-heart surgery that is now so commonplace should be read by anyone who has read this chapter. Of equal impact are the thoughts offered by the discussants, who include some of the more prominent figures in the field of cardiac surgery. Having read this paper, one will have a better understanding of the historical debt that is owed to those individuals with the insight and creativity to tackle the problems of open cardiac surgery.

Vobecky, S. J., Williams, W. G., Trusler, G. A., Coles, J. G., Rebeyka, I. M., Smallhorn, J., Burrows, P., Gow, R., and Freedom, R. M.: Survival analysis of infants under age 18 months presenting with tetralogy of Fallot. Ann. Thorac. Surg., 56:944, 1993.

Results for 270 patients with TOF are presented over a 10-year period at the Hospital for Sick Children in Toronto. Patients were treated by a protocol of palliation (with aortopulmonary shunts) if they were younger than 18 months old and with total correction if they were 18 months or older. Survival was tracked from the time of diagnosis, and the authors provide outstanding outcome data for patients born with TOF who are treated by a protocol of early palliation. Although they found that the surgical mortality for those patients who eventually came to surgery was only 3.2%, there were 15 patients who died before surgical correction, either as a result of palliation or as an outcome following palliation. Along with an excellent "companion" invited commentary from Aldo Castañeda (Boston Children's Hospital), this study demonstrates the risks of palliation versus early total correction. The authors also found that palliation, in the form of aortopulmonary shunts, was particularly hazardous for those infants with small (<2 mm.) pulmonary arteries—the very patients who might most require a palliative procedure to increase pulmonary blood flow.

REFERENCES

1. Albert, J. D., Bishop, D. A., Fullerton, D. A., Campbell, D. N., and Clarke, D. R.: Conduit reconstruction of the right ventricular outflow tract: Lessons learned in a twelve-year experience. J. Thorac. Cardiovasc. Surg., 106:228, 1993.

2. Arciniegas, E., Blackstone, E. H., Pacifico, A. D., and Kirklin, J. W.: Classic shunting operations as part of two-stage repair for tetralogy of Fallot. Ann. Thorac. Surg., 27:514, 1979.

3. Barratt-Boyes, B. G., and Neutze, J. M.: Primary repair of tetralogy of Fallot in infancy using profound hypothermia with circulatory arrest and limited cardiopulmonary bypass: A comparison with conventional two-stage management. Ann. Surg., 178:406, 1973.

4. Bellinger, D. C., Jonas, R. A., Rappaport, L. A., Wypij, D., Wernovsky, G., Kuban, K. C. K., Barnes, P. D., Holmes, G. L., Hickey, P. R., Strand, R. D., Walsh, A. Z., and Helmers, S. L.: Developmental and neurologic status of children after heart surgery with hypothermic circulatory arrest or low-flow cardiopulmonary bypass. N. Engl. J. Med., 332:549, 1995.

5. Blackstone, E. H., Kirklin, J. W., Bertranou, E. G., Labrosse, C. J., Soto, B., and Bargeron, L. M., Jr.: Preoperative prediction from cineangiograms of postrepair right ventricular pressure in tetralogy of Fallot. J. Thorac. Cardiovasc. Surg., 78:542, 1979.

6. Blalock, A., and Taussig, H. B.: The surgical treatment of malformations of the heart in which there is pulmonary stenosis or pulmonary atresia. JAMA, 128:189, 1945.

7. Borow, K. M., Green, L. H., Castañeda, A. R., and Keane, J. F.: Left ventricular function after repair of tetralogy of Fallot and its relationship to age at surgery. Circulation, 61:1150, 1980.

8. Boucek, M. M., Webster, H. E., Orsmond, G. S., and Ruttenberg, H. D.: Balloon pulmonary valvotomy: Palliation for cyanotic heart disease. Am. Heart J., 115:318, 1988.

9. Castañeda, A. R.: Invited commentary to article by Vobecky, et al. Ann. Thorac. Surg., 56:949, 1993.

10. Castañeda, A. R., and Mayer, J.: Tetralogy of Fallot. In Stark, J., and de Leval, M. [Eds.]: Surgery for Congenital Heart Defects, 2nd ed. Philadelphia, W. B. Saunders, 1994, pp. 405–416.

11. Castañeda, A. R., Mayer, J. E. J., Jonas, R. A., and Hanley, F.: Cardiac Surgery of the Neonate and Infant. Philadelphia, W. B. Saunders, 1994.

12. Cullen, S., Shore, D., and Redington, A.: Characterization of right ventricular diastolic performance after complete repair of tetralogy of Fallot: Restrictive physiology predicts slow postoperative recovery. Circulation, 91:1782, 1995.

13. Donahoo, J. S., Roland, J. M., Kan, J, Gardner, T. J., and Kidd, B. S.: Prostaglandin E₁ as an adjunct to emergency cardiac operations in neonates. J. Thorac. Cardiovasc. Surg., 81:227, 1981.

14. Elzenga, N. J., von Suylen, R. J., Frohn-Mulder, I., et al.: Juxtaductal pulmonary artery coarctation: An underestimated cause of branch pulmonary artery stenosis in patients with pulmonary atresia or stenosis and a ventricular septal defect. J. Thorac. Cardiovasc. Surg., 100:416, 1990.

15. Fallot, E. L. A.: Contribution á fanatomic pathologique de la maladie bleue (cyanose cardiaque). Marseille Med., 25:77, 138, 207, 270, 341, 403, 1888.

16. Fort, L., III, Morrow, A. G., Pierce, G. E., Saigusa, M., and McLaughlin, J. S.: The distribution of pulmonary blood flow after subclavian-pulmonary anastomosis: An experimental study. J. Thorac. Cardiovasc. Surg., 50:671, 1965.

17. Freed, M. D., Heymann, M. A., and Lewis, A. B.: Prostaglandin E₁ in infants with ductus arteriosus–dependent congenital heart disease. Circulation, 64:899, 1981.

18. Garson, A., Nihill, M. R., McNamara, D. G., and Cooley, D. A.: Status of the adult and adolescent after repair of tetralogy of Fallot. Circulation, 59:1232, 1979.

19. Gatzoulis, M. A., Clark, A. L., Cullen, S., Newman, C. G. H., and Redington, A. N.: Right ventricular diastolic function 15 to 35 years after repair of tetralogy of Fallot: Restrictive physiology predicts superior exercise performance. Circulation, 91:1775, 1995.

20. Greeley, W. J., Stanley, T. E., Ungerleider, R. M., and Kisslo, J. A.: Intraoperative hypoxemic spells in tetralogy of Fallot: An echocardiographic analysis of diagnosis and treatment. Anesth. Analg., 68:815, 1989.

21. Groh, M. A., Meliones, J. N., Bove, E. L., Kirklin, J. W., Blackstone, E. H., Lupinetti, F. M., Snider, A. R., and Rosenthal, A.: Repair of tetralogy of Fallot in infancy: Effect of pulmonary artery size on outcome. Circulation, 84(Suppl. III):206, 1991.

22. Harris, A. M., Segel, N., Biship, J. M.: Blalock-Taussig anastomosis for tetralogy of Fallot: A ten- to fifteen-year follow-up. Br. Heart J., 26:266, 1964.

23. Horneffer, P. J., Zahka, K. G., Rowe, S. A., Manolio, T. A., Gott, V. L., Reitz, B. A., Gardner, T. J.: Long-term results of total repair of tetralogy of Fallot in childhood. Ann. Thorac. Surg., 50:179, 1990.

24. Jonsson, H., Ivert, T., Jonasson, R., Wahlgren, H., Holmgren, A., Bjork, V. O.: Pulmonary function thirteen to twenty-six years after repair of tetralogy of Fallot. J. Thorac. Cardiovasc. Surg., 108:1002, 1994.

25. Karl, T. R., Sano, S., Pornviliwan, S., Mee, R. B. B.: Tetralogy of Fallot: Favorable outcome of nonneonatal transatrial, transpulmonary repair. Ann. Thorac. Surg., 54:903, 1992.

26. Kirklin, J. K., Kirklin, J. W., Blackstone, E. H., Milano, A., and Pacifico, A. D.: Effect of transannular patching on outcome after repair of tetralogy of Fallot. Ann. Thorac. Surg., 48:783, 1989.

27. Kirklin, J. W., Barratt-Boyes, B. G.: Cardiac Surgery, 2nd ed. New York, Churchill Livingstone, 1993, p. 1779.

28. Kirklin, J. W., Blackstone, E. H., Jonas, R. A., Shimazaki, Y., Kirklin, J. K., Mayer, J. E., Pacifico, A. D., and Castañeda, A. R.: Morphologic and surgical determinants of outcome events after repair of tetralogy of Fallot and pulmonary stenosis: A two institution study. J. Thorac. Cardiovasc. Surg., 103:706, 1992.

29. Klein, M. D., Shaheen, K. W., Whittlesey, G. C., Pinsky, W. W., and Arciniegas, E.: Extracorporeal membrane oxygenation for the circulatory support of children after repair of congenital heart disease. J. Thorac. Cardiovasc. Surg., 100:498, 1990.

30. Kvelselis, D. A., Rocchini, A. P., Snider, A. R., and Rosenthal, A.: Results of balloon valvuloplasty in the treatment of congenital valvar pulmonary stenosis in children. Am. J. Cardiol., 56:527, 1985.

31. Lodge, F. A., Lamberti, J. J., Goodman, A. H., Kirkpatrick, S. E., George, L., Mathewson, J. W., and Waldman, J. D.: Vascular consequences of subclavian artery transection for the treatment of congenital heart disease. J. Thorac. Cardiovasc. Surg., 86:18, 1983.

32. Marino, B., Corno, A., and Pasquini, L.: Indication for systemic-pulmonary artery shunts guided by two-dimensional and Doppler echocardiography: Criteria for patient selection. Ann. Thorac. Surg., 44:495, 1987.

33. Mavroudis, C., and Backer, C.: Pediatric Cardiac Surgery, 2nd ed. St. Louis, C. V. Mosby, 1994.

34. Meliones, J. N., Ungerleider, R. M., Kern, F. H., Greeley, W. J., Schulman, S. R., and Stockwell, J.: Perioperative management of patients with congenital heart disease: An approach based on physiology. In Moylan, J. (Ed.): Surgical Critical Care. Philadelphia, J. B. Lippincott, 1994.

35. Mendelsohn, A. M., Bove, E. L., Lupinetti, F. M., Crowley, D. C., Lloyd, T. R., Fedderly, R. T., and Beekman, R. H., III: Intraoperative and percutaneous stenting of congenital pulmonary artery and vein stenosis. Circulation, 88:II-210, 1993.

36. Miura, T., Nakano, S., Shimazaki, Y., Kobayashi, J., Hirose, H., Sano, T., Matsuda, H., and Kawashima, Y.: Evaluation of right ventricular function by regional wall motion analysis in patients after correction of tetralogy of Fallot: Comparison of transventricular and nontransventricular repairs. J. Thorac. Cardiovasc. Surg., 104:917, 1992.

37. Muhiudeen, I. A., Roberson, D. A., Silverman, N. H., Haas, G., Turley, K., and Cahalan, M. K.: Intraoperative echocardiography in infants and children with congenital cardiac shunt lesions: Transesophageal versus epicardial echocardiography. J. Am. Coll. Cardiol., 16:1687, 1990.

38. Murphy, J. D., Freed, M. D., Keane, J. F.: Hemodynamic results after intracardiac repair of tetralogy of Fallot by deep hypothermia and cardiopulmonary bypass. Circulation, 62(Suppl. I):168, 1980.

39. O'Laughlin, M. P., Slack, M. C., Grifka, R. G., Perry, S. B., Lock, J. E., and Mullins, C. E.: Implantation and intermediate-term follow-up of stents in congenital heart disease. Circulation, 88:605, 1993.

40. Pacifico, A. D., Sand, M. E., Bargeron, L. M., Jr., and Colvin, E. C.: Transatrial-transpulmonary repair of tetralogy of Fallot. J. Thorac. Cardiovasc. Surg., 93:919, 1987.

41. Papagiannis, J., Kanter, R. J., Armstrong, B. E., Greeley, W. J., and Ungerleider, R. M.: Intraoperative epicardial echocardiography during repair of tetralogy of Fallot. J. Am. Soc. Echocardiog., 6:366, 1993.

42. Pridjian, A. K., Pearce, F. B., Culpepper, W. S., Williams, L. C., Van Meter,

C. H., and Ochsner, J. L.: Atrioventricular valve competence after takedown to improve exposure during ventricular septal defect repair. J. Thorac. Cardiovasc. Surg., 106:1122, 1993.

43. Rosenberg, H. G., Williams, W. G., and Trusler, G. A.: Structural composition of central pulmonary arteries: Growth potential after surgical shunts. J. Thorac. Cardiovasc. Surg., 94:498, 1987.

44. Shimazake, Y., Blackstone, E. H., Kirklin, J. W., Jonas, R. A., Mandell, B., and Colvin, E. V.: The dimensions of the right ventricular outflow tract and pulmonary arteries in tetralogy of Fallot and pulmonary stenosis. J. Thorac. Cardiovasc. Surg., 103:692, 1992.

45. Silverman, N. H.: Pediatric Echocardiography. Baltimore, Williams & Wilkins, 1993.

46. Sreeram, N., Saleem, M., Jackson, M., Peart, I., McKay, R., Arnold, R., and Walsh, K.: Results of balloon pulmonary valvuloplasty as a palliative procedure in tetralogy of Fallot. J. Am. Coll. Cardiol., 18:159, 1990.

47. Stark, J., and de Leval, M.: Surgery for Congenital Heart Defects. Philadelphia, W. B. Saunders, 1994.

48. Starnes, V. A., Luciani, G. B., Latter, D. A., and Griffin, M. L.: Current surgical management of tetralogy of Fallot. Ann. Thorac. Surg., 58:211, 1994.

49. Touati, G. D., Vouhe, P. R., Amodeo, A., Pouard, P., Mauriat, P., Leca, F., Neveux, J. Y., and Castañeda, A. R.: Primary repair of tetralogy of Fallot in infancy. J. Thorac. Cardiovasc. Surg., 99:396, 1990.

50. Ungerleider, R. M.: Right ventricular function after transatrial versus transventricular repair of tetralogy of Fallot (Invited Letter). J. Thorac. Cardiovasc. Surg., 104:1173, 1992.

51. Ungerleider, R. M., Greeley, W. J., Kanter, R. J., and Kisslo, J. A.: The learning curve for intraoperative echocardiography during congenital heart surgery. Ann. Thorac. Surg., 54:691, 1992.

52. Ungerleider, R. M., Greeley, W. J., Sheikh, K. H., Kern, F. H., Kisslo, J. A., and Sabiston, D. C., Jr.: The use of intraoperative echo with Doppler color flow imaging to predict outcome after repair of congenital cardiac defects. Ann. Surg., 201:526, 1989.

53. Ungerleider, R. M., Greeley, W. J., Sheikh, K. H., Philips, J., Pearce, F. B., Kern, F. H., and Kisslo, J. A.: Routine use of intraoperative epicardial echo and Doppler color flow imaging to guide and evaluate repair of congenital heart lesions: A prospective study. J. Thorac. Cardiovasc. Surg., 100:297, 1990.

54. Uva, M. S., Lacour-Gayet, F., Komiya, T., Serraf, A., Bruniaux, J., Touchot, A., Roux, D., Petit, J., and Planche, C.: Surgery for tetralogy of Fallot at less than six months of age. J. Thorac. Cardiovasc. Surg., 107:1291, 1994.

55. Vobecky, S. J., Williams, W. G., Trusler, G. A., Coles, J. G., Rebeyka, I. M., Smallhorn, J., Burrows, P., Gow, R., and Freedom, R. M.: Survival analysis of infants under age 18 months presenting with tetralogy of Fallot. Ann. Thorac. Surg., 56:944, 1993.

56. Zahka, K. G., Manolio, T. A., Rykiel, M. J. F., Abel, D. L., Neill, C. A., and Kidd, L.: Handgrip strength after the Blalock-Taussig shunt: 14- to 34-year follow-up. Clin. Cardiol., 11:627, 1988.

57. Zhao, H. X., Miller, D. C., Reitz, B. A., and Shumway, N. E.: Surgical repair of tetralogy of Fallot: Long-term follow-up with particular emphasis on late death and reoperation. J. Thorac. Cardiovasc. Surg., 89:204, 1985.

VIII ———————————————————————

DOUBLE OUTLET RIGHT VENTRICLE

Albert D. Pacifico, M.D., and Henry L. Walters III, M.D.

Double outlet right ventricle (DORV) is a congenital cardiac anomaly in which both the aorta and the pulmonary arteries arise wholly or in large part from the right ventricle.[15] A ventricular septal defect (VSD) represents the only outlet from the morphologic left ventricle. In DORV, the connections of the atria to the ventricles are usually normal. These connections of the right atrium to the right ventricle and the left atrium to the left ventricle are called atrioventricular (AV) concordance. In rare cases the AV connections are discordant: the right atrium connects to the left ventricle, and the left atrium connects to the right ventricle. DORV is also rarely associated with connection of the atria to a single ventricle (univentricular atrioventricular connection)[11] or absence (atresia) of one of the atrioventricular valves.

HISTORICAL ASPECTS

Peacock and Rokitansky first documented cases of DORV in the mid-nineteenth century. Braun[2] was the first to use the term *double outlet ventricle* in 1952. The first correct intraoperative recognition and surgical repair of DORV was undertaken by Kirklin at the Mayo Clinic in May 1957. Unfortunately this 18-month-old male infant died 2 hours postoperatively.

HEARTS WITH AV CONCORDANCE
Definition and Morphology

The precise morphologic definition of DORV is controversial. The authors consider DORV to be present when more than 50% of the aorta and pulmonary artery arise from the morphologic right ventricle.[15] An exception to this rule is found in defects that also have severe obstruction of the right ventricular outflow tract, which are categorized as tetralogy of Fallot until more than 90% of the aorta arises from the right ventricular cavity. When more than 90% of the aorta arises from the right ventricular cavity, these lesions are called DORV with pulmonary stenosis.[10, 30] The subset of DORV hearts with the VSD located beneath the pulmonary valve (subpulmonary VSD) is classified as the Taussig-Bing malformation of DORV when less than 90% of the pulmonary trunk arises from the left ventricle. When greater than 90% of the pulmonary trunk arises from the left ventricle, these heart lesions are classified as transposition of the great arteries with VSD.[10, 30]

Controversies. This definition of DORV is based solely on the origin of the great arteries. In normal hearts there is a fibrous connection between the aortic valve and the anterior leaflet of the mitral valve (aortic-mitral continuity). Often, in hearts with DORV, there is muscle interposed between these two valves that separates them from direct contact with each other (aortic-mitral discontinuity). This muscle interposed between a semilunar (aortic or pulmonary) and an AV (mitral or tricuspid) valve is called a conus. The presence of this conus between the aortic and mitral valves producing aortic-mitral discontinuity is sometimes used in the basic definition of DORV. Because not all hearts with DORV possess this feature, this anatomic variant should not be an essential part of the definition. In point of fact, hearts with DORV may have a muscular conus located beneath both the aorta and the pulmonary artery (bilateral conus), a single conus beneath one of these structures, or no conus at all.

AV Connections. Approximately 86% of patients with DORV have concordant AV connections; AV discordance is present in 11%.

VSD. The VSD, which represents the only outflow tract for the left ventricle, is usually unrestrictive to flow. In 10% of cases the VSD is restrictive.[3, 20] In 13% of cases of DORV the VSDs are multiple.[11]

Relationships. Because the hemodynamics, clinical course, and specific type of operation employed depend on the relationship of the VSD to either great artery and the relationship of these great vessels to each other, knowledge of the precise location of all of these structures is important. It is surgically useful to describe the commitment of the VSD to either or both great arteries as suggested by Lev and colleagues.[15] In hearts in which the aorta is to the right and either side by side with or posterior to the pulmonary artery (i.e., great arteries more or less in their normal relationship to each other), the VSD may be subaortic, doubly committed, or noncommitted (Fig. 54–73).

Subaortic VSD. The subaortic VSD lies immediately beneath the aortic annulus or its subaortic muscular conus. It is usually perimembranous and extends to the commissure between the septal and anterior tricuspid valve leaflets. The subaortic VSD is the most common type and occurs in approximately 50% of surgical patients with DORV.[10, 21] These perimembranous VSDs can extend inferiorly from the perimembranous region to lie partly beneath the septal leaflet of the tricuspid valve (inlet extension).[37]

Doubly Committed VSD. The doubly committed VSD lies immediately beneath both the aorta and the pulmonary artery, which, in these hearts, are often in a side-by-side and contiguous relationship. This VSD occurs in approximately 10% of surgical series of DORV.[10, 21]

Noncommitted VSD. The noncommitted VSD has no extension into the perimembranous or outlet septum and thus is far removed from the great vessels.[12, 18] This defect occurs in 10% to 20% of patients in surgical series.[10, 21] It may be located

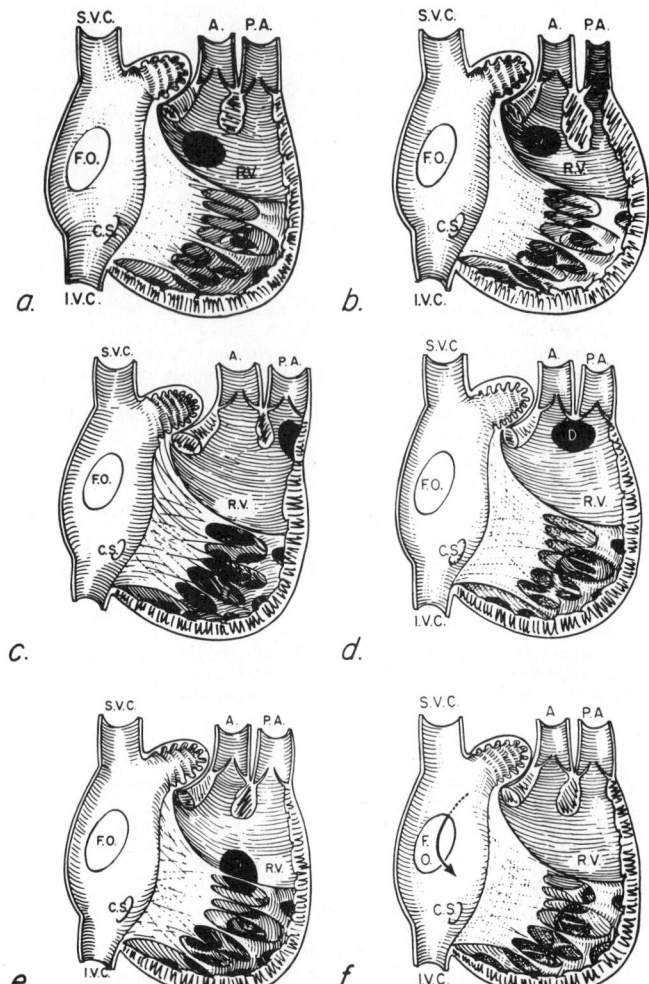

Figure 54–73. The relationship of the VSD to the great arteries in DORV. *a,* Subaortic VSD without pulmonary stenosis. *b,* Subaortic VSD with pulmonary stenosis. *c,* Subpulmonary VSD (Taussig-Bing malformation). *d,* Doubly committed VSD. *e,* Noncommitted (remote) VSD. *f,* Intact interventricular septum. A, aorta; CS, coronary sinus; D, ventricular septal defect; FO, foramen ovale; IVC, inferior vena cava; PA, pulmonary artery; RV, right ventricle; SVC, superior vena cava. (Adapted from Zamora, R., Moller, J. H., and Edwards, J. E.: Double-outlet right ventricle. Chest, *68:*672, 1975.)

in the inlet portion of the ventricular septum beneath the septal leaflet of the tricuspid valve or in the apical-trabecular portions of the muscular septum. When DORV is associated with a complete AV canal defect, the VSD usually includes the perimembranous septum and is subaortic, although less commonly it is unrelated to either great artery and is noncommitted.

Taussig-Bing Malformation. The Taussig-Bing malformation consists of hearts with DORV in which the VSD is subpulmonary. This anomaly occurs in approximately 30% of patients in surgical series of DORV.[10, 21] The VSD is either directly adjacent to the pulmonary valve or is separated from it by a subpulmonary conus. The aorta is usually to the right and is slightly anterior to or side by side with the pulmonary artery. These two great arteries are usually parallel to each other in that they do not spiral around each other as in the normal heart.

L-Malposition. DORV can exist in hearts with the aorta to the left (l-malposition) and anterior to the pulmonary artery. In this rare malformation the VSD is usually subaortic.[16] This type of DORV with l-malposition of the aorta has also been described with a subpulmonary, noncommitted, and doubly committed VSD.

AV Canal-Type Defects. Although most hearts with AV concordance and DORV have separate and distinct AV valves, this malformation may also exist in the presence of a common valve between the atria and the ventricles (AV canal-type defect).

Conduction Tissue. The AV node in DORV with AV concordant connections is located in the normal position. The bundle of His lies along the posteroinferior margin of the VSD in lesions that are perimembranous, whether the defect is subaortic, doubly committed, or subpulmonary. When muscle is interposed between the defect and the tricuspid valve, this muscle protects the bundle, which no longer runs along the posteroinferior free margin of the defect. This knowledge usually permits the placement of sutures away from the conduction tissue to avoid the creation of surgical heart block during surgical repair.

Associated Lesions. DORV exists with or without valvular and/or subvalvular pulmonary stenosis; this is an important determinant of both clinical course and choice of operation (see Fig. 54–73). Other important associated anomalies include mitral stenosis and atresia, coarctation and aortic arch interruption, and valvular or subvalvular aortic stenosis. The various forms of left ventricular outflow tract obstruction are most commonly associated with the Taussig-Bing malformation.[6] DORV has also been associated with straddling mitral or tricuspid valves.[24]

Pathophysiology

Subaortic, Doubly Committed, and Noncommitted VSDs Without Pulmonary Stenosis. The clinical course of patients with DORV depends primarily on the relationship of the VSD to the great arteries and the presence and severity, or absence, of pulmonary stenosis. Patients with large subaortic, doubly committed, or noncommitted VSDs without pulmonary stenosis present with congestive heart failure due to excessive pulmonary blood flow. They remain acyanotic because of streaming of oxygenated left ventricular blood into the aorta, and their presentation is indistinguishable from patients with an isolated and large VSD. Severe pulmonary vascular disease may develop within the first 2 years of life due to the large left-to-right shunt.

Subpulmonary VSD Without Pulmonary Stenosis. In contrast, patients with a subpulmonary VSD and no pulmonary stenosis have a course more similar to that of patients with transposition of the great arteries with VSD. Cyanosis is present, usually from birth, because streaming directs the desaturated systemic venous return toward the aorta and the oxygenated left ventricular blood into the pulmonary artery. These patients tend to develop early congestive heart failure or severe pulmonary vascular disease and are usually symptomatic within the first few months of life.

Effects of Pulmonary Stenosis. Pulmonary stenosis is usually present in hearts with subaortic VSDs and usually absent in those with subpulmonary defects.[15] Although pulmonary stenosis protects the lungs from pulmonary vascular disease, these patients exhibit varying degrees of cyanosis due to restricted pulmonary blood flow and their clinical course often resembles that of patients with tetralogy of Fallot.

Diagnosis

Cardiac Catheterization and Angiocardiography. High-quality angiocardiograms, using axial projections after separate injection of contrast media into the left and right ventricles, offer the greatest diagnostic reliability. These data, coupled with hemodynamic information obtained during cardiac catheterization, provide knowledge of the great artery relationships, size and location of the VSD, functional and anatomic status of each AV valve, and the presence and severity, or absence, of pulmonary stenosis.[36]

Echocardiography. Two-dimensional echocardiography, particularly with color-flow mapping, is very useful in the noninvasive diagnosis of DORV and has eliminated much of the variable reliability previously found with M-mode echocardiography.

Natural History

The natural history of DORV with a subaortic, doubly committed, or noncommitted VSD without pulmonary stenosis is similar to that of a large, isolated VSD except that spontaneous closure of the VSD in DORV, a fatal event, is extremely rare. The natural history of patients with pulmonary stenosis is similar to that of patients with tetralogy of Fallot. The natural history of patients with DORV and subpulmonary VSD is similar to that of patients with transposition of the great arteries and VSD except for the tendency of the patients with Taussig-Bing malformation to develop pulmonary vascular disease earlier in life.[11]

Surgical Methods, Timing, and Results

The goals of corrective surgery are to relieve pulmonary stenosis, to provide separate and unobstructed outflow pathways from each ventricle to the correct great vessel, and to separate the pulmonary and systemic circulation. In general, the timing of surgical intervention depends on the symptomatic state of the patient and the anatomy of, and other cardiac anomalies associated with, the DORV itself. Anatomic repair of DORV can be contraindicated by the presence of ventricular hypoplasia, serious abnormalities of either AV valve, the presence of very remote and/or multiple VSDs, and the presence of irreversible pulmonary vascular disease.

Subaortic or Doubly Committed VSD Without Pulmonary Stenosis. The repair for this subset of patients with subaortic or doubly committed VSDs without pulmonary stenosis (Fig. 54–74) consists of connecting the left ventricle to the aorta with an intracardiac tunnel.[5] When the VSD is restrictive, it must be enlarged anteriorly to avoid the conduction tissue. In some hearts the tricuspid valve is so positioned that it interferes with construction of this tunnel and alternative methods are required.[26]

As a group these patients tend to develop pulmonary vascular disease within the first few years of life; hence, if operation is unduly delayed, the risk of late death increases. These conditions advise repair by 6 months of age or sooner if poorly controlled heart failure is present.

In the current era, the risk of death early after repair of DORV with subaortic or doubly committed VSD without pulmonary stenosis approaches 0%. The actuarial 15-year survival, including hospital death, is 96%. In an earlier era younger age was a risk factor for death after repair; however, currently this risk factor has been neutralized. Older age has remained a significant risk factor over time, possibly owing to the presence of increasing pulmonary vascular disease with age.[10, 17]

Subaortic or Doubly Committed VSDs with Pulmonary Stenosis. In patients with subaortic or doubly committed VSDs with coexisting pulmonary stenosis, the techniques of repair are similar to those described for repair of tetralogy of Fallot, except the VSD is connected to the aorta with the tunnel technique rather than with a straight patch.[27] If it is thought that an intracardiac repair can be performed, primary repair is generally advised in symptomatic patients or at 6 to 12 months of age, whichever comes first.

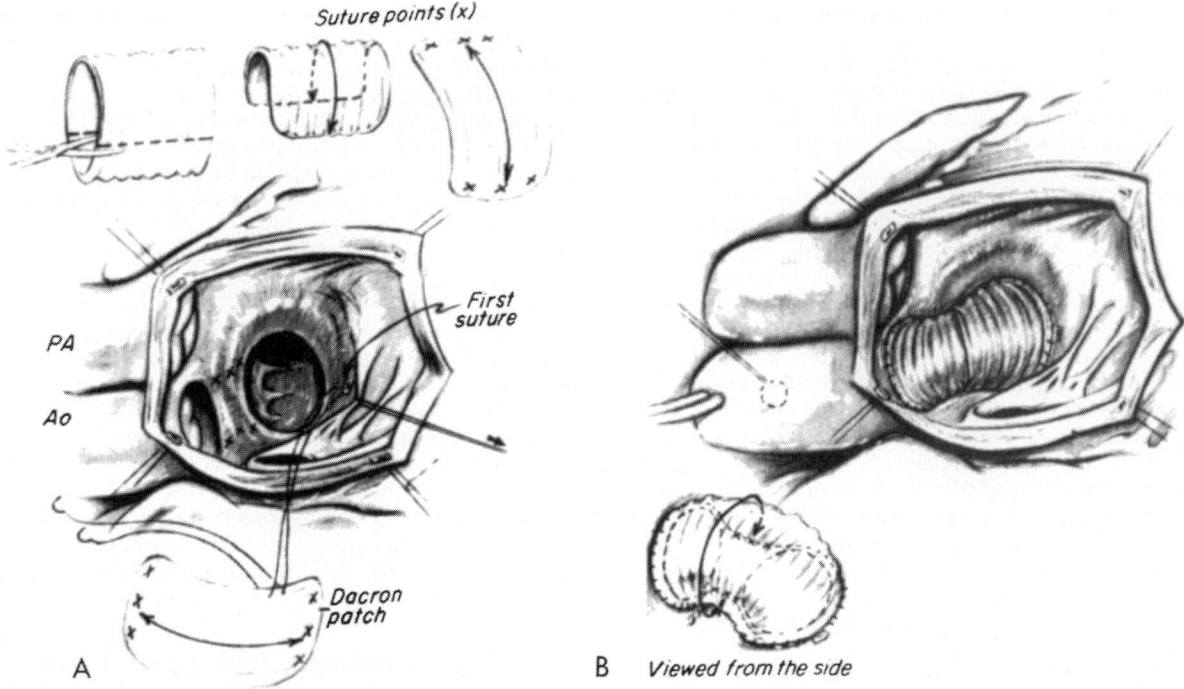

Figure 54–74. Construction of an intraventricular tunnel connecting VSD to aorta (Ao) is depicted in a heart with DORV and subaortic VSD. *A*, The patch is tailored from a woven Dacron tube that forms the anterior two thirds of the tunnel. Its proper geometry and orientation during repair are essential to avoid subaortic stenosis. The first suture is placed well away from the edge of the VSD to avoid injury to conduction tissue. *B*, The completed repair is demonstrated leaving an unobstructed path through right ventricle to pulmonary artery (PA). (From Stewart, R. W., Kirklin, J. W., Pacifico, A. D., et al.: Repair of double outlet right ventricle: An analysis of 62 cases. J. Thorac. Cardiovasc. Surg., 78:502, 1979.)

The use of palliative systemic-to-pulmonary artery shunts should be minimized but may be required in patients with severe pulmonary artery hypoplasia or in patients in whom an extracardiac conduit may be required for the repair. A cryopreserved homograft extracardiac conduit connecting the right ventricle to the pulmonary artery to bypass the right ventricular outflow tract obstruction must be used when a coronary artery crossing the right ventricular outflow tract prevents the placement of a transannular patch. The most common example of such a coronary anomaly is origin of the left anterior descending coronary artery from the right coronary artery.

The functional status of survivors of repair of DORV with subaortic or doubly committed VSDs and pulmonary stenosis is excellent. The early and late survival of this group of patients is similar to that described earlier for patients without pulmonary stenosis if the repair of the pulmonary stenosis does not require the placement of an extracardiac conduit or a transannular patch. In these latter two groups of patients the risks of early and late death are higher than when simpler forms of relief of right ventricular outflow tract obstruction are used.[10]

The Taussig-Bing Malformation Without Pulmonary Stenosis. Repair of the Taussig-Bing type of DORV is more complex, and many approaches have been proposed.[40] Because the streaming of blood in these patients is similar to that found in transposition of the great arteries with VSD, an initial balloon atrial septostomy is performed in the catheterization laboratory to improve the admixture of systemic and pulmonary venous blood. The result of this improved mixing is to raise the arterial oxygen saturations to acceptable levels.

The presence or absence of pulmonary stenosis and the relationship of the great arteries to each other and to the interventricular septum affect the choice of operation in this malformation. The position and interrelations of the VSD, the aortic and pulmonary valves, the tricuspid valve and its tensor apparatus, and the infundibular septum are carefully assessed through the right atrium at the time of surgical repair.

Kawashima Repair. The most attractive surgical option is a totally intraventricular repair without the need for an arterial switch or for the use of an extracardiac conduit. This Kawashima repair[9, 25] can be best accomplished when the great arteries are in a more or less side-by-side relationship, with the aorta to the right of the pulmonary artery. The infundibular septum must first be generously resected to provide an unobstructed pathway from the VSD to the aorta. The VSD, and hence the left ventricle, is then connected directly to the aorta by an intraventricular tunnel that runs posterior to the pulmonary artery.

Series of the Kawashima operation are small; however, Kawashima's most recent report documents 10 patients in whom the average follow-up was 8 years.[9] There were no early or late deaths, and reoperation was required in only one patient for residual pulmonary stenosis.

Arterial Switch Procedure. The most common approach to the repair of DORV with subpulmonary VSD is the arterial switch procedure combined with connection of the VSD to the pulmonary artery with a tunnel.[7, 8, 31] Although this technique is best suited for hearts in which the aorta is more-orless anterior to the pulmonary artery, it has been successfully employed for the repair of Taussig-Bing hearts with any arrangement of the great arteries. In this technique, connection of the VSD to the adjacent pulmonary artery creates transposition of the great arteries with an intact interventricular septum. The arterial switch procedure then establishes ventriculoarterial concordance. In one series of this technique of repair,[21] the hospital mortality was 14.3% and there were no late deaths at the time of follow-up. One patient underwent reoperation for a residual VSD.

Patients with the Taussig-Bing malformation in the absence of pulmonary stenosis tend to develop severe congestive heart failure or pulmonary vascular disease early in life. This poor natural history mandates operation within the first 3 months of life.

Taussig-Bing Malformation with Pulmonary Stenosis. When pulmonary stenosis is present in patients with the Taussig-Bing malformation, repair may be accomplished by one of the three following techniques.

"Rastelli-Type" Repair. One option consists of constructing a tunnel that connects the VSD with the origin of the aorta (and includes the origin of the pulmonary artery because it is usually directly posterior to the aorta), closing the pulmonary artery, and using a valved extracardiac conduit to restore continuity between the right ventricle and the pulmonary artery. This is similar to the operation described by Rastelli and associates for repair of transposition, VSD, and pulmonary stenosis.[32]

Réparation à l'Étage Ventriculaire. The réparation à l'étage ventriculaire (REV) repair[14, 33, 34, 38] is similar to the Rastelli-type repair in that it consists of aggressive resection of the infundibular septum, connection of the VSD (and hence the left ventricle) to the aorta with an intraventricular tunnel, and closure of the pulmonary artery orifice. It differs in that right ventricular to pulmonary artery continuity is established by connecting the main pulmonary artery directly to a vertical incision in the right ventricular outflow tract rather than using an extracardiac conduit. The hospital mortality was 18% in a series of 50 patients with anomalies of ventriculoarterial connection and VSD who underwent the REV procedure. This series was not limited to patients with DORV.[1]

Nikaidoh Procedure. The Nikaidoh aortic translocation and biventricular outflow tract reconstruction technique[22] can also be applied to this subset of patients. This radical technique involves detaching the aortic root from its right ventricular origin, transection of the pulmonary artery with excision of the pulmonary valve, division of the pulmonary root into the VSD, posterior translocation of the aorta, closure of the VSD to the translocated aorta, and connection of the main pulmonary artery to the right ventricle with a generous pericardial patch. To date the Nikaidoh procedure has been performed in 11 children with no deaths. One patient has poor right ventricular function due to infarction.[23]

Choice of Procedure. Given its increased complexity there is no compelling indication to use the Nikaidoh procedure over the Rastelli-type or REV procedures in patients with the Taussig-Bing malformation and pulmonary stenosis. A disadvantage of the Rastelli-type repair, not inherent to the REV procedure, is the need to perform future conduit replacements. However, the long-term effects of pulmonary insufficiency after the REV procedure in this subset of patients is not known and may balance the relative disadvantages of these two techniques.

Timing of Repair. There is no general consensus as to the best timing for surgical repair of patients with the Taussig-Bing malformation and pulmonary stenosis. An initial systemic-to-pulmonary artery shunt may be advisable in symptomatic patients in whom eventual repair will include the placement of an extracardiac conduit. This allows the placement of an initially larger conduit when the child is 2 to 3 years of age and possibly reduces the number of future obligatory conduit replacements. There are no definite guidelines concerning the optimal age for performance of the REV procedure. In Lecompte's experience, it has been performed as early as 4 months of age and as late as 13 years of age. It would seem reasonable to perform the REV procedure in symptomatic patients or at 6 to 12 months of age, whichever comes first.

Noncommitted VSD. Repair of hearts with DORV and noncommitted VSD can be accomplished by constructing an intraventricular tunnel (or Dacron patch partition) connecting the VSD (which usually must be enlarged anterosuperiorly) with the aorta, closing the pulmonary artery, and placing a valved extracardiac conduit from the right ventricle to the pulmonary artery.[37] Alternative techniques consist of patch closure of the VSD, closure of the pulmonary artery, placement of a valved extracardiac conduit from the left ventricle to the pulmonary artery, and construction of an intra-atrial transposition of venous return (Senning or Mustard procedure).[10] Additionally, repair including an arterial switch operation has been successfully accomplished.[31] Alternatively, when appropriate anatomic and hemodynamic criteria exist, repair can be accomplished by a modification of the operation described by Fontan.[19] Repair of this complex malformation has generally been associated with a higher hospital mortality.[10, 12, 21, 30, 37]

Timing of Repair. Patients with DORV and noncommitted VSD without pulmonary stenosis should have pulmonary artery banding in the first 6 months of life to control heart failure and to prevent the development of advanced pulmonary vascular disease. When pulmonary stenosis is present, an initial systemic-to-pulmonary artery shunt is performed to relieve cyanosis in patients younger than approximately 2 years of age. Repair in this subset of patients usually requires a valved extracardiac conduit or a modification of the Fontan procedure and should be delayed until 2 to 3 years of age.

Complete AV Canal. DORV associated with complete AV canal has been repaired by tunneling the VSD to the aorta with a comma-shaped patch along with concomitant repair of the common AV valve.[28] Although early results were associated with high hospital mortality, more recently results have improved.[29] Alternative methods of repair include mitral and tricuspid valve replacement with closure of the atrial and ventricular septal defects and placement of a valved extracardiac conduit from the left ventricle to the aorta, or a modification of the Fontan procedure.

Timing of Repair. When it is possible to repair the defects of these patients using an intraventricular tunnel technique and pulmonary stenosis is absent, operation should be undertaken by 4 to 6 months of age to avoid the development of severe pulmonary vascular disease. When pulmonary stenosis is present, the timing of surgical intervention is similar to that in patients with tetralogy of Fallot. When the interventricular communication is not related to the aorta and there is an absence of pulmonary stenosis, a pulmonary artery band should be placed in early infancy in anticipation of performing a repair with a valved extracardiac conduit at 2 to 3 years of age. When pulmonary stenosis is present in this subgroup, a systemic-to-pulmonary artery shunt may be necessary to treat severe cyanosis before complete repair with a valved extracardiac conduit at 2 to 3 years of age.

Late Sudden Death After Repair of DORV. It is interesting to note that Shen and colleagues[35] found an 18% incidence of late sudden death when they analyzed 89 survivors of repair of DORV. Older age at the time of operation, perioperative or postoperative ventricular tachyarrhythmias, and third-degree AV block were significant risk factors for late sudden death. This high incidence of late sudden death has not been reported in more recent surgical series of DORV.

HEARTS WITH AV DISCORDANCE

Morphology

DORV is less common in hearts with AV discordant connections. All of these patients have VSDs; the majority have associated pulmonary stenosis; and most have situs solitus of the atria and viscera with dextrocardia. In this defect, usually the right atrium lies to the right and connects to a morphologic left ventricle that is right sided. The only outlet for this ventricle is a VSD that leads to the left-sided morphologic right ventricle that also receives blood from the left atrium. Both great arteries arise from the morphologic right ventricle; and although the relationship of each great artery is variable, the aorta is most commonly anterior and to the left (l-malposition) of the pulmonary artery. The VSD is usually in a subpulmonary position in those with l-malposition of the aorta and in a subaortic position when the aorta is to the right (d-malposition) or directly anterior to the pulmonary artery. The bundle of His and specialized conduction tissue are abnormally located, and, in some, abnormalities of the left AV valve exist, similar to patients with corrected transposition of the great arteries.[39]

Surgical Repair

Kiser and associates first described the surgical repair of this entity in 1968 using a solely intraventricular technique connecting the VSD to the pulmonary artery in two patients. In one patient, they closed the VSD and pulmonary artery followed by placement of a nonvalved extracardiac conduit from the left ventricle to the pulmonary artery.[13] The latter type of repair with the use of a valved extracardiac conduit from the left ventricle to the pulmonary artery is probably preferable, because it avoids an incision in the systemic (right) ventricle, can be used regardless of the location of the VSD, and avoids residual pulmonary stenosis.[4] The incidence of surgically induced complete heart block is high, approaching 30%, and hospital mortality is approximately 15%.[13]

SELECTED REFERENCES

Kawashima, Y., Matsuda, H., Yagihara, T., Shimazaki, Y., Yamamoto, F., Nishigaki, K., Miura, T., and Uemura, H.: Intraventricular repair for Taussig-Bing anomaly. J. Thorac. Cardiovasc. Surg., *105*:591, 1993.
This report of 10 patients with the Taussig-Bing malformation and a side-by-side relationship of the great arteries describes the technique and results for an entirely intraventricular tunnel repair. There were no operative deaths, and after a mean follow-up of 6 years only one reoperation was required. The postoperative left ventricular outflow tract gradients were less than 19 mm. Hg.

Kirklin, J. W., Pacifico, A. D., Blackstone, E. H., Kirklin, J. K., and Bargeron, L. M., Jr.: Current risks and protocols for operations for double outlet right ventricle. J. Thorac. Cardiovasc. Surg., *92*:913, 1986.
This report of 127 patients who underwent repair of various types of DORV during an 18-year period thoroughly describes early and late results using various surgical methods. Results of tunnel repair of DORV with subaortic or doubly committed VSD were excellent, and reoperation was required in only 1 of 56 patients. Predicted survival rates for intraventricular tunnel repair currently performed in a 6-month-old infant was 99% at 2 weeks and 97% at 10 years. Early and late results in patients with DORV and subpulmonary VSD were poor when an arterial switch operation was part of the repair. Results were least good in the subset of DORV with noncommitted VSD.

Lecompte, Y., Batisse, A., and Duccio, D.: Double-outlet right ventricle: A surgical synthesis. Adv. Cardiac Surg., *4*:109, 1993.
This paper describes the réparation à l'étage ventriculaire (REV) repair for DORV. It is a technique similar to the Rastelli-type repair in that it consists of aggressive resection of the infundibular septum, connection of the VSD (and hence the left ventricle) to the aorta with an intraventricular tunnel, and closure of the pulmonary artery orifice. It differs from the Rastelli-type repair in that right ventricular-to-pulmonary artery continuity is established by connecting the main pulmonary artery directly to a vertical incision in the right ventricular outflow tract rather than to an extracardiac conduit. The detailed preoperative evaluation of the patient with DORV and the indications for the use of the REV procedure are described. The intraoperative assessment and surgical technique are also outlined for this procedure.

Lev, M., Bharati, S., Meng, C. C. L., Liberthson, R. R., Paul, M. H., and Idriss, F.: A concept of double-outlet right ventricle. J. Thorac. Cardiovasc. Surg., *64*:271, 1972.
This classic article analyzes in detail the anatomic features of 91 hearts with DORV. The relation of each specific type of VSD to the great arteries is discussed, and the precise intracardiac anatomic details are presented. The differentiation of DORV with subaortic VSD and pulmonary stenosis from tetralogy of Fallot is considered.

Musumeci, F., Shumway, S., Lincoln, C., and Anderson, R. H.: Surgical treat-

ment for double-outlet right ventricle at the Brompton Hospital, 1973 to 1986. J. Thorac. Cardiovasc. Surg., *96*:278, 1988.
Surgical results were thoroughly analyzed for 120 consecutive patients who underwent repair of various types of DORV. Best results were obtained when the VSD was subaortic or doubly committed, and the arterial switch operation was demonstrated to be the optimal approach when a subpulmonary VSD exists.

Sondheimer, H. M., Freedom, R. M., and Olley, P. M.: Double outlet right ventricle: Clinical spectrum and prognosis. Am. J. Cardiol., *39*:709, 1977.
This paper reviews the natural history of 80 children with various types of DORV observed over a 19-year period at the Hospital for Sick Children in Toronto. Patients were grouped according to the location of the VSD and the presence or absence of pulmonary stenosis. Prognosis was significantly influenced by the associated presence of coarctation of the aorta or severe mitral valve abnormalities. The effect of palliative or corrective surgery on the prognosis of each group is presented.

Tabry, I. F., McGoon, D. C., Danielson, G. K., Wallace, R. B., Davis, Z., and Maloney, J. D.: Surgical management of double-outlet right ventricle associated with atrioventricular discordance. J. Thorac. Cardiovasc. Surg., *76*:336, 1978.
A surgical series with 20 corrective operations performed for DORV with atrioventricular discordant connections is discussed. The various methods employed, the early and late results, and the abnormal location of the conduction system determined by electrophysiologic mapping are presented.

REFERENCES

1. Borromee, L., Lecompte, Y., Batisse, A., et al.: Anatomic repair of anomalies of ventriculoarterial connection associated with ventricular septal defect: II. Clinical results in 50 patients with pulmonary outflow tract obstruction. J. Thorac. Cardiovasc. Surg., *95*:96, 1988.
2. Braun, K., DeVries, A., Feingold, D. S., et al.: Complete dextroposition of the aorta, pulmonary stenosis, interventricular septal defect, and patent foramen ovale. Am. Heart J., *43*:773, 1952.
3. Daicoff, G. R., and Kirklin, J. W.: Surgical correction of Taussig-Bing malformation: Report of three cases (Abstract). Am. J. Cardiol., *19*:125, 1967.
4. Fox, L. S., Kirklin, J. W., Pacifico, A. D., et al.: Intracardiac repair of cardiac malformations with atrioventricular discordance. Circulation, *54*:123, 1976.
5. Gomes, M. M. R., Weidman, W. H., McGoon, D. C., and Danielson, G. K.: Double-outlet right ventricle with pulmonic stenosis: Surgical considerations and results of operation. Circulation, *43*:889, 1971.
6. Goor, D. A., and Ebert, P. A.: Left ventricular outflow tract obstruction in Taussig-Bing malformation: Anatomic and surgical implications. J. Thorac. Cardiovasc. Surg., *70*:69, 1975.
7. Kanter, K. R., Anderson, R. H., Lincoln, C., et al.: Anatomic correction for complete transposition and double outlet right ventricle. J. Thorac. Cardiovasc. Surg., *90*:690, 1985.
8. Kanter, K. R., Anderson, R., Lincoln, C., et al.: Anatomic correction of double-outlet right ventricle with subpulmonary ventricular septal defect (the "Taussig-Bing" anomaly). Ann. Thorac. Surg., *41*:287, 1986.
9. Kawashima, Y., Matsuda, H., Yagihara, T., et al.: Intraventricular repair for Taussig-Bing anomaly. J. Thorac. Cardiovasc. Surg., *105*:591, 1993.
10. Kirklin, J. W., Pacifico, A. D., Blackstone, E. H., et al.: Current risks and protocols for operations for double-outlet right ventricle. J. Thorac. Cardiovasc. Surg., *92*:913, 1986.
11. Kirklin, J. W., and Barratt-Boyes, B. G.: Double outlet right ventricle. *In* Cardiac Surgery, 2nd ed. New York, Churchill Livingstone, 1993, p. 1470.
12. Kirklin, J. K., and Castañeda, A. R.: Surgical correction of double-outlet right ventricle with noncommitted ventricular septal defect. J. Thorac. Cardiovasc. Surg., *73*:399, 1977.
13. Kiser, J. C., Ongley, P. A., Kirklin, J. W., et al.: Surgical treatment of dextrocardia with inversion of ventricles and double-outlet right ventricle. J. Thorac. Cardiovasc. Surg., *55*:6, 1968.
14. Lecompte, Y., Batisse, A., and DiCarlo, D.: Double-outlet right ventricle: A surgical synthesis. *In* Advances in Cardiac Surgery, vol. 4. St. Louis, C. V. Mosby, 1993.
15. Lev, M., Bharati, S., Meng, C. C. L., et al.: A concept of double-outlet right ventricle. J. Thorac. Cardiovasc. Surg., *64*:271, 1972.
16. Lincoln C., Anderson R. H., Shinebourne, E. A., et al.: Double outlet right ventricle with l-malposition of the aorta. Br. Heart J., *37*:453, 1975.
17. Luber, J. M., Castañeda, A. R., Lang, P., et al.: Repair of double-outlet right ventricle: Early and late results. Circulation, *68*:144, 1983.
18. Luisi, V. S., Verunelli, F., and Eufrate, S.: Double outlet right ventricle, noncommitted ventricular septal defect and pulmonic stenosis: Anatomical and surgical considerations. J. Thorac. Cardiovasc. Surg., *28*:368, 1980.
19. Marin-Garcia, J., Neches, W. H., Park, S. C., et al.: Double-outlet right ventricle with restrictive ventricular septal defect. J. Thorac. Cardiovasc. Surg., *76*:853, 1978.
20. Matsuoka, Y., Akimoto, K., Sennari, E., et al.: Double outlet right ventricle with severe left ventricular outflow tract obstruction due to small ventricular septal defect and anomalous adherence of the mitral valve to the ventricular septum. Jpn. Circ. J., *51*:1335, 1987.
21. Musumeci, F., Shumway, S., Lincoln, C., et al.: Surgical treatment for double-outlet right ventricle at the Brompton Hospital, 1973 to 1986. J. Thorac. Cardiovasc. Surg., *96*:278, 1988.
22. Nikaidoh, H.: Aortic translocation and biventricular outflow tract recon-

struction: A new surgical repair for transposition of the great arteries associated with ventricular septal defect and pulmonary stenosis. J. Thorac. Cardiovasc. Surg., 88:365, 1984.

23. Nikaidoh, H.: Personal communication, April 1993.
24. Pacifico, A. D., Soto, B., and Bargeron, L. M., Jr.: Surgical treatment of straddling tricuspid valves. Circulation, 60:655, 1979.
25. Pacifico, A. D., Kirklin, J. K., Colvin, E. V., et al.: Intraventricular tunnel repair for Taussig-Bing heart and related cardiac anomalies. Circulation, 74(Suppl. I):153, 1986.
26. Pacifico, A. D., Kirklin, J. W., and Bargeron, L. M., Jr.: Complex congenital malformations: Surgical treatment of double-outlet right ventricle and double-outlet left ventricle. In Kirklin, J. W. (Ed.): Advances in Cardiovascular Surgery. New York, Grune & Stratton, 1973, p. 57.
27. Pacifico, A. D., Kirklin, J. W., and Blackstone, E. H.: Surgical management of the pulmonary stenosis in the tetralogy of Fallot. J. Thorac. Cardiovasc. Surg., 74:382, 1977.
28. Pacifico, A. D., Kirklin, J. W., and Bargeron, L. M., Jr.: Repair of complete atrioventricular canal associated with tetralogy of Fallot or double outlet right ventricle: Report of 10 cases. Ann. Thorac. Surg., 29:351, 1980.
29. Pacifico, A. D., Ricchi, A., Bargeron, L. M., Jr., et al.: Corrective repair of complete atrioventricular canal defects and major associated cardiac anomalies. Ann. Thorac. Surg., 46:645, 1988.
30. Piccoli, G., Pacifico, A. D., Kirklin, J. W., et al.: Changing results and concepts in the surgical treatment of double-outlet right ventricle: Analysis of 137 operations in 126 patients. Am. J. Cardiol., 52:549, 1983.
31. Quaegebeur, J. M., Rohmer, J., Ottenkamp, J., et al.: The arterial switch operation: An eight-year experience. J. Thorac. Cardiovasc. Surg., 92:365, 1986.

32. Rastelli, G. C., McGoon, D. C., and Wallace, R. B.: Anatomic correction of transposition of the great arteries with ventricular septal defect and subpulmonic stenosis. J. Thorac. Cardiovasc. Surg., 58:545, 1969.
33. Rubay, J., Lecompte, Y., Batisse, A., et al.: Anatomic repair of anomalies of ventriculo-arterial connection (REV). Eur. J. Cardiothorac. Surg., 2:305, 1988.
34. Sakata, R., Lecompte, Y., Batisse, A., et al.: Anatomic repair of anomalies of ventriculoarterial connection associated with ventricular septal defect: I. Criteria of surgical decision. J. Thorac. Cardiovasc. Surg., 95:90, 1988.
35. Shen, W. K., Holmes, D. R., Porter, C. J., et al.: Sudden death after repair of double outlet right ventricle. Circulation, 81:128, 1990.
36. Sridaromont, S., Ritter, D. G., Feldt, R. H., et al.: Double-outlet right ventricle: Anatomic and angiocardiographic correlations. Mayo Clin. Proc., 53:555, 1978.
37. Stewart, R. W., Kirklin, J. W., Pacifico, A. D., et al.: Repair of double outlet right ventricle: An analysis of 62 cases. J. Thorac. Cardiovasc. Surg., 78:502, 1979.
38. Vouhe, P. R., Tamisier, D., Leca, F., et al.: Transposition of the great arteries, ventricular septal defect and pulmonary outflow tract obstruction: Rastelli or Lecompte procedure? J. Thorac. Cardiovasc. Surg., 103:428, 1992.
39. Waldo, A. L., Pacifico, A. D., Bargeron, L. M., Jr., et al.: Electrophysiological delineation of the specialized A-V conduction system in patients with corrected transposition of the great vessels and ventricular septal defect. Circulation, 52:435, 1975.
40. Walters, H. L., and Pacifico, A. D.: Double outlet ventricles. In Mavroudis, C., and Backer, C. L. (Eds.): Pediatric Cardiac Surgery. St. Louis, Mosby–Year Book, 1994, p. 321.

IX

TRICUSPID ATRESIA

Erle H. Austin III, M.D.

Tricuspid atresia is a congenital heart defect in which there is no direct communication between the right atrium and the right ventricle. Systemic venous blood reaches the pulmonary vascular bed by passing through an interatrial communication, mixing with pulmonary venous blood, entering the left ventricle, and then passing through a ventricular septal defect into the outlet portion of a diminutive right ventricle. The obligatory right-to-left shunt at the atrial level results in cyanosis, which is especially severe in those whose pulmonary blood flow is restricted. Tricuspid atresia represents 1.4% of all congenital malformations of the heart, occurring at a rate of approximately 1 in 10,000 live births.[30] Behind tetralogy of Fallot and transposition of the great arteries, it is the third most common cyanotic congenital heart defect. Without surgical intervention, 90% of patients with tricuspid atresia and significant obstruction to pulmonary blood flow are dead by the age of 1 year. Patients with normal or increased pulmonary blood flow may survive several years with only mild cyanosis, but survival beyond 10 years of age is uncommon, even in this favorable group.[12, 16]

Surgical therapy significantly improves the outlook of patients with tricuspid atresia by providing controlled pulmonary blood flow in the infant and optimizing single-ventricle physiology in the older child. Lessons learned from the surgical treatment of tricuspid atresia have favorably impacted on the management of other complex heart defects that present as univentricular anatomy and physiology, such as hypoplastic left heart syndrome.

HISTORICAL ASPECTS

The pathologic anatomy of tricuspid atresia was described by Kuhne in 1906.[22] Its clinical features were well described in the 1930s by Bellet and Stewart[1] and Taussig.[37] Surgical palliation became possible with the development of the sys-

temic-pulmonary arterial shunt by Blalock and Taussig in 1945.[2] In 1958, Glenn reported anastomosis of the superior vena cava to the right pulmonary artery as a specific treatment for tricuspid atresia.[17] Clinical success with this technique was based on much preliminary experimental work by Glenn and Patino[18] as well as on similar studies by Carlon and associates[4] and Robicsek and associates[31] that showed that systemic venous pressure was adequate to provide pulmonary blood flow. The first successful correction of tricuspid atresia with separation of the pulmonary and systemic circulations was performed in 1968 by Fontan and Baudet.[14] This original Fontan procedure included a superior vena cava to right pulmonary artery (Glenn) anastomosis, closure of the atrial communication, insertion of an aortic allograft valve into the opening of the inferior vena cava, anastomosis of the right atrial appendage to the proximal end of the divided right pulmonary artery, and ligation of the main pulmonary artery. Fontan's clinical success was preceded by experimental studies by Starr and co-workers in 1943[34] and Rodbard and Wagner in 1949[32] that demonstrated the feasibility of bypassing the right ventricle.

ANATOMY

Tricuspid atresia is characterized by an absent connection between the right atrium and the right ventricle. In over 85% of cases, the atresia is muscular with only a small dimple noted within the right atrium at the expected site of the atrioventricular valve. Less commonly, the atresia is membranous with what appears to be an imperforate valve membrane. Rarely, this imperforate valve displays characteristics of an Ebstein malformation.

The right atrium is typically enlarged and thickened, and the atrial septal defect is usually large and unrestrictive. The left atrium, mitral valve, and left ventricle are enlarged because both systemic and pulmonary circulations must pass through them. A ventricular septal defect is almost always present and provides the only access of blood to the right ventricle. The hypoplastic right ventricle lacks an inlet portion and usually consists of a small trabecular segment and a tubular outlet portion. When the great arteries are normally related, the right ventricle is commonly connected to a hypoplastic pulmonary anulus, although atresia or a normal pulmonary valve may occur at this point. Obstruction to pulmonary blood flow may occur at any point between the left ventricle and the main pulmonary artery, including the ventricular septal defect, the right ventricular infundibulum, and the pulmonary valve. In those cases with pulmonary atresia, pulmonary blood flow is entirely dependent on a patent ductus arteriosus.

In approximately 30% of cases, the great arteries are transposed. In these cases, the systemic blood flow may be restricted with excessive flow to the pulmonary circulation. Aortic arch obstruction (coarctation or arch interruption) is seen in as many as 30% of patients with tricuspid atresia and transposition of the great arteries.

Although several classification systems have been devised for tricuspid atresia, the system most commonly employed was described by Tandon and Edwards[36] (Fig. 54–75) and is based on the most common anatomic and physiologic presentations. All cases with normally related great vessels are classified as Type I, while those with transposition of the great arteries are Type II. Each of these groups is further subdivided on the basis of the degree of obstruction to pulmonary blood flow, with *a* indicating pulmonary atresia, *b* indicating pulmonary stenosis, and *c* indicating a normal pulmonary valve without obstruction. Because natural history and preferred treatment options are determined by the underlying pathophysiology, this classification permits a rational therapeutic approach to all patients.

PATHOPHYSIOLOGY

In tricuspid atresia, the left ventricle must provide blood flow to both the systemic and pulmonary circulations. The venous returns from both circulations mix in the left atrium, and this admixture is then distributed by the left ventricle to the lungs and the body. The pathophysiology of this single ventricle circulation is determined by the relative resistances to flow into the systemic and pulmonary circulations. If blood flow to the lungs is severely obstructed, inadequate pulmonary blood flow results in marked cyanosis. If blood flow to the body is obstructed, inadequate systemic perfusion results in hypotension and metabolic acidosis. Thus, a balanced delivery to both circulations is desirable.

In patients with tricuspid atresia and normally related great vessels (Type I), pulmonary blood flow is commonly restricted (Ia and Ib). If the restriction is such that pulmonary blood flow is inadequate, the delivery of oxygen to the tissues is limited by the low content of oxygen in the blood, not by the volume of blood delivered. If pulmonary blood flow is not increased by directing more of the left ventricular outflow to the lungs, the patient will not survive. If restriction to pulmonary blood flow is only moderate, a relatively normal volume of blood is delivered to the pulmonary vascular bed and the volume and oxygen content of blood delivered to the body permits satisfactory oxygen delivery. In some patients with tricuspid atresia, this favorable balance exists at birth, but as the normal postnatal reduction of pulmonary vascular resistance occurs, pulmonary blood flow increases and systemic blood decreases. The progressive volume load on the left ventricle leads to congestive heart failure and pulmonary edema. If these patients do not succumb to progressive heart failure, an increase in pulmonary vascular resistance occurs as a result of the development of obstructive pulmonary vascular disease.

TYPE I

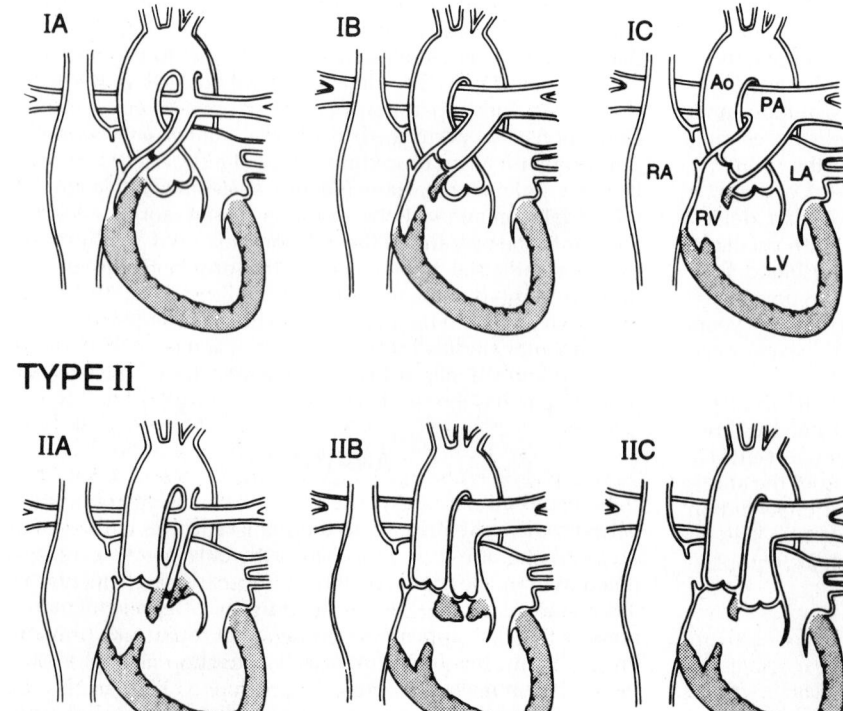

TYPE II

Figure 54–75. Tandon and Edwards classification of tricuspid atresia. Type I: normally related great vessels; Type II: transposition of the great arteries; (A) pulmonary atresia; (B) pulmonary stenosis; (C) normal unobstructed pulmonary valve. Ao, aorta; PA, pulmonary artery; LA, left atrium; RA, right atrium; LV, left ventricle. (From Kopf, G. S.: Tricuspid atresia. *In* Mavroudis, C., and Backer, C. L. [Eds.]: Pediatric Cardiac Surgery, 2nd ed. St. Louis, C. V. Mosby, 1994.)

The pathophysiology in patients with tricuspid atresia and transposition of the great arteries (Type II) is often less favorable, because restriction to systemic blood flow is likely to coexist with unobstructed pulmonary blood flow. Even in patients with well-balanced flows, the chronic effects of volume overload and persistent cyanosis result in impaired left ventricular function over time.

Surgical techniques employed in tricuspid atresia are applied to optimize the physiology of the single ventricle. Systemic-to-pulmonary arterial shunts increase pulmonary blood flow and minimize cyanosis. Pulmonary artery banding diminishes pulmonary blood flow and prevents pulmonary edema and obstructive pulmonary vascular disease. The superior cavopulmonary (Glenn) anastomosis provides adequate pulmonary blood flow without volume overloading the left ventricle. The Fontan procedure eliminates the volume overload and chronic hypoxia imposed by parallel and unseparated circulations.

CLINICAL FEATURES

Tricuspid atresia occurs in males and females with equal frequency. Most patients with tricuspid atresia and normally related great arteries have restricted blood flow (Ib) and present in the first stage of life with cyanosis and a loud systolic ejection murmur. When pulmonary atresia exists (Ia), the severity of hypoxia may become life threatening as the ductus arteriosus closes. A small portion of patients with tricuspid atresia and normally related great arteries have no obstruction to pulmonary blood flow (Ic) and are more likely to present in the first 4 to 6 weeks of life with signs and symptoms of congestive heart failure. When tricuspid atresia and transposition of the great arteries coexist (Type II), signs and symptoms of excessive pulmonary blood flow are likely to present earlier. In fact, those with coexistent aortic obstruction will present in the first days of life with congestive failure and metabolic acidosis from poor systemic perfusion.

Chest radiography reflects the level of pulmonary blood flow, most commonly displaying a decrease in pulmonary vascular markings. Electrocardiography usually demonstrates tall, notched P waves from right atrial hypertrophy and left-axis deviation from left ventricular hypertrophy.

Definitive diagnosis is made with two-dimensional echocardiography. The absence of the right atrioventricular valve is the prime diagnostic feature. The relation of the great vessels, the size of the right ventricle, and any obstruction to systemic or pulmonary flow can be determined with this noninvasive technique. Cardiac catheterization and angiography are usually performed to delineate the pulmonary arteries as well as confirm the echocardiographic findings.

SURGICAL MANAGEMENT

Early Palliation

Initial surgical management is tailored to the pathophysiology at presentation and is designed to prepare the patient for a successful Fontan procedure at between 2 and 4 years of age. Initial palliation involves manipulating pulmonary blood flow to achieve adequate systemic oxygen delivery without excessive volume load to the left ventricle.

For newborns with severe cyanosis, pulmonary blood flow is increased by creating a systemic artery to pulmonary artery shunt. At present, the Blalock-Taussig shunt is preferred for this purpose, because it is unlikely to provide excessive pulmonary blood flow. A commonly used modification of this technique involves the insertion of a 4- or 5-mm. polytetrafluoroethylene tube graft from the side of the subclavian artery to the side of the ipsilateral pulmonary artery. Al-

though the shunt can be performed on either side, placing it on the left preserves the right side for a possible Glenn shunt as an intermediate step toward Fontan correction. Skillful performance of the Blalock-Taussig shunt is essential to avoid pulmonary artery distortion and possible unsuitability for Fontan operation.

Infants with tricuspid atresia and congestive heart failure from excessive pulmonary blood flow may require limitation of pulmonary blood flow by pulmonary artery banding. Most infants with tricuspid atresia and transposition of the great arteries (Type IIc) require this procedure to manage the congestive heart failure and to prevent the development of pulmonary vascular disease. Pulmonary artery banding is best avoided, however, in patients with normally related great vessels and increased pulmonary blood flow (Type Ic), because progressive narrowing of the ventricular septal defect or infundibular obstruction will usually begin to limit pulmonary blood flow in the first months of life.

A superior cavopulmonary (Glenn) anastomosis is a valuable palliative procedure for tricuspid atresia[38] but is not suitable for infants younger than 3 months of age because of the high pulmonary vascular resistance of the neonate. However, after 3 months of age, the Glenn shunt provides palliation superior to that of a systemic-to-pulmonary artery shunt because it provides pulmonary blood flow without placing a volume load on the left ventricle. Although the classic Glenn shunt achieves satisfactory palliation, it has the disadvantage of directing one third of the systemic venous return to the right lung, which makes up almost two thirds of total pulmonary volume. A modified version (bidirectional Glenn) is now commonly performed by anastomosing the divided superior vena cava end-to-side into the upper aspect of the right pulmonary artery (Fig. 54–76). Either the classic or the bidirectional Glenn can be incorporated into an eventual Fontan operation.

Definitive Palliation—The Fontan Procedure

Satisfactory early palliation of tricuspid atresia should balance systemic and pulmonary blood flow and permit survival into the first decade of life. However, the persistent effects of volume overload and cyanosis lead to impaired function of the left ventricle over time. Furthermore, the admixture of venous returns imposes a continued risk of embolic stroke and the development of brain abscess. By separating the pulmonary and systemic circulations and diverting all of the systemic venous return to the lungs, the Fontan procedure improves arterial saturation and reduces the volume workload on the left ventricle. Thus, to maximize survival in tricuspid atresia, performance of the Fontan procedure should be considered between 2 and 4 years of age, before left ventricular function begins to deteriorate.

Patient Selection. Proper selection of candidates is essential for the short- and long-term success of the Fontan procedure. Paramount to a successful Fontan procedure are low pulmonary vascular resistance and good left ventricular function. Ideally, pulmonary vascular resistance should be less than 2 Woods units and pulmonary artery pressure less than 15 mm. Hg. Pulmonary vascular resistance greater than 4 Woods units and/or a pulmonary artery pressure greater than 25 mm. Hg may likely result in high systemic venous pressures and low cardiac output. Ideal measurements for left ventricular function would include an ejection fraction greater than 45% and a left ventricular end-diastolic pressure of less than 10 mm. Hg. An ejection fraction as low as 30% or a left ventricular end-diastolic pressure as high as 15 mm. Hg, however, may be acceptable if pulmonary vascular resistance is low. Other relative risk factors for the Fontan procedure include mitral insufficiency and pulmonary artery dis-

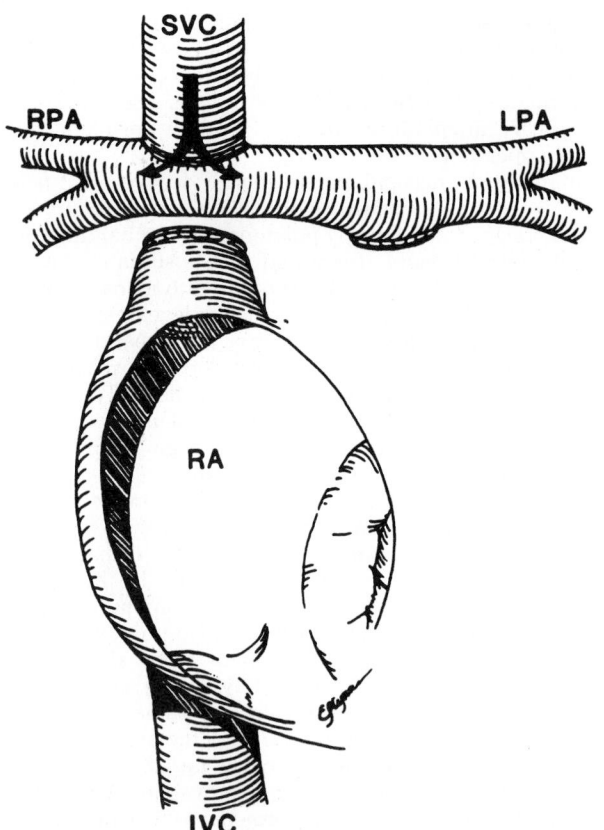

Figure 54–76. A bidirectional cavopulmonary anastomosis is created by performing an end-to-side anastomosis of the superior vena cava (SVC) to the superior aspect of the right pulmonary artery (RPA). The junction of the SVC with the right atrium (RA) is oversewn. This technique maintains continuity between the right and left pulmonary arteries. IVC, inferior vena cava; LPA, left pulmonary artery. (Reproduced with permission from Bridges, N. D., Jonas, R. A., Mayer, J. E., Flanagan, M. F., Keane, J. F., and Castañeda, A. R.: Bidirectional cavopulmonary anastomosis as interim palliation for high-risk Fontan candidates: Early results. Circulation, 82[Suppl. IV]:IV-170, 1990. Copyright 1990, American Heart Association.)

tortion. If these problems are mild, they usually can be corrected at the time of the Fontan operation. Should either problem be severe, however, it should be corrected and combined with a bidirectional Glenn anastomosis, leaving the completion of the Fontan procedure as a later stage.

Although early recommendations suggested that the Fontan procedure not be done in patients younger than 4 years of age,[5] increasing experience has reduced the lower limit to

1½ to 2 years.[21, 29] Because postponing the Fontan procedure past 4 years of age only prolongs the exposure of the left ventricle to volume overload and cyanosis, the window between 2 and 4 years of age represents the best time for physiologic correction.

Operative Procedure. The technical aspects of performing a Fontan correction have changed considerably since Fontan's first success.[6] Experience over the past two decades has indicated that valves, valved conduits, and irregularly shaped venous reservoirs (like the right atrium) along the pathway from the systemic veins to the pulmonary arteries result in turbulence and significant energy loss in addition to introducing potential for reoperation for obstruction. Currently, the preferred technique for Fontan correction is referred to as a lateral tunnel with total cavopulmonary anastomosis (Fig. 54–77).[8, 20, 35] With this technique, a piece of polytetrafluoroethylene is inserted as a partition within the right atrium to create a tunnel from the orifice of the inferior vena cava to the orifice of the superior vena cava. The superior vena cava is divided with the cardiac end anastomosed end-to-side into the inferior aspect of the right pulmonary artery. The cephalad end is anastomosed end-to-side into the superior aspect of the right pulmonary artery as in a bidirectional Glenn anastomosis. This results in a direct pathway of systemic venous return into the pulmonary arteries without turbulence. Furthermore, most of the right atrium remains at low pressure, diminishing the likelihood of atrial distention and supraventricular arrhythmias.

RESULTS

Reports on initial palliation for tricuspid atresia indicate an operative mortality of between 5% and 10% for the Blalock-Taussig shunt,[13] 10% to 20% for pulmonary artery banding,[13] and 5% to 10% for the bidirectional Glenn shunt.[3, 33] Unfortunately, even if early palliation is successful, attainment of a Fontan correction is not ensured. In a study of 237 consecutive infants with tricuspid atresia, Franklin and colleagues[16] noted that after palliation almost 10% of patients died suddenly and another 16% became unsuitable candidates for a Fontan procedure owing to the development of left ventricular dysfunction, subaortic stenosis, or pulmonary artery distortion.

For patients with tricuspid atresia undergoing Fontan correction, operative mortality has improved significantly in the past decade. At the Mayo Clinic, mortality decreased from 17% before 1980 to 8% between 1981 and 1989.[23] Mortality rates of less than 5% are now being reported, especially in low-risk patient groups.[19, 25, 26] A common early complication after the Fontan procedure is the development of pleural

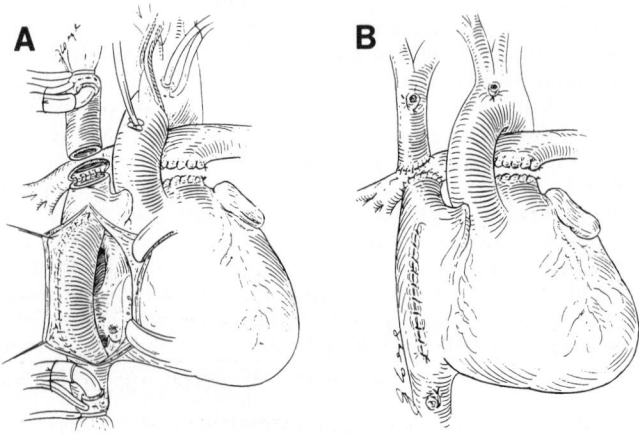

Figure 54–77. Modification of the Fontan procedure referred to as lateral tunnel with total cavopulmonary anastomosis. *A,* A polytetrafluoroethylene patch is inserted within the right atrium, creating a tunnel of uniform diameter between the orifices of the superior and inferior venae cavae. The main pulmonary artery is transected and oversewn proximally and distally. The superior vena cava is divided, and each end is anastomosed end-to-side into the right pulmonary artery. *B,* The completed total cavopulmonary connection. (From Stein, D. G., Laks, H., Drinkwater, D. C., Permut, L. C., Louie, H. W., Pearl, J. M., George, B. L., and Williams, R. G.: Results of total cavopulmonary connection in the treatment of patients with a functional single ventricle. J. Thorac. Cardovasc. Surg., 102:280, 1991.)

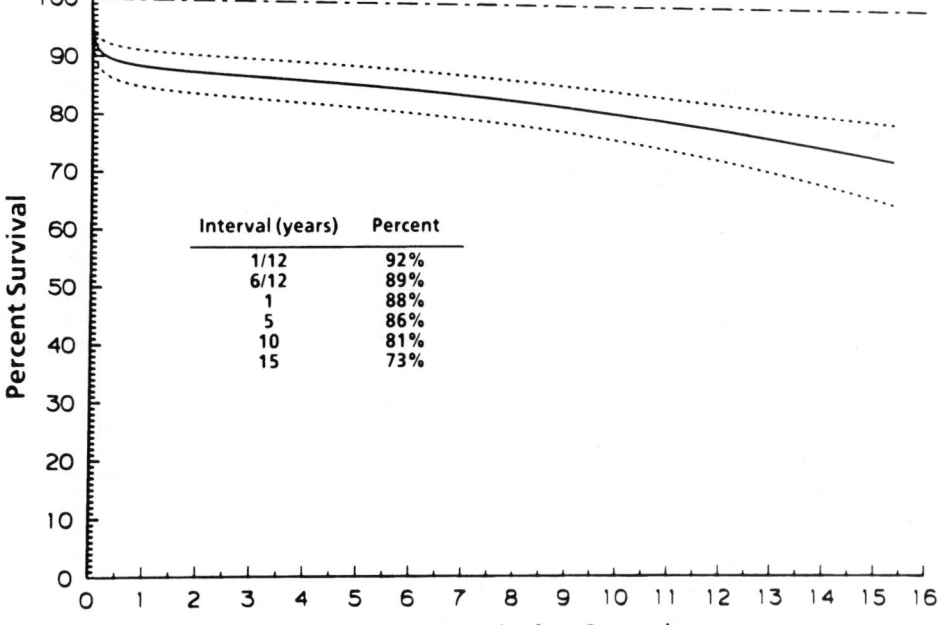

Figure 54–78. Predicted survival after a "perfect Fontan operation" performed under ideal circumstances. This curve was derived from a multivariate analysis of risk factors in a group of 334 patients undergoing Fontan correction between 1968 and 1988. An equation for a nomogram of risk of death over time was derived. When optimal values for each risk factor were entered, this predicted survival curve was derived. (Reproduced with permssion from Fontan, F., Kirklin, J. W., Fernandez, G., Costa, F., Naftel, D. C., Tritto, F., and Blackstone, E. H.: Outcome after a "perfect" Fontan operation. Circulation, 81:1520, 1990. Copyright 1990, American Heart Association.)

Interval (years)	Percent
1/12	92%
6/12	89%
1	88%
5	86%
10	81%
15	73%

effusions, which can persist for greater than a week in as many as 30% of patients.[27]

After a successful Fontan procedure, exercise tolerance and cardiorespiratory responses to exercise are significantly improved over the preoperative state but do not attain normal levels.[9] Over 85% of patients classify themselves as in good to excellent condition with minimal or no physical limitations.[24] Long-term follow-up is now available past 15 years.[10, 15, 23] In a heterogeneous group of patients, Fontan and associates[15] reported 69% 5-year, 63% 10-year, and 52% 15-year survival. Normalizing for optimal risk factors they predicted an 86% 5-year, 81% 10-year, and 73% 15-year survival (Fig. 54–78). The causes of death included arrhythmia, heart failure, sud-

den unexplained deaths, and problems associated with reoperation for conduit or allograft obstruction.[11] Other long-term complications include protein-losing enteropathy[7] and pulmonary arteriovenous fistulas.[28] After the Fontan procedure over 85% of patients are in New York Heart Association functional Class I, but with time the percentage of patients in Class I diminishes (Fig. 54–79). The late and slow-rising risk of death and diminished functional capacity noted by Fontan and associates is probably related to the Fontan physiology itself, emphasizing the limitations of a single ventricle even when cyanosis and volume overload have been minimized. These long-term results, however, are based on strategies and techniques that were applied over 10 years ago.

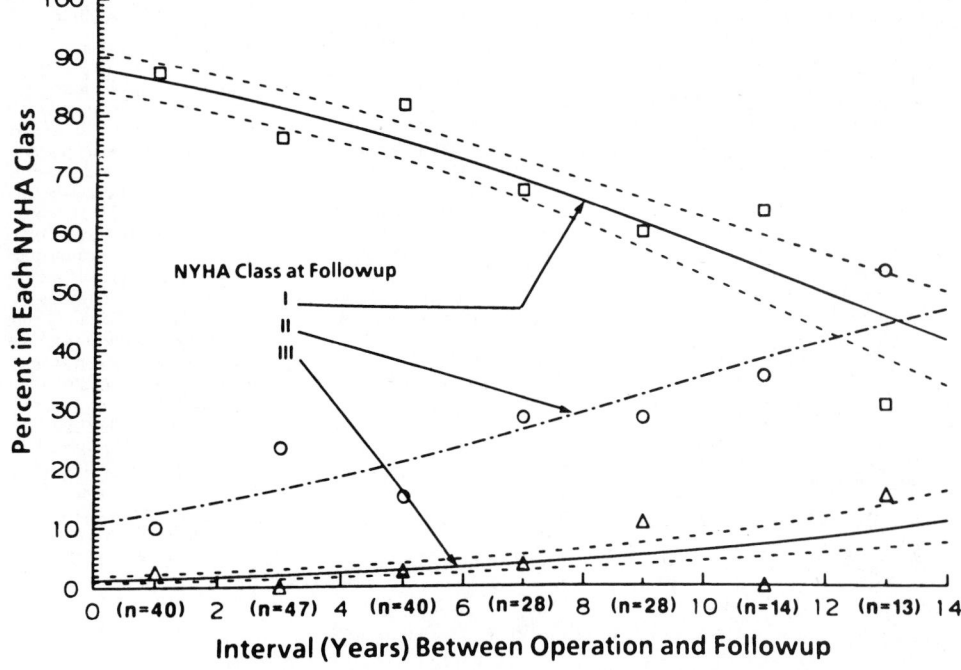

Figure 54–79. Per cent of patients in each New York Heart Association (NYHA) functional class after the Fontan operation. The solid lines show parametrically determined percentages for classes I and III with dashed lines encompassing 70% confidence intervals. The squares, circles, and triangles represent actual percentages. (Reproduced with permission from Fontan, F., Kirklin, J. W., Fernandez, G., Costa, F., Naftel, D. C., Tritto, F., and Blackstone, E. H.: Outcome after a "perfect" Fontan operation. Circulation, 81:1520, 1990. Copyright 1990, American Heart Association.)

Newer strategies that minimize exposure of the myocardium to cyanosis and volume overload as well as technical modifications that improve the efficiency of the Fontan circulation should further improve the longevity and functional status of patients born with tricuspid atresia.

SELECTED REFERENCES

Cowgill, L. D.: The Fontan procedure: A historical review. Ann. Thorac. Surg., 51:1026, 1991.
This is an interesting discussion of the experimental background leading to the clinical application of the Fontan procedure. Modifications in the operation that have occurred over the last 20 years are reviewed.

Fontan, F., Kirklin, J. W., Fernandez, G., Costa, F., Naftel, D. C., Tritto, F., and Blackstone, E. H.: Outcome after a "perfect" Fontan operation. Circulation, 81:1520, 1990.
This important study recognizes the limited long-term results of the Fontan procedure.

Franklin, R. C., Spiegelhalter, D. J., Sullivan, I. D., Anderson, R. H., Thoele, D. G., Shinebourne, E. A., and Deanfield, J. E.: Tricuspid atresia presenting in infancy: Survival and suitability for the Fontan operation. Circulation, 87:427, 1993.
A comprehensive evaluation of 237 consecutive infants with tricuspid atresia that presented between 1972 and 1987 was done. The accumulating incidence of adverse events resulting in death or unsuitability for Fontan correction argues for performing the procedure in patients younger than 4 years of age.

Mair, D. D., Hagler, D. J., Puga, F. J., Schaff, H. V., and Danielson, G. K.: Fontan operation in 176 patients with tricuspid atresia: Results and a proposed new index for patient selection. Circulation, 82(Suppl. 5):IV-164, 1990.
In this most recent update of the Mayo Clinic's extensive experience with the Fontan procedure for tricuspid atresia, a significant improvement in hospital mortality was noted.

REFERENCES

1. Bellet, S., and Stewart, H. L.: Congenital heart disease, atresia of tricuspid orifice. Am. J. Dis. Child., 45:1247, 1933.
2. Blalock, A., and Taussig, H. B.: The surgical treatments of malformations of the heart in which there is pulmonary stenosis or pulmonary atresia. JAMA, 132:627, 1946.
3. Bridges, N. D., Jonas, R. A., Mayer, J. E., Flanagan, M. F., Keane, J. F., and Castañeda, A. R.: Bidirectional cavopulmonary anastomosis as interim palliation for high-risk Fontan candidates: Early results. Circulation, 82:(Suppl. IV):IV-170, 1990.
4. Carlon, C. A., Mondini, P. G., and De Marchi, R.: Surgical treatment of some cardiovascular diseases. J. Int. Coll. Surg., 16:1, 1951.
5. Choussat, A., Fontan, F., Besse, P., Vallot, F., Chauve, A., and Bricaud, H.: Selection criteria for Fontan procedure. In Anderson R. H., and Shinebourne, E. A. (Eds.): Paediatric Cardiology. Edinburgh, Churchill Livingstone, 1978, pp. 559–566.
6. Cowgill, L. D.: The Fontan procedure: A historical review. Ann. Thorac. Surg., 51:1026, 1991.
7. Crupi, G., Locatelli, G., Tiraboschi, R., et al.: Protein-losing enteropathy after Fontan operation for tricuspid atresia (imperforate tricuspid valve). Thorac. Cardiovasc. Surg., 28:359, 1980.
8. de Leval, M. R., Kilner, P., Gewillig, M., Bull, C., and McGoon, D. C.: Total cavopulmonary connection: A logical alternative to atriopulmonary connection for complex Fontan operations. J. Thorac. Cardiovasc. Surg., 96:682, 1988.
9. Driscoll, D. J., Danielson, G. K., Puga, F. J., Schaff, H. V., Heise, C. T., and Statts, B. A.: Exercise tolerance and cardiorespiratory response to exercise after the Fontan operation for tricuspid atresia or functional single ventricle. J. Am. Coll. Cardiol., 7:1087, 1986.
10. Driscoll, D. J., Offord, K. P., Feldt, R. H., Schaff, H. V., Puga, F. J., and Danielson, G. K.: Five- to fifteen-year follow-up after Fontan operation. Circulation, 85:469, 1992.
11. Fernandez, G., Costa, F., Fontan, F., Naftel, D. C., Blackstone, E. H., and Kirklin, J. W.: Prevalence of reoperation for pathway obstruction after Fontan operation. Ann. Thorac. Surg., 48:654, 1989.
12. Fesslova, V., Hunter, S., Stark, J., and Taylor, J. F.: Long-term clinical outcome of patients with tricuspid atresia: I. "Natural history." J. Cardiovasc. Surg., 30:262, 1989.
13. Fesslova, V., Hunter, S., Stark, J., and Taylor, J. F.: The long-term clinical

outcome of patients with tricuspid atresia: II. Influence of surgical procedures. J. Cardiovasc. Surg., 32:225, 1991.
14. Fontan, F., and Baudet, E.: Surgical repair of tricuspid atresia. Thorax, 26:240, 1971.
15. Fontan, F., Kirklin, J. W., Fernandez, G., Costa, F., Naftel, D. C., Tritto, F., and Blackstone, E. H.: Outcome after a "perfect" Fontan operation. Circulation, 81:1520, 1990.
16. Franklin, R. C., Spiegelhalter, D. J., Sullivan, I. D., Anderson, R. H., Thoele, D. G., Shinebourne, E. A., and Deanfield, J. E.: Tricuspid atresia presenting in infancy: Survival and suitability for the Fontan operation. Circulation, 87:427, 1993.
17. Glenn, W. W. L.: Circulatory bypass of the right side of the heart: II. Shunt between superior vena cava and distal right pulmonary artery—report of a clinical application. N. Engl. J. Med., 259:117, 1958.
18. Glenn, W. W. L., and Patino, J. F.: Circulatory bypass of the right heart: I. Preliminary observations on the direct delivery of vena caval blood into the pulmonary arterial circulation: Azygos vein-pulmonary artery shunt. Yale J. Biol. Med., 27:147, 1954.
19. Jacobs, M. L., and Norwood, W. I.: Fontan operation: Influence of modifications on morbidity and mortality. Ann. Thorac. Surg., 58:945, 1994.
20. Jonas, R. A., and Castañeda, A. R.: Modified Fontan procedure: Atrial baffle and systemic venous to pulmonary artery anastomotic techniques. J. Card. Surg., 3:91, 1988.
21. Kirklin, J. K., Blackstone, E. H., Kirklin, J. W., Pacifico, A. D., and Bargeron, L. M., Jr.: The Fontan operation: Ventricular hypertrophy, age, and date of operation as risk factors. J. Thorac. Cardiovasc. Surg., 92:1049, 1986.
22. Kuhne, M.: Uber zwei Falle kongenitaler Atresie des Ostium venosum dextrum. Jahrb. Kinderheilkd. Phys. Erziehung, 63:235, 1906.
23. Mair, D. D., Hagler, D. J., Puga, F. J., Schaff, H. V., and Danielson, G. K.: Fontan operation in 176 patients with tricuspid atresia: Results and a proposed new index for patient selection. Circulation, 82(Suppl. 5):IV-164, 1990.
24. Mair, D. D., Puga, F. J., and Danielson, G. K.: Late functional status of survivors of the Fontan procedure performed during the 1970s. Circulation, 86(Suppl. II):II-106, 1992.
25. Malm, T., Pawade, A., Karl, T. R., and Mee, R. B.: Recent results with the modified Fontan operation. Scand. J. Thorac. Cardiovasc. Surg., 27:65, 1993.
26. Mayer, J. E., Jr., Bridges, N. D., Lock, J. E., Hanley, F. L., Jonas, R. A., and Castañeda, A. R.: Factors associated with marked reduction in mortality for Fontan operations in patients with single ventricle. J. Thorac. Cardiovasc. Surg., 103:444, 1992.
27. Mayer, J. E., Jr., Helgason, H., Jonas, R. A., et al.: Extending the limits for modified Fontan procedures. J. Thorac. Cardiovasc. Surg., 92:1021, 1986.
28. Moore, J. W., Kirby, W. C., Madden, W. A., and Gaither, N. S.: Development of pulmonary arteriovenous malformations after modified Fontan operation. J. Thorac. Cardiovasc. Surg., 92:1021, 1989.
29. Pearl, J. M., Laks, H., Drinkwater, D. C., Capouya, E. R., George, B. L., and Williams, R. G.: Modified Fontan procedure in patients less than 4 years of age. Circulation, 86:(Suppl. II):II-100, 1992.
30. Rao, P. S.: Demographic features of tricuspid atresia. In Rao, P. S. (Ed.): Tricuspid Atresia, 2nd ed. Mount Kisco, N. Y., Futura Publishing, 1992, p. 26.
31. Robicsek, R., Temesvari, A., and Kadar, R. L.: A new method for the treatment of congenital heart disease associated with impaired pulmonary circulation. Acta Med. Scand., 154:151, 1956.
32. Rodbard, S., and Wagner, D.: Bypassing the right ventricle. Proc. Soc. Exp. Biol. Med., 71:69, 1949.
33. Salmon, A. P., Sethia, B., Silove, E. D., Goh, D., Mitchell, I., Alton, H., De Giovanni, J. V., Wright, J. G. C., and Abrams, L. D.: Cavopulmonary anastomosis as long-term palliation for patients with tricuspid atresia. Eur. J. Cardiothorac. Surg., 3:494, 1989.
34. Starr, L., Jeffers, W. A., and Meade, R. H., Jr.: The absence of conspicuous increments of venous pressure after severe damage to the right ventricle of the dog, with a discussion of the relation between clinical congestive failure and heart disease. Am. Heart J., 26:291, 1943.
35. Stein, D. G., Laks, H., Drinkwater, D. C., Permut, L. C., Louie, H. W., Pearl, J. M., George, B. L., and Williams, R. G.: Results of total cavopulmonary connection in the treatment of patients with a functional single ventricle. J. Thorac. Cardiovasc. Surg., 102:280, 1991.
36. Tandon, R., and Edwards, J. E.: Tricuspid atresia: A re-evaluation and classification. J. Thorac. Cardiovasc. Surg., 67:530, 1974.
37. Taussig, H. B.: The clinical and pathological findings in congenital malformation of the heart due to defective development of the right ventricle associated with tricuspid atresia or hypoplasia. Bull. Johns Hopkins Hosp., 59:435, 1936.
38. Trusler, G. A., Williams, W. G., Cohen, A. J., Rabinovitch, M., Moes, C. A. F., Smallhorn, J. F., Coles, J. G., Lightfoot, N. E., and Freedom, R. M.: The cavopulmonary shunt: Evolution of a concept. Circulation, 82(Suppl. IV):IV-131, 1990.

X _____

HYPOPLASTIC LEFT HEART SYNDROME

Erle H. Austin III, M.D.

Hypoplastic left heart syndrome comprises a group of cardiac anomalies characterized by an inadequately developed left ventricle and a hypoplastic ascending aorta. The spectrum of defects ranges from aortic valve stenosis with a left ventricle incapable of supporting the systemic circulation to combined aortic and mitral atresia with complete absence of the left ventricle. In this syndrome the right ventricle is the only effective ventricle and must, in addition to providing pulmonary blood flow, also provide systemic blood flow through a patent ductus arteriosus. Hypoplastic left heart syndrome is the most common form of univentricular heart and the most common cardiac malformation resulting in death of the neonate.[51] It occurs in about 0.15 per 1000 live births, making up 4% to 9% of congenital heart defects presenting in the neonate.[8, 23, 25, 32] Approximately two thirds of affected infants are male. Without intervention, 70% of these infants die within the first week of life and over 90% are dead within the first month. Despite the lethal nature of this cardiac defect, the majority of these children are otherwise well developed without associated extracardiac anomalies.[23, 32]

Before the early 1980s, hypoplastic left heart syndrome was considered an untreatable condition, and virtually all neonates diagnosed with this defect were allowed to die without intervention. During the 1980s, however, hope for survival of these otherwise doomed infants arrived with two independently derived surgical strategies. In Boston and Philadelphia, Norwood developed a staged reconstructive approach culminating in the application of the Fontan procedure. Almost concurrently, in Loma Linda, California, Bailey demonstrated the feasibility of cardiac transplantation in infants born with this fatal condition.

HISTORICAL ASPECTS

The pathologic components of hypoplastic left heart syndrome were described in the early 1900s, but it was not until 1952 that Lev recognized the interrelationships of the left-sided and aortic complexes.[28] The pathophysiology and natural history were described by Taussig in 1947.[49] The term *hypoplastic left heart syndrome* was coined in 1958 by Noonan and Nadas[34] in a comprehensive review describing the spectrum of abnormalities. The first successful surgical palliation was reported by Cayler and associates in 1970.[13] Several other authors reported variations on this technique.[18, 29, 37] The potential for physiologic correction of patients born with a solitary ventricle was realized with the report of Fontan and Baudet[21] in 1971 describing an operation for tricuspid atresia. In 1983, Norwood and associates reported the first successful Fontan procedure to follow surgical palliation of hypoplastic left heart syndrome.[38] The recognition that surgical palliation could permit infants with this anomaly to survive to successful Fontan correction encouraged other surgeons to attempt Norwood's procedure. Most early series, however, demonstrated a very high mortality.[44] As another potential solution for hypoplastic left heart syndrome, Bailey and associates introduced neonatal heart transplantation in 1984.[5] The first attempt received international attention because the donor heart was taken from a baboon. Although success in this case was short lived and the use of a nonhuman donor controversial, it brought much attention to the plight of infants born with this fatal condition. Within months Bailey

successfully transplanted a human heart into another neonate with hypoplastic left heart syndrome.[4]

PATHOLOGIC ANATOMY

As the name implies, hypoplastic left heart syndrome represents a spectrum of malformations in which the left ventricle is markedly undersized and the aortic and/or mitral valves are stenotic or atretic. Over 60% of cases have aortic valve atresia, and the majority of these also have mitral valve atresia (Fig. 54–80). The next most common subgroup has severe aortic stenosis and mitral stenosis. In cases with aortic atresia, the ascending aorta is very small (2–3 mm. in diameter), because it only provides a retrograde pathway for coronary blood flow. Cases with aortic stenosis have somewhat larger ascending aortas (4–5 mm.). In most cases of hypoplastic left heart syndrome, the aortic arch is also hypoplastic (3–5 mm.). In contrast to the tiny ascending aorta, the main pulmonary artery is large (11–15 mm.). The ductus arteriosus, which appears as a direct extension from the main pulmonary artery, curves posteriorly to join the proximal descending aorta. At this junction, a coarctation shelf commonly

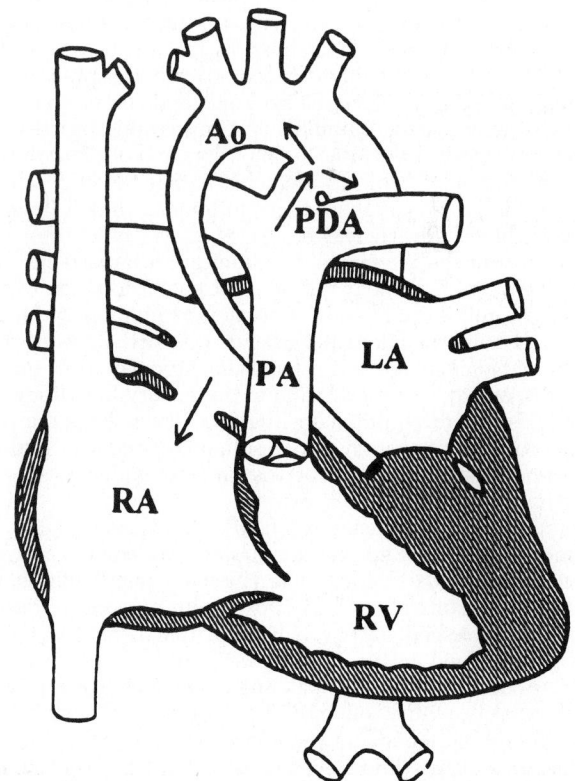

Figure 54–80. Hypoplastic left heart syndrome with aortic atresia, mitral atresia, and marked hypoplasia of the left ventricle. The right ventricle (RV) provides blood flow through the pulmonary artery (PA) to the lungs and through a patent ductus arteriosus (PDA) to the body. The tiny ascending aorta (Ao) serves as a conduit for retrograde flow to the coronary arteries. Pulmonary venous return must pass from the left atrium (LA) to the right atrium (RA) through a patent foramen ovale or atrial septal defect. (From Zahka, K. G., Spector, M., and Hanisch, D.: Hypoplastic left heart syndrome: Norwood operation, transplantation, or compassionate care. Clin. Perinatol., 20:145, 1993.)

exists. The diminutive aortic arch often looks more like a small branch of the ductus than what would be expected for the most proximal portion of the aorta.

PATHOPHYSIOLOGY

The absence of a functional left ventricle causes a major alteration in circulation, with the right ventricle solely responsible for propelling blood and a patent ductus arteriosus the only route to the systemic circulation. Prenatally, oxygenation is derived from the placenta, and this oxygenated blood is delivered by the right ventricle through the patent ductus arteriosus to the body. Flow in the aortic arch and the ascending aorta is retrograde, providing blood to the upper body and coronary circulation. Cardiac output and the delivery of oxygen to the tissues is usually adequate *in utero,* such that most infants survive full-term pregnancy and are usually born at a normal birth weight. At birth, pulmonary blood flow and venous return become important because the oxygenated blood returning from the lungs must pass through an interatrial communication to join the desaturated blood that has returned from the body to the right atrium. The relative contributions of pulmonary and systemic venous blood that mix in the right atrium result in a hypoxemic cardiac output from the right ventricle that must provide parallel blood flow to the lungs through the branch pulmonary arteries and to the body through the ductus arteriosus. The balance between pulmonary and systemic blood flow is determined by the relative ratio of vascular resistances in the pulmonary and systemic circulations. At birth, these resistances are similar; but within hours pulmonary vascular resistance begins to decrease, and a greater proportion of the cardiac output is directed to the lungs with a diminishing proportion to the body. Moreover, as the ductus arteriosus begins to close, the shift of blood toward the pulmonary circulation and away from the systemic (and coronary) circulation is accentuated. Without intervention, this process results in progressive acidosis, hypotension, and death. Arterial oxygen saturation typically demonstrates increasing values during this process as the ratio of pulmonary blood flow to systemic blood flow increases.

The size of the interatrial communication importantly affects the pathophysiology. The typical patent foramen ovale imposes a mild-to-moderate restriction to pulmonary blood flow and helps maintain the balance of blood flow toward the systemic circulation. If a large unrestrictive atrial septal defect exists, the only restriction to pulmonary blood flow is what exists at the pulmonary arteriolar level. Thus the potential for overcirculation to the pulmonary bed and undercirculation to the systemic bed is greatest under these circumstances. At the other extreme, a severely restrictive communication between the left and right atria results in pulmonary venous hypertension, pulmonary edema, and inadequate pulmonary blood flow. The inadequate pulmonary blood flow results in severe hypoxia with inadequate tissue delivery of oxygen despite a balance that favors systemic delivery of blood.

After successful surgical palliation, single-ventricle physiology persists, with a solitary right ventricle providing blood flow to both systemic and pulmonary circulations. With the ductus arteriosus eliminated, unobstructed right ventricular output is directed into the systemic circulation, and pulmonary blood flow is limited by the insertion of a small (3.5 mm.) conduit from the systemic arterial to pulmonary arterial system. Pulmonary venous hypertension is avoided, and mixing of pulmonary and systemic venous blood is improved by complete excision of atrial septal tissue. At this point a satisfactory balance between pulmonary and systemic circulation is affected by the relative vascular resistances of these two circulations. As in the preoperative condition, supplemental oxygen tends to decrease pulmonary vascular resistance, whereas elevated levels of Pco_2 tend to increase it. Recognition of these effects permits optimal balance of pulmonary and systemic blood flow (Q_P/Q_S) at presentation as well as after initial palliative reconstruction.

CLINICAL PRESENTATION

Infants with hypoplastic left heart syndrome are typically born after a full-term pregnancy and are normal in birth weight. Apgar scores are usually normal at birth. In most cases the child appears completely normal at first, but within 24 to 48 hours tachypnea and mild cyanosis are noted. As the ductus arteriosus closes, the infant becomes pale, lethargic, and poorly perfused. Oliguria and metabolic acidosis develop and, without intervention, death often ensues within hours.

Cardiac examination reveals a dominant right ventricular impulse and a loud single S_2. A soft systolic murmur may be heard at the left sternal border. Chest radiography usually demonstrates cardiomegaly and increased pulmonary blood flow. Electrocardiography reveals right ventricular hypertrophy. Oximetric measures of peripheral oxygen saturation range from 70% to 95%. The higher the saturation the more likely the infant will be poorly perfused. Any neonate who presents with tachypnea, mild cyanosis, cardiomegaly, pulmonary plethora, and marginal peripheral perfusion should be assumed to have hypoplastic left heart syndrome and appropriate measures (prostaglandin E_1; avoidance of oxygen) instituted before the diagnosis is confirmed.

Definitive diagnosis is made by two-dimensional echocardiography. The tiny ascending aorta is characteristically identified along with a very large pulmonary artery. Furthermore, a large dominant right ventricle with a diminutive (or even absent) left ventricle is seen. Cardiac catheterization rarely adds additional information and is only performed in cases when echocardiography suggests an atypical pattern.

The increasing application of ultrasonography in obstetrics has led to the field of fetal echocardiography. At present, hypoplastic left heart syndrome can be reliably diagnosed prenatally.[1] Prenatal diagnosis is especially valuable in hypoplastic left heart syndrome because it allows parents time to understand and prepare for the birth. Planning on delivery at or near a facility experienced in caring for infants with hypoplastic left heart syndrome permits proper management from the moment of birth and avoids circulatory instability with its potential for organ (liver and kidney) damage.

INITIAL MANAGEMENT

Initial management must be individualized but follows general principles. Intravenous infusion of prostaglandin E_1 (0.05 to 0.1 µg./kg./min.) is started immediately to ensure ductal patency and systemic blood flow. Supplemental oxygen is strictly avoided except in the rare patient with severe hypoxemia (O_2 sat $< 65\%$) from inadequate pulmonary blood flow. Placement of an umbilical arterial catheter permits arterial blood pressure monitoring and blood sampling. The placement of an umbilical venous catheter may also be valuable to provide central venous access for reliable delivery of prostaglandin E_1 and for monitoring systemic venous saturations in the inferior vena cava. Further management is directed at achieving a balance between pulmonary and systemic blood flow ($Q_P/Q_S \cong 1$). Evidence of optimal balance are *ideal* arterial blood gases with a pH of 7.40, a Pco_2 of 40 to 45 mm. Hg, and a Po_2 of 40 mm. Hg. How this balance is achieved is determined by the condition of the infant at presentation. In general, patients can be divided into three

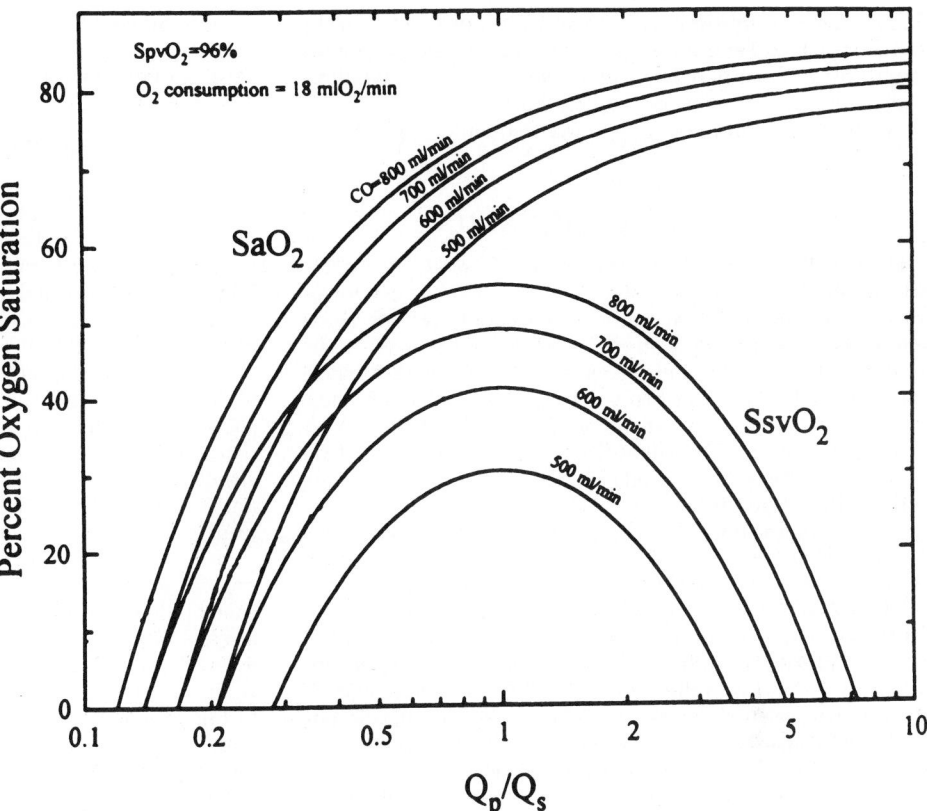

Figure 54–81. Per cent oxygen saturation of systemic arterial (SaO$_2$) and venous (SsvO$_2$) blood as a function of the pulmonary/systemic flow ratio (Q$_P$/Q$_S$) for different values of cardiac output (CO) in hypoplastic left heart syndrome. The SaO$_2$ curve flattens as the Q$_P$/Q$_S$ exceeds 2, making additional increases in this value insensitive to major increases in pulmonary blood flow. Concomitant measurement of systemic venous oxygen saturation (SsvO$_2$) allows recognition of a significant imbalance in systemic and pulmonary blood flow. SpvO$_2$, per cent oxygen saturation of pulmonary venous blood. (From Barnea, O., Austin, E. H., Richman, B., and Santamore, W. B.: Balancing the circulation: Theoretic optimization of pulmonary/systemic flow ratio in hypoplastic left heart syndrome. J. Am. Coll. Cardiol., *24*:1376, 1994. Reprinted with permission from the American College of Cardiology.)

groups: (1) those with nearly balanced circulations as a consequence of a relatively restrictive interatrial septum; (2) those with torrential pulmonary blood flow from an unrestricted atrial septal defect; and (3) those with insufficient pulmonary blood flow due to an inadequate interatrial communication.

Patients presenting with balanced circulations can be managed expectantly. They should only require intubation and mechanical ventilation if apnea develops as a result of the prostaglandin E$_1$ infusion. Patients with torrential pulmonary blood flow usually present with metabolic acidosis (base deficits of 8 or greater) from systemic hypoperfusion. To compensate for the acidosis, these infants hyperventilate to lower the arterial PCO$_2$. Unfortunately this creates a further reduction in pulmonary vascular resistance, a greater shift of blood flow away from the systemic circulation, and a progressively worse metabolic acidosis. Although intravenous administration of sodium bicarbonate may be effective in some of these patients, many require tracheal intubation, neuromuscular blockade, and mechanical ventilation, allowing the PCO$_2$ to rise to 40 to 45 mm. Hg. Again, supplemental oxygen must be avoided. Other techniques to increase pulmonary vascular resistance to redirect a greater proportion of the cardiac output to the systemic circulation include the addition of positive end-expiratory pressure, the dilution of room air with nitrogen to decrease the FIO$_2$ to as low as 0.16, and the addition of CO$_2$ into the inspired gas mixture.[19, 26] In addition to regular evaluation of arterial blood gases, continuous monitoring of peripheral arterial saturations with pulse oximetry allows continuous estimation of Q$_P$/Q$_S$. A peripheral arterial saturation between 70% and 80% is usually associated with a Q$_P$/Q$_S$ in the range of 1:1 to 2:1. When peripheral arterial saturations exceed 80% to 85%, each incremental increase in arterial saturation is associated with a progressively greater increase in Q$_P$/Q$_S$. Thus, when peripheral arterial saturations are consistently greater than 85%, it is useful to have access to systemic venous oxygen satura-

tions (Fig. 54–81).[6, 42] Blood sampled from the inferior vena cava through an umbilical venous catheter or a continuous readout from an oximetric catheter (5F) positioned in the inferior vena cava permits direct calculation of Q$_P$/Q$_S$* and allows reliable assessment of the effects of ventilatory and pharmacologic manipulations on the distribution of blood between the two circulations. Systemic venous saturations consistent with satisfactory oxygen delivery to the tissues usually exceed 40% and for an individual patient can be expected to reach a peak value when Q$_P$/Q$_S$ is equal to 1.[6]

Because most infants with hypoplastic left heart syndrome can be stabilized satisfactorily with these techniques, the small group with inadequate interatrial flow must be expeditiously treated with tracheal intubation, mechanical ventilation, supplemental oxygen, and emergency relief of the pulmonary venous obstruction. This can be done transvenously in the cardiac catheterization laboratory with a limited atrial septostomy or, if conditions are suitable, by proceeding immediately to surgery for a Norwood procedure.

The majority of infants can be stabilized within 24 to 48 hours of presentation. During that period the next course of action is decided after thorough discussions between the medical caregivers and the infant's parents. If staged reconstruction or transplantation is elected, it is important that any major organ dysfunction (e.g., hepatic, renal) resulting from the initial circulatory collapse be allowed to resolve before surgical intervention is initiated. If transplantation is elected, it is preferable for the infant to be weaned off me-

---

*Q$_P$/Q$_S$ is calculated using a Fick equation: Q$_P$/Q$_S$ = Ao sat $-$ M̄vO$_2$ sat/P̄v sat $-$ PA sat, where Ao sat = systemic arterial O$_2$ saturation, M̄vO$_2$ = mixed venous O$_2$ saturation, P̄v sat = pulmonary venous O$_2$ saturation, and PA sat = pulmonary artery O$_2$ saturation. For these patients pulmonary artery O$_2$ saturations and systemic arterial O$_2$ saturations are the same. Pulmonary venous O$_2$ saturation is assumed to be 96%.

chanical ventilatory support, maintained on prostaglandin E$_1$ and room air, and started on enteral nutrition. The placement of a Broviac central line is advisable for infants awaiting transplantation so that prostaglandin E$_1$ infusion can be maintained without interruption and frequent peripheral intravenous insertions are avoided.

SURGICAL MANAGEMENT

The development of the Norwood procedure and the introduction of neonatal heart transplantation have clearly introduced hope for children born with hypoplastic left heart syndrome. Unfortunately, they have also introduced a dilemma for the parents and physicians. Staged reconstruction and neonatal heart transplantation are themselves in their infancy. The long-term outcomes of children treated with either approach remain unknown. This uncertainty must be conveyed to the parents along with the relative advantages and disadvantages of the two procedures. Because long-term success cannot be reliably predicted, at most institutions compassionate care (no treatment) remains an option for these infants. In the current state of experience, a consensus regarding the best treatment approach has not been reached. Some centers recommend compassionate care, some are committed to transplantation,[15] others are committed to staged reconstruction,[24, 35] and yet others try to provide both approaches.[47] If well-informed physicians who deal with hypoplastic left heart syndrome on a regular basis cannot reach a consensus, how can a parent who has just learned about the defect be expected to know what to do? Thus, while hope has been extended to these families, much uncertainty and many unanswered questions remain. Parents must be given time to understand the diagnosis and prognosis, as well as the treatment options. A compassionate physician must honestly explain the options and expected results without imposing personal bias. If the family chooses compassionate care, the prostaglandin E$_1$ is discontinued and the family is allowed to comfort the infant until death. If treatment is chosen, ductal patency is maintained with prostaglandin E$_1$ until surgical palliation or heart transplantation is performed.

Staged Reconstruction

Surgery for hypoplastic left heart syndrome is based on the understanding that one functional ventricle must provide blood flow to both the systemic and pulmonary circulations in a balanced and efficient fashion. In older children, the Fontan procedure makes the most efficient use of a single ventricle by placing the two circulations in series and employing the single ventricle to provide the solitary propulsive force to propel blood through two successive resistances. Unfortunately, high pulmonary vascular resistance precludes successful application of the Fontan procedure in the neonate.[17] If, however, univentricular cardiac output can be constructed to provide parallel and equal blood flow to the body and lungs, satisfactory hemodynamics can permit survival until pulmonary vascular resistance decreases to a level that permits placing the two circulations in series. The Norwood procedure is such a construction, designed to mimic the more easily palliated conditions of tricuspid atresia and pulmonary atresia. The essential principles of the Norwood procedure include (1) creation of an unobstructed pathway from the right ventricle to the systemic circulation; (2) provision of pulmonary blood flow sufficient for adequate tissue oxygenation but regulated to avoid volume overload on the ventricle and the development of pulmonary vascular obstructive disease; and (3) excision of the interatrial septum to prevent pulmonary venous hypertension.

The Norwood procedure requires cardiopulmonary bypass as well as deep hypothermic circulatory arrest. Once the circulation is arrested, the interatrial septum is excised and the branch pulmonary arteries are separated from the circulation by ligation and division of the ductus arteriosus and transection of the main pulmonary artery. With a gusset of

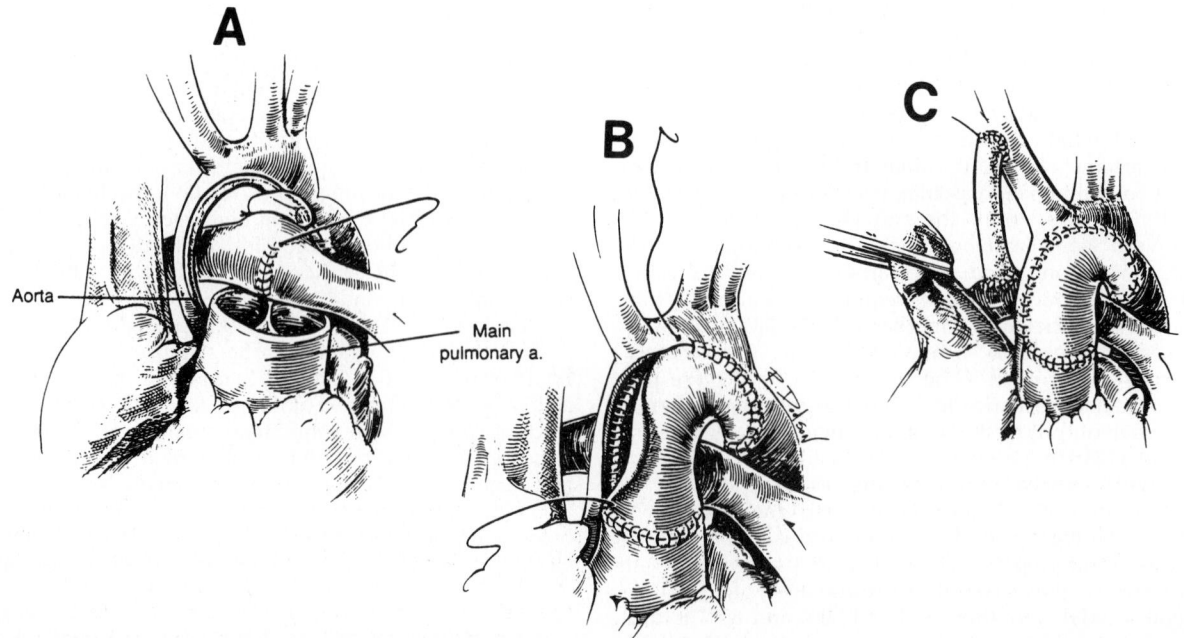

Figure 54–82. First-stage reconstruction of hypoplastic left heart syndrome: the Norwood procedure. *A,* The main pulmonary artery is divided just proximal to the bifurcation, the ductus arteriosus is ligated and divided, and the aortic arch is opened from the level of the divided pulmonary artery to at least 1 cm. distal to the entry site of the ductus. *B,* A gusset of pulmonary or aortic allograft is used to create an unobstructed anastomosis between the proximal divided main pulmonary artery and the ascending aorta, aortic arch, and proximal descending aorta. *C,* A 3.5-mm. polytetrafluoroethylene tube graft is placed between the innominate artery and the right pulmonary artery. An atrial septectomy is also performed during the period of circulatory arrest. (From Castañeda, A. R., Jonas, R. A., Mayer, J. E., and Hanley, F. L.: Cardiac Surgery of the Neonate and Infant. Philadelphia, W. B. Saunders, 1994.)

pulmonary homograft material, the proximal main pulmonary artery is anastomosed to the underside of the aortic arch and proximal descending aorta (Fig. 54–82). Cardiopulmonary bypass is reinstituted; and as rewarming progresses, a 3.5-mm. polytetrafluoroethylene tube graft is interposed from the innominate artery to the proximal right pulmonary artery. Cardiopulmonary bypass is discontinued at 37° C. At this point significant hypoxemia (oxygen saturations of 60%–65%) is common as a result of the effects of cardiopulmonary bypass on the lungs, the relatively high pulmonary vascular resistance of the neonate, and the restriction of pulmonary blood flow imposed by the shunt. An FIO_2 of 1.0 and vigorous ventilation to minimize PCO_2 to 25 to 35 mm. Hg are usually necessary initially. Within the first minutes to hours after the procedure, peripheral oxygen saturations begin to increase and the FIO_2 and ventilation are decreased appropriately. Continuous monitoring of peripheral arterial oxygen saturations and systemic venous saturations provides reliable feedback during the first 24 to 48 hours when abrupt alterations in the balance between pulmonary and systemic flows are most likely to occur.[6, 42] Sedation and paralysis with fentanyl and vecuronium are maintained for this period of time, and any manipulations such as endotracheal suctioning and weighing are minimized to avoid initiating pulmonary hypertensive crises. By 48 hours, paralysis is discontinued and sedation and mechanical ventilation are weaned to extubation. Oral feeding is begun along with regular doses of digoxin and furosemide. Hospital discharge is usually achieved 2 to 3 weeks postoperatively.

Regular and frequent cardiovascular evaluations are important up until the next stage. Complications that develop after the Norwood procedure include restriction at the atrial septum, pulmonary artery distortion, and aortic arch obstruction.[27] Arch obstruction after the Norwood procedure imposes a concomitant volume and pressure load on the right ventricle that can result in significant deterioration in ventricular function. This complication should be meticulously investigated with upper and lower extremity blood pressures and thorough echocardiography with pulsed Doppler interrogation of the reconstructed aorta. Significant arch obstruction warrants early reoperation or balloon dilation. If no problems are detected during routine evaluation, cardiac catheterization is performed between 3 and 6 months of age to confirm an unobstructed aortic arch as well as to evaluate the pulmonary arteries and ventricular function. Aortic arch obstruction and pulmonary artery distortion can be addressed at the second-stage procedure. A poorly contractile right ventricle, however, usually precludes further staged reconstruction, leaving cardiac transplantation as the only alternative.[9]

The initial treatment strategy developed by Norwood involved primary palliation followed by a Fontan procedure at 18 months of age. The attrition of patients between initial palliation and Fontan procedure, as well as a relatively high mortality for the Fontan in these patients, encouraged Norwood to change to a three-stage approach. The second stage is performed between 3 and 9 months of age and consists of changing the systemic-to-pulmonary artery shunt to a bidirectional superior cavopulmonary anastomosis (also referred to as a bidirectional Glenn procedure) (Fig. 54–83).[14, 41] With this technique, the systemic venous return from the upper body provides pulmonary blood flow and the volume load imposed on the ventricle by the previous shunt is eliminated. Because pulmonary and systemic venous returns continue to mix in the right atrium, cyanosis with saturations of 70% to 75% persist after the bidirectional Glenn procedure, but the diminished workload on the right ventricle tends to result in stable hemodynamics, allowing satisfactory survival and growth to some time between 18 months and 3 years,

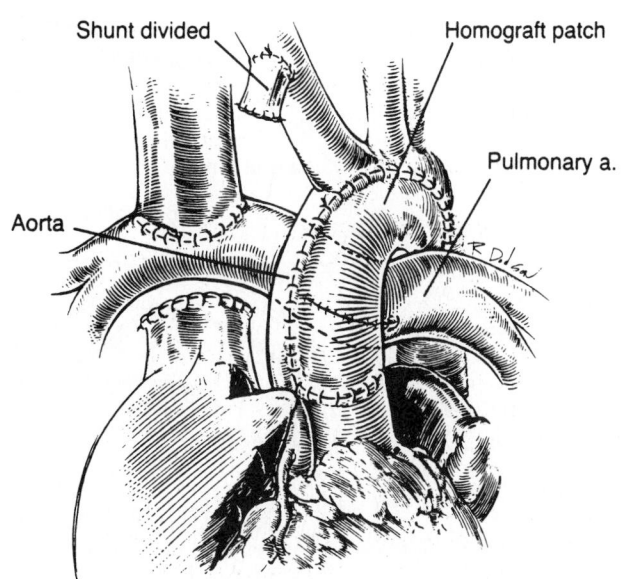

Figure 54–83. Second-stage reconstruction of hypoplastic left heart syndrome: The bidirectional Glenn shunt. The divided superior vena cava is anastomosed to the site of the distal anastomosis of the previous systemic to pulmonary artery shunt. (From Castañeda, A. R., Jonas, R. A., Mayer, J. E., and Hanley, F. L.: Cardiac Surgery of the Neonate and Infant. Philadelphia, W. B. Saunders, 1994.)

when the final stage (modified Fontan procedure) is performed. In this final stage, the systemic and pulmonary venous returns are separated by directing the inferior vena caval flow directly to the underside of the pulmonary artery (Fig. 54–84). The placement of a small fenestration in the baffle that separates the two venous returns diminishes the systemic venous pressure and augments the cardiac output at the expense of a small decrement in arterial saturation. This fenestration appears to ameliorate the postoperative course and diminish the incidence of postoperative effusions.[30]

Results of Staged Reconstruction. Early results of staged reconstruction for hypoplastic left heart syndrome were disappointing, with high mortality at initial palliation (37.5%–54%),[31, 33] a high incidence of interim deaths and complications, and a high mortality at Fontan correction (34%–50%).[20, 31] Based on the experience with staged reconstruction at the University of Michigan between 1983 and 1989, Meliones and colleagues[31] reported an estimated survival of only 34% at 6 months, 27% at 1 year, and 24% at 2 years. As experience has accrued, however, remarkable improvements in operative mortality and actuarial survival have been reported. At Children's Hospital of Philadelphia, operative mortality decreased from 37.5% (1985–1989) to 19% (1991–1992),[33, 36] while at the University of Michigan it decreased from 54% (1983–1989) to 15% (1990–1993).[24, 31] Reports from centers performing fewer procedures indicate that a mortality of approximately 15% can be achieved for the initial palliation.[42, 47] Conversion to a three-stage approach has also significantly diminished the operative risk of the Fontan procedure for these patients and improved the overall actuarial survival. At Children's Hospital of Philadelphia the hospital mortality for a modified Fontan procedure in hypoplastic left heart syndrome has decreased from 34% (1984–1989) to 5% (1991–1992).[20, 36] Based on their most recent results with a three-stage approach, the University of Michigan group is now able to report actuarial survivals of 76% at 6 months, 69% at 1 year, and 69% at 2 years.[24]

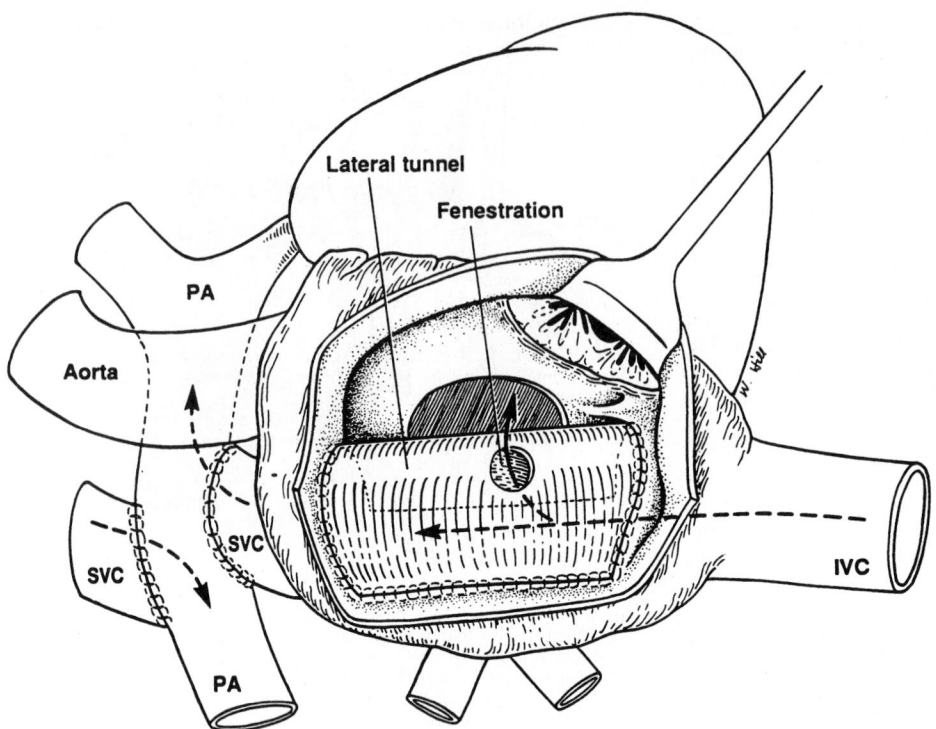

Figure 54–84. Final-stage reconstruction of hypoplastic left heart syndrome: The fenestrated Fontan procedure. Using a polytetrafluoroethylene patch, a tunnel is created in the lateral wall of the right atrium to direct inferior vena cava (IVC) flow to the superior vena cava (SVC) that is anastomosed to the pulmonary artery (PA). A 4- to 5-mm. fenestration in the baffle diminishes systemic venous pressure and improves cardiac output at the expense of a small decrease in systemic arterial oxygen saturation. (From Kopf, G. S., Kleinman, C. S., Hijazi, Z. M., Fahey, J. T., Dewar, M. L., and Hellenbrand, W. E.: Fenestrated Fontan operation with delayed transcatheter closure of atrial septal defect: Improved results in high-risk patients. J. Thorac. Cardiovasc. Surg., *103*:1039, 1992.)

Cardiac Transplantation

After initial hemodynamic stabilization, infants considered for transplantation undergo thorough screening to rule out genetic and neurologic malformations. Prostaglandin E_1 maintained by Broviac catheter is carefully weaned to a low dose (0.0125 μg./kg./min.) to minimize side effects. Infection must be assiduously avoided by minimizing endotracheal intubations and urinary and intravenous catheters. Enteral nutrition is started early, and adequate caloric intake is maintained. If blood transfusion is required, only irradiated, cytomegalovirus-negative, and white blood cell–filtered red blood cells are used.

Donor availability is the primary limitation to heart transplantation in neonates.[48] Most potential donors are victims of trauma or asphyxia. Although heightened awareness of the need for donor organs has increased organ donation, more centers are placing neonates on the waiting list. When the wait begins to exceed several weeks, problems with intercurrent infections and progressive heart failure lead to death in some infants before a donor heart becomes available. Some centers are proceeding to staged reconstruction if a donor does not become available within several weeks of life.[47] Other centers have employed interim palliative procedures, including transvenous atrial septostomy and the insertion of a ductal stent to permit longer survival until a donor is found.[43, 46] Such long waits, however, impose a significantly higher risk for the development of pulmonary vascular disease.

When a potential donor is identified, the donor heart is carefully evaluated by two-dimensional echocardiography. A shortening fraction of 35% or greater and the absence of mitral insufficiency is verified. At donor harvest, ventricular distention is avoided by widely incising the donor inferior vena cava and left atrium when the aortic cross-clamp is applied. Care should also be taken to include the donor arch. The recipient procedure (Fig. 54–85) requires cardiopulmonary bypass and a period of deep hypothermic circulatory arrest. By using two separate venous cannulas, the period of arrest can be limited to the time it takes to widely excise the

ductus arteriosus and perform a long anastomosis of the donor aortic arch onto the underside of the diminutive recipient aortic arch.[2] The atrial and pulmonary artery anastomoses can be performed during cardiopulmonary bypass. After rewarming, cardiopulmonary bypass is discontinued with the patient on low-dose dobutamine and isoproterenol. Because the donor's right ventricle is unaccustomed to high pressure, pulmonary hypertension must be carefully avoided. For this reason, prostaglandin E_1 is continued postoperatively (0.05 μg./kg./min.) and acidosis is rigorously avoided.

Immunosuppression consists of triple-drug therapy, which includes cyclosporine, azathioprine, and prednisone. In most centers,[3, 11, 16] cyclosporine is begun several hours before transplantation, stopped during cardiopulmonary bypass, then resumed and adjusted according to blood levels. Intravenous

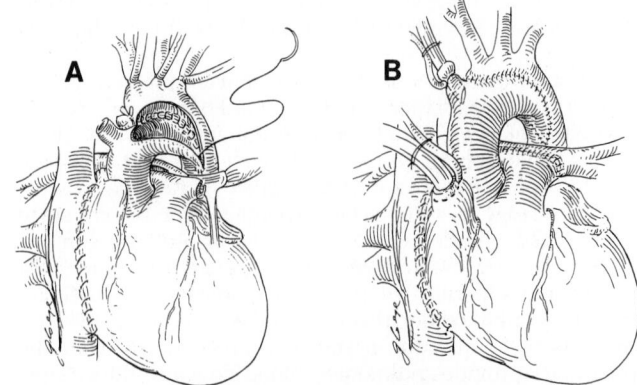

Figure 54–85. Cardiac transplantation for hypoplastic left heart syndrome. *A,* Under deep hypothermic circulatory arrest the donor aortic arch is widely anastomosed to the underside of the recipient aortic arch that has been incised from the innominate artery to the descending aorta beyond the junction of the ductus arteriosus. *B,* The completed implantation before decannulation. (From Haas, G. S., Bailey, L., and Pennington, D. G.: Pediatric cardiac transplantation. *In* Baue, A. E. [Ed.]: Glenn's Thoracic and Cardiovascular Surgery, 5th ed. Norwalk, Conn., Appleton & Lange, 1991.)

administration is changed over to oral administration as soon as feeding is tolerated. Methylprednisolone is administered on cardiopulmonary bypass and every 12 hours for four doses. Azathioprine is also administered at the time of transplantation and on a daily basis at a dose that keeps the white blood cell count between 4000 and 7000 per cu. mm. Some centers also employ induction therapy with monoclonal (OKT-3)[10] or polyclonal antibodies (antilymphocyte globulin).

Most patients are weaned off the ventilator in 2 to 4 days and are ready for discharge between 2 and 4 weeks after the transplant procedure. Triple-drug therapy is continued after discharge, decreasing the dose of corticosteroids until they are discontinued between 6 to 12 months post transplant.[12] Careful monitoring for infection, rejection, and side effects of immunosuppressive agents must be maintained. Thorough clinical evaluation and routine echocardiography generally permit reliable monitoring without the morbidity of routine endocardial biopsy.[7] However, when rejection is suspected, endocardial biopsy is performed to confirm the diagnosis. When rejection is diagnosed, a pulse of corticosteroids is administered over 4 days and tapered over 2 weeks. Rejection that is unresponsive to the corticosteroid pulse is treated with OKT-3 or antithymocyte globulin.

Results of Cardiac Transplantation. The largest experience with transplantation for hypoplastic left heart syndrome was reported in 1993 by the Loma Linda group[15] and includes 111 infants who entered their transplantation protocol between 1985 and 1991. Twenty-seven (24%) infants died while waiting for a donor heart. Eighty-four infants (76%) received transplants, with an operative mortality of 13%. The waiting period averaged 26 days (range: 1 to 111 days). Late death occurred in only 4 infants (5%). Based on this experience, survival probability for transplantation for hypoplastic left heart syndrome was 86% at 1 month, 64% at 6 months, and 61% at 1 and 5 years. Of those who survived to transplant and survived the procedure, survival was 99% at 6 months and 95% at 1 and 5 years. Favorable results have been published by other centers,[3, 11, 50] but few match the success of the Loma Linda group.

Staged Reconstruction or Transplantation?

Which treatment approach is best for patients with hypoplastic left heart syndrome remains controversial. Each technique has its own set of advantages and disadvantages. Transplantation permits establishment of normal circulatory physiology without the need for subsequent surgical procedures. Unfortunately, the wait for an appropriate donor heart imposes its own morbidity and mortality. Furthermore, the length of graft survival that can be achieved is unknown.[45] In addition to the risks of rejection and infection, the specter of posttransplant coronary artery disease looms for all heart transplant patients, including neonates.[39] The registry of the International Society of Heart Transplantation reported an incidence of hypertension of 39%, renal dysfunction of 17%, graft atherosclerosis of 8%, and malignancy of 3% in a group of 362 children undergoing heart transplantation for a variety of reasons, including hypoplastic left heart syndrome.[40] Staged reconstruction can be applied to most infants with hypoplastic left heart syndrome waiting only for hemodynamic stability and organ recovery. Two additional surgical procedures, however, must be performed, each with its own risk. Recent improvements in operative risks for all phases of the staged approach have renewed interest in this method, especially when early actuarial survival at some centers[24] begins to match or even exceed what has been reported for transplantation. The long-term results of Fontan correction, however, predict a late phase of mortality for even the strongest candidates.[22] Thus, the best approach to hypoplastic left

heart syndrome remains to be determined. Nevertheless, because of both techniques, children and infants are alive today who would otherwise not have survived. Further observation of these children will provide much needed insight into the benefits and shortcomings of each treatment modality.

SELECTED REFERENCES

Bailey, L. L., Nehlsen-Cannarella, S. L., Doroshow, R. W., et al.: Cardiac allotransplantation in neonates as therapy for hypoplastic left heart syndrome. N. Engl. J. Med., 315:949, 1986.
The initial experience with neonatal cardiac transplantation at Loma Linda University Hospital is described.

Chiavarelli, M., Gundry, S. R., Razzouk, A. J., and Bailey, L. L.: Cardiac transplantation for infants with hypoplastic left-heart syndrome. JAMA, 270:2944, 1993.
All patients with hypoplastic left heart syndrome registered at Loma Linda University Hospital for cardiac transplantation from the inception of the program in 1985 through 1991 are analyzed. The results presented in this paper represent a benchmark for other centers to emulate. The study does, however, point out the problem of donor availability and the significant mortality (24%) that occurs while awaiting a donor heart.

Iannettoni, M. D., Bove, E. L., Mosca, R. S., Lupinetti, F. M., Dorostkar, P. C., Ludominsky, A., Crowley, D. C., Kulik, T. J., and Rosenthal, A.: Improving results with first-stage palliation for hypoplastic left heart syndrome. J. Thorac. Cardiovasc. Surg., 107:934, 1994.
This report documents the significant improvements in results that can be achieved with staged palliation for hypoplastic left heart syndrome. Based on the authors' recent experience with a three-staged approach, initial actuarial survival matches or exceeds that reported by Loma Linda University Hospital for heart transplantation.

Jonas, R. A.: Management of hypoplastic left heart syndrome. Semin. Thorac. Cardiovasc. Surg., 6:28, 1994.
This recent update and summary describes the evolution of technical modifications at each stage of the surgical palliation of hypoplastic left heart syndrome. The author describes his complete personal experience with 78 consecutive patients at Boston Children's Hospital.

Noonan, J. A., and Nadas, A. S.: The hypoplastic left heart syndrome: An analysis of 101 cases. Pediatr. Clin. North Am., 5:1029, 1958.
This classic paper describes the spectrum of anomalies first referred to by these authors as the hypoplastic left heart syndrome.

Norwood, W. I., Jr., Jacobs, M. L., and Murphy, J. D.: Fontan procedure for hypoplastic left heart syndrome. Ann. Thorac. Surg., 54:1025, 1992.
Norwood and colleagues' experience with 138 consecutive patients treated with some modification of the Fontan procedure after initial palliative reconstruction for hypoplastic left heart syndrome at The Children's Hospital of Philadelphia from 1985 through 1991 is reviewed. Results, technical details, and rationale for changing to a three-staged approach are discussed.

Norwood, W. I., Jr., Lang, P., and Hansen, D.: Physiologic repair of aortic atresia—hypoplastic left heart syndrome. N. Engl. J. Med., 308:23, 1983.
This was the first report of an infant with hypoplastic left heart syndrome achieving physiologic correction with a modified Fontan procedure. The patient is known to be clinically well more than 10 years after this operation.

REFERENCES

1. Allen, L. D., Chita, S. K., Sharland, G. K., Fagg, N., Anderson, R. H., and Crawford, D. C.: The accuracy of fetal echocardiography in the diagnosis of congenital heart disease. Int. J. Cardiol., 25:279, 1989.
2. Backer, C. L., Idriss, F. S., Zales, V. R., and Mavroudis, C.: Cardiac transplantation for hypoplastic left heart syndrome: A modified technique. Ann. Thorac. Surg., 50:894, 1990.
3. Backer, C. L., Zales, V. R., Idriss, F. S., Lynch, P., Crawford, S., Benson, D. W., Jr., and Mavroudis, C.: Heart transplantation in neonates and in children. J. Heart Lung Transplant, 11:311, 1992.
4. Bailey, L. L., Nehlsen-Cannarella, S. L., Doroshow, R. W., et al.: Cardiac allotransplantation in newborns as therapy for hypoplastic left heart syndrome. N. Engl. J. Med., 315:949, 1986.
5. Bailey, L. L., Nehlsen-Cannarella, S. L., Concepcion, W., and Jolley, W. B.: Baboon-to-human cardiac xenotransplantation in a neonate. JAMA, 254:3321, 1985.
6. Barnea, O., Austin, E. H., Richman, B., and Santamore, W. P.: Balancing the circulation: Theoretic optimization of pulmonary/systemic flow ratio in hypoplastic left heart syndrome. J. Am. Coll. Cardiol., 24:1376, 1994.
7. Boucek, M. M., Mathis, C. M., Boucek, R. J., Jr., Hodgkin, D. D., Kanakriyeh, M. S., McCormack, J., Gundry, S. R., and Bailey, L. L.: Prospective evaluation of echocardiography for primary rejection surveillance after infant heart transplantation: Comparison with endomyocardial biopsy. J. Heart Lung Transplant, 12:66, 1994.
8. Boughman,, J. A., Berg, K. A., Astemboski, J. A., et al.: Familial risks of

congenital heart disease assessed by a population-based epidemiologic study. Am. J. Med. Genet., 26:839, 1987.

9. Bove, E. L.: Transplantation after first-stage reconstruction for hypoplastic left heart syndrome. Ann. Thorac. Surg., 52:701, 1991.

10. Brown, J. W., Turrentine, M. W., Kesler, K. A., Mahomed, Y., Darragh, R., Evans, K., Thompson, L., and Caldwell, R.: Triple-drug immunosuppression for heart transplantation in infants and children. J. Heart Lung Transplant, 12:S265, 1993.

11. Canter, C. E., Saffitz, J. E., Moorhead, S., et al.: Early results after pediatric cardiac transplantation with triple immunosuppression therapy. Am. J. Cardiol., 71:971, 1993.

12. Canter, C. E., Moorhead, S., Saffitz, J. E., Huddleston, C. B., and Spray, T. L.: Steroid withdrawal in the pediatric heart transplant recipient initially treated with triple immunosuppression. J. Heart Lung Transplant, 13:74, 1994.

13. Cayler, G. G., Smeloff, E. A., and Miller, G. E., Jr.: Surgical palliation of hypoplastic left side of the heart. N. Engl. J. Med., 282:780, 1970.

14. Chang, A. C., Hanley, F. L., Wernovsky, G., Rosenfeld, H. M., Wessel, D. L., Jonas, R. A., Mayer, J. E., Jr., Lock, J. E., and Castañeda, A. R.: Early bidirectional cavopulmonary shunt in young infants: Postoperative course and early results. Circulation, 88(Suppl. II):149, 1993.

15. Chiavarelli, M., Gundry, S. R., Razzouk, A. J., and Bailey, L. L.: Cardiac transplantation for infants with hypoplastic left-heart syndrome. JAMA, 270:2944, 1993.

16. Chinnock, R. E., Baum, M. F., Larsen, R., and Bailey, L.: Rejection management and long-term surveillance of the pediatric heart transplant recipient: The Loma Linda experience. J. Heart Lung Transplant, 12:S255, 1993.

17. Doty, D. B., and Knott, H. W.: Hypoplastic left heart syndrome: Experience with an operation to establish functionally normal circulation. J. Thorac. Cardiovasc. Surg., 74:624, 1977.

18. Doty, D. B., Marvin, W. J., Schieken, R. M., and Lauer, R. M.: Hypoplastic left heart syndrome: Successful palliation with a new operation. J. Thorac. Cardiovasc. Surg., 80:148, 1980.

19. Emery, J. R.: Strategies for prolonged survival before heart transplantation in the neonatal intensive care unit. J. Heart Lung Transplant, 12:S162, 1992.

20. Farrell, P. E., Jr., Chang, A. C., Murdison, K. A., Baffa, J. M., Norwood, W. I., and Murphy, J. D.: Outcome and assessment after the modified Fontan procedure for hypoplastic left heart syndrome. Circulation, 85:116, 1992.

21. Fontan, F., and Baudet, E.: Surgical repair of tricuspid atresia. Thorax, 26:240, 1971.

22. Fontan, F., Kirklin, J. W., Fernandez, G., Costa, F., Naftel, D. C., Tritto, F., and Blackstone, E. H.: Outcome after a "perfect" Fontan operation. Circulation, 81:1520, 1990.

23. Fyler, D. C., Buckley, L. P., Hellenbrand, W. E., et al.: Report of the New England Regional Infant Cardiac Program. Pediatrics, 65:377, 1980.

24. Iannettoni, M. D., Bove, E. L., Mosca, R. S., Lupinetti, F. M., Dorostkar, P. C., Ludominsky, A., Crowley, D. C., Kulik, T. J., and Rosenthal, A.: Improving results with first-stage palliation for hypoplastic left heart syndrome. J. Thorac. Cardiovasc. Surg., 107:934, 1994.

25. Izukawa, T., Mulholland, H. D., Rowe, R. D., et al.: Structural heart disease in the newborn: Changing profile: Comparison of 1975 and 1965. Arch. Dis. Child., 54:281, 1979.

26. Jobes, D. R., Nicolson, S. C., Steven, J. M., Miller, M., Jacobs, M. L., and Norwood, W. I., Jr.: Carbon dioxide prevents pulmonary overcirculation in hypoplastic left heart syndrome. Ann. Thorac. Surg., 54:150, 1992.

27. Jonas, R. A.: Intermediate procedures after first-stage Norwood operation facilitate subsequent repair. Ann. Thorac. Surg., 52:696, 1991.

28. Lev, M.: Pathologic anatomy and interrelationship of hypoplasia of the aortic tract complexes. Lab. Invest., 1:61, 1952.

29. Litwin, S. B., Van Praagh, R., and Bernhard, W. F.: A palliative operation for certain infants with aortic arch interruption. Ann. Thorac. Surg., 14:369, 1972.

30. Mayer, J. E., Jr., Bridges, N. D., Lock, J. E., Hanley, F. L., Jonas, R. A., and Castañeda, A. R.: Factors associated with marked reduction in mortality for Fontan operations in patients with single ventricle. J. Thorac. Cardiovasc. Surg., 103:444, 1992.

31. Meliones, J. N., Snider, A. R., Bove, E. L., Rosenthal, A., and Rosen, D. A.: Longitudinal results after first-stage palliation for hypoplastic left heart syndrome. Circulation, 82(Suppl. IV):151, 1990.

32. Morris, C. D., Outcalt, J., and Menashe, V. D.: Hypoplastic left heart syndrome: Natural history in a geographically defined population. Pediatrics, 85:977, 1990.

33. Murdison, K. A., Baffa, J. M., Farrell, P. E., Jr., Chang, A. C., Barber, G., Norwood, W. J., and Murphy, J. D.: Hypoplastic left heart syndrome: Outcome after initial reconstruction and before modified Fontan procedure. Circulation, 82(Suppl. IV):199, 1990.

34. Noonan, J. A., and Nadas, A. S.: The hypoplastic left heart syndrome: An analysis of 101 cases. Pediatr. Clin. North Am., 5:1029, 1958.

35. Norwood, W. I., Jr.: Hypoplastic left heart syndrome. Ann. Thorac. Surg., 52:688, 1991.

36. Norwood, W. I., Jr., Jacobs, M. L., and Murphy, J. D.: Fontan procedure for hypoplastic left heart syndrome. Ann. Thorac. Surg., 54:1025, 1992.

37. Norwood, W. I., Jr., Kirklin, J. K., and Sanders, S. P.: Hypoplastic left heart syndrome: Experience with palliative surgery. Am. J. Cardiol., 45:87, 1980.

38. Norwood, W. I., Jr., Lang, P., and Hansen, D.: Physiologic repair of aortic atresia—hypoplastic left heart syndrome. N. Engl. J. Med., 308:23, 1983.

39. Pahl, E., Zales, V. R., Fricker, F. J., and Addonizio, L. J.: Post-transplant coronary artery disease in children: A multicenter national survey. Circulation, 90:II-56, 1994.

40. Pennington, D. G., Noedel, N., McBride, L. R., Naunheim, K. S., and Ring, W. S.: Heart transplantation in children: An international survey. Ann. Thorac. Surg., 52:710, 1991.

41. Pridjian, A. K., Mendelsohn, A. M., Lupinetti, F. M., Beekman, R. H., III, Dick, M., II, Serwer, G., and Bove, E. L.: Usefulness of the bidirectional Glenn procedure as staged reconstruction for the functional single ventricle. Am. J. Cardiol., 71:959, 1993.

42. Rossi, A. F., Sommer, R. J., Lotvin, A., Gross, R. P., Steinberg, L. G., Kipel, G., Golinko, R. J., and Griepp, R. B.: Usefulness of intermittent monitoring of mixed venous oxygen saturation after stage I palliation for hypoplastic left heart syndrome. Am. J. Cardiol., 73:1118, 1994.

43. Ruiz, C. E., Zhang, H. P., and Larsen, R. L.: The role of interventional cardiology in pediatric heart transplantation. J. Heart Lung Transplant, 12:S164, 1992.

44. Sade, R. M., Crawford, F. A., Jr., and Fyfe, D. A.: Symposium on hypoplastic left heart syndrome (Letter). J. Thorac. Cardiovasc. Surg., 91:937, 1986.

45. Sarris, G. E., Smith, J. A., Bernstein, D., Griffin, M. L., Pitlick, P. T., Baum, D., Billingham, M. E., Oyer, P. E., Stinson, E. B., Starnes, V. A., Shumway, N. E., and Reitz, B. A.: Pediatric cardiac transplantation: The Stanford experience. Circulation, 90:II-51, 1994.

46. Stack, M. C., Kirby, W. C., Towbin, J. A., Denfield, S. W., Grifka, R. R., Bricker, J. T., Ott, D. A., and Frazier, O. H.: Stenting of the ductus arteriosus in hypoplastic left heart syndrome as an ambulatory bridge to cardiac transplantation. Am. J. Cardiol., 74:636, 1994.

47. Starnes, V. A., Griffin, M. L., Pitlick, P. T., Bernstein, D., Baum, D., Ivens, K., and Shumway, N. E.: Current approach to hypoplastic left heart syndrome: Palliation, transplantation, or both. J. Thorac. Cardiovasc. Surg., 104:189, 1992.

48. Stuart, A. G., Wren, C., Sharples, P. M., et al.: Hypoplastic left heart syndrome: More potential transplant recipients than suitable donors. Lancet, 20:957, 1991.

49. Taussig, H. B.: Congenital Malformations of the Heart. New York, The Commonwealth Fund, 1947.

50. Turrentine, M. W., Kesler, K. A., Caldwell, R., et al.: Cardiac transplantation in infants and children. Ann. Thorac. Surg., 57:546, 1994.

51. Watson, D. G., and Rowe, R. D.: Aortic valve atresia: Report of 43 cases. JAMA, 179:14, 1962.

XI

TRUNCUS ARTERIOSUS

Richard A. Hopkins, M.D., and Robert B. Wallace, M.D.

HISTORICAL ASPECTS

Truncus arteriosus is a rare but important congenital cardiac malformation constituting between 1% and 4% of congenital cardiac defects in autopsy series. The condition is characterized by a single arterial vessel arising from the heart, receiving blood from both ventricles, and supplying blood to the aorta, lungs, and coronary arteries. The pathologic anatomy was first described by Taruffi in 1875.[31] In 1949, Collett and Edwards classified the defect according to anatomic types, which is the basis for the surgical classification used today.[9] In 1968, McGoon and associates reported the first successful repair of truncus arteriosus.[19] They employed the work of Rastelli and associates in which a conduit consisting of a homograft of the ascending aorta and aortic valve was used to construct a pulmonary artery.[25] Subsequently, Bowman and co-workers suggested that a Dacron graft containing a porcine valve be used as the conduit.[6] Modifications of this technique represent the current definitive treatment for truncus arteriosus.[24, 32]

ANATOMY AND CLASSIFICATION

Truncus arteriosus is due to a lack of partitioning of the embryonic conus during the first few weeks of fetal development and is almost always associated with a ventricular septal defect (VSD). Collett and Edwards classified truncus arteriosus into four types, based on the origin of the pulmonary arteries (Fig. 54–86).[9] A VSD immediately beneath the truncal valve has been present in all patients with truncus arteriosus except two reported by Van Praagh and Van Praagh.[33] The truncus most commonly overrides the ventricular septum or arises to the left of the plane of the septum. Collet and Edwards reported a 25% incidence of a common ventricle, although this was not present in any of Van Praagh and Van Praagh's series and in only one of the 80 specimens studied by Bharati and associates.[3] The truncal valve may have from two to six cusps, although most valves have three cusps. Four cusps have been noted in approximately 25% of valves and two cusps in 5%. Truncal valve incompetence is severe in 5% to 10%, moderate in 30%, and absent or minimal in two thirds of patients who undergo operation. The aortic arch is to the right in approximately 20% of patients with truncus arteriosus, and an interruption of the aortic arch occurs in 10% to 15%. The left or right pulmonary artery was shown to be absent in 2% of Van Praagh and Van Praagh's series and in 4.5% of Bharati and associates' series.

Other defects of surgical significance occurring with truncus arteriosus include patent ductus arteriosus in 15% to 30%, persistent left superior vena cava in 10% to 15%, and an atrial septal defect in 20%. The location and level of the coronary ostia are different than in the normal aortic root, whereas the epicardial courses are usually typical, with the coronary arteries being normally distributed in 95% of hearts with truncus arteriosus; in up to 10% of cases, the coronary arterial orifices are at risk for damage during excision of the pulmonary arteries from the common arterial trunk.[4, 30] The relationship of the conduction system to the VSD follows the usual rules. When the VSD is perimembranous, then the atrioventricular bundle is close to the VSD, running along the inferoposterior border. In those cases in which the VSD is anterior and separated from the membranous septum by muscle, the atrioventricular bundle is far away from the VSD and unlikely to be damaged during VSD closure.[2] By definition, the infundibular septum is absent in truncus arteriosus.[1]

HEMODYNAMICS

All the blood from both the left and the right ventricles is ejected into the truncus arteriosus. The systemic and pulmonary venous blood mixes, and the degree of arterial oxygen saturation depends on the amount of pulmonary blood flow. Pulmonary blood flow may be limited by stenosis of the pulmonary arteries, but this is uncommon. In most instances, pulmonary blood flow (and thus arterial oxygen saturation) is determined by the resistance to flow in the pulmonary vascular bed. As with isolated VSD, the pulmonary vascular bed in truncus arteriosus is exposed to high flow at systemic pressure, a condition that may lead to progressive changes of pulmonary vascular obstructive disease.[17]

SYMPTOMS AND DIAGNOSIS

The symptoms associated with truncus arteriosus are related primarily to the amount of pulmonary blood flow. During the first few weeks of life, when pulmonary vascular resistance is normally increased, symptoms are usually absent unless there is associated significant truncal valve incompetence.[11] With maturation of the fetal pulmonary vascular bed, associated with a decrease in pulmonary vascular resistance and an increase in pulmonary blood flow, symptoms of congestive heart failure may develop. These include dyspnea, excessive perspiration, and failure to thrive. Cyanosis is not usually apparent, because the arterial oxygen saturation is generally greater than 85%. With the progressive development of pulmonary vascular obstructive disease and the associated decrease in pulmonary blood flow, cyanosis becomes more evident. The condition then resembles tetralogy of Fallot or VSD with severe pulmonary vascular obstructive disease.

Physical examination usually reveals a systolic thrill and murmur over the left third and fourth intercostal spaces parasternally. The apical impulse is prominent, and there are signs of cardiomegaly. The second heart sound is single and accentuated. When truncal valve incompetence is present, a diastolic murmur follows the second heart sound.

Chest roentgenography shows cardiomegaly with biventricular enlargement (Fig. 54–87). The aortic arch is to the right in 20% of patients, and the left pulmonary artery may be elevated from the normal position. The peripheral pulmonary vasculature is increased, unless there is advanced pulmonary vascular obstructive disease. The electrocardiogram is nonspecific and usually indicates biventricular hypertrophy.

Heart catheterization (Fig. 54–88) and angiocardiographic studies are indicated in all patients suspected of having truncus arteriosus to establish the diagnosis, define the anatomy, and determine the pulmonary vascular resistance. Ventricular pressures are equal, and in the absence of pulmonary artery stenosis there are equal pressures in the ventricles, truncus, and pulmonary arteries. Oxygen saturation studies indicate bidirectional shunting at the ventricular level, the predominant shunt being left to right. Pulmonary flow and resistance should be determined by measurement of pressures and oxygen saturations in both pulmonary arteries.

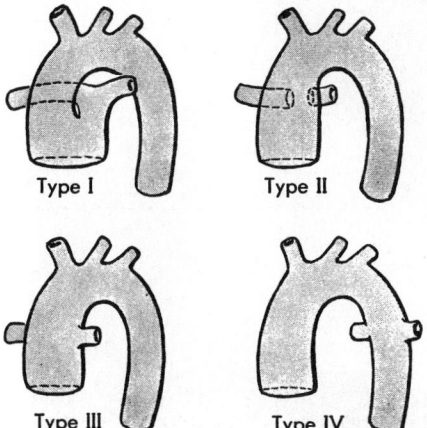

Figure 54–86. Anatomic types of truncus arteriosus. Collett and Edwards' classification. (Reprinted with the permission of Simon & Schuster from HEART DISEASE IN INFANCY AND CHILDHOOD, 3/e by JD Keith, RD Rowe, P Vlad. Copyright © 1958, 1967, 1978 Macmillan Publishing Company.)

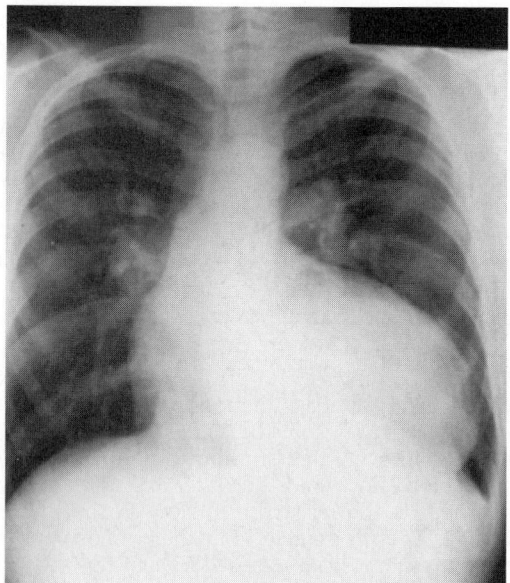

Figure 54–87. Chest roentgenogram of patient with truncus arteriosus showing cardiomegaly, increased pulmonary vasculature, and elevation of the left pulmonary artery relative to the right. (From Hallermann, F. J., Kincaid, O. W., Tsakiris, A. G., Ritter, D. G., and Titus, J. L.: Persistent truncus arteriosus: A radiographic and angiocardiographic study. AJR, *107*:827, 1979, © American Roentgenology Society.)

PROGNOSIS

Most patients with persistent truncus arteriosus die of congestive heart failure in early infancy. Only 3 patients in Van Praagh and Van Praagh's autopsy series of 57 cases lived beyond 6 months of age. In Keith and associates' review of 89 patients, 22% survived beyond 6 months of age and 10 patients survived to the second or third decade.[15] The causes of death for those who survived the first 2 years of life were generally related to pulmonary vascular obstructive disease and decreased pulmonary blood flow.[13]

Medical therapy is directed toward the treatment of congestive heart failure, the prevention of bacterial endocarditis, and, in older patients with pulmonary vascular obstructive disease, the complications of right-to-left shunts and the associated polycythemia.

TREATMENT AND RESULTS
Pulmonary Artery Banding

Banding of the pulmonary artery was proposed by Müller and Dammann[20] to decrease pulmonary artery pressure and flow, in an attempt to control congestive heart failure and to limit the progression of pulmonary vascular obstructive disease in patients with large left-to-right shunts. This procedure has been used in truncus arteriosus, as reported by Smith and associates,[26] Oldham and co-workers,[21] and Stark and associates.[28] Although the mortality has been high in the reported series, a number of patients have been successfully palliated, and this has enabled them to undergo complete repair at a later age. It is currently reserved for patients with severe concomitant diseases (e.g., necrotizing enterocolitis) or with more complex forms of truncus arteriosus (e.g., multiple VSDs).

Complete Surgical Repair

Technique. The operation is performed through a median sternotomy, using total cardiopulmonary bypass and deep hypothermia, either with total circulatory arrest or low flow. Myocardial protection is provided by cold cardioplegic arrest during aortic cross-clamping. Arterial cannulation is in the ascending aorta. The left ventricle is vented with a catheter introduced through the foramen ovale (Figs. 54–89 and 54–90).

The pulmonary arteries can be excised from the truncus as a single segment, even in Type II truncus. This occasionally can be facilitated by a short anterior aortotomy or division of the truncal root.[22] In smaller infants, the posterior defect is usually closed with a patch to avoid distortion of the semilunar valve pillars. The incision in the right ventricle is made high in the ventricle in the planned direction of the conduit. The aortic cross-clamp is temporarily released after air has been removed from the aortic root, and the competency of the valve is assessed. If incompetence is severe, valve replacement or repair must be considered. A patch is used to close the VSD. An appropriately sized valved Dacron

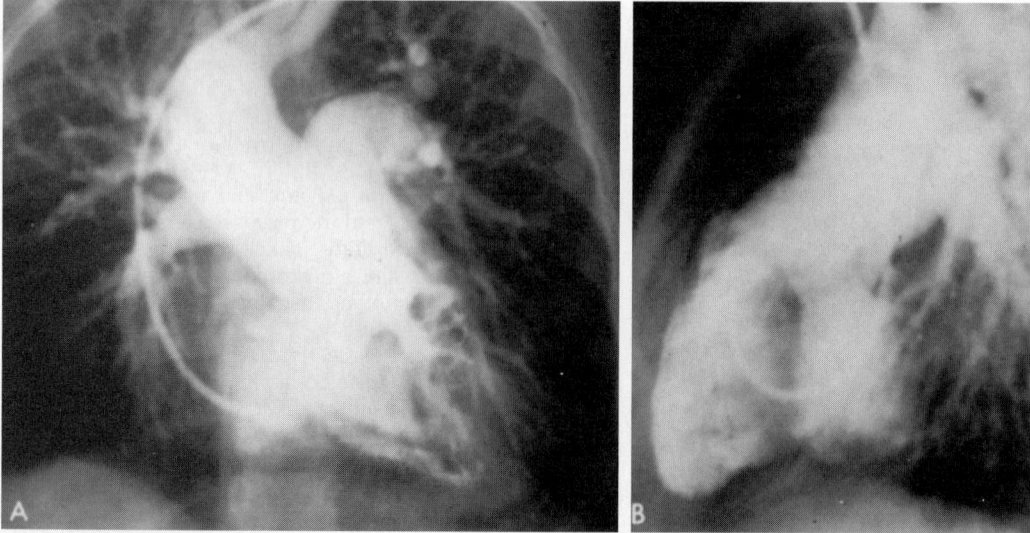

Figure 54–88. Angiocardiograms. Anteroposterior view *(A)* and left lateral view *(B)* after injection of contrast material into right ventricle. Both ventricles are enlarged; ventricular septal defect is present immediately beneath truncus. Right ventricular infundibulum is absent, and pulmonary arteries arise from truncus. (From Hallermann, F. J., Kincaid, O. W., Tsakiris, A. G., Ritter, D. G., and Titus, J. L.: Persistent truncus arteriosus: A radiographic and angiocardiographic study. AJR, *107*:827, 1979, © American Roentgenology Society.)

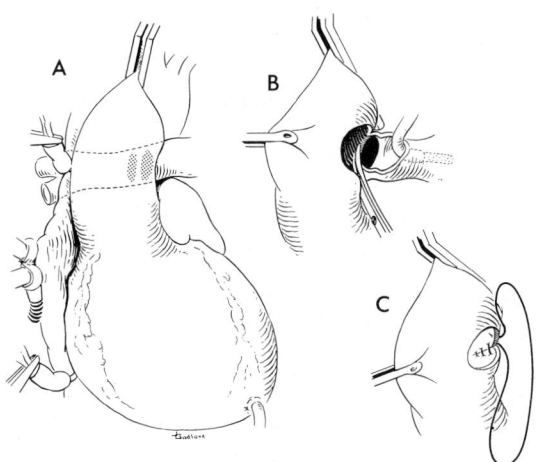

Figure 54–89. Surgical repair. *A*, Cardiopulmonary bypass, left ventricle vented at apex, aorta cross-clamped. *B*, Origin of pulmonary arteries excised from truncus. *C*, Closure of defect in truncus. (From Wallace, R. B., Rastelli, G. C., Ongley, P. A., Titus, J. L., and McGoon, D. C.: Complete repair of truncus arteriosus defects. J. Thorac. Cardiovasc. Surg., *57*:95, 1969; by permission of C. V. Mosby Company.)

or homograft conduit is cut to proper length and used to establish continuity between the right ventricle and the pulmonary arteries. The course of the conduit should be such that kinking is avoided and the closed sternum does not compress the conduit.

Although repairs have been performed successfully with valveless conduits for connection of the right ventricle to the pulmonary arteries,[27] most authorities recommend a valved conduit when there is high or reactive pulmonary vascular

resistance, which also protects right ventricular function.[14] The 12-mm. porcine valved conduit has been used successfully for this reconstruction,[7] but the technical ease of insertion and perhaps greater durability of the homograft supports its use when available (Fig. 54–91).[5, 8, 14, 16]

In patients in whom a previous pulmonary artery banding has been performed, the pulmonary arteries usually need to be incised to a point distal to the area of banding to relieve the stenosis produced by the band.[23] The distal end of the conduit is then tailored to produce an angioplastic enlargement of the pulmonary arteries (Fig. 54–92).

Results. The Mayo Clinic experience with 167 patients with Type I and Type II truncus arteriosus who underwent surgical repair between 1965 and 1982 has been reported.[18] There were 48 hospital deaths (28.7%). The most significant risk factors in this series included age younger than 2 years at operation and a postrepair right ventricular/left ventricular pressure ratio greater than 0.8. The operative mortality was 70% for patients younger than 2 years of age, and 5 of 6 patients under 6 months of age died. During this period, truncus arteriosus in children younger than 2 years of age was repaired only when medical management failed. Late follow-up of the 119 hospital survivors ranged from 1.1 to 15.4 years, with a mean of 7 years, and revealed a 5-year survival of 84.4% and a 10-year survival of 68.8%. Thirty-six patients (30%) required reoperation during the follow-up period; and in 32 an obstructive valve conduit was replaced. Nine of the patients required truncal valve replacement be-

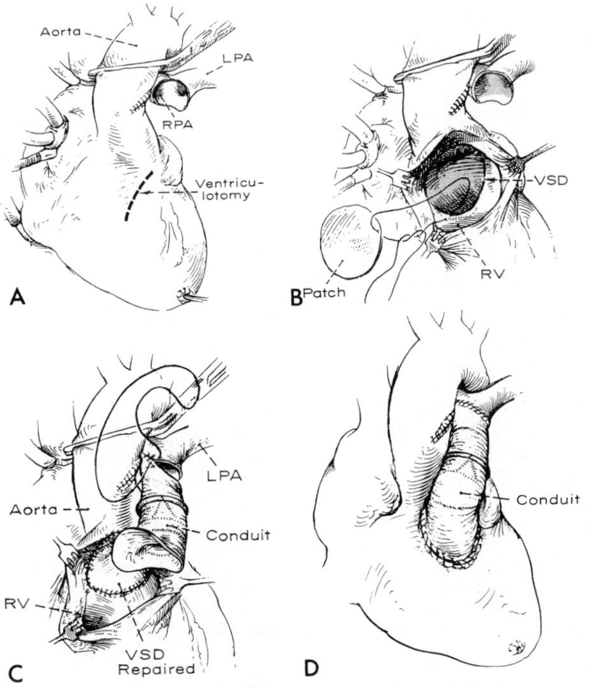

Figure 54–90. Surgical repair *(continued)*. *A*, Incision made high in right ventricle. *B*, Ventricular septal defect closed with Teflon patch. *C*, Dacron graft with porcine valve sutured to pulmonary arteries. *D*, Proximal end of graft anastomosed to right ventricle. LPA, left pulmonary artery; RPA, right pulmonary artery; VSD, ventricular septal defect; RV, right ventricle. (From Wallace, R. B.: Truncus arteriosus. *In* Sabiston, D. C., Jr., and Spencer, F. C. [Eds.]: Gibbon's Surgery of the Chest, 3rd ed. Philadelphia, W. B. Saunders, 1976.)

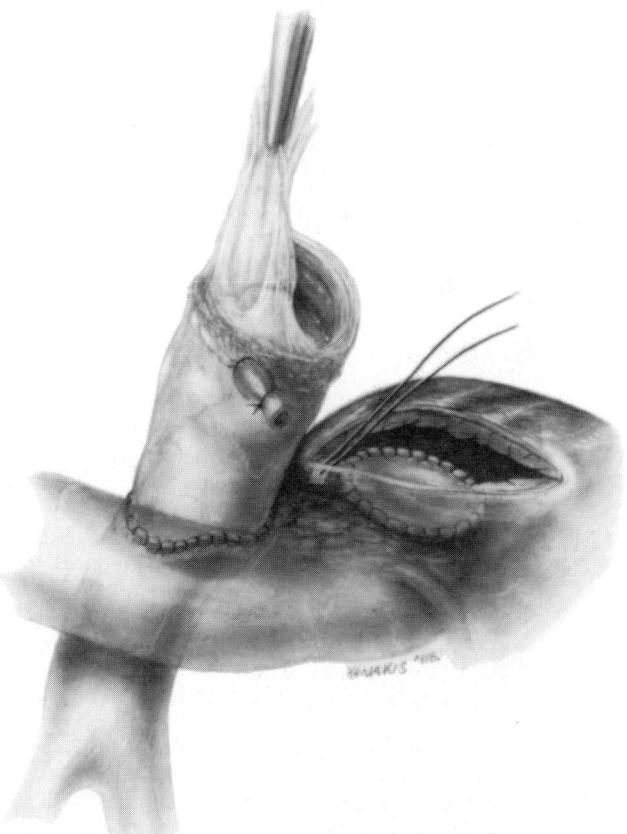

Figure 54–91. Homograft sutured to right ventriculotomy above VSD closure. There is minimum muscular tissue in this region because the infundibular septum is absent in truncus arteriosus. Thus the VSD patch is usually sutured to the edge of the ventriculotomy. It is often helpful to use a pledget at the start of the proximal conduit anastomosis to the ventriculotomy with the sutures incorporating the edge of the VSD patch. (From Hopkins, R. A.: Cardiac Reconstructions with Allograft Valves. New York, Springer-Verlag, 1989, p. 164; by permission.)

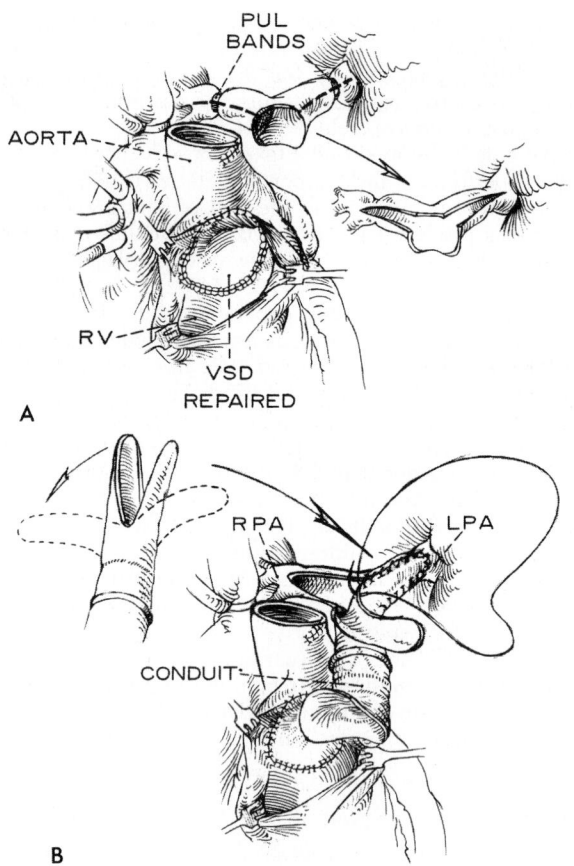

Figure 54–92. Complete repair with previous pulmonary artery banding. *A,* Pulmonary arteries are incised through areas of banding. *B,* Distal end of conduit tailored to enlarge the pulmonary arteries. (LPA, left pulmonary artery; RPA, right pulmonary artery; RV, right ventricle; VSD, ventricular septal defect.) (From Parker, R. K., McGoon, D. C., Danielson, G. K., Wallace, R. B., and Mair, D. D.: Repair of truncus arteriosus in patients with prior banding of the pulmonary artery. Surgery, *78:*761, 1975; by permission of C. V. Mosby Company.)

cause of progressive valve incompetence. Of the 90 patients alive at the end of the follow-up period, 59 (66%) were in functional New York Heart Association Class I, 28 (31%) in Class II, and 3 (3%) in Class III.

Reported experiences from institutions in which elective repair in infancy has been performed indicate that this can be accomplished at an acceptable mortality.[8, 29] Ebert and co-workers reported an 11% hospital mortality in 100 consecutive patients who underwent correction when younger than 6 months of age; 86 patients were alive at 16 months to 8 years postoperatively, and 55 of the survivors required conduit replacement (accomplished with no deaths).[10] At the time of follow-up, no survivors had evidence of pulmonary vascular disease. Bove and colleagues have reported neonatal repairs in 11 patients, with a 9% mortality.[5] Hanley and colleagues have reported 63 patients undergoing surgical repair in the first 3 months of life.[12] They examined 30 variables as potential risk factors for death and morbidity and found that only severe truncal valve regurgitation, associated interrupted aortic arch anatomy, coronary artery anomalies, and age of repair *greater* than 100 days were important risk factors for perioperative death. In their 33 patients without these risk factors, early survival was 100%, while the other 30 patients with one or more of these characteristics had only a 63% survival. Their series demonstrated that earlier operation (i.e., before 30 days of age) was associated with a shorter course in an intensive care unit with fewer complications, especially those of pulmonary hypertensive crises and prolonged ventilator dependence. Thus, the preferred timing for surgical correction is now in the neonatal period, preferably after the initial fall in pulmonary vascular resistance, which usually occurs between the first and third weeks of life.

Indications for Operation

Definitive treatment for truncus arteriosus is complete repair. Operation is ideally performed during the first 30 days of life. The alternative of nonsurgical management results in at least an 80% mortality by 6 months. Neonatal operation not only protects against the development of pulmonary vascular obstructive disease but also reduces the severity of postoperative reactive pulmonary hypertension. The right ventricular outflow reconstruction should include a valved conduit, which is preferably a homograft, but successful use of the Dacron conduit containing a porcine valve has also been demonstrated. The use of the valve mitigates the obligatory right ventricular dysfunction. The Boston group has also emphasized the importance of leaving at least a partially patent foramen ovale to provide cardiovascular stability postoperatively if severe right ventricular failure occurs.[12] Although pulmonary artery banding can reduce pulmonary blood flow and protect against the development of pulmonary vascular obstructive disease without increasing operative mortality at the time of complete repair, the results achieved by performing complete repair in early infancy clearly establish this as the current standard of practice.

SELECTED REFERENCES

Collett, R. W., and Edwards, J. E.: Persistent truncus arteriosus: A classification according to anatomic types. Surg. Clin. North Am., *8:*1245, 1949.
Anatomy, embryology, and criteria for diagnosis of truncus arteriosus based on 80 cases from the literature and the authors' material were reviewed. The embryologic discussion emphasized the development of the septal system that divides the ventricles, the conus arteriosus, and the truncus arteriosus to form two separate circulations. Two absolute criteria for the pathologic diagnosis of persistent truncus arteriosus were established: (1) that there be only one main arterial trunk leaving the base of the heart with no remnant of an atretic pulmonary trunk or aorta and (2) that this single arterial trunk supply branches to the coronary, pulmonary, and systemic circulations.

Hanley, F. L., Heinemann, M. K., Jonas, R. A., Cook, N. R., Wessel, D. L., and Castañeda, A. R.: Repair of truncus arteriosus in the neonate. J. Thorac. Cardiovasc. Surg., *6:*1047, 1993.
This report describes an experience with 63 patients in which univariate and multivariate analytic techniques were used to assess risk factors for perioperative death and postoperative morbidity. This series establishes the superiority of neonatal repair. It also demonstrates that reoperation for right ventricular outflow tract obstruction can be performed at low mortality (0%) and morbidity. Risk factors for death after primary repair of truncus arteriosus in early infancy included interrupted aortic arch, severe truncal valve insufficiency, coronary anomalies, and repair later than 100 days of age. In the absence of these risk factors, truncus arteriosus was repaired with a 100% survival.

Pearl, J. M., Hillel, L., Drinkwater, D. C., Jr., Milgalter, E., Charas, O-A., Giacobetti, F., George, B., and Williams, R.: Repair of truncus arteriosus in infancy. Ann. Thorac. Surg., *52:*780, 1991.
The authors review their experience with 32 patients younger than age 12 months undergoing surgical correction of truncus arteriosus. Early mortality for the entire group was 15.6% and appeared related to associated complex defects. In this series, both Dacron porcine-valve conduits and homografts were used. In the former, 71% of patients required conduit replacement secondary to obstruction (at a mean follow-up of 73 months), while only 14% of the patients with homografts had required replacements secondary to obstruction at a mean follow-up of 36 months.

REFERENCES

1. Anderson, R. H., and Thiene, G.: Categorization and description of hearts with a common arterial trunk. Eur. J. Cardiothorac. Surg., *3:*481, 1989.
2. Bharati, S., Karp, R., and Lev, M.: The conduction system in truncus arteriosus and its surgical significance. J. Surg. Res., *104:*954, 1992.

3. Bharati, S., McAllister, H. A., Jr., Rosenquist, G. C., Miller, R. A., Tatooles, C. J., and Lev, M.: The surgical anatomy of truncus arteriosus communis. J. Thorac. Cardiovasc. Surg., 67:501, 1974.

4. Bogers, A. J. J. C., Bartelings, M. M., Bokenkamp, R., et al.: Common arterial trunk, uncommon coronary arterial anatomy. J. Thorac. Cardiovasc. Surg., 106:1133, 1993.

5. Bove, E. L., Beekman, R. H., Snider, A. R., et al.: Repair of truncus arteriosus in the neonate and young infant. Ann. Thorac. Surg., 47:499, 1989.

6. Bowman, F. O., Jr., Hancock, W. D., and Malm, J. R.: A valve-containing Dacron prosthesis: Its use in restoring pulmonary artery–right ventricular continuity. Arch. Surg., 107:724, 1973.

7. Boyce, S. W., Turley, K., Yee, E. S., Verrier, E. D., and Ebert, P. A.: The fate of the 12-mm. porcine valved conduit from the right ventricle to the pulmonary artery: A ten-year experience. J. Thorac. Cardiovasc. Surg., 95:201, 1988.

8. Castañeda, A. R.: Truncus arteriosus. Ann. Thorac. Surg., 47:491, 1989.

9. Collett, R. W., and Edwards, J. E.: Persistent truncus arteriosus: A classification according to anatomic types. Surg. Clin. North Am., 8:1245, 1949.

10. Ebert, P. A., Turley, K., and Stanger, P.: Surgical treatment of truncus arteriosus in the first six months of life. Ann. Surg., 200:451, 1984.

11. Gelband, H., Van Meter, S., and Gersony, W. M.: Truncal valve abnormalities in infants with persistent truncus arteriosus: A clinicopathologic study. Circulation, 45:397, 1972.

12. Hanley, F. L., Heinemann, M. K., Jonas, R. A., et al.: Repair of truncus arteriosus in the neonate. Cardiovasc. Surg., 105:1047, 1993.

13. Heath, D., and Edwards, J. E.: The pathology of hypertensive pulmonary vascular disease: A description of six grades of structural changes in the pulmonary arteries with special reference to congenital cardiac septal defects. Circulation, 18:533, 1958.

14. Hopkins, R. A.: Right ventricular outflow tract reconstructions: The role of valves in the viable allograft era. Ann. Thorac. Surg., 45:593, 1988.

15. Keith, J. D., Rowe, R. D., and Vlad, P.: Heart Disease in Infancy and Childhood. New York, Macmillan, 1958, p. 521.

16. Kirklin, J. W., Blackstone, E. H., Maehara, T., et al.: Intermediate-term fate of cryopreserved allograft and xenograft valved conduits. Ann. Thorac. Surg., 44:598, 1989.

17. Mair, D. D., Ritter, D. G., Davis, G. D., Wallace, R. B., Danielson, G. K., and McGoon, D. C.: Selection of patients with truncus arteriosus for surgical correction: anatomic and hemodynamic considerations. Circulation, 49:144, 1974.

18. Marcelletti, C., McGoon, D. C., Danielson, G. K., Wallace, R. B., and Mair, D. D.: Early and late results of surgical repair of truncus arteriosus. Circulation, 55:636, 1977.

19. McGoon, D. C., Rastelli, G. C., and Ongley, P. A.: An operation for the correction of truncus arteriosus. JAMA, 205:69, 1968.

20. Müller, W. H., Jr., and Dammann, J. F.: The treatment of certain congenital malformations of the heart by the creation of pulmonic stenosis to reduce pulmonary hypertension and excessive pulmonary blood flow: A preliminary report. Surg. Gynecol. Obstet., 95:213, 1952.

21. Oldham, N. H., Jr., Kakos, G. S., Jarmakani, M. M., and Sabiston, D. C., Jr.: Pulmonary artery banding in infants with complex congenital heart defects. Ann. Thorac. Surg., 13:342, 1972.

22. Ott, D. A., Eren, E. E., Huhta, J. C., and Gutgesell, H. P.: Surgical treatment for the type II and III truncus: Complete division of the truncal root with primary repair using absorbable suture. Ann. Thorac. Surg., 40:201, 1985.

23. Parker, R. K., McGoon, D. C., Danielson, G. K., Wallace, R. B., and Mair, D. D.: Repair of truncus arteriosus in patients with prior banding of the pulmonary artery. Surgery, 78:761, 1975.

24. Pearl, J. M., Laks, H., Drinkwater, D. C., et al.: Repair of truncus arteriosus in infancy. Ann. Thorac. Surg., 52:780, 1991.

25. Rastelli, G. C., Titus, J. L., and McGoon, D. C.: Homograft of ascending aorta and aortic valve as a right ventricular outflow: An experimental approach to the repair of truncus arteriosus. Arch. Surg., 95:698, 1967.

26. Smith, G. W., Thompson, W. M., Jr., Dammann, J. F., Jr., and Muller, W. H., Jr.: Use of the pulmonary artery banding procedure in treating type II truncus arteriosus. Circulation, 29(Suppl. I):108, 1964.

27. Spicer, R. L., Behrendt, D., Crowley, D. C., et al.: Repair of truncus arteriosus in neonates with the use of a valveless conduit. Circulation, 70(Suppl. I):I-26, 1984.

28. Stark, J., Aberdeen, E., Waterston, D. J., Bonham-Carter, R. E., and Tynan, M.: Pulmonary artery constriction (banding): A report of 146 cases. Surgery, 65:808, 1969.

29. Stark, J., Gandhi, D., de Leval, M., Macartney, F., and Taylor, J. F. N.: Surgical treatment of persistent truncus arteriosus in the first year of life. Br. Heart J., 40:1280, 1978.

30. Suzuki, A., Ho, S. Y., Anderson, R. H., and Deanfield, J. E.: Coronary arterial and sinusal anatomy in hearts with a common arterial trunk. Ann. Thorac. Surg., 48:792, 1989.

31. Taruffi, C.: Sulle malattie congenite e sulle anomalie del cuore. Mem. Soc. Med. Chir. Bologna, 8:215, 1875.

32. Turley, K.: Current method of repair of truncus arteriosus. J. Card. Surg., 1:1, 1992.

33. Van Praagh, R., and Van Praagh, S.: The anatomy of common aorticopulmonary trunk (truncus arteriosus communis) and its embryologic implications: A study of 57 necropsy cases. Am. J. Cardiol., 16:406, 1965.

XII

TRANSPOSITION OF THE GREAT ARTERIES

Thomas L. Spray, M.D.

Complete transposition of the great arteries ([S,D,D], TGA, or D-TGA) is a congenital cardiac defect in which there is anatomic reversal of the relationship of the great arteries: the aorta arises entirely or largely from the right ventricle, and the pulmonary artery arises entirely or largely from the left ventricle (ventriculoarterial discordant connection). The lesion is incompatible with life without surgical intervention because the resulting physiologic abnormality is of separate pulmonary and systemic circulations existing in parallel instead of in series. Survival depends on mixing between the pulmonary and systemic circulation. In spite of the severity of this cardiac defect, surgical therapy has now become standardized such that anatomic and physiologic repair can be accomplished in the first few weeks of life in the majority of affected children.

TGA may coexist with other cardiac lesions. The discussion here is confined to patients with complete transposition with intact ventricular septum (50% of patients), complete transposition with ventricular septal defect (VSD) (25%), and complete transposition with VSD and functional or anatomic left ventricular outflow tract obstruction (pulmonary stenosis)

(25%). Common associated anomalies include coarctation of the aorta and patent ductus arteriosus.

Although reference was made to malposition of the aorta and pulmonary artery by Steno in 1672 and Morgagni in 1761, the anatomic description of TGA is credited to Baillie in 1797.[1] It was Farre in 1814 who introduced the term *transposition of aorta and pulmonary artery*, meaning that the aorta and pulmonary artery are displaced across the ventricular septum.[2] An attempt to classify the various types of transposition was reported by Rokitansky, and the first clinical recognition of TGA in life was noted by Fanconi in 1932.[3, 4] In 1938, Taussig described the pathologic anatomy and hemodynamic and clinical characteristics of the cardiac defect.[5] Ferguson, in 1960, and Ferenz, in 1966, noted the rapid appearance of pulmonary vascular disease in patients with TGA even when the ventricular septum was intact.[6, 7]

ANATOMY

Complete TGA is characterized by connection of the atria to their appropriate ventricles with inappropriate ventriculoarterial connections. The aorta and pulmonary artery are therefore misplaced across the ventricular septum, resulting in atrioventricular (AV) concordance and ventriculoarterial discordance (S,D,D). Although some have used the term *transposition* to describe a discordant ventriculoarterial connection, other authors have used transposition to describe any heart in which the aorta is anterior to the pulmonary artery. Use of the term TGA is confused by the use of this definition in some patients with double inlet ventricle or absent AV connection and in patients with nonlateralized atrial arrangements (some heterotaxy syndromes). *D-TGA* has also been used to describe a concordant AV and discordant ventriculoarterial arrangement, but this nomenclature does not adequately describe patients in whom the aorta is anterior and to the *left* of the pulmonary artery. Thus, in this section complete TGA is defined as normal atrial solitus, AV concordance, and ventriculoarterial discordance.

Several theories have been postulated regarding the morphogenesis of the abnormal relationship between the great arteries and the ventricles in TGA. It has been suggested that the subaortic conus persists and develops during normal looping of the ventricles while the subpulmonary conus undergoes absorption and thus establishes eventual fibrous continuity between the mitral and pulmonary valves, the reverse of the normal situation.[8] In the normal heart the subaortic conus does not grow, and dominant growth of the pulmonary conus forces the pulmonary valve anterior, superior, and to the left. Therefore, differential growth of the subaortic conus in transposition pushes the aorta anteriorly and disrupts the aortic valve continuity. If the subpulmonary conus fails to develop, the pulmonary artery will maintain a posterior location and pulmonary-to-mitral-valve continuity will occur. As a consequence of this relationship, the aortic valve becomes anterior to the pulmonary valve, permitting both semilunar valves to connect with the distal great vessels without the rotation that is hypothesized to occur in normal cardiac development. Because conal development determines rotation of the truncus arteriosus, the great arteries are similar in relationship at the semilunar valves as they are at the arch, resulting in no twist in the great arteries.

Anatomic variations are often encountered, although the heart is left sided, with atrial situs solitus in 95% of patients. Left-to-right juxtaposition of the atrial appendages signals the presence of other intracardiac anomalies. A true ostium secundum atrial septal defect is present in 10% to 20% of cases; however, the majority of atrial communications are through a patent foramen ovale. Right aortic arch is present in 4% of patients with intact ventricular septum and up to 16% of those with VSD.[9] Up to 50% of patients with TGA have an associated VSD, many of which spontaneously close.[10] The VSDs are commonly perimembranous (conoventricular), although they may be found anywhere in the ventricular septum. Pulmonary stenosis or atresia, overriding or straddling AV valves, coarctation of the aorta, and interruption of the aortic arch have all been noted in association with transposition and VSD.

The spatial relationship of the great vessels is quite variable; however, the aorta is most frequently to the right and anterior to the pulmonary artery. In almost all cases, the sinuses of Valsalva and the coronary artery ostia face the corresponding pulmonary arterial sinuses of Valsalva (Fig. 54–93). This situation is favorable for transfer of the coronary arteries with the arterial switch operation. Only a small number of patients who have origin of a coronary artery from a nonfacing coronary sinus pose a problem for arterial switch reconstruction. The most common coronary pattern in D-TGA (68%) consists of the left main coronary arising from the leftward coronary sinus, giving rise to the left anterior descending and circumflex coronary arteries.[11] The right coro-

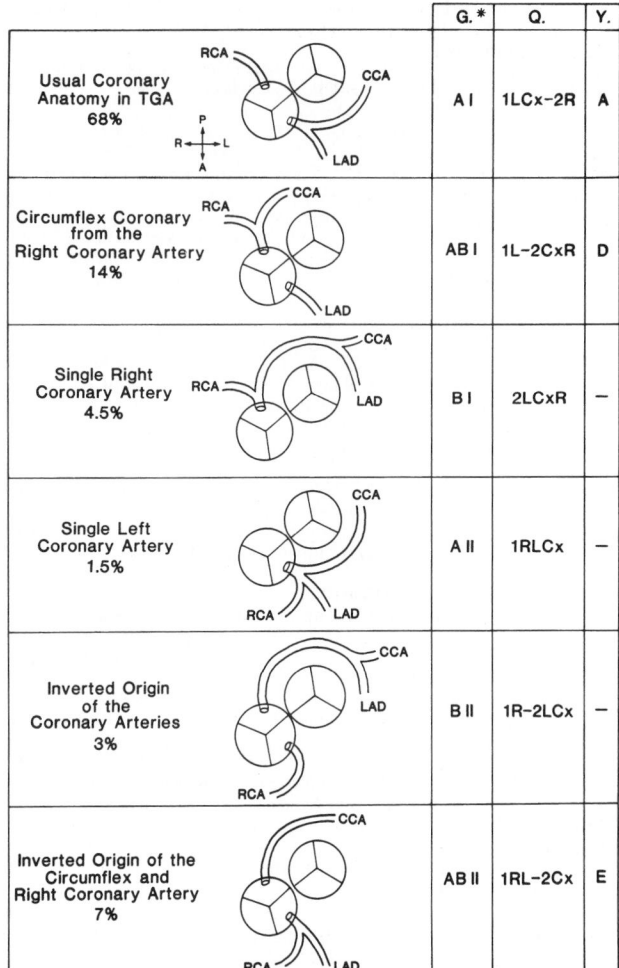

Figure 54–93. Diagram of the six most common types of coronary artery anatomy in TGA. Descriptive classification is on the left, and three simplified classification codes are described on the right. (From DiDonato, R. M., and Castañeda, A. R.: Anatomic correction of transposition of the great arteries at the arterial level. *In* Sabiston, D. C., Jr., and Spencer, F. C. [Eds.]: Surgery of the Chest, 5th ed. Philadelphia, W. B. Saunders, 1990, pp. 1435–1451.)

nary arises as a separate ostium from the rightward posterior-facing sinus. Occasionally, there is no true circumflex coronary artery but separate branches arise from the left coronary to supply the corresponding portion of the left ventricle. In up to 20% of cases, the circumflex coronary arises from the right coronary artery off the rightward posterior-facing sinus and passes behind the pulmonary artery. The left anterior descending artery then arises from a separate coronary ostium off the left coronary sinus. More rare coronary patterns involve a single right coronary artery from the rightward posterior sinus (4.5%) or a single left coronary artery from the leftward coronary sinus (1.5%).[12] Intramural coronary arteries that proceed in the aortic wall for a distance before exiting to the epicardial surface have been described and commonly occur at the commissural attachment of the atrioventricular valve.[13] Single coronary ostium or separate ostia close together arising from a single sinus have also been described. Abnormal coronary anatomies are more commonly seen in transposition with associated VSD than in the intact septum variety.

Important left ventricular outflow tract obstruction is unusual in association with TGA but has significant implications for the management of these neonates. The most common type of left ventricular outflow tract obstruction is dynamic, developing in patients with TGA and an intact ventricular septum as a result of leftward displacement of the muscular ventricular septum secondary to the development of higher systemic right ventricular pressures. The septum may then narrow the outflow tract, resulting in abnormal systolic anterior mitral leaflet motion and a situation similar to that noted in hypertrophic obstructive cardiomyopathy. Occasionally, subvalvular obstruction may be produced by a subvalvular fibrous ridge. Posterior malalignment of the ventricular septum may produce a more tunnel-type obstruction. In addition, fibrous tags arising from the mitral apparatus or membranous septum may result in significant subvalvular obstruction, more commonly when a VSD is present. Valvular stenosis is uncommon, although a bicuspid pulmonary valve has frequently been noted. In rare cases, aortic arch obstruction with coarctation or true interruption of the aortic arch has been observed in patients with TGA, left ventricular outflow tract obstruction, and VSD.[14]

PATHOPHYSIOLOGY

TGA is a relatively common form of congenital heart disease, accounting for 9.9% of infants with congenital heart disease in one New England study.[15] This incidence represents a frequency of 0.206 per 1000 live births. A distinct male predominance is noted, with a 2:1 male-to-female ratio that increases to 3.3:1 when the ventricular septum is intact.[16] In complex forms of transposition, a sexual predominance has not been noted. If TGA is not treated, 90% of children with D-TGA and intact septum will die by 1 year of age.

In complete TGA the pulmonary and systemic circulations exist in parallel instead of in series. This results in nonoxygenated venous blood passing through the right ventricle to the aorta while the oxygenated pulmonary venous blood passes through the left ventricle back to the pulmonary arterial circulation. Mixing between the pulmonary and systemic circulations at the atrial, ventricular, or great vessel level through a patent foramen ovale or atrial septal defect, a VSD, or a patent ductus arteriosus, respectively, is mandatory for survival. Patients with TGA and an intact ventricular septum survive initially because of aortopulmonary flow through a patent ductus arteriosus. After birth, both ventricles are relatively noncompliant, and infants with TGA often have an increased pulmonary blood flow, which causes enlargement of the left atrium and functional incompetence of the foramen ovale, resulting in atrial-level mixing of oxygenated and nonoxygenated blood. Inadequacy of this mixing, however, may result in only marginal tissue oxygenation, which does not improve with oxygen administration. Atrial balloon septostomy results in improved admixture and an improved tissue oxygen delivery in these patients.

Patients with TGA and significant VSD often have higher oxygen saturations by virtue of greater pulmonary blood flow and greater mixing at both atrial and ventricular level. In children with high pulmonary blood flow, pulmonary resistance may progressively increase throughout infancy. Ferenz has observed significant histologic changes in children older than 2 years of age with TGA, and children as young as 1 month of age have had intimal fibrosis noted in the pulmonary arteries.[7] This early development of severe pulmonary vascular disease in children with TGA is exacerbated in patients with associated VSD. Thus, early important pulmonary vascular disease can occur in patients with TGA regardless of the presence of a VSD. The rapidity of development of pulmonary obstructive disease has been suggested to be related to hypoxemia associated with increased sympathetic activity and in association with excessive pulmonary blood flow.[17]

Although neonatal pulmonary vascular resistance is normal in infants with TGA, the resistance falls progressively during the neonatal period with associated changes in the pulmonary and systemic ventricular compliance. Shortly after birth in the normal infant there is an increase in the left ventricular volume load and pressure load and a decrease in right ventricular volume and pressure load. These physiologic changes result in a rapid increase in the left ventricular myocardial mass.[18] This normal development of the left ventricle is lost in infants with D-TGA where the left ventricle ejects to the low-resistance pulmonary vascular bed (Fig. 54–94). Thus, the left ventricle does not increase muscle mass relative to the right ventricle; and within a few weeks it loses the ability to maintain adequate cardiac output against significant afterload. This change occurs despite the fact that the left ventricle still maintains a volume load in patients with transposition and intact ventricular septum. When, however, a VSD or large patent ductus arteriosus is present, both volume and pressure overload of the left ventricle is maintained, and in D-TGA with left ventricular outflow tract obstruction without a VSD a ventricular pressure load is imposed without a significant volume load. These physiologic changes in the neonatal heart are important for the consideration of surgical approaches because after a few weeks of postuterine life, the left ventricle in D-TGA with intact ventricular septum takes on the characteristics and wall thickness of a pulmonary ventricle and may not be adequate to support the systemic circulation.

CLINICAL FEATURES

The most common clinical finding in the infant with TGA is cyanosis (arterial PO$_2$ of 25 to 40 mm. Hg), which will vary in degree depending on associated anomalies. Typically, the cyanosis is more pronounced when the ventricular septum is intact and is often present at birth. The development of cyanosis later in infancy is usually associated with the pres-

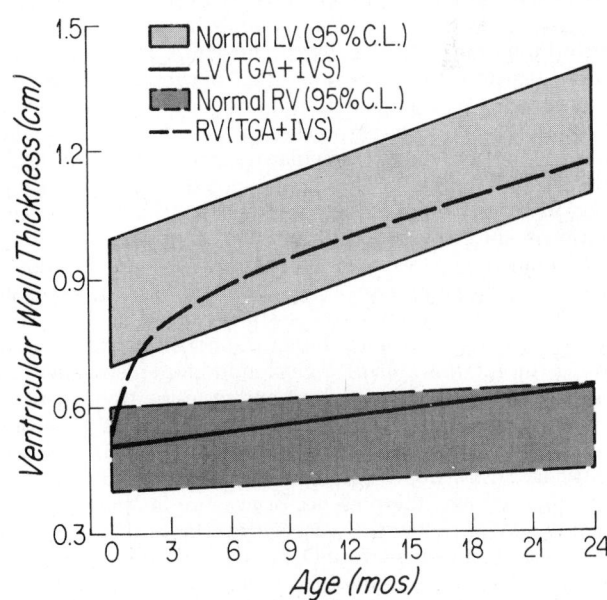

Figure 54–94. Graft describing the normal left ventricular wall thickness in TGA at birth. The solid line shows the decreased development of left ventricular muscle mass in TGA that results from a rapid decrease in pulmonary vascular resistance and drop in left ventricular pressure. The upper bar shows increase in left ventricular thickness and normally related great arteries. The dashed line shows the similar increase in right ventricular muscle mass in TGA with time. From Castañeda, A. R., Jonas, R. A., Mayer, J. E., Jr., and Hanley, F. L.: D-transposition of the great arteries. In: Cardiac Surgery of the Neonate and Infant. Philadelphia, W. B. Saunders, 1994, pp 409–438.)

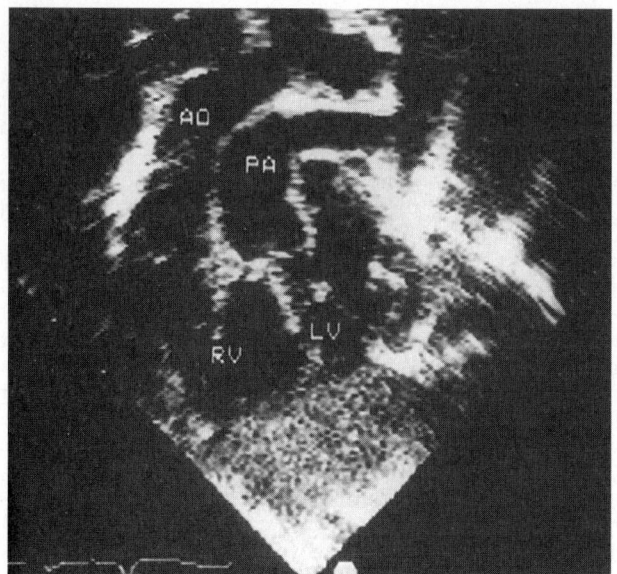

Figure 54–95. Subcostal sagittal view of the heart in D-TGV and intact ventricular septum. The anterior great vessel (AO) is the aorta, and the posterior great vessel that bifurcates is the pulmonary artery (PA). LV, left ventricle; RV right ventricle. (From Mavroudis, C., and Backer, C. L.: D-transposition of the great arteries. *In* Mavroudis, C., and Backer, C. L. [Eds.]: Pediatric Cardiac Surgery, 2nd ed. St. Louis, C. V. Mosby, 1994, pp. 339–366.)

ence of a significant VSD. Congestive heart failure may be the predominant clinical finding in patients with large VSD or patent ductus arteriosus, and the combination of cyanosis and increased pulmonary blood flow is almost pathognomonic of TGA in the infant. Symptoms of cardiac failure, however, are rarely present in the first week of life but commonly appear by 1 month of age, as pulmonary vascular resistance decreases and pulmonary blood flow becomes excessive, even in the patient with an intact ventricular septum.

Cardiac examination typically reveals a mildly overactive precordium, and 75% of patients with TGA and intact ventricular septum have a soft systolic murmur. The second heart sound is typically single and loud due to the proximity of the aorta to the anterior chest wall, which may make assessment of pulmonary vascular resistance difficult.[17] End-diastolic gallop rhythms are often noted in patients with associated VSD. In the presence of a large patent ductus arteriosus, the femoral pulses are often bounding. The liver may be enlarged in patients with a large systemic-to-pulmonary shunt and may be associated with tachypnea, intercostal retractions, and inability to successfully nurse. Children with significant valvular or subvalvular pulmonary stenosis often have a cardiac murmur of a crescendo/decrescendo nature along the left sternal border transmitted to the right clavicular area. The electrocardiogram may be normal at birth but over time shows signs of increasing right ventricular or biventricular hypertrophy. Electrocardiographic findings vary depending on age, the presence or absence of VSD, and the development of pulmonary vascular resistance. The axis may be normal in patients with VSD, but typically right-axis deviation is noted in children with an intact ventricular septum. Chest x-ray findings in D-TGA include an egg-shaped cardiac configuration, narrow superior mediastinum, and increased pulmonary markings with cardiomegaly. Asymmetry of pulmonary blood flow due to preferential right pulmonary arterial flow may result in right-sided congestive changes. The chest roentgenogram may be normal at birth, although progressive development of prominent pulmonary markings usually occurs along with progressive cardiomegaly.

MANAGEMENT

The widespread use of fetal ultrasound techniques has resulted in the common antenatal diagnosis of TGA. This fact and the fact that the majority of children with TGA are cyanotic in the first week of life has led to the initiation of treatment at a very early age in these patients. While in the past cardiac catheterization was generally necessary to confirm the diagnosis of TGA and to confirm the position of the cardiac chambers and the associated lesions, echocardiography has now generally supplanted cardiac catheterization in the majority of patients with simple complete transposition. Cardiac catheterization is now often indicated only in infants in whom inadequate shunting is noted or infants with associated intracardiac or extracardiac abnormalities that require clarification. Echocardiographic views confirming a posterior great vessel that divides into right and left pulmonary arteries and arises from the left ventricle in association with an anterior aorta arising from a right ventricle confirms the diagnosis of TGA (Fig. 54–95). The intracavitary shunts can be determined by Doppler echocardiography techniques, and several echo views can determine the size and location of VSDs with reference to the infundibular septum, the nature and size of atrial communications, the anatomy of the AV valves, and the presence and location of significant degrees of subpulmonary stenosis. In addition, in the majority of cases the origins and anatomic distributions of the coronary arteries can be adequately visualized by echocardiography to preclude cardiac catheterization (Fig. 54–96). Because the majority of coronary arterial variations can be successfully addressed at operation, identification of the origins of the coronary arteries is usually sufficient by echocardiography to permit operation without catheterization intervention.

Cardiac catheterization is reserved for those patients with significant clinical instability to improve the degree of intracavitary shunting by enlarging the interatrial septal commu-

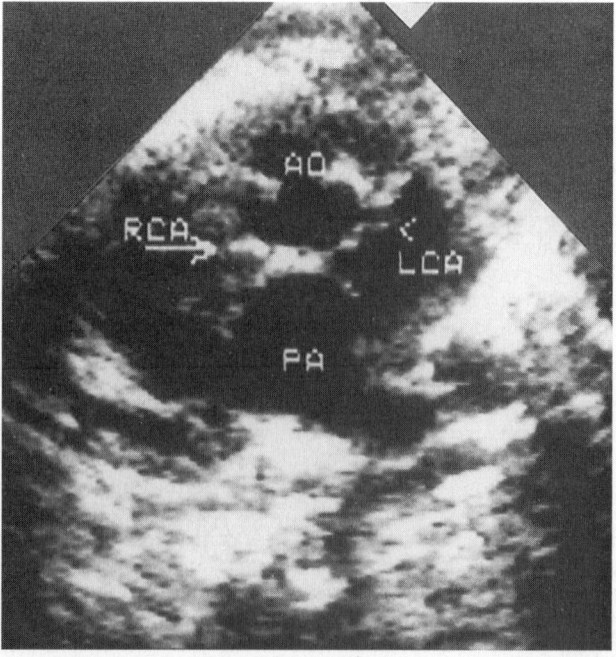

Figure 54–96. Parasternal short-axis view of the heart in D-TGA and intact ventricular septum with usual coronary anatomy. Coronary arteries are noted to arise from the left and right coronary cusps, and the pulmonary artery is posterior. AO, aorta; LCA, left coronary artery; PA, pulmonary artery; RCA, right coronary artery. (From Mavroudis, C., and Backer, C. L.: D-transposition of the great arteries. *In:* Mavroudis, C., and Backer, C. L. [Eds.]: Pediatric Cardiac Surgery, 2nd ed. St. Louis, C. V. Mosby, 1994, pp. 339–366.)

nication. At catheterization, the left atrial pressure is usually greater than the right atrial pressure and the pressure in the pulmonary (left) ventricle is dependent on the presence or absence of VSD, valvular or subvalvular stenosis, and the age of the patient and magnitude of elevation of pulmonary vascular resistance.

If inadequate interatrial shunting is noted and results in clinical instability (acidemia, severe hypoxemia), the mainstay of management has been a Rashkind balloon atrial septostomy.[19] A balloon-tipped catheter is passed through the systemic veins, through the right atrium and foramen ovale, and into the left atrium; the balloon is inflated and pulled vigorously across the atrial septum to tear the foramen ovale, improving admixture of pulmonary and systemic venous blood. Although this procedure is usually used at catheterization, it may be performed in the intensive care unit with echocardiographic guidance in children whose conditions are unstable. Performance of a Rashkind atrial septostomy results in decompression of the left ventricle and therefore may result in poor left ventricular performance if a subsequent arterial switch procedure is delayed. Therefore, patients who are good anatomic candidates for an arterial switch procedure who have acceptable arterial oxygen saturations are generally referred for early arterial switch without intervening atrial septostomy if the clinical condition permits. Prostaglandin E_1, however, is usually administered to maintain ductal patency and increase pulmonary blood flow and improve stabilization of patients before early operative repair. In addition, relative dehydration may decrease the degree of interatrial shunting and volume infusions may improve hemodynamics in infants presenting with TGA and intact septum early in life.

HISTORY OF SURGICAL REPAIR

Initial surgical therapy for TGA involved creation of an atrial septal defect using a closed technique to increase the mixing between systemic venous and pulmonary venous circulations by Blalock and Hanlon in 1950.[20] Although the early mortality was high with this operative approach, successful creation of an atrial septal defect resulted in significant palliation in many of these children. Initial attempts to reverse the transposed vessels by both Mustard and Bailey and their colleagues were frustrated by their inability to maintain coronary perfusion and by poor function of the anatomic left ventricle.[21, 22] Thus, initial surgical therapy was directed toward atrial transposition of pulmonary and systemic venous returns. In 1952, Lillehei and Varco transferred the right-sided pulmonary veins to the right atrium and connected the inferior vena cava to the left atrium.[23] A successful modification of this technique using an allograft to connect the inferior vena cava to the left atrium was described by Baffes in 1956.[24]

Multiple attempts were made at both atrial and arterial repairs of TGA during the 1950s, and in 1954 Albert suggested the concept of switching the atrial septum so that caval return was directed to the left ventricle and pulmonary venous return to the right ventricle at the atrial level.[25] This atrial switch concept was first successfully accomplished by Senning in 1959, using an ingenious technique for relocating the walls of the right atrium and the atrial septum.[26] Many of the early attempts at atrial repair were frustrated by the fact that operation was performed in children between 1 and 2 years of age, and significant pulmonary vascular obstructive disease had already developed in many of these children. In 1964, Mustard described an alternate procedure for intraatrial repair excising the atrial septum and creating a large interatrial baffle of pericardium to redirect pulmonary and systemic venous blood.[27] This repair resulted in larger atrial

size than the Senning operation. Early results with the Mustard operation were markedly improved over the previously reported Senning repairs and reflected the significant patient population in Toronto who had had successful Blalock-Hanlon atrial septectomies early in life.

A major development in the surgical treatment of TGA occurred in 1966 when Rashkind and Miller reported the use of a balloon catheter technique to enlarge the atrial septal defect in patients with TGA, causing improved early physiologic stability and decreasing the need for operative atrial septectomy.[19] Over the decade of the 1960s, the Mustard operation became the most commonly performed procedure for transposition, and it became clear that repair in the first few months of life could be accomplished with a low operative mortality and improved results compared with repair at a later age, as techniques of cardiovascular surgery became improved over this decade. In 1970, the Senning procedure re-emerged as the persistent problems of baffle obstruction and arrhythmias following the Mustard operation became well defined, and the ability to use autologous tissue for the atrial reconstruction became a preferred approach.

The success with the atrial switch operations for TGA with intact septum did not translate to repair of transposition with large VSD. Disappointing results with VSD closure and atrial repair in this group of patients continued to be a stimulus for development of an arterial switch procedure that was first successfully performed by Jatene and colleagues in 1975.[28] Yacoub shortly thereafter reported additional successful cases.[29] The success of arterial switch procedure with reimplantation of the coronary arteries in some patients with TGA and VSD led to reintroduction of this technique for patients with intact ventricular septum. Yacoub's initial attempts in patients with TGA and an intact ventricular septum were unsuccessful in 1972; however, additional reports by 1976 suggested that such repair was possible in infancy.[29] Early mortality with the arterial switch in infancy was related to the fact that the pulmonary left ventricle was not prepared to sustain systemic pressure. Therefore, initial approaches included pulmonary arterial banding as a first stage, followed by arterial switch at a later time.[30] However, Yacoub, Quagebeur, Brawn, and Castañeda and their associates have subsequently demonstrated the ability to repair simple transposition in the first few days of life by arterial switch operation while the pulmonary ventricle has relatively high pressure.[29, 31–33] The rapidly decreasing mortality for arterial switch operations has resulted in this surgical approach becoming the standard corrective surgical procedure at the present time and results in both an anatomic and physiologic reconstruction of this cardiac defect.

Operative approaches to TGA, VSD, and significant left ventricular outflow tract obstruction were less successful in the early period of cardiac surgery. In 1969, Rastelli suggested combination of an intraventricular tunnel repair, closing the VSD and baffling the pulmonary venous blood from the left ventricle to the aorta, closing the pulmonary artery exit from the left ventricle and creating an extracardiac conduit from the anatomic right ventricle to the pulmonary bifurcation, resulting in an anatomic repair for TGA/VSD and left ventricular outflow tract obstruction.[34] Obstruction of the reconstructed left ventricular outflow tract remains a common complication of the Rastelli type repair and has led to recommendation of a variation of intraventricular repair by Lecompte (the REV procedure).[34]

OPERATIVE INTERVENTION
Palliative Operations

The advent of the balloon atrial septostomy by Rashkind and Miller has essentially eliminated the need for the Blalock-Hanlon operative atrial septectomy. Infants with associated cardiac abnormalities and a thick atrial septum who are considered for later atrial baffle repair may benefit from the Blalock-Hanlon technique, although the safety of cardiopulmonary bypass has resulted in the common use of open atrial septectomy in these patients. Pulmonary arterial banding has been used for palliation in patients with TGA and VSD in young infants who have intractable congestive heart failure until operative repair at 3 to 6 months of age. As the results with arterial switch procedure and VSD closure in infancy have improved, banding in most instances is unnecessary because complete repair can be effected in infancy. Therefore, banding of the pulmonary artery has now been limited to very small neonates who might benefit from delay in corrective operation and those patients with TGA and intact ventricular septum who present late for arterial switch repair and require *training* of the left ventricle to work at a higher pressure to become the systemic ventricle. For similar reasons, pulmonary arterial banding is used in patients with TGA who develop right ventricular dysfunction and failure after atrial baffle operations as a component of staged conversion to an arterial switch repair. Pulmonary arterial banding in TGA is a delicate procedure, because limitation of pulmonary blood flow results in significant hypoxia and metabolic acidosis, and loose banding results in inadequate protection of the pulmonary vascular bed and poor development of the left (pulmonary) ventricle. Thus, in most situations where preparation of the left ventricle is undertaken for conversion to an arterial switch procedure, banding must be associated with creation of an aortopulmonary shunt to maintain adequate pulmonary blood flow and prevent hypoxemia and ventricular dysfunction.

Surgical Correction

Satisfactory correction of TGA results in rerouting of systemic venous blood to the pulmonary circulation and the pulmonary venous blood into the systemic arterial circulation. This may be accomplished at the atrial, the ventricular, or the great arterial level. The earliest repairs of TGA involve rerouting of the systemic and pulmonary venous returns at the atrial level, resulting in an adequate physiologic repair but not an anatomic repair because the morphologic right ventricle continues to be the systemic ventricle. Both ventricular (Rastelli) and great arterial (arterial switch) repairs are more-anatomic corrections, resulting in a morphologic left ventricle as the systemic ventricle.

Atrial Repairs

The first successful rerouting of venous flow at the atrial level was described by Senning in 1959.[26] In this operation, pulmonary and systemic venous return was rerouted by incising and realigning the atrial septum over the pulmonary veins and using the free right atrial wall to create a pulmonary venous baffle (Fig. 54–97). The Senning operation, while brilliant in concept, was not associated with high survival in its early use because of its difficulty and the fact that many patients had associated VSD and developed progressive pulmonary vascular obstructive disease. In 1964, Mustard described an operation accomplishing the same goals as the Senning operation but using a large interatrial baffle of either autologous pericardium or synthetic tissue.[27] As a preliminary to the Mustard operation, creation of a virtual common atrium is necessary with resection of the atrial septum and the ridge of tissue between the superior vena caval entrance and the superior aspect of the atrial septum. Inadequate resection of the atrial septum has resulted in the occurrence of baffle obstruction of the systemic venous return to the heart (Fig. 54–98). While the Mustard operation supplanted the Senning technique early in the history of repair of TGA because of its technical simplicity, the tendency for obstruction of the pulmonary venous or systemic venous sides of the baffle and the development of atrial arrhythmias after this procedure led to reassessment of the Senning technique. Reintroduction of the Senning operation in infancy after successful balloon atrial septostomy resulted in the use of autologous atrial tissue rather than synthetic baffles and appeared to be associated with a lower incidence of atrial arrhythmias and caval obstruction, and thus became the preferred technique in many centers. As techniques improved, the use of either Senning- or Mustard-type repairs in infancy was noted

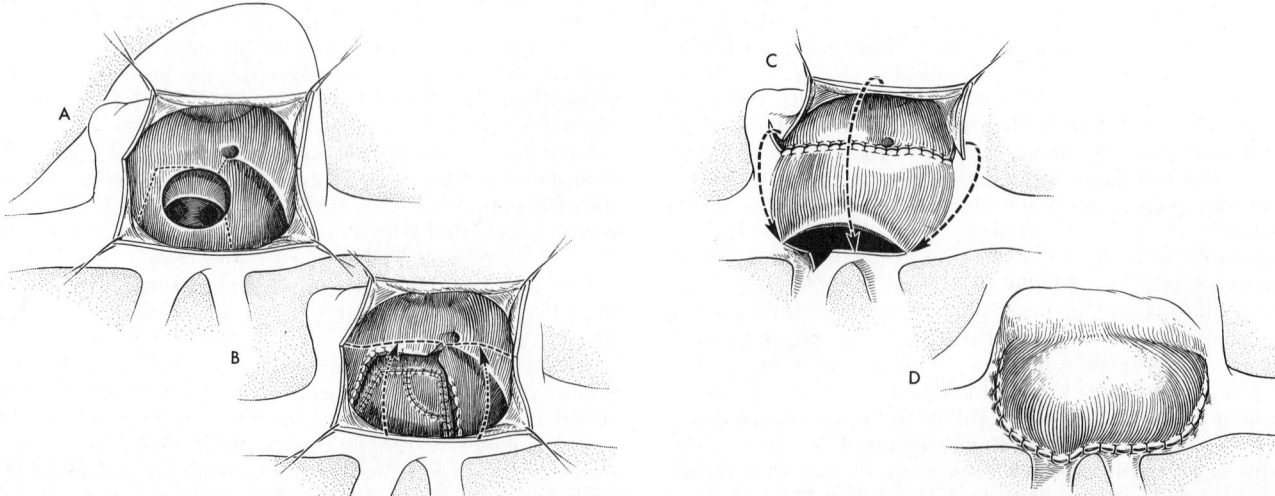

Figure 54–97. The Senning operation. *A,* View from the right atrium showing incision lines (dashed lines) to create a flap of the posterior atrial septum and an incision into the base of the coronary sinus. *B,* The posterior flap of atrial septum is augmented with a piece of pericardium and sutured inferiorly over the origins of the pulmonary veins in the left atrium. The posterior wall of the right atrium is then sutured to the anterior portion of the atrial septum, baffling the vena caval return across the septum to the mitral valve. *C,* After completion of the venous baffle, the anterior wall of the right atrium is sutured to an opening made in the left atrium posterior to the interatrial septum at the entrance point of the right pulmonary veins, baffling the pulmonary venous blood over the systemic venous pathway into the right ventricle. *D,* Completed suture line showing repair with autologous tissue. (From Mavroudis, C., and Backer, C. L.: D-transposition of the great arteries. *In* Mavroudis, C., and Backer, C. L. [Eds.]: Pediatric Cardiac Surgery, 2nd ed. St. Louis, C. V. Mosby, 1994, pp. 339–366.)

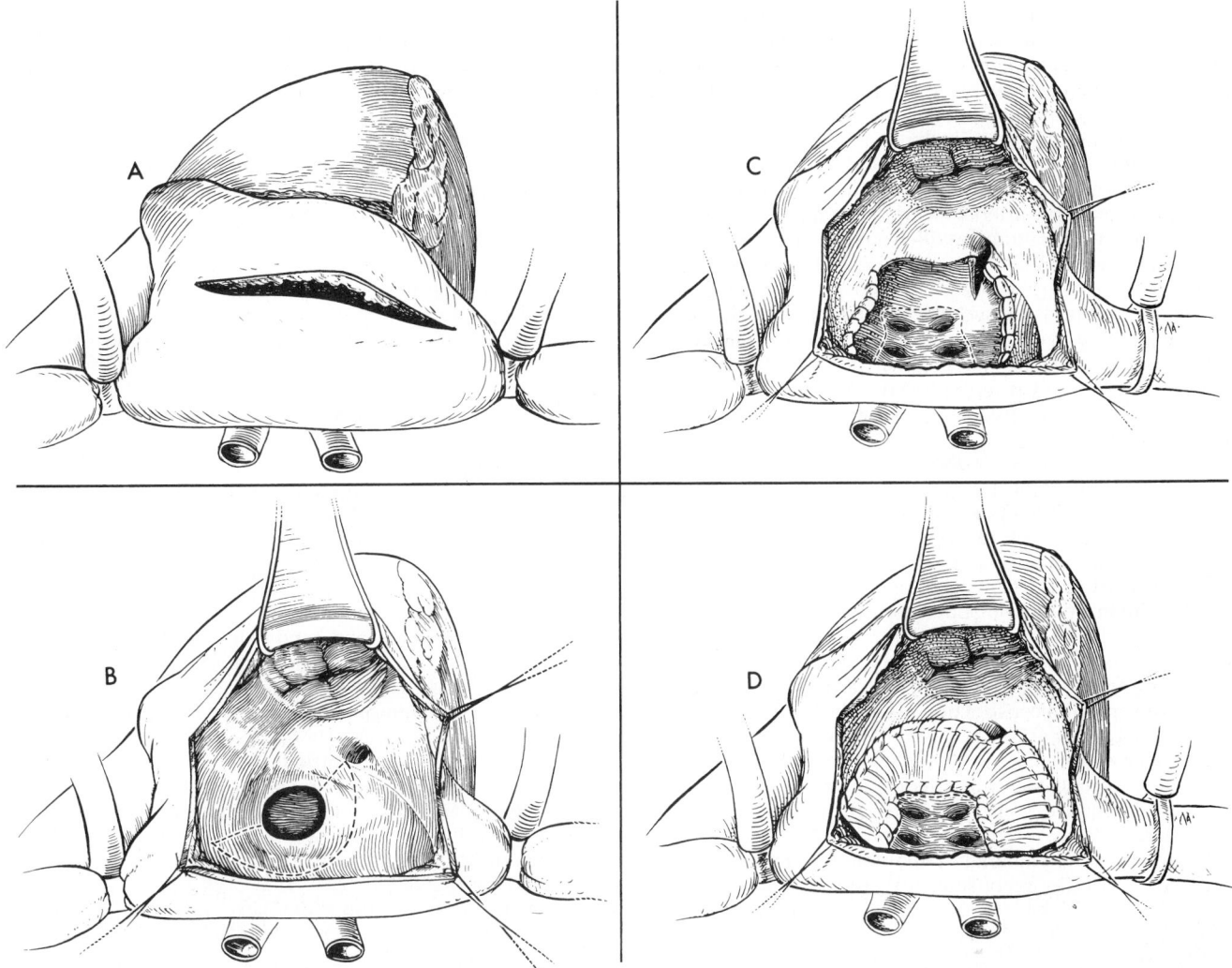

Figure 54–98. The Mustard operation. *A,* A longitudinal incision is made in the right atrium away from the sinus node. *B,* The posterior aspect of the atrial septum is excised, creating a wide opening for baffling the venous blood into the left atrium (dotted lines). *C,* The coronary sinus is cut back into the left atrium to avoid suturing near the atrioventricular node. Raw margins of atrial septum may be oversewn. The suture line for the placement of the baffle around the pulmonary veins is noted with the dotted line. *D,* A baffle of Dacron or pericardium is used to baffle the vena caval blood flow to the left atrium across the mitral valve. Completion of this baffle allows venous blood to enter the right atrium and cross the tricuspid valve to the aorta. (From Trusler, G. A., and Freedom, R. M.: Transposition of the great arteries: The Mustard procedure. *In* Sabiston, D. C., Jr., and Spencer, F. C. [Eds.]: Gibbons Surgery of the Chest. Philadelphia, W. B. Saunders, 1983, p. 1138.)

to be associated with a lower incidence of cerebral thrombosis and hypoxic injury due to cyanosis and peripheral emboli from right-to-left shunting. Thus, a standard approach using balloon atrial septostomy in infancy followed by the elective repair in infants between the ages of 3 and 8 months resulted in excellent survival of as high as 95%.[36] Some series reported only a 1% or 2% operative mortality even in early infancy with the Senning-type repair.[37]

Arterial Repairs

In spite of the excellent results with the atrial switch operations, by either the Mustard or the Senning technique, both operations are associated with physiologic and not anatomic correction. The morphologic right ventricle remains the systemic ventricle in these patients, and although many patients have had many years of successful function of the right ventricle as the systemic ventricle, there remain concerns about the long-term function of a morphologic right ventricle in the systemic circulation. The right ventricle is typically thin walled and heavily trabeculated, and the geometric configuration of the ventricle is different from a morphologic

left ventricle. The tricuspid atrioventricular valve also is not anatomically designed to maintain competency at systemic pressure as is the mitral valve. Although it may not be inevitable that systemic morphologic right ventricles will fail with time, a considerable number of patients have now returned after an atrial baffle operation with complications of intractable atrial arrhythmias and right ventricular failure. Thus, there has been increasing interest in the more anatomic correction of the arterial switch operation in hopes of preventing late ventricular dysfunction and arrhythmias.

The first successful use of an arterial reconstruction in TGA was by Jatene in 1975.[28] The principles of successful anatomic correction involve dividing the aorta and pulmonary artery and excising the origins of the coronary arteries with a button of aortic wall and repositioning the coronary arteries to the posterior great vessel (pulmonary artery). The defects in the aorta from which the coronary arteries have been excised are reconstructed with additional tissue, and then the posterior great vessel is anastomosed to the distal aorta and the anterior great vessel is anastomosed to the pulmonary arterial bifurcation. Initially, the Jatene arterial switch procedure was used in infants and children with VSD and TGA who had an adequately prepared left ventricle for use as a systemic ventricle. Early mortality, however, was high in these patients owing to the development of pulmonary vascular obstructive disease and the complexity of the operation. However, improvements in infant operations have permitted the application of this technique routinely in infants with TGA and intact septum or VSD, and the arterial switch procedure is now the procedure of choice for correction of TGA. Successful application of the arterial switch technique to infants with intact ventricular septum results from the fact that elevated pulmonary vascular resistance is present at birth and the left ventricle is therefore at relatively high pressure and able to adequately support the systemic circulation after the operation. In addition, improvements in the techniques of coronary transfer, myocardial protection, and neonatal vessel reconstruction have resulted in improved survival statistics in the arterial switch procedure that now rival the results with atrial baffle operations.

The basic techniques of the arterial switch operation involve transection of the great arteries, transfer of the coronary arterial origins, and repositioning of the great vessels (Fig. 54–99). The details of the operative techniques, however, vary from one institution to another. The procedures are performed with a median sternotomy incision and the use of cardiopulmonary bypass and hypothermia, although hypothermic circulatory arrest is used for the procedure in varying degrees in many institutions. After the median sternotomy is made, a portion of the anterior pericardium is excised for autologous patch reconstruction of the defects in the anterior great vessel. The pericardium may be used fresh or fixed in glutaraldehyde to make it easier to manipulate during the operation. The ligamentum arteriosum or ductus arteriosus is dissected out and branches of the right and left pulmonary arteries mobilized to the bifurcation of the vessels in the hilum of the lung bilaterally. It is important to mobilize the pulmonary arteries freely so as to permit anterior relocation of the pulmonary bifurcation without distortion of the pulmonary artery or aorta. The aorta is typically cannulated for bypass distally to allow room for manipulation of the proximal aorta during the reconstruction. After bypass is established, the ductus arteriosus is ligated and divided and the aortic end and pulmonary arterial end oversewn as necessary. The aorta is then clamped close to the aortic cannula and cardioplegia administered into the aortic root.

If a VSD is present, it is approached either through the right atrium across the tricuspid valve or occasionally through the anterior great vessel. The aorta is then transected above the level of the coronary ostia and the pulmonary artery transected just below the bifurcation, with care not to carry the incision into the left pulmonary artery. The ductus arteriosus is divided and the pulmonary artery bifurcation brought anterior to the aorta (the Lecompte maneuver). The coronary ostia are examined and excised from the anterior great vessel with a button of aortic wall extending down into the base of the sinuses of Valsalva. The epicardial course of the coronaries is then mobilized adequately to allow turning the coronary ostia to the posterior great vessel without kinking of the epicardial course. On occasion, the small conal branches of the coronaries may need to be sacrificed to permit adequate mobilization. An incision is then made in the posterior great vessel at the site for reattachment of the coronary ostia, and a medially based flap incision is created to allow takeoff of the coronary ostia without tension or kinking. The coronary ostia are then sewn to the incisions in the posterior great vessel using an absorbable suture to allow for maximum growth. The distal aorta is then anastomosed to the posterior great vessel to which the coronary arteries have been transferred. Additional cardioplegia may be administered at this time to check for hemostasis of the suture

lines and to confirm that good myocardial perfusion without kinking of the coronary anastomoses is present. The defects in the anterior great vessels from which the coronary arteries have been excised is then repaired with a generous portion of glutaraldehyde-fixed pericardium. The anterior great vessel is then sutured to the pulmonary artery bifurcation, with care being taken to avoid tension on the pulmonary arteries that may interfere with symmetrical pulmonary blood flow. Finally, the atrial septal defect is either closed primarily or with a small patch of pericardial material and the atrium is closed.

In the situation in which the great vessels are side to side rather than anteroposterior, it may be advisable to leave the pulmonary confluence posterior to the aorta and open the right pulmonary artery, closing the pulmonary bifurcation to transpose the opening in the pulmonary artery more to the right than usual. This may facilitate reconstruction to the right ventricle.

After completion of the repair, left atrial and right atrial lines are placed for postoperative monitoring and temporary pacemaker wires applied. The infants are weaned from bypass, maintaining a systemic pressure of approximately 60 mm. Hg to prevent distention of the newly systemic left ventricle.

Continuous sedation and neuromuscular blockade with mechanical ventilation and moderate inotropic support are usually used in the first 18 hours post repair, as in other infants undergoing complex congenital heart repair.

Infants with significant left ventricular outflow tract obstruction represent a small proportion of children presenting with TGA. Because left ventricular outflow tract obstruction is often dynamic, the relative contributions of the dynamic components of obstruction and the more fixed components such as subvalvular fibrous rings and mitral valve leaflet tags are often difficult to ascertain. Although it may be possible to resect fixed forms of left ventricular outflow tract obstruction with exposure across the pulmonary valve at the time of arterial switch operation, complete relief of obstruction is not often possible. However, in the majority of cases, moderate relief of left ventricular outflow tract obstruction can be well tolerated after the arterial switch procedure because the pulmonary ventricle has been preconditioned to elevated intracavitary pressure. In the rare forms of severe left ventricular outflow tract obstruction presenting in infancy, creation of an interatrial communication and a systemic-to-pulmonary arterial shunt may be the best early approach, followed by later repair, although in some centers early complete repair is preferred. Repair is by the Rastelli operation, in which pulmonary venous blood is directed through a patch through the VSD across to the aorta and a valved conduit placed from the right ventricle to the distal pulmonary arteries (Fig. 54–100). In patients with an intact ventricular septum and significant left ventricular outflow tract obstruction, atrial baffle repair and creation of a conduit from the left ventricular cavity to the pulmonary bifurcation may also be considered. More recently, patients with significant VSD and TGA with left ventricular outflow tract obstruction may have a more anatomic repair by use of Lecompte's réparation à l'etage ventriculaire (REV) procedure, which results in transposition of the aorta to a more normal location over the left ventricular outflow tract and in some cases may preclude the need for a valved conduit from the right ventricle to the pulmonary bifurcation and the subsequent necessity for replacement of this nonviable conduit (Fig. 54–101).

SURGICAL RESULTS
Atrial Repairs

The results of either a Mustard or Senning operative repair have generally been good, with survival rates of 80% to 95%

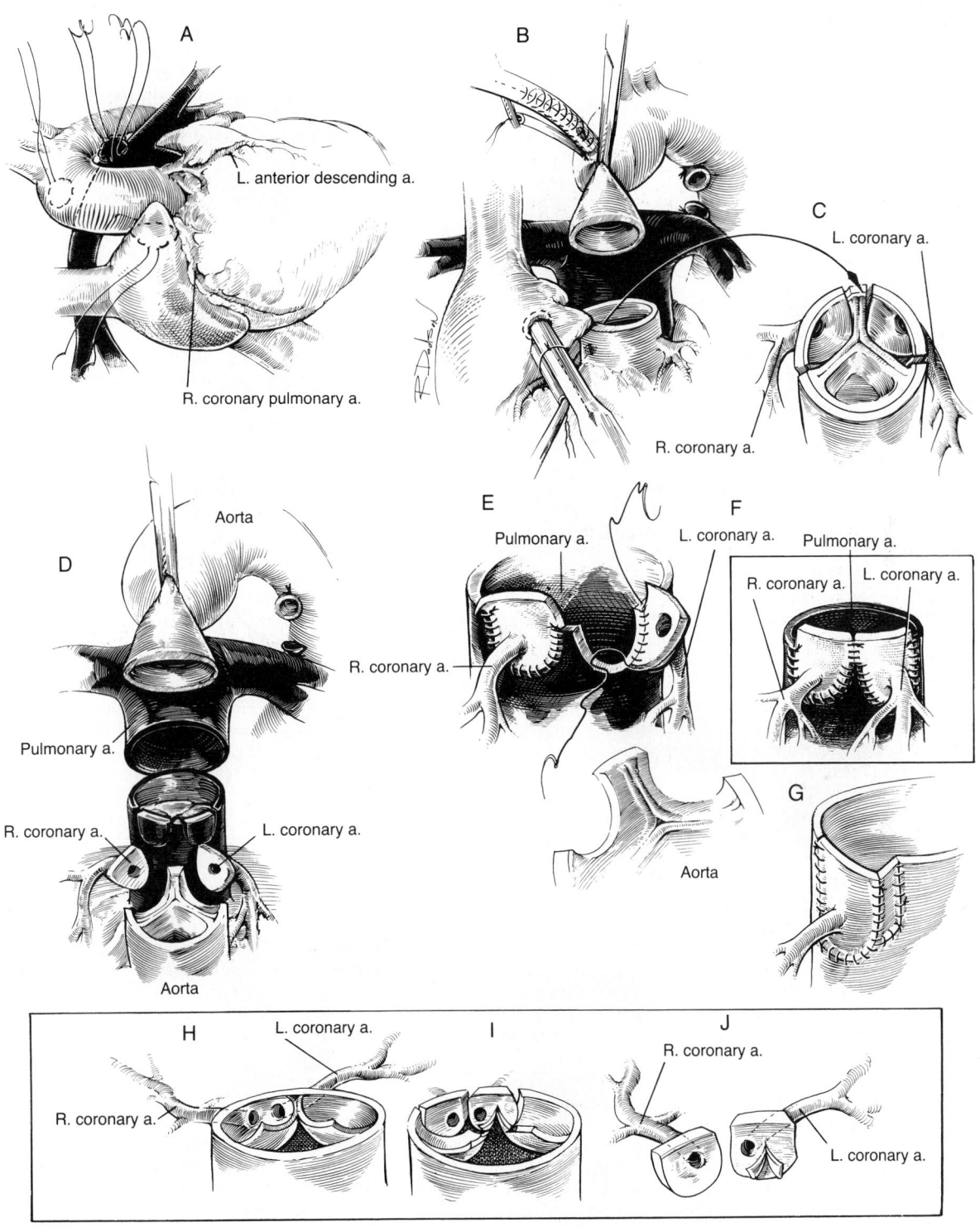

Figure 54–99. *A,* Cannulation sites for cardiopulmonary bypass in the arterial switch operation. Single atrial cannulation can be performed or bicaval venous cannulation utilized. The ductus arteriosus is ligated and divided between sutures. *B,* Division of the ductus arteriosus and ascending aorta after initiation of cardioplegic arrest. *C,* Excision of the left and right coronary ostia with a button of aortic wall. *D,* Excision of corresponding segments of the posterior great vessel wall to which the coronary arteries will be reimplanted. Alternatively, medially based flap incisions can be used. *E,* Suturing of the coronary ostial buttons to the posterior great vessel. *F,* Completed anastomoses of the reimplanted coronary arteries. In some cases, the coronary buttons can be approximated together in the midline. *G,* Augmentation of the medial aspect of the anastomosis to prevent kinking is occasionally necessary, although less common if medially based flap incisions are used for coronary reimplantation. *H,* If juxtacommissural origins of either or both coronary arteries from the facing sinuses are present, excision of a portion of the native aortic valve may be necessary to allow mobilization. *I* and *J,* Separation of the coronary arteries is done if possible to prevent distortion and provide easier implantation. (From Castañeda, A. R., Jonas, R. A., Mayer, J. E., Jr., and Hanley, F. L.: D-transposition of the great arteries. *In:* Cardiac Surgery of the Neonate and Infant. Philadelphia, W. B. Saunders, 1994, pp. 409–438.)

Illustration continued on following page

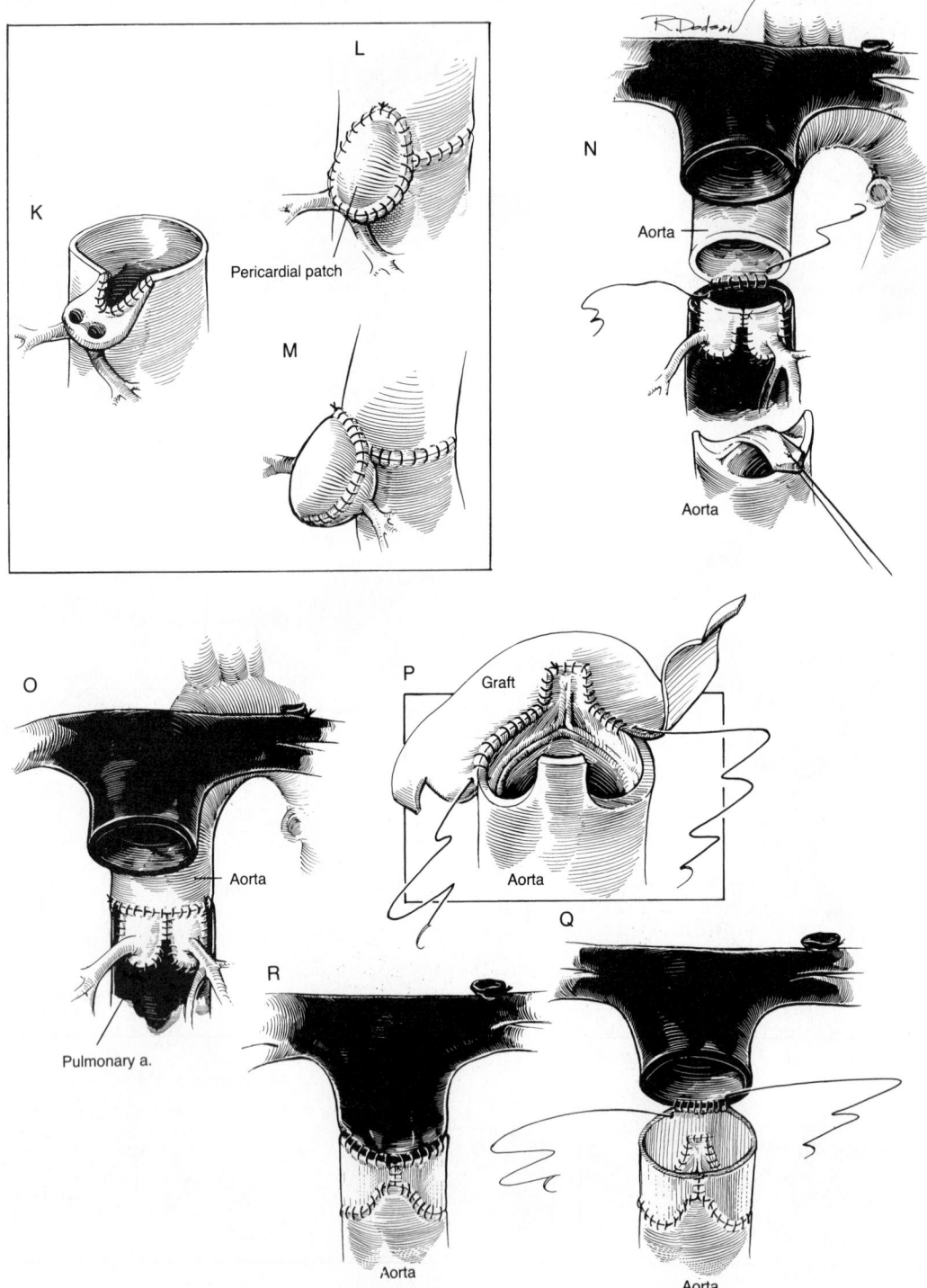

Figure 54–99 *Continued K,* If right and left intramural coronary arteries are present, the aortic coronary flap is left in place and sutured along the cephalic border to an incision in the anterior neoaorta. *L* and *M,* A pericardial patch is then used to provide unrestricted entrance of blood into the coronary ostia. *N,* After completion of the coronary transfer, the distal aorta is anastomosed to the neoaorta. *O,* The pulmonary bifurcation is brought anterior to the aorta in the Lecompte maneuver. *P,* The defects in the aorta from which the coronary arteries have been excised is augmented with a pantaloon-shaped patch of pericardium. *Q,* The pulmonary bifurcation is then anastomosed to the augmented aorta. In most cases the pericardium is not sutured completely around the aorta to create a complete pericardial tube. *R,* Completed anastomosis of the pulmonary artery anterior to the new aorta. (From Castañeda, A. R., Jonas, R. A., Mayer, J. E., Jr., and Hanley, F. L.: D-transposition of the great arteries. *In:* Cardiac Surgery of the Neonate and Infant. Philadelphia, W. B. Saunders, 1994, pp. 409–438.)

reported for infants with intact ventricular septum. A large series of 329 infants and children undergoing atrial repair procedures at the Hospital for Sick Children in Toronto had a 10.5% operative mortality that included the entire experience but only a 0.9% mortality in the decade beginning in 1974. Ten-year actuarial survival was 93.7% in the last 223 patients in the series.[36] Similarly, excellent results have been noted in the more recent collected series of the Senning operation for transposition with intact septum.[37] Complications of the atrial operations, however, have been a high incidence of sinus node dysfunction or other atrial dysrhythmias and the development of dynamic left ventricular outflow tract obstruction from the systemic right ventricular pressure load. The Senning operation has been associated with improved rates of sinus rhythm, although atrial arrhythmias remain not uncommon with this approach. The incidence of late deterioration in right ventricular function is unknown but may approach as high as 10% of patients. Results with atrial correction appear to be improved with early repair before the development of significant pulmonary vascular obstructive disease, and age alone does not appear to be a significant independent predictor of operative risk.

Results of Arterial Repairs

Perhaps the largest series of arterial repairs for TGA has been reported by the group at Boston Children's Hospital. A recent report of 470 patients undergoing an arterial switch operation indicated a survival rate at 1 month and 1, 5, and 8 years of 93%, 92%, 91%, and 91%, respectively.[38] Significant risk factors for death after repair included abnormal coronary artery patterns and longer duration of circulatory arrest during operation. Twenty-eight of the 470 patients required a reintervention to relieve right ventricular or pulmonary artery stenosis. Additional studies by the same group have shown that left ventricular size, mass, functional status, and contractility continue to be normal on follow-up with no evidence of deterioration.[39] In addition, careful follow-up of atrial and ventricular arrhythmias after the arterial switch operation has shown a 96% incidence of sinus rhythm on electrocardiogram and 99% during Holter monitor studies a mean of 2.1 years after the procedure.[40] These results represent marked improvement over the long-term results with the atrial operations, although additional follow-up is necessary. The results of these careful studies have confirmed the superiority of the anatomic arterial switch procedure over atrial repairs. Therefore, despite evolution of the manage-

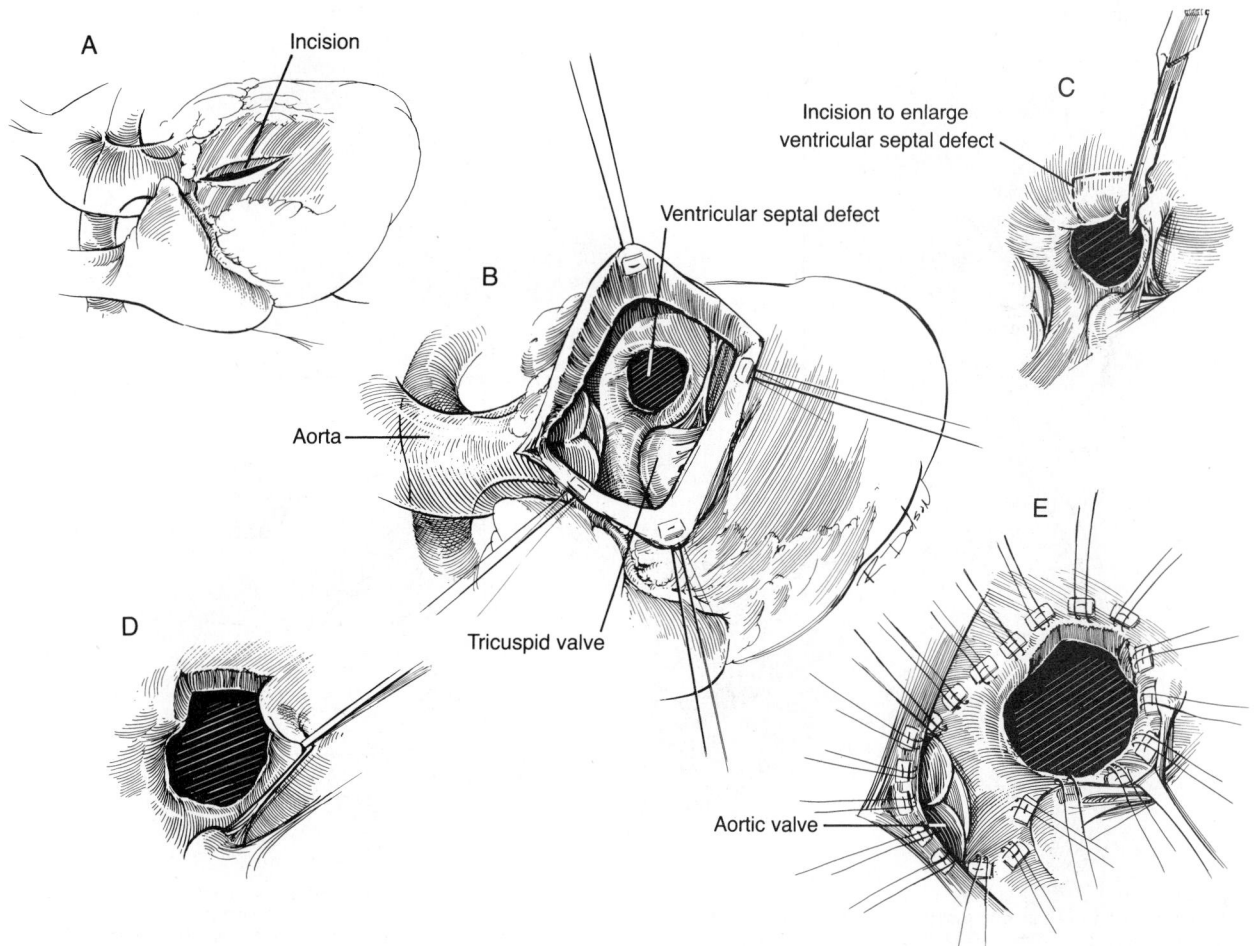

Figure 54–100. The Rastelli operation for TGA with VSD and left ventricular outflow tract obstruction. *A,* An incision is made in the right ventricular muscle, avoiding major coronary branches. *B,* The VSD is exposed through the right ventricle. *C* and *D,* Excision of the anterior-superior limb of the septal band enlarges the VSD to provide unobstructed flow from the left ventricle to the aorta. *E,* Mattress sutures are used to place the VSD patch, baffling blood across the defect to the anteriorly located aorta. (From Castañeda, A. R., Jonas, R. A., Mayer, J. E. Jr., and Hanley, F. L.: D-transposition of the great arteries. *In:* Cardiac Surgery of the Neonate and Infant. Philadelphia, W. B. Saunders, 1994, pp. 409–438.)

Illustration continued on following page

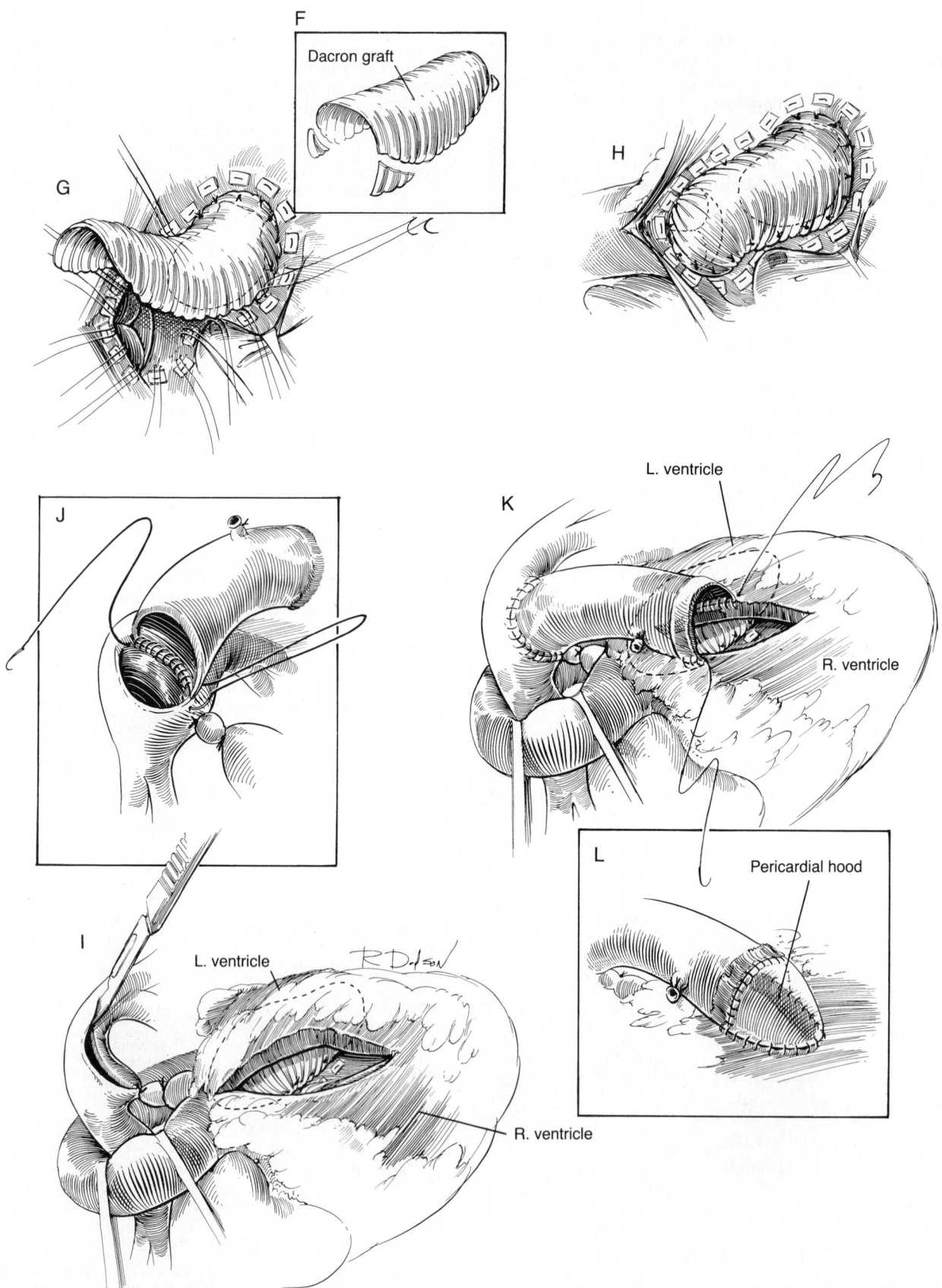

Figure 54–100 *Continued F*, A baffle is created from a Dacron graft to prevent compression against the conal muscle and obstruction of the outflow tract and secured in place with the previous sutures *(G)*. *H*, Completed VSD closure with the Dacron baffle. *I* and *J*, Ligation of the main pulmonary artery proximal to the bifurcation and suturing of a homograft conduit to the pulmonary artery bifurcation. *K*, Proximal anastomosis of the homograft valve containing conduit to the incision in the right ventricle. *L*, Augmentation of the takeoff of the pulmonary homograft with a pericardial hood to prevent compression and obstruction. (From Castañeda, A. R., Jonas, R. A., Mayer, J. E., Jr., and Hanley, F. L.: D-transposition of the great arteries. *In:* Cardiac Surgery of the Neonate and Infant. Philadelphia, W. B. Saunders, 1994, pp. 409–438.)

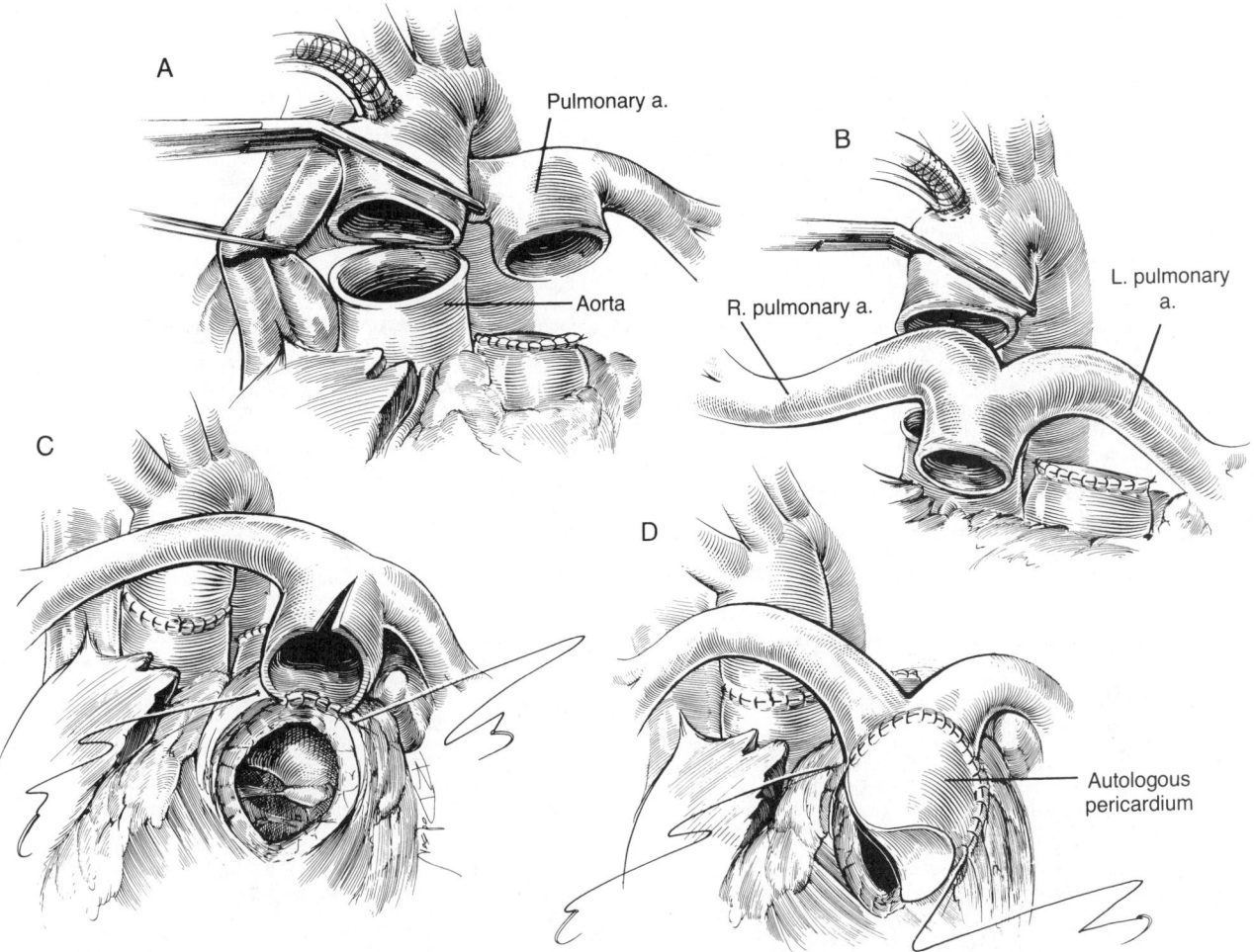

Figure 54–101. Lecompte's REV procedure (réparation à l'etage ventriculaire). *A,* Division of ascending aorta and pulmonary artery. The pulmonary artery is oversewn, eliminating the egress of blood from the left ventricle. The VSD is closed as in a Rastelli operation, baffling blood to the aorta. B, The Lecompte maneuver is performed, bringing the pulmonary artery bifurcation anterior to the great vessels. *C,* The aorta is reconstructed after anterior translocation of the pulmonary bifurcation, and the pulmonary bifurcation is sewn to an incision in the right ventricular infundibulum. *D,* Completion of the repair with augmentation of the outflow tract with autologous pericardium prevents outflow tract with autologous pericardium prevents outflow tract obstruction. (From Castañeda, A. R., Jonas, R. A., Mayer, J. E., Jr., and Hanley, F. L.: D-transposition of the great arteries. *In:* Cardiac Surgery of the Neonate and Infant. Philadelphia, W. B. Saunders, 1994, pp. 409–438.)

ment of patients with TGA, current surgical techniques have resulted in favorable long-term clinical outcomes for these children.

Selected References

Castañeda, A. R., Trusler, G. A., et al.: Congenital Heart Surgeons Society: The early results of treatment of simple transposition in the current era. J. Thorac. Cardiovasc. Surg., 95:14, 1988.
This landmark study describes a multi-institutional comparison of treatment of neonates with TGA. Neonates were entered into a protocol leading to arterial switch operation, Mustard atrial repair, or Senning atrial repair. Although survival was 81% at 1 year, neither the arterial or atrial switch protocol was a risk factor for death in the study. This paper established that arterial switch operation could be safely performed in neonates with results equivalent or superior to the atrial operation.

Colan, S. D., Boutin, C., Castañeda, A. R., and Wernovsky, G.: Status of the left ventricle after arterial switch operation for transposition of the great arteries: Hemodynamic and echocardiographic evaluation. J. Thorac. Cardiovasc. Surg., 109:311, 1995.
Additional analysis of a very large series of arterial switch operations performed at Children's Hospital in Boston demonstrates that left ventricular size, mass, functional status, and contractility remain normal with no evidence of time-related deterioration after arterial switch reconstruction in the neonate. A two-stage arterial switch operation to prepare the left ventricle in older patients has been associated with mild impairment in myocardial mechanics late after operation, confirming the desirability of early complete correction.

Rhodes, L. A., Wernovsky, G., Keane, J. F., et al.: Arrhythmias and intracardiac conduction after the arterial switch operation. J. Thorac. Cardiovasc. Surg., 109:303, 1995.
Early and late analysis of conduction in a large series of 390 infants who underwent arterial switch procedures at Boston Children's Hospital has confirmed the theoretical advantage of arterial switch over atrial operations for TGA. Sinus node function was preserved, and a very low incidence of clinical significant arrhythmias was identified at a mean follow-up of 2.1 years after the operation.

Wernovsky, G., Mayer, J. E., Jr., Jonas, R. A., Hanley, F. L., Blackstone, E. H., Kirklin. J. W., and Castañeda, A. R.: Factors influencing early and late outcome of the arterial switch operation for transposition of the great arteries. J. Thorac. Cardiovasc. Surg., 109:289, 1995.
This study of a large series of 470 patients undergoing arterial switch operation with intact septum or VSD showed excellent survivals of 93% at 1 month and 91% at 8 years after surgery. This represents the largest single series of arterial switch operations and has described incremental risk factors of multiple ventricular septal defects, a rapid two-stage arterial switch, and the single coronary pattern as significant indicators of early mortality.

REFERENCES

1. Baillie, M.: The Morbid Anatomy of Some of the More Important Parts of the Human Body. London, Johnson & Nichol, 1797, p. 38.
2. Farre, J. R.: Pathological Researches. Essay 1: On Malformations of the Human Heart. London, Longman, Hurst, Rees, Orme, Brown, 1814, p. 28.
3. Von Rokitansky, C.: Die Defekte der Scheidewande der Herzens. Vienna, Braumuller, 1875.
4. Fanconi, G.: Die Transposition der grossen Gefuse (das Charakteristische Rontgenbild). Arch. Kinderheilkd., 95:202, 1932.

5. Taussig, H. B.: Complete transposition of the great vessels. Am. Heart J., 16:728, 1938.
6. Ferguson, D. J., Adams, P., and Watson, D.: Pulmonary arteriosclerosis in transposition of the great vessels. Am. J. Dis. Child., 99:653, 1960.
7. Ferencz, C.: Transposition of the great vessels: Pathophysiologic considerations based upon a study of the lungs. Circulation, 33:232, 1966.
8. Van Praagh, R., and Van Praagh, S.: Isolated ventricular inversion: A consideration of the morphogenesis, definition and diagnosis of nontransposed and transposed great arteries. Am. J. Cardiol., 17:395, 1966.
9. Mathew, R., Rosenthal, A., and Fellows, K. E.: The significance of right aortic arch in d-transposition of the great arteries. Am. Heart J., 87:314, 1974.
10. Moene, R. J., Oppenheimer-Dekker, A., Wenink, A. C. G., et al.: Morphology of ventricular septal defect in complete transposition of the great arteries. Am. J. Cardiol., 55:1566, 1985.
11. Gittenberger-de Groot, A. C., Sauer, U., Oppenheimer-Dekker, A., et al.: Coronary arterial anatomy in transposition of the great arteries: A morphologic study. Pediatr. Cardiol. (Suppl.)4:15, 1983.
12. DiDonato, R. M., and Castañeda, A. R.: Anatomic correction of transposition of the great arteries at the arterial level. In Sabiston, D. C., Jr., and Spencer, F. C. (Eds.): Surgery of the Chest, 5th ed. Philadelphia, W. B. Saunders, 1990, pp. 1435–1451.
13. Kurasawa, H., Imai, Y., and Kawada, M.: Coronary arterial anatomy in regard to the arterial switch procedure. Cardiol. Young, 1:54, 1991.
14. Castañeda, A. R., Jonas, R. A., Mayer, J. E., Jr., and Hanley, F. L.: D-transposition of the great arteries. In Cardiac Surgery of the Neonate and Infant. Philadelphia, W. B. Saunders, 1994, pp. 409–438.
15. Fyler, D. C.: Report of the New England Regional Infant Cardiac Program. Pediatrics, 65:375, 1980.
16. Liebman, J., Cullum, L., and Belloc, N. B.: Natural history of transposition of the great arteries: Anatomy and birth and death characteristics. Circulation, 40:237, 1969.
17. Ebert, P. A.: Transposition of the great arteries. In Sabiston, D. C., Jr., (Ed): Textbook of Surgery, 14th ed. Philadelphia, W. B. Saunders, 1986, pp. 2249–2259.
18. Bano-Rodrigo, A., Quero-Jimenez, M., and Moreno-Granado, F.: Wall thickness of ventricular chambers in transposition of the great arteries: Surgical implications. J. Thorac. Cardiovasc. Surg., 79:592, 1980.
19. Rashkind, W. J., and Miller, W. W.: Creation of an atrial septal defect without thoracotomy: A palliative approach to complete transposition of the great arteries. JAMA, 96:991, 1966.
20. Blalock, A., and Hanlon, C. R.: The surgical treatment of complete transposition of the aorta and pulmonary artery. Surg. Gynecol. Obstet., 90:1, 1950.
21. Mustard, W. T., Chute, A. L., Keith, J. D., et al: A surgical approach to transposition of the great vessels with extracorporeal circuit. Surgery, 36:39, 1954.
22. Bailey, C. P., Cookson, B. A., Downing, D. F., and Neptune, W. B.: Cardiac surgery under hypothermia. J. Thorac. Cardiovasc. Surg., 27:73, 1954.
23. Lillehei, C. W., and Varco, R. L.: Certain physiologic, pathologic and surgical features of complete transposition of the great vessels. Surgery, 34:376, 1953.
24. Baffes, T. G.: A new method for surgical correction of transposition of the aorta and pulmonary artery. Surg. Gynecol. Obstet., 102:227, 1956.
25. Albert, H. M.: Surgical correction of transposition of the great arteries. Surg. Forum, 5:74, 1954.
26. Senning, A.: Surgical correction of transposition of the great vessels. Surgery, 45:966, 1959.
27. Mustard, W. T.: Successful two-stage correction of transposition of the great vessels. Surgery, 55:469, 1964.
28. Jatene, A., Fontes, V. F., Paulista, P. P., Souza, L. C. B., Neger, F., Galantier, M., and Souza, J. E. M. R.: Anatomic correction of transposition of the great vessels. J. Thorac. Cardiovasc. Surg., 72:364, 1976.
29. Yacoub, M. H., Radley-Smith, R., and Hilton, C. J.: Anatomical correction of complete transposition of the great arteries and ventricular septal defect in infancy. Br. Med. J., 1:1112, 1976.
30. Yacoub, M. H., Radley-Smith, R., and MacLaurin, R.: Two-stage operation for anatomical correction of transposition of the great arteries with intact interventricular septum. Lancet, 1:1275, 1977.
31. Quaegebeur, J. M., Rohmer, J., Ottenkamp, J., Buis, T., Kirklin, J. W., Blackstone, E. H., and Brom, A. G.: The arterial switch operation. J. Thorac. Cardiovasc. Surg., 92:361, 1986.
32. Brawn, W. J., and Mee, R. B. B.: Early results for anatomic correction of transposition of the great arteries and for double-outlet right ventricle with subpulmonary ventricular septal defect. J. Thorac. Cardiovasc. Surg., 95:230, 1988.
33. Castañeda, A. R., Trusler, G. A., Paul, M. H., et al.: Congenital Heart Surgeons Society: The early results of treatment of simple transposition in the current era. J. Thorac. Cardiovasc. Surg., 95:14, 1988.
34. Rastelli, G. C., Wallace, R. B., and Ongley, P. A.: Complete repair of transposition of the great arteries with pulmonary stenosis: A review and report of a case corrected by using a new surgical technique. Circulation, 39:83, 1969.
35. Lecompte, Y.: Réparation à l'etage ventriculaire—the REV procedure: Technique and clinical results. Cardiol. Young, 1:63, 1991.
36. Trusler, G. A., Williams, W. G., Duncan, K. F., Hesslein, P. S., Benson, L. M., Freedom, R. M., Izukawa, T., and Olley, P. M.: Results with the Mustard operation in simple transposition of the great arteries. Ann. Surg., 206:251, 1987.
37. Pacifico, A. D.: Concordant transposition: Senning operation. In Stark, J., and DeLeval, M. (Eds.): Surgery for Congenital Heart Defects. New York, Grune & Stratton, 1983, pp. 345–361.
38. Wernovsky, G., Mayer, J. E., Jr., Jonas, R. A., Hanley, F. L., Blackstone, E. H., Kirklin, J. W., and Castañeda, A. R.: Factors influencing early and late outcome of the arterial switch operation for transposition of the great arteries. J. Thorac. Cardiovasc. Surg., 109:289, 1995.
39. Colan, S. D., Boutin, C., Castañeda, A. R., Wernovsky, G.: Status of left the ventricle after arterial switch operation for transposition of the great arteries: Hemodynamic and echocardiographic evaluation. J. Thorac. Cardiovasc. Surg., 109:311, 1995.
40. Rhodes, L. A., Wernovsky, G., Keane, J. F., et al.: Arrhythmias and intracardiac conduction after the arterial switch operation. J. Thorac. Cardiovasc. Surg., 109:303, 1995.

XIII

CONGENITAL AORTIC STENOSIS

Erle H. Austin III, M.D.

Congenital aortic stenosis refers to a group of malformations that cause obstruction of blood flow from the left ventricle to the aorta. Stenosis occurs most commonly at the level of the aortic valve but may also occur above or below it (Fig. 54–102). Aortic stenosis is one of the most common congenital heart defects, representing 5% to 10% of congenital cardiac anomalies.[30, 38] A broad spectrum of lesions exist, ranging from a mildly stenotic bicuspid valve producing an asymptomatic systolic murmur in the older child to a marginally perforate unicommissural valve creating life-threatening heart failure in the neonate.

HISTORICAL ASPECTS

Although pathologic descriptions of aortic stenosis in the adult had been made as early as the seventeenth century, the first report of congenital aortic stenosis was made by Chevers in 1842 in a patient with discrete subvalvular aortic stenosis.[9] Two years later, Paget described a congenitally obstructed bicuspid aortic valve.[61] Supravalvular aortic stenosis was not recognized pathologically until it was reported by Mencarelli in 1930.[52] The first suggestion that supravalvular aortic stenosis could be part of a familial syndrome was made by Williams and associates in 1961.[91] Accurate pathologic description of muscular subaortic stenosis (hypertrophic obstructive cardiomyopathy [HOCM]; idiopathic hypertrophic subaortic stenosis [IHSS]) was made by Teare in 1958.[81] The first successful aortic valvotomy was performed by Tuffier in 1913 in an adult with calcific aortic stenosis.[82] The first successful surgical treatment of congenital aortic stenosis was reported in 1955 by Marquis and associates,[48] who opened the valve by inserting dilators through the left ventricular apex. Successful

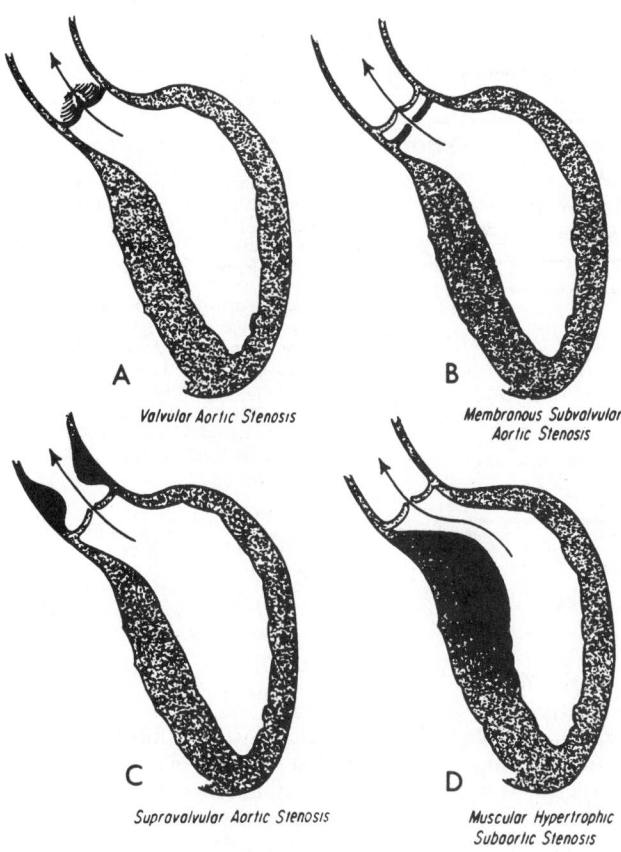

Figure 54–102. *A* to *D*, Schematic representation of the types of congenital aortic stenosis.

Valvular Aortic Stenosis

Membranous Subvalvular Aortic Stenosis

Supravalvular Aortic Stenosis

Muscular Hypertrophic Subaortic Stenosis

open valvotomy using surface cooling and inflow occlusion was reported independently by Swan and Lewis in that same year.[45, 80] Reports of open valvotomy with cardiopulmonary bypass (CPB) followed shortly.[22, 75] Transventricular dilatation of discrete subvalvular aortic stenosis was reported by Brock in 1956.[4] Subsequent application of CPB permitted direct excision of this lesion.[76] Supravalvular aortic stenosis was first successfully treated by Kirklin and colleagues in 1956 by enlarging the noncoronary sinus of Valsalva with a patch.[49] The first surgical attempt to treat muscular subaortic stenosis was performed by Cleland in 1960 and consisted of incising the anterior ridge of the muscular septum (myotomy).[27] Other authors preferred an excision of septal muscle (myectomy).[36, 37]

PATHOPHYSIOLOGY

Aortic stenosis, regardless of the level of obstruction, causes systolic left ventricular hypertension and a compensatory concentric increase in left ventricular mass. Systolic function may be preserved by this hypertrophy, but left ventricular compliance is decreased and higher end-diastolic pressures are required to achieve adequate ventricular filling. When the hypertrophy is severe, the combination of high systolic wall tension and increased myocardial mass may cause subendocardial ischemia. Symptoms of congestive heart failure develop as left ventricular end-diastolic pressure rises. Symptoms of angina or syncope begin to occur during exertion when myocardial oxygen demands are increased. The degree of hypertrophy correlates with the severity of stenosis, which is graded on the basis of the pressure gradient measured across the obstruction. For mild stenoses, the systolic outflow gradient is less than 50 mm. Hg. In moderate stenoses, the

gradient is between 50 and 75 mm. Hg. Any gradient greater than 75 mm. Hg represents severe stenosis.

VALVULAR AORTIC STENOSIS

In 70% of cases of congenital aortic stenosis, the primary obstruction occurs at the level of the valve. Stenosis at this level is more common in males than females by a factor of 3 to 1. Approximately 10% of patients with valvular aortic stenosis present in the neonatal period, with a clinical course much different from that seen in patients presenting after 1 year of age.

Critical Aortic Stenosis in the Neonate

Pathologic Anatomy. Neonatal presentation is associated with significant deformity of the aortic valve characterized by fusion of the valve leaflets often resulting in only one or two recognizable commissures. The leaflet tissue is usually thickened with irregular edges and myxomatous excrescences and nodules. The annular opening itself may be stenotic or hypoplastic in association with an underdeveloped left ventricle, thus passing into the spectrum of hypoplastic left heart syndrome. Endocardial fibroelastosis often occurs in association with a hypoplastic left ventricle, a narrowed aortic anulus, and critical aortic valvular stenosis. Coarctation of the aorta, patent ductus arteriosus, and mitral stenosis are other significant lesions associated with both hypoplastic left heart syndrome and critical aortic stenosis.

Clinical Features. Neonates with critical aortic stenosis present in the first weeks of life with irritability, difficulty feeding, poor weight gain, and progressive tachypnea. Pallor, poor peripheral perfusion, and diminished peripheral pulses all indicate a low cardiac output. Cyanosis may be noted in patients with a patent ductus arteriosus and right-to-left shunting. A systolic ejection murmur is usually present but may be diminished in intensity if cardiac output is marginal. Other signs of congestive failure, including hepatomegaly, may be present.

Chest radiography usually demonstrates cardiomegaly, and electrocardiography displays left ventricular hypertrophy. Both of these studies, however, can be normal in the presence of severe aortic stenosis. Usually, the most significant laboratory abnormality is a metabolic acidosis caused by compromised oxygen delivery to the tissues. Two-dimensional echocardiography provides definitive diagnosis of aortic stenosis, and Doppler flow studies permit estimation of the transvalvular gradient. Echocardiography also allows evaluation of the left ventricular size and aortic annular diameter, as well as the presence of any associated cardiac anomalies. Cardiac catheterization may also be employed but is usually unnecessary unless performed as a prelude to balloon valvotomy.

Natural History. The presentation of aortic stenosis in the neonate signifies a severe obstruction that almost uniformly results in progressive circulatory failure and death within days or weeks of presentation (Fig. 54–103). Any chance of survival depends on adequate relief of the valvular obstruction, assuming the left ventricle is of adequate size. Rhodes and colleagues determined that an adequate left ventricle exists when (1) the ratio of the left ventricular long axis to the heart long axis is greater than 0.8; (2) the aortic root diameter is greater than 3.5 cm. per sq. m.; (3) the mitral valve area is greater than 4.75 sq. cm. per sq. m.; and (4) the left ventricular mass is greater than 35 gm. per sq. m. Valvotomy in patients failing two or more of these criteria resulted in 100% mortality, compared with only 8% in patients with only one or no risk factors.[64] In a separate study, Leung and colleagues found that patients with a left ventricular inflow

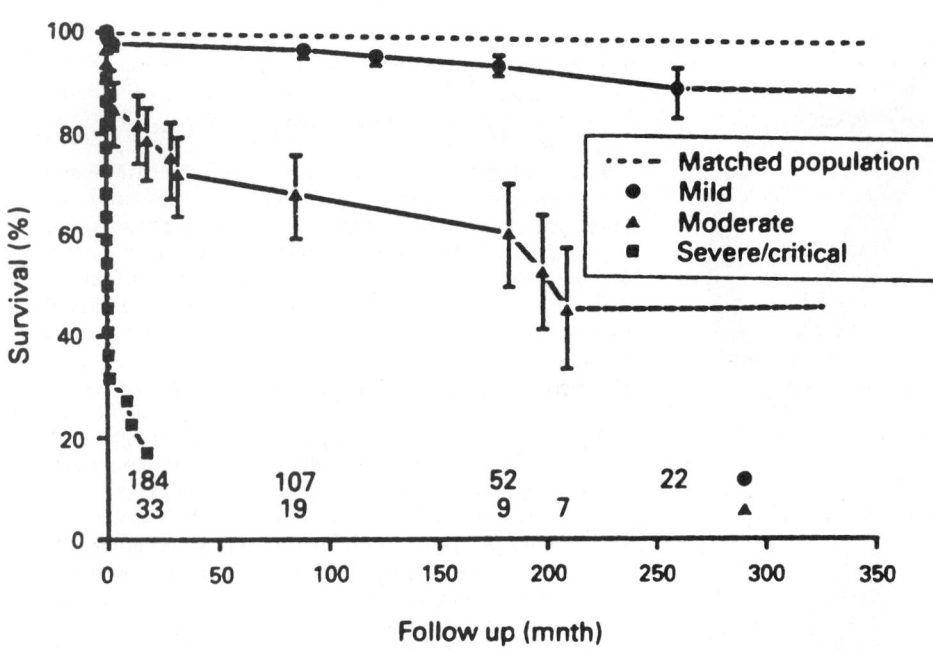

Figure 54–103. Actuarial survival from the time of presentation in patients with valvular aortic stenosis. Prognosis is markedly limited in neonates with critical aortic stenosis. On the other hand, survival in older children with mild aortic stenosis approaches that seen in a matched population. (From Kitchiner, D. J., Jackson, M., Walsh, K., Peart, I., and Arnold, R.: Incidence and prognosis of congenital aortic valve stenosis in Liverpool [1960–1990]. Br. Heart J., 69:71, 1993.)

dimension (the distance from the posterior mitral anulus to the left ventricular apex) of less than 25 mm., an aortic anulus of less than 5 mm. in diameter, and a mitral valve orifice of less than 9 mm. in diameter were unlikely to survive aortic valvotomy.[44] Thus, should these echocardiographically determined measurements indicate an inadequate left ventricle, aortic valvotomy should be avoided and the patient managed according to treatment protocols for hypoplastic left heart syndrome.

Initial Management. Management of the neonate with critical aortic stenosis should include expeditious diagnosis, resuscitation, stabilization, and urgent relief of obstruction. Administration of prostaglandin E_1 (0.1 μg./kg./min.) is begun immediately to achieve and maintain ductal patency and allow the right ventricle to assist with systemic cardiac output.[33, 43] Metabolic acidosis is corrected with sodium bicarbonate or tromethamine (THAM). Intubation and mechanical ventilation as well as intravenous inotropic support help stabilize these critically ill infants. If echocardiography indicates the left ventricle is adequate to sustain systemic circulation, preparation should be made for urgent aortic valvotomy.

Valvotomy Techniques. A variety of techniques for surgical valvotomy have been described. Among these techniques are open valvotomy using inflow occlusion and closed valvotomy with a dilator inserted through the left ventricular apex. Both of these approaches can be performed without CPB. Experience, however, suggests that CPB may be advantageous in these patients because of the circulatory stabilization that it provides. Once CPB is established, the valve can be opened with either an open or closed technique. If an open technique is preferred, the aorta is cross-clamped and the heart is arrested with a cold cardioplegic solution. The aorta is opened, and under direct vision a precise valvotomy is performed. Careful division of the fused commissures is performed to within 1 mm. of the aortic wall (Fig. 54–104). Commissures must be distinctly differentiated from false raphes, because division of the latter will result in severe valvular insufficiency. Dysplastic nodules that appear to be obstructive should also be carefully excised.

Although many surgeons prefer an open technique because of the precision it provides, satisfactory valvotomy may also be achieved with a closed method. The concomitant use

of CPB permits initial stabilization, correction of metabolic acidosis and electrolyte abnormalities, and improved renal perfusion. Through a pursestring suture placed in the left ventricular apex, Bakes or Hegar dilators of progressively larger size are introduced and carefully guided through the aortic orifice. Having the infant on CPB ensures continuous cerebral blood flow during the valvotomy. Because aortic

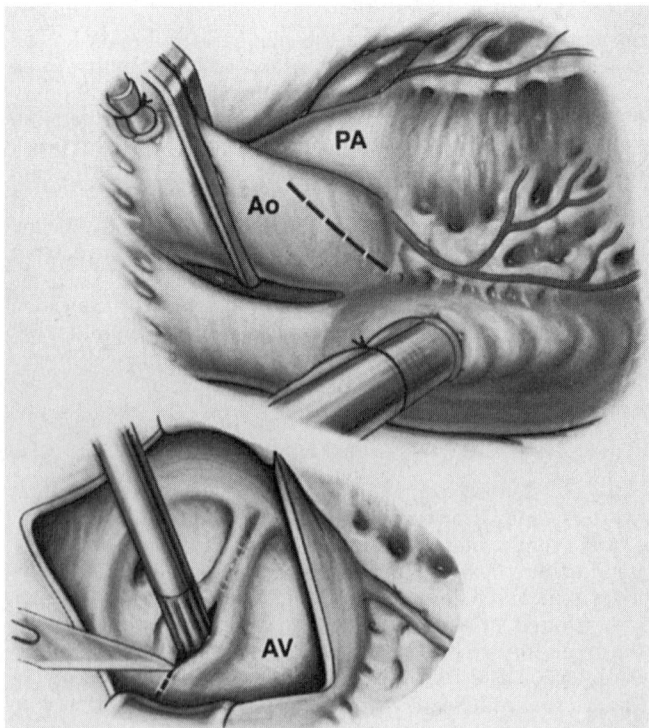

Figure 54–104. Valvular aortic stenosis as seen during an open aortic valvotomy. This procedure is performed on cardiopulmonary bypass with the aorta (Ao) crossclamped and cardioplegic arrest. The fused commissures are incised up to within 1 mm. of the aortic wall. PA, pulmonary artery; AV, aortic valve. (From deLeval, M.: Surgery of the left ventricular outflow tract. In Stark, J., and deLeval, M. [Eds.]: Surgery for Congenital Heart Defects, 2nd ed. Philadelphia, W. B. Saunders, 1994, p. 517.)

cross-clamping is not performed, myocardial ischemia is avoided. The valve is dilated up to the diameter of the anulus as measured by echocardiography. An opening of at least 6 mm. is desired, but overzealous attempts to stretch a smaller anulus should be avoided. Although this approach does not provide the surgeon with the visual feedback obtained with an open technique, it has provided good relief of obstruction with minimal valvular insufficiency.[56, 83]

Percutaneous transluminal balloon valvotomy has also been successfully applied to critical aortic stenosis in the neonate and has become the procedure of choice in some centers experienced with interventional catheter techniques.[2, 95] In small neonates, however, the need to introduce a large catheter through a small artery has produced a relatively high incidence of arterial complications.[65] Use of the umbilical artery for arterial access has decreased these problems to some extent.

Results. Before 1980, reported mortality for surgical valvotomy in neonates with critical aortic stenosis ranged from 50% to 70%.[19, 41, 69] By avoiding valvotomy in patients with inadequately developed left ventricles, and with improvements in preoperative and intraoperative support, the mortality for operative valvotomy in these critically ill infants has fallen to approximately 10%. As early as 1984, Messina and colleagues reported a 9% mortality in neonates undergoing open valvotomy with CPB. Several patients in that report developed ventricular fibrillation at the beginning of the procedure and were unlikely to have survived if CPB had not been employed.[53] A more recent study presented the combined results of three separate institutions. Hospital mortality was 12.5% (5/40) with no differences between institutions nor between open or closed techniques. Cardiopulmonary bypass, however, was used in all patients at all three institutions.[83] Mortality as low as 0% has been reported for neonates with isolated critical aortic stenosis, but patients requiring concomitant repair of other cardiac lesions (such as coarctation, atrial septal defect, or ventricular septal defect) may experience operative mortality approaching 50%.[34] The presence of endocardial fibroelastosis, although commonly associated with a small left ventricle, may be an independent risk factor significantly elevating the risk of valvotomy.[28, 84]

Results of balloon dilatation for aortic stenosis are improving as more experience is acquired, but the incidence of complications from the technique is particularly high in infants younger than 1 month of age. In a 1990 report of 204 infants and children undergoing balloon aortic valvuloplasty, major life-threatening complications occurred in 8 of 22 infants who were younger than 1 month of age, with 3 of the 8 dying as a direct result of the complication and another requiring emergency open-heart surgery.[65] Although some institutions experienced with balloon angioplasty have reported early results comparable to those of surgical valvotomy,[95] an open or closed aortic valvotomy with CPB is the preferred method at most centers for relieving critical aortic stenosis in the infant younger than 1 month of age.

Reports of long-term follow-up after valvotomy for neonatal aortic stenosis are sparse, but a study by Ettedgui and colleagues[20] concluded that infants fortunate enough to survive the initial operation had a good long-term prognosis with a 90% chance of being free from reoperation at 10 years. The structural integrity of the valves in these children, however, will never be normal, and as they reach the second, third, and fourth decades of life the potential for recurrent stenosis or progressive insufficiency may be realized. Lifelong follow-up and antibiotic prophylaxis for dental and invasive procedures should be standard for these patients.

Valvular Aortic Stenosis in the Older Child

The greatest proportion of patients with congenital left ventricular outflow tract obstruction are children with valvu-

lar aortic stenosis. In contrast to the severely ill neonate, these patients are more likely to be asymptomatic and the stenosis discovered during a routine physical examination. Although the prognosis is much more favorable in this group (see Fig. 54–103), optimal medical and surgical management requires thoughtful assessment and a carefully planned and applied treatment strategy.

Pathologic Anatomy. Seventy percent of stenotic aortic valves in older children are bicuspid with fusion at one or both commissures. One of the leaflets, usually the left one, is typically larger and displays a central ridge (false raphe) representing a rudimentary commissure. Thirty percent of congenitally stenotic aortic valves are trileaflet with three clearly recognizable commissures with varying degrees of fusion. The valve leaflets may be thickened, but calcification is uncommon in the child. In contrast to neonatal aortic stenosis, the leaflet edges are usually smooth without dysplasia or myxomatous excrescences. The aortic anulus is usually normal.

Clinical Features. These patients present most commonly with an asymptomatic systolic murmur. A review of symptoms may elicit easy fatigability or dyspnea upon exertion, but the majority do not express physical complaints or limitations. Angina or syncope can occur, however, and usually signifies the presence of a severe degree of stenosis. Expeditious evaluation and treatment should be applied to the truly symptomatic child to avoid the risk of sudden death.

A loud crescendo-decrescendo systolic murmur with a prominent systolic ejection click is the most consistent physical finding. A diastolic murmur of aortic insufficiency may also be present. Cardiac size is usually normal on chest radiography. Electrocardiography demonstrates left ventricular hypertrophy. Two-dimensional echocardiography with Doppler flow studies provides a definitive diagnosis and reliably determines a transvalvular gradient. Cardiac catheterization is usually only necessary to confirm the degree of gradient and to assess other defects.

Natural History and Indications for Surgery. Natural history correlates with the degree of stenosis. Patients with mild stenosis (peak gradient < 50 mm. Hg) exhibit an actuarial survival close to that of a matched population (see Fig. 54–103) with only 15% coming to surgical intervention. Patients presenting with moderate stenosis (peak gradient between 50–75 mm. Hg), however, demonstrate a diminished actuarial survival (see Fig. 54–103) requiring aortic valvotomy or valve replacement in at least two thirds of cases.

A history of syncope, angina, or congestive failure with a transvalvular gradient greater than 50 mm. Hg is a clear-cut indication for operation. If these symptoms do not exist and there is no electrocardiographic evidence of left ventricular strain or ischemia at rest or during exercise, a gradient of 75 mm. Hg is generally required before surgical treatment is recommended.

Techniques of Aortic Valvotomy. The majority of patients with congenital aortic stenosis can be successfully treated with aortic valvotomy. Only a small proportion require valve replacement as an initial procedure. Aortic valvotomy is performed routinely with CPB, aortic cross-clamping, cardioplegic arrest, and direct visualization of the aortic valve. As in the neonate, the fused commissures are carefully incised to within 1 mm. of the aortic wall (see Fig. 54–104). Ilbawi and associates described extending this incision in a circumferential fashion beyond the commissure into the aortic wall.[31] This technique achieved a lower transvalvular gradient in Ilbawi's patients without increasing the incidence of valvular insufficiency.[31] It should be cautioned, however, that in most cases it is better to err on the side of leaving residual stenosis than to create valvular insufficiency. An early requirement for aortic valve replacement is more likely to result from aortic insufficiency than mild residual aortic stenosis.

Presently, at most institutions, satisfactory aortic valvotomy is being achieved with percutaneous balloon dilatation and may be the procedure of choice for children older than 1 year of age. As with surgical valvotomy, care must be taken to avoid excessive dilatation and the creation of significant aortic insufficiency.

Aortic Valve Replacement in Children. Because of the long-term limitations of valve replacement devices and the potential need to reoperate to place larger prostheses in growing children, aortic valve replacement is undertaken only when lesser operations cannot achieve satisfactory aortic valve function. This situation occurs most commonly when significant aortic insufficiency develops at some time after a primary valvotomy.

When isolated valve replacement is performed in a child with an adequate aortic anulus, the procedure is performed as it is in an adult. Xenograft valves, however, are not used because of their very limited durability in the young. Mechanical valves are preferred by many surgeons because of their long-term durability and ease of implantation. Unfortunately, they are a source of long-term thromboembolic complications and require life-long anticoagulation.

As a compromise between the xenograft valve and the mechanical valve, the aortic valve allograft has been used successfully in children. The allograft does not calcify as rapidly as the xenograft and does not require anticoagulation. It does not achieve the durability of a mechanical valve but can be expected to endure for 10 to 15 years before a replacement is necessary. Aortic allografts exhibit excellent hemody-

namics in relatively small sizes and are more resistant to infection than standard valve prostheses. Allografts can be inserted either free-hand within the native aortic root or as a complete aortic root replacement with reimplantation of the coronary arteries.

Most recently the pulmonary valve autograft technique has been applied to children and young adults requiring aortic valve replacement.[21, 40, 70] This method, originally described by Ross[68] and often referred to as the Ross procedure, involves removing the patient's own pulmonary valve and transferring it to the aortic position and replacing the patient's pulmonary valve with an allograft pulmonary valve (Fig. 54–105). Thus a normal trileaflet semilunar valve made up of the patient's own tissue is used as the aortic valve replacement. The less ideal allograft valve is placed on the pulmonary side of the circulation where it is less burdened and where stenosis or insufficiency is far better tolerated.

When performing aortic valve replacement in infants and children, the surgeon may need to enlarge the aortic anulus.[32] By incising the anulus posteriorly, either at the commissure between the left and the noncoronary cusps or through the noncoronary cusp, the annular diameter can be increased 2 to 4 mm.[47, 59] If a more radical enlargement is required, an anterior incision is made between the right and left coronary ostia extending into the right ventricular outflow tract and through the interventricular septum (Fig. 54–106). The defect in the anulus, septum, and aortic root is then filled with a Dacron patch. A piece of pericardium is placed to close the right ventricular outflow tract. This aortoventriculoplasty is often called the Konno-Rastan procedure after its original describers.[39, 62]

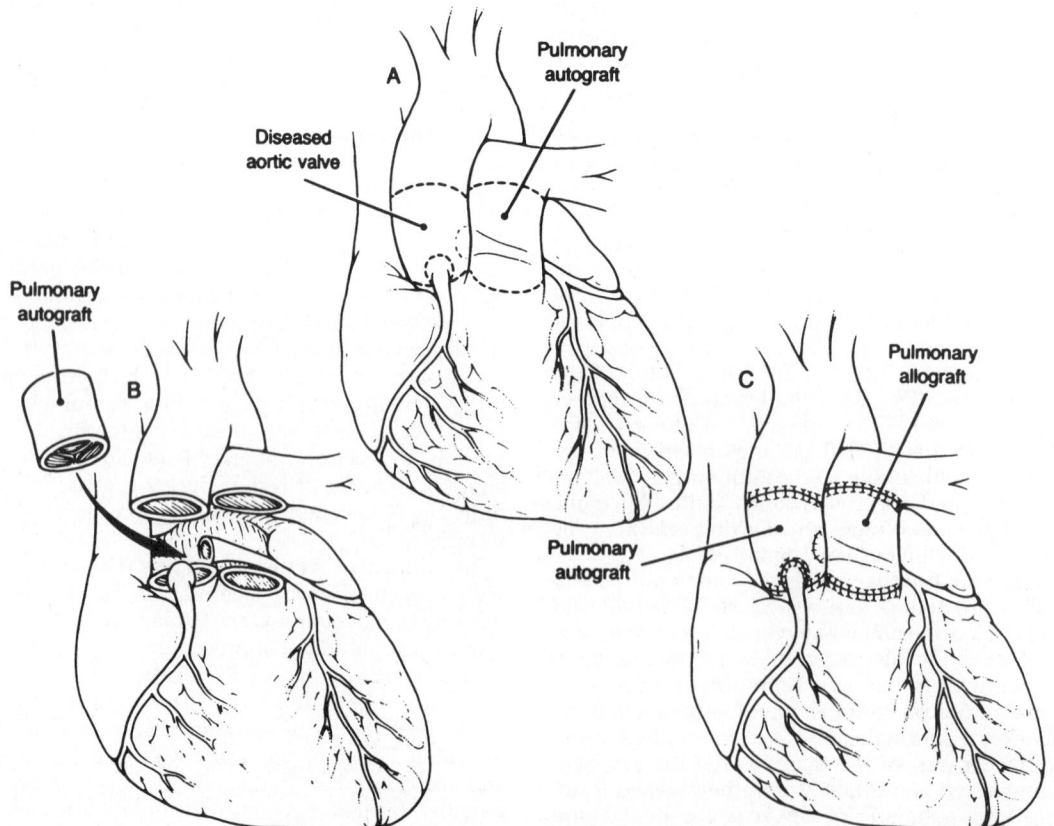

Figure 54–105. *A* to *C*, The pulmonary autograft for aortic valve replacement. The aortic valve and adjacent aorta are excised preserving buttons of aortic tissue around the coronary ostia. The pulmonary valve and main pulmonary artery are excised and transferred to the aortic position. The coronary buttons are then attached to the neoaortic root. A pulmonary allograft is inserted to re-establish the right ventricular outflow tract. (From Kouchoukos, N. T., Davila-Roman, V. G., Spray, T. L., Murphy, S. F., and Perrillo, J.: Replacement of the aortic root with a pulmonary autograft in children and young adults with aortic-valve disease. N. Engl. J. Med., *330*:1, 1994. Copyright 1994, Massachusetts Medical Society. Reprinted with permission of The New England Journal of Medicine.)

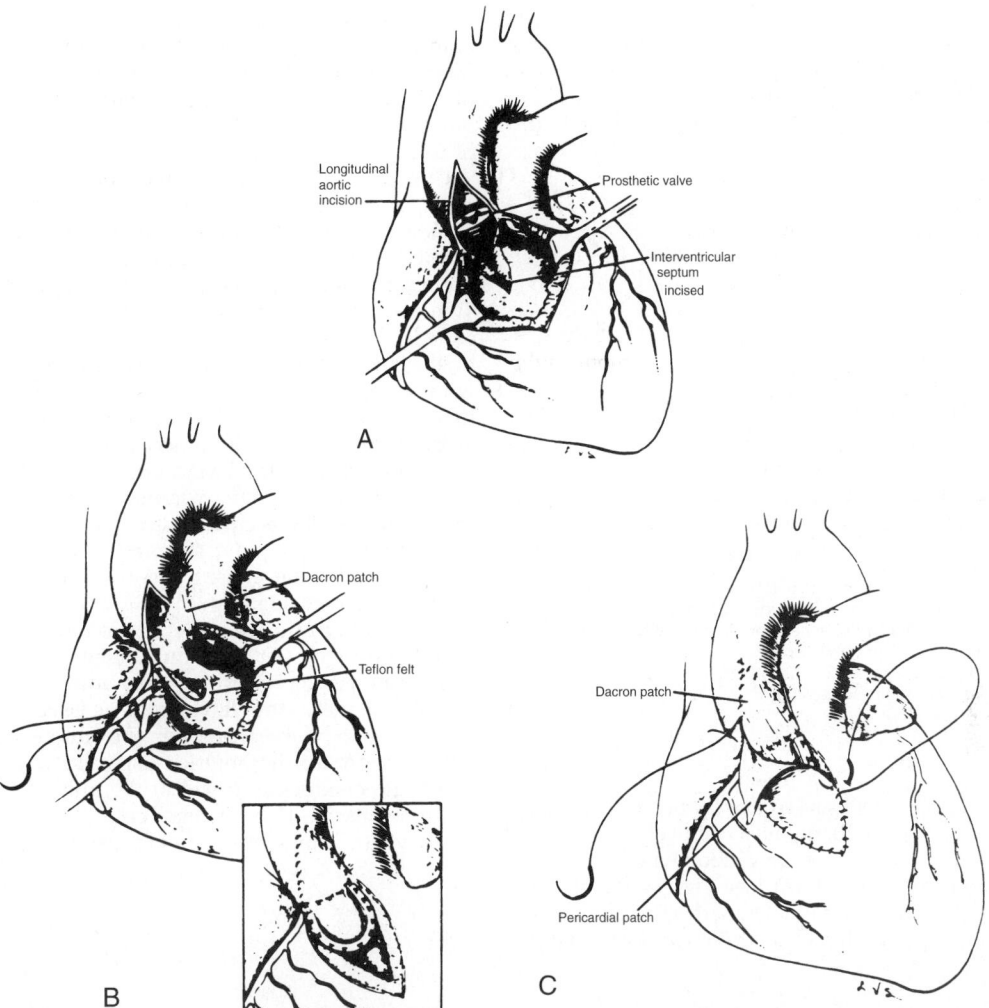

Figure 54–106. The Konno-Rastan aortoventriculoplasty permits significant enlargement of the aortic anulus and subaortic region. *A,* A vertical aortotomy is made to the left of the right coronary artery and extended into the right ventricular outflow tract. After excising the aortic valve the interventricular septum is incised and an aortic valve prosthesis is secured within the enlarged anulus. *B,* A Dacron patch that is attached to the sewing ring of the prosthesis closes the interventricular septum and the aortotomy. *C,* A separate pericardial patch closes the right ventriculotomy. (From Misbach, G. A., Turley, K., Ullyot, D. J., and Ebert, P. A.: Left ventricular outflow enlargement by the Konno procedure. J. Thorac. Cardiovasc. Surg., *84:*696, 1982.)

When the complexity of left ventricular outflow obstruction precludes reconstruction using standard methods, a valved conduit can be placed from the left ventricular apex to the aorta.[6, 16] Although this technique provides excellent palliative relief of left ventricular outflow obstruction, the incidence of late complications and the high risk of reoperation have relegated it to only a few select situations.[26]

Results. For children older than 1 year of age, the hospital mortality for operative aortic valvotomy is currently less than 1%. Actuarial survival is 94% at 5 years and 77% at 22 years after valvotomy (Fig. 54–107).[29] The probability of reoperation at 5 years is only 2% but increases to 44% at 22 years.[29] Causes of late mortality include sudden death, bacterial endocarditis, and death at reoperation.[13, 35] Recurrent stenosis or aortic insufficiency are the main reasons for reoperation with valve replacement necessary in the majority of cases.

Early results of balloon dilatation indicate satisfactory relief of obstruction with a mortality of less than 1% in children older than 1 year of age.[60, 65, 88] Femoral artery thrombosis or damage is infrequent in these older children. The development of new aortic insufficiency after balloon dilatation, however, ranges from 26% to 72% of patients.[60, 72, 93] Thus in the short-term, percutaneous balloon valvotomy compares favorably with surgical valvotomy. Data are not yet available for the long term, but concerns exist that the high incidence of new aortic insufficiency resulting from balloon dilatation may accelerate the need for valve replacement.

Aortic valve replacement in children is performed at an operative risk of 1% to 3%. This risk increases to 20% when complex techniques such as aortoventriculoplasty (the Konno-Rastan procedure) are required.[67] Children receiving mechanical valves experience a continuing risk of thromboembolism and anticoagulant-related bleeding. Allograft replacement of the aortic valve in children older than 3 years of age has demonstrated good valve function through 5 years of follow-up.[11] Significant early allograft degeneration, however, has been recognized in children younger than 3 years of age.[11] Early and intermediate follow-up of the pulmonary autograft technique suggests that this may be the procedure of choice for children and young adults requiring aortic valve replacement.[21, 40, 70, 78]

SUBVALVULAR AORTIC STENOSIS

Ten to 20% of patients with left ventricular outflow tract obstruction exhibit stenosis below the valve.[30, 63] The fixed

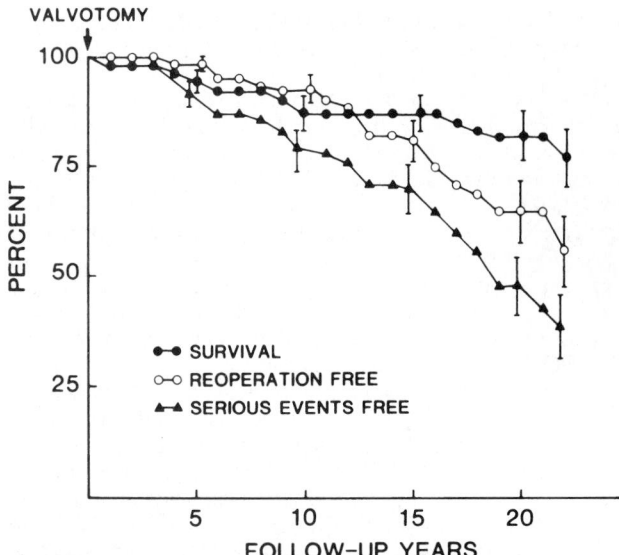

Figure 54–107. Actuarial survival after aortic valvotomy in patients older than 1 year of age at time of operation. Reoperation includes all types of aortic valve surgery. Serious events include death, reoperation, and bacterial endocarditis. Bars represent ± standard error. (From Hsieh, K., Keane, J. F., Nadas, A. S., Bernhard, W. F., and Castēneda, A. R.: Long-term follow-up of valvotomy before 1968 for congenital aortic stenosis. Am. J. Cardiol., *58*:338, 1986. Copyright 1986 by Excerpta Medica Inc.)

fibrous form of subaortic stenosis can exist either as a discrete membrane (see Fig. 54–102B) or as a diffusely narrowed tunnel. These fixed lesions should be differentiated from the dynamic and purely muscular form (see Fig. 54–102D) that is usually referred to as idiopathic hypertrophic subaortic stenosis (IHSS) or hypertrophic obstructive cardiomyopathy (HOCM).

Fixed Subvalvular Aortic Stenosis (Discrete and Diffuse)

Because of its rarity in neonates and its documented development in patients with previously unobstructed left ventricular outflow tracts, fibrous subvalvular aortic stenosis is thought to be an *acquired* and progressive lesion.[24, 42] It is commonly associated with other cardiac defects, including ventricular septal defects and coarctation of the aorta. It does not appear to be genetically inherited but may originate as a nidus of subtle aortic obstruction in fetal life that develops over time into a discrete subvalvular membrane. It has also been noted to occur in patients with atrioventricular canal defects, often only becoming manifest at some time after surgical repair.[15] Hemodynamic factors, such as increased or turbulent flow across the left ventricular outflow tract, are thought to play a major role in the development of this lesion. Further evidence of its progressive nature is the well-documented progression from a simple membrane to a fibromuscular tunnel. The rate of progression, however, is variable, with some patients with minimal gradients remaining stable for years.[25] Even in these patients, aortic insufficiency may develop over time as a result of a high-velocity jet of blood traumatizing the aortic leaflets.[7, 94]

Pathologic Anatomy. Terminology used to describe this type of left ventricular outflow tract obstruction is variable and includes discrete, membranous, fibrous, and fixed subaortic stenosis. A spectrum of pathology exists, but it is most useful to separate these patients into two categories. The most common form, *discrete subaortic stenosis*, consists of a thin crescent-shaped or circular fibrous shelf, 0.5 to 1 cm.

below the aortic valve extending from the muscular septum onto the aortic leaflet of the mitral valve. The less common form is termed *diffuse (or tunnel) subaortic stenosis* and consists of a tubular fibromuscular narrowing of the left ventricular outflow tract. The aortic anulus is abnormally small in many of these patients.

Clinical Features. As in children with valvular aortic stenosis, symptoms are uncommon. A loud crescendo-decrescendo murmur without an ejection click is the most typical physical sign. The chest radiograph is usually normal, and the electrocardiogram displays left ventricular hypertrophy. Two-dimensional echocardiography clearly demonstrates the subaortic shelf of the discrete lesion or the narrowed collar of the diffuse form. An outflow gradient can be estimated with Doppler flow interrogation. Unless they are needed to evaluate associated lesions, cardiac catheterization and angiography are usually unnecessary. In most cases, the progressive nature of the lesion and its potential untoward effects on the aortic valve warrant preceding to operation once the diagnosis has been made. If, however, the Doppler-derived gradient is low (< 40 mm. Hg), the operation can be postponed and the patient observed with subsequent echocardiographic evaluations.

Surgical Techniques. Relief of discrete subaortic stenosis is performed using CPB and cardioplegic arrest. The subaortic membrane is exposed through an aortotomy and careful retraction of the aortic valve leaflets. Using sharp and blunt dissection, the surgeon excises the fibrous ring, taking care not to perforate the anterior leaflet of the mitral valve or injure the conduction tissue in the area of the membranous septum (Fig. 54–108). In most cases, a portion of hypertrophied ventricular septum should also be excised. This myec-

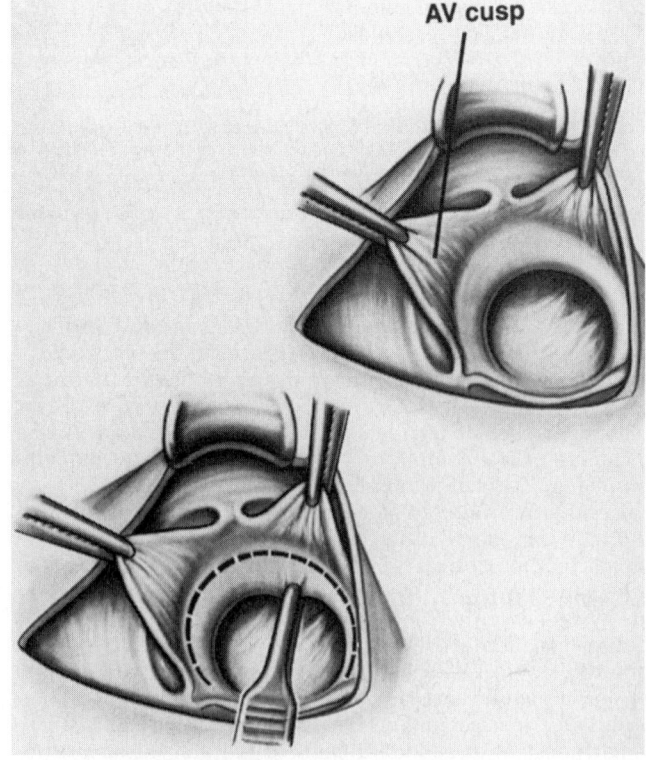

Figure 54–108. Transaortic excision of discrete subaortic stenosis. On cardiopulmonary bypass the aorta is crossclamped and the heart arrested with cardioplegia. The aorta is opened and the aortic valve leaflets are carefully retracted to expose the subaortic membrane. The membrane is excised circumferentially. (From deLeval, M.: Surgery of the left ventricular outflow tract. *In* Stark, J. and deLeval, M. [Eds.]: Surgery for Congenital Heart Defects, 2nd ed. Philadelphia, W. B. Saunders, 1994, p. 525.)

tomy is performed by placing one incision beneath the commissure between the left and right coronary cusp and another incision beneath the nadir of the right coronary cusp. The muscle between these two incisions is then excised (Fig. 54–109).

When diffuse subaortic stenosis exists, localized resection rarely provides adequate relief of obstruction and a more aggressive surgical approach is required. The technique preferred by many surgeons is a modification of the Konno-Rastan procedure. With this technique, the interventricular septum is approached through an incision in the right ventricular outflow tract. The septum is then incised longitudinally, and the left ventricular outflow tract is opened superiorly to within 1 or 2 mm. of the nadir of the right aortic cusp. The fibromuscular tissue is then excised, and a Dacron patch is inserted to enlarge the left ventricular outflow tract. With this modification, the native aortic valve is preserved. In cases of diffuse subaortic stenosis with concomitant aortic valve pathology or a narrowed aortic anulus, a standard Konno-Rastan procedure with a mechanical valve prosthesis is performed. Complete aortic root replacement with an aortic allograft or a pulmonary autograft may also be applied in these difficult cases.[10, 78]

Results. Hospital mortality for excision of a discrete subaortic membrane with or without a myectomy ranges from 0% to 3%.[1, 8, 18, 46, 57, 86] Postoperative complete heart block occurs in 0% to 8% of cases.[8, 46, 86] The major long-term risk in these patients, recurrence requiring reoperation, has been reported to occur in 4% to 36% of cases.[1, 46, 79, 86] Most studies indicate that the rate of recurrence is significantly diminished by adding septal myectomy to resection of the subvalvular membrane (Fig. 54–110).[8, 46, 86]

For patients with diffuse subaortic stenosis, hospital mortalities approximating 10% have been reported with the standard and modified Konno-Rastan procedures.[14, 89] The incidence of complete heart block ranges from 0% to 20%. Little long-term follow-up data exist for these patients.

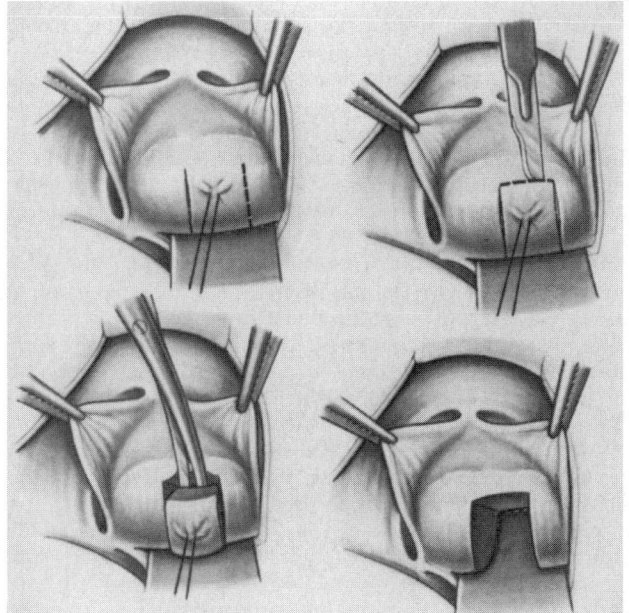

Figure 54–109. Transaortic septal myectomy. This procedure is performed as an adjunct to excision of discrete subaortic stenosis and as the primary procedure for hypertrophic obstructive cardiomyopathy. If the muscular excision is kept to the left of the midpoint of the right aortic leaflet, injury to the conduction tissue is avoided. (From deLeval, M.: Surgery of the left ventricular outflow tract. In Stark, J. and deLeval, M. [Eds.]: Surgery for Congenital Heart Defects, 2nd ed. Philadelphia, W. B. Saunders, 1994, p. 525.)

Dynamic Subvalvular Aortic Stenosis: Hypertrophic Obstructive Cardiomyopathy

An uncommon but important form of subaortic stenosis results from muscular hypertrophy of the interventricular septum creating a dynamic obstruction of the left ventricular outflow tract (see Fig. 54–102D). This entity appears to be a primary disease of cardiac muscle characterized by ventricular hypertrophy and myocardial fiber disarray primarily affecting the ventricular septum. It has been referred to as muscular subaortic stenosis, asymmetric septal hypertrophy (ASH), idiopathic hypertrophic subaortic stenosis (IHSS), and the currently favored term, *hypertrophic obstructive cardiomyopathy (HOCM)*. This disease is genetically determined and is transmitted as an autosomal dominant trait. Advances in genetic analysis now permit identification of affected family members before the disease becomes clinically evident.[66]

Pathologic Anatomy. The muscular hypertrophy of hypertrophic obstructive cardiomyopathy primarily involves the left ventricle and varies in severity. The ventricular septum is usually most thickened at the level of the free edge of the anterior mitral leaflet. Microscopic examination of the hypertrophied septum reveals foci of disarrayed myocytes interspersed among areas of hypertrophied but normally aligned cells. The endocardial surface of this muscular bulge is usually covered with a thickened fibrous plaque. The anterior leaflet of the mitral valve is often also thickened at this point. Within the septum and left ventricular free wall, areas of fibrosis are commonly present, suggesting the presence of localized areas of ischemia and infarction. The epicardial coronary arteries are usually normal, but in areas of marked hypertrophy intramural coronary branches are often narrowed.[77]

Pathophysiology. The obstructive effect of hypertrophic obstructive cardiomyopathy differs somewhat from the stenosis imposed by fixed lesions. The degree of obstruction created by the septal bulge is dynamic and related to the size of the left ventricular cavity. Conditions that encourage a larger left ventricular volume, such as increased preload, increased afterload, or diminished contractility, tend to increase the dimension of the left ventricular outflow tract and decrease the degree of obstruction. Conversely, the opposite conditions tend to increase the outflow obstruction. In addition, in hypertrophic obstructive cardiomyopathy the free edge of the anterior leaflet of the mitral valve moves anteriorly during systole, further obstructing ejection. Although the mechanism of this systolic anterior motion is debated, its degree correlates with the severity of obstruction and permits definitive diagnosis by echocardiography.

Clinical Features. Hypertrophic obstructive cardiomyopathy can present at any age but is most commonly identified in the adolescent or young adult. Symptoms are uncommon but include dyspnea on exertion, easy fatigability, and exertional chest pain. Syncope is an ominous and important symptom, suggesting the potential for sudden death.

Physical findings include a late-onset systolic ejection murmur that increases in intensity with a Valsalva maneuver and decreases in intensity with squatting. There is no ejection click. The left ventricular apical impulse is double, and the arterial pulse is jerky with a rapid upstroke. The electrocardiogram is more likely to show left ventricular strain than hypertrophy, and chest radiography may show mild to moderate cardiomegaly. The definitive diagnosis is made with M-mode and two-dimensional echocardiography by demonstrating asymptomatic septal hypertrophy and systolic anterior motion of the mitral valve.

The natural history of hypertrophic obstructive cardiomyopathy is variable and unpredictable. The severity of symptoms and the degree of obstruction do not necessarily corre-

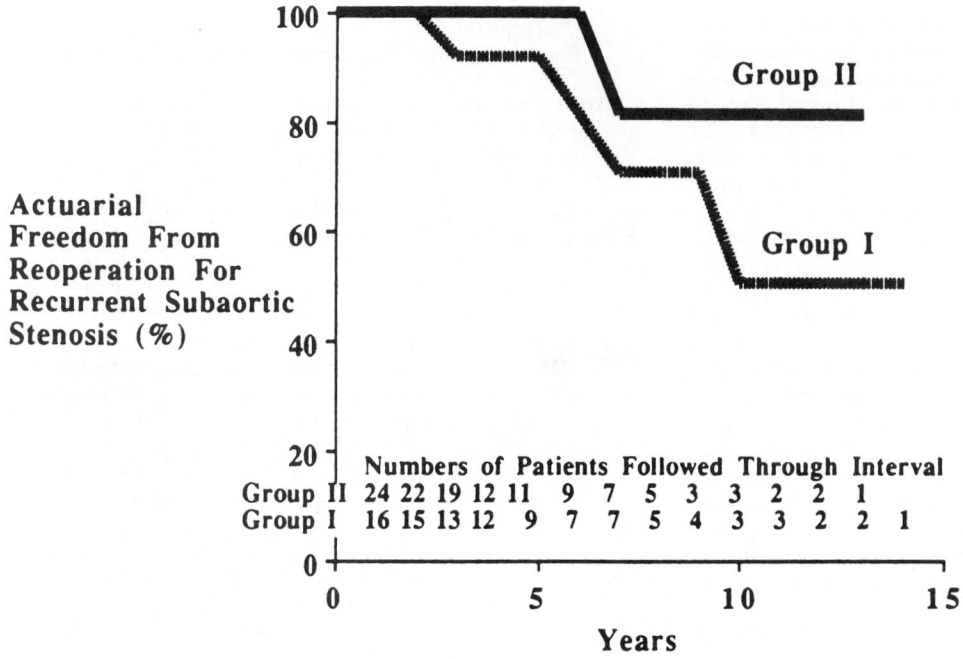

Figure 54–110. Actuarial freedom from reoperation for recurrent subaortic stenosis. Patients in Group I underwent excision of the subaortic membrane alone and those in Group II underwent membrane excision combined with septal myectomy. (From Lupinetti, F. M., Pridjian, A. K., Callow, L. B., Crowley, D. C., Beekman, R. H., and Bove, E. L.: Optimum treatment of discrete subaortic stenosis. Ann. Thorac. Surg., *54*:467, 1992. Reprinted with permission from the Society of Thoracic Surgeons [The Annals of Thoracic Surgery].)

late, although virtually all patients with gradients above 100 mm. Hg are symptomatic.[73] Actuarial survival after diagnosis and without surgery is approximately 85% at 5 years and 75% at 10 years in patients diagnosed as adults. Prognosis is significantly worse when the diagnosis is made in childhood, with a 10-year survival of only 52%.[51] The most common cause of mortality is sudden death.[73]

At present, most patients with hypertrophic obstructive cardiomyopathy are treated medically with beta blockers, such as propranolol, and calcium channel blockers, such as verapamil and nifedipine. Diuretics, digoxin, and vasodilators are avoided because these agents tend to worsen the degree of obstruction.

Surgery. Surgery is considered for symptomatic patients who fail to respond to optimal medical therapy or develop side effects from these medications. The procedure most commonly used is a transaortic myectomy similar to that illustrated in Figure 54–109. With this technique a generous wedge of septal muscle is excised, taking care to avoid conduction tissue.[55] Because the mitral valve has been implicated in the pathophysiology of this condition, mitral valve replacement has been applied in some cases.[90] The technical ease of transaortic myectomy and the long-term adverse effects of valve prostheses, however, have dissuaded most surgeons from using mitral valve replacement for hypertrophic obstructive cardiomyopathy. On the other hand, there has been enthusiasm for performing mitral valve plication in combination with septal myectomy to minimize the redundancy of the anterior mitral leaflet and decrease the potential for systolic anterior motion of the mitral valve postoperatively.[12, 50]

As an alternative to open-heart surgery for patients refractory to medical treatment, dual-chamber permanent pacing has been evaluated.[23] This approach is based on the concept that pre-exciting the ventricular septum with atrioventricular sequential pacing can prompt the septum to move away from the left ventricular wall during systole and open the left ventricular outflow tract. Initial reports have documented a significant reduction of symptoms and left ventricular outflow tract gradients with this technique. Experience so far, however, is too limited to determine the effect of dual-chamber pacing on long-term survival.

Results. Septal myectomy is performed with a hospital mortality between 1% and 5%.[54, 92] Preoperative symptoms of syncope are relieved in approximately 95% of patients, and symptoms of dyspnea and angina are relieved in 80%.[54] Long-term follow-up also suggests that longevity is extended with myectomy, although the risk of sudden death is not eliminated.[71]

SUPRAVALVULAR AORTIC STENOSIS

Supravalvular aortic stenosis is the rarest form of congenital aortic stenosis. The stenosis is most often localized at the level of the aortic commissures, but the narrowing can involve the entire ascending aorta and extend into the brachiocephalic arteries. Idiopathic hypercalcemia, abnormal vitamin D and calcium metabolism, and rubella have all been implicated as possible etiologic factors. Supravalvular aortic stenosis is the major cardiovascular component of William's syndrome, which is characterized by a variable level of mental retardation and an *elfin* facies.[91] Peripheral pulmonary artery stenoses also occur in both the familial and sporadic forms of this syndrome.

Pathologic Anatomy. Congenital supravalvular aortic stenosis occurs in two forms: discrete and diffuse. Approximately 85% of patients who come to surgery have the discrete form, which is characterized by thickening of the aortic media and an external narrowing at the level of the sinotubular junction. This results in a typical *hourglass* appearance. The intima may also be thickened, creating an intimal shelf at the top of the commissural posts. In some cases, the aortic valve leaflets can be adherent to the intimal shelf and obstruct coronary blood flow. In the much less common diffuse form of supravalvular stenosis, marked thickening of the aortic wall with associated luminal narrowing extends from the sinotubular junction to involve the entire ascending aorta with variable extension into the aortic arch and its branches.

Pathologic changes in the coronary arteries and myocardium have been noted in patients as young as 2 years of age who have died of both the discrete and diffuse form of the disease.[87] Because the coronary arteries are located proximal to the area of obstruction, they are exposed to abnormally high pressures and are at increased risk for developing intimal hyperplasia, medial hypertrophy, and luminal obstruction. The combination of coronary artery dysplasia and left ventricular hypertrophy with patients with this disease increases the risk of developing myocardial ischemia.

Clinical Features. As with other childhood forms of aortic stenosis, a systolic murmur is often discovered before symptoms are realized. When symptoms do develop, they include decreased exercise tolerance, dyspnea on exertion, and angina. Although the diagnosis can often be made with two-dimensional echocardiography, cardiac catheterization and angiography should be performed to determine the degree and extent of obstruction and identify any associated anomalies.

Surgery. Because of the progressive nature of this disease, the presence of symptoms or a gradient of 50 mm. Hg are sufficient indications for operative relief. Repair is performed with CPB and cardioplegic arrest. For the discrete form of the disease, the aorta is opened above the valve and an incision is extended down into the noncoronary sinus of Valsalva. Any intimal shelf is carefully excised, and a tear-shaped patch of pericardium is inserted in the incision to enlarge the aortic diameter (Fig. 54–111). Doty and associates have recommended extending the incision into both the noncoronary and the right coronary sinuses and inserting a pantaloon-shaped patch (Fig. 54–112).[17] One technique that results in the most anatomic reconstruction requires transection of the aorta at the level of the stenosis and incisions into all three sinuses of Valsalva. Each sinus is then enlarged with a triangular piece of pericardium[5] or by advancing flaps of the ascending aorta (Fig. 54–113).[58]

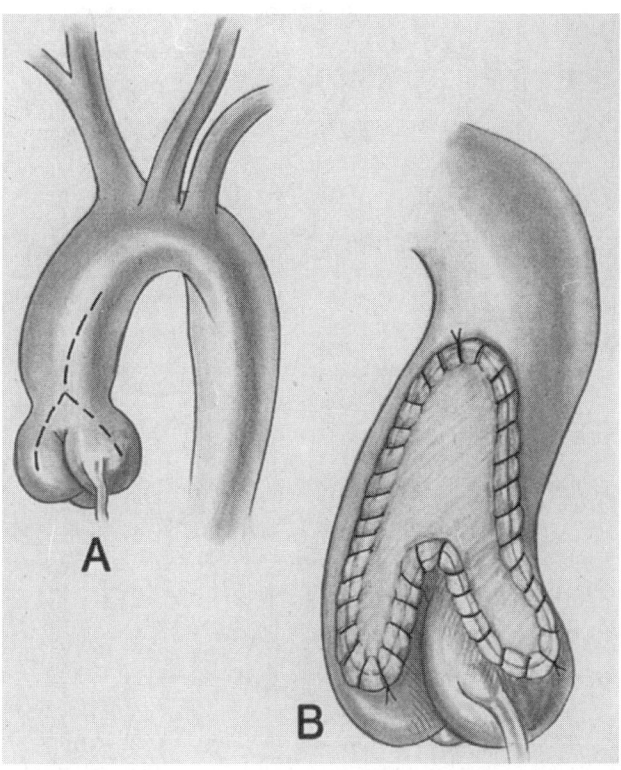

Figure 54–112. Pantaloon patch repair of discrete supravalvular aortic stenosis. *A,* The aortotomy is extended into both the noncoronary and right coronary sinuses of Valsalva. *B,* After the supravalvular ridge is excised, an inverted "Y" pantaloon-shaped patch of autologous pericardium is sutured in place. (From van Son, J. A. M., Danielson, G. K., Puga, F. J., Schaff, H. V., Rastogi, A., Edwards, W. D., and Feldt, R. H.: Supravalvular aortic stenosis: Long-term results of surgical treatment. J. Thorac. Cardiovasc. Surg., *107*:103, 1994.)

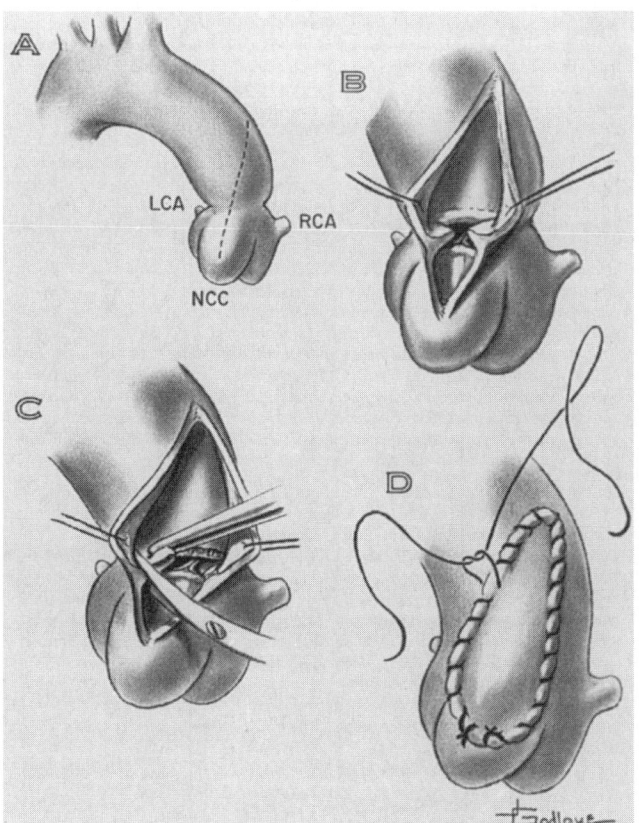

Figure 54–111. Single patch repair of the discrete form of supravalvular aortic stenosis. *A,* The aortotomy is extended into the noncoronary sinus of Valsalva. *B* and *C,* The supravalvular ridge is exposed and excised. *D,* A teardrop-shaped patch of autologous pericardium is sutured in place. (From van Son, J. A. M., Danielson, G. K., Puga, F. J., Schaff, H. V., Rastogi, A., Edwards, W. D., and Feldt, R. H.: Supravalvular aortic stenosis: Long-term results of surgical treatment. J. Thorac. Cardiovasc. Surg., *107*:103, 1994.)

For the diffuse form of supravalvular aortic stenosis, the operative approach must be individualized to the extent of obstruction. At the level of the aortic root an incision is made into the noncoronary sinus of Valsalva. This incision is then extended up the ascending aorta and, if necessary, into the aortic arch and brachiocephalic vessels. Extension into the arch and head vessels must be done using a brief period of total circulatory arrest after core cooling on CPB to a temperature of 18° C. A large patch of Dacron is inserted to increase the diameter of the aortic root, ascending aorta, and arch branches. In some cases, a tube graft between the ascending and descending aorta with side branches to the head vessels must be performed.

Results. Operative results for discrete supravalvular aortic stenosis are good, with a hospital mortality of less than 1% and actuarial survival exceeding 90% at 20 years.[85] Most patients are in functional Class I or II and rarely need reoperation unless associated aortic valve disease is also present.[74, 85] Although newer methods[4, 58] provide more symmetric and anatomic reconstruction of the aortic root, it remains to be seen if these more complex procedures can improve on the excellent results already achieved with single or pantaloon patch techniques.

Hospital mortality for surgical relief of diffuse supravalvular aortic stenosis was initially 50% to 60%[3] but has improved to 15% or less with newer techniques.[74, 85] Long-term survival in operative survivors of this group was similar to that seen for patients with discrete supravalvular aortic stenosis in the report by van Son and associates.[85] Other reports, however, indicate that the diffuse form of the disease is a significant risk factor for late mortality.[74]

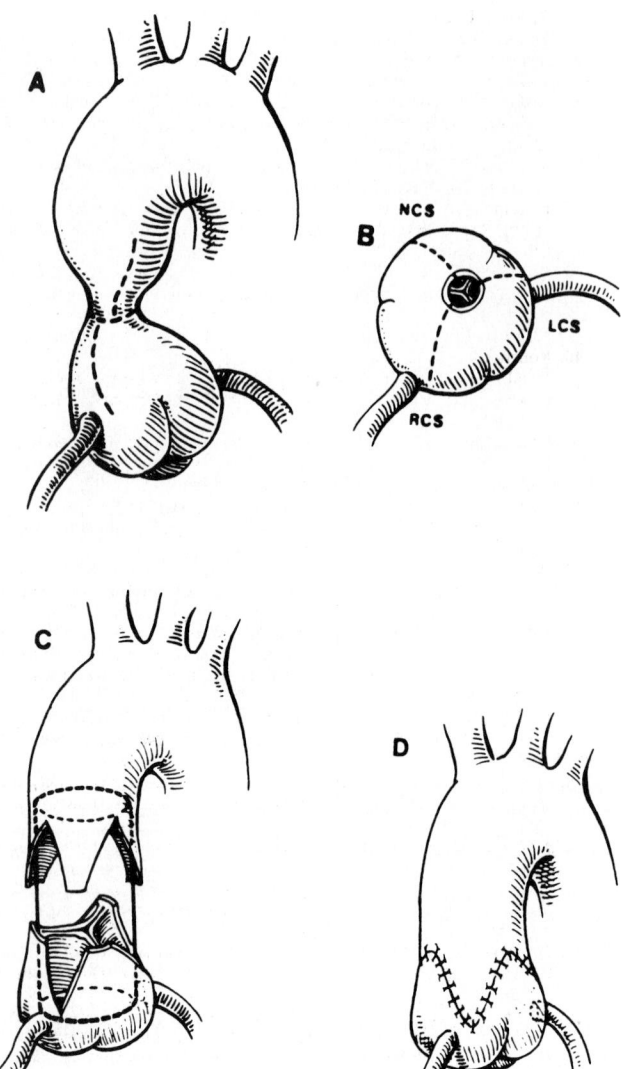

Figure 54–113. Aortic root reconstruction for discrete supravalvular aortic stenosis. *A,* The aorta is divided at the level of the stenosis. *B,* Incisions are extended into each sinus of Valsalva. *C,* Counterincisions in the distal ascending aorta are extended cephalad until the diameter of the aorta equals that of the aortic root. *D,* Normal aortic root geometry is achieved by sewing the three flaps of distal aorta into the corresponding sinuses of Valsalva. (From Myers, J. L., Waldhausen, J. A., Cyran, S. E., Gleason, M. M., Weber, H. S., and Baylen, B. G.: Results of surgical repair of congenital supravalvular aortic stenosis. J. Thorac. Cardiovasc. Surg., *105*:281, 1993.)

SELECTED REFERENCES

Elkins, R. C., Santangelo, K., Randolph, J. D., Knott-Craig, C. J., Stelzer, P., Thompson, W. M., Razook, J. D., Ward, K. E., and Overholt, E. D.: Pulmonary autograft replacement in children: The ideal solution? Ann. Surg., 216:363, 1992.
  Dr. Elkins deserves the credit for revitalizing the operation originally described by Ross in 1967. In this report, 51 patients between 1.8 and 21 years of age are reviewed. There was only one operative death and no late deaths. Actuarial freedom from reoperation was 93% ± 5.5 at 5.6 years. The value of this technique for children requiring aortic valve replacement is strongly supported by these data.

Hsieh, K. S., Keane, J. F., Nadas, A. S., Bernhard, W. F., and Castāneda, A. R.: Long-term follow-up of valvotomy before 1968 for congenital aortic stenosis. Am. J. Cardiol., 58:338, 1986.
  This study reviews the clinical course of 59 children who underwent aortic valvotomy for aortic stenosis before 1968. All patients were older than 1 year of age at the time of operation. Actuarial analysis demonstrated 94% survival at 5 years and 77% survival at 22 years. Probability of reoperation increased from 2% at 5 years to 44% at 22 years. This analysis revealed the palliative nature of valvotomy and the necessity for life-long follow-up in these patients.

Jonas, R. A.: Radical aortic root enlargement in the infant and child. J. Card. Surg., 9(Suppl. 2):165, 1994.
  In this review Dr. Jonas discusses the numerous surgical options employed for relief of all levels of left ventricular outflow tract obstruction. He emphasizes the desirability of preserving the child's own aortic valve, whenever possible, and maintaining growth potential to diminish the need for repeat operations.

Kitchiner, D. J., Jackson, M., Walsh, K., Peart, I., and Arnold, R.: Incidence and prognosis of congenital aortic valve stenosis in Liverpool (1960–1990). Br. Heart J., 69:71, 1993.
  This is a thorough analysis of the incidence and prognosis of all cases of congenital valvular aortic stenosis presenting within a defined population over a 30-year period. Valvular aortic stenosis occurred in 5.7% of patients with congenital heart disease. Sixty-one percent of the patients had mild stenosis, and of these only 15% came to operation. Fourteen percent had moderate stenosis with 67% requiring operation. Nine percent presented as neonates with critical aortic stenosis, and of these over half died before surgery could be performed and only 30% of those undergoing operation survived.

Mohr, R., Schaff, H. V., Danielson, G. K., Puga, F., Pluth, F. R., and Tajik, A. J.: The outcome of surgical treatment of hypertrophic obstructive cardiomyopathy. J. Thorac. Cardiovasc. Surg., 97:666, 1989.
  This report describes the Mayo Clinic experience with the surgical treatment of hypertrophic obstructive cardiomyopathy. From 1972 through 1987, 115 patients between the ages of 1 and 83 years underwent operation. Operative mortality rate was 1.2% in patients younger than 65 years of age. Septal myectomy resulted in a decrease in systolic gradient from 70 ± 38 mm. Hg to 9 ± 11 mm. Hg. Preoperative symptoms were relieved or improved in over 90% of patients. Late mortality was associated with residual systolic gradients greater than 15 mm. Hg and age greater than or equal to 65.

Myers, J. L., Waldhausen, J. A., Cyran, S. E., Gleason, M. M., Weber, H. S., and Baylen, B. G.: Results of surgical repair of congenital supravalvular aortic stenosis. J. Thorac. Cardiovasc. Surg., 105:281, 1993.
  Dr. Myers and associates describe the evolution of techniques applied to the discrete form of supravalvular aortic stenosis at the Milton S. Hershey Medical Center. A new technique that employs all autologous aortic tissue and results in a geometrically restored aortic root is described.

Turley, K., Bove, E. D., Amato, J. J., Iannettoni, M., Yeh, J., Cotroneo, J. V., and Galdieri, R. J.: Neonatal aortic stenosis. J. Thorac. Cardiovasc. Surg., 99:679, 1990.
  This multicenter study presents recent results of surgical valvotomy for neonatal aortic stenosis. An approach of stabilization with CPB followed by aortic valvotomy was applied to 40 neonates between 1983 and 1989 at three institutions. Hospital survival was 87.5% without significant differences between institutions or between open or transventricular valvotomy. The benefit of CPB for stabilization and support during valvotomy is emphasized in this study.

van Son, J. A. M., Danielson, G. K., Puga, F. J., Schaff, H. V., Rastogi, A., Edwards, W. D., and Feld, R. H.: Supravalvular aortic stenosis: Long-term results of surgical treatment. J. Thorac. Cardiovasc. Surg., 107:103, 1994.
  The entire Mayo Clinic experience with this rare lesion is described in this report. Sixty-seven patients with discrete and 13 patients with diffuse supravalvular aortic stenosis are reviewed. There was no operative mortality in those with discrete supravalvular stenosis undergoing aortic root enlargement with either a teardrop-shaped patch (n = 61) or a pantaloon-shaped patch (n = 6). Late reoperation or death occurred only in those patients who also had associated aortic valvular pathology. Operative mortality among the patients with diffuse supravalvular aortic stenosis was 15%, occurring early in the experience when the patch enlargement was confined to the root and proximal ascending aorta. Two survivors of this early approach required reoperation for persistent gradients exceeding 75 mm. Hg. The subsequent experience using patch extension into and beyond the ascending aorta resulted in no further mortality or need for reoperation.

van Son, J. A. M., Schaff, H. V., Danielson, G. K., Hagler, D. J., and Puga, F. J.: Surgical treatment of discrete and tunnel subaortic stenosis. Late survival and risk of reoperation. Circulation, 88(5 pt. 2):II-159, 1993.
  The complete experience of the Mayo Clinic from 1957 through 1992 with fixed subaortic stenosis is described. Among 108 patients undergoing operation for discrete lesions, operative mortality was 4.6%. The risk of reoperation and/or late development of aortic insufficiency was greater in those undergoing isolated membranectomy compared with those undergoing combined membranectomy and septal myectomy. Among 21 patients with discrete subaortic stenosis at initial operation who required reoperation for recurrent stenosis, 19 (92%) were found to have tunnel (diffuse) obstruction at reoperation. Ten-year survival was 91% in the group with discrete subaortic stenosis. Among 61 patients with tunnel subaortic stenosis, operative mortality was 4.9% and 10-year survival was 79%.

REFERENCES

1. Ashraf, H., Dhar, N., Gingell, R., Roland, M., Pieroni, D., and Subramanian, S.: Long-term results after excision of fixed subaortic stenosis. J. Thorac. Cardiovasc. Surg., 90:864, 1985.
2. Beekman, R. H., Rocchini, A. P., and Andes, A.: Balloon valvuloplasty for critical aortic stenosis in the newborn: Influence of new catheter technology. J. Am. Coll. Cardiol., 17:1172, 1991.
3. Bernhard, W. F., Keane, J. F., Fellows, K. E., Litwin, S. B., and Gross, R. E.:

Progress and problems in surgical management of congenital aortic stenosis. J. Thorac. Cardiovasc. Surg., 66:404, 1973.

4. Brock, R., and Fleming, P. R.: Aortic subvalvar stenosis: A report of 5 cases diagnosed during life. Guys Hosp. Rep., 105:391, 1956.

5. Brom, A. G.: Obstruction to the left ventricular outflow tract. In Khonsari, S. (Ed.): Cardiac Surgery: Safeguards and Pitfalls in Operative Technique. Rockville, MD, Aspen, 1988, pp. 276–280.

6. Brown, J. W., Girod, D. A., Hurwitz, R. A., et al.: Apicoaortic valved conduits for complex left ventricular outflow obstruction: Technical considerations and current status. Ann. Thorac. Surg., 38:162, 1984.

7. Brown, J., Stevens, L., Lynch, L., Caldwell, R., Girod, D., Hurwitz, R., Mahony, L., and King, H.: Surgery for discrete subvalvular aortic stenosis: Actuarial survival, hemodynamic results, and acquired aortic regurgitation. Ann. Thorac. Surg., 40:151, 1985.

8. Cain, T., Campbell, D., Paton, B., and Clarke, D.: Operation for discrete subvalvular aortic stenosis. J. Thorac. Cardiovasc. Surg., 87:366, 1984.

9. Chevers, N.: Observations on the diseases of the orifice and valves of the aorta. Guys Hosp. Rep., 1842, p. 387.

10. Clarke, D. R.: Extended aortic root replacement for treatment of left ventricular outflow tract obstruction. J. Card. Surg., 1(Suppl.):121, 1987.

11. Clarke, D. R., Campbell, D. N., Hayward, A. R., and Bishop, D. A.: Degeneration of aortic valve allografts in young recipients. J. Thorac. Cardiovasc. Surg., 105:934, 1993.

12. Cooley, D. A.: Surgical techniques for hypertrophic left ventricular obstructive myopathy including mitral valve plication. J. Card. Surg., 6:29, 1991.

13. De Boer, D. A., Robbins, R. C., Maron, B. J., McIntosh, C. L., and Clark, R. E.: Late results of aortic valvotomy for congenital valvar aortic stenosis. Ann. Thorac. Surg. 50:69, 1990.

14. DeLeon, S. Y., Ilbawi, M. N., Roberson, D. A., Arcilla, R. A., Thilenius, O. G., Wilson, W. R., Duffy, E. C., and Quinones, J. A.: Conal enlargement for diffuse subaortic stenosis. J. Thorac. Cardiovasc. Surg., 10:814, 1991.

15. DeLeon, S. Y., Ilbawi, M. N., Wilson, W. R., Jr., Arcilla, R. A., Thilenius, O. G., Bharati, S., Lev, M., and Idriss, F. S.: Surgical options in subaortic stenosis associated with endocardial cushion defects. Ann. Thorac. Surg., 52:1076, 1991.

16. DiDonato, R. M., Danielson, G. K., McGoon, D. C., Driscoll, D. J., Julsrud, P. R., and Edwards, W. D.: Left ventricle-aortic conduits in pediatric patients. J. Thorac. Cardiovasc. Surg., 88:82, 1984.

17. Doty, D. B., Polansky, D. B., and Jenson, C. B.: Supravalvular aortic stenosis. J. Thorac. Cardiovasc. Surg., 74:362, 1977.

18. Douville, E. C., Sade, R. M., Crawford, F. A., Jr., and Wiles, H. B.: Subvalvar aortic stenosis: Timing of operation. Ann. Thorac. Surg., 50:29, 1990.

19. Edmonds, L. H., Wagner, H. R., and Heyman, M. A.: Aortic valvulotomy in neonates. Circulation, 61:421, 1980.

20. Ettedgui, J. A., Tallman-Eddy, T., Neches, W. H., Pahl, E., Zuberbuhler, J. R., Fischer, D. R., Beerman, L. B., and Siewers, R. D.: Long-term results of survivors of surgical valvotomy for severe aortic stenosis in early infancy. J. Thorac. Cardiovasc. Surg., 104:1714, 1992.

21. Elkins, R. C., Santangelo, K., Randolph, J. D., et al.: Pulmonary autograft replacement in children: The ideal solution? Ann. Surg., 3:363, 1992.

22. Ellis, F. H., Jr., and Kirklin, J. W.: Congenital valvular aortic stenosis: Anatomic findings and surgical techniques. J. Thorac. Cardiovasc. Surg., 43:199, 1962.

23. Fananapazir, L., Cannon, R. O., Tripodi, D., and Panza, J. A.: Impact of dual-chamber permanent pacing in patients with obstructive hypertrophic cardiomyopathy with symptoms refractory to verapamil and β-adrenergic blocker therapy. Circulation, 85:2149, 1992.

24. Firpo, C., Maitre-Azcarte, M. J., Quero-Jimenez, M., and Saravalli, O.: Discrete subaortic stenosis (DSS) in childhood: A congenital or acquired disease? Follow-up in 65 patients. Eur. Heart J., 11:1033, 1990.

25. Freedom, R. M., Pelech, A., Brand, A., Vogel, M., Olley, P. M., Smallhorn, J., and Rowe, R. D.: The progressive nature of subaortic stenosis in congenital heart disease. Int. J. Cardiol., 8:137, 1985.

26. Frommelt, P. C., Rochini, A. P., and Bove, E. L.: Natural history of apical left ventricular to aortic conduits in pediatric patients. Circulation, 84(Suppl. III):III-213, 1991.

27. Goodwin, J. F., Hollman, A., Cleland, W. P., and Teare, D.: Obstructive cardiomyopathy simulating aortic stenosis. Br. Heart J., 22:403, 1960.

28. Gundry, S. R., and Behrendt, D. M.: Prognostic factors in valvotomy for critical aortic stenosis in infancy. J. Thorac. Cardiovasc. Surg., 92:747, 1986.

29. Hsieh, K. S., Keane, J. F., Nadas, A. S., Bernhard, W. F., and Castañeda, A. R.: Long-term follow-up of valvotomy before 1968 for congenital aortic stenosis. Am. J. Cardiol., 58:338, 1986.

30. Hoffman, J. E. I., and Christianson, R.: Congenital heart disease in a cohort of 19,502 births with long-term follow-up. Am. J. Cardiol., 42:641, 1978.

31. Ilbawi, M. N., De Leon, S. Y., Wilson, W. R., Jr., Roberson, D. A., Husayni, T. S., Quinones, J. A., and Arcilla, R. A.: Extended aortic valvuloplasty: A new approach for the management of congenital valvar aortic stenosis. Ann. Thorac. Surg., 52:663, 1991.

32. Jonas, R. A.: Radical aortic root enlargement in the infant and child. J. Card. Surg., 9(Suppl. 2):165, 1994.

33. Jonas, R. A., Lang, P., Mayer, J. E., and Castēneda, A. R.: The importance of prostaglandin E_1 in resuscitation of the neonate with critical aortic stenosis (Letter). J. Thorac. Cardiovasc. Surg., 89:314, 1985.

34. Karl, T. R., Sano, S., Brawn, W. J., and Mee, R. B. B.: Critical aortic stenosis in the first month of life: Surgical results in 26 infants. Ann. Thorac. Surg., 50:105, 1990.

35. Keane, J. F., Driscoll, D. J., Gersony, W. M., Hayes, C. J., Kidd, L., O'Fallon, W. M., Pieroni, D. R., Wolfe, R. R., and Weidman, W. H.: Second natural history study of congenital heart defects: Results of treatment of patients with aortic valvar stenosis. Circulation, 87(Suppl. 2):116, 1993.

36. Kelly, D. T., Barratt-Boyes, B. G., and Lowe, J. B.: Results of surgery and hemodynamic observations in muscular subaortic stenosis. J. Thorac. Cardiovasc. Surg., 51:353, 1966.

37. Kirklin, J. W., and Ellis, F. J., Jr.: Surgical relief of diffuse subvalvular aortic stenosis. Circulation, 24:739, 1961.

38. Kitchiner, D. J., Jackson, M., Walsh, K., Peart, I., and Arnold, R.: Incidence and prognosis of congenital aortic valve stenosis in Liverpool (1960–1990). Br. Heart J. 69:71, 1993.

39. Konno, S., Imai, Y., Iida, Y., Nakajima, M., Tatsuno, K.: A new method for prosthetic valve replacement in congenital aortic stenosis associated with hypoplasia of the aortic valve ring. J. Thorac. Cardiovasc. Surg., 70:909, 1975.

40. Kouchoukos, N. T., Davila-Roman, V. G., Spray, T. L., Murphy, S. F., and Perrill, J. B.: Replacement of the aortic root with a pulmonary autograft in children and young adults with aortic-valve disease. N. Engl. J. Med., 330:1, 1994.

41. Lakier, J. B., Lewis, A. B., Heymann, M. A., Stanger, P., Hoffman, J. I. E, and Rudolph, A. M.: Isolated aortic stenosis in the neonate: Natural history and hemodynamic considerations. Circulation, 50:801, 1974.

42. Leichter, D. A., Sullivan, I., and Gersony, W. M.: "Acquired" discrete subvalvular aortic stenosis: Natural history and hemodynamics. J. Am. Coll. Cardiol., 14:1539, 1989.

43. Leoni, F., Huhta, J. C., Douglas, J., MacKay, R., deLeval, M. R., Macartney, F. J., and Stark, J.: Effect of prostaglandin on early surgical mortality in obstructive lesions of the systemic circulation. Br. Heart J., 52:654, 1984.

44. Leung, M. P., MacKay, R., Smith, A., Anderson, R. H., and Arnold, R.: Critical aortic stenosis in early infancy: Anatomic and echocardiographic substrates of successful open valvotomy. J. Thorac. Cardiovasc. Surg., 101:526, 1991.

45. Lewis, F. J., Shumway, N. E., and Niazi, S. A.: Aortic valvulotomy under direct vision during hypothermia. J. Thorac. Cardiovasc. Surg., 32:481, 1956.

46. Lupinetti, F. M., Pridjian, A. K., Callow, L. B., Crowley, D. C., Beekman, R. H., and Bove, E. L.: Optimum treatment of discrete subaortic stenosis. Ann. Thorac. Surg., 54:467, 1992.

47. Manouguian, S., and Seybold-Epting, W.: Patch enlargement of the aortic valve ring by extending the aortic incision into the anterior mitral leaflet: New operative technique. J. Thorac. Cardiovasc. Surg., 78:402, 1979.

48. Marquis, R. M., and Logan, R.: Congenital aortic stenosis and its surgical treatment. Br. Heart J., 17:373, 1955.

49. McGoon, D. C., Mankin, H. T., Vlad, P., and Kirklin, J. W.: The surgical treatment of supravalvular aortic stenosis. J. Thorac. Cardiovasc. Surg., 41:125, 1961.

50. McIntosh, C. L., Maron, B. J., Cannon, R. O., and Klues, H. G.: Initial results of combined anterior mitral leaflet plication and ventricular septal myotomy-myectomy for relief of left ventricular outflow obstruction in patients with hypertrophic cardiomyopathy. Circulation, 86(Suppl II):II-60, 1992.

51. McKenna, W., Deanfield, J., Farugui, A., England, D., Oakley, C., and Goodwin, J.: Prognosis in hypertrophic cardiomyopathy: Role of age and clinical electrocardiographic and hemodynamic features. Am. J. Cardiol., 47:532, 1981.

52. Mencarelli, L.: Stenosis sopravalvolare aortica e anello. Arch. Ital. Anat. Istol. Patol., 1:829, 1930.

53. Messina, L. M., Turley, K., Stanger, P., Hoffman, J. I., and Ebert, P. A.: Successful aortic valvotomy for severe congenital valvular aortic stenosis in the newborn infant. J. Thorac. Cardiovasc. Surg., 88:92, 1984.

54. Mohr, R., Schaff, H. V., Danielson, G. K., Puga, F., Pluth, F. R., and Tajik, A. J.: The outcome of surgical treatment of hypertrophic obstructive cardiomyopathy. J. Thorac. Cardiovasc. Surg., 97:666, 1989.

55. Morrow, A. G., Reitz, B. A., Epstein, S. E., Henry, W. L., Conkle, D. M., Itscoitz, S. B., and Redwood, D. R.: Operative treatment in hypertrophic subaortic stenosis: Techniques and the results of pre- and post-operative assessments in 83 patients. Circulation, 52:88, 1975.

56. Mosca, R. S., Iannettoni, M. D., Schwartz, S. M., Ludomirsky, A., Beekman, T. H., III, Lloyd, T., and Bove, E. L.: Critical aortic stenosis in the neonate: A comparison of balloon valvuloplasty and transventricular dilation. J. Thorac. Cardiovasc. Surg., 109:147, 1995.

57. Moses, R. D., Barnhart, G. R., and Jones, M.: The late prognosis after localized resection for fixed (discrete and tunnel) left ventricular outflow tract obstruction. J. Thorac. Cardiovasc. Surg., 87:410, 1984.

58. Myers, J. L., Waldhausen, J. A., Cyran, S. E., Gleason, M. M., Weber, H. S., and Baylen, B. G.: Results of surgical repair of congenital supravalvular aortic stenosis. J. Thorac. Cardiovasc. Surg., 105:281, 1993.

59. Nicks, R., Cartmill, T., Bernstein, L.: Hypoplasia of the aortic root: The problem of aortic valve replacement. Thorax, 25:339, 1970.

60. O'Connor, B. K., Beekman, R. H., Rocchini, A. P., and Rosenthal, A.: Intermediate-term effectiveness of balloon valvuloplasty for congenital aortic stenosis: A prospective follow-up study. Circulation, 84:732, 1991.

61. Paget, J.: On obstructions of the branches of the pulmonary artery. Med. Chir. Trans., 27:162, 1844.

62. Rastan, H., Abu-Aishah, N., Rastan, D., et al.: Results of aortoventricu-

loplasty in 21 consecutive patients with left ventricular outflow tract obstruction. J. Thorac. Cardiovasc. Surg., 75:659, 1978.

63. Roberts, W. C.: Valvular, subvalvular and supravalvular aortic stenosis: Morphologic features. Cardiovasc. Clin., 5:97, 1973.

64. Rhodes, L. A., Colan, S. D., Perry, S. B., Jonas, R. A., and Sanders, S. P.: Predictors of survival in neonates with critical aortic stenosis. Circulation, 84:2325, 1991.

65. Rocchini, A. P., Beekman, R. H., Ben Shachar, G., Benson, L., Schwartz, D., and Kan, J. S.: Balloon aortic valvuloplasty: Results of the Valvuloplasty and Angioplasty of Congenital Anomalies Registry. Am. J. Cardiol., 65:784, 1990.

66. Rosenzweig, A., Watkins, H., Hwang, D. S., et al.: Preclinical diagnosis of familial hypertrophic cardiomyopathy by genetic analysis of blood lymphocytes. N. Engl. J. Med., 325:1753, 1991.

67. Ross, D. B., Trusler, G. A., Coles, J. G., Rebeyka, I. M., Smallhorn, J., Williams, W. G., and Freedom, R. M.: Small aortic root in childhood: Surgical options. Ann. Thorac. Surg., 58:1617, 1994.

68. Ross, D. N.: Replacement of the aortic and mitral valves with a pulmonary autograft. Lancet 2:956, 1967.

69. Sandor, G. G. S., Olley, P. M., Trusler, G. A., Williams, W. G., Rowe, R. D., and Morch, J. E.: Long-term follow-up of patients after valvotomy for congenital valvular aortic stenosis in children. J. Thorac. Cardiovasc. Surg., 80:171, 1980.

70. Schoof, P. H., Cromme-Dijkhuis, A. H., Bogers, J. J. C., Thijssen, E. J. M., Witsenburg, M., Hess, J., and Boss, E.: Aortic root replacement with pulmonary autograft in children. J. Thorac. Cardiovasc. Surg., 107:367, 1994.

71. Seiler, C., Hess, O. M., Schoenbeck, M., et al: Long-term follow-up of medical versus surgical therapy for hypertrophic cardiomyopathy: A retrospective study. J. Am. Coll. Cardiol., 17:634, 1991.

72. Shaddy, R. E., Boucek, M. M., Sturtevant, J. E., Ruttenberg, H. D., and Orsmond, G. S.: Gradient reduction, aortic valve regurgitation and prolapse after balloon aortic valvuloplasty in 32 consecutive patients with congenital aortic stenosis (see comments). J. Am. Coll. Cardiol., 16:451, 1990.

73. Shah, P. M., Adelman, A. G., Wigle, E. D., Gobel, F. L., Burchell, H. B., Hardarson, T., Curiel, R., de la Calzada, C., Oakley, C. M., and Goodwin, J. F.: The natural (and unnatural) history of hypertrophic obstructive cardiomyopathy: A multicenter study. Circ. Res., 34/35(Suppl. II):179, 1974.

74. Sharma, B. K., Fujiwara, H., Hallman, G. L., Ott, D. A., Reul, G. J., and Cooley, D. A.: Supravalvar aortic stenosis: A 29-year review of surgical experience. Ann. Thorac. Surg., 51:1031, 1991.

75. Spencer, F. C., Neill, C. A., and Bahnson, H. T.: The treatment of congenital aortic stenosis with valvotomy during cardiopulmonary bypass. Surgery, 44:109, 1958.

76. Spencer, F. C., Neill, C. A., Sank, L., and Bahnson, H. T.: Anatomical variations in 46 patients with congenital aortic stenosis. Am. Surg., 26:204, 1960.

77. Spray, T. L., Maron, B. J., Morrow, A. G., Epstein, S. E., and Roberts, W. C.: Clinical pathologic conference: A discussion on hypertrophic cardiomyopathy. Am. Heart J., 95:511, 1978.

78. Stelzer, P., Jones, D. J., and Elkins, R. C.: Aortic root replacement with pulmonary autograft. Circulation, 87:(Suppl. III):III-209, 1989.

79. Stewart, J. R., Merrill, W. H., Hammon, J. W., Jr., Graham, T. P., and Bender, H. W.: Reappraisal of localized resection for subvalvar aortic stenosis. Ann. Thorac. Surg., 50:197, 1990.

80. Swan, H., and Kortz, A: Direct vision trans-aortic approach to the aortic valve during hypothermia: Experimental observations and report of a successful clinical case. Ann. Surg., 144:205, 1956.

81. Teare, R. D.: Asymmetrical hypertrophy of the heart in young adults. Br. Heart J., 20:1, 1958.

82. Tuffier, T.: Etat actuel de la chirurgie intrathoracique. Trans. Int. Cong. Med., London, 1914.

83. Turley, K., Bove, E. D., Amato, J. J., Iannettoni, M., Yeh, J., Cotroneo, J. V., and Galdieri, R. J.: Neonatal aortic stenosis. J. Thorac. Cardiovasc. Surg., 99:679, 1990.

84. Tveter, K. J., Foker, J. E., Moller, J. H., Ring, W. S., Lillehei, C. W., and Varco, R. L.: Long-term evaluation of aortic valvotomy for congenital aortic stenosis. Ann. Surg., 206:496, 1987.

85. van Son, J. A. M., Danielson, G. K., Puga, F. J., Schaff, H. V., Rastogi, A., Edwards, W. D., and Feld, R. H.: Supravalvular aortic stenosis: Long-term results of surgical treatment. J. Thorac. Cardiovasc. Surg., 107:103, 1994.

86. van Son, J. A. M., Schaff, H. V., Danielson, G. K., Hagler, D. J., and Puga, F. J.: Surgical treatment of discrete and tunnel subaortic stenosis: Late survival and risk of reoperation. Circulation, 88(5 Pt. 2):II-159, 1993.

87. van Son, J. A. M., Edwards, W. D., and Danielson, G. K.: Pathology of coronary arteries, myocardium, and great arteries in supravalvular aortic stenosis. J. Thorac. Cardiovasc. Surg., 108:21, 1994.

88. Vogel, J., Benson, L. N., Burrows, P., Smallhorn, J. F., and Freedom, R. M.: Balloon dilatation of congenital aortic valve stenosis in infants and children: Short-term and intermediate results. Br. Heart J., 62:148, 1989.

89. Vouhe, P. R., and Neveux, J. Y.: Surgical management of diffuse subaortic stenosis: An integrated approach. Ann. Thorac. Surg., 52:654, 1991.

90. Walker, W. S., Reid, K. G., Cameron, E. W. J., Walbaum, P. R., and Kitchin, A. H.: Comparison of ventricular septal surgery and mitral valve replacement for hypertrophic obstructive cardiomyopathy. Ann. Thorac. Surg., 48:528, 1989.

91. Williams, J. C. P., Barratt-Boyes, B. G., and Lowe, J. B.: Supravalvular aortic stenosis. Circulation, 24:1311, 1961.

92. Williams, W. G., Wigle, E. D., Rakowski, H., Smallhorn, J., LeBlanc, J., and Trusler, G. A.: Results of surgery for hypertrophic obstructive cardiomyopathy. Circulation, 76(Suppl. V):V-104, 1987.

93. Witsenburg, M., Cromme-Dijkhuis, A. H., Frohn-Mulder, I. M., and Hess, J.: Short- and midterm results of balloon valvuloplasty for valvular aortic stenosis in children. Am. J. Cardiol., 69:945, 1992.

94. Wright, G. B., Keane, J. F., Nadas, A. S., et al.: Fixed subaortic stenosis in the young: Medical and surgical course in 83 patients. Am. J. Cardiol., 52:830, 1983.

95. Zeevi, B., Keane, J. F., Castañeda, A. R., Perry, S. B., and Lock, J. E.: Neonatal critical valvar aortic stenosis: A comparison of surgical and balloon dilation therapy. Circulation, 80:831, 1989.

XIV

THE CORONARY CIRCULATION

R. Duane Davis, Jr., M.D., and David C. Sabiston, Jr., M.D.

In certain cases of angina pectoris, when the mouth of the coronary arteries is calcified, it would be useful to establish a complementary circulation for the lower part of the arteries.

ALEXIS CARREL, 1910

Atherosclerotic coronary artery disease (CAD) continues to be the leading cause of death and lost life expectancy in the United States. It has been estimated that over one third of the population eventually will die of CAD, and 20% will develop symptoms when younger than age 60 years. Approximately 7 million Americans have symptomatic CAD, 1.5 million experience myocardial infarction annually, and more than 500,000 die each year of related complications. The annual direct and indirect economic cost of CAD in the United States is estimated to exceed 80 billion dollars, and similar data are available for most of the western world.[27]

The age-adjusted mortality attributable to CAD per unit population of the United States has been decreasing since 1965, and the absolute incidence continues to increase.[49] If one assumes constant risk factors and therapeutic efficacies, epidemiologic models predict that aging of the population of the United States, and especially maturation of the post–World War II baby-boom generation, will increase *absolute* CAD prevalence, annual incidence, total mortality, and economic cost by 40% to 50% by the year 2010 (Table 54–5). Thus, the medical significance of coronary atherosclerosis and the number of patients presenting for surgical intervention will, in all likelihood, continue to increase in coming decades. In this discussion, basic principles of coronary atherosclerosis and myocardial ischemia are reviewed, current techniques for surgical coronary revascularization are described, and the prognostic efficacy of contemporary surgical therapy is delineated as precisely as possible.

TABLE 54–5. Projections of Absolute Coronary Heart Disease Incidence, Prevalence, Mortality, and Cost

Year	Incidence	Prevalence	Mortality	Cost*
1980	692,117	5,977,405	432,613	31.9
1985	729,235	6,700,639	486,428	35.3
1990	759,583	7,230,904	540,557	37.8
1995	792,006	7,625,001	567,798	39.9
2000	834,522	7,973,869	596,777	42.0
2005	888,438	8,385,046	608,434	44.4
2010	953,750	8,939,816	632,304	47.4

*Billions of 1980 dollars, direct cost only.

From Weinstein, M. C., et al.: Forecasting coronary heart disease incidence, mortality, and cost: The Coronary Heart Disease Policy Model. Am. J. Public Health, 77:1417, 1987.

ANATOMY OF THE CORONARY ARTERIES

The first branches of the aorta are the right and left coronary arteries and arise from the sinuses of Valsalva. The right coronary artery passes deep in the right atrioventricular groove and proceeds over the anterior surface of the heart. At the superior end of the acute margin of the heart, the vessel turns posteriorly toward the crux and usually terminates as the posterior descending coronary artery in the posterior interventricular groove. The right coronary artery initially provides a number of small vessels, which anastomose on the anterior ventricle in the pulmonary conus region with corresponding branches from the left coronary artery (the arterial circle of Vieussens). It next supplies multiple right ventricular branches and the sinus node artery (the latter may arise from the left circumflex artery). Along the acute right border of the heart, the right marginal artery takes origin. In the 90% of patients with *right coronary dominance,* the right coronary artery terminates in the posterior descending artery and, by an extension to the crux, branches into an atrioventricular node artery and several terminal posterolateral left ventricular branches.

The left main coronary artery is usually about 1 cm. in length and gives rise to the left anterior descending (LAD) and left circumflex coronary arteries. The LAD provides branches to the arterial circle of Vieussens and several diagonal branches to the anterior left ventricular wall. As it proceeds distally in the anterior interventricular groove, the LAD provides a number of anterior perforating branches to the interventricular septum and, in most patients, wraps the apex of the heart, anastomosing with the posterior descending artery. Thus, the LAD is *usually* the largest and most important of the coronary arteries, supplying the anterior wall of the left ventricle, the left margin of the right ventricle, the apex of the heart, and the majority of the interventricular septum.

The left circumflex artery lies in the left atrioventricular groove and proceeds laterally and posteriorly around the left lateral aspect of the left ventricle, usually terminating in several left marginal arteries. In the 10% of patients with *left coronary dominance,* the circumflex system provides the posterior descending coronary artery. The first branch of the circumflex artery is usually the auricular anastomotic artery (Kugel's artery).

The venous drainage of the heart is through superficial and deep circuits. The superficial veins conduct most of the venous blood and accompany the respective coronary arteries. The surface coronary veins empty either into the coronary sinus (which drains into the right atrium) or into the anterior cardiac veins, the latter emptying individually into the right atrium. The deep veins communicate with both the atrial and ventricular cavities through thebesian and sinusoidal and channels.

NORMAL PHYSIOLOGY

Coronary blood flow delivers oxygen and metabolic substrates to the myocardium and simultaneously removes carbon dioxide and metabolic byproducts by transcapillary exchange. Normal coronary blood flow approximates 0.7 to 0.9 ml. per gm. of myocardium per minute and delivers 0.1 ml. of oxygen per gm. per minute to the heart; this is an extreme rate of energy utilization, compared with the rest of the body. The extraction of oxygen in the coronary bed is high, averaging 75% under normal conditions and increasing to nearly 100% during stress. Coronary artery blood flow occurs primarily during diastole because systolic myocardial contraction increases intramyocardial vascular resistance.[45] Normally, mean coronary resistance is three to six times the totally vasodilated value, implying an extreme degree of vasodilatory reserve. During stress, increasing oxygen delivery is provided primarily by vasodilation because of the high baseline oxygen extraction. If adequate perfusion pressure is assumed, total and regional myocardial blood flow under normal conditions is determined by autoregulation of regional arteriolar resistance modulated by local metabolic demand.

The metabolic activity of heart muscle transfers the chemical energy provided by myocardial oxygen and substrate utilization into mechanical energy in the form of circulatory pressure and flow. With electrical depolarization of the myocardial cell membrane, ionized calcium fluxes into the cytoplasm, causing the myosin molecule to hydrolyze adenosine triphosphate (ATP) into adenosine diphosphate and inorganic phosphate. When ATP is split, a considerable amount of chemical energy is released from the ATP molecule and transferred into a conformational change in the myosin crossbridge. This chemomechanical alteration in the crossbridge produces sliding of myosin filaments relative to actin and shortening of the sarcomere.[47] Over the physiologic range of sarcomere lengths (1.6 to 2.0 μm.), the surface area of available crossbridge interactions and, therefore, the metabolic energy transferred into mechanical work during sarcomere contraction are directly proportional to end-diastolic sarcomere length. This length dependency of crossbridge interaction at the sarcomere level constitutes the fundamental basis for the Frank-Starling relationship. As a final step in the process, calcium is removed from the cell by active transport of the cytoplasmic reticulum and ATP is generated at the mitochondrial level by aerobic metabolism of oxygen and substrates.

The ventricles appear to function as an integrated sum of their component sarcomeres. Mechanical energy production, in the form of external pressure and flow generation (stroke work), is a direct linear function of end-diastolic volume and is not influenced significantly by physiologic changes in afterload.[18] Therefore, short-term alterations in myocardial inotropism (defined as load-independent intrinsic myocardial performance) can be assessed by the slope of the stroke work/end-diastolic volume relationship. This fundamental Frank-Starling property of the heart is probably directly reflective of sarcomere and myosin crossbridge dynamics.

Cardiac metabolic activity over time can be assessed by myocardial oxygen consumption. Each milliliter of oxygen utilized by the heart provides 2.02 J. of energy to the contractile apparatus through aerobic metabolic pathways and ATP. Thus, oxygen consumption can be used for quantification of myocardial *energy utilization.* Myocardial *energy expenditure* has two components: (1) external energy, which is stroke work or the integral of the ventricular pressure (P)-volume

(V) loop; and (2) internal energy, which is the thermodynamic cost of maintaining systolic ventricular pressure at a given volume.[35] Internal energy expenditure can be estimated at the product of ventricular mean ejection pressure (PME) × end-diastolic volume (VED) and constitutes the sole mechanical energy production during isovolumic contraction. Total mechanical energy expenditure (TME) for each cardiac cycle can be calculated as:

$$TME = \int PdV + (PME \cdot VED)$$

where PdV is the product of pressure with the derivative of volume. Because 1 mm. Hg × ml. is equivalent to 1.333×10^{-4} J., total mechanical energy expenditure can be compared with metabolic energy utilization for obtaining a measure of metabolic to mechanical energy transfer efficiency. Oxygen consumption is tightly coupled to mechanical energy expenditure, both on a steady-state and beat-to-beat basis.

PATHOLOGIC ANATOMY

A progressive disease, coronary atherosclerosis may begin early in life and has been seen microscopically in infants. The earliest lesions consist of rupture, degeneration, and regeneration of the internal elastic membrane, together with deposition of mucopolysaccharide and proliferation of endothelial cells and fibroblasts. At this early stage, such lesions are quite minimal and solely microscopic. However, gross lesions subsequently appear within a few years in the form of small yellow deposits of lipoid material visible beneath the intima. These lesions are present in half the hearts examined at autopsy during the second decade of life. The presence of extensive coronary atherosclerosis in otherwise healthy young males was emphasized in routine autopsies on young military casualties in the Korean conflict, which demonstrated that 77% had gross evidence of coronary atherosclerosis and 10% showed advanced disease, with 70% or greater occlusion of one or more major arteries.[11] In a community study, coronary atherosclerosis (from 24% to complete occlusion of one or more major arteries) was present in three fourths of the entire population. These figures indicate the extreme prevalence of the disorder; but, unfortunately, its presence is usually not made manifest until serious symptoms appear. In the final stages of the disease, rupture of an intimal atherosclerotic plaque appears to be a dominant mechanism of worsening symptoms, with deposition of platelets and thrombus progressing to thrombotic occlusion and acute myocardial infarction. Subtotal occlusions by *dynamic* thrombotic lesions appear to be of major importance in the pathogenesis of unstable angina.

Pathologic studies assessing the incidence and degree of atherosclerosis in each of the major coronary arteries have shown that the anterior descending coronary artery is the most frequently involved, followed in incidence by the right coronary artery, the left circumflex artery, the left main artery, and, least frequently of all, the right posterior descending coronary artery (Table 54–6). The more severe changes occur in the proximal third or half of the coronary arteries. The most common sites of obstruction noted for each of the three major coronary vessels are shown in Figure 54–114.

ISCHEMIC PATHOPHYSIOLOGY

The mechanisms of myocardial ischemia are complex. Reduction in myocardial oxygen supply during ischemia, or increasing oxygen demand during hemodynamic stress, produces regulatory coronary vasodilation. With decreasing arteriolar resistance, diastolic intramyocardial pressure becomes a more important determinant of mean myocardial perfusion. In the presence of adequate arterial pressure and low diastolic cavitary pressure, the modest transmural gradient of

TABLE 54–6. Frequency of Obstructive Lesions in the Coronary Arteries Due to Atherosclerosis as Found in a Series of 300 Consecutive Patients with Coronary Atherosclerosis

Coronary Artery	No. of Cases	Percentage
Right	165	28.4
Left main	26	4.5
Left anterior descending	251	43.4
Left circumflex	134	23.7
Total	576	100.0

From Berger, R. L., and Stary, J. C.: Anatomic assessment of operability by the saphenous-vein bypass operation in coronary artery disease. N. Engl. J. Med., 285:248, 1971. Copyright 1971, Massachusetts Medical Society. Reprinted by permission of The New England Journal of Medicine.

diastolic intramyocardial pressure has little effect on regional myocardial blood flow through the dilated vascular bed. However, transmural blood flow becomes pressure dependent, and if aortic perfusion pressure decreases or diastolic intracavitary pressure increases, coronary perfusion may be redistributed away from the subendocardium where intramural compressive forces are the highest. This redistribution of flow can induce subendocardial ischemia, even in the presence of normal coronary arteries.

When an atherosclerotic plaque in a proximal coronary artery decreases the cross-sectional area by 75% or more, the resistance to flow caused by the plaque becomes significant. The dominant point of coronary vascular resistance then becomes the critical stenosis that can limit myocardial perfusion to a fixed value. Whereas flow may be adequate at rest, exercise or other factors that increase myocardial oxygen demand can produce relative ischemia, a fall in the coronary pressure distal to the stenosis, and redistribution of blood flow away from the subendocardium. This appears to be the mechanism of exercise-induced angina pectoris and associated transient myocardial dysfunction. Superimposed on the phenomenon, coronary vasospasm and unstable thrombotic plaques can compound the obstructive physiologic process.

Acute coronary occlusion produces an almost immediate decrement in myocardial segment shortening and work. When full reperfusion is accomplished after a 15-minute period of reversible ischemia, dysfunction can be prolonged, requiring up to 24 to 48 hours for complete recovery. Ischemic myocardial dysfunction in this setting is characterized by a diminished slope of the stroke work/end-diastolic segment length relationship together with a rightward shift of the x-

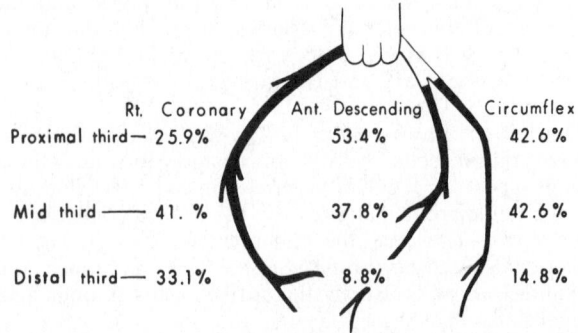

Figure 54–114. Localization of stenotic lesions in the three major coronary trunks. Each coronary artery is divided into three equal segments, and the percentage of the total number of lesions in each third is noted. In the anterior descending and circumflex arteries the obstructions tend to be in the proximal two thirds, whereas the primary involvement is in the distal two thirds of the right coronary artery. (From Berger, R. L., and Stary, H. C.: Anatomic assessment of operability by the saphenous-vein bypass operation in coronary artery disease. N. Engl. J. Med., 285:248, 1971. Copyright 1971, Massachusetts Medical Society. Reprinted by permission of The New England Journal of Medicine.)

intercept ($\int_o$), termed *diastolic creep*.[20] With reperfusion, the slope recovers rapidly but $\int_o$ remains overstretched, diminishing the work capacity at any given preload. Subsequent recovery of systolic function occurs slowly and is associated with a reversal of creep. Catecholamine infusion, increasing afterload, or a second ischemic event during early reperfusion can worsen dysfunction and prolong recovery.

Postischemic systolic dysfunction and diastolic creep can be correlated at an ultrastructural level with sarcomere overstretching, increased Z-band separation, and widening of the I-bands (Fig. 54–115). It appears that the sarcomeres become stretched beyond their normal working range, and disengagement of actin filaments from the M-band may reduce the number of possible crossbridge interactions and potentially be responsible for the mechanical findings.

CORONARY COLLATERAL CIRCULATION

Extensive studies have been made of the coronary collateral circulation in both experimental animals and in man. The

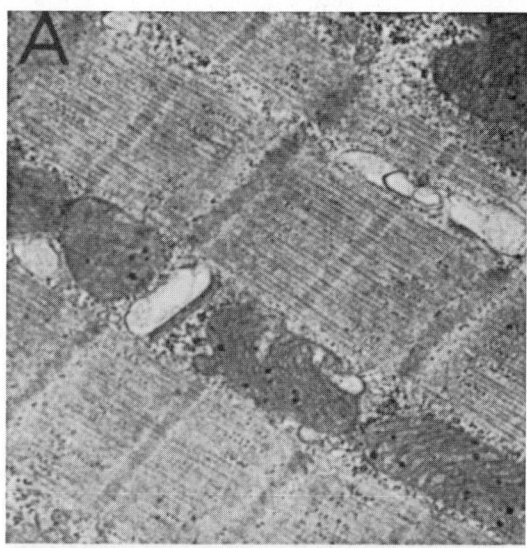

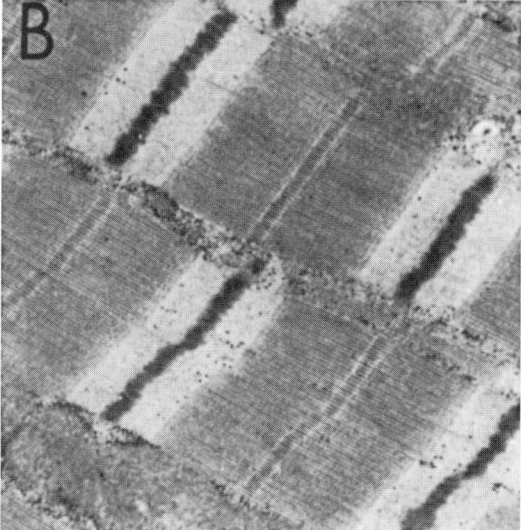

Figure 54–115. Typical electron micrographs of nonischemic *(A)* and ischemic *(B)* myocardium after 15 minutes of coronary occlusion. Ischemic tissue displays myofilament relaxation with increased Z-band separation and widening of bands. (From Glower, D. D., Schaper, J., Kabas, J. S., et al.: Relation between reversal of diastolic creep and recovery of systolic function after ischemic myocardial injury in conscious dogs. Circ. Res., *60*:850, 1987.)

human heart has few natural collateral vessels of sufficient diameter for delivering a significant quantity of blood in the event of a major coronary occlusion. It is for this reason that sudden occlusion of an otherwise normal coronary artery is such a hazardous event. A number of collateral vessels the size of 200 μm or less are present in most hearts, but these channels require enlargement over a period of time, usually stimulated by the development of favorable pressure differentials to become functionally significant.

A slowly occluding obstructing device (ameroid constrictor) can be placed on a major coronary artery in animals and used for total occlusion of the vessel occurring over a period of weeks. Under these circumstances, the pressure and flow through the involved coronary artery are slowly reduced, during which time the natural collateral vessels concomitantly enlarge. As a result, the distal pressure after slow occlusion may progressively rise to essentially that of the preocclusion value. In the human, however, the coronary collateral circulation is usually less reliable and effective.

Stenotic lesions of 90% or greater are required for production of significant collateral vessels in man. Under these circumstances, the mean back-pressure at the time of operation for totally occluded arteries varies from 30 to 40 mm. Hg; and for those arteries with less than a 90% stenosis, the average is only 18 to 20 mm. Hg. These findings indicate only marginal function, at best, of human collateral vessels. Angiographically defined coronary collaterals can appear and regress rapidly according to myocardial nutritional needs and pressure gradients, as may occur with the insertion of a bypass graft or its subsequent occlusion.

Some patients experience myocardial infarction with minimal or even absent coronary narrowing. Coronary arterial spasm may be responsible for this phenomenon (Prinzmetal's variant or atypical angina). Spasm can cause myocardial infarction in the absence of atherosclerotic lesions or can be superimposed on standard atherosclerotic stenoses, contributing to unstable pain patterns. Experience with the clinical spectrum of coronary spasms has indicated that patients with insignificant atherosclerosis are best managed by medical therapy (usually calcium channel blocking agents) and those with coronary lesions by angioplasty or coronary artery bypass.

Myocardial ischemia is most often made manifest by retrosternal chest pain, or angina pectoris, produced by a reduction in coronary blood flow. The discomfort is generally substernal and is often described by the patient as a pressure, choking sensation, or tightness. Early in the symptomatic course, a number of factors, such as exercise, cold exposure, eating, and emotional stress, can initiate the symptoms. The pain frequently radiates down the left arm and into the left neck and occasionally to the right arm or mandible. The severity of chest pain can be graded by the New York Heart Association (NYHA) classification, with Class I indicating no symptoms; Class II, symptoms with severe exertion; Class III, chest pain with mild exertion; and Class IV, angina occurring at rest. Whereas minimal anginal symptoms are often easily tolerated and compatible with a fairly normal lifestyle (stable angina), the occurrence of an increasing NYHA class over a short period of time (progressive angina) worsens the clinical prognosis. In the late stages, ischemia occurs at rest and is refractory to medical therapy (unstable angina). Unstable pain patterns signify a poor outlook, with an excessive early infarction and death rate. Significantly, a large proportion of patients do not follow the classic symptomatic progression and present initially with acute myocardial infarction or sudden death. Still others experience no symptoms during ischemia (silent myocardial ischemia), and coronary artery disease is discovered only in the late stage of congestive heart failure after severe ventricular damage has occurred.

The physical examination is frequently unremarkable, but a fourth heart sound can occasionally be heard on auscultation, reflecting an increase in the amplitude of the atrial systolic filling sound of the left ventricle. Although cardiac enlargement may be evident in patients with more advanced disease, the chest radiograph is normal in the majority of patients. Left ventricular aneurysms can sometimes be detected radiographically as an isolated prominence of the left border of the heart. Although the electrocardiogram is within normal limits in at least half the patients, abnormal findings can be useful in establishing the diagnosis. Myocardial ischemia may be manifested by the presence of inverted T waves on the resting electrocardiogram or, alternatively, by transient ST-segment and T-wave changes during the course of an anginal episode. ST-segment elevation or depression is an especially reliable sign and, if not present at rest, may be elicited by an exercise stress test. Exercise testing using electrocardiography, echocardiography, and nuclear cardiography is useful in assessing the functional significance in a patient with CAD. Although stress testing may be used as a screening technique for the presence of CAD, false-negative and false-positive responses occur. Importantly, exercise testing provides useful information regarding prognosis. Patients with early positive studies are likely to have severe CAD and are more likely to suffer acute myocardial infarction and cardiac death. Particularly, the left ventricular ejection fraction measured during exercise is a powerful predictor of survival.[31]

Coronary arteriography is essential in defining the presence and extent of coronary atherosclerotic lesions. A trend has favored early coronary arteriography in most patients with suspected CAD to define, as precisely as possible, individual prognostic characteristics. This approach has allowed a more objective application of medical therapy to low-risk subsets and selection of patients at high medical risk for elective surgical intervention. At angiography, the major anatomic predictors of coronary death, such as the number of coronary vessels diseased and the resting left ventricular ejection fraction, are documented. Although the extent of disease can be underestimated in up to 10% of patients, coronary arteriography has the highest sensitivity and specificity of any test available. Coronary angiography is clearly more precise, and even perhaps more cost-effective, than are other approaches. In patients with borderline anatomic indications for coronary bypass, physiologic assessment with radionuclide exercise ventriculography or stress thallium scanning can be useful in operative selection.

MEDICAL MANAGEMENT

If hypertension is present, it should be controlled; and smoking should be avoided because the vasoconstrictive effects of nicotine and its influence on the coronary circulation are well established. It has also been demonstrated that cessation of smoking in patients with myocardial infarction tends to prevent reinfarction. Hyperlipidemias have a major role in the pathogenesis of coronary atherosclerosis, and clinical efforts should be directed toward aggressive management of lipid abnormalities by use of either dietary or pharmacologic means. After bypass grafting, risk factor modification and continued medical management are especially important, because atherosclerotic involvement of saphenous vein grafts is a major long-term risk.

When the choice is being made between medical and surgical therapy, the natural history of angina pectoris should be recalled. One study of the natural history of coronary atherosclerosis was obtained at a time when coronary arteriography was well established in the diagnosis of this disorder but when surgical therapy was rarely employed.[40] In a series of patients with proven coronary arterial lesions observed for 10 years, it was shown that the annual mortality was lowest in those with single-vessel disease, next lowest in those with double-vessel disease, and highest in patients with triple-vessel and left main coronary artery disease. The degree of impairment in left ventricular function was also important. In current practice, adverse prognostic characteristics that might suggest abandoning medical treatment and referral for coronary revascularization include severe or progressive angina on medical therapy, significant left main coronary disease, multivessel coronary obstruction (especially with proximal LAD involvement), ventricular impairment with a reduced ejection fraction, and evidence of exercise-induced ischemia. Although this topic is controversial and the decision in each patient has to be individualized, each of these factors, individually or in combination, significantly reduces survival with medical therapy and predicts improved longevity after coronary bypass grafting, as subsequently discussed.

In patients with low-risk coronary anatomy, it is generally agreed that medical management is the treatment of choice, if anginal symptoms and exercise capacity can be maintained satisfactorily.

Beta-adrenergic blocking agents, such as propranolol, atenolol, and timolol, are highly effective and safe in the chronic management of angina pectoris. These drugs act by lowering myocardial oxygen requirement through a reduction in heart rate with secondary effects on arterial blood pressure and myocardial contractility. Calcium channel blocking agents such as nifedipine, diltiazem, and verapamil are well established in clinical practice and are effective in anginal management. There is evidence, however, that the symptomatic efficacy of these drugs may not be directly associated with an improvement in ultimate patient prognosis. Angiotension converting enzyme inhibitors have been shown to improve survival in patients with impaired ventricular function and those after myocardial infarction. Antiplatelet agents, such as aspirin, have a definite therapeutic role and have been shown to decrease coronary events significantly. Likewise, short-term heparinization has been effective in preventing coronary thrombosis and infarction in patients with unstable angina.

SURGICAL MANAGEMENT

To establish the appropriate management of patients with CAD, one should carefully assess the relative risk of an adverse myocardial event, including acute myocardial infarction, death, and the severity of symptoms. The natural history of patients with CAD indicates that survival is decreased with the increasing amount of myocardium at risk for ischemia. Arterial obstruction occurring proximally, as compared with distally, involving the LAD as compared with the right coronary artery, and involving the left main artery or three-vessel disease as compared with two-vessel or single-vessel disease is associated with impaired survival. Further risk is associated with an increase in the severity of symptoms, impaired left ventricular function, and ischemia inducible by low levels of exercise.

The influence of treatment modality on survival has been demonstrated in certain groups of patients with CAD. An advantage in survival in patients treated with coronary artery bypass grafting (CABG) has been demonstrated in a number of randomized clinical trials in the following patient groups: patients with more than 75% stenosis of the left main artery; patients with three-vessel or two-vessel disease with proximal LAD involvement, and in association with one of the following: moderate to severe anginal symptoms (NYHA

Class III-IV), impaired left ventricular ejection fraction (LVEF <50%), or easily inducible ischemia with exercise. Therefore, CABG is recommended as therapy in these patients, although some may be amenable to treatment with percutaneous transluminal coronary angioplasty (PTCA). In randomized trials comparing revascularization with PTCA or CABG, there was no survival advantage at 3 years of follow-up, but there were fewer repeat interventions in those treated with CABG.[20, 23, 30] In the Bypass Angioplasty Revascularization Investigation (BARI) trial, there were no differences in survival or myocardial infarction between nondiabetic patients treated with CABG or PTCA. In diabetic patients, there was a significant survival advantage and fewer myocardial infarctions in those treated with CABG. In a study comparing long-term survival benefits based on different treatment of CAD, those patients with greater severity of disease benefited more from CABG (Fig. 54–116).[29] Patients with three-vessel and two-vessel disease with greater than or equal to 95% proximal LAD stenosis benefited from bypass surgery campared with angioplasty. All patients with single-vessel disease, except those with greater than or equal to 95% proximal LAD stenosis benefited from angioplasty as compared with bypass surgery. Patients with two-vessel disease without severe proximal LAD involvement or those with isolated severe proximal LAD disease were treated equally well with CABG or PTCA. CABG is indicated in patients with diabetes mellitus and those with anginal symptoms refractory to medical management, particularly when the anatomy is not appropriate for PTCA, and also in those patients with three-vessel disease and those with two-vessel disease with severe proximal LAD involvement.

Patients who are assessed to have low-risk coronary events are managed medically. The pharmacologic agents that have been effective in either reducing the frequency of anginal episodes or preventing acute myocardial infarction or cardiac death include nitrates, beta-blockers, calcium channel blockers, and aspirin. In addition, modification of known risk factors associated with CAD should be initiated, including cessation of tobacco use, control of hypertension, reduction of serum lipids, and, when appropriate, weight reduction. Successful diminution of these risk factors has been shown to decrease the incidence of acute myocardial infarction, lead to regression of atherosclerosis, and, in patients having undergone CABG, improve graft patency.

Those patients who initially have unstable angina should be managed medically. Because of the strong association of complicated plaques with the development of unstable angina, heparin and aspirin are effective agents. Early coronary arteriography is indicated in patients who continue to have angina. Approximately 80% of patients have multivessel or left main occlusive disease. The incidence of adverse myocardial events is increased over the initial months after presentation, particularly in patients with multivessel disease, rest pain, complex lesion morphology, intracoronary thrombi, or ischemia demonstrated during Holter monitoring or those who are elderly. If angina persists, an intra-aortic balloon pump (IABP) is efficacious. Revascularization using PTCA or CABG is frequently indicated, although the risk of a periprocedural myocardial infarction or mortality is approximately twice that of elective procedures.

Clinical evidence has reinforced the importance of obtaining myocardial reperfusion as early as possible. Thrombolytics have been shown to decrease mortality, decrease infarct size, and preserve ventricular function. The benefit is greatest when given early after onset of pain. Less benefit is achieved when given more than 6 hours after the onset of pain. The adjuvant use of heparin and aspirin has limited reocclusion and reinfarction rates. Patients not achieving reperfusion with thrombolytic therapy who have a contraindication to thrombolytic therapy, or who have recurrent ischemia benefit from reperfusion using PTCA. Less than 25% of patients with acute myocardial infarction receive thrombolytic therapy due to delays in presentation after the onset of pain and delays in diagnosis. Those at a high risk for subsequent cardiac events should undergo cardiac catheterization, and those with multivessel disease with proximal LAD involvement have survival benefit with revascularization.

Complications of acute myocardial infarction occur due to tearing of myocardial tissue, and these include rupture of the ventricular free wall, ventricular septal defect, and rupture of a papillary muscle with severe mitral regurgitation. Echocardiography can establish the diagnosis. They occur less frequently in patients treated with thrombolytic agents and more frequently in those taking corticosteroids or nonsteroidal anti-inflammatory drugs and the elderly. The mortality in patients treated medically with these complications exceeds 90%.

Rupture of the ventricular free wall causes hemopericardium and resulting tamponade. This accounts for 10% of hospital deaths due to acute myocardial infarction. Pericardiocentesis can confirm the diagnosis and provide temporary hemodynamic relief. Urgent surgical therapy with ventricular reconstruction can lead to survival.

Postinfarction ventricular septal defect is manifest by the new onset of a harsh holosystolic murmur, often associated with a thrill. Hemodynamic compromise with ventricular failure occurs early. In addition to color-flow echocardiography, right-sided heart catheterization demonstrating an oxygen saturation step-up at the level of the right ventricle can establish the diagnosis. Except in moribund patients, correction by patch closure of the ventricular septal defect and bypass grafting should be undertaken. Rarely, the patient's condition may be stable, and the operation can be delayed, allowing the infarct tissue to heal. Better results are obtained in these patients, with survival approaching 90%. In the majority of patients, urgent operation is required. Use of an IABP provides hemodynamic support. Emergency coronary bypass and patch closure of the septal defect are then performed to prevent the consequences of intractable acute right ventricular overload and/or multiorgan failure.

The defects are often irregular, ragged tracts through the anterior apical septum with occlusion of the LAD artery or through the posterior septum in cases with right coronary occlusion. In the latter, right ventricular infarction may compound the problem. Multiple defects are present in approximately one third of patients. Cardiopulmonary bypass is

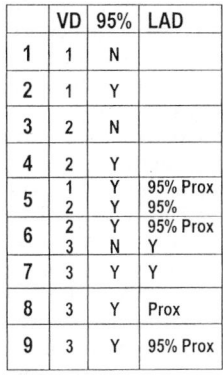
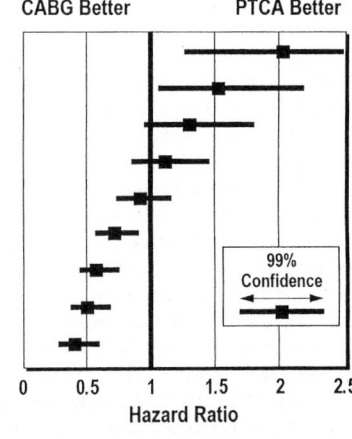

	VD	95%	LAD
1	1	N	
2	1	Y	
3	2	N	
4	2	Y	
5	1 / 2	Y / Y	95% Prox / 95%
6	2 / 3	Y / N	95% Prox / Y
7	3	Y	Y
8	3	Y	Prox
9	3	Y	95% Prox

Figure 54–116. CABG vs. PTCA hazard ratios. Comparison of the benefit of the two interventional treatments shows effectiveness of angioplasty in the first two groups. Groups 3 and 4 are not statistically different but tend toward benefit from angioplasty. Group 5 patients have equivalent outcomes. Patients in groups 6 to 9 benefit from bypass compared with angioplasty.

institued with bicaval cannulation, although a single right atrial cannula can be used for simple anterior defects. After cardioplegic arrest, an incision is made in the area of infarction and good exposure of the interiors of both the left and right ventricles is obtained. A portion of the necrotic edge of the defect is resected, and a double-patch technique is used for repair. For posterior defects, an identical procedure is performed with the apex elevated and the incision in the posterior interventricular groove. Coronary bypass grafts are constructed to all diseased vessels, including the right coronary artery in cases of right ventricular infarction. Fifty to 80% of patients should survive the operative procedure, depending on the severity of preoperative shock and multiorgan failure.

Rupture of the papillary muscle leads to severe mitral regurgitation and rapid development of pulmonary edema and hypotension. A holosystolic murmur is usually present. Echocardiography is diagnostic. Unlike postinfarction ventricular septal defect, papillary muscle rupture is often associated with a limited infarction size. Frequently, limited circumflex or right coronary artery disease is present. IABP use provides hemodynamic support. Early operative therapy with mitral valve repair when possible or mitral valve replacement in conjunction with bypass grafting is indicated. Survival is reported as 50% to 70%.

Preoperative Preparation

It is essential that the goals and anticipated results of CABG are explained in detail to both the patient and family before the procedure. Potential risks and complications should be reviewed in a manner designed to be factual and yet to minimize fear and anxiety. All aspects of the physical examination, cardiac catheterization, and other special procedures should be reviewed, with emphasis on a full knowledge of cardiac anatomy and dynamics. Any neurologic deficits, including the presence of carotid bruits, should be fully evaluated; and respiratory status, renal function, and blood coagulation should be assessed. Aspirin should be discontinued, if possible, for 1 to 2 weeks before operation. In many patients, especially those with unstable angina, this may not be practical; and the increased risk of postoperative bleeding associated with aspirin must be accepted.[13] Antianginal agents, including beta-blocking compounds, calcium channel blocking drugs, isosorbide dinitrate, and nitroglycerin ointment, should be continued until the procedure. If further pharmacologic therapy is required for recurring angina, an intravenous nitroglycerin infusion can be employed. The IABP can be particularly effective for preoperative stabilization of patients with unstable angina in the coronary care unit. Prophylactic broad-spectrum antibiotics are administered intravenously immediately before anesthetic induction and for 24 hours postoperatively.

Procedures

The majority of patients who are candidates for surgical management are treated with simple bypass of the obstructed coronary vessels by use of either the internal mammary artery or reversed segments of the saphenous vein. After a median sternotomy has been performed, the left internal mammary artery is dissected from the chest wall in the majority of patients. The procedure is conducted with extracorporeal circulation and cold potassium cardioplegia. Aortic arch cannulation is almost uniformly employed. For most coronary bypass procedures, single venous cannulation is used through the right atrial appendage and direct cardiac venting is avoided. Cardiopulmonary bypass is initiated with mild hypothermia (28° C. to 34° C.), distal coronary grafting

sites are visualized, and internal mammary artery flow is measured. A cardioplegia cannula is inserted into the proximal ascending aorta, and a retrograde cannula may be inserted into the coronary sinus through the right atrium if retrograde cardioplegia is to be used. A myocardial temperature needle may be placed in the interventricular septum to ensure adequate myocardial hypothermia. In addition, iced saline slush is applied topically; and a rapid reduction in myocardial temperature, well below 15° C., is usually achieved. If myocardial hypothermia is inadequate, additional volumes of cardioplegia solution are infused for attaining the desired temperature. A side arm on the cardioplegia cannula is used for venting the aorta and left ventricle during aortic occlusion. The coronary bypass procedure is then performed, and additional 200- to 500-ml. volumes of cardioplegia solution are infused every 20 to 30 minutes for maintenance of myocardial temperature below 15° C. Five to 10 minutes before aortic unclamping, full rewarming is begun and a 200-mg. dose of lidocaine is administered into the oxygenator for diminishing reperfusion arrhythmias. After aortic unclamping, additional procedures such as proximal aorta-vein graft anastomoses may be completed; and cardiopulmonary bypass is discontinued after adequate rewarming.

All coronary arteries 1.5 mm. or greater in diameter with more than 60% luminal narrowing are generally selected for bypass of all significant vessels in over 90% of cases. If a major vessel, such as the LAD, is completely occluded or diffusely diseased, an attempt at distal revascularization is still performed by use of single or sequential mammary artery grafting, intraoperative balloon dilation, or other techniques. Coronary endarterectomy is used when necessary, although there is an appreciable incidence of distal intimal flaps and perioperative infarction. Three to four grafts are usually inserted per patient, which reflects a philosophy of complete revascularization together with the tendency to reserve surgical therapy for symptomatic patients with multivessel disease. In general, the internal mammary artery and adjunctive saphenous vein grafts are used for additional vessels. Although the indications for multiple internal mammary artery procedures are not fully defined, conservative criteria include patients with limited or diseased saphenous veins, younger patients with extended life expectancy,[32] reoperative cases with previous early vein graft failure, and extensive atherosclerotic calcification of the ascending aorta precluding proximal vein graft anastomoses.

A standard method for distal saphenous vein–coronary artery anastomosis is illustrated in Figure 54–117. As a routine, the veins are dissected from the lower legs by use of gentle technique and care is taken to prevent overdistention during preparation. For distal anastomosis, a running 7-0 polypropylene suture and 8 to 12 stitches are employed, depending on the size of the vein graft and coronary artery. With the "toe" of the vein suspended by the first assistant, the anastomosis is begun on the side opposite the surgeon, and a continuous suture line is constructed around the "heel" of the vein. After the middle suture on the surgeon's side is placed, the suture line is tightened, pulling the vein onto the arteriotomy. With slight traction on the graft, the toe of the arteriotomy is exposed. which facilitates placement of the final sutures. Whereas deeper bites are performed on the sides for anchoring the vein, the toe and heel sutures are placed superficially so that no narrowing occurs. The polypropylene suture is sometimes tied with an appropriately sized probe lying within the vessel for elimination of the possibility of anastomotic narrowing. Cardioplegia solution can be infused directly into the completed vein graft so that adequate myocardial hypothermia beyond severely obstructed coronary lesions is ensured.

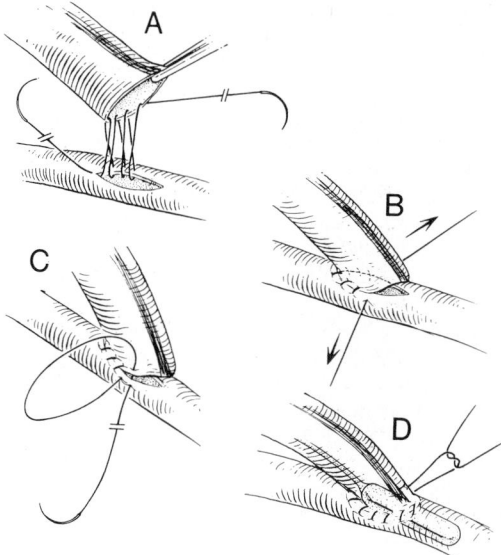

Figure 54–117. *A* to *D* from a standard method for distal vein graft anastomosis with use of a running suture technique. See text for details.

A method for performing the aortic anastomosis is illustrated in Figure 54–118; a 6-0 polypropylene suture is usually employed. The beveled vein is sutured to a 4.5-mm. circular aortotomy by circumference around the heel with the vein suspended. After tightening of the suture line, the toe sutures are completed. Care is taken to obtain optimal graft lengths, where the graft is under no tension and makes a gentle curve to the coronary vessel without kinking. Although the aortic anastomoses are often performed after release of the aortic cross clamp using partial occluding vascular clamps, performing these anastomoses during a single aortic clamping may be associated with fewer adverse neurologic events, particularly in elderly patients and those patients with aortic atherosclerosis.

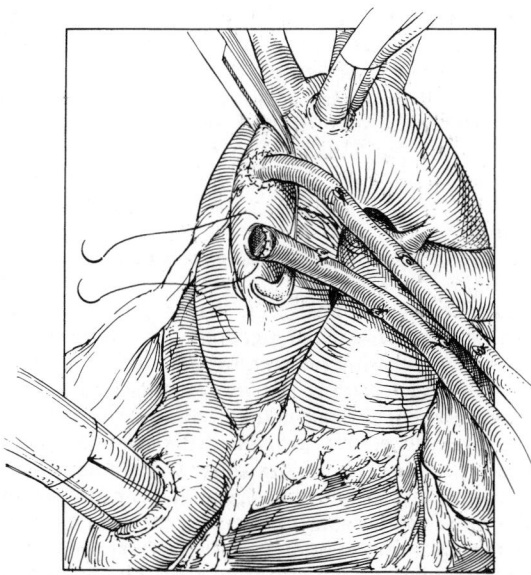

Figure 54–118. Method for performing proximal saphenous vein anastomoses to the aorta. A portion of the aorta is excluded by use of a partial occlusion clamp, and the vein grafts are anastomosed to circular aortotomies with running 6-0 polypropylene sutures. (Modified from Oschner, J. L., and Mills, N. L.: Coronary Artery Surgery. Philadelphia, Lea & Febiger, 1978.)

With increasing evidence of superior long-term mammary artery patency, at least one internal mammary graft is employed in most patients. In over 95% of cases, mammary arteries are suitable; and in contrast to previous experiences, mammary grafts are used for emergency procedures, in patients with poor ventricular function, and in the elderly. Because many venous grafts and a lesser number of internal mammary artery grafts become stenotic or occluded, severe isolated coronary lesions may be amenable to endarterectomy. Endarterectomy for isolated left main coronary artery stenosis has been reported to be the preferred procedure under these circumstances, because the long-term results have been quite favorable. For example, a patient with a severe left main lesion (95%) and unstable angina, who was operated on emergently in 1964 using this technique, is alive 32 years later without return of symptoms of myocardial ischemia. The coronary arteriogram and procedure performed are shown in Figures 54–119 to 54–121.

In all but the most hemodynamically unstable patients, the

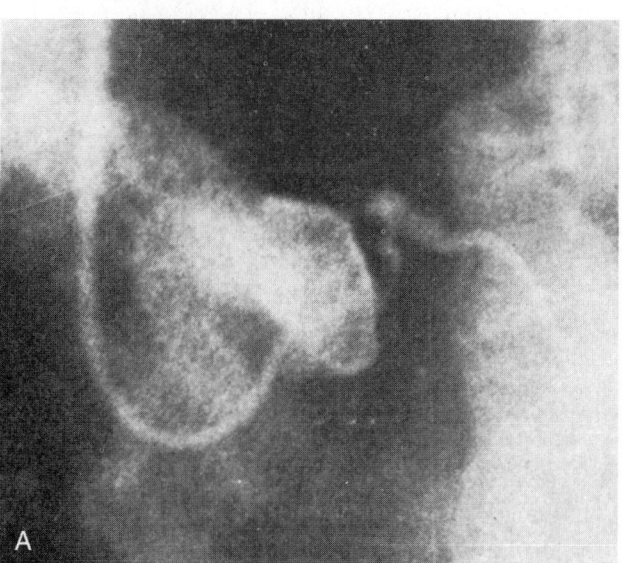

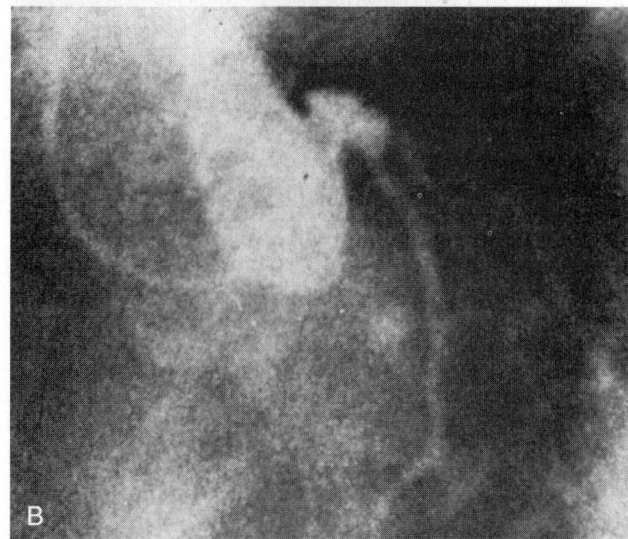

Figure 54–119. *A,* Preoperative coronary arteriogram shows severe stenosis of left coronary artery at aortic origin. *B,* Coronary arteriogram 5 months after operation shows patent left main coronary artery with good filling of anterior descending and circumflex branches. (*A* and *B* from Sabiston, D. C., Jr., Ebert, P. A., Friesinger, G. C., Ross, R. S., and Sinclair-Smith, B.: Proximal endarterectomy, arterial reconstruction for coronary occlusion at aortic origin. Arch. Surg., *91:*758–764, 1965. Copyright 1965, American Medical Association.)

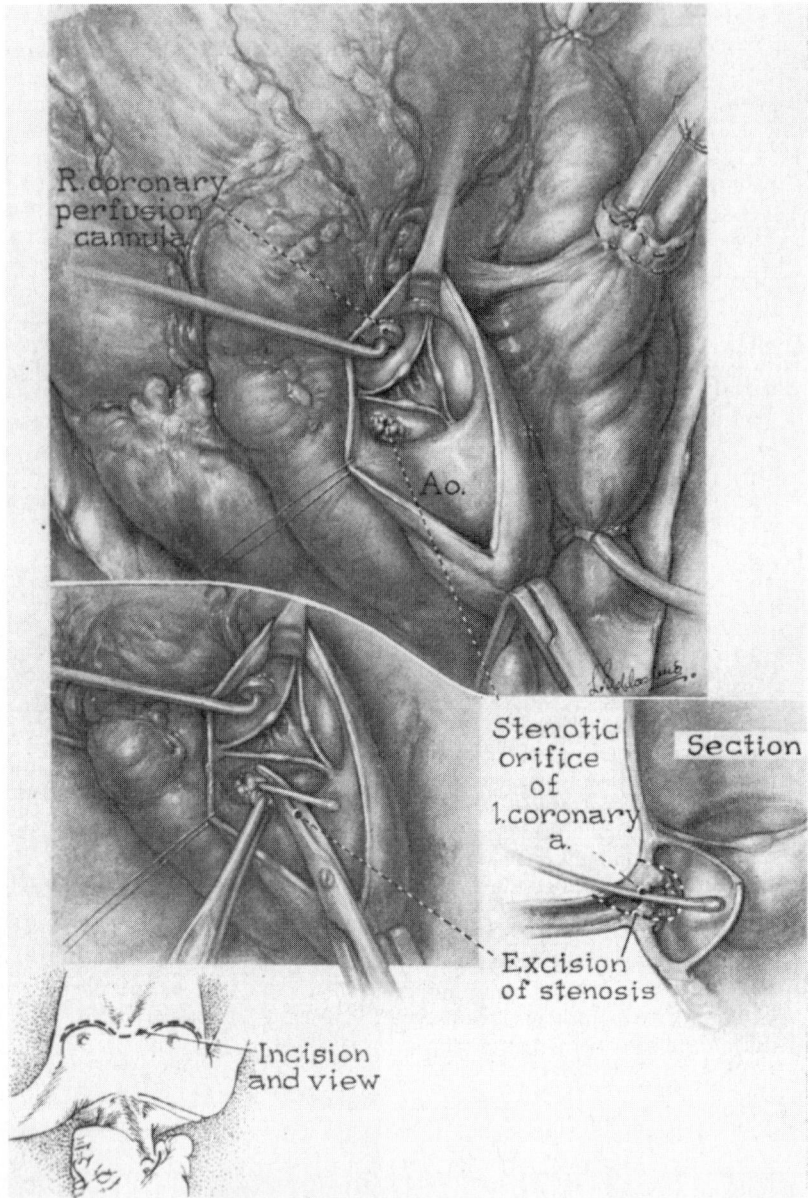

Figure 54–120. Illustration of marked stenosis of left coronary artery as seen from within aorta during open correction. Right coronary artery is being perfused continuously through cannula. Probe is inserted from left coronary artery into aortic lumen, and stenosis at the orifice of left coronary artery is excised. (From Sabiston, D. C., Jr., Ebert, P. A., Friesinger, G. C., Ross, R. S., and Sinclair-Smith, B.: Proximal endarterectomy, arterial reconstruction for coronary occlusion at aortic origin. Arch. Surg., *91*:758–764, 1965. Copyright 1965, American Medical Association.)

left internal mammary artery is gently dissected from the chest wall in a narrow pedicle by use of the low-current electrocautery. Arterial spasm is prevented by topical application of papaverine solution, and the distal coronary anastomosis is constructed with a technique similar to vein grafts. The pedicle is transected sharply at an appropriate length, and adequate flow capacity is documented on cardiopulmonary bypass before the heart is arrested. The pedicle rather than the graft is held with forceps by the first assistant, and the arterial wall is never grasped; a no-touch technique is used. After completion of the suture line with 7-0 or 8-0 polypropylene suture, the graft is opened, the suture is tied, and the pedicle is fixed to the epicardium for stabilization. If an important coronary artery beyond the reach of the in situ mammary artery needs to be grafted, extra length can be obtained by disconnecting the graft from its origin and suturing the proximal aspect to the aorta (free mammary grafting).

Postoperative Management

Monitoring

The postoperative care of patients after coronary bypass procedures is of primary importance and is assuming a greater role as increasingly ill patients are selected for surgical therapy. Whereas most patients have a smooth and uncomplicated course, 5% to 10% experience postoperative problems. A number of parameters are monitored for warning of developing complications. Standard measurements include radial arterial blood pressure, central venous pressure, urinary output, a continuous electrocardiographic tracing, and periodic determinations of arterial blood gases (PO_2, PCO_2, and pH). In most patients, cardiac function is assessed with measurements of cardiac output and pulmonary capillary wedge pressure, as provided by a thermodilution Swan-Ganz catheter. Appropriate hematologic and blood chemistry

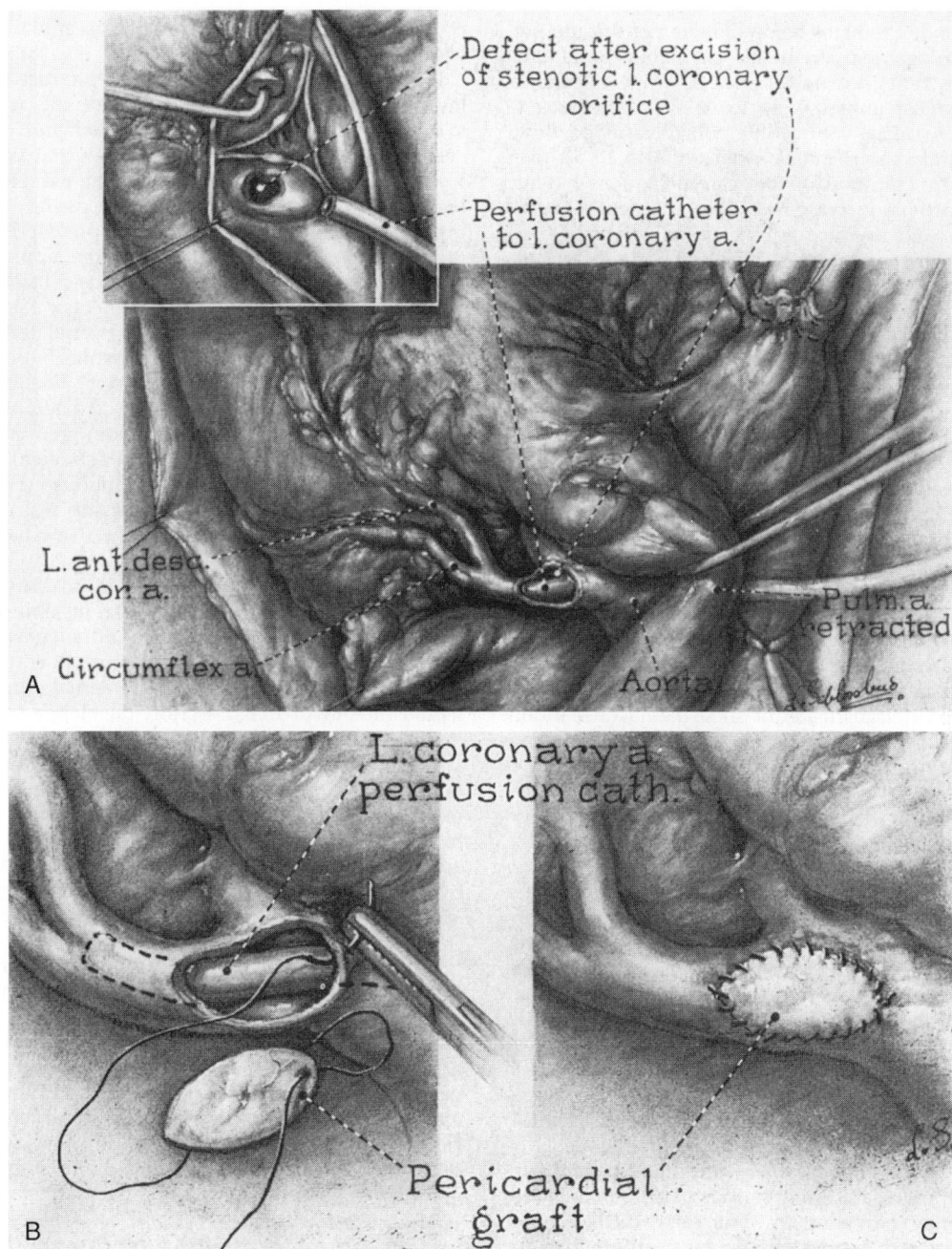

Figure 54–121. *A*, Opening made into anterior surface of left main coronary artery at site of stenosis. Catheter is introduced from aorta and passed into distal left main coronary artery for continuous arterial perfusion while reconstruction of left main coronary artery is accomplished. *B*, Placement of pericardial autograft at site of previous stenosis of left main coronary artery. Perfusion cannula is seen in place. *C*, Pericardial graft sutured in place with reconstruction of left main coronary artery and relief of stenosis. (*A* to *C* from Sabiston, D. C., Jr., Ebert, P. A., Friesinger, G. C., Ross, R. S., and Sinclair-Smith, B.: Proximal endarterectomy, arterial reconstruction for coronary occlusion at aortic origin. Arch. Surg., *91*:758–764, 1965. Copyright 1965, American Medical Association.)

studies, as well as chest radiographs, are obtained periodically. Body weight is recorded daily for monitoring potential fluid retention.

Postoperative Complications

With improving surgical techniques, and especially the introduction of cold potassium cardioplegia, postoperative low cardiac output is now uncommon in most centers. When it is encountered, however, all possible etiologic factors should be specifically considered, including hypovolemia, cardiac tamponade, concealed bleeding, dysrhythmias, myocardial insufficiency, and acidosis. If filling pressures are inadequate, appropriate volumes of crystalloid solutions, col-

loid-containing solution, or blood components are infused for raising pulmonary capillary wedge or left atrial pressure toward 15 mm. Hg. If low cardiac output persists despite adequate filling, optimization of afterload, or arterial blood pressure, should be considered by means of a continuous infusion of sodium nitroprusside. This agent acts directly on vascular smooth muscle for production of vasodilation independent of the autonomic nervous system. Infusion rates of up to 10 μg. per kg. per minute may be used transiently for treatment of hypertension, although potential complications such as methemoglobinemia should be borne in mind. Additionally, the mean arterial blood pressure should not be reduced below 65 to 75 mm. Hg for a prolonged period of time because of the possibility of multiorgan underperfusion.

If the cardiac index remains below 2 liters per minute per sq. m., pharmacologic support of the circulation is usually indicated. At this time, dopamine is the first-line catecholamine chosen in most units, owing to its simultaneous enhancement of myocardial contractility and renal blood flow. Continuous central venous infusion rates of 3 to 10 μg. per kg. per minute are employed. Other catecholamines having beta-adrenergic activity increase heart rate, augment myocardial contractility, and produce arterial vasodilation. In contrast, pure alpha-adrenergic drugs do not influence heart rate or myocardial contractility but primarily produce peripheral vasoconstriction. Most adrenergic agents have varying degrees of mixed alpha and beta action, and drug selection should be based on the desired physiologic effect. The relative merits to be considered in the selection of inotropic agents are discussed elsewhere. If circulatory insufficiency persists despite inotropic stimulation, placement of an IABP can be lifesaving.

Cardiac tamponade can produce postoperative low cardiac output, and the characteristic hemodynamic finding is elevated and equalized central venous and pulmonary wedge pressures, usually in the setting of excessive mediastinal bleeding. The chest radiograph may demonstrate mediastinal widening or blood collection, but if a significant question of tamponade exists, reoperation should be considered. Excessive *mediastinal bleeding* in the setting of stable hemodynamics is managed by correction of clotting defects with blood component therapy. Autotransfusion of shed mediastinal blood may be used.[10] Early reoperation is performed if bleeding remains excessive.

Atrial dysrhythmias are common after coronary revascularization. Premature atrial contractions, atrial fibrillation, or atrial flutter reflects postoperative atrial irritability and occurs in 10% to 30% of patients. If atrial tachycardia occurs, control of ventricular response is achieved with intravenous digoxin, followed by attempts at pharmacologic cardioversion with atenolol, procainamide, or calcium channel blocking agents or sotelol. Rapid atrial pacing or direct-current cardioversion can sometimes be effective in atrial flutter after initial drug therapy. Although transient atrial dysrhythmias are usually well tolerated, significant low cardiac output or systemic thromboembolism can occur.

Ventricular irritability manifested by frequent or multifocal premature ventricular contractions, ventricular tachycardia, or ventricular fibrillation is managed by intravenous lidocaine and/or procainamide together with direct-current cardioversion when necessary. Short periods of closed-chest cardiac massage may be necessary, but early cardioversion should be emphasized. Serious ventricular dysrhythmias are usually a manifestation of significant myocardial ischemia, and problems with the quality or revascularization should be considered. Beta-blocking agents and/or oral procainamide are used for long-term management of persistent ventricular ectopy.

After uncomplicated elective operations, most patients can be removed from ventilatory support and extubated within a few hours. After anesthetic recovery, criteria for early extubation include good pulmonary gas exchange, adequate ventilatory mechanics, a clear chest radiograph, absence of dysrhythmias and excess bleeding, and stable cardiac and neurologic function. Occasional patients exhibit prolonged *pulmonary dysfunction,* requiring controlled ventilation, positive end-expiratory pressure, diuresis, and transiently increased fractional inspired oxygen. If pulmonary infection is suggested by radiographic infiltrates, high white blood cell counts, or positive sputum cultures, appropriate antibiotic coverage is added. As the period of required ventilatory support through an endotracheal tube approaches 2 weeks, tracheostomy should be considered. Tracheostomy is especially useful for clearing pulmonary secretions and assisting ventilatory weaning.

Postoperative *renal dysfunction* can produce transient elevations in blood urea nitrogen and creatinine, with progression to oliguria or total renal shutdown. Ischemic renal injury can occur in the setting of low cardiac output or if excessively low perfusion pressures are encountered on cardiopulmonary bypass or perioperatively. Pre-existing renal artery stenosis or arteriolar nephrosclerosis predisposes certain patients to renal hypoperfusion. In the appropriate clinical setting, developing sepsis must also be considered as a cause of worsening renal performance. Therapy for renal dysfunction consists of maintaining higher arterial perfusion pressure (especially in patients with pre-existing hypertension), low-dose intravenous dopamine infusion, adequate free water hydration, and general support of cardiac output. Fluid balance and potassium intake are monitored carefully for the prevention of overhydration or hyperkalemia. If dialysis is required, peritoneal lavage or continuous venovenous hemodialysis is favored because patient survival associated with a policy of aggressive intermittent hemodialysis has been disappointing.

Sternal wound infection occurs in 1% to 2% of patients after coronary bypass. Developing sternal instability, fever, leukocytosis, and wound drainage should suggest the diagnosis. Severity varies from a superficial subcutaneous infection with a stable sternum to an isolated sternal infection with no mediastinal involvement to fully developed septic mediastinitis. At the first suspicion of a major wound infection, broad-spectrum antibiotics should be instituted and cultures obtained. The combination of diabetes and bilateral internal mammary artery harvesting may predispose some patients to sternal infection. Infections producing sternal disruption are treated with a brief course of open wound care followed by wound closure with pectoral or omental pedicle flaps.[25] Mortality using this approach has been reduced to less than 10%, although morbidity remains high.

With improvements in myocardial protection and coronary grafting techniques, perioperative myocardial infarction should occur in only 1% to 4% of patients. The etiology varies from subclinical closure of an ungrafted small secondary coronary artery to failure of a major coronary bypass leading to cardiogenic shock. Therefore, the cause should be carefully evaluated, and most cases produce little clinical morbidity or deterioration of global ventricular function. Conversely, the development of serious problems might suggest early angiography or reintervention if it is deemed clinically feasible.

SURGICAL RESULTS
Analytic Methods

Clinical investigation of treatment efficacy is important in all areas of surgical therapy but is especially critical to the subject of coronary bypass. Survival analysis has been widely applied for this purpose and is a form of inductive reasoning with its origins in the philosophical discipline of logic. Prognostic analysis is useful in determining operative risk for each individual patient, as well as the appropriateness of surgical therapy in various patient subsets. Two methods generally have been employed: prospective randomized clinical trials[6, 12, 38] and retrospective observational analysis.[3] Both have advantages and limitations for a given question and require proper interpretation within the limits of clinical practice.

Risk Factors Influencing Surgical Results

Numerous risk factors are associated with increased early mortality after coronary revascularization, including emergency operation, increasing age, redo operation, decreased ejection fraction, female sex, and left main coronary artery disease. Other risk factors that are present less commonly but have been shown to adversely affect early survival are listed in Table 54–7.

The overall operative mortality averages 2%, with a 92% 4-year survival. Better-risk patients undergoing an elective operation, who are younger than 65 years of age or with an ejection fraction greater than 0.40, experience an operative mortality of approximately 1% with a 4-year survival exceeding 95%. Only 0.9% have required reoperation to an average of 43 years of follow-up. When the serious baseline illness profile displayed by these patients is considered, the long-term results are surprisingly good and represent the standard with which other emerging therapies must be compared.

In current series, the number of vessels diseased and female gender are only of marginal significance, whereas diabetes is a risk factor for late cardiac death possibly due to accelerated vein graft atherosclerosis. Most analyses have suggested that performing one internal mammary artery graft independently reduces the probability of late cardiac death and reoperation.[6, 32] The use of a mammary artery to bypass a severe stenosis in the left anterior descending coronary artery appears to be a more important predictor of survival than the progression of native coronary atherosclerosis.[4a] However, consistent data demonstrating an additional survival advantage of multiple internal mammary artery grafting are not available at present.

Therapeutic Efficacy

The effects of bypass grafting on the clinical course of patients with coronary atherosclerosis can be assessed in several ways. Improvement in anginal symptoms is observed in the majority of patients in the first several postoperative years, and the rate of improvement is significantly better than that observed with medical therapy. In most series, long-term complete relief of angina is achieved in over two thirds of patients. In one experience, 92% of patients had significant improvement in angina and 62% were completely pain free at an average of 20 months postoperatively. In addition, the incidence of subsequent myocardial infarction is significantly reduced for many years in patients who undergo surgical therapy. However, 7 to 10 years postoperatively, the rate again increases, probably as a result of progression of the original disease or involvement of the vein grafts with atherosclerosis.

TABLE 54–7. Risk Factors for Early Mortality After Coronary Artery Bypass Grafting

Major Factors

Emergency operation
Increasing age
Redo operation
Decreased ejection fraction
Female sex
Left main coronary artery disease

Minor Factors

History of myocardial infarction
Life-threatening ventricular dysrhythmia
Congestive heart failure
Mitral regurgitation
Diabetes mellitus
Cerebrovascular disease
Peripheral vascular disease
Renal insufficiency
Chronic obstructive lung disease

Whereas conflicting data have been reported in the past, consensus now exists that a primary physiologic effect of coronary revascularization is maintenance or augmentation of left ventricular function.[13] Hemodynamic improvement can be demonstrated by comparison of preoperative and postoperative contrast medium–enhanced ventriculograms or noninvasive radionuclide angiocardiograms obtained at rest, in which an increased ejection fraction, higher cardiac output, decreased diastolic volume, and improved left ventricular wall motion can be demonstrated in a significant proportion of patients. Moreover, improvement in exercise ventricular function has been demonstrated as early as 1 week postoperatively.[1] Clinical stabilization of exercise tolerance noted by the majority of patients after coronary bypass further supports the concept of improved ventricular function after revascularization.

Anatomic quality of revascularization can be assessed by angiographic studies of graft patency. With improvements in operative technique, saphenous vein graft patency in the first postoperative year should approximate 92% and 85% of patients should have all grafts patent. A slow attrition rate then occurs over the next decade because of the development of graft atherosclerosis, so that 10-year vein graft patency averages approximately 50%. Up to half of the patent vein grafts at 10 years are involved with the atherosclerotic process; thus, functional patency is somewhat less than 50%. Persistent hyperlipidemias are a major risk factor for the development of vein graft atherosclerosis,[45] and aggressive lipid management is indicated postoperatively along with general risk factor modification. Evidence exists that pharmacologic therapy for hyperlipidemias can improve long-term graft patency and reduce the incidence of subsequent coronary events.[2] Aspirin is also administered indefinitely for its beneficial effects on graft patency.[19]

The long-term patency of internal mammary artery grafts is better.[22, 34] In modern series, the early patency of these grafts, including the more complex sequential grafts, is 95% to 99%.[42] Because late atherosclerotic involvement of these grafts is rare, 10-year patency averages 85% to 90%, which translates into better survival, less anginal recurrence, and fewer reoperations.[4, 6, 8] It is for this reason that routine utilization of at least one internal mammary artery graft has been standard surgical policy in most medical centers since the early 1980s.

Whereas patient symptoms are important, perhaps the most objective measure of surgical outcome is long-term survival. As described in the preceding section, several methods exist for evaluating the survival benefits of coronary bypass procedures, from randomized prospective trials to retrospective observational statistical analysis. These techniques have demonstrated consistent survival advantages in patients treated with bypass surgery who have severe coronary artery disease. Although the overall mortality rate for patients undergoing bypass surgery at most centers has been unchanged, this represents increasingly more high-risk patients having CABG. The risk-adjusted mortality for patients undergoing CABG continues to decrease.

The exact cause of the selective improvement in surgical survival cannot be precisely determined but may be due to a number of reasons. Refinements in surgical technique may be the most important factor, including improved myocardial preservation, more complete coronary revascularization, improved methods of graft construction producing enhanced graft patency, and better intraoperative support.

With the development of coronary balloon angioplasty and interventional cardiology, the focus of cardiologic practice appears to have shifted toward acute coronary care. However, it is important to bear in mind the excellent long-term results that are now possible with elective referral for coronary bypass grafting. Patients with high-risk coronary lesions should be considered for early referral for elective coronary bypass so that the best early and late therapeutic results can be achieved.

REFERENCES

1. Austin, E. H., Oldham, H. N., Jr., and Jones, R. H.: Early assessment of rest and exercise left ventricular function following coronary artery surgery. Ann. Thorac. Surg., 35:159, 1983.
2. Blankenhorn, D. H., Nessim, S. A., Johnson, R. L., Sanmarco, M. E., Azen, S. P., and Cashin-Hemphill, L.: Beneficial effects of combined colestipol-niacin therapy on coronary atherosclerosis and coronary venous bypass grafts. JAMA, 257:3233, 1987.
3. Califf, R. M., Harrell, F. E., Lee, K. L., et al.: The evolution of medical and surgical therapy for coronary artery disease: A 15-year perspective. JAMA, 261:2077, 1989.
4. Cameron, A., Davis, K. B., Green, G. E., et al.: Clinical implications of internal mammary artery bypass grafts: The Coronary Artery Surgery Study experience. Circulation, 77:815, 1988.
4a. Cameron, A., Davis, K. B., Green, G., and Schaff, H. V.: Coronary bypass surgery with internal thoracic artery grafts: Effects on survival over a 15-year period. N. Engl. J. Med., 334:216, 1996.
5. Carrel, A.: On the experimental surgery of the thoracic aorta and the heart. Ann. Surg., 52:83, 1910.
6. Coronary Artery Surgery Study (CASS) Principal Investigators: Coronary artery bypass surgery: Survival data. Circulation, 68:939, 1983.
7. Cosgrove, D. M., Amiot, D. M., and Meserko, J. J.: An improved technique for autotransfusion of shed mediastinal blood. Ann. Thorac. Surg., 40:519, 1985.
8. Cosgrove, D. M., Loop, F. D., Lytle, B. W., et al.: Predictors of reoperation after myocardial revascularization. J. Thorac. Cardiovasc. Surg., 92:811, 1986.
9. Dilsizian, V., Bonow, R. O., Cannon, R. O., Tracy, C. M., Vitale, D. F., McIntosh, C. L., Clark, R. E., Bacharach, S. L., and Green, M. V.: The effect of coronary artery bypass grafting on left ventricular systolic function at rest: Evidence for preoperative subclinical myocardial ischemia. Am. J. Cardiol., 61:1248, 1988.
10. Dinerman, J. L., and Mehta, J. L.: Endothelial, platelet and leukocyte interactions in ischemic heart disease: Insights into potential mechanisms and their clinical relevance. J. Am. Coll. Cardiol., 16:207, 1990.
11. Enos, W. F., Holmes, R. H., and Beyer, J.: Coronary disease among United States soldiers killed in action in Korea. Preliminary report. JAMA, 152:1090, 1953.
12. European Coronary Surgery Study Group: Prospective randomized study of coronary artery bypass surgery in stable angina pectoris. Lancet, 2:491, 1980.
13. Ferraris, V. A., Ferraris, S. P., Lough, F. C., and Berry, W. R.: Preoperative aspirin ingestion increases operative blood loss after coronary artery bypass grafting. Ann. Thorac. Surg., 45:71, 1988.
14. Foster, E. D., Fisher, L. D., Kaiser, G. C., and Myers, W. O.: Comparison of operative mortality and morbidity for initial and repeat coronary artery bypass grafting: The Coronary Artery Surgery Study (CASS) registry experience. Ann. Thorac. Surg., 38:563, 1984.
15. Franch, R. H., et al.: Techniques of cardiac catheterization including coronary arteriography. In Hurst, J. W. (Ed.): The Heart, 5th ed. New York, McGraw-Hill, 1982.
16. Garrett, H. E., Dennis, E. W., and DeBakey, M. E.: Aortocoronary bypass with saphenous vein graft. JAMA, 223:792, 1973.
17. Glower, D. D., Spratt, J. A., Snow, N. D., et al.: Linearity of the Frank-Starling relationship in the intact heart: The concept of preload recruitable stroke work. Circulation, 71:994, 1985.
18. Glower, D. D., Schaper, J., Kabas, J. S., et al.: Relation between reversal of diastolic function after ischemic myocardial injury in conscious dogs. Circ. Res., 60:859, 1987.
19. Goldman, S., Copeland, J., Moritz, T., Henderson, W., Zadina, K., Ovitt, T., Doherty, J., Reed, R., Chesler, E., Sako, Y., et al.: Saphenous vein graft patency 1 year after coronary artery bypass surgery and effects of antiplatelet therapy: Results of Veterans Administration Cooperative Study. Circulation, 80:1190, 1989.
20. Goy, J. J., et al.: Coronary angioplasty versus left internal mammary artery grafting for isolated proximal left anterior descending artery stenosis. Lancet, 343:1449, 1994.
21. Green, G. E., Stertzer, S. H., Gordon, R. B., and Tice, D. A.: Anastomosis of the internal mammary artery to the distal left anterior descending artery. Circulation, 41 (Suppl. II):79–85, 1970.
22. Grondon, C. M., Campeau, L., Lesperance, J., Enjalbert, M., and Bourassa, M. G.: Comparison of late changes in internal mammary artery and saphe-

nous vein grafts in two consecutive series of patients 10 years after operation. Circulation, 70(Suppl. I):I-208, 1984.
23. Ham, C. W., et al.: A randomized study of coronary angioplasty compared with bypass surgery in patients with symptomatic multivessel coronary disease: German Angioplasty Bypass Surgery Investigation (GABI). N. Engl. J. Med., 331:1037, 1994.
24. Hearse, D. J., Braimbridge, M. V., and Jynge, P.: Protection of the Ischemic Myocardium: Cardioplegia. New York, Raven Press, 1981.
25. Herrera, H. R., and Ginsberg, M. E.: The pectoralis major myocutaneous flap and omental transposition for closure of infected median sternotomy wounds. Plast. Reconstr. Surg., 70:465, 1982.
26. Herrick, J. B.: Clinical features of sudden obstruction of the coronary arteries. JAMA, 59:2015, 1912.
27. Higgins, M. W., and Luepker, R. V. (Eds.): Trends in Coronary Heart Disease Mortality: The Influence of Medical Care. New York, Oxford University Press, 1988.
28. Johnson, W. D., Flemma, R. J., Lepley, D., Jr., and Ellison, E. H.: Extended treatment of severe coronary artery disease: A total surgical approach. Ann. Surg., 170:460, 1969.
29. Jones, R. H., Kessler, K., Phillips, H. R., Mark, D. B., Smith, P. K., Nelson, C. L., Newman, M. F., Reves, J. G., Anderson, R. W., Califf, R. M. Long-term survival benefit of CABG and PTCA in patients with coronary artery disease. J. Thorac. Cardiovasc. Surg. (In Press).
30. King, S. B., III, et al.: A randomized trial comparing coronary angioplasty with coronary bypass surgery: Emory Angioplasty versus Surgery Trial (EAST). N. Engl. J. Med., 331:1044, 1994.
31. Lee, K. L., Pryor, D. B., Pieper, K. S., Harrell, F. E., Califf, R. M., Mark, D. B., Hlatky, M. A., Coleman, R. E., Cobb, F. R., and Jones, R. H.: Prognostic value of radionuclide angiography in medically treated patients with coronary artery disease. Circulation, 82:1705, 1990.
32. Loop, F. D., Lytle, B. W., Cosgrove, D. M., et al.: Influence of the internal mammary artery graft on 10-year survival and other cardiac events. N. Engl. J. Med., 314:1, 1986.
33. Lytle, B. W., Kramer, J. R., Golding, L. R., et al.: Young adults with coronary atherosclerosis: 10 year results of surgical myocardial revascularization. J. Am. Coll. Cardiol., 4:445, 1984.
34. Lytle, B. W., Loop, F. D., Cosgrove, D. M., Ratliff, N. B., Easley, K., and Taylor, P. C.: Long-term (5–12 years) serial studies of internal mammary artery and saphenous vein coronary bypass grafts. J. Thorac. Cardiovasc. Surg., 89:248, 1985.
35. Lytle, B. W., Loop, F. D., Cosgrove, D. M., et al.: Fifteen hundred coronary reoperations. J. Thorac. Cardiovasc. Surg., 93:847, 1987.
36. Maier, G. W., Owen, C. H., Feneley, M. P., et al.: The mechancal determinants of myocardial oxygen consumption in the conscious dog. Circulation, 73:II-67, 1988.
37. Muhlbaier, L. H., Pryor, D. B., Rankin, J. S., Smith, L. R., Mark, D. B., Jones, R. H., Glower, D. D., Harrell, F. E., Lee, K. L., Califf, R. M., and Sabiston, D. C.: Observation comparison of event-free survival with medical and surgical therapy in patients with coronary artery disease. Circulation, 86(Suppl. II):II-198, 1992.
38. Murphy, M., Hultgren, H., Detre, K., et al.: Treatment of chronic stable angina: A preliminary report of survival data of the Randomized Veterans Administration Cooperation Study. N. Engl. J. Med., 297:621, 1977.
39. Parisi, A. F., Folland, E. D., and Hartigan, P.: A comparison of angioplasty with medical therapy in the treatment of single-vessel coronary artery disease: Veterans Affairs ACME Investigators. N. Engl. J. Med., 326:10, 1992.
40. Proudfit, W. L., Bruschke, A. V. G., and Sones, F. M., Jr.: Natural history of obstructive coronary artery disease: Ten-year study of 601 non-surgical cases. Prog. Cardiovasc. Dis., 21:53, 1978.
41. Pryor, D. B., Harrell, F. E., Rankin, J. S., et al.: The changing survival benefits of coronary revascularization over time. Circulation, 76:V-13, 1987.
42. Rankin, J. S., Newman, G. E., Bashore, T. M., et al.: Clinical and angiographic assessment of complex mammary artery bypass grafting. J. Thorac. Cardiovasc. Surg., 92:832, 1986.
43. Ryan, T. J., Faxon, D. P., Gunnar, R. M., et al.: Guidelines for percutaneous transluminal angioplasty: A report of the American Cardiology/American Heart Association task force on assessment of diagnostic and therapeutic cardiovascular procedures. J. Am. Coll. Cardiol., 13:529, 1988.
44. Sabiston, D. C., Jr.: The coronary circulation: The Wlliam F. Reinhoff, Jr. Lecture. Johns Hopkins Med. J., 134:314, 1974.
45. Snellen, H. A.: A Disorder of the Breast. Rotterdam, Kooyker Scientific Publications, 1976.
46. Solymoss, B. C., Nadeau, P., Millette, D., and Campeau, L.: Late thrombosis of saphenous vein coronary bypass grafts related to risk factors. Circulation, 78:II-40, 1988.
47. Squire, J.: The Structural Basis of Muscular Contraction. New York, Plenum Press, 1981.
48. Weinstein, M. C., Coxson, P. G., Williams, L. W., et al.: Forecasting coronary heart disease incidence, mortality, and cost: The coronary heart disease policy model. Am. J. Public Health, 77:1417, 1987.

SURGICAL MANAGEMENT OF FAILED ANGIOPLASTY

Peter Van Trigt III, M.D.

Percutaneous transluminal coronary angioplasty (PTCA) has gained increasing popularity as a primary treatment for coronary atherosclerotic heart disease. Since 1977, when PTCA was an investigational technique in humans,[17] the number of procedures performed has dramatically increased. It is estimated that more than 400,000 PTCA procedures are performed annually in the United States.[35, 38]

The development of PTCA as a therapeutic modality has been associated with a concomitant rise in the need for emergency surgical myocardial revascularization for acute coronary angioplasty failure. Emergency coronary artery bypass grafting (CABG) in the setting of acute myocardial ischemia secondary to vessel dissection, thrombosis, or spasm (recoil) causes significant morbidity and definite mortality. It is reasonable to assume that mortality and morbidity from failed angioplasty will increase as the procedure is extended to patients with multivessel disease, more complex lesions, and decreased left ventricular function.[29] Reports indicate a definite trend toward management of increasingly complex lesions by angioplasty, including diseased stenotic vein grafts.[26] This progression appears inevitable, even though a decline in the need for emergency CABG has been documented as experience with angioplasty is acquired. The current incidence of failed PTCA requiring emergency CABG is reported at 4% to 5% by most centers performing high-volume angioplasty.[9, 11, 30]

This discussion reviews the role of CABG after failed PTCA and examines determinants of risk in this patient population. Strategies to minimize ischemic injury to the myocardium after failed coronary angioplasty are also outlined.

PREDICTORS OF ACUTE CLOSURE AFTER CORONARY ANGIOPLASTY

PTCA uses intracoronary balloon inflation to approximately 4 atm. of pressure to produce localized trauma to the coronary artery wall; the intended result is atheroma fracture and arterial expansion that produces an increase in luminal area. Unfortunately, balloon inflation or guide wire and catheter manipulation can cause more extensive arterial wall damage with medial dissection and creation of an occlusive intimal flap. Thrombosis and spasm may also occur at the dilation site. In the absence of a well-developed collateral circulation, acute coronary occlusion causes severe myocardial ischemia and evolving myocardial infarction.

In a review of approximately 5000 PTCA procedures between 1982 and 1986,[12] a multivariate analysis found seven independent predictors of increased risk of vessel closure during PTCA: (1) stenosis length of two or more luminal diameters, (2) female gender, (3) stenosis at a bend point of the vessel, (4) stenosis at a branch point, (5) thrombus at the site of stenosis, (6) other stenoses in the same vessel, and (7) multivessel disease. Although an estimation of risk for vessel closure can be made before PTCA, the most powerful predictors can be assessed only during the procedure (intimal tear after PTCA, persistent stenosis or gradient after PTCA, and requirement for prolonged heparin infusion after angioplasty).

If coronary occlusion occurs, recrossing the occluded segment and repeating prolonged balloon inflation or using

TABLE 54–8. Techniques to Minimize Ischemic Injury After Failed PTCA

Within Catheterization Laboratory

Coronary vasodilators
Intracoronary thrombolytic therapy
Repeat balloon inflations
Prolonged balloon inflation with perfusion balloon catheter
Reperfusion catheter placed across lesion
Insertion of intra-aortic balloon pump
Placement of coronary intraluminal stent
Rescue atherectomy of intimal flap
Placement on percutaneous cardiopulmonary bypass

Within Operating Room

Expeditious placement on cardiopulmonary bypass
Systemic hypothermia
Hyperkalemic hypothermic cardioplegic arrest (warm blood reperfusion)
Internal mammary artery or saphenous vein bypass grafts
Rapid revascularization

intracoronary thrombolytic or vasodilator agents can occasionally re-establish coronary artery patency and relieve ischemia (Table 54–8). However, prolonged maneuvers to this end are absolutely contraindicated because they inevitably delay emergency surgical revascularization. Rapid surgical revascularization after failed PTCA is the *only option* to reduce the associated mortality and morbidity.

USE OF THE REPERFUSION CATHETER AND INTRA-AORTIC BALLOON PUMP

The intracoronary reperfusion catheter has been introduced as a means of sustaining coronary flow past an occlusion after failed angioplasty.[13, 18] The device, a 4.3-French catheter with 30 side holes over its distal 10 cm., can maintain vessel flow in patients awaiting emergency coronary bypass surgery after failed coronary angioplasty. This causes reversal of active myocardial ischemia and can significantly contribute to clinical stabilization of the patient, allowing transport of the patient to the operating room under more controlled conditions. The utility of the reperfusion catheter to maintain coronary flow through a vessel closed during PTCA is illustrated in Figures 54–122 to 54–124. A preangioplasty arte-

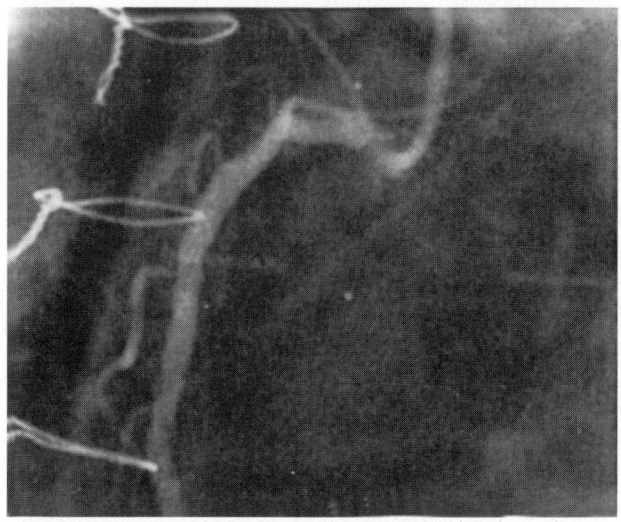

Figure 54–122. Angiogram made before angioplasty demonstrating 95% ostial lesion of the right coronary artery.

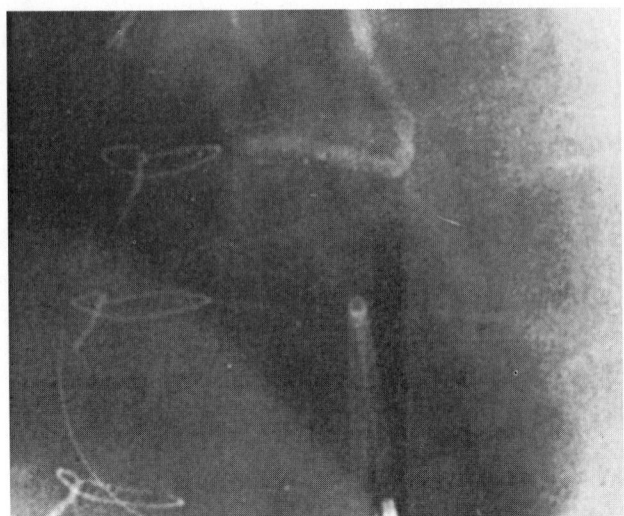

Figure 54–123. Angiogram made after angioplasty. The right coronary artery was dissected, which caused total distal occlusion.

riogram demonstrating a 95% right ostial lesion is shown in Figure 54–122. The angioplasty caused dissection of the right coronary artery (see Fig. 54–123). After placement of the reperfusion catheter across the lesion, blood flow is restored to the ischemic myocardium (see Fig. 54–124). Electrocardiographic changes following successful placement of a reperfusion catheter after PTCA and closure of a left anterior descending lesion are shown in Figure 54–125. Re-establishment of coronary flow through the reperfusion catheter and reduction of the duration of acute occlusion have a direct influence on reducing the extent of myocardial infarction that occurs in 30% to 40% of angioplasty failures despite successful later surgical revascularization.[31, 32] Reversal of acute ischemia also allows time to harvest the internal mammary artery for use in surgical revascularization.[13, 14, 21] An additional advantage of the reperfusion catheter is that cardioplegia can be delivered through the device after aortic cross-clamping directly to ischemic myocardium. The reperfusion catheter is then withdrawn through the aortic cross clamp, into the descending thoracic aorta, and then out the femoral artery sheath.

Routine use of the intra-aortic balloon pump (IABP) after

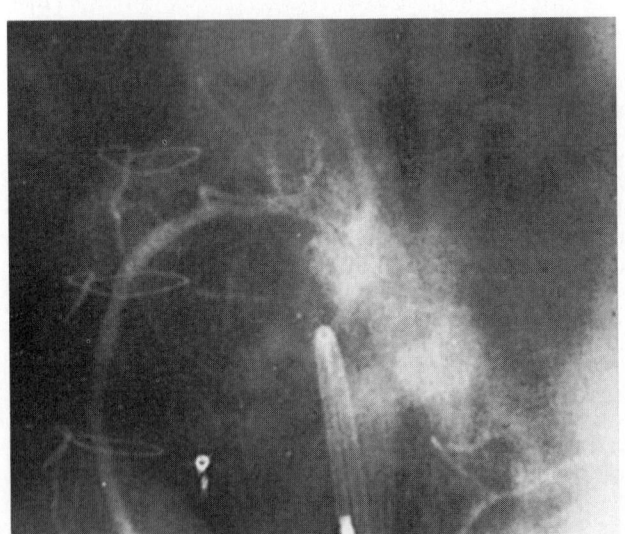

Figure 54–124. Angiogram performed after placement of the reperfusion catheter across the lesion. Blood flow was restored to the ischemic myocardium.

Pre PTCA

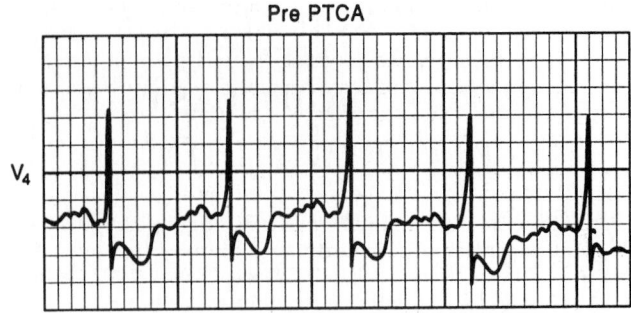

During Occlusion

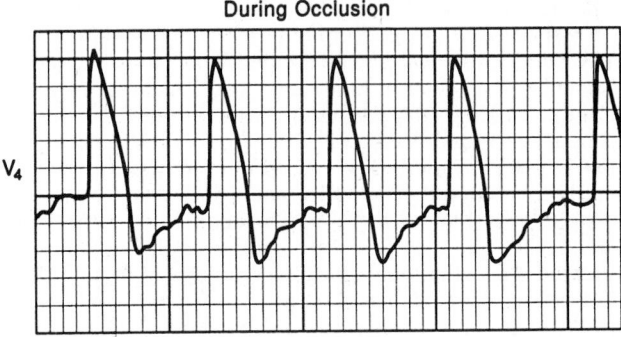

With RPC

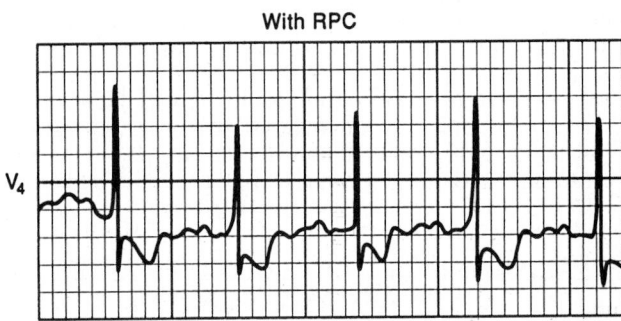

Figure 54–125. Total occlusion of the left anterior descending coronary artery after PTCA in lead V₄. *Top,* before PTCA; *middle,* during total occlusion; *bottom,* after placement of reperfusion catheter.

failed PTCA was advocated in two studies published in 1984.[2, 27] The IABP was applied to patients with ST-segment elevation after PTCA failure, and this intervention reduced the eventual development of Q-wave infarction after emergency CABG (although not a statistically significant reduction). Despite these reports, the IABP has not been used routinely in management of angioplasty failure, with its role limited to patients with hemodynamic instability. Balloon insertion does not greatly alter blood flow through diastolic augmentation to infarcting muscle, nor does afterload reduction reduce injury to ischemic, nonreperfused myocardium. If hemodynamic instability exists, then balloon insertion should be performed expeditiously with efforts directed toward the *main* priority of surgical revascularization.[4]

OTHER STRATEGIES AVAILABLE IN THE CARDIAC CATHETERIZATION LABORATORY

New direct approaches to failed angioplasty strategy employed in the catheterization laboratory by the angioplasty operator include laser welding of the dissected intimal flap, placement of an endoluminal stent, and use of the atherectomy device to excise the intimal flap *(rescue atherectomy).*[38] Rescue atherectomy has been shown to be effective in selected patients with short segment dissection and vessel closure but not for long segment spiral dissections.[25]

New indirect techniques applied in the interventional cardiac catheterization laboratory to improve myocardial perfusion and function include synchronized coronary venous retroperfusion *(back door perfusion)* through the coronary sinus[20] and percutaneous femoral-to-femoral cardiopulmonary bypass (CPB). The goal of CPB is to provide systemic perfusion and unload the left ventricle to lower myocardial oxygen consumption during periods of decreased coronary flow.

In general, these newer techniques have a very narrow range of clinical applicability, and continued attempts to reopen a damaged artery produce increased amounts of myocardial damage. The main goal should be expeditious transfer of the patient to the operating room for CABG.

SURGICAL CONSIDERATIONS

When the patient leaves the catheterization laboratory, with or without a reperfusion catheter or IABP, expeditious placement on CPB with systemic cooling is the primary goal (see Table 54–8). By converting the heart from a normothermic ejecting environment to a hypothermic empty beating state, oxygen demands are reduced significantly. The internal thoracic artery should be harvested if the patient has been stable and shows no evidence of ischemia by electrocardiographic or other clinical criteria. This can be readily done after the patient is placed on CPB and the myocardial oxygen demands are minimized. In one series of surgically treated angioplasty failures, the internal mammary artery was harvested and used as a graft conduit in 50% of patients.[14] In a more recent report, the internal mammary artery was used in 87% (27/32) of patients undergoing emergency CABG after failed PTCA without added mortality, especially in hemodynamically stable patients.[8]

Hypothermic hyperkalemic cardioplegia is then delivered into the aortic root through the reperfusion catheter, if one has been placed while the patient was in the catheterization laboratory. In the situation in which multiple grafts are required and no reperfusion catheter has been inserted preoperatively, the vessel occluded during PTCA should be the first vessel grafted and the cardioplegia delivered through the vein graft after distal coronary anastomosis.

The efficiency of normothermic blood cardioplegia given on induction and just before reperfusion has been examined in two series, which demonstrate some benefits provided by the technique in terms of reduction of perioperative myocardial infarction and restoration of regional function. In a series of 163 consecutive patients undergoing emergency CABG for acute coronary occlusion (94% after failed angioplasty), the clinical outcomes were compared in four different cohorts grouped by time periods using four different techniques of myocardial protection.[5] Despite the higher risk of patients undergoing emergency CABG in the contemporary group (older age, greater number of diseased vessels, poorer left ventricular function, a higher incidence of preoperative cardiogenic shock), a decreased hospital mortality was associated with *maximal protection* of the ischemic myocardium with the use of preoperative IABP, combined antegrade and retrograde substrate enhanced cardioplegia, warm induction, and warm controlled reperfusion.[5] In addition, the group with this type of myocardial protection regained regional contractility to a greater degree. In 19 patients receiving warm blood cardioplegia during emergency CABG after failed PTCA, a decrease in perioperative myocardial infarction from 65% (cold blood cardioplegia) to 26% (warm

blood cardioplegia) was demonstrated. The authors suggest normothermic blood cardioplegia provides a *salvage effect* for ischemic myocardium in the setting of failed PTCA.[7]

In approximately 10% of patients with angioplasty failure and acute coronary occlusion, the vessel has sustained a distal dissection, which requires special technical considerations. Extreme care is necessary in performing the arteriotomy, which when possible should be placed distal to the hematoma surrounding the vessel. Intracoronary probes should be avoided, and the vessel dissection is repaired in the course of performing the distal anastomosis by careful reapproximation of the intima to the media and adventitial layers of the coronary vessel.

In patients with multivessel coronary disease, other *major* vessels with greater than 50% stenosis documented by preoperative catheterization should be grafted at the time of operation.

MORTALITY AND MORBIDITY ASSOCIATED WITH EMERGENCY CABG AFTER FAILED ANGIOPLASTY

Most recent series of coronary angioplasty document an early failure rate of 4% to 5%. This contrasts remarkably to a 14% incidence of emergency CABG required for PTCA failure in Grüntzig's first 50 patients.[17] Despite improved strategies developed to manage patients with acute myocardial ischemia after PTCA failure (intracoronary thrombolysis, reperfusion catheter placement), the operative mortality, although usually less than 5%, is still approximately three times the mortality for elective CABG at most centers.[1, 6, 15, 22, 33, 37] Just as significant is a perioperative infarction incidence of over 30% (Table 54–9). This infarction rate is consistent in nearly all series, despite successful surgical revascularization of the vessel occluded during PTCA.[36] This appears to be the result of the necessary time (approximately 120 minutes) required to transport the patient from the catheterization laboratory to the operating room, place the patient on CPB, and establish surgical revascularization. If ischemia was present on the presurgical electrocardiogram after failed PTCA, the postoperative myocardial infarction rate was 57% in one study.[15] In those patients without ischemia, the rate of perioperative infarction was reduced to 10%. In 10 patients in whom CPB was established within 25 minutes of the onset of symptoms after PTCA failure, no perioperative deaths or infarctions were reported.[34] The predictors of operative mortality in patients undergoing emergency CABG for failed PTCA include prior coronary bypass surgery, presence of multiple vessel disease, age greater than 70, and cardiogenic shock.[22]

The effect of vessel closure requiring emergency CABG after elective coronary angioplasty versus emergent PTCA for acute myocardial infarction was reviewed in 1988.[14] Between 1984 and 1986, 1350 angioplasties were performed, 393 of these for acute myocardial infraction. Twenty-one patients (Group I) required emergency CABG after unsuccessful elective PTCA (failure rate 2.2%), and 32 patients (Group II) underwent emergency CABG after unsuccessful emergent angioplasty (failure rate 8.1%). All patients treated in Group II received thrombolytic therapy, and a reperfusion catheter was used in over half the patients in each group. There was no difference in mortality between the groups (4.7% after elective PTCA failure versus 6.2% after emergency PTCA failure, p = NS), and half of the patients in each group required postoperative inotropic support. The incidence of perioperative myocardial infarction was 24% in Group I and 34% in Group II. The internal mammary artery was used for grafting in 50% of patients in each group, and both groups had similar bypass times and number of vessels bypassed. Hemorrhagic complications were significantly greater in the

TABLE 54–9. Emergency Revascularization for Failed Angioplasty

Author	Years of Study	Year Reported	No. of Patients	Operative Mortality (%)	Perioperative Infarction (%)
Talley	1980–1986	1989	202	5 (2.5)	27.0
Ferguson	1984–1986	1988	18	0 (0.0)	23.8
Barner	1986–1987	1989	31	1 (3.2)	48.4
Naunheim	1984–1987	1989	79	4 (5.1)	35.9
Golding	1981–1985	1986	79	0 (0.0)	44.3
Page	1981–1985	1985	26	2 (7.7)	22.2
Killen	1980–1984	1985	75	3 (4.0)	43.5
Pellitier	1980–1983	1985	30	0 (0.0)	28.6
Akins	1978–1983	1984	11	0 (0.0)	9.1
Cowley	1977–1982	1984	202	13 (6.4)	41.0
Murphy	1981–1983	1984	32	0 (0.0)	53.0
Reul	1979–1983	1984	63	1 (1.4)	30.0
Craver	1980–1990	1992	699	22 (3.1)	18.0
Borkon	1989–1991	1992	91	11 (12.1)	29.0
Pragliola	1989–1992	1994	114	2 (1.7)	21.0

emergent PTCA failure group, in which 15.6% of patients required re-exploration for bleeding versus none in Group I. The effects of thrombolytic therapy have been shown to affect operative morbidity up to 12 hours after administration.[24] This study concludes that emergency CABG can be performed when necessary in the setting of emergent failed PTCA, with results comparable to CABG after failed elective angioplasty.

The in-hospital mortality and morbidity of patients who had failed elective PTCA and then underwent emergent or elective CABG was reviewed in a large series of 316 patients between 1980 and 1986.[37] Emergency coronary bypass surgery was performed in 202 (64%) of the patients, with a 2.5% operative mortality and a 27% perioperative incidence of myocardial infarction. The internal mammary artery was used in only 20% of the emergency CABG patients, and the IABP was used preoperatively in 24% of the patients. These clinical parameters in the emergency CABG group were compared with 114 patients who underwent elective surgical revascularization after failed PTCA during the same hospitalization (Table 54–10). Although operative mortality in the elective CABG group was not statistically different from the elective CABG group, the perioperative myocardial infarction incidence was only 4% in the patients requiring elective surgical revascularization.

A more recent review examined a 10-year experience with emergency bypass surgery in 699 patients (of 12,000 PTCA) after failed elective angioplasty.[10] The overall operative mortality was 3.1%, the incidence of new Q-wave myocardial infarction was 18%, and actuarial 5-year survival was 91%. Interestingly, when the most recent 3-year cohort of patients was examined, a significantly higher hospital death rate was found (7.1%). This increase in operative mortality occurred even though fewer patients in the group presented with

refractory myocardial ischemia. The authors thought this increase in hospital mortality in the recent cohort of patients was due to more clinical characteristics associated with poor outcome of CABG (older age, multivessel disease, diabetes, decreased left ventricular ejection fraction, prior CABG). Additionally, because this group had a higher incidence of multivessel disease, a more extensive CABG procedure was required. When these older patients died after CABG, they seemed to die not from cardiac failure but from complications in other systems due to insults related to the ischemic, hypotensive episode. The presence of multivessel disease, age older than 60 years, and active ischemia at the time of emergency CABG produced the highest risk of hospital death.

In another study examining operative management of failed coronary angioplasty between 1981 and 1986, 81 patients required emergency operative revascularization within 24 hours of failed PTCA (4.4% of the total PTCA population).[15] There were two early deaths in the series (2.5% mortality) and a 43% incidence of perioperative myocardial infarction. A significantly higher incidence of postoperative complications was encountered in this group of patients (Table 54–11), compared with a group of patients undergoing elective revascularization during the same time period.

A review of 53 patients undergoing emergency CABG after failed angioplasty in the late 1980s noted the differences in outcome between patients having single-vessel versus those with multivessel disease.[16] The patients requiring emergency CABG after failed PTCA with multivessel disease had a higher mortality (6% vs. 0%), higher requirement for postoperative IAPB support (25% vs. 5%), higher perioperative incidence of myocardial infarction (56% vs. 43%), and higher incidence of postoperative complications (28% vs. 5%).

It is possible that a patient with multivessel disease may be more predisposed to higher rates of myocardial infarction

TABLE 54–10. Surgical Management of Failed PTCA (at Emory University Medical Center)

Clinical Characteristics	Total Population (%)	Emergency CABG (%)	Elective CABG (%)	p
Patients	316	202	114	
Intra-aortic balloon pump	50 (16)	48 (24)	2 (2)	<.05
Internal mammery artery	75 (24)	39 (20)	36 (32)	<.05
Inotropic therapy	106 (34)	84 (42)	22 (20)	<.05

Data from Craver, J. M., Weintraub, W. S., Jones, E. L., Guyton, R. A., and Hatcher, C. R., Jr.: Emergency coronary artery bypass surgery for failed percutaneous angioplasty: A 10-year experience. Ann. Surg., 215:425, 1992.

TABLE 54–11. Emergency CABG After Failed PTCA: Postoperative Morbidity (at Cleveland Clinic)

	Emergency CABG (n = 81)	Elective CABG (n = 5000)
Myocardial infarction	43%	0.7%
Postoperative hemorrhage	11%	3.5%
Postoperative respiratory failure	9%	2.5%

Data from Golding, L. A. R., Loop, F. D., Hollman, J. L., Franco, I., Borsh, J., Stewart, R. W., and Lytle, B. W.: Early results of emergency surgery after coronary angioplasty. Circulation, 74(Suppl. III):III-26, 1986.

and other complications after failure of angioplasty, owing to inadequate collateral circulation secondary to the presence of stenosis of other major vessels after total occlusion of the culprit vessel during PTCA.

The change in clinical characteristics of patients undergoing PTCA and its influence on outcome after emergency CABG for PTCA failure was reported in 1992.[23] Two groups of PTCA failure were compared: 1980–1985 and 1986–1988. Despite increases in risk factors associated with Group II, there was no increase in incidence of myocardial infarction (39%), mortality (11%), or complications after emergency CABG. The findings were attributed to early detection of myocardial ischemia in the catheterization laboratory, use of the reperfusion catheter, and a high use of preoperative IABP (70%).

The devastating effect of cardiogenic shock occurring in a patient after PTCA failure has been reported in a series of 53 patients having emergency CABG after PTCA failure.[19] Cardiogenic shock was present in 25%, and in this group the mortality was 50%. Identifying PTCA failure before the presence of cardiogenic shock, with early surgical intervention, was recommended.

A possible late complication of percutaneous coronary angioplasty not reported in other series was noted in 1985.[15] In a group of 286 patients undergoing coronary bypass grafting for restenosis after PTCA, 7 patients had documented occurrence of severe left main stenosis during the interval between the initial PTCA and subsequent CABG. In 6 of the 7 patients, the interval was less than 1 year; and in 4 patients less than 6 months passed between the time of angioplasty and development of left main coronary artery stenosis. It is postulated that PTCA manipulations through the left main coronary artery cause arterial damage that leads to development of coronary stenosis. In each of the patients who developed left main coronary artery stenosis, lesions in the left coronary arterial circulation had been dilated but disease in the left main coronary artery at that time was only minimal. The mechanism may be similar to one that has been postulated in the evolution of left main coronary artery stenosis after cannulation and direct perfusion of the left coronary artery at the time of aortic valve replacement.

Management of the patient who has sustained a failed coronary angioplasty and requires emergent CABG requires careful strategies to minimize myocardial ischemia after vessel closure before surgical revascularization can be accomplished. Of paramount importance is rapid surgical revascularization, which requires well-coordinated cardiac anesthesia and surgical services working with the cardiac catheterization laboratory. Current experience has shown that operative mortality can be reduced to a low level (although not equivalent to elective surgical coronary mortality). However, the in-hospital morbidity remains quite high, specifically, a perioperative myocardial infarction rate of approximately 30%. Further attempts to reduce this rate of

perioperative infarction must involve intervention techniques to restore perfusion to the ischemic region preoperatively or to protect the myocardium from injuries associated with reperfusion.[3]

SELECTED REFERENCES

Borkon, A. M., Failing, T. L., Piehler, J. M., Killen, D. A., Hoskins, M. L., and Reed, W. A.: Risk analysis of operative intervention for failed coronary angioplasty. Ann. Thorac. Surg., 54:884, 1992.
A series of 91 patients undergoing emergency CABG after failed angioplasty was compared with a matched cohort of patients undergoing elective CABG. The operative mortality in the emergency CABG group was 12.1% versus 1.0%, with emergency CABG patients requiring more postoperative inotropes and IABP support; they had a higher incidence of perioperative myocardial infarction and an increased length of hospital stay. The presence of multivessel disease or use of a reperfusion catheter had no influence on clinical outcome in the emergency CABG group.

Craver, J. M., Weintraub, W. S., Jones, E. L., Guyton, R. A., and Hatcher, C. R.: Emergency coronary artery bypass surgery for failed percutaneous coronary angioplasty. Ann. Surg., 215:425, 1992.
This is an excellent review of 699 patients undergoing emergency CABG after failed PTCA from 1980 to 1990. Patients with ongoing, refractory ischemia at the time of CABG had an increased mortality (3.7% vs. 0.8%), increased incidence of perioperative myocardial infarction (21% vs. 2.4%), and increased use of IABP (19% versus 0.8%). Multivariate analysis of preoperative characteristics showed predictors of hospital mortality to include age older than 65 years, multivessel disease, and refractory myocardial ischemia.

Ferguson, T. B., Muhlbaier, L. H., Salai, D. L., and Wechsler, A. S.: Coronary bypass grafting after failed elective and failed emergent percutaneous angioplasty-relative risks of emergent surgical intervention. J. Thorac. Cardiovasc. Surg., 95:761, 1988.
The authors compared clinical outcome of patients requiring emergency CABG after failed angioplasty in the setting of elective PTCA (21 patients) versus PTCA for acute myocardial infarction (32 patients). All patients in the acute myocardial infarction group received thrombolytic therapy, and a reperfusion catheter was used in over half the patients in each group. The internal mammary artery was used as a conduit in 50% of patients in each group. The operative mortality was no different in the two groups (5%), and the perioperative myocardial infarction rates were also not significantly different. The authors conclude that emergency CABG can be performed in the setting of failed emergent PTCA with results comparable to coronary bypass after failed elective PTCA.

REFERENCES

1. Akins, C. W.: Early and late results following emergency myocardial revascularization during hypothermic fibrillatory arrest. Ann. Thorac. Surg., 43:131, 1987.
2. Akins, C. W., and Block, P.C.: Surgical intervention for failed percutaneous transluminal coronary angioplasty. Am. J. Cardiol., 53:108c, 1984.
3. Allen, B. S., Okamoto, F., Buckberg, G. D., Bugyi, H., Young, H., Leaf, J., Beyersdorf, F., Sjostrand, F., and Maloney, J. V., Jr.: Immediate functional recovery after six hours of regional ischemia by careful control of conditions of reperfusion and composition of reperfusate. J. Thorac. Cardiovasc. Surg., 92:621, 1986.
4. Barner, H. B., Lea, J. W., IV, Naunheim, K. S., and Stoney, W. S., Jr.: Emergency coronary bypass not associated with preoperative cardiogenic shock in failed angioplasty, after thrombolysis, and for acute myocardial infarction. Circulation, 79(Suppl. I):I-152, 1989.
5. Beyersdorf, F., Mitrev, Z., Sarai, K., Eckel, L., Klepzig, H., Maul, F. D., Ihnken, K., and Satter, P.: Changing patterns of patients undergoing emergency surgical revascularization for acute coronary occlusion: Importance of myocardial protection techniques. J. Thorac. Cardiovasc. Surg., 106:137, 1993.
6. Borkon, A. M., Failing, T. L., Piehler, J. M., Killen, D. A., Hoskins, M. L., and Reed, W. A.: Risk analysis of operative intervention for failed coronary angioplasty. Ann. Thorac. Surg., 54:884, 1992.
7. Bottner, R. L., Wallace, R. B., Visner, J. S., Stark, K. S., Recientes, E., Katz, N. M., Hopkins, R. A., Patrissi, G. A., and Kent, K. M.: Reduction of myocardial infarction after emergency coronary artery bypass grafting for failed coronary angioplasty with use of a normothermic reperfusion cardioplegia protocol. J. Thorac. Cardiovasc. Surg., 101:1069, 1991.
8. Caes, F. L., and Van Nooten, G. J.: Use of internal mammary artery for emergency grafting after failed coronary angioplasty. Ann. Thorac. Surg., 57:1295, 1994.
9. Cowley, M. J., Dorros, G., Kelsey, S. F., Raden, M. V., and Detre, K. M.: Emergency coronary bypass surgery after coronary angioplasty: The National Heart, Lung, and Blood Institute's percutaneous transluminal coronary angioplasty registry experience. Am. J. Cardiol., 53:22c, 1985.
10. Craver, J. M., Weintraub, W. S., Jones, E. L., Guyton, R. A., and Hatcher, C. R., Jr.: Emergency coronary artery bypass surgery for failed percutaneous coronary angioplasty: A 10-year experience. Ann. Surg., 215:425, 1992.

11. Detre, K., Holubkov, R., Kelsey, S., et al.: Percutaneous transluminal coronary angioplasty in 1985–1986 and 1977–1981. The National Heart, Lung, and Blood Institute Registry. N. Engl. J. Med., 318:265, 1988.

12. Ellis, S. G., Roubin, G. S., King, S. B., III, Douglas, J. S., Jr., Weintraub, W. S., Thomas, R. G., and Cox, W. R.: Angiographic and clinical predictors of acute closure after native vessel coronary angioplasty. Circulation, 77:372, 1988.

13. Ferguson, T. B., Hinohara, T., Simpson, J., Stack, R. S., and Wechsler, A. S.: Catheter reperfusion to allow optimal coronary bypass grafting following failed coronary angioplasty. Ann. Thorac. Surg., 42:399, 1986.

14. Ferguson, T. B., Muhlbaier, L. H., Salai, D. L., and Wechsler, A. S.: Coronary bypass grafting after failed elective and failed emergent percutaneous angioplasty. J. Thorac. Cardiovasc. Surg., 95:761, 1988.

15. Golding, L. A. R., Loop, F. D., Hollman, J. L., Franco, I., Borsh, J., Stewart, R. W., and Lytle, B. W.: Early results of emergency surgery after coronary angioplasty. Circulation, 74(Suppl. III):III-26, 1986.

16. Greene, M. A., Gray, L. A., Jr., Slater, A. D., Ganzel, B. L., and Mavroudis, C.: Emergency aortocoronary bypass after failed angioplasty. Ann. Thorac. Surg., 51:194, 1991.

17. Grüntzig, A. R., Senning, A., and Seigenthaler, W. E.: Nonoperative dilatation of coronary-artery stenosis: Percutaneous transluminal coronary angioplasty. N. Engl. J. Med., 301:61, 1979.

18. Hinohara, T., Simpson, J. B., Phillips, H. R., and Stack, R. S.: Transluminal intracoronary reperfusion catheter: A device to maintain coronary perfusion between failed coronary angioplasty and emergency coronary bypass surgery. J. Am. Coll. Cardiol., 11:977, 1988.

19. Hochberg, M. S., Gregory, J. J., McCullough, J., Gielchinsky, I., and Parsonnet, V.: Early emergent coronary bypass after failed angioplasty. Del. Med. J., 65(12):775, 1993.

20. Kar, S., Drury, J. K., Hajduczki, I., Eigler, N., Wakida, Y., Litvack, F., Buchbinder, N., Marcus, H., Nordlander, R., and Corday, E.: Synchronized coronary venous retroperfusion for support and salvage of ischemic myocardium during elective and failed angioplasty. J. Am. Coll. Cardiol., 18:271, 1991.

21. Kereiakas, J. R.: Emergent internal thoracic artery grafting following failed PTCA. Am. Heart J., 113:1018, 1987.

22. Killen, D. A., Hamaker, W. R., and Reed, W. A.: Coronary artery bypass following percutaneous transluminal coronary angioplasty. Ann. Thorac. Surg., 40:133, 1985.

23. Lazar, H. L., Faxon, D. P., Paone, G., Rajaii-Khorasani, A., Jacobs, A. K., Fallon, M. P., and Shemin, R. J.: Changing profiles of failed coronary angioplasty patients: Impact on surgical results. Ann. Thorac. Surg., 53:269, 1992.

24. Lee, K. F., Mandell, J., Rankin, J. S., Muhlbaier, L. H., and Wechsler, A. S.: Immediate versus delayed coronary grafting after streptokinase treatment. J. Thorac. Cardiovasc. Surg., 95:216, 1988.

25. McCluskey, E. R., Cowley, M., and Whitlow, P. L.: Multicenter clinical experience with rescue atherectomy for failed angioplasty. Am. J. Cardiol., 72:42E, 1993.

26. Morrison, D. A., Crowley, S. T., Veerakul, G., Barbiere, C., and Grover, F.: Percutaneous transluminal angioplasty of saphenous vein graft lesions for medically refractory rest angina. J. Am. Coll. Cardiol., 23:1066, 1994.

27. Murphy, D. A., Carver, J. M., Jones, E. L., et al.: Surgical management of acute myocardial ischemia following percutaneous transluminal coronary angioplasty: Role of the intra-aortic balloon pump. J. Thorac. Cardiovasc. Surg., 87:332, 1984.

28. Naunheim, K. S., Fiore, A. C., Fagan, D. C.,, McBride, L. R., Barner, H. B., Pennington, D. G., Willman, V. L., Kern, M. J., Deligonul, U., Vandormael, M. C., and Kaiser, G. C.: Emergency coronary artery bypass grafting for failed angioplasty: Risk factors and outcome. Ann. Thorac. Surg., 47:816, 1989.

29. O'Keefe, J. H., Allan, J. J., McCallister, B. D., McConahay, D. R., Vacek, J. L., Piehler, J. M., Ligon, R., and Hartzler, G. O.: Angioplasty versus bypass surgery for multivessel coronary artery disease with left ventricular ejection fraction ≤ 40%. Am. J. Cardiol., 71:897, 1993.

30. Page, W. S., Okies, J. E., Colburn, L. Q., et al.: Percutaneous transluminal angioplasty: A growing surgical problem. J. Thorac. Cardiovasc. Surg., 92:847, 1985.

31. Pellitier, L. C., Pardini, A., Renkin, J., David, P. R., Hebert, Y., and Bourassa, M. G.: Myocardial revascularization after failure of percutaneous transluminal coronary angioplasty. J. Thorac. Cardiovasc. Surg., 90:265, 1985.

32. Phillips, S. J., Kongtahworn, C., Zeff, R. H., Skinner, J. R., Toon, R. S., Grignon, A., Spector, M., and Iannone, L. A.: Disrupted coronary artery caused by angioplasty: Supportive and surgical considerations. Ann. Thorac. Surg., 47:880, 1989.

33. Pragliola, C., Kootstra, G., J., Lanzillo, G., Rose, P. A., Quafford, M., and Uitdenhaag, G.: Current results of coronary bypass surgery after failed angioplasty. J. Cardiovasc. Surg., 35:365, 1994.

34. Reul, G. J., Cooley, D. A., Hallman, G. L., Duncan, J. M., Livesay, J. J., Frazier, O. H., Ott, D. A., Angelini, P., Massumi, A., and Mathur, V. S.: Coronary artery bypass for unsuccessful percutaneous transluminal coronary angioplasty. J. Thorac. Cardiovasc. Surg., 88:685, 1984.

35. Ryan, T. J., et al.: Guidelines for percutaneous transluminal coronary angioplasty. J. Am. Coll. Cardiol., 12:529, 1988.

36. Spencer, F. C.: A critique of emergency and urgent operations for complications of coronary artery disease. Circulation, 79(Suppl. I):I-160, 1989.

37. Talley, J. D., Jones, E. L., Weintraub, W. S., and King, S. B., III: Coronary artery bypass surgery after failed elective percutaneous transluminal coronary angioplasty. Circulation, 79(Suppl. I):I-126, 1989.

38. Topol, E. J.: Emerging strategies for failed percutaneous transluminal coronary angioplasty. Am. J. Cardiol., 63:249, 1989.

REOPERATIVE CORONARY SURGERY

Stanley A. Gall, Jr., M.D.

EPIDEMIOLOGY

As more numbers of patients undergo coronary artery bypass grafting (CABG), more numbers of patients are surviving longer after CABG, and technical and technologic advances have reduced the risk of reoperative coronary surgery, this procedure has gained importance in the treatment of coronary artery disease. In 1994, more than 250,000 CABG procedures are estimated to have been accomplished, with 7% to 15% of these as reoperative cases. As coronary revascularization has evolved over the three decades since its conception in this country, the reoperative patient population, the conduct of the procedure, and the indications for operative procedures have changed. Since 1970, the average interval to reoperation has lengthened from 58 to 110 months.[26] Reoperation will be accomplished in a cumulative 3% to 3.4% of patients after 5 years, 5.5% to 11% after 10 years, and 17% after 12 years after CABG.[10, 44] The annual risk of requiring reoperation increases markedly after 5 to 7 years, with the yearly incidence of reoperation increasing from 1.1% at five years after primary CABG to 3.2% and 3.9% at 10 and 12 years, respectively.[10]

The group of patients who present for coronary reoperation differ significantly from those undergoing primary CABG.[26, 43, 44] These reoperative patients are older, have more diffuse coronary artery disease, and have diminished ventricular function. One third of patients lose ventricular function between procedures.[27] Patients undergoing reoperation now are also significantly different from those patients undergoing reoperation in past decades. The time between procedures has lengthened.[1, 26] Patients are now older at the time of both procedures, more likely to have left main coronary artery or three-vessel disease, more likely to have a further diminished ejection fraction, and more likely to present with failure of their bypass grafts.[1, 29] Formerly, native vessel disease progression was the angiographic indication in 55% of patients; now the majority of patients (82%) present with angiographic indications of both vein graft stenosis and progression of native vessel disease.[31] Reoperative candidates are older and more medically infirm than the group undergoing primary CABG, factors that impact on postoperative survival and morbidity.

The process of atherosclerosis continues in the native coronary circulation and develops in the saphenous vein grafts (SVGs) after CABG. The internal mammary artery (IMA) is rarely afflicted with atherosclerosis, which occurs in only 1% to 3% of IMAs in autopsy or angiographic studies.[34, 47] This resistance to atherosclerosis continues after the vessel is implanted as a bypass conduit. The IMA-to-coronary-artery anastomosis, however, is subject to errors in technique, resulting in stenosis at the anastomosis. SVG failure may be arbitrarily divided into early and late failure, with early failure defined as occurring sooner than 5 years postoperatively. SVGs occlude most frequently in the first year after surgery, at a rate of 15% to 25%.[7, 49] The cause of early SVG failure is most often imperfect technique in performing anastomoses or selecting recipient vessels of poor quality or limited outflow. Vein graft occlusion thereafter occurs at an annual rate of 0.5% to 3.0% for years 2 to 7 after grafting.[50] Vein grafts will develop fibrous hyperplasia, which results in an intimal thickening. This process is usually adaptive, resulting in an SVG lumen that more closely matches the size of the recipient coronary vessel. Rare patients may have an exaggerated hyperplastic response that can result in premature closure of grafts in the first weeks or months after bypass. Intimal fibroplasia may also affect the distal anastomosis of vein or IMA grafts. Late failure of SVGs is secondary to atherosclerotic degeneration of the vein graft. Atherosclerosis is morphologically different in vein grafts than coronary arteries, developing as a diffuse, usually concentric lesion, with no overlying fibrous cap.[50] This process of atherosclerotic involvement accelerates in grafts that are more than 7 years old, resulting in occlusion of 6% to 10% of grafts annually.[50] Graft atherosclerosis is one factor increasing the risk of graft thrombosis. Late thrombosis is also more likely with increased graft age, continued smoking, and hypercholesterolemia.

The risk of occlusion is difficult to define for any individual graft. SVGs that were stenotic at 1 year after CABG progressed to occlusion in 30% at 10 years, for a cumulative 10-year patency of 60%. Examination of the grafts that remain patent revealed significant involvement with atherosclerosis in 46%.[7] When a population of patients who underwent reoperation were examined, explanted grafts demonstrated late thrombosis in 69% of all grafts and in 80% of atherosclerotic grafts.[49] A lower incidence of saphenous vein occlusion was noted in patients who had angiographic determination of SVG disease 5.1 and 11.0 years after CABG but did not undergo reoperation. In this selected group of patients, of those SVGs that had stenoses less than 35% or were normal 5.1 years after placement, 53% remained normal or minimally diseased at 11-year follow-up. Twenty-one percent of these grafts were occluded, and an additional 8% had hemodynamically significant stenosis. Minimally diseased grafts had a similar progression as grafts without disease, demonstrating a patency of 79% five years after initial postoperative assessment.[8] Continued patency of SVGs cannot be considered to be reliable after 7 years because atherosclerosis, the major determinant of occlusion or thrombosis, has its most marked effect at this time.

The effect of these SVG lesions is to limit survival. Patients with SVG stenoses of 20% to 99% identified more than 5 years after primary CABG had a diminished survival compared with patients with no SVG disease.[30] For the first 2 years after catheterization, patients with vein grafts having 20% to 49% stenoses did as well as those with less severe stenoses and then suffered from much worse survival. Early SVG stenosis had no survival advantage when treated surgically. The medically managed patients were highly selected, however, and many subsequently did undergo revascularization. Late stenosis of SVG to the left anterior descending (LAD) coronary artery had a much different prognosis, significantly reducing survival, reoperation-free survival, and event-free survival. The risk of sudden death in this group was highest when an SVG to the LAD artery demonstrated stenosis greater than 50%. Lesions in the vein grafts to the circumflex or right coronary systems did not carry such a morbid prognosis. In subgroups with SVG stenoses, survival was adversely affected by decreased left ventricular function, three-vessel or left main coronary artery disease, and increased age. Progression of native coronary artery atherosclerosis also occurs, with 47% of previously involved vessels demonstrating worsened stenosis and 47% of vessels previously normal developing new lesions. These native vessel lesions, even when involving the LAD artery, have less impact on survival than stenosis in a SVG to the LAD artery.

This stenosis confers a mortality of 30% over 2 years as compared with 3% for a comparable LAD artery stenosis. Stenoses in an existing conduit are now the most important reason for reoperation. Even grafts that are minimally diseased 6 years after CABG will show severe stenosis or occlusion in 29% over 5 years, subjecting these patients to an increased risk of requiring reoperation. This progression of disease is the leading reason to consider replacement of patent SVGs at the time of reoperation.

Multivariate analysis demonstrates that the factors that increase the risk of requiring reoperation include the absence of an IMA graft, younger age, incomplete revascularization, congestive heart failure, and New York Heart Association (NYHA) Class III or IV angina.[10] Single- or double-vessel disease and normal ventricular function were also risk factors for reoperation but probably identify patients who are younger and more likely to be selected for further interventions. Younger age (age <50 years) is likely a surrogate marker for more severe, aggressive atherosclerosis, which will progress and require further treatment. This study did not include percutaneous transluminal coronary angioplasty (PTCA) after CABG or other cardiac events as endpoints with reoperation. An evaluation using all cardiac events—death, myocardial infarction, PTCA, or reoperations—as endpoints demonstrated that diabetes mellitus, severe angina, systolic hypertension, and diminished ejection fraction were predisposing risk factors for any intervention.[55] This population did not have placement of IMA grafts. Despite the higher likelihood of repeated interventions, the younger patients still had a superior survival compared with the group older than age 70 years. Placement of an IMA graft at the time of the first operation was critically important, neutralizing the adverse effects of elevated serum cholesterol, hypertension, and smoking on reoperation-free survival.[10] Conversely, patients with these characteristics had markedly worse survival when an IMA graft was not employed. The benefit of IMA use extended across all age groups. Patients with an IMA graft placed at primary CABG were better candidates for reoperation because they had better-preserved left ventricular function at the time of reoperation. Although the risk of damaging an intact IMA during reoperation is 3% to 5%, the benefits of a functioning IMA are so great that the presence of this graft does not pose a risk factor for reoperative morbidity or mortality.[9, 32] Maximal survival and freedom from reoperation can be achieved in patients after CABG only by aggressive treatment of hypertension, diabetes mellitus, hypercholesterolemia, and smoking.

Anginal symptoms recur at a rate of 3.5% to 7.2% per year, placing 17% to 36% of patients at risk for recurrent angina within 5 years of primary CABG. Those patients surviving to 10 years have a 40% to 50% incidence of angina. Medical management of recurrent angina after CABG includes appropriate afterload reduction, coronary vasodilators, and beta-adrenergic blockade. Percutaneous angioplasty techniques have been used to reduce stenosis of isolated, symptomatic lesions in native coronary vessels, the IMA, and SVGs. Angioplasty catheters may traverse an SVG with minimal disease or the IMA to access some native vessel lesions or sites of anastomotic stenosis. Angioplasty of SVG stenoses is angiographically successful in 85% to 95% of vessels; however, complications such as atheroembolism into the distal coronary vasculature, perforation, myocardial infarction, or rupture of the graft occur in 4% to 7% of cases.[13, 41] The complication rate increases with graft age. Lesions of the body of SVGs are at the highest risk for restenosis, which occurs in 50% to 60% of lesions within 6 months. Endovascular stenting has slightly improved initial success rates but has not affected restenosis rates. Angioplasty of native vessels, accessed through graft conduit or through the native circulation, has a similar success rate as PTCA performed as a primary procedure. Access to lesions distal to the anastomosis may be limited by progression of proximal lesions in the native circulation; by soft, friable, atherosclerotic lesions in vein grafts; or by excessive graft tortuosity. Anastomotic stenoses of SVGs or the IMA may result from technical errors in construction or from intimal fibroplasia. Regardless of etiology, these lesions are amenable to catheter-based therapy. Angioplasty of anastomotic stenosis of the IMA or SVG has a high initial success rate of 82% to 100%.[36, 40, 48] However, restenosis of these lesions is less frequent, occurring in 8% to 14% of IMA anastomoses and 26% of SVG anastomoses. Long-term patency is approximately 80%. Lesions of the body or ostium of the IMA are very unusual and may be treated by stenting or direct bypass to the IMA itself.[18]

INDICATIONS

Indications for reoperative coronary surgery generally follow the indications for primary CABG. Strong indications for a surgical procedure include the acute complications of vessel dissection or perforation at catheterization or angioplasty, left main coronary artery equivalent anatomy, unstable angina, or postinfarction angina. Patients who are unable to control symptoms medically, those who have symptoms of congestive heart failure, those who have a positive exercise tolerance test after myocardial infarction, or those who have silent ischemia with a large proportion of myocardium at risk should also be considered for reoperation. Patients with an intact IMA graft are less likely to require reoperation, but if stenosis distal to the IMA or disease in other vein grafts has progressed or a large portion of myocardium is at risk, reoperation is recommended.[31] Patients with angiographic findings of a stenosed SVG to the LAD artery, even with stable Class I or Class II angina, have a higher mortality when managed medically and therefore should be offered reoperative revascularization. These indications suppose that vessels technically adequate for bypass are available.

CONTRAINDICATIONS

Accepting a patient for reoperative CABG involves an assessment of benefit and of the patient's risk of mortal and morbid events. Such factors as evolving myocardial infarction, cardiogenic shock, and concurrent sepsis are strong contraindications to surgery, as is poor medical condition. Patients with marked obesity, dialysis-dependent chronic renal failure, severe chronic obstructive pulmonary disease, advanced age, metastatic carcinoma, or a bleeding diathesis are poor candidates for reoperation. Patients who are unstable, in congestive heart failure, or evolving a myocardial infarction should be treated medically. Maximal medical treatment, including the use of intra-aortic balloon counterpulsation, is continued until a physiologically stable state is achieved and end-organ dysfunction is reversed or stabilized. Emergent revascularization can technically be accomplished but has poor immediate and long-term results, including a higher mortality and earlier return of anginal symptoms.[21, 24] After stabilization, the appropriateness of reoperation may be reconsidered. Poor left ventricular function is a relative contraindication to reoperation, but the presence of a prior IMA graft is not a contraindication to reoperation. Patients with intact IMA grafts sustained a lower mortality, blood use, and cerebrovascular accident rate at reoperation.[3] Although harvesting bilateral IMAs does not consistently subject the patient to an increased risk of mediastinal infection or sternal dehiscence, this risk is magnified in the elderly, female, and diabetic populations. The sequential use of the contralateral IMA in successive coronary procedures does not predispose

to sternal healing complications.[17] A history of prior mediastinal irradiation or existing cardiac cachexia significantly increases the risk of sternal re-entry and is a contraindication to reoperation. Prior pericarditis or mediastinitis severely increases the difficulty of dissection and may preclude identification of graftable vessels.

Adequate conduit for bypass grafting must be ensured. If the greater saphenous vein is no longer available, lesser saphenous vein and alternative arterial conduits should be considered. Although arm vein is a potential conduit, patency rates of 47% to 57% at a mean of 4.6 years was less than the patency of SVGs (77%) or IMA grafts (93%).[51, 56] This conduit should be considered only when no autologous lower limb vein or alternate arterial conduits are available. Cryopreserved saphenous vein, even if ABO matched, has a markedly diminished patency of 0% to 41% at 7 to 24 months[23, 46] and appropriately is relegated to a very limited role as a coronary bypass conduit. Use of both IMAs and of the gastroepiploic, radial, and superior epigastric arteries are preferable options. Careful inquiry into the patient's past surgical history is critically important to verify that prior procedures have not jeopardized use of these vessels.

COMORBIDITIES/RISK FACTORS

Technical factors that increase the difficulty of reoperative CABG in comparison to primary CABG include a longer time to initiate cardiopulmonary bypass, more advanced native vessel disease, longer cross-clamp time, longer cross-clamp time per graft, and an increased blood loss. The risk factors, by multivariate analysis, for heightened morbidity and mortality after reoperative CABG include advanced age, diminished ventricular function, absence of an IMA graft at either primary or reoperative CABG, and diabetes mellitus. Additional risk factors including sex and emergency procedure are not as consistently identified. An interval between operation of greater than 10 years appears to increase operative risk.[43, 44] Although the presence of left main coronary artery disease (stenosis >50%) is associated with early mortality, particularly increasing mortality if perioperative myocardial infarction occurs, left main coronary artery disease has no effect on late mortality.[29]

OPERATIVE TECHNIQUES

Although access to the mediastinum through the previous sternal incision is the most commonly employed approach for reoperation, in select patients alternative incisions may be employed. For patients with limited grafting requirements, the heart may be exposed through either a left or right thoracotomy.[53, 54] A thoracotomy approach avoids the IMA graft and although it decreases the risk of damaging existing vein grafts, these SVGs may not be accessible for elective replacement. Lesions in the right coronary artery distribution are amenable to an approach through a right thoracotomy. The ascending aorta or femoral artery provides arterial access, and the atrium provides access for venous return for cardiopulmonary bypass. From a right thoracotomy, aortic cross clamp and cardioplegic arrest may be accomplished.

A left thoracotomy approach may be employed for lesions of the circumflex distribution but may not consistently provide exposure to the left anterior coronary artery distribution. The descending aorta or femoral artery provides arterial access; however, venous return for cardiopulmonary bypass is best accomplished through a long catheter advanced through the femoral vein into the right atrium. Although a left thoracotomy limits access to the ascending aorta, precluding aortic cross-clamping and thus cardioplegic arrest, fibrillation can be induced. Aortic insufficiency limits the usefulness of fibrillatory arrest from either hemithorax. In combination with systemic hypothermia and ventricular venting through the pulmonary veins or left atrial appendage as needed, fibrillation provides a still field for completion of coronary anastomoses. Temporary occlusion of the coronary artery facilitates accurate construction of the distal anastomoses. The ipsilateral IMA may be harvested by either of these approaches. Proximal anastomoses may be accomplished using the subclavian vessels or descending aorta if the ascending aorta is not available or cannot be exposed. When disease in the LAD artery distribution or lesions in both the right and left coronary distributions are present that require bypass, a reentry sternotomy is required.

Careful preoperative preparation facilitates safe sternal reentry. The operative report from the primary CABG should be examined, as well as reports from other procedures that may have affected the epigastric, radial, or gastroepiploic vessels, should inadequate saphenous vein be available. Ultrasonography may be used to map remaining greater saphenous vein or lesser saphenous vein. The lateral chest radiograph will demonstrate the relationship between the heart and the posterior sternum. The lateral view of the IMA graft obtained during cardiac catheterization will demonstrate its course in relation to the sternum. In the operating room, complete invasive monitoring should be accomplished. Adhesive defibrillation patches are placed, one anteriorly that may be sterile and one posteriorly, to provide a means for defibrillation if adequate access by internal paddles is not possible. Rapid transfusion access must be ensured. Several factors are believed to increase the risk of sternal re-entry: recent sternotomy, adhesion of the right ventricle or the IMA to the sternum, ascending aortic aneurysm, right ventricular hypertrophy, multiple prior sternal entries, or a history of mediastinitis. In these high-risk patients, consideration should be given to different levels of preparation for cardiopulmonary bypass: exposure of the femoral vessels, cannulation of the femoral vessels, or even initiating cardiopulmonary bypass through the femoral vessels before sternotomy. Cardiopulmonary bypass may decompress a dilated right ventricle or large, aneurysmal aorta before sternal entry. Additionally, bypass allows hypothermia to be induced early and blood that is lost in the event of entry into a cardiac chamber or great vessel may be returned to the pump circuit to avoid fatal exsanguination. After incision of the skin and overlying soft tissues, existing sternal wires are removed. Whereas the reciprocating saw can be used for re-entry sternotomy, the oscillating saw allows improved control. The oscillating saw is used to first divide the anterior sternal table over the entire length of the sternum, then to carefully divide the posterior table, taking care not to injure underlying structures. The structures most often damaged are the right ventricle, the aorta, the right atrium, the innominate vein, SVGs, and prior IMA grafts. A right IMA graft to the LAD artery is at particular risk for injury. Catastrophic hemorrhage during sternal re-entry occurs in 2% to 6% of reoperations and carries an overall 37% mortality.[14] Mortality is greatest after division of an aortocoronary bypass graft (56%) and slightly less after entry into the innominate vein (13%). The temptation to immediately improve exposure after entry into one of these structures, by rapid completion of the median sternotomy, must be resisted. This maneuver results in tearing of cardiac chambers or great vessels with mortal consequences. Bleeding should be controlled by gauze packing or by approximation of the sternal halves with towel clips. The patient is anticoagulated and femoral-femoral cardiopulmonary bypass instituted, and then controlled completion of sternal division may be accomplished. Institution

of anticoagulation and cardiopulmonary bypass also allows return of any lost blood to the pump circuit.

The conduct of reoperative coronary procedure has been modified as the frequency of this procedure has increased. The evolution of the technique to the current state, whereby minimal dissection is performed until cardiopulmonary bypass and cardioplegic arrest can be induced and retrograde cardioplegia supplements antegrade delivery, is believed by several authors to be responsible for the stable or improving outcome results despite a progressively higher risk population of reoperative candidates.[28, 31, 45] The sternal halves are separated very gently by use of bone hooks and the mediastinal structures sharply dissected free from the sternum for a distance of several centimeters on either side. A small chest retractor may then be inserted to allow further dissection. The innominate vein frequently is a limiting factor to further opening of the sternal retractor; this structure must be dissected free from the sternum as well. Dissection of any IMAs to be used as grafts should then be accomplished. After the IMA graft or grafts are available or when not used, the aorta must be the first structure sought in the mediastinum, particularly if the femoral vessels have not been exposed or cannulated. Once the ascending aorta is identified and isolated, arterial cannulation should be accomplished. Aortic cannulation affords optimal access for transfusion and for rapid institution of cardiopulmonary bypass in the event of uncontrolled entry into the heart or great vessels during subsequent dissection. Choosing a site distal to the prior cannulation site will leave more space on the proximal aorta for proximal anastomoses and a cardioplegia cannula. A minimal but adequate portion of the right atrium is then dissected to allow placement of venous return and retrograde cardioplegia cannulae. Tightly adherent pericardium at the site of prior cannulation may be left and dissection continued in an extrapericardial plane, if care is taken to avoid damage to the phrenic nerve. After cardiopulmonary bypass is initiated, systemic hypothermia is induced to 28° C. or 26° C. The IMA is dissected only enough so that a light clamp may be applied to limit cardiac warming during arrest. An antegrade cardioplegia cannula placed in the aorta allows the initial dose of cardioplegia to be given antegrade, which provides cardioplegia to regions subtended by patent grafts. A myocardial temperature probe will guide initial and subsequent cardioplegia administration to maintain septal myocardial temperature less than 12° C to 14° C. Dissection of the heart and SVGs is continued under cardioplegic arrest. Patent SVGs are divided at the distal anastomosis to limit embolism from friable atheromatous debris. Further cardioplegia is administered through the retrograde coronary sinus catheter, which may help to float atheromatous debris from the coronary arteries and also provide cardioplegia to regions with limited coronary arterial perfusion. Distal and proximal anastomoses are then constructed. If retrograde cardioplegia is not used, then antegrade cardioplegia may be administered after each distal anastomosis is completed. Sequential construction of distal and proximal anastomoses allows delivery of antegrade cardioplegia to be administered to each region of the heart supplied by the newly completed grafts. The IMA anastomosis is completed; and after exclusion of air from the ascending aorta, the cross clamp is removed. Constructing the proximal anastomoses during a single period of aortic cross clamp limits manipulation of the aorta, allows perfusion of cardioplegia into each graft as it is constructed, and allows immediate perfusion of myocardium after removing the aortic cross clamp. The risk for embolization of aortic atheromatous debris and subsequent neurologic morbidity may be decreased. The cross-clamp time is longer, but with retrograde cardioplegia morbidity and mortality have not been increased despite application to a higher risk population.[28, 45]

Retrograde cardioplegia has been developed to the point of being a routine adjunct, particularly with the use of the coronary sinus catheter. Although cardioplegic arrest may be accomplished by retrograde infusion solely,[20] some authors believe that a combination of antegrade and retrograde cardioplegia is optimal.[28, 42] The controversial topic of cardioplegia temperature and composition is beyond the scope of this discussion. Although reoperative CABG can be accomplished without the use of cardiopulmonary bypass,[15] use of this technique is limited to a very few patients who may be candidates.[12] Limitations include the safety of sternal re-entry without availability of cardiopulmonary bypass, management of patent SVGs, the requirement of large target vessels, and possible inadequacy of myocardial protection.

PATENT GRAFTS

Patent SVGs present a particular danger in reoperative procedures. These conduits may be injured during sternal re-entry, may be a source of atheroembolism, and are at risk for later stenosis or thrombosis if not replaced. Untimely division of patent grafts forces a period of normothermic ischemia, and, in patients totally dependent on graft flow because of total occlusion of the native circulation, coronary flow interruption represents a grave event. The risk of myocardial infarction in the presence of patent vein grafts is as high as 19%, which may be due in part to graft atheroembolism. This is a frequently discussed event, however, and emboli have been less frequently documented.[19, 22, 39] It is logical to consider early division of grafts that will be replaced to limit this risk of embolization. Although division before the first dose of antegrade cardioplegia has been recommended to limit embolization, this practice has little demonstrated benefit and has the disadvantage of limiting initial cardioplegia delivery, subsequent cooling, and cardiac arrest. A more critical decision concerns the replacement of a patent SVG. There is little question that most SVGs that are patent and have critical stenoses should be replaced. Because actual atherosclerotic involvement of SVGs is much worse than the angiographic appearance, some authors recommend replacing all SVGs regardless of age or angiographic appearance.[33] Still others recommend that only SVGs with demonstrable stenoses greater than 20% be replaced. Stenoses in SVGs progress at a much more rapid pace than lesions in the native coronary circulation, particularly later than 5 years postoperatively. Because this is the period that atherosclerosis affects SVG, angiographic assurance of normality may give a false sense of security. Despite angiographic evidence that 53% of SVGs patent with minimal disease at 6 years remain so at follow-up 5 years thereafter, 39% demonstrate greater than 35% stenosis and 29% have occlusion or stenosis greater than 70%. Most authors recommend that SVGs older than 5 years be replaced.

A specific problem is the presence of a stenosed SVG to a totally occluded LAD artery. In patients in whom the SVG was replaced by the IMA, 16% to 19% developed a hypoperfusion syndrome in the anterior circulation.[37, 52] This syndrome is diagnosed by the presence of anterior ischemia, sudden hypotension, elevated filling pressures, diminished contractility, and ventricular dysrhythmias.[37] Patients with this syndrome who were managed medically had an extremely high mortality, whereas those patients returned to the operating room for placement of an additional SVG to the LAD artery or replacement of the IMA with an SVG had no mortality. To decide optimal management of a stenotic SVG to an occluded LAD artery, the outcome of patients with this anatomy were compared. Treatment was either replacement of the stenotic, patent vein graft with a new SVG, an IMA and SVG, or an IMA alone or placement of an IMA graft without disturbing the original stenotic SVG. The lowest mortality and myocardial infarction rates occurred in the group of patients where the stenotic SVG is left in place and a distal IMA anastomosis constructed. This approach presumably gives the IMA time to hypertrophy or dilate as the SVG stenoses farther and does not predispose the IMA to early closure. Twenty of 22 IMAs were patent at a mean of 58 months.[52]

RESULTS

The mortality of reoperative coronary surgery has progressively improved over time but still exceeds that of primary CABG.[26, 43] Mortality varies by institution, with lower mortality achieved by greater experience. Mortality for reoperative CABG ranges from 2.9% to 9.7% for all patients. In comparison to primary CABG in which mortality was most often the result of end organ failure, mortality after reoperation (78% to 82%) occurs almost exclusively as a result of cardiac causes. Mortality in a group of patients defined as high risk, by the postoperative requirement of intra-aortic balloon counterpulsation, was 9.5%, whereas mortality in the group in whom no balloon counterpulsation was required was 0.9%.

Morbid events occurring after reoperative bypass were more likely in patients with NYHA Class III/IV symptoms, in patients undergoing emergent procedures, and in the presence of left main coronary artery or three-vessel disease. These complications include a greater volume of shed mediastinal blood, a higher rate of intra-aortic balloon counterpulsation (4.5% to 8%), a higher risk of requiring reoperation for mediastinal bleeding or tamponade, and higher myocardial infarction and pulmonary complication rates in comparison to primary CABG.[3, 26, 43] Bleeding is increased because of the greater raw surface area exposed during lysis of adhesions and mobilization of the heart and because of the longer cardiopulmonary bypass times. Reinfusion of shed mediastinal blood postoperatively is beneficial in reducing transfusion of bank blood products.[35] Adhering to defined transfusion indications, tolerance of relative anemia, combining hemodilution with use of autologous donation in the operating room before anticoagulation, limiting preoperative aspirin use, reinfusion of intraoperative shed blood, and use of medical adjuncts are further methods of reducing transfusion requirements.[35, 38] The serine protease inhibitor aprotinin has a demonstrated benefit in reducing chest tube output, total donor exposures, and total transfusion requirements after reoperative coronary procedure.[4, 11, 25] This medication remains very expensive but may be cost effective in reoperative cases in which the risk of requiring transfusion is known to be higher.

The increased incidence of myocardial infarction in reoperations (2.1% to 6.9%) may result from inadequate myocardial protection during aortic cross clamping, atheroembolism, or incomplete revascularization. Myocardial infarction is twice as prevalent in reoperations as in primary coronary procedures.[26, 44] Myocardial creatine kinase is also more markedly elevated after reoperation.[44] Myocardial protection may be compromised by cardiac warming through enhanced noncoronary cardiac collateral blood flow, the presence of a patent IMA graft, and more diffuse disease limiting cardioplegia delivery. Retrograde cardioplegia techniques have reduced the incidence of myocardial infarction and requirements for intra-aortic balloon counterpulsation.[20, 28, 42] Complete revascularization is less likely in reoperative cases as compared with primary procedures (75% vs. 90%). Pericardial reaction from the first procedure and more diffuse coronary artery disease limit the number and identification of adequate bypass targets.[29] Atheroembolism from patent, atherosclerotic vein grafts has an unknown true incidence. Studies examining this phenomenon are limited by the small number of patients examined, the inability to determine the etiology of myocardial infarction in living patients, and the inability to assign a period of maximal risk for embolization during the perioperative period. Necropsy examination of 27 patients who had postoperative myocardial infarction demonstrated no distal embolization.[32] Perioperative myocardial infarction after primary CABG increases the risk for further cardiac events when combined with poor left ventricular function or incomplete revascularization and diminishes event-free survival.[16] The effect of perioperative myocardial infarction on survival from reoperation has not been elucidated.

Survival and freedom from angina are diminished after reoperative coronary bypass surgery in comparison to primary CABG. Survival is 66% to 90% at 5 years and 35% to 88% at 10 years.[2, 6, 26, 29, 32, 52] Survival is significantly enhanced by construction of an IMA to LAD artery anastomosis and good preoperative ventricular function. The factors that decrease survival 10 years after operation include advanced age (>65), more severe anginal symptoms, left main coronary artery occlusion, poor left ventricular function, angiographic indications for surgery of native vessel disease and graft failure, and an absence of an IMA graft placed at either primary or repeat operation.

Return of angina occurs at a rate of 47% for the first year after reoperation, much greater than the 20% rate for primary CABG.[6] Anginal symptoms recur thereafter at an annual rate similar to primary CABG (2.8% vs. 2.7%). The cumulative rate of return of angina is 66% and 75% after 5 and 10 years, respectively.[6, 44] Patients who have Class I-II angina preoperatively are likely to maintain their low level of symptoms. Patients who have severe angina (Class III-IV) preoperatively are more likely to have return of severe angina postoperatively.[26] Evaluation of SVGs after primary CABG reveals hypercholesterolemia and hypertension as particularly important determinants of graft failure. Appropriate risk factor modification may ameliorate the effects of these disease processes.

Repeat reoperation may be accomplished in a select subset of patients. Severe ischemia must be documented by a functional study. Mortality in this group was higher (12%) than either primary or first-reoperation CABG and was the result of cardiac causes in 78% of one series of 150 patients.[5] These patients are at higher risk for injury of vital structures during sternal re-entry (10%). This population is likewise at high risk for incomplete revascularization given their greater propensity for diffuse coronary disease. The requirement of multiple endarterectomies confirmed the diffuse nature of these patients' native disease and was a risk factor for postoperative mortality. Additional risk factors for mortality were similar to initial reoperation and include ejection fraction less than 40% and age greater than 65. Morbid events of pulmonary complications and reoperation for postoperative bleeding were higher in this group than after primary or initial reoperation. The 5-year survival of 76% in this difficult group of patients indicates that repeat reoperation can be accomplished, but with a further increment in the risk of morbidity and mortality above that of initial coronary reoperation.

SELECTED REFERENCES

Coltharp, W. H.: Internal mammary artery graft at reoperation: Risks, benefits, and methods of preservation. Ann. Thorac. Surg., 52:225, 1991.
This analysis of over 400 patients details the advantages of use of the internal mammary artery as a coronary artery bypass graft at reoperation. A prior internal

mammary graft did not increase the risk of reoperation and better preserved left ventricular function.

Cosgrove, D. M.: Predictors of reoperation after myocardial revascularization. J. Thorac. Cardiovasc. Surg., 92:811, 1986.
This series from the Cleveland Clinic details the predictors of survival and reoperation in 8000 patients with 99.5% follow-up.

Lytle, B. W.: Coronary reoperations. Coron. Artery Dis., 4:703, 1993.
This report reviews the current approach of the Cleveland Clinic, reviewing indications, myocardial protection, and treatment of patent saphenous vein grafts.

Savage, E. B.: "No touch" dissection, antegrade-retrograde blood cardioplegia, and single aortic cross-clamp significantly reduce operative mortality of reoperative CABG. Circulation, 90:II–140, 1994.
This report details the effect of institution of a number of techniques on the mortality of reoperation in a consecutive series of 131 patients.

Weintraub, W. S.: Frequency of repeat coronary bypass or coronary angioplasty after CABG using saphenous venous grafts. Am. J. Cardiol., 73:103, 1994.
This report of nearly 3500 patients examines the predictors of cardiac events and reoperation after saphenous vein only CABG. The critical effect of risk factors for atherosclerosis on graft function and survival is demonstrated. Highly detailed tables and figures are presented with subset analysis and 12-year follow-up.

REFERENCES

1. Akins, C. W., Buckley, M. J., Daggett, W. M., Hilgenberg, A. D., Vlahakes, G. J., Torchiana, D. F., and Austen, W. G.: Reoperative coronary grafting: Changing patients profiles, operative indication, techniques, and results. Ann. Thorac. Surg., 58:359, 1994.
2. Akl, E. S., Ozdogan, E., Ohri, S. K., Barbir, M., Kiti-Chei, Gaer, J. A. R., Mitchell, A. G., and Yacoub, M. H.: Early and long term results of reoperation for coronary artery disease. Br. Heart J., 68:176, 1992.
3. Baillot, R. G., Loop, F. D., Cosgrove, D. M., and Lytle, B. W.: Reoperation after previous grafting with the internal mammary artery: Technique and early results. Ann. Thorac. Surg., 40:271, 1985.
4. Bidstrup, B. P., Harrison, J., Royston, D., Taylor, K. M., and Treasure, T.: Aprotinin therapy in cardiac operations: A report on use in 41 cardiac centers in the United Kingdom. Ann. Thorac. Surg., 55:971, 1993.
5. Brenowitz, J. B., Johnson, W. D., Kayser, K. L., Saedi, S. F., Dorros, G., and Schley, L.: Coronary artery bypass grafting for the third time or more. Circulation, 78:II–166, 1988.
6. Cameron, A., Kemp, H. G., and Green, G. E.: Reoperation for coronary artery disease: 10 years of clinical follow-up. Circulation, 78:I–158, 1988.
7. Campeau, L., Enjalbert, M., Lesperance, J., Bourassa, M. G., Kwiterovich, P., Wacholder, S., and Sniderman, A.: The relation of risk factors to the development of atherosclerosis in saphenous-vein bypass grafts and the progression of disease in the native circulation. N. Engl. J. Med., 311:1329, 1984.
8. Campos, E. E., Cinderella, J. A., and Farhi, E. R.: Long-term angiographic follow-up of normal and minimally diseased saphenous vein grafts. J. Am. Coll. Cardiol., 21:1175, 1993.
9. Coltharp, W. H., Decker, M. D., Lea, J. W., Petracek, M. R., Galssford, D. M., Thomas, C. S., Burrus, G. R., Alford, W. C., and Stoney, W. S.: Internal mammary artery graft at reoperation: Risks, benefits, and methods of preservation. Ann. Thorac. Surg., 52:225, 1991.
10. Cosgrove, D. M., Loop, F. D., Lytle, B. W., Gill, C. C., Golding, L. A. R., Gibson, C., Stewart, R. W., Taylor, P. C., and Goormastic, M.: Predictors of reoperation after myocardial revascularization. J. Thorac. Cardiovasc. Surg., 92:811, 1986.
11. Cosgrove, D. M., Heric, B., Lytle, B. W., Taylor, P. C., Novoa, R., Golding, L. A. R., Stewart, R. W., McCarthy, P. M., and Loop, F. D.: Aprotinin therapy for reoperative myocardial revascularization: A placebo-controlled study. Ann. Thorac. Surg., 54:1031, 1992.
12. Cosgrove, D. M.: Is coronary reoperation without the pump an advantage? Ann. Thorac. Surg., 55:329, 1993.
13. deFeyter, P., van Suylen, R. J., deJaegere, P. P. T., Topol, E. J., and Serruys, P. W.: Balloon angioplasty for the treatment of lesions in saphenous vein bypass grafts. J. Am. Coll. Cardiol., 21:1539, 1993.
14. Dobell, A. R. C., and Jain, A. K.: Catastrophic hemorrhage during redo sternotomy. Ann. Thorac. Surg., 37:273, 1984.
15. Fanning, W. J., Kakos, G. S., and Williams, T. E.: Reoperative coronary artery bypass grafting without cardiopulmonary bypass. Ann. Thorac. Surg., 55:486, 1993.
16. Force, T., Hibberd, P., Weeks, G., Kemper, A. J., Bloomfield, P., Tow, D., Josa, M., Khuri, S., and Parisi, A. F.: Perioperative myocardial infarction after coronary artery bypass surgery: Clinical significance and approach to risk stratification. Circulation, 82:903, 1990.
17. Galbut, D. L., Traad, E. A., Dorman, M. J., DeWitt, P. L., Larsen, P. B., Durlansky, P. A., Button, J. H., Ally, J. M., and Gentsh, T. O.: Bilateral internal mammary artery grafts in reoperative and primary coronary bypass surgery. Ann. Thorac. Surg., 52:20, 1991.
18. Gall, S. A., Owen, C. H., Clements, F. M., and McCann, R. L.: Revascularization of the internal mammary artery after coronary artery bypass grafting. Ann. Thorac. Surg., 60:186, 1995.

19. Grondin, C. M., Pomar, J. L., Hebert, Y., Bosch, X., Santos, J. M., Enjalbert, M., and Campeau, L.: Reoperation in patients with patent atherosclerotic coronary vein grafts. J. Thorac. Cardiovasc. Surg., 87:379, 1984.
20. Gundry, S. R., Razzouk, A. J., Vigesaa, R. E., Wang, N., and Bailey, L. L.: Optimal delivery of cardioplegic solution for "redo" operations. J. Thorac. Cardiovasc. Surg., 103:896, 1992.
21. Kahn, J. K., Rutherford, B. D., McConahay, D. R., Johnson, W. L., Giorgi, L. V., Shimshak, T. M., and Hartzler, G. O.: Outcome following emergency coronary artery bypass grafting for failed elective balloon coronary angioplasty in patients with prior coronary bypass. Am. J. Cardiol., 66:285, 1990.
22. Keon, W. J., Heggtveit, H. A., and Leduc, J.: Perioperative myocardial infarction caused by atheroembolism. J. Thorac. Cardiovasc. Surg., 84:849, 1982.
23. Laub, G. W., Muralidharan, S., Clancy, R., Eldredge, W. J., Chen, C., Adkins, M. S., Fernandez, J., Anderson, W. A., and McGrath, L. B.: Cryopreserved allograft veins as alternative coronary artery bypass conduits: Early phase results. Ann. Thorac. Surg., 54:826, 1992.
24. Lemmer, J. H., Ferguson, D. W., Rakei, B. A., and Rossi, N. P.: Clinical outcome of emergency repeat coronary artery bypass surgery. J. Cardiovasc. Surg., 31:492, 1990.
25. Lemmer, J. H., Stanford, W., Bonney, S. L., Breen, J. F., Chomka, E. V., Eldredge, W. J., Holt, W. W., Karp, R. B., Laub, G. W., Lipton, J. J., Schaff, H. V., Tatooles, C. J., and Rumberger, J. A.: Aprotinin for coronary bypass operations: Efficacy, safety, and influence on early saphenous vein graft patency. J. Thorac. Cardiovasc. Surg., 107:543, 1994.
26. Loop, F. D., Lytle, B. W., Cosgrove, D. M., Woods, E. L., Stewart, R. W., Golding, L. A. R., Goormastic, M., and Taylor, P. C.: Reoperation for coronary atherosclerosis. Ann. Surg., 212:378, 1990.
27. Loop, F. D., Lytle, B. W., and Cosgrove, D. M.: Bilateral internal thoracic artery grafting in reoperations. Ann. Thorac. Surg., 52:3, 1991.
28. Loop, F. D., Higgins, T. L., Panda, R., Pearce, G., and Estafanous, F. G.: Myocardial protection during cardiac operations. J. Thorac. Cardiovasc. Surg., 104:608, 1992.
29. Lytle, B. W., Loop, F. D., Cosgrove, D. M., Taylor, P. C., Goormastic, M., Peper, W., Gill, C. C., Golding, L. A. R., and Stewart, R. W.: Fifteen hundred coronary reoperations: Results and determinants of early and late survival. J. Thorac. Cardiovasc. Surg., 93:847, 1987.
30. Lytle, B. W., Loop, F. D., Taylor, P. C., Simpfendorfer, C., Kramer, J. R., Ratliff, N. B., Goormastic, M., and Cosgrove, D. M.: Vein graft disease: The clinical impact of stenoses in saphenous vein bypass grafts to coronary arteries. J. Thorac. Cardiovasc. Surg., 103:831, 1992.
31. Lytle, B. W.: Coronary reoperations. Coron. Artery Dis., 4:703, 1993.
32. Lytle, B. W., McElroy, D., McCarthy, P., Loop, F. D., Taylor, P. C., Goormastic, M., Stewart, R. S., and Cosgrove, D. M.: Influence of arterial coronary bypass grafts on the mortality in coronary reoperations. J. Thorac. Cardiovasc. Surg., 107:675, 1994.
33. Marshall, W. G., Saffitz, J., and Kouchoukos, N. T.: Management during reoperation of aortocoronary saphenous vein grafts with minimal atherosclerosis by angiography. Ann. Thorac. Surg., 42:163, 1986.
34. Mestres, C. A., Rives, A., Igual, A., Vehi, C., and Murtra, M.: Atherosclerosis of the internal mammary artery: Histopathological analysis and implications on its results in coronary artery bypass graft surgery. Thorac. Cardiovasc. Surg., 34:356, 1986.
35. Morris, J. J., and Tan, Y. S.: Autotransfusion: Is there a benefit in a current practice of aggressive blood conservation? Ann. Thorac. Surg., 58:502, 1994.
36. Najm, H. K., Leddy, D., Hendry, P. J., Marquis, J. F., Richardson, D., and Keon, W. J.: Postoperative symptomatic internal thoracic artery stenosis and successful treatment with PTCA. Ann. Thorac. Surg., 59:323, 1995.
37. Navia, D., Cosgrove, D. M., Lytle, B. W., Taylor, P. C., McCarthy, P. M., Stewart, R. W., Rosenkranz, E. R., and Loop, F. D.: Is the internal thoracic artery the conduit of choice to replace a stenotic vein graft? Ann. Thorac. Surg., 57:40, 1994.
38. Paone, G., Spencer, T., and Silverman, N. A.: Blood conservation in coronary artery surgery. Surgery, 115:672, 1994.
39. Perrault, L., Carrier, M., Cartier, R., LeClerc, Y., Hebert, Y., Diaz, O. S., and Pelletier, C.: Morbidity and mortality of reoperation for coronary artery bypass grafting: Significance of atheromatous vein grafts. Can. J. Cardiol., 7:427, 1991.
40. Popma, J. J., Cooke, R. H., Leon, M. B., Start, K., Satler, L. F., Kent, K. M., Hunn, D., and Prichard, A. D.: Immediate procedural and long-term clinical results of internal mammary artery angioplasty. Am. J. Cardiol., 69:1237, 1992.
41. Reeves, F., Bonan, R., Cote, G., Crepeau, J., deGuise, P., Gosselin, G., Campeau, L., and Lesperance, J.: Long-term angiographic follow-up after angioplasty of venous coronary bypass grafts. Am. Heart J., 122:620, 1991.
42. Rosengart, T. K., Krieger, K., Lang, S. J., Gold, J. P., Altorki, N., Roussel, M., Debois, W. J., and Isom, O. W.: Reoperative coronary artery bypass surgery: Improved preservation of myocardial function with retrograde cardioplegia. Circulation, 88:II–330, 1993.
43. Rosengart, T. K.: Risk analysis of primary versus reoperative coronary artery bypass grafting. Ann. Thorac. Surg., 56:S–74, 1993.
44. Salomon, N. W., Page, U. S., Bigelow, J. C., Krause, A. H., Okies, J. E., and Metzdorff, M. T.: Reoperative coronary surgery. J. Thorac. Cardiovasc. Surg., 100:250, 1990.
45. Savage, E. B., and Cohn, L. H.: "No touch" dissection, antegrade-retrograde blood cardioplegia, and single aortic cross-clamp significantly reduce operative mortality of reoperative CABG. Circulation, 90:II–140, 1994.
46. Sellke, F. W., Stanford, W., and Rossi, N. P.: Failure of cryopreserved saphenous vein allografts following coronary artery bypass surgery. J. Cardiovasc. Surg., 32:820, 1991.
47. Sisto, T., and Isola, J.: Incidence of atherosclerosis in the internal mammary artery. Ann. Thorac. Surg., 47:884, 1989.
48. Sketch, M. H., Quigley, P. J., Perez, J. A., Davidson, C. J., Muhlestein, J. B., Herndon, J. E., Glower, D. D., Philips, H. R., Califf, R. M., and Stack, R. S.: Angiographic follow-up after internal mammary artery graft angioplasty. Am. J. Cardiol., 70:401, 1992.
49. Solymoss, B. C., Nadeau, P., Millette, D., and Campeau, L.: Late thrombosis of saphenous vein coronary bypass grafts related to risk factors. Circulation, 78:I–140, 1988.
50. Solymoss, B. C., Leung, T. K., Pelletier, L. C., and Campeau, L.: Pathologic changes in coronary artery saphenous vein grafts and related etiologic factors. Cardiovasc. Clin., 21:45, 1991.
51. Stoney, W. S., Alford, W. C., Burrus, G. R., Glassford, D. M., Petracek, M. R., and Thomas, C. S.: The fate of arm veins used for aorto-coronary bypass grafts. J. Thorac. Cardiovasc. Surg., 88:522, 1984.
52. Turner, F. E., Lytle, B. W., Navia, D., Loop, F. D., Taylor, P. C., McCarthy, P. M., Stewart, R. W., Rosenkranz, E. R., and Cosgrove, D. M.: Coronary reoperation: Results of adding an internal mammary artery graft to a stenotic vein graft. Ann. Thorac. Surg., 58:1353, 1994.
53. Uppal, R., Mills, N. L., Wechsler, A. S., and Smith, P. K. 1993 Update: Left thoracotomy for reoperative coronary artery bypass procedures. Ann. Thorac. Surg., 55:1275, 1993.
54. Uppal, R., Wolfe, W. G., Lowe, J. E., and Smith, P. K.: Right thoracotomy for reoperative right coronary artery bypass procedures. Ann. Thorac. Surg., 57:123, 1994.
55. Weintraub, W. S., Jones, E. L., Carver, J. M., and Guyton, R. A.: Frequency of repeat coronary bypass or coronary angioplasty after coronary artery bypass surgery using saphenous venous grafts. Am. J. Cardiol., 73:103, 1994.
56. Wijnberg, D. S., Boeve, W. J., Ebels, T., van Gelder, I. C., van den Toren, E. W., Lie, K. I., and van der Heide, J. N. H.: Patency of arm vein grafts used in aorto-coronary bypass surgery. Eur. J. Cardiothorac. Surg., 4:510, 1990.

RADIONUCLIDE EVALUATION OF CORONARY ARTERY DISEASE

Robert H. Jones, M.D.

HISTORICAL ASPECTS

The first use of radioactive tracers to assess any biologic process in man was for evaluation of blood flow. More than 60 years ago, Blumgart and associates injected radon gas into the veins of normal subjects and patients with a variety of cardiac disorders to measure transit times throughout the cardiovascular system.[3] The crude technology then available for detecting radiation and lack of an apparent clinical use for these measurements caused this early insightful work to lapse into obscurity. In 1948, Prinzmetal and colleagues used newly developed single-probe detectors to quantitate passage of a bolus of radioactive sodium through the heart and named this rediscovered procedure radiocardiography.[21] Continued improvement in technology renewed interest in use of radionuclide indicator-dilution curves for calculation of cardiac output and measurement of intracardiac shunts in patients.[20] Soon after their development, gamma cameras were used to image individual cardiac chambers as tracer flowed through the heart.[2] The potential was soon recognized for these instruments to be interfaced with computers to obtain data with sufficient anatomic resolution to provide indicator-dilution curves from individual cardiac chambers.[13, 17]

BASIC PRINCIPLES
Cardiac Function Measurements

Initial transit radionuclide angiocardiography has evolved as a useful clinical modality applied primarily to measure left

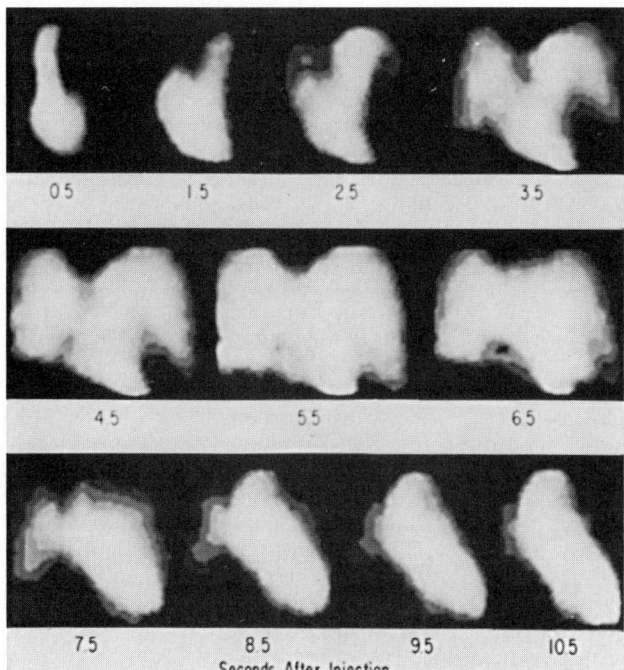

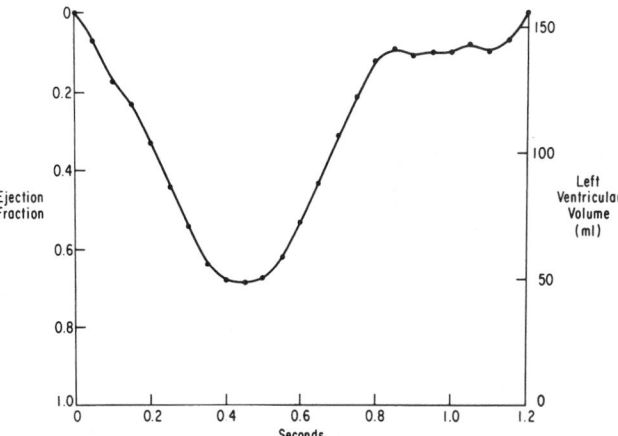

Figure 54–128. A representative cardiac cycle was constructed from radionuclide data obtained during several individual contractions during the initial passage of tracer through the left ventricle. The volume changes are expressed as fractional changes. In addition, planimetry of the end-diastolic image provides an end-diastolic volume in milliliters, so that the volume curve can also be calibrated as an absolute change in volume relative to time. The rapid increase in volume during end diastole reflects left atrial contraction.

Figure 54–126. Serial 1-second images each composed of 20 0.05-second data frames depict the progression of the tracer bolus through the central circulation in the anterior view. The rapid transit through the heart is apparent by the almost complete clearance of counts from the right ventricle during the time when count rates are maximal in the left ventricle.

ventricular function.[14, 27] This technique requires intravenous injection of a single bolus of radioactive tracer using a high-sensitivity gamma camera for precordial counting at brief intervals, usually 25 milliseconds. Dynamic counting images blood flow through the right side of the heart, lungs, and left side of the heart (Fig. 54–126). To construct left ventriculograms, computer processing combines phasically related counts from within the left ventricle during several cardiac cycles into an averaged cardiac beat that has greater spatial and temporal resolution than the individual beats (Fig. 54–127). After subtraction of background counts arising outside the left ventricle, the remaining left ventricular count changes reflect relative left ventricular volume changes during the cardiac cycle (Fig. 54–128). Geometric assumptions commonly used to derive cardiac volumes from contrast medium–enhanced ventriculograms can also be applied to radionuclide images to calculate absolute left ventricular volumes. Radionuclide measurements of ejection fraction and cardiac chamber volumes and volumetric cardiac output compare favorably with contrast medium–enhanced ventriculogram measurements. Technology for performing initial-transit radionuclide angiocardiography has been well standardized and is commercially available. Newer instrumentation is portable and can be taken into the operating room and intensive care units to measure cardiac function in surgical patients. Moreover, introduction of a high-fidelity micromanometer into the left ventricle to record pressure simultaneously during radionuclide volume measurement permits the construction of pressure-volume loops that more completely characterize systolic and diastolic left ventricular function than use of either pressure or volume parameters alone (Fig. 54–129).[23]

Standard gamma cameras do not have sufficient counting sensitivity to image the heart from data recorded during the 5 to 10 cardiac beats when an injected tracer bolus first passes through the heart. An alternate approach of gated cardiac imaging acquires data after injected labeled red blood cells reach equilibrium within the blood pool. A simultaneous electrocardiogram synchronizes acquisition of radionuclide data with the appropriate phase of each of the 100 to 300 heartbeats as counts are added to form a single averaged cardiac beat, which is used to image cardiac motion and calculate ejection fraction. An advantage of gated equilibrium over initial transit cardiac imaging is that it does not require specific instrumentation or a discrete bolus injection. However, the 2 to 3 minutes required to acquire the gated image makes the approach less well suited than the initial transit

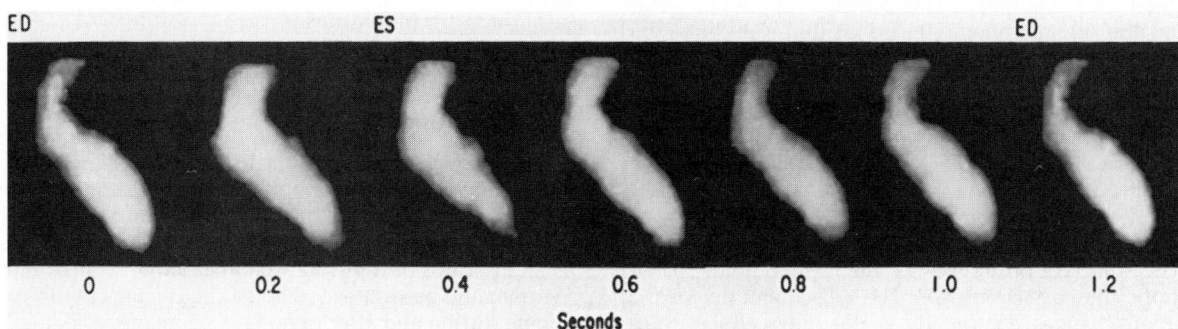

Figure 54–127. Serial images of the spatial distribution of counts taken from the representative cardiac cycle in Figure 54–128 depict normal left ventricular wall motion.

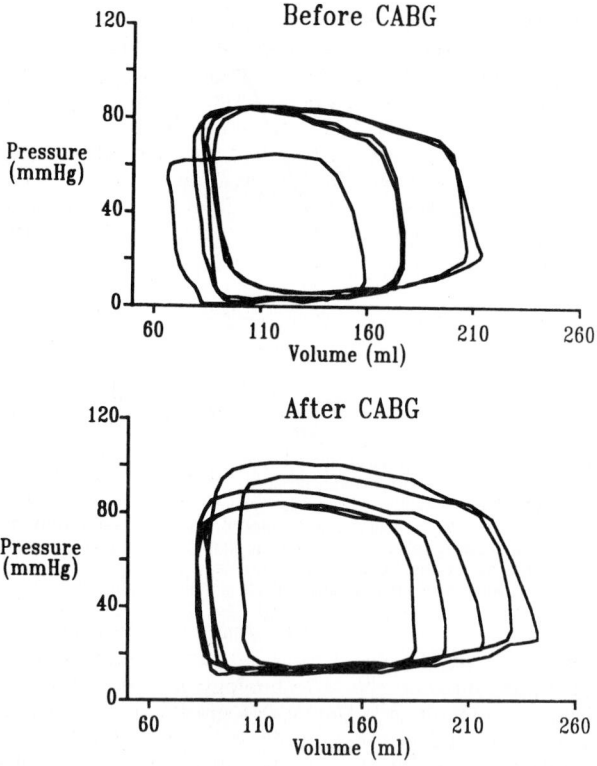

Figure 54–129. Pressure-volume loops obtained at different levels of filling before and immediately after coronary artery bypass grafting show minimal depression of left ventricular function immediately after myocardial revascularization.

technique for measuring cardiac function during periods of rapid change in cardiac function, such as during exercise or pharmacologic intervention. Moreover, cardiac volume calculations are less accurate and reproducible using the gated technique because of higher background, which results when tracer is at equilibrium in the blood pool. Measurement of cardiac volumes using the gated equilibrium technique also requires withdrawal of a blood sample at equilibrium to relate observed counts to absolute cardiac volumes, and this step is not required using the initial transit approach.

Myocardial Perfusion and Metabolism Measurements

Radionuclide methods for noninvasive regional myocardial blood flow measurement are based on the observation of Saperstein that tissue content of any tracer with a high extraction rate during initial capillary transit is primarily determined by blood flow.[25] This principle applies to potassium and the similar cationic tracers cesium, rubidium, and thallium, which accumulate in myocardium proportional to blood flow after intravenous injection. Love first reported use of rubidium-86 in dogs and humans for estimation of myocardial perfusion. Currently, the potassium analog thallium-201 with a half-life of 73 hours and photon energy of about 69 and 83 keV. is the most widely used radionuclide for evaluation of regional myocardial perfusion.

After intravenous injection, thallium-201 attains a high initial myocardial concentration as the initial bolus passes through the coronary circulation. The subsequent myocardial distribution changes continually as the intracellular tracer exchanges with that remaining in the blood pool. Therefore, the distribution of thallium-201 during the first few minutes

after injection closely reflects regional myocardial blood flow but several hours after injection more closely resembles the potassium content of the heart. This characteristic of thallium-201 is used to obtain exercise and delayed redistribution images from a single tracer injection. A large clinical experience with thallium-201 has documented the value and limitations of myocardial scintigraphy in patients with myocardial infarction and ischemia.[7] Technetium-99m–labeled myocardial perfusion agents with superior physical characteristics for imaging are growing in popularity over thallium-201 for measuring the distribution of coronary blood flow.[5]

The interaction of specific radiopharmaceuticals with the heart may be used to study regional myocardial metabolism. During myocardial infarction, calcium ions accumulate within injured myocardial cells. The affinity of technetium-99m pyrophosphate for calcium results in a high accumulation of this tracer in infarcted myocardium.[4] More recently, labeled monoclonal antibodies that react with myosin and fibrin have been developed that show promise for detecting myocardial cell breakdown and intravascular thrombosis.[10] Cyclotron production of positron-emitting radiopharmaceuticals containing radioisotopes of carbon, oxygen, nitrogen, and fluorine now permit investigation of the full array of biochemical pathways in the myocardium.[26] In addition to measurement of blood flow, regional myocardial accumulation and utilization of glucose, fatty acids, and amino acids can be assessed. Future application of these techniques is certain to enhance understanding of abnormal cardiac metabolism in patients with cardiac disorders.

Images of the distribution of a radioactive tracer in the heart detected by a gamma camera represent two-dimensional projections of counts arising from three dimensions of the cardiac volume. Simultaneous interpretation of several images obtained from different projections offers reasonable approximation of the three-dimensional counts distribution in the heart. The most quantitative approach now available for imaging three-dimensional cardiac counts is single photon emission computed tomography (SPECT). During SPECT imaging, the gamma camera detector encircles the patient and data from these multiple projections are later reconstructed into a three-dimensional representation of counts. These counts matrices can be quantitated by comparison with normal standards or visually interpreted as a series of heart slice images. The accurate regional quantitation of counts provided by SPECT imaging adds objectivity to radionuclide measurements of regional perfusion and metabolism.

Positron emission tomography (PET) is a technique that also uses a number of detectors encircling a patient to image positron emitting tracers. Positron decay emits high-energy photons in opposite directions simultaneously, and this characteristic is used to accurately position the three-dimensional location of the original event. PET requires more expensive and complicated technology than SPECT imaging, and present applications are primarily for cardiac metabolism research.

Applications of Radionuclide Techniques in Patients with Coronary Artery Disease

Myocardial ischemia can be detected clinically by angina pectoris, electrocardiographically by ST-segment depression, and functionally by regional perfusion abnormalities and segmental contraction abnormalities with associated hemodynamic alterations. Reversible left ventricular dysfunction as an indicator of ischemia was first demonstrated in man by Herman and associates,[11] who studied patients with unstable angina during and after periods of spontaneous pain. Sharma and associates,[28] in 1976, used contrast angiography to demonstrate reversible alterations of regional left ventricular function induced by exercise and cardiac pacing. Exercise-induced left ventricular dysfunction is a very sensitive marker of ischemia, which commonly occurs before electrocardiographic abnormality as ischemia progressively increases in an individual patient (Fig. 54–130).[29] Radionuclide techniques measuring ventricular function and myocardial perfusion reflect similar biologic processes because of the close link between myocardial integrity and blood flow. Therefore, perfusion defects on myocardial scintigraphy performed during exercise, which disappear after an interval adequate for thallium-201 redistribution, are also sensitive markers of ischemia. Myocardial infarction with subsequent fibrosis decreases resting regional and global ventricular function and also results in a resting perfusion defect because of loss of myocardial mass and the lower tissue blood flow rate of fibrotic myocardium.

Soon after introduction of radionuclide tests for detecting exercise-induced perfusion defects and functional abnormalities as indicators of myocardial ischemia, enthusiastic reports suggested that the procedures were highly accurate for diagnosis of coronary artery disease. Further experience with broader populations of patients shows that rest/exercise perfusion and function tests have an accuracy that ranges between 0.75 and 0.85 for the prediction of coronary disease.[16, 24] Therefore, the severity of coronary artery disease

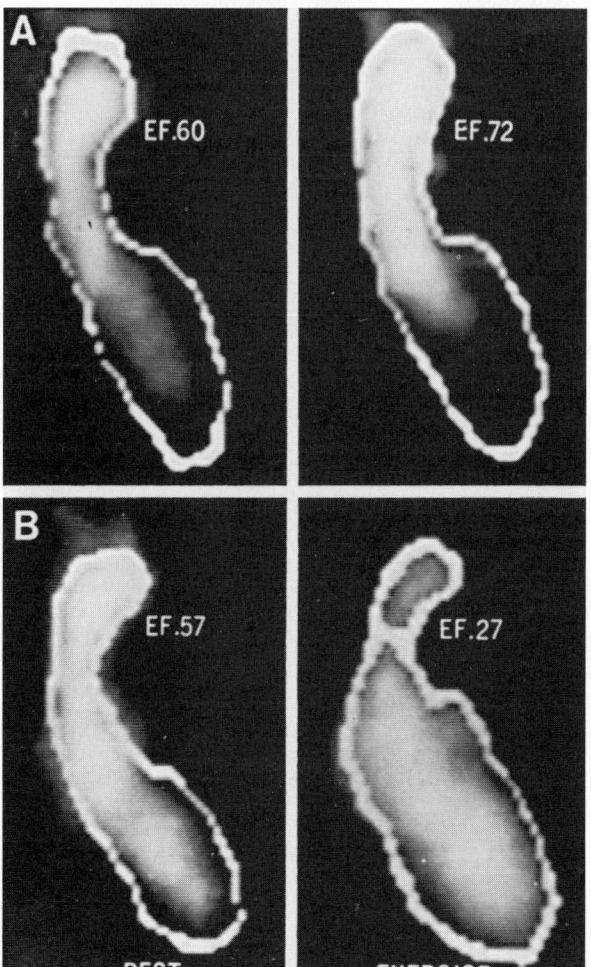

Figure 54–130. End-diastolic outlines and end-systolic images demonstrating wall motion at rest and at exercise in a normal subject *(A)* and a patient with coronary artery disease *(B)*. Patients with myocardial ischemia show marked cardiac dilatation and global hypokinesis with acute exercise.

reflected by the anatomic information from the coronary arteriogram correlates with that suggested by ischemia assessment of radionuclide stress tests in patient groups. However, consistent discrepancy occurs between the two approaches of assessment in 15% to 25% of patients with coronary artery disease. The early disappointment in lack of complete agreement between radionuclide tests and coronary angiograms has more recently come to be interpreted as a benefit, because the two forms of information appear to be complementary but independent.

Prognosis in Patients with Coronary Artery Disease

Radionuclide tests appear particularly well suited for screening large groups of patients, and individuals with the most severe abnormalities can be selected for cardiac catheterization and possible further intervention, whereas those defined to be very low risk would require catheterization in only special circumstances. In a study of 100 medically treated patients without prior myocardial infarction observed for a mean of 3.7 years, a cardiac event rate of 3% in patients with a normal thallium test and of 33% in patients with three or more defects was documented.[6] In 1689 consecutive patients with suspected coronary artery disease observed for 1 year, three variables provided independent prognostic information: (1) the number of reversible thallium defects, an extent variable; (2) the magnitude of initial reversible defect, a severity variable; and (3) the maximal heart rate achieved during exercise.[18] Combining these variables into a prognostic model categorized risk of cardiac event from a low cardiac event rate of less than 1% in patients with a normal exercise thallium study to a high event rate of 78% in patients developing severe and extensive reversible defects at a low achieved heart rate.

Multivariate analysis identified radionuclide variables related to later myocardial infarction or cardiovascular death in 386 medically treated patients.[22] The exercise ejection fraction was the most important radionuclide variable providing prognostic information in patients with coronary artery disease. These early observations have been extended in 571 medically treated patients observed for up to 10 years.[19] This analysis documented that the radionuclide angiocardiogram alone had as much prognostic information as the cardiac catheterization and added significant prognostic information even when all clinical and catheterization information was known. The exercise ejection fraction was the single most important radionuclide variable that contained 80% of the prognostic information of the test. The amount of increase in heart rate and measurement of cardiac volume provided the remaining prognostic information. Analysis of the entire population of patients undergoing radionuclide angiocardiography for evaluation of coronary artery disease, including patients undergoing and not undergoing cardiac catheterization, demonstrated equivalent prognostic power in both patient populations.[15] Curves describing survival as a function of the exercise ejection fraction showed that patients with exercise ejection fractions greater than 0.50 have a low risk of cardiac death and that risk increases progressively as ejection fraction falls below 0.50 (Fig. 54–131).

Measurement of cardiac function during exercise, and especially documentation of the exercise ejection fraction, appears to provide a very sensitive index of the magnitude of myocardial ischemia. The amount of potential myocardial ischemia is the main determinant of survival in individual patients with coronary artery disease. Interventional therapy, which is devised to reverse ischemia, can only be expected to benefit patients with a significant amount of ischemic potential. Definition of the pathologic anatomy of the coro-

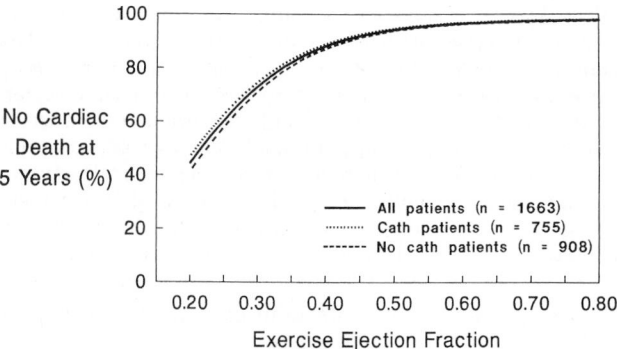

Figure 54–131. Comparison of probability of survival 5 years after radionuclide angiocardiogram as a function of exercise ejection fraction in 1663 patients evaluated for coronary artery disease, including 908 patients without and 755 patients with cardiac catheterization.

nary arterial tree by angiography is indispensable for the planning of interventional procedures and provides some insight regarding the magnitude of myocardium at potential risk. However, radionuclide measurements of ventricular function during exercise provide important independent prognostic information useful in identifying patients likely to benefit from interventional therapy.

Use of Radionuclide Angiocardiography to Document Outcome of Coronary Artery Bypass Grafting

Not every patient who survives coronary artery bypass grafting (CABG) has an optimal functional result. Even the absence of angina after surgery cannot be used as a valid endpoint, because either denervation of the heart or perioperative infarction of previously ischemic myocardium may decrease or obliterate anginal pain.

Patients with good anatomic results documented by angiography after CABG also improve exercise-induced myocardial dysfunction and perfusion deficits after successful bypass. However, coronary blood flow at rest and potential for flow augmentation during exercise cannot always be predicted from the coronary angiogram. Graft and vessel patency on arteriogram does not always correlate with improvements in regional function and perfusion. Therefore, as before operation, radionuclide tests provide important data, which are complementary but do not always duplicate the information obtained from coronary angiography. Radionuclide procedures appear useful to objectively document improvement in myocardial perfusion and function to judge effectiveness of operative outcome and predict the future clinical course of individual patients.

Radionuclide measurements of resting left ventricular function before and after CABG show 10% to 20% of patients to have a significant decrease in left ventricular function.[8] This documented loss in function is permanent and often occurs without clinical symptoms or changes suggestive of infarction on the electrocardiogram. A prospective study of 104 patients showed a surprising lack of relationship between QRS complex change on an electrocardiogram and left ventricular function after CABG.[9] Loss of left ventricular function did not relate to the duration of hypothermic cardioplegic arrest, and the etiology of this functional result probably relates to multiple causative factors that are now poorly understood. Ten to 20% of patients have significantly improved resting function after myocardial revascularization, suggesting that reversible resting ischemic dysfunction was

present before operation in the absence of resting pain. Although resting improvement in left ventricular function is modest in most patients, in some patients quite abnormal function observed before operation dramatically normalized after revascularization.

Physiologic improvement after myocardial revascularization is most consistently documented by radionuclide studies of myocardial function and perfusion during exercise. As early as 8 days after surgery, patients have been shown to greatly improve exercise left ventricular ejection fraction, and this improvement persists on later studies.[1] This early documentation of reversal of myocardial ischemia provides a useful baseline for patients who later become symptomatic. Subsequent radionuclide studies can quantify the amount of return of ischemia associated with disease progression or graft occlusion and provide a rational basis for selection of patients who might profit from repeat catheterization and consideration of another revascularization procedure.

SELECTED REFERENCE

AHA/ACC Task Force Report:. Guidelines for Clinical Use of Cardiac Radionuclide Imaging: A report of the American Heart Association/American College of Cardiology Task Force on Assessment of Diagnostic and Therapeutic Cardiovascular Procedures, Committee on Radionuclide Imaging, developed in collaboration with the American Society of Nuclear Cardiology. Circulation, 91:1278, 1995.
These comprehensive guidelines devised jointly by the American Heart Association and the American College of Cardiology summarize current indications for use of radionuclide studies in patients with cardiac disorders.

REFERENCES

1. Austin, E. H., Oldham, H. N., Jr., Sabiston, D. C., Jr., and Jones, R. H.: Early assessment of rest and exercise left ventricular function following coronary artery surgery. Ann. Thorac. Surg., 35:159, 1983.
2. Bender, M. A., and Blau, M.: The autofluoroscope. Nucleonics, 21:52, 1963.
3. Blumgart, H. L., and Weiss, S.: Clinical studies on the velocity of blood flow: The pulmonary circulation time, the velocity of venous blood flow to the heart and related aspects fo the circulation in patients with cardiovascular disease. J. Clin. Invest., 4:343, 1927.
4. Bonte, F. J., Parkey, R. W., Graham, K. D., Moore, J., and Stokely, E. M.: A new method for radionuclide imaging of myocardial infarcts. Radiology, 110:473, 1974.
5. Borges-Neto, S., Coleman, R. E., and Jones, R. H.: Perfusion and function at rest and treadmill exercise using Tc-99 sestamibi: Comparison of one- and two-day protocols in normal volunteers. J. Nucl. Med., 31:1128, 1990.
6. Brown, K. A., Boucher, C. A., Okada, R. D., Guiney, T. E., Newell, J. B., Strauss, H. W., and Pohost, G. M.: Prognostic value of exercise thallium-201 imaging in patients presenting for evaluation of chest pain. J. Am. Coll. Cardiol., 4:994, 1983.
7. Detrano, R., Janosi, A., Lyons, K. D., Marcondes, G., Abbassi, N., and Froelicher, V. F.: Factors affecting sensitivity and specificity of a diagnostic test: The exercise thallium scintigram. Am. J. Med., 84:699, 1988.
8. Floyd, R. D., Sabiston, D. C., Jr., Lee, K. L., and Jones, R. H.: The effect of duration of hypothermic cardioplegia on ventricular function. J. Thorac. Cardiovasc. Surg., 85:606, 1983.
9. Floyd, R. D., Wagner, G. S., Austin, E. H., Sabiston, D. C., Jr., and Jones, R. H.: Relation between QRS changes and left ventricular function after coronary artery bypass grafting. Am. J. Cardiol., 52:943, 1983.
10. Haber, E.: *In vivo* diagnostic and therapeutic uses of monoclonal antibodies in cardiology. Ann. Rev. Med., 37:249, 1986.
11. Herman, M. V., Heinle, R. A., Klein, M. D., and Gorlin, R.: Localized disorders in myocardial contraction: Asynergy and its role in congestive heart failure. N. Engl. J. Med., 277:222, 1967.
12. Jones, R. H., Floyd, R. D., Austin, E. H., and Sabiston, D. C., Jr.: The role of radionuclide angiocardiography in the preoperative prediction of pain relief and prolonged survival following coronary artery bypass grafting. Ann. Surg., 197:743, 1983.
13. Jones, R. H., Goodrich, J. K., and Sabiston, D. C., Jr.: Radioactive lung scanning in the diagnosis and management of pulmonary disorders. J. Thorac. Cardiovasc. Surg., 54:520, 1967.
14. Jones, R. H., Goodrich, J. K., and Sabiston, D. C., Jr.: Quantitative radionuclide angiocardiography in evaluation of cardiac function. Surg. Forum., 22:128, 1971.
15. Jones, R. H., Johnson, S. H., Bigelow, C., Pieper, K. S., Coleman, R. E., Cobb, F. R., Pryor, D. B., and Lee, K. L.: Exercise radionuclide angiocardiography

predicts cardiac death in patients with coronary artery disease. Circulation, *84*(Suppl. I):I-52, 1991.

16. Jones, R. H., McEwan, P., Newman, G. E., Port, S., Rerych, S. K., Scholz, P. M., Upton, M. T., Peter, C. A., Austin, E. H., Leong, K., Gibbons, R. J., Cobb, F. R., Coleman, R. E., and Sabiston, D. C., Jr.: The accuracy of diagnosis of coronary artery disease by radionuclide measurement of left ventricular function during rest and exercise. Circulation, *64*:586, 1981.

17. Jones, R. H., Sabiston, D. C., Jr., Bates, B. B., Morris, J. J., Anderson, P. A. W., and Goodrich, J. K.: Quantitative radionuclide angiocardiography for determination of chamber-to-chamber transit times. Am. J. Cardiol., *30*:855, 1972.

18. Ladenheim, M. L., Pollock, B. H., Rozanski, A., Berman, D. S., Staniloff, H. M., Forrester, J. S., and Diamond, G. S.: Extent and severity of myocardial hypoperfusion as predictors of prognosis in patients with suspected coronary artery disease. J. Am. Coll. Cardiol., *7*:464, 1986.

19. Lee, K. L., Pryor, D. B., Pieper, K. S., Harrell, F. E., Jr., Califf, R. M., Mark, D. B., Hlatky, M. A., Coleman, R. E., Cobb, F. R., and Jones, R. H.: The prognostic value of radionuclide angiography in medically-treated patients with coronary artery disease: A comparison with clinical and catheterization variables. Circulation, *82*:1705, 1990.

20. MacIntyre, W. J., Pritchard, W. H., Eckstein, R. W., and Friedell, H. L.: The determination of cardiac output by a continuous recording system utilizing iodinated (I-131) human serum albumin: I. Animal studies. Circulation, *4*:552, 1951.

21. Prinzmetal, M., Corday, E., Bergman, H. C., Schwartz, L., and Spritzler, R. J.: Radiocardiography: A new method for studying the blood flow through the chambers of the heart in human beings. Science, 108:340, 1948.

22. Pryor, D. B., Harrell, F. E., Jr., Lee, K. L., Califf, R. M., and Rosati, R. A.: An improving prognosis over time in medically treated patients with coronary artery disease. Am. J. Cardiol., *52*:444, 1983.

23. Purut, C. M., Sell, T. L., and Jones, R. H.: A new method to determine left ventricular pressure-volume loops in the clinical setting. J. Nucl. Med., *29*:1492, 1988.

24. Rozanski, A., and Berman, D. S.: The efficacy of cardiovascular nuclear medicine exercise studies. Semin. Nucl. Med., *17*:104, 1987.

25. Saperstein, L. A.: Regional blood flow by fractional distribution of indicators. Am. J. Physiol., *193*:161, 1958.

26. Schelbert, H. R., and Buxton, D.: Insights into coronary artery disease gained from metabolic imaging. Circulation, *78*:496, 1988.

27. Scholz, P. M., Rerych, S. K., Moran, J. F., Newman, G. E., Douglas, J. M., Jr., Sabiston, D. C., Jr., and Jones, R. H.: Quantitative radionuclide angiocardiography. Cathet. Cardiovasc. Diagn., *6*:265, 1980.

28. Sharma, B., Goodwin, J. F., Raphael, M. J., Steiner, R. E., Rainbow, R. G., and Taylor, S. H.: Left ventricular angiography on exercise: A new method of assessing left ventricular function in ischaemic heart disease. Br. Heart. J., *38*:59, 1976.

29. Upton, M. T., Rerych, S. K., Newman, G. E., Port, S., Cobb, F. R., and Jones, R. H.: Detecting abnormalities in left ventricular function during exercise before angina and ST-segment depression. Circulation, *62*:341, 1980.

VENTRICULAR ANEURYSM

William A. Gay, Jr., M.D.

The majority of ventricular aneurysms are due to acute transmural myocardial infarction with its resultant muscle necrosis followed by scar formation. Rarely, however, aneurysms may follow trauma or congenital cardiac defects.[17, 18] There are also false aneurysms, which may be due to previous surgical procedures,[35] trauma,[6] and bacterial endocarditis.[36] The typical ventricular aneurysm has been described as "a thinned-out transmural scar that has completely lost its trabecular pattern ... always clearly delineated from the surrounding muscle."[23] Although this accurate description of ventricular aneurysms was given by John Hunter in the eighteenth century, it was more than 150 years later that the relationship of this entity with coronary occlusive disease was appreciated.[40] Moreover, it remained for Tennant and Wiggers to demonstrate the deleterious effects of acute coronary arterial occlusion on regional myocardial contractile function in 1935.[42]

In 1931, the famed German surgeon Sauerbruch accidentally entered an aneurysm of the right ventricle during the course of exploration of a patient believed to have a mediastinal tumor. He was able to resect the aneurysm sac and successfully suture its neck.[37] Beck, in 1944, used a fascia lata stent to reinforce the left ventricular wall of a patient with a ventricular aneurysm that was accurately diagnosed preoperatively.[4] In 1954, Bailey successfully resected a ventricular aneurysm by placing a large vascular clamp about its neck, excising the aneurysm, and oversewing the neck.[3] The use of cardiopulmonary bypass in operations for ventricular aneurysm was first described by Cooley in 1958.[8] The practice of simultaneous coronary revascularization became popular as direct coronary arterial operations became commonplace in the late 1960s and early 1970s.[17] Jatene, in 1985, described a technique for the geometric reconstruction of the left ventricle after aneurysmectomy with a significant reduction in operative mortality and improved postoperative ventricular performance.[25] Since that time others have been more attentive to reconstructive techniques, with similar improvements in results.[9, 13, 29, 30]

CLINICAL MANIFESTATIONS

The precise incidence of left ventricular aneurysm formation after acute myocardial infarction is not known. Retrospective clinical and autopsy analyses indicate an incidence of 10% to 15%.[1, 38] These figures were generated before the era of prompt interventional therapy for acute myocardial infarction, such as thrombolysis and/or angioplasty or bypass surgery. It is hoped that the use of one or more of these therapeutic interventions combined with better hemodynamic and arrhythmia control has lowered the incidence of aneurysm formation.

Although the relationship between coronary occlusion and aneurysm formation has been well established, until recently it was poorly understood why some infarctions caused aneurysms whereas others did not. A review of patients suffering their first myocardial infarction, all anterior, revealed that the absence of significant collateral circulation concomitant with total occlusion of the left anterior descending coronary artery was a significant determinant of aneurysm formation.[19] Another report evaluating the effectiveness of early reperfusion after myocardial infarction concluded that although collateral circulation to an area of anterior infarction did not improve global ventricular function in the absence of successful reperfusion, it did lower the incidence of left ventricular aneurysm.[22] Thus, it would seem that the presence of significant collateral circulation in the distribution of an acutely occluded coronary artery may lessen the likelihood of development of an aneurysm.

Before the establishment of special care units and use of sophisticated monitoring and aggressive therapy, many patients who developed left ventricular aneurysms succumbed in the early peri-infarction period. The typical patient who develops a left ventricular aneurysm has a turbulent post-infarction course, usually marked by overt or borderline congestive heart failure or recurring arrhythmias. In the absence of other hemodynamic lesions, such as mitral valve insufficiency or ventricular septal defect, the occurrence of congestive heart failure usually indicates that 20% or more of the left ventricular mass is involved and that aneurysm formation is not unlikely. The most common symptom in patients with ventricular aneurysm is dyspnea, with frequently associated palpitations and angina. Manifestations of peripheral embolization occur rarely (Table 54–12). Many patients have more than one symptom.

Although the presence of a ventricular aneurysm may be suspected from the previously described clinical course, substantiation of the diagnosis and therapeutic decision-making depend on further evaluation. An abnormal cardiac impulse is usually detectable at the apex, and a ventricular gallop (S_3)

TABLE 54–12. Symptoms in 80 Patients with Ventricular Aneurysm

Symptom	Number	Percentage
Dyspnea	61	75
Palpitations	36	45
Angina	32	40
Emboli	1	~1

is often audible. The aneurysm produces no cardiac murmurs, but coexisting valvular dysfunction produces characteristic findings when present.

The persistence of elevated ST segments after acute myocardial infarction is very suggestive of a developing left ventricular aneurysm, but this finding has not proved sufficiently reliable to be diagnostic.[7, 20, 21] Chest films most often reveal enlargement of the left ventricle and pulmonary congestion. Cardiac fluoroscopy may reveal systolic expansion (paradox) in the area of the aneurysm. The demonstration of abnormalities in segmental left ventricular wall motion using ultrasound and/or gated blood pool ventriculography is helpful in identifying patients for whom further study is indicated.[5, 12, 14, 34] Whereas the diagnosis of left ventricular aneurysm may be confirmed by means of these minimally invasive techniques, left ventriculography and selective coronary arteriography most accurately outline the extent of the aneurysm, the presence of mural thrombus, the existence of valvular dysfunction, and the localization of coronary occlusive lesions.

TREATMENT

The treatment of left ventricular aneurysm is aneurysmectomy combined with correction of any significant valvular abnormalities and bypass of major coronary obstructive lesions. Operation is indicated in patients whose aneurysms cause symptoms. Additionally, those patients whose aneurysms were discovered during the course of coronary arteriography in anticipation of coronary bypass surgery should have aneurysmectomy at the time of bypass operation. Whereas the 3-year mortality after uncomplicated myocardial infarction is 15% to 20%, this figure rises to 70% to 75% in patients with aneurysms and to nearly 90% after 5 years.[32, 38]

Operation for left ventricular aneurysm is best done through a midline sternotomy incision. One or more internal mammary arteries and/or saphenous veins should be prepared if coronary artery bypass grafting is planned as a part of the procedure. Cardiopulmonary bypass is begun, and the core body temperature is lowered to 26° to 28° C. Venting of the left ventricle is probably unnecessary but, if done, should be undertaken with extreme care so as not to dislodge any existing thrombotic material. Whereas most cardiac surgeons currently utilize aortic cross-clamping and myocardial protection with cold cardioplegia, Akins[2] has had success in a large series of operations using hypothermia and induced ventricular fibrillation without aortic cross-clamping. Shapira and associates[39] have reported on repair of a left ventricular aneurysm using a left posterolateral thoracotomy in a patient with patent coronary bypass grafts. Moderate hypothermia and induced ventricular fibrillation were used without aortic cross-clamping.

One method of aneurysm repair is illustrated in Figure 54–132. The importance of geometric reconstruction of the left ventricle was emphasized by Hutching and Brawley[24] and made practical by Jatene.[25] The techniques have been modified by Dor and associates[18] and by Cooley[9] with steadily improving results. First, the aneurysm is opened and any

mural thrombus is carefully and completely removed. The sac of the aneurysm is then inspected and followed back to its junction with healthy myocardium. This process allows identification of a circular or oval defect with a fibrous rim (see Fig. 54–132B). A patch is then trimmed to approximate the size and shape of the defect and sewn into place with a continuous nonabsorbable suture (2-0 or 3-0 polypropylene). The aneurysm sac is then trimmed (see Fig. 54–132C) and closed (see Fig. 54–132D) over the repair. The use of buttressing strips or pledgets is usually not necessary. Although experience with this type of repair is not yet extensive, the improved functional results reported appear to justify its use wherever possible.[9, 30, 31] A recently described procedure involved a tailored scar excision, which removes the nonfunc-

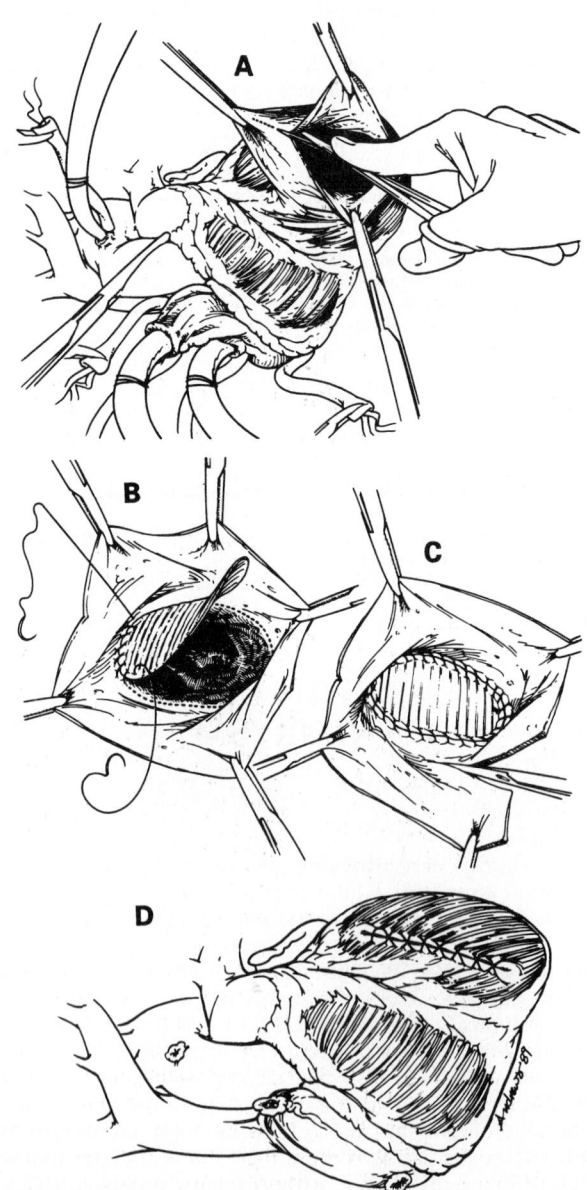

Figure 54–132. Steps for aneurysmectomy and reconstruction of the left ventricle. *A,* The aneurysm is opened and any mural thrombus carefully and completely removed. *B,* The fibrous rim of the aneurysm is identified from within the aneurysm and is closed using a patch fashioned to approximate the size of the defect. *C,* The remaining aneurysm sac is trimmed. *D,* The aneurysm sac is closed over the repair, usually without buttresses or pledgets. (From Cooley, D. A.: Ventricular endoaneurysmorrhaphy: Results of an improved method of repair. Tex. Heart Inst. J., *16:*72, 1989. Drawn by Bill Andrews.)

tioning wall and restores left ventricular geometry without the use of an internal patch.[30] Follow-up studies demonstrated an acceptable survival up to 5 years, improved ejection fraction, and reduction of valvular regurgitation, when present. Moreover, no difference in survival, functional classification, or ejection fraction was found between patients having linear versus circular, or patch, closure of resected aneurysms in other studies.[16, 21] Follow-up studies of a tailored scar excision that removes the nonfunctioning wall and restores left ventricular geometry without the use of an internal patch demonstrated acceptable survival up to 5 years, improved ejection fraction, and reduction of valvular regurgitation, when present.[30] Moreover, other groups[16, 26] have found no difference in survival, functional classification, or ejection fraction between patients having linear versus circular, or patch, closure of resected aneurysms.

The operative mortality for elective excision of left ventricular aneurysm is about 5%, even when combined with other procedures. Moreover, it has been found that 80% of the survivors are alive 4 years later. Factors influencing early mortality include advanced age (over 65 years), emergent operation, left main coronary disease, history of cardiogenic shock, renal failure, and New York Heart Association Class IV status.[10, 28] Factors that negatively affect long-term survival include left main coronary disease and poor left ventricular function (ejection fraction < 20%).[27] Intraoperative echocardiography used in seven patients who had aneurysmectomy without geometric reconstruction caused no improvement in end-systolic function[33]; elimination of paradox apparently increased mechanical efficiency after aneurysmectomy and was responsible for the observed clinical improvement. A study of 42 patients with radionuclide ventriculography before aneurysmectomy and again 10 months later found that global ejection fraction, both at rest and after exercise, had improved.[29] The inherent inaccuracy of using global ejection fraction as an index of ventricular performance after aneurysmectomy has been well substantiated.[15, 41] Perhaps application of more sophisticated technology, such as multiple-gated acquisition scanning, intraoperative transesophageal echocardiography, and magnetic resonance imaging will improve the objectivity of perioperative evaluations.[16]

Although aneurysms of the posterior and basilar aspects of the left ventricle are less common than those of the anterior and apical portions, they do occur. Resection and primary closure would cause significant distortion of ventricular geometry. This distortion in the posterobasal area, in addition to producing a disturbed and less effective contractile pattern, would probably lead to significant mitral valvular incompetence. Use of an adynamic patch is most often required to repair aneurysms in this area.[11]

COMPLEX VENTRICULAR ANEURYSMS

Some patients require consideration of operation soon after myocardial infarction because of hemodynamic deterioration producing refractory heart failure or, in some instances, cardiogenic shock. Whereas many of these critically ill patients die because the amount of residual functioning myocardium is inadequate to sustain circulation, in some patients operative intervention may prove lifesaving. In these patients, the plan of choice is temporary circulatory cardiac assistance with a device such as the intra-aortic balloon pump and evaluation of operability by ventriculography and coronary arteriography. Acute, discrete left ventricular aneurysm, ruptured or dysfunctional papillary muscle causing acute mitral valve incompetence, and rupture of the interventricular septum represent lesions for which operative intervention is warranted. When there is no discrete area of ventricular dyskinesia, no ventricular septal defect, or no mitral incom-

petence or when the shock state has been prolonged so as to produce prolonged anuria or when the ventricle fails to respond even minimally to inotropic stimulation, operation is not indicated. For patients in this category, long-term ventricular support and/or cardiac transplantation represents the most favorable likelihood of survival.

Because of the severity of illness and the frequent presence of associated dysfunction of other organ systems, mortality is much higher in this group of patients than in those undergoing elective aneurysmectomy. If, however, hemodynamic improvement follows operation, many of these individuals who otherwise would not have survived may go on to a full recovery.

SELECTED REFERENCES

Cosgrove, D. M., Lytle, B. W., Taylor, P. C., Stewart, R. W., Golding, L. A. R., Mahfood, S., Goormastic, M., and Loop, F. D.: Ventricular aneurysm resection: Trends in surgical risk. Circulation, 79:I-97, 1989.
This is a retrospective analysis of 1183 patients operated on at the Cleveland Clinic over a 15-year period. Significant risk factors included emergent procedures, advanced age (older than 65 years), left main coronary artery disease, and congestive heart failure. Despite advancing patient age and the presence of more extensive coronary disease, operative mortality for ventricular aneurysm has remained in the 5% to 10% range.

Forman, M. B., Collins, H. W., Kapelman, H. A., Vaughan, W. K., Parry, J. M., Virmani, R., and Friesinger, G. C.: Determinants of left ventricular aneurysm formation after anterior myocardial infarction: A clinical and angiographic study. J. Am. Coll. Cardiol., 8:1256, 1986.
This group studied 79 patients who experienced a transmural anterior infarction as their myocardial infarction. Total occlusion of the left anterior descending coronary artery in the absence of collateral circulation was found to be a significant factor in the formation of a left ventricular aneurysm after anterior myocardial infarction.

Jatene, A. D.: Left ventricular aneurysmectomy: Resection or reconstruction. J. Thorac. Cardiovasc. Surg., 89:321, 1985.
By applying novel reconstructive techniques that cause less distortion of the normal ventricular geometry, this group of surgeons was able to reduce early operative mortality from 11.6% to 4.3%. More important, attention was called to the desirability of geometric reconstruction after aneurysmectomy.

Mills, N. L., Everson, C. T., and Hockmuth, D. R.: Technical advances in the treatment of left ventricular aneurysm. Ann. Thorac. Surg., 55:792, 1993.
The authors review the major technical advances that have taken place over the past 50 years in repair of left ventricular aneurysm. The techniques are nicely illustrated and described. Geometric reconstruction with preservation and bypass of the left anterior descending artery is preferred.

REFERENCES

1. Abrams, D. L., Edelist, A., Luria, M. H., and Miller, A. S.: Ventricular aneurysm: A reappraisal based on a study of sixty-five consecutive autopsied cases. Circulation, 27:164, 1963.
2. Akins, C. W.: Resection of left ventricular aneurysm during hypothermic fibrillatory arrest without aortic occlusion. J. Thorac. Cardiovasc. Surg., 91:610, 1986.
3. Bailey C. P., Holton, H. E., and Nichols, H.: Ventriculoplasty for cardiac aneurysm. J. Thorac. Cardiovasc. Surg., 35:37, 1958.
4. Beck, C. S.: Operation for aneurysm of the heart. Ann. Surg., 120:34, 1944.
5. Borer, J. S., Jacobstein, J. G., Bacharach, S. L., and Green, M. V.: Detection of left ventricular aneurysm and evaluation of effects of surgical repair: The role of radionuclide cineangiography. Am. J. Cardiol., 45:1103, 1980.
6. Candell, J., Valle, V., Paya, J., Cortadellas, J., Esplugas, E., and Ruis J.: Posttraumatic coronary occlusion and early left ventricular aneurysm. Am. Heart J., 97:509, 1979.
7. Cokkinos, D. V., Hallman, G. L., Cooley, D. A., Zamalloa, O., and Leachman, R. C.: Left ventricular aneurysm: Analysis of electrocardiographic features and postresection changes. Am. Heart J., 82:149, 1971.
8. Cooley, D. A., Colling, H. A., Morris, C. G., and Chapman, D. W.: Ventricular aneurysm after myocardial infarction: Surgical excision with use of temporary cardiopulmonary bypass. J.A.M.A., 167:557, 1958.
9. Cooley, D. A., Frazier, O. H., Duncan, J. M., Reul, G. J., and Krajeer, Z.: Intracavitary repair of ventricular aneurysm and regional dyskinesia. Ann. Surg., 215:417, 1992.
10. Cosgrove, D. A., Lytle, B. W., Taylor, P. C., Stewart, R. W., Golding, L. A. R., Mahfood, S., Goormastic, M., and Loop, F. D.: Ventricular aneurysm resection: Trends in surgical risk. Circulation, 79:i97, 1989.
11. Daggett, W. M.: Surgical technique for early repair of posterior ventricular septal rupture. J. Thorac. Cardiovasc. Surg., 84:306, 1982.
12. Dillon, J., Feigenbaum, H., Weyman, A., Peskoe, S., and Chang, S.: Echocardiography in the evaluation of patients for aneurysmectomy (abstract). Circulation, 52(Suppl. II):135, 1975.

13. Dor, V., Saab, M., Coste, P., Kornaszewska, M., and Montiglio, F.: Left ventricular aneurysm: A new surgical approach. J. Thorac. Cardiovasc. Surg., 37:11, 1989.

14. Dymond, D. S., Jarritt, P. H., Britton, K. E., and Spurrell, R. A. J.: Detection of postinfarction aneurysms by first-pass radionuclide ventriculography using a multicrystal gamma camera. Br. Heart J., 41:68, 1979.

15. Edmunds, L. H., Jr.: Discussion of Komeda, M., et al. Ann. Thorac. Surg., 53:22, 1992.

16. Elefteriades, J. A., Solomon, L. W., Salazar, A. M., Batsford, W. P., Baldwin, J. C., and Kopf, G. S.: Linear left ventricular aneurysmectomy: Modern imaging studies reveal improved morphology and function. Ann. Thorac. Surg., 56:242, 1993.

17. Favaloro, R. G., Effler, D. B., Groves, L. K., Wescott, R. N., Saurez, E., and Lozada, J.: Ventricular aneurysm—Clinical experience. Ann. Thorac. Surg., 6:227, 1968.

18. Flemma, R. J., Marx, L., Litwin, S. B., and Gallen, W. J.: Left ventricular aneurysmectomy in a child. Ann. Thorac. Surg., 19:457, 1975.

19. Forman, M. B., Collins, H. W., Kapelman, H. A., Vaughan, W. K., Parry, J. M., Virmani, R., and Friesinger, G. C.: Determinants of left ventricular aneurysm formation after anterior myocardial infarction: A clinical and angiographic study. J. Am. Coll. Cardiol., 8:1256, 1986.

20. Gorlin, R., Klein, M. D., and Sullivan, J. M.: Prospective correlative study of ventricular aneurysm: Mechanic concept and clinical recognition. Am. J. Med., 42:512, 1967.

21. Groden, B. M., and James, W. B.: Significance of persistent R-ST elevation after acute myocardial infarction. Br. Heart J., 31:34, 1969.

22. Hirai, T., Fujita, M., Nakajima, H., Asamoi, H., Yamanishi, K., Ohno, A., and Sasayama, S.: Clinical investigation: Importance of collateral circulation for prevention of left ventricular aneurysm formation in acute anterior myocardial infarction. Circulation, 79:791, 1989.

23. Hunter, J.: An account of the dissection of morbid bodys. London, Library of the Royal College of Surgeons, 32:30, 1757.

24. Hutching, G. M., and Brawley, R. K.: The influence of cardiac geometry on the result of ventricular aneurysm repair. Am. J. Pathol., 99:221, 1980.

25. Jatene, A. D.: Left ventricular aneurysmectomy: Resection or reconstruction. J. Thorac. Cardiovasc. Surg., 89:321, 1985.

26. Kesler, K. A., Fiore, A. C., Naunheim, K. S., Sharp, T. G., Mahomed, Y., Zollinger, T. W., Sawada, S. G., Brown, J. W., Labovitz, A. J., and Barner, H. B.: Anterior wall left ventricular aneurysm repair. J. Thorac. Cardiovasc. Surg., 103:841, 1992.

27. Komeda, M., David, T. E., Malik, A., Ivanov, J., and Sun, Z.: Operative risks and long-term results of operation for left ventricular aneurysm. Ann. Thorac. Surg., 53:22, 1992.

28. Magovern, G. J., Sakert, T., Simpson, K., Laug, G. W., Park, S. B., Liebler, G., Burkholder, J., Maher, T., Benkart, D., and Magovern, G. J., Jr.: Surgical therapy for left ventricular aneurysms—A ten year experience. Circulation, 79:i-102, 1989.

29. Mangschau, A., Forfang, K., Rootwelt, K., and Froysaker, T.: Improvement in cardiac performance and exercise tolerance after left ventricular aneurysm surgery—A prospective study. J. Thorac. Cardiovasc. Surg., 36:320, 1988.

30. Mickleborough, L. L., Maruyanma, H., Liu, P., and Mohamed, S.: Results of left ventricular aneurysmectomy with a tailored scar excision and primary closure technique. J. Thorac. Cardiovasc. Surg., 107:690, 1994.

31. Mills, N. L., Everson, C. T., and Hockmuth, D. R.: Technical advances in the treatment of left ventricular aneurysm. Ann. Thorac. Surg., 55:792, 1993.

32. Nagle, R. E., and Williams, D. O.: Natural history of ventricular aneurysm without surgical treatment. Br. Heart J., 36:1037, 1974.

33. Nicolosi, A. C., and Spotnitz, H. M.: Clinical investigation: Quantitative analysis of regional systolic function with left ventricular aneurysm. Circulation, 78:856, 1988.

34. Rakowski, R., Martin, R. P., Schapira, J. N., Wexler, L., Silverman, J. F., Cipriano, P. R., Guthaner, D. F., and Popp, R. L.: Left ventricular aneurysm: Detection and determination of resectability by two-dimensional ultrasound. Circulation, 55/56(Suppl. III):153, 1977.

35. Rittenhouse, E. A., Sauvage, L. R., Mansfield, P. R., Smith, J. C., Davis, C. C., and Hall, D. G.: False aneurysm of the left ventricle: Report of four cases and review of the surgical management. Ann. Surg., 189:409, 1979.

36. Sapsford, R. N., Fitchett, D. H., Tarin, D., and Anderson, R. H.: Aneurysm of the left ventricle secondary to bacterial endocarditis. J. Thorac. Cardiovasc. Surg., 78:79, 1979.

37. Sauerbruch, F.: Erfolgreiche operative Beseitigung cines Aneurysm ab der rechten Herzkammer. Arch. Klin. Chir., 167:586, 1931.

38. Schlichter, J., Hellerstein, H. K., and Katz, L. N.: Aneurysm of the heart: A correlative study of one hundred and two proved cases. Medicine, 33:43, 1954.

39. Shapira, O. M., Aldea, G. S., Carr, T. G., and Shemin, R. J.: Thoracotomy for repair of left ventricular aneurysm in a patient with patent coronary bypass grafts. Ann. Thorac. Surg., 58:1536, 1994.

40. Sternberg, M.: Das chronische partielle Herzaneurysma. Vienna and Leipsig, Franz Deutlicke, 1914.

41. Stoney, W. S., Jr.: Discussion of Komeda, M., et al. Ann. Thorac. Surg., 53:28, 1992.

42. Tennant, R., and Wiggers, C. J.: Effect of coronary occlusion on myocardial contraction. Am. J. Physiol., 112:351, 1935.

KAWASAKI'S DISEASE

Thomas A. D'Amico, M.D.

Kawasaki's disease, a vasculitic disorder of undetermined etiology, is the leading cause of acquired heart disease in children in the United States; approximately 2000 cases are reported annually. The acute illness, as first described by Kawasaki, is characterized by fever, conjunctivitis, rash, and cervical lymphadenopathy.[17] Various causative agents have been proposed, but the etiology of Kawasaki's disease is still unclear. Although usually indolent and self-limiting, in its advanced stage the syndrome is characterized by the development of multiple coronary artery aneurysms.

Kawasaki's disease predominately affects infants and children. Eighty percent of cases involve children younger than 5 years of age, and the highest incidence is at 12 to 16 months. In the United States, the overall incidence in children younger than 5 years of age is 6 to 9 per 100,000 population, equivalent to the incidence of acute rheumatic fever.[35] The pathophysiology has been well described, but the infrequent progression to severe cardiovascular manifestations is not well understood. Increased awareness of the potential severity of Kawasaki's disease has contributed to more prompt diagnosis and the earlier institution of therapy. Current management consists of antiplatelet and anti-inflammatory agents; surgical intervention is reserved for patients with advanced disease. An ideal treatment that ameliorates the early inflammatory symptoms, arrests the vasculitic progression, and prevents the formation of coronary aneurysms has not been discovered.

ETIOLOGY

The pathogenesis of Kawasaki's disease has not yet been completely described. Many clinical aspects of the syndrome imply a communicable causative factor. The acute presentation of fever, rash, conjunctivitis, and lymphadenopathy in children suggests an infectious disease. Kawasaki's disease exclusively affects children, and recurrences are uncommon, suggesting a mechanism of acquired immunity. Epidemiologic evidence supports the theory of an infectious etiology. In addition to geographic areas where it appears to be endemic, such as Japan, seasonal epidemic outbreaks are common.

The search for a single etiologic agent has been unsuccessful. Possibilities include rickettsiae, spirochetes, bacteria, viruses (particularly Epstein-Barr virus), and superantigens, all without confirmation.[19] The lack of evidence for person-to-person transmissibility has made it difficult to isolate a single causative factor. Variable immunity or low communicability could explain this phenomenon. Investigation of peripheral lymphocytes isolated from the blood during the acute stage of Kawasaki's disease has demonstrated increased helper T-lymphocytic activity and decreased suppressor T-lymphocyte activity, which suggests a retroviral component in the etiology of Kawasaki's disease.[31] That Kawasaki's disease is recurrent in 3% of patients suggests a cell-associated agent, persistently infecting lymphocytes.[22] Reverse transcriptase, which synthesizes DNA from a template of RNA, is the hallmark of retroviral activity. Analysis of supernatants from lymphocyte cultures of patients with Kawasaki's disease showed significantly increased reverse transcriptase activity compared with controls. Although this finding has been confirmed in multiple laboratories, there has been no conclusive evidence of a specific viral agent.[2, 32]

CLINICAL MANIFESTATIONS

The original description of the clinical features of the syndrome by Kawasaki has been consistently supported by others. The diagnosis of Kawasaki's disease is secured by the presence of five of the six major criteria (Table 54–13). The presentation of this syndrome is acute, and the symptoms evolve during a period of a few days, a stereotypical clinical pattern that leads to certain diagnosis. However, various reports of atypical presentations suggest that a high index of suspicion is required to prevent delayed diagnosis and late recognition of cardiovascular complications.

The principal presenting symptom is fever, which usually has an abrupt onset, is generally high and spiking, and does not respond to antibiotics.[4] The fever lasts from 7 to 14 days but may persist in more severe cases. Kawasaki's disease should be considered in the differential diagnosis of any child with prolonged unexplained fever. The appearance of fever is often accompanied by the presence of bilateral and sterile congested conjunctivae. After the appearance of conjunctivitis, several changes in the lips and oral cavity occur. Commonly, there is a reddening of the lips, which may then become dry and fissured. The tongue may appear prominently, with protuberant papillae *(strawberry tongue)*, or there may be only diffuse reddening of the oropharyngeal mucosa.[30] By the third day of the illness, a polymorphous macular erythematous rash appears. The rash begins with reddening of the palms and soles; individual lesions may coalesce as the rash progresses proximally to spread over the trunk, usually over 48 hours. As the rash resolves, secondary changes in digits appear. A unique desquamation begins at the junction of the nails and the skin on the tips of the digits. In approximately 50% of patients, nonpurulent cervical lymphadenopathy develops. Cervical lymphadenopathy is considered a principal finding when at least one lymph node is greater than 1.5 cm. in diameter. The lymphadenopathy is usually unilateral, and the nodes are firm and mildly tender but not fluctuant. Associated findings of Kawasaki's disease may include arthralgia, arthritis, aseptic meningitis, diarrhea, hydrops of the gallbladder, jaundice, proteinuria, and urethritis.

The differential diagnosis of Kawasaki's disease includes measles, scarlet fever, Stevens-Johnson syndrome, Rocky Mountain spotted fever, juvenile rheumatoid arthritis, and other febrile viral exanthems.[4]

Cardiovascular manifestations are prominent in the acute phase of the illness and are the leading cause of morbidity and mortality. Examination of the heart may reveal tachycardia, distant heart sounds, or a gallop, suggestive of myocarditis or congestive failure; a holosystolic murmur signifies mitral valve insufficiency. Palpation of the peripheral arteries, especially in the axillary and inguinal regions, may reveal an aneurysm. Palpation of the abdomen may show congestive hepatomegaly or right upper quadrant tenderness, secondary

to hydrops of the gallbladder. Although infrequent, the presence of peritoneal signs suggests vascular compromise in the mesenteric arteries. Auscultation of the abdomen may reveal the bruit of an aneurysm of the renal, celiac, mesenteric, or iliac arteries. Examination of the neck often yields prominent cervical lymphadenopathy, an early finding that precedes other classic findings.

LABORATORY STUDIES

Leukocytosis is invariably present and is often accompanied by a leftward shift in the differential. Anemia and thrombocytosis may be present. Other findings include an increase in interleukin-6, interleukin-8, tumor necrosis factor-alpha, erythrocyte sedimentation rate, C-reactive protein, factor VII concentration, and fibrinogen level.[21, 30] The electrocardiogram is abnormal in 70% of patients. The most common findings are sinus tachycardia, prolonged PQ and QR intervals, second-degree atrioventricular block, decreased voltage, ST-segment changes, and T-wave changes.

The radiographic studies are often abnormal. Chest films may reveal cardiomegaly or pleural effusion, and echocardiograms are positive in 45% of patients, providing early objective evidence of cardiovascular dysfunction.[3] Pericardial effusion may be detected by echocardiography in 30% of patients yet rarely progresses to tamponade.[5]

NATURAL HISTORY

Kawasaki's disease is the progression of a nonspecific vasculitis that involves the microvasculature of the aorta and its major branches, manifested by endarteritis of the vasa vasorum of the coronary, brachiocephalic, celiac, renal, and iliofemoral systems. As the inflammatory process of the intima and adventitia progresses, aneurysms form in these vessels and lead to stenosis, thromboembolism, ischemia, rupture, or healing.

Kawasaki's disease may be divided into three clinical stages. The *acute* phase lasts approximately 10 days, during which fever and the development of the characteristic rash predominate. The *subacute* phase then ensues, during which the cardiac complications commonly occur; and the *convalescent* phase is defined as the period during which the erythrocyte sedimentation rate remains elevated.

A spectrum of cardiovascular manifestations may occur in Kawasaki's disease but are usually self-limited; cardiac fatalities occur in less than 1% of patients. Myocarditis is present in as many as 50% of patients. In the acute phase, myocarditis may cause exercise intolerance, congestive heart failure, or death. Mitral regurgitation occurs in only 5% of patients; however, in patients with coronary aneurysms, the incidence is 25%.[15] Ischemia to the papillary muscles secondary to coronary artery involvement is responsible for most cases, although diffuse myocarditis and anular dilatation may also contribute.[34] Myocardial ischemia is due to profound fibrotic changes or is secondary to multiple stenotic lesions. Myocardial infarction, a rare complication of Kawasaki's disease, may occur after diffuse ischemia or a thromboembolic event. The presence of collateral circulation usually preserves ventricular function, despite multiple stenotic lesions; however, left ventricular hypertrophy associated with diffuse hypokinesia sometimes develops.

The most serious complication of Kawasaki's disease is the formation of coronary artery aneurysms, which has an incidence of 10% to 40% (Fig. 54–133).[1, 11] Coronary artery aneurysms are responsible for at least 85% of the mortality associated with Kawasaki's disease. The mortality among boys with Kawasaki's disease is twice that among healthy boys, and most deaths occur within 2 months of the diagno-

TABLE 54–13. Criteria for the Diagnosis of Kawasaki's Disease

Fever of at least 5 days' duration
Presence of four of the following:
    Sterile conjunctivitis
    Changes in the mouth and oral cavity (dry, fissured, or reddened lips; prominent reddened tongue; diffuse reddening of the oral mucosa)
    Changes of the extremities (reddening of the palms or soles; indurative edema of the hands or feet; desquamation)
    Polymorphous truncal rash
    Cervical adenopathy

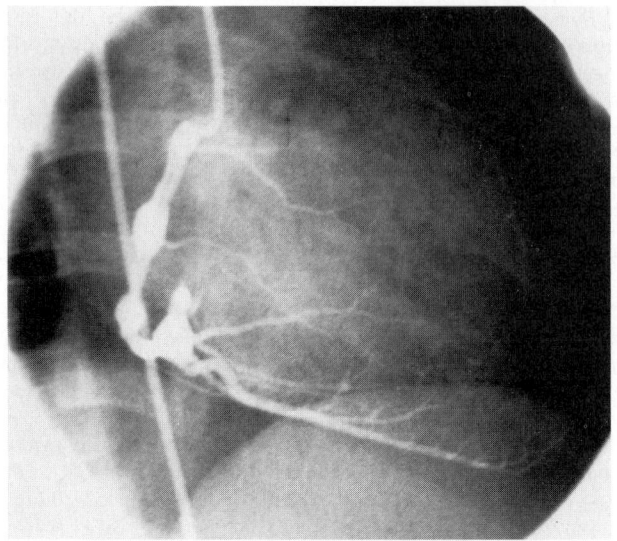

Figure 54–133. Coronary arteriogram demonstrating three aneurysms of the right coronary artery in a 10-year-old boy with Kawasaki's disease.

TABLE 54–14. Risk Factors for the Development of Coronary Aneurysms in Kawasaki's Disease

Male sex
Age younger than 1 year
Duration of fever greater than 16 days
White blood cell count greater than 30 × 10⁹/L.
Erythrocyte sedimentation rate greater than 100 mm./h.
Elevated C-reactive protein
Thrombocytosis

complications.[27] The major risk factors for the development of coronary aneurysms are listed in Table 54–14. Selective coronary angiography is reserved for patients with complications of known coronary aneurysms. Analysis of retrospective studies has demonstrated groups of patients who are most likely to develop aneurysms and who require serial coronary echocardiograms, selective coronary angiography, and surgical intervention.[18, 26] The indications for cardiac catheterization are shown in Table 54–15.

TREATMENT

Therapy During the Acute Stage. Originally the mortality of Kawasaki's disease was 1% to 2%. Since 1976, the mortality has decreased to approximately 0.5%, owing to earlier diagnosis and the evolution of effective therapy, including surgical intervention. Early diagnosis and recognition of the appearance of cardiovascular complications are critical in the successful management of patients with Kawasaki's disease, because death may occur in the first week of the illness.

The goal of initial therapy for Kawasaki's disease is the reduction of inflammation, including coronary and myocardial inflammation. After the diagnosis of Kawasaki's disease is confirmed, patients are treated with intravenous gamma-globulin and high doses of aspirin.[5] Gamma-globulin (2 gm./kg.) is administered as a single infusion over 12 hours. Treatment with intravenous immune globulin has been shown to decrease the duration of fever, to decrease the prevalence of cardiovascular complications,[23] and to prevent the progression to giant coronary aneurysms.[29] In addition, immune globulin therapy improves cardiac function in patients with wall motion abnormalities secondary to myocarditis.[28] Proposed mechanisms to explain the efficacy of intravenous immune globulin therapy include competition for endothelial cell receptors, negative feedback on the B-cell lymphocyte system, and direct neutralization of a viral agent.[20]

High-dose aspirin therapy contributes to the resolution of the acute manifestations of Kawasaki's disease. When Kawasaki's disease is diagnosed, children are given a regimen of aspirin (100 mg./kg./day), which is continued until defervescence. Thereafter, they are maintained on low-dose aspirin (3 to 5 mg./kg./day) for 8 weeks. In children who develop aneurysms, low-dose aspirin therapy may be continued indefinitely[7]; the risk of associated salicylate complications, including Reye's syndrome, is low. The goal of aspirin ther-

sis.[27] Echocardiographic studies have demonstrated that coronary arterial wall changes occur in all patients, which progress to dilatation in half and to true aneurysms in over one fourth of patients.[8] The aneurysms may be asymptomatic or may not become symptomatic until years later, whereas other aneurysms present initially with myocardial infarction, cardiogenic shock, or sudden death.[7]

Serial angiographic studies have shown resolution of aneurysms that are discovered as early as the second week; several studies have demonstrated resolution of 50% of coronary aneurysms 1 year after initial presentation.[3, 10] Pathologic analysis has shown that angiographic resolution may be caused by intimal proliferation rather than by healing, which leaves these arteries at further risk for stenosis and thromboembolism.[27]

Aneurysms of the coronary arteries follow inflammatory changes in the intima and adventitia, caused by perivasculitis of the major coronary arteries. As in atherosclerotic coronary artery disease, the most common locations for lesions are at the bifurcation of the left anterior descending and circumflex vessels (found in 74% of patients with coronary aneurysms) and at the origin of the right coronary artery (48%).[25] Most patients are found to have multiple aneurysms, but only aneurysms that reach 4 mm. in diameter are considered clinically significant. Patients with giant coronary aneurysms (greater than 8 mm.) have the worst prognosis, and this group constitutes nearly all the late deaths from Kawasaki's disease. Within the aneurysm, turbulence and stagnation produce platelet aggregation and thrombosis. Advanced thrombosis causes critical stenoses in the coronary arteries, the most common indication for surgical intervention. Thromboembolic phenomena are also common and may produce acute myocardial infarction.

The diagnosis of Kawasaki's disease should be accompanied routinely by echocardiography, which has demonstrated a sensitivity of greater than 90% in detecting coronary aneurysms. However, echocardiography is not effective in detecting stenotic lesions. To reduce the mortality of Kawasaki's disease, early detection and treatment of coronary lesions are necessary. To ensure prompt institution of therapy, evaluation of the severity of the disease in a particular patient is required at a stage before most aneurysms can be detected by echocardiography. Thus, many clinicians have developed a scoring system, using risk factors, to anticipate major cardiac

TABLE 54–15. Indications for Cardiac Catheterization in Kawasaki's Disease

Severe symptoms at onset
Symptoms of ischemic heart disease
Symptoms of congestive heart failure
Mitral regurgitation
Coronary calcifications evident on chest films
Persistent coronary aneurysms

apy is the amelioration of symptoms and the prevention of the thrombotic and embolic complications of Kawasaki's disease. Aspirin does not decrease the risk of the development of coronary aneurysms, nor does it prevent the obstruction of giant aneurysms.

Long-term Management. The long-term follow-up of patients with Kawasaki's disease depends on the degree of coronary involvement. Repeat echocardiography examination is performed at 8-week intervals after the acute onset of the febrile period. Serial echocardiographic examinations should document the progression or regression of coronary aneurysms. Thrombus formation may be observed in patients with giant coronary aneurysms, and these patients require more frequent follow-up. Patients with no evidence of aneurysm or ectasia 1 year after the diagnosis is made do not require further echocardiographic examinations.[5]

Patients with no coronary changes on echocardiography at any stage of the illness require no pharmacologic therapy after the acute phase of the illness resolves. Patients with single coronary aneurysms (small to medium) are maintained on low-dose aspirin until the abnormalities resolve. Annual echocardiographic follow-up is performed throughout the first decade of life.[5]

Patients with multiple coronary aneurysms or with one or more giant coronary aneurysms are maintained on low-dose aspirin indefinitely. In addition to annual evaluation with echocardiography, electrocardiograms are performed at 6-month intervals. Coronary arteriography is performed if other studies suggest the presence of coronary stenoses. Patients with coronary artery obstruction confirmed by angiography are also maintained on low-dose aspirin therapy. Repeated cardiac catheterization and coronary angiography are performed when new-onset or progressive myocardial ischemia is suggested by noninvasive testing or clinical presentation.

Surgical Management. Advanced cardiovascular complications require surgical intervention. The operative indications for coronary bypass grafting are shown in Table 54–16.[33] The first use of coronary artery bypass grafting (CABG) for obstructive coronary aneurysms in Kawasaki's disease was reported in 1976.[17] General problems with CABG became apparent with experience. Homologous and autologous saphenous vein grafts (SVGs) showed frequent early occlusion. In many patients, the distal coronary arteries appeared to be too small to accept vein grafts. The potential for SVGs to grow as the thoracic cavity expands is unknown.

In 1985 the first use of the internal mammary artery (IMA) to treat patients with Kawasaki's disease was described,[16] and subsequent studies have demonstrated the superiority of the IMA graft for revascularization. In one study,[17] the authors reported 100% early and late patency (more than 1 year) of the IMA, compared with 90% early patency and 50% late patency of the SVG. In children younger than 8 years of age, patency of the SVG was 65%; in older children, the patency was 87%.

TABLE 54–16. Criteria for Coronary Artery Bypass Grafting in Kawasaki's Disease

Progressive coronary lesions with no distal coronary aneurysms or stenoses
Localized aneurysm with significant stenosis in the left main coronary artery
Progressive stenosis in the left anterior descending coronary artery
Significant stenosis in two coronary arteries
Collateral vessels arising from a coronary artery with a proximal aneurysm
Presence of left ventricular aneurysm

A retrospective multicenter study analyzing the long-term outcome of myocardial revascularization in patients with Kawasaki's disease has recently been completed.[13] Of 168 patients in the study, 54 underwent CABG with SVG alone and 114 received at least one IMA graft to the left anterior descending artery. The operative mortality was similar in the two groups, but the late cardiac death rate was significantly higher in the SVG group than in the IMA group (13% vs. 1%). Actuarial analysis demonstrated a significantly higher survival at 90 months after operation in the IMA group than in the SVG group (99% vs. 82%). Finally, the actuarial patency rate was significantly higher for the arterial grafts than for the vein grafts (81% vs. 38%). The IMA has been demonstrated to be the graft of choice for myocardial revascularization for children with Kawasaki's disease.

SUMMARY

A disorder with many cardiovascular manifestations, Kawasaki's disease has several unexplained features, including etiology, selectivity for children, and ability to progress to severe stages in view of its usually benign and self-limited nature. The initial therapy for Kawasaki's disease is directed toward reducing coronary artery and myocardial inflammation. Therapy in the later stages for the disease is designed to prevent coronary thrombosis by inhibiting platelet aggregation. Specific therapy for Kawasaki's disease awaits the discovery of the etiologic agent.

REFERENCES

1. Akagi T., Rose V., Benson L. N., et al.: Outcome of coronary artery aneurysms after Kawasaki disease. J. Pediatr., 121:689, 1992.
2. Burns, J. C., Wiggins, J. W., Jr., Toews, W. H., et al.: Clinical spectrum of Kawasaki disease in infants younger than 6 months of age. J. Pediatr., 109:759, 1986.
3. Chung, K. J., Fulton, D. R., Lapp, R., et al.: One-year follow-up of cardiac and coronary artery disease in infants and children with Kawasaki disease. Am. Heart. J., 115:1263, 1988.
4. Dajani, A. S., Taubert, K. A., Gerber, M. A., et al.: Diagnosis and therapy of Kawasaki disease in children. Circulation, 87:1776, 1993.
5. Dajani, A. S., Taubert, K. A., Takahashi, M., et al.: Guidelines for long-term management of patients with Kawasaki disease: Report from the Committee on Rheumatic Fever, Endocarditis, and Kawasaki Disease, Council on Cardiovascular Disease in the Young, American Heart Association. Circulation, 89:916, 1994.
6. Furusho, K., Kamiya, T., Nakano, H., et al.: Japanese gamma globulin trials for Kawasaki disease. Prog. Clin. Biol. Res., 250:425, 1987.
7. Gersony, W. M.: Long-term issues in Kawasaki disease. J. Pediatr., 121:731, 1992.
8. Kamiya, T., and Suzuki, A.: Ischemic heart disease in Kawasaki disease. Prog. Clin. Biol. Res., 250:347, 1987.
9. Kato, H.: Cardiovascular involvement in Kawasaki disease. Prog. Clin. Biol. Res., 250:277, 1987.
10. Kato, H., Ichinose, E., Yoshioka, F., et al.: Fate of coronary aneurysms in Kawasaki disease: Serial coronary angiography and long-term follow-up study. Am. J. Cardiol., 49:1758, 1982.
11. Kato, H., Ichinose, E., and Kawasaki, T.: Myocardial infarction in Kawasaki disease: Clinical analysis in 195 cases. J. Pediatr., 108:923, 1986.
12. Kawasaki, T.: Acute febrile mucocutaneous syndrome with lymphoid involvement with specific desquamation of the fingers and toes in children. Jpn. J. Allerg., 16:178, 1967.
13. Kitamura, S., Kameda, Y., Seki, T., et al.: Long-term outcome of myocardial revascularization in patients with Kawasaki coronary artery disease: A multicenter cooperative study. J. Thorac. Cardiovasc. Surg., 107:663, 1994.
14. Kitamura, S., Kawashima, Y., Fujita, T., et al.: Aortocoronary bypass grafting in a child with coronary artery obstruction due to mucocutaneous lymph node syndrome. Circulation, 53:1035, 1976.
15. Kitamura, S., Kawashima, Y., Kawachi, K., et al.: Severe mitral regurgitation due to coronary arteritis of mucocutaneous lymph node syndrome: A new surgical entity. J. Thorac. Cardiovasc. Surg., 80:629, 1980.
16. Kitamura, S., Kawachi, K., Oyama, C., et al.: Severe Kawasaki heart disease treated with an internal mammary artery graft in pediatric patients: A first successful report. J. Thorac. Cardiovasc. Surg., 89:860, 1985.
17. Kitamura, S., Seki, S., Kawachi, K., et al.: Excellent patency and growth potential of internal mammary artery grafts in pediatric coronary artery bypass surgery: New evidence for a "live" conduit. Circulation, 78 (Suppl.):I-129, 1988.

18. Koren, G., Lavi, S., Rose, V., et al.: Kawasaki disease: Review of risk factors for coronary artery aneurysms. J. Pediatr., 108:388, 1986.
19. Leung, D. Y. M.: Kawasaki disease. Curr. Opin. Rheum., 5:41, 1993.
20. Leung, D. Y., Burns, J. D., Newburger, J. W., et al.: Reversal of lymphocyte activation in vivo in the Kawasaki syndrome by intravenous gammaglobulin. J. Clin. Invest., 79:468, 1987.
21. Lin, C. Y., Lin, C. C., and Hwang, B.: Serial changes of serum interleukin-6, interleukin-8, and tumor necrosis factor alpha among patients with Kawasaki disease. J. Pediatr., 121:924, 1992.
22. Marchette, N. J., Ho, D., Kihara, S., et al.: Search for retrovirus etiology of Kawasaki syndrome. Prog. Clin. Biol. Res., 250:131, 1987.
23. Nagashima, M., Matasushima, M., Matsuoka, H., et al.: High-dose gamma-globulin therapy for Kawasaki disease. J. Pediatr., 110:710, 1987.
24. Nakamura, Y., Yanagawa, H., and Kawasaki, T.: Mortality among children with Kawasaki disease in Japan. N. Engl. J. Med., 326:1246, 1992.
25. Nakanishi, T., Takao, A., Nakazawa, M., et al.: Mucocutaneous lymph node syndrome: Clinical and angiographic features of coronary obstructive disease. Am. J. Cardiol., 55:662, 1985.
26. Nakano, H., Ueda, K., Saito, A., et al.: Repeated quantitative angiograms in coronary arterial aneurysms in Kawasaki disease. Am. J. Cardiol., 56:846, 1985.
27. Nakano, H., Ueda, K., Saito, A., et al.: Scoring method for identifying patients with Kawasaki disease at high risk of coronary artery aneurysms. Am. J. Cardiol., 58:739, 1986.
28. Newburger, J. W., Sanders, S. P., Burns, J. C., et al.: Left ventricular contractility in Kawasaki syndrome: Effect of intravenous gamma-globulin. Circulation, 79:1237, 1989.
29. Rowley, A. H., and Shulman, S. T.: What is the status of intravenous gamma-globulin for Kawasaki syndrome in the United States and Canada? Pediatr. Infect. Dis. J., 7:463, 1988.
30. Rowley, A. H., Gonzalez-Crussi, F., and Shulman, S. T.: Kawasaki syndrome. Rev. Infect. Dis., 10:1, 1988.
31. Shulman, S. T., and Rowley, A. H.: Does Kawasaki disease have a retroviral etiology? Lancet, 2:545, 1986.
32. Shulman, S. T., Rowley, A. H., Fresco, R., et al.: The etiology of Kawasaki disease: Retrovirus? Prog. Clin. Biol. Res., 250:117, 1987.
33. Suzuki, A., Kamiya, T., Ono, Y., et al.: Indication of aortocoronary bypass for coronary arterial obstruction due to Kawasaki disease. Heart Vessels, 1:94, 1985.
34. Takao, A., Niwa, K., Kondo, C., et al.: Mitral regurgitation in Kawasaki disease. Prog. Clin. Biol. Res., 250:311, 1987.
35. Taubert, K. A., Rowley, A. H., and Shulman, S. T.: A nationwide survey of Kawasaki disease and acute rheumatic fever. J. Pediatr., 119:279, 1991.

XV

EBSTEIN'S ANOMALY

Theodore C. Koutlas, M.D.

Ebstein's anomaly is an uncommon heart defect, occurring with a frequency of approximately 1 in 20,000 live births. It accounts for less than 1% of all congenital heart disease. The malformation is characterized by the downward displacement of the septal and posterior leaflets of the tricuspid valve into the chamber of the right ventricle. Ebstein's anomaly encompasses a broad spectrum of clinical presentations, owing to the morphologic variability of the defect and the presence of other cardiac malformations.

HISTORICAL ASPECTS

In 1866, Wilhelm Ebstein, a physician in Breslau (Prussia), reported his findings of a congenital heart lesion found during an autopsy performed 2 years earlier. The patient was a 19-year-old male laborer who was hospitalized for dyspnea and palpitations. He was noted to be profoundly cyanotic on examination and died of pulmonary edema 8 days after admission. Ebstein described with great detail the unusual findings of his postmortem cardiac examination.[18] A review of the world's literature in 1937 found a total of 16 cases, all diagnosed post mortem.[49] The first case of Ebstein's anomaly diagnosed during life, reported in 1949, used the aid of cardiac catheterization.[46] Early surgical approaches to this defect were palliative, either simple repair of the atrial septal defect alone or creation of a Blalock-Taussig or Glenn shunt, and had exceedingly high mortality rates.[47] Hunter and Lillihei proposed a method of complete repair of Ebstein's anomaly in 1958, which combined plication of the atrialized right ventricle, tricuspid anuloplasty, and closure of the atrial septal defect.[26] Hardy and colleagues reported the first successful application of this technique in 1964.[23] Tricuspid valve replacement for this defect was first successfully performed in 1962 by Christiaan Barnard.[5]

EMBRYOLOGY

The leaflets of the tricuspid valve are thought to be derived embryologically from the inner right ventricle. Delamination or undermining of the right ventricular wall occurs during fetal development, forming a muscular skirt of tissue that later develops into the valve apparatus. Openings form in the lower portion of the skirt, leaving the remaining tissue to form the papillary muscles and chordae tendinae. The anterior leaflet of the tricuspid valve is formed relatively early in development, while the septal and posterior cusps are still not fully formed by 3 months' gestation. The development of Ebstein's anomaly may be explained by an abnormality in the undermining process. The septal and posterior leaflets, formed later in development, are thus rudimentary and arise from the right ventricular wall. In addition, the underlying right ventricular myocardium does not develop normally and is usually thin or fibrotic.[10] Exposure of the fetus to lithium carbonate during the first trimester of pregnancy has been implicated in the etiology of Ebstein's anomaly, although this is controversial.[50] A familial association of the malformation has also been reported.[14, 47]

ANATOMY

The primary pathology in Ebstein's anomaly is the inferior displacement of the tricuspid valve apparatus into the right ventricle. Although there is significant variability of tricuspid valve structure with the malformation, the basic pattern of displacement is relatively constant.[2, 31] The anterior leaflet is attached normally to the anulus, and only the attachments of the septal and posterior leaflets are displaced into the ventricle. The commissure between these two leaflets is usually the point of maximum displacement. The degree of displacement and the morphology of the displaced valve leaflets are highly variable in these patients. The leaflets, especially the septal leaflet, are usually dysplastic and adherent to the ventricular wall. Whereas the anterior leaflet is not displaced, it is by no means normal. It is usually described as large, redundant, and *sail-like* and has abnormal attachments from its free edge to the ventricular wall. Uncommonly, a continuous attachment from the leaflet edge to the apex of the right ventricle occurs, with only perforations in the leaflet to allow blood through to the infundibulum. The papillary muscles are often anomalous and malpositioned. The abnormal tricuspid valve in Ebstein's anomaly divides the right ventricle into two parts: The inlet portion of the right ventricle located between the true anulus and the displaced leaflets is referred to as the *atrialized* ventricle, while the trabecular and outlet regions make up the *true* or functional ventricle. The atrialized ventricle is characteristically thinner than the functional ventricle, often fibrotic and occasionally devoid of any muscle tissue (Fig. 54–134). Although the atrialized ventricle is invariably thin and often aneurysmal, in up to two thirds of patients the distal functional ventricle is dilated as well, possibly due to an abnormal decrease in the number of myocardial fibers.[2, 10] Nearly all patients with Ebstein's anomaly have an associated atrial septal defect or patent foramen ovale.[15] The anatomy of the coronary arteries is similar to that of a normal heart with the exception of the right coronary artery, which is displaced superiorly and posteriorly by the dilated atrialized ventricle. Similarly, the conduction system, including both the sinoatrial node and the atrioventricular node, is normally situated in these hearts.

Although this malformation typically involves the right atrioventricular valve, left-sided Ebstein's anomaly has been described, usually in patients with atrioventricular discordance. In fact, Ebstein's anomaly occurs in up to 75% of patients with corrected transposition of the great arteries.[1] Although the nature of the valve displacement is similar to right-sided Ebstein's anomaly, the anterior leaflet is typically smaller and often cleft. Atrial septal defects are uncommonly seen, in contrast to right-sided Ebstein's anomaly. Left-sided Ebstein's anomaly of the mitral valve in the absence of corrected transposition may occur, but it is rare.[2] Also, Ebstein's anomaly may rarely occur simultaneously in both the tricuspid and mitral valves.

The most common cardiac abnormalities found to occur with Ebstein's anomaly are pulmonary stenosis or atresia (10% to 20%) and ventricular septal defects (5%). Less common associated cardiac defects include patent ductus arteriosus, anomalous pulmonary venous drainage, tetralogy of Fallot, coarctation of the aorta, and right-sided aortic arch.[15, 31, 47] Rarely, Ebstein's anomaly is seen in combination with a common atrioventricular canal defect.[13] The coexistence of Ebstein's anomaly and Wolff-Parkinson-White syndrome was described as early as 1955.[30] Accessory pathways are typically the atrioventricular type and are localized to either the right ventricular free wall or the posterior interventricular septum (Kent bundles).[43] Left-sided accessory pathways are seen only

in those patients with left-sided Ebstein's anomaly and corrected transposition of the great vessels.

PATHOPHYSIOLOGY

The tricuspid valve in Ebstein's anomaly is usually regurgitant, but occasionally it may be stenotic or even imperforate. Functional outflow obstruction of the true right ventricle may be caused by the large anterior leaflet. During atrial systole the atrialized portion of the right ventricle functions as a reservoir, allowing less blood to fill the functional ventricle. The atrialized ventricle then contracts during ventricular systole, and this, in turn, impedes atrial filling. The small chamber size of the functional right ventricle also contributes to the right ventricular dysfunction. The impaired filling of the functional right ventricle and pulmonary circulation results in systemic venous hypertension, leading to dilation and hypertrophy of the right atrium. The right atrium may become enormous, exacerbating any tricuspid regurgitation that may be present, and this results in further atrial dilation. In most cases the high right atrial pressure leads to right-to-left shunting through the defect in the atrial septum, resulting in cyanosis. Factors that may impede right ventricular filling or cause pulmonary hypertension may lead to worsened cyanosis or exacerbate symptoms. These include tachycardias or atrial arrhythmias, right ventricular outflow tract obstruction, pulmonary emboli, and aneurysmal formation of the atrialized ventricle.

Despite the apparently isolated involvement of the right ventricle in Ebstein's anomaly, significant changes in both left ventricular function and geometry have been described.[7] These appear to correlate with both the displacement of the tricuspid valve and the size of the right ventricle and may be due to paradoxical motion of the interventricular septum during systole. Over 90% of patients have abnormalities in contraction on cineangiogram, and mitral valve prolapse is present in up to a third of patients.

CLINICAL MANIFESTATIONS

As mentioned previously, Ebstein's anomaly is an uncommon abnormality that represents 0.4% to 1.0% of congenital heart disease.[25] The malformation occurs in both sexes equally. Extracardiac defects consist of craniofacial, central nervous system, and limb malformations but are uncommon. Ebstein's anomaly may be diagnosed prenatally by ultrasonography, and severe forms may be fatal.[10, 40] Although early studies showed only 5% to 10% of patients presented in infancy with the defect,[47] in more recent studies nearly 40% of patients presented when younger than 1 month of age.[25, 40] This change most likely reflects the development of echocardiography as a screening tool for congenital heart disease. Patients initially presenting in their late 20s or 30s are still not uncommon, and one patient was diagnosed at 80 years of age.[22] The majority of patients present with dyspnea, fatigue, and cyanosis, although asymptomatic patients may be found due to murmur on physical examination or to abnormalities on routine electrocardiography or chest x-ray. Paradoxical embolism has also been reported with Ebstein's anomaly.[19, 40] Growth and development are generally normal in patients with Ebstein's anomaly, although asymmetry of the chest may be present. Paroxysmal supraventricular arrhythmias occur in 25% to 40% of patients, mostly in adolescents or adults.[25, 47] Ventricular dysrhythmias are also common and have been shown to originate in the atrialized right ventricle. Wolff-Parkinson-White syndrome has been documented in 10% to 18% of patients.[25, 47] Sudden death due to arrhythmias is not uncommon and may occur in up to 7% of patients.[25] Exercise tolerance is markedly abnormal in

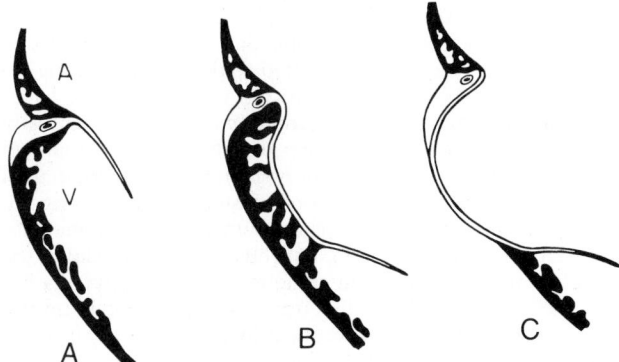

Figure 54–134. Section through the right atrioventricular junction. *A,* Normal heart. A, right atrium; V, right ventricle. *B,* Mild degree of Ebstein's anomaly. *C,* Severe Ebstein's anomaly. Note in *B* and *C* the apparent displacement of the tricuspid valve. (From Van Mierop, L. H. S., Kutsche, L. M., and Victoria, B. E.: Ebstein's anomaly. *In* Adams, F. H., Emmanoulides, G. C., and Riemenschneider, T. A. [Eds.]: Moss' Heart Disease in Infants, Children, and Adolescents, 4th ed. Baltimore, Williams & Wilkins, 1987, p. 362.)

children and adults with Ebstein's anomaly, and maximum oxygen uptake during exercise has been shown to be less than half the predicted amount.[3]

Findings of physical examination include a v wave in the jugular venous pulse due to tricuspid regurgitation. Both first and second heart sounds are widely split, and a soft systolic murmur of tricuspid regurgitation may be present along the left sternal border. Occasionally, a soft diastolic murmur of tricuspid stenosis may be heard. Both murmurs intensify during inspiration. In patients with pulmonary outflow obstruction, the second heart sound may be diminished and a systolic murmur may be heard in the second interspace. Hepatomegaly is often present, especially in infants, but ascites and peripheral edema are uncommon.

The electrocardiogram in Ebstein's patients is always abnormal. Right-axis deviation and right bundle branch block are the most common findings. P-wave morphology is characteristic of right atrial enlargement, and the PR interval is often prolonged. The Wolff-Parkinson-White pattern, usually type B, may be seen on an electrocardiogram in a small percentage of patients. Both atrial and ventricular arrhythmias are a common problem in patients with Ebstein's anomaly. Twenty-four-hour ambulatory electrocardiographic monitoring should be performed on patients with a significant history of arrhythmias or palpitations. Electrophysiologic studies are recommended for those patients with documented ventricular pre-excitation, wide-complex tachycardia or history of syncope.

The findings on chest radiography in patients with Ebstein's anomaly range from normal to massive cardiomegaly, with cardiothoracic ratios greater than 0.90.[10, 22] Typically, the vascular pedicle of the heart is narrow due to a small aorta and main pulmonary artery. The heart assumes a globular shape owing to right atrial enlargement, and the dilated right ventricular outflow tract produces an upward and lateral displacement of the left border of the heart. The apex of the heart is often elevated from the diaphragm. Pulmonary vascularity is either normal or decreased, and the finding of increased vascular markings should cause one to question the diagnosis.

Echocardiography has emerged over the past decade as the primary diagnostic tool for Ebstein's anomaly and many other cardiac defects. Excellent correlation of echocardiographic findings with surgical and autopsy specimens has been well documented.[41] Echocardiography allows precise determination of the tricuspid valve morphology, including leaflet displacement, dysplasia, and tethering. In addition, size, thickness, and function of both ventricles is assessed. Echocardiography is also useful in identifying coexisting cardiac defects. The development of color-flow Doppler analysis now permits better quantification of valvular incompetence or stenosis and of blood flow across the atrial septum. In those cases in which echocardiography is inadequate or indeterminate, both cine computed tomography and magnetic resonance imaging have demonstrated diagnostic capabilities in Ebstein's anomaly.[33]

Cardiac catheterization, historically the definitive method for diagnosing Ebstein's anomaly, has essentially been replaced by echocardiography. Early studies demonstrated a 30% risk of inciting arrhythmias during catheterization, and the mortality rate for catheterization was 3%.[47] More recent studies have shown a dramatic decrease in catheterization-related morbidity, but arrhythmias still occur infrequently.[10] Catheterization findings include elevated right atrial pressures, with normal right ventricular and pulmonary artery pressures. A large v wave may be seen if tricuspid incompetence is present; a prominent a wave is present if the tricuspid valve is stenotic. The demonstration of right atrial pressures in the proximal right ventricle is diagnostic of Ebstein's anomaly. In addition, oximetry is useful in identifying the presence and degree of atrial shunting. Angiography reveals right atrial enlargement with abnormal positioning of the tricuspid valve anulus. The origin of the displaced tricuspid valve leaflets are seen as an indentation on the inferior wall of the right ventricle, and contrast medium may be seen moving back and forth between the ventricle and the atrium. Currently, cardiac catheterization is reserved for patients with Ebstein's anomaly who have additional cardiac abnormalities, previous systemic-pulmonary or cavopulmonary shunts, or suspected pulmonary artery hypoplasia.

NATURAL HISTORY

The natural history of Ebstein's anomaly has been well established in the literature despite the rarity of the defect. Neonates diagnosed with this disorder are almost always cyanotic, and those patients with associated right ventricular outflow tract obstruction usually present early in life.[10] In addition, the elevated pulmonary vascular resistance present in neonates may create a functional pulmonary atresia, which worsens the tricuspid regurgitation and right-to-left shunting. Over 75% of infants present with New York Heart Association Class IV congestive heart failure, and the mortality rate for infants diagnosed with Ebstein's anomaly may be as high as 50%, half of whom die during the neonatal period.[22, 47] Cardiac failure is the common cause of early death, while sudden death accounts for an increased proportion of late deaths. Factors that may predispose to early mortality include right ventricular dysplasia or fibrosis, tethering of the distal attachments of the anterior leaflet, left ventricular compression, and the combined right atrial and atrialized ventricle area being greater than the combined areas of the functional right ventricle, left atrium, and left ventricle.[40]

If patients survive beyond the neonatal period, pulmonary vascular resistance decreases, and they may become relatively free of symptoms. This is reflected in the actuarial survival curve for Ebstein's anomaly, which is 67% at 1 year of age and 59% at age 10.[10] The majority of patients diagnosed after infancy are functional Class I or II, and late follow-up has demonstrated that up to 40% remain in that functional class.[22] Over time the functional impairment of the right ventricle worsens, as does the tricuspid regurgitation; and over half of patients progress to functional Class III or IV. The British cooperative study demonstrated a 15% mortality in 346 patients ages 1 to 25, with half of these patients dying of cardiac failure and 20% of sudden death.[47] Patients older than age 25 had a mortality rate of 18%, but the number of deaths from cardiac failure and sudden death were equal. Risk factors for early death in Ebstein's anomaly include presentation in infancy, functional Class III or IV symptoms, severe cyanosis, and severe cardiomegaly (cardiothoracic ratio > 0.65).[10, 20, 25]

Pregnancy in women with Ebstein's anomaly is generally well tolerated, although cyanotic women have been shown to have infants with significantly lower birth weight than acyanotic women.[14] The incidence of offspring with congenital heart disease is higher for both men and women with Ebstein's anomaly. Children with this disorder should be restricted from competitive athletics, and prophylaxis for subacute bacterial endocarditis is recommended when undergoing any dental or surgical procedures.

TREATMENT

Treatment of Ebstein's anomaly must be individualized owing to the variability of the defect, concomitant cardiac defects, and wide range of clinical manifestations. In general, surgical intervention is required in most patients and the medical treatment of Ebstein's anomaly is reserved for fluid management and control of arrhythmias. Indications for surgery include functional Class III or IV symptoms, significant cyanosis, severe cardiomegaly (cardiothoracic ratio > 0.65), right ventricular outflow tract obstruction, history of paradoxical emboli, or evidence of ventricular pre-excitation. Patients with mild forms of the anomaly, functional Class I or II, are observed closely and may not require treatment.

Neonates diagnosed with Ebstein's anomaly have a high mortality rate, and the management goal is palliation through the early neonatal period until pulmonary vascular resistance decreases. Prostaglandin E_1 infusion has been shown to improve the severe cyanosis seen in these infants.[27] Extracorporeal membrane oxygenation, used extensively in infants with persistent fetal circulation, has also been successfully applied in several cases of neonatal Ebstein's anomaly.[37] Early attempts at palliative surgery for infants with this disorder were uniformly unsuccessful.[47] Starnes and colleagues have described an approach to critically ill neonates with Ebstein's anomaly that has been successful in a small number of patients.[44] The procedure combines closure of the tricuspid orifice with autologous pericardium or Gore-Tex, atrial septectomy, and placement of a systemic-pulmonary shunt, thus creating a single ventricle physiology (Fig. 54–135). These infants are then staged to either a Glenn shunt or modified Fontan procedure at 2 years of age. The modified Fontan procedure alone has also been used successfully in children with severe tricuspid stenosis due to Ebstein's anomaly.[29] Orthotopic heart transplantation has been reported in infants with severe disease.[34]

The preferential surgical treatment of Ebstein's anomaly is repair of the tricuspid valve. Danielson and colleagues at the Mayo Clinic have pioneered this approach and have the largest experience in the literature. In their latest series of 189 patients, they have been able to repair the tricuspid valve in 60% of these patients.[15] The repair consists of plication of the free wall of the atrialized right ventricle, posterior tricuspid anuloplasty, patch repair of the atrial septal defect, and excision of redundant right atrium (Fig. 54–136). Repair of coexisting defects (ventricular septal defects or pulmonary outflow obstruction) is carried out at the same time. Thus the goal of the repair is to create a functional monocuspid valve using the anterior leaflet. Postoperatively, the majority of patients have only trivial or mild tricuspid regurgitation,

and long-term follow-up has shown reoperation for tricuspid valve replacement necessary in only 3% of patients. Operative mortality was 7.3%, with most of the deaths due to ventricular arrhythmias or low cardiac output. Danielson subsequently recommended the prophylactic use of intravenous lidocaine in all patients for the first 48 hours postoperatively, with conversion to oral procainamide, which is then discontinued in 3 months if no further ventricular ectopy is seen. Echocardiography has been useful preoperatively in predicting patients who are candidates for tricuspid valve repair, and the presence of a tethered anterior valve leaflet or small functional right ventricle is a strong indicator of the need for valve replacement.[42]

Carpentier described his technique for tricuspid valve repair in Ebstein's anomaly in 1988.[9] The procedure involves detachment of the anterior leaflet and adjacent portion of the posterior leaflet from the anulus, followed by longitudinal plication of the atrialized right ventricle, with plication of the tricuspid anulus and right atrium (Fig. 54–137). The anterior and posterior leaflets are then resuspended on the tricuspid anulus, followed by placement of a prosthetic ring. Repair was possible in 13 of 14 patients, with an operative mortality of 14%. Significant tricuspid regurgitation was present in 1 patient, while 77% had minimal or no insufficiency. All surviving patients were functional Class I or II, with a mean follow-up of 3 years. Quaegebeur and colleagues have subsequently reported their experience with this repair in 10 patients, with no operative deaths and similar long-term results.[39]

Whereas the recent trend has been toward repair of the tricuspid valve, tricuspid valve replacement has been the traditional treatment of Ebstein's anomaly and is still frequently necessary. Long-term survivors without reoperation have been reported up to 28 years after surgery.[28] Early studies reported the use of mechanical valves[40, 48]; however, the significant risk of bleeding and thromboembolic complications (especially in teenage patients who may be noncompliant) has led to the preferential use of bioprosthetic valves.[45] Valve failure due to thrombosis has also been seen with mechanical prostheses in the tricuspid position.[24] Several studies have demonstrated excellent durability of bioprosthetic valves in the tricuspid position,[17, 21] although accelerated degeneration due to valve calcification has been reported in children.[36] Tricuspid valve replacement is usually

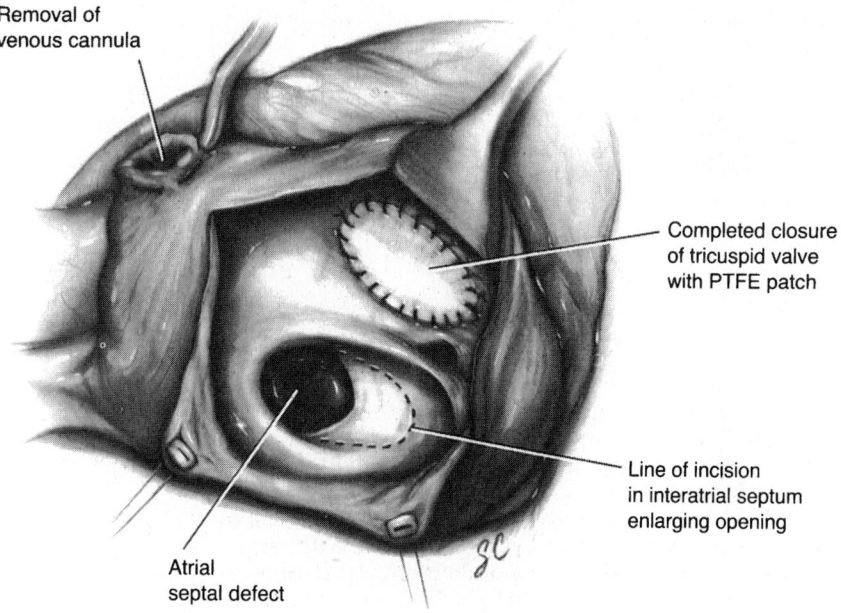

Figure 54–135. Repair of Ebstein's anomaly in neonates. The atrial septal defect is enlarged by excising the remaining septum primum to produce an unrestrictive atrial communication. The tricuspid valve is closed with a patch of Gore-Tex placed through the leaflet material along the septal region to limit the risk of damage to the conduction tissue. A Gore-Tex shunt (usually 4.0 mm.) is placed between the innominate artery and the right pulmonary artery later in the procedure (not shown). (From Sabiston, D. C., Jr. [Ed.]: The Atlas of Cardiothoracic Surgery. Philadelphia, W. B. Saunders, 1995, p. 373.)

Removal of
venous cannula

Completed closure
of tricuspid valve
with PTFE patch

Line of incision
in interatrial septum
enlarging opening

Atrial
septal defect

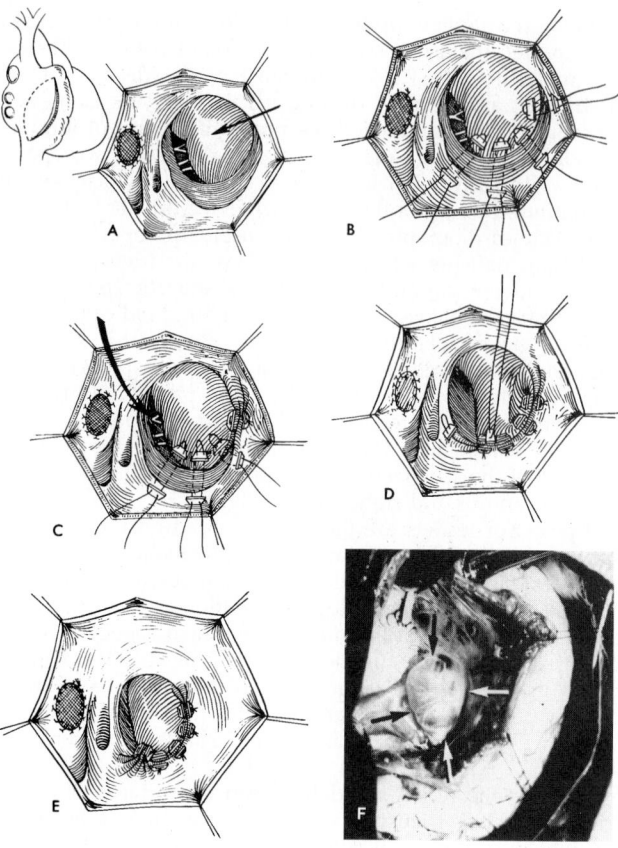

Figure 54–136. Diagram of surgical repair. *A, left,* The right atrium is incised from the appendage to the inferior vena cava. The redundant portion of the right atrium is excised (broken line). *A, right,* Atrial septal defect is closed with a patch. The large anterior leaflet is indicated by the arrow. The posterior leaflet is displaced down from the anulus. The septal leaflet is hypoplastic and is not seen in this view. *B,* Mattress sutures passed through pledgets of Teflon felt are used to pull the tricuspid anulus and tricuspid valve together. Sutures are placed in the atrialized portion of the right ventricle (as shown) so that when they are subsequently tied, the atrialized ventricle is plicated and the aneurysmal cavity is obliterated. *C,* Sutures are tied down sequentially. Hypoplastic, markedly displaced septal leaflet is now visible (arrow). *D,* Posterior anuloplasty is done to narrow the diameter of the tricuspid anulus. Coronary sinus marks the posterior–left-sided extent of the anuloplasty, which is terminated there to avoid injury to the conduction bundle. *E,* Completed repair, which allows the anterior leaflet to function as a monocuspid valve. *F,* Operative photograph of the completed repair. Large anterior leaflet forms competent monocuspid valve (arrows). (From Danielson, G. K., Maloney, J. D., and Devloo, R. A. E.: Surgical repair of Ebstein's anomaly. Mayo Clin. Proc., *54:*185, 1979.)

combined with closure of the atrial septal defect. The prosthesis is sutured above the coronary sinus to avoid injury to the atrioventricular node (Fig. 54–138). Plication of the atrialized right ventricle during valve replacement is controversial, with small retrospective series supporting either method.[6, 8, 36, 48] In general, plication is performed if the atrialized right ventricle is significantly dilated, thin, or hypocontractile. Op-

erative mortality reported for tricuspid valve replacement in Ebstein's anomaly ranges from 5.8% to 20%.[4, 15, 48]

In patients with preoperatively documented ventricular pre-excitation, intraoperative electrophysiologic mapping should be included in the procedure. Identification and interruption of accessory pathways is performed before valve repair or replacement. There is no increase in morbidity

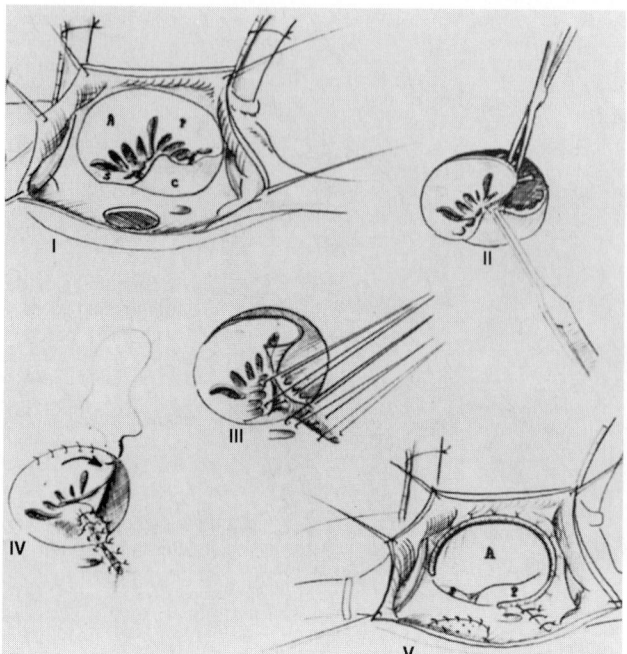

Figure 54–137. Surgical technique. *I,* Operative view: anterior leaflet (A); posterior leaflet (P); septal leaflet (S); atrialized chamber (C). *II,* Anterior leaflet and adjacent portion of posterior leaflet are detached from anulus. Leaflet time is mobilized by cutting fibrous bands attached to ventricular wall. Interchordal spaces are fenestrated if obliterated. *III,* Longitudinal plication of right ventricle by simple sutures passed through septal and posterior leaflet remnants. The tricuspid anulus and right atrium are plicated. *IV,* Anterior and posterior leaflets are sutured to the tricuspid anulus after clockwise rotation (arrow) to cover entire orifice area. *V,* Prosthetic ring is inserted for remodeling the orifice and reinforcing repair. The atrial septal defect is closed. (From Carpentier, A., Chauvaud, S., Mace, L., Relland, J., Mihaileanu, S., Marino, J. P., Abry, B., and Guibourt, P.: A new reconstructive operation for Ebstein's anomaly of the tricuspid valve. J. Thorac. Cardiovasc. Surg., *96:*95, 1988.)

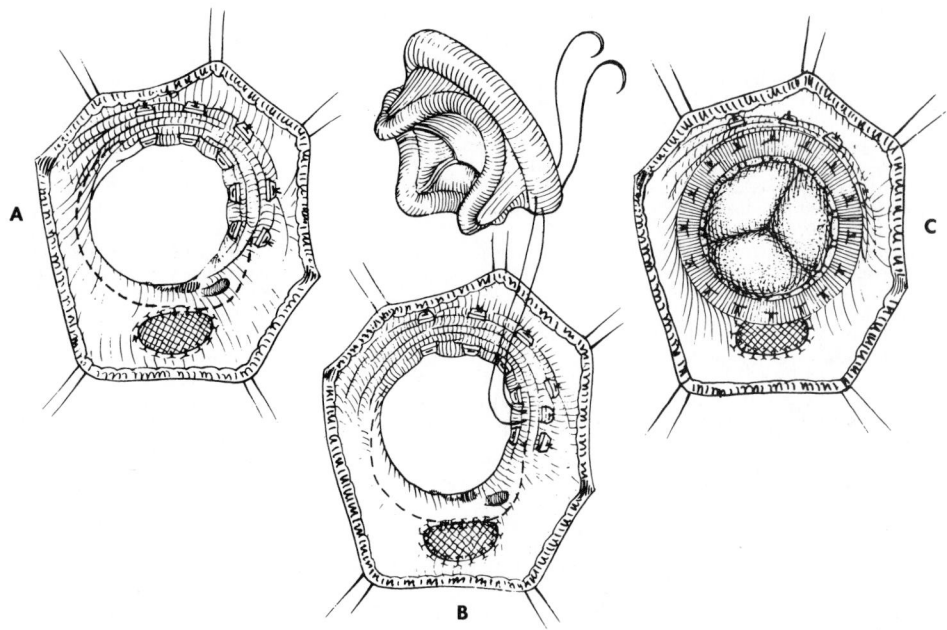

Figure 54–138. Diagram of technique for tricuspid valve replacement in Ebstein's anomaly. *A*, If the atrialized right ventricle is dilated, thin, and hypocontractile, it is plicated. *B*, The suture line is placed on the atrial side of the coronary sinus and AV node to avoid injury to the conduction mechanism. *C*, The sutures are tied with the heart perfused and beating to ensure that a conducted rhythm is preserved. (From Danielson, G. K.: Ebstein's anomaly of the tricuspid valve. *In* Mavroudis, C., and Backer, C. L. [Eds.]: Pediatric Cardiac Surgery, 2nd ed. St. Louis, Mosby–Year Book, 1994, p. 421.)

associated with combined valve repair and pathway ablation, and long-term results are excellent, with up to 90% of patients reporting minimal or no symptoms of arrhythmias on follow-up.[38] In asymptomatic patients with Ebstein's anomaly (functional Class I or II) and atrioventricular accessory pathways, radiofrequency ablation is a useful alternative to operative treatment.[32]

Long-term results with the surgical treatment of Ebstein's anomaly are excellent. Over 90% of survivors are functional Class I or II, and reduction of cardiomegaly frequently occurs.[15] Improvement in resting and exercise arterial oxygen saturation and exercise tolerance has also been well documented.[16] In addition, only one third of patients with preoperative paroxysmal supraventricular tachycardias continued to have symptomatic arrhythmias postoperatively.[35] The late mortality rate for surgical repair of Ebstein's anomaly is approximately 6%, with sudden death occurring in half of these patients.

SELECTED REFERENCES

Celermajer, D. S., Bull, C., Till, J. A., Cullen, S., Vassillikos, V. P., Sullivan, I. D., Allan, L., Nihoyannopoulos, P., Somerville, J., and Deanfield, J. E.: Ebstein's anomaly: Presentation and outcome from fetus to adult. J. Am. Coll. Cardiol., 23:170, 1994.
This is a current review of the natural history of 220 patients presenting over the past 35 years to a number of hospitals in the United Kingdom. This review focuses on a large subset of patients diagnosed during infancy, while most older reports include mainly adolescents and adults. Patient characteristics and diagnostic and management strategies are also discussed.

Danielson, G. K., Driscoll, D. J., Mair, D. D., Warnes, C. A., and Oliver, W. C.: Operative treatment of Ebstein's anomaly. J. Thorac. Cardiovasc. Surg., 104:1195, 1992.
The latest report from the Mayo Clinic is the largest series in the literature of the surgical treatment of Ebstein's anomaly. Techniques in tricuspid valve repair and replacement are discussed, and postoperative and long-term follow-up results are summarized.

Schiebler, G. L., Gravenstein, J. S., and Van Mierop, L. H.: Ebstein's anomaly of the tricuspid valve: Translation of original description with comments. Am. J. Cardiol., 22:867, 1968.
This is the English translation of Ebstein's classic paper. It is complete with the original drawings of Ebstein's autopsy findings, along with his hypothesis regarding the pathophysiology of the defect.

Starnes, V. A., Pitlick, P. T., Bernstein, D., Griffin, M. L., Choy, M., and Shumway, N. E.: Ebstein's anomaly appearing in the neonate: A new surgical approach. J. Thorac. Cardiovasc. Surg., 101:1082, 1991.
An innovative approach to severely ill infants with Ebstein's anomaly is described.

The pathophysiology of the defect characteristically seen in the neonatal period is well documented by the report. Late follow-up was obtained, and most patients were staged to either a Glenn shunt or Fontan procedure as their definitive palliative procedure.

REFERENCES

1. Allwork, S. P., Bentall, H. H., Becker, A. E., Cameron, H., Gerlis, L. M., Wilkinson, J. L., and Anderson, R. H.: Congenitally corrected transposition of the great arteries: Morphologic study of 32 cases. Am. J. Cardiol., 38:910, 1976.
2. Anderson, K. R., Zuberbuhler, J. R., Anderson, R. H., Becker, A. E., and Lie, J. T.: Morphologic spectrum of Ebstein's anomaly of the heart. Mayo Clin. Proc., 54:174, 1979.
3. Barber, G., Danielson, G. K., Heise, C. T., and Driscoll, D. J.: Cardiorespiratory response to exercise in Ebstein's anomaly. Am. J. Cardiol., 56:509, 1985.
4. Barbero-Marcial, B., Verginelli, G., Awad, M., Ferreira, S., Ebaid, M., and Zerbini, E. J.: Surgical treatment of Ebstein's anomaly: Early and late results in twenty patients subjected to valve replacement. J. Thorac. Cardiovasc. Surg., 78:416, 1979.
5. Barnard, C. N., and Schrire, V.: Surgical correction of Ebstein's malformation with prosthetic tricuspid valve. Surgery, 54:302, 1963.
6. Behl, P. R., and Blesovsky, A.: Ebstein's anomaly: Sixteen years' experience with valve replacement without plication of the right ventricle. Thorax, 39:8, 1984.
7. Benson, L. N., Child, J. S., Schwaiger, M., Perloff, J. K., and Schelbert, H. R.: Left ventricular geometry and function in adults with Ebstein's anomaly of the tricuspid valve. Circulation, 75:353, 1987.
8. Bove, E. L., and Kirsch, M. M.: Valve replacement for Ebstein's anomaly of the tricuspid valve. J. Thorac. Cardiovasc. Surg., 78:229, 1979.
9. Carpentier, A., Chauvaud, S., Mace, L., Relland, J., Mihaileanu, S., Marino, J. P., Abry, B., and Guibourt, P.: A new reconstructive operation for Ebstein's anomaly of the tricuspid valve. J. Thorac. Cardiovasc. Surg., 96:92, 1988.
10. Celermajer, D. S., Bull, C., Till, J. A., Cullen, S., Vassillikos, V. P., Sullivan, I. D., Allan, L., Nihoyannopoulos, P., Somerville, J., and Deanfield, J. E.: Ebstein's anomaly: Presentation and outcome from fetus to adult. J. Am. Coll. Cardiol., 23:170, 1994.
11. Celermajer, D. S., Cullen, S., Sullivan, I. D., Spiegelhalter, D. J., Wyse, R. K., and Deanfield, J. E.: Outcome in neonates with Ebstein's anomaly. J. Am. Coll. Cardiol., 19:1041, 1992.
12. Celermajer, D. S., Dodd, S. M., Greenwald, S. E., Wyse, R. K., and Deanfield, J. E.: Morbid anatomy in neonates with Ebstein's anomaly of the tricuspid valve: Pathophysiologic and clinical implications. J. Am. Coll. Cardiol., 19:1049, 1992.
13. Choe, K., McConnell, M. E., Mesa, J., and Soto, B.: Atrioventricular septal defect and Ebstein's malformation. Am. J. Cardiol., 65:939, 1990.
14. Connolly, H. M., and Warnes, C. A.: Ebstein's anomaly: Outcome of pregnancy. J. Am. Coll. Cardiol., 23:1194, 1994.
15. Danielson, G. K., Driscoll, D. J., Mair, D. D., Warnes, C. A., and Oliver, W. C.: Operative treatment of Ebstein's anomaly. J. Thorac. Cardiovasc. Surg., 104:1195, 1992.
16. Driscoll, D. J., Mottram, C. D., and Danielson, G. K.: Spectrum of exercise

intolerance in 45 patients with Ebstein's anomaly and observations on exercise tolerance in 11 patients after surgical repair. J. Am. Coll. Cardiol., *11*:831, 1988.

17. Dunn, J. M.: Porcine valve durability in children. Ann. Thorac. Surg., *32*:357, 1981.

18. Ebstein, W.: Ueber einen sehr seltenen Fall von Insufficiency der Valvula Tricuspidalis, bedengt durch eine angeborene hochgradige Missbildung derselben. Arch. Anat. Physiol. Wissenschaft. Med., 238, 1866.

19. Fornace, J., Rozanski, L. T., and Berger, B. C.: Right heart thromboembolism and suspected paradoxical embolism in Ebstein's anomaly. Am. Heart J., *114*:1520, 1987.

20. Gentles, T. L., Calder, A. L., Clarkson, P. M., and Neutze, J. M.: Predictors of long-term survival with Ebstein's anomaly of the tricuspid valve. Am. J. Cardiol., *69*:377, 1992.

21. Glower, D. D., White, W. D., Hatton, A. C., Smith, L. R., Young, W. G., Wolfe, W. W., and Lowe, J. E.: Determinants of reoperation after 960 valve replacements with Carpentier-Edwards prostheses. J. Thorac. Cardiovasc. Surg., *107*:381, 1994.

22. Giuliani, E. R., Fuster, V., Brandenburg, R. O., and Mair, D. D.: The clinical features and natural history of Ebstein's anomaly of the tricuspid valve. Mayo Clin. Proc., *54*:163, 1979.

23. Hardy, K. L., May, I. A., Webster, C. A., and Kimball, K. G.: Ebstein's anomaly: A functional concept and successful definitive repair. J. Thorac. Cardiovasc. Surg., *48*:927, 1964.

24. Harjula, H., Kupari, M., Ventila, M., and Mattila, S.: Failure of mechanical valves in Ebstein's malformation. Int. J. Cardiol., *11*:265, 1986.

25. Hong, Y. M., and Moller, J. H.: Ebstein's anomaly: A long-term study of survival. Am. Heart J., *125*:1419, 1993.

26. Hunter, S. W., and Lillihei, C. W.: Ebstein's malformation of the tricuspid valve: Study of a case together with suggestion of a new form of surgical therapy. Dis. Chest, *33*:297, 1958.

27. Ivy, D., Loehr, J., and Schaffer, M.: Usefulness of prolonged prostaglandin infusion in neonates with Ebstein's anomaly. Am. J. Cardiol., *72*:1327, 1993.

28. Kirklin, J. K.: Christaan Barnard's contribution to the surgical treatment of Ebstein's malformation. Ann. Thorac. Surg., *51*:147, 1991.

29. Leung, M. P., Lee, J., Lo, R. N., and Mok, C. K.: Modified Fontan procedure for severe Ebstein's malformation with predominant tricuspid stenosis. Ann. Thorac. Surg., *54*:523, 1992.

30. Lev, M., Gibson, S., and Miller, R. A.: Ebstein's disease with Wolff-Parkinson-White syndrome: Report of a case with a histopathologic study of possible conduction pathways. Am. Heart J., *49*:724, 1955.

31. Lev, M., Liberthson, R. R., Joseph, R. H., Seten, C. E., Kunske, R. D., Eckner, F. A., and Miller, R. A.: The pathologic anatomy of Ebstein's disease. Arch. Pathol., *90*:334, 1970.

32. Levine, J. C., Walsh, E. P., and Saul, J. P.: Radiofrequency ablation of accessory pathways associated with congenital heart disease including heterotaxy syndrome. Am. J. Cardiol., *72*:689, 1993.

33. Link, K. M., Herrera, M. A., D'Souza, V. J., and Formanek, A. G.: MR imaging of Ebstein anomaly: Results in four cases. AJR, *150*:363, 1988.

34. Mayer, J. E., Perry, S., O'Brien, P., Perez-Atayde, A., Jonas, R. A., Castaneda, A. R., and Parness, I. A.: Orthotopic heart transplantation for complex congenital heart disease. J. Thorac. Cardiovasc. Surg., *99*:484, 1990.

35. Oh, J. K., Holmes, D. R., Hayes, D. L., Porter, C. J., and Danielson, G. K.:

Cardiac arrhythmias in patients with surgical repair of Ebstein's anomaly. J. Am. Coll. Cardiol., *6*:1351, 1985.

36. Pasque, M., Williams, W. G., Coles, J. G., Trusler, G. A., and Freedom, R. M.: Tricuspid valve replacement in children. Ann. Thorac. Surg., *44*:164, 1987.

37. Plowden, J. S., Kimball, T. R., Bensky, A., Savani, R., Flake, A. W., Warner, B. W., von Allmen, D., and Ryckman, F. C.: The use of extracorporeal membrane oxygenation in critically ill neonates with Ebstein's anomaly. Am. Heart J., *121*:619, 1991.

38. Pressley, J. C., Wharton, J. M., Tang, A. S., Lowe, J. E., Gallagher, J. J., and Prystowsky, E. N.: Effect of Ebstein's anomaly on short- and long-term outcome of surgically treated patients with Wolff-Parkinson-White syndrome. Circulation, *86*:1147, 1992.

39. Quaegebeur, J. M., Sreeram, N., Fraser, A. G., Rogers, J. J., Stumper, O. F., Hess, J., Bos, E., and Sutherland, G. R.: Surgery for Ebstein's anomaly: The clinical and echocardiographic evaluation of a new technique. J. Am. Coll. Cardiol., *17*:722, 1991.

40. Roberson, D. A., and Silverman, N. H.: Ebstein's anomaly: Echocardiographic and clinical features in the fetus and neonate. J. Am. Coll. Cardiol., *14*:1300, 1989.

41. Shiina, A., Seward, J. B., Edwards, W. D., Hagler, D. J., and Tajik, A. J.: Two-dimensional echocardiographic spectrum of Ebstein's anomaly: Detailed anatomic assessment. J. Am. Coll. Cardiol., *3*:356, 1984.

42. Shiina, A., Seward, J. B., Tajik, A. J., Hagler, D. J., and Danielson, G. K.: Two-dimensional echocardiographic-surgical correlation in Ebstein's anomaly: Preoperative determination of patients requiring tricuspid valve plication vs. replacement. Circulation, *68*:534, 1983.

43. Smith, W. M., Gallagher, J. J., Kerr, C. R., Sealy, W. C., Benson, D. W., Jr., Reiter, M. J., Sterba, R., and Grant, A. O.: The electrophysiologic basis and management of symptomatic recurrent tachycardia in patients with Ebstein's anomaly of the tricuspid valve. Am. J. Cardiol., *49*:1223, 1982.

44. Starnes, V. A., Pitlick, P. T., Bernstein, D., Griffin, M. L., Choy, M., and Shumway, N. E.: Ebstein's anomaly appearing in the neonate: A new surgical approach. J. Thorac. Cardiovasc. Surg., *101*:1082, 1991.

45. Stewart, S., Cianciotta, D., Alexson, C., and Manning, J.: The long-term risk of warfarin sodium therapy and the incidence of thromboembolism in children after prosthetic cardiac valve replacement. J. Thorac. Cardiovasc. Surg., *93*:551, 1987.

46. Tourniaire, A., Deyrieux, F., and Tartulier, M.: Maladie d'Ebstein: Essai de diagnostic clinique. Arch. Mal. Coeur, *42*:1211, 1949.

47. Watson, H.: Natural history of Ebstein's anomaly of tricuspid valve in childhood and adolescence: An international co-operative study of 505 cases. Br. Heart J., *36*:417, 1974.

48. Westaby, S., Karp, R. B., Kirklin, J. W., Waldo, A. L., and Blackstone, E. H.: Surgical treatment of Ebstein's malformation. Ann. Thorac. Surg., *34*:388, 1982.

49. Yater, W. M., and Shapiro, M. J.: Congenital displacement of the tricuspid valve (Ebstein's disease): Review and report of a case with electrocardiographic abnormalities and detailed histologic study of the conduction system. Ann. Intern. Med., *11*:1043, 1937.

50. Zalzstein, E., Koren, G., Einarson, T., and Freedom, R. M.: A case-control study on the association between first trimester exposure to lithium and Ebstein's anomaly. Am. J. Cardiol., *65*:817, 1990.

XVI

CONGENITAL LESIONS OF THE CORONARY CIRCULATION

James E. Lowe, M.D., James D. St. Louis, M.D., and David C. Sabiston, Jr., M.D.

Although congenital coronary arterial malformations have long been recognized, the introduction of selective coronary arteriography by Sones and Shirey[30] in 1959 greatly increased the number discovered. In a review of 224 patients with coronary malformations, Ogden proposed three basic classifications: (1) major anomalies, in which there is an abnormal communication between an artery and a cardiac chamber or abnormal origin of a major coronary artery from the pulmonary artery; (2) minor anomalies, in which there is variation of the origin of the vessels from the aorta but the distal circulation is normal; and (3) secondary anomalies, in which

the coronary arterial variation probably represents a circulatory response of the primary intracardiac pathologic defect.[22]

Lesions amenable to surgical correction include congenital coronary fistulas, the anomalous origin of either the left or right coronary artery from the pulmonary artery, congenital aneurysms of the coronary arteries, and congenital membranous obstruction of the ostium of the left main coronary artery. Minor anomalies, in which there is variation in the origin of the coronary arteries from the aorta with normal distal circulation, and secondary anomalies, associated with congenital heart defects, such as transposition of the great vessels, truncus arteriosus, and tetralogy of Fallot, seldom require surgical intervention.

It is recommended that most patients with major congenital coronary arterial malformations be considered candidates for surgical correction. The natural history of these lesions is associated with a reduced life expectancy in the majority of these patients, with the possible exception of patients with congenital origin of the right coronary artery from the pulmonary artery. Because these malformations can be safely corrected with excellent long-term results, surgical intervention should be strongly recommended when a precise diagnosis has been established.

CORONARY ARTERY FISTULAS

More than 400 patients have been reported in the literature with coronary artery fistulas since Krause first described the first case in 1865. The number is steadily increasing with the widespread use of cardiac catheterization and selective coronary arteriography in the evaluation of various cardiac problems.

Fistulas represent the most common of the congenital coronary malformations. They are characterized by normal origin of the involved coronary artery from the aorta with a fistulous communication with the atria or ventricles or with the pulmonary artery, coronary sinus, or superior vena cava without any interposed capillary bed. Coronary artery fistulas are found with no sex predilection in 1 of every 50,000 patients with congenital heart disease and in 1 of every 500 patients who have coronary arteriography.

Clinical Manifestations. Whereas it was previously commonly believed that most patients with coronary artery fistulas were asymptomatic, it is now recognized that some 55% are symptomatic at the time of presentation.[18] Because the underlying pathophysiology is essentially that of a left-to-right cardiac shunt, the most common manifestation is congestive heart failure. Angina pectoris is another common symptom of the defect secondary to a steal of coronary arterial flow through the fistulous communication.[4] Bacterial endocarditis, anemia, and glomerulonephritis in the same patient have been reported.[28] Infants and children with this lesion may demonstrate a failure to thrive. Less commonly, patients present with acute myocardial infarction, aneurysm formation with subsequent rupture of embolization, or symptoms secondary to pulmonary hypertension.

In asymptomatic patients, the diagnosis is usually made after coronary angiography is performed for evaluation of asymptomatic murmurs, mild cardiomegaly discovered on routine chest film, or persistent electrocardiographic abnormalities.

A continuous murmur over the site of the abnormal communication is the most common clinical finding. The murmur may closely resemble that of a patent ductus arteriosus, and the first patient on whom closure was performed was operated on by Bjork and Crafoord in 1947 for a presumed patent ductus. Because a patent ductus was not found, the pericardium was opened and a coronary artery fistula draining into the pulmonary artery was identified and obliterated. The differential diagnosis of coronary artery fistulas, in addition to a patent ductus arteriosus, includes congenital aortic-pulmonary fistula, sinus of Valsalva fistula, ventricular septal defect with aortic insufficiency, pulmonary arteriovenous malformation, and fistulas of systemic vessels such as the subclavian and internal mammary arteries connecting to veins of the chest wall or to the lung.

In congenital coronary artery fistulas the right coronary artery is most often involved (56%) and most often communicates with a chamber of the right side of the heart. The fistula usually involves the right ventricle (39%), followed closely

in incidence by drainage into the right atrium (33%), including the coronary sinus and superior vena cava or the pulmonary artery (20%). Left coronary artery fistulas are less common but usually drain into the right ventricle or right atrium. Rarely, coronary artery fistulas may drain into the left atrium or left ventricle.

Evaluation. Surgical management of patients with congenital coronary artery fistulas depends on a thorough preoperative evaluation that precisely defines the anatomy and pathophysiology of the anomaly. Although echocardiography and computed chest tomography have been used noninvasively to identify coronary fistulas, the precise diagnosis requires arteriographic demonstration of the involved coronary artery, the recipient cardiac chamber, and the exact site of communication. In patients with a large fistula, injection of contrast medium into the aortic root may clearly delineate the lesion (Fig. 54–139). In patients with a smaller fistulous communication from both coronary arteries, selective coronary arteriography is preferable and may be essential to establish the diagnosis.

Spontaneous closure of a coronary fistula is rare, and only three documented cases have been reported. The ideal time for elective surgical closure is before the development of symptoms and major pathologic changes in the heart, the coronary arteries, and the pulmonary circulation. As shown by Liberthson and associates,[16] most patients with congenital coronary artery fistula develop both symptoms and fistula-related complications with increased age and care subject to increased morbidity and mortality when the operation is done later in life.

Surgical Management. Because patients with coronary artery fistulas have a precise and detailed angiographic examination showing the involved coronary artery, the recipient cardiac chamber, and the exact site of communication, it can often be anticipated preoperatively whether cardiopulmonary bypass (CPB) is required. Patients with a single communication that is easily dissected usually do not require CPB for suture obliteration. However, in patients with multiple communications or large tortuous, draining channels, the fistula is best obliterated by opening the recipient cardiac chamber with the patient on CPB to completely close all fistulous tracts (Fig. 54–140).[18] Finally, if fistula obliteration in any way jeopardizes distal coronary arterial flow, a saphenous vein or internal mammary bypass graft should be placed under hypothermic potassium cardioplegic arrest. These procedures should be planned with pump standby, because the majority are now done using CPB.

Results. Thirty-eight patients with congenital coronary fistulas have been evaluated at the Duke University Medical Center. These patients were between 6 weeks and 76 years of age, with a mean of 32 years and equal distribution between males and females. Half of the patients came to surgical attention because of symptoms such as congestive heart failure, angina, or failure to thrive. The remainder were asymptomatic and came to operation after evaluation of asymptomatic heart murmurs or cardiomegaly found on routine chest film. Thirty-one of these patients have had operative repair. All procedures were done through a median sternotomy, and 14 patients had suture obliteration of the fistula without bypass (48%). Seventeen patients had CPB to open recipient cardiac chamber and successfully occlude multiple draining fistulous tracts (52%). The mean time of follow-up for these 31 patients has been 10 years. There were no operative deaths, and all patients are well and do not have evidence of recurrent fistula formation, although one patient with a complex fistula of the circumflex coronary artery to the right ventricle has a small residual shunt. Similar surgical results in 56 patients have been reported from the Texas Heart Institute with an overall survival of 98.3%.[36]

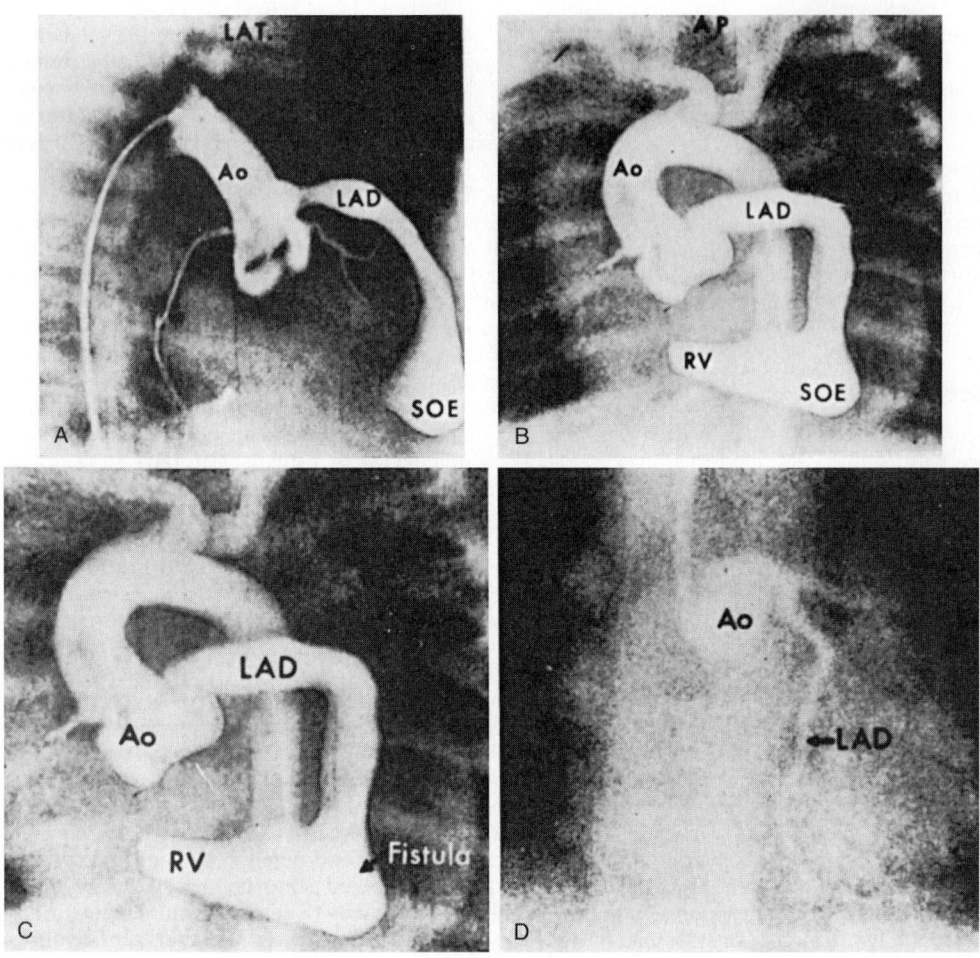

Figure 54–139. Ascending aortogram (lateral [A] and anteroposterior [B] views) in a 6-week-old infant who presented with severe congestive heart failure. The aortogram shows a left coronary artery–right ventricular fistula. Ao, aorta; LAD, left anterior descending coronary artery; SOE, site of entry of the fistula into the right ventricle; RV, incompletely opacified right ventricle. C, Preoperative aortogram of patient in A (RV, right ventricle). D, Repeat aortogram 1 year after successful surgical obliteration of the fistula. The left anterior descending coronary artery has returned to normal size. (A to D from Daniel, T. M., Graham, T. P., and Sabiston, D. C., Jr.: Coronary artery-right ventricular fistula with congestive heart failure: Surgical correction in the neonatal period. Surgery, 67:985, 1970.)

A recent update of their series further documents excellent long-term results in 93 patients.[10]

CONGENITAL ORIGIN OF THE LEFT CORONARY ARTERY FROM THE PULMONARY ARTERY

Origin of the left coronary artery from the pulmonary artery is a rare but important cause of congestive heart failure, mitral insufficiency, and left ventricular infarction in infants and children. It has been reported to occur once in every 300,000 live births. Without surgical intervention, it has been estimated that 95% of patients with the left coronary artery originating from the pulmonary artery die within the first years of life. Thus, its early recognition and proper treatment are essential.

Abbott was the first to report a left coronary artery originating from the pulmonary artery in 1908. Abrikossoff later described a 5-month-old infant who died of congestive heart failure and was found to have an aneurysm of the left ventricle at autopsy. Photomicrographs of the ventricle revealed infarction, including areas of calcification. Bland and associates[2] integrated clinical and pathologic data and recorded an electrocardiogram in a 3-year-old infant with this condition, showing that a diagnosis during life was possible.

It was thought for many years that symptoms resulted from poorly oxygenated blood from the pulmonary artery flowing into the left coronary artery under low pressure. Numerous studies of postmortem specimens clearly reveal the presence of many collateral vessels originating from the right coronary artery and connecting to the left coronary artery. In fact, if the right coronary artery is injected in postmortem specimens, branches of the artery rapidly fill in significant amounts. At the time of operation, occlusion of the left coronary artery at its origin causes an increase in pressure within the coronary artery, suggesting that flow originates from the right coronary artery by collateral vessels.[26, 27] Of additional significance is the fact that blood withdrawn from the coronary artery at the time of operation is fully saturated with oxygen. This is clear evidence that this blood originates from a systemic arterial source rather than the pulmonary artery and that the direction of blood flow is from the right coronary artery by collateral vessels into the left coronary artery and then into the pulmonary artery. The resultant symptoms and clinical manifestations are secondary to the left ventricular myocardial ischemia, which follows inadequate collateral flow from the right coronary artery to the left coronary artery or a steal of adequate collateral flow into the low-pressure pulmonary artery system.

Clinical Manifestations. Most patients (90% or more) with anomalous origin of the left coronary artery from the pulmonary artery develop symptoms during infancy. The infant usually appears normal at birth, because the pulmonary artery pressure at this age is elevated and allows perfusion of the left coronary artery from the pulmonary artery for a brief period of time. Symptoms may be present at birth, especially if there are associated cardiac defects. Symptoms are most likely to occur during the first several months of life as left ventricular ischemia becomes more pronounced. When symptoms appear, there is generally a course of progressive deterioration; progressive left ventricular dysfunction occurs, and unless operative therapy is undertaken, death ensues.

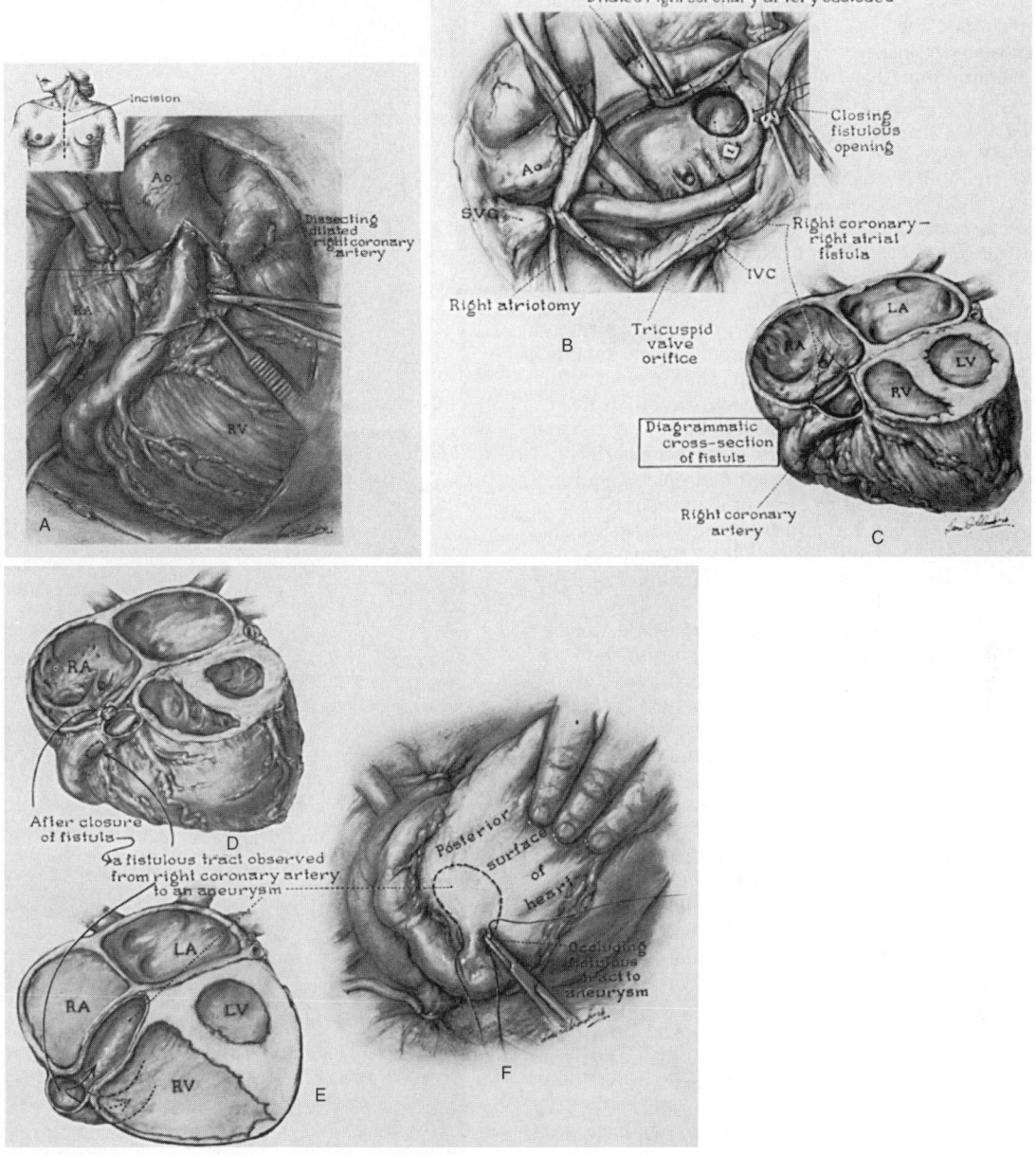

Figure 54–140. *A*, Right coronary–right atrial congenital coronary fistula as seen at operation in a 76-year-old woman who presented with severe congestive heart failure. Through a median sternotomy, the patient was placed on cardiopulmonary bypass with separate venous return cannulas placed in the superior and inferior venae cavae. *B*, Tapes are secured around the superior (SVC) and inferior (IVC) venae cavae to eliminate venous return to the right atrium. The heart is then fibrillated and the right atrium is opened. The large fistulous opening is identified and closed by using interrupted nonabsorbable pledgeted sutures. The site of entry into the right coronary fistula is shown in *C*. After closure of the site of entry into the right atrium, a second fistulous tract was found entering an aneurysm over the posterior surface of the heart (*D* and *E*). This fistulous tract was closed by using multiple transfixion sutures *(F)*. (*A* to *F* from Lowe, J. E., and Sabiston, D. C., Jr.: Congenital coronary malformations. *In* Cohn, L. [Ed]: Modern Technics in Surgery: Cardiac-Thoracic Surgery. Mt. Kisco, NY, Futura, 1981.)

Nevertheless, some patients survive to adult life with few if any symptoms. In a collected review, Harthorne and associates,[12] in 1966, reported 28 adults with this malformation and provided long-term follow-up after surgical correction. Purut and Sabiston[24] described the oldest patient with this malformation, a 61-year-old woman who underwent surgical repair. Of interest, only 7 patients older than the age of 50 at the time of diagnosis have been reported.

Symptoms. It has been shown that blood flow in the left coronary artery is retrograde from the right coronary artery through collateral vessels into the left coronary artery and subsequently into the pulmonary artery. Symptoms occur either from poor collateral flow from the pulmonary artery

or secondary to a *steal* phenomenon of blood passing through well-developed collateral vessels into the left coronary arterial system with drainage into the pulmonary artery.[18] Because of the low pressure in the pulmonary artery, blood flow is selectively shunted into the pulmonary system instead of perfusing the left ventricular myocardium. The chief symptoms are intimately associated with the onset of heart failure and include dyspnea and tachycardia. Wheezing respirations, cough, and cyanosis usually follow. "Angina of feeding" is an interesting finding described as episodes of pain and distress during or immediately after feeding. Paroxysms of distress with pallor, sweating, and dyspnea have also been reported and are also thought to be anginal. Often on presentation, the infant may have a respiratory tract infection that serves to precipitate the heart failure and often delays the proper diagnosis.

Physical Examination. The infant usually has rapid respiratory rate, tachycardia, and cardiac enlargement. A murmur is not usually present early in life, and congenital origin of the left coronary artery from the pulmonary artery is one of the few malformations that in infancy can cause congestive heart failure without a murmur. Evidence of a respiratory tract infection is commonly present with fever, cough, nasal discharge, or rales in the chest. In older infants and children, mitral regurgitation develops secondarily either to left ventricular dilatation or to chronic ischemia or infarction, which results in papillary muscle dysfunction. The liver is characteristically enlarged, and the spleen is palpable in a smaller number of patients. Occasionally, patients first present with signs of cardiovascular collapse and shock similar to those manifested by adults with sudden coronary artery occlusion.

Evaluation. Review of the chest film demonstrates cardiomegaly, predominantly involving the left ventricle. Aneurysmal dilatation may be present as a result from marked thinning of the left ventricular wall; and in many instances the left border of the heart extends to the lateral rib margin. As a result of left ventricular failure, the pulmonary vascular markings are usually exaggerated.

Emphasis has been placed on the characteristic electrocardiographic changes that can establish the diagnosis. The first description of myocardial ischemia on the electrocardiogram of an infant with this condition was made in 1933 by Bland and associates. Based on the work, congenital origin of the left coronary artery from the pulmonary artery has also been referred to as Bland-White-Garland syndrome. Generally, it is possible to make a relatively firm diagnosis on the basis of electrocardiographic changes. Tachycardia is almost always present. The T waves are characteristically inverted in the standard limb leads, and slight ST-segment elevation may be noted in lead I. The T waves in the precordial leads, especially V_5 and V_6, are usually inverted, and deep Q waves are frequently present. The body surface potential distribution has also been helpful in diagnosis and providing evidence of improved coronary blood flow after operation.

Assessment by noninvasive tests is being used more frequently in the diagnosis and evaluation of anomalous origin of the left coronary artery from the pulmonary artery. Two-dimensional echocardiography, thallium scans, pulsed-wave Doppler echocardiography, and, most recently, magnetic resonance imaging are diagnostic modalities that have been used to evaluate patients with an anomalous left coronary artery. Experience with these techniques is limited, but preliminary reports suggest that although these serve as valuable adjuvants in the diagnosis of an anomalous left coronary artery, they do not obviate the need for preoperative cardiac catheterization. Additionally, noninvasive studies can be used to assess the patient intraoperatively and accurately assess and monitor patients after the operation. The right side of the heart is usually normal on the angiogram. The pulmonary vasculature may show subpectoral engorgement and enlargement. The most striking feature is enlargement of the left atrium and left ventricle. The wall of the left ventricle may be quite thin, especially on its anterolateral aspect near the apex. A true ventricular aneurysm with paradoxical pulsations may be present, and mitral insufficiency is quite common.

Injection of contrast medium into a catheter placed in the proximal aorta (or, when possible, directly into the right coronary ostium) demonstrates the classic findings (Fig. 54–141). Contrast medium enters the right coronary artery as it originates from the aorta and passes through dilated collateral vessels that communicate with the left coronary artery.

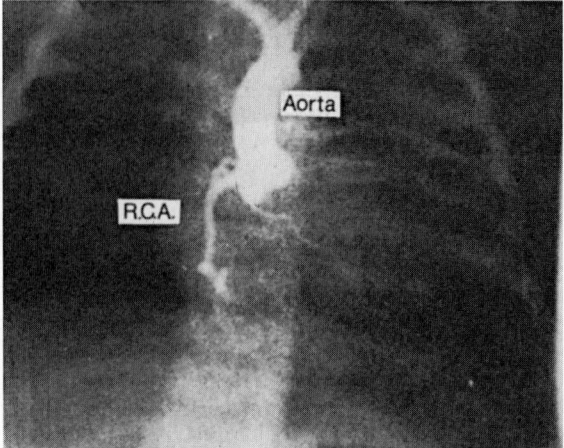

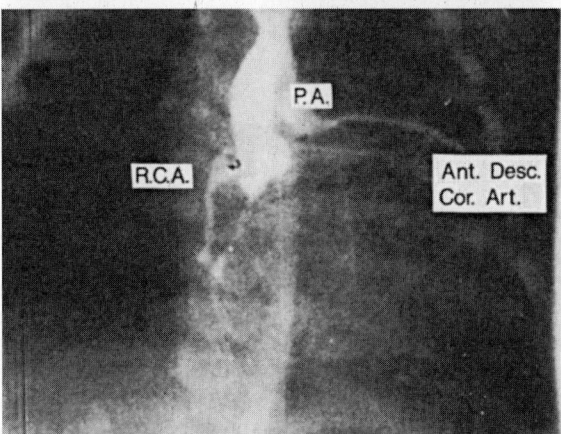

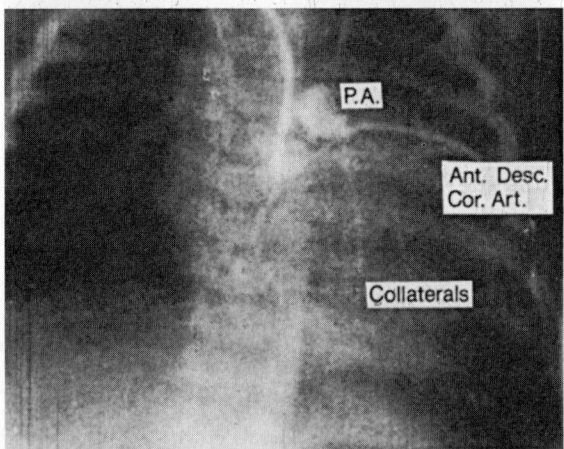

Figure 54–141. Several cine frames taken from a series illustrating coronary arterial filling during aortography. *Top,* Filling of the right coronary artery as it arises normally from the aorta. Note that its size is slightly greater than normal. *Middle,* Filling of the branches of the left coronary artery through collateral vessels from the right coronary artery. *Bottom,* Filling of the pulmonary artery by retrograde flow from the left coronary artery. (From Sabiston, D. C., Jr., and Orme, S. K.: Congenital origin of the left coronary artery from the pulmonary artery. J Cardiovasc. Surg., *9:*543, 1968.)

The contrast medium can then be followed into the left anterior descending and circumflex coronary arteries where it converges to enter the left main coronary artery, with ultimate drainage into the pulmonary artery. Thus, retrograde flow of blood in the left coronary artery can be convincingly demonstrated in such a study, conclusively establishing the diagnosis.

Cardiac catheterization is also helpful because the right

ventricular and pulmonary artery pressures may be elevated. Moreover, it is usually possible to demonstrate left-to-right shunt at the pulmonary artery level by contrast medium. Although the oxygen saturation may at times show a significant increase from the right ventricle to the pulmonary artery, this is not always present, even when it can be demonstrated that the left coronary artery arises from the pulmonary artery. The ejection fraction in patients with anomalous origin of the left coronary artery was determined in eight preoperative patients in whom it varied between 0.13 and 0.72. Among those who died, the ejection fraction was less than 0.36, whereas in survivors the ejection fraction was more than 0.55.

Pathology. The major pathologic features of this condition are apparent at the time of operation. The left ventricle is characteristically greatly dilated, and the wall is thin. The left coronary artery is larger than normal, and numerous collateral vessels connect the right and left coronary arteries. These are usually tortuous and thin walled. The right coronary artery arises in its normal position and is also enlarged. Its branches tend to be more tortuous than usual because they emit various collateral vessels. Over time, and especially in adults, the right coronary artery may become quite large and increasingly tortuous. Similarly, the left coronary artery may also enlarge, up to 10 mm. or more in diameter, at its origin. The left coronary artery arises from the left or posterior cusp of the pulmonary artery. The branches and course of the anterior descending and circumflex branches are usually otherwise normal. When sectioned, the left ventricle may be very thin and in areas totally replaced by scar tissue. Various degrees of subendocardial fibroelastosis may also be present. Calcification is often present in the fibrotic portion of the left ventricle. Infarction of the ventricle may involve the papillary muscles, producing mitral insufficiency. If the left ventricle is dilated, the mitral ring may be sufficiently enlarged to prevent normal coaptation of the valve leaflets, also causing mitral insufficiency.

Surgical Management. The objective of surgical correction in anomalous origin of the left coronary artery from the pulmonary artery is to establish adequate blood flow in the left coronary artery and its branches. Historically, several surgical procedures were advocated to accomplish this: Mustard's left common carotid artery anastomosis to the left coronary artery, Potts' aortopulmonary anastomosis, and the pulmonary artery banding of Case. Disappointing results, however, led to the abandonment of these procedures. In the modern era, two basic approaches are used in the surgical treatment of this malformation: (1) simple ligation at the site of origin of the anomalous left coronary artery and (2) the establishment of a two-coronary artery system.

Ligation at the site of origin from the pulmonary artery is an effective treatment if enough collateral vessels from the right coronary exist to supply the left coronary system adequately. Ligation prevents the *coronary steal* into the pulmonary artery, increases the coronary artery pressure, and improves myocardial blood flow.[28] Long-term follow-up of patients undergoing this procedure has demonstrated the beneficial effects of simple ligation with relief of symptoms and decrease in heart size.[17]

Ligation alone, however, has led to high mortality, owing to the variability in the number of intercoronary collateral vessels and to the inability of simple ligation to produce immediate and sufficient improvement in left ventricular myocardial perfusion in all patients. Survivors of this procedure are left with a single-coronary artery system, which is theoretically less physiologic and at greater risk for arteriosclerosis. It has also been shown that the incidence of sudden death is higher in patients who have undergone simple ligation compared with those who have had a two-coronary artery system established. Poorer performance on treadmill exercise testing and higher late mortality (not due to sudden death) have also been reported in patients with simple ligature of nonfunctioning grafts (ligature equivalent) compared with those with two coronary artery systems. It is therefore recommended that simple ligation be reserved only for those critically ill patients in whom it may be lifesaving[17] and creation of a two-coronary artery system can be accomplished later in life.

Re-establishment of the two-coronary artery system is the treatment of choice for an anomalous left coronary artery arising from the pulmonary artery.[38] The surgical alternatives include left subclavian–left coronary artery anastomosis[15] or connection of the left coronary artery to the aorta. The latter can be performed by direct implantation, autologous artery,[20] or venous bypass grafting,[15] or more recently by intrapulmonary tunneling. This transpulmonary aorta–left coronary artery continuity has been accomplished by using a flap of anterior pulmonary wall,[32] autogenous pericardium,[11] a free segment of left subclavian artery, or polytetrafluoroethylene (PTFE, Gore-Tex) to connect a side-to-side aortopulmonary window to the left coronary ostium within the lumen of the pulmonary artery (Figs. 54–142 to 54–144).

A two-coronary artery system can be reconstructed using saphenous vein graft[39] (Fig. 54–145) or internal mammary bypass grafting in older children and adults. These methods are technically difficult in infants and small children. Moreover, graft occlusion in infants is a problem. Combined with its inability to grow with the child, bypass grafting with veins is considered an unsatisfactory method of reconstruction of a two-coronary-vessel circulation in infants.

Direct implantation of the anomalous left coronary artery into the root of the aorta is a method of establishing a two-coronary-vessel circulation by re-creating the normal anatomy. Excellent patency rates of 100% have been reported in

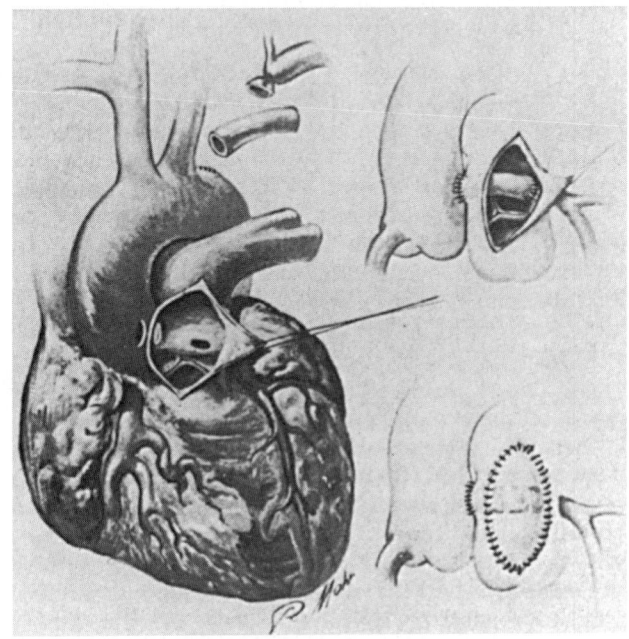

Figure 54–142. Transpulmonary arterial aortocoronary bypass grafting is performed with a free segment of the left subclavian artery (LSCA). A 4-mm. aortopulmonary window is constructed, and the LSCA segment is sutured within the pulmonary artery to the aortopulmonary anastomosis and around the ostium of the anomalous left coronary artery. A pericardial angioplasty prevents luminal compromise of the pulmonary artery containing the transpulmonary arterial bypass graft. (From Arciniegas, E. A., Farooki, Z. Q., Hakimi, M., and Green, E. W.: Management of anomalous left coronary artery from the pulmonary artery. Circulation, 62[Suppl. I]:180, 1980. Copyright 1980, American Heart Association.)

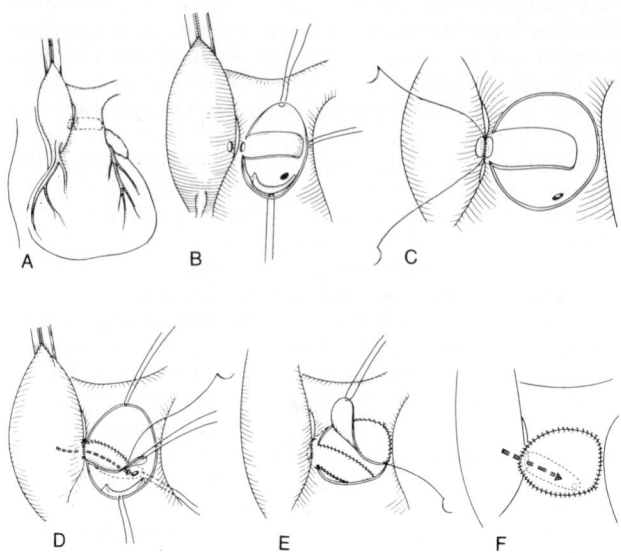

Figure 54–143. After institution of hypothermic cardiopulmonary bypass, the aorta is cross-clamped and the heart is arrested by infusion of cold potassium cardioplegia. An aortopulmonary window is created, and a flap of the anterior pulmonary wall is sutured to the aortopulmonary window (*A* to *C*). By using the pulmonary arterial flap, a tunnel is created in the pulmonary artery between the aortopulmonary window and the anomalous left coronary ostium by suturing the pulmonary arterial flap to the posterior wall of the pulmonary trunk. The defect in the anterior wall of the pulmonary artery is then repaired using a pericardial patch (*D* to *F*). (From Takeuchi, S., Imamura, H., Katsumoto. K., et al.: New surgical methods for repair of anomalous left coronary artery from the pulmonary artery. J. Thorac. Cardiovasc. Surg., *78*:7, 1979.)

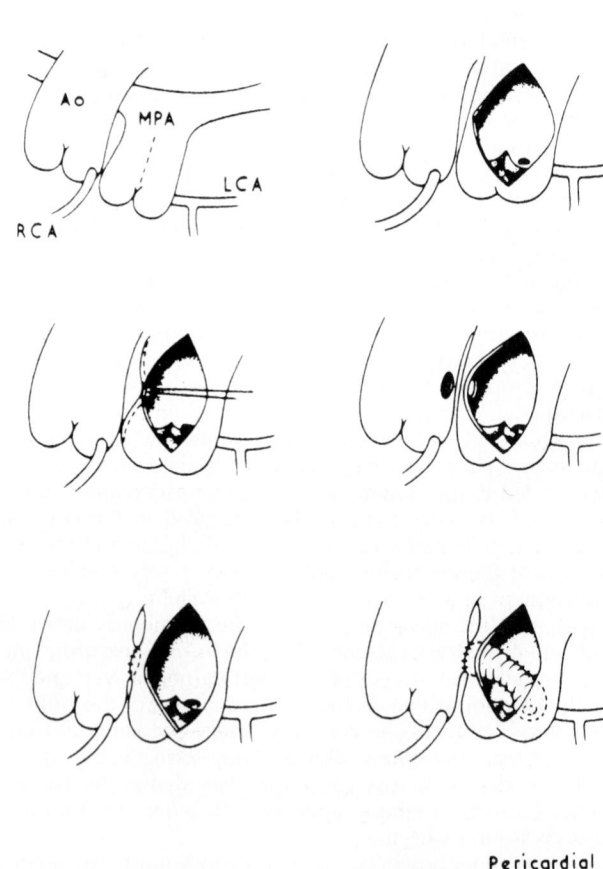

Figure 54–144. An opening is made in the pulmonary artery and an aortopulmonary window is created. A pericardial tunnel is then constructed and connecting the aortopulmonary window within the pulmonary artery to the anomalous origin of the left main coronary artery from the pulmonary artery. The defect in the anterior pulmonary arterial wall is repaired using a Dacron patch. (From Hamilton, D. E., Ghosh, P. K., and Donnelly, R. J.: An operation for anomalous origin of the left coronary artery. Br. Heart J., *41*:121, 1979.)

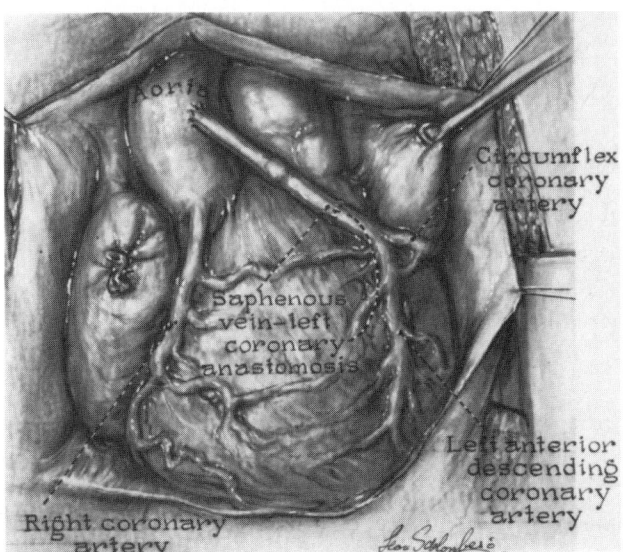

Figure 54–145. Congenital origin of the left coronary from the pulmonary artery can also be managed by division of the left coronary artery at its site of origin and reconstruction of a two-coronary system using a saphenous vein graft. Through a median sternotomy, and with a patient on cardiopulmonary bypass, the saphenous vein graft is attached to the ascending aorta using a partial occlusion clamp. The left coronary is then divided at its site of origin from the pulmonary artery. The saphenous vein graft is then anastomosed in end-to-end fashion to the left coronary artery using interrupted 7-0 nonabsorbable sutures. (From Lowe, J. E., and Sabiston, D. C., Jr.: Surgical correction of congenital malformation of the coronary circulation. South. Med. J., *75:*1508, 1982. Reprinted by permission from the SOUTHERN MEDICAL JOURNAL.)

patients who survived direct aortic reimplantation,[34, 38] but operative mortality remains prohibitively high, especially in patients younger than 1 year old. Technical difficulties with the inability to mobilize adequate length may also preclude the use of this technique. Moreover, reimplantation alters both the shape of the left coronary orifice and the angle it subtends with the aorta.[29] The clinical significance of these changes awaits further follow-up of survivors and detailed study of coronary blood flow and ventricular function in these infants.

The technique of subclavian–left coronary anastomosis was first described by Apley, Horton, and Wilson in 1951.[1] Meyer first performed this successfully in 1968 (Fig. 54–146).[19] This procedure can be performed through a left posterolateral thoracotomy without CPB or with CPB through a median sternotomy or bilateral anterior thoracotomies with transverse sternotomy. Excellent results have been reported using this procedure in 6 patients between the ages of 2 and 76 months.[31] Transpulmonary arterial bypass is now considered by some to be the procedure of choice in infants because it is associated with low mortality and good patency rates.

Whereas the best form of surgical treatment for this disorder is unknown, the establishment of a two-coronary-vessel circulation is most desirable. Simple ligation should be reserved for neonates whose critical illness precludes a lengthy CPB procedure. Direct switch of the left coronary artery from the pulmonary artery to the ascending aorta restores normal coronary anatomy and is a useful procedure (Fig. 54–147). In older children and adults, a two-coronary-artery system can be reconstructed by using saphenous vein or internal mammary artery grafts. In young children, infants, and neonates, the surgical alternatives include direct implantation of the anomalous coronary artery into the aorta, intrapulmonary conduits, and left subclavian–left coronary artery anastomosis. Bypass grafting with venous autograft is not a satisfactory option in this group because of technical difficulty and poor graft patency. Intrapulmonary artery conduits are being

used increasingly. Long-term results in significant numbers of patients, however, are still to be established.

Results. The authors have evaluated 40 patients with anomalous origin of the left coronary artery from the pulmonary artery, and 30 have been managed surgically. Twenty-two patients had severe congestive heart failure, 6 had angina, and 2 infants had failure to thrive. The remaining 10 patients were evaluated for murmurs of uncertain cause, cardiomegaly on physical examination or chest films, and unexplained dyspnea. The 10 patients not operated on all died within several hours to several months after diagnosis. Of the 30 patients undergoing repair, 17 had simple ligation at the origin of the left coronary artery from the pulmonary artery, with six operative deaths (35%) and one additional death 4 months postoperatively. Seven patients had ligation of the left coronary artery followed by saphenous vein or left internal mammary artery grafting. There were no operative deaths, and all 7 have been well 4 to 14 years after operation. Five of seven grafts were closed on repeat angiography done 4 months to 2 years postoperatively. One patient treated with ligation of the left coronary artery at its origin had left subclavian–left coronary artery anastomosis at 14 months of age and is now a teenaged gymnast. Two patients underwent a pulmonary artery tunnel procedure, and one died 1 hour postoperatively. Although the overall operative mortality was 30%, because there is a 95% to 100% mortality in those treated nonoperatively, surgical treatment should be recommended.

ORIGIN OF THE RIGHT CORONARY ARTERY FROM THE PULMONARY ARTERY

St. John Brooks in 1886 first described this rare malformation in two cadavers studied in the anatomic dissection laboratory at the University of Dublin. Both lesions occurred in adults, neither of whom had evidence of heart disease. Brooks noted dilated collateral vessels from the left coronary artery feeding the right coronary artery and correctly postulated, based on this observation, that flow in the right coronary artery might actually be retrograde into the pulmonary artery.

Clinical Manifestations. The clinical manifestations of this condition are usually minimal or absent. In 17 cases collected from the literature,[33] the abnormal artery was discovered in individuals whose age ranged from 17 to 90 years. The malformation was thought to have been associated with death in only two cases. One of these was a 17-year-old girl who died suddenly. Autopsy showed complete occlusion of the left coronary artery by thrombus with evidence of left ventricular infarction. The only other death occurred in a 55-year-old woman who presented with angina and congestive heart failure. In three additional patients, the anomaly was found in association with other congenital malformations.

Although origin of the right coronary artery from the pulmonary artery is a rare anomaly with a benign natural history in most patients, it can lead to myocardial ischemia, infarction, congestive heart failure, and myocardial fibrosis.[37] Because it can be safely corrected when diagnosed, operative correction is indicated.

Evaluation. In the rare patient with this condition who comes to medical attention, the diagnosis is established by aortography and selective coronary arteriography. The left coronary artery is found to be dilated and large intercoronary collateral vessels feed the right coronary artery. As Brooks correctly suggested, flow in the right coronary artery is retrograde, emptying into the pulmonary artery. In contrast to patients who have the more frequently occurring malformation of origin of the left coronary artery from the pulmonary artery, there are usually no electrocardiographic or radio-

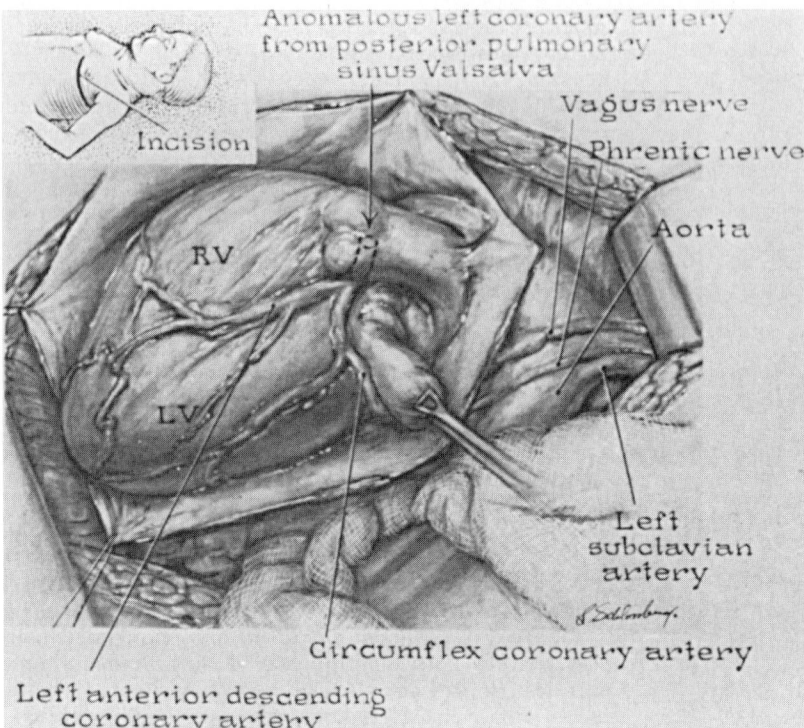

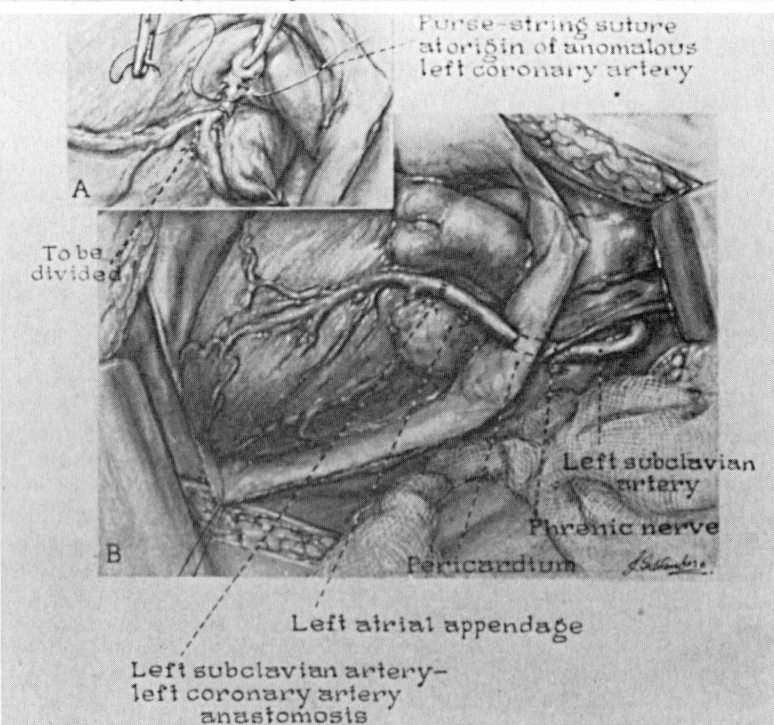

Figure 54–146. For congenital origin of the left coronary artery from the pulmonary artery, through a left anterior third interspace thoracotomy, the left coronary artery is occluded at its site of origin with suture ligatures and then is divided. The left subclavian artery is then anastomosed to the left coronary artery in end-to-end fashion with interrupted 7-0 nonabsorbable sutures. (From Lowe, J. E., and Sabiston, D. C., Jr.: Surgical correction of congenital malformation of the coronary circulation. South. Med. J., *75*:1508, 1982. Reprinted by permission form the SOUTHERN MEDICAL JOURNAL.)

graphic abnormalities. The diagnosis is therefore established only in those who have selective coronary arteriography. Two-dimensional echocardiography has been used to diagnose this malformation, which was confirmed later by coronary arteriography.[40]

Surgical Management and Results. Tingelstad and colleagues[33] reported an interesting case of a 12-year-old boy who was asymptomatic but had a to-and-fro systolic and diastolic murmur along the left sternal border in the third intercostal space. The chest film showed slight cardiac enlargement and normal pulmonary vasculature. Mild left ventricular hypertrophy was shown by a solar electrocardio-

gram. An aortogram revealed a dilated left coronary artery arising normally from the left sinus of Valsalva of the aorta, and the right coronary artery was filled through tortuous intercoronary anastomosis from the left coronary artery and drained into the main pulmonary artery. At operation, a narrow rim of tissue from the pulmonary artery was removed with the origin of the right coronary artery, and this was successfully reimplanted into the ascending aorta. This represents the ideal form of surgical management and has also been done successfully by others.[37] Other alternatives include simple ligation at the site of anomalous origin with or without saphenous vein bypass grafting.[25]

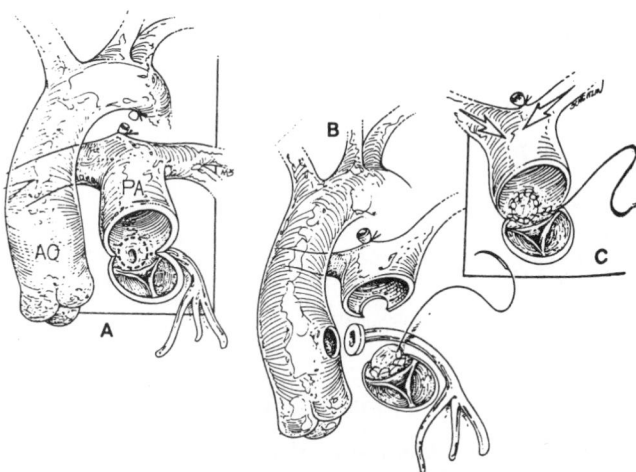

Figure 54–147. Direct aortic reimplantation of anomalous origin of the left coronary artery from the pulmonary artery (PA) is becoming the procedure of choice by many surgeons for both infants and adults. *A,* Excision of the anomalous origin of the left coronary ostium from the pulmonary artery. Ao, aorta. *B,* Aortic reimplantation of the coronary ostium to the aorta using an 8-0 absorbable continuous suture. Mobilization of the pulmonary bifurcation and division of the ligamentum arteriosum allow end-to-end reconstruction of the PA in most patients. However, when compression of the reimplanted left coronary artery is apparent, a patch of autologous pericardium is used to close the defect created in the pulmonary wall. *C,* Reconstruction of the pulmonary artery. (A to C, From Vouhe, P. R., Tamisier, D., Sidi, D., et al.: Anomalous left coronary artery from the pulmonary artery: Results of isolated aortic reimplantation. Ann. Thorac. Surg., *54*:621, 1992. Reprinted with permission from the Society of Thoracic Surgeons.)

ORIGIN OF BOTH CORONARY ARTERIES FROM THE PULMONARY ARTERY

Twenty-five infants in whom both coronary arteries arose from the pulmonary artery have been reviewed in detail by Heifetz and colleagues.[13] The survival time ranged from 9 hours to 7 years. The patient who lived to the age of 7 years was able to do so because of severe pulmonary hypertension secondary to a ventricular septal defect and congenital mitral stenosis. The pressure in the pulmonary artery was sufficient to force blood into the myocardial capillary bed, and the child lived for an amazingly long time. This malformation has been diagnosed by cardiac catheterization, and surgical repair has been attempted.[21] Most recently, Urcelay and associates performed the first successful repair of this malformation in two infants.[35] Both procedures were accomplished by reimplantation of a single coronary trunk into the ascending aorta. One-year follow-up reveals both infants to be in good general health.

ANEURYSMS OF THE CORONARY ARTERIES

Bougon first reported an aneurysm of the coronary arteries in 1812. These lesions have been reported from infancy to adult life. Congenital aneurysms of the coronary arteries are rare and constituted only 15% of the coronary artery aneurysms in 89 patients reported by Daoud and associates.[6] Other causes of aneurysms of the coronary arteries include atherosclerosis, mycotic aneurysms, syphilis, rheumatic heart disease, and mucocutaneous lymph node syndrome (Kawasaki's disease).

These lesions are most often asymptomatic until complications occur. Complications include thrombosis or embolization with subsequent myocardial ischemia or infarction or actual rupture of aneurysm. An example of a congenital coronary artery aneurysm involving the left circumflex vessels is shown in Figure 54–148A. In this patient, a mural thrombus occurred in the aneurysm; it embolized and produced acute myocardial infarction (see Fig. 54–148B). The aneurysm was resected, and a saphenous vein autograft was inserted (see Fig. 54–148C). Surgical management of a coronary artery aneurysm is indicated if the aneurysm is symptomatic, especially if there is evidence of emboli arising from the aneurysm, producing myocardial ischemia in the distal coronary bed.

MEMBRANOUS OBSTRUCTION OF THE OSTIUM OF THE LEFT MAIN CORONARY ARTERY

Atresia of the coronary arteries in infancy and childhood has been reported and usually causes severe impairment of ventricular function and sudden death. Congenital atresia of the left main coronary artery had been reported in nine patients, all of whom presented with signs and symptoms

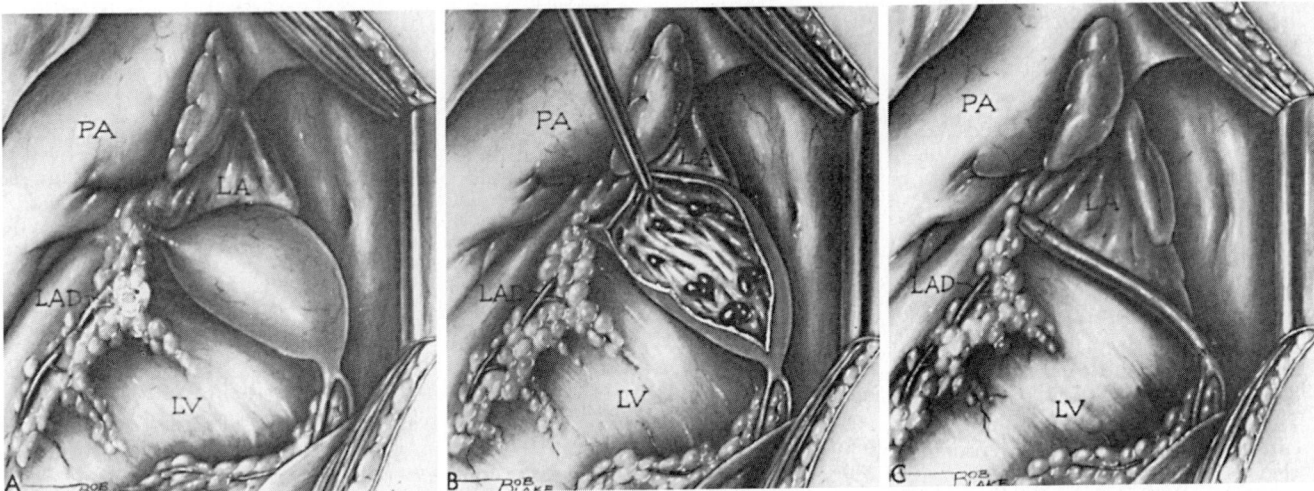

Figure 54–148. *A,* Congenital aneurysm of the left circumflex coronary artery as seen at operation on a 31-year-old woman who presented with an acute myocardial infarction with subsequent disabling angina. PA, pulmonary artery; LAD, left anterior descending coronary artery; LV, left ventricle; LA, left atrium. *B,* Numerous small fresh thrombi are shown adherent to the rough, irregular surface of the aneurysm. The proximal opening into the aneurysm was a discrete, mildly dilated vessel of good quality and normal-appearing intima. The distal branches of the circumflex coronary artery were of normal size. *C,* The entire aneurysm was excised, and an interposition graft of saphenous vein was placed. There was only minimal discrepancy in the size of a saphenous vein graft and the ends of the circumflex coronary artery. A continuous 7-0 nonabsorbable suture was used at each anastomosis. (From Ebert, P. A., Peter, R. H., Gunnells, J. C., and Sabiston, D. C., Jr.: Resecting and grafting of coronary artery aneurysm. Circulation, *43*:593, 1971. Copyright 1971, American Heart Association.)

of myocardial ischemia, congestive heart failure, or both. Histopathologic studies in these patients showed that the left main coronary artery had been replaced by fibromuscular tissue and that the left coronary ostium was absent. These conditions are not surgically correctable. However, three patients have been reported with membranous obstruction at the ostium of the left main coronary artery, associated with a normal distal coronary artery. The first patient was a 6-month-old infant who died after myocardial infarction and the diagnosis was established at the time of autopsy. Josa and associates reported two cases diagnosed at the time of operation.[14] One patient, a 2-year-old child being operated on for congenital aortic stenosis, was found to have a membrane markedly obstructing the ostium of the left main coronary artery. The second patient was an 8-year old boy with Type I truncus arteriosus who also had membranous obstruction of the ostium of the left main coronary artery at operation. Both of these patients showed evidence of myocardial ischemia preoperatively, and after excision of the membrane at operation the symptoms were totally relieved. Grossly, the membranous structure appeared to be continuous with the aortic intima, and histologic studies revealed that its structure was similar to that of normal aortic root media. These two examples indicated the importance of careful evaluation of the origin and distribution of the coronary arteries in patients with congenital heart disease, especially when the signs and symptoms of ischemia and heart failure are disproportionate to the congenital lesion being evaluated.[14]

SELECTED REFERENCES

Ebert, P. A., Peter, R. H., Gunnells, J. C., and Sabiston, D. C., Jr.: Resecting and grafting of coronary artery aneurysm. Circulation, 43:593, 1971.
A congenital aneurysm of the circumflex coronary artery containing a thrombus that later embolized and produced myocardial infarction is reported. A review of the problem, the clinical manifestations, and management are discussed.

Heifetz, S. A., Robinowitz, M., Mueller, K. H., and Virmani, R.: Total anomalous origin of the coronary arteries from the pulmonary artery. Pediatr. Cardiol., 7:11, 1986.
Four patients with total anomalous origin of the coronary arteries from the pulmonary artery are presented and compared with 21 previously reported patients. Of the 19 patients in whom a clinical history was available, 16 were symptomatic before 3 days of age. All patients died, 60% before 2 weeks of age. Longer survival was associated with additional cardiovascular malformations that caused pulmonary hypertension, increased oxygen saturation, or both. Cardiomegaly was present in 56% of patients, and most had myocardial fibrosis or infarction. Surgical correction has been attempted in 2 patients, but both attempts failed secondary to severe pre-existent myocardial injury.

Lowe, J. E., and Sabiston, D. C., Jr.: Congenital coronary malformations. *In* Cohn, L. (Ed.): Modern Technics in Surgery: Cardiac-Thoracic Surgery. Mt. Kisco, N. Y., Futura Publishing, 1981.
This review presents the surgical techniques used to correct congenital coronary artery fistulas, anomalous origin of the left or right coronary artery from the pulmonary artery, and congenital coronary artery aneurysms. The details of the preoperative evaluation, anesthetic management, and postoperative care are also reviewed.

Lowe, J. E., Oldham, N. H., Jr., and Sabiston, D. C., Jr.: Surgical management of congenital coronary artery fistulas. Ann. Surg., 194:371, 1981.
This paper reports the clinical manifestations of 28 patients with congenital coronary artery fistulas seen at one institution and summarizes the results of surgical management in 22 patients. An additional 258 patients reported earlier are also reviewed. The natural history and pathophysiology of coronary fistulas are discussed, and the reason for early surgical intervention is presented.

Sabiston, D. C., Jr., and Orme, S. K.: Congenital origin of the left coronary artery from the pulmonary artery. J. Cardiovasc. Surg., 9:543, 1968.
In this report, 23 patients with origin of the left coronary artery from the pulmonary artery are described. The youngest patient was 1 day of age and the oldest patient was 31 years of age. The natural history, clinical findings, laboratory data, and ultimate course are presented.

Stephenson, L. W., Edmunds, L. H., Jr., Friedman, S., et al: Subclavian–left coronary artery anastomosis (Meyer operation) for anomalous origin of the left coronary artery from the pulmonary artery. Circulation, 64(Suppl. II):130, 1981.
Six patients, age 2 to 76 months had subclavian to coronary artery anastomosis for anomalous origin of the left coronary artery from the pulmonary artery. Five of the patients had congestive heart failure and ongoing ischemia. All six had cardiomegaly, and preoperative left ventricular ejection fractions averaging 0.46 ± 0.171.

Five patients survived operation and were alive at 8 to 92 months after operation, and four of the five anastomoses were patent at postoperative cardiac catheterization. None of the surviving patients have required cardiac medications, and all of them are symptom free at follow-up. In addition to subclavian–left coronary anastomosis, multiple other surgical options including intrapulmonary shunts are discussed in detail.

Wei, J., and Wang, D.: A giant congenital aneurysm of the right coronary artery. Ann. Thorac. Surg., 41:322, 1986.
The authors report a 26-year-old patient who presented with shortness of breath and a chronic cough. A chest film showed a huge mass on the right ventricular border, and the patient was admitted with a tentative diagnosis of mediastinal tumor. Coronary arteriography showed a giant coronary aneurysm arising from the right coronary artery. At the time of operation, the aneurysm measured 15 cm. in diameter. The aneurysm was resected, and histologic examination of the aneurysmal wall showed no evidence of atheromatous change. The patient recovered and symptoms resolved completely.

REFERENCES

1. Apley, J., Horton, R. E., and Wilson, M. G.: The possible role of surgery in the treatment of anomalous left coronary artery. Thorax, 12:28, 1951.
2. Bland, E. F., White, P. D., and Garland, J.: Congenital anomalies of coronary arteries: Report of an unusual case associated with cardiac hypertrophy. Am. Heart J., 8:787, 1933.
3. Brooks, H. St. J.: Two cases of an abnormal coronary artery of the heart arising from the pulmonary. J. Anat. Physiol., 20:26, 1886.
4. Cason, B. A., and Gordon, H. J.: Coronary steal caused by a coronary artery fistula. J. Cardiothorac. Vasc. Anesth., 6:65, 1992.
5. Daniel, T. M., Graham, T. P., and Sabiston, D. C., Jr.: Coronary artery–right ventricular fistula with congestive heart failure: Surgical correction in the neonatal period. Surgery, 67:985, 1970.
6. Daoud, A. S., Pankin, D., Tulgan, H., and Florentin, R. A.: Aneurysms of the coronary artery. Am. J. Cardiol., 11:228, 1963.
7. De Salazar, A. O., Juanena, C., Aramendi, J. I., Castellanos, E., Cabrera, A., and Agosti, J.: Anomalous origin of the left coronary artery from the pulmonary artery: Surgical alternatives depending on the age of the patient. J. Cardiovasc. Surg., 31:801, 1990.
8. Ebert, P. A., Peter, R. H., Gunnells, J. C., and Sabiston, D. C., Jr.: Resecting and grafting of coronary artery aneurysm. Circulation, 43:593, 1971.
9. Edwards, J. E.: Anomalous coronary arteries with special reference to arteriovenous-like communications. Circulation, 17:1001, 1958.
10. Fernandes, E. D., Kadivar, H., Hallman, G. L., Reul, G. J., Ott, D. A., and Cooley, D. A.: Congenital malformation of the coronary arteries: The Texas Heart Institute experience. Ann. Thorac. Surg., 54:732, 1992.
11. Hamilton, D. E., Ghosh, P. K., and Donnelly, R. J.: An operation for anomalous origin of left coronary artery. Br. Heart J., 41:121, 1979.
12. Harthorne, J. W., Scannell, J. G., and Dinsmore, R. E.: Anomalous origin of the left coronary artery: Remediable cause of sudden death in adults. N. Engl. J. Med., 275:660, 1966.
13. Heifetz, S. A., Robinowitz, M., Mueller, K. H., and Virmani, R.: Total anomalous origin of the coronary arteries from the pulmonary artery. Pediatr. Cardiol., 7:11, 1986.
14. Josa, M., Danielson, G. K., Weidman, W. H., and Edwards, W. D.: Congenital ostial membrane of left main coronary artery. J. Thorac. Cardiovasc. Surg., 81:338, 1981.
15. Kessler, K. A., Pennington, G., Nouri, S., et al.: Left subclavian–left coronary artery anastomosis for anomalous origin of the left coronary artery: Long-term follow-up. J. Thorac. Cardiovasc. Surg., 98:25, 1989.
16. Liberthson, R. R., Sagar, K., Behocoben, J. P., et al.: Congenital coronary arteriovenous fistula. Circulation, 59:849, 1979.
17. Lowe, J. E., and Sabiston, D. C., Jr.: Congenital coronary malformation. *In* Cohn, L. (Ed.): Modern Technics in Surgery: Cardiac-Thoracic Surgery. Mt. Kisco, N. Y., Futura Publishing, 1981.
18. Lowe, J. E., and Sabiston, D. C., Jr.: Surgical correction of congenital malformations of the coronary circulation. South. Med. J., 75:1508, 1982.
19. Meyer, W., Stefanik, G., Stiles, Q. R., et al.: A method of definitive surgical treatment of anomalous origin of left coronary artery. J. Thorac. Cardiovasc. Surg., 56:104, 1968.
20. Neches, W. H., Mathews, R. A., Pack, S. C., et al.: Anomalous origin of the left coronary artery from the pulmonary artery. Circulation, 50:582, 1974.
21. Ogasawara, K., Aizawa, T., Fijii, J., et al.: A case with fistulas from both coronary arteries and the left bronchial artery to the pulmonary artery. Jpn. Heart J., 26:597, 1985.
22. Ogden, J. A.: Congenital anomalies of the coronary arteries. Am. J. Cardiol., 25:474, 1970.
23. Pinsky, W. W., Fagan, L. R., Kraeger, R. R., et al.: Anomalous left coronary artery. J. Thorac. Cardiovasc. Surg., 65:810, 1973.
24. Purut, C. M., and Sabiston, D. C., Jr.: Origin of the left coronary artery from the pulmonary artery in older adults. J. Thorac. Cardiovasc. Surg., 102:566, 1991.
25. Rowe, G. G., and Young, W. P.: Anomalous origin of the coronary arteries with special reference to surgical treatment. J. Thorac. Cardiovasc. Surg., 39:777, 1960.
26. Sabiston, D. C., Jr., and Orme, S. K.: Congenital origin of the coronary artery from the pulmonary artery. J. Cardiovasc. Surg., 9:543, 1968.
27. Sabiston, D. C., Jr., Floyd, W. L., and MacIntosh, H. D.: Anomalous origin

of the left coronary artery from the pulmonary artery in adults: Surgical management. Arch. Surg., *97*:963, 1968.

28. Sabiston, D. C., Jr., Ross, R. S., Criley, J. M., et al.: Surgical management of congenital lesions of the coronary circulation. Ann. Surg., *157*:908, 1963.

29. Smith, A., Arnold, R., Anderson, R. H., et al.: Anomalous origin of the left coronary artery from the pulmonary trunk: Anatomic findings in relation to pathophysiology and surgical repair. J. Thorac. Cardiovasc. Surg., *98*:16, 1989.

30. Sones, F. M., and Shirey, E. K.: Collateral arterial channels in living human with coronary artery disease. Circulation, *22*:815, 1960.

31. Stephenson, L. W., Edmunds, L. H., Friedman, S., et al.: Subclavian–left coronary artery anastomosis (Meyer operation) for anomalous origin of the left coronary artery from the pulmonary artery. Circulation, *64*(Suppl. II):130, 1981.

32. Takeucki, S., Imamura, H., Katsumoto, K., et al.: New surgical method for repair of anomalous left coronary artery from pulmonary artery. J. Thorac. Cardiovasc. Surg., *78*:7, 1979.

33. Tingelstad, J. B., Lower, R. R., and Eldredge, W. J.: Anomalous origin of the right coronary artery from the main pulmonary artery. Am. J. Cardiol., *30*:670, 1972.

34. Tkebuchava, T., Carrel, T., von Segesser, L., Real, R., Jenni, R., and Turina,

M.: Repair of anomalous origin of the left coronary artery from the pulmonary artery without early and late mortality in 9 patients. J. Cardiovasc. Surg., *33*:479, 1992.

35. Urcelay, G. E., Iannettoni, M. D., Ludomirsky, A., Mosca, R. S., Cheatham, J. P., Danford, D. A., and Bove, E. L.: Origin of both coronary arteries from the pulmonary artery. Circulation, *90*:2379, 1994.

36. Urrutia-S, C. O., Falaschi, G., Ott, D. A., and Cooley, D. A.: Surgical management of 56 patients with congenital coronary artery fistulas. Ann. Thorac. Surg., *35*:300, 1983.

37. Vairo, U., Marino, B., De Simone, G., and Marcelletti, C.: Early congestive heart failure due to origin of the right coronary artery from the pulmonary artery. Chest, *102*:1610, 1992.

38. Vouhé, P. R., Tamisier, D., Sidi, D., Vernant, F., Mauriat, P., Pouard, P., and Leca, F.: Anomalous left coronary artery from the pulmonary artery: Results of isolated aortic reimplantation. Ann. Thorac. Surg., *54*:621, 1992.

39. Wilson, C. L., Dlabol, P. W., HoleyField, R. W., et al.: Anomalous origin of left coronary artery from pulmonary artery: Case report and review of literature concerning teenagers and adults. J. Thorac. Cardiovasc. Surg., *73*:887, 1977.

40. Worsham, C., Sanders, S. P., and Burger, B. M.: Origin of the right coronary artery from the pulmonary trunk: Diagnosis by two-dimensional echocardiography. Am. J. Cardiol., *55*:232, 1985.

XVII

ACQUIRED DISORDERS OF THE AORTIC VALVE AND SUBAORTIC VALVE

David A. Fullerton, M.D., and Alden H. Harken, M.D.

ACQUIRED DISEASE OF THE AORTIC VALVE

Historical Aspects. The first investigator to appreciate an association between aortic valve disease and heart failure was Cowper, who described thickened nonpliable aortic valves with calcific vegetations at autopsy of several patients dying of congestive heart failure in 1706.[10] Surgical attempts to correct aortic stenosis began in the early twentieth century. In 1912, Tuffier attempted transaortic digital dilatation of a stenotic aortic valve.[32] In 1947, Smithy, who died of mitral stenosis at age 43, and Parker described an experimental model of aortic valvotomy.[33] Three years later, Bailey reported successful aortic valvotomy in patients by insertion of a mechanical dilator across the stenotic valve of patients to open fused commissures (Fig. 54–149).[1] In 1952, Hufnagel and Harvey placed the first prosthetic ball valve prosthesis into the descending aorta of a patient with aortic insufficiency.[13] The development of cardiopulmonary bypass by Gibbon in 1954 allowed surgeons to open the aorta and operate directly on the aortic valve. Initially, open aortic valve operations were limited to aortic valve commissurotomy and débridement of calcified aortic valve leaflets. But in 1960, Harken[12] and, in 1963, Starr[35] reported replacement of the aortic valve with a ball valve prosthesis. In 1962, Ross successfully performed orthotopic homograft valve replacement.[30] In the mid 1960s, stent-mounted porcine aortic valves were implanted, but these formaldehyde-fixed valves rapidly degenerated. In 1974, Carpentier reported superior longevity of the glutaraldehyde-preserved porcine valve.[7]

Surgical Anatomy of the Aortic Valve. The normal aortic valve is composed of three thin, pliable leaflets, or cusps, attached to the heart at the junction of the aorta and the left ventricle. The leaflets are attached within the three sinuses of Valsalva of the proximal aorta and join together in three commissures, which create the shape of a coronet. Because the coronary arteries arise from two of the three sinuses of

Valsalva, the aortic leaflets are named after their respective sinuses as the left coronary leaflet, the right coronary leaflet, and the noncoronary leaflet. There are two important surgical landmarks. First, the commissure between the left and noncoronary leaflets is positioned over the anterior leaflet of the mitral valve. Second, the commissure between noncoronary and right coronary leaflet is positioned over the left bundle of His. Injury to this conduction bundle during aortic valve surgery may create heart block (Fig. 54–150).

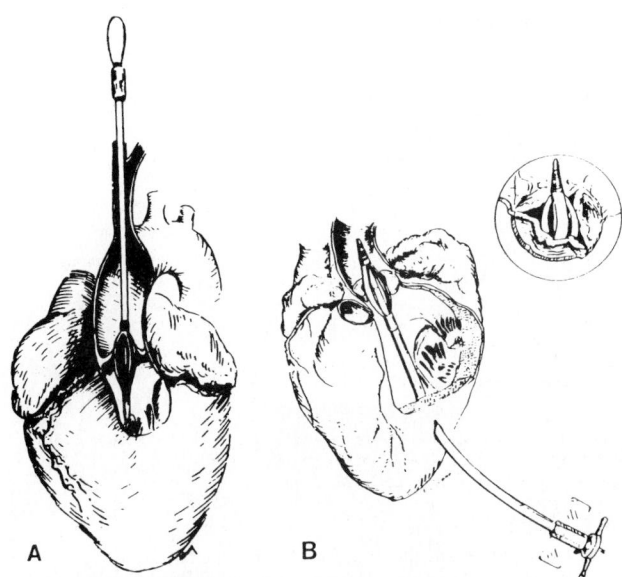

Figure 54–149. Instrument used by Bailey for mechanical dilatation of the stenotic aortic valve. The instrument was inserted through either the left ventricle or the aorta. (From Larzelere, G., and Bailey, C. P.: New instrument for cardiac valvular commissurotomy. J. Thorac. Surg., *25*:66, 1953.)

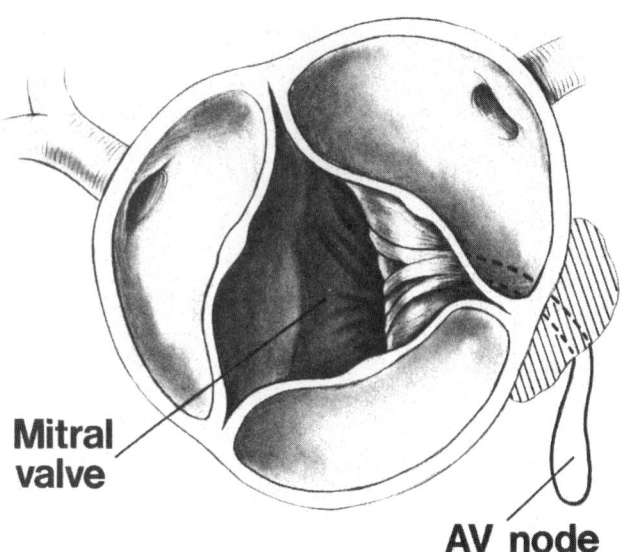

Figure 54–150. Surgical anatomy of the aortic valve. The commissure between the noncoronary and left coronary leaflets lies anterior to the left bundle of His. Injury to this conduction tissue during aortic valve surgery may result in heart block.

AORTIC STENOSIS

Pathologic Anatomy. Aortic stenosis may be congenital or acquired (Fig. 54–151). Congenital valvular abnormalities may be clinically significant immediately after birth, as with unicuspid and dome-shaped valves. However, congenitally bicuspid valves, usually asymptomatic at birth, generally lead to symptomatic stenosis in the sixth to eighth decades.[28] The bicuspid valve produces turbulent flow across the leaflets, leading to fibrosis, calcification, and stiffening. Acquired aortic stenosis usually results from rheumatic fever or from degeneration of the valve leaflets.[28] In rheumatoid aortic stenosis, inflammation produces adhesions and fusion of the commissures and leaflets with thickening and calcification (Fig. 54–152). Retraction of the leaflets often makes these valves both regurgitant and stenotic. The inflammatory process of rheumatic fever rarely involves the aortic valve alone, usually involving the mitral valve as well. In degenerative

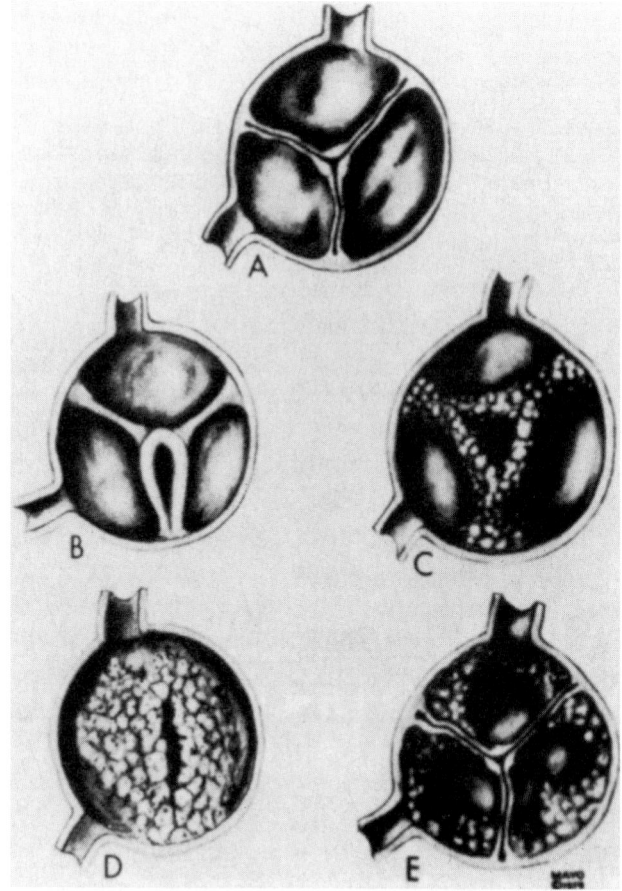

Figure 54–152. Types of aortic valve stenosis. *A,* Normal aortic valve. *B,* Congenital aortic stenosis. *C,* Rheumatic aortic stenosis. *D,* Calcific aortic stenosis. *E,* Calcific senile aortic stenosis. (From Brandenburg, R. O., et al.: Valvular heart disease—when should the patient be referred? Pract. Cardiol., 5:50, 1979.)

or senile aortic stenosis, grossly normal leaflets become calcified as a result of normal leaflet stress at the flexion points, causing leaflet immobility. This calcification may extend down onto the anterior mitral valve leaflet or upward along the aorta, occasionally causing coronary ostial stenosis.

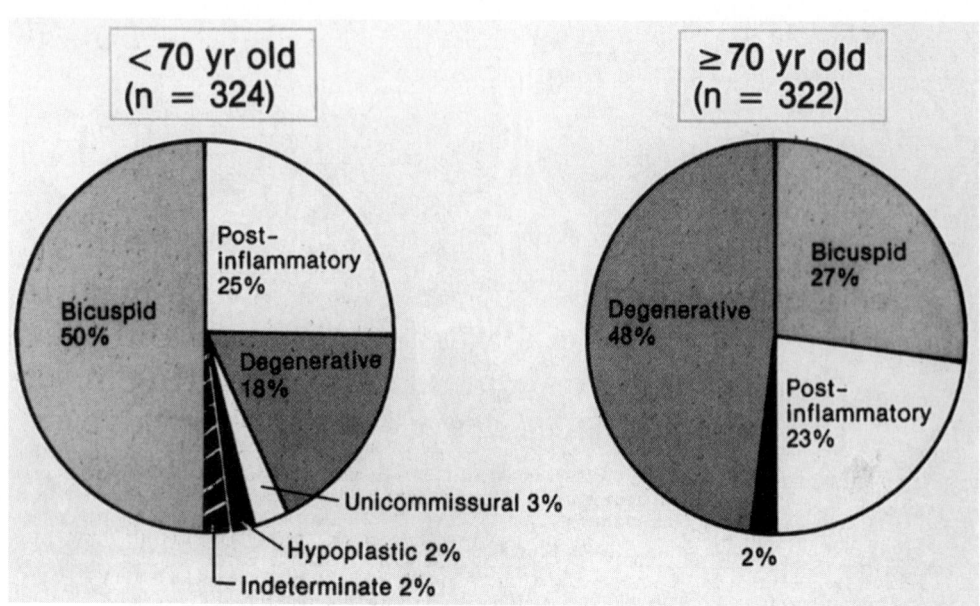

Figure 54–151. Causes of aortic stenosis as a function of age. (From Passik, C. S., et al.: Temporal changes in the causes of aortic stenosis: A surgical pathologic study of 646 cases. Mayo Clin. Proc., 62:119, 1987.)

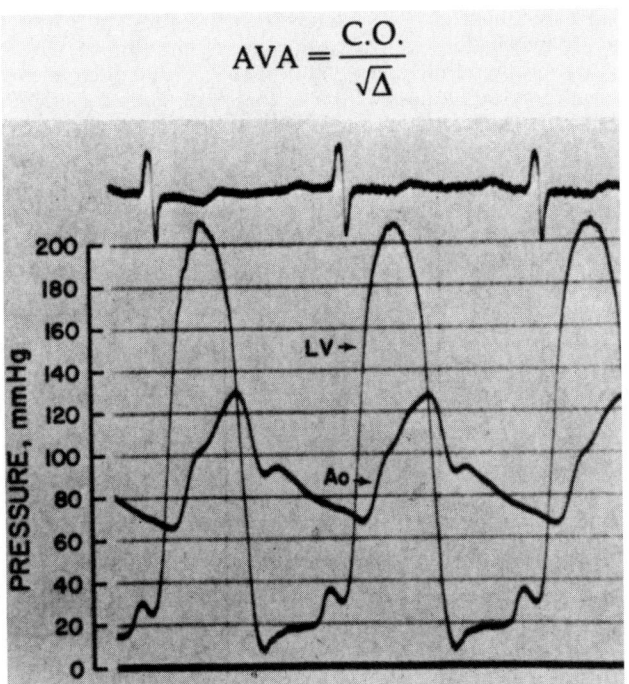

$$AVA = \frac{C.O.}{\sqrt{\Delta}}$$

Figure 54–153. Pressure-time curve of simultaneous left ventricular (LV) and aortic pressure (Ao). Note that in this patient with severe aortic stenosis, a peak-to-peak gradient of 80 mm. Hg is present, suggesting a severely compromised aortic valve area. Also note the prolonged and delayed aortic upstroke ("parvus et tardus"). The A wave in the LV trace represents atrial contraction with filling of a noncompliant ventricle. (From Grossman, W.: Cardiac Catheterization, Angiography, and Intervention, 4th ed. Philadelphia, Lea & Febiger, 1991.)

Pathophysiology. In acquired aortic stenosis there is a chronic, progressive narrowing of the aortic valve. As the valve narrows, the appropriate compensatory response of the left ventricle is hypertrophy. As the ventricle hypertrophies, it becomes more stiff as its compliance decreases; a higher left ventricular end-diastolic pressure is needed to maintain the same volume of cardiac output (Fig. 54–153). To achieve a sufficiently high left ventricular end-diastolic pressure (diastolic loading), the heart becomes increasingly dependent on the atrial kick; loss of the atrial kick, as occurs with atrial fibrillation, may result in a significant decline in cardiac output and acute hemodynamic decompensation.[36]

Although left ventricular hypertrophy is an appropriate biologic response to an increasing afterload, it has detrimental effects. The combined effects of greater left ventricular muscle mass, decreased left ventricular compliance producing greater ventricular wall tension, higher systolic ventricular pressure, and longer systolic ejection time culminate in increased myocardial oxygen demand. At the same time coronary artery blood flow is compromised by increased wall tension compressing the vessels and higher left ventricular diastolic pressure, which lowers the coronary artery perfusion pressure. These factors contribute to inadequate coronary arterial perfusion of the subendocardium, leading to chronic ischemia. In turn, chronic ischemia leads to cell death and fibrosis.[8]

Left ventricular hypertrophy may allow the heart to achieve a normal cardiac output under resting conditions. But as the aortic valve area becomes smaller, the gradient across the valve from left ventricle to aorta increases. This relationship of flow across the valve, valve area, and transvalvular pressure gradient is expressed in the Gorlin formula[11]:

$$AVA = \frac{\text{Aortic valve flow}}{C \times \sqrt{\text{aortic valve mean systolic gradient}}}$$

where aortic valve flow equals cardiac output (ml./min.)/ systolic ejection period (sec./min.), AVA is the aortic valve area in square centimeters, and C is the empirical orifice constant 44.5. For quick calculations this simplifies to:

$$AVA = \frac{\text{Cardiac output}}{\sqrt{\text{Mean pressure gradient}}}$$

The relationship of flow across the aortic valve and the transvalvular pressure gradient is shown in Figure 54–154. As the valve area decreases to 1 sq. cm., there is little change in the transvalvular gradient needed to generate the same flow, and patients frequently experience no symptoms. With a valve area of 0.7 sq. cm., patients are invariably symptomatic.[38]

Diagnosis. Auscultation of the patient with aortic stenosis reveals a systolic murmur, best heard at the base of the heart, that radiates into the carotid arteries and to the cardiac apex. This murmur is associated with a slow, prolonged rise in the arterial pulse, "pulsus parvus et tardus." The electrocardiogram is notable for left ventricular hypertrophy in 85% and evidence of left atrial enlargement in 80% of patients.[5] T-wave inversion and ST-segment depression are common. The chest roentgenogram is usually normal but may reveal post-stenotic dilation of ascending aorta or calcification of the aortic valve. The severity of aortic stenosis may be estimated by echocardiography. The peak transvalvular gradient may be calculated from velocity of blood traversing the valve by the following formula:

$$\Delta = 4V^2$$

where Δ is the peak ventriculoaortic gradient and V is the maximal measured blood velocity (measured in meters/second) across the valve.[39] The most accurate measure of aortic stenosis is determined by cardiac catheterization. A catheter may be pulled back from the left ventricle to the aorta to determine the transvalvular pressure gradient. However, simultaneous aortic and ventricular pressure measurements are more precise and, in fact, are mandatory when the patient is in atrial fibrillation.

Clinical Course. The natural history of aortic stenosis was reported by Ross and Braunwald.[31] When the aortic valve area diminishes from the normal 3 to 4 sq. cm. to less than 1

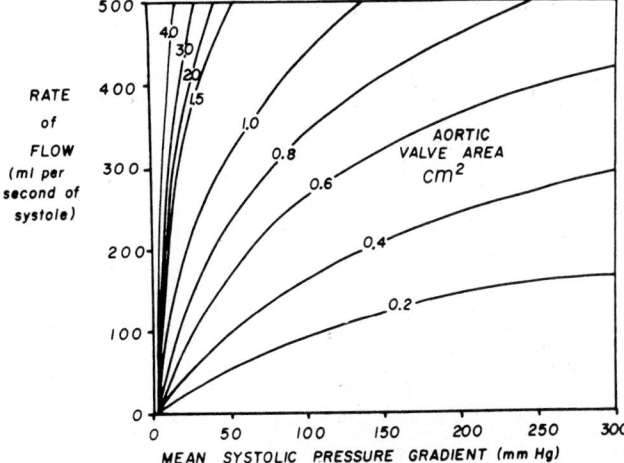

Figure 54–154. Chart illustrating the relation between mean systolic pressure gradient across the aortic valve and the rate of flow across the aortic valve per second of systole, as predicted by the Gorlin formula. As the valve area is reduced to about 0.7 sq. cm., little increase in flow is achieved despite marked increases in mean gradient, thus defining "critical" aortic stenosis. (From Hurst, J. W., Logue, R. B., Schlant, R. C., and Wenger, N. K. [Eds.]: Hurst's The Heart: Arteries and Veins, 3rd edition. New York, McGraw-Hill, 1974, p. 811. Reproduced with permission of the McGraw-Hill Book Companies.)

sq. cm., patients are usually symptomatic.[17] Once symptomatic, patient survival is limited. The three principal symptoms of aortic stenosis are angina, syncope, and congestive heart failure (Fig. 54–155).[14] Angina is usually the earliest symptom, and the mean survival of a patient with aortic stenosis and angina is 4.7 years. When a patient experiences syncope, survival is typically less than 3 years. Patients with dyspnea and congestive failure, in keeping with their associated left ventricular dysfunction, have a mean survival of 1 to 2 years.[31] Congestive heart failure is the presenting symptom in nearly one third of patients.[15]

Management. Aortic stenosis is a mechanical obstruction to flow from the left ventricle. The only effective therapy is operative intervention. The existence of symptoms is an indication for valve replacement. Angina and syncope warrant elective surgical therapy, whereas congestive heart failure mandates urgent intervention. The issue of aortic valve replacement in the asymptomatic patient with aortic stenosis is unanswered. The risk of sudden death in asymptomatic patients with a transvalvular gradient greater than or equal to 50 mm. Hg or a valve area less than 0.5 sq. cm. is approximately 4% per year.[4] In one study of 113 asymptomatic patients with critical aortic stenosis, 38 became symptomatic within 2 years. There were no sudden cardiac deaths in 118 patient-years of follow-up.[29] Surgical therapy should be recommended to the symptomatic patient with evidence of left ventricular decompensation.

In patients with good ventricular function, aortic valve replacement is associated with an operative mortality of 2% to 8%.[15] Independent perioperative risk factors include age, left ventricular function, New York Heart Association class, and pulmonary function. After aortic valve replacement, the projected 5-year survival is 80% to 85%.[15] Symptoms are relieved in nearly all patients; however, improvement in ejection fraction and resolution of ventricular hypertrophy may require months to occur. Surgical mortality increases exponentially with decreasing left ventricular ejection fraction. Aortic valve replacement in patients with congestive heart failure has a mortality reported up to 24%.[15] In patients with aortic stenosis and coronary artery disease, valve replacement and myocardial revascularization should be performed concurrently. Perioperative mortality is higher in those patients who do not undergo simultaneous coronary artery bypass grafting.[22]

Percutaneous aortic balloon valvuloplasty is an alternative in the treatment of aortic stenosis. In this procedure, either one or two balloon catheters are passed through the aortic orifice and then inflated in an effort to *crack* the calcium that is retarding leaflet motion. The patient population considered eligible for percutaneous aortic balloon valvuloplasty consists of those patients not thought to be surgical candidates. The immediate results show an increase in the aortic valve area of only 50%, with a 3% to 10% mortality. The long-term results are even more disappointing, with an expected 1-year mortality of at least 25% and a 30% to 35% recurrence rate of symptoms within 6 months. There is a recurrence of symptoms, death, aortic valve restenosis, or a combination of these in over 50% of patients within 6 months.[19] The only potential role of aortic balloon valvuloplasty may be in the aged, frail, and possibly senile patient whose long-term survival is poor.

AORTIC INSUFFICIENCY

Pathologic Anatomy. Aortic insufficiency may result from disease of the valve leaflets or of the aortic root. Rheumatic fever may affect the leaflets by shortening the distance from the leaflet free edge to the aortic annulus rather than by leading to commissural fusion. This prevents coaptation of the leaflets during diastole and causes a central leak (Fig. 54–156). Annuloaortic ectasia may produce valvular incompetence despite normal leaflet morphology. This may commonly result from cystic medial necrosis of the ascending aorta and may be associated with Marfan's syndrome. As the sinuses of Valsalva and the proximal aorta dilate, diastolic coaptation of the leaflets is precluded, resulting in valvular insufficiency. Congenital bicuspid aortic valves typically lead to aortic stenosis but may become regurgitant if a leaflet prolapses. Similarly, myxoid degeneration of the aortic valve leaflets, as seen in Marfan's syndrome, Ehlers-Danlos syndrome, and cystic medial necrosis, may lead to redundancy, progressive prolapse, and regurgitation. Infective endocarditis with bacterial destruction of the valve leaflets or scarring with leaflet retraction may cause valvular insufficiency. Trauma or dissection of the aortic wall may produce aortic regurgitation if it leads to loss of commissural suspension and leaflet prolapse.

Pathophysiology. The aortic valve leaks during diastole, which lowers diastolic pressure and widens the pulse pressure (Fig. 54–157). Because coronary blood flow occurs primarily in diastole, the lower diastolic blood pressure lowers

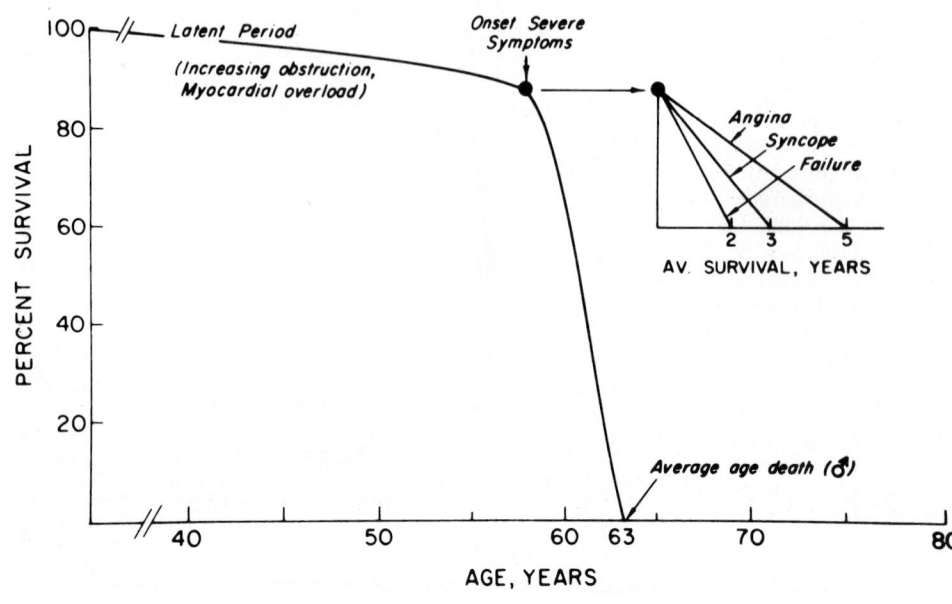

Figure 54–155. The natural history of medically treated aortic stenosis. One can understand the difficulty in deciding to operate on the asymptomatic patient (latent period). However, with the onset of symptoms, the issue becomes clear. (From Ross, J., and Braunwald, E.: Aortic stenosis. Circulation, *37*:V61, 1968. Copyright 1968, American Heart Association.)

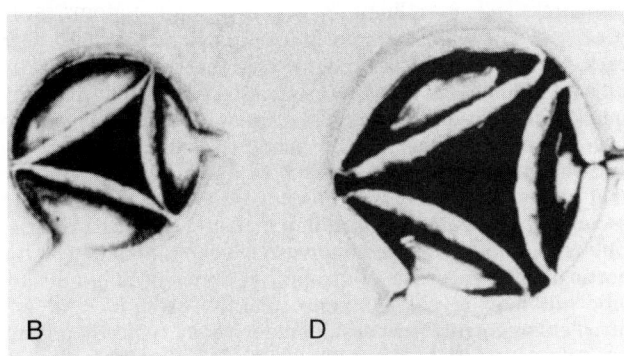

Figure 54–156. Variations in the aortic valve, leading to aortic regurgitation. *A,* Normal valve. *B,* Shortening of the cusps characteristic of rheumatic aortic regurgitation. The caliber of the aorta is normal. *C,* Dilatation of aorta, as occurs in syphilitic aortitis and annuloaortic ectasia. *D,* In addition to the features shown in *C,* there is atherosclerosis of the aorta, as occurs in syphilitic aortitis, with consequent coronary ostial narrowing. (From Roberts, W. C.: Valvular, subvalvular and supravalvular aortic stenosis: Morphologic features. *In* Edwards, J. E., Jr. [Ed.]: Clinical-Pathologic Correlations, 2nd ed. Philadelphia, F. A. Davis, 1973, p. 133.)

coronary perfusion pressure. Unlike aortic stenosis, in which the pathologic process is left ventricular pressure overload, the pathophysiology in aortic insufficiency derives from left ventricular volume overload. The increased left ventricular end-diastolic volume (preload) results from filling via the mitral valve as well as the incompetent aortic valve. Patients with chronic aortic insufficiency may have the greatest left ventricular end-diastolic volume of any form of heart disease. But because left ventricular compliance is often increased, left ventricular end-diastolic pressure may not be elevated. With left ventricular dilatation, normal forward stroke volume and ejection fraction may be maintained by increased left ventricular end-diastolic and end-systolic volumes. Ac-

cording to the law of Laplace, this left ventricular dilatation increases the left ventricular wall tension required to develop systolic pressure.[5] Such increased wall stress not only increases myocardial oxygen demand but also initiates left ventricular hypertrophy and increases left ventricular wall mass. Ultimately, myocardial fibrosis occurs.

With well-compensated aortic insufficiency, exercise may be tolerated because peripheral vascular resistance declines, lowering left ventricular afterload and increasing effective forward flow. At the same time heart rate increases, which shortens diastolic time, thereby decreasing the regurgitant flow. But as the ventricle ultimately decompensates, the left ventricular end-diastolic volume increases even without an

Figure 54–157. Simultaneous left ventricular and aortic pressure-time curves in a patient with severe aortic insufficiency. Note that in this trace the aortic and left ventricular end-diastolic pressures nearly equalize, suggesting the magnitude of this patient's regurgitant volume. (From Grossman, W.: Cardiac Catheterization, Angiography, and Intervention, 4th ed. Philadelphia, Lea & Febiger, 1991.)

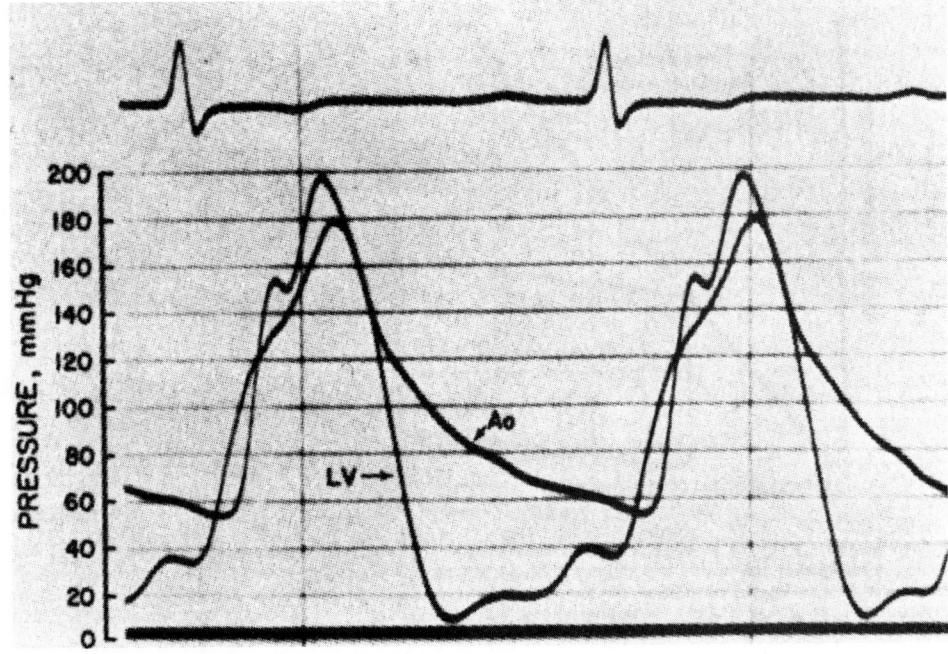

increase in aortic regurgitant volume. The end-systolic volume increases as the forward stroke volume declines because ventricular emptying is impaired; the ventricle fails (Fig. 54–158).

In severe aortic regurgitation, increased myocardial oxygen demand exceeds myocardial oxygen supply, causing ischemia despite normal coronary arteries. Increased left ventricular mass and wall tension occur concurrently with low diastolic pressures (low coronary perfusion pressure). Consequently, and particularly with exercise when the diastolic period shortens, coronary blood flow may not meet demand.

Diagnosis. The physical examination of patients with aortic regurgitation is distinctive because of the wide pulse pressure. The peripheral pulses rise and fall abruptly (Corrigan's or water-hammer pulse), the head may bob with each systole (de Musset's sign), and the capillaries visibly pulsate (Quincke's sign). Auscultation reveals a high-frequency decrescendo diastolic regurgitant murmur. A mid- to late-diastolic rumble may be heard (Austin-Flint murmur) and represents rapid antegrade flow across the mitral valve that closes prematurely because of rapid ventricular filling secondary to the aortic regurgitation. Doppler echocardiography is the most accurate noninvasive technique to determine aortic insufficiency. The electrocardiogram is usually nonspecific but may reveal left ventricular hypertrophy and left atrial enlargement. The chest roentgenogram typically reveals an enlarged cardiac silhouette with an enlarged left atrial shadow and chronic aortic regurgitation, although the cardiac size may not be enlarged with acute aortic regurgitation. The severity of the aortic regurgitation may be visualized angiographically at cardiac catheterization or may be delineated by transthoracic or transesophageal echocardiography.

Clinical Course. Because of the compensatory mechanisms discussed earlier, patients with chronic aortic regurgitation may be asymptomatic for long periods of time (Fig. 54–159). In fact, patients with mild to moderate aortic regurgitation have an excellent long-term prognosis; 10-year survival after diagnosis is 85% to 95%.[27] Studies in which patients with severe aortic regurgitation have been included revealed a 70% 10-year survival and a 50% 20-year survival.[27]

However, once these compensatory mechanisms begin to fail, left ventricular dysfunction becomes manifest. Symptoms, generally the result of an elevation of left atrial pressure, include dyspnea on exertion, orthopnea, and paroxysmal nocturnal dyspnea. Nocturnal angina occurs occasionally as a result of a slow heart rate and an exceedingly low diastolic pressure, with resultant poor coronary flow. Once symptoms of congestive heart failure occur, survival is markedly decreased. Almost 50% of patients with left ventricular failure die within 2 years.[5]

Management. Patients with symptomatic aortic insufficiency require surgical therapy, because their prognosis, if treated medically, is only a few years. However, optimal timing of surgical intervention in the asymptomatic or mildly symptomatic patient may be a very difficult clinical decision. Such patients may be successfully managed with diuretics and afterload reduction for long periods of time. Significant irreversible left ventricular systolic dysfunction may develop before clinical evidence of congestive heart failure. These patients should be carefully followed noninvasively with serial echocardiography or radionuclide ventriculography for evidence of systolic dysfunction or decreasing ejection fraction. An end-systolic dimension greater than 55 mm. estimated by echocardiography has been associated with irreversible left ventricular dysfunction, even after aortic valve replacement.[27] Aortic valve replacement should be performed before this degree of left ventricular dilatation. At cardiac catheterization, the end-systolic volume may help in determining management of these asymptomatic patients. When end-systolic volume is less than 30 ml. per sq. m., prognosis after surgical therapy is excellent. Progressive systolic dysfunction with end-systolic volumes greater than 90 ml. per sq. m. have intermediate short- and long-term results.[3] When left ventricular dysfunction is noted in patients with diminished ejection fraction and good exercise tolerance, elective operation is recommended. Persistent medical management of these patients severely jeopardizes surgical outcome and ultimate prognosis.[2]

The mortality associated with aortic valve replacement for aortic insufficiency is 4% to 6%.[15] Long-term survival is de-

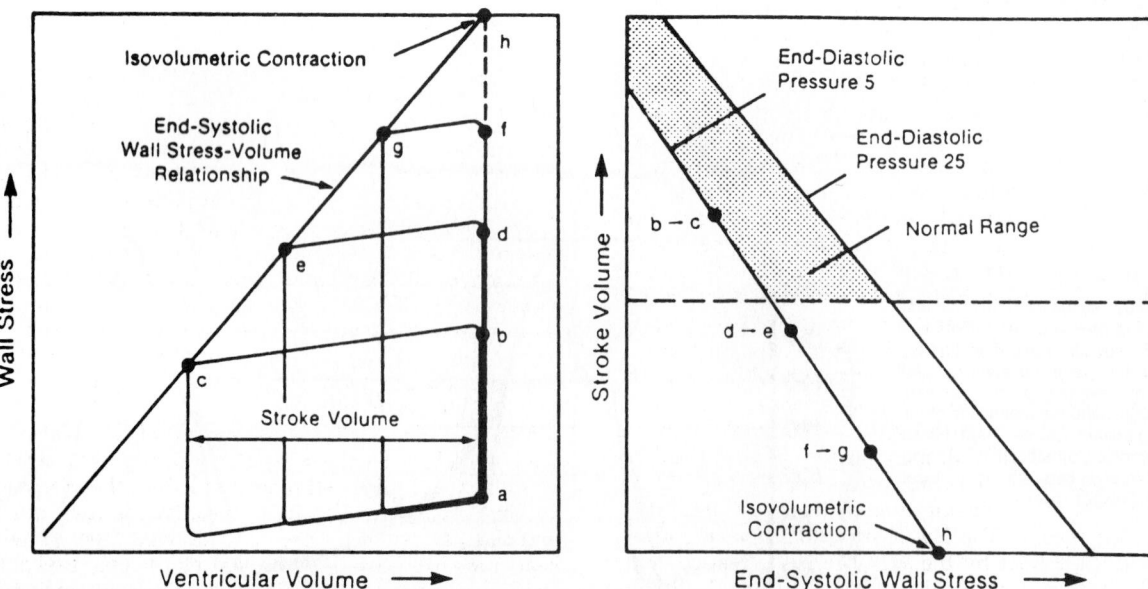

Figure 54–158. On the left a series of stress-volume loops is shown. As afterload is progressively increased, wall stress is increased such that ejection, which initially occurred at b, now occurs at d and then f. Stroke volume diminishes from b–c to d–e, and then f–g. At maximal wall stress h, there is no stroke volume but rather simply isovolumetric contraction. On the right, the inverse relationship between stroke volume and end-systolic wall stress is portrayed. The two negative slopes represent families of stroke volumes generated with an LVEDP of 5 mm. Hg. (From Weber, K. T., et al.: The mechanics of ventricular function. Hosp. Pract., *18*:113, 1983.)

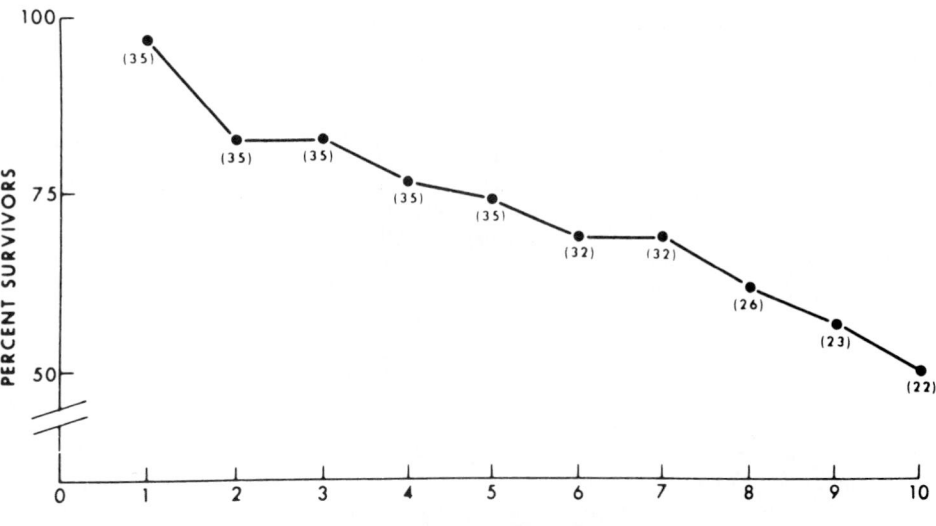

Figure 54–159. The natural history of medically treated aortic insufficiency. This curve is not too dissimilar from the result of surgically treated patients, although the two groups are not at all comparable. However, it supports the concept that the decision to operate on the asymptomatic patient with aortic insufficiency cannot be taken lightly. (From Rapport, E.: Natural history of aortic and mitral disease. Am. J. Cardiol., *35*:221, 1975.)

pendent on preoperative left ventricular function. Both early and late results are improved when surgical intervention precedes left ventricular decompensation.

HYPERTROPHIC OBSTRUCTIVE CARDIOMYOPATHY

Historical Aspects. In 1957, Brock suggested that hypertrophy of the interventricular septum could produce obstruction of the left ventricular outflow tract and performed resection of the septum through a closed transventricular approach.[6] Teare's association of septal hypertrophy with sudden death was published in 1958 after his review of the autopsy findings of seven patients who died suddenly.[37] In 1961, Kirklin and Ellis described a combined transaortic and transventricular technique for myectomy,[16] and Morrow and Brockenbrough described the technique of transaortic myectomy, which has become the standard surgical procedure.[25] In 1971, Cooley reported relief of left ventricular outflow tract obstruction by mitral valve replacement.[9]

Pathologic Anatomy and Physiology. Hypertrophic obstructive cardiomyopathy (HOCM) is associated with a marked increase in myocardial mass with greater involvement of the left than the right ventricle. The hypertrophy is asymmetrical and most pronounced in the basilar portion of the interventricular septum, creating a muscular prominence in the subaortic left ventricular outflow tract. Left ventricular ejection into the aorta is impeded, but the exact mechanism of this obstruction to flow is disputed. Three factors contributing to this impediment include the mechanical obstruction to flow created by the subaortic muscular hypertrophy, the increased systolic function of the left ventricle, which creates a dynamic obstruction of the already narrowed left ventricular outflow tract, and systolic anterior motion of the mitral valve (SAM).[24, 34] Although SAM is a consistent finding in obstructive forms of HOCM, its pathogenesis is unclear. It is commonly held that the prominent septal hypertrophy causes anterior displacement of the anterior mitral valve leaflet during systole. The leaflet is further drawn into the subaortic outflow tract by the Venturi effect created by the flow of blood during systole through the narrowed subaortic outflow tract, even further impeding left ventricular emptying. Not only does SAM contribute to the obstruction to flow from the left ventricle but it frequently results in mitral regurgitation.

Diagnosis. HOCM is usually identified in patients in the third and fourth decades of life, although the majority of patients are asymptomatic.[34] When symptoms are present, they are typically angina, dyspnea on exertion, and syncope. Unfortunately, the first clinical manifestation may be sudden death, which has been associated with exercise in patients with HOCM.

On physical examination, a harsh crescendo-decrescendo systolic murmur is present. The intensity of the murmur increases with provocative maneuvers, which either decrease left ventricular preload (Valsalva, standing), increase left ventricular contractility, or reduce left ventricular afterload (nitrovasodilators). Conversely, the murmur is diminished by maneuvers that increase left ventricular afterload (squatting) or decrease contractility (beta-blockade). The electrocardiogram is abnormal and reveals left ventricular hypertrophy and ST-segment and T-wave abnormalities. The chest roentgenogram may reveal cardiac enlargement but is more often normal. The echocardiogram is diagnostic and reveals the asymmetrical septal hypertrophy and left ventricular outflow tract obstruction.

Clinical Course. The annual mortality rate is approximately 3% for adults and 6% in children.[20] Aside from sudden death, clinical deterioration is slow. As in aortic stenosis, the onset of atrial fibrillation is poorly tolerated and quickly produces symptoms. Death from HOCM is usually sudden, often in previously asymptomatic patients. Risk factors for sudden death include age younger than 30 years and family history of sudden death from HOCM. Nonsustained ventricular tachycardia detected on ambulatory electrocardiographic monitoring is associated with an increased mortality. Surprisingly, neither the severity of left ventricular outflow gradient nor the presence of symptoms correlate with risk of death.[21] Although unconfirmed, sudden death is thought to be due to ventricular dysrhythmia.

Management. Medical management of HOCM is based on the use of beta blockade and/or calcium antagonists. Beta blockade was initially employed to reduce the left ventricular outflow tract obstruction by its negative inotropic effects, but its principal benefit is probably derived from slowing the heart rate. Verapamil has proven efficacious, probably as a result of improving diastolic function and as a negative inotrope. Disopyramide and amiodarone have been successfully used to control symptoms in patients in whom beta blockade and calcium antagonists have failed. Exercise should be avoided because of the risk of sudden death.

Surgical intervention is indicated in symptomatic patients with a left ventricular outflow tract gradient greater than 50 mm. Hg refractory to medical therapy. The most commonly performed procedure, myotomy-myectomy, entails a limited resection of the hypertrophied septum as exposed retrograde through the aortic valve (Fig. 54–160).[26] Approximately 70% of patients reported symptomatic improvement for up to 25 years after surgery.[23] The potential risks of the procedure include complete heart block (5%) and iatrogenic ventricular septal defect. Based on the premise that SAM contributes significantly to the pathophysiology of HOCM, mitral valve replacement has been performed as primary surgical therapy and has successfully relieved symptoms.[18] However, it is usually reserved for recurrent symptoms after septal myot-omy-myectomy or if the thickness of the basal interventricular septum is less than 2 cm. and therefore not amenable to effective myotomy-myectomy.

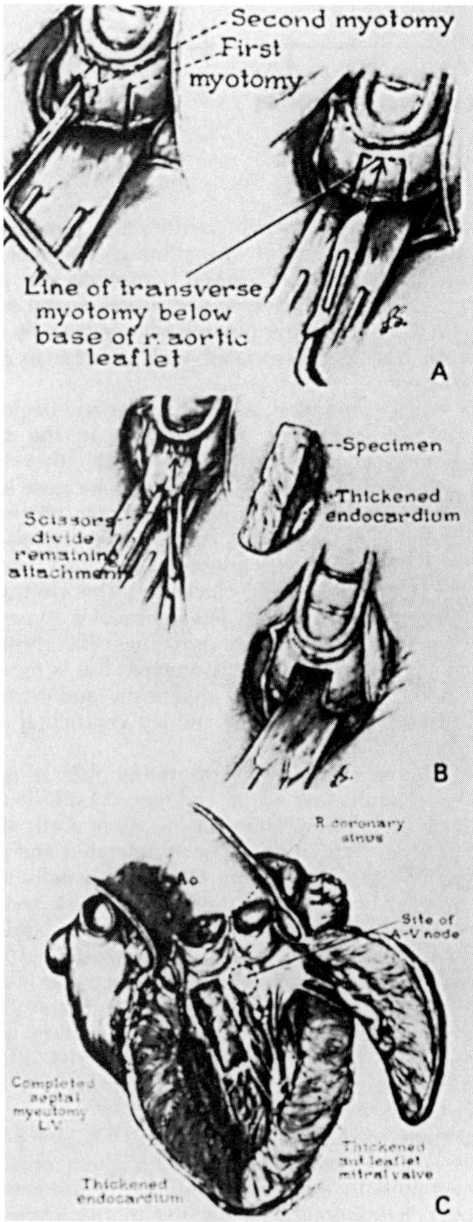

SELECTED REFERENCES

Morrow, A. G.: Hypertrophic subaortic stenosis. J. Thorac. Cardiovasc. Surg., 76:423, 1978.
  In masterful detail, Morrow instructs the reader in the operative technique of myotomy-myectomy for relief of hypertrophic obstructive cardiomyopathy.

Ross, J. Jr., and Braunwald, E.: Aortic stenosis. Circulation, 38:V61, 1968.
  This remains the classic article documenting the natural history of untreated aortic stenosis. The authors identified the precipitous decline in survival after the onset of the symptoms of angina, syncope, or congestive heart failure.

REFERENCES

1. Bailey, C. P., Glover, R. P., O'Neill, T. J. E., and Redondo-Ramirez, H. P.: Surgical relief of aortic stenosis. J. Thorac. Surg., 20:516, 1950.
2. Bonow, R. O., Picone, A. L., McIntosh, C. L., et al.: Survival and functional results after valve replacement for aortic regurgitation from 1976 to 1983: Impact of preoperative left ventricular function. Circulation, 72:1244, 1985.
3. Borow, K., Green, L. H., Mann, T., et al.: End-systolic volume overload from valvular regurgitation. Am. J. Med., 68:655, 1980.
4. Braunwald, E.: On the natural history of severe aortic stenosis. J. Am. Coll. Cardiol., 15:1018, 1990.
5. Braunwald, E.: Valvular heart disease. In Braunwald, E. (Ed.): Heart Disease: A Textbook of Cardiovascular Medicine. Philadelphia, W. B. Saunders, 1992, pp. 1035–1053.
6. Brock, R. C.: Functional obstruction of the left ventricle: Acquired subvalvar stenosis. Guy's Hosp. Rep., 106:221, 1957.
7. Carpentier, A., Deloche, A., Relland, J., et al.: Six-year follow-up of glutaraldehyde-preserved heterografts. J. Thorac. Cardiovasc. Surg., 68:771, 1974.
8. Cheitlin, M. D.: The timing of surgery in mitral and aortic valve disease. Curr. Prob. Cardiol., 12:115, 1987.
9. Cooley, D. A., Leachman, R. D., Hallman, G. L., Gerami, S., and Hall, R. D.: Idiopathic hypertrophic subaortic stenosis: Surgical treatment including mitral valve replacement. Arch. Surg., 103:606, 1971.
10. Cowper, W.: "Of ossifications or petrifications in the coats of arteries, particularly in valves of the great artery." Philos. Trans. R. Soc. (Lond.), 1706, Chap. 24.
11. Gorlin, R., and Gorlin, S. G.: Hydraulic formula for calculation of area of stenotic mitral valve, other cardiac valves, and central circulatory shunts. Am. Heart J., 41:1, 1951.
12. Harken, D. E., Soroff, H. S., Taylor, W. J., et al.: Partial and complete prostheses in aortic insufficiency. J. Thorac. Cardiovasc. Surg., 40:744, 1960.
13. Hufnagel, C. A., and Harvey, W. P.: The surgical correction of aortic regurgitation: A preliminary report. Bull. Georgetown U. Med. Cntr., 6:60, 1952.
14. Kennedy, K. D., Nishimura, R. A., Holmes, D. R., et al.: Natural history of moderate aortic stenosis. J. Am. Coll. Cardiol., 17:313, 1991.
15. Kirklin, J. W., and Barratt-Boyes, B. G.: Aortic valve disease. In: Cardiac Surgery. New York, Churchill Livingstone, 1993, pp. 491–571.
16. Kirklin, J. W., and Ellis, F. H.: Surgical relief of diffuse subvalvular aortic stenosis. Circulation, 24:739, 1961.
17. Lombard, J. T., and Selzer, A.: Valvular aortic stenosis: Clinical and hemodynamic profile of patients. Ann. Intern. Med., 106:292, 1987.
18. McIntosh, M. C., Greenberg, G. J., Maron, B. J., et al.: Clinical and hemodynamic results after mitral valve replacement in patients with obstructive hypertrophic cardiomyopathy. Ann. Thorac. Surg., 47:236, 1989.
19. McKay, R. G.: The Mansfield Scientific Aortic Valvuloplasty Registry: Overview of acute hemodynamic results and procedural complications. J. Am. Coll. Cardiol., 17:485, 1991.
20. McKenna, W. J.: The natural history of hypertrophic cardiomyopathy. Cardiovasc. Clin., 19:135, 1988.
21. McKenna, W. J., and Camm, A. J.: Sudden death in hypertrophic cardiomyopathy: Assessment of patients at high risk. Circulation, 80:1489, 1989.
22. Miller, D. C., Sinson, E. B., Oyer, P. E., Rossiter, S. J., Reitz, B. A., and Shumway, N. E.: Surgical implications and results of combined aortic valve replacement and myocardial revascularization. Am. J. Cardiol., 43:494, 1979.
23. Molar, R., Schaff, H. V., Danielson, G. K., Puga, F. J., Pluth, J. R., and Rafik, A. J.: The outcome of surgical treatment of hypertrophic obstructive cardiomyopathy. J. Thorac. Cardiovasc. Surg., 97:666, 1989.
24. Moran, B. J., Bonow, R. O., Cannon, R. O., et al.: Hypertrophic cardiomyopathy: Interrelations of clinical manifestations, pathophysiology, and therapy. I and II. N. Engl. J. Med., 316:780 and 844, 1987.
25. Morrow, A. G., and Brockenbrough, E. C.: Surgical treatment of idiopathic hypertrophic subaortic stenosis: Technic and hemodynamic results of subaortic ventriculotomy. Ann. Surg., 154:181, 1961.
26. Morrow, A. G., Reitz, B. A., Epstein, S. E., et al.: Operative treatment in hypertrophic subaortic stenosis: Techniques, and the results of pre- and post-operative assessment in 83 patients. Circulation, 52:88, 1975.

Figure 54–160. Septal myotomy-myectomy for hypertrophic cardiomyopathy. *A,* The aortic valve is retracted, and two parallel cuts are made in the ventricular septum. *B,* The portion of septum between the two incisions is excised, leaving a rectangular channel in the outflow tract. *C,* View of the open left ventricle and aorta demonstrating the relationships between the site of the myectomy, the aortic valve leaflets, and the conduction tissue. (From Morrow, A. G.: Operative methods utilized to relieve left ventricular outflow obstruction. J. Thorac. Cardiovasc. Surg., 76:423, 1978.)

27. Nishimura, R. A., McGoon, M. D., Schaff, H. V., and Giuliani, E. R.: Chronic aortic regurgitation: Indications for operation—1988. Mayo Clin. Proc., 63:270, 1988.
28. Passik, C. S., Adkermann, D. N., Pluth, J. R., and Edwards, W. D.: Temporal changes in the causes of aortic stenosis: A surgical pathologic study of 646 cases. Mayo Clin. Proc., 62:119, 1987.
29. Pellikka, P. A., Nishimura, R. A., Bailey, K. R., and Tajik, A. J.: The natural history of adults with asymptomatic hemodynamically significant aortic stenosis. J. Am. Coll. Cardiol., 15:1012, 1990.
30. Ross, D. N.: Homograft replacement of the aortic valve. Lancet, 2:877, 1962.
31. Ross, J., Jr., and Braunwald, E.: Aortic stenosis. Circulation, 38:V61, 1968.
32. Shumacker, H. B., Jr.: The Evolution of Cardiac Surgery. Bloomington, Indiana University Press, 1992, pp. 115–116.
33. Smithy, H. G., and Parker, E. F.: Experimental aortic valvulotomy: A preliminary report. Surg. Gynecol. Obstet., 84:625, 1947.
34. Spirito, P., Chiarella, F., Carratino, L., et al.: Clinical course and prognosis of hypertrophic cardiomyopathy in an outpatient population. N. Engl. J. Med., 320:749, 1989.
35. Starr, A., Edwards, M. L., McCord, C. W., and Griswold, H. E.: Aortic replacement: Clinical experience with a semirigid ball-valve prosthesis. Circulation, 27:779, 1963.
36. Stott, D. K., Marpose, D. G. F., Bristow, J. D., et al.: The role of left atrial transport in aortic and mitral stenosis. Circulation, 41:1031, 1970.
37. Teare, D.: Asymmetrical hypertrophy of the heart in young adults. Br. Heart J., 20:1, 1958.
38. Wallace, A. G.: Pathophysiology of cardiovascular disease. In Smith, L. H., Jr., and Thier, S. O. (Eds.): Pathophysiology: The Biological Principles of Disease. Philadelphia, W. B. Saunders, 1981, p. 1200.
39. Yeager, M., Yock, P. G., and Popp, R. L.: Companion of Doppler derived pressure gradient to that determined at cardiac catheterization in adults with aortic valve stenosis: Implications for management. Am. J. Cardiol., 57:644, 1986.

XVIII

MITRAL AND TRICUSPID VALVE DISEASE

Donald D. Glower, M.D.

NORMAL ANATOMY AND PHYSIOLOGY

The normal mitral valve consists of two leaflets—anterior and posterior (Fig. 54–161). The posterior leaflet attaches to roughly twice the anular circumference, as does the broader anterior leaflet, but the net surface areas of the anterior and posterior leaflets are similar. The anterior and posterior leaflets meet at the anterolateral and posteromedial commissures, which sit directly over the anterolateral and posteromedial papillary muscles, and the anterior and posterior leaflets each attach to both papillary muscles by means of fibrous chordae tendineae. First-order chordae originate at the tips of the papillary muscles and insert into the mitral valve leaflet edges; secondary chordae insert from the papillary muscle tips to the ventricular undersurface of the mitral valve leaflets; and tertiary chordae insert from the ventricular walls to the basal aspects of the leaflets. When the mitral valve is closed, the point of leaflet coaptation is generally 1 to 3 mm. from the actual leaflet free edge.

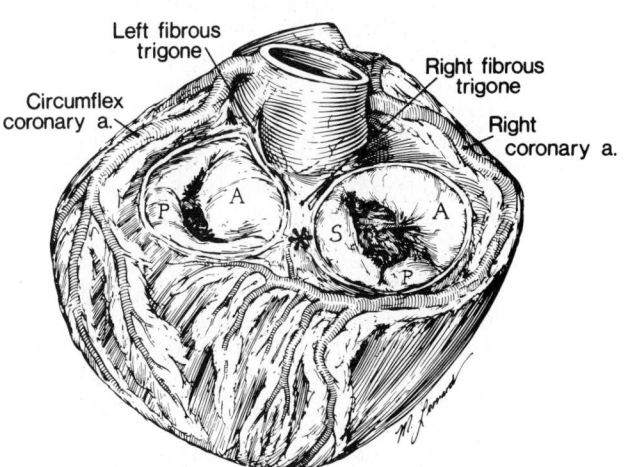

Figure 54–161. Anatomic interrelationships of the atrioventricular valves: Anterior leaflet (A); posterior leaflet (P); septal leaflet (S); the asterisk represents the area of the bundle of His. (Redrawn from McAlpine, W. A.: Heart and Coronary Arteries. New York, Springer-Verlag, 1975.)

The tricuspid valve is composed of three leaflets—anterior, posterior, and septal. As in the mitral valve, the tricuspid valve leaflets are attached to multiple papillary muscles by anterior, inferior, and septal chordae. Although the mitral and tricuspid valve leaflets consist of fibrous and elastic tissue, which is relatively avascular, the anterolateral and posteromedial papillary muscles of the mitral valve derive blood supply from the anterolateral and posterolateral branches of the coronary arteries, respectively.

During systole, the tricuspid and mitral valves normally close to prevent regurgitation of blood into the atria. Factors contributing to normal valve closure during systole include blood flow deceleration, ring vortices of blood flow returning from the ventricular apex toward the base, and rise of left ventricular pressure during systole. During diastole, the tricuspid and mitral valves open because of several factors, including the fall in left ventricular pressure, the rise in left atrial pressure during atrial systole, and active ventricular restorative forces during myocardial relaxation in the left ventricle.

Evidence has demonstrated that the mitral valve apparatus does make an important contribution to left ventricular function by maintaining continuity between the left ventricular papillary muscles and the mitral valve anulus through the chordae tendineae.[10, 36, 38] The mitral valve anulus does contract and deform slightly during systole, yet restriction of this motion appears to impair left ventricular function minimally, if at all.[16] Although viability of the papillary muscles had been thought to be important for normal closure of the mitral valve and in preventing mitral regurgitation due to *papillary muscle dysfunction,* experimental evidence suggests that papillary muscle necrosis contributes little to mitral regurgitation.[35] Instead, abnormal contraction of the left ventricular wall underlying each of the papillary muscles is probably more important than dysfunction of the papillary muscles in producing mitral regurgitation.

MITRAL STENOSIS

Pathophysiology. Worldwide, rheumatic fever remains the most common cause of mitral stenosis and is often associated with group A streptococcal pharyngitis. Other causes of mitral stenosis include calcific degeneration, malignant carcinoid disease, and congenital mitral stenosis. Acute rheumatic fever often produces an inflammatory myocarditis characterized histologically by Aschoff nodules, which may remain detectable for years after an acute episode of rheumatic fever. In rheumatic fever, an acute inflammatory infiltrate forms on one or more of the cardiac valves, which then heal by fibrosis with fusion of the valvular commissures, loss of leaflet pliability, thickening and fusion of the chordae, and, ultimately, calcification of the leaflets and subvalvular apparatus. Symptoms of mitral stenosis secondary to rheumatic fever may be absent until the third or fourth decade of life. The increased pressure gradient across the mitral valve increases left atrial pressure with resultant left atrial dilation, onset of atrial fibrillation, and often formation of left atrial thrombi, which may embolize. In turn, pulmonary artery pressures may rise over time and produce irreversible pulmonary arteriosclerosis and right ventricular failure. Cardiac output falls owing to right ventricular failure and inadequate filling of the left ventricle.

Patients with mitral stenosis may develop symptoms of exertional dyspnea, followed by dyspnea at rest or orthopnea. Reduced cardiac output may produce easy fatigability and cardiac cachexia over a prolonged period. In addition, patients may complain of hoarseness due to compression of the left recurrent laryngeal nerve by the left pulmonary artery or dysphasia due to encroachment on the esophagus by the left atrium. Paradoxically, the onset of severe pulmonary hypertension may actually protect the pulmonary capillaries from pulmonary edema due to sudden rises in left atrial pressure. Patients ultimately develop right ventricular failure with peripheral edema, hepatic congestion, cirrhosis, and anasarca. Patients with long-standing mitral stenosis can die of pulmonary edema, hemoptysis, arterial embolism, or endocarditis.

Natural History. In the United States, the average age that rheumatic fever occurs has been reported to be 8 to 12 years, with the onset of clinical mitral stenosis occurring 10 years after illness. The mean age at onset of symptoms of mitral stenosis is 31 years.[32] Patients with asymptomatic mitral stenosis may have a mean survival of 15 to 20 years, whereas patients with increasing symptoms of mitral stenosis have a life expectancy of 2 to 7 years, depending on the degree of symptoms (Fig. 54–162).[28] The onset of atrial fibrillation commonly exacerbates symptoms due to increased heart rate

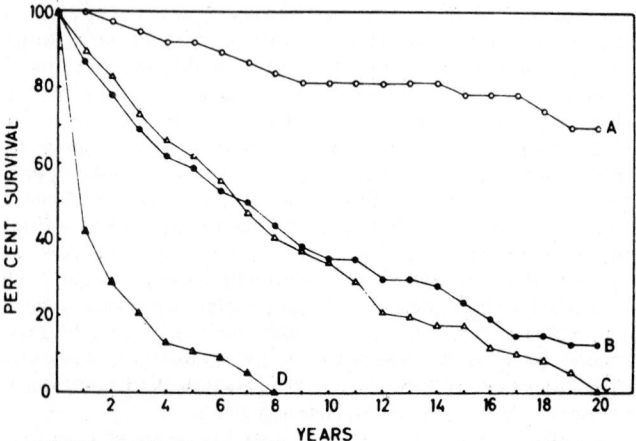

Figure 54–162. Survival in mitral stenosis after first observation. Group A is patients with sinus rhythm and Class II symptoms. Group B represents sinus rhythm and Class III symptoms. Group C is atrial fibrillation with Class II or Class III symptoms. Group D is Class IV symptoms. (From Olesen, K. H.: The natural history of 271 patients with mitral stenosis under medical treatment. Br. Heart J., *24*:349, 1962.)

and loss of atrial contraction to aid in transmitral blood flow. Embolic events may occur in 10% to 19% of patients with untreated mitral stenosis.[28, 32]

Diagnosis. On examination, the patient with chronic mitral stenosis may be thin and cachectic with peripheral cyanosis and *mitral facies* characterized by ruddy cheeks. Jugular venous distention may be present, along with pedal edema. The presence of right-sided heart failure may produce ascites and hepatojugular reflux demonstrated by jugular venous distention on pressing over the right upper quadrant. On cardiac examination, the pulse may be irregular. The first heart sound may be accentuated in early mitral stenosis and may be diminished with severe valvular thickening. The second heart sound may be accentuated by pulmonary hypertension, and an opening mitral snap may be audible in diastole, with the snap occurring earlier in diastole as left atrial pressure increases. A mid-diastolic rumble may be audible and may occur during 50% or more of diastole in severe mitral stenosis (Fig. 54–163). In normal sinus rhythm, presystolic accentuation of the diastolic rumble may be present. A sternal heave may indicate right ventricular enlargement and pulmonary hypertension.

The chest radiograph may demonstrate left atrial enlargement with prominence of the left atrial appendage, elevation of the left mainstem bronchus, double density of the central heart shadow over the right atrium, cephalization of pulmonary blood flow, and occasionally the presence of Kerley B-lines, or even pulmonary edema (Fig. 54–164). Right atrial and right ventricular enlargement may be present in association with right ventricular failure.

The electrocardiogram of patients in sinus rhythm may show a prominent p-wave, termed *p mitrale*. Atrial fibrillation, right ventricular hypertrophy, and right-axis deviation may also be present. Two-dimensional echocardiography may demonstrate mitral leaflet thickening and calcification, leaflet immobility, and thickening of the subvalvular mitral apparatus. Doppler echocardiography may quantify the mitral valve gradient during diastole and provide an estimate of mitral valve orifice area.

The gold standard for quantifying the severity of mitral stenosis is left- and right-sided heart catheterization. Additional indications for cardiac catheterization include age older than 35 years or the presence of risk factors for coronary artery disease in patients likely to need an operation. Left atrial pressure can be measured directly by puncture of the interatrial septum, or the pulmonary capillary wedge pressure may be used as an estimate of left atrial pressure. A resting mitral valve pressure gradient at end diastole of 10 mm. Hg indicates significant mitral stenosis. The mitral valve orifice area (MVA), measured in square centimeters, is calculated from the Gorlin formula using the mean diastolic mitral gradient (ΔP), measured in millimeters of mercury, and the average diastolic mitral flow (F), measured in milliliters per second, determined by thermodilution or Fick measurement of cardiac output and measurement of the duration of diastole.

$$MVA = \frac{F}{38\sqrt{\Delta P}}$$

The normal mitral valve has an orifice area of 3 sq. cm. per sq. m. of body surface area. Significant mitral stenosis is considered to be present when the mitral valve area is 1 sq. cm. per sq. m. or less. Calculation of mitral valve orifice area is subject to error due to valvular regurgitation and inaccurate determination of pressure gradients.

Treatment. Medical treatment of mitral stenosis includes prophylaxis for bacterial endocarditis, diuretics, use of antiarrhythmic agents and/or electrical cardioversion to convert atrial fibrillation to sinus rhythm, and use of digitalis, beta blocking agents, or calcium channel blocking agents to con-

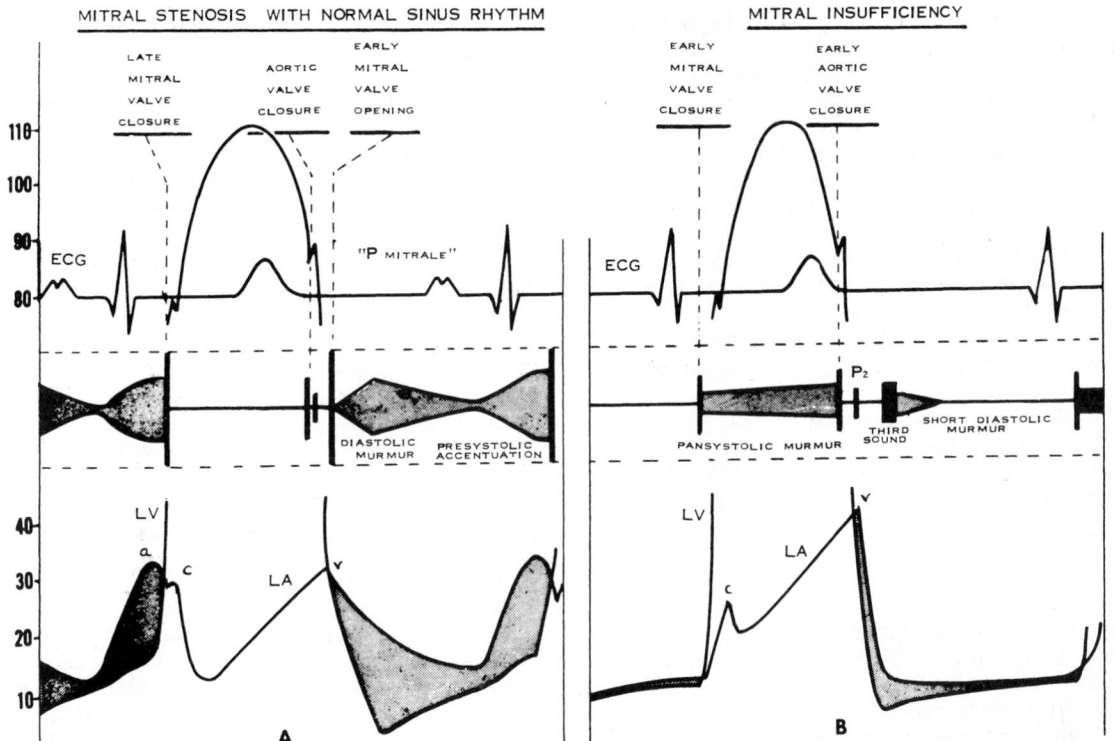

Figure 54–163. Classic illustration of clinical and hemodynamic features of mitral stenosis and regurgitation. *A,* Mitral stenosis in sinus rhythm. *B,* Mitral insufficiency in atrial fibrillation. (From Glover, R. P., and Davilla, J. C.: The Surgery of Mitral Stenosis. New York, Grune & Stratton, 1961.)

trol heart rate in atrial fibrillation. Electrical cardioversion of atrial fibrillation may be effective if atrial fibrillation has been present for less than 6 to 12 months and if the left atrial diameter does not exceed 5 cm. Three to 4 weeks of anticoagulation with digitalis and antiarrhythmic therapy should be instituted before cardioversion. Chronic anticoagulation may be indicated in patients with a history of embolism, with known left atrial thrombus, or in selected patients with chronic atrial fibrillation.

Current indications for percutaneous or operative treatment of mitral stenosis include the presence of at least moderate mitral stenosis with a calculated valve area of 1 sq. cm. per sq. m. and with New York Heart Association (NYHA) Class III or Class IV symptoms or the onset of atrial fibrillation. Additional indications for intervention include worsening pulmonary hypertension, systemic embolization, or bacterial endocarditis.

Percutaneous balloon mitral valvotomy has been in clinical use since 1984; and for institutions where balloon valvotomy is available, this procedure is preferred for most patients with significant mitral stenosis. With balloon valvotomy, the stenotic mitral valve may be dilated, with one or two balloons passed retrograde through the aortic valve or transseptally from the femoral vein. Balloon valvotomy may increase mitral valve area to roughly 2 sq. cm. in selected patients with an echocardiographic score of 8 or less.[27] The presence of left atrial thrombus, 2+ or greater mitral regurgitation, significant leaflet thickening or calcification, or significant scarring of the subvalvular apparatus all constitute relative contraindications to percutaneous balloon mitral valvotomy. Complications of percutaneous balloon mitral valvotomy include arterial embolism, acute mitral regurgitation, and cardiac perforation, each occurring in less than 1% to 2% of properly selected patients.[26] Roughly 66% of patients are free from subsequent intervention 3 years after percutaneous balloon mitral valvotomy.[7]

Although percutaneous balloon mitral valvotomy has become more frequent than operative management of mitral stenosis in many institutions, operative management of mitral stenosis remains indicated in those patients where percutaneous balloon mitral valvotomy is relatively contraindicated or at institutions where percutaneous balloon mitral valvotomy is not available. Several operative techniques are available for treatment of mitral stenosis. Closed mitral commissurotomy without use of cardiopulmonary bypass may provide excellent long-term results but has been largely supplanted by percutaneous balloon mitral valvotomy at those institutions where percutaneous techniques are available to avoid the morbidity of general anesthesia and a thoracotomy incision. In the United States, most patients going to operation for mitral stenosis undergo open mitral commissurotomy on cardiopulmonary bypass because of the advantages of being able to visualize and remove left atrial thrombus as well as assess and repair valvular pathology more precisely than is possible with a closed mitral commissurotomy. Finally, mitral valve replacement is indicated for significant mitral stenosis coincident with 2+ or greater mitral regurgitation or with severe leaflet or subvalvular calcification or fibrosis not amenable to repair. Patients requiring open mitral valve repair for rheumatic mitral stenosis are more likely to need reoperation than are patients undergoing repair for mitral regurgitation or mitral valve replacement using modern prostheses for mitral stenosis.[7, 14] Strong consideration should be given to mitral valve replacement for those patients with severe mitral valvular disease and no contraindications to long-term anticoagulation.

Results. Percutaneous balloon mitral valvotomy, open mitral commissurotomy, and mitral valve replacement carry hospital mortalities of 1% to 2%, 1% to 5%, and 4% to 10%, respectively, and over 90% of patients initially revert to NYHA Class I or Class II symptoms. After mitral commissurotomy or percutaneous balloon mitral valvotomy, the likeli-

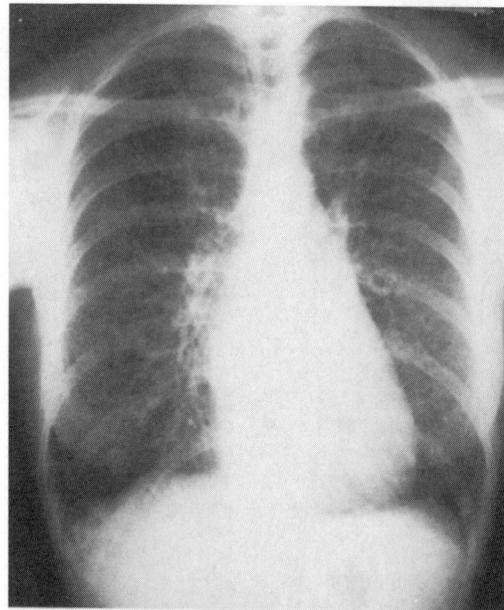

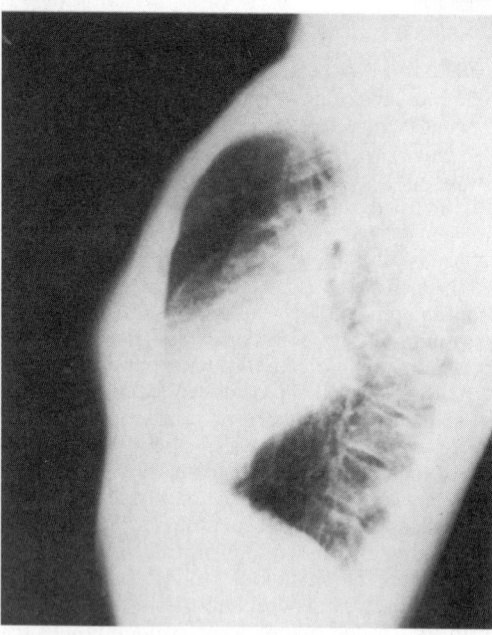

Figure 54–164. Posteroanterior and lateral chest radiographs of a patient with moderate mitral stenosis. Minimal overall cardiac enlargement is present, even though the left atrium is severely displaced toward the spine in the lateral view. A suggestion of a "double density" on the right border of the heart, right ventricular enlargement, and Kerley B lines in the right costophrenic angle are evident. (Courtesy of James T. T. Chen, M.D.)

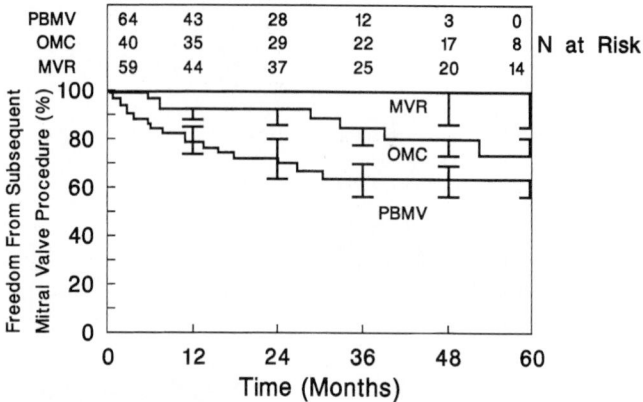

Figure 54–165. Freedom from subsequent mitral valve procedures ± standard error after percutaneous balloon mitral valvuloplasty (PBMV), open mitral commissurotomy (OMC), or mitral valve replacement (MVR) for mitral stenosis. (From Cohen, J. M., Glower, D. D., Harrison, J. K., et al.: Comparison of balloon valvuloplasty with operative treatment for mitral stenosis. Reprinted with permission from the Society of Thoracic Surgeons [The Annals of Thoracic Surgery, 1993;56:1254].)

MITRAL REGURGITATION

Pathophysiology and Natural History. The causes of mitral regurgitation are many and include rheumatic fever, mitral valve prolapse (myxomatous valve degeneration, Barlow's syndrome), chordal rupture, bacterial endocarditis, calcific valvular degeneration, hypertrophic cardiomyopathy, and myocardial infarction or ischemia. Carpentier classified the mechanical causes of mitral regurgitation as anular dilation, leaflet prolapse, and leaflet restriction (Fig. 54–167). In rheumatic heart disease, leaflet thickening and shortening of the subvalvular chordae prevent full coaptation of the leaflet edges during systole. Mitral valve prolapse is present in 2% to 5% of the adult population and is occasionally associated with a midsystolic click and late systolic murmur. Approximately 5% of patients with mitral valve prolapse ultimately develop mitral regurgitation due to chordal elongation, chordal rupture, or leaflet redundancy, each preventing adequate coaptation of the mitral valve leaflet edges. Chordal rupture may occur due to myxomatous degeneration, endocarditis, or chest trauma; and bacterial endocarditis may produce leaflet perforation in addition to chordal rupture. Like rheumatic heart disease, mitral valve calcification can restrict

hood of requiring a repeat mitral valve procedure increases over 3 to 10 years (Fig. 54–165).[7] With current prostheses such as the St. Jude valve, freedom from reoperation at 10 years or more after mitral valve replacement for mitral stenosis is 95%.[20] Even after percutaneous or operative correction of mitral stenosis, the likelihood of chronic atrial fibrillation increases over time, and 36% of patients undergoing biologic mitral valve replacement required anticoagulation 4 years after mitral valve replacement in the series of Louagie.[22] Ten-year survival after open commissurotomy or mitral valve replacement is roughly 80% or 60%, respectively.[20, 31] Risk factors for diminished survival after operative management of mitral stenosis include increased age, coronary artery disease, and other valvular heart disease (Fig. 54–166).[20]

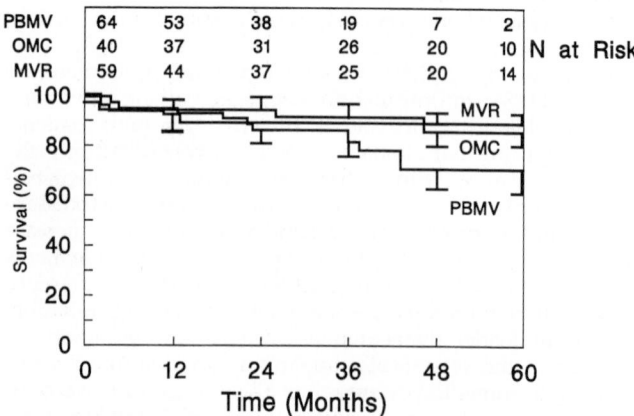

Figure 54–166. Patient survival ± standard error after percutaneous balloon mitral valvuloplasty (PBMV), open mitral commissurotomy (OMC), or mitral valve replacement (MVR) for mitral stenosis. (From Cohen, J. M., Glower, D. D., Harrison, J. K., et al.: Comparison of balloon valvuloplasty with operative treatment for mitral stenosis. Reprinted with permission from the Society of Thoracic Surgeons [The Annals of Thoracic Surgery, 1993;56:1254].)

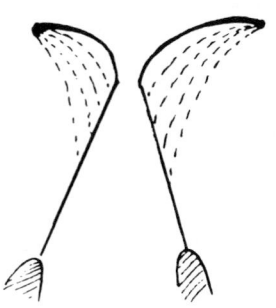 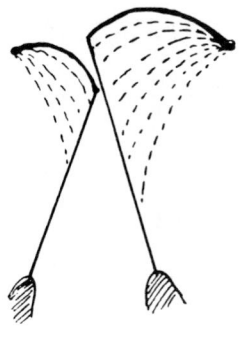 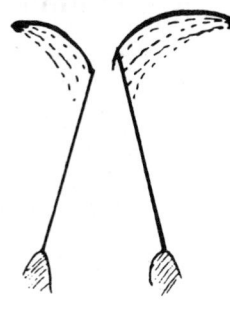

TYPE I
NORMAL LEAFLET MOTION

TYPE II
LEAFLET PROLAPSE

TYPE III
RESTRICTED LEAFLET MOTION

Figure 54–167. Carpentier classification of mitral regurgitation pathophysiology. Dotted lines represent the motion of the leaflets between opening and closing positions. (From Carpentier, A.: Cardiac valve surgery—the "French Correction." J. Thorac. Cardiovasc. Surg., *86*:323, 1983.)

leaflet motion and produce mitral regurgitation. Hypertrophic obstructive cardiomyopathy may produce mitral regurgitation due to abnormal insertion and movement of the papillary muscles. Papillary muscle rupture with resultant mitral regurgitation can occur 3 to 7 days after relatively small myocardial infarctions of the posterior ventricular wall. Myocardial ischemia or infarction may produce mitral regurgitation by papillary-anular dysfunction when abnormal motion of the posterior left ventricular wall prevents normal coaptation of the mitral valve leaflet edges during systole owing to abnormal ventricular wall motion. Myocardial infarction or ischemia may also produce mitral regurgitation caused by generalized dilation of the posterior mitral valve anulus, which prevents coaptation of the leaflet edges during systole.

All forms of mitral regurgitation cause an abnormal v wave in the left atrial and pulmonary capillary wedge pressure tracings. The resultant increase in left atrial pressure may produce dyspnea or pulmonary edema; and secondary pulmonary arterial hypertension, right ventricular failure, and tricuspid regurgitation may ultimately follow. Because the left atrium presents a low-pressure afterload to the left ventricle, left ventricular ejection fraction may initially rise after onset of mitral regurgitation and then progressively fall as the left ventricle dilates because of the increased diastolic filling and wall stress. As left ventricular dilation occurs, compensatory left ventricular hypertrophy (eccentric hypertrophy) also results. As in mitral stenosis, atrial fibrillation may be caused by left atrial dilation. Ultimately, left ventricular failure, pulmonary edema, and right ventricular failure may produce death. The time course from onset of mitral regurgitation to onset of symptoms and death is highly variable depending on the cause of the mitral regurgitation. Patients with acute mitral valve perforation due to endocarditis or acute papillary muscle rupture may die of cardiogenic shock and pulmonary edema within 2 to 5 days, whereas patients with mitral regurgitation due to mitral valve prolapse may tolerate mitral regurgitation for decades. Once mitral regurgitation becomes moderate (3+ on a scale of 0 to 4+), clinical symptoms and deterioration of left ventricular function tend to progress more rapidly.

Diagnosis. Patients with mitral regurgitation may develop exertional dyspnea, fatigue, orthopnea, paroxysmal nocturnal dyspnea, peripheral edema, and angina pectoris. On physical examination, jugular venous distention and an irregular pulse may be present. Cardiac examination will generally demonstrate a holosystolic murmur heard best at the apex, with radiation into the axilla (see Fig. 54–163). The first heart sound may be less prominent, and the second heart sound may have increased splitting. An S₃ gallop may correlate with depressed left ventricular function. Pulmonary rales may be audible, and pedal edema may coincide with right ventricular failure.

On the chest radiograph, left atrial and left ventricular enlargement, Kerley B-lines, and pulmonary edema may be present. The electrocardiogram may demonstrate p-mitrale, left ventricular or biventricular hypertrophy, or atrial fibrillation.

The mitral valve apparatus is best visualized by echocardiography, which may detect mitral valve prolapse, ruptured chordae, vegetations, leaflet thickening, and calcification of the mitral valve leaflet or anulus. Doppler echocardiography can quantify the severity of regurgitation based on the velocity, width, and length of the regurgitant jet. Echocardiography can also estimate left ventricular ejection fraction and detect left atrial or left ventricular enlargement.

Left- and right-sided heart catheterization is indicated to evaluate mitral regurgitation, ventricular function, and coronary anatomy in most patients with symptomatic mitral regurgitation likely to need operation if the patient is older than 35 years old or if risk factors for coronary artery disease are present. At cardiac catheterization, the severity of mitral regurgitation is quantified on a 1+ to 4+ scale based on the amount of regurgitant dye within the left atrium. Left ventricular ejection fraction, left ventricular volume, right-sided heart pressures, and cardiac output all should be evaluated at catheterization.

Treatment. Medical treatment for mitral regurgitation includes prophylaxis for endocarditis, diuretics, vasodilators to reduce left ventricular afterload and to increase cardiac output, and use of digoxin, beta blockade, or calcium channel blockade to control heart rate in atrial fibrillation.

Indications for operation include 3+ or greater mitral regurgitation with NYHA Class III or Class IV symptoms of heart failure or angina, onset of atrial fibrillation, or evidence of impaired left ventricular function (reduced ejection fraction or left ventricular enlargement) either at rest or with exercise.[34] In patients with endocarditis, additional relative indications for mitral valve operation may include persistent sepsis, intracardiac abscess, recurrent embolism, fungal endocarditis, or staphylococcal prosthetic valve endocarditis. Given the morbidity associated with chronic atrial fibrillation and the improved results from mitral valve repair in appropriate patients, patients with at least moderate mitral regurgitation are being referred for mitral valve repair at earlier stages, such as onset of intermittent atrial fibrillation, any ventricular enlargement, or ventricular dysfunction.[34] Even patients with poor ventricular function may benefit from operation. Patients likely to do poorly include those with ejection fraction significantly less than 40% and those with a depressed relationship between end-systolic stress and end-systolic volume index.[4]

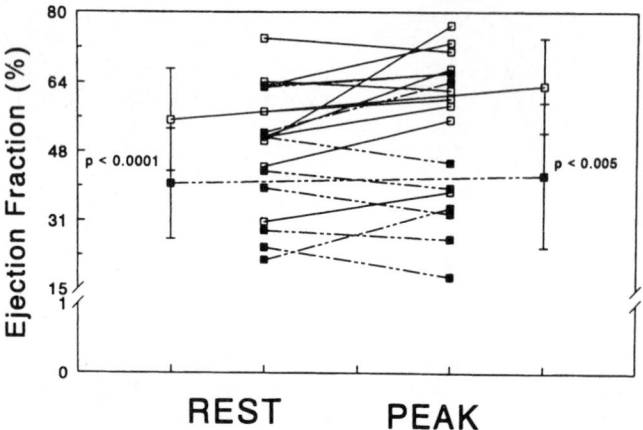

Figure 54–168. Demonstration of superior left ventricular ejection fraction at rest and at peak exercise in patients with mitral valve repair (white squares) versus mitral valve replacement (black squares). (Reproduced with permission from Tischler, M. D., Cooper, K. A., Rowen, M., and LeWinter, M. M.: Mitral valve replacement versus mitral valve repair: A Doppler and quantitative stress echocardiographic study. Circulation, *89*:132, 1994. Copyright 1994 American Heart Association.)

In those patients in whom mitral valve pathology is amenable to an effective and long-lasting repair, mitral valve repair is the procedure of choice for mitral regurgitation. A relative indication for mitral valve replacement instead of repair is significant fibrosis or calcification of the mitral valve leaflets or subvalvular apparatus. Mitral valve repair has several advantages over mitral valve replacement: less impairment of left ventricular function by maintaining papillary-anular continuity (Fig. 54–168)[10, 19, 36, 38]; potentially eliminating the need for chronic anticoagulation; and improving durability relative to biologic prostheses.[11] In those patients in whom mitral valve repair is likely to be ineffective or less durable than available mechanical prostheses, mitral valve replacement is indicated, particularly in those patients already in chronic atrial fibrillation. Mitral valve replacement is also indicated in patients with significant mitral regurgitation produced by hypertrophic cardiomyopathy with obstruction of the left ventricular outflow tract by the anterior leaflet of the mitral valve.

Results. Operative mortality from isolated mitral valve repair has generally been 2% to 5%,[11, 14] as compared with

4% to 10% mortality after mitral valve replacement.[20] Incremental risk factors for mortality with mitral valve repair or replacement include older age, left ventricular dysfunction, worse NYHA functional class, other comorbid disease, and the presence of coronary artery disease.[14] Long-term survival after mitral repair or replacement is roughly 60% at 10 years (Fig. 54–169). Especially in those patients with diminished left ventricular function preoperatively, the left ventricular ejection fraction may fall after mitral valve repair or replacement due to two factors. First, correction of mitral regurgitation also corrects the abnormally low left ventricular afterload caused by low left atrial pressure relative to aortic pressure.[18] Second, mitral valve replacement with loss of papillary-anular continuity may directly impair left ventricular contractility.[10, 19, 29, 38] Studies now suggest improved preservation of left ventricular function with mitral valve repair versus replacement (see Fig. 54–168),[10, 36] but newer techniques of mitral valve replacement that preserve papillary-anular continuity[9, 13] may minimize differences in left ventricular function after mitral valve repair versus replacement (Fig. 54–170).[10, 19, 29, 38] The incidence of thromboembolism after mitral valve repair is low (less than 1% per patient-year) and generally less than after mitral valve replacement.[11, 12] Freedom from reoperation after mitral valve replacement with modern mechanical prostheses may be as high as 95% at 10 years.[20] After mitral valve repair, freedom from reoperation may approach 87% at 15 years but is less for rheumatic valve disease relative to myxomatous or degenerative disease (Fig. 54–171).[11, 14]

TRICUSPID VALVE DISEASE

Pathophysiology and Natural History. Tricuspid regurgitation may be caused by either functional or organic abnormalities of the tricuspid valve. Functional tricuspid regurgitation is by far the most common form of tricuspid valve disease and generally results from tricuspid anular dilation due to right-sided heart failure and long-standing pulmonary hypertension. Organic tricuspid regurgitation is more unusual but may occur after rheumatic fever, carcinoid heart disease, bacterial endocarditis, and trauma. Tricuspid stenosis is uncommon but may be caused by rheumatic heart disease, carcinoid heart disease, congenital defects, or cardiac tumors. Both tricuspid stenosis and regurgitation elevate right atrial pressures and may produce pedal edema, ascites, hepatic congestion, hepatic failure, and renal failure. Correction of

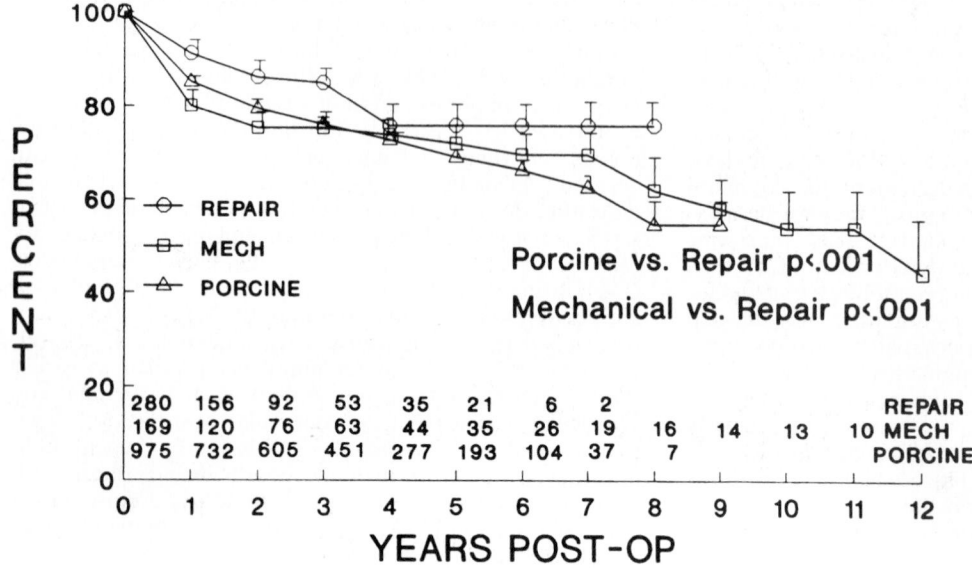

Figure 54–169. Actuarial survival after mitral valve repair versus mitral valve replacement. (From Galloway, A. C., Colvin, S. B., Baumann, F. G., et al.: A comparison of mitral valve reconstruction with mitral valve replacement: Intermediate-term results. Reprinted with permission from the Society of Thoracic Surgeons [The Annals of Thoracic Surgery, 1989;47:655].)

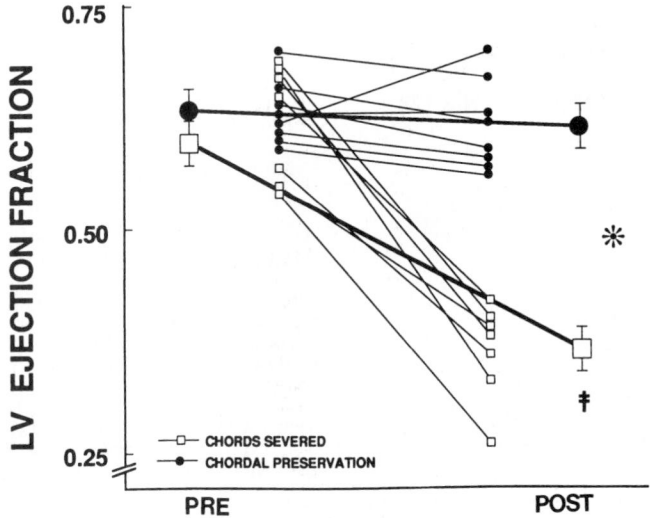

Figure 54–170. Preoperative (pre) and postoperative (post) left ventricular (LV) ejection fraction for patients undergoing mitral valve replacement with chordae tendineae preserved (closed circles) or severed (open squares). *p < .05 chordal preservation vs. chords severed. ‡ p < .05 pre vs. post mitral valve replacement. (Reproduced with permission from Rozich, J. D., Carabello, B. A., Usher, B. W., Kratz, J. M., Bell, A. G., and Zile, M. R.: Mitral valve replacement with and without chordal preservation in patients with chronic mitral regurgitation. Circulation, *86*:1718, 1992. Copyright 1992 American Heart Association.)

atrial a wave, right ventricular hypertrophy, or atrial fibrillation. Right atrial and/or right ventricular enlargement and occasional bilateral pleural effusions may be present on the chest radiograph. Echocardiography can readily visualize thickening or deformity of the tricuspid valve leaflets along with enlargement of the right ventricle and right atrium. The degree of tricuspid regurgitation and stenosis can be quantified using Doppler echocardiography. Right-sided heart catheterization may confirm the diagnosis of tricuspid valve dysfunction and allow direct measurement of diastolic gradients across the tricuspid valve in tricuspid stenosis, with a 5-mm. Hg gradient being significant and a 3-mm. Hg gradient occasionally producing symptoms. In tricuspid regurgitation, a right atrial v wave will be present and right ventriculography can quantify tricuspid regurgitation on a scale of 1+ to 4+. Left-sided heart catheterization may be employed in operative candidates who are older than the age of 35 years or have other risk factors for coronary disease.

Treatment. Medical management of tricuspid stenosis or regurgitation includes endocarditis prophylaxis along with the use of diuretics, and furosemide in combination with spironolactone may be particularly effective. Indications for operation for tricuspid valve disease include moderate tricuspid stenosis or regurgitation concurrent with other valvular disease requiring operation, severe symptomatic tricuspid stenosis or regurgitation, or moderate tricuspid disease with onset of atrial fibrillation. Because most patients requiring reoperation for tricuspid valve replacement had previous operation on the mitral valve alone, relatively aggressive treatment of tricuspid regurgitation is indicated at the time of operation for aortic or mitral valve disease.[16] Available procedures include tricuspid anuloplasty for functional tricuspid regurgitation, tricuspid valve repair for tricuspid stenosis, tricuspid valve replacement, and tricuspid valvectomy for patients with isolated tricuspid valve endocarditis and a high likelihood of returning to intravenous drug abuse.[1]

Results. Survival and freedom from reoperation have been similar after either tricuspid valve repair or tricuspid valve replacement (Figs. 54–172 and 54–173).[25] Operative mortality from isolated tricuspid valve replacement is 5% to 15%, whereas mortality for tricuspid valve repair or replacement in general approaches 20% because most tricuspid valve op-

the underlying cause of right-sided heart failure may often reverse functional tricuspid regurgitation. Long-standing tricuspid regurgitation may produce left ventricular dysfunction by leftward shift of the interventricular septum, with resultant decrease in septal fiber preload.

Diagnosis. On physical examination, jugular venous distention may be noted along with hepatic enlargement, ascites, and pedal edema. Tricuspid regurgitation may produce a pulsatile liver along with hepatojugular reflex and a holosystolic murmur augmented by inspiration. In tricuspid stenosis, an opening snap may be present along with a mid-diastolic murmur accentuated by inspiration.

The electrocardiogram may demonstrate enlarged right

Figure 54–171. Freedom from mitral valve reoperation after mitral valve replacement or mitral valve repair for rheumatic or nonrheumatic disease. (From Galloway, A. C., Colvin, S. B., Baumann, F. G., et al.: A comparison of mitral valve reconstruction with mitral valve replacement: Intermediate-term results. Reprinted with permission from the Society of Thoracic Surgeons [The Annals of Thoracic Surgery, 1989;47:655].)

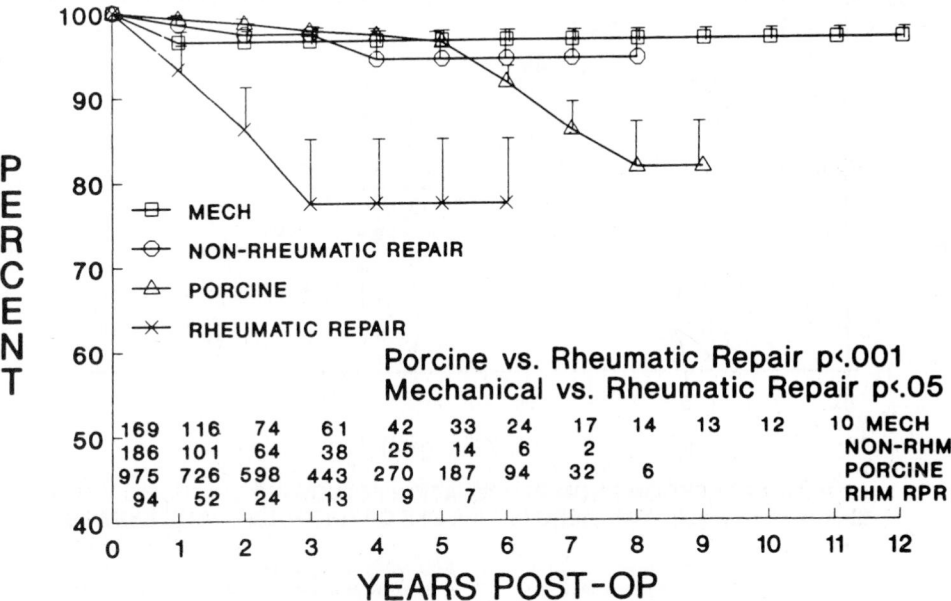

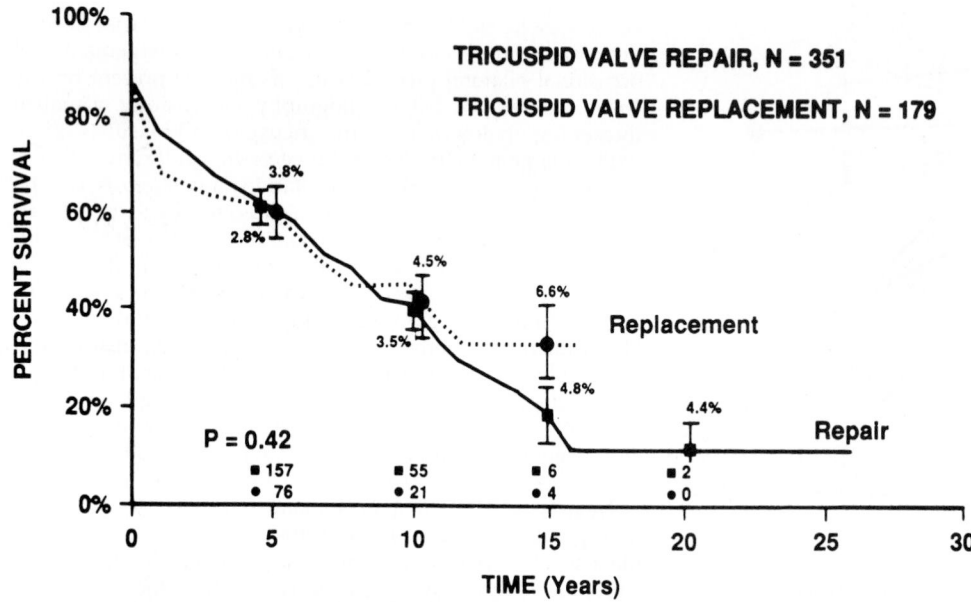

Figure 54–172. Actuarial survival after tricuspid valve replacement or repair. (From McGrath, L. B., Gonzalez-Lavin, L., Bailey, B. M., Grunkemeier, G. L., Fernandez, J., and Laub, G. W.: Tricuspid valve operations in 530 patients: Twenty-five-year assessment of early and late phase events. J. Thorac. Cardiovasc. Surg., *99*:124, 1990.)

erations are performed at the same time as operation on other cardiac valves. Survival 10 years after tricuspid valve repair or replacement is about 50% because of long-standing cardiac disease present in most patients.[16, 25] Long-term complications from tricuspid valve repair or replacement can include thrombosis of mechanical valves, heart block (2% for repair, 2%–5% for replacement), and endocarditis. Of patients undergoing tricuspid valvectomy for endocarditis and intravenous drug abuse, 11% will ultimately require tricuspid valve replacement for symptomatic tricuspid regurgitation.[1]

OPERATIVE TECHNIQUE

The mitral valve and the tricuspid valve are generally approached through a median sternotomy. Exposure of the tricuspid or mitral valve through a right anterolateral thoracotomy in the fourth or fifth intercostal space may be indicated to avoid mediastinal adhesions from a previous median sternotomy or to avoid patent coronary grafts when access to the aortic valve or coronary arteries is not required.[2] A right anterolateral thoracotomy is greatly facilitated by the

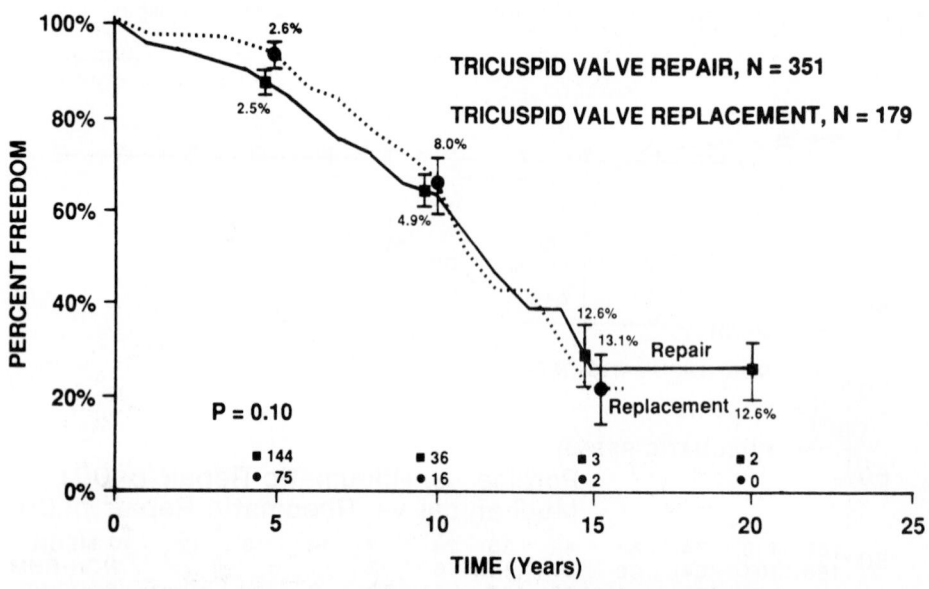

Figure 54–173. Actuarial freedom from reoperation after tricuspid valve replacement or repair. (From McGrath, L. B., Gonzalez-Lavin, L., Bailey, B. M., Grunkemeier, G. L., Fernandez, J., and Laub, G. W.: Tricuspid valve operations in 530 patients: Twenty-five-year assessment of early and late phase events. J. Thorac. Cardiovasc. Surg., *99*:124, 1990.)

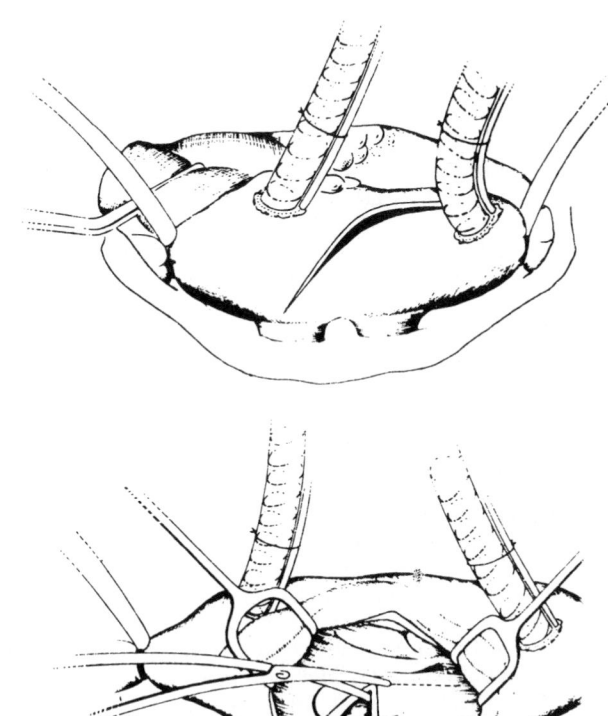

Figure 54–174. Transseptal approach to the mitral valve. *Top,* The right atrial incision extends from the right superior pulmonary vein to the medial inferior caval cannula. *Bottom,* The septal incision follows the dotted line from the right superior pulmonary vein toward the inferior cava. (From Deloche, A., Acar, C. Jebara, V, Fabiani, J. N., and Carpentier, A.: Biatrial transseptal approach in case of difficult exposure to the mitral valve. Reprinted with permission from the Society of Thoracic Surgeons [The Annals of Thoracic Surgery, 1990;50:318].)

use of the dual-lumen endotracheal tube, cannulation of the right femoral artery, and cannulation of the right femoral vein and the right atrium.

Open Mitral Commissurotomy. Open mitral commissurotomy is generally performed through a median sternotomy using cardiopulmonary bypass (CPB) with cannulation of the ascending aorta and the superior and inferior venae cavae. The heart may be arrested with cardioplegic solution, or the operation may be performed without clamping the aorta and utilizing hypothermic left ventricular fibrillation at 28° C. A mitral valve retractor (Carpentier or Cosgrove) may aid

exposure, as may use of additional adjuncts such as a transseptal approach to the mitral valve (Fig. 54–174), vena caval mobilization, and wide opening of the left pleural space. After the left atrium is opened, any left atrial thrombus is débrided, and the mitral valve is inspected for pathologic processes such as fusion of the commissures, leaflet thickening or calcification, and fibrosis or calcification of the subvalvular apparatus. The fused commissures are identified and opened sharply to within 2 to 3 mm. of the mitral valve anulus (Fig. 54–175). Small amounts of calcium may be débrided, and fused mitral valve chordae may occasionally

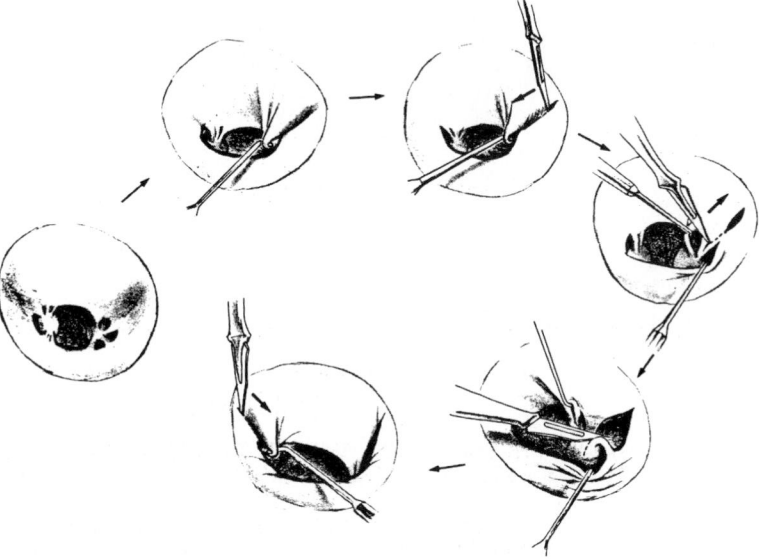

Figure 54–175. Operative technique of open mitral commissurotomy with leaflet retraction to demonstrate the commissural fold and sharp incision of the commissure to 3 to 4 mm. from the anulus. (From Carpentier, A.: Cardiac valve surgery—the "French Correction." J. Thorac. Cardiovasc. Surg., *86*:323, 1983.)

be mobilized. Significant mitral regurgitation or significant calcification and fibrosis of the leaflets or subvalvular apparatus should prompt consideration of mitral valve replacement. After testing the mitral valve for competence by injecting cold saline into the left ventricle, and after venting air from the left ventricle and atrium, the atriotomy is closed, and residual intracardiac air is aspirated from the ascending aorta. The aortic cross-clamp is released, the patient is rewarmed, and CPB is discontinued. Transesophageal echocardiography is useful in assessing mitral valve function after repair.

Mitral Valve Repair. Many techniques have been described for repairing regurgitant mitral valves. Many of the simpler and older techniques such as commissural anuloplasty have the advantage of requiring less operative time but providing a greater likelihood of recurrent anular dilation and mitral regurgitation. The most commonly practiced techniques of mitral valve repair today involve mitral anuloplasty with prosthetic material as originally described by Carpentier, Duran, and others.[5]

After achieving CPB with cannulation of the ascending aorta and superior and inferior venae cavae, the patient is cooled to 26° C. and ventricular fibrillation is induced. The mitral valve is carefully inspected through a left atriotomy for any prolapse of the leaflet edges, ruptured chordae, or restriction of leaflet motion. The aorta is then clamped, and the heart is arrested with cardioplegic solution. Placement of a cardioplegic catheter into the coronary sinus (Fig. 54–176) before CPB may facilitate repeated doses of cardioplegia without loss of mitral valve exposure during a long clamp

time. Prolapse of the posterior mitral valve leaflet is generally treated by quadrangular resection of the prolapsed segment (Fig. 54–177). Prolapse of the anterior leaflet may be treated by chordal or papillary muscle shortening (Fig. 54–178), insertion of artificial polytetrafluoroethylene chordae to the anterior mitral valve leaflet (Fig. 54–179), or transfer of chordae from a resected portion of the posterior leaflet.[33] The resected defect in the posterior leaflet is then closed either by anular plication or by a sliding leaflet plasty (see Fig. 54–177). In patients with papillary muscle rupture and an intact underlying ventricular wall, the papillary muscle head may occasionally be reattached with pledgeted sutures. Mitral valve replacement should be considered for papillary muscle rupture with extensive necrosis of the underlying myocardium. As a general rule, to prevent recurrent mitral regurgitation, all mitral valve repairs should employ an anuloplasty ring secured to the mitral valve anulus using interrupted 2-0 horizontal mattress sutures (see Fig. 54–177). The valve may now be inspected for competence by injecting cold saline into the left ventricle. When an adequate result is observed, the patient is rewarmed, the atriotomy is closed after evacuating air from the heart, the cross-clamp is removed, and the patient is removed from CPB. Transesophageal echocardiography is quite useful in assessing mitral valve abnormalities before CPB and in assessing the final result after CPB.

Mitral Valve Replacement. If mitral valve replacement is planned through a median sternotomy, CPB at 28° C. is initiated by cannulating the ascending aorta and the superior and inferior venae cavae. The ascending aorta is clamped,

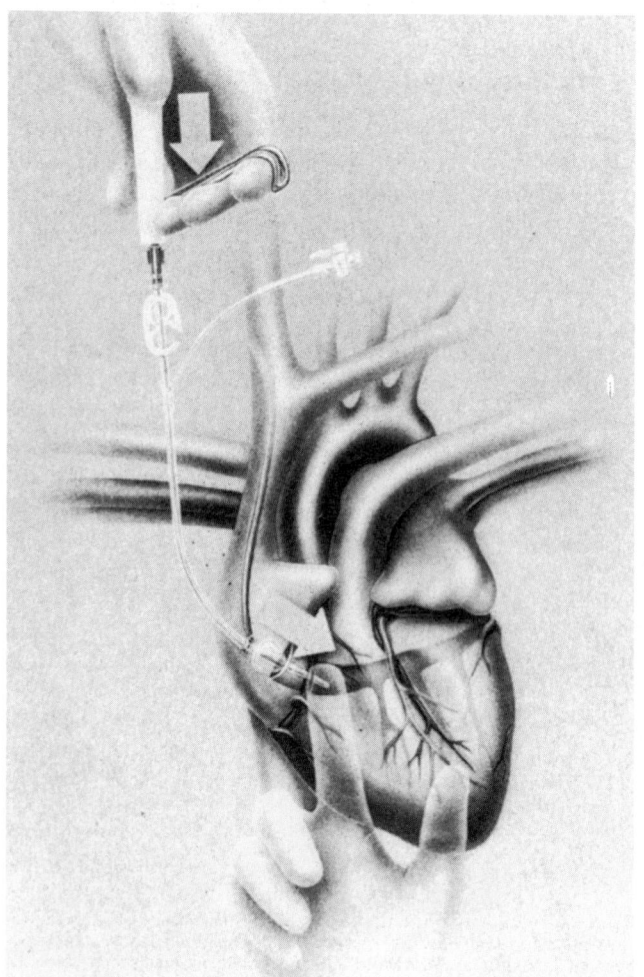

Figure 54–176. Technique of insertion of retrograde cardioplegia cannula through a small pursestring in the right atrium into the coronary sinus. One hand manipulates the catheter while the other hand palpates the catheter tip in the coronary sinus. (From Drinkwater, D. C., Laks, H., and Buckberg, G. D.: A new simplified method of optimizing cardioplegic delivery without right heart isolation. J. Thorac. Cardiovasc. Surg., *100*:56, 1990.)

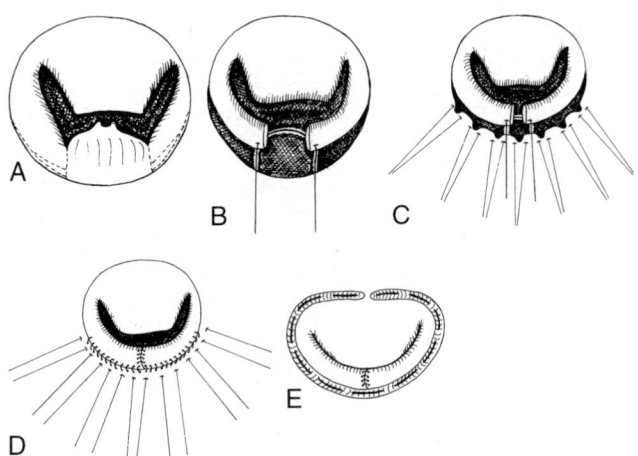

Figure 54–177. Quadrangular resection of the posterior leaflet with reconstruction using sliding plasty of the posterior leaflet. *A* and *B,* Quadrangular resection of posterior leaflet with mobilization of remaining posterior leaflet from anulus. *C* and *D,* Plication of posterior anulus and reconstruction of posterior leaflet. *E,* Reinforcement with anuloplasty ring. (From Perier, P., Clausnizer, B., and Mistarz, K.: Carpentier "sliding leaflet" technique for repair of the mitral valve: early results. Reprinted with permission from the Society of Thoracic Surgeons [The Annals of Thoracic Surgery, 1994;57:383].)

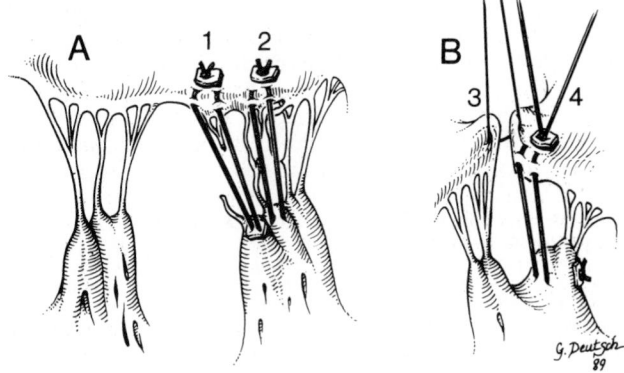

Figure 54–179. *A,* Use of PTFE suture to replace ruptured chordae (1) or elongated chordae unsuitable for shortening (2). Sutures are anchored in the papillary muscle with one or two autogenous pericardial pledgets, then sutures are passed through the free leaflet edge and tied on a pericardial pledget. *B,* Use of a temporary suture (3) to keep chordae taut while the chordae are tied (4). (Reproduced with permission from Frater, R. W. M., Vetter, H. O., Zussa, C., and Dahm, M.: Chordal replacement in mitral valve repair. Circulation, *82*:IV-125, 1990. Copyright 1990 American Heart Association.)

and the heart is arrested with cardioplegic solution. A retrograde coronary sinus cardioplegia catheter placed before cannulating the atrium can be quite useful to allow repeated cardioplegia administration without loss of mitral valve exposure. A left atriotomy is performed, and the mitral valve is inspected. Efforts should be made to preserve all mitral valve chordae that do not leave sufficiently bulky tissue to prevent placement of a functioning prosthesis. Preservation of chordal integrity during mitral valve replacement[9, 13] appears to improve postoperative left ventricular function (see Fig. 54–170) and diminish the incidence of postoperative ventricular-anular disruption.[10, 19, 29, 38] If both anterior and posterior leaflets along with their chordae do need resection, consideration may be given to placement of artificial polytetrafluoroethylene chordae from each of the papillary muscles to the mitral valve anulus (Fig. 54–180).[9] If the anterior leaflet can be preserved, the anterior leaflet may be detached

from the anterior anulus and secured intact to the posterior anulus, or may in fact be split in the middle and attached to the lateral aspects of the posterior anulus (Fig. 54–181). Failure to detach or debulk the anterior leaflet can result in left ventricular outflow tract obstruction.[37] Placement of 2-0 horizontal mattress sutures with supra-anular pledgets is done circumferentially about the anulus, taking care to fix preserved leaflet tissue securely to the anulus with the free ends of the sutures passing through the free edges of the preserved leaflets (see Fig. 54–181). Sutures are passed through the sewing ring of the prosthesis and then secured.

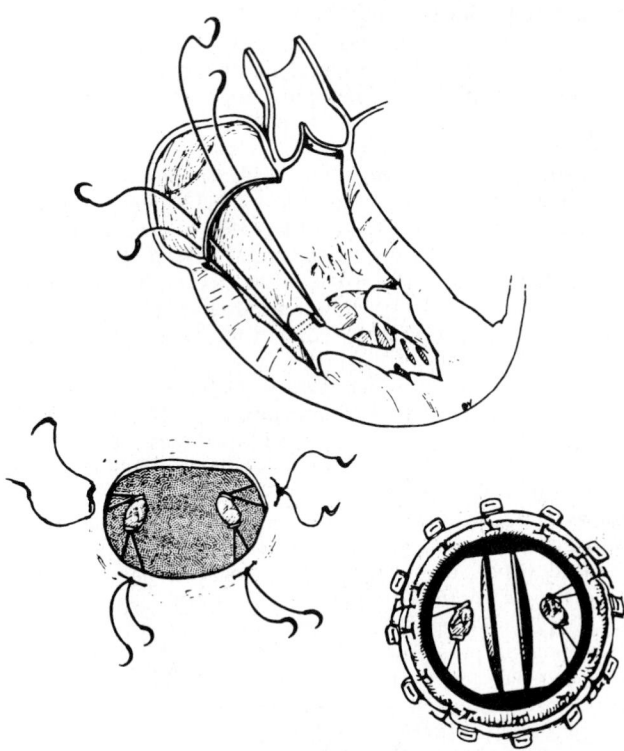

Figure 54–180. Replacement of the mitral valve maintaining papillary-anular continuity with 4-0 PTFE sutures anchored to the papillary muscles, then tied to the mitral valve anulus. (From David, T. E.: Papillary muscle-anular continuity: Is it important? J. Card. Surg., *9*(Suppl.):252, 1994.)

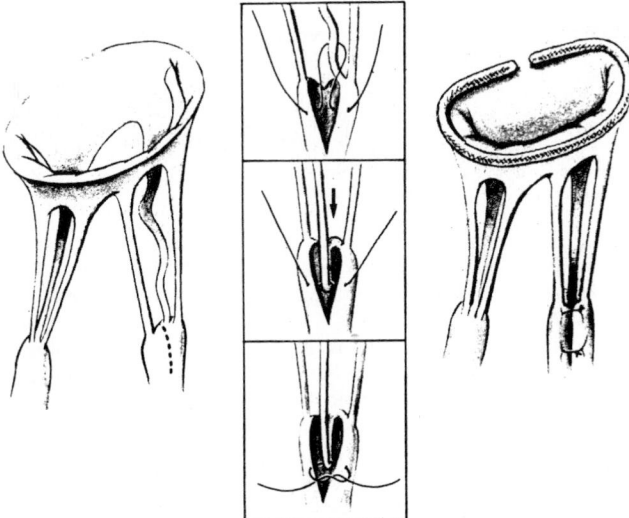

Figure 54–178. Repair of anterior leaflet prolapse due to chordal elongation by shortening plasty of the chordae followed by reinforcement with an anuloplasty ring. (From Carpentier, A.: Cardiac valve surgery—the "French Correction." J. Thorac. Cardiovasc. Surg., *86*:323, 1983.)

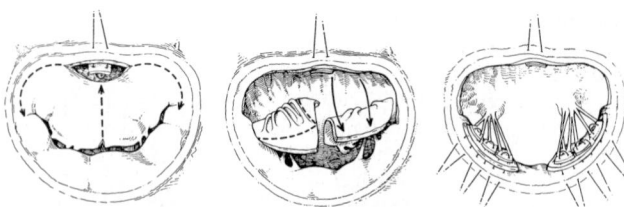

Figure 54–181. Replacement of the mitral valve with preservation of anterior and posterior leaflet chordae. The anterior leaflet is detached from the anulus *(left)*, débrided of excess leaflet tissue *(middle)*, then secured to the posterior anulus with subanular or supra-anular pledgeted sutures *(right)*. The posterior leaflet may be plicated by passing anular sutures through the free edge of the posterior leaflet. (From Feikes, H. L., Daugharthy, J. B., Perry, J. G., Bell, J. H., Hieb, R. E., and Johnson, G. H.: Preservation of all chordae tendineae and papillary muscle during mitral valve replacement with a tilting disc valve. J. Card. Surg., 5:81, 1990.)

The valve is inspected for unimpeded opening, a catheter is placed across the mitral valve to vent the left ventricle, the left atrium is closed after venting air from the heart, and the cross-clamp is removed with evacuation of remaining cardiac air from the ascending aorta.

Tricuspid Valve Repair or Replacement. The tricuspid valve may be approached through a median sternotomy with cannulation of the ascending aorta and cannulation of the inferior and superior venae cavae. Although tricuspid valve operation may be performed under cardioplegic arrest, tricuspid valve anuloplasty performed concurrently with other valvular procedures is often performed after removal of the aorta cross-clamp and during rewarming on CPB. The right atrium is opened, and the tricuspid valve is inspected. Tricuspid stenosis due to fused commissures may be treated by commissurotomy. Functional tricuspid regurgitation due to anular dilation may be repaired by tricuspid anuloplasty using one of several techniques, including placement of a rigid tricuspid ring, tricuspid leaflet bicuspidization, or a DeVega anuloplasty (Fig. 54–182). The DeVega procedure may be more rapid and less expensive than the rigid ring anuloplasty, but the DeVega anuloplasty may carry increased risk of recurrent tricuspid regurgitation, especially if preoperative tricuspid regurgitation or pulmonary hypertension is severe or of long standing.

For tricuspid valve replacement, obstructing leaflet tissue may be excised and remaining chords and leaflets preserved. First, 2-0 horizontal mattress sutures with supra-anular pledgets are placed into the valve anulus, except that sutures pass only through leaflet tissue in the area of the conduction system on the septal leaflet. Sutures are then passed through the valve sewing ring and tied, and the atriotomy is closed after evacuating air.

Valve Selection. Prosthetic devices for mitral and tricuspid valve replacement fall into the two general categories of biologic prostheses and mechanical prostheses (Fig. 54–183). Biologic prostheses have advantages of low rates of thromboembolism (1.0% to 2.0% per patient-year) and generally do not require anticoagulation.[12] Biologic valves have the disadvantage of lesser durability than mechanical prostheses. Mechanical valves require anticoagulation and have a higher incidence of thromboembolism (1.5% to 2.5% per patient-year with anticoagulation)[12] but have a greater durability than biologic prostheses. Choice of mechanical versus biologic prostheses should be based on the ability of the patient to comply with anticoagulation, likelihood of hemorrhagic complications, expected patient longevity, valve position, and match of the prosthesis to the valvular anulus.[21]

Most biologic prostheses available today are either glutaraldehyde-fixed porcine heterografts (Carpentier-Edwards, Hancock), glutaraldehyde-fixed bovine pericardium (Carpen-

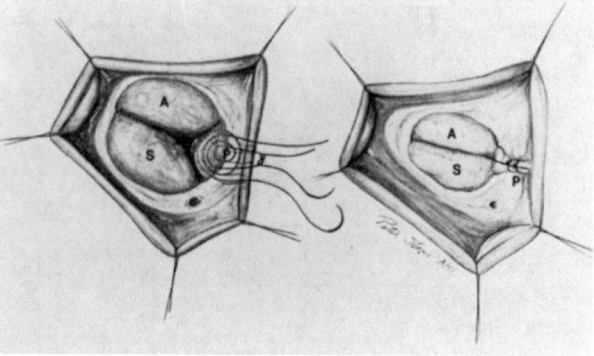

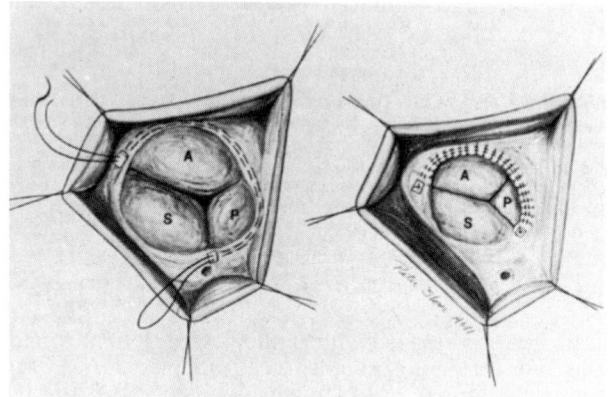

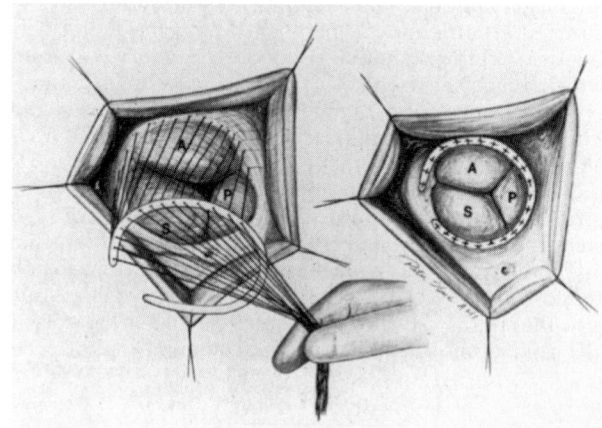

Figure 54–182. Tricuspid anuloplasty with valve bicuspidization and plication of the posterior leaflet *(top)*, DeVega anuloplasty with a 2-0 pledgeted polypropylene suture *(middle)*, or use of a Carpentier tricuspid anuloplasty ring *(bottom)*. (From Rackley, C. E., Wallace, R. B., Edwards, J. E., and Katz, N. M.: Tricuspid and pulmonary valve disease. *In* Schlant, R. C., and Alexander, R. W.: Hurst's The Heart, 8th ed. New York, McGraw-Hill, 1994; Reproduced with permission of McGraw-Hill, Inc.)

tier-Edwards pericardial), or occasionally stented heterograft tissue (see Fig. 54–183). Hemolysis and valve thrombosis are rare with biologic prostheses.[12] Pericardial valves for the mitral position are not available in the United States. Biologic valves in the mitral position have less durability than similar biologic valves in the aortic or tricuspid positions.[15] The durability of biologic valves is a continuous function of patient age, with older patients experiencing greater durability of biologic prostheses.[15] Although case reports of premature valve calcification have caused many to consider dialysis-dependent renal failure to contraindicate a biologic prosthesis, recent data suggest that biologic valves may avoid the troublesome hemorrhagic complications of mechanical valves in dialysis patients while providing a low incidence of pre-

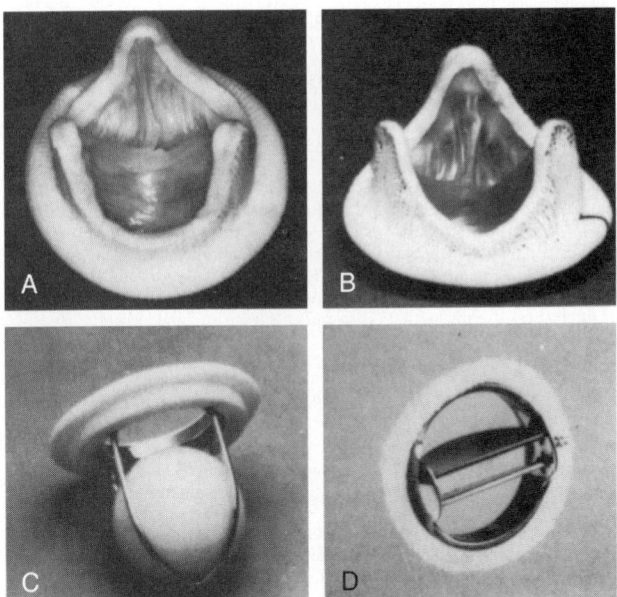

Figure 54–183. Commonly used prosthetic mitral valves. *A*, Hancock valve. (*A*, Reprinted with permission from Medtronic, Inc. © Medtronic, Inc., 1996.) *B*, Carpentier-Edwards valve. *C*, Starr-Edwards 6120 valve (*B* and *C*, Courtesy of Baxter Healthcare Corp., Irvine, CA). *D*, St. Jude Medical Valve. (*D*, Courtesy of St. Jude Medical, St. Paul, MN.)

mature calcification.[23] Patients receiving biologic and mechanical prostheses generally have a similar likelihood of developing endocarditis.

For patients with mechanical prostheses, the rate of anticoagulant-related hemorrhage has been reduced in recent years to 4% to 6% per patient-year using lower levels of anticoagulation with an international normalized ratio (INR) of 2.5 to 3.5, often in conjunction with low-dose aspirin.[30] Mechanical failure of currently available mechanical prostheses is quite rare. Causes of reoperation on mechanical valves include prosthetic endocarditis, valve thrombosis, and leaflet entrapment by surrounding tissues.

Because of the high incidence of thrombosis of mechanical prostheses in the tricuspid position, biologic prostheses are generally used for tricuspid valve replacement, but the St. Jude prosthesis may be considered in selected young patients.[16] Specific indications for biologic prostheses may include young women desiring pregnancy without the hemorrhagic or teratogenic risks of anticoagulation. In patients with limited life expectancy, such as patients older than 70 years of age undergoing isolated mitral valve replacement or older than age 65 years undergoing mitral valve replacement and coronary bypass grafting, biologic prostheses should be considered if the patient is in normal sinus rhythm.[21] Because without anticoagulation atrial fibrillation increases the risk of thromboembolism for mitral bioprostheses,[12] chronic atrial fibrillation is a relative indication for placement of a mechanical prosthesis. Procedures are being developed to potentially convert atrial fibrillation to a sinus or paced rhythm in selected patients undergoing mitral valve repair,[8] but the relative risks of atrial fibrillation versus operation to correct atrial fibrillation remain unclear. Patients undergoing operation on multiple valves generally should receive mechanical prostheses due to the increased likelihood of one of several biologic valves failing and requiring reoperation.

POSTOPERATIVE CARE

All patients receiving mechanical prostheses in the mitral or tricuspid positions should be maintained on chronic war-

farin anticoagulation with an INR of 2.5 to 3.5.[30] Consideration should be given to use of low-dose aspirin in addition to warfarin. Patients in normal sinus rhythm undergoing mitral valve repair or replacement with a biologic prosthesis may adequately be managed with postoperative aspirin alone without even short-term anticoagulation, unless other risk factors for thromboembolism are present.[3] Patients in atrial fibrillation undergoing mitral valve repair or mitral valve replacement with a biologic prosthesis should probably receive anticoagulation for the first 6 to 9 weeks, if not indefinitely, as long as they remain in atrial fibrillation and do not have contraindications to anticoagulation. The mortality rate associated with chronic warfarin therapy is 0.5% to 1.3% per patient-year.[12] Roughly 5% of patients undergoing mitral valve repair may develop systolic anterior motion of the mitral valve with dynamic left ventricular outflow obstruction. This problem generally resolves after 6 to 8 weeks but may require beta blockade and hydration in the early postoperative period.[17]

SELECTED REFERENCES

Carpentier, A.: Cardiac valve surgery—the "French Correction." J. Thorac. Cardiovasc. Surg., 86:323, 1983.
This paper remains the most authoritative work regarding techniques for mitral valve repair and the anatomic basis for mitral valve dysfunction. Many lucid illustrations of operative technique are provided.

Cobanoglu, A., and Ott, G. Y.: Tricuspid valve surgery: Indications, methods, and results. Cardiovasc. Clin., 23:265, 1993.
The authors provide a concise review of the diagnosis and treatment of tricuspid valve disease. The techniques of tricuspid valve repair and replacement are presented along with clinical results.

Jamieson, W. R. E.: Modern cardiac valve devices—bioprostheses and mechanical prostheses: State of the art. J. Card. Surg., 8:89, 1993.
A current overview is provided of the many valvular prostheses available along with the relative indications for choosing mechanical versus biologic prostheses.

Yun, K. L., and Miller, D. C.: Mitral valve repair versus replacement. Cardiol. Clin., 9:315, 1991.
This paper thoroughly reviews clinical and experimental evidence comparing mitral valve repair to mitral valve replacement in terms of the effects on left ventricular function and the clinical outcomes of survival and reoperation.

REFERENCES

1. Arbulu, A., Holmes, R. J., and Asfaw, I.: Tricuspid valvulectomy without replacement: Twenty years' experience. J. Thorac. Cardiovasc. Surg., 102:917, 1991.
2. Balasundarum, S. G., and Duran, C.: Surgical approaches to the mitral valve. J. Card. Surg., 5:163, 1990.
3. Blair, K. L., Hatton, A. C., White, W. D., et al.: Comparison of anticoagulation regimens after Carpentier-Edwards aortic or mitral valve replacement. Circulation, 90(Suppl. II):214, 1994.
4. Carabello, B. A., Williams, H., Gash, A. K., et al.: Hemodynamic predictors of outcome in patients undergoing valve replacement. Circulation, 74:1309, 1986.
5. Carpentier, A.: Cardiac valve surgery—the "French Correction." J. Thorac. Cardiovasc. Surg., 86:323, 1983.
6. Castro, L. J., Moon, M. R., Rayhill, S. C., et al.: Annuloplasty with flexible or rigid ring does not alter left ventricular systolic performance, energetics, or left ventricular-arterial coupling in conscious dogs. J. Thorac. Cardiovasc. Surg., 105:643, 1993.
7. Cohen, J. M., Glower, D. D., Harrison, J. K., et al.: Comparison of balloon valvuloplasty with operative treatment for mitral stenosis. Ann. Thorac. Surg., 56:1254, 1993.
8. Cox, J. L.: The surgical treatment of atrial fibrillation. J. Thorac. Cardiovasc. Surg., 101:584, 1991.
9. David, T. E.: Papillary muscle-annular continuity: Is it important? J. Card. Surg., 9(Suppl.):252, 1994.
10. David, T. E., Bos, J., and Rakowski, H.: Mitral valve repair by replacement of chordae tendineae with polytetrafluoroethylene sutures. J. Thorac. Cardiovasc. Surg., 101:495, 1991.
11. Deloche, A., Jebara, V. A., Relland, J. Y. M., et al.: Valve repair with Carpentier techniques. J. Thorac. Cardiovasc. Surg., 99:990, 1990.
12. Edmunds, L. H., Jr.: Thrombotic and bleeding complications of prosthetic heart valves. Ann. Thorac. Surg., 44:430, 1987.
13. Feikes, H. L., Daugharthy, J. B., Perry, J. E., Bell, J. H., Hieb, R. E., and Johnson, G. H.: Preservation of all chordae tendinae and papillary muscle

during mitral valve replacement with a tilting disc valve. J. Card. Surg., 5:81, 1990.

14. Galloway, A. C., Colvin, S. B., Baumann, F. G., et al.: A comparison of mitral valve reconstruction with mitral valve replacement: Intermediate-term results. Ann. Thorac. Surg., 47:655, 1989.

15. Glower, D. D., White, W. D., Hatton, A. C., et al.: Determinants of reoperation after 960 valve replacements with Carpentier-Edwards prostheses. J. Thorac. Cardiovasc. Surg., 107:381, 1994.

16. Glower, D. D., White, W. D., Smith, L. R., et al.: In-hospital and long-term outcome after porcine tricuspid valve replacement. J. Thorac. Cardiovasc. Surg. 109:877, 1995.

17. Grossi, E. A., Galloway, A. C., Parish, M. A., et al.: Experience with 28 cases of systolic anterior motion after Carpentier mitral valve reconstruction. J. Thorac. Cardiovasc. Surg., 103:466, 1992.

18. Harpole, D. H., Jr., Rankin, J. S., Wolfe, W. G., et al.: Effects of standard mitral valve replacement on left ventricular function. Ann. Thorac. Surg., 49:866, 1990.

19. Horskotte, D., Schulte, H. D., Bircks, W., and Strauer, B. E.: The effect of chordal preservation on late outcome after mitral valve replacement: A randomized study. J. Heart Valve. Dis., 2:148, 1993.

20. Ibrahim, M., O'Kane, H., Cleland, J., Gladstone, D., Sarsam, M., and Patterson, C.: The St. Jude Medical prosthesis: A thirteen year experience. J. Thorac. Cardiovasc. Surg., 108:221, 1994.

21. Jamieson, W. R. E.: Modern cardiac valve devices—bioprostheses and mechanical prostheses: state of the art. J. Card. Surg., 8:89, 1993.

22. Louagie, Y., Noirhomme, P., Aranguis, E., et al.: Use of the Carpentier-Edwards porcine bioprosthesis: Assessment of a patient selection policy. J. Thorac. Cardiovasc. Surg., 104:1013, 1992.

23. Lucke, J. C., Samy, R. N., Atkins, B. Z., et al.: Results of valve replacement with mechanical versus biological prostheses in patients on chronic renal dialysis. J. Am. Coll. Cardiol. Suppl.:429A, 1995.

24. MacArthur, K. J., Bain, W. H., Turner, M. A., et al.: Mechanical versus biological heart valves: A ten-year comparison in a single centre. Eur. J. Cardiothorac. Surg., 2:143, 1988.

25. McGrath, L. B., Gonzales-Levin, L., Bailey, B. M., Grunkemeier, G. L., Fernandez, J., and Laub, G. W.: Tricuspid valve operations in 530 patients: Twenty-five-year assessment of early and late phase results. J. Thorac. Cardiovasc. Surg., 99:124, 1990.

26. National Heart, Lung and Blood Institute Balloon Valvuloplasty Registry: Complications and mortality of percutaneous balloon mitral commissurotomy. Circulation, 85:2014, 1992.

27. Palacios, I. F., Block, P. C., Wilkins, G. T., and Weyman, A. E.: Follow-up of patients undergoing mitral balloon valvotomy: Analysis of factors determining restenosis. Circulation, 79:573, 1989.

28. Rowe, J. C., Bland, E. F., Sprague, H. B., and White, P. D.: The course of mitral stenosis without surgery: Ten- and twenty-year perspectives. Ann. Intern. Med., 52:741, 1960.

29. Rozich, J. D., Carabello, B. A., Usher, B. W., Kratz, J. M., Bell, A. E., and Zile, M. R.: Mitral valve replacement with and without chordal preservation in patients with chronic mitral regurgitation: Mechanisms for differences in postoperative ejection performance. Circulation, 86:1718, 1992.

30. Saour, J. N., Sieck, J. O., Mamo, L. A. R., and Gallus, A. S.: Trial of different intensities of anticoagulation in patients with prosthetic heart valves. N. Engl. J. Med., 322:428, 1990.

31. Scalia, D., Rizzoli, G., Campanile, F., et al.: Long-term results of mitral commissurotomy. J. Thorac. Cardiovasc. Surg., 105:633, 1993.

32. Selzer, A., and Cohn, K. E.: Natural history of mitral stenosis: A review. Circulation, 45:878, 1972.

33. Sousa Uva, M., Grare, P., Jebara, V., et al.: Transposition of chordae in mitral valve repair: Mid-term results. Circulation, 88(Suppl. II):35, 1993.

34. Stewart, W. J.: Choosing the "golden moment" for mitral valve repair. J. Am. Coll. Cardiol., 24:1544, 1994.

35. Taylor, D. E. M., Wade, J. D., and Hider, C. F.: Experimental study of mitral valve incompetence and mitral valve lesions following papillary muscle inactivation in the dog. Cardiovasc. Res., 4:319, 1970.

36. Tischler, M. D., Cooper, K. A., Rowen, M., and LeWinter, M. M.: Mitral valve replacement versus mitral valve repair: A Doppler and quantitative stress echocardiographic study. Circulation, 89:132, 1994.

37. Waggoner, A. D., Perez, J. E., Barzilai, B., Rosenbloom, M., Eaton, M. H., and Cox, J. L.: Left ventricular outflow obstruction resulting from insertion of mitral prostheses leaving the native leaflets intact: Adverse clinical outcome in seven patients. Am. Heart J., 122:483, 1991.

38. Yun, K. L., Rayhill, S. C., Niczyporuk, M. A., et al.: Mitral valve replacement in dilated canine hearts with chronic mitral regurgitation: Importance of the mitral subvalvular apparatus. Circulation, 84:III-112, 1991.

XIX

SURGICAL TREATMENT OF CARDIAC ARRHYTHMIAS

James L. Cox, M.D.

The knowledge gained from surgery to correct cardiac arrhythmias during the past quarter-century has contributed in large part to the endocardial catheter techniques that are now used to cure most refractory arrhythmias.[1, 2] The contemporary therapy for cardiac arrhythmias, including antiarrhythmic drugs, catheter ablation, and surgery, is capable of curing essentially all supraventricular and ventricular tachyarrhythmias. When these therapeutic interventions fail, or when surgery is contraindicated, antitachycardia pacemaker-cardioverter-defibrillators may provide substantial benefit. Although the indications for surgical intervention have narrowed during the past 5 years, surgery remains an important therapeutic modality for the treatment of cardiac arrhythmias, especially for the most common of all arrhythmias, atrial fibrillation.

ATRIAL FIBRILLATION

Atrial fibrillation is present in 0.4% to 2.0% of the general population[3–7] and in approximately 10% of the population older than the age of 60 years,[8–11] making it the most common of all sustained cardiac arrhythmias. Although atrial fibrillation is frequently considered to be an innocuous arrhythmia, it is associated with significant morbidity and mortality because of its three detrimental sequelae: (1) an irregular heartbeat, which causes patient discomfort and anxiety; (2) loss of synchronous atrioventricular (AV) contraction, which compromises cardiac hemodynamics resulting in varying levels of congestive heart failure; and (3) stasis of blood flow in the left atrium, which increases the vulnerability to thromboembolism.

Historical Aspects. Until recently, elective His bundle ablation, either by open-heart surgery or by endocardial catheter techniques, was the only effective means of treating atrial fibrillation nonpharmacologically. However, because these procedures do not actually ablate atrial fibrillation, they control only the ventricular rate and rhythm during atrial fibrillation. Unfortunately, His bundle ablation does not protect the patient from the other detrimental effects of atrial fibrillation (i.e., loss of the atrial *kick* and the increased vulnerability to thromboembolism). Despite that fact, the most common indication for endocardial catheter ablation of the His bundle is atrial fibrillation.[12]

The left atrial isolation procedure was first introduced experimentally in 1980[13] and clinically in 1982.[14] This procedure is capable of confining atrial fibrillation associated with mitral valve disease to the left atrium, but because the left atrium continues to fibrillate postoperatively, it was elected not to apply it routinely to control the detrimental effects of atrial fibrillation clinically. In 1985, Guiraudon introduced the *corridor procedure,* in which a strip of atrial septum between the sinoatrial (SA) node and AV node was isolated from the remainder of the atrial myocardium in patients with atrial fibrillation.[15] Although this procedure has now been performed in several patients, it unfortunately alleviates only the rapid, irregular ventricular response to atrial fibrillation, but it does not restore AV synchrony, nor does it reduce the vulnerability of patients with atrial fibrillation to the development of thromboembolic problems.[16]

In 1991, the author and colleagues described the first surgical procedure designed specifically to cure atrial fibrillation, the so-called maze procedure.[17-20] The maze procedure is now considered to be the surgical treatment of choice for medically refractory atrial fibrillation.[21-29]

Anatomic-Electrophysiologic Basis. Three theories have been proposed to explain the mechanism of atrial activation during atrial fibrillation: (1) a single automatic ectopic focus in the atrium, firing at an extremely rapid rate; (2) multiple automatic foci in the atria, firing independently throughout the atria; and (3) intra-atrial re-entry in which multiple re-entrant wavelets are present in the atria. This last multiple wavelet theory was originally proposed by Moe[30] and was subsequently verified by the studies of Boineau and colleagues[31, 32] and Allessie and associates.[33] Those authors demonstrated that atrial geometry, local refractory distribution, and the resultant local conduction velocity of the atrial tissues determined whether re-entry occurred, how many wavelets formed, and whether the process was sustained. During the past few years, we have employed epicardial template electrodes on the atria, both experimentally[34, 35] and clinically.[36, 37] The results of our studies documented complete re-entrant loops in some instances and partial loops in others and demonstrated that the re-entrant wavefronts could move through the septum around the pulmonary veins, inferior vena cava, or superior vena cava. The more complex patterns in which complete re-entrant loops were not documented were consistent with the multiple wavelet hypothesis of Moe[30] and the experimental data of Allessie and associates.[33] Although anatomic obstacles, such as the pulmonary veins, inferior vena cava, and superior vena cava, were frequently involved in the re-entrant loops, complete re-entrant circuits were frequently recorded in the absence of these anatomic obstacles. These re-entrant loops rotated around areas of functional conduction block, the most common site being along the sulcus terminalis. Our studies confirmed that as atrial size increases, the number of wavefronts during atrial fibrillation and the duration of atrial fibrillation increase. As the cycle lengths decrease and become more variable, various regions of the atria are completely dissociated from one another. The importance of these experimental and clinical studies lies in the fact that they have documented unequivocally that atrial flutter and atrial fibrillation are due to intra-atrial re-entry as first suggested by Moe and that the concept of multifocal automaticity is not operative in the genesis or perpetuation of atrial fibrillation in man.

Surgical Indications and Contraindications. The major indication for surgery is intolerance of the arrhythmia. Major symptoms in the group with paroxysmal (intermittent) atrial fibrillation include dyspnea on exertion, easy fatigability, lethargy, malaise, and a general sense of impending doom during the periods of atrial flutter/fibrillation. Patients with chronic (continuous) atrial fibrillation are usually better adapted to the sensation of an irregular heartbeat, but the majority complain of exercise limitations, dyspnea on exertion, and easy fatigability. In addition, they frequently express concern over the possibility of having a stroke.

All patients who are considered for surgery must have failed the maximum amount of tolerable drug therapy preoperatively. In addition, approximately one fourth of the pa-

tients in the series had experienced at least one episode of cerebral thromboembolism that resulted in significant temporary or permanent neurologic deficit. Documented cerebral thromboembolism in a patient with paroxysmal or chronic atrial fibrillation, in the absence of other demonstrable etiologies, is considered an absolute indication for surgery, because anticoagulation does not protect such patients from a *second* stroke.[38-40] Despite that fact, it should be emphasized that the *threat* of thromboembolism should not be considered to be an indication for surgery in patients who have not previously experienced a transient ischemic attack or frank stroke due to atrial fibrillation. The author and colleagues have pursued this policy because the *incidence* of stroke as a result of atrial fibrillation in an individual patient with no history of transient ischemic attack and no associated anomalies is considered to be less than the risk of the operation.

Contraindications to the maze procedure include the presence of significant left ventricular dysfunction, not attributable to the arrhythmia itself, and concomitant cardiac or noncardiac disease that constitutes an excessive surgical risk.

Preoperative Electrophysiology Evaluation. A preoperative endocardial catheter electrophysiology study is routinely performed in all patients with atrial flutter and in patients with *paroxysmal* atrial fibrillation. The primary purpose of the preoperative study is to document the function of the SA node, particularly in patients with atrial fibrillation, and to determine both SA node function and the site of the re-entrant circuit in patients with atrial flutter. Preoperative electrophysiology studies are not performed in patients with *chronic* atrial fibrillation since the SA node cannot be evaluated without electrical cardioversion, which would introduce too great a risk of thromboembolism.

Surgical Technique. The original maze-I procedure (Fig. 54–184)[17-20] was modified to the maze-II procedure (Fig. 54–185)[27] in an effort to improve long-term sinus node chronotropic function and to decrease postoperative interatrial conduction time, which caused apparent left atrial dysfunction in a substantial number of patients. Although the maze-II procedure represented an improvement,[41] it was an unusually difficult procedure to perform technically. As a result, it was further modified to the maze-III procedure (Fig. 54–186),[27, 41, 42] which is now considered to be the surgical technique of choice for the treatment of medically refractory atrial flutter and atrial fibrillation.

Surgical Results. Between September 25, 1987, and June 25, 1994, 32 patients had the maze-I procedure, 15 had the maze-II procedure, and 76 had the maze-III procedure for the treatment of atrial flutter and/or atrial fibrillation. Approximately 45% of all patients experienced perioperative atrial fibrillation within the first 3 months after the operation. These early postoperative arrhythmias invariably disappeared, and they had no correlation with long-term results of the operation. Once the atrium healed from surgery (3 months), the recurrent arrhythmia rate has been less than 10% overall and 0% in patients having the maze-III procedure. Thus, 90% of patients were cured of atrial fibrillation by the operation alone and 9% of patients were cured with a combination of operation and postoperative medicine, an overall postoperative cure rate of 99%. In the patients who had the maze-III procedure, 75% returned to a normal sinus rhythm postoperatively and 25% required a permanent atrial pacemaker for sick sinus syndrome. The maze procedure itself resulted in injury of the sinus node in only two patients in the author and his colleagues' entire series.

Twenty-five percent of patients experienced a thromboembolic episode before the surgical procedure. However, there has been only one transient ischemic attack in any patient postoperatively and there have been no strokes related to the surgical procedure, recurrent atrial fibrillation, or anticoagu-

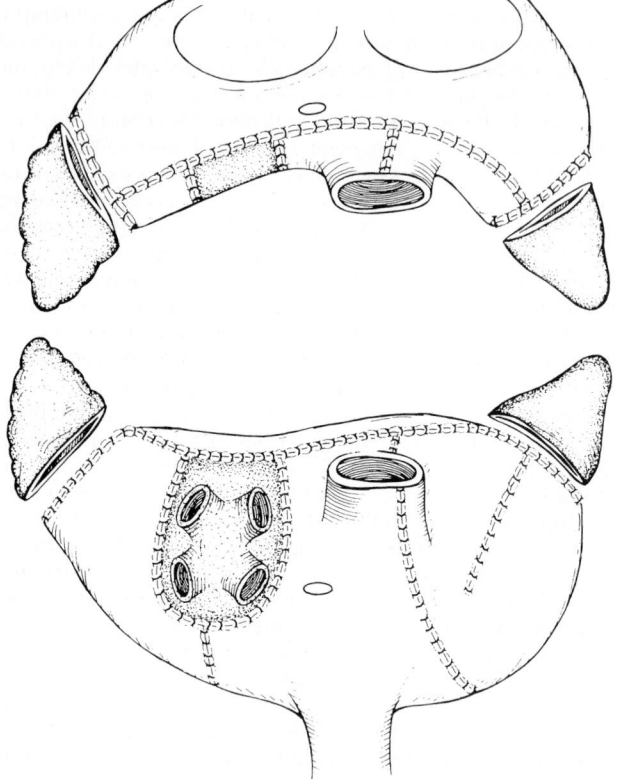

ity. Because these patients also have a normal bundle of His that connects the atria to the ventricles electrically, they have two routes by which an electrical impulse may travel between the atria and ventricles. For tachycardia to occur, antegrade (from the atrium to the ventricle) conduction across the accessory pathway must first be blocked. When antegrade block occurs in the accessory pathway with the patient in normal sinus rhythm, the sinus impulse still activates the atria normally. The electrical activity propagates through the AV node–His bundle complex normally and activates the ventricles normally. However, when the electrical activity reaches the AV groove at the base of the heart it encounters a bundle of muscle, the accessory pathway, that has not yet been depolarized. As a result, the electrical activity simply propagates across the accessory pathway retrogradely (from the ventricle to the atrium) and quickly reactivates the atria. The atrial activation wavefront then passes normally through the AV node–His bundle complex again and reactivates the ventricle. In this manner, a macro-re-entrant circuit is established around which electrical activity can propagate as fast as 4 times per second or 240 times a minute.

Historical Aspects. Gaskell was the first to demonstrate that electrical activity propagated from the atrium to the ventricle through myocardial tissue rather than nerves, with his studies on the turtle heart being reported in 1883.[43] Kent identified muscular connections between the atria and ventricles of mammals in 1893 but erroneously concluded that these connections were multiple and that they represented

Figure 54–184. Original maze procedure: This is a schematic depiction of the atria viewed from posteriorly (below) with the corresponding anterior portion of the atria flipped up and depicted above. Both the right and left atrial appendages are excised. The pulmonary veins are completely encircled and, therefore, do not participate in either the electrical or mechanical activity of the atrium postoperatively. Note the short incision just anterior to the junction of the superior vena cava and right atrium. This short incision passes directly through the "sinus tachycardia" area of the right atrium. Also note that there is a transverse incision extending from the base of the excised right atrial appendage to the base of the excised left atrial appendage. This "dome" incision interfered with conduction of sinus impulses from the right atrium to the left atrium. (From Cox, J. L.: Evolving applications of the maze procedure for atrial fibrillation [Invited Editorial]. Ann. Thorac. Surg., 55:578, 1993. Reprinted with permission from the Society of Thoracic Surgeons.)

lation. Indeed, the patients are not anticoagulated postoperatively except under unusual circumstances.

Finally, all patients were documented to have both right atrial and left atrial transport function in the immediate postoperative period that contributed to forward cardiac output. On late follow-up evaluation, all patients have continued to have right atrial transport function and 74 of 76 patients with the maze-III procedure have had documented left atrial function as well.

WOLFF-PARKINSON-WHITE SYNDROME

Anatomic-Electrophysiologic Basis. The introduction of endocardial catheter techniques utilizing radiofrequency energy has had its most dramatic impact on the treatment of supraventricular arrhythmias due to the Wolff-Parkinson-White (WPW) syndrome.[1] Nevertheless, occasional patients still present for surgery, thus requiring cardiac surgeons to maintain an understanding of the anatomy, physiology, and surgical techniques related to this abnormality.

The WPW syndrome is characterized by the presence of an abnormal muscular connection between the atrium and ventricle ("accessory atrioventricular connection" or "accessory pathway") that is capable of conducting electrical activ-

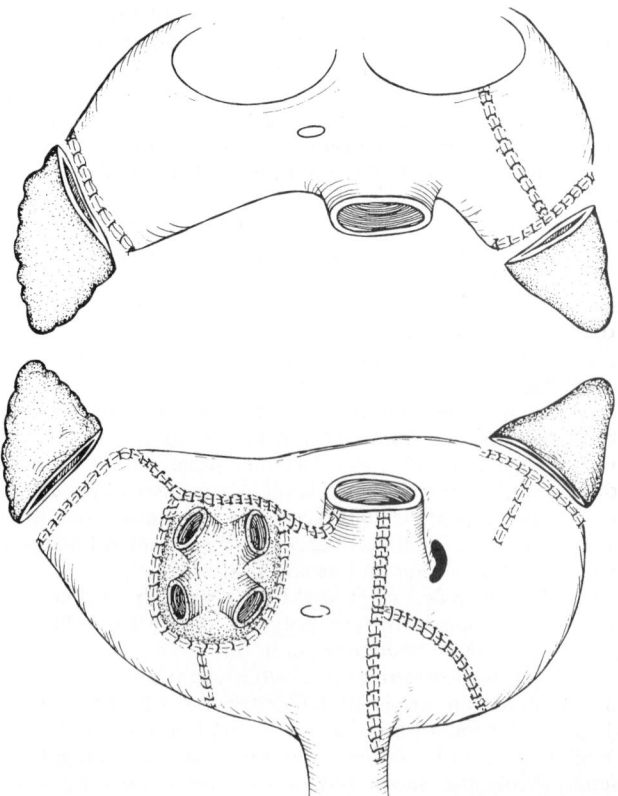

Figure 54–185. First modification of the maze procedure (maze-II). Same view as in Figure 54–184. Note that the "dome" incision has been moved more posteriorly and now intersects with the superior vena cava on its left side rather than anteriorly. The short incision that previously passed through the sinus tachycardia area has been deleted entirely. To prevent re-entry around the base of the right atrium, an anterior incision from the base of the excised atrial appendage to the anterior tricuspid valve has been added. (From Cox, J. L.: Evolving applications of the maze procedure for atrial fibrillation [Invited Editorial]. Ann. Thorac. Surg., 55:578, 1993. Reprinted with permission from the Society of Thoracic Surgeons.)

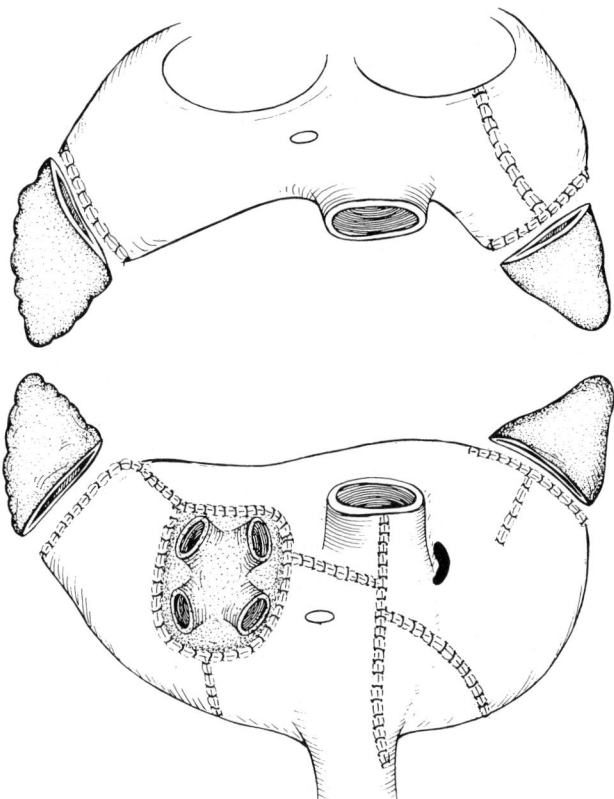

Figure 54–186. Second modification of the maze procedure (maze-III). The right end of the "dome incision" has now been moved posterior to the superior vena cava. This made the maze-III procedure much easier to perform technically than either the maze-I or maze-II procedure. In addition, it moves the "dome" incision even farther posteriorly, thereby interfering even less with the conduction of impulses from the sinus node to the left atrium. (From Cox, J. L.: Evolving applications of the maze procedure for atrial fibrillation [Invited Editorial]. Ann. Thorac. Surg., 55:578, 1993. Reprinted with permission from the Society of Thoracic Surgeons.)

the normal pathways of AV conduction.[44] Despite this misconception, his name serves as the eponym for the accessory AV connections responsible for the WPW syndrome (Kent bundles).

Perhaps the most important work delineating the specialized conduction system of the heart was reported in 1906 when Tawara, working in Aschoff's laboratory in Germany, identified and characterized the AV node, His bundle, bundle branches, and the Purkinje system.[45] In the same year, Keith and Flack identified the sinoatrial node as the heart's normal pacemaker.[46]

During the 1920s, Paul Dudley White, one of the great teachers and clinical cardiologists of this century, noted that a small group of young, apparently normal patients with ventricular pre-excitation on their standard electrocardiograms (ECGs) had frequent bouts of paroxysmal tachycardia. During a trip to London, he discovered that John Parkinson, an English physician, had collected a similar series of patients. White suggested that Louis Wolff, one of White's fellows, combine their series of patients and report their observations, which Wolff did in 1930.[47] Neither the ventricular pre-excitation nor the bouts of tachycardia were explained, however, until Wolferth and Wood reported a patient with the same clinical syndrome in 1933 and suggested that the ECG abnormalities were due to accessory pathways between the atrium and ventricle similar to those previously described by Kent. Although they accepted Kent's erroneous hypothesis that these accessory pathways were normal and

occurred on the right free wall, Wolferth and Wood directed their attention to that region in a patient with the syndrome who died and, fortuitously, they were able to document an accessory pathway histologically at autopsy, which they reported in 1943.[48]

Although the basis for the WPW syndrome was suspected, the issue remained controversial for many years. The picture became somewhat clearer in 1967, however, when Dirk Durrer of Amsterdam, the generally acknowledged father of modern clinical electrophysiology, performed intraoperative mapping in a patient with the WPW syndrome and demonstrated electrical conduction across the AV groove in the region of ventricular pre-excitation.[49] In the same year Howard Burchell of the Mayo Clinic performed intraoperative mapping in a patient with the WPW syndrome who was undergoing surgery for closure of an atrial septal defect. After identifying the suspected site of the accessory pathway on the right free wall, Burchell was able to abolish ventricular pre-excitation by injecting procainamide into the AV groove at that site.[50] Although the pre-excitation returned postoperatively, this procedure demonstrated for the first time that a surgical technique might be capable of permanently interrupting conduction across an accessory pathway, thereby curing the WPW syndrome. The first surgical attempt at permanent ablation followed several months later on May 28, 1968, when Will Sealy of Duke University successfully divided a right free-wall accessory pathway in a 31-year-old man.[51]

Indications for Surgery. The major contemporary indication for surgical intervention in the WPW syndrome is failure of radiofrequency catheter ablation (RFCA). Between 1980 and 1991, when RFCA became the procedure of choice for the treatment of the WPW syndrome, approximately 500 patients underwent surgery for the WPW syndrome on the author's service. The dramatic change from surgical therapy to catheter ablative therapy can be appreciated by noting that during the past 45 months, the author and his colleagues have operated on only 15 patients for the WPW syndrome, all of whom had failed multiple attempts at RFCA of the accessory pathway(s). Nevertheless, these patients represent a relatively large group in terms of patients who have undergone surgery only after failed RFCA and they are instructive in terms of what surgeons can expect in the future.

Only a third of these patients were completely free of some type of associated anomaly capable of making RFCA either more difficult or totally impossible to accomplish successfully. The other patients had various anatomic abnormalities or variations in normal anatomy, including an anomalous coronary sinus, Ebstein's anomaly, cardiac hypertrophy, mitral regurgitation, coronary artery disease, catheter perforation of the right ventricle, or a small heart due to age.

At the time of the operation, several patients had severe scarring in the dissection planes of the AV groove, making surgical dissection both difficult and hazardous. The patients who had Ebstein's anomaly frequently demonstrated a heavy muscle layer encompassing the coronary sinus that extended directly down to the posterior ventricular septum as a thick (6–8 mm.) band of muscle fibers, representing the accessory pathway. It would have been technically impossible in these patients to ablate the accessory pathway with current RFCA technology.

This surgical experience with failed RFCA suggests that if one cannot ablate an accessory pathway in a reasonable period of time, it is highly probable that some type of anatomic abnormality exists that precludes one from doing so. Thus, electrophysiologists should exercise common sense in knowing when to terminate their attempts at RFCA, since too much local radiofrequency trauma and injury can render a patient surgically incurable.

Preoperative Electrophysiologic Evaluation. Patients who are now subjected to surgery for the WPW syndrome have first undergone an endocardial catheter electrophysiologic study in association with their failed attempt at RFCA. The most important information for the surgeon to know before surgery is the location of the accessory pathway, the technique and number of ablative attempts employed by the electrophysiologist during the attempted RFCA, and the associated (if any) anatomic abnormalities to be encountered during surgery.

Intraoperative Electrophysiologic Mapping. Computerized mapping systems have obviated the need to use cardiopulmonary bypass for the intraoperative mapping of patients with the WPW syndrome.[52] Epicardial pacing and sensing electrodes are sutured onto the atrium and ventricle near the suspected site of the accessory pathway. A band electrode is placed around the ventricular side of the AV groove, and electrograms are recorded during normal sinus rhythm and during atrial pacing.[53] The electrogram recorded from the electrode located nearest the site of the ventricular insertion of the accessory pathway shows the earliest activation. The band electrode is then moved to the atrial side of the AV groove, and reciprocating tachycardia is induced with programmed electrical stimulation. Atrial electrograms are recorded from the bipolar electrodes on the band. This display of the atrial data is especially important because it demonstrates unsuspected concealed accessory pathways that had gone undetected until this point in the mapping procedure. When reciprocating tachycardia cannot be induced, the retrograde atrial map is performed during ventricular pacing.

These antegrade and retrograde computerized mapping techniques are capable of detecting not only free-wall pathways but also anterior and posterior septal accessory pathways. However, if either is detected during the computerized mapping procedure, the patient is placed on cardiopulmo-nary bypass, a right atriotomy is performed, and endocardial mapping of the right atrium and atrial septum is completed using a hand-held single-point mapping system before proceeding with surgical dissection.

Surgical Techniques and Results. Accessory AV connections may be located anywhere around the anulus fibrosis of the heart except between the right and left fibrous trigones (Fig. 54–187). However, from a surgical standpoint, their locations are classified, in decreasing order of frequency, as left free-wall, posterior septal, right free-wall, and anterior septal.[52] Twenty percent of the patients in the author's series have had multiple (two, three, or four) accessory pathways.

Two surgical approaches are commonly employed to divide accessory AV connections (Fig. 54–188). The endocardial technique is designed to divide the ventricular end of the accessory pathway, and the epicardial technique is directed toward division of the atrial end of the pathway. The results with both approaches are excellent with virtual assurance of surgical cure of the abnormality.[52, 54–56]

PAROXYSMAL SUPRAVENTRICULAR TACHYCARDIA

Paroxysmal supraventricular tachycardia (PSVT) is a contemporary term for what has previously been called paroxysmal atrial tachycardia. PSVT is a clinical condition in which supraventricular tachycardia occurs suddenly in a patient who otherwise has a normal ECG. There are two abnormalities that account for essentially all PSVT: (1) a concealed accessory AV connection and (2) AV node re-entry.

Concealed Accessory Pathway. Accessory AV connections may be *manifest* or *concealed*. If an accessory pathway is capable of conducting in the antegrade (atrial-to-ventricular) direction, thereby causing a delta wave on the standard ECG,

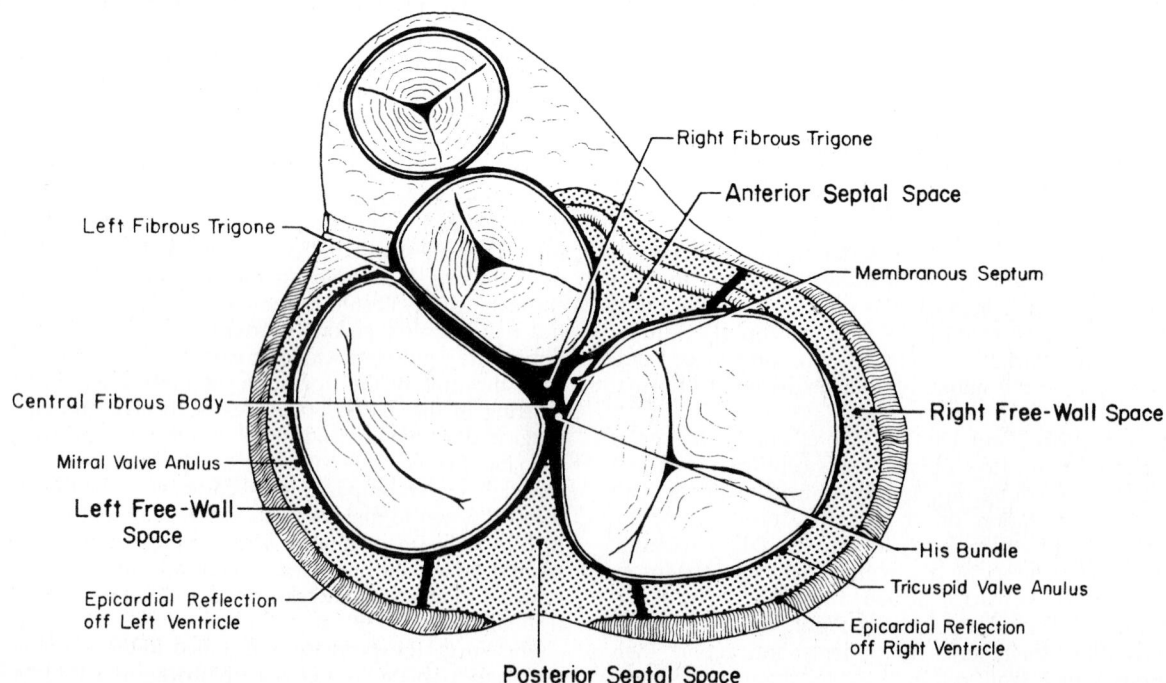

Figure 54–187. Diagram of the superior view of the heart with the atria cut away demonstrating the boundaries of each of the four anatomic areas where accessory pathways can occur in the Wolff-Parkinson-White syndrome. The boundaries of the *left free-wall space* are the mitral valve anulus and the ventricular epicardial reflection extending from the left fibrous trigone to the posterior septum. The boundaries of the *posterior septal space* are the tricuspid valve anulus, the mitral valve anulus, the posterior-superior process of the left ventricle, and the ventricular epicardial reflection. The boundaries of the *right free-wall space* are the tricuspid valve anulus and the epicardial reflection extending from the posterior septum to the anterior septum. The boundaries of the *anterior septal space* are the tricuspid valve anulus, the membranous portion of the interatrial septum, and the ventricular epicardial reflection. All accessory atrioventricular connections must insert into the ventricle somewhere within these anatomic boundaries. (From Cox, J. L., Gallagher, J. J., and Cain, M. E.: Experience with 118 consecutive patients undergoing surgery for the Wolff-Parkinson-White syndrome. J. Thorac. Cardiovasc. Surg., *90*:490, 1985.)

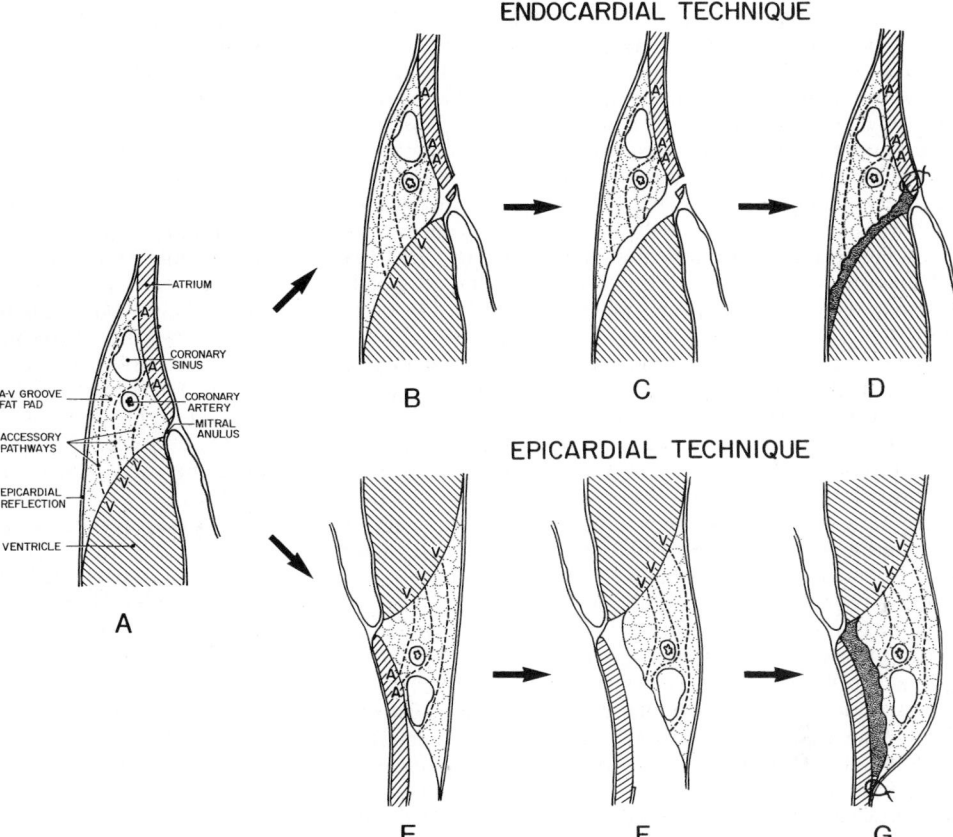

Figure 54–188. Diagrammatic representation of a cross-section of the posterior left side of the heart showing the different depths at which left free-wall pathways can be located in relation to the mitral anulus and epicardial reflection (*A*). The endocardial surgical technique is depicted in *B* to *D* and the epicardial technique in *E* to *G*. See text for further discussion.

it is said to be manifest, that is, its presence is apparent electrocardiographically. The retrograde (ventricular-to-atrial) conduction characteristics of such a pathway determine the heart rate and frequency of occurrence of the associated reciprocating tachycardia. Some patients harbor accessory AV connections that are capable of conducting in the retrograde direction only. Because antegrade conduction across the accessory pathway does not occur, the ventricles are activated only through the normal AV node–His bundle complex and the standard ECG is normal. Therefore, such accessory pathways are said to be concealed. Because these accessory pathways are capable of conducting in the retrograde direction, however, reciprocating tachycardia can occur just as it does in the classic WPW syndrome. Thus, from a clinical standpoint, the only difference between patients with manifest accessory pathways and those with concealed accessory pathways is the appearance of the standard ECG during normal sinus rhythm. The former have ECGs characteristic of the WPW syndrome, and the latter have normal ECGs.

In patients with a concealed accessory pathway, the absence of antegrade conduction across the pathway precludes the necessity of performing antegrade ventricular mapping intraoperatively. Thus, only retrograde atrial mapping is performed, and these maps are recorded during ventricular pacing or during induced reciprocating tachycardia. The surgical technique employed to divide concealed accessory pathways is the same as for patients with the classic WPW syndrome.

AV NODE RE-ENTRY TACHYCARDIA

Historical Aspects. In 1926, Scherf and Shookhoff first observed reciprocating beats of AV nodal re-entry,[57] but it was not until 30 years later that Moe first characterized discontinuous AV node conduction over *fast* and *slow* pathways and associated this finding with reciprocating (echo) beats in response to premature stimulation.[58] In 1971, Goldreyer and Damato first inferred that AV node re-entry tachycardia was due to a re-entrant mechanism involving the AV node.[59] The role of AV node re-entry as a mechanism for PSVT in humans was subsequently confirmed by Bigger and Goldreyer[60, 61] and Denes.[62] Subsequent studies showed this to be the most common mechanism for PSVT in humans.[63–66]

During the 1970s, a few patients with medically refractory AV node re-entry tachycardia underwent surgical interruption of the His bundle, either by surgical dissection or by the application of cryolesions directly to the AV node–His bundle complex.[67] The objective of elective His bundle ablation was to protect the ventricles from the AV node re-entry. However, because the surgical block was created below the level of the AV node, AV node re-entry could persist at the atrial level. Thus, elective His bundle ablation represented perhaps the first surgical isolation procedure designed to control the detrimental effects of a medically refractory cardiac arrhythmia without actually ablating the arrhythmia. Because the procedure resulted in complete heart block, however, a permanent ventricular pacemaker was required postoperatively in all patients.

In 1982, Scheinman described a technique for ablating the His bundle by introducing an electrical shock through a catheter placed adjacent to the His bundle.[68] This closed-chest procedure immediately replaced the open-heart surgical method for interrupting the His bundle for obvious reasons. However, since the catheter fulguration technique of Scheinman also created complete heart block, all of these patients also required permanent pacemaker systems.

Although both the surgical technique and the catheter ablative technique for His bundle interruption ameliorated the unpleasant and detrimental effects of AV node re-entry tachycardia, both procedures replaced one type of arrhythmia (tachycardia) with another (heart block). No specific attempt at curing AV node re-entry tachycardia was made until a fortuitous occurrence in 1979.[69] During attempted surgical division of the His bundle in a patient with incessant AV node re-entry tachycardia, the tachycardia suddenly terminated but the patient maintained normal AV conduction. After observation of the patient for some time, the surgical procedure was terminated with the patient having normal AV conduction, and the patient subsequently remained free of tachycardia. This stimulated evaluation of the possibility of attaining this fortuitous result on a reproducible basis. After several years of animal experimentation using a discrete perinodal cryosurgical technique,[70-72] the first clinical cure of AV node re-entry tachycardia was attained with this cryosurgical technique (Fig. 54–189) on August 13, 1982.[14] Ross and colleagues[73] and Guiraudon and associates[74] subsequently reported the cure of AV node re-entry tachycardia using surgical dissection of the perinodal tissues.

Anatomic-Electrophysiologic Basis. AV node re-entry tachycardia is caused by a re-entrant circuit that is confined to the AV node or to the perinodal tissues of the lower atrial septum. The anatomic-electrophysiologic basis for this re-entrant circuit is the presence of two functional conduction pathways, one slow and one fast, through the AV node, the so-called dual AV node conduction pathways. The fast AV nodal pathway manifests rapid conduction but relatively long refractoriness. The slow AV nodal pathway manifests slow conduction but relatively short refractoriness. Although the complete dimensions of the re-entrant circuit have not been elucidated, the micro-re-entrant circuit is confined to the region of the AV node. During supraventricular tachycardia, antegrade conduction proceeds through the slow pathway and retrograde conduction proceeds through the fast pathway, owing to proximal antegrade block in the fast pathway.

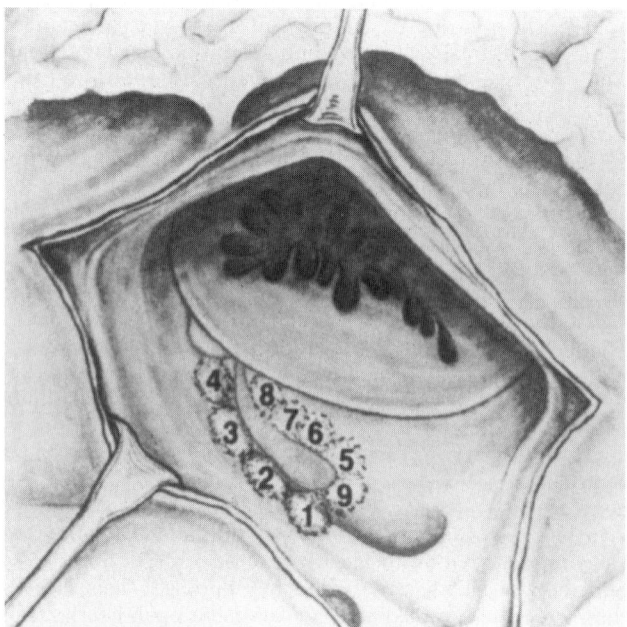

Figure 54–189. Discrete cryosurgical procedure for the treatment of AV node re-entry tachycardia. Multiple cryolesions are placed around the periphery of the AV node beginning along the tendon of Tadaro. During application of these cryolesions, the AV conduction time is continuously monitored on a beat-to-beat basis. See text for further discussion. (Reported with permission from Cox, J. L., Holman, W. L., and Cain, M. E.: Cryosurgical treatment of atrioventricular node reentry tachycardia. *Circulation, 76*:1329, 1987. Copyright 1987, American Heart Association.)

This results in nearly simultaneous activation of the ventricles and atria.

Surgical Indications and Contraindications. The surgical techniques designed to cure AV node re-entry tachycardia enjoyed excellent results. There were no operative deaths in any of the three major series reported. After the perinodal cryosurgical procedure, smooth AV node conduction curves through the remaining single conduction pathway were demonstrated in all patients in our series and none of the patients had inducible AV node re-entry tachycardia postoperatively.[75] Moreover, all patients maintained normal conduction through the AV node–His bundle complex with no recurrent AV node re-entry tachycardia. The surgical dissection techniques were associated with a low incidence of permanent complete heart block and a low incidence of recurrent AV node re-entry tachycardia.[73, 76] Presently, however, RFCA techniques have replaced surgery as the procedure of choice for AV node re-entry tachycardia.[1, 2]

AUTOMATIC ATRIAL TACHYCARDIAS

Historical Aspects. Automatic atrial tachycardias were first described by Sir Thomas Lewis in 1909.[77] In 1973, Goldreyer and colleagues reported the first electrophysiologic demonstration of automatic atrial tachycardia in man.[78] Because of the frequent suppression of the automatic atrial tachycardias by general anesthesia intraoperatively and the inability to induce the arrhythmias by pacing techniques, the most frequent surgical approach applied in the 1970s was His bundle ablation and insertion of a permanent pacemaker system.[67] However, because many of these tachycardias originate in the body of the left atrium, the concept of surgically isolating only the left atrium (Fig. 54–190) was introduced, leaving the remainder of the heart in normal sinus rhythm.[79] Because the sinus node, AV node, His bundle, and bundle branches are all located in the right atrium, atrial septum, or ventricular septum, surgical isolation of the left atrium does not interfere with the normal cardiac conduction system. Therefore, no pacemaker system is necessary postoperatively. The left atrial isolation procedure was first performed clinically for automatic left atrial tachycardia in 1982.[14] Currently, excision procedures, cryoablative procedures, and isolation procedures can be employed for automatic atrial tachycardias arising in the right or left atrium with excellent results.

Anatomic-Electrophysiologic Basis. Automatic atrial tachycardia is caused by an automatic focus of arrhythmogenic tissue lying outside the region of the normal anatomic SA node. Histologic examination of the atrial tissue excised at the site of origin of automatic atrial tachycardias has not revealed a specific finding common to all patients. In Lowe's excellent review of the world literature on this subject,[80] it was noted that a variety of pathologic findings have been identified. Monocytic infiltrates, focal myocyte hypertrophy, islets of fatty tissue, fibrous tissue foci, proliferation of abnormal cells, and small atrial wall aneurysms have been documented in the excised atrial myocardium responsible for the automatic atrial tachycardias.

Surgical Indications and Contraindications. Automatic atrial tachycardias frequently occur in pediatric patients in whom the tachycardia may be asymptomatic or may present as vomiting and epigastric pain. Adult patients more commonly present with palpitations, presyncope, syncope, or symptoms of congestive heart failure. One of the most common manifestations of automatic atrial tachycardia is cardiomegaly and congestive heart failure, with the overall incidence being 54% to 63%.[81-84] Damiano and coworkers demonstrated experimentally that chronic atrial tachycardia may lead to significant left ventricular enlargement and dysfunction and that restoration of normal rhythm after termina-

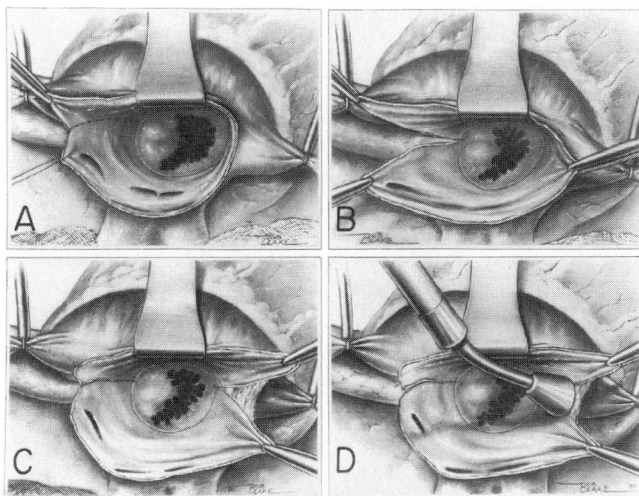

Figure 54–190. Left atrial isolation procedure. *A*, After a standard left atriotomy incision, the interatrial septum is retracted gently and the atriotomy is extended anteriorly (dashed line) across Bachmann's bundle to the level of the mitral valve anulus just to the left of the right fibrous trigone. *B*, The anterior extension of the standard left atriotomy has been completed. The base of the aorta and its juxtaposition with the anterior leaflet of the mitral valve are demonstrated. Note that the anterior atriotomy extends across the mitral valve anulus. The main body of the left atrium has been separated anteriorly from the remainder of the heart. *C*, The transmural left atriotomy is extended posteriorly to the level of the coronary sinus. The remaining portion of the incision is made through the endocardium and extends across the mitral valve anulus posteriorly just to the left of the interatrial septum. At this point, electrical activity continues to be propagated in a 1:1 fashion between the right and left atria because of the presence of interatrial muscular connections accompanying the coronary sinus. *D*, A cryoprobe is positioned over the endocardial aspect of the posterior atriotomy, and its temperature is decreased to −60° C. for 2 minutes. This cryolesion ablates the endocardial interatrial fibers accompanying the coronary sinus. A similar cryolesion is created on the epicardial aspect of the AV groove on the opposite side of the coronary sinus to ablate all remaining interatrial epicardial connections. The left atriotomy is closed with a continuous 4-0 nonabsorbable suture. (From Williams, J. M., Ungerleider, R. M., Lofland, G. K., and Cox, J. L.: Left atrial isolation: New technique for treatment of supraventricular arrhythmias. J. Thorac. Cardiovasc. Surg., *80*:373, 1980.)

tion of the atrial tachycardia results in restoration of normal ventricular function.[85] Thus, the indications for surgical intervention in patients with automatic atrial tachycardias include medical refractoriness, intolerable side effects of antiarrhythmic drugs, poor patient compliance, patient preference to medical therapy, tachycardia-induced ventricular dysfunction, and congestive heart failure.

Preoperative Electrophysiologic Evaluation. In patients with automatic atrial tachycardia, the standard ECG demonstrates a P-wave morphologic pattern that is different from that seen in sinus rhythm, suggesting the presence of an ectopic focus remote from the sinus node. Preoperative endocardial catheter electrophysiologic studies typically fail to initiate or terminate the tachycardia by programmed electrical stimulation techniques. However, either premature atrial extrastimuli or direct-current countershock usually will reset, rather than terminate, the tachycardia.[86] Rapid atrial pacing may result in overdrive suppression of the underlying automatic atrial tachycardia, being manifested by a pause after termination of pacing or slowing of the automatic atrial tachycardia, which then accelerates to its previous rate.

Lowe noted that of the 125 patients with automatic atrial tachycardia reported to date, the location of the automatic focus was specified in 89 patients.[80] Sixty-one (68%) were located in the right atrial free wall, 5 (6%) within the atrial septum, and the remaining 23 (26%) within the left atrium.

Intraoperative Mapping. If only a single-point, hand-held mapping system is available, it may be virtually impossible to identify the site of origin of an automatic atrial tachycardia

intraoperatively because of the vulnerability of the tachycardia to suppression by general anesthesia.[87] However, the introduction of computerized multipoint mapping systems has alleviated this problem, because only one beat of an automatic tachycardia is necessary to localize its site of origin using such mapping systems. The author employs three epicardial electrode templates containing a total of 156 bipolar electrode pairs. These templates, fashioned of silicone rubber, are designed to conform to the epicardial surfaces of the atria. The templates are attached to the epicardial surfaces of the atria by sutures placed at their periphery to avoid interference with data acquisition. As mentioned, once these electrode templates have been positioned on the atria, only a single beat of the automatic tachycardia is necessary to localize its site of origin.

Surgical Technique. If the site of origin of an automatic atrial tachycardia can be localized precisely by intraoperative mapping, the arrhythmogenic focus may be either excised or cryoablated. Automatic foci located in the free wall of the left atrium or in either of the atrial appendages are ideal for excision or cryoablation. Automatic atrial tachycardias arising near the orifices of the pulmonary veins are best treated either by pulmonary vein isolation or by left atrial isolation.

Theoretically, if intraoperative mapping properly localizes automatic foci in the free wall of the body of the right atrium, those foci can be either excised or cryoablated. However, automatic right atrial tachycardias are frequently multifocal, and the ablation or excision of one automatic focus may be followed by the appearance of another at some later date. Thus, the recurrence rate after local excision or cryoablation of automatic right atrial tachycardias is unacceptably high, and, as a result, the author prefers to perform a right atrial isolation procedure, even though the site of origin of the tachycardia may be well defined by intraoperative computerized mapping. The right atrial isolation procedure has now been performed in six patients, with uniform success and no recurrences during an 8-year follow-up period.

Surgical Results. Lowe reported that electrophysiologically guided operative procedures have been performed in 63 of the 125 patients available for review.[80] Fifty-six (89%) have been completely cured without the need for permanent pacemaker implantation or postoperative antiarrhythmic therapy. One perioperative death occurred in a patient with severe congestive heart failure and dilated cardiomyopathy who had cardiac arrest during the induction of anesthesia.

IDIOPATHIC VENTRICULAR TACHYCARDIA

An arrhythmia may occur in patients in whom the only clinical manifestation of cardiac disease is the ventricular arrhythmia. Both the macroscopic appearance of the heart at operation and the pathologic data acquired at the time of autopsy in such patients fail to show any evidence of primary cardiac disease. The only abnormality noted has been global dilatation of the heart secondary to functional post-tachycardia heart failure. If these patients require surgery, they first undergo intraoperative electrophysiologic mapping during ventricular tachycardia in an effort to localize the apparent site of origin of the arrhythmia. Initial surgical approaches included simple ventriculotomy, exclusion procedures, and cryoablation, but the results were poor, primarily because many of these arrhythmias arise within the ventricular septum. More recent approaches have included local isolation procedures if the site of origin is in the right ventricular free wall and multipoint map-guided cryoablation if it is in the septum.[89]

NONISCHEMIC CARDIOMYOPATHY

A small group of patients have been shown to have ventricular tachycardia due to cardiomyopathy unassociated with ischemic heart disease. This group comprises patients with angiographic and catheter data indicating some type of abnormal myocardial contractility associated with recurrent ventricular tachycardia. These patients usually show a diffuse dilatation of both ventricles with widespread patchy myocardial fibrosis. These tachyarrhythmias frequently arise in the right ventricle, and the author's approach to such patients has been to employ a combination of surgical isolation and cryoablation of the apparent site of origin of the arrhythmia.

ARRHYTHMOGENIC RIGHT VENTRICULAR DYSPLASIA

Fontaine and associates described a previously unrecognized form of cardiomyopathy localized to the right ventricle that they termed *arrhythmogenic right ventricular dysplasia*.[88] This syndrome is a congenital cardiomyopathy characterized by transmural infiltration of adipose tissue resulting in weakness and aneurysmal bulging of the infundibulum, apex, and/or posterior basilar region of the right ventricle. The syndrome is characterized clinically by intractable ventricular tachycardia originating from one or all of the three pathologic areas of the right ventricle. Because the origin of the tachycardia is in the right ventricle, the standard electrocardiogram shows a pattern consistent with left bundle branch block during the tachycardia. Right ventricular angiography should be performed in all patients who exhibit ventricular tachycardia with a left bundle branch block pattern. In patients with arrhythmogenic right ventricular dysplasia, the right ventricle appears enlarged; ventricular bulges or frank aneurysms are seen in the infundibulum, the apex, and/or the basal portion of the inferior wall; and right ventricular contractility is usually markedly decreased. Hypertrophic muscular bands in the infundibulum and anterior right ventricular wall result in apparent pseudodiverticula, the so-called feathering appearance of the right ventricular outflow tract. The author's approach to such patients employs a transmural encircling ventriculotomy that effectively isolates the arrhythmogenic myocardium from the remainder of the heart (Fig. 54–191).[89]

Although Fontaine's original description of arrhythmogenic right ventricular dysplasia suggested that the cardiomyopathy was confined to three discrete areas of the right ventricle, intraoperative mapping of these patients has suggested that the entire right ventricular free wall may be arrhythmogenic in certain cases. In the author's experience, there may be as many as seven different sites of origin of tachycardia in these patients, each site giving rise to a different morphologic type of ventricular tachycardia. Computerized intraoperative mapping systems are able to localize these tachycardias only if each of them can be induced at the time of surgery, an unrealistic expectation. As a result of these problems, the author has had to resort to surgical isolation of the entire right ventricular free wall on occasion to relieve the life-threatening sequelae of arrhythmogenic dysplasia (Fig. 54–192).[14] Although the follow-up of these patients documents excellent control of their tachycardia, the right ventricle may undergo progressive dilatation postoperatively. Nevertheless, the patients in whom this procedure has been performed have remained in excellent functional status for over 13 years.

UHL'S SYNDROME

Uhl's syndrome is a rare congenital cardiomyopathy that, from the anatomic point of view, may be considered to be a more complete form of arrhythmogenic right ventricular dysplasia. The right ventricle is extremely dilated, but the

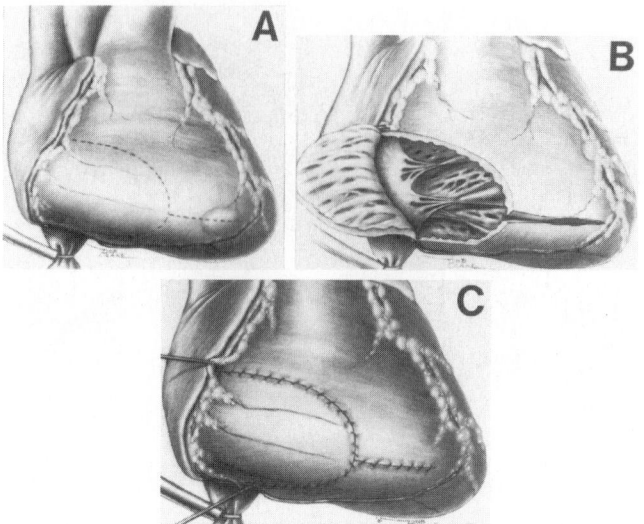

Figure 54–191. *A,* Appearance of the right ventricle in a patient with arrhythmogenic right ventricular dysplasia. Note the three coronary arteries coursing from the AV groove across the surface of the right ventricle. The acute margin of the right ventricle corresponded to the location of the middle coronary artery shown in this drawing. An area approximately 2 × 3 cm. near the upper coronary artery was electrically silent. Epicardial mapping during ventricular tachycardia showed the earliest site of activation to be located near the lower edge of this electrically silent region just below the midsegment of the middle coronary region on the posterior basilar region of the right ventricle. A transmural ventriculotomy was placed around the electrically silent area and included the apparent site of origin of the ventricular tachycardia on the posterior basilar region of the heart (broken line). The two ends of this incision were based at the AV groove, where cryolesions were applied to ensure isolation of the arrhythmogenic region of myocardium from the remainder of the heart. In addition, a second transmural incision was made from the apex of the semicircular incision to the apex of the right ventricle to include the small saccular aneurysm in that region. *B,* The isolated pedicle of right ventricular myocardium containing the electrically silent area and the apparent site of origin of the ventricular tachycardia has been reflected to show the internal anatomy of the right ventricle. Note the extension of the incision to the right ventricular apex to open the small aneurysm located in that region. *C,* The transmural encircling ventriculotomy around the arrhythmogenic region of the right ventricle and the simple ventriculotomy through the right ventricular apical aneurysm have been closed with a continuous 3-0 nonabsorbable suture. After completion of this procedure for arrhythmogenic right ventricular dysplasia, the isolated pedicle was paced at a rapid rate, but the paced impulses were not conducted to the remainder of the heart. In addition, the remainder of the right ventricle was then paced rapidly, but those paced impulses were not conducted into the isolated pedicle, confirming total isolation of the arrhythmogenic right ventricular myocardium from the remainder of the heart. (From Cox, J. L.: Surgery for cardiac arrhythmias. Curr. Prob. Cardiol., 8[4]:7, 1983.)

tricuspid valve remains in a normal position, thus differentiating it from Ebstein's anomaly. The main characteristic of Uhl's syndrome is the complete absence of myocardium in the right ventricular free wall, resulting in the endocardial and epicardial layers being in direct contact without interposition of myocardial fibers. Since Uhl's description of this cardiomyopathy in 1952,[90] the descriptive term *parchment heart* has been applied to the abnormality. Although Uhl's syndrome usually leads to rapid cardiac failure in the first month or years of life, an adult form of this condition occurs in which associated ventricular tachycardia is the dominant feature.

LONG QT SYNDROME

In 1957, Jervell and Lange-Nielsen described a clinical entity consisting of a long QT interval, congenital deafness, and syncopal attacks due to ventricular fibrillation occurring after emotional or physical stresses.[91] The absence of congenital deafness characterizes the otherwise identical Romano-Ward syndrome.[92, 93] Ventricular tachycardia that occurs in associa-

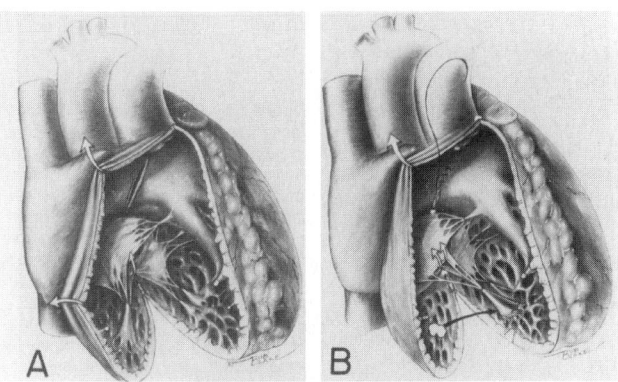

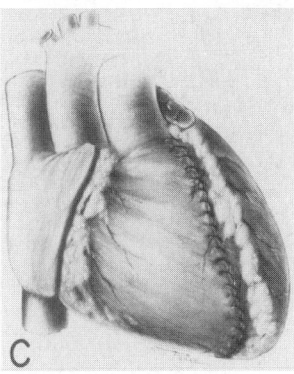

Figure 54–192. Right ventricular disconnection procedure. *A,* A transmural right ventriculotomy is placed parallel to and 5 mm. from the interventricular septum extending from just across the pulmonic valve anulus anteriorly to the tricuspid valve posteriorly. It is necessary to divide several large infundibular muscular bundles and to divide the moderator band of the right ventricle. Although the entire incision is transmural, special care must be taken to avoid injury to the right coronary artery lying in the AV groove at the posterior extent of this incision. After identification of the location of the His bundle and right bundle branch, a second transmural incision is placed from the posterior pulmonic valve anulus to the anterior medial tricuspid valve anulus, exposing the underlying aortic root. If the tricuspid portion of this incision is placed too far anteriorly, the bundle of His may be inadvertently divided. *B,* After completion of the two transmural incisions, the papillary muscle attached to the anterior leaflet of the tricuspid valve is divided at its base and reimplanted on the lower ventricular septum using interrupted 3-0 pledgeted Prolene sutures. Cryolesions are placed at each end of the anterior-posterior ventriculotomy and at each end of the ventriculotomy between the posterior pulmonic valve anulus and the anterior medial suture followed by closure of the long free-wall ventriculotomy with continuous 3-0 nonabsorbable sutures *(C).* (From Cox, J. L.: Surgery for cardiac arrhythmias. Curr. Probl. Cardiol., 8[4]:7, 1983.)

tion with the long QT syndrome is frequently of a distinct type called *torsades de pointes.* This term is derived from the appearance of the ventricular tachycardia on a standard electrocardiogram on which the polarity of the tachycardia is inconstant. One of the most frequent causes of torsades de pointes is the administration of medications that prolong ventricular repolarization, particularly quinidine.[94]

These observations support the concept that torsades de pointes represents an abnormality in myocardial *repolarization,* as opposed to most other types of ventricular tachycardia, which are thought to be abnormalities in myocardial *depolarization.* As a result, the surgical treatment of recurrent ventricular tachycardia associated with long QT syndrome has centered around efforts to modify cardiac innervation. Left stellate ganglion resection has been reported to abolish symptoms in many patients with the long QT syndrome.[95–98] However, the author's experience[99] and that of others[100] have been characterized by early success and late failure.

ISCHEMIC VENTRICULAR TACHYCARDIA

Historical Aspects. Sir Thomas Lewis was apparently the first to recognize the relationship between ventricular aneu-

rysm and ventricular tachycardia in 1909 when he suggested the need for a controlled method of inducing tachycardia so that it could be studied in a systematic fashion.[101] In the absence of such a technique even 50 years later, Couch and associates performed a simple aneurysmectomy specifically for the treatment of intractable ventricular tachycardia.[102] In 1967, Dirk Durrer and Hein Wellens of Amsterdam and their associates[103] and Phillipe Coumel of Paris and his colleagues[104] described the technique of programmed electrical stimulation, precisely the tool desired by Lewis to induce and terminate tachycardia in a reproducible manner for purposes of diagnosis and evaluation of interventional therapy.

Experimental studies in the mid and late 1960s documented the heterogeneity of tissue injury in acute myocardial infarction,[105] and the re-entrant basis of ischemic ventricular tachyarrhythmias was confirmed.[106–112] Thus, with the advent of coronary bypass surgery in the late 1960s, it seemed apparent that ischemic ventricular tachycardia would be easily corrected by this new procedure, because the basis for the arrhythmia (myocardial ischemia) could be alleviated by myocardial revascularization. During the 1970s, however, it became apparent that neither revascularization nor resection of the injured myocardium resulted in acceptable cure rates and, in addition, the operative mortality rates reported when these procedures were performed primarily for ventricular tachycardia control were prohibitively high.[113] Although the demonstration that ischemic ventricular tachyarrhythmias occurred on a re-entrant basis improved the concept of the arrhythmia, there remained a profound ignorance of the uncharted interplay between the autonomic nervous system, endogenous humoral stimulants, intracellular electrophysiology, extracellular electrophysiology, the specialized conduction system, coronary artery disease, myocardial ischemia and infarction, and normal myocardial conduction, all of which undoubtedly play a role in the genesis and perpetuation of ischemic ventricular tachyarrhythmias.

Because of the lack of efficacy of myocardial revascularization and/or resection in controlling ischemic ventricular tachycardia, several groups began to approach the problem in a more direct surgical manner. In 1969, Daniel and associates[114] and Kaiser and coworkers[115] independently reported intraoperative mapping in patients with ischemic heart disease to localize the area of ischemic injury. Fontaine and associates performed intraoperative mapping before performing a standard aneurysmectomy in 1974,[116] but Wittig and Boineau[117] and Gallagher and colleagues[118] first reported the use of intraoperative mapping specifically to guide the attempted surgical ablation of ischemic ventricular tachycardia. In 1978, Guiraudon described the encircling endocardial ventriculotomy (Fig. 54–193), a procedure he had successfully employed to ablate ventricular tachycardia in five patients.[119] Shortly thereafter, Harken and associates[120] described the endocardial resection procedure, modifications of which remain the mainstay of surgery for the treatment of ischemic ventricular tachycardia to the present time. In recent years, Jatene[121] and Dor and coworkers[122] have independently described surgical techniques for *repairing* left ventricular aneurysms that have the unexpected side-effect of curing most associated ventricular tachycardia.

Anatomic-Electrophysiologic Basis. The arrhythmogenic regions of most re-entrant ischemic ventricular tachycardias are located in the endocardium and subendocardium, especially at the periphery of myocardial infarcts or ventricular aneurysms.[105, 123] Re-entrant ischemic ventricular arrhythmias result from a complex interplay among a nonuniform (heterogeneous) state of repolarization, slow desynchronized conduction over abnormal myocardial pathways created by fibrotic or ischemic discontinuity, and ventricular ectopy.[109] Slow desynchronized conduction is a hallmark of myocardial

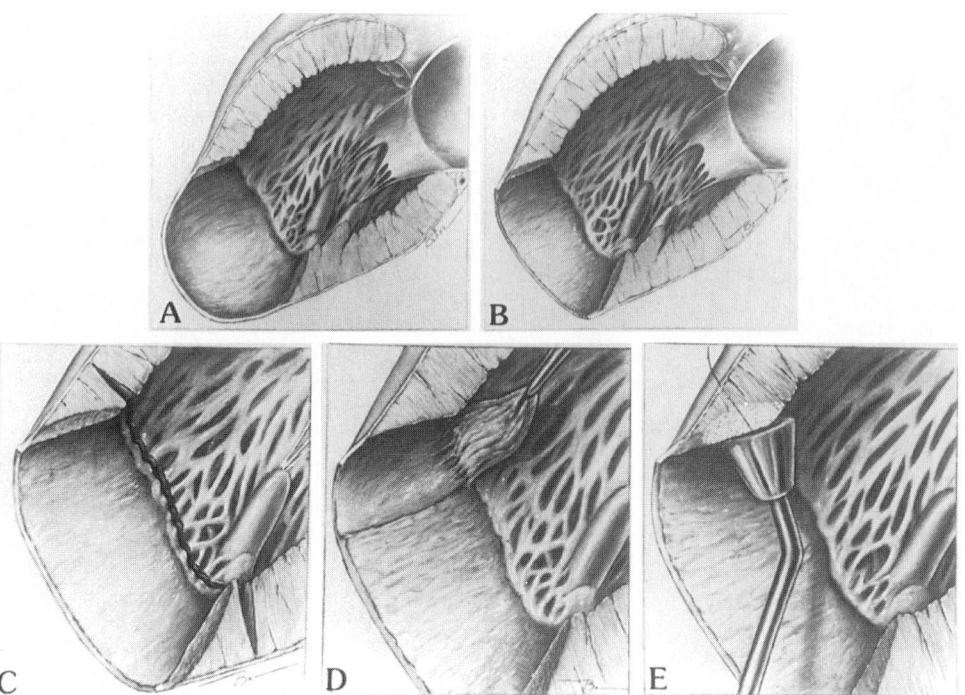

Figure 54-193. Diagrammatic cross-section of an anterior left ventricular aneurysm showing more proximal extension of the associated fibrosis at the endocardial level than at the epicardial level (A). Because the re-entrant circuits responsible for ischemic ventricular tachycardia occur most commonly at the junction of this endocardial fibrosis and normal myocardium, a standard left ventricular aneurysm resection (B) does not ablate or remove them. The encircling endocardial ventriculotomy (C), localized endocardial (or "subendocardial") resection (D), and endocardial cryoablation (E) were all introduced specifically to ablate ventricular tachycardia associated with left ventricular aneurysms or infarcts. (Modified from Cox, J. L.: Anatomic-electrophysiologic basis for the surgical treatment of refractory ischemic ventricular tachycardia. Ann. Surg., *198*:119, 1983.)

injury or fibrosis. Conduction velocity is dependent on the synchrony of the activation process. Because fibrosis is nonuniform at the borders of infarcts, it produces complex interdigitations between normal myocardium and scar. A synchronous wavefront, on approaching such an area, may become desynchronized, fragmenting into many individual wavelets. A slowing of conduction time accompanies the desynchronization.

Electrical activity is thought to be identifiable as part of the re-entrant tachycardia circuit if it precedes the onset of ventricular depolarization evident on the surface ECG and is required for the initiation and perpetuation of the tachycardia. The site of origin of the tachycardia is believed to be the area exhibiting the earliest presystolic electrical activity in the latter half of diastole and represents the region of myocardium that must be identified and removed at the time of surgery to prevent the arrhythmias.[124]

Preoperative Electrophysiologic Evaluation. All patients who are to undergo surgical therapy for ventricular tachyarrhythmias should first undergo an endocardial catheter electrophysiology study. The objectives of the preoperative study are to confirm that the arrhythmia is ventricular rather than supraventricular; demonstrate that the ventricular arrhythmia can be induced and terminated by programmed electrical stimulation techniques (i.e., that it is a re-entrant arrhythmia); and localize the region of origin of the ventricular tachycardia by *catheter mapping* when possible. In addition to the preoperative electrophysiology study, patients with ventricular tachyarrhythmias routinely undergo cardiac catheterization and coronary angiography before surgical intervention.

Surgical Indications and Contraindications. Decisions regarding surgical intervention for ischemic ventricular tachycardia are based on a variety of clinical factors and must be individualized for each patient. Because no surgical technique exists for the ablation of primary ventricular fibrillation, an internal cardioverter-defibrillator (ICD) device can be implanted in all patients with this unusual problem. However, even though ventricular fibrillation may be the primary diagnosis in a given patient who has been resuscitated from an episode of sudden death, an electrophysiology study will usually confirm that the episode of fibrillation is preceded

by at least a short run of ventricular tachycardia, most commonly of the polymorphic type. Such patients are considered to have primary ventricular tachycardia, not ventricular fibrillation, which is believed to be a secondary problem that will be alleviated if the ventricular tachycardia can be controlled.

Perhaps the major contraindication to surgery is left ventricular dysfunction so severe that it precludes any reasonable possibility of surviving an operative procedure. Before availability of ICDs, there was no viable alternative to surgery in such patients if their arrhythmia could not be controlled pharmacologically. However, it is now preferred to implant an ICD in such patients because of the lower operative mortality rate associated with this relatively simple procedure. One benefit of this *selection* of patients who will not undergo ventricular tachycardia surgery has been an improvement in the operative mortality rate of the remaining patients who now undergo direct surgery.

Intraoperative Electrophysiologic Mapping. In patients undergoing surgery for ventricular tachyarrhythmias, the first step intraoperatively is to perform detailed electrophysiologic mapping procedures to guide the specific surgical technique to be employed. During the past few years, a new method of intraoperative electrophysiologic mapping called potential distribution mapping has been used.[125-129] Form-fitting, molded endocardial electrode arrays are inserted across the mitral and tricuspid valves to obtain three-dimensional potential distribution electrophysiologic maps of the endocardium. This type of mapping is much more conducive to computerization, and, as a result, it is quicker and more accurate than the standard activation time mapping.

Surgical Technique

Map-Guided Surgery. The site(s) of origin of the ventricular tachycardia is localized as described previously. Then with the heart in the normothermic beating state, preferably during ventricular tachycardia, the ventricle is opened through the infarct or aneurysm and all of the associated endocardial fibrosis is resected except that which extends onto the base of the papillary muscles (Fig. 54-194). After resecting all visible endocardial fibrosis, endocardial cryolesions are applied to the site(s) of origin of the tachycardia as determined

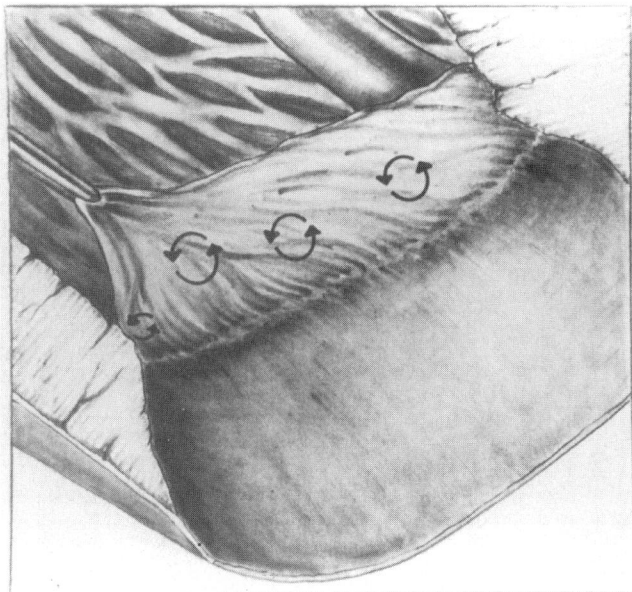

Figure 54–194. Diagrammatic sketch of an extended endocardial resection procedure (EERP) in an anterior left ventricular aneurysm. The principle involved in this procedure is the same as that for a localized ERP (see Fig. 54–193*D*), but in this procedure *all* of the endocardial fibrosis associated with the aneurysm is resected except that involving the papillary muscles. (From Cox, J. L.: Surgical treatment of ischemic and nonischemic ventricular tachyarrhythmias. *In* Cohn, L. H. [Ed.]: Modern Technics in Surgery. Mount Kisco, N.Y., Futura Publishing, 1985.)

by the intraoperative mapping (Fig. 54–195). The cryothermia is applied only after removal of the endocardial scar because approximately 10% of patients will still have inducible ventricular tachycardia intraoperatively after removal of all visible endocardial fibrosis. This would indicate that the actual

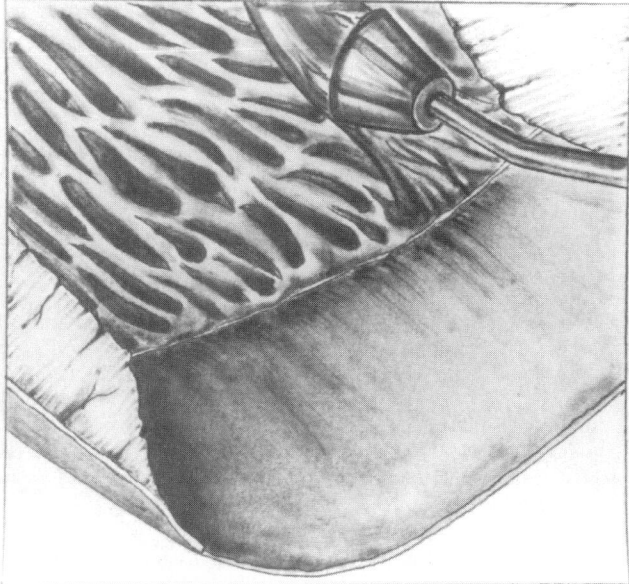

Figure 54–195. After all of the endocardial scar is resected as a preliminary measure, endocardial cryolesions are placed at the site or sites of origin of the ventricular tachycardia as determined by intraoperative mapping. In addition, any remaining scar on the papillary muscle is cryoablated as shown. (From Cox, J. L.: Surgical treatment of ischemic and nonischemic ventricular tachyarrhythmias. *In* Cohn, L .H. [Ed.]: Modern Technics in Surgery. Mount Kisco, N.Y., Futura Publishing, 1985.)

site of origin of the tachycardia in these patients is deeper in the myocardium than the visible border of the endocardial fibrosis and that, therefore, the myocardium underneath the fibrosis must be destroyed to ablate the tachycardia. In those cases in which one site of origin is a scarred papillary muscle, one or more cryolesions are placed directly on the base of the involved papillary muscle without removing the scar. More than 100 papillary muscles have been cryoablated without a single instance of mitral valve regurgitation. This experience would argue strongly against the practice of resecting papillary muscles for ventricular tachycardia as has been reported in the past.[130]

Once the extended endocardial resection and subsequent endocardial cryoablation have been completed, programmed electrical stimulation is applied in an attempt to reinduce the arrhythmia. If ventricular tachycardia is still inducible, it is again mapped and the remaining arrhythmogenic myocardium is cryoablated. If the arrhythmia is no longer inducible, one can be confident that it has been permanently ablated. If other procedures are to be performed, such as coronary bypass grafting, they are then carried out under cardioplegic arrest. Cardioplegia is not administered until the ventricular tachycardia has been ablated. The reason for this strict approach is that the cardioplegia itself may temporarily alter the delicate re-entry circuits causing the tachycardia, and, therefore, if the antitachycardia procedure is performed under cardioplegic arrest, it is impossible to determine intraoperatively whether the surgical procedure has ablated the arrhythmia. It is this point that is so often ignored when considering the factors that predispose to postoperative recurrences, and it emphasizes the importance of the manner in which the operative procedure is conducted. The practice of performing ventricular tachycardia surgery under cardioplegic arrest is the major reason for the high reinducibility rates at the time of the postoperative electrophysiology study reported in most series.

Repair of Left Ventricular Aneurysms Without Map Guidance. During the past few years, two entirely new surgical techniques have been developed for the surgical resection and *repair* of left ventricular aneurysms.[121, 122] Both of these techniques attempt to restore the normal contour of the left ventricle, eliminate the adverse effects of the septal component of the aneurysm, and realign the myofibrils of the left ventricular free wall to restore their optimal contractile function. The *functional* improvement of the left ventricle after either of these two procedures has been dramatic and remarkable when compared with the old technique of simply resecting the aneurysm and closing the ventricle. Of great interest is the unexpected observation that both of these procedures appear to cure any ventricular tachyarrhythmias associated with the aneurysm. The surgical results include an operative mortality rate of 2% to 3% (comparable to that of ICDs), even in higher-risk patients, and a ventricular tachycardia cure rate of approximately 98%. The reason that the operative mortality rate is so much lower, even in higher-risk patients, is threefold: (1) for the first time, a major and immediate improvement in left ventricular function can be attained; (2) the residual postoperative detrimental effects of septal aneurysmal involvement are eliminated; and (3) cardiopulmonary bypass time is reduced substantially because the procedures are not only quick and relatively easy to perform but also require no intraoperative mapping. Because these techniques are apparently capable of eliminating ventricular tachycardia and restoring cardiac function with operative mortality and recurrence rates comparable to those attained with ICDs, it is expected that the window of indications for the surgical treatment of ventricular tachycardia may again broaden.

SELECTED REFERENCES

Boineau, J. P., and Cox, J. L.: Slow ventricular activation in acute myocardial infarction: A source of re-entrant premature ventricular contractions. Circulation, 48:702, 1973.
This paper is the first to document experimentally that ventricular arrhythmias following a myocardial infarction occur on the basis of a re-entrant mechanism.

Cobb, F. R., Blumenschein, S. D., Sealy, W. C., Boineau, J. P., Wagner, G. S., and Wallace, A. G.: Successful surgical interruption of the bundle of Kent in a patient with Wolff-Parkinson-White syndrome. Circulation, 38:1018, 1968.
This is the first description of the successful surgical treatment of the Wolff-Parkinson-White syndrome. Although current surgical techniques differ significantly from those described in this original article, this paper represents a milestone in the surgical treatment of cardiac arrhythmias.

Cox, J. L., Schuessler, R. B., and Boineau, J. P.: The surgical treatment of atrial fibrillation: I. Summary of the current concepts of the mechanisms of atrial flutter and atrial fibrillation. J. Thorac. Cardiovasc. Surg., 101:402, 1991.
Cox, J. L., Canavan, T. E., Schuessler, R. B., Cain, M. E., Lindsay, B. D., Stone, C., et al.: The surgical treatment of atrial fibrillation: II. Intraoperative electrophysiologic mapping and description of the electrophysiologic basis of atrial flutter and atrial fibrillation. J. Thorac. Cardiovasc. Surg., 101:406, 1991.
Cox, J. L., Schuessler, R. B., D'Agostino, H. J., Jr., Stone, C. M., Chang, B. C., and Cain, M. E.: The surgical treatment of atrial fibrillation: III. Development of a definite surgical procedure. J. Thorac. Cardiovasc. Surg. 101:569, 1991.
Cox, J. L.: The surgical treatment of atrial fibrillation: IV. Surgical technique. J. Thorac. Cardiovasc. Surg., 101:584, 1991.
These four sequential papers describe the electrophysiologic basis of atrial flutter and fibrillation and the surgical technique developed to treat these arrhythmias.

Cox, J. L., McLaughlin, V. W., Flowers, N. C., and Horan, L. G.: The ischemic zone surrounding acute myocardial infarction: Its morphology as detected by dehydrogenase staining. Am. Heart J., 76:650, 1968.
This is the first anatomic documentation and characterization of the ischemic zone surrounding an acute myocardial infarction.

Cox, J. L.: Patient selection criteria and results of surgery from refractory ischemic ventricular tachycardia. Circulation, 79(Suppl. I):I-163, 1989.
This is a comprehensive review of the first 10 years' experience with the direct surgical procedures for refractory ischemic ventricular tachycardia. The surgical results are analyzed in detail, and the roles of intraoperative mapping, surgical technique, and the automatic internal cardioverter-defibrillator are discussed. An algorithm is then presented for the treatment of these arrhythmias based on the accumulated clinical experience.

REFERENCES

1. Jackman, W. M., Wang, X. Z., Friday, K. J., Roman, C. A., Moulton, K. P., Beckman, K. J., et al.: Catheter ablation of accessory atrioventricular pathways (Wolff-Parkinson-White syndrome) by radiofrequency current. N. Engl. J. Med., 324:1605, 1991.
2. Lee, M. A., Morady, F., Kadish, A., Schamp, D. J., Chin, M. C., Scheinman, M. M., et al.: Catheter modification of the atrioventricular junction with radiofrequency energy for control of atrioventricular nodal reentry tachycardia. Circulation, 83:827, 1991.
3. Savage, D. D., Garrison, R. J., Castelli, W. P., et al.: Prevalence of submitral (anular) calcium and its correlates in a general population-based sample (the Framingham study). Am. J. Cardiol., 51:1375, 1983.
4. Diamantopoulos, E. J., Anthopoulos, L., Nanas, S., Maliaras, G., Chrisos, D., and Moulopoulos, S. D.: Detection of arrhythmias in a representative sample of the Athens population. Eur. Heart J., 8(Suppl. D):17, 1987.
5. Onundarson, P. T., Thorgeirsson, G., Jonmundsson, E., Sigfusson, N., and Hardarson, T.: Chronic atrial fibrillation: Epidemiologic features and 14-year follow-up: A case control study. Eur. Heart J., 8:521, 1987.
6. Hirosawa, K., Sekiguchi, M., Kasanuki, H., et al.: Natural history of atrial fibrillation. Heart Vessels, Suppl. 2:14, 1987.
7. Cameron, A., Schwartz, M. J., Kronmal, R. A., and Kosinski, A. S.: Prevalence and significance of atrial fibrillation in coronary artery disease (CASS Registry). Am. J. Cardiol., 61:714, 1988.
8. Tammaro, A. E., Ronzoni, D., Bonaccorso, O., et al.: Le aritmie nell'anziano. Minerva Med., 74:1313, 1983.
9. Cobler, J. L., Williams, M. E., and Greenland, P.: Thyrotoxicosis in institutionalized elderly patients with atrial fibrillation. Arch. Intern. Med., 144:1758, 1984.
10. Martin, A., Benbow, L. J., Butrous, G. S., Leach, C., and Camm, A. J.: Five-year follow-up of 101 elderly subjects by means of long-term ambulatory cardiac monitoring. Eur. Heart J., 5:592, 1984.
11. Treseder, A. S., Sastry, B. S., Thomas, T. P., Yates, M. A., and Pathy, M. S.: Atrial fibrillation and stroke in elderly hospitalized patients. Age Aging, 15:89, 1986.
12. Scheinman, M. M., and Evans-Bell, T: Catheter ablation of the atrioventricular junction: A report of the percutaneous mapping and ablation registry. Circulation, 70:1024, 1984.
13. Williams, J. M., Ungerleider, R. M., Lofland, G. K., and Cox, J. L.: Left atrial isolation: New technique for the treatment of supraventricular arrhythmias. J. Thorac. Cardiovasc. Surg., 80:373, 1980.
14. Cox, J. L.: Surgery for cardiac arrhythmias. Curr. Prob. Cardiol., 8(4):7, 1983.
15. Guiraudon, G. M., Campbell, C. S., Jones, D. L., McLellan, J. L., and MacDonald, J. L.: Combined sino-atrial node atrio-ventricular node isolation: A surgical alternative to His' bundle ablation in patients with atrial fibrillation. Circulation, 72(Suppl. 3):220, 1985.
16. Cox, J. L.: Discussion of Defauw, J. J. A. M. T., Guiraudon, G. M., van Hemel, N. M., Vermeulen, F. E. E., Kingma, J. H., and de Bakker, J. M. T.: Surgical therapy of paroxysmal atrial fibrillation with the "Corridor" operation. Ann. Thorac. Surg., 53:571, 1992.
17. Cox, J. L., Schuessler, R. B., and Boineau, J. P.: The surgical treatment of atrial fibrillation: I. Summary of the current concepts of the mechanisms of atrial flutter and atrial fibrillation. J. Thorac. Cardiovasc. Surg., 101:402, 1991.
18. Cox, J. L., Canavan, T. E., Schuessler, R. B., Cain, M. E., Lindsay, B. D., Stone, C., et al.: The surgical treatment of atrial fibrillation: II. Intraoperative electrophysiologic mapping and description of the electrophysiologic basis of atrial flutter and atrial fibrillation. J. Thorac. Cardiovasc. Surg., 101:406, 1991.
19. Cox, J. L., Schuessler, R. B., D'Agostino, H. J., Jr, Stone, C. M., Chang, B. C., and Cain, M. E.: The surgical treatment of atrial fibrillation: III. Development of a definite surgical procedure. J. Thorac. Cardiovasc. Surg., 101:569, 1991.
20. Cox, J. L.: The surgical treatment of atrial fibrillation: IV. Surgical technique. J. Thorac. Cardiovasc. Surg., 101:584, 1991.
21. Cox, J. L., Boineau, J. P., Schuessler, R. B., Ferguson, T. B., Jr., Cain, M. E., Lindsay, B. D., Corr, P. B., Kater, K. M., and Lappas, D. G.: Successful surgical treatment of atrial fibrillation. JAMA, 266:1976, 1991.
22. Cox, J. L.: Surgical treatment of atrial fibrillation (Letter Reply). J. Thorac. Cardiovasc. Surg., 104:1492, 1992.
23. Blitz, A., McLoughlin, D., Gross, J., Schwartz, D. S., Fisher, J. D., Kim, S. G., Frame, R., and Brodman, R. F.: Combined maze procedure and septal myectomy in a septuagenarian. Ann. Thorac. Surg., 54:364, 1992.
24. Bonchek, L. I., Burlingame, M. W., Worley, S. J., Vazales, B. E., and Lundy, E. F.: Cox/maze procedure for atrial septal defect with atrial fibrillation: Management strategies. Ann. Thorac. Surg., 55:607, 1993.
25. Hioki, M., Ikeshita, M., Iedokoro, Y., Nitta, T., Harada, A., Asano, T., Tanaka, S., and Shoji, T.: Successful combined operation for mitral stenosis and atrial fibrillation. Ann. Thorac. Surg., 55:776, 1993.
26. Cox, J. L., Boineau, J. P., Scheussler, R. B., Kater, K. M., and Lappas, D. M.: Five-year experience with the maze procedure for atrial fibrillation. Ann. Thorac. Surg., 56:814, 1993.
27. Cox, J. L.: Evolving applications of the maze procedure for atrial fibrillation (Invited Editorial). Ann. Thorac. Surg., 55:578, 1993.
28. Kosakai, Y., Kawaguchi, A. T., Isobe, F., Sasako, Y., Kito, Y., and Kawashima, Y.: Cox-maze procedure for chronic atrial fibrillation associated with mitral valve disease, J. Thorac. Cardiovasc. Surg., 108:1049, 1994.
29. Cox, J. L., Boineau, J. P., Schuessler, R. B., Kater, K. M., Ferguson, T. B., Jr., Cain, M. E., Lindsay, B. D., Smith, J. M., Corr, P. B., Hogue, C. B., and Lappas, D. G.: The electrophysiologic basis, surgical development, and clinical results of the Maze procedure for atrial flutter and atrial fibrillation. In Karp, R. E. (Ed.): Advances in Cardiac Surgery. Chicago, Mosby–Year Book, 1994.
30. Moe, G. K.: On the multiple wavelet hypothesis of atrial fibrillation. Arch. Int. Pharmacodyn., 140:183, 1962.
31. Boineau, J. P., Mooney, C., Hudson, R., Hughes, D., Erdin, R., and Wylds, A.: Observations on re-entrant excitation pathways and refractory period distribution in spontaneous and experimental atrial flutter in the dog. In Kulbertus, H. E. (Ed.): Re-entrant Arrhythmias. Baltimore, University Park Press, 1977, pp. 79–98.
32. Boineau, J. P., Schuessler, R. B., Mooney, C. R., Miller, C. B., Wylds, A. C., Hudson, R. D., Borremans, J. M., and Brockus, C. W.: Natural and evoked atrial flutter due to circus movement in dogs. Am. J. Cardiol., 45:1167, 1980.
33. Allessie, M. A., Lammers, W. J. E. P., Bonke, I. M., and Hollen, J.: Intra-atrial reentry as a mechanism for atrial flutter induced by acetylcholine and rapid pacing in the dog. Circulation, 70:123, 1984.
34. D'Agostino, H. J., Jr., Harada, A., Schuessler, R. B., Boineau, J. P., and Cox, J. L.: Global epicardial mapping of atrial fibrillation in a canine model of chronic mitral regurgitation. Circulation, 76(Suppl. IV):IV–165, 1987.
35. Yamauchi, S., Sato, S., Schuessler, R. B., Boineau, J. P., Matsunaga, Y., and Cox, J. L.: Induced atrial arrhythmias in a canine model of left atrial enlargement. PACE, 13:556, 1990.
36. Canavan, T. E., Schuessler, R. B., Boineau, J. P., Corr, P. B., Cain, M. E., and Cox, J. L.: Computerized global electrophysiological mapping of the atrium in patients with Wolff-Parkinson-White syndrome. Ann. Thorac. Surg., 46:223, 1988.
37. Canavan, T. E., Schuessler, R. B., Cain, M. E., Lindsay, B. D., Boineau, J. P., Corr, P. B., and Cox, J. L.: Computerized global electrophysiological mapping of the atrium in a patient with multiple supraventricular tachyarrhythmias. Ann. Thorac. Surg., 46:232, 1988.
38. Petersen, P., Boysen, G., Godtfredsen, J., et al.: Placebo-controlled, randomized trial of warfarin and aspirin for prevention of thromboembolic complications in chronic atrial fibrillation: The Copenhagen AFASAK study. Lancet, 1:175, 1989.
39. Stroke Prevention in Atrial Fibrillation Study Group Investigators: Prelim-

inary report of the Stroke Prevention in Atrial Fibrillation study. N. Engl. J. Med., 322:863, 1990.

40. Boston Area Anticoagulation Trial in Atrial Fibrillation Investigators: The effect of low dose warfarin on the risk of stroke in patients with nonrheumatic atrial fibrillation. N. Engl. J. Med., 323:1505, 1990.

41. Cox, J. L., Schuessler, R. B., Boineau, J. P., and Lappas, D. G.: Modification of the maze procedure for atrial flutter and atrial fibrillation: I. Rationale and surgical results. J. Thorac. Cardiovasc. Surg., 110:485, 1995.

42. Cox, J. L., Jaquiss, R. D. B., Schuessler, R. B., and Boineau, J. P.: Modification of the maze procedure for atrial flutter and atrial fibrillation: II. Surgical technique of the maze-III procedure. J. Thorac. Cardiovasc. Surg., 110:485, 1995.

43. Gaskell, W. H.: On the innervation of the heart, with especial reference to the heart of the tortoise. J. Physiol., 4:43, 1883.

44. Kent, A. F. S.: Researches on structure and function of mammalian heart. J. Physiol., 14:233, 1893.

45. Aschoff, K. A. L.: A discussion on some aspects of heart-block. BMJ, 2:1103, 1906.

46. Keith, A., and Flack, M.: The form and nature of the muscular connections between the primary divisions of the vertebrate heart. J. Anat. Physiol., 41:172, 1906–1907.

47. Wolff, L., Parkinson, J., and White, P. D.: Bundle branch block with short PR interval in healthy young people prone to paroxysmal tachycardia. Am. Heart J. 5:685, 1930.

48. Wood, F. C., Wolferth, C. C., and Geckler, G. D.: Histologic demonstration of accessory muscular connections between auricle and ventricle in a case of short P-R interval and prolonged QRS complex. Am. Heart J., 25:454, 1943.

49. Durrer, D., and Roos, J. P.: Epicardial excitation of the ventricles in a patient with Wolff-Parkinson-White syndrome (type B): Temporary ablation at surgery. Circulation, 35:15, 1967.

50. Burchell, H. B., Frye, R. L., Anderson, M. W., et al.: Atrial-ventricular and ventricular-atrial excitation in Wolff-Parkinson-White syndrome (type B): Temporary ablation at surgery. Circulation, 36:663, 1967.

51. Cobb, F. R., Blumenschein, S. D., Sealy, W. C., Boineau, J. P., Wagner, G. S., and Wallace, A. G.: Successful surgical interruption of the bundle of Kent in a patient with Wolff-Parkinson-White syndrome. Circulation, 38:1018, 1968.

52. Cox, J. L., Gallagher, J. J., and Cain, M. E.: Experience with 118 consecutive patients undergoing surgery for the Wolff-Parkinson-White syndrome. J. Thorac. Cardiovasc. Surg., 90:490, 1985.

53. Kramer, J. B., Corr, P. B., Cox, J. L., Witkowski, F. X., and Cain, M. E.: Arrhythmia and conduction disturbances: Simultaneous computer mapping to facilitate intraoperative localization of accessory pathways in patients with Wolff-Parkinson-White syndrome. Am. J. Cardiol., 56:571, 1985.

54. Klein, G. J., Guiraudon, G. M., Perkins, D. G., Jones, D. L., Yee, R., and Jarvis, E.: Surgical correction of the Wolff-Parkinson-White syndrome in the closed heart using cryosurgery: A simplified approach. J. Am. Coll. Cardiol., 3:405, 1984.

55. Guiraudon, G. M., Klein, G. J., Sharma, A. D., Jones, D. L., and McLellan, D. G.: Surgical ablation of posterior septal accessory pathways in the Wolff-Parkinson-White syndrome by a closed heart technique. J. Thorac. Cardiovasc. Surg., 92:406, 1986.

56. Guiraudon, G. M., Klein, G. J., Sharma, A. D., Milstein, S., and McLellan, D. G.: Closed-heart technique for Wolff-Parkinson-White syndrome: Further experience and potential limitations. Ann. Thorac. Surg., 42:651, 1986.

57. Scherf, D., and Shookhoff, C.: Experimentalle Untersuchung über die Umkehrextrasystole. Wien Arch. Int. Med., 12:501, 1926.

58. Moe, G. K., Preston, J. B., and Burlington, H.: Physiologic evidence for a dual A-V transmission system. Circ. Res., 4:357, 1956.

59. Goldreyer, B. N., and Damato, A. N.: The essential role of atrioventricular and conduction delay in the initiation of paroxysmal supraventricular tachycardia. Circulation, 43:679, 1971.

60. Bigger, J. T., and Goldreyer, B. N.: The mechanism of supraventricular tachycardia. Circulation, 42:673, 1970.

61. Goldreyer, B. N., and Bigger, J. T.: Site of reentry in paroxysmal supraventricular tachycardia in man. Circulation, 43:15, 1971.

62. Denes, P., Delon, W., Dhingra, R. C., Chuquimia, R., and Rosen, K. M.: Demonstration of dual AV nodal pathways in patients with paroxysmal supraventricular tachycardia. Circulation, 48:549, 1973.

63. Akhtar, M.: Atrioventricular nodal reentry. Circulation, 75:26, 1987.

64. Denes, P., Delon, W., Dhingra, R. C., Chuquimia, R., and Rosen K. M.: Demonstration of dual AV nodal pathways in patients with paroxysmal supraventricular tachycardia. Circulation, 48:549, 1973.

65. Josephson, M. E., and Kastor, J. A.: Paroxysmal supraventricular tachycardia: Is the atrium a necessary link? Circulation, 54:430, 1976.

66. Wu, D., Denes, P., Amat-y-Leon, F., Dhingra, R., Wyndham, C. R. C., Baurnfeind, R., Latif, P., and Rosen, K. M.: Clinical electrocardiographic and electrophysiologic observations in patients with paroxysmal supraventricular tachycardia. Am. J. Cardiol., 41:1045, 1978.

67. Sealy, W. C., Gallagher, J. J., and Kasell, J. H.: His bundle interruption for control of inappropriate ventricular responses to atrial arrhythmias. Ann. Thorac. Surg., 32:429, 1981.

68. Scheinman, M. M., Morady, F., Hess, D. S., and Gonzalez, R.: Catheter-induced ablation of the atrioventricular junction to control refractory supraventricular arrhythmias. JAMA, 248:851, 1982.

69. Pritchett, E. L. C., Anderson, R. W., Benditt, D. G., Kasell, J., Harrison, L., Wallace, A. G., Sealy, W. C., and Gallagher, J. J.: Reentry within the atrioventricular node: Surgical cure with preservation of atrioventricular conduction. Circulation, 60:440, 1979.

70. Holman, W., Ikeshita, M., Lease, J., Smith, P., Ferguson, T., and Cox, J.: Elective prolongation of atrioventricular conduction by multiple discrete cryolesions: A new technique for the treatment of paroxysmal supraventricular tachycardia. J. Thorac. Cardiovasc. Surg., 84:554, 1982.

71. Holman, W. L., Ikeshita, M., Lease, J. G., Ferguson, T. B., Jr., Lofland, G. K., and Cox, J. L.: Alteration of antegrade atrioventricular conduction by cryoablation of periatrioventricular nodal tissue. J. Thorac. Cardiovasc. Surg., 88:67, 1984.

72. Holman, W. L., Ikeshita, M., Lease, J. G., Smith, P. K., Lofland, G. K., and Cox, J. L.: Cryosurgical modification of retrograde atrioventricular conduction: Implications for the surgical treatment of atrioventricular node reentry tachycardia. J. Thorac. Cardiovasc. Surg., 91:826, 1986.

73. Ross, D. L., Johnson, D. C., Denniss, A. R., Cooper, M. J., Richards, D. A., and Uther, J. B.: Curative surgery for atrioventricular junctional ("A-V nodal") reentrant tachycardia. J. Am. Coll. Cardiol., 6:1383, 1985.

74. Guiraudon, G. M., Klein, G. K., Sharma, A. D., Yee, R., Kaushik, R. R., and Fujimura, O.: Skeletonization of the atrioventricular node for AV node reentrant tachycardia: Experience with 32 patients. Ann. Thorac. Surg., 49:565, 1990.

75. Cox, J. L., Holman, W. L., and Cain, M. E.: Cryosurgical treatment of atrioventricular node reentry tachycardia. Circulation, 76:1329, 1987.

76. Fujimara, O., Guiraudon, G. M., Yee, R., et al.: Operative therapy of atrioventricular node reentry and results of an anatomically guided procedure. Am. J. Cardiol., 64:1327, 1989.

77. Lewis, T.: Paroxysmal tachycardia, the result of ectopic impulse formation. Heart, 1:262, 1909–1910.

78. Goldreyer, B. N., Gallagher, J. J., and Damato, A. N.: The electrophysiologic demonstration of atrial ectopic tachycardia in man. Am. Heart J., 85:205, 1973.

79. Williams, J. M., Ungerleider, R. M., Lofland, G. K., and Cox, J. L.: Left atrial isolation: New technique for the treatment of supraventricular arrhythmias. J. Thorac. Cardiovasc. Surg., 80:373, 1980.

80. Lowe, J. E., Hendry, P. J., Packer, D. L., and Tang, A. S.: Surgical management of chronic ectopic atrial tachycardia. Semin. Thorac. Cardiovasc. Surg., 1:58, 1989.

81. Borggrefe, M., and Breithardt, G.: Ectopic atrial tachycardia after transvenous catheter ablation of a posteroseptal accessory pathway. J. Am. Coll. Cardiol., 8:441, 1986.

82. Garson, G., and Gillette, P. C.: Electrophysiologic studies of supraventricular tachycardia in children: I. Clinical-electrophysiologic correlations. Am. Heart J., 102:223, 1981.

83. Giorgi, L. V., Hartzler, G. O., and Hamaker, W. R.: Incessant focal atrial tachycardia: A surgically remediable cause of cardiomyopathy. J. Thorac. Cardiovasc. Surg., 87:466, 1984.

84. Packer, D. L., Bardy, G. H., Worley, S. J., et al.: Tachycardia-induced cardiomyopathy: A reversible form of left ventricular dysfunction. Am. J. Cardiol., 57:563, 1986.

85. Damiano, R. J., Tripp, H. F., Asano, T., et al.: Left ventricular dysfunction and dilatation resulting from chronic supraventricular tachycardia. J. Thorac. Cardiovasc. Surg., 94:135, 1987.

86. Cain, M. E., and Lindsay, B. D.: The preoperative electrophysiologic study. In Cox, J. L. (Ed.): Cardiac Surgery: State of the Art Reviews. Philadelphia, Hanley & Belfus, 1990, pp. 53–91.

87. Gallagher, J. J., Kasell, J. H., Cox, J. L., Smith, W. M., Ideker, R. E., and Smith, W. M.: The techniques of intraoperative electrophysiologic mapping. Am. J. Cardiol., 49:221, 1982.

88. Fontaine, G., Guiraudon, G., and Frank, R.: Management of chronic ventricular tachycardia. In Narula, O. S. (Ed.): Innovations in Diagnosis and Management of Cardiac Arrhythmias. Baltimore, Williams & Wilkins, 1979.

89. Cox, J. L., Bardy, G. H., Damiano, R. J., et al.: Right ventricular isolation procedures for non-ischemic ventricular tachycardia. J. Thorac. Cardiovasc. Surg., 90:212, 1985.

90. Uhl, H. S.: A previously undescribed malformation of the heart: Almost total absence of the myocardium of the right ventricle. Bull. Johns Hopkins Hosp., 91:197, 1952.

91. Jervell, A., and Lange-Nielsen, F.: Congenital deaf-mutism, functional heart disease with prolongation of the Q-T interval, and sudden death. Am. Heart J., 54:59, 1957.

92. Romano, C., Gemme, G., and Pongiglione, R.: Aritmie cardiacherare dell'eta pediatrica. Clin. Pediatr., 45:656, 1963.

93. Ward, O. C.: New familial cardiac syndrome in children. J. Irish Med. Assoc., 54:103, 1964.

94. Kulbertus, H. E.: The arrhythmogenic effects of anti-arrhythmic agents. In Befeler, B. (Ed.): Selected Topics in Cardiac Arrhythmias. Mount Kisco, N. Y., Futura Publishing, 1980, p. 113.

95. Moss, A. J., and McDonald, J.: Unilateral cervicothoracic sympathetic ganglionectomy for the treatment of long Q-T interval syndrome. N. Engl. J. Med., 285:903, 1971.

96. Schwartz, P. J., Periti, M., and Malliani, A.: The long Q-T syndrome. Fund. Clin. Cardiol., 89:378, 1975.

97. Smith, W., and Gallagher, J. J.: Q-T prolongation syndromes. Pract. Cardiol., 5:118, 1979.

98. Malliani, A., Schwartz, P. J., and Zanchetti, A.: Neural mechanisms and life-threatening arrhythmias. Am. Heart J., *100*:705, 1980.

99. Benson, D. W., Jr., and Cox, J. L.: Surgical treatment of cardiac arrhythmias. *In* Roberts, N. K., and Gelband, H. (Eds.): Cardiac Arrhythmias in the Neonate, Infant and Child, 2nd ed. New York, Appleton-Century-Crofts, 1982, pp. 341–366.

100. Bhandari, A. K., Scheinman, M. M., Morady, F., Svinarich, J., Mason, J., and Winkle, R.: Efficacy of left cardiac sympathectomy in the treatment of patients with the long QT syndrome. Circulation, *70*:1018, 1984.

101. Lewis, T.: The experimental production of paroxysmal tachycardia and the effects of ligation of the coronary arteries. Heart, *1*:98, 1909.

102. Couch, O. A., Jr.: Cardiac aneurysm with ventricular tachycardia and subsequent excision of aneurysm. Circulation, *20*:251, 1959.

103. Durrer, D., Schoo, L., Schuilenburg, R. M., and Wellens, H. J. J.: The role of premature beats in the initiation and the termination of supraventricular tachycardia in the Wolff-Parkinson-White syndrome. Circulation, *36*:644, 1967.

104. Coumel, P., Cabarol, C., Fabiato, A., Gourgon, R., and Slama, R.: Tachycardia permanente par rythme reçiproque. Arch. Mal. Coeur, *60*:1830, 1967.

105. Cox, J. L., McLaughlin, V. W., Flowers, N. C., and Horan, L. G.: The ischemic zone surrounding acute myocardial infarction: Its morphology as detected by dehydrogenase staining. Am. Heart J., *76*:650, 1968.

106. Cox, J. L., Daniel, T. M., Sabiston, D. C., Jr., and Boineau, J. P.: Desynchronized activation in myocardial infarction: A re-entry basis for ventricular arrhythmias (Abstract). Circulation, *39*(Suppl. 3):63, 1969.

107. Han, J., Gael, B. G., and Hansen, C. S.: Re-entrant beats induced in the ventricle during coronary occlusion. Am. Heart J., *80*:778, 1970.

108. Durrer, D., van Dam, R. T., Freud, G. E., and Janse, M. J.: Re-entry and ventricular arrhythmias in local ischemia and infarction of the intact dog heart. Proc. K. Ned. Akad. Wet. Series C. (Biol. Med.), *74*:321, 1971.

109. Boineau, J. P., and Cox, J. L.: Slow ventricular activation in acute myocardial infarction: A source of re-entrant premature ventricular contractions. Circulation, *48*:702, 1973.

110. Waldo, A. L., and Kaiser, G. A.: A study of ventricular arrhythmias associated with acute myocardial infarction in the canine heart. Circulation, *47*:1222, 1973.

111. Scherlag, B. J., El-Sherif, N., Hopen, R. R., and Lazzara, R.: Characterization and localization of ventricular arrhythmias resulting from myocardial ischemia and infarction. Circ. Res., *35*:372, 1974.

112. El-Sherif, N., Scherlag, B. J., Lazzara, R., and Hopen, R. R.: Re-entrant ventricular arrhythmias in the late myocardial infarction period: I. Conduction characteristics of the infarction zone. Circulation, *55*:686, 1977.

113. Boineau, J. P., and Cox, J. L.: Rationale for a direct surgical approach to control ventricular arrhythmias. Am. J. Cardiol., *49*:381, 1982.

114. Daniel, T. M., Cox, J. L., Sabiston, D. C., Jr., and Boineau, J. P.: Epicardial and intramural mapping activation of the human heart: A technique for localizing infarction and ischemia of the myocardium (Abstract). Circulation, *40*(Suppl. III):III-66, 1969.

115. Kaiser, G. A., Waldo, A. L., Harris, P. D., Bowman, F. O., Jr., Hoffman, B. F., and Malm, J. R.: New method to delineate myocardial damage at surgery. Circulation, *39*(Suppl. I):83, 1969.

116. Fontaine, G., Frank, R., and Guiraudon, G.: Surgical treatment of resistant re-entrant ventricular tachycardia by ventriculotomy: A new application of epicardial mapping (Abstract). Circulation, *50*(Suppl. III):III-82, 1974.

117. Wittig, J. H., and Boineau, J. P.: Surgical treatment of ventricular arrhythmias using epicardial transmural and endocardial mapping. Ann. Thorac. Surg., *20*:117, 1975.

118. Gallagher, J. J., Oldham, H. N., Jr., Wallace, A. G., Peter, R. H., and Kasell, J.: Ventricular aneurysm with ventricular tachycardia: Report of a case with epicardial mapping and successful resection. Am. J. Cardiol., *35*:696, 1975.

119. Guiraudon, G., Fontaine, G., Frank, R., Escande, G., Etievent, P., and Cabrol, C.: Encircling endocardial ventriculotomy: A new surgical treatment of life-threatening ventricular tachycardias resistant to medical treatment following myocardial infarction. Ann. Thorac. Surg., *26*:438, 1978.

120. Josephson, M. E., Harken, A. H., and Horowitz, L. N.: Endocardial excision—a new surgical technique for the treatment of recurrent ventricular tachycardia. Circulation, *60*:1430, 1979.

121. Jatene, A. D.: Left ventricular aneurysmectomy: Resection or reconstruction. J. Thorac. Cardiovasc. Surg., *89*:321, 1985.

122. Dor, V., Saab, M., Coste, P., Kornaszewska, M., and Montiglio, F.: Left ventricular aneurysm: A new surgical approach. Thorac. Cardiovasc. Surg., *37*:11, 1989.

123. Horowitz, L. N., Josephson, M. E., and Harken, A. H.: Epicardial and endocardial activation during sustained ventricular tachycardia in man. Circulation, *61*:1227, 1980.

124. Miller, J. M., Kienzle, M. G., Harken, A. H., and Josephson, M. E.: Subendocardial resection for ventricular tachycardia: Predictors of surgical success. Circulation, *70*:624, 1984.

125. Harada, A., D'Agostino, H. J., Jr., Schuessler, R. B., Boineau, J. P., and Cox, J. L.: Potential distribution mapping: A new method for precise localization of the intramural septal origin of ventricular tachycardia. Circulation, *78*:III-137, 1988.

126. Harada, A., Tweddell, J., Schuessler, R. B., Branham, B. H., Boineau, J. P., and Cox, J. L.: Computerized potential distribution mapping: A new intraoperative mapping technique for ventricular tachycardia surgery. Ann. Thorac. Surg., *49*:649, 1990.

127. Tweddell, J. S., Harada, A., Schuessler, R. B., Stone, C. M., Rokkas, C. K., Branham, B. H., Boineau, J. P., and Cox, J. L.: Computerized potential distribution mapping for rapid localization of ventricular tachycardia of septal origin. Surg. Forum, *39*:257, 1988.

128. Tweddell, J. S., Branham, B. H., Harada, A., Stone, C. M., Rokkas, C. K., Schuessler, R. B., Boineau, J. P., and Cox, J. L.: Potential mapping in septal tachycardia: Evaluation of a new intraoperative mapping technique. Circulation, *80*(Suppl. I):I-97, 1989.

129. Tweddell, J. S., Branham, B. H., Stone, C. M., Schuessler, R. B., Boineau, J. P., and Cox, J. L.: Focal cryoablation guided solely by intraoperative potential mapping ablates ventricular tachycardia of endocardial origin. Surg. Forum, *40*:216, 1989.

130. Moran, J. M., Kehoe, R. F., Loeb, J. M., Frederickson, J. W., Zheutlin, T. A., Sanders, J. H., Jr., and Michaelis, L. L.: The role of papillary muscle resection and mitral valve replacement in the control of refractory ventricular arrhythmia. Circulation, *68*:II-154, 1983.

131. Cox, J. L.: Anatomic-electrophysiologic basis for the surgical treatment of refractory ischemic ventricular tachycardia. Ann. Surg., *198*:119, 1983.

132. Cox, J. L.: Surgical treatment of ischemic and non-ischemic ventricular tachyarrhythmias. *In* Cohn, L. H. (Ed.): Modern Technics in Surgery. Mount Kisco, N.Y., Futura Publishing, 1985.

XX

CARDIAC NEOPLASMS

Norman A. Silverman, M.D., and David C. Sabiston, Jr., M.D.

INCIDENCE AND CLINICAL PRESENTATION

The rarity of primary cardiac tumors is evidenced by an autopsy incidence ranging between 0.002% and 0.33%. In the Armed Forces Institute of Pathology's series of over 500 tumors,[19] 80% are benign, with myxoma being by far the most common. The malignant tumors are predominantly various forms of sarcoma. However, this incidence varies with age, with malignant neoplasms constituting less than 10% of primary cardiac tumors in children. In contrast, tumors metastatic to the heart and pericardium are 20 to 30 times more common than primary lesions, because 10% to 20% of patients with known malignancy have secondary involvement at autopsy.[27, 28]

The clinical manifestations of cardiac tumors are protean.[6] Cardiac performance can be compromised when an intracavitary tumor obstructs flow through the cardiac chambers or interferes with valvular function, when an intramural tumor infiltrates and destroys ventricular myocardium, or when neoplastic pericarditis causes effusion with tamponade or constriction. Systemic emboli from left-sided heart lesions, especially left atrial myxoma, are common, but right-sided heart tumors may embolize the pulmonary arteries. Particularly in the pediatric age group, cardiac tumors may cause recurrent supraventricular or ventricular arrhythmias or, less often, infiltrate the conduction system, causing heart block and sudden death.[11, 14] Most intriguing are the systemic constitutional symptoms of fever, malaise, weight loss, polymyo-

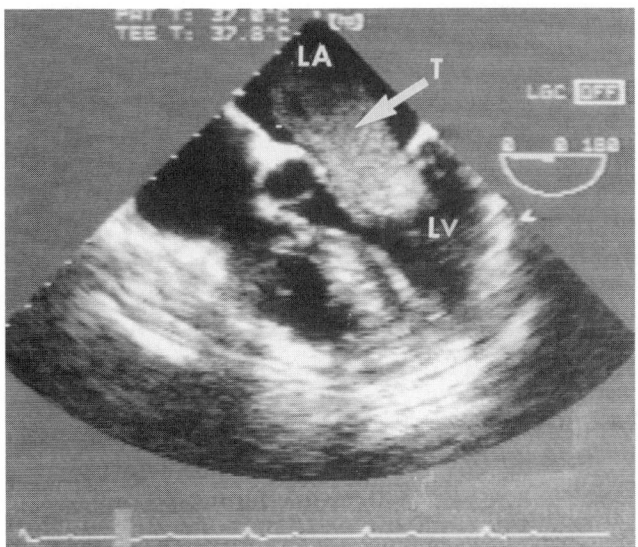

Figure 54–196. Two-dimensional echocardiogram shows a large intracavitary tumor (T) obstructing the mitral orifice. At surgery, this was the myxoma shown in Figure 54–200*A.* LA, left atrium; LV, left ventricle. (Courtesy of Moshin Alam, M.D., Henry Ford Hospital.)

sitis, hepatic dysfunction, Raynaud's phenomenon, hyperglobulinemia, and elevated erythrocyte sedimentation rate that have been noted, particularly with left atrial myxomas. That such manifestations may reflect an autoimmune response is suspected by the recent demonstration of both tumor-specific and histocompatibility antigens on surgically extirpated cardiac myxoma tissue.[18] Whatever the exact immunopathology, these systemic symptoms promptly abate after tumor resection.

DIAGNOSTIC MODALITIES

Echocardiography is the technique of choice in the initial evaluation of an intracardiac tumor. It is widely available at the bedside as well as in the laboratory, rapidly performed, noninvasive, and relatively inexpensive. Although the M-mode technique was introduced first, improved accuracy for real-time imaging of all cardiac chambers and more precise quantitation of tumor size, shape, location, consistency, and mobility is afforded by two-dimensional echocardiography

(Fig. 54–196).[4] Transesophageal probe placement is well suited for intraoperative usage but does not provide sufficient improvement in diagnostic accuracy to warrant routine application because of patient discomfort and potential morbidity compared with transthoracic imaging. Concomitant Doppler color-flow imaging techniques can assess valvular dysfunction caused by tumor encroachment. Findings suggestive of intracavitary tumor occur in 95% of patients examined by echocardiography and provide sufficient information to pre-empt the need, risk, and expense of further diagnostic studies before surgical intervention.[6] Whereas previously cardiac catheterization and angiography were used to visualize intracavitary defects, these invasive procedures have been supplanted by noninvasive imaging, and patients are no longer subjected to the inherent risk of tumor embolization associated with intracardiac manipulation. Unresolved is the need for coronary angiography before surgical therapy for asymptomatic patients at risk for occult coronary artery disease.

For certain patients, additional diagnostic studies are warranted. Excessive mitral valvular calcifications and lipomatous atrial septal hypertrophy can mimic an intracavitary mass. Intramural tumors are nonechogenic, and extracavitary origin or extension may not be seen in their entirety by ultrasonic imaging. With the introduction of electrocardiographic gating and ultrafast scanners, computed tomography is an alternative for imaging cardiac tumors. Contrast medium enhancement allows cardiac and intracardiac structures to be differentiated from blood, and image reconstruction reveals cardiac anatomy in three dimensions. Computed tomography is best used for showing the myocardial and intrapericardial extension of tumor (Fig. 54–197). Magnetic resonance imaging is a newer technique that also enables high-resolution tomography in three dimensions. Unlike computed tomography, magnetic resonance imaging is nonionizing and generates tissue contrast without the need for injecting contrast medium (Fig. 54–198). However, the expense and limited availability of this technology preclude usage as the primary diagnostic modality despite its potent and reliable imaging ability.

BENIGN TUMORS

Approximately 50% of benign primary cardiac tumors are *myxomas.* The typical patient is a middle-aged woman (70%) with a solitary, left atrial tumor (75%). The right atrium is the other common site for myxomas (20%). The majority of

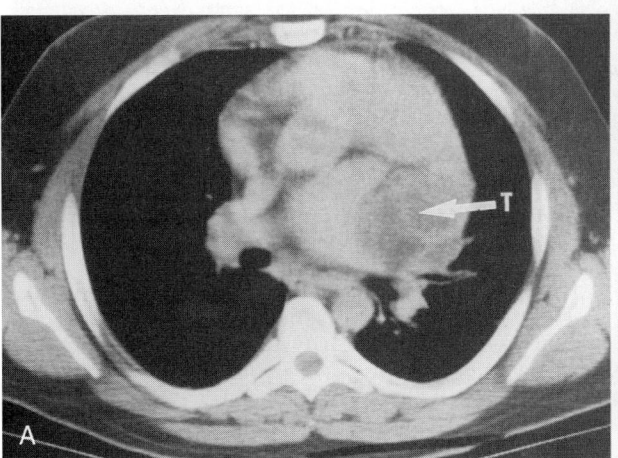

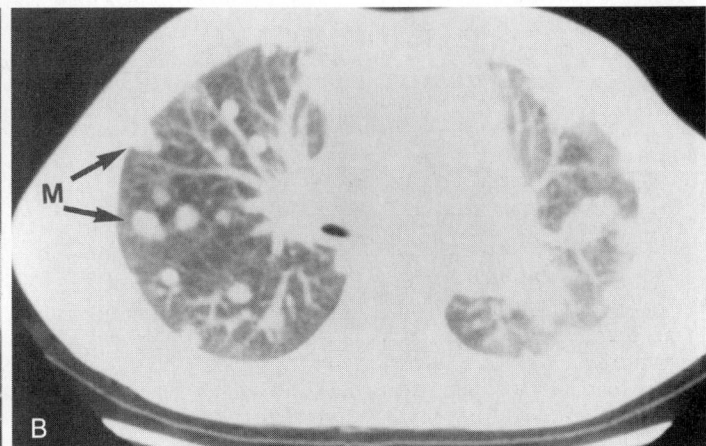

Figure 54–197. *A,* Computed tomographic scan with contrast medium enhancement of a malignant tumor (T) encroaching on the left atrium. Biopsy specimen showed angiosarcoma. *B,* Multiple pulmonary metastases (M) were present at initial clinical presentation. (*A* and *B* courtesy of David Spizarny, M.D., Henry Ford Hospital.)

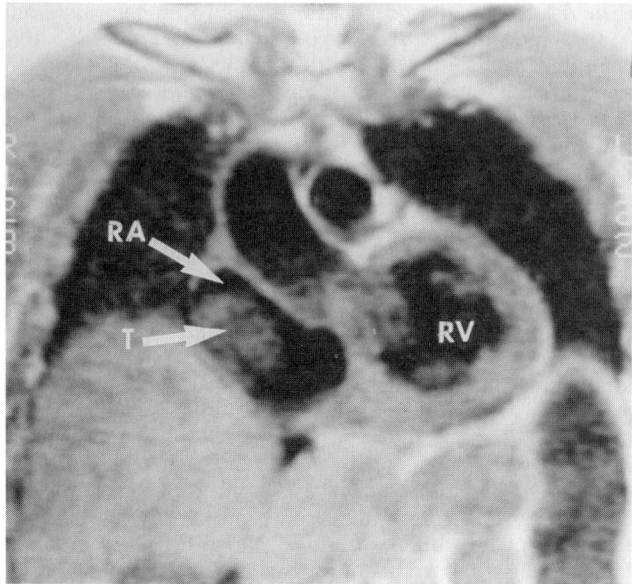

Figure 54–198. Magnetic resonance image of a tumor (T) obstructing the tricuspid orifice. This proved to be a myxoma. RA, right atrium; RV, right ventricle. (Courtesy of David Spizarny, M.D., Henry Ford Hospital.)

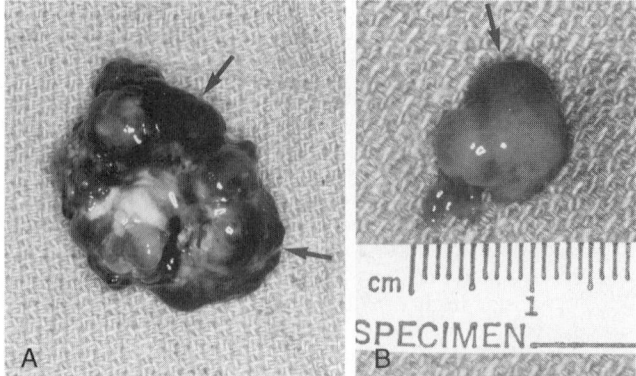

Figure 54–200. Gross appearance of typical myxoma. A, Large multilobulated tumor. B, Small, smooth-surfaced left ventricular tumor. Arrows point to area of hemorrhage.

atrial lesions arise from the interatrial septum in the region of the fossa ovalis but may arise from the lateral or posterior walls (Fig. 54–199). Ventricular myxomas are rare and arise from the outflow tract or interventricular septum. Exceptions to these generalizations are the predilection for young children (those younger than 5 years of age) to have right atrial tumors[8] and patients with a familial, complex myxomatous syndrome.[30] Fifteen families have been described whose members have the inheritable constellation of cutaneous and cardiac myxomas, lentiginosis, and multiple endocrine neoplasms, including pituitary, adrenal, and testicular tumors. This younger, predominantly male cohort of patients often

has multicentric intracardiac tumors occurring in unusual locations and prone to recurrence. The aggressive biologic behavior of these *syndrome* myxomas may be explained by abnormal DNA tetraploid patterns noted by flow cytometry of excised tumor tissue.[20]

Most myxomas are friable, multilobulated masses attached to the endocardial surface by a fibrovascular stalk that permits tumor mobility during the cardiac cycle. However, smaller tumors may have a smooth surface (Fig. 54–200). Of surgical significance is the fact that myxomas rarely extend deeper than the endocardium but enlarge, filling the cardiac chamber. All have a gelatinous consistency, with frequent areas of hemorrhage and necrosis seen on cut section. Microscopically, polyhedral cells with small, round nuclei are separated by an afibrillar, eosinophilic acid mucopolysaccharide. Although benign tumors, myxomas have been reported to undergo malignant degeneration with systemic metastases.[27]

Because they often obstruct the mitral orifice and produce systemic emboli, left atrial myxomas frequently masquerade as rheumatic mitral stenosis. Up to one half of patients have

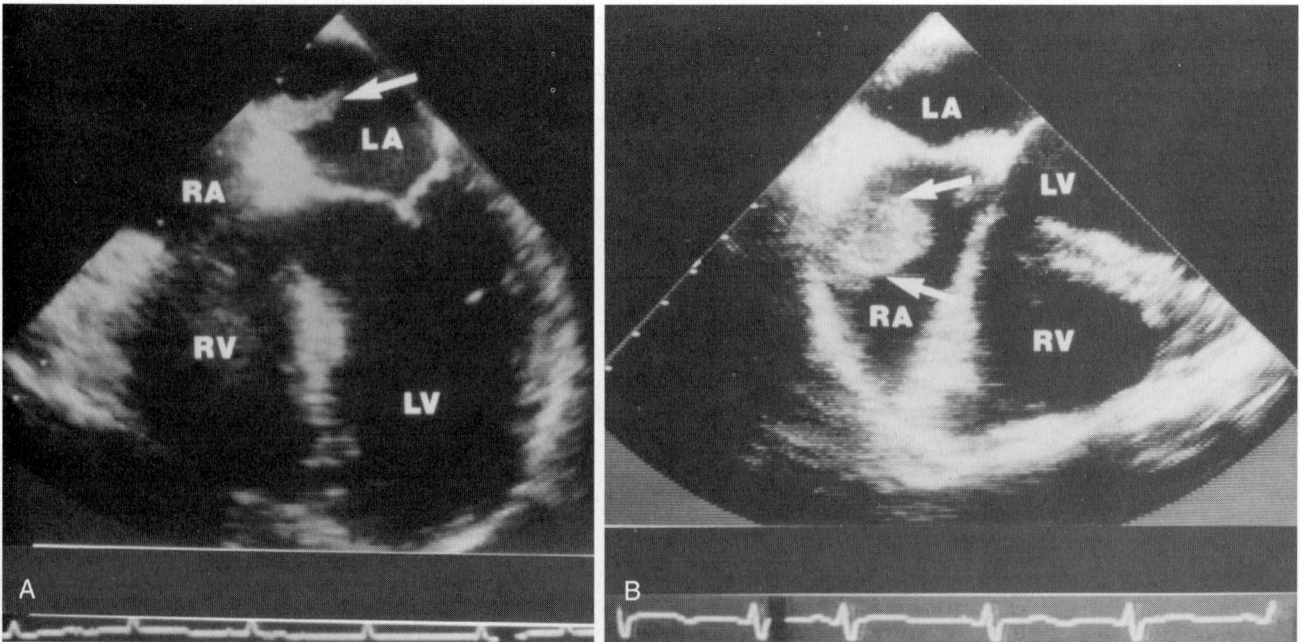

Figure 54–199. A, Transesophageal echocardiogram of small left atrial myxoma (arrow) originating from atrial septum. RA, right atrium; RV, right ventricle; LV, left ventricle. B, Right atrial myxoma (arrows) originating from lateral wall as imaged by intraoperative transesophageal echocardiography. LA, left atrium; LV, left ventricle; RA, right atrium; RV, right ventricle. (B courtesy of Moshin Alam, M.D., Henry Ford Hospital.)

some form of systemic emboli, most often to the brain, kidneys, and lower extremities. Therefore, any specimen surgically extracted from the arterial system should be sent for pathologic examination, because this is often the presenting manifestation of a cardiac myxoma. In addition, any patient younger than 40 years of age who has evidence of arterial embolism and is in sinus rhythm should be screened for myxoma by echocardiography, regardless of the presence or absence of precordial murmurs. When constitutional symptoms predominate, infective endocarditis, collagen vascular disease, and occult malignancy or infection enter the differential diagnosis. Right atrial myxomas produce signs and symptoms by obstructing vena caval return or the tricuspid valve. Less often, tumor embolization to the pulmonary vasculature causes chest pain, cough, and dyspnea. The differential diagnosis includes rheumatic tricuspid valve disease, constrictive pericarditis, myocardiopathy, Ebstein's anomaly, and carcinoid heart disease. The rare ventricular myxomas may induce syncope due to transient obstruction of ventricular ejection or cause embolization. Ventricular lesions must be differentiated from other causes of valvular or subvalvular stenosis.

Rhabdomyoma is a congenital, glycogen-rich hamartoma that is the most common cardiac tumor of childhood and accounts for 20% of all benign primary cardiac tumors.[19] Most often manifested in infancy, one half of the patients have tuberous sclerosis. The lesions are most often multicentric, ventricular masses that cause recurrent tachyarrhythmias. Because of their usual multiplicity, poor encapsulation, and deep myocardial location, rhabdomyomas are most often unresectable by standard surgical techniques. For most patients, the prognosis is poor and survival beyond infancy is unusual. However, electrophysiologic mapping has allowed cryoablation of arrhythmogenic foci in a small selected series of infants.[14] Similarly, the rare cardiac *fibromas* are amenable to surgical cure when limited to the right ventricular chamber.[24, 31] *Mesothelioma* is a lethal congenital tumor that selectively destroys the atrioventricular node, resulting in sudden death.[11] *Lipoma* is classically an epicardial tumor easily approached without the need for cardiopulmonary bypass, but an intracavitary location has been reported. Hemangioma, lymphangioma, teratoma, chemodectoma, neurilemmoma, nerve sheath and nerve cell tumors, and granular cell myoblastoma have also been reported to arise from the heart. Lambl's excrescences and simple cysts can arise from the cardiac valves but rarely are of physiologic consequence.[7] In contrast, intracardiac papillary fibroelastoma on either left-sided heart valve does embolize and is an uncommon source of occult cerebral emboli.[13, 21]

MANAGEMENT

The diagnosis of a primary cardiac tumor mandates prompt operative intervention. Minimal tumor manipulation during cannulation and before aortic cross-clamping is critical to prevent perioperative tumor dislodgment and embolization. Antegrade rather than retrograde cardioplegic delivery may be preferable for similar reasons. Right-sided myxomas are approached through the appropriate chamber. Left atrial myxomas can be approached through a standard left atriotomy posterior to the interatrial groove, biatrial incision or transseptal incision guided by intraoperative transesophageal echocardiography, depending on atrial size and tumor location.[6, 12] Adequate excision includes a margin of normal atrial septum around the tumor stalk to prevent local recurrence. An aortotomy with retraction of the aortic valve is the preferable access for removal of left ventricular lesions. In addition, these lesions can be approached through the mitral valve. Ventriculotomy through normal myocardium

should be avoided. All resections should be complete, but zealous removal of normal myocardium or trauma to intrinsically normal valvular apparatus should be avoided. Rarely, extensive reconstruction of the right atrial wall and prosthetic valve replacement are necessary for curative excision of large tumors,[23] and cardiac transplantation is a feasible alternative for an otherwise unresectable tumor.

In studies comprising over 300 patients, operative mortality was less than 2% for excision of benign tumors.[5, 6, 17, 22, 23, 26] The most common postoperative complication is atrial dysrhythmia; however, permanent rhythm disturbances are rare. After complete tumor resection, the prognosis is excellent, with less than 1% recurrence, except in patients with complex or familial myxoma, which have a significantly worse prognosis.

MALIGNANT TUMORS

Malignant tumors are almost always some variant of sarcoma that originates from the right atrium or less frequently from the right ventricle and rapidly grows to infiltrate all layers of the heart, invade adjacent mediastinal structures, and metastasize widely.[6, 27] Systemic metastases are present in 80% of patients at the time of diagnosis. Sudden death or rapid vena caval obstruction is not uncommon. Angiosarcoma and rhabdomyosarcoma are the usual histologic types, but a precise histologic classification is not only difficult but also of little practical significance because the clinical picture and prognosis are comparable with progressive, unrelenting congestive heart failure, chest pain, fever, and hemopericardium. When the diagnosis is made at exploratory surgery, the growth pattern of these lesions most often makes them unresectable (see Fig. 54–197). Recent reviews document a median survival of less than 1 year despite surgical intervention, if feasible, and postoperative chemotherapy and/or irradiation.[1, 3, 10, 25]

METASTATIC TUMORS

An increase in cardiac metastases has occurred and relates to prolonged survival from prior surgical intervention and combined-modality therapy. Tumors that most frequently metastasize to the heart include lung and breast carcinoma, as well as leukemia, lymphoma, and melanoma.[28] Twenty-five to 50% of these patients have cardiac involvement at autopsy. The myocardium and pericardium are involved with equal frequency by embolic hematogenous and retrograde lymphatic spread of tumor (Fig. 54–201). The pericardium can also be invaded by direct extension of adjacent intrathoracic malignancies, in particular, bronchogenic carcinoma. Myocardial metastases often cause rhythm disturbances or congestive heart failure if extensive infiltration of myocardial mass by tumor has occurred. Pericardial metastases produce inflammation, hemorrhagic effusion, tamponade, or cardiac constriction. Noninvasive imaging by echocardiography, or, more recently, computed tomography, is helpful to delineate the feasibility of surgical intervention, to establish a tissue diagnosis, or to decompress symptomatic pericardial effusion. Relief of tamponade is easily accomplished by a subxiphoid approach. Aggressive debulking of constrictive or bulky pericardial tumor is unwarranted and ineffective. Unfortunately, pericardial involvement heralds limited survival. However, in carefully selected patients, surgical resection of solitary metastases to the right ventricular outflow tract has provided worthwhile survival.[15] In contrast, operative intervention for tumors metastatic to the heart is best reserved for intra-atrial extensions of hypernephroma or Wilms' tumor. Although some surgeons have utilized profound hypothermia and circulatory arrest for cavoatrial tumor thrombec-

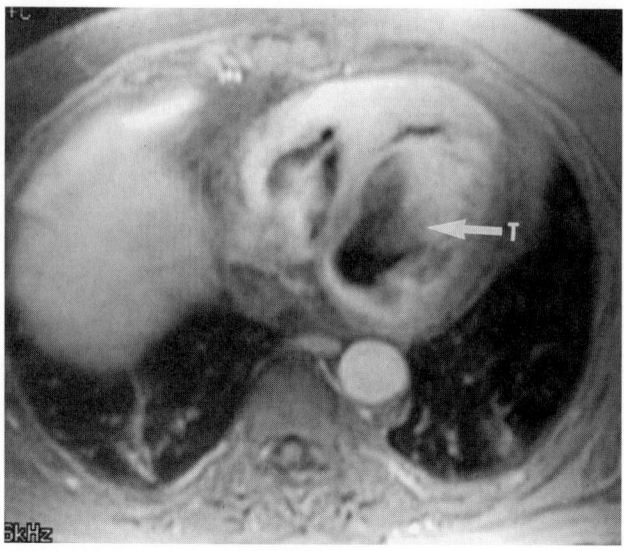

Figure 54–201. Magnetic resonance image of a tumor (T) infiltrating left ventricular wall and encroaching on the chamber cavity. This is a metastatic renal cell carcinoma. (Courtesy of David Spizarny, M.D., Henry Ford Hospital.)

tomy, standard cardiopulmonary bypass provides satisfactory visualization and avoids the potential deleterious complications of cerebral and renal dysfunction associated with total circulatory arrest.[29]

SELECTED REFERENCES

Chitwood, W. R.: Cardiac neoplasms: Current diagnosis, pathology and therapy. J. Cardiac. Surg., 3:119, 1988.

This is a comprehensive review of all aspects of benign and malignant cardiac tumors. The illustrations are superb, and the references are comprehensive and still valuable. The newer imaging modalities are emphasized, and operative techniques are detailed.

Edwards, F. H., Hale, D., Cohen, A., Thompson, L., Pezella, A. T., and Virmani, R.: Primary cardiac valve tumors. Ann. Thorac. Surg., 52:1127, 1991.

This multi-institutional experience is the largest report of the clinical characteristics of primary valve tumors. Although previous anecdotal papers suggested the pathological curiosity of these lesions, this paper emphasizes the propensity of valve tumors to result in serious clinical sequelae and the fact that they constitute a clinical entity with more important differences than extravalvular cardiac tumors.

McAllister, A., and Fenoglio, J. J.: Tumors of the cardiovascular system. In: Atlas of Tumor Pathology. Washington, D.C., Armed Forces Institute of Pathology, 1978, 2nd series, fascicle 15.

This classic article remains the largest published modern series of benign and malignant primary neoplasms in adults and children. Data are derived from the collection of cardiac tumors at the Armed Forces Institute of Pathology. The authors are leading authorities on the subject, and this article is one of the definitive works on tumor pathology.

Miralles, A., Bracamonte, L., Soncul, H., del Castillo, R. D., Akhtar, R., Bors, V., Pavie, A., Gandjbackhch, I., and Cabrol, C.: Cardiac tumors: Clinical experience and surgical results in 74 patients. Ann. Thorac. Surg. 52:886, 1991.

This article details a large clinical experience in the modern era of both diagnostics and therapeutics with long-term follow-up of both benign and malignant lesions. A wide spectrum of lesions are reported, not just myxomas. The excellent results with benign tumors after resection and the limited success with malignancies despite combined modality therapy are documented.

Murphy, M. C., Sweeney, M. S., Putnam, J. B., Walker, W. E., Frazier, O. H., Ott, D. A., and Cooley, D. A.: Surgical treatment of cardiac tumors: A 25-year experience. Ann. Thorac. Surg., 49:612, 1990.

This is the largest series of surgically treated patients reported, comprising 133 patients. All forms of operative therapy are described, ranging from biopsy to complete excision. The use of hypothermic circulatory arrest and cardiac autotransplantation for selected patients is outlined.

REFERENCES

1. Antunes, M. J., Vanderdonck, K. M., Andrade, C. M., and Rebelo, L. S.: Primary cardiac leiomyosarcomas. Ann. Thorac. Surg., 51:999, 1991.
2. Aufiero, T. X., Pae, W. E., Jr., Clemson, B. S., Pawlush, D. G., and Davis, D.: Heart transplantation for tumor. Ann. Thorac. Surg., 56:1171, 1993.
3. Bear, P. A., and Moodie, D. S.: Malignant primary cardiac tumors. Chest, 92:858, 1987.
4. Bogren, H. G., DeMaria, A. N., and Mason, D. T.: Imaging procedures in the detection of cardiac tumors with emphasis on echocardiography: A review. Cardiovasc. Intervent. Radiol., 3:107, 1980.
5. Bortolotti, U., Maraglino, G., Rubino, M., Santini, F., Mazzucco, A., Milano, A., Fasoli, G., Livi, U., Thiene, G., and Gallucci, V.: Surgical excision of intracardiac myxomas: A 20-year follow-up. Ann. Thorac. Surg., 49:449, 1990.
6. Chitwood, W. R.: Cardiac neoplasms: Current diagnosis, pathology and therapy. J. Cardiac. Surg., 3:119, 1988.
7. Edwards, F. H., Hale, D., Cohen, A., Thompson, L., Pezella, A. T., and Virmani, R.: Primary cardiac valve tumors. Ann. Thorac. Surg., 52:1127, 1991.
8. Ergina, P. L., Kochamba, G. S., Tchervenkov, C. I., and Gibbons, J. E.: Atrial myxomas in young children: An alternative surgical approach. Ann. Thorac. Surg., 56:1180, 1993.
9. Freedberg, R. S., Kronzon, I., Rumancik, W. M., and Liebeskind, D.: The contribution of magnetic resonance imaging to the evaluation of intracardiac tumors diagnosed by echocardiography. Circulation, 77:96, 1988.
10. Herrmann, M. A., Shankerman, R. A., Edwards, W. D., Shub, C., and Schaff, H. V.: Primary cardiac angiosarcoma: A clinicopathologic study of six cases. J. Thorac. Cardiovasc. Surg., 103:655, 1992.
11. James, T. N., and Galakhov, I.: De Subitaneis Mortibus XXVI. Fatal electrical instability of the heart associated with benign congenital polycystic tumor of the atrioventricular node. Circulation, 56:667, 1977.
12. Kabbani, S. S., Jokhadar, M., Meada, R., Hisham, J., Abdun, F., Sandouk, A., and Nabhani, F.: Atrial myxoma: Report of 24 operations using the biatrial approach. Ann. Thorac. Surg., 58:483, 1994.
13. Kasarskis, E. J., O'Connor, W., and Earle, G.: Embolic stroke from cardiac papillary fibroelastomas. Stroke, 19:1171, 1988.
14. Kearney, D. L., Titus, J. L., Hawkins, E. P., Ott, D. A., and Garson, A.: Pathologic features of myocardial hamartomas causing childhood tachyarrhythmias. Circulation, 75:705, 1987.
15. Labib, S. B., Schick, E. C., Jr., and Isner, J. M.: Obstruction of right ventricular outflow tract caused by intracavitary metastatic disease: Analysis of 14 cases. J. Am. Coll. Cardiol., 19:1664, 1992.
16. Larsson, S., Lepore, V., and Kennergren, C.: Atrial myxomas: Results of 25 years' experience and review of the literature. Surgery, 105:695, 1989.
17. Lazarra, R. R., Park, S. B., and Magovern, G. J.: Cardiac myxomas: Results of surgical treatment. J. Cardiovasc. Surg., 32:824, 1991.
18. Magee, M. J., Pham, S. M., Sapun, S., Zeevi, A., and Hattler, B. G.: Characterization of the immune response to cardiac myxomas. Surg. Forum., 44:218, 1993.
19. McAllister, A., and Fenoglio, J. J.: Tumors of the cardiovascular system. In: Atlas of Tumor Pathology, Washington, D.C., Armed Forces Institute of Pathology, 1978, 2nd series, fascicle 15.
20. McCarthy, P. M., Schaff, H. V., Winkler, H. Z., Lieber, M. M., and Carney, J. A.: Deoxyribonucleic acid ploidy pattern of cardiac myxomas. J. Thorac. Cardiovasc. Surg., 98:1083, 1989.
21. McFadden, P. M., and Lacy, J. R.: Intracardiac papillary fibroelastoma: An occult cause of embolic neurologic deficit. Ann. Thorac. Surg., 43:667, 1987.
22. Miralles, A., Bracamonte, L., Soncul, H., del Castillo, R. D., Akhtar, R., Bors, V., Pavie, A., Gandjbackhch, I., and Cabrol, C.: Cardiac tumors: Clinical experience and surgical results in 74 patients. Ann. Thorac. Surg., 52:886, 1991.
23. Murphy, M. C., Sweeney, M. S., Putnam, J. B., Jr., Walker, W. E., Frazier, O. H., Ott, D. A., and Cooley, D. A.: Surgical treatment of cardiac tumors: A 25-year experience. Ann. Thorac. Surg., 49:612, 1990.
24. Parmley, L. F., Salley, R. K., Williams, J. P., and Head, G. B., III: The clinical

spectrum of cardiac fibroma with diagnostic and surgical considerations: Noninvasive imaging enhances management. Ann. Thorac. Surg., 45:455, 1988.

25. Putnam, J. B., Jr., Sweeney, M. S., Colon, R., Lanza, L. A., Frazier, O. H., and Cooley, D. A.: Primary cardiac sarcomas. Ann. Thorac. Surg., 51:906, 1991.

26. Sellke, F. W., Lemmer, J. H., Jr., Vandenberg, B. F., and Ehrenhaft, J. L.: Surgical treatment of cardiac myxomas: Long-term results. Ann. Thorac. Surg., 50:557, 1990.

27. Silverman, N. A.: Primary cardiac tumors. Ann. Surg., 191:127, 1980.

28. Stark, R. M., Perloff, J. K., Glick, J. H., Hirshfield, J. W., Jr., and Devereux, R. B.: Clinical recognition and management of cardiac metastatic disease. Am. J. Med., 63:653, 1977.

29. Stewart, J. R., Carey, J. A., McCall, W. S., Merrill, W. H., Koch, M. O., and Bender, H. W., Jr.: Cavoatrial tumor thrombectomy using cardiopulmonary bypass without circulatory arrest. Ann. Thorac. Surg., 51:717, 1991.

30. van Gelder, H. M., O'Brien, D. J., Staples, E. D., and Alexander, J. A.: Familial cardiac myxoma. Ann. Thorac. Surg., 53:419, 1992.

31. Yamaguchi, M., Hosokawa, Y., Ohashi, H., Imai, M., Oshima, Y., and Minamiji, K.: Cardiac fibroma. J. Thorac. Cardiovasc. Surg., 103:140, 1992.

XXI

CARDIAC PACEMAKERS

James E. Lowe, M.D.

FUNCTIONAL ANATOMY OF THE NORMAL CARDIAC CONDUCTION SYSTEM

The sinoatrial (SA) node is a group of specialized cells located subepicardially at the lateral junction of the superior vena cava within the right atrium, although some anatomic variation may occur with extension of the node anteriorly across the caval-atrial junction. The SA node extends for several centimeters along the crista terminalis to the mid-high posterolateral right atrium. It is especially vulnerable to surgical trauma because of its location. Three types of cells can be found in the human SA node, in addition to supporting elements of fibrocytes, nerves, and vessels. Pacemaker or polygonal cells are polyhedral and contain prominent nuclei and sparse numbers of contractile elements. These cells are believed to be the site of impulse formation in the SA node, although electrophysiologic confirmation in humans is lacking. Transitional cells are found surrounding pacemaker cells and interposed between nodal cells and atrial myocardium. These cells have some features of both nodal cells and myocardial cells, with larger numbers of contractile elements. Atrial myocardial cells with prominent longitudinally oriented myofibrils may also be found in SA node tissue.

The atrioventricular (AV) node is located subendocardially in the triangle of Koch, an anatomic region on the medial wall of the right atrium formed by the tendon of Todaro, the eustachian valve of the coronary sinus, and the tricuspid anulus. The AV node is composed of a transitional zone and a compact zone. Transitional cells gradually merge into the compact zone that rests along the most inferior portion of the interatrial septum. Three distinct inputs of transitional cells into the AV node have been identified—posterior, right septal, and left septal inputs.

There are probably three preferential pathways of interatrial conduction between the SA node and the AV node.[25] The posterior internodal pathway, which is the crista terminalis, extends from the SA node to merge with the posterior input to the AV node in the region of the coronary sinus ostium. The middle and anterior preferential interatrial pathways extend from the SA node across the posterior and anterior interatrial septum to provide the right septal input to the AV node. Although the orientation of atrial muscle fibers appears to produce preferential pathways of conduction, evidence for functionally distinct conduction pathways across the atrium from the SA node is lacking in humans.

The compact AV nodal cells can be identified along the length of Koch's triangle, with the greatest proportion anteriorly. From the anular side of the small compact AV nodal cells, large, linear Purkinje cells gradually emerge and coalesce to form the penetrating bundle of His within the central fibrous body. The His bundle courses a short distance along the crest of the muscular interventricular septum below the membranous septum to branch into the right and left bundle branches. The right bundle branch is a discrete fascicle that runs along the endocardial surface of the right ventricular septum to the moderator band where initial branches to the apical septum exit. The right bundle then provides a dense network of Purkinje fibers across the right ventricular endocardium. The left bundle branch is occasionally a discrete fascicle of approximately 1 cm. in length, but more usually there is no discrete left bundle. Instead, a complex, interdigitating network of left-sided Purkinje fascicles fan out from the bifurcation at the distal His bundle to run across the left ventricular endocardium.[77] Although electrocardiographic (ECG) patterns of left anterior and left posterior fascicles conduction block have been defined and have clinical utility, discrete left anterior and posterior fascicles cannot be identified anatomically in most patients.

Decremental conduction, a characteristic feature of conduction through the AV node, is the normal slowing of conduction that occurs as the rate of impulse transmission to the AV node increases. In the absence of changes in autonomic tone as the atrial rate increases, the AV nodal conduction time likewise increases to the point that physiologic block (Wenckebach's or Mobitz I second-degree AV block) occurs. This usually occurs at rates of 150 to 170 beats per minute. However, conduction through the AV node depends heavily on autonomic tone. Withdrawal of vagal tone due to exercise or administration of atropine results in accelerated AV conduction, whereas increased vagal tone results in slower AV conduction or transient AV block. Increased sympathetic tone likewise improves conduction through the AV node. Thus, during exercise or stress, autonomic changes improve AV nodal conduction concomitantly with increases in heart rate, allowing maintenance of AV conduction.

The delay in conduction that occurs in the AV node is responsible for the majority of the PR interval of the standard ECG as well as the atrial-His interval of the bundle of His recording. Normal conduction times across the AV node are between 60 and 120 msec., whereas conduction from the SA node to the AV node is 30 to 40 msec. and from the His bundle to ventricle 35 to 45 msec.

Conduction of impulses may proceed retrogradely from ventricle to atrium across the AV node. Retrograde conduction has been estimated to be intact in two thirds of normal humans. Retrograde AV block often occurs in or below the bundle of His, compared with antegrade conduction block that normally occurs in the AV node.

INDICATIONS FOR PACEMAKER THERAPY

Artificial pacing has clearly prolonged and improved the lives of thousands of patients with symptomatic bradyarrhythmias. The recognition of this impact on patient care has steadily increased pacemaker implantations worldwide. In the United States, approximately 360 pacemakers are inserted annually per million population, and this has been increasing at a rate of about 19 implants per million per year. Analysis of trends since 1975 indicates an increasing awareness of the benefits of pacing in patients with sinus node dysfunction. Implantation of a pacemaker for sinus node dysfunction accounted for 23% of primary implants in 1975 and 48% by 1989. AV node and His-Purkinje conduction disturbances were indications for pacing in 45% of patients in 1989, drug-induced bradycardia was the reason in 4%, with tachyarrhythmias in 2%. Furthermore, there has been an increasing dependence on dual-chamber pacing in a number of clinical conditions as the multiple benefits of this pacing modality are demonstrated. Over 30% of pacemakers implanted today are dual-chamber devices, and this percentage is anticipated to increase further in the next decade. In addition, the availability of various sensors to increase the pacemaker rate during periods of physiologic stress have improved exercise capabilities in patients receiving pacemakers. Single-chamber, rate-responsive devices now account for another third of all pacemakers implanted. As pacemaker technology continues to improve, new indications for pacemakers are identified, and the percentage of the elderly in the population increases, it is anticipated that the need for permanent pacemakers will continue to increase.

Although there is still some controversy regarding indications for permanent cardiac pacing as well as the type of pacing system chosen, most physicians would agree with the following guidelines.

Indications for Permanent Pacing

Implantation of a permanent pacemaker commits the patient to a lifetime with an implantable device and its associated costs, inconveniences, and potential complications. Therefore, the decision to implant a permanent pacemaker must weigh both the benefits and the risks and complications associated with its use. Fortunately, pacemaker and lead technology and implantation techniques have been so greatly improved that the acute and long-term risk associated with permanent pacemakers is small. Nonetheless, the decision to implant a permanent pacemaker needs to be made with the aim of improving the patient's quality of life and longevity.

Because controversy exists about appropriate indications for implantation of a permanent pacemaker, guidelines have been written by a task force of the American College of Cardiology and American Heart Association (Committee of Pacemaker Implantation, 1991). Indications for permanent pacemaker implantation have been grouped in this report into three classifications:

Class I: Conditions for which there is general agreement that a permanent pacemaker should be implanted.
Class II: Conditions for which permanent pacemakers are frequently used but in which there may be a divergence of opinion with respect to the necessity of their implantation.
Class III: Conditions in which there is general agreement that permanent pacemaker implantation is not indicated.

Thus, Class I and II indications are those in which the patient definitely or probably benefits from implantation of a permanent pacemaker, whereas in Class III indications, there is no or minimal potential benefit to the patient. The ACC/AHA guidelines for implantation of permanent pace-

makers in different clinical situations are listed in Table 54–17.

Acquired AV Block in Adults

Before permanent pacemakers were available, 50% of patients with complete heart block died within 1 year.[15, 26] The most common cause of acquired complete heart block is sclerodegenerative disease of the cardiac skeleton and AV conduction system. Other causes of complete heart block include ischemic heart disease, cardiomyopathic processes, Chagas' disease, and traumatic injury. Permanent pacemaker implantation is indicated in any patient with symptomatic complete, high-grade, or second-degree AV block. Symptoms include congestive heart failure, altered mental status, or other end-organ failure, particularly if it can be shown that temporary pacing improves the symptom. Permanent pacing is usually recommended for surgically induced complete heart block that persists more than 1 week after the operation. Symptomatic complete or high-grade AV block in the setting of atrial fibrillation or other atrial tachyarrhythmias is also an indication unless the AV block is caused by digitalis or other drugs and these drugs are not necessary for the patient's management. In patients with second-degree AV block, symptoms should be shown to be related to the episodes of AV block. Patients with asymptomatic Mobitz Type II are frequently considered to benefit from permanent pacing, given the high risk for development of complete heart block in these patients. Patients with Wenckebach (Mobitz Type I) second-degree AV block shown to be caused by a block in or below the His bundle during electrophysiologic testing are also candidates for permanent pacing because their risk for developing complete heart block is similar to that of patients with classic Mobitz Type II second-degree AV block. Patients with Wenckebach second-degree AV block due to intra- or infra-Hisian Wenckebach conduction patterns usually have associated bundle branch block. Wenckebach second-degree AV block with a narrow QRS complex is almost always due to AV nodal block, and three fourths of the cases associated with bundle branch block are also due to AV nodal block and thus are not indications for permanent pacemaker implantation.[37]

AV Block After Myocardial Infarction

Unlike those for acquired AV block in other conditions, indications for permanent pacemaker implantation in the setting of recent myocardial infarction do not necessarily require the presence of symptoms. Patients with persistent complete or high-grade AV block after myocardial infarction, whether associated with symptoms or not, should be permanently paced given their poor prognosis. In addition, patients with transient complete heart block during acute myocardial infarction who have persistent bundle branch block have been shown in some studies to have a high risk of late complete heart block and thus should be permanently paced. Because alternating bundle branch blocks have high rates of progression to complete heart block, they also should be permanently paced, even if episodes of transient complete or high-grade AV block have not been documented.[47]

Chronic Bifascicular and Trifascicular Block

Bifascicular and trifascicular block suggest extensive damage to the His bundle and bundle branches. Although the overall risk for progression to permanent or symptomatic complete heart block is low, certain patients with bifascicular and trifascicular blocks are at considerably higher risks. Patients with bifascicular or trifascicular block with intermittent

TABLE 54–17. Indications for Permanent Pacing (Guidelines of the ACC/AHA Task Force)

Indications for Permanent Pacing in Acquired Atrioventricular Block in Adults

Class I

A. Complete heart block, permanent or intermittent, at any anatomic level, associated with any one of the following complications:
1. Symptomatic bradycardia. In the presence of complete heart block, symptoms must be presumed to be due to the heart block unless proved otherwise
2. Congestive heart failure
3. Ectopic rhythms and other medical conditions that require drugs that suppress the automaticity of escape pacemakers and result in symptomatic bradycardia
4. Documented periods of asystole ≥ 3.0 seconds or any escape rate < 40 beats per minute in symptom-free patients
5. Confusional states that clear with temporary pacing
6. Post AV junction ablation, myotonic dystrophy
B. Second-degree AV block, permanent or intermittent, regardless of the type or the site of block, with symptomatic bradycardia
C. Atrial fibrillation, atrial flutter or rare cases of supraventricular tachycardia with complete heart block or advanced AV block, bradycardia, and any of the conditions described under A. The bradycardia must be unrelated to digitalis or drugs known to impair AV conduction

Class II

A. Asymptomatic complete heart block, permanent or intermittent, at any anatomic site, with ventricular rates of 40 beats per minute or faster
B. Asymptomatic Type II second-degree AV block, permanent or intermittent
C. Asymptomatic Type I second-degree AV block at intra-His or infra-His levels

Class III

A. First-degree AV block
B. Asymptomatic Type I second-degree AV block at the supra-His (AV node) level

Indications for Permanent Pacing After Myocardial Infarction

Class I

A. Persistent advanced second-degree AV block or complete heart block after acute myocardial infarction with block in the His-Purkinje system (bilateral bundle branch block)
B. Patients with transient advanced AV block and associated bundle branch block

Class II

A. Patients with persistent advanced block in the AV node

Class III

A. Transient AV conduction disturbances in the absence of intraventricular conduction defects
B. Transient AV block in the presence of isolated left anterior hemiblock
C. Acquired left anterior hemiblock in the absence of AV block
D. Patients with persistent first-degree AV block in the presence of bundle branch block not demonstrated previously

Indications for Permanent Pacing in Bifascicular and Trifascicular Block

Class I

A. Bifascicular block with intermittent complete heart block associated with symptomatic bradycardia (as defined)
B. Bifascicular or trifascicular block with intermittent Type II second-degree AV block without symptoms attributable to the heart block

Class II

A. Bifascicular or trifascicular block with syncope that is not proved to be due to complete heart block, but other possible causes for syncope are not identifiable
B. Markedly prolonged HV (> 100 ms.)
C. Pacing-induced infra-His block

Class III

A. Fascicular block without AV block or symptoms
B. Fascicular block with first-degree AV block without symptoms

Indications for Permanent Pacing in Sinus Node Dysfunction

Class I

A. Sinus node dysfunction with documented symptomatic bradycardia; in some patients this will occur as a consequence of long-term (essential) drug therapy of a type and dose for which there are no acceptable alternatives

Class II

A. Sinus node dysfunction, occurring spontaneously or as a result of necessary drug therapy, with heart rates < 40 beats per minute when a clear association between significant symptoms consistent with bradycardia and the actual presence of bradycardia has not been documented

Class III

A. Sinus node dysfunction in asymptomatic patients, including those in whom substantial sinus bradycardia (heart rate < 40 beats per minute) is a consequence of long-term drug treatment
B. Sinus node dysfunction in patients in whom symptoms suggestive of bradycardia are clearly documented not to be associated with a slow heart rate

Indications for Permanent Pacing in Hypersensitive Carotid Sinus and Neurovascular Syndromes

Class I

A. Recurrent syncope associated with clear, spontaneous events provoked by carotid sinus stimulation; minimal carotid sinus pressure induces asystole of > 3 seconds' duration in the absence of any medication that depresses the sinus node or AV conduction

Class II

A. Recurrent syncope without clear, provocative events and with a hypersensitive cardioinhibitory response
B. Syncope with associated bradycardia reproduced by a head-up tilt with or without isoproterenol or other forms of provocative maneuvers and in which a temporary pacemaker and a second provocative test can establish the likely benefits of a permanent pacemaker

Class III

A. A hyperactive cardioinhibitory response to carotid sinus stimulation in the absence of symptoms
B. Vague symptoms, such as dizziness, lightheadedness, or both, with a hyperactive cardioinhibitory response to carotid sinus stimulation
C. Recurrent syncope, lightheadedness, or dizziness in the absence of a cardioinhibitory response

From Sabiston, D. C., Jr., and Spencer, F. C. (Eds.): Surgery of the Chest, 6th ed. Philadelphia, W. B. Saunders, 1996.

complete heart block, high-grade AV block, or Mobitz Type II second-degree AV block represent such a high-risk group and should undergo permanent pacemaker implantation. Because syncope is the usual symptom associated with transient complete or high-grade AV block, patients with syncope and bifascicular or trifascicular block should undergo electrophysiologic testing to determine if infra-Hisian block can be induced by pacing, in which case a pacemaker should be implanted. It has also been suggested that even asymptomatic patients with a markedly prolonged infranodal conduction time (Hisian-ventricular interval > 100 msec.) should undergo prophylactic permanent pacing, given their high risk for progression to complete heart block. Even in the absence of pacing induced infra-Hisian block or a markedly prolonged Hisian-ventricular interval, patients with syncope and bifascicular or trifascicular block in whom a cause for syncope cannot be identified with extensive testing should receive a permanent pacemaker, given the high probability that their syncope was secondary to a high-grade although transient conduction disturbance and their potential increased risk of death from a bradyarrhythmia. Although patients with bifascicular and trifascicular disease have a relatively high mortality rate, this is largely due to the underlying heart disease that caused the conduction disorder, not to the development of complete heart block. Thus, routine implantation of pacemakers in asymptomatic patients with bifascicular and trifascicular block is not indicated.

Sinus Node Dysfunction

Patients with sinus node dysfunction may develop a number of arrhythmias, such as inappropriate sinus bradycardia, chronotropic incompetence, SA exit block, and sinus arrest. This group of rhythm disorders typically occurs in older patients with or without underlying heart disease and is collectively known as the sick sinus syndrome. In addition, many patients with sick sinus syndrome have associated atrial tachyarrhythmias, particularly atrial fibrillation. This association of atrial tachyarrhythmias in patients with the sick sinus syndrome is called the tachycardia-bradycardia (or tachy-brady) syndrome. Patients with symptomatic bradycardia not incurred by reversible causes are candidates for permanent pacing. In addition, patients with the tachycardia-bradycardia syndrome frequently require digitalis, other AV nodal blocking agents, or antiarrhythmic drugs to control atrial tachyarrhythmias, which cause an exaggerated suppression of sinus node function. If these drugs are not avoidable in this situation, then permanent pacing will be needed to protect against drug-induced bradycardia. Some patients with intermittent symptoms suggestive of bradycardia and documented bradycardias with rates less than 40 beats per minute, but in whom the symptoms have not been documented to occur with bradycardia, may be candidates for permanent pacing. However, a concerted effort should be made to confirm the presence of bradycardia with symptoms.

Neurovascular Syndromes

Several neurovascular syndromes cause exaggerated parasympathetic tone with resultant sinus bradycardia, asystole, and transient high-grade AV block (cardioinhibitory effect). In addition, reflex withdrawal of sympathetic tone may further exacerbate the bradyarrhythmias and also cause profound vasodilation (vasodepressor effect), sometimes without significant bradyarrhythmias. The most common of these syndromes is the carotid sinus hypersensitivity syndrome when it is associated with a significant cardioinhibitory response and syncope. In these patients, mild carotid sinus massage will cause significant asystole (> 3 sec.). Some individuals, however, may have a hypersensitive response to carotid sinus massage and remain asymptomatic. For this reason, it is useful to document significant bradyarrhythmia during a spontaneous episode of syncope or near-syncope in patients suspected of having carotid sinus hypersensitivity syndrome. However, in some patients with recurrent syncope, clear documentation of bradycardia during a spontaneous episode is not possible, although demonstration of a hypersensitive response to carotid massage suggests the diagnosis. The most common neurovascular syndrome is the neurally mediated syncope syndrome, which occurs after an exaggerated Bezold-Jarisch reflex induced when relative hypovolemia and increased sympathetic tone create left ventricular chamber obliteration during systole. Some patients may have palliation of symptoms with permanent pacing to alleviate the bradycardia component of the Bezold-Jarisch reflex if temporary pacing demonstrates improvement in symptoms during provocative tilt-table testing.

Tachyarrhythmias

Permanent pacing can be useful in some cases of medically refractory supraventricular and ventricular tachycardia if pacing the atria or ventricles, respectively, at tolerated rates above the intrinsic heart rate prevents arrhythmia recurrence (overdrive suppression). However, a prolonged period of overdrive suppression using a temporary pacemaker should be tried before implanting a permanent pacemaker to demonstrate the efficacy of this approach. Patients with symptoms and torsades de pointes can be effectively treated with overdrive pacing if reversible causes are not found.[9] Permanent pacemakers have been designed to detect and terminate with pacing both supraventricular and ventricular tachycardias. With the advent of highly effective catheter ablation techniques for treatment of paroxysmal supraventricular tachycardias, the use of pacemakers for overdrive suppression or termination of supraventricular tachycardias is rarely needed. Pacemakers that only pace terminate ventricular tachycardia can accelerate the tachycardia to a poorly tolerated ventricular tachycardia or fibrillation. These have been incorporated as part of implantable defibrillators to administer high-energy shocks if pacing causes degeneration of an initially hemodynamically stable arrhythmia.

Intractable Congestive Heart Failure and Cerebral or Renal Insufficiency Benefitted by Temporary Pacing

Patients with refractory congestive heart failure and decreased perfusion causing cerebral or renal insufficiency may be improved occasionally by increasing heart rate with temporary pacing. If temporary pacing has proved to be effective under these conditions and long-term therapy is indicated, permanent pacing should be considered. Most of these patients require atrial contraction to improve cardiac output. Therefore, dual-chamber atrial synchronous pacing is usually indicated in this subgroup. Studies have suggested that AV sequential pacing with relatively short AV intervals may improve left ventricular function in patients with dilated cardiomyopathies without overt bradycardia,[23] but further evaluation of this phenomenon is needed before this indication can be recommended. Patients with hypertrophic obstructive cardiomyopathy are also favorably influenced by ventricular pacing, presumably because of the asyneresis induced by pacing the ventricular apex that partially alleviates outflow tract obstruction.[12]

THE IMPULSE GENERATOR

An implantable cardiac pacemaker consists of an impulse generator, lead wire, and electrode. The impulse generator

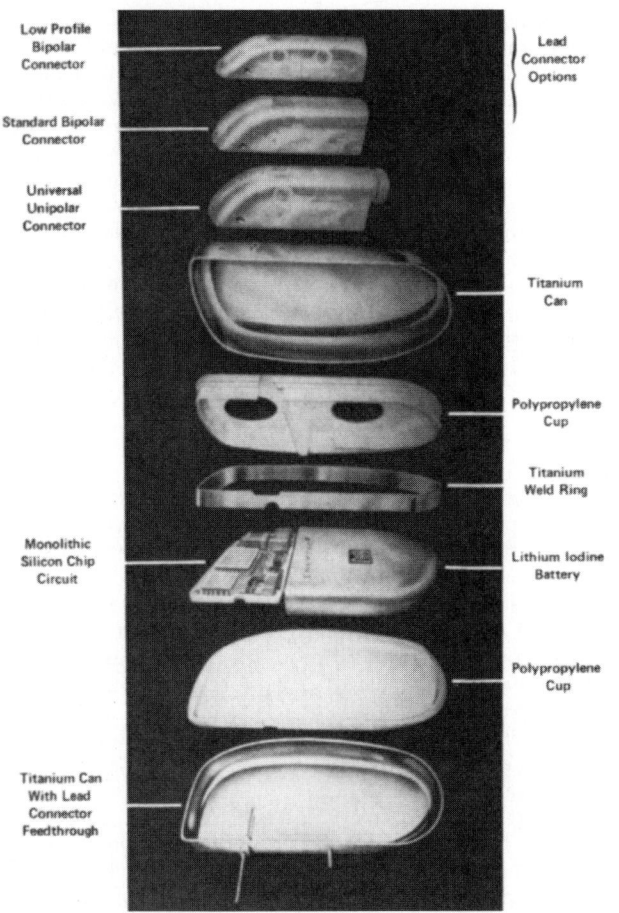

Low Profile
Bipolar
Connector

Standard Bipolar
Connector

Universal
Unipolar
Connector

Monolithic
Silicon Chip
Circuit

Titanium Can
With Lead
Connector
Feedthrough

Lead
Connector
Options

Titanium
Can

Polypropylene
Cup

Titanium
Weld Ring

Lithium Iodine
Battery

Polypropylene
Cup

Figure 54–202. Exploded view of a modern multiprogrammable impulse generator. Various lead connectors are available to accept a variety of epicardial and transvenous leads. The battery and pacemaker electronics are enclosed in a titanium metal case. Hybrid circuit technology allows all components of the circuit including semiconductors, resistors, and capacitors to be diffused into a substrate to produce what is called a monolithic silicon chip. As shown, the major advantage of the silicon chip circuit is its extremely small size. This technology combined with the improved lithium power source has allowed modern multiprogrammable pacemakers to be much smaller, lighter, and more reliable than earlier pacemakers. (Courtesy of Paul Craven, Joe Hitselberger, and Gene Boone, Medtronic, Inc.)

contains a power source or battery, hybrid circuits, and a lead connector (Fig. 54–202). All of these components are kept in a hermetically sealed metal container. The size and weight of the impulse generator depend on the size of the battery and the number of electronic components. Impulse generators are usually kept in rectangular or oval packages with rounded edges and weigh between 20 and 50 gm.

Power Sources

The power source used in a totally implantable pacemaker may be biologic, rechargeable, nuclear, or chemical. Biologic power sources convert mechanical or chemical energy of the body into electrical energy using piezoelectric crystals, biogalvanic cells, or biofuel cells. Theoretically, these power sources can be renewed potentially for the patient's lifetime, but they have not been developed to a point at which they are clinically practical. In 1973, a highly reliable, hermetically sealed, nickel-cadmium rechargeable pacemaker was developed at Johns Hopkins University and introduced commercially by Pacesetter, Inc.[13] The useful battery life of such a rechargeable pacemaker has been calculated to be 70 to 80 years. Rechargeable pacemakers, although reliable, are not

widely used, primarily because of the necessity for weekly recharging. Nuclear-powered impulse generators have been implanted in more than 3000 patients worldwide. Their longevity is predicted to be longer than 20 years; however, nuclear generators are no longer used because of cost, the improved longevity of newer chemical power sources, legislative restrictions, and concerns about the risk of chronic low-level radiation exposure. Chemical power sources continue to be the primary component of power cells in implantable pacemakers.

The modern power cell or battery is composed of an anode, a cathode, and an electrolyte. The power cell is generally named for the material used in the anode and cathode (e.g., lithium-iodine). Current solid-state cells have a dry, crystalline electrolyte between the anode and cathode. Electric current is produced by ionization of the anode, resulting in the migration of positively charged metallic ions through the electrolyte toward the cathode. Electrons are left behind on the anode, which becomes negatively charged relative to the cathode. When the anode and cathode are connected by a conductive pathway, a flow of electrons passes from the anode to the cathode. The higher the resistance in the conductor, the slower the flow of electrons and the longer the power cell will last. In the modern lithium-iodine power cell, the migrating or positively charged ions are lithium, which combines with iodine from the cathode to form a lithium-iodide electrolyte barrier. Most currently available lithium-powered pacemakers contain a single power cell, unlike the original mercury-zinc generators, which were powered by multiple-cell batteries.

Lithium power cells are available in five chemical types: (1) lithium-iodine (polyvinyl pyridine); (2) lithium-lead sulfide; (3) lithium-silver chromate; (4) lithium-copper sulfide; and (5) lithium-thionyl chloride.[45] All of these lithium power sources have been extremely reliable and durable when compared with the earlier mercury-zinc systems. Most current pacemaker implants worldwide contain a solid-state lithium-iodine cell, which appears to be the power source of choice. Overall, pulse generator performance based on the type of power source is shown in Figure 54–203. The results with rechargeable impulse generators are essentially parallel to those of the nuclear power sources. The power source lon-

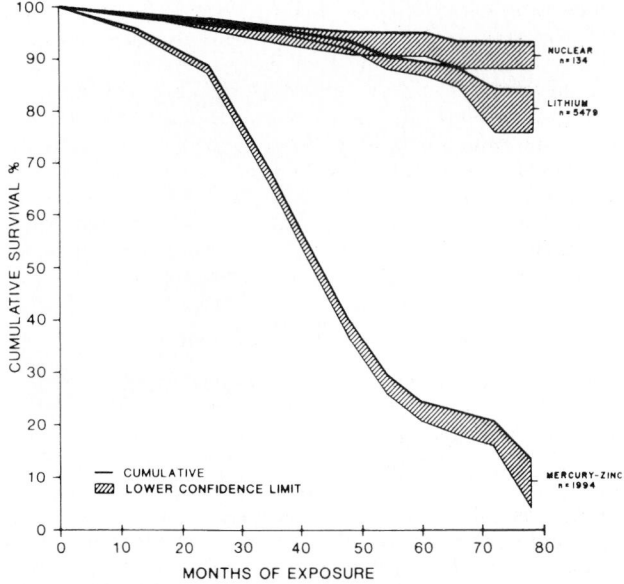

Figure 54–203. Impulse generator performance based on the type of power source. (From Bilitch, M., Hauser, R. G., Goldman, B. S., et al.: Performance of cardiac pacemaker pulse generators. PACE, 4:254, 1981.)

gevity of lithium pacemakers is estimated to be 10 to 12 years. However, battery longevity is determined by a number of factors, including percentage of time the generator is pacing; requirements for single- or dual-chamber pacing; lead impedance; programmed voltage and pulse width; and power drainage from monitoring, sensor, and special-function circuits. Because of wound, lead-electrode, and functional problems relating to pacing and sensing, it appears that fewer than 10% of patients have required reoperation 4 to 5 years after implantation of a lithium-powered pacemaker.[20] Therefore, it is unwise to suggest to a patient that the life of the pacemaker is governed only by the predicted life expectancy of the power cell. Even modern lithium-powered pacemakers have been associated with a small incidence of random failure.

Pacemaker Electronics

The first implantable pacemakers contained individual or discrete components, including resistors, capacitors, diodes, transistors, reed switches, and wire coils for induction. These individual components were mounted on or between printed circuit boards. A major advance in pacemaker electronics has been the development of hybrid circuits. Hybrid technology allows all components of the circuit, including semiconductors, resistors, and capacitors, to be diffused into a substrate to produce a monolithic silicon chip (Fig. 54–204). The major advantage of the single-chip circuit is its small size. Customized digital, silicon, large-scale integrated circuits are used in almost all multiprogrammable pacemakers and may include as many as 40,000 transistors on a 4-sq. mm. wafer. This technology combined with the improved lithium power source has allowed modern multiprogrammable pacemakers to be much smaller, lighter, and more reliable than earlier, simpler pacemakers. The lithium-powered pacemaker containing a custom-integrated circuit design is exceptionally reliable and capable of providing both multiprogrammable and physiologic pacing functions and extensive monitoring

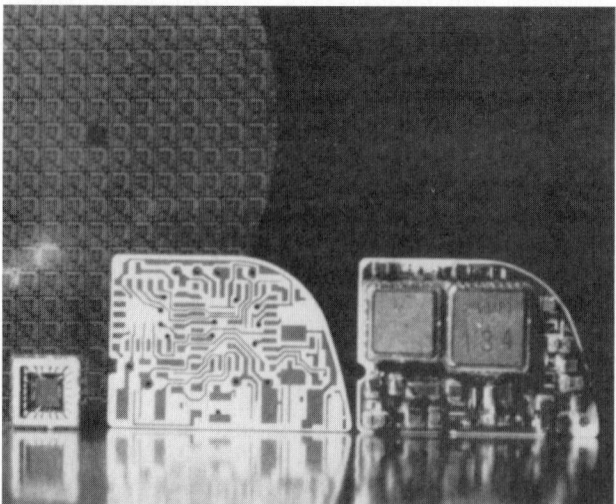

Figure 54–204. A highly magnified view of a modern hybrid circuit. Hybrid technology allows all components of the circuit including semiconductors, resistors, and capacitors to be diffused into a substrate to produce a monolithic silicon chip. The obvious advantage of the single chip circuit is its small size. Such hybrid circuits are used in almost all multiprogrammable pacemakers and may include as many as 40,000 transistors on a 4-sq. mm. wafer. Such a hybrid circuit is exceptionally reliable and capable of providing both multiprogrammable and physiologic pacing functions. However, its capacity for monitoring and data processing is limited and it may be replaced in the future by single chip microcomputers. (From Sabiston, D. C., Jr., and Spencer, F. C. [Eds.]: Surgery of the Chest, 6th ed. Philadelphia, W. B. Saunders, 1996.)

capabilities. Future pacemakers will most likely use low-current-drain, custom microcomputers consisting of a central processing unit, a memory unit, and an input-output circuit.[3] Pacemakers containing microcomputers are now capable of monitoring various physiologic changes to control in online manner pacemaker function. Physiologic changes that can be monitored include cardiac output requirements as determined by online measurement of temperature, QT interval, oxygen saturation, right ventricular pressure change, depolarization gradient, body motion, and respiratory rate. Moreover, microcomputer-based pacemakers can automatically select an appropriate pacing technique for the control of various arrhythmias. Future pacemakers will be able to automatically detect loss of capture due to threshold changes and adjust their output accordingly.

Hermetic Seal

The electronics and power source of the first totally implantable pacemakers were protected by epoxy resins and silicone rubber.[45] Gradually, however, moisture gained access to the interior of the pacemaker, causing short circuits, sudden cessation of pacing, battery explosion, pacemaker runaway, and occasionally even ventricular fibrillation.[44] Fluid infiltration problems were responsible for the massive recalls that eventually terminated the use of mercury-zinc, epoxy-enclosed pacemakers.[44]

The modern pacemaker is hermetically enclosed, rendering it airtight and fluid-tight. Pacemaker manufacturers determine the quality of the hermetic seal in terms of a leak rate for an inert gas under standard conditions.[45] For example, an acceptable helium leak rate of 10^{-8} ml. per second at 1 atm. involves the passage of less than 0.01 ml. of helium per 24 hours. Permeability to fluid is many orders of magnitude lower. Hermetic seal is now achieved by encasing the power source and electronics in a sealed metal container, which usually requires laser welding. The materials chosen for enclosure have included stainless steel, Haynes' alloy, and titanium. Most modern pacemakers are enclosed in titanium.

Lead Connector

Impressive advances have been made in leads and electrodes and in pacemaker power sources and circuitry. As described by Tyers in 1981, the ideal pacemaker connector should be tangential to reduce electrode stress, universal to accept all available leads without adapters, simple, and short-circuit proof.[45] A standard coaxial bipolar connector that has been developed is an industry standard that eliminates incompatibilities among various leads and pacemakers. This universal lead connector is referred to as the VS-1 (voluntary standard) and is a 3.2-mm. diameter connector designed to fit potentially all bipolar pacemakers as well as to reduce the size of the connector itself.

LEAD-ELECTRODE

A pacemaker lead is an insulated wire used to connect the pacemaker impulse generator to the heart. The electrode is the uninsulated, electrically active metal tip that is in contact with the myocardium (Fig. 54–205). The lead-electrode system in a demand pacemaker has two equally important functions: it conducts the electric stimulus from the impulse generator to the myocardium and transmits an endocardial electrogram from the heart to the pacemaker. In unipolar systems, only the cathode is in the heart and the indifferent electrode, or anode, which is a part of the metallic pacemaker case, is in soft tissue. In a bipolar system, a double wire runs from the pacemaker to the heart and the two electrodes are

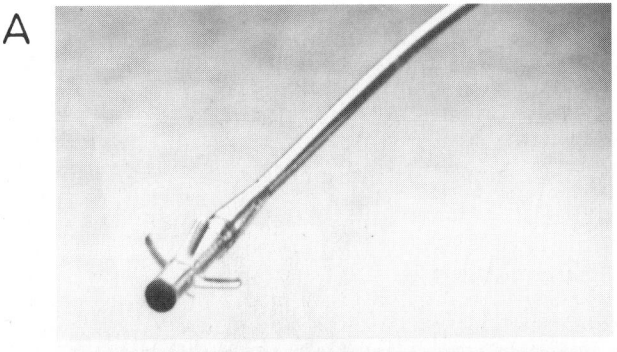

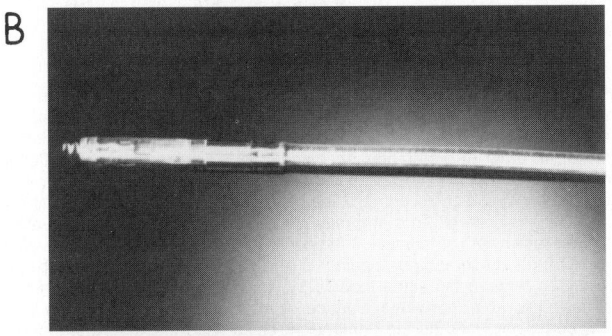

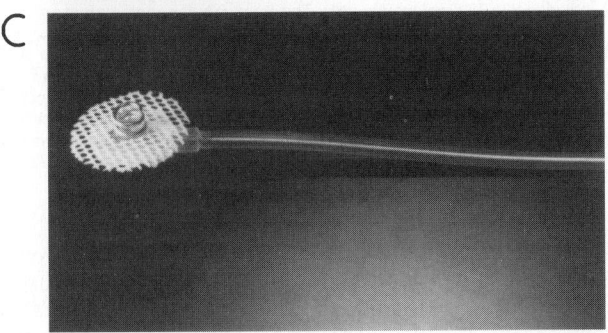

Figure 54–205. Examples of a passive-fixation (tined) bipolar endocardial pacing lead *(A)*, an active-fixation (retractable helical screw) bipolar endocardial lead *(B)*, and a screw-in epicardial pacing lead *(C)*. (A to C Reprinted with permission from Medtronic, Inc., © Medtronic, Inc., 1996.)

most common and may be either porous or solid. Steroid-eluding lead tips improve chronic sensing and pacing function by decreasing scar formation at the tip as it heals into place. Studies have suggested that porous-tipped, steroid-eluding suture-on epicardial leads also have improved chronic sensing and pacing thresholds in pediatric patients.

Two general types of lead-electrode systems exist. The most common are the systems passed transvenously to embed within the subendocardium of the right atrium or right ventricle or both. The second group are those placed transthoracically; they are directly attached to the myocardium of any chamber. These leads have been referred to as *epicardial leads,* but this term is a misnomer because they are actually embedded within the myocardium and not just within the epicardium. Transthoracic leads are used primarily in small infants and children, after repeated failure of the transvenous approach, and sometimes when the chest is already open, such as after cardiac surgical procedures. Generally, transvenous lead-electrode systems are preferred because of their improved chronic thresholds and decreased incidence of lead fracture.

Transvenous lead systems are referred to as active or passive. Passive leads have a small flanged expansion just proximal to the exposed distal electrode or have short, flexible tines. These tined leads are designed to catch beneath trabeculae and reduce the incidence of dislodgment, which should be less than 1%. Currently used active fixation leads contain sharpened screws that may be remotely activated and retracted (see Fig. 54–205). Active fixation leads are used in the ventricular location when the right ventricle is smooth walled, when there is significant tricuspid regurgitation, or when a site other than the right ventricular apex is needed. Active fixation of the atrial lead is typically performed in the setting of a markedly dilated right atrium or in patients who have undergone prior cardiopulmonary bypass with resultant trauma to the right appendage. Passive leads designed primarily for placement in the atrial appendage by the transvenous route differ from ventricular leads in that when the stylet is withdrawn they assume a J shape, which allows them to be positioned well up into the atrial appendage.

As mentioned earlier, pacing lead systems are either bipolar or unipolar. Possible advantages of unipolar systems include smaller lead diameter with an attendant slight decreased risk of right ventricular perforation, increased stimulus artifact size, allowing easier identification of pacemaker function, and simpler connection. Earlier concerns about better sensing and pacing function have been eliminated by improvements in bipolar lead design. Advantages of bipolar pacing include reduced risk of skeletal muscle stimulation, lower susceptibility to electromagnetic interference, elimination of pacemaker inhibition by skeletal muscle myopotential sensing, decreased risk of cross-talk between atrial and ventricular stimuli, and greater range of location for placement of the pulse generator without concern for skeletal muscle stimulation (e.g., submuscular implantation). With the advent of programmable polarity of both sensing and pacing functions, the use of bipolar leads allows programming of either unipolar or bipolar leads whereas unipolar pacing leads restrict options to unipolar modes only. Although personal preferences vary, the increased benefits of bipolar pacing leads make them preferable to unipolar leads in most cases.

To a certain extent, decreasing electrode tip size results in lower thresholds, both at the time of implant as well as chronically because of higher current density. However, better sensing function is directly related to electrode area and is adversely affected by small electrode size. Therefore, a compromise between pacing and sensing efficiency is re-

separated by approximately 1 cm. within the heart. The lead wire is most often a continuous helical coil that is resistant to fracture caused by repeated flexion.

In the past, the lead was most commonly insulated with silicone rubber. Polyurethane insulation has been introduced because of its greater elasticity and tensile strength, which allows lead diameter to be reduced. Furthermore, polyurethane has a smoother surface, which improves handling characteristics during multilead placement. However, several models of bipolar polyurethane leads have been shown to increase the risk of compression fracture of the polyurethane coating, causing early lead failure.[21] Similarly constructed bipolar silicone rubber leads have been much less likely to demonstrate insulation breaks. This argues strongly for the continued use of silicone rubber insulation, at least for bipolar leads. Newer polymers of polyurethane with greater compression strength are now being used on some polyurethane leads, but whether these newer polymers prevent the increased risk of insulation fracture awaits long-term follow-up in a large number of patients.

The uninsulated, electrically active metal tip of the lead in contact with the myocardium is the electrode. This exposed tip is usually made of platinum, iridium, nickel alloys, or activated carbon. Platinum-iridium electrodes are now the

quired. Typical electrode surface areas for pacing are between 8 and 10 sq. mm. The effective surface area for sensing is increased many times through the use of microporous electrodes. These porous-tip electrodes improve sensing for a given electrode size because the interstices increase the sensing area without increasing overall electrode size and subsequent stimulation energy requirements. Techniques such as platinization of the electrode or use of activated carbon result in lower stimulation thresholds by reducing polarizing currents at the electrode surface.

OPERATIVE TECHNIQUES AND EVALUATION OF PACEMAKER FUNCTION
Operative Techniques

Implantation of a permanent impulse generator and lead-electrode system should be done in a fluoroscopic unit or a cardiac catheterization laboratory under sterile conditions. Various impulse generators and lead electrodes as well as a pacing system analyzer should be readily available. Most commonly, the pacemaker lead-electrode is passed transvenously under local anesthesia to become embedded within the subendocardium of the right atrium or right ventricle. Transthoracic leads are used primarily in small infants and children, after repeated failure of the transvenous approach, and sometimes after cardiac procedures when a permanent pacemaker is indicated. In general, for elective permanent pacemakers, transvenous leads are preferred because of their improved chronic sensing and pacing thresholds and decreased incidence of lead fracture.

Preoperatively, patients receive a therapeutic dose of an antistaphylococcal antibiotic based on the proven beneficial effects of prophylactic antibiotic administration in general and thoracic surgical procedures. Antibiotics are discontinued 24 hours postoperatively. Regardless of the planned approach for implantation, the entire anterior chest from the chin to the umbilicus should be prepared and draped as a sterile field. This wide field of preparation allows conversion from one transvenous approach to another and permits a limited anterior thoracotomy without interruption of the procedure.

Based on the work of Lagergren and Johansson in 1963 in Sweden and by Furman and Schwedel in 1959 and Chardack and colleagues in 1965 in the United States, the transvenous approach under local anesthesia is now used in more than 90% of patients requiring pacemakers. The venous anatomy of the anterior chest wall is particularly well suited for implantation of pacing leads (Fig. 54–206). Generally, the pacemaker pocket is placed over the anterior side of the chest beneath the junction of the inner and middle thirds of the clavicle on the patient's nondominant side. The cephalic or subclavian veins are the preferred venous approaches for lead introduction. Implantation through the external or internal jugular veins requires a separate neck incision, and the lead must be tunneled over or under the clavicle to reach the pacemaker pocket and generator. Passing the lead over the clavicle predisposes to skin erosion and lead fracture; tunneling beneath the clavicle increases the risk of hemorrhage due to vascular injury.

An oblique incision on the anterior chest wall inferior to the deltopectoral groove provides excellent exposure of the cephalic vein and also allows introducer cannulation of the subclavian vein (Fig. 54–207). The pacemaker pocket should be as far medial as is comfortable for the patient to minimize pectoral stimulation. It should be made only slightly larger than the impulse generator so that migration laterally, which tends to follow the curvature of the chest wall, is minimized. Small arterial and venous bleeding vessels are ligated or

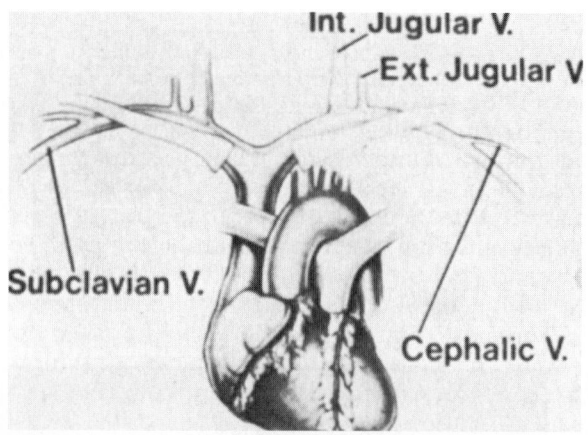

Figure 54–206. Anatomy for preferred venous approaches. Any vein in the neck, chest, or shoulder may be used for a permanent transvenous lead, but it is preferable to expose the vein through the same incision used for making the pocket. In order of preference, acceptable veins are as follows: (1) Cephalic vein, a tributary of the subclavian vein. It lies in the deltopectoral groove and is usually large enough to admit a lead up to No. 7- or 8-French. In 10% of patients, it is quite delicate and may not be usable. It is occasionally absent. (2) Subclavian vein or tributary. If the cephalic vein cannot be used, it is always possible to expose another tributary of the subclavian vein or the subclavian vein itself through the same incision by freeing the pectoralis major from its lateral origin from the inferior surface of the clavicle. The subclavian vein is now commonly used as the primary choice for lead insertion with introducer techniques. (3) External jugular vein. This is usually the most prominent visible vein in the neck, although it may be absent in 10% of patients. Because of the necessity of tunneling the electrode over or under the clavicle, with an increased incidence of fracture and erosion, this is a poor choice for permanent pacing. (4) Internal jugular vein. This is also a poor choice, unless purulent infections exist at every other potential site or an unusually large electrode is required as for an implantable defibrillator. (From Parsonnet, V.: Implantation of Transvenous Pacemakers. Tarpon Springs, FL, Tampa Tracings, 1972.)

electrocoagulated to avoid postoperative hematoma formation. The pacemaker generator pocket should be just superficial to the pectoralis major in thick-chested individuals or beneath the premuscular fascia or muscle itself in thin-chested patients.

Several techniques have evolved for cannulating the venous system for insertion of permanent pacing leads. With the cephalic vein approach, the lead is directly inserted into

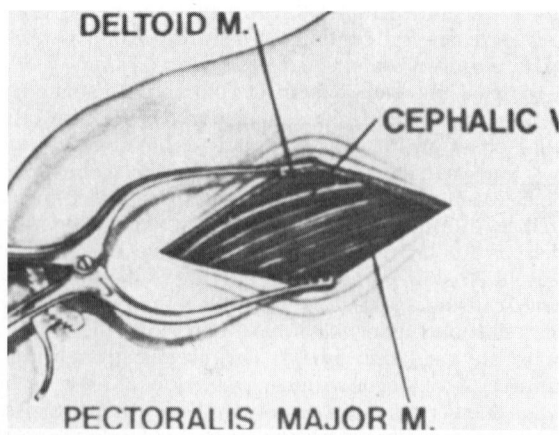

Figure 54–207. Cephalic vein approach. After the incision is made below the clavicle, the deltopectoral groove is identified. The cephalic vein is usually found with ease in the fat pad that fills the groove. Division of a few fibers of the pectoralis major from the clavicle will allow dissection of the vein proximally, and if gentle traction is applied, the angle of entrance of the cephalic vein into the subclavian vein can be made more oblique. Passage of the electrode toward the heart rather than into the axilla is facilitated. (From Parsonnet, V.: Implantation of Transvenous Pacemakers. Tarpon Springs, FL, Tampa Tracings, 1972.)

the small incision made in the vein (Fig. 54–208). There are two subclavian vein approaches. In the commonly performed intrathoracic approach, the subclavian vein is cannulated with a thin wall introducer needle underneath the middle portion of the clavicle within the thoracic cavity (Fig. 54–209). Care should be taken to approach the subclavian vein as laterally as possible, because more medial subclavian vein approaches are more likely to create lead compression between the first rib and clavicle and soft tissue entrapment in the subclavius muscle, which may cause lead fracture. Recently, an extrathoracic approach for subclavian vein cannulation has been described. In this approach, the subclavian vein is cannulated with the thin wall needle as it crosses the first rib before entering the thoracic cavity underneath the clavicle (Fig. 54–210). The vein is located in this position by maneuvering the thin wall needle posteriorly along the first rib until the vein is punctured. The extrathoracic approach may be better than the intrathoracic approach because of the decreased risk of pneumothorax and avoidance of lead fracture due to compression between the first rib and clavicle seen with the more medial intrathoracic approach.

After the subclavian vein is cannulated, a guide wire is initially placed into the venous system through the thin wall needle. A lead introducer sheath is then advanced over the guide wire into the venous system to the superior vena cava. The guide wire and dilator to the sheath are removed, and the pacing lead is advanced through the sheath to the level of the right atrium. The sheath can then be peeled away from the lead to remove it from the body while leaving the pacing lead in the vein. The flexible pacing lead is made more steerable by use of an internal stylet to give the lead some rigidity. Once the lead is in the right atrium, the standard straight stylet is exchanged for one with a J tip, which allows the lead to be passed across the tricuspid valve (Fig. 54–211). The lead is then advanced across the pulmonic valve to confirm that the right ventricle has been cannulated, not the

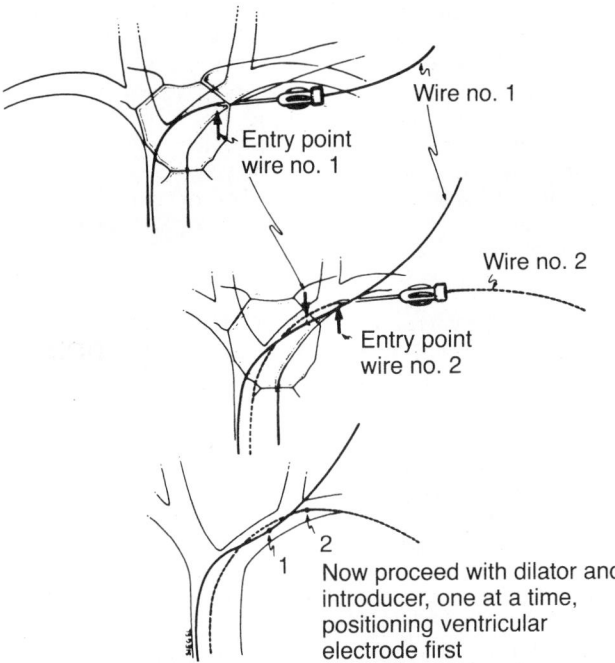

Figure 54–209. Two-entry point dual-lead introducer technique. Method for inserting separate guide wires, introducers, and sheaths with a small distance between the electrode entrance sites. (From Parsonnet V., Werres, R., Atherley, T., et al.: Transvenous insertion of double set of permanent electrodes: Atraumatic technique for atrial synchronous and atrial ventricular sequential pacemakers. JAMA, *243*:62, 1980. Copyright 1980, American Medical Association.)

coronary sinus. The lead is then withdrawn into the cavity of the right ventricle, and the curved stylet is replaced with a straight one. The lead is then gradually withdrawn until the electrode falls and points toward the apex of the right ventricle. The stylet is then withdrawn a few millimeters, and the lead is gently maneuvered to lodge the pacing and sensing electrode beneath right ventricular trabeculae (see Fig. 54–211). If a dual-chamber procedure is planned, ventricular lead placement is accomplished first, followed by placement of an atrial J lead, which is designed to lodge in the right atrial appendage. If stable positioning of an atrial J

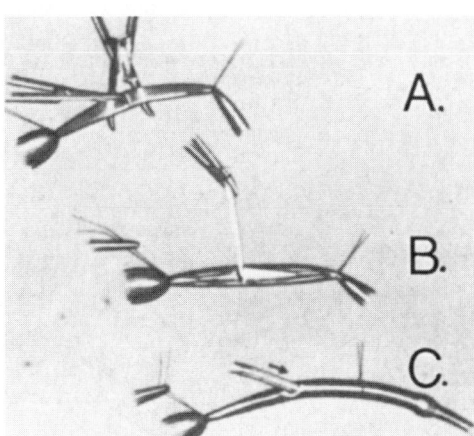

Figure 54–208. Small vein introduction technique. If the vein is large, an electrode can be inserted simply by any standard method. When the vein is small, gentle handling and care permit insertion of an electrode that at first may seem to be much larger than the vein. The vein is ligated distally; a loose, nonabsorbable suture is placed proximally; and a transverse incision is made one third of the way across the anterior wall of the vessel (A). A plastic inserter (present in the lead packages from many manufacturers) is carefully slipped into the opening (B). With upward traction on the inserter, which is concave on its inferior surface, the electrode can be passed underneath the inserter, which is not withdrawn until the tip of the electrode has passed medially a centimeter or so. As the electrode is advanced, the proximal ligature is loosened and then tightened to prevent bleeding. Countertraction on the distal ligature is maintained to assist passage into the subclavian vein (C). Traction on the distal ligature is easily maintained by pulling it over a self-retaining retractor by placing a straight hemostat across it, with the tip of the hemostat underneath the ratchet of the retractor. (A–C from Parsonnet, V.: Implantation of Transvenous Pacemakers. Tarpon Springs, Fla., Tampa Tracings, 1972.)

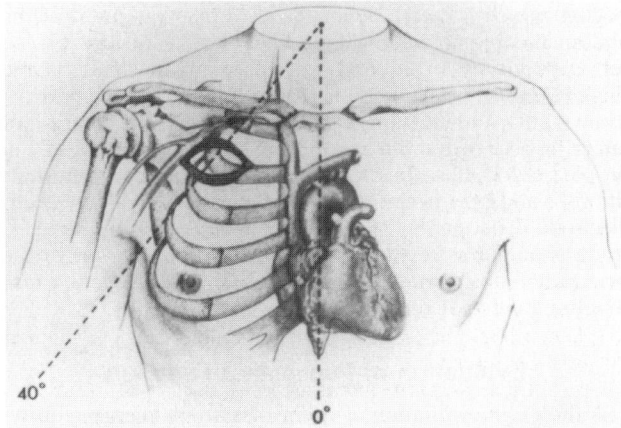

Figure 54–210. Extrathoracic approach to subclavian vein cannulation. The thin-walled introducer needle is shown inserted into the subclavian vein outside the thoracic cavity as the vein crosses over the first rib. The introducer needle is initially advanced to the anterior portion of the first rib and then advanced more posteriorly by a series of partial insertions and withdrawals along the body of the first rib until the subclavian vein is cannulated. (From Byrd, C. L.: Safer introducer technique for pacemaker lead implantation. PACE, *15*:262, 1992.)

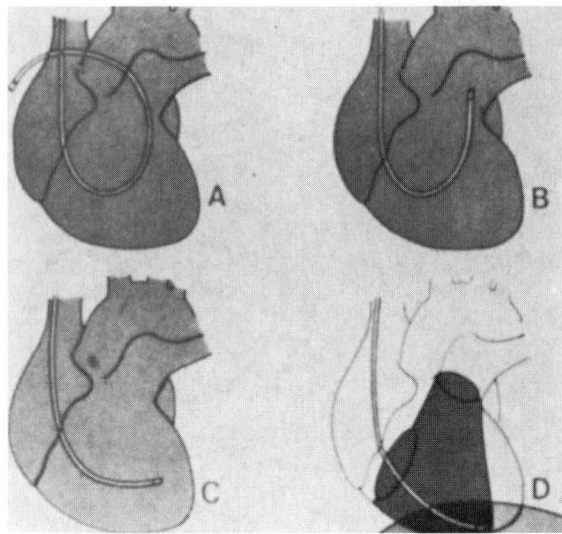

Figure 54–211. Right ventricular lead positioning technique. If the catheter is advanced into the pulmonary artery *(A)*, which is easily confirmed by seeing the tip in the lung fields, there can be no question that on slow withdrawal of the electrode tip *(B)*, it will fall into the ventricle *(C)*, assuming the absence of ventricular septal defects. *D,* The shaded area reflects the approximate shape of the right ventricle. Note that the apex is far lateral and that the electrode usually lies below the dome of the left diaphragm as seen fluoroscopically. (*A–D* from Parsonnet, V.: Implantation of Transvenous Pacemakers. Tarpon Springs, Fla., Tampa Tracings, 1972).

lead cannot be accomplished, an endocardial screw-in lead is placed into the wall of the right atrium. After transvenous positioning and testing of thresholds, the lead is anchored at the fascial or venous exit site to prevent dislodgment by tying a suture around the movable sewing ring provided on the pacing lead. Tying directly onto the pacing lead will frequently cause fracture of the lead's insulation and subsequent lead malfunction. The wound is irrigated with a diluted bacitracin-saline solution. The pacing lead is then connected to the impulse generator, which is then positioned in its pocket, and the wound is closed in layers by using absorbable suture.

Permanent transthoracic leads can be placed through either a small left anterior thoracotomy or subxiphoid mediastinotomy. Generally, sutureless screw-in or hook leads are used and tunneled beneath the costal margin to the pacemaker pocket, which is created over the left upper quadrant of the abdomen well above the belt line or occasionally placed retroperitoneally in either lower quadrant in small infants (Fig. 54–212). The electrode is placed by opening the pericardium and by identifying a fat-free area on the anterior or lateral aspect of the left ventricle. The electrode should not be placed too close to the apex of the heart because of its thinness and because increased motion in this area may cause electrode dislodgment or lead fracture. In addition, the electrode should not be placed in myocardium adjacent to the pericardial course of the phrenic nerve, which could cause diaphragmatic pacing.

Evaluation of Pacemaker Function

A thorough evaluation of pacing threshold energy requirements, atrial and ventricular endocardial electrograms, and impulse generator parameters should be done at the time of initial pacemaker implantation as well as at the time of replacement. A pacing system analyzer simulates the function of the pacemaker's output and sensing circuits and is also capable of evaluating the integrity of the impulse generator itself. The pacemaker's energy output and sensing cir-

cuits communicate with the myocardium through the implanted lead at the electrode-myocardial interface. The pacemaker impulse generator delivers an electrical discharge, which passes through its output circuit into the lead, to the electrode-myocardial interface, and back through body tissue to an indifferent electrode. This system is a simple series electrical circuit described by Ohm's law (resistance = voltage ÷ current).

The electrical pulse discharged by the impulse generator's output circuit is designed to initiate cardiac depolarization. The pacing threshold of the electrode-myocardial interface can be expressed in terms of energy, current, or voltage. The electrical energy discharged by the impulse generator is defined as follows: energy = voltage × current × time. This electrical energy has both an amplitude (voltage or current) and a time component (pulse width or duration). The lowest voltage or current that is delivered to the heart at a given pulse width and that results in cardiac depolarization is referred to as the stimulation threshold. A strength-duration curve (Fig. 54–213) is a graphic plot that shows the stimulation threshold for each pulse width. Any amplitude–pulse width combination on or above the strength-duration curve is sufficient to initiate cardiac depolarization. As shown in Figure 54–213, the amplitude component approaches an infinite value at very short pulse widths, such as less than 0.1 msec., and it approaches a minimal value at long pulse widths, such as greater than 1.5 msec. As can be seen from the strength-duration curve, at a short pulse width the stimulation threshold may exceed the output of the pacemaker and result in loss of pacing. Conversely, excessively long

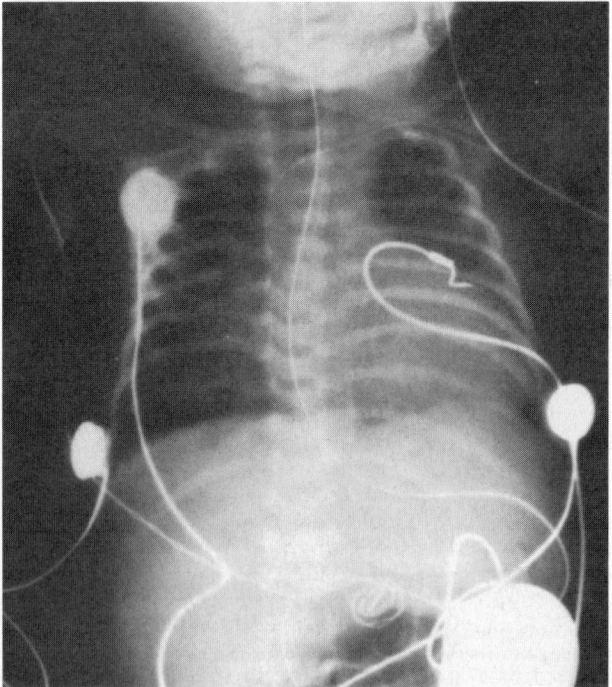

Figure 54–212. Chest film of a 36-hour-old infant born with congenital complete heart block. A fish-hook lead-electrode (Medtronic, Inc., model 4951) was embedded over the lateral aspect of the left ventricle. The lead was then tunneled beneath the musculature of the anterior abdominal wall down to the left lower quadrant. A left lower quadrant incision was made, and the anterior abdominal wall musculature was split. The peritoneum was identified and swept down and medially to create a retroperitoneal pacemaker pocket. The lead was connected to a Pacesetter Programalith III unipolar impulse generator. Most children who require pacemakers do not require a retroperitoneal pocket because of the small size of current impulse generators. However, in the extremely small infant, it is occasionally necessary to place the impulse generator in a retroperitoneal position. (From Sabiston, D. C., Jr., and Spencer, F. C. [Eds.]: Surgery of the Chest, 6th ed. Philadelphia, W. B. Saunders, 1996.)

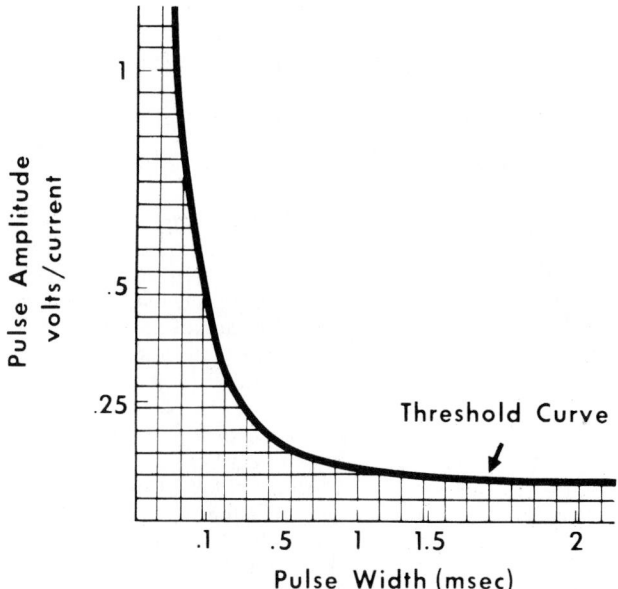

Figure 54–213. Strength-duration curve. A strength-duration curve demonstrates the relationship between the pulse amplitude (volts and current) and the pulse width. Each point on the curve is the stimulation threshold for that respective pulse amplitude and pulse width. The area above the strength-duration curve represents the pulse amplitude and pulse width combinations that will stimulate an endocardial depolarization. The area below the curve represents the combinations of pulse amplitude and pulse width insufficient to stimulate a depolarization. (From Samet, P., and El-Sherif, N. [Eds.]: Cardiac Pacing, 2nd ed. New York, Grune & Stratton, 1980).

pulse widths do not lower the pacing threshold and waste energy. In right ventricular implants using currently available transvenous electrodes, a pulse width of at least 0.5 msec. is usually used acutely to obtain a voltage threshold of less than or equal to 0.5 V. Generally, an acute threshold greater than 1 V. is unsatisfactory. Atrial pacing thresholds are usually comparable with ventricular thresholds but may be slightly higher. Atrial thresholds greater than 2 V. are unsatisfactory. In general, a low acute threshold provides a substantial safety margin because acute thresholds generally rise to higher values during the first several weeks and then decline slightly to their chronic levels secondary to maturation of the electrode-myocardial interface.

In addition to measuring pulse amplitude (voltage and current) and pulse width, resistance is also determined. As described by Ohm's law, resistance is calculated by dividing voltage by current. Resistance calculations are made at a voltage near that of the pacemaker's output. The calculated resistance at 5 V. should range from 300 to 800 Ω. Low resistances cause higher currents and are unsatisfactory for pacing. An unsatisfactorily low resistance can develop secondary to location of the electrode in the ventricular chamber or because of a separate competing electrical pathway (parallel circuit). If a competing pathways exists, current flows through a stimulating and nonstimulating pathway. The current flow through the nonstimulating pathway lowers the resistance and represents wasted energy. This phenomenon can be seen with poorly positioned endocardial electrodes as well as with epicardial electrodes. Very low acute resistances are unsatisfactory because current is wasted and battery life is shortened, which results in a potential for exit block or an increased incidence of muscle stimulation due to increased current. Conversely, excessively high resistances (>800 Ω) increase battery life but decrease the current delivered to the heart for both constant-voltage and constant-current pacemakers. For example, current flow from a 5-V battery

through a resistance greater than 1000 Ω is reduced below 5 mA., which is an inadequate safety margin to compensate for eventual chronic threshold elevation.

In addition to measuring stimulation thresholds and resistance, the sensing circuit of the pacemaker must be evaluated. The sensing circuit monitors spontaneous myocardial depolarizations. The voltage change at the electrode caused by cardiac depolarization (P wave or R wave) is transmitted through the lead to the sensing circuit of the impulse generator. The sensing circuit is designed to detect electrical signals above a particular amplitude within the frequency range of endocardial electrograms. Measurements of amplitude and frequency are essential to ensure proper operation of the sensing circuit. As shown in Figure 54–214, an endocardial waveform has both an amplitude and a frequency component. The frequency component of the endocardial signal is approximated by the slew rate for the measured portion of the waveform. The slew rate represents the maximum rate of change electrogram amplitude with respect to time and is expressed as millivolts per millisecond (or, more simply, volts per second). As shown in Figure 54–214, the amplitude of the atrial or ventricular electrogram is measured in millivolts. As this waveform passes through the sensing circuit of the pacemaker, both the amplitude and the slew rate (rate of amplitude rise or frequency) must be acceptable for the signal to be detected. In general, ventricular endocardial electrograms should be at least 6 mV., and atrial endocardial electrograms greater than 2.0 mV. in amplitude can be detected and provide a safety margin over time. A slew rate of 0.5 or greater is sufficient for detection of both types of signal. Although these values of electrogram amplitude and slew rate represent acceptable minimum values, every effort should be made at the time of lead placement to maximize these parameters to ensure appropriate chronic sensing.

A pacing system analyzer that is capable of simulating the function of a given pacemaker's output and sensing circuits is provided by each pacemaker manufacturer. In addition, the pacing system analyzer is used to evaluate the pacemaker's rate, interval, pulse width, voltage, current, sensitivity, refractory period, and AV interval in dual-chamber devices. After complete testing of threshold energy requirements, atrial and ventricular endocardial signals, and pacemaker parameters, high-voltage settings are used to detect diaphragmatic or phrenic nerve stimulation, which require lead repositioning. The patient is then asked to do deep-breathing and coughing exercises to attempt to produce electrode dislodgment before securing the pacemaker leads and implanting the generator.

PHYSIOLOGY OF PACING

Pacing Modes

Perhaps the most dramatic example of the advancement in pacemaker technology is the various ways in which the heart can be paced. The way in which an impulse generator functions is referred to as the pacing mode. An accurate description of pacing mode must convey not only the chamber of the heart that is being paced but also the chamber sensed by the pacemaker and the manner in which the pacemaker responds to sensed activity. Simple descriptive terms, such as *ventricular-demand pacemaker*, sufficed well for single-chamber devices but have become more awkward as the complexity of pacemakers increases. Devices that pace and sense both atrial and ventricular activity are now frequently implanted. To meet the need for a uniform method of describing pacemaker function, the Intersociety Commission for Heart Disease Resources (ICHD) recommended a five-letter code that succinctly and accurately describes various pacing modes.[34]

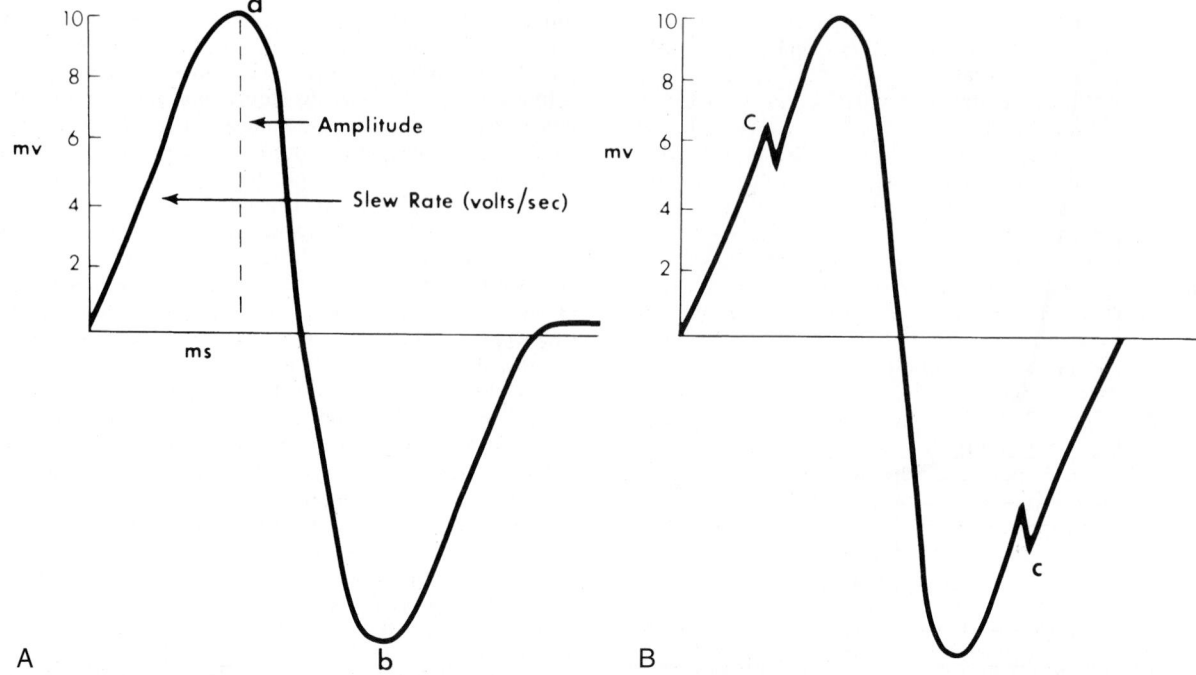

Figure 54–214. Endocardial waveform analysis. *A,* An endocardial waveform, as demonstrated on an electrogram, consists of deflections above and below the baseline. The pacemaker sensing circuit evaluates these deflections by rapidly determining the slew rate (rate of change of the amplitude with respect to time) and amplitude of that deflection. The amplitude is defined by a sensing circuit as the maximal uninterrupted excursion of the wave deflection at a constant slew rate (point a and point b). *B,* A change in the slew rate for a deflection such as a notch (point c) on the wave will be interpreted as a point of maximal excursion (the amplitude or peak for that deflection). Modern sensing circuits can determine not only the peak deflections (points a, b, and c) from the baseline but also the peak-to-peak deflections across the base line (point a to point b). The sensing circuit samples only a small portion of the waveform to determine the slew rate and amplitude. The slew rate obtained from a peak deflection above and below the baseline or a peak-to-peak analysis can be extrapolated into a frequency measurement assuming the entire waveform has that slew rate. (From Samet, P., and El-Sherif, N. [Eds.]: Cardiac Pacing, 2nd ed. New York, Grune & Stratton, 1980).

This code was updated in 1987 to accommodate newer pacemakers (Table 54–18).[4]

The ICHD code uses the letters A and V for atrium and ventricle. The letter D stands for *dual,* indicating both chambers, or when indicating a mode of response, more than one mode. The two traditional response modes to sensed activity, either inhibition or triggering, are indicated by I and T. When no function or response is possible, the letter O is used. In the three-letter code system, the first letter designates the chamber(s) paced, the second letter the chamber(s) sensed, and the third letter the mode of response of the pacemaker to sensed activity. Thus, a pacemaker that paces only the ventricle, senses ventricular activity when intrinsic beats are present, and responds to the sensed activity by inhibiting its output (the well-known ventricular-demand pacemaker) is designated VVI in the ICHD code. An asynchronous ventricular pacemaker that does not sense but that paces at a constant rate regardless of intrinsic cardiac rhythm would be designated VOO (the ventricle is paced, neither chamber is sensed, and there is therefore no response mode to sensed events). In the case of the standard AV sequential pacemaker in which both the atrium and ventricle are paced but only ventricular activity is sensed, the designation is DVI.

The five-letter code has a tremendous advantage in describing not only a certain pacemaker but also various possible modes of function incorporated into a single programma-

TABLE 54–18. NBG (NASPE/BPEG) Generic Pacemaker Code

Position/ Category	I Chamber(s) Paced	II Chamber(s) Sensed	III Response to Sensing	IV Programmability, Rate Modulation	V Antitachyarrhythmia Function(s)
	O = None	O = None	O = None	O = None	O = None
	V = Ventricle	V = Ventricle	T = Triggers pacing	P = Simple programmable	P = Pacing (antitachy-arrhythmia)
Letter Codes	A = Atrium	A = Atrium	I = Inhibits pacing	M = Multiprogrammable	S = Shock
	D = Dual (A + V)	D = Dual (A + V)	D = Dual (T + I)	C = Communicating (telemetry)	D = Dual (P + S)
				R = Rate modulation	

NOTE: Positions I through III are used exclusively for antibradyarrhythmia pacing
Manufacturers may use "S" in positions I and II to indicate single chamber (A or V)
A minimum of four positions is required to describe a pacemaker

Adapted from Bernstein, A. D., Camm, A. J., Fletcher, R. D., et al.: The NASPE/BPEG Genetic Pacemaker Code for antibradyarrhythmia and adaptive-rate pacing and antitachyarrhythmia devices. PACE, *10*:794, 1987.
NASPE, North American Society of Pacing and Electrophysiology; BPEG, British Pacing and Electrophysiology Group.

ble pacemaker. The magnet mode of a pacemaker may also be described. This is the test mode in which a pacemaker functions when the internal reed switch is closed by the external application of a strong magnet. Thus, a VVI pacemaker generally functions in the VOO (asynchronous) mode when an external magnet is applied. Likewise, a sophisticated DDD pacemaker, discussed later, may be programmed to function in one of many modes, including DVI, VVI, AAI, AOO, VDD, and many more.

Fourth and fifth letters are used to denote programmability and antitachycardia capabilities, respectively (see Table 54–18). In this system, the letter P in the fourth position indicates the ability to program one or two parameters and the letter M represents multiprogrammability. However, because all modern pacemakers have multiple programmable features, the M is usually omitted. The letter R in the fourth position is used to designate a rate-modulated pacemaker (e.g., VVI-R); an O in the fourth position indicates a nonprogrammable pacemaker. In the fifth position, various antitachycardia functions may be indicated, including P for pacing, S for shock, and D (for both pacing and shock). These modes are discussed later in detail.

Multiple pacing modes are potentially feasible, although only seven modes have real significance in clinical practice. Of these, two (VVI and DDD) comprise the majority of pacing applications (Table 54–19).

VVI Pacing

Single-chamber ventricular pacing has been the main type of cardiac pacing but is being replaced by more physiologic pacing modes. This mode, often referred to as ventricular-demand pacing, is the simplest of the routinely used pacing modes. As the ICHD code states, the pacemaker senses intrinsic ventricular activity and is inhibited when this activity exceeds the standby or escape rate of the pacemaker. When the intrinsic ventricular rate falls below the escape rate of the pulse generator, the pacemaker begins to function at its programmed rate. The escape rate and the automatic rate (pacing rate) may be identical or may be different if hysteresis is programmed into the pacemaker.

Potential disadvantages of VVI pacing are the lack of AV synchrony and the inability to increase heart rate with physiologic stress. Loss of coordinated contraction of the atria and ventricles may cause unpleasant symptoms due to atrial contraction against a closed tricuspid valve and may produce symptoms of low cardiac output, referred to as the pacemaker syndrome. The magnet code for VVI pacemakers (VOO) allows the function of the pacemaker to be observed even when an intrinsic rhythm is present that would otherwise inhibit pacemaker function.

Asynchronous ventricular pacing was used clinically before units capable of inhibition were available. Because of the potential dangers of asynchronous pacemaker function, with paced beats falling in the T wave of preceding spontaneous beats and inducing ventricular arrhythmias, VOO pacing is now relegated to the rare situation in which oversensing results in inappropriate inhibition that cannot be corrected by reprogramming.

AAI Pacing

Atrial pacing is potentially of great benefit in patients with intact AV conduction and sinus bradycardia, as in the sick sinus syndrome. Until recently, atrial pacing was not used extensively because of technical problems related to stability of endocardial atrial leads. In addition to achieving stable pacing, the atrial electrode must be able to sense an adequate atrial electrogram to avoid asynchronous atrial pacing, which can induce atrial fibrillation. Advances in electrode technology have resulted in preformed J-shaped atrial tined leads that may be placed in position in the atrial appendage and active fixation leads that can be screwed into the atrial endocardium in other locations. These leads are capable of providing reliable atrial pacing in most patients.

Single-Chamber Rate-Modulated Pacing

Single-chamber rate-modulated pacing (VVI-R or AAI-R) has become an important and frequently used pacing mode with the commercial availability of pacemakers using various sensors to regulate the pacing rate. In rate-modulated pacing, the pacing rate is determined by a physiologic parameter, other than atrial rate, that is measured by a special sensor in the pacemaker or pacing lead. During exertion, the required increase in cardiac output is obtained mostly by the increase in heart rate, although increased venous filling and maintenance of AV synchrony are also important contributors. Currently, the most commonly used physiologic parameters used in rate-modulated pacemakers are body motion and minute ventilation. Other parameters that are less commonly used or under evaluation include QT interval, venous blood temperature, mixed venous oxygen saturation, contractility, stroke volume, pH, and the paced depolarization gradient. Although the commonly used body motion sensors increase heart rate (and thus cardiac output) with exercise, the newer physiologic sensors can theoretically respond to a wider variety of physiologic states. However, whether more physiologic sensors improve the quality of life of patients compared with body motion sensors remains controversial. One particular problem with some special sensors is that they require specialized pacing leads to detect the physiologic parameters, such as an oxygen or pH detector on the distal portion of the lead. Whether such specialized leads are more prone to premature lead or sensor failure remains to be determined.

Patients who have chronic or intermittent atrial fibrillation and in whom atrial synchronous pacing is impossible may be able to maintain normal heart rate responses to exercise through the use of ventricular-rate-modulated pacing. In patients with normal AV conduction and sinus bradycardia that does not respond to exercise, rate-modulated atrial pacing may be indicated.

DVI Pacing

Dual-chamber pacing provides an important improvement over simple ventricular pacing in patients in whom optimal cardiac function depends on the atrial contribution to cardiac output. Before the development of atrial synchronous pacing, *bifocal* or AV sequential pacing was the only modality available.

TABLE 54–19. Commonly Used Pacing Modes

ICHD Code	Description
VVI	Ventricular demand
VOO	Ventricular asynchronous
AAI	Atrial demand
AOO	Atrial asynchronous
DVI	AV sequential fixed rate
VDD	Atrial synchronous
DDD	AV "universal"
VVI-R	Ventricular rate modulated

ICHD, Inter-Society Commission for Heart Disease.
From Sabiston, D. C., Jr., and Spencer, F. C. (Eds.): Surgery of the Chest, 6th ed. Philadelphia, W. B. Saunders, 1996.

In this mode, both the atrium and the ventricle are paced, with an artificial AV delay programmed between the atrial and ventricular impulses. In other respects, these devices function similarly to VVI pacemakers. Only ventricular activity is sensed, thus atrial stimulation is asynchronous if the spontaneous atrial rate exceeds the paced rate. DVI pacemakers may be of two varieties: committed or noncommitted. Committed systems are those in which the ventricular output must be delivered when the atrial pulse has occurred. In these systems, a QRS complex appearing in the AV interval will not inhibit ventricular output, and the ventricular pulse will fall in the QRS or ST segment (Fig. 54–215). The advantage of the committed system is that false inhibition of the ventricular output due to cross-talk from the atrial channel cannot result in inappropriate failure to pace. In noncommitted systems, ventricular activity occurring in the AV interval produces inhibition of the ventricular output. Cross-talk from the atrial channel is prevented by means of a blanking period of 20 to 30 msec. after atrial output, during which the ventricular sensing circuits are closed. Some systems have used a compromise between these two modes, in which sensed ventricular activity after the atrial output causes a paced beat with a shortened AV interval; this provides protection from failure to pace and diminishes the chance that the paced beat will fall in the vulnerable period, causing an arrhythmia.

VDD Pacing

One of the primary limitations of DVI pacing is its fixed rate and the need for pacing at a rate faster than the patient's intrinsic sinus rate if the benefits of AV synchrony are to be

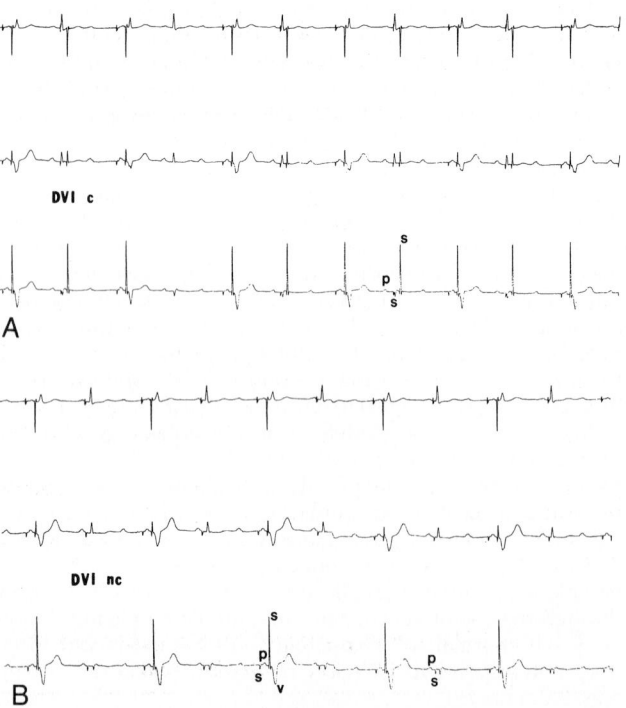

DVI c

A

DVI nc

B

Figure 54–215. *A*, Simultaneous three-channel rhythm strip showing a normally functioning DVI pacemaker in the committed mode. Even though a normally conducted QRS occurs in the AV interval (second, sixth, eighth, and tenth complexes), a ventricular pacing output occurs after the QRS. Note that there is no atrial sensing in the DVI mode. The pacemaker is completely inhibited only when a QRS occurs sufficiently early to inhibit both atrial and ventricular outputs (fourth complex). *B*, A normally functioning noncommitted DVI pacemaker. P waves are not sensed in the DVI mode (second, fourth, sixth, eighth, and tenth complexes) and atrial pacing artifacts occur in the PR interval. Conducted QRS complexes that follow these P waves inhibit the ventricular output. (From Sabiston, D. C., Jr., and Spencer, F. C. [Eds.]: Surgery of the Chest, 6th ed. Philadelphia, W. B. Saunders, 1996.)

maintained. Atrial synchronous pacing allows the ventricle to be pacing after sensed atrial activity (Fig. 54–216). This method has the advantage of preserving AV synchrony and allowing the ventricular rate to vary as the sinus rate varies. VDD pacing is differentiated from an earlier form of atrial synchronous pacing (VAT) in which the ventricle was paced synchronously with atrial activity but without sensing in the ventricle.

Older VDD pacemakers required both an atrial and a ventricular lead and had no advantage over DDD units. However, advancements in lead technology have allowed the development of a single-lead VDD pacemaker.[2] A single lead is placed into the right ventricle for pacing and sensing. However, unlike traditional pacing leads, the lead also has a sensing electrode located several centimeters proximal to the ventricular leads in the right atrial chamber. This proximal electrode can sense atrial activity remotely, although the lack of contact with atrial myocardium precludes atrial pacing. Single-lead VDD pacemakers allow many of the advantages of two-lead DDD units but obviate the difficulties of placing an atrial lead. However, because a VDD pacemaker cannot pace the atrium when the atrial rate decreases below the programmed lower rate limit, VVI pacing results, with its potential disadvantages. Furthermore, failure to sense the atrium will cause ventricular pacing at the lower rate, despite the faster atrial activity.

DDD and DDD-R Pacing

Universal or DDD pacing increasingly has been shown to have many benefits over other pacing modalities, including the ability to track the intrinsic sinus rate, pace the atrium and ventricle, maintain AV synchrony, and avoid the pacemaker syndrome. Recognition of these benefits has steadily increased the use of DDD pacemakers in the past decade. Studies have suggested that the overall impact on the quality of life in patients with pacemakers may be greater than previously recognized.[41] Thus, DDD pacing is the preferred pacing modality in most patients unless chronic or frequent atrial tachyarrhythmias are present or the anticipated frequency of pacing is expected to be minimal. If chronotropic incompetence is present intrinsically or if drugs suppressing sinus node automaticity must be, or are anticipated to be, used, then a rate-modulated dual-chamber pacemaker (DDD-R) should be selected.

The primary difference between early DDD pacemakers and VDD pacemakers was the ability to pace the atrium at the lower rate limit. Thus, instead of VVI pacing at the low rate, AV synchrony was maintained by DVI pacing. DDD pacemakers can be programmed to almost every pacing mode conceivable in addition to DDD, including AAI, VVI, DVI, and VOO. Thus, another benefit of DDD pacemakers is flexibility in programmable options. With newer DDD-R pacemakers, rate-modulated options for each available pacing mode are available (e.g., AAI and AAI-R or VVI and VVI-R). Such flexibility in programmable options allows the greatest freedom to change pacing function as the patient's condition changes over time.

With atrial rates above the lower limit of the DDD pacemaker, the atrial output is inhibited and the pacemaker tracks atrial activity and responds with ventricular pacing after the programmed AV delay if intrinsic ventricular activation is not detected before completion of the AV interval. The ability of the pacemaker to track intrinsic atrial activity provides a range of rates between the lower and upper programmed rate limits. Dual-chamber pacemakers (both VDD and DDD) have a programmable upper rate limit or an atrial rate, beyond which the pacemaker does not continue to track atrial activity. This is a programmable function that can be set

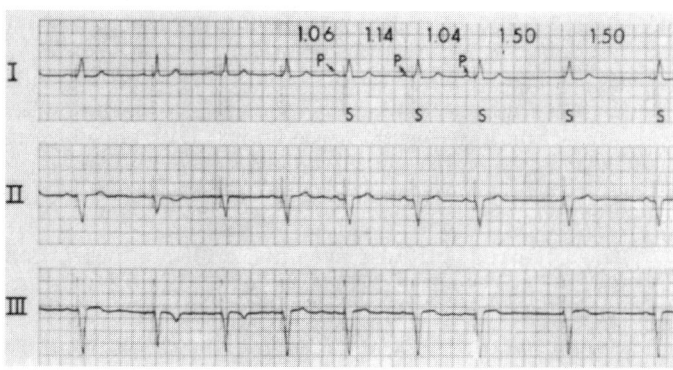

Figure 54–216. A normally functioning VDD pacemaker. Spontaneous atrial activity is sensed and followed by paced ventricular beats, resulting in slight variation in cycle length. When the atrial activity falls below the lower rate limit of the pacemaker, in this case a rate of 40 beats per minute (RR interval of 1.5 second), ventricular pacing results. In the case of a DDD device, DVI pacing would be present at the lower rate. (From Sabiston, D. C., Jr., and Spencer, F. C. [Eds.]: Surgery of the Chest, 6th ed. Philadelphia, W. B. Saunders, 1996.)

according to the patient's needs and to avoid excessive paced rates in the event of rapid atrial arrhythmias.

Two responses to rapid atrial rates can be seen, and these depend on how the pacemaker is programmed. If atrial activity exceeds the programmed upper rate limit before encountering programmed refractoriness of the pacemaker to sense atrial activity, the pacemaker maintains a fixed upper ventricular rate. This produces an apparent Wenckebach sequence, with gradual lengthening of the AV intervals before an atrial beat occurs in the atrial refractory period of the pacemaker and creates a *nonconducted* atrial beat (Fig. 54–217). The total atrial refractory period (TARP) is the sum of two programmed intervals: the AV interval and the postventricular atrial refractory period (PVARP). The PVARP is the interval after a paced or sensed ventricular event, during which the pacemaker does not respond to sensed atrial complexes. For Wenckebach behavior to occur, the TARP must be less than the upper rate interval (i.e., 60,000 msec./min.$^{-1}$/upper rate min.$^{-1}$ = upper rate interval [in milliseconds]). In other words, atrial rates exceeding the upper rate limit do not encounter refractoriness of the pacemaker to sense atrial activity. When the upper rate interval is programmed to a value less than TARP and the atrial rate is faster than that allowed by the TARP, then alternating P waves fall during the pacemaker's period of atrial refractoriness and the pacemaker will track only every other P wave (the 2:1 block point). Thus, in programming VDD and DDD pacemakers, TARP should be programmed at less than the upper rate interval. Injudicious programming of the atrial refractory period may cause an abrupt conversion to 2:1 conduction by the pacemaker at or near the upper rate limit, and the patient will have an abrupt and frequently symptomatic decrease in heart rate.

Programmability

Programmability is defined as the ability to change permanently and noninvasively one or more of the operating characteristics of an implanted pacemaker. The advantages of modifying pacemaker function after implantation have been apparent for a long time. Early devices were made with the capability of changing rate by inserting a transcutaneous needle that turned a potentiometer in the pacemaker. Noninvasive programming was made possible originally through the use of an external magnet that activated a switch inside the pacemaker and changed its rate in incremental steps.

Almost all pacemakers now implanted have multiprogrammable functions. The use of programmability in terms of avoiding reoperation for pacing system malfunction and in improving the patient's tolerance of the pacemaker has been documented.[5] No indications exist for the implantation of nonprogrammable pacemakers. Simple programmability usually includes the ability to change rate, pulse width, mode (usually from inhibited to asynchronous), and refractory period. The ability to change many parameters is called multiprogrammability (Table 54–20). The various programmable functions found on current devices are discussed in detail later in this section.

To effect programming of an implanted pacemaker, a signal must be sent from a programmer to the pacemaker (Fig. 54–218). In practical terms, a programmer must be placed relatively close to the pacemaker to transmit coded information to the pacemaker that is specific for the change desired. The pacemaker must be able to reject inappropriate signals from the environment or from other programmers that could potentially cause unwanted changes in pacemaker function. The pacemaker may respond by returning a signal to the programmer, indicating acceptance of the programming instructions.

Programming features that are desirable include the ability of the programmer to interrogate the pacemaker to retrieve three kinds of information: the programmed settings of the

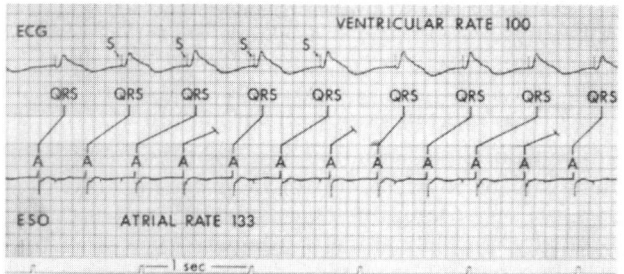

Figure 54–217. An atrial synchronous pacemaker functioning at the upper rate limit. The atrial rate is 133 beats per minute, and the upper rate limit of the pacemaker has been programmed to 100 beats per minute. The interval between sensed atrial activity recorded from an esophageal lead and the pacing stimulus progressively lengthens until a P wave cannot be "tracked," which results in a dropped beat. (From Sabiston, D. C., Jr., and Spencer, F. C. [Eds.]: Surgery of the Chest, 6th ed. Philadelphia, W. B. Saunders, 1996.)

TABLE 54–20. Commonly Programmable Functions of a Multiprogrammable Pulse Generator

Mode	Hysteresis
Rate	Polarity
Pulse width	AV interval*
Output	Upper rate limit*
Sensitivity	Lower rate limit*
Refractory period	

*Dual-chamber devices only.

From Sabiston, D. C., Jr., and Spencer, F. C. (Eds.): Surgery of the Chest, 6th ed. Philadelpia, W. B. Saunders, 1996.

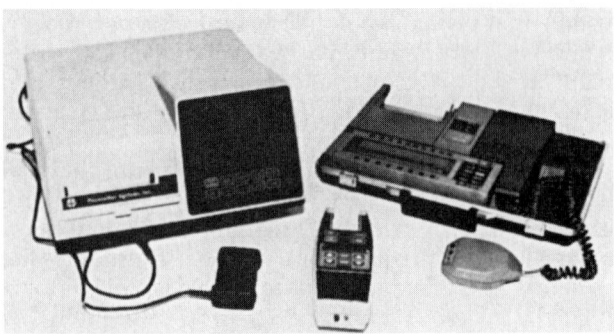

Figure 54–218. Three programmers currently in use, showing the range of complexity and size. *Left,* The programmer for Pacesetter Systems, Inc., models 281, 283, and 285 pacemakers. The programming head is placed over the pacemakers for programming or interrogation. *Center,* A portable hand-held programmer that can perform many of the same functions as the larger unit on the left. The programming head is incorporated into the device itself. *Right,* The Medtronic model 9710 programmer with printer and programming head. This device is compatible with all programmable Medtronic pulse generators.

pacemaker (i.e., what the pacemaker is supposed to be doing); measured data from the pacemaker that indicate what the pacemaker is actually doing, what kind of sensed electrograms the pacemaker is receiving, lead impedance and the battery status; and an increasing variety of stored monitoring data, such as the percentage of time spent at various heart rates and the percentage of paced or sensed beats.

Most pacemakers now use radiofrequency signals to transmit coded information to and from the pacemaker. The functions that can be programmed in a given pacemaker vary considerably, depending on the manufacturer and model. Obviously, the functions subject to programmability depend a great deal on the type of pacemaker (e.g., VVI, DDD-R). The most important functions for programmability are generally considered to be rate, pulse width, pulse amplitude, and sensitivity. Most of the potentially correctable problems encountered with implanted pacemakers can be managed by using these functions. Other functions that can be programmed in various models include refractory period, mode, and hysteresis. In dual-chamber pacemakers, the AV interval, upper and lower rate limits, and the mode of response to upper rate limit may be programmed. In sophisticated units, the pacemaker may actually be programmed off; blanking periods on atrial and ventricular channels can be changed; polarity can be programmed from bipolar to unipolar; and the pacemaker can even be programmed to respond or not respond to an external magnet.

Rate Programmability

The ability to change the rate of an implanted pacemaker is the single most useful programmable function. In patients with chronic cardiac disease, cardiac output may be highly rate dependent. The ability to increase rate allows the individual patient's heart rate to be changed to accommodate temporary changes in physical condition (e.g., cardiac procedures, heart failure, angina pectoris). Some patients develop an unpleasant sensation during pacemaker function or may actually have adverse hemodynamic effects from ventricular pacing. These situations may be remedied by lowering the pacing rate to allow more time in sinus rhythm. The ability to change rate also allows one pacemaker model to be used in all patient age groups, obviating the need for different models for use in pediatric patients who may require higher rates. In most pacemakers, rate can be programmed in steps from 40 to 150 pulses per minute. In rate-responsive pacemakers, the upper sensor drive rate can often be pro-

grammed even higher (150 to 180 pulses per minute). In some rate-responsive DDD units, the upper rate limit for tracking intrinsic atrial activity can be programmed to different values than the upper rate drive by the sensor.

Output Programmability

The output of the pacemaker in terms of total pacing energy is a function of both voltage and pulse width. The energy consumed varies by the square of the voltage but linearly with pulse width; thus, when possible, it is preferable to adjust pulse width rather than amplitude for changes in stimulation threshold. Standard lithium-iodine batteries have an output of approximately 2.5 V. The nominal voltage output of most pacemakers is 5 V., achieved by the use of a voltage multiplier circuit. The ability to program the voltage output down to the lower value may help greatly in prolonging the battery life when chronic lead thresholds permit a lower stimulation energy. In addition, some models have the capability of increasing voltage output to the 7- to 10-V. range, thus accommodating unusually high pacing thresholds, although substantially shortening the longevity of the impulse generator.

Pulse width programmability also allows the output of the pacemaker to be lowered to prolong battery life. Lowering pulse width below 0.3 msec. is not generally recommended, because very high stimulation voltages may be required. Unfortunately, as evident from the strength-duration curve, increasing the pulse width beyond approximately 1 msec. does little to lower the stimulation threshold; thus, raising pulse width in situations of high threshold has little value (see Fig. 54–213).

Sensitivity Programmability

The sensitivity setting of the pacemaker determines the amplitude of the patient's intrinsic cardiac activity required for proper sensing to occur. A balance must be reached among settings that are oversensitive and may allow inhibition by extraneous signals such as myopotentials or T waves and settings that are too insensitive and cause failure to sense intrinsic electrograms. Most pacemakers have a ventricular R wave sensitivity ranging from 1.25 to 8 mV. (the lower value representing the highest sensitivity). In the atrium, sensitivity values of 0.5 to 4.0 mV. are usual. Whether a given electrogram is sensed by a pacemaker depends not only on the actual amplitude of the electrogram but also on the slew rate or change in voltage per time (dV/dt). Thus, the programmed sensitivities do not necessarily guarantee adequate sensing of an electrogram based on its peak-to-peak amplitude. The ability to program sensitivity frequently corrects sensing problems that might otherwise require lead repositioning. Failure to sense premature ventricular contractions is a common example of a situation in which failure to sense may develop, despite proper sensing of sinus beats.

Refractory Period Programmability

The refractory period of the pacemaker is the interval after a sensed or paced event, during which the pacemaker does not respond to sensed electrical activity. This feature prevents inappropriate inhibition of the pacemaker due to artifacts from the stimulus and prevents sensing of other waveforms of the ECG, such as the T wave. When electrodes are implanted in the atrium for AAI pacing, the refractory period should be extended to prevent sensing of farfield R waves. The PVARP of DDD pacemakers should be programmed so that retrograde atrial activation generated by premature ventricular contractions falls within the PVARP. If the retrograde atrial activation is sensed and triggers the pacemaker to pace the ventricle, retrograde atrial activation may again occur, and the process may continue to repeat itself to generate a pacemaker-mediated tachycardia (endless loop tachycardia). Dual-chamber pacemakers frequently have a programmable or fixed PVARP extension in which the PVARP is automatically prolonged when two consecutive ventricular events occur without an intervening atrial event, such as occurs with premature ventricular contractions.

Hysteresis

Hysteresis is a feature that has more theoretical appeal than practical applicability. Hysteresis is usually expressed in terms of the number of pulses per minute below the programmed rate required to initiate pacing. Thus, the escape interval is longer than the automatic or pacing interval. A pacemaker programmed to pace at a rate of 60 pulses per minute with a hysteresis rate of 40 pulses per minute would remain inhibited until a sensed rate of 40 pulses per minute was present, at which time the pacemaker would begin to pace at a rate of 60 pulses per minute. The theoretical advantage of this function is that the patient is allowed to remain in sinus rhythm at intermediate rates between 40 and 60 beats per minute; but when pacing is required, the heart rate is maintained at the faster rate. A problem often encountered with hysteresis is that the patient's intrinsic rate must exceed the automatic rate to inhibit the pacemaker again. For patients who tend to maintain slow rates, hysteresis works well on the front end of the loop, but when pacing is initiated, patients may be unable to elevate their heart rate sufficiently to once again inhibit the pacemaker.

Physiologic Pacing

Physiologic pacing is a term used to describe pacing modes that attempt to duplicate normally conducted sinus rhythm.[42] This concept assumes an understanding of the physiologic relationships between the conduction of the cardiac impulse and the hemodynamic events it initiates and implies that duplication of this physiology can be achieved with an artificial pacemaker. At best, current artificial pacemakers are only crude substitutes for normal sinus rhythm; therefore, the term *physiologic pacing* must be considered to be an oversimplification. Physiologic pacing has also been recognized as synonymous with dual-chamber pacing, although this is not necessarily true.

It has been well established that AV synchrony (i.e., the contraction of the atria and the ventricles with normal sequence and timing) provides some margin of improved cardiac output when compared with ventricular pacing alone at comparable rates.[33, 42] Appropriately timed atrial contraction has been shown to increase cardiac output by as much as 25%. This difference may be even greater during exercise or in certain pathologic states. The deleterious effects of AV dissociation due to ventricular pacing vary greatly from one patient to another and depend on the heart's ability to compensate for a fixed rate, the presence of retrograde ventriculoatrial (VA) conduction, and the patient's overall level of activity.

The ability to increase heart rate to meet increased metabolic demand is also an important feature of normal cardiac conduction. Cardiac output is related directly to heart rate and stroke volume and, when cardiac disease impairs the ability to increase stroke volume, increased heart rate is the only mechanism remaining to increase cardiac output. Therefore, a physiologic pacing system has two aspects: the maintenance of AV synchrony and the preservation of rate variation. AV synchrony is maintained by atrial pacing in the presence of intact AV conduction or dual-chamber pacing in the presence of heart block. Preservation of rate variation is achieved either by pacemakers that track sinus rhythm or imitate normal rate variation using sensors to artificially modulate heart rate.

The pacing modes that offer some preservation of normal physiologic relationships include AAI-R, DVI, VVI-R, DDD, and DDD-R. AAI-R pacing has the advantages of maintaining normal AV conduction, requiring only one electrode, and offering rate variation. It is used in patients with chronic sinus bradycardia with intact AV conduction. DVI obviates the concern for AV conduction but has the limitation of fixed rate (no atrial tracking) and has been replaced by DDD and DDD-R pacing. In patients with chronic atrial fibrillation, VVI-R pacemakers allow more physiologic increases in heart rate with stress. DDD pacing offers both rate variation and AV synchrony and is the optimal form of pacing when sinus node function is normal. DDD-R pacing is preferable when sinus node dysfunction is present or medications blunting sinus node function are necessary. Because DDD-R pacemakers can be programmed to the DDD mode, it can be argued that all candidates for DDD pacemakers should receive a DDD-R unit, so that the rate response option is available for use in the future should it be required.

The acute benefits of AV sequential or atrial synchronous pacing compared with ventricular pacing have been well documented. Numerous studies have also substantiated a sustained hemodynamic benefit of physiologic pacing modalities compared with fixed-rate ventricular pacing. Improvement in acute and chronic exercise capacity, symptoms (dyspnea and fatigue), and even survival have been attributed to rate-modulated and dual-chamber atrial synchronous pacing when compared with simple ventricular pacing.

The AV interval is an important programmable feature of DDD and DDD-R pacemakers. The optimal AV interval must be defined in relationship to the pacing rate, because AV conduction shortens with increasing heart rate under physiologic stresses. Thus, a shorter AV interval may be needed during exercise than at rest. Many modern DDD pacemakers have a function called rate adaptive AV delay in which the AV interval is shortened as the intrinsic or sensor-driven rate increases. Besides potential hemodynamic benefits, the shortening of the AV delay allows higher programmable upper rate limits by decreasing the total atrial refractory period. Studies have suggested that optimal programming of the AV interval allows timing between left atrial and left ventricular contraction rather than between right atrial and right ventricular contraction.[46] In the setting of prolonged intra-atrial conduction, relatively normal programmed AV intervals (e.g., 150 msec.) may not allow sufficient time for left atrial activation before left ventricular activation and may cause left-sided AV dyssynchrony with its potential for adverse hemodynamic sequelae. Other investigators have seen improvement in hemodynamic parameters in patients with severe cardiomyopathies when programmed to short AV intervals, presumably due to prolonged intraventricular conduction.[23] Optimal selection of an AV interval in any patient may depend on monitoring blood pressure during dual-chamber pacing at a number of AV intervals and choosing the interval associated with the best hemodynamic response. A final consideration of the AV interval is that the latency from the atrial stimulus to the onset of atrial systole creates a longer AV interval during atrial pacing than occurs when ventricular pacing follows a sensed atrial event. Newer pacemakers have the feature of different programmable AV intervals for sensed and paced events to adjust for this problem.

It might be held that patients with normal cardiac function and potentially high levels of normal activity should benefit the most from physiologic pacing systems, whereas patients with limited exercise capacity should benefit the least. However, the former patients are probably best able to compensate for a fixed-rate ventricular pacing system through an increase in stroke volume, whereas patients with cardiac disease may depend completely on an increase in heart rate to increase their cardiac output.

An aspect of pacing that may also have significance in terms of physiologic pacing is the pacing site. Normal ventricular contraction is related to the sequence of myocardial depolarization. Ventricular dyssynergy is present during artificial ventricular pacing. This may cause an increase in myocardial oxygen consumption, inefficient ventricular emptying, and abnormal mitral valve function. The deleterious effects of artificial ventricular stimulation may depend on pacing site and are present even when AV synchrony is maintained with dual-chamber pacing. Thus, in patients with intact AV conduction and sinus bradycardia, atrial pacing can be expected to be superior to both VVI and DDD pacing.

INDICATIONS FOR PACING MODES

AAI Pacing. Atrial fixed-rate pacing may be indicated in patients with resting sinus bradycardia and intact AV conduction. Patients with the sick sinus syndrome may be included in this category; however, the potential effects of antiarrhythmic drugs on AV conduction must be considered before an atrial pacing system is implanted. Likewise, the intermittent occurrence of atrial fibrillation would render this pacing mode ineffective. AAI-R (rate-modulated) pacing is indicated when a normal increase in sinus rate with exercise is absent.

Technical problems with atrial lead stability have been mainly overcome with the use of tined J leads as well as the availability of endocardial screw-in leads. These active fixation leads make atrial pacing possible in patients who have had cardiac procedures with cannulation of the right atrial appendage. Screw-in leads may also be useful in other patients in whom a stable pacing site cannot be found in the atrial appendage. Atrial pacing from the coronary sinus has also been an effective method.

VVI Pacing. VVI pacing is indicated for patients with chronic atrial fibrillation and symptomatic bradycardia and for patients with infrequent and intermittent symptoms and who have sinus rhythm. VVI pacemakers should not be implanted in patients with sick sinus syndrome and frequent pacing requirements because of the increased risk of atrial fibrillation, embolic events, and heart failure in addition to the pacemaker syndrome. VVI pacing systems should not be implanted in patients who would benefit from dual-chamber units because of unfamiliarity with these units or difficulties with atrial lead placement. VVI-R pacing is indicated when dual-chamber pacing is not possible because of atrial arrhythmias and when normal chronotropic response to exercise is not present.

DDD Pacing. Over the past decade, there has been an increasing use of dual-chambered pacemakers for several reasons. First, dual-chamber pacing maintains normal AV synchrony with its hemodynamic benefits. Patients with compromised cardiac systolic function and/or diastolic dysfunction are particularly likely to benefit from maintaining AV synchrony. Second, overt pacemaker syndrome occurs relatively frequently in patients with ventricular pacing and intact VA conduction (Fig. 54–219). Patients with the pacemaker syndrome classically present with fatigue, lightheaded spells, decreased exercise capacity, dyspnea, headaches, pulsations in the abdomen or neck, chest pain, syncope, and other vague symptoms. It may be difficult to prove a causal relationship between nonspecific symptoms such as fatigue

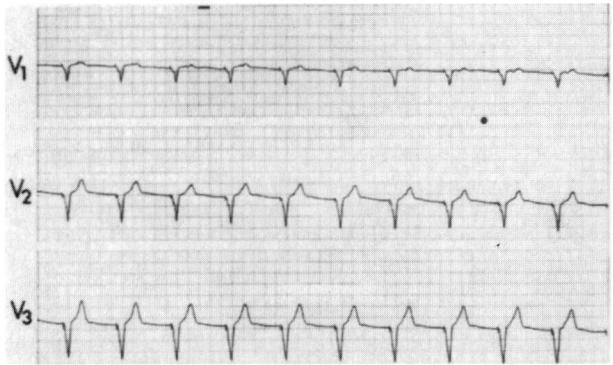

Figure 54–219. VVI pacing at a rate of 60 beats per minute with retrograde conduction. A retrograde P wave can be seen in the ST segment of each paced beat. This patient had symptoms of low cardiac output due to pacemaker syndrome. (From Sabiston, D. C., Jr., and Spencer, F. C. [Eds.]: Surgery of the Chest, 6th ed. Philadelphia, W. B. Saunders, 1996.)

or decreased exercise capacity and the presence of ventricular pacing, although careful monitoring and correlation of symptoms with periods of ventricular pacing can be helpful. However, VA conduction and thus symptoms may be intermittent during ventricular pacing. It has been demonstrated that many patients who do not report symptoms of pacemaker syndrome feel substantially better when their pacemaker is upgraded to a dual-chamber device.[41] Thus, many patients with a single-chamber ventricular pacemaker actually have a subclinical pacemaker syndrome that is not manifested unless dual-chamber pacing is initiated.

Another benefit of DDD pacing is that it decreases the risk of atrial fibrillation in selected patients. Several large studies have demonstrated that VVI pacing in the sick sinus syndrome is associated with a severalfold increased risk of development of atrial fibrillation, strokes, peripheral emboli, heart failure, and possibly death compared with dual-chamber (or atrial) pacing. The increased risk of these events with VVI pacing may be due to the adverse hemodynamic effects of this pacing modality. In addition to maintaining AV synchrony, DDD pacing (or AAI pacing with intact AV conduction) prevents atrial bradycardia, which may allow the escape of atrial arrhythmias. Finally, between 20% and 50% of patients with sick sinus syndrome or heart block have some evidence of chronotropic incompetence, and thus these patients would best be treated with a DDD-R device to maximize exercise capacity. Furthermore, DDD-R pacemakers, because of their wide range of programmable options, can be programmed to VVI-R should refractory atrial fibrillation or atrial lead malfunction occur.

For these reasons, DDD or DDD-R pacemakers are the preferable options for most patients with symptomatic bradycardias and an underlying sinus rhythm. The numerous benefits that have been well documented in patients with sick sinus syndrome appear to extend to the patients with heart block as well. Dual-chamber pacing is also the preferable mode of pacing in patients with carotid sinus hypersensitivity and neurally mediated syncope, given the greater attenuation of hypotension if a vasodepressor component is present.

An algorithm for choosing pacing modes based on the presence of atrial arrhythmias and AV conduction is shown in Figure 54–220.

COMPLICATIONS

As summarized in Table 54–21, pacemaker complications can be divided into four categories: immediate surgical complications, wound problems, delayed complications, and

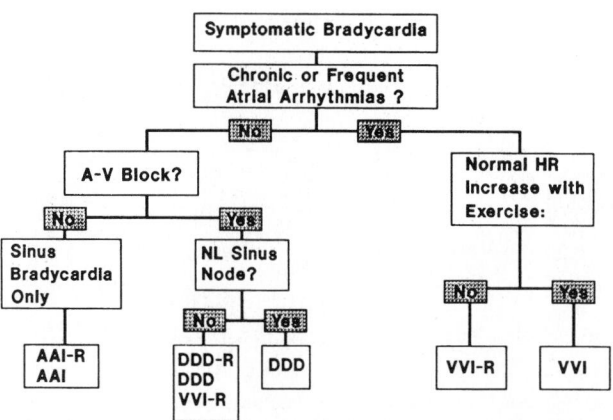

Figure 54–220. Algorithm for choosing pacing mode. Patients with frequent atrial arrhythmias are generally not considered to be candidates for dual-chamber systems but may do well with a rate-modulated pacemaker if their heart rate does not increase with exercise. Patients with an insufficient heart rate response to exercise and AV conduction abnormalities are candidates for the newer DDD-R pacemakers. Atrial pacing alone should be used only when AV conduction is known to be reliably intact. (From Sabiston, D. C., Jr., and Spencer, F. C. [Eds.]: Surgery of the Chest, 6th ed. Philadelphia, W. B. Saunders, 1996.)

pacemaker malfunctions. Fortunately, all are relatively uncommon, making pacemaker insertion an exceptionally safe procedure when performed by experienced surgeons.

Immediate Surgical Complications

As described earlier, perhaps the safest way of inserting a permanent transvenous lead-electrode system is through the cephalic vein. The risk of pneumothorax, vascular injury, air embolism, and air entrapment within the pacing pocket is increased when the subclavian vein access route is chosen. Air entrapment within the pacemaker pocket secondary to either pneumothorax, with subcutaneous emphysema, or to air entrapped during pacemaker pocket closure, can cause pacemaker failure in unipolar systems secondary to insulation of the unipolar anodal plate (indifferent electrode) from the subcutaneous tissues.[22, 28, 29] Neural injury to both the phrenic and recurrent laryngeal nerves has been reported when the lead-electrode system is introduced through the

internal jugular vein. Regardless of the venous access route chosen, cardiac perforation can occur but fortunately rarely leads to hemopericardium and tamponade (Fig. 54–221). A final complication is immediate electrode dislodgment. The risk of this complication can be reduced by doing provocative maneuvers such as coughing and deep breathing at the time of initial implantation. Transvenous electrode dislodgment problems have not been significantly increased in patients with congenitally corrected transposition of the great vessels, although this would have been expected because of the decreased trabeculation of the embryologic left ventricle, which is where the pacing lead lies.[11]

Wound Problems

Perhaps the most common wound problem associated with permanent pacemaker implantation is a hematoma. Obviously, this complication can be prevented by strict attention to hemostasis at the time of implantation. In patients who require impulse generator change, the pacemaker pocket should be débrided of excess pseudocapsule to prevent the formation of a sterile seroma. Fortunately, wound infection is a rare problem prevented by meticulous operative technique and the appropriate use of prophylactic antibiotics. In general, when infection occurs, the entire pacing system, including the impulse generator and lead-electrode system, should be removed, the patient should be treated with appropriate intravenous antibiotics, and a temporary pacemaker should be used for an interim period. When infection has completely cleared, a new pacemaker system is implanted through another access site. Skin erosion by either the impulse generator or lead can be prevented by proper positioning of pacemaker hardware deep within the subcutaneous tissues or beneath the fascia of the pectoralis major muscle. Unipolar impulse generators can cause muscle stimulation if placed immediately adjacent to skeletal muscle. However, bipolar impulse generators can be placed either in the subcutaneous tissue or beneath muscle. Migration of the impulse generator most commonly occurs in infraclavicular pacemaker pockets. Migration tends to follow the curvature of the chest wall, and the impulse generator tends to migrate laterally. This can be prevented by creating an anteromedial pocket sufficiently large to contain the impulse generator and lead. In susceptible individuals, the impulse generator can be further secured to the chest wall to prevent migration.

Delayed Complications

Unusual delayed complications associated with transvenous pacemakers include thrombosis of the superior vena cava with resultant superior vena caval syndrome, axillary vein thrombosis with upper-extremity edema, cerebral venous sinus thrombosis, and right atrial and right ventricular thrombosis. Pulmonary thromboembolism has also been recognized as a rare but lethal complication that occurs most often in patients with low cardiac output and underlying right atrial or right ventricular thrombi. Constrictive pericarditis has been reported in patients who have received both transvenous and transthoracic electrodes.[14, 40] Tricuspid insufficiency is rare, is usually asymptomatic, and is secondary to either lead placement or lead removal. Electrode dislodgment and lead fracture can be caused by unconscious or habitual *twiddling* of the impulse generator (Fig. 54–222). Twiddler's syndrome has been reported most commonly in patients with transvenous pacing systems but has also been reported in those with transmediastinal pacing systems.[38] An uncommon late complication is an allergic reaction to the pacemaker, usually to the titanium components. This can be confirmed by skin testing to various pacemaker components. However,

TABLE 54–21. Pacemaker Complications

Immediate Surgical Complications	Delayed Complications
Pneumothorax	Venous thrombosis
Vascular injury	Pulmonary embolism
Air embolism	Twiddler's syndrome
Cardiac perforation	Constrictive pericarditis
Tamponade	Tricuspid insufficiency
Lead-electrode dislodgment	Pacemaker syndrome
Neural injury—phrenic, recurrent laryngeal	**Pacemaker Malfunctions**
Air entrapment in pocket	Radiation damage
Wound Problems	Runaway pacemaker
Hematoma	Pacemaker-induced ventricular fibrillation
Infection	Irregular pacing
Skin erosion	Failure of sensing
Migration of impulse generator	Failure of capture
Skeletal muscle stimulation	Electrode fracture
	Knotting of lead
	Inhibition of pacemaker by skeletal myopotentials
	Electromagnetic interference

From Sabiston, D. C., Jr., and Spencer, F. C. (Eds.): Surgery of the Chest, 6th ed. Philadelphia, W. B. Saunders, 1996.

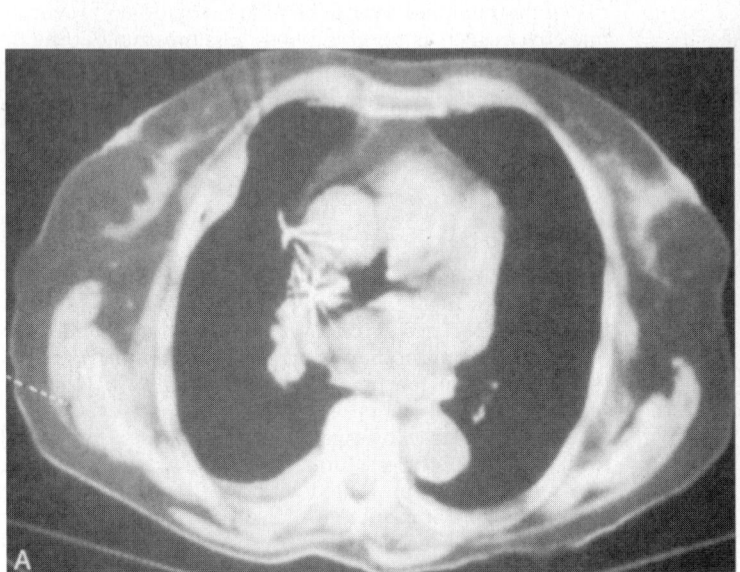
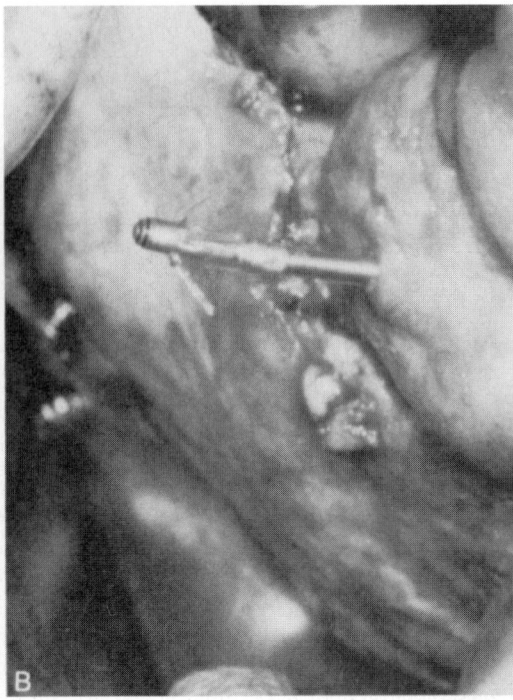

Figure 54–221. Transvenous atrial lead perforation. An 80-year-old woman was referred to Duke University Medical Center several months after implantation of a DDD pacemaker system. The patient initially had done well but was referred for evaluation of a recent syncopal episode. During evaluation, she was noted to have hiccups that coincided with atrial pacing. An electrocardiogram demonstrated atrial pacing without atrial capture. The admission chest film showed a new right pleural effusion and suggested displacement of the atrial lead outside the cardiac silhouette. A repeat echocardiogram could not show the position of the atrial lead, but a chest computed tomographic scan (A) clearly showed that the atrial lead perforated the atrium. A pneumomediastinum was also noted. The patient was taken to the operating room and underwent a right anterior thoracotomy (B) for removal of the lead and atrial repair under direct visualization. An atrial epicardial lead was placed and tunneled across the chest subcutaneously to the chronic left pectoral pacemaker pocket where the ventricular endocardial lead was still attached. The patient recovered uneventfully. This case demonstrates that unlike ventricular perforations, which often seal with retraction of the pacing wire, the thin-walled atrium may not and indeed, as in this case, may require surgical repair. (A and B from Irwin, J. M., Greer, G. S., Lowe, J. E., et al.: Atrial lead perforation: A case report. PACE, 10:1378, 1987.)

many cases of pacemaker allergic reactions are actually smoldering pocket infections with nonvirulent bacteria and should be treated as outlined earlier.

Pacemaker Malfunctions

Most pacemaker system malfunctions are caused by abnormalities of the pacing lead or lead-tissue interface. Primary pacemaker generator malfunction is uncommon, because biomedical engineering improvements have produced exceptionally durable and reliable permanent pacemakers. The possibility of pacemaker generator and lead malfunction and failure emphasizes the need for appropriate long-term follow-up. Pacemaker system malfunction may cause failure to capture the myocardium, oversensing and undersensing, alterations in the preset pacing rate (either acceleration or slowing), and various combinations of these events. These abnormalities may be either persistent or intermittent, the latter presenting a diagnostic challenge to confirm if it occurs infrequently.

When patients present with presumed pacemaker malfunction, they should be extensively monitored to detect periods of inappropriate pacemaker function. A chest film sometimes helps detect lead fracture or displacement (Fig. 54–223). However, the most useful information usually comes from a careful and methodical interrogation of the pacemaker to assess whether the pacemaker is sensing and/or pacing appropriately. Intermittent lead malfunction can sometimes be manifested by stressing the lead with direct compression of the lead at the clavicle or by having the patient raise the arms over the head. Usually detailed evaluation of the patient will uncover the nature of the pacemaker malfunction.

Failure of the pacemaker to capture the myocardium may be persistent or intermittent. Pacing failure may be due to a number of factors, but most commonly these are lead problems, including displacement, perforation, fracture, insulation disruption, and poor generator-lead connection. An increased stimulation threshold, which may also cause failure to capture, may simply be related to the increase in pacing requirements seen in new leads as they heal into place or to other factors, such as acute inferior myocardial infarction, hyperkalemia, hypokalemia, or drug effect/toxicity (especially with antiarrhythmic drugs such as amiodarone or flecanide). Measurement of telemetered lead impedance may help define the cause of pacing failure. If the lead impedance is high ($>1000 \Omega$), a lead discontinuity is present such as is seen in a lead fracture. If the impedance is low ($<300 \Omega$), an insulation break is probably present. A normal lead impedance suggests a stimulation threshold problem; however, the lead impedance may also be normal in the setting of intermittent fractures or insulation disruption. If none of these factors are present, the impulse generator itself may be malfunctioning.

Inappropriate sensing by the pacemaker may result from either undersensing or oversensing of electrical signals. The most common cause of failure to sense appropriate signals is caused by poor initial positioning of the lead electrode or to lead dislodgment. Disruption of insulation around the lead elements and primary pacemaker malfunction may also cause undersensing. Oversensing refers to the detection of electrical signals that were not meant to be detected by the pacemaker. Such signals could be generated by the T wave, by electrical noise from motion at a lead fracture or other source, by myopotentials generated by the pectoral muscles

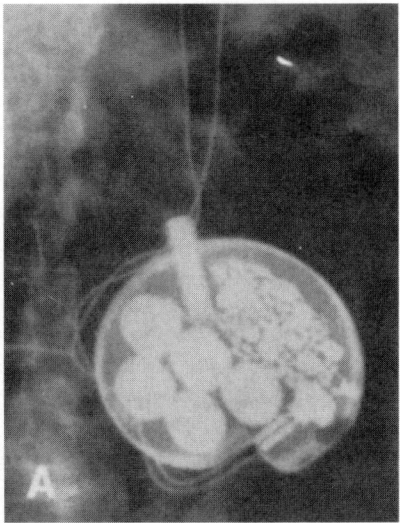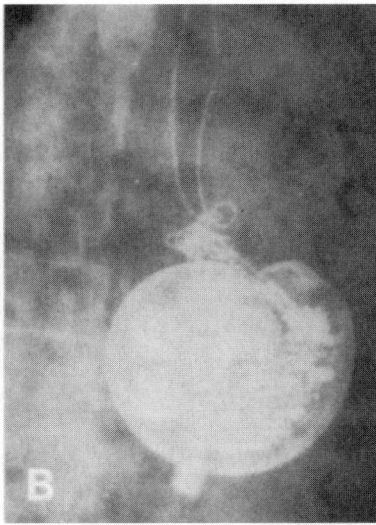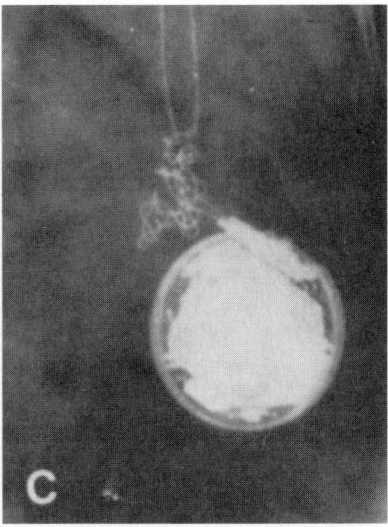

Figure 54–222. Abdominal films. *A,* Film 1 year after initial implant shows normal relationship between the wires and the impulse generator. *B,* Film 2 years later shows rotation of impulse generator 180° and twisting of wires close to the generator. *C,* Six months after implantation of a new impulse generator, additional twisting is evident. (*A–C* from Rodan, B. A., Lowe, J. E., and Chen, J. T. T.: Abdominal twiddler's syndrome. AJR, *131*:1084, 1978. Copyright 1978 by Williams & Wilkins Company.)

(with unipolar pacemakers), or by far-field, high-voltage sources such as electrocautery. Most modern pacemakers can record intracardiac electrograms or event markers, which permits direct documentation of undersensing and oversensing.

Sudden accelerations in the paced rate may be due to several factors. With DDD pacemakers, the most common cause is the development of an atrial tachyarrhythmia, which is tracked by the pacemaker to produce ventricular pacing near the upper rate limit. Application of the magnet typically places the pacemaker in the asynchronous pacing mode and allows detection or termination of the underlying atrial arrhythmia. Recording intracardiac atrial electrograms or event markers also allows the diagnosis to be made. Rate-responsive pacemakers may have erratic fluxes in rate if the sensor is programmed too sensitively; this can be corrected by reprogramming. Motion sensors respond to vibration to cause accelerations in paced rate, as exemplified by very rapid paced rates in patients with activity sensor–driven pacemakers transported by helicopters. Acutely, this can be corrected by magnet applications to deactivate sensor activity or by eliminating the source of vibration.

Pacemaker-mediated tachycardia (PMT) occurs in the setting of intact VA conduction. Typically, premature ventricular contractions may be conducted retrogradely through the AV conduction system and cause retrograde activation of the atrium. If this retrograde atrial activation occurs after completion of the PVARP, the atrial event is sensed by the DDD pacemaker and evokes a paced ventricular event that may cause further VA conduction. If each ventricularly paced event results in retrograde atrial activation sensed by the pacemaker, PMT (or endless loop tachycardia) will be generated. Because PMT is caused by sensing of retrograde atrial activation, placement of the pacemaker in the asynchronous mode by application of the magnet or programming will terminate the tachycardia. Another alternative is to reprogram the PVARP to a large value so that retrograde atrial activation occurs during the refractory period of the pacemaker and cannot be sensed to continue tachycardia. Prevention of further episodes of PMT can be achieved by prolonging the PVARP or using PVARP extension. Some newer pacemakers have programmable options to terminate possible PMT episodes, such as dropping ventricular paced events intermittently when the pacemaker reaches maximum atrial tracking rates. Occasionally, drugs that block AV nodal conduction must be used to prevent retrograde atrial activation after premature ventricular contractions.

Primary pacemaker malfunction may abruptly accelerate the pacing rate, the so-called runaway pacemaker, which creates pacemaker-induced ventricular tachycardia. Fortunately, runaway pacemaker is rarely encountered with modern pacemaker generators. Runaway pacemaker is a medical emergency that should be treated by immediate replacement of the malfunctioning pacemaker. Persistent slowing of the pacemaker rate below the programmed lower rate may be

Figure 54–223. Chest film of a patient who presented with pacing and sensing malfunction. Note the fracture of the outer coil of the pacing lead at the junction of the clavicle. Lead fracture probably occurred at this location because of compression between the clavicle and the first rib. (From Sabiston, D. C., Jr., and Spencer, F. C. [Eds.]: Surgery of the Chest, 6th ed. Philadelphia, W. B. Saunders, 1996.)

an indication that the pacemaker's battery is nearly depleted. Knowledge of the pacing rates that suggest generator end-of-life is important for recognition of this problem. Electrical interference, such as with electrocautery during surgical procedures, may alter the paced rate in some pacemakers (the *noise reversion mode*). Oversensing the T wave can also result in apparent slowing of the paced rate.

Environmental Interactions

Electrocautery may have a number of adverse effects on pacemaker function, depending on the amplitude of the radiofrequency current used and its proximity to the pacing lead and pacemaker generator. In general, unipolar pacemakers are more likely to be affected by electrocautery, given their increased sensitivity to detect noncardiac electrical events. If the pacemaker senses electrocautery potentials of sufficient amplitude, this may inhibit the pacing output. Atrial sensing of electrocautery in DDD pacemakers may produce rapid pacing of the ventricles. Electrocautery can also cause pacemaker reprogramming, fall-back to noise reversion mode, permanent pacemaker generator damage, and permanent or temporary pacing or sensing abnormalities by damaging the myocardium adjacent to the lead electrodes. Patients with pacemakers who are scheduled for surgical procedures in which electrocautery is used should probably be programmed to asynchronous modes to avoid inhibition or oversensing, or they should have the magnet placed over the pacemaker to obtain asynchronous pacing during periods of electrocautery.

PACEMAKER FOLLOW-UP

An organized follow-up program for pacemaker patients should be provided by every clinic engaged in implanting permanent pacemakers. An adequate follow-up program must do more than merely document normal or abnormal function of a pacemaker, and the purpose of pacemaker follow-up is not just to detect pacemaker failure. Instead, a comprehensive program should provide preimplant and postimplant teaching, continued reassurance for the patient and family, transtelephonic monitoring of both the pacemaker and the patient's spontaneous rhythm, office or clinic visits when necessary, and assistance when admission to the hospital is required for complications, for routine battery changes, or for reasons not related to the pacemaker directly.

A properly designed follow-up program should not only provide support for the patient with a pacemaker but should also be capable of providing important information concerning the patient's pacemaker for the physicians who are involved in the patient's care. The functions of the pacemaker follow-up program may be summarized as involving the education of both the patient and physician; documenting normal and abnormal pacemaker function; detecting complications (surgical and related to pacemaker functions); facilitating efficient medical care for the patient with the pacemaker; and storing critical data regarding the pacemaker and electrodes for each patient in an organized system so that it is available to any physician who takes care of the patient. Commercial services can provide transtelephonic ECG tracings and monitor pacemaker function, but these services cannot substitute for a program that involves the medical personnel involved in pacemaker implantation and patient follow-up.

Although commonly thought to involve primarily transtelephonic ECG recording, pacemaker follow-up should be an integrated system of postimplant teaching, clinic visits, and telephone transmissions. The purposes of teaching the patient when the pacemaker is implanted are to allay the patient's and family's concerns about the pacemaker, to inform the patient about the normal function of the pacemaker, and to teach the patient how to use the telephone transmission equipment. A schedule of call-in times should be arranged before discharge, and the use of the transmitter should be practiced with the personnel who will receive the calls. Baseline recordings should be made of the ECG with and without magnet and an overpenetrated chest film obtained to document lead position.

The patient should be examined as an outpatient at 6 weeks after implantation, at which time a noninvasive assessment of pacing threshold should be made. This assessment is performed in different ways, depending on the model and manufacturer of the pacemaker. Pulse generator output can be decreased in a stepwise manner by shortening pulse width in some generators and by lowering output voltage in others. By observing the point at which capture is lost, an estimation of the chronic pacing threshold can be obtained and the pacemaker's output programmed down to lower levels to prolong battery life. A margin of safety of at least 3:1 over the capture threshold should be maintained. Because pacing thresholds may rise during the first few weeks after implantation, decreasing pacing output, either by reprogramming pulse width or voltage, should not be done earlier than 4 to 6 weeks after implantation. The return visit also provides an opportunity to carefully examine the surgical site for signs of excessive skin tension, inflammation, or improper wound healing.

Telephone transmissions should begin immediately after discharge and are done weekly for the first 4 weeks to document proper function. Subsequent telephone transmissions should be made regularly, but at longer intervals. In most patients, transmissions are probably not required more frequently than every 2 to 3 months in the absence of symptoms. At the time of the telephone transmission, recordings should be made of the spontaneous rhythm and then with the application of the external magnet. Readings of pulse width and AV interval (for dual-chamber devices) can also be obtained. These data are recorded in the follow-up files so that proper pacemaker function can be documented and future malfunctions ascertained.

The response of the pacemaker to application of the magnet varies with the manufacturer, and model number and the appropriate magnet response of each patient's pacemaker should be noted in the records. Application of the magnet usually converts the pacemaker to an asynchronous functional mode, typically VOO for a VVI pacemaker and DOO for a DDD pacemaker, although this rule has exceptions. The pacing rate with application of the magnet usually relays information about battery status, with predefined decreases in rate indicating either approaching or imminent battery depletion. Some pacemakers demonstrate an increase in the pulse width above the programmed value as the battery approaches its end-of-life. When rate changes or pulse width increases suggest approaching battery depletion, transtelephonic follow-up should be increased in frequency to at least once a month to monitor for the occurrence of an elective replacement indicator. Magnet application also allows assessment of the pacing function of the pacemaker during asynchronous pacing, even if the intrinsic rhythm is more rapid. Some pacemakers perform threshold tests during application of the magnet. The most commonly encountered method is the threshold margin test, in which three pulses are generated at a relatively rapid rate by the pacemaker on application of the magnet, with the last of the three pulses being 25% of the programmed pulse width. If the third pulse does not capture the appropriate chamber and the previous pulses do, the safety margin for capture is too small and pacing outputs need to be programmed to higher values. Some pacemakers are placed in the vario mode with magnet application, during which the rate is accelerated slightly for 16 beats and the voltage output is decreased by 1/15 between each beat. By calculating the number of complexes that capture the paced chamber, one can ascertain the relative safety margin for pacing.

Finally, records of any reprogramming should be maintained in the follow-up files so that changes in pacemaker function that appear on routine tracings can be properly interpreted.

FUTURE TRENDS

Future trends in cardiac pacing will undoubtedly continue to follow the advances in technology that have characterized the field during the past 10 years. Improvements in lead-electrode technology can be expected to produce smaller leads and improved electrodes, with lower chronic pacing thresholds resulting in lower energy requirements and longer battery life. The ability to pace with less energy output may permit the use of smaller batteries and thus smaller pulse generators.

One of the predictable areas of continued progress is the field of antitachycardia pacing. Devices that can terminate supraventricular tachycardia are being refined. Successful treatment of ventricular tachycardia requires the development of devices that incorporate both antitachycardia pacing and backup defibrillation.

The proliferation of programmable pacemakers has required pacemaker centers to stock an increasingly large number of different manufacturers' programmers. At present, there is no compatibility between the various programmers. Unfortunately, it is unlikely that a device will be devised to program all existing pacemakers. In the future, it would seem to be in the best interests of efficiency and cost reduction to work toward a universal system for pacemaker programmability.

Finally, continued advances in physiologic pacing devices can also be expected. Among these advances will be pacemakers that respond to various physiologic parameters and allow changes in heart rate that correspond with the patient's physiologic needs.

With further technological advances in the field of physiologic pacing, improved ways of determining which patients will benefit from these devices will be necessary. This can be accomplished only through clinical databases located at centers that implant and closely monitor large numbers of patients with pacemakers.

SELECTED REFERENCES

Benditt, D. G. (Ed.): Rate-Adaptive Pacing. Boston, Blackwell Scientific, 1993.
The area of rate-adaptive pacing is rapidly changing. This text reviews in detail the specifics of the hemodynamic and clinical benefits of rate-adaptive pacing and discusses advances in rate-adaptive pacing technology. There are excellent chapters reviewing each of the sensors presently being evaluated for use in rate-adaptive pacemakers.

Committee on Pacemaker Implantation: Guidelines for implantation of cardiac pacemakers and antiarrhythmia devices. J. Am. Coll. Cardiol., 18:1, 1991.
These are the most recent published guidelines for implantation of permanent pacemakers, antitachycardia pacemakers, and implantable cardioverter-defibrillators, as established by a joint committee of the American Heart Association and the American College of Cardiology. These guidelines provide practical information on acceptable and unacceptable indications for pacemaker and defibrillator implantation, and they provide useful clinical background information supporting the indications. This should be read in detail by anyone prescribing or implanting pacemakers or defibrillators.

Naccarelli, G. V., and Veltri, E. P. (Eds.): Implantable Cardioverter-Defibrillators. Boston, Blackwell Scientific, 1993.
This well-written, multiauthored text concerns technical and clinical aspects of the implantable cardioverter-defibrillators. It provides practical information for individuals involved in the care of patients with implantable cardioverter-defibrillators.

The preoperative evaluation, intraoperative testing, and postoperative management of patients with defibrillators are discussed.

REFERENCES

1. Allen, P., and Lillehei, C. W.: Use of induced cardiac arrest in open heart surgery: Results in seventy patients. Minn. Med., 40:672, 1957.
2. Antonioli, G. E., Anscani, L., Barbieri, D., et al.: Single-lead VDD pacing. *In* Barold, S. S., and Mugica, J. (Eds.): New Perspectives in Cardiac Pacing 2. Mt. Kisco, N.Y., Futura, 1993, pp. 359–381.
3. Barold, S. S., and Mugica, J.: Advances in technology and clinical applications. *In* Barold, S. S. (Ed.): The Third Decade of Cardiac Pacing. Mt. Kisco, N.Y., Futura Publishing, 1982.
4. Bernstein, A. D., Camm, A. J., Fletcher, R. D., et al.: The NASPE/BPEG generic pacemaker code for antibradyarrhythmia and adaptive-rate pacing and antitachyarrhythmia devices. PACE, 10:794, 1987.
5. Billhardt, R. A., Rosenbush, S. W., and Hauser R. G.: Successful management of pacing system malfunctions without surgery: The role of programmable pulse generators. PACE, 5:675, 1982.
6. Brockman, S. K., Webb, R. C., Jr., and Bahnson, H. T.: Monopolar ventricular stimulation for the control of acute surgically produced heart block. Surgery, 44:910, 1958.
7. Chardack, W. M., Gage, A. A., and Greatbatch, W.: A transistorized self-contained, implantable pacemaker for the long-term correction of heart block. Surgery, 48:643, 1960.
8. Ekestrom, S., Johansson, L., and Lagergren, H.: Behandling av Adams-Stokes Syndrom med en intracardiell Pacemaker elektrod. Opusc. Med., 7:1, 1962.
9. Eldar, M., Griffin, J. C., Van Hare, G. F., et al.: Combined use of beta-adrenergic blocking agents and long-term cardiac pacing for patients with the long QT syndrome. J. Am. Coll. Cardiol., 20:830, 1992.
10. Elmquist, R., and Senning, A.: Implantable pacemaker for the heart. *In* Smyth, C. N. (Ed.): Medical Electronics. Proceedings on the Second International Conference on Medical Electronics. Paris, June 1959. London, Iliffe & Sons, Ltd., 1960.
11. Estes, N. A. M., III, Salem, D. N., Isner, J. M., and Gamble, W. J.: Permanent pacemaker therapy in corrected transposition of the great arteries: Analysis of site of lead placement in 40 patients. Am. J. Cardiol., 52:1091, 1983.
12. Fananapazir, L., Cannon, R. O., Tripodi, D., and Panza, J. A.: Impact of dual-chamber permanent pacing in patients with obstructive hypertrophic cardiomyopathy with symptoms refractory to verapamil and β-adrenergic blocker therapy. Circulation, 85:2149, 1992.
13. Fischell, R. E., Lewis, K. B., Schulman, J. H., et al.: A long-lived, reliable, rechargeable cardiac pacemaker. *In* Schaldach, M. (Ed.): Advances in Pacemaker Technology, New York, Springer-Verlag, 1975, p. 357.
14. Foster, C. J.: Constrictive pericarditis complicating an endocardial pacemaker. Br. Heart J., 47:497, 1982.
15. Friedberg, C. K., Donoso, E., and Stein, W. G.: Nonsurgical acquired heart block. Ann. N.Y. Acad. Sci., 111:835, 1964.
16. Furman, S., Escher, D. J. W., Solomon, N., et al.: Electrocardiographic manifestation of standby pacing. J. Thorac. Cardiovasc. Surg., 54:723, 1967.
17. Furman, S., and Robinson, G.: Stimulation of the ventricular endocardial surface in control of complete heart block. Ann. Surg., 150:841, 1959.
18. Glenn, W. W. L., Mauro, A., Longo, E., et al.: Remote stimulation of the heart by radiofrequency transmission: Clinical application to a patient with Stokes-Adams syndrome. N. Engl. J. Med., 261:948, 1959.
19. Goetz, R. H., Dormandy, J. A., and Berkovits, B.: Pacing on demand in the treatment of atrioventricular conduction disturbances of the heart. Lancet, 2:599, 1966.
20. Gross, J. N., Moser, S., Benedek, Z. M., et al.: DDD pacing mode survival in patients with a dual-chamber pacemaker. J. Am. Coll. Cardiol., 19:1536, 1992.
21. Hayes, D. L., Graham, K. J., Irwin, M., et al.: A multicenter experience with a bipolar tined polyurethane ventricular lead. PACE, 15:1033, 1992.
22. Hearne, S. F., and Maloney, J. D.: Pacemaker system failure secondary to air entrapment within the pulse generator pocket: A complication of subclavian venipuncture for lead placement. Chest, 82:651, 1982.
23. Hochleitner, M., Hortnagl, H., Hortnagl, H., et al.: Long-term efficacy of physiologic dual-chamber pacing in the treatment of end-stage idiopathic dilated cardiomyopathy. Am. J. Cardiol., 70:1320, 1992.
24. Hyman, A. S.: Resuscitation of the stopped heart by intracardial therapy. II: Experimental use of an artificial pacemaker. Arch. Intern. Med., 50:283, 1932.
25. James, T. N.: The connecting pathways between the sinus node and AV node and between the right and left atrium in the human heart. Am. Heart J., 66:498, 1963.
26. Johansson, B. W.: Longevity in complete heart block. Ann. N.Y. Acad. Sci., 167:1031, 1969.
27. Kantrowitz, A., Cohen, R., Raillard, H., et al.: The treatment of complete heart block with an implanted, controllable pacemaker. Surg. Gynecol. Obstet., 115:415, 1962.
28. Kreis, D. J., Jr., Licalzi, L., and Shaw, R. K.: Air entrapment as a cause of transient cardiac pacemaker malfunction. PACE, 2:641, 1979.
29. Lasala, A. F., Fieldman, A., Diana, D. J., and Humphrey, C. B.: Gas pocket causing pacemaker malfunction. PACE, 2:183, 1979.

30. Leatham, A., Cook, P., and Davies, J. G.: External electric stimulator for treatment of ventricular standstill. Lancet, 2:1185, 1956.
31. Lemberg, L., Castellanos, A., Jr., and Berkovits, B.: Pacing on demand in AV block. JAMA, 191:12, 1965.
32. Nicks, R., Stening, G. F., and Hulme, E. C.: Some observations on the surgical treatment of heart block in degenerative heart disease. Med. J. Aust., 49:857, 1962.
33. Ogawa, S., Dreifus, L. S., Shenoy, P. N., et al.: Hemodynamic consequences of atrioventricular and ventriculoatrial pacing. PACE, 1:8, 1978.
34. Parsonnet, V., Furman, S., and Smyth, N. P.: A revised code for pacemaker identification. PACE, 4:400, 1981.
35. Parsonnet, V., Zucker, I. R., Gilbert, L., et al.: An intracardiac bipolar electrode for interim treatment of complete heart block. Am. J. Cardiol., 10:261, 1962.
36. Parsonnet, V., Zucker, I. R., Gilbert, L., et al.: Clinical use of an implantable standby pacemaker. JAMA, 196:784, 1966.
37. Peuch, P., Grolleau, R., and Guimond, C.: Incidence of different types of AV block and their localization by His bundle recordings. In Wellens, H. J. J., Lie, K. I., Janse, M. J. (Eds.): The Conduction System of the Heart. Lieden, H. E. Stenfert Kroese, 1976, pp. 467–484.
38. Rodan, B. A., Lowe, J. E., and Chen, J. T. T.: Abdominal twiddler's syndrome. AJR, 131:1084, 1978.
39. Schechter, D. C.: Exploring the Origins of Electrical Cardiac Stimulation. Minneapolis, Medtronic, Inc., 1983, p. 91.
40. Schwartz, D. J., Thanavaro, S., Kleiger, R. E., et al.: Epicardial pacemaker complicated by cardiac tamponade and constrictive pericarditis. Chest, 76:226, 1979.
41. Sulke, N., Dritsas, A., Bostock, J., et al.: "Subclinical" pacemaker syndrome: A randomized study of symptom free patients with ventricular demand (VVI) pacemakers upgraded to dual chamber devices. Br. Heart J., 67:57, 1992.
42. Sutton, R., Perrins, J., and Citron, P.: Physiological cardiac pacing. PACE, 3:207, 1980.
43. Sutton, R., Perrins, J., Morley, C., and Chen, S. L.: Sustained improvement in exercise tolerance following physiological cardiac pacing. Eur. Heart. J., 4:781, 1983.
44. Tyers, G. F. O., and Brownlee, R. R.: The non-hermetically sealed pacemaker myth, or, Navy-Ribicoff 22,000-FDA-Weinberger. J. Thorac. Cardiovasc. Surg., 71:253, 1976.
45. Tyers, G. F. O., and Brownlee, R. R.: Power pulse generators, electrodes and longevity. Prog. Cardiovasc. Dis., 23:421, 1981.
46. Wish, M., Fletcher, R. D., Gottdiener, J. S., and Cohen, A. I.: Importance of left atrial timing in the programming of dual-chamber pacemakers. Am. J. Cardiol., 60:566, 1987.
47. Wu, D., Denes, P., Dhingra, R. C., et al.: Electrophysiological and clinical observations in patients with alternating bundle branch block. Circulation, 53:456, 1976.
48. Zoll, P. M.: Resuscitation of the heart in ventricular standstill by external electric stimulation. N. Engl. J. Med., 247:768, 1952.
49. Zoll, P. M., Frank, J. A., Zarsky, L. R. N., et al.: Long-term electric stimulation of the heart for Stokes-Adams disease. Ann. Surg., 154:330, 1961.

XXII

THE USE OF CARDIOVASCULAR PHARMACOLOGIC AGENTS IN SURGICAL PATIENTS

Jeffrey H. Lawson, M.D., Ph.D., and Robert W. Anderson, M.D.

Recent advances in medical care have led to a change in the population of patients who are now referred for surgical treatment. Many patients are now older and have multiple medical problems, which often include cardiovascular disease. Optimal preoperative and postoperative care of these patients requires that the surgeon know the basic principles of cardiovascular pharmacology. Advances in cardiovascular pharmacology are outlined here so that appropriate treatment plans can be formed for these patients during the perioperative period.

EVALUATION OF OPERATIVE RISK: CARDIOVASCULAR FACTORS

Operative risk is defined as the probability of morbidity or mortality from preoperative preparation, anesthesia, the surgical procedure, or postoperative convalescence. The decision as to whether to proceed with any therapeutic intervention, either medical or surgical, must be determined by the potential risks and benefits of the intervention as contrasted to the natural history of the disorder. The cardiovascular system is particularly important in this evaluation, because myocardial infarction, stroke, and congestive heart failure are among the most common complications that occur in surgical patients.

In most cardiac patients undergoing noncardiac surgical procedures, the greatest potential risk arises from coronary artery disease. Historical data from three large series that included 46,000 patients show the risk of perioperative myocardial infarction is 0.15% in patients without prior clinical evidence of heart disease.[16, 33, 41] In those with a prior myocardial infarction, the incidence of reinfarction during a major noncardiac operation increases to approximately 6%.

The risk of perioperative infarction is inversely related to the time between the preoperative myocardial infarction and the noncardiac surgical procedure. This risk follows a nonlinear relationship in which a noncardiac surgical procedure performed within 3 months after an acute infarction is associated with a reinfarction rate of approximately 30%, whereas at 3 to 6 months after an infarction the corresponding rate is approximately 14% and after 6 months the reinfarction rate drops to under 4%. Furthermore, Rao and colleagues[33] demonstrated a significant decrease in reinfarction rates with the implementation of aggressive and perioperative cardiovascular management that was guided by noninvasive hemodynamic monitoring. However, in spite of major advances in intraoperative and postoperative care, the mortality from perioperative myocardial infarction remains high and averages approximately 50%. The risk of cardiac death from reinfarction less than 6 months after a preoperative myocardial infarction is significantly greater than that observed after 6 months, at which time the risk of death is similar to that in patients with no history of cardiac disease who have a perioperative infarction. Factors that appear to be particularly important in evaluating the status of the patient with cardiac disease who is being considered for a major surgical procedure are outlined in Table 54–22.[13]

Obtaining a thorough cardiovascular history is vital for noncardiac surgical procedures, and the findings must be correlated with the chest x-ray and electrocardiogram. A history of prior myocardial infarction should be sought and evidence of left ventricular dysfunction carefully investigated. Close attention should also be paid to the presence, severity, and pattern of angina pectoris and the effectiveness of the current medical program. Exercise stress testing may

TABLE 54–22. Cardiac Risk Factors in Noncardiac Surgical Patients

Historical Factors

Myocardial infarction (especially within the past 3 months)
Congestive heart failure (especially if refractory)
Angina pectoris
Poorly controlled hypertension
Symptomatic cardiac rhythm disturbance

Physical Examination Findings

Presence of third heart sound gallop or venous distention
Abnormal cardiac rhythm
Pulmonary rales
Significant valvular murmur
Hypertension

Laboratory Findings

Cardiomegaly on chest film
Ischemic changes on electrocardiogram (rest or stress)
Ventricular ectopy on electrocardiogram
Abnormal cardiac rhythm

---

be useful in determining the functional limitation of a patient with suspected ischemic heart disease. Even if minimal symptoms of ischemic heart disease are present, stress testing should be undertaken before a major abdominal, intrathoracic, or peripheral vascular surgical procedure if the patient gives a prior history of myocardial infarction, demonstrates symptomatic left ventricular dysfunction, or has diabetes mellitus. If the patient's condition limits the ability of the patient to perform adequately during an exercise stress test, a stress thallium test should be performed, which will chemically induce the heart to a work state in which subtle cardiac disease may be unmasked. Coronary arteriography should be done if the patient demonstrates an early positive stress test or is unable to tolerate the increased cardiac workload of either exercise or chemical stress tests because of ischemic symptoms. In such a situation, coronary revascularization must be considered before the noncardiac surgical procedure. If severe valvular heart disease is identified on physical examination, the cause and severity of valvular heart disease should be investigated. The specific nature of cardiac valvular disease can usually be clarified by echocardiography, but cardiac catheterization may be required in certain cases.

CARDIOVASCULAR DRUGS: MANAGEMENT IN THE PERIOPERATIVE PERIOD

During the past decade, there has been a substantial decrease noted in the mortality from cardiovascular diseases. Although there is a great deal of speculation as to the reasons for this decline, no definitive data are available to explain this phenomenon. Modifications in dietary habits and an increasing awareness of physical fitness are most frequently cited as the reasons for the improvement in cardiovascular health. However, a variety of studies have provided excellent evidence that the use of modern pharmacologic therapy that controls hypertension, modifies the effects of ischemic heart disease, and alters the hemostatic mechanism are important in lowering cardiovascular disease mortality. As a consequence, a larger number of patients are surviving the ravages of cardiovascular disease and are seen by surgeons for problems requiring surgical therapy. These patients often have associated illnesses, and operative risks must be carefully considered in the design of their overall surgical management plan.

Many drugs are used for the management of cardiovascular diseases. Six general categories encompass the majority of commonly used agents: (1) antihypertensives and diuretics; (2) agents for the management of chronic congestive heart failure; (3) antianginal drugs; (4) inotropic drugs; (5) antiarrhythmics; and (6) anticoagulants. Therapeutic overlap exists among many of these drugs, and their indications for use may include several of the broader categories cited. Both the drug and the disease for which it is prescribed will influence the course of anesthetic and surgical management.

Antihypertensives and Diuretics

Hypertension is a common problem, and the number of patients being treated for this disorder has increased substantially during the past 2 decades. In approximately 95% of patients in whom hypertension is diagnosed, no single cause for the elevation in blood pressure can be identified. Although there are many popular theories to explain the increased vascular resistance that seems to occur invariably in hypertension, the possibility that a single defect is responsible for all essential hypertension appears unlikely.

Despite an incomplete understanding of the pathophysiology of essential hypertension, there has been rapid growth in the use of pharmacologic agents to control blood pressure. It is well recognized from a number of therapeutic trials that many of the vascular complications occurring as a result of hypertension can be decreased by pharmacologic intervention. Five general classes of antihypertensive drugs are available for clinical use in the United States: (1) diuretics, (2) adrenergic inhibitors, (3) vasodilators, (4) angiotensin-converting enzyme inhibitors, and (5) calcium channel antagonists. A summary of these antihypertensive agents is presented in Table 54–23. Although the list of drugs is far from complete and new antihypertensive agents are constantly being introduced into clinical practice, certain precautions related to each of the various classes of antihypertensive agents should be observed in surgical patients. In many instances, hypertension is most effectively controlled by a combination of two or more of these drugs, each of which may act by a different mechanism. Although the antihypertensive drugs are commonly used and play an important role

---

TABLE 54–23. Antihypertensive Agents

Diuretics

Thiazides and related drugs
Loop diuretics (furosemide and ethacrynic acid)
Potassium-sparing diuretics (spironolactone and triamterene)

Adrenergic Inhibitors

Peripheral (reserpine and guanethidine)
Central (methyldopa and clonidine)
Beta-receptor (propranolol, atenolol, nadolol, etc.)
Alpha-receptor (prazosin, phenoxybenzamine, phentolamine)

Vasodilators

Hydralazine
Minoxidil
Nitroprusside

Angiotensin-Converting Enzyme Inhibitors

Captopril
Enalapril
Lisinopril

Calcium Antagonists

Nifedipine
Verapamil
Diltiazem
Nicardipine

in current medical therapy, they are all potentially toxic and work by inhibiting or modifying normal physiologic regulatory mechanisms. For this reason they may be particularly troublesome and potentially dangerous in surgical patients in whom the stress of disease and the use of anesthetic agents may unmask potentially hazardous reactions and physiologic responses.

Diuretics. The thiazide agents and furosemide are the antihypertensive agents most commonly employed for the treatment of mild or moderate hypertension. Thiazides act at the distal convoluted renal tubule to inhibit sodium transport,[43] whereas furosemide acts at the ascending limb of the loop of Henle to inhibit chloride transport.[17] Because both of these drugs increase urinary excretion of salt and water, hypovolemia secondary to dehydration may occur in surgical patients. This results in tachycardia and a predisposition to hypotension when anesthetics are administered that blunt the normal homeostatic responses to decreasing blood pressure. In this setting, what might be considered a trivial loss in blood volume during an operative procedure may cause profound hypotension if pre-existing intravascular and extracellular fluid deficits are not corrected. By obtaining a careful medication history and searching for clinical signs of volume depletion, such as orthostatic hypotension, appropriate measures to restore intravascular volume before operation can be undertaken and such problems can be avoided.

Because both furosemide and the thiazides increase delivery of sodium to the distal renal tubule where aldosterone-dependent sodium-potassium exchange occurs, potassium loss and hypokalemia may occur after chronic administration of these agents.[39] In the presence of hypokalemia, the arrhythmogenic effects of digitalis or anesthetic agents that sensitize the myocardium may result in severe disturbances of cardiac rhythm. This may produce hemodynamic compromise or even fatal ventricular fibrillation. Such problems can be avoided or minimized by repleting diminished potassium stores before undertaking any extensive surgical procedure. Although serum potassium levels will generally indicate that hypokalemia exists, this value does not always reflect the severity of intracellular deficits after long-standing diuretic therapy. Repletion of diminished total body potassium stores before major surgical procedures, particularly cardiac operations, is essential to diminish cardiac rhythm disturbances, particularly if alkalosis or digitalis therapy coexists.

Adrenergic Inhibitors. Antihypertensive drugs that act pharmacologically by inhibiting function of the sympathetic nervous system are common and are classified according to the site at which they inhibit the sympathetic reflex arc. Each class of drug exhibits different forms of potential adverse side effects and may produce problems in the surgical patient. The peripherally acting agents such as reserpine and guanethidine are capable of producing profound sympathoplegia by blocking or inhibiting biogenic amine functions in both peripheral and central neurons. Although these actions account for the success of the drugs in controlling hypertension, the potential problems of depressed cardiac output and hypotension due to blunted sympathetic responses in the presence of volume depletion or exposure to anesthetic agents are often seen in surgical patients. For this reason, it is generally advisable to discontinue peripherally acting adrenergic blocking drugs for a period of time before an elective surgical procedure. The substitution of a more rapidly acting and easily managed agent may be required.

The centrally acting adrenergic inhibitors such as clonidine and methyldopa reduce sympathetic outflow from vasopressor centers in the brain stem. Because they allow these centers to retain their sensitivity to baroreceptor control, they do not depress normal cardiovascular reflexes and thus do not depress cardiac output or produce the orthostatic hypoten-

sion seen with the peripherally acting agents. Abrupt withdrawal of clonidine may result in severe hypertension and increased sympathetic activity. Thus, this drug should be continued throughout the perioperative period or gradually withdrawn while other antihypertensive therapy is substituted.

Although beta-blocking agents were initially employed in the treatment of angina pectoris, these agents are also extremely effective for treating a variety of other disorders, such as hypertension, thyrotoxicosis, migraine, arrhythmias, and glaucoma.[8] Most treatment programs in patients with mild or moderately severe hypertension include one of the beta-blockers. There was initially a great reluctance to administer a general anesthetic to a patient taking one of the beta-blocking drugs because of the frequent occurrence of bradycardia or hypotension secondary to a depression of cardiac output, but it is now generally considered safer to continue these agents throughout the surgical procedure and to utilize a specific beta-agonist or atropine if hypotension or bradycardia develops. The beta-blockers appear to be well tolerated in cardiac surgical patients and offer a significant degree of protection from postoperative rhythm disturbance if continued without interruption throughout the perioperative period. Although there has been much discussion regarding the *cardiac selectivity* of certain beta-blocking drugs, the clinical differences among the various beta-blockers are of minor importance from a surgical standpoint, and all are generally well tolerated. The most prudent policy may, therefore, be to continue administering these drugs during the perioperative period unless the dosage is very high, in which case it should be tapered to a normal recommended dosage. Abrupt withdrawal of beta-blockers has been associated with acute myocardial infarction and should be avoided.

The alpha-receptor antagonists are rarely used for the management of uncomplicated hypertension. The most commonly employed agent is prazosin, which antagonizes stimulation of the vascular alpha-receptors and appears to cause both arteriolar and venous vasodilation.[34] Surgical patients who have been taking prazosin may develop a relative volume loss that may require preoperative fluid replacement. A similar problem may be encountered with the other alpha-receptor antagonists, phenoxybenzamine and phentolamine. When possible, it is preferable to discontinue alpha-receptor antagonists before performing any elective surgical procedure unless specific indications exist for continuing the use of these agents, such as in a patient with a pheochromocytoma in whom phenoxybenzamine or phentolamine may be important in the preoperative preparation. However, careful management of the patient's fluid volume status is mandatory or profound hypotension may occur.

Vasodilators. Peripheral vasodilators are usually employed in the management of hypertension when a diuretic and/or adrenergic blocker do not control the blood pressure. Hydralazine is the only drug employed routinely as an oral agent. It is usually reserved for patients with severe hypertension and is given in combination with a diuretic and beta-blocker. If given alone, hydralazine commonly elicits a number of reflex responses such as tachycardia that are troublesome and limit its usefulness. Other vasodilating agents used in the management of hypertension include minoxidil, which is usually reserved for the management of very severe hypertension in patients with renal insufficiency, and diazoxide and nitroprusside, two intravenous agents reserved for the management of malignant hypertension or hypertensive emergencies. These latter two agents act very rapidly and may need to be employed in patients with severe and refractory hypertension. These drugs should only be used under carefully monitored circumstances because of their rapid onset of action and propensity for inducing hypotension and tachycardia. Nitroprusside is the agent of choice for the control of acute hypertension in the operating room or during the postoperative period due to its rapid onset of action. Its ease of titration under conditions of proper monitoring allows for the prompt detection and correction of perioperative fluid deficits.

Angiotensin-Converting Enzyme Inhibitors. Captopril, enalapril, and lisinopril are inhibitors of angiotensin-converting enzyme, which converts inactive angiotensin I to the pressor peptide angiotensin II.[30, 31] These agents are very potent and specific antihypertensive agents that lower total peripheral vascular resistance and cause little change in cardiac output, heart rate, and pulmonary wedge pressure.[11] They are particularly effective in hypertensive patients with elevated renin levels. These compounds do not appear to interfere with normal cardiovascular homeostatic responses, even when simultaneously administered with a diuretic. However, if significant volume depletion occurs as a result of a concomitantly administered diuretic, hypotension may develop. Abrupt withdrawal of these agents may result in severe hypertension that is difficult to manage; therefore, these drugs should be continued throughout the perioperative period.

Calcium Antagonists. Calcium channel blockers are a class of compounds that selectively antagonize calcium ion movement across intracellular membranes by specifically blocking the transmembrane calcium ion channels.[22] These agents are widely used in the control of hypertension and cardiac arrhythmias and in the treatment of angina. Their broad range of activities in both cardiac and smooth muscle have extended their use to include the treatment of asthma, migraine headaches, arterial disease, and cardiomyopathy. The most common calcium channel blockers used in surgical patients are nifedipine, diltiazem, and verapamil. Nifedipine has the strongest peripheral vasodilatory effect of the calcium channel blockers and has become popular in the treatment of hypertension due to the extended-release form of the drug, which makes once-a-day dosing of the agent convenient for most patients. For minor surgical procedures, it is reasonable to keep most patients on their regular dose of nifedipine through the perioperative period. For major noncardiac surgical procedures it is best to discontinue the agent the morning of surgery and closely monitor the patient's hemodynamic status in the perioperative period. Postoperatively, the patient can be started on small (10 mg.) doses of nifedipine sublingually as needed to control blood pressure, and once the patient has had full return of gastrointestinal tract function the routine dose of calcium channel blocker can be resumed. For patients who require aggressive calcium channel blockade in the immediate postoperative period, a new intravenous calcium channel blocker, nicardipine, is available.[21] This agent has a similar hemodynamic profile to nifedipine but can easily be titrated to control blood pressure by constant intravenous infusion. It is recommended to start nicardipine at 5 mg. per hour and to increase the dose 2.5 mg. per hour each 15 minutes to a limit of 15 mg. per hour or until blood pressure control is achieved. Because of the rapid onset and the potent action of this agent, its use is recommended only in the intensive care unit setting with continous blood pressure monitoring.

Although certain antihypertensive agents may cause problems in surgical patients because of their particular mode of action, uncontrolled hypertension in the surgical patient is a very serious problem. It is, therefore, essential that a rational plan for the management and control of blood pressure in the operating room and postoperative period be formulated before any form of antihypertensive therapy is discontinued. After the period of hemodynamic instability surrounding the immediate operative period has passed, the patient's normal antihypertensive regimen should be reinstituted to make the perioperative management less complex. Rapid-acting agents such as intravenous nitroprusside and nicardipine are preferred for treatment of severe hypertension during the intraoperative or immediate postoperative period. These agents must be administered only under carefully monitored conditions because of their ability to produce profound hypotension.

Agents for the Management of Congestive Heart Failure

Traditional treatment for patients with evidence of cardiac failure has consisted of salt restriction, diuretics, and the administration of a digitalis preparation for cardiac rate control and an inotropic effect. It is now recognized that an increase in impedance to left ventricular ejection is an important factor in producing the left ventricular dysfunction that characterizes cardiac failure states. This increased impedance to ejection is the result of a complex series of peripheral vascular events produced by increased activity of the sympathetic system and the renin-angiotensin system.[5, 9] The final result of this abnormal activity is narrowing of the arterioles, decreased arterial compliance, and a reduction in venous compliance that shifts blood into the central circulation and increases cardiac filling. Thus, current management strategies have changed from vigorously stimulating the failing heart with inotropic agents to attempting to reduce the cardiac load by means of vasodilators. The concept of afterload reduction by pharmacologic means is well established for the treatment of hypertension and has now been extended to other disease states, including severe congestive heart failure (particularly if due to hypertension), aortic or mitral valve incompetence, ischemic heart disease with accompanying congestive heart failure, and all of the cardiomyopathic states that produce cardiac failure.[5, 6] Although it would appear illogical for the body to respond to a failing myocardium by increasing the work of the ventricle, this seems to be the case. An increased level of peripheral vascular resistance and aortic impedance to ejection is characteristic of heart failure, and this reflex vasoconstriction, which probably was intended to deal with volume depletion, becomes a deleterious feedback mechanism in the patient with cardiac failure due to impaired left ventricular function. Neuroendocrine responses are activated in congestive heart failure, as demonstrated by the striking variation in plasma norepinephrine and renin levels observed in patients with this disorder, but the levels of these substances do not correlate well with the level of cardiac failure or the form of therapy employed.[5]

Drugs that produce vasodilation of vascular smooth muscle can favorably affect the performance of the heart in two ways.[4, 35] By decreasing the peripheral vascular resistance through the mechanism of arteriolar relaxation the ventricular ejection fraction improves, stroke volume improves, and end-systolic volume decreases. In addition, the relaxation of venous smooth muscle shifts blood from the central circulation into the peripheral venous capacitance bed, thereby decreasing the preload or end-diastolic volume. This redistribution of volume results in the following physiologic effects: (1) a reduction in myocardial wall stress and consequent lowering of myocardial oxygen requirements; (2) a shift to the more effective portion of the diastolic pressure-volume curve, which allows for increasing amounts of volume with lesser increases in diastolic pressure; (3) a decrease in end-diastolic pressure in the left ventricle with a consequent decrease in pulmonary venous pressure and relief of pulmonary congestion; and (4) improved diastolic perfusion of the myocardium caused by the lowered transmyocardial pressure gradient between epicardial and endocardial blood vessels. The improvement of ventricular emptying leading to enhancement of stroke volume is the fundamental objective of any form of therapy for congestive heart failure secondary to cardiac dysfunction. Clinical trials evaluating the use of vasodilators for congestive heart failure have demonstrated that this approach to management of heart failure is physiologically rational.[6]

The surgical management of patients with evidence of congestive heart failure has been greatly improved by the addition of vasodilator drugs to the therapeutic armamentarium. This has been particularly evident in cardiac surgical patients, who can now be stabilized hemodynamically preoperatively and then brought to the operating room in a much more stable condition than was previously possible. The deleterious effects of uncontrolled hypertension are well recognized, and currently available drugs allow for improved regulation of cardiac function and blood pressure both preoperatively and intraoperatively. Although many vasodilating agents are available, only a few are commonly employed clinically (Table 54–24).

Any patient with cardiac disease severe enough to produce symptoms of congestive heart failure represents a substantial risk for any major surgical operation. A comprehensive evaluation of the patient's underlying cardiac disorder, the institution or continuation of appropriate therapy, and the judicious use of intraoperative monitoring of cardiac function are mandatory if surgical risk is to be reduced to an acceptable level. In almost all instances, pharmacologic agents that have successfully controlled symptoms of cardiac failure before surgery should be continued or more appropriate agents utilized throughout the preoperative, operative, and postoperative periods. The vasodilator drugs discussed previously are generally short-acting and can usually be easily employed in the adequately monitored patient. However, abrupt termination of most of these drugs in the patient with severe cardiac compromise may result in significant hemodynamic instability and subsequent congestive heart failure.

Antianginal Drugs

Operative mortality and morbidity are significantly increased among patients with coronary artery disease. The optimal management of these patients is predicated on identifying those at significant risk, assessing their cardiac reserve and ability to withstand the stress of anesthesia and surgical therapy, and instituting suitable treatment before surgery in an effort to minimize risk.

The most important cardiovascular risk factor in evaluating a patient for a major surgical procedure is the history of a recent myocardial infarction. Many institutions require a comprehensive cardiac evaluation, including stress testing and coronary angiography if indicated, for patients with a history of recent myocardial infarction or severe angina pectoris before performing any major elective noncardiac surgical procedure. Although no definitive study has been reported that documents the ability of this plan to prevent myocardial infarction or cardiac death, there are isolated uncontrolled reports of the success of such an approach. In any event, patients undergoing major surgical procedures who have any history of ischemic cardiac disease must be optimally managed from a cardiac standpoint. Many patients with symptomatic angina take medication to control symptoms; however, other patients may have equally severe coronary disease despite minimal clinical symptoms. Patients with severe peripheral vascular disease have been found angiographically to have an incidence of coronary artery disease as high as 95%. In nearly half of these patients, no symptoms of coronary artery disease are present. A well-planned course of management should include either a surgical or a pharmacologic approach for the control of ischemic heart disease.

Three general classes of pharmacologic agents are specifically used for the treatment of angina pectoris: nitrates, beta-blockers, and calcium antagonists. A more complete list of the commonly used antianginal agents is presented in Table 54–25.

The short- and long-acting nitrates present no particular surgical problems and can be continued up to the time of operation. Either transdermal or intravenous nitroglycerin can be used at the time of operation if evidence of ischemic change is noted on the electrocardiogram or if signs of congestive heart failure develop. Patients who have been taking nitrates for a prolonged period of time may develop serious cardiac ischemia if the drugs are abruptly withdrawn; therefore, suitable precautions must be taken to prevent this occurrence.

Unless patients show evidence of profound beta-blockade with a very low resting heart rate, have a history of physical findings suggesting congestive heart failure, show evidence of a low cardiac output, or are having pulmonary symptoms such as wheezing, it is generally advisable to continue beta-blocking drugs up to the time of operation and then to reinstitute them immediately after operation. Abrupt withdrawal of beta-blockers may lead to evidence of ischemia during the stresses of anesthesia and operation that may cause serious arrhythmias or other ischemic complications. If problems develop during the operative period that appear to be due to excessive beta-blockade, specific treatment should be instituted. Profound bradycardia can usually be managed with atropine (1 to 2 mg. intravenously). Failure to increase

TABLE 54–24. Vasodilator Drugs

Drug	Afterload Reduction	Preload Reduction	Indications
Nitroprusside (intravenous)	+ + +	+ +	Acute hypertension Cardiac failure Valvular insufficiency
Nitrates (intravenous, oral, patch)	+	+ + +	Ischemic failure
Hydralazine (oral or intravenous)	+ + +	0	Chronic cardiac failure
Prazosin (oral)	+ +	+ +	Hypertensive failure Pulmonary hypertension Chronic cardiac failure
Captopril (oral)	+ +	+	Chronic cardiac failure
Nifedipine (sublingual)	+ +	0	Acute left ventricular failure
Nicardipine (intravenous)	+ +	0	Acute hypertension

+, present.

TABLE 54–25. Antianginal Drugs

Agent	Route of Administration and Usual Dosage
Short-acting Nitrates	
Nitroglycerin	Sublingual, 0.3–0.6 mg.
	Intravenous, 0.6–12 mg./min.
Isosorbide dinitrate	Sublingual, 2.5–5 mg.
Long-acting Nitrates	
Isosorbide dinitrate	Oral, 10–40 mg., every 4–6 hr.
Nitroglycerin capsules	Oral, 2.5–9 mg., every 6–12 hr.
Nitroglycerin paste	Skin, ½–2 inches, every 6–12 hr.
Nitroglycerin patch	Transdermal, 5–10 mg., daily
Beta-blocking Agents	
Noncardioselective	
Propranolol	Oral, 20–80 mg., every 6–8 hr.
	Intravenous, 0.5–5 mg., slow infusion
Nadolol	Oral, 100 mg., daily
Timolol	Oral, 5–15 mg., three times/day
Pindolol	Oral, 2.5–7.5 mg., three times/day
Cardioselective	
Atenolol	Oral, 100 mg., daily
Metoprolol	Oral, 50–100 mg., three times/day
Calcium Antagonists	
Verapamil	Oral, 80–120 mg., every 8 hr.
Nifedipine	Oral, 10–40 mg., every 6–8 hr.; extended release 30–120 mg. daily
Diltiazem	Oral, 30–90 mg., every 6 hr.

the heart rate with atropine or evidence of a low cardiac output or hypotension secondary to these agents can be managed by the intravenous infusion of glucagon (2.5 to 5 mg./hr.). This agent is the drug of choice because it stimulates formation of cyclic adenosine monophosphate by a route that bypasses the occupied beta receptor.[27] The competitive beta-blockade may also be overcome by infusing dopamine or dobutamine. Isoproterenol would be a specific agonist but is not a good choice in patients with ischemic heart disease because of its peripheral vasodilating effect, which may produce severe hypotension. Temporary transvenous cardiac pacing may be required in rare instances when pharmacologic therapy fails.

The calcium antagonists or calcium channel blockers are an important group of agents used in the treatment of angina pectoris that also have antihypertensive and antiarrhythmic properties.[19, 28] Unlike beta-blockers, which cause constriction of smooth muscle, the calcium antagonists cause vasodilation and therefore are not associated with side effects such as bronchospasm. Thus, they are useful antianginal agents in patients with chronic obstructive pulmonary disease. The antianginal properties of the calcium channel blockers have been ascribed to three basic mechanisms: (1) an increase in coronary blood flow due to direct vasodilation of coronary arteries; (2) a decrease in myocardial oxygen demand as a result of a decrease in systolic ventricular wall stress or afterload and an improvement in diastolic relaxation; and (3) a cardioprotective effect during periods of transient ischemia.[26] Some evidence also suggests that the calcium channel antagonists inhibit platelet aggregation and help improve myocardial oxygen delivery.[28]

Although all of the calcium antagonists possess antianginal properties, their structural differences involve varying sites and modes of action.[24] Verapamil has its most prominent effect on the atrioventricular (AV) node, slowing both antegrade and retrograde conduction through this node. As such, verapamil is also useful in the treatment of supraventricular

tachycardias. Diltiazem also decreases AV nodal conduction and, like verapamil, may be used in the management of supraventricular tachycardia. Nifedipine has very little effect on the AV node. It is most noted for its potent peripheral vasodilating effect and thus may be used in patients with both ischemic heart disease and hypertension. Although all were initially thought to have profound negative inotropic effects, it has since become apparent that in the usual clinical dosages their myocardial depressant properties are not great unless they are given in combination with a beta-blocker or in the presence of pre-existing left ventricular dysfunction.

The calcium antagonists may, however, produce several problems in the surgical patient. Because of their peripheral vasodilating effects, these agents may unmask latent hypovolemia and lead to profound hypotension after relatively minor amounts of volume loss. This is a particularly troublesome side effect of nifedipine, which has the strongest peripheral vascular vasodilating properties of the calcium channel blockers. Thus, careful hemodynamic monitoring with attention to volume status must be undertaken in surgical patients who are maintained on these agents. Another problem that may be encountered is severe myocardial depression due to the combined use of beta-blockers and calcium channel antagonists, a combination often used in patients with angina pectoris. The combination of agents may result in cardiac depression by blunting the normal reflex sympathetic responses to the depressant effects of the calcium antagonist and may be compounded by the use of inhalational anesthetic agents, which may have negative inotropic effects on the myocardium. For these reasons, it is usually prudent to discontinue the calcium antagonist and continue the beta-blocker before major cardiac or general surgical procedures. This is particularly true for patients with evidence of severe myocardial dysfunction on the basis of ischemic, valvular, or nonspecific myopathic disease. The interaction between digitalis preparations and the calcium antagonists is safe in the absence of digitalis toxicity, but lethal AV blockage may result if these drugs are administered in the presence of digitalis toxicity. Verapamil should be administered very cautiously to patients receiving a beta-blocker because of the sinus AV nodal slowing that is commonly observed when these agents are administered simultaneously.

At present, nitrates remain the first-line treatment for the relief or prevention of angina in patients with coronary artery disease. These agents present little problem for the surgical patient, because they have few serious limiting side effects and may be administered safely throughout the patient's operative course.

Inotropic Drugs

Inotropic drugs offer the most direct approach for improving cardiac performance. If a new pump (cardiac transplantation) is considered as a form of improving systolic or diastolic dysfunction, it is quite clear that the multiple abnormalities that develop as a result of heart failure (activation of the renin-angiotensin system, increased sympathetic nervous system activity, increased secretion of arginine) are reversible. The ideal myocardial-stimulating drug should improve myocardial contractile force without greatly increasing myocardial oxygen demand or producing excessive afterload for the heart to work against by causing peripheral vasoconstriction. Additionally, it should not stimulate tachycardia or other cardiac arrhythmias. Unfortunately, none of the currently available inotropic agents fulfill these criteria.[7, 27] Nonetheless, inotropic drugs continue to play an important role in the management of patients with heart failure and are particularly important in the management of surgical patients with cardiovascular instability on the basis of either primary cardiac dysfunction or peripheral vascular disease. The agents commonly employed for inotropic stimulation include the digitalis compounds, the sympathomimetic amines, and the phosphodiesterase inhibitors. The pharmacologic properties of these three classes of agents and potential problems that may arise after their administration are vastly different and are therefore discussed separately.

Digitalis Compounds. Digitalis has multiple direct and indirect cardiovascular effects that are both therapeutic and potentially toxic. At the molecular level, the digitalis compounds inhibit the membrane-bound sodium-potassium adenosine triphosphatase.[10] This inhibition causes a loss of potassium from the myocardial cell and an increase in calcium released to the contractile proteins at the time of excitation-contraction coupling. The net result is an increase in myocardial contractility. The alterations in the mechanical and metabolic properties of the cardiac cell are accompanied by changes in the electrical properties that may cause rhythm disturbances as secondary toxic side effects. These same electrophysiologic properties of the digitalis compounds may also be employed therapeutically for the control of cardiac rhythm disturbances that are supraventricular.

Because it has a moderately consistent inotropic effect and can be administered orally, digitalis is, in theory, a very useful agent for the management of cardiac failure. However, there has been increasing controversy as to whether the proposed benefits of the drug outweigh its narrow therapeutic index.[27] The indications for digitalis are diminishing, particularly for the treatment of acute heart failure. Currently, the major indication for the administration of digitalis is the combination of congestive heart failure and atrial fibrillation.[29] Congestive heart failure in the presence of sinus rhythm may be more safely managed by diuretics or a combination of diuretics and a vasodilator, and acute left ventricular failure is generally treated by more potent inotropic drugs such as dopamine or dobutamine, a diuretic, and vasodilators before digitalis is considered. The issue of using digitalis to treat chronic congestive heart failure remains questionable, but because it appears that some patients are substantially improved by the administration of this agent, the challenge is to develop better methods of identifying those patients who have a good response and are at minimal risk for development of troublesome side effects.

Intraoperative conditions may arise that predispose the surgical patient to toxic manifestations (usually arrhythmias) of the digitalis compounds. Both acute hypoxemia and hypokalemia increase susceptibility to digitalis-induced ventricular arrhythmias, and these disturbances require prompt and specific correction. Hypercalcemia, cardiac ischemia, certain anesthetic agents, and myocardial infarction are also responsible for a heightened sensitivity to the digitalis compounds. It is generally best to withhold digitalis compounds for a period of time before any surgical procedure and use safer pharmacologic agents throughout the operative and immediate postoperative period for the management of cardiac failure or rhythm disturbances.

Sympathomimetic Amines. The catecholamines increase contractility by stimulating cardiac beta-receptors with subsequent augmentation of calcium availability to the contractile system and enhancement of myocardial contractility.[29] The beta$_1$-receptors normally respond to norepinephrine, which is released by cardiac sympathetic nerves. The norepinephrine stores in these nerves are depleted in chronic heart failure, and the sympathomimetic drugs that act by releasing norepinephrine stores may be ineffective. The receptors, however, are intact and may respond to exogenously administered catecholamines.

The sympathomimetic drugs available in the United States

as inotropic agents are all delivered intravenously, and their overall effect on the circulatory system is influenced by their relative stimulatory effect on receptors other than those in the heart. The alpha-receptors in the peripheral circulation produce vasoconstriction, and the beta$_2$-receptors in the lungs and peripheral circulation produce bronchodilation and peripheral vasodilation.

Epinephrine and norepinephrine are prototypes of the class of sympathomimetic amines. Both drugs have potent beta$_1$-receptor–stimulating properties and therefore are powerful cardiac stimulants. As a result of beta$_1$-receptor stimulation, both drugs increase heart rate and myocardial oxygen consumption, which could prove to be detrimental to patients with coronary artery disease. In addition to the beta-receptor stimulation, both agents posses alpha-adrenergic effects and subsequently cause peripheral vasoconstriction at relatively low dosages. Renal blood flow is reduced because of the vasoconstrictive properties, and if these drugs are used for supporting the failing heart, an alpha-adrenergic blocking drug should be administered simultaneously for minimizing the vasoconstriction. Because of these potential limitations, epinephrine and norepinephrine are usually employed in patients with refractory hypotension and low cardiac output, as may be seen in various shock states.

Isoproterenol is a synthetic catecholamine with dominant beta-adrenergic activity. Because its beta-receptor effects are largely unopposed by any alpha-receptor stimulation, isoproterenol produces significant peripheral vasodilation, which may be a very desirable feature in patients with severe vasoconstriction; but this same property could produce hypotension and limit its clinical usefulness. The most limiting feature of isoproterenol is that it increases myocardial oxygen demand, which may precipitate ischemia in patients with significant coronary artery disease. For this reason, isoproterenol should be used only in patients without evidence of ischemic disease.

Dopamine has become the drug of choice for patients with myocardial failure who require inotropic support for maintenance of hemodynamic stability. It is an intermediate compound in the synthesis of epinephrine and norepinephrine and also releases norepinephrine stores from nerve endings in the heart.[15] It has both beta- and alpha-adrenergic effects; however, these effects are seen at different dosages. At the lower dosages of 2 to 10 µg. per kg. per minute, it increases cardiac contractility by beta-stimulation while causing widespread peripheral vasodilation and improving renal blood flow by selective stimulation of dopaminergic receptors.[27] It is less likely than other catecholamine drugs to produce ventricular irritability, tachycardia, or excessive increase in myocardial oxygen demands. In dosages greater than 10 µg. per kg. per minute, the alpha-stimulating properties of dopamine become more prominent, and the resultant vasoconstriction may prove to be deleterious to the failing heart. Thus, vasodilators may be required for reversal of some of the vasoconstricting properties of the drug. The combination of dopamine and nitroprusside has proved to be particularly useful in the management of patients after cardiac surgery who demonstrate a persistent low cardiac output that is unresponsive to volume therapy alone.

Dobutamine is a synthetic analog of dopamine that acts directly on beta$_1$-adrenergic receptors, thus causing a stronger inotropic than chronotropic effect.[27] Although it has alpha$_1$-agonist effects, the beta$_2$-adrenergic effects tend to override these, producing a mild peripheral vasodilation. In contrast to dopamine, dobutamine does not release norepinephrine, nor does it stimulate the dopaminergic receptors in the kidneys. Because it does not rely on norepinephrine release for its inotropic action, dobutamine may be more effective than is dopamine in patients with long-standing myocardial failure in whom endogenous catecholamine levels are depressed. Dobutamine has been shown to decrease myocardial oxygen consumption by decreasing wall stress; thus, it is a useful inotropic agent in patients with coronary artery disease undergoing general or cardiac surgical procedures.

Phosphodiesterase Inhibitors. These agents function by inhibiting intracellular phosphodiesterase type III, which increases intracellular levels of cyclic adenosine monophosphate.[12] These drugs possess strong inotropic effects as well as direct arterial and venous vasodilatory properties.[25] The prototypical agent in this class of drugs is amrinone, which is available in intravenous form for the treatment of congestive heart failure. Amrinone produces an increase in cardiac output while reducing peripheral vascular resistance and left-sided heart filling pressures. It has essentially no effect on heart rate or blood pressure. Because of its afterload-reducing properties, amrinone is useful in patients with low cardiac output and mitral or aortic insufficiency, because it tends to decrease regurgitant volume during systole, thus increasing forward flow. It has also been used with success in patients with the low output syndrome after cardiac surgery. One important side effect with relatively long-term amrinone use is a nonimmunologic-mediated thrombocytopenia, which could prove to be deleterious in the preoperative or postoperative setting.

Milrinone is 20 times more potent than amrinone with a similar mechanism of action in addition to a prominent vasodilatory component.[23] When milrinone is given acutely, its inotropic and vasodilatory effect is combined with an increase in heart rate. When it is given chronically, only some patients benefit and there is risk of arrhythmias. Although amrinone in the oral form is no longer used, the intravenous preparation with its major inotropic and vasodilator effects should be especially useful in patients with beta-receptor downgrading, such as those in severe congestive heart failure or with prior prolonged therapy with dobutamine or other beta$_1$-stimulants. Milrinone is available in oral form, but its efficacy remains undetermined.[7]

Antiarrhythmic Agents

The perioperative management of patients with cardiac arrhythmias and conduction disturbances is an important part of patient care. A knowledge of the preoperative drug ingestion history, electrocardiographic status, and cardiovascular history is mandatory and must be combined with an understanding of the intraoperative and postoperative factors that facilitate the occurrence of cardiac rhythm disturbances. A number of factors may be encountered perioperatively that predispose to the development of arrhythmias: (1) ventilatory problems that produce hypoxia or respiratory alkalosis, (2) hypokalemia and other electrolyte abnormalities, (3) toxicity to cardioactive anesthetics and other drugs, (4) hypotension, (5) hypertension, (6) reduced cardiac output, (7) anemia, (8) myocardial infarction, and (9) cardiac trauma and pericarditis. These factors must always be considered in the evaluation of a surgical patient with cardiac rhythm disturbance, and initial treatment should always be directed toward correction of these abnormalities. Thus, the aim of modern antiarrhythmia therapy is to reduce the ectopy of pacemaker activity and to modify impaired conduction, either by improving it in an area of depressed conduction or by suppressing it entirely.

Investigators have categorized antiarrhythmic compounds by their effects on the fast sodium current, the sympathetic activity of the heart, the repolarization current, and the slow inward calcium current.[1, 20] The sodium channel blockers are the most important group of agents and are similar to local anesthetics in that they exhibit membrane-stabilizing proper-

ties. This group is referred to as Class I agents and includes lidocaine, quinidine, procainamide, disopyramide, phenytoin, and the newer agents mexiletine, aprindine, tocainide, and encainide. These drugs are effective in the treatment of ventricular and supraventricular arrhythmias.[40] All these agents are capable of causing a variety of severe toxic side effects that either may directly affect the heart conduction system or may cause extracardiac manifestations.

Class II agents are the beta-antagonist drugs and include propranolol and similar drugs that have antiarrhythmic properties by virtue of their adrenergic receptor blocking action and direct membrane effects. The relative contributions of the beta-blocking and direct membrane effects are unknown. These agents have also been shown in clinical trials to lower the incidence of recurrent infarction and sudden death in patients recovering from myocardial infarction.[14] In addition, beta-adrenergic blocking drugs are particularly effective in suppressing ventricular premature beats and ventricular tachycardia that are increased by or occur from exercise or are associated with mitral valve prolapse syndrome.

Class III agents function by widening the duration of the action potential. Recent clinical experience suggests that this group of drugs will emerge as the most significant for control of cardiac arrhythmias.[42] The Class III agents available in the United States are amiodarone and bretylium. Both are effective in the management of atrial flutter and fibrillation in association with the Wolff-Parkinson-White syndrome, and amiodarone has been used extensively in the treatment of sustained ventricular tachycardia refractory to other antiarrhythmic agents.[32] There are reports of adverse effects of long-term amiodarone treatment, and the most common side effects are corneal microdeposits, liver function abnormalities, and pulmonary fibrosis. Amiodarone noncompetitively blocks both alpha- and beta-adrenergic receptors *in vivo*. It increases coronary blood flow but reduces cardiac work and oxygen consumption, as well as peripheral vascular resistance. Small intravenous doses in man do not affect cardiac contractility; however, with larger doses, contractility is depressed and the left ventricular end-diastolic pressure is increased.

Class IV agents are the calcium channel blockers. The prototype Class IV drug is verapamil, which has become the agent of choice for the control of supraventricular arrhythmias because of its ability to slow conduction through the AV node with very few side effects and a low incidence of toxicity.[38] Verapamil, however, should not be used for treatment of atrial fibrillation in patients with the Wolff-Parkinson-White syndrome, because conduction across the accessory pathway may increase as a result of inhibition of AV conduction, and this may cause hemodynamic collapse.[18]

From a practical standpoint, the indications for the use of antiarrhythmic drugs in surgical patients must be based on a knowledge of the natural history of the rhythm disturbance and whether it is of physiologic significance in the overall management of the patient. Careful documentation and precise diagnosis of the type of rhythm disturbance are essential. There is a limited role for the prophylactic use of drug therapy in an attempt to prevent the development of arrhythmias, because all antiarrhythmic drugs have proarrhythmic effects and, therefore, may precipitate a rhythm disturbance.[20] In general, all cardiac rhythm disturbances that are potentially life threatening, that can be shown to cause hemodynamic compromise, or that cause symptoms should be precisely diagnosed and specifically treated. Patients with no known structural heart disease usually do not require specific drug therapy for benign rhythm disturbances, such as sinus tachycardia, premature atrial beats, or unifocal premature ventricular beats. The most prudent approach may be to define underlying etiologic factors such as fever, hypoxia, or anxiety, and attempt to eliminate them. In some patients, the presence of heart disease may complicate the use of antiarrhythmic therapy. Heart failure and conduction problems are the most serious. Most of the antiarrhythmic drugs depress left ventricular function to a variable and dose-related degree, and patients with left ventricular dysfunction may tolerate these agents poorly. Drug therapy for patients with AV nodal disease or with conduction disease below the level of the AV node should be carefully monitored because of the potential for serious side effects and profound depression of cardiac conduction.

Anticoagulants

Many surgical patients with underlying cardiac risk factors, cardiac dysrhythmias, or angina pectoris are treated with some form of anticoagulant therapy to decrease their risk of coronary artery thrombosis or systemic cardiac embolism. The most common of these agents are aspirin and warfarin (Coumadin). Aspirin has become widely used in patients with signs or symptoms of coronary artery disease due to its antiplatelet effects, and it has now become rare to see elderly patients with documented coronary artery disease who are not on low-dose aspirin therapy. Warfarin is widely used in patients with atrial dysrythmias, mechanical heart valves, and a history of deep venous thrombosis.

Aspirin functions as an inhibitor of arachidonic acid metabolism and irreversibly inhibits platelet activation.[37] For minor surgical procedures in patients with severe coronary artery disease, it is reasonable to continue aspirin therapy during the surgical procedure, with careful attention to surgical hemostasis during the operative procedure. For more extensive surgical procedures it may be necessary to stop aspirin therapy 7 days before the procedure and, if the patient is at severe risk for coronary artery thrombosis, heparin therapy should be started preoperatively. This will allow the operation to proceed during a heparin window where the level of anticoagulation can be easily titrated or reversed using protamine. After completion of the surgical procedure, aspirin therapy should be restarted as soon as the gastrointestinal tract can tolerate oral medication. Furthermore, patients who are treated with aspirin and undergo the stress of surgical intervention should be treated with some form of antacid (H$_2$ blocker) therapy to decrease the risk of perioperative gastroduodenal ulcer formation.

Warfarin is an anticoagulant that inhibits the vitamin K–dependent carboxylation of clotting factors II, VII, IX, X, protein C, and protein S.[2] This inhibition of clotting factors renders them functionally inactive in their normal hemostatic function by blocking their ability to form functional procoagulant complexes. Patients who require elective surgical intervention and are treated with warfarin for underlying cardiac or hypercoagulable states should discontinue therapy with warfarin before the operative procedure. In most patients, warfarin should be stopped 5 days before surgery and the prothrombin time (PT) should be checked. As the PT international normalized ratio (INR) level drops below 2.0, heparin therapy should be started and the activated partial thromboplastin time (aPTT) should be monitored to keep the aPTT twice the control value. The best hemostatic control is achieved when the patient's PT has normalized and the aPTT is well regulated with heparin. If intraoperative bleeding becomes a problem, the heparin can be abruptly stopped and protamine can be given to reverse the heparin anticoagulant effect. Postoperatively the patient should be kept on heparin until gastrointestinal function returns, at which time the patient's warfarin therapy can be resumed. As soon as the patient's PT INR is 2.0 or greater, the heparin may be discontinued.

When postoperative bleeding develops in a patient with severe coronary artery disease or in a patient who has a history of deep venous thrombosis, the balance between the patient's risk for further bleeding and the potential for thrombosis must be assessed. If there is no obvious technical reason that the patient is continuing to bleed, reversal of anticoagulant therapy should be considered. As noted earlier, protamine can be given to block the anticoagulant effect of circulating heparin. If bleeding persists, then one must consider using fresh frozen plasma (to provide more clotting factors) or platelets. Vitamin K may be given in 10-mg. doses, but this will only help ensure that the new clotting factors that are being synthesized in the liver are properly carboxylated and will do little to help with the immediate postoperative bleeding problem. Other agents such as the antifibrinolytics aminocaproic acid (Amicar) and aprotinin may be helpful in acute postoperative bleeding, but their exact role in patients who were originally on anticoagulant therapy due to cardiac or hypercoagulable states remains to be determined.

PHARMACOLOGIC MANAGEMENT OF SPECIFIC CARDIOVASCULAR PROBLEMS IN THE SURGICAL PATIENT
Arrhythmias and Conduction Disturbances

Bradyarrhythmias. Sinus bradycardia in the surgical patient is usually caused by increased vagal tone related to direct stimulation of the carotid sinus, stimulation of the vagus nerves, or pain. Myocardial ischemia should always be excluded as a cause for sudden cardiac slowing.

Bradycardia is best treated by administering atropine intravenously in 0.5-mg. boluses up to 2 mg. over a 30-minute period. If atropine therapy is unsuccessful, a continuous infusion of isoproterenol may be administered at a rate of 1 to 10 μg. per minute titrated to the heart rate responses. If pharmacologic therapy is unsuccessful, a temporary pacemaker should be placed.

Ventricular Arrhythmias. The treatment of ventricular arrhythmias is a complex and changing area that cannot readily be simplified. The criteria for instituting therapy are not clear cut, although patients with sustained ventricular tachycardia and those with symptomatic or hemodynamically compromising ventricular dysrhythmia require treatment.

Intraoperative or postoperative ventricular ectopy is often precipitated by hypoxia, hypercarbia, hypokalemia, anxiety, fever, or drug excess, and correction of these problems often resolves the ectopy without resorting to specific drug therapy. Ventricular ectopic activity that occurs in the absence of clinical heart disease or electrocardiographic abnormalities is generally benign and well tolerated.

Ventricular ectopic activity in the form of frequent multifocal ventricular beats or ventricular couplets in patients with a history of ischemic heart disease or with electrocardiographic or clinical evidence of perioperative ischemia or infarction requires that lidocaine therapy should be administered. An initial 100-mg. intravenous bolus of lidocaine should then be followed by a continuous infusion at a rate 1 to 3 mg. per minute titrated for control of the ectopy. If lidocaine fails to stabilize the cardiac rhythm, procainamide can be used as a second-line drug, and, in severe cases, bretylium may be required when cardiac dysrhythmias are refractory to more conventional drugs.

Supraventricular Tachyarrhythmias. The development of supraventricular tachyarrhythmias in the surgical patient is usually associated with certain identifiable risk factors, such as myocardial infarction or ischemia, congestive heart failure, electrolyte derangements, hypoxia, pulmonary embolism, the administration of arrhythmogenic drugs such as catecholamines, or fever associated with a major infection. Correction of these problems obviates the need for specific drug therapy in about one third of the patients.

Atrial fibrillation is the most common supraventricular arrhythmia observed in surgical patients. The first goal of treatment is control of the rapid ventricular response rate, which is usually best done by administering digoxin. For patients who have not previously taken digoxin or any other digitalis agent, a total intravenous loading dose of 1 mg. should be administered over a 6- to 12-hour period, usually beginning with 0.5 mg. intravenously and then repeating 0.25-mg. doses at 2-hour intervals to lower the ventricular rate below 90 beats per minute. In patients with a rapid ventricular response to atrial fibrillation and no evidence of depressed ventricular function, verapamil can be administered in doses of 2.5 to 5 mg. intravenously every 15 minutes until a total dose of 10 mg. is given. For severe cardiac compromise due to tachycardia, synchronized cardioversion remains the treatment of choice.

Treatment of the underlying medical problems and rate control of the ventricular response to atrial fibrillation often result in spontaneous conversion to normal sinus rhythm. If the patient remains in atrial fibrillation for 48 hours despite adequate control of the ventricular response, a specific antiarrhythmic drug such as procainamide or quinidine should be administered in an attempt to achieve conversion into sinus rhythm.

Control of the ventricular rate in patients with atrial flutter is often more difficult than in those with atrial fibrillation. Although the treatment approach has traditionally been to *digitalize* the patient, there is good clinical evidence suggesting that the use of verapamil as the first drug may be more efficacious. Also, it is well known that atrial flutter is uniquely susceptible to cardioversion, and this form of treatment should be employed if there is any evidence of hemodynamic compromise.

Other forms of supraventricular tachyarrhythmia, including AV nodal re-entry tachycardia, sinus node re-entry tachycardia, intra-atrial tachycardia, automatic junctional tachycardia, or a re-entrant conduction pathway, may occur in surgical patients and may require pharmacologic treatment. In many instances, these arrhythmias may be terminated by vagotonic maneuvers, but if this is unsuccessful, intravenous verapamil in the same dosage recommended for atrial fibrillation is the agent of choice. Verapamil should be successful in about 80% of cases, but in those patients in whom rate reduction is not achieved, the administration of propranolol is indicated.

Esmolol is an ultra-short-acting cardioselective beta blocker that is rapidly converted to inactive metabolites by blood esterases, allowing full recovery from beta blockade within 30 minutes in patients with a normal cardiovascular system. Esmolol is indicated in situations where rapid beta blockade and termination are desired, such as in supraventricular tachycardia, perioperative tachycardia, or perioperative hypertension.[3] The dose range is 50 to 400 µg. per kg. per minute intravenously. Due to the rapid onset of esmolol action, it should only be used in the setting of continuous hemodynamic monitoring.

Low Cardiac Output Syndrome

The low cardiac output syndrome in surgical patients must be recognized and promptly treated before severe cellular and organ damage occurs. The syndrome represents a state of inadequate perfusion at the tissue level and may occur for a number of reasons. The clinical pattern is characterized by evidence of decreased organ perfusion with decreasing urinary output and an altered mental status in the awake patient. Acidosis is often noted and is due to decreased tissue perfusion.

A low cardiac output state in a surgical patient can best be managed by a methodical and physiologic approach. Careful clinical observation and serial monitoring of hemodynamic parameters such as heart rate, arterial blood pressure, cardiac filling pressures, and cardiac output are mandatory. The metabolic status of the patient should be evaluated by serial arterial blood gas measurements and mixed venous oxygen content analysis. Electrolyte abnormalities should be assessed and corrected as required.

The most common cause of the low cardiac output state in surgical patients is hypovolemia, which follows uncorrected blood or extracellular fluid losses that occur as a result of both the underlying disease process and the losses incurred at the time of any surgical procedure. Typical features in these patients are low cardiac output and reduced filling pressures, particularly as noted from the measurement of pulmonary artery diastolic pressure or pulmonary capillary wedge pressure, which reflect left-sided filling pressures. Because of sympathetic compensatory efforts, the peripheral circulation is profoundly vasoconstricted and the peripheral vascular resistance is elevated.

The management of the low cardiac output state secondary to hypovolemia is straightforward and involves controlling blood and fluid loss while judiciously replacing deficits with appropriate solutions or blood products. Therapy should be carefully guided by the measurements of left-sided cardiac filling pressures and repeated determinations of cardiac output.

Another cause of the low cardiac output syndrome is primary myocardial dysfunction, which is the result of the heart's failure to perform as a competent pump. The usual cause of primary myocardial dysfunction in noncardiac surgical patients is ischemic heart disease, with regional dysfunction due to severe ischemia or infarction. The development of a dysfunctional state that produces a low cardiac output syndrome suggests that at least 40% of the ventricle is disabled. This type of injury may be related to pre-existing cardiac disease, recent myocardial infarction, or the residual effects of prolonged ischemia that may occur after cardiac surgical procedures in which preservation of the myocardium is unsuccessful in preventing injury to the myocardial muscle. Regardless of the etiologic factor, the principles of diagnosis and the approach to management are the same. The filling pressures of the ventricular chambers must be carefully optimized to promote peak performance of the ventricles without causing pulmonary edema. Cardiac rate and the normal synchrony between atrium and ventricle are important factors in the maintenance of cardiac pump function, and every attempt should be made to normalize them, including the use of pacing devices.

It is widely recognized that the impaired myocardium will function best if the afterload or systolic wall stress against which it must function is reduced. This afterload reduction is best achieved by the use of short-acting peripheral vasodilators such as nitroprusside or nitroglycerin. Both drugs are administered intravenously under carefully monitored conditions and are titrated for maintenance of a systemic vascular resistance in the low-normal range. Additional support for the poorly functioning myocardium can be achieved by the use of an inotropic agent that improves cardiac contractility without producing a pronounced increase in cardiac rate or significant increases in peripheral vascular resistance. The inotropic agents that appear to best achieve these goals are dopamine, dobutamine, and amrinone, used either alone or in combination.[36] In the patient with a chronically diseased and failing heart, epinephrine in small doses is occasionally beneficial. If pharmacologic and fluid therapy are unsuccessful in restoring myocardial function, mechanical support with a device such as the intra-aortic balloon pump or ventricular assist device must be considered.

An increasingly common cause of the low cardiac output syndrome in surgical patients is the presence of systemic sepsis. A wide range of microbial agents can cause profound cardiovascular alterations, leading to shock and death. The treatment of septic low-flow states is much more controversial than that of either hypovolemic or cardiogenic shock, and the mortality remains greater than 50% in almost all reported series.

The most important factors in the management of the septic surgical patient are prompt recognition of the problem and careful monitoring of the hemodynamic status while a thorough search for the source of sepsis is begun. Surgical drainage of sources of infection and the institution of antibiotics are crucial. In many instances, intravascular volume deficits are present and should be corrected. The hemodynamic interventions instituted in septic shock should augment cardiac output when demands for increased perfusion exist.

When perfusion cannot be improved further by expanding the intravascular volume and increasing the preload, afterload reduction and inotropic intervention with pharmacologic agents should be considered. In some forms of septic shock, the primary hemodynamic alteration appears to be intense peripheral vasoconstriction that eventually produces tissue and organ damage unless treated. In this setting, the use of a vasodilator such as nitroprusside or nitroglycerin is indicated under conditions of careful monitoring. A fall in blood pressure commonly occurs when these agents are used despite a rise in cardiac output. Some degree of hypotension is usually well tolerated by younger patients without preexisting coronary artery or cerebrovascular disease, but the fixed and stenotic lesions often present in the coronary and cerebral circulation of older patients place them at substantial risk for myocardial infarction or stroke.

When afterload reduction fails to improve cardiac output, inotropic pharmacologic agents should be considered. The sympathomimetic agents dopamine, dobutamine, epinephrine, isoproterenol, and amrinone can provide inotropic support in association with the dose-related peripheral vascular effects previously discussed.

Patients with the hyperdynamic form of septic shock appear to have a unique problem and present a dilemma in management, because their cardiac output is usually more than sufficient to meet the peripheral metabolic demands of the body for the delivery of oxygen and substrate. Patients in this category are often refractory to pharmacologic interventions and, by sustaining a very high cardiac output, may eventually exhaust their cardiac reserves. The use of a vasoconstricting agent would appear to be physiologically appropriate, but this type of intervention usually severely depresses cardiac output and is not recommended. Treatment in this group of patients remains controversial, but the best available evidence suggests that therapies should be directed toward correction of the metabolic abnormalities that appear to be the cause of this particular problem.

Acute Congestive Heart Failure and Pulmonary Edema

Therapy for the management of congestive heart failure with associated pulmonary edema is a curious blend of the application of physiologic principles and the results of successful clinical trials. This situation reflects incomplete understanding of the pathophysiology of congestive heart failure and the mechanisms by which currently accepted therapeutic agents effect improvement.

When congestive heart failure becomes evident, acid-base assessment, along with determination of blood gases, serum electrolytes, and calcium and glucose levels, must be rapidly performed. Inotropic drug infusions may be started and titrated, and associated problems such as hypothermia and rhythm disturbances need to be aggressively corrected. In the case of cardiac arrest, standard recommendations for cardiopulmonary resuscitation must be instituted with recovery of reasonably stable cardiac rhythm and evidence of an adequate cardiac output.

Acute pulmonary edema in the surgical setting is often the result of fluid overload in the presence of chronically compromised cardiac function or the occurrence of a recent myocardial infarction. Basic therapy involves the use of oxygen and an intravenous diuretic such as furosemide, which also acts as a vasodilator. Morphine, a narcotic possessing vasodilatory properties, may be of benefit and may alleviate the anxiety often seen in awake patients. In some situations, it may be necessary to aid the failing ventricle by the use of intravenous vasodilators such as nitroprusside or nitroglycerin.

In the event that a rapid diuresis occurs, aggressive replacement of potassium is necessary for preventing hypokalemia. This is best accomplished by the intravenous route; however, care must be taken to avoid hyperkalemia, which may also cause life-threatening arrhythmias. For patients who develop pulmonary edema in association with marked renal insufficiency, the use of low-dose dopamine (2 to 3 μg./kg./min.) may improve renal blood flow and aid in diuresis. In those situations in which dopamine fails, aggressive fluid removal with ultrafiltration or dialysis may be required.

SELECTED REFERENCES

Freeman, W. K., Gillons, R. J., and Shub, C.: Preoperative assessment of cardiac patients undergoing noncardiac surgical procedures. Mayo Clin. Proc., 64:1105, 1989.
Emphasis in this excellent review of the entire problem of assessing patients with all forms of cardiac disease and their management in the preoperative, operative, and postoperative period is placed on the physiologic assessment of such patients. An extensive bibliography covering all aspects of the problem is included.

Opie, L. H.: Drugs for the Heart. Philadelphia, W. B. Saunders, 1991.
A concise and up-to-date review of the major cardiovascular drugs employed in clinical practice is presented. An extensive bibliography covers all areas of modern cardiovascular clinical pharmacology.

Waldhausen, J. A., and Biebuyck, J. F.: Surgery in the cardiac patient. Surg. Clin. North Am., 63:985, 1983.
The cardiovascular effects of surgical therapy and anesthesia on patients and particularly those with known cardiac risk factors are discussed. The discussion concerning interaction of drugs and anesthesia on the patient with cardiac disease is particularly helpful.

REFERENCES

1. Arnsdorf, M. F., and Wasserstrom, J. A.: Mechanisms of action of antiarrhythmic drugs: A matrical approach. *In* Fozzard, H. A., Haher, E., Jennings, R. B., Katz, A. M., and Morgan, H. E. (Eds.): The Heart and Cardiovascular System: Scientific Foundations, vol. 2. New York, Raven Press, 1986, pp. 1259–1316.
2. Bovill, E. G., Lawson, J. H., Sadowski, J. A., and Mann, K. G.: Biochemistry of vitamin K: Implications for warfarin therapy. *In* Ezekowitz, M.D. (Ed.): Systemic Cardiac Embolism. New York, Marcel Dekker, 1994.
3. Byrd, R. C., Sung, R. J., Marks, J., and Parmley, W. W.: Safety and efficacy of esmolol (ASL-8052: an ultra short-acting beta-adrenergic blocking agent) for control of ventricular rate in supraventricular tachycardias. J. Coll. Cardiol., 3:394, 1984.
4. Chatterjee, K., and Parmley, W. W.: Vasodilator therapy for acute myocardial infarction and chronic congestive heart failure. J. Am. Coll. Cardiol., 1:133, 1983.
5. Cohn, J. N.: Physiologic basis of vasodilator therapy for heart failure. Am. J. Med., 71:135, 1982.
6. Cohn, J. N., Archibald, D. G., Phil, M., et al.: Effect of vasodilator therapy

on mortality and chronic congestive heart failure. N. Engl. J. Med., *314*:1547, 1986.

7. Colucci, W. S., Wright, R. F., and Braunwald, E.: New positive inotropic agents in the treatment of congestive heart failure. N. Engl. J. Med., *314*:290, 349, 1986.

8. Cruickshank, J. M., and Prichard, B. N. C.: Beta-blockers in clinical practice. New York, Churchill Livingstone, 1994.

9. Curtiss, C., Cohn, J. N., Vrobel, T., and Franciosa, J. A.: Role of the renin angiotensin system in the vasoconstriction of congestive heart failure. Circulation, *58*:763, 1978.

10. Deitmer, J. W., and Ellis, D.: The intracellular sodium activity of cardiac Purkinje fibers during inhibition and reactivation of the Na-K pump. J. Physiol. (Lond.), *284*:241, 1978.

11. Edwards, C. R. W., and Padfield, P. L.: Angiotensin-converting enzyme inhibitors: Past, present and bright future. Lancet, *1*:30, 1985.

12. Farah, A. E., Alousi, A. A., and Schwarz, R. P., Jr.: Positive inotropic agents. Annu. Rev. Pharmacol. Toxicol., *24*:275, 1984.

13. Freeman, W. K., Gibbons, R. J., and Shub, C.: Preoperative assessment of cardiac patients undergoing noncardiac surgical procedures. Mayo Clin. Proc., *64*:1105, 1989.

14. Friedman, L. M., Byington, R. P., Capone, R. J., et al.: Effect of propranolol in patients with myocardial infarction and ventricular arrhythmia. J. Am. Coll. Cardiol. 7:1, 1986.

15. Goldberg, L. I., and Rajfer, S. I.: Dopamine receptors: Applications in clinical cardiology. Circulation, *72*:245, 1985.

16. Goldman, D., Cardera, D., Nussbaum, S., et al.: Multifactorial index of cardiac risk in noncardiac surgical procedures. N. Engl. J. Med., *297*:845, 1977.

17. Greger, R., and Wangemann, P.: Loop diuretics. Renal Physiol., *10*:174, 1987.

18. Gulamhusein, S., Ko, P., Carruthers, S. G., et al.: Acceleration of the ventricular response during atrial fibrillation in the Wolff-Parkinson-White syndrome after verapamil. Circulation, *65*:348, 1982.

19. Halperin, A. K., and Cubeddu, L. X.: The role of calcium channel-blockers in the treatment of hypertension. Am. Heart J., *111*:363, 1986.

20. Harrison, D. C.: Antiarrhythmic drug classification: New science and practical applications. Am. J. Cardiol., *56*:185, 1985.

21. Hasegawa, G. R.: Nicardipine, nitrendipine and bepridil: New calcium antagonists for cardiovascular disorders. Clin. Pharm., *7*:97, 1988.

22. Henrey, P. D.: Mechanisms of action of calcium antagonists in cardiac and smooth muscle. *In* Stone, P. H., and Antman, E. M. (Eds.): Calcium Channel Blocking Agents in the Treatment of Cardiovascular Disorders. Mount Kisco, N.Y., Futura Publishing, 1983, pp. 107–154.

23. Holmes, J. R., Kubo, S. H., Cody, R. J., et al.: Milrinone in congestive heart failure: Observations on ambulatory ventricular arrhythmias. Am. Heart J., *110*:800, 1985.

24. Kates, R. E.: Calcium antagonists: Pharmacokinetic properties. Drugs, *25*:113, 1983.

25. Konstam, M. A., Cohen, S. R., Weiland, D. S., et al.: Relative contribution of inotropic and vasodilator effects to amrinone-induced hemodynamic improvement in congestive heart failure. Am. J. Cardiol. *57*:242, 1986.

26. Low, R. I., Takeda, P., Mason, D. T., and DeMaria, A. N.: The effects of calcium channel blocking agents on cardiovascular function. Am J. Cardiol., *49*:547, 1982.

27. Opie, L. H.: Drugs for the Heart. Philadelphia, W.B. Saunders, 1991.

28. Opie, L. H.: Calcium ions, drug action and the heart with special reference to calcium antagonist drugs. Pharmacol. Ther., *25*:271, 1984.

29. Opie, L. H.: Drugs and the heart: V. Digitalis and sympathomimetic stimulants. Lancet, *1*:912, 1980.

30. Opie, L. H.: Angiotensin Converting Enzyme Inhibitors. New York, Wiley-Liss, 1992.

31. Petrillo, E. W., Jr., and Ondetti, M. A.: Angiotensin converting enzyme inhibitors: Medicinal chemistry and biological actions.: Med. Res. Rev. 2:1, 1982.

32. Podrid, P. J., and Lowin, B.: Amiodarone therapy in symptomatic, sustained refractory atrial and ventricular tachyarrhythmias. Am. Heart J., *101*:374, 1981.

33. Rao, T. L. K., Jacobs, K. H., and El-Etr, A. A.: Reinfarction following anesthesia in patients with myocardial infarction. Anesthesiology, *59*:499, 1983.

34. Rawlins, M. D., Lund-Johansen, P., and Laurie, T. D. (Eds.). Prazosin: Pharmacology, Hypertension and Congestive Heart Failure. New York, Grune & Stratton, 1981.

35. Ribner, H. S., Bresnahan, D., and Hsieh, A. M.: Acute hemodynamics responses to vasodilator therapy in congestive heart failure. Prog. Cardiovasc. Dis., *25*:1, 1982.

36. Richard, D., Ricome, J. L., Rimailho, A., et al.: Combined hemodynamic effects of dopamine and dobutamine in cardiogenic shock. Circulation, *67*:620, 1983.

37. Roth, G. J., Stanford, N., and Majerus, P. W.: Acetylation of prostaglandin synthase by aspirin. Proc. Natl. Acad. Sci. USA, *72*:3073, 1975.

38. Singh, B., Ellrodt, G., and Peter, C. T.: Verapamil: A review of its pharmacological properties and therapeutic use. Drugs, *15*:169, 1978.

39. Stewart, D. E., Ikram, H., Espiner, E. A., et al.: Arrhythmogenic potential of diuretic induced hypokalemia in patients with mild hypertension and ischemic heart disease. Br. Heart J., *54*:290, 1985.

40. Swiryn, S., Palileo, E., and Rosen, K. M.: Prediction of response to Class I antiarrhythmic drugs during electrophysiologic study of ventricular tachycardia. Am. Heart J., *104*:43, 1982.

41. Tarhan, S., Moffitt, E. A., Taylor, W. F., et al.: Myocardial infarction after general anesthesia. JAMA, *220*:1451, 1972.

42. Torres, V., Tepper, D., Flowers, D., et al.: QT prolongation and the antiarrhythmic efficacy of amiodarone. J. Am. Coll. Cardiol., *7*:142, 1986.

43. Valazquez, H.: Thiazide diuretics. Renal Physiol., *10*:184, 1987.

XXIII

CARDIOPULMONARY BYPASS FOR CARDIAC SURGERY

William L. Holman, M.D., David C. McGiffin, M.D., and James K. Kirklin, M.D.

PUMP OXYGENATOR APPARATUS

The precise apparatus available for cardiopulmonary bypass (CPB) changes frequently, but the basic components remain constant. A *venous reservoir* is usually present and is positioned to provide adequate siphonage of blood by gravity. This provides storage of excess volume and allows escape of any air bubbles returning with venous blood.

The *oxygenator* provides oxygen to the blood and allows elimination of carbon dioxide. Currently, bubble oxygenators, membrane oxygenators, and microporous hollow-fiber oxygenators are available for clinical use. In bubble oxygenators gas is bubbled into the venous blood, and gas exchange occurs at the blood-gas interface. Antifoaming agents then cause the small bubbles to burst, and the gas escapes through exhaust portals. Membrane oxygenators utilize a semipermeable membrane between layers of blood and gas, across

which gas transfer occurs. The advantage of this type of oxygenator is the potential avoidance of the damaging effects of CPB related to the direct blood-gas interface of the bubble oxygenator. However, under most clinical conditions no clear-cut advantage of the membrane oxygenator has been demonstrated. Microporous hollow-fiber oxygenators contain a mass of 50,000 to 60,000 hollow fibers to provide a surface for gas exchange. The fibers have a diameter of 200 μm. and are generally made of polypropylene or Teflon, with an average pore size of 0.1 to 0.5 μm. The microporous hollow-fiber oxygenators share many of the theoretical advantages of the nonporous membrane oxygenating devices.

An efficient *heat exchanger* is necessary for control of the perfusate temperature to achieve systemic cooling and rewarming during CPB. Most heat-exchanging devices are included as an integral part of the pump oxygenator.

The *arterial pump* is usually a roller pump, which should

be adjusted before each perfusion to be slightly nonocclusive. The pump tubing is either Silastic or latex, which, unlike the Tygon tubing, does not become stiff at low temperatures. The arterial pump should be calibrated at frequent intervals so that accurate perfusion rates can be established. Although several nonocclusive vortex pumps are also available, their use is generally restricted to extracorporeal membrane oxygenator (ECMO) or ventricular assist device (VAD) circuits.

The arterial line pressure in the pump oxygenator must be continuously monitored. When this pressure exceeds 300 mm. Hg, the risk of disruption of the arterial line or cavitation in the region of the arterial cannula increases. These risks are minimized by a properly positioned and adequately sized arterial cannula.

An arterial bubble trap may be used as a safety device to remove air that enters the arterial line. A low-porosity filter may be placed in the arterial perfusion line to remove solid and gaseous microemboli.

PHYSIOLOGIC RESPONSE TO CARDIOPULMONARY BYPASS

Many complex physiologic changes occur when a patient is temporarily supported by means of an oxygenator system. The term *total CPB* indicates that nearly all of the systemic venous blood is returned to the oxygenator. *Partial CPB* implies that some of the systemic venous blood returns to the heart and is ejected into the aorta. Two main types of physiologic variables exist during CPB: *externally controlled variables*, which are controlled by the surgeon and perfusionist, and *patient variables*, which are less easily regulated.

Externally Controlled Variables

The *perfusion flow rate* is controlled by the perfusionist but should be actively established by the surgeon. At normothermia, lactic acidosis regularly occurs at flows of less than 1.6 liters per minute per sq. m.. Experimental and clinical data indicate that normothermic perfusion flow rates of 1.7 liters per minute per sq. m. or greater are usually acceptable, but flow rates of 2.0 to 2.5 liters per minute per sq. m. provide a more secure margin of safety for organ perfusion. For large patients (body surface area $\geq$ 2.0 sq. m.) a flow rate of 1.8 to 2.0 liters per minute per sq. m. is selected to avoid the potential risks of exceeding the oxygenating capability of the pump oxygenator, exceeding the flow capacity of the venous cannulas, and increasing the damage to blood elements.

Because of the inherent individual variability of response to CPB, no absolute criteria exist for safe flow rates at a given temperature. Furthermore, the lowest blood hemoglobin concentration during CPB that is safe cannot be predicted for an individual patient. Organ damage appears least likely to occur when the blood hemoglobin concentration is above 7 gm. per 100 ml. and the microcirculation is perfused at flows that maintain nearly normal tissue oxygen levels and maximal oxygen consumption. During hypothermic CPB, maximal perfusion of the microcirculation probably occurs near the asymptote of the temperature-specific curve relating flow to oxygen consumption ($\dot{V}O_2$) (Fig. 54–224).[18]

The *temperature of the perfusate*, and secondarily of the patient, is controlled by the perfusionist by means of the heat exchanger. This is one of the most important decisions to be made about each patient during CPB. Particularly in small infants, moderate and profound hypothermic perfusion allows the safe, temporary reduction in flow that is advantageous for the accurate intracardiac repair of many malformations (see section on low flow perfusion). The authors use some degree of hypothermic perfusion for nearly all cardiac operations, because hypothermia provides an element of

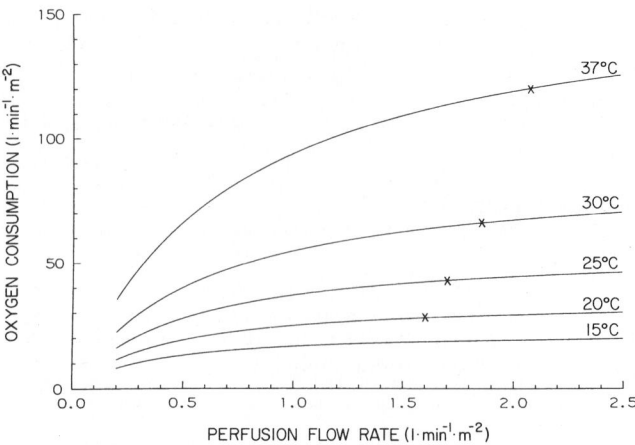

Figure 54–224. Nomogram of an equation expressing the relation of oxygen consumption ($\dot{V}O_2$) to perfusion flow rate ($\dot{Q}$) and temperature (T). The small x's represent the perfusion flow rates used by the authors at these temperatures. The equation is

$$1/(\dot{V}O_2) = 0.168 \cdot 10^{-387\,T} + 0.0378\,\dot{Q}^{-1}\,10^{-0.0253\,T}$$

(From Kirklin, J. W., et al.: Cardiopulmonary bypass for cardiac surgery. *In* Sabiston, D. C., Jr., and Spencer, F. C. [Eds.]: Surgery of the Chest, 5th ed. Philadelphia, W. B. Saunders, 1990.)

safety if a mechanical pump oxygenator failure requires a brief period of total circulatory arrest while the apparatus is being repaired. The commonly used roller pump provides nonpulsatile flow. Pulsatile flow during CPB can be achieved with pulsatile arterial pumps, the patient's own cardiac ejection, or the intra-aortic balloon pump.

The systemic venous pressure is directly proportional to systemic blood flow and blood viscosity and is inversely proportional to venous cannula size, venous line diameter, and venous line suction. The systemic venous pressure should be maintained as close to 0 mm. Hg as possible during CPB and should certainly not exceed 10 mm. Hg because of the increased potential for cerebral edema and accumulation of extracellular fluid with high venous pressures. It is therefore advisable to use the largest venous cannulas consistent with satisfactory operation conditions. If a smaller than desired venous cannula must be used, the adverse effect on venous pressure can be overcome by reducing the perfusion flow rate.

Pulmonary venous pressure (left atrial pressure) should also be maintained near 0 mm. Hg during total CPB. High pulmonary venous pressure during CPB may result from excessive pulmonary collateral blood flow, an unrecognized extracardiac left-to-right shunt (e.g., patent ductus arteriosus), or incomplete venous drainage leading to increased pulmonary blood flow. Marked and prolonged elevation in pulmonary venous pressure during CPB promotes accumulation of extravascular lung water and probably contributes to postoperative pulmonary dysfunction.

The *hematocrit* of the patient-oxygenator system is determined by the body size and hematocrit of the patient, the composition and amount of the initial priming volume of the pump oxygenator, the amount of blood lost, and the composition and volume of solutions infused during CPB. The initial priming volume is determined by the volume required for the oxygenator and its reservoir, the pump lines, the bubble trap, and the cardioplegia apparatus.

At normothermia, a hematocrit of 30% to 40% appears optimal for oxygen transport and preserves the appropriate blood rheologic properties. Higher hematocrits result in increased oxygen content at the expense of increased viscosity and decreased blood flow.

During hypothermia, a lower hematocrit appears desirable because of the lower resultant viscosity and lower shear rates, theoretically providing improved perfusion of the microcirculation. Excessive hemodilution, however, is probably deleterious because of inadequate blood oxygen content and the greater extravascular extravasation of fluid secondary to the decreased intravascular osmotic pressure. Because most pediatric and adult cardiac surgical patients are operated on with hypothermic perfusion, it is probably advisable to maintain the "patient-machine" hematocrit between 25% and 30% to take advantage of both of these effects.

Before operation, a calculation is made of the mixed patient-machine hematocrit that would result if the pump oxygenator is primed with an asanguinous solution. The equation used is shown below:

$$Hct_{pm} = \frac{[\text{Body weight (kg.)} \cdot f \cdot 1000] \, [Hct_p]}{[\text{Body weight (kg.)} \cdot f \cdot 1000] + \text{machine BV}}$$

where Hct_{pm} = hematocrit of combined patient-machine blood volume, Hct_p = patient hematocrit, BV = blood volume, f = 0.08 in infants and children (younger than age 12 years), and f = 0.065 in older patients (older than age 12 years).

If the hematocrit is in the desired range, an asanguinous prime is used with approximately 20% of the prime as 5% dextrose and 80% as a balanced salt solution with enough human albumin added to make it colloidally isosmotic. If the calculated hematocrit is too low, an appropriate amount of blood or packed cells is added. In that instance an additional equation is used:

$$Hct = \frac{\begin{array}{c}\text{Patient red cell vol. (ml.)} + \\ \text{machine red cell vol. (ml.)}\end{array}}{\text{Patient BV} + \text{machine BV (ml.)}}$$

If possible, packed red cells less than 5 days old are generally used. Because the blood is calcium free and acidotic, heparin, calcium, and buffer are added (Table 54–26).

The *glucose concentration* is increased in the priming solution (about 350 mg. per 100 ml.) to provide an energy source as well as to promote an osmotic diuresis during and soon after CPB.

Arterial oxygen levels are usually maintained between 100 and 250 mm. Hg with current bubble and membrane oxygenators. Hypothermic perfusion produces a decrease in Vo_2 and an increase in mixed venous oxygen pressure ($P\bar{v}o_2$), both of which result in an increased Pao_2. During rewarming, the increasing Vo_2 results in relatively low $P\bar{v}o_2$ levels and a decreased Pao_2. This is the period of maximal demand on oxygenator reserves.

The *arterial carbon dioxide pressure* ($Paco_2$) is determined by the ratio of gas flow to blood flow in the oxygenator, with higher ratios resulting in a lower $Paco_2$. A $Paco_2$ of 30 to 40 mm. Hg (measured at 37° C.) is considered optimal during CPB. The optimal $Paco_2$ during profound hypothermia remains controversial. Reeves and Rahn[33] have emphasized

that at low temperatures ionic neutrality is associated with a higher pH than at normothermia because of the change in the dissociation constant of water. Thus, in a patient with a temperature of 20° C., the $Paco_2$ measured at 37° C. should be 30 to 40 mm. Hg, which is a $Paco_2$ of 14 to 20 mm. Hg at 20° C., and a pH at 20° C. of about 7.6.

Patient Variables

The body's physiologic response to CPB is extremely complex and only partially understood. *Systemic vascular resistance* falls abruptly with the onset of CPB. Thereafter, it gradually increases throughout the period of bypass, although there is considerable variation among patients. The importance of maintaining a certain level of mean arterial perfusion pressure during bypass is controversial. Although some clinical and experimental studies suggest that decreased cerebral blood flow is associated with a mean perfusion pressure less than about 50 to 60 mm. Hg, experience indicates that pharmacologic manipulation of the resistance during hypothermic bypass is usually not necessary. During rewarming, however, it seems rational to increase arterial blood pressure pharmacologically if it persists at a level less than 50 to 55 mm. Hg, both to ensure adequate cerebral perfusion and to optimize coronary perfusion. Because of the theoretical potential for intracerebral bleeding with very high arterial perfusion pressures during bypass, it is probably desirable to reduce the mean arterial perfusion pressure pharmacologically if it exceeds 100 mm. Hg.

Total body Vo_2 and $P\bar{v}o_2$ levels are both partially controlled by the perfusion flow rate and the patient's temperature. Although individual variation occurs, it is generally assumed that the microcirculation is being effectively perfused if the mixed venous oxygen levels during bypass are 30 to 40 mm. Hg with a mixed venous oxygen saturation of 60% to 70%.

Metabolic acidosis is almost always present during bypass, but lactate levels should not exceed 5 mEq. per liter if adequate perfusion flow rates are maintained. CPB is also associated with a massive release of epinephrine (primarily from the adrenal medulla). Plasma epinephrine levels rise in nearly all patients shortly after the onset of CPB and begin to fall after bypass.

Changes in *body composition* also occur. During and after CPB, extracellular fluid is increased. The major shift of fluid is from the intravascular space to the interstitial space, resulting in increased interstitial fluid pressure and decreased plasma volume. The magnitude of the increase in extravascular fluid volume is directly related to the duration of CPB, and it is further increased with hemodilution. The amount of exchangeable potassium is decreased, whereas exchangeable sodium is increased. The increase in microvascular permeability during CPB probably results from an increase in the size of large pores in capillary walls. These large pores allow diffusion of macromolecules into the extravascular space, which reduces the colloid osmotic pressure gradient and promotes movement of fluid out of the microvasculature.

DAMAGING EFFECTS OF CPB

Safe CPB is characterized by the absence of structural or functional damage after the perfusion. The vast majority of patients suffer no clinically apparent ill effects from CPB; however, an occasional patient develops severe multiorgan dysfunction despite an otherwise accurate and complete intracardiac repair.

In its most severe form, the *postperfusion syndrome* is characterized by a diffuse whole-body inflammatory reaction, with elements of increased capillary permeability, extravascular extravasation of plasma, increased interstitial fluid, leukocy-

TABLE 54–26. Additives to a Unit of CPD Blood for the Pump Oxygenator

CPD Blood	500 ml.
Heparin	3 ml. (3000 units; mean 6 units/ml. of blood)
NaHCO₃	10 ml.
CaCl₂	5 ml. (added last)
	518 ml.

CPD, citrate phosphate dextrose.
From Kirklin, J. W., et al.: *In* Sabiston, D. C., Jr., and Spencer, F. C. (Eds.): Surgery of the Chest, 5th ed. Philadelphia, W. B. Saunders, 1990.

tosis, fever, peripheral vasoconstriction, breakdown of red blood cells, and a diffuse bleeding diathesis. The fact that most patients convalesce normally after CPB attests not to the absence of these ill effects but rather to the ability of the organism to tolerate them. Much of the residual mortality and morbidity after CPB is related to these damaging effects.

Some incremental risk factors for an adverse clinical response to CPB have been identified, but the precise nature and magnitude of their effects have not been quantified. One is the *duration of bypass*. In most adults the probability of structural or functional damage seems to increase as the perfusion time extends beyond approximately 3 hours, and it probably sharply increases after 4 hours. Another incremental risk factor is *age*. The susceptibility to organ dysfunction after CPB appears to increase in neonates. The very elderly also appear less tolerant of the damaging effects of CPB, particularly in the presence of pre-existing renal dysfunction. These two risk factors undoubtedly interact, making the safe time constraints more rigid in the very young and the very old patient.

Other factors undoubtedly interact, including the type of oxygenator, the composition of the perfusate, the perfusion flow rate, the presence or absence of pulsatile flow, and the patient's temperature. Certain cardiac malformations, particularly cyanotic congenital heart disease, may also be incremental risk factors. Although the importance of each of these factors has not yet been clarified, further research and development will likely lead to modifications of the bypass circuit that will improve its safety, particularly in high-risk situations.

The mechanisms for damage after CPB are most likely *altered arterial blood flow patterns and exposure of blood to abnormal events*, with the exposure of blood to abnormal events being the more powerful determinant (Fig. 54–225).

Altered Arterial Blood Flow Patterns

The standard roller pump for CPB produces nonpulsatile flow while the heart is empty on full bypass. This represents a marked deviation from the normal physiologic conditions, in which the arterial pulse pressure is about one third of the systolic pressure. *Pulsatile* perfusion during full bypass has been noted to provide lower vascular resistance, less red cell aggregation, improved renal function, and less cellular hypoxia than nonpulsatile flow during CPB. However, clinical studies comparing pulsatile to nonpulsatile flow during CPB have been inconclusive. Some studies suggest a beneficial effect of pulsatile flow, while other studies indicate no advantage over nonpulsatile perfusion.

Exposure of Blood to Abnormal Events

During CPB the exposure of blood to abnormal events includes exposure to shear stresses, incorporation of abnormal substances, and, perhaps most important, exposure to unphysiologic (*nonendothelial*) surfaces.

Blood is a complex substance composed of both formed and unformed elements. The formed elements include red blood cells, white blood cells, and platelets. Among the unformed elements in blood, the plasma proteins seem particularly vulnerable during CPB. Plasma proteins include those proteins with primary osmotic effects (albumin), those acting as carrier vehicles for other blood-borne substances (albumin, lipoproteins, and immunoglobulin), and those constituting the humoral amplification system (coagulation, fibrinolytic, complement, and kallikrein cascades). *Shear stresses* are generated by blood pumps, by suction devices, and by cavitation around the end of the arterial cannula. Leukocytes appear to be particularly sensitive to shear stresses, which cause destruction of leukocytes or functional impairments such as decreased aggregation, decreased chemotactic migration, and impaired phagocytosis in surviving leukocytes. During CPB, an initial leukopenia develops that returns to baseline values after approximately 2 hours of CPB. This increase occurs in part secondary to active movement of leukocytes out of the vascular space. Immediately after CPB a leukocytosis is present and continues for several days.

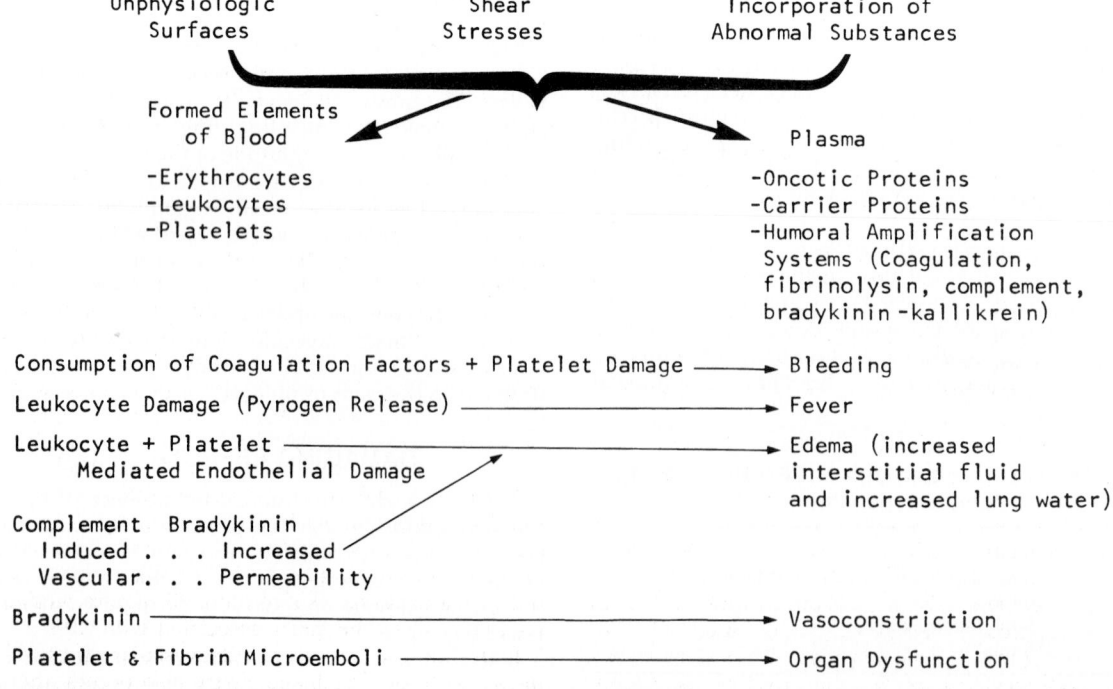

Figure 54–225. Schematic representation of a current concept of the damaging effects of cardiopulmonary bypass related to the exposure of blood to abnormal events. (From Kirklin, J. K., Kirklin, J. W., and Pacifico, A. D.: Cardiopulmonary bypass. *In* Arciniegas, E. [Ed.]: Pediatric Cardiac Surgery. Chicago, Year Book Medical Publishers, 1985.)

Lymphocytes, including both B cells and T cells, are decreased after CPB, and T-cell function is depressed. This depression of cellular immunity is specifically due to CPB and appears to resolve more rapidly in patients *not* exposed to blood transfusions.[25] Methods to restore cell-mediated immunity after CPB are under development.[29]

During CPB, red blood cells are damaged mainly by shear stresses. The result is either immediate hemolysis with release of free hemoglobin or a shortened red blood cell life span with delayed hemolysis. Hemolysis is less evident when an oxygenator is not in the system, and bubble oxygenators generally produce more hemolysis than membrane oxygenators. The intracardiac suction lines are particularly damaging to red blood cells. Levels of free hemoglobin have been noted to increase fourfold within 10 minutes after initiating CPB, and the decreased red blood cell survival time after CPB results in a progressive loss of red cell mass during the first 3 or 4 postoperative days.

The *incorporation of abnormal substances* during CPB includes air bubbles, fibrin, tissue debris, and platelet thrombi, as well as defoaming agents. Thromboplastinogen is activated when blood makes contact with injured tissues, and this may contribute to intravascular coagulation and the formation of thrombin and platelet emboli. High circulating levels of plasticizing agents leached from polyvinyl chloride surfaces have been documented in patients undergoing operations that include CPB, and evidence for cerebral microembolization during CPB has been obtained from humans and animals.

It is the *exposure to unphysiologic surfaces* that produces the greatest damage during bypass. The most critical surfaces are probably those of the oxygenating device. The unphysiologic surface is gas in bubble, disk, and screen oxygenators and the membrane in a membrane oxygenator. The proportion of blood exposed to an unphysiologic surface is relatively small in the reservoirs, tubes, and cannulas. The effect on platelets is to promote platelet aggregation,[14] resulting in platelet emboli as well as decreased platelet number and function after CPB. Fibrinogen is rapidly adsorbed to the surfaces within the CPB circuit. Platelet surface glycoproteins (e.g., GPIIb-IIIa complex) then bind to these sites, producing platelet activation.[23]

A portion of platelets exposed to the CPB circuit undergo degranulation and are irreversibly damaged, whereas other platelets undergo partial degranulation and reversible aggregation. The precise sequence of events and proportions of impaired and destroyed platelets remain controversial.[23, 44] There is evidence to suggest that the platelet function defect after CPB is actually not intrinsic to the platelet itself. Instead, it may be related to deficiencies in activators of platelet function that are extrinsic to the platelet.[26]

Methods to protect platelet function during CPB are under development. Methods that attenuate platelet damage during CPB include protein *passivation* of oxygenator surfaces[23] and rendering platelets reversibly nonfunctional during CPB using prostanoids.[1] Aprotinin is a serine protease inhibitor that is available for clinical use. A known inhibitor of plasmin and kallikrein, it also appears to preserve platelets during CPB.[38] The effect of aprotinin on platelets has not yet been completely defined, but the results of several studies demonstrate markedly improved hemostasis using this drug.[2, 38] Adverse effects from aprotinin may exist,[37, 42] but they remain controversial.[34]

Denaturation of carrier proteins occurs during CPB, with breakdown of lipoproteins and generation of fat emboli. Protein denaturation increases plasma viscosity and promotes clumping of erythrocytes; however, this effect can be attenuated by hemodilution.

The *humoral amplification system* is a complex system of plasma proteins that responds to a local stimulus with a self-perpetuating and expanding series of reactions. These normally involve an inflammatory reaction in a localized area of the body. The components of the humoral amplification system include the *coagulation cascade*, the *fibrinolytic cascade*, the *kallikrein system*, and the *complement system*. The authors believe that the damaging effects of CPB are related in large degree to the humoral amplification system, which initiates a whole-body inflammatory response during CPB.[7]

Hageman factor (factor XII) is activated almost immediately after the onset of CPB by the massive contact of blood with nonendothelial surfaces. This results in activation of the coagulation cascade and also other cascades. Even with appropriate heparinization during CPB, there is evidence of ongoing microcoagulation with consumption of clotting factors. Surface activation may be attenuated by coating the surfaces of the pump oxygenator with heparin,[16, 24] although at this time potential adverse consequences of this treatment must still be considered.[15]

The fibrinolytic cascade is also activated with the onset of CPB. Increased levels of serum plasmin (the active fibrinolytic agent) have been detected shortly after initiation of CPB. Plasmin itself may serve as an activator of prekallikrein, the complement system, and possibly Hageman factor.

The kallikrein cascade may be activated by Hageman factor, resulting in the production of bradykinin. Bradykinin increases vascular permeability, dilates arterioles, initiates smooth muscle contraction, and elicits pain. Kallikrein can itself activate Hageman factor and activate plasminogen to form plasmin, again demonstrating the complex interaction between these amplification systems. High levels of bradykinin are present during CPB. Since bradykinin is metabolized mainly in the lungs, exclusion of the pulmonary circulation during CPB acts to sustain circulating bradykinin levels. In addition, very young infants appear to be less able to eliminate bradykinin.

The complement system is composed of a group of circulating glycoproteins and forms a basic part of the body's response to immunologic, traumatic, or foreign-body insult. Two pathways exist for activation of the complement sequence (Fig. 54–226).[30] The classical pathway is usually initiated through interaction with antigen-antibody complexes. The alternative or properdin pathway is activated by exposure of blood to foreign surfaces, and it is this pathway that is initially activated during CPB,[40] with later activation of the classical pathway during protamine administration after CPB.[27]

In 1972, Parker and colleagues[32] noted that complement was consumed during CPB, and they hypothesized that the complement system may promote the increases in capillary permeability that are frequently seen after CPB. Chenoweth and colleagues[9] at the University of Alabama at Birmingham and Scripps Institute have demonstrated that the complement anaphylatoxin C3a is increased shortly after the onset of CPB, with continuing production throughout the duration of bypass (Fig. 54–227). In contrast, patients undergoing cardiac operations without CPB have normal levels of C3a at the end of the operation.[27] The anaphylatoxins C5a and C3a have physiologic effects similar to those observed in many patients after CPB, including vasoconstriction and increased capillary permeability.[3] Inhibition of complement activation during CPB in experimental animals attenuates, but does not eliminate, this organ injury.[21, 22] The other arms of the whole-body inflammatory response to CPB require modification to effectively block the injury associated with CPB.

In addition to the direct microvascular effects of complement, neutrophil-mediated injury also occurs after complement activation (Fig. 54–228). There are specific C5a receptor sites on human neutrophils. Activation of the alternative

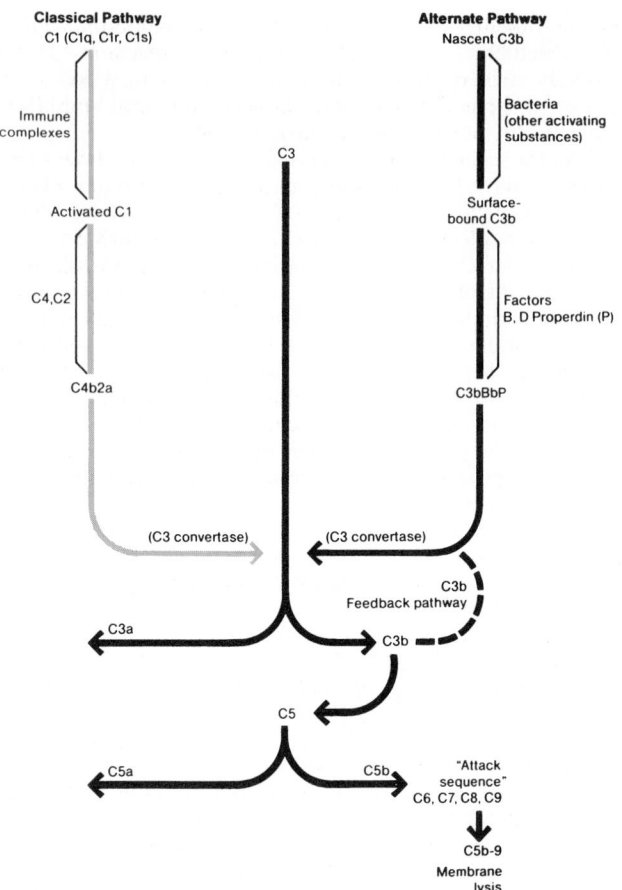

Figure 54–226. Pathways of complement activation. (From Goldstein, I. M.: Complement in infectious diseases. Current Concepts, The Upjohn Company, 1980.)

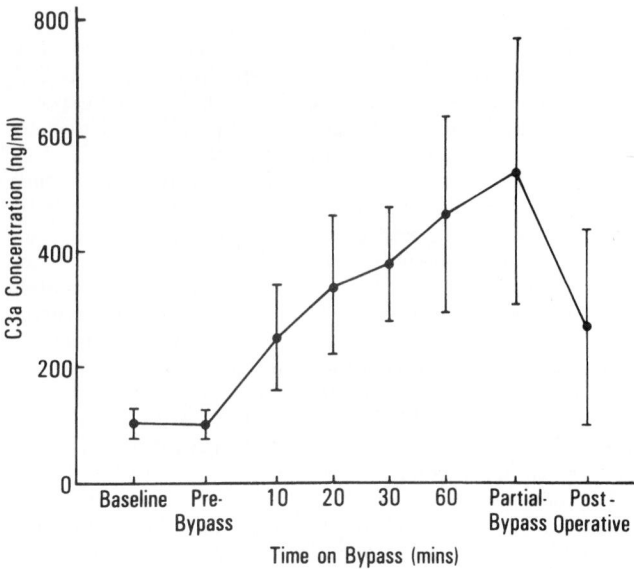

Figure 54–227. Plasma levels of C3a in patients undergoing cardiopulmonary bypass. (From Chenoweth, D. E., et al.: Complement activation during cardiopulmonary bypass: Evidence for generation of C3a and C5a anaphylatoxins. N. Engl. J. Med., *304*:497, 1981. Copyright 1981, Massachusetts Medical Society. Reprinted by permission of The New England Journal of Medicine.)

Blood Conservation

During the past decade, efforts have been directed toward conservation of blood and avoidance of nonautologous transfusions in patients undergoing CPB. Autotransfusion of shed mediastinal blood after cardiac operations has been shown to be a safe and effective method for minimizing postoperative transfusion requirements, although large-volume autotransfusion is probably deleterious.[13] Red blood cells aspirated from the operative field can be separated by centrifugation and washing before reinfusion. Intraoperative ultrafiltration of blood using hollow-fiber hemofilters may also be used to conserve blood. Studies by Boldt and associates[4] and Solem and coworkers[36] have demonstrated that hemofiltration conserves the plasma fraction as well as the red blood cells. Hemofiltration or cell separation techniques can be used to conserve the blood that remains in the oxygenator after the termination of CPB. Autologous blood donated before cardiac operations has been shown to reduce the need for ho-

pathway produces C5a that is rapidly bound to neutrophils, which are then deposited in the lungs as well as other organs.[11] Neutrophil activation and degranulation during CPB have been demonstrated in humans[41] and may be responsible for some of the deleterious effects of CPB. Endothelial cell damage by oxygen radicals produced by complement-stimulated granulocytes has been demonstrated.[36] Several groups[5, 12] have demonstrated associations during CPB between the generation of peroxidation products and pulmonary neutrophil sequestration, as well as between oxygen free radical generation and complement activation.[8] It is hypothesized that a portion of the pulmonary dysfunction after CPB is caused by complement activation, with the elaboration of C3a and C5a. C5a then promotes pulmonary leukosequestration and release of superoxides and lysosomal enzymes, which in turn produce direct endothelial damage and alterations in permeability (see Fig. 54–228). Cytokines are also activated in this process and likely are important contributors to endothelial injury.[19]

Studies at the University of Alabama at Birmingham have correlated cardiac, pulmonary, renal, and hematologic dysfunction after CPB with higher levels of C3a after bypass, longer elapsed times of bypass, and younger age at operation.[28] An increased understanding of complement activation during CPB allows the development of methods to attenuate complement activation and diminish the deleterious effects of CPB. This may be achieved by designing oxygenator systems that produce less complement activation[39] or developing pharmacologic methods to inhibit complement activation during CPB.[40]

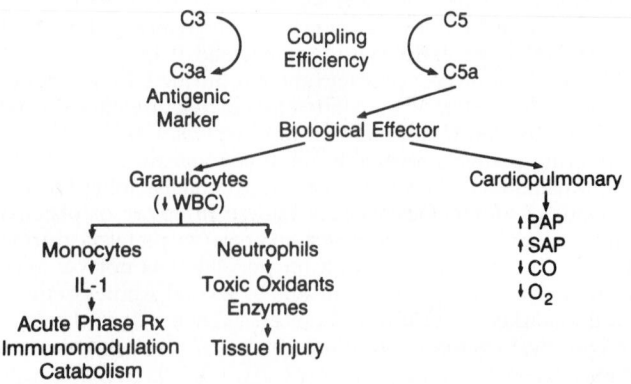

Figure 54–228. Diagram outlining the two modes of action for the human anaphylatoxins C3a and C5a produced during complement activation. The coupling efficiency refers to the relative quantity of C5a produced as compared with C3a. The coupling efficiency varies according to the activating or nonactivating character of the foreign surface in contact with blood. (From Leonard, E. F., Turitto, V. T., and Vroman, L. [Eds.]: Blood in Contact with Natural and Artificial Surfaces. New York, The New York Academy of Sciences, 1987.)

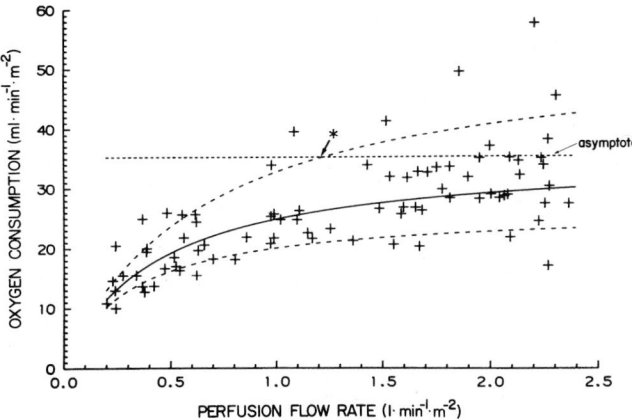

Figure 54–229. Relationship of oxygen consumption ($\dot{V}O_2$) to perfusion flow rate ($\dot{Q}$) during nonpulsatile cardiopulmonary bypass at 20° C. Plus signs represent individual measurements. The solid line is the nomogram of the hyperbolic equation

$$\dot{V}O_2 = 35 \pm 2.03 \, (\dot{Q}/[\dot{Q} + 0.42 \pm 0.055])$$

The significance levels of coefficients are less than 0.0001. The dashed lines, also derived from the regression analysis, are the 70 per cent confidence limits for the observations (± 1 SD). The dotted line is the asymptote (35.3) representing the estimate of maximal $\dot{V}O_2$. The asterisk indicates the flow rate (1.2 liters per minute per sq. m.) above which the upper 70 per cent confidence limit overlaps the asymptote. (From Fox, L. S., et al.: Relationship of whole body oxygen consumption to perfusion flow rate during hypothermic cardiopulmonary bypass. J. Thorac. Cardiovasc. Surg., *83*:239, 1982.)

mologous transfusion, whereas the harvesting of platelet-rich plasma remains unproven as a means to improve post-CPB hemostasis.[43]

Low-Flow Perfusion

Particularly during infant intracardiac surgery, a nearly bloodless field can usually be achieved with hypothermic low-flow perfusion for a portion of the repair. At a nasopharyngeal temperature of 20° C., a flow rate of 1.2 to 1.6 liters per minute per sq. m. is well tolerated. A large clinical experience indicates that at 20° C. nasopharyngeal temperature, the perfusion flow rate can be safely reduced to 0.5 liter per minute per sq. m. for 30 to 45 minutes.

Oxygen consumption ($\dot{V}O_2$) is an important indicator of the adequacy of perfusion to the microcirculation. The decrease in $\dot{V}O_2$ during low-flow perfusion probably results from the closing down of portions of the microcirculation. The relationship between $\dot{V}O_2$ and the perfusion flow rate during hypothermic CPB (20° C.) is such that $\dot{V}O_2$ decreases rapidly only after flow is reduced below 1.0 liter per minute per sq. m. (Fig. 54–229).[18]

A series of hyperbolic curves can be generated from various experimental and clinical studies that describe the rela-

tionship between $\dot{V}O_2$ and flow at various temperatures during CPB (see Fig. 54–224). Maximal perfusion of the microcirculation probably occurs near the asymptote of the curve, and from this a minimal safe flow rate at a given temperature can be selected during CPB.

The adequacy of cerebral perfusion during low-flow hypothermic perfusion has been examined in animal experiments.[17] Cerebral $\dot{V}O_2$ is well maintained as flow is reduced from 1.5 to 0.5 liters per minute per sq. m. on CPB at 20° C. (Table 54–27). In addition, calculated vascular resistance in the brain remains constant while overall systemic vascular resistance progressively increases as flow is reduced from 1.5 to 0.5 liters per minute per sq. m. (Table 54–28). The contribution of autoregulation to the maintenance of cerebral perfusion during hypothermic low-flow perfusion has been confirmed in adult human studies.[6] In infants, low-flow CPB is associated with less early postoperative neurologic morbidity than total circulatory arrest.[31] However, the longer-term outcomes of these perfusion strategies remain under investigation.

Clinical Methodology in CPB

CPB should be used as a flexible clinical tool, recognizing its physiologic limitations, risks, and damaging effects. Some degree of hypothermia is utilized for nearly all operations performed on CPB. Whenever possible, part of the repair is performed during the rewarming phase if hypothermia is used. An important advantage of hypothermia is that it allows a safe transient period of low-flow perfusion (0.5 to 1.0 liter per minute per sq. m.) if improved visibility is desired or a brief period of safe circulatory arrest if repair of an oxygenator malfunction is required.

The size of arterial (Table 54–29) and venous cannulas (Table 54–30) is determined primarily by the selected total perfusion flow rate. At any given patient size, there is an acceptable range of perfusion rates, which allows somewhat smaller cannulas to be used if the anatomic situation dictates. An arterial cannula is generally selected that provides a gradient across the cannula of 100 mm. Hg or less to minimize the risks of a high arterial line pressure (see Pump Oxygenator Apparatus). The constituents of the priming solution are reviewed with the perfusionist, and a decision is made regarding the addition of blood to the prime, depending on the desired *patient machine* hematocrit (see Externally Controlled Variables).

After performing a median sternotomy and opening and tacking up the pericardium, the external cardiac anatomy is carefully assessed. Any dissection before CPB is usually accomplished before heparin is administered. Pursestring sutures are placed for arterial and venous cannulation and placement of the cardioplegic needle. The initial heparin dose is 3000 units per kg., and adequate anticoagulation is verified by an activated clotting time greater than 8 minutes.

TABLE 54–27. Oxygen Consumption During Profoundly Hypothermic, Nonpulsatile, Hemodiluted CPB in Monkeys

Organ	Oxygen Consumption (ml. /min.[-1]/100 gm.[-1])			
	1.5*	1.0*	0.5*	*p*
Whole body	0.119 ± 0.0077 (17.3 ± 1.16)†	0.086 ± 0.0045 (12.5 ± 0.65)	0.056 ± 0.0029 (8.3 ± 0.44)	<.0001
Brain	0.51 ± 0.095	0.47 ± 0.076	0.45 ± 0.113	.5
Whole body minus brain	0.114 ± 0.0074	0.081 ± 0.0085	0.0518 ± 0.00176	<.0001

*Perfusion flow rate (L./min.[-1]/m.[-2]).
†The numbers in parentheses are the whole-body oxygen consumption expressed as ml./min./sq. m.
From Fox, L. S., et al.: Relationship of brain blood flow and oxygen consumption to perfusion flow rate during profoundly hypothermic cardiopulmonary bypass: An experimental study. J. Thorac. Cardiovasc. Surg., *87*:658, 1984.

TABLE 54–28. Resistance to Blood Flow in the Brain and Remainder of the Body at Various Perfusion Rates During CPB in Monkeys

Organ	Resistance (units/100 gm.)						
	1.75*	1.5*	1.25*	1.0*	0.5*	0.25*	p
Brain	1.2±0.51	0.80±0.080	0.8±0.22	0.78±0.126	0.80±0.117	1.02±0.173	.4
Whole body minus brain	2.8±0.157	3.3±0.22	3.3±1.21	3.9±0.24	5.1±0.49	9.5±0.70	<.0001

*Perfusion flow rate (L./min.$^{-1}$/m.$^{-2}$).

From Fox, L. S., et al.: Relationship of brain blood flow and oxygen consumption to perfusion flow rate during profoundly hypothermic cardiopulmonary bypass: An experimental study. J. Thorac. Cardiovasc. Surg., *87*:658, 1984.

Arterial Cannulation

The ascending aorta is generally used for arterial cannulation. The femoral artery is used under special circumstances, such as in patients undergoing resection of aneurysms or dissection of the ascending aorta.

The aortic cannula should be inserted proximal to the takeoff of the innominate artery, and only a short length of cannula is introduced so that its tip cannot inadvertently enter a brachiocephalic vessel or lie near its orifice. The tapered plastic cannula is fitted for each patient with a small collar adjusted so that just the proper short length of cannula is beyond the collar. Care must be taken to ensure that enough cannula is beyond the collar to prevent inadvertent creation of an aortic dissection secondary to perfusion within the layers of the aortic wall rather than into its lumen. The cannula is inserted up to the collar. Alternatively, a long segment of the aortic cannula may be inserted into the aortic lumen, with the tip directed away from the orifice of the innominate artery.

The authors generally place two concentric pursestring sutures in the aortic adventitia and media at the proposed site of cannulation. The aorta is then incised with a stab wound within the pursestring stitch, and the arterial cannula is directly inserted. The ends of the inner pursestring stitch have previously been threaded through a long narrow rubber or plastic tube, and the tube is tucked down snugly and secured as a tourniquet and then tied to the cannula. After the cannula is connected to the arterial line in such a way as to exclude or remove any air bubbles, the line and cannula are secured so that the end of the cannula lies freely within the aortic lumen and the beveled end faces downstream, the surgical field is uncluttered, and the line from the pump oxygenator is free from kinks.

As the cannula is removed after CPB, the assistant crosses the outer pursestring suture for hemostasis and the surgeon ties the inner one. The outer pursestring suture is then tied. Rarely is anything further required to establish hemostasis.

Venous Cannulation

In infants and children, two angled, metal-tipped venous cannulas, which are inserted directly into each vena cava, are used for most operations, particularly if working through the right atrium or right ventricle. A single venous cannula is often used if working through the left atrium, left ventricle, or ascending aorta and occasionally through the high right ventricle (e.g., changing a valved external conduit). A single venous cannula is also employed in those neonates in whom the entire repair is performed under total circulatory arrest.

In adults, a single large cavoatrial (two-stage) venous cannula with additional holes that come to lie in the right atrium while the tip is in the inferior vena cava, may be used for coronary bypass grafting, aortic valve operations, mitral valve operations, and combinations of these. When working in the right atrium, two venous cannulas are employed.

When a single venous cannula is used, a pursestring suture is placed around the right atrial appendage. When two venous cannulas are employed, tapes or large strings are placed around the superior or inferior venae cavae. The superior vena caval pursestring suture is placed in an elliptical fashion to avoid narrowing the superior vena cava when it is tied. The inferior vena caval pursestring suture is placed near the junction of the inferior vena cava with the diaphragm.

Conduct of Cardiopulmonary Bypass

After the patient is heparinized, cannulation is effected and CPB is established. The initial perfusate temperature is 30° C. to 34° C., which usually allows for effective cardiac action if CPB needs to be discontinued abruptly because of an oxygenator system malfunction. The perfusion flow is gradually increased to about 2.2 liters per minute per sq. m., after which perfusion cooling is begun by decreasing the water temperature in the heat exchanger, either by decrements (to avoid ventricular fibrillation) or by direct reduction

TABLE 54–29. Arterial Cannula Flow Chart: Pressure Gradient in Millimeters of Mercury (mm. Hg)

	Flow in Liters per Minute							
	0.5	1.0	1.5	2.0	2.5	3.0	3.5	4.0
10	60	175	350					
12	40	100	225	325				
14	25	60	140	240	350			
16		25	50	90	150	200	260	
18		20	40	60	80	120	150	200
20			25	40	60	80	100	120
22			25	40	50	60	75	90
24				40	50	60	70	80

TABLE 54–30. Venous Cannula Chart

Total Flow (L./min.)	Single Tygon	Single USCI*	Two-Angled Metal	
			SVC	IVC
<0.9	3/16 in.	20-Fr.	16-Fr.	20-Fr.
0.9–1.2	4/16 in.	24-Fr.	20-Fr.	20-Fr.
1.2–1.6			20-Fr.	24-Fr.
1.6–1.75			24-Fr.	24-Fr.
1.75–2.2		28-Fr.	24-Fr.	28-Fr.
2.2–3.2	5/16 in.		28-Fr.	28-Fr.
3.2–3.7	6/16 in.		28-Fr.	32-Fr.
>3.7	7/16 in.		32-Fr.	32-Fr.

*In adults, at the University of Alabama at Birmingham, USCI "two-stage" single cannula is used (46-French, tapering to 34-French).

to 4° C. In operations performed through the right atrium or right ventricle in infants and small children, the left atrium is usually vented through the sump sucker placed across the atrial septum through the foramen ovale. In older children and adults undergoing aortic operations, a vent is generally placed directly into the left atrium through a pursestring stitch positioned in the base of the right superior pulmonary vein.

The intracardiac portion of the operation is generally performed with the aorta cross-clamped and with cardioplegic-induced cardiac arrest. The precise perfusate temperature selected depends on the expected duration of the ischemic period as well as on the anticipated needs for low perfusion flow rates or total circulatory arrest. In the absence of total circulatory arrest, perfusate temperature is generally maintained at 25° C. to 30° C. during the repair. When the nasopharyngeal temperature is reduced to 25° C. to 28° C., the perfusion flow rate can safely be reduced to 1.8 liters per minute per sq. m. When total circulatory arrest is planned, the nasopharyngeal temperature is reduced to 15° C. or less.

Approximately 5 minutes before removing the aortic cross-clamp, rewarming is initiated by increasing the flow rate to 2.0 to 2.5 liters per minute per sq. m. and raising the temperature of the water in the heat exchanger to 42° C. The arterial line blood temperature should not exceed 39° C. to prevent heat damage to the blood elements. Air is evacuated from the cardiac chambers by needle aspiration or saline injection before the cross-clamp is removed. Suction is placed on the aortic needle vent as the cross-clamp is removed, and this is continued until CPB is discontinued. When the cardiac action is vigorous, the venous line is partially occluded to elevate the left atrial pressure to 10 to 14 mm. Hg to promote effective cardiac ejection for debubbling the heart. With strong suction on the aortic needle vent, the heart is gently massaged, and the left atrial appendage is gently inverted as the anesthesiologist inflates the lungs to force any residual air out of the pulmonary veins. CPB is then gradually discontinued when the cardiac action is vigorous and the nasopharyngeal temperature reaches 37° C. A polyvinyl catheter is usually placed in the left and right atria to facilitate postoperative hemodynamic management, and atrial and ventricular temporary pacing wires are usually placed for postoperative pacing and management of arrhythmias.

SELECTED REFERENCES

Butler, J., Rocker, G. M., and Westaby, S.: Inflammatory response to cardiopulmonary bypass. Ann. Thorac. Surg., 55:552, 1993.
The authors review information currently available to describe inflammation that occurs following CPB. Post-CPB inflammation is a multifaceted response that includes complement and neutrophil activation, among other events. Attenuation or blockade of this response may obviate the adverse consequences of CPB, which are currently accepted as usual clinical phenomena.

Clowes, G. H. A.: Extracorporeal maintenance of circulation and respiration. Physiol. Rev., 40:826, 1960.
This paper reviews the development of devices for CPB and was written shortly after completion of the basic research and development of extracorporeal pump oxygenators and their successful clinical application. The author notes that "the single greatest factor in tissue damage during perfusion of the whole organism is no longer one of metabolic homeostasis, but rather, one of damage to blood elements, which adversely affects the circulation and function of the various organs of the body."

Gibbon, J. H.: Application of a mechanical heart and lung apparatus to cardiac surgery. Minn. Med., 37:171, 1954.
This classic paper described the first successful use of a heart-lung machine in man to entirely support the circulation during open-heart surgery, with the closure of an atrial septal defect. The author discusses the physiologic response to CPB, including hemolysis, adequate tissue perfusion, and the problems of cardiac distention and air emboli. Gibbon concluded, "It seems to me that there will always be a place for an extracorporeal blood circuit because it permits a longer safe interval for opening the heart than can ever be obtained by any of the hypothermic methods."

Kirklin, J. K., Westaby, S., Blackstone, E. H., Kirklin, J. W., Chenoweth, D. E.,

and Pacifico, A. D.: Complement and the damaging effects of cardiopulmonary bypass. J. Thorac. Cardiovasc. Surg., 86:845, 1983.
This prospective clinical study is one of the first rigorous attempts to identify those factors associated with CPB that contribute to organ system dysfunction after cardiac surgery. Complement levels remained normal in patients undergoing cardiac operations without CPB, in contrast to the marked complement activation that occurred during CPB. Cardiac, renal, pulmonary, and hemostatic dysfunction increased with higher levels of the complement anaphylatoxin C3a after bypass, younger age at operation, and longer time on bypass. The authors suggest that a more complete understanding of the biologic response to CPB may eventually lead to the neutralization of the damaging effects.

Moore, F. D., Jr.: Therapeutic regulation of the complement system in acute injury states. Adv. Immunol., 56:267, 1994.
Dr. Moore has written an excellent review that provides a synopsis of complement activation as it is currently understood and reviews the methodology used to assess complement activation. A variety of clinical syndromes, including postperfusion organ injury, is placed in the perspective of acute complement activation or the failure of intrinsic regulation of complement activation. Note that the therapeutic use of soluble complement receptor type 1 to attenuate complement activation has recently been examined in animals.[21]

REFERENCES

1. Addonizio, V. P., Macarak, E. J., Niewiarowski, S., Colman, R. W., and Edmunds, L. H.: Preservation of human platelets with prostaglandin E1 during *in vitro* simulation of cardiopulmonary bypass. Circ. Res., 44:350, 1979.
2. Bidstrup, B. P., Royston, D., Sapsford, R. N., Taylor, K. M., and Cosgrove, D. M.: Reduction in blood loss and blood use after cardiopulmonary bypass with high dose aprotinin (Trasylol). J. Thorac. Cardiovasc. Surg., 97:364, 1989.
3. Bjork, J., Hugli, T. E., and Smedegard, G.: Microvasculature effects on anaphylatoxins C3a and C5a. J. Immunol., 134:1115, 1985.
4. Boldt, J., Kling, D., vonBormann, B., Zuge, M., Scheld, H., and Hempelmann, G.: Blood conservation in cardiac operations. J. Thorac. Cardiovasc. Surg., 97:832, 1989.
5. Braude, S., Nolop, K. B., Fleming, J. S., Krausz, T., Taylor, K. M., and Royston, D.: Increased pulmonary transvascular protein flux after canine cardiopulmonary bypass. Am. Rev. Respir. Dis., 134:867, 1986.
6. Brusino, F. G., Reves, J. G., Smith, R., Prough, D. S., Stump, D. A., and McIntyre, R. W.: The effect of age on cerebral blood flow during hypothermic cardiopulmonary bypass. J. Thorac. Cardiovasc. Surg., 97:541, 1989.
7. Butler, J., Rocker, G. M., and Westaby, S.: Inflammatory response to cardiopulmonary bypass. Ann. Thorac. Surg., 55:552, 1993.
8. Cavarocchi, N. C., England, M. D., Schaff, H. V., et al.: Oxygen free radical generation during cardiopulmonary bypass: Correlation with complement activation. Circulation, 74:130, 1986.
9. Chenoweth, D. E., Cooper, S. W., Hugli, T. E., Stewart, R. W., Blackstone, E. J., and Kirklin, J. W.: Complement activation during cardiopulmonary bypass: Evidence for generation of C3a and C5a anaphylatoxins. N. Engl. J. Med., 304:497, 1981.
10. Clowes, G. H. A.: Extracorporeal maintenance of circulation and respiration. Physiol. Rev., 40:826, 1960.
11. Craddock, P. R., Fehr, J., Brigham, K. L., Kronenberg, R. S., and Jacob, H. S.: Complement and leukocyte-mediated pulmonary dysfunction in hemodialysis. N. Engl. J. Med., 296:769, 1977.
12. Davies, S. W., Duffy, J. P., Wickens, D. G., et al.: Time-course of free radical activity during coronary artery operations with cardiopulmonary bypass. J. Thorac. Cardiovasc. Surg., 105:979, 1993.
13. de Haan, J., Schonberger, J., Haan, J., van Oeveren, W., and Eijgelaar, A.: Tissue-type plasminogen activator and fibrin monomers synergistically cause platelet dysfunction during retransfusion of shed blood after cardiopulmonary bypass. J. Thorac. Cardiovasc. Surg., 106:1017, 1993.
14. Edmunds, L. H.: Invited letter concerning: Blood platelets and bypass. J. Thorac. Cardiovasc. Surg., 97:470, 1989.
15. Edmunds, L. H., Jr.: Surface-bound heparin—panacea or peril? Ann. Thorac. Surg., 58:285, 1994.
16. Fosse, E., Moen, O., Johnson, E., et al.: Reduced complement and granulocyte activation with heparin-coated cardiopulmonary bypass. Ann. Thorac. Surg., 58:472, 1994.
17. Fox, L. S., Blackstone, E. H., Kirklin, J. W., and Bishop, S. P.: Relationship of brain blood flow and oxygen consumption to perfusion flow rate during profoundly hypothermic cardiopulmonary bypass: An experimental study. J. Thorac. Cardiovasc. Surg., 87:658, 1984.
18. Fox, L. S., Blackstone, E. H., Kirklin, J. W., Steward, R. W., and Samuelson, P. N.: Relationship of whole body oxygen consumption to perfusion flow rate during hypothermic cardiopulmonary bypass. J. Thorac. Cardiovasc. Surg., 83:239, 1982.
19. George, J. F.: Invited letter concerning: Cytokines and mechanisms of capillary leakage after cardiopulmonary bypass. J. Thorac. Cardiovasc. Surg., 106:566, 1993.
20. Gibbon, J. H.: Application of a mechanical heart and lung apparatus to cardiac surgery. Minn. Med., 37:171, 1954.
21. Gillinov, A. M., DeValeria, P. A., Winkelstein, J. A., et al.: Complement

inhibition with soluble complement receptor type 1 in cardiopulmonary bypass. Ann. Thorac. Surg., 55:619, 1993.

22. Gillinov, A. M., Redmond, J. M., Winkelstein, J. A., et al.: Complement and neutrophil activation during cardiopulmonary bypass: A study in the complement-deficient dog. Ann. Thorac. Surg., 57:345, 1994.

23. Gluszko, P., Rucinski, B., Musial, J., et al.: Fibrinogen receptors in platelet adhesion to surfaces of extracorporeal circuit. Am. J. Physiol., 252:H615, 1987.

24. Gu, Y. J., van Oeveren, W., Akkerman, C., Boonstra, P. W., Huyzen, R. J., Wildevuur, C. R. H.: Heparin-coated circuits reduce the inflammatory response to cardiopulmonary bypass. Ann. Thorac. Surg., 55:917, 1993.

25. Hisatomi, K., Isomura, T., Kawara, T., et al.: Changes in lymphocyte subsets, mitogen responsiveness, and interleukin-2 production after cardiac operations. J. Thorac. Cardiovasc. Surg., 98:580, 1989.

26. Kestin, A. S., Valeri, C. R., Khuri, S. F., et al.: The platelet function defect of cardiopulmonary bypass. Blood, 82:107, 1993.

27. Kirklin, J. K., Chenoweth, D. E., Naftel, D. C., et al.: Effects of protamine administration after cardiopulmonary bypass on complement, blood elements, and the hemodynamic state. Ann. Thorac. Surg., 41:193, 1986.

28. Kirklin, J. K., Westaby, S., Blackstone, E. H., Kirklin, J. W., Chenoweth, D. E., and Pacifico, A. D.: Complement and the damaging effects of cardiopulmonary bypass. J. Thorac. Cardiovasc. Surg., 86:845, 1983.

29. Markewitz, A., Faist, E., Lang, S., Endres, S., Fuchs, D., and Reichart, B.: Successful restoration of cell-mediated immune response after cardiopulmonary bypass by immunomodulation. J. Thorac. Cardiovasc. Surg., 105:15, 1993.

30. Moore, F. D., Jr.: Therapeutic regulation of the complement system in acute injury states. Adv. Immunol., 56:267, 1994.

31. Newburger, J. W., Jonas, R. A., Wernovsky, G., et al.: A comparison of the perioperative neurologic effects of hypothermic circulatory arrest versus low-flow cardiopulmonary bypass in infant heart surgery. N. Engl. J. Med., 329:1057, 1993.

32. Parker, D. J., Cantrell, J. W., Karp, R. B., Stroud, R. M., and Digerness, S. B.: Changes in serum complement and immunoglobulins following cardiopulmonary bypass. Surgery, 71:824, 1972.

33. Rahn, H., Reeves, R. B., and Howell, B. J.: Hydrogen ion regulation temperature and evolution. Am. Rev. Resper. Dis., 112:165, 1975.

34. Royston, D.: Intraoperative coronary thrombosis: Can aprotinin be incriminated? J. Cardiothorac. Vasc. Anesth., 8:137, 1994.

35. Sacks, T., Moldow, C. F., Craddock, P. R., Bowers, T. K., and Jacob, H. S.: Oxygen radicals mediate endothelial cell damage by complement stimulated granulocytes. Am. Soc. Clin. Invest., 21:1161, 1978.

36. Solem, J. O., Tengborn, L., Steen, S., and Luhrs, C.: Cell saver versus hemofilter for concentration of oxygenator blood after cardiopulmonary bypass. Thorac. Cardiovasc. Surg., 35:42, 1987.

37. Sundt, T. M., III, Kouchoukos, N. T., Saffitz, J. E., Murphy, S. F., Wareing, T. H., and Stahl, D. J.: Renal dysfunction and intravascular coagulation with aprotinin and hypothermic circulatory arrest. Ann. Thorac. Surg., 55:1418, 1993.

38. vanOeveren, W., Janson, N. J. G., Bidstrup, B. P., et al.: Effects of aprotinin on hemostatic mechanisms during cardiopulmonary bypass. Ann. Thorac. Surg., 44:640, 1987.

39. Vibeke, V., Fosse, E., Mollnes, T. E., Ellingsen, O., Pedersen, T., and Karlsen, H.: Different oxygenators for cardiopulmonary bypass lead to varying degrees of human complement activation in vitro. J. Thorac. Cardiovasc. Surg., 97:764, 1989.

40. Volanakis, J. E.: Invited letter concerning: Complement activation caused by different oxygenators. J. Thorac. Cardiovasc. Surg., 98:292, 1989.

41. Wachtfogel, Y. T., Kucich, U., Greenplate, J., et al.: Human neutrophil degranulation during extracorporeal circulation. Blood 69:324, 1987.

42. Westaby, S.: Aprotinin in perspective. Ann. Thorac. Surg., 55:1033, 1993.

43. Wong, C. A., Franklin, M. L., and Wade, L. D.: Coagulation tests, blood loss, and transfusion requirements in platelet-rich plasmapheresed versus nonpheresed cardiac surgery patients. Anesth. Analg., 78:29, 1994.

44. Zilla, P., Fasol, R., Groscurth, P., Klepetko, W., Reichenspurner, H., and Wolner, E.: Blood platelets in cardiopulmonary bypass operations. J. Thorac. Cardiovasc. Surg., 97:379, 1989.

XXIV

INTRA-AORTIC BALLOON COUNTERPULSATION: PHYSIOLOGY, INDICATIONS, AND TECHNIQUES

W. Randolph Chitwood, Jr., M.D., and Joseph R. Elbeery, M.D.

PHYSIOLOGIC EFFECTS OF INTRA-AORTIC BALLOON PUMPING

Major determinants of myocardial oxygen consumption in intact hearts include pulse rate, transmural wall stress, and intrinsic contractile properties. Myocardial oxygen consumption relates linearly to peak systolic wall stress and is influenced by intraventricular pressure, afterload, end-diastolic volume, and wall thickness. Sarnoff and colleagues[43] first fully appreciated this relationship between ventricular work and myocardial energetics. They determined that pressure work, as indicated by a tension-time index (TTI), influenced myocardial oxygen demands more than preload, heart rate, or left ventricular stroke work. Because intra-aortic balloon pumping (IABP) can modify left ventricular ejection pressure significantly, and therefore afterload, determinants of transmural wall stress become diminished.[39] To compare these energy requirements with oxygen and substrate supply, the diastolic pressure-time index (DPTI), or difference between the area under the diastolic aortic and left ventricular pressure curves, was derived as a hemodynamic correlate of coronary perfusion.[5] Figure 54–230 suggests how IABP can decrease the TTI while increasing the DPTI favorably in compromised hearts, causing improved cardiac function.[5] Thus, DPTI and TTI help illustrate the supply and demand components of myocardial metabolism during IABP. The majority of ventricular oxygen requirements occur during isovolumic systole when wall stresses are maximal. During periods of cardiac failure, both ventricular dilation and afterload augmentation result in concomitant increases in intramural wall tension. Under these conditions, oxygen requirements have been shown to be significantly higher than in normal hearts. During counterpulsation, rapid collapse of the balloon reduces impedance to aortic flow in the proximal aorta by creating an instant abyss. Thus, the aortic valve is allowed to open at a 10% to 15% lower systolic pressure, reducing myocardial work and simultaneous oxygen utilization (Fig. 54–231).[5]

In damaged hearts, many of the benefits of IABP also probably result from coronary flow augmentation, which occurs during the DPTI supply phase (see Fig. 54–230). When adequate pharmacologic afterload reduction causes intolerable hypotension, IABP support can be instituted to maintain efficient myocardial perfusion. In most clinical situations, abnormal metabolic demands ablate coronary autoregulation and transmural ventricular blood flow becomes almost entirely pressure dependent. The effects of progressive diastolic hypotension become compounded by a rising left ventricular end-diastolic pressure, effectively reducing transmural coronary perfusion even further. Additive effects result in spiraling failure secondary to enhanced myocardial demands, decreased cardiac output, and ventricular dilation at a time

EFFECTS OF IABP ON MYOCARDIAL OXYGEN SUPPLY (DPTI) AND DEMAND (TTI)

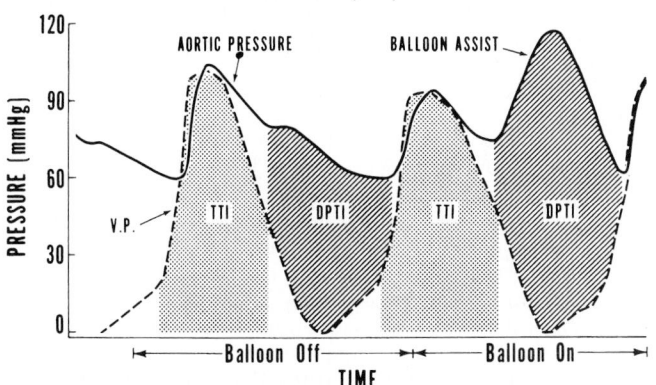

Figure 54–230. Effects of intra-aortic balloon pumping on myocardial oxygen supply and demand. DPTI, diastolic perfusion time index; TTI, tension time index; VP, ventricular pressure. During diastole, balloon assistance produced an elevated DPTI, suggesting an increase in myocardial oxygen supply. At the same time, ventricular work (TTI) decreased significantly. (From Bolooki, H.: Clinical Applications of the Intra-aortic Balloon Pump. Mount Kisco, N.Y., Futura Publishing, 1984.)

when blood supply continues to diminish. Under these conditions, the IABP reduces left ventricular end-diastolic pressure, effectively augmenting the transmural coronary driving pressure.[5] In a classic study, Powell showed that the balloon pump enhances coronary flow more in the presence of failure than in normal hearts.[39] Clinically, the diastolic pressure may increase up to 90% with the IABP. The additive effects of afterload reduction and coronary flow augmentation usually eventuate in decreases in ischemia and left ventricular end-diastolic pressure with an elevated cardiac output of 20% to 50%.[4] Secondary benefits include a decreased heart rate and diminished peripheral vascular tone. These and other physiologic benefits of IABP in clinical situations have been detailed by others and are summarized in Table 54–31.[5, 40, 45]

TABLE 54–31. Physiologic Effects of Intra-aortic Balloon Pumping

Aortic systolic pressure	↓ ↓
Aortic diastolic pressure	↑ ↑
Left ventricular systolic pressure	↓
Left ventricular end-diastolic pressure	↓
Cardiac output	↑
Cardiac afterload	↓ ↓
Cardiac preload	↓
Left ventricular wall tension	↓
Left ventricular volume	↓
Left ventricular stroke work	↓
Coronary blood flow	↑
Renal blood flow	↑

INDICATIONS FOR INTRA-AORTIC BALLOON PUMPING

Current major indications (Table 54–32) for IABP include (1) intractable cardiac failure after a cardiac surgical procedure (35% to 40%); (2) refractory angina, despite maximal medical management (15% to 25%); (3) perioperative treatment of the complications of myocardial infarction (10%), including acute ventricular septal defects, acute mitral regurgitation, arrhythmias, and ventricular aneurysms; (4) failed percutaneous coronary angioplasty and support during complex angioplasties; and (5) as a bridge to cardiac transplantation. Compared with former years, IABP is almost never used to treat postinfarction cardiogenic shock unless the potential of coronary angioplasty or surgical revascularization exists. Moreover, with the evolution of newer monitoring and anesthetic techniques, prophylactic usage of IABP before coronary surgery has declined markedly. Conversely, counterpulsation has been expanded to use in children, patients with isolated right ventricular failure, and more pretransplant patients.

Myocardial Infarction and Cardiogenic Shock. As mentioned earlier, the major earlier indication for IABP was re-

Figure 54–231. *Left,* With balloon augmentation both aortic peak systolic and end-diastolic pressures decrease, suggesting a reduction in ventricular afterload. At the same time the diastolic (D) aortic pressure is enhanced (B). AO, aortic pressure; PC, pulmonary capillary wedge; V, ventricular wave; a, atrial wave. *Right,* In a failing heart, the left ventricular end-diastolic pressure (EdP) markedly decreases with balloon pumping. LV, left ventricular pressure. (From Bolooki, H. K.: Clinical Applications of the Intra-aortic Balloon Pump. Mt. Kisco, N.Y., Futura Publishing, 1984.)

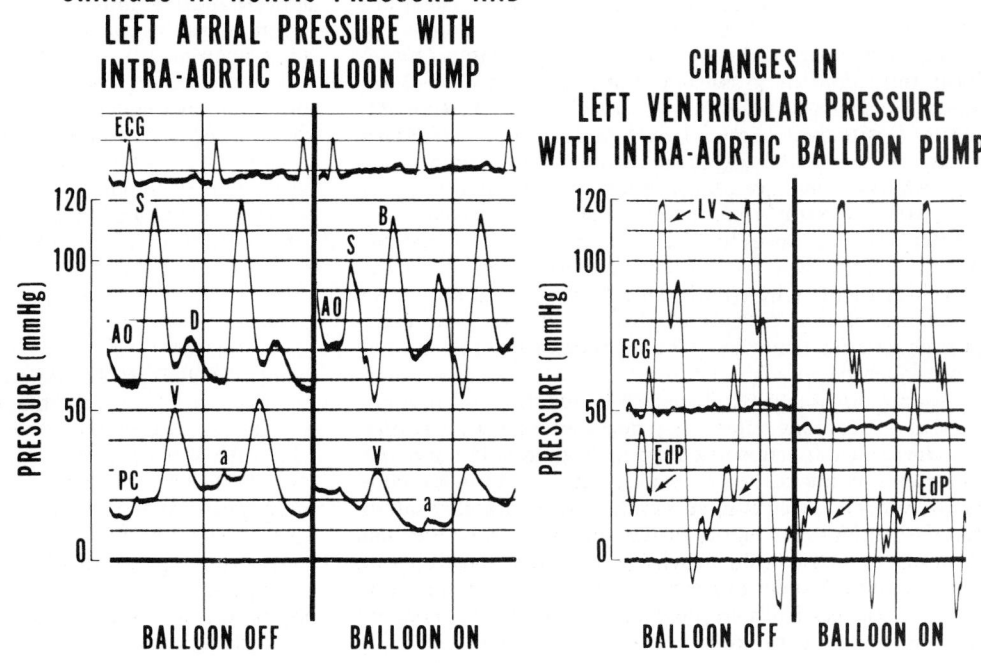

TABLE 54–32. General Indications for IABP Support

Unstable angina
    Medically refractory or post-infarction
Postcardiotomy cardiac failure
Angioplasty
    Failure: Precoronary surgery
    Complex angioplasty support
Complications of myocardial infarction
    Acute mitral insufficiency
    Acute ventricular septal defect
    Refractory arrhythmias
    Ventricular aneurysm
Cardiogenic shock
    Only before surgery or angioplasty
Precardiac transplantation
Occasional prophylactic use
    Poor ventricular function
    Severe left main coronary stenosis
    Very severe multivessel disease
Rarely high-risk noncardiac surgery

fractory cardiogenic shock after myocardial infarction.[5, 6] Although some patients with profound ventricular failure improve transiently, only 15% to 20% of patients not being revascularized can be weaned from IABP. Moreover, the long-term survival for these few individuals only ranges between 10% and 30%.[3] Although earlier studies suggest postinfarction survival to be unaffected by IABP, Ohman and associates[33] found in a randomized trial that counterpulsation markedly benefits infarct-related vessel patency after angioplasty and/or thrombolysis. Kern and coworkers[23] showed independently that diastolic flow velocity increases significantly, however, only after the angioplasty has opened the vessel. Thus, patients usually improve with IABP after thrombolysis or angioplasty so that they may undergo surgical revascularization or a more complete angioplasty with safety. Patients having postinfarction angina without shock benefit significantly from IABP as well.[24] The notion that IABP alone can modify an infarct size still remains controversial.[34]

Refractory Angina. The intra-aortic balloon pump has been very effective for treating patients with pharmacologically refractory angina who are being readied for interventional or surgical revascularization.[25, 46] When persistent angina occurs in the presence of ineffective doses of intravenous nitroglycerin, IABP enables angiography/angioplasty to be done more safely. In this setting, IABP has been shown to decrease myocardial ischemia and improve left ventricular function significantly.[31] At least 80% of patients obtain pain relief from IABP. Survival in patients with medically refractory angina has been excellent using IABP support followed by surgical revascularization.[10, 25, 46]

After Cardiac Surgery. IABP remains very helpful for weaning refractory patients from cardiopulmonary bypass.[32, 35] Patients who require intraoperative insertion of an intra-aortic balloon pump have either sustained ventricular damage preoperatively and experience deleterious additional ischemia or begin with relatively normal cardiac function and experience severe, but reversible, myocardial stunning intraoperatively. The latter group does better postoperatively, because cardiac function often improves gradually if a major infarction has not occurred. Despite attention to intraoperative myocardial protection and maximal pharmacologic support, 3% to 6% of patients still require IABP to be weaned from cardiopulmonary bypass.[32] Norman and associates have outlined indices reflecting survival for postcardiotomy patients requiring IABP.[32] At the Cleveland Clinic, 2.8% of patients having isolated coronary bypass surgery require

balloon counterpulsation.[13] In general, 75% to 85% of postcardiotomy IABP patients can be weaned effectively from balloon support.[32] Between 50% and 80% of this group leave the hospital, and a majority of these have a significant long-term survival.[5, 32] Specific guidelines have been established to aid in instituting IABP during or after operative procedures (Table 54–33).

Although efficacious for postcardiotomy ventricular failure, IABP should be added to vasodilator and inotropic drug therapy for maximal reduction in peripheral vascular resistance with enhanced coronary perfusion pressure. However, larger infusions of dopamine, epinephrine, and norepinephrine are associated with both increased contractility and afterload, and resultant ischemia may promote additional myocardial damage. Optimal coronary perfusion with minimal myocardial energy expenditure remains the curative goal. Thus, selection of counterpulsation before infusing large doses of inotropic agents is more physiologic and early IABP treatment appears a more reasonable alternative for these patients than massive inotropic support.

In past years, IABP in children and infants was considered impractical. However, recently IABP has been used to wean children from infancy to 18 years old from cardiopulmonary bypass after congenital heart surgery.[17, 36–38] Although smaller balloon catheters have allowed insertion of balloons in children, IABP survival has not been as satisfactory (40%) as in adults after cardiac surgery. These disappointing results may relate to either intrinsic physiologic characteristics related to IABP in younger patients or simply the differences that congenital cardiac conditions and operations impose. In infants and children, balloon catheters are available in volumes from 2.5 to 20 ml. on 4.5- to 7.0-French catheters, all of which must be inserted under direct vision. Extreme care must be used, especially in infants, to position these devices correctly because occlusion of intra-abdominal vessels may occur more easily. In children and infants with congestive failure, markedly elevated heart rates (190 to 200 beats per minute) may make timing and diastolic augmentation difficult. Significant aortic elasticity in children has been implicated as impeding effective counterpulsation. Here much of the energy during balloon filling may be transferred to the expansile aorta rather than being converted to retrograde diastolic flow.

Complications of Myocardial Infarction. After myocardial infarction, circulatory deterioration may occur rapidly from either papillary muscle rupture or dysfunction, producing severe mitral insufficiency. Moreover, the development of an acute ventricular septal defect after an infarction may cause intractable failure. Patients with either of these conditions require immediate surgical repair and benefit from early IABP support. In these circumstances, IABP counterpulsation is preferable to pharmacologic afterload reduction, which may augment hypotension.

Acute mitral insufficiency after a myocardial infarction often results in pulmonary edema, hypotension, and low cardiac output. Most commonly, papillary muscle ruptures

TABLE 54–33. Indications for IABP During Cardiac Surgery

Inability to discontinue bypass: multiple interventions
Inadequate hemodynamics: after ↑ ↑ inotropic support
    ↓ ↓ Systolic blood pressure ↓ 80 mm. Hg
    ↓ ↓ Cardiac index ↓ 2.0 L./min./sq. m.
    ↑ ↑ Left atrial pressure ↑ 20 mm. Hg
    ↑ ↑ Vascular resistance ↑ 2500 dynes/sec./cm.$^{-5}$
Large doses of multiple inotropic drugs
Continued refractory ventricular arrhythmias

occur after an inferior myocardial infarction. Mitral regurgitation may produce cardiogenic shock, even in patients with minimal impairment of left ventricular function. Patients having both severe left ventricular dysfunction and acute mitral insufficiency have a poor prognosis. In this clinical setting, accurate quantitation of preoperative cardiac function becomes impossible because of retrograde ejection. Treatment with systemic vasopressors may augment afterload, causing even more shunting into the lower resistance left atrium. Initiation of the IABP decreases cardiac afterload and usually augments left ventricular ejection, lessening the regurgitant fraction.[11] Under these conditions the balloon pump effects significant decreases in both pulmonary capillary wedge and left atrial pressures. At the same time, mean arterial pressure and cardiac output become increased (Fig. 54–232).[11, 41] Counterpulsation should be instituted relatively early in patients who are beginning to decompensate. In one review, long-term survival of patients undergoing mitral valve replacement was 78% if the preoperative ejection fraction was greater than 35% but only 38% if it was less.[41] Because the salutary effects of IABP may be short lived after stabilization

of patients with ischemic mitral regurgitation and ventricular septal rupture, catheterization and surgery should proceed rapidly.[11, 41]

Ventricular septal rupture occurs in 1% to 3% of patients with acute myocardial infarctions. Rapid hemodynamic deterioration occurs in approximately 60% of patients. Without surgery, nearly 80% of the remainder die within 2 months of the infarction. Thus, nearly all patients should undergo immediate surgical repair.[42] Use of the IABP combined with early repair has eventuated in an operative mortality as low as 30%. In operative patients surviving repair, long-term survival has been approximately 70% if remaining left ventricular function was good.

As with mitral regurgitation, an acute ventricular septal defect that eventuates in shock may occur in the presence of moderate to good left ventricular function. Many of the unphysiologic effects may occur after severe right ventricular failure induced by increased left-to-right shunting. Stabilization with the IABP markedly reduces both shunting and the pulmonary capillary wedge pressure with a concomitant increase in cardiac output and mean arterial pressure (see

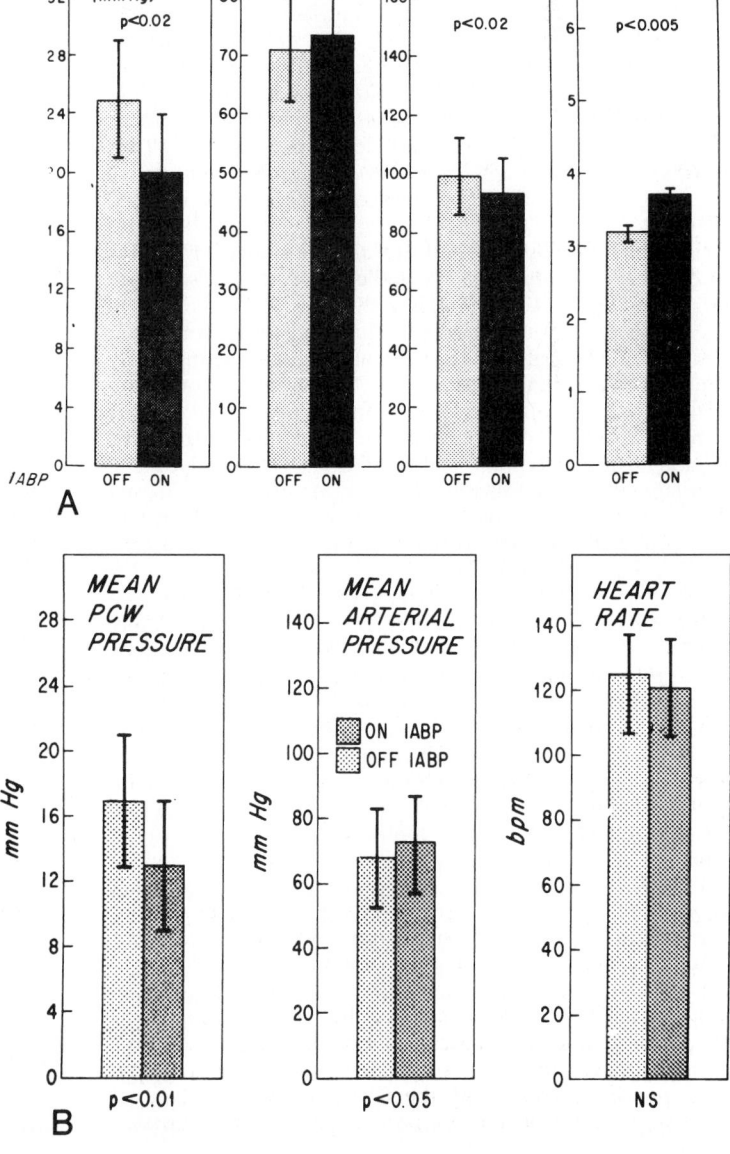

Figure 54–232. *A,* Patients with acute mitral insufficiency showed a significant decrease in pulmonary capillary wedge pressure and an increase in cardiac output after introduction of balloon counterpulsation. *B,* In patients with an acute ventricular septal rupture, balloon pumping decreased the mean pulmonary capillary wedge pressure (PCW) while increasing mean arterial pressure. At the same time, abnormal shunting across the septal defect decreased significantly. (From Gold, H. K., Leinbach, R. C., Sanders, C. A., Buckley, M. J., Mundth, E. D., and Austen, W. G.: Intra-aortic balloon pumping for ventricular septal defect or mitral regurgitation complicating acute myocardial infarction. Circulation, *47:*1191, 1973. Copyright 1973, American Heart Association.)

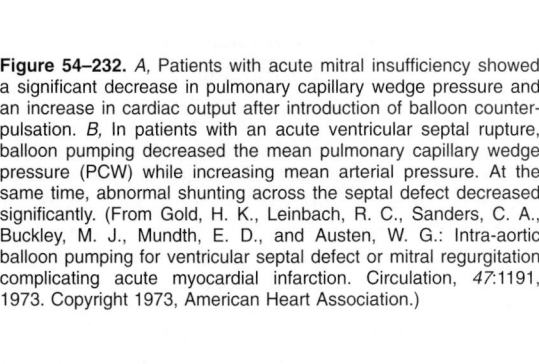

Fig. 54–232).[11, 40] These improvements occur largely from afterload reduction, which provides less resistance to systemic ejection. Also, enhanced coronary perfusion may help reduce ischemic ventricular dysfunction simultaneously. Most clinicians institute balloon pumping as early as possible after diagnosis and one hopes before cardiac decompensation.

Significant ventricular arrhythmias occur in 10% to 50% of patients after an acute myocardial infarction. The majority are well controlled with antiarrhythmic medications, cardioversion, and pacing. However, patients with sustained refractory ventricular irritability have a very poor prognosis.[15] Both continuing ischemia and altered myocardial substrate can propagate problematic arrhythmias. When ischemia persists as the major etiology, institution of counterpulsation effectively controls ventricular irritability in most patients. Hanson found an 86% improvement in ischemic patients with a 55% resolution of arrhythmias after institution of IABP.[15] In contrast, when myocardial fibrosis causes arrhythmogenicity, IABP is less effective; and endocardial resection, either alone or combined with coronary artery bypass grafting, and implantation of an automatic internal defibrillator should be considered.

Ventricular aneurysms develop in up to 20% of patients after a myocardial infarction.[3] Patients with acute ventricular aneurysms are much more difficult to manage than those who develop chronic aneurysms. Ventricular irritability occurs in the former group in 7% to 40% of cases; however, only 7% to 10% require surgical intervention because of arrhythmias. In these surgical candidates, hemodynamic improvement usually results from the additive salutary effects of the IABP on heart failure and electrical irritability. When a chronic aneurysm results in severe failure, preoperative insertion of an IABP may be protective because of reduced afterload.

Coronary Angioplasty Failures and Supported Complex Angioplasty. In patients being readied for emergent coronary surgery after a failed angioplasty, the IABP has been shown to provide optimal stabilization.[44] This is especially important in the presence of multivessel coronary disease or markedly impaired ventricular function, when ischemia in other regions may become additive, resulting in cardiogenic shock. In most instances, cardiologists can accomplish intra-aortic balloon insertion rapidly using guide wires placed during the diagnostic catheterization. Modern reperfusion or *bail out* catheters may allow the counterpulsed IABP waveform to reach the distal segment of the jeopardized coronary artery. Small portable balloon consoles and dual-lumen balloon catheters with continuous central aortic pressure monitoring enable transport to the operating room with greater safety and speed. By minimizing ischemia after a failed angioplasty and early institution of cardiopulmonary bypass, many patients can be revascularized with safety using the internal mammary artery instead of all vein grafts. Kahn and coworkers have advocated the prophylactic insertion of the intra-aortic balloon pump before complex multivessel or left main coronary artery angioplasty.[18] This type of supported angioplasty may be helpful in selected patients.

Bridge to Cardiac Transplantation. Thirteen to 29% of end-stage cardiomyopathy patients awaiting transplantation need mechanical support.[26] The importance of IABP support has increased with the declining donor heart supply. The waiting period now approaches 2 to 3 months before a donor heart is available. A balloon pump may provide sufficient afterload reduction and obviate the need for a more invasive left ventricular assist device, for which the benefits may be more short lived. In these patients there has been no difference in long-term survival between those supported with the IABP compared with individuals transplanted electively.[26]

Other Indications. Previously, prophylactic IABP before cardiac surgery was popular in patients with left main coronary artery disease, unstable angina, poor left ventricular function, and severe aortic stenosis. Presently, most cardiac surgeons and anesthesiologists believe that very few patients require prophylactic IABP. Patients with either poor left ventricular function or severe left main coronary artery disease, who develop chest pain or become hypotensive in the operating room, may require IABP. However, nearly all of these patients can undergo induction of anesthesia safely using newer monitoring and pharmacologic techniques. Additionally, use of IABP for protection during noncardiac operations is indicated rarely. However, for patients either with inoperable coronary artery disease or requiring emergent surgery for other reasons, IABP has been employed with success. Other infrequent indications published include septic shock and massive pulmonary emboli.

CONTRAINDICATIONS TO IABP

With severe aortic insufficiency, IABP enhances left ventricular regurgitation and cardiac failure. However, patients with mild aortic insufficiency still may be improved by IABP. Although the presence of an aortic aneurysm may be a relative contraindication to IABP insertion, fluoroscopic or emergency intraoperative introduction may be necessary in specific situations. IABP catheter sheaths can be inserted through aortoiliac grafts, with few complications. Most patients with coronary artery disease have some degree of diffuse atherosclerosis. In past years, this precluded insertion through the femoral artery in 10% to 25% of patients. However, fluoroscopic percutaneous guidance has aided in positioning IABP catheters even with diffuse atherosclerosis and tortuous vessels. Recently, retrograde axillary artery and transthoracic introduction has rejuvenated the possibility of using IABP in patients with totally occluded aortas. The previous administration of thrombolytic agents or anticoagulants has not proposed any contraindication to IABP, but local hemorrhage control may be necessary.

INSERTION TECHNIQUES
Percutaneous Insertion

In the majority of patients, IABP catheters can be inserted percutaneously through the femoral artery using a modified Seldinger technique.[2, 9, 35] This method precludes the necessity of either an arteriotomy closure, patch closure, or a stump of graft material left attached to the artery. Currently, the smallest dual-lumen (inner guide wire and arterial pressure channel) percutaneous catheter with a standard 40-ml. balloon has an outside diameter of 9.0-French. For single-lumen catheters, 8.5-French is the smallest with a 40-ml. balloon. For smaller patients, catheters designed for surgical insertion also are available with balloon sizes ranging between 20 and 30 ml. Surgical balloons ranging between 2.5 and 20 ml. are manufactured for children and infants. Figure 54–233 compares an 8.5-French (40 ml.) percutaneous balloon to an older

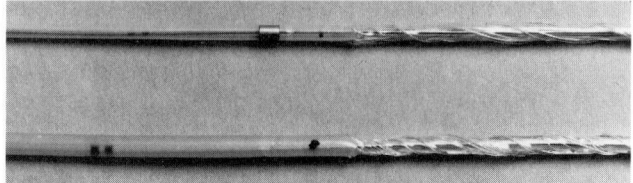

Figure 54–233. Size comparison of an 8.5-French percutaneous intra-aortic balloon catheter to an older 10.5-French model.

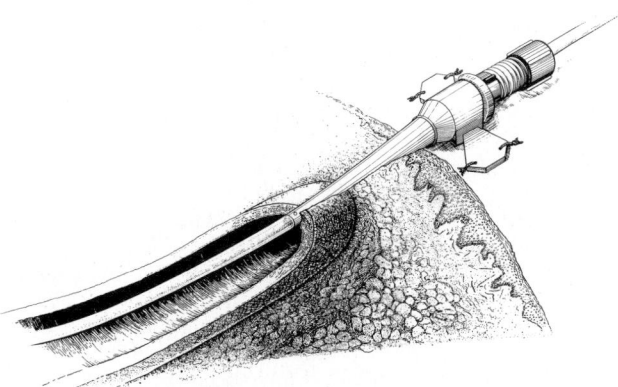

Figure 54–234. Sheathless introduction of a percutaneous balloon catheter. The catheter has been passed over a guide wire into a non-atherosclerotic femoral artery. Insertion through calcified vessels or graft material usually requires an introducer technique; however, the sheathless method helps to obviate limb ischemia.

12-French catheter. Smaller catheters may minimize limb ischemia while providing a balloon volume adequate for counterpulsation; however, an overall decrease in complications with smaller catheters has not been seen.[9] In patients with noncalcified femoral arteries, IABP catheters often can be inserted over a guide wire by the *sheathless* technique, in which the catheter is introduced immediately after percutaneous dilation (Fig. 54–234). The ratio between catheter size and balloon volume remains the limiting factor for helium exchange. Thus, development of small catheters with large

balloons has become limited. Overall, adult IABP catheters are approximately 70 cm. long with a 25-cm. long balloon at the tip. Variable catheter lengths matched for patient heights are available from some manufacturers. With percutaneous balloons the internal lumen allows the guide wire to be threaded to the thoracic aorta for control during difficult insertion. After balloon introduction, the guide wire channel provides a means for central aortic pressure measurement and sequence timing.

The recommended method for percutaneous intra-aortic balloon insertion is illustrated in Figure 54–235. For proper positioning immediately distal to the subclavian artery origin, the prewrapped catheter should be measured from the groin insertion site to the sternal notch. First, a Cournand needle, inserted at a 45-degree angle to the skin, is used to puncture the common femoral artery just below the inguinal ligament (see Fig. 54–235A). After pulsatile arterial flow returns, a guide wire should be passed to above the iliac arterial bifurcation and the needle withdrawn (see Fig. 54–235B). A coaxial vessel dilator then is positioned over the wire and passed into the arterial lumen (see Fig. 54–235C). If the sheathless method is used, a prewrapped IABP catheter is threaded over the wire and into the dilated artery and passed to the subclavian level over the wire before inflation. Figure 54–235D shows the standard sheath introduction technique. The introducer sheath is threaded over a larger dilator, and together the two are passed over the wire and into the arterial lumen with a clockwise twisting motion. Long sheaths are available to make insertion with severely diseased or tortuous vessels easier. As shown in Figure 54–235E, the dilator should be removed, leaving the guide wire and

Figure 54–235. Percutaneous insertion technique. *A* and *B,* The Seldinger technique is used to insert guide wire into the femoral artery. *C* and *D,* Subsequently, a dilator and introducing sheath are inserted over the guide wire and into the femoral artery. *E* and *F,* The guide wire and dilator are then removed, and the prewrapped catheter is inserted with a clockwise twisting motion until the balloon is passed to the premeasured length just distal to the subclavian artery.

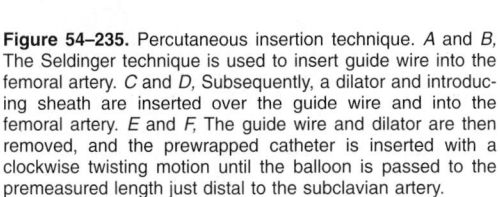

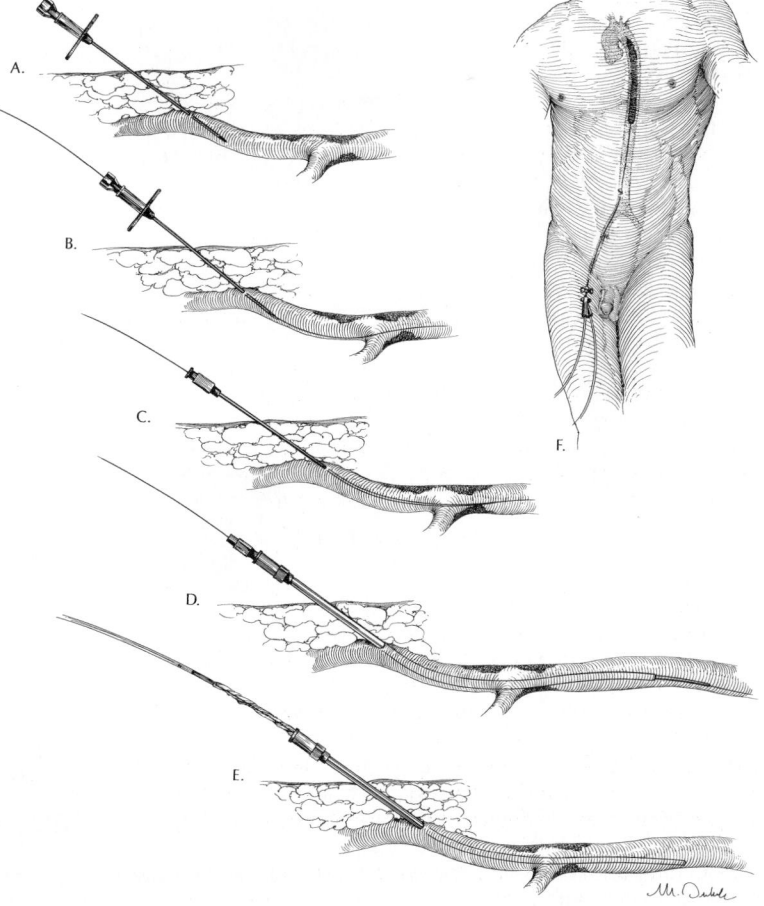

sheath in the artery. When a dual-lumen balloon catheter is selected, it should be passed into the proximal aorta over the wire. Single-lumen catheters are smaller but require removal of the guide wire before introduction. With a clockwise twisting motion, the prewrapped balloon should be placed in the sheath and advanced to the premeasured length (see Fig. 54–235E). Care must be taken not to force the balloon against any obstruction because iliac or aortic perforation may occur. Most balloons will unwrap spontaneously either from pulsatile aortic flow or after the first inflation. Balloon augmentation then can be timed appropriately from cutaneous electrocardiographic leads, a ventricular electrogram, or the arterial pressure tracing. Ventricular pacing wires may provide an excellent source for electrocardiographic timing when all else fails.

Introducer sheaths should be withdrawn slightly to help prevent iliac obstruction. Some catheters have a sterile positioning sleeve, which becomes helpful for repositioning after the surgical field is removed. After insertion, extremity arterial pulses, skin temperature and color, as well as motor and sensory function should be assessed and documented frequently. In general, patients undergoing IABP should be anticoagulated with heparin. However, immediately after surgery heparin may be withheld for at least 24 hours because most balloon catheters are made of antithrombogenic material.

Surgical Insertion: Femoral, Axillary, and Transthoracic

Formerly, balloon catheters were inserted through a 10-mm. Dacron/PTFE graft sewn onto the femoral artery. Although rarely required today, femoral surgical insertion techniques may become necessary. The lack of a palpable femoral pulse during nonpulsatile cardiopulmonary bypass may make percutaneous insertion difficult. Balloon catheters can be introduced surgically through a Dacron side graft sewn to a longitudinal iliac arteriotomy (Fig. 54–236). At present, when an open technique is required, many surgeons obviate side-grafting the artery and simply place a pledgeted suture around a small arteriotomy and insert surgical balloons directly. This method is preferred for placement of catheters in children and very small adults.

Balloon catheters can be inserted into the axillary artery and passed retrograde toward the left subclavian artery and down the aorta. Some transplant surgeons have used this method to enable ambulation of patients requiring cardiac assist who are awaiting a donor heart. This method could provide access in the presence of an occluded aorta. As mentioned earlier, aortic occlusion or diffuse atherosclerosis may prevent retrograde femoral insertion of balloon catheters requisite for weaning from cardiopulmonary bypass. In this situation the transthoracic approach may be required (Fig. 54–237).[27, 35] Balloon catheters may be inserted into the as-

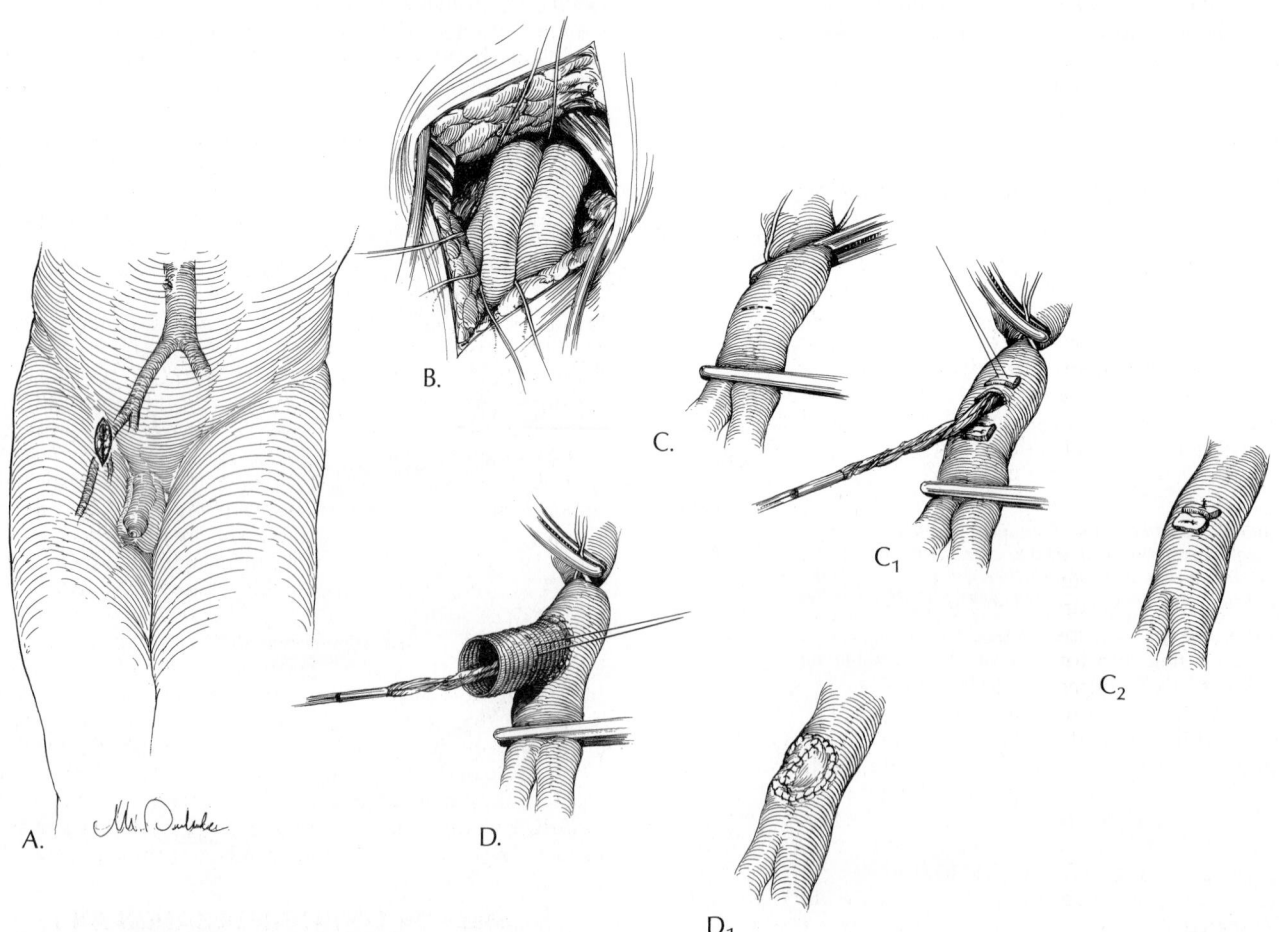

Figure 54–236. Surgical insertion technique. *A* and *B,* The common femoral artery is exposed just below the inguinal ligament. The profunda femoris artery should be identified. *C* and *C₁,* A sheathless balloon catheter is passed via a small artery subtended by a pledgeted suture. *C₂,* After balloon removal, the arteriotomy is closed in the intensive care unit with a second suture. Thrombectomy may be required should a good pulse not return. *D* and *D₁,* An alternate and older technique is to sew a graft onto the common femoral artery for graft insertion. After catheter removal, a stump of graft can be oversewn to effect rapid removal in the intensive care unit.

Figure 54–237. *A* to *C*, Transthoracic balloon catheter insertion. Intraoperatively, intra-aortic balloon catheters may be inserted into the ascending aorta and passed retrograde into the descending aorta with good flow augmentation resulting. The catheter is inserted either directly or by means of the Seldinger technique described in Figure 54–236. The catheter is passed first through the chest wall and then into the ascending aorta. Removal can be done in an intensive care unit equipped for meticulous sterile technique; however, most surgeons do this in the operating room.

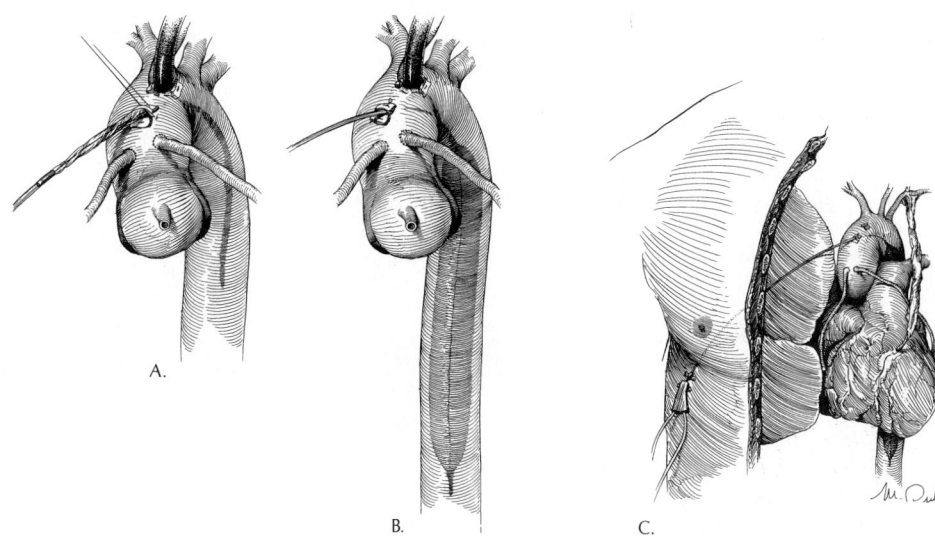

A.

B.

C.

cending aortic arch through either an attached 10-mm. Dacron/PTFE graft or a pursestring suture. Alternately, an introducer sheath can be placed through the opened chest wall and a balloon passed over a wire by the Seldinger method. Direct visualization of the insertion site remains paramount. Surgeons should be careful not to thread the IABP catheter into an arch vessel. After aortic introduction, the sheath should be withdrawn through the chest wall, and a pursestring suture placed around the aortic entrance site to prevent leakage. Usually, removal of the balloon catheter requires return to the operating room; however, removal has been done in unstable patients in sterile intensive care unit facilities.

BALLOON CATHETER REMOVAL

Generally, removal should be done as soon as possible, but only after inotropic support has been weaned to moderate levels. Should the extremity become ischemic and the hemodynamic status remain unstable, then the balloon should be removed and another inserted in the contralateral femoral artery. Before balloon catheter removal, heparin should be stopped at least 6 hours in advance. Both the platelet count and coagulation factors should be determined and corrected if necessary. Surgical femoral balloons may be removed in the intensive care unit if an appropriate sterile environment is available. Before removal of these catheters, the balloon should be evacuated totally to reduce catheter size and minimize trauma at the entrance site. During surgical removal, embolectomy catheters should be passed both proximally and distally to ensure arterial patency. After withdrawal of percutaneous balloons, constant point-pressure should be applied to the groin for at least 30 minutes. During occlusive pressure, distal pulses should be monitored by Doppler ultrasonography to ensure distal flow and prevent arterial thrombosis. Although methods have been reported that allow withdrawal of transthoracic balloon catheters through a long graft, returning to the operating room for removal of the balloon may be preferred. Leaky balloons may develop an internal thrombosis, which can prevent achieving a minimal diameter during deflation. Thrombosed catheters should be removed in the operating room where vascular repair can be facilitated.

COMPLICATIONS OF BALLOON PUMPING

Major complications associated with insertion and use of intra-aortic balloon catheters have been reported in 9% to 30% of patients and include (1) limb ischemia from primary thrombosis, emboli, or vascular dissection; (2) intra-abdominal and intrathoracic hemorrhage from vascular perforation and/or dissection; (3) groin hematomas, lymph drainage, and femoral artery false aneurysms; (4) local wound infections and systemic sepsis; (5) renal failure and bowel infarction from balloon malposition; (6) device malfunction in IABP-dependent patients; (7) neurologic complications, including paraplegia; and (8) hematologic complications, including IABP and heparin-induced thrombocytopenia as well as primary hemolysis. Kantrowitz, Barnett, and Eltchaninoff and their colleagues have independently reviewed IABP complications in over 1400 patients, and their reviews should be consulted.[2, 9, 22] In up to 25% of patients requiring this support, the balloon catheter cannot be advanced because of an atherosclerotic obstruction.[12, 16] Complications of difficult insertions result in 10% to 35% of patients and significant vascular problems occur in approximately 15%.[1] Between 2% and 10% of the latter group will require vascular repair, which may include either patch or femoral-femoral bypass grafting. Morbidity has remained relatively stable for percutaneous balloon catheters; however, the IABP is being used more liberally, eventuating in more aggregate complications. Concurrently, major complications including aortic dissection and perforation, limb amputation, and the need for vascular grafting have decreased as have IABP-related deaths.[1, 2] Diabetes, peripheral vascular disease, female gender, and time period of counterpulsation appear to be major variables relating to limb ischemia.[9] The incidence of major IABP complications has been reported to be higher with percutaneous balloon catheters (20%) versus surgical insertion (4%).[12] Figure 54–238 illustrates how a balloon catheter may enter the aortic wall at an ulcerated plaque, creating a retrograde dissection.[16] In most situations, ischemic complications can be obviated by sheathless insertion, early removal of the balloon catheter, or partial withdrawal of the introducer sheath. Smaller balloon catheters (8.5- and 9.0-French) with 40- and 50-ml. volumes appear beneficial in smaller patients. As noted previously, sheathless percutaneous balloon insertion has been used widely and should have promise for these patients.

TIMING OF COUNTERPULSATION AND WEANING

After the intra-aortic balloon pump has been advanced to a satisfactory position, inflation and deflation must be timed carefully with either an electrocardiographic or arterial pres-

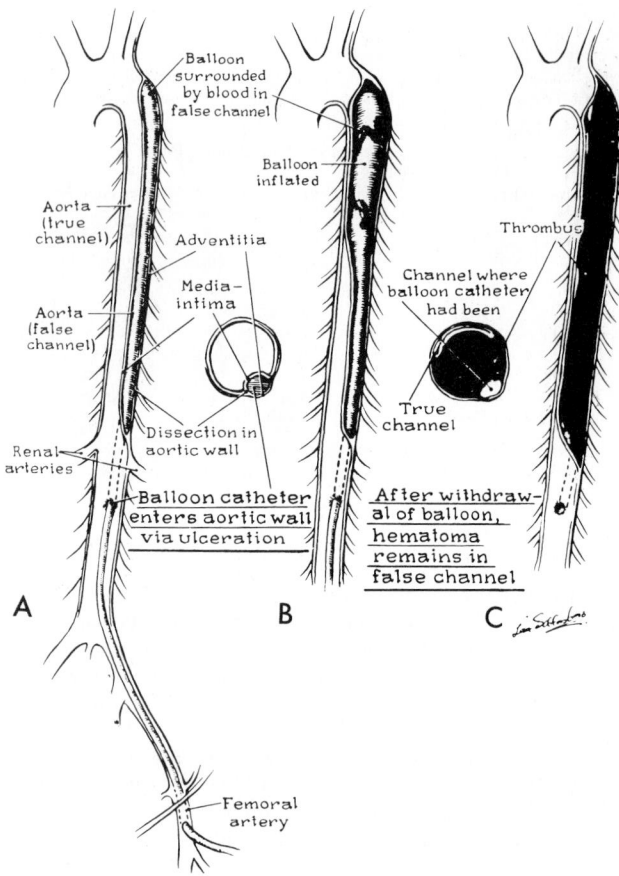

Figure 54–238. *A* to *C*, A major complication can occur when a balloon catheter enters the aortic wall at an ulcerated plaque creating a dissection and ultimate aortic occlusion. Fluoroscopic insertion may help obviate this dangerous complication. (From Isner, J. M., Cohen, S. R., Virmani, R., Lawrinson, W., and Roberts, W. C.: Complications of the intra-aortic balloon counterpulsation device: Clinical and morphologic observations in 45 necropsy patients. Am. J. Cardiol., *45*:260, 1980.)

sure tracing.[5] The central aortic pressure channel in dual-lumen percutaneous balloon catheters enables optimal timing because inflation delays of 50 to 120 msec. may occur with peripheral arterial monitoring catheters. Radial arterial vasoconstriction, accompanying low cardiac output, vasopressor infusions, and hypothermia, may enhance timing problems.

As shown in Figure 54–239, the balloon should inflate about 40 msec. before the arterial dicrotic notch (the ascending T-wave) and deflate during early isovolumic contraction (after the P wave).[5] Total deflation must occur before ejection or the R wave. Usually, this provides excellent diastolic augmentation and optimal afterload reduction as reflected by a significant decrease in both the aortic systolic and end-diastolic pressures. Early inflation results in premature closure of the aortic valve with reduced stroke volume, and late inflation causes inadequate diastolic pressure augmentation. Early deflation effects poor afterload reduction, and late deflation impedes systole, resulting in increased cardiac work.

With either the initiation of electrical pacing or the development of atrial or ventricular arrhythmias, intra-aortic balloon timing may become difficult, resulting in inefficient augmentation. During pacing, a decrease in the pacer artifact amplitude may lessen the tendency for balloon pump dual sensing. Most newer pump consoles have good electrocautery suppression and pacemaker sensing capabilities. Timing from ventricular pacing wires placed during surgery may provide an improved timing signal in difficult situations.

Some prefer to wean the majority of inotropic medications before balloon catheter removal unless limb ischemia or bleeding problems prevail. Before establishing a 1:2 pumping ratio, dopamine or dobutamine infusions have usually been decreased to below 5.0 μg. per kg. per minute, and no other vasopressors are usually present. Thereafter, the balloon pump inflation ratio and remaining inotropic support are weaned simultaneously. Counterpulsation also can be weaned by decreasing the balloon inflation volume gradually. Some motion and balloon volume must be maintained while in the aorta to prevent thrombosis and emboli.

ADVANTAGES OF IABP COMPARED WITH OTHER ASSIST DEVICES

When ventricular mechanical assistance is required, IABP is preferred. However, if complete cardiac chamber decompression is necessary, either axial flow pumps (Hemopump) or more complete ventricular bypass pumps (Novocor, Thoratec) should be selected. These devices provide superior ventricular decompression to the IABP but with more complexity. At present many of the ventricular assist pumps still require institutional approval and operational protocols. IABP support is more economical and has less overall hematologic and bleeding complications. Lastly, IABP technology is well established and can be used with facility by the nursing and perfusion personnel.

HELICOPTER, AIR AMBULANCE, AND MOBILE INTENSIVE CARE UNIT BALLOON SUPPORT

Smaller balloon consoles are optimal in the catheterization laboratory, operating room, and for air or ground transport (Fig. 54–240). Many have been tested for flight and mobile conditions but may have different power requirements, purging characteristics, and Federal Aviation Administration requirements for motion security. These devices will fit in a variety of helicopters and mobile intensive care units. Helicopters usually fly below 10,000 feet and are not pressurized. However, during fixed-wing air transport, intra-aortic balloon characteristics will be altered by aircraft pressurization. Because of constant balloon gas expansion and contraction (1.5 ml./1000 feet of altitude), it is recommended that the IABP operator be apprised constantly of changes in altitude to effect proper purging of the device. Mertlich and Quaal[28] have outlined these changes as well as in-flight instructions

Arterial Waveform Variations During IABP Therapy

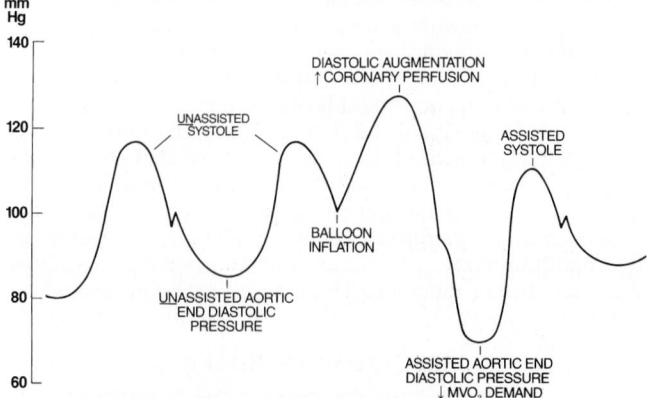

Figure 54–239. Correct timing of an intra-aortic balloon pressure tracing is shown. Diastolic augmentation should begin with closure of the aortic valve and proceed until isovolumic systole. (Courtesy of Datascope Corp., Paramus, N.J.)

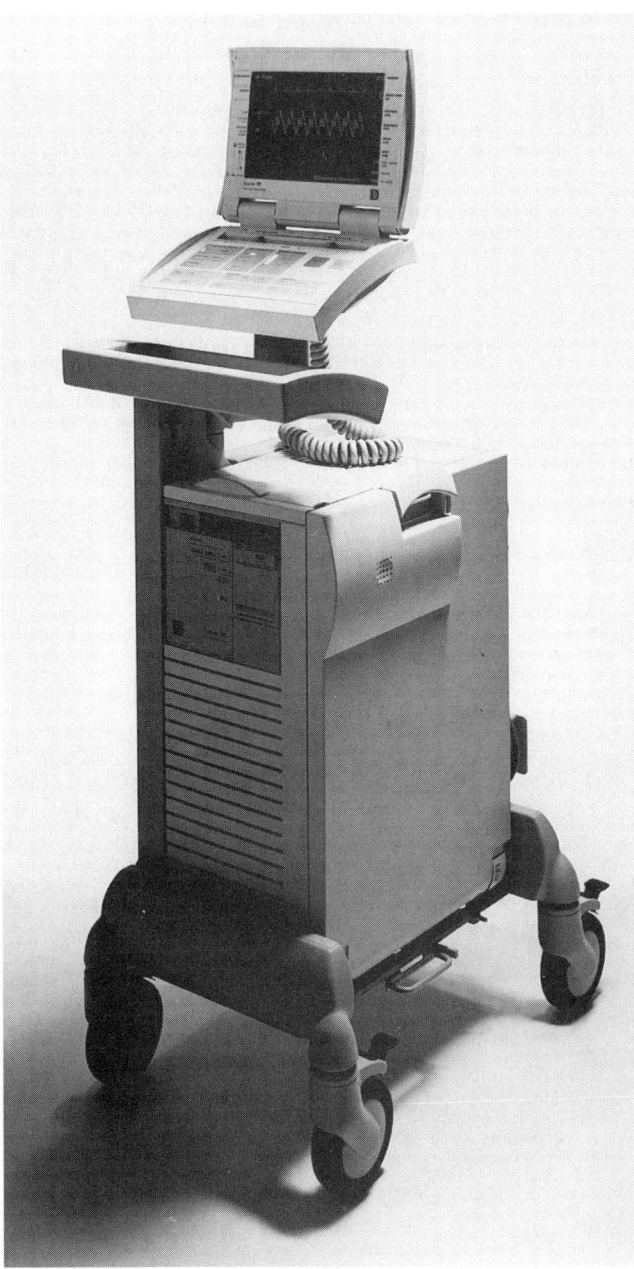

Figure 54–240. One of the newest and more mobile IABP consoles. Most manufacturers now provide portability when designing these devices because air and ground transport of balloon pump dependent patients is now needed. (Courtesy of Datascope Corp., Paramus, N.J.)

for IABP users. At the University Medical Center of Eastern Carolina, balloon pump patients are transported routinely from regional hospitals with safety by specially equipped helicopters and mobile intensive care units, staffed by cardiac intensive care unit–trained transport nurses. During transport, intensive care unit monitoring as well as complete IABP and pharmacologic support are maintained by an intensive care unit nurse who can consult with a physician by radio.

SELECTED REFERENCES

Barnett, M. G., Swartz M. T., Peterson, G. J., Naunheim, K. S., Pennington, D. G., Vaca, K. J., Fiore, A. C., McBride, L. R., Peigh, P., Willman, V. L., and Kaiser, G. C.: Vascular complications from intra-aortic balloons: Risk analysis. J. Vasc. Surg., *19*:8, 1994.

In this paper a retrospective risk analysis for vascular complications was performed in 580 cardiac surgical patients who required intra-aortic balloons. The incidence of vascular complications was unchanged since 1983: however, the severity of complications had decreased significantly. Smoking, the presence of peripheral vascular disease, female sex, and postoperative balloon pump insertion were independent risk factors for complications.

Bolooki, H.: Clinical Application of Intra-aortic Balloon Pump. Mount Kisco, N.Y., Futura Publishing, 1984.

This textbook gives a comprehensive overview of intra-aortic balloon counterpulsation. It details the technical aspects of surgical insertion as well as complications of this technique. This work represents a major reference from a pioneering author and illustrates the clinical indications and physiologic advantages of balloon pumping.

Kantrowitz, A., Wasfie, T., Freed, P. S., Rubenfire, M., Wajszuzuk, W., and Schork, M. A.: Intra-aortic balloon pumping 1967 through 1982: Analysis of complications in 733 patients. Am. J. Cardiol., *57*:976, 1986.

This paper analyzes complications relating to balloon counterpulsation in 733 patients over a 15-year period. The author is the progenitor of the technique as an assist device. This work should be consulted for a comprehensive understanding of problems associated with IABP usage.

Pennington, D. G., Swartz, M., Codd, J. E., Merjavy, J. P., and Kaiser, G. C.: Intra-aortic balloon pumping in cardiac surgical patients: A nine year experience. Ann. Thorac. Surg., *36*:125, 1983.

This is a recent review of 378 patients requiring intra-aortic balloon pumping during cardiac surgery. Preoperative indications included unstable angina (5%) and cardiogenic shock (9%). In 252 patients (67%) intra-aortic balloon pumping was required because of hemodynamic deterioration after surgery. The overall survival rate in this group was 53%, and the incidence of complications was 11.6%. The article is an excellent overview of clinical indications, complications, and benefits of intra-aortic balloon pumping.

Radford, M. J., Johnson, R. A., Daggett, W. M., Fallon, J. T., Buckley, M. J., Gold, H. K., and Leinbach, R. C.: Ventricular septal rupture: A review of clinical and physiologic features and an analysis of survival. Circulation, *64*:545, 1981.

This paper is an excellent review of 41 patients developing post-infarction ventricular septal rupture. Cardiac shock developed in 55% of these patients and intra-aortic balloon pumping was used before operative repair in 18 of the 22 patients having cardiogenic shock. This paper emphasizes the physiologic benefits of balloon pumping in preparing these patients for reparative cardiac surgery.

REFERENCES

1. Alderman, J. D., Gabliani, G. I., McCabe, C. H., Brewer, C. C., Lorell, B. H., Pasternak, R. C., Skillman, J. J., Steer, M. L., and Biam, D. S.: Incidence and management of limb ischemia with percutaneous wire-guided intraaortic balloon catheters. J. Am. Coll. Cardiol., *9*:524, 1987.
2. Barnett, M. G., Swartz, M. T., Peterson, G. J., Naunheim, K. S., Pennington, D. G., Vaca, K. J., Fiore, A. C., McBride, L. R., Peigh, P., Willman, V. L., and Kaiser, G. C.: Vascular complications from intra-aortic balloons: Risk analysis. J. Vasc. Surg., *19*:8, 1994.
3. Baudet, M., Rigaud, M., Rocha, P., Bardet, J., and Bourdarias, J. P.: Treatment of early postinfarction ventricular aneurysm by intra-aortic balloon pumping and surgery. J. Thorac. Cardiovasc. Surg., *78*:445, 1979.
4. Bolooki, H., Williams, W., Thurer, R. J., Vargas, A., Kaiser, G. A., Mack, F., and Chahramani, A. R.: Clinical and hemodynamic criteria for use of the intra-aortic balloon pump in patients requiring cardiac surgery. J. Thorac. Cardiovasc. Surg., *72*:756, 1976.
5. Bolooki, H.: Clinical Application of Intra-aortic Balloon Pump. Mt. Kisco, N.Y., Futura Publishing, 1984.
6. Buckley, M. J., Craver, J. M., Gold, H. K., Mundth, E. D., Daggett, W. M., and Austen, W. G.: Intra-aortic balloon assist for cardiogenic shock after cardiopulmonary bypass. Circulation, *48*(Suppl. 3):III–90, 1973.
7. Clauss, R. H., Birtwell, W. C., Albertal, G., Lunzer, S., Taylor, W. J., Fosberg, A. M., and Harken, D. E.: Assisted circulation: The arterial counterpulsator. J. Thorac. Cardiovasc. Surg., *41*:447, 1961.
8. Daggett, W. M., Guyton, R. A., Mundth, E. D., Buckley, M. J., McEnany, M. T., Gold, H. K., Leinbach, R. C., and Austen, W. G.: Surgery for postmyocardial infarct ventricular septal defect. Ann. Surg., *186*:260, 1977.
9. Eltchaninoff, H., Dimas, A. P., and Whitlow, P. L.: Complications associated with percutaneous placement and use of intraaortic balloon counterpulsation. Am. J. Cardiol., *71*:328, 1993.
10. Gold, H. K., Leinbach, R. C., Buckley, M. J., Mundth, E. D., Daggett, W. M., and Austen, W. G.: Refractory angina pectoris: Follow-up after intra-aortic balloon pumping and surgery. Circulation, *54*(Suppl. 3):41, 1976.
11. Gold, H. K., Leinbach, R. C., Sanders, C. A., Buckley, M. J., Mundth, E. D., and Austen, W. G.: Intra-aortic balloon pumping for ventricular septal defect or mitral regurgitation complicating acute myocardial infarction. Circulation, *47*:1191, 1973.
12. Goldberg, M. J., Rubenfire, M., Kantrowitz, A., Goodman, G., Freed, P. S., Hallen, L., and Reimann, P.: Intraaortic balloon pump insertion: A randomized study comparing percutaneous and surgical techniques. J. Am. Coll. Cardiol., *9*:515, 1987.
13. Golding, L. A. R.: Postcardiotomy mechanical support. Semin. Thorac. Cardiovasc. Surg., *3*:29, 1991.

14. Grotz, R. L., and Yeston, N. S.: Intra-aortic balloon counterpulsation in high-risk cardiac patients undergoing noncardiac surgery. Surgery, 106:1, 1989.
15. Hanson, E. C., Levine, F. H., Kay, H. R., Leinbach, R. C., Gold, H. K., Daggett, W. M., Austen, W. G., and Buckley, M. J.: Control of postinfarction ventricular irritability with the intraaortic balloon pump. Circulation, 62(Suppl. 1):130, 1980.
16. Isner, J. M., Cohen, S. R., Virmani, R., Lawrinson, W., and Roberts, W. C.: Complications of the intraaortic balloon counterpulsation device: Clinical and morphologic observations in 45 necropsy patients. Am. J. Cardiol., 45:260, 1980.
17. Jensen, C., and Hill, C. S.: Mechanical support for congestive heart failure in infants and children. Crit. Care Nurs. Clin. North Am., 6:165, 1994.
18. Kahn, J. K., Rutherford, B. D., McConahay, D. R., Johnson, W. L., Giorgi, L. V., and Hartzler, G. O.: Supported high risk coronary angioplasty using intra-aortic balloon pump counterpulsation. J. Am. Coll. Cardiol., 15:1151, 1990.
19. Kantrowitz, A.: Initial clinical experience with intra-aortic balloon pumping in cardiogenic shock. JAMA, 203:113, 1968.
20. Kantrowitz, A., and Kantrowitz, A.: Experimental augmentation of coronary blood flow by retardation of arterial pressure pulse. Surgery, 34:678, 1953.
21. Kantrowitz, A., Tjonneland, S., Krakauer, J. S., Phillips, S. J., Freed, P. S., and Butner, A. N.: Mechanical intraaortic cardiac assistance in cardiogenic shock. Arch. Surg., 97:1000, 1968.
22. Kantrowitz, A., Wasfie, T., Freed, P. S., Rubenfire, M., Wajszuzuk, W., and Schork, M. A.: Intraaortic balloon pumping 1967 through 1982: Analysis of complications in 733 patients. Am. J. Cardiol., 57:976, 1986.
23. Kern, M. J., Ahuirre, F., Bach, R., Donohue, T., Siegel, R., and Segal, J.: Augmentation of coronary blood flow by intra-aortic balloon pumping in patients after coronary angioplasty. Circulation, 87:500, 1993.
24. Leinbach, R. C., Gold, H. K., Harper, R. W., Buckley, M. J., and Austen, W. G.: Early intraaortic balloon pumping for anterior myocardial infarction without shock. Circulation, 58:204, 1978.
25. Levine, F. H., Gold, H. K., Leinbach, R. C., Daggett, W. M., Austen, W. G., and Buckley, M. J.: Management of acute myocardial ischemia with intraaortic balloon pumping and coronary bypass surgery. Circulation, 58(Suppl. 1):69, 1978.
26. Marks, J. D., Karawande, S. V., Richenbacher, W. E., Jones, K. W., Doty, D. B., Millar, R. C., O'Connell, J. B., Renlund, D. G., Bristow, M. R., Panatalos, G. M., and Gay, W. A.: Perioperative mechanical circulatory support for transplantation. J. Heart Lung Transplant, 11:117, 1992.
27. McGeehin, W., Sheikh, F., Donahoo, J. S., Lechman, M. J., and MacVaugh, H.: Transthoracic intraaortic balloon pump support: Experience in 39 patients. Ann. Thorac. Surg., 44:26, 1987.
28. Mertlich, G., and Quaal, S. J.: Air transport of the patient requiring intra-aortic balloon pumping. Crit. Care Nurs. Clin. North Am., 1:443, 1989.
29. Moulopoulos, S. D., Topaz, S., and Kolff, W. J.: Diastolic balloon pumping (with carbon dioxide) in the aorta: A mechanical assistance of the failing circulation. Am. Heart J., 63:669, 1962.
30. Mundth, E. D., Yurchak, P. M., Buckley, M. J., and Austen, W. G.: Circulatory assistance and emergency direct artery surgery for shock complicating myocardial infarction. N. Engl. J. Med., 283:1383, 1970.
31. Nichols, A. B., Pohost, G. M., Gold, H. K., Leinbach, R. C., Beller, G. A.,

McKusick, K. A., Strauss, H. W., and Buckley, M. J.: Left ventricular function during intra-aortic balloon pumping assessed by multigated cardiac blood pool imaging. Circulation, 58(Suppl. 1):I–176, 1978.
32. Norman, J. C., Cooley, D. A., Igo, S. R., Hibbs, C. W., Johnson, M. D., Bennett, J. G., Fuqua, J. M., Trono, R., and Edmonds, C. H.: Prognostic indices for survival during postcardiotomy intra-aortic balloon pumping: Methods of scoring and classification, with implications for left ventricular assist device utilization. J. Thorac. Cardiovasc. Surg., 74:709, 1977.
33. Ohman, E. M., George, B. S., White, C. J., Kern, M. J., Gurbel, P. A., Freedman, R. J., Lundergren, C., Hartmann, J. R., Talley, J. D., Frey, M. J., Taylor, G., Leimberger, J. D., Owens, P. M., Lee, K. L., Stack, R. S., and Califf, R. M.: Use of aortic counterpulsation to improve sustained coronary artery patency during acute myocardial infarction: Results of a randomized trial. Circulation, 90:792, 1994.
34. O'Rourke, M. F., Norris, R. M., Campbell, T. J., Chang, V. P., and Sammel, N. L.: Randomized controlled trial of intra-aortic balloon counterpulsation in early myocardial infarction with acute heart failure. Am. J. Cardiol., 47:815, 1981.
35. Pennington, D. G., Swartz, M., Codd, J. E., Merjavy, J. P., and Kaiser, G. C.: Intraaortic balloon pumping in cardiac surgical patients: A nine year experience. Ann. Thorac. Surg., 36:125, 1983.
36. Pennington, D. G., and Swartz, M. T.: Circulatory support in infants and children. Ann. Thorac. Surg., 55:233, 1993.
37. Phillips, S. J.: Percutaneous cardiopulmonary bypass and innovations in clinical counterpulsation. Crit. Care Clin., 2:297, 1986.
38. Pollock, J. C., Charlton, M., Williams, W. G., Edmonds, J. F., and Trusler, G. A.: Intraaortic balloon pumping in children. Ann. Thorac. Surg., 29:522, 1980.
39. Powell, M. J., Daggett, W. M., Magro, A. E., Bianco, J. A., Buckley, M. J., Sanders, C. A., Kantrowitz, A. R., and Austen, W. G.: Effects of intra-aortic balloon counterpulsation on cardiac performance, oxygen consumption, and coronary blood flow in dogs. Circ. Res. 26:753, 1970.
40. Quall, S. J.: Comprehensive Intra-aortic Balloon Pumping. St. Louis, C. V. Mosby, 1984.
41. Radford, M. J., Johnson, R. A., Buckley, M. J., Daggett, W. M., Leinbach, R. C., and Gold, H. K.: Survival following mitral valve replacement for mitral regurgitation due to coronary artery disease. Circulation, 60(Suppl. 1):39, 1979.
42. Radford, M. J., Johnson, R. A., Daggett, W. M., Fallon, J. T., Buckley, M. J., Gold, H. K., and Leinbach, R. C.: Ventricular septal rupture: A review of clinical and physiologic features and an analysis of survival. Circulation.
43. Sarnoff, S. J., Braunwald, E., Welch, G. H., Case, R. B., Stainsby, W. N., and Macruz, R.: Hemodynamic determinants of oxygen consumption of the heart with special reference to the tension-time index. Am. J. Physiol., 192:148, 1958.
44. Talley, J. D., Jones, E. L., Weintraub, W. S., and King, S. B.: Coronary artery bypass surgery after failed elective percutaneous transluminal coronary angioplasty. Circulation, 79(Suppl.):I–126, 1989.
45. Weber, K. T., and Janicki, J. S.: Intraaortic balloon counterpulsation: A review of physiological principles, clinical results and device safety. Ann. Thorac. Surg., 17:602, 1974.
46. Weintraub, R. M., Aroesty, J. M., Paulin, S., Levine, F. H., Markis, J. E., LaRaia, P. J., Cohen, S. F., and Kurland, G. F.: Medically refractory unstable angina pectoris: Long term follow-up of patients undergoing intra-aortic balloon counterpulsation and operation. Am. J. Cardiol., 43:877, 1979.

XXV

THE ARTIFICIAL HEART

William S. Pierce, M.D.

The heart-lung machine was first used in successful clinical application by Gibbon in 1953. It was developed to provide temporary support of the systemic circulation and lung function during intracardiac operations. The device is large, and full anticoagulation is required. The components were designed with the primary goals of safety and reliability but not small size and weight. Many modifications were made to the initial Gibbon machine. Among those pioneers involved in the early heart-lung machine was the Dutch physician-scientist who had developed the artificial kidney, Dr. William Kolff. Kolff believed that intrathoracic replacement of the heart might be possible and, in 1959, with Akutsu,

published an article describing their initial attempt to replace the dog's heart. Early models of the artificial heart used a small electric motor, but these were difficult to control; detrimental and often lethal suction was applied during the ventricle filling phase. Furthermore, the dog proved to be a difficult model; associated thromboembolic complications were common. Kolff's group, and subsequently DeBakey and colleagues, found that artificial hearts having separate left and right ventricles to simplify control, pneumatic power systems with low vacuum to aid pump filling, and the use of the calf model with a large chest size and more compatible coagulation mechanism improved the survival time. Indeed, by 1970, the 100-hour barrier had been broken and, a decade later, survival of animals with artificial hearts had exceeded 200 days.

THE PNEUMATIC ARTIFICIAL HEART

Pneumatic artificial hearts consist of separate right and left ventricles powered by separate right and left pneumatic power units with fail-safe back-up units and a control mechanism. Great care has been exercised in the design of the implanted ventricles to minimize tissue reaction and to avoid thrombus formation. Inert metal and plastic components are used, all of which have a long-functioning life. Each prosthetic ventricle consists of a rigid outer shell with a flexible polyurethane sac having hydrodynamic flow characteristics. Air pulses from the pneumatic power unit enter the space between the cases and compress the sac (Fig. 54–241). A control diaphragm may be used to control the compression of the sac. Inlet and outlet valves, either of a mechanical or xenograft type, ensure unidirectional flow. Each ventricle is attached to the native remnant atrium with an atrial suture cuff, while the outlet port is attached to the aorta or pulmonary artery by a conventional vascular graft. The pneumatic power units provide a systolic pressure as high as 100 mm./Hg for the right ventricle and 300 mm./Hg for the left ventricle, and vacuum ranges from 0 to 70 mm./Hg to aid in ventricle filling. Independent rate control, from 50 to 150 beats per minute, provides needed flexibility. Either manual or automatic control can be employed to balance the output of the two ventricles and to increase cardiac output when required. Pneumatic artificial hearts for human use provide a stroke volume of about 70 ml. and cardiac output from 4 to 8 liters per minute (Fig. 54–242). The artificial heart is of such a size that a body weight of at least 150 lbs. is required to ensure that compression of the atria will not occur when the chest is closed.

Artificial heart implantation is performed in a similar manner as heart transplantation (Fig. 54–243). Full cardiopulmonary bypass is employed with bicaval cannulation. The aorta is cross clamped, and the great arteries are divided. The atria are then divided at the atrioventricular junction. The

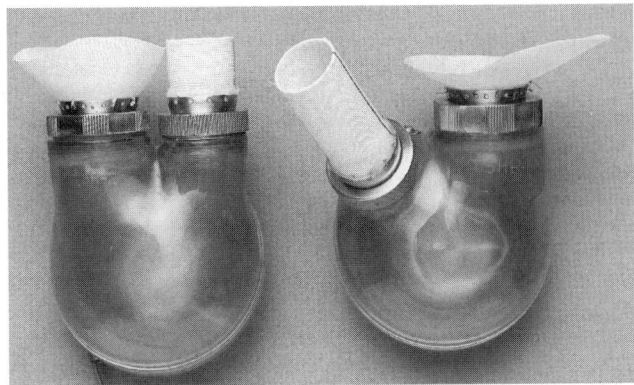

Figure 54–242. This photograph shows the artificial heart developed at Pennsylvania State University. The prosthetic left ventricle *(left)* and the prosthetic right ventricle *(right)* each have a sewing cuff or flange for anastomosis to the respective atria and Dacron grafts for anastomosis to the great vessels. The connectors are attached to the prosthetic ventricles by means of union nut connectors. The design is representative of other pneumatic hearts that have been developed.

prosthetic atrial cuffs and arterial grafts are sewn into place. The ventricles are attached using union nut–type quick connects. De-airing is accomplished. Two six-foot pneumatic lines pass through the chest wall to the pneumatic power unit. Weaning from the heart-lung machine is performed with mild vacuum (10–20 mm./Hg) and systolic drive pressures sufficient to empty the blood sacs. Control in the steady state requires that the arterial pressure be maintained in a

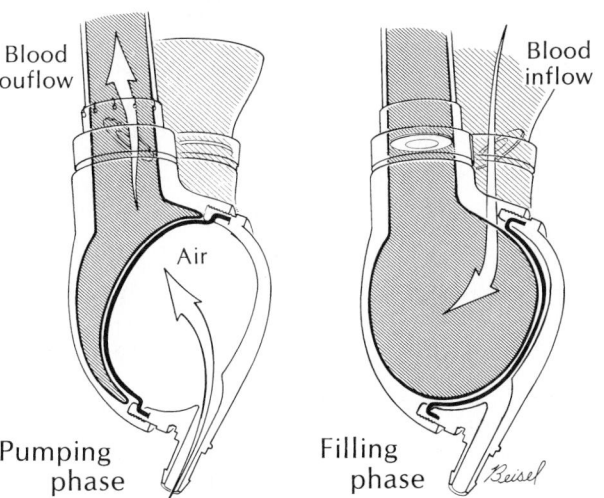

Figure 54–241. The ventricle of a pneumatic heart is shown in the pumping or systolic phase *(left)* and in the filling or diastolic phase *(right)*. Considerable effort has been expended in the development of artificial hearts to ensure highly smooth surfaces, adequate ejection fraction, and high surface shear rates. The inlet and outlet valves are passive and function in a similar manner as prosthetic heart valves. (From Pierce, W. S., Rosenberg, G., Snyder, A. J., Pae, W. E., and Waldhausen, J. A.: An electric artificial heart for clinical use. Ann. Surg., *212*:339, 1990.)

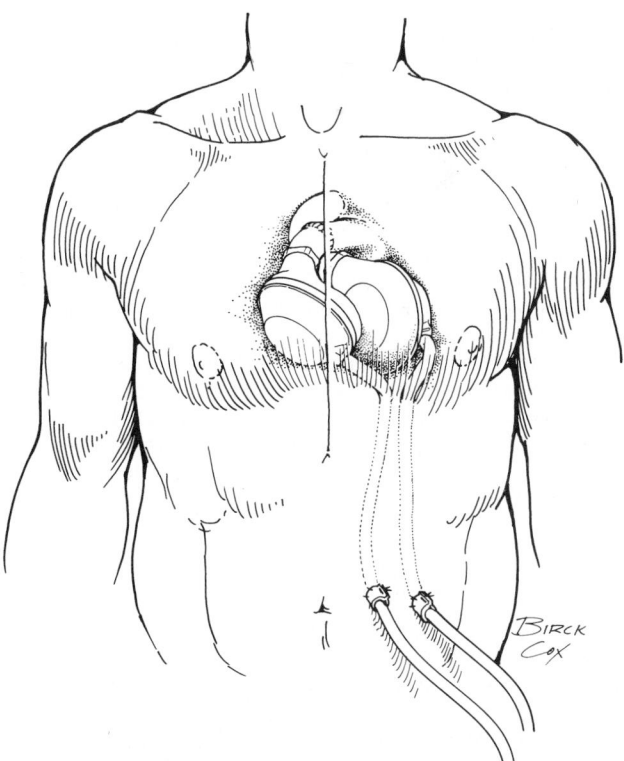

Figure 54–243. This schematic diagram shows the position of the pneumatic heart in the chest after the heart has been removed. The implantation operation is very similar to that of a heart transplantation. Separate left and right drive lines exit the body through skin tunnels and are connected to the pneumatic power unit. Patients have lived with pneumatic hearts for over 1 year. (From Richenbacher, W. E., Pae, W. E., Jr., and Pierce, W. S.: Artificial heart implantation for end-stage cardiac disease. J. Card. Surg., *1*:3, 1986.)

normal range and that sufficient cardiac output be provided (about 2.4 L./min./sq. m.).

Two control techniques have been employed: manual or automatic control. In manual or Starling law control, the systolic pressure is set to completely empty the sac; rate and diastolic vacuum are set to incompletely fill the pump during the diastolic period provided. Any increase in atrial pressure, as may occur during exercise, increases pump filling. Because the pump always ejects completely, stroke volume is automatically increased. If required, greater increases in cardiac output can be achieved by manually increasing ventricle beat rate.

Automatic control has been successfully employed to control pneumatic artificial hearts. Using this method, the bioengineer sets the left ventricle to pump a full stroke with each beat and at a rate sufficient to maintain the arterial pressure within a normal range. The right ventricle is set to maintain a left atrial pressure within a normal range (5–12 mm./Hg). Any decrease in arterial blood pressure automatically increases left ventricle rate while a decrease in left atrial pressure results in an increase in right pump rate. The control system has been employed in calf and human implants and works well.

The Pneumatic Artificial Heart as a Bridge Device

Whereas the pneumatic artificial heart was originally developed as a permanent cardiac substitute, the advent of heart transplantation led to the need for a temporary (days to weeks) cardiac substitute for critically ill patients awaiting heart transplantation. In 1969, and again in 1981, Cooley used a pneumatic heart for several days while donor hearts were identified. The artificial hearts were said to function satisfactorily, but long-term survival was not achieved. In the mid 1980s, the Jarvik pneumatic heart, a product of the Kolff laboratory, became commercially available and was employed in nearly 200 applications as a bridge to transplantation. Considerable success was reported. However, the best results were obtained when the device was employed for less than 1 week. Infection and thromboembolism were frequent complications and ultimately resulted in withdrawal of the Jarvik heart from the commercial market. Although some cardiac surgical groups continue to employ the pneumatic artificial heart as a bridge device, most agree that better results have been obtained with univentricular or biventricular assist systems.

In a multicenter clinical evaluation, a left ventricular assist device (HeartMate) was inserted, and the results showed it to be effective as a bridge to cardiac transplantation. Survivors had very few thromboembolic events. This pump may also be placed intraperitoneally and has been implanted by the preperitoneal approach.

The Pneumatic Artificial Heart as a Permanent Cardiac Substitute

By 1983, the University of Utah Artificial Heart Program, directed by Kolff, had developed the pneumatic heart to a point where the device was reliable and calf survival of 3 to 4 months was routinely achieved. Rapid growth of the animals made longer survival uncommon. The group requested and received approval from the Food and Drug Administration to implant their Jarvik artificial heart in a series of patients who had end-stage heart disease but who were not transplantation candidates. During a historic operation, the Jarvik heart was implanted in the chest of Dr. Barney Clark by Dr. William DeVries. Dr. Clark had a stormy course but was able to leave the bed and walk for a period of time. He died of

an infection 112 days after operation. DeVries subsequently moved to Louisville where he employed the heart in three additional patients, one of whom survived more than 600 days. Again, strokes and infection were major problems and the study was subsequently terminated. Nevertheless, these studies were of considerable importance. They showed that the available artificial hearts would fit in the chest of an appropriately sized patient, would provide an adequate cardiac output, and could maintain cardiovascular pressures within a physiologic range. In these critically ill patients, the problems of infection and thromboembolism appeared to be more problematic than had been predicted from animal implant studies. Moreover, the use of the pneumatic heart, with the requisite tubes (1–2 cm. in diameter passing through the chest wall) and the bulky power unit seemed undesirable if a better alternative is potentially available. That alternative is the electrical motor-driven artificial heart.

THE MOTOR-DRIVEN ARTIFICIAL HEART

The past three decades have produced unprecedented advances in electronics. Taking advantage of these develop-

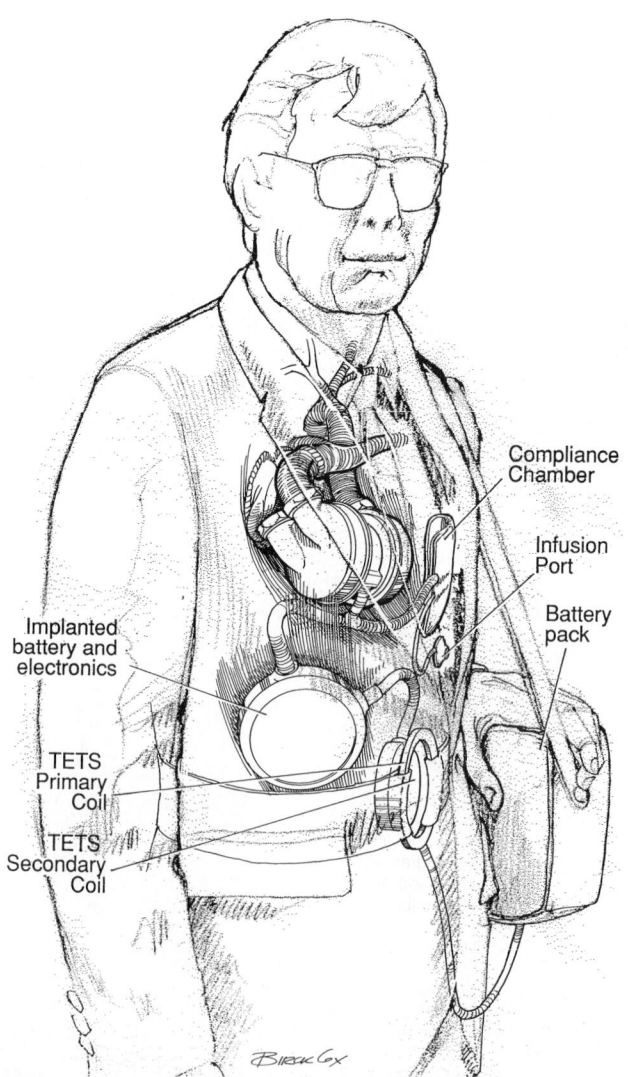

Figure 54–244. This schematic diagram shows the position of the electric heart within the chest. Components required for proper function of the electric heart include an implanted battery and electronics canister, a compliance chamber and its associated infusion port, and a secondary coil. The external battery pack provides power to the primary coil. (From Rosenberg, G., Pae, W. E., Jr., and Pierce, W. S.: The totally implantable electric artificial heart: The Penn State experience. Card. Surg., 4:530, 1990.)

Compliance Chamber

Infusion Port

Battery pack

Implanted battery and electronics

TETS Primary Coil

TETS Secondary Coil

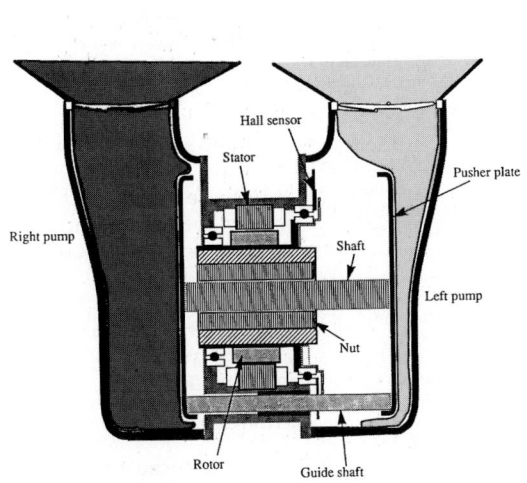

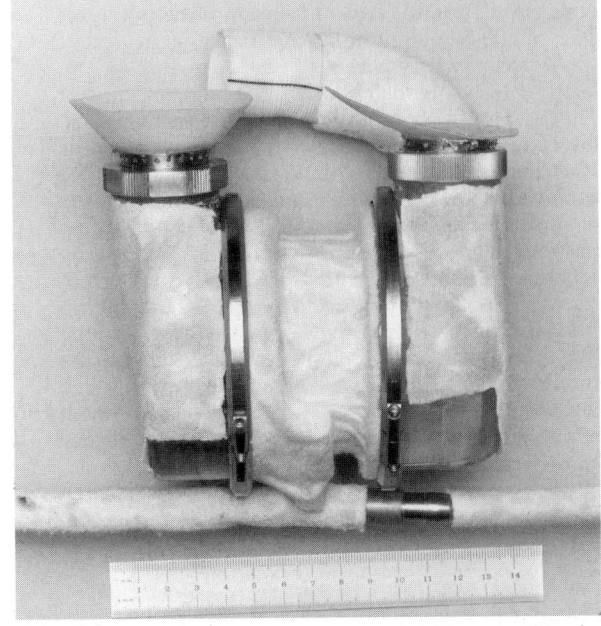

Figure 54–245. The electric artificial heart being developed at Pennsylvania State University consists of a right and left ventricle with the motor-motion translation unit positioned between the two ventricles. *Left,* This schematic diagram shows the position of the planetary roller screw (nut and shaft) positioned within the motor (rotor and stator). The pusher plates move to and fro and create an alternating pumping action. A Hall sensor provides important position information to the control system while the guide shaft ensures that rotary motion of the motor is not transmitted to the pusher plate. *Right,* A photograph of the unit with the suture cuffs in place. The artificial heart is covered with a thin layer of a velour fabric to allow tissue ingrowth, improve fixation, and reduce the incidence of infection. (From Pierce, W. S.: The artificial heart–1986: Partial fulfillment of a promise. ASAIO Trans., *32*:5, 1986.)

ments, the bioengineer can control the function of an electric motor in ways that allow the development of a compact, implantable heart. The electric motor can directly drive pusher plates, compressing the blood sacs, or it can pressurize a working fluid that alternately compresses the right and left blood sac. However, in contrast to a pacemaker, the artificial heart cannot be continuously powered by an implanted battery because the power requirements are so much greater. Importantly, the risks of infection and discomfort associated with having a wire cross the chest wall can be obviated by the use of wireless energy transmission by inductive coupling. This is the principle underlying the electrical transformer. However, when the primary and secondary coils are parallel with skin interposed rather than interlocking as in a transformer, the efficiency decreases from 99% to about 70%.

The National Institutes of Health are funding three groups to develop an electrically powered artificial heart (Fig. 54–244). Each group is composed of a medical and industrial partnership: Abiomed and the Texas Health Institute; Nimbus, Inc., and the Cleveland Clinic Foundation; and Penn State University with 3M (Fig. 54–245). The implantable hearts have features similar to the pneumatic devices in having valved polyurethane sacs. The sacs are actuated by pusher plates or by hydraulic fluid. In addition, each system has an implanted battery that provides 30 to 45 minutes of pump function in the event that the external battery coil system is removed. As indicated previously, each system has

Figure 54–246. The electric artificial heart is being developed in the calf model. This schematic diagram shows the electric artificial heart with the associated components, including the electronics canister, the compliance chamber and infusion port, and the transcutaneous energy transfer coils (T.E.T.S.). The battery pack is positioned within a saddle bag. LA, left atrium; RA, right atrium; Ao, aorta; PA, pulmonary artery. (From Rosenberg, G., Pae, W. E., Jr., and Pierce, W. S.: The totally implantable electric artificial heart: The Penn State experience. J. Card. Surg., *4*:532, 1990.)

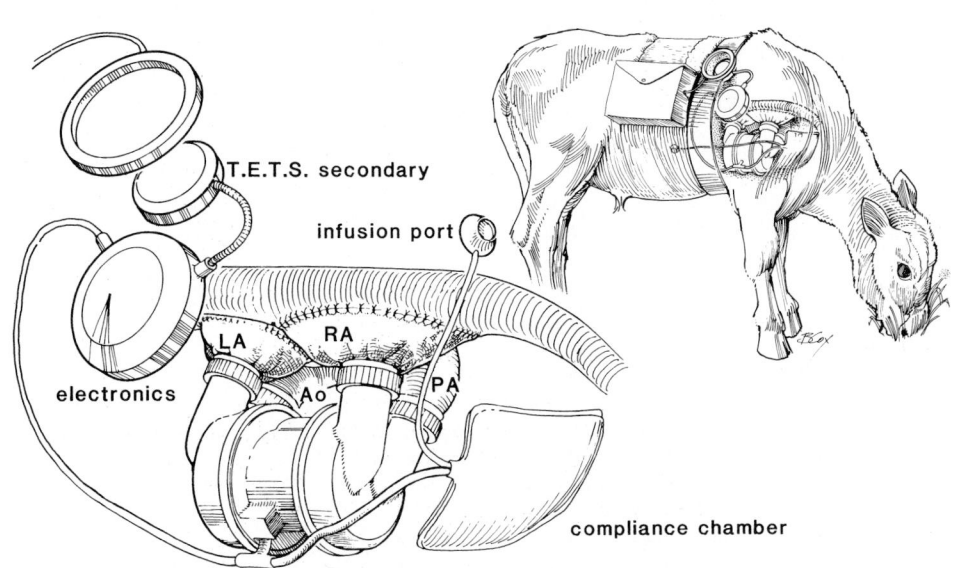

a complex electronic control system to balance the output of the two pumps and to permit automatic increases in cardiac output in association with exercise.

The electric hearts are being evaluated in calf implant studies (Fig. 54–246). Although relatively early in the development stage, one animal has already survived for 13 months with an electric heart. The implantation technique is similar to that employed with the pneumatic heart. Animals generally stand within a few hours after operation, and many do well. However, bleeding, pneumonia, and a variety of electromechanical problems are still all too frequent. Current research is designed to improve the survival rate and to increase the reliability of the device. As outlined by the National Institutes of Health, completion of design of the devices should be performed by 1995 and extensive mock look testing and animal implant studies should be completed over the next 5 years. Clinical implantation should occur shortly after the year 2000.

SELECTED REFERENCES

DeVries, W. C.: The permanent artificial heart: Four case reports. JAMA, 259:849, 1988.
   Dr. DeVries pioneered the use of an artificial heart as a permanent heart substitute. Pneumatic devices were implanted into four patients not considered suitable for heart transplantation. This classic article describes the thinking surrounding these historic operations.

Johnson, K. E., Liska, M. B., Joyce, L. D., and Emery, R. W.: Use of Total Artificial Hearts: Summary of World Experience, 1969–1991. ASAIO J., 38:M486, 1992.
   This article summarizes the experience with 230 pneumatic artificial hearts used as a bridge to transplantation or as a permanent heart substitute. Long-term results and complications of this relatively new technology are clearly described.

Pierce, W. S.: An electric artificial heart for clinical use. Ann. Surg., 212(3):339, 1990.
   The electric heart under development obviates problems associated with the pneumatic hearts. In place of the bulky pneumatic power unit, the electric heart requires only an external battery power source. No percutaneous tubes or wires, generally considered sources of sepsis, are required by the electric heart.

REFERENCES

1. Akutsu, T., Houston, C. S., and Kolff, W. J.: Artificial heart inside the chest, using small electromotors. Trans. Am. Soc. Artif. Intern. Organs, 6:299, 1960.
2. Akutsu, T., and Kolff, W. J.: Permanent substitute for valves and hearts. Trans. Am. Soc. Artif. Intern. Organs, 4:230, 1958.
3. DeVries, W. C.: The permanent artificial heart. JAMA, 259:849, 1988.
4. Farrar, D. S., and Hill, J. D.: Univentricular and biventricular Thoratec VAD support as a bridge-to-transplantation. Ann. Thorac. Surg., 55:276, 1993.
5. Gibbon, J. H., Jr.: Application of a mechanical heart and lung apparatus in cardiac surgery. Minn. Med., 37:171, 1954.
6. Griffith, B. P., Hardesty, R. L., Kormos, R. L., et al.: Temporary use of the Jarvik-7 total artificial heart before transplantation. N. Engl. J. Med., 316:130, 1987.
7. Griffith, B. P., Kormos, R. L., Dummer, J. S., and Hardesty, R. L.: The artificial heart: Infection-related morbidity and its effect on transplantation. Ann. Thorac. Surg., 45:409, 1988.
8. Himley, S. C., Butler, K. C., Massiello, A., et al.: Development of the E4T electrohydraulic total artificial heart. ASAIO Trans., 36:M234, 1990.
9. Jarvik, R. K., Smith, L. M., Lawson, J. H., et al.: Comparison of pneumatic and electrically powered total artificial heart *in vivo*. Trans. Am. Soc. Artif. Intern. Organs, 24:593, 1978.
10. Kawaguchi, A. T., Cabrol, C., Pavie, A., et al.: Survival prediction in staged heart transplantation using Jarvik-7 artificial heart. Circulation, 86:II–311, 1992.
11. Kirby, C. K., Pierce, W. S., Burney, R. G., et al.: The development of an artificial intrathoracic heart. Surgery, 56:719, 1964.
12. Klain, M., Mrava, G. L., Tajima, K., et al.: Can we achieve over 100 hours' survival with a total mechanical heart? Trans. Am. Soc. Artif. Intern. Organs, 17:437, 1971.
13. Kwan-Gett, C. S., Wu, Y., Collan, R., Jacobsen, S., and Kolff, W. J.: Total replacement artificial heart and driving system with inherent regulation of cardiac output. Trans. Am. Soc. Artif. Intern. Organs, 15:245, 1969.
14. Landis, D. L., Pierce, W. S., Rosenberg, G., et al.: Long-term *in vivo* automatic electronic control of the artificial heart. Trans. Am. Soc. Artif. Intern. Organs, 23:519, 1977.
15. Nosé, Y., Topaz, S., SenGupta, A., et al.: Artificial hearts inside the pericardial sac in calves. Trans. Am. Soc. Artif. Intern. Organs, 11:255, 1965.
16. Pierce, W. S., Rosenberg, G., Snyder, A. J., Pae, W. E., and Waldhausen, J. A.: An electric artificial heart for clinical use. Ann. Surg., 212:339, 1990.
17. Richenbacher, W. E., Pae, W. E., Jr., and Pierce, W. S.: Artificial heart implantation for end-stage cardiac disease. J. Card. Surg., 1:3, 1986.
18. Ross, N. J., Jr., Akers, W. W., O'Bannon, W., et al.: Problems encountered during the development and implantation of the Baylor-Rice orthotopic cardiac prosthesis. Trans. Am. Soc. Artif. Intern. Organs, 18:168, 1972.
19. Shaffer, L. J., Donachy, J. H., Rosenberg, G., Phillips, W. M., Landis, D. L., Prophet, G. A., Olsen, E. K., Arrowood, J. A., and Pierce, W. S.: Total artificial heart implantation in calves with pump of an angled port design. Trans. Am. Soc. Artif. Intern. Organs, 25:254, 1979.
20. Snyder, A. J., Rosenberg, G., Reibson, J., Donachy, J. H., Prophet, G. A., Arenas, J., Daily, W., McGary, S., Kawaguchi, O., Quinn, R., and Pierce, W. S.: An electrically powered total artificial heart: Over 1 year survival in the calf. ASAIO J., 38:M707, 1992.
21. Weiss, W. J., Rosenberg, G., Snyder, A. J., et al.: *In vivo* performance of a transcutaneous energy transmission system with the Penn State motor-driven ventricular assist device. Trans. Am. Soc. Artif. Intern. Organs, 35:284, 1989.
22. Yu, L. S., Finnegan, M., Vaughan, S., Ochs, B., Parnis, S., Frazier, O. H., Kung, R. T. V.: A compact and noise-free electrohydraulic total artificial heart (TAH). ASAIO J., 39:M386, 1993.

APPENDIX

Laboratory Reference Values of Clinical Importance

William Z. Borer, M.D.

REFERENCE INTERVALS FOR THE INTERPRETATION OF LABORATORY TESTS

Most of the tests performed in a clinical laboratory are quantitative in nature. That is, the amount of a substance present in blood or serum is measured and reported in terms of concentration, activity (e.g., enzyme activity) or counts (e.g., blood cell counts). The laboratory must provide reference values to assist the clinician in the interpretation of laboratory results. These reference ranges comprise the physiologic quantities of substance (concentrations, activities, or counts) to be expected in healthy people. Deviation above or below the reference range may be associated with a disease process, and the severity of the disease process may be associated with the magnitude of the deviation. Unfortunately there is rarely a sharp demarcation between physiologic and pathological values, and the transition between these two is often gradual as the disease process progresses.

The terms *normal* and *abnormal* have been used to describe the laboratory values that fall inside or outside of the reference range respectively. Use of these terms is now discouraged because it is virtually impossible to define normality and because normal may be confused with the statistical term *Gaussian*. Reference ranges are established from statistical studies in groups of healthy volunteers. Although these study subjects must be free of disease, they may have lifestyles or habits that produce subtle variations in their laboratory values. Examples of these variables include diet, body mass, exercise, and geographic location. Age and gender may also affect reference values. When the data from a large cohort of healthy subjects fit a Gaussian distribution, the usual statistical approach is to define the reference limits as two standard deviations above and below the mean. By definition, the reference range excludes the highest and the lowest 2.5% of the population. Non-Gaussian distributions are handled by different statistical methods, but the result is similar in that the reference range is defined by the central 95% of the population. In other words, the odds are 1 in 20 that a healthy person will have a laboratory result that falls outside the reference range. If 12 laboratory tests are performed, the odds increase to about 1 in 2 that at least one of the results is outside the reference range. This means that all healthy people are likely to have a few laboratory results that are unexpected. The clinician must then integrate these data with other clinical information, such as the history and physical examination, to arrive at the appropriate clinical decision. The reference range for many tests (especially enzyme and immunochemical measurements) varies with the method used. It is important that each laboratory establish reference ranges appropriate for the methods that it employs.

SI Units

During the 1980s a concerted effort was made to introduce SI units (le Système International d'Unités). The rationale for conversion to SI units is sound. Laboratory data are scientifically more informative when the units are based on molar concentration rather than mass concentration. For example, the conversion of glucose to lactate and pyruvate or the binding of a drug to albumin is more easily understood in units of molar concentration. Another example is illustrated as follows:

Conventional Units

1.0 gram of hemoglobin
Combines with 1.37 ml of oxygen
Contains 3.4 mg of iron
Forms 34.9 mg of bilirubin

SI Units

4.0 mmol of hemoglobin
Combines with 4.0 mmol of oxygen
Contains 4.0 mmol of iron
Forms 4.0 mmol of bilirubin

The international use of SI units would also enhance the standardization of nomenclature to facilitate global communication of medical and scientific information. The units, symbols, and prefixes employed in the International System are shown in Appendix Tables 1, 2, and 3.

TABLE 1. Base SI Units

Property	Base Unit	Symbol
Length	meter	m
Mass	kilogram	kg
Amount of substance	mole	mol
Time	second	s
Thermodynamic temperature	kelvin	K
Electric current	ampere	A
Luminous intensity	candela	cd
Catalytic amount	katal	kat

Adapted from Rakel, R. E.: Conn's Current Therapy. Philadelphia, W. B. Saunders Company, 1996.

TABLE 2. Derived SI Units and Non-SI Units Retained for Use with the SI

Property	Unit	Symbol
Area	square meter	m^2
Volume	cubic meter	m^3
	liter	L
Mass concentration	kilogram/cubic meter	kg/m^3
	gram/liter	g/L
Substance concentration	mole/cubic meter	mol/m^3
	mole/liter	mol/L
Temperature	degree Celsius	$°C = °K - 273.15$

Unfortunately, problems have arisen with the implementation of SI units in the United States. Their introduction in 1987 prompted many medical journals to report laboratory values in both SI and conventional units in anticipation of complete conversion to SI units in the early 1990s. The lack of a coordinated effort toward this goal has forced a retrenchment on the issue. Physicians continue to think and practice using laboratory results expressed in conventional units, and few if any American hospitals or clinical laboratories exclusively use SI units. It is not likely that complete conversion to SI units will occur in the foreseeable future, yet most medical journals will probably continue to publish both sets of units. For this reason, the tables of reference ranges in this appendix are given in both conventional units and SI units.

TABLE 3. Standard Prefixes

Prefix	Multiplication Factor	Symbol
yocto	10^{-24}	y
zepto	10^{-21}	z
atto	10^{-18}	a
femto	10^{-15}	f
pico	10^{-12}	p
nano	10^{-9}	n
micro	10^{-6}	u
milli	10^{-3}	m
centi	10^{-2}	c
deci	10^{-1}	d
deca	10^{1}	da
hecto	10^{2}	h
kilo	10^{3}	k
mega	10^{6}	M
giga	10^{9}	G
tera	10^{12}	T

SELECTED REFERENCES

Tietz, N. W., Conn, R. B., and Pruden, E. L. (Eds.): Applied Laboratory Medicine. Philadelphia, W.B. Saunders Company, 1992.

Composed of case studies, this volume provides practical instruction in the use of the laboratory.

Henry, J. B.: Clinical Diagnosis and Management by Laboratory Methods, 18th ed. Philadelphia, W. B. Saunders Company, 1991.
This comprehensive textbook provides detailed information on laboratory methodology and clinical utility.

Speicher, C. E.: The Right Test: A Physician's Guide to Laboratory Medicine, 2nd ed. Philadelphia, W. B. Saunders Company, 1993.
A portable paperback, this focused guide offers the physician a concise, information-packed, user-friendly approach to the selection of laboratory tests.

Tietz, N. W., (Ed.): Clinical Guide to Laboratory Tests, 2nd ed. Philadelphia, W. B. Saunders Company, 1990.
Tables of laboratory tests comprise this handbook, which provides a broad range of information on specimen requirements, reference ranges, and test interferences.

REFERENCES

1. Bick, RL (Ed.): Hematology: Clinical and Laboratory Practice. St. Louis, Mosby–Year Book, Inc., 1993.
2. Borer, W. Z.: Selection and use of laboratory tests. *In* Tietz, NW., Conn, R.B., and Pruden, E. L. (Eds): Applied Laboratory Medicine. Philadelphia, W. B. Saunders Company, 1992, pp. 1–5.
3. Campion, E. W.: A retreat from SI units. N. Engl. J. Med., 327:49, 1992.
4. Drug Evaluations Annual, Chicago, American Medical Association, 1994.
5. Friedman, R.B. and Young, D. S.: Effects of Disease on Clinical Laboratory Tests, 2nd ed. Washington, D.C., AACC Press, 1989.
6. Henry, J. B.: Clinical Diagnosis and Management by Laboratory Methods, 18th ed. Philadelphia, W. B. Saunders Company, 1991.
7. Hicks, J. M., and Young, D. S.: DORA '92–93: Directory of Rare Analyses. Washington, D.C., AACC Press, 1992.
8. Jacobs, D. S., Kasten, B. L, Demott, W. R. and Wolfson, W. L: Laboratory Test Handbook, 2nd ed. Baltimore, Williams & Wilkins Company, 1990.
9. Kaplan, L. A., and Pesce, A.J.: Clinical Chemistry: Theory, Analysis, and Correlation, 2nd ed. St. Louis, C.V. Mosby, 1989.
10. Kjeldsberg, C. R., and Knight J. A.: Body Fluids: Laboratory Examination of Amniotic, Cerebrospinal, Seminal, Serous, and Synovial fluids, 3rd ed. Chicago, ASCP Press, 1993.
11. Laposata, M.: SI Unit Conversion Guide. Boston, NEJM Books, 1992.
12. Scully, R. E., McNeely, W. F., Mark, E. J., and McNeely, B. U: Normal Reference Laboratory Values. N. Engl. J.: Med., 327:718–724, 1992.
13. Speicher, C. E.: The Right Test: A Physician's Guide to Laboratory Medicine, 2nd ed. Philadelphia, W. B. Saunders Company, 1993.
14. Tietz, N. W. (Ed.): Clinical Guide to Laboratory Tests, 2nd ed. Philadelphia, W. B. Saunders Company, 1990.
15. Wallach, J.: Interpretation of Diagnostic Tests: A Synopsis of Laboratory Medicine, 5th ed. Boston, Little, Brown and Company, 1992.
16. Young, D. S.: Determination and validation of reference intervals. Arch. Pathol. Lab. Med., 116:704–709, 1992.
17. Young, D.S : Effects of Drugs on Clinical Laboratory Tests, 3rd ed. Washington, D.C., AACC Press, 1990.
18. Young, D. S.: Implementation of SI units for clinical laboratory data. Ann. Intern. Med., 106:114–129, 1987.

Some of the values included in the tables have been established by the Clinical Laboratories at Thomas Jefferson University Hospital, Philadelphia, Pennsylvania, and have not been published elsewhere. Other values have been compiled from the sources cited in the Reference List. These tables are provided for information and educational purposes only. They are intended to complement data derived from other sources, including the medical history and physical examination. Users must exercise individual judgment when employing the information provided in this appendix.

REFERENCE VALUES FOR HEMATOLOGY

	Conventional Units	SI Units
Acid hemolysis (Ham test)	No hemolysis	No hemolysis
Alkaline phosphatase, leukocyte	Total score 14–100	Total score 14–100
Cell counts		
Erythrocytes		
Males	4.6–6.2 million/mm³	$4.6–6.2 \times 10^{12}$/L
Females	4.2–5.4 million/mm³	$4.2–5.4 \times 10^{12}$/L
Children (varies with age)	4.5–5.1 million/mm³	$4.5–5.1 \times 10^{12}$/L
Leukocytes, total	4500–11,000/mm³	$4.5–11.0 \times 10^{9}$/L
Leukocytes, differential counts*	*Per Cent*	*Absolute Count*
Myelocytes	0	0/L
Band neutrophils	3–5	$150–400 \times 10^{6}$/L
Segmented neutrophils	54–62	$3000–5800 \times 10^{6}$/L
Lymphocytes	25–33	$1500–3000 \times 10^{6}$/L
Monocytes	3–7	$300–500 \times 10^{6}$/L
Eosinophils	1–3	$50–250 \times 10^{6}$/L
Basophils	0–1	$15–50 \times 10^{6}$/L
Platelets	150,000–400,000/mm³	$150–400 \times 10^{9}$/L
Reticulocytes	25,000–75,000/mm³ (0.5–1.5% of erythrocytes)	$25–75 \times 10^{9}$/L
Coagulation tests		
Bleeding time (template)	2.75–8.0 min	2.75–8.0 min
Coagulation time (glass tube)	5–15 min	5–15 min
D-dimer	<0.5 ug/mL	<0.5 mg/L
Factor VIII and other coagulation factors	50–150% of normal	0.5–1.5 of normal
Fibrin split products (Thrombo-Welco test)	<10 ug/mL	<10 mg/L
Fibrinogen	200–400 mg/dL	2.0–4.0 g/L
Partial thromboplastin time (PTT)	20–35 sec	20–35 s
Prothrombin time (PT)	12.0–14.0 sec	12.0–14.0 s
Coombs' test		
Direct	Negative	Negative
Indirect	Negative	Negative
Corpuscular values of erythrocytes		
Mean corpuscular hemoglobin (MCH)	26–34 pg/cell	26–34 pg/cell
Mean corpuscular volume (MCV)	80–96 μm³	80–96 fL
Mean corpuscular hemoglobin concentration (MCHC)	32–36 g/dL	320–360 g/L
Haptoglobin	20–165 mg/dL	0.20–1.65 g/L
Hematocrit		
Males	40–54 mL/dL	0.40–0.54
Females	37–47 mL/dL	0.37–0.47
Newborns	49–54 mL/dL	0.49–0.54
Children (varies with age)	35–49 mL/dL	0.35–0.49
Hemoglobin		
Males	13.0–18.0 g/dL	8.1–11.2 mmol/L
Females	12.0–16.0 g/dL	7.4–9.9 mmol/L
Newborn	16.5–19.5 g/dL	10.2–12.1 mmol/L
Children (varies with age)	11.2–16.5 g/dL	7.0–10.2 mmol/L
Hemoglobin, fetal	<1.0% of total	<0.01 of total
Hemoglobin A_{1C}	3–5% of total	0.03–0.05 of total
Hemoglobin A_2	1.5–3.0% of total	0.015–0.03 of total
Hemoglobin, plasma	0.0–5.0 mg/dL	0.0–3.2 μmol/L
Methemoglobin	30–130 mg/dL	19–80 μmol/L
Sedimentation rate (ESR)		
Wintrobe, Males	0–5 mm/hr	0–5 mm/hr
Females	0–15 mm/hr	0–15 mm/hr
Westergren, Males	0–15 mm/hr	0–15 mm/hr
Females	0–20 mm/hr	0–20 mm/hr

*Conventional units are percentages; SI units are absolute counts.

REFERENCE VALUES* FOR CLINICAL CHEMISTRY (BLOOD, SERUM, AND PLASMA)

	Conventional Units	SI Units
Acetoacetate plus acetone		
Qualitative	Negative	Negative
Quantitative	0.3–2.0 mg/dL	30–200 μmol/L
Acid phosphatase, serum	0.1–0.6 U/L	0.1–0.6 U/L
(Thymolphthalein monophosphate substrate)		
ACTH (see corticotropin)		
Alanine aminotransferase (ALT, SGPT), serum	1–45 U/L	1–45 U/L
Albumin, serum	3.3–5.2 g/dL	33–52 g/L
Aldolase, serum	0.0–7.0 U/L	0.0–7.0 U/L
Aldosterone, plasma		
Standing	5–30 ng/dL	140–830 pmol/L
Recumbent	3–10 ng/dL	80–275 pmol/L
Alkaline phosphatase (ALP), serum		
Adult	35–150 U/L	35–150 U/L
Adolescent	100–500 U/L	100–500 U/L
Child	100–350 U/L	100–350 U/L
Ammonia nitrogen, plasma	10–50 μmol/L	10–50 μmol/L
Amylase, serum	25–125 U/L	25–125 U/L
Anion gap, serum, calculated	8–16 mEq/L	8–16 mmol/L
Ascorbic acid, blood	0.4–1.5 mg/dL	23–85 μmol/L
Aspartate aminotransferase (AST, SGOT), serum	1–36 U/L	1–36 U/L
Base excess, arterial blood, calculated	0 ± 2 mEq/L	0 ± 2 mmol/L
Bicarbonate		
Venous plasma	23–29 mEq/L	23–29 mmol/L
Arterial blood	21–27 mEq/L	21–27 mmol/L
Bile acids, serum	0.3–3.0 mg/dL	0.8–7.6 μmol/L
Bilirubin, serum		
Conjugated	0.1–0.4 mg/dL	1.7–6.8 μmol/L
Total	0.3–1.1 mg/dL	5.1–19.0 μmol/L
Calcium, serum	8.4–10.6 mg/dL	2.10–2.65 mmol/L
Calcium, ionized, serum	4.25–5.25 mg/dL	1.05–1.30 mmol/L
Carbon dioxide, total, serum or plasma	24–31 mEq/L	24–31 mmol/L
Carbon dioxide tension (P_{CO_2}), blood	35–45 mm Hg	35–45 mm Hg
Beta-carotene, serum	60–260 μg/dL	1.1–8.6 μmol/L
Ceruloplasmin, serum	23–44 mg/dL	230–440 mg/L
Chloride, serum or plasma	96–106 mEq/L	96–106 mmol/L
Cholesterol, serum or EDTA plasma		
Desirable range	<200 mg/dL	<5.20 mmol/L
LDL cholesterol	60–180 mg/dL	1.55–4.65 mmol/L
HDL cholesterol	30–80 mg/dL	0.80–2.05 mmol/L
Copper	70–140 μg/dL	11–22 μmol/L
Corticotropin (ACTH), plasma, 8 A.M.	10–80 pg/mL	2–18 pmol/L
Cortisol, plasma		
8:00 A.M.	6–23 μg/dL	170–630 nmol/L
4:00 P.M.	3–15 μg/dL	80–410 nmol/L
10:00 P.M.	<50% of 8:00 A.M. value	<50% of 8:00 A.M. value
Creatine, serum		
Males	0.2–0.5 mg/dL	15–40 μmol/L
Females	0.3–0.9 mg/dL	25–70 μmol/L
Creatine kinase (CK), serum		
Males	55–170 U/L	55–170 U/L
Females	30–135 U/L	30–135 U/L
Creatine kinase MB	<5% of total CK activity	<5% of total CK activity
isoenzyme, serum	<5% ng/mL by immunoassay	<5% ng/mL by immunoassay
Creatinine, serum	0.6–1.2 mg/dL	50–110 μmol/L
Estradiol-17β, adult		
Males	10–65 pg/mL	35–240 pmol/L
Females		
Follicular phase	30–100 pg/mL	110–370 pmol/L
Ovulatory phase	200–400 pg/mL	730–1470 pmol/L
Luteal phase	50–140 pg/mL	180–510 pmol/L
Ferritin, serum	20–200 ng/mL	20–200 μg/L
Fibrinogen, plasma	200–400 mg/dL	2.0–4.0 g/L

REFERENCE VALUES* FOR CLINICAL CHEMISTRY (BLOOD, SERUM, AND PLASMA)
Continued

	Conventional Units	SI Units
Folate, serum	2.0–9.0 ng/mL	4.5–20.4 nmol/L
erythrocytes	170–700 ng/mL	385–1590 nmol/L
Follicle-stimulating hormone (FSH), plasma		
Males	4–25 mU/mL	4–25 U/L
Females, premenopausal	4–30 mU/mL	4–30 U/L
Females, postmenopausal	40–250 mU/mL	40–250 U/L
Gamma-glutamyltransferase (GGT), serum	5–40 U/L	5–40 U/L
Gastrin, fasting, serum	0–10 pg/mL	0–110 mg/L
Glucose, fasting, plasma or serum	70–115 mg/dL	3.9–6.4 nmol/L
Growth hormone (hGH), plasma, adult, fasting	0–6 ng/mL	0–6 μg/L
Haptoglobin, serum	20–165 mg/dL	0.20–1.65 g/L
Immunoglobulins, serum (see Immunologic Procedures)		
Insulin, fasting, plasma	5–25 μU/mL	36–179 pmol/L
Iron, serum	75–175 μg/dL	13–31 μmol/L
Iron binding capacity, serum		
Total	250–410 μg/dL	45–73 μmol/L
Saturation	20–55%	0.20–0.55
Lactate		
Venous whole blood	5.0–20.0 mg/dL	0.6–2.2 mmol/L
Arterial whole blood	5.0–15.0 mg/dL	0.6–1.7 mmol/L
Lactate dehydrogenase (LD, LDH), serum	110–220 U/L	110–220 U/L
Lipase, serum	10–140 U/L	10–140 U/L
Lutropin (LH), serum		
Males	1–9 U/L	1–9 U/L
Females		
Follicular phase	2–10 U/L	2–10 U/L
Midcycle peak	15–65 U/L	15–65 U/L
Luteal phase	1–12 U/L	1–12 U/L
Postmenopausal	12–65 U/L	12–65 U/L
Magnesium, serum	1.3–2.1 mg/dL	0.65–1.05 mmol/L
Osmolality	275–295 mOsm/kg water	275–295 mOsm/kg water
Oxygen, blood, arterial, room air		
Partial pressure (PaO_2)	80–100 mm Hg	80–100 mm Hg
Saturation (SaO_2)	95–98%	95–98%
pH, arterial blood	7.35–7.45	7.35–7.45
Phosphate, inorganic, serum		
Adult	3.0–4.5 mg/dL	1.0–1.5 mmol/L
Child	4.0–7.0 mg/dL	1.3–2.3 mmol/L
Potassium		
Serum	3.5–5.0 mEq/L	3.5–5.0 mmol/L
Plasma	3.5–4.5 mEq/L	3.5–4.5 mmol/L
Progesterone, serum, adult		
Males	0.0–0.4 ng/mL	0.0–1.3 mmol/L
Females		
Follicular phase	0.1–1.5 ng/mL	0.3–4.8 mmol/L
Luteal phase	2.5–28.0 ng/mL	8.0–89.0 mmol/L
Prolactin, serum		
Males	1.0–15.0 ng/mL	1.0–15.0 μg/L
Females	1.0–20.0 ng/mL	1.0–20.0 μg/L
Protein, serum, electrophoresis		
Total	6.0–8.0 g/dL	60–80 g/L
Albumin	3.5–5.5 g/dL	35–55 g/L
Globulins		
Alpha$_1$	0.2–0.4 g/dL	2.0–4.0 g/L
Alpha$_2$	0.5–0.9 g/dL	5.0–9.0 g/L
Beta	0.6–1.1 g/dL	6.0–11.0 g/L
Gamma	0.7–1.7 g/dL	7.0–17.0 g/L
Pyruvate, blood	0.3–0.9 mg/dL	0.03–0.10 mmol/L
Rheumatoid factor	0.0–30.0 IU/mL	0.0–30.0 kIU/L
Sodium, serum or plasma	135–145 mEq/L	135–145 mmol/L
Testosterone, plasma		
Males, adult	300–1200 ng/dL	10.4–41.6 nmol/L
Females, adult	20–75 ng/dL	0.7–2.6 nmol/L
Pregnant females	40–200 ng/dL	1.4–6.9 nmol/L

Table continued on following page

REFERENCE VALUES* FOR CLINICAL CHEMISTRY (BLOOD, SERUM, AND PLASMA)
Continued

	Conventional Units	SI Units
Thyroglobulin	3–42 ng/mL	3–42 µg/L
Thyrotropin (hTSH), serum	0.4–4.8 µIU/mL	0.4–4.8 mIU/L
Thyrotropin-releasing hormone (TRH)	5–60 pg/mL	5–60 ng/L
Thyroxine (FT$_4$), free, serum	0.9–2.1 ng/dL	12–27 pmol/L
Thyroxine (T$_4$), serum	4.5–12.0 µg/dL	58–154 nmol/L
Thyroxine-binding globulin (TBG)	15.0–34.0 µg/mL	15.0–34.0 mg/L
Transferrin	250–430 mg/dL	2.5–4.3 g/L
Triglycerides, serum, 12–hr fast	40–150 mg/dL	0.4–1.5 g/L
Triiodothyronine (T$_3$), serum	70–190 ng/dL	1.1–2.9 nmol/L
Triiodothyronine uptake, resin (T$_3$RU)	25–38%	0.25–0.38
Urate		
Males	2.5–8.0 mg/dL	150–480 µmol/L
Females	2.2–7.0 mg/dL	130–420 µmol/L
Urea, serum or plasma	24–49 mg/dL	4.0–8.2 nmol/L
Urea nitrogen, serum or plasma	11–23 mg/dL	8.0–16.4 nmol/L
Viscosity, serum	1.4–1.8 × water	1.4–1.8 × water
Vitamin A, serum	20–80 µg/dL	0.70–2.80 µmol/L
Vitamin B$_{12}$, serum	180–900 pg/mL	133–664 pmol/L

*Reference values may vary, depending on the method and sample source used.

REFERENCE VALUES FOR THERAPEUTIC DRUG MONITORING (SERUM)

	Therapeutic Range	Toxic Concentrations	Proprietary Names
Analgesics			
Acetaminophen	10–20 µg/mL	>250 µg/mL	Tylenol Datril
Salicylate	100–250 µg/mL	>300 µg/mL	Aspirin Ascriptin Bufferin
Antibiotics			
Amikacin	25–30 µg/mL	Peak >35 µg/mL Trough >10 µg/mL	Amikin
Chloramphenicol	10–20 µg/mL	>25 µg/mL	Chloromycetin
Gentamicin	5–10 µg/mL	Peak >10 µg/mL Trough >2 µg/mL	Garamycin
Tobramycin	5–10 µg/mL	Peak >10 µg/mL Trough >2 µg/mL	Nebcin
Vancomycin	5–10 µg/mL	Peak >40 µg/mL Trough >10 µg/mL	Vancocin
Anticonvulsants			
Carbamazepine	5–12 µg/mL	>15 µg/mL	Tegretol
Ethosuxamide	40–100 µg/mL	>150 µg/mL	Zarontin
Phenobarbital	15–40 µg/mL	40–100 ng/mL (varies widely)	Luminal
Phenytoin	10–20 µg/mL	>20 µg/mL	Dilantin
Primidone	5–12 µg/mL	>15 µg/mL	Mysoline
Valproic acid	50–100 µg/mL	>100 µg/mL	Depakene
Antineoplastics and Immunosuppressives			
Cyclosporine	50–400 ng/mL	>400 ng/mL	Sandimmune
Methotrexate high dose, 48 hr	Variable	>1 µmol/L 48 hr after dose	Mexate Folex
Tacrolimus (FK-506), whole blood	3–10 µg/L	>15 µg/L	Prograf
Bronchodilators and Respiratory Stimulants			
Caffeine	3–15 ng/mL	>30 ng/mL	Aerolate
Theophylline (Aminophylline)	10–20 µg/mL	>20 µg/mL	Elixophyllin Quibron Theobid

REFERENCE VALUES FOR THERAPEUTIC DRUG MONITORING (SERUM) *Continued*

	Therapeutic Range	Toxic Concentrations	Proprietary Names
Cardiovascular Drugs			
Amiodarone	1.0–2.0 μg/mL	>2.0 μg/mL	Cordarone
(Obtain specimen more than 8 hr after last dose)			
Digitoxin	15–25 ng/mL	>35 ng/mL	Crystodigin
(Obtain specimen 12–24 hr after last dose)			
Digoxin	0.8–2.0 ng/mL	>2.4 ng/mL	Lanoxin
(Obtain specimen more than 6 hr after last dose)			
Disopyramide	2–5 μg/mL	>7 μg/mL	Norpace
Flecainide	0.2–1.0 ng/mL	>1 ng/mL	Tambocor
Lidocaine	1.5–5.0 μg/mL	>6 μg/mL	Xylocaine
Mexiletine	0.7–2.0 μg/mL	>2 ng/mL	Mexitil
Procainamide	4–10 μg/mL	>12 μg/mL	Pronestyl
Procainamide + NAPA	8–30 μg/mL	>30 μg/mL	
Propranolol	50–100 ng/mL	Variable	Inderal
			Cardioquin
Quinidine	2–5 μg/mL	>6 μg/mL	Quinaglute
Tocainide	4–10 ng/mL	>10 ng/mL	Tonocard
Psychopharmacologic Drugs			
Amitriptyline	120–150 ng/mL	>500 ng/mL	Amitril
			Elavil
			Triavil
Bupropion	25–100 ng/mL	Not applicable	Wellbutrin
Desipramine	150–300 ng/mL	>500 ng/mL	Norpramin
			Pertofrane
Imipramine	125–250 ng/mL	>400 ng/mL	Tofranil
			Janimine
Lithium	0.6–1.5 mEq/L	>1.5 mEq/L	Lithobid
(Obtain specimen 12 hr after last dose)			
Nortriptyline	50–150 ng/mL	>500 ng/mL	Aventyl
			Pamelor

REFERENCE VALUES* FOR CLINICAL CHEMISTRY (URINE)

	Conventional Units	SI Units
Acetone and acetoacetate, qualitative	Negative	Negative
Albumin		
Qualitative	Negative	Negative
Quantitative	10–100 mg/24 hr	0.15–1.5 μmol/day
Aldosterone	3–20 μg/24 hr	8.3–55 nmol/day
Delta-aminolevulinic acid (delta-ALA)	1.3–7.0 mg/24 hr	10–53 μmol/day
Amylase	<17 U/hr	<17 U/hr
Amylase/creatinine clearance ratio	0.01–0.04	0.01–0.04
Bilirubin, qualitative	Negative	Negative
Calcium (regular diet)	<250 mg/24 hr	<6.3 nmol/day
Catecholamines		
Epinephrine	<10 μg/24 hr	<55 nmol/day
Norepinephrine	<100 μg/24 hr	<590 nmol/day
Total free catecholamines	4–126 μg/24 hr	24–745 nmol/day
Total metanephrines	0.1–1.6 mg/24 hr	0.5–8.1 μmol/day
Chloride (varies with intake)	110–250 mEq/24 hr	110–250 mmol/day
Copper	0–50 μg/24 hr	0.0–0.80 μmol/day
Cortisol, free	10–100 μg/24 hr	27.6–276 nmol/day
Creatine		
Males	0–40 mg/24 hr	0.0–0.30 mmol/day
Females	0–80 mg/24 hr	0.0–0.60 mmol/day
Creatinine	15–25 mg/kg/24 hr	0.13–0.22 mmol/kg/day
Creatinine clearance (endogenous)		
Males	110–150 mL/min/1.73 m²	110–150 mL/min/1.73 m²
Females	105–132 mL/min/1.73 m²	105–132 mL/min/1.73 m²
Cystine or cysteine	Negative	Negative

Table continued on following page

REFERENCE VALUES* FOR CLINICAL CHEMISTRY (URINE) *Continued*

	Conventional Units	SI Units
Dehydroepiandrosterone		
Males	0.2–2.0 mg/24 hr	0.7–6.9 μmol/day
Females	0.2–1.8 mg/24 hr	0.7–6.2 μmol/day
Estrogens, total		
Males	4–25 μg/24 hr	14–90 nmol/day
Females	5–100 μg/24 hr	18–360 nmol/day
Glucose (as reducing substance)	<250 mg/24 hr	<250 mg/day
Hemoglobin and myoglobin, qualitative	Negative	Negative
Homogentisic acid, qualitative	Negative	Negative
17–Ketogenic Steroids		
Males	5–23 mg/24 hr	17–80 μmol/day
Females	3–15 mg/24 hr	10–52 μmol/day
17–Hydroxycorticosteroids		
Males	3–9 mg/24 hr	8.3–25 μmol/day
Females	2–8 mg/24 hr	5.5–22 μmol/day
5–Hydroxyindoleacetic acid		
Qualitative	Negative	Negative
Quantitative	2–6 mg/24 hr	10–31 μmol/day
17–Ketosteroids		
Males	8–22 mg/24 hr	28–76 μmol/day
Females	6–15 mg/24 hr	21–52 μmol/day
Magnesium	6–10 mEq/24 hr	3–5 mmol/day
Metanephrines	0.05–1.2 ng/mg creatinine	0.03–0.70 mmol/mmol creatinine
Osmolality	38–1400 mOsm/kg H_2O	38–1400 mOsm/kg H_2O
pH	4.6–8.0	4.6–8.0
Phenylpyruvic acid, qualitative	Negative	Negative
Phosphate	0.4–1.3 g/24 hr	13–42 mmol/day
Prophobilinogen		
Qualitative	Negative	Negative
Quantitative	<2 mg/24 hr	<9 μmol/day
Porphyrins		
Coproporphyrin	50–250 μg/24 hr	77–380 nmol/day
Uroporphyrin	10–30 μg/24 hr	12–36 nmol/day
Potassium	25–125 mEq/24 hr	25–125 mmol/day
Pregnanediol		
Males	0.0–1.9 mg/24 hr	0.0–6.0 μmol/day
Females		
Proliferative phase	0.0–2.6 mg/24 hr	0.0–8.0 μmol/day
Luteal phase	2.6–10.6 mg/24 hr	8–33 μmol/day
Postmenopausal	0.2–1.0 mg/24 hr	0.6–3.1 μmol/day
Pregnanetriol	0.0–2.5 mg/24 hr	0.0–7.4 μmol/day
Protein, total		
Qualitative	Negative	Negative
Quantitative	10–150 mg/24 hr	10–150 mg/day
Protein/creatinine ratio	<0.2	<0.2
Sodium (regular diet)	60–260 mEq/24 hr	60–260 mmol/day
Specific gravity		
Random specimen	1.003–1.030	1.003–1.030
24-hour collection	1.015–1.025	1.015–1.025
Urate (regular diet)	250–750 mg/24 hr	1.5–4.4 mmol/day
Urobilinogen	0.5–4.0 mg/24 hr	0.6–6.8 μmol/day
Vanillylmandelic acid (VMA)	1.0–8.0 mg/24 hr	5–40 μmol/day

*Reference values may vary depending upon the method used.

REFERENCE VALUES FOR TOXIC SUBSTANCES

	Conventional Units	SI Units
Arsenic, urine	<130 μg/24 hr	<1.7 μmol/day
Bromides, serum, inorganic	<100 mg/dL	<10 mmol/L
Toxic symptoms	140–1000 mg/dL	14–100 mmol/L
Carboxyhemoglobin, blood	*Per Cent Saturation*	*Saturation*
Urban environment	<5%	<0.05
Smokers	<12%	<0.12
Symptoms		
Headache	>15%	>0.15
Nausea and vomiting	>25%	>0.25
Potentially lethal	>50%	>0.50
Ethanol, blood	<0.05 mg/dL	<1.0 mmol/L
	<0.005%	
Intoxication	>100 mg/dL	>22 mmol/L
	>0.1%	
Marked intoxication	300–400 mg/dL	65–87 mmol/L
	0.3–0.4%	
Alcoholic stupor	400–500 mg/dL	87–109 mmol/L
	0.4–0.5%	
Coma	>500 mg/dL	>109 mmol/L
	>0.5%	
Lead, blood		
Adults	<25 μg/dL	<1.2 μmol/L
Children	<15 μg/dL	<0.7 μmol/L
Lead, urine	<80 μg/24 hr	<0.4 μmol/day
Mercury, urine	<30 μg/24 hr	<150 nmol/day

REFERENCE VALUES FOR CEREBROSPINAL FLUID

	Conventional Units	SI Units
Cells	<5/mm³; all mononuclear	<5 × 10⁶/L, all mononuclear
Protein electrophoresis	Albumin predominant	Albumin predominant
Glucose	50–75 mg/dL (20 mg/dL less than in serum)	2.8–4.2 mmol/L (1.1 mmol less than in serum)
Immunoglobulin G (IgG)		
Children <14 yr. of age	<8% of total protein	<0.08% of total protein
Adults	<14% of total protein	<0.14% of total protein
IgG index $\left(\dfrac{\text{CSF/serum IgG ratio}}{\text{CSF/serum albumin ratio}} \right)$	0.3–0.6	0.3–0.6
Oligoclonal banding on electrophoresis	Absent	Absent
Pressure, opening	70–180 mmH₂O	70–180 mm H₂O
Protein, total	15–45 mg/dL	150–450 mg/L

REFERENCE VALUES FOR TESTS OF GASTROINTESTINAL FUNCTION

	Conventional Units
Bentiromide	6-hr urinary arylamine excretion >57% excludes pancreatic insufficiency
Beta-carotene, serum	60–250 ng/dL
Fecal fat estimation	
Qualitative	No fat globules seen by high-power microscope
Quantitative	<6 g/24 hr (>95% coefficient of fat absorption)
Gastric acid output	
Basal	
Males	0.0–10.5 mmol/hr
Females	0.0–5.6 mmol/hr
Maximum (after histamine or pentagastrin)	
Males	9.0–48.0 mmol/hr
Females	6.0–31.0 mmol/hr
Ratio: basal/maximum	
Males	0.0–0.31
Females	0.0–0.29
Secretin test, pancreatic fluid	
Volume	>1.8 mL/kg/hr
Bicarbonate	>80 mEq/L
D-Xylose absorption test, urine	>20% of ingested dose excreted in 5 hr

REFERENCE VALUES FOR IMMUNOLOGIC PROCEDURES

	Conventional Units	SI Units
Complement, serum		
C3	85–175 mg/dL	0.85–1.75 g/L
C4	15–45 mg/dL	150–450 mg/L
Total hemolytic (CH_{50})	150–250 U/mL	150–250 U/mL
Immunoglobulins, serum, adult		
IgG	640–1350 mg/dL	6.4–13.5 g/L
IgA	70–310 mg/dL	0.70–3.1 g/L
IgM	90–350 mg/dL	0.90–3.5 g/L
IgD	0.0–6.0 mg/dL	0.0–60 mg/L
IgE	0.0–430 ng/dL	0.0–430 μg/L

Lymphocyte subsets, whole blood, heparinized

Antigen	Cell Type	Percentage	Absolute
CD3	Total T cells	56–77	860–1880
CD19	Total B cells	7–17	140–370
CD3 and CD4	Helper-inducer cells	32–54	550–1190
CD3 and CD8	Suppressor-cytotoxic cells	24–37	430–1060
CD3 and DR	Activated T cells	5–14	70–310
CD2	E rosette T cells	73–87	1040–2160
CD16 and CD56	Natural killer (NK) cells	8–22	130–500

Helper/suppressor ratio: 0.8–1.8.

REFERENCE VALUES FOR SEMEN ANALYSIS

	Conventional Units	SI Units
Volume	2–5 mL	2–5 mL
Liquefaction	Complete in 15 min	Complete in 15 min
pH	7.2–8.0	7.2–8.0
Leukocytes	Occasional or absent	Occasional or absent
Spermatozoa		
Count	$60–150 \times 10^6$/mL	$60–150 \times 10^6$/mL
Motility	>80% motile	>0.80 motile
Morphology	80–90% normal forms	>0.80–0.90 normal forms
Fructose	>150 mg/dL	>8.33 mmol/L

INDEX

SABISTON

WBS

5887-3

ISBN 0-7216-5887-3

90071

9 780721 658872